Williams
Hematology

Williams
Hematology
Ninth Edition

Kenneth Kaushansky, MD, MACP
Senior Vice President for Health Sciences
Dean, School of Medicine
SUNY Distinguished Professor
Stony Brook University
Stony Brook, New York

Josef T. Prchal, MD
Professor of Medicine, Pathology, and Genetics
Hematology Division
University of Utah
Salt Lake City, Utah
Department of Pathophysiology
First Faculty of Medicine
Charles University in Prague
Prague, Czech Republic

Oliver W. Press, MD, PhD
Acting Director, Clinical Research Division
Dr. Penny E. Peterson Memorial Chair for Lymphoma
  Research
Fred Hutchinson Cancer Research Center
Professor of Medicine and Bioengineering
University of Washington
Seattle, Washington

Marshall A. Lichtman, MD
Professor of Medicine and of Biochemistry and Biophysics
University of Rochester Medical Center
Rochester, New York

Marcel Levi, MD, PhD
Professor of Medicine
Dean, Faculty of Medicine
Academic Medical Center
University of Amsterdam
Amsterdam, The Netherlands

Linda J. Burns, MD
Professor of Medicine
Division of Hematology, Oncology and Transplantation
University of Minnesota
Minneapolis, Minnesota

Michael A. Caligiuri, MD
Director, Comprehensive Cancer Center
CEO, James Cancer Hospital and Solove Research Institute
Professor of Medicine
The Ohio State University
Columbus, Ohio

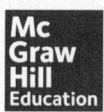

New York   Chicago   San Francisco   Athens   London   Madrid   Mexico City
Milan   New Delhi   Singapore   Sydney   Toronto

Williams HEMATOLOGY, Ninth Edition

Copyright © 2016, by McGraw-Hill Education. All rights reserved. Printed in United States of America. Except as permitted under the United States Copyright Act of 1976, no part of this publication may be reproduced or distributed in any form or by any means, or stored in a data base or retrieval system, without the prior written permission of the publisher.

1 2 3 4 5 6 7 8 9 0   DOW/DOW   20 19 18 17 16 15

ISBN 978-0-07-183300-4
MHID 0-07-183300-5

This book was set in Minion Pro by Cenveo® Publisher Services
The editors were Karen Edmonson and Harriet Lebowitz.
The production supervisor was Richard Ruzycka.
Project management was provided by Harleen Chopra, Cenveo Publisher Services.
Production services were provided by Cenveo Publisher Services.
The designer was Eve Siegel.
The cover designer was Dreamit, Inc.
RR Donnelley was printer and binder.

This book is printed on acid-free paper.

Library of Congress Cataloging-in-Publication Data

Williams hematology / editors, Kenneth Kaushansky, Marshall A. Lichtman, Josef T. Prchal, Marcel Levi, Oliver W. Press, Linda J. Burns, Michael A. Caligiuri.—Ninth edition.
    p. ; cm.
  Hematology
  Preceded by Williams hematology / editors, Kenneth Kaushansky . . . [et al.]. 8th ed. c2010.
  Includes bibliographical references and index.
  ISBN 978-0-07-183300-4 (alk. paper)—ISBN 0-07-183300-5
  I. Kaushansky, Kenneth, editor.   II. Title: Hematology.
  [DNLM: 1. Hematologic Diseases.   2. Hematology—methods.   WH 100]
  RC633
  616.1′5—dc23
                                                    2015020062

McGraw-Hill Education books are available at special quantity discounts to use as premiums and sales promotions, or for use in corporate training programs. To contact a representative please visit the Contact Us pages at www.mhprofessional.com.

CONTENTS

Contributors ix

Preface xxi

PART I

Clinical Evaluation of the Patient

1. Initial Approach to the Patient: History and Physical Examination. 3
   Marshall A. Lichtman and Linda J. Burns

2. Examination of Blood Cells. 11
   Daniel H. Ryan

3. Examination of The Marrow 27
   Daniel H. Ryan

4. Consultative Hematology. 41
   Rondeep S. Brar and Stanley L. Schrier

PART II

The Organization of the Lymphohematopoietic Tissues

5. Structure of the Marrow and the Hematopoietic Microenvironment 53
   Utpal P. Davé and Mark J. Koury

6. The Organization and Structure of Lymphoid Tissues 85
   Aharon G. Freud and Michael A. Caligiuri

PART III

Epochal Hematology

7. Hematology of the Fetus and Newborn. 99
   James Palis and George B. Segel

8. Hematology during Pregnancy 119
   Martha P. Mims

9. Hematology in Older Persons 129
   William B. Ershler, Andrew S. Artz, and Bindu Kanapuru

PART IV

Molecular and Cellular Hematology

10. Genetic Principles and Molecular Biology 145
    Lynn B. Jorde

11. Genomics. 155
    Lukas D. Wartman and Elaine R. Mardis

12. Epigenetics. 165
    Bradley R. Cairns

13. Cytogenetics and Genetic Abnormalities 173
    Lucy A. Godley, Madina Sukhanova, Gordana Raca, and Michelle M. Le Beau

14. Metabolism of Hematologic Neoplastic Cells. 191
    Zandra E. Walton, Annie L. Hsieh, and Chi V. Dang

15. Apoptosis Mechanisms: Relevance to the Hematopoietic System. 203
    John C. Reed

16. Cell-Cycle Regulation and Hematologic Disorders 213
    Yun Dai, Prithviraj Bose, and Steven Grant

17. Signal Transduction Pathways. 247
    Kenneth Kaushansky

18. Hematopoietic Stem Cells, Progenitors, and Cytokines 257
    Kenneth Kaushansky

19. The Inflammatory Response 279
    Jeffrey S. Warren and Peter A. Ward

20. Innate Immunity. 293
    Bruce Beutler

21. Dendritic Cells and Adaptive Immunity 307
    Madhav Dhodapkar, Crystal L. Mackall, and Ralph M. Steinman

PART V

Therapeutic Principles

22. Pharmacology and Toxicity of Antineoplastic Drugs 315
    Benjamin Izar, Dustin Dzube, James M. Cleary, Constantine S. Mitsiades, Paul G. Richardson, Jeffrey A. Barnes, and Bruce A. Chabner

23. Hematopoietic Cell Transplantation 353
    Andrew R. Rezvani, Robert Lowsky, and Robert S. Negrin

24. Treatment of Infections in The Immunocompromised Host. 383
    Lisa Beutler and Jennifer Babik

25. Antithrombotic Therapy 393
    Gregory C. Connolly and Charles W. Francis

26. Immune Cell Therapy. 409
    Carolina Berger and Stanley R. Riddell

27. Vaccine Therapy 421
    Katayoun Rezvani and Jeffrey J. Molldrem

28. Therapeutic Apheresis: Indications, Efficacy, and Complications 427
    Robert Weinstein

29. Gene Therapy for Hematologic Diseases. 437
    Hua Fung and Stanton Gerson

30. Regenerative Medicine: Multipotential Cell Therapy for Tissue Repair 447
    Jakub Tolar, Mark J Osborn, Randy Daughters, Anannya Banga, and John Wagner

PART VI

The Erythrocyte

31. Structure and Composition of the Erythrocyte 461
    Narla Mohandas

32. Erythropoiesis 479
    Josef T. Prchal and Perumal Thiagarajan

33. Erythrocyte Turnover. 495
    Perumal Thiagarajan and Josef Prchal

34. Clinical Manifestations and Classification of Erythrocyte Disorders 503
    Josef T. Prchal

35. Aplastic Anemia: Acquired and Inherited............... 513
George B. Segel and Marshall A. Lichtman

36. Pure Red Cell Aplasia................................. 539
Neal S. Young

37. Anemia of Chronic Disease 549
Tomas Ganz

38. Erythropoietic Effects of Endocrine Disorders............ 559
Xylina T. Gregg

39. The Congenital Dyserythropoietic Anemias............... 563
Achille Iolascon

40. Paroxysmal Nocturnal Hemoglobinuria 571
Charles J. Parker

41. Folate, Cobalamin, and Megaloblastic Anemias........... 583
Ralph Green

42. Iron Metabolism 617
Tomas Ganz

43. Iron Deficiency and Overload......................... 627
Tomas Ganz

44. Anemia Resulting from Other Nutritional Deficiencies 651
Ralph Green

45. Anemia Associated with Marrow Infiltration.............. 657
Vishnu VB Reddy and Josef T. Prchal

46. Erythrocyte Membrane Disorders 661
Theresa L Coetzer

47. Erythrocyte Enzyme Disorders........................ 689
Wouter W. van Solinge and Richard van Wijk

48. The Thalassemias: Disorders of Globin Synthesis 725
David J. Weatherall

49. Disorders of Hemoglobin Structure: Sickle Cell
    Anemia and Related Abnormalities.................... 759
Kavita Natrajan and Abdullah Kutlar

50. Methemoglobinemia and Other Dyshemoglobinemias 789
Archana M. Agarwal and Josef T. Prchal

51. Fragmentation Hemolytic Anemia..................... 801
Kelty R. Baker and Joel Moake

52. Erythrocyte Disorders as a Result of Chemical
    and Physical Agents 809
Paul C. Herrmann

53. Hemolytic Anemia Resulting from Infections
    with Microorganisms 815
Marshall A. Lichtman

54. Hemolytic Anemia Resulting from Immune Injury........ 823
Charles H. Packman

55. Alloimmune Hemolytic Disease of the Fetus
    and Newborn...................................... 847
Ross M. Fasano, Jeanne E. Hendrickson, and Naomi L. C. Luban

56. Hypersplenism and Hyposplenism..................... 863
Jaime Caro and Srikanth Nagalla

57. Primary and Secondary Erythrocytoses 871
Josef T. Prchal

58. The Porphyrias..................................... 889
John D. Phillips and Karl E. Anderson

59. Polyclonal and Hereditary Sideroblastic Anemias......... 915
Prem Ponka and Josef T. Prchal

PART VII

Neutrophils, Eosinophils, Basophils, and Mast Cells

60. Structure and Composition of Neutrophils,
    Eosinophils, and Basophils 925
C. Wayne Smith

61. Production, Distribution, and Fate of Neutrophils 939
C. Wayne Smith

62. Eosinophils and Related Disorders.................... 947
Andrew J. Wardlaw

63. Basophils, Mast Cells, and Related Disorders............. 965
Stephen J. Galli, Dean D. Metcalfe, Daniel A. Arber, and Ann M. Dvorak

64. Classification and Clinical Manifestations of
    Neutrophil Disorders 983
Marshall A. Lichtman

65. Neutropenia and Neutrophilia 991
David C. Dale and Karl Welte

66. Disorders of Neutrophil Function 1005
Niels Borregaard

PART VIII

Monocytes and Macrophages

67. Structure, Receptors, and Functions of Monocytes and
    Macrophages 1045
Steven D. Douglas and Anne G. Douglas

68. Production, Distribution, and Activation of Monocytes and
    Macrophages 1075
Steven D. Douglas and Anne G. Douglas

69. Classification and Clinical Manifestations of Disorders
    of Monocytes and Macrophages 1089
Marshall A. Lichtman

70. Monocytosis and Monocytopenia 1095
Marshall A. Lichtman

71. Inflammatory and Malignant Histiocytosis 1101
Kenneth L. McClain and Carl E. Allen

72. Gaucher Disease and Related Lysosomal Storage Diseases.. 1121
Ari Zimran and Deborah Elstein

PART IX

Lymphocytes and Plasma Cells

73. The Structure of Lymphocytes and Plasma Cells 1137
Natarajan Muthusamy and Michael A. Caligiuri

74. Lymphopoiesis..................................... 1149
Christopher S. Seet and Gay M. Crooks

75. Functions of B Lymphocytes and Plasma Cells in
    Immunoglobulin Production 1159
Thomas J. Kipps

76. Functions of T Lymphocytes: T-Cell Receptors
    for Antigen 1175
Fabienne McClanahan and John Gribben

77. Functions of Natural Killer Cells 1189
Giorgio Trinchieri, Richard W. Childs, and Lewis L. Lanier

78. Classification and Clinical Manifestations of
    Lymphocyte and Plasma Cell Disorders 1195
Yvonne A. Efebera and Michael A. Caligiuri

79. Lymphocytosis and Lymphocytopenia 1199
Sumithira Vasu and Michael A. Caligiuri

80. Immunodeficiency Diseases 1211
Hans D. Ochs and Luigi D. Notarangelo

81. Hematologic Manifestations of Acquired Immunodeficiency
Syndrome 1239
Virginia C. Broudy, Robert D. Harrington

82. Mononucleosis Syndromes 1261
Robert F. Betts

PART X

Malignant Myeloid Diseases

83. Classification and Clinical Manifestations of the
Clonal Myeloid Disorders 1275
Marshall A. Lichtman

84. Polycythemia Vera 1291
Jaroslav F. Prchal and Josef T. Prchal

85. Essential Thrombocythemia 1307
Philip A. Beer and Anthony R. Green

86. Primary Myelofibrosis 1319
Marshall A. Lichtman and Josef T. Prchal

87. Myelodysplastic Syndromes. 1341
Rafael Bejar and David P. Steensma

88. Acute Myelogenous Leukemia 1373
Jane L. Liesveld and Marshall A. Lichtman

89. Chronic Myelogenous Leukemia and Related Disorders . . . 1437
Jane L. Liesveld and Marshall A. Lichtman

PART XI

Malignant Lymphoid Diseases

90. Classification of Malignant Lymphoid Disorders. 1493
Robert A. Baiocchi

91. Acute Lymphoblastic Leukemia 1505
Richard A. Larson

92. Chronic Lymphocytic Leukemia 1527
Farrukh T. Awan and John C. Byrd

93. Hairy Cell Leukemia. 1553
Michael R. Grever and Gerard Lozanski

94. Large Granular Lymphocytic Leukemia 1563
Pierluigi Porcu and Aharon G. Freud

95. General Considerations for Lymphomas: Epidemiology,
Etiology, Heterogeneity, and Primary Extranodal Disease . . 1569
Oliver W. Press and Marshall A. Lichtman

96. Pathology of Lymphomas. 1587
Randy D. Gascoyne and Brian F. Skinnider

97. Hodgkin Lymphoma. 1603
Oliver W. Press

98. Diffuse Large B-Cell Lymphoma and Related Diseases. 1625
Stephen D. Smith and Oliver W. Press

99. Follicular Lymphoma 1641
Oliver W. Press

100. Mantle Cell Lymphoma 1653
Martin Dreyling

101. Marginal Zone B-Cell Lymphomas 1663
Pier Luigi Zinzani and Alessandro Broccoli

102. Burkitt Lymphoma 1671
Andrew G. Evans and Jonathan W. Friedberg

103. Cutaneous T-Cell Lymphoma (Mycosis Fungoides
and Sézary Syndrome) 1679
Larisa J. Geskin

104. Mature T-Cell and Natural Killer Cell Lymphomas. 1693
Neha Mehta, Alison Moskowitz, and Steven Horwitz

105. Plasma Cell Neoplasms: General Considerations. 1707
Guido Tricot, Siegfried Janz, Kalyan Nadiminti, Erik Wendlandt, and
Fenghuang Zhan

106. Essential Monoclonal Gammopathy 1721
Marshall A. Lichtman

107. Myeloma. 1733
Elizabeth O'Donnell, Francesca Cottini, Noopur Raje, and
Kenneth Anderson

108. Immunoglobulin Light-Chain Amyloidosis 1773
Morie A. Gertz, Taimur Sher, Angela Dispenzieri, and
Francis K. Buadi

109. Macroglobulinemia. 1785
Steven P. Treon, Jorge J. Castillo, Zachary R. Hunter, and
Giampaolo Merlini

110. Heavy-Chain Disease 1803
Dietlind L. Wahner-Roedler and Robert A. Kyle

PART XII

Hemostasis and Thrombosis

111. Megakaryopoiesis and Thrombopoiesis. 1815
Kenneth Kaushansky

112. Platelet Morphology, Biochemistry, and Function. 1829
Susan S. Smyth, Sidney Whiteheart, Joseph E. Italiano Jr.,
Paul Bray, and Barry S. Coller

113. Molecular Biology and Biochemistry of the
Coagulation Factors and Pathways of Hemostasis. 1915
Mettine H. A. Bos, Cornelis van 't Veer, and Pieter H. Reitsma

114. Control of Coagulation Reactions 1949
Laurent O. Mosnier and John H. Griffin

115. Vascular Function in Hemostasis 1967
Katherine A. Hajjar, Aaron J. Marcus, and
William Muller

116. Classification, Clinical Manifestations, and
Evaluation of Disorders of Hemostasis 1985
Marcel Levi, Uri Seligsohn, and Kenneth Kaushansky

117. Thrombocytopenia 1993
Reyhan Diz-Küçükkaya and José A. López

118. Heparin-Induced Thrombocytopenia 2025
Adam Cuker and Mortimer Poncz

119. Reactive Thrombocytosis. 2035
Kenneth Kaushansky

120. Hereditary Qualitative Platelet Disorders 2039
A. Koneti Rao and Barry S. Coller

121. Acquired Qualitative Platelet Disorders 2073
Charles S. Abrams, Sanford J. Shattil, and Joel S. Bennett

122. The Vascular Purpuras 2097
Doru T. Alexandrescu and Marcel Levi

123. Hemophilia A and Hemophilia B 2113
Miguel A. Escobar and Nigel S. Key

124. Inherited Deficiencies of Coagulation Factors II, V,
V+VIII, VII, X, XI, and XIII 2133
Flora Peyvandi and Marzia Menegatti

125. Hereditary Fibrinogen Abnormalities 2151
Marguerite Neerman-Arbez and Philippe de Moerloose

126. von Willebrand Disease 2163
Jill Johnsen and David Ginsburg

127. Antibody-Mediated Coagulation Factor Deficiencies 2183
Sean R. Stowell, John S. (Pete) Lollar, and Shannon L. Meeks

128. Hemostatic Alterations in Liver Disease and Liver
Transplantation 2191
Frank W.G. Leebeek and Ton Lisman

129. Disseminated Intravascular Coagulation 2199
Marcel Levi and Uri Seligsohn

130. Hereditary Thrombophilia. 2221
Saskia Middeldorp and Michiel Coppens

131. The Antiphospholipid Syndrome 2233
Jacob H. Rand and Lucia Wolgast

132. Thrombotic Microangiopathies 2253
J. Evan Sadler

133. Venous Thrombosis 2267
Gary E. Raskob, Russell D. Hull, and Harry R. Buller

134. Atherothrombosis: Disease Initiation, Progression,
and Treatment 2281
Emile R. Mohler III and Andrew I. Schafer

135. Fibrinolysis and Thrombolysis 2303
Katherine A. Hajjar and Jia Ruan

PART XIII

Transfusion Medicine

136. Erythrocyte Antigens and Antibodies 2329
Marion E. Reid and Christine Lomas-Francis

137. Human Leukocyte and Platelet Antigens 2353
Myra Coppage, David Stroncek, Janice McFarland, and Neil Blumberg

138. Blood Procurement and Red Cell Transfusion. 2365
Jeffrey McCullough, Majed A. Refaai, and Claudia S. Cohn

139. Preservation and Clinical Use of Platelets 2381
Terry Gernsheimer and Sherrill Slichter

Index 2393

CONTRIBUTORS

Charles S. Abrams, MD [121]
Professor of Medicine, Pathology and Laboratory Medicine
Vice Chair for Research & Chief Scientific Officer
Department of Medicine
University of Pennsylvania School of Medicine
Philadelphia, Pennsylvania

Archana M. Agarwal, MD [50]
Department of Pathology
University of Utah/ARUP Laboratories
Salt Lake City, Utah

Doru T. Alexandrescu, MD [122]
Department of Medicine
Division of Dermatology
University of California, San Diego
VA San Diego Health Care System
San Diego, California

Carl E. Allen, MD, PhD [71]
Associate Professor of Pediatrics
Texas Children's Cancer Center/Hematology
Baylor College of Medicine
Houston, Texas

Karl E. Anderson, MD, FACP [58]
Professor, Departments of Preventative Medicine and Community
Health, Internal Medicine, and Pharmacology and Toxicology
University of Texas Medical Branch
Galveston, Texas

Kenneth Anderson, MD [107]
Dana-Farber Cancer Institute
Boston, Massachusetts

Daniel A. Arber, MD [63]
Ronald F. Dorfman, MBBch, FRCPath Professor in Hematopathology
Professor of Pathology
Stanford University School of Medicine
Stanford University Medical Center
Stanford, California

Andrew S. Artz, MD, MS [9]
Associate Professor of Medicine
University of Chicago
Chicago, Illinois

Farrukh T. Awan, MD [92]
Associate Professor of Internal Medicine
Division of Hematology
Department of internal Medicine
The Ohio State University Comprehensive Cancer Center
Columbus, Ohio

Jennifer Babik, MD, PhD [24]
Division of Infectious Diseases
Department of Medicine
University of California
San Francisco, California

Robert A. Baiocchi, MD, PhD [90]
Associate Professor of Medicine
Division of Hematology
Department of Internal Medicine
The Ohio State University
Columbus, Ohio

Kelty R. Baker, MD [51]
Clinical Assistant Professor
Baylor College of Medicine
Houston, Texas

Anannya Banga, PhD, [30]
Assistant Professor
Department of Genetics
Cell Biology, and Development, Stem Cell Institute
University of Minnesota
Minneapolis, Minnesota

Jeffrey A. Barnes [22]
Instructor in Medicine
Dana-Farber Cancer Institute
Harvard Medical School
Boston, Massachusetts

Philip A. Beer, MRCP, FRCPath, PhD [85]
Wellcome Trust Sanger Institute
    Wellcome Trust Genome Campus, Hinxton
Cambridge, United Kingdom

Rafael Bejar, MD, PhD [87]
Division of Hematology and Oncology
Moores Cancer Center
University of California San Diego
La Jolla, California

Joel S. Bennett, MD [121]
Professor of Medicine
Division of Hematology-Oncology
University of Pennsylvania School of Medicine
Philadelphia, Pennsylvania

Carolina Berger, MD [26]
Fred Hutchinson Cancer Research Center
Seattle, Washington

Robert F. Betts, MD [82]
Professor of Medicine, Emeritus
Division of Infectious Diseases
University of Rochester Medical Center
Rochester, New York

Bruce Beutler, MD [20]
Regental Professor and Director
Center for the Genetics of Host Defense
Raymond and Ellen Willie Distinguished Chair in Cancer Research in
    Honor of Laverne and Raymond Willie Sr.
University of Texas Southwestern Medical Center
Dallas, Texas

Lisa Beutler, MD, PhD [24]
Department of Medicine
UCSF School of Medicine
San Francisco, California

Neil Blumberg, MD [137]
Professor and Director, Clinical Laboratories and Transfusion
    Medicine
Department of Pathology and Laboratory Medicine
University of Rochester
Rochester, New York

Niels Borregaard, MD, PhD [66]
Professor of Hematology
Department of Hematology
University of Copenhagen
Copenhagen, Denmark

Prithviraj Bose, MD [16]
Assistant Professor
Department of Leukemia
University of Texas MD Anderson Cancer Center
Houston, Texas

Rondeep S. Brar, MD [4]
Clinical Assistant Professor of Medicine (Hematology and Oncology)
Stanford University School of Medicine
Stanford, California

Paul Bray, MD [112]
Professor
Director, Division of Hematology
Jefferson University
Philadelphia, Pennsylvania

Alessandro Broccoli, MD [101]
Institute of Hematology "L. e A. Seràgnoli"
University of Bologna
Bologna, Italy

Virginia C. Broudy, MD [81]
Professor of Medicine
Scripps Professor of Hematology
University of Washington
Seattle, Washington

Francis K. Buadi, MD [108]
Division of Hematology
Mayo Clinic
Rochester, Minnesota

Harry R. Buller, MD [133]
Professor of Medicine,
Department of Vascular Medicine
Academic Medical Center
Amsterdam, The Netherlands

Linda J. Burns, MD [1]
National Marrow Donor Program/Be The Match
Vice President and Medical Director
Health Services Research
Minneapolis, Minnesota

John C. Byrd, MD [92]
D. Warren Brown Chair of Leukemia Research
Professor of Medicine, Medicinal Chemistry, and Veterinary
    Biosciences
Director, Division of Hematology
Department of Medicine
The Ohio State University
Columbus, Ohio

Bradley R. Cairns, PhD [12]
Howard Hughes Medical Institute
Professor and Chair
Department of Oncological Sciences
Huntsman Cancer Institute
University of Utah School of Medicine
Salt Lake City, Utah

Michael A. Caligiuri, MD [6, 73, 78, 79]
Professor and Director, The Ohio State University Comprehensive
    Cancer Center
CEO, James Cancer Hospital and Solove Research Institute
The Ohio State University
Columbus, Ohio

Jaime Caro, MD [56]
Professor of Medicine
Department of Medicine
Thomas Jefferson University
Cardeza Foundation for Hematologic Research
Philadelphia, Pennsylvania

Jorge J. Castillo, MD [109]
Assistant Professor of Medicine
Dana-Farber Cancer Institute
Harvard Medical School
Boston, Massachusetts

Bruce A. Chabner, MD [22]
Professor of Medicine
Massachusetts General Hospital Cancer Center
Harvard Medical School
Boston, Massachusetts

Richard W. Childs, MD [77]
Clinical Director, NHLBI
Chief, Section of Transplantation Immunotherapy
National Heart, Lung, and Blood Institute, NIH
Bethesda, Maryland

James M. Cleary, MD, PhD [22]
Instructor in Medicine
Dana-Farber Cancer Institute
Harvard Medical School
Boston, Massachusetts

Theresa L Coetzer, MD [46]
Head: Red Cell Membrane Unit
Department of Molecular Medicine and Haematology
National Health Laboratory Service
University of the Witwatersrand
Wits Medical School
Johannesburg, South Africa

Claudia S. Cohn, MD [138]
Assistant Professor, Laboratory Medicine and Pathology
University of Minnesota
Minneapolis, Minnesota

Barry S. Coller, MD [112, 120]
Head
Allen and Frances Adler Laboratory of Blood and Vascular Biology
Physician-in-Chief
Vice President for Medical Affairs
The Rockefeller University
New York, New York

Gregory C. Connolly, MD [25]
Department of Medicine
Lipson Cancer Center
Rochester Regional Health System
Rochester, New York

Myra Coppage [137]
Associate Professor of Laboratory Medicine
Department of Pathology and Laboratory Medicine
University of Rochester
Rochester, New York

Michiel Coppens, MD, PhD [130]
Department of Vascular Medicine
Academic Medical Center
Amsterdam, The Netherlands

Francesca Cottini, MD [107]
Dana-Farber Cancer Institute
Boston, Massachusetts

Gay M. Crooks, MB, BS, FRACP [74]
Professor
Departments of Pathology & Laboratory Medicine and Pediatrics
David Geffen School of Medicine
University of California, Los Angeles
Los Angeles, California

Adam Cuker, MD, MS [118]
Assistant Professor of Medicine & of Pathology and Laboratory Medicine
Perelman School of Medicine at the University of Pennsylvania
Philadelphia, Pennsylvania

Yun Dai, MD [16]
Associate Professor of Medicine
Department of Medicine
Massey Cancer Center
Virginia Commonwealth University
Richmond, Virginia

David C. Dale, MD [65]
Professor of Medicine
Department of Medicine
University of Washington
Seattle, Washington

Chi V. Dang, MD, PhD [14]
Professor and Director
Abramson Cancer Center
University of Pennsylvania
Philadelphia, Pennsylvania

Utpal P. Davé, MD [5]
Division of Hematology/Oncology
Department of Medicine
Vanderbilt University Medical Center
Nashville, Tennessee

Randy Daughters, PhD [30]
Assistant Professor
Department of Genetics
Cell Biology, and Development, Stem Cell Institute
University of Minnesota
Minneapolis, Minnesota

Philippe de Moerloose, MD [125]
Professor
Division of Angiology and Haemostasis
University of Geneva Faculty of Medicine
Geneva, Switzerland

Madhav Dhodapkar, MBBS [21]
Arthur H. and Isabel Bunker Professor of Medicine (Hematology) and Professor of Immunobiology
Chief, Section of Hematology, Department of Internal Medicine
Clinical Research Program Leader, Hematology Program
Yale Cancer Center
New Haven, Connecticut

Angela Dispenzieri, MD [108]
Division of Hematology
Mayo Clinic
Rochester, Minnesota

Reyhan Diz-Küçükkaya, MD [117]
Associate Professor
Department of Internal Medicine
Division of Hematology
Istanbul University
Istanbul Faculty of Medicine
Istanbul, Turkey

Anne G. Douglas, BA [67, 68]
Student, Perelman School of Medicine
University of Pennsylvania (Class of 2017)
Philadelphia, Pennsylvania

Steven D. Douglas, MD [67, 68]
Professor and Associate Chair
Department of Pediatrics
Perelman School of Medicine
University of Pennsylvania
Children's Hospital of Philadelphia
Philadelphia, Pennsylvania

Martin Dreyling, MD [100]
Department of Internal Medicine III
Medical Center of the University of Munich
Munich, Germany

Ann M. Dvorak, MD [63]
Senior Pathologist, Professor of Pathology
Department of Pathology
Beth Israel Deaconess Medical Center
Harvard Medical School
Boston, Massachusetts

Dustin Dzube, MD [22]
Resident Physician
Massachusetts General Hospital
Harvard Medical School
Boston, Massachusetts

Yvonne A. Efebera, MD, MPH [78]
Associate Professor of Internal Medicine
Division of Hematology
Department of Internal Medicine
The Ohio State University
Columbus, Ohio

Deborah Elstein, PhD [72]
Gaucher Clinic
Shaare Zedek Medical Center
Jerusalem, Israel

William B. Ershler, MD [9]
Scientific Director
Institute for Advanced Studies in Aging and Geriatrics
Falls Church, Virginia

Miguel A. Escobar, MD [123]
Professor of Medicine and Pediatrics
Division of Hematology
University of Texas Health Science Center at Houston
Director, Gulf States Hemophilia and Thrombophilia Center
Houston, Texas

Andrew G. Evans, MD, PhD [102]
Assistant Professor
Department of Pathology and Laboratory Medicine
University of Rochester Medical Center
Rochester, New York

Ross M. Fasano, MD [55]
Assistant Professor
Emory University School of Medicine
Departments of Pathology and Pediatric Hematology
Assistant Director, Children's Healthcare of Atlanta Transfusion
    Services
Associate Director, Grady Health System Transfusion Service
Atlanta, Georgia

Charles W. Francis, MD [25]
Hematology/Oncology Division
University of Rochester Medical Center
Rochester, New York

Aharon G. Freud, MD, PhD [6, 94]
Assistant Professor
Department of Pathology
The Ohio State University
Columbus, Ohio

Jonathan W. Friedberg, MD [102]
Samuel Durand Professor of Medicine
Director, Wilmot Cancer Institute
University of Rochester Medical Center
Rochester, New York

Hua Fung, MD [29]
Case Western Reserve University
University Hospital of Cleveland
Cleveland, Ohio

Stephen J. Galli, MD [63]
Mary Hewitt Loveless, MD, Professor
Professor of Pathology and of Microbiology and Immunology
Chair, Department of Pathology
Stanford University School of Medicine
Stanford University Medical Center
Stanford, California

Tomas Ganz, MD, PhD [37, 42, 43]
Departments of Medicine and Pathology, David Geffen School of
    Medicine
University of California, Los Angeles
Los Angeles, California

Randy D. Gascoyne, MD, FRCPC [96]
Clinical Professor of Pathology
Research Director, Centre for Lymphoid Cancers
Departments of Pathology and Advanced Therapeutics British
Columbia Cancer Agency, the BC Centre Research Center and
University of British Columbia
Vancouver, British Columbia, Canada

Terry B. Gernsheimer, MD [139]
Professor of Medicine
Department of Medicine, Division of Hematology
University of Washington School of Medicine
Seattle Cancer Care Alliance
Seattle, Washington

Stanton Gerson, MD [29]
Director, Case Comprehensive Cancer, Seidman Cancer Center
& National Center for Regenerative Medicine
Distinguished University Professor
Case Western Reserve University
University Hospital of Cleveland
Cleveland, Ohio

Morie A. Gertz, MD, MACP [108]
Division of Hematology
Mayo Clinic
Rochester, Minnesota

Larisa J. Geskin, MD, FAAD [103, 105]
Associate Professor of Dermatology and Medicine
Director, Division of Cutaneous Oncology and Comprehensive Skin
    Cancer Center
Department of Dermatology
Columbia University
New York, New York

David Ginsburg, MD [126]
Professor, Department of Internal Medicine, Human Genetics and
    Pediatrics
Investigator, Howard Hughes Medical Institute
Life Sciences Institute
University of Michigan
Ann Arbor, Michigan

Lucy A. Godley, MD, PhD [13]
Section of Hematology/Oncology
Department of Medicine and The University of Chicago
    Comprehensive Cancer Center
The University of Chicago
Chicago, Illinois

Steven Grant, MD [16]
Professor of Medicine and Biochemistry
Shirley and Sture Gordon Olsson Professor of Oncology
Associate Director
Translational Research, Massey Cancer Center
Virginia Commonwealth University Health Sciences Center
Richmond, Virginia

Anthony R. Green, PhD, FRCP, FRCPath, FMedSci [85]
Professor of Haematology
Cambridge Institute for Medical Research and Stem Cell Institute
University of Cambridge
Cambridge, United Kingdom

Ralph Green, MD, PhD, FRCPath [41, 44]
Professor of Pathology and Medicine
University of California Davis Medical Center
Sacramento, California

Xylina T. Gregg, MD [38]
Director of Laboratory Services
Utah Cancer Specialists
Salt Lake City, Utah

Michael R. Grever, MD [93]
Chair and Professor
Department of Internal Medicine
Bertha Bouroncle MD and Andrew Pereny Chair in Medicine
The Ohio State University
Columbus, Ohio

John Gribben, MD, DSc, FRCP, FRCPath, FMedSci [76]
Chair of Medical Oncology
Barts Cancer Institute
Centre for Haemato-Oncology
Queen Mary University of London
London, United Kingdom

John H. Griffin, PhD [114]
Professor
Department of Molecular and Experimental Medicine
The Scripps Research Institute
La Jolla, California

Katherine A. Hajjar, MD [115, 135]
Professor of Pediatrics
Brine Family Professor, Department of Cell and Developmental
    Biology
Professor of Medicine
Well Cornell Medical College
Attending Pediatrician
New York Presbyterian Hospital
New York, New York

Robert D. Harrington, MD [81]
Professor of Medicine
University of Washington
Seattle, Washington

Jeanne E. Hendrickson, MD [55]
Associate Professor
Departments of Laboratory Medicine and Pediatrics
Yale University School of Medicine
New Haven, Connecticut

Paul C. Herrmann, MD, PhD [52]
Associate Professor and Chair
Department of Pathology and Human Anatomy
Loma Linda University School of Medicine
Loma Linda, California

Steven Horwitz, MD [104]
Department of Medicine
Memorial Sloan Kettering Cancer Center
New York, New York

Annie L. Hsieh, MD [14]
Department of Pathology
Johns Hopkins University, School of Medicine
Baltimore, Maryland

Zachary R. Hunter, PhD [109]
Bing Center for Waldenstrom's Macroglobulinemia
Dana-Farber Cancer Institute
Instructor of Medicine, Harvard Medical School
Boston, Massachusetts

Russell D. Hull, MD [133]
Professor
Department of Medicine
University of Calgary
Active Staff
Department of Internal Medicine
Foothills Hospital
Calgary, Alberta, Canada

Achille Iolascon, MD, PhD [39]
Professor of Medical Genetics
Dept. of Molecular Medicine and Medical Biotechnologies
University Federico II of Naples
Naples, Italy

Joseph E. Italiano Jr., PhD [112]
Associate Professor of Medicine
Brigham and Women's Hospital
Harvard Medical School
Boston, Massachusetts

Benjamin Izar, MD, PhD [22]
Post-doctoral Scientist
Dana-Farber Cancer Institute and Broad Institute
Associate Physician, Brigham and Women's Hospital
Harvard Medical School
Boston, Massachusetts

Siegfried Janz, MD, DSc [105]
Division of Hematology/Oncology & Blood and Marrow Transplantation
Department of Pathology, Carver College of Medicine
University of Iowa Health Care
Iowa City, Iowa

Jill M. Johnsen, MD [126]
Assistant Member, Research Institute
Bloodworks Northwest
Puget Sound Blood Center
Assistant Professor, Division of Hematology
Department of Medicine
University of Washington
Seattle, Washington

Lynn B. Jorde, PhD [10]
H. A. and Edna Benning Presidential Professor
Department of Human Genetics
University of Utah School of Medicine
Salt Lake City, Utah

Bindu Kanapuru, MD [9]
Institute for Advanced Studies in Aging and Geriatrics
Falls Church, Virginia

Kenneth Kaushansky, MD, MACP [17, 18, 111, 116, 119]
Senior Vice President, Health Sciences
Dean, School of Medicine
SUNY Distinguished Professor
Stony Brook Medicine
State University of New York
Stony Brook, New York

Nigel S. Key, MB, ChB, FRCP [123]
Harold R. Roberts Distinguished Professor of Medicine
Director, University of North Carolina Hemophilia and Thrombosis
    Center
Chapel Hill, North Carolina

Thomas J. Kipps, MD, PhD [75]
Evelyn and Edwin Tasch Chair in Cancer Research
Professor of Medicine
Division of Hematology/Oncology
Deputy Director for Research Operations
Moores UCSD Cancer Center
University of California, San Diego
La Jolla, California

Mark J. Koury, MD [5]
Division of Hematology/Oncology
Department of Medicine
Vanderbilt University Medical Center
Nashville, Tennessee

Abdullah Kutlar, MD [49]
Professor of Medicine
Georgia Sickle Cell Center
Medical College of Georgia
Sickle Cell Center
Augusta, Georgia

Robert A. Kyle, MD [110,]
Professor of Medicine
Laboratory Medicine and Pathology
Mayo Clinic
Rochester, Minnesota

Lewis L. Lanier, PhD [77]
Professor
Department of Microbiology and Immunology
University of California, San Francisco
San Francisco, California

Richard A. Larson, MD [91]
Section of Hematology/Oncology
Department of Medicine and the Comprehensive Cancer Center
University of Chicago
Chicago, Illinois

Michelle M. Le Beau, PhD [13]
Section of Hematology/Oncology
Department of Medicine and the Center Research Center
University of Chicago
Chicago, Illinois

Frank W.G. Leebeek, MD, PhD [128]
Professor of Hematology
Department of Hematology
Erasmus University Medical Center
Rotterdam, The Netherlands

Marcel Levi, MD, PhD [116, 122, 129]
Department of Medicine/Vascular Medicine
Academic Medical Center
University of Amsterdam
Amsterdam, The Netherlands

Marshall A. Lichtman, MD [1, 35, 53, 64, 69, 70, 83, 86, 88, 89, 95, 106]
Professor of Medicine and of Biochemistry and Biophysics
University of Rochester Medical Center
Rochester, New York

Jane L. Liesveld, MD [88, 89]
Professor of Medicine (Hematology-Oncology)
James P. Wilmot Cancer Institute
University of Rochester Medical Center
Rochester, New York

Ton Lisman, PhD [128]
Professor of Experimental Surgery
Surgical Research Laboratory and Section of Hepatobiliary Surgery and Liver Transplantation
Department of Surgery
University Medical Center, Groningen
Groningen, The Netherlands

John S. (Pete) Lollar III, MD [127]
Aflac Cancer Center and Blood Disorders Services
Department of Pediatrics
Emory University
Atlanta, Georgia

Christine Lomas-Francis, MSc, FIBMS [136]
Technical Director
Laboratory of Immunohematology and Genomics
New York Blood center
New York, New York

José A. Lópéz, MD [117]
Chief Scientific Officer
Bloodworks Northwest
Professor of Medicine and Biochemistry
University of Washington
Seattle, Washington

Robert Lowsky, MD [23]
Division of Blood and Marrow Transplantation
Stanford University
Stanford, California

Gerard Lozanski, MD [93]
Director, Hematopathology
Medical Director
Flow Cytometry Laboratory
Associate Professor—Clinical
Department of Pathology
The Ohio State University
Columbus, Ohio

Naomi L. C. Luban, MD [55]
Professor, Pediatrics and Pathology
George Washington University Medical Center
Division Chief, Laboratory Medicine
Director, Transfusion Medicine/Donor Center
Children's National Medical Center
Washington, D.C.

Crystal L. Mackall, MH [21]
Head, Immunology Section and
Chief, Pediatric Oncology Branch
National Cancer Institute
Bethesda, Maryland

Aaron J. Marcus, MD* [115]
Professor of Medicine
Weill Cornell Medical College
Attending Physician
New York Harbor Healthcare System
New York, New York

Elaine R. Mardis, PhD [11]
Robert E. and Louise F. Dunn Distinguished Professor of Medicine
Co-director, The Genome Institute, Division of Genomics and Bioinformatics, Department of Medicine, Washington University School of Medicine
Siteman Cancer Center, Washington University School of Medicine
Saint Louis, Missouri

Fabienne McClanahan, MD, PhD [76]
Barts Cancer Institute
Centre for Haemato-Oncology
Queen Mary University of London
London, United Kingdom

Kenneth L. McClain, MD, PhD [71]
Professor of Pediatrics
Texas Children's Cancer Center/Hematology
Baylor College of Medicine
Houston, Texas

Jeffrey McCullough, MD [138]
Professor
Department of Laboratory Medicine and Pathology
American Red Cross Professor, Transfusion Medicine
University of Minnesota Medical School
Minneapolis, Minnesota

Janice McFarland, MD [137]
Blood Center of Southeast Wisconsin
Milwaukee, Wisconsin

Shannon L. Meeks, MD [127]
Aflac Cancer Center and Blood Disorders Services
Department of Pediatrics
Emory University
Atlanta, Georgia

*Deceased

Neha Mehta, MD [104]
Department of Medicine
Memorial Sloan Kettering Cancer Center
New York, New York

Marzia Menegatti, MD [124]
Angelo Bianchi Bonomi Hemophilia and Thrombosis Center
Fondazione IRCCS Ca' Granda Ospedale Maggiore Policlinico
University of Milan
Milan, Italy

Giampaolo Merlini, MD [109]
Director, Center for Research and Treatment of Systematic
    Amyloidoses
University Hospital Policlinico San Matteo
Professor, Department of Medicine
University of Pavia
Pavia, Italy

Dean D. Metcalfe, MD [63]
Chief, Laboratory of Allergic Diseases
Chief, MCBS/LAD
NAID/National Institute of Health
Bethesda, Maryland

H. A. Mettine Bos, HA, PhD [113]
Assistant Professor
Division of Thrombosis and Hemostasis
Einthoven Laboratory for Experimental Vascular Medicine
Leiden University Medical Center
Leiden, The Netherlands

Saskia Middeldorp, MD, PhD [130]
Department of Vascular Medicine
Academic Medical Center
Amsterdam, The Netherlands

Martha P. Mims, MD, PhD [8]
Professor of Medicine
Section Chief, Section of Hematology/Oncology
Baylor College of Medicine
Houston, Texas

Constantine S. Mitsiades, MD, PhD [22]
Assistant Professor of Medicine
Dana-Farber Cancer Institute
Harvard Medical School
Boston, Massachusetts

Joel Moake, MD [51]
Senior Research Scientist and Associate Director
Biomedical Engineering Laboratory
Rice University
Houston, Texas

Narla Mohandas, D.Sc [31]
Red Cell Physiology Laboratory
New York Blood Center
New York, New York

Emile R. Mohler III, MD [134]
Director, Vascular Medicine
Professor of Medicine
Division of Cardiovascular Medicine
Perelman School of Medicine at the University of Pennsylvania
Philadelphia, Pennsylvania

Jeffrey J. Molldrem, MD [27]
Professor of Medicine
Stem Cell Transplantation and Cellular Therapy,
MD Anderson Cancer Center
Houston, Texas

Alison Moskowitz, MD [104]
Department of Medicine
Memorial Sloan Kettering Cancer Center
New York, New York

Laurent O. Mosnier, PhD [114]
Associate Professor
Department of Molecular and Experimental Medicine
The Scripps Research Institute
La Jolla, California

William A. Muller, MD, PhD [115]
Magerstadt Professor and Chair
Department of Pathology
Feinberg School of Medicine
Northwestern University
Chicago, Illinois

Natarajan Muthusamy, DVM, PhD [73]
Professor of Medicine
Division of Hematology
Department of Internal Medicine
The Ohio State University
Columbus, Ohio

Kalyan Nadiminti, MD [105]
Division of Hematology/Oncology & Blood and Marrow Transplantation
Department of Pathology, Carver College of Medicine
University of Iowa Health Care
Iowa City, Iowa

Srikanth Nagalla, MBBS, MS [56]
Assistant Professor of Medicine
Division of Hematology
Cardeza Foundation for Hematologic Research
Thomas Jefferson University
Philadelphia, Pennsylvania

Kavita Natrajan, MBBS [49]
Associate Professor of Medicine
Division of Hematology/Oncology
Georgia Regents University
Augusta, Georgia

Marguerite Neerman-Arbez, PhD [125]
Professor
Department of Genetic Medicine and Development
University of Geneva Faculty of Medicine
Geneva, Switzerland

Robert S. Negrin, MD [23]
Division of Blood and Marrow Transplantation
Stanford University
Stanford, California

Luigi D. Notarangelo, MD [80]
Professor of Pediatrics and Pathology
Harvard Medical School
Jeffrey Modell Chair of Pediatric Immunology Research
Division of Immunology, Children's Hospital Boston
Boston, Massachusetts

Hans D. Ochs, MD [80]
Professor of Pediatrics
Jeffrey Modell Chair of Pediatric Immunology Research
Division of Immunology
Seattle Children's Research Hospital
Department of Pediatrics
University of Washington
Seattle, Washington

Elizabeth O'Donnell, MD [107]
Massachusetts General Hospital
Boston, Massachusetts

Mark J. Osborn, PhD [30]
Assistant Professor
Pediatrics
Blood and Marrow Transplantation, Stem Cell Institute
University of Minnesota
Minneapolis, Minnesota

Charles H. Packman, MD [54]
Professor of Medicine
University of North Carolina School of Medicine
Levine Cancer Institute, Hematologic Oncology and Blood Disorders
Charlotte, North Carolina

James Palis, MD [7]
Professor of Pediatrics
University of Rochester Medical Center
Rochester, New York

Charles J. Parker, MD [40]
Professor of Medicine
Division of Hematology and Bone Marrow Transplantation
University of Utah School of Medicine
Salt Lake City, Utah

Flora Peyvandi, MD [124]
Angelo Bianchi Bonomi Hemophilia and Thrombosis Center
Fondazione IRCCS Ca' Granda Ospedale Maggiore Policlinico
University of Milan
Milan, Italy

John D. Phillips, PhD [58]
Associate Professor of Medicine
Division of Hematology
University of Utah School of Medicine
Salt Lake City, Utah

Mortimer Poncz, MD [118]
Jane Fishman Grinberg Professor of Pediatrics
Perelman School of Medicine at the University of Pennsylvania
Children's Hospital of Philadelphia
Philadelphia, Pennsylvania

Prem Ponka, MD [59]
Professor of Physiology and Medicine
Lady Davis Institute
McGill University
Montreal, Quebec, Canada

Pierluigi Porcu, MD [94]
Professor of Internal Medicine
Division of Hematology, and Comprehensive Cancer Center
The Ohio State University
Columbus, Ohio

Jaroslav F. Prchal, MD [84]
Director, Department of Oncology
St. Mary's Hospital
Montreal, Quebec, Canada

Josef T. Prchal, MD [32, 33, 34, 45, 50, 57, 59, 84, 86]
The Charles A. Nugent, M.D., and Margaret Nugent Professor
Division of Hematology, Pathology, and Genetics
University of Utah
Salt Lake City, Utah
Department of Pathophysiology
First Faculty of Medicine
Charles University
Prague, Czech Republic

Oliver W. Press, MD, PhD [95, 97, 98, 99]
Acting Senior Vice President, Fred Hutchinson Cancer Research Center
Acting Director, Clinical Research Division, FHCRC
Recipient, Dr. Penny E. Peterson Memorial Chair for Lymphoma Research
Professor of Medicine and Bioengineering
University of Washington
Seattle, Washington

Gordana Raca, MD, PhD [13]
Section of Hematology/Oncology
Department of Medicine and The University of Chicago Comprehensive Cancer Center
University of Chicago
Chicago, Illinois

Noopur Raje, MD [107]
Massachusetts General Hospital
Boston, Massachusetts

Jacob H. Rand, MD [131]
Professor of Pathology and Medicine
Director of Hematology Laboratory
Montefiore Medical Center
The University Hospital for the Albert Einstein College of Medicine
Bronx, New York

A. Koneti Rao, MD [120]
Sol Sherry Professor of Medicine
Director of Benign Hematology, Hemostasis and Thrombosis
Co-Director, Sol Sherry Thrombosis Research Center
Temple University School of Medicine
Philadelphia, Pennsylvania

Gary E. Raskob, PhD [133]
Dean, College of Public Health
Regents Professor, Epidemiology and Medicine
The University of Oklahoma Health Science Center
Oklahoma City, Oklahoma

Vishnu VB Reddy, MD [45]
Department of Pathology,
University of Alabama in Birmingham,
Birmingham, Alabama

John C. Reed, MD, PhD [15]
Pharmaceutical Research & Early Development
Roche Innovation Center-Basel
Basel, Switzerland

Majed A. Refaai, MD [138]
Associate Professor
Department of Pathology and Laboratory Medicine
University of Rochester Medical Center
Rochester, New York

Marion E. Reid, PhD, DSc (Hon.) [136]
(Retired)
New York Blood Center
New York, New York

Pieter H. Reitsma, PhD [113]
Professor in Experimental Molecular Medicine
Division of Thrombosis and Hemostasis
Einthoven Laboratory for Experimental Vascular Medicine
Leiden University Medical Center
Leiden, The Netherlands

Andrew R. Rezvani, MD [23]
Division of Blood and Marrow Transplantation
Stanford University
Stanford, California

Katayoun Rezvani, MD [27]
Professor of Medicine
Stem Cell Transplantation and Cellular Therapy
MD Anderson Cancer Center
Houston, Texas

Paul G. Richardson, MD [22]
Professor of Medicine
Dana-Farber Cancer Institute
Harvard Medical School
Boston, Massachusetts

Stanley R. Riddell, MD [26]
Member, Clinical Research Division
Fred Hutchinson Cancer Research Center
Seattle, Washington

Jia Ruan, MD, PhD [135]
Associate Professor
Department of Medicine
Weill Cornell Medical College
Associate Attending Physician
New York Presbyterian Hospital
New York, New York

Daniel H. Ryan, MD [2, 3]
Professor Emeritus
Department of Pathology and Laboratory Medicine
University of Rochester Medical Center
Rochester, New York

J. Evan Sadler, MD, PhD [132]
Ira M. Lang Professor of Medicine
Washington University School of Medicine
St. Louis, Missouri

Andrew I. Schafer, MD [134]
Professor of Medicine,
Director, The Richard T. Silver Center for Myeloproliferative
    Neoplasms,
Weill Cornell Medical College
New York, New York

Stanley L. Schrier, MD [4]
Professor of Medicine (Hematology)
Active emeritus
Division of Hematology
Stanford University School of Medicine
Stanford, California

Christopher S. Seet, MD [74]
Department of Medicine
Division of Hematology/Oncology
David Geffen School of Medicine
University of California
Los Angeles, California

George B. Segel, MD [7, 35]
Professor of Pediatrics, Emeritus
Professor of Medicine
University of Rochester Medical Center
Rochester, New York

Uri Seligsohn, MD [116, 129]
Professor of Hematology and Director
Amalia Biron Research Institute of Thrombosis and Hemostasis
Sheba Medical Center
Tel-Hashomer and Sackler Faculty of Medicine
Tel Aviv University
Tel Aviv, Israel

Sanford J. Shattil, MD [121]
Professor and Chief, Division of Hematology-Oncology
Department of Medicine
University of California, San Diego
Adjunct Professor of Molecular and Experimental Medicine
The Scripps Research Institute
La Jolla, California

Taimur Sher, MD [108]
Division of Hematology/Oncology
Mayo Clinic
Jacksonville, Florida

Brian F. Skinnider, MD [96]
Clinical Associate Professor
Department of Pathology
Vancouver General Hospital, British Columbia Cancer Agency, and
    University of British Columbia
Vancouver, British Columbia, Canada

Sherrill J. Slichter, MD [139]
Professor of Medicine
Department of Medicine, Division of Hematology
University of Washington School of Medicine
Bloodworks Northwest
Seattle, Washington

C. Wayne Smith, MD [60, 61]
Professor and Head, Section of Leukocyte Biology
Department of Pediatrics
Baylor College of Medicine
Houston, Texas

Stephen D. Smith, MD [98]
Associate Professor, Internal Medicine Division of Medical Oncology
University of Washington
Seattle, Washington

Susan S. Smyth, MD, PhD [112]
Jeff Gill Professor of Cardiology
Chief, Division of Cardiovascular Medicine
Medical Director, Gill Heart Institute
University of Kentucky
Lexington, Kentucky

David P. Steensma, MD [87]
Department of Medical Oncology
Division of Hematological Malignancies
Dana-Farber Cancer Institute
Boston, Massachusetts

Sean R. Stowell, MD, PhD [127]
Department of Pathology and Laboratory Medicine
Emory University
Atlanta, Georgia

David Stroncek [137]
Department of Transfusion Medicine
National Institutes of Health
Bethesda, Maryland

Madina Sukhanova, PhD [13]
Section of Hematology/Oncology
Department of Medicine and the Center Research Center
University of Chicago
Chicago, Illinois

Perumal Thiagarajan, MD [32, 33]
Professor of Medicine and Pathology
Baylor College of Medicine
Director, Blood Bank and Hematology Laboratory
Michael E. DeBakey VA Medical Center
Houston, Texas

Jakub Tolar, MD, PhD [30]
Professor, Department of Pediatrics
Blood and Marrow Transplantation, Stem Cell Institute
University of Minnesota
Minneapolis, Minnesota

Steven P. Treon [109]
Director, Bing Center for Waldenstrom's Macroglobulinemia
Dana-Farber Cancer Institute
Associate Professor, Harvard Medical School
Boston, Massachusetts

Guido Tricot, MD, PhD [105]
Division of Hematology/Oncology & Blood and Marrow
    Transplantation
Department of Pathology, Carver College of Medicine
University of Iowa Health Care
Iowa City, Iowa

Giorgio Trinchieri, MD [77]
Director, Cancer and Inflammation Program
Chief, Laboratory of Experimental Immunology
Center for Cancer Research, NCI, NIH
Bethesda, Maryland

Wouter W. van Solinge, PhD [47]
Professor of Laboratory Medicine
Head of Department
Chair and Medical Director Division Laboratories and Pharmacy
Department of Clinical Chemistry and Haematology
University Medical Center Utrecht
Utrecht, The Netherlands

Cornelis van 't Veer, PhD [113]
Associate Professor
Center for Experimental and Molecular Medicine
Academic Medical Center
Amsterdam, The Netherlands

Richard van Wijk, PhD [47]
Associate professor
Department of Clinical Chemistry and Haematology
Division Laboratories and Pharmacy
University Medical Center Utrecht
Utrecht, The Netherlands

Sumithira Vasu, MBBS [79]
Assistant Professor
Medical Director, Cell Therapy Lab
Blood and Marrow Transplantation Section
Division of Hematology
The Ohio State University
Columbus, Ohio

John Wagner, MD [30]
Professor, Department of Pediatrics
Blood and Marrow Transplantation, Stem Cell Institute
University of Minnesota
Minneapolis, Minnesota

Dietlind L. Wahner-Roedler, MD [110]
Professor of Medicine
Mayo Clinic
Rochester, Minnesota

Zandra E. Walton [14]
Abramson Family Cancer Research Institute
Perelman School of Medicine
University of Pennsylvania
Philadelphia, Pennsylvania

Peter A. Ward, MD [19]
Godfrey D. Stobbe Professor of Pathology
Department of Pathology
University of Michigan Medical School
Ann Arbor, Michigan

Andrew J. Wardlaw, MD, PhD [62]
Institute for Lung Health
Department of Infection
Immunity and Inflammation
Leicester University Medical School
Leicester, United Kingdom

Jeffrey S. Warren, MD [19]
Aldred S. Warthin Professor of Pathology
Department of Pathology
University of Michigan Medical School
Ann Arbor, Michigan

Lukas D. Wartman, MD [11]
Assistant Professor, Section of Stem Cell Biology
Division of Oncology, Department of Medicine, Washington
    University School of Medicine
Siteman Cancer Center, Washington University School of Medicine
Assistant Director, Section of Cancer Genomics
The Genome Institute, Washington University School of Medicine
St. Louis, Missouri

Sir David J. Weatherall, MD [48]
Professor
Weatherall Institute of Molecular Medicine
John Radcliffe Hospital
Headington, Oxford, United Kingdom

Robert Weinstein, MD [28]
Professor of Medicine and Pathology
University of Massachusetts Medical School
Chief, Division of Transfusion Medicine
UMass Memorial Medical Center
Worcester, Massachusetts

Karl Welte, MD [65]
Senior-Professor
Department of Pediatrics
University of Tübingen
Tübingen, Germany

Erik Wendlandt, PhD [105]
Division of Hematology/Oncology & Blood and Marrow
    Transplantation
Department of Pathology, Carver College of Medicine
University of Iowa Health Care
Iowa City, Iowa

Sidney Whiteheart, PhD [112]
Professor
Molecular and Cellular Biochemistry
University of Kentucky College of Medicine
Lexington, Kentucky

Lucia Wolgast, MD [131]
Assistant Professor of Pathology (Clinical)
Director, Clinical Laboratories, Moses Division
Associate Director, Hematology Laboratories
Montefiore Medical Center/Albert Einstein College of Medicine
Department of Pathology
Bronx, New York

Neal S. Young, MD [36]
Hematology Branch
National Heart, Lung, and Blood
National Institutes of Health
Bethesda, Maryland

Fenghuang Zhan, MD, PhD [105]
Division of Hematology/Oncology & Blood and Marrow
    Transplantation
Department of Pathology, Carver College of Medicine
University of Iowa Health Care
Iowa City, Iowa

Ari Zimran, MD [72]
Gaucher Clinic
Shaare Zedek Medical Center
Jerusalem, Israel

Pier Luigi Zinzani, MD, PhD [101]
Professor
Institute of Hematology "L. e A. Seràgnoli"
University of Bologna
Bologna, Italy

PREFACE

The first edition of *Williams Hematology* (né *Hematology*) was published in 1972. This, our 9th edition, will represent our continued efforts over nearly one-half century to provide the most current concepts of the pathophysiology and treatment of hematologic diseases.

The rate of growth in our understanding of diseases of blood cells and coagulation pathways provides a challenge for editors of a comprehensive textbook of hematology. The sequencing of individual genomes, analysis of the "dark DNA" and noncoding RNAs, advances in knowledge in proteomics, metabolomics, and other "-omics" fields, as applied to hematologic disorders, have accelerated the understanding of the pathogenesis of the diseases of our interest. The rate at which basic knowledge in molecular and cellular biology and immunology has been translated into improved diagnostic and therapeutic methods is equally impressive. Specific molecular targets for therapy in several hematologic disorders have become reality, and it is not hyperbole to state that hematology is the poster child for the rational design of therapeutics applicable to other fields of medicine.

This edition of *Williams Hematology* includes changes designed to facilitate ease of access to information, both within the book and its associated links, and has been modestly reorganized to reflect our greater understanding of the origins of hematologic disorders. Each chapter has been revised or rewritten to provide current information. Four new chapters have been added and other notable changes have been made. Chapter 4 "Consultative Hematology" is new to this edition. The chapter "Epigenetics and Genomics" has been divided into separate chapters to reflect the growth of knowledge in those disciplines. Chapter 14, "Metabolism of Hematologic Neoplastic Cells" is new, as this topic has become the basis of multiple potential drug targets for hematologic disease. A section on "Autophagy" has been added to Chap 15 "Apoptosis Mechanisms: Relevance to the Hematopoietic System," as the topic is becoming increasingly important for understanding of the physiology of blood cell development; and an independent chapter "Heparin-Induced Thrombocytopenia" (Chap 118) has been created to reflect both its pathophysiologic and clinical importance. Recognizing that at the heart of diagnostic hematology is blood and marrow cell morphology, we have continued our incorporation of informative color images of the relevant disease topics in each chapter, allowing easy access to illustrations of cell morphology important to diagnosis.

The 9th edition of *Williams Hematology* is also available online, as part of the excellent www.accessmedicine.com website. With direct links to a comprehensive drug therapy database and to other important medical texts, including *Harrison's Principles of Internal Medicine* and *Goodman and Gilman's The Pharmacological Basis of Therapeutics*, *Williams Hematology Online* is part of a powerful resource covering all disciplines within medical education and practice. The online edition of *Williams Hematology* also includes PubMed links to journal articles cited in the references.

In addition, *Williams Manual of Hematology* will be revised to reflect the diagnostic and therapeutic advances incorporated in the 9th edition of *Williams Hematology*. The convenient *Manual* features the most clinically salient content from the parent text, and is useful in time-restricted clinical situations. The *Manual* will be available for iPhone™ and other mobile formats.

The readers of the 9th edition of *Williams Hematology* will note a "changing of (some of) the guard" of our editorial group; Drs. Marcel Levi (a member of the 8th edition of *Williams Manual of Hematology* editorial group), Oliver Press, Linda Burns, and Michael Caligiuri have joined continuing editors Drs. Kenneth Kaushansky, Marshall Lichtman, and Josef Prchal in the 9th edition.

The production of this book required the timely cooperation of 101 contributors for the production of 139 chapters. We are grateful for their work in providing this comprehensive and up-to-date text. Despite the growth of both basic and clinical knowledge and the passion that each of our contributors brings to the topic of their chapter, we have been able to maintain the text in a single volume through scrupulous attention to chapter length.

Each editor has had expert administrative assistance in the management of the manuscripts for which they were primarily responsible. We thank Susan Madden in Salt Lake City, Utah; Nancy Press and Deborah Lemon in Seattle, Washington; and Annie Thompson, Rebecca Posey, and Kimberly Morley in Columbus, Ohio for their very helpful participation in the production of the book. Special thanks go to Susan Daley in Rochester, New York, and Marie Brito in Stony Brook, New York, who were responsible for coordinating the management of 139 chapters, including many new figures and tables, and managing other administrative matters, a challenging task that Ms. Daley and Ms. Brito performed with skill and good humor. The editors also acknowledge the interest and support of our colleagues at McGraw-Hill, including James F. Shanahan, Publisher, Medical Publishing; Karen Edmonson, Senior Editor for Williams Hematology; and Harriet Lebowitz, Senior Project Development Editor for *Williams Hematology*.

Kenneth Kaushansky
Marshall A. Lichtman
Joseph T. Prchal
Marcel Levi
Oliver W. Press
Linda J. Burns
Michael A. Caligiuri

Part I Clinical Evaluation of the Patient

1. Initial Approach to the Patient: History and Physical Examination.   3

2. Examination of Blood Cells   11

3. Examination of the Marrow.   27

4. Consultative Hematology   41

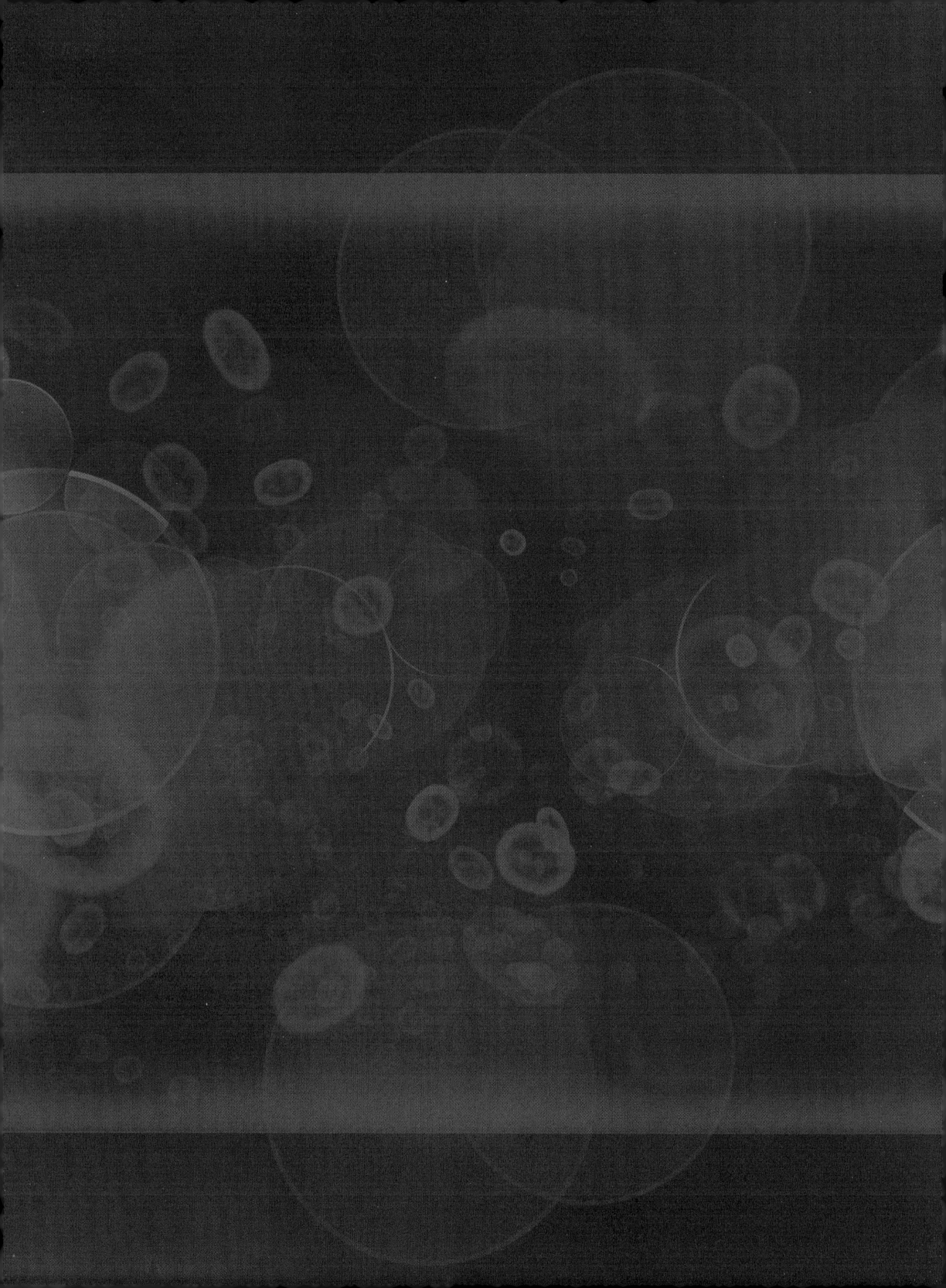

CHAPTER 1
INITIAL APPROACH TO THE PATIENT: HISTORY AND PHYSICAL EXAMINATION

Marshall A. Lichtman and Linda J. Burns

SUMMARY

The care of a patient with a suspected hematologic abnormality begins with a systematic attempt to determine the nature of the illness by eliciting an in-depth medical history and performing a thorough physical examination. The physician should identify the patient's symptoms systematically and obtain as much relevant information as possible about their origin and evolution and about the general health of the patient by appropriate questions designed to explore the patient's recent and remote experience. Reviewing previous records may add important data for understanding the onset or progression of illness. Hereditary and environmental factors should be carefully sought and evaluated. The use of drugs and medications, nutritional patterns, and sexual behavior should be considered. The physician follows the medical history with a physical examination to obtain evidence for tissue and organ abnormalities that can be assessed through bedside observation to permit a careful search for signs of the illnesses suggested by the history. Skin changes and hepatic, splenic, or lymph nodal enlargement are a few findings that may be of considerable help in pointing toward a diagnosis. Additional history is obtained during the physical examination, as findings suggest an additional or alternative consideration. Thus, the history and physical examination should be considered as a unit, providing the basic information with which further diagnostic information is integrated: blood and marrow studies, imaging studies, and biopsies.

Primary hematologic diseases are common in the aggregate, but hematologic manifestations secondary to other diseases occur even more frequently. For example, the signs and symptoms of anemia and the presence of enlarged lymph nodes are common clinical findings that may be related to a hematologic disease but occur frequently as secondary manifestations of disorders not considered primarily hematologic. A wide variety of diseases may produce signs or symptoms of hematologic illness. Thus, in patients with a connective tissue disease, all the signs and symptoms of anemia may be elicited and lymphadenopathy may be notable, but additional findings are usually present that indicate primary involvement of some system besides the hematopoietic (marrow) or lymphopoietic (lymph nodes or other lymphatic sites). In this discussion, emphasis is placed on the clinical findings resulting from either primary hematologic disease or the complications of hematologic disorders so as to avoid presenting an extensive catalog of signs and symptoms encountered in general clinical medicine.

Acronyms and Abbreviations: Ig, immunoglobulin; IL, interleukin; POEMS, polyneuropathy, organomegaly, endocrinopathy, monoclonal gammopathy, and skin changes; PS, performance status.

In each discussion of specific diseases in subsequent chapters, the signs and symptoms that accompany the particular disorder are presented, and the clinical findings are covered in detail. In this chapter, a more general systematic approach is taken.

● THE HEMATOLOGY CONSULTATION

Table 1–1 lists the major abnormalities that result in the evaluation of the patient by the hematologist. The signs indicated in Table 1–1 may reflect a primary or secondary hematologic problem. For example, immature granulocytes in the blood may be signs of myeloid diseases such as myelogenous leukemia, or, depending on the frequency of these cells and the level of immaturity, the dislodgment of cells resulting from marrow metastases of a carcinoma. Nucleated red cells in the blood may reflect the breakdown in the marrow–blood interface seen in primary myelofibrosis or the hypoxia of congestive heart failure. Certain disorders have a propensity for secondary hematologic abnormalities; renal, liver, and connective tissue diseases are prominent among such abnormalities. Chronic alcoholism, nutritional fetishes, and the use of certain medications may be causal factors in blood cell or coagulation protein disorders. Pregnant women and persons of older age are prone to certain hematologic disorders: anemia, thrombocytopenia, or intravascular coagulation in the former case, and hematologic malignancies, pernicious anemia and the anemia of aging in the latter. The history and physical examination can provide vital clues to the possible diagnosis and also to the rationale choice of laboratory tests.

● THE HISTORY

In today's technology- and procedure-driven medical environment, the importance of carefully gathering information from patient inquiry and examination is at risk of losing its primacy. The history (and physical examination) remains the vital starting point for the evaluation of any clinical problem.[1-3]

GENERAL SYMPTOMS AND SIGNS

Performance status (PS) is used to establish semiquantitatively the extent of a patient's disability. This status is important in evaluating patient comparability in clinical trials, in determining the likely tolerance to cytotoxic therapy, and in evaluating the effects of therapy. Table 1–2 presents a well-founded set of criteria for measuring PS.[4] An abbreviated version sometimes is used, as proposed by the Eastern Cooperative Oncology Group (Table 1–3).[5]

Weight loss is a frequent accompaniment of many serious diseases, including primary hematologic malignancies, but it is not a prominent accompaniment of most hematologic diseases. Many "wasting" diseases, such as disseminated carcinoma and tuberculosis, cause anemia, and pronounced emaciation should suggest one of these diseases rather than anemia as the primary disorder.

Fever is a common early manifestation of the aggressive lymphomas or acute leukemias as a result of pyrogenic cytokines (e.g., interleukin [IL]-1, IL-6, and IL-8) released as a reflection of the disease itself. After chemotherapy-induced cytopenias or in the face of accompanying immunodeficiency, infection is usually the cause of fever. In patients with "fever of unknown origin," lymphoma, particularly Hodgkin lymphoma, should be considered. Occasionally, primary myelofibrosis, acute leukemia, advanced myelodysplastic syndrome, and other lymphomas may also cause fever. In rare patients with severe pernicious

TABLE 1–1. Findings That May Lead to a Hematology Consultation

Decreased hemoglobin concentration (anemia)

Increased hemoglobin concentration (polycythemia)

Elevated serum ferritin level

Leukopenia or neutropenia

Immature granulocytes or nucleated red cells in the blood Pancytopenia

Granulocytosis: neutrophilia, eosinophilia, basophilia, or mastocytosis

Monocytosis

Lymphocytosis

Lymphadenopathy

Splenomegaly

Hypergammaglobulinemia: monoclonal or polyclonal

Purpura

Thrombocytopenia

Thrombocytosis

Exaggerated bleeding: spontaneous or trauma related

Prolonged partial thromboplastin or prothrombin coagulation times

Venous thromboembolism

Thrombophilia

Obstetrical adverse events (e.g., recurrent fetal loss, stillbirth, and HELLP syndrome)

HELLP, *h*emolytic anemia, *e*levated *l*iver enzymes, and *l*ow *p*latelet count.

TABLE 1–2. Criteria of Performance Status (Karnofsky Scale)[4]

Able to carry on normal activity; no special care is needed.

100%	Normal; no complaints, no evidence of disease
90%	Able to carry on normal activity; minor signs or symptoms of disease
80%	Normal activity with effort; some signs or symptoms of disease

Unable to work; able to live at home, care for most personal needs; a varying amount of assistance is needed.

70%	Cares for self; unable to carry on normal activity or to do active work
60%	Requires occasional assistance but is able to care for most personal needs
50%	Requires considerable assistance and frequent medical care

Unable to care for self; requires equivalent of institutional or hospital care; disease may be progressing rapidly.

40%	Disabled; requires special care and assistance
30%	Severely disabled; hospitalization is indicated though death not imminent
20%	Very sick; hospitalization necessary; active supportive treatment necessary
10%	Moribund; fatal processes progressing rapidly
0%	Dead

Adapted with permission from Mor V, Laliberte L, Morris JN, Wiemann M: The Karnofsky performance status scale: An examination of its reliability and validity in a research setting *Cancer* 1984 May 1; 53(9):2002–2007.

TABLE 1–3. Eastern Cooperative Oncology Group Performance Status[5]

Grade	Activity
0	Fully active, able to carry on all predisease performance without restriction
1	Restricted in physically strenuous activity but ambulatory and able to carry out work of a light or sedentary nature, e.g., light housework, office work
2	Ambulatory and capable of all self-care but unable to carry out any work activities; up and about more than 50% of waking hours
3	Capable of only limited self-care, confined to bed or chair more than 50% of waking hours
4	Completely disabled; cannot carry on any self-care; totally confined to bed or chair
5	Dead

Oken MM, Creech RH, Tormey DC, et al: Toxicity and response criteria of the Eastern Cooperative Oncology Group. *Am J Clin Oncol.*

anemia or hemolytic anemia, fever may be present. *Chills* may accompany severe hemolytic processes and the bacteremia that may complicate the immunocompromised or neutropenic patient. *Night sweats* suggest the presence of low-grade fever and may occur in patients with lymphoma or leukemia.

Fatigue, malaise, and *lassitude* are such common accompaniments of both physical and emotional disorders that their evaluation is complex and often difficult. In patients with serious disease, these symptoms may be readily explained by fever, muscle wasting, or other associated findings. Patients with moderate or severe anemia frequently complain of fatigue, malaise, or lassitude and these symptoms may accompany the hematologic malignancies. Fatigue or lassitude may occur also with iron deficiency even in the absence of sufficient anemia to account for the symptom. In slowly developing chronic anemias, the patient may not recognize reduced exercise tolerance, or other loss of physical capabilities except in retrospect, after a remission or a cure has been induced by appropriate therapy. Anemia may be responsible for more symptoms than has been traditionally recognized, as suggested by the remarkable improvement in quality of life of most uremic patients treated with erythropoietin.

Weakness may accompany anemia or the wasting of malignant processes, in which cases it is manifest as a general loss of strength or reduced capacity for exercise. The weakness may be localized as a result of neurologic complications of hematologic disease. In vitamin B_{12} deficiency (e.g., pernicious anemia), there may be weakness of the lower extremities, accompanied by numbness, tingling, and unsteadiness of gait. Peripheral neuropathy also occurs with monoclonal immunoglobulinemias. Weakness of one or more extremities in patients with leukemia, myeloma, or lymphoma may signify central or peripheral nervous system invasion or compression as a result of vertebral collapse, a paraneoplastic syndrome (e.g., encephalitis), or brain or meningeal involvement. Myopathy secondary to malignancy occurs with the hematologic malignancies and is usually manifest as weakness of proximal muscle groups. Foot drop or wrist drop may occur in lead poisoning, amyloidosis, systemic autoimmune diseases, or as a complication of vincristine therapy. Paralysis may occur in acute intermittent porphyria.

SPECIFIC SYMPTOMS OR SIGNS

Nervous System

Headache may be the result of a number of causes related to hematologic diseases. Anemia or polycythemia may cause mild to severe headache.

Invasion or compression of the brain by leukemia or lymphoma, or opportunistic infection of the central nervous system by *Cryptococcus* or *Mycobacterium* species, may also cause headache in patients with hematologic malignancies. Hemorrhage into the brain or subarachnoid space in patients with thrombocytopenia or other bleeding disorders may cause sudden, severe headache.

Paresthesias may occur because of peripheral neuropathy in pernicious anemia or secondary to hematologic malignancy or amyloidosis. They may also result from therapy with vincristine.

Confusion may accompany malignant or infectious processes involving the brain, sometimes as a result of the accompanying fever. Confusion may also occur with severe anemia, hypercalcemia (e.g., myeloma), thrombotic thrombocytopenic purpura, or high-dose glucocorticoid therapy. Confusion or apparent senility may be a manifestation of pernicious anemia. Frank psychosis may develop in acute intermittent porphyria or with high-dose glucocorticoid therapy.

Impairment of consciousness may be a result of increased intracranial pressure secondary to hemorrhage or leukemia or lymphoma in the central nervous system. It may also accompany severe anemia, polycythemia, hyperviscosity secondary, usually, to an immunoglobulin (Ig) M monoclonal protein (uncommonly IgA or IgG) in the plasma, or a leukemic hyperleukocytosis syndrome, especially in chronic myelogenous leukemia.

Eyes
Conjunctival plethora is a feature of polycythemia and pallor a result of anemia. Occasionally blindness may result from retinal hemorrhages secondary to severe anemia and thrombocytopenia or blurred vision resulting from severe hyperviscosity resulting from macroglobulinemia or extreme hyperleukocytosis of leukemia. Partial or complete visual loss can stem from retinal vein or artery thrombosis. Diplopia or disturbances of ocular movement may occur with orbital tumors or paralysis of the third, fourth, or sixth cranial nerves because of compression by tumor, especially extranodal lymphoma, extramedullary myeloma, or myeloid (granulocytic) sarcoma.

Ears
Vertigo, tinnitus, and "roaring" in the ears may occur with marked anemia, polycythemia, hyperleukocytic leukemia, or macroglobulinemia-induced hyperviscosity. Ménière disease was first described in a patient with acute leukemia and inner ear hemorrhage.

Nasopharynx, Oropharynx, and Oral Cavity
Epistaxis may occur in patients with thrombocytopenia, acquired or inherited platelet function disorders, and von Willebrand disease. *Anosmia* or *olfactory hallucinations* occur in pernicious anemia. The nasopharynx may be invaded by a granulocytic sarcoma or extranodal lymphoma; the symptoms are dependent on the structures invaded. The paranasal sinuses may be involved by opportunistic organisms, such as fungus in patients with severe, prolonged neutropenia. *Pain or tingling in the tongue* occurs in pernicious anemia and may accompany severe iron deficiency or vitamin deficiencies. *Macroglossia* occurs in amyloidosis. *Bleeding gums* may occur with bleeding disorders. Infiltration of the gingiva with leukemic cells occurs notably in acute monocytic leukemia. *Ulceration* of the tongue or oral mucosa may be severe in the acute leukemias or in patients with severe neutropenia. *Dryness of the mouth* may be caused by hypercalcemia, secondary, for example, to myeloma. *Dysphagia* may be seen in patients with severe mucous membrane atrophy associated with chronic iron-deficiency anemia.

Neck
Painless swelling in the neck is characteristic of lymphoma but may be caused by a number of other diseases as well. Occasionally, the enlarged lymph nodes of lymphomas may be tender or painful because of secondary infection or rapid growth. Painful or tender lymphadenopathy is usually associated with inflammatory reactions, such as infectious mononucleosis or suppurative adenitis. *Diffuse swelling* of the neck and face may occur with obstruction of the superior vena cava due to lymphomatous compression.

Chest and Heart
Both *dyspnea* and *palpitations,* usually on effort but occasionally at rest, may occur because of anemia or pulmonary embolism. *Congestive heart failure* may supervene, and *angina pectoris* may become manifest in anemic patients. The impact of anemia on the circulatory system depends in part on the rapidity with which it develops, and chronic anemia may become severe without producing major symptoms; with severe acute blood loss, the patient may develop shock with a nearly normal hemoglobin level, prior to compensatory hemodilution. *Cough* may result from enlarged mediastinal nodes compressing the trachea or bronchi. *Chest pain* may arise from involvement of the ribs or sternum with lymphoma or multiple myeloma, nerve-root invasion or compression, or herpes zoster; the pain of herpes zoster usually precedes the skin lesions by several days. Chest pain with inspiration suggests a pulmonary infarct, as does *hemoptysis. Tenderness of the sternum* may be quite pronounced in chronic myelogenous or acute leukemia, and occasionally in primary myelofibrosis, or if intramedullary lymphoma or myeloma proliferation is rapidly progressive.

Gastrointestinal System
Dysphagia has already been mentioned under "Nasopharynx, Oropharynx, and Oral Cavity" above. *Anorexia* frequently occurs but usually has no specific diagnostic significance. Hypercalcemia and azotemia cause anorexia, nausea, and vomiting. A variety of ill-defined gastrointestinal complaints grouped under the heading "indigestion" may occur with hematologic diseases. *Abdominal fullness, premature satiety, belching,* or *discomfort* may occur because of a greatly enlarged spleen, but such splenomegaly may also be entirely asymptomatic. *Abdominal pain* may arise from intestinal obstruction by lymphoma, retroperitoneal bleeding, lead poisoning, ileus secondary to therapy with the *vinca* alkaloids, acute hemolysis, allergic purpura, the abdominal crises of sickle cell disease, or acute intermittent porphyria. *Diarrhea* may occur in pernicious anemia. It also may be prominent in the various forms of intestinal malabsorption, although significant malabsorption may occur without diarrhea. In small-bowel malabsorption, steatorrhea may be a notable feature. Malabsorption may be a manifestation of small-bowel lymphoma. *Gastrointestinal bleeding* related to thrombocytopenia or other bleeding disorder may be occult but often is manifest as *hematemesis* or *melena. Hematochezia* can occur if a bleeding disorder is associated with a colonic lesion. *Constipation* may occur in the patient with hypercalcemia or in one receiving treatment with the *vinca* alkaloids.

Genitourinary and Reproductive Systems
Impotence or *bladder dysfunction* may occur with spinal cord or peripheral nerve damage caused by one of the hematologic malignancies or with pernicious anemia. Priapism may occur in hyperleukocytic leukemia, essential thrombocythemia, or sickle cell disease. *Hematuria* may be a manifestation of hemophilia A or B. *Red urine* may also occur with intravascular hemolysis (hemoglobinuria), myoglobinuria, or porphyrinuria. Injection of anthracycline drugs or ingestion of drugs such as phenazopyridine (Pyridium) regularly causes the urine to turn red. The use of deferoxamine mesylate (Desferal) may result in rust colored urine. *Amenorrhea* may also be induced by certain drugs, such as antimetabolites or alkylating agents. *Menorrhagia* is a common cause of iron deficiency, and care must be taken to obtain a history of the

number of prior pregnancies and an accurate assessment of the extent of menstrual blood loss. Semiquantification can be obtained from estimates of the number of days of heavy bleeding (usually <3), the number of days of any bleeding (usually <7), number of tampons or pads used (requirement for double pads suggests excessive bleeding), degree of blood soaking, and clots formed, and inquiries such as, "Have you experienced a gush of blood when a tampon is removed?" However, an objective distinction between menorrhagia (loss of more than 80 mL blood per period) and normal blood loss can best be made by a visual assessment technique using pictorial charts of towels or tampons.[6] Menorrhagia may occur in patients with bleeding disorders.

Back and Extremities

Back pain may accompany acute hemolytic reactions or be a result of involvement of bone or the nervous system in acute leukemia or aggressive lymphoma. It is one of the most common manifestations of myeloma.

Arthritis or *arthralgia* may occur with gout secondary to increased uric acid production in patients with hematologic malignancies, especially acute lymphocytic leukemia in childhood, myelofibrosis, myelodysplastic syndrome, and hemolytic anemia. They also occur in the plasma cell dyscrasias, acute leukemias, and sickle cell disease without evidence of gout, and in allergic purpura. Arthritis may accompany hemochromatosis, although the association has not been carefully established. In the latter case the arthritis starts typically in the small joints of the hand (second and third metacarpal joints), and episodes of acute synovitis may be related to deposition of calcium pyrophosphate dehydrate crystals. Hemarthroses in patients with severe bleeding disorders cause marked joint pain. Autoimmune diseases may present as anemia and/or thrombocytopenia, and arthritis appears as a later manifestation. *Shoulder pain* on the left may be a result of infarction of the spleen and on the right of gall bladder disease associated with chronic hemolytic anemia such as hereditary spherocytosis. *Bone pain* may occur with bone involvement by the hematologic malignancies; it is common in the congenital hemolytic anemias, such as sickle cell anemia, and may occur in myelofibrosis. In patients with Hodgkin lymphoma, ingestion of alcohol may induce pain at the site of any lesion, including those in bone. *Edema* of the lower extremities, sometimes unilateral, may occur because of obstruction to veins or lymphatics by lymphomatous masses or from deep venous thrombosis. The latter can also cause edema of the upper extremities.

Skin

Skin manifestations of hematologic disease may be of great importance; they include changes in texture or color, itching, and the presence of specific or nonspecific lesions. The skin in iron-deficient patients may become dry, the hair dry and fine, and the nails brittle. In hypothyroidism, which may cause anemia, the skin is dry, coarse, and scaly. *Jaundice* may be apparent with pernicious anemia or congenital or acquired hemolytic anemia. The skin of patients with pernicious anemia is said to be "lemon yellow" because of the simultaneous appearance of jaundice and pallor. Jaundice may also occur in patients with hematologic malignancies, especially lymphomas, as a result of liver involvement or biliary tract obstruction. *Pallor* is a common accompaniment of anemia, although some severely anemic patients may not appear pale. Erythromelalgia may be a troublesome complication of polycythemia vera. Patchy plaques or widespread *erythroderma* occur in cutaneous T-cell lymphoma (especially Sézary syndrome) and in some cases of chronic lymphocytic leukemia or lymphocytic lymphoma. The skin is often involved, sometimes severely, in graft-versus-host disease following hematopoietic cell transplantation. Patients with hemochromatosis may have bronze or grayish pigmentation of the skin. *Cyanosis* occurs

with methemoglobinemia, either hereditary or acquired; sulfhemoglobinemia; abnormal hemoglobins with low oxygen affinity; and primary and secondary polycythemia. Cyanosis of the ears or the fingertips may occur after exposure to cold in individuals with cryoglobulins or cold agglutinins.

Itching may occur in the absence of any visible skin lesions in Hodgkin lymphoma and may be extreme. Mycosis fungoides or other lymphomas with skin involvement may also present as itching. A significant number of patients with polycythemia vera will complain of itching after bathing.

Petechiae and *ecchymoses* are most often seen in the extremities in patients with thrombocytopenia, nonthrombocytopenic purpura, or acquired or inherited platelet function abnormalities and von Willebrand disease. Unless secondary to trauma, these lesions usually are painless; the lesions of psychogenic purpura and erythema nodosum are painful. *Easy bruising* is a common complaint, especially among women, and when no other hemorrhagic symptoms are present, usually no abnormalities are found after detailed study. This symptom may, however, indicate a mild hereditary bleeding disorder, such as von Willebrand disease or one of the platelet disorders. *Infiltrative lesions* may occur in the leukemias (leukemia cutis) and lymphomas (lymphoma cutis) and are sometimes the presenting complaint. Monocytic leukemia has a higher frequency of skin infiltration than other forms of leukemia. *Necrotic lesions* may occur with intravascular coagulation, purpura fulminans, and warfarin-induced skin necrosis, or rarely with exposure to cold in patients with circulating cryoproteins or cold agglutinins.

Leg ulcers are a common complaint in sickle cell anemia and occur rarely in other hereditary anemias.

DRUGS AND CHEMICALS

Drugs

Drug therapy, either self-prescribed or ordered by a physician, is extremely common in our society. Drugs often induce or aggravate hematologic disease, and it is therefore essential that a careful history of drug ingestion, including beneficial and adverse reactions, should be obtained from all patients. Drugs taken regularly, including nonprescription medications, often become a part of the patient's way of life and are forgotten or are not recognized as "drugs."

Agents such as aspirin, laxatives, tranquilizers, medicinal iron, vitamins, other nutritional supplements, and sedatives belong to this category. Furthermore, drugs may be ingested in unrecognized form, such as antibiotics in food or quinine in tonic water. Specific, persistent questioning, often on several occasions, may be necessary before a complete history of drug use is obtained. It is very important to obtain detailed information on alcohol consumption from every patient. The four "CAGE" questions—about needing to **c**ut down, being **a**nnoyed by criticism, having **g**uilt feelings, and requiring a drink as a morning **e**ye-opener—provide an effective approach to the history of alcohol use. Patients should also be asked about the use of recreational drugs. The use of "alternative medicines" and herbal medicines is common, and many patients will not consider these medications or may actively withhold information about their use. Nonjudgmental questioning may be successful in identifying agents in this category that the patient is taking. Some patients equate the term "drugs," as opposed to "medicines," with illicit drugs. Establishing that the examiner is interested in all forms of ingestants—prescribed drugs, self-remedies, alternative remedies, etcetera—is important to ensure getting the information required.

Chemicals

In addition to drugs, most people are exposed regularly to a variety of chemicals in the environment, some of which may be potentially harmful agents and result in a deleterious hematologic effect, such as anemia or leukopenia. An occupational history should explore exposure to potentially harmful chemicals. This information should be supplemented by inquiries about hobbies and other interests that result in work with chemicals, such as glues and solvents. When a toxin is suspected, the patient's daily activities and environment should be carefully reviewed, as significant exposure to toxic chemicals may occur incidentally.

VACCINATION

Vaccinations can be complicated by acute immune thrombocytopenia. In infants, this is most notable after measles, mumps, rubella (MMR) vaccine. This occurrence is approximately 1 in 25,000 children vaccinated, occurs within 6 weeks of vaccination, and in the majority of occurrences is self-limited. There is no evidence that children with antecedent immune thrombocytopenia are at risk of recurrence after MMR vaccination.[7] Analysis, thus far, shows rare cases in following administration of other vaccines (hepatitis A, diphtheria-pertussis-tetanus, or varicella) administered to older children and adolescents and significant risk has not been ascertained.[8]

NUTRITION

Children who are breastfed without iron supplementation may develop iron-deficiency anemia. Nutritional information can be useful in deducing the possible role of dietary deficiency in anemia. The avoidance of certain food groups, as might be the case with vegetarians, or the ingestion of uncooked fish can be clues to the pathogenesis of megaloblastic anemia.

FAMILY HISTORY

A carefully obtained family history may be of great importance in the study of patients with hematologic disease (Chap. 10). In the case of hemolytic disorders, questions should be asked regarding jaundice, anemia, and gallstones in relatives. In patients with disorders of hemostasis or venous thrombosis, particular attention must be given to bleeding manifestations or venous thromboembolism in family members. In the case of autosomal recessive disorders such as pyruvate kinase deficiency, the parents are usually not affected, but a similar clinical syndrome may have occurred in siblings. It is particularly important to inquire about siblings who may have died in infancy, as these may be forgotten, especially by older patients. When sex-linked inheritance is suspected, it is necessary to inquire about symptoms in the maternal grandfather, maternal uncles, male siblings, and nephews. In patients with disorders with dominant inheritance, such as hereditary spherocytosis, one may expect to find that one parent and possibly siblings and children of the patient have stigmata of the disease. Ethnic background may be important in the consideration of certain diseases such as α- and β-thalassemia, sickle cell anemia, glucose-6-phosphate dehydrogenase deficiency, hemoglobin E, and other inherited disorders that are prevalent in specific geographic areas, such as the Mediterranean basin or Southeast Asia.

SEXUAL HISTORY

Because of the frequency of infections with the human immunodeficiency viruses, it is important to ascertain the sexual behavior of the patient, especially risk factors for transmission of HIV.

PREVENTIVE HEMATOLOGY

Ideally, the physician's goal is to prevent illness, and opportunities exist for hematologists to prevent the development of hematologic disorders. These opportunities include identification of individual genetic risk factors and avoidance of situations that may make a latent disorder

manifest. Prophylactic therapy, as for example in avoiding venous stasis in patients heterozygous for protein C deficiency or administering prophylactic heparin at the time of major surgery, is a more immediate aspect of prevention because it depends on the physician's intervention. Hematologists may also prevent disease by reinforcing community medicine efforts. Examples include fostering the elimination of sources of environmental lead that may result in childhood anemia. Prenatal diagnosis can provide information to families as to whether a fetus is affected with a hematologic disorder.

● PHYSICAL EXAMINATION

A detailed physical examination should be performed on every patient, with sufficient attention paid to all systems so as to obtain a full evaluation of the general health of the individual. The skin, eyes, tongue, lymph nodes, skeleton, spleen and liver, and nervous system are especially pertinent to hematologic disease and therefore deserve special attention.

SKIN

Pallor and Flushing

The color of the skin is a result of the pigment contained therein and to the blood flowing through the skin capillaries. The component of skin color related to the blood may be a useful guide to anemia or polycythemia, as pallor may result when the hemoglobin level is reduced, and redness when the hemoglobin level is increased. The amount of pigment in the skin modifies skin color and can mislead the clinician, as in individuals with pallor resulting from decreased pigment, or make skin color useless as a guide because of the intense pigmentation present.

Alterations in blood flow and in hemoglobin content may change skin color; this, too, can mislead the clinician. Thus emotion may cause either pallor or blushing. Exposure of the skin to cold or heat may similarly cause pallor or blushing. Chronic exposure to wind or sun may lead to permanent redness of the skin, and chronic ingestion of alcohol to a flushed face. The degree of erythema of the skin can be evaluated by pressing the thumb firmly against the skin, as on the forehead, so that the capillaries are emptied, and then comparing the color of the compressed spot with the surrounding skin immediately after the thumb is removed.

The mucous membranes and nail beds are usually more reliable guides to anemia or polycythemia than the skin. The conjunctivae and gums may be inflamed, however, and therefore not reflect the hemoglobin level, or the gums may appear pale because of pressure from the lips. The gums and the nail beds may also be pigmented and the capillaries correspondingly obscured. In some individuals, the color of the capillaries does not become fully visible through the nails unless pressure is applied to the fingertip, either laterally or on the end of the nail.

The palmar creases are useful guides to the hemoglobin level and appear pink in the fully opened hand unless the hemoglobin is 7 g/dL or less. Liver disease may induce flushing of the thenar and hypothenar eminences of the palm, even in patients with anemia.

Cyanosis

The detection of cyanosis, like the detection of pallor, may be made difficult by skin pigmentation. Cyanosis is a function of the total amount of reduced hemoglobin, methemoglobin, or sulfhemoglobin present. The minimum amounts of these pigments that cause detectable cyanosis are approximately 5 g/dL blood of reduced hemoglobin, 1.5 to 2.0 g/dL of methemoglobin, and 0.5 g/dL of sulfhemoglobin.

Jaundice

Jaundice may be observed in the skin of individuals who are not otherwise deeply pigmented or in the sclerae or the mucous membranes.

The patient should be examined in daylight rather than under incandescent or fluorescent light, because the yellow color of the latter masks the yellow color of the patient. Jaundice is a result of actual staining of the skin by bile pigment, and bilirubin glucuronide (direct-reacting or conjugated bilirubin) stains the skin more readily than the unconjugated form. Jaundice of the skin may not be visible if the bilirubin level is below 2 to 3 mg/dL. Yellow pigmentation of the skin may also occur with carotenemia, especially in young children.

Petechiae and Ecchymoses

Petechiae are small (1 to 2 mm), round, red or brown lesions resulting from hemorrhage into the skin and are present primarily in areas with high venous pressure, such as the lower extremities. These lesions do not blanch on pressure, and this can be readily demonstrated by compressing the skin with a glass microscope slide or magnifying lens. Petechiae may occasionally be elevated slightly, that is, palpable; this finding suggests vasculitis. Ecchymoses may be of various sizes and shapes and may be red, purple, blue, or yellowish green, depending on the intensity of the skin hemorrhage and its age. They may be flat or elevated; some are painful and tender. The lesions of hereditary hemorrhagic telangiectasia are small, flat, nonpulsatile, and violaceous. They blanch with pressure.

Excoriation

Itching may be intense in some hematologic disorders, such as Hodgkin lymphoma, even in the absence of skin lesions. Excoriation of the skin from scratching is the only physical manifestation of this severe symptom.

Leg Ulcers

Open ulcers or scars from healed ulcers are often found in the region of the internal or external malleoli in patients with sickle cell anemia, and, rarely, in other hereditary anemias.

Nails

Detection of pallor or rubor by examining the nails was discussed earlier. The fingernails in chronic, severe iron-deficiency anemia may be ridged longitudinally and flattened or concave rather than convex. The latter change is referred to as *koilonychia* and is uncommon in present practice.

Eyes

Jaundice, pallor, or *plethora* may be detected from examination of the eyes. Jaundice is usually more readily detected in the sclerae than in the skin. Ophthalmoscopic examination is also essential in patients with hematologic disease. *Retinal hemorrhages* and *exudates* occur in patients with severe anemia and thrombocytopenia. These hemorrhages are usually the typical "flame-shaped" hemorrhages, but they may be quite large and elevate the retina so that they may appear as a darkly colored tumor. Round hemorrhages with white centers are also often seen. *Dilatation of the veins* may be seen in polycythemia; in patients with macroglobulinemia, the veins are engorged and segmented, resembling link sausages.

Mouth

Pallor of the mucosa has already been discussed (see "Pallor and Flushing" above). *Ulceration* of the oral mucosa occurs commonly in neutropenic patients. In leukemia there may also be infiltration of the gums with swelling, redness, and bleeding. *Bleeding* from the mucosa may occur with a hemorrhagic disease. A dark line of lead sulfide may be deposited in the gums at the base of the teeth in lead poisoning. The *tongue* may be completely smooth in pernicious anemia and iron-deficiency anemia. Patients with an upper dental prosthesis may also have

papillary atrophy, presumably on a mechanical basis. The tongue may be smooth and red in patients with nutritional deficiencies. This may be accompanied by fissuring at the corners of the mouth, but fissuring may also be caused by ill-fitting dentures. An enlarged tongue, abnormally firm to palpation, may indicate the presence of primary amyloidosis.

Lymph Nodes

Lymph nodes are widely distributed in the body, and in disease, any node or group of nodes may be involved. The major concern on physical examination is the detection of enlarged or tender nodes in the cervical, supraclavicular, axillary, epitrochlear, inguinal, or iliofemoral regions. Under normal conditions in adults, the only readily palpable lymph nodes are in the inguinal region, where several firm nodes 0.5 to 2.0 cm long are normally attached to the dense fascia below the inguinal ligament and in the femoral triangle. In children, multiple small (0.5 to 1.0 cm) nodes may be palpated in the cervical region as well. Supraclavicular nodes may sometimes be palpable only when the patient performs the Valsalva maneuver.

Enlarged lymph nodes are ordinarily detected in the superficial areas by palpation, although they are sometimes large enough to be seen. Palpation should be gentle and is best performed with a circular motion of the fingertips, using slowly increasing pressure. Tender lymph nodes usually indicate an inflammatory etiology, although rapidly proliferative lymphoma may be tender to palpation.

Nodes too deep to palpate may be detected by specific imaging procedures, including computerized tomography, magnetic resonance imaging, ultrasound studies, gallium scintography, and positron emission tomography.[9,10]

Chest

Increased rib or sternal tenderness is an important physical sign often ignored. Increased bone pain may be generalized, as in leukemia, or spotty, as in plasma cell myeloma or in metastatic tumors. The superficial surfaces of all bones should be examined thoroughly by applying intermittent firm pressure with the fingertips to locate potential areas of disease.

Spleen

The normal adult spleen is usually not palpable on physical examination, but occasionally the tip may be felt.[11] Palpability of the normal spleen may be related to body habitus, but there is disagreement on this point. Percussion, palpation, or a combination of these two methods may detect enlarged spleens.[12] Some enlarged spleens may be visible by protrusion of the abdominal wall.

The normal spleen weighs approximately 150 g and lies in the peritoneal cavity against the diaphragm and the posterolateral abdominal wall at the level of the lower three ribs. As it enlarges it remains close to the abdominal wall, while the lower pole moves downward, anteriorly, and to the right. Spleens enlarged only 40 percent above normal may be palpable, but significant splenic enlargement may occur and the organ still not be felt on physical examination. A good but imperfect correlation has been reported between spleen size estimated from radioisotope scanning or ultrasonography and spleen weight determined after splenectomy or at autopsy.[13] Although it is common to fail to palpate an enlarged spleen on physical examination, palpation of a normal-sized spleen is unusual, and therefore a palpable spleen is usually a significant physical finding.

An enlarged spleen lies just beneath the abdominal wall and can be identified by its movement during respiration. The splenic notch may be evident if the organ is moderately enlarged. During the examination the patient lies in a relaxed, supine position. The examiner, standing on the patient's right, lightly palpates the left upper abdomen with the right hand while exerting pressure forward with the palm of the left hand placed over the lower ribs posterolaterally. This action permits the spleen to descend and be felt by the examiner's fingers. If nothing is felt, the palpation should be performed repeatedly, moving the examining hand approximately 2 cm toward the inguinal ligament each time. It is often advantageous to carry out the examination initially with the patient lying on the right side with left knee flexed and to repeat it with the patient supine.

It is not always possible to be sure that a left upper quadrant mass is spleen; masses in the stomach, colon, kidney, or pancreas may mimic splenomegaly on physical examination. When there is uncertainty regarding the nature of a mass in the left upper quadrant, imaging procedures will usually permit accurate diagnosis.[13–15]

Liver

Palpation of the edge of the liver in the right upper quadrant of the abdomen is commonly used to detect hepatic enlargement, although the inaccuracies of this method have been demonstrated. It is necessary to determine both the upper and lower borders of the liver by percussion in order to properly assess liver size.[16,17] The normal liver may be palpable as much as 4 to 5 cm below the right costal margin but is usually not palpable in the epigastrium. The height of liver dullness is best measured in a specific line 8, 10, or 12 cm to the right of the midline. Techniques should be standardized so that serial measurements can be made. The vertical span of the normal liver determined in this manner will range approximately 10 cm in an average-size man and approximately 2 cm smaller in a woman. Because of variations introduced by technique, each physician should determine the normal area of liver dullness by the physician's own procedure. Correlation of radioisotope imaging data with results from routine physical examinations indicates that often a liver of normal size is considered enlarged on physical examination and an enlarged liver is considered normal. Ultrasonography and computed tomography measurements are useful in determining size and demonstrating localized infiltrative lesions.[18–20]

Nervous System

A thorough evaluation of neurologic function is necessary in many patients with hematologic disease. Vitamin B_{12} deficiency impairs cerebral, olfactory, spinal cord, and peripheral nerve function, and severe chronic deficiency may lead to irreversible neurologic degeneration. Leukemic meningitis is often manifested by headache, visual impairment, or cranial nerve dysfunction. Tumor growth in the brain or spinal cord compression may be caused by malignant lymphoma or plasma cell myeloma. A variety of neurologic abnormalities may develop in patients with leukemias, lymphomas, and myeloma as a consequence of tumor infiltration, bleeding, infection, or a paraneoplastic syndrome. Essential monoclonal gammopathy is associated with several types of sensory and motor neuropathies. Polyneuropathy is a feature of POEMS, a syndrome marked by polyneuropathy, organomegaly, endocrinopathy, monoclonal gammopathy, and skin changes.

Joints

Deformities of the knees, elbows, ankles, shoulders, wrists, or hips may be the result of repeated hemorrhage in patients with hemophilia A, hemophilia B, or severe factor VII deficiency. Often, a target joint is prominently affected.

REFERENCES

1. Bickley LS: *Bates Guide to Physical Examination and History Taking*, 11th ed. Lippincott Williams & Wilkins, Philadelphia, 2012.
2. Sackett DL: A primer on the precision and accuracy of the clinical examination. *JAMA* 267:2638, 1992.
3. Williams ME: *Geriatric Physical Diagnosis: A Guide to Observation and Assessment.* McFarland & Company, Jefferson, NC, 2008.
4. Mor V, Laliberte L, Morris JN, Wiemann M: The Karnofsky performance status scale: An examination of its reliability and validity in a research setting. *Cancer* 53:2002, 1984.
5. Oken MM, Creech RH, Tormey DC, et al: Toxicity and response criteria of the Eastern Cooperative Oncology Group. *Am J Clin Oncol* 5:649, 1982.
6. Janssen CAH, Scholten PC, Heintz APM: A simple visual assessment technique to discriminate between menorrhagia and normal menstrual blood loss. *Obstet Gynecol* 85:977, 1995.
7. Black C, Kaye JA, Jick H: MMR vaccine and idiopathic thrombocytopaenic purpura. *Br J Clin Pharmacol* 55:107, 2003.
8. O'Leary ST, Glanz JM, McClure DL, et al: The risk of immune thrombocytopenic purpura after vaccination in children and adolescents. *Pediatrics* 129:248, 2012.
9. Grubnic S, Vinnicombe SJ, Norman AR, Husband JE: MR evaluation of normal retroperitoneal and pelvic lymph nodes. *Clin Radiol* 57:193, 2002.
10. Atula TS, Varpula MJ, Kurki TJI, et al: Assessment of cervical lymph node status in head and neck cancer patients: Palpation, computed tomography and low-field magnetic resonance imaging compared with ultrasound-guided fine needle aspiration cytology. *Eur J Radiol* 25:152, 1997.
11. Arkles LB, Gill GD, Nolan MP: A palpable spleen is not necessarily enlarged or pathological. *Med J Aust* 145:15, 1986.
12. Barkun AN, Camus M, Green L, et al: The bedside assessment of splenic enlargement. *Am J Med* 91:512, 1991.
13. Benter T, Klühs L, Teichgräber U. Sonography of the spleen. *J Ultrasound Med* 30:1281, 2011.
14. Lamb PM, Lund A, Kanagasbay RR, et al: Spleen size: How well do linear ultrasound measurements correlate with three-dimensional CT volume assessments? *Br J Radiol* 75:573, 2002.
15. Palas J, Matos AP, Ramalho M. The spleen revisited: An overview on magnetic resonance imaging. *Radiol Res Pract* 2013:219297, 2013.
16. Castell DO, O'Brien KD, Muench H, Chalmers TC: Estimation of liver size by percussion in normal individuals. *Ann Intern Med* 70:1183, 1969.
17. Tucker WN, Saab S, Rickman LS, Mathews WC: The scratch test is unreliable for detecting the liver edge. *J Clin Gastroenterol* 25:410, 1997.
18. Bennett WF, Dova JG: Review of hepatic imaging and a problem-oriented approach to liver masses. *Hepatology* 12:761, 1990.
19. Barloon TJ, Brown BP, Abu-Yousef MM, et al: Teaching physical examination of the adult liver with the use of real-time sonography. *Acad Radiol* 5:101, 1998.
20. Elstein D, Hadas-Halpern I, Azuri Y, et al: Accuracy of ultrasonography in assessing spleen and liver. *J Ultrasound Med* 16:209, 1997.

CHAPTER 2
EXAMINATION OF BLOOD CELLS

Daniel H. Ryan

SUMMARY

Determining a patient's blood cell counts and examining the appearance of cells on a blood film is central to the diagnosis of blood cell diseases and can give important information about numerous other degenerative, inflammatory, and neoplastic diseases that are reflected in quantitative or qualitative changes of blood cells. The quantity and quality of blood cells reflects the aggregate function of the major blood forming tissue, the marrow, and is thus an essential component of diagnosis and followup of primary hematological disorders. The decision to perform a marrow examination, and the types of special studies required, follow from a careful analysis of blood cells. Currently available automated blood cell analyzers continue to evolve and are the mainstay of blood cell counting, providing an increasing array of novel quantitative parameters, and flagging of abnormal samples that need manual microscopic review. The blood provides a unique example of a tissue that can be readily analyzed with a degree of quantitative detail unavailable in any other organ system.

INTRODUCTION

The blood is examined so as to answer these questions: Is the marrow producing appropriate numbers of mature cells in the major hematopoietic lineages? Is the development of each hematopoietic lineage qualitatively normal? Are there abnormal (e.g., leukemia or lymphoma) cells in the blood? Quantitative measures available from automated cell counters are reliable and provide a rapid and cost-effective way to screen for primary or secondary disturbances of hematopoiesis. Light microscopic observation of the blood film is essential to confirm certain quantitative results and to investigate qualitatively abnormal differentiation of the hematopoietic lineages. Based on examination of the blood, the physician is directed toward a more focused assessment of marrow function or to systemic disorders that secondarily involve the hematopoietic system.

Acronyms and Abbreviations: CHr, reticulocyte-specific hemoglobin content; EDTA, ethylenediaminetetraacetic acid; fl, femtoliter; FRC, fragmented red cell counts; Hct, hematocrit; HYPO%, percentages of red cells falling below a cutoff for hemoglobin concentration; %HypoHe, percentages of red cells falling below a cutoff for hemoglobin content; Ig, immunoglobulin; MCH, mean cell hemoglobin; MCHC, mean cell hemoglobin concentration; MCV, mean cell volume; MPV, mean platelet volume; NHANES, National Health and Nutrition Examination Survey; NK, natural killer; PDW, platelet volume distribution width; RBC, red blood cell; RDW, red cell distribution width; RET-He, reticulocyte-specific hemoglobin content.

The complete blood count is a necessary part of the diagnostic evaluation in a broad variety of clinical conditions. Similarly, the leukocyte differential count and examination of the blood film, in spite of limitations as a screening test for occult disease, is important in initial consideration of the differential diagnosis in most ill patients. Although quantitative and qualitative (morphologic) examination of the cells of the blood are considered separately in this chapter, the distinction between these two is not absolute, and measures once considered "qualitative" become quantitative as technology advances.

QUANTITATIVE MEASURES OF CELLS IN THE BLOOD

PRINCIPLES OF AUTOMATED BLOOD CELL ANALYSIS

Automated blood cell analysis is the cornerstone of the modern hematology laboratory, allowing rapid, cost-effective, and accurate analysis of the cells of the blood, including new parameters with diagnostic utility. The morphologic and functional complexity of blood cells requires direct microscopic examination of a stained blood film by a trained observer. However, it is possible to use automated techniques to analyze and report on the majority of samples, using defined criteria ("flags") to select those that need further microscopic review. Automated hematology analyzers typically incorporate multiple proprietary software flags based on acceptability criteria related to pattern recognition in the multiparameter displays or comparison of different detection modes for the same cell type. These are frequently updated in software or when new models are introduced to improve sensitivity and specificity. In this way, instruments identify samples that contain cells or abnormalities the instrument cannot definitively identify, so that a skilled morphologist can visually evaluate that specimen. Some of these flags can be adjusted or suppressed by the user to achieve an appropriate balance that minimizes both false positives and false negatives. The optimum balance is dependent on the patient population examined. Guidelines for manual smear review based on comparative data have been published, based on instruments then in common use.[1] Protocols for evaluating and adjusting flagging criteria within an individual laboratory have been described.[2] Manual review may consist of a scan of the blood film, a more detailed blood film examination including leukocyte differential count, or a physician's review, based on laboratory defined criteria.[3] The proportion of samples requiring manual blood film review differs among instruments and the type of patient population tested. Studies show a 10 to 30 percent manual review rate,[4-6] with a false negative rate (i.e., abnormal samples that were not flagged for review) varying from approximately 3 percent[1] to 10–14 percent.[4] Most of the false negatives with current instrumentation are related to red cell and platelet morphology with relatively limited diagnostic significance.[4] Continued improvement in methodology and increased sophistication of data analysis will result in further reduction of unnecessary manual smear reviews. Depending on workload and space considerations, laboratories may choose to link automated hematology analyzers with automated blood film preparation and automated image analyzers to facilitate manual morphologic review of cells by traditional light microscopy or online review of digitized images.[7] These instruments can provide a provisional differential count with good accuracy,[8] although typically final classification of problematic cells is performed by a technologist or physician.

The characteristics of automated hematology analyzer systems have been reviewed.[9] A detailed description of individual instruments is beyond the scope of this chapter, but the general principles employed by state-of-the-art instrumentation are summarized below. The major analytical challenges are the frequency of the different cell types, which vary over many orders of magnitude, from red cells (millions per μL) to basophils (dozens per μL), and the complexity of the structure of normal and abnormal blood cells. Over the past several decades, instruments have become increasingly sophisticated with the use of multiple parameters to produce more precise results in the great majority of patient samples. In a typical automated hematology analyzer, the blood sample is aspirated and separated into different fluidic streams. The streams are mixed with various buffers that accomplish specific purposes in the analysis, for instance, using differential lysis to distinguish subsets of leukocytes, reagents to measure hemoglobin or detect myeloperoxidase containing leukocytes, and various fluorescent dyes. Measurements of each fluidic stream are made in flow as the sample passes through a series of detectors in what are essentially modified flow cytometers (Chap. 3). Commonly used principles include light scatter at various angles, electrical impedance and conductivity, and fluorescence or light absorption of cells stained in flow. Light scatter yields information about cell size (using scatter at low-incident angles), nuclear lobulation, and cytoplasmic granularity (using high-angle light scatter) and refractive index, with polarization of the scattered light as an additional parameter. If red cells are converted to spherocytes by the buffer solution to eliminate the variability of cell shape, light scatter at different angles can provide information about hemoglobin content, as well as size of individual red cells. Cell size is also estimated by measuring change in electrical resistance, which is proportional to cell size as cells enter a narrow orifice through which a direct current is maintained, the original Coulter principle, named for Wallace Coulter who developed the electronic particle counter.[10] Radiofrequency capacitance measurement yields additional intracellular structural information that complements the direct current measurement. Differential lysis with detergents of varying strength or pH is used to separate certain leukocyte types, such

as basophils and immature granulocytic cells, from the major normal blood cell types. In addition, nucleic-acid-binding fluorescent dyes incorporated into the lysis buffer measure total RNA plus DNA in the cells and are used in some analyzers to help differentiate leukocyte types. Fluorescence measurements after staining with RNA binding dyes are commonly used to detect and subclassify reticulocytes and platelets. Light absorption is the principle used for hemoglobin measurement and in some instruments for identifying peroxidase-positive granulocytes. Instruments rely on a combination of techniques for accuracy and precision[11] (Fig. 2–1). Complex algorithms are invoked to determine whether the distribution of variables for a specific result or for the specimen as a whole fit sufficiently within an expected variable space so that the results can be reported with high confidence, or whether the specimen should be "flagged" for further analysis or manual blood film review (Fig. 2–2). There is significant overlap in methodology between automated hematology analyzers and flow cytometers (flow cytometers are discussed in Chap. 3). The latter are distinguished by extensive use of fluorochrome tagged antibodies to identify cell subtypes. These instruments have replaced laborious manual work, but also demand increasing interpretation skills on the part of laboratory technologists. Automated blood analyzers have been adapted to accurately count the smaller numbers of blood cells typically found in body fluids,[12] but accurate differential counts[13] and detection of blast cells in fluids of patients[14] remains a challenge.

Point of care "bedside" testing is far more challenging in hematology than for typical clinical chemistry analytes for many of the reasons described above. Instruments have been described for bedside measurement of hemoglobin, total leukocytes, three-part leukocyte differential count, malaria parasitemia, and CD4+ T-cell count, mainly targeting clinical settings with limited access to standard laboratory testing. More work remains to be done to demonstrate the reliability and clinical impact of such testing strategies.[15]

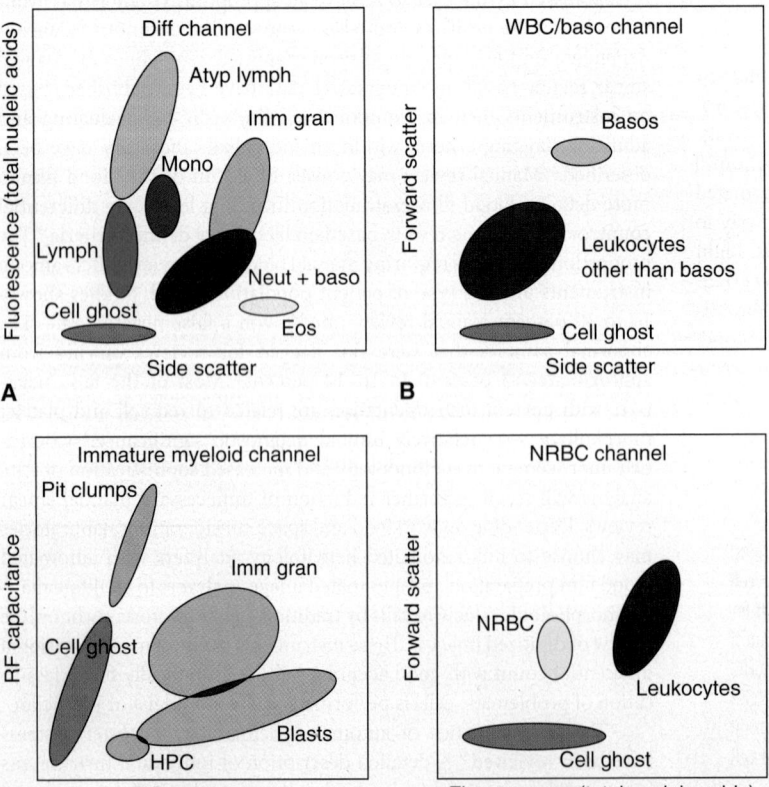

Figure 2–1. Schematic of multiparameter cell discrimination in an automated hematology analyzer. The Sysmex XE-2100 is used as an example, in which leukocytes are discriminated by **(A)** DNA/RNA fluorescence using a polymethine dye versus high-angle (side) light scatter in lysed blood; **(B)** side scatter versus low-angle (forward) light scatter after acidic lysis in a separate aliquot that preserves basophil structure; and **(C)** direct current (DC) impedance versus radio frequency (RF) capacitance of cells subjected to a lysis reagent that relatively preserves immature cells with lower membrane lipid content. Nucleated red blood cells (NRBC) are distinguished **(D)** in a lysed sample stained with nucleic acid dye where leukocyte nuclei have detectably higher DNA/RNA content than red cell nuclei. Atyp Lymph, atypical lymphocytes; Baso, basophils; Blasts, blast cells; Diff Channel, differential count channel; Eos, eosinophils; HPC, hematopoietic progenitor cells; Imm Gran, immature granulocytes; Lymph, lymphocytes; Mono, monocytes; Neut + Baso, neutrophils + basophils; Plt Clumps, platelet clumps; WBC, white blood cells.

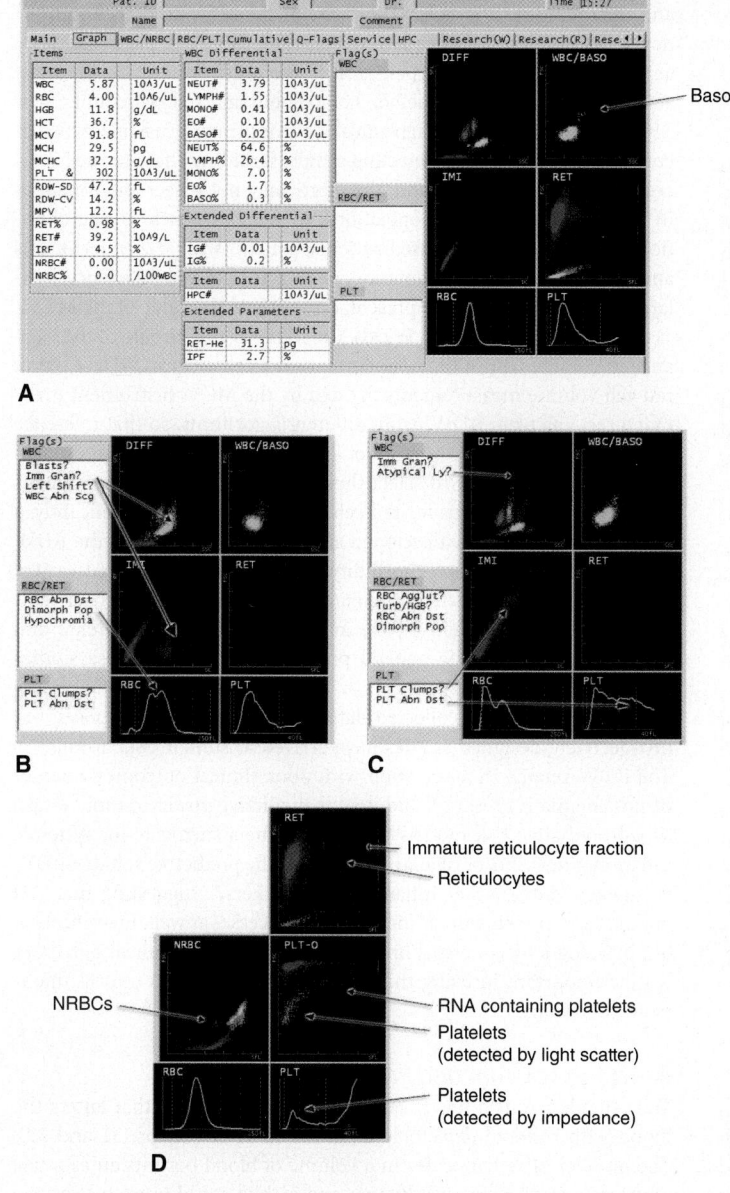

Figure 2–2. Examples of how samples containing various abnormal findings are flagged for manual review. **A.** Normal sample showing how the major variables and results are displayed. **B.** Immature granulocytes appearing on the DIFF (leukocyte differential count) and IMI (immature myeloid) histograms, as well as a dimorphic red cell population. **C.** Multiple flags, including cells in the area of atypical lymphocytes, and platelet clumps with abnormal platelet volume distribution. **D.** Appearance of nucleated red blood cells (NRBCs), reticulocytes, and reticulated platelets on a different set of parameters. This figure is not intended as a comprehensive illustration of the technical details, but serves to demonstrate that differential lysing reactions coupled with multiparameter light-scatter, impedance, capacitance, and fluorescence measurements are used to analyze blood cells in current high-throughput instruments.

AUTOMATED ANALYSIS OF RED CELLS

Some red cell parameters (for instance, mean cell volume [MCV], red cell number, hemoglobin concentration, red cell distribution width [RDW]) are directly measured, while others (for instance, hematocrit, mean cell hemoglobin [MCH], mean cell hemoglobin concentration [MCHC]) are derived from these primary measurements.

Measurement of the Red Cell Count and Hematocrit

In electronic instruments, the hematocrit (Hct; fractional volume of blood occupied by erythrocytes) is calculated from the product of direct measurements of the erythrocyte count and the MCV: (Hct [μL/100 μL] = RBC [$\times 10^{-6}$ /μL] $\times$ MCV [fl]/10). Falsely elevated MCV and decreased red cell counts can be observed when red cell autoantibodies are present and retain binding capability at room temperature (cold agglutinins and some cases of autoimmune hemolytic anemia). This causes red cells to clump and affects the accuracy of both the red blood cell (RBC) count and MCV, as well as the resultant hematocrit.

The hematocrit may also be determined by subjecting the blood to sufficient centrifugal force to pack the cells while minimizing trapped extracellular fluid. This approach was traditionally done in capillary tubes filled with blood and centrifuged at very high speed in a small tabletop centrifuge, and the technique was referred to as the "microhematocrit" or informally as a "spun crit." Before standardized methods for hemoglobin quantification were available, the hematocrit was the simplest and most accurate method for determining the fractional volume of red cells in blood and by inference the hemoglobin. However, this is a manual procedure not well adapted to routine processing in a high-volume clinical laboratory, and is affected by varying amounts of plasma trapped between red cells in the packed cell volume,[16] typically about 2 to 3 percent of the packed volume.[17] The hematocrit from polycythemic samples or blood containing abnormal erythrocytes (sickle cells, thalassemic red cells, iron-deficient red cells, spherocytes, macrocytes) is increased because of enhanced plasma trapping associated with increased red cell rigidity.[17] Therefore, although automated hematocrit values are adjusted to be equivalent to spun hematocrit for normal samples, in abnormal samples, the spun hematocrit may be spuriously elevated (up to 6 percent in microcytosis).[18] The hemoglobin determination now is preferred to the hematocrit, because it is measured directly and is the best indicator of the oxygen-carrying capacity of the blood.

Measurement of Hemoglobin

Hemoglobin is intensely colored, and this property has been used in methods for estimating its concentration in blood. Erythrocytes contain a mixture of hemoglobin, oxyhemoglobin, carboxyhemoglobin, methemoglobin, and minor amounts of other forms of hemoglobin. To determine hemoglobin concentration in the blood, red cells are lysed and hemoglobin variants are converted to the stable compound cyanmethemoglobin for quantification by absorption at 540 nm. All forms of hemoglobin are readily converted to cyanmethemoglobin except sulfhemoglobin, which is rarely present in significant amounts. In automated blood cell counters, hemoglobin is usually measured by a modified cyanmethemoglobin or an alternate lauryl sulphate method. In practice, the major interference with this measurement is chylomicronemia, but newer instruments identify and minimize this interference. Noninvasive transcutaneous monitoring of total hemoglobin concentration, as well as methemoglobin and carboxyhemoglobin, using multiwavelength pulse oximetry has become available.[19] Although these instruments offer the opportunity to track hemoglobin concentration trends in patients subject to blood loss and fluid shifts,[20] it is not yet clear that they have sufficient precision to guide transfusion decisions.[21,22] Such hemoglobin measurements may be unreliable under conditions of peripheral circulatory hypoperfusion.

The hemoglobin level varies with age (Table 2–1). Chapter 7 discusses changes in hemoglobin in the neonatal period. After the first week or two of extrauterine life, the hemoglobin falls from levels of approximately 17 g/dL to levels of approximately 12 g/dL by 2 months of age. Thereafter, the levels remain relatively constant throughout the first year of life. Any child with a hemoglobin level below 11 g/dL should be considered anemic.[23] Chapter 8 discusses changes in hemoglobin concentration with pregnancy and Chap. 9 discusses changes in hemoglobin levels in older persons.

Standard Red Cell Indices

The size and hemoglobin content of erythrocytes (red cell indices), based on population averages, have traditionally been used to assist in the differential diagnosis of anemia.[24] A variety of newer indices based on size and hemoglobinization characteristics of red cell subpopulations are discussed in the section "Novel Red Cell and Reticulocyte Indices".

Mean Cell Volume Automated blood counters measure the MCV directly by either electrical impedance or light scatter measurements of individual red cells. The MCV has been used to guide the diagnostic workup in patients with anemia; for example, testing patients with microcytic anemia for iron deficiency or thalassemia, and those with macrocytic anemia for folate or vitamin B_{12} deficiency. This approach has practical value, but also limitations[25]; for instance, MCV may be normal in some older patients with pernicious anemia,[26] or in advanced pernicious anemia with severe red cell fragmentation,[27] while one-third of older patients have an elevated MCV without an evident cause.[28] Mathematical manipulations of various red cell indices take advantage of the trend toward relatively more severe microcytosis than hypochromia in thalassemia trait versus iron-deficiency anemia to assist in the differential diagnosis of these disorders,[29] particularly in high-prevalence populations where laboratory resources are limited,[30] but their usefulness has been questioned.[31]

Mean Cell Hemoglobin The MCH, the amount of hemoglobin per red cell, increases or decreases in parallel with the red cell volume (i.e., MCV) and generally provides similar diagnostic information, although because this parameter is affected by both hypochromia and microcytosis, it is as least sensitive as the MCV in detecting iron-deficiency states.[32] Another advantage of the MCH is the consistency across different analyzer types, as it is derived from two of the most accurately measured parameters: hemoglobin and red cell count.[33] The MCHC is not used much diagnostically, and is primarily useful for quality control purposes, such as detecting sample turbidity. These red cell indices are average quantities and, therefore, may not detect abnormalities in blood with mixed-cell populations. In situations such as sideroblastic anemia, recently transfused patients, patients with severe pernicious anemia with red cell fragmentation, and folate plus iron deficiency, both large and small red cells are present, diminishing the value of the MCV.

Red Cell Distribution Width The RDW is an estimate of the variance in volume within the population of red cells, expressed as 1 SD of red cell volume measurements divided by the MCV. Instrument manufacturers calculate RDW using different algorithms, so that reference ranges vary according to analyzer model. The RDW can be used in the laboratory as a flag to select those samples that should have manual review of blood films for red cell morphology. More significantly, a large literature has now developed around the evidence that the RDW is a biomarker predicting morbidity and mortality in a broad variety of clinical settings,[34] such as angina/myocardial infarction,[35] heart failure, trauma, pneumonia, sepsis, intensive care treatment, renal and liver disease, and in the general population.[36] Most of these studies are retrospective, observational, or cohort-based studies, often using databases of routinely collected data gathered for other purposes, but prospectively designed studies have arrived at similar conclusions.[37,38] The RDW retains its association with poor clinical outcomes whether or not anemia is present,[39] and it adds predictive power to more established predictive risk models.[40] RDW may be a surrogate for systemic inflammation[41] and/or oxidative stress, but the predictive value of RDW is independent of other inflammatory markers,[40] suggesting that this biomarker is tracking other mechanistic processes as well. Identification of physiologic mechanisms linking RDW to adverse clinical outcomes will be important in using this predictive biomarker to inform therapeutic decisions.[34]

Reticulocyte Count and RNA Content

The reticulocyte is a newly released anucleate red cell that enters the blood with residual detectable amounts of RNA (Chaps. 31 and 32). The number of reticulocytes in a volume of blood permits an estimate of marrow erythrocyte production and is thus useful in evaluating the pathogenesis of anemia by distinguishing inadequate production from accelerated destruction (Chap. 32). The manual method for enumerating reticulocytes by placing a sample of blood in a tube containing new methylene blue and preparing a blood film to enumerate the proportion of cells that show blue beaded precipitates (residual ribosomes) has largely been replaced by automated methods, which are incorporated into high-volume hematology analyzers.[42] Reticulocytes are identified by direct fluorescence measurement after staining with RNA-binding dyes or light scatter measurements to detect staining if nonfluorescent RNA-binding dyes are used. Various proprietary combinations of light scatter and other parameters are used to minimize interferences such as nucleated red cells, nuclear remnants (Howell-Jolly bodies), malaria parasites, or platelet clumps.

Automated reticulocyte counts are typically reported in absolute numbers (reticulocytes per μL or per L of blood), obviating the need to correct for a reduced red cell count (anemia), if present. However, one may still consider the effect of elevated erythropoietin levels secondary to severe anemia, which results in premature release of reticulocytes persisting in the circulation for more than the usual 1 day, correspondingly inflating estimates of daily marrow reticulocyte production based

TABLE 2-1. Reference Ranges for Leukocyte Count, Differential Count, and Hemoglobin Concentration in Children*

Age	Leukocytes Total (× 10³/μL)	Neutrophils Total	Band	Segmented	Eosinophils	Basophils	Lymphocytes	Monocytes	Hemoglobin g/dL Blood
12 mo	11.4(6.0–17.5)	3.5(1.5–8.5)	0.35(0–1.0)	3.2(1.0–8.5)	0.30(0.05–0.70)	0.05(0–0.20)	7.0(4.0–10.5)	0.55(0.05–1.1)	12.6(11.1–14.1)
		31	*3.1*	*28*	*2.6*	*0.4*	*61*	*4.8*	
4 yr	9.1(5.5–15.5)	3.8(1.5–8.5)	0.27(0–1.0)	3.5(1.5–7.5)	0.25(0.02–0.65)	0.05(0–0.2)	4.5(2.0–8.0)	0.45(0–0.8)	12.7(11.2–14.3)
		42	*3.0*	*39*	*2.8*	*0.6*	*50*	*5.0*	
6 yr	8.5(5.0–14.5)	4.3(1.5–8.0)	0.25(0–1.0)	4.0(1.5–7.0)	0.23(0–0.65)	0.05(0–0.2)	3.5(1.5–7.0)	0.40(0–0.8)	13.0(11.4–14.5)
		51	*3.0*	*48*	*2.7*	*0.6*	*42*	*4.7*	
10 yr	8.1(4.5–13.5)	4.4(1.8–8.0)	0.24(0–1.0)	4.2(1.8–7.0)	0.20(0–0.60)	0.04(0–0.2)	3.1(1.5–6.5)	0.35(0–0.8)	13.4(11.8–15.0)
		54	*3.0*	*51*	*2.4*	*0.5*	*38*	*4.3*	
21 yr	7.4(4.5–11.0)	4.4(1.8–7.7)	0.22(0–0.7)	4.2(1.8–7.0)	0.20(0–0.45)	0.04(0–0.2)	2.5(1.0–4.8)	0.30(0–0.8)	M: 15.5(13.5–17.5) F: 13.8(12.0–15.6)
		59	*3.0*	*56*	*2.7*	*0.5*	*34*	*4.0*	

*The means and ranges are in thousands of cells per mL. This table is provided as a guide. Normal ranges should be validated by the clinical laboratory for the specific methods in use. The number in *italic* is mean percentage of total leukocytes.

For leukocyte and differential count, see Altman PL, Dittmer DS (eds): *Blood and Other Body Fluids.* Federation of American Societies for Experimental Biology, Washington, DC, 1961.

For hemoglobin concentration, see Rudolph AM, Hoffman JI (eds): *Pediatrics*, 18th ed, pp 1011, 1012. Appleton and Lange, Norwalk, CT, 1987.

on the reticulocyte count (Chap. 32). The correlation between manual and automated methods of reticulocyte enumeration is good, but reference ranges differ slightly among the methods, given the different dyes and conditions used and the continuous nature of the variables separating reticulocytes from mature red cells.

Many hematology analyzers now report some quantitative measure of reticulocyte RNA content. Increase in the immature (highest RNA content) reticulocyte fraction is an early sign of marrow recovery from cytotoxic therapy[43] or treatment for nutritional anemias, usually preceding the rise in total reticulocyte count. A limitation at present is that the methods lack standardization and reference ranges for these parameters are instrument dependent.[44]

Additional Red Cell and Reticulocyte Indices

Current high-end automated cell counters measure unique properties of mature red cells and reticulocytes on a cell-by-cell basis, not just as population averages. The result is a plethora of new indices that are in many cases specific to an instrument manufacturer, presenting new diagnostic opportunities but also a confusing nomenclature and a potential lack of comparability. Some examples of parameters that have been studied include %HypoHe, %MicroR, RET-He (available on Sysmex instruments), CHr, HYPO% (Siemens), RSf, LHD% (Beckman-Coulter), and FRC (fragmented red cells; Sysmex and Siemens).

New formulas for distinguishing causes of microcytosis based on several novel red cell indices function about as well[45] or somewhat better[46] than traditional formulas for differentiating iron deficiency from thalassemia trait. More sophisticated mathematical modeling of individual cell-based volume and hemoglobin content data available in current analyzers has been used in a systems biology approach to demonstrate latent iron deficiency and to distinguish causes of microcytosis.[47,48] The ability of new automated analyzers to measure parameters specifically in reticulocytes on a cell-by-cell basis also opens up the possibility of reticulocyte-specific indices. The theoretical advantage is that acute changes in red cell function would be detected more rapidly and reliably in the reticulocyte fraction as opposed to the total red cell population.

Estimates of reticulocyte-specific hemoglobin content (CHr and RET-He, which are comparable) by light-scatter measurements of reticulocytes are closely related to adequacy of iron availability to erythroid precursors during the preceding 24 to 48 hours, and have been described as diagnostically useful in detecting functional iron deficiency in complex clinical settings, such as chronic inflammation[49] and chronic renal disease.[50] The increase in serum ferritin as an acute phase reactant combined with the physiologic variation of serum iron and iron-binding capacity limits the value of conventional parameters in these settings. The CHr may be a better predictor of depleted marrow iron stores than traditional serum iron parameters in nonmacrocytic patients,[51] and is a more sensitive predictor of iron deficiency than hemoglobin for screening infants[52] and adolescents for iron deficiency. Estimates of percentages of red cells falling below a cutoff for hemoglobin concentration (HYPO%) or hemoglobin content (%HypoHe) may provide greater sensitivity than the corresponding mean values averaged over all red cells, for instance with respect to iron deficiency in renal disease.[53] Four of the newer parameters (HYPO%, %HypoHe, CHr, RetHe) similarly outperformed transferrin saturation and ferritin in hemodialysis patients[54] for diagnosis of iron deficiency. However, both the CHr and RET-He are less effective than the MCH in screening elderly patients for iron-deficiency anemia.[55] The RSf (square root of MCV times MRV [mean reticulocyte volume]) and LHD% (a mathematical transformation of the MCHC) have similar diagnostic utility as RET-He.[56] Fragmented red cell (FRC) counts by automated analyzers, based on better methods of separating small red cells from platelets, appear to lack specificity and their clinical role is not yet defined.

These parameters have the advantage of ready access in the context of an automated blood count, but the availability of differently derived and calculated parameters from various instrument makers is a challenge to remember and compare across laboratories.

Other Red Cell Findings

Nucleated Red Cells Nucleated red cells are present in newborns, particularly if physiologically stressed, and in a variety of disorders, including hypoxic states (congestive heart failure), severe hemolytic anemia, primary myelofibrosis, and infiltrative disease of the marrow (Chap. 45). Most modern automated hematology analyzers are capable of detecting and quantitating nucleated red blood cells, which were a source of spuriously elevated leukocyte counts in earlier instruments, at a level of 1 to 2 nucleated red cells per 100 leukocytes.

Malarial Parasites Malarial parasites can also be detected by some current analyzers, based on detecting parasite infected red cells or neutrophils containing ingested hemozoin in regions of the multiparameter display that are not characteristically populated in normal blood (sometimes causing spurious eosinophilia[57]). Some reports indicate high sensitivity and specificity with certain instrumentation,[58] a useful consideration in endemic areas where access to technologists with morphologic expertise may not be consistent. Careful attention to instrument characteristics and limitations as well as the relative prevalence of disorders causing instrument flags in the laboratory's patient population is essential in fine tuning instrument review criteria to provide reasonable sensitivity and specificity.

Other Abnormalities Not Detected by Automation Some disorders, such as immune and hereditary spherocytosis (Chaps. 46 and 54), hemoglobin C disease (Chap. 49), elliptocytosis (Chap. 46), inherited granule abnormalities (Chap. 66), and malaria and other parasitic diseases (Chap. 53), may not be reliably detected by the various flagging strategies on automated analyzers, and morphologic findings such as basophilic stippling (Chap. 31), toxic granulation (Chap. 60), siderocytes (Chap. 31), and pathologic rouleaux (Chap. 109) are only detectable by microscopic examination of the blood film.

AUTOMATED ANALYSIS OF LEUKOCYTES

Leukocyte Count

Leukocyte counts are performed by automated cell counters on blood samples appropriately diluted with a solution that lyses the erythrocytes (e.g., an acid or a detergent), but preserves leukocyte integrity. Manual counting of leukocytes is used only when the instrument reports a potential interference or the count is beyond instrument linearity limits. Manual counts are subject to much greater technical variation than automated counts because of technical and statistical factors, and with modern instrumentation, need to be done infrequently. Instruments that perform an automated 5-part differential can measure absolute neutrophil counts accurately down to $100/\mu L$.[59] Automated leukocyte counts may be falsely elevated as a result of cryoglobulins or cryofibrinogen, clumped platelets or fibrin from an inadequately anticoagulated or mixed sample, ethylenediaminetetraacetic acid (EDTA)–induced platelet aggregation, nucleated red blood cells, or nonlysed red cells, and falsely decreased because of EDTA-induced neutrophil aggregation. This potential interference is instrument dependent, and current analyzers use a variety of algorithms to minimize their effect and flag those rare samples on which accurate automated analysis cannot be performed.

Leukocyte Differential

Leukocytes in the blood serve different functions and arise from different hematopoietic lineages, so it is important to evaluate each of the major leukocyte types separately. Modern automated instruments use multiple parameters to identify and enumerate the five major morphologic leukocyte types in blood: neutrophils, basophils, eosinophils, lymphocytes, and monocytes, as well as indicate the possible presence of immature or abnormal cell. Customarily, both absolute (cells per μL) and relative (percent of leukocytes) counts are reported in the leukocyte differential. It is the absolute values that relate to pathologic states, and percentages are sometimes misleading (e.g., absolute neutropenia appearing as a relative lymphocytosis) if the absolute values are not carefully examined. Some have proposed to eliminate the reporting of differential count percentages entirely for this reason.[60] "Band" neutrophils cannot be identified as such by automated analyzers, although they will usually trigger a manual review flag if present in increased numbers. Current high-throughput instruments can perform an accurate automated "five-part" differential count with a false-positive rate (i.e., unnecessarily flagged for review) of 2 to 15 percent in samples from a medical center patient population.[61] Eosinophils are accurately counted by current state-of-the-art instruments, but automated basophil counts remain imprecise.[11] Small numbers of abnormal cells can escape detection by either automated or manual methods. The false-negative rate for detection of abnormal cells varies from 1 to 20 percent, depending on the instrument, type of abnormal cell examined, and the detection limit desired (1–5 percent abnormal cells).[62-64] Careful attention to use of flagging criteria designed to prompt manual review, which are linked to instrument-specific methodology, is essential to insure that optimum workflow strategies are used to detect samples containing abnormal cells with a manageable rate of manual review. Many instruments have "blast" flags designed to pick up leukemic blasts, but the sensitivity of such flags alone varied from 65 to 94 percent in a recent study,[11] and is lower in leukopenic patients.[65] One must rely not only on the specifically designed "blast" flags, but also on other abnormalities identified in the automated blood count, including other flags, to select samples for manual morphologic smear review. Lymphoma cells and reactive lymphocytes are the most difficult for both automated instruments and the human observer to identify. If one needs to search for infrequent abnormal cells or evaluate leukocyte morphology, there is still no substitute for microscopic examination of a properly stained blood film by a trained observer. The variability of morphologic quantification of band neutrophils is so high that some have advocated ceasing quantitative reporting of band cells.[66] In spite of instrumentation that permits automated analysis of a majority of clinical samples, the leukocyte differential count is still labor intensive relative to other high-volume laboratory tests, and its value as a cause-finding tool in screening of asymptomatic patients has been questioned.[67]

The normal differential leukocyte count varies with age. As described in Chap. 7, polymorphonuclear neutrophils are predominant in the first few days after birth, but thereafter lymphocytes account for the majority of leukocytes. This pattern persists up to approximately 4 to 5 years of age, when the polymorphonuclear leukocyte again becomes the predominant cell and remains so throughout the rest of childhood and adult life. Chapter 9 discusses the leukocyte count in older persons. The leukocyte count may decrease slightly in older subjects because of a fall in the lymphocyte count with age. Neutrophil counts are lower in individuals of African descent, and in some Middle Eastern populations than in persons of European descent.[68]

AUTOMATED ANALYSIS OF PLATELETS

Platelet Count

Platelets are usually counted electronically by enumerating particles in the unlysed sample within a specified volume window (e.g., 2–20 fl), where volume may be measured by electrical impedance or light scatter.[69] The platelet count was more difficult to automate than the red cell count because of the small size, tendency to aggregate, and potential overlap of platelets with more numerous smaller red cells and cellular debris. Current instruments typically construct a platelet volume histogram based on platelet size within a reliably measured platelet volume window and mathematically extrapolate this histogram to account for platelets whose size overlaps with debris (smaller) or small red cells (larger). This works because platelet volumes in health or disease follow a log-normal distribution. Some analyzers compare platelet counts determined by different methods (e.g., impedance, light scatter, or fluorescence staining) to improve accuracy, especially useful for low platelet counts. Based on analysis of volume-distribution histograms of platelets and red cells and comparison of optical and impedance-based platelet counts, suspect samples are flagged for microscopic review. Automated platelet counting by current instrumentation is accurate and far more precise than manual methods. At very low platelet counts (less than 20×10^9/L), results are less precise[70] and there is a method-dependent tendency to overestimate platelet counts.[71] Conversely, platelet activation in disorders such as disseminated intravascular coagulation (DIC) and acute leukemia may result in systematic slight undercounting of platelets.[72] Advances in instrumentation, such as fluorescent dyes to more specifically identify platelets in thrombocytopenic[73] and microcytic[74] samples, should improve accuracy. When reviewing the blood film, platelet count may be roughly estimated as 2000 times the number of platelets in 10 consecutive oil immersion (1000×) fields.[75]

Falsely Decreased Platelet Counts Causes of falsely decreased platelet counts include incomplete anticoagulation of the sample (sometimes accompanied by small clots in the specimen or fibrin strands on the stained film) and platelet clumping (pseudothrombocytopenia) or "satellitism" (adherence of platelets to neutrophils), caused by aggregation induced by nonpathogenic antibodies recognizing platelet adhesion molecule epitopes exposed as a result of chelation of divalent cations in the anticoagulated sample.[69] Platelet clumping occurs in approximately 0.1 percent of hospitalized patients.[76] The same phenomenon may occur to a lesser degree in citrate, which is often used to obtain platelet count in such cases. Magnesium EDTA, as compared to sodium EDTA, anticoagulant is reported to more effectively inhibit platelet aggregation in these patients and provide an accurate platelet count.[77] Classical causes of falsely elevated platelet count include severe microcytosis, cryoglobulins, and leukocyte cytoplasmic fragmentation.[69] Infrequently, it may be necessary to confirm automated results by a microscopic (phase contrast) platelet count or platelet estimate from the blood film, bearing in mind that these methods are imprecise.

Mean Platelet Volume The mean platelet volume (MPV) has been proposed as a useful clinical tool in the differential diagnosis of thrombocytopenias, and is associated with cardiovascular risk, stroke, and metabolic disease. Increased MPV may be related in a complex way to thrombopoietic stimuli that affect megakaryocyte ploidy, and not platelet age per se. A platelet volume distribution width (PDW) can be calculated just as the RDW, and is correlated with platelet count and MPV.[78] However, platelet size parameters are difficult to accurately quantify and use diagnostically because of the wide physiologic variation of the MPV in normal subjects, lack of standardization of automated measurement techniques and instability of platelet size parameters in the presence of commonly used anticoagulants.[79]

Newly Released (Reticulated) Platelets Newly released platelets contain RNA, as do newly released red cells, and are functionally more active, with enhanced expression of adhesion molecules and bound coagulation factors.[80] The number of platelets with high RNA content (sometimes termed *reticulated platelets* or *immature platelet fraction*, measured by flow cytometry with RNA-binding fluorescent dyes, or by certain automated analyzers[81]) is a marker of marrow megakaryocytopoiesis and is proposed as a way of differentiating decreased production of platelets from circulatory destruction or removal as a cause of thrombocytopenia, in an analogous fashion to the use of the reticulocyte count. The percentage of reticulated platelets is increased in destructive thrombocytopenias, but remains within the reference range in hypoproductive states.[82] Reticulated platelet number or RNA content correlates with imminent platelet recovery after chemotherapy.[83] Reticulated platelet number is correlated with risk of death in patients with acute coronary syndrome[84] and DIC,[85] and with hyporesponsiveness to platelet function inhibitors[86] or aspirin.[87]

REFERENCE RANGES

The use of reference ranges for quantitative hematology measurements deserves some additional comment. The physiologic variation of certain blood cell counts is notably higher than usually found in blood chemistry analytes. This is a reflection of the adaptive responsiveness of the marrow and other tissues to cytokine and hormonal signaling. For instance, the leukocyte and differential counts are affected by stress, diurnal variation, tobacco smoking, and ethnic origin. With increasing globalization of clinical research and therapy, ethnic characterization of populations used for reference ranges is critical to data interpretation of clinical studies.[88] Platelet count and MPV show substantial ethnic variation.[89]

The platelet and absolute neutrophil counts are lower in individuals of African ethnic origin.[68] American men and women of African descent have lower hemoglobin concentrations than do men and women of European descent, a difference that is reduced by half, but still significant, when subjects with iron deficiency, thalassemia, sickle trait, and renal disease are excluded.[90] Important clinical consequences may result from these differences; for instance, reduced neutrophil counts in Americans of African descent result in lower-dose intensity of treatment in early stage breast cancer, which may be related to survival outcome disparities.[91] Beutler and West[90] summarize the situation well: "The problem cannot be solved by simply establishing different ranges for different ethnic groups, especially since all represent some degree of admixture. Thus, it is basically information that the physician must possess that becomes one of the many factors that we designate as clinical judgment." With these caveats in mind, reference ranges for children, and African American, Hispanic, and white adults are presented in Tables 2–1 and 2–2. As with all laboratory parameters, clinical interpretation of patient results should be based on laboratory specific reference ranges. Therefore, these tables are not presented to guide interpretation of specific laboratory results, but to indicate the challenges facing laboratories and physicians in constructing and interpreting reference ranges of even standard and traditional assays.

TABLE 2–2. Published Reference Ranges for Key Blood Variables

	NORIP[107]	Wakeman[92]	Cheng[93]			Bain[106]	
Date	2003	2004	1994	1994	1994	1996	1996
Ethnicity	Nordic	U.K.	U.S. European descent	U.S. African descent	U.S. Mexican descent	U.K. European descent	U.K. African descent
No.	1800	250	3125	1712	1735	200	115
Hgb (g/dL) (M)	13.4–17.0	13.7–17.2	13.2–16.9	12.0–16.2	13.1–16.7	NA	NA
(F)	11.7–15.3	12.0–15.2	10.7–15.1	10.2–14.4	11.4–15.0		
Hct (%) (M)	40–50	40–50	39–50	36–48	39–50	NA	NA
(F)	35–46	37–46	34–45	32–43	33–45		
MCV (fl)	82–98	83–98 (M)	79–97 (M)	75–97 (M)	83–96 (M)	NA	NA
		85–98 (F)	77–97 (F)	75–97 (F)	81–98 (F)		
WBC (× 10⁹/L)	3.5–8.8	3.6–9.2	4.1–11.7 (M)	3.5–9.5 (M)	4.6–10.6 (M)	3.6–9.2 (M)	2.8–7.2 (M)
			4.3–12.0 (F)	3.4–10.5 (F)	4.3–11.3 (F)	3.5–10.8 (F)	3.2–7.8 (F)
Neutrophils (× 10⁹/L)	NA	1.7–6.2	2.7–8.1 (M)	1.5–7.4 (M)	2.2–6.6 (M)	1.7–6.1 (M)	0.9–4.2 (M)
			2.5–6.9 (F)	1.5–8.4 (F)	2.5–7.9 (F)	1.7–7.5 (F)	1.3–4.2 (F)
Lymphocytes (× 10⁹/L)	NA	1.0–3.4	1.1–3.7 (M)	1.1–3.6 (M)	1.3–3.4 (M)	1.0–2.9 (M)	1.0–3.2 (M)
			1.2–3.7 (F)	1.3–3.9 (F)	1.3–3.9 (F)	1.0–3.5 (F)	1.1–3.6 (F)
Monocytes (× 10⁹/L)	NA	0.2–0.8	0.13–0.86 (M)	0.11–0.72 (M)	0.14–0.70 (M)	0.18–0.62 (M)	0.15–0.58 (M)
			0.11–0.78 (F)	0.12–0.83 (F)	0.12–0.79 (F)	0.14–0.61 (F)	0.15–0.39 (F)
Platelets (× 10⁹/L) (M)	145–348	140–320	161–385	161–381	166–388	143–332	115–290
(F)	165–387	180–380	178–434	178–452	171–411	169–358	125–342

F, female; Hct, hematocrit; Hgb, hemoglobin; M, male; MCV, mean cell; NORIP, Nordic Reference Interval Project; U.K., United Kingdom; U.S., United States; WBC, white blood cell count; NA, measurement not available.

*Ranges calculated from adult (>18 years) data, assuming equal contribution of subjects from each of multiple adult age groups, derived from the National Health and Nutrition Examination Survey (NHANES) III.

This table is provided as a guide. Normal ranges should be validated by the clinical laboratory for the specific methods in use.

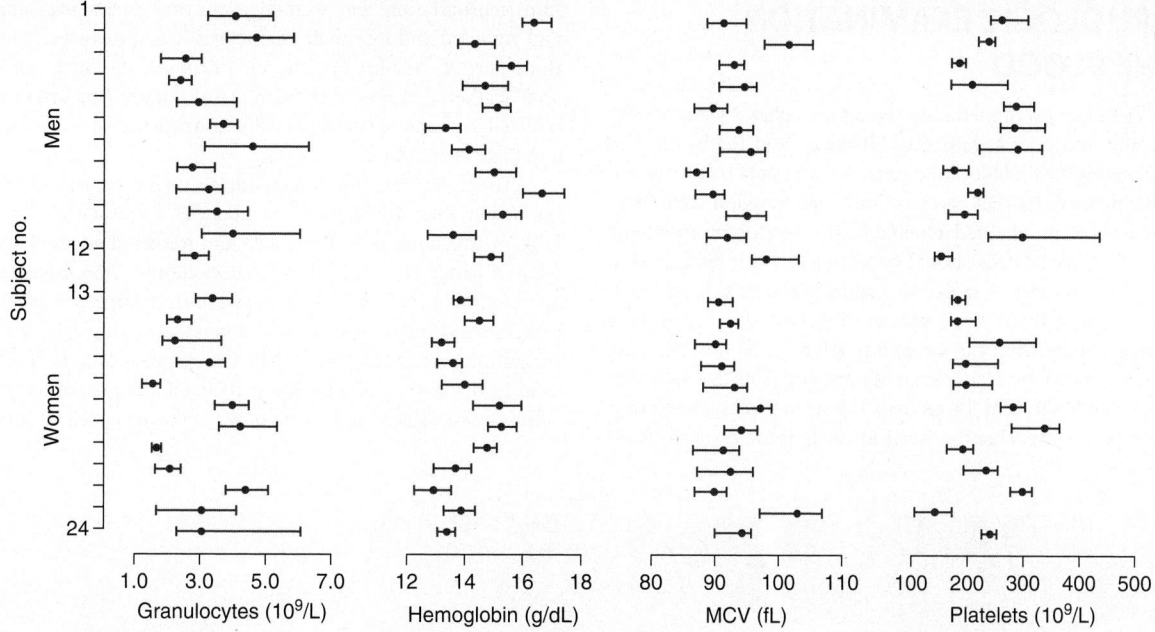

Figure 2–3. Absolute neutrophil count, hemoglobin, mean cell volume (MCV), and platelet count determined repeatedly by automated hematology analyzer on 24 healthy elderly subjects. Fasting (7–9 AM) blood samples were obtained 9 to 10 times at 14-day intervals from seated elderly subjects with minimal stasis by the same phlebotomist and performed in duplicate on the morning specimen collection. Subjects had no chronic medical conditions requiring therapy and were not taking drugs. The mean and range for each patient is shown separately for each assay. This is an illustration of the relatively narrow range within which most variables are maintained in an individual, whereas there are striking differences in both mean and variance between subjects. Reference ranges need to encompass at least 95% of values from all healthy individuals, placing limits on diagnostic sensitivity in detecting progressive change in a hematologic variable, previously maintained in a homeostatic range. *(Adapted with permission from Fraser CG, Wilkinson SP, Neville RG, et al: Biologic variation of common hematologic laboratory quantities in the elderly. Am J Clin Pathol 92(4):465–470. 1989.)*

Note the variation in reference ranges obtained from different studies. The major variability is likely population selection, especially the degree to which chronic illness or asymptomatic iron deficiency are excluded, and physiologic factors, such as diurnal variation, are considered. For example, the Wakeman study[92] exclusively used early morning samples, hence the upper limit of leukocyte count is lower because of diurnal physiologic variation. The National Health and Nutritional Examination Surveys (NHANES) III national database has the advantage of being a very large broad nationwide sampling, which, as used by Cheng and colleagues,[93] excluded any subjects with history of smoking, alcohol consumption, contraceptive use, and a variety of chronic diseases (excluding 60 percent of the tested subjects). However, those with asymptomatic iron deficiency were not excluded, so hemoglobin tends to be lower than in studies that may have been weighted toward groups of individuals in which undiagnosed iron deficiency and other asymptomatic disorders are less common. α- and β-thalassemia traits are also quite common in healthy individuals of certain ethnic groups, and inclusion of subjects with these disorders will also affect reference ranges. Normal lower limits for hemoglobin have been determined in U.S. subjects of different ethnic backgrounds carefully screened for occult disease.[94] Such considerations also affect determination of the upper (97.5th percentile) limit of normal hematocrit and hemoglobin in relation to a possible diagnosis of polycythemia, where one has to carefully weigh the likelihood that a "normal-range" study has adequately excluded iron-deficient subjects.[95,96] Biomedical parameters are also subject to historical trends, such as the observed improvement in hemoglobin levels in the post–folic-acid-fortification era.[97] Finally, when one observes significant changes in reference ranges based on age (e.g., glomerular filtration rate, lipid parameters, hemoglobin), there is the question of whether this is physiologic or a result of increased prevalence of undiagnosed occult disease.

Most hematologic variables show more stability within an individual than between individuals, illustrating one reason for the lack of sensitivity and specificity of any test "cutoff," which is typically designed for a population rather than for an individual person. A study of repeated analyses of blood variables from older subjects[98] graphically demonstrates this phenomenon. Some normal subjects have a normal steady-state platelet count between $170 \times 10^9/L$ and $200 \times 10^9/L$, whereas others have one between $280 \times 10^9/L$ and $310 \times 10^9/L$ (Fig. 2–3). For the latter group, a progressive fall in platelet count because of marrow failure may not be detected as quickly as the former group. The same observations are shown for absolute neutrophil count, hemoglobin, and MCV, among others. In normal subjects, the ratio of between subject to within subject variation ranges from about two times for absolute neutrophil count[99] to four to six times for hemoglobin, platelet count, absolute reticulocyte count, and MCV.[100] Data from a large clinical trial's central laboratory show similar findings for hemoglobin in study subjects with various disease states. In this report bayesian methods were used to construct a (narrower) personalized reference range using progressive accumulation of baseline measurements to achieve greater sensitivity to perturbations following treatment.[101] Circadian variations in hematologic laboratory values, including hematocrit, total leukocyte count, serum iron, and serum folate have been described.[102] Some have proposed to customize reference ranges for time of sample collection, so that reference ranges aren't inflated by the need to accommodate circadian variation.[103] Genetic loci affect quantitative hematologic traits (such as hemoglobin, MCH, platelet count, leukocyte count, etc.) in normal subjects of European, African, and South Asian ancestry.[104,105] The loci contain many candidate genes known to be involved in hematopoiesis, but known genetic influences identified in such studies only explain a small proportion (4–9 percent) of the observed phenotypic heterogeneity of these variables.

●MORPHOLOGIC EXAMINATION OF THE BLOOD

Microscopic examination of the blood spread on a glass slide or cover-slip yields useful information regarding all the cells of the blood. The process of preparing a thin blood film causes mechanical trauma to the cells, introducing artifacts that can be minimized by good technique. The optimal part of the stained blood film to use for morphologic examination of the blood cells should be sufficiently thin that a small proportion of erythrocytes in a ×1000 magnification field touch each other, but not so thin that no red cells are touching. Figure 2–4 is a composite image taken from the optimal portion of the film showing the five major leukocyte types, normal red cells, and platelets. Selection of a portion of the blood film for analysis that is too thick or too thin for proper morphologic evaluation is the most common error in blood film interpretation. For example, leukemic blasts may appear dense and rounded and lose their characteristic features when viewed in the thick part of the film. For specific purposes, the thick portion or side and "feathered" edges of the film are of interest (for instance, to detect microfilariae and malarial parasites or to search for large abnormal cells and platelet clumps).

The blood film is first scanned at low magnification (×200) to confirm reasonably even distribution of leukocytes and to check for abnormally large or immature cells in the side and feathered edges of the film. The feathered edge is examined for platelet clumps. Abnormal cells, red cell aggregation or rouleaux, background bluish staining consistent with para-proteinemia, and parasites are all findings that can be suggested by medium magnification examination (×400). The optimal portion of the film is then examined at high magnification (×1000, oil immersion) to systematically assess the size, shape, and morphology of the major cell lineages.

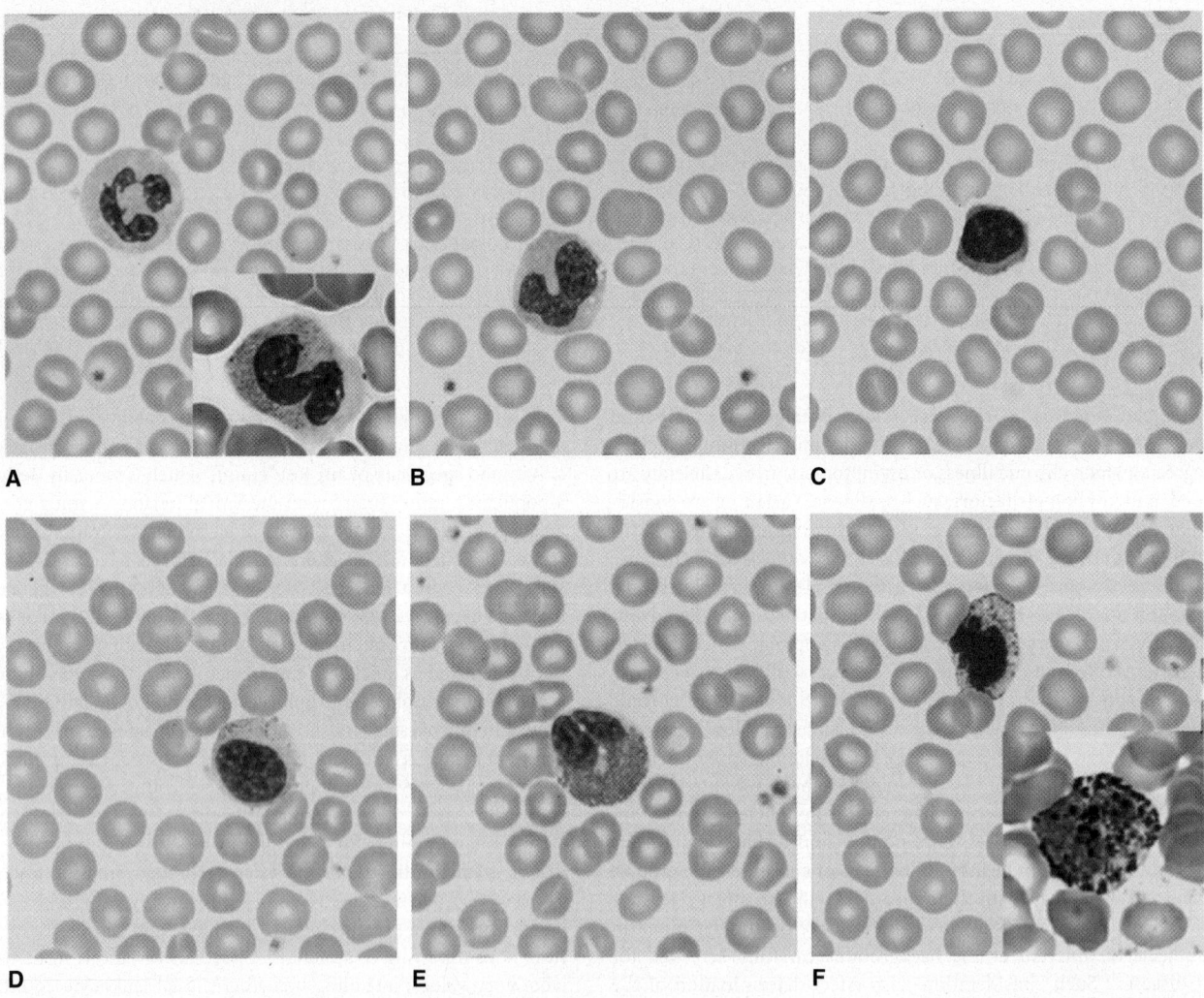

Figure 2–4. Images from a normal blood film showing major leukocyte types. The red cells are normocytic (normal size) and normochromic (normal hemoglobin content) with normal shape. The scattered platelets are normal in frequency and morphology. **A.** A platelet caught sitting in the biconcavity of the red cell in the preparation of the blood film. This normal finding should not be mistaken for a red cell inclusion. Images are taken from the optimal portion of the blood film for morphologic analysis. Image shows a **(A)** segmented (polymorphonuclear) neutrophil and in the inset a band neutrophil; **(B)** monocyte; **(C)** small lymphocyte; **(D)** large granular lymphocyte, note larger size than lymphocyte in **(C)** and increased amount of cytoplasm containing scattered eosinophilic granules; and **(E)** eosinophil. Virtually all normal blood eosinophils are bilobed and filled with relatively large (compared to the neutrophil) eosinophilic granules. **F.** Basophil and in inset a basophil that was less degranulated during film preparation, showing relatively large basophilic granules. The eosinophilic and basophilic granules are readily resolvable by light microscopy (×1000), whereas the neutrophilic granule is not resolvable but in the aggregate imparts a faint tan coloration to the neutrophil cytoplasm, quite distinctly different from the blue-gray cytoplasmic coloring of the monocyte and lymphocyte.

RED CELL MORPHOLOGY

Normal erythrocytes on dried films are nearly uniform in size, with a mean diameter of approximately 7.5 μm (normal and abnormal red cells are described in more detail in Chap. 31). The normal-sized erythrocyte is about the diameter of the nucleus of a small lymphocyte. The MCV is a more sensitive measure of red cell volume than the red cell diameter; however, an experienced observer should be able to recognize abnormalities in average red cell size when the MCV is significantly elevated or decreased. *Anisocytosis* is the term that describes variation in erythrocyte size, and is the morphologic correlate of the RDW. *Macrocytes* and *microcytes* are red cells larger or smaller than normal, and their presence consistent with the measured MCV suggests certain diagnostic possibilities. Early ("shift" or "stress") *reticulocytes* (i.e., those with the most residual RNA) appear in stained films as large, slightly bluish cells, referred to as *polychromatophilic* cells (Chap. 32). These cells are roughly the morphologic counterpart of the immature reticulocyte fraction identified by automated instruments.

The normal erythrocyte on a blood film is circular with central pallor. *Poikilocytosis* is a term used to describe variations in the shape of erythrocytes. The predominant appearance of a specific abnormality in red cell shape can be an important diagnostic clue in patients with anemia (Fig. 2–5). Erythrocytes with evenly spaced spikes (echinocytes or crenated cells) can be an artifact caused by prolonged storage, or may reflect metabolic erythrocyte abnormalities.

The normal erythrocyte appears as a disc with a rim of hemoglobin and a clear central area, which normally occupies less than one-half the cell diameter. Increased central pallor *(hypochromia)* is associated with disorders characterized by diminished hemoglobin synthesis, such as iron deficiency (Chap. 42). Evaluation of red cell hemoglobin content, as well as red cell size, is dependent on examining the proper part of the blood film. Cells at the far "feathered edge" will always be large and lack central pallor, whereas cells in the thick part of the film will look small and rounded and will also lack central pallor. A sharp refractile border demarcating the central area of pallor is an artifact secondary to inadequate drying of the film before staining (associated with high humidity, and more common in anemic samples). *Spherocytes* are more densely stained and appear smaller because of their rounded shape, and show decreased or absent central pallor. A red cell with a spot or disc of hemoglobin within the central pale area is a *target cell,* in reality a cup-shaped cell that distorts as it is flattened on the glass slide. These cells are typically found in disorders of hemoglobin synthesis (e.g., thalassemia), liver disease, and postsplenectomy where the cell-surface-to-cell-volume ratio is high. Chapter 31 describes the inclusions that may be observed in erythrocytes on blood films.

Erythrocytes are usually distributed evenly throughout the blood film. In some cases the cells become aligned in overlapping stacks, referred to as rouleaux (Chap. 109), resembling overlapping rows of coins. Rouleaux are normal in the thick part of the film, but when found in the optimal viewing portion of the film, suggest a pathologic increase in immunoglobulin (Ig), particularly IgM-macroglobulinemia. Occasionally, high concentrations of IgA or IgG in patients with myeloma may also produce rouleaux.

The blood film is also useful to identify red cells with basophilic stippling (evidence of dyserythropoiesis), siderotic granules (evidence of sideroblastic erythropoiesis), Heinz bodies (evidence of unstable hemoglobins), and Howell-Jolly bodies (nuclear remnants). Microorganisms other than malaria parasites also may be found in or attached to red cells (Chap. 53).

PLATELET MORPHOLOGY

Platelets appear in normal stained blood film as small blue or colorless bodies with red or purple granules (see Fig. 2–4). Normal platelets average approximately 1 to 2 μm in diameter, but show wide variation in shape, from round to elongated, cigar-shaped forms. In improperly prepared films, platelets may form large aggregates in some areas and appear to be diminished or absent in others. The frequent occurrence of giant platelets or platelet masses may indicate a myeloproliferative neoplasm or improper collection of the blood specimen. The latter circumstance can occur when venipuncture technique is faulty and platelets become activated before the blood sample is thoroughly mixed with anticoagulant. These platelet masses are apparent typically in the thin "feathered edge" of the film, with corresponding fewer platelets elsewhere.

	Name	Characteristic of	Also seen in
●	Spherocyte (Chaps. 31, 46, 54)	Hereditary spherocytosis, immune hemolytic anemia	Clostridial perfringens septicemia, Wilson disease
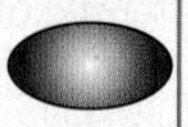 ◕	Elliptocyte (Chaps. 31, 46)	Hereditary elliptocytosis (HE)	Iron deficiency, megaloblastic anemia, thalassemia, myelofibrosis, MDS
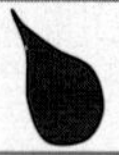 ◣	Dacryocyte (teardrop) (Chaps. 31, 86)	Myelofibrosis	Severe iron deficiency, megaloblastic anemia, thalassemia, MDS
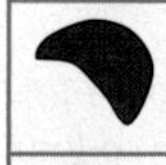 ◣	Schistocyte (Chaps. 31, 51, 129, 132)	Microangiopathic, mechanical hemolytic anemia	Occasional schistocytes are seen in many disorders affecting red cells.
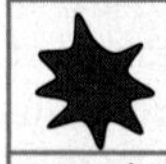 ✦	Echinocyte (Chaps. 31, 37)	Renal failure, malnutrition	Common *in vitro* artifact after storage
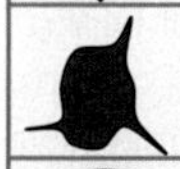 ◣	Acanthocyte (Chaps. 31, 56)	Spur cell anemia, abetalipoproteinemia	Postsplenectomy
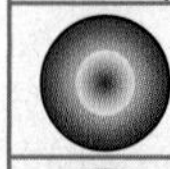 ◉	Target cell (Chaps. 31, 48)	Cholestasis, Hgb C disease	Iron deficiency, thalassemia
◖	Stomatocyte (Chaps. 31, 46)	Hereditary stomatocytosis	Alcoholism

Figure 2–5. Disorders associated with certain red cell morphologic changes. *Poikilocytosis* is a general term used to indicate the presence of abnormally shaped red cells, such as dacryocytes (teardrop-shaped red cells), schistocytes (fragmented red cells), and elliptocytes, as is found in the most extreme form in hereditary pyropoikilocytosis (Chap. 46). MDS, myelodysplastic syndromes (Chap. 87).

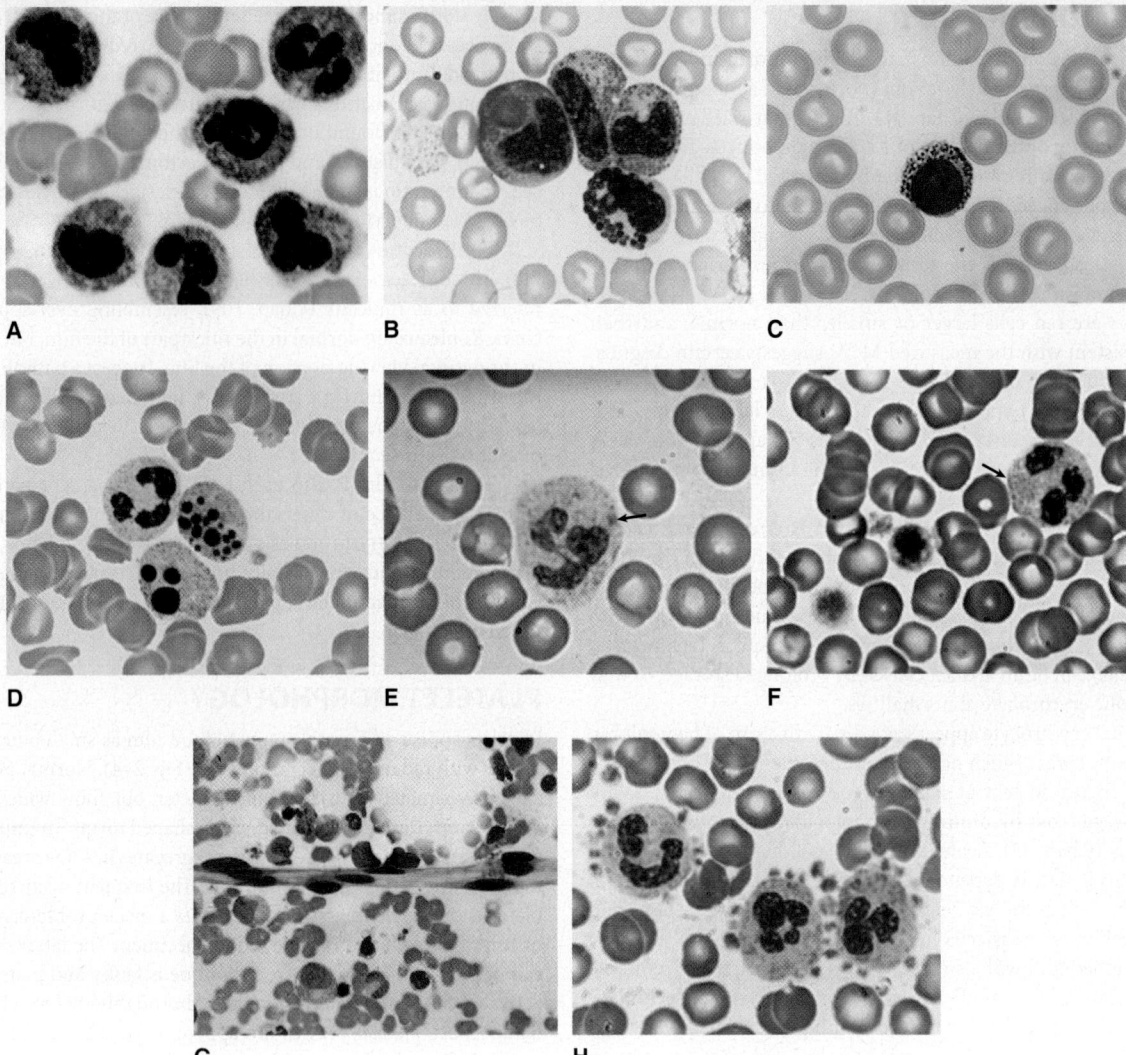

Figure 2–6. Blood films. **A.** Toxic granules in neutrophils. In inflammatory states the neutrophil may develop overt purplish granules as shown in this example of reactive neutrophilia. **B.** Chédiak-Higashi disease. Note the giant eosinophilic granule in the monocyte and the numerous enlarged granules in the lymphocyte (Chap. 66). **C.** Hurler syndrome. Note characteristic prominent dense cytoplasmic inclusions in the mononuclear cell. These inclusions are accumulations of glycosaminoglycans resulting from a deficiency of α-L-iduronidase in leukocytes and other tissues. **D.** Examples of apoptosis of two neutrophils in normal anticoagulated blood during standing at room temperature. Nuclear condensation and fragmentation are evident. A normal neutrophil is also present. **E.** Döhle bodies. These RNA remnants of rough endoplasmic reticulum appear as blue rod-shaped structures (*arrow* points to one) in neutrophils involved in inflammatory reactions. **F.** May-Hegglin disease. The large blue-gray inclusions (*arrow*) represent precipitates of nonmuscle myosin heavy chain type IIA. Note also the two macrothrombocytes (the size of red cells) characteristic of this disorder (Chap. 120). The neutrophil inclusions stain with fluorescent antibodies to nonmuscle myosin heavy chain type IIA. **G.** Marrow film. A strand of endothelial cells derived from vascular tissue caught on the biopsy needle. Individual endothelial cells may be found, rarely in a blood film. **H.** Platelet satellitism. Three neutrophils surrounded by adherent platelets. This blood film was prepared from an EDTA-anticoagulated sample. *(Reproduced with permission from Lichtman's Atlas of Hematology, www.accessmedicine.com.)*

Platelet clumping throughout the blood film, or platelet "satellitism" (adherence of platelets to neutrophils), may be a result of platelet agglutinins (Fig. 2–6). A platelet will occasionally overlie an erythrocyte, where it may be mistaken for an inclusion body or a parasite. The differentiation depends on the observation of a halo around the platelet, determination that it lies above the plane of the erythrocyte, and observation of the characteristics of a normal platelet in the "inclusion."

LEUKOCYTE MORPHOLOGY

The cells normally found in blood are mature neutrophils, lymphocytes, and monocytes, with smaller numbers of eosinophils and basophils

(see Fig. 2–4). *Neutrophils* are round cells ranging from 10 to 14 μm in diameter on a blood film. The nucleus is lobulated, with two to four lobes connected by a thin chromatin thread. The defining feature of the mature neutrophil is the round lobes with condensed chromatin, because the chromatin thread may overlie the nucleus and not be visible. The chromatin stains purple and is coarse and arranged in clumps. The nucleus of 1 to 16 percent of the neutrophils from females may have an appendage that is shaped like a drumstick and is attached to one lobe by a strand of chromatin. It represents the inactive X chromosome of the pair. The cytoplasm is diffusely pale pink and contains many small, tan to pink granules distributed evenly throughout the cell. *Bands* are identical in appearance to mature neutrophils except that the nucleus is not segmented but is sausage-shaped or U-shaped (see Fig. 2–4). Nuclear chromatin is slightly less condensed than the mature neutrophil (Chap. 60).

Eosinophils are on the average slightly larger than neutrophils (Chap. 62). The nucleus usually has two lobes (see Fig. 2–4). The chromatin pattern is the same as that of the neutrophil, but the nucleus tends to be more lightly stained. The differentiating characteristic of these cells is the presence of many refractile, orange-red granules that are distributed evenly throughout the cell and may be visible overlying the nucleus. These granules are larger than those in the neutrophil and are more uniform in size. Occasionally, some of the granules in eosinophils stain light blue rather than orange-red.

Basophils are similar to the other polymorphonuclear cells and are slightly smaller than neutrophils (Chap. 63). The nucleus may stain more faintly and usually is less segmented and has less distinct chromatin condensation than is the case in neutrophils. The large deeply basophilic granules of basophils are fewer in number and less regular in size and shape than in the eosinophil. The granules are visible overlying the nucleus and, in some cells, almost completely obscure the lightly stained nuclear chromatin. Because the granular constituents are water soluble, some granules may stain only faintly or not at all or may be lost from the cell during preparation (see Fig. 2–4).

Lymphocytes on blood films are usually smaller than other leukocytes, approximately 10 μm in diameter, but large lymphocytes up to 20 μm in diameter occasionally are seen (see Fig. 2–4). The small lymphocyte, the predominant type in normal blood, is round and contains a relatively large, round, densely stained nucleus (Chap. 73). The cytoplasm is scanty and stains pale to dark blue. In the large lymphocytes, the nuclear-to-cytoplasmic ratio is lower and the chromatin is slightly less condensed than in the small lymphocytes. The nucleus is usually round but may be oval or indented. The cytoplasm is abundant and may contain a few azurophilic granules. *Large granular lymphocytes* contain azurophilic granules and relatively abundant cytoplasm, and generally represent cytotoxic T or natural killer (NK) cells (Chap. 94). *Reactive lymphocytes*, as seen in viral infections caused by Epstein-Barr virus, cytomegalovirus, adenovirus, or other organisms, are large with indented nuclei and abundant blue cytoplasm (Chap. 82). Nuclear chromatin condensation is variable, and nucleoli may be evident. A low nuclear-to-cytoplasmic ratio and greater degree of chromatin condensation distinguishes them from neoplastic cells.

Monocytes are the largest normal cells in the blood, usually measuring from 15 to 22 μm in diameter (see Fig. 2–4). The nucleus is of various shapes—round, kidney-shape, oval, or lobular—and frequently appears to be folded (Chap. 67). The lacy chromatin is arranged in fine strands with sharply defined margins. The cytoplasm is light gray, contains variable numbers of fine lilac or purple granules, and is often vacuolated. The gray (as opposed to blue) color of monocyte cytoplasm is a result of fine granules (staining pink) seen on the background of RNA-containing cytoplasm (staining blue), and helps to distinguish between monocytes and reactive lymphocytes. The monocyte nuclear chromatin contains a fine, string-like structure as opposed to the smudgy-appearing clumps of the lymphoid chromatin. Nuclear shape and cytoplasmic vacuolization are less reliable for distinguishing features between monocytic and lymphoid cells.

LEUKOCYTE INCLUSIONS

Abnormal Granules

In a systemic inflammatory reaction, neutrophil granules may appear larger than normal and stain more darkly, often assuming a dark blue-black color. This has been called *toxic granulation* (see Fig. 2–6). These granules if unusually prominent can be confused with the larger granules of basophils. In *mucopolysaccharidoses*, coarse, dark granules may be found in the neutrophils, and large azurophilic granules in some lymphocytes and monocytes (see Fig. 2–6). Huge misshapen granules are found in the neutrophils, and giant azurophilic granules are present in the lymphocytes of patients exhibiting the *Chédiak-Higashi* anomaly (see Fig. 2–6; Chap. 66). *Auer rods* are sharply outlined, red-staining rods found in the cytoplasm in blast cells, and occasionally in more mature leukemic cells, in the blood of some patients with acute myelogenous leukemia or myelodysplastic syndromes (Chap. 88).

Abnormal Neutrophil Inclusions

Light blue round or oval *Döhle bodies,* approximately 1 to 2 μm in diameter, may be seen in the cytoplasm of neutrophils of patients with infections, burns, and other inflammatory states (see Fig. 2–6). The blue staining is caused by RNA of the rough-surfaced endoplasmic reticulum contained in Döhle bodies. These bodies are thought to be a reflection of accelerated maturation of neutrophils with residual endoplasmic reticulum from the promyelocyte stage. They usually occur in circumstances in which toxic granulation may be present. *May-Hegglin* anomaly is one of several MYH9 disorders, autosomal dominant macrothrombocytopenias secondary to defective megakaryocyte maturation and fragmentation, with leukocyte inclusion bodies (also Fechtner, Sebastian, Epstein, and Alport-like syndromes; Chap. 112). The leukocytic inclusions, pale blue-stained, irregularly shaped inclusions are precipitates of nonmuscle myosin heavy chains (see Fig. 2–6). Neutrophil function is normal.

LEUKOCYTE ARTIFACTS

Damaged ("Smudge," "Basket") and Apoptotic Cells

During film preparation, leukocytes may be damaged, resulting in an enlarged nucleus with homogeneous, slightly reddish chromatin strands with a large blue nucleolus. There is no specific association with disease other than chronic lymphocytic leukemia (Chap. 92), where increased cell fragility commonly results in variable numbers of smudge cells, which connote a favorable prognosis. Eosinophils and basophils often are partially or largely degranulated in preparation film with the granules scattered beside the cell. Occasional neutrophils may be seen in stages of apoptosis after standing in anticoagulated blood at room temperature (see Fig. 2–6).

Radial Nuclear Segmentation

This refers to abnormal segmentation of the nuclei of leukocytes on the blood film, in which the lobes appear to radiate from a single point, giving a cloverleaf or cartwheel picture. This change is common in cytocentrifuged preparations (i.e., from a body fluid), EDTA anticoagulated blood after excessive storage, and samples collected in oxalate.

Vacuolization

Vacuoles may develop in the nucleus and cytoplasm of leukocytes, especially monocytes and neutrophils, with prolonged storage in EDTA anticoagulated blood. Vacuoles may be associated with swelling of the nuclei and loss of granules from the cytoplasm. In blood films prepared without anticoagulation, vacuoles in neutrophils suggest sepsis.

Endothelial Cells

If the blood film is prepared from the first drop of blood issuing from fingerstick, endothelial cells may be present singly, in clumps, or as strings of attached cells (see Fig. 2–6). These cells en face may simulate the appearance of abnormal cells and may be misinterpreted as blasts or metastatic tumor cells.

REFERENCES

1. Barnes PW, McFadden SL, Machin SJ, Simson E: The international consensus group for hematology review: Suggested criteria for action following automated CBC and WBC differential analysis. *Lab Hematol* 11:83–90, 2005.
2. Sireci A, Schlaberg R, Kratz A: A method for optimizing and validating institution-specific flagging criteria for automated cell counters. *Arch Pathol Lab Med* 134: 1528–1533, 2010.
3. Gulati G, Song J, Florea AD, Gong J: Purpose and criteria for blood smear scan, blood smear examination, and blood smear review. *Ann Lab Med* 33:1–7, 2013.
4. Kim SJ, Kim Y, Shin S, et al: Comparison study of the rates of manual peripheral blood smear review from 3 automated hematology analyzers, Unicel DxH 800, ADVIA 2120i, and XE 2100, using international consensus group guidelines. *Arch Pathol Lab Med* 136:1408–1413, 2012.
5. Hur M, Cho JH, Kim H, et al: Optimization of laboratory workflow in clinical hematology laboratory with reduced manual slide review: Comparison between Sysmex XE-2100 and ABX Pentra DX120. *Int J Lab Hematol* 33:434–440, 2011.
6. Hotton J, Broothaers J, Swaelens C, Cantinieaux B: Performance and abnormal cell flagging comparisons of three automated blood cell counters: Cell-Dyn Sapphire, DxH-800, and XN-2000. *Am J Clin Pathol* 140:845–852, 2013.
7. Ceelie H, Dinkelaar RB, van Gelder W: Examination of peripheral blood films using automated microscopy; evaluation of Diffmaster Octavia and Cellavision DM96. *J Clin Pathol* 60:72–79, 2007.
8. Smits SM, Leyte A: Clinical performance evaluation of the CellaVision Image Capture System in the white blood cell differential on peripheral blood smears. *J Clin Pathol* 67:168–172, 2014.
9. Buttarello M, Plebani M: Automated blood cell counts: state of the art. *Am J Clin Pathol* 130:104–116, 2008.
10. Coulter WH: High speed automatic blood cell counter and cell size analyzer. *Proc Natl Elect Conf* 12:1034, 1956.
11. Meintker L, Ringwald J, Rauh M, Krause SW: Comparison of automated differential blood cell counts from Abbott Sapphire, Siemens Advia 120, Beckman Coulter DxH 800, and Sysmex XE-2100 in normal and pathologic samples. *Am J Clin Pathol* 139:641–650, 2013.
12. Lippi G, Cattabiani C, Benegiamo A, et al: Evaluation of the fully automated hematological analyzer Sysmex XE-5000 for flow cytometric analysis of peritoneal fluid. *J Lab Autom* 18:240–244, 2013.
13. Perne A, Hainfellner JA, Womastek I, et al: Performance evaluation of the Sysmex XE-5000 hematology analyzer for white blood cell analysis in cerebrospinal fluid. *Arch Pathol Lab Med* 136:194–198, 2012.
14. Paris A, Nhan T, Cornet E, et al: Performance evaluation of the body fluid mode on the platform Sysmex XE-5000 series automated hematology analyzer. *Int J Lab Hematol* 32:539–547, 2010.
15. Briggs C, Kimber S, Green L: Where are we at with point-of-care testing in haematology? *Br J Haematol* 158:679–690, 2012.
16. England JM, Walford DM, Waters DA: Re-assessment of the reliability of the haematocrit. *Br J Haematol* 23:247–256, 1972.
17. Fairbanks VF: Nonequivalence of automated and manual hematocrit and erythrocyte indices. *Am J Clin Pathol* 73:55, 1980.
18. England JM: *Blood Cell Sizing.* Churchill Livingstone, New York, 1991.
19. Shamir MY, Avramovich A, Smaka T: The current status of continuous noninvasive measurement of total, carboxy, and methemoglobin concentration. *Anesth Analg* 114:972–978, 2012.
20. Lindner G, Exadaktylos AK: How noninvasive haemoglobin measurement with pulse co-oximetry can change your practice: An expert review. *Emerg Med Int* 2013:701529, 2013.
21. Dewhirst E, Naguib A, Winch P, et al: Accuracy of noninvasive and continuous hemoglobin measurement by pulse co-oximetry during preoperative phlebotomy. *J Intensive Care Med* 29:238–242, 2013.
22. Rice MJ, Gravenstein N, Morey TE: Noninvasive hemoglobin monitoring: How accurate is enough? *Anesth Analg* 117:902–907, 2013.
23. Dallman PR, Siimes MA: Percentile curves for hemoglobin and red cell volume in infancy and childhood. *J Pediatr* 94:26, 1979.
24. Wintrobe MM: Anemia: Classification and treatment on the basis of differences in the average volume and hemoglobin content of the red corpuscles. *Arch Intern Med* 54:256, 1934.
25. Seward SJ, Safran C, Marton KI, Robinson SH: Does the mean corpuscular volume help physicians evaluate hospitalized patients with anemia? *J Gen Intern Med* 5: 187–191, 1990.
26. Carmel R: Pernicious anemia. The expected findings of very low serum cobalamin levels, anemia, and macrocytosis are often lacking. *Arch Intern Med* 148:1712–1714, 1988.
27. Sekhar J, Stabler SP: Life-threatening megaloblastic pancytopenia with normal mean cell volume: Case series. *Eur J Intern Med* 18:548–550, 2007.
28. Mahmoud MY, Lugon M, Anderson CC: Unexplained macrocytosis in elderly patients. *Age Ageing* 25:310–312, 1996.
29. Eldibany MM, Totonchi KF, Joseph NJ, Rhone D: Usefulness of certain red blood cell indices in diagnosing and differentiating thalassemia trait from iron-deficiency anemia. *Am J Clin Pathol* 111:676–682, 1999.
30. Rathod DA, Kaur A, Patel V, et al: Usefulness of cell counter-based parameters and formulas in detection of beta-thalassemia trait in areas of high prevalence. *Am J Clin Pathol* 128:585–589, 2007.
31. Lafferty JD, Crowther MA, Ali MA, Levine M: The evaluation of various mathematical RBC indices and their efficacy in discriminating between thalassemic and non-thalassemic microcytosis. *Am J Clin Pathol* 106:201–205, 1996.
32. Jolobe OM: Mean corpuscular haemoglobin, referenced and resurrected. *J Clin Pathol* 64:833–834, 2011.
33. Brugnara C, Mohandas N: Red cell indices in classification and treatment of anemias: From M.M. Wintrobe's original 1934 classification to the third millennium. *Curr Opin Hematol* 20:222–230, 2013.
34. Patel A, Brett SJ: Identifying future risk from routine tests? *Crit Care Med* 42: 999–1000, 2014.
35. Gul M, Uyarel H, Ergelen M, et al: The relationship between red blood cell distribution width and the clinical outcomes in non-ST elevation myocardial infarction and unstable angina pectoris: A 3-year follow-up. *Coron Artery Dis* 23:330–336, 2012.
36. Patel KV, Semba RD, Ferrucci L, et al: Red cell distribution width and mortality in older adults: A meta-analysis. *J Gerontol A Biol Sci Med Sci* 65:258–265, 2010.
37. Hunziker S, Stevens J, Howell MD: Red cell distribution width and mortality in newly hospitalized patients. *Am J Med* 125:283–291, 2012.
38. Zorlu A, Bektasoglu G, Guven FM, et al: Usefulness of admission red cell distribution width as a predictor of early mortality in patients with acute pulmonary embolism. *Am J Cardiol* 109:128–134, 2012.
39. Lam AP, Gundabolu K, Sridharan A, et al: Multiplicative interaction between mean corpuscular volume and red cell distribution width in predicting mortality of elderly patients with and without anemia. *Am J Hematol* 88:E245–E249, 2013.
40. Wang F, Pan W, Pan S, et al: Red cell distribution width as a novel predictor of mortality in ICU patients. *Ann Med* 43:40–46, 2011.
41. Lippi G, Targher G, Montagnana M, et al: Relation between red blood cell distribution width and inflammatory biomarkers in a large cohort of unselected outpatients. *Arch Pathol Lab Med* 133:628–632, 2009.
42. Piva E, Brugnara C, Chiandetti L, Plebani M: Automated reticulocyte counting: State of the art and clinical applications in the evaluation of erythropoiesis. *Clin Chem Lab Med* 48:1369–1380, 2010.
43. Noronha JF, De Souza CA, Vigorito AC, et al: Immature reticulocytes as an early predictor of engraftment in autologous and allogeneic bone marrow transplantation. *Clin Lab Haematol* 25:47–54, 2003.
44. Buttarello M, Bulian P, Farina G, et al: Five fully automated methods for performing immature reticulocyte fraction: Comparison in diagnosis of bone marrow aplasia. *Am J Clin Pathol* 117:871–879, 2002.
45. Urrechaga E, Borque L, Escanero JF: The role of automated measurement of RBC subpopulations in differential diagnosis of microcytic anemia and beta-thalassemia screening. *Am J Clin Pathol* 135:374–379, 2011.
46. Schoorl M, Schoorl M, Linssen J, et al: Efficacy of advanced discriminating algorithms for screening on iron-deficiency anemia and beta-thalassemia trait: A multicenter evaluation. *Am J Clin Pathol* 138:300–304, 2012.
47. Higgins JM, Mahadevan L: Physiological and pathological population dynamics of circulating human red blood cells. *Proc Natl Acad Sci U S A* 107:20587–20592, 2010.
48. Weatherall DJ: Systems biology and red cells. *N Engl J Med* 364:376–377, 2011.
49. Thomas L, Franck S, Messinger M, et al: Reticulocyte hemoglobin measurement—comparison of two methods in the diagnosis of iron-restricted erythropoiesis. *Clin Chem Lab Med* 43:1193–1202, 2005.
50. KDOQI; National Kidney Foundation: KDOQI clinical practice guidelines and clinical practice recommendations for anemia in chronic kidney disease. *Am J Kidney Dis* 47(5 Suppl 3):S11–S145, 2006.
51. Mast AE, Blinder MA, Lu Q, et al: Clinical utility of the reticulocyte hemoglobin content in the diagnosis of iron deficiency. *Blood* 99:1489–1491, 2002.
52. Ullrich C, Wu A, Armsby C, et al: Screening healthy infants for iron deficiency using reticulocyte hemoglobin content. *JAMA* 294:924–930, 2005.
53. Urrechaga E, Borque L, Escanero JF: Erythrocyte and reticulocyte indices in the assessment of erythropoiesis activity and iron availability. *Int J Lab Hematol* 35: 144–149, 2013.
54. Buttarello M, Pajola R, Novello E, et al: Diagnosis of iron deficiency in patients undergoing hemodialysis. *Am J Clin Pathol* 133:949–954, 2010.
55. Joosten E, Lioen P, Brusselmans C, et al: Is analysis of the reticulocyte haemoglobin equivalent a useful test for the diagnosis of iron deficiency anaemia in geriatric patients? *Eur J Intern Med* 24:63–66, 2013.
56. Osta V, Caldirola MS, Fernandez M, et al: Utility of new mature erythrocyte and reticulocyte indices in screening for iron-deficiency anemia in a pediatric population. *Int J Lab Hematol* 35:400–405, 2013.
57. Yoo JH, Song J, Lee KA: Automated detection of malaria-associated pseudoeosinophilia and abnormal WBC scattergram by the Sysmex XE-2100 hematology analyzer: A clinical study with 1,801 patients and real-time quantitative PCR analysis in vivax malaria-endemic area. *Am J Trop Med Hyg* 82:412–414, 2010.
58. Lee HK, Kim SI, Chae H, et al: Sensitive detection and accurate monitoring of *Plasmodium vivax* parasites on routine complete blood count using automatic blood cell analyzer (DxH800(TM)). *Int J Lab Hematol* 34:201–207, 2012.
59. Amundsen EK, Urdal P, Hagve TA, et al: Absolute neutrophil counts from automated hematology instruments are accurate and precise even at very low levels. *Am J Clin Pathol* 137:862–869, 2012.

60. Zwick DL: Time to drop routine reporting of differential percentage values from CBC reports. *Lab Hematol* 16:1–2, 2010.
61. Bourner G, Dhaliwal J, Sumner J: Performance evaluation of the latest fully automated hematology analyzers in a large, commercial laboratory setting: A 4-way, side-by-side study. *Lab Hematol* 11:285–297, 2005.
62. Aulesa C, Pastor I, Naranjo D, Galimany R: Application of receiver operating characteristics curve (ROC) analysis when definitive and suspect morphologic flags appear in the new Coulter LH 750 analyzer. *Lab Hematol* 10:14–23, 2004.
63. Rabizadeh E, Pickholtz I, Barak M, et al: Acute leukemia detection rate by automated blood count parameters and peripheral smear review. *Int J Lab Hematol* 37;44–49, 2015.
64. Barnes PW, Eby CS, Shimer G: Blast flagging with the UniCel DxH 800 Coulter Cellular Analysis System. *Lab Hematol* 16:23–25, 2010.
65. Eilertsen H, Vollestad NK, Hagve TA: The usefulness of blast flags on the Sysmex XE-5000 is questionable. *Am J Clin Pathol* 139:633–640, 2013.
66. van der Meer W, van Gelder W, de Keijzer R, Willems H: Does the band cell survive the 21st century? *Eur J Haematol* 76:251–254, 2006.
67. Atwater S, Corash L: Advances in leukocyte differential and peripheral blood stem cell enumeration. *Curr Opin Hematol* 3:71–76, 1996.
68. Lim EM, Cembrowski G, Cembrowski M, Clarke G: Race-specific WBC and neutrophil count reference intervals. *Int J Lab Hematol* 32:590–597, 2010.
69. Zandecki M, Genevieve F, Gerard J, Godon A: Spurious counts and spurious results on haematology analysers: A review. Part I: platelets. *Int J Lab Hematol* 29:4–20, 2007.
70. Lozano M, Mahon A, van der Meer PF, et al: Counting platelets at transfusion threshold levels: Impact on the decision to transfuse. A BEST Collaborative-UK NEQAS(H) International Exercise. *Vox Sang* 106:330–336, 2014.
71. De la Salle BJ, McTaggart PN, Briggs C, et al: The accuracy of platelet counting in thrombocytopenic blood samples distributed by the UK National External Quality Assessment Scheme for General Haematology. *Am J Clin Pathol* 137:65–74, 2012.
72. Kim SY, Kim JE, Kim HK, et al: Accuracy of platelet counting by automated hematologic analyzers in acute leukemia and disseminated intravascular coagulation: Potential effects of platelet activation. *Am J Clin Pathol* 134:634–647, 2010.
73. Schoorl M, Schoorl M, Oomes J, van Pelt J: New fluorescent method (PLT-F) on Sysmex XN2000 hematology analyzer achieved higher accuracy in low platelet counting. *Am J Clin Pathol* 140:495–499, 2013.
74. Pan LL, Chen CM, Huang WT, Sun CK: Enhanced accuracy of optical platelet counts in microcytic anemia. *Lab Med* 45:32-36, 2014.
75. Nosanchuk JS, Chang J, Bennett JM: The analytic basis for the use of platelet estimates from peripheral blood smears. Laboratory and clinical applications. *Am J Clin Pathol* 69:383–387, 1978.
76. Bartels PC, Schoorl M, Lombarts AJ: Screening for EDTA-dependent deviations in platelet counts and abnormalities in platelet distribution histograms in pseudothrombocytopenia. *Scand J Clin Lab Invest* 57:629–636, 1997.
77. Schuff-Werner P, Steiner M, Fenger S, et al: Effective estimation of correct platelet counts in pseudothrombocytopenia using an alternative anticoagulant based on magnesium salt. *Br J Haematol* 162:684–692, 2013.
78. Osselaer JC, Jamart J, Scheiff JM: Platelet distribution width for differential diagnosis of thrombocytosis. *Clin Chem* 43:1072–1076, 1997.
79. Leader A, Pereg D, Lishner M: Are platelet volume indices of clinical use? A multidisciplinary review. *Ann Med* 44:805–816, 2012.
80. Fager AM, Wood JP, Bouchard BA, et al: Properties of procoagulant platelets: Defining and characterizing the subpopulation binding a functional prothrombinase. *Arterioscler Thromb Vasc Biol* 30:2400–2407, 2010.
81. Hoffmann JJ: Reticulated platelets: analytical aspects and clinical utility. *Clin Chem Lab Med* 52:1107–1117, 2014.
82. Kurata Y, Hayashi S, Kiyoi T, et al: Diagnostic value of tests for reticulated platelets, plasma glycocalicin, and thrombopoietin levels for discriminating between hyperdestructive and hypoplastic thrombocytopenia. *Am J Clin Pathol* 115:656–664, 2001.
83. Chaoui D, Chakroun T, Robert F, et al: Reticulated platelets: A reliable measure to reduce prophylactic platelet transfusions after intensive chemotherapy. *Transfusion* 45:766–772, 2005.
84. Cesari F, Marcucci R, Gori AM, et al: Reticulated platelets predict cardiovascular death in acute coronary syndrome patients. Insights from the AMI-Florence 2 Study. *Thromb Haemost* 109:846–853, 2013.
85. Hong KH, Kim HK, Kim JE, et al: Prognostic value of immature platelet fraction and plasma thrombopoietin in disseminated intravascular coagulation. *Blood Coagul Fibrinolysis* 20:409–414, 2009.
86. Ibrahim H, Nadipalli S, DeLao T, et al: Immature platelet fraction (IPF) determined with an automated method predicts clopidogrel hyporesponsiveness. *J Thromb Thrombolysis* 33:137–142, 2012.
87. Cesari F, Marcucci R, Gori AM, et al: High platelet turnover and reactivity in renal transplant recipients patients. *Thromb Haemost* 104:804–810, 2010.
88. Eller LA, Eller MA, Ouma B, et al: Reference intervals in healthy adult Ugandan blood donors and their impact on conducting international vaccine trials. *PLoS One* 3: e3919, 2008.
89. Peng L, Yang J, Lu X, et al: Effects of biological variations on platelet count in healthy subjects in China. *Thromb Haemost* 91:367–372, 2004.
90. Beutler E, West C: Hematologic differences between African-Americans and whites: The roles of iron deficiency and alpha-thalassemia on hemoglobin levels and mean corpuscular volume. *Blood* 106:740–745, 2005.
91. Hershman D, Weinberg M, Rosner Z, et al: Ethnic neutropenia and treatment delay in African American women undergoing chemotherapy for early-stage breast cancer. *J Natl Cancer Inst* 95:1545–1548, 2003.
92. Wakeman L, Al-Ismail S, Benton A, et al: Robust, routine haematology reference ranges for healthy adults. *Int J Lab Hematol* 29:279–283, 2007.
93. Cheng CK, Chan J, Cembrowski GS, van Assendelft OW: Complete blood count reference interval diagrams derived from NHANES III: Stratification by age, sex, and race. *Lab Hematol* 10:42–53, 2004.
94. Beutler E, Waalen J: The definition of anemia: What is the lower limit of normal of the blood hemoglobin concentration? *Blood* 107:1747–1750, 2006.
95. Fairbanks VF, Tefferi A: Normal ranges for packed cell volume and hemoglobin concentration in adults: Relevance to "apparent polycythemia". *Eur J Haematol* 65: 285–296, 2000.
96. Pearson TC: Correspondence: Normal ranges for packed cell volume and hemoglobin concentration in adults: Relevance to "apparent polycythemia." *Eur J Haematol* 67: 56–59, 2001.
97. Ganji V, Kafai MR: Hemoglobin and hematocrit values are higher and prevalence of anemia is lower in the post-folic acid fortification period than in the pre-folic acid fortification period in US adults. *Am J Clin Nutr* 89:363–371, 2009.
98. Fraser CG, Wilkinson SP, Neville RG, et al: Biologic variation of common hematologic laboratory quantities in the elderly. *Am J Clin Pathol* 92:465–470, 1989.
99. Tang H, Jing J, Bo D, Xu D: Biological variations of leukocyte numerical and morphologic parameters determined by UniCel DxH 800 hematology analyzer. *Arch Pathol Lab Med* 136:1392–1396, 2012.
100. Zhang P, Tang H, Chen K, et al: Biological variations of hematologic parameters determined by UniCel DxH 800 hematology analyzer. *Arch Pathol Lab Med* 137:1106–1110, 2013.
101. Sottas PE, Kapke GF, Vesterqvist O, Leroux JM: Patient-specific measures of a biomarker for the generation of individual reference intervals: Hemoglobin as example. *Transl Res* 158:360–368, 2011.
102. Sennels HP, Jorgensen HL, Hansen AL, et al: Diurnal variation of hematology parameters in healthy young males: The Bispebjerg study of diurnal variations. *Scand J Clin Lab Invest* 71:532–541, 2011.
103. Braude S, Beck A: Complete blood counts with differential: More accurate reference ranges based on circadian leukocyte trafficking. *J Clin Pathol* 66:909–910, 2013.
104. Soranzo N, Spector TD, Mangino M, et al: A genome-wide meta-analysis identifies 22 loci associated with eight hematological parameters in the HaemGen consortium. *Nat Genet* 41:1182–1190, 2009.
105. van der Harst P, Zhang W, Mateo Leach I, et al: Seventy-five genetic loci influencing the human red blood cell. *Nature* 492:369–375, 2012.
106. Bain BJ: Ethnic and sex differences in the total and differential white cell count and platelet count. *J Clin Pathol* 49:664, 1996.
107. Gerdes U, Johnsson JJ, Kairisto V, et al: Nordic Reference Interval Project [unpublished observations].

CHAPTER 3
EXAMINATION OF THE MARROW

Daniel H. Ryan

SUMMARY

Microscopic examination of the marrow is a mainstay of hematologic diagnosis. Even with the advent of specialized biochemical and molecular assays that capitalize on advances in our understanding of the cell biology of hematopoiesis, the primary diagnosis of hematologic malignancies and many nonneoplastic hematologic disorders relies upon examination of the cells in the marrow. An aspirate and biopsy of the marrow can be obtained with minimal risk and only minor discomfort and are quickly and easily processed for examination. The marrow should be examined when the clinical history, blood cell counts, blood film, or laboratory test results suggest the possibility of a primary or secondary hematologic disorder for which morphologic analysis or special studies of the marrow would aid in the diagnosis. Leukopenia or thrombocytopenia may require a marrow examination for diagnosis. Nonhemolytic anemia that is not readily diagnosed by blood cell examination and supporting laboratory tests often requires a marrow examination. Abnormal cells in the blood, such as nucleated red cells, white cell precursors, abnormal lymphocytes not explained by concurrent infection, and blast cells, usually require a marrow examination. In addition to determining the cellularity and morphology of precursor cells, or infiltration by nonhematopoietic cells, the study provides marrow cells for immunophenotyping, cytogenetic, molecular and genomic studies, culture of infectious organisms, and storage of marrow cells for further analysis.

HISTORY OF THE MARROW EXAMINATION

The first recorded examinations of marrow in living patients occurred in the first decades of the 20th century, first using the tibia as the source of marrow and then surgical bone biopsies. Neither technique led to routine examination of the marrow, because in the former case the tibia was usually hypocellular in adults, and in the latter case, because of the invasiveness of an open procedure and the discomfort and risk of infection and bleeding. In 1923, Arinkin devised the marrow aspiration technique,[1] which was the prototype for our current aspiration procedure. Thirty years passed before the suggestion that the pelvis might

Acronyms and Abbreviations: CD, cluster of differentiation; CLL, chronic lymphocytic leukemia; CML, chronic myelogenous leukemia; DMSO, dimethylsulfoxide; EDTA, ethylenediaminetetraacetic acid; FISH, fluorescence *in situ* hybridization; GPI, glycosylphosphatidylinositol; MDS, myelodysplastic syndrome; M:E, myeloid-to-erythroid cell ratio; MRD, minimal residual disease; PCR, polymerase chain reaction.

be preferable to the sternum gained hold, and another 10 years passed before a practical marrow biopsy instrument was put to use. Regular use of the posterior iliac crest for aspiration and biopsy and regular use of biopsy to complement aspiration did not occur until the 1970s, when staging of lymphoma made biopsy a frequent procedure and new simpler biopsy instruments became readily available.

INDICATIONS FOR MARROW ASPIRATE OR BIOPSY

The International Council for Standardization in Hematology has published guidelines for marrow aspirate and biopsy to promote consistency in performance and reporting.[2] Although marrow aspiration and biopsy techniques are safe, they should be performed with a clear idea as to how the results will help distinguish the differential diagnoses under consideration or provide followup of treatment.[3-5] In many hematologic disorders, such as most cases of iron-deficiency anemia, thalassemia, and acquired and inherited hemolytic anemia, examination of the blood and specialized laboratory tests usually suffice to make the diagnosis without the need for a marrow examination.

When examination of the marrow is indicated, the decision as to whether an aspirate or an aspirate plus biopsy is desired should be made. Aspiration is always attempted because of the superior morphology offered by examination of the aspirate smear. However, a marrow biopsy is superior to the aspirate in quantifying marrow cellularity and diagnosing infiltrative diseases of the marrow and should be performed when these conditions are part of the differential diagnosis.[6,7] Marrow biopsy is useful for diagnosing and following the course of disorders that are commonly associated with reticulin fibrosis, such as megakaryoblastic leukemia, hairy cell leukemia, and the chronic myeloproliferative neoplasms.[8] In myelodysplastic syndromes, marrow biopsy is useful for evaluating abnormal localization of immature precursor cells and abnormal megakaryocytes. Marrow necrosis and gelatinous transformation are more readily detected in marrow sections than in aspirate films. Marrow aspirate alone may be appropriate in some clinical settings where the diagnostic question is very targeted, such as diagnosis of childhood immune thrombocytopenia purpura or surveillance followup of leukemia patients in apparent remission.

Depending on the diagnostic question, availability of material, and expected frequency of the abnormal cells, an appropriate selection of specialized diagnostic methods may be needed to support the clinical diagnosis. Morphology of marrow cells is still the gold standard for diagnosis of hematologic malignancy and allows construction of a good differential diagnosis for nonmalignant disorders. Immunocytochemistry provides excellent phenotype–morphology correlation on an individual cell basis, but is limited to epitopes that resist destruction by fixation, decalcification, and paraffin embedding. Flow cytometry allows study of almost any surface or intracellular protein, with the added ability to detect important quantitative changes in cellular proteins and simultaneous determination of multiple proteins within the same cell. However, flow cytometry requires that cells be viable and dissociated from tissue. Gene expression arrays allow analysis of complex patterns of RNA expression by sophisticated mathematical algorithms to discover diagnostic patterns based on gene expression. These studies may point the way to a smaller more practical set of proteins that can be studied by immunocytochemistry or immunofluorescence. Molecular assays target oncogenic DNA sequence alterations from the chromosome to the nucleotide, and include classic metaphase cytogenetics, fluorescence *in situ* hybridization (FISH), reverse transcriptase polymerase chain reaction (PCR), and targeted or whole-genome sequencing.

● MARROW ASPIRATION TECHNIQUE

At birth, all bones contain hematopoietic marrow. Fat cells begin to replace hemopoietic marrow in the extremities in the fifth to seventh year. By adulthood, the hemopoietic marrow is limited to the axial skeleton and the proximal portions of the extremities (Chaps. 5 and 9). Fatty marrow appears yellow, whereas hematopoietic marrow is red. Red marrow contains fat, however, and fat droplets are visible grossly in aspirated marrow specimens. Histologically, yellow marrow consists almost entirely of fat cells and supporting connective tissue. Red marrow contains an abundance of hematopoietic cells, fat cells, and connective tissue. The marrow fills the spaces between the trabeculae of bone in the marrow cavity. Marrow is soft and friable and can be readily aspirated or biopsied with a needle.

The posterior iliac crest (Fig. 3–1) is the preferred site for marrow aspiration and biopsy. In adults, the anterior iliac crest and rarely the sternum have been used (Fig. 3–2). The sternum should be used for aspiration only. The anterior iliac crest is less preferred than the posterior crest in adults because of its thick cortical bone. The anteromedial surface of the tibia is an option for infants younger than 1 year old (particularly newborns), but the posterior iliac crest is still the preferred site. Serious adverse outcomes after marrow aspiration or biopsy are rare, occurring in less than 0.05 percent. One direct fatality and three

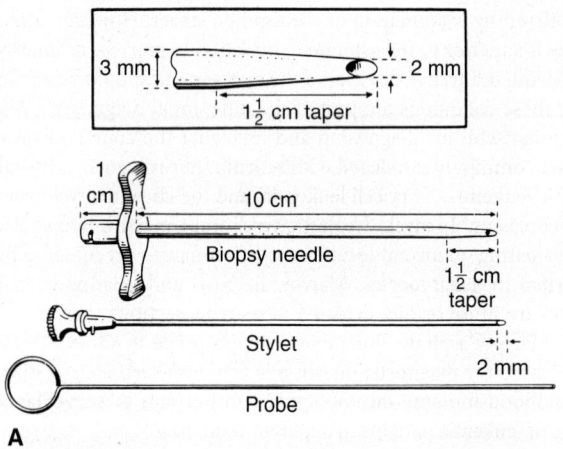

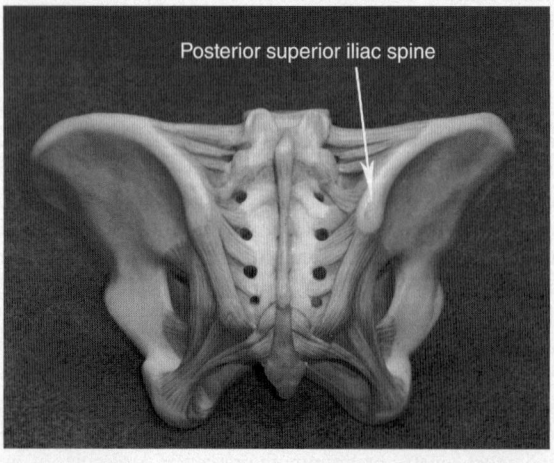

Figure 3–1. A. Jamshidi biopsy instrument. **B.** Site of marrow biopsy.[96]
(A, reproduced with permission from Jamshidi K, Swaim WR: Bone marrow biopsy with unaltered architecture: A new biopsy device. J Lab Clin Med 77(2):335–342, 1971.)

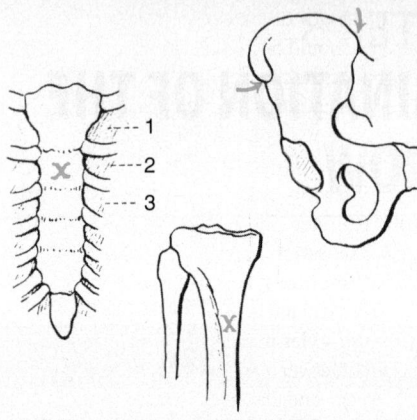

Figure 3–2. Sites used for marrow aspiration. *(Modified with permission from Schwartz SO, Hartz WH Jr, Robbins JH: Hematology in Practice. New York, NY: McGraw-Hill; 1961.)*

episodes of prolonged but not permanent disability were reported in nearly 55,000 marrow biopsies.[9] Morbidity most frequently involved hemorrhage, which was associated more with platelet function impairment than thrombocytopenia or coagulation factor defects.[9] Infection and reactions to anesthetic agents are other infrequent complications. Penetration of the bone with damage to the underlying structures is possible with all marrow aspirations, but the hazard is greatest in sternal aspirations because the sternum at the second interspace is only approximately 1 cm thick in adults, and the distance from posterior sternal cortex to the ascending aorta varies greatly and may be as little as 4 to 5 mm,[10] giving rise to the rare but dramatic consequence of aortal wall tear. To prevent this, a guard should be in place on the needle if a sternal aspirate needs to be done.

For either a marrow biopsy or aspiration, sedation minimizes anxiety and pain,[11] particularly in children,[12] for whom propofol, with or without fentanyl, administered under carefully controlled conditions[13] with monitoring of oxygen saturation, blood pressure, and vital signs, is frequently used. Midazolam (Versed) is a popular choice for conscious sedation of adult patients, although a variety of other premedications have been used. There is a relative lack of empirical research and consensus guidelines on the subject of pain reduction during adult marrow procedures.[14,15] The experience of marrow procedures from the patient's point of view is worth reading.[16] The only significant correlates with severe/unbearable pain (experienced by 4 percent of patients) during marrow examination were quality of the information about the procedure provided before the examination and previous painful experiences.[17] Marrow biopsies and aspirations for lymphoma staging purposes often can be performed while the patient is under anesthesia for other procedures. Several different types of needles are available for marrow aspiration.[3] For adults, a 16-gauge needle is sufficiently large to permit aspiration of adequate specimens; larger needles are unnecessary. The patient is prone or in the left or right lateral decubitus position. Sterile precautions must be observed. The skin over the puncture site is shaved if necessary and cleansed with a disinfectant solution. The skin, subcutaneous tissues, and periosteum are infiltrated with a local anesthetic solution, such as 1 percent lidocaine. Adequate infiltration of the anesthetic at the periosteal surface is important to minimize severe pain during the procedure, but no more than 20 mL of 1 percent lidocaine should be used in an adult.[18] Adequate anesthesia can be achieved with much less lidocaine in virtually all cases. An air gun can be used to anesthetize the skin surface prior to application of anesthetic to the periosteal surface by injection. After the anesthesia has taken effect, usually in 3 to 5 minutes, the marrow needle is inserted through the skin, subcutaneous tissue, and cortex of the bone using a slight twisting motion. In obese patients, the length of the needle must be sufficient to reach the iliac crest. The stylet should be locked into place on the hub of the needle to prevent plugging of the needle with tissue prior to needle entry into the marrow cavity. Penetration of the cortex can be sensed by a slight, rapid forward movement accompanied by a sudden increase in the ease of advancing the needle. The stylet of the needle is removed promptly, the hub is attached to a 10- or 20-mL syringe, and approximately 0.5 to 1.5 mL of fluid is aspirated. The actual aspiration of the marrow causes a transient painful sensation for most patients. If additional specimen volume is required, another syringe is fitted on the marrow needle, the syringe and needle is rotated and an adjacent area is entered and marrow is aspirated. The stylet may be reinserted and the marrow needle slightly repositioned between aspirations. When aspiration is complete, the stylet is reinserted and the needle immediately removed from the bone. Pressure is applied to the skin over the aspiration site for at least 5 minutes to minimize bruising at the site. If platelet number or function is decreased, firm pressure should be applied for at least 10 to 15 minutes. The bloody fluid that is aspirated contains light-colored particles of marrow approximately 0.5 to 1 mm in diameter. They often are readily visible in the syringe, but may not be detected until the syringe contents are discharged on glass slides for film preparation.

If nothing enters the syringe when aspiration is performed, the needle may not be properly placed in the marrow cavity. The needle can be cautiously advanced 1 to 2 mm after reinsertion of the stylet and aspiration attempted again, or the needle can be removed from the bone and reinserted in a nearby site in the anesthetized area. The thickness of the bone must be considered when the needle is being adjusted in the bone. Occasionally the needle must be rotated on its longitudinal axis, or in a larger orbit, in order to loosen the marrow mechanically before the marrow can be aspirated. If a small amount of blood has been aspirated, a new needle should be used because of the probability of clotting the aspirate when it finally is obtained. Aspiration with a 50-mL syringe may succeed if use of a smaller syringe fails. Fibrotic or densely packed leukemic marrow may resist all attempts at aspiration, in which case a biopsy is necessary. The most common cause of failure to obtain marrow is faulty positioning of the needle, and a second attempt at aspiration usually succeeds. A specimen preparation checklist used at the time of procedure to verify presence of spicules, length of biopsy, and other protocol items has been found to increase biopsy specimen length and decrease frequency of non-diagnostic samples.[19]

NEEDLE BIOPSY TECHNIQUE

Needle biopsy usually is performed with the Jamshidi needle, using the same preparation as described above. The Jamshidi instrument (see Fig. 3–1) consists of a cylindrical needle with constant bore, except for a concentrically tapered distal portion ending in a sharp, beveled cutting tip. The stylet fits precisely inside the opening at the tapered tip, interlocks at the hub of the needle, and extends 1 to 2 mm beyond the end of the needle. An 11-gauge needle is most commonly used in the United States. After the skin and the periosteum of the biopsy site are anesthetized, a 3-mm incision is made in the skin. The needle, with obturator in place, is inserted into the skin incision and through the subcutaneous tissue to the cortex of the bone. The needle is directed toward the posterior iliac spine and advanced with a twisting motion. Penetration of the cortex is sensed by a decreased resistance to forward movement of the needle. The obturator is removed, and the needle is slowly advanced with reciprocal clockwise–counterclockwise twisting motions around the long axis. After sufficient penetration of the bone (up to approximately 3 cm), the needle is rotated several times on its axis and withdrawn approximately 2 to 3 mm. Some needles now come with a "trap" that snares the biopsy so that the needle can be directly

removed. The needle is reinserted to the original depth at a slightly different angle, taking care not to bend the needle, and rotated several times to free the specimen from attachments in the marrow cavity. The needle is slowly withdrawn, with the same twisting motion used during insertion. The core of marrow inside the needle is removed by inserting the probe through the cutting tip and extruding the specimen through the hub of the needle. The smaller size of the cutting aperture relative to the bore of the shaft of the Jamshidi instrument yields a specimen that fits loosely inside the needle and therefore is less subject to compression, distortion, or fragmentation. The technique reliably produces good quality biopsy specimens. Marrow biopsy should be performed before marrow aspiration is attempted (or in a slightly different site on the iliac crest) to avoid hemorrhage and distorted marrow architecture in the biopsy core. With the availability of the biopsy needles described in this section, open (surgical) biopsies rarely are necessary but may be performed, for example, for diagnosis of deeply situated bone lesions or at the time of a surgical procedure performed for a related indication (e.g., staging). An FDA-approved battery-powered drill that inserts a biopsy needle into the posterior iliac bone of adult patients provides more consistent and longer biopsy cores and shortens procedure time.[20]

PREPARATION OF MARROW SPECIMENS FOR STUDY

Several types of preparations can be made from the marrow aspirate to maximize use of the diagnostic material. Most important is the *direct film*, which is made immediately from a drop of marrow suspension from the unmanipulated aspirate. This preparation is the best for evaluating cellular morphology and differential counts of the marrow. The *particle film* is best for estimating marrow cellularity and megakaryocyte abundance, but morphology is obscured in the thicker parts of the film. A *concentrate film*, which is prepared from a concentrate of nucleated cells (marrow buffy coat) achieved by centrifugation of a small volume of anticoagulated marrow, is sometimes used for detecting low-abundance cells when the marrow is hypocellular. The relative proportions of cell lineages are not maintained in the concentrate film preparation (often erythroid precursors are relatively enriched). In addition, this preparation is subject to anticoagulant-induced changes in nuclear morphology or cytoplasmic vacuolization. The *touch imprint* from the biopsy is quite valuable and sometimes diagnostically necessary for evaluating cellular morphology when the aspirate is hypocellular.[21]

MARROW FILMS

After aspiration, approximately 0.5 mL of marrow is placed on a glass slide; the rest is mixed into a tube containing ethylenediaminetetraacetic acid (EDTA) solution. The marrow specimen is examined to ensure the presence of "spicules" or particles of marrow containing bony or fatty pieces, indicating successful aspiration of the marrow cavity. Direct marrow films are immediately prepared by transferring drops of the unanticoagulated marrow pool to fresh slides and making push films with coverslips. Sufficient films should be made for special stains. Heparinization of the aspirate is not necessary if the operator works rapidly and should be avoided because heparinization may introduce artifacts. Formalin vapor artifact that can distort morphology can be avoided by making sure formalin containers are not opened until aspirate smears are prepared and put away.

A useful technique is preparing a thick film of marrow by discharging a drop or two of the aspirate on a slide, covering the aspirate with a second slide, gently pressing the slides together to express most of the blood into a gauze sponge, and then pulling the slides apart longitudinally. Such preparations may contain an increased number of broken cells if too much pressure is applied, but they provide a large number of particles from which marrow cellularity can be estimated and which are useful for estimating the amount of hemosiderin present. Broken cells may be minimized using a squash technique with coverslips instead of glass slides, which compared favorably to push (wedge) films in achieving representative distribution of intact cells derived from marrow particles.[22]

The EDTA-anticoagulated sample may be centrifuged (1500 g for 10 minutes) in a Wintrobe tube to concentrate the cellular elements of the marrow. After centrifugation, the fatty layer and plasma are removed, and the "buffy coat" is mixed with an equal amount of plasma. Multiple films of this preparation are made. All smears should be thoroughly air-dried, which can take longer in a humid environment, before staining to avoid artifacts.

TOUCH PREPARATIONS

After a biopsy specimen is obtained using the Jamshidi needle, the specimen should be extruded through the hub of the needle and then gently rolled across a glass slide (using an applicator stick to move the specimen) before it is placed in fixative, taking care to avoid crushing. The touch preparations are allowed to dry and are stained in the same manner as films.

SPECIAL STUDIES

It is essential to formulate the diagnostic question before performing a marrow aspiration to ensure an adequate sample is obtained for all the special studies that may be needed to make the correct diagnosis, while avoiding aspiration of more marrow than is needed, which can lead to dilution of the sample.[23] A sterile anticoagulated sample containing viable unfixed cells in single-cell suspension is the best substrate for nearly all special studies. Specifically, flow cytometry is best performed on EDTA- or heparin-anticoagulated aspirate specimens, which are stable for at least 24 hours at room temperature. For cytogenetic or cell culture analysis, preservative-free heparin-anticoagulated marrow should be added to tissue culture medium and analyzed as soon as possible to maintain optimal cell viability. Cytogenetic samples are generally not adversely affected by overnight incubation.[24] In cases where the marrow aspirate is dry, a duplicate biopsy specimen can be disaggregated to produce a cell suspension for morphology, flow cytometry, and cytogenetic studies.[25] FISH for detection of chromosomal deletions, duplications, and translocations can be performed in marrow biopsies when EDTA-based decalcification protocols are used.[26]

For molecular analysis of fresh specimens, sample storage should be minimized, and storage at 4°C is preferable. EDTA is the preferred anticoagulant because heparin can interfere with some molecular assays. DNA is relatively stable, but RNA has a variable half-life in an intact cell and is degraded rapidly (on the order of seconds to minutes) in a cell lysate by ubiquitous ribonucleases. Sample storage prior to RNA isolation should be minimized.[27] Collection tubes have been designed for stabilization of RNA, but for maximal RNA recovery, samples should be transported to the laboratory immediately, where cell suspensions (typically buffy coat or mononuclear cell preparations) can be prepared and nucleic acids extracted under conditions that inhibit ribonucleases. DNA and messenger RNA can be extracted and analyzed from paraffin-embedded tissue sections[28] and dried stained films,[29] with variable degree of degradation dependent on the length of sequence required.

Archival storage of marrow specimens is important in light of advances in molecular diagnosis that may necessitate validation studies using samples of known origin or retrospective testing of diagnostic material. Isolated DNA or RNA can be stored for long periods at −70°C, whereas viable, intact cells can be reliably preserved only by controlled rate freezing in dimethylsulfoxide (DMSO) and storage in liquid nitrogen.

HISTOLOGIC SECTIONS

A variety of techniques for preparing aspirated material for histologic study have been advocated. All of the techniques are designed to collect a sufficient number of marrow particles in a small volume so that adequate sections can be prepared. This goal can be accomplished by discharging the marrow aspirate onto a glass slide, allowing the particles to settle for a few seconds, and then gently tilting the slide so that the excess blood runs off. The particles then are pushed together with an applicator stick, and the remaining blood is allowed to clot. The clot is promptly fixed, typically in buffered formalin, for tissue processing and sectioning. An alternative method using filtration of the anticoagulated aspirate specimen has been described.[30]

The core marrow biopsy specimen is processed for histologic examination typically by fixation in neutral buffered formalin, followed by decalcification and embedding in paraffin. Decalcification can be accomplished with acid reagents or EDTA, the latter of which is preferred as it provides better preservation of nucleic acid and protein antigens. Sections of high quality cut at 3 μm and stained with hematoxylin and eosin are satisfactory for routine work. Refinements in fixation and embedding techniques have enabled use of many immunologic markers in decalcified paraffin-embedded marrow biopsy specimens. Fixation in neutral-buffered formalin and embedding without decalcification in plastic resin has the advantage of superior morphology,[31] but is less frequently used as the potential for immunostaining and molecular assays is more restricted.

● MORPHOLOGIC INTERPRETATION OF MARROW PREPARATIONS

OVERVIEW

The Wright-Giemsa–stained direct marrow aspirate film should be examined as quickly as possible to provide a preliminary assessment of the marrow morphology and allow setup of specialized testing based on this preliminary evaluation while the sample is fresh. Final interpretation of the marrow biopsy and aspirate should be integrated with results from the clinical history, blood film, cell counts, laboratory data, cell marker studies, and molecular or cytogenetic data. No other histologic specimen exists in which a state-of-the-art interpretation is dependent on such an array of supportive data. The challenge for the hematopathologist and hematologist is to understand the advantages and limitations of each diagnostic approach so that results can be reconciled and placed into perspective. Some common pitfalls in preparation and interpretation of marrow aspirates[4] and biopsies[5] have been reviewed.

ADEQUACY OF THE MARROW SAMPLE

The first question in interpreting the marrow is whether the sample is adequate for diagnosis. At the time of the procedure, the presence of marrow particles in the aspirate is the best indicator that the needle entered the medullary cavity and marrow was successfully withdrawn. Marrow particles are bony with a glistening appearance caused by fat in the particles. Specimens containing cortical bone, muscle, or other tissue with little or no medullary bone are inadequate for marrow interpretation. Samples with extensive crush artifact or hemorrhage are suboptimal, underscoring the importance of proper technique in obtaining a useful sample. An unspoken assumption is that the piece of marrow provided for diagnostic evaluation is representative of the marrow as a whole. Based on reproducibility of bilateral biopsies, this more likely is true in leukemia and myeloma than in lymphoma and metastatic tumor.[32] A biopsy specimen should contain at least a 0.5-cm length of marrow cavity. However, for detection of lymphoma or metastatic tumor, current recommendations suggest a biopsy length of 1.6 to 2.0 cm.[33] A significant proportion of biopsies obtained in routine practice may fall short of this recommended length.[34]

The marrow cavity was entered if the aspirate contains marrow particles or hematopoietic precursors (e.g., megakaryocytes, nucleated red cells) not found in the blood film. However, this finding does not ensure the specimen is adequate for diagnosis, because the amount of marrow actually aspirated can vary significantly in disease states. Also, some cell types, notably fibroblasts and metastatic tumor cells, are not as readily removed from the marrow space by aspiration as are normal precursors. Lack of particles or precursor cells does not prove the marrow cavity was not entered, because marrow packed with leukemic cells or infiltrated with fibroblasts may yield few cells ("dry tap").[35] Marrow aspirations resulting in a dry tap usually are a consequence of significant pathology (only 7 percent show normal histology on biopsy[35]) and indicate the need to examine a biopsy specimen, which should include a touch imprint.[21]

MARROW CELLULARITY

The "gold standard" for overall marrow cellularity is examination of an adequate marrow biopsy specimen.[36] The normal cellularity percentage of marrow space occupied by hematopoietic cells as opposed to fatty and nonhematopoietic tissue of iliac crest marrow decreases from a mean of 80 percent in early childhood to 50 percent by age 30 years, with further decreases after age 70 years.[37] Consequently, marrow cellularity should be evaluated with reference to normal individuals of the same age as the patient.[38] When evaluating cellularity, consider that the marrow spaces directly adjacent to cortical bone frequently are fatty and are not representative of the cellularity of the deeper marrow spaces. A grid can be used to estimate marrow cellularity of a biopsy.[39]

Cellularity assessment by examination of the direct marrow aspirate film is more difficult because of loss of histologic structure and mixture with blood. The aspirate may suggest the marrow is more hypocellular than indicated by the biopsy.[40] Marrow particles (seen in the direct film or a particle preparation) are the best indicators of cellularity. These particles are like "mini-biopsies" and contain sufficient hematopoietic and fatty elements to give some idea of marrow cellularity. Cellularity estimates based on careful examination of particles in the aspirate preparation agree well with cellularity estimated from the marrow biopsy.[38]

The degree of dilution of marrow aspirate specimens with blood during the aspiration is variable and may affect interpretation of marrow cellularity. Adult marrows with greater than 30 percent lymphocytes plus monocytes likely are substantially admixed with blood, as shown by cytokinetic studies of paired marrow aspirate and biopsy preparations.[41] A higher-than-expected proportion of mature neutrophils in the marrow differential is another clue to a hemodilute marrow aspirate. In patients with hematologic disease, from 6 to 93 percent of the nucleated cells were derived from the blood.[42] The greatest admixture was observed in patients with leukemia. Substantial dilution with blood may occur in difficult aspirates or when multiple draws were taken from the same puncture site. For instance, contamination of marrow aspirates with blood cells was only 8 percent in the first 1 mL, but 20 percent in subsequent draws.[43]

Cellularity of individual lineages is best assessed by examination of the biopsy specimen. Erythroid cells typically are arranged in clusters, whereas megakaryocytes are scattered throughout the biopsy. Erythroid and megakaryocytic cellularity is best appreciated at low power. In the aspirate, a myeloid-to-erythroid (M:E) ratio frequently is calculated to give some impression of the relative cellularity of these two major lineages. As a rule of thumb, the M:E ratio normally should be between 2:1 and 4:1 (Table 3–1 lists the normal ranges in men and women). The relative proportions of cell types should be assessed only on the direct marrow film, biopsy imprint, or particle preparation, not a concentrate film, which has been manipulated by centrifugation. A decreased M:E ratio can be interpreted as either myeloid hypocellularity or erythroid hyperplasia, depending on the overall marrow cellularity. Megakaryocyte numbers can be assessed from the direct marrow aspirate film, where at least five megakaryocytes should be present in the optimal portion of the film. In the particle preparation, most large particles should contain one or more megakaryocytes. Megakaryocyte number varies markedly in direct marrow aspirate films of normal subjects and depends on the degree of admixture of the specimen with blood. Megakaryocytes are enriched at the feathered edge of concentrate films.

INFILTRATIVE DISEASES OF THE MARROW
Malignant Neoplasms
Metastatic nonhematopoietic tumor in the marrow biopsy is characterized by disruption of the marrow architecture with groups of cytologically abnormal cells. Assessment of the tissue of origin is primarily based on morphology, clinical history, and immunocytochemical staining. The tendency of carcinoma cells to form tightly adherent clusters frequently is helpful in recognizing these neoplasms (Chap. 45). The clumps can appear on the marrow aspirate, but the aspirate is less sensitive than the biopsy for detecting metastatic tumor. Tumor clumps may occur only on side or feathered edges of the film, or only in the concentrate preparation. These tumor clumps must be distinguished from clumps of damaged hematopoietic cells, which commonly appear in aspirate preparations, especially the concentrate film. The distinction is best accomplished by examining cells at the periphery of the clumps to determine if the cells show the morphology of hematopoietic precursors or are cytologically atypical cells. Isolated nonhematopoietic tumor cells are seen infrequently in aspirate preparations, even when tumor is obvious in the biopsy, because of the adherent nature of most nonhematopoietic tumors. Examination of multiple films may be necessary to find isolated tumor cell clumps.[44] Methods for identifying rare micrometastatic tumor cells (disseminated tumor cells) in marrow aspirates and blood have continued to evolve, but have not yet found an established role in guiding clinical prognosis or therapy.[45,46]

Myeloma[47] and lymphomas[48] are nonhomogeneously distributed and more reliably detected on the biopsy preparation. Abnormal lymphoid aggregates should be distinguished from lymphoid aggregates found in reactive conditions or in older patients. Neoplastic aggregates show cytologic atypia and a monomorphous cellular population, and they often are adjacent to bony trabeculae, but the distinction can be difficult in some cases. The cellular morphology often can be better appreciated on the marrow aspirate, but the key histologic features are lost. Lymphoma cells do not form the tight clusters seen in nonhematopoietic tumors on the marrow aspirate film. In hairy cell leukemia (Chap. 93), the hematopoietic cells are sufficiently adherent to each other and the marrow matrix with variably increased collagen matrix that the aspirate specimen is often markedly hypocellular (dry tap), whereas biopsy specimens show extensive infiltration with hairy

TABLE 3–1. Normal Values for Marrow Differential Cell Count at Different Ages (Percent of Cells)

| Type of Cell | Rosse[64] et al: Infants Tibial Marrow | | | Glaser[97] et al: Subjects Age 1–20 Years, Sternal Marrow, 1 mL Aspirated | Bain[98]: Subjects Age 21–56 Years, Iliac Marrow, 0.1–0.2 mL Aspirated, Men (n = 30), Women (n = 20) |
	<1 month (n = 57)	1 month (n = 7)	18 months (n = 19)		
Myeloblast	–	–	–	1.2 (0–3)	1.4 (0–3.0)
Promyelocyte	0.79 ± 0.91	0.76 ± 0.65	0.64 ± 0.59	1.8 (0–4)	7.8 (3.2–12.4)
Myelocyte	3.95 ± 2.93	2.50 ± 1.48	2.49 ± 1.39	16.5 (8–25)	
Neutrophilic					7.6 (3.7–10.0)
Eosinophilic					1.3 (0–2.8)
Basophilic					
Metamyelocyte	19.37 ± 4.84	11.34 ± 3.59	12.42 ± 4.15	23 (14–34)	4.1 (2.3–5.9)
Band form	28.89 ± 7.56	14.10 ± 4.63	14.20 ± 5.63	–	**
Segmented					
Neutrophil	7.37 ± 4.64	3.64 ± 2.97	6.31 ± 3.91	12.9 (4.5–29)	Men: 32.1 (21.9–42.3); women: 37.4 (28.8–4.9)
Eosinophil	2.70 ± 1.27	2.61 ± 1.40	2.70 ± 2.16	–	2.2 (0.3–4.2)
Basophil	0.12 ± 0.20	0.07 ± 0.16	0.10 ± 0.12	–	0.1 (0–0.4)
Lymphocyte	14.42 ± 5.54	47.05 ± 9.24	43.55 ± 8.56	16 (5–36)	13.1 (6.0–20.0)
Monocyte	0.88 ± 0.85	1.01 ± 0.89	2.12 ± 1.59	–	1.3 (0–2.6)
Plasma cell	0.00 ± 0.02	0.02 ± 0.06	0.06 ± 0.08	–	0.6 (0–1.2)
Proerythroblast	0.02 ± 0.06	0.10 ± 0.14	0.08 ± 0.13	0.5 (0–1.5)	
Erythroblast					Men: 28.1 (16.2–40.1)[§]; women: 22.5 (13.0–32.0)[§]
Basophilic	0.24 ± 0.25	0.34 ± 0.33	0.50 ± 0.34	1.7 (0–5)	
Polychromatophilic	13.06 ± 6.78	6.90 ± 4.45	6.97 ± 3.56	18 (5–34)	
Orthochromatic	0.09 ± 0.73	0.54 ± 1.88	0.44 ± 0.49	2.7 (0–8)	
Megakaryocyte	0.06 ± 0.15	0.05 ± 0.09	0.07 ± 0.12	–	31 (6–77)[†]
Macrophage					0.4 (0–1.3)
Others					¶
Transitional cells*	1.18 ± 1.13	1.95 ± 0.94	1.99 ± 1.00	–	
Broken cell	5.79 ± 2.78	5.50 ± 2.46	5.05 ± 2.15	–	
M:E ratio	4.4	4.4	4.8	2.9 (1–5)	Men: 2.1 (1.1–4.1); women: 2.8 (1.6–5.2)

*Immature lymphoid cells.

**Bands included in segmented neutrophil count.

§All erythroblast forms (basophilic, polychromatophilic, orthochromatic) grouped together.

†Number of megakaryocytes near the advancing edge of the film (mean, range).

¶Osteoclasts noted in 8 of 50 subjects, osteoblasts in 5 of 50 subjects, no mast cells observed.

cells. Immunohistochemistry is useful in the differential diagnosis of plasma cell myeloma and other lymphoproliferative disorders, as is flow cytometry when the abnormal cells are sufficiently represented in the aspirated material. Demonstration of immunoglobulin light-chain restriction in B-cell lymphoma is not possible by immunohistochemistry, but *in situ* hybridization for κ versus λ light-chain messenger RNA may be successful. Detection of clonal immunoglobulin gene rearrangements by PCR amplification of messenger RNA transcripts may be used for this purpose, but clinical interpretation of the results can be problematic, and morphology remains the standard in evaluating marrow involvement by lymphoma.[49] Positron emission tomography using [18F]fluorodeoxyglucose (FDG-PET) has been recommended to replace staging marrow biopsy in Hodgkin lymphoma,[50,51] and in many patients with diffuse large B-cell lymphoma.[52]

Fibrosis

Marrow fibrosis typically is recognizable only on a marrow biopsy specimen; the aspirate merely shows reduced or absent recovery of hematopoietic cells. Early stages of fibrosis are characterized by increased stainable marrow reticulin fibers (Chap. 86). Fibrosis may accompany either primary hematopoietic disorders (e.g., myelofibrosis) or infiltrative diseases such as metastatic tumor.

Storage Diseases

Storage disorders, such as Gaucher and Niemann-Pick diseases (Chap. 72), are characterized by abnormal macrophages containing stored material in various forms seen in aspirate or biopsy.[53] Reactive cells, such as the histiocytes with "sea-blue" inclusion granules (Chap. 72) or pseudo-Gaucher cells associated with chronic myelogenous leukemia (CML) (Chap. 89),[53] can resemble the cells seen in storage disorders.

Amyloidosis

Amyloid refers to extracellular proteins that become insoluble as a result of alteration in secondary structure to form beta pleated sheets. Amyloid light-chain amyloidosis may result from a plasma cell neoplasm, and is associated with nephrotic syndrome, restrictive cardiomyopathy, neuropathy and other tissue involvement. Amyloid deposits can be identified in the marrow by characteristic birefringence or fluorescence of deposits when stained with Congo Red.[54]

INFECTIONS

Infectious organisms with an intracellular location, such as *Leishmania*, *Histoplasma*, and *Toxoplasma*,[55] can be visualized in monocytic cells by morphologic examination of the marrow (Fig. 3–3). Identification of mycobacterial organisms in the marrow by acid-fast staining lacks sensitivity but allows early diagnosis in one-third of cases with HIV-related *Mycobacterium avium* complex infection.[56] Microscopic examination and culture of the marrow are the most sensitive diagnostic tests for disseminated leishmaniasis.[57] Mycobacteria, also, may be cultured from marrow. Marrow morphology also is a sensitive diagnostic tool for detecting disseminated histoplasmosis.[58] However, marrow culture has a low diagnostic yield in the workup of fever of unknown origin in nonimmunosuppressed patients.[59] Definitive diagnoses arising from marrow examination in this setting are usually hematologic malignancies.[59,60] The presence of marrow granulomas, recognizable

only on biopsy specimens, necessitates examination by special stains for fungal and mycobacterial organisms, but the differential diagnosis is extensive.[53,61]

NECROSIS AND GELATINOUS TRANSFORMATION

Marrow necrosis may occur in a variety of disorders, particularly sickle cell disease and neoplastic processes involving the marrow.[62] Aspirates of necrotic marrow stained with polychrome stains contain cells with indistinct margins and smudged basophilic nuclei surrounded by acidophilic material. Marrow sections stained with hematoxylin and eosin show loss of normal marrow architecture, indistinct cellular margins, and a background of amorphous eosinophilic material. Patients with severe weight loss may develop gelatinous transformation of the marrow, characterized by amorphous extracellular material (proteoglycans), fat atrophy, and marrow hypoplasia.[63]

● MORPHOLOGIC DIFFERENTIATION OF HEMATOPOIETIC LINEAGES

OVERVIEW

Marrow aspirate films should be examined under low-power magnification to assess the cellularity of particles and estimate the number of megakaryocytes, plasma cells, and mast cells. Low-power examination may also permit detection of malignancy or abnormal storage cells. The entire film should be examined, including the particles, and higher magnification should be used to study any abnormalities discovered. Similarly, biopsy sections are examined at low power to assess adequacy, overall cellularity, presence of infiltrative disease, and cellularity of the major hematopoietic lineages.

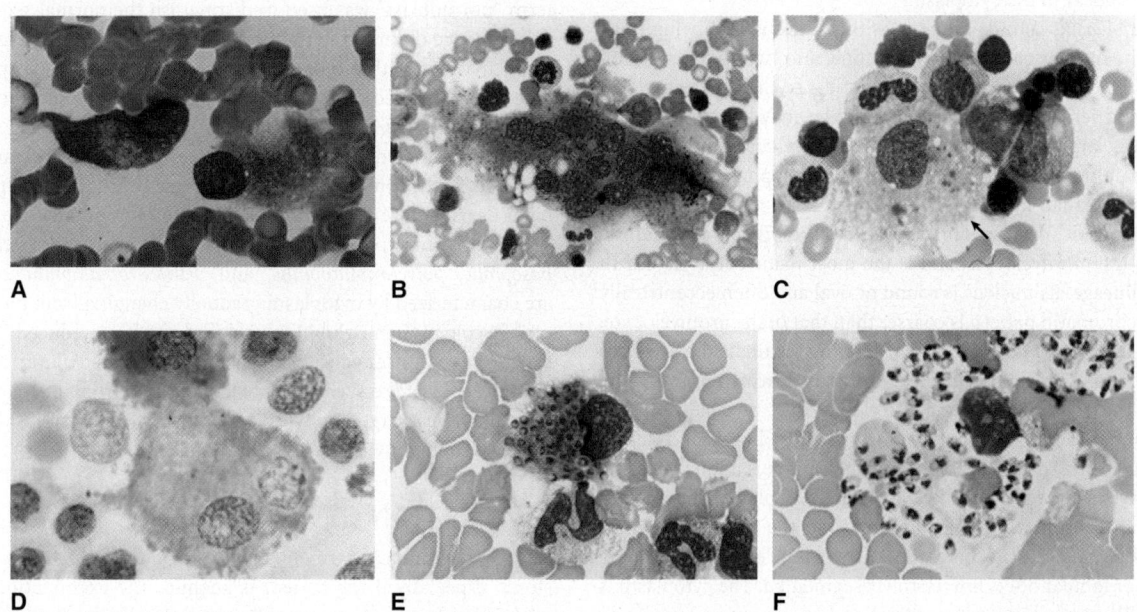

Figure 3–3. Marrow findings. **A.** Two osteoblasts are in this field. Elongated ovoid cells with nucleus at extreme end, a morphology which characteristically looks like the nucleus is falling out of the cell. A clear area is apparent spaced at an interval from the nucleus. **B.** Osteoclast. Multinucleated giant cell. The nuclei are characteristically scattered throughout the cell, appearing separate. **C.** Macrophage *(arrow)*, relatively large cell with circular nucleus and abundant cytoplasm. Ingested debris and few vacuoles. **D.** Macrophage (two). Prussian blue stain. Relatively large cell with circular nuclei. One binucleate. Each macrophage is full of iron as indicated by blue reaction product of stain. **E.** Macrophage engorged with *Histoplasma capsulatum*. **F.** Macrophage engorged with amastigote forms of *Leishmania donovani*. *(Reproduced with permission from* Lichtman's Atlas of Hematology, *www.accessmedicine.com.)*

After the low-power survey, the films should be examined at higher power and under oil-immersion magnification to determine the various hemopoietic cell types present and assess adequacy of differentiation in each hematopoietic lineage. For most diagnostic questions, careful and systematic visual examination of the marrow is sufficient to assess differentiation, but a marrow differential cell count can be performed to quantify blasts or other abnormal cells. Based on the diagnostic question at issue, the marrow differential count may require examination of 300 to 500 nucleated cells. Table 3–1 lists the normal values for these determinations, including data for infants from birth to age 18 months.[64] Between birth and age 1 month, lymphocytes increase and erythroid and granulocytic precursors decrease. After 1 month, the marrow differential count varies little to age 18 months, the duration of the study.[64] The proportion of segmented neutrophils increases with large volumes of aspirate, probably because of dilution of marrow cells by mature granulocytes in the blood.[65] The range of normal for all cell types is broad, and differential counts and M:E ratios should be considered rough guides to the character of the marrow as a whole.

Progenitors of all lineages typically are unremarkable cells without distinctive morphologic attributes. Precursors and mature cells of the hematopoietic lineages show characteristic diagnostic morphologic changes as described below. Further details of the morphology of these cells are discussed in the relevant specific chapters of this book as referenced below.

GRANULOCYTES

Granulocytes are precursors or mature forms of leukocytes characterized by neutrophilic, eosinophilic, or basophilic granules in their cytoplasm in the more mature stages of development. This series sometimes is referred to as the *myeloid series* (Chap. 60). The overall trend is a gradual decrease in nuclear size and enhanced clumping of nuclear chromatin as cells lose proliferative capacity, while granules of varying types progressively appear in the cytoplasm.

The *myeloblast* is round and large, with a nucleus occupying most of the cell. The nuclear chromatin is very fine, and two to five nucleoli are present. The cytoplasm is basophilic, but less so than the cytoplasm of the erythroid series. Few azurophilic granules may be present.[66] The *promyelocyte* is larger than the myeloblast, with a coarser chromatin, but still containing nucleoli. The cytoplasm is basophilic with a clear Golgi area and a small number of prominent, large red granules—the primary, nonspecific, or azurophilic granules. The *myelocyte* is slightly smaller than the promyelocyte, and is the most mature mitotic cell in the myeloid lineage. Its nucleus is round or oval and often eccentrically located. The chromatin pattern is coarser than that of the promyelocyte, and nucleoli usually are not visible. The defining feature is the presence of specific granules in the perinuclear cytoplasm, which identify the cell lineage. The granules may be neutrophilic (fine, variable size, lilac color), eosinophilic (larger, round, orange–red), or basophilic (larger still, irregular in size, deep blue). The *metamyelocyte* is about the same size as the myelocyte and resembles it closely, except that the nucleus is indented, the chromatin is more coarse, and the cytoplasm is less basophilic. The *band cell* is characterized by a nucleus that is horseshoe shaped or lobular but is not narrowly segmented. The cytoplasm is yellowish–pink or nearly colorless with abundant lineage specific granules. *Segmented (polymorphonuclear) granulocytes* differ from band cells by the multilobed character of the nucleus. At least two separate lobes are defined by a complete rounded shape, whether or not the thin filament joining them is seen. Nuclear chromatin is very dense. The mature eosinophil typically has only two lobes, whereas the nuclei of most neutrophils have two to four lobes. Basophil nuclei may be obscured by the abundant basophilic granules.

MONOCYTES

Monocytes in normal marrow are identical morphologically to those in the blood. Promonocytes (Chap. 67) have delicate lace-like chromatin similar to a monoblast, but with indented or convoluted nuclear outline.[67] These are important cells to identify as they are considered blast equivalents in the evaluation of myelodysplastic syndrome (MDS) and acute leukemia.

MACROPHAGES (HISTIOCYTES)

These cells are derived from monocytes but are larger, reaching 20 to 30 μm in the longest dimension (Chap. 67). The nucleus is oval with delicate reticular chromatin and one or two small nucleoli. The cytoplasm ranges from blue-gray to pale and colorless, and often contains phagocytosed cells, degenerating cell debris, and vacuoles. Normally, intact red cells are rarely visible inside marrow macrophages. Erythrophagocytic macrophages are a feature of autoimmune hemolytic anemia, hemophagocytic lymphohistiocytosis (HLH), a severe uncontrolled hyperinflammatory reaction that can occur in a variety of clinical settings, such as infection, neoplasia, and autoimmune disorders (where it is termed *macrophage activation syndrome*), in addition to certain rare genetic disorders of cytotoxic granule function or immunodeficiency states[68] (Chap. 71).

ERYTHROID CELLS

During erythroid differentiation, the nucleus progressively becomes smaller and nuclear chromatin more condensed, as the cell's proliferative capacity decreases. The cytoplasm gradually loses the bluish color imparted by RNA, which is replaced by the pink-staining hemoglobin. Cells in the erythroid series are termed *erythroblasts* (previously the term "normoblast" was used to distinguish the normal sequence from the sequence observed in megaloblastic anemia). These stages are arbitrary divisions within a continuum of differentiation. Chapter 31 provides more detailed descriptions of normal red cell precursors.

The *proerythroblast* is a large, round cell measuring from 15 to 20 μm in diameter. The nucleus occupies most of the cell and contains nucleoli. The chromatin is present in a fine reticular or stippled pattern but is usually more densely stained than the chromatin of the myeloblast. The cytoplasm typically is more basophilic than the myeloblast. The *basophilic, polychromatophilic,* and *orthochromatophilic erythroblasts* are characterized by cytoplasm gradually changing from blue to gray to pink in color as hemoglobin is produced and RNA reduced. The *erythrocyte* is the mature anucleate red cell. *Polychromatophilic erythrocytes* are mature anucleate red cells that are just released from the marrow (corresponding to early reticulocytes) and still have sufficient residual RNA to impart a slight grayish tinge to the cytoplasm (Chap. 32).

EVALUATION OF IRON STORES

Marrow examination often should include evaluation of the iron stores, especially if the patient is anemic. The examination is accomplished by staining a marrow film or section by the Prussian blue technique. Because decalcification of marrow biopsy specimens results in decreased recovery of stainable iron,[69] a nondecalcified specimen or aspirate should be stained when evaluating iron stores in the differential diagnosis of anemia. Marrow macrophages (seen best in the aspirate particle preparation) are evaluated for storage iron (see Fig. 3–3), and erythroblasts (best evaluated in the direct film or concentrate) are examined for the presence of iron granules in the cytoplasm (sideroblasts). Late erythroblasts are readily identified by their small size and the size, shape, and chromatin pattern of the nucleus. The proportion of normal late erythroblasts that contain one to four small Prussian blue granules is extremely variable (3–69 percent) in normal subjects.[70] Pathologic ring sideroblasts are characterized by an increased number of iron granules arranged in a ring encircling at least 1/3 of the nucleus, reflecting accumulation of iron in mitochondria (Chap. 87).

MEGAKARYOCYTES

Chapter 111 discusses the megakaryocyte in detail. Megakaryocytes are large cells (30–150 μm) with darkly stained, irregularly lobed nuclei. The cytoplasm is blue "cotton candy" textured, and the more mature cells contain many azurophilic granules.

LYMPHOCYTES

In normal marrow, lymphocytes similar to those found in the blood occur in variable numbers, depending on the degree of blood contamination of the marrow (Chap. 73). Immature lymphoid cells with a high nuclear-to-cytoplasmic ratio and moderately dense, but finely distributed, chromatin ("hematogones") often are seen in marrow aspirates of children, and mostly represent B-cell precursors.[71] These cells may cause diagnostic difficulty in some clinical settings, such as the "rebound" lymphocytosis that occurs after cessation of maintenance chemotherapy for acute lymphoblastic leukemia.

PLASMA CELLS

Normal plasma cells vary in size but usually are 12 to 16 μm in diameter when spread on a slide. They are round or oval. The nucleus is small, round, eccentrically placed, and stained densely purple. The chromatin is coarse and clumped. Nucleoli are not visible. The cytoplasm is deep blue, often with a paranuclear clear zone (Chap. 73). Binucleate forms may be found in normal marrow.

OTHER CELL TYPES

Mast cells are readily recognized by their content of dark-blue granules, which usually completely fill the cytoplasm and may obscure the nucleus (Chap. 63). The cells are round or spindle-shaped and often are located deep in the particles, frequently lying along blood vessels. The nucleus often is not visible but when seen is round or oval with a vesicular chromatin pattern.

Osteoclasts and *osteoblasts* are uncommon, and are more likely seen in hypocellular marrow or marrow obtained from children and from adults with hyperparathyroidism or osteoblastic reactions to tumors. *Osteoclasts* are large cells and may be larger than 100 μm in diameter (see Fig. 3–3). They superficially resemble megakaryocytes but contain multiple separated nuclei that have a moderately fine chromatin pattern with nucleoli. The cytoplasm varies from slightly basophilic to intensely acidophilic because of the content of acidophilic granules. Osteoclasts may contain coarse basophilic debris. *Osteoblasts* usually are oval cells up to 30 μm in the longest diameter (see Fig. 3–3). They often occur in groups. The nucleus usually is quite eccentric and may seem to be spilling out of the cell. The chromatin pattern is uniform, and one to three nucleoli are present. The cytoplasm is light blue and may contain a few red granules. Osteoblasts may be mistaken for plasma cells. In osteoblasts, the pale centrosomal region of the cytoplasm is separated from the nucleus, in contrast to that of the plasma cell, in which the centrosomal region directly abuts the nucleus.

● PRINCIPLES OF FLOW CYTOMETRY INTERPRETATION

Immunophenotyping is complementary to morphology in the contemporary practice of marrow cell identification. Flow cytometers use similar principles to the automated hematology analyzers discussed in Chap. 2, with the notable difference that fluorescence-labeled monoclonal antibodies directed toward cluster of differentiation (CD) antigens are the primary diagnostic tool. As described in the World Health Organization classification of hematologic malignancies,[72] immunophenotypic data (expression of cell surface, intracytoplasmic, and nuclear antigens) are key determinants of diagnosis and classification of hematopoietic malignancies. The principle of immunophenotyping is to diagnose and follow neoplastic cell populations by virtue of differential patterns of protein expression. Only the basic principles of flow cytometry analysis are described in this chapter, so that the reader has the basis for understanding the phenotypic characteristics associated with the hematopoietic disorders described in greater detail in other chapters of this book.

METHODOLOGY

Flow cytometers are automated hematology analyzers that use principles of light scatter and fluorescence to define cellular populations in which to analyze expression of proteins typically identified by fluorescent tagged antibodies. A single-cell suspension is aspirated into a laminar flow of isotonic diluent that passes in front of one or more laser beams. Light scatter and fluorescence data are collected using specific photomultiplier tubes with appropriate filtration to collect scattered light (same wavelength as the incident laser light) or fluorescence emitted light (at a longer wavelength determined by the dye used). Multiple detectors with different filtration coupled with single or multiple lasers are used to collect highly multiplexed data. As with automated hematology analyzers, light scatter information is collected at a low angle (correlates with cell size) and 90-degree angle (correlates with cellular granularity and nuclear complexity; Chap. 2, Fig. 2–1). The latter measurement is especially useful in separating developing myeloid progenitors, monocytes, and mature granulocytes from lymphoid cells and blasts.

Immunophenotyping can be achieved by using monoclonal antibodies specific to certain cell surface proteins, most of which have CD designations as defined by international workshops. A primary requirement for flow cytometry analysis is that cells must be viable and in single-cell suspension prior to staining, which is why this method is used largely for hematopoietic malignancies and immunologic disorders, and not for analysis of solid tumors. This consideration also explains differences in results between flow cytometry and morphologic or immunohistochemical observations when samples with highly adherent neoplastic cells are analyzed. For instance, in multiple myeloma or large cell lymphoma the proportion of malignant cells is typically lower (or absent) by flow cytometry compared with marrow biopsy. In a well-equipped and appropriately staffed clinical laboratory, preliminary information often can be provided within 3 to 4 hours after the initial sample collection, thereby facilitating institution of appropriate therapy (e.g., in the case of newly diagnosed acute leukemias).

Clinical laboratories typically use four- to six-color analysis, plus side and forward light scatter, for routine diagnostic panels. For research studies, simultaneous analysis of up to 20 simultaneous fluorochromes is possible, by excitation with up to 5 lasers and separate collection of the emitted light produced by interaction with each laser. At present, routine use of that many simultaneously measured markers is not necessary for clinical diagnosis. An important consideration is that analysis with more simultaneous colors places greater demand on resources for development, maintenance and ongoing quality assurance. Most clinically important phenotypic markers are analyzed as cell surface proteins by directly adding conjugated antibodies to cell suspension, followed by washing and lysis of red cells.[73] Assessment of intracytoplasmic and nuclear-associated proteins is accomplished after staining for surface makers by then fixing cells in suspension and adding the relevant antibodies in conjunction with a membrane-permeabilizing agent. Some lineage-specific markers (CD3 in precursor T cells; CD79a and CD22 in B cells; myeloperoxidase in granulocyte lineage; cyclin D1 in mantle cell lymphoma) are expressed only in the cytoplasm at certain stages of development. Fluorescence and light scatter data are stored electronically as list mode data files that can be archived and later reanalyzed using appropriate software. As the number of parameters collected on individual cells increases, standard ways of looking at multiple two-parameter histograms of gated cell populations become more difficult. Data analysis techniques and automation appropriate to discovery and interpretation of multidimensional data sets such as those generated by various "-omics" analyses may become part of the multiparameter flow cytometry workflow.[74,75] Computational methods for identifying cell populations in highly multidimensional data sets have been shown to be more effective in reliable and consistent identification of clinically relevant cell populations in multicolor flow cytometry than manual gating and analysis,[76] particularly in the context of a consensus approach using an ensemble of algorithms, as is commonly done today in weather forecasting.

GATING STRATEGIES

In heterogeneous specimens such as marrow, in which the relevant clinical population (such as blasts) may be a minor population overall, a strategy for specifically identifying the population(s) of interest is necessary. As discussed in Chap. 2, this is accomplished for blood cells by very complex cluster analysis using multiple physical parameters. Because the flow cytometer has a much more sophisticated analytical capability at the back end with the fluorescent markers, the front-end selection of cells is not intended to be definitive, but should include the cells of interest and exclude nonrelevant cells, particularly those that may create an interpretive problem if included in the analysis. This process, referred to as *gating*, is typically accomplished by a combination of CD45 (common leukocyte antigen) and 90-degree light scatter (side scatter). As shown in Figure 3–4, lymphocytes, monocytes, myeloid precursors, and blast cells can be reasonably distinguished in marrow using this method. It is important to exclude monocytes, if they are not the cells one wishes to phenotype, as they express high-affinity Fc receptors that nonspecifically bind antibodies and may cause false-positive fluorescence signals. Individual lineages, such as eosinophils, basophils, and neutrophils, or stages of neutrophilic maturation, are not distinguished as automated hematology analyzers do for blood, but this is not necessary for the diagnostic questions usually asked by flow cytometry. The "blast gate," defined by dim CD45 expression and low to intermediate side scatter, is a helpful region within which to identify and phenotype blast cells using more specific markers (only a minority of cell in this gate may be blasts,[77] but many cells with confounding immunophenotypes are excluded). Care must be taken to look for cells with unusual light scatter patterns not fitting in the usual "gates" to make sure the abnormal cells are not "hiding" in these regions. In particularly complex clinical circumstances, several fluorescent markers can be used just to identify a rare or subtly defined neoplastic subset, which can then be more definitively phenotyped in additional tubes containing those "backbone" markers to define the cells of interest plus additional markers to phenotype them. This strategy benefits from the ability to simultaneously measure up to 8 fluorescent markers in currently available clinical

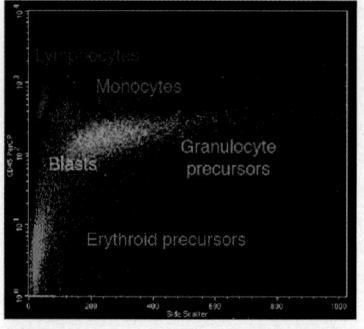

A

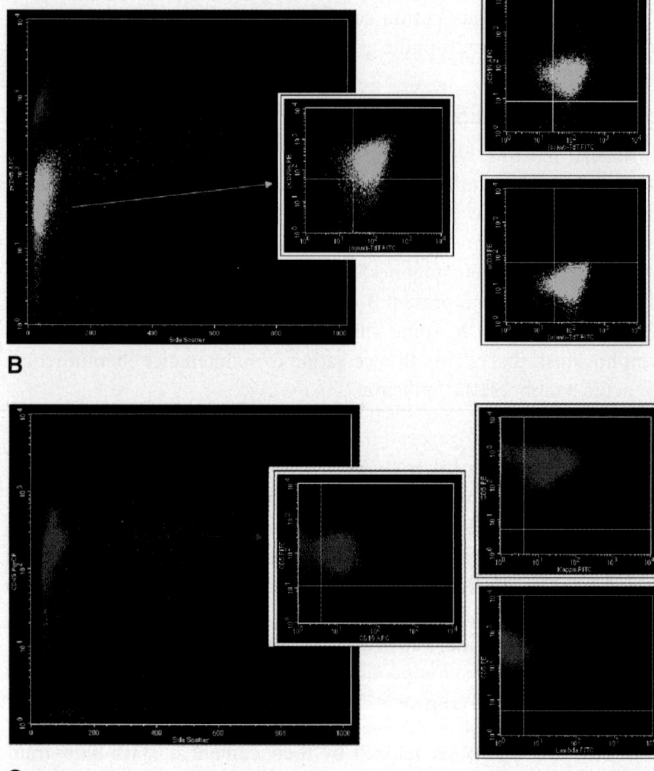

B

C

Figure 3–4. Flow cytometry examples: **A.** Normal marrow showing CD45 versus side scatter, which identifies major cell populations as indicated. **B.** Acute lymphoid leukemia, in which an expanded blast population is evident in the CD45 versus side scatter histogram (shown in *green*). Those cells with dim CD45 and negative side scatter (*green*) are then gated, so that expression of cell markers on this population only can be analyzed, as shown in the three histograms to the right, where the population is shown to be CD19+/CD79a+ (B cell), terminal deoxynucleotidyl transferase (TdT)+ (immature lymphoid), and CD3– (not T cell), hence B-precursor lymphoblastic leukemia. **C.** Chronic lymphocytic leukemia (CLL), in which an expanded lymphocyte population is evident on the CD45 versus side scatter histogram (shown in *red*), with coexpression of CD5 and CD19 (consistent with CLL), and expression of only surface immunoglobulin light-chain κ isotype on the CD5+ cells, showing that the population is monoclonal.

systems.[75] For samples with low cell viability, gating strategies based on light scatter and/or vital exclusion dyes, such as 7α-actinomycin-D, to limit analysis to the viable cell population only, may be used.[73] Strategies are commonly used to exclude cell doublets, for instance, based on the relationship of the pulse width (duration of signal) to pulse height of the forward light scatter signal. Immunocytochemistry of a marrow biopsy specimen is the preferred method for phenotyping solid tumors and is highly complementary to flow cytometry in diagnosis of lymphoid infiltrates.

COMMON FLOW CYTOMETRY APPLICATIONS IN HEMATOLOGY

Often the diagnostic question involves characterizing an expanded blast population or detection and analysis of a clonal lymphoid population (see Fig. 3–4). These determinations can be achieved by examining lineage-specific or maturation stage-specific markers. For instance, in marrow, immature cell populations can be identified by expression of antigens such as CD34 and CD117. In some instances, the stage of differentiation can be determined using combinations of markers that are expressed only during certain phases of differentiation (e.g., dual expression of CD4 and CD8 in an immature T-precursor population). Stage-specific phenotypes are sometimes valuable clues to clinically relevant diagnoses, such as the characteristic lack of human leukocyte antigen-D related (HLA-DR) expression in promyelocytic leukemia, a phenotype that mimics the normal loss of this antigen in promyelocytes. Among lymphoid leukemia/lymphomas, chronic lymphocytic leukemia (CLL)/small cell lymphoma, mantle cell lymphoma, hairy cell leukemia, and B- or T-precursor lymphoblastic leukemia, among others, have distinctive immunophenotypes. Methodologic advances such as multicolor analysis (6 or more simultaneous fluorescence colors) have allowed flow cytometers to detect and analyze diagnostically important rare subpopulations such as Reed-Sternberg cells in classical Hodgkin lymphoma.[78] Aberrant phenotype combinations suggestive of malignancy, such as coexpression of high levels of CD56 or CD117 on plasma cells in plasma cell myeloma, or loss of the T-cell markers CD7 or CD26 in a mature phenotype T cell in T-cell lymphoma, are diagnostically useful. Expression intensity is a frequent clue to diagnosis; for example, the weak surface immunoglobulin and weak CD20 expression in CLL. In reporting flow cytometry immunophenotyping results, the summary immunophenotype of the relevant population(s) should be described, rather than simply a listing of the percentage of cells positive for each marker, with subpopulations noted as observed.

Immunophenotyping of marrow by flow cytometry is a useful adjunct to established morphologic and cytogenetic criteria in diagnosing MDS,[79] and is predictive of later development of overt MDS in the diagnostically challenging group of cytopenic patients with initially morphologically equivocal marrow findings.[80] Abnormalities in MDS marrow include an increase in the percentages of CD34+ cells even when blasts are not morphologically increased; decreased CD34+ B progenitors; aberrant antigen expression by myeloid progenitors, mature granulocytic cells, or monocytes; and decreased side scatter of mature granulocytic cells. A simplified scoring system (so-called Ogata score) has been validated for use in an interlaboratory study,[81] and international guidelines for a more extensive scoring panel have been published by the International/European Leukemia Net Working Group for Flow Cytometry in MDS.[82] Immunophenotyping may provide therapeutically relevant prognostic information independent of existing risk factors incorporated in the commonly used (and recently revised) International Prognosis Scoring System (IPSS) score.[83]

Clonality of immunoglobulin-expressing B-cell malignancies involving marrow (e.g., CLL and lymphoplasmacytic lymphoma) can be determined by simultaneous assessment of surface κ and λ immunoglobulin light-chain expression on the surface of B cells, often in combination with a characteristic neoplastic immunophenotype, such as CD5 expression in CLL B cells. Technical considerations are important to minimize nonspecific binding of serum monoclonal immunoglobulins to the surface of lymphocytes. Cytoplasmic κ and λ identification,

in conjunction with aberrant surface immunophenotype, can also be useful in establishing the clonality of plasma cell neoplasms in marrow. T-cell clonality is not as easily demonstrated, because there are dozens of Vβ specificities expressed by T cells, and antibodies exist only to identify approximately 70 percent of these. Analysis of Vβ repertoire of the $\alpha\beta$ T-cell antigen receptor in cells with an atypical immunophenotype, can identify clonal populations of T cells at diagnosis and posttherapy,[84] but this methodology is less-routinely used in clinical laboratories.

Presence of minimal residual disease (MRD) measured by either detection of a molecular target using PCR or aberrant immunophenotype using multicolor flow cytometry is increasingly used as a prognostic marker, often in the setting of clinical trials, in a variety of hematopoietic neoplasms, including acute leukemia, plasma cell myeloma, and CLL. In some settings, such as chronic phase CML, MRD monitoring by molecular assay is standard practice. In others, both flow cytometry and molecular methods for MRD detection are used successfully, each having their own advantages and limitations.[85] Flow cytometry assays for MRD are considerably more complex than standard diagnostic phenotyping and need to be designed for this specific purpose,[86] with collection of large numbers of events, multicolor strategies for detecting different types of subtle aberrant phenotypes, consistent data interpretation protocols, and confirmation of absence of "background" cells in noninvolved (but otherwise comparable; e.g., posttherapy) marrows expressing each aberrant phenotype to be tested. Immunophenotypic evidence of MRD can be sought by detection of specific leukemia associated immunophenotype, or by observation of a population in multidimensional space shifted significantly from any corresponding normal population ("different from normal" approach). Immunophenotypic shifts can occur during treatment, so identification of more than one aberrant phenotype to be tested is advisable when possible. Interpretation of MRD assays is dependent on type of neoplasia, timing of testing, treatment regimen, and standardization of assay methods. Standardization of flow cytometry MRD assays is a challenge that will need to be resolved as these assays move into more routine clinical practice. In acute leukemia, where MRD testing by flow cytometry has been most intensively studied, the assays provide posttreatment prognostic information, but the translation of this information into therapeutic decision making based on MRD risk stratification is further advanced in pediatric leukemia and acute promyelocytic than in adult acute myelogenous leukemia (AML).[87] MRD detection by either flow cytometry or PCR is standard clinical practice in pediatric acute lymphocytic leukemia (ALL),[85,86] where nearly all patients have leukemia associated targets suitable for either molecular or flow cytometry MRD assays. Detection of MRD in AML is more challenging because half of patients lack a molecular target suitable for MRD testing, but the majority of AML patients have a leukemia-associated phenotype that can be detected at the 0.1 percent level or below by multicolor flow cytometry. MRD detection in chronic lymphocytic leukemia (CLL)[88,89] and plasma cell myeloma[90] is also possible by flow cytometry and molecular techniques, and is becoming a relevant clinical issue now that therapeutic options in these malignancies are rapidly improving.

Flow cytometry is used to enumerate CD34+ progenitors when evaluating the adequacy of blood stem cell collections (Chaps. 23 and 28), with several routine assay kits available.[91] Flow cytometry offers the potential to incorporate other markers defining clinically relevant progenitor and stem cell subpopulations.[92] Lymphocyte subset quantitation is diagnostically important in acquired and congenital immunodeficiency states. Flow cytometry analysis of glycosylphosphatidylinositol (GPI) linked proteins in multiple blood cell types is the gold standard for diagnosis of paroxysmal nocturnal hemoglobinuria (Chap. 40).[93] Flow cytometry detection of paroxysmal nocturnal hemoglobinuria (PNH) clones is facilitated by using FLAER (fluorescently labeled inactive variant of the bacterial protein aerolysin), which binds to all (GPI) linked structures thus sensitively detecting GPI-linked protein expression in multiple cell lineages. Guidelines for standardized PNH flow assays have been published[94] and these assays are readily set up in clinical laboratories.

REFERENCES

1. Arinkin M: Die intravital Untersuchungsmethodik des Knockenmarks. *Folia Haematol (Frankf)* 38:233, 1929, reproduced in Lichtman MA, Spivak JL, Boxer LA, et al: *Hematology: Landmark Papers of the Twentieth Century.* English translation p 824. Academic Press, New York, 2000.
2. Lee SH, Erber WN, Porwit A, et al: ICSH guidelines for the standardization of bone marrow specimens and reports. *Int J Lab Hematol* 30:349–364, 2008.
3. Riley RS, Hogan TF, Pavot DR, et al: A pathologist's perspective on bone marrow aspiration and biopsy: I. Performing a bone marrow examination. *J Clin Lab Anal* 18:70–90, 2004.
4. Bain BJ, Bailey K: Pitfalls in obtaining and interpreting bone marrow aspirates: To err is human. *J Clin Pathol* 64:373–379, 2011.
5. Wilkins BS: Pitfalls in bone marrow pathology: Avoiding errors in bone marrow trephine biopsy diagnosis. *J Clin Pathol* 64:380–386, 2011.
6. Sabharwal BD, Malhotra V, Aruna S, Grewal R: Comparative evaluation of bone marrow aspirate particle smears, imprints and biopsy sections. *J Postgrad Med* 36:194–198, 1990.
7. Pasquale D, Chikkappa G: Comparative evaluation of bone marrow aspirate particle smears, biopsy imprints, and biopsy sections. *Am J Hematol* 22:381–389, 1986.
8. Bartl R, Frisch B, Wilmanns W: Potential of bone marrow biopsy in chronic myeloproliferative disorders (MPD). *Eur J Haematol* 50:41, 1993.
9. Bain BJ: Bone marrow biopsy morbidity and mortality. *Br J Haematol* 121:949–951, 2003.
10. Inoue H, Nakasato T, Yamauchi K, et al: Risk factors concerning sternal bone marrow aspiration and patient safety in Japan. *Intern Med* 49:1089–1095, 2010.
11. Dunlop TJ, Deen C, Lind S, et al: Use of combined oral narcotic and benzodiazepine for control of pain associated with bone marrow examination. *South Med J* 92:477–480, 1999.
12. Hertzog J, Dalton H, Anderson B: Prospective evaluation of propofol anesthesia in the pediatric intensive care unit for elective oncology procedures in ambulatory and hospitalized children. *Pediatrics* 106:742, 2000.
13. Reeves ST, Havidich JE, Tobin DP: Conscious sedation of children with propofol is anything but conscious. *Pediatrics* 114:e74-e76, 2004.
14. Watmough S, Flynn M: A review of pain management interventions in bone marrow biopsy. *J Clin Nurs* 20:615–623, 2011.
15. Hjortholm N, Jaddini E, Halaburda K, Snarski E: Strategies of pain reduction during the bone marrow biopsy. *Ann Hematol* 92:145–149, 2013.
16. McGrath P, Rawson-Huff N, Holewa H: Procedural care for adult bone marrow aspiration and biopsy: Qualitative research findings from Australia. *Cancer Nurs* 36:309–316, 2013.
17. Degen C, Christen S, Rovo A, Gratwohl A: Bone marrow examination: A prospective survey on factors associated with pain. *Ann Hematol* 89:619–624, 2010.
18. Cannell H: Evidence for safety margins of lignocaine local anaesthetics for peri-oral use. *Br Dent J* 181:243–249, 1996.
19. Odejide OO, Cronin AM, DeAngelo DJ, et al: Improving the quality of bone marrow assessment: Impact of operator techniques and use of a specimen preparation checklist. *Cancer* 119:3472–3478, 2013.
20. Voigt J, Mosier M: A powered bone marrow biopsy system versus manual methods: A systematic review and meta-analysis of randomised trials. *J Clin Pathol* 66:792–796, 2013.
21. James L, Stass S, Schumacher H: Value of imprint preparation of bone marrow biopsies in hematologic diagnosis. *Cancer* 46:173, 1980.
22. Lewandowski K, Kowalik MM, Pawlaczyk R, et al: Microscopic examination of bone marrow aspirate in healthy adults—comparison of two techniques of slide preparation. *Int J Lab Hematol* 34:254–261, 2012.
23. Helgestad J, Rosthoj S, Johansen P, et al: Bone marrow aspiration technique may have an impact on therapy stratification in children with acute lymphoblastic leukaemia. *Pediatr Blood Cancer* 57:224–226, 2011.
24. Tomkins DJ, Scheid EE: Effect of sample holding, cryopreservation, and storage on the human lymphocyte cytogenetic test. *Am J Ind Med* 9:385–390, 1986.
25. Novotny JR, Schmucker U, Staats B, Duhrsen U: Failed or inadequate bone marrow aspiration: A fast, simple and cost-effective method to produce a cell suspension from a core biopsy specimen. *Clin Lab Haematol* 27:33–40, 2005.
26. Neat MJ, Moonim MT, Dunn RG, et al: Fluorescence in situ hybridisation analysis of bone marrow trephine biopsy specimens; an additional tool in the diagnostic armoury. *J Clin Pathol* 66:54–57, 2013.
27. Breit S, Nees M, Schaefer U, et al: Impact of pre-analytical handling on bone marrow mRNA gene expression. *Br J Haematol* 126:231–243, 2004.
28. Bock O, Lehmann U, Kreipe H: Quantitative intra-individual monitoring of BCR-ABL transcript levels in archival bone marrow trephines of patients with chronic myeloid leukemia. *J Mol Diagn* 5:54–60, 2003.
29. Akoury DA, Seo JJ, James CD, Zaki SR: RT-PCR detection of mRNA recovered from archival glass slide smears. *Mod Pathol* 6:195–200, 1993.
30. Hyun BH, Stevenson AJ, Hanau CA: Fundamentals of bone marrow examination. *Hematol Oncol Clin North Am* 8:651–663, 1994.
31. Moosavi H, Lichtman MA, Donnelly JA, Churukian CJ: Plastic-embedded human marrow biopsy specimens: improved histochemical methods. *Arch Pathol Lab Med* 105:269–273, 1981.
32. Wang J, Wiess L, Chang K, et al: Diagnostic utility of bilateral bone marrow examination: Significance of morphologic and ancillary technique study in malignancy. *Cancer* 94:1522–1531, 2002.
33. Cheson B, Horning S, Coiffier B, et al: Report of an international workshop to standardize response criteria for non-Hodgkin's lymphomas. NCI Sponsored International Working Group. *J Clin Oncol* 17: 1244, 1999.
34. Bishop PW, McNally K, Harris M: Audit of bone marrow trephines. *J Clin Pathol* 45:1105–1108, 1992.
35. Humphries J: Dry tap bone marrow aspiration: Clinical significance. *Am J Hematol* 35:247–250, 1990.
36. Ozkaynak MF, Scribano P, Gomperts E, et al: Comparative evaluation of the bone marrow by the volumetric method, particle smears, and biopsies in pediatric disorders. *Am J Hematol* 29:144–147, 1988.
37. Hartsock RJ, Smith EB, Petty CS: Normal variations with aging of the amount of hemopoietic tissue in bone marrow from the anterior iliac crest. *Am J Clin Pathol* 43:326, 1965.
38. Tuzuner N, Cox C, Rowe JM, Bennett JM: Bone marrow cellularity in myeloid stem cell disorders: Impact of age correction. *Leuk Res* 18:559–564, 1994.
39. Tuzuner N, Bennett JM: Reference standards for bone marrow cellularity. *Leuk Res* 18:645–647, 1994.
40. Gruppo RA, Lampkin BC, Granger S: Bone marrow cellularity determination: Comparison of the biopsy, aspirate, and buffy coat. *Blood* 49:29–31, 1977.
41. Abrahamsen JF, Lund-Johansen F, Laerum OD, et al: Flow cytometric assessment of peripheral blood contamination and proliferative activity of human bone marrow cell populations. *Cytometry* 19:77–85, 1995.
42. Holdrinet, RSG, Egmond J, Wessels, JMC, Haanen C: A method for quantification of peripheral blood admixture in bone marrow aspirates. *Exp Hematol* 8:103, 1980.
43. Batinic D, Marusic M, Pavletic Z, et al: Relationship between differing volumes of bone marrow aspirates and their cellular composition. *Bone Marrow Transplant* 6:103–107, 1990.
44. Atac B, Lawrence C, Goldberg S: Metastatic tumor: The complementary role of the marrow aspirate and biopsy. *Am J Med Sci* 302:211, 1991.
45. Janni W, Rack B, Kasprowicz N, et al: DTCs in breast cancer: Clinical research and practice. *Recent Results Cancer Res* 195:173–178, 2012.
46. Falck AK, Bendahl PO, Ingvar C, et al: Analysis of and prognostic information from disseminated tumour cells in bone marrow in primary breast cancer: A prospective observational study. *BMC Cancer* 12:403, 2012.
47. Terpstra W, Lokhorst H, Blomjous F: Comparison of plasma cell infiltration in bone marrow biopsies and aspirates in patients with multiple myeloma. *Br J Haematol* 82:46, 1992.
48. Montserrat E, Villamor N, Reverter JC, et al: Bone marrow assessment in B-cell chronic lymphocytic leukaemia: Aspirate or biopsy? A comparative study in 258 patients. *Br J Haematol* 93:111–116, 1996.
49. Kang Y, Park C, Seo E, et al: Polymerase chain reaction-based diagnosis of bone marrow involvement in 170 cases of non-Hodgkin lymphoma. *Cancer* 94:3073–3082, 2002.
50. El-Galaly TC, d'Amore F, Mylam KJ, et al: Routine bone marrow biopsy has little or no therapeutic consequence for positron emission tomography/computed tomography-staged treatment-naive patients with Hodgkin lymphoma. *J Clin Oncol* 30:4508–4514, 2012.
51. Hofman MS: Fluorodeoxyglucose positron emission tomography/computed tomography for evaluation of bone marrow involvement in lymphoma: When is it superior to biopsy? *Leuk Lymphoma* 53:349–351, 2012.
52. Khan AB, Barrington SF, Mikhaeel NG, et al: PET-CT staging of DLBCL accurately identifies and provides new insight into the clinical significance of bone marrow involvement. *Blood* 122:61–67, 2013.
53. Chang KL, Gaal KK, Huang Q, Weiss LM: Histiocytic lesions involving the bone marrow. *Semin Diagn Pathol* 20:226–236, 2003.
54. Marcus A, Sadimin E, Richardson M, et al: Fluorescence microscopy is superior to polarized microscopy for detecting amyloid deposits in Congo red-stained trephine bone marrow biopsy specimens. *Am J Clin Pathol* 138:590–593, 2012.
55. Brouland JP, Audouin J, Hofman P, et al: Bone marrow involvement by disseminated toxoplasmosis in acquired immunodeficiency syndrome: The value of bone marrow trephine biopsy and immunohistochemistry for the diagnosis. *Hum Pathol* 27:302–306, 1996.
56. Hussong J, Peterson LR, Warren JR, Peterson LC: Detecting disseminated *Mycobacterium avium* complex infections in HIV-positive patients. The usefulness of bone marrow trephine biopsy specimens, aspirate cultures, and blood cultures. *Am J Clin Pathol* 110:806–809, 1998.
57. Agostoni C, Dorigoni N, Malfitano A, et al: Mediterranean leishmaniasis in HIV-infected patients: Epidemiological, clinical, and diagnostic features of 22 cases. *Infection* 26:93–99, 1998.
58. Neubauer MA, Bodensteiner DC: Disseminated histoplasmosis in patients with AIDS. *South Med J* 85:1166–1170, 1992.

59. Hot A, Jaisson I, Girard C, et al: Yield of bone marrow examination in diagnosing the source of fever of unknown origin. *Arch Intern Med* 169:2018–2023, 2009.

60. Ben-Baruch S, Canaani J, Braunstein R, et al: Predictive parameters for a diagnostic bone marrow biopsy specimen in the work-up of fever of unknown origin. *Mayo Clin Proc* 87:136–142, 2012.

61. Eid A, Carion W, Nystrom JS: Differential diagnoses of bone marrow granuloma. *West J Med* 164:510–515, 1996.

62. Norgard MJ, Carpenter JTJ, Conrad ME: Bone marrow necrosis and degeneration. *Arch Intern Med* 139:905, 1979.

63. Seaman JP, Kjeldsberg CR, Linker A: Gelatinous transformation of the bone marrow. *Hum Pathol* 9:685, 1978.

64. Rosse C, Krauner MJ, Dillon TL, et al: Bone marrow cell populations of normal infants: The predominance of lymphocytes. *J Lab Clin Med* 89:1225, 1977.

65. Dresch C, Faille A, Poirier O, Kadouche J: The cellular composituon of the granylocyte series in the normal human bone marrow according to the volume of the sample. *J Clin Pathol* 27:106, 1974.

66. Mufti GJ, Bennett JM, Goasguen J, et al: Diagnosis and classification of myelodysplastic syndrome: International Working Group on Morphology of myelodysplastic syndrome (IWGM-MDS) consensus proposals for the definition and enumeration of myeloblasts and ring sideroblasts. *Haematologica* 93:1712–1717, 2008.

67. Goasguen JE, Bennett JM, Bain BJ, et al: Morphological evaluation of monocytes and their precursors. *Haematologica* 94:994–997, 2009.

68. Janka GE, Lehmberg K: Hemophagocytic syndromes—an update. *Blood Rev* 28:135–142, 2014.

69. DePalma L: The effect of decalcification and choice of fixative on histiocytic iron in bone marrow core biopsies. *Biotech Histochem* 71:57–60, 1996.

70. Bain BJ: The bone marrow aspirate of healthy subjects. *Br J Haematol* 94:206–209, 1996.

71. Longacre TA, Foucar K, Crago S, et al: Hematogones: A multiparameter analysis of bone marrow precursor cells. *Blood* 73:543–552, 1989.

72. Jaffe ES, Harris NL, Stein H: *WHO Classification of Tumours of Haematopoietic and Lymphoid Tissue (IARC WHO Classification of Tumours)*, 4th ed. The International Agency for Research on Cancer, Lyon, France, 2008.

73. Stelzer GT, Marti G, Hurley A, et al: U.S.–Canadian Consensus recommendations on the immunophenotypic analysis of hematologic neoplasia by flow cytometry: Standardization and validation of laboratory procedures. *Cytometry* 30:214–230, 1997.

74. Zare H, Bashashati A, Kridel R, et al: Automated analysis of multidimensional flow cytometry data improves diagnostic accuracy between mantle cell lymphoma and small lymphocytic lymphoma. *Am J Clin Pathol* 137:75–85, 2012.

75. Sewell WA, Smith SA: Polychromatic flow cytometry in the clinical laboratory. *Pathology* 43:580–591, 2011.

76. Aghaeepour N, Finak G, Hoos H, et al: Critical assessment of automated flow cytometry data analysis techniques. *Nat Methods* 10:228–238, 2013.

77. Harrington AM, Olteanu H, Kroft SH: A dissection of the CD45/side scatter "blast gate." *Am J Clin Pathol* 137:800–804, 2012.

78. Fromm JR, Wood BL: A six-color flow cytometry assay for immunophenotyping classical Hodgkin lymphoma in lymph nodes. *Am J Clin Pathol* 141:388–396, 2014.

79. Tang G, Jorgensen LJ, Zhou Y, et al: Multi-color CD34(+) progenitor-focused flow cytometric assay in evaluation of myelodysplastic syndromes in patients with post cancer therapy cytopenia. *Leuk Res* 36:974–981, 2012.

80. Truong F, Smith BR, Stachurski D, et al: The utility of flow cytometric immunophenotyping in cytopenic patients with a non-diagnostic bone marrow: A prospective study. *Leuk Res* 33:1039–1046, 2009.

81. Della Porta MG, Picone C, Pascutto C, et al: Multicenter validation of a reproducible flow cytometric score for the diagnosis of low-grade myelodysplastic syndromes: results of a European LeukemiaNET study. *Haematologica* 97:1209–1217, 2012.

82. Porwit A, van de Loosdrecht AA, Bettelheim P, et al: Revisiting guidelines for integration of flow cytometry results in the WHO classification of Myelodysplastic Syndromes-proposal from the International/European LeukemiaNet Working Group for Flow Cytometry in MDS (IMDSFlow). *Leukemia* 28:1793–1798, 2014.

83. Alhan C, Westers TM, Cremers EM, et al: High flow cytometric scores identify adverse prognostic subgroups within the revised international prognostic scoring system for myelodysplastic syndromes. *Br J Haematol* 167:100–109, 2014.

84. Tembhare P, Yuan CM, Xi L, et al: Flow cytometric immunophenotypic assessment of T-cell clonality by Vbeta repertoire analysis: detection of T-cell clonality at diagnosis and monitoring of minimal residual disease following therapy. *Am J Clin Pathol* 135:890–900, 2011.

85. Schrappe M: Minimal residual disease: Optimal methods, timing, and clinical relevance for an individual patient. *Hematology Am Soc Hematol Educ Program* 2012:137–142, 2012.

86. Campana D: Should minimal residual disease monitoring in acute lymphoblastic leukemia be standard of care? *Curr Hematol Malig Rep* 7:170–177, 2012.

87. Paietta E: Minimal residual disease in acute myeloid leukemia: Coming of age. *Hematology Am Soc Hematol Educ Program* 2012:35–42, 2012.

88. Ghia P: A look into the future: Can minimal residual disease guide therapy and predict prognosis in chronic lymphocytic leukemia? *Hematology Am Soc Hematol Educ Program* 2012:97–104, 2012.

89. Strati P, Keating MJ, O'Brien SM, et al: Eradication of bone marrow minimal residual disease may prompt early treatment discontinuation in CLL. *Blood* 123:3727–3732, 2014.

90. Hart AJ, Jagasia MH, Kim AS, et al: Minimal residual disease in myeloma: Are we there yet? *Biol Blood Marrow Transplant* 18:1790–1799, 2012.

91. Preti RA, Chan WS, Kurtzberg J, et al: Multi-site evaluation of the BD Stem Cell Enumeration Kit for CD34 cell enumeration on the BD FACSCanto II and BD FACSCalibur flow cytometers. *Cytotherapy* 16:1558–1574,2014.

92. Beksac M, Preffer F: Is it time to revisit our current hematopoietic progenitor cell quantification methods in the clinic? *Bone Marrow Transplant* 47:1391–1396, 2012.

93. Preis M, Lowrey CH: Laboratory tests for paroxysmal nocturnal hemoglobinuria. *Am J Hematol* 89:339–341, 2014.

94. Borowitz MJ, Craig FE, Digiuseppe JA, et al: Guidelines for the diagnosis and monitoring of paroxysmal nocturnal hemoglobinuria and related disorders by flow cytometry. *Cytometry B Clin Cytom* 78:211–230, 2010.

95. Jamshidi K, Swaim WR: Bone marrow biopsy with unaltered architecture: A new biopsy device. *J Lab Clin Med* 77:335, 1971.

96. Ellis LD, Jensen WN, Westerman MP: Needle biopsy of bone marrow: An experience with 1,445 biopsies. *Arch Intern Med* 114:213, 1964.

97. Glaser K, Limarzi LR, Poncher HG: Cellular composition of the bone marrow in normal infants and children. *Pediatrics* 6:789, 1950.

98. Bain BJ: Ethnic and sex differences in the total and differential white cell count and platelet count. *J Clin Pathol* 49:664–666, 1996.

CHAPTER 4
CONSULTATIVE HEMATOLOGY

Rondeep S. Brar and Stanley L. Schrier

SUMMARY

Hematology is a unique science in that its complexity is readily accessible via the examination of blood and marrow. The ease with which a complete blood count (CBC) may be obtained also leads to frequent observation of values which fall outside the reference range. Such perturbations may be the sign of something as ominous as acute leukemia, or as inconsequential as the common cold. That such changes might generate considerable anxiety, both for patients and providers, is not surprising given the plethora of life-threatening diseases that often manifest classic CBC findings.

This ever-increasing dependence on labs as screening tools generates a seemingly endless supply of "abnormal" results, often triggering hematologic consultation. Electronic medical records (EMRs), as repositories for this ever-growing data, serve as invaluable tools in evaluating the chronicity and trend of such findings.

Acronyms and Abbreviations: AC, anticoagulation; ACD, anemia of chronic disease; ADAMTS13, a disintegrin and metalloprotease with a thrombospondin type 1 motif member 13; ALC, absolute lymphocyte count; ALL, acute lymphoblastic leukemia; ANC, absolute neutrophil count; APS, antiphospholipid antibody syndrome; BCR-Abl, breakpoint cluster region-Abelson; CBC, complete blood count; CD, clonal designator; CLL, chronic lymphocytic leukemia; CML, chronic myelogenous leukemia; CMML, chronic myelomonocytic leukemia; CNL, chronic neutrophilic leukemia; CRP, C-reactive protein; DIC, disseminated intravascular coagulation; DVT, deep venous thrombosis; EDTA, ethylenediaminetetraacetic acid; EMR, electronic medical record; EPO, erythropoietin; ER, emergency room; ESR, erythrocyte sedimentation rate; ET, essential thrombocythemia; HELLP, hemolysis, elevated liver enzymes, low platelet count; HHT, hereditary hemorrhagic telangiectasia; HIT, heparin-induced thrombocytopenia; HUS, hemolytic uremic syndrome; ITP, immune thrombocytopenia; JAK2, Janus kinase 2; LDH, lactate dehydrogenase; LGL, large granular lymphocytic; LMWH, low-molecular-weight heparin; MCH, mean corpuscular hemoglobin; MCV, mean corpuscular volume; MDS, myelodysplastic syndrome; MGUS, monoclonal gammopathy of undetermined significance; MPN, myeloproliferative neoplasm; MTHFR, methylenetetrahydrofolate reductase; nRBC, nucleated red blood cell; NSAID, nonsteroidal antiinflammatory drug; p50, partial pressure required to achieve 50 percent saturation; PCR, polymerase chain reaction; PE, pulmonary embolism; PFA, platelet function analysis; PMN, polymorphonuclear neutrophil; PNH, paroxysmal nocturnal hemoglobinuria; PT, prothrombin time; PTT, partial thromboplastin time; PV, polycythemia vera; RBC, red blood cell; RIPA, ristocetin-induced platelet aggregation; RT, reptilase time; SPEP, serum protein electrophoresis; TT, thrombin time; TTP, thrombotic thrombocytopenic purpura; UPEP, urine protein electrophoresis; VWD, von Willebrand disease; WBC, white blood cell.

In this chapter, we outline our approach to dealing with these common queries. The individual epidemiology, pathogenesis, and treatment of such disorders are covered comprehensively and with clarity within their corresponding chapters and are not repeated here. Rather, what we describe is our thought process in approaching such questions and narrowing the broad differential to that which is reasonable and probable.

● LEUKOPENIA

Detection of a low white blood cell (WBC) count is a common reason for hematologic consultation. Clinicians and patients are attentive to early signs of marrow pathology, such as myelodysplastic syndrome (MDS), although such diseases are found only in a minority of referrals. Nevertheless, the severity of potential pathology mandates leukopenia be taken seriously and approached thoughtfully.

One begins by determining if the predominant finding is neutropenia, lymphopenia, monocytopenia, or all of the above.

NEUTROPENIA

The potential causes of neutropenia are diverse and include congenital disorders, autoimmune disorders, infections, nutritional deficiencies, medications, and, of course, hematolymphoid neoplasias. These are discussed in detail in Chap. 65.

Degrees of neutropenia may be broadly classified as mild (absolute neutrophil count [ANC] 1000–1500 cells/μL), moderate (ANC 500–1000 cells/μL), or severe (ANC <500 cells/μL).

The three most important historical details are the degree of neutropenia, acuity of onset, and presence or absence of associated symptoms. Each is considered individually and within the context of other findings.

The degree of neutropenia is informative. There is no specific ANC threshold that mandates evaluation. In general, mild neutropenia with preservation of other lineages in the asymptomatic patient may be observed, whereas moderate or severe neutropenia increases the risk of infection and probability of underlying pathology. The degree of neutropenia is not *a priori* a measure of its potential consequences. For example, patients with chronic idiopathic neutropenia may have blood neutrophil counts approaching zero with no symptoms or increased risk of infection.

The acuity of neutropenia is quite helpful, and the advent of the electronic medical record (EMR) allows for the rapid evaluation of such trends. In acute onset neutropenia, it is useful to inquire about recent infections and new medications. The latter is often an important clue. The number of medications that might cause neutropenia is vast, and some representative agents are shown in Chap. 65, Table 65–1. The temporal association of new medications with cytopenias is often the strongest evidence of causality. If there is suspicion for drug-induced neutropenia, the offending medication should be discontinued. If this is not possible, switching to a congener with a different chemical structure should be strongly considered.

In cases of chronic neutropenia, one should explore possibilities such as congenital neutropenia, chronic idiopathic neutropenia, infection particularly hepatitis and HIV, and autoimmune disorders. With respect to the latter, systemic lupus erythematosus is important to be cognizant of, as nearly half of such patients will be leukopenic. Thus symptoms of photosensitivity, arthralgia, and recurrent pregnancy morbidity should trigger rheumatologic consultation.

Hematolymphoid neoplasias may present with either acute or chronic cytopenias. When considering the presence of malignancy, one should attempt to identify other concerning findings, such as other cytopenias, adenopathy, fever, organomegaly, or unintentional weight loss, in addition to isolated neutropenia.

LYMPHOPENIA

Lymphopenia, defined as an absolute lymphocyte count (ALC) less than 1500 cells/μL, may be seen in a variety of settings. One should begin by assessing the chronicity and severity of lymphopenia, along with a thorough physical examination. The latter should focus on any evidence of splenomegaly, adenopathy, or evidence of fungal infection, such as oral candidiasis. The numerous inherited and acquired causes of lymphopenia are noted in Chap. 79.

Notably HIV infection should be excluded in the lymphopenic patient. Similarly, a concomitant infection with a number of viral or bacterial pathogens may result in lymphopenia. One of the most common iatrogenic causes of lymphopenia is the use of glucocorticoids. Alcoholism may also result in lymphopenia.

MONOCYTOPENIA

Although monocytopenia is described in a number of settings (Chap. 70), the most notable entity to exclude is hairy cell leukemia. Although rare, this B-cell lymphoproliferative disorder presents with constitutional symptoms, splenomegaly, and the majority of patients are monocytopenic as well as neutropenic (Chap. 93). Thus, in a patient with compatible symptoms and monocytopenia, even without classic hairy cells on the blood film, it is worthwhile performing flow cytometry with attention to hairy cell markers, including clonal designator (CD) 11c and CD103.

Severe monocytopenia may rarely be seen in the MonoMAC (monocytopenia and mycobacterial infection) syndrome. Described in 2010, it is associated with extreme monocytopenia or amonocytosis, may be associated with mycobacterial and viral infections and results from a mutation in the *GATA-2* gene. It has a high risk of progressing to MDS or acute myelogenous leukemia (Chap. 70).

● ANEMIA

The underlying pathophysiology of the anemia must be identified. We use three interacting analytic tools:

1. Standard hematologic indices, particularly mean corpuscular volume (MCV) and mean corpuscular hemoglobin (MCH).
2. Kinetic analysis (Chaps. 32 and 33) seeking to determine if the underlying cause is a defect in red blood cell (RBC) production, an increase in RBC destruction (hemolysis), or blood loss. Humans replace 1 percent of their RBCs per day (Chap. 32). Any decrease in hemoglobin greater than 1 percent/day implies the patient is bleeding, hemolyzing, or both.
3. An awareness of patient demographics. For example, a pediatric practice may place hemoglobinopathies high on the differential, whereas a geriatric internal medicine practice will commonly encounter anemia of chronic disease and iron deficiency.

The history and medical records are important tools in identifying the severity and duration of anemia. The timeline of development is crucial: if it has been lifelong, congenital causes are likely. If not, then the events surrounding the development of anemia may also provide clues, as well as indicate if additional abnormalities in the other cell lines are present.

The physical should be a comprehensive exam with particular attention to lymphadenopathy, liver/spleen size, and assessment of cardiovascular status. Laboratory analysis requires a current complete blood count (CBC) and a blood film. Critically, one cannot rely on an isolated hemoglobin value without the remainder of the CBC. An absolute reticulocyte count, corrected for the degree of anemia, is also required. A comprehensive metabolic panel as well, including renal and liver function tests, is useful in narrowing the differential.

If the anemia is of recent origin with a normal MCV and a low corrected absolute reticulocyte count (meaning there is a production defect), then anemia of chronic disease (ACD) (Chap. 37) is likely. Additional labs evaluating inflammatory activity, such as ferritin, erythrocyte sedimentation rate (ESR), and C-reactive protein (CRP), may be helpful. If there is a RBC production defect, but no evidence of inflammatory disease, it is important to exclude renal dysfunction. In this setting, we evaluate serum creatinine and erythropoietin levels.

One must maintain a high suspicion for iron deficiency, even in the setting of a normal MCV and blood film (Chap. 43). Useful items include a ferritin, transferrin saturation, and clinical evaluation for blood loss. Conversely, consider a patient in which the hemoglobin is 10.5 g/dL, MCV 64 fL, MCH 19 pg, and absolute reticulocyte count is elevated to 180,000. The blood film shows microcytic, hypochromic RBCs with occasional target cells. Although iron levels should be determined, thalassemia will be much more likely (Chap. 48).

If the MCV is greater than 100 fL and the reticulocyte count suggests a production defect, examine both the WBC and platelet number and morphology. If either is abnormal, then primary marrow disorders such as MDS become more likely than nutritional deficiencies such as vitamin B_{12} or folate. A marrow biopsy should be performed in this setting.

If the rate of hemoglobin fall is greater than 1 percent/day, and the corrected reticulocyte count is elevated, bleeding or hemolysis is occurring. One should search for specific RBC morphologic anomalies on the blood film. If spherocytes, fragmented cells, or Heinz bodies (Chaps. 2 and 31) are present, then hemolysis is likely. We obtain a haptoglobin, indirect bilirubin, lactate dehydrogenase (LDH), and a direct Coombs study. The history is informative. If the hemolysis is lifelong, then RBC intracorpuscular defects (either of hemoglobin, membrane, or enzymes [Chaps. 46, 47, and 49]) are likely. If the hemolysis is recent, then acquired extracorpuscular causes, such as autoimmune hemolysis, parasitic disease, renal/hepatic disease, or hypersplenism, are likely (Chaps. 51 to 54 and 56).

If the anemia is persistent, symptomatic, and the aforementioned workup has not provided a diagnosis, then marrow biopsy and aspiration are indicated.

● THROMBOCYTOPENIA

Whereas the consultative approach to thrombocytosis is relatively straightforward, the opposite is true for thrombocytopenia. The clinical situation may be urgent and the differential diagnosis, upon which management is based, is huge (Chap. 117). It is helpful to think of the underlying cause(s) mechanistically:

- *Platelet production is low:* The marrow is replaced (leukemia, lymphoma), empty (aplastic anemia), or ineffective (MDS, vitamin B_{12} deficiency).
- *Platelets are being rapidly removed from circulation:* Thrombotic microangiopathy (thrombotic thrombocytopenic purpura [TTP], hemolytic uremic syndrome [HUS], disseminated intravascular

coagulation [DIC], hemolysis, elevated liver enzymes, low platelet count [HELLP]) or autoimmune platelet removal (immune thrombocytopenia [ITP], drug-induced thrombocytopenia, heparin-induced thrombocytopenia [HIT]).

- *Platelets are being sequestered:* Massive splenomegaly or hemangiomas.

If one encounters a new finding of severe thrombocytopenia, one must immediately review the blood film for the presence of microangiopathy. If present, concern is raised for TTP, and immediate intervention is required (Chap. 132).

The history provides key information. Comorbid autoimmune and lymphoproliferative diseases may be associated with ITP. Culprit drugs, such as heparin or quinidine, must be explored. Hepatic disease is a common cause of thrombocytopenia and should be queried. The EMR should be used to explore the temporal nature of the thrombocytopenia and other associated CBC anomalies. The physical exam should pay special attention to petechiae, oral blood blisters, ecchymoses, adenopathy, and organomegaly. In reviewing the blood film, one should exclude *spurious thrombocytopenia* (Chap. 117) that may include ethylenediaminetetraacetic acid (EDTA)-induced platelet clumping (pseudothrombocytopenia), presence of megathrombocytes that are too large to be recognized as such by automatic cell counters, or adherence of platelets to neutrophils (platelet satellitism) which can be ameliorated by using sodium citrate as an anticoagulant. Next, one should check for the presence of microangiopathy which, if present, would lead to consideration for TTP, HUS, or DIC. Spherocytes and polychromasia would raise the possibility of combined ITP and autoimmune hemolytic anemia, otherwise known as Evans syndrome. Giant hypogranulated platelets raise consideration of MDS, and more than six lobed polymorphonuclear neutrophils (PMNs) associated with an MCV >115 suggest vitamin B_{12} or folate deficiency (Chap. 41). In a patient with newly developed isolated thrombocytopenia, megathrombocytes, platelets greater in diameter than one-third of a red cell diameter (>2.5 μM), are the parallel of the reticulocyte count. More than 10 percent such platelets are suggestive of immune platelet destruction with a compensatory increase in thrombopoiesis.

In the case of isolated thrombocytopenia, the most common cause is autoimmune thrombocytopenia. ITP may also be drug-induced. An important feature of autoimmune thrombocytopenia is the absence of splenomegaly, thus an enlarged spleen points to other diagnoses such as lymphoproliferative disease, hypersplenism, or lupus. Approximately 25 percent of patients with the antiphospholipid antibody syndrome have mild thrombocytopenia (50 to 130 × 10^9/L). Bleeding is not a feature of this phenomenon and it may be confused with autoimmune thrombocytopenia. HIT is an event seen in hospitalized patients or those receiving heparin through home care (Chap. 118). The thrombocytopenia can be mild (e.g., 20 to 100 × 10^9/L) and bleeding is unusual. It usually occurs 5 to 10 days after exposure to heparin and is associated with both venous and arterial thrombosis. Often, the patient may be quite ill, postoperative, and have other plausible explanations for thrombosis, thus requiring a high index of suspicion. It is less frequent with low-molecular-weight heparin (LMWH) preparations, but still can occur in that setting. The specifics of diagnostic tests and management are discussed in Chap. 118.

With baseline data from history, exam, and routine labs, a preliminary analysis should be performed to focus subsequent specialized testing. For example, in a patient with CNS symptoms, microangiopathic hemolysis, and an elevated serum creatinine, a disintegrin and metalloprotease with a thrombospondin type 1 motif member 13 (ADAMTS13) activity level should be ordered in addition to instituting prompt plasmapheresis for the tentative diagnosis of TTP. In a patient who received heparin 5 days prior during cardiac surgery, HIT is considered and an immunoassay for antiplatelet factor 4 obtained.

PANCYTOPENIA

The presentation of a patient with new-onset pancytopenia requires immediate medical attention. In formulating an approach to a patient who presents with a combination of anemia, thrombocytopenia, and leukopenia it is useful to think of the pathophysiology in mechanistic terms. It is also important in constructing a differential diagnosis to determine whether the leukopenia is balanced, neutropenia, or lymphopenia.

The blood counts may be low because the normal hematopoietic marrow has been replaced (fibrosis, infiltrative malignancy), is absent (aplastic anemia), or is ineffective (MDS, vitamin B_{12} deficiency). Hypersplenism can also result in the rapid removal of cells from the blood, for example in the context of a malignant lymphoma.

The history provides several critical pieces of information: How severe is the pancytopenia? How long has it been present? Is it getting better or worse? What was going on when it began? Was there an infection at onset, or has the patient had any new medications or occupational exposures? Symptoms of anemia (fatigue, shortness of breath), thrombocytopenia (mucosal bleeding, bruising), and leukopenia (recurrent infections, stomatitis) are important to determine, as are risk factors for hepatic disease (as cirrhosis commonly results in pancytopenia).

The physical exam should be comprehensive with a particular focus on organomegaly and adenopathy.

If the MCV is greater than 100 fL, consider MDS. Chemistry panels are obtained to evaluate for evidence of renal or hepatic dysfunction. An increase in MCV of greater than 115 fL is more common in megaloblastic anemia than in MDS. Folate deficiency may be seen in settings of alcohol abuse or celiac sprue. Pernicious anemia is an important consideration for vitamin B_{12} deficiency because it is treatable with cobalamin and, if unrecognized, may proceed to severe neurologic impairment. Uncommonly, the latter may be the presenting feature (in addition to the cognitive abnormalities known as megaloblastic madness; Chap. 41).

As always, a critical review of the blood film may suggest the diagnosis, including the presence of dysplasia (MDS), hypersegmented neutrophils (vitamin B_{12} and folate deficiency), and myelophthisic features (leukoerythroblastic findings such as nucleated RBCs and teardrops) that might suggest primary myelofibrosis (Chap. 86) or a marrow-replacing process (Chap. 45). The presence of abnormal or neoplastic cells in the blood may be diagnostic, such as leukemic blasts, hairy cells, or circulating lymphoma cells.

With this information one can decide on a further diagnostic strategy. Occasionally one sees patients where the pancytopenia is mild and resolves spontaneously within 1 month, which may represent a viral infection with transient suppression of hematopoiesis.

If, in a patient with pancytopenia, the reticulocyte count is very low, aplastic anemia becomes a primary consideration. Other malignant causes of severe cytopenias, such as acute leukemia or MDS, are uncommonly associated with reticulocyte counts less than 0.4 percent. An enlarged spleen is not a feature of aplastic anemia, and its presence would argue against the diagnosis.

Nearly all patients with unexplained severe and persistent pancytopenia will require a diagnostic marrow aspirate and biopsy.

LEUKOCYTOSIS

An elevated leukocyte count often raises concern for marrow pathology, but may be seen in nearly any systemic disorder. There is no numeric cutoff that reliably distinguishes between primary hematolymphoid and secondary causes of leukocytosis. Rather, a thorough history, physical, and focused laboratory evaluation is required.

Leukocytosis refers to an elevated total leukocyte count. When combined with an elevated ANC, the term *neutrophilic leukocytosis* is used. If an elevated ANC is present without leukocytosis, the term *neutrophilia* is applied. The same terminology holds for elevations of the lymphocyte, monocyte, eosinophil, and basophil compartments. In practice, however, these distinctions are rarely made, nor do they have a major impact on diagnostic evaluations, and thus we use them interchangeably.

NEUTROPHILIA

Neutrophilia may be seen in a variety of settings as outlined in Chap. 65. Primary marrow disorders include chronic myelogenous leukemia (CML), other myeloproliferative neoplasms, neutrophilic leukemia, and sickle cell disease. Secondary disorders include infection, inflammation, smoking, stress (both physical and emotional), asplenia, and medications. With respect to the latter, common offenders include corticosteroids, lithium, and exogenous growth factors such as granulocyte colony-stimulating factor. Rare cases of dramatic neutrophilia (usually accompanied by mild anemia) can be associated with granulocyte colony-stimulating factor–secreting tumors (e.g., bronchogenic carcinoma). In a patient with persistent neutrophilia of unclear etiology, it is generally advisable to exclude CML with a qualitative breakpoint cluster region-Abelson (BCR-Abl) polymerase chain reaction (PCR) analysis. The other classic myeloproliferative neoplasms (MPNs), such as polycythemia vera (PV), essential thrombocythemia (ET), and myelofibrosis, will typically have other manifestations suggesting the diagnosis, such as erythrocytosis, thrombocytosis, organomegaly, and/or a leukoerythroblastic blood film. Chronic neutrophilic leukemia (CNL), though often considered by clinicians, is a rare disorder. The WBC should be greater than 25,000/μL of which greater than 80 percent are neutrophils to consider this entity.

Smokers commonly demonstrate a mild neutrophilia, and if this has been longstanding in an otherwise asymptomatic patient, further measures other than smoking cessation are typically unnecessary. Similarly, mild neutrophilic leukocytosis may be seen in obese patients, perhaps reflective of an underlying inflammatory state. It is rarely useful to perform a marrow examination for neutrophilia during times of systemic infection or critical illness in the intensive care unit, except for the rare instance in which neutrophilia is felt to be the proximate illness, as in CNL.

LYMPHOCYTOSIS

The diverse causes of lymphocytosis are listed in Chap. 79. Primary marrow disorders include chronic lymphocytic leukemia (CLL), acute lymphoblastic leukemia (ALL), and hairy cell leukemia. Reactive lymphocytosis may be seen in viral infection (classically infectious mononucleosis), HIV, bacterial infection, smokers, and autoimmune disorders (such as rheumatoid arthritis).

Lymphocyte morphology is generally more informative than is the case in neutrophilia. If the lymphocytes display coarse, clumped chromatin, suspicion is raised for CLL. Readily identifiable lymphoblasts suggest ALL. An excess of large granular lymphocytes, particularly in a patient with autoimmune disease such as rheumatoid arthritis, suggest large granular lymphocytic (LGL) leukemia. The presence of lymphocytes with villous projections might suggest splenic marginal zone lymphoma or hairy cell leukemia. Larger lymphocytes with cleaved nuclei may be seen in follicular lymphoma, and cells with cerebriform nuclei might represent the malignant T cells of Sézary syndrome. Hence, examination of the blood film is a critical component of the lymphocytosis evaluation. The laboratory evaluation might also include flow cytometric analysis, as the immunophenotype of atypical lymphocytes often leads to significant narrowing of the differential diagnosis.

EOSINOPHILIA

Eosinophilia has a daunting differential, as discussed in Chap. 62. On initial screen, we seek to identify patients with moderate (>1500 cells/μL) or greater eosinophilia, or those with evidence of end organ damage, as these groups are more likely to have serious pathology. The history should include assessment of B symptoms, rash, diarrhea, allergic symptoms, travel history, and food intake. Ingestion of raw or undercooked meat, especially pork, increases the chance of parasitic infection with *Trichinella spiralis,* which may be accompanied by significant eosinophilia, periorbital edema, myositis, and fever. This infestation usually occurs at festivities where a pig is roasted and served. Pork from abattoirs involves mixing of meat from a large number of pigs, diluting the *Trichinella* organisms that might have infected a rare animal. The geographic location and lifestyle of the patient determines if consideration of another parasitic infestation is a high probability. In underdeveloped countries, helminthic infections are the most common cause of eosinophilia (see Chap. 62, Table 62–5 for causes of helminthic-induced eosinophilia). Signs of adrenal insufficiency (fatigue, hypotension, hyperpigmentation) a rare cause of eosinophilia, may be subtle. Rhinosinusitis, asthma, and eosinophilia should trigger screening for eosinophilic granulomatosis with polyangiitis (Churg-Strauss syndrome). Mast cell disorders are also associated with eosinophilia, and should be kept in mind in patients with a rash suggestive of urticaria pigmentosa or symptoms of mediator release with identified triggers. Patients with extreme eosinophilia are often critically ill and nearly always require hospitalization because of the high probability of malignancy or infection, in addition to risks for life-threatening damage to the cardiac, respiratory, nervous, and gastrointestinal systems.

BASOPHILIA AND MONOCYTOSIS

Disorders associated with basophilia and monocytosis are more limited, and are listed in Chaps. 63 and 70, respectively. In the absence of an obvious infectious/inflammatory insult, basophilia should always trigger evaluation for CML and PV. Unexplained monocytosis, particularly in elderly patients with other cytopenias, should reflex concern for myeloid malignancies such as MDS and chronic myelomonocytic leukemia (CMML) and generally warrants examination of the marrow.

● ERYTHROCYTOSIS/POLYCYTHEMIA

As opposed to hematologic consultation for the cytopenias, evaluation for polycythemia generally has a more limited differential diagnosis (Chaps. 57 and 84). Technically, "polycythemia" refers to increases in RBC, WBC, and platelets, while "erythrocytosis" more specifically refers to increases in RBCs alone. We are aware, however, that in common hematologic parlance the term *polycythemia* is frequently used to indicate erythrocytosis and here we use them interchangeably. The disorders that may cause polycythemia are diverse and have widely varying treatments. Attention to detail is critical.

First, the distinction between absolute and relative polycythemia should be made. The former refers to a true elevation of the red cell mass, whereas the latter refers to an apparent increase in hemoglobin caused by a contracted plasma volume. Reduced plasma volumes might be seen in patients who are dehydrated and are also reported in chronic smokers. However, smokers are more often polycythemic by virtue of their cardiopulmonary disease, so this distinction is difficult to make.

When evaluating a referral for elevated RBC, hemoglobin, or hematocrit, one begins by determining which measure is elevated. Although definitions vary, one may assume polycythemia is present if the hemoglobin is greater than 18.5 g/dL in men or greater than 16.5 g/dL in women.

If a referral is received for an elevated RBC count in the absence of true erythrocytosis, a major consideration is thalassemic trait. Additional clues for this would include a normal or low hemoglobin in addition to severe microcytosis, and a blood film showing targets, as well as hypochromia and microcytosis.

The history is critical in evaluation of erythrocytosis (Chap. 57). Key items after determining if the abnormality is acquired or congenital include:

- History of pulmonary disease or chronic hypoxia
- Risk factors for renal, hepatic, or CNS tumors
- History of obstructive sleep apnea
- Family history of polycythemia
- Use of androgens or anabolic steroids
- Surreptitious erythropoietin (EPO) injection (particularly in competitive athletes)
- Presence of symptoms related to polycythemia

Primary polycythemia refers to autonomous marrow production of erythrocytes, as in PV, whereas secondary polycythemia refers to increased erythrocyte production from stimulation by EPO (Chap. 57). Elevated EPO levels may be a compensatory response to hypoxia or produced in excess by malignancy. Secondary causes of polycythemia are discussed at length in Chap. 57.

Historical symptoms related to polycythemia should also be elicited, including headache, fatigue, visual changes, and shortness of breath. Symptoms of pruritus, erythromelalgia, or intolerance of hot water might be more suggestive of PV.

Clues during the physical exam include:

1. Digital clubbing, which might suggest pulmonary disease
2. Splenomegaly, which might suggest PV
3. Hepatomegaly, which might suggest PV or a hepatic tumor
4. Facial plethora, which is often seen in PV, although can be seen in erythrocytosis of any cause

The laboratory evaluation should include a CBC, EPO level, and venous blood gas measurement. The latter is useful in that it allows indirect calculation of the partial pressure required to achieve 50 percent saturation (p50) (reduced in high-affinity hemoglobinopathies, which should be considered in cases of familial polycythemia) and also provides information regarding carboxyhemoglobin (elevated in smokers or in carbon monoxide poisoning) and methemoglobin levels.

The combination of polycythemia and a low EPO level is highly suggestive of PV. This should trigger reflex mutational testing for $JAK2^{V617F}$ (exon 14), and, if negative, Janus kinase 2 (JAK2) exon 12 mutation. These two mutations capture nearly all cases of PV, and if negative, should trigger the diagnosis to be reconsidered and/or tertiary referral.

More commonly, the EPO level is found to be normal or elevated. This makes PV less likely, although certainly not exclusory. If the patient has symptoms suggestive of PV or otherwise unexplained polycythemia, JAK2 mutational testing should still be obtained.

If the EPO level is high normal/elevated and there are no PV-related symptoms, a thorough evaluation for secondary polycythemia should be performed. In the absence of cardiopulmonary disease or obvious offending medications, polycythemia with a significantly elevated EPO level should trigger evaluation for malignancy.

Although rare, familial polycythemia should always be in the differential, particularly if the family history is suggestive. The various mutations in regulators of erythropoiesis and hypoxia-sensing, and are discussed in detail in Chap. 57.

A diagnostic algorithm for erythrocytosis is shown in Chap. 57, Fig. 57–6.

● THROMBOCYTOSIS

When evaluating thrombocytosis, one must generally determine whether it is reactive or the manifestation of a MPN (Chaps. 84 to 86).

Historical details should include: When were the platelets first elevated? Is the elevation intermittent or constant? Have the platelets ever exceeded 1,000,000/μL? Has there been any thrombosis? Has there been paradoxical bleeding suggestive of acquired von Willebrand disease (VWD)? Causes of reactive thrombocytosis (Chap. 119), such as inflammatory disease, infection, recent splenectomy, iron deficiency, and malignancy, should be explored.

The physical exam should include evaluation for organomegaly, given this may be seen in a variety of MPNs.

In reviewing the CBC, a concomitant elevation of the hemoglobin and platelets might suggest PV. Neutrophilia, myeloid immaturity, or basophilia might suggest CML or myelofibrosis.

If there is significant suspicion for a MPN, such as organomegaly, persistent thrombocytosis, polycythemia, or neutrophilia, additional evaluation might include molecular testing for BCR-Abl, JAK2, and/or calreticulin mutations (Chaps. 84–86).

● PREGNANCY

Hematologic issues arising during pregnancy are a common cause for consultation. In contrast to the nonpregnant patient, the consultant must consider both the patient and the fetus (Chaps. 7 and 8). In this section we will not consider hematologic disorders of the fetus such as hemolytic disease of the newborn and neonatal alloimmune thrombocytopenia (Chaps. 8 and 55).

During the transition from the second to third trimester, the plasma volume increases by approximately 1.0 L while the RBC mass increases by approximately 0.25 L. This partial hemodilution can cause a drop in hemoglobin values below the normal 12 g/dL for women. There are further complicating issues. The growing fetus requires approximately 500 mg of iron from the mother, and if the mother is already iron deficient and/or not taking adequate iron supplements, iron-deficiency anemia will develop. In mothers with thalassemia intermedia, the marrow is already stressed and providing close to maximum compensatory erythropoiesis at baseline. The marrow cannot provide the additional 0.25 L of RBC mass during pregnancy, causing hemoglobin levels to fall where both the patient and fetus may be stressed. Supportive transfusions are often necessary in this case.

One is often asked to consult because of a neutrophilic leukocytosis occurring during the second and third trimesters. This is typically physiologic and the film may show myeloid immaturity with bands, metamyelocytes, and even myelocytes. Observation is recommended.

Other than the variations noted above, the approach to anemia and WBC abnormalities is essentially identical to the nonpregnant patient.

Thrombocytopenia as low as 50,000 to 70,000/μL may be seen as a normal consequence of pregnancy and is termed *gestational thrombocytopenia*. It requires no specific management. Nongestational thrombocytopenia, however, requires particular care because the differential is broader in pregnancy and because of the risk of both maternal and fetal hemorrhage. For example, when treating patients with ITP, there is concern that the causative antiplatelet antibody will cross the placenta and cause fetal thrombocytopenia. The distortion of the fetus, particularly of the cranium during delivery, raises concern about intracranial hemorrhage if the neonate is thrombocytopenic. Newborns of mothers with ITP should generally have serial platelet counts over the first week of life as thrombocytopenia may be delayed as splenic function develops.

The appearance of low platelets along with hypertension in the third trimester raises concern for preeclampsia. Perhaps a more-severe variant of preeclampsia is the HELLP syndrome (Chaps. 8 and 51), an emergency where low platelets are accompanied by microangiopathic hemolysis and hepatic dysfunction. The blood film and liver function tests are essential in making this diagnosis.

Disorders of hemostasis/coagulation include placental abruption and retained products of conception. These two conditions are unique to pregnancy and release large amounts of necrotic tissue into the circulation, leading to DIC (Chap. 129). The consultant is often called because of severe bleeding from many sites, including the vagina, vascular access sites, and surgical incisions. Laboratory findings often demonstrate profound anemia and thrombocytopenia, and the blood film shows microangiopathy. The coagulation panel demonstrates a prolonged prothrombin time (PT) and partial thromboplastin time (PTT), low fibrinogen, and significantly elevated D-dimer. If assayed, virtually all coagulation factors will be low. The key to management is prompt recognition, establishment of adequate IV access, and massive replacement of RBCs, platelets, and coagulation factors, along with removal of the uterine contents.

Two disorders have a specific predilection for the immediate postpartum period: appearance of a factor VIII inhibitor and postpartum TTP. Patients with a factor VIII inhibitor will show a long PTT and mixing studies will identify and quantify the inhibitor. Patients with postpartum TTP will have a clinical presentation like other TTP patients: microangiopathic hemolysis, thrombocytopenia, and potentially CNS and renal involvement.

● BLEEDING

Clinical bleeding is a common request for hematologic consultation. The setting and context provide important clues about the diagnosis. Requests arising from the ICU or emergency room (ER) usually relate to a specific event like trauma or surgery. These requests may involve hemodynamic compromise and often mandate a rapid response. Conversely, complaints about "easy bruising" can be equally ominous, but often don't rise to the same level of acuity.

The conventional wisdom is that mucosal and skin bleeding is likely to be caused by platelet abnormalities (qualitative or quantitative), vascular disorders, or VWD, whereas deep tissue or joint bleeding is caused by coagulation factor deficiencies. This is generally accurate, although there is substantial overlap caused by factors like age and comorbid medications (including aspirin, nonsteroidal antiinflammatory drugs [NSAIDs], and anticoagulants).

As expected, the history is critical. One must inquire about bleeding length, duration, and context. A long duration and early onset suggest a hereditary disorder. Bleedings that occurs after dental extractions or surgery are clues for mild hemophilia or VWD. If the bleeding always occurs at one site, there may well be a local issue, whereas bleeding at multiple sites points to a systemic disorder. Drug history is critical, not only for anticoagulant drugs, but also for the many agents that cause drug-induced platelet functional abnormalities (Chap. 121). A history of alcohol abuse, hepatic disease, or renal disease is relevant.

The exam should be used to identify petechiae, oral blood blisters, ecchymoses, hematomas, giant hemangiomas, hemarthroses, and liver/spleen size.

Laboratory analysis should include a blood film, CBC, and chemistry panel. A basic coagulation panel containing a PT, PTT, fibrinogen, D-dimer, thrombin time (TT), and reptilase time (RT) is also important (Chaps. 114 and 116). The PT and PTT screen both the intrinsic and extrinsic pathways. The fibrinogen and D-dimer provide useful information about DIC and fibrinolysis, while a discrepancy between the RT and TT can determine whether there is *in vivo* presence of heparin.

Before deciding that a prolonged PT or PTT is because of a factor deficiency, consider the possibility of an inhibitor by ordering a mixing study. If an inhibitor is ruled out, then one can determine whether specific factor assays are warranted. A prolonged PTT might also be the result of a lupus anticoagulant, which generally poses a risk for thrombosis rather than hemorrhage.

If there is recurrent mucosal bleeding and a family history of bleeding, we generally obtain screening for VWD. A platelet function analysis (PFA) is a highly sensitive test for VWD. Additional tests, such as a von Willebrand antigen, ristocetin cofactor activity, and factor VIII levels can be used to confirm the diagnosis. More expensive studies, such as multimer analysis and ristocetin-induced platelet aggregation (RIPA) are generally not needed if screening studies are negative. A variety of disorders are associated with acquired VWD, including cardiac valvular disorders, extreme thrombocytosis, paraproteinemias, and autoimmune disorders (Chap. 126).

Mucosal or posttraumatic bleeding might also suggest a platelet functional defect. Screening with a PFA is often useful before launching into more detailed studies, such as formal platelet aggregometry.

A low fibrinogen and markedly elevated D-dimer points to DIC, which can be seen in a variety of systemic illnesses and is associated with both bleeding and thrombosis.

Of course, not all bleeding is related to disorders of coagulation factors and platelets. One should not forget vasculitis or other vascular defects, such as hereditary hemorrhagic telangiectasia (HHT), when evaluating a patient with recurrent mucosal bleeding and epistaxis. Vitamin C deficiency (scurvy) can rarely be encountered in alcoholics or severely malnourished individuals and results in bruising and gingival bleeding because of defective collagen synthesis.

Pathologic fibrinolysis may also result in bleeding and is not easily assessed by standard coagulation panels (Chap. 135).

We have used thromboelastography to evaluate global hemostasis on an individualized basis, although this study lacks broad clinical utility.

Finally, preoperative consultations for bleeding can be frustrating because there are no generally accepted guidelines. The most important tool is the history including family and personal history of bleeding. The type, site, and timing of prior episodes of bleeding, whether postoperative, traumatic, or spontaneous, provide the requisite information upon which to base further testing as discussed above.

● THROMBOSIS

VENOUS THROMBOSIS

Consultations regarding deep venous thrombosis (DVT) may be daunting. The decision to commit a young patient to indefinite anticoagulation (AC), or to cease AC in an older patient at increased risk for recurrence often gives the physician pause.

Here we discuss some of the highlights of our approach to venous thromboembolism. The individual components are discussed at length in other chapters, including principles of AC (Chap. 25), DVT (Chap. 133), hereditary thrombophilia (Chap. 130), and the antiphospholipid antibody syndrome (APS; Chap. 131).

Patients often have significant anxiety after a thrombotic event. Although considerable progress has been made in the safety and convenience of AC, the process still poses serious risk and may impair the patient's quality of life. It is important to communicate that AC management is inherently complex, therapeutic approaches must be individualized, and, ultimately, no approach is without risk, including life-threatening bleeding and/or thrombosis.

One should begin the evaluation of a new DVT by defining the context of the event. Critical questions include:

1. Were there any risk factors, such as surgery, immobility, trauma, indwelling catheters, cirrhosis, nephrotic syndrome, inflammatory disorders, or systemic estrogen therapy (Chap. 133)?
2. If present, are those risk factors modifiable and might they have reasonably provoked the event?
3. If dealing with a reoccurrence while on AC, had the patient been compliant with therapy?
4. Are there historical or physical clues that might suggest malignancy, APS, or a hereditary thrombophilia?

When probing hard enough, one is often able to identify a "risk factor" for thrombosis. This alone is insufficient to label an event "provoked"; rather, that risk factor must be thought to have reasonably caused the event. Attribution of causality is arduous and ultimately subjective.

When dealing with recurrent events in patients on AC, compliance must be probed at length. Labeling a patient as having "failed" therapy has significant consequences. First, this might suggest an underlying thrombophilia, such as malignancy or APS. Second, the lack of clear superiority data of one agent over another makes management decisions murky.

The physical exam must of necessity focus on the affected extremity. However, a comprehensive exam may provide valuable clues. Adenopathy or temporal wasting might suggest malignancy. Arthritis and malar rash might suggest an autoimmune diathesis such as lupus. Organomegaly and erythromelalgia should trigger concern for an MPN such as PV or ET. Spontaneous upper-extremity events might suggest thoracic outlet syndrome whereas unprovoked left iliofemoral DVT, particularly in young women, may represent May-Thurner syndrome.

Screening for underlying hereditary thrombophilias is often pursued although the general utility of this approach is not clear. This is discussed at length in Chap. 130. In general, such screening rarely changes management and has the potential for error if performed at the incorrect time. For example, levels of antithrombin III, protein C, and protein S may be falsely low in the acute setting. Functional protein S levels might be reduced when the factor V Leiden mutation is present, leading to erroneous diagnosis. Anticardiolipin antibodies require sustained elevation over 12 weeks to satisfy criteria for APS. Pregnancy and hepatic disease can also affect the serum levels of various pro- and anticoagulants and confound diagnosis.

The decision regarding the duration of therapy is complex (Chap. 133). These decisions must incorporate the risk of recurrence, risk of bleeding, and patient preferences. Generally, patients with either a provoked or distal DVT may be treated for a finite course, generally three months. Patients with unprovoked DVT/pulmonary embolism (PE), APS, recurrent thromboses, or active malignancy are often considered for indefinite therapy should the bleeding risk be acceptable.

In patients with unprovoked events who discontinue AC after a finite course, efforts aimed at risk stratification via D-dimer assays appear to be useful. Thromboprophylaxis with aspirin, has shown promise. However these approaches are not standardized. The American College of Chest Physicians publishes evidence-based antithrombotic guidelines that provide specific recommendations for a variety of scenarios and are a useful resource.

The availability of new, oral anticoagulants has dramatically changed AC management from both the patient and physician perspectives. Dabigatran, a direct thrombin inhibitor, and rivaroxaban, a factor Xa inhibitor, are FDA approved for the treatment of venous thromboembolism, with the former requiring an initial 5 to 10 days of parenteral AC. Both agents are oral, require adequate renal function, and produce a reliable anticoagulant effect that need not be monitored or titrated. They lack reliable antidotes in the event of bleeding, although such products are in development. It should be noted that patients with poor warfarin compliance are equally poor candidates for these agents. Because of their short half-life, skipped doses will result in a prompt loss of AC and increased risk of recurrent thrombosis.

In general, there is insufficient information regarding the superiority of one anticoagulant over another. There is abundant experience with warfarin (Coumadin) and LMWH. The latter is often preferred in patients with malignancy, although high-quality evidence in its support is lacking. Dabigatran and rivaroxaban lack specific data in hereditary thrombophilias, malignancy, and APS, and therefore caution should be exercised in these settings. Dabigatran showed an excess risk of bleeding and thrombosis when compared to Coumadin in patients with mechanical heart valves, exemplifying the potential peril in assuming anticoagulants are of equal efficacy in different settings.

Decisions regarding AC touch upon every aspect of a patient's life and are not taken lightly. They are not as black and white as standardized chemotherapy regimens and require an understanding of the patient's lifestyle, values, and risk of recurrence. Such assessment is difficult in the modern time-constrained environment. Furthermore, such decisions should not be made in a single-instance and then followed indefinitely. Rather, the decision to continue (or withdraw) AC is dynamic and should be revisited serially depending on the tolerance of therapy and other medical comorbidities.

ARTERIAL THROMBOSIS

Consultation is often requested in patients with arterial thrombosis, such as myocardial infarction, cerebrovascular accident, or acute limb ischemia. In the vast majority of cases, however, this is related to underlying atherosclerosis with local inflammation rather than a primary hypercoagulable state. Risk factors, mechanisms, and treatment of atherothrombosis are discussed in Chap. 134.

In rare cases where underlying risk factors for atherothrombosis are absent or there is a strong family history of thrombosis, particularly at young ages, we perform a limited hypercoagulable evaluation, including studies for the APS. Paroxysmal nocturnal hemoglobinuria (PNH) and MPNs may rarely result in arterial thromboses. We rarely find it helpful to obtain studies for protein C, protein S, or antithrombin III deficiency, and do not obtain studies for factor V Leiden or prothrombin 20210A mutations as these do not have a meaningful effect on management. Furthermore, routine screening for the thermolabile variant of the methylenetetrahydrofolate reductase (MTHFR) should be discouraged as there is no evidence of benefit in reducing plasma homocysteine levels.

Hence, broad hypercoagulable evaluations are not useful in isolated arterial thrombosis, as most findings are likely incidental rather than causal, and do not have a direct impact on patient management.

● IMMATURE CELLS ON THE BLOOD FILM

Consultations may arise from the discovery of incidental abnormalities on the blood film. Nucleated RBCs (nRBCs) and immature myeloid cells are relatively common.

NUCLEATED RED BLOOD CELLS

The clinical lab may report the finding of nRBCs, which is often reported in the differential as #nRBC/100 WBC.

Although there are several causes for the appearance of nRBCs, two predominate: stress erythropoiesis and extramedullary hematopoiesis.

Stress erythropoiesis occurs as a response to severe anemia. The marrow attempts to compensate by increasing erythropoiesis (Chaps. 32 and 33) and discharges reticulocytes of increasingly younger age to the blood. If the anemic stress is not ameliorated or deepens further, nRBCs, usually late normoblasts, leave the marrow. The blood film often shows abundant polychromasia, skip macrocytes, and late normoblasts.

Extramedullary hematopoiesis can occur if the normal marrow is replaced by fibrosis or cancer or if somatic mutation such as seen in primary myelofibrosis decreases stem cell adherence (Chap. 86). The hematopoietic stem cells travel through the blood to find suitable alternative sites for growth, often settling in the spleen. However, the sinusoidal structure there is not identical to that of the marrow. Hence, blood cells, particularly nRBCs, are released in an uncoordinated manner.

A leukoerythroblastic smear (nRBCs, teardrop RBCs, myeloid immaturity, giant platelets) is a significant clue. If clinically indicated, biopsy of the marrow will usually confirm the diagnosis.

IMMATURE MYELOID CELLS

The clinical lab may report the presence of metamyelocytes, myelocytes, promyelocytes, or blasts on the blood film. The differential is enormous, ranging from normal pregnancy to myeloid malignancies (Chaps. 61–63). One begins with a thorough history, CBC, and blood film. We inquire about recent stressors and the use of glucocorticoids. In patients with normal blood counts and rare metamyelocytes, observation is generally appropriate. The presence of peripheral blasts, particularly in association with cytopenias, is never normal and mandates examination of the marrow. A full spectrum of myeloid maturity, particularly in association with basophilia, should raise concern for CML.

● LYMPHADENOPATHY

On occasion, consultation is requested for lymphadenopathy without a tissue diagnosis. The differential diagnosis is vast, including benign adenopathy, viral infections, autoimmune disorders, and malignant lymphomas. A thorough history is critical (Chap. 1). Laboratory studies should include a CBC and blood film.

Generally with this information, the diagnostic studies can be focused and lymph node biopsy is not always required. For example, in adolescents with fever, pharyngitis, and cervical adenopathy, tests for infectious mononucleosis are pursued. If there is an accompanying lymphocytosis, the diagnosis might be established via flow cytometry of the blood, as in CLL. If the patient is well appearing, asymptomatic, and the nodes are minimally enlarged, a short period of observation is often prudent.

In patients with cytopenias, B symptoms, and organomegaly without obvious infections, lymph node biopsy is nearly always indicated. Fine-needle aspirates, although often more convenient, are discouraged because the lack of lymph node architecture impairs pathologic analysis. If a diagnosis of malignant lymphoma is suspected, treatment with glucocorticoids prior to tissue diagnosis is also discouraged as it may impair diagnostic sensitivity.

● SPLENOMEGALY

Referrals for splenomegaly open up an immense differential, including hemoglobinopathies, infection, liver disease, heart failure, autoimmune disorders, and malignant leukemia or lymphoma (Chap. 56).

Critical diagnostic elements include personal history, family history, CBC, and the blood film. Has the diagnosis been made on physical exam or was it detected incidentally on an imaging procedure? If prior studies are available for comparison, one may be able to use the EMR to determine how long the spleen has been enlarged. On exam, is the spleen tip barely palpable or does it extend into the pelvis and cross the midline as might be the case with primary myelofibrosis (Chap. 86)?

Evidence of cirrhosis or heart failure might suggest congestive splenomegaly. Erythrocytosis and pruritus would raise concern for PV.

A blood film showing basophilia and myeloid immaturity might indicate CML. If risk factors are present, HIV testing is appropriate. Thalassemia can readily be identified via the blood film. Because the diagnostic possibilities are innumerable, it is critical to avoid a shotgun approach, identify the likely diagnostic possibilities, and focus the workup accordingly. It is almost never necessary to do a diagnostic splenectomy.

● MONOCLONAL GAMMOPATHY

Monoclonal gammopathies are increasingly detected given the wide availability of comprehensive metabolic panels and the subsequent use of serum protein electrophoresis (SPEP) as a screening tool. Referring physicians often have already requested a SPEP in cases of suspected myeloma, anemia, unexplained renal failure, or neuropathy. The finding of elevated serum protein or globulin fractions, or the report of extensive rouleaux formation on blood film may also trigger a request for SPEP. The SPEP can demonstrate the presence of a monoclonal protein whereas immunofixation defines the heavy-chain isotype and light-chain restriction.

Rouleaux formation reported on a CBC is not synonymous with a monoclonal protein. Rouleaux simply describes visible stacked red cells, either as a result of poor smear preparation, inappropriate viewing in the "thick" area of the slide, or as a consequence of increased plasma proteins, such as immunoglobulins and fibrinogen. Although rouleaux may result from a monoclonal gammopathy, it may also be seen in chronic infections, autoimmune disorders, and liver disease.

When seeing referrals for monoclonal gammopathies, one should obtain a CBC, renal and liver function studies, blood film, immunoglobulin panel, free light-chain ratio, urine protein electrophoresis (UPEP) with immunofixation, and skeletal survey. This analysis seeks to identify any evidence of end organ damage attributable to the monoclonal population, such as hypercalcemia, anemia, renal dysfunction, or lytic bone disease. The physical exam focuses on the presence of adenopathy or organomegaly that might suggest a lymphoproliferative disorder.

If there is no clear evidence of end organ damage, the term *monoclonal gammopathy of undetermined significance* (MGUS) is often applied, and observation is pursued. The natural history, risk stratification, and prognosis of such patients in discussed in Chaps. 106 and 107. Monoclonal proteins may also be seen in association with several disorders, including plasma cell dyscrasias, lymphoproliferative disorders, infections, and various autoimmune diseases. Notably, it is important to identify patients with signs concerning for immunoglobulin light-chain amyloidosis (nephrotic range proteinuria, macroglossia, neuropathy). In cases of immunoglobulin (Ig) M paraproteins, look for evidence of Waldenström macroglobulinemia (adenopathy, constitutional symptoms, organomegaly, bleeding). Although rare, in patients with anemia and IgM κ paraproteins, one should inquire about cold sensitivity and seek to exclude cold agglutinin hemolysis.

One is often faced with an elderly patient with multiple comorbidities, such as chronic renal dysfunction, peripheral neuropathy, diabetes mellitus, and osteoporosis in conjunction with a systemic paraprotein.

In most cases, if these findings have been chronic and longstanding, they are thought to be unrelated to the paraprotein, and ongoing observation is appropriate rather than cytotoxic chemotherapy. In some cases, particularly those in which historical labs are unavailable, this distinction is more difficult to make, and marrow exam may be useful to assess the degree of marrow effacement. In younger patients with monoclonal proteins greater than 1.5 g/dL, non-IgG isotypes, or abnormal free light-chain ratios, we often obtain marrow biopsies given the higher likelihood of progression and potential intervention for patients with high-risk smoldering myeloma.

ADVICE TO REFERRING PHYSICIANS

A good relationship and open line of communication between hematologists and referring physicians are imperative. A few points to keep in mind:

- The clinical history is invaluable. If there is lack of clarity, we recommend a quick phone call to the referring physician focusing on the salient features of the patient's medical history and the reason for consultation. Much like pathologists, this information helps us place the labs and blood film in appropriate context and aids the diagnostic evaluation, particularly in cases with broad differentials such as anemia or leukopenia. The importance of the history and physical exam also reinforces the need for the attending hematologist to personally review the blood film, rather than relying solely on hematopathologists or laboratory technicians.
- Avoid the laboratory "shotgun" approach. For example, exhaustive hypercoagulable studies in patients with provoked thromboses are not particularly useful and can create patient anxiety. Patients have concerns about their "genetic disease," and hematologists have a hard time explaining the implications of tests they would not typically order. The consulting hematologist should direct the laboratory evaluation to avoid unnecessary, duplicate, and/or costly tests.
- The increasing variety of molecular and genetic diagnostics, in addition to the evolving complexity of hematopathology, mandates one be aware of the resources of their local hematologist. For example, rare disorders such as systemic mastocytosis, CNL, severe eosinophilia, and atypical CML are often best evaluated in a tertiary center. Once the diagnosis is made and a treatment plan established, care should then be transitioned to local physicians, with intermittent input from an academic center if required. Value should always be placed on avoiding repeat marrow examinations.
- With rare exception, diagnoses should not be made off scant marrow specimens. Terms such as "aspiculate aspirate" and "subcortical biopsy" should trigger concern for an inadequate specimen. In such cases, a repeat biopsy should be obtained by an experienced provider rather than making diagnostic assumptions from a poor specimen.
- A referral to a hematologist, "cancer center," or hematologist/oncologist often generates considerable patient anxiety, even if not verbalized. The waiting period of several days to weeks to see such a provider can cause significant distress. Unless the diagnosis is clear, it is useful to counsel patients that such a referral does not imply the presence of "cancer" or "leukemia" but rather a request for more information.

Part II The Organization of the Lymphohematopoietic Tissues

5. Structure of the Marrow and the Hematopoietic Microenvironment...... 53

6. The Organization and Structure of Lymphoid Tissues 85

CHAPTER 5
STRUCTURE OF THE MARROW AND THE HEMATOPOIETIC MICROENVIRONMENT

Utpal P. Davé and Mark J. Koury*

SUMMARY

The marrow, located in the medullary cavity of bone, is the site of hematopoiesis in humans. The marrow produces approximately 6 billion cells per kilogram of body weight per day. Hematopoietically active (red) marrow regresses after birth until late adolescence, after which it is focused in the lower skull, vertebrae, shoulder and pelvic girdles, ribs, and sternum. Fat cells (yellow marrow) replace hematopoietic cells in the bones of the hands, feet, legs, and arms. Fat comprises approximately 50 percent of red marrow in the adult. Further fatty replacement of the red marrow continues slowly with aging, but hematopoiesis can be expanded when demand for blood cells is increased.

Acronyms and Abbreviations: AGM, aorta-gonad-mesonephros; ALCAM, activated leukocyte adhesion molecule; bFGF, basic fibroblast growth factor; BFU-E, burst-forming unit−erythroid; BMP, bone morphogenetic protein; CAR, CXCL 12−abundant reticular cells; CD, cluster of differentiation; C/EBP, CCAAT/enhancer-binding protein; CFU-E, colony forming unit−erythroid; CFC-G, colony-forming cell-granulocyte; CXCL12/SDF1, stromal cell-derived factor; dpc, days postcoitum; EBI, erythroblastic island; ECM, extracellular matrix; ELAM, endothelial leukocyte adhesion molecule; EPO, erythropoietin; FN, fibronectin; GAG, glycosaminoglycan; G-CSF, granulocyte colony-stimulating factor; GM-CSF, granulocyte-macrophage colony-stimulating factor; GMP, granulocyte-macrophage progenitor; HGF, hepatocyte growth factor; HIF, hypoxia-inducible factor; HSC, pluripotent hematopoietic stem cell; ICAM, intercellular adhesion molecule; IHH, Indian hedgehog family of proteins; IL, interleukin; LFA, lymphocyte function antigen; MAdCAM, mucosal addressin cell adhesion molecule; M-CSF, macrophage colony-stimulating factor; MEP, megakaryocytic-erythroid progenitor; MIP, macrophage inflammatory protein; MMP, matrix metalloproteinase; MPP, multipotential pluripotential progenitor; MSC, mesenchymal stem cell; NFAT, nuclear factor of activated T cells; NK, natural killer; OPG, osteoprotegerin; PDGF, platelet-derived growth factor; PECAM, platelet endothelial cell adhesion molecule; PPAR, peroxisome proliferator-activated receptor; ProEBs, proerythroblasts; PSGL, P-selectin glycoprotein ligand; RANK, receptor activator of nuclear factor-κB; Rb, retinoblastoma tumor-suppressor protein; SCF, stem cell factor; Siglecs, sialic acid-binding immunoglobulin (Ig)-like lectins; SP, side population; TGF-β, transforming growth factor-β; TLR, toll-like receptor; TNF-α, tumor necrosis factor-α; TPO, thrombopoietin; TRAP, tartrate-resistant acid phosphatase; TSP, thrombospondin; VCAM, vascular cell adhesion molecule; VEGF, vascular endothelial growth factor; VLA, very-late antigen.

*Marshall A. Lichtman was an author of this chapter in the previous six editions, and some material from those editions, including all illustrations, has been retained.

The marrow stroma consists principally of a network of sinuses that originate at the endosteum from cortical capillaries and terminate in collecting vessels that enter the systemic venous circulation. The trilaminar sinus wall is composed of endothelial cells; a thin basement membrane; and adventitial reticular cells that are progenitors of chondrocytes, osteoblasts and adipocytes. Stem cells can leave and reenter marrow as part of their normal circulation.

Hematopoiesis, the proliferation and differentiation of stem cells and their progeny in the intersinus spaces, is controlled by a complex array of stimulatory and inhibitory cytokines, cell−cell contacts, and interactions with the extracellular matrix. In this unique environment, lymphohematopoietic stem cells differentiate into all the blood cell lineages. Mature cells are produced and released to maintain steady-state blood cell levels. The hematopoietic system also can respond to meet increased demands for additional cells as a result of blood loss, hemolysis, inflammation, immune cytopenias, and other causes.

● HISTORY AND GENERAL CONSIDERATIONS

The marrow, one of the largest organs in the human body, is the principal site for blood cell formation. In the normal adult, daily marrow production amounts to approximately 2.5 billion red cells, 2.5 billion platelets, and 1 billion granulocytes per kilogram of body weight. The rate of production adjusts to actual needs and can vary from a basal rate to several times normal. Until the late 19th century, blood cell formation was thought to be the prerogative of the lymph nodes or the liver and spleen. In 1868, Neuman[1] and Bizzozero[2] independently observed nucleated blood cells in material squeezed from the ribs of human cadavers and proposed that the marrow is the major source of blood cells.[3] The first *in vivo* marrow biopsy probably was done in 1876 by Mosler,[4] who used a wood drill to obtain marrow particles from a patient with leukemia. Studies by Arinkin[5] in 1929 established marrow aspiration as a safe, easy, and useful technique (Chap. 3).

Kinetic studies of marrow cells, using radioisotopes and *in vitro* cultures, have shown that cell lineages consist mainly of maturing cells with a finite functional life span. On the other hand, sustained cellular production depends on pools of primordial cells capable of both differentiation and self-replication.[6] The most primitive pool consists of pluripotential lymphohematopoietic stem cells with the capacity for continuous self-renewal, that is, hematopoietic stem cells (HSCs). The more mature pools consist of differentiating progenitor cells, with their maturation restricted to single or limited numbers of cell lineages and more restricted capacities for self-renewal (Chap. 18). The proliferative activity of these pools involves humoral feedback from peripheral target tissues[7] and cell−cell and cell−matrix interactions within the microenvironment of the marrow.[8] The marrow stroma and nearby hematopoietic cells provide unique structural and chemical environments (niches) that support the survival, differentiation, and proliferation of pluripotential HSCs. HSC interactive niches[9] have been identified at the structural and molecular[10] levels and are dynamically controlled by bone morphogenetic proteins (BMPs)[11] and factors regulating intramedullary osteoblastic cells and their progenitors.[12] Early stem cells can be identified and isolated using a unique array of surface antigen-receptor expressions (CD34+/−, Thy1,[lo] KIT+, CD38−, CD33−, vascular endothelial [VE]-cadherin+, KDR/FLK1+, FLK2−/FLT3−, CD133+/−)[13–18] and have a unique molecular signature.[19,20] The ability to efflux specific chemical dyes has also been used to provide enriched populations of HSC.[21–24] Isolated cell populations enriched in HSC can be quantified

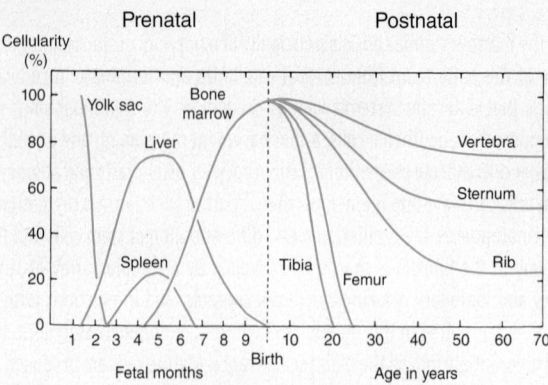

Figure 5–1. Expansion and recession of hematopoietic activity in extramedullary and medullary sites. For details regarding the nature of yolk sac and hepatic hematopoiesis, see "Sites of Hematopoiesis: Embryogenesis and Early Stem Cell Development." Chapter 7 provides a more comprehensive treatment of this topic (see Fig. 7–1 in Chap. 7).

using *in vitro* long-term progenitor assays and surrogate *in vivo* repopulating assays in severely immunodeficient mice and xenogeneic animal models (Chap. 18).

● SITES OF HEMATOPOIESIS

EMBRYOGENESIS AND EARLY STEM CELL DEVELOPMENT

As shown in Fig. 5–1, the marrow is the last in a series of anatomical sites of hematopoiesis that change several times during embryonic and fetal development.[25–28] The earliest hematopoietic cells develop in the blood islands of the extraembryonic yolk sac during late gastrulation and form the primitive hematopoietic system. This primitive hematopoiesis is transient, lasting from the appearance of the blood islands at embryonic days 7.5 days postcoitum (dpc) in mice and 19 dpc in humans through the final cellular divisions in the circulating embryonic blood at 13.5 dpc in mice and week 6 in humans.[28,29] The large majority of primitive blood cells produced are erythrocytes that enucleate after release into the circulation, and their hemoglobin contains the embryonic α- and β-globin chains. Primitive hematopoietic cells also give rise to macrophages and megakaryocytes. Overlapping with this transient primitive hematopoiesis is definitive hematopoiesis that gives rise to all of the blood cell types found in the adult (Chap. 7).

Transplantation experiments in hematopoietically ablated mice have demonstrated that definitive hematopoietic cells arise on 8.5 to 11.5 dpc in mice and weeks 4 to 6 in humans in three different embryonic locations: the yolk sac blood islands, the anterior portion of the aorta-gonad-mesonephros (AGM) region, and the allantoic portion of the developing placenta.[26–28] The definitive murine erythroid cells circulating on 8.5 to 11.5 dpc appear to be descendent from a transient population of erythroid/myeloid progenitors derived from the yolk sac, rather than being derived from HSCs that arise in the placenta and AGM as occurs at later times in the fetus and adult.[30] Serial transplantation in irradiated mice demonstrated that the earliest appearance of the intraembryonic human HSCs is in the AGM at week 5.[31] HSCs migrate through the blood to the fetal liver where they seed and mature into all of the cellular elements of the blood.[25–28] Erythrocytes, the predominant cell produced by definitive hematopoiesis during prenatal development, are smaller than the primitive erythrocytes, and their hemoglobin contains the fetal and adult globin chains. In mid-gestation, the HSCs that have migrated to the fetal liver undergo an exponential expansion and

display a specific integrin (Mac-1) that is not found in marrow HSCs.[32] In the last third of gestation, the HSCs and early hematopoietic progenitor cells migrate from the fetal liver through the circulation seeding the spleen and marrow. Fetal liver hematopoiesis declines steadily as the spleen and marrow become the major hematopoietic sites. At birth, the marrow is the major hematopoietic site in humans, while the spleen remains a prominent but decreasing site in the mouse (Chap. 7).

Visceral endoderm is in close proximity to the mesoderm formed by gastrulation in those sites where HSCs are generated in the embryo. This proximity is important in that the endoderm appears to induce both endothelial and blood cell development in the adjacent mesoderm through secretion of Indian hedgehog (IHH), a member of the hedgehog family of proteins.[33] IHH, in turn, upregulates the expression of BMP4 in the developing mesodermal cells.[33] BMP4 upregulation is important for the development of both the endothelial cells that form blood vessels and the HSCs located within these vessels.[33,34] Developing endothelial cells and hematopoietic cells in the vessels formed by these endothelial cells are found in each site of primitive and definitive hematopoiesis. The close association of these two cell types in the developing embryo has led to the proposal for their having a common precursor, the hemangioblast.[35,36] Important proteins involved in the development of the hemangioblasts are BMP4, VE growth factor receptor KDR/Flk-1, transcription factor TAL1, and TAL1's binding partner LMO2.[35,36]

Marked endothelial cells in mice give rise to the HSCs.[37] Imaging studies in zebrafish[38,39] and mice[40] indicate that specialized hemogenic endothelial cells in the ventral part of the aorta can transform without mitosis into HSCs. The differentiation of HSCs from hemangioblasts and/or hemogenic endothelium requires the signaling protein Notch1 and the transcription factors GATA-2, MYB, and Runx1.[35,36,41,42] The mechanism driving this earliest expansion of HSC is not well-defined, but two factors that also play roles later, KIT ligand/stem cell factor (SCF) and interleukin (IL)-3, are important in the embryo. BMP4, in addition to its role in the induction of hematopoietic and endothelial differentiation, increases proliferative and self-renewal of HSCs[33,34] as it differentially upregulates KIT (SCF receptor) in the HSCs, but not in adjacent endothelial cells.[43] Expansion of the earliest definitive HSC is also mediated by Notch signaling as it induces the Runx1 transcription factor[41,42] and one of its targets, the IL-3 gene.[44]

STEM CELL AND MESENCHYMAL CELL PLASTICITY

Primitive stem cells from human fetal liver or marrow reconstitute all lymphohematopoietic-derived cells and part of the stromal microenvironment in *in vivo* repopulation assays.[45] These observations are consistent with the early derivation of hematopoietic, vascular, and stromal cells from a CD34–, KDR/Flk-1+, multipotential mesenchymal stem cell.[14–16,46] Identification of AC133+, CD34–, CD7– HSCs[47] and demonstration of endothelial precursors in AC133+ progenitor cells[48] underscore the crosstalk between hematopoiesis and angiogenesis signaling pathways and establish the functional role of hemangioblasts in ontogeny.[49–51] As early fetal hematopoiesis is established, the yolk sac vascular networks remain active sites of progenitor production and hematopoiesis.[28] Long-term reconstituting HSCs express two members of the ATP-binding cassette genes (ABCG-2 and P-glycoprotein), allowing the efflux of mitochondrial vital dyes such as Hoechst 33342 and rhodamine 123 and their isolation by multiparameter flow cytometry based on their low side scatter (side population [SP] cells).[21–24] Enrichment of the SP population for HSC has been achieved in both adult marrow[52] and fetal liver[53] populations by using the signaling lymphocyte and activation markers (SLAMs) to select cells with the specific phenotype

(CD150+, CD244−, CD48−). Nearly half of the individual cells in the CD150+, CD244−, CD48− population provide long-term hematopoietic reconstitution in irradiated mice.[52]

Derivation of hematopoietic cells from adult tissue (muscle, liver) is attributed to resident marrow-derived stem cells in these tissues.[54,55] A role for adult marrow-derived mesenchymal stem cells in the repair and regeneration of nonmarrow organs has been described, including cardiac and smooth muscle, liver, and brain.[56,57] However, these marrow-derived mesenchymal stem cells function mainly by providing a microenvironment through various cytokines that induce cell growth and stimulate vascularization or by fusing with local cells, rather than by transdifferentiation into specific differentiated cells of the organ undergoing repair (Chap. 18).[56,57]

HISTOGENESIS

Stroma and Hematopoietic Tissue

The formation of the marrow in the third trimester of mammalian prenatal development involves the circulation and chemotaxis of HSCs, which have greatly expanded their numbers in the fetal liver, to the newly developed marrow niche (see "Marrow Structure" below). The release of HSC from the murine fetal liver coincides with the progressive loss of two adhesion proteins, CD144 (VE-cadherin) and CD41 (integrin α_{2b}).[58,59] In mice, the seeding of the marrow with HSCs is first detected at 17.5 dpc,[60] but the formation of the marrow niches for the HSCs and their progeny occurs in the preceding 3 days in sites of endochondral bone formation.[61] Differentiation of a clonal skeletal progenitor stem cell results in cell populations that form cartilage, bone, or marrow niches that either support HSCs or the differentiating progeny of HSCs.[62] The specific cells supported by a niche depend upon the expressions of endoglin, Thy1, and aminopeptidase A by the mesenchymal descendants of the skeletal progenitor stem cell. The migration of the circulating HSCs to their supporting marrow niches, which are formed by cells expressing aminopeptidase A but not endoglin or Thy1,[62] is directed by the synergistic action of the chemokines CXCL12 and SCF for which the HSCs display the respective receptors, CXCR4 and KIT.[60] Other chemotactic factors and adhesion molecules contribute to HSC migration from the fetal liver to the developing bone where their seeding and differentiation initiates marrow hematopoietic function in mammals.[58–60]

Cavities within bone occur in the human being at about the fifth fetal month and soon become the exclusive site for granulocytic and megakaryocytic proliferation. Erythropoietic activity at the time is confined to the liver. The microenvironment in the marrow becomes supportive of erythroblasts only toward the end of the last trimester (see Fig. 5–1). The formation of the marrow cavities in the developing mouse bones appear at a relatively later time in the prenatal life of mice than humans, and it involves an IHH-regulated[63] synchronized maturation of osteoblast progenitors arising from mesenchymal stem cells and osteoclast progenitors arising from HSCs in the areas of mineralized cartilage of the fetal bones.[64] Most of the marrow spaces form in the endochondral bones but some marrow develops in the intramembranous bones of the cranium and scapulae. As these respective progenitors differentiate *in situ* they acquire the phenotype of osteoblasts with expression of osteopontin, osteonectin, bone sialoprotein, and macrophage colony-stimulating factor (M-CSF), and of osteoclasts with expression of tartrate-resistant acid phosphatase (TRAP), calcitonin receptors, and c-FMS (M-CSF receptor).[64] In the human, marrow hematopoiesis begins at the 11th week of gestation in specialized mesodermal structures termed *primary logettes*.[65] The logettes are composed of mesenchymal cells and fibers that surround a central artery and protrude into the venous sinuses of the developing marrow cavities. The myeloid and erythroid hematopoietic cells that populate the logettes are derived not from HSCs but rather from later-committed progenitors.[65] Just after birth the HSCs are found in the marrow, and hematopoiesis is evident throughout the marrow cavity.

Adipose Tissue

By the fourth year of life, a significant number of fat cells have appeared in the diaphysis of the human long bones.[66] These cells slowly replace hematopoietic elements and expand centripetally until, at approximately 18 years of age, hematopoietic marrow is found only in the vertebrae, ribs, skull, pelvis, and proximal epiphyses of the femora and humeri. Direct measurements of the volume of bone cavities reveal increases from 1.4 percent of body weight at birth to 4.8 percent in the adult,[66] whereas blood volume decreases from 8 percent of body weight in the newborn to approximately 7 percent in the adult.[67] Expansion of marrow space continues throughout life, resulting in a further gradual increase in the amount of fatty tissue in all bone cavities, especially in the long bones.[68,69] Although the quantity of adipose tissue in the head and trochanteric parts of the femur varies in individuals, the fat content of this area of hematopoietic marrow progressively increases as adult humans age.[70] The preference of hematopoietic tissue for centrally located bones has been ascribed to higher central tissue temperature with greater vascularity.[71] In mice, an increased prevalence of adipose tissue in tail vertebrae as opposed to the more central thoracic vertebrae is associated with fewer HSCs and hematopoietic progenitors.[72] Genetic absence of adipose tissue or chemical inhibition of adipocyte generation was associated with improved posttransplant hematopoietic regeneration, suggesting that marrow adipocytes are negative regulators in the hematopoietic microenvironment.[72]

● MARROW STRUCTURE

VASCULATURE

The blood supply to the marrow comes from two major sources. The nutrient artery, the principal source, penetrates the cortex through the nutrient canal. In the marrow cavity, the nutrient artery bifurcates into ascending and descending central or medullary arteries from which radial branches travel to the inner face of the cortex. After repenetrating the endosteum, the radial vessels diminish in caliber to structures of capillary size that course within the canalicular system of the cortex. In the canalicular system, arterial blood from the nutrient artery mixes with blood that enters the cortical capillary system from the periosteal capillaries derived from muscular arteries.[73] After reentering the marrow cavity, the cortical capillaries form a sinusoidal network (Fig. 5–2). Hematopoietic cells are located in the intersinusoidal tissue spaces. Some arteries have specialized, thin-walled segments that arise abruptly as continuations of arteries with walls of normal thickness.[74] These vessels give off nearly perpendicular branches analogous to the arterial branching observed in the spleen and kidney, permitting volume compensation for changes in intramedullary pressure. In the marrow cavity, blood flows through a highly branching network of medullary sinuses. These sinuses collect into a large central sinus from which the blood enters the systemic venous circulation through emissary veins. Histomorphic studies of normal murine marrow demonstrate that all hematopoietic cells are within 18 μm or less than 3 cell diameters of a blood vessel.[75]

Vascular networks consisting of cells expressing CD31, CD34, and CD105 (endoglin) but lacking intercellular adhesion molecule (ICAM)-1, ICAM-2, ICAM-3, or endothelial leukocyte adhesion molecule (ELAM)-1 (E-selectin) can form within the stroma of long-term marrow cultures. These findings underscore the intimate relationship of

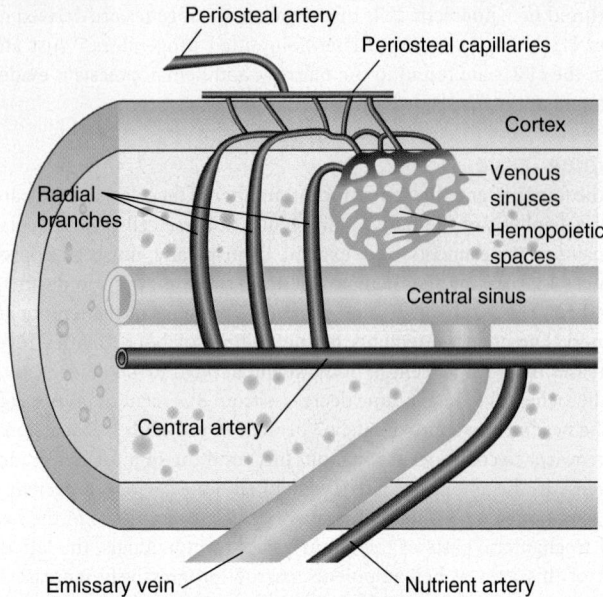

Figure 5–2. Schematic of the marrow circulation (see "Marrow Structure" for further explanation). *(Used with permission of Lichtman MA, University of Rochester.)*

blood vessels to hematopoietic activity.[76] A study of early hematopoiesis of human marrow from long bones (ages 6–28 weeks) has shown an absence of CD34+ hematopoietic progenitors before onset of hematopoiesis, a predominance of CD68+ cells mediating chondrolysis, and CD34+ endothelial cells developing into specific vascular structures organized by endothelial cells and myoid cells.[77] Vascular endothelial growth factor (VEGF) receptors found on CD34+ cells[16] and AGM primitive stem cells underscore the common ontogeny.[78] Subsets of CD34+ cells expressing the AC133 antigen and the human VEGF receptor-2 (KDR/FLK1) define the functional endothelial precursor phenotype.[79] Endothelial progenitors residing in the CD34+, CD11b+ subsets are capable of producing and binding angiopoietins,[80] and fibronectin (FN) enhances VEGF-induced CD34 cell differentiation into endothelial cells.[81] Growth and remodeling of bone, marrow space, and the vasculature that supplies them with nutrients and oxygen are closely linked by the relative hypoxia of the marrow and surrounding bone.[82] The transcription factors, hypoxia-inducible factor (HIF)-1α and -2α, are stabilized by hypoxia and increase *VEGF* expression in osteoblasts, and lead to regulated, coupled growth by endothelial cells and osteoblasts, both of which have VEGF receptors.[82] The expansion of erythropoiesis in response to erythropoietin (EPO) in mice is associated with a reciprocal decrease in the vasculature.[83]

INNERVATION

Myelinated and nonmyelinated nerve fibers are present in periarterial sheaths in the marrow,[84] where they are believed to regulate arterial vessel tone. Nerve terminals are distributed between layers of periarterial adventitial cells or localize next to arterial smooth muscle cells.[85] Nonmyelinated fibers terminate in the hematopoietic spaces, implying that neurohumors elaborated from free-nerve terminals affect hematopoiesis. Intimate cell–cell communication between sympathetic nerve cells and structural elements within the marrow sinuses occurs at less than 5 percent of nerve terminals that terminate within the hematopoietic parenchyma or on sinus walls. This anatomical unit, termed a *neuroreticular complex*, consists of efferent (autonomic) nerves and marrow stromal cells connected by gap junctions.[85] The marrow is

highly innervated along the arterioles and less frequently along capillaries, where neurologic control of blood flow and angiogenesis appear to be mediated via neurokinin A and substance P.[86]

SINUS ARCHITECTURE, NONHEMATOPOIETIC CELL ORGANIZATION AND NICHE FORMATION

In mammals, hematopoiesis occurs in the extravascular spaces between marrow sinuses. The marrow sinus wall is composed of a luminal layer of endothelial cells and an abluminal coat of adventitial reticular cells, which forms an incomplete outer lining (Fig. 5–3). A thin, interrupted basement lamina is present between the cell layers. Circulating HSCs move across the sinus endothelium into the extravascular space where they proliferate and differentiate into mature cells, which move across the sinus endothelium and circulate in the blood. Nonhematopoietic cells and extracellular matrix in the extravascular space form the marrow stroma. Stromal cells obtained from animal or human marrow can be studied in cultures,[87] are derived from fibroblasts, and have unique phenotypic and functional characteristics that allow them to nurture hematopoietic development in highly specialized microenvironmental niches.[88] However, newer studies with mutant mice and mice with specific cells that can be identified by direct fluorescence microscopy[89] have led to an understanding of the spatial orientation of the stroma and the localization of hematopoietic niches that they form in the marrow.

The hematopoietic niche concept was originally described for an operationally defined murine multipotential pluripotential progenitor (MPP) in the spleen,[90] but it has been extended to various marrow hematopoietic subpopulations, including physically demonstrated niches of HSCs,[91] lymphoid cells,[92,93] and erythroid cells.[93,94] The cellular components of these hematopoietic areas of the marrow include several types of nonhematopoietic cells including: (1) the sinus endothelial cells, (2) mesenchymal stem cells (MSCs) that form the skeletal elements of bone and marrow space such as chondrocytes, osteoblasts, osteocytes, fibroblasts, and adipocytes, and (3) terminally differentiated cells of hematopoietic origin such as macrophages, lymphocytes, and plasma cells. Experiments in both mice[61] and humans[95] have demonstrated by heterotopic bone formation that host marrow sinusoidal endothelial cells and hematopoietic cells will infiltrate and develop within microenvironment provided by a transplanted MSCs and its progeny. In mice, these MSCs are identified by a CD105+, Thy1−, 6C3− phenotype, which can support specific hematopoietic populations as their progeny develop Thy1 and 6C3 expression.[62] In humans, these MSCs are identified as CD45−, CD146+ adventitial reticular cells with fibroblast colony forming capacity that can interconvert between this MSC status and CD146− chondrocytes.[96]

Studies localizing marrow areas that support murine HSCs and their early progeny the hematopoietic progenitor cells (HPCs) have led to the concept of two niches for these hematopoietic cells: an endosteal niche that promotes HSC quiescence and a vascular/perivascular niche that is associated with self-replicating HSCs.[97] Studies combining vascular and endosteal imaging demonstrate that HSC/HPCs localized in the endosteal areas were also within a few cell diameters of VE cells.[75,98] The hypoxic status of HSC/HPCs, in terms of HIF expression, is unrelated to their proximity to blood vessels,[98] the flow rate of blood in the marrow vessels in the vicinity of HSCs appears to be very low,[99] and the lowest oxygen tension directly measured in the marrow is in the perivascular areas of microvessels.[100] These results suggest that the functional status of microvessels has a larger role in HSC niche activity than the proximity of the potential niche to its vascular supply.

Endothelial Cells

Endothelial cells are broad flat cells that completely cover the inner surface of the sinus.[101] They form a major barrier and control the system

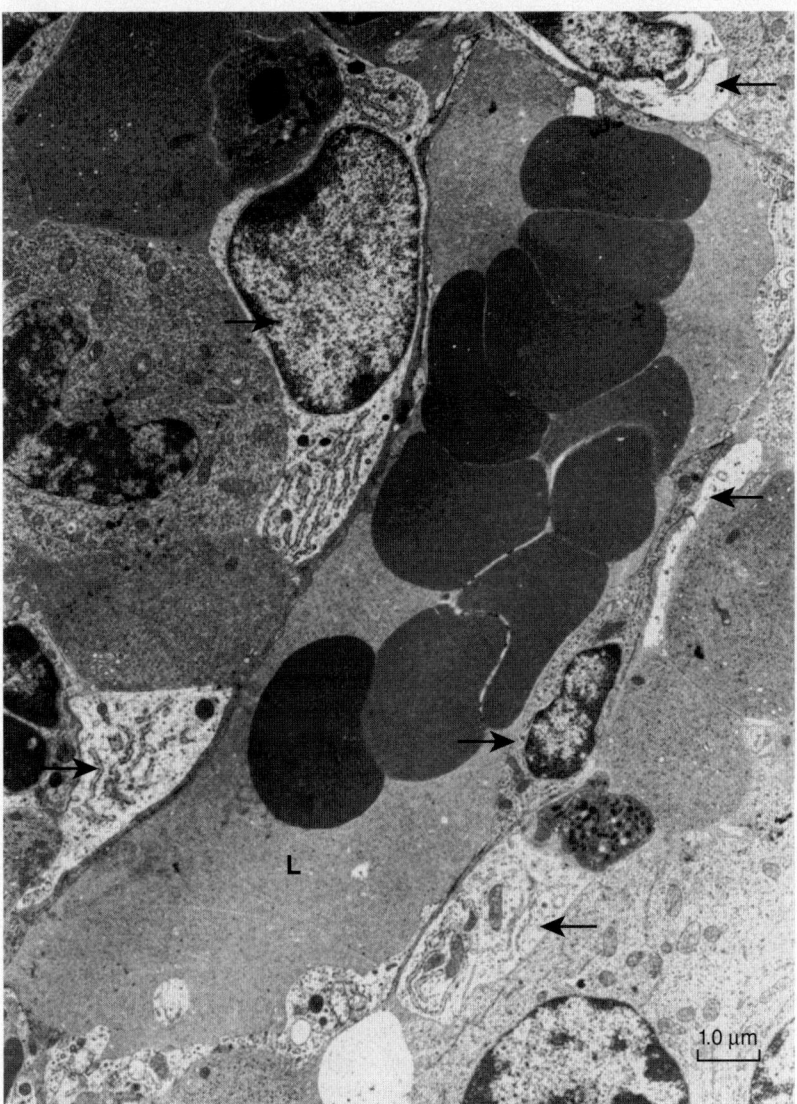

Figure 5–3. Transmission electron micrograph of a mouse marrow sinus. The *small arrow* in the sinus lumen (*L*) indicates the perikaryon of an endothelial cell. Several endothelial cell junctions are present along the circumference of the sinus endothelial wall. Thus, the wall is composed of the cytoplasm of endothelial cells that overlap or interdigitate. Two adventitial reticular cell bodies are identified by *arrows* at the top and upper left of the sinus. The cytoplasm of the adventitial reticular cells is discontinuous as it is followed around the sinus. Three cytoplasmic processes of adventitial reticular cells are indicated by *arrows*. Other, smaller processes of reticular cell cytoplasm are found upon close inspection of the sinus periphery and the hematopoietic spaces. The scattered rough endoplasmic reticulum and dense bodies are characteristic of the reticular cell cytoplasm. *(Reproduced with permission from Lichtman MA: The ultrastructure of the hemopoietic environment of the marrow: A review. Exp Hematol 9:391, 1981.)*

for chemicals and particles entering and leaving the hematopoietic spaces, with overlapping or interdigitating unions permitting volume expansion.[102] The endothelium of marrow sinusoids is actively endocytic and contains clathrin-coated pits, clathrin-coated vesicles, lysosomes, phagosomes, transfer tubules, and diaphragmed fenestrae.[103,104] Marrow endothelial cells express von Willebrand factor protein,[105] type IV collagen, and laminin.[106] They also constitutively express adhesion molecules: ICAM-3,[107] vascular cell adhesion molecule (VCAM)-1, and E-selectin,[108] all of which regulate HSC proliferation.[109] The distribution of sialic acid and other carbohydrates on the luminal surface of marrow sinus endothelium is discontinued at diaphragmed fenestrae and coated pits, suggesting such glycosylation plays a role in endothelial membrane function and cellular interactions.[110] *In vivo*, the conditional deletion in endothelial cells of gp130, the common receptor component for several cytokines, including IL-6, leads to a hypocellular marrow as mice age.[111] The loss of gp130 from marrow endothelial cells affects the progenitor cell populations rather than the HSC leading to a lethal anemia, a leukocytosis, but normal platelets.[108]

Marrow endothelial cells via direct cell–cell contacts and secreted peptides uniquely influence osteoprogenitor cell differentiation[112] and regulate hematopoiesis.[113] Marrow microvascular endothelium has major roles in osteogenesis through its physiologic production of the VEGF164 isoform as well as multiple cytokines that are usually associated with inflammation.[114] Other marrow endothelial cell cytokines that affect hematopoiesis include SCF,[115] angiopoietin-like protein 3,[116] IL-5,[117] thymosin β_4, AcSDKP,[118] and B-type natriuretic peptide.[119] Endothelial cells also regulate cellular trafficking into and out of the marrow sinusoidal spaces by altering their permeability and reorganizing their cytoskeleton by ICAM-3, by VE-cadherin–mediated cell–cell contacts,[107,120] and via specialized heparin sulfate proteoglycans,[121] CXCL12 bound to surface proteoglycans,[122] and other chemokines/chemokine receptors,[123,124] such as fractalkine, a membrane-bound chemokine with a mucin stalk expressed in activated vascular beds.[125] Marrow sinusoidal endothelium specifically expresses hyaluron and sialylated CD22 ligands, which are homing receptors for recirculating HSCs[75] and B lymphocytes,[126] respectively.

Adventitial Reticular Cells

The abluminal or adventitial surface of the vascular sinus is composed of reticular cells.[101,127,128] The reticular cell bodies are contiguous with the sinus, forming part of its adventitial coat (see Fig. 5–3). Their extensive branching cytoplasmic processes envelop the outer wall of the sinus to form an adventitial sheath. The sheath is interrupted and is estimated to cover approximately two-thirds of the abluminal surface area of sinuses.

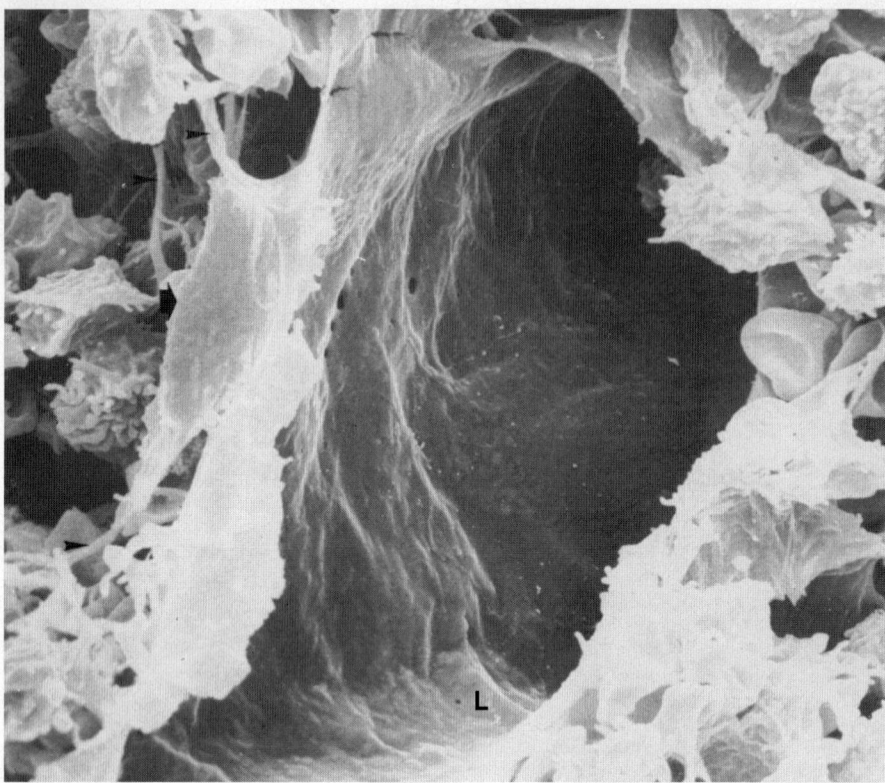

Figure 5–4. Scanning electron micrograph of rat marrow sinus. The floor of the lumen (*L*) is indicated. The *arrow on the left* indicates the cell body of an adventitial reticular cell, which is just beneath the endothelial cell layer. Reticular cell processes can be seen coursing between the sinus wall and the hematopoietic compartment *(small arrows).(Reproduced with permission from Lichtman MA: The ultrastructure of the hemopoietic environment of the marrow: A review.* Exp Hematol *9:391, 1981.)*

The reticular cells synthesize reticular (argentophilic) fibers that, with their cytoplasmic processes, extend into the hematopoietic compartments and form a meshwork on which hematopoietic cells rest (Figs. 5–4 and 5–5). The cell bodies, their broad processes, and their fibers constitute the reticulum of the marrow.

Adventitial reticular cells can differentiate along the smooth muscle pathway and contain α smooth-muscle actin, vimentin, laminin, FN, and collagens I, III, and IV.[129,130] More specialized contractile reticular "barrier cells" have been described in mouse marrow after hematopoietic stress.[131] Barrier cells increase in number and seem to enclose small

vessels and extend the venous sinuses so that release of precursors is restrained while accommodating an increased entry of mature cells into the circulation.[131]

Studies in both mice and humans have identified subsets of adventitial reticular cells as MSCs with adipocytic-osteogenic potential that in mice appear to have significant overlap: (1) CXCL12–abundant reticular (CAR) cells,[132] (2) adventitial reticular cells expressing the intermediate filament protein Nestin and displaying the surface proteins platelet-derived growth factor (PDGF) receptor-α and CD51 (Nestin+, PDGFRα+, CD51+),[133] and (3) adventitial reticular cells

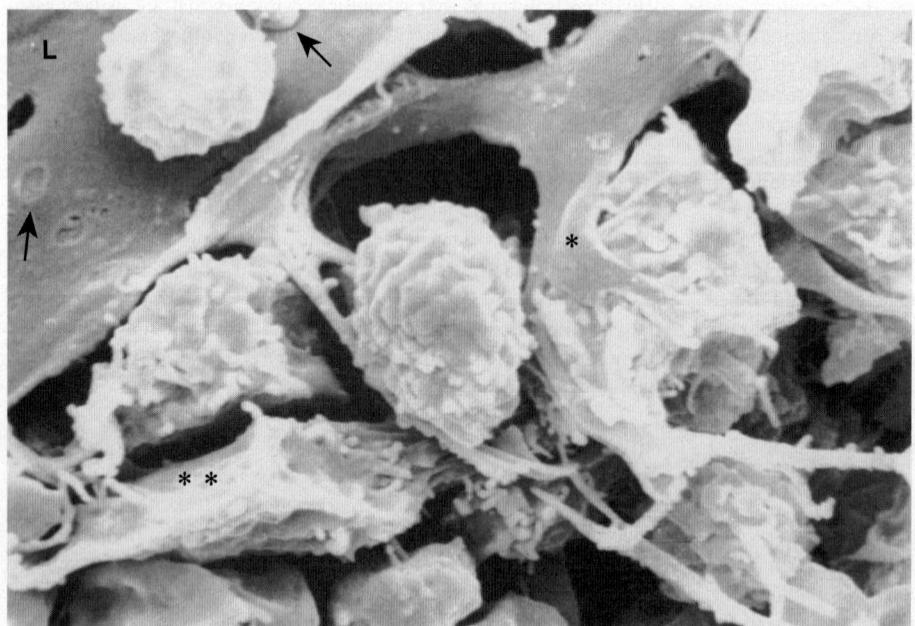

Figure 5–5. Scanning electron micrograph of rat femoral marrow sinus. The lumen (*L*) of an exposed sinus that has been cut open is indicated. The *single asterisk* indicates the process of an adventitial reticular cell and the intimate contact it makes with a hematopoietic cell. To the left of this process are adventitial reticular cell fibers, which form a scaffold for hematopoietic cells. The *double asterisk* identifies a portion of a reticular cell. The hole in the sinus floor is an artifact of preparation or a migration channel bereft of the emigrating cell. Empty spaces between cells and fibers are artifacts of preparation. The *arrow to the left* points to thin-walled fenestrae in the endothelial cytoplasm. The *arrow to the right* identifies the portion of a reticulocyte that may be penetrating the sinus wall, early in egress (see Fig. 5–8A). (*Used Lichtman MA, University of Rochester.*)

expressing leptin receptors.[115,134] The human equivalents are a population of CD45−, CD146+ adventitial reticular cells that have smaller subsets that express Nestin, PDGFRα, and CD51.[133] A major proportion of these subsets are restricted to the perivascular area, but have some cells scattered throughout the hematopoietic marrow. However, because these adventitial reticular subsets are also the major sources of CXCL12 and SCF in the marrow, they have important roles in establishing the HSC niche near the marrow microvasculature while their progeny establish the endosteum and its associated hematopoietic niche in the marrow.

The majority of CAR cells are in close association with the sinusoidal endothelial cells but some are also associated with the endosteum. Like the Nestin+ MSCs, CAR cells appear to be progenitors of osteoblasts and adipocytes while producing major amounts of CXCL12 and SCF.[135] Development of CAR cells and their production of CXCL12 and SCF is associated with the expression of the transcription factor Fox1c.[136] CAR cells and the niches that they create in the marrow are required for the normal development of HSC, various differentiation stages of B-lymphocytes, natural killer cells, and the plasmacytoid dendritic cells that are all found in close physical association with CAR cells.[137]

Autonomic neurons innervate the perivascular Nestin+, PDG-FRα+, CD51+ adventitial reticular cells which maintain the HSC niche by several surface-displayed and/or secreted products including IL-7 and VCAM-1, in addition to SCF and CXCL12.[138] β-Adrenergic neurotransmission inhibits the expression of these proteins so that mice with specific denervation have decreased marrow cellularity and increased circulating hematopoietic progenitors.[139] The sympathetic nervous system controls circadian fluctuations in circulating HSC numbers though its effect on MSC expression of the chemokine CXCL12 in the marrow.[140] Studies in mice with defective myelinization and mice treated with adrenergic antagonists or agonists indicate that the adrenergic nervous system in the marrow also regulates mobilization of HSCs by granulocyte colony-stimulating factor (G-CSF).[141] However, the non-myelinating Schwann cells associated with the autonomic nerves of the marrow secrete transforming growth factor-β (TGF-β) and thereby maintain the HSC quiescence.[142]

Adipocytes

Adipocytes in the marrow develop by lipogenesis in fibroblast-like cells (Fig. 5–6). Reticular cells in mouse and human marrow can undergo transformation to fat cells *in vitro* and can revert into fibroblasts in culture by lipolysis,[101,143] and the Nestin+ MSCs[138] and CAR MSCs can differentiate into adipocytes. A reciprocal relationship between adipocyte and osteoblast differentiation of MSCs appears to be controlled by multiple transcription factors, with both peroxisome proliferator-activated receptor-γ2 (PPARγ2)[144] and CCAAT/enhancer binding protein (C/EBP)[145] promoting adipocyte differentiation. Marrow fat cells are relatively resistant to lipolysis during starvation, and their phenotype is consistent with both white and brown fat.[146,147] Although the proportion of saturated fatty acids is lower than in other fat deposits, marrow fat composition depends on whether it is located in the red, hematopoietically active, or the yellow, hematopoietically inactive, marrow. Human marrow adipocytes support the differentiation of late-stage, committed, myeloid and lymphoid hematopoietic cells, but they are unable to support earlier progenitor stages.[148] Quantification of immature hematopoietic cells including HSCs shows reduced numbers in human marrows with increased fat,[70] and in vivo studies in mice confirm that marrow adipocytes create a negative hematopoietic microenvironment that reduces development of HSCs and early-stage common hematopoietic progenitors.[72]

Bone Cells

Osteoblasts, osteoclasts, and elongated flat cells with a spindle-shaped nucleus form the marrow endosteal lining.[149] These endosteal cells and the closely associated microvascular cells participate in a dynamic process in which endochondral bone formation proceeds with removal of calcified cartilage and connective tissues by macrophages while new bone is formed by osteoblasts and remodeled by specialized osteoclasts.[114,150] Osteoblasts that become embedded in the bone matrix proteins are termed *osteocytes*, a terminally differentiated cell that has secretory capacity and influences the activities of osteoblasts, osteoclasts, and hematopoietic cells. Resting endosteal cells express vimentin, tenascin, α smooth-muscle actin, osteocalcin, CD51, and CD56. They

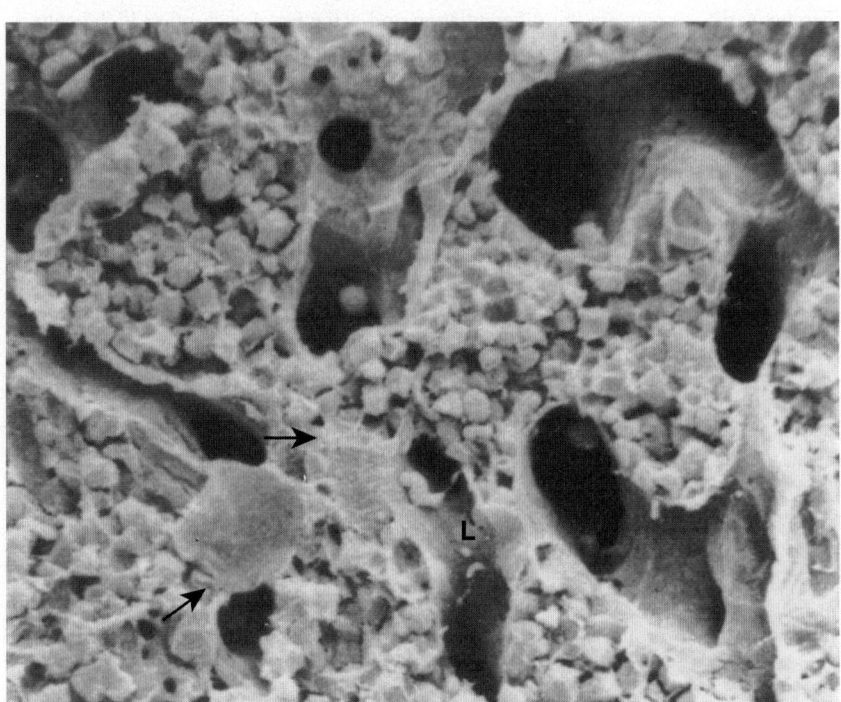

Figure 5–6. Scanning electron micrograph of rat femoral marrow. Several sinuses and the intervening hematopoietic cords are evident. The exposed lumen (*L*) of one branching sinus is indicated. The sinus, just above the *L*, contains a bean-shaped proplatelet with an attenuated strand connected to a separating smaller proplatelet fragment. Smaller proplatelet fragments are below the *L*. The *short horizontal arrow* points to the cytoplasm of a transected megakaryocyte. The *lower arrow* points to a fat cell. The rat femoral marrow contains a modest number of fat cells. Spaces in the hematopoietic cords are artifacts resulting from transecting the femur. *(Reproduced with permission from Lichtman MA: The ultrastructure of the hemopoietic environment of the marrow: A review.* Exp Hematol 9:391, 1981.)

do not react with antibodies to CD3, CD15, CD20, CD34, CD45, CD68, or CD117.[151] Enriched CD56+, CD45−, CD34− endosteal cells grown in the presence of cytokines (insulin growth factor I, basic fibroblast growth factor [bFGF], SCF, IL-3, granulocyte-macrophage colony-stimulating factor [GM-CSF]) do not give rise to hematopoietic cells, which suggests they are not totipotent MSCs.[151] In the next sections, the two major types of cells responsible for endosteal activity, osteoblasts and osteoclasts, are considered in terms of their potential roles in maintaining the hematopoietic niche.

Osteoblasts

Osteoblasts have three major functions: formation of new bone by regulating the secretion of the bone matrix proteins, regulation of bone resorption via osteoclast activity, and regulation of the hematopoietic environment mainly by secretion of cytokines. Bone-forming osteoblast progenitor cells, like stromal precursors, reside in the CD34−, STRO-1+ nonadherent marrow cell population.[152,153] The differentiation of mesenchymal cells into either osteoblasts or adipocytes is related to the relative activities of Runx2 and PPARγ, respectively.[154] With aging, the sensitivity to PPARγ appears to increase, contributing to the increase in adipose tissue in the marrow found with older age.[154] BMP2,[155] bFGF,[156] hepatocyte growth factor (HGF),[157] parathyroid hormone[12] and endothelin-1[158] promote osteoblast growth, whereas the cytokine TGF-β[159] and the transcription factor osterix[160] promote differentiation. Osteoblasts increase early hematopoietic progenitor survival in long-term cultures and secrete hematopoietic growth factors such as M-CSF, G-CSF, GM-CSF, IL-1, and IL-6.[161,162] Osteoblasts also produce various cytokines such as hematopoietic cell-cycle inhibitory factors TGF-β,[163] osteopontin,[164] and CXCL12,[12] as well as cell-cycle stimulatory factor Dickkopf-1,[165] all of which contribute to stem cell regulation within the marrow microenvironment. Direct cell–cell communication has been shown in the marrow and in osteoblastic cell networks,[166] indicating a potential regulatory role for anatomical gap junctions in hematopoiesis.[167,168] The size of stem cell niches increases after osteoblastic expansion and Notch activation in transgenic models.[11,12] In another model, intramedullary hematopoiesis and stem cell numbers are severely diminished following *in vivo* ablation of osteoblasts,[169] underscoring the importance of this cell type to the marrow hematopoietic inductive microenvironment. The lymphoid niches for early lymphoid progenitors and differentiating B cells are located adjacent to the endosteal surface.[92,93] Osteocytes, which are terminally differentiated osteoblasts trapped in the bony matrix, secrete cytokines into the marrow space that act in a negative feedback manner on new bone formation. Specifically, the osteoblast and stromal cell surface protein receptor activator of nuclear factor-κB ligand (RANKL) activates osteoclasts,[170] while the cytokine sclerostin suppresses osteoblast activity.[171] Disruption of the signaling mechanism of G-protein receptors in osteocytes leads to an expansion of myelopoiesis that is mediated by secreted myelopoietic cytokines, most likely G-CSF.[172]

Osteoclasts

Mature osteoclasts are multinucleated giant cells derived from fusion of progenitor cells of the monocyte/macrophage lineage of the HSC.[173] The mature osteoclasts resorb and remodel bone, regulate osteoblast activity, and help control the HSC entry into and exit from the marrow.[174,175] The osteoclasts have motile and resorptive phases. They require the Wiskott-Aldrich syndrome protein during clustering and fusion of actin-based adhesion structures named *podosomes*.[176] Podosomes are involved in the formation of specific structures termed *sealing zones* in which actin rings surround an area of ruffled plasma membrane at the face of the endosteal bone. Within these sealing zones, osteoclasts secrete hydrochloric acid and digestive enzymes that resorb bone.

Osteoclasts also can be derived from pro-B cells, as shown by Pax-5 knockout mice, which have increased osteoclasts and severe osteopenia.[177] When osteoclast activity or number are reduced or eliminated in mice through null mutations or homologous recombination, the marrow cavities fail to form resulting in osteopetrosis. Based on studies of osteopetrotic mice, proteins required for osteoclast differentiation include the macrophage transcription factor PU.1; the secreted and surface displayed cytokine M-CSF of stromal cells and its receptor c-FMS on osteoclasts; the transcription factor c-FOS; the cytokine RANKL; its osteoclast receptor RANK, the signaling transducer tumor necrosis factor-α (TNF-α) receptor-associated factor 6 (TRAF 6); the downstream transcription factor nuclear factor (NF)-κB, and nuclear factor of activated T cells (NFAT).[175,178,179] Other osteopetrotic mice strains have deficiency of proteins required for the bone resorption function of osteoclasts. These proteins include the β_3 component of the $\alpha_v\beta_3$ integrin (vitronectin receptor) required for binding of the osteoclast sealing zone to bone; c-Src signaling protein; the proton transporting H+ adenosine triphosphatase (ATPase) and chloride channel protein required for HCl secretion; and the secreted osteoclast proteins cathepsin K, matrix metalloproteinases, and TRAP that digest the bone matrix.[174,175,179]

Osteoblast/stromal cells regulate differentiation of osteoclasts through intimate cell–cell contacts. They are found in direct apposition to osteoclasts with coated pit formation, suggesting accumulation of receptor–ligand complexes in endocytic vesicles.[180,181] The recruitment of the osteoblasts and osteoclasts appears to be through capillaries associated with the remodeling compartment.[182] A major regulatory mechanism by which osteoblasts and osteoclasts interact is the RANK/RANKL/osteoprotegerin (OPG) system of signaling.[182] Osteoclast differentiation and maturation require the signaling cascade from RANK on the cell surface through TRAF 6, NF-κB, and NFAT.[180] Osteoblasts and their progenitor cells display RANKL on their surfaces, and binding of RANKL to the RANK on the osteoclasts and their progenitors promotes differentiation and activation of the osteoclasts. Osteoblasts also secrete OPG, a decoy receptor for RANKL, which inactivates RANKL by binding to the active site of RANKL, thereby preventing its binding to RANK. As a result, osteoclastic activity is decreased when OPG concentrations are high and increased when they are low.[183] Another signaling mechanism by which osteoclasts and osteoblasts reciprocally regulate the differentiation and activities of each other is the ephrin-B2-EphB4 signaling system.[184] Osteoclasts express ephrinB2 on their surfaces while the osteoblasts express EphB4, a member of the receptor tyrosine kinase (RTK) family, which is the receptor for ephrinB2. Binding of ephrinB2-EphB4 results in bidirectional signaling in which osteoclast differentiation is decreased though suppression of the c-FOS–NFATc1 activity, whereas osteoblast differentiation is increased by EphB4 signaling.[184]

Osteoclasts produce HGF and express c-Met, the HGF receptor, implying a paracrine and autocrine regulatory pathway between them and adjoining osteoblasts.[157,185] Similarly, blocking expression of cadherin-6 interferes with heterotypic interactions between osteoclasts and stromal cells, impairing their ability to support osteoclast formation.[186] CD9, a tetraspanin transmembrane adhesion protein on stromal cells,[187] influences myelopoiesis in long-term marrow cultures.[188] Inhibition of stromal cell CD9-mediated signaling by a blocking antibody reduces osteoclast differentiation factor transcription, leading to reduced osteoclastogenesis.[189] Macrophage-stimulating protein, a HGF-like protein, signals through the stem cell-derived tyrosine kinase, a member of the HGF receptor family. It also stimulates osteoclast bone-resorbing activity by enhanced cytoskeletal reorganization without affecting proliferation of osteoclast precursors.[190,191] Osteoclast differentiation is influenced by monocytes expressing ADAM-8 (CD156), a protein of the disintegrin and metalloproteinase family,[192] and eosinophil chemotactic factor-L (ECFL),[193] characterizing complex cell–cell, cell adhesion protein, stromal cell cytokine, and chemokine signals within the marrow microenvironment.

LYMPHOCYTES

Lymphocytes, including T, natural killer (NK), B, and plasma cells, and macrophages, including monocyte-derived, antigen-presenting dendritic cells, arise from the HSCs and undergo part of their differentiation in the marrow. They then circulate and, in the case of the lymphoid cells, reside and further differentiate in other organs such as the thymus, spleen or lymph nodes, before returning to the marrow, where they terminally differentiate and form part of the marrow microenvironment by producing growth factors (IL-3, CCL3) and participating in cell–cell interactions with developing progenitors.[84,101,194] Monocytic/macrophage progenitor cells can enter the circulation and later enter many different tissues where they differentiate into macrophages. In the marrow, the monocytic/macrophage progenitors can differentiate into macrophages or fuse and become osteoclasts. Lymphocytes and macrophages concentrate around arterial vessels, near the center of the hematopoietic cords. B cells also cluster near the osteal surface.[92,93] Mature B and T lymphocytes in the marrow are in contact with a specific set of monocyte-derived, antigen-presenting dendritic cells that are clustered around the blood vessels.[195]

Lymphocytic differentiation begins as HSCs that have committed to differentiation as multipotent HPCs (MPPs) lose their potential to become megakaryocytic-erythroid progenitors (MEPs) and granulocyte-macrophage (GM) progenitors; this change in differentiation potential is detectable as the upregulation of lymphoid-specific transcripts, that is, they are lymphoid-primed multipotent progenitors (LMPPs). The commitment of LMPPs to lymphoid differentiation in these early-stage HPCs is reinforced by progressive expression of FMS-like tyrosine kinase 3 (Flt-3), IL-7 receptors (IL-7R), and recombination activating genes-1/2 (Rag-1/2) proteins.[196,197] These early lymphoid progenitors (ELPs) require a microenvironment provided by MSCs and their osteogenic progeny which supplies VCAM-1, CXCL12, Flt-3 ligand, and IL-7.[198,199] The ELPs enter the blood with transit to the thymus where they undergo differentiation into T cells. In addition, to its role as site of early T-lymphocyte development, the marrow acts a secondary organ for the proliferation of mature CD8 and CD4 memory T lymphocytes. Although no specific organized structure or niche has been found for these T lymphocytes, they can represent up to 4 percent of nucleated cells in the marrow that they reenter by migrating through the sinusoidal endothelium from the blood.[200] Alternatively, LMPPs can remain in the marrow and differentiate into common lymphocyte progenitors (CLPs) that give rise to NK progenitor cells, which differentiate in the marrow, or prepro-B cells that mature to the pro-B cells, which migrate from the marrow to the lymph nodes or spleen where they differentiate further.[196,197]

Marrow stromal cells facilitate the maturation of NK cells,[201] an effect likely mediated by stromal-derived Flt-3 ligand and IL-15.[202] Within the marrow, both NK cells and CD8+ memory T cells require the coordinated expression of secreted IL-15 and surface IL-15 receptors by other marrow cells for their survival and development.[203] The marrow MSCs and their osteogenic progeny also create a microenvironment for proliferation and differentiation of ELPs through the later sequential lymphoid stages of CLPs, prepro-B cells, pro-B cells, and pre-B cells via the provision of osterix and galectin-1.[198]

The differentiation stages subsequent to the pro-B cells occur after the cells enter the blood and seed the lymphoid follicles of the secondary lymphoid organs, mainly spleen and lymph nodes. From these lymphoid organs, the cells reenter the blood as B lymphocytes or immature plasma cells. The immature plasma cells that have differentiated in the spleen and will become the long-lived plasma cells return home to the marrow, where they are located in contact with CXCL12-producing stromal cells. A negative feedback is completed as the mature plasma cells either compete with the prepro-B cells for sites on the CXCL12-producing stromal cells or directly induce apoptosis of the prepro-B cells.[204] Marrow blood vessel-associated dendritic cells produce macrophage migration-inhibition factor, a cytokine required for survival of mature B lymphocytes that have matured in secondary lymphoid organs and recirculated to the marrow.[195]

MACROPHAGES

Hematopoietic progenitors restricted to monocyte/macrophage differentiation are characterized by expression of M-CSF receptors (FMS), membrane-activating complex-1 (CD11b), and F4/80 antigen, and give rise to monocytes that enter the blood.[205] These nondividing monocytes can then enter various organs, including a subset with high Ly6C that reenter the marrow where they become macrophages and antigen-presenting dendritic cells.[205,206] Although they are both descendants of similar M-CSF–dependent monocytic progenitors, macrophages differ from osteoclasts by their single nucleus and, in mice, expression of F4/80 antigen as well as lack of TRAP and calcitonin receptors.[206] Marrow macrophage phenotype[207] is regulated by adjoining stromal cell–accessory cell–derived colony-stimulating factors and cytokines,[208] such as M-CSF–induced upregulation of $\alpha_4\beta_1$- and $\alpha_5\beta_1$-integrin expression[209] and Flt-3 ligand-promoting macrophage outgrowth with B-cell-associated antigens.[210] Macrophages are an integral component of the local microenvironment and regulate hematopoiesis via a complex array of dual-acting stem cell stimulatory and inhibitory factors, such as IL-1, CCL3, TNF-α, and TGF-β.[211-213] Macrophages respond to PDGF by upregulating IL-1 secretion and thereby activating primitive hematopoietic cells.[214] Macrophages also modulate the structure and composition of the extracellular matrix (ECM) and its FN content.[215]

Specialized macrophages termed *osteomacs* form a canopy over the active osteoblasts and osteoclasts on the endosteal surface, where the macrophages coordinate the bone-forming activity of osteoblasts and bone-resorbing activity of osteoclasts.[206] Another subset of macrophages, which are identified by CD169 (sialoadhesin/Siglec-1 [sialic acid-binding immunoglobulin-like lectin-1]), act to retain in the marrow those HSCs and early progenitor cells that are capable of circulation in the blood.[216] CD169-expressing macrophages also comprise the central macrophages of erythroblastic islands that interact directly with erythroid cells,[217] enhancing their proliferation and differentiation. Similarly, mature B and T lymphocytes in the marrow are supported in the specific microenvironment provided by monocyte-derived, antigen-presenting dendritic cells that are clustered around the blood vessels.[195]

EXTRACELLULAR MATRIX

Mesenchymal cells forming the cellular stroma in the marrow create a network of ECM proteins, such as proteoglycans or glycosaminoglycans (GAGs), FN, tenascin, collagen, laminin, and thrombospondin (TSP).[218-221] Localizing signals are provided by stromal–ECM and hematopoietic cell adhesive interactions[222,223] in concert with chemokines[224] and cytokines bound to heparin-like structures in the GAGs.[225] The binding of specific cytokines may enhance the activity of a cytokine if the GAG-binding site does not interfere with the site that binds the cytokine receptor, whereas GAG-binding sites that overlap or interfere with a cytokine receptor-binding site can inhibit the cytokine function.[225] Table 5–1 lists the cytokines that are presented on the surface of stromal cells and matrix-binding chemokines and cytokines.[225-238]

TABLE 5–1. Cell Membrane Presentation and Matrix Association of Cytokines and Chemokines

Cell Membrane	Matrix Association
Chemokine	*Chemokine*
Fractalkine	RANTES, PF-4, IP-10, IL-8
	Macrophage inflammatory proteins (MIP-1α, MIP-1β)
	CXCL12/stromal cell-derived growth factor-1 (SDF-1α, SDF-1β)
	Monocyte chemoattractant protein-1 (MCP-1)
Cytokine	*Cytokine*
c-KIT ligand	Granulocyte-macrophage colony-stimulating factor
Tumor necrosis factor-α (TNF-α)	Interferon-γ (IFN-γ)
Interleukin-1 (IL-1)	Leukemia inhibitory factor (LIF)
Macrophage colony-stimulating factor (M-CSF)	Interleukins (IL-1α, IL-1β, IL-2, IL-3, IL-4, IL-5, IL-6, IL-7, IL-12)
	Basic fibroblast growth factor (bFGF)
Transforming growth factor-α (TGF-α)	Hepatocyte growth factor (HGF)
	Transforming growth factor-β (TGF-β; binding to endoglin and heparan sulfate)

IP-10, interferon-inducible protein 10; PF-4, platelet factor 4; RANTES, regulated upon activation normal T-cell expressed and secreted.

In addition to its supply of hematopoietic growth factors, the ECM provides noncellular binding partners for surface adhesion molecules of the hematopoietic and mesenchymal cells. The marrow microelasticity, which is a function of cellular density and ECM composition, varies more than 100-fold from the soft central areas to the much stiffer endosteal areas.[239] This microelasticity determines the differentiation of MSCs,[240] and the fate of HSCs and committed hematopoietic cells.[241] In HSCs and HPCs, the activities of two nonmuscle myosin isozymes are regulated in response to the elasticity of the ECM. The increased relative activity of nonmuscle myosin II B that mediates asymmetric cell division and self-renewal is greatest in the stiffer ECM of endosteal areas, whereas increased relative activity of non-muscle myosin IIA in the areas of softer ECM mediates symmetric cell division and differentiation.[239]

Proteoglycans

Proteoglycans are polyanionic macromolecules (heparan sulfate, dermatan, chondroitin sulfate, hyaluronic acid) that are distributed on the surface of adventitial reticular cells and within the ECM.[218,242] Heparan sulfate is the main cell-surface GAG in long-term marrow cultures, and chondroitin sulfate is the major secreted species.[243] D-xylosides, which stimulate artificial sulfated GAG synthesis, increase chondroitin sulfate synthesis and hematopoietic cell production.[243] Hyaluronic acid and chondroitin sulfate-containing proteoglycans are prominent in the adherent and nonadherent compartments of long-term marrow cultures.[242] Heparin-containing and heparan sulfate-containing proteoglycans interact with laminin and type IV collagen[244] and may play a role in cell–cell interactions, cytokine presentation, and cell

differentiation.[245-247] They also mediate progenitor cell binding to other ECM molecules such as FN.[248–250]

Agrin, a proteoglycan associated with neuromuscular junctions, is produced in the marrow by MSCs, osteoblasts and monocytes, and interacts through α-dystroglycan receptors on HSCs[251] and their progeny as they differentiate along the monocyte/macrophage lineage.[252] Agrin-deficient mice have hypocellular marrows as a result of decrease in all marrow hematopoietic cell lineages[251] as well as specific inhibition of numbers and phagocytic function of monocytes and macrophages.[252] An important hematopoietic cell proteoglycan, CD44, has hyaluronate as a major matrix ligand. The CD44–hyaluronate interaction is greatly enhanced by various cytokines, and it promotes other matrix and cellular interactions by hematopoietic cells.[253] Cytokines (GM-CSF, IL-3, SCF) rapidly induce CD44 expression and increase CD44-mediated adhesion of CD34+ hematopoietic progenitors to hyaluronan.[254] Lymphocyte CD44 has a binding site on the carboxy-terminal heparin-binding domain of FN,[255] and neutralizing antibodies to CD44 inhibit hematopoiesis in long-term marrow cultures.[256] Chondroitin sulfates A and B mediate monocyte and B-cell activation via a CD44-dependent pathway.[257] Hyaluronate binding enhances hematopoiesis by releasing IL-1 in a CD44-dependent manner and IL-6 by a CD44-independent pathway.[258] In humans, a specific CD44 isoform displayed on hematopoietic cells is a ligand for E- and L-selectins and plays a role in HSC homing and integrin-mediated transendothelial migration in the marrow.[259]

Heparan sulfate mediates IL-7–dependent lymphopoiesis[235] and modulates hematopoiesis and stromal cell–matrix remodeling[260] by anchoring HGF[236,261] and bFGF.[260,262,263] On the surface of marrow stromal cells, the main heparan sulfate-containing proteoglycans are syndecan-3, syndecan-4, and glypican-1. In the ECM, the most prevalent form is perlecan.[264] Syndecan-3 is expressed by marrow stromal cells as a variant form with a core protein of 50 to 55 kDa, suggesting syndecan-3 plays a role in hematopoiesis.[264] Perlecan promotes bFGF receptor binding and mitogenesis, and can bind GM-CSF.[257,265] Heparan sulfate expression is induced on the cell surface in early erythroid differentiation of multipotential HSC.[266] Glypican-4, another member of this family, is found on marrow stromal cells and progenitor cells.[267] Syndecan-1 expression in B lymphoid cells is reduced by IL-6, which implies similar regulatory pathways in other cell types.[268] Biglycan, a matrix glycoprotein, with homology to osteonectin, and the molecule SIM, a transmembrane protein, selectively increase IL-7–dependent proliferation of B cells.[269] Interactions of B cells with other components of the immune system are mediated by syndecan-4, which facilitates the formation of dendritic processes[270] and regulates focal adhesion, stress fiber formation, and cell migration.[271]

Fibronectin

FN localizes at sites of attachment of hematopoietic cells and marrow stromal cells *in vitro*[219,272] and at sites of interaction between these cells and developing granulocytes or monocytes.[273] Early erythroid progenitors bind FN through their integrin receptors $\alpha_5\beta_1$ and $\alpha_4\beta_1$.[274,275] Adhesion of HPCs to stroma is partly mediated by FN.[248,276] The alternatively spliced form of FN (type III connecting segment [IIICS]), which is expressed uniquely within the marrow microenvironment, associates with the $\alpha_4\beta_1$-integrin receptor on HSC.[277] Additional IIICS FN variants have been detected in marrow stroma, providing for finely controlled progenitor–stem cell interactions based on messenger RNA splicing.[278] FN adhesion to peptide domains, such as the CS1 domain (which activates α_4 integrins) or stromal cells, can have dual effects of stimulation and inhibition of hematopoietic progenitor growth.[279-282]

The very-late antigens (VLA)-4 and VLA-5 ($\alpha_4\beta_1$ and $\alpha_5\beta_1$) and CD44 cooperate to promote FN adhesive interactions.[279,282-284] Cytokines such as IL-3, SCF, and thrombopoietin (TPO) augment the magnitude of FN-mediated HPC adhesion and migration.[285-288] Functional effects of FN within the marrow ECM include decreased erythroblast FN adhesion as differentiation progresses[274,283] with modulation of erythroid cell differentiation dependent upon competing binding of $\alpha_4\beta_1$ integrin with FN in the ECM and with central macrophages in erythroblastic islands.[289] Binding of collagen I in the marrow ECM by megakaryocytes leads to their spreading and inhibition of proplatelet formation by a mechanism involving FN induction and secretion with polymerization via cosecreted factor XIII-A.[290] FN is required for expression of gelatinase in macrophages[291] and regulates cytokine release by M-CSF–activated macrophages[292] and chondrocytes.[293]

Tenascin

The fibrillar glycoprotein tenascin-C is found in the microenvironment surrounding maturing hematopoietic cells.[218,294] Tenascin-C has distinct functional domains that promote hematopoietic cell adhesion to ECM proteins or mediate a strong mitogenic signal to marrow mononuclear cells.[295] Although tenascin-C–deficient mutant mice appear to have normal steady-state hematopoiesis, colony-forming capacity of marrow is markedly decreased,[296] marrow regeneration capacity after cytoreductive agents is decreased,[297] and retention of T-lymphocyte progenitors is impaired.[297] This last effect is mediated through the $\alpha_9\beta_1$ integrin on T-lymphocytes progenitors, but effects on HSCs and early hematopoietic progenitors is mediated by a different mechanism.[297] Mutant tenascin-C–deficient animals also display decreased FN in their marrow, suggesting a possible mechanistic interaction between tenascin-C and FN in the marrow microenvironment.[298]

Collagen

Collagen types I and III are associated with microvascular walls, whereas collagen type IV is confined to basal lamina beneath endothelial cells.[160,299] Marrow-derived capillary networks grow in collagen gel cultures,[300] inhibition of collagen synthesis reduces hematopoiesis in vitro,[301] and collagen-based scaffolds are most effective for in vitro three-dimensional models of the hematopoietic microenvironment.[302] Marrow-derived fibroblasts and stromal cells synthesize collagens I, III, IV, V, and VI.[303] Collagen VI binds von Willebrand factor and is a strong cytoadhesive component of the marrow microenvironment.[304] Erythroid and granulocytic progenitors adhere to collagen type I in vitro.[305] Collagen type XIV, another fibril-associated collagen, promotes hematopoietic cell adhesion of myeloid and lymphoid cell lines.[306] In situ immunolocalization of ECM proteins in murine marrow shows that collagen types I and IV and FN localize to the endosteum.[307] Megakaryocyte binding to collagen I that induces FN secretion and polymerization[290] enhances the $\alpha_2\beta_1$-mediated collagen binding by megakaryocytes, permitting increased megakaryocyte adhesion and migration,[308] which are also mediated by other megakaryocytic collagen receptors including glycoprotein VI and discoid domain receptor 1(DDR1).[309]

Laminin

Laminins, multidomain glycoproteins with mitogenic and adhesive sites, are major components of the ECM and basement membranes.[310] Laminin interactions with collagen type IV and basement membrane components such as proteoglycans and entactin[311] regulate leukocyte chemotaxis.[312,313] CD34+ granulocytic progenitors,[314] mature monocytes,[315] and neutrophils[316] adhere to laminins. The role of laminins within the cytomatrix may be to strengthen adhesive interactions with $\alpha_6\beta_1$ (VLA-5) and $\alpha_6\beta_1$ (VLA-6) on hematopoietic cells.[316] In combination with FN in vitro, laminins can expand both HSCs and several more differentiated progenitors.[317] Laminins are composed of α, β, and γ polypeptides with expression of laminin-2 ($\alpha_2\beta_1\gamma_1$), laminin-8 ($\alpha_4\beta_1\gamma_1$),

and laminin-10 ($\alpha_5\beta_1\gamma_1$) in the marrow.[318] Stromal cells in cultures and cytokine-expanded CD34+cells also express laminin β_2, which is found in the pericellular space in marrow and intracellularly in megakaryocytes.[319] Laminin-γ_2 chain expression, which is unique to marrow-derived stromal cells, colocalizes with α smooth-muscle actin in marrow and is not expressed in endothelial cells or megakaryocytes.[320]

Integrins $\alpha_6\beta_1$ and $\alpha_6\beta_4$ are receptors for laminin-10/11 and laminin-8.[314] Laminin-10/11 ($\alpha_5\beta_1\gamma_1/\gamma_5\beta_2\gamma_1$) and FN bind CD34+ and CD34+ CD38–progenitors, whereas laminin-8 ($\alpha_4\beta_1\gamma_1$) and laminin-10/11 facilitate CXCL12–mediated transmigration of CD34+ cells.[314] In mouse repopulation studies, antibodies that block the α_6 components of laminin receptors decreased the homing of HSCs and colony-forming units–granulocyte-macrophage (CFU-GM).[321] When combined with antibodies to the α_4 component of integrins, antibodies that block the α_6 components synergistically decreased marrow homing of the short-term, multipotent repopulating cells. In contrast to this role of these integrin receptors in the homing of HSCs, a 67-kDa, nonintegrin laminin receptor is upregulated in HSCs following G-CSF stimulation and plays a significant role in their mobilization.[322] This 67-kDa nonintegrin receptor for laminin also has a role in the marrow homing of burst-forming units–erythroid (BFU-Es), early-stage erythroid progenitors that circulate in the blood.[323] On the other hand, the Lutheran blood group glycoproteins serve as receptors for the α_5 integrin component of laminins on the late-stage erythroid cells.[324] Laminin promotes the M-CSF–dependent proliferation of marrow-derived macrophages via the α_6-integrin subunit,[325] and $\alpha_6\beta_1$ mediates mast cell adhesion to laminin.[326]

Thrombospondin

The TSPs are secreted matrix glycoproteins that modulate cell function by altering cell–matrix interactions.[327] TSP1, a multifunctional ECM protein initially identified in platelet α granules, has domains that interact with collagen and FN and may participate in HSC lodgment.[328] TSP activates TGF-β[329] which results in a stimulatory effect on NK cells.[330] TSP binds to matrix heparan sulfates[178] and inhibits osteogenic differentiation.[331,332] Receptors on hematopoietic and nonhematopoietic cells can interact with TSP, including CD36[333] and the cutaneous lymphocyte antigen-1 protein of the CD36/LIMP II gene family.[334] CD36 is expressed during erythroid and megakaryocytic maturation.[335] TSP stimulates matrix metalloproteinase-9 activity in endothelial cells[336] and is chemotactic to monocytes.[337] A 140-kDa fragment of TSP1 binds bFGF, and TSP1 acts as a scavenger for matrix-associated angiogenic factors (fibroblast growth factor 2, VEGF, HGF), underscoring its antiangiogenic properties.[338,339] Mice deficient in TSP2 demonstrate that TSP2 is taken up in an integrin-dependent manner within the marrow and is necessary for the release of functionally competent platelets by megakaryocytes.[340] The 21-amino acid, C-terminal peptide of TSP4 stimulates proliferation of multiple types of early hematopoietic progenitors through the regulator of differentiation 1 (ROD1) nuclear receptor and increases erythropoiesis in mice.[341]

Vitronectin

Vitronectin, a major cytoadhesive glycoprotein, is present in plasma and the interstitial matrix of tissues. It interacts with a vast number of ECM components, cytokines, growth factors and proteolytic enzymes in vitro and in vivo.[342] Vitronectin also binds to several α_v-containing integrins,[342] including the integrin $\alpha_v\beta_3$ receptor (CD51) on fibroblasts, endothelial cells, osteoclasts,[343,344] and mature hematopoietic cells, including megakaryocytes, platelets,[345] and mast cells.[346] The integrin $\alpha_v\beta_3$ is expressed on monocyte-macrophages and neutrophils and mediates their transendothelial migration.[347,348] The vitronectin receptor cooperates with TSP and CD36 in the recognition and phagocytosis of apoptotic cells by neutrophils, macrophages, and dendritic cells.[349-351] Vitronectin-deficient mice have normal blood cell counts,[352] but thrombogenesis, new microvessel formation and tissue repair capacity are impaired,[353] most likely due to failure of inflammatory and thrombotic mechanisms. Thus, in the marrow ECM, vitronectin functions mainly in the coordination of apoptotic cell clearance, cellular migration, bone remodeling, and angiogenesis.

Other Matrix Proteins

Osteopontin, a glycoprotein produced by osteoblasts and hematopoietic cells in the marrow, binds to FN and collagen.[354,355] The predominant form of osteopontin in the marrow is thrombin-cleaved, and its N-terminal peptide is the active ligand for the $\alpha_9\beta_1$ and $\alpha_4\beta_1$ integrins on HSCs and circulating hematopoietic progenitors that plays a role in their attraction to and binding in the marrow.[356] Osteopontin can bind numerous integrins and CD44, and its binding through β_1-integrin results in suppression of proliferation and maintenance of quiescence in HSCs.[354,355] Conversely, the same osteopontin–β_1-integrin pathway induces proliferation in erythroblasts.[357] Osteopontin also plays a role in the development of NK cells[358,359] and T lymphocytes.[355] The fibulins are proteins secreted by the stromal cells of marrow, including osteoblasts and endothelial cells.[360,361] The metalloproteinase-resistant fibulin-1 accumulates in the ECM where it binds to a specific site on FN,[360,361] thereby disrupting HSC binding to FN with resultant decreases in HSC proliferation and differentiation.[361] Thus, fibulin-1 can act as a negative regulator that can maintain the quiescence of HSCs in the marrow.

HEMATOPOIETIC CELL ORGANIZATION

Erythroblasts

Erythroid progenitor cells arise from MPPs via the activity of the transcription factor GATA-1, which promotes differentiation toward the bipotent MEP that can subsequently differentiate into either erythroblasts or megakaryocytes (Chap. 32).[362] MEP fate is determined by the relative activities of two competing transcription factors, KLF-1, which directs differentiation toward the erythroid lineage, and Fli-1, which directs differentiation toward the megakaryocytic lineage.[362,363] The earliest progenitor cells committed solely to erythroid differentiation, BFU-Es,[364] which are defined by production of large colonies or bursts of erythroblasts after weeks in tissue culture, can circulate in the blood and reenter the marrow. When a BFU-E or one of its progeny, the colony-forming units–erythroid (CFU-Es),[364] associates with a marrow macrophage, they form the precursor of the basic unit of terminal erythropoiesis, the erythroblastic island (EBI).[94] Under the influence of the KLF-1 in both the macrophage and the erythroid cells,[365,366] an EBI develops as a central macrophage surrounded by as many as 30 adherent erythroblasts at various stages of differentiation from CFU-E through enucleating orthochromatic erythroblast. At least five cell-surface protein pairs contribute to adherence between macrophages and erythroblasts in EBIs[94]: (1) VCAM-1 on macrophages and $\alpha_4\beta_1$ integrin (VLA-4) on erythroblasts; (2) α_v component of integrins on macrophages and ICAM-4 on erythroblasts; (3) erythroblast-macrophage protein (EMP), on both erythroblasts and macrophages via a homophilic reaction; (4) CD169/Siglec-1 on macrophages and sialylated glycoproteins on erythroblasts; and (5) hemoglobin-haptoglobin receptor (CD163) on macrophages and an unknown binding partner on erythroblasts.

Differentiating erythroblasts are defined as basophilic, polychromatophilic, and orthochromatic erythroblasts by their morphologic appearances in Giemsa-stained films of aspirated marrows. However, CFU-Es and their immediate progeny, the proerythroblasts (ProEBs), as well as the morphologically defined, later erythroblast stages can be purified and defined by flow cytometry. Murine erythroid cells from

CFU-Es through ProEBs, are identified by flow cytometric expression patterns of transferrin receptor (CD71) and the erythroid-specific membrane glycoprotein Ter119,[367] or of CD44 and forward light scatter.[368] Likewise, expression patterns of glycophorin A, Band 3, and the α_4 component of integrin permit identification of the same stages in human erythroid differentiation.[369]

In EBIs, CFU-Es lose SCF dependence that had been present throughout their differentiation from HSCs, and CFU-Es, ProEBs, and early basophilic erythroblasts develop a dependence upon EPO to prevent apoptosis.[370] The level of EPO, the principal regulator of erythropoiesis, is regulated by tissue oxygen delivery in the kidney, and is dependent on both blood oxygen levels and red cell numbers.[370] However, during hypoxic stress, CFU-Es and ProEBs can be increased without differentiation in response to circulating glucocorticoid hormones[371,372] and BMP4 from central macrophages of EBIs.[373] EPO prevents apoptosis by decreasing expression of Fas, a membrane protein of the TNF-α receptor family that is prominently expressed on CFU-E, ProEBs and early basophilic stage erythroblasts. Fas activation triggers a series of caspases, a family of intracellular proteases that cleave other caspase members in sequential fashion, ultimately inducing apoptosis.[374] Fas-ligand, which binds and activates Fas, is produced mainly by immature erythroblasts in mice[375] and by mature erythroblasts in humans.[376] EPO also suppresses apoptosis in late-stage erythroblasts by inducing the antiapoptotic protein Bcl-X$_L$, which stabilizes mitochondria, preventing the activation of caspases other than those activated by Fas.[377] As a result of the Fas/Fas-ligand negative feedback within the EBI, differentiating erythroblasts can modulate the rate of CFU-E/ProEB apoptosis and provide regulated control rates of erythrocyte production commensurate with erythropoietic demand.

In EBIs, differentiation events include: (1) hemoglobin production in differentiating erythroblasts, (2) formation of the erythrocyte plasma membrane and underlying membrane skeleton, (3) cell size decrease associated with the terminal 4 to 5 cell divisions being a result of decreased duration of the G$_1$ phase of erythroblasts attached to central macrophages,[378] and (4) nuclear condensation,[379] stiffening,[380] and extrusion.[381] Erythroblast enucleation requires nonmuscle myosin IIB[382] and filamentous actin[381] to produce a membrane-enveloped nucleus and a nascent reticulocyte. The central macrophage sends out extensive slender membranous processes that envelop each erythroblast and phagocytize defective erythroblasts and extruded nuclei.[383] The extruded nuclei display phosphatidylserine on their plasma membranes that leads to rapid phagocytosis by the central macrophage.[384] Phagocytosis of extruded nuclei with recycling of the DNA components is essential in that deoxyribonuclease II–deficient mice die from an underproduction anemia with fetal liver macrophages filled with extruded erythroid nuclei.[385] The irregularly shaped, maturing reticulocytes can interact directly with the central macrophages before entering the blood through the venous sinuses.[94]

Megakaryocytes

During thrombopoiesis, HSC in the subcortical regions of the hematopoietic cords generate megakaryocytes by sequential, overlapping expressions of specific transcription factors. First HSCs differentiate to common myeloid progenitors (CMPs) via the influence of PU.1 and GATA-1, next to MEPs via GATA-1/FOG, then to megakaryocytic progenitors via Fli-1, and finally to megakaryocytes via NF-E2 (Chap. 111).[362,386] The microenvironmental factors that control survival and differentiation of megakaryocytes and their progenitors include a similar pattern of dependence to that of erythroid progenitors, with an overlapping decrease in dependence on SCF and an increasing dependence upon a physiologically regulated cytokine, TPO in the case of megakaryocytes, which ceases before the completion of differentiation.[386,387]

TPO concentrations are reciprocally related to the circulating platelet mass, which is the major site of metabolism of the hormone.[388] As the major regulator of megakaryocyte development, TPO acts in concert with several synergistic cytokines, including IL-11, IL-3, and IL-6.[386,387] TPO induces endomitosis in terminally differentiating megakaryocytes by inhibiting cytokinesis through reduced function of the contractile ring of filamentous actin and suppression of nonmuscle myosin expression.[389,390] However, DNA replication and accumulation of cytoplasmic proteins continues during six to seven of these endomitotic cell cycles. The resultant polyploid nucleus and abundant cytoplasm characterize the mature megakaryocyte which can account for 2 percent of marrow hematopoietic cell volume.[93]

Mature megakaryocytes lie directly outside the marrow vascular sinus wall[391] because of their translocation during differentiation under the influence of platelet endothelial cell adhesion molecule (PECAM)-1 (CD31) expressed on endothelial cells[392,393] and an autocrine pathway of VEGF-A and its receptor Flt-1 stimulating CXCR4 (receptor for CXCL12) expression on megakaryocytes.[394] This migration of maturing megakaryocytes is associated with the development of podosomes, actin-based extensions that bind to and remodel the local ECM.[395] The podosomes not only direct the megakaryocytes through the marrow to the sinus wall, but they also extend through the sinus basement membrane into the circulation.[395] Terminal differentiation of megakaryocytes involves the development of branching cytoplasmic protrusions, the proplatelets. Proplatelets are formed around a microtubular core that both provides a sliding mechanism that elongates and extends them into the vascular sinus lumen, but also provides a conduit for the redistribution of cytoplasmic granules from the megakaryocytes to bulbous formations at the distal ends of the proplatelets.[389]

Granulocytes

Granulocytes are mature myeloid cells comprised of neutrophils, eosinophils, and basophils originating from stem cells and myeloid progenitor cells concentrated in the subcortical regions of the hematopoietic cords (Chap. 18).[396] Granulocytes are terminally differentiated from common granulocyte-macrophage progenitor (GMP) cells which arise from MPPs through the expression of multiple transcription factors (Chap. 61). The transcription factor PU.1 promotes the development of the GMP phenotype and antagonizes the activity of GATA-1, which promotes MEP differentiation.[397,398] The myeloid commitment of GMPs is reinforced by C/EBPα, which promotes myeloid differentiation while suppressing the B-lymphoid transcription factor Pax5.[398,399] The further activity of C/EBPα is associated with granulocytic differentiation, whereas increased PU.1 activity is associated with monocytic differentiation.[400] The progression of myeloid differentiation beyond the promyelocyte stage, including the formation of secondary and tertiary granules, requires both C/EBP and the GFI-1 transcription factors.[400,401] GFI-1 also antagonizes the activity of the Egr-1 and Egr-2 transcription factors that are associated with monocytic differentiation.[400] The timing of expression and relative ratios of C/EBPα and GATA-2 transcription factors regulate differentiation of the GMP into a mature neutrophil, eosinophil, basophil, or mast cell.[399] Increased C/EBPα activity at this stage promotes a differentiation pathway toward neutrophils and eosinophils, whereas increased GATA-2 activity promotes differentiation toward basophils and mast cells.[399] Cells differentiating along the neutrophil and/or eosinophil pathway will follow a terminal neutrophil path when only C/EBPα is expressed, and a terminal eosinophil path when both C/EBPα and GATA-2 are expressed. Those cells differentiating along the basophil/mast cell pathway will follow a terminal mast cell path when only GATA-2 is active and a terminal basophil path when both GATA-2 and C/EBPα are active.

A group of hematopoietic growth factors, including SCF, GM-CSF, G-CSF, IL-6, and IL-5, support granulocytic progenitor/precursor viability and proliferation. In some cases, these growth factors can mobilize of these progenitors/precursors and their mature progeny from the marrow. These growth factors are produced in sites of inflammation in peripheral tissues, although some such as SCF and M-CSF are normally produced in the marrow stroma. Two hematopoietic growth factors have lineage-specific late-stage granulocytic cells as targets: IL-5 for eosinophil progenitors and G-CSF for neutrophilic progenitors. IL-5 is produced mainly by the T-helper type 2 (Th2) lymphocytes in response to allergens (Chap. 62).[402,403] Eosinophilic progenitor cells display an IL-5α receptor protein that when associated with the common β receptor (CSF2RB), binds IL-5, leading to their survival and proliferation.[402] Mature eosinophils have survival and chemotactic responses to IL-5, which mediates their entry into the circulation and accumulation in sites of allergic inflammation. GM-CSF, G-CSF, IL-3, and IL-6 all stimulate granulopoiesis *in vivo*, but only the deficiency of G-CSF results in severe neutropenia, making it the likely regulator of normal circulating granulocyte numbers.[404] Under normal steady-state conditions, 1 to 2 percent of neutrophils circulate transiently in the blood, while the majority remains in the marrow unless mobilized by inflammation in other areas of the body.

Models of G-CSF regulation of granulopoiesis and circulating neutrophils under normal conditions and during inflammatory states have been proposed.[405,406] Newly formed neutrophils have low expression of CXCR4 and can exit the marrow by migration through sinusoidal endothelial cells. As they age in the circulation they express more CXCR4 and are attracted back to the marrow by stromal CXCL12, the CXCR4 ligand.[405] After reentering the marrow, the senescent neutrophils undergo apoptosis and are phagocytosed by macrophages that, in turn, produce G-CSF stimulating more granulopoiesis.[405] Cells at sites of inflammation produce both G-CSF and chemokines, including KC chemokine (CXCL1), and macrophage inhibitory protein (MIP)-2 (CXCL2). The secreted G-CSF acts on the marrow mobilizing neutrophils by its ability to reduce both marrow CXCL12 production and neutrophilic CXCR4 expression. G-CSF, however, does not recruit the neutrophils to sites of inflammation from the blood.[405] By their chemotactic properties, CXCL1 and CXCL2 also induce rapid mobilization from the marrow into the blood and to sites of inflammation.[405] Another model involves similar migration of neutrophils from the marrow that depends on G-CSF downregulating CXCL12 production and neutrophilic CXCR4 expression, but the feedback that decreases G-CSF occurs in the peripheral tissues.[406] In this model, macrophages that phagocytose apoptotic neutrophils in the peripheral tissues decrease IL-23 production, which decreases IL-17 production by a subset of T-lymphocytes that, in turn, results in decreased G-CSF in the marrow.

● CELL ADHESION AND HOMING

After their initial migration from the yolk sac, AGM, or placenta to the marrow, the HSCs are located in specific sites in the marrow through interactions with other types of cells and with matrix proteins. HSCs do not remain permanently in the marrow because a small percentage of them are continuously entering the blood through the venous sinusoids, circulating briefly, and then reentering the marrow.[407,408] In addition to the HSCs, the more differentiated progenitor cells, such as the short-term repopulating cells and the primitive BFU-Es, can circulate in a similar manner. When circulating, the HSCs can either reenter the marrow or they can enter other organs. After entering the interstitium of a peripheral organ, the HSCs can give rise to myeloid progeny and/or they enter the lymphatic drainage of the organ and circulate through lymphatic vessels and thoracic duct before reentering the blood.[409] HSCs display multiple adhesion and cytokine receptors that allow them to attach to cellular and matrix components within the marrow sinusoidal spaces.[275,277,410–412] Such attachments facilitate HSC homing and lodgment in the marrow and provide the cell–cell contacts required for HSC survival and steady-state proliferation,[413] as shown by membrane-bound SCF regulation of HSC lodgment in the endosteal marrow region.[414]

In most lineages, differentiated cells are released from the marrow, circulate in the blood, and eventually home to the marrow. In some cell types, the circulating cells will differentiate further in peripheral organs such as B lymphocytes in the lymph nodes and spleen, monocytes in the tissues, and T lymphocytes in the thymus. After a period of residence in these secondary lymphoid organs, some lymphocytes travel through the lymph and blood, homing to the marrow, where they become functioning mature cells, such as plasma cells and CD4 and CD8 mature T lymphocytes.[199,200,204] Mature and band forms of neutrophils exit the marrow, circulate in the blood and, if not recruited to a site of inflammation, home as senescent cells to the marrow by the CXCL12/CXCR4 mechanism described in the preceding "Granulocytes" section.[405] Senescent erythrocytes are also removed from circulation through a mechanism that involves binding surface ICAM-4 to integrin $\alpha_L\beta_2$ (lymphocyte function-associated antigen [LFA]-1) on macrophages in the spleen and marrow.[415] Mature leukocytes that participate in inflammatory reactions, such as the lymphocytes, monocytes/macrophages, and eosinophils, exit the circulation in areas of infection, allergic reactions, or injury. Table 5–2 lists the adhesive receptors and their ligands present on HSCs, progenitor cells, and components of the hematopoietic microenvironment, but receptor–ligand interactions that regulate the trafficking of mature leukocytes are not exhaustively listed.[416,417]

INTEGRINS

Integrins mediate important cellular functions, including embryonic development, cell differentiation, and adhesive interactions between hematopoietic cells and inflammatory cells and surrounding vascular and stromal microenvironments.[411,412,418] Integrins are divalent cation-requiring heterodimeric proteins (18 α subunits and 8 β subunits) subdivided by the β-chain component. Table 5–2 indicates that α-chains can associate with more than one β-chain subunit. The principal integrin receptors of the β_1 subgroup involved in HSC-endothelial and HSC-stromal interactions are $\alpha_4\beta_1$ (VLA-4), $\alpha_5\beta_1$ (VLA-5), and $\alpha_L\beta_2$ (LFA-1) of the β_2 subgroup. $\alpha_4\beta_1$-based stromal adhesion events regulate erythropoiesis in the stages after EPO dependence.[419] Granulopoiesis is stimulated by $\alpha_4\beta_1$ activation by marrow stromal cells in cooperation with PECAM-1 (CD31), an immunoglobulin superfamily member.[420] Antibodies against α_4 or small molecule antagonists can mobilize hematopoietic stem and progenitor cells into the peripheral circulation.[421] The high expression of $\alpha_4\beta_1$ in granulocytic precursor cells and newly formed granulocytes has an important role in their adherence to VCAM-1 in the marrow, whereas the downregulation of $\alpha_4\beta_1$ in the more mature neutrophils works in concert with CXCL12/CXCR4 for their release into the blood.[422] The $\alpha_4\beta_1$ integrin on B lymphocytes is important for interactions with the VCAM-1 on the stromal cells in the B-lymphocyte niche, both in early B-lymphocyte development prior to migration out of the marrow and in later development of plasma cell precursors that have reentered the marrow.[199] An acquired defect in stromal function, characterized by a deficiency in VCAM-1 and IL-7 expression,[423–425] accounts for the delayed B-lymphoid reconstitution seen after marrow transplantation. During thrombopoiesis, CXCL12 induces VCAM-1 in the marrow sinusoid endothelial cells[426] that mediates the binding of the megakaryocytes to the endothelium.[427] Integrin $\alpha_4\beta_7$ and its receptor, mucosal addressin cell adhesion molecule

(MAdCAM)-1, like the integrin $\alpha_4\beta_1$/VCAM-1 receptor pair, contribute equally to the homing of HSC to the marrow.[428,429]

Integrins are signaling molecules.[430] After engaging their ligands, or subsequent to activation by monoclonal antibodies, multiple events (tyrosine phosphorylation of focal adhesion kinase, paxillin, and ERK-2) are triggered (outside–in signaling), culminating with Ras activation.[431,432] Integrin receptor crosstalk[433] with other adhesive receptor members, such as the immunoglobulin superfamily (NK cell–T cell [$\alpha_1\beta_2$/DYNAM-1], CD34+endothelial cell PECAM-1,[434–436] or selectins,[437] also results from outside–in signaling events that regulate receptor-binding affinity[438,439] and mediates inhibitory signals for erythroid, myeloid, and lymphoid progenitor growth.[440–443] Integrin binding of their respective receptors, such as $\alpha_4\beta_1$/VCAM-1 or $\alpha_4\beta_1$/FN, in early CD34+ progenitors enhances viability and preserves their long-term repopulating ability.[444] In studies of isolated SP cells, high expression of the vitronectin receptor $\alpha_v\beta_3$ (CD51/CD61) is associated with quiescence and long-term repopulating ability.[445] Conversely, expression of the α_2 integrin is associated with only short-term repopulating capacity.[446]

IMMUNOGLOBULIN SUPERFAMILY

The immunoglobulin superfamily designates a group of molecules containing one or more amino acid repeats also found in immunoglobulins and includes PECAM-1 (CD31), ICAM-3/R (CD50) and ICAM-1 (CD54), LFA-3 (CD58), ICAM-2 (CD102), VCAM-1 (CD106), KIT (CD117), and LW/ICAM-4 (CD242) (see Table 5–2).[447–461] VCAM-1 is upregulated by inflammatory cytokines, IL-4 and IL-13.[462,463] Immunoglobulin-like adhesion molecules also include NCAM, a neural cell-adhesion molecule that binds lymphocytes but not hematopoietic progenitors; Thy1, a stem cell antigen; major histocompatibility complex classes I and II; and CD2, CD4, and CD8 (see Table 5–2).[247] LW/ICAM-4 on erythroblasts binds the α_v component of integrins on macrophages in EBIs,[94] whereas the normal function of Lutheran red blood cell antigen, Lu/B-CAM (CD239), which binds the α_5 component of laminin and is expressed late in erythroblast differentiation, is uncertain.[461] The sialic acid-binding immunoglobulin-like lectins (Siglecs) are a family of surface proteins found on lymphocytes and myeloid cells that bind sialic acid residues of glycoproteins.[464] Some Siglecs are evolutionarily conserved, such as Siglec-1 (sialoadhesin), which is highly expressed on macrophages, including the central macrophages of EBIs, and CD22, a coreceptor on B-lymphocytes. The remaining Siglecs, which are phylogenetically evolving rapidly, include CD33, which is expressed in lymphocytes and in all stages of myeloid cells where it is a commonly used marker for acute myeloid leukemia.

LECTINS (SELECTINS)

Homing of stem cells requires lectin receptors with galactosyl and mannosyl specificities.[465,466] The selectins are a family of adhesion molecules, each containing type C lectin structures.[467] The leukocyte selectin (L-selectin, CD62L) is expressed on hematopoietic stem and progenitor cells and mediates adhesive interactions with other receptors (addressins), such as the CD34 sialomucin present on specialized endothelium, using sialylated fucosyl-glucoconjugates (see Table 5–2).[259] The CD34 receptor on stem cells, however, does not bind L-selectin,[259] as a putative L-selectin ligand may exist on these cells but is yet to be defined. The selectin family also contains CD62E, an E-selectin constitutively expressed on the marrow sinusoidal endothelium that regulates transmigration of leukocytes and CD34+ stem cell homing. The third member of this family is P-selectin, which is found on platelets. P-selectin can bind HSCs using a mucin receptor, CD162 also known as

TABLE 5–2. Hematopoietic and Microenvironment Adhesion Receptors and Their Ligands

Receptor Subgroups	Receptor	Cellular Distribution	Ligand
INTEGRINS			
β_1 subgroup (CD29)	CD49d, $\alpha_4\beta_1$ (VLA-4)	CD34+ cells (erythroid, and lympho-myeloid progenitors)	VCAM-1 (CD106), FN, TSP
	CD49e, $\alpha_5\beta_1$ (VLA-5)	CD34+ cells, bone cells	FN, laminin
	CD49f, $\alpha_6\beta_1$ (VLA-6)	Rare CD34+ cells, monocytes	Collagen, laminin
β_2 subgroup (CD18)	CD11a/CD18, $\alpha_L\beta_2$ (LFA-1)	CD34+ cell subsets, not on repopulating stem cells	ICAM-1, ICAM-2, ICAM-3, DNAM-1
	CD11b/CD18, $\alpha_M\beta_2$ (Mac-1)	CD34+ subsets, monocytes	ICAM-1, ICAM-2, iC3b, fibrinogen
β_3 subgroup	Vβ_3 (VNR)	Megakaryocytes, osteoclast	FN, TSP, CD31
β_7 subgroup	$\alpha_4\beta_7$ (LPAM-1)	Lymphoid and myeloid progenitor cells, mature myeloid cells	MAdCAM-1, VCAM-1, FN
IMMUNOGLOBULINS			
	CD31 (PECAM-1)	ECs, CD34+ cells, monocytes	CD31 homophilic adhesion, $\alpha_V\beta_3$ (VNR), CD38
	CD50 (ICAM-3, ICAM-R)	CD34+ cells, monocytes	$\alpha_L\beta_2$ (LFA-1), CD11d/CD18 ($\alpha_D\beta_2$)
	CD54 (ICAM-1)	CD34+ cells, stroma, activated ECs	$\alpha_L\beta_2$ (LFA-1), $\alpha_M\beta_2$ (Mac-1)
	CD58 (LFA-3)	CD34+ progenitors, stroma, ECs	CD2
	CD102 (ICAM-2)	ECs, monocytes	$\alpha_L\beta_2$ (LFA-1)
	CD106 (VCAM-1)	Stroma, activated ECs	$\alpha_4\beta_1$ (VLA-4), $\alpha_4\beta_7$ (LPAM-1)
	CD117 (c-KIT)	CD34+ progenitors	Membrane KIT ligand
	CD242 (ICAM-4)	Erythroid cells	α_V-Integrins
	PRR2 (related to CD155, the poliovirus receptor)	CD34+, CD33+, CD41+, myelomonocytic cells, megakaryocytic cells, ECs	PRR2 homophilic adhesion
LECTINS			
	CD62L (L-selectin)	Stroma, CD34+ cells	GlyCAM-1, MAdCAM-1, CD162, CD34, sLe^x, PCLP1
	CD62E (E-selectin)	Activated ECs, (marrow ECs express CD62E constitutively)	CD15, sLe^a, CD162, CLA, sLe^x
	CD62P (P-selectin)	Activated ECs	CD162, sLe^x, CD24 (HSA)
SIALOMUCINS			
	CD34	CD34+ cells, ECs	Selectins, other ligands?
	CD43	CD34+, monocytes, NK cells	CD54 (ICAM-1)
	CD162 (PSGL-1)	CD34+ cells, ECs	CD62L, CD62E, CD62P
	CD164 (MGC-24v)	CD34+ cells, stroma, monocytes	Unknown
	CD166 (HCA, ALCAM)	CD34+ cells, stromal cells, ECs	CD6, CD166
HYALADHERIN			
	CD44	CD34+ cells, broad distribution	Hyaluronan, bFGF, HGF
OTHER			
	CD38	CD34+ subsets, early T and B cells, plasma cells, thymocytes	CD31, hyaluronan
	CD144 (VE-cadherin)	CFU-E, stromal cells, ECs	E-cadherin
	CD157 (BST-1)	Stroma, T and B cells, myeloid cells	Unknown

ALCAM, activated leukocyte adhesion molecule; bFGF, basic fibroblast growth factor; BST, bone marrow stroma; CD, cluster designation; CFU-E, colony forming unit–erythroid; CLA, cutaneous lymphocyte antigen; DNAM-1, DNAX accessory Molecule-1; EC, endothelial cell; FN, fibronectin; GlyCAM, glycosylation-dependent cell adhesion molecule; HCA, hematopoietic cell antigen; HGF, hepatocyte growth factor; HSA, heat-stable antigen; ICAM, intercellular adhesion molecule; iC3b, inactive complement 3b complex; KIT, tyrosine-protein kinase; LFA, lymphocyte function-associated antigen; LPAM, lymphocyte Peyer patch-specific adhesion molecule; MAdCAM, mucosal addressin cell adhesion molecule; MGC-24, multiglycosylated core of 24 kDa; NK, natural killer; PCLP, podocalyxin-like protein; PECAM, platelet/endothelial cell adhesion molecule; PRR2, poliovirus receptor-related protein 2; PSGL-P, selectin glycoprotein ligand; sLe, sialyl Lewis; TSP, thrombospondin; VCAM, vascular cell adhesion molecule; VE, vascular endothelial; VLA, very-late antigen; VNR, vitronectin receptor.

the P-selectin glycoprotein ligand (PSGL)-1, which binds to all three selectins (see Table 5–2). These proteins are responsible for leukocyte rolling over endothelial surfaces and tethering, thereby allowing integrin-mediated firm adhesion to the endothelium and mediating cellular homing events using specialized high endothelial venule lymphocyte homing sites.[140,467,468] In addition to their role in HSC homing in the marrow, E-selectin and P-selectin can promote quiescence in HSC and induce apoptosis of late-stage myeloid progenitors while promoting the expansion (P-selectin) or differentiation (E-selectin) of short-term repopulating cells.[469]

SIALOMUCINS

Three members of the CD34 family—CD34, podocalyxin, and endoglycan—are expressed on vascular endothelium, HSCs, and various hematopoietic cell lineages.[470] When expressed on lymphoid high endothelial venules, these sialomucins are receptors for L-selectin, but their differential glycosylation in hematopoietic cells prevents L-selectin binding and results in their reducing nonspecific adhesion and potentially enhancing mobility. Although its function has not been determined, endomucin is another CD34-like sialomucin expressed in endothelium and in HSCs.[471] In T lymphocytes, where it affects mobility, CD43 (leukosialin) acts in concert with PSGL-1 and binds both P-selectin and E-selectin.[472,473] CD43 in neutrophils can foster adhesion when binding to E-selectin on endothelial cells, but it inhibits adhesion in most instances.[473] CD43 can also regulate hematopoietic progenitor survival.[474] CD162 (PSGL-1), a sialomucin that binds all three selectins, is important in leukocyte trafficking and stem cell homing.[467,468,470] CD164 (endolyn), another sialomucin receptor displayed on HSCs, forms a complex with CXCR4, VLA-4, and VLA-5 on the leading edge of migrating HSCs after exposure to FN-bound CXCL12, indicating a role for CD164 in the homing of HSCs.[475] CD166 (hematopoietic cell antigen [HCA], activated leukocyte adhesion molecule [ALCAM]) is expressed on HSCs and osteoblasts and is required for long-term engraftment potential of donor HSCs in murine transplantation models, probably through homophilic interaction.[476–478] CD166's only other ligand is CD6.[477,479]

HYALADHERINS

The fifth subgroup listed in Table 5–2 is the cartilage-related proteoglycan, CD44, also known as the *lymphocyte homing cell adhesion molecule* (HCAM). This adhesion receptor, which binds the hyaluronic acid in the marrow matrix and can be a receptor for E-selectin, is expressed on neutrophils, lymphocytes, erythroblasts, and HSC.[467,468] CD44 displayed on HSCs facilitates their homing and adhesion to the marrow and plays a role in their mobilization in response to G-CSF.[467,468,480] Studies with CD44-deficient mice show no defects in HSC homing and growth, and no decrease in hematopoiesis, suggesting that another hyaladherin receptor may compensate for the absence of CD44.[481] The other hyaladherin receptor on HSC is the receptor for hyaluron-mediated mobility (CD168/RHAMM),[467,481] which does provide hyaluronic acid binding by neutrophils under inflammatory conditions in CD44 deficiency.[482] Thus, CD44 and CD168/RHAMM may provide redundant hyaluronic acid binding in HSC.

OTHER ADHESION MOLECULES

CD38 is an adhesion receptor that binds the CD31 receptor and matrix hyaluronan. It is expressed on early T and B cells and subsets of CD34+ hematopoietic progenitors.[483] Similar to CD38, the stromal adhesion receptor BST-1 (CD157) is an adenosine diphosphate-ribosyl cyclase that is involved in regulation of intracellular calcium concentrations.

CD157 is expressed on marrow stroma, T and B cells, and myeloid cells. It promotes pre–B-cell adhesion and growth.[483] Cadherins are large molecules involved in cell–cell junctions and vascular integrity. CD144 (VE-cadherin) is expressed on CD34+ hematopoietic and endothelial progenitor cells and is an important molecule for trafficking of HSCs in fetal tissues and for the maintenance of HSC self-renewal.[115,484,485] Downregulation of VE-cadherin is associated with crosslinking of VCAM-1, resulting in enhanced transendothelial migration of CD34+ cells in response to CXCL12.[120] Although N-cadherin expression by both HSC and osteoblasts has been proposed to play a role in their interactions, experimental results in knockout mice do not support such a role.[11,486]

● CELLULAR HOMING

Leukocyte trafficking and migration have been central to understanding mechanisms of tissue homing. One of the best studied processes is lymphocyte homing to secondary lymphoid organs via specialized high endothelial venules (HEVs). Generally, leukocytes home to areas of inflammation by adhering to the endothelium and migrating between intercellular spaces by a sequence of specific events that begins with tethering of the leukocytes to the luminal surface of the endothelial cells.[487] In the secondary lymphoid organs, tethering is mediated by L-selectin/CD62L receptor on the surface of naïve lymphocytes that binds a complex carbohydrate determinant, 6-sulfo-sialyl Lewis X, on glycoproteins called peripheral node addressins, such as CD34, podocalyxin, and endomucin.[488,489] P-selectin and E-selectin are upregulated on the endothelial cell surface in response to various inflammatory cytokines, where they bind their respective receptors, PSGL-1 and CD44 on leukocytes.[466,490] Tethering results in rolling of the leukocytes along the endothelial surface. Interactions of VLA-4 and $\alpha_4\beta_7$ integrin on the surface of lymphocytes with their respective ligands VCAM-1 and MAdCAM-1 on HEVs may also mediate rolling.[467] Rolling of neutrophils is slowed further by PSGL-1 and L-selectin activation of other adhesion molecules that include the β_2 integrins $\alpha_L\beta_2$ (LFA-1) and $\alpha_M\beta_2$ (Mac-1).[490–492] These β_2 integrins, in turn, bind ICAM-1 on endothelial cells. The rolling leukocytes also receive signals through surface G-protein–coupled receptors that bind chemokines in the heparan sulfate proteoglycans on the endothelial cells.[490–492]

The interaction of PSGL-1, L-selectin, integrins, and G-protein–coupled receptors with their endothelial ligands leads to cytoskeletal changes with arrest of rolling and adhesion to the endothelium. The adherent leukocytes undergo a rapid diapedesis, with migration either through or between the endothelial cells into the abluminal interstitium. At the interface with the adherent leukocyte, ICAM-1 and VCAM-1 in the endothelial cell are concentrated in a cup-like, caveolin-rich structure that internalizes ICAM-1.[492–494] This caveolin-rich structure is linked to the endothelial cell cytoskeleton through vimentin. The internalization of the ICAM caveolae leads to the formation of a channel through the cell to the abluminal surface. When leukocytes follow a paracellular route through the endothelium, they require the coordinated activity of multiple adhesion proteins. These include PECAM-1, CD99, JAM proteins, and VE-cadherin, each of which mediates homophilic interactions at intercellular junctions between endothelial cells, and ICAM-2.[492–494] Although the roles of these proteins are uncertain, antibody inhibition and knockout mice demonstrate that they are necessary for the unidirectional migration of the leukocyte through the endothelium. PECAM-1, CD99, and JAM-C are expressed on leukocytes and may be involved in homophilic interactions between the migrating leukocyte and the endothelial junction. LFA-1 and Mac-1 on leukocytes can bind and interact with ICAM-2 and JAM-A on endothelium, whereas leukocyte VLA-4 can interact with endothelial JAM-B.

The driving force for the migration and homing of leukocytes is the expression of chemoattractants at the site of inflammation or areas of constitutive production, such as the secondary lymphoid organs or the marrow. Bacterial peptides, complement components, and cytokines are produced in inflammatory sites. More than 40 different, but structurally related, chemotactic cytokines (chemokines) can be produced by leukocytes in inflammatory sites.[495,496] Chemokines accumulate on cell surfaces or in extracellular matrices through their binding to GAGs.[495-497] Concentrations and chemotactic activities of each cytokine are related to production rate, binding affinities to GAGs, presence of decoy chemokines that can compete with chemotactic activity, and modulation by metalloproteinases that enhance or diminish activities of substrate chemokines.[495]

Based on the location of one or two cysteine residues in the amino terminus, chemokines are divided into four subfamilies.[224,495,496] One large subfamily comprises the CXC ligand (CXCL) chemokines (e.g., platelet factor 4, IL-8, melanocyte growth-stimulating activity/GROα, neutrophil activating protein-2, granulocyte chemotactic protein-2), which mediate neutrophil migration and activation. The other large subfamily comprises the CC ligand (CCL) chemokines (e.g., CCL3 [MIP-1α], CCL4 [MIP-1β], [CCL5] RANTES [regulated on activation, normal T-cell expressed, presumed secreted], MCP-1 through MCP-5), which mediate mostly monocyte, and in some cases lymphocyte, chemotaxis.[497] A chemokine with CXXXCL structure is fractalkine, an endothelial transmembrane mucin–chemokine hybrid molecule that mediates the rapid capture, firm adhesion, and activation under physiologic flow of circulating monocytes, resting or IL-2–activated CD8 lymphocytes, and NK cells.[498] The cytokines TNF-α and IL-1 upregulate fractalkine, in keeping with the need to rapidly recruit effector cells at sites of inflammation. The chemokine receptors on the surface of leukocytes are coupled to G proteins that initiate signaling for chemotaxis upon chemokine ligand binding.[495,496] The chemokine receptors for the two large subfamilies bind those members such that CXCLs bind CXCRs and CCLs bind CCRs. However, within these two subfamilies is significant redundancy and promiscuity in chemokine-receptor binding. Table 5–3 gives a detailed listing of chemokine receptors and the cellular targets and ligands interacting with each receptor subgroup.

A major exception to this redundant and promiscuous chemokine-receptor interaction is the specific binding of CXCL12/stromal cell-derived factor (SDF)-1α to its receptor CXCR4, which is associated with homeostatic maintenance of cell populations, including HSCs and their progeny in the marrow.[496,499] CXCL12 can bind to one other chemokine receptor (CXCR7), but mouse knockout experiments show that CXCL12 null and CXCR4 null mice have embryonic lethal phenotypes that are markedly similar whereas CXCR7 null mice have postnatal lethality due to cardiovascular defects; CXCR7 may have a role in ligand sequestration but not in hematopoiesis.[496,500-502] CXCL12 is produced by the bone, endothelial, perivascular reticular cells and some hematopoietic cells in the marrow, and its receptor CXCR4 is expressed on various hematopoietic and mature blood cells.[468,499,503] The murine gene Cxcl12 was floxed, allowing conditional deletion by various Cre transgenics expressed in mesenchymal progenitor cells. Conditional deletion of Cxcl12 in mineralizing osteoblasts resulted in no obvious phenotype whereas deletion in Osterix-Cre–expressing reticular (CAR cells) and osteoblast cells resulted in constitutive HSC mobilization and loss of B-lymphoid progenitor cells.[504,505] The Cre transgenics that delete floxed Cxcl12 alleles have complicated patterns of expression and current evidence supports a more important role for the perivascular niche in the homing of HSCs.[505] Hence, mouse genetics and pharmacologic inhibition show that CXCL12 and CXCR4 are involved in the trafficking of HSCs, committed progenitor cells, and mature cells, including neutrophils, dendritic cells, NK cells, and T and B lymphocytes.[404,405,421,499,503] The cellular specificity of the homing, localization, and mobilization that are driven by CXCL12 and CXCR4 are regulated by additional chemokines, adhesion proteins, and metalloproteinases associated with specific hematopoietic cell types and/or the organs to which they home, in which they reside, and from which they are mobilized.[499,503] In the case of HSCs homing from the peripheral tissues through which they migrate, their initial entry into the lymphatic vessels is driven by the lipid chemoattractant sphingosine-1-phosphate (S-1-P).[409] HSC display S-1-P receptors that respond to high levels in the lymph compared to the peripheral tissues where S-1-P is degraded.

For the HSCs and the marrow, multiple experiments using inhibitors and antibodies with stem cell transplantation in mice and humans, parabiotic experiments with mice, and transplantation of human HSCs into immunocompromised mice (e.g., nonobese diabetic [NOD]/severe combined immunodeficiency [SCID] strains) have contributed to an understanding of some interactions of these multiple factors that influence HSCs within the marrow.[506] Two adhesion mechanisms that play major roles in CXCL12-mediated HSCs homing to the marrow are the binding and activation of $\alpha_4\beta_1$ integrin and selectin ligands, particularly PSGL-1,[140,468,507] on HSCs to their respective receptors, VCAM-1, and P- and E-selectins on the marrow sinusoidal endothelium.[428,508] Although $\alpha_4\beta_1$ integrin appears to be the major integrin on HSCs involved in the first step of homing, other integrins have been implicated as having supporting roles, including $\alpha_5\beta_1$, $\alpha_4\beta_7$, and $\alpha_6\beta_1$ or $\alpha_6\beta_4$ integrin that bind to FN, MAdCAM-1, and laminins in the marrow.[321,421] Similarly, a coordinated action between CXCR4 that has bound CXCL12 and the CD44 isoform on HSCs,[509] or another hyaladherin such as RHAMM,[481] may provide a source of adhesion for HSCs to hyaluronic acid on marrow endothelial cells in the homing process. In cord blood cells enriched for HSCs, the colocalization and cooperative activity of the endolyn with CXCR4, $\alpha_4\beta_1$, and $\alpha_5\beta_1$ integrin appears to enhance HSCs homing to the marrow in response to CXCL12.[475] CXCR4 has also been colocalized in lipid rafts on HSCs with Rac-1, a member of the receptor-associated RhoGTPases.[510] The RhoGTPases have two members, Rac-2 and RhoH, that are hematopoietic specific and, with other more widely expressed members such as Rac-1, Cdc42, and Rho A, are downstream effectors of CXCR4, β_1-integrin, and KIT signaling in HSCs.[511] The various RhoGTPases modulate actin polymerization and lead to cytoskeletal changes that are required for survival, proliferation, homing, and mobilization of HSCs and their progeny. In the homing of HSCs, the RhoGTPase-mediated signaling provided by the coordinated action of CXCR4, β_1 integrins, and CD44 leads to the rolling, arrest, and transmigration of the marrow sinus endothelial cells.

Once the HSCs have migrated across the sinusoidal endothelial cells, they migrate further within the marrow in response to CXCL12. Using fluorescent SLAM-labeled markers for the identification of HSC in murine transplantation experiments, the homing of HSCs in the marrow cavity is associated with reticular cells that harbor the highest numbers of CAR cells in the marrow.[132] The majority of CAR cells are in the perivascular areas to which the HSCs home.[52] Another factor that may contribute to perivascular homing, especially following stress, such as lethal irradiation, is the ability of the marrow sinusoidal endothelial cells that express CXCR4 that binds circulating CXCL12 and transports it into the perivascular areas of the marrow.[503,512] A second area in the marrow to which HSC home is the endosteal niche because of the proximity of these endosteal areas to perivascular areas,[512] as well as the abundant CXCL12 production by osteoblasts and osteoclasts.[134,165] Thus, two HSC niches are recognized in the marrow—perivascular and endosteal—with HSCs in the perivascular areas more likely to proliferate, differentiate, and mobilize into the blood than HSCs in the endosteal areas.[75,150,512]

TABLE 5–3. Chemokine Receptors, Interacting Chemokine Ligands, and Cellular Specificity

Receptors	Receptor Expression	Chemokine Ligands
CXCR1	Neutrophils, monocytes	CXCL2 (GROβ), CXCL3 (GROγ), CXCL5 (ENA78), CXCL6 (GCP-2), CXCL8 (IL-8)
CXCR2	Neutrophils, IL-5–primed Eos, monocytes	CXCL1,2,3 (GROα/β/γ), CXCL5 (ENA78), CXCL6, CXCL7 (NAP-2), CXCL8(IL-8),
CXCR3	Activated memory and naïve T cells, NK cells; T (preferentially Th1) cells, B cells	CXCL9 (MIG), CXCL10 (IP-10), CXCL11 (I-TAC)
CXCR4	Neutrophils, monocytes, megakaryocytes, CD34+ and pre–B-cell precursors, resting and activated T cells, DCs	CXCL12 (SDF-1α, SDF-1β)
CXCR5	B lymphocytes, T lymphocytes	CXCL13 (BCA-1/BLC)
CXCR6	T lymphocytes	CXCL16 (SR-PSOX)
CXCR7	B lymphocyte, T lymphocytes, Basos, monocytes, NK cells	CXCL11 (I-TAC), CXCL12 (SDF-1α)
CX3CR1	Monocytes, DCs, CD34+ cells, NK cells; in nodal tissues activated T-helper lymphocytes, activated B cells, and follicular DCs	CX3CL1 (fractalkine/neurotactin)
XCR1	Resting T cells, NK cells	XCL1 (lymphotactin/SCM-1α/ATAC), XCL2 (SCM-1β)
CCR1	Monocytes, EOS, basophils, activated Neu and T cells, CD34+ cells, immature DCs	CCL3 (MIP-1α), CCL5 (RANTES), CCL7 (MCP-3), CCL8 (MCP-2), CCL13 (MCP-4), CCL22 (MDC), CCL23 (MPIF-1)
	Monocytes, T cells (not Neu, EOS, or B cells)	CCL14 (HCC-1), CCL15 (HCC-2/MIP-5), CCL16 (HCC-4/LEC)
CCR2	Monocytes, basophils, DCs, T cells, activated memory CD4 T cells, NK cells	CCL2(MCP-1), CCL7 (MCP-3), CCL8 (MCP-2), CCL13 (MCP-4)
CCR3	Eos, thymocytes, basophils, DCs, activated memory CD4 T cells	CCL5 (RANTES), CCL7 (MCP-3), CCL8 (MCP-2), CCL11 (Eotaxin-1), CCL13 (MCP-4), CCL15 (HCC-2/MIP-5), CCL24 (Eotaxin-2/MPIF-2), CCL26 (Eotaxin-3)
CCR4	Activated T cells, immature DCs	CCL17 (TARC)
	Monocyte-derived DCs, activated NK cells	CCL22 (MDC)
	Thymocytes (CD3+, CD4+, CD8low)	CCL22 (MDC)
CCR5	Monocytes, activated memory CD4 T cells	CCL5 (RANTES), CCL8 (MCP-2), CCL13 (MCP-4), CCL14 (HCC-1)
	Immature DCs, CD34+ cells, NK cells	CCL3 (MIP-1α), CCL4 (MIP-1β)
	Human thymocytes	CCL4 (MIP-1β)
CCR6	T cells, CD34+–derived dendritic cells	CCL20 (MIP-3α/LARC/exodus-1)
CCR7	Activated T (naïve and memory T cells) > B lymphocytes, NK cells subsets, CD34+ macrophage progenitors, mature DCs	CCL19 (MIP-3β/ELC/exodus-3), CCL21 (SLC/exodus-2/6Ckine) (6Ckine inactive on B cells)
CCR8	Monocytes, T (Th2) cells, NK cells	CCL1 (I309), CCL17 (TARC)
CCR9	Thymocytes (CD4+/CD8+, CD4+/CD8–), activated macrophages	CCL25 (TECK)
CCR10	Skin-homing memory T cells, CD4/CD8 cells	CCL26 (Eotaxin-3), CCL27 (CTACK/ILC/ESkine), CCL28 (MEC)
CCR1 and CCR3	Neutrophils, monocytes, lymphocytes	CCL15 (HCC-2/MIP-5)
Not known	Resting T cells	CCL18 (DC-CK1/PARC)
CCR3/CCR10	Memory lymphocytes, Eos, IgA plasmablasts	CCL28 (MEC)

6Ckine, chemokine with 6 cysteines; ATAC, activation-induced, chemokine-related molecule; Baso, basophil; BCA, B-cell attracting chemokine; BLC, B-cell homing chemokine that activates Burkitt lymphoma receptor 1 (BLR1); CTACK, cutaneous T-cell–attracting chemokine; DC, dendritic cell; ELC, EBI1-ligand chemokine; ENA, epithelial neutrophil-activating protein; EOS, eosinophil; ESkine, embryonal stem cell chemokine; GCP, granulocyte chemotactic protein; GRO, growth-related oncogene; HCC, human C-C chemokine; IgA, immunoglobulin A; IL-8 is also chemotactic for a specific subset of (CD3+, CD8+, CD56+, CD26–) T cells; IP, interferon-inducible protein; I-TAC, interferon-inducible T-cell α chemoattractant; LARC, liver and activation-regulated chemokine; LEC, liver-expressed chemokine; MCP, monocyte chemoattractant protein; MDC, macrophage-derived chemokine, MDC is chemotactic to eosinophils, in a CCR3- and CCR4-independent manner; MEC, mucosae-associated epithelial chemokine; MIG, monokine induced by interferon-γ; MIP, macrophage inflammatory protein; MPIF, myeloid progenitor inhibitory factor; NAP, neutrophil-activating peptide; NK, natural killer; PARC, pulmonary and activation-regulated chemokine; RANTES, regulated on activation, normal T-cell expressed and secreted; SCM, single-C motif; SDF, stromal cell-derived factor; SLC, secondary lymphoid tissue chemokine, also known as exodus-2 and 6Ckine; SR-PSOX, scavenger receptor for phosphatidylserine and oxidized lipoprotein; TARC, thymus and activation-regulated chemokine; TECK, thymus-expressed chemokine; Th2, T-helper cell type 2.

In the marrow, multiple mechanisms act to stabilize and reinforce the lodgment of HSC, that is, to maintain the HSC in niches. One prominent mechanism is the binding of SCF, either secreted in and adherent to the marrow matrix or displayed on stromal cells. The absence of either KIT or SCF results in embryonic failure of hematopoiesis as a result of impaired homing of HSCs to the fetal liver where SCF acts cooperatively with CXCL12 as a chemoattractant, and to impaired retention of HSCs in the marrow[513] where KIT upregulates HSC expression of integrins $\alpha_4\beta_1$ and $\alpha_5\beta_1$.[514] The β_1 integrins of the HSCs also bind osteopontin, which, in turn, is bound to other matrix proteins, such as FN and collagen. Similarly, CD44 on HSCs binds to hyaluronic acid, FN, and collagen the marrow matrix.[164] Two receptors on HSCs that contribute specifically to endosteal niche retention are the calcium-sensing receptor,[515] which is needed for effective binding to collagen, and the Tie family receptor kinases, specifically Tie-2 receptor, which mediates HSC integrin binding to FN after engaging its ligand, angiopoitein-1, that is expressed by osteoblasts.[516,517] Marrow SP cells enriched with long-term repopulating quiescent HSCs display high expression of β_3-integrin, most likely as the vitronectin receptor $\alpha_v\beta_3$, suggesting another integrin–matrix protein interaction that supports HSC retention.[445,518] One mechanism of retention in the endosteal niche is the long-term maintenance of HSCs by TPO produced by adjacent osteoblasts.[519,520] The binding of TPO by its receptor induces HSC quiescence, whereas the absence of TPO leads to active cell cycling and to a protracted and progressive depletion of HSCs.[519,520]

● CELLULAR RELEASE

Cell migration from the marrow occurs between adventitial cells and through endothelial cell channels that develop at the time of cell transit. Electron micrographs of leukocytes partially translocated across endothelium indicate that marked deformation of these cells occurs as they penetrate the cytoplasm of the endothelial cell and enter the sinus lumen (Fig. 5–7).[391] As with reticulocytes, egress occurs adjacent to junctions of endothelial cells.[383] The nucleus of the granulocyte, usually segmented, does not require as marked a deformation to traverse the migration pore as do the nuclei of monocytes and lymphocytes.[391] This transendothelial migration is likely to be related to leukocyte migration from the blood and into areas of inflammation described in the section on adhesion and homing because the marrow sinusoidal endothelial cells constitutively express adhesion proteins that are upregulated in inflammation, including VCAM-1, ICAM-1, and E- and P-selectin.[405] Immature granulocytes in the marrow are anchored to adventitial reticular cells through lectin-like adhesion molecules. Gradual loss of these molecules (e.g., shedding of L-selectin) during maturation or after activation could permit movement toward the sinus wall.[521] Transient changes in surface glycoproteins (upregulation of α-2,6-sialylation of CD11b and CD18) of maturing marrow myeloid cells lead to decreased stromal and FN adhesion and may favor contact with endothelium and cell egress.[522] The complement component C5a and G-CSF administration recruit neutrophils by altering integrins (low CD11a with G-CSF) and decreased L-selectin expression (with both agents).[523,524] Similar findings obtained in mice lacking two or all three selectins underscore the essential role of selectins in neutrophil recruitment.[525] Mature leukocytes retain their nuclei as they enter the marrow venous sinuses and circulate in the blood, but erythroid and megakaryocytic cells release anucleate cells and their residual nuclei are rapidly phagocytosed by marrow macrophages.[94,384,526] Occasional immature granulocytes and megakaryocyte nuclei or whole megakaryocytes are present in cell concentrates of normal blood.[527] Restrictions on the release of immature myeloid cells, erythroblasts, and megakaryocytes are associated with the relative stiffness of their nuclei because of the ratio of nuclear lamin isotypes in erythroid and immature myeloid precursors and increased total lamins in megakaryocytes.[380]

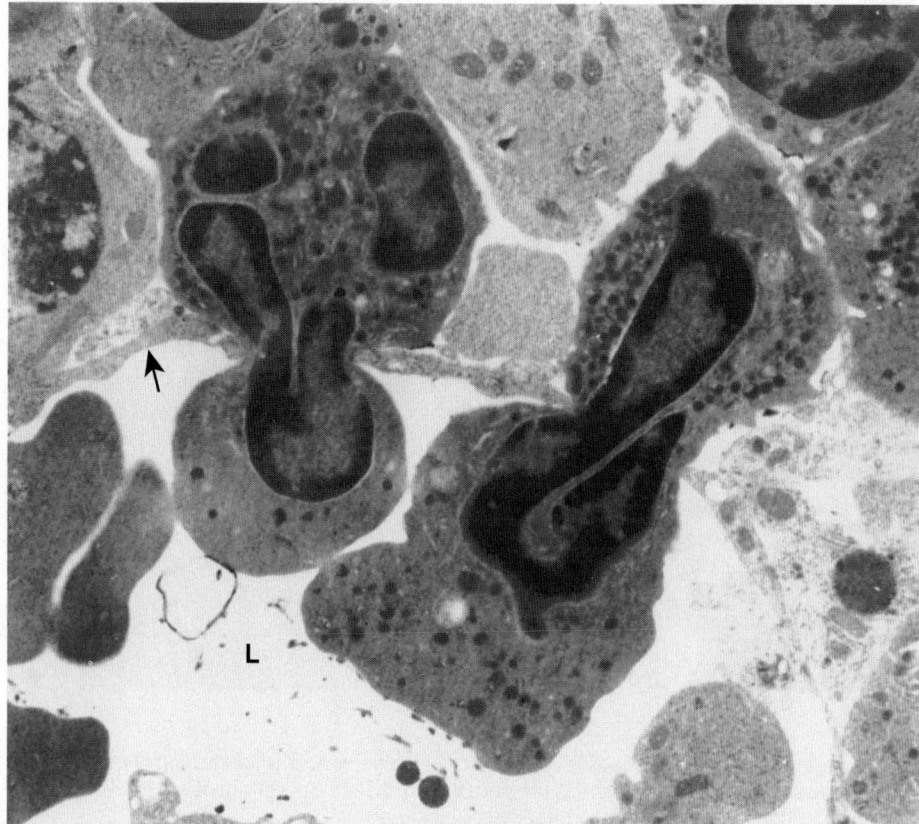

Figure 5–7. Transmission electron micrograph of mouse femoral marrow. The lumen (*L*) of a sinus is indicated. Endothelial cell cytoplasm separates the sinus lumen from the hematopoietic spaces (*arrow*). Two neutrophils are evident traversing the sinus wall. Note deformation of the cell producing a narrow waist where the cell passes through endothelium. The luminal portion of the migrating cells is granule-poor. The remainder of the cytoplasm is granule-rich, possibly reflecting gel-sol transformation during pseudopod formation. (*Used with permission of Lichtman MA, University of Rochester.*)

A number of releasing factors are implicated in the initiation of marrow granulocyte egress, including G-CSF,[528,529] GM-CSF,[530] the C3e component of complement,[531] zymosan-activated plasma-containing complement fragments,[532] glucocorticoid hormones,[533] androgenic steroids,[534] and endotoxin.[535] Neutrophils residing in the marrow venous sinusoids are rapidly released into the circulation by IL-8.[536] In a rat model in which releasing factors can be given through the femoral artery and neutrophils collected from the femoral vein, chemokines CXCL2 (MIP-2) and CXCL1 (KC) that are produced at sites of inflammation induce rapid, selective neutrophil migration from the marrow compartment into the blood.[537,538] Blocking or inhibiting the α_4-integrin component, β_2-integrin component, or the sheddase that catalyzes the proteolysis of L-selectin on migrating HSCs indicates that the interaction of the highly expressed VLA-4 on neutrophils with VCAM-1 on the sinusoidal endothelial cells is required for transendothelial migration, whereas shedding of L-selectin has no effect, and β_2-integrin binding helps retain the neutrophils in the marrow.[537] Blocking the neutrophil enzyme matrix metalloproteinase-9 (MMP-9) had no effect on the chemokine-induced neutrophil migration.[538] CXCL2- and CXCL1-induced migration is synergistic with the rapid, selective neutrophil migration from the marrow induced by G-CSF,[539] which is mediated by interrupting the interaction of CXCL12 in the marrow and CXC4R on neutrophils.[540] In a similar hind-leg model in guinea pigs, IL-5 and eotaxin, both of which are produced in sites of allergic inflammation, induce the rapid, selective migration of eosinophils from the marrow to blood with a synergistic effect when both are administered.[541] CCL11 (eotaxin) alone induces the migration of both eosinophil progenitor cells and mature eosinophils.[541] The route of migration is transendothelial, and blocking experiments demonstrate that β_2-integrin binding enhances eosinophil migration from the marrow to the blood, whereas α_4-integrin binding helps retain eosinophils in the marrow.[542] Prostaglandin D$_2$ (PGD$_2$ is produced by mast cells in sites of allergic inflammation, and it induces rapid, selective migration of eosinophils from the marrow to the blood in the guinea pig model.[543] The eosinophils respond via two PGD$_2$ receptors, chemoattractant receptor-homologous molecule on Th2 (CRHTH2) and D-type prostanoid (DP) receptors.[543]

Releasing factors for reticulocytes have been difficult to identify. Adventitial reticular cell cytoplasm is a barrier to the reticulocytes on the abluminal surface of the endothelium.[544] Phlebotomy, phenylhydrazine-induced hemolytic anemia, and EPO result in marked reduction of the adventitial cell cover of the sinus, a process that is thought to facilitate cell egress through the endothelium.[545] Immature reticulocytes have much less deformability than more mature ones,[546] suggesting that active migration by nascent reticulocytes through the endothelial cells is relatively unlikely, and release is via a passive mechanism. Thus, reticulocytes appear to require a pressure gradient to cross the venous endothelium and enter the blood as shown in Fig. 5–8.[544,545] The pressures within the marrow sinuses are pulsatile, and pressures sufficient to cause egress may be transient.[547] Another force that may contribute to reticulocyte egress is provided by the increasing numbers of erythroblasts proliferating in the EBIs that displace the more mature reticulocytes peripherally toward the venous sinuses.[548]

Platelet release by the megakaryocyte requires both actin-based podosomes and microtubulin-based proplatelets that extend through of the marrow sinus endothelium into the blood as described in the "Megakaryocytes" section of this chapter. The proplatelets can be separated from the megakaryocyte in the marrow, but the fate of these separated proplatelets is not certain, and they may not give rise to platelets.[549] In normal thrombopoiesis, increased concentrations of S-1-P in the circulating blood activate the S-1-P receptor on the megakaryocytes, thereby, promoting proplatelet extension into the vascular sinus.[550] The proplatelets extend through the endothelium (Fig. 5–9) and into the lumen of the venous sinus (see Figs. 5-6 and 5–10) producing elongated bean-shaped proplatelets.[389,391] The formation of platelets also requires S-1-P and its receptor[550] combined with the shear force of the blood flow,[549] which releases both individual platelets or proplatelets themselves that later fragment in the circulation.

Under homeostatic conditions, the migration of HSCs from the marrow into the blood is a rare but steady process.[408,409,551] With the stress of chemotherapeutic agents or pharmacologic doses of G-CSF administration, many HSCs are recruited into active cell cycle,[551] and they migrate into the blood before homing again to the marrow.[408] The

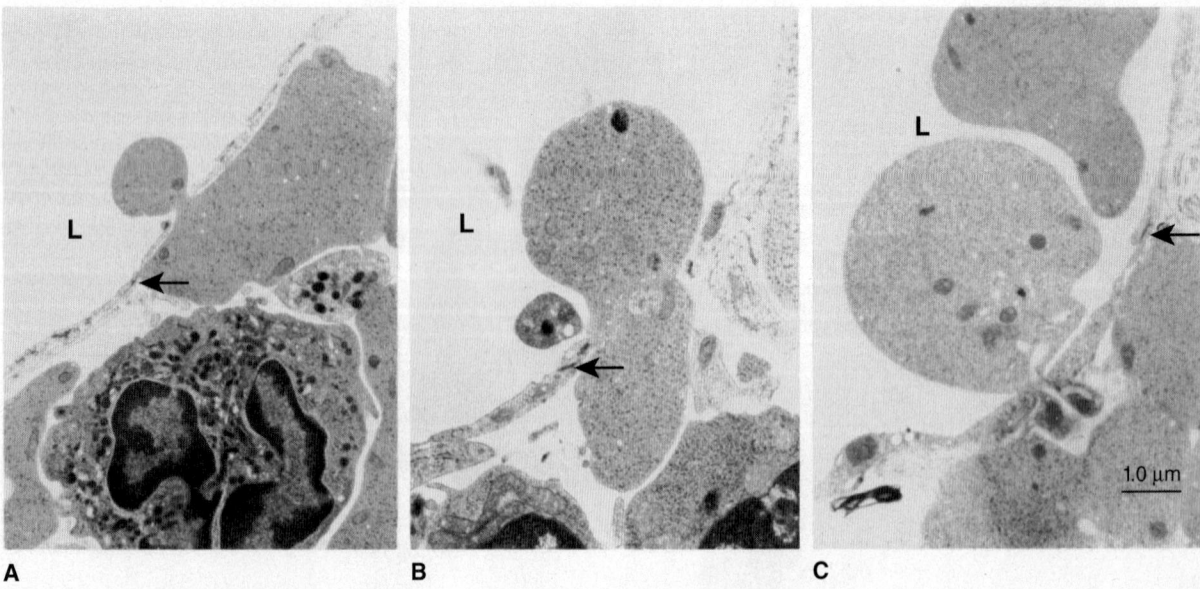

Figure 5–8. Transmission electron micrograph of mouse femoral marrow. Composite of reticulocytes in egress. **A.** Small protrusion of marrow reticulocyte into sinus lumen (*L*). **B.** Reticulocyte in egress, with approximately half the cell in the sinus lumen. **C.** Reticulocyte virtually in the sinus. Egress occurs through a migration pore that is parajunctional in position (*arrows* point to endothelial cell junctions).

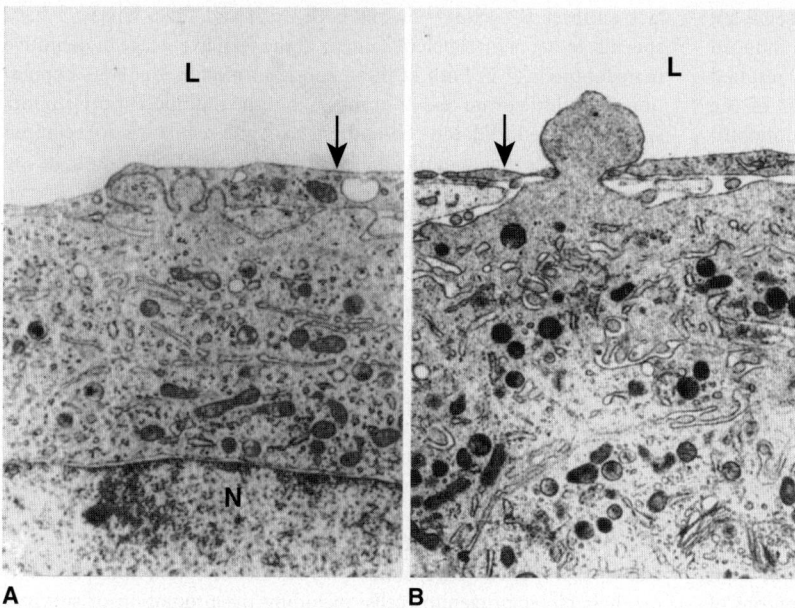

Figure 5–9. Transmission electron micrograph of mouse femoral marrow. **A.** The lumen (*L*) of a marrow sinus is indicated. The *arrow* points to the thin endothelial cytoplasmic lining of the sinus. The nucleus of a megakaryocyte (*N*) is indicated, with the cytoplasm of the megakaryocyte invaginating the endothelial cell cytoplasm in three places below the lumen. **B.** The *arrow* indicates the thin endothelial cell cytoplasmic lining of the sinus. The endothelium is attenuated to a double membrane in two places. A small process of megakaryocyte cytoplasm has formed a pore in the endothelial cell and has entered the sinus lumen (*L*). Cytoplasm flows through such pores and delivers proplatelets to the sinus lumen. *(Used with permission of MA Lichtman, University of Rochester.)*

stress of moderate blood loss also increases the cell cycling of the HSCs, but those cycling HSCs cannot be detected in the blood,[552] indicating that the migration of HSCs in response to stress is very likely related to the inflammatory/injury component of the stress. This relationship between inflammation/injury and HSC migration has been used experimentally to understand the mechanisms of HSC migration into the blood and clinically to mobilize the HSCs into the blood for collection for use in stem cell transplantation. Not surprisingly, these studies demonstrate that much of the regulation of HSC migration involves the reversal or inhibition of the mechanisms by which the HSCs home to the marrow and develop quiescence.

Many hematopoietic growth factors can mobilize HSCs from the marrow to the blood, but the best understood and most used clinically is G-CSF.[480,506,553] Similar to other growth factors, the G-CSF mobilization of HSCs requires several days for maximal effect. A major determinant in both the homing to and migration from the marrow is the interaction of CXCR4 on HSCs with its ligand CXCL12 in the marrow. G-CSF induces stem cell mobilization by decreasing CXCL12 signaling.[554] CXCR4 knockout mice do not mobilize HSCs with G-CSF, but they mobilize HSCs in response to VLA-4 ($\alpha_4\beta_1$ integrin) antagonists.[555] Inhibitor studies originally identified the mobilization mechanism as

the degradation of CXCL12 by neutrophil-associated enzymes such as neutrophil elastase, cathepsin G, and MMP-9 or the HSC enzyme CD26/dipeptidylpeptidase, but mice genetically null for the proteases or treated with other protease inhibitors still show the G-CSF–induced decrease of CXCL12 mRNA and protein.[480,553,556,557] Multiple mechanisms for CXCL12 modulation have been proposed, including the adrenergic nervous system suppressing MSC production of CXCL12 and direct G-CSF suppression of osteoblast lineage cells in the marrow.[140,141,557,558] The successful development of small antagonists of CXCR4, such as plerixafor (formerly AMD3100), has provided a rapid means to mobilize HSCs and is used clinically for those patients that fail to mobilize with G-CSF.[421] Similarly, blocking α_4-integrin binding or genetic deletion of the α_4-integrin component leads to HSC mobilization within 1 or 2 days under both homeostatic or G-CSF–induced conditions.[421] This mobilization appears to be mainly mediated through disruption of VLA-4 activity and is further enhanced by blocking other adhesion mediators such as the β_2-integrins or E-selectin, neither of which has an effect when used alone.[421,559] Some of β_2-integrin's synergistic effects may be indirect through the action on other cells.[560] HSC mobilization with antibodies against the α_4 component of integrin[561] is replicated by potent and selective small molecule antagonists.[562] The results of interfering

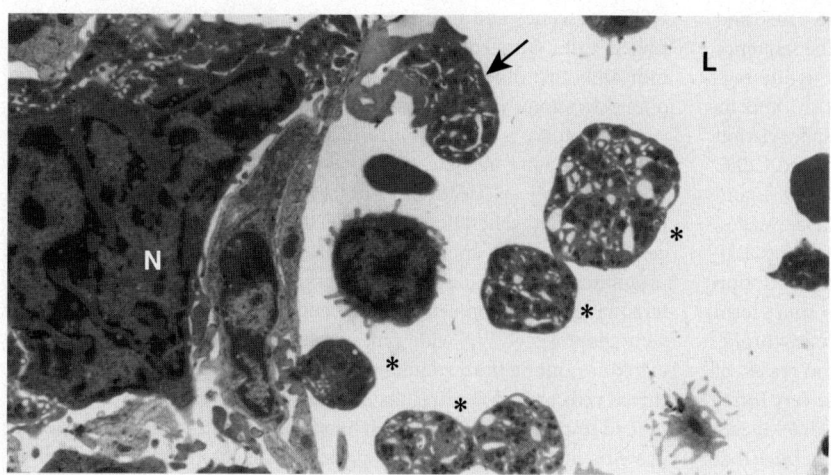

Figure 5–10. Transmission electron micrograph of mouse femoral marrow. The marrow sinus lumen (*L*) and a megakaryocyte nucleus (*N*) virtually denuded of cytoplasm are indicated. The megakaryocyte nucleus abuts the nucleus of an adventitial reticular cell; the latter is separated from the lumen by the very thin endothelial cell cytoplasm. A portion of residual megakaryocyte cytoplasm (proplatelet) can be seen streaming into the lumen *(arrow)*. The lumen contains several proplatelets *(asterisks)*. Compare the size of the proplatelets to that of lymphocyte in the sinus. The bean-shaped, three-dimensional appearance of the proplatelets can be seen in the scanning micrograph shown in Fig. 5–6. *(Used with permission of MA Lichtman, University of Rochester.)*

with two other adhesion mediators of HSC homing, CD44 and SCF, are unclear in that antibodies to CD44 or administration of SCF induced HSC mobilization while genetic deficiencies of CD44 or KIT resulted in decreased G-CSF mobilization.[480] Two chemokine ligands of the CXCR2 receptor, IL-8 and GRO-β (KC in mice), induce HSC mobilization within minutes to hours and can synergize with G-CSF, but their action is more complex in that it is mediated through neutrophils and their enzymes including MMP-9.[480,563]

CELL PROLIFERATION, APOPTOSIS, AND MATURATION

Irrespective of their location during the postnatal period, HSCs undergo continued self-renewal divisions, but at 3 to 4 weeks of age in mice (corresponding to 2 to 4 years in humans), they switch to their characteristic cell-cycle quiescence found in adult HSCs.[564,565] This switch appears to be an intrinsic event that also decreases the myeloid differentiation potential of the HSCs.[564] In the marrow endosteal niche, HSCs have multiple stimuli that induce cell-cycle quiescence. These stimuli include high concentrations of CXCL12 binding CXCR4[499,503]; low concentrations of CD34, podocalyxin, and endoglycan; TPO binding by MPL[519,520]; variable binding to matrix proteins such as osteopontin, FN, and fibulin, that depend upon angiopoietin-1/Tie-2, and SCF/KIT activities.[355,514,516] Compared to HSCs located outside the endosteal niche, HSCs that are closely associated with to the endosteum have greater quiescence, marrow homing, and long-term reconstitution capacity.[566]

In murine transplantation studies, cell-cycle status significantly impacts the rate of engraftment and donor hematopoiesis with HSCs in G_0 phase providing maximal long-term reconstitution, whereas HSCs in G_1, S, G_2, or M phases provide minimal engraftment or long-term reconstitution.[551,564,567] In long-term *in vivo* labeling with bromodeoxyuridine (BrdU), murine HSC immunophenotypically defined as Lin−, Sca-1+, KIT+, CD150+, CD48−, and CD34− have the greatest reconstitution capacity and are located in both endosteal and central areas of the marrow.[551] These HSCs are extremely quiescent, dormant, with an estimated division rate of only four or five times over the life of the adult mouse. However, the large majority of them are able to enter cell cycle and are mobilized within a day or two of stressful stimuli, including G-CSF or 5-fluorouracil (5-FU) administration.[551] Dormancy or quiescence is resumed upon homing and reestablishing marrow residence, indicating that the long-term reconstituting HSCs provide a large reserve that is able to respond, but only under situations of stress.[551]

Dormant or quiescent HSCs are determined to be in G_0 based on lower RNA content and diploid genomic DNA content.[567,568] Entry into the cell cycle induces cells into the G_1 phase where a restriction (R) point is encountered beyond which further progression to S phase and subsequent transit through G_2 to M phases is irreversible. The sequence of events and in particular transit through the R point is tightly regulated by the retinoblastoma tumor-suppressor protein (Rb) and its paralogs (p107, and p130).[569,570] Rb is regulated by phosphorylation that is catalyzed by cyclin-dependent kinases, Cdk2, Cdk4, and Cdk6. Cdk4 and Cdk6 are regulated by D-type cyclins (D1, D2, D3), and Cdk2 is regulated by E-type cyclins (E1 and E2), at early and late stages, respectively, of the G_1 phase. Hyperphosphorylated Rb releases E2F transcription factors that promote entry into S phase by transcription of multiple genes required for replication.[571,572] MPPs, the short-term repopulating cells and the colony-forming unit–granulocyte-erythroid-monocyte-macrophage (CFU-GEMM), have relatively low rates of proliferation, but they are greatly increased compared to the very infrequent cell divisions of HSC. The D cyclins and Cdk4 and Cdk6 kinases are important in these early progenitor cells because knockout mice that lack all three D cyclins[573] or lack both Cdk4 and Cdk6 kinases[574] have specific, lethal hematopoietic failures at the fetal liver stage of definitive hematopoiesis.[572] In both of these knockout models, the HSC populations have little or no loss of numbers, but the multipotent progenitors are severely reduced, indicating these cell cycle regulators are required for the process that commits the HSC to increased proliferation during differentiation.[573,574]

As they divide, MPPs have progressively restricted lineage potential, which is regulated by various transcription factors as described above in the sections on the individual cell types in the marrow. The single-lineage progenitors further increase the percentages of their populations in active cell cycle so that by the later stages of CFU-E, CFC-G, and more mature hematopoietic precursor cell development, the majority are in the S, G_2, and M phases.[575] The two potential sources of extracellular stimuli that increase hematopoietic cell division are soluble hematopoietic cytokines and local interactions of the progenitors with other cells and matrix in the marrow. Hematopoietic cytokines include those produced either in remote organs, such as EPO, or those produced in a wide variety of organs, including the marrow, such as TPO, GM-CSF, and G-CSF.[576] These latter hematopoietic cytokines have multiple effects on their target progenitor cells, including the promotion of survival, maturation, and migration, that are important for the increased production and recruitment of the mature cells to sites of inflammation.[576] Among the cytokines, M-CSF is mitogenic, that is, it promotes progression from G_1 to S phase, in macrophages and their precursors.[577] The signaling from FMS (CSF1R), the M-CSF receptor, which leads to S-phase progression, is mediated by both cyclin D1 and the transcription factor MYC.[578] Among the various cellular interactions of late progenitors and precursors, attachment to central macrophages of EBIs promotes the G_1 to S phase transition in erythroid progenitors/precursors.[378] This mitogenic effect of macrophage-erythroid cell interaction is unrelated to the antiapoptotic effect of EPO on the erythroid cells during these stages of erythroid differentiation.[378]

Mature hematopoietic cells cease cell division prior to their release from the marrow, but the mechanisms that signal cell cycle arrest in hematopoietic cells as they mature are uncertain. Among the potential mediators of this cell-cycle arrest are Rb and several intracellular inhibitors of the cyclin-dependent kinases, specifically the INK4 proteins (p15, p16, p18, p19) that inhibit Cdk4 and Cdk6 and the CIP/KIP family of Cdk2 inhibitors (p21, p27, and p57).[575] Rb knockout mice have a lethal anemia during fetal liver hematopoiesis that is associated with persistent progression through cell cycle, but the erythroblast apoptosis appears to be related to failure of mitochondrial biogenesis.[570] Understanding the activity of p16[INK4a] in regulating cell cycle is complicated by its potential role in senescence and apoptosis of HSC.[579] Although p21 and p27 proteins are proposed as having roles in the TGF-β–induced HSC quiescence and in the increased proliferation of later progenitor stages, Cdk2 knockout mice do not have impaired hematopoiesis,[580] indicating that other cell-cycle mediators are required for the cessation of proliferation that accompanies terminal differentiation.

Apoptosis is the major regulator of cellular populations in the marrow. Because of the exponential expansion of cells in a proliferating population, cell death has a dramatic effect on the numbers of cells in subsequent generations.[581] Thus, the regulation of hematopoietic cell populations by apoptosis provides a mechanism for dramatic and prompt changes in blood cell production. During various stages of differentiation, hematopoietic cells depend upon specific cytokines to prevent apoptosis.[576,581] A wide range of sensitivities to the hematopoietic cytokines among the dependent cells, as has been demonstrated for erythroid cells and EPO,[582] results in differential survival that allows for a graded response. Experiments in knockout mice have identified specific proteins in the Bcl-2 family as principal regulators of the intrinsic or mitochondrial apoptosis pathway in the homeostasis of the hematopoietic cells populations in the marrow.[583,584] Antiapoptotic members of the Bcl-2 family (Bcl-2, Bcl-X$_L$, Mcl-1, and A1) stabilize the mitochondrial membranes by preventing mitochondrial depolarization by the pore-forming family members, Bax and Bak.[585] The antiapoptotic members are also opposed by the proapoptotic, regulatory family members that consist of the BH3-only domain, such as Bim, Bid, Nix, and Puma.

In HSC and multipotent progenitors, Mcl-1 is required to prevent apoptosis, and SCF stimulation increases the Mcl-1 expression.[586,587] In the later stages of single-lineage progenitors, Mcl-1 continues to be required for survival of neutrophil and B and T lymphocytes, but it is antagonized by the expression of Bim and Puma in these progenitors, providing a means to eliminate specific cells, such as autoreactive B and T lymphocytes.[583,584] A1 is required for normal neutrophil survival.[588] In the erythroid lineage, Bcl-X$_L$ is required to prevent apoptosis at the late erythroblast stage,[589] and the proapoptotic Nix protein is also expressed.[590] The sequential proapoptotic and antiapoptotic stimuli that regulate erythropoiesis demonstrate overlapping and cooperative interactions that affect erythroid cell homeostasis by both survival and differentiation. Following moderate blood loss, an increased percentage of HSC enter cell cycle and self-renewal.[552] In the BFU-E through CFU-E stages, SCF and glucocorticoids act in concert to upregulate proliferation according to the erythropoietic requirements.[591] However, because CFU-E depends upon EPO, SCF and EPO act together, enhancing the proliferation and survival, respectively, of CFU-E.[592] EPO prevents apoptosis of CFU-E through basophilic erythroblast stages by decreasing Fas expression,[374,375] but its upregulation of Bcl-X$_L$ prevents the apoptosis of the late-stage hemoglobin-producing erythroblasts.[589] Expression of proapoptotic Nix in very late erythroblasts and reticulocytes plays a major role in targeting mitochondria for nontoxic elimination by autophagy.[593,594]

Various mathematical models have been constructed to explain the production rates for each cell type during homeostasis and during periods of increased and decreased production. A model of homeostatic human marrow has been based upon marrow films and sections relating differential counts of marrow samples to their content of injected radioactive iron. A number of assumptions and approximations are made,[595] but the summary data (Table 5–4) agree well with many other observations on the cellular content and kinetics of normal marrows. Under pathologic conditions such as infection, inflammation, or hematopoietic dysplasia, the proliferation and differentiation of hematopoietic progenitors may be affected by microbial products, cytokines, and cellular interactions that do not have a role in normal hematopoietic development. Infections, for example, can lead to increased myelopoiesis

without the involvement of the hematopoietic cytokines. HSC and their myeloid and lymphoid progeny have multiple toll-like receptors (TLRs) which bind specific bacterial or viral molecules.[596,597] The activation of TLRs leads to increased myelopoietic proliferation and differentiation, especially of the monocyte/macrophage lineage, and differentiation of lymphoid cells toward the dendritic cell phenotype.[596,598] Although increased hematopoietic cytokines are produced by TLR activation, a direct response to TLR activation in hematopoietic cells changes the prevalent myeloid transcription factor from C/EBPα, which mediates homeostasis by hematopoietic cytokines, to C/EBPβ, which mediates the emergency responses to TLR activation.[599] In response to the activation of TLRs, mature neutrophils have decreased apoptosis as a result of increased Mcl-1 and decreased Bad activity.[600] This may be a result of direct ligation of TLR receptors on LT-HSC, ST-HSC, and MPP that are then stimulated to secrete cytokines such as IL-6, GM-CSF, and TNF-α.[601,602] An alternative path to apoptosis in hematopoietic cells is the activation of specific death-domain receptors for the ligands such as FAS ligand, TNF-α, and TRAIL (tumor necrosis factor–related apoptosis-inducing ligand). Although these ligands are most commonly associated with pathologic states where they may play a role in the anemias of chronic disease, they have also been proposed to have a regulatory role in normal erythropoiesis.[603]

REFERENCES

1. Neuman E: Ueber die Bedeutung des Knochenmarks für die Blutbildung. *Cbl Med Wiss* 6:689, 1868.
2. Bizzozero G: Sulla funzione ematopoietica del midollo delle ossa. *Gazz Med Ital Lomb* 1:381, 1868.
3. Neuman E: Du Role de la möelle des os dans la formation du sang. *C R Acad Sci Paris* 68:1112, 1869.
4. Mosler F: Klinische Symptome und Therapie der medullären Leukämie. *Berl Klin Wochenschr* 49:701, 1876.
5. Arinkin MJ: Die intravitale Untersuchungsmethodik des Knochenmarks. *Folia Haematol Int Mag Klin Morphol Blutforsch* 38:233, 1929.
6. Lajatha L: The common ancestral cell, in *Blood Pure and Eloquent*, edited by M Wintrobe, p 81. McGraw-Hill, New York, 1980.
7. Erslev AJ: Feedback circuits in the control of stem cell differentiation. *Am J Pathol* 65:629, 1971.
8. Trentin JJ: Determination of bone marrow stem cell differentiation by stromal hemopoietic inductive microenvironments (HIM). *Am J Pathol* 65:621, 1971.
9. Lemischka IR, Moore KA: Stem cells: Interactive niches. *Nature* 425:778, 2003.
10. Hackney JA, Charbord P, Brunk BP, et al: A molecular profile of a hematopoietic stem cell niche. *Proc Natl Acad Sci U S A* 99:13061, 2002.
11. Zhang J, Niu C, Ye L, et al: Identification of the haematopoietic stem cell niche and control of the niche size. *Nature* 425:836, 2003.
12. Calvi LM, Adams GB, Weibrecht KW, et al: Osteoblastic cells regulate the haematopoietic stem cell niche. *Nature* 425:841, 2003.
13. Weissman IL, Anderson DJ, Gage F: Stem and progenitor cells: Origins, phenotypes, lineage commitments, and transdifferentiations. *Annu Rev Cell Dev Biol* 17:387, 2001.
14. Dao MA, Arevalo J, Nolta JA: Reversibility of CD34 expression on human hematopoietic stem cells that retain the capacity for secondary reconstitution. *Blood* 101:112, 2003.
15. Kuci S, Wessels JT, Buhring HJ, et al: Identification of a novel class of human adherent CD34-stem cells that give rise to SCID-repopulating cells. *Blood* 101:869, 2003.
16. Ziegler BL, Valtieri M, Almeida-Porada G, et al: KDR receptor: A key marker defining hematopoietic stem cells. *Science* 285:1553, 1999.
17. Christensen JL, Weissman IL: Flk-2 is a marker in hematopoietic stem cell differentiation: A simple method to isolate long-term stem cells. *Proc Natl Acad Sci U S A* 98:14541, 2001.
18. Bhatia M: AC133 expression in human stem cells. *Leukemia* 15:1685, 2001.
19. Steidl U, Kronenwett R, Rohr U-P, et al: Gene expression profiling identifies significant differences between the molecular phenotypes of bone marrow-derived and circulating human CD34+ hematopoietic stem cells. *Blood* 99:2037, 2002.
20. Ivanova NB, Dimos JT, Schaniel C, et al: A stem cell molecular signature. *Science* 298:601, 2002.
21. Nadin BM, Goodell MA, Hirschi KK: Phenotype and hematopoietic potential of side population cells throughout embryonic development. *Blood* 102:2436, 2003.
22. Scharenberg CW, Harkey MA, Torok-Storb B: The ABCG2 transporter is an efficient Hoechst 33342 efflux pump and is preferentially expressed by immature human hematopoietic progenitors. *Blood* 99:507, 2002.
23. Pearce DJ, Ridler CM, Simpson C, Bonnet D: Multiparameter analysis of murine bone marrow side population cells. *Blood* 103:2541, 2004.

TABLE 5–4. Normal Precursor Cell Kinetics

Cell Type	Marrow		
	Number (cells/kg)	Transit Time (days)	Production Rate (cells/kg/day)
I. Red cells			
Erythroblasts	5.3×10^9	~5.0	3.0×10^9
Reticulocytes	8.2×10^9	2.8	3.0×10^9
II. Megakaryocytes	15.0×10^6	~7.0	2.0×10^6
III. Granulocytes			
Proliferation pool	2.1×10^9	~5.0	0.85×10^9
Postmitotic pool	5.6×10^9	6.6	0.85×10^9

Reproduced with permission from Finch CA, Harker LA, Cook JD: Kinetics of the formed elements of human blood. *Blood* 50(4): 699–707, 1977.

24. Eaker SS, Hawley TS, Ramezani A, Hawley RG: Detection and enrichment of hematopoietic stem cells by side population phenotype. *Methods Mol Biol* 263:161, 2004.

25. Baron MH: Embryonic origins of mammalian hematopoiesis. *Exp Hematol* 31:1160, 2003.

26. Mikkola HKA, Gekas C, Orkin SH, Dieterlen-Lievre F: Placenta as a site for hematopoietic stem cell development. *Exp Hematol* 33:1048, 2005.

27. Dieterlen-Lievre F: Emergence of haematopoietic stem cells during development. *C R Biol* 330:504, 2007.

28. McGrath K, Palis J: Ontogeny of erythropoiesis in the mammalian embryo. *Curr Top Dev Biol* 82:1, 2008.

29. Migliaccio G, Migliaccio AR, Petti S, et al: Human embryonic hemopoiesis. Kinetics of progenitors and precursors underlying the yolk sac—liver transition. *J Clin Invest* 78:51, 1986.

30. McGrath KE, Frame JM, Fromm GJ, et al: A transient definitive erythroid lineage with unique regulation of the β-globin locus in the mammalian embryo. *Blood* 117:4600, 2011.

31. Ivanovs A, Rybtsov S, Welch L, et al: Highly potent human hematopoietic stem cells first emerge in the intraembryonic aorta-gonad-mesonephros region. *J Exp Med* 208:2417, 2011.

32. Morrison SJ, Hemmati HD, Wandycz AM, Weissman IL: The purification and characterization of fetal liver hematopoietic stem cells. *Proc Natl Acad Sci U S A* 92:10302, 1995.

33. Snyder A, Fraser ST, Baron MH: Bone morphogenetic proteins in vertebrate hematopoietic development. *J Cell Biochem* 93:224, 2004.

34. Durand C, Robin C, Bollerot K, et al: Embryonic stromal clones reveal developmental regulators of definitive hematopoietic stem cells. *Proc Natl Acad Sci U S A* 104:20838, 2007.

35. Nishikawa SI: A complex linkage in the developmental pathway of endothelial and hematopoietic cells. *Curr Opin Cell Biol* 13:673, 2001.

36. Jaffredo T, Nottingham W, Liddiard K, et al: From hemangioblast to hematopoietic stem cell: An endothelial connection? *Exp Hematol* 33:1029, 2005.

37. Zovein AC, Hofmann JJ, Lynch M, et al: Fate tracing reveals the endothelial origin of hematopoietic stem cells. *Cell Stem Cell* 3:625, 2008.

38. Bertrand JY, Chi NC, Santoso B, et al: Haematopoietic stem cells derive directly from aortic endothelium during development. *Nature* 464:108, 2010.

39. Kissa K, Herbomel P: Blood stem cells emerge from aortic endothelium by a novel type of cell transition. *Nature* 464:112, 2010.

40. Boisset J-C, van Cappellen W, Andrieu-Soler C, et al: In vivo imaging of haematopoietic cells emerging from the mouse aortic endothelium. *Nature* 464:116, 2010.

41. Burns CE, Traver D, Mayhall E, et al: Hematopoietic stem cell fate is established by the Notch-Runx pathway. *Genes Dev* 19:2331, 2005.

42. Nakagawa M, Ichikawa M, Kumano K, et al: AML1/Runx1 rescues Notch1-null mutation-induced deficiency of para-aortic splanchnopleural hematopoiesis. *Blood* 108:3329, 2006.

43. Marshall CJ, Sinclair JC, Thrasher AJ, Kinnon C: Bone morphogenetic protein 4 modulates c-Kit expression and differentiation potential in murine embryonic aorta-gonad-mesonephros haematopoiesis in vitro. *Br J Haematol* 139:321, 2007.

44. Robin C, Ottersbach K, Durand C, et al: An unexpected role for IL-3 in the embryonic development of hematopoietic stem cells. *Dev Cell* 11:171, 2006.

45. Almeida-Porada GD, Hoffman R, Manalo P, et al: Detection of human cells in human/sheep chimeric lambs with in vitro human stroma-forming potential. *Exp Hematol* 24:482, 1996.

46. Zanjani ED, Almeida-Porada G, Livingston AG, et al: Reversible expression of CD34 by adult human bone marrow long-term engrafting hematopoietic stem cells. *Exp Hematol* 31:406, 2003.

47. Gallacher L, Murdoch B, Wu DM, et al: Isolation and characterization of human CD34(−)Lin(−) and CD34(+)Lin(−) hematopoietic stem cells using cell surface markers AC133 and CD7. *Blood* 95:2813, 2000.

48. Gehling UM, Ergün S, Schumacher U, et al: In vitro differentiation of endothelial cells from AC133-positive progenitor cells. *Blood* 95:3106, 2000.

49. Takakura N, Watanabe T, Suenobu S, et al: A role for hematopoietic stem cells in promoting angiogenesis. *Cell* 102:199, 2000.

50. Cogle CR, Wainman DA, Jorgensen ML, et al: Adult human hematopoietic cells provide functional hemangioblast activity. *Blood* 103:133, 2004.

51. Bailey AS, Jiang S, Afentoulis M, et al: Transplanted adult hematopoietic stems cells differentiate into functional endothelial cells. *Blood* 103:13, 2004.

52. Kiel MJ, Yilmaz OH, Iwashita T, et al: SLAM family receptors distinguish hematopoietic stem and progenitor cells and reveal endothelial niches for stem cells. *Cell* 121:1109, 2005.

53. Kim I, He S, Yilmaz OH, et al: Enhanced purification of fetal liver hematopoietic stem cells using SLAM family receptors. *Blood* 108:737, 2006.

54. Geiger H, True JM, Grimes B, et al: Analysis of the hematopoietic potential of muscle-derived cells in mice. *Blood* 100:721, 2002.

55. Issarachai S, Priestley GV, Nakamoto B, Papayannopoulou T: Cells with hemopoietic potential residing in muscle are itinerant bone marrow-derived cells. *Exp Hematol* 30:366, 2002.

56. Zipori D: The stem state: Mesenchymal plasticity as a paradigm. *Curr Stem Cell Res Ther* 1:95, 2006.

57. Phinney DG, Prockop DJ: Concise review: Mesenchymal stem/multipotent stromal cells: The state of transdifferentiation and modes of tissue repair—current views. *Stem Cells* 25:2896, 2007.

58. Mazo IB, Massberg S, von Andrian UH: Hematopoietic stem and progenitor cell trafficking. *Trends Immunol* 32:493, 2011.

59. Ciriza J, Thompson H, Petrosian R, et al: The migration of hematopoietic progenitors from the fetal liver to the fetal bone marrow: Lessons learned and possible clinical applications. *Exp Hematol* 41:411, 2013.

60. Christensen JL, Wright DE, Wagers AJ, Weissman IL: Circulation and chemotaxis of fetal hematopoietic stem cells. *PLoS Biol* 2:E75, 2004.

61. Chan CKF, Chen C-C, Luppen CA, et al: Endochondral ossification is required for haematopoietic stem-cell niche formation. *Nature* 457:490, 2009.

62. Chan CKF, Lindau P, Jiang W, et al: Clonal precursor of bone, cartilage, and hematopoietic niche stromal cells. *Proc Natl Acad Sci U S A* 110:12643, 2013.

63. Colnot C, de la Fuente L, Huang S, et al: Indian hedgehog synchronizes skeletal angiogenesis and perichondrial maturation with cartilage development. *Development* 132:1057, 2005.

64. Cecchini MG, Hofstetter W, Halasy J, et al: Role of CSF-1 in bone and bone marrow development. *Mol Reprod Dev* 46:75, 1997.

65. Tavian M, Péault B: The changing cellular environments of hematopoiesis in human development in utero. *Exp Hematol* 33:1062, 2005.

66. Custer RP, Ahlfeldt FE: Studies on the structure and function of the bone marrow. *J Lab Clin Med* 17 951, 1932.

67. Gregersen MI, Rawson RA: Blood volume. *Physiol Rev* 39:307, 1959.

68. Christy M: Active marrow distribution as a function of age in humans. *Phys Med Biol* 26:389, 1981.

69. Babyn PS, Ranson M, McCarville ME: Normal bone marrow: Signal characteristics and fatty conversion. *Magn Reson Imaging Clin N Am* 6:473, 1998.

70. Tuljapurkar SR, McGuire TR, Brusnahan SK, et al: Changes in human bone marrow fat content associated with changes in hematopoietic stem cell numbers and cytokine levels with aging. *J Anat* 219:574, 2011.

71. Huggins C, Blocksom BH: Changes in outlying bone marrow accompanying a local increase of temperature within physiological limits. *J Exp Med* 64:253, 1936.

72. Naveiras O, Nardi V, Wenzel PL, et al: Bone-marrow adipocytes as negative regulators of the haematopoietic microenvironment. *Nature* 460:259, 2009.

73. Brookes M: *The Blood Supply of Bone*. Butterworth, London, 1971.

74. Tavassoli M: Arterial structure of bone marrow in the rabbit with special reference to the thin-walled arteries. *Acta Anat (Basel)* 90:608, 1974.

75. Ellis SL, Grassinger J, Jones A, et al: The relationship between bone, hemopoietic stem cells, and vasculature. *Blood* 118:1516, 2011.

76. Wilkins BS, Jones DB: Vascular networks within the stroma of human long-term bone marrow cultures. *J Pathol* 177:295, 1995.

77. Charbord P, Tavian M, Humeau L, Péault B: Early ontogeny of the human marrow from long bones: An immunohistochemical study of hematopoiesis and its microenvironment. *Blood* 87:4109, 1996.

78. Huber TL, Kouskoff V, Fehling HJ, et al: Haemangioblast commitment is initiated in the primitive streak of the mouse embryo. *Nature* 432:625, 2004.

79. Peichev M, Naiyer AJ, Pereira D, et al: Expression of VEGFR-2 and AC133 by circulating human CD34(+) cells identifies a population of functional endothelial precursors. *Blood* 95:952, 2000.

80. Hildebrand P, Cirulli V, Prinsen RC, et al: The role of angiopoietins in the development of endothelial cells from cord blood CD34+ progenitors. Blood. *Blood* 104:2010, 2004.

81. Wijelath ES, Rahman S, Murray J, et al: Fibronectin promotes VEGF-induced CD34 cell differentiation into endothelial cells. *J Vasc Surg* 39:655, 2004.

82. Schipani E, Maes C, Carmeliet G, Semenza GL: Regulation of osteogenesis-angiogenesis coupling by HIFs and VEGF. *J Bone Miner Res* 24:1347, 2009.

83. Singbrant S, Russell MR, Jovic T, et al: Erythropoietin couples erythropoiesis, B-lymphopoiesis, and bone homeostasis within the bone marrow microenvironment. *Blood* 117:5631, 2011.

84. Lichtman MA: The ultrastructure of the hemopoietic environment of the marrow: A review. *Exp Hematol* 9:391, 1981.

85. Yamazaki K, Allen TD: Ultrastructural morphometric study of efferent nerve terminals on murine bone marrow stromal cells, and the recognition of a novel anatomical unit: The "neuro-reticular complex." *Am J Anat* 187:261, 1990.

86. Pelletier L, Angonin R, Regnard J, et al: Human bone marrow angiogenesis: In vitro modulation by substance P and neurokinin A. *Br J Haematol* 119:1083, 2002.

87. Lichtman MA: The relationship of stromal cells to hemopoietic cells in marrow, in *Long-Term Bone Marrow Culture*, edited by DG Wright, JS Greenberger, p 3. Liss, New York, 1984.

88. Seshi B, Kumar S, Sellers D: Human bone marrow stromal cell: Coexpression of markers specific for multiple mesenchymal cell lineages. *Blood Cells Mol Dis* 26:234, 2000.

89. Mazo IB, Gutierrez-Ramos JC, Frenette PS, et al: Hematopoietic progenitor cell rolling in bone marrow microvessels: Parallel contributions by endothelial selectins and vascular cell adhesion molecule 1. *J Exp Med* 188:465, 1998.

90. Schofield R: The relationship between the spleen colony-forming cell and the haemopoietic stem cell. *Blood Cells* 4:7, 1978.

91. Wang L, Benedito R, Bixel MG, et al: Identification of a clonally expanding haematopoietic compartment in bone marrow. *EMBO J* 32:219, 2013.

92. Ding L, Morrison SJ: Haematopoietic stem cells and early lymphoid progenitors occupy distinct bone marrow niches. *Nature* 495:231, 2013.

93. Takaku T, Malide D, Chen J, et al: Hematopoiesis in 3 dimensions: Human and murine bone marrow architecture visualized by confocal microscopy. *Blood* 116:e41, 2010.

94. Chasis JA, Mohandas N: Erythroblastic islands: Niches for erythropoiesis. *Blood* 112:470, 2008.

95. Sacchetti B, Funari A, Michienzi S, et al: Self-renewing osteoprogenitors in bone marrow sinusoids can organize a hematopoietic microenvironment. *Cell* 131:324, 2007.

96. Serafini M, Sacchetti B, Pievani A, et al: Establishment of bone marrow and hematopoietic niches in vivo by reversion of chondrocyte differentiation of human bone marrow stromal cells. *Stem Cell Res* 12:659, 2014.

97. Ehninger A, Trumpp A: The bone marrow stem cell niche grows up: Mesenchymal stem cells and macrophages move in. *J Exp Med* 208:421, 2011.

98. Nombela-Arrieta C, Pivarnik G, Winkel B, et al: Quantitative imaging of haematopoietic stem and progenitor cell localization and hypoxic status in the bone marrow microenvironment. *Nat Cell Biol* 15:533, 2013.

99. Winkler IG, Barbier V, Wadley R, et al: Positioning of bone marrow hematopoietic and stromal cells relative to blood flow in vivo: Serially reconstituting hematopoietic stem cells reside in distinct nonperfused niches. *Blood* 116:375, 2010.

100. Spencer JA, Ferraro F, Roussakis E, et al: Direct measurement of local oxygen concentration in the bone marrow of live animals. *Nature* 508:269, 2014.

101. Abboud CN, Liesveld JL, Lichtman MA: The architecture of marrow and its role in hematopoietic cell lodgement, in *The Hematopoietic Microenvironment*, edited by MW Long, MS Wicha, p 2. Johns Hopkins University Press, Baltimore, MD, 1993.

102. Tavassoli M, Shaklai M: Absence of tight junctions in endothelium of marrow sinuses: Possible significance for marrow cell egress. *Br J Haematol* 41:303, 1979.

103. Bankston PW, De Bruyn PP: The permeability to carbon of the sinusoidal lining cells of the embryonic rat liver and rat bone marrow. *Am J Anat* 141:281, 1974.

104. Lichtman MA, Packman CH, Constine LS: Molecular and cellular traffic across the marrow sinuses, in *Handbook of the Hemopoietic Microenvironment*, edited by M Tavassoli, p 87. Humana Press, Clifton, NJ, 1989.

105. Hasthorpe S, Bogdanovski M, Rogerson J, Radley JM: Characterization of endothelial cells in murine long-term marrow culture. Implication for hemopoietic regulation. *Exp Hematol* 20:476, 1992.

106. Perkins S, Fleischman RA: Stromal cell progeny of murine bone marrow fibroblast colony-forming units are clonal endothelial-like cells that express collagen IV and laminin. *Blood* 75:620, 1990.

107. van Buul JD, Mul FPJ, van der Schoot CE, Hordijk PL: ICAM-3 activation modulates cell-cell contacts of human bone marrow endothelial cells. *J Vasc Res* 41:28, 2004.

108. Schweitzer KM, Dräger AM, van der Valk P, et al: Constitutive expression of E-selectin and vascular cell adhesion molecule-1 on endothelial cells of hematopoietic tissues. *Am J Pathol* 148:165, 1996.

109. Winkler IG, Barbier V, Nowlan B, et al: Vascular niche E-selectin regulates hematopoietic stem cell dormancy, self renewal and chemoresistance. *Nat Med* 18:1651, 2012.

110. Kataoka M, Tavassoli M: Identification of lectin-like substances recognizing galactosyl residues of glycoconjugates on the plasma membrane of marrow sinus endothelium. *Blood* 65:1163, 1985.

111. Yao L, Yokota T, Xia L, et al: Bone marrow dysfunction in mice lacking the cytokine receptor gp130 in endothelial cells. *Blood* 106:4093, 2005.

112. Guillotin B, Bourget C, Remy-Zolgadri M, et al: Human primary endothelial cells stimulate human osteoprogenitor cell differentiation. *Cell Physiol Biochem* 14:325, 2004.

113. Kobayashi H, Butler JM, O'Donnell R, et al: Angiocrine factors from Akt-activated endothelial cells balance self-renewal and differentiation of haematopoietic stem cells. *Nat Cell Biol* 12:1046, 2010.

114. Maes C: Role and regulation of vascularization processes in endochondral bones. *Calcif Tissue Int* 92:307, 2013.

115. Ding L, Saunders TL, Enikolopov G, Morrison SJ: Endothelial and perivascular cells maintain haematopoietic stem cells. *Nature* 481:457, 2012.

116. Zheng J, Huynh H, Umikawa M, et al: Angiopoietin-like protein 3 supports the activity of hematopoietic stem cells in the bone marrow niche. *Blood* 117:470, 2011.

117. Mohle R, Salemi P, Moore MA, Rafii S: Expression of interleukin-5 by human bone marrow microvascular endothelial cells: Implications for the regulation of eosinophilopoiesis in vivo. *Br J Haematol* 99:732, 1997.

118. Huang WQ, Wang QR: Bone marrow endothelial cells secrete thymosin beta4 and AcS-DKP. *Exp Hematol* 29:12, 2001.

119. Bordenave L, Georges A, Bareille R, et al: Human bone marrow endothelial cells: A new identified source of B-type natriuretic peptide. *Peptides* 23:935, 2002.

120. van Buul JD, Voermans C, van den Berg V, et al: Migration of human hematopoietic progenitor cells across bone marrow endothelium is regulated by vascular endothelial cadherin. *J Immunol* 168:588, 2002.

121. Netelenbos T, van den Born J, Kessler FL, et al: In vitro model for hematopoietic progenitor cell homing reveals endothelial heparan sulfate proteoglycans as direct adhesive ligands. *J Leukoc Biol* 74:1035, 2003.

122. Netelenbos T, van den Born J, Kessler FL, et al: Proteoglycans on bone marrow endothelial cells bind and present SDF-1 towards hematopoietic progenitor cells. *Leukemia* 17:175, 2003.

123. Hillyer P, Mordelet E, Flynn G, Male D: Chemokines, chemokine receptors and adhesion molecules on different human endothelia: Discriminating the tissue-specific functions that affect leucocyte migration. *Clin Exp Immunol* 134:431, 2003.

124. Yun H-J, Jo D-Y: Production of stromal cell-derived factor-1 (SDF-1)and expression of CXCR4 in human bone marrow endothelial cells. *J Korean Med Sci* 18:679, 2003.

125. Imai T, Hieshima K, Haskell C, et al: Identification and molecular characterization of fractalkine receptor CX3CR1, which mediates both leukocyte migration mand adhesion. *Cell* 91:521, 1997.

126. Nitschke L, Floyd H, Ferguson DJ, Crocker PR: Identification of CD22 ligands on bone marrow sinusoidal endothelium implicated in CD22-dependent homing of recirculating B cells. *J Exp Med* 189:1513, 1999.

127. Weiss L, Chen LT: The organization of hemopoietic cords and vascular sinuses in bone marrow. *Blood Cells* 1:617, 1975.

128. Leblond PF, Chamberlain JK, Weed RI: Scanning electron microscopy of erythropoietin-stimulated bone marrow. *Blood Cells* 1:639, 1975.

129. Galmiche MC, Koteliansky VE, Brière J, et al: Stromal cells from human long-term marrow cultures are mesenchymal cells that differentiate following a vascular smooth muscle differentiation pathway. *Blood* 82:66, 1993.

130. Dennis JE, Charbord P: Origin and differentiation of human and murine stroma. *Stem Cells* 20:205, 2002.

131. Weiss L, Geduldig U: Barrier cells: Stromal regulation of hematopoiesis and blood cell release in normal and stressed murine bone marrow. *Blood* 78:975, 1991.

132. Sugiyama T, Kohara H, Noda M, Nagasawa T: Maintenance of the hematopoietic stem cell pool by CXCL12-CXCR4 chemokine signaling in bone marrow stromal cell niches. *Immunity* 25:977, 2006.

133. Pinho S, Lacombe J, Hanoun M, et al: PDGFRalpha and CD51 mark human nestin+ sphere-forming mesenchymal stem cells capable of hematopoietic progenitor cell expansion. *J Exp Med* 210:1351, 2013.

134. Greenbaum A, Hsu YM, Day RB, et al: CXCL12 in early mesenchymal progenitors is required for haematopoietic stem-cell maintenance. *Nature* 495:227, 2013.

135. Omatsu Y, Sugiyama T, Kohara H, et al: The essential functions of adipo-osteogenic progenitors as the hematopoietic stem and progenitor cell niche. *Immunity* 33:387, 2010.

136. Omatsu Y, Seike M, Sugiyama T, et al: Foxc1 is a critical regulator of haematopoietic stem/progenitor cell niche formation. *Nature* 508:536, 2014.

137. Nagasawa T, Omatsu Y, Sugiyama T: Control of hematopoietic stem cells by the bone marrow stromal niche: The role of reticular cells. *Trends Immunol* 32:315, 2011.

138. Mendez-Ferrer S, Michurina TV, Ferraro F, et al: Mesenchymal and haematopoietic stem cells form a unique bone marrow niche. *Nature* 466:829, 2010.

139. Afan AM, Broome CS, Nicholls SE, et al: Bone marrow innervation regulates cellular retention in the murine haemopoietic system. *Br J Haematol* 98:569, 1997.

140. Mendez-Ferrer S, Lucas D, Battista M, Frenette PS: Haematopoietic stem cell release is regulated by circadian oscillations. *Nature* 452:442, 2008.

141. Katayama Y, Battista M, Kao W-M, et al: Signals from the sympathetic nervous system regulate hematopoietic stem cell egress from bone marrow. *Cell* 124:407, 2006.

142. Yamazaki S, Ema H, Karlsson G, et al: Nonmyelinating Schwann cells maintain hematopoietic stem cell hibernation in the bone marrow niche. *Cell* 147:1146, 2011.

143. Tavassoli M: Fatty evolution of marrow and the role of adipose tissue in hematopoiesis, in *Handbook of the Hemopoietic Microenvironment*, edited by M Tavassoli, p 157. Humana Press, Clifton, NJ, 1989.

144. Sadie-Van Gijsen H, Hough FS, Ferris WF: Determinants of bone marrow adiposity: The modulation of peroxisome proliferator-activated receptor-gamma2 activity as a central mechanism. *Bone* 56:255, 2013.

145. Nuttall ME, Shah F, Singh V, et al: Adipocytes and the regulation of bone remodeling: A balancing act. *Calcif Tissue Int* 94:78, 2014.

146. Krings A, Rahman S, Huang S, et al: Bone marrow fat has brown adipose tissue characteristics, which are attenuated with aging and diabetes. *Bone* 50:546, 2012.

147. Poloni A, Maurizi G, Serrani F, et al: Molecular and functional characterization of human bone marrow adipocytes. *Exp Hematol* 41:558, 2013.

148. Corre J, Planat-Benard V, Corberand JX, et al: Human bone marrow adipocytes support complete myeloid and lymphoid differentiation from human CD34 cells. *Br J Haematol* 127:344, 2004.

149. Miller SC, de Saint-Georges L, Bowman BM, Jee WS: Bone lining cells: Structure and function. *Scanning Microsc* 3:953, 1989.

150. Bianco P: Bone and the hematopoietic niche: A tale of two stem cells. *Blood* 117:5281, 2011.

151. Sillaber C, Walchshofer S, Mosberger I, et al: Immunophenotypic characterization of human bone marrow endosteal cells. *Tissue Antigens* 53:559, 1999.

152. Long MW, Robinson JA, Ashcraft EA, Mann KG: Regulation of human bone marrow-derived osteoprogenitor cells by osteogenic growth factors. *J Clin Invest* 95:881, 1995.

153. Gronthos S, Zannettino AC, Graves SE, et al: Differential cell surface expression of the STRO-1 and alkaline phosphatase antigens on discrete developmental stages in primary cultures of human bone cells. *J Bone Miner Res* 14:47, 1999.

154. Moerman EJ, Teng K, Lipschitz DA, Lecka-Czernik B: Aging activates adipogenic and suppresses osteogenic programs in mesenchymal marrow stroma/stem cells: The role of PPAR-gamma2 transcription factor and TGF-beta/BMP signaling pathways. *Aging Cell* 3:379, 2004.

155. Hanada K, Dennis JE, Caplan AI: Stimulatory effects of basic fibroblast growth factor and bone morphogenetic protein-2 on osteogenic differentiation of rat bone marrow-derived mesenchymal stem cells. *J Bone Miner Res* 12:1606, 1997.

156. Blanquaert F, Delany AM, Canalis E: Fibroblast growth factor-2 induces hepatocyte growth factor/scatter factor expression in osteoblasts. *Endocrinology* 140:1069, 1999.

157. Grano M, Galimi F, Zambonin G, et al: Hepatocyte growth factor is a coupling factor for osteoclasts and osteoblasts in vitro. *Proc Natl Acad Sci U S A* 93:7644, 1996.

158. Yin JJ, Mohammad KS, Käkönen SM, et al: A causal role for endothelin-1 in the pathogenesis of osteoblastic bone metastases. *Proc Natl Acad Sci U S A* 100:10954, 2003.

159. Erlebacher A, Filvaroff EH, Ye JQ, Derynck R: Osteoblastic responses to TGF-beta during bone remodeling. *Mol Biol Cell* 9:1903, 1998.

160. Nakashima K, Zhou X, Kunkel G, et al: The novel zinc finger-containing transcription factor osterix is required for osteoblast differentiation and bone formation. *Cell* 108:17, 2002.

161. Taichman RS, Emerson SG: The role of osteoblasts in the hematopoietic microenvironment. *Stem Cells* 16:7, 1998.

162. Ahmed N, Khokher MA, Hassan HT: Cytokine-induced expansion of human CD34+ stem/progenitor and CD34+CD41+ early megakaryocytic marrow cells cultured on normal osteoblasts. *Stem Cells* 17:92, 1999.

163. Robey PG, Young MF, Flanders KC, et al: Osteoblasts synthesize and respond to transforming growth factor-type beta (TGF-beta) in vitro. *J Cell Biol* 105:457, 1987.

164. Haylock DN, Nilsson SK: Osteopontin: A bridge between bone and blood. *Br J Haematol* 134:467, 2006.

165. Frisch BJ, Porter RL, Calvi LM: Hematopoietic niche and bone meet. *Curr Opin Support Palliat Care* 2:211, 2008.

166. Civitelli R, Beyer EC, Warlow PM, et al: Connexin43 mediates direct intercellular communication in human osteoblastic cell networks. *J Clin Invest* 91:1888, 1993.

167. Dorshkind K, Green L, Godwin A, Fletcher WH: Connexin-43-type gap junctions mediate communication between bone marrow stromal cells. *Blood* 82:38, 1993.

168. Montecino-Rodriguez E, Leathers H, Dorshkind K: Expression of connexin 43(Gx43) is critical for normal hematopoiesis. *Blood* 96:917, 2000.

169. Visnjic D, Kalajzic Z, Rowe DW, et al: Hematopoiesis is severely altered in mice with an induced osteoblast deficiency. *Blood* 103:3258, 2004.

170. Nakashima T, Hayashi M, Fukunaga T, et al: Evidence for osteocyte regulation of bone homeostasis through RANKL expression. *Nat Med* 17:1231, 2011.

171. van Bezooijen RL, Roelen BA, Visser A, et al: Sclerostin is an osteocyte-expressed negative regulator of bone formation, but not a classical BMP antagonist. *J Exp Med* 199:805, 2004.

172. Fulzele K, Krause DS, Panaroni C, et al: Myelopoiesis is regulated by osteocytes through Gsalpha-dependent signaling. *Blood* 121:930, 2013.

173. Matayoshi A, Brown C, DiPersio JF, et al: Human blood-mobilized hematopoietic precursors differentiate into osteoclasts in the absence of stromal cells. *Proc Natl Acad Sci U S A* 93:10785, 1996.

174. Edwards CM, Mundy GR: Eph receptors and ephrin signaling pathways: A role in bone homeostasis. *Int J Med Sci* 5:263, 2008.

175. Askmyr MK, Fasth A, Richter J: Towards a better understanding and new therapeutics of osteopetrosis. *Br J Haematol* 140:597, 2008.

176. Calle Y, Jones GE, Jagger C, et al: WASp deficiency in mice results in failure to form osteoclast sealing zones and defects in bone resorption. *Blood* 103:3552, 2004.

177. Horowitz MC, Lorenzo JA: The origins of osteoclasts. *Curr Opin Rheumatol* 16:464, 2004.

178. Dai X-M, Zong X-H, Sylvestre V, Stanley ER: Incomplete restoration of colony-stimulating factor 1 (CSF-1) function in CSF-1-deficient Csf1op/Csf1op mice by transgenic expression of cell surface CSF-1. *Blood* 103:1114, 2004.

179. Asagiri M, Takayanagi H: The molecular understanding of osteoclast differentiation. *Bone*. 40:251, 2007.

180. Udagawa N, Takahashi N, Yasuda H, et al: Osteoprotegerin produced by osteoblasts is an important regulator in osteoclast development and function. *Endocrinology* 141:3478, 2000.

181. Domon T, Yamazaki Y, Fukui A, et al: Ultrastructural study of cell-cell interaction between osteoclasts and osteoblasts/stroma cells in vitro. *Ann Anat* 184:221, 2002.

182. Takahashi N, Udagawa N, Suda T: A new member of tumor necrosis factor ligand family, ODF/OPGL/TRANCE/RANKL, regulates osteoclast differentiation and function. *Biochem Biophys Res Commun* 256:449, 1999.

183. Shalhoub V, Faust J, Boyle WJ, et al: Osteoprotegerin and osteoprotegerin ligand effects on osteoclast formation from human peripheral blood mononuclear cell precursors. *J Cell Biochem* 72:251, 1999.

184. Zhao C, Irie N, Takada Y, et al: Bidirectional ephrinB2-EphB4 signaling controls bone homeostasis. *Cell Metab* 4:111, 2006.

185. Jimi E, Nakamura I, Amano H, et al: Osteoclast function is activated by osteoblastic cells through a mechanism involving cell-to-cell contact. *Endocrinology* 137:2187, 1996.

186. Mbalaviele G, Nishimura R, Myoi A, et al: Cadherin-6 mediates the heterotypic interactions between the hemopoietic osteoclast cell lineage and stromal cells in a murine model of osteoclast differentiation. *J Cell Biol* 141:1467, 1998.

187. Hayashi S, Miyake K, Kincade PW: The CD9 molecule on stromal cells. *Leuk Lymphoma* 38:265, 2000.

188. Oritani K, Wu X, Medina K, et al: Antibody ligation of CD9 modifies production of myeloid cells in long-term cultures. *Blood* 87:2252, 1996.

189. Tanio Y, Yamazaki H, Kunisada T, et al: CD9 molecule expressed on stromal cells is involved in osteoclastogenesis. *Exp Hematol* 27:853, 1999.

190. Iwama A, Yamaguchi N, Suda T: STK/RON receptor tyrosine kinase mediates both apoptotic and growth signals via the multifunctional docking site conserved among the HGF receptor family. *EMBO J* 15:5866, 1996.

191. Kurihara N, Tatsumi J, Arai F, et al: Macrophage-stimulating protein (MSP) and its receptor, RON, stimulate human osteoclast activity but not proliferation: Effect of MSP distinct from that of hepatocyte growth factor. *Exp Hematol* 26:1080, 1998.

192. Choi SJ, Han JH, Roodman GD: ADAM8: A novel osteoclast stimulating factor. *J Bone Miner Res* 16:814, 2001.

193. Oba Y, Chung HY, Choi SJ, Roodman GD: Eosinophil chemotactic factor-L (ECF-L): A novel osteoclast stimulating factor. *J Bone Miner Res* 18:1332, 2003.

194. Crocker PR, Morris L, Gordon S: Novel cell surface adhesion receptors involved in interactions between stromal macrophages and haematopoietic cells. *J Cell Sci Suppl* 9:185, 1988.

195. Sapoznikov A, Pewzner-Jung Y, Kalchenko V, et al: Perivascular clusters of dendritic cells provide critical survival signals to B cells in bone marrow niches. *Nat Immunol* 9:388, 2008.

196. Ye M, Graf T: Early decisions in lymphoid development. *Curr Opin Immunol* 19:123, 2007.

197. Ichii M, Shimazu T, Welner RS, et al: Functional diversity of stem and progenitor cells with B-lymphopoietic potential. *Immunol Rev* 237:10, 2010.

198. Panaroni C, Wu JY: Interactions between B lymphocytes and the osteoblast lineage in bone marrow. *Calcif Tissue Int* 93:261, 2013.

199. Tokoyoda K, Egawa T, Sugiyama T, et al: Cellular niches controlling B lymphocyte behavior within bone marrow during development. *I Immunity.* 20:707, 2004.

200. Di Rosa F, Pabst R: The bone marrow: A nest for migratory memory T cells. *Trends Immunol* 26:360, 2005.

201. Tsuji JM, Pollack SB: Maturation of murine natural killer precursor cells in the absence of exogenous cytokines requires contact with bone marrow stroma. *Nat Immunol* 14:44, 1995.

202. Yu H, Fehniger TA, Fuchshuber P, et al: Flt3 ligand promotes the generation of a distinct CD34(+) human natural killer cell progenitor that responds to interleukin-15. *Blood* 92:3647, 1998.

203. Burkett PR, Koka R, Chien M, et al: Coordinate expression and trans presentation of interleukin (IL)-15Ralpha and IL-15 supports natural killer cell and memory CD8+ T cell homeostasis. *J Exp Med* 200:825, 2004.

204. Fairfax KA, Kallies A, Nutt SL, Tarlinton DM: Plasma cell development: From B-cell subsets to long-term survival niches. *Semin Immunol* 20:49, 2008.

205. Varol C, Yona S, Jung S: Origins and tissue-context-dependent fates of blood monocytes. *Immunol Cell Biol* 87:30, 2009.

206. Pettit AR, Chang MK, Hume DA, Raggatt LJ: Osteal macrophages: A new twist on coupling during bone dynamics. *Bone* 43:976, 2008.

207. Baldus SE, Wickenhauser C, Stefanovic A, et al: Enrichment of human bone marrow mononuclear phagocytes and characterization of macrophage subpopulations by immunoenzymatic double staining. *Histochem J* 30:285, 1998.

208. Wijffels JF, de Rover Z, Kraal G, Beelen RH: Macrophage phenotype regulation by colony-stimulating factors at bone marrow level. *J Leukoc Biol* 53:249, 1993.

209. Shima M, Teitelbaum SL, Holers VM, et al: Et al: Macrophage-colony-stimulating factor regulates expression of the integrins alpha 4, beta 1 and alpha 5, beta 1 by murine marrow macrophages. *Proc Natl Acad Sci U S A* 92:5179, 1995.

210. Dannaeus K, Johannisson A, Nilsson K, Jönsson JI: Flt3 ligand induces the outgrowth of Mac-1+B220+ mouse bone marrow progenitor cells restricted to macrophage differentiation that coexpress early B cell-associated genes. *Exp Hematol* 27:1646, 1999.

211. Wright EG, Pragnell IB: Stem cell proliferation inhibitors. *Baillieres Clin Haematol* 5:723, 1992.

212. Su S, Mukaida N, Wang J, et al: Inhibition of immature erythroid progenitor cell proliferation by macrophage inflammatory protein-1alpha by interacting mainly with a C-C chemokine receptor, CCR1. *Blood* 90:605, 1997.

213. Jacobsen SE, Ruscetti FW, Dubois CM, Keller JR: Tumor necrosis factor alpha directly and indirectly regulates hematopoietic progenitor cell proliferation: Role of colony-stimulating factor receptor modulation. *J Exp Med* 175:1759, 1992.

214. Yan XQ, Brady G, Iscove NN: Platelet-derived growth factor (PDGF) activates primitive hematopoietic precursors (pre-CFCmulti) by up-regulating IL-1 in PDGF receptor-expressing macrophages. *J Immunol* 150:2440, 1993.

215. Lerat H, Lissitzky JC, Singer JW, et al: Role of stromal cells and macrophages in fibronectin biosynthesis and matrix assembly in human long-term marrow cultures. *Blood* 82:1480, 1993.

216. Chow A, Lucas D, Hidalgo A, et al: Bone marrow CD169+ macrophages promote the retention of hematopoietic stem and progenitor cells in the mesenchymal stem cell niche. *J Exp Med* 208:261, 2011.

217. Chow A, Huggins M, Ahmed J, et al: CD169(+) macrophages provide a niche promoting erythropoiesis under homeostasis and stress. *Nat Med* 19:429, 2013.

218. Klein G: The extracellular matrix of the hematopoietic microenvironment. *Experientia* 51:914, 1995.

219. Bentley SA, Tralka TS: Fibronectin-mediated attachment of hematopoietic cells to stromal elements in continuous bone marrow culture. *Exp Hematol* 11:129, 1983.

220. Campbell AD, Long MW, Wicha MS: Haemonectin, a bone marrow adhesion protein specific for cells of granulocyte lineage. *Nature* 329:744, 1987.

221. Lawler J: The structural and functional properties of thrombospondin. *Blood* 67:1197, 1986.

222. Simmons PJ, Levesque JP, Zannettino AC: Adhesion molecules in haemopoiesis. *Baillieres Clin Haematol* 10:485, 1997.

223. Verfaille CM: Adhesion receptors as regulators of the hematopoietic process. *Blood* 92:2609, 1998.

224. Broxmeyer HE, Kim CH: Regulation of hematopoiesis in a sea of chemokine family members with a plethora of redundant activities. *Exp Hematol* 27:1113, 1999.

225. Coombe DR: Biological implications of glycosaminoglycan interactions with haemopoietic cytokines. *Immunol Cell Biol* 86:598, 2008.

226. Hoogewerf AJ, Kuschert GS, Proudfoot AE, et al: Glycosaminoglycans mediate cell surface oligomerization of chemokines. *Biochemistry* 36:13570, 1997.

227. Luster AD, Greenberg SM, Leder P: The IP-10 chemokine binds to a specific cell surface heparan sulfate site shared with platelet factor 4 and inhibits endothelial cell proliferation. *J Exp Med* 182:219, 1995.

228. Tanaka Y, Adams DH, Hubscher S, et al: T-cell adhesion induced by proteoglycan-immobilized cytokine MIP-1 beta. *Nature* 361:79, 1993.

229. Chakravarty L, Rogers L, Quach T, et al: Lysine 58 and histidine 66 at the C-terminal alpha-helix of monocyte chemoattractant protein-1 are essential for glycosaminoglycan binding. *J Biol Chem* 273:29641, 1998.

230. Spillman D, Witt D, Lindahl U: Defining the interleukin-8-binding domain of heparan sulfate. *J Biol Chem* 273:15487, 1998.

231. Koopman W, Ediriwickrema C, Krangel MS: Structure and function of the glycosaminoglycan binding site of chemokine macrophage-inflammatory protein-1 beta. *J Immunol* 163:2120, 1999.

232. Amara A, Lorthioir O, Valenzuela A, et al: Stromal cell derived factor-1 alpha associates with heparan sulfates through the first beta-strand of the chemokine. *J Biol Chem* 274:23916, 1999.

233. Wolff EA, Greenfield B, Taub DD, et al: Generation of artificial proteoglycans containing glycosaminoglycan-modified CD44. Demonstration of the interaction between rantes and chondroitin sulfate. *J Biol Chem* 274:2518, 1999.

234. Lipscombe RJ, Nakhoul AM, Sanderson CJ, Coombe DR: Interleukin-5 binds to heparin/heparan sulfate. A model for an interaction with extracellular matrix. *J Leukoc Biol* 63:342, 1998.

235. Borghesi LA, Yamashita Y, Kincade PW: Heparan sulfate proteoglycans mediate interleukin-7-dependent B lymphopoiesis. *Blood* 93:140, 1999.

236. Lyon M, Deakin JA, Mizuno K, et al: Interaction of hepatocyte growth factor with heparan sulfate. Elucidation of the major heparan sulfate structural determinants. *J Biol Chem* 269:11216, 1994.

237. Kiefer MC, Stephans JC, Crawford K, et al: Ligand-affinity cloning and structure of a cell surface heparan sulfate proteoglycan that binds basic fibroblast growth factor. *Proc Natl Acad Sci U S A* 87:6985, 1990.

238. Robledo MM, Ursa MA, Sánchez-Madrid F, Teixidó J: Associations between TGF-beta1 receptors in human bone marrow stromal cells. *Br J Haematol* 102:804, 1998.

239. Shin JW, Buxboim A, Spinler KR, et al: Contractile forces sustain and polarize hematopoiesis from stem and progenitor cells. *Cell Stem Cell* 14:81, 2014.

240. Engler AJ, Sen S, Sweeney HL, Discher DE: Matrix elasticity directs stem cell lineage specification. *Cell* 126:677, 2006.

241. Holst J, Watson S, Lord MS, et al: Substrate elasticity provides mechanical signals for the expansion of hemopoietic stem and progenitor cells. *Nat Biotechnol* 28:1123, 2010.

242. Wight TN, Kinsella MG, Keating A, Singer JW: Proteoglycans in human long-term bone marrow cultures: Biochemical and ultrastructural analyses. *Blood* 67:1333, 1986.

243. Allen TD, Dexter TM, Simmons PJ: Marrow biology and stem cells. *Immunol Ser* 49:1, 1990.

244. Yurchenco PD, Schittny JC: Molecular architecture of basement membranes. *FASEB J* 4:1577, 1990.

245. Keating A, Gordon MY: Hierarchical organization of hematopoietic microenvironments: Role of proteoglycans. *Leukemia* 2:766, 1988.

246. Gordon MY, Riley GP, Clarke D: Heparan sulfate is necessary for adhesive interactions between human early hemopoietic progenitor cells and the extracellular matrix of the marrow microenvironment. *Leukemia* 2:804, 1988.

247. Bruno E, Luikart SD, Long MW, Hoffman R: Marrow-derived heparan sulfate proteoglycan mediates the adhesion of hematopoietic progenitor cells to cytokines. *Exp Hematol* 23:1212, 1995.

248. Minguell JJ, Hardy C, Tavassoli M: Membrane-associated chondroitin sulfate proteoglycan and fibronectin mediate the binding of hemopoietic progenitor cells to stromal cells. *Exp Cell Res* 201:200, 1992.

249. Han ZC, Bellucci S, Shen ZX, et al: Glycosaminoglycans enhance megakaryocytopoiesis by modifying the activities of hematopoietic growth regulators. *J Cell Physiol* 168:97, 1996.

250. Gordon MY, Lewis JL, Marley SB, et al: Stromal cells negatively regulate primitive haemopoietic progenitor cell activation via a phosphatidylinositol-anchored cell adhesion/signalling mechanism. *Br J Haematol* 96:647, 1997.

251. Mazzon C, Anselmo A, Cibella J, et al: The critical role of agrin in the hematopoietic stem cell niche. *Blood* 118:2733, 2011.

252. Mazzon C, Anselmo A, Soldani C, et al: Agrin is required for survival and function of monocytic cells. *Blood* 119:5502, 2012.

253. Lewinsohn DM, Nagler A, Ginzton N, et al: Hematopoietic progenitor cell expression of the H-CAM (CD44) homing-associated adhesion molecule. *Blood* 75:589, 1990.

254. Legras S, Levesque JP, Charrad R, et al: CD44-mediated adhesiveness of human hematopoietic progenitors to hyaluronan is modulated by cytokines. *Blood* 89:1905, 1997.

255. Jalkanen S, Jalkanen M: Lymphocyte CD44 binds the COOH-terminal heparin-binding domain of fibronectin. *J Cell Biol* 116:817, 1992.

256. Miyake K, Medina KL, Hayashi S, et al: Monoclonal antibodies to Pgp-1/CD44 block lympho-hemopoiesis in long-term bone marrow cultures. *J Exp Med* 171:477, 1990.

257. Rachmilewitz J, Tykocinski ML: Differential effects of chondroitin sulfates A and B on monocyte and B-cell activation: Evidence for B-cell activation via a CD44-dependent pathway. *Blood* 92:223, 1998.

258. Khaldoyanidi S, Moll J, Karakhanova S, et al: Hyaluronate-enhanced hematopoiesis: Two different receptors trigger the release of interleukin-1beta and interleukin-6 from bone marrow macrophages. *Blood* 94:940, 1999.

259. Sackstein R: Expression of an L-selectin ligand on hematopoietic progenitor cells. *Acta Haematol* 97:22, 1997.

260. Sternberg D, Peled A, Shezen E, et al: Control of stroma-dependent hematopoiesis by basic fibroblast growth factor: Stromal phenotypic plasticity and modified myelopoietic functions. *Cytokines Mol Ther* 2:29, 1996.

261. Weimar IS, Miranda N, Muller EJ, et al: Hepatocyte growth factor/scatter factor (HGF/SF) is produced by human bone marrow stromal cells and promotes proliferation, adhesion and survival of human hematopoietic progenitor cells (CD34+). *Exp Hematol* 26:885, 1998.

262. Pivak-Kroizman T, Lemmon MA, Dikic I, et al: Heparin-induced oligomerization of FGF molecules is responsible for FGF receptor dimerization, activation, and cell proliferation. *Cell* 79:1015, 1994.

263. Ratajczak MZ, Ratajczak J, Skorska M, et al: Effect of basic (FGF-2) and acidic (FGF-1) fibroblast growth factors on early haemopoietic cell development. *Br J Haematol* 93:772, 1996.

264. Schofield KP, Gallagher JT, David G: Expression of proteoglycan core proteins in human bone marrow stroma. *Biochem J* 343 Pt 3:663, 1999.

265. Klein G, Conzelmann S, Beck S, et al: Perlecan in human bone marrow: A growth-factor-presenting, but anti-adhesive, extracellular matrix component for hematopoietic cells. *Matrix Biol* 14:457, 1995.

266. Drzeniek Z, Stöcker G, Siebertz B, et al: Heparan sulfate proteoglycan expression is induced during early erythroid differentiation of multipotent hematopoietic stem cells. *Blood* 93:2884, 1999.

267. Siebertz B, Stöcker G, Drzeniek Z, et al: Expression of glypican-4 in haematopoietic-progenitor and bone-marrow-stromal cells. *Biochem J* 344:937, 1999.

268. Reijmers RM, Spaargaren M, Pals ST: Heparan sulfate proteoglycans in the control of B cell development and the pathogenesis of multiple myeloma. *FEBS J* 280:2180, 2013.

269. Oritani K, Kincade PW: Identification of stromal cell products that interact with pre-B cells. *J Cell Biol* 134:771, 1996.

270. Yamashita Y, Oritani K, Miyoshi EK, et al: Syndecan-4 is expressed by B lineage lymphocytes and can transmit a signal for formation of dendritic processes. *J Immunol* 162:5940, 1999.

271. Longley RL, Woods A, Fleetwood A, et al: Control of morphology, cytoskeleton and migration by syndecan-4. *J Cell Sci* 112:3421, 1999.

272. Zuckerman KS, Wicha MS: Extracellular matrix production by the adherent cells of long-term murine bone marrow cultures. *Blood* 61:540, 1983.

273. Sorrel JM: Ultrastructural localization of fibronectin in bone marrow of the embryonic chick and its relationship to granulopoiesis. *Cell Tissue Res* 252:565, 1988.

274. Vuillet-Gaugler MH, Breton-Gorius J, Vainchenker W, et al: Loss of attachment to fibronectin with terminal human erythroid differentiation. *Blood* 75:865, 1990.

275. Rosemblatt M, Vuillet-Gaugler MH, Leroy C, Coulombel L: Coexpression of two fibronectin receptors, VLA-4 and VLA-5, by immature human erythroblastic precursor cells. *J Clin Invest* 87:6, 1991.

276. Liesveld JL, Winslow JM, Kempski MC, et al: Adhesive interactions of normal and leukemic human CD34+ myeloid progenitors: Role of marrow stromal, fibroblast, and cytomatrix components. *Exp Hematol* 19:63, 1991.

277. Williams DA, Rios M, Stephens C, Patel VP: Fibronectin and VLA-4 in haematopoietic stem cell-microenvironment interactions. *Nature* 352:438, 1991.

278. Schofield KP, Humphries MJ: Identification of fibronectin IIICS variants in human bone marrow stroma. *Blood* 93:410, 1999.

279. Verfaillie CM, Benis A, Iida J, et al: Adhesion of committed human hematopoietic progenitors to synthetic peptides from the C-terminal heparin-binding domain of fibronectin: Cooperation between the integrin alpha 4 beta 1 and the CD44 adhesion receptor. *Blood* 84:1802, 1994.

280. Hassan HT, Sadovnikova E, Drize NJ, et al: Fibronectin increases both non-adherent cells and CFU-GM while collagen increases adherent cells in human normal long-term bone marrow cultures. *Haematologia (Budap)* 28:77, 1997.

281. Yokota T, Oritani K, Mitsui H, et al: Growth-supporting activities of fibronectin on hematopoietic stem/progenitor cells in vitro and in vivo: Structural requirement for fibronectin activities of CS1 and cell-binding domains. *Blood* 91:3263, 1998.

282. Hurley RW, McCarthy JB, Verfaillie CM: Direct adhesion to bone marrow stroma via fibronectin receptors inhibits hematopoietic progenitor proliferation. *J Clin Invest* 96:511, 1995.

283. Goltry KL, Patel VP: Specific domains of fibronectin mediate adhesion and migration of early murine erythroid progenitors. *Blood* 90:138, 1997.

284. van der Loo JC, Xiao X, McMillin D, et al: VLA-5 is expressed by mouse and human long-term repopulating hematopoietic cells and mediates adhesion to extracellular matrix protein fibronectin. *J Clin Invest* 102:1051, 1998.

285. Schofield KP, Rushton G, Humphries MJ, et al: Influence of interleukin-3 and other growth factors on alpha4beta1 integrin-mediated adhesion and migration of human hematopoietic progenitor cells. *Blood* 90:1858, 1997.

286. Levesque JP, Haylock DN, Simmons PJ: Cytokine regulation of proliferation and cell adhesion are correlated events in human CD34+ hemopoietic progenitors. *Blood* 88:1168, 1996.

287. Cui L, Ramsfjell V, Borge OJ, et al: Thrombopoietin promotes adhesion of primitive human hemopoietic cells to fibronectin and vascular cell adhesion molecule-1: Role of activation of very late antigen (VLA)-4 and VLA-5. *J Immunol* 159:1961, 1997.

288. Schofield KP, Humphries MJ, de Wynter E, et al: The effect of alpha4 beta1-integrin binding sequences of fibronectin on growth of cells from human hematopoietic progenitors. *Blood* 91:3230, 1998.

289. Spring FA, Griffiths RE, Mankelow TJ, et al: Tetraspanins CD81 and CD82 facilitate alpha4beta1-mediated adhesion of human erythroblasts to vascular cell adhesion molecule-1. *PLoS One* 8:e62654, 2013.

290. Malara A, Gruppi C, Rebuzzini P, et al: Megakaryocyte-matrix interaction within bone marrow: New roles for fibronectin and factor XIII-A. *Blood* 117:2476, 2011.

291. Xie B, Laouar A, Huberman E: Fibronectin-mediated cell adhesion is required for induction of 92-kDa type IV collagenase/gelatinase (MMP-9) gene expression during macrophage differentiation. The signaling role of protein kinase C-beta. *J Biol Chem* 273:11576, 1998.

292. Kremlev SG, Chapoval AI, Evans R: Cytokine release by macrophages after interacting with CSF-1 and extracellular matrix proteins: Characteristics of a mouse model of inflammatory responses in vitro. *Cell Immunol* 185:59, 1998.

293. Yonezawa I, Kato K, Yagita H, et al: VLA-5-mediated interaction with fibronectin induces cytokine production by human chondrocytes. *Biochem Biophys Res Commun* 219:261, 1996.

294. Chiquet-Ehrismann R, Matsuoka Y, Hofer U, et al: Tenascin variants: Differential binding to fibronectin and distinct distribution in cell cultures and tissues. *Cell Regul* 2:927, 1991.

295. Seiffert M, Beck SC, Schermutzki F, et al: Mitogenic and adhesive effects of tenascin-C on human hematopoietic cells are mediated by various functional domains. *Matrix Biol* 17:47, 1998.

296. Ohta M, Sakai T, Saga Y, et al: Suppression of hematopoietic activity in tenascin-C-deficient mice. *Blood* 91:4074, 1998.

297. Nakamura-Ishizu A, Okuno Y, Omatsu Y, et al: Extracellular matrix protein tenascin-C is required in the bone marrow microenvironment primed for hematopoietic regeneration. *Blood* 119:5429, 2012.

298. Mackie EJ, Tucker RP: The tenascin-C knockout revisited. *J Cell Sci* 112:3847, 1999.

299. Bentley SA: Collagen synthesis by bone marrow stromal cells: A quantitative study. *Br J Haematol* 50:491, 1982.

300. Mori M, Sadahira Y, Kawasaki S, et al: Formation of capillary networks from bone marrow cultured in collagen gel. *Cell Struct Funct* 14:393, 1989.

301. Zuckerman KS, Rhodes RK, Goodrum DD, et al: Inhibition of collagen deposition in the extracellular matrix prevents the establishment of a stroma supportive of hematopoiesis in long-term murine bone marrow cultures. *J Clin Invest* 75:970, 1985.

302. Leisten I, Kramann R, Ventura Ferreira MS, et al: 3D co-culture of hematopoietic stem and progenitor cells and mesenchymal stem cells in collagen scaffolds as a model of the hematopoietic niche. *Biomaterials* 33:1736, 2012.

303. Chichester CO, Fernández M, Minguell JJ: Extracellular matrix gene expression by human bone marrow stroma and by marrow fibroblasts. *Cell Adhes Commun* 1:93, 1993.

304. Klein G, Muller CA, Tillet E, et al: Collagen type VI in the human bone marrow microenvironment: A strong cytoadhesive component. *Blood* 86:1740, 1995.

305. Koenigsmann M, Griffin JD, DiCarlo J, Cannistra SA: Myeloid and erythroid progenitor cells from normal bone marrow adhere to collagen type I. *Blood* 79:657, 1992.

306. Klein G, Kibler C, Schermutzki F, et al: Cell binding properties of collagen type XIV for human hematopoietic cells. *Matrix Biol* 16:307, 1998.

307. Nilsson SK, Debatis ME, Dooner MS, et al: Immunofluorescence characterization of key extracellular matrix proteins in murine bone marrow in situ. *J Histochem Cytochem* 46:371, 1998.

308. Malara A, Gruppi C, Pallotta I, et al: Extracellular matrix structure and nano-mechanics determine megakaryocyte function. *Blood* 118:4449, 2011.

309. Abbonante V, Gruppi C, Rubel D, et al: Discoidin domain receptor 1 protein is a novel modulator of megakaryocyte-collagen interactions. *J Biol Chem* 288:16738, 2013.

310. Kleinman HK, Weeks BS: Laminin: Structure, functions and receptors. *Curr Opin Cell Biol* 1:964, 1989.

311. Senior RM, Gresham HD, Griffin GL, et al: Entactin stimulates neutrophil adhesion and chemotaxis through interactions between its Arg-Gly-Asp (RGD) domain and the leukocyte response integrin. *J Clin Invest* 90:2251, 1992.

312. Bryant G, Rao CN, Brentani M, et al: A role for the laminin receptor in leukocyte chemotaxis. *J Leukoc Biol* 41:220, 1987.

313. Lundgren-Akerlund E, Olofsson AM, Berger E, Arfors KE: CD11b/CD18-dependent polymorphonuclear leucocyte interaction with matrix proteins in adhesion and migration. *Scand J Immunol* 37:569, 1993.

314. Gu YC, Kortesmaa J, Tryggvason K, et al: Laminin isoform-specific promotion of adhesion and migration of human bone marrow progenitor cells. *Blood* 101:877, 2003.

315. Tobias JW, Bern MM, Netland PA, Zetter BR: Monocyte adhesion to subendothelial components. *Blood* 69:1265, 1987.

316. Bohnsack JF: CD11/CD18-independent neutrophil adherence to laminin is mediated by the integrin VLA-6. *Blood* 79:1545, 1992.

317. Bohnsack JF, Akiyama SK, Damsky CH, et al: Human neutrophil adherence to laminin in vitro. Evidence for a distinct neutrophil integrin receptor for laminin. *J Exp Med* 171:1221, 1990.

318. Gu Y, Sorokin L, Durbeej M, et al: Characterization of bone marrow laminins and identification of alpha5-containing laminins as adhesive proteins for multipotent hematopoietic FDCP-Mix cells. *Blood* 93:2533, 1999.

319. Vogel W, Kanz L, Brugger W, et al: Expression of laminin beta2 chain in normal human bone marrow. *Blood* 94:1143, 1999.

320. Siler U, Rousselle P, Muller CA, Klein G: Laminin gamma2 chain as a stromal cell marker of the human bone marrow microenvironment. *Br J Haematol* 119:212, 2002.

321. Qian H, Tryggvason K, Jacobsen SE, Ekblom M: Contribution of alpha6 integrins to hematopoietic stem and progenitor cell homing to bone marrow and collaboration with alpha4 integrins. *Blood* 107:3503, 2006.

322. Selleri C, Ragno P, Ricci P, et al: The metastasis-associated 67-kDa laminin receptor is involved in G-CSF-induced hematopoietic stem cell mobilization. *Blood* 108:2476, 2006.

323. Bonig H, Chang K-H, Nakamoto B, Papayannopoulou T: The p67 laminin receptor identifies human erythroid progenitor and precursor cells and is functionally important for their bone marrow lodgment. *Blood* 108:1230, 2006.

324. El Nemer W, Gane P, Colin Y, et al: The Lutheran blood group glycoproteins, the erythroid receptors for laminin, are adhesion molecules. *J Biol Chem* 273:16686, 1998.

325. Ohki K, Kohashi O: Laminin promotes proliferation of bone marrow-derived macrophages and macrophage cell lines. *Cell Struct Funct* 19:63, 1994.

326. Fehlner-Gardiner C, Uniyal S, von Ballestrem C, et al: Integrin VLA-6 (alpha 6 beta 1) mediates adhesion of mouse bone marrow-derived mast cells to laminin. *Allergy* 51:650, 1996.

327. Bornstein P: Thrombospondins as matricellular modulators of cell function. *J Clin Invest* 107:929, 2001.

328. Long MW, Dixit VM: Thrombospondin functions as a cytoadhesion molecule for human hematopoietic progenitor cells. *Blood* 75:2311, 1990.

329. Crawford SE, Stellmach V, Murphy-Ullrich JE, et al: Thrombospondin-1 is a major activator of TGF-beta1 in vivo. *Cell* 93:1159, 1998.

330. Pierson BA, Gupta K, Hu WS, Miller JS: Human natural killer cell expansion is regulated by thrombospondin-mediated activation of transforming growth factor-beta 1 and independent accessory cell-derived contact and soluble factors. *Blood* 87:180, 1996.

331. Delany AM, Hankenson KD: Thrombospondin-2 and SPARC/osteonectin are critical regulators of bone remodeling. *J Cell Commun Signal* 3:227, 2009.

332. Bailey Dubose K, Zayzafoon M, Murphy-Ullrich JE: Thrombospondin-1 inhibits osteogenic differentiation of human mesenchymal stem cells through latent TGF-beta activation. *Biochem Biophys Res Commun* 422:488, 2012.

333. Li WX, Howard RJ, Leung LL: Identification of SVTCG in thrombospondin as the conformation-dependent, high affinity binding site for its receptor, CD36. *J Biol Chem* 268:16179, 1993.

334. Calvo D, Vega MA: Identification, primary structure, and distribution of CLA-1, a novel member of the CD36/LIMPII gene family. *J Biol Chem* 268:18929, 1993.

335. Nakahata T, Okumura N: Cell surface antigen expression in human erythroid progenitors: Erythroid and megakaryocytic markers. *Leuk Lymphoma* 13:401, 1994.

336. Qian X, Wang TN, Rothman VL, et al: Thrombospondin-1 modulates angiogenesis in vitro by up-regulation of matrix metalloproteinase-9 in endothelial cells. *Exp Cell Res* 235:403, 1997.

337. Mansfield PJ, Suchard SJ: Thrombospondin promotes chemotaxis and haptotaxis of human peripheral blood monocytes. *J Immunol* 153:4219, 1994.

338. Taraboletti G, Belotti D, Borsotti P, et al: The 140-kilodalton antiangiogenic fragment of thrombospondin-1 binds to basic fibroblast growth factor. *Cell Growth Differ* 8:471, 1997.

339. Margosio B, Marchetti D, Vergani V, et al: Thrombospondin 1 as a scavenger for matrix-associated fibroblast growth factor 2. *Blood* 102:4399, 2003.

340. Kyriakides TR, Rojnuckarin P, Reidy MA, et al: Megakaryocytes require thrombospondin-2 for normal platelet formation and function. *Blood* 101:3915, 2003.

341. Sadvakassova G, Dobocan MC, Difalco MR, Congote LF: Regulator of differentiation 1 (ROD1) binds to the amphipathic C-terminal peptide of thrombospondin-4 and is involved in its mitogenic activity. *J Cell Physiol* 220:672, 2009.

342. Leavesley DI, Kashyap AS, Croll T, et al: Vitronectin—master controller or micromanager? *IUBMB Life* 65:807, 2013.

343. Boissy P, Machuca I, Pfaff M, et al: Aggregation of mononucleated precursors triggers cell surface expression of alphavbeta3 integrin, essential to formation of osteoclast-like multinucleated cells. *J Cell Sci* 111:2563, 1998.

344. Mbalaviele G, Jaiswal N, Meng A, et al: Human mesenchymal stem cells promote human osteoclast differentiation from CD34+ bone marrow hematopoietic progenitors. *Endocrinology* 140:3736, 1999.

345. Poujol C, Nurden AT, Nurden P: Ultrastructural analysis of the distribution of the vitronectin receptor (alpha v beta 3) in human platelets and megakaryocytes reveals an intracellular pool and labelling of the alpha-granule membrane. *Br J Haematol* 96:823, 1997.

346. Shimizu Y, Irani AM, Brown EJ, et al: Human mast cells derived from fetal liver cells cultured with stem cell factor express a functional CD51/CD61 (alpha v beta 3) integrin. *Blood* 86:930, 1995.

347. Weerasinghe D, McHugh KP, Ross FP, et al: A role for the alphavbeta3 integrin in the transmigration of monocytes. *J Cell Biol* 142:595, 1998.

348. Rainger GE, Buckley CD, Simmons DL, Nash GB: Neutrophils sense flow-generated stress and direct their migration through alphaVbeta3-integrin. *Am J Physiol* 276:H858, 1999.

349. Savill J, Hogg N, Ren Y, Haslett C: Thrombospondin cooperates with CD36 and the vitronectin receptor in macrophage recognition of neutrophils undergoing apoptosis. *J Clin Invest* 90:1513, 1992.

350. Fadok VA, Warner ML, Bratton DL, Henson PM: CD36 is required for phagocytosis of apoptotic cells by human macrophages that use either a phosphatidylserine receptor or the vitronectin receptor (alpha v beta 3). *J Immunol* 161:6250, 1998.

351. Rubartelli A, Poggi A, Zocchi MR: The selective engulfment of apoptotic bodies by dendritic cells is mediated by the alpha(v)beta3 integrin and requires intracellular calcium and extracellular calcium. *Eur J Immunol* 27:1893, 1997.

352. Zheng X, Saunders TL, Camper SA, et al: Vitronectin is not essential for normal mammalian development and fertility. *Proc Natl Acad Sci U S A* 92:12426, 1995.

353. Jang YC, Tsou R, Gibran NS, Isik FF: Vitronectin deficiency is associated with increased wound fibrinolysis and decreased microvascular angiogenesis in mice. *Surgery* 127:696, 2000.

354. Nilsson SK, Johnston HM, Whitty GA, et al: Osteopontin, a key component of the hematopoietic stem cell niche and regulator of primitive hematopoietic progenitor cells. *Blood* 106:1232, 2005.

355. Stier S, Ko Y, Forkert R, et al: Osteopontin is a hematopoietic stem cell niche component that negatively regulates stem cell pool size. *J Exp Med* 201:1781, 2005.

356. Grassinger J, Haylock DN, Storan MJ, et al: Thrombin-cleaved osteopontin regulates hemopoietic stem and progenitor cell functions through interactions with alpha9beta1 and alpha4beta1 integrins. *Blood* 114:49, 2009.

357. Kang JA, Zhou Y, Weis TL, et al: Osteopontin regulates actin cytoskeleton and contributes to cell proliferation in primary erythroblasts. *J Biol Chem* 283:6997, 2008.

358. Chung JW, Kim MS, Piao ZH, et al: Osteopontin promotes the development of natural killer cells from hematopoietic stem cells. *Stem Cells* 26:2114, 2008.

359. Diao H, Iwabuchi K, Li L, et al: Osteopontin regulates development and function of invariant natural killer T cells. *Proc Natl Acad Sci U S A* 105:15884, 2008.

360. Gu YC, Nilsson K, Eng H, Ekblom M: Association of extracellular matrix proteins fibulin-1 and fibulin-2 with fibronectin in bone marrow stroma. *Br J Haematol* 109:305, 2000.

361. Hergeth SP, Aicher WK, Essl M, et al: Characterization and functional analysis of osteoblast-derived fibulins in the human hematopoietic stem cell niche. *Exp Hematol* 36:1022, 2008.

362. Mancini E, Sanjuan-Pla A, Luciani L, et al: FOG-1 and GATA-1 act sequentially to specify definitive megakaryocytic and erythroid progenitors. *EMBO J* 31:351, 2012.

363. Siatecka M, Bieker JJ: The multifunctional role of EKLF/KLF1 during erythropoiesis. *Blood* 118:2044, 2011.

364. Gregory CJ, Eaves AC: Human marrow cells capable of erythropoietic differentiation in vitro: Definition of three erythroid colony responses. *Blood* 49:855, 1977.

365. Porcu S, Manchinu MF, Marongiu MF, et al: Klf1 affects DNase II-alpha expression in the central macrophage of a fetal liver erythroblastic island: A non-cell-autonomous role in definitive erythropoiesis. *Mol Cell Biol* 31:4144, 2011.

366. Xue L, Galdass M, Gnanapragasam MN, et al: Extrinsic and intrinsic control by EKLF (KLF1) within a specialized erythroid niche. *Development* 141:2245, 2014.

367. Socolovsky M, Nam H, Fleming MD, et al: Ineffective erythropoiesis in Stat5a(−/−)5b(−/−) mice due to decreased survival of early erythroblasts. *Blood* 98:3261, 2001.

368. Chen K, Liu J, Heck S, et al: Resolving the distinct stages in erythroid differentiation based on dynamic changes in membrane protein expression during erythropoiesis. *Proc Natl Acad Sci U S A* 106:17413, 2009.

369. Hu J, Liu J, Xue F, et al: Isolation and functional characterization of human erythroblasts at distinct stages: Implications for understanding of normal and disordered erythropoiesis in vivo. *Blood* 121:3246, 2013.

370. Koury MJ: Abnormal erythropoiesis and the pathophysiology of chronic anemia. *Blood Rev* 28:49, 2014.

371. Panzenbock B, Bartunek P, Mapara MY, Zenke M: Growth and differentiation of human stem cell factor/erythropoietin-dependent erythroid progenitor cells in vitro. *Blood* 92:3658, 1998.

372. Bauer A, Tronche F, Wessely O, et al: The glucocorticoid receptor is required for stress erythropoiesis. *Genes Dev* 13:2996, 1999.

373. Millot S, Andrieu V, Letteron P, et al: Erythropoietin stimulates spleen BMP4-dependent stress erythropoiesis and partially corrects anemia in a mouse model of generalized inflammation. *Blood* 116:6072, 2010.

374. Rubiolo C, Piazzolla D, Meissl K, et al: A balance between Raf-1 and Fas expression sets the pace of erythroid differentiation. *Blood* 108:152, 2006.

375. Liu Y, Pop R, Sadegh C, et al: Suppression of Fas-FasL coexpression by erythropoietin mediates erythroblast expansion during the erythropoietic stress response in vivo. *Blood* 108:123, 2006.

376. De Maria R, Testa U, Luchetti L, et al: Apoptotic role of Fas/Fas ligand system in the regulation of erythropoiesis. *Blood* 93:796, 1999.

377. Koulnis M, Porpiglia E, Porpiglia PA, et al: Contrasting dynamic responses in vivo of the Bcl-xL and Bim erythropoietic survival pathways. *Blood* 119:1228, 2012.

378. Rhodes MM, Kopsombut P, Bondurant MC, et al: Adherence to macrophages in erythroblastic islands enhances erythroblast proliferation and increases erythrocyte production by a different mechanism than erythropoietin. *Blood* 111:1700, 2008.

379. Popova EY, Krauss SW, Short SA, et al: Chromatin condensation in terminally differentiating mouse erythroblasts does not involve special architectural proteins but depends on histone deacetylation. *Chromosome Res* 17:47, 2009.

380. Shin JW, Spinler KR, Swift J, et al: Lamins regulate cell trafficking and lineage maturation of adult human hematopoietic cells. *Proc Natl Acad Sci U S A* 110:18892, 2013.

381. Koury ST, Koury MJ, Bondurant MC: Cytoskeletal distribution and function during the maturation and enucleation of mammalian erythroblasts. *J Cell Biol* 109:3005, 1989.

382. Ubukawa K, Guo YM, Takahashi M, et al: Enucleation of human erythroblasts involves non-muscle myosin IIB. *Blood* 119:1036, 2012.

383. Lichtman MA, Waugh RE: Red cell egress from the marrow: Ultrastructural and biophysical aspects, in *Regulation of Erythropoiesis* edited by ED Zanjani, M Tavassoli, J Ascencao, p 15. PMA Literary and Film Management, Great Neck, NY, 1989.

384. Yoshida H, Kawane K, Koike M, et al: Phosphatidylserine-dependent engulfment by macrophages of nuclei from erythroid precursor cells. *Nature* 437:754, 2005.

385. Kawane K, Fukuyama H, Kondoh G, et al: Requirement of DNase II for definitive erythropoiesis in the mouse fetal liver. *Science* 292:1546, 2001.

386. Deutsch VR, Tomer A: Advances in megakaryocytopoiesis and thrombopoiesis: From bench to bedside. *Br J Haematol* 161:778, 2013.

387. Hitchcock IS, Kaushansky K: Thrombopoietin from beginning to end. *Br J Haematol* 165:259, 2014.

388. Scheding S, Bergmann M, Shimosaka A, et al: Human plasma thrombopoietin levels are regulated by binding to platelet thrombopoietin receptors in vivo. *Transfusion* 42:321, 2002.

389. Machlus KR, Italiano JE Jr: The incredible journey: From megakaryocyte development to platelet formation. *J Cell Biol* 201:785, 2013.

390. Lordier L, Bluteau D, Jalil A, et al: RUNX1-induced silencing of non-muscle myosin heavy chain IIB contributes to megakaryocyte polyploidization. *Nat Commun* 3:717, 2012.

391. Lichtman MA, Chamberlain JK, Simon W, Santillo PA: Parasinusoidal location of megakaryocytes in marrow: A determinant of platelet release. *Am J Hematol* 4:303, 1978.

392. Wu Y, Welte T, Michaud M, Madri JA: PECAM-1: A multifaceted regulator of megakaryocytopoiesis. *Blood* 110:851, 2007.

393. Dhanjal TS, Pendaries C, Ross EA, et al: A novel role for PECAM-1 in megakaryocytokinesis and recovery of platelet counts in thrombocytopenic mice. *Blood* 109:4237, 2007.

394. Pitchford SC, Lodie T, Rankin SM: VEGFR1 stimulates a CXCR4-dependent translocation of megakaryocytes to the vascular niche, enhancing platelet production in mice. *Blood* 120:2787, 2012.

395. Schachtner H, Calaminus SD, Sinclair A, et al: Megakaryocytes assemble podosomes that degrade matrix and protrude through basement membrane. *Blood* 121:2542, 2013.

396. Lambertsen RH, Weiss L: A model of intramedullary hematopoietic microenvironments based on stereologic study of the distribution of endocloned marrow colonies. *Blood* 63:287, 1984.

397. Rosenbauer F, Tenen DG: Transcription factors in myeloid development: Balancing differentiation with transformation. *Nat Rev Immunol* 7:105, 2007.

398. Rosmarin AG, Yang Z, Resendes KK: Transcriptional regulation in myelopoiesis: Hematopoietic fate choice, myeloid differentiation, and leukemogenesis. *Exp Hematol* 33:131, 2005.

399. Iwasaki H, Akashi K: Myeloid lineage commitment from the hematopoietic stem cell. *Immunity* 26:726, 2007.

400. Hock H, Orkin SH: Zinc-finger transcription factor Gfi-1 Versatile regulator of lymphocytes, neutrophils and hematopoietic stem cells. *Curr Opin Hematol* 13.1:1, 2006.

401. Friedman AD: Transcriptional control of granulocyte and monocyte development. *Oncogene* 26:6816, 2007.

402. Mori Y, Iwasaki H, Kohno K, et al: Identification of the human eosinophil lineage-committed progenitor: Revision of phenotypic definition of the human common myeloid progenitor. *J Exp Med* 206:183, 2009.

403. Rosenberg HF, Phipps S, Foster PS: Eosinophil trafficking in allergy and asthma. *J Allergy Clin Immunol* 119:1303, 2007.

404. Christopher MJ, Link DC: Regulation of neutrophil homeostasis. *Curr Opin Hematol* 14:3, 2007.

405. Furze RC, Rankin SM: Neutrophil mobilization and clearance in the bone marrow. *Immunology* 125:281, 2008.

406. Stark MA, Huo Y, Burcin TL, et al: Phagocytosis of apoptotic neutrophils regulates granulopoiesis via IL-23 and IL-17. *Immunity* 22:285, 2005.

407. Wright DE, Wagers AJ, Gulati AP, et al: Physiological migration of hematopoietic stem and progenitor cells. *Science* 294:1933, 2001.

408. Abkowitz JL, Robinson AE, Kale S, et al: Mobilization of hematopoietic stem cells during homeostasis and after cytokine exposure. *Blood* 102:1249, 2003.

409. Massberg S, Schaerli P, Knezevic-Maramica I, et al: Immunosurveillance by hematopoietic progenitor cells trafficking through blood, lymph, and peripheral tissues. *Cell* 131:994, 2007.

410. Kerst JM, Sanders JB, Slaper-Cortenbach IC, et al: Alpha 4 beta 1 and alpha 5 beta 1 are differentially expressed during myelopoiesis and mediate the adherence of human CD34+ cells to fibronectin in an activation-dependent way. *Blood* 81:344, 1993.

411. Hynes RO: Integrins: Versatility, modulation, and signaling in cell adhesion. *Cell* 69:11, 1992.

412. Hynes RO: Integrins: Bidirectional, allosteric signaling machines. *Cell* 110:673, 2002.

413. Naito K, Tamahashi N, Chiba T, et al: The microvasculature of the human bone marrow correlated with the distribution of hematopoietic cells. A computer-assisted three-dimensional reconstruction study. *Tohoku J Exp Med* 166:439, 1992.

414. Driessen RL, Johnston HM, Nilsson SK: Membrane-bound stem cell factor is a key regulator in the initial lodgment of stem cells within the endosteal marrow region. *Exp Hematol* 31:1284, 2003.

415. Ihanus E, Uotila LM, Toivanen A, et al: Red-cell ICAM-4 is a ligand for the monocyte/macrophage integrin CD11c/CD18: Characterization of the binding sites on ICAM-4. *Blood* 109:802, 2007.

416. Kishimoto TK, Baldwin ET, Anderson DC: The role of β_2 integrins in inflammation, in *Inflammation Basic Principles and Clinical Correlates*, 3rd ed, edited by JI Gallin, R Snyderman, DT Fearon, BF Haynes, C Nathan, p 537. Lippincott, Williams and Wilkins, Philadelphia, 1999.

417. Lasky LA: Selectin-carbohydrate interactions and the initiation of the inflammatory response. *Annu Rev Biochem* 64:113, 1995.

418. Takada Y, Ye X, Simon S: The integrins. *Genome Biol* 8:215, 2007.

419. Eshghi S, Vogelezang MG, Hynes RO, et al: Alpha4beta1 integrin and erythropoietin mediate temporally distinct steps in erythropoiesis: Integrins in red cell development. *J Cell Biol* 177:871, 2007.

420. Iguchi A, Okuyama R, Koguma M, et al: Selective stimulation of granulopoiesis in vitro by established bone marrow stromal cells. *Cell Struct Funct* 22:357, 1997.

421. Rettig MP, Ansstas G, DiPersio JF: Mobilization of hematopoietic stem and progenitor cells using inhibitors of CXCR4 and VLA-4. *Leukemia* 26:34, 2012.

422. Petty JM, Lenox CC, Weiss DJ, et al: Crosstalk between CXCR4/stromal derived factor-1 and VLA-4/VCAM-1 pathways regulates neutrophil retention in the bone marrow. *J Immunol* 182:604, 2009.

423. Dittel BN, LeBien TW: Reduced expression of vascular cell adhesion molecule-1 on bone marrow stromal cells isolated from marrow transplant recipients correlates with a reduced capacity to support human B lymphopoiesis in vitro. *Blood* 86:2833, 1995.

424. Funk PE, Stephan RP, Witte PL: Vascular cell adhesion molecule 1-positive reticular cells express interleukin-7 and stem cell factor in the bone marrow. *Blood* 86:2661, 1995.

425. Galotto M, Berisso G, Delfino L, et al: Stromal damage as consequence of high-dose chemo/radiotherapy in bone marrow transplant recipients. *Exp Hematol* 27:1460, 1999.

426. Avecilla ST, Hattori K, Heissig B, et al: Chemokine-mediated interaction of hematopoietic progenitors with the bone marrow vascular niche is required for thrombopoiesis. *Nat Med* 10:64, 2004.

427. Avraham H, Cowley S, Chi SY, et al: Characterization of adhesive interactions between human endothelial cells and megakaryocytes. *J Clin Invest* 91:2378, 1993.

428. Priestley GV, Ulyanova T, Papayannopoulou T: Sustained alterations in biodistribution of stem/progenitor cells in Tie2Cre+ alpha4(f/f) mice are hematopoietic cell autonomous. *Blood* 109:109, 2007.

429. Katayama Y, Hildalgo A, Peired A, Frenette PS: Integrin alpha4beta7 and its counterreceptor MAdCAM-1 contribute to hematopoietic progenitor recruitment into bone marrow following transplantation. *Blood* 104:2020, 2004.

430. Campbell ID, Humphries MJ: Integrin structure, activation, and interactions. *Cold Spring Harb Perspect Biol* 3, 2011.

431. Aplin AE, Howe A, Alahari SK, Juliano RL: Signal transduction and signal modulation by cell adhesion receptors: The role of integrins, cadherins, immunoglobulin-cell adhesion molecules, and selectins. *Pharmacol Rev* 50:197, 1998.

432. Shen B, Delaney MK, Du X: Inside-out, outside-in, and inside–outside-in: G protein signaling in integrin-mediated cell adhesion, spreading, and retraction. *Curr Opin Cell Biol* 24:600, 2012.

433. Porter JC, Hogg N: Integrin cross talk: Activation of lymphocyte function-associated antigen-1 on human T cells alters alpha4beta1- and alpha5beta1-mediated function. *J Cell Biol* 138:1437, 1997.

434. Shibuya K, Lanier LL, Phillips JH, et al: Physical and functional association of LFA-1 with DNAM-1 adhesion molecule. *Immunity* 11:615, 1999.

435. Rodriguez-Fernandez JL, Gomez M, Luque A, et al: The interaction of activated integrin lymphocyte function-associated antigen 1 with ligand intercellular adhesion molecule 1 induces activation and redistribution of focal adhesion kinase and proline-rich tyrosine kinase 2 in T lymphocytes. *Mol Biol Cell* 10:1891-1907, 1999.

436. Leavesley DI, Oliver JM, Swart BW, et al: Signals from platelet/endothelial cell adhesion molecule enhance the adhesive activity of the very late antigen-4 integrin of human CD34+ hemopoietic progenitor cells. *J Immunol* 153:4673, 1994.

437. Vestweber D, Blanks JE: Mechanisms that regulate the function of the selectins and their ligands. *Physiol Rev* 79:181, 1999.

438. Oostendorp RA, Dörmer P: VLA-4-mediated interactions between normal human hematopoietic progenitors and stromal cells. *Leuk Lymphoma* 24:423, 1997.

439. Gotoh A, Ritchie A, Takahira H, Broxmeyer HE: Thrombopoietin and erythropoietin activate inside-out signaling of integrin and enhance adhesion to immobilized fibronectin in human growth-factor-dependent hematopoietic cells. *Ann Hematol* 75:207, 1997.

440. Liesveld JL, Winslow JM, Frediani KE, et al: Expression of integrins and examination of their adhesive function in normal and leukemic hematopoietic cells. *Blood* 81:112, 1993.

441. Ryan DH, Nuccie BL, Abboud CN: Inhibition of human bone marrow lymphoid progenitor colonies by antibodies to VLA integrins. *J Immunol* 149:3759, 1992.

442. Sugahara H, Kanakura Y, Furitsu T, et al: Induction of programmed cell death in human hematopoietic cell lines by fibronectin via its interaction with very late antigen 5. *J Exp Med* 179:1757, 1994.

443. Oostendorp RA, Spitzer E, Reisbach G, Dörmer P: Antibodies to the beta 1-integrin chain, CD44, or ICAM-3 stimulate adhesion of blast colony-forming cells and may inhibit their growth. *Exp Hematol* 25:345, 1997.

444. Dao MA, Nolta JA: Cytokine and integrin stimulation synergize to promote higher levels of GATA-2, c-myb, and CD34 protein in primary human hematopoietic progenitors from mouse marrow. *Blood* 109:2373, 2007.

445. Umemoto T, Yamato M, Shiratsuchi Y, et al: Expression of Integrin beta3 is correlated to the properties of quiescent hemopoietic stem cells possessing the side population phenotype. *J Immunol* 177:7733, 2006.

446. Wagers AJ, Weissman IL: Differential expression of alpha2 integrin separates long-term and short-term reconstituting Lin-/loThy1.1(lo)c-kit+ Sca-1+ hematopoietic stem cells. *Stem Cells* 24:1087, 2006.

447. Makgoba MW, Sanders ME, Ginther Luce GE, et al: ICAM-1 a ligand for LFA-1-dependent adhesion of B, T and myeloid cells. *Nature* 331:86, 1988.

448. Woodfin A, Voisin MB, Nourshargh S: PECAM-1: A multi-functional molecule in inflammation and vascular biology. *Arterioscler Thromb Vasc Biol* 27:2514, 2007.

449. Arkin S, Naprstek B, Guarini L, et al: Expression of intercellular adhesion molecule-1 (CD54) on hematopoietic progenitors. *Blood* 77:948, 1991.

450. Gunji Y, Nakamura M, Hagiwara T, et al: Expression and function of adhesion molecules on human hematopoietic stem cells: CD34+ LFA-1- cells are more primitive than CD34+ LFA-1+ cells. *Blood* 80:429, 1992.

451. Rao SG, Chitnis VS, Deora A, et al: An ICAM-1 like cell adhesion molecule is responsible for CD34 positive haemopoietic stem cells adhesion to bone-marrow stroma. *Cell Biol Int* 20:255, 1996.

452. Staunton DE, Dustin ML, Springer TA: Functional cloning of ICAM-2, a cell adhesion ligand for LFA-1 homologous to ICAM-1. *Nature* 339:61, 1989.

453. Fawcett J, Holness CL, Needham LA, et al: Molecular cloning of ICAM-3, a third ligand for LFA-1, constitutively expressed on resting leukocytes. *Nature* 360:481, 1992.

454. Campanero MR, Sánchez-Mateos P, del Pozo MA, Sánchez-Madrid F: ICAM-3 regulates lymphocyte morphology and integrin-mediated T cell interaction with endothelial cell and extracellular matrix ligands. *J Cell Biol* 127:867, 1994.

455. Nielsen M, Gerwien J, Geisler C, et al: MHC class II ligation induces CD58 (LFA-3)-mediated adhesion in human T cells. *Exp Clin Immunogenet* 15:61, 1998.

456. Le Guiner S, Le Dréan E, Labarrière N, et al: LFA-3 co-stimulates cytokine secretion by cytotoxic T lymphocytes by providing a TCR-independent activation signal. *Eur J Immunol* 28:1322, 1998.

457. Itzhaky D, Raz N, Hollander N: The glycosylphosphatidylinositol-anchored form and the transmembrane form of CD58 are released from the cell surface upon antibody binding. *Cell Immunol* 187:151, 1998.

458. Kirby AC, Cahen P, Porter SR, Olsen I: LFA-3 (CD58) mediates T-lymphocyte adhesion in chronic inflammatory infiltrates. *Scand J Immunol* 50:469, 1999.

459. De Waele M, Renmans W, Jochmans K, et al: Different expression of adhesion molecules on CD34+ cells in AML and B-lineage ALL and their normal bone marrow counterparts. *Eur J Haematol* 63:192, 1999.

460. Kinashi T, Springer TA: Regulation of cell-matrix adhesion by receptor tyrosine kinases. *Leuk Lymphoma* 18:203, 1995.

461. Toivanen A, Ihanus E, Mattila M, et al: Importance of molecular studies on major blood groups—intercellular adhesion molecule-4, a blood group antigen involved in multiple cellular interactions. *Biochim Biophys Acta* 1780:456, 2008.

462. McCarty JM, Yee EK, Deisher TA, et al: Interleukin-4 induces endothelial vascular cell adhesion molecule (VCAM-1) by an NF-kappa b-independent mechanism. *FEBS Lett* 372:194, 1995.

463. Bochner BS, Klunk DA, Sterbinsky SA, et al: IL-13 selectively induces vascular cell adhesion molecule-1 expression in human endothelial cells. *J Immunol* 154:799, 1995.

464. Crocker PR, Redelinghuys P: Siglecs as positive and negative regulators of the immune system. *Biochem Soc Trans* 36:1467, 2008.

465. Aizawa S, Tavassoli M: In vitro homing of hemopoietic stem cells is mediated by a recognition system with galactosyl and mannosyl specificities. *Proc Natl Acad Sci U S A* 84:4485, 1987.

466. Tavassoli M, Hardy CL: Molecular basis of homing of intravenously transplanted stem cells to the marrow. *Blood* 76:1059, 1990.

467. Sperandio M: Selectins and glycosyltransferases in leukocyte rolling in vivo. *FEBS J* 273:4377, 2006.

468. Chute JP: Stem cell homing. *Curr Opin Hematol* 13:399, 2006.

469. Eto T, Winkler I, Purton LE, Lévesque J-P: Contrasting effects of P-selectin and E-selectin on the differentiation of murine hematopoietic progenitor cells. *Exp Hematol* 33:232, 2005.

470. Nielsen JS, McNagny KM: Novel functions of the CD34 family. *J Cell Sci* 121:3683, 2008.

471. Matsubara A, Iwama A, Yamazaki S, et al: Endomucin, a CD34-like sialomucin, marks hematopoietic stem cells throughout development. *J Exp Med* 202:1483, 2005.

472. Stockton BM, Cheng G, Manjunath N, et al: Negative regulation of T cell homing by CD43. *I Immunity.* 8:373, 1998.

473. Matsumoto M, Shigeta A, Miyasaka M, Hirata T: CD43 plays both antiadhesive and proadhesive roles in neutrophil rolling in a context-dependent manner. *J Immunol* 181:3628, 2008.

474. Bazil V, Brandt J, Chen S, et al: A monoclonal antibody recognizing CD43 (leukosialin) initiates apoptosis of human hematopoietic progenitor cells but not stem cells. *Blood* 87:1272, 1996.

475. Forde S, Tye BJ, Newey SE, et al: Endolyn (CD164) modulates the CXCL12-mediated migration of umbilical cord blood CD133+ cells. *Blood* 109:1825, 2007.

476. Jeannet R, Cai Q, Liu H, et al: Alcam Regulates Long-Term Hematopoietic Stem Cell Engraftment and Self-Renewal. *Stem Cells* 31:560, 2013.

477. Ohneda O, Ohneda K, Arai F, et al: ALCAM (CD166): Its role in hematopoietic and endothelial development. *Blood* 98:2134, 2001.

478. Chitteti B, Kobayashi M, Cheng Y, et al: CD166 regulates human and murine hematopoietic stem cells and the hematopoietic niche. *Blood* 2014.

479. Bowen MA, Aruffo A: Adhesion molecules, their receptors, and their regulation: Analysis of CD6-activated leukocyte cell adhesion molecule (ALCAM/CD166) interactions. *Transplant Proc* 31:795, 1999.

480. Greenbaum AM, Link DC: Mechanisms of G-CSF-mediated hematopoietic stem and progenitor mobilization. *Leukemia* 25:211, 2011.

481. Oostendorp RA, Ghaffari S, Eaves CJ: Kinetics of in vivo homing and recruitment into cycle of hematopoietic cells are organ-specific but CD44-independent. *Bone Marrow Transplant* 26:559, 2000.

482. Nedvetzki S, Gonen E, Assayag N, et al: RHAMM, a receptor for hyaluronan-mediated motility, compensates for CD44 in inflamed CD44-knockout mice: A different interpretation of redundancy. *Proc Natl Acad Sci U S A* 101:18081, 2004.

483. Malavasi F, Deaglio S, Funaro A, et al: Evolution and function of the ADP ribosyl cyclase/CD38 gene family in physiology and pathology. *Physiol Rev* 88:841, 2008.

484. Turel KR, Rao SG: Expression of the cell adhesion molecule E-cadherin by the human bone marrow stromal cells and its probable role in CD34(+) stem cell adhesion. *Cell Biol Int* 22:641, 1998.

485. Butler JM, Nolan DJ, Vertes EL, et al: Endothelial Cells Are Essential for the Self-Renewal and Repopulation of Notch-Dependent Hematopoietic Stem Cells. *Cell Stem Cell* 6:251, 2010.

486. Kiel MJ, Acar M, Radice GL, Morrison SJ: Hematopoietic stem cells do not depend on N-cadherin to regulate their maintenance. *Cell Stem Cell* 4:170, 2009.

487. Springer TA: Traffic signals for lymphocyte recirculation and leukocyte emigration: The multistep paradigm. *Cell* 76:301, 1994.

488. Butcher EC, Williams M, Youngman K, et al: Lymphocyte trafficking and regional immunity. *Adv Immunol* 72:209, 1999.

489. Girard J-P, Moussion C, Forster R: HEVs, lymphatics and homeostatic immune cell trafficking in lymph nodes. *Nat Rev Immunol* 12:762, 2012.

490. Zarbock A, Ley K: Neutrophil adhesion and activation under flow. *Microcirculation* 16:31, 2009.

491. Pals ST, de Gorter DJJ, Spaargaren M: Lymphoma dissemination: The other face of lymphocyte homing. *Blood* 110:3102, 2007.

492. Petri B, Bixel MG: Molecular events during leukocyte diapedesis. *FEBS J* 273:4399, 2006.

493. Garrido-Urbani S, Bradfield PF, Lee BPL, Imhof BA: Vascular and epithelial junctions: A barrier for leucocyte migration. *Biochem Soc Trans* 36:203, 2008.

494. Hordijk PL: Endothelial signalling events during leukocyte transmigration. *FEBS J* 273:4408, 2006.

495. Pease JE, Williams TJ: The attraction of chemokines as a target for specific anti-inflammatory therapy. *Br J Pharmacol* 147(Suppl 1):S212, 2006.

496. Watt SM, Forde SP: The central role of the chemokine receptor, CXCR4, in haemopoietic stem cell transplantation: Will CXCR4 antagonists contribute to the treatment of blood disorders? *Vox Sang* 94:18, 2008.

497. Bruserud Ø, Kittang AO: The chemokine system in experimental and clinical hematology. *Curr Top Microbiol Immunol* 341:3, 2010.

498. Fong AM, Robinson LA, Steeber DA, et al: Fractalkine and CX3CR1 Mediate a Novel Mechanism of Leukocyte Capture, Firm Adhesion, and Activation under Physiologic Flow. *J Exp Med* 188:1413, 1998.

499. Broxmeyer HE: Chemokines in hematopoiesis. *Curr Opin Hematol* 15:49, 2008.

500. Gerrits H, van Ingen Schenau DS, Bakker NEC, et al: Early postnatal lethality and cardiovascular defects in CXCR7-deficient mice. *Genesis* 46:235, 2008.

501. Sierro F, Biben C, Martínez-Muñoz L, et al: Disrupted cardiac development but normal hematopoiesis in mice deficient in the second CXCL12/SDF-1 receptor, CXCR7. *Proc Natl Acad Sci U S A* 104:14759, 2007.

502. Boldajipour B, Mahabaleshwar H, Kardash E, et al: Control of chemokine-guided cell migration by ligand sequestration. *Cell* 132:463, 2008.

503. Dar A, Kollet O, Lapidot T: Mutual, reciprocal SDF-1/CXCR4 interactions between hematopoietic and bone marrow stromal cells regulate stem cell migration and development in NOD/SCID chimeric mice. *Exp Hematol* 34:967, 2006.

504. Greenbaum A, Hsu Y-MS, Day RB, et al: CXCL12 in early mesenchymal progenitors is required for haematopoietic stem-cell maintenance. *Nature* 495:227, 2013.

505. Morrison SJ, Scadden DT: The bone marrow niche for haematopoietic stem cells. *Nature* 505:327, 2014.

506. Bonig H, Papayannopoulou T: Hematopoietic stem cell mobilization: Updated conceptual renditions. *Leukemia* 27:24, 2013.

507. Nabors LK, Wang LD, Wagers AJ, Kansas GS: Overlapping roles for endothelial selectins in murine hematopoietic stem/progenitor cell homing to bone marrow. *Exp Hematol* 41:588, 2013.

508. Scott LM, Priestley GV, Papayannopoulou T: Deletion of alpha4 integrins from adult hematopoietic cells reveals roles in homeostasis, regeneration, and homing. *Mol Cell Biol* 23:9349, 2003.

509. Avigdor A, Goichberg P, Shivtiel S, et al: CD44 and hyaluronic acid cooperate with SDF-1 in the trafficking of human CD34+ stem/progenitor cells to bone marrow. *Blood* 103:2981, 2004.

510. Wysoczynski M, Reca R, Ratajczak J, et al: Incorporation of CXCR4 into membrane lipid rafts primes homing-related responses of hematopoietic stem/progenitor cells to an SDF-1 gradient. *Blood* 105:40, 2005.

511. Williams DA, Zheng Y, Cancelas JA: Rho GTPases and regulation of hematopoietic stem cell localization. *Methods Enzymol* 439:365, 2008.

512. Kiel MJ, Morrison SJ: Uncertainty in the niches that maintain haematopoietic stem cells. *Nat Rev Immunol* 8:290, 2008.

513. Czechowicz A, Kraft D, Weissman IL, Bhattacharya D: Efficient transplantation via antibody-based clearance of hematopoietic stem cell niches. *Science* 318:1296, 2007.

514. Levesque JP, Leavesley DI, Niutta S, et al: Cytokines increase human hemopoietic cell adhesiveness by activation of very late antigen (VLA)-4 and VLA-5 integrins. *J Exp Med* 181:1805, 1995.

515. Adams GB, Chabner KT, Alley IR, et al: Stem cell engraftment at the endosteal niche is specified by the calcium-sensing receptor. *Nature* 439:599, 2006.

516. Arai F, Hirao A, Ohmura M, et al: Tie2/angiopoietin-1 signaling regulates hematopoietic stem cell quiescence in the bone marrow niche. *Cell* 118:149, 2004.

517. Puri MC, Bernstein A: Requirement for the TIE family of receptor tyrosine kinases in adult but not fetal hematopoiesis. *Proc Natl Acad Sci U S A* 100:12753, 2003.

518. Umemoto T, Yamato M, Ishihara J, et al: Integrin-αvβ3 regulates thrombopoietin-mediated maintenance of hematopoietic stem cells. *Blood* 119:83, 2012.

519. Qian H, Buza-Vidas N, Hyland CD, et al: Critical role of thrombopoietin in maintaining adult quiescent hematopoietic stem cells. *Cell Stem Cell* 1:671, 2007.

520. Yoshihara H, Arai F, Hosokawa K, et al: Thrombopoietin/MPL signaling regulates hematopoietic stem cell quiescence and interaction with the osteoblastic niche. *Cell Stem Cell* 1:685, 2007.

521. van Eeden SF, Miyagashima R, Haley L, Hogg JC: Possible role for L-selectin in the release of polymorphonuclear leukocytes from bone marrow. *Am J Physiol* 272:H1717, 1997.

522. Le Marer N, Skacel PO: Up-regulation of alpha2,6 sialylation during myeloid maturation: A potential role in myeloid cell release from the bone marrow. *J Cell Physiol* 179:315, 1999.

523. Jagels MA, Chambers JD, Arfors KE, Hugli TE: C5a- and tumor necrosis factor-alpha-induced leukocytosis occurs independently of beta 2 integrins and L-selectin: Differential effects on neutrophil adhesion molecule expression in vivo. *Blood* 85:2900, 1995.

524. Stroncek DF, Jaszcz W, Herr GP, et al: Expression of neutrophil antigens after 10 days of granulocyte-colony-stimulating factor. *Transfusion* 38:663, 1998.

525. Jung U, Ley K: Mice lacking two or all three selectins demonstrate overlapping and distinct functions for each selectin. *J Immunol* 162:6755, 1999.

526. Radley JM, Haller CJ: Fate of senescent megakaryocytes in the bone marrow. *Br J Haematol* 53:277, 1983.

527. Efrati P, Rozenszajn L: The morphology of buffy coats in normal human adults. *Blood* 16: 1012, 1960.

528. Ulich TR, del Castillo J, Souza L: Kinetics and mechanisms of recombinant human granulocyte-colony stimulating factor-induced neutrophilia. *Am J Pathol* 133:630, 1988.

529. Yong KL: Granulocyte colony stimulating factor (G-CSF) increases neutrophil migration across vascular endothelium independent of an effect on adhesion: Comparison with granulocyte-macrophage colony-stimulating factor (GM-CSF). *Br J Haematol* 94:40, 1996.

530. DiPersio JF, Abboud CN: Activation of neutrophils by granulocyte-macrophage colony-stimulating factor. *Immunol Ser* 57:457, 1992.

531. Ghebrehiwet B, Müller-Eberhard HJ: C3e: An acidic fragment of human C3 with leuko-cytosis-inducing activity. *J Immunol* 123:616, 1979.

532. Kubo H, Graham L, Doyle NA, et al: Complement fragment-induced release of neutrophils from bone marrow and sequestration within pulmonary capillaries in rabbits. *Blood* 92:283, 1998.

533. Deinard AS, Page AR: A study of steroid-induced granulocytosis in a patient with chronic benign neutropenia of childhood. *Br J Haematol* 28:333, 1974.

534. Vogel JM, Yankee RA, Kimball HR, et al: The effect of etiocholanolone on granulocyte kinetics. *Blood* 30:474, 1967.

535. Cybulsky MI, McComb DJ, Movat HZ: Neutrophil leukocyte emigration induced by endotoxin. Mediator roles of interleukin 1 and tumor necrosis factor alpha 1. *J Immunol* 140:3144, 1988.

536. Terashima T, English D, Hogg JC, van Eeden SF: Release of polymorphonuclear leukocytes from the bone marrow by interleukin-8. *Blood* 92:1062, 1998.

537. Burdon PCE, Martin C, Rankin SM: The CXC chemokine MIP-2 stimulates neutrophil mobilization from the rat bone marrow in a CD49d-dependent manner. *Blood* 105:2543, 2005.

538. Burdon PCE, Martin C, Rankin SM: Migration across the sinusoidal endothelium regulates neutrophil mobilization in response to ELR + CXC chemokines. *Br J Haematol* 142:100, 2008.

539. Wengner AM, Pitchford SC, Furze RC, Rankin SM: The coordinated action of G-CSF and ELR + CXC chemokines in neutrophil mobilization during acute inflammation. *Blood* 111:42, 2008.

540. Suratt BT, Petty JM, Young SK, et al: Role of the CXCR4/SDF-1 chemokine axis in circulating neutrophil homeostasis. *Blood* 104:565, 2004.

541. Palframan RT, Collins PD, Williams TJ, Rankin SM: Eotaxin induces a rapid release of eosinophils and their progenitors from the bone marrow. *Blood* 91:2240, 1998.

542. Palframan RT, Collins PD, Severs NJ, et al: Mechanisms of acute eosinophil mobilization from the bone marrow stimulated by interleukin 5: The role of specific adhesion molecules and phosphatidylinositol 3-kinase. *J Exp Med* 188:1621, 1998.

543. Schratl P, Royer JF, Kostenis E, et al: The role of the prostaglandin D2 receptor, DP, in eosinophil trafficking. *J Immunol* 179:4792, 2007.

544. Chamberlain JK, Weiss L, Weed RI: Bone marrow sinus cell packing: A determinant of cell release. *Blood* 46:91, 1975.

545. Waugh RE, Sassi M: An in vitro model of erythroid egress in bone marrow. *Blood* 68:250, 1986.

546. Chasis JA, Prenant M, Leung A, Mohandas N: Membrane assembly and remodeling during reticulocyte maturation. *Blood* 74:1112, 1989.

547. Dabrowski Z, Szyguła Z, Miszta H: Do changes in bone marrow pressure contribute to the egress of cell from bone marrow? *Acta Physiol Pol* 32:729, 1981.

548. Eymard N, Bessonov N, Gandrillon O, et al: The role of spatial organization of cells in erythropoiesis. *J Math Biol* 2014. 70:71, 2015.

549. Junt T, Schulze H, Chen Z, et al: Dynamic visualization of thrombopoiesis within bone marrow. *Science* 317:1767, 2007.

550. Zhang L, Orban M, Lorenz M, et al: A novel role of sphingosine 1-phosphate receptor S1pr1 in mouse thrombopoiesis. *J Exp Med* 209:2165, 2012.

551. Wilson A, Laurenti E, Oser G, et al: Hematopoietic stem cells reversibly switch from dormancy to self-renewal during homeostasis and repair. *Cell* 135:1118, 2008.

552. Cheshier SH, Prohaska SS, Weissman IL: The effect of bleeding on hematopoietic stem cell cycling and self-renewal. *Stem Cells Dev* 16:707, 2007.

553. Nervi B, Link DC, DiPersio JF: Cytokines and hematopoietic stem cell mobilization. *J Cell Biochem* 99:690, 2006.

554. Petit I, Szyper-Kravitz M, Nagler A, et al: G-CSF induces stem cell mobilization by decreasing bone marrow SDF-1 and up-regulating CXCR4. *Nat Immunol* 3:687, 2002.

555. Christopher MJ, Liu F, Hilton MJ, et al: Suppression of CXCL12 production by bone marrow osteoblasts is a common and critical pathway for cytokine-induced mobilization. *Blood* 114:1331, 2009.

556. Levesque J-P, Liu F, Simmons PJ, et al: Characterization of hematopoietic progenitor mobilization in protease-deficient mice. *Blood* 104:65, 2004.

557. Semerad CL, Christopher MJ, Liu F, et al: G-CSF potently inhibits osteoblast activity and CXCL12 mRNA expression in the bone marrow. *Blood* 106:3020, 2005.

558. Christopher MJ, Link DC: Granulocyte colony-stimulating factor induces osteoblast apoptosis and inhibits osteoblast differentiation. *J Bone Miner Res* 23:1765, 2008.

559. Papayannopoulou T, Priestley GV, Nakamoto B, et al: Synergistic mobilization of hemopoietic progenitor cells using concurrent beta1 and beta2 integrin blockade or beta2-deficient mice. *Blood* 97:1282, 2001.

560. Velders GA, Pruijt JFM, Verzaal P, et al: Enhancement of G-CSF-induced stem cell mobilization by antibodies against the beta 2 integrins LFA-1 and Mac-1. *Blood* 100:327, 2002.

561. Ramirez P, Rettig MP, Uy GL, et al: BIO5192, a small molecule inhibitor of VLA-4, mobilizes hematopoietic stem and progenitor cells. *Blood* 114:1340, 2009.

562. Leone DR, Giza K, Gill A, et al: An assessment of the mechanistic differences between two integrin α4β1 inhibitors, the monoclonal antibody TA-2 and the small molecule BIO5192, in rat experimental autoimmune encephalomyelitis. *J Pharmacol Exp Ther* 305:1150, 2003.

563. Pruijt JFM, Verzaal P, van Os R, et al: Neutrophils are indispensable for hematopoietic stem cell mobilization induced by interleukin-8 in mice. *Proc Natl Acad Sci U S A* 99:6228, 2002.

564. Bowie MB, Kent DG, Dykstra B, et al: Identification of a new intrinsically timed developmental checkpoint that reprograms key hematopoietic stem cell properties. *Proc Natl Acad Sci U S A* 104:5878, 2007.

565. Pietras EM, Warr MR, Passegué E: Cell cycle regulation in hematopoietic stem cells. *J Cell Biol* 195:709, 2011.

566. Haylock DN, Williams B, Johnston HM, et al: Hemopoietic stem cells with higher hemopoietic potential reside at the bone marrow endosteum. *Stem Cells* 25:1062, 2007.

567. Passegué E, Wagers AJ, Giuriato S, et al: Global analysis of proliferation and cell cycle gene expression in the regulation of hematopoietic stem and progenitor cell fates. *J Exp Med* 202:1599, 2005.

568. Shapiro HM: Flow cytometric estimation of DNA and RNA content in intact cells stained with Hoechst 33342 and pyronin Y. *Cytometry* 2:143, 1981.

569. Dick FA, Rubin SM: Molecular mechanisms underlying RB protein function. *Nat Rev Mol Cell Biol* 14:297, 2013.

570. Walkley CR, Sankaran VG, Orkin SH: Rb and hematopoiesis: Stem cells to anemia. *Cell Div* 3:13, 2008.

571. Narasimha A, Kaulich M, Shapiro G, et al: Cyclin D activates the Rb tumor suppressor by mono-phosphorylation. *Elife* 3, 2014.

572. Sherr CJ, Roberts JM: Living with or without cyclins and cyclin-dependent kinases. *Genes Dev* 18:2699, 2004.

573. Kozar K, Ciemerych MA, Rebel VI, et al: Mouse development and cell proliferation in the absence of D-cyclins. *Cell* 118:477, 2004.

574. Malumbres M, Sotillo R, Santamaría D, et al: Mammalian cells cycle without the D-type cyclin-dependent kinases Cdk4 and Cdk6. *Cell* 118:493, 2004.

575. Steinman RA: Cell cycle regulators and hematopoiesis. *Oncogene* 21:3403, 2002.

576. Metcalf D: Hematopoietic cytokines. *Blood* 111:485, 2008.

577. Tushinski RJ, Stanley ER: The regulation of mononuclear phagocyte entry into S phase by the colony stimulating factor CSF-1. *J Cell Physiol* 122:221, 1985.

578. Roussel MF, Theodoras AM, Pagano M, Sherr CJ: Rescue of defective mitogenic signaling by D-type cyclins. *Proc Natl Acad Sci U S A* 92:6837, 1995.

579. Oguro H, Iwama A: Life and death in hematopoietic stem cells. *Curr Opin Immunol* 19:503, 2007.

580. Berthet C, Rodriguez-Galan MC, Hodge DL, et al: Hematopoiesis and thymic apoptosis are not affected by the loss of Cdk2. *Mol Cell Biol* 27:5079, 2007.

581. Koury MJ: Programmed cell death (apoptosis) in hematopoiesis. *Exp Hematol* 20:391, 1992.

582. Kelley LL, Koury MJ, Bondurant MC, et al: Survival or death of individual proerythroblasts results from differing erythropoietin sensitivities: A mechanism for controlled rates of erythrocyte production. *Blood* 82:2340, 1993.

583. Opferman JT: Life and death during hematopoietic differentiation. *Curr Opin Immunol* 19:497, 2007.

584. Reed JC: Bcl-2-family proteins and hematologic malignancies: History and future prospects. *Blood* 111:3322, 2008.

585. Llambi F, Green DR: Apoptosis and oncogenesis: Give and take in the BCL-2 family. *Curr Opin Genet Dev* 21:12, 2011.

586. Kaisho T, Ishikawa J, Oritani K, et al: BST-1, a surface molecule of bone marrow stromal cell lines that facilitates pre-B-cell growth. *Proc Natl Acad Sci U S A* 91:5325, 1994.

587. Opferman JT, Iwasaki H, Ong CC, et al: Obligate role of anti-apoptotic MCL-1 in the survival of hematopoietic stem cells. *Science* 307:1101, 2005.

588. Hamasaki A, Sendo F, Nakayama K, et al: Accelerated neutrophil apoptosis in mice lacking A1-a, a subtype of the bcl-2-related A1 gene. *J Exp Med* 188:1985, 1998.

589. Rhodes MM, Kopsombut P, Bondurant MC, et al: Bcl-x(L) prevents apoptosis of late-stage erythroblasts but does not mediate the antiapoptotic effect of erythropoietin. *Blood* 106:1857, 2005.

590. Aerbajinai W, Giattina M, Lee YT, et al: The proapoptotic factor Nix is coexpressed with Bcl-xL during terminal erythroid differentiation. *Blood* 102:712, 2003.

591. von Lindern M, Schmidt U, Beug H: Control of erythropoiesis by erythropoietin and stem cell factor: A novel role for Bruton's tyrosine kinase. *Cell Cycle* 3:876, 2004.

592. Muta K, Krantz SB, Bondurant MC, Wickrema A: Distinct roles of erythropoietin, insulin-like growth factor I, and stem cell factor in the development of erythroid progenitor cells. *J Clin Invest* 94:34, 1994.

593. Sandoval H, Thiagarajan P, Dasgupta SK, et al: Essential role for Nix in autophagic maturation of erythroid cells. *Nature* 454:232, 2008.

594. Schweers RL, Zhang J, Randall MS, et al: NIX is required for programmed mitochondrial clearance during reticulocyte maturation. *Proc Natl Acad Sci U S A* 104:19500, 2007.

595. Finch CA, Harker LA, Cook JD: Kinetics of the formed elements of human blood. *Blood* 50:699, 1977.

596. Nagai Y, Garrett KP, Ohta S, et al: Toll-like receptors on hematopoietic progenitor cells stimulate innate immune system replenishment. *Immunity* 24:801, 2006.

597. Yáñez A, Goodridge HS, Gozalbo D, Gil ML: TLRs control hematopoiesis during infection. *Eur J Immunol* 43:2526, 2013.

598. Sioud M, Fløisand Y, Forfang L, Lund-Johansen F: Signaling through toll-like receptor 7/8 induces the differentiation of human bone marrow CD34+ progenitor cells along the myeloid lineage. *J Mol Biol* 364:945, 2006.

599. Hirai H, Zhang P, Dayaram T, et al: C/EBPbeta is required for "emergency" granulopoiesis. *Nat Immunol* 7:732, 2006.

600. McGettrick AF, O'Neill LAJ: Toll-like receptors: Key activators of leucocytes and regulator of haematopoiesis. *Br J Haematol* 139:185, 2007.

601. Zhao JL, Ma C, O'Connell RM, et al: Conversion of danger signals into cytokine signals by hematopoietic stem and progenitor cells for regulation of stress-induced hematopoiesis. *Cell Stem Cell* 14:445, 2014.

602. Welner Robert S, Kincade Paul W: 9-1-1: HSCs respond to emergency calls. *Cell Stem Cell* 14:415, 2014.

603. Testa U: Apoptotic mechanisms in the control of erythropoiesis. *Leukemia* 18:1176, 2004.

CHAPTER 6
THE ORGANIZATION AND STRUCTURE OF LYMPHOID TISSUES

Aharon G. Freud and Michael A. Caligiuri*

SUMMARY

The lymphoid tissues can be divided into primary and secondary lymphoid organs. Primary lymphoid tissues are sites where lymphocytes develop from progenitor cells into functional and mature lymphocytes. The major primary lymphoid tissue is the marrow, the site where all lymphocyte progenitor cells reside and initially differentiate. This organ is discussed in Chap. 5. The other primary lymphoid tissue is the thymus, the site where progenitor cells derived from the marrow differentiate into mature thymus-derived (T) cells. Secondary lymphoid tissues are sites where lymphocytes undergo additional maturation and also interact with each other and with nonlymphoid cells to generate immune responses to antigens. These tissues include the spleen, lymph nodes, and mucosa-associated lymphoid tissues such as tonsils. The structure of these tissues provides insight into how the immune system discriminates between self-antigens and foreign antigens and develops the capacity to orchestrate a variety of specific and nonspecific defenses against invading pathogens.

● THE THYMUS

The thymus is the site for development of thymic-derived lymphocytes, or T cells. In this organ, developing T cells, called *thymocytes*, differentiate from lymphoid stem cells derived from the marrow into functional, mature T cells.[1] It is here that T cells acquire their repertoire of specific antigen receptors to cope with the antigenic challenges received throughout one's life span. Once they have completed their maturation, the T cells leave the thymus and circulate in the blood and through secondary lymphoid tissues.

Acronyms and Abbreviations: *AIRE,* autoimmune regulatory gene; APECED, autoimmune polyendocrinopathy-candidiasis-ectodermal dystrophy; CT, computed tomography; GALT, gastrointestinal-associated lymphoid tissue; Ig, immunoglobulin; IL, interleukin; ILC, innate lymphoid cell; MALT, mucosa-associated lymphoid tissue; MHC, major histocompatibility complex; NK, natural killer; PALS, periarteriolar lymphoid sheath; PGA syndrome, polyglandular autoimmune syndrome; r, correlation coefficient; T, thymus-derived; TCR, T-cell receptor.

*This chapter was prepared by Thomas J. Kipps in the 8th edition and much of the text has been retained.

THYMIC ANATOMY

The thymus is located in the superior mediastinum, overlying, in order, the left brachiocephalic (or innominate) vein, the innominate artery, the left common carotid artery, and the trachea. It overlaps the upper limit of the pericardial sac below and extends into the neck beneath the upper anterior ribs. It receives its blood supply from the internal thoracic arteries. Venous blood from the thymus drains into the brachiocephalic and internal thoracic veins, which communicate above with the inferior thyroid veins.

Arising from the third and fourth branchial pouches as an epithelial organ populated by lymphoid cells and endoderm-derived thymic epithelial cells, the thymus develops at about the eighth week of gestation.[2] The thymus increases in size through fetal and postnatal life and remains ample into puberty,[3] when it weighs approximately 40 g. Thereafter, the size progressively decreases with aging as a consequence of thymic involution.[4] The cause of thymic involution is likely in part a result of the influence of glucocorticoid hormones.[5] Nonetheless, there is evidence that T lymphocytes continue to develop throughout life, potentially including in some extrathymic sites.[6]

The volume of the thymus can be estimated by sonography. In one study of 149 healthy term infants within 1 week of birth, there was a significant correlation between the estimated thymic volume and the weight of the infant.[3,7] However, no correlation was apparent between the estimated thymic volume and the infant's sex, length, or gestational age. Also, there was no apparent correlation between estimated volume and the proportions of CD4+ T cells or CD8+ T cells found in the blood. The estimated thymic volume of healthy infants increases from birth to 4 and 8 months of age and then decreases.[3] Most of the individual variation at 4 and 10 months of age appears to correlate with breastfeeding status, body size, and, to a lesser extent, illness. Breastfed infants at 4 months of age have significantly larger estimated thymic volumes than do age-matched formula-fed infants with similar thymic volumes at birth.[8]

THYMIC ARCHITECTURE

A longitudinal fissure divides the thymus into two asymmetrical lobes, a larger right and a smaller left, that are derived from the right and left branchial pouches, respectively. These two developmentally separate parts of the thymus are easily separated from each other by blunt dissection.

Each lobe of the thymus is divided into multiple lobules by fibrous septa that extend inward from an outer capsule. Each lobule consists of an outer cortex and an inner medulla (Fig. 6–1). The cortex contains dense collections of thymocytes (developing immature T cells) that cytologically appear as lymphocytes of slightly variable size with scattered, rare mitoses. The lighter-staining medulla is loosely arranged and more sparsely populated by mature thymocytes and characteristic tightly packed whorls of squamous-appearing epithelial cells, called *thymic* or *Hassall corpuscles* (Fig. 6–2). These appear to be remnants of degenerating cells and are rich in high-molecular-weight cytokeratins. Hassall's corpuscles are thought to serve a critical role in the development of regulatory T cells.[9]

The thymus contains several important cell types that serve a variety of functions including supporting the maturation of thymocytes into mature T cells. There are several types of specialized epithelial cells within the thymus.[10] The three main categories of thymic epithelial cells are the medullary epithelial cells, which are organized into clusters; the cortical epithelial cells, which form an epithelial network; and the epithelial cells of the outer cortex. The epithelial cells in the cortex and medulla often have a stellate shape, display desmosomal intercellular connections, and likely function as support cells to developing thymocytes by providing important growth factors such

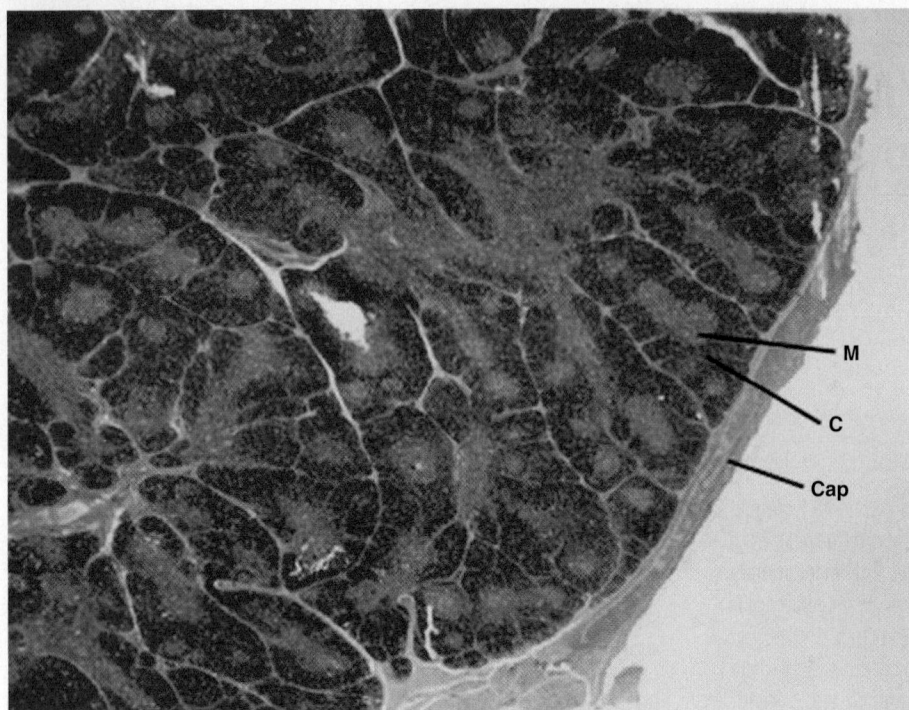

Figure 6–1. Normal human infant thymus. The thymus is surrounded by dense connective tissue capsule *(Cap)*. It is organized into adjacent lobules separated by capsular connective tissue extensions or trabeculae. The lobules each have a dense cortex *(C)* and a lighter staining medulla *(M)*. The medulla is a continuous tissue surrounded by the cortex that extends throughout the thymus, and it cannot be appreciated in a single section. *(Reproduced with permission from Lichtman's Atlas of Hematology, www.accessmedicine. com.)*

as interleukin (IL)-7.[11] In addition, at primarily the corticomedullary junction, the thymus contains marrow-derived antigen-presenting cells, mostly interdigitating dendritic cells and macrophages. Scattered B cells are also present in the thymus, and these interact with maturing thymocytes and potentially regulate T-cell development.[12,13]

After puberty, thymic involution begins within the cortex. This region may disappear completely with aging, while medullary remnants persist throughout life. Glucocorticoids also may induce atrophy of the cortex secondary to glucocorticoid-induced apoptosis of cortical thymocytes.[5] This also may be seen in conditions that are associated with increases in circulating glucocorticoid hormones, for example, pregnancy or stress.[14,15]

THYMIC IMMUNE FUNCTION

The thymus is the site of T-cell development. The importance of the thymus is underscored by patients with DiGeorge syndrome, or chromosome 22q11.2 deletion syndrome, who lack the genes required for

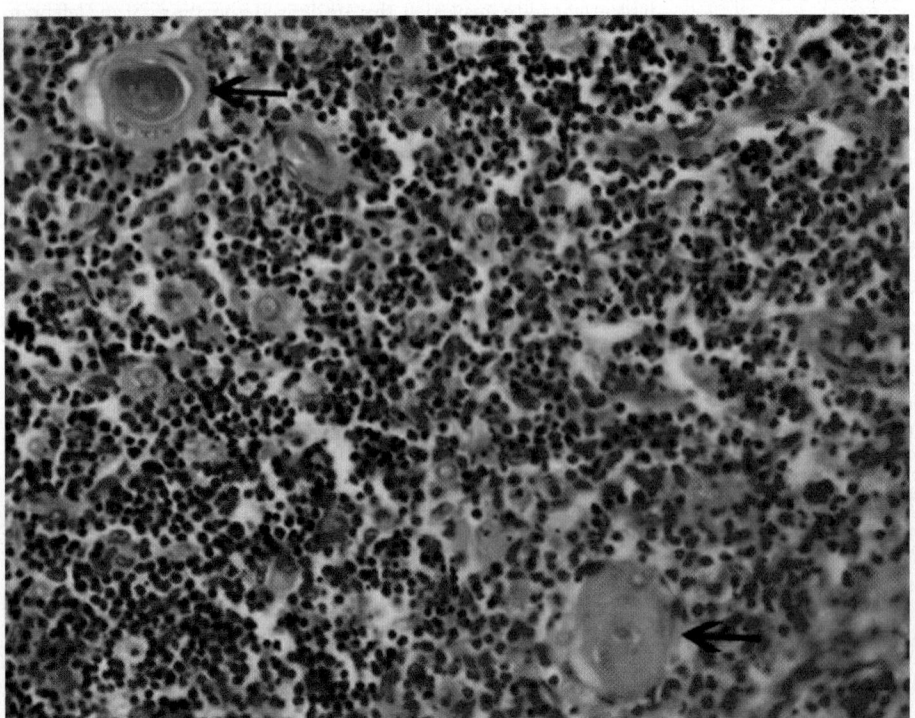

Figure 6–2. Normal human infant thymus. Higher magnification. Medulla. The *arrows* indicate thymic corpuscles (synonymous with Hassall corpuscles). They are composed of tightly packed, concentrically arranged, type IV endothelioreticular cells with flattened nuclei. The central mass is composed of keratinized cells. In addition to thymic corpuscles and the mass of small densely stained T lymphocytes, the medulla contains scattered, larger, type V epithelioreticular cells with their light nuclei, dark nucleolus, and eosinophilic cytoplasm, evident on this section. *(Reproduced with permission from Lichtman's Atlas of Hematology, www.accessmedicine.com.)*

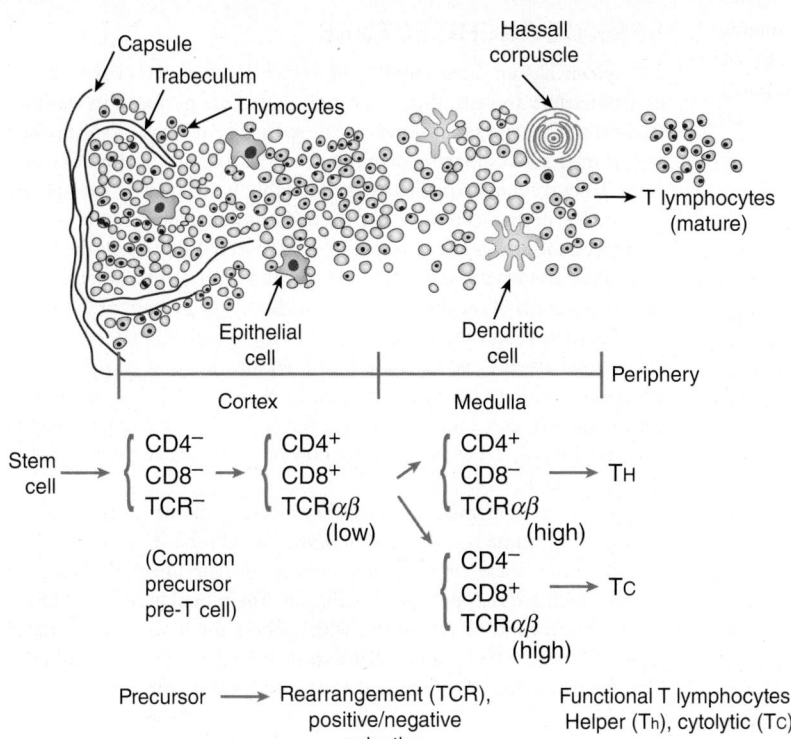

Figure 6-3. Structure of the thymus. The top half of the figure provides a cross section of a thymic lobule, indicating the outer cortex *(left)*, inner medulla *(center)*, and periphery *(far right)*. The *arrows* indicate various structures and cell types. As thymocytes mature, they migrate from the cortex toward the medullary region and acquire phenotypic features that are outlined at the bottom of the figure, as described in the text (Chap. 74).

thymic development.[16] These patients do not develop T cells and hence have profound immune deficiency.

Prothymocytes originate in the marrow and migrate to the thymus, where they mature into T cells (Chap. 76). Maturation of T cells is accompanied by the sequential acquisition of various T-cell markers including CD2, CD3, CD4 or CD8, CD5, and the T-cell receptor (TCR) (Fig. 6-3).[17] Terminal deoxynucleotidyl transferase (TdT) is found in prothymocytes and immature thymocytes but is absent in mature T cells. TdT facilitates the successful rearrangement of TCR genes in immature thymocytes.[18]

T-cell precursors can be found in distinct microenvironments within the thymus. Marrow-derived CD34+ pre-T cells enter the cortex via small blood vessels and are double-negative for CD4 and CD8 antigens.[1] One of the earliest identifiable T-cell membrane antigens is CD2. As the thymocytes proliferate and differentiate in the cortex, they acquire CD4 and CD8 antigens. They subsequently acquire the CD3 antigen and the TCR for antigen as they migrate toward the medulla. In the cortex, the thymocytes are induced to express the chemokine receptor, CCR7, which directs their migration to CCL19- and CCL21-producing cells in the thymic medulla where they undergo further maturation.[19]

Positive and negative selection of maturing T cells takes place in the thymus.[20] Double-positive (CD4+ and CD8+) thymocytes undergo an initial positive selection step that is mediated exclusively by thymic cortical epithelium to ensure that developing T cells can recognize peptides in the context of self major histocompatibility complex (MHC) molecules.[21] Thymocytes that have TCRs capable of interacting with self MHC molecules expressed by thymic cortical epithelial cells undergo expansion, whereas thymocytes with defective TCR undergo apoptosis.[22-24] As these positively selected cells migrate toward the medulla, they experience negative selection through their interaction with thymic medullary epithelial cells in order to ensure that any T cells that react too strongly to self MHC molecules are deleted. These thymic medullary epithelial cells uniquely express the autoimmune regulatory

gene *(AIRE)*. *AIRE* encodes a transcriptional regulator that promotes ectopic expression of a large repertoire of transcripts encoding proteins that ordinarily are restricted to differentiated organs residing in the periphery.[25] This allows the thymic medullary epithelial cells to express many different self-antigens, which are presented to developing thymocytes. Those thymocytes that have TCR that react too vigorously with the MHC molecules of the medullary epithelium will undergo apoptosis.[23] Most of the developing thymocytes are destroyed. In this way, only those T cells that have the appropriate level of affinity for self-MHC molecules yet are not reactive against self antigens will reach the medulla to undergo the final maturation stages and eventually exit the thymus via efferent lymphatics as functionally competent naïve CD4+ and CD8+ single-positive T cells.

Patients with the rare disease *autoimmune polyendocrinopathy-candidiasis-ectodermal dystrophy* (APECED) or *polyglandular autoimmune* (PGA) syndrome type I (PGA I) underscore the importance of negative selection of thymocytes by thymic medullary epithelial cells. APECED, or PGA I, is characterized by chronic mucocutaneous candidiasis, hypoparathyroidism, and adrenal insufficiency. In addition, most patients also have a number of other autoimmune manifestations, including thyroiditis, type 1 diabetes, ovarian failure, alopecia, and/or hepatitis.[26] These patients have genetic defects in *AIRE*,[27] which precludes their thymic epithelial cells from expressing the large variety of tissue differentiation self-antigens required for the negative selection of self-reactive thymocytes and the generation of central T-cell tolerance.[25,28]

● THE SPLEEN

The spleen is a specialized abdominal organ serving multiple functions in erythrocyte clearance, innate and adaptive immunity, and the regulation of blood volume. In general the spleen contains two structurally and functionally distinct components: white and red pulp. The white pulp of the spleen consists of secondary lymphoid tissue that provides an environment in which the cells of the immune system can interact with one another to mount adaptive immune responses to bloodborne antigens. The splenic red pulp contains macrophages that are responsible for clearing the blood of unwanted foreign substances and senescent erythrocytes, even in the absence of specific immunity. Thus, it acts as a filter for the blood.

SPLENIC ANATOMY

The spleen is located within the peritoneum in the left upper quadrant of the abdomen between the fundus of the stomach and the diaphragm. It receives its blood supply from the systemic circulation via the splenic artery, which branches off the celiac trunk, and the left gastroepiploic artery.[29] The blood returning from the spleen drains into the portal circulation via the splenic vein. Therefore, the spleen can become congested with blood and increase in size when there is portal vein hypertension (Chap. 56).

Approximately 10 percent of individuals have one or more accessory spleens. Accessory spleens are usually 1 cm in diameter and resemble lymph nodes. However, they usually are covered with peritoneum, as is the spleen itself. Accessory spleens typically lie along the course of the splenic artery or its gastroepiploic branch, but they may be elsewhere.[30] The commonest location is near the hilus of the spleen, but approximately 1 in 6 accessory spleens can be found embedded in the tail of the pancreas, where they may be occasionally mistaken for a pancreatic mass lesion.[31]

The average weight of the spleen in the adult human is 135 g (range: 100 to 250 g). However, when emptied of blood it weighs only approximately 80 g. On autopsy of 539 subjects with normal spleens, there was a positive correlation between the spleen weight and both the degree of acute splenic congestion and the subject's height and weight, but not with the subject's sex or age.[32]

The splenic volume can be estimated by computed tomography (CT) of the abdomen.[33] In one study, the splenic volume was calculated from the linear and the maximal cross-sectional area measurements of the spleen, using the following formula: splenic volume = 30 cm³ + 0.58 (the product of the width, length, and thickness of the spleen measured in centimeters).[34] Using this formula, the mean value of the calculated splenic volume for 47 normal subjects was 214.6 cm³, with a range of 107.2 to 314.5 cm³. The calculated splenic volume did not appear to vary significantly with the subject's age, gender, height, weight, body mass index, or the diameter of the first lumbar vertebra, the latter being considered representative of body habitus on CT.

The splenic volume also can be estimated by sonography, which provides good correlation with volumes measured by helical abdominal CT or actual volume displaced by the excised organ. In one study of 50 patients, the linear measurement by sonography that correlated most closely with CT volume was the spleen width measured on a longitudinal section with the patient in the right lateral decubitus position (correlation coefficient [r] = 0.89, p <0.001). There was also good correlation between splenic length measured in the right lateral decubitus position and CT volume (r = 0.86, p <0.001). In another postmortem analysis of 32 normal adult spleens, the ultrasonogram measurements of maximal height, width, and breadth of the spleen were compared with the actual volume displaced by the excised organ.[35] The mean actual splenic volume was approximately 148 cm³ (±81 cm³ SD), whereas mean splenic volume estimated from ultrasonography was 284 cm³ (±168 cm³ SD). Despite the differences between the actual and estimated volumes, these investigators did find a roughly linear correlation between actual splenic volume and the estimated splenic volume measured by ultrasound. However, there may be operator-to-operator variation in measurement of the estimated splenic volume, making the use of sonography in longitudinal studies technically demanding.

SPLENIC ARCHITECTURE

The spleen has an open circulation, which lacks endothelial continuity from artery to vein. When isolated spleens are perfused in washout studies, erythrocytes that appear in the splenic vein appear to be flushed out from three compartments. The red cells that are flushed out first come from a compartment that presumably is formed by the splenic vessels. The erythrocytes that are flushed out next come from a second compartment, where they presumably are loosely held within the filtration beds. The erythrocytes that are flushed out last presumably were adherent to cells of the filtration beds. Although 90 percent of the blood flow passes through the splenic vessels, only approximately 10 percent of the total splenic red cells are found within this first compartment. The second compartment is perfused by 9 percent of the total inflow yet contains 70 percent of the splenic red cells. The last compartment is perfused by only 1 percent of the inflow but contains 20 percent of the splenic red cells.

These compartments reflect the anatomy of the spleen and its stroma. The stroma is composed of branched, fibroblast-like cells called reticular cells. These cells produce slender collagen fibers, the reticular fibers, which are rich in type III collagen. The reticular cells and fibers form a meshwork, or reticulum, which filters the blood. Three major types of filtration beds can be distinguished by their structure and content: the white pulp, the marginal zone, and the red pulp.

White Pulp

The white pulp contains the lymphocytes and other mononuclear cells that surround the arterioles branching off the splenic artery. After the splenic artery pierces the splenic capsule at the hilum, it divides into progressively smaller branches. Each branch is called a central artery because it runs through the central longitudinal axis of a distinctive filtration bed that surrounds each central artery (Fig. 6–4). This is composed of a cuff of lymphocytes called the periarteriolar lymphoid sheath (PALS). The PALS is composed mostly of T lymphocytes, about two-thirds of which are CD4+ T cells. The PALS around white pulp arterioles of the human spleen is not continuous.[36] Indeed, segments of the central arterioles might not be surrounded by T cells in areas where they run through lymphoid follicles containing pale areas of activated B lymphocytes interspersed with large, pale macrophages and dendritic cells.[1] The migration of T cells to the PALS is governed by stromal cell production of chemokines, primarily CCL19 and CCL21, which interact with the chemokine receptor CCR7 that is expressed by naïve T cells.[37] Stromal production of these chemokines can be stimulated by certain cytokines, such as lymphotoxin.[38]

On gross inspection of the surface of a freshly cut spleen, these follicles appear as white dots referred to as malpighian corpuscles (Fig. 6–5). These corpuscles contain a germinal center and have the same anatomic features and functions as secondary follicles in the lymph node. Branches coming off the central artery deliver disproportionate amounts of plasma and lymphocytes to the rim of the PALS (Fig. 6–6). These branches tend to run at acute angles, leading to a selective loss of plasma from the blood, a phenomenon referred to as "skimming." After becoming relatively depleted of plasma, the arterioles then carry plasma-reduced blood into the filtration beds of the red pulp and marginal zone. As a result, the red pulp and marginal zone beds contain relatively high concentrations of red cells.

The Marginal Zone

The marginal zone surrounds the PALS and follicles. It is composed of a reticulum, which forms a finely meshed filtration bed, serving as a vestibule for much of the blood that flows through the spleen. The marginal zone surrounds the white pulp and merges with the red pulp. It contains more lymphocytes than the red pulp. These are primarily B cells and

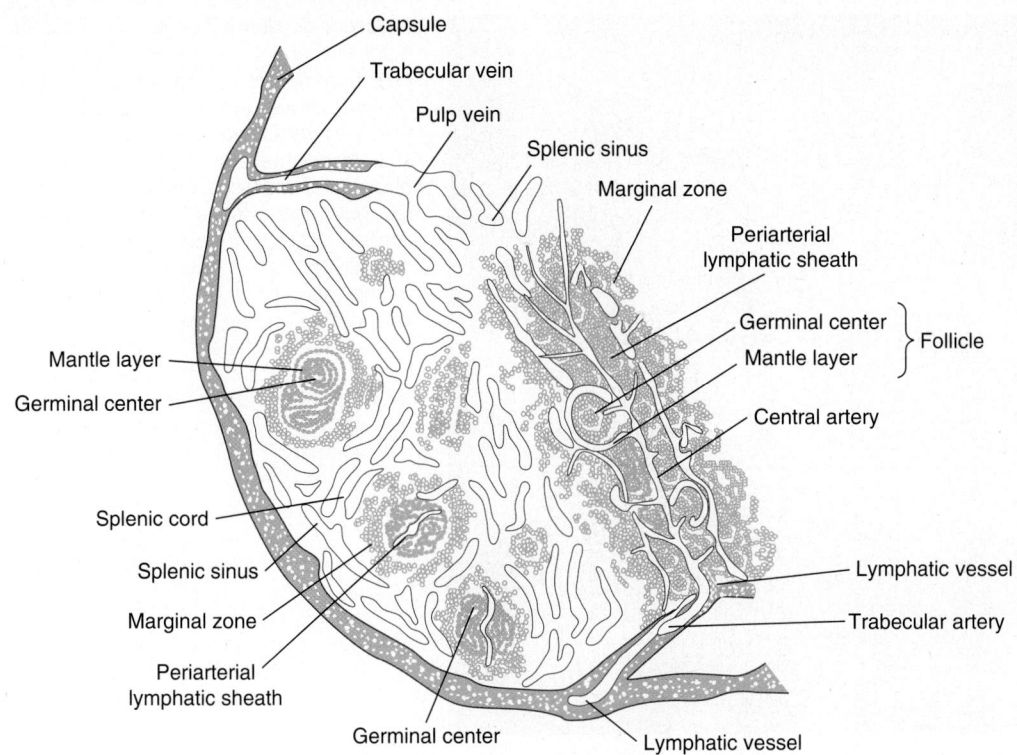

Figure 6–4. Structure of the spleen. A branch of the splenic artery enters the pulp and becomes a central artery. Surrounding the central artery is a periarterial lymphoid sheath (PALS). At the circumference of the PALS is the marginal zone, which generally separates the white pulp of the PALS from the red pulp. Follicles of B cells with occasional germinal centers (malpighian corpuscles) are located at the outer margins of the PALS for the depicted central artery and the PALS of central arteries that are in a different plane from that of the figure.

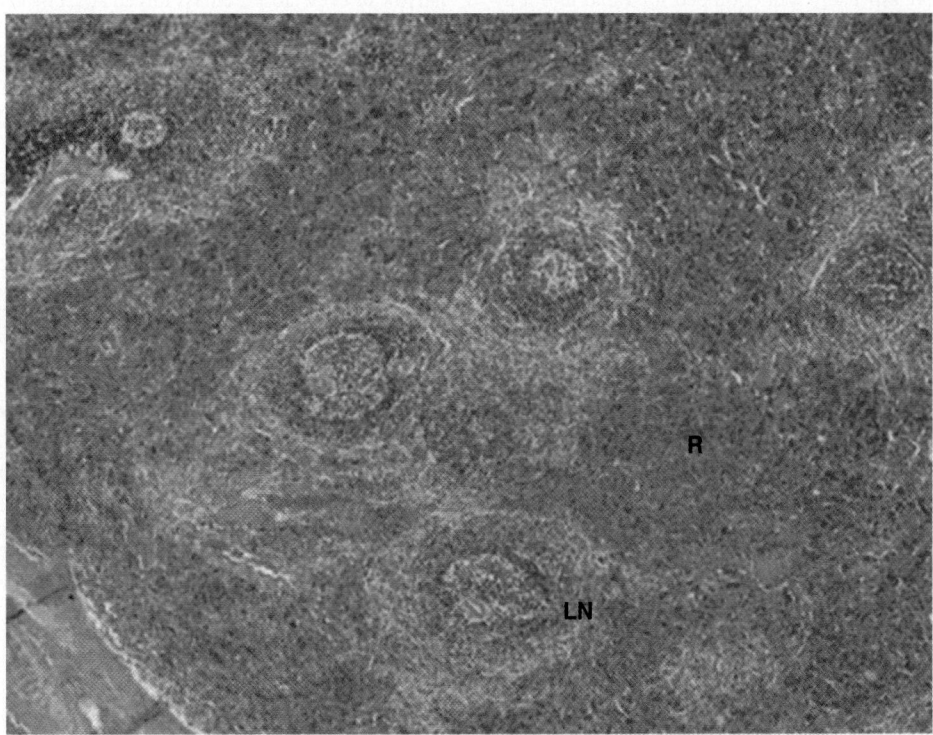

Figure 6–5. Normal human spleen. The splenic tissue is composed of red and white pulp. The red pulp *(R)*, shown here as masses of red cells, is imparted a red color in living tissue as a result of the natural color of hemoglobin in red cells and in stained sections as a result of the intensified red (eosinophilic) stain taken up by hemoglobin. The red pulp contains venous sinuses separated by cords of red cells (cords of Billroth), which cannot be seen in a light micrograph. The white pulp is composed of spherical aggregates of lymphocytes (lymphatic nodule *[LN]*) with a lighter staining germinal center and an outer, relatively thin, darker stained marginal zone, which separates white pulp from red pulp. Thick-walled central arteries are usually evident penetrating the white pulp. The central artery is cut obliquely in the white pulp at the upper left. Two arteries are seen penetrating the nodule in the center-left of the field and a single artery penetrating the white pulp in the lower-center of the field. The central artery is often seen in the lymphatic nodule in an eccentric position. Other nodules do not show a vessel in this plane of section. *(Reproduced with permission from Lichtman's Atlas of Hematology, www.accessmedicine.com.)*

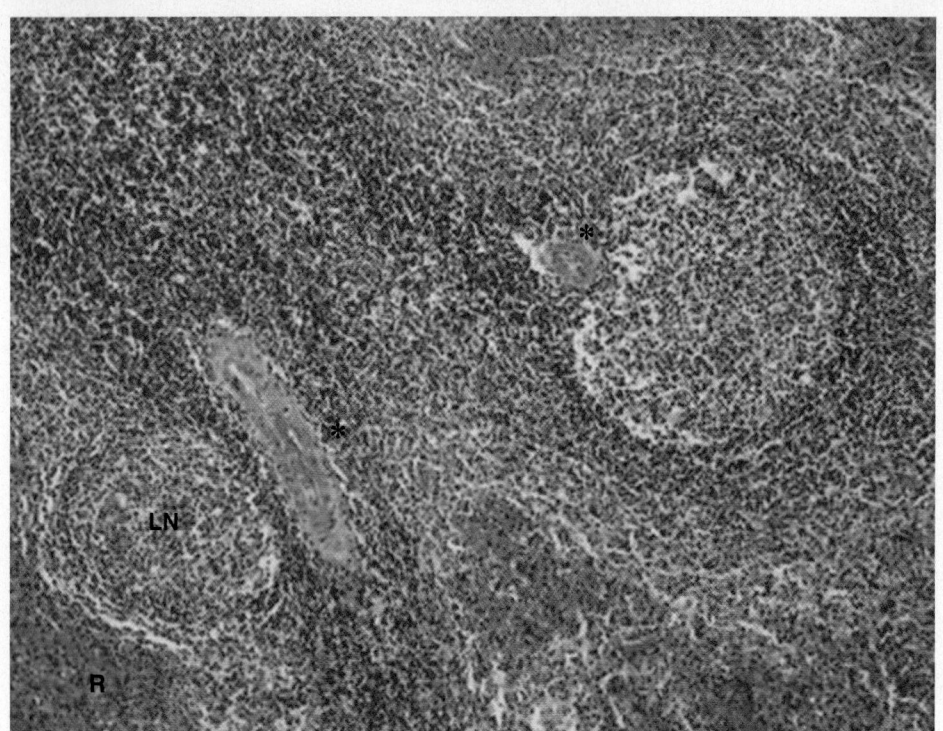

Figure 6–6. Normal human spleen (higher magnification of white pulp). The white pulp is composed of spherical aggregates of lymphocytes (lymphatic nodules [LN]) with a lighter staining germinal center and an outer, relatively thin, darker stained marginal zone, which separates white pulp from red pulp. The lymphatic nodules largely consist of B lymphocytes. Thick-walled central arteries are usually evident penetrating the white pulp, often in an eccentric position as noted by the asterisks. The T-cell–rich periarteriolar lymphoid sheath surrounds the central artery, which is cut longitudinally in the lymphatic nodule at the left. A single central artery penetrating the lymphatic nodule in the upper-right part of the field is in a characteristically eccentric position. R, red pulp. (*Reproduced with permission from* Lichtman's Atlas of Hematology, *www.accessmedicine.com.*)

CD4+ T cells that appear especially well equipped for rapid antibody immune responses to bloodborne antigens.[39–41] However, like the red pulp, the marginal zone may become congested and remove damaged and senescent red cells and parasites.

The Red Pulp

The splenic red pulp is composed of a reticular meshwork, called the splenic cords of Billroth, and splenic sinuses.[42] This region predominantly contains erythrocytes but also has large numbers of macrophages and dendritic cells as well as fewer numbers of granulocytes, cytolytic CD8+ T cells, and natural killer (NK) cells.

As the central arteries branch and decrease in size, the PALS also branches and decreases in diameter to but a few cells surrounding the arteriole. The small arteriole finally emerges from its sheath and then terminates in either the marginal zone or the red pulp. Here these vessels are suspended and anchored by adventitial reticular cells in the periarterial beds. They often terminate abruptly as arteriolar capillaries or as vessels with a trumpet-like flare with widened slits called interendothelial slits. The blood flows through these slits into filtration beds composed of large-meshed loculi that open to one another.

The blood in the red pulp and marginal zone drains into venous sinuses that form anastomosing, blind-ending vessels. These venous sinuses actually are specialized postcapillary venules. The endothelial cells are shaped as tapered rods that are stiffened by basal, longitudinal, intermediate cytoskeletal filaments and contractile filaments of actin and myosin. These intracellular contractile filaments can shorten the vein, causing the endothelium to buckle and form interendothelial gaps, favoring transmural passage.

The endothelial cells are attached to a basement membrane. Although this appears to be fashioned of fibers, the basement membrane actually is an extracellular membranous wall with large, regular defects that expose considerable basal endothelial surface. This includes the interendothelial slits through which blood may flow from the filtration bed and into the vein. Ordinarily the interendothelial slits are

narrow or even closed unless forced apart by cells in transmural transit or by endothelial contraction.

Splenic arterioles terminate at varied distances from the walls of venous vessels. Blood flowing from arterioles that terminate at the venous vessel wall may flow directly into the splenic vein. However, blood flowing from arterioles that terminate at a distance from a vein must traffic through the spleen. In so doing, the blood either may pass quickly through a nonsinusoidal venous aperture or slowly through sinusoidal interendothelial slits and the fibroblast stroma.

The fibroblast stroma contains reticular cells and myofibroblast cells, which are also called barrier cells. The latter may fuse with each other to form a syncytial membrane that connects the arterial terminals with venous interendothelial slits or apertures. Like other myofibroblasts, these cells contain actin and myosin and may contract, thereby approximating splenic arterial and venous vessels with one another. Thus, the fibroblast stroma may affect the relative proportion of blood that flows through the stroma or the sinusal interendothelial slits. Such redistribution might occur during periods of acute physiologic stress, allow for increased expulsion of red cells from the spleen, and account for some of the increase in hematocrit observed during strenuous exercise.[43]

SPLENIC FUNCTION

Red Cell Clearance

Mixed within the stroma of the red pulp and marginal zone are monocytes and macrophages. As the blood passes through the stroma, monocytes adhere to the stroma, where the microenvironment is conducive to their maturation into macrophages and large, dendritic, lysosome-rich phagocytes. These cells assist the reticular cells in mechanical filtration. More importantly, these cells have phagocytic activity that allows them to ingest imperfect erythrocytes, store platelets, and remove infectious agents, such as plasmodia, from the circulation.[44] In addition, the monocytes and macrophages have nonphagocytic functions, such as the presentation of antigens to T cells or the elaboration of immunomodulatory cytokines.

Collectively, the anatomy of the spleen allows the marginal zone and red pulp to cull defective erythrocytes. As the blood passes slowly through the sinusoidal interendothelial slits and the fibroblast stroma, the erythrocytes must undergo alterations in shape to squeeze through the mechanical barrier generated by this filtration compartment. Normal red cells that are supple may pass through readily because the interendothelial slits can open to approximately 0.5 μm. However, erythrocytes containing large, rigid inclusions, such as plasmodium-containing erythrocytes, are delayed or sequestered.[45] Antibody-coated red cells, as present in autoimmune hemolytic anemia, are also recognized and removed by macrophages in the splenic red pulp. Polymorphisms of FcγRII (CD32) or FcγRIII (CD16) that affect immunoglobulin (Ig) G binding *in vitro* can alter the efficiency of clearance of antibody-coated red cells *in vivo*.[46]

When these filtration beds sequester imperfect red cells, the blood pools inside the spleen, causing stasis and congestion. This stimulates sphincter-like contraction of the distal vein, resulting in proximal plasma transudation that produces a viscous luminal mass of high-hematocrit blood. During episodes of enhanced red cell sequestration, as occurs during malarial crises or hemolytic episodes in a small proportion of patients with sickle cell disease, the splenic volume and weight may increase 10- to 20-fold (Chap. 56).[47] Although the white pulp may enlarge, particularly in germinal centers, the marginal zones and red pulp become greatly widened with pooled erythrocytes and macrophages in this setting.

Regulation of Blood Volume

The spleen also can play a role in modulating blood volume. Release of high-hematocrit blood through splenic contraction occurs in response to activation of the baroreflex, which also may be activated during conditions of decreased blood pressure and cardiac output.[48,49] On the other hand, physiologic agents such as atrial natriuretic peptide, nitric oxide, and adrenomedullin can induce fluid extravasation from the splenic circulation into lymphatic reservoirs.[50] Excessive splenic extravasation can contribute to the inability to maintain adequate intravascular volume during septic shock. There also is evidence that the splenic afferent and renal sympathetic nerves play a role in maintaining renal microvascular tone.[50] This splenorenal reflex can influence blood pressure and, during septic shock, help promote renal sodium and water reabsorption and release of the vasoconstrictor angiotensin II. On the other hand, in portal hypertension, the splenorenal reflex can promote renal sodium and water retention and possibly play a role in the hemodynamic complications of portal hypertension through neurohormonal modulation of the mesenteric vascular bed.

Splenic Immune Function

The spleen and its responses to antigens are similar to those of lymph nodes, the major difference being that the spleen is the major site of immune responses to bloodborne antigens, while lymph nodes are involved in responses to antigens in the lymph.[42] Antigens and lymphocytes enter the spleen through the vascular sinuses, because the spleen lacks high endothelial venules. Upon entry, the lymphocytes home to the white pulp. T cells, which express the chemokine receptor CCR7, migrate to the PALS in response to CCL19 and CCL21, and B cells, which express CXCR5, migrate to the lymphoid follicles in response to CXCL13.[37,51] Dendritic cells also express CCR7 and hence migrate to the same area as do naïve T cells. T and B cells migrate within these compartments for about 5 and 7 hours, respectively. In the absence of an immune response, these cells migrate through a reticulum arranged around the circumference of the central artery.

Upon immune activation in response to antigen, the lymphocytes may remain in the spleen to sustain a primary or secondary immune response. Activation of B cells is initiated in the marginal zones that are adjacent to CD4+ T cells in the PALS. Activated B cells then migrate into germinal centers or into the red pulp.[52] Lymphoid nodules appear and expand by recruiting lymphocytes from the blood and the peripheral zone of the follicles, termed the mantle zone. These cells then proliferate and differentiate in the center of a lymphoid nodule, forming a germinal center.[53] In their path from the marginal zone to the follicles, B cells pass into the PALS, where they remain in contact with T lymphocytes for a few hours, allowing ample time for T- and B-cell interaction in response to antigens. If they are not recruited in an immune response to antigen, both T and B lymphocytes exit the spleen via deep efferent lymphatics, not the splenic veins.

These efferent lymphatics are not distinguished as separate structures within the PALS, being quite thin-walled and often packed with efferent lymphocytes. However, they are important in moving nonreactive lymphocytes out of the spleen and in producing high-hematocrit pulp blood. After leaving the spleen, the efferent lymphocytes become the afferent lymphatics of the perisplenic mesenteric lymph nodes or empty into the thoracic duct. This duct empties into the left subclavian vein, thus returning the lymphocytes to the venous circulation.

●LYMPH NODES

The lymphoid nodes are secondary lymphoid tissues. They form part of a network that filters antigens from the interstitial tissue fluid and lymph during its passage from the periphery to the thoracic duct. Thus, the lymph nodes are the primary sites of immune response to tissue antigens.

LYMPH NODE ANATOMY

The lymph nodes are round or kidney-shaped clusters of mononuclear cells that normally are less than 1 cm in diameter (Fig. 6–7). A collagenous capsule surrounds a typical lymph node and has an indentation called the hilus where blood vessels enter and leave.

Lymph nodes typically are present at the branches of the lymphatic vessels and form part of the extensive network of lymphatic channels that extends throughout the body. Several afferent lymphatic channels that drain lymph from regional tissues into the lymph node perforate the capsule of each lymph node. The lymph draining from the node leaves through one efferent lymphatic vessel at the hilus. The lymph from the node, in turn, empties into efferent lymphatic vessels that eventually drain into larger lymphatic channels leading eventually to the thoracic duct. The thoracic duct, in turn, drains into the left subclavian vein, thus returning lymph into the systemic circulation.

Clusters of lymph nodes are located strategically in areas that drain various superficial and deep regions of the body, such as the neck, axillae, groin, mediastinum, and abdominal cavity. The lymph nodes that receive lymph that drains from the skin, termed somatic nodes, are superficial. The lymph nodes that receive their lymph from the mucosal surface of the respiratory, digestive, or genitourinary tract, termed visceral nodes, are usually deep within body cavities.

LYMPH NODE STRUCTURE

Beneath the collagenous capsule is the subcapsular sinus, into which the afferent lymphatic channels drain (Fig. 6–8). This sinus is lined with phagocytic cells. Fibrous trabeculae radiate from the medulla adjacent to the hilus of the node to the subcapsular sinus, thus breaking the node into several follicles, called cortical follicles. These trabeculae, together

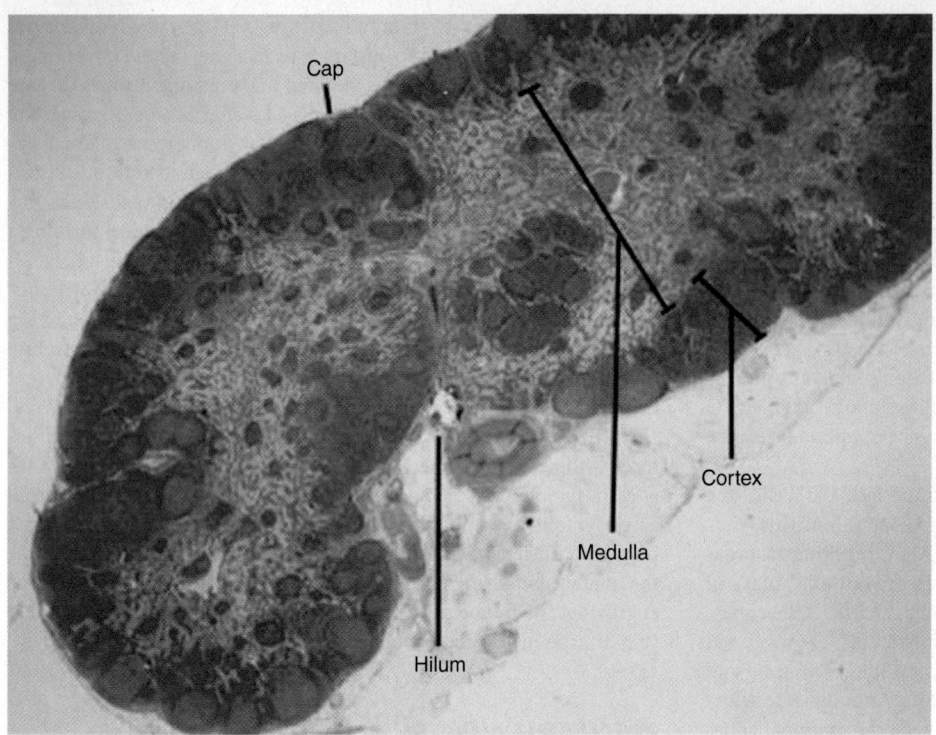

Cap

Cortex

Medulla

Hilum

Figure 6–7. Normal human lymph node. Low power. Capsule *(Cap)* is a thin connective tissue covering. Below the capsule is the subcapsular sinus. Lymphatics penetrate the capsule and enter the subcapsular sinus. The cortex is composed of adjacent lymphatic nodules, usually with fine connective tissue trabecula extending from the capsule separating the nodules. The nodule has a germinal center that stains lighter than the outer mantle zone because of the proliferating medium-sized and large lymphocytes with less dense staining properties. The medulla is composed of interconnecting medullary cords composed of lymphocytes and interspersed light staining channels, the medullary sinuses. Lymph flows from the subcapsular sinus down the trabecular sinuses and into the medullary sinuses and exits the node via efferent lymphatics at the hilum. *(Reproduced with permission from* Lichtman's Atlas of Hematology, *www.accessmedicine.com.)*

with the capsule and a network of reticulin fibers, support the various cellular components of the node and serve as the scaffolding for lymphatic spaces, namely, the subcapsular and cortical sinuses. These lymphatic spaces are continuous with medullary sinuses and the solitary efferent lymphatic channel exiting the hilus.

Each cortical follicle contains dense collections of small, mature, recirculating lymphocytes. These consist of a B-cell area (cortex), a T-cell–rich area (paracortex), and a central medulla with cellular cords that contain T cells, B cells, plasma cells, and macrophages.[1] Some follicles contain lightly staining areas of 1- to 2-mm in diameter, called germinal centers. Germinal centers are the specialized sites for the

generation of memory B cells and antibody affinity maturation via the process of immunoglobulin variable-region somatic hypermutation.[54] Follicles without germinal centers are called primary follicles, and those with germinal centers are called secondary follicles. Primary lymphoid follicles contain nodules that consist predominantly of small, mature, recirculating B lymphocytes.

Within 1 week after antigenic stimulation, secondary follicles develop a germinal center that contains proliferating B cells and macrophages.[55,56] The small, nonreactive B cells are apparently forced to the periphery of the follicle, where they form a dense follicular mantle. The B cells within the germinal center, on the other hand, are highly

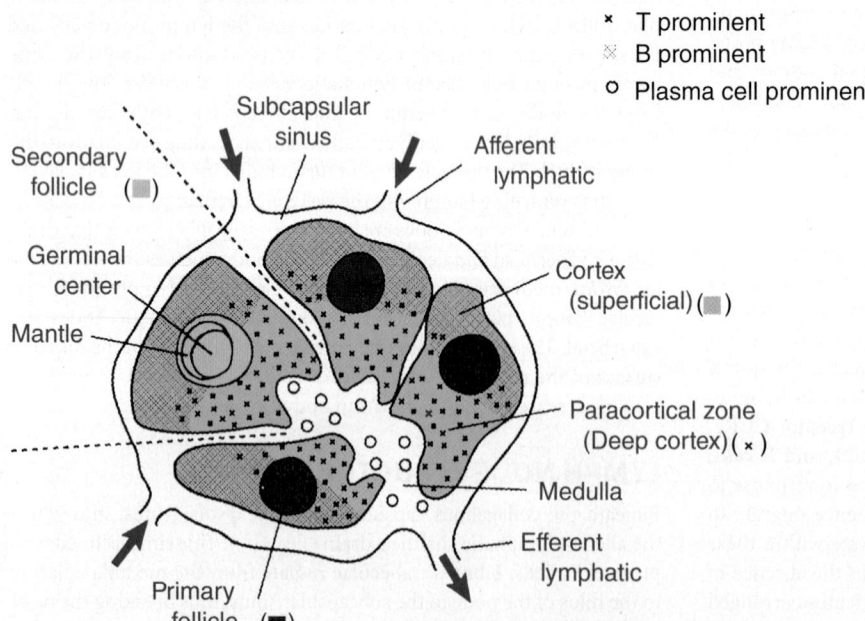

× T prominent
B prominent
o Plasma cell prominent

Secondary follicle (▣)

Subcapsular sinus

Afferent lymphatic

Germinal center

Mantle

Cortex (superficial) (▣)

Paracortical zone (Deep cortex) (×)

Medulla

Efferent lymphatic

Primary follicle (■)

Figure 6–8. Structure of the lymph node. The lymph enters via afferent lymphatic channels and exits via the efferent lymphatic channel. The *large arrows* indicate the direction of the lymphatic flow into and out of the lymph node. The legend shows the symbols used for the T-cell zone *(x)* and the B-cell zone *(shade)* of each follicle. The follicle in the lower left part of the node contains a primary follicle lacking a germinal center. The follicle immediately above this follicle contains a germinal center. Thus, the entire follicle delineated by the dashed lines is a secondary follicle. The cortex, paracortical area, and medulla are also shown.

activated, typically forming blasts that have abundant cytoplasm and round, cleaved, or convoluted shapes. Follicular dendritic cells also are found within the germinal centers. These cells can trap and retain antigens for months, possibly in the form of immune complexes.[57] The germinal centers of the secondary follicle may gradually regress after the antigenic stimulus is eliminated.

Surrounding the lymphoid follicles of the superficial cortex are sheets of lymphocytes that extend to the deep cortex, the paracortex, that blend into medullary cords of cells. The paracortical zones are formed mostly of T cells. The ratio of T cells to B cells in these zones is approximately 3:1. The medulla, however, contains scattered B cells, dendritic cells, macrophages, rare NK cells, and, during an immune response, plasma cells. The superficial cortex and medulla of the lymph nodes are the thymic-independent areas, while the deep cortex is particularly enriched with T cells, forming an area that sometimes is referred to as the thymic-dependent area. The major T-cell population found within the lymph node consists of CD4+ T cells. The scattering of CD4+ T cells in the follicles, and in more prominent numbers in the interfollicular zones, reveals the proximity of CD4+ T and B cells important for T-B cooperation during proliferation and maturation of antigen-stimulated B cells.[58]

The T-cell–rich paracortex is also relatively enriched with specialized NK cells and other innate lymphoid cell (ILC) populations that likely have roles in shaping innate and adaptive immune responses in lymph nodes, as well as other secondary lymphoid tissues (SLT), through the production of immunomodulatory cytokines. The NK cell population present in the lymph node paracortex is predominantly composed of the CD56[bright] subset that can rapidly produce cytokines, such as interferon-γ and tumor necrosis factor-α, in response to monocyte-derived cytokines (IL-12, IL-15, and IL-18).[59,60] However, these NK cells show relatively weak cytotoxicity in comparison to CD56[dim] NK cells that predominate in the blood (Chap. 77).[61] There is accumulating evidence that CD56[bright] NK cells represent the immediate precursors to CD56[dim] NK cells and likely differentiate into the latter just prior to their egress from lymph nodes.[62–64] Moreover, CD34+CD45RA+ hematopoietic progenitor cells capable of giving rise to CD56[bright] NK cells are also enriched in the lymph node paracortex indicating that these tissues are also likely sites of NK cell development.[65–67]

Lymphocytes primarily enter lymphatic tissues from the blood by migrating across the tall, active endothelium of specialized postcapillary venules called *high endothelial venules*.[68] Cellular adhesion molecules and various chemokines, including CXCL13, CCL19, and CCL21, are responsible for the pattern of lymphocyte trafficking and determine the associations among stromal (e.g., reticular and endothelial) and parenchymal (e.g., T and B lymphocytes, dendritic cells, and macrophages) cells in the lymphoid tissues.[54,69]

LYMPH NODE FUNCTION

The lymph node is the site where different types of lymphocytes, macrophages, and dendritic cells can interact with one another to generate an immune response to antigens carried within the lymph. As the lymph passes across the nodes from afferent to efferent lymphatic vessels, particulate antigens are removed by the phagocytic cells and transported into the lymphoid tissue of the lymph node.[1] Abnormal cells within the lymph, such as neoplastic cells, also can be trapped within the lymph node.

Within the lymph node, antigen is presented to T cells as processed peptides by MHC molecules of antigen-presenting cells (Chap. 76). Various T-cell subsets comprise a network of interactive cells. CD4+ and CD8+ cell-mediated contacts, as well as T-cell–derived soluble factors, induce and regulate the immune response. T-cell recognition

is mediated by the TCR for antigen. Which T cells are activated is determined by the specificity of the TCRs, the structure of MHC molecules, and the nature of antigen-presenting cells, including the dendritic reticular cells, macrophages, and B cells.

Along with TCR recognition of processed antigen presented in the MHC of the antigen-presenting cell, adequate T-cell activation requires secondary signals, or costimulation, delivered through accessory molecules, such as CD28.[70] Without these secondary signals, T cells may become anergic or specifically nonresponsive to antigen stimulation.[71] This specific suppression is thought to play an important regulatory role in the maintenance of self-tolerance.[72,73]

T-cell recognition of specific antigen may induce release of soluble factors, such as interleukins, that can activate the T cells themselves or have paracrine effects on other neighboring leukocytes.[74] Also, activated T cells express surface molecules, such as CD40-ligand (CD154), that also can activate B cells, dendritic cells, or macrophages.[75,76]

The T-dependent immune response includes the formation of early germinal centers within days after antigen exposure. There is a mixture of B cells and activated CD4+ T cells in the lymphoid follicles. T-B cooperation involves the accessory B-cell antigen CD40 and the CD154 antigen expressed on activated T cells (Chap. 76). Activated B cells differentiate and take on the cytomorphologic characteristics of centroblasts and comprise the largest numbers of cells in the early germinal center.[56] Subsequently, centroblasts give rise to smaller B cells, the centrocytes. B cells undergo affinity maturation within the germinal center. During this process, the genes encoding the surface immunoglobulin of B cells undergo high rates of mutation, called somatic hypermutation.[53,77] B cells that express immunoglobulin with little or no affinity for antigen undergo apoptosis.[78] The resulting cellular debris is tingible, or capable of being stained, and is found prominently within macrophages specifically designated tingible body macrophages. On the other hand, B cells expressing surface immunoglobulin with high affinity for antigen are selected to proliferate and differentiate to memory B cells or plasma cells.[54] As well as promoting activation of B cells, CD4+ T cells, and CD8+ T cells may give rise to circulating memory T cells.[79,80]

Following the release of specific antibody, antigen–antibody complexes may form and become sequestered on the surface of follicular dendritic cells within the germinal centers. These antigen–antibody complexes produce a coating of small, bead-like, immune complex-coated bodies called *iccosomes*. Iccosomes may be presented to CD4+ T cells by B cells and dendritic cells. Iccosomes also appear to assist in anamnestic recall following reentry of antigen in the host.[81] T- and B-cell memory functions depend upon persistence of antigen.[82]

PERIPHERAL LYMPHOID TISSUES

MUCOSA-ASSOCIATED LYMPHOID TISSUES

The mucosa-associated lymphoid tissues (MALTs) are diffusely organized aggregates of lymphocytes that protect the respiratory and gastrointestinal epithelium.[83] The lymphoid aggregates associated with the respiratory epithelium are sometimes referred to as the bronchial-associated lymphoid tissue. The lymphoid aggregates associated with the intestinal epithelium are sometimes referred to as the gut-associated lymphoid tissue (GALT). Lymphocytes in the GALT are located in three main regions: within the epithelial layer, scattered through the lamina propria, and clustered in organized collections in the lamina propria. The latter includes the tonsils, adenoids, appendix, and specialized structures called Peyer patches found in the ileum (Fig. 6–9). Most intraepithelial lymphocytes are CD8+ T cells, 10 percent of which express the γ/δ form of the TCR (Chap. 76). On the other hand, the intestinal lamina propria contains a mixed population of cells, including

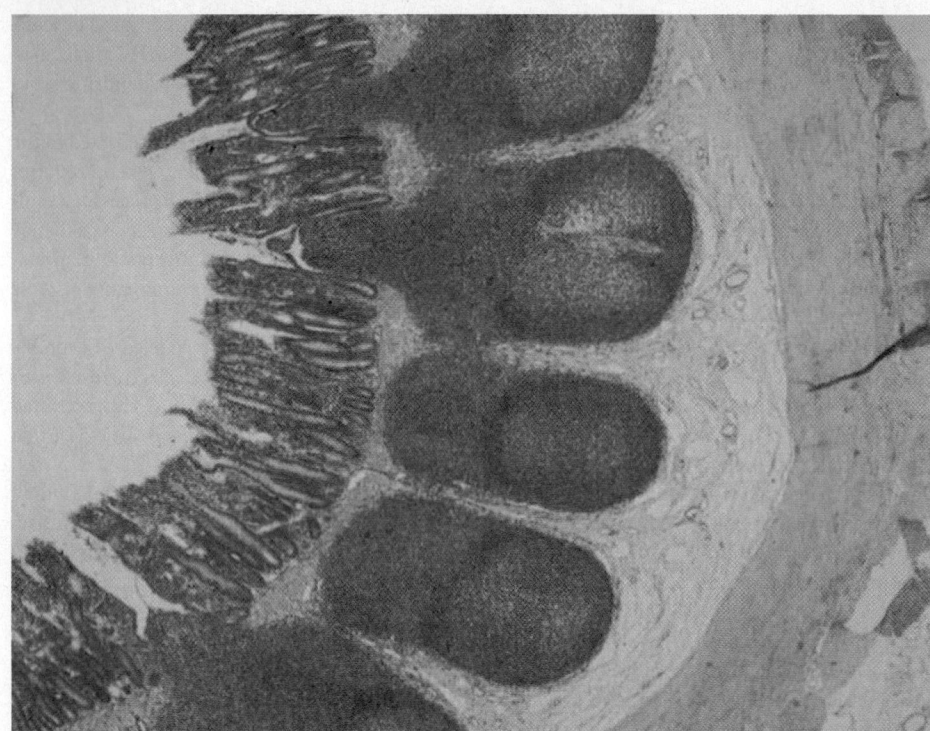

Figure 6–9. A cross-section of human terminal ileum. The columnar epithelium shown to the left is organized into villi. A series of lymphatic nodules in the mucosa extending from the lamina propria to the submucosa is part of the gastrointestinal-associated lymphoid tissue (GALT). In the ileum, this highly organized lymphatic tissue is referred to as Peyer patches. They each contain a germinal center. The GALT is a subset of the mucosa-associated lymphatic tissue. Scattered lymphatic nodules may also be seen in the mucosa of other parts of the small bowel and colon but they are usually isolated single nodules. *(Reproduced with permission from* Lichtman's Atlas of Hematology, *www.accessmedicine.com.)*

activated CD4+ T cells as well as a recently described and heterogeneous population of ILC. ILCs are now known to be key players in mucosal immunity; they release immunomodulatory cytokines, and a subset also produces IL-22 which supports epithelial homeostasis.[84] Similar to the lymphoid follicles of the spleen and lymph nodes, the mucosal follicles in the lamina propria contain mostly B cells, which sometimes are organized into germinal centers.

Solitary lymph nodules with follicular and germinal center structures occur in the mucosa and submucosa of the respiratory tract, the gastrointestinal tract (particularly within the ileum), the urinary tract, and the vagina. Microfolds overlying specialized epithelial cells in the gut transport antigenic material by pinocytosis, with potential subsequent activation of the immune response. During states of chronic inflammation, lymphoid nodules may form as a localized center of lymphocytes with marked follicular activity. The Waldeyer ring of pharyngeal lymphoid tissues and Peyer patches in the ileum contain prominent aggregated nodular lymphoid tissue. No capsule or efferent or afferent lymphatic vessels are present in these accessory lymphoid tissues.

The MALT are rich in plasma cells and eosinophils. The plasma cells are a source of secretory immunoglobulin that is transferred into the lumina of the bronchi and gastrointestinal tract. The majority of plasma cells in the mucosa of the bronchi and gut contain IgA.[85] IgA is released from the plasma cell and then combines with a secretory piece synthesized within the mucosal epithelium to become secretory IgA (Chap. 75). Secretory IgA then is secreted across the microvilli of mucosal epithelium into the lumen, where it may prevent colonization of mucosal membranes by pathogens. Lymphoid nodules along mucosa-lined tracts serve as precursors of IgA-producing cells. These nodules form a barrier against many microorganisms and antigens.[86]

Peyer Patches

Peyer patches are the most important and highly organized of the GALT.[83] They are found in the lamina propria of the ileum (near the ileocolonic junction) and consist of up to 50 or more lymphoid nodules covered by a single layer of columnar epithelium (see Fig. 6–9). They are well developed in youth and regress with age. Antigens from the intestinal epithelium are collected by specialized epithelial cells called M cells, allowing for generation of specific immune responses against intestinal pathogens.[87] Peyer patches are the sites at which B cells differentiate in response to these antigens into the plasma cells found within the intestine.[88]

Tonsils

The tonsils are the major component of the Waldeyer ring of pharyngeal lymphoid tissues. They are covered by variable epithelial surfaces that have deep, branching depressions called crypts. Fused lymphatic nodules lie adjacent to the crypts, and germinal centers are prominent. A pseudocapsule of condensed connective tissue surrounds the tonsils, and septae within the structures form lobulations. Together with the other lymphoid tissues of the Waldeyer ring, the tonsils provide the initial barrier to pathogens entering the oral pharynx.

REFERENCES

1. Crivellato E, Vacca A, Ribatti D: Setting the stage: An anatomist's view of the immune system. *Trends Immunol* 25:210–217, 2004.
2. Blackburn CC, Manley NR: Developing a new paradigm for thymus organogenesis. *Nat Rev Immunol* 4:278–289, 2004.
3. Hasselbalch H, Jeppesen DL, Ersboll AK, et al: Thymus size evaluated by sonography. A longitudinal study on infants during the first year of life. *Acta Radiol* 38:222–227, 1997.
4. Linton PJ, Dorshkind K: Age-related changes in lymphocyte development and function. *Nat Immunol* 5:133–139, 2004.
5. Cifone MG, Migliorati G, Parroni R, et al: Dexamethasone-induced thymocyte apoptosis: Apoptotic signal involves the sequential activation of phosphoinositide-specific phospholipase c, acidic sphingomyelinase, and caspases. *Blood* 93:2282–2296, 1999.
6. McClory S, Hughes T, Freud AG, et al: Evidence for a stepwise program of extrathymic T cell development within the human tonsil. *J Clin Invest* 122:1403–1415, 2012.
7. Hasselbalch H, Jeppesen DL, Ersboll AK, et al: Sonographic measurement of thymic size in healthy neonates. Relation to clinical variables. *Acta Radiol* 38:95–98, 1997.

8. Hasselbalch H, Jeppesen DL, Engelmann MD, et al: Decreased thymus size in formula-fed infants compared with breastfed infants. *Acta Paediatr* 85:1029–1032, 1996.

9. Watanabe N, Wang YH, Lee HK, et al: Hassall's corpuscles instruct dendritic cells to induce CD4+CD25+ regulatory T cells in human thymus. *Nature* 436:1181–1185, 2005.

10. Rezzani R, Bonomini F, Rodella LF: Histochemical and molecular overview of the thymus as site for T-cells development. *Prog Histochem Cytochem* 43:73–120, 2008.

11. Alves NL, Richard-Le Goff O, Huntington ND, et al: Characterization of the thymic IL-7 niche in vivo. *Proc Natl Acad Sci U S A* 106:1512–1517, 2009.

12. Fujihara C, Williams JA, Watanabe M, et al: T cell-B cell thymic cross-talk: Maintenance and function of thymic B cells requires cognate CD40-CD40 ligand interaction. *J Immunol* 193:5534–5544, 2014.

13. Walters SN, Webster KE, Daley S, Grey ST: A role for intrathymic B cells in the generation of natural regulatory T cells. *J Immunol* 193:170–176, 2014.

14. Ayala A, Herdon CD, Lehman DL, et al: Differential induction of apoptosis in lymphoid tissues during sepsis: Variation in onset, frequency, and the nature of the mediators. *Blood* 87:4261–4275, 1996.

15. Rijhsinghani AG, Thompson K, Bhatia SK, Waldschmidt TJ: Estrogen blocks early T cell development in the thymus. *Am J Reprod Immunol* 36:269–277, 1996.

16. Sullivan KE: Chromosome 22q11.2 deletion syndrome: Digeorge syndrome/velocardiofacial syndrome. *Immunol Allergy Clin North Am* 28:353–366, 2008.

17. Hale LP: Histologic and molecular assessment of human thymus. *Ann Diagn Pathol* 8:50–60, 2004.

18. Kronenberg M, Siu G, Hood LE, Shastri N: The molecular genetics of the T-cell antigen receptor and T-cell antigen recognition. *Annu Rev Immunol* 4:529–591, 1986.

19. Kwan J, Killeen N: CCR7 directs the migration of thymocytes into the thymic medulla. *J Immunol* 172:3999–4007, 2004.

20. Starr TK, Jameson SC, Hogquist KA: Positive and negative selection of T cells. *Annu Rev Immunol* 21:139–176, 2003.

21. Laufer TM, Glimcher LH, Lo D: Using thymus anatomy to dissect T cell repertoire selection. *Semin Immunol* 11:65–70, 1999.

22. Blackman M, Kappler J, Marrack P: The role of the T cell receptor in positive and negative selection of developing T cells. *Science* 248:1335–1341, 1990.

23. Muller-Hermelink HK, Wilisch A, Schultz A, Marx A: Characterization of the human thymic microenvironment: Lymphoepithelial interaction in normal thymus and thymoma. *Arch Histol Cytol* 60:9–28, 1997.

24. Nikolich-Zugich J, Slifka MK, Messaoudi I: The many important facets of T-cell repertoire diversity. *Nat Rev Immunol* 4:123–132, 2004.

25. Mathis D, Benoist C: Aire. *Annu Rev Immunol* 27:287–312, 2009.

26. De Martino L, Capalbo D, Improda N, et al: APECED: A paradigm of complex interactions between genetic background and susceptibility factors. *Front Immunol* 4:331, 2013.

27. Vogel A, Strassburg CP, Obermayer-Straub P, et al: The genetic background of autoimmune polyendocrinopathy-candidiasis-ectodermal dystrophy and its autoimmune disease components. *J Mol Med (Berl)* 80:201–211, 2002.

28. Mathis D, Benoist C: Back to central tolerance. *Immunity* 20:509–516, 2004.

29. Romero-Torres R: The true splenic blood supply and its surgical applications. *Hepatogastroenterology* 45:885–888, 1998.

30. Paul R, Bielmeier J, Breul J, et al: [Accessory spleen of the spermatic cord] [in German]. *Urologe A* 36:262–264, 1997.

31. Lauffer JM, Baer HU, Maurer CA, et al: Intrapancreatic accessory spleen. A rare cause of a pancreatic mass. *Int J Pancreatol* 25:65–68, 1999.

32. Sprogoe-Jakobsen S, Sprogoe-Jakobsen U: The weight of the normal spleen. *Forensic Sci Int* 88:215–223, 1997.

33. Watanabe Y, Todani T, Noda T, Yamamoto S: Standard splenic volume in children and young adults measured from CT images. *Surg Today* 27:726–728, 1997.

34. Prassopoulos P, Daskalogiannaki M, Raissaki M, et al: Determination of normal splenic volume on computed tomography in relation to age, gender and body habitus. *Eur Radiol* 7:246–248, 1997.

35. Rodrigues Junior AJ, Rodrigues CJ, Germano MA, et al: Sonographic assessment of normal spleen volume. *Clin Anat* 8:252–255, 1995.

36. Steiniger B, Ruttinger L, Barth PJ: The three-dimensional structure of human splenic white pulp compartments. *J Histochem Cytochem* 51:655–664, 2003.

37. Muller G, Hopken UE, Lipp M: The impact of CCR7 and CXCR5 on lymphoid organ development and systemic immunity. *Immunol Rev* 195:117–135, 2003.

38. Schneider K, Potter KG, Ware CF: Lymphotoxin and light signaling pathways and target genes. *Immunol Rev* 202:49–66, 2004.

39. Mebius RE, Nolte MA, Kraal G: Development and function of the splenic marginal zone. *Crit Rev Immunol* 24:449–464, 2004.

40. Steiniger B, Timphus EM, Barth PJ: The splenic marginal zone in humans and rodents: An enigmatic compartment and its inhabitants. *Histochem Cell Biol* 126:641–648, 2006.

41. Weill JC, Weller S, Reynaud CA: Human marginal zone B cells. *Annu Rev Immunol* 27:267–285, 2009.

42. Kraus MD: Splenic histology and histopathology: An update. *Semin Diagn Pathol* 20:84–93, 2003.

43. Stewart IB, McKenzie DC: The human spleen during physiological stress. *Sports Med* 32:361–369, 2002.

44. Chotivanich K, Udomsangpetch R, McGready R, et al: Central role of the spleen in malaria parasite clearance. *J Infect Dis* 185:1538–1541, 2002.

45. Suwanarusk R, Cooke BM, Dondorp AM, et al: The deformability of red blood cells parasitized by *Plasmodium falciparum* and *P. vivax*. *J Infect Dis* 189:190–194, 2004.

46. Kumpel BM, De Haas M, Koene HR, et al: Clearance of red cells by monoclonal IgG3 anti-D in vivo is affected by the VF polymorphism of Fcgamma RIIIa (CD16). *Clin Exp Immunol* 132:81–86, 2003.

47. Smith NC, Fell A, Good MF: The immune response to asexual blood stages of malaria parasites. *Chem Immunol* 70:144–162, 1998.

48. Bakovic D, Eterovic D, Saratlija-Novakovic Z, et al: Effect of human splenic contraction on variation in circulating blood cell counts. *Clin Exp Pharmacol Physiol* 32:944–951, 2005.

49. Palada I, Eterovic D, Obad A, et al: Spleen and cardiovascular function during short apneas in divers. *J Appl Physiol* 103:1958–1963, 2007.

50. Hamza SM, Kaufman S: Role of spleen in integrated control of splanchnic vascular tone: Physiology and pathophysiology. *Can J Physiol Pharmacol* 87:1–7, 2009.

51. Forster R, Davalos-Misslitz AC, Rot A: CCR7 and its ligands: Balancing immunity and tolerance. *Nat Rev Immunol* 8:362–371, 2008.

52. Rizzo LV, Secord EA, Tsiagbe VK, et al: Components essential for the generation of germinal centers. *Dev Immunol* 6:325–330, 1998.

53. Hollowood K, Goodlad JR: Germinal centre cell kinetics. *J Pathol* 185:229–233, 1998.

54. Klein U, Dalla-Favera R: Germinal centres: Role in B-cell physiology and malignancy. *Nat Rev Immunol* 8:22–33, 2008.

55. Dunn-Walters DK, Isaacson PG, Spencer J: Analysis of mutations in immunoglobulin heavy chain variable region genes of microdissected marginal zone (MGZ) B cells suggests that the MGZ of human spleen is a reservoir of memory B cells. *J Exp Med* 182:559–566, 1995.

56. Tarlinton D: Germinal centers: Form and function. *Curr Opin Immunol* 10:245–251, 1998.

57. Burton GF, Masuda A, Heath SL, et al: Follicular dendritic cells (FDC) in retroviral infection: Host/pathogen perspectives. *Immunol Rev* 156:185–197, 1997.

58. Gulbranson-Judge A, Casamayor-Palleja M, MacLennan IC: Mutually dependent T and B cell responses in germinal centers. *Ann N Y Acad Sci* 815:199–210, 1997.

59. Cooper MA, Fehniger TA, Turner SC, et al: Human natural killer cells: A unique innate immunoregulatory role for the CD56(bright) subset. *Blood* 97:3146–3151, 2001.

60. Fehniger TA, Cooper MA, Nuovo GJ, et al: CD56bright natural killer cells are present in human lymph nodes and are activated by T cell-derived IL-2: A potential new link between adaptive and innate immunity. *Blood* 101:3052–3057, 2003.

61. Cooper MA, Fehniger TA, Caligiuri MA: The biology of human natural killer-cell subsets. *Trends Immunol* 22:633–640, 2001.

62. Ferlazzo G, Thomas D, Lin SL, et al: The abundant NK cells in human secondary lymphoid tissues require activation to express killer cell Ig-like receptors and become cytolytic. *J Immunol* 172:1455–1462, 2004.

63. Huntington ND, Legrand N, Alves NL, et al: IL-15 trans-presentation promotes human NK cell development and differentiation in vivo. *J Exp Med* 206:25–34, 2009.

64. Romagnani C, Juelke K, Falco M, et al: CD56brightCD16- killer Ig-like receptor- NK cells display longer telomeres and acquire features of CD56dim NK cells upon activation. *J Immunol* 178:4947–4955, 2007.

65. Freud AG, Becknell B, Roychowdhury S, et al: A human CD34(+) subset resides in lymph nodes and differentiates into CD56bright natural killer cells. *Immunity* 22:295–304, 2005.

66. Freud AG, Yokohama A, Becknell B, et al: Evidence for discrete stages of human natural killer cell differentiation in vivo. *J Exp Med* 203:1033–1043, 2006.

67. Freud AG, Yu J, Caligiuri MA: Human natural killer cell development in secondary lymphoid tissues. *Semin Immunol* 26:132–137, 2014.

68. Butcher EC, Williams M, Youngman K, et al: Lymphocyte trafficking and regional immunity. *Adv Immunol* 72:209–253, 1999.

69. Warnock RA, Askari S, Butcher EC, von Andrian UH. Molecular mechanisms of lymphocyte homing to peripheral lymph nodes. *J Exp Med* 187:205–216, 1998.

70. Greenfield EA, Nguyen KA, Kuchroo VK: CD28/B7 costimulation: A review. *Crit Rev Immunol* 18:389–418, 1998.

71. Schwartz RH: T cell anergy. *Annu Rev Immunol* 21:305–334, 2003.

72. Malvey EN, Telander DG, Vanasek TL, Mueller DL: The role of clonal anergy in the avoidance of autoimmunity: Inactivation of autocrine growth without loss of effector function. *Immunol Rev* 165:301–318, 1998.

73. Van Parijs L, Abbas AK: Homeostasis and self-tolerance in the immune system: Turning lymphocytes off. *Science* 280:243–248, 1998.

74. Seder RA, Gazzinelli RT: Cytokines are critical in linking the innate and adaptive immune responses to bacterial, fungal, and parasitic infection. *Adv Intern Med* 44:353–388, 1999.

75. Grewal IS, Flavell RA: CD40 and CD154 in cell-mediated immunity. *Annu Rev Immunol* 16:111–135, 1998.

76. Ranheim EA, Kipps TJ: Activated T cells induce expression of B7/BB1 on normal or leukemic B cells through a CD40-dependent signal. *J Exp Med* 177:925–935, 1993.

77. Vora KA, Ravetch JV, Manser T: Insights into the mechanisms of antibody-affinity maturation and the generation of the memory B-cell compartment using genetically altered mice. *Dev Immunol* 6:305–316, 1998.

78. Liu YJ, de Bouteiller O, Fugier-Vivier I. Mechanisms of selection and differentiation in germinal centers. *Curr Opin Immunol* 9:256–262, 1997.

79. Callan MF, Annels N, Steven N, et al: T cell selection during the evolution of CD8+ T cell memory in vivo. *Eur J Immunol* 28:4382–4390, 1998.

80. Doherty PC, Topham DJ, Tripp RA: Establishment and persistence of virus-specific CD4+ and CD8+ T cell memory. *Immunol Rev* 150:23–44, 1996.

81. Liu YJ, Grouard G, de Bouteiller O, Bancherau J: Follicular dendritic cells and germinal centers. *Int Rev Cytol* 166:139–179, 1996.

82. Freitas AA, Rocha B: Peripheral T cell survival. *Curr Opin Immunol* 11:152–156, 1999.

83. MacDonald TT: The mucosal immune system. *Parasite Immunol* 25:235–246, 2003.

84. Spits H, Artis D, Colonna M, et al: Innate lymphoid cells—A proposal for uniform nomenclature. *Nat Rev Immunol* 13:145–149, 2013.

85. Macpherson AJ, McCoy KD, Johansen FE, Brandtzaeg P: The immune geography of IgA induction and function. *Mucosal Immunol* 1:11–22, 2008.

86. Mason KL, Huffnagle GB, Noverr MC, Kao JY: Overview of gut immunology. *Adv Exp Med Biol* 635:1–14, 2008.

87. Clark MA, Jepson MA: Intestinal m cells and their role in bacterial infection. *Int J Med Microbiol* 293:17–39, 2003.

88. Dunn-Walters DK, Isaacson PG, Spencer J: Sequence analysis of human IgVH genes indicates that ileal lamina propria plasma cells are derived from peyer's patches. *Eur J Immunol* 27:463–467, 1997.

Part III Epochal Hematology

7. Hematology of the Fetus and
   Newborn 99

8. Hematology during Pregnancy 119
9. Hematology in Older Persons. 129

CHAPTER 7
HEMATOLOGY OF THE FETUS AND NEWBORN

James Palis and George B. Segel

SUMMARY

During embryogenesis, hematopoiesis occurs in spatially and temporally distinct sites, including the extraembryonic yolk sac, the fetal liver, and the preterm marrow. The development of primitive erythroblasts in the yolk sac is critical for embryonic survival. Primitive erythroblasts differentiate within the vascular network rather than in the extravascular space and circulate as nucleated cells. Although it is widely assumed that primitive red cells remain nucleated throughout their life span, primitive erythroblasts ultimately enucleate upon terminal differentiation. After 7 weeks of gestation, hematopoietic progenitors are no longer detected in the yolk sac. Hematopoietic stem cells emerge from major arterial vessels at 5 weeks of gestation. The liver serves as the primary source of red cells from the 9th to the 24th week of gestation. Like primitive erythropoiesis in the yolk sac, definitive erythropoiesis in the fetal liver is necessary for continued survival of the embryo. In contrast to the yolk sac, where hematopoiesis is restricted to maturing primitive erythroid, macrophage, and megakaryocytic cells, hematopoiesis in the fetal liver consists of definitive erythroid, megakaryocyte, and multiple myeloid, as well as lymphoid lineages. Hematopoietic cells are first seen in the marrow of the 10- to 11-week embryo, and they remain confined to the diaphyseal regions of long bones until 15 weeks of gestation. Lymphopoiesis is present in the lymph plexuses and the thymus beginning at 9 weeks of gestation. Yolk sac stem cells were first thought to seed the liver and eventually the marrow. However, later experiments in avian and amphibian embryos indicate that the hematopoietic stem cells that seed the marrow arise within the body of the embryo proper rather than from the yolk sac. The aorta-gonad-mesonephros (AGM) region generates hematopoietic stem cells that seed the liver and the marrow to provide lifelong hematopoiesis. Hemoglobin (Hgb) Gower-1 ($\zeta_2\varepsilon_2$) is the major hemoglobin in embryos younger than 5 weeks. Hgb F ($\alpha_2\gamma_2$) is the major hemoglobin of fetal life. The fetal hemoglobin concentration in blood decreases after birth by approximately 3 percent per week and is generally less than 2 to 3 percent of the total hemoglobin by 6 months of age. The mean hemoglobin level in cord blood at term is 16.8 g/dL, with 95 percent of the values falling between 13.7 and 20.1 g/dL. The red cells of the newborn are macrocytic, with a mean cell volume in excess of 110 fL/cell. The red cell, hemoglobin, and hematocrit values decrease only slightly during the first week after birth, but decline more rapidly in the following 5 to 8 weeks, producing the physiologic anemia of the newborn. The absolute number of neutrophils in the blood of term and premature infants is usually greater than that found in older children. Segmented neutrophils are the predominant leukocytes in the first few days after birth. As their number decreases, the lymphocyte becomes the most numerous cell type and remains so during the first 4 years of life. Phagocytosis of bacteria by neutrophils from premature and term infants is normal. Bactericidal activity varies according to the conditions of testing and the clinical status of the neonates. The platelet counts in term and preterm infants are between 150 and 400 × 10⁹/L, comparable to adult values. The absolute number of lymphocytes in the newborn is equivalent to that in older children, with lower values in premature infants at birth. The absolute number of CD3+ and CD4+ (helper/inducer phenotype) T-cell subsets in blood of newborns is significantly higher than in adults. Humoral (B-cell) immunity also develops early in gestation, but it is not fully active until after birth. In the newborn, approximately 15 percent of lymphocytes have immunoglobulin on their surface, with all immunoglobulin isotypes represented. The term newborn has reduced mean plasma levels (<60 percent of adult levels) of factors II, IX, X, XI, and XII, prekallikrein, and high-molecular-weight kininogen. In contrast, the plasma concentration of factor VIII is similar and von Willebrand factor is increased compared to older children and adults.

Acronyms and Abbreviations: ADP, adenosine diphosphate; AGM, aorta-gonad-mesonephros; ATP, adenosine triphosphate; ATPase, adenosine triphosphatase; BFU-E, burst-forming unit–erythroid; BPG, bisphosphoglycerate; BPI, bacterial permeability-increasing protein; cAMP, cyclic adenosine monophosphate; CFU-E, colony-forming unit–erythroid; CFU-GEMM, colony-forming unit–granulocyte-erythroid-monocyte-macrophage; CFU-GM, colony-forming unit–granulocyte-monocyte; CFU-Meg, colony-forming unit–megakaryocyte; G-CSF, granulocyte colony-stimulating factor; GM-CSF, granulocyte-monocyte colony-stimulating factor; IL, interleukin; MCV, mean cell volume; NBT, nitroblue tetrazolium; NK, natural killer; RDW, red cell distribution width; SIDS, sudden infant death syndrome; TNF, tumor necrosis factor; TPO, thrombopoietin.

FETAL HEMATOLYMPHOPOIESIS

PRODUCTION OF EMBRYONIC AND FETAL HEMATOPOIETIC CELLS

During embryogenesis, hematopoiesis occurs in spatially and temporally distinct sites, including the extraembryonic yolk sac, the fetal liver, the thymus, and the preterm marrow. The origin of hematopoietic cells is closely tied to gastrulation, the formation of mesoderm cells, and to the emergence of the endothelial lineage. Hematopoiesis is first established soon after implantation of the blastocyst, with the appearance of primitive erythroid cells in blood islands of the yolk sac beginning at day 18 of gestation.[1] The spatial and temporal association of embryonic red cells and endothelial cells in these blood islands suggests that the transient erythromyeloid potential of the yolk sac arises from hemangioblast precursors that also contain endothelial potential.[2] This concept is supported by *in vitro* studies of human embryonic stem cells cultured as embryoid bodies.[3,4] Hematopoietic stem cells, containing erythromyeloid and lymphoid potential, subsequently arise from intraembryonic vasculature, particularly the aorta (Fig. 7–1). These hematopoietic stem cells provide for fetal and long-term postnatal blood cell production. The ontogeny of the hematopoietic system remains a topic of active research using mammalian and several nonmammalian model systems.

Yolk Sac Hematopoiesis

"Primitive" red cells derived from the yolk sac constitute a distinct transient erythroid lineage that differs from "definitive" red cells that subsequently mature in the fetal liver and marrow. The development of primitive erythroblasts is critical for embryonic survival. In the mouse, targeted disruption of the transcription factors SCL (TAL1), LM02

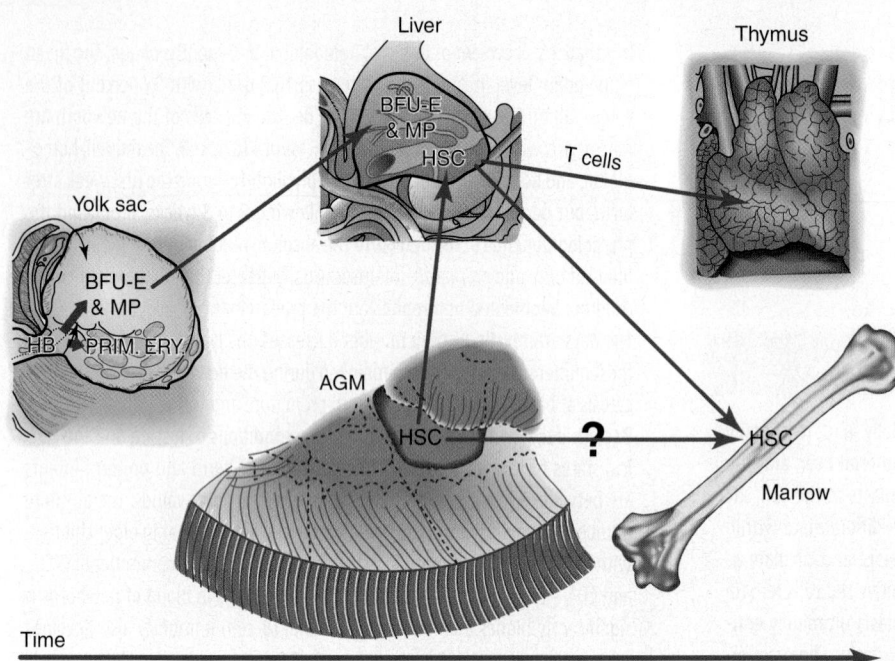

Figure 7–1. Hypothetical model of human hematopoietic ontogeny based on amphibian, avian, murine, and human developmental data. The yolk sac provides two transient populations of committed progenitors that are thought to arise from a mesoderm-derived hemangioblast (HB) precursor. The first wave of progenitors produces primitive erythroblasts (*PRIM. ERY.*) (see text). The second wave produces burst-forming unit–erythroid (*BFU-E*) and several myeloid progenitors (*MP*) that seed the liver. Long-term hematopoietic stem cells (*HSCs*) arise later in the aortagonad-mesonephros (*AGM*) region that subsequently populate the liver and ultimately the marrow to generate the full panoply of definitive hematopoiesis. The HSCs from liver also provide naïve lymphoid cells to the thymus, and T-lineage maturation occurs there.

(RBTN2), and GATA-1 abrogates primitive erythropoiesis in the yolk sac and leads to early embryonic death.[5–7] In the human, primitive erythroblasts begin to enter the embryo proper at days 21 to 22 of gestation with the onset of cardiac contractions[8] and circulate until approximately 12 weeks of gestation. Yolk sac erythroblasts have several characteristics that distinguish them from their later definitive counterparts. Primitive erythroblasts circulate as nucleated cells, accumulating embryonic hemoglobins and completing terminal differentiation within the vascular network.[9] Because of their extremely large size, with an estimated MCV of >400 fL/cell, yolk sac erythroblasts have been termed *megaloblasts*. Although it is widely assumed that primitive red cells remain nucleated throughout their life span, human primitive erythroblasts, like their murine counterparts, ultimately enucleate upon terminal differentiation.[10–12]

In the mouse, primitive red cells are derived from a transient population of primitive erythroid progenitors that is confined to the yolk sac.[13] Ultrastructural examination of the human yolk sac reveals the presence, not only of primitive erythroblasts, but also of macrophage cells and megakaryocytes.[11] These findings are consistent with hematopoietic progenitor studies in the mouse embryo and in human embryonic stem cells differentiated *in vitro*, which support the concept that "primitive" hematopoiesis in the yolk sac consists of primitive erythroid, macrophage, and megakaryocyte lineages.[13–15]

The initial wave of primitive erythroid progenitors is followed by a second wave of yolk sac–derived definitive erythroid progenitors, termed *burst forming units–erythroid* (BFU-E). BFU-E are present in the human yolk sac as early as 4 weeks' gestation and are found in the fetal liver by 5 weeks' gestation.[16] These findings suggest that the fetal liver is initially seeded by hematopoietic progenitors derived from the yolk sac (see Fig. 7–1).[17] Erythroid and nonerythroid progenitors are evident also in the nonliver regions of the embryo proper.[18] After 7 weeks' gestation, hematopoietic progenitors are no longer detected in the yolk sac.[19]

Hepatic Hematopoiesis

The liver serves as the primary source of red cells from the 9th to the 24th weeks of gestation. Between 7 and 15 weeks' gestation, 60 percent of the liver cells are hematopoietic.[20] Erythroid cells differentiate in close

physical association with macrophages and extrude their nuclei prior to entering the blood. These fetal-liver–derived definitive "macrocytes" are smaller than yolk sac–derived primitive megaloblasts and contain one-third the amount of hemoglobin. Differentiation of murine erythroid cells in the fetal liver is critically dependent on erythropoietin signaling through its receptor and the Janus kinase 2 (JAK2) pathway.[21,22] Fetal-liver–derived erythroid progenitors can differentiate *in vitro* with erythropoietin alone, in contrast to adult marrow-derived BFU-E, which requires erythropoietin plus interleukin (IL)-3 or stem cell factor.[23,24] Erythropoietin transcripts are present during the first trimester in the liver, which remains a primary site of erythropoietin transcription throughout fetal life.[25] Erythropoietin transcripts also are present in the developing human kidney as early as 17 weeks' gestation and increase after 30 weeks.[25] Like primitive erythropoiesis in the yolk sac, definitive erythropoiesis in the fetal liver is necessary for continued survival of the embryo. Targeted disruption of the c-myb transcription factor in the mouse blocks fetal liver erythropoiesis and leads to fetal death.[26] This mutation does not affect primitive erythropoiesis, indicating fundamental differences in the transcriptional regulation of these distinct forms of erythropoiesis.

In contrast to the yolk sac, where hematopoiesis is restricted primarily to erythromyeloid lineages, hematopoiesis in the fetal liver eventually will consist of definitive erythroid, megakaryocyte, multiple myeloid, as well as, lymphoid lineages. Megakaryocytes are present in the liver by 6 weeks' gestation. Platelets are first evident in the circulation at 8 to 9 weeks' gestation.[20] Granulopoiesis is present in the liver parenchyma as early as 7 weeks' gestation and small numbers of circulating leukocytes are present at the 11th week of gestation. Despite the low number and immature appearance of hepatic neutrophils, the fetal liver contains abundant hematopoietic progenitor cells, including the multipotential colony-forming unit–granulocyte-erythroid-monocyte-macrophage (CFU-GEMM) and colony-forming unit–granulocyte-monocyte (CFU-GM).[27] CFU-GM growth depends upon several cytokines, including granulocyte colony-stimulating factor (G-CSF), granulocyte-monocyte colony-stimulating factor (GM-CSF), and interleukins. When compared to adult marrow-derived myeloid progenitors, these fetal liver-derived myeloid progenitors have a similar dose–response *in vitro* to G-CSF.[28] G-CSF is expressed by hepatocytes at 14 weeks' gestation.[29]

Lymphopoiesis

Lymphopoiesis is present in the lymph plexuses and the thymus beginning at 9 weeks' gestation.[20] B cells with surface immunoglobulin (Ig) M are present in the liver, and circulating lymphocytes also are seen at 9 weeks' gestation. T lymphocytes are found only rarely before 12 weeks' gestation.[30] Lymphocyte subpopulations are detected by 13 weeks' gestation in fetal liver.[31] Absolute numbers of major lymphoid subsets in 20- to 26-week-old fetuses, as defined by the antigens CD2, CD3, CD4, CD8, CD16, CD19, and CD20, are similar to those in newborns (see "Neonatal Lymphopoiesis" below).[32,33]

Marrow Hematopoiesis

Hematopoietic cells are first seen in the marrow of the 10- to 11-week embryo,[1] and they remain confined to the diaphyseal regions of long bones until 15 weeks' gestation.[34] Initially, there are approximately equal numbers of myeloid and erythroid cells in the fetal marrow. However, myeloid cells predominate by 12 weeks' gestation, and the myeloid-to-erythroid ratio approaches the adult level of 3:1 by 21 weeks' gestation.[20] Macrophage cells in the fetal marrow, but not in the fetal liver, express the lipopolysaccharide receptor CD14.[29] The marrow becomes the major site of hematopoiesis after the 24th week of gestation and remains so throughout the remainder of fetal life.

ONTOGENY OF HEMATOPOIETIC STEM CELLS

The reconstitution of the entire hematopoietic system by transplantation with cord blood indicates that hematopoietic stem cells are circulating in the blood at birth.[35] The immunologic reconstitution of an immunodeficient human fetus with fetal-liver-derived cells also indicates that hematopoietic stem cells exist in the late gestation fetal liver.[36] It was first postulated that hematopoietic stem cells originate independently in each hematopoietic site (yolk sac, liver, and marrow) of the embryo.[37] However, experiments in the mammalian embryo indicate that the liver rudiment, like the marrow, is seeded by exogenous hematopoietic cells.[38,39] It was initially thought that the liver, and eventually the marrow, were seeded by yolk sac–derived hematopoietic stem cells.[40] However, experiments in avian and amphibian embryos indicate that the hematopoietic stem cells that ultimately provide for long-term adult hematopoiesis arise within the body of the embryo proper rather than from the yolk sac.[41,42] Subsequent investigations in the mouse embryo indicate that stem cells capable of engrafting myeloablated adult recipients originate in the aorta-gonad-mesonephros (AGM) region of the embryo proper.[43] Cells capable of long-term engraftment of immunodeficient mice also first originate at 35 days of gestation in the aorta region of human embryos.[44] This correlates anatomically with the transient appearance of clusters of CD34+ blood cells closely associated with the ventral wall of the aorta in several mammalian species, including the 5 weeks' gestation human embryo.[45,46] These findings, as well as direct visualization of developing zebrafish embryos,[47] support the concept that hematopoietic stem cells arise from "hemogenic" aortic endothelium through an endothelial-to-hematopoietic transition and then seed the liver, and eventually the marrow, to provide lifelong hematopoiesis (see Fig. 7–1). Studies in the murine embryo indicate that the placenta also serves as a site of hematopoietic stem cell origin and expansion.[48] It is not known if the placenta serves a similar function during human development. The underlying relationship of the transient erythromyeloid hematopoiesis derived from the yolk sac to long-term hematopoietic stem cell–derived intraembryonic hematopoiesis remains unclear. However, studies in the mouse indicate that resident macrophage populations in multiple organs of the adult, particularly microglia in the brain, are ultimately derived from the yolk sac of the embryo and undergo limited maintenance after birth from hematopoietic stem cells.[49,50]

SYNTHESIS OF FETAL HEMOGLOBINS

Human hemoglobin (Hgb) is a tetramer composed of two α-type and two β-type globin chains (Table 7–1). The α-globin gene cluster is located on chromosome 16 and contains the ζ gene 5′ to the pair of α-globin genes. The β-globin gene cluster is located on chromosome 11 and contains five globin genes oriented 5′ to 3′ as ε-γ^A-γ^G-δ-β.[51] During embryogenesis the genes on both chromosomes are activated sequentially from the 5′ to the 3′ end. This globin "switching" is related not only to the relative positions of the globin genes within their respective chromosomal clusters, but also to interacting upstream "locus control regions."[52]

Hgb Gower-1 ($\zeta_2\varepsilon_2$) is the major hemoglobin in embryos younger than 5 weeks' gestation (see Table 7–1).[53] Hgb Gower-2 ($\alpha_2\varepsilon_2$) has been found in embryos with a gestational age as young as 4 weeks and is absent in embryos older than 13 weeks.[54] Hgb Portland ($\zeta_2\gamma_2$) is found in young embryos, but persists in infants with homozygous α-thalassemia (Chap. 48). Synthesis of the ζ and ε chains decreases as those of the α and γ chains increase (Fig. 7–2). The ζ-to-α-globin switch precedes the ε-to-γ-globin switch as the liver replaces the yolk sac as the main site of erythropoiesis.[9,55]

Hgb F ($\alpha_2\gamma_2$) is the major hemoglobin of fetal life (see Fig. 7–2).[56] Synthesis of Hgb A can be demonstrated in fetuses as young as 9 weeks' gestation.[57] In fetuses of 9 to 21 weeks' gestation, the amount of Hgb A ($\alpha_2\beta_2$) rises from 4 to 13 percent of the total hemoglobin.[57] These levels of Hgb A have enabled the antenatal diagnosis of β-thalassemia using globin-chain synthesis. After 34 to 36 weeks' gestation the percentage of Hgb A rises, whereas that of Hgb F decreases (see Fig. 7–2). The mean synthesis of Hgb F in term infants was 59.0 ± 10 percent (1 SD) of total hemoglobin synthesis as assessed by ^{14}C-leucine uptake.[58] The amount of Hgb F in blood varies in term infants from 53 to 95 percent of total hemoglobin.[59]

The fetal hemoglobin concentration in blood decreases after birth by approximately 3 percent per week and is generally less than 2 to 3 percent of the total hemoglobin by 6 months of age. This rate of decrease in Hgb F production is closely related to the gestational age of the infant and is not affected by the changes in environment and oxygen tension that occur at the time of birth.[60] Hgb A₂ ($\alpha_2\delta_2$) has not been detected in fetuses. Normal adult levels of Hgb A₂ are achieved by 4 months of age.[61] Increased proportions of Hgb F at birth have been reported in infants who are small for gestational age, who have experienced chronic intrauterine hypoxia, who have trisomy 13, or who have died from sudden infant death syndrome (SIDS).[62-66] Decreased levels of Hgb F at birth are found in trisomy 21.[67]

TABLE 7–1. Embryonic Hemoglobins

Hemoglobin	Chain Composition	Primary Site	Appearance
Gower-1	$\zeta_2\varepsilon_2$	Yolk sac	<5–6 weeks
Gower-2	$\alpha_2\varepsilon_2$	Yolk sac	4–13 weeks
Portland	$\zeta_2\gamma_2$	Yolk sac	4–13 weeks
Fetal (F)	$\alpha_2\gamma_2$	Liver	Early, 53–95% at term
Adult (A)	$\alpha_2\beta_2$	Marrow	9 weeks, 5–45% at term

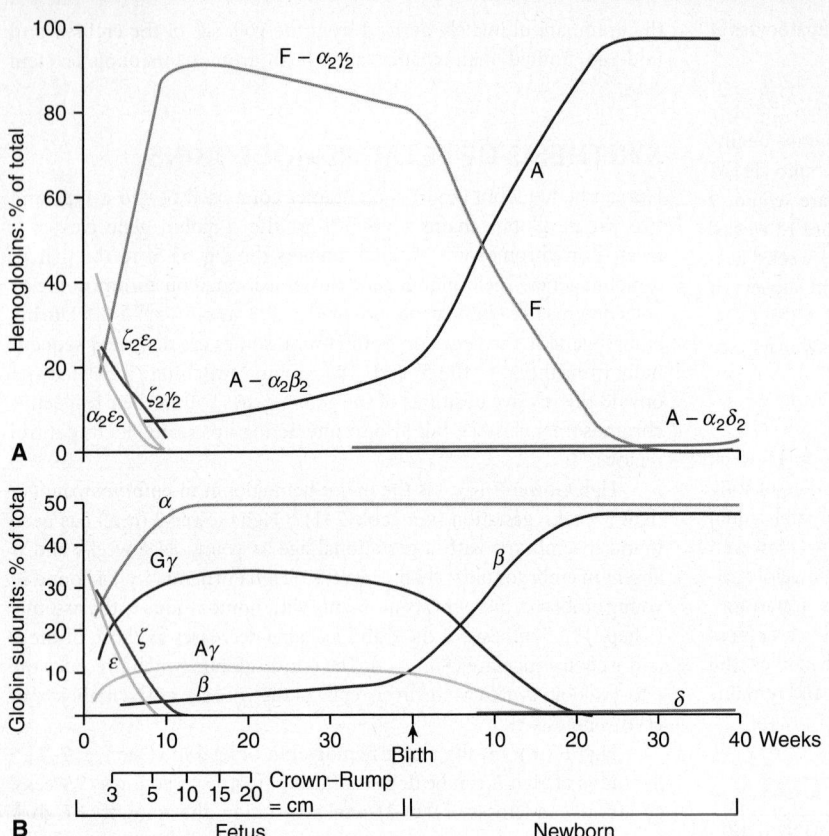

Figure 7–2. Changes in hemoglobin tetramers **(A)** and in globin subunits **(B)** during human development from embryo to early infancy. *(Reproduced with permission from Bunn HF, Forget BG: Hemoglobin: Molecular, Genetic and Clinical Aspects. Philadelphia, PA: WB Saunders; 1986.)*

FETAL BLOOD

The cellular composition of fetal blood changes markedly during the second and third trimesters. The mean blood hemoglobin concentration in fetuses progressively increases from 9.0 ± 2.8 g/dL at age 10 weeks to 16.5 ± 4.0 g/dL at age 39 weeks.[68] There is a concomitant decrease in the MCV of fetal red cells from a mean of 134 fL/cell at 18 weeks' gestation to 118 fL/cell at 30 weeks' gestation.[69] The total white blood cell count averages 2×10^9/L between 10 and 17 weeks of gestation,[31] and increases during the middle trimester to between 4.0 and 4.5×10^9/L, with an 80 to 85 percent preponderance of lymphocytes and 5 to 10 percent neutrophils.[69] The percentage of circulating nucleated red cells decreases from a mean of 12 percent at 18 weeks to 4 percent at 30 weeks.[69] The platelet count remains greater than 150,000/μL from 15 weeks' gestation to term.[69,70]

Large numbers of committed hematopoietic progenitors circulate in the fetal blood. Blood samples obtained by fetoscopy at 12 to 19 weeks' gestation reveal a mean of 20,450 BFU-E/mL and 12,490 CFU-GM/mL.[71] This is in striking contrast to adult blood, which contains many fewer erythroid progenitors and 30 to 250 CFU-GM/mL.[70,72] Most (70–80%) circulating hematopoietic progenitors at 26 to 28 weeks' gestation are cycling.[72] In contrast, adult-marrow-derived progenitors in the bloodstream are relatively quiescent with only 0 to 5 percent cycling.

● NEONATAL HEMATOPOIESIS

NEONATAL ERYTHROPOIESIS AND RED CELLS

Hemoglobin, Hematocrit, and Indices

The mean hemoglobin level in cord blood at term is 16.8 g/dL, with 95 percent of the values falling between 13.7 and 20.1 g/dL.[73] This variation reflects perinatal events, particularly asphyxia,[74] and also the amount

of blood transferred from the placenta to the infant after delivery. Early cord clamping appears to heighten the occurrence of anemia at 2 months and to impair cardiopulmonary adaptation.[75] Delay of cord clamping may increase the blood volume and red cell mass of the infant by as much as 55 percent.[76,77] This results in fewer transfusions and fewer days requiring oxygen and ventilation in preterm infants.[75] The mean total blood volume after birth is 86 mL/kg for the term infant and 89 mL/kg for the premature infant.[78] The blood volume per kilogram decreases over the ensuing weeks, reaching a mean value of approximately 65 mL/kg by 3 to 4 months of age.

Normally the hemoglobin and hematocrit values rise in the first several hours after birth because of the movement of plasma from the intravascular to the extravascular space.[79] A venous hemoglobin concentration of less than 14 g/dL in a term infant and/or a fall in hemoglobin or hematocrit level in the first postnatal day are abnormal. Table 7–2 shows the normal red cell values from capillary blood samples for term infants in the first 12 weeks after birth.[80] Capillary hematocrit values in newborns are higher than those in simultaneous venous samples, particularly during the first postnatal days, and the capillary-to-venous ratio is approximately 1.1:1.[81] This difference reflects circulatory factors and is greater in preterm and sick infants.

The red cells of the newborn are macrocytic, with an MCV in excess of 110 fL/cell. The MCV begins to fall after the first week, reaching adult values by the ninth week (see Table 7–2).[80,82] The blood film from a newborn infant shows macrocytic normochromic cells, polychromasia, and a few nucleated red blood cells. Even in healthy infants there may be mild anisopoikilocytosis.[83] Three to 5 percent of the red cells may be fragments, target cells, or otherwise distorted. By 3 to 5 days after birth, nucleated red blood cells are not found normally in the blood of term or premature infants, but they may be present in markedly elevated numbers in the presence of hemolysis or hypoxic stress. As

TABLE 7–2. Red Cell Values for Term Infants during the First 12 Weeks after Birth*

Age	Hbg, g/dL ± SD	RBC × 10^{12}/L ± SD	Hematocrit, % ± SD	MCV, fL ± SD	MCHC, g/dL ± SD	Reticulocytes, % ± SD
DAYS						
1	19.3 ± 2.2	5.14 ± 0.7	61 ± 7.4	119 ± 9.4	31.6 ± 1.9	3.2 ± 1.4
2	19.0 ± 1.9	5.15 ± 0.8	60 ± 6.4	115 ± 7.0	31.6 ± 1.4	3.2 ± 1.3
3	18.8 ± 2.0	5.11 ± 0.7	62 ± 9.3	116 ± 5.3	31.1 ± 2.8	2.8 ± 1.7
4	18.6 ± 2.1	5.00 ± 0.6	57 ± 8.1	114 ± 7.5	32.6 ± 1.5	1.8 ± 1.1
5	17.6 ± 1.1	4.97 ± 0.4	57 ± 7.3	114 ± 8.9	30.9 ± 2.2	1.2 ± 0.2
6	17.4 ± 2.2	5.00 ± 0.7	54 ± 7.2	113 ± 10.0	32.2 ± 1.6	0.6 ± 0.2
7	17.9 ± 2.5	4.86 ± 0.6	56 ± 9.4	118 ± 11.2	32.0 ± 1.6	0.5 ± 0.4
WEEKS						
1–2	17.3 ± 2.3	4.80 ± 0.8	54 ± 8.3	112 ± 19.0	32.1 ± 2.9	0.5 ± 0.3
2–3	15.6 ± 2.6	4.20 ± 0.6	46 ± 7.3	111 ± 8.2	33.9 ± 1.9	0.8 ± 0.6
3–4	14.2 ± 2.1	4.00 ± 0.6	43 ± 5.7	105 ± 7.5	33.5 ± 1.6	0.6 ± 0.3
4–5	12.7 ± 1.6	3.60 ± 0.4	36 ± 4.8	101 ± 8.1	34.9 ± 1.6	0.9 ± 0.8
5–6	11.9 ± 1.5	3.55 ± 0.2	36 ± 6.2	102 ± 10.2	34.1 ± 2.9	1.0 ± 0.7
6–7	12.0 ± 1.5	3.40 ± 0.4	36 ± 4.8	105 ± 12.0	33.8 ± 2.3	1.2 ± 0.7
7–8	11.1 ± 1.1	3.40 ± 0.4	33 ± 3.7	100 ± 13.0	33.7 ± 2.6	1.5 ± 0.7
8–9	10.7 ± 0.9	3.40 ± 0.5	31 ± 2.5	93 ± 12.0	34.1 ± 2.2	1.8 ± 1.0
9–10	11.2 ± 0.9	3.60 ± 0.3	32 ± 2.7	91 ± 9.3	34.3 ± 2.9	1.2 ± 0.6
10–11	11.4 ± 0.9	3.70 ± 0.4	34 ± 2.1	91 ± 7.7	33.2 ± 2.4	1.2 ± 0.7
11–12	11.3 ± 0.9	3.70 ± 0.3	33 ± 3.3	88 ± 7.9	34.8 ± 2.2	0.7 ± 0.3

MCHC, mean corpuscular hemoglobin concentration; MCV, mean corpuscular volume; RBC, red blood cell.

*Capillary blood samples. The RBC count and MCV measurements were made on an electronic counter.

Adapted with permission from Matoth Y, Zaizor R, Varsano I: Postnatal changes in some red cell parameters. *Acta Paediatr Scand* 60(3):317–323, 1971.

expected from these findings, the red cell distribution width (RDW) is markedly elevated in the newborn period.[84]

There are significant numbers of circulating progenitor cells in cord blood.[85–87] Cord blood BFU-E and colony-forming unit–erythroid (CFU-E) differentiate more rapidly than their adult counterparts.[88] Furthermore, the proportion of cord blood hematopoietic progenitors in the mitotic cycle is approximately 50 percent, intermediate between the proportions found in fetal and adult progenitor cells.[72,86]

In several,[89,90] but not all,[91] studies, premature infants at birth had lower hemoglobin levels, higher reticulocyte counts, and higher nucleated red cell counts than did the term infants. The reticulocyte counts of premature infants are inversely proportional to their gestational age, with a mean of 8 percent reticulocytes evident at 32 weeks' gestation and 4 to 5 percent at term.[92] Infants who are small for their gestational ages have higher red cell counts, hematocrit levels, and hemoglobin concentrations as compared with infants whose size is appropriate for their gestational age.[90,93]

Erythropoietin and Physiologic Anemia of the Newborn Erythropoietin is the primary regulator of erythropoiesis (Chaps. 32 and 33). Although erythropoietin is present in cord blood, it falls to undetectable levels after birth in healthy infants.[94] Subsequently, the reticulocyte count falls to less than 1 percent by the sixth day after birth.[80,95] The red cell, hemoglobin, and hematocrit values decrease only slightly during the first week, but decline more rapidly in the following 5 to 8 weeks (see Table 7–2),[80] producing the physiologic anemia of the newborn. The lowest hemoglobin values in the term infant occur at approximately

2 months of age.[82] When the hemoglobin concentration falls below 11 g/dL, erythropoietic activity begins to increase. Erythropoietin can be measured after the 60th postnatal day,[96] corresponding to the recovery from physiologic anemia. If there is sufficient stimulus, such as hemolytic anemia or cyanotic heart disease, the newborn infant is able to produce erythropoietin prior to the 60th postnatal day.[94]

The fall in hemoglobin level is more pronounced in the premature infant. In one study of premature infants, the mean hemoglobin level at 2 months was 9.4 g/dL, with a 95 percent range of 7.2 to 11.7 g/dL.[97] In healthy premature infants erythropoietin becomes detectable when the hemoglobin level falls to approximately 12 g/dL. In infants with a lower percentage of Hgb F (as from transfusion) and, consequently, better oxygen delivery, erythropoietin does not rise until the hemoglobin falls to approximately 9.5 g/dL.[98] The mean values for iron-sufficient premature infants reached those of term infants by 4 months for red cell count, 5 months for hemoglobin level, and 6 months for mean corpuscular volume and mean corpuscular hemoglobin.[97]

Blood Viscosity The viscosity of blood increases logarithmically in relation to the hematocrit.[99,100] Hyperviscosity was found in 5 percent of infants,[101] and in 18 percent of infants who were small for gestational age.[102] Newborn infants with hematocrit values of greater than 65 to 70 percent may become symptomatic because of increased viscosity.[103] In one study of infants with documented hyperviscosity and a mean hematocrit greater than 65 percent, 38 percent displayed symptoms of irritability, hypotonia, tremors, or poor suck reflex.[104] Partial plasma exchange transfusion reduced blood viscosity, improved cerebral blood flow, and relieved the symptoms. However, cerebral blood flow was normal in the asymptomatic infants with hyperviscosity, and, consequently, there was no benefit from exchange transfusion.[104] Studies of neurodevelopmental status do not show any clear long-term benefits for the use of partial exchange transfusions in asymptomatic neonates.[105]

Red Cell Antigens The blood group antigens on neonatal red cells differ from those of the older child and adult. The i antigen is expressed strongly, whereas the I antigen and the A and B antigens are expressed only weakly on neonatal red cells. The i antigen is a straight-chain carbohydrate that is replaced by the branched-chain derivative, I antigen, as a result of the developmental acquisition of a glycosyltransferase.[106] By 1 year of age the i antigen is undetectable, and the ABH antigens increase to adult levels by age 3 years (Chap. 136). The ABH, Kell, Duffy, and Vel antigens can be detected on the cells of the fetus in the first trimester and are present at birth.[107] The Lu^a and Lu^b antigens also are detectable on fetal red cells and are more weakly expressed at birth, increasing to adult levels by age 15 years.[107] The Xg antigen is variably expressed in the fetus and is weaker on newborn than on adult red cells. Moreover, particularly poor expression of Xg has been noted in newborns with trisomy 13, 18, and 21.[107] The Lewis group (Le^a/Le^b) antigens are adsorbed on the red cell membrane and become detectable within 1 to 2 weeks after birth as the receptor sites develop. Anti-A and anti-B isohemagglutinins develop during the first 6 postnatal months, reaching adult levels by 2 years of age.

Red Cell Life Span The life span of the red cells in the newborn infant is shorter than that of red cells in the adult (Chap. 33). The average of several studies of mean half-life of newborn red cells is 60 to 80 days.[108] The reasons for this shortened survival are unclear, but the known susceptibility to oxidant injury of newborn red cells may be a contributing factor.

Iron and Transferrin The serum iron level in cord blood of the normal infant is elevated compared to maternal levels. The mean value is approximately 150 ± 40 mcg/dL (1 SD).[109] Infants on an iron-supplemented diet have a median serum iron level of 125 mcg/dL at 1 month of age and of approximately 75 mcg/dL at 6 months of age. The total iron-binding capacity rises throughout the first year. The median transferrin saturation falls from almost 65 percent at 2 weeks to 25 percent at 1 year, and saturations as low as 10 percent may be observed in the absence of iron deficiency.[110] The mean serum ferritin levels in iron-sufficient infants are high at birth, 160 mcg/L, rise further during the first month, and then fall to a mean of 30 mcg/L by 1 year of age.[111] The amount of stainable iron in the marrow at birth is small but increases in both term and premature infants during the first weeks after birth. Stainable marrow iron begins to decrease after 2 months and is gone by 4 to 6 months in term infants and earlier in premature infants.[112] Iron is preferentially allocated to erythropoiesis if the availability of iron is limited.[113] This makes the availability of adequate iron particularly important to avoid iron lack in the brain, heart, and skeletal muscle.

Red Cell Functions

Oxygen Delivery The oxygen affinity of cord blood is greater than that of maternal blood, because the affinity of Hgb F for 2,3-bisphosphoglycerate (2,3-BPG) is less than that of Hgb A.[114] Levels of 2,3-BPG are lower in newborn red cells than in adult cells and even more decreased in the red cells of premature infants,[115] and this low 2,3-BPG level further heightens the oxygen affinity of newborn red cells. Consequently, the red cell oxygen equilibrium curve of the newborn is shifted to the left of that of the adult (Fig. 7–3). The mean partial pressure of oxygen (pO_2) at which hemoglobin is 50 percent saturated with oxygen at 1 day of age in term infants is 19.4 ± 1.8 torr, as compared with the normal adult value of 27.0 ± 1.1 torr.[116] This results in a decrease in the oxygen released at the tissue level, as shown in Fig. 7–3. As the partial pressure of oxygen

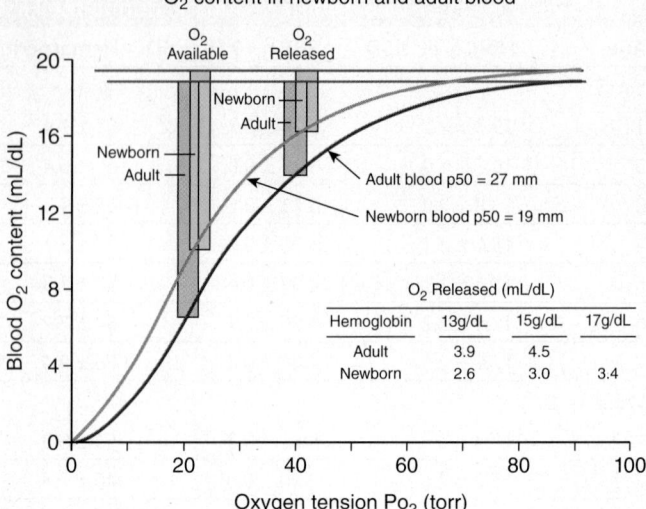

Figure 7–3. The oxygen equilibrium curves are based on the assumption that the Hgb concentration is 15 g/dL and that there is full O_2 saturation of Hgb at a partial pressure of arterial oxygen (Pao_2) of 100 torr. The O_2 released is the difference in O_2 content between a Pao_2 of 90 torr and the mixed venous Pao_2 of 40 torr. The O_2 available is the difference in O_2 content between a Pao_2 of 90 torr and a mixed venous Pao_2 of 20 torr. This is the maximum O_2 available without evoking compensatory mechanisms such as increased cardiac output.

(Po_2) falls from 90 torr in arterial to 40 torr in the venous blood, 3.0 mL/dL of oxygen are released from newborn blood, whereas 4.5 mL/dL are released from adult Hgb A-containing blood. The shift to the left of the oxygen equilibrium curve is even more pronounced in the premature infant, requiring a larger fall in Po_2 to release an equivalent amount of oxygen. After birth the oxygen equilibrium curve shifts gradually to the right, reaching the position of the adult curve by 6 months of age. The position of the curve in the premature infant correlates with gestational age rather than with postnatal age,[116] and its shift to the adult position is more gradual.

Metabolism Many differences have been found between the metabolism of the red cells of newborn infants and that of adults.[117,118] Some of the differences may be explained by the younger mean cell age in the newborn, but others seem to be properties of the fetal cell. The glucose consumption in newborn red cells is lower than that in adult red cells.[119] Elevated levels of glucose phosphate isomerase, glyceraldehyde-3-phosphate dehydrogenase, phosphoglycerate kinase, and enolase beyond those explainable by the young cell age have been found in neonatal cells.[115,120] The level of phosphofructokinase is low in red cells of term and premature infants.[115,120,121] The pentose phosphate shunt is active in red cells of term and premature infants,[122] but glutathione instability leads to a heightened susceptibility to oxidant injury. The result of oxidant stress is depletion of adenosine triphosphate (ATP) and adenine nucleotides leading to iron release, denaturing of membrane proteins, and hemoglobin and membrane peroxidation.[123] The levels of ATP and adenosine diphosphate (ADP) are higher in the red cells of term and preterm infants,[121] but may merely reflect the younger age of the erythrocyte population. Finally, lower-than-adult activities have been found for several other red cell enzymes, including cytochrome B_5 reductase[124] and glutathione peroxidase.[125]

Membrane The membrane of the newborn red cell also is different from that of the adult red cell. Ouabain-sensitive adenosine triphosphatase (ATPase) is decreased,[126] and active potassium influx is significantly less in neonatal red cells.[127] Newborn cells are more

TABLE 7–3. The White Cell Count and the Differential Count during the First 2 Weeks after Birth*

Age	Leukocytes	Neutrophils			Eosinophils	Basophils	Lymphocytes	Monocytes
		Total	Segmented	Bands				
BIRTH								
Mean	18.0	11.0	9.4	1.6	0.40	0.10	5.5	1.05
Range	9.0–30.0	6.0–26.0	—	—	0.02–0.85	0–0.64	2.0–11.0	0.4–3.1
Mean %	—	61	52	9	2.2	0.6	31	5.8
7 DAYS								
Mean	12.2	5.5	4.7	0.83	0.50	0.05	5.0	1.1
Range	5.0–21.0	1.5–10.0	—	—	0.07–1.1	0–0.25	2.0–17.0	0.3–2.7
Mean %	—	45	39	6	4.1	0.4	41	9.1
14 DAYS								
Mean	11.4	4.5	3.9	0.63	0.35	0.05	5.5	1.0
Range	5.0–20.0	1.0–9.5	—	—	0.07–1.0	0–0.23	2.0–17.0	0.2–2.4
Mean %	—	40	34	5.5	3.1	0.4	48	8.8

*All white cell counts are expressed as cells $\times 10^9$/L.

Data from Altman PL, Dittmer DS: *Blood and Other Body Fluids.* Federation of American Societies for Experimental Biology, Washington, DC, 1961 and Dallman PR: Pediatrics, 16th edition. New York, NY: Appleton-Century-Crofts, 1977.

sensitive to osmotic hemolysis and to oxidant injury than are adult cells. Newborn red cell membranes have higher total lipid, phospholipid, and cholesterol per cell than adult red cells.[128,129] The patterns of phospholipid and phospholipid fatty acid composition also differ from those in adult red cells. Red cells of newborns have the same pattern of membrane proteins on polyacrylamide gel electrophoresis[130] and the same rate of mobility in an electric field[131] as do red cells from adults. After trypsin treatment of newborn and adult cells, however, there is a difference in electrophoretic mobility, indicating that the surface trypsin-resistant proteins are different.[131] The relationship of the metabolic and membrane alterations in neonatal red cells to their shorter life span is not clear.

WHITE CELLS

Granulocytopoiesis and Monocytopoiesis

Colony-Stimulating Factors and Granulomonopoiesis The absolute number of neutrophils in the blood of term and premature infants usually is greater than that found in older children (Table 7–3).[132] The neutrophil count tends to be lower in the premature than in the term infant, and the proportion of myelocytes and band neutrophils is higher.[133] Serum and urinary colony-stimulating activity are elevated during the period of neutrophilia.[134] When granulopoiesis was studied in cord blood, blood, and marrow of infants, the macrophage colony-forming unit was predominant despite the clinical neutrophilia, and this pattern was not altered by different sources of colony-stimulating factors.[135,136] The endogenous cytokines produced by mononuclear cells from cord or systemic venous blood support the growth of neutrophil colonies in assays using marrow from adults.[135] However, there is diminished GM-CSF, G-CSF, and IL-3 production in stimulated newborn compared to adult mononuclear cells,[137–139] which may limit the response to bacterial infection in the newborn. Furthermore, preterm infants have a reduced neutrophil storage pool and a restricted capacity to increase their progenitor proliferation, and their neutrophil count may fall precipitously with neonatal bacterial infection.[140] Dysregulation, as well as

diminished capacity of neonatal granulopoiesis, may impair the neonatal response to infection.[141] Smaller numbers of CFU-GM colonies were observed in the blood of sick infants, who also have diminished endogenous production of colony-stimulating factors in culture.[136] The clinical use of cytokines to treat neonatal sepsis remains controversial,[142] but circulating neutrophils are increased in preterm infants treated with recombinant G-CSF, and the infants' length of stay in the neonatal intensive care unit is shortened.[143]

White Cell and Differential Counts Table 7–3 gives the values for the white cell and differential counts during the first 2 weeks after birth. The absolute number of segmented neutrophils rises in both term and premature infants in the first 24 hours.[144] In term infants, the mean value increases from 8×10^9/L to a peak of 13×10^9/L and then falls to 4×10^9/L by 72 hours of age, remaining at this level through the following 7 days. In the premature infant, the mean values for neutrophils are 5×10^9/L at birth, 8×10^9/L at 12 hours, and 4×10^9/L at 72 hours. The mean count then falls gradually to 2.5×10^9/L by the 28th postnatal day. The level after the first 72 hours is very stable for an individual infant, whether term or premature. Immature forms, including an occasional promyelocyte and blast cell, may be seen in the blood of healthy infants in the first few days after birth and are more frequent in premature infants than in term infants.[144] Segmented granulocytes are the predominant cells in the first few days after birth. As their number decreases, the lymphocyte becomes the most numerous cell and remains so during the first 4 years of life. An absolute eosinophil count of greater than 0.7×10^9/L was found in 76 percent of premature infants at 2 to 3 weeks of age. The onset of the eosinophilia coincided with the establishment of steady weight gain in the infants.[145] It is increased by the use of total parenteral nutrition, endotracheal intubation, and blood transfusions.

Phagocyte Functions

Bacterial infections are a major cause of morbidity and mortality in the newborn period.[146] The infections frequently are caused by organisms of low virulence in normal children and adults, including *Staphylococcus* and Lancefield group B β-hemolytic streptococci, but, also, by

Pseudomonas, and other Gram-negative bacilli. Cellular defense mechanisms and humoral immunity of the newborn differ from those found later in life, and these undoubtedly contribute to the unusual susceptibility to infection noted in the neonatal period.[146]

Opsonins and Complement Engulfment and destruction of bacteria by neutrophils depend on opsonic activity of the plasma and on chemotaxis, phagocytosis, and the bacteriocidal capacity of the leukocyte. The serum factors necessary for optimal phagocytosis (opsonins) include the immunoglobulins and complement components. In term infants, opsonic activity is normal for *Staphylococcus aureus*,[147,148] but it is low for yeast[149] and *Escherichia coli*.[147,148] Diminished opsonic antibody is associated with group B streptococcal infection and represents one risk factor for neonatal infection.[150]

In premature infants, opsonic activity is low for *S. aureus* and *Serratia marcescens*,[147] but is normal for *Pseudomonas aeruginosa*.[151] When serum concentrations of fibronectin and IgG subclasses C3 and C4 were measured at birth, 1 month, 3 months, and 6 months, early gestational age was correlated with lower initial levels.[152] The decreased opsonic activity for some organisms in premature infants is attributed to diminished IgG levels, because additional IgG will correct the opsonic defect both *in vivo* and *in vitro*.[147] The added IgG improves bacterial opsonization by serum of premature infants in part because complement consumption and deposition of C3 on the bacterial surface are augmented.[153,154]

Complement components appear in fetal blood before 20 weeks' gestation and increase markedly during the third trimester. However, in many newborns both the classical and alternative complement pathways are decreased in activity and in levels of individual components.[155] The mean level of C3, the first common component of the two pathways of complement activation, is approximately 65 percent of that in normal adults.[156-158] There is no transplacental transfer of this protein, and levels in infants are lower than those in their mothers.[156] Total serum hemolytic complement (CH_{50}) and alternative pathway activity (PH_{50}) in newborns are lower than in adults, as are mean levels of C1q, C2–C9, properdin, and factors B, I, and H.[157-159] In general, the mean levels in full-term infants are greater than 50 percent of those in normal adult controls and may be somewhat less in premature infants. There is considerable overlap, however, between levels in infants and in controls. A functional deficiency in the alternative pathway has been detected in infants.[160]

Fibronectin mediates more efficient interactions between phagocytes and infectious agents. Fibronectin, a 450-kDa glycoprotein found in plasma and in the intercellular matrix, promotes the attachment of staphylococci to neutrophils[161] and enhances opsonic activity of antibodies against group B streptococci.[162] Because both these bacteria are common pathogens for neonates, the deficiency in fibronectin observed in neonates[163] may further compromise opsonic capacity and hence bactericidal activity in the neonate.

The administration of intravenous IgG may be useful in the treatment or prophylaxis of infection in preterm infants based on the reduced placental transfer of maternal antibody and the restricted endogenous synthesis of IgG.[164] IgG administered to septic neonates appears to enhance serum opsonic capacity as well as to increase the quantity of circulating neutrophils.[165] In premature neonates, added IgG heightens granulocyte phagocytosis.[165,166] Intravenous IgG has been reported to effectively treat infected premature neonates, but these reports involved small numbers of subjects.[167,168] The clinical efficacy of IgG prophylaxis against neonatal pathogens is not firmly established.[169,170] New IgG preparations with consistent, adequate levels of antibodies directed against neonatal pathogens can be achieved by selection of sera with high levels of functional antibodies,[171] or potentially by the addition of monoclonal antibodies, and these may prove more effective.

Chemotaxis Chemotactic function of leukocytes is low in neonates, whereas random motility is normal.[172-174] Neonatal serum does not generate as much chemotactic factor as does adult serum, even after the addition of purified C3. The defect in chemotaxis may be related to decreased granulocyte deformability and impaired capping of cell surface receptors.[175] The role of observed cyclic adenosine monophosphate (cAMP) and membrane potential alterations in the defective chemotaxis is not clear.[175] The ability of neutrophils to roll along the blood vessel endothelium also is impaired in neonates. Diminished upregulation and surface migration of β_2 integrins and fewer L-selectin receptors reduce the ability of neonatal neutrophils to interact with adhesion molecules on the endothelium.[139]

The densities of the C3bi receptor (CD11b/CD18) and of the low-affinity receptor for immunoglobulin, FcRIII (CD16), are decreased on neutrophils of premature infants, whereas term infants' cells show a lesser impairment.[176-178] The deficient upregulation of C3bi correlates with decreased adherence and chemotaxis by neonatal neutrophils.[179] Low FcRIII is associated with impaired chemotaxis of neonatal neutrophils,[180] although decreased FcRIII might also be responsible for subtle defects in adherence and subsequent phagocytosis of opsonized[171] and unopsonized[181] organisms by neutrophils.

Adherence Neutrophil cell adhesion molecules are central to the bonding of neutrophils to the vascular endothelium, and reduction of these molecules diminishes the capacity of neonatal neutrophils to properly adhere and migrate (Chap. 19).[182] Although L-selectin, a key adhesion molecule, is expressed at high levels on hematopoietic progenitor cells, it decreases markedly during the first 3 days of life and remains low compared to adult levels during the first weeks, impairing the neutrophil's ability to "roll" as part of the adhesion process. Also, there are defects in expression of CD18/CD11b, which are members of the β_2-integrin family of adhesion molecules.[183] These characteristics likely contribute to the newborn susceptibility to bacterial infections.

Phagocytic and Bactericidal Activity Phagocytosis of bacteria and latex granules by neutrophils from premature and term infants is normal.[147,151,184] Bactericidal activity varies according to the conditions of testing and the clinical status of the neonates. The intracellular killing of *S. aureus* and *S. marcescens* in cells from most term and low-birth-weight infants is normal,[147,185] as is that of *E. coli* in term infants.[148] Similar studies have shown defective bactericidal activity against *S. aureus* in some infants in the first 12 hours after birth,[183] *P. aeruginosa* in cells from premature infants,[151] and *Candida albicans* in granulocytes from term and premature infants.[186] With bacteria-to-neutrophil ratios of 1:1, newborn cells kill *S. aureus* and *E. coli* as effectively as controls; however, at the higher ratio of 100:1, killing and oxidative responses as measured by chemiluminescence are markedly depressed, although phagocytosis is normal.[184] Depressed activity also has been found in cells from newborns who have had clinical stress, either from infection or other disorders, shown both as decreased chemiluminescence and impaired bactericidal activity against *S. aureus*, *E. coli*, and group B streptococci.[187-189] The decreased granulocyte function shown in these studies also is found in liquid culture, where neutrophils from newborns do not survive as long as those from adults, perhaps because of decreased resistance to autoxidation.[188] Although superoxide dismutase levels are normal and superoxide production is normal or increased in neutrophils from newborns, glutathione peroxidase and catalase levels are decreased.[189,190] The relationship of these *in vitro* cellular defects to bacterial infections in the newborn is still not clear.

Antimicrobial proteins and peptides are present in neutrophil cytoplasmic granules. Bacterial permeability-increasing protein (BPI), located in the primary granules, is markedly lower in newborns, particularly preterm newborns.[191,192] BPI is an antimicrobial protein that binds and neutralizes endotoxin. Other granule components, such as myeloperoxidase (bacterial killing) and defensins (antimicrobial proteins), are not diminished.

Monocytes from newborn infants have normal nitroblue tetrazolium (NBT) reduction,[193] normal antibody-dependent cellular cytotoxicity,[194] and normal *in vitro* killing of *S. aureus* and *E. coli*.[195] However, they are slower than monocytes from adults in phagocytosis of polystyrene spheres,[196] and they have reduced ATP production.[197] Furthermore, chemotaxis to serum-derived factors is decreased, as is monocyte appearance in skin windows.[198] These functional aspects may contribute to the observed susceptibility of newborns to a variety of infectious agents.

Cytokine Effects on Neonatal Phagocytic Function There is a complex interaction between cytokines produced by lymphocytes and macrophages, and the activation status of neutrophils during infection. There is decreased production of interferon-γ by neonatal leukocytes.[199,200] Interferon-γ causes the upregulation of the C3bi receptor and induces the surface expression of the high-affinity immunoglobulin receptor FcRI (CD64)[201] on neutrophils. C3bi is required for adherence and efficient chemotaxis by neutrophils. Low levels of this receptor also impair complement-mediated phagocytosis and oxidative metabolism. FcRI also mediates oxidative responses, and appears on neutrophils of adults during infection. The diminished production of G-CSF and GM-CSF by neonatal mononuclear cells[137–139] may not only limit progenitor colony growth, but may also impair neonatal neutrophil functions, including chemotaxis, superoxide production, and C3bi expression, which are enhanced by these factors.[202,203] Tumor necrosis factor (TNF)-α and IL-4, cytokines that modulate neutrophil functions, also may be produced at lower levels in neonates.[204]

THROMBOPOIESIS AND PLATELETS

The platelet counts in term and preterm infants are between 150 and 400×10^9/L (150,000 to 400,000/μL), comparable to adult values.[205,206] Thrombocytopenia of fewer than 100×10^9/L (100,000/μL) may occur in high-risk infants with respiratory distress or sepsis,[207] small-for-date infants,[208] and newborns with trisomy syndromes.[209] Even normal newborns are unable to regulate thrombopoiesis and myelopoiesis in a wholly effective manner.[210] Although committed megakaryocyte progenitors (colony-forming unit–megakaryocyte [CFU-Meg]) are increased in the marrow and cord blood of newborns, they are less able to produce adequate numbers of platelets when severely stressed. Reduced levels of G-CSF, GM-CSF, and IL-3 may play a role in the impaired response.[211] Thrombopoietin (TPO) is a major regulator of platelet production in adults. TPO transcripts have been detected as early as 6 weeks postconception and the primary source of TPO in the fetus and neonate is thought to be the liver.[212] Serum TPO levels are higher in preterm and term neonates compared to adults. However, thrombocytopenic newborns do not increase serum TPO levels as robustly as thrombocytopenic adults, which may contribute to the high incidence of thrombocytopenia seen in sick infants.[212]

Platelet Functions

Bleeding Time and Closure Time The expected inverse relationship between the platelet count and bleeding time has been described in term and preterm newborns.[213] However, the bleeding time often is longer than would be predicted by the platelet count because of sepsis or respiratory distress resulting in impaired platelet function, aggravating the effects of thrombocytopenia.

The bleeding time reflects platelet function and capillary integrity, as well as the platelet count, and traditionally has been used to assess these parameters. However, there are technical difficulties in applying a technique for measuring bleeding time to neonates or preterm infants because of the need for venous occlusion of the forearm, where the test

normally is performed, and for a minimal incision to avoid scarring of the skin. Bleeding times were measured using an automatic device to minimize trauma in normal neonates, with venous occlusion of 20 torr for infants who weigh less than 1000 g, 25 torr for those who weigh 1000 to 2000 g, and 30 torr for those who weigh more than 2000 g. In 82 observations, 97 percent of the measurements were below 3.5 minutes, which was suggested as the upper limit for normal in these infants.[214] A similar upper limit (200 seconds) for the bleeding time of normal infants has been obtained using an automated device and vertical incisions.[215] Generally, newborn infants have shorter bleeding times than do children and adults, which may reflect their higher hematocrit, increased concentration of von Willebrand factor, and higher proportion of high-molecular-weight multimers of von Willebrand factor.[216] Children have longer bleeding times than either adults or newborns,[217] and the upper limit measured with an automated pediatric device may be as high as 13 minutes before age 10 years, compared to an upper limit of 7 minutes in adults measured with the same device.[217]

The bleeding times in newborns may be prolonged for a variety of reasons, including neonatal infection and respiratory distress syndrome, which do not necessarily result in thrombocytopenia.[218] Platelets from healthy newborns are relatively deficient in phospholipid metabolism, granule secretion, and aggregation,[219] but there is heightened platelet adhesion because of increased large von Willebrand multimers. The result of these differences is shortened bleeding and closure times in normal neonates (see below).

The use of indomethacin for treatment of patent ductus arteriosus in preterm infants has been questioned because this agent interferes with prostaglandin metabolism and the production of thromboxane A_2, an important initiator of platelet aggregation. Although bleeding times are prolonged from a normal 3.5 minutes to approximately 9 minutes in indomethacin-treated patients,[220] indomethacin did not result in an increase in periventricular or intraventricular hemorrhage in preterm infants treated for patent ductus arteriosus.

The closure time to assess platelet function may replace the bleeding time, particularly for neonates and young children in whom bleeding times are difficult to perform and interpret. Newborn infants have closure times that are shorter than those of adults, likely related to their higher hematocrits, increased von Willebrand multimers and hence ristocetin cofactor, and higher leukocyte counts.[221–223] The normal adult value for collagen-epinephrine closure time is less than 164 seconds, and for collagen-ADP closure time is less than 116 seconds. However, each laboratory must determine its own normal range for these tests.

Platelet Aggregation and Metabolism A variety of differences have been described in the platelet function of neonates. These include decreases in ADP release, in platelet factor 3 activity, in platelet adhesiveness, and in platelet aggregation in response to ADP, epinephrine, collagen, or thrombin.[224,225] These defects result from intrinsic differences in neonatal compared to adult platelets.[226] Paradoxically, these insufficiencies have little effect on the bleeding time of neonates. The *in vitro* findings do not appear related to a significant defect in prostaglandin synthesis or to storage pool deficiency of adenine nucleotides.[224] Furthermore, electron micrographs of neonatal platelets do not differ from those of platelets from normal adults.[227] This leaves unexplained the *in vitro* observations in neonatal platelets, which may be related to platelet membrane immaturity. These *in vitro* abnormalities may aggravate the impairment in platelet function and the predisposition to bleeding that result from neonatal diseases, particularly respiratory distress syndrome and sepsis.

Maternal aspirin ingestion also results in abnormalities in platelet aggregation in the newborn in response to collagen.[228,229] However, aspirin has been studied extensively in patients with preeclampsia, and there is no significant bleeding in the fetus or newborn.[230,231]

Newborn infants commonly have petechiae, particularly on the head, neck, and shoulders, after vertex deliveries. They are presumably caused by trauma associated with passage through the birth canal and disappear within a few days. Petechiae usually are not present in infants delivered by cesarean section.

Platelet Antigens and Glycoproteins The glycoprotein complex GPIIb/IIIa represents approximately 15 percent of platelet surface protein and exhibits two allelic forms, Pl[A1] and Pl[A2].[232] The Pl[A1] antigen can be identified on fetal platelets by 16 weeks' gestation.[233] Pl[A1] antigen is observed in a higher percentage of fetuses between 18 and 26 weeks' gestation than in adults. Approximately 2 percent of the population in the United States of European descent is homozygous for Pl[A2] and thus are Pl[A1]-negative. The complete expression of the Pl[A1] antigen during early gestation likely permits sensitization in women who are Pl[A1]-negative even during their first pregnancy.[233] The membrane glycoprotein GPIb, as well as the GPIIb/IIIa complex, is expressed by 18 weeks of gestation.[233] The difference between Pl[A1] and Pl[A2] is a leucine 33–proline 33 amino acid polymorphism in glycoprotein IIIA.[232] Prenatal diagnosis of the glycoprotein genotype using DNA from amniocytes and the polymerase chain reaction can establish the potential for neonatal alloimmune thrombocytopenia,[234] as well as the diagnosis of Glanzmann thrombasthenia. Rarely, other fetal platelet antigens, such as Pl[E2], DUZO[a], Ko[a], and Bak[a] have caused maternal sensitization and neonatal alloimmune thrombocytopenia.[235] The gestational ages for expression of these antigens have not been defined but are sufficiently early to permit sensitization.

NEONATAL LYMPHOPOIESIS

T-Lymphocyte Functions—Cellular Immunity

The absolute number of lymphocytes in the newborn is equivalent to that in older children, ages 6 months to 2 years, with lower values in premature infants at birth. Thymus-derived cells (T cells) develop early in gestation.[236] Tables 7–4 and 7–5 show the various lymphocyte subsets in infants and children.[237,238] The absolute number of CD3+ and CD4+

TABLE 7–4. Blood Lymphocyte Subsets: Infants Age 1 to 3 Days

Lymphocyte Subsets	Median (10th–90th percentile range)	
	Infants (1–3 Days)	Adults
Lymphocytes × 10⁹/L	3.1×10^9/L (3.1–6.8)	___
CD3+ % of lymphocytes	83% (72–90)	77 (69–84)
Count × 10⁹/L	3.7 (2.6–5.8)	___
CD3–/CD19+ % of lymphocytes	14% (6–22)	14 (8–18)
Count × 10⁹/L	0.58 (0.23–1.2)	___
NK (CD3–/CD16+ or CD56+) % of Lymphocytes	4% (2–8)	11 (6–17)
Count × 10⁹/L	0.2 (0.06–0.38)	___
CD3+/CD4+ % of lymphocytes	63% (52–72)	46 (37–55)
Count × 10⁹/L	2.7 (2.0–4.4)	___
CD3+/CD8+ % of lymphocytes	23% (16–29)	28 (20–34)
Count × 10⁹/L	1.1 (0.55–1.9)	___

Data from O'Gorman MRG, Millard DD, Lowder JN, et al: Lymphocyte subpopulations in 1–3 day old infants. *Cytometry* 34:235, 1998.

(helper/inducer phenotype) T-cell subsets in blood of newborns is higher than in adults.[239] This is a result of an increased total lymphocyte count in neonates (and older children) as compared with adults.[240] The percentages of major lymphoid subsets (CD2, CD3, CD4, CD8, CD19) and natural killer (NK) cells are not markedly different in neonates, children, and adults when measured by flow cytometry methods.[241,242] However, functional defects are present in the NK cell population.[242] Furthermore, the responses of T-helper type 1 (Th1 cell-mediated immunity) and T-helper type 2 (Th2-assisted humoral immunity) differ in newborns and adults in response to various antigens such as vaccines, infectious agents, and environmental antigens.[243] The numbers of T and B lymphocytes are sustained or increased during the first 2 postnatal months.[244] There is a trend toward increased CD4 and decreased CD8 lymphocytes in newborns and children, resulting in an increased CD4:CD8 ratio.[245,246] In spite of this, T-cell suppressor activity may be increased in newborns.[247] Most responses of the cellular immunity system, such as antigen recognition and binding, antibody-dependent cytotoxicity, and graft-versus-host reactivity are present in the newborn,[247] although some are decreased in comparison with adults.[248] The *in vitro* response to phytohemagglutinin of cord blood lymphocytes is increased,[249,250] but the response of the newborn to 2,4-dinitrofluorobenzene, a potent inducer of delayed hypersensitivity, is not as consistent as that seen in older children.[251] Impaired T-cell production of interferon-γ and other lymphokines may be related to immature macrophage rather than to T-lymphocyte function, because intercellular cooperation is a requisite for these processes.[252] Furthermore, cord blood T lymphocytes form a functional IL-2 receptor complex and have normal IL-2 receptors, but they do not upregulate interferon-γ in response to IL-2.[253]

B-Lymphocyte Functions–Humoral Immunity

Humoral (B-cell) immunity also develops early in gestation,[236] but it is not fully active until after birth. In the newborn, approximately 15 percent of lymphocytes have immunoglobulin on their surface, with all immunoglobulin isotypes represented.[254] A percentage of these cells are CD5+ B cells (B-1 cells), which produce polyreactive autoantibodies whose function is yet unclear.[255] The proportion of CD5+ B cells is markedly higher in the fetus compared to adults. The percentages of B cells expressing specific immunoglobulin isotypes are not related to the plasma levels of those isotypes. Variation in antibody response to specific antigens relates to the interaction of macrophages, T cells, and B cells. B lymphocytes are well represented in newborns, but T-lymphocyte–independent B-lymphocyte responses are limited during the first year.[256] T-lymphocyte–dependent B-lymphocyte antibody production matures much earlier.[256]

Fetal lymphocytes synthesize little immunoglobulin, presumably because of the sheltered environment *in utero*. Animals kept germ-free after birth have few plasma cells and markedly decreased production of immunoglobulins.[257] IgG levels of term infants are similar to maternal levels because of transplacental transfer.[258] IgM, IgD, and IgE do not cross the placenta,[258,259] and the levels of these immunoglobulins and of IgA are low or not detectable at birth. Breastfeeding provides some transfer of antibodies, particularly secretory IgA, lysozyme, and lactoferrin. Large numbers of lymphocytes and monocytes (10⁶ cells/mL) are found in colostrum and milk during the first 2 months postpartum.[260] These may provide local gastrointestinal protection against infection,[261,262] and there is some evidence for absorption of immunoglobulin and transfer of tuberculin sensitivity to the infant.

Although the newborn infant can produce specific IgG antibody,[263] only small amounts of IgG are usually produced by the fetus. IgG levels in premature infants are reduced in relation to gestational age because of the low placental transport early in pregnancy.[264-266] The ability of the fetus to produce IgM and IgA with appropriate stimuli is indicated by

TABLE 7–5. Blood Lymphocyte Subsets: Infants and Children to Age 18 Years

Lymphocyte Subsets	0–3 Months	3–6 Months	6–12 Months	1–2 Years	2–6 Years	6–12 Years	12–18 Years
WBC × 10⁹/L	10.60 (7.20–18.00)	9.20 (6.70–14.00)	9.10 (6.40–13.00)	8.80 (6.40–12.00)	7.10 (5.20–11.00)	6.50 (4.40–9.50)	6.00 (4.40–8.10)
Lymphocytes × 10⁹/L	5.40 (3.40–7.60)	6.30 (3.90–9.00)	5.90 (3.40–9.00)	5.50 (3.60–8.90)	3.60 (2.30–5.40)	2.70 (1.90–3.70)	2.20 (1.40–3.30)
CD3+ % of lymphocytes	73% (53–84)	66% (51–77)	65% (49–76)	65% (53–75)	66% (56–75)	69% (60–76)	73% (56–84)
Count × 10⁹/L	3.68 (2.50–5.50)	3.75 (2.50–5.60)	3.93 (1.90–5.90)	3.55 (2.10–6.20)	2.39 (1.40–3.70)	1.82 (1.20–2.60)	1.48 (1.00–2.20)
CD19+ % of lymphocytes	15% (06–32)	25% (11–41)	24% (14–37)	25% (16–35)	21% (14–33)	18% (13–27)	14% (06–23)
Count × 10⁹/L	0.73 (0.30–2.00)	1.55 (0.43–3.00)	1.52 (0.61–2.60)	1.31 (0.72–2.60)	0.75 (0.39–1.40)	0.48 (0.27–0.86)	0.30 (0.11–0.57)
CD16+/CD56+ % of lymphocytes	8% (04–18)	6% (03–14)	7% (03–15)	7% (03–15)	9% (04–17)	9% (04–17)	9% (03–22)
Count × 10⁹/L	0.42 (0.17–1.10)	0.42 (0.17–0.83)	0.40 (0.16–0.95)	0.36 (0.18–0.92)	0.30 (0.13–0.72)	0.23 (0.10–0.48)	0.19 (0.07–0.48)
CD4+ % of lymphocytes	52% (35–64)	46% (35–56)	46% (31–56)	41% (32–51)	38% (28–47)	37% (31–47)	41% (31–52)
Count × 10⁹/L	2.61 (1.60–4.00)	2.85 (1.80–4.00)	2.67 (1.40–4.30)	2.16 (1.30–3.40)	1.38 (0.07–2.20)	0.98 (0.65–1.50)	0.84 (0.53–1.30)
CD8+ % of lymphocytes	18% (12–28)	16% (12–23)	17% (12–24)	20% (14–30)	23% (16–30)	25% (18–35)	26% (18–35)0
Count × 10⁹/L	0.98 (0.56–1.70)	1.05 (0.59–1.60)	1.04 (0.50–1.70)	1.04 (0.62–2.00)	0.84 (0.49–1.30)	0.68 (0.37–1.10)	0.53 (0.33–0.92)

WBC, white blood cells.

Data from Shearer WT, Rosenblatt HM, Gelman RS, et al: Lymphocyte subsets in healthy children from birth through 18 years of age: The Pediatric AIDS Clinical Trials Group P1009 Study. *J Allergy Clin Immunol* 112:973, 2003.

the presence of these antibodies in many newborn infants who have had prenatal infections[267] and by the presence of IgM isohemagglutinins in more than half of term newborn infants.[268] In human newborns and in fetal animals, the IgM response is predominant, and the appearance of IgG after exposure to specific antigens is delayed. These differences from the adult may relate to functional immaturity of B and T lymphocytes,[269-271] to increased activity of suppressor T cells,[258,269] and perhaps to altered macrophage function.[272]

Newborns also may have relative splenic hypofunction, suggested by the large number of "pocked" red cells seen in the blood films of neonates, particularly premature infants. These "pocks" represent residual intraerythrocyte inclusions, which remain because of monocyte and macrophage hypofunction.[273,274]

COAGULATION IN THE NEONATE

Plasma Coagulation Factors

When the term newborn is compared to older children and adults, several differences in the coagulation and fibrinolytic systems are apparent.[275-281] A comprehensive evaluation of the developmental changes in the levels of clotting factors and coagulation tests in preterm and term infants has been published.[282,283] The term newborn has reduced mean plasma levels (<60 percent of adult levels) of factors II, IX, X, XI, XII, prekallikrein, and high-molecular-weight kininogen (Table 7–6). This is not a result of impaired mRNA expression, at least in the case of factors II and X.[284] In contrast, the plasma concentration of factor VIII is similar and von Willebrand factor is increased compared to that of older

children and adults. In spite of the lower levels of factors, the functional tests (prothrombin and partial thromboplastin times) are only slightly prolonged compared to adult normal values (Table 7–6). Although different coagulation factors show different postnatal patterns of maturation, near-adult values are achieved for most components by 6 months of age.[278]

Factors II (prothrombin), VII, IX, and X require vitamin K for the final γ-glutamyl carboxylation step in their synthesis.[285] These factors decrease during the first 3 to 4 days after birth. This fall may be lessened by administration of vitamin K,[286] effectively preventing classic, early occurring (first few days after birth) hemorrhagic disease of the newborn. Inactive prothrombin molecules have been found in the plasma of some newborns, but they disappear after administration of vitamin K.[287] Early occurring hemorrhagic disease is most often associated with maternal administration of medications such as phenytoin (Dilantin)[288] and warfarin,[289] which reduce the vitamin K–dependent factors. In rare cases, no contributing factor is found.

A hemorrhagic diathesis also may occur later, 2 to 12 weeks after birth, as a result of lack of vitamin K, and is called *late hemorrhagic disease of the newborn* or *acquired prothrombin complex deficiency.*[290,291] The etiology of the vitamin K lack is unclear but may result from poor dietary intake, particularly related to breastfeeding, alterations in liver function with cholestasis and decreased vitamin K absorption, or a toxic or infectious impairment of hepatic utilization.[290] Unfortunately, intracranial hemorrhage frequently is the presenting event in this condition. This problem can be prevented by parenteral or oral vitamin K, but the preferred route of administration remains controversial.[292] The

TABLE 7-6. Reference Values for Coagulation Tests in Preterm and Full-Term Infants*

Coagulation Test	Preterm 28–31-Week Infants Day 1	Preterm 30–36-Week Infants			Full-Term Infants			Adults
		Day 1	Day 30	Day 180	Day 1	Day 30	Day 180	
PT(s)	15.4 (14.6–16.9)	13.0 (10.6–16.2)	11.8 (10.0–13.6)	12.5 (10.0–15.0)	13.0 (10.1–15.9)	11.8 (10.0–14.3)	12.3 (10.7–13.9)	12.4 (10.8–13.9)
INR	1.0 (0.61–1.70)	1.00 (0.53–1.62)	0.79 (0.53–1.11)	0.91 (0.53–1.48)	1.00 (0.53–1.26)	0.79 (0.53–1.26)	0.88 (0.61–1.17)	0.89 (0.64–1.17)
APTT(s)	108 (80.0–168)	53.6 (27.5–79.4)	44.7 (26.9–62.5)	37.5 (27.2–53.5)	42.9 (31.3–54.5)	40.4 (32.0–55.2)	35.5 (28.1–42.9)	33.5 (26.6–40.3)
TCT(s)	24.8 (19.2–30.4)	24.4 (18.3–29.9)	25.2 (18.9–31.5)	23.5 (19.0–28.3)	24.3 (19.4–29.2)	25.5 (19.8–31.2)	25.0 (19.7–30.3)	
Fibrinogen (g/L)	2.56 (1.60–5.50)	2.43 (1.50–3.73)	2.54 (1.50–4.14)	2.28 (1.50–3.60)	2.83 (1.67–3.99)	2.70 (1.62–3.78)	2.51 (1.50–3.87)	2.78 (1.56–4.00)
II (U/mL)	0.31 (0.19–0.54)	0.45 (0.20–0.77)	0.57 (0.36–0.95)	0.87 (0.51–1.23)	0.48 (0.26–0.70)	0.68 (0.34–1.02)	0.88 (0.60–1.16)	1.08 (0.70–1.46)
V (U/mL)	0.65 (0.43–0.80)	0.88 (0.41–1.44)	1.02 (0.48–1.56)	1.02 (0.58–1.46)	0.72 (0.34–1.08)	0.98 (0.62–1.34)	0.91 (0.55–1.27)	1.06 (0.62–1.50)
VII (U/mL)	0.37 (0.24–0.76)	0.67 (0.21–1.13)	0.83 (0.21–1.45)	0.99 (0.47–1.51)	0.66 (0.28–1.04)	0.90 (0.42–1.38)	0.87 (0.47–1.27)	1.05 (0.67–1.43)0
VIII (U/mL)	0.79 (0.37–1.26)	1.11 (0.50–2.13)	1.11 (0.50–1.99)	0.99 (0.50–1.87)	1.00 (0.50–1.78)	0.91 (0.50–1.57)	0.73 (0.50–1.09)	0.99 (0.50–1.49)
VWF (U/mL)	1.41 (0.83–2.23)	1.36 (0.78–2.10)	1.36 (0.66–2.16)	0.98 (0.54–1.58)	1.53 (0.50–2.87)	1.28 (0.50–2.46)	1.07 (0.50–1.97)	0.92 (0.50–1.58)
IX (U/mL)	0.18 (0.17–0.20)	0.35 (0.19–0.65)	0.44 (0.13–0.80)	0.81 (0.50–1.20)	0.53 (0.15–0.91)	0.51 (0.21–0.81)	0.86 (0.36–1.36)	1.09 (0.55–1.63)
X (U/mL)	0.36 (0.25–0.64)	0.41 (0.11–0.71)	0.56 (0.20–0.92)	0.77 (0.35–1.19)	0.40 (0.12–0.68)	0.59 (0.31–0.87)	0.78 (0.38–1.18)	1.06 (0.70–1.52)
XI (U/mL)	0.23 (0.11–0.33)	0.30 (0.08–0.52)	0.43 (0.15–0.71)	0.78 (0.46–1.10)	0.38 (0.10–0.66)	0.53 (0.27–0.79)	0.86 (0.49–1.34)	0.97 (0.67–1.27)
XII (U/mL)	0.25 (0.05–0.35)	0.38 (0.10–0.66)	0.43 (0.11–0.75)	0.82 (0.22–1.42)	0.53 (0.13–0.93)	0.49 (0.17–0.81)	0.77 (0.39–1.15)	1.08 (0.52–1.64)
PK (U/mL)	0.26 (0.15–0.32)	0.33 (0.09–0.57)	0.59 (0.31–0.87)	0.78 (0.40–1.16)	0.37 (0.18–0.69)	0.57 (0.23–0.91)	0.86 (0.56–1.16)	1.12 (0.62–1.62)
HK (U/mL)	0.32 (0.19–0.52)	0.49 (0.09–0.89)	0.64 (0.16–1.12)	0.83 (0.41–1.25)	0.54 (0.06–1.02)	0.77 (0.33–1.21)	0.82 (0.36–1.28)	0.92 (0.50–1.36)
XIIIa (U/mL)	0.70 (0.32–1.08)		0.99 (0.51–1.47)	1.13 (0.65–1.61)	0.79 (0.27–1.31)	0.93 (0.39–1.47)	1.04 (0.46–1.62)	1.05 (0.55–1.55)
XIIIb (U/mL)	0.81 (0.35–1.27)		1.07 (0.57–1.57)	1.15 (0.67–1.63)	0.76 (0.30–1.22)	1.11 (0.50–1.70)	1.10 (0.50–1.70)	0.97 (0.57–1.37)

APTT, activated partial thromboplastin time; HK, high-molecular-weight kininogen; INR, international normalized ratio; PK, prekallikrein; PT, prothrombin time; TCT, thrombin clotting time; VWF, von Willebrand factor.

*All factors except fibrinogen are expressed as units per milliliter (U/mL), where pooled plasma contains 1.0 U/mL. All values are expressed as the mean of 40 to 77 samples for each population. The range of values encompassing 95 percent of the population is shown in parentheses.

Data from Andrew M, Paes B, Milner B, et al: Development of the human coagulation system in the full-term infant. *Blood* 70:165, 1987 and Monagle P, Massicotte P: Developmental haemostasis: Secondary haemostasis. *Sem in Fetal and Neonatal Medicine* 16:294–300, 2011.

parenteral route may result rarely in neuromuscular complications,[293] and an association of intramuscular vitamin K prophylaxis and cancer in infancy was suggested but not substantiated. Oral administration, however, appears less reliable and may require repeated doses.[290] The current recommendation of the American Academy of Pediatrics suggests that vitamin K_1, 0.5 to 1.0 mg, be administered intramuscularly at birth.[294] Even the lower (0.5 mg) parenteral dose may be excessive for preterm (<32 weeks' gestation) infants, although no toxic effects have been reported as a result of very high plasma values.[295] Recent data suggest that 0.2 mg vitamin K may be appropriate prophylaxis for infants delivered at fewer than 32 weeks' gestation, but additional oral supplementation is needed when feeding is established.[296] A mixed micellar vitamin K_1 preparation is particularly well absorbed and may permit prophylaxis with a single oral dose,[297] but the efficacy and safety of oral prophylaxis require further study.

Table 7–6 shows the values for coagulation factors in healthy 30 to 36 weeks' gestation premature infants. More prominent decreases in factors IX, XI, and XII are noted, which tend to prolong the partial thromboplastin time. Table 7–6 also shows the values for coagulation factors in 28 to 31 weeks' gestation infants. All of the coagulation factors are lower at earlier gestational ages.

There are no significant differences in mean prothrombin time determinations between 30 and 36 weeks' gestation premature and full-term infants who have not received vitamin K.[298] Premature infants given vitamin K have a longer mean prothrombin time than do term infants similarly treated. In some small infants there is no improvement in prothrombin time or levels of prothrombin, and factors VII and X after the intramuscular administration of vitamin K.[286,299] These results suggest a greater degree of "immaturity" of the liver in the small infants.

Bleeding and Thrombosis

Significant bleeding occurs more often in low-birth-weight infants than in term newborn infants. Increased capillary fragility is frequently found in premature infants in the first 2 days after birth and is not associated with thrombocytopenia.[286] Bleeding under the scalp or in other superficial areas may be caused by trauma at birth coupled with increased capillary fragility. The more serious disorders of periventricular–intraventricular hemorrhage and pulmonary hemorrhage probably are not caused by coagulation disorders, although such disorders may increase the bleeding.[300] Hypoxia seems to affect the clotting status of low-birth-weight infants.[301] Many infants with markedly abnormal prothrombin times have had hypoxia during delivery or shortly thereafter.[296] Cardiovascular collapse seen with episodes of cardiac arrest or with profound shock may cause disseminated intravascular coagulation and generalized bleeding. In many sick premature infants, a combination of shock, sepsis, liver immaturity, hypoxia, and other factors may contribute to the pathogenesis of coagulation abnormalities.

Arterial and venous thromboses are relatively frequent in newborns as compared to other age groups, but greater than 90 percent of arterial and greater than 80 percent of venous clots are related to catheters. Spontaneous thromboses are much less common, and most involve the renal veins or, rarely, the pulmonary vasculature.[302] Relative hypercoagulability in the newborn could result from a difference in the vascular endothelium, activation of the coagulation cascade, diminished coagulation inhibitor activity, or a defect in fibrinolysis. Inhibitors of coagulation include antithrombin, heparin cofactor II, protein C, and protein S.[283,303] The levels of proteins C and S, which are vitamin K dependent, as well as antithrombin and heparin cofactor II, are low in the newborn; they are in a range associated with thrombotic episodes in adults with inherited deficiencies.[303] In addition, the presence of factor V Leiden may occur in as many as 6 percent of newborns.[304] This produces resistance to the action of protein C and may heighten the susceptibility to thrombosis (Chap. 130). Hyperprothrombinemia caused by the 20210A allele prothrombin gene may affect 1 percent of the population,[305] but the elevated prothrombin level predisposing to thrombosis occurs in older patients.[306] The combined deficiency of these anticoagulant proteins may further intensify the thrombotic risk. However, the precise role of these inhibitors of coagulation in newborn hypercoagulability is uncertain because a proportionate decrease in vitamin K–dependent procoagulant factors (II, VII, IX, X) also is present, and an additional inhibitor, α_2-macroglobulin, is increased (Chap. 130). Table 7–7 shows the values for plasma inhibitors of coagulation in premature and term infants.

TABLE 7–7. Reference Values for Inhibitors of Coagulation in Preterm and Full-Term Infants*

Inhibitor Levels	Day 1	Day 30	Day 180	Day 1	Day 30	Day 180	Adults
AT (U/mL)	0.38 (0.14–0.62)	0.59 (0.37–0.81)	0.90 (0.52–1.28)	0.63 (0.39–0.87)	0.78 (0.48–1.08)	1.04 (0.84–1.24)	1.05 (0.79–1.31)
α_2M (U/mL)	1.10 (0.56–1.82)	1.38 (0.72–2.04)	2.09 (1.10–3.21)	1.39 (0.95–1.83)	1.50 (1.06–1.94)	1.91 (1.49–2.33)	0.86 (0.52–1.20)
C_1E-INH (U/mL)	0.65 (0.31–0.99)	0.74 (0.40–1.24)	1.40 (0.96–2.04)	0.72 (0.36–1.08)	0.89 (0.47–1.31)	1.41 (0.89–1.93)	1.01 (0.71–1.31)
α_1AT (U/mL)	0.90 (0.36–1.44)	0.76 (0.38–1.12)	0.82 (0.48–1.16)	0.93 (0.49–1.37)	0.62 (0.36–0.88)	0.77 (0.47–1.07)	0.93 (0.55–1.31)
HCII (U/mL)	0.32 (0.10–0.60)	0.43 (0.15–0.71)	0.89 (0.45–1.40)	0.43 (0.10–0.93)	0.47 (0.10–0.87)	1.20 (0.50–1.90)	0.96 (0.66–1.26)
Protein C (U/mL)	0.28 (0.12–0.44)	0.37 (0.15–0.59)	0.57 (0.31–0.83)	0.35 (0.17–0.53)	0.43 (0.21–0.65)	0.59 (0.37–0.81)	0.96 (0.64–1.28)
Protein S (U/mL)	0.26 (0.14–0.38)	0.56 (0.22–0.90)	0.82 (0.44–1.20)	0.36 (0.12–0.60)	0.63 (0.33–0.93)	0.87 (0.55–1.19)	0.92 (0.60–1.24)

α_1AT, α_1-antitrypsin; α_2M, α_2-macroglobulin; AT, antithrombin; C_1E-INH, C_1 esterase inhibitor; HCII, heparin cofactor II.

*All values are expressed in units per milliliter (U/mL) where pooled plasma contains 1.0 U/mL. All values are expressed as the mean of 40 to 75 samples for each population. The range of values encompassing 95 percent of the population is shown in parentheses.

Data from Andrew M, Paes B, Milner B, et al: Development of the human coagulation system in the full-term infant. *Blood* 70:165, 1987 and Monagle P, Massicotte P: Developmental haemostasis: Secondary haemostasis. *Sem in Fetal and Neonatal Medicine* 16:294–300, 2011.

TABLE 7–8. Hematologic Effects of Maternal Drugs on the Fetus and Newborn

Drug	Effect	Certainty*	Mechanism	Reference
Antiretroviral agents in combination	Decreased hemoglobin	Established	Unknown—only seen with combination of zidovudine, lamivudine + nelfinavir	318
Aspirin	Bleeding; kernicterus	Established; potential	Interference with platelet function	123, 224, 228
			Displacement of bilirubin from albumin	317
Diazoxide	Bleeding	Questionable	Thrombocytopenia	307
Nalidixic acid	Hyperbilirubinemia	Potential	Oxidant damage to hemoglobin	315
Nitrofurantoin	Hyperbilirubinemia	Potential	Oxidant damage to hemoglobin	314, 316
Phenytoin (Dilantin/ phenobarbital)	Bleeding	Suspected	Depletion of vitamin K–dependent coagulation factors by hepatic enzyme induction and factor degradation	288
Rifampin/isoniazid	Bleeding	Suspected	Depletion of vitamin K–dependent coagulation factors	313
Sulfonamides	Kernicterus	Established	Displacement of bilirubin from albumin	317
Thiazides	Bleeding	Suspected	Thrombocytopenia	308, 309
Warfarin (Coumadin)	Bleeding	Established	Known depletion of vitamin K–dependent coagulation factors by blocking carboxylation	288, 289

*Certainty reflects the level of confidence in the data, assigned in increasing order from potential through questionable, suspected, and established.

Data from Haley TJ, Berndt WO: *Handbook of Toxicology*. Washington, DC: Hemisphere Publishing; 1987.

HEMATOLOGIC EFFECTS OF MATERNAL DRUGS ON THE FETUS AND NEWBORN

Hemostatic Effects

A number of maternally administered pharmacologic agents have been implicated in hematologic abnormalities of the fetus or newborn (Table 7–8). Maternal aspirin ingestion results in impaired platelet aggregation but does not foster neonatal bleeding. Other agents taken by the mother, including diazoxide and thiazides, might be associated with neonatal thrombocytopenia.[307–309]

The newborn's plasma coagulation factors may be depressed by maternal warfarin ingestion.[289] This drug is best avoided during pregnancy because it is teratogenic (first trimester) and may cause growth retardation of the fetus as well as bleeding.[289] In contrast, heparin does not cross the placenta, and maternal treatment with heparin appears to be safe for the fetus.[310]

Phenytoin (Dilantin) and/or phenobarbital also may reduce the newborn's vitamin K–dependent factors, possibly by microsomal enzyme induction, which enhances their degradation.[287] Furthermore, phenytoin may depress the platelet count as a result of prenatal exposure[311] and cause teratogenic effects, for example, the fetal hydantoin syndrome.[312] The decision to use this agent during pregnancy should reflect an assessment of the need for this specific drug, and also the risk of maternal seizures to the fetus and mother versus the potential side effects of treatment. Newborns of mothers taking rifampin and isoniazid also may have depressed vitamin K–dependent factors.[313]

Hyperbilirubinemia and Kernicterus

Nitrofurantoin and nalidixic acid may cause oxidant injury to the red cell membrane and hemoglobin.[314,315] If there is glucose-6-phosphate dehydrogenase deficiency, or if reduced glutathione is diminished, as in newborn red cells, these drugs have the potential to induce hemolysis and heighten neonatal hyperbilirubinemia (Chap. 47). Although this problem has not been documented by transplacental transfer of nitrofurantoin or nalidixic acid, hemolysis has occurred in glucose-6-phosphate

dehydrogenase-deficient infants who acquired the drugs from breast milk.[315,316] Alternatively, sulfonamides may cause displacement of bilirubin bound to albumin and heighten the risk of kernicterus.[317] Salicylates, phenylbutazone, and naproxen may have a similar effect at very high plasma concentrations.[317] Ideally, all these medications should be avoided during pregnancy unless their indication outweighs the potential risk to the fetus and newborn.

REFERENCES

1. Bloom W, Bartelmez GW: Hematopoiesis in young human embryos. *Am J Anat* 67:21, 1940.
2. Huber TL, Kouskoff V, Fehling HJ, et al: Haemangioblast commitment is initiated in the primitive streak of the mouse embryo. *Nature* 432:625, 2004.
3. Zambidis ET, Peault B, Park TS, et al: Hematopoietic differentiation of human embryonic stem cells progresses through sequential hematoendothelial, primitive, and definitive stages resembling human yolk sac development. *Blood* 106:860, 2005.
4. Kennedy M, D'Souza SL, Lynch-Kattman, et al: Development of the hemangioblast defines the onset of hematopoiesis in human ES cell differentiation cultures. *Development* 109:2679, 2007.
5. Shivdasani RA, Mayer EL, Orkin SH: Absence of blood formation in mice lacking T-cell leukemia oncoprotein tal-1/SCL. *Nature* 373:432, 1995.
6. Warren AJ, Colledge WH, Carlton MBL, et al: The oncogenic cysteine-rich LIM domain protein is essential for erythroid development. *Cell* 78:45, 1994.
7. Fujiwara Y, Browne CP, Cuniff K, Goff SC, Orkin SH: Arrested development of embryonic red cell precursors in mouse embryos lacking transcription factor GATA-1. *Proc Natl Acad Sci U S A* 93:12355, 1996.
8. Tavian M, Hallais M-F, Peault B: Emergence of intraembryonic hematopoietic precursors in the pre-liver human embryo. *Development* 126:793, 1999.
9. Peschle C, Mavilio F, Care A, et al: Haemoglobin switching in human embryos: Asynchrony of zeta→alpha and epsilon→gamma-globin switches in primitive and definite erythropoietic lineage. *Nature* 313:235, 1985.
10. Fukuda T: Fetal hemopoiesis. I. Electron microscopic studies on human yolk sac hemopoiesis. *Virchows Arch B Cell Pathol* 14:197, 1973.
11. Kingsley PD, Malik J, Fantauzzo KA, Palis J: Yolk sac derived primitive erythroblasts enucleate during mammalian embryogenesis. *Blood* 104:19, 2004.
12. Van Handel B, Prashad SL, Hassanzadeh-Kiabi N, et al: The first trimester human placenta is a site for terminal maturation of primitive erythroid cells. *Blood* 116:3321, 2010.
13. Palis J, Robertson S, Kennedy M, Wall C, Keller G: Development of erythroid and myeloid progenitors in the yolk sac and embryo proper of the mouse. *Development* 126:5073, 1999.

14. Tober J, Koniski A, McGrath KE, et al: The megakaryocyte lineage originates from hemangioblast precursors and is an integral component both of primitive and definitive hematopoiesis. *Blood* 109:1433, 2007.

15. Paluru P, Hudock KM, Cheng X, et al: The negative impact of wnt signaling on megakaryocyte and primitive erythroid progenitors derived from human embryonic stem cells. *Stem Cell Res* 12:41, 2014.

16. Migliaccio G, Migliaccio AR, Petti S, et al: Human embryonic hemopoiesis. Kinetics of progenitors and precursors underlying the yolk sac–liver transition. *J Clin Invest* 78:51, 1986.

17. Tavian M, Peault B: Embryonic development of the human hematopoietic system. *Int J Dev Biol* 49:243, 2005.

18. Huyhn A, Dommergues M, Izac B, et al: Characterization of hematopoietic progenitors from human yolk sacs and embryos. *Blood* 86:4474, 1995.

19. Dommergues M, Aubeny E, Dumez Y, et al: Hematopoiesis in the human yolk sac: Quantitation of erythroid and granulopoietic progenitors between 3.5 and 8 weeks of development. *Bone Marrow Transplant* 9:23, 1992.

20. Keleman E, Calvo W, Fliedner TM: *Atlas of Human Hemopoietic Development.* Springer-Verlag, Berlin, 1979.

21. Lin C-S, Lim S-K, D'Agati V, Constantini F: Differential effects of an erythropoietin receptor gene disruption on primitive and definitive erythropoiesis. *Genes Dev* 10:154, 1996.

22. Neubauer H, Cumano A, Muller M, et al: Jak2 deficiency defines an essential developmental checkpoint in definitive hematopoiesis. *Cell* 93:397, 1998.

23. Valtieri M, Gabbianelli M, Pelosi E, et al: Erythropoietin alone induces erythroid burst formation by human embryonic but not adult BFU-E in unicellular serum-free culture. *Blood* 74:460, 1989.

24. Emerson SG, Shanti T, Ferrara JL, Greenstein JL: Developmental regulation of erythropoiesis by hematopoietic growth factors: Analysis on populations of BFU-E from bone marrow, peripheral blood, and fetal liver. *Blood* 74:49, 1989.

25. Dame C, Fahnenstich H, Feitag P, et al: Erythropoietin mRNA expression in human fetal and neonatal tissue. *Blood* 92:3218, 1998.

26. Mucenski ML, McLain K, Kier AB, et al: A functional c-myb gene is required for normal murine fetal hepatic hematopoiesis. *Cell* 65:677, 1991.

27. Hann IM, Bodger MP, Hoffbrand AV: Development of pluripotent hematopoietic progenitor cells in the human fetus. *Blood* 62:118, 1983.

28. Ohls RK, Li Y, Abdel-Mageed A, et al: Neutrophil pool sizes and granulocyte colony-stimulating factor production in human mid-trimester fetuses. *Pediatr Res* 37:806, 1995.

29. Slayton WB, Juul SE, Calhoun DA, et al: Hematopoiesis in the liver and marrow of human fetuses at 5 to 16 weeks postconception: Quantitative assessment of macrophage and neutrophil populations. *Pediatr Res* 43:774, 1998.

30. Pahal GS, Jauniaux E, Kinnon C, et al: Normal development of human hematopoiesis between eight and seventeen weeks' gestation. *Am J Obstet Gynecol* 183:1029, 2000.

31. Gupta S, Pahwa R, O'Reilly R, et al: Ontogeny of lymphocyte subpopulation in human fetal liver. *Proc Natl Acad Sci U S A* 73:919, 1976.

32. Rainaut M, Pagniez M, Hercend T, et al: Characterization of mononuclear cell subpopulations in normal fetal peripheral blood. *Hum Immunol* 18:331, 1987.

33. Hann IM, Gibson BES, Letsky EA: *Fetal and Neonatal Hematology.* Baillaire Tindale, Philadelphia, 1991.

34. Charbord P, Tavian M, Humeau L, Peault B: Early ontogeny of the human marrow from long bones: An immunohistochemical study of hematopoiesis and its microenvironment. *Blood* 87:4109, 1996.

35. Cairo MS, Wagner JE: Placental and/or umbilical cord blood: An alternative source of hematopoietic stem cells for transplantation. *Blood* 90:4665, 1997.

36. Touraine JL, Raudrant D, Laplace S: Transplantation of hemopoietic cells from the fetal liver to treat patients with congenital diseases postnatally or prenatally. *Transplant Proc* 29:712, 1997.

37. Maximow AA: Relation of blood cells to connective tissues and endothelium. *Physiol Rev* IV(4):532, 1924.

38. Houssaint E: Differentiation of the mouse hepatic primordium. II. Extrinsic origin of the haemopoietic cell line. *Cell Differ* 10:243, 1981.

39. Cudennec CA, Thiery J-P, Le Douarin N-M: *In vitro* induction of adult erythropoiesis in early mouse yolk sac. *Proc Natl Acad Sci U S A* 78:2412, 1981.

40. Moore MAS, Owen JJT: Stem-cell migration in developing myeloid and lymphoid systems. *Lancet* i:658, 1967.

41. Dieterlen-Lievre F: On the origin of hematopoietic stem cells in the avian embryo: An experimental approach. *J Embryol Exp Morphol* 33:607, 1975.

42. Carpenter KL, Turpen JB: Experimental studies on hemopoiesis in the pronephros of *Rana pipiens*. *Differentiation* 14:167, 1979.

43. Muller AM, Medvinsky A, Strouboulis J, et al: Development of hematopoietic stem cell activity in the mouse embryo. *Immunity* 1:291, 1994.

44. Ivanovs A, Rybtsov S, Welch L, et al: Highly potent human hematopoietic stem cells first emerge in the intraembryonic aorta-gonad-mesonephros region. *J Exp Med* 208:2417, 2011.

45. Smith RA, Glomski CA: "Hemogenic endothelium" of the embryonic aorta: Does it exist? *Dev Comp Immunol* 6:359, 1982.

46. Tavian M, Coulombel L, Luton D, et al: Aorta-associated CD-34+ hematopoietic cells in the early human embryo. *Blood* 87:67, 1996.

47. Bertrand JY, Chi NC, Santoso B, et al: Haematopoietic stem cells derive directly from aortic endothelium during development. *Nature* 464:108, 2010.

48. Gekas C, Dieterlen-Lièvre F, Orkin SH, Mikkola HK: The placenta is a niche for hematopoietic stem cells. *Dev Cell* 8:297, 2005.

49. Alliot F, Godin I, Pessac B: Microglia derive from progenitors, originating from the yolk sac, and which proliferate in the brain. *Brain Res Dev Brain Res* 117:145, 1999.

50. Schulz C, Gomez Perdiguero E, et al: A lineage of myeloid cells independent of Myb and hematopoietic stem cells. *Science* 336:86, 2012.

51. Proudfoot NJ, Shander MH, Manley JL, et al: Structure and in vitro transcription of human globin genes. *Science* 209:1329, 1980.

52. Grosveld F, Van Assendelft GB, Greaves DR, Kolias B: Position independent, high-level expression of the human globin gene in transgenic mice. *Cell* 51:975, 1987.

53. Hecht F, Motulsky AG, Lemire RJ, et al: Predominance of hemoglobin Gower 1 in early human embryonic development. *Science* 152:91, 1966.

54. Huehns ER, Dance N, Beaven GH, et al: Human embryonic hemoglobins. *Cold Spring Harb Symp Quant Biol* 29:327, 1964.

55. Gale RE, Clegg JB, Huehns ER: Human embryonic haemoglobins Gower 1 and Gower 2. *Nature* 280:162, 1979.

56. Pataryas HA, Stomatoyannopoulos G: Hemoglobins in human fetuses: Evidence of adult hemoglobin production after the 11th gestational week. *Blood* 39:688, 1972.

57. Kazazian HH, Woodhead AP: Hemoglobin A synthesis in the developing fetus. *N Engl J Med* 289:58, 1973.

58. Bard H: The effect of placental insufficiency on fetal and adult hemoglobin synthesis. *Am J Obstet Gynecol* 120:67, 1974.

59. Armstrong D, Schroeder WA, Fenninger W: A comparison of the percentage of fetal hemoglobin in human umbilical cord blood as determined by chromatography and by alkali denaturation. *Blood* 22:554, 1963.

60. Bard H: Postnatal fetal and adult hemoglobin synthesis in early preterm newborn infants. *J Clin Invest* 60:1789, 1973.

61. Metaxotou-Mavromati AD, Antonopoulou HK, Laskari SA, et al: Developmental changes in hemoglobin F levels during the first two years of life in normal and heterozygous beta-thalassemia infants. *Pediatrics* 69:734, 1982.

62. Bard H, Makowski EL, Meschia G, et al: The relative rates of synthesis of hemoglobins A and F in red cells of newborn infants. *Pediatrics* 45:766, 1970.

63. Bromberg YN, Abrahamov A, Salzberger M: The effect of maternal anoxemia on the foetal haemoglobin of the newborn. *J Obstet Gynaecol Br Commonw* 63:875, 1956.

64. Huehns ER, Hecht F, Keil JV, et al: Developmental hemoglobin anomalies in a chromosomal triplication. *Proc Natl Acad Sci U S A* 51:89, 1964.

65. Lee CSN, Boyer SH, Bowen P, et al: The D1 trisomy syndrome: Three subjects with unequally advancing development. *Johns Hopkins Med J* 118:374, 1966.

66. Giulian GG, Gilbert EF, Moss RL: Elevated fetal hemoglobin levels in sudden infant death syndrome. *N Engl J Med* 316:1122, 1987.

67. Wilson MG, Schroeder WA, Graves DA: Postnatal change of hemoglobins F and A2 in infants with Down's syndrome (G trisomy). *Pediatrics* 42:349, 1968.

68. Brown MS: Fetal and neonatal erythropoieses, in *Developmental and Neonatal Hematology*, edited by JA Stockman, III, C Pochedly, p 39. Raven Press, New York, 1988.

69. Forestier F, Daffos F, Galacteros F, et al: Haematological values of 163 normal fetuses between 18 and 30 weeks of gestation. *Pediatr Res* 20:342, 1986.

70. Millar DS, Davis LR, Rodich CH, et al: Normal blood cell values in the early midtrimester fetus. *Prenat Diagn* 5:367, 1985.

71. Linch DC, Knott LJ, Rodech CH, et al: Studies of circulating hemopoietic progenitor cells in human fetal blood. *Blood* 59:976, 1982.

72. Christensen RD: Hematopoiesis in the fetus and neonate. *Pediatr Res* 26:531, 1989.

73. Marks J, Gairdner D, Roscoe JD: Blood formation in infancy. III. Cord blood. *Arch Dis Child* 30:117, 1955.

74. Linderkamp O, Versmold HT, Messow-Zahn K, et al: The effect of intrapartum and intra-uterine asphyxia on placental transfusion in premature and full-term infants. *Eur J Pediatr* 127:91, 1978.

75. Mercer JS: Current best evidence: A review of the literature on umbilical cord clamping. *J Midwifery Womens Health* 46:402, 2001.

76. Yao AC, Hirvensalo M, Lind J: Placental transfusion rate and uterine contraction. *Lancet* i:380, 1968.

77. Usher R, Shepard M, Lind J, et al: The blood volume of the newborn and placental transfusion. *Acta Paediatr* 52:497, 1963.

78. Bratteby LE: Studies on erythro-kinetics in infancy. XI. The change in circulating red cell volume during the first five months of life. *Acta Paediatr Scand* 57:215, 1968.

79. McCue CM, Garner FB, Hurt WG, et al: Placental transfusion. *J Pediatr* 72:15, 1968.

80. Matoth Y, Zaizor R, Varsano I: Postnatal changes in some red cell parameters. *Acta Paediatr Scand* 60:317, 1971.

81. Linderkamp O, Versmold HT, Strohhacker I, et al: Capillary-venous hematocrit differences in newborn infants. *Eur J Pediatr* 127:9, 1977.

82. Saarinen UM, Simmes MA: Developmental changes in red blood cell counts and indices of infants after exclusion of iron deficiency by laboratory criteria and continuous iron supplementation. *J Pediatr* 92:412, 1978.

83. Zipursky A, Brown E, Palko J, et al: The erythrocyte differential count in newborn infants. *Am J Pediatr Hematol Oncol* 5:45, 1983.

84. Alter BP, Goldberg JD, Berkowitz RL: Red cell size heterogeneity during ontogeny. *Am J Pediatr Hematol Oncol* 10:279, 1988.

85. Shannon KM, Naylor GS, Torkildson JC, et al: Circulating erythroid progenitors in the anemia of prematurity. *N Engl J Med* 317:728, 1987.

86. Christensen RD: Circulating pluripotent hematopoietic progenitor cells in neonates. *J Pediatr* 11:622, 1987.

87. Clapp DW, Baley JE, Gerson SL: Gestational age dependent changes in circulating hematopoietic stem cells in newborn infants. *J Lab Clin Med* 113:422, 1989.

88. Holbrook SR, Christensen RD, Rothstein G: Erythroid colonies derived from fetal blood display different growth patterns from those derived from adult marrow. *Pediatr Res* 24:605, 1988.

89. Burman D, Morris AF: Cord hemoglobin in low birth weight infants. *Arch Dis Child* 49:382, 1974.

90. Meberg A: Haemoglobin concentrations and erythropoietin levels in appropriate and small for gestational age infants. *Scand J Haematol* 24:162, 1980.

91. Zaizov R, Matoth Y: Red cell values on the first postnatal day during the last 16 weeks of gestation. *Am J Hematol* 1:275, 1976.

92. Lockridge S, Pass R, Cassidy G: Reticulocyte counts in intrauterine growth retardation. *Pediatrics* 47:919, 1971.

93. Humbert JR, Abelson H, Hathaway WE, et al: Polycythemia in small for gestational age infants. *J Pediatr* 75:1812, 1969.

94. Halvorsen S, Finne PH: Erythropoietin production in the human fetus and newborn. *Ann N Y Acad Sci* 149:576, 1968.

95. Seip M: The reticulocyte level and the erythrocyte production judged from reticulocyte studies in newborn infants during the first week of life. *Acta Paediatr Scand* 44:355, 1955.

96. Mann DL, Sites ML, Donati RM, et al: Erythropoietic stimulating activity during the first ninety days of life. *Proc Soc Exp Biol Med* 118:212, 1965.

97. Lundstrom U, Simmes MA: Red blood cell values in low-birth-weight infants: Ages at which values become equivalent to those of term infants. *J Pediatr* 96:1040, 1980.

98. Stockman JA III, Garcia JF, Oski FA: The anemia of prematurity: Factors governing the erythropoietin response. *N Engl J Med* 296:647, 1977.

99. MackIntosh TF, Walker CHM: Blood viscosity in the newborn. *Arch Dis Child* 48:547, 1973.

90. Bergqvist G: Viscosity of the blood in the newborn infant. *Acta Paediatr Scand* 63:858, 1974.

101. Wirth FH, Goldberg WR, Lubchenco L: Neonatal hyperviscosity. I. Incidence. *Pediatrics* 63:833, 1979.

102. Hakanson DO, Oh W: Hyperviscosity in the small-for-gestational age infant. *Biol Neonate* 37:190, 1980.

103. Ramamurthy RS, Berlanga M: Postnatal alteration in hematocrit and viscosity in normal and polycythemic infants. *J Pediatr* 110:929, 1987.

104. Bada HS, Korones SB, Pourcyrous M, et al: Asymptomatic syndrome of polycythemic hyperviscosity: Effect of partial plasma exchange transfusion. *J Pediatr* 120:579, 1992.

105. Sarkar S, Rosenkrantz TS: Neonatal polycythemia and hyperviscosity. *Semin Fetal Neonatal Med* 13:248, 2008.

106. Bierhuizen MF, Mattei MG, Fukuda M: Expression of the developmental I antigen by a cloned human cDNA encoding a member of a beta-1,6-N-acetylglucosaminyltransferase gene family. *Genes Dev* 7:468, 1993.

107. Race RR, Sanger R: *Blood Groups in Man*, 6th ed. Blackwell Scientific, London, 1975.

108. Pearson HA: Life-span of the fetal red blood cell. *J Pediatr* 70:166, 1967.

109. Weipple G, Pantlitschko M, Bauer P, et al: Normal values and distribution of serum iron in cord blood. *Clin Chim Acta* 44:147, 1973.

110. Saarinen UM, Siimes MA: Developmental changes in serum iron, total iron-binding capacity, and transferrin saturation in infancy. *J Pediatr* 91:875, 1977.

111. Saarinen UM, Siimes MA: Serum ferritin in assessment of iron nutrition in healthy infants. *Acta Paediatr Scand* 67:745, 1978.

112. Seip M, Halvorsen S: Erythrocyte production and iron stores in premature infants during the first months of life. The anemia of prematurity—Etiology, pathogenesis, iron requirement. *Acta Paediatr Scand* 45:600, 1956.

113. Rao R, Georgieff MK: Perinatal aspects of iron metabolism. *Acta Paediatr Suppl* 91:124, 2002.

114. Bauer C, Ludwig I, Ludwig M: Different effects of 2,3-diphosphoglycerate and adenosine triphosphate on oxygen affinity of adult and fetal hemoglobin. *Life Sci* 7:1339, 1968.

115. Oski FA: Red cell metabolism in the newborn infant. V. Glycolytic intermediates and glycolytic enzymes. *Pediatrics* 44:84, 1969.

116. Oski FA, Delivoria-Papadopoulos M: The red cell, 2,3-diphosphoglycerate, and tissue oxygen release. *J Pediatr* 77:941, 1970.

117. Zipursky A: The erythrocytes of the newborn infant. *Semin Hematol* 2:167, 1965.

118. Oski FA, Komazawa M: Metabolism of the erythrocytes of the newborn infant. *Semin Hematol* 12:209, 1975.

119. Oski FA, Smith CA: Red cell metabolism in the premature infant. III. Apparent inappropriate glucose consumption for cell age. *Pediatrics* 41:473, 1968.

120. Konrad PN, Valentine WN, Paglia DE: Enzymatic activities and glutathione content of erythrocytes in the newborn: Comparison with red cells of older normal subjects and those with comparable reticulocytosis. *Acta Haematol* 48:193, 1972.

121. Gross RT, Schroeder EAR, Brounstein SA: Energy metabolism in the erythrocytes of premature infants compared to full term newborn infants and adults. *Blood* 21:755, 1963.

122. Oski FA: Red cell metabolism in the premature infant. II. The pentose phosphate pathway. *Pediatrics* 39:689, 1967.

123. Bracci R, Perrone S, Buonocore G: Oxidant injury in neonatal erythrocytes during the neonatal period. *Acta Paediatr Suppl* 91:130, 2002.

124. Ross JD: Deficient activity of DPNH-dependent methemoglobin diaphorase in cord blood erythrocytes. *Blood* 21:51, 1963.

125. Gross RT, Bracci R, Rudolph N, et al: Hydrogen peroxide toxicity and detoxification in erythrocytes of newborn infants. *Blood* 29:481, 1967.

126. Whaun JM, Oski FA: Red cell stromal adenosine triphosphatase (ATPase) of newborn infants. *Pediatr Res* 3:105, 1969.

127. Blum SF, Oski FA: Red cell metabolism in the newborn infant. IV. Transmembrane potassium flux. *Pediatrics* 43:396, 1969.

128. Crowley J, Ways P, Jones JW: Human fetal erythrocyte and plasma lipids. *J Clin Invest* 44:989, 1965.

129. Neerhout RC: Erythrocyte lipids in the neonate. *Pediatr Res* 2:172, 1968.

130. Shapiro DL, Pasqualini P: Erythrocyte membrane proteins of premature and full-term infants. *Pediatr Res* 12:176, 1978.

131. Kosztolanyi G, Jobst K: Electrokinetic analysis of the fetal erythrocyte membrane after trypsin digestion. *Pediatr Res* 14:138, 1980.

132. Altman PL, Dittmer DS: *Blood and Other Body Fluids*. Federation of American Societies for Experimental Biology, Washington, DC, 1961.

133. Coulombel L, Dehan M, Tchernia G, et al: The number of polymorphonuclear leukocytes in relation to gestational age in the newborn. *Acta Paediatr Scand* 68:709, 1979.

134. Laver J, Duncan E, Abboud M, et al: High levels of granulocyte and granulocyte-macrophage colony-stimulating factors in cord blood of normal full-term neonates. *J Pediatr* 116:627, 1990.

135. Ijima H, Suda T, Miura Y: Predominance of macrophage-colony formation in human cord blood. *Exp Hematol* 10:234, 1982.

136. Prindull G, Ben-Ishay Z, Gabriel M, et al: A comparison of spontaneous and CSF added CFU-GM colony formation in healthy, sick and hypotrophic pre-term infants. *Blut* 45:167, 1982.

137. Satwani P, Morris R, van de Ven C, et al: Dysregulation of expression of immunoregulatory and cytokine genes and its association with the immaturity in neonatal phagocytic and cellular immunity. *Biol Neonate* 88:214, 2005.

138. English BK, Hammond WP, Lewis DB, et al: Decreased granulocyte-macrophage colony-stimulating factor production by human neonatal blood mononuclear cells and T cells. *Pediatr Res* 31:211, 1992.

139. Cairo MS, Suen Y, Knoppel E, et al: Decreased G-CSF and IL-3 production and gene expression from mononuclear cells of newborn infants. *Pediatr Res* 31:574, 1992.

140. Carr R: Neutrophil production and function in newborn infants. *Br J Haematol* 110:18, 2000.

141. Rosenthal J, Cairo MS: The role of cytokines in modulating neonatal myelopoiesis and host defense. *Cytokines Mol Ther* 1:165, 1995.

142. Banerjea MC, Speer CP: The current role of colony-stimulating factors in prevention and treatment of neonatal sepsis. *Semin Neonatol* 7:335, 2002.

143. Kucukoduk S, Sezer T, Yildiran A, et al: Randomized, double-blinded, placebo-controlled trial of early administration of recombinant human granulocyte colony-stimulating factor to non-neutropenic preterm newborns between 33 and 36 weeks with presumed sepsis. *Scand J Infect Dis* 34:893, 2002.

144. Xanthou M: Leucocyte blood picture in healthy full-term and premature babies during neonatal period. *Arch Dis Child* 45:242, 1970.

145. Gibson EL, Vaucher Y, Corrigan JJ Jr: Eosinophilia in premature infants. Relationship to weight gain. *J Pediatr* 95:99, 1979.

146. Koenig JM and Yoder MC: Neonatal neutrophils: The good, the bad and the ugly. *Clin Perinatol* 31:39, 2004.

147. Forman ML, Stiehm ER: Impaired opsonic activity but normal phagocytosis in low-birth-weight infants. *N Engl J Med* 281:926, 1969.

148. Dossett JH, Williams RC Jr, Quie PG: Studies on interaction of bacteria, serum factors and polymorphonuclear leukocytes in mothers and newborns. *Pediatrics* 44:49, 1969.

149. Miller ME: Phagocytosis in the newborn infant: Humoral and cellular factors. *J Pediatr* 74:255, 1969.

150. Hill HR, Shigeoka AO, Pincus S, Christensen RD: Intravenous IgG in combination with other modalities in the treatment of neonatal infection. *Pediatr Infect Dis* 5:180, 1986.

151. Cocchi P, Marianelli L: Phagocytosis and intracellular killing of *Pseudomonas aeruginosa* in premature infants. *Helv Paediatr Acta* 22:110, 1967.

152. Drossou V, Kanakoudi F, Diamanti E, et al: Concentrations of main serum opsonins in early infancy. *Arch Dis Child* 72:F172, 1995.

153. Yang KD, Bathras JM, Shigeoka AO, et al: Mechanisms of bacterial opsonization by immune globulin: Intravenous correlation of complement consumption with opsonic activity and protective efficacy. *J Infect Dis* 159:701, 1989.

154. Shaio MF, Yang KD, Bohnsack JF, Hill HR: Effect of immune globulin intravenous on opsonization of bacteria by classic and alternative complement pathways in premature serum. *Pediatr Res* 25:634, 1989.

155. Hill H: Host defenses in the neonate: Prospects for enhancement. *Semin Perinatol* 9:2, 1985.

156. Alper CA: C3 synthesis in the human fetus and lack of transplacental passage. *Science* 162:672, 1968.

157. Johnston RB Jr, Altenburger KM, Atkinson AW Jr, et al: Complement in the newborn infant. *Pediatr* 64:781, 1979.

158. Strunk RC, Fenton LJ, Gaines JA: Alternative pathway of complement activation in full term and premature infants. *Pediatr Res* 13:641, 1979.

159. Davis CA, Vallota EH, Forristal J: Serum complement levels in infancy: Age related changes. *Pediatr Res* 13:1043, 1979.

160. Mills EL, Bjorksten B, Quie PG: Deficient alternative complement pathway activity in newborn sera. *Pediatr Res* 13:1341, 1979.

161. Proctor RA, Prendergast E, Mosher DF: Fibronectin mediates attachment of *Staphylococcus aureus* to human neutrophils. *Blood* 59:681, 1982.

162. Hill HR, Shigeoka AO, Augustine NH, et al: Fibronectin enhances the opsonic and protective activity of monoclonal and polyclonal antibody against group B streptococci. *J Exp Med* 159:1618, 1984.

163. Harris MC, Levitt J, Douglas SD, et al: Effect of fibronectin on adherence of neutrophils from newborn infants. *J Clin Microbiol* 21:243, 1985.

164. Hill HR, Shigeoka AO, Gonzales LA, Christensen RD: Intravenous immune globulin use in newborns. *J Allergy Clin Immunol* 84:617, 1989.

165. Christensen RD, Brown MS, Hall DC, et al: Effect on neutrophil kinetics and serum opsonic capacity of intravenous administration of immune globulin to neonates with clinical signs of early-onset sepsis. *J Pediatr* 118:606, 1991.

166. Fujiwara T, Taniuchi S, Hattori K, et al: Effect of immunoglobulin therapy on phagocytosis by polymorphonuclear leucocytes in whole blood of neonates. *Clin Exp Immunol* 107:435, 1997.

167. Weisman LE, Stoll BJ, Kueser TJ, et al: Intravenous immune globulin therapy for early-onset sepsis in premature neonates. *J Pediatr* 121:434, 1992.

167. 8chreiber JR, Berger M: Intravenous immune globulin therapy for sepsis in premature neonates. *J Pediatr* 121:401, 1992.

169. Baker CJ, Melish ME, Hall RT, et al: Intravenous immune globulin for the prevention of nosocomial infection in low-birth-weight infants. *N Engl J Med* 327:213, 1992.

170. Suri M, Harrison L, Van de Ven C, et al: Immunotherapy in the prophylaxis of neonatal sepsis. *Curr Opin Pediatr* 15:155, 2003.

171. Fischer GW, Weisman LE, Hemming VG: Directed immune globulin for the prevention or treatment of neonatal group B streptococcal infections: A review. *Clin Immunol Immunopathol* 62:S92, 1992.

172. Miller ME: Chemotactic function in the neonate. Humoral and cellular aspects. *Pediatr Res* 5:487, 1971.

173. Klei RB, Fischer TJ, Gard SE, et al: Decreased mononuclear and polymorphonuclear chemotaxis in human newborns, infants, and young children. *Pediatrics* 60:467, 1977.

174. Tono-oka T, Nakayama M, Uehara H, et al: Characteristics of impaired chemotactic function in cord blood leukocytes. *Pediatr Res* 13:148, 1979.

175. Hill HR, Augustine NH, Newton JA, et al: Correction of a developmental defect in neutrophil activation and movement. *Am J Pathol* 128:307, 1987.

176. Bruce MC, Baley JE, Medvik KA, et al: Impaired surface membrane expression of C3bi but not C3b receptors on neonatal neutrophils. *Pediatr Res* 21:306, 1987.

177. Anderson DC, Freeman KLB, Heerdt B, et al: Abnormal stimulated adherence of neonatal granulocytes: Impaired induction of surface MAC-1 by chemotactic factors or secretagogues. *Blood* 70:740, 1987.

178. Carr R, Davies JM: Abnormal PcRIII expression by neutrophils from very preterm neonates. *Blood* 76:607, 1990.

189. Anderson DC, Rothlein R, Marlin SD, et al: Impaired transendothelial migration by neonatal neutrophils: Abnormalities of Mac-1(CD11b/CD18)-dependent adherence reactions. *Blood* 76:2613, 1990.

180. Masuda K, Kinoshita Y, Kobayashi Y: Heterogeneity of Fc expression in chemotaxis and adherence of neonatal neutrophils. *Pediatr Res* 25:6, 1989.

181. Tosi MF, Berger M: Functional differences between the 40 kDa and 50 kDa IgG Fc receptors on human neutrophils revealed by elastase treatment and antireceptor antibodies. *J Immunol* 141:2097, 1988.

182. Koenig JM, Yoder MC: Neonatal neutrophils: The good, the bad and the ugly. *Clin Perinatol* 31:39-51, 2004.

183. Kim SK, Keeney SE, Alpard SK: Comparison of L-selectin and CD11b on neutrophils of adults and neonates during the first month of life. *Pediatr Res* 53:132-136, 2003.

184. Mills EL, Thompson T, Bjorksten B, et al: The chemiluminescence response and bactericidal activity of polymorphonuclear neutrophils from newborns and their mothers. *Pediatrics* 63:429, 1979.

185. Park BH, Holmes B, Good RA: Metabolic activities in leukocytes of newborn infants. *J Pediatr* 76:237, 1970.

186. Xanthou M, Valassi-Adam E, Kintronidou E, et al: Phagocytosis and killing ability of Candida albicans by blood leucocytes of healthy term and preterm babies. *Arch Dis Child* 50:72, 1975.

187. Shigeoka AO, Charette RP, Wyman ML, et al: Defective oxidative metabolic responses of neutrophils from stressed neonates. *J Pediatr* 98:392, 1981.

188. Strauss RG, Snyder EL: Neutrophils from human infants exhibit decreased viability. *Pediatr Res* 15:794, 1981.

189. Strauss RG, Snyder EL, Wallace PO, et al: Oxygen-detoxifying enzymes in neutrophils of infants and their mothers. *J Lab Clin Med* 95:897, 1980.

190. Yamazaki M, Matsuoka T, Yasui K, et al: Increased production of superoxide anion by neonatal polymorphonuclear leukocytes stimulated with a chemotactic peptide. *Am J Hematol* 27:169, 1988.

191. Levy O: Impaired innate immunity at birth: Deficiency of bacteriocidal/permeability-increasing protein (BPI) in the neutrophils of newborns. *Pediatr Res* 51:667, 2002.

192. Neupponen I, Turunen R, Nevalainen T, et al: Extracellular release of bactericidal/permeability increasing protein in newborn infants. *Pediatr Res* 51:670, 2002.

193. Kretschmer RR, Papierniak CK, Stewardson-Krieger P, et al: Quantitative nitroblue tetrazolium reduction by normal newborn monocytes. *J Pediatr* 91:306, 1977.

194. Milgrom H, Shore SL: Assessment of monocyte function in the normal newborn infant by antibody-dependent cellular cytotoxicity. *J Pediatr* 91:612, 1977.

195. Orlowski JP, Sieger L, Anthony BF: Bactericidal capacity of monocytes of newborn infants. *J Pediatr* 89:797, 1976.

196. Schuit KE, Powell DA: Phagocytic dysfunction in monocytes of normal newborn infants. *Pediatrics* 65:501, 1980.

197. Das M, Henderson T, Feig SA: Neonatal mononuclear cell metabolism: Further evidence for diminished monocyte function in the neonate. *Pediatr Res* 13:632, 1979.

198. Mills EL: Mononuclear phagocytes in the newborn: Their relation to the state of relative immunodeficiency. *Am J Pediatr Hematol Oncol* 5:189, 1983.

199. Bryson YJ, Winter HS, Gard SE, et al: Deficiency of immune interferon production by leukocytes of normal newborns. *Cell Immunol* 55:191, 1987.

200. Frenkel L, Bryson YJ: Ontogeny of phytohemagglutinin-induced gamma interferon by leukocytes of healthy infants and children: Evidence for decreased production in infants younger than 2 months of age. *J Pediatr* 111:97, 1987.

201. Perussia B, Dayton ET, Lazarus R, et al: Immune interferon induces the receptor for monomeric IgG on human monocytic and myeloid cells. *J Exp Med* 158:1092, 1983.

202. Cairo MS: Review of G-CSF and GM-CSF effects on neonatal neutrophil kinetics. *Am J Pediatr Hematol Oncol* 11:238, 1989.

203. Cairo MS, VandeVen C, Toy C, et al: GM-CSF primes and modulates neonatal PMN motility: Up-regulation of C3bi (Mol) expression with alteration in PMN adherence and aggregation. *Am J Pediatr Hematol Oncol* 13:249, 1991.

204. Sautois B, Fillet G, Beguin Y: Comparative cytokine production by in vitro stimulated mononucleated cells from cord blood and adult blood. *Exp Hematol* 25:103, 1997.

205. Fogel BJ, Arais D, Kung F: Platelet counts in healthy premature infants. *J Pediatr* 73:108, 1968.

206. Sell EJ, Corrigan JJ: Platelet counts, fibrinogen concentrations and factor V and factor VIII levels in healthy infants according to gestational age. *J Pediatr* 82:1028, 1973.

207. Mehta P, Vasa R, Neumann L, Karpatkin M: Thrombocytopenia in the high-risk infant. *J Pediatr* 97:791, 1980.

208. Meberg A, Halvorsen S, Orstavik I: Transitory thrombocytopenia in small-for-dates infants, possibly related to maternal smoking. *Lancet* 2:303, 1977.

209. Thuring W, Tonz O: Neonatale thrombozytenwerte be: Kindern mit Down-Syndrom und anderen autosomalen trisomien. *Helv Paediatr Acta* 34:545, 1979.

210. Cairo, MS: The regulation of hematopoietic growth factor production from cord mononuclear cells and its effect on newborn rat hematopoiesis. *J Hematother* 2:217, 1993.

211. Suen Y, Chang M, Lee SM, et al: Regulation of interleukin-11 protein and mRNA expression in neonatal and adult fibroblasts and endothelial cells. *Blood* 84:4125, 1994.

212. Murray NA, Watts TL, Roberts IAG: Thrombopoietin in the fetus and neonate. *Early Hum Dev* 59:1, 2000.

213. Feusner JH: Normal and abnormal bleeding times in neonates and young children utilizing a fully standardized template technic. *Am J Clin Pathol* 74:73, 1980.

214. Rennie JM, Gibson T, Cooke RWI: Micromethod for bleeding time in the newborn. *Arch Dis Child* 60:51, 1985.

215. Andrew M, Paes B, Bowker J, Vegh P: Evaluation of an automated bleeding time device in the newborn. *Am J Hematol* 35:275, 1990.

216. Weinstein MJ, Blanchard R, Moake JL, et al: Fetal and neonatal von Willebrand factor (vWF) is unusually large and similar to the vWF in patients with thrombotic thrombocytopenic purpura. *Br J Haematol* 72:68, 1989.

217. Andrew M, Vegh P, Johnston M, et al: Maturation of the hemostatic system during childhood. *Blood* 80:1988, 1992.

218. Andrew M, Castle V, Saigal S, et al: Clinical impact of neonatal thrombocytopenia. *J Pediatr* 110:457, 1987.

219. Israels SJ, Rand ML, Michelson AD: Neonatal platelet function [review]. *Semin Thromb Hemost* 29:363, 2003.

220. Corazza MS, Davis RF, Merritt TA, et al: Prolonged bleeding time in preterm infants receiving indomethacin for patent ductus arteriosus. *J Pediatr* 105:292, 1984.

221. Israels SJ, Cheang T, McMillan-Ward EM, et al: Evaluation of primary hemostasis in neonates with a new in vitro platelet function analyzer. *J Pediatr* 138:116, 2001.

222. Knofler R, Weissbach G, Kuhlisch E: Platelet function tests in childhood. Measuring aggregation and release reaction in whole blood. *Semin Thromb Hemost* 24:513, 1998.

223. Saxonhouse MA, Sola MC: Platelet function in term and preterm neonates. *Clin Perinatol* 31:15, 2004.

224. Stuart MJ: Platelet function in the neonate. *Am J Pediatr Hematol Oncol* 1:227, 1979.

225. Israels SJ, Daniels M, McMillan EM: Deficient collagen-induced activation in the newborn platelet. *Pediatr Res* 27:337, 1990.

226. Rajasekhar D, Kestin AS, Bednarek FJ, et al: Neonatal platelets are less reactive than adult platelets to physiological agonists in whole blood. *Thromb Haemost* 72:957, 1994.

227. Ts'ao C, Green D, Schultz K: Function and ultrastructure of platelets of neonates: enhanced ristocetin aggregation of neonatal platelets. *Br J Haematol* 32:225, 1976.

228. Blieyer WA, Breckenridge RT: Studies on the detection of adverse drug reactions in the newborn. II. The effects of prenatal aspirin on newborn hemostasis. *JAMA* 213:2049, 1970.

229. Corby DG, Schulman I: The effects of antenatal drug administration on aggregation of platelets of newborn infants. *J Pediatr* 79:307, 1971.

230. Hauth JC, Goldenberg RL, Parker CR Jr, et al: Low-dose aspirin: Lack of association with an increase in abruptio placentae or perinatal mortality. *Obstet Gynecol* 85:1055, 1995.

231. Sibai BM, Caritis SN, Thom E, et al: Low-dose aspirin in nulliparous women: Safety of continuous epidural block and correlation between bleeding time and maternal-neonatal bleeding complications. National Institute of Child Health and Human Developmental Maternal–Fetal Medicine Network. *Am J Obstet Gynecol* 172:1553, 1995.

232. Newman PJ, Derbes RS, Aster RH: The human platelet alloantigens, PLA1 and PLA2, are associated with a leucine 33/proline 33 amino acid polymorphism in membrane glycoprotein IIIa, and are distinguishable by DNA typing. *J Clin Invest* 83:1778, 1989.

233. Gruel Y, Boizard B, Daffos F, et al: Determination of platelet antigens and glycoproteins in the human fetus. *Blood* 68:488, 1986.

234. McFarland JG, Aster RH, Bussel JB, et al: Prenatal diagnosis of neonatal alloimmune thrombocytopenia using allele-specific oligonucleotide probes. *Blood* 78:2276, 1991.

235. Shulman NR, Jordan JV Jr: Platelet immunology, in *Hemostasis and Thrombosis: Basic Principles and Clinical Practice*, 2nd ed, edited by RW Colman, J Hirsh, VJ Marder, EW Salzman, pp 476–483. JB Lippincott, Philadelphia, 1987.

236. Pabst HF: Ontogeny of the immune response as a basis of childhood diseases. *J Pediatr* 97:519, 1980.

237. O'Gorman MRG, Millard DD, Lowder JN, et al: Lymphocyte subpopulations in 1–3 day old infants. *Cytometry* 34:235 1998.

238. Shearer WT, Rosenblatt HM, Gelman RS, et al: Lymphocyte subsets in healthy children from birth through 18 years of age: The Pediatric AIDS Clinical Trials Group P1009 Study. *J Allergy Clin Immunol* 112:973, 2003.

239. De Waele M, Foulon W, Renmans W, et al: Hematologic values and lymphocyte subsets in fetal blood. *Am J Clin Pathol* 89:742, 1988.

240. Hicks MJ, Jones JF, Minnich LL, et al: Age-related changes in T- and B-lymphocyte subpopulations in the peripheral blood. *Arch Pathol Lab Med* 107:518, 1983.

241. Kotylo PA, Baenzinger JC, Yoder MC, et al: Rapid analysis of lymphocyte subsets in cord blood. *Am J Clin Pathol* 93:263, 1990.

242. Kohl S: Human neonatal natural killer cell cytotoxicity function. *Pediatr Infect Dis J* 18:635, 1999.

243. Adkins B. Neonatal T cell function. *J Pediatr Gastroenterol Nutr* 40:S5, 2005.

244. Comans-Bitter WM, de Groot R, van den Beemd R, et al: Immunophenotyping of blood lymphocytes in childhood. Reference values for lymphocyte subpopulations. *J Pediatr* 130:388, 1997.

245. Slukvin II, Chernishov VP: Two-color flow cytometric analysis of natural killer and cytotoxic T-lymphocyte subsets in peripheral blood of normal human neonates. *Biol Neonate* 61:156, 1992.

246. Neubert R, Delgado I, Abraham K, et al: Evaluation of the age-dependent development of lymphocyte surface receptors in children. *Life Sci* 62:1099, 1998.

247. Miller ME: Immune-inflammatory response in the human neonate. *Am J Pediatr Hematol Oncol* 3:199, 1981.

248. Stiehm ER, Winter HS, Bryson YF: Cellular (T cell) immunity in the human new-born. *Pediatrics* 64:814, 1979.

249. Carr MC, Stites DP, Fudenberg HH: Cellular immune aspects of the human fetal-maternal relationship. I. In vitro response of cord blood lymphocytes to phytohemagglutinin. *Cell Immunol* 5:21, 1972.

250. Papiernick M: Comparison of human foetal with child blood lymphocytic kinetics. *Biol Neonate* 19:163, 1971.

251. Uhr JW, Dancis J, Newmann CG: Delayed-type hypersensitivity in premature neonatal humans. *Nature* 187:1130, 1960.

252. Blaese RM, Poplack DG, Muchmore AV: The mononuclear phagocyte system: Role in expression of immunocompetence in neonatal and adult life. *Pediatrics* 64(Suppl):829, 1979.

253. Von Freeden U, Zessack N, Van Valen F, Burdach S: Defective interferon gamma production in neonatal T cells is independent of interleukin-2 receptor binding. *Pediatr Res* 30:270, 1991.

254. Sterm CMM: Changes in lymphocytes subpopulations in the blood of healthy and sick newborn infants. *Pediatr Res* 13:792, 1979.

255. Raveche ES: Possible immunoregulatory role for CD5+ B cells. *Clin Immunol Immunopathol* 56:135, 1990.

256. Wilson CB, Kollmann TR: Induction of antigen specific immunity in human neonates and infants [review]. *Nestle Nutr Workshop Ser Pediatr Program* 61:183 2008.

257. Gustafsson BE, Laurell CB: Gamma globulin production in germ free rats after bacterial contamination. *J Exp Med* 110:675, 1959.

258. Gitlin D: The differentiation and maturation of specific immune mechanisms. *Acta Paediatr Scand* 172(Suppl):60, 1967.

259. Stiehm ER: Fetal defense mechanisms. *Am J Dis Child* 129:438, 1975.

260. Goldman AS, Garza C, Nichols BL, Goldblum RM: Immunological factors in human milk during the first year of lactation. *J Pediatr* 100:563, 1982.

261. Goldman AS, Ham Pong AJ, Goldblum RM: Host defenses: Development and maternal contributions. *Adv Pediatr* 32:71, 1985.

262. Newburg DS, Walker WA: Protection of the neonate by the innate immune system of developing gut and of human milk. *Pediatr Res* 61:2 2007.

263. Rothberg RM: Immunoglobulin and specific antibody synthesis during the first weeks of life of premature infants. *J Pediatr* 75:391, 1969.

264. Harworth JC, Norris M, Dilling L: A study of the immunoglobulins in premature infants. *Arch Dis Child* 40:243, 1965.

265. Thom H, McKay E, Gray DWG: Protein concentrations in the umbilical cord plasma of premature and mature infants. *Clin Sci* 33:433, 1967.

266. Yeung CY, Hoffs JR: Serum gamma-G-globulin levels in normal, premature, postmature, and "small-for-dates" newborn babies. *Lancet* 1:1167, 1968.

267. Sever JH: Immunological responses to perinatal responses to perinatal infections. *J Pediatr* 75:1111, 1969.

268. Thomaidis T, Agathopoulos A, Matsaniotis N: Natural isohemagglutinin production by the fetus. *J Pediatr* 74:39, 1969.

269. Morito T, Bankhurst AD, Williams RC Jr: Studies of human cord blood and adult lymphocyte interactions with in vitro immunoglobulin production. *J Clin Invest* 64:990, 1979.

270. Miyagawa Y, Sugita K, Komiyama A, et al: Delayed in vitro immunoglobulin production by cord lymphocytes. *Pediatrics* 65:497, 1980.

271. Ferguson AC, Cheung SC: Modulation of immunoglobulin M and G synthesis by monocytes and T lymphocytes in the newborn infant. *J Pediatr* 98:385, 1981.

272. Blaese RM, Poplack DG, Muchmore AV: The mononuclear phagocyte system: Role in expression of immunocompetence in neonatal and adult life. *Pediatrics* 64:829, 1977.

273. Holroyde CP, Oski FA, Gardner FH: The "pocked" erythrocyte. *N Engl J Med* 281:516, 1969.

274. Freedman RM, Johnston D, Mahoney MJ, et al: Development of splenic reticuloendothelial function in neonates. *J Pediatr* 96:466, 1980.

275. Gross SJ, Stuart MJ: Hemostasis in the premature infant. *Clin Perinatol* 4:259, 1977.

276. Barnard DR, Hathaway WE: Neonatal thrombosis. *Am J Pediatr Hematol Oncol* 1:235, 1979.

277. Bleyer WA, Hakami N, Shepard TH: The development of hemostasis in the human fetus and newborn infant. *J Pediatr* 79:838, 1971.

278. Andrew M, Paes B, Milner B, et al: Development of the human coagulation system in the full-term infant. *Blood* 70:165, 1987.

279. Andrew M, Paes B, Milner R, et al: Development of the human coagulation system in the healthy premature infant. *Blood* 72:1651, 1988.

280. Corrigan JJ Jr: Neonatal thrombosis and the thrombolytic system: Pathophysiology and therapy. *Am J Pediatr Hematol Oncol* 10:83, 1988.

281. Monagle P, Massicotte P: Developmental haemostasis: Secondary haemostasis. *Semin Fetal Neonatal Med* 16:294, 2011.

282. Andrew M, Paes B, Johnston M: Development of the hemostatic system in the neonate and young infant. *Am J Pediatr Hematol Oncol* 12:95, 1990.

283. Andrew M: The relevance of developmental hemostasis to hemorrhagic disorders of newborns. *Semin Perinatol* 21:70, 1997.

284. Karpatkin M, Lee M, Cohen L, et al: Synthesis of coagulation proteins in the fetus and neonate. *J Pediatr Hematol Oncol* 22:276, 2000.

285. Furie B, Furie BC: Molecular basis of gamma-carboxylation. Role of the propeptide in the vitamin K-dependent proteins. *Ann N Y Acad Sci* 614:1, 1991.

286. Aballi AJ, deLamerens S: Coagulation changes in the neonatal period and in early infancy. *Pediatr Clin North Am* 9:785, 1962.

287. Muntean W, Petek W, Rosanelli K, et al: Immunologic studies of prothrombin in newborns. *Pediatr Res* 13:1262, 1979.

288. Lane PA, Hathaway WE: Vitamin K in infancy. *J Pediatr* 106:351, 1985.

289. Stevenson RE, Burton OM, Ferlauto GJ, et al: Hazards of oral anticoagulants during pregnancy. *JAMA* 243:1549, 1980.

290. Shearer MJ: Annotation: Vitamin K and vitamin K-dependent proteins. *Br J Haematol* 75:156, 1990.

291. von Kries R, Hanawa Y: Neonatal vitamin K prophylaxis. Report of Scientific and Standardization Subcommittee on Perinatal Haemostasis. *Thromb Haemost* 69:293, 1993.

292. Sutor AH, Gobel U, Kries RV, et al: Vitamin K prophylaxis in the newborn. *Blut* 60:275, 1990.

293. Hathaway WE, Isarangkura PB, Mahasandana C, et al: Comparison of oral and parenteral vitamin K prophylaxis for prevention of late hemorrhagic disease of the newborn. *J Pediatr* 119:461, 1991.

294. Blackmon L, Batton DG, Bell EF, et al: Controversies concerning vitamin K and the newborn. American Academy of Pediatrics Policy Statement. *Pediatrics* 112:191, 2003.

295. Costakos DT, Porte M: Did "controversies concerning vitamin K and the newborn" cover all the controversies? *Pediatrics* 113:1466, 2004.

296. Clarke P, Mitchell SJ, Wynn R, et al: Vitamin K prophylaxis for preterm infants: A randomized, controlled trial of three regimens. *Pediatrics* 118:1657, 2006.

297. Amadee-Manesme O, Labert WE, Alagille D, De Leenheer AP: Pharmacokinetics and safety of a new solution of vitamin K1(20) in children with cholestasis. *J Pediatr Gastroenterol Nutr* 14:160, 1996.

298. Aballi AJ: The action of vitamin K in the neonatal period. *South Med J* 58:48, 1965.

299. Gray OP, Ackerman A, Fraser AJ: Intracranial haemorrhage and clotting in low-birth-weight infants. *Lancet* 1:545, 1968.

300. Volpe JJ: Neonatal intraventricular hemorrhage. *N Engl J Med* 304:886, 1981.

301. Appleyard WJ, Cottom DG: Effect of asphyxia on Thrombotest values in low birthweight infants. *Arch Dis Child* 45:705, 1970.

302. Schmidt B, Zipursky A: Thrombotic disease in newborn infants. *Clin Perinatol* 2:461, 1984.

303. Rodgers GM, Shuman MA: Congenital thrombotic disorders. *Am J Hematol* 21:419, 1986.

304. Sifontes MT, Nuss R, Hunger SP, et al: Correlation between the functional assay for activated protein C resistance and factor V Leiden in the neonate. *Pediatr Res* 42:776, 1997.

305. Leroyer C, Mercier B, Oger E, et al: Prevalence of 20210 A allele of the prothrombin gene in venous thromboembolism patients. *Thromb Haemost* 80:49, 1998.

306. Poort SR, Rosendaal FR, Reitsma PH, Bertina RM: A common genetic variation in the 3′-untranslated region of the prothrombin gene is associated with elevated plasma prothrombin levels and an increase in venous thrombosis. *Blood* 88:3698, 1996.

307. Miller RK, Kellogg CR, Saltzman RA: Reproductive and perinatal toxicology, in *Handbook of Toxicology*, edited by TJ Haley, WO Berndt, pp 195–309. Hemisphere Publishing, Washington, DC, 1987.

308. Gray MJ: Use and abuse of thiazides in pregnancy. *Clin Obstet Gynecol* 11:568, 1968.

309. Leikin SL: Thiazide and neonatal thrombocytopenia. *N Engl J Med* 271:161, 1964.

300. Ginsberg JS, Kowalchuk G, Hirsh J, Brill-Edwards P, Burrows R: Heparin therapy during pregnancy. *Arch Intern Med* 149:2233, 1989.

311. Page TE, Hoyme HE, Markarian M, et al: Neonatal hemorrhage secondary to thrombocytopenia: An occasional effect of prenatal hydantoin exposure. *Birth Defects Orig Artic Ser* 18:47, 1982.

312. Hanson JW, Buehler BA: Fetal hydantoin syndrome: Current status. *J Pediatr* 101:816, 1982.

313. Eggermont E, Logghe N, van de Casseye W, et al: Haemorrhagic disease of the newborn in the offspring of rifampin and isoniazid treated mothers. *Acta Paediatr Belg* 29:87, 1976.

314. Powell RD, DeGowin RL, Alving AS, et al: Nitrofurantoin-induced hemolysis. *J Lab Clin Med* 62:1002, 1963.

315. Belton EM, Jones RV: Haemolytic anaemia due to nalidixic acid. *Lancet* 2:691, 1965.

316. Varsano I, Fischl J, Tikvah P, et al: The excretion of orally ingested nitrofurantoin in human milk. *J Pediatr* 82:886, 1973.

317. Brodersen R: Prevention of kernicterus, based on recent progress in bilirubin chemistry. *Acta Paediatr* 66:625, 1977.

318. El Beitune P, Duarte G: Antiretroviral agents during pregnancy: Consequences on hematologic parameters in HIV-exposed, uninfected newborn infants. *Eur J Obstet Gynecol Reprod Biol* 128:59, 2006.

CHAPTER 8
HEMATOLOGY DURING PREGNANCY

Martha P. Mims

SUMMARY

Normal pregnancy involves many changes in maternal physiology, including alterations in hematologic parameters. These changes include expansion in maternal plasma volume. The increase in plasma volume is relatively larger than the increase in red cell mass resulting in a decrease in hemoglobin concentration. An increase in the levels of some plasma proteins alters the balance of coagulation and fibrinolysis. Worldwide, the predominant cause of anemia in pregnancy is iron deficiency. Fetal requirements for iron are met despite maternal deficiency, but maternal iron deficiency has a number of adverse consequences including an increased frequency of preterm delivery and low-birth-weight infants. Bleeding disorders in pregnancy are a common reason for hematologic consultation and evoke concern for both the mother and child. Life-threatening bleeding caused by disseminated intravascular coagulation is seen with some complications unique to pregnancy, including placental abruption, retained dead fetus, and amniotic fluid embolism. von Willebrand disease is the commonest inherited bleeding disorder, but because of increases in factor VIII level and von Willebrand factor during pregnancy, excessive bleeding at delivery is rarely a problem in such patients. Factor levels fall rapidly postpartum, and serious hemorrhage can occur during this period. Carriers of hemophilia A and B should be monitored during pregnancy to determine if factor levels will be adequate for delivery at term. Caution should be exercised at delivery and during the first few days of life with offspring of hemophilia carriers until hemophilia testing is completed and the infant's status is known. Acquired hemophilia as a result of factor VIII autoantibodies is rare, but can occur during pregnancy or the puerperium. Thrombocytopenia is not uncommon in pregnancy, and its causes include several conditions that are unique to pregnancy, such as preeclampsia. Idiopathic thrombocytopenic purpura (ITP) is common, it is often exacerbated in pregnancy, and is managed conservatively if possible; close followup of newborns of mothers with ITP is essential. HELLP (hemolysis, elevated liver enzymes, and low platelet count) syndrome and TTP (thrombotic thrombocytopenic purpura)/hemolytic uremic syndrome are also seen in pregnancy and the puerperium. HELLP syndrome is managed by immediate delivery, if possible, whereas TTP, usually, can be managed with plasma exchange. Inherited and acquired prothrombotic conditions can be exacerbated by pregnancy and can result in adverse reproductive outcomes as well as maternal venous thromboembolism. The strongest evidence for an association between a thrombophilia and recurrent fetal loss exists for antiphospholipid antibody syndrome; however, evidence is mounting for a connection between inherited thrombophilias and the severity of some complications of pregnancy. These thrombophilias increase the risk of maternal venous thromboembolism in pregnancy and the puerperium. Treatment of hematologic malignancies in pregnancy can present a difficult dilemma both in terms of staging studies and management. In many cases of Hodgkin lymphoma, treatment can be delayed safely until after delivery. In contrast, in aggressive lymphomas and acute leukemias rapid initiation of chemotherapy is often necessary to save the life of the mother. In general, the teratogenic effects of chemotherapy are greatest in the first trimester; however, care must be taken in later trimesters to avoid cytopenias of both mother and fetus at delivery. Hemorrhagic and thrombotic complications associated with pregnancy in females with essential thrombocythemia and polycythemia vera present a unique challenge because of the lack of controlled trials in these situations.

Acronyms and Abbreviations: DDAVP, desmopressin acetate, a synthetic analogue of the pituitary hormone vasopressin; DIC, disseminated intravascular coagulation; ESR, erythrocyte sedimentation rate; ET, essential thrombocythemia; HELLP, hemolysis, elevated liver enzymes, low platelets syndrome; ITP, idiopathic thrombocytopenic purpura; PNH, paroxysmal nocturnal hemoglobinuria; PT, prothrombin time; PTT, partial thromboplastin time; PV, polycythemia vera; TTP, thrombotic thrombocytopenic purpura; VTE, venous thromboembolism; VWD, von Willebrand disease; VWF, von Willebrand factor.

● BLOOD VOLUME, ERYTHROPOIETIN LEVEL, AND HEMOGLOBIN CONCENTRATION

Maternal blood volume increases by an average of 40 to 50 percent above the nonpregnant level.[1] Plasma volume begins to rise early in pregnancy, with most of the escalation taking place in the second trimester and prior to week 32 of gestation.[2] Red cell mass increases significantly beginning in the second trimester and continues to expand throughout pregnancy, but to a lesser extent than plasma volume.[2] Erythropoietin levels increase throughout pregnancy, reaching approximately 150 percent of their prepregnancy levels at term.[3,4] The overall effect of these changes in most women is a slight drop in hemoglobin concentration, which is most pronounced at the end of the second trimester and slowly improves approaching term.

PLATELET AND WHITE CELL COUNTS

The effect of pregnancy on maternal platelet count is somewhat more controversial; some studies demonstrate a mild decline in platelet count over the course of gestation,[5] whereas others do not.[6] In general, white cell counts rise during pregnancy with the occasional appearance of myelocytes or metamyelocytes in the blood.[7] During labor and the early puerperium, there is a rise in the leukocyte count. Leukocytosis appears to be linearly related to the duration of labor.[8]

PLASMA PROTEINS

The levels of some plasma proteins also increase during pregnancy. In particular, C-reactive protein concentration is higher in pregnant women and rises even further during labor.[9] Erythrocyte sedimentation rate (ESR) rises during pregnancy, and is affected by both hemoglobin concentration and gestational age.[10] The rise in ESR during pregnancy, in large part a result of an increase in levels of plasma globulins and fibrinogen, makes its use as a marker of inflammation difficult. The levels of many of the procoagulant factors increase during pregnancy whereas activity of the fibrinolytic system diminishes in preparation for the hemostatic challenge of delivery. Plasma levels of von Willebrand factor (VWF), fibrinogen, and factors VII, VIII, and X all increase markedly, whereas factors II, V, IX, and XII are essentially unchanged and factor XIII declines.[11] Levels of protein C and antithrombin remain stable throughout pregnancy whereas total and free protein S fall with increasing gestational age.[12] Fibrinolysis is also impaired by increases in plasminogen activator inhibitors I and II, the latter a product of the placenta.[13]

ANEMIA IN PREGNANCY

IRON DEFICIENCY

Worldwide, the contribution of anemia to maternal and fetal morbidity and mortality is well recognized; in some parts of Africa, more than 75 percent of pregnant women are anemic, and there is a significant correlation between maternal mortality and anemia.[14] It has been suggested that iron deficiency may protect against placental malaria, but epidemiologic studies have not been conducted to verify this supposition.[15] In pregnant women, anemia is defined as a hemoglobin concentration of less than 11 g/dL in the first and third trimesters, and less than 10.5 g/dL in the second trimester.[15] In both the industrialized and the developing world, iron-deficiency anemia (Chap. 43) is the commonest cause of anemia.[16] On average approximately 1 g of iron is required during a normal pregnancy; 300 mg of iron are required by the fetus and the placenta, whereas expansion of the maternal red cell mass requires 500 mg, and 200 mg are lost via excretion.[17] These requirements exceed the iron storage of most young women and in general cannot be met by the diet. Even in cases of maternal iron deficiency, the fetal requirements for iron are always met; thus there is no correlation between the hemoglobin of the fetus and that of the mother.[18]

Iron-deficiency anemia during the first two trimesters of pregnancy is associated with a twofold increased risk for preterm delivery and a threefold increased risk for delivery of a low-birth-weight infant.[19] However, a large randomized trial comparing routine iron prophylaxis in pregnancy versus iron supplementation given only as needed demonstrated no significant differences in adverse maternal or fetal outcomes.[20] As in nonpregnant individuals, iron-deficiency anemia can generally be diagnosed using laboratory values such as serum ferritin, and transferrin saturation levels (Chap. 43). *Pica*, the ingestion of non-nutritive substances, is said to be more common among iron-deficient pregnant women than among other populations with iron deficiency. Ice, clay or dirt, and starch are the most frequent substances ingested (Chap. 43); to some extent, however, the choice appears to be cultural and much more widespread than most practitioners realize.[21]

FOLATE AND VITAMIN B$_{12}$ DEFICIENCY

Apart from iron deficiency, folate deficiency is the next most frequent nutritional deficiency leading to anemia in pregnant women. In the United States, where foodstuffs are supplemented with folate and the level of awareness of the association between folate deficiency and neural tube defects in the embryo is high, folate deficiency is relatively unusual. Folate requirements in pregnancy are roughly twice those in the nonpregnant state (800 mcg/day vs. 400 mcg/day), and if diet is insufficient may exceed the body's stores of folate (5–10 mg) relatively quickly.[22] Anemia related to folate deficiency most often presents in the third trimester and responds to folate supplementation with reticulocytosis within 24 to 72 hours.[16] Reports of severe pancytopenia and even states resembling the HELLP (hemolysis, elevated liver enzymes, and low platelet count) syndrome as a result of folate deficiency in pregnancy have appeared in the literature.[23,24] Despite these case reports, a review of 21 trials measuring the effect of folate supplementation on biochemical and hematologic parameters and pregnancy outcome

(excluding neural tube defects) revealed improvement in low hemoglobin level in late pregnancy, but had no measurable effect on any substantive measures of pregnancy outcome (Chap. 41).[25]

Vitamin B$_{12}$ (cobalamin) deficiency during pregnancy is rare, in part because deficiency of this vitamin leads to infertility. Serum cobalamin levels are known to fall during pregnancy.[26] A shift from the serum to tissue stores is proposed to account for the drop in serum B$_{12}$ levels. However, values less than 180 pmol/L usually are not observed in healthy women, and these low-normal levels are not accompanied by increased levels of methylmalonic acid, an indicator of cellular deficiency of cobalamin (Chap. 41).[27]

RED CELL APLASIA

A rare cause of anemia in pregnancy is pure red cell aplasia (Chap. 36). In pure red cell aplasia, anemia tends to occur early in pregnancy and often resolves within weeks of delivery. The pathogenic mechanism leading to red cell aplasia does not appear to be transferred to the fetus, but does tend to recur in subsequent pregnancies.[28,29] Conservative treatment, if feasible, is probably best until delivery; successful prenatal treatments with glucocorticoids and with intravenous immunoglobulin have been reported.[30,31]

BLEEDING DISORDERS AND CAUSES OF THROMBOCYTOPENIA

Bleeding disorders in pregnancy require consideration of maternal bleeding and hemorrhagic complications in the newborn. Data on the fetus are often lacking, and the practitioner must base decisions on past experience and the mother's previous reproductive history.

DISSEMINATED INTRAVASCULAR COAGULATION

Life-threatening bleeding is seen with some pregnancy-unique complications, resulting in disseminated intravascular coagulation (DIC). Because of the changes in coagulation factor levels, D-dimer, and platelet count during pregnancy, the normal range for tests routinely used to diagnose DIC in a nonpregnant state cannot be extrapolated directly to DIC in pregnancy. Serial measurement of the prothrombin time (PT), partial thromboplastin time (PTT), D-dimer, and fibrinogen are likely to be more helpful than measuring a single value.[32] The DIC score developed by the International Society on Thrombosis and Hemostasis has been modified for pregnancy and this score may be more useful in identifying DIC.[33]

Complications of pregnancy that lead to DIC include placental abruption, a retained dead fetus, and amniotic fluid embolism (Chap. 129). Although amniotic fluid embolism is a significant cause of maternal death in developed countries, the mortality decreased from 86 percent in 1979 to less than 30 percent in 1994 and 1995, perhaps from a better supportive therapy.[34] Amniotic fluid embolism is most likely to occur in older multiparous women whose pregnancies have gone beyond the 40th week and during tumultuous labor. Amniotic fluid enters the maternal circulation through tears in the chorioamniotic membranes, injury to the uterine veins, or uterine rupture. Its onset is heralded by maternal vascular collapse with dyspnea, hypotension, and cardiac arrhythmias followed by DIC that is manifested by oozing from intravenous lines, hematuria, hemoptysis, and excessive uterine bleeding. Atypical presentations have also been reported in which there is rapid deterioration of the fetus, followed by maternal respiratory and cardiovascular deterioration with development of DIC.[35]

In amniotic fluid embolism, DIC appears to involve an abnormal host response to exposure to various foreign antigens with the subsequent release of endogenous mediators which drive the clinical manifestations.[36] Treatment is not significantly different than in other cases of DIC with bleeding (Chap. 129); however, there are some reports of successful management with uterine artery embolization.[37]

Placental abruption has also led to development of DIC, and the spectrum of hemostatic failure is broad and appears to be related to the degree of placental separation.[38] Volume resuscitation, delivery of the fetus, and infusion of blood products to correct the maternal coagulation defect are indicated. Regional anesthesia is contraindicated because of the risk of bleeding in the epidural space and of the pooling of blood in the lower limb vascular bed, which could worsen hypovolemia.[38] Fetal trophoblast cells have distinct properties which may activate coagulation including expression of tissue factor, suppression of fibrinolysis, and exposure of anionic phospholipids.[39] Finally, intrauterine fetal death can also lead to DIC. Thromboplastic substances and specifically tissue factor released from dead fetal tissues into the maternal circulation are thought to trigger DIC; however, this is not usually detectable by laboratory tests until 3 or 4 weeks after fetal demise. Overt DIC is present in approximately 50 percent of women who retain a dead fetus for 5 weeks or longer.[40]

VON WILLEBRAND DISEASE

Although von Willebrand disease (VWD) is transmitted in an autosomal dominant fashion, women appear to be disproportionately affected with bleeding symptoms, primarily menorrhagia and postpartum hemorrhage (Chap. 126). In normal women and in types 1 and 2 (but not type 3) VWD patients, levels of factor VIII and VWF rise during pregnancy, with the most pronounced increase in the third trimester.[39] As a result, prophylactic administration of VWF-containing factor concentrates at delivery is often unnecessary in type 1 and type 2 VWD patients; however, the risk of postpartum hemorrhage is significant (13–29 percent) as levels fall rapidly after birth.[41] Thus in type 1 patients, factor VIII levels should be tested not only late in the third trimester, but also for 1 to 2 weeks postpartum. These patients should be monitored for increases in menstrual blood flow for at least 1 month. Risk of bleeding appears to be minimal when factor VIII levels are greater than 50 U/dL. There are several reports of severe thrombocytopenia developing late in pregnancy in patients with type 2B VWD,[42,43] and at least one of these patients developed a pulmonary embolus while receiving cryoprecipitate for postpartum hemorrhage. Despite the possible risk of thrombosis, these patients may require treatment with plasma-derived VWF-containing concentrates at delivery or postpartum if there is abnormal bleeding, and with platelets if thrombocytopenic bleeding is not controlled with infusion of VWF concentrate. Type 3 VWD patients require infusion of a plasma-derived VWF-containing concentrate at delivery, typically 40 to 80 IU/kg, followed by doses of 20 to 40 IU/kg daily for a week then tapered over the next few weeks.[44] Use of desmopressin acetate (DDAVP) antepartum is controversial because of the theoretical risk of vasoconstriction and placental insufficiency and the risk of maternal hyponatremia. Guidelines for management of VWD at delivery and during the puerperium have been published and are also reviewed in Chap. 126.[45,46]

COAGULATION FACTOR DEFICIENCIES

Carriers of hemophilia A and B generally have factor levels approximately 50 percent of normal; however, a wide range of values have been reported as a result of random inactivation of the X chromosome (Chaps. 10 and 123).[47,48] Ideally, carriers are identified before pregnancy when prenatal counseling can be offered. Baseline factor levels should be tested at the first visit during pregnancy and again in the third trimester, but it should be noted that factor IX levels generally do not rise during the course of the pregnancy.[47] The sex of the fetus should be determined to guide the obstetrician at delivery. With the recognition that maternal serum contains cell free fetal DNA, genomic strategies have been developed to determine fetal gender as early as 7 weeks of gestation. Similarly, strategies to determine whether a male fetus is affected by hemophilia based on testing of maternal blood have now been developed and will doubtless enter the clinical arena in the near future.[49] Cranial hemorrhage is the commonest site of bleeding in newborns with severe hemophilia, and has the highest potential for long-term serious sequelae. Risk factors for cranial hemorrhage include prolonged labor and use of instruments during delivery.[48] To protect a potentially affected or known hemophiliac fetus, vacuum extraction should be avoided at delivery and forceps should be used only with caution. All intramuscular injections should be withheld from the newborn until hemophilia testing is completed. If an infant's hemophilia status is not known, testing should be done on cord blood to avoid potential bleeding or bruising after a blood draw.[48] The mother's factor level should be followed for a few days after delivery and menstrual bleeding should be monitored to ensure adequate hemostasis.

There is also an association between pregnancy and acquired hemophilia caused by factor VIII autoantibodies (Chap. 127). This condition usually appears 1 to 4 months postpartum, but emerges during pregnancy in up to 14 percent of patients.[50] In general, the Bethesda titer of the inhibitor is low and in most cases the inhibitor disappears spontaneously. Inhibitors can recur in subsequent pregnancies.[51]

Rarely, pregnant women with factor deficiencies other than factors VIII and IX may be identified. The most important of these to recognize is deficiency of factor XIII, which is associated with habitual hemorrhagic abortions and postpartum hemorrhage. In rare pregnancies reaching term, bleeding complications, including intracranial hemorrhage in the infant, have been observed.[52,53] Treatment of this deficiency with fresh-frozen plasma, cryoprecipitate, or plasma-derived factor XIII concentrates (now available in the United States) prevents abortion in women, although there are no controlled studies.[54] Most authorities recommend more frequent prophylactic therapy during pregnancy (every 3 weeks vs. every 5–6 weeks) with booster doses during labor or before cesarean section to ensure a level of 5 percent or greater.[55] Although rare, congenital afibrinogenemia, hypofibrinogenemia, and dysfibrinogenemia (Chap. 125) can cause hemorrhagic and thrombotic pregnancy complications. Most experts recommend fibrinogen replacement (using cryoprecipitate or fibrinogen concentrate) to maintain a level of 60 to 100 mg/dL during pregnancy and for 6 weeks postpartum.[56]

CAUSES OF THROMBOCYTOPENIA

Thrombocytopenia in pregnancy is relatively common, with up to 5 percent of all pregnant women exhibiting asymptomatic thrombocytopenia.[57] Many causes of thrombocytopenia in pregnancy are identical to those seen in the nonpregnant state, with some predisposing to bleeding whereas others predispose to clotting. However, there are several conditions leading to thrombocytopenia that are unique to pregnancy, including gestational thrombocytopenia, preeclampsia/HELLP syndrome/eclampsia, and acute fatty liver of pregnancy.

Gestational and Immune Thrombocytopenia

Gestational thrombocytopenia and idiopathic thrombocytopenic purpura (ITP) are best discussed together as they can be difficult to differentiate and, in fact, may be two extremes of a spectrum of disease. In general, gestational thrombocytopenia is asymptomatic and is said to occur later in pregnancy and be less severe than ITP. Most sources suggest that gestational thrombocytopenia occurs in the second and third trimesters, with platelet counts rarely falling below 70,000/μL.[58] Gestational thrombocytopenia can sometimes be diagnosed with certainty only after delivery; usually there is no past history of low platelets, except perhaps with previous pregnancies, the platelet count returns to normal after delivery, and there is no association with fetal thrombocytopenia. It is not clear whether or not gestational thrombocytopenia is a variant of immune-mediated platelet destruction (Chap. 117).[58]

In contrast to gestational thrombocytopenia, ITP can occur at any point in pregnancy and the fall in platelet count can be severe. Diagnosis is essentially the same as it would be in any patient in that alternative causes of thrombocytopenia must be ruled out. As in other cases, treatment of ITP in pregnancy must take into account the severity of the thrombocytopenia and the presence or absence of symptoms. In general, platelet counts less than 10,000/μL require treatment regardless of the trimester; platelet counts of 30,000 to 50,000/μL without bleeding require no treatment, and platelet counts of 10,000 to 30,000/μL in later trimesters or in the presence of bleeding require treatment. Although glucocorticoid and intravenous immunoglobulin are safe in pregnancy, they may have no effect on fetal counts and should only be used to treat the mother.[59] Splenectomy for ITP in pregnancy is best done in the second trimester if platelet counts are extremely low and unresponsive to treatment.[58] One small study evaluated the safety of anti-D antibodies during pregnancy; all 10 of the women studied achieved a platelet count greater than 30,000/μL, but larger studies are needed before this intervention can be recommended.[60] Similarly, there are case reports of rituximab administration for treatment of refractory ITP in pregnancy; at least one report demonstrated transient inhibition of neonatal B-lymphocyte development.[61] There are no adequate and well-controlled studies of either eltrombopag or romiplostim in pregnant women and both are considered pregnancy category C drugs. In animal studies, both drugs crossed the placental and fetal effects included thrombocytosis, postimplantation loss, increase in fetal mortality, but no major structural malformations were reported.[62] Case reports describing the use of romiplostim in pregnancy have appeared and in one report the newborn had severe thrombocytopenia at birth complicated by intracranial hemorrhage.[63] Maternal platelet counts of greater than 50,000/μL usually are safe for both vaginal and cesarean delivery. In most cases, spinal anesthesia should not be used if the platelet count is less than 75,000/μL.[64] Less than 5 percent of babies born to mothers with ITP have platelet counts less than 20,000/μL, although there does seem to be some correlation between very severely depressed maternal platelet count and severe thrombocytopenia in the newborn.[65] No clear recommendations can be given for measuring fetal platelet count prior to or at delivery as measurements are fraught with error; however, if the fetal platelet count is known to be less than 20,000/μL, cesarean section is probably reasonable. Newborns of mothers with ITP should be monitored for 5 to 7 days after delivery to ensure that the platelet count does not drop (Chap. 117).

Eclampsia and HELLP Syndrome

The spectrum of hypertensive disorders of pregnancy ranging from preeclampsia to severe preeclampsia and HELLP syndrome to eclampsia (see Chap. 51) may also result in thrombocytopenia, although thrombosis is more of an issue than is bleeding. There is some debate in the literature as to whether thrombocytopenia can be diagnosed in preeclampsia without HELLP syndrome; however, data from one large study[57] indicated that approximately 15 percent of cases of preeclampsia are complicated by thrombocytopenia. In general, the symptoms of preeclampsia, including hematologic manifestations, resolve with delivery; however, in a small proportion of cases they persist, worsen, or even develop immediately postpartum. When symptoms persist postpartum,

the differentiation from thrombotic thrombocytopenic purpura (TTP)/hemolytic uremic syndrome becomes more difficult. Some data suggest that maternal recovery from the HELLP syndrome is accelerated by administration of intravenous dexamethasone[66]; however, a meta-analysis demonstrated no clear advantage to the use of glucocorticoids to decrease maternal or perinatal morbidity or mortality.[67] A collaborative randomized controlled trial of glucocorticoids in HELLP syndrome (COHELLP) is underway to determine the effectiveness of dexamethasone to accelerate the postpartum recovery of patients with class I HELLP syndrome.[68] Observation or treatment of HELLP with glucocorticoids alone postpartum should probably not persist beyond the third postpartum day. If the patient is not clearly improving, plasma exchange should be initiated as one would do for thrombotic thrombocytopenic purpura (TTP).[69,70] Although not associated with hypertension, acute fatty liver of pregnancy is another rare disorder that can present in the third trimester with severe liver dysfunction, but thrombocytopenia, if present, is generally mild and does not require treatment (Chaps. 51, 117, and 129).

●THROMBOPHILIA

FETAL LOSS AND COMPLICATIONS

Pregnancy is a prothrombotic state. Inherited prothrombotic conditions contribute to 50 percent of the cases of venous thromboembolism and pulmonary embolism, as well as to stroke in pregnancy and the puerperium. Hereditary thrombophilias (Chap. 130) may also predispose to fetal loss through placental vascular disorders. The best evidence for an association between a thrombophilia, albeit acquired, and recurrent fetal loss exists for antiphospholipid antibody syndrome in which the association between the antibodies and pregnancy loss has been recognized for more than 20 years.[71] As many as 20 percent of women with recurrent fetal loss have antiphospholipid antibodies,[72] and studies show that without treatment up to 90 percent will experience fetal loss.[73] One study suggests that poor pregnancy outcomes occur more frequently in primary antiphospholipid syndrome when patients have more than one positive laboratory test (lupus anticoagulant, immunoglobulin [Ig] G/IgM anticardiolipin, IgG/IgM antihuman β_2-glycoprotein I antibodies).[74] In a randomized controlled trial including 90 women with a history of recurrent miscarriage associated with phospholipid antibodies (or antiphospholipid antibodies), lupus anticoagulant, and cardiolipin antibodies (or anticardiolipin antibodies), the rate of live births with low-dose aspirin (75 mg/day) and unfractionated heparin (5000 U subcutaneously twice per day) was 71 percent (32 of 45 pregnancies) and 42 percent (19 of 45 pregnancies) with low-dose aspirin alone (odds ratio: 3.37 [95% confidence interval: 1.40 to 8.10]).[75] A rarer acquired cause of fetal loss and thrombosis in pregnancy is paroxysmal nocturnal hemoglobinuria (PNH; Chap. 40). Though no clinical trials data exist, recommendations are to provide prophylactic or intermediate-dose low-molecular-weight heparin antepartum and for 6 weeks postpartum. Eculizumab should be consider both prior to and following delivery.[76]

Although an association between inherited thrombophilias and pregnancy loss has been elusive and there are inconsistencies between studies, there is an association between factor V Leiden and recurrent fetal loss.[77,78] Less-convincing data exist for prothrombin 20210A, but there is no clear association with homozygous methylene tetrahydrofolate reductase C677T polymorphism (hyperhomocysteinemia).[79] Clinical trials examining the use of low-molecular-weight heparins or aspirin to prevent adverse pregnancy outcomes in women with inherited thrombophilias have been criticized for lack of an untreated control group.[80–82] Pregnancy outcomes from a large ongoing trial conducted with a no-treatment control have yet to be published.[83] Studies evaluating a role for inherited thrombophilias in preeclampsia and intrauterine growth retardation indicate that these factors may not be causative, but may contribute to disease severity.[80,81]

THROMBOEMBOLIC EVENTS

Risk Factors

Estimates place the relative risk of arterial and venous thromboembolism (VTE) in pregnant women (Chaps. 133 and 134) at two to six times that of nonpregnant women.[11,82] Factors specific to pregnancy that increase the risk of VTE include obstruction of venous return by the gravid uterus, acquired prothrombotic changes in hemostatic proteins, and venous atonia caused by hormonal factors.[84] Additional risk factors include cesarean section (especially emergency), obesity, and increasing age. Approximately 80 percent of deep vein thromboses in pregnancy occur in the iliofemoral veins on the left, probably as a consequence of compression of the left iliac vein by the right iliac and ovarian arteries.[85,86] Rates of VTE immediately postpartum are difficult to assess as many occur after the patient is discharged; one large study estimates rates as much as 5 times higher in postpartum women than pregnant women.[87] Inherited thrombophilias (Chap. 130) are associated with more than half of VTE in pregnancy. Factor V Leiden and the prothrombin gene mutation are the commonest abnormalities associated with VTE in pregnancy, accounting for 44 and 17 percent, respectively. In general 1 in 500 factor V Leiden heterozygotes and 1 in 200 heterozygous carriers of the prothrombin 20210 gene mutation will have a VTE in pregnancy. Homozygosity for either of these mutations increases risk about fourfold. Based on recent studies, the risk for VTE during pregnancy is 1 in 113 for protein C deficiency, approximately 1 in 3 for type I antithrombin deficiency, and 1 in 42 for type II antithrombin deficiency. Risk for carriers of protein S deficiency is similar to that for protein C deficiency.[88-90]

Diagnostic Methods

Diagnosis of VTE in pregnancy is complicated both because the presenting complaints—leg edema, back pain, and chest pain—are common in pregnancy, and because radiologic studies used to make the diagnosis in nonpregnant individuals are relatively contraindicated in pregnant women. Compression ultrasonography is the initial test of choice in pregnant women. If this test is nondiagnostic, several other tests may be considered. If pulmonary embolus is suspected, lung ventilation perfusion scanning, which gives relatively low-dose radiation, may be used. Magnetic resonance imaging or magnetic resonance venography are also informative if available. Measurement of D-dimers is a useful adjunct in nonpregnant patients to rule out VTE (D-dimers are sensitive, but not specific, for VTE). However, D-dimer levels rise over the course of normal pregnancy[91,92] and with several complications of pregnancy, including preterm labor, hypertension, and placental abruption,[93] and thus may not be useful in excluding VTE.

Prophylaxis

Prophylaxis for VTE is a controversial issue as only a few prospective studies have been done to assess the risk of use.[94,95] There is general agreement, however, that because of its teratogenic potential, warfarin should not be used during pregnancy and that low-molecular-weight heparins are the anticoagulant of choice because they do not cross the placenta and have a lower risk of osteoporosis and heparin-induced thrombocytopenia than unfractionated heparin.[96] Most experts now agree that risk assessment should be based on both personal and family history of VTE as well as the presence of a known hypercoagulable state. Based on the most recent Chest Guidelines,[97] all women with prior history of VTE should be offered postpartum prophylaxis with

prophylactic or intermediate dose low molecular weight heparin for 6 weeks. For pregnant women with a low risk of recurrence (e.g., a single VTE with a transient risk factor unrelated to pregnancy or estrogen use) surveillance is recommended antepartum, whereas those with higher risk should receive prophylactic or intermediate dose low molecular weight heparin prior to delivery. Women with no prior VTE are divided into four categories. Those with higher risk of VTE in pregnancy including Factor V Leiden or Prothrombin 20210 homozygotes or compound heterozygotes with a family history of VTE should receive prophylactic or intermediate dose low molecular weight heparin antepartum and postpartum prophylaxis with prophylactic or intermediate dose low molecular weight heparin for 6 weeks. Factor V Leiden or Prothrombin 20210 homozygotes or compound heterozygotes without a family history of VTE should undergo surveillance antepartum and should receive postpartum prophylaxis with prophylactic or intermediate dose low molecular weight heparin for 6 weeks. Pregnant women with no personal history of VTE with any other thrombophilia and a family history of VTE should undergo surveillance antepartum and should be offered postpartum prophylaxis with prophylactic or intermediate-dose low-molecular-weight heparin for 6 weeks. Finally, women with lower risk thrombophilias and no personal or family history of VTE should be offered surveillance post antepartum and postpartum. Patients with two or more episodes of VTE should probably be treated throughout pregnancy and the puerperium.[98-102] As noted above, women who meet the criteria for antiphospholipid antibody syndrome should receive antepartum prophylactic or intermediate dose unfractionated or prophylactic low molecular weight heparin and low dose aspirin throughout pregnancy. Treatment of VTE in pregnancy should be with full-dose low-molecular-weight heparin. Ideally, women on treatment doses of heparin have elective induction of labor. Heparin is usually discontinued 24 hours prior to induction; however, women deemed to be at very high risk of recurrent VTE can then receive intravenous heparin up to 4 to 6 hours prior to delivery.[100,101] Great care should be taken with epidural anesthesia, and it should be avoided if there is any question of a significant anticoagulant effect. Heparins and warfarin are safe postpartum, even when breastfeeding.[103]

●TREATMENT OF HEMATOLOGIC MALIGNANCIES IN PREGNANCY

Although not common, leukemias and lymphomas do occur in pregnancy and present problems with proper diagnosis, staging, and treatment (Chaps. 88–90). The literature suggests that the incidence of Hodgkin lymphoma is 1:1000 to 1:6000 pregnancies, whereas the incidence of non-Hodgkin lymphoma is manyfold lower.[104] Leukemia in pregnancy is uncommon.

HODGKIN LYMPHOMA

Neither the histology nor the outcome of patients who present during pregnancy is worse than that of other patients.[104] Diagnosis, usually by biopsy of a lymph node, is usually not problematic, but staging can be difficult. Posterior–anterior chest films with abdominal shielding and marrow biopsy (in the presence of B symptoms, leukopenia, or thrombocytopenia) should be done and present little risk to the fetus. Laboratory studies, including blood counts, liver functions tests, and ESR, should be done, but care should be taken in interpreting the alkaline phosphatase and ESR measurements, which both rise during the course of a normal pregnancy. Evaluation for the presence of abdominopelvic disease is difficult because computed tomography imaging is contraindicated in pregnant women. Abdominal ultrasonograms are safe, but provide limited information. If necessary, magnetic resonance imaging scans can probably be done safely in pregnancy; however, this is rarely necessary and most experts recommend waiting until after the first trimester. The toxicities of treatment and the risks of delaying treatment until later in pregnancy or postpartum need to be considered carefully in each case. Fetal risks of chemotherapy are greatest in the first trimester during the period of organogenesis, with folate antagonists and antimetabolites carrying the largest risk.[105] Despite the changes in physiology that occur during pregnancy, there is no evidence that dosing should be changed. If chemotherapy is indicated, it should be delayed until the second trimester; however, single-agent vinblastine has been given in the first trimester with a low incidence of fetal abnormalities.[106] Treatment should be timed so that there is the maximum amount of time possible between the last dose of chemotherapy and delivery to avoid cytopenias in either the mother or the fetus. In some cases, radiotherapy may be a feasible alternative in the second and third trimesters of pregnancy. Of 16 patients who received radiotherapy for supradiaphragmatic Hodgkin lymphoma (clinical stages IA and IIA) during pregnancy, 11 received full mantle irradiation, and all patients had lead shielding of the uterus.[107] All 16 pregnancies were carried to completion with full-term deliveries of normal infants. However, a review of the records of 382 women treated with radiotherapy for Hodgkin lymphoma suggests that the risk of breast cancer after radiation therapy is nearly sevenfold greater with irradiation around the time of pregnancy.[108] Additional studies are needed to confirm these findings, but this potential risk should be borne in mind by the clinician when making therapeutic decisions.[109] Relapse of Hodgkin lymphoma usually occurs within the first 2 years following treatment, and patients are counseled to avoid pregnancy during this period. Vigilance for second cancers in these patients is also advised as is monitoring for hypothyroidism in those who receive radiation therapy, especially during subsequent pregnancies when hypothyroidism could have profound maternal and fetal effects.

NON-HODGKIN LYMPHOMA

As compared with Hodgkin lymphoma, other lymphomas (Chap. 95) are less frequent in pregnancy, tend to present with a higher stage disease, and have a poorer prognosis.[110] Burkitt or Burkitt-like lymphoma can involve the breasts of young pregnant or lactating women and typically behaves aggressively.[111,112] A recent review of more than 100 cases of Non-Hodgkin lymphoma in pregnancy, 75 percent of the patients had stage IV disease at diagnosis and nearly half had involvement of reproductive organs, primarily the breast. Very few cases of placental or fetal involvement were observed.[113] In patients with high-grade lymphomas, chemotherapy often cannot be delayed and difficult decisions must be made. However, in one report of 16 pregnant patients who received aggressive chemotherapy for non-Hodgkin lymphoma during their pregnancies, all survived to delivery.[114] Half of the 16 patients received chemotherapy in their first trimester and all 16 delivered healthy infants despite episodes of myelosuppression during the pregnancies. In a subsequent report, the health of 84 children born to mothers who received chemotherapy for hematologic malignancies during pregnancy revealed no abnormalities in physical or cognitive development and no increase in cancers at a median followup of 18.7 years.[115] Rituximab in pregnancy, both as a single agent and in combination with chemotherapy, has not been associated with abnormalities of the newborn when given in the first, second, or third trimester[116]; however, there is one report of prolonged lymphopenia in a neonate whose mother received rituximab in pregnancy.[61,116,117] A retrospective study of 231 pregnancies associated with maternal rituximab exposure identified 153 pregnancies with known outcomes. Among these pregnancies there were 90 live births, 22 of which were premature. There were four neonatal infections and two congenital malformations.[118]

ACUTE LEUKEMIA

Leukemia is distinctly uncommon in pregnancy; estimates derived from studies beginning in the 1950s place the incidence at approximately 1:75,000 pregnancies (Chaps. 88 and 91).[119,120] Acute leukemias make up nearly 90 percent of the total, followed by chronic myeloid leukemia, which comprises an additional 10 percent; chronic lymphocytic leukemia is extremely rare.[121] The acute leukemias require urgent treatment, and while pregnancy itself does not alter the course of the leukemia, the outcome is much worse if treatment is delayed.[122] A summary of data on 96 pregnant women reported in the literature from 1983 to 1995 who were treated with cytotoxic chemotherapy for leukemias (most of which were acute) revealed that most patients received regimens that included multiple drugs and were not different from those given to nonpregnant patients.[123] Nearly one-third of patients were treated in the first trimester of pregnancy. Among the 96 pregnancies, there were 2 maternal deaths, 2 children were stillborn, 2 therapeutic abortions were performed, 1 child had chromosomal abnormalities, and 8 had congenital defects. Seven of the eight children born with congenital defects were born to mothers who had been treated in the first trimester. It was not possible to identify a drug (or drugs) that was most likely responsible for adverse outcomes. Treatment in the first trimester carries a high risk of fetal anomaly or miscarriage. For patients with acute myelogenous leukemia (AML) receiving a standard induction regimen of cytarabine and an anthracycline, it is probably best to avoid idarubicin, which is more lipophilic with elevated placental transfer. Doxorubicin has been extensively studied in pregnancy women with breast cancer and is probably the anthracycline of choice in pregnant patients with AML.[124] Although few cases of fetal cardiotoxicity related to anthracyclines have been reported, fetal cardiac function should be monitored in pregnancy. Very few data exist for consolidation therapy in pregnancy. Case reports of treatment of acute promyelocytic leukemia in pregnancy with all-*trans*-retinoic acid[125-127] suggest that it may be safe after the first trimester. Arsenic trioxide is not recommended for use at any stage of pregnancy because of its high potential for embryotoxicity.[128] For patients who require chemotherapy postpartum, breastfeeding is not recommended so as to avoid exposure of the newborn to cytotoxic drugs in the breast milk.[129] Patients with chronic myeloid leukemia have been successfully treated in pregnancy with interferon-α, hydroxyurea, leukapheresis, and even busulfan.[130-132] A review of 125 women treated with imatinib mesylate during pregnancy revealed that most pregnancies had successful outcomes; however, 12 infants had abnormalities, 3 of which involved complex malformations.[133]

Supportive treatment with antiemetics, including ondansetron, aprepitant and metoclopramide, is safe, and these agents do not cause congenital malformations.[134] Little data exist for the effects of growth factors including granulocyte colony-stimulating factors, but there are no reports of teratogenic effects.[135] Care should be taken with prescribing antibiotics and quinolones in specific should be avoided in pregnancy as should sulfonamides. When antifungal therapy is required, amphotericin may be the drug of choice as there have been no reports of teratogenicity with this agent. Fluconazole appears to be safe at doses less than 150 mg per day, but ketoconazole and voriconazole can cause fetal malformations and should avoided altogether.[136]

● ESSENTIAL THROMBOCYTHEMIA

The management of pregnant patients with essential thrombocythemia (ET) is a challenge because thrombosis is the main complication of ET (Chap. 85) and is accentuated by the prothrombotic state of pregnancy. In addition, of all the myeloproliferative neoplasms, ET has the highest proportion of affected females of child-bearing age. One study reviewed 155 pregnancies in 86 women with ET, and only 59 percent of these pregnancies resulted in a live neonate.[137] First-trimester abortion was seen in 31 percent of pregnancies, the main cause being placental infarction. Maternal thrombotic or hemorrhagic complications were infrequent, but were more common than in normal pregnancy. Pregnancy did not appear to adversely affect the course and prognosis of ET.

A meta-analysis revealed a benefit for aspirin treatment, whereas the benefit of heparin prophylaxis has not been established, but may have a role in selected cases.[138] If cytoreductive therapy becomes necessary, interferon-α is the drug of choice. A similar incidence of pregnancy complications in patients with ET was reported in a series from the Mayo clinic.[139] Another large single institution study of 68 young ET patients demonstrated that for both polycythemia vera (PV) and ET, most thromboses in young patients occurred at the time of diagnosis and also suggested, but did not prove, the benefit of aspirin.[140] The most detailed analysis was published by the Italian Society of Hematology in its guidelines.[138] The Society's report analyzed pooled outcome data from 461 pregnancies in women with ET. The mean age of the pregnant patients was 29 years, and the mean platelet count at the beginning of pregnancy was 1000×10^9/L, which declined to 400×10^9/L in the second trimester. This decrease in the platelet count during pregnancy documented for the first time the anecdotal observation that some women with ET spontaneously normalize their platelet count during their pregnancy. (The authors of this chapter have rarely observed this phenomenon; however, in one of their ET patients a spontaneous, but transient, ET remission occurred in the first pregnancy, but not in the following pregnancy.) The Italian study found that 44 percent of pregnancies were unsuccessful in women with ET, a figure that is threefold higher than in the general population. Among the 461 pregnancies there were 13 pre- or postpartum significant bleeding events. The median duration of gestation was 38 weeks because of abortions and preterm deliveries. Cesarean section was necessary in 15 percent of the patients. The platelet count at the beginning of pregnancy did not predict pregnancy outcome. Placental infarctions were reported in 18 pregnancies and these were associated with intrauterine fetal growth retardation (11 pregnancies). Placental abruption was reported in 3.6 percent of ET pregnancies compared to 1 percent in the non-ET population. Preeclampsia was seen at a rate equal to that seen in non-ET pregnancies. Postpartum thrombotic episodes were reported in 5.2 percent of the pregnancies and included venous thrombosis, pulmonary embolism, sagittal sinus thrombosis, transient ischemic attacks, and Budd-Chiari syndrome (rates for all problems were significantly higher than in non-ET pregnancies). The impact of therapy was difficult to evaluate because management of ET pregnancies was heterogeneous; no specific therapy for ET was given in 48 percent of the pregnancies. Aspirin therapy at doses ranging from 75 to 500 mg per day was used in 106 pregnancies, low-molecular-weight heparin (pre-/postpartum) was used in 26 pregnancies, interferon-α was used in 19 pregnancies, and a handful of patients had various chemotherapies and radioactive phosphorus. When the outcome of the ET pregnancies was reviewed, 74 percent of patients treated with aspirin during pregnancy had successful pregnancies, whereas 55 percent of the patients not receiving aspirin had successful pregnancies. Based on the detailed analyses of all variables, this panel of experts felt that there was no direct evidence of the efficacy of aspirin in pregnant ET women, but that "it seems possible that aspirin increases the rate of successful pregnancies." The panel also recommended that ET patients with a thrombotic episode (peripheral or placental) during pregnancy should receive low-molecular-weight heparin at therapeutic doses and oral anticoagulant therapy (PT international normalized ratio 2 to 3) for at least 6 weeks postpartum. Longer periods of anticoagulation were recommended for patients with familial thrombophilia. Pregnant women deemed candidates for platelet-lowering therapy (a history

of major thrombosis, or of major bleeding, platelet count greater than 1000×10^9/L, familial thrombophilia or cardiovascular risk factors) were recommended to receive interferon. The Italian panel also recommended avoidance of anagrelide in pregnancy because of uncertainty about its teratogenic potential; however, several normal infants have been born to women who inadvertently took this drug during pregnancy (FDA documents submitted by the manufacturer). Although the risk of congenital anomalies among infants of women treated with hydroxyurea during pregnancy was thought to be substantial, of 15 infants born to women treated with hydroxyurea at conception and/or during pregnancy, no malformations were observed, and only one stillbirth was reported in a woman who also had eclampsia. At least one publication has identified the presence of the *JAK2* V617F mutation as a risk factor for pregnancy complications; however, to date there is no consensus on whether to manage these patients differently.[141] A review of 158 young women with ET experiencing 237 pregnancies demonstrated that pregnancy complications are associated with higher risk of subsequent thrombosis.[142]

POLYCYTHEMIA VERA

Although there is significant overlap in the clinical features of PV and ET, there are some noteworthy differences (Chap. 84). In PV, the number of reported pregnancies is low because most PV patients are past childbearing age, and comorbid conditions are more frequent. One authoritative review suggests maintaining the hematocrit below 45 percent[141] in pregnancy, and another recommends using interferon-α when myelosuppression is indicated.[143] Another noted authority in PV recommends that the hematocrit be kept lower than 35 percent in pregnancy.[144] However, because of a dearth of data and controlled studies, optimal management of PV pregnancies is poorly defined and agreed upon protocols are not available. None of the available information allows definite therapeutic recommendations; however, some authorities recommend that, at a minimum, all pregnant patients with PV be treated with low-dose aspirin.[144]

HEMOGLOBINOPATHIES

SICKLE SYNDROMES

Although pregnancy in patients with sickle cell trait is typically uneventful, these patients probably have an increased risk for urinary tract infection.[145] Earlier studies suggested an increased risk for preeclampsia in patients with sickle cell trait, but a large study demonstrated that sickle cell trait is not an independent risk factor for preeclampsia (Chap. 49).[146]

Patients with sickle cell anemia should receive at least 1 mg of folate per day; however, they should not receive iron supplementation until a ferritin level is checked and iron deficiency is documented.[147] Because of the risk of fetal malformation, hydroxyurea should be discontinued at least 3 months before pregnancy. However, successful outcomes have been reported in sickle cell disease patients who were exposed to the drug while pregnant.[148] Women with sickle cell anemia and their fetuses have an increased risk of complications during pregnancy. A large study of more than 17,000 deliveries to women with sickle cell anemia compared with controls demonstrated that infectious complications, including pneumonia, systemic inflammatory response syndrome, and sepsis, were more common in the women with sickle cell anemia. Furthermore, thrombotic complications such as cerebral vein and deep vein thrombosis and pregnancy complications including preeclampsia, eclampsia, abruption and antepartum bleeding were significantly more common in patients with sickle cell anemia. As in previous reports, rates of intrauterine growth retardation and preterm labor, as well as rates of maternal mortality, were higher in mothers with sickle cell anemia.[149] The issue of prophylactic versus need-based transfusion in sickle cell patients is controversial. A Cochrane Review identified only two small randomized studies conducted in the United States in the 1980s addressing this issue. These studies demonstrated no difference in perinatal outcome between the offspring of mothers with sickle cell disease who were assigned to treatment with prophylactic transfusions and those who were not.[1,150]

Although the incidence of cesarean section in sickle cell patients is reported to be as high as 36 percent,[151] delivery can generally be accomplished vaginally. Most experts recommend avoiding induction of labor as this can lead to sickle crisis.[152] Epidural anesthesia is reported to be safe and to decrease the risk of peripartum painful crises.[153]

THALASSEMIA SYNDROMES

β-Thalassemia Syndromes

Preconception evaluation of patients with β-thalassemia syndromes is recommended and should include assessment of transfusion needs, chelation therapy, body iron status and organ function, and the presence of antibodies to red cell antigens.[154] Patients with β-thalassemia minor generally tolerate pregnancy well; however, doses of at least 4 mg of folate per day are recommended in the preconception period and the first trimester as there is some data to suggest an increased risk of neural tube defects in their offspring.[155] Transfusion and iron chelation therapy has improved both life expectancy and fertility in patients with β-thalassemia intermedia and major, and successful pregnancies have been reported in both disorders.[156] A high rate of maternal mortality is reported in women with thalassemia and cardiac iron overload emphasizing the need for aggressive management of iron status prior to undertaking a pregnancy.[157] During pregnancy, regular transfusions are recommended to keep the hemoglobin level at 10 mg/dL and transfusion requirements often increase as compared to prepregnancy values.[158] Iron-chelation therapy with deferoxamine in pregnancy is controversial and most authorities recommend a hiatus during pregnancy; however, no fetal abnormalities have been reported in pregnancies in which it was continued (Chap. 48).[159]

α-Thalassemia Syndromes

Patients with the silent carrier state or α-thalassemia trait have no increase in pregnancy complications; however, identification of patients with heterozygous α-thalassemia trait is important in assessing the risk of having a fetus that has hemoglobin H or hemoglobin Bart. Although women with hemoglobin H are generally able to have successful pregnancies, the chronic anemia often worsens, requiring blood transfusion. Patients with hemoglobin H are sensitive to oxidizing compounds and medications, which should be borne in mind, particularly during pregnancy (Chap. 48).

REFERENCES

1. Pritchard JA: Changes in the blood volume during pregnancy and delivery. *Anesthesiology* 26:393, 1965.
2. Scott DE: Anemia in pregnancy. *Obstet Gynecol Annu* 1:219, 1972.
3. Harstad TW, Mason RA, Cox SM: Serum erythropoietin quantitation in pregnancy using an enzyme-linked immunoassay. *Am J Perinatol* 9:233, 1992.
4. McMullin MF, White R, Lappin T, et al: Haemoglobin during pregnancy: Relationship to erythropoietin and haematinic status. *Eur J Haematol* 71:44, 2003.
5. Pitkin RM, Witte DL: Platelet and leukocyte counts in pregnancy. *JAMA* 242:2696, 1979.
6. van Buul EJA SE, Johnsman HW, et al: Haematological and biochemical profile of uncomplicated pregnancy in nulliparous women: A longitudinal study. *Neth J Med* 46:73, 1995.
7. England JM, Bain BJ: Total and differential leucocyte count. *Br J Haematol* 33:1, 1976.
8. Acker DB, Johnson MP, Sachs BP, et al: The leukocyte count in labor. *Am J Obstet Gynecol* 153:737, 1985.
9. Watts DH, Krohn MA, Wener MH, et al: C-reactive protein in normal pregnancy. *Obstet Gynecol* 77:176, 1991.
10. van den Broe NR, Letsky EA: Pregnancy and the erythrocyte sedimentation rate. *BJOG* 108:1164, 2001.
11. Greer IA: Thrombosis in pregnancy: Maternal and fetal issues. *Lancet* 353:1258, 1999.
12. Clark P, Brennand J, Conkie JA, et al: Activated protein C sensitivity, protein S and coagulation in normal pregnancy. *Thromb Haemost* 79:1166, 1998.
13. Halligan A BJ, Sheppard B, et al: Haemostatic, fibrinolytic and endothelial variables in normal pregnancies and pre-eclampsia. *Br J Obstet Gynaecol* 101:448, 1992.
14. Brabin BJ, Hakimi M, Pelletier D: An analysis of anemia and pregnancy-related maternal mortality. *J Nutr* 131:604S, 2001.
15. Centers for Disease Control (CDC): CDC criteria for anemia in children and childbearing-aged women. *MMWR Morb Mortal Wkly Rep* 38:400, 1989.
16. Sifakis S, Pharmakides G: Anemia in pregnancy. *Ann N Y Acad Sci* 900:125, 2000.
17. FAO/WHO: *Joint Expert Consultation Report: Requirements of Vitamin A, Iron, Folate, and Vitamin B12*. FAO Food and Nutrition Series 23. FAO, Rome, 1988.
18. Harthoorn-Lasthuizen EJ, Lindemans J, Langenhuijsen MM: Does iron-deficient erythropoiesis in pregnancy influence fetal iron supply? *Acta Obstet Gynecol Scand* 80:392, 2001.
19. Scholl TO, Hediger ML, Fischer RL, et al: Anemia vs iron deficiency: Increased risk of preterm delivery in a prospective study. *Am J Clin Nutr* 55:985, 1992.
20. Hemminki E, Rimpela U: A randomized comparison of routine versus selective iron supplementation during pregnancy. *J Am Coll Nutr* 10:3, 1991.
21. Horner RD, Lackey CJ, Kolasa K, et al: Pica practices of pregnant women. *J Am Diet Assoc* 91:34, 1991.
22. Shojania AM: Folic acid and vitamin B12 deficiency in pregnancy and in the neonatal period. *Clin Perinatol* 11:433, 1984.
23. Van de Velde A, Van Droogenbroeck J, Tjalma W, et al: Folate and Vitamin B(12) deficiency presenting as pancytopenia in pregnancy: A case report and review of the literature. *Eur J Obstet Gynecol Reprod Biol* 100:251, 2002.
24. Walker SP, Wein P, Ihle BU: Severe folate deficiency masquerading as the syndrome of hemolysis, elevated liver enzymes, and low platelets. *Obstet Gynecol* 90:655, 1997.
25. Mahomed K: Folate supplementation in pregnancy. *Cochrane Database Syst Rev* (2):CD000183, 2000.
26. Bruinse HW, van den Berg H: Changes of some vitamin levels during and after normal pregnancy. *Eur J Obstet Gynecol Reprod Biol* 61:31, 1995.
27. Frenkel EP, Yardley DA: Clinical and laboratory features and sequelae of deficiency of folic acid (folate) and vitamin B12 (cobalamin) in pregnancy and gynecology. *Hematol Oncol Clin North Am* 14:1079, 2000.
28. Aggio MC, Zunini C: Reversible pure red-cell aplasia in pregnancy. *N Engl J Med* 297:221, 1977.
29. Baker RI, Manoharan A, de Luca E, et al: Pure red cell aplasia of pregnancy: A distinct clinical entity. *Br J Haematol* 85:619, 1993.
30. Makino Y, Nagano M, Tamura K, et al: Pregnancy complicated with pure red cell aplasia: A case report. *J Perinat Med* 31:530, 2003.
31. Mant MJ: Chronic idiopathic pure red cell aplasia: Successful treatment during pregnancy and durable response to intravenous immunoglobulin. *J Intern Med* 236:593, 1994.
32. Thachil J, Toh C-H: Disseminated intravascular coagulation in obstetric disorders and its acute haematological management. *Blood Rev* 23: 167, 2009.
33. Erez O, Novack L, Beer-Weisel R, et al: DIC score in pregnant women—a population based modification of the International Society on Thrombosis and Hemostasis score. *PLoS One* 9:e93240, 2014.
34. Tuffnell DJ: Amniotic fluid embolism. *Curr Opin Obstet Gynecol* 15:119, 2003.
35. Awad IT, Shorten GD: Amniotic fluid embolism and isolated coagulopathy: Atypical presentation of amniotic fluid embolism. *Eur J Anaesthesiol* 18:410, 2001.
36. Clark SL: Amniotic Fluid Embolism. *Obstet Gynecol* 123:337, 2014.
37. Goldszmidt E, Davies S: Two cases of hemorrhage secondary to amniotic fluid embolus managed with uterine artery embolization. *Can J Anaesth* 50:917, 2003.
38. Letsky EA: Disseminated intravascular coagulation. *Best Pract Res Clin Obstet Gynaecol* 15:623, 2001.
39. Rodeghiero F: Von Willebrand disease: Pathogenesis and management. *Thromb Res* 131 Suppl 1:S47, 2013.
40. Romero R, Copel JA, Hobbins JC: Intrauterine fetal demise and hemostatic failure: The fetal death syndrome. *Clin Obstet Gynecol* 28:24, 1985.
41. Batlle J, Noya MS, Giangrande P, et al: Advances in the therapy of von Willebrand disease. *Haemophilia* 8:301, 2002.
42. Mathew P, Greist A, Maahs JA, et al: Type 2B vWD: The varied clinical manifestations in two kindreds. *Haemophilia* 9:137, 2003.
43. Rick ME, Williams SB, Sacher RA, et al: Thrombocytopenia associated with pregnancy in a patient with type IIB von Willebrand's disease. *Blood* 69:786, 1987.
44. Foster PA: The reproductive health of women with von Willebrand Disease unresponsive to DDAVP: Results of an international survey. On behalf of the Subcommittee on von Willebrand Factor of the Scientific and Standardization Committee of the ISTH. *Thromb Haemost* 74:784, 1995.
45. Nichols WL, Hultin MB, James AH, et al: von Willebrand disease (VWD): Evidence-based diagnosis and management guidelines, the National Heart, Lung, and Blood Institute (NHLBI) Expert Panel report (USA). *Haemophilia* 14:171, 2008.

46. Peyvandi F, Bidlingmaier C, Garagiola I. Management of pregnancy and delivery in women with inherited bleeding disorders. *Semin Fetal Neonatal Med* 16:311, 2011.
47. Briet E, Reisner HM, Blatt PM: Factor IX levels during pregnancy in a women with hemophilia B. *Haemostasis* 11:87, 1982.
48. Giangrande PL: Management of pregnancy in carriers of haemophilia. *Haemophilia* 4:779, 1998.
49. Tsui NB, Kadir RA, Chan KC, et al: Noninvasive prenatal diagnosis of hemophilia by microfluidic digital PCR analysis of maternal plasma DNA. *Blood* 117:3684, 2011.
50. Michiels JJ, Hamulyak K, Nieuwenhuis HK, et al: Acquired haemophilia A in women postpartum: Management of bleeding episodes and natural history of the factor VIII inhibitor. *Eur J Haematol* 59:105, 1997.
51. Solymoss S: Postpartum acquired factor VIII inhibitors: Results of a survey. *Am J Hematol* 59:1, 1998.
52. Kobayashi T, Terao T, Kojima T, et al: Congenital factor XIII deficiency with treatment of factor XIII concentrate and normal vaginal delivery. *Gynecol Obstet Invest* 29:235, 1990.
53. Rodeghiero F, Castaman GC, Di Bona E, et al: Successful pregnancy in a woman with congenital factor XIII deficiency treated with substitutive therapy. Report of a second case. *Blut* 55:45, 1987.
54. Burrows RF, Ray JG, Burrows EA: Bleeding risk and reproductive capacity among patients with factor XIII deficiency: A case presentation and review of the literature. *Obstet Gynecol Surv* 55:103, 2000.
55. Anwar R, Miloszewski KJ: Factor XIII deficiency. *Br J Haematol* 107:468, 1999.
56. Bornikova L, Peyvandi F, Allen G, et al: Fibrinogen replacement therapy for congenital fibrinogen deficiency. *J Thromb Haemost* 9:1687, 2011.
57. Burrows RF, Kelton JG: Fetal thrombocytopenia and its relation to maternal thrombocytopenia. *N Engl J Med* 329:1463, 1993.
58. George JN, Woolf SH, Raskob GE, et al: Idiopathic thrombocytopenic purpura: A practice guideline developed by explicit methods for the American Society of Hematology. *Blood* 88:3, 1996.
59. Kaplan C, Daffos F, Forestier F, et al: Fetal platelet counts in thrombocytopenic pregnancy. *Lancet* 336:979, 1990.
60. Cromwell C, Tarantino M, Aledort LM: Safety of anti-D during pregnancy. *Am J Hematol* 84:261, 2009.
61. Klink DT, van Elburg RM, Schreurs MW, van Well GT: Rituximab administration in third trimester of pregnancy suppresses neonatal B-cell development. *Clin Dev Immunol* 2008:271363, 2008.
62. http://www.accessdata.fda.gov/drugsatfda_docs/label/2014/022291Orig1s011lbl.pdf, http://www.accessdata.fda.gov/drugsatfda_docs/label/2014/125268s141lbl.pdf
63. Patil AS, Dotters-Katz SK, Metjian AD, et al: Use of a thrombopoietin mimetic for chronic immune thrombocytopenic purpura in pregnancy. *Obstet Gynecol* 122:483, 2013.
64. van Veen JJ, Nokes TJ, Makris M: The risk of spinal haematoma following neuraxial anaesthesia or lumbar puncture in thrombocytopeic individuals. *Br J Haematol* 148:15, 2010.
65. Valat AS, Caulier MT, Devos P, et al: Relationships between severe neonatal thrombocytopenia and maternal characteristics in pregnancies associated with autoimmune thrombocytopenia. *Br J Haematol* 103:397, 1998.
66. Martin JN Jr, Perry KG Jr, Blake PG, et al: Better maternal outcomes are achieved with dexamethasone therapy for postpartum HELLP (hemolysis, elevated liver enzymes, and thrombocytopenia) syndrome. *Am J Obstet Gynecol* 177:1011, 1997.
67. Woudstra DM, Chandra S, Hofmeyr GJ, Dowswell T: Corticosteroids for HELLP (hemolysis, elevated liver enzymes, low platelets) syndrome in pregnancy. *Cochrane Database Syst Rev* (9):CD008148, 2010.
68. Katz L, Amorim M, Souza JP, et al: COHELLP: Collaborative randomized controlled trial on corticosteroids in HELLP syndrome. *Reprod Health* 10:28, 2013.
69. Martin JN Jr, Blake PG, Perry KG Jr, et al: The natural history of HELLP syndrome: Patterns of disease progression and regression. *Am J Obstet Gynecol* 164:1500, 1991.
70. Martin JN Jr, Files JC, Blake PG, et al: Postpartum plasma exchange for atypical preeclampsia-eclampsia as HELLP (hemolysis, elevated liver enzymes, and low platelets) syndrome. *Am J Obstet Gynecol* 172:1107, 1995.
71. Rouget JP, Goudemand J, Ducloux G, et al: [Circulating anticoagulant, recurrent abortions and venous thrombosis: A new entity or a pre-lupus syndrome? 2 cases] [in French]. *Ann Med Interne (Paris)* 134:111, 1983.
72. Kutteh WH: Antiphospholipid antibodies and reproduction. *J Reprod Immunol* 35:151, 1997.
73. Rai RS, Clifford K, Cohen H, et al: High prospective fetal loss rate in untreated pregnancies of women with recurrent miscarriage and antiphospholipid antibodies. *Hum Reprod* 10:3301, 1995.
74. Pengo V, Banzato A, Bison E, et al: What have we learned about antiphospholipid syndrome from patients and antiphospholipid carrier cohorts? *Semin Thromb Hemost* 38:322, 2012.
75. Rai R, Cohen H, Dave M, et al: Randomised controlled trial of aspirin and aspirin plus heparin in pregnant women with recurrent miscarriage associated with phospholipid antibodies (or antiphospholipid antibodies). *BMJ* 314:253, 1997.
76. Brodsky RA: How I treat paroxysmal nocturnal hemoglobinuria. *Blood* 113:6522, 2009.
77. Martinelli I, Taioli E, Cetin I, et al: Mutations in coagulation factors in women with unexplained late fetal loss. *N Engl J Med* 343:1015, 2000.
78. Ridker PM, Miletich JP, Buring JE, et al: Factor V Leiden mutation as a risk factor for recurrent pregnancy loss. *Ann Intern Med* 128:1000, 1998.
79. Rey E, Kahn SR, David M, et al: Thrombophilic disorders and fetal loss: A meta-analysis. *Lancet* 361:901, 2003.
80. Greer IA: Thrombophilia: Implications for pregnancy outcome. *Thromb Res* 109:73, 2003.
81. Morrison ER, Miedzybrodzka ZH, Campbell DM, et al: Prothrombotic genotypes are not associated with pre-eclampsia and gestational hypertension: Results from a large population-based study and systematic review. *Thromb Haemost* 87:779, 2002.
82. Gerhardt A, Scharf RE, Beckmann MW, et al: Prothrombin and factor V mutations in women with a history of thrombosis during pregnancy and the puerperium. *N Engl J Med* 342:374, 2000.
83. Grandone E, Tomaiuolo M, Colaizzo D, et al: Role of thrombophilia in adverse obstetric outcomes and their prevention using antithrombotic therapy. *Semin Thromb Hemost* 35:630, 2009.
84. Macklon NS, Greer IA, Bowman AW: An ultrasound study of gestational and postural changes in the deep venous system of the leg in pregnancy. *Br J Obstet Gynaecol* 104:191, 1997.
85. Cockett FB, Thomas ML: The iliac compression syndrome. *Br J Surg* 52:816, 1965.
86. Ginsberg JS, Brill-Edwards P, Burrows RF, et al: Venous thrombosis during pregnancy: Leg and trimester of presentation. *Thromb Haemost* 67:519, 1992.
87. Conard J, Horellou MH, Van Dreden P, et al: Thrombosis and pregnancy in congenital deficiencies in AT III, protein C or protein S: Study of 78 women. *Thromb Haemost* 63:319, 1990.
88. Battinelli EM, Marshall A, Connors JM: The role of thrombophilia in pregnancy. *Thrombosis* 2013:516420, 2013.
89. Robertson L, Wu O, Langhorne P, et al: Thrombophilia in pregnancy: A systematic review. *Br J Haematol* 132:171, 2006.
90. Benedetto C, Marozio L, Tavella AM, et al: Coagulation disorders in pregnancy: Acquired and inherited thrombophilias. *Ann N Y Acad Sci* 1205:106, 2010.
91. Chabloz P, Reber G, Boehlen F, et al: TAFI antigen and D-dimer levels during normal pregnancy and at delivery. *Br J Haematol* 115:150, 2001.
92. Paniccia R, Prisco D, Bandinelli B, et al: Plasma and serum levels of D-dimer and their correlations with other hemostatic parameters in pregnancy. *Thromb Res* 105:257, 2002.
93. Kobayashi T, Tokunaga N, Sugimura M, et al: Coagulation/fibrinolysis disorder in patients with severe preeclampsia. *Semin Thromb Hemost* 25:451, 1999.
94. Brill-Edwards P, Ginsberg JS, Gent M, et al: Safety of withholding heparin in pregnant women with a history of venous thromboembolism. Recurrence of Clot in This Pregnancy Study Group. *N Engl J Med* 343:1439, 2000.
95. Pabinger I, Grafenhofer H, Kyrle PA, et al: Temporary increase in the risk for recurrence during pregnancy in women with a history of venous thromboembolism. *Blood* 100:1060, 2002.
96. Ageno W, Crotti S, Turpie AG: The safety of antithrombotic therapy during pregnancy. *Expert Opin Drug Saf* 3:113, 2004.
97. Bates SM, Greer IA, Middeldorp S, et al: Venous thromboembolism, thrombophilia antithrombotic therapy, and pregnancy. American College of Chest Physicians Evidence-Based Clinical Practice Guidelines (9th ed.). *Chest* 141(2 Suppl):e691S, 2012.
98. Bauer KA: Management of thrombophilia. *J Thromb Haemost* 1:1429, 2003.
99. Bowles L, Cohen H: Inherited thrombophilias and anticoagulation in pregnancy. *Best Pract Res Clin Obstet Gynaecol* 17:471, 2003.
100. Ginsberg JS, Bates SM: Management of venous thromboembolism during pregnancy. *J Thromb Haemost* 1:1435, 2003.
101. Kearon C, Crowther M, Hirsh J: Management of patients with hereditary hypercoagulable disorders. *Annu Rev Med* 51:169, 2000.
102. Schafer AI, Levine MN, Konkle BA, et al: Thrombotic disorders: Diagnosis and treatment. *Hematology Am Soc Hematol Educ Program* 520, 2003.
103. Clark SL, Porter TF, West FG: Coumarin derivatives and breast-feeding. *Obstet Gynecol* 95:938, 2000.
104. Ward FT, Weiss RB: Lymphoma and pregnancy. *Semin Oncol* 16:397, 1989.
105. Doll DC, Ringenberg QS, Yarbro JW: Antineoplastic agents and pregnancy. *Semin Oncol* 16:337, 1989.
106. Nisce LZ, Tome MA, He S, et al: Management of coexisting Hodgkin's disease and pregnancy. *Am J Clin Oncol* 9:146, 1986.
107. Woo SY, Fuller LM, Cundiff JH, et al: Radiotherapy during pregnancy for clinical stages IA-IIA Hodgkin's disease. *Int J Radiat Oncol Biol Phys* 23:407, 1992.
108. Chen J, Lee RJ, Tsodikov A, et al: Does radiotherapy around the time of pregnancy for Hodgkin's disease modify the risk of breast cancer? *Int J Radiat Oncol Biol Phys* 58:1474, 2004.
109. Kal HB, Struikmans H. Radiotherapy during pregnancy: Fact and fiction. *Lancet Oncol* 6:328, 2005.
110. Gelb AB, van de Rijn M, Warnke RA, et al: Pregnancy-associated lymphomas. A clinicopathologic study. *Cancer* 78:304, 1996.
111. Bobrow LG, Richards MA, Happerfield LC, et al: Breast lymphomas: A clinicopathologic review. *Hum Pathol* 24:274, 1993.
112. Brogi E, Harris NL: Lymphomas of the breast: Pathology and clinical behavior. *Semin Oncol* 26:357, 1999.
113. Horowitz NA, Benyamini N, Wohlfart K: Reproductive organ involvement in non-Hodgkin lymphoma during pregnancy: A systematic review. *Lancet Oncol* 14:e275, 2013.
114. Aviles A, Diaz-Maqueo JC, Talavera A, et al: Growth and development of children of mothers treated with chemotherapy during pregnancy: Current status of 43 children. *Am J Hematol* 36:243, 1991.

115. Aviles A, Neri N: Hematological malignancies and pregnancy: A final report of 84 children who received chemotherapy in utero. *Clin Lymphoma* 2:173, 2001.
116. Herold M, Schnohr S, Bittrich H: Efficacy and safety of a combined rituximab chemotherapy during pregnancy. *J Clin Oncol* 19:3439, 2001.
117. Kimby E, Sverrisdottir A, Elinder G: Safety of rituximab therapy during the first trimester of pregnancy: A case history. *Eur J Haematol* 72:292, 2004.
118. Chakravarty EF, Murray ER, Kelman A, Farmer P: Pregnancy outcomes after maternal exposure to rituximab. *Blood* 117:1499, 2011.
119. Catanzarite VA, Ferguson JE, 2nd: Acute leukemia and pregnancy: A review of management and outcome, 1972–1982. *Obstet Gynecol Surv* 39:663, 1984.
120. Yahia C, Hyman GA, Phillips LL: Acute leukemia and pregnancy. *Obstet Gynecol Surv* 13:1, 1958.
121. Pavlidis NA: Coexistence of pregnancy and malignancy. *Oncologist* 7:279, 2002.
122. Kawamura S, Yoshiike M, Shimoyama T, et al: Management of acute leukemia during pregnancy: From the results of a nationwide questionnaire survey and literature survey. *Tohoku J Exp Med* 174:167, 1994.
123. Ebert U, Loffler H, Kirch W: Cytotoxic therapy and pregnancy. *Pharmacol Ther* 74:207, 1997.
124. Cardonick E, Iacobucci A: Use of chemotherapy during human pregnancy. *Lancet Oncol* 5:283, 2004.
125. Delgado-Lamas JL, Garces-Ruiz OM: Malignancy: Case report: Acute promyelocytic leukemia in late pregnancy. Successful treatment with all-*trans*-retinoic acid (ATRA) and chemotherapy. *Hematology* 4:415, 2000.
126. Giagounidis AA, Beckmann MW, Giagounidis AS, et al: Acute promyelocytic leukemia and pregnancy. *Eur J Haematol* 64:267, 2000.
127. Lipovsky MM, Biesma DH, Christiaens GC, et al: Successful treatment of acute promyelocytic leukaemia with all-*trans*-retinoic-acid during late pregnancy. *Br J Haematol* 94:699, 1996.
128. Gupta D, Bagel B, Gujral S: Parenthood in patients of acute promyelocytic leukemia after treatment with arsenic trioxide: A case series. *Leuk Lymphoma* 53:2192, 2012.
129. Pejovic T, Schwartz PE: Leukemias. *Clin Obstet Gynecol* 45:866, 2002.
130. Baer MR, Ozer H, Foon KA: Interferon-alpha therapy during pregnancy in chronic myelogenous leukaemia and hairy cell leukaemia. *Br J Haematol* 81:167, 1992.
131. Bazarbashi MS, Smith MR, Karanes C, et al: Successful management of Ph chromosome chronic myelogenous leukemia with leukapheresis during pregnancy. *Am J Hematol* 38:235, 1991.
132. Delmer A, Rio B, Bauduer F, et al: Pregnancy during myelosuppressive treatment for chronic myelogenous leukemia. *Br J Haematol* 82:783, 1992.
133. Gleevec package insert. Novartis Pharmaceuticals, East Hanover, NJ, 2001.
134. Asker C, Norstedt Wikner B, Kallen B. Use of antiemetic drugs during pregnancy in Sweden. *Eur J Clin Pharmacol* 61: 899, 2005.
135. Cottle TE, Fier CJ, Donadieu J, Kinsey SE: Risk and benefit of treatment of severe chronic neutropenia with granulocyte colony-stimulating factor. *Semin Hematol* 39:134, 2002.
136. Milojkovic D, Apperley JF: How I treat leukemia during pregnancy. *Blood* 123:974, 2014.
137. Griesshammer M, Grunewald M, Michiels JJ: Acquired thrombophilia in pregnancy: Essential thrombocythemia. *Semin Thromb Hemost* 29:205, 2003.
138. Barbui T, Barosi G, Grossi A, et al: Practice guidelines for the therapy of essential thrombocythemia. A statement from the Italian Society of Hematology, the Italian Society of Experimental Hematology and the Italian Group for Bone Marrow Transplantation. *Haematologica* 89:215, 2004.
139. Elliott MA, Tefferi A: Thrombocythaemia and pregnancy. *Best Pract Res Clin Haematol* 16:227, 2003.
140. Randi ML, Rossi C, Fabris F, et al: Essential thrombocythemia in young adults: Major thrombotic complications and complications during pregnancy—A follow-up study in 68 patients. *Clin Appl Thromb Hemost* 6:31, 2000.
141. Griesshammer M, Bergmann L, Pearson T: Fertility, pregnancy and the management of myeloproliferative disorders. *Baillieres Clin Haematol* 11:859, 1998.
142. Randi ML, Bertozzi I, Rumi E et al: Pregnancy complications predict thrombotic events in young women with essential thrombocythemia. *Am J Hematol* 89:306, 2014.
143. Silver RT: Interferon alfa: Effects of long-term treatment for polycythemia vera. *Semin Hematol* 34:40, 1997.
144. Spivak JL: Polycythemia vera: Myths, mechanisms, and management. *Blood* 100:4272, 2002.
145. Pastore LM, Savitz DA, Thorp JM Jr: Predictors of urinary tract infection at the first prenatal visit. *Epidemiology* 10:282, 1999.
146. Stamilio DM, Sehdev HM, Macones GA: Pregnant women with the sickle cell trait are not at increased risk for developing preeclampsia. *Am J Perinatol* 20:41, 2003.
147. Thinkhamrop J, Apiwantanakul S, Lumbiganon P, et al: Iron status in anemic pregnant women. *J Obstet Gynaecol Res* 29:160, 2003.
148. Diav-Citrin O, Hunnisett L, Sher GD, et al: Hydroxyurea use during pregnancy: A case report in sickle cell disease and review of the literature. *Am J Hematol* 60:148, 1999.
149. Villers MS, Jamison MG, DeCastro LM, James AH: Morbidity associated with sickle cell disease in pregnancy. *Am J Obstet Gynecol* 199:125.e1, 2008.
150. Okusanya BO, Oladapo OT: Prophylactic versus selective blood transfusion for sickle cell disease in pregnancy. *Cochrane Database Syst Rev* 12:CD010378, 2013.
151. Koshy M, Burd L: Management of pregnancy in sickle cell syndromes. *Hematol Oncol Clin North Am* 5:585, 1991.
152. Rappaport VJ, Velazquez M, Williams K: Hemoglobinopathies in pregnancy. *Obstet Gynecol Clin North Am* 31:287, 2004.
153. Finer P, Blair J, Rowe P: Epidural analgesia in the management of labor pain and sickle cell crisis—A case report. *Anesthesiology* 68:799, 1988.
154. Aessopos A, Karabatsos F, Farmakis D, et al: Pregnancy in patients with well-treated beta-thalassemia: Outcome for mothers and newborn infants. *Am J Obstet Gynecol* 180:360, 1999.
155. Ibba RM, Zoppi MA, Floris M, et al: Neural tube defects in the offspring of thalassemia carriers. *Fetal Diagn Ther* 18:5, 2003.
156. Tamakoudis P, Tsatalas C, Mamopoulos M, et al: Transfusion-dependent homozygous beta-thalassemia major: Successful pregnancy in five cases. *Eur J Obstet Gynecol Reprod Biol* 74:127, 1997.
157. Rachmilewitz EA, Giardina PJ: How I treat thalassemia. *Blood* 118:3479, 2011.
158. Kumar RM, Rizk DE, Khuranna A: Beta-thalassemia major and successful pregnancy. *J Reprod Med* 42:294, 1997.
159. Singer ST, Vichinsky EP: Deferoxamine treatment during pregnancy: Is it harmful? *Am J Hematol* 60:24, 1999.

CHAPTER 9
HEMATOLOGY IN OLDER PERSONS

William B. Ershler, Andrew S. Artz, and Bindu Kanapuru

SUMMARY

This chapter presents a current appraisal of our understanding of aging followed by a more detailed description of age-associated changes in hematopoiesis and their clinical consequences. Those who are older than the age of 75 years comprise a rapidly growing segment of the population. Marrow, like other organs, undergoes characteristic changes with advancing age, and many of these changes are evident by standard examination. For example, within the marrow space, hematopoietic cells occupy approximately one-half the volume at mid-life, with adipose tissue making up the difference. Yet, in the absence of disease, blood counts are generally maintained within a range established as normal for younger individuals. This is possible because hematopoietic stem cells increase in number with age and are of sufficient functional capacity to respond to homeostatic signals. Older people are more likely to have chronic diseases that may produce additional stress on marrow reserve. Anemia, for example, is present in just over 10 percent of community-dwelling individuals older than age 65 years; for those residing in nursing homes, the prevalence is closer to 50 percent. One distinction between anemias in older people compared with younger people is that for approximately one-third of older anemic patients, a specific cause for the anemia cannot be determined. This "unexplained anemia" is likely the result of multiple factors, including inappropriately low erythropoietin response, inflammatory cytokines, androgen deficiency, and, in some persons, incipient myelodysplasia. Platelet and neutrophil changes with age have been incompletely characterized but are likely to be subtle and of little clinical consequence. There is a well-characterized, age-associated involution of the thymus gland that precedes the histologic changes within the marrow, and marrow-derived T- and B-cell precursors are affected. Older people have fewer naïve, reactive T cells and an increase in relatively inert memory T cells. Thus, the capacity to react to new antigenic challenges is reduced and there is an increased susceptibility to certain infections and vaccines. Also evident are deficient regulatory functions, which may explain the observed increase in autoantibody, paraproteins, and inflammatory cytokines in those of advanced age. In the absence of disease, however, these alterations are of little consequence. In the presence of chronic debilitating disease, they are likely to become more pronounced and as such, contribute to an exaggerated decline in overall function. Similar conclusions can be drawn regarding

Acronyms and Abbreviations: EPESE, Established Populations for the Epidemiological Study of the Elderly; HSCs, hematopoietic stem cells; IADL, independent activities of daily living; IL, interleukin; NHANES III, National Health and Nutrition Examination Survey III; PAI-1, plasminogen activating inhibitor-I; TNF, tumor necrosis factor; UA, unexplained anemia; WHO, World Health Organization.

dysregulated inflammatory pathways and coagulation. In balance, advancing age is associated with a procoagulant profile that may be of clinical importance in the presence of underlying atherosclerotic vascular disease.

A PRIMER ON AGING

The world's population is aging at an unprecedented rate and the implications for health care delivery are profound.[1-4] Over the next several decades, the percentage of the population older than age 65 years will nearly double.[5] In anticipation, an increased research effort is being made to better understand the basic biology of aging and the mechanisms whereby individuals become susceptible to disease.[6,7]

A central dogma of gerontology is that aging is not a disease. Yet, intrinsic biologic aging is the major risk factor for virtually all major diseases of developed societies, including cancer, diabetes, atherosclerotic cardiovascular and cerebrovascular disease, diabetes, neurodegenerative diseases (e.g., Alzheimer and Parkinson), osteoporosis and infection. Examination of the mechanisms by which biologic aging contributes to the pathogenesis of these diseases has now become recognized in the mainstream of scientific inquiry over a broad range of disciplines.[7] However, from a biogerontologist's perspective, there remain certain features of aging that transcend the more discipline-focused investigations.

One of these common features of aging is heterogeneity. For example, for any measureable variable, the range of values among normal older individuals is much wider than the range of normal among younger individuals.[8,9] This variation is particularly relevant for hematologists consulted to examine older, but otherwise healthy, individuals with laboratory values outside the "normal range."

Although functional declines that accompany normal aging have been well characterized,[10,11] in general these are not of sufficient magnitude to account for symptoms or be mistaken for disease. For example, that kidney function declines with age is well recognized,[12,13] and, in fact, has proven to be a useful biologic marker of aging. Yet, clinical consequences of this change in renal function, in the absence of a disease or the exposure to an exogenous nephrotoxic agent, do not occur commonly. Similarly, the marrow changes with age. Marrow stem cells increase in number and proliferative capacity, yet the *in vitro* proliferative potential of progenitor cells is less.[14-16] Although clinically significant cytopenias do not occur in the absence of disease, mild to moderate anemia that has not been fully characterized occurs with increasing frequency, especially in the frail elderly.[17-20] Furthermore, in frail individuals even a mild reduction in hemoglobin level is associated with untoward clinical outcomes.[19,21,22]

Certain immune functions decrease with age,[23-25] but these may be of only marginal clinical significance. For example, whether the laboratory-observed declines in immune function contribute to a heightened susceptibility to infection is a subject of debate, but data support an association of age-associated qualitative change in lymphocyte function and susceptibility to reactivation of tuberculosis[26,27] or herpes zoster[28,29] and diminished response to influenza vaccine.[30-33] There is compelling evidence that a profound decline in immunity is causally related to certain malignancies,[34] but there remains debate over whether the more modest decline associated with normal aging is sufficient to account for the observed increased rate of cancer in the elderly.[35,36] In fact, there is some evidence that cancer incidence is even lower in frail elderly;[37] a population known to be functionally immunodeficient.[38] Similarly, development of autoantibodies appear with increasing frequency with advancing age, but these are considered markers of an acquired humoral immune dysregulation, and with regard to autoantibody, not of clinical importance.[39] In contrast, essential monoclonal gammopathy, a clonal B lymphocyte expansion that increases in frequency with age and that stabilizes at a clone size that does not impair normal immunoglobulin synthesis or inhibit hematopoiesis, does have a probability of undergoing clonal evolution to a B-cell malignancy, such as myeloma, lymphoma, or monoclonal light-chain amyloidosis at a rate of 1 percent per year (Chap. 106).[40]

THEORIES OF AGING

Providing a rational, unifying explanation for the aging process has been the subject of a great number of theoretical expositions. Yet, no single proposal suffices to account for the complexities observed (Table 9–1).

Genetic Effects

That genetic controls are involved seems obvious when one considers that lifespan is highly species-specific. For example, mice generally live approximately 30 months and humans approximately 90 years. However, the aging phenomenon is not necessarily a direct consequence of primary DNA sequence. For example, mice and bats have 0.25 percent difference in their primary DNA sequence, but bats live for 25 years, 10 times longer than mice. Thus, regulation of gene expression seems likely to be the major source of species longevity differences.

Progeria Syndromes Gerontologists have long been intrigued by the concept of accelerated aging and by examining those rare individuals who are so affected. From work with invertebrate models a number of genes have been identified that associate with longevity. Yet, the identification and functional analysis of analogous genes in humans remains elusive. With regard to genetic examples of accelerated aging, two syndromes have been well characterized: Hutchison-Guilford syndrome (early-onset progeria) and Werner syndrome (adult-onset progeria).[41,42] Although neither these nor other progeria syndromes manifest a complete phenotype of advanced age, the identification of the genes responsible for these particular syndromes is beginning to pay dividends by providing clues to the molecular mechanisms involved in the aging process. For example, Werner syndrome is now defined by mutations in a single gene on chromosome 8 that encodes a protein containing a helicase-like domain.[43,44] The activity of the Werner protein helps to maintain telomere structure and homology-dependent recombination.[45] Similarly, a mutation in the lamin A (*LMNA*) gene localized to chromosome 1 has been causally related to the Hutchison-Guilford syndrome.[46] The product of the mutated *LMNA* gene (termed *progerin*) accumulates, producing a variety of nuclear distortions of which telomere dysfunction and associated replicative senescence are notable.[47]

Examination of aging in yeast has also been informative with regard to the genetic controls of aging. These single-cell organisms follow the replicative limits of mammalian cells and it has been observed that "life span" is related to silencing large chromosomal regions. Mutations in these silencing genes lead to increased longevity.[48]

Thus, if there are certain genes that regulate normal aging, or at least are associated with the development of an aged phenotype, it stands to reason that acquired mutations of those genes might influence the rate of aging. Over the years several theories have been proposed that relate to this supposition. In general, they hypothesize a random or stochastic accumulation of damage, either to DNA or protein that leads eventually to dysfunctional cells, cell death and subsequent organ dysfunction, and ultimately death. Prominent among these is the *somatic mutation* theory,[49] which predicts that genetic damage from background radiation, for example, accumulates and produces mutations that ultimately result in functional decline. A variety of refinements have been suggested to this theory, invoking the importance of mutational interactions,[50] transposable elements,[51] and changes in DNA methylation status.[52]

A related hypothesis is Burnet's *intrinsic mutagenesis* theory,[53] which proposes that spontaneous or endogenous mutations occur at different rates in different species and that this accounts for the variability observed in life span. Closely related to this notion is the *DNA repair* theory.[54] Initially, there was great excitement about this idea as it was found that long-lived animals had demonstrably more active DNA repair mechanisms than shorter-lived species.[54] However, longitudinal studies within a species have not revealed a consistent decline in repair mechanisms with age. This, of course, does not rule out the possibility that repair of certain specific and critical DNA lesions is altered with advancing age. We now understand that there are multiple DNA repair mechanisms, including base excision repair, transcription-coupled repair, and even mitochondrial DNA repair mechanisms. Disorders involving one or a subset of repair mechanisms could lead to accumulation of DNA damage and dysfunction.

In yet another intrinsic/stochastic model, Orgel[55] proposed the *error catastrophe* theory in which he suggested that random errors in protein synthesis occur and when the proteins involved are those responsible for DNA or RNA synthesis, there is resultant DNA damage and the consequences thereof to daughter cells. Although this model has appeal, there has been no reported evidence for impaired or inaccurate protein synthesis machinery with advancing age. However, a candidate protein that may eventually be shown to be so affected is telomerase. This critical enzyme is necessary for maintaining telomere length and cell replicative potential. *In vitro* cellular senescence is associated with diminished telomerase activity,[56] but whether this relates to aging of the organism as a whole remains controversial.[57]

Posttranslational Effects

Evidence that exogenous factors are involved in the acquisition of age-associated damage to DNA and protein is derived from a number of observations, many of which are circumstantial or correlative, but nonetheless provocative. It now appears that the accumulation of abnormal protein within senescent cells, as predicted by the *error catastrophe* theory, actually reflects posttranslational events, such as oxidation or glycation, and resultant crosslinking. There is theoretic appeal to the concept that key proteins, such as collagen or other extracellular matrix proteins, and DNA become dysfunctional with age as a consequence of the impairment produced by these crosslinks.[58-60]

Glycation One mechanism producing crosslinks is called *glycation*, the nonenzymatic reaction of glucose with the amino groups of proteins. Presumably, glycation would occur more readily in the presence of higher serum levels of glucose, and, thus, this theory fits well with the observed, age-associated dysregulation of glucose metabolism and prevalent hyperglycemia in geriatric populations. Of course, these

TABLE 9–1. Theories of Aging	
Intrinsic-stochastic	Somatic mutation[50,51]
	Intrinsic mutagenesis[55]
	Impaired DNA repair[56]
	Error catastrophe[58]
Extrinsic-stochastic	Ionizing radiation[50,51,53,58]
	Free radical[63,64]
Genetically determined	Neuroendocrine[298]
	Immune[77]

findings also point out the theory's deficiency as a unifying mechanism, as there is no question that individuals with well-maintained glucose levels throughout their life span will still be subject to the acquired changes typical of aging.

Free Radical Hypothesis

Another mechanism held responsible for crosslinking is the damage produced by free radicals, which forms the basis of the *free radical hypothesis* initially promoted by Harman.[61,62] This theory offers that aging is the result of DNA and protein damage (e.g., mutagenesis or crosslinking) by atoms or molecules that contain unpaired electrons (free radicals). These highly reactive species are produced as byproducts of a variety of metabolic processes and are normally inhibited by intrinsic cellular antioxidant defense mechanisms. Nitrate-based free radicals are also generated by *in vivo* processes and another set of nitrogen free-radical scavenging mechanisms are in place. If free radical generation increases with age, or the defense mechanisms that scavenge free radicals (e.g., glutathione) or repair free radical damage decline, the accumulated free radical damage may account for altered DNA and protein function. Evidence to support this widely held notion is incomplete. It is known that free radical generation in mammals correlates inversely with longevity[63] and, similarly, the level of free radical inhibiting enzymes, such as superoxide dismutase were higher in those species with longer life spans.[63] However, efforts at enhancing antioxidant mechanisms with dietary vitamin E have resulted in only a modest enhancement of median survival in mice and no effect on maximum life span.[64–66]

Much attention has been focused on mitochondrial function in the context of free radical damage because the bulk of oxidative metabolism and the production of reactive oxygen species occur in these organelles. Although mitochondrial DNA codes for antioxidant enzymes in addition to enzymes involved in energy production, it is currently believed that energy production declines with age as a result of mitochondrial DNA damage by those reactive products. Indeed, mitochondrial damage increases with age in experimental models,[67–69] and the shortened survival of knockout mice deficient in mitochondrial antioxidant enzymes has supported the potential importance of this mechanism.[70]

The most compelling data to date in support of the free radical hypothesis come from experiments in which transgenic *Drosophila* producing enhanced levels of superoxide dismutase and catalase had a maximum survival 33 percent greater than controls.[26] Furthermore, it is known that flies produce high levels of free radicals associated with their impressive metabolic requirements, and that survival is enhanced dramatically when the ability to fly is experimentally hindered.[65] However, the generalizability of these findings has been questioned. It has been noted that transgenic mice overexpressing free radical scavenging enzymes have produced very modest effects on life span.[71] Thus, the conclusion that augmentation of free radical scavenging mechanisms increases longevity in mammalian species is not established.

Neuroendocrine Theory

From a different perspective, very good evidence implicates a nonrandom, perhaps genetically regulated endogenous mechanism involved in aging. For example, the *neuroendocrine* theory suggests that the decrements in neuronal and associated hormonal function are central to aging. It has been suggested that age-associated decline of hypothalamic–pituitary–adrenal axis function results in a physiologic cascade leading, ultimately, to the "frail" phenotype. This hypothesis is appealing because it is well established that this neuroendocrine axis regulates much of development and also the involution of ovarian and testicular function. Furthermore, age-associated declines in growth hormone and related factors,[72] dehydroepiandrosterone,[73] and secondary sex steroids[74]

are implicated in age-associated impairments, including a reduction in lean body mass and bone density. Furthermore, pharmacologic reconstitution using these or related hormones has met with some success at reversing age-associated functional decline.[75,76]

Immunologic Theory

Similarly, it has been argued that involution of the thymus gland and subsequent decline in immune function discussed below is a key regulator of aging.[77] The argument is based upon the observation that the decline in immune function occurs in all mammalian species, but occurs later in those with longer survival.[78] Furthermore, dietary restriction is associated with maintained thymic mass and measurable immune function as well as prolonged survival, suggesting an association of a decline in immunity with primary aging processes.

The possibility is highlighted by the observation that differences in maximum survival of different mouse strains has been associated with specific alleles in the major histocompatibility complex, which, in turn, code for immunologic determinants.[79] This hypothesis, although not without its appeal, is not widely accepted as a major explanation for aging. Perhaps this relates to the fact that biologic aging is a universal phenomenon and certain features are held in common, even in organisms with primitive or no immune function. (The same could also be said for the neuroendocrine theory.) It is obvious that the immune system is of great importance in minimizing the chance of early death, particularly from infectious diseases. However, immunologic reconstitution of middle aged or old animals has not been shown to prolong survival.[80]

LIFE SPAN: MEDIAN AND MAXIMUM SURVIVAL

From the perspective of those who study aging, an important distinction is made between median (life expectancy) and maximum life span. Over the past century, a dramatic increase in median survival has been mostly attributable to modern sanitation and refrigeration, as well as public health measures, including vaccination and antibiotics.[81] Early deaths have been diminished and more individuals are reaching old age. In the United States today, expected survival from birth is approximately 80 years.[82] Median survival is what concerns public health officials and healthcare providers. In contrast, maximum survival is the focus of those gerontologists interested in the biology of aging and longevity.

The oldest human being alive today is approximately 120 years old. It is intriguing that the oldest age limit has remained stable, unchanged by the public health initiatives mentioned above. In the laboratory, limits on age have been established for a variety of species. *Drosophila*, free of predators, disease or fly swatters, can live 30 days, whereas C57BL/6 mice in a laboratory environment and allowed to eat a healthy diet *ad libitum*, may survive 40 months. Unlike health-related interventions in humans, certain experimental interventions in lower species are associated with a prolongation of maximum survival. In *Drosophila*, for example, transgenic offspring producing extra copies of the free radical scavenging enzymes superoxide dismutase and catalase survive approximately 33 percent longer than controls.[83] In nutritional intervention studies involving lower species, controlled restriction of dietary intake (dietary restriction) has become a common experimental paradigm exploited in the investigation of primary processes of aging and maximum survival.[84,85]

Dietary Restriction

Dietary restriction typically involves a reduction of 30 to 40 percent in caloric intake with careful attention to the provision of adequate amounts of essential nutrients. It is associated with both a delay in the acquisition of age-related diseases (including cancer) and a reduction in the rate of achieving certain established biomarkers of aging (i.e., a retardation in primary aging). The critical questions remain: What is the mechanism of the effect of dietary restriction, and will it be applicable to higher species? With regard to the latter, there are now comprehensive and interactive studies within the United States in which dietary restriction is being examined in nonhuman primates[86,87] and human studies are also underway.[88,89] Although it appears that the calorie restricted monkeys in these studies are assuming a more youthful phenotype in a variety of physiologic measures,[86,90,91] it remains too early to predict whether maximum survival will be affected.

CELLULAR SENESCENCE AND ORGANISMAL AGING

After a finite number of divisions, normal somatic cells invariably enter a state of irreversibly arrested growth, a process termed *replicative senescence*.[92] In fact, it has been proposed that escape from the regulators of senescence is what oncologists term *malignant transformation*. However, the role of replicative senescence as an explanation of organismal aging remains the subject of vigorous debate (for review, see references 93 and 94). The controversy relates, in part, to the fact that certain organisms (e.g., *Drosophila, Cunninghamella elegans*) undergo an aging process, yet all of their adult cells are postreplicative.

What is clear is that the loss of proliferative capacity of human cells in culture is intrinsic to the cells and not dependent on environmental factors or even culture conditions.[92] Unless transformation occurs, cells age with each successive division. The number of divisions turns out to be more important than the actual amount of time passed. Thus, cells held in a quiescent state for months, when allowed back into a proliferative environment, will continue approximately the same number of divisions as those that were allowed to proliferate without a quiescent period.[95] The question remains whether this *in vitro* phenomenon is relevant to animal aging.[95] Although when various species are compared, replicative potential is directly and significantly related to life span,[96] within an organism there is great variability in proliferative capacity from tissue to tissue and organ to organ. As such, age-associated changes in the marrow or gut might relate to replicative senescence, whereas in muscle or brain other processes most certainly are involved. But, added to this heterogeneity within an individual, is that fact that certain commonly employed models of aging (e.g., *Drosophila, C. elegans*) undergo an aging process despite a long held belief that all of their adult cells were post replicative.[94,97,98] However, this notion has been countered by the demonstration of multipotent intestinal stem cells within the midgut near the intestinal basement membrane of *Drosophila*.[99] Unlike intestinal stem cells in vertebrates that interact with stromal cells within a niche, analogous cells within *Drosophila* reside on the surface of the basement membrane and interact directly with daughter cells. Nevertheless, the presence of such cells has rekindled an interest in *Drosophila* as a model for stem cell biology, cancer, and whole-animal aging.[100,101]

CELLULAR SENESCENCE AND CANCER

A feature of cellular senescence is diminished proliferative capacity. In fact, it is now understood that genes considered tumor suppressors (e.g., p53, RB [retinoblastoma gene]) prevent cancer by inducing programmed cell death (apoptosis), particularly in cells at risk for neoplastic transformation. Alternatively, they can prevent potential cancer cells from proliferating by inducing permanent withdrawal from the cell cycle (cellular senescence). Although little is known about how cells choose between apoptotic and senescence responses, both are crucial for suppressing cancer[102,103] and both are highly relevant to functional decline and longevity.[104]

There are a multitude of oncogenic stimuli that may result in either cancerous transformation or cellular senescence.[105,106] Epigenetic changes within chromatin, histones, or nucleic acids may be caused by pharmacologic agents or altered expression of proteins.[107-109] Such changes can alter the expression of protooncogenes or tumor-suppressor genes and are a frequent occurrence among malignant tumors. Thus the senescence response aborts the uncontrolled proliferative response an assortment of potentially oncogenic stimuli.

Although diverse stimuli can induce a senescence response, they appear to converge on one or both of the two pathways that establish and maintain the senescence growth arrest. These pathways are governed by the gatekeeper tumor-suppressor proteins p53 and pRB.[104,110,111] Furthermore, the senescence response to dysfunctional telomeres requires the integrity of the p53 pathway.[112,113] Overexpression of the *RAS* gene may also trigger a p53-dependent damage response by producing high levels of reactive oxygen species.[113-115] However, oncogenic RAS can also induce p16, an activator of the pRB pathways, which provides a second barrier to the proliferation of potentially oncogenic cells. There is an emerging consensus that senescence occurs through one pathway or the other, with the p53 pathway mediating senescence primarily as a result of telomere dysfunction and DNA damage and p16/pRB pathway–mediating senescence primarily as a result of oncogenes, chromatin disruption, and various stresses.

A more speculative, but potentially important consequence of cellular senescence may be its impact on stem cells.[116] Embryonic stem cells, whether human or rodent, express a high level of telomerase and thus are considered resistant to replicative senescence.[117,118] However, mammalian adult stem cells or progenitor cells do not proliferate indefinitely.[119-122] The ability of stem cells to undergo senescence and apoptosis is likely to be an important mechanism for preventing cancer.[123,124]

● AGING AND HEMATOPOIESIS

Aging is a universal phenomenon that affects all normal cells, tissues, organ systems, and organisms. Accordingly, the marrow undergoes changes with age. Age-related hematologic changes are reflected by a decline in marrow cellularity, an increased risk of clonal myeloid neoplams[125] and anemia,[17,126-130] and a decline in adaptive immunity.[131-134]

MARROW: ANATOMIC CHANGES

The percentage of marrow space occupied by the hematopoietic tissue declines from 90 percent at birth to a level of approximately 50 percent at age 30 years and 30 percent at age 70 years.[135,136] A similar change occurs in the thymus, where involution begins at an earlier age and is reflected anatomically by a reduction in lymphoid mass with an increase in fat[137] and functionally by a steady decrease in the production of naïve T cells.[80,138] Fat infiltration into the marrow and thymus results in a diminished volume of hematopoietic tissue.

Although age-related change in the marrow is well described, the exact mechanisms that regulate these changes remains speculative.[139] For example, it remains unclear whether the age-associated expansion of marrow fat is a cause or an effect of aging and whether the changes seen in marrow and histologically similar changes within the thymus are intrinsically related. Because of the intricate association of hematologic and immune functions and these common histologic patterns of change with age, both changes in blood and innate immunity are discussed below in the sections on Blood Cell Changes with Age and Aging and Immunity.

MARROW: STEM CELLS

The ontogeny of hematopoietic stem cells is the focus of much attention.[140,141] In fetal development the manufacture of blood cells occurs in several organs, but after birth this function is subsumed by the marrow.[142–148] The process of embryonic and fetal hematopoiesis is described in Chap. 7. Hematopoietic cells appear in the medullary cavities of bone around 14 weeks of gestation,[149] and by birth the marrow is the primary site of hematopoiesis.

Unlike the commonly held notion that stem cell compartments diminish either in number or function with age ultimately resulting in an inability to meet homeostatic demands, age-related hematopoietic stem cell (HSC) changes appear to be an exception, at least for murine species in which this question has been most directly addressed.[150,151] Early work demonstrated that marrow serially transplanted could reconstitute hematopoietic function for an estimated 15 to 20 life spans.[152] Furthermore, the capacity for old marrow to reconstitute proved superior to that of young.[153] Subsequently, a number of investigators using a variety of techniques have concluded that HSC frequency in old mice and humans is approximately 2 to 10 times greater than in the young.[16,150,151,154–156] Some evidence suggests that the intrinsic function of HSCs changes somewhat with age, most notably in a shift in lineage potential from lymphoid to myeloid development. This may contribute to an observed relative increase in neutrophils and decrease in lymphocytes in the blood of older people.[157]

There is an intrinsic change in HSCs with age, most notably resulting in a shift in lineage potential from lymphoid to myeloid development. This may contribute to a relative increase in neutrophils and decrease in lymphocytes in the blood of older persons.[157] As HSCs age, they accumulate genotypic (mutational) and phenotypic alterations. Indeed, human stem-progenitor cells from healthy volunteers were found to accumulate 13 exonic (private) mutations per year of age.[157a] Current opinion is that such changes are responsible for the development of immune senescence and that such changes are responsible for the development of immune senescence, as well as the increased occurrence of age-associated diseases such as myelodysplasia and leukemia. Thus, the process of "immunosenescence," as it affects the innate and adaptive immune system, may result from HSC aging. For example, an age-related decrease in the provision of B-cell precursors may be the result of HSC aging.[148]

MARROW DURING ADULT LIFE

The most apparent change seen in the marrow with aging is decreased cellularity (Fig. 9–1).[135] Under normal circumstances, the marrow is the only site of hematopoiesis. Foci of extramedullary hematopoiesis may occur in the liver, spleen, or lymph nodes in pathologic states, but they are not of functional consequence. Until puberty the entire skeleton remains hematopoietically active, but by age 18 years only the vertebrae, ribs, sternum, skull, pelvis, proximal epiphyseal regions of humerus and femur remain active sites of blood production, with other medullary sites infiltrated with fatty tissue. By age 40 years, the marrow in sternum, ribs, pelvis and vertebrae is composed of equal amounts of hematopoietic tissue and fat and cellularity declines gradually thereafter. By age 65 years, marrow cellularity is estimated to be approximately 30 percent,[135,136] with a corresponding increase in marrow fat. Age-associated imbalanced bone remodeling and osteoporosis results in decreased trabecular bone which itself may contribute to diminished hematopoiesis.[158] The presence of fat correlates with the occurrence and severity of osteoporosis, both of which are evident with aging.[159] Several age-related qualitative changes have been identified in hematopoietic cells, including skewed X-chromosome inactivation, telomere shortening,[160–162] accumulation of mitochondrial DNA mutations,[163,164] and

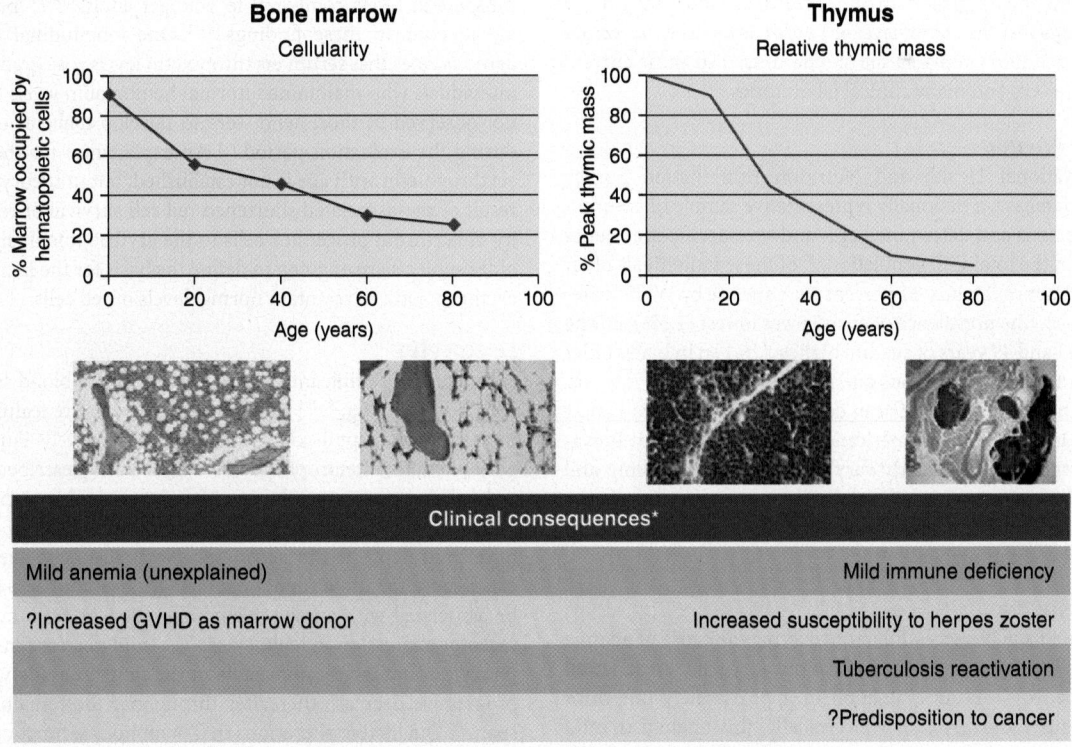

Figure 9–1. Aging of marrow and thymus. Marrow cellularity declines from birth in a manner comparably to thymic mass. This is reflected histologically by the increased presence of fat. The clinical consequences of these age-associated changes, in the absence of disease, are a mild anemia and immune deficiency. The latter is reflected by an increased predisposition to certain infections (e.g., herpes zoster or reactivation of latent tuberculosis) and possibly to the increased predisposition to cancer. GVHD, graft-versus-host disease.

micronuclei formation,[165] any of which could result in cellular dysfunction. Furthermore, growth hormone production declines with age, and this, too, is linked with deposition of fat within the marrow.[166] Administration of growth hormone to old rats reduces marrow fat and increases hematopoietic tissue.[167]

BLOOD CELL CHANGES WITH AGE

Red Cells

Anemia is a significant health problem in the elderly because of a high prevalence and significant associated morbidity, including reduced quality of life, clinical depression, falls, functional impairment, slower walking speed, reduced grip strength, loss of mobility, worsening comorbidities, and mortality.[168,169]

In older men and women, anemia defined using the World Health Organization (WHO) criteria of hemoglobin levels less than 13 g/dL for men and 12 g/dL for women[170] is associated with an increase in mortality.[171-176] It has been pointed out that the WHO criteria do not take into account inherent ethnic variations, particularly with respect to Americans of African descent who have lower levels of hemoglobin without significant adverse outcomes.[177,178] In a study that analyzed 1018 Americans of African descent and 1583 Americans of European descent adults aged 71 to 82 years, anemia defined by the WHO criteria was associated with increased mortality in those of European descent but not those of African descent.[177,178] The reasons for these ethnic differences are undefined. However, the difference is one of degree. In general, the impact of anemia on functional status and mortality in Americans of African descent becomes apparent at hemoglobin levels approximately 1 g/dL lower than in whites. The issue of establishing criteria for the diagnosis of anemia is relevant in the context of age, as well. Older women, for example, have better physical performance and function at hemoglobin values between 13 and 15 g/dL than at between 12.0 and 12.9 g/dL,[179] suggesting perhaps that the cut off level of 12 g/dL is too low. Nevertheless, the WHO definition remains the standard used in most current epidemiologic surveys and many clinical laboratories.

Prevalence of Anemia

In the third National Health and Nutrition Examination Survey (NHANES III) database, a nationally representative sample of community-dwelling persons and determined age- and sex-specific prevalence rates of anemia in the total U.S. population,[127] of those individuals older than age 65 years approximately 11 percent were anemic by WHO criteria (see Table 9–1). The prevalence of anemia was lowest (1.5%) among males between 17 and 49 years of age and highest (26.1%) in males older than 85 years. Among those 65 years and older, the prevalence rate was notably higher in Americans of African descent as compared to Americans of European descent and Americans of Hispanic descent. Prevalence rates of anemia in the elderly vary in community-dwelling and institutionalized populations. Also, anemia is more common among frail elderly. In the nursing home, for example, anemia prevalence approaches 50 percent or higher.[126,180-182]

Unexplained Anemia

Hematologists are usually successful in uncovering the cause of anemia in young adults. However, in older populations a specific explanation cannot be defined by routine evaluation in approximately one-third of anemic patients (Table 9–2).[20,183,184] Typically, this anemia is mild (hemoglobin concentration in the 10–12 g/dL range), normocytic, and hypoproliferative (low reticulocyte index). It has been postulated that the cause relates to a number of factors including declining testosterone level,[185] occult inflammation,[186] impaired renal function with inappropriately low serum erythropoietin,[187] or incipient myelodysplasia.[188] Likely, unexplained anemia represents an amalgam of these and perhaps

TABLE 9–2. Anemia Prevalence in the Elderly Using the WHO* Criteria

Study	Age (Years)	Population	Prevalence
Guralnik, 2004[127]	≥65	Community-dwelling elderly American	10.6%
Ferrucci, 2007[299]	≥70	Community-dwelling elderly Italian	11%
Denny[300]	≥71	Community dwelling	24%
Joosten[128]	≥65	Hospitalized	24% (defined as hemoglobin <11.5 g/dL)
Artz[126]	Most ≥65	Nursing home	48%
Robinson[182]	≥65	Nursing home	59.6%

*World Health Organization anemia criteria; hemoglobin <13 g/dL for adult men and <12 g/dL for adult women.

other factors, such as shortened red cell survival, refractoriness of the erythroid precursors to erythropoietin stimulation, and/or the presence of as yet undiagnosed illness.

Serum Erythropoietin and Aging

Data on erythropoietin levels in nonanemic older persons are inconsistent. Some suggest that nonanemic older persons have higher erythropoietin levels compared to younger adults,[189-191] but other studies fail to confirm these findings.[10-12] One longitudinal analysis clearly demonstrates that serum erythropoietin levels rose gradually in healthy individuals who maintained normal hemoglobin levels but the rise was not observed in those who were to develop diabetes or hypertension during the evaluation period.[192] An explanation for the rise in serum erythropoietin with age is not established, but in theory, it could be the result of age-associated shortened red cell survival or reduced sensitivity of erythroid progenitor cells to the erythropoietin signal. Studies in older subjects are ongoing to define the basis for the increasing need for erythropoietin to maintain normal levels of red cells.

Leukocytes

Although no significant change is seen in the blood leukocyte count with normal aging,[193,191] among those who acquire features of frailty, an increased neutrophil count may be observed.[157,195] Furthermore, several qualitative neutrophil defects have been described. For example, a decreased respiratory burst response to soluble signals,[193] defective phagocytosis,[194] and impaired neutrophil migration to sites of stress[196] have been described in accordance with advanced age. Although the exact cause for these functional changes has not been clarified, it may be associated with an age-related alteration in actin cytoskeleton and receptor expression in leukocytes.[197] A mild decrease in the blood lymphocyte count is first noticeable in the fourth decade with a gradually progressive decrease thereafter throughout the remainder of the lifespan.[198] Qualitative alterations in T-lymphocyte function in the elderly have also been demonstrated.[199]

Platelets

At present, knowledge about the influence of age on platelet counts has been limited to cross-sectional data derived from selected populations. From those data, no or very limited changes in platelet number are noted with age.[200–203] To date, a longitudinal data set describing alterations in platelet number with advancing age has not been produced nor are there conclusive studies describing age-associated changes in platelet function.

AGING AND COAGULATION

Coagulation Factors and Aging

A number of proteins critical to clot formation and fibrinolysis change in characteristic ways with advancing age.[204–206] Plasma concentrations of factor VII coagulant activity and antigen,[204–208] and factor VIIIC,[191,206,209] as well as von Willebrand factor,[191,209] fibrinogen,[191,206,208,210] fibrinopeptide A,[191,206,207] and tissue plasminogen activator antigen[191,211–213] increase with age. In healthy centenarians, levels of activated factor VII, activation peptides of prothrombin, factors IX and X, and thrombin–antithrombin complex concentration were increased, which are signs of higher-than-expected coagulation enzyme activity.[206] Age-associated increases in levels of protein C occur in both sexes. Aging is also associated with increasing levels of free protein S.[204] In contrast, antithrombin tends to decrease with age in males and increases with age in females following menopause.[214] Higher D-dimer and plasmin–antiplasmin complexes indicate an accompanying increase in fibrinolytic activity.[206,215] In contrast, plasma tissue-plasminogen activator inhibitor levels increase with increasing age, as do levels of thrombin-activatable fibrinolysis inhibitor in women[216] and its proenzyme form, procarboxypeptidase U, in both sexes.[217] These latter findings are suggestive of a possible age-dependent compromise in fibrinolytic activity.[218] Thus, procoagulant and, in some studies, fibrinolytic activities appear to be increased in older subjects by both *in vitro*[206,219,220] and *in vivo* studies,[190,221] but the changes in fibrinolytic activity are inconsistent. Older patients may show an exaggerated anticoagulant response to warfarin.[222]

Aging as a Prothrombotic State

Activation of the coagulation system and increase in procoagulant markers are associated with the pathogenesis of atherosclerosis.[223,224] However, procoagulant markers, most notably D-dimer,[225] fibrinogen, and factor VIII,[226] also increase with advancing age, and may, in fact, correlate better with aging than with cardiovascular disease.[223,224] In a study examining 1729 participants age 70 years and older in the Established Populations for the Epidemiological Study of the Elderly (EPESE) cohort, increasing age was associated with high D-dimer levels. For example, 23 percent of the participants age 90 to 99 years had high D-dimer levels (>600 mcg/L) compared to 13 percent in the 80- to 89-year-old age group and 7 percent in the 70- to 79-year-old age group.[215] Investigators measured fibrinogen concentrations in healthy subjects ages 19 to 96 years and found levels to be significantly higher in participants older than age 60 years when compared to younger subjects.[227] Healthy individuals across the life span had fibrinogen levels increased by 25 mg/dL per decade of life, and levels as high as 320 mg/dL were found in more than 80 percent of people older than 65 years of age.[228] Other markers of activated coagulation, such as plasminogen activating inhibitor-I (PAI-1) and factor VIII also increased with age.[209,229,230] Thus, it is now apparent that aging is associated with markers of activated coagulation. In this context, it is notable that the incidence of venous thrombosis and pulmonary emboli increases dramatically in geriatric populations.[231,232] Bleeding complications from anticoagulation therapy are also increased in older patients. No interventional study has identified an at-risk population of normal-age subjects without prior thrombosis in whom prophylactic anticoagulation is of value.

Coagulation and Functional Decline

In the EPESE study, increases in D-dimer and interleukin (IL)-6 were related to increases in both morbidity and mortality.[215] In fact, the correlation for adverse outcomes was stronger with D-dimer than IL-6.[233] In this, and other studies,[234–236] D-dimer and other markers of activated coagulation were associated with limitation in a wide variety of functional domains, including independent activities of daily living (IADL), lower-extremity function, and performance on cognitive testing. The age-associated changes in coagulation markers occur earlier than other aging biomarkers, and hence it has been argued that they could be early predictors of those elderly at increased risk for functional decline.[237]

This age-associated prominence of coagulation factors has also been reproduced in animals. For example, when stress associated with physical restraint was compared in aged versus young C57BL/6J mice, significantly increased expression of PAI-1 mRNA was noted in almost all the tissues in older mice.[238] Similar results were seen for expression of tissue factor mRNA in aged mice.[238] In both these experimental models an increase in microthrombi was noted with clots distributed through multiple organ systems in the older mice.

In humans, both the presence of depression and/or psychological stress are associated with increased coagulation[239–241] and decreased fibrinolytic activity.[242] In elderly subjects without cardiovascular disease, physical exhaustion, a characteristic frequently used to distinguish frail from nonfrail individuals, was associated with significant increases in both inflammatory and coagulation factors as assessed by fibrinogen, C-reactive protein, and white cell levels.[239] Frail and prefrail subjects from the Cardiovascular Health Study had significantly higher levels of fibrinogen, factor VIII, and D-dimer levels as compared to the nonfrail group. The association with frailty persisted even after adjusting for the presence of cardiovascular disease and diabetes.[243] Frailty is also associated with increased risk of venous thromboembolism when compared to nonfrail individuals of the same age, especially in association with increased factor VIII levels.[244]

AGING AND IMMUNITY

Whether related to primary processes of aging or not, the thymus gland undergoes a very characteristic pattern of involution beginning well in advance of other phenotypic changes attributed to aging (see Figs. 9–1 and 9–2; Chap. 6).[245] Among the consequences are a decreased generation of naïve T cells.[246] Despite this, the total lymphocyte count does not decline greatly because peripheral T cells are capable of expanding to fill the T-cell niche in the absence of generation of new T cells. However, when they do so, the repertoire for antigen recognition becomes less comprehensive. Thymic involution may result from the aging T-cell progenitor population,[247] from the defects in rearrangement of T-cell receptor β genes,[248,249] from loss of self-peptide expressing thymic epithelium,[250] and/or from the loss of thymic trophic cytokines.[251] Thymic epithelial cells produce a variety of colony-stimulating factors and hematopoietic cytokines, such as IL-1, IL-3, IL-6, IL-7, transforming growth factor-β, oncostatin M, and leukemia inhibitory factor,[252–254] which influence the complex process of T-cell production. It is proposed that thymic atrophy and decreased thymopoiesis is an active process and mediated by the upregulation of thymosuppressive cytokines (leukemia inhibitory factor, IL-6, and oncostatin M), which results in the altered peripheral lymphatic tissue T-lymphocyte function with aging.[255]

There is a notable shift in the overall blood T-cell population toward lymphocytes with memory T-cell markers,[256] and many of these are thought to have attained replicative senescence.[257] With the decreasing numbers of naïve T cells in the peripheral lymphatic tissue and increasing memory T cells reaching senescence, elderly persons have difficulties responding to old and new antigens and demonstrate impaired reactions to vaccinations. The decreased efficacy of vaccines

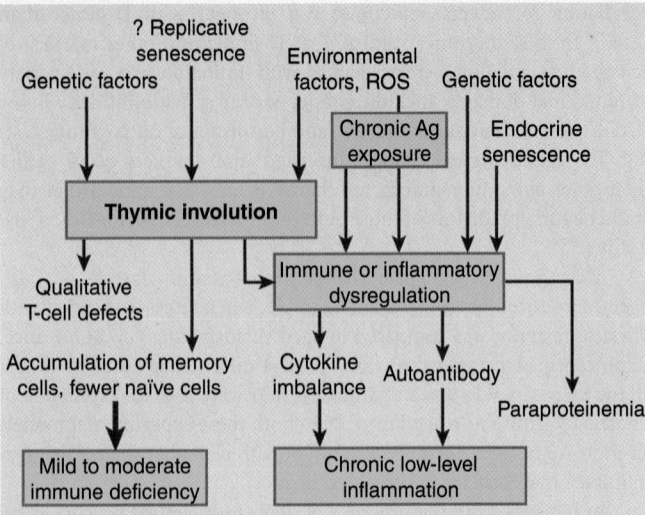

Figure 9–2. Immunity and aging. A variety of factors have been associated with thymic involution, the consequence of which is a mild to moderate immune deficiency. Dysregulated inflammatory pathways are also observed with advancing age and these may be of greater clinical importance. Ag, antigen; ROS, reactive oxygen species.

may also be a result of alterations in antigen presentation with age. Within the T-helper cell fraction there is a shift to the T-helper (Th) type 2 subset and away from Th1,[258] thereby influencing cytokine production and overall immune response.

In addition to the anatomic changes within marrow and thymus (see Figs. 9–1 and 9–2), similar age-associated morphologic changes within the paracortical and medullary zones of secondary lymphoid tissues (spleen, and lymph nodes) occur, including a decline in the paracortical and medullary zones and increased deposition of fat within the germinal centers.[259,260] It remains unclear to what extent these changes contribute to the overall change in immune function with age.

A wide range of lymphocyte functional changes have been described in the context of aging; however, cataloguing these would be beyond the scope of this chapter. Such changes are detailed in several excellent reviews.[24,261-264] Briefly stated, there is a shift in the T-cell population toward memory T cells,[256] which attain replicative senescence in response to repeated antigen exposures.[257] With the relative and absolute decrease in numbers of naïve T cells in the peripheral lymphatic tissue and the accumulation of functionally diminished memory senescent T cells, primary and secondary immune responses are reduced in elderly persons.

Coincident with the age-related changes in lymphocyte function is the increase in levels of circulating proinflammatory cytokines, measureable in some, even in the absence of definable inflammatory disease. IL-6 is the prototype in this regard. In young adults, expression of IL-6 is tightly regulated and serum levels are usually unmeasurable or very low in the absence of inflammatory conditions. Animal studies reveal an increased production of IL-6[265,266] from mononuclear cells and lymphoid cells after stimulation with lipopolysaccharide or other mitogens. Similarly, in humans serum IL-6 levels increase significantly with age.[267-271] Other inflammatory proteins, including tumor necrosis factor-α (TNF-α) and C-reactive protein are also seen at higher levels in the elderly.[272-274] Visceral adipose tissue from older mice express greater levels of both IL-6 and TNF-α mRNA than tissue from younger mice,[275] and thus, some of the age-associated rise in IL-6 may be the consequence of those metabolic shifts mentioned above.

CLINICAL CONSEQUENCES

Marrow Aging

Although a number of measureable changes occur in the marrow, not the least of which is a reduction in cellularity, apparent compensatory stem cell changes allow the sustenance of normal or near-normal blood counts throughout the life span. It is notable from transplant experience that even when marrow is donated from a 65-year-old person to an human leukocyte antigen (HLA)-matched younger recipient, the donor marrow supports hematopoiesis for the life of the recipient, although allogeneic marrow from older donors has a greater chance of being associated with graft-versus-host disease.[276]

Unexplained Anemia

To the extent that marrow contains continuously repopulating cell lines, it is quite remarkable that changes attributable to aging alone (i.e., in the absence of disease) are quite subtle. Nonetheless "unexplained anemia" (UA) accounts for up to one-third of cases of anemia in older patients and its frequency increases with advancing age.[20]

UA is usually mild, with hemoglobin levels approximately 1 g/dL lower than the WHO standard. The red cells are typically of normal size and examination of the blood film reveals no evidence for intravascular destruction or morphologic features suggestive of myelodysplasia. Although inflammatory cytokine levels may be elevated, the intensity of inflammation is insufficient to produce increased levels of hepcidin; thus, UA has a distinct pathogenesis from the anemia of chronic disease (Chap. 37). Because UA is typically mild, it is likely to be overlooked. In fact, in one population-based cohort that included elderly patients with even more significant anemia, the medical records of affected individuals did not mention anemia as a problem in 75 percent of the cases.[171] However, there is now evidence that this casual acceptance of lower hemoglobin levels in older populations may not be advisable.[168] Not only can a decline in important functional measures be related to mild anemia,[172,277-280] but longitudinal studies demonstrate increased mortality among individuals with even mild anemia.[174,179,281] Furthermore, a retrospective cohort study of the U.S. Veterans Administration National Surgical Quality Improvement database, indicated that of 310,311 subjects age 65 years and older who underwent noncardiac surgery, the 30-day mortality and cardiac event rates increased by 1.6 percent for each 1 percent decrease in hematocrit below the level of 39 percent.[275] Thus, although in younger individuals mild anemia may be well tolerated, in many older individuals it is associated with important negative consequences. That stated, it remains to be established whether the correction of anemia for those with UA will result in improved quality of life, physical function, or survival.

For elderly patients with UA, the presence of macrocytosis; thrombocytopenia; neutropenia; splenomegaly; or unexplained constitutional findings of fever, chills, or weight loss; or symptoms of early satiety; or bone pain should prompt consideration of a marrow examination to rule out myelodysplasia or other diseases affecting marrow function, most of which occur with increasing frequency with advancing age.

Immune Senescence

The complex alterations in immune function with age have been described comprehensively in several reviews.[261-264] The changes may explain an age-associated predisposition to certain infections (herpes zoster, tuberculosis reactivation) and perhaps a failure to mount a sufficient vaccine response (e.g., influenza hemagglutinin[282-286]). The more profound immune deficiency commonly observed in older people most often reflects the debilitating effects of concurrent diseases, most of which occur more commonly with age, and side effects of the medicines used to manage those diseases.

Inflammation/Coagulation Dysregulation and Frailty

Presumably on the basis of chronic inflammatory stimuli, there is an age-associated activation of coagulation[232] and fibrinolytic[287] pathways that favor thrombus formation. Fibrinogen levels are typically high with more than 80 percent of those age 65 years and older having levels above 320 mg/dL.[227] Similarly an analysis of D-dimer levels in the EPESE, including 1727 community elderly, revealed an age-associated increase that correlated with declining overall physical function.[215] Furthermore, when combining D-dimer and IL-6 levels, those individuals who had elevations of both were at greatest risk for mortality over a 4-year interval.[233] In the Cardiovascular Health Study, which included relatively healthy elderly, higher fibrinogen and factor VIII levels were associated with a greater risk for cardiovascular disease and mortality, even after adjustment for other cardiovascular risk factors.[232,288] Summarizing what has now become a robust literature, higher IL-6, TNF-α, D-dimer, and C-reactive protein are each associated with negative physiologic consequences, including reduced lower-extremity muscle mass and strength,[289,290] cognitive decline,[291] insulin resistance,[292] subclinical and clinical cardiovascular disease,[293,294] renal insufficiency,[295] loss of bone mineral density,[296] depression,[297] anemia,[186] dementia,[235] and mortality.[289] As a result, a general consensus has emerged that activated inflammatory mediators are, at least in part, contributing to the physiology of aging, and to the extent that these pathways are dysregulated, important functional outcomes are impaired.

REFERENCES

1. Kinsella KG: Future longevity-demographic concerns and consequences. *J Am Geriatr Soc* 53(9 Suppl):S299–S303, 2005.
2. Olshansky SJ, Goldman DP, Zheng Y, Rowe JW: Aging in America in the twenty-first century: Demographic forecasts from the MacArthur Foundation Research Network on an Aging Society. *Milbank Q* 87(4):842–862, 2009.
3. Blakely T, Atkinson J, Kvizhinadze G, et al: Health system costs by sex, age and proximity to death, and implications for estimation of future expenditure. *N Z Med J* 127(1393):12–25, 2014.
4. Pallin DJ, Espinola JA, Camargo CA Jr: US population aging and demand for inpatient services. *J Hosp Med* 9(3):193–196, 2014.
5. Kinsella K, Velkoff VA: *An Aging World.* US Government Printing Office, Washington, DC, 2001.
6. Walston J, Hadley EC, Ferrucci L, et al: Research agenda for frailty in older adults: Toward a better understanding of physiology and etiology: Summary from the American Geriatrics Society/National Institute on Aging Research conference on frailty in older adults. *J Am Geriatr Soc* 54(6):991–1001, 2006.
7. Martin GM: The biology of aging: 1985–2010 and beyond. *FASEB J* 25(11):3756–3762, 2011.
8. Huber KR, Mostafaie N, Stangl G, et al: Clinical chemistry reference values for 75-year-old apparently healthy persons. *Clin Chem Lab Med* 44(11):1355–1360, 2006.
9. Milman N, Pedersen AN, Ovesen L, Schroll M: Hemoglobin concentrations in 358 apparently healthy 80-year-old Danish men and women. Should the reference interval be adjusted for age? *Aging Clin Exp Res* 20(1):8–14, 2008.
10. Shock NW, Gueulich RC, Andres R: *Normal human aging: The Baltimore Longitudinal Study of Aging.* NIH Publication No. 84–2450. 1984.
11. Harada CN, Natelson Love MC, Triebel KL: Normal cognitive aging. *Clin Geriatr Med* 29(4):737–752, 2013.
12. Lindeman RD: Overview: Renal physiology and pathophysiology of aging. *Am J Kidney Dis* 16(4):275–282, 1990.
13. Wiggins JE: Aging in the glomerulus. *J Gerontol A Biol Sci Med Sci* 67(12):1358–1364, 2012.
14. Gazit R, Weissman IL, Rossi DJ: Hematopoietic stem cells and the aging hematopoietic system. *Semin Hematol* 45(4):218–224, 2008.
15. Rossi DJ, Bryder D, Zahn JM, et al: Cell intrinsic alterations underlie hematopoietic stem cell aging. *Proc Natl Acad Sci U S A* 102(26):9194–9199, 2005.
16. Sudo K, Ema H, Morita Y, Nakauchi H: Age-associated characteristics of murine hematopoietic stem cells. *J Exp Med* 192(9):1273–1280, 2000.
17. Beghe C, Wilson A, Ershler WB: Prevalence and outcomes of anemia in geriatrics: A systematic review of the literature. *Am J Med* 116 Suppl 7A:3S-10S, 2004.
18. Pautas E, Siguret V, Kim TM, et al: Anemia in the elderly: Usefulness of an easy and comprehensive laboratory screen. *Ann Biol Clin (Paris)* 70(6):643–647, 2012.
19. Artz AS: Anemia and the frail elderly. *Semin Hematol* 45(4):261–266, 2008.
20. Makipour S, Kanapuru B, Ershler WB: Unexplained anemia in the elderly. *Semin Hematol* 45(4):250–254, 2008.
21. Chaves PHM: Functional outcomes of anemia in older adults. *Semin Hematol* 45(4):255–260, 2008.
22. Thein M, Ershler WB, Artz AS, et al: Diminished quality of life and physical function in community-dwelling elderly with anemia. *Medicine (Baltimore)* 88(2):107–114, 2009.
23. Pawelec G, Larbi A: Immunity and ageing in man: Annual review 2006/2007. *Exp Gerontol* 43(1):34–38, 2008.
24. Longo DL: Immunology of aging, in *Fundamental Immunology*, 5th ed, edited by WE Paul, pp 1043–1075. Lippincott, Williams and Wilkins, Philadelphia, 2003.
25. Fulop T, Witkowski JM, Pawelec G, et al: On the immunological theory of aging. *Interdiscip Top Gerontol* 39:163–176, 2014.
26. Dubrow EL: Reactivation of tuberculosis: A problem of aging. *J Am Geriatr Soc* 24(11):481–487, 1976.
27. Nagami PH, Yoshikawa TT: Tuberculosis in the geriatric patient. *J Am Geriatr Soc* 31(6):356–363, 1983.
28. Arvin A: Aging, immunity, and the varicella-zoster virus. *N Engl J Med* 352(22):2266–2267, 2005.
29. Schmader K: Herpes zoster in older adults. *Clin Infect Dis* 32(10):1481–1486, 2001.
30. Arden NH, Patriarca PA, Kendal A: Experiences in the use and efficacy of inactivated influenza vaccine in the nursing home, in *Options for the Control of Influenza*, edited by A Kendal, P Patriarca, pp 155–168. Alan Liss, New York, 1986.
31. Deng Y, Jing Y, Campbell AE, Gravenstein S: Age-related impaired type 1 T cell responses to influenza: Reduced activation ex vivo, decreased expansion in CTL culture in vitro, and blunted response to influenza vaccination in vivo in the elderly. *J Immunol* 172(6):3437–3446, 2004.
32. Hilleman MR: Realities and enigmas of human viral influenza: Pathogenesis, epidemiology and control. *Vaccine* 20(25–26):3068–3087, 2002.
33. Powers DC, Sears SD, Murphy BR, et al: Systemic and local antibody responses in elderly subjects given live or inactivated influenza A virus vaccines. *J Clin Microbiol* 27(12):2666–2671, 1989.
34. Corthay A: Does the immune system naturally protect against cancer? *Front Immunol* 5:197, 2014.
35. Kaesberg PR, Ershler WB. The importance of immunesenescence in the incidence and malignant properties of cancer in hosts of advanced age. *J Gerontol* 44(6):63–66, 1989.
36. Miller RA: The cell biology of aging: Immunological models. *J Gerontol* 44(1):B4–B8, 1989.
37. Kanapuru B, Simonsick EM, Ershler WB: Is cancer incidence decreased in the frail elderly? Evidence from a prospective cohort study. *J Geriatr Oncol* 4(1):19–25, 2013.
38. Chan TC, Hung IF, Luk JK, et al: Functional status of older nursing home residents can affect the efficacy of influenza vaccination. *J Gerontol A Biol Sci Med Sci* 68(3):324–330, 2013.
39. Radl J: Age-related monoclonal gammapathies: Clinical lessons from the aging C57BL mouse. *Immunol Today* 11(7):234–236, 1990.
40. Korde N, Kristinsson SY, Landgren O: Monoclonal gammopathy of undetermined significance (MGUS) and smoldering multiple myeloma (SMM): Novel biological insights and development of early treatment strategies. *Blood* 117(21):5573–5581, 2011.
41. Martin GM: The genetics of aging. *Hosp Pract (1995)* 32(2):47–50, 55–56, 59–61 passim, 1997.
42. Burtner CR, Kennedy BK: Progeria syndromes and ageing: What is the connection? *Nat Rev Mol Cell Biol* 11(8):567–578, 2010.
43. Yu CE, Oshima J, Fu YH, et al: Positional cloning of the Werner's syndrome gene. *Science* 272(5259):258–262, 1996.
44. Yu CE, Oshima J, Wijsman EM, et al: Mutations in the consensus helicase domains of the Werner syndrome gene. Werner's Syndrome Collaborative Group. *Am J Hum Genet* 60(2):330–341, 1997.
45. Kudlow BA, Kennedy BK, Monnat RJ Jr: Werner and Hutchinson-Gilford progeria syndromes: Mechanistic basis of human progeroid diseases. *Nat Rev Mol Cell Biol* 8(5):394–404, 2007.
46. Eriksson M, Brown WT, Gordon LB, et al: Recurrent de novo point mutations in lamin A cause Hutchinson-Gilford progeria syndrome. *Nature* 423(6937):293–298, 2003.
47. Cao K, Blair CD, Faddah DA, et al: Progerin and telomere dysfunction collaborate to trigger cellular senescence in normal human fibroblasts. *J Clin Invest* 121(7):2833–2844, 2011.
48. Kennedy BK, Guarente L: Genetic analysis of aging in Saccharomyces cerevisiae. *Trends Genet* 12(9):355–359, 1996.
49. Szilard L: On the nature of the aging process. *Proc Natl Acad Sci U S A* 45(1):30–45, 1959.
50. Morley AA: Is ageing the result of dominant and co-dominant mutations? *J Theor Biol* 98(3):469–474, 1982.
51. Cummings DJ: Mitochondrial DNA in Podospora anserina. A molecular approach to cellular senescence. *Monogr Dev Biol* 17:254–266, 1984.
52. Fairweather DS, Fox M, Margison GP: The in vitro lifespan of MRC-5 cells is shortened by 5-azacytidine-induced demethylation. *Exp Cell Res* 168(1):153–159, 1987.
53. Burnet M: *Intrinsic Mutagenesis: A Genetic Approach for Aging.* Wiley, New York, 1974.
54. Hart RW, Setlow RB: Correlation between deoxyribonucleic acid excision-repair and life-span in a number of mammalian species. *Proc Natl Acad Sci U S A* 71(6):2169–2173, 1974.
55. Orgel LE: The maintenance of the accuracy of protein synthesis and its relevance to ageing. *Proc Natl Acad Sci U S A* 49:517–521, 1963.
56. Allsopp RC, Vaziri H, Patterson C, et al: Telomere length predicts replicative capacity of human fibroblasts. *Proc Natl Acad Sci U S A* 89(21):10114–10118, 1992.

57. Longo DL: Telomere dynamics in aging: much ado about nothing? J Gerontol A Biol Sci Med Sci 64(9):963–964, 2009.

58. Bjorkstein J: Cross linkage and the aging process, in *Theoretical Aspects of Aging,* edited by M Rothstein, pp 43–56. Academic Press, New York, 1974.

59. Kohn RR: *Principles of Mammalian Aging,* 2nd ed. Prentice Hall, Englewood Cliffs, NJ, 1978.

60. Kreisle RA, Stebler BA, Ershler WB: Effect of host age on tumor-associated angiogenesis in mice. J Natl Cancer Inst 82(1):44–47, 1990.

61. Harman D: Aging: A theory based on free radical and radiation chemistry. J Gerontol 11(3):298–300, 1956.

62. Harman D: The aging process. Proc Natl Acad Sci U S A 78(11):7124–7128, 1981.

63. Sohal RS, Svensson I, Sohal BH, Brunk UT: Superoxide anion radical production in different animal species. Mech Ageing Dev 49(2):129–135, 1989.

64. Sohal RS, Sohal BH, Brunk UT: Relationship between antioxidant defenses and longevity in different mammalian species. Mech Ageing Dev 53(3):217–227, 1990.

65. Sohal RS, Weindruch R: Oxidative stress, caloric restriction, and aging. Science 273(5271):59–63, 1996.

66. Perez VI, Van Remmen H, Bokov A, et al: The overexpression of major antioxidant enzymes does not extend the lifespan of mice. Aging Cell 8(1):73–75, 2009.

67. Lee CM, Chung SS, Kaczkowski JM, et al: Multiple mitochondrial DNA deletions associated with age in skeletal muscle of rhesus monkeys. J Gerontol 48(6):B201–B205, 1993.

68. Melov S, Shoffner JM, Kaufman A, Wallace DC: Marked increase in the number and variety of mitochondrial DNA rearrangements in aging human skeletal muscle. Nucleic Acids Res 23(20):4122–4126, 1995.

69. Schwarze SR, Lee CM, Chung SS, et al: High levels of mitochondrial DNA deletions in skeletal muscle of old rhesus monkeys. Mech Ageing Dev 83(2):91–101, 1995.

70. Li Y, Huang TT, Carlson EJ, et al: Dilated cardiomyopathy and neonatal lethality in mutant mice lacking manganese superoxide dismutase. Nat Genet 11(4):376–381, 1995.

71. Epstein CJ, Avraham KB, Lovett M, et al: Transgenic mice with increased Cu/Zn-superoxide dismutase activity: Animal model of dosage effects in Down syndrome. Proc Natl Acad Sci U S A 84(22):8044–8048, 1987.

72. Harris TB, Kiel D, Roubenoff R, et al: Association of insulin-like growth factor-I with body composition, weight history, and past health behaviors in the very old: The Framingham Heart Study. J Am Geriatr Soc 45(2):133–139, 1997.

73. Birkenhager-Gillesse EG, Derksen J, Lagaay AM: Dehydroepiandrosterone sulphate (DHEAS) in the oldest old, aged 85 and over. Ann N Y Acad Sci 719:543–552, 1994.

74. Rudman D, Drinka PJ, Wilson CR, et al: Relations of endogenous anabolic hormones and physical activity to bone mineral density and lean body mass in elderly men. Clin Endocrinol (Oxf) 40(5):653–661, 1994.

75. Hobbs CJ, Plymate SR, Rosen CJ, Adler RA: Testosterone administration increases insulin-like growth factor-I levels in normal men. J Clin Endocrinol Metab 77(3):776–779, 1993.

76. Rudman D, Feller AG, Nagraj HS, et al: Effects of human growth hormone in men over 60 years old. N Engl J Med 323(1):1–6, 1990.

77. Walford R: *The Immunological Theory of Aging.* Williams and Wilkins, Baltimore, 1969.

78. Makinodan T, Kay MM: Age influence on the immune system. Adv Immunol 29:287–330, 1980.

79. Smith GS, Walford RL: Influence of the main histocompatibility complex on ageing in mice. Nature 270(5639):727–729, 1977.

80. Hirokawa K: Understanding the mechanism of the age-related decline in immune function. Nutr Rev 50(12):361–366, 1992.

81. Christensen K, Vaupel JW: Determinants of longevity: Genetic, environmental and medical factors. J Intern Med 240(6):333–341, 1996.

82. Population Division, Department of Economic and Social Affairs, United Nations: *World Population Prospects: The 2006 Revision.* http://www.un.org/esa/population/ordering.htm.

83. Orr WC, Sohal RS: Extension of life-span by overexpression of superoxide dismutase and catalase in Drosophila melanogaster. Science 263(5150):1128–1130, 1994.

84. Anderson RM, Shanmuganayagam D, Weindruch R: Caloric restriction and aging: Studies in mice and monkeys. Toxicol Pathol 37(1):47–51, 2009.

85. Mattson MP. Dietary factors, hormesis and health. Ageing Res Rev 7(1):43–48, 2008.

86. Ramsey JJ, Colman RJ, Binkley NC, et al: Dietary restriction and aging in rhesus monkeys: The University of Wisconsin study. Exp Gerontol 35(9–10):1131–1149, 2000.

87. Lane MA, Roth GS, Ingram DK: Caloric restriction mimetics: A novel approach for biogerontology. Methods Mol Biol 371:143–149, 2007.

88. Heilbronn LK, de Jonge L, Frisard MI, et al: Effect of 6-month calorie restriction on biomarkers of longevity, metabolic adaptation, and oxidative stress in overweight individuals: A randomized controlled trial. JAMA 295(13):1539–1548, 2006.

89. Redman LM, Martin CK, Williamson DA, Ravussin E. Effect of caloric restriction in non-obese humans on physiological, psychological and behavioral outcomes. Physiol Behav 94(5):643–648, 2008.

90. Fowler CG, Chiasson KB, Hart DB, et al: Tympanometry in rhesus monkeys: Effects of aging and caloric restriction. Int J Audiol 47(4):209–214, 2008.

91. Raman A, Ramsey JJ, Kemnitz JW, et al: Influences of calorie restriction and age on energy expenditure in the rhesus monkey. Am J Physiol Endocrinol Metab 292(1):E101–E106, 2007.

92. Hayflick L: The limited in vitro lifetime of human diploid cell strains. Exp Cell Res 37:614–636, 1965.

93. Partridge L: The new biology of ageing. Philos Trans R Soc Lond B Biol Sci 365(1537):147–154, 2010.

94. Partridge L: Some highlights of research on aging with invertebrates, 2010. Aging Cell 10(1):5–9, 2011.

95. Cristofalo VJ, Lorenzini A, Allen RG, et al: Replicative senescence: A critical review. Mech Ageing Dev 2004;125(10–11):827–848, 2007.

96. Rohme D: Evidence for a relationship between longevity of mammalian species and life spans of normal fibroblasts in vitro and erythrocytes in vivo. Proc Natl Acad Sci U S A 78(8):5009–5013, 1981.

97. Schaffitzel E, Hertweck M: Recent aging research in Caenorhabditis elegans. Exp Gerontol 41(6):557–563, 2006.

98. D'Angelo MA, Raices M, Panowski SH, Hetzer MW: Age-dependent deterioration of nuclear pore complexes causes a loss of nuclear integrity in postmitotic cells. Cell 136(2):284–295, 2009.

99. Ohlstein B, Spradling A: The adult Drosophila posterior midgut is maintained by pluripotent stem cells. Nature 439(7075):470–474, 2006.

100. Marianes A, Spradling AC. Physiological and stem cell compartmentalization within the Drosophila midgut. Elife 2:e00886, 2013.

101. Sun Y, Yolitz J, Wang C, et al: Aging studies in Drosophila melanogaster. Methods Mol Biol 1048:77–93, 2013.

102. Campisi J: Cellular senescence as a tumor-suppressor mechanism. Trends Cell Biol 11(11):S27–S31, 2001.

103. Green DR, Evan GI: A matter of life and death. Cancer Cell 1(1):19–30, 2002.

104. Campisi J. Cellular senescence and apoptosis: How cellular responses might influence aging phenotypes. Exp Gerontol 2003;38(1–2):5–11, 2001.

105. Hasty P, Campisi J, Hoeijmakers J, et al: Aging and genome maintenance: Lessons from the mouse? Science 299(5611):1355–1359, 2003.

106. Samper E, Nicholls DG, Melov S: Mitochondrial oxidative stress causes chromosomal instability of mouse embryonic fibroblasts. Aging Cell 2(5):277–285, 2003.

107. Bandyopadhyay D, Medrano EE: The emerging role of epigenetics in cellular and organismal aging. Exp Gerontol 38(11–12):1299–1307, 2003.

108. Narita M, Lowe SW: Executing cell senescence. Cell Cycle 3(3):244–246, 2004.

109. Neumeister P, Albanese C, Balent B, et al: Senescence and epigenetic dysregulation in cancer. Int J Biochem Cell Biol 34(11):1475–1490, 2002.

110. Bringold F, Serrano M: Tumor suppressors and oncogenes in cellular senescence. Exp Gerontol 35(3):317–329, 2000.

111. Lundberg AS, Hahn WC, Gupta P, Weinberg RA: Genes involved in senescence and immortalization. Curr Opin Cell Biol 12(6):705–709, 2000.

112. Itahana K, Dimri G, Campisi J: Regulation of cellular senescence by p53. Eur J Biochem 268(10):2784–2791, 2001.

113. Serrano M, Lin AW, McCurrach ME, et al: Oncogenic ras provokes premature cell senescence associated with accumulation of p53 and p16INK4a. Cell 88(5):593–602, 1997.

114. Ferbeyre G, de Stanchina E, Querido E, et al: PML is induced by oncogenic ras and promotes premature senescence. Genes Dev 14(16):2015–2027, 2000.

115. Pearson M, Carbone R, Sebastiani C, et al: PML regulates p53 acetylation and premature senescence induced by oncogenic Ras. Nature 406(6792):207–210, 2000.

116. Rossi D, Cerri M, Capello D, et al: Biological and clinical risk factors of chronic lymphocytic leukaemia transformation to Richter syndrome. Br J Haematol 142(2):202–215, 2008.

117. Miura T, Mattson MP, Rao MS: Cellular lifespan and senescence signaling in embryonic stem cells. Aging Cell 3(6):333–343, 2004.

118. Odorico JS, Kaufman DS, Thomson JA: Multilineage differentiation from human embryonic stem cell lines. Stem Cells 19(3):193–204, 2001.

119. Chen J: Senescence and functional failure in hematopoietic stem cells. Exp Hematol 32(11):1025–1032, 2004.

120. Geiger H, Van Zant G: The aging of lympho-hematopoietic stem cells. Nat Immunol 3(4):329–333, 2002.

121. Park IK, Morrison SJ, Clarke MF: Bmi1, stem cells, and senescence regulation. J Clin Invest 113(2):175–179, 2004.

122. Villa A, Navarro-Galve B, Bueno C, et al: Long-term molecular and cellular stability of human neural stem cell lines. Exp Cell Res 294(2):559–570, 2004.

123. Boulanger CA, Smith GH: Reducing mammary cancer risk through premature stem cell senescence. Oncogene 20(18):2264–2272, 2001.

124. Serakinci N, Guldberg P, Burns JS, et al: Adult human mesenchymal stem cell as a target for neoplastic transformation. Oncogene 23(29):5095–5098, 2004.

125. Lichtman MA, Rowe JM: The relationship of patient age to the pathobiology of the clonal myeloid diseases. Semin Oncol 31(2):185–197, 2004.

126. Artz AS, Fergusson D, Drinka PJ, et al: Prevalence of anemia in skilled-nursing home residents. Arch Gerontol Geriatr 39(3):201–206, 2004.

127. Guralnik JM, Eisenstaedt RS, Ferrucci L, et al: Prevalence of anemia in persons 65 years and older in the United States: Evidence for a high rate of unexplained anemia. Blood 104(8):2263–2268, 2004.

128. Joosten E, Pelemans W, Hiele M, et al: Prevalence and causes of anaemia in a geriatric hospitalized population. Gerontology 38(1–2):111–117, 1992.

129. Cesari M, Penninx BW, Lauretani F, et al: Hemoglobin levels and skeletal muscle: Results from the InCHIANTI study. J Gerontol A Biol Sci Med Sci 59(3):249–254, 2004.

130. Cesari M, Penninx BW, Pahor M, et al: Inflammatory markers and physical performance in older persons: The InCHIANTI study. J Gerontol A Biol Sci Med Sci 59(3):242–248, 2004.

131. Hakim FT, Gress RE: Immunosenescence: Deficits in adaptive immunity in the elderly. Tissue Antigens 70(3):179–189, 2007.

132. Linton PJ, Dorshkind K: Age-related changes in lymphocyte development and function. *Nat Immunol* 5(2):133–139, 2004.

133. Haq K, McElhaney JE: Immunosenescence: Influenza vaccination and the elderly. *Curr Opin Immunol* 29C:38–42, 2014.

134. Pritz T, Weinberger B, Grubeck-Loebenstein B: The aging bone marrow and its impact on immune responses in old age. *Immunol Lett* 162(1 Pt B):310–315, 2014.

135. Hartsock RJ, Smith EB, Petty CS: Normal variations with aging of the amount of hematopoietic tissue in bone marrow from the anterior iliac crest. A study made from 177 cases of sudden death examined by necropsy. *Am J Clin Pathol* 43:326–331, 1965.

136. Ricci C, Cova M, Kang YS, et al: Normal age-related patterns of cellular and fatty bone marrow distribution in the axial skeleton: MR imaging study. *Radiology* 177(1):83–88, 1990.

137. Steinmann GG, Klaus B, Muller-Hermelink HK: The involution of the ageing human thymic epithelium is independent of puberty. A morphometric study. *Scand J Immunol* 22(5):563–575, 1985.

138. Haynes BF, Sempowski GD, Wells AF, Hale LP: The human thymus during aging. *Immunol Res* 22(2–3):253–261, 2000.

139. Woolthuis CM, de Haan G, Huls G: Aging of hematopoietic stem cells: Intrinsic changes or micro-environmental effects? *Curr Opin Immunol* 23(4):512–517, 2011.

140. Geiger H, Denkinger M, Schirmbeck R: Hematopoietic stem cell aging. *Curr Opin Immunol* 2014;29C:86–92.

141. Van Zant G, Liang Y: Concise review: Hematopoietic stem cell aging, life span, and transplantation. *Stem Cells Transl Med* 1(9):651–657, 2012.

142. Golub R, Cumano A: Embryonic hematopoiesis. *Blood Cells Mol Dis* 51(4):226–231, 2013.

143. Baron MH, Vacaru A, Nieves J: Erythroid development in the mammalian embryo. *Blood Cells Mol Dis* 51(4):213–219, 2013.

144. Bigas A, Guiu J, Gama-Norton L: Notch and Wnt signaling in the emergence of hematopoietic stem cells. *Blood Cells Mol Dis* 51(4):264–270, 2013.

145. Kurtzberg J, Denning SM, Nycum LM, et al: Immature human thymocytes can be driven to differentiate into nonlymphoid lineages by cytokines from thymic epithelial cells. *Proc Natl Acad Sci U S A* 86(19):7575–7579, 1989.

146. Fowlkes BJ, Pardoll DM: Molecular and cellular events of T cell development. *Adv Immunol* 44:207–264, 1989.

147. Rothenberg EV: The development of functionally responsive T cells. *Adv Immunol* 51:85–214, 1992.

148. Geiger H, de Haan, G, Florian MC: The ageing of the haematopoietic stem cell compartment. *Nat Immunol* 13:376–389, 2013.

149. Charbord P, Tavian M, Humeau L, Peault B: Early ontogeny of the human marrow from long bones: An immunohistochemical study of hematopoiesis and its microenvironment. *Blood* 87(10):4109–4119, 1996.

150. Kuranda K, Vargaftig J, de la Rochere P, et al: Age-related changes in human hematopoietic stem/progenitor cells. *Aging Cell* 10(3):542–546, 2011.

151. Pang WW, Price EA, Sahoo D, et al: Human bone marrow hematopoietic stem cells are increased in frequency and myeloid-biased with age. *Proc Natl Acad Sci U S A* 108(50):20012–20017, 2011.

152. Harrison DE, Astle CM: Loss of stem cell repopulating ability upon transplantation. Effects of donor age, cell number, and transplantation procedure. *J Exp Med* 156(6):1767–1779, 1982.

153. Harrison DE: Long-term erythropoietic repopulating ability of old, young, and fetal stem cells. *J Exp Med* 157(5):1496–1504, 1983.

154. Rossi DJ, Bryder D, Zahn JM, et al: Cell intrinsic alterations underlie hematopoietic stem cell aging. *Proc Natl Acad Sci U S A* 102(26):9194–9199, 2005.

155. Beerman I, Maloney WJ, Weissmann IL, Rossi DJ: Stem cells and the aging hematopoietic system. *Curr Opin Immunol* 22:500–506, 2010.

156. Liang Y, Van Zant G, Szilvassy SJ: Effects of aging on the homing and engraftment of murine hematopoietic stem and progenitor cells. *Blood* 106(4):1479–1487, 2005.

157. Leng SX, Hung W, Cappola AR, et al: White blood cell counts, insulinlike growth factor-1 levels, and frailty in community-dwelling older women. *J Gerontol A Biol Sci Med Sci* 2009;64A(4):499–502.

157a. Welch JS, Ley, TJ, Link DC, et al: The origin and evolution of mutations in acute myeloid leukemia. *Cell* 150:264–278, 2012.

158. Justesen J, Stenderup K, Ebbesen EN, et al: Adipocyte tissue volume in bone marrow is increased with aging and in patients with osteoporosis. *Biogerontology* 2(3):165–171, 2001.

159. Verma S, Rajaratnam JH, Denton J, et al: Adipocytic proportion of bone marrow is inversely related to bone formation in osteoporosis. *J Clin Pathol* 55(9):693–698, 2002.

160. De Meyer T, De Buyzere ML, Langlois M, et al: Lower red blood cell counts in middle-aged subjects with shorter peripheral blood leukocyte telomere length. *Aging Cell* 7(5):700–705, 2008.

161. Greider CW: Telomeres and senescence: The history, the experiment, the future. *Curr Biol* 8(5):R178–81.

162. Frenck RW Jr, Blackburn EH, Shannon KM: The rate of telomere sequence loss in human leukocytes varies with age. *Proc Natl Acad Sci U S A* 95(10):5607–5610, 1998.

163. Gattermann N: Mitochondrial DNA mutations in the hematopoietic system. *Leukemia* 18(1):18–22, 2004.

164. Kadenbach B, Munscher C, Frank V, et al: Human aging is associated with stochastic somatic mutations of mitochondrial DNA. *Mutat Res* 338(1–6):161–172, 1995.

165. Bolognesi C, Abbondandolo A, Barale R, et al: Age-related increase of baseline frequencies of sister chromatid exchanges, chromosome aberrations, and micronuclei in human lymphocytes. *Cancer Epidemiol Biomarkers Prev* 6(4):249–256, 1997.

166. Lamberts SW, van den Beld AW, van der Lely AJ: The endocrinology of aging. *Science* 278(5337):419–424, 1997.

167. French RA, Broussard SR, Meier WA, et al: Age-associated loss of bone marrow hematopoietic cells is reversed by GH and accompanies thymic reconstitution. *Endocrinology* 143(2):690–699, 2002.

168. Nissenson AR, Goodnough LT, Dubois RW: Anemia: Not just an innocent bystander? *Arch Intern Med* 163(12):1400–1404, 2003.

169. Balducci L, Ershler WB, Bennett JM, editors: *Anemia in the Elderly*. Springer, New York, 2007.

170. Blanc B, Finch CA, Hallberg L: Nutritional anaemias. Report of a WHO Scientific Group. *World Health Organ Tech Rep Ser* 405:1–40, 1968.

171. Ania BJ, Suman VJ, Fairbanks VF, et al: Incidence of anemia in older people: An epidemiologic study in a well-defined population. *J Am Geriatr Soc* 45(7):825–831, 1997.

172. Chaves PH, Ashar B, Guralnik JM, Fried LP: Looking at the relationship between hemoglobin concentration and prevalent mobility difficulty in older women. Should the criteria currently used to define anemia in older people be reevaluated? *J Am Geriatr Soc* 50(7):1257–1264, 2002.

173. Culleton BF, Manns BJ, Zhang J, et al: Impact of anemia on hospitalization and mortality in older adults. *Blood* 107(10):3841–3846, 2006.

174. Izaks GJ, Westendorp RG, Knook DL: The definition of anemia in older persons. *JAMA* 281(18):1714–1717, 1999.

175. Zakai NA, Katz R, Hirsch C, et al: A prospective study of anemia status, hemoglobin concentration, and mortality in an elderly cohort: The Cardiovascular Health Study. *Arch Intern Med* 165(19):2214–2220, 2005.

176. Penninx BW, Pahor M, Woodman RC, Guralnik JM: Anemia in old age is associated with increased mortality and hospitalization. *J Gerontol A Biol Sci Med Sci* 61(5):474–479, 2006.

177. Beutler E, West C: Hematologic differences between African-Americans and whites: The roles of iron deficiency and alpha-thalassemia on hemoglobin levels and mean corpuscular volume. *Blood* 106(2):740–745, 2005.

178. Patel KV, Harris TB, Faulhaber M, et al: Racial variation in the relationship of anemia with mortality and mobility disability among older adults. *Blood* 109(11):4663–4670, 2007.

179. Chaves PH, Xue QL, Guralnik JM, et al: What constitutes normal hemoglobin concentration in community-dwelling disabled older women? *J Am Geriatr Soc* 52(11):1811–1816, 2004.

180. Gaskell H, Derry S, Andrew Moore R, McQuay HJ: Prevalence of anaemia in older persons: Systematic review. *BMC Geriatr* 8:1, 2008.

181. Pandya N, Bookhart B, Mody SH, et al: Study of anemia in long-term care (SALT): Prevalence of anemia and its relationship with the risk of falls in nursing home residents. *Curr Med Res Opin* 24(8):2139–2149, 2008.

182. Robinson B, Artz AS, Culleton B, et al: Prevalence of anemia in the nursing home: Contribution of chronic kidney disease. *J Am Geriatr Soc* 55(10):1566–1570, 2007.

183. Artz AS, Thirman MJ: Unexplained anemia predominates despite an intensive evaluation in a racially diverse cohort of older adults from a referral anemia clinic. *J Gerontol A Biol Sci Med Sci* 66(8):925–932, 2011.

184. Price EA, Mehra R, Holmes TH, Schrier SL. Anemia in older persons: Etiology and evaluation. *Blood Cells Mol Dis* 46(2):159–165, 2011.

185. Ferrucci L, Maggio M, Bandinelli S, et al: Low testosterone levels and the risk of anemia in older men and women. *Arch Intern Med* 166(13):1380–1388, 2006.

186. Ferrucci L, Guralnik JM, Woodman RC, et al: Proinflammatory state and circulating erythropoietin in persons with and without anemia. *Am J Med* 118(11):1288, 2005.

187. Artz AS, Fergusson D, Drinka PJ, et al: Mechanisms of unexplained anemia in the nursing home. *J Am Geriatr Soc* 52(3):423–427, 2004.

188. Strom SS, Velez-Bravo V, Estey EH: Epidemiology of myelodysplastic syndromes. *Semin Hematol* 45(1):8–13, 2008.

189. Mori M, Murai Y, Hirai M, et al: Serum erythropoietin titers in the aged. *Mech Ageing Dev* 1988;46(1–3):105–109, 2005.

190. Kario K, Matsuo T, Nakao K: Serum erythropoietin levels in the elderly. *Gerontology* 37(6):345–348, 1991.

191. Kario K, Matsuo T, Kodama K, Nakao K, Asada R: Reduced erythropoietin secretion in senile anemia. *Am J Hematol* 41(4):252–257, 1992.

192. Ershler WB, Sheng S, McKelvey J, et al: Serum erythropoietin and aging: A longitudinal analysis. *J Am Geriatr Soc* 53(8):1360–1365, 2005.

193. Lipschitz DA, Udupa KB, Milton KY, Thompson CO: Effect of age on hematopoiesis in man. *Blood* 63(3):502–509, 1984.

194. Nagel JE, Pyle RS, Chrest FJ, Adler WH: Oxidative metabolism and bactericidal capacity of polymorphonuclear leukocytes from normal young and aged adults. *J Gerontol* 37(5):529–534, 1982.

195. Leng SX, Xue QL, Tian J, et al: Inflammation and frailty in older women. *J Am Geriatr Soc* 55(6):864–871, 2007.

196. MacGregor RR, Shalit M: Neutrophil function in healthy elderly subjects. *J Gerontol* 45(2):M55–M60, 1990.

197. Rao KM, Currie MS, Padmanabhan J, Cohen HJ: Age-related alterations in actin cytoskeleton and receptor expression in human leukocytes. *J Gerontol* 47(2):B37–B44, 1992.

198. MacKinney AA Jr: Effect of aging on the peripheral blood lymphocyte count. *J Gerontol* 33(2):213–216, 1978.

199. Pawelec G, Akbar A, Caruso C, et al: Human immunosenescence: Is it infectious? *Immunol Rev* 205:257–268, 2005.

200. Lugada ES, Mermin J, Kaharuza F, et al: Population-based hematologic and immunologic reference values for a healthy Ugandan population. *Clin Diagn Lab Immunol* 11(1):29–34, 2004.

201. Nilsson-Ehle H, Jagenburg R, Landahl S, et al: Haematological abnormalities and reference intervals in the elderly. A cross-sectional comparative study of three urban Swedish population samples aged 70, 75 and 81 years. *Acta Med Scand* 224(6):595–604, 1988.

202. Lee SJ, Lindquist K, Segal MR, Covinsky KE: Development and validation of a prognostic index for 4-year mortality in older adults. *JAMA* 295(7):801–808, 2006.

203. Takubo T, Tatsumi N. [Reference values for hematologic laboratory tests and hematologic disorders in the aged] [in Japanese]. *Rinsho Byori* 48(3):207–216, 2000.

204. Haverkate F, Thompson SG, Duckert F: Haemostasis factors in angina pectoris; relation to gender, age and acute-phase reaction. Results of the ECAT Angina Pectoris Study Group. *Thromb Haemost* 73(4):561–567, 1995.

205. Kario K, Matsuo T, Kobayashi H: Close relationship between hemostatic factors and acute-phase reaction as normal aging process. *J Am Geriatr Soc* 44(5):614–615, 1996.

206. Mari D, Mannucci PM, Coppola R, et al: Hypercoagulability in centenarians: The paradox of successful aging. *Blood* 85(11):3144–3149, 1995.

207. Scarabin PY, Van Dreden P, Bonithon-Kop C, et al: Age-related changes in factor VII activation in healthy women. *Clin Sci (Lond)* 75(4):341–343, 1988.

208. Balleisen L, Bailey J, Epping PH, et al: Epidemiological study on factor VII, factor VIII and fibrinogen in an industrial population: I. Baseline data on the relation to age, gender, body-weight, smoking, alcohol, pill-using, and menopause. *Thromb Haemost* 54(2):475–479, 1985.

209. Conlan MG, Folsom AR, Finch A, et al: Associations of factor VIII and von Willebrand factor with age, race, sex, and risk factors for atherosclerosis. The Atherosclerosis Risk in Communities (ARIC) Study. *Thromb Haemost* 70(3):380–385, 1993.

210. Ernst E, Resch KL: Fibrinogen as a cardiovascular risk factor: A meta-analysis and review of the literature. *Ann Intern Med* 118(12):956–963, 1993.

211. Cadroy Y, Daviaud P, Saivin S, et al: Distribution of 16 hemostatic laboratory variables assayed in 100 blood donors. *Nouv Rev Fr Hematol* 32(4):259–264, 1990.

212. Gudnason T, Hrafnkelsdottir T, Wall U, et al: Fibrinolytic capacity increases with age in healthy humans, while endothelium-dependent vasodilation is unaffected. *Thromb Haemost* 89(2):374–381, 2003.

213. Sundell IB, Nilsson TK, Ranby M, et al: Fibrinolytic variables are related to age, sex, blood pressure, and body build measurements: A cross-sectional study in Norsjo, Sweden. *J Clin Epidemiol* 42(8):719–723, 1989.

214. Dolan G, Neal K, Cooper P, et al: Protein C, antithrombin III and plasminogen: Effect of age, sex and blood group. *Br J Haematol* 86(4):798–803, 1994.

215. Pieper CF, Rao KM, Currie MS, et al: Age, functional status, and racial differences in plasma D-dimer levels in community-dwelling elderly persons. *J Gerontol A Biol Sci Med Sci* 55(11):M649–M657, 2000.

216. Juhan-Vague I, Renucci JF, Grimaux M, et al: Thrombin-activatable fibrinolysis inhibitor antigen levels and cardiovascular risk factors. *Arterioscler Thromb Vasc Biol* 20(9):2156–2161, 2000.

217. Schatteman KA, Goossens FJ, Scharpe SS, et al: Assay of procarboxypeptidase U, a novel determinant of the fibrinolytic cascade, in human plasma. *Clin Chem* 45(6 Pt 1):807–813, 1999.

218. Mehta J, Mehta P, Lawson D, Saldeen T: Plasma tissue plasminogen activator inhibitor levels in coronary artery disease: Correlation with age and serum triglyceride concentrations. *J Am Coll Cardiol* 9(2):263–268, 1987.

219. Eliasson M, Evrin PE, Lundblad D: Fibrinogen and fibrinolytic variables in relation to anthropometry, lipids and blood pressure. The Northern Sweden Monica study. *J Clin Epidemiol* 47(5):513–524, 1994.

220. Cawkwell RD: Patient's age and the activated partial thromboplastin time test. *Thromb Haemost* 39(3):780–781, 1978.

221. Bauer KA, Weiss LM, Sparrow D, et al: Aging-associated changes in indices of thrombin generation and protein C activation in humans. Normative Aging Study. *J Clin Invest* 80(6):1527–1534, 1987.

222. Gurwitz JH, Avorn J, Ross-Degnan D, et al: Aging and the anticoagulant response to warfarin therapy. *Ann Intern Med* 116(11):901–904, 1992.

223. Deguchi K, Deguchi A, Wada H, Murashima S: Study of cardiovascular risk factors and hemostatic molecular markers in elderly persons. *Semin Thromb Hemost* 26(1):23–27, 2000.

224. Scarabin PY, Aillaud MF, Amouyel P, et al: Associations of fibrinogen, factor VII and PAI-1 with baseline findings among 10,500 male participants in a prospective study of myocardial infarction—the PRIME Study. Prospective Epidemiological Study of Myocardial Infarction. *Thromb Haemost* 80(5):749–756, 1998.

225. Hager K, Platt D: Fibrin degeneration product concentrations (D-dimers) in the course of ageing. *Gerontology* 41(3):159–165, 1995.

226. Tracy RP, Bovill EG, Fried LP, et al: The distribution of coagulation factors VII and VIII and fibrinogen in adults over 65 years. Results from the Cardiovascular Health Study. *Ann Epidemiol* 2(4):509–519, 1992.

227. Laharrague PF, Cambus JP, Fillola G, Corberand JX: Plasma fibrinogen and physiological aging. *Aging (Milano)* 5(6):445–449, 1993.

228. Hager K, Felicetti M, Seefried G, Platt D: Fibrinogen and aging. *Aging (Milano)* 6(2):133–138, 1994.

229. Takeshita K, Yamamoto K, Ito M, et al: Increased expression of plasminogen activator inhibitor-1 with fibrin deposition in a murine model of aging, "Klotho" mouse. *Semin Thromb Hemost* 28(6):545–554, 2002.

230. Tofler GH, Massaro J, Levy D, et al: Relation of the prothrombotic state to increasing age (from the Framingham Offspring Study). *Am J Cardiol* 96(9):1280–1283, 2005.

231. Cushman M, Yanez D, Psaty BM, et al: Association of fibrinogen and coagulation factors VII and VIII with cardiovascular risk factors in the elderly: The Cardiovascular Health Study. Cardiovascular Health Study Investigators. *Am J Epidemiol* 143(7):665–676, 1996.

232. Tracy RP, Arnold AM, Ettinger W, et al: The relationship of fibrinogen and factors VII and VIII to incident cardiovascular disease and death in the elderly: Results from the cardiovascular health study. *Arterioscler Thromb Vasc Biol* 19(7):1776–1783, 1999.

233. Cohen HJ, Harris T, Pieper CF: Coagulation and activation of inflammatory pathways in the development of functional decline and mortality in the elderly. *Am J Med* 114(3):180–187, 2003.

234. McDermott MM, Greenland P, Green D, et al: D-dimer, inflammatory markers, and lower extremity functioning in patients with and without peripheral arterial disease. *Circulation* 107(25):3191–3198, 2003.

235. Wilson CJ, Cohen HJ, Pieper CF: Cross-linked fibrin degradation products (D-dimer), plasma cytokines, and cognitive decline in community-dwelling elderly persons. *J Am Geriatr Soc* 51(10):1374–1381, 2003.

236. Rafnsson SB, Deary IJ, Smith FB, et al: Cognitive decline and markers of inflammation and hemostasis: The Edinburgh Artery Study. *J Am Geriatr Soc* 55(5):700–707, 2007.

237. McDermott MM, Ferrucci L, Liu K, et al: D-dimer and inflammatory markers as predictors of functional decline in men and women with and without peripheral arterial disease. *J Am Geriatr Soc* 53(10):1688–1696, 2005.

238. Yamamoto K, Shimokawa T, Yi H, et al: Aging and obesity augment the stress-induced expression of tissue factor gene in the mouse. *Blood* 100(12):4011–4018, 2002.

239. Kop WJ, Gottdiener JS, Tangen CM, et al: Inflammation and coagulation factors in persons > 65 years of age with symptoms of depression but without evidence of myocardial ischemia. *Am J Cardiol* 89(4):419–424, 2002.

240. Panagiotakos DB, Pitsavos C, Chrysohoou C, et al: Inflammation, coagulation, and depressive symptomatology in cardiovascular disease-free people; the ATTICA study. *Eur Heart J* 25(6):492–499, 2004.

241. von Kanel R, Dimsdale JE, Mills PJ, et al: Effect of Alzheimer caregiving stress and age on frailty markers interleukin-6, C-reactive protein, and D-dimer. *J Gerontol A Biol Sci Med Sci* 61(9):963–969, 2006.

242. von Kanel R, Mills PJ, Fainman C, Dimsdale JE: Effects of psychological stress and psychiatric disorders on blood coagulation and fibrinolysis: A biobehavioral pathway to coronary artery disease? *Psychosom Med* 63(4):531–544, 2001.

243. Walston J, McBurnie MA, Newman A, et al: Frailty and activation of the inflammation and coagulation systems with and without clinical comorbidities: Results from the Cardiovascular Health Study. *Arch Intern Med* 162(20):2333–2341, 2002.

244. Folsom AR, Boland LL, Cushman M, et al: Frailty and risk of venous thromboembolism in older adults. *J Gerontol A Biol Sci Med Sci* 62(1):79–82, 2007.

245. Chinn IK, Blackburn CC, Manley NR, Sempowski GD: Changes in primary lymphoid organs with aging. *Semin Immunol* 24(5):309–320, 2012.

246. Aspinall R: Longevity and the immune response. *Biogerontology* 1(3):273–278, 2000.

247. Tyan ML: Age-related decrease in mouse T cell progenitors. *J Immunol* 118(3):846–851, 1977.

248. Aspinall R: Age-associated thymic atrophy in the mouse is due to a deficiency affecting rearrangement of the TCR during intrathymic T cell development. *J Immunol* 158(7):3037–3045, 1997.

249. Lacorazza HD, Guevara Patino JA, Weksler ME, et al: Failure of rearranged TCR transgenes to prevent age-associated thymic involution. *J Immunol* 163(8):4262–4268, 1999.

250. Hartwig M, Steinmann G: On a causal mechanism of chronic thymic involution in man. *Mech Ageing Dev* 75(2):151–156, 1994.

251. Plum J, De Smedt M, Leclercq G, et al: Interleukin-7 is a critical growth factor in early human T-cell development. *Blood* 88(11):4239–4245, 1996.

252. Le PT, Kurtzberg J, Brandt SJ, et al: Human thymic epithelial cells produce granulocyte and macrophage colony-stimulating factors. *J Immunol* 141(4):1211–1217, 1988.

253. Le PT, Lazorick S, Whichard LP, et al: Human thymic epithelial cells produce IL-6, granulocyte-monocyte-CSF, and leukemia inhibitory factor. *J Immunol* 145(10):3310–3315, 1990.

254. Le PT, Tuck DT, Dinarello CA, et al: Human thymic epithelial cells produce interleukin 1. *J Immunol* 138(7):2520–2526, 1987.

255. Gruver AL, Hudson LL, Sempowski GD: Immunosenescence of ageing. *J Pathol* 211(2):144–156, 2007.

256. Cakman I, Rohwer J, Schutz RM, et al: Dysregulation between TH1 and TH2 T cell subpopulations in the elderly. *Mech Ageing Dev* 87(3):197–209, 1996.

257. Hodes RJ: Aging and the immune system. *Immunol Rev* 160:5–8, 1997.

258. Perussia B, Kobayashi M, Rossi ME, et al: Immune interferon enhances functional properties of human granulocytes: Role of Fc receptors and effect of lymphotoxin, tumor necrosis factor, and granulocyte-macrophage colony-stimulating factor. *J Immunol* 138(3):765–774, 1987.

259. Sokolov VV, Kaplunova OA, Ovseenko TE: [Age factors in architectonics of the splenic arterial vessels] [in Russian]. *Morfologiia* 124(4):57–60, 2003.

260. Luscieti P, Hubschmid T, Cottier H, et al: Human lymph node morphology as a function of age and site. *J Clin Pathol* 33(5):454–461, 1980.

261. Effros RB, Cai Z, Linton PJ: CD8 T cells and aging. *Crit Rev Immunol* 23(1–2):45–64, 2003.

262. Globerson A, Effros RB: Ageing of lymphocytes and lymphocytes in the aged. *Immunol Today* 21(10):515–521, 2000.

263. Grubeck-Loebenstein B, Wick G: The aging of the immune system. *Adv Immunol* 80:243–284, 2002.

264. Vallejo AN: Age-dependent alterations of the T cell repertoire and functional diversity of T cells of the aged. *Immunol Res* 36(1–3):221–228, 2006.

265. Mascarucci P, Taub D, Saccani S, et al: Age-related changes in cytokine production by leukocytes in rhesus monkeys. *Aging (Milano)* 13(2):85–94, 2001.

266. Mascarucci P, Taub D, Saccani S, et al: Cytokine responses in young and old rhesus monkeys: Effect of caloric restriction. *J Interferon Cytokine Res* 22(5):565–571, 2002.

267. Daynes RA, Araneo BA, Ershler WB, et al: Altered regulation of IL-6 production with normal aging. Possible linkage to the age-associated decline in dehydroepiandrosterone and its sulfated derivative. *J Immunol* 150(12):5219–5230, 1993.

268. Fagiolo U, Cossarizza A, Scala E, et al: Increased cytokine production in mononuclear cells of healthy elderly people. *Eur J Immunol* 23(9):2375–2378, 1993.

269. Kania DM, Binkley N, Checovich M, et al: Elevated plasma levels of interleukin-6 in postmenopausal women do not correlate with bone density. *J Am Geriatr Soc* 43(3):236–239, 1995.

270. Straub RH, Konecna L, Hrach S, et al: Serum dehydroepiandrosterone (DHEA) and DHEA sulfate are negatively correlated with serum interleukin-6 (IL-6), and DHEA inhibits IL-6 secretion from mononuclear cells in man in vitro: Possible link between endocrinosenescence and immunosenescence. *J Clin Endocrinol Metab* 83(6):2012–2017, 1998.

271. Young DG, Skibinski G, Mason JI, James K: The influence of age and gender on serum dehydroepiandrosterone sulphate (DHEA-S), IL-6, IL-6 soluble receptor (IL-6 sR) and transforming growth factor beta 1 (TGF-beta1) levels in normal healthy blood donors. *Clin Exp Immunol* 117(3):476–481, 1999.

272. Chorinchath BB, Kong LY, Mao L, McCallum RE: Age-associated differences in TNF-alpha and nitric oxide production in endotoxic mice. *J Immunol* 156(4):1525–1530, 1996.

273. O'Mahony L, Holland J, Jackson J, et al: Quantitative intracellular cytokine measurement: Age-related changes in proinflammatory cytokine production. *Clin Exp Immunol* 113(2):213–219, 1998.

274. Roubenoff R, Harris TB, Abad LW, et al: Monocyte cytokine production in an elderly population: Effect of age and inflammation. *J Gerontol A Biol Sci Med Sci* 53(1):M20–M26, 1998.

275. Wu WC, Schifftner TL, Henderson WG, et al: Preoperative hematocrit levels and postoperative outcomes in older patients undergoing noncardiac surgery. *JAMA* 297(22):2481–2488, 2007.

276. Kollman C, Howe CW, Anasetti C, et al: Donor characteristics as risk factors in recipients after transplantation of bone marrow from unrelated donors: The effect of donor age. *Blood* 98(7):2043–2051, 2001.

277. Penninx BW, Guralnik JM, Onder G, et al: Anemia and decline in physical performance among older persons. *Am J Med* 115(2):104–110, 2003.

278. Penninx BW, Kritchevsky SB, Newman AB, et al: Inflammatory markers and incident mobility limitation in the elderly. *J Am Geriatr Soc* 52(7):1105–1113, 2004.

279. Penninx BW, Pahor M, Cesari M, et al: Anemia is associated with disability and decreased physical performance and muscle strength in the elderly. *J Am Geriatr Soc* 52(5):719–724, 2004.

280. Penninx BW, Pluijm SM, Lips P, et al: Late-life anemia is associated with increased risk of recurrent falls. *J Am Geriatr Soc* 53(12):2106–2111, 2005.

281. Ezekowitz JA, McAlister FA, Armstrong PW: Anemia is common in heart failure and is associated with poor outcomes: Insights from a cohort of 12 065 patients with new-onset heart failure. *Circulation* 107(2):223–225, 2003.

282. Bernstein E, Kaye D, Abrutyn E, et al: Immune response to influenza vaccination in a large healthy elderly population. *Vaccine* 17(1):82–94, 1999.

283. Gross PA, Quinnan GV Jr, Weksler ME, et al: Relation of chronic disease and immune response to influenza vaccine in the elderly. *Vaccine* 7(4):303–308, 1989.

284. McElhaney JE, Meneilly GS, Lechelt KE, et al: Antibody response to whole-virus and split-virus influenza vaccines in successful ageing. *Vaccine* 11(10):1055–1060, 1993.

285. Murasko DM, Bernstein ED, Gardner EM, et al: Role of humoral and cell-mediated immunity in protection from influenza disease after immunization of healthy elderly. *Exp Gerontol* 2002;37(2–3):427–439, 1998.

286. Muszkat M, Friedman G, Dannenberg HD, et al: Response to influenza vaccination in community and in nursing home residing elderly: Relation to clinical factors. *Exp Gerontol* 38(10):1199–1203, 2003.

287. Yamamoto K, Takeshita K, Shimokawa T, et al: Plasminogen activator inhibitor-1 is a major stress-regulated gene: Implications for stress-induced thrombosis in aged individuals. *Proc Natl Acad Sci U S A* 99(2):890–895, 2002.

288. Tracy RP, Bovill EG, Yanez D, et al: Fibrinogen and factor VIII, but not factor VII, are associated with measures of subclinical cardiovascular disease in the elderly. Results from The Cardiovascular Health Study. *Arterioscler Thromb Vasc Biol* 15(9):1269–1279, 1995.

289. Harris TB, Ferrucci L, Tracy RP, et al: Associations of elevated interleukin-6 and C-reactive protein levels with mortality in the elderly. *Am J Med* 106(5):506–512, 1999.

290. Taaffe DR, Harris TB, Ferrucci L, et al: Cross-sectional and prospective relationships of interleukin-6 and C-reactive protein with physical performance in elderly persons: MacArthur studies of successful aging. *J Gerontol A Biol Sci Med Sci* 55(12):M709–M715, 2000.

291. Yaffe K, Lindquist K, Penninx BW, et al: Inflammatory markers and cognition in well-functioning African-American and white elders. *Neurology* 61(1):76–80, 2003.

292. Abbatecola AM, Ferrucci L, Grella R, et al: Diverse effect of inflammatory markers on insulin resistance and insulin-resistance syndrome in the elderly. *J Am Geriatr Soc* 52(3):399–404, 2004.

293. Cesari M, Leeuwenburgh C, Lauretani F, et al: Frailty syndrome and skeletal muscle: Results from the Invecchiare in Chianti study. *Am J Clin Nutr* 83(5):1142–1148, 2006.

294. Pai JK, Pischon T, Ma J, et al: Inflammatory markers and the risk of coronary heart disease in men and women. *N Engl J Med* 351(25):2599–2610, 2004.

295. Shlipak MG, Fried LF, Crump C, et al: Elevations of inflammatory and procoagulant biomarkers in elderly persons with renal insufficiency. *Circulation* 107(1):87–92, 2003.

296. Ding C, Parameswaran V, Udayan R, et al: Circulating levels of inflammatory markers predict change in bone mineral density and resorption in older adults: A longitudinal study. *J Clin Endocrinol Metab* 93(5):1952–1958, 2008.

297. Spranger J, Kroke A, Mohlig M, et al: Inflammatory cytokines and the risk to develop type 2 diabetes: Results of the prospective population-based European Prospective Investigation into Cancer and Nutrition (EPIC)-Potsdam Study. *Diabetes* 52(3):812–817, 2003.

298. Finch CE, Landfield PW: Neuroendocrine and autonomic functions in aging mammals, in *Handbook of the Biology of Aging*, edited by CE Finch, EL Schenider, pp 567–595. Van Nostrand Reinhold, New York, 1985.

299. Ferrucci L, Guralnik JM, Bandinelli S, et al: Unexplained anaemia in older persons is characterised by low erythropoietin and low levels of pro-inflammatory markers. *Br J Haematol* 136(6):849–855, 2007.

300. Denny SD, Kuchibhatla MN, Cohen HJ: Impact of anemia on mortality, cognition, and function in community-dwelling elderly. *Am J Med* 119(4):327–334, 2006.

Part IV **Molecular and Cellular Hematology**

10. Genetic Principles and Molecular
    Biology 145

11. Genomics. 155

12. Epigenetics 165

13. Cytogenetic and Genetic
    Abnormalities 173

14. Metabolism of Hematologic Neoplastic
    Cells. 191

15. Apoptosis Mechanisms: Relevance to
    the Hematopoietic System 203

16. Cell-Cycle Regulation and Hematologic
    Disorders 213

17. Signal Transduction Pathways 247

18. Hematopoietic Stem Cells, Progenitors,
    and Cytokines 257

19. The Inflammatory Response. 279

20. Innate Immunity. 293

21. Dendritic Cells and Adaptive
    Immunity. 307

CHAPTER 10
GENETIC PRINCIPLES AND MOLECULAR BIOLOGY

Lynn B. Jorde*

SUMMARY

The understanding of hematology is dependent upon an appreciation of genetic principles and the tools that can be used to study genetic variation. All the genetic information that makes up an organism is encoded in the DNA. This information is transcribed into mRNA, and then the triplet code of those mRNAs is translated into protein. Changes that affect the DNA or RNA sequence or its expression, either in the germline or acquired after birth, can cause hematologic disorders. These may be mutations that change the DNA sequence, including single base changes, deletions, insertions, and duplications, or they may be epigenetic changes that affect gene expression without any change in the DNA sequence.

The detection of mutations that cause a variety of diseases is now possible and has become a routine method for the diagnosis of some disorders. Large-scale DNA sequencing can be used to identify disease-causing genes and to carry out genetic testing. The development of methods to disrupt or prevent expression of specific genes has made it possible to produce mouse models of human hematologic diseases, and such models have the potential to serve as means to better understand pathophysiology and to study treatment strategies.

Inheritance patterns depend upon the biologic effect and chromosomal location of the mutation. Common autosomal recessive hematologic diseases include sickle cell disease, the thalassemias, and Gaucher disease. Hereditary spherocytosis, thrombophilia caused by factor V Leiden, most forms of von Willebrand disease, and acute intermittent porphyria are characterized by autosomal dominant inheritance. Mutations that cause glucose-6-phosphate dehydrogenase deficiency, hemophilias A and B, and the most common form of chronic granulomatous disease, are all carried on the X chromosome and, therefore, manifest X-linked inheritance, with transmission of the disease state from a heterozygous mother to her son. Understanding the genetics of a disorder is necessary for accurate genetic counseling.

Acronyms and Abbreviations: BACs, bacterial artificial chromosomes; bp, base pairs; cDNA, complementary DNA; CNV, copy number variant; CpG, cytosine phosphate guanine; ENU, N-ethyl-N-nitrosourea; G6PD, glucose-6-phosphate dehydrogenase; HNPCC, hereditary nonpolyposis colorectal cancer; lncRNA, long noncoding RNA; miRNA, microribonucleic acid; mRNA, messenger ribonucleic acid; mtDNA, mitochondrial DNA; NADH, nicotinamide adenine dinucleotide (reduced form); PACs, P1-derived artificial chromosomes; PCR, polymerase chain reaction; RISC, RNA-induced silencing complex; RNAi, RNA interference; rRNA, ribosomal ribonucleic acid; RT-PCR, reverse transcriptase polymerase chain reaction; SCID, severe combined immunodeficiency; siRNA, small interfering ribonucleic acid; SNP, single nucleotide polymorphism; STR, short tandem repeat; tRNA, transfer ribonucleic acid; YAC, yeast artificial chromosome.

*In the previous edition, this chapter was written by Ernest Beutler and portions of that chapter have been retained.

● GENETICS AND HEMATOLOGIC DISORDERS

Many of the hematologic diseases described in this text have a genetic basis. Often the disease is caused by a mutation in a single gene. Some of these disorders, such as sickle cell disease (Chap. 49), thalassemia (Chap. 48), glucose-6-phosphate dehydrogenase (G6PD) deficiency (Chap. 47), and factor V Leiden (Chap. 130), are common, whereas others, such as congenital dyserythropoietic anemia type I (Chap. 39), chronic granulomatous disease (Chap. 66), and afibrinogenemia (Chap. 125), are rare. All are caused by mutations in a gene that result in the formation of a defective protein or an insufficient amount of a normal protein. The principal focus of this chapter is such genetic disorders. However, a number of acquired hematologic diseases, including lymphomas, leukemias, and other clonal hematologic diseases, are the consequence of acquired damage to the genetic apparatus. Understanding these diseases requires an appreciation of how the genetic apparatus functions.

All of the information required for the development of a complete adult organism is encoded in the DNA of a single cell—the zygote. This information, designated the *genome*, includes the data needed for the synthesis of all enzymes; all the plasma proteins, including the clotting factors, complement components, and the transport proteins; all the membrane proteins, including receptors; and all of the cytoskeletal proteins. The units of information into which the genome is organized are the *genes*, which are composed of sequences of DNA. By serving as the blueprints of proteins in the body, genes ultimately influence all aspects of body structure and function. There are approximately 21,000 protein-coding genes and an additional 10,000 genes that do not encode proteins but affect the regulation of genes.[1] An error in one of these genes often leads to a recognizable genetic disease. To date, more than 20,000 genetic traits and diseases have been identified and cataloged.

DNA, RNA, AND PROTEINS: HEREDITY AT THE MOLECULAR LEVEL

DNA

DNA has three basic components: the pentose sugar molecule, deoxyribose; a phosphate molecule; and four types of nitrogenous bases. Two of the bases, *cytosine* and *thymine*, are single carbon-nitrogen rings called *pyrimidines*. The other two bases, *adenine* and *guanine*, are double carbon-nitrogen rings called *purines*. The four bases are commonly represented by their first letters: A, C, T, and G.

Watson and Crick demonstrated how these molecules are physically assembled together as DNA, proposing the *double-helix model*, in which DNA appears like a twisted ladder with chemical bonds as its rungs (Fig. 10–1).[2,3] The two sides of the ladder are made up of the sugar and phosphate molecules, held together by strong phosphodiester bonds. Projecting from each side of the ladder, at regular intervals, are the nitrogenous bases. The base projecting from one side is bound to the base projecting from the other by a weak hydrogen bond. Therefore, the nitrogenous bases form the rungs of the ladder; adenine pairs with thymine, and guanine pairs with cytosine. Each DNA subunit—consisting of one deoxyribose molecule, one phosphate group, and one base—is called a *nucleotide*.

DNA directs the synthesis of all the body's proteins. Proteins are composed of one or more *polypeptides* (intermediate protein compounds), which are, in turn, composed of sequences of *amino acids*. The body contains 20 different types of amino acids, which are specified by the four nitrogenous bases. To specify (code for) 20 different amino acids with only four bases, different combinations of bases, occurring in groups of three, are used. These triplets of bases are known as *codons*. Each codon specifies a single amino acid in a corresponding protein.

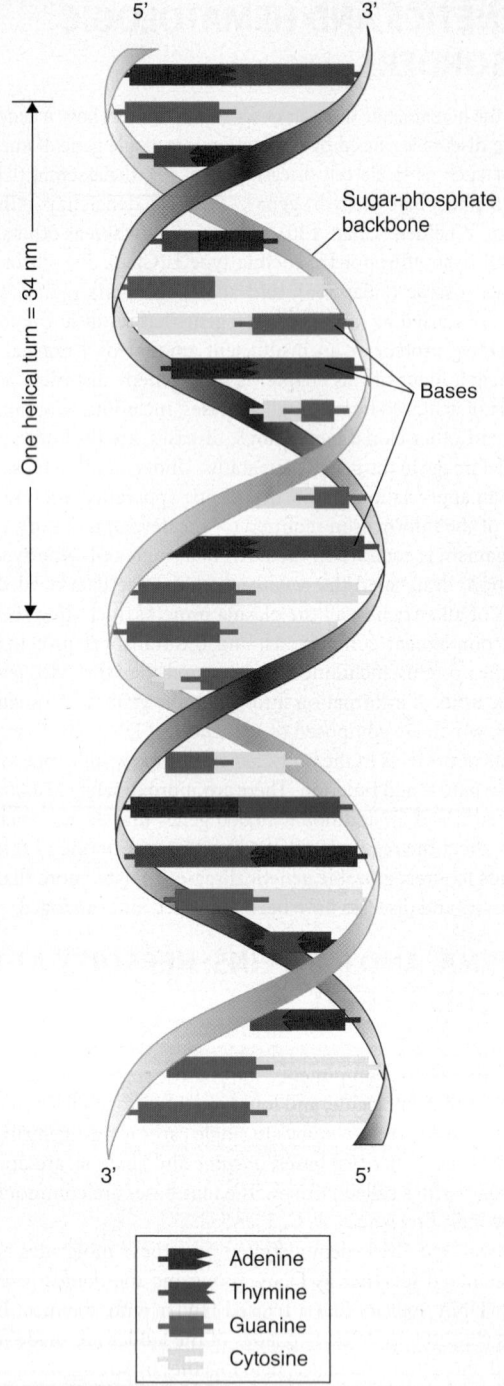

5'   3'

One helical turn = 34 nm

Sugar-phosphate
backbone

Bases

3'   5'

➤ Adenine
➤ Thymine
■ Guanine
▦ Cytosine

Figure 10–1. Watson-Crick model of the DNA molecule. The DNA structure illustrated here is based on that published by James Watson and Francis Crick in 1953. Note that each side of the DNA molecule consists of alternating sugar and phosphate groups. Each sugar group is united to the sugar group opposite it by a pair of nitrogenous bases (adenine-thymine or cytosine-guanine). The sequence of these pairs constitutes a genetic code that determines the structure and function of a cell. *(Reproduced with permission from Patton KT, Thibodeau GA: Anatomy & physiology, 8th edition. St. Louis, MO:Mosby/Elsevier, 2013.)*

Because there are 64 ($4 \times 4 \times 4$) possible codons but only 20 amino acids, there are many cases in which several codons correspond to the same amino acid.

The genetic code is universal: All living organisms use precisely the same DNA codes to specify proteins except for mitochondria, the cytoplasmic organelles in which cellular respiration takes place—they have their own extranuclear DNA. Several codons of mitochondrial DNA encode different amino acids than do the same nuclear DNA codons.

DNA replication consists of breaking the weak hydrogen bonds between the bases, leaving a single strand with each base unpaired. The consistent pairing of adenine with thymine and of guanine with cytosine, known as *complementary base pairing,* is the key to accurate replication. The unpaired base attracts a free nucleotide only if the nucleotide has the proper complementary base. When replication is complete, a new double-stranded molecule identical to the original is formed. The single strand is said to be a *template,* or molecule on which a complementary molecule is built, and is the basis for synthesizing the new double strand.

Several different proteins are involved in DNA replication. The most important of these proteins is an enzyme known as *DNA polymerase.* This enzyme travels along the single DNA strand, adding the correct nucleotides to the free end of the new strand and checking to make sure that its base is actually complementary to the template base. This mechanism of DNA proofreading substantially enhances the accuracy of DNA replication.

MUTATIONS

A *mutation* is any inherited alteration of genetic material. Mutations may cause disease or be subtle, silent substitutions that do not change amino acids. A base pair change that alters a single amino acid is termed a *missense* mutation, and a base pair change that produces a premature stop codon is termed a *nonsense* mutation. Because they typically result in a complete loss of gene product, nonsense mutations usually produce a more-severe disease phenotype than do missense mutations. For example, nonsense mutations in the factor VIII gene are much more likely to produce severe hemophilia A than are missense mutations. This is an example of a *genotype-phenotype* correlation, which can be useful in predicting the severity of disease. A *frameshift* mutation involves the insertion or deletion of one or more base pairs of the DNA molecule. These mutations change the entire "reading frame" of the DNA sequence because the deletion or insertion is not a multiple of three base pairs (bp; the number of base pairs in a codon). Frameshift mutations can thus greatly alter the amino acid sequence and typically lead to a premature stop codon downstream of the mutation. ("In-frame" insertions or deletions, in which a multiple of three bases is inserted or lost, tend to have less-severe disease consequences than do frameshift mutations.) *Splice-site* mutations describe alterations of the DNA sequence at intron–exon boundaries (see section on Genes to Proteins above). These result in a mature mRNA transcript that contains introns or lacks exons. Table 10–1 gives examples of hematologic diseases caused by different types of mutations.

Mutations are rare events. The rate of *spontaneous mutations* (those occurring in the absence of exposure to known mutagens) in humans is approximately 10^{-4} to 10^{-6} per gene per generation. This rate varies from one gene to another, with larger mutation rates for larger genes. At the nucleotide level, the human mutation rate is approximately 10^{-8} per nucleotide per generation.[4,5] Certain DNA sequences have particularly high mutation rates and are known as *mutational hot spots.* In particular, sequences consisting of a cytosine base followed by a guanine base (CpG) are highly susceptible to mutation and are known to account for a disproportionately large percentage of disease-causing mutations.

FROM GENES TO PROTEINS

DNA is formed and replicated in the cell nucleus, but protein synthesis takes place in the cytoplasm. The DNA code is transported from nucleus to cytoplasm, and subsequent protein is formed through two basic processes: transcription and translation. These processes are mediated by RNA, which is chemically similar to DNA except that the sugar molecule is ribose rather than deoxyribose, and uracil rather than thymine is one of the four bases. The other bases of RNA, as in DNA, are adenine, cytosine, and guanine. Uracil is structurally similar to thymine, so it also can pair with adenine. Whereas DNA usually occurs as a double strand, RNA usually occurs as a single strand.

In *transcription*, RNA is synthesized from a DNA template, forming *messenger RNA (mRNA)*. *RNA polymerase* binds to a *promoter* site, a sequence of DNA that specifies the beginning of a gene. RNA polymerase then separates a portion of the DNA, exposing unattached DNA bases. One DNA strand then provides the template for the sequence of mRNA nucleotides.

The sequence of bases in the mRNA is thus complementary to the template strand, and except for the presence of uracil instead of thymine, the mRNA sequence is identical to the other DNA strand. Transcription continues until a *termination sequence* is reached. Then the RNA polymerase detaches from the DNA, and the transcribed mRNA is freed to move out of the nucleus and into the cytoplasm.

When the mRNA is first transcribed from the DNA template, it reflects exactly the base sequence of the DNA. In eukaryotes, many RNA sequences are removed by nuclear enzymes, and the remaining sequences are spliced together to form the functional mRNA that migrates to the cytoplasm. The excised sequences are called *introns*, and the sequences that are left to code for proteins are called *exons*.

In *translation*, RNA directs the synthesis of a polypeptide, interacting with *transfer RNA (tRNA)*, a cloverleaf-shaped strand of approximately 80 nucleotides. The tRNA molecule has a site where an amino acid attaches. The three-nucleotide sequence at the opposite side of the cloverleaf is called the *anticodon*. It undergoes complementary base pairing with an appropriate codon in the mRNA, which specifies the sequence of amino acids through tRNA.

The site of actual protein synthesis is in the *ribosome*, which consists of roughly equal parts of protein and *ribosomal RNA (rRNA)*. During translation, the ribosome first binds to an initiation site on the mRNA sequence and then binds to its surface, so that base pairing can occur between tRNA and mRNA. The ribosome then moves along the mRNA sequence, processing each codon and translating an amino acid by way of the interaction of mRNA and tRNA.

The ribosome provides an enzyme that catalyzes the formation of covalent peptide bonds between the adjacent amino acids, resulting in a growing polypeptide. When the ribosome arrives at a termination signal on the mRNA sequence, translation and polypeptide formation cease; the mRNA, ribosome, and polypeptide separate from one another; and the polypeptide is released into the cytoplasm to perform its required function.

All cells receive the same complement of genes. Nonetheless, some proteins are tissue-specific. Several circumstances can account for this. Some enzymes that appear to perform the same function are encoded by different genes in different tissues. For example, the pyruvate kinase of leukocytes and that of erythrocytes are under separate genetic control (Chap. 47). In other cases, alternative splicing of the primary mRNA can produce different polypeptides, a phenomenon that is particularly prominent with some of the red cell membrane proteins. Differences in posttranslational processing, including proteolysis and glycosylation of the same polypeptide by different enzymes in different tissues, can lead to different final products. However, in most instances a mutation that affects an enzyme in one type of blood cell will also affect the same enzyme in other blood cells, in liver, in brain, and in other tissues.

MENDELIAN GENETICS

Traits caused by single genes are called mendelian traits (after Gregor Mendel). Each gene occupies a position along a chromosome known as a *locus*. The genes at a particular locus can take different forms (i.e., they can be composed of different nucleotide sequences) called *alleles*. A locus that has two or more alleles that each occurs with an appreciable frequency (classically defined as 1%) in a population is said to be *polymorphic* (or a *polymorphism*). Polymorphisms that involve a single nucleotide are termed *single nucleotide polymorphisms (SNPs)*, while those that involve the presence or absence of larger pieces of DNA are termed *copy number variants (CNVs)*.[6,7] Sometimes genetic variants, such as the alleles responsible for sickle cell disease, thalassemia, or G6PD deficiency, reach polymorphic levels because the deleterious effects that they may have are counterbalanced by beneficial effects on survival, such as increased resistance to malaria.[8] They are known as *balanced polymorphisms*. *Short tandem repeats (STRs)* are a special form of polymorphism consisting of differing numbers of repeating units of one to six nucleotides, for example, ATATATATAT. Such sequences are unstable in evolution of a species and tend to be very polymorphic. Instead of only two possible genotypes, as in the case of most SNPs, there may be 5, 10, or more different numbers of repeats at a given locus in different individuals. As a result, STRs are very useful in genetic mapping and in forensic analysis.[9] In addition, an expanded number of repeat copies of some STRs located within or near genes is an important cause of inherited disease.[10]

Because humans are diploid organisms, each chromosome is represented twice, with one member of the chromosome pair contributed by the father and one by the mother. At a given locus, an individual has one allele whose origin is paternal and one whose origin is maternal. When the two alleles are identical, the individual is *homozygous* at that locus. When the alleles are not identical, the individual is *heterozygous* at that locus. The composition of genes at a given locus is known as the *genotype*. The outward appearance of an individual, which is the result of both genotype and environment, is the *phenotype*.

DOMINANCE AND RECESSIVENESS

In his experiments with garden peas, Gregor Mendel established that many traits can be either *dominant* or *recessive*. In dominant traits, such as von Willebrand disease or porphyria cutanea tarda type II, one copy of a disease-causing allele is sufficient for disease causation, so heterozygotes are typically affected. In recessive traits, such as β-thalassemia, two copies of the disease-causing allele must be present, so the affected individual is a homozygote. A *carrier* is an individual who has a disease gene but is phenotypically normal. Many alleles for a recessive disease occur in heterozygotes that carry one copy of the gene but do not express the disease. When recessive alleles are lethal in the homozygous state, they are eliminated from the population when they occur in homozygotes. By "hiding" in carriers, however, recessive genes for diseases are passed on to the next generation (the word "recessive" comes from the Latin for "hidden").

GENE DUPLICATION

Crossing over during meiosis usually occurs with great precision. Homologous genes pair with each other, and although genes that were together on the chromosome before meiosis may now be on opposite chromosomes of the pair, each chromosome still contains a complete set of genes (see Fig. 10–1). Occasionally, however, an error occurs and pairing during meiosis is imperfect. Under these circumstances—unequal crossing over (see Fig. 10–5)—one of the daughter chromosomes contains a duplicated gene, while the other one exists with a gene deleted. Once a duplication has occurred, further duplications occur more readily, because pairing of the first of the duplicate genes on one chromosome with the second gene of the duplicate on the other produces one chromosome with a triplicated gene and one with a single gene (Chap. 48). Duplication has probably played a very important role in the course of evolution[11] because the presence of two genes with the same function allows experiments of nature: Mutations can accumulate on one of the genes while the original function is still provided by the duplicate. Examples of the results of gene duplication abound in hematology, particularly with respect to the hemoglobin loci. The γ-chain loci are duplicated, and there are also two nearly identical copies of the α-chain locus (Chap. 48). Furthermore, the close similarity of their amino acid sequence and the fact that they are tightly linked indicate that the β, γ, and δ loci represent the result of duplication of a single ancestral gene. The process of unequal crossing over takes place not only between genes, but also within genes. When this occurs, one would anticipate that a portion of the amino acid sequence of a protein is represented twice on one chromosome and is missing on the other. The Lepore hemoglobins, leading to a thalassemic clinical state, are an example of this type of unequal crossing over (Fig. 48–8). These abnormal hemoglobins have the amino acid sequence of the δ chain at the amino end, and the sequence of the β chain at the carboxyl end. The complement to this kind of abnormality, the "anti-Lepore" hemoglobin, also has also been found (Chap. 49). Similarly, a mutation of the glucocerebrosidase gene causing Gaucher disease has been found to be the result of a crossover between the active gene and the pseudogene.[12] The two types of haptoglobin represent an ancestral gene and one in which a major part of that gene has been duplicated.[13]

● TRANSMISSION OF GENETIC DISEASES

The known single-gene diseases can be classified into four major modes of inheritance: autosomal dominant, autosomal recessive, X-linked dominant, and X-linked recessive.[14] The first two types involve genes known to occur on the 22 pairs of autosomes. The last two types occur on the X chromosome; very few disease-causing genes are found on the Y chromosome.

The *pedigree* chart summarizes family relationships and shows which members of a family are affected by a genetic disease (Fig. 10–2).[15] Generally, the pedigree begins with one individual in the family, the *proband*. This individual is usually the first person in the family diagnosed or seen in a clinic.

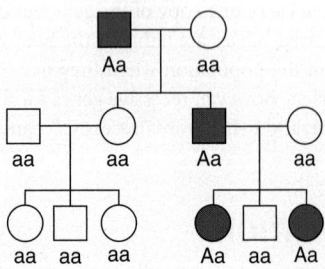

Figure 10–2. Pedigree for an autosomal dominant disease. (*Reproduced with permission from Jorde LB, Carey JC, Barnshad MJ: Medical Genetics, 4th edition. Philadelphia, PA: Mosby/Elsevier, 2010.*)

AUTOSOMAL DOMINANT INHERITANCE

Diseases caused by autosomal dominant genes are rare, with the most common occurring in fewer than 1 in 500 individuals. Therefore, it is uncommon for two individuals who are both affected by the same autosomal dominant disease to produce offspring together. Affected offspring are usually produced by the union of a normal parent with an affected heterozygous parent. The affected parent can pass either a disease gene or a normal gene to the next generation. On average, half the children will be heterozygous and will express the disease, and half will be normal.

The pedigree in Fig. 10–2 shows the transmission of an autosomal dominant trait or disease. Several important characteristics of this pedigree support the conclusion that the trait is inherited in autosomal dominant fashion:

1. The two sexes exhibit the trait in approximately equal proportions, and males and females are equally likely to transmit the trait to their offspring.
2. No generations are skipped. If an individual has the trait, one parent must also have it. If neither parent has the trait, none of the children have it (with the exception of new mutations, as discussed later in this section).
3. Affected heterozygous individuals transmit the trait to approximately half their children, and because gamete transmission is subject to chance fluctuations, all or none of the children of an affected parent may have the trait. When large numbers of matings of this type are studied, however, the proportion of affected children closely approaches one-half.

The probability that an at-risk individual (e.g., someone with a positive family history) will develop a genetic disease is termed the *recurrence risk*. When one parent is affected by an autosomal dominant disease (and is a heterozygote) and the other is unaffected, the recurrence risk for each child is one-half.

An important principle is that each birth is an independent event, much like a coin toss. Thus, even though parents may have already had a child with the disease, their recurrence risk remains one-half. Even if they have had several children, all affected (or all unaffected) by the disease, the law of independence dictates that the probability that their next child will have the disease is still one-half. Parents' misunderstanding of this principle is a common problem encountered in genetic counseling.

If a child is born with an autosomal dominant disease and there is no history of the disease in the family, the child is probably the product of a new (or *de novo*) mutation.[16] The gene transmitted by one of the parents has thus undergone a mutation from a normal to a disease-causing allele. The genes at this locus in most of the parent's other germ cells are still normal. In this situation the recurrence risk for the parent's subsequent offspring is not greater than that of the general population. The offspring of the affected child, however, will have a recurrence risk of one-half. Because these diseases often reduce the potential for reproduction, many autosomal dominant diseases result from new mutations.

Occasionally, two or more offspring have symptoms of an autosomal dominant disease when there is no family history of the disease. Because mutation is a rare event, it is unlikely that this disease would be a result of multiple mutations in the same family. The mechanism most likely responsible is termed *germline mosaicism*.[17] During the embryonic development of one of the parents, a mutation occurred that affected all or part of the germline, but few or none of the somatic cells of the embryo. Thus, the parent carries the mutation in the parent's germline but does not actually express the disease. As a result, the unaffected parent can transmit the mutation to multiple offspring. This phenomenon, although relatively rare, can have significant effects on recurrence risks.[18]

AUTOSOMAL RECESSIVE INHERITANCE

Like autosomal dominant diseases, diseases caused by autosomal recessive genes are rare in populations, although there can be numerous carriers. Sickle cell disease is seen in approximately 1 in 600 Americans of African descent, but it occurs in the heterozygote state in approximately 1 in 12 members of this population.[19] Under most circumstances, carriers are phenotypically normal. Like autosomal dominant diseases, many autosomal recessive diseases are characterized by incomplete penetrance and variable expressivity.

Figure 10–3 shows a pedigree for an autosomal recessive condition such as sickle cell disease. The important criteria for discerning autosomal recessive inheritance include the following:

1. Males and females are affected in equal proportions.
2. Consanguinity (marriage between related individuals) is sometimes present, especially for rare recessive diseases.
3. The disease may be seen in siblings of affected individuals, but usually not in their parents.
4. On average, one-fourth of the offspring of carrier parents will be affected.

In most cases of recessive disease, both of the parents of affected individuals are heterozygous carriers. On average, one-fourth of their offspring will be normal homozygotes, one-half will be phenotypically normal carrier heterozygotes, and one-fourth will be homozygotes with the disease. Thus, the recurrence risk for the offspring of carrier parents is 25 percent. However, in any given family, there are chance fluctuations.

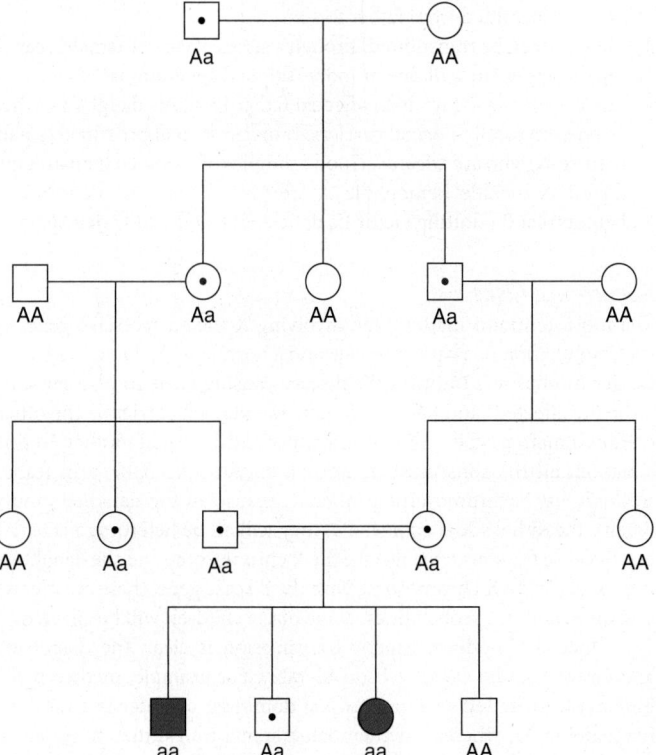

Figure 10–3. Pedigree for sickle cell disease. The double bar denotes a consanguineous mating. Because sickle cell disease is relatively common in some populations, most cases do not involve consanguinity. *(Reproduced with permission from Jorde LB, Carey JC, Barnshad MJ: Medical Genetics, 4th edition. Philadelphia, PA: Mosby/Elsevier, 2010.)*

If two parents both have a recessive disease, they each must be homozygous for the disease. Therefore, all their children also must be affected. This distinguishes recessive from dominant inheritance because two parents both affected by a dominant gene are nearly always both heterozygotes and thus one-fourth of their children will be unaffected.

Because carrier parents usually are unaware that they both carry the same recessive allele, they often produce an affected child before knowing of their condition. Carrier detection tests can identify heterozygotes by measuring the reduced amount of a critical enzyme. This enzyme is totally lacking in a homozygous recessive individual, but a carrier, although phenotypically normal, will typically have half the normal enzyme level. Increasingly, carriers are now detected by direct examination of their DNA to reveal a mutation. Carrier detection tests are available for many hematologic recessive diseases, including sickle cell disease, α- and β-thalassemia, Gaucher disease, and hemochromatosis.[20-22]

PENETRANCE AND EXPRESSIVITY

The *penetrance* of a trait is the percentage of individuals with a specific genotype who also exhibit the expected phenotype. Incomplete penetrance means that individuals who have the gene disease-causing genotype may not exhibit the disease phenotype at all, even though the genotype and the associated disease may be transmitted to the next generation. Penetrance can increase with age, and it can differ between the sexes. For example, the penetrance of hemochromatosis, an autosomal recessive condition, increases with age as iron accumulates in organs such as the heart and liver. The penetrance of the hemochromatosis genotype is higher in males than females because females deplete their iron supplies by menstruation, childbirth, and lactation.[23]

Expressivity is the extent of variation in phenotype associated with a particular genotype. If the expressivity of a disease is variable, penetrance may be complete but the severity of the disease can vary greatly. Many hematologic conditions, including sickle cell disease and β-thalassemia, have variable expressivity. This can be a result of the effects of other genes *(modifier loci)*, an example of which is variants in the *BCL11A* gene that increase fetal hemoglobin levels and attenuate the effects of sickle cell disease.[24] Similarly, the factor V Leiden variant is more likely to produce thrombophilia if a second mutation of a gene encoding another coagulation factor, such as protein C, is coinherited.[25] In addition, different mutations at a locus can cause variation in severity. For example, a mutation that alters only one amino acid of the factor VIII gene usually produces a mild form of hemophilia A, whereas a "stop" codon (premature termination of translation) usually produces a more-severe form of this clotting disorder.[26,27] Nongenetic ("environmental") factors can also influence expression, as in hemochromatosis, where alcohol abuse can increase the severity of expression.[28]

X-LINKED INHERITANCE

Some genetic conditions are caused by mutations in genes located on the sex chromosomes, and that mode of inheritance is termed *sex linked*. Only a few diseases are known to be inherited as X-linked dominant or Y chromosome traits, so only the more common X-linked recessive diseases are discussed here.

Because females receive two X chromosomes, one from the father and one from the mother, they can be homozygous for a disease allele at a given locus, homozygous for the normal allele at the locus, or heterozygous. Males, having only one X chromosome, are *hemizygous* for genes on this chromosome. If a male inherits a recessive disease gene on the X chromosome, he will be affected by the disease because the

Y chromosome does not carry a normal allele to counteract the effects of the disease gene. Because a single copy of an X-linked recessive gene will cause disease in a male, whereas two copies are required for disease expression in females, more males are affected by X-linked recessive diseases than are females.

X INACTIVATION

In the late 1950s, Mary Lyon proposed that one X chromosome in the somatic cells of females is permanently inactivated, a process termed *X inactivation* (Fig. 10–4).[29-33] This proposal, the Lyon hypothesis, explains why most gene products coded by the X chromosome are present in equal amounts in males and females, even though males have only one X chromosome and females have two X chromosomes. This phenomenon is called *dosage compensation*. The inactivated X chromosomes are observable in many interphase cells as highly condensed intranuclear chromatin bodies, termed *Barr bodies* (after Barr and Bertram, who discovered them in the late 1940s). Normal females have one Barr body in each somatic cell, whereas normal males have no Barr bodies.

X-inactivation occurs very early in embryonic development—approximately 7 to 14 days after fertilization. In each somatic cell, one of the two X chromosomes is inactivated. In some cells, the inactivated X chromosome is the one contributed by the father; in other cells it is the one contributed by the mother. Once the X chromosome has been inactivated in a cell, all the descendants of that cell have the same chromosome inactivated. Thus inactivation is said to be random but *fixed*.

Some individuals do not have the normal number of X chromosomes in their somatic cells. For example, males with Klinefelter syndrome typically have two X chromosomes and one Y chromosome. These males do have one Barr body in each cell. Females whose cell nuclei have three X chromosomes have two Barr bodies in each cell, and females whose cell nuclei have four X chromosomes have three Barr bodies in each cell. Females with Turner syndrome have only one X chromosome and no Barr bodies. Thus, the number of Barr bodies is always one less than the number of X chromosomes in the cell. All but one X chromosome are always inactivated.

Persons with abnormal numbers of X chromosomes, such as those with Turner syndrome or Klinefelter syndrome, are not physically normal. This situation presents a puzzle because they presumably have only one active X chromosome, just as individuals with normal numbers of chromosomes do. This is probably because the distal tips of the short and long arms of the X chromosome, as well as several other regions on the chromosome arm, are not inactivated. Thus, X inactivation is also known to be *incomplete*.

Although the mechanisms underlying X inactivation are only partially understood, the gene responsible for initiating X inactivation, *XIST*, has been identified.[34] This gene encodes a *long noncoding RNA (lncRNA)* that coats one of the X chromosomes, which is then inactivated (it is estimated that the human genome contains approximately 9000 lncRNA genes[1]). Methylation of X chromosome DNA, a process in which DNA is inactivated when cytosine bases are enzymatically converted to 5-methylcytosine, occurs on the inactivated X chromosome. Inactive X chromosomes can be at least partially reactivated *in vitro* by administering 5-azacytidine, a demethylating agent.

Characteristics of Pedigrees

X-linked pedigrees show distinctive modes of inheritance. The most striking characteristic is that females seldom are affected. To express an X-linked recessive trait, a female must be homozygous: either both her parents are affected, or her father is affected and her mother is a carrier. Such matings are rare.

The following are important principles of X-linked recessive inheritance:

1. The trait is seen much more often in males than in females.
2. Because a father can give a son only a Y chromosome, the trait is never transmitted from father to son.
3. The gene can be transmitted through a series of carrier females, causing the appearance of one or more "skipped generations."
4. The gene is passed from an affected father to all his daughters, who, as phenotypically normal carriers, transmit it to approximately half their sons, who are affected. Good examples of X-linked hematologic disorders include hemophilia A (clotting factor VIII deficiency), hemophilia B (clotting factor IX deficiency), and G6PD deficiency.

Recurrence Risks

The most common mating type involving X-linked recessive genes is the combination of a carrier female and a normal male. On average, the carrier mother will transmit the disease-causing allele to half her sons (who are affected) and half her daughters (who are carriers). The other common mating type is an affected father and a normal mother. In this situation, all the sons must be normal because the father can transmit only his Y chromosome to them. Because all the daughters must receive the father's X chromosome, they will all be heterozygous carriers. Because the sons *must* receive the Y chromosome and the daughters *must* receive the X chromosome with the disease gene, these are precise outcomes and not probabilities. None of the children will be affected.

Once the mode of genetic transmission is clear, the diagnostic alternatives can be narrowed considerably. For example, methemoglobinemia transmitted as an autosomal dominant disorder is a result of hemoglobin M, whereas methemoglobinemia transmitted as an autosomal recessive disorder is a result of cytochrome b5 reductase (the reduced form of nicotinamide adenine dinucleotide [NADH] diaphorase) deficiency (Chap. 49). Hemolytic anemia with autosomal dominant transmission is likely to be a result of hereditary spherocytosis, but sex-linked transmission of the hemolytic state suggests a deficiency of G6PD or, more rarely, phosphoglycerate kinase. A bleeding disorder that is transmitted in an X-linked fashion may be caused by a deficiency

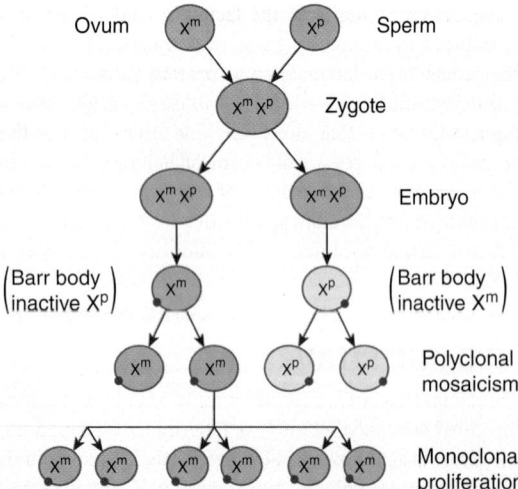

Figure 10–4. The X inactivation process. At fertilization, the female zygote inherits one maternal chromosome (X^m) and one paternal X chromosome (X^p). At some time early in embryogenesis, one X in each cell is inactivated at random and condenses to form the Barr body. The active X remains active not only for the lifetime of that cell but for the lifetime of all of its progeny. A tumor with a clonal origin will consist entirely of cells in all of which either X^m or X^p is active. A tumor with a multicentric origin may contain both X^m and X^p cells.

of factor VIII or factor IX, but autosomal recessive inheritance should suggest to the physician a deficiency of other clotting factors, such as factor X, XI, or V. Careful analysis of the family history not only will make possible more appropriate genetic counseling to the patient and family, but also will shorten the road to a correct diagnosis.

EPIGENETICS AND GENOMIC IMPRINTING

Although this chapter focuses on DNA sequence variation and its consequence for disease, there is increasing evidence that the same DNA sequence can produce dramatically different phenotypes because of chemical modifications that alter the *expression* of genes (these modifications are collectively termed *epigenetic*; Chap. 12). Epigenetic alteration of gene activity can have important disease consequences. For example, a major cause of one form of inherited colon cancer (termed *hereditary nonpolyposis colorectal cancer [HNPCC]*) is the methylation of a gene whose protein product repairs damaged DNA.[35] When this gene becomes inactive, damaged DNA accumulates eventually resulting in colon tumors.[36]

LINKAGE ANALYSIS AND GENE IDENTIFICATION

Locating genes on specific regions of chromosomes has been one of the most important goals of human genetics. The location and identification of a gene can tell much about the function of the gene, its interaction with other genes, and the likelihood that certain individuals will develop a genetic disease.

Mendel's second law, the principle of independent assortment, states that an individual's genes will be transmitted to the next generation independently of one another. This law is only partly true, however, because genes located close together on the same chromosome do tend to be transmitted together to the offspring. Thus Mendel's principle of independent assortment holds true for most pairs of genes but not those that occupy the same region of a chromosome. Such loci demonstrate *linkage* and are said to be linked.

During the first meiotic stage, the arms of homologous chromosome pairs intertwine and sometimes exchange portions of their DNA (Fig. 10–5) in a process known as *crossover*. During crossover, new combinations of alleles can be formed. For example, two loci on a chromosome have alleles *A* and *a* and alleles *B* and *b*. Alleles *A* and *B* are located together on one member of a chromosome pair, and alleles *a* and *b* are located on the other member. The genotype of this individual is denoted as *AB/ab*.

As Fig. 10–5A shows, the allele pairs *AB* and *ab* would be transmitted together when no crossover occurs. However, when crossover occurs (Fig. 10–5B), all four possible pairs of alleles can be transmitted to the offspring: *AB*, *aB*, *Ab*, and *ab*. The process of forming such new arrangements of alleles is called *recombination*. Crossover does not necessarily lead to recombination, however, because double crossover between two loci can result in no actual recombination of the alleles at the loci (Fig. 10–5).

The analysis of recombination in families is used to determine the locations of disease-causing genes.[37] Millions of SNPs have been identified in the human genome, and their chromosome locations

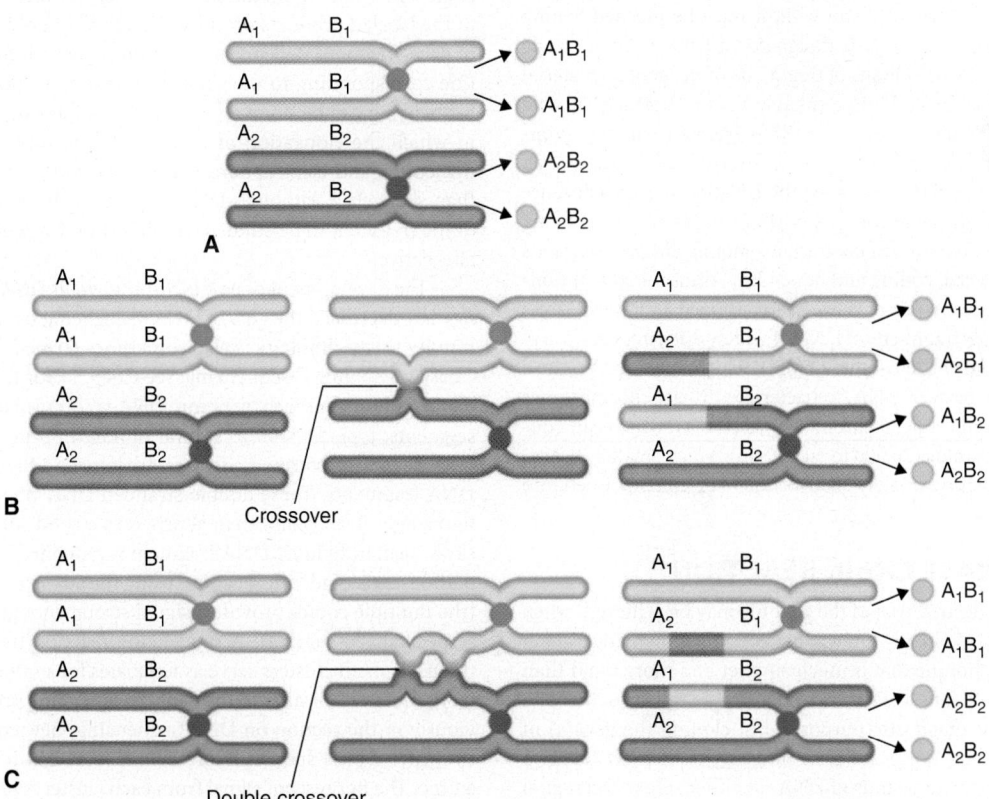

Figure 10–5. Genetic results of crossing over. **A.** No crossing over. **B.** Crossing over with recombination. **C.** Double crossing over, resulting in no recombination. *(Reproduced with permission from McCance KL, Huether SE, Brashers VL, et al: Pathophysiology: The biologic basis for disease in adults and children, 6th edition. St. Louis, MO:Mosby/Elsevier, 2010.)*

are known.[38] If a SNP demonstrates close linkage with a disease phenotype in a family or a series of families, then the disease-causing locus must be located near the SNP. This establishes the approximate location of the disease-causing locus. Linkage can be used in some cases to help diagnose genetic disease in family members by determining whether a parent who has a disease-causing allele has transmitted a linked SNP allele to their offspring.

The Human Genome Project was initiated in 1990 and completed in 2003. Its main goals were to discover polymorphisms useful for linkage throughout the genome (the "gene map") and to determine the entire human DNA sequence.[39–41] These goals have been accomplished, and DNA sequencing has become far cheaper and more efficient in recent years (Chap. 11). Consequently, many thousands of individuals have now been sequenced, and the genes responsible for approximately 4000 mendelian conditions have been identified.[14,42,43] This has greatly increased our understanding of the mechanisms that underlie many diseases and has permitted more accurate genetic testing and diagnosis.

● THE METHODS OF MOLECULAR BIOLOGY

CLONING DNA

The sequencing of DNA and the preparation of probes requires that a fragment of DNA is amplified manyfold to provide a relatively pure sample for study. The classical method by which this is achieved, *cloning*, is a central technique of molecular biology.[3] It is generally accomplished by inserting the DNA into a vector, a bacteriophage or plasmid, that normally replicates within a bacterial cell. When such a phage or plasmid contains a foreign DNA fragment, the fragment also undergoes replication and can then be purified in greatly amplified form. If the DNA is not available in pure form to begin with, it must be purified from a collection of DNA fragments that is designated a *library*. An adequate genomic library consists of millions of fragments of the genetic material of a cell that have been ligated into a suitable vector. Another valuable type of library is made by transcribing mRNA from a tissue into complementary DNA (cDNA) using the enzyme reverse transcriptase. Such a cDNA library is particularly useful for the isolation of genes because in it are represented only the intron-free portions of genes that are being actively transcribed in a tissue. In contrast, a genomic library represents all of the genetic material, coding and noncoding, transcribed and nontranscribed. Many different vectors have been designed and they possess the capacity to replicate fragments of DNA of widely differing sizes, varying from yeast artificial chromosomes (YACs), which may incorporate a million or more base pairs of DNA, to bacterial artificial chromosomes (BACs) and P1-derived artificial chromosomes (PACs), which can contain 100,000 bp, to cosmids (20,000 to 30,000 bp). Much smaller inserts, ranging in size from approximately 3000 to 12,000 bp can be cloned into bacteriophages.

THE POLYMERASE CHAIN REACTION

Amplification of the desired part of the genome may be achieved, when some of the sequence is already known, by using the polymerase chain reaction (PCR), a technique that is much simpler and more rapid than cloning.[44] For example, one may wish to determine the sequence of a portion of a gene for diagnostic purposes, but cloning the gene(s) of interest is too time-consuming and labor intensive to be practical. Two primers matching opposite strands of DNA on either side of the region of interest are used to amplify the intervening specific segment of DNA by more than a million-fold. Successive cycles of DNA synthesis from the primers and chain separation by heating between the cycles are the basis of this powerful technique.

PCR can be carried out just a few nanograms of DNA, as opposed to the micrograms required for cloning. The amount of DNA in a several-year-old blood stain, a single hair, or even the back of a licked postage stamp is often sufficient for analysis. PCR is so sensitive that under optimal conditions the DNA from a single cell may be amplified. Moreover, the stability of DNA is such that very old preserved material may be used. Thus, it is possible to amplify the DNA from blood films, mummies, and other ancient biologic material.[45] In addition, because it does not require cloning, the procedure is much faster than older techniques. Genetic testing for sickle cell disease, for example, can be done in a single day with PCR.

Amplifying by PCR cDNA produced by reverse-transcribing mRNA in tissue extracts (reverse transcriptase polymerase chain reaction [RT-PCR]) provides a very sensitive means for measuring the expression of genes in tissues.[46] In the early cycles of PCR, the rate of amplification is a function of the amount of template; thus it allows for quantification of mRNA or DNA. For this purpose, a housekeeping mRNA is also measured and the ratio of this reference mRNA to tested mRNA is used. Thus, the slope of the curve can be used to measure the amount of mRNA or DNA in a specimen. This process, which has been designated *real-time PCR*, has been automated by using fluorescent probes that are destroyed during the amplification process or a dye that binds only to double-stranded DNA.

DNA SEQUENCING

The chain termination technique has traditionally been used to determine the sequence of DNA.[47] It depends upon synthesizing a labeled strand of DNA, with the DNA to be sequenced serving as the template. The mixture of nucleotides used contains a nucleotide analogue that results in chain termination when incorporated. Gel electrophoresis of the labeled products produces "ladders" of polynucleotides. The size of each fragment depends on the point at which there exists a nucleotide corresponding to the chain terminating analogue in the mixture. Sequencing can be done rapidly and accurately by automated methods in which the elongation of the strand is terminated by a fluorescent nucleotide and electrophoresis is carried out in capillary tubes rather than slab gels.[48] Although DNA sequencing formerly required cloning of the fragment to be studied, amplification by PCR serves as a simpler alternative.

The development of new *high-throughput DNA sequencing* technology has decreased the cost of DNA sequencing by many orders of magnitude (this technology is also sometimes termed "next-generation" or "massively parallel" sequencing; see Chap. 11 for further details).[49–51] In one common approach, genomic DNA is chopped at random into small segments, typically 100 to several hundred bp in size. Short synthetic DNA sequences, termed *adapters*, are joined to the ends of the genomic DNA fragments. These double-stranded DNA fragments are separated into single strands and then attached to a solid surface, such as a glass slide. Each individual DNA fragment is amplified by PCR into a cluster of thousands of identical copies, using the adapters as primer sequences (the multiple copies provide a signal strong enough to be visualized by a specilialized camera). A sequencing reaction then occurs, in which these fragment clusters serve as templates for synthesizing complementary sequences. Similar to the Sanger sequencing process described previously in the section on DNA sequencing, new complementary bases (to which a base-specific fluorescent label is attached) are added one at a time. The fluorescent signal from each cluster is recorded by a camera, revealing the base-pair sequence of each fragment. The key advantage of this approach is that millions of different DNA fragments are sequenced simultaneously, in contrast to older methods in which only a few dozen fragments are sequenced at a time.

INTERFERENCE WITH GENE EXPRESSION

Antisense RNA and DNA

It is possible to interdict the expression of a gene at several different levels. The translation of mRNA can be inhibited and the mRNA degraded by *antisense* RNA or DNA, molecules that have a sequence complementary to the mRNA that is to be inactivated. When such oligonucleotides are present, they inhibit gene expression through a variety of mechanisms. For example, they form a double strand with the RNA, just as two complementary strands of DNA will hybridize to form the normal double-stranded form of DNA. Because the double-stranded form cannot be translated and is probably degraded rapidly, the production of its protein product is inhibited specifically. In experimental systems, antisense DNA or stable DNA analogues, such as the methylphosphonates, can be transfected directly into cells or the RNA can be made off of a plasmid with the appropriate DNA template and a promoter. Originally this approach was used, for example, to suppress lymphoma growth with DNA oligonucleotides antisense to introns of the oncogene c-myc, to suppress marrow cells from patients with chronic myelogenous leukemia by antisense DNA directed at the BCR-ABL junction, or to suppress BCL-2–positive lymphoma cells in culture by BCL-2 antisense.[64] Because antisense RNA can be produced *in vivo* by transcribing the complementary strand of a gene, it may represent a natural regulatory mechanism.

Interfering RNA

RNA plays a much broader role in the physiologic regulation of genes than merely the formation of antisense mRNAs. siRNAs (small interfering ribonucleic acids) and the closely related miRNAs (microribonucleic acids) represent a mechanism for silencing of genes, through a process known as RNA interference (RNAi[52,53]). In the case of siRNA, double-stranded RNA is cleaved by the "dicer" enzyme into approximately 22 bp segments that trigger the destruction through the RNA-induced silencing complex (RISC) of the homologous targeted mRNA. Although siRNAs tend to operate through RISC and slice the targeted mRNA, the miRNAs that represent endogenous duplexes can decrease the amount of target mRNA(s) or can also posttranscriptionally regulate gene expression by complexing with the same RISC and interfering with the targeted mRNA translation. miRNAs may play an important role in hematopoietic differentiation[54] and seem to be widely used as a gene regulatory and antiviral measure. The use of siRNA has become very useful to molecular biologists as a powerful method for the downregulation of genes in experimental systems.

Ribozymes

Cleaving RNA at defined sequences, much as restriction endonucleases cleave DNA, is one of the known enzymatic functions of RNA, and this function provides a means by which the expression of a gene can be interdicted in experimental systems. This *ribozyme* approach has been used, for example, in preventing replication of the HIV-1 virus[55] and by cleaving BCR-ABL fusion transcript with a view to developing a treatment for chronic myelogenous leukemia.[56]

Transgenic and Knockout Animal Models

The insertion of DNA fragments into the nucleus of a fertilized ovum provides a means for altering the genetic constitution of animals. Animals that have been engineered in this manner are referred to as *transgenic*. The use of promoters that are inducible or tissue specific permits studies of the effect of a gene product that might be lethal if expressed in all tissues or at all times during embryogenesis. Transgenic mice that carry the human sickle β-globin gene have been produced and when superimposed on a murine thalassemic genotype produce high enough levels of human hemoglobin S to have some potential as an animal model of sickle disease (Chaps. 48 and 49).[57] Another valuable technique for the study of gene function is targeted disruption ("knocking out") of genes. In this technique, a DNA construct that contains regions homologous to the gene being targeted and selectable markers is transfected into an embryonic mouse stem cell. Once a cell in which recombination has occurred within a gene is found, it can be implanted into a blastocyst, with the hope that some of the progeny of the implanted cell will become germ cells. If this does occur, the knockout can be propagated and homozygous animals bred. The value of the technique is often limited by the fact that the knockout may be lethal (e.g., G6PD75 deficiency and Gaucher disease) or may not have any abnormal phenotype. But in some diseases, such as hemochromatosis,[58] knockout models of various forms of the disease are valuable resources. In situations in which a knockout proves to be lethal, or where it would be useful to limit the deficiency to a single-organ system, the Cre/LoxP site-specific recombination system has proven to be very useful.[59] The LoxP sequence, a 13-bp inverted repeat, is inserted so that it flanks the gene that is to be removed. Site specific recombination is catalyzed by the P-1 bacteriophage Cre recombinase, excising the intervening DNA targeted by the LoxP sequence and ligating the remaining 5′ and 3′ DNA. Tissue-specific excision can be achieved by inserting the Cre-recombinase downstream from a tissue-specific promoter. Random mutagenesis with agents such as N-ethyl-N-nitrosourea (ENU) can identify functions of genes whose role in a metabolic pathway was unsuspected. For example, a mutation in a membrane serine protease of unknown function revealed that it was a negative regulator of hepcidin, and subsequent investigations revealed that mutations of this gene caused hereditary iron deficiency in humans.[60]

● GENE THERAPY

In somatic cell *gene therapy*, the DNA of a specific set of a patient's somatic cells is altered. It is also possible to carry out germline therapy, which affects all cells, including reproductive cells, but for technical and ethical reasons this is not being pursued in humans. Most commonly, somatic cell therapy is used for conditions in which a mutation has caused the absence of a gene product in a cell (e.g., adenosine deaminase in T cells, which leads to an autosomal recessive form of severe combined immunodeficiency [SCID]).[61] A vector is used to carry a normal copy of the mutated gene into the patient's cells. These vectors are usually viruses, such as retroviruses or adenoviruses, which have been genetically modified so that they contain the normal human gene and cannot make copies of themselves (otherwise they could cause a viral infection). Once inside the patient's cells, the normal human gene begins to encode the missing gene product. For diseases caused by a gain of function, techniques such as antisense DNA or RNA and RNAi (discussed in the section on Interference with Gene Expression.) are being used.

Gene therapy has faced a number of technical hurdles, including immune responses against the vector, limited efficiency of antisense and RNAi approaches, and difficulties in producing sufficient quantities of a desired gene product. In one case, an immune response against an adenoviral vector proved fatal, and several cases of leukemia have resulted from the insertion of a modified retrovirus near an oncogene.[62] Nevertheless, gene therapy has now been successful in treating a number of inherited conditions, including X-linked and ADA SCID, β-thalassemia, hemophilia B, and X-linked adrenoleukodystrophy.[63–66] In addition to the treatment of hereditary diseases, gene therapy is being used to alter tumor cells in the treatment of various types of cancer. It is hoped that further research will lead to safe, efficient and cost-effective treatment of many human diseases through gene therapy.

REFERENCES

1. Harrow J, Frankish A, Gonzalez JM, et al: GENCODE: The reference human genome annotation for The ENCODE Project. *Genome Res* 22:1760–1774, 2012.
2. Watson JD, Crick FHC: Molecular structure of nucleic acids: A structure for deoxyribose nucleic acid. *Nature* 171:737, 1953.
3. Lewin B: *Genes VIII*. Prentice Hall, Englewood Cliffs, NJ, 2003.
4. Roach JC, Glusman G, Smit AF, et al: Analysis of genetic inheritance in a family quartet by whole-genome sequencing. *Science* 328:636–639, 2010.
5. Campbell CD, Eichler EE: Properties and rates of germline mutations in humans. *Trends Genet* 29:575–584, 2013.
6. Sudmant PH, Kitzman JO, Antonacci F, et al: Diversity of human copy number variation and multicopy genes. *Science* 330:641–646, 2010.
7. Mills RE, Walter K, Stewart C, et al: Mapping copy number variation by population-scale genome sequencing. *Nature* 470:59–65, 2011.
8. Taylor SM, Cerami C, Fairhurst RM: Hemoglobinopathies: Slicing the Gordian knot of *Plasmodium falciparum* malaria pathogenesis. *PLoS Pathog* 9:e1003327, 2013.
9. Kayser M, de Knijff P: Improving human forensics through advances in genetics, genomics and molecular biology. *Nat Rev Genet* 12:179–192, 2011.
10. Nelson DL, Orr HT, Warren ST: The unstable repeats—Three evolving faces of neurological disease. *Neuron* 77:825–843, 2013.
11. Stankiewicz P, Lupski JR: Structural variation in the human genome and its role in disease. *Annu Rev Med* 61:437–455, 2010.
12. Zimran A, Gelbart T, Beutler E: Linkage of the PvuII polymorphism with the common Jewish mutati. *Am J Hum Genet* 46:902–905, 1990.
13. Manoharan A: Congenital haptoglobin deficiency. *Blood* 90:1709, 1997.
14. Jorde LB, Carey JC, Bamshad MJ: *Medical Genetics*, 4th ed. Mosby-Elsevier, St. Louis, 2010.
15. Bennett RL, French KS, Resta RG, Doyle DL: Standardized human pedigree nomenclature: Update and assessment of the recommendations of the National Society of Genetic Counselors. *J Genet Couns* 17:424–433, 2008.
16. Veltman JA, Brunner HG: De novo mutations in human genetic disease. *Nat Rev Genet* 13:565–575, 2012.
17. Biesecker LG, Spinner NB: A genomic view of mosaicism and human disease. *Nat Rev Genet* 14:307–320, 2013.
18. Zlotogora J: Germ line mosaicism. *Hum Genet* 102:381–386, 1998.
19. Rees DC, Williams TN, Gladwin MT: Sickle-cell disease. *Lancet* 376:2018–2031, 2010.
20. Khoury MJ, McCabe LL, McCabe ER: Population screening in the age of genomic medicine. *N Engl J Med* 348:50–58, 2003.
21. Bell CJ, Dinwiddie DL, Miller NA, et al: Carrier testing for severe childhood recessive diseases by next-generation sequencing. *Sci Transl Med* 3:65ra4, 2011.
22. Bodurtha J, Strauss JF: Genomics and perinatal care. *N Engl J Med* 366:64–73, 2012.
23. Allen KJ, Gurrin LC, Constantine CC, et al: Iron-overload-related disease in HFE hereditary hemochromatosis. *N Engl J Med* 358:221–230, 2008.
24. Lettre G, Sankaran VG, Bezerra MA, et al: DNA polymorphisms at the BCL11A, HBS1L-MYB, and beta-globin loci associate with fetal hemoglobin levels and pain crises in sickle cell disease. *Proc Natl Acad Sci U S A* 105:11869–11874, 2008.
25. Lane DA, Grant PJ: Role of hemostatic gene polymorphisms in venous and arterial thrombotic disease. *Blood* 95:1517–1532, 2000.
26. Bolton-Maggs PHB, Pasi KJ: Haemophilias A and B. *Lancet* 361:1801–1809, 2003.
27. Graw J, Brackmann HH, Oldenburg J, et al: Haemophilia A: From mutation analysis to new therapies. *Nat Rev Genet* 6:488–501, 2005.
28. Adams PC, Barton JC: Haemochromatosis. *Lancet* 370:1855–1860, 2007.
29. Lyon MF: X chromosomes and dosage compensation. *Nature* 320:313–330, 1986.
30. Lyon MF: Some milestones in the history of X-chromosome inactivation. *Annu Rev Genet* 26:17–28, 1992.
31. Wutz A, Gribnau J: X inactivation Xplained. *Curr Opin Genet Dev* 17:387–393, 2007.
32. Lee JT, Bartolomei MS: X-inactivation, imprinting, and long noncoding RNAs in health and disease. *Cell* 152:1308–1323, 2013.
33. Deng X, Berletch JB, Nguyen DK, Disteche CM: X chromosome regulation: Diverse patterns in development, tissues and disease. *Nat Rev Genet* 15:367–378, 2014.
34. Ballabio A, Willard HF: Mammalian X-chromosome inactivation and the XIST gene. *Curr Opin Genet Dev* 2:439–447, 1992.
35. Esteller M: Epigenetics in cancer. *N Engl J Med* 358:1148–1159, 2008.
36. Lynch HT, de la Chapelle A: Hereditary colorectal cancer. *N Engl J Med* 348:919–932, 2003.
37. Altshuler D, Daly MJ, Lander ES: Genetic mapping in human disease. *Science* 322:881–888, 2008.
38. Durbin RM, Abecasis GR, Altshuler DL, et al: A map of human genome variation from population-scale sequencing. *Nature* 467:1061–1073, 2010.
39. Lander ES: Initial impact of the sequencing of the human genome. *Nature* 470:187–197, 2011.
40. Lander ES, Linton LM, Birren B, et al: Initial sequencing and analysis of the human genome. *Nature* 409:860–921, 2001.
41. Venter JC, Adams MD, Myers EW, et al: The sequence of the human genome. *Science* 291:1304–1351, 2001.
42. Davies K: The era of genomic medicine. *Clin Med* 13:594–601, 2013.
43. Yang Y, Muzny DM, Reid JG, et al: Clinical whole-exome sequencing for the diagnosis of mendelian disorders. *N Engl J Med* 369:1502–1511, 2013.
44. White TJ, Arnheim N, Erlich HA: The polymerase chain reaction. *Trends Genet* 5:185–190, 1989.
45. Callaway E: Ancient DNA reveals secrets of human history. *Nature* 476:136–137, 2011.
46. VanGuilder HD, Vrana KE, Freeman WM: Twenty-five years of quantitative PCR for gene expression analysis. *Biotechniques* 44:619–626, 2008.
47. Sanger F, Nicklen S, Coulson AR: DNA sequencing with chain-terminating inhibitors. *Proc Natl Acad Sci U S A* 74:5463–5467, 1977.
48. Mardis ER: A decade's perspective on DNA sequencing technology. *Nature* 470:198–203, 2011.
49. Metzker ML: Sequencing technologies-the next generation. *Nat Rev Genet* 11:31–46, 2010.
50. Hayden EC: Technology: The $1,000 genome. *Nature* 507:294–295, 2014.
51. Koboldt DC, Steinberg KM, Larson DE, et al: The next-generation sequencing revolution and its impact on genomics. *Cell* 155:27–38, 2013.
52. Downward J: RNA interference. *BMJ* 328:1245–1248, 2004.
53. Marsden PA: RNA interference as potential therapy—not so fast. *N Engl J Med* 355:953–954, 2006.
54. Chen CZ, Li L, Lodish HF, Bartel DP: MicroRNAs modulate hematopoietic lineage differentiation. *Science* 303:83–86, 2004.
55. Heidenreich O, Eckstein F: Hammerhead ribozyme-mediated cleavage of the long terminal repeat RNA of human immunodeficiency virus type 1. *J Biol Chem* 267:1904–1909, 1992.
56. Soda Y, Tani K, Bai Y, et al: A novel maxizyme vector targeting a bcr-abl fusion gene induced specific cell death in Philadelphia chromosome-positive acute lymphoblastic leukemia. *Blood* 104:356–363, 2004.
57. Beuzard Y: Mouse models of sickle cell disease. *Transfus Clin Biol* 15:7–11, 2008.
58. Zhou XY, Tomatsu S, Fleming RE, et al: HFE gene knockout produces mouse model of hereditary hemochromatosis. *Proc Natl Acad Sci U S A* 95:2492–2497, 1998.
59. Yu Y, Bradley A: Engineering chromosomal rearrangements in mice. *Nat Rev Genet* 2:780–790, 2001.
60. Melis MA, Cau M, Congiu R, et al: A mutation in the TMPRSS6 gene, encoding a transmembrane serine protease that suppresses hepcidin production, in familial iron deficiency anemia refractory to oral iron. *Haematologica* 93:1473–1479, 2008.
61. Cavazzana-Calvo M, Fischer A, Hacein-Bey-Abina S, Aiuti A: Gene therapy for primary immunodeficiencies: Part 1. *Curr Opin Immunol* 24:580–584, 2012.
62. Wirth T, Parker N, Yla-Herttuala S: History of gene therapy. *Gene* 525:162–169, 2013.
63. Kay MA: State-of-the-art gene-based therapies: The road ahead. *Nat Rev Genet* 12:316–328, 2011.
64. Nathwani AC, Tuddenham EGD, Rangarajan S, et al: Adenovirus-associated virus vector-mediated gene transfer in hemophilia B. *N Engl J Med* 365:2357–2365, 2011.
65. High KA: The gene therapy journey for hemophilia: Are we there yet? *Blood* 120:4482–4487, 2012.
66. Ginn SL, Alexander IE, Edelstein ML, et al: Gene therapy clinical trials worldwide to 2012—An update. *J Gene Med* 15:65–77, 2013.

CHAPTER 11
GENOMICS

Lukas D. Wartman and Elaine R. Mardis

SUMMARY

The introduction of next-generation sequencing platforms, coincident with genome-scale preparatory and analytical approaches and the completion of the Human Genome Reference, has ushered in the era of genomics. This chapter introduces the fundamentals of next-generation sequencing methods, provides an overview of the basics of data analysis, and explores the myriad applications developed to exploit the scale and throughput of next-generation sequencing toward questions of biomedical importance. Specifics of cancer genomics, complex disease genomics, and how they pertain to hematologic basic science and clinical practice are discussed, along with the modern-day realities of the consenting process.

HISTORY OF GENOMICS: SANGER SEQUENCING

The scientific discipline known as genomics has dramatically changed since the publication of the Human Reference Genome in 2003, primarily as a result of the introduction and broad-based implementation of new sequencing technologies.[1] Prior to the mid-2000s, Sanger sequencing was the predominant DNA sequencing approach, and was used to complete the sequencing of the first human reference genome. Frederick Sanger and his colleagues developed Sanger or "chain termination" sequencing in the late 1970s.[2] In their original method, four reactions were used to accomplish chain termination by incorporating separate di-deoxynucleoside triphosphates (ddNTPs), each included with a mix of three unmodified deoxynucleoside triphosphates (dNTPs) and a

fourth, radiolabeled dNTP. Each reaction consisted of the DNA template to be sequenced in a mixture containing a DNA primer, a DNA polymerase, a mixture of four dNTPs, and one of the four ddNTPs. Here, the chemistry of ddNTPs, which lack the 3′ hydroxyl group present in a native dNTP, resulted in chain termination when incorporated into a growing DNA chain, as DNA polymerase cannot add another nucleoside without the 3′ hydroxyl group present. With multiple rounds of primer elongation, the ddNTPs incorporate randomly in the newly synthesized strands according to the complementary nucleotides of the DNA template. By denaturing the newly synthesized strands from the DNA templates and resolving each of the four DNA fragment mixtures on separate lanes by gel electrophoresis, one could read out the sequence of the DNA template from the resulting autoradiograph. Significant improvements to the original Sanger sequencing protocol included the use of fluorescently labeled ddNTPs to allow for sequencing to occur in one reaction rather than four,[3] improved thermally stable DNA polymerases that permitted temperature cycling ("cycled sequencing"), and the use of capillary electrophoresis rather than standard gel electrophoresis for automated separation matrix filling between samples.[4-7] Modern Sanger capillary sequencers typically generate DNA sequencing reads in the range of 400 to 900 base pairs (bp). The main limitation of Sanger sequencing is that the sequencing reaction is decoupled from the electrophoretic separation and detection steps. To piece together the sequence for a large segment of DNA or entire genome, genomic DNA must be randomly fragmented and subcloned into a bacterial vector, with each cloned DNA isolated and sequenced. The resulting sequencing reads are assembled computationally to recreate larger fragments that recapitulate the starting DNA nucleotide sequence. This process is expensive, time-consuming, and laborious. However, with the availability of robotic DNA isolation and sequencing reactions, coupled with high-throughput capillary sequencers, the human genome, among the genomes of many other organisms, was decoded. Currently, Sanger sequencing is still in use to complete smaller scale sequencing projects and to validate findings from next-generation sequencing studies.

MODERN GENOMICS: NEXT-GENERATION SEQUENCING

OVERVIEW OF NEXT-GENERATION SEQUENCING

The method for next-generation sequencing (NGS), or massively parallel digital sequencing, is distinct from Sanger sequencing in that the sequencing reactions alternate with cycles of signal detection to provide the data readout at a significantly accelerated scale.[8,9] The use of NGS in the years after the completion of the Human Genome Project has greatly increased the use of genomics and has significantly impacted the pace of biomedical research.[10] Although there are several different NGS platforms offered commercially, they are methodologically quite similar. Unlike Sanger sequencing, NGS does not require subcloning of DNA, propagation in a bacterial host, and isolation of individual templates prior to sequencing. Instead, DNA is randomly fragmented into a pool of small pieces (generally 100 to 500 bp) and then ligated with specific synthetic DNA linkers (or adaptors) at the fragment ends to generate a NGS "library." The library fragments are subsequently amplified by a process that isolates individual library fragments to a specific location prior to amplification. In general, this *in situ* amplification occurs on a covalently modified surface (a bead or flat silicon surface) with complementary linkers covalently attached to it, using a specific dilution of library fragments as input. In this step, the individual library fragment amplification permits sufficient signal output for detection

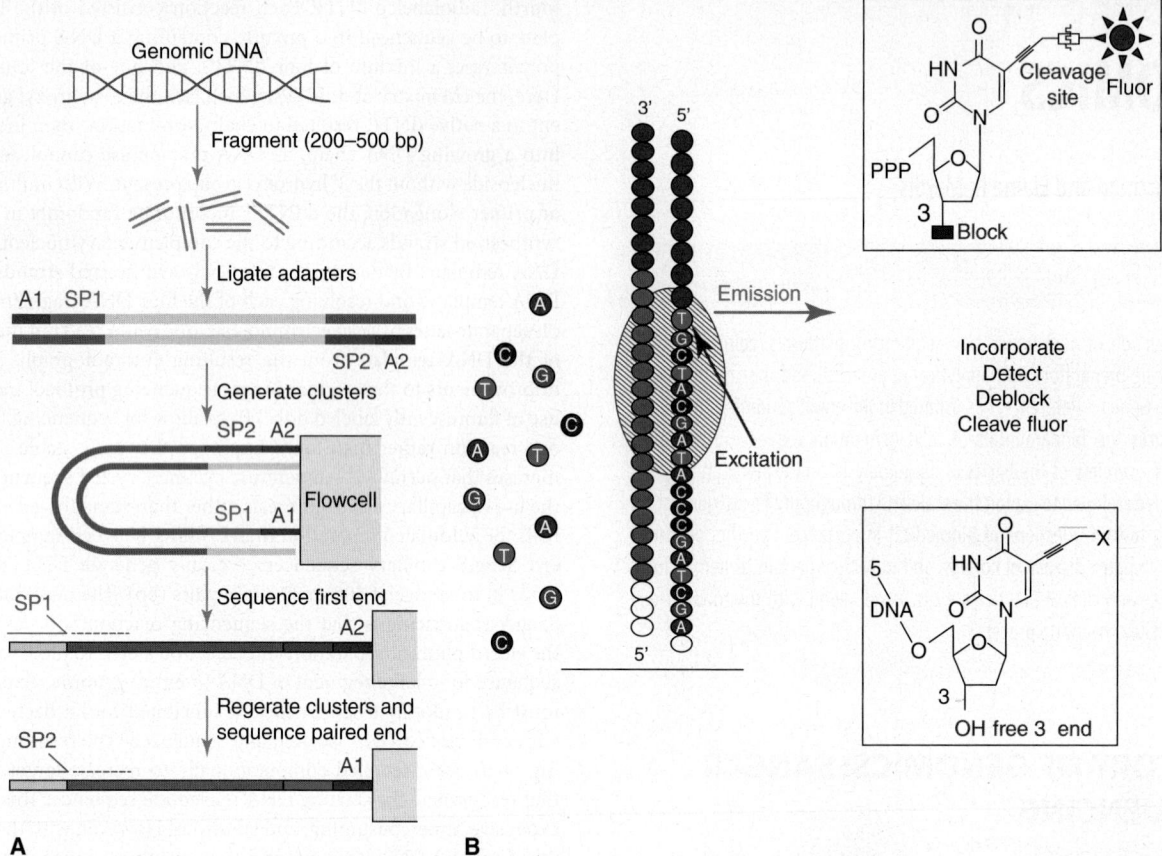

Figure 11–1. Illumina library construction and sequencing process. Panel **A** represents the library construction process whereby high-molecular-weight genomic DNA is fragmented, ligated with adaptors, and amplified on a solid support prior to annealing of adaptor-complementary primers. Panel **B** represents the stepwise sequencing process whereby reagents are introduced to extend the primed fragments, the incorporated fluorescent nucleotides are detected, the 3′ end is deblocked, and the fluorescent groups on the incorporated nucleotides removed prior to the next stepwise sequencing-by-synthesis series. *(Reproduced with permission from Mardis, ER: Next-generation sequencing platforms. Annu Rev Anal Chem (Palo Alto Calif) 6:287–303, 2013.)*

during the sequencing steps that follow. Because each sequencing read derived from an amplified library fragment originates from that single unique fragment, NGS data are digital in nature. This fact underlies an important concept for digital sequencing methods: the number of specific sequencing reads generated is directly proportional to the amount of input nucleic acid, accurately reflecting amplified regions of a genome, for example. However, as the generation of libraries and the amplification of fragments involve polymerase chain reaction (PCR) amplification, inaccuracies can result via amplification biases or from PCR enzyme substitution errors in which the wrong base is incorporated during amplification.

SEQUENCING BY SYNTHESIS: THE ILLUMINA PLATFORM

Currently, there are two commercially available NGS platforms in common use. One uses an approach called *sequencing by synthesis* that occurs in the microfluidic channels of a silicon-derived "flow cell" device (Fig. 11–1).[11] Here, enzymatic amplification of library fragments on the flow cell surface results in hundreds of millions of DNA clusters, and the sequencing of each cluster occurs in parallel with all of the other clusters by a stepwise series of events. Solexa marketed the first commercially available sequencer using this technology in 2006, and was acquired by Illumina in 2007. Illumina offers a variety of different

sequencing machines with varying run times (from hours to days), sequencing capacities (from 25 million reads to nearly 3 billion reads per flow cell), and overall output (from approximately 0.5 gigabase (Gb) to greater than 1.5 terabase (Tb) of sequenced bases per run).

SEQUENCING BY SYNTHESIS: OVERVIEW OF METHODOLOGY

As in Sanger sequencing, the sequencing-by-synthesis steps begin with annealing sequencing primers complementary to the adaptors to the amplified library fragments on the flow cell surface. Then, a solution containing DNA polymerases and fluorescently-labeled, chemically modified dNTPs are added to the flow cell to begin an incorporation step. The DNA polymerases incorporate the complementary dNTP onto the 3′ ends of the primed fragments in each cluster. Each incorporation reaction is terminated after a dNTP is added, because of a blocking group at the 3′ position. After a cycle of dNTP incorporation on the flow cell, a laser-based detection system scans the flow cell surfaces to excite the incorporated fluorescent groups and to collect the unique light emission of each of the four fluorescently labeled dNTPs. Chemical deblocking steps follow to (1) remove the fluorophore by cleavage (the fluorescently-labeled dNTPs are known as "reversible dye terminators") and (2) unblock the 3′ hydroxyl group to permit the next cycle of incorporation, detection and blocking.

Unlike Sanger sequencing, Illumina's sequencing-by-synthesis method generates relatively short read lengths, typically 100 to 300 bp. The limitations on read length are primarily a signal-to-noise issue, where increasing numbers of steps in the sequencing-by-synthesis approach produces increasing noise at each step that competes with true signal detection. Hence, the data quality of Illumina reads tends to decrease with increasing step numbers. Illumina error rates are low, in the 0.1 to 0.3 percent range, and the predominant error type is base substitution.[12] Ultimately, a complex, repetitive genome such as the human genome cannot be assembled from 300-bp read lengths, so algorithms were developed to align reads to the reference genome as a first step toward data interpretation.[13] One approach by which Illumina has improved read mapping is by enabling paired-end sequencing that permits the sequence read off first one end and then the other of each amplified fragment cluster on the flow cell. Paired end reads of this type physically are linked and defined by the fragment size, permitting their accurate placement onto the reference genome by alignment, and effectively permitting more reads to contribute to coverage from a given sequencer run (when compared to single-end reads).[14] Furthermore, as described later, the expected read placement onto the reference genome, when not met, is a source of information used to interpret structural variation.

SEQUENCING BY PH CHANGE SENSING: THE ION TORRENT PLATFORM

The second type of NGS platform in common use is the sequencing by pH sensing method that is marketed by Life Technologies (now a part of Thermo Fisher) as their Ion Torrent platform (Fig. 11–2). Life Technologies acquired Ion Torrent in 2010.[15] The sequencing by pH-sensing method involves similar steps of library construction as described for sequencing by synthesis. However, the library DNA fragments are diluted and combined with (1) individual micron-scale beads that have covalently attached complementary adaptors on their surface and (2) PCR reagents, including DNA polymerase, into an emulsion PCR reaction. In emulsion PCR, one generates individual aqueous micelles that permit bead-based amplification of library fragments prior to sequencing. The emulsion PCR process generates beads carrying copies of identical DNA fragments suitable for sequencing. The DNA-coated beads are purified from the emulsion, enriched for those beads with amplified DNA on their surfaces, and then deposited into individual wells of a specifically constructed semiconductor plate, known as an Ion Chip. Sequencing primers (complementary to the adaptors) are annealed to the bead-amplified fragments, and then the sequencing process is initiated by the addition of DNA polymerase and flow of a single

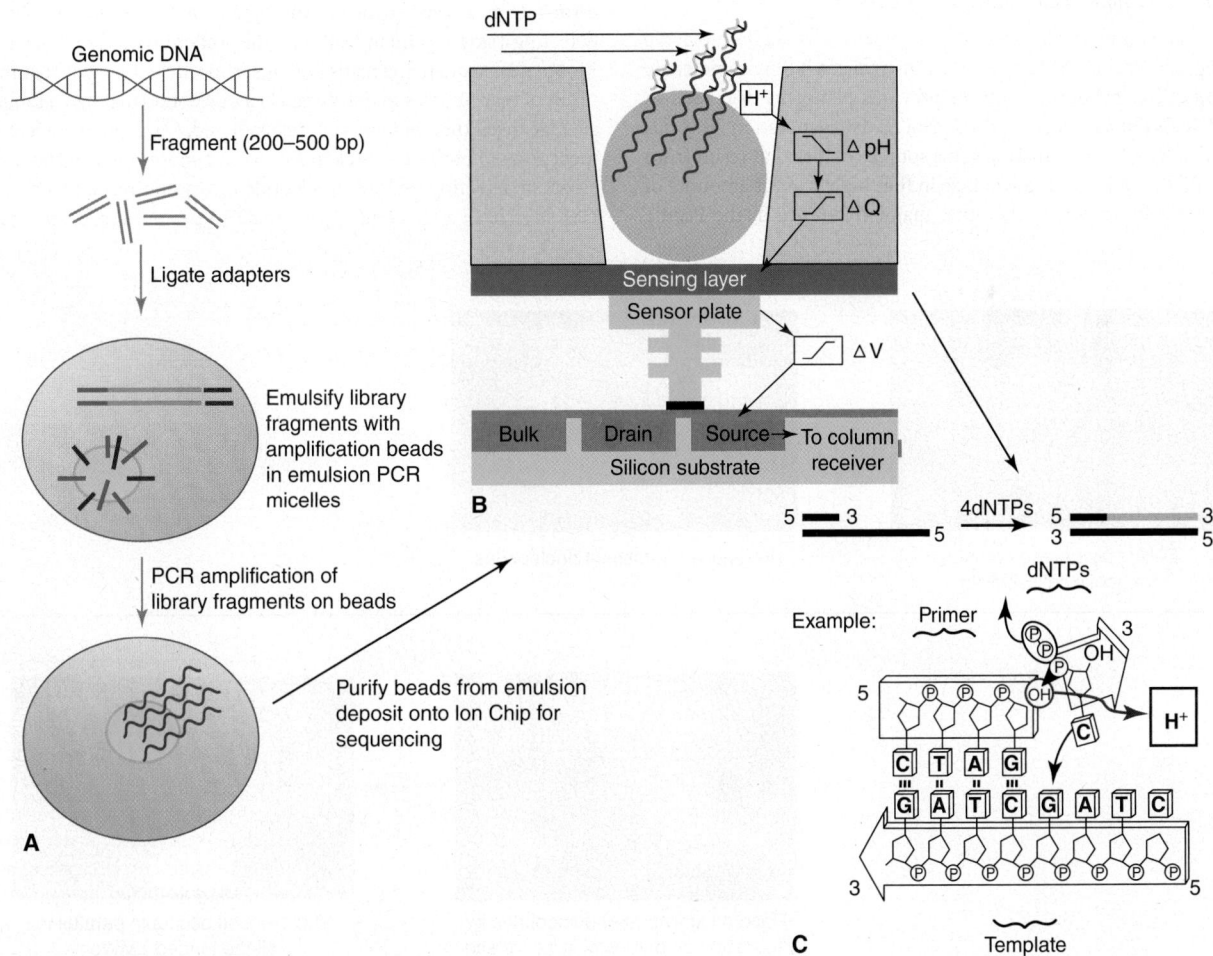

Figure 11–2. Ion Torrent library construction and sequencing process. Panel **A** represents the specifics of the Ion Torrent library amplification process, which requires an emulsion PCR amplification on the surface of a bead with covalently attached adaptor-complementary primers, followed by emulsion breaking and bead addition to the Ion Chip for sequencing. The sequencing process, illustrated in panel **B**, flows sequential high-purity dNTP solutions across the chip surface for incorporation. Upon incorporation, there is a release of hydrogen ions that are detected by the pH-sensing capability of the chip, detected in panel **C**. (Used with permission from Thermo Fisher Scientific.)

dNTP-containing buffer solution across the Ion Chip surface. The flow of the four nucleotides occurs in a stepwise fashion, with a detection step and an intervening wash. When a specific dNTP is incorporated into the elongating strands of DNA fragments on a specific bead, hydrogen ions are released, and a highly sensitive pH sensor built into the Ion Chip can read out the subsequent change in pH for the well containing that bead. If no dNTP is incorporated at that cycle, no change in pH is registered for that well. This approach follows for all wells containing beads on the Ion Chip, resulting in massively parallel sequencing. As with the Illumina technology, read lengths are short, in the 100 to 400 bp range. Unlike the Illumina platform that uses paired-end reads, Ion Torrent sequencing reads are single-end reads. The source of most sequencing errors generated by the Ion Torrent platform are insertion/deletion errors in stretches of identical bases on the template strand as a result of the difficulty of discerning the pH change ratio associated with incorporation of the same nucleotide above four consecutive identical nucleotides.[16] Advantages of the Ion Torrent are that run times are very short (in the 2- to 7-hour range), and the cost per run is relatively inexpensive. The output, read length, run time, and cost vary by the Ion Chip type used (up to 2 Gb).

NEXT-GENERATION SEQUENCING TECHNOLOGY IN DEVELOPMENT: SINGLE-MOLECULE SEQUENCING

There is one commercially available platform for single-molecule sequencing, the Pacific Biosciences RSII instrument.[17] Single-molecule sequencing differs primarily from the previous platforms discussed in that no PCR amplification is required prior to data generation. This has obvious advantages in eliminating some sources of bias that result from the use of PCR, but has a disadvantage in that higher input amounts of DNA are typically required. The other major difference in the Pacific Biosciences approach is in the read length obtained, which ranges according to the template type but can exceed 50,000 bases with the input of very long molecules to the library construction.

The Pacific Biosciences approach couples primed DNA library fragments with DNA polymerase molecules that are specifically engineered for the sequencing system (Fig. 11–3). These complexes are introduced to the surface of a SMRTCell, a nanofabricated sequencing device, which consists of 150,000 zero-mode waveguides (ZMWs). In effect, the loading of complexes aims to place one DNA polymerase/DNA template complex into each ZMW in preparation for sequencing. The ZMW is a nanofabricated pore that focuses the laser excitation and detection optics at the bottom of the ZMW where the DNA polymerase complex is bound, isolating the detection area to the active site of the polymerase. The sequencing process initiates with the introduction of fluorescent nucleotides and buffers, and is continuously monitored by the excitation/detection optics during the run time. As fluorescently tagged nucleotides sample into the active site, they can be detected with sufficient dwell time upon their incorporation into the synthesized strand. Because each fluorescent group is specific to the nucleotide identity, the sequence is read out based on the detected emission wavelength. The fluorescent group is attached to the phosphate portion of the nucleotide, so incorporation removes it by cleavage during the phosphodiester bond formation, and it diffuses out of the ZMW focus.

Single-molecule sequencing has, by definition, an inherently higher error rate as a consequence of the signal-to-noise ratio associated with detecting a single event in real time. The predominant error type in Pacific Biosciences sequencing reads is an insertion/deletion error that may be a result of inaccuracies in detecting (1) a nucleotide that had a longer than average dwell time but was not incorporated, (2) a single nucleotide that incorporated but was mistaken for two (or more) nucleotides, or (3) by errors in detecting multiple nucleotide incorporations into a homopolymer stretch. In spite of an approximate 15 percent error rate, the errors

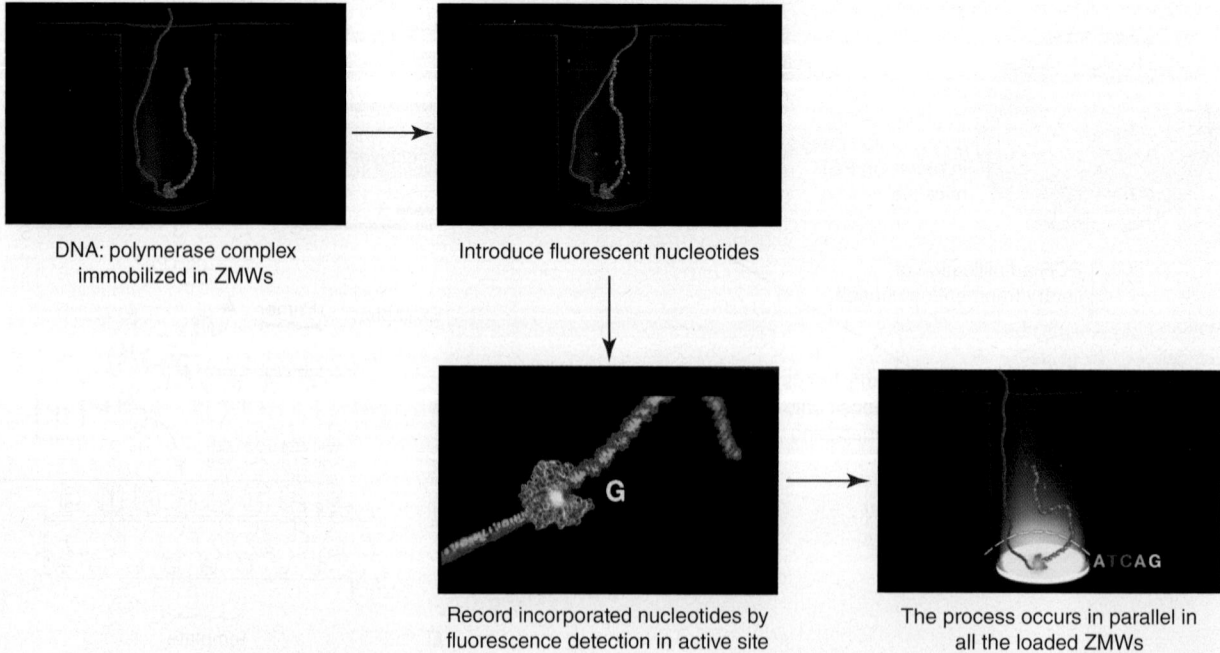

DNA: polymerase complex immobilized in ZMWs

Introduce fluorescent nucleotides

Record incorporated nucleotides by fluorescence detection in active site

The process occurs in parallel in all the loaded ZMWs

Figure 11–3. Pacific Biosciences real-time sequencing and detection process. The primed library fragments are complexed to DNA polymerases and applied to the surface of a SMRTCell, where they locate into zero-mode waveguides (ZMWs). After providing fluorescently labeled nucleotides and buffer, the sequencing process is monitored by real time detection, whereby incorporated nucleotides are detected in the active site of each ZMW-isolated polymerase complex by the laser/detection optics of the instrument. Here, the fluorescence events are recorded for each active ZMW throughout a preset duration, resulting in the final sequencing read data for each single DNA molecule. *(Used with permission from Pacific Biosciences.)*

are essentially random, which means that oversampling (or "coverage") of the sequence of interest can correct most errors, resulting in a cumulative error rate of around 0.1 percent following read assembly.[18] The very long read lengths possible on this platform enable read assembly, rather than read alignment needed in short read platform data analysis. Assembly has obvious advantages in its ability to represent novel content in a genome and to provide long-range haplotyping information.

Emerging DNA sequencing technologies are being developed around the central concept of translocating DNA molecules through nanopores, which can be either biologic or nanofabricated pores.[19] In nanopore sequencing, detection of the nucleotide sequences occurs during nanopore translocation events that are sensed by changes in electrical current that correlate to sequence, or by laser-based detection of incorporated fluorescent nucleotides. Nanopore sequencing, while still somewhat theoretical, may offer rapid sequencing with very long read lengths.

TARGETED NEXT-GENERATION SEQUENCING: FROM GENE PANELS TO EXOMES AND BEYOND

Initially, NGS platforms were used for whole-genome sequencing of organisms with relatively small genomes, such as bacteria or model organisms (*Caenorhabditis elegans*, *Drosophila melanogaster*, etc.), or for combining large numbers of PCR products into a single sequencing run. As the throughput per run improved, larger genomes, including human genomes, were studied, including the first cancer genome.[20,21] However, the cost and complexity of analysis for whole human genome studies, along with the difficulty of interpretation of variants identified

outside of the known genes, inspired the development of methods to focus sequencing onto these loci. In particular, hybrid capture techniques were developed that provided either a subset of known genes (all kinases, for example), or all the known genes (the "exome") by a series of selective steps that led directly to NGS data generation (Fig. 11–4).[22] At its essence, hybrid capture relies on synthetic DNA probes that are complementary to sequences of the known exons of genes in the genome of interest.[23,24] In typical current protocols, the probes have covalently attached biotin moieties that enable downstream selection by streptavidin-coated magnetic particles. By combining a whole-genome library with the hybrid capture probes under conditions that favor hybridization (stoichiometry of probes to targets, temperature, and buffer conditions), probe:library fragment hybrids are formed. Following their selection by streptavidin magnetic bead binding and application of a magnetic force to isolate the beads, the noncaptured library fragments are removed, washes performed and the hybridized fragments eluted by denaturation from the probes. The resulting fragments are PCR amplified, quantitated, and sequenced by NGS. At present, the throughput of genome-scale NGS platforms permits the combination or "multiplexing" of the resulting fragments from several hybrid capture reactions into a sequencing run. Multiplexing is enabled by the inclusion of DNA barcodes that are synthesized onto the library adapters, and demultiplexing of the sequencing reads occurs downstream of the instrument run using the appropriate bioinformatics program. Although exome sequencing costs about one-tenth of whole-genome sequencing, it is important to note that typical yields from hybrid capture range from 85 to 90 percent of the targeted regions being covered at sufficient depth to confidently predict variants. Furthermore, the range of variant types

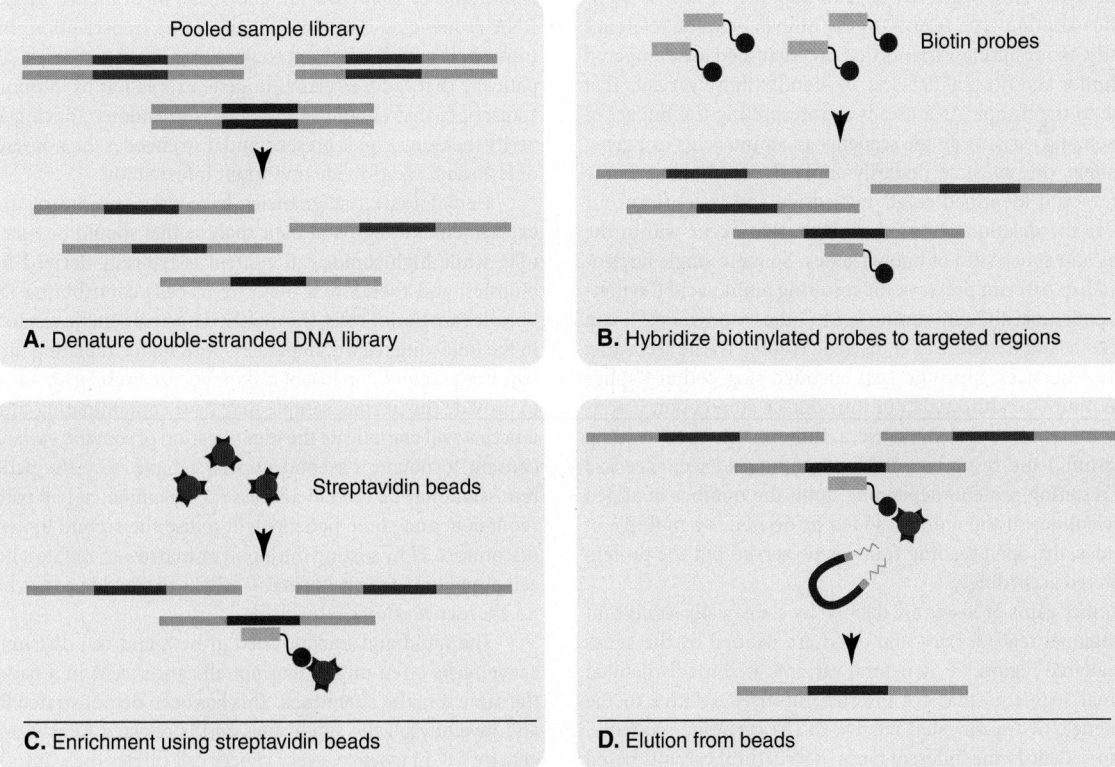

A. Denature double-stranded DNA library

Pooled sample library

B. Hybridize biotinylated probes to targeted regions

Biotin probes

C. Enrichment using streptavidin beads

Streptavidin beads

D. Elution from beads

Figure 11–4. Overview of hybrid capture preparation for sequencing. This illustration presents a generalized overview of the process for hybrid capture selection prior to DNA or RNA sequencing. In general, probes are designed for the targeted regions of interest, which can constitute a small number of genes or hotspot loci, up to the full exome (all annotated genes in a genome). Following hybrid capture, the probe:library duplexes are isolated from solution by streptavidin magnetic beads. Release of the library fragments by denaturation is followed by amplification, quantitation, and sequencing. *(Used with permission from Illumina, Inc.)*

detected by hybrid capture is often limited. Single nucleotide variants and short insertion/deletion variants can be detected, but copy number and structural variants are difficult to detect reliably, especially if they are not anticipated by the addition of specially designed probes to capture them and by the specialized analyses required to detect them.

OVERVIEW OF NEXT-GENERATION DNA SEQUENCING ANALYSIS

It can be easily argued that the relative ease of performing biomedical experimentation imparted by NGS-based methods has conversely required more complicated analytical approaches to accurately interpret the resulting data.[25] As mentioned earlier, this is partly a result of the complexities of the human genome and the requirement for short reads to be aligned to the reference sequence as a first step for data analysis. It also is a result of computational infrastructure and software pipeline requirements to align and analyze data because of the sheer magnitude of data generated in a single experiment, which is exacerbated by multiple samples, multiple time points, and the need to integrate data of different types for the correlative analyses that are desired.

Most cancer-focused analyses have as a central goal the identification of DNA variants that are unique to the tumor cells ("somatic") as compared to the inherited ("constitutional" or "germline") genome. In practice, the desired comparison (whether the sequencing platform is a targeted gene panel, exome, or whole genome) is achieved by first aligning sequencing reads from the tumor library and from the matched normal library against the human genome reference sequence as separate entities. Algorithms that have specialized logic to identify different types of variation (single nucleotide, or "point" mutations, small insertions or deletions, copy number, or structural alterations) then are used to separately examine each set of read alignments and to identify the specific variation type relative to the human genome reference sequence. Lastly, the resulting variants that are identified are compared between the tumor and normal datasets, to identify those variants that appear unique to the tumor. As a means of interpreting the impact of all identified somatic variants on the sequence of amino acids in a given gene, for example, one must secondarily apply the annotation of the human genome onto identified single nucleotide and indel (term for the *in*sertion or the *del*etion of bases) variants that occur within the coding regions and splice sites of known genes. Somatic single nucleotide variants (Chap. 10) can preserve the resulting amino acid ("synonymous"); can encode a different amino acid ("nonsynonymous"); can abolish a splice site and therefore alter the gene reading frame according to the intronic sequences up to the next encoded stop codon ("splice site"); and can omit ("readthrough") or introduce a stop codon ("nonsense"). Indel mutations typically cause a shift in the open reading frame ("frameshift") and result in a different amino acid sequence and length of the resulting protein, depending upon the number of added or deleted nucleotides. If the number added or deleted is a multiple of three nucleotides, the open reading frame is preserved but the protein sequence is altered accordingly.

Copy number gains or losses are defined by statistically significant variation in regional read density, and often are defined by the genes that lie in the altered region.[26,27] Structural variants are broadly defined as chromosomal segments that are inserted, inverted relative to the germline sequence, or translocated relative to the germline sequence. Here, algorithms identify the different types of structural variants based on multiple read alignments that are spaced farther apart than expected defined by the insert size of the sequencing library used ("insertions"); or are spaced more closely than expected ("deletions"); or have the incorrect orientation of read direction for the read pairs aligned to the same chromosome ("inversions"); or have the forward and reverse reads of multiple read pairs on different chromosomes ("translocations"). Insertions and inversions may result in a fusion protein by virtue of juxtaposition of exons from two genes on either the same (inversion) or different (insertion) chromosomes. Translocations also can result in gene fusions but involve juxtaposed exons from genes present on different chromosomes in the germline. There are multiple examples of gene fusions that result in proteins with a demonstrated role in oncogenesis.[28]

Genetic susceptibility to hematologic malignancies can occur either by inheritance or by *de novo* mutations in genes, such as BRCA1/2, TP53, and others. Here, variants in the germline can be identified from aligned sequence read data to the human reference sequence, followed by annotation of the known cancer susceptibility genes. The pathogenicity of a given variant can be evaluated relative to databases of previously catalogued variants in these genes, if available. Identification of these variants typically will require consenting the patient and family members to a genetic counseling session to communicate the information about the germline susceptibility and its possible consequences for siblings and children (discussed below in "Next-Generation Sequencing as a Clinical Assay: Implications for the Practicing Hematologist").

There are a variety of data analyses that integrate NGS data from different starting materials such as DNA and RNA from the same tumor, or across large groups of tumors (either from the same or different disease site). One example of data integration is evaluating RNA sequencing data to support a specific variant identified initially from tumor to normal DNA comparisons such as for a predicted fusion gene. In this example, the confirmed detection of the gene fusion in RNA provides confidence that the structural variant algorithm has identified a true positive. Such a result can also confirm cytogenetic results from conventional diagnostic assays. Similarly, the identification of a DNA level mutation that appears to introduce a protein truncating variant (frameshift or splice site mutation) can be evaluated by examining the RNA sequencing data for evidence of its transcription. Because these transcripts are often subject to nonsense-mediated decay (a surveillance pathway that reduces errors in gene expression by eliminating mRNA transcripts that contain premature stop codons), having RNA data to verify the transcript is present, and if so encodes the nonsense mutation, or is absent, can provide important information.

Hematologic malignancies have very specific considerations in experimental design and data analysis that should be noted. In particular, while high tumor cell content is typically derived from marrow biopsies, and therefore a majority of cells contributing DNA to NGS libraries are tumor cells, the matched normal sample can be problematic in the following regard. In patients with high circulating tumor cell content in the blood, the use of a skin, buccal swab, or mouthwash sample to provide the normal sample may have contaminating tumor cell content that will complicate the identification of somatic variants. Although consent to obtain a second normal sample once the patient achieves remission may be used to address this dilemma, not all patients achieve remission, and some patients will refuse the second biopsy because of discomfort. Flow sorting the blood or marrow to isolate a nonmalignant cell population (often normal T cells) can provide a matched normal if no alternative source is available.

The rapid and uncontrolled growth and cell division inherent to cancer cells often means that not all cancer cells in a patient will have the same somatic alterations. This has been demonstrated for leukemias and myelodysplastic syndromes and is referred to as genomic heterogeneity.[29-36] In essence, every cancer cell carries the same set of founder mutations (sometimes referred to as "truncal"), but subclones can exist in the tumor cell population, each of which carries additional mutations unique to that subclone. As yet, the importance of heterogeneity has not been definitively demonstrated in the context of outcome, likelihood to relapse, resistance to therapy, or other possible clinical attributes. Tumor subclones can be defined by their somatic mutational landscape from high depth NGS, where the digital nature of the NGS data is exploited by algorithmic clustering of mutations that share the same variant allele fraction (VAF). In particular, the VAF of any mutation is defined as the fraction of sequencing reads that contain the somatic variant (as compared to the germline or inherited nucleotide at that locus). Changes in the heterogeneity of cancer cell populations can be studied by comparing data from temporal sampling of a patient, such as at diagnosis and disease relapse.

NEXT-GENERATION SEQUENCING–BASED COMPREHENSIVE GENOMICS: FROM STUDIES OF THE TRANSCRIPTOME TO DNA METHYLATION TO CHROMATIN ACCESSIBILITY AND MODIFICATIONS

The study of modern genomics by NGS methods is not limited to the sequencing of genomic DNA but also can include (1) the characterization of RNA transcripts, (2) the physical structure of genomes including chromatin organization and protein-DNA interactions, and (3) the identification of specific chemical modifications to nucleotides and histones.[37]

Analysis of the Transcriptome: RNA Sequencing

RNA sequencing (RNA-seq) involves the conversion of RNA into complementary DNA (cDNA) by reverse transcription followed by NGS library construction.[38] RNA-seq uses the digital nature of NGS technology to quantify levels of RNA transcripts. Previously, microarrays (designed with a fixed content of gene-specific probes) were used to assay gene expression by hybridization to reverse-transcribed RNA isolates. By contrast, RNA-seq offers the advantages of comprehensive and less-biased data analysis, with a broader dynamic range for detection of high and low abundance transcripts. With the single base resolution provided by RNA-seq, one can determine the expression of specific mutant alleles present in the germline or in cancer samples, which may be highly relevant for implementing a small molecule or immunotherapy-based targeted therapeutic. RNA-seq data can be analyzed to detect the expression of alternatively spliced isoforms of transcribed genes or to detect the transcriptional product(s) of gene fusions in cancer cells. RNA-seq can be produced as either single- or paired-end reads, where the latter are better suited to detect alternative splicing and gene fusions. Additionally, RNA-seq data can identify strand specificity of the DNA template, wherein RNA derived from the antisense strand may play an important role in regulating gene expression. Finally, the insert size of the RNA-seq libraries can be targeted to enrich for different subsets of the transcriptome. Small fragment size libraries (approximately 15 to 70 bp) enrich for microRNA (miRNA), short-interfering RNA (siRNA) and PIWI-interacting RNA (piRNA), intermediate size libraries (approximately 70 to 200 bp) enrich for small nuclear (snRNA) and small nucleolar RNA (snoRNA), and larger fragment libraries (excluding fragments less than 200 bp) enrich for messenger RNA (mRNA) and long noncoding RNA (lncRNA).

There are many protocols for RNA-seq, including different commercially available kits that exploit the aforementioned experimental focus areas. For example, protocols to study the "transcriptome," which is defined as all the expressed RNA from a given cell or cell population, are often optimized to preferentially target one (or more) types of RNA that are pertinent to a particular area of clinical or research interest. Thus, a researcher interested only in detecting gene expression of annotated mRNA transcripts would choose either an RNA-seq protocol that included ribosomal RNA (rRNA) depletion (rRNA may

represent up to 60 percent of transcripts in a cell) or one that used an initial poly-A enrichment step (as rRNAs are not polyadenylated). By comparison, noncoding RNAs play a role in many cellular processes but are not polyadenylated, so even though poly-A enrichment would not be applied, a protocol that preserves strand specificity should be.

RNA is a less-stable molecule than DNA and hence assessing the quality of the isolated RNA prior to creating a sequencing library is of paramount importance. The source for the RNA may be fresh tissue, fresh-frozen tissue, or formalin-fixed, paraffin-embedded (FFPE) tissue, and each of these sources may influence the quality of the resulting RNA. RNA derived from FFPE tissue is often at least partially degraded because of formalin crosslinks with the RNA backbone that result in breakage. Similarly, the amount of RNA available from clinical specimens is often quite limited, making necessary the use of RNA amplification prior to library construction, or the use of hybrid capture probes to enrich the on-gene yield of sequencing data from low input sources.[39]

As the analysis of RNA-seq data is distinct in many ways compared to DNA sequencing data analysis, multiple software tools are available to characterize differential gene expression, differential splicing, gene fusion detection, and allele-specific expression.[40,41] In regard to cancer-specific analyses of RNA, a paired "normal" comparator from adjacent nonmalignant cells is often not available (or even understood), which complicates the analysis and interpretation of RNA-seq data. However, efforts are now cataloguing expression in normal human tissues and providing these results in public databases for comparison purposes.

Next-Generation Sequencing–Based Studies of Chromatin Modifications

Chromatin immunoprecipitation followed by NGS-based whole-genome sequencing is known as ChIP-seq.[42] When studying chromatin modifications (Chap. 12), the targets are often transcription factors or specific histone modifications (such as methylation or acetylation) that may be important for regulation of gene expression. In brief, ChIP-seq begins with standard chromatin immunoprecipitation: protein and DNA are crosslinked in growing cell culture, the fixed and crosslinked DNA–protein complexes are fragmented, immunoprecipitated with an antibody specific for the protein of interest, and the DNA isolated from the precipitated material. After DNA isolation, a standard NGS library is prepared by adapter ligation and sizing, and the DNA is sequenced by standard NGS methods. Given the digital nature of NGS, the number of reads aligning to a particular area of the genome is directly proportional to the amount of input DNA from that region. Thus, one can determine "peaks" with a statistically significant increased number of aligned reads and infer that the genomic regions underlying the peaks are the specific areas where the protein of interest was bound to the DNA.[43,44] Antibody specificity and avidity remain key determinants for the validity of ChIP-seq data, as does identifying the appropriate coverage cutoff value that determines a "peak."

Next-Generation Sequencing–Based Studies of Chromatin Accessibility

The interaction of DNA and proteins to form chromatin plays an increasingly recognized role in the study of genomics and epigenomics (Chap. 12). Several methods using NGS-based approaches can interrogate the physical structure of DNA. These methods, which fragment DNA based on the accessibility of chromatin, allow for the determination of nucleosome positioning and inferred protein–DNA binding sites. Although these studies are not a direct method for determining specific protein–DNA binding sites, one can use sequence from the inferred protein–DNA binding sites as an indirect method for assaying global transcription factor binding genome-wide without the limitations of ChIP-seq described above. NGS-based protocols used to determine chromatin accessibility differ in the approach to the DNA fragmentation step. Three commonly used protocols are DNase-seq, MNase-seq, and ATAC-seq. DNase-seq uses DNase I to fragment DNA based on DNase I hypersensitive sites as a marker of chromatin accessibility.[45] MNase-seq uses micrococcal nuclease (MNase) to cleave the DNA at accessible sites.[46] ATAC-seq uses the hyperactive Tn5 transposase to simultaneously fragment (with minimal sequence bias) and add sequencing adaptors to accessible DNA.[47] Another approach to studying chromatin accessibility is known as FAIRE-seq, which involves formalin crosslinking of DNA to proteins prior to random fragmentation via sonication.[48] A variation of this protocol, called chromosome conformational capture (or "3C"), in which chromatin domains are crosslinked, sequenced, and analyzed to determine higher-order structural associations, can provide details into the spatial organization of a genome.[49]

Next-Generation Sequencing-Based Studies of Chemical Modifications to DNA: DNA Methylation and Hydroxy-methylation

Unless otherwise specified, DNA methylation is generally synonymous with cytosine methylation. Cytosine can undergo methylation or hydroxymethylation at its C5 position to form 5-methylcytosine (5-mC) or 5-hydroxymethylcytosine (5-hmC). Both cytosine methylation and 5-hydroxymethylation typically occur when a 5′ cytosine is positioned directly adjacent to a downstream guanine (known as a CpG dinucleotide). There are approximately 26 million CpGs in the human genome. The first genome-wide platforms to detect DNA methylation changes at base pair resolution were microarrays designed to hybridize targeted CpGs across the genome (current methylation microarrays target approximately 500,000 CpGs). However, the design of CpG representation on a microarray was often biased toward gene promoters or other areas of predetermined interest.

Many protocols exist for differential fragmentation of a genome based on DNA methylation prior to array capture. For example, methylated cytosines are protected from cleavage by particular restriction enzymes: HpaII will cleave C-C-G-G but not C-5mC-G-G, whereas MspI will cleave both sites. By creating separate fragmentation libraries using each individual enzyme and then hybridizing each library to a separate array, differentially methylated sites can be determined.[50] Alternatively, one can perform DNA methylation studies using the sodium bisulfite conversion of cytosine to uracil (which is read as a thymidine). Both 5-mC and 5-hmC do not undergo bisulfite conversion and are read out as cytosine in a downstream assay. Microarrays that were designed for bisulfite-treated DNA have distinct paired probe sets that are designed to capture specific differentially methylated CpGs. NGS has enabled the direct sequencing of bisulfite converted DNA for unbiased evaluation of methylation and hydroxymethylation genome-wide.[51] In whole-genome bisulfite sequencing (WGBS), a standard sequencing library is prepared with methylated C–containing adaptors, followed by the bisulfite conversion of the library. WGBS is complicated by numerous factors, including (1) the large amount of input DNA necessary for sequencing (bisulfite conversion results in DNA degradation), (2) incomplete conversion of cytosine to uracil, and (3) the analytic challenge of determining accurately which sequencing reads have been converted because of the presence of cytosine methylation or hydroxymethylation. To determine if cytosines are methylated versus hydroxymethylated, researchers have designed alternative protocols with an added chemical or enzyme-mediated conversion step or antibody-mediated differential capture of 5-mC and 5-hmC prior to sequencing.[52,53] Capture-based methods can also be used to target only

5-mC prior to library preparation and sequencing, which may allow for genome-wide methylation studies at base pair resolution using smaller amounts of input DNA than WGBS.[54] A new transposase-based tagmentation method, similar to the approach used for ATAC-seq, also allows for WGBS with very small amounts of input DNA.[55]

APPROACHES TO DNA SEQUENCING FOR RESEARCH PURPOSES

The study of genomics for research purposes has also shifted as a result of NGS technology. Prior to the broad availability of NGS platforms, most genomics research studies were genome-wide association studies (GWASs) that used a microarray platform to assay for significant changes in allele frequency from the panel of single nucleotide polymorphisms (SNPs) included on the array (modern arrays often have probes to detect the genotype of more than 1 million SNPs).[56] GWASs require large numbers of samples (cases and controls), and are powered to identify SNPs that are in linkage disequilibrium with an associated condition.[57] It is unlikely that the true pathologic variant will be discovered via a GWAS. Instead, the results of a GWAS could provide the basis for a targeted sequencing study to determine the pathologic alteration(s). In the era of decreasing cost and broad availability of NGS, most genomics studies have shifted to a more inclusive discovery platform, such as whole-genome sequencing or exome sequencing. Using a platform with single-base resolution rather than a defined content microarray increases the power to identify a pathologic variant, and the number of samples may decrease. However, for complex genetic diseases, in which multiple genes may play a causative role, the number of samples required remains large and can be cost prohibitive. In these situations, investigators often use a combination of GWAS methods (with cheaper microarrays) to perform the initial discovery work followed by region-specific NGS discovery sequencing.

Several ethical issues complicate the NGS-based study of human genomes. First, sequencing data may be potentially "identifiable," meaning that one could potentially determine another person's identity based on sequencing results obtained by a genomic study, when compared to data from a second genotyping assay (such as for diagnostic or criminal purposes). The Genetic Information Nondiscrimination Act (GINA) of 2008 made it illegal in the United States for employers and health insurance providers to discriminate based on the results of genetic findings. However, persons enrolling into genomics research trials must be informed of this theoretical risk of identifiability and be properly consented. Another consequence of genomics studies is that researchers must consider the return of genetic results to patients. The return of results is divided into two general categories: incidental findings and findings pertinent to the condition being studied. There is no standard approach for return of results as the approach varies on a case-by-case basis, depending on the sequencing study and the result to be communicated; however, new guidelines are emerging.[58] There is general consensus in the genomics research community that these issues, and how they will be handled for the particular study, must be clearly presented in the study protocol and the informed consent documentation.

The sequencing of cancer genomes, whether by whole-genome sequencing, exome sequencing, or multigene panels, is also associated with several specific considerations. Proper informed consent is again paramount. Proper sample banking is critical to avoid degradation of nucleic acids prior to their isolation, as high-quality DNA or RNA increases the likelihood of successful sequencing independent of the NGS platform used. For DNA sequencing studies of a cancer sample, a matched "normal" sample is often also sequenced to discern the somatic versus germline status of any identified alterations.

NEXT-GENERATION SEQUENCING AS A CLINICAL ASSAY: IMPLICATIONS FOR THE PRACTICING HEMATOLOGIST

Using NGS as a clinical assay platform offers many opportunities for new clinical tests and potential therapeutic interventions. Clinical sequencing requires the same high standards regarding sample banking, nucleic acid isolation and proper informed consent. Moreover, clinical sequencing must be done in an appropriately certified clinical laboratory environment. As the depth of coverage increases for NGS-based platforms, the statistical power to detect variation will increase up until the point that it is outweighed by the intrinsic error associated with the sequencing platform. For clinical NGS-based diagnostic tests, these error metrics must be predetermined for each protocol, whether it be whole-genome sequencing, a specific exome reagent, or a specific gene panel test.

NGS-based diagnostics have specific potential applications for both hematologic malignancies and nonmalignant hematologic conditions. For leukemias, lymphomas, myelodysplastic syndromes (MDS), myeloproliferative neoplasms and other hematologic malignancies (or premalignant conditions), the use of clinical sequencing can be employed to determine the spectrum of mutations that are driving the particular malignancy. For any given tumor, comprehensive sequencing may identify an "actionable" mutation that could lead to the use of a targeted therapy.

In the past, a clinician may have ordered a single gene test to determine if a particular molecular abnormality were present in a tumor sample, such as testing for *FLT3* internal tandem duplications (*FLT3*-ITD) in patients with acute myeloid leukemia (AML). The presence of such an alteration has prognostic implications and may have therapeutic significance pending the results of ongoing clinical studies with FLT3 inhibitors. A single-gene or single "hot spot" assay that is designed to detect a specific alteration has several limitations that are now leading to wider use of NGS-based approaches to clinical diagnostics. To continue using *FLT3*-ITD alterations in AML as an example, the use of a more comprehensive sequencing platform could be used to discern the subclonal architecture of the cancer tissue. If the *FLT3*-ITD mutation was present only in a subclone but not in the founding clone, one would predict that a FLT3 inhibitor would only be active in eradicating the subclone. Therefore, clinicians would need to incorporate another therapy to eradicate the founding clone, so as to achieve remission or prevent disease relapse. Ideally, the choice of this therapy would be determined based on the other mutations identified in the founding clone.

As clinicians better understand the mutational drivers of any particular tumor, they may be able to use targeted therapies directed at particular pathways rather than individual gene mutations. For example, researchers may be able to develop a drug that is effective if a patient with AML or MDS harbors a mutation in any of the genes involved in the spliceosome complex or associated proteins. A similar scenario could be envisioned targeting mutations in genes in the cohesin complex (protein complex that regulates the separation of sister chromatids in cell division) or genes that alter the hydroxymethylation of cytosine in DNA. Clinical trials built around these concepts will be necessary to establish their validity. Additionally, comprehensive sequencing can identify somatic mutations that result in the formation of neo-antigens expressed on the tumor cells. Clinicians could then use tumor-specific immunotherapy to target the malignancy.[59,60]

Researchers are using NGS-based technology to detect minimal residual disease (MRD) in hematologic malignancies.[61-63] An advantage of NGS-based methods of MRD detection is that the data not only provide information regarding the presence or absence of MRD but

also may reveal the clonal architecture of persistent disease from the mutations detected. Finally, clinicians could use knowledge gained by sequencing an individual's genome to determine the choice of therapy, whether for a malignant or non-malignant hematologic disease. In one such example, a therapy choice could be optimized based on pharmacogenomic studies in which the response or toxicity of a given drug is associated with underlying inherited genetic variation in the patient.[64] In a second example, a genomic assay might identify a somatic alteration corresponding to a targeted therapy that might help a patient with residual MRD to achieve remission. These examples are illustrative of the translational potential of NGS from research tool into clinical care.

REFERENCES

1. International Human Genome Sequencing Consortium: Finishing the euchromatic sequence of the human genome. *Nature* 431(7011):931–945, 2004.
2. Sanger F, Nicklen S, Coulson AR: DNA sequencing with chain-terminating inhibitors. *Proc Natl Acad Sci U S A* 74(12):5463–5467, 1977.
3. Prober JM, Trainor GL, Dam RJ, et al: A system for rapid DNA sequencing with fluorescent chain-terminating dideoxynucleotides. *Science* 238(4825):336–341, 1987.
4. Smith LM, Sanders JZ, Kaiser RJ, et al: Fluorescence detection in automated DNA sequence analysis. *Nature* 321(6071):674–679, 1986.
5. Tabor S, Huber HE, Richardson CC: *Escherichia coli* thioredoxin confers processivity on the DNA polymerase activity of the gene 5 protein of bacteriophage T7. *J Biol Chem* 262(33):16212–16223, 1987.
6. Huber HE, Tabor S, Richardson CC: *Escherichia coli* thioredoxin stabilizes complexes of bacteriophage T7 DNA polymerase and primed templates. *J Biol Chem* 262(33):16224–16232, 1987.
7. Heller C: Principles of DNA separation with capillary electrophoresis. *Electrophoresis* 22(4):629–643, 2001.
8. Metzker ML: Sequencing technologies-the next generation. *Nat Rev Genet* 11(1):31–46, 2010.
9. Mardis ER: Next-generation sequencing platforms. *Annu Rev Anal Chem (Palo Alto Calif)* 6:287–303, 2013.
10. Mardis ER: A decade's perspective on DNA sequencing technology. *Nature* 470 (7333):198–203, 2011.
11. Bentley DR, Balasubramanian S, Swerdlow HP, et al: Accurate whole human genome sequencing using reversible terminator chemistry. *Nature* 456(7218):53–59, 2008.
12. Dohm JC, Lottaz C, Borodina T, Himmelbauer H: Substantial biases in ultra-short read data sets from high-throughput DNA sequencing. *Nucleic Acids Res* 36(16):e105, 2008.
13. Flicek, P, Birney E: Sense from sequence reads: Methods for alignment and assembly. *Nat Methods* 6(11 Suppl):S6–S12, 2009.
14. Fullwood MJ, Wei CL, Liu ET, Ruan Y: Next-generation DNA sequencing of paired-end tags (PET) for transcriptome and genome analyses. *Genome Res* 2009;19(4):521–532, 2008.
15. Rothberg JM, Hinz W, Rearick TM, et al: An integrated semiconductor device enabling non-optical genome sequencing. *Nature* 475(7356):348–352, 2011.
16. Bragg LM, Stone G, Butler MK, et al: Shining a light on dark sequencing: Characterising errors in Ion Torrent PGM data. *PLoS Comput Biol* 9(4):e1003031, 2013.
17. Eid J, Fehr A, Gray J, et al: Real-time DNA sequencing from single polymerase molecules. *Science* 323(5910):133–138, 2009.
18. Ross MG, Russ C, Costello M, et al: Characterizing and measuring bias in sequence data. *Genome Biol* 14(5):R51, 2013.
19. Branton D, Deamer DW, Marziali A, et al: The potential and challenges of nanopore sequencing. *Nat Biotechnol* 26(10):1146–1153, 2008.
20. Wheeler DA, Srinivasan M, Egholm M, et al: The complete genome of an individual by massively parallel DNA sequencing. *Nature* 452(7189):872–876, 2008.
21. Ley TJ, Mardis ER, Ding L, et al: DNA sequencing of a cytogenetically normal acute myeloid leukaemia genome. *Nature* 456(7218):66–72, 2008.
22. Ng SB, Turner EH, Robertson PD, et al: Targeted capture and massively parallel sequencing of 12 human exomes. *Nature* 461(7261):272–276, 2009.
23. Mamanova L, Coffey AJ, Scott CE, et al: Target-enrichment strategies for next-generation sequencing. *Nat Methods* 7(2):111–118, 2010.
24. Altmuller J, Budde BS, Nurnberg P: Enrichment of target sequences for next-generation sequencing applications in research and diagnostics. *Biol Chem* 395(2):231–237, 2014.
25. Koboldt DC, Steinberg KM, Larson DE, et al: The next-generation sequencing revolution and its impact on genomics. *Cell* 155(1):27–38, 2013.
26. Alkan C, Coe BP, Eichler EE: Genome structural variation discovery and genotyping. *Nat Rev Genet* 12(5):363–376, 2011.
27. Koboldt DC, Larson DE, Chen K, et al: Massively parallel sequencing approaches for characterization of structural variation. *Methods Mol Biol* 838:369–384, 2012.
28. Mitelman F, Johansson B, Mertens F: The impact of translocations and gene fusions on cancer causation. *Nat Rev Cancer* 7(4):233–245, 2007.
29. Landau DA, Carter SL, Getz G, Wu CJ: Clonal evolution in hematological malignancies and therapeutic implications. *Leukemia* 28(1):34–43, 2014.

30. Greaves M, Maley CC: Clonal evolution in cancer. *Nature* 481(7381):306–313, 2012.

31. Landau DA, Carter SL, Stojanov P, et al: Evolution and impact of subclonal mutations in chronic lymphocytic leukemia. *Cell* 152(4):714–726, 2013.

32. Cancer Genome Atlas Research Network: Genomic and epigenomic landscapes of adult de novo acute myeloid leukemia. *N Engl J Med* 368(22):2059–2074, 2013.

33. Welch JS, Ley TJ, Link DC, et al: The origin and evolution of mutations in acute myeloid leukemia. *Cell* 150(2):264–278, 2012.

34. Ding L, Ley TJ, Larson DE, et al: Clonal evolution in relapsed acute myeloid leukaemia revealed by whole-genome sequencing. *Nature* 481(7382):506–510, 2012.

35. Walter MJ, Shen D, Ding L, et al: Clonal architecture of secondary acute myeloid leukemia. *N Engl J Med* 366(12):1090–1098, 2012.

36. Walter MJ, Shen D, Shao J, et al: Clonal diversity of recurrently mutated genes in myelodysplastic syndromes. *Leukemia* 27(6):1275–1282, 2013.

37. ENCODE Project Consortium: An integrated encyclopedia of DNA elements in the human genome. *Nature* 489(7414):57–74, 2012.

38. Mortazavi A, Williams BA, McCue K, et al: Mapping and quantifying mammalian transcriptomes by RNA-Seq. *Nat Methods* 5(7):621–628, 2008.

39. Cabanski CR, Magrini V, Griffith M, et al: CDNA hybrid capture improves transcriptome analysis on low-input and archived samples. *J Mol Diagn* 16(4):440–451, 2014.

40. Trapnell C, Hendrickson DG, Sauvageau M, et al: Differential analysis of gene regulation at transcript resolution with RNA-seq. *Nat Biotechnol* 31(1):46–53, 2013.

41. Trapnell C, Roberts A, Goff L, et al: Differential gene and transcript expression analysis of RNA-seq experiments with TopHat and Cufflinks. *Nat Protoc* 7(3):562–578, 2012.

42. Park PJ: ChIP-seq: Advantages and challenges of a maturing technology. *Nat Rev Genet* 10(10):669–680, 2009.

43. Bailey T, Krajewski P, Ladunga I, et al: Practical guidelines for the comprehensive analysis of ChIP-seq data. *PLoS Comput Biol* 9(11):e1003326, 2013.

44. Landt SG, Marinov GK, Kundaje A, et al: ChIP-seq guidelines and practices of the ENCODE and modENCODE consortia. *Genome Res* 2012;22(9):1813–1831, 2013.

45. He HH, Meyer CA, Hu SS, et al: Refined DNase-seq protocol and data analysis reveals intrinsic bias in transcription factor footprint identification. *Nat Methods* 11(1):73–78, 2014.

46. Cui K, Zhao K: Genome-wide approaches to determining nucleosome occupancy in metazoans using MNase-Seq. *Methods Mol Biol* 833:413–419, 2012.

47. Buenrostro JD, Giresi PG, Zaba LC, et al: Transposition of native chromatin for fast and sensitive epigenomic profiling of open chromatin, DNA-binding proteins and nucleosome position. *Nat Methods* 10(12):1213–1218, 2013.

48. Yang CC, Buck MJ, Chen MH, et al: Discovering chromatin motifs using FAIRE sequencing and the human diploid genome. *BMC Genomics* 14:310, 2013.

49. Jin F, Li Y, Dixon JR, et al: A high-resolution map of the three-dimensional chromatin interactome in human cells. *Nature* 503(7475):290–294, 2013.

50. Oda M, Greally JM: The HELP assay. *Methods Mol Biol* 507:77–87, 2009.

51. Krueger F, Kreck B, Franke A, Andrews SR: DNA methylome analysis using short bisulfite sequencing data. *Nat Methods* 9(2):145–151, 2012.

52. Booth MJ, Branco MR, Ficz G, et al: Quantitative sequencing of 5-methylcytosine and 5-hydroxymethylcytosine at single-base resolution. *Science* 336(6083):934–937, 2012.

53. Booth MJ, Ost TW, Beraldi D, et al: Oxidative bisulfite sequencing of 5-methylcytosine and 5-hydroxymethylcytosine. *Nat Protoc* 8(10):1841–1851, 2013.

54. Lee EJ, Luo J, Wilson JM, Shi H: Analyzing the cancer methylome through targeted bisulfite sequencing. *Cancer Lett* 340(2):171–178, 2013.

55. Wang Q, Gu L, Adey A, et al: Tagmentation-based whole-genome bisulfite sequencing. *Nat Protoc* 8(10):2022–2032, 2013.

56. McCarthy MI, Abecasis GR, Cardon LR, et al: Genome-wide association studies for complex traits: Consensus, uncertainty and challenges. *Nat Rev Genet* 9(5):356–369, 2008.

57. Risch N, Merikangas K: The future of genetic studies of complex human diseases. *Science* 273(5281):1516–1517, 1996.

58. Green RC, Berg JS, Grody WW, et al: ACMG recommendations for reporting of incidental findings in clinical exome and genome sequencing. *Genet Med* 15(7):565–574, 2013.

59. Li L, Goedegebuure P, Mardis ER, et al: Cancer genome sequencing and its implications for personalized cancer vaccines. *Cancers (Basel)* 3(4):4191–4211, 2011.

60. Linette GP, Carreno BM: Dendritic cell-based vaccines: Shining the spotlight on signal 3. *Oncoimmunology* 2(11):e26512, 2013.

61. Salipante SJ, Fromm JR, Shendure J, et al: Detection of minimal residual disease in NPM1-mutated acute myeloid leukemia by next-generation sequencing. *Mod Pathol* 27(11):1438–1446, 2014.

62. Ladetto M, Brüggemann M, Monitillo L, et al: Next-generation sequencing and real-time quantitative PCR for minimal residual disease detection in B-cell disorders. *Leukemia* 28(6):1299–1307, 2014.

63. Thol F, Kölking B, Damm F, et al: Next-generation sequencing for minimal residual disease monitoring in acute myeloid leukemia patients with FLT3-ITD or NPM1 mutations. *Genes Chromosomes Cancer* 51(7):689–695, 2012.

64. Relling MV, Altman RB, Goetz MP, Evans WE: Clinical implementation of pharmacogenomics: Overcoming genetic exceptionalism. *Lancet Oncol* 11(6):507–509, 2010.

CHAPTER 12
EPIGENETICS

Bradley R. Cairns

SUMMARY

Epigenetics involves a heritable change in phenotype without a change in genotype—with the inheritance of particular chromatin and transcription states often underlying the mechanism. Chromatin regulates gene expression by controlling the density and positioning of nucleosomes, and by the use of histone- and DNA-modifying enzymes. Chromatin and transcription factors drive proper differentiation decisions through their coregulation of key factors in development and proliferation. Of particular interest to hematologists are instances when misregulation/mutation of chromatin factors drives hematologic malignancies and myeloproliferative disorders. Here, fusion proteins that involve the mistargeting of chromatin regulators have been known for decades. More recently, high-throughput sequencing and other genomics approaches have revealed mutations in many types of chromatin regulators in hematologic malignancies, including mutations in chromatin remodelers, DNA methylation regulators, histone modification enzymes, and metabolic enzymes affecting epigenetic cofactors. Overall, these studies reveal a consistent theme: epigenetic and genetic mutations confer both variation and plasticity to the transcriptome, and when combined with selection, arrive at transcriptomes that promote proliferation, survival, and adaptability. This chapter addresses these mechanistic principles of chromatin, and their misregulation in hematologic malignancies, as well as emerging therapeutic approaches.

Acronyms and Abbreviations: AF, ALL1-fused gene; ALL, acute lymphocytic leukemia; AML, acute myeloid leukemia; BAF, BRG/BAF-associated factors; BCL, B-cell lymphoma family of regulator proteins that regulate cell death; BET, bromo and extraterminal; CHD, chromodomain remodeler; CMML, chronic myelomonocytic leukemia; DNAme, DNA methylation; DNMT, DNA methyltransferase; DOT1, a histone H3 methyltransferase; EGR1, early growth response protein 1; EZH2, enhancer of zeste homologue 2; H3, histone H3; HAT, histone acetyltransferase; HDAC, histone deacetylase; HIF, hypoxia-inducible transcription factor; 5hmC, 5-hydroxymethylcytosine; HMT, histone methyltransferase; HSC, hematopoietic stem cell; IDH, isocitrate dehydrogenase; Ifng promoter, interferon-γ promoter; ISWI, imitation SWI remodeler; MBD, methyl-domain binding; 5mC, 5-methylcytosine; MLL, mixed lineage leukemia; MTA, metastasis-associated; NuRD, nucleosome remodeling and deacetylation factor; NURF, nucleosome remodeling factor; 2OG, 2-oxoglutarate; PRC2, polycomb repressive complex 2; R-2HG, (R)-2-hydroxyglutarate; RAR, retinoic acid receptor; RNAP II, RNA polymerase II; SDH, succinate dehydrogenase; SRF, serum response factor; SWI/SNF, switch and sucrose nonfermenting remodeler; TDG, thymine DNA glycosylase; UHRF1, ubiquitin-like with PHD and ring finger domains; UTX, X-chromosome encoded ubiquitously transcribed tetratricopeptide repeat.

DEFINITION AND OVERVIEW

Epigenetics is defined as a heritable change in phenotype without a change in genotype. Although epigenetic mechanisms vary, this chapter focuses on the most common mechanism: chromatin. Changes in chromatin/epigenetics accompany many steps in transcription, replication, and recombination. However, the aspects of highest interest and relevance involve examples where epigenetic factors and enzymes *drive* differentiation decisions, and where misregulation/mutation of these factors *drives* pathologies, such as hematologic malignancies. This decision making must be precise, as differentiation along the lymphoid and myeloid lineages involves the regulated generation of multiple cell types in temporal order and proper proportion. Decisions are arrived through collaboration among signaling systems, transcription factors, and chromatin regulators-which together regulate the key genes governing self-renewal, differentiation, and survival. This chapter focuses on chromatin factors with central roles in these processes: ATP-dependent remodelers, DNA methylation (DNAme)/demethylation enzymes, and histone modification enzymes. As a complete treatment is beyond the scope of this chapter, the focus here will be conceptual, with particular examples provided to create a framework for understanding the many instances where chromatin factors influence decision-making.

Beyond their roles in normal blood cell development, misregulation of chromatin factors is now known to be common in hematologic malignancies. Indeed, high-throughput whole-genome and/or exome sequencing of leukemias and lymphomas has revealed mutations in many types of chromatin regulators, including mutations in chromatin remodelers, DNA methyltransferases (DNMT), and histone modification enzymes, as well as revealing fusion proteins that involve chromatin regulators.[1] In certain instances, modeling in the mouse supports these epigenetic mutations as the main drivers of the cancer phenotype. In other instances, epigenetic mutations cooperate with (and likely enable) additional genetic mutations, which cooperate to impact proliferation, survival, and plasticity, which can enable both cancer progression and therapy resistance. However, as many chromatin regulators are enzymes, they may be more targetable than mutations in DNA binding transcription factors, providing new therapeutic approaches.[2] This chapter expands on these concepts, addressing the mechanistic basis of chromatin misregulation in hematologic malignancies, as well as emerging therapeutic approaches.

CHROMATIN REMODELING AND DNA ACCESS

CHROMATIN REGULATES TRANSCRIPTION FACTOR BINDING

Chromatin has a major impact on gene expression, mediated through interplay with transcription factors. Sequence-specific DNA-binding transcription factors are the most important factors in defining whether and when a gene is transcribed, and also define the locations and character of chromatin regions, as they target chromatin remodeling and modifying proteins. However, the initial chromatin landscape can control whether transcription factors have access to the DNA at a particular gene/region. Access to DNA is deterred by nucleosomes, the main repeating unit of chromatin structure, which can block the binding sites of transcription factors to chromatin.[3] Likewise, DNAme can also block the binding of transcription factors, many of which will not bind DNA if the cytosine in their binding site is methylated (DNAme is discussed more extensively in the section "DNA Methylation and Demethylation").

Thus, the nucleosome and DNAme landscape together define the initial "open versus closed" chromatin state of a region with which the current repertoire of transcription factors within that cell type must contend. However, this landscape is dynamic, as signaling systems can modify transcription factors and chromatin components, altering their activity and the landscape both through their binding, and through their recruitment of nucleosome remodelers and chromatin modifiers.[3-5]

CHROMATIN REMODELERS CONTROL GENOME ACCESS

ATP-dependent chromatin remodeling complexes (termed hereafter *remodelers*) conduct central roles in regulating nucleosome occupancy and positioning (Fig. 12–1).[3-5] For example, *remodelers* specialized for chromatin assembly (such as imitation SWI *remodeler* [ISWI]-family and chromodomain *remodeler* [CHD]-family *remodelers*) utilize ATP hydrolysis to facilitate tight-packed nucleosomes that lead to the occlusion of sites for site-specific DNA binding proteins, such as transcription factors. Access to chromatin at enhancers, promoters and other loci can be enabled by *remodelers* such as the switch and sucrose non-fermenting *remodeler* (SWI/SNF) complex, also termed the BRG/BAF-associated factors (BAF) complex, which can slide or eject the histone octamer, using the energy of ATP hydrolysis (Fig. 12–1). Notably, SWI/SNF can interact with (and facilitate the binding of) DNA-binding activators or repressors and can, therefore, help facilitate either activation or repression.[3-5] Here, the ability of activators or repressors to interact with SWI/SNF complexes can be influenced by signaling cascades, which impart covalent modifications that enable or disable protein interactions. Taken together, ISWI and CHD *remodelers* often act to silencing genes via site blockage at enhancers and promoters, whereas SWI/SNF *remodelers* promote site exposure at those locations (Fig. 12–1), which is important for gene activation.

● CHROMATIN REMODELING COMPLEXES IN BLOOD CELL DIFFERENTIATION

Clear roles for *remodelers* in blood cell differentiation are emerging. For example, SWI/SNF components affect the pool size of fetal hematopoietic stem cells (HSCs), and also impact HSC (and progenitor) proliferation and survival.[6] SWI/SNF complex is also used for myeloid differentiation to granulocytes and for multiple steps in thymocyte development. More specifically, in mice SWI/SNF binds the interferon-γ (*Ifng*) promoter, and is required for its full transcription. Furthermore, mutations in the adenosine triphosphatase (ATPase) function of SWI/SNF are known to reduce β-globin expression and to prevent erythroid differentiation.[7] Notably, B-cell lymphoma (BCL) factors BCL7A and BCL11B, which are considered members of SWI/SNF complex in many cell types, are common in hematologic malignancies; for example, mutations in BCL7A are found in approximately 20 percent of non-Hodgkin lymphoma and multiple myeloma cases, and mutations in BCL11B are found in 6 to 12 percent of T-cell acute lymphocytic leukemias (ALLs).[8]

Roles for ISWI- and CHD-family *remodelers* include roles for the well-characterized CHD-family *remodeler* nucleosome remodeling and deacetylation factor (NuRD), which interacts with histone deacetylase (HDAC) enzymes to silence genes. The metastasis-associated (MTA) subunits of NuRD help target NuRD subtypes to particular genes through their interaction with transcription factors and chromatin modifications.[9] For example, in B-lymphocytes, MTA3 interacts with BCL6, a major regulator of B-cell differentiation, targeting NuRD repression and preventing terminal differentiation into plasma cells.[10] Remarkably, expressing BCL6 in plasma cells while MTA3 is functional results in a reversion of the cell fate and reprogramming into

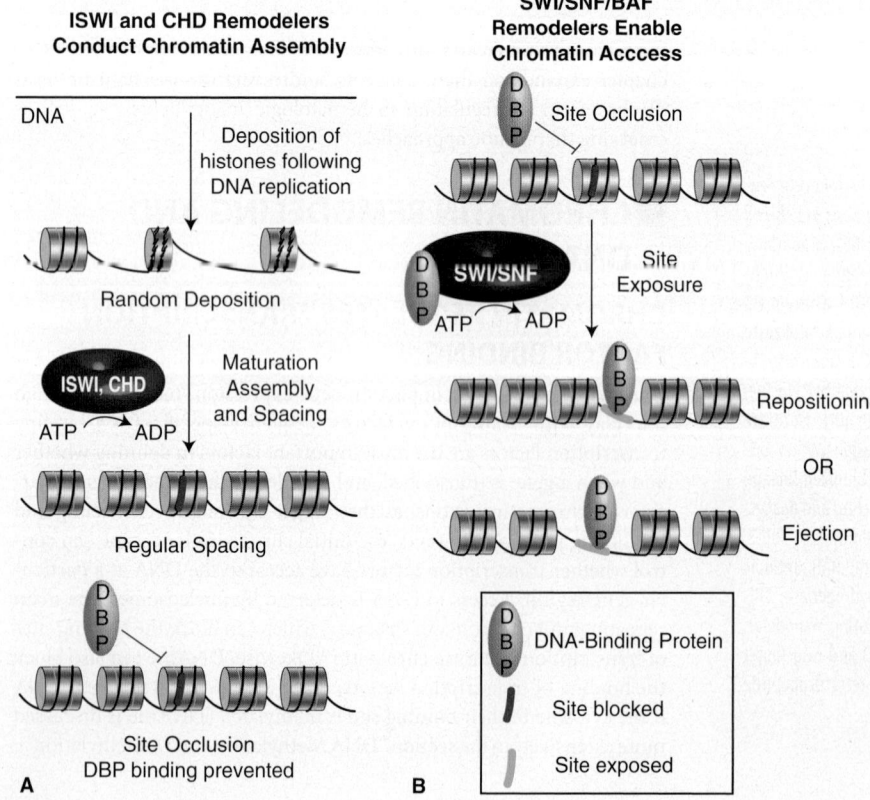

Figure 12–1. Roles for ATP-dependent chromatin remodelers in chromatin assembly or chromatin access. Imitation SWI *remodelers* (ISWI)- and chromodomain *remodelers* (CHD)-family *remodelers* are involved in chromatin assembly genome-wide, and also interact with site-specific repressors to organize nucleosome spacing at genes, which can occlude sites for DNA-binding proteins. Switch and sucrose nonfermenting *remodelers* (SWI/SNF)-family *remodelers* conduct both nucleosome repositioning/sliding as well as ejection to expose DNA to DNA-binding proteins.

ISWI and CHD Remodelers Conduct Chromatin Assembly

DNA

Deposition of histones following DNA replication

Random Deposition

ISWI, CHD

ATP → ADP

Maturation Assembly and Spacing

Regular Spacing

Site Occlusion DBP binding prevented

A

SWI/SNF/BAF Remodelers Enable Chromatin Acccess

DBP — Site Occlusion

SWI/SNF

ATP → ADP

Site Exposure

DBP — Repositioning

OR

DBP — Ejection

B

DBP — DNA-Binding Protein

Site blocked

Site exposed

B lymphocytes.[10] Furthermore, the recruitment of the ISWI-family complex nucleosome remodeling factor (NURF) to the early growth response protein 1 (EGR1) locus (important for thymocyte maturation) involves interaction with the transcription factor serum response factor (SRF) by the NURF subunit BPTF, enabling its stable binding to promoters.[11] Notably, Ikaros (which drives lymphoid differentiation) acts to inhibit both the ATP-dependent remodeling and HDAC activities of NuRD at target genes to enable activation rather than silencing.[12] Taken together, these and other examples illustrate the use of *remodeler* function and recruitment to activate or repress key genes in blood differentiation.

● PRINCIPLES OF HISTONE MODIFICATION

HISTONE MODIFICATION CONCEPTS: WRITE, READ, ERASE

The process of transcriptional regulation is accompanied by the ordered placement of particular histone modifications at enhancers, promoters, and coding regions. There are dozens of different modifications that occur on histones, with the most common modifications

being acetylation, methylation, ubiquitylation, and phosphorylation. An inventory and functional analysis of all of these modifications, the enzymes that place and remove these modifications, is beyond the scope of this chapter; however, more important are the concepts, which can then be applied widely to various contexts.

First, the vast majority of histone modifications occur either on the extended aminoterminal "tails" of histones, whereas a minority also occur on the histone octamer "core."[13] The core of the histone octamer wraps the DNA, whereas histone tails serve as platforms for the regulated binding of proteins, and covalent modifications can either enhance or deter binding of chromatin *remodelers*, chromatin modifiers, and transcription factors, and help to orchestrate protein associations during transcription (Fig. 12–2). For example, methylation on histone H3 (H3) H3K4me can deter interaction with DNMTs and therefore cause passive DNA demethylation; in contrast, H3K4me3 can facilitate interaction with RNA polymerase II (RNAP II) machinery.[14] Second, histone modifiers are typically targeted by site-specific DNA binding proteins (see Fig. 12–2), which are themselves responsive to developmental and environmental/metabolic signaling. Third, some histone modifiers are targeted or regulated by other histone modifications, which underlies (in part) why certain sets of histone modifications are coincident in regions.[13]

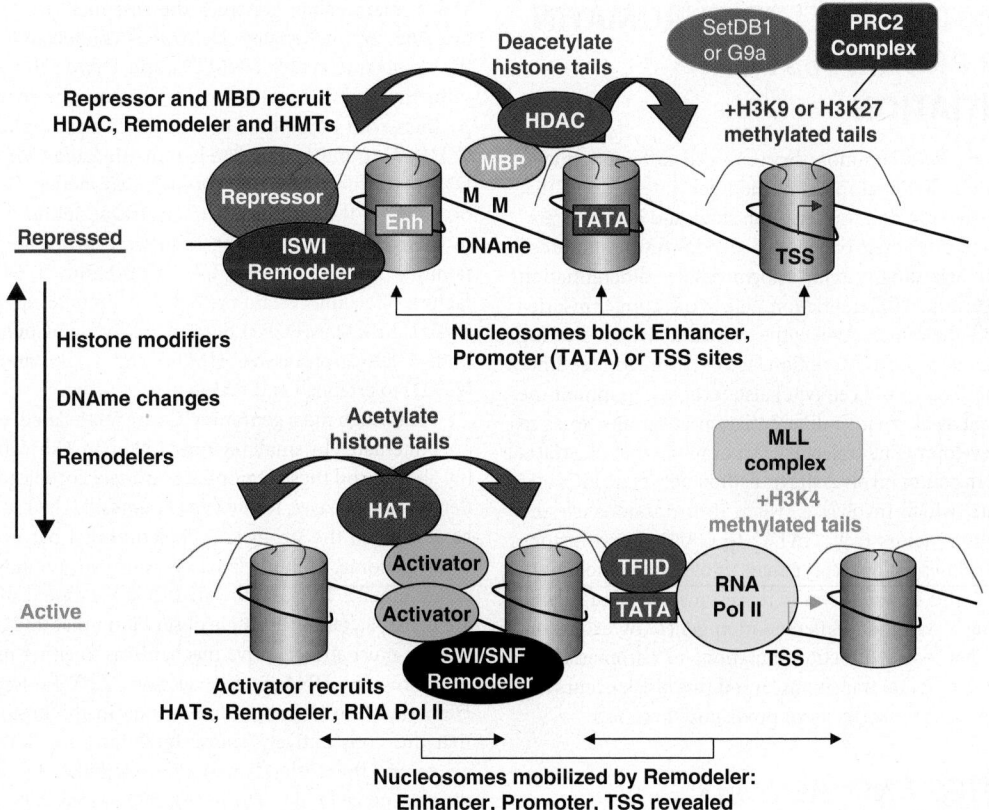

Figure 12–2. Chromatin changes that accompany the transition from a repressed to an active state. Repression *(top)* is enforced by site-specific DNA-binding repressors which recruit factors such as histone deacetylates (HDACs), histone methyltransferases (HMTs; for H3K9me or H3K27me), and DNA methyltransferases (not shown), which are used to methylate the DNA (M). Methyl-binding domain proteins (MBDs) bind to DNA methylation (DNAme) and also recruit a similar set of chromatin modifiers. These repressors also recruit imitation SWI remodeler (ISWI)-family *remodelers*, which help position nucleosomes on important *cis*-controlling elements like enhancers (Enh), the TATA box, or the transcription start site (TSS). The transition from the repressed state to the active state involves the modification and repositioning of nucleosomes, as well as DNA demethylation by passive or active modes. Nucleosomes are modified by histone acetyltransferases (HATs), and activating HMTs (mixed-lineage leukemia [MLL] complex, specific for H3K4me). Such modifications are believed to be recognized by the bromodomains present on *remodelers*, which then mobilize modified nucleosomes, allowing the transcription machinery to bind. Components of the transcription machinery, such as TFIID, can also detect histone modifications.

A major concept in histone modification biology is dynamic reversibility, termed *write, read, erase*.[1,15,16] "Writing" involves the enzymatic *addition* of a covalent modification to an amino acid, within a particular protein sequence context. "Reading" involves the ability of a second protein/domain to bind that modification, within a particular protein sequence context, defining the *impact* of the modification. "Erasing" involves the *removal* of the covalent modification, within a particular sequence context, regenerating the prior/initial state. These concepts are actually quite general, and can be applied widely in protein signal transduction biology, with this terminology simply having become popularized in the chromatin field. Nevertheless, these terms are quite useful for framing histone modification cycles that accompany transcription cycles. One illustrative example is the addition of histone acetylation by histone acetyltransferase (HAT) enzymes, the binding of acetylated histone tails by the bromodomain (present in SWI/SNF *remodelers* and certain chromatin modifiers),[17,18] and the removal of acetylation by HDAC enzymes.[19] Finally, although this chapter discusses histone modifications and modifiers, histone modifiers often also modify additional chromatin proteins, including proteins that contain "histone mimic" regions. Although beyond the scope of this chapter, those chromatin modifications often go through similar "write, read, erase" cycles to enable additional layers of protein recruitment and release within a chromatin process.

TRANSCRIPTION FACTOR-CHROMATIN MODIFIER PROGRAMS FOR DIFFERENTIATION

Within the context above, a common theme in cell differentiation is waves of transcription factor–chromatin modifier interactions that define the current chromatin and transcription state, and also help prepare the enhancers and promoters of genes needed for future states/cell types (see Fig. 12–2). Signaling systems inform cellular differentiation decisions, and define the next differentiation state by affecting transcription factor activity and their interaction with chromatin factors, creating a forward loop. Quite often, the transcription factor–chromatin modifier interactions of the new state (and cell type) also feedback to inhibit the prior program, as well as alternative differentiation programs, so as to ensure the proper developmental trajectory. An example that illustrates part of this program in action involves the transition between HSCs and erythroid progenitors, which involves a switch in the abundance and activity of transcription factors (e.g., GATA2 to GATA1) and histone methyltransferase (HMT) paralogs (e.g., enhancer of zeste homologue 2 [EZH2] to EZH1).[20,21] This switch serves to repress a set of stem-related genes while activating a set of pro-differentiation genes. By extension, many studies show that loss-of-function mutations in chromatin factors can prevent developmental transitions, and if this block occurs at a highly proliferative progenitor stage, it can predispose to cancer.

EPIGENETICS AND MEMORY: TRAINED IMMUNITY

Trained immunity refers to a type of memory in the innate immune system where genes that have been activated in the past (via infection or vaccination, termed *stimulation*) are "primed" for a more rapid and/or robust future response. Here, prior to initial stimulation, monocytes and macrophages bear "latent" enhancers neighboring proinflammatory genes, which lack histone modifications. Following stimulation, these latent enhancers acquire histone modifications (e.g., H3K4me and H3K27ac) that are correlated with gene activation and maintain those

modifications for days following withdrawal of the initial stimulus.[22] Importantly, the retention of these modifications is correlated with a more robust or rapid activation in response to a second stimulus. Thus, chromatin states can confer a memory of prior transcriptional states that shapes future response. Here, one can infer within Fig. 12–2 that following activation, this system does not return to the initial repressed state, but rather to an intermediate "poised" state where histone modifications are retained at the enhancer.

DNA METHYLATION AND DEMETHYLATION PRINCIPLES

DNA METHYLATION

DNAme is a major component of epigenetic regulation in mammals, with central roles in gene and transposon silencing, imprinting, and X-chromosome inactivation.[23] Furthermore, DNAme can predispose to cancer by at least two routes: first, through the improper placement of focal DNAme, leading to the silencing of tumor-suppressor genes; second, through hypomethylation of the genome, causing genome instability.[2] Here, basic principles of DNAme and demethylation are first discussed, with a later section "Epigenetic and Hematologic Malignancies" focusing on their misregulation in hematologic malignancies.

DNAme primarily involves cytosine methylation in a CpG context, and in mammalian genomes the vast majority (>85 percent) of such cytosines are methylated. DNAme is conducted by DNMTs, involving the *de novo* enzymes DNMT3a and DNMT3b (which can methylate unmethylated regions) or by the maintenance enzyme DNMT1, which partners with ubiquitin-like with PHD and ring finger domains factor (UHRF1) to fully methylate hemimethylated CGs during replication.[24] DNAme confers silencing through two modes. First, DNAme inhibits or prevents the binding of many transcription factors with CG sites in their consensus binding sequence, including cMyb,[25] cMyc, E2F-family,[26] nuclear factor-κB,[27] CREB-family,[28] ETS-family, and AP2 factors.[29] Second, certain methyl-domain binding (MBD) proteins (e.g., MBD1, MBD2, MECP2) bind to methylated CpG sites and can recruit both HDAC, repressive HMTs, and CHD-family *remodelers* (e.g., NuRD) to establish and maintain repression.[30]

Although most genomic CGs are methylated, mammalian genomes are punctuated by small regions (250 bp to 2 kb) where DNAme is notably absent, and these regions are strongly correlated with a high relative density of CG bases, termed *CpG islands*.[31] (CpG islands are regions that have avoided the strong CG depletion that has occurred over the rest of the genome, as methylated cytosine can spontaneously deaminate to create uracil). Thus, methylated CGs are absent in regions where CGs are dense, a counterintuitive observation that underscores that CG-rich regions must attract active mechanisms to either prevent DNMT activity or remove DNAme (see section "TET Proteins and Active DNA Demethylation"). CpG islands reside in the promoters of most genes that are constitutively transcribed, such as housekeeping/metabolic genes, and these islands remain unmethylated under virtually all conditions and cell types. However, CpG islands vary in size and composition; those of intermediate CG density are often found at developmental genes; notably, these intermediate CpG islands are typically unmethylated in stem cells, but undergo developmentally regulated DNAme to confer silencing in cell types where their expression might confer alternative fates.[32] Notably, CpG islands often contain binding sites for transcription factors; for those transcription factors that display methylation-sensitive binding (listed above), a lack of DNAme in these regions can permit their binding, whereas CpG island methylation can prevent binding. Taken together, proper regulation of DNAme is critical, as the improper placement of focal DNAme can lead to gene silencing.

TET PROTEINS AND ACTIVE DNA DEMETHYLATION

DNAme is chemically highly stable, and therefore very useful in stable propagation of epigenetic states, even through germline inheritance. Although stable, DNA demethylation can occur, and does so mainly through two routes: (1) "passive" demethylation (dilution of DNAme by the failure to conduct maintenance DNAme after DNA replication), and (2) "active" demethylation, mainly involving proteins of the TET family. TET proteins are dioxygenase enzymes that oxidize the methyl group of 5-methylcytosine (5mC) to 5-hydroxymethylcytosine[33,34] (5hmC) and additional oxidized intermediates (not addressed further). Here, 5hmC and other intermediates cause DNA demethylation by one of two modes: first, following replication the maintenance DNMT1 and its partner, UHRF1, do not recognize these oxidized products as 5mC, leading to passive demethylation.[24] Second, glycosylases with roles in DNA repair (e.g., thymine DNA glycosylase [TDG]) can remove 5-hydroxymethylcytosine (5hmC) and similar oxidized intermediates, which are then replaced with an unmodified cytosine by base-excision repair systems.[35] An important aspect of TET-family dioxygenases is their use of iron and 2-oxoglutarate (2OG) as cofactors during the oxidation reaction; a feature that renders TET enzymes sensitive to concentrations of these metabolites and related compounds, which can act as inhibitors during metabolic dysregulation (see section "Misregulation of Dna Methylation/ Demethylation In Hematologic Malignancies").

EPIGENETICS AND HEMATOLOGIC MALIGNANCIES

CONCEPTS IN CANCER EPIGENETICS

Misregulation of epigenetic factors is common in cancer, and a higher level of understanding is achieved by recognizing recurring themes. Epigenetic factors are often misregulated by one of three modes: fusion, loss-of-function (via mutation or expression changes), or gain-of-function (via mutation or expression changes). Notably, each mode impacts the genome and transcriptome in a particular manner, as described below:

Theme 1: Fusion Proteins

Fusion proteins are commonly observed in hematologic malignances, and are often the product of reciprocal chromosomal translocations. Common configurations involve fusions of DNA-binding proteins to chromatin modifiers, or proteins that interact with chromatin modifiers. This creates a dominant gain-of-function protein that targets chromatin-modifying activity to genes important for proliferation, development, or survival. A well-studied and conceptually informative example involves fusion of the aminoterminal portion of the HMT mixed-lineage leukemia (MLL) protein to other proteins that interact with chromatin modifiers.[36,37] Oncogenic MLL fusions are typically driven by the endogenous MLL promoter and retain the DNA-binding domain and additional regions present in the MLL aminoterminus, but omit the catalytic HMT domain normally present at the MLL C-terminus. MLL is normally part of a large complex that methylates histones (H3K4me3) at the promoters of active genes. Oncogenic MLL-fusion proteins can dimerize with normal full-length MLL, and retain the ability to bind DNA binding and also the ability to interact with chromatin and DNA-binding factors.

As previewed above, the fusion partner of MLL is often a protein that interacts with and recruits chromatin modifiers, providing a route to aberrant/constitutive recruitment of chromatin modifiers to particular loci. The most common MLL fusions involve fusion of the MLL

N-terminus to the ALL1-fused (AF) genes (AF9) and AF4 proteins (partial internal tandem duplications are also leukemogenic, which likely also affect interactions with chromatin modifiers). Interestingly, the AF9 and AF4 partners are themselves members of more than one chromatin and transcription complex,[38,39] and therefore capable of recruiting a range of chromatin modifiers, including a H3 methyltransferase, DOT1 (which methylates histone H3K79),[40–42] or TIP60, CBP, and EP300 (which acetylate histones H3 and H4). AF4 is also a member of a complex important for transcriptional elongation,[38,39] which interacts with acetylated histone tails via a bromo and extraterminal (BET)-family bromodomain present in the BRD4 subunit. MLL fusions also involve direct fusion to a chromatin modifier, including fusion to the HAT enzymes CBP or EP300. (Fusion of MLL to TET proteins are covered separately in the context of DNAme in the section "Misregulation of Dna Methylation/Demethylation In Hematologic Malignancies").

Regarding mechanism, current thinking supports the targeting of MLL fusions to constitutively activate key genes involved in blood development, causing a block in differentiation. This block (and continued proliferation) provides the opportunity for other genetic and epigenetic events that enhance proliferation and survival. Confirmed targets for MLL fusions include *HoxA9* and the *Meis1* gene in mouse, where the fusion contributes to their transcriptional activation.[41] However, it is likely that a larger repertoire of target genes is involved, as ectopic expression of *HoxA9* and *Meis1* in mice is effective at inducing leukemias only under certain contexts. Finally, it is important to note that MLL fusions represent one particular class and mechanism; in contrast, fusions involving the retinoic acid receptor (RAR) (e.g., RAR-PLZF) are known to block differentiation through the constitutive recruitment of repressive chromatin modifiers (e.g., HDACs), conferring repression of genes important for activation.[43,44] Thus, as illustrated in Fig. 12–3, proper differentiation involves waves of transcription that involve activating a new program and silencing the former program.

The involvement of multiple enzymes in MLL fusions has inspired therapeutic approaches based on enzyme inhibition.[2] For example,

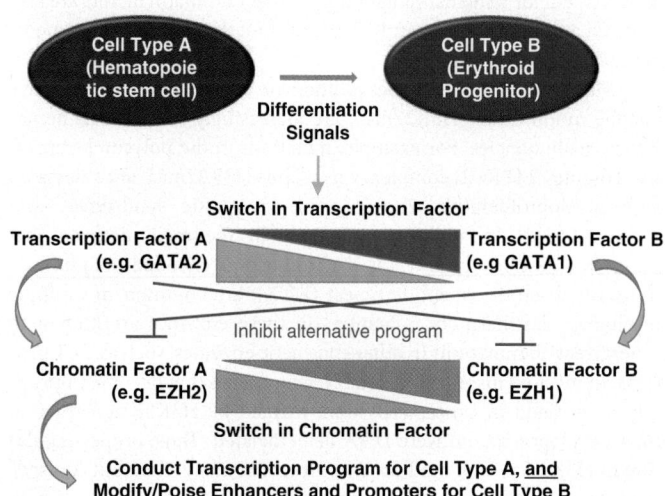

Figure 12–3. Conceptual model for a developmental switch involving transcription factors, chromatin modifiers, and a feedback loop. Here signals for differentiation alter transcription factor and chromatin modifier abundance and activity. This collaboration defines the current chromatin and transcription state and helps prepare the enhancers and promoters of genes needed for future states/cell types, with an example given related to HSC-to-erythroid transition.[21] Furthermore, the transcription factor-chromatin modifier interactions of the new state (cell type) can feed back to inhibit the prior program, ensuring the proper developmental trajectory.

DOT1 (a histone H3 methyltransferase) inhibitors have proven useful in mouse models of MLL-fusion–induced leukemia (and in cell lines),[45] and have entered phase I clinical trials (NCT01684150). Notably, the involvement of BRD4 in this system, along with its known importance in transcriptional activation in MYC-driven cancers, provides additional therapeutic possibilities. Here, inhibitors of BET-family bromodomains (JQ1 and others) have proven very effective in cell lines from patients, laying the foundation for clinical trials.[46–49]

Theme 2: Loss-of-Function Mutations in Chromatin Modifiers

Loss-of-function mutations in chromatin modifiers are now very common in many cancers. The key concept in this theme is that the loss of epigenetic control confers both gene-specific and genome-wide epigenetic variation, eliciting transcriptome variation and plasticity. As a result, individual cells with transcriptomes that promote growth, survival, and/or metastasis can be selected from a diverse population. For example, this epigenetic variation can allow cells to sample a transcriptome that promotes invasion and later convert to a transcriptome that favors colonization. One mode involves the aberrant epigenetic silencing of tumor-suppressor proteins, either by the acquisition of "silencing" histone modifications, DNAme, or both. Epigenetic variation and selection are themselves powerful tools; however, they can also combine with genetic mutations to provide a further fitness benefit and reinforce oncogenic properties.

Examples of mutations in epigenetic factors in hematologic malignancies are numerous; even a partial list of factors and their impact is beyond the scope of this chapter.[1] However, mutations in certain factors are found in many hematologic malignancies and help to illustrate the concepts above; consequently, they are treated further here. One example that builds on an earlier section "Epigenetics and Hematologic Malignancies" involves mutations in MLL genes. MLL is actually a family of five similar genes; however, whereas MLL1 is most commonly involved in leukemogenic fusion proteins (discussed earlier), mutations in MLL2 are very common in lymphomas, with mutation rates as high as 89 percent for follicular lymphoma.[50] Other chromatin factors are also mutated at high frequency in BCLs, including the HAT complex members EP300 and CREBBP.[50]

Mutations that affect the addition or removal of the repressive histone modification H3K27me3, are increasingly common in hematologic malignancies. For example, mutations in the polycomb repressive complex 2 (PRC2) complex, which adds H3K27me3, are associated with myeloproliferative diseases, myelodysplastic syndromes, and T-cell ALL.[51–53] In addition, mutations in the main enzyme that removes H3K27me3, known as X-chromosome encoded ubiquitously transcribed tetratricopeptide repeat (UTX), are common in multiple myeloma.[54] Furthermore, mutations in these enzymes are known to synergize with mutations in other epigenetic enzymes, such as TET proteins, in myeloid disorders.[51] Notably, many genes that become improperly methylated in cancer cells were marked by H3K27me earlier in their development and were DNA demethylated. Thus, proper regulation of H3K27me3—a modification present at many silent but "poised" developmental genes—appears critical for tumor prevention.

Theme 3: Gain-of-Function Mutations in Chromatin Modifiers

Gain-of-function of epigenetic enzymes typically occurs either through upregulation of expression (through copy number variation or promoter fusions) or via mutations that upregulate the activity of the enzyme. The main concept in this theme is that high levels and/or the inability to turn off an epigenetic enzyme can lead to sustained activation or silencing of target loci, depending on the main function of the modification. Among many examples is EZH2, the main enzyme for H3K27me addition, which is either greatly overexpressed or hyperactivated (via mutation) in various hematologic malignancies.[55] For example, EZH2 is highly expressed in mantle cell lymphomas, whereas activating mutations (conferred by amino acid substitutions in the catalytic domain) are common in diffuse large B-cell and follicular lymphomas.[56] This hyperactivity has led to therapeutic strategies involving selective competitive inhibitors that mimic the cofactor S-adenosyl-methionine, the methyl donor for the EZH2 enzyme, which have proven effective in mouse xenografts.[56]

● MISREGULATION OF DNA METHYLATION/DEMETHYLATION IN HEMATOLOGIC MALIGNANCIES

Over the past several years, several studies have made striking links between hematologic malignancies and the misregulation of DNAme. High-throughput sequencing of leukemias and lymphomas have revealed three different types of mutations: (1) loss-of-function mutations in the de novo DNMT3a enzyme; (2) loss-of-function mutations in particular TET proteins; and (3) gain-of-function mutations in the metabolic enzymes isocitrate dehydrogenase (IDH)1 and IDH2, which create small molecule inhibitors of TET proteins (expanded below in this section). To begin, hypomorphic mutations in DNMT3a are common in acute myeloid leukemias (AMLs),[57] although precisely how a reduction in DNMT3a activity promotes leukemia is not yet understood. Of the three TET-family genes, particular TET genes are mutated at high frequency in hematologic malignancies. Strikingly, mutations in TET2 are found in almost half of chronic myelomonocytic leukemias (CMML)[58,59] and are also common in certain T-cell lymphomas. The key emerging concept is that defects in DNA demethylation by TET2 mutations may lead to increases in DNAme at certain CpG island regions (including those bearing H3K27me),[60] which may confer gene silencing of developmental and/or tumor-suppressor type genes; however, clear cause-and-effect links have not yet been made. Consistent with this mechanism, TET2 mutations are often found with mutations in EZH2, which catalyzes H3K27me addition.[51,59]

Of particular interest are recent links between metabolic dysregulation, hematologic malignancies, and gliomas. Remarkably, gain-of-function mutations in the TCA cycle enzymes IDH1 and IDH2 are oncogenic.[61–66] Normally, IDH1/2 convert isocitrate to 2OG (also known as α-ketoglutarate), a cofactor for both TET enzymes and JmjC-class lysine demethylases. Notably, oncogenic IDH1/2 mutations create proteins that additionally convert 2OG to (R)-2-hydroxyglutarate (R-2HG).[66,67] This both depletes the normal cofactor for TETs and JmjC demethylases and further creates a potent "oncometabolite" inhibitor of TET enzymes and prolyl hydroxylases (which regulate hypoxia-inducible transcription factor [HIF] proteins). Additionally, mutations in other Krebs cycle enzymes (e.g., succinate dehydrogenase [SDH]) accumulate succinate, which can likewise inhibit TET, JmjC, and prolyl hydroxylases[68]; notably, SDH mutations and HIF mutations are both common in neuroendocrine tumors.[68] These observations have inspired multiple therapeutic approaches, including: (1) reversing the impact of these oncometabolites on the epigenome (e.g., via DNMT, HDAC or HMT inhibitors); (2) implementing selective inhibitors of these gain-of-function IDH mutant proteins to prevent (R)-2HG production; (3) using selective inhibitors of prolyl-hydroxylases; and (4) the use of ascorbic acid (vitamin C), which can enhance TET protein activity by affecting the reduction-oxidation (redox) state of iron, an essential cofactor for TET enzymes.

REFERENCES

1. Dawson MA, Kouzarides T: Cancer epigenetics: From mechanism to therapy. *Cell* 150(1):12–27, 2012.
2. Baylin SB, Jones PA: A decade of exploring the cancer epigenome-biological and translational implications. *Nat Rev Cancer* 11(10):726–734, 2011.
3. Clapier CR, Cairns BR: The biology of chromatin remodeling complexes. *Annu Rev Biochem* 78:273–304, 2009.
4. Narlikar GJ, Fan HY, Kingston RE: Cooperation between complexes that regulate chromatin structure and transcription. *Cell* 108(4):475–487, 2002.
5. Lessard JA, Crabtree GR: Chromatin regulatory mechanisms in pluripotency. *Annu Rev Cell Dev Biol* 26(1):503–532, 2010.
6. Krasteva V, Buscarlet M, Diaz-Tellez A, et al: The BAF53a subunit of SWI/SNF-like BAF complexes is essential for hemopoietic stem cell function. *Blood* 120(24):4720–4732, 2012.
7. Bultman SJ, Gebuhr TC, Magnuson T: A Brg1 mutation that uncouples ATPase activity from chromatin remodeling reveals an essential role for SWI/SNF-related complexes in beta-globin expression and erythroid development. *Genes Dev* 19(23):2849–2861, 2005.
8. Kadoch C, Hargreaves DC, Hodges C, et al: Proteomic and bioinformatic analysis of mammalian SWI/SNF complexes identifies extensive roles in human malignancy. *Nat Genet* 45(6):592–601, 2013.
9. Nair SS, Li DQ, Kumar R: A core chromatin remodeling factor instructs global chromatin signaling through multivalent reading of nucleosome codes. *Mol Cell* 49(4):704–718, 2013.
10. Fujita N, Jaye DL, Geigerman C, et al: MTA3 and the Mi-2/NuRD complex regulate cell fate during B lymphocyte differentiation. *Cell* 119(1):75–86, 2004.
11. Landry JW, Banerjee S, Taylor B, et al: Chromatin remodeling complex NURF regulates thymocyte maturation. *Genes Dev* 25(3):275–286, 2011.
12. Zhang J, Jackson AF, Naito T, et al: Harnessing of the nucleosome-remodeling-deacetylase complex controls lymphocyte development and prevents leukemogenesis. *Nat Immunol* 13(1):86–94, 2012.
13. Kouzarides T: Chromatin modifications and their function. *Cell* 128(4):693–705, 2007.
14. Vermeulen M, Mulder KW, Denissov S, et al: Selective anchoring of TFIID to nucleosomes by trimethylation of histone H3 lysine 4. *Cell* 131(1):58–69, 2007.
15. Yun M, Wu J, Workman JL, Li B: Readers of histone modifications. *Cell Res* 21(4):564–578, 2011.
16. Strahl BD, Allis CD: The language of covalent histone modifications. *Nature* 403(6765):41–45, 2000.
17. Dhalluin C, Carlson JE, Zeng L, et al: Structure and ligand of a histone acetyltransferase bromodomain. *Nature* 399(6735):491–496, 1999.
18. Zeng L, Zhou MM: Bromodomain: An acetyl-lysine binding domain. *FEBS Lett* 513(1):124–128, 2002.
19. Li Carey BM, Workman JL: The role of chromatin during transcription. *Cell* 128(4):707–719, 2007.
20. Shen X, Liu Y, Hsu YJ, et al: EZH1 mediates methylation on histone H3 lysine 27 and complements EZH2 in maintaining stem cell identity and executing pluripotency. *Mol Cell* 32(4):491–502, 2008.
21. Xu J, Shao Z, Li D, et al: Developmental control of polycomb subunit composition by GATA factors mediates a switch to non-canonical functions. *Mol Cell* 57(2):304–316, 2015.
22. Ostuni R, Piccolo V, Barozzi I, et al: Latent enhancers activated by stimulation in differentiated cells. *Cell* 152(1–2):157–171, 2013.
23. Goll MG, Bestor TH: Eukaryotic cytosine methyltransferases. *Annu Rev Biochem* 74:481–514, 2005.
24. Bostick M, Kim JK, Estève PO, et al: UHRF1 plays a role in maintaining DNA methylation in mammalian cells. *Science* 317(5845):1760–1764, 2007.
25. Klempnauer KH: Methylation-sensitive DNA binding by v-myb and c-myb proteins. *Oncogene* 8(1):111–115, 1993.
26. Campanero MR, Armstrong MI, Flemington EK: CpG methylation as a mechanism for the regulation of E2F activity. *Proc Natl Acad Sci U S A* 97(12):6481–6486, 2000.
27. Kirillov A, Kistler B, Mostoslavsky R, et al: A role for nuclear NF-kappaB in B-cell-specific demethylation of the Igkappa locus. *Nat Genet* 13(4):435–441, 1996.
28. Weih F, Nitsch D, Reik A, et al: Analysis of CpG methylation and genomic footprinting at the tyrosine aminotransferase gene: DNA methylation alone is not sufficient to prevent protein binding *in vivo*. *EMBO J* 10(9):2559–2567, 1991.
29. Comb M, Goodman HM: CpG methylation inhibits proenkephalin gene expression and binding of the transcription factor AP-2. *Nucleic Acids Res* 18(13):3975–3982, 1990.
30. Hendrich B, Bird A: Identification and characterization of a family of mammalian methyl-CpG binding proteins. *Mol Cell Biol* 18(11):6538–6547, 1998.
31. Bogdanovic O, Veenstra GJ: DNA methylation and methyl-CpG binding proteins: Developmental requirements and function. *Chromosoma* 118(5):549–565, 2009.
32. Baylin S, Bestor TH: Altered methylation patterns in cancer cell genomes: Cause or consequence? *Cancer Cell* 1(4):299–305, 2002.
33. Tahiliani M, Koh KP, Shen Y, et al: Conversion of 5-methylcytosine to 5-hydroxymethylcytosine in mammalian DNA by MLL partner TET1. *Science* 324(5929):930–935, 2009.
34. Ito S, Shen L, Dai Q, et al: Tet proteins can convert 5-methylcytosine to 5-formylcytosine and 5-carboxylcytosine. *Science* 333(6047):1300–1303, 2011.
35. He YF, Li BZ, Li Z, et al: Tet-mediated formation of 5-carboxylcytosine and its excision by TDG in mammalian DNA. *Science* 333(6047):1303–1307, 2011.
36. Meyer C, Kowarz E, Hofmann J, et al: New insights to the MLL recombinome of acute leukemias. *Leukemia* 23(8):1490–1499, 2009.
37. Corral J, Lavenir I, Impey H, et al: An Mll-AF9 fusion gene made by homologous recombination causes acute leukemia in chimeric mice: A method to create fusion oncogenes. *Cell* 85(6):853–861, 1996.
38. Yokoyama A, Lin M, Naresh A, et al: A higher-order complex containing AF4 and ENL family proteins with P-TEFb facilitates oncogenic and physiologic MLL-dependent transcription. *Cancer Cell* 17(2):198–212, 2010.
39. Lin C, Smith ER, Takahashi H, et al: AFF4, a component of the ELL/P-TEFb elongation complex and a shared subunit of MLL chimeras, can link transcription elongation to leukemia. *Mol Cell* 37(3):429–437, 2010.
40. Bernt KM, Zhu N, Sinha AU, et al: MLL-rearranged leukemia is dependent on aberrant H3K79 methylation by DOT1L. *Cancer Cell* 20(1):66–78, 2011.
41. Okada Y, Feng Q, Lin Y, et al: HDOT1L links histone methylation to leukemogenesis. *Cell* 121(2):167–178, 2005.
42. Nguyen AT, Taranova O, He J, Zhang Y: DOT1L, the H3K79 methyltransferase, is required for MLL-AF9-mediated leukemogenesis. *Blood* 117(25):6912–6922, 2011.
43. Grignani F, De Matteis S, Nervi C, et al: Fusion proteins of the retinoic acid receptor-alpha recruit histone deacetylase in promyelocytic leukaemia. *Nature* 391(6669):815–818, 1998.
44. Lin RJ, Nagy L, Inoue S, et al: Role of the histone deacetylase complex in acute promyelocytic leukaemia. *Nature* 391(6669):811–814, 1998.
45. Daigle SR, Olhava EJ, Therkelsen CA, et al: Selective killing of mixed lineage leukemia cells by a potent small-molecule DOT1L inhibitor. *Cancer Cell* 20(1):53–65, 2011.
46. Zuber J, Shi J, Wang E, et al: RNAi screen identifies Brd4 as a therapeutic target in acute myeloid leukaemia. *Nature* 478(7370):524–528, 2011.
47. Fiskus W, Sharma S, Qi J, et al: Highly active combination of BRD4 antagonist and histone deacetylase inhibitor against human acute myelogenous leukemia cells. *Mol Cancer Ther* 13(5):1142–1154, 2014.
48. Dawson MA, Prinjha RK, Dittmann A, et al: Inhibition of BET recruitment to chromatin as an effective treatment for MLL-fusion leukaemia. *Nature* 478(7370):529–533, 2011.
49. Delmore JE, Issa GC, Lemieux ME, et al: BET bromodomain inhibition as a therapeutic strategy to target c-Myc. *Cell* 146(6):904–917, 2011.
50. Morin RD, Mendez-Lago M, Mungall AJ, et al: Frequent mutation of histone-modifying genes in non-Hodgkin lymphoma. *Nature* 476(7360):298–303, 2011.
51. Muto T, Sashida G, Oshima M, et al: Concurrent loss of Ezh2 and Tet2 cooperates in the pathogenesis of myelodysplastic disorders. *J Exp Med* 210(12):2627–2639, 2013.
52. Nikoloski G, Langemeijer SM, Kuiper RP, et al: Somatic mutations of the histone methyltransferase gene EZH2 in myelodysplastic syndromes. *Nat Genet* 42(8):665–667, 2010.
53. Ernst T, Chase AJ, Score J, et al: Inactivating mutations of the histone methyltransferase gene EZH2 in myeloid disorders. *Nat Genet* 42(8):722–726, 2010.
54. van Haaften G, Dalgliesh GL, Davies H, et al: Somatic mutations of the histone H3K27 demethylase gene UTX in human cancer. *Nat Genet* 41(5):521–523, 2009.
55. Bejar R, Stevenson K, Abdel-Wahab O, et al: Clinical effect of point mutations in myelodysplastic syndromes. *N Engl J Med* 364(26):2496–2506, 2011.
56. McCabe MT, Ott HM, Ganji G, et al: EZH2 inhibition as a therapeutic strategy for lymphoma with EZH2-activating mutations. *Nature* 492(7427):108–112, 2012.
57. Itzykson R, Kosmider O, Renneville A, et al: Prognostic score including gene mutations in chronic myelomonocytic leukemia. *J Clin Oncol* 31(19):2428–2436, 2013.
58. Tefferi A, Lim KH, Abdel-Wahab O, et al: Detection of mutant TET2 in myeloid malignancies other than myeloproliferative neoplasms: CMML, MDS, MDS/MPN and AML. *Leukemia* 23(7):1343–1345, 2009.
59. Grossmann V, Kohlmann A, Eder C, et al: Molecular profiling of chronic myelomonocytic leukemia reveals diverse mutations in >80% of patients with TET2 and EZH2 being of high prognostic relevance. *Leukemia* 25(5):877–879, 2011.
60. Wu H, D'Alessio AC, Ito S, et al: Genome-wide analysis of 5-hydroxymethylcytosine distribution reveals its dual function in transcriptional regulation in mouse embryonic stem cells. *Genes Dev* 25(7):679–684, 2011.
61. Figueroa ME, Abdel-Wahab O, Lu C, et al: Leukemic IDH1 and IDH2 mutations result in a hypermethylation phenotype, disrupt TET2 function, and impair hematopoietic differentiation. *Cancer Cell* 18(6):553–567, 2010.
62. Kats LM, Reschke M, Taulli R, et al: Proto-oncogenic role of mutant IDH2 in leukemia initiation and maintenance. *Cell Stem Cell* 14(3):329–341, 2014.
63. Losman JA, Looper RE, Koivunen P, et al: (R)-2-hydroxyglutarate is sufficient to promote leukemogenesis and its effects are reversible. *Science* 339(6127):1621–1625, 2013.
64. Lu C, Ward PS, Kapoor GS, et al: IDH mutation impairs histone demethylation and results in a block to cell differentiation. *Nature* 483(7390):474–478, 2012.
65. Sasaki M, Knobbe CB, Munger JC, et al: IDH1(R132H) mutation increases murine haematopoietic progenitors and alters epigenetics. *Nature* 488(7413):656–659, 2012.
66. Dang Jin LS, Su SM: IDH mutations in glioma and acute myeloid leukemia. *Trends Mol Med* 16(9):387–397, 2010.
67. Ye D, Ma S, Xiong Y, Guan KL: R-2-hydroxyglutarate as the key effector of IDH mutations promoting oncogenesis. *Cancer Cell* 23(3):274–276, 2013.
68. Xiao M, Yang H, Xu W, et al: Inhibition of α-KG-dependent histone and DNA demethylases by fumarate and succinate that are accumulated in mutations of FH and SDH tumor suppressors. *Genes Dev* 26(12):1326–1338, 2012.

CHAPTER 13
CYTOGENETICS AND GENETIC ABNORMALITIES

Lucy A. Godley, Madina Sukhanova, Gordana Raca,
and Michelle M. Le Beau

SUMMARY

Cytogenetic and genetic analysis provides pathologists and clinicians with a powerful tool for the diagnosis and classification of hematologic malignant diseases. The detection of an acquired, somatic mutation establishes the diagnosis of a neoplastic disorder and rules out hyperplasia, dysplasia, or morphologic changes from toxic injury or vitamin deficiency. Specific cytogenetic and genetic abnormalities have been identified that are very closely, and sometimes uniquely, associated with morphologically distinct subsets of leukemia or lymphoma, enabling clinicians to predict their clinical course and likelihood of responding to particular treatments. The detection of one of these recurring abnormalities is helpful in establishing the diagnosis and adds information of prognostic importance. In many cases, the prognostic information derived from cytogenetic and genetic analysis is independent of that provided by other clinical features. Patients with favorable genetic prognostic features benefit from standard therapies with a well-known spectra of toxicities, whereas those with less-favorable clinical and cytogenetic or genetic characteristics may be better treated with more intensive or investigational therapies. Pretreatment cytogenetic analysis also can be useful in choosing between post-remission therapies that differ widely in cost, acute and chronic morbidity, and effectiveness. The appearance of new abnormalities in the karyotype of a patient under observation often signals clonal evolution and more aggressive behavior. The disappearance of a chromosomal abnormality present at diagnosis is an important indicator of complete remission following treatment, and its reappearance may herald disease recurrence.

Acronyms and Abbreviations ALCL, anaplastic large cell lymphoma; ALL, acute lymphocytic or lymphoblastic leukemia; AML, acute myeloid leukemia; AMML, acute myelomonocytic leukemia; APL, acute promyelocytic leukemia; CDS, commonly deleted segment; CLL, chronic lymphocytic leukemia; CMA, chromosome microarray analysis; CML, chronic myeloid leukemia; del, deletion; DLBCL, diffuse large B-cell lymphoma; EBV, Epstein-Barr virus; FAB, French-American-British; FISH, fluorescence *in situ* hybridization; FLT3, FMS-like tyrosine kinase; HSC, hematopoietic stem cell; IGH, immunoglobulin heavy chain; inv, inversion; ITD, internal tandem duplication; JAK, Janus kinase; LOH, loss of heterozygosity; MALT, mucosa-associated lymphoid tissue; MAPK, mitogen-activated protein kinase; MDS, myelodysplastic syndrome; Ph, Philadelphia chromosome; PI3K, phosphatidylinositide 3'-kinase; qRT-PCR, quantitative reverse transcriptase polymerase chain reaction; RA, refractory anemia; RAEB, refractory anemia with excess blasts; RARa, retinoic acid receptor-a; RARS, refractory anemia with ring sideroblasts; RARS-t, refractory anemia with ringed sideroblasts and thrombocytosis; RCMD, refractory cytopenia with multilineage dysplasia; SNP, single nucleotide polymorphism; STAT, signal transducer and activator of transcription; t, translocation; t-, therapy-related; TKI, tyrosine kinase inhibitor; WHO, World Health Organization.

GENETIC CONSEQUENCES OF GENOMIC REARRANGEMENTS

Over the past two decades, the genes that are located at the breakpoints of a number of the recurring chromosomal translocations have been identified. Alterations in the expression of the genes or in the properties of the encoded proteins resulting from the rearrangement play an integral role in the process of malignant transformation.[1,2] The altered genes fall into several functional classes, including tyrosine or serine protein kinases, cell surface receptors, growth factors and, the largest class, transcription factors. These latter proteins are involved in the induction or repression of gene transcription, often functioning in a tissue-specific fashion to regulate cell growth and differentiation.

There are two general mechanisms by which chromosomal translocations result in altered gene function. The first is deregulation of gene expression (Chap. 10). This mechanism is characteristic of the translocations in lymphoid neoplasms that involve the immunoglobulin genes in B-lineage tumors and the T-cell receptor genes in T-lineage tumors. These rearrangements result in the inappropriate or constitutive expression of an oncogene. The second mechanism is the encoding and expression of a novel fusion protein, resulting from the juxtaposition of coding sequences from two genes that are normally located on different chromosomes. Such chimeric proteins are "tumor specific" in that the fusion gene typically does not exist in nonmalignant cells. Thus, the detection of such a fusion gene or protein product can be important in diagnosis and in the detection of residual disease or early relapse. Moreover, they may also be appropriate targets for tumor-specific therapies. An example is the chimeric BCR-ABL1 protein resulting from the t(9;22) in chronic myeloid leukemia (CML) (see "Methods of Cell Preparation" below). All of the translocations cloned to date in the myeloid leukemias result in a fusion protein.

Chromosomal translocations result in the activation of genes in a dominant fashion. A number of human tumors result from homozygous, recessive mutations. These mutations lead to the absence of a functional protein product, suggesting that these genes function as "suppressor" genes, whose normal role(s) is to limit cellular proliferation. The hallmark of tumor suppressor genes is the loss of genetic material in malignant cells, resulting from chromosomal loss or deletion, as well as by other genetic mechanisms (Chap. 10).[1] A subset of tumor suppressor genes act by haploinsufficiency, whereby loss of one allele results in a reduction in the level of the protein product by half, thereby perturbing normal cellular processes. This mechanism is common in the recurring deletions in myeloid neoplasms (Chap. 83).

Extensive experimental evidence indicates that more than one mutation is required for the pathogenesis of hematologic malignancies. That is, expression of translocation-specific fusion genes or deregulated expression of oncogenes is required, but insufficient to induce leukemia. Thus, an important aspect of leukemia biology is the elucidation of the spectrum of chromosomal and molecular mutations that cooperate in the pathways leading to leukemogenesis. Where known, we describe the cooperating mutations associated with specific cytogenetic subsets of leukemia or lymphoma.

METHODS OF CELL PREPARATION

Cytogenetic analysis of malignant diseases should be based upon the study of the tumor cells themselves. In leukemia, the specimen is usually obtained by marrow aspiration and is typically cultured for 24 to 72 hours. When a marrow aspirate cannot be obtained, a marrow biopsy (bone core specimen) or a blood sample for patients who have circulating immature myeloid or lymphoid cells, can often be processed successfully. An involved lymph node or tumor mass specimen may be examined for the analysis of lymphoma cells.

For specimen collection, 1 to 5 mL of marrow are aspirated aseptically into a syringe coated with preservative-free sodium heparin and transferred to a sterile 15-mL centrifuge tube containing 5 mL of culture medium (RPMI 1640, 100 units sodium heparin). The use of Vacutainer tubes containing heparin as an anticoagulant should be avoided, as the heparin contains preservatives that suppress cell growth. If a marrow aspirate cannot be obtained, a marrow biopsy may be taken and placed into the collection tube. Approximately 75 percent of marrow biopsies can be minced to generate suspension of cells that will yield adequate numbers of metaphase cells for complete analysis. For blood specimens, 10 mL are drawn aseptically by venipuncture into a syringe coated with preservative-free heparin. To avoid loss of cell viability, it is critical that the specimen be transported at room temperature to the cytogenetics laboratory without delay. Overnight shipment of specimens frequently results in loss of cell viability, and most laboratories experience a high proportion (25–50 percent) of inadequate analyses using such specimens. For optimally handled specimens, approximately 95 percent of all cases should be adequate for cytogenetic analysis. Those cases that are inadequate generally represent samples from patients with hypocellular marrows.

CHROMOSOME NOMENCLATURE

Chromosomal abnormalities are described according to the International System for Human Cytogenetic Nomenclature (Table 13–1).[3] To describe the chromosomal complement, the total chromosome number is listed first, followed by the sex chromosomes, and numerical and structural abnormalities in ascending order. The observation of at least two cells with the same structural rearrangement, for example, translocations, deletions or inversions, or gain of the same chromosome, or three cells each showing loss of the same chromosome, is considered evidence for the presence of an abnormal clone. However, one cell with a normal karyotype is considered evidence for the presence of a normal cell line. Patients whose cells show no alteration or nonclonal (single cell) abnormalities are considered to be normal. An exception to this is a single cell characterized by a recurring structural abnormality. In such instances, it is likely that this represents the karyotype of the mutated subclone in that particular patient.

METHODS THAT COMPLEMENT KARYOTYPE ANALYSIS

FLUORESCENCE *IN SITU* HYBRIDIZATION

Cytogenetic analysis of human tumors is often technically difficult because of the presence of multiple abnormalities and requires highly skilled personnel. These factors have led investigators to seek alternative methods for identifying chromosomal abnormalities, such as fluorescence *in situ* hybridization (FISH).[4] The FISH technique is based on the same principle as Southern blot analysis, namely, the ability of single-stranded DNA to anneal to complementary DNA.[4] FISH can be performed on marrow or blood films, or fixed and sectioned tissue, as it does not require dividing cells. The target DNA is the nuclear DNA of interphase cells, or the DNA of metaphase chromosomes that are affixed to a glass microscope slide. Commercial probes are now available for the most common abnormalities, and are directly labeled with fluorochrome, which simplifies the technique by eliminating the probe preparation and detection steps. With the development of dual- and triple-pass filters, most laboratories now have the capacity to hybridize and detect two to three probes simultaneously. Table 13–1 summarizes

the most frequently used commercially available FISH probes. Several types of probes can be used to detect chromosomal abnormalities by FISH. Hybridization of centromere-specific probes has been used to detect monosomy, trisomy, and other aneuploidies in both leukemias and solid tumors, as well as the sex chromosome complement in the transplant setting (Fig. 13–1).

Translocations and deletions can also be identified in interphase or metaphase cells by using genomic probes that are derived from the breakpoints of recurring translocations or within the deleted segment (see Fig. 13–1). In some cases, FISH analysis provides more sensitivity, in that cytogenetic abnormalities have been identified by FISH in samples that appeared to be normal by conventional cytogenetic analyses. Advantages of FISH include (1) the rapid nature of the method and the ability to analyze large numbers of cells; (2) its high sensitivity and specificity; and (3) the ability to obtain cytogenetic data from samples with a low mitotic index or from terminally differentiated cells. A further increase in sensitivity in cases with a low percentage of malignant cells can be achieved by performing FISH analysis on samples that have been enriched previously for specific subpopulations of cells. For example, the use of FISH in combination with plasma cell enrichment techniques is routinely applied in the clinical setting to maximize the detection rate of specific chromosome rearrangements in myeloma.[5,6] The major disadvantage of FISH testing is the inability to interrogate more than a few abnormalities. FISH is most powerful when the analysis is targeted toward those abnormalities that are known to be associated with a particular tumor or disease. In a clinical setting, cytogenetic analysis could be performed at the time of diagnosis to identify the chromosomal abnormalities in an individual patient's malignant cells. Thereafter, FISH with the appropriate probes could be used to detect residual disease or early relapse, and to assess the efficacy of therapeutic regimens. For example, the use of FISH to detect the t(9;22) in CML patients following therapy with an oral tyrosine kinase inhibitor, or sex chromosome determination after a sex-mismatched transplant, is widespread. Material from patients newly presenting are often analyzed most efficiently by conventional cytogenetic analysis, combined with quantitative reverse transcriptase polymerase chain reaction (qRT-PCR) analysis if a specific chromosome rearrangement is suspected, for example, a BCR-ABL1 fusion. Molecular qRT-PCR monitoring of the blood and marrow of CML patients is now part of the recommended testing for patient followup.[7]

MICROARRAY ANALYSIS

Several microarray-based technologies play an important role in the diagnosis and experimental analysis of hematologic malignancies, including high-density copy number/single nucleotide polymorphism (SNP) array testing (also known as chromosomal microarray analysis [CMA]), microarray-based gene expression profiling, and high-throughput SNP genotyping. CMA allows genome-wide detection of copy number abnormalities (deletions and duplications) at a much higher resolution than karyotyping; it also enables detection of loss of heterozygosity (LOH) that occurs without concurrent changes in the gene copy number, that is, uniparental disomy (UPD) (Chap. 10), and can be attributed to somatic mitotic recombination (also referred to as copy-neutral LOH) (Fig. 13–2). CMA is clinically available as an adjunct test to karyotyping and FISH, and it facilitates detection of genomic abnormalities in a substantial proportion of patients with myelodysplastic syndromes (MDSs) and leukemia with a normal karyotype; it can also be used as a cost-effective alternative to large panels of FISH probes, and as a very useful tool to characterize chromosomal abnormalities of uncertain significance. Microarray-based gene expression profiling has been applied to study a variety of hematopoietic

TABLE 13-1. Glossary of Cytogenetic Terminology

Aneuploidy—An abnormal chromosome number because of either gain or loss of chromosomes.

Banded chromosomes—Chromosomes with alternating dark and light segments as a result of special stains or pretreatment with enzymes before staining. Each chromosome pair has a unique pattern of bands.

Breakpoint—A specific site on a chromosome containing a DNA break that is involved in a structural rearrangement, such as a translocation or deletion.

Centromere—The chromosome constriction that is the site of the spindle fiber attachment. The position of the centromere determines whether chromosomes are *metacentric* (X-shaped, e.g., chromosomes 1–3, 6–12, X, 16, 19, 20) or *acrocentric* (inverted V-shaped, e.g., chromosomes 13–15, 21, 22, Y). During mitosis, the two exact copies of the DNA in each chromosome are separated by shortening of the spindle fibers attached to opposite sides of the dividing cell.

Clone—In the cytogenetic sense, this is defined as two cells with the same additional or structurally rearranged chromosome, or three cells with loss of the same chromosome.

Deletion—A segment of a chromosome is missing as the result of two breaks and loss of the intervening piece (interstitial deletion). Molecular studies of many recurring deletions have shown that, in each case, the deletions were interstitial, rather than terminal (single break with loss of the terminal segment).

Diploid—Normal chromosome number and composition of chromosomes.

Fluorescence *in situ* hybridization (FISH)—A molecular-cytogenetic technique based on the visualization of fluorescently-labeled DNA probes hybridized to complementary DNA sequences from metaphase or interphase cells, used to detect numerical and structural abnormalities. A short nomenclature description is used to describe the results of in situ hybridization. For interphase FISH, the abbreviation "nuc ish" is followed immediately by the locus designation in parentheses (or multiple loci separated by a comma), a multiplication symbol, and the number of signals observed. The number of cells scored is placed in brackets. For example, normal results for the *BCR-ABL1* probe are described as "nuc ish (ABL1, BCR)×2[400]." A case with the t(9;22) resulting in the *BCR-ABL1* fusion analyzed using a dual-color, dual-fusion probe would be described as "nuc ish (ABL1×3), (BCR×3), (ABL1 con BCR×2)[400]."

Haploid—Only one-half the normal complement, i.e., 23 chromosomes.

Hyperdiploid—Additional chromosomes; therefore, the modal number is 47 or greater.

Hypodiploid—Loss of chromosomes with a modal number of 45 or less.

Inversion—Two breaks occur in the same chromosome with rotation of the intervening segment. If both breaks were on the same side of the centromere, it is called a paracentric inversion. If they were on opposite sides, it is called a pericentric inversion.

Isochromosome—A chromosome that consists of identical copies of one chromosome arm with loss of the other arm. Thus, an isochromosome for the long arm of No. 17 [i(17)(q10)] contains two copies of the long arm (separated by the centromere) with loss of the short arm of the chromosome.

Karyotype—Arrangement of chromosomes from a particular cell according to an internationally established system such that the largest chromosomes are first and the smallest ones are last. A normal female karyotype is described as 46, XX and a normal male karyotype is 46, XY. An *idiogram* is an idealized representation (diagram) of the chromosomes.

Pseudodiploid—A diploid number of chromosomes accompanied by structural abnormalities.

Recurring Abnormality—A numerical or structural abnormality noted in multiple patients who have a similar neoplasm. Such abnormalities are characteristic or diagnostic of distinct subtypes of leukemia and lymphoma that have unique morphologic and/or immunophenotypic features. Recurring abnormalities represent genetic mutations that are involved in the pathogenesis of the corresponding diseases; many recurring abnormalities have prognostic significance.

Translocation—A break in at least two chromosomes with exchange of material. In a reciprocal translocation, there is no obvious loss of chromosomal material. Translocations are indicated by t; the chromosomes involved are noted in the first set of brackets and the breakpoints in the second set of brackets. The Ph translocation is t(9;22)(q34.1;q11.2).

Nomenclature symbols:

p—Short arm

q—Long arm

+—If before the chromosome, indicates a gain of a whole chromosome (e.g., +8)

−—If before the chromosome, indicates a loss of a whole chromosome (e.g., −7) and if after the chromosome indicates loss of part of the chromosome (e.g., 5q−, loss of part of the long arm of chromosome 5)

?—Indicates uncertainty about the identity of the chromosome or band listed just after the ?

t—translocation

del—deletion

inv—inversion

i—isochromosome

mar—marker chromosome

r—ring chromosome

Data from Rowley JD: Chromosome abnormalities in human cancer. In De Vita VT, Hellman S, Rosenberg S (eds): *Practice and Principles of Oncology* 3rd ed. Philadelphia, PA: Lippincott Williams & Wilkins; 1991.

malignancies, often revealing complex but unique expression signatures for each disease subtype. For example, gene expression profiling has shown that diffuse large B-cell lymphoma (DLBCL) comprises at least three different subtypes—germinal center B-cell (GCB)-like, activated B-cell (ABC)-like, and primary mediastinal B-cell lymphoma (PMBL)—each with a distinct oncogenic mechanism, prognosis, and response to therapies (Chap. 98).[8] Expression profiling studies led to the recognition of a novel genetic subtype of high-risk B-cell acute lymphocytic or lymphoblastic leukemia (ALL), which has a similar expression signature as Ph-chromosome-positive ALL (Chap. 91).[9,10] High-throughput array-based SNP genotyping, enabling the analysis of large numbers of cases and controls, has facilitated genome-wide association studies for the identification of disease susceptibility loci.[11] Future diagnostic evaluation, identification of high-risk cases and management decisions will be

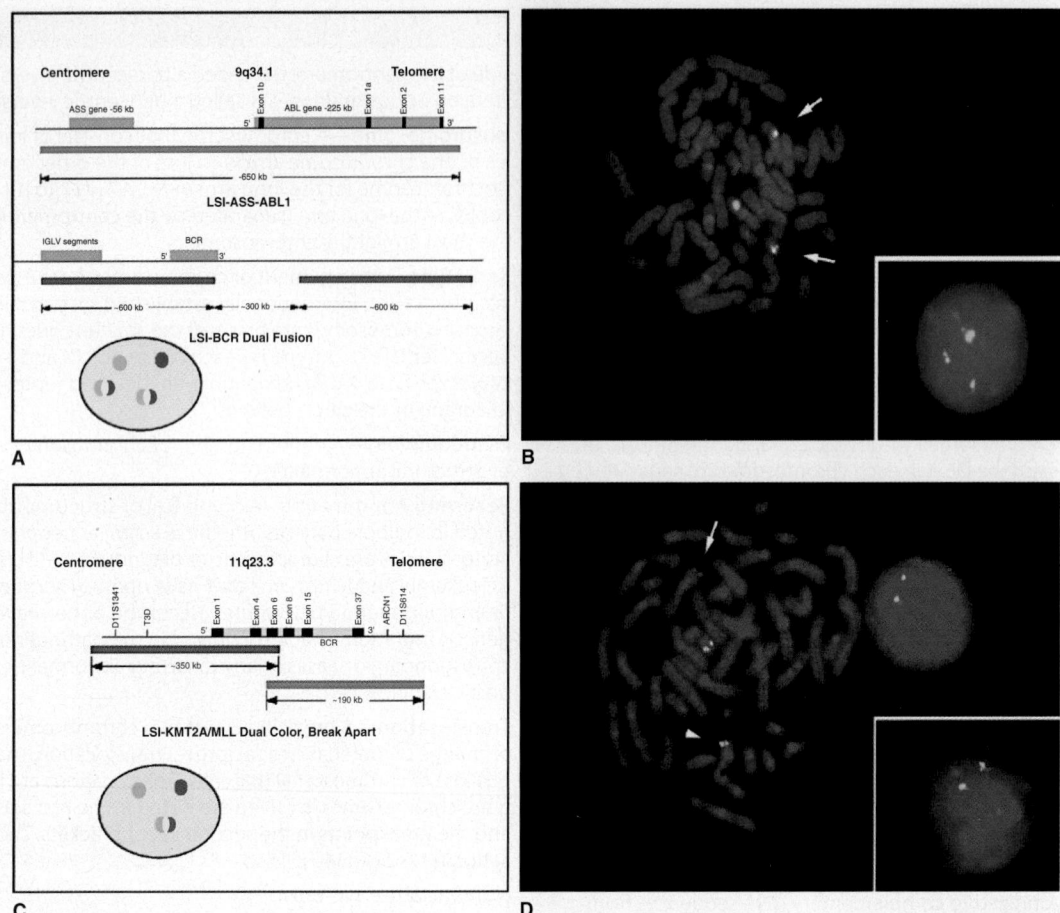

Figure 13–1. Fluorescence *in situ* hybridization (FISH) analysis. Panels **B** and **D** illustrate images of metaphase and interphase cells following FISH; the cells are counterstained with 4,6-diamidino-2-phenylindole-dihydrochloride (DAPI). **A.** Schematic of the *BCR* and *ABL1* loci, location of the *BCR* and *ABL1* dual fusion probe (Vysis, Inc), and configuration of signals in interphase cells. **B.** Hybridization of the *BCR-ABL1* dual fusion probe to metaphase and interphase cells with the t(9;22). In cells with the t(9;22), only one green and one red signal is observed on the normal 9 and 22 homologs, and two yellow fusion signals *(arrows)* are observed on the der(9) and the der(22) (Ph) chromosomes as a result of the juxtaposition of the *ABL1* and *BCR* sequences. **C.** Schematic of the *KMT2A/MLL* gene, location of the *KMT2A* break-apart probe (Vysis, Inc.), and configuration of signals in interphase cells. **D.** Hybridization of the *KMT2A* break-apart probe to metaphase and interphase cells with a t(11q23.3). In cells with a *KMT2A* translocation, a yellow fusion signal is observed for the germline configuration on the normal chromosome 11 homolog, a green signal is observed in the der(11) chromosome, and a red signal is observed on the partner chromosome.

increasingly based on genomic and even proteomic profiling of patients' germline and tumor samples, which will likely utilize a combination of array-based and next-generation sequencing–based technologies.

●SPECIFIC CLONAL DISORDERS

CHRONIC MYELOID LEUKEMIA

The first consistent chromosomal abnormality in any malignant disease was identified in CML (Chap. 89). The Philadelphia (Ph) chromosome results from a translocation involving chromosomes 9 and 22, t(9;22) (q34.1;q11.2), (Fig. 13–3), and arises in a pluripotential stem cell that gives rise to both lymphoid and myeloid lineage cells. The standard t(9;22) is identified in approximately 92 percent of CML patients, whereas 6 to 8 percent have variant translocations that involve a third chromosome in addition to chromosomes 9 and 22 (see Chap. 89, Fig. 89–8). The genetic consequences of the t(9;22) or the complex translocations are to move a segment of the Abelson (*ABL1*) oncogene on chromosome 9 next to a segment of the *BCR* gene on 22. Analyses of leukemia cells from rare patients with typical CML lacking the t(9;22)

has revealed a rearrangement involving *ABL1* and *BCR* that is detectable only at the molecular level (1 to 2 percent of cases).[12]

The t(9;22) and resultant *BCR-ABL1* fusion is the *sine qua non* of CML.[12] The BCR-ABL1 fusion protein is located on the cytoplasmic surface of the cell membrane and acquires a novel function in transmitting growth-regulatory signals to the nucleus via the RAS/MAPK, phosphatidylinositide 3′-kinase (PI3K)/AKT, and Janus kinase (JAK)/signal transducer and activator of transcription (STAT) signal transduction pathways. The tyrosine kinase activity of the BCR-ABL1 fusion protein can be specifically inhibited by several commercially available oral tyrosine kinase inhibitors (TKIs): imatinib mesylate (Gleevec/STI571, Novartis Pharmaceuticals, East Hanover, NJ), dasatinib (Sprycel, BMS-354825, Bristol-Myers Squibb, Princeton, NJ), and nilotinib (Tasigna, AMN107, Novartis Pharmaceuticals, East Hanover, NJ) (Chap. 89). Additional oral agents are also being tested in clinical trials.[13,14] The *BCR-ABL1* translocation can be detected by cytogenetic and FISH analysis, qRT-PCR, and Southern blot analysis to diagnose the disease and detect residual disease. Studies of patients treated with TKIs show a strong correlation between *BCR-ABL1* levels as measured in the blood by qRT-PCR and the percentage of Ph+ cells in the marrow.

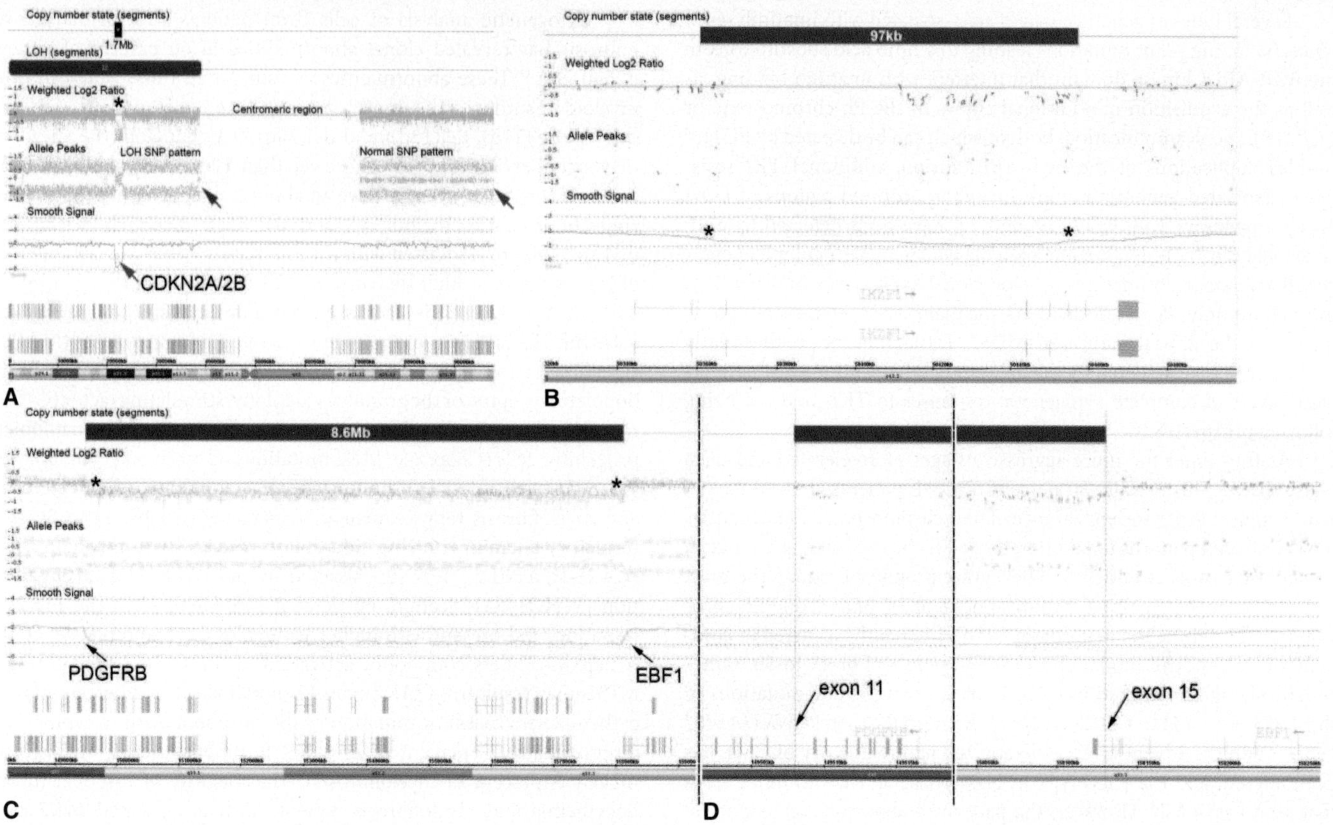

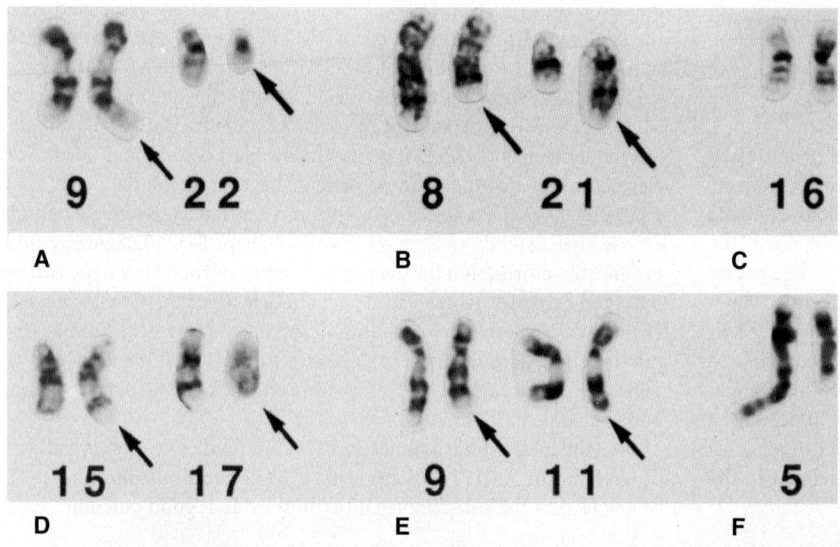

Figure 13–2. Representative results for three B-cell ALL samples illustrating detection of submicroscopic deletions and LOH by CMA. **A.** A 1.7-Mb deletion affecting the *CDKN2A* and *CDKN2B* tumor suppressor genes at 9p (shown by the *dark bar* on the top and the *red arrow*). The deletion is accompanied by an extended region of a copy-number neutral LOH affecting the entire short arm of chromosome 9 (indicated by the *purple bar*) and resulting in biallelic loss of *CDKN2A* and *CDKN2B*. The normal SNP pattern is indicated with a *blue arrow*, whereas the abnormal pattern associated with LOH is identified by the *purple arrow*. **B.** *IKZF1* deletion detected by SNP array is associated with an adverse treatment outcome of pediatric B-cell ALL patients. **C.** Array plot showing 5q32-q33.3 deletion that fuses the *PDGFRB* and *EBF1* genes in a case of Ph+-like ALL **(D)**.

Figure 13–3. Partial karyotypes from trypsin-Giemsa-banded metaphase cells depicting recurring chromosomal rearrangements observed in myeloid leukemias. The rearranged chromosomes are identified with *arrows*. **A.** t(9;22)(q34.1;q11.2), CML. **B.** t(8;21)(q22;q22.3), AML-M2. **C.** inv(16)(pl3.1q22), AMMoL-M4Eo. **D.** t(15;17)(q24.1;q21.1), APL. **E.** t(9;11)(p21.3;q23.3), AMoL-M5. **F.** del(5)(q13q33), t-AML.

Several types of genetic changes are associated with imatinib resistance, including point mutations leading to amino acid substitutions in the BCR-ABL1 kinase domain that interfere with imatinib binding, as well as the acquisition of additional copies of the Ph chromosome or *BCR-ABL1* gene amplification, both of which can be detected by FISH.[14] Besides duplications of the *BCR-ABL1* fusion, additional TKI resistance-associated genomic lesions, including acquired regions of LOH on chromosomes 1, 8, 9, 17, 19, and 22, have been detected by SNP array analysis.[15] Although some patients who achieve a complete cytogenetic response on imatinib develop clonal karyotypic abnormalities, most commonly +8, −7, or del(20q), the majority of them do not go on to develop the clinical features of MDS.[16] The significance of these early findings will be elucidated by the analysis of a large number of patients who have had complete cytogenetic responses to TKIs and are being followed prospectively.

As they enter the more aggressive stages of accelerated and blast phase disease, historically 80 percent of CML patients showed karyotypic evolution with the appearance of new chromosomal abnormalities in very distinct patterns in addition to the Ph chromosome. A change in the karyotype was considered to be a grave prognostic sign.[17] The most common changes, a gain of chromosomes 8 or 19, or a second Ph chromosome (by gain of the first), or an i(17q), frequently occurred in combination to produce modal chromosome numbers of 47 to 50. Other genetic changes identified in CML in blast crisis include mutations in the *TP53, RB1, MYC, CDKN2A (p16), KRAS/NRAS,* or *RUNX1/AML1* genes. With the advent of TKI therapy, the natural history of CML has been altered, and the karyotype in blast phase appears to differ from that seen previously. However, the pattern of abnormalities is not yet well described.

Rarely, marrow biopsies from patients will appear similar to those patients with CML, but will lack a Ph chromosome or the *BCR-ABL1* fusion. Most often these patients have a MDS or myeloproliferative neoplasm (MPN), most commonly chronic myelomonocytic leukemia, refractory anemia with excess blasts (RAEB), or the poorly understood disorder of "atypical CML." Some of the latter have *JAK2*[V617F] mutations and a phenotype consistent with *chronic neutrophilic leukemia* (Chaps. 84 and 89). Cytogenetic analysis of marrow biopsies from these patients commonly have a normal karyotype, +8, +13, del(20q), or i(17q). These patients have a substantially shorter survival than do those whose cells have the t(9;22). Because each of the oral TKIs blocks kinase activities in addition to BCR-ABL1, they have proven to be effective in other disorders, including chronic MPNs with platelet-derived growth factor receptor (PDGFR)-β rearrangements, a myeloproliferative variant of hypereosinophilic syndrome that expresses the FIP1L1-PDGFRA fusion protein, and in patients with mast cell malignancies that express an activating point mutation in *KIT* (Chap. 89).[18]

OTHER MYELOPROLIFERATIVE NEOPLASMS

A cytogenetically abnormal clone is present in 15 percent of untreated polycythemia vera patients compared with 40 percent of treated patients (Table 13–2).[19] When the disease transforms to acute myeloid leukemia (AML), almost 100 percent have a cytogenetically abnormal clone. The presence of a chromosome abnormality at diagnosis does not necessarily predict a short survival or the development of leukemia. However, a change in the karyotype may be an ominous sign. Marrow cells frequently contain additional chromosomes (+8 or +9). Trisomy 8 and 9 may occur together which is otherwise rare.[19] Structural rearrangements most often involve a del(13q) or del(20q), noted in 30 percent of patients. Loss of chromosome 7 (20 percent) and del(5q) (40 percent) are often observed in the leukemic phase, and may be related to the prior treatment received by these patients (Chap. 84).

Cytogenetic analysis of cells from patients with primary myelofibrosis has revealed clonal abnormalities in 60 percent of patients (Chap. 86).[19] These abnormalities are similar to those noted in other myeloid disorders. The most common anomalies are +8, −7, or a del(7q), del(11q), del(13q), and del(20q).[19] A change in the karyotype may signal evolution to AML. Fewer than 10 percent of patients with essential thrombocythemia have an abnormal clone (Chap. 85). Recurring abnormalities include +8 and del(13q). Although del(5q) and inv(3)/t(3;3) are associated with thrombocytosis, they are characteristic of MDS or AML, rather than essential thrombocythemia.

Mutant *JAK2*[V617F] is a constitutively active tyrosine kinase that activates the STAT, PI3Ks, and mitogen-activated protein kinases (MAPKs) signalling pathways downstream of the erythropoietin receptor, thrombopoietin receptor, or the granulocyte colony-stimulating factor (G-CSF) receptor to promote proliferation and transformation of hematopoietic progenitor cells (Chap. 84). *JAK2* mutations occur in polycythemia vera (95 percent), essential thrombocythemia (approximately 50 percent), and myelofibrosis (approximately 50 percent) (Chaps. 84 to 86).[20] In refractory anemia with ring sideroblasts (RARS) with thrombocytosis (RARS-t), a MDS/MPN, unclassified by the World Health Organization (WHO) classification, 60 percent of patients have the *JAK2*[V617F] mutation, and present with higher white blood cell and platelet counts (Chap. 87).[21] Less commonly, activation of the JAK-STAT pathway in MPNs may result from *JAK2* exon 12 mutations (1 to 2 percent of polycythemia vera cases) or mutation of the thrombopoietin receptor, *MPL* (approximately 2 percent of essential thrombocythemia and approximately 5 percent of myelofibrosis). The majority of essential thrombocythemia and myelofibrosis patients with nonmutated *JAK2* carry somatic mutations in the calreticulin gene (*CALR*) (Chaps. 85 and 86).[22,23]

MYELODYSPLASTIC SYNDROMES

The MDSs are a heterogeneous group of neoplasms, including refractory cytopenia with unilineage dysplasia, RARS, refractory cytopenia with multilineage dysplasia (RCMD), RAEB–1,2, MDS with isolated del(5q), MDS unclassifiable, and childhood MDS, including refractory cytopenia of childhood (Chap. 87).[24] Clonal chromosome abnormalities can be detected in marrow cells of approximately 50 percent of patients with primary MDS at diagnosis (refractory anemia [RA], 25 percent; RARS, 10 percent; RCMD, 50 percent; RAEB –1,2, 50 to 70 percent; MDS with isolated del (5q), 100 percent) (see Table 13–2).[25,26] The proportion varies with the risk that a subtype will transform to AML, which is highest for RCMD and RAEB. The common chromosome changes, +8, del(5q), −7/del(7q), and del(20q), are similar to those seen in AML *de novo*. The recurring translocations that are closely associated with the distinct morphologic subsets of AML *de novo* are almost never seen in MDS. With the exception of MDS with isolated del(5q), the chromosome changes show no close association with the specific subtypes of MDS. MDS with isolated del(5q) occurs in a subset of older patients, frequently women, with RA, generally low blast counts, and normal or elevated platelet counts.[27] These patients have an interstitial deletion of 5q, typically as the sole abnormality, and can have a relatively benign course that extends over several years (Chap. 87).[27] Diagnostic and prognostic information for the patients with a normal karyotype can be provided by CMA, which can detect abnormalities in 10 to 15 percent of these cases. Some abnormalities detectable by CMA, including submicroscopic microdeletions in 4q24 affecting the *TET2* gene, as well as LOH 7q, LOH 11q, and LOH 17p, were shown to be associated with a poor outcome in MDS.[28,29]

Cytogenetic abnormalities in MDS are predictive of survival and progression to AML.[26] Patients with a "very good outcome" have −Y or del(11q) as the sole abnormality; those with a "good outcome" have

TABLE 13–2. Recurring Chromosome Abnormalities in Malignant Myeloid Diseases

Disease	Chromosome Abnormality	Frequency	Involved Genes*		Consequence
CML	t(9;22)(q34.1;q11.2)	~99%†	ABL1	BCR	Fusion protein–altered cytokine signaling pathways, genomic instability
CML blast phase	t(9;22) with +8, +der(22) t(9;22), +19, or i(17q)	~70%			
PV	+8	20% (all abnormalities combined)			
	+9				
	del(20q)				
	del(13q)				
	partial trisomy 1q				
PMF	+8	30% (all abnormalities combined)			
	+9				
	−7/del(7q)				
	del(5q)/t(5q)				
	del(20q)				
	del(13q)				
	partial trisomy 1q				
AML	t(8;21)(q22;q22.3)	10%	RUNX1T1/ETO	RUNX1/AML1	Fusion protein–altered transcriptional regulation
	t(15;17)(q24.1;q21.1)	9%	PML	RARA	Fusion protein–altered transcriptional regulation
	inv(16)(p13.1q22) or t(16;16)(p13.1;q22)	5%	MYH11	CBFB	Fusion protein–altered transcriptional regulation
	t(9;11)(p21.3;q23.3)	5–8% for all t(11q23.3)	MLLT3/AF9	KMT2A/MLL	KMT2A histone methyltransferase fusion proteins–altered chromatin structure and transcriptional regulation
	t(10;11)(p12;q23.3)		MLLT10/AF10	KMT2A	
	t(11;17)(q23.3;q25)		KMT2A	MLLT6/AF17	
	t(11;19)(q23.3;p13.3)		KMT2A	MLLT1/ENL	
	t(11;19)(q23.3;p13.1)		KMT2A	ELL	
	t(6;11)(q27;q23.3)		MLLT4/AF6	KMT2A	
	Other t(11q23.3)		KMT2A		
	del(11)(q23)				
	+8	8%			
	+11	1–2%	KMT2A		Internal tandem duplication
	−7 or del(7q)	14%			
	del (5q)/t(5q)	12%			
	t(6;9)(p23;q34.1)	1%	DEK	NUP214/CAN	Overexpression of MECOM
	inv(3)(q21.3q26.2) or t(3;3)	2%	MECOM/EVI1		
	del(20q)	5%			
	t(12p) or del(12p)	2%			
Therapy-related MDS/AML	−7 or del(7q)	45%			
	del(5q)/t(5q)	40%			
	der(1;7)(q10;p10)	2%			
	dic(5;17)(q11.1–13;p11.1–13)	5%		TP53	Loss of function–DNA damage response
	t(9;11)(p21.3;q23.3)/t(11q23)	3%	MLLT3	KMT2A	KMT3A histone methyltransferase fusion proteins–altered transcriptional regulation
	t(11;16)(q23.3;p13.3)	2% (t-MDS)	KMT2A	CREBBP	
	t(21q22.3)	2%	RUNX1/AML1		Overexpression of MECOM
	t(3;21)(q26.2;q22.3)	3%	MECOM	RUNX1	

(continued)

TABLE 13–2. Recurring Chromosome Abnormalities in Malignant Myeloid Diseases (Continued)

Disease	Chromosome Abnormality	Frequency	Involved Genes*		Consequence
MDS	+8	10%			
(Unbalanced)	−7/del(7q)‡	12%			
	del(5q)/t(5q)‡	15%			
	del(20q)	5–8%			
	−Y	5%			Loss of function, DNA damage response
	i(17q)/t(17p)‡	3–5%	TP53		
	−13/del(13q)‡	3%			
	del(11q)‡	3%			
	del(12p)/t(12p)‡	3%			
	del(9q)‡	1–2%			
	idic(X)(q13)‡	1–2%			
(Balanced)	t(1;3)(p36.3;q21.2)‡	1%	MMEL1	RPN1	Deregulation of MMEL1–transcriptional activation?
	t(2;11)(p21;q23.3)/t(11q23.3)‡	1%		KMT2A	KMT2A fusion protein-altered transcriptional regulation
	inv(3)(q21.3q26.2)/t(3;3)‡	1%	RPN1	MECOM/EVI1	Altered transcriptional regulation by MECOM
	t(6;9)(p23;q34.1)‡	1%	DEK	NUP214	Fusion protein-nuclear pore protein
CMML	t(5;12)(q32;p13.2)	~2%	PDGFRB	ETV6/TEL	Fusion protein–altered signaling pathways

AML, acute myeloid leukemia; CML, chronic myeloid leukemia; CMML, chronic myelomonocytic leukemia; MDS, myelodysplastic syndrome; PMF, primary myelofibrosis; PV, polycythemia vera.

*Genes are listed in order of citation in the karyotype; e.g., for CML, ABL1 is at 9q34.1 and BCR at 22q11.2.

†Rare patients with CML have an insertion of ABL1 adjacent to BCR in a normal-appearing chromosome 22.

‡Cytogenetic abnormalities considered in the WHO 2008 Classification as presumptive evidence of MDS in patients with persistent cytopenias(s), but with no dysplasia or increased blasts.

normal karyotypes, del(5q) alone, or with one additional abnormality, del(12p) alone, or del(20q) alone; those with an "intermediate outcome" have del(7q), +8, +19, i(17q), or any other single or double abnormality; those with a "poor outcome" have −7, inv(3q)/t(3;3), double abnormalities, including −7/del(7q), and complex karyotypes with 3 abnormalities; and those with a "very poor outcome" have complex karyotypes with more than three abnormalities, typically with abnormalities of chromosome 5.[26] With larger data sets, the inclusion of additional rare recurring cytogenetic abnormalities has facilitated a refinement of the cytogenetic risk groups, and provided the clinician with more information to predict the expected outcome for their patient.[30,31]

ACUTE MYELOID LEUKEMIA *DE NOVO*

Clonal chromosomal abnormalities are detected in 80 to 90 percent of patients with AML. The most frequent abnormalities are +8 and −7, which are seen in most subtypes of AML.[1] Specific rearrangements are closely associated with particular subtypes of AML as recognized by the WHO and French-American-British (FAB) classification schemes (see Table 13–2; Chap. 88).[32]

Translocation 8;21

The 8;21 translocation [t(8;21)(q22;q22.3)], described in 1973, was the first translocation identified in AML (see Fig. 13–3). The t(8;21) is common and is observed in 5 to 10 percent of all patients with AML with an abnormal karyotype and in 10 percent of patients with AML with maturation. This translocation is the most frequent abnormality in children with AML and occurs in 15 to 20 percent of karyotypically abnormal cases. Loss of a sex chromosome (−Y in males, −X in females), or a del(9q) with loss of 9q22, accompanies the t(8;21) in 75 percent of cases. The presence of the t(8;21) identifies a morphologically and clinically distinct subset of AML, and most cases with the t(8;21) are classified as AML with maturation. AML with the t(8;21) has a favorable prognosis in adults (overall 5-year survival of 70 percent), but the outcome in children is poor.[33] At the molecular level, the t(8;21) involves the RUNX1/AML1 gene, which encodes a transcription factor, also known as core-binding factor, that is essential for hematopoiesis. The RUNX1 gene on chromosome 21 is fused to the RUNX1T1/ETO gene on chromosome 8 and results in a RUNX1-RUNX1T1 chimeric protein. Transformation by RUNX1-RUNX1T1 likely results from transcriptional repression of normal RUNX1 target genes via aberrant recruitment of nuclear transcriptional corepressor complexes.[33]

Inversion 16 and Translocation 16;16

Another clinical–cytogenetic association involves acute myelomonocytic leukemia (AMML) with abnormal eosinophils, including large and irregular basophilic granules, and positive reactions with periodic acid–Schiff and chloroacetate esterase. Most patients have an inversion of chromosome 16, inv(16)(p13.1q22) (see Fig. 13–3), but some have a t(16;16)(p13.1;q22), and the WHO classification system now recognizes these as a distinct form of AML (Chap. 88). These aberrations are relatively common, occurring in 5 percent of AML and 25 percent of AMML patients.[1] These patients have a good response to intensive chemotherapy with a complete remission rate of approximately 90 percent and an overall 5-year survival of 60 percent.[33] The breakpoint at 16q22 occurs within the *CBFB* gene, which encodes one subunit of the RUNX1/CBFB transcription factor. Thus, like the t(8;21), the inv(16) disrupts the RUNX1/AML1 pathway regulating hematopoiesis. Secondary cooperating mutations of *KIT, KRAS,* and *NRAS* are common in core-binding factor-associated leukemias, although only *KIT* mutations confer a poor prognosis.[33]

Translocation 15;17

The t(15;17)(q24.1;q21.1) (see Fig. 13–3) is specific for acute promyelocytic leukemia (APL) and has not been found in any other disease.[34] Rare variant translocations, which occur in less than 2 percent of cases, include the t(11;17)(q23.2;q21.1) and t(5;17)(q35.1;q21.1), which result in the ZBTB16 (PLZF)-RARA and NPM1-RARA fusion proteins, respectively. Establishing the diagnosis of APL with the typical t(15;17) is important, because this disease is sensitive to therapy with all-*trans* retinoic acid, whereas other cases of AML and some of the APL-like disorders associated with the variant translocations do not respond to this treatment (Chap. 88). The t(15;17) results in a fusion retinoic acid receptor-α protein (PML-RARA). The oncogenic potential of the APL fusion proteins appears to result from the aberrant repression of RARA-mediated gene transcription through histone deacetylase (HDAC)-dependent chromatin remodeling. Genetic mutations that cooperate with PML-RARA include *FLT3* internal tandem duplications (ITDs), observed in 35 percent of patients.

Translocations Involving 11q

Recurring translocations involving 11q23.3 are seen in approximately 35 percent of acute monocytic leukemia patients and are of great interest in acute leukemia for at least three reasons.[1,35] First, there are more than 50 different recurring rearrangements that involve 11q23.3 and, thus, along with 14q32.3, 11q23.3 is one of the bands most frequently involved in rearrangements in human tumor cells.[35,36] The most common breakpoints in the translocation partners include 1p32, 4q21.3, and 19p13.3 in ALL (Chap. 91), and 1q21, 2q21, 6q27, 9p21.3, 10p12, 17q25, 19p13.3, and 19p13.1 in AML (Chap. 88). Second, these translocations occur in both lymphoid and myeloid leukemias. One common translocation in infants, t(4;11)(q21.3;q23.3), has a lymphoblastic phenotype, whereas other translocations, such as the t(9;11)(p21.3;q23.3) (see Fig. 13–3) and t(11;19)(q23.3;p13.1), are common in acute monocytic leukemias. Finally, translocations involving 11q23.3 have a very unusual age distribution, comprising about three-quarters of the chromosome abnormalities in leukemia cells of children younger than 1 year of age.[35] With the exception of the t(9;11) which may have an intermediate outcome, translocations of 11q23.3 are associated with a poor outcome.[32] Translocations of 11q23.3 involve *KMT2A/MLL*, a very large gene (>100 kb) with multiple transcripts of 12 to 15 kb. KMT2A protein is a histone methyltransferase that assembles in protein complexes that regulate gene transcription via chromatin remodeling.[36] All of the *KMT2A* translocations identified to date result in fusion proteins.

Trisomy 11

Trisomy 11 is a rare abnormality, noted as a sole aberration in 1 to 2 percent of MDS or AML, and confers an unfavorable outcome.[37] It is notable that an ITD of the *KMT2A* gene is detected in 90 percent of AMLs with +11 as the sole abnormality and in 10 percent of AML cases with a normal karyotype. The rearrangement is the result of a duplication of

KMT2A exons 2 to 6 or 2 to 8 mediated by recombination between *Alu* repetitive elements and may produce a partially duplicated protein.

Inversion 3 and t(3;3)

Each of the other recurring rearrangements in AML occurs in fewer than 3 percent of patients. A unique feature of abnormalities involving the long arm of chromosome 3 [inv(3)(q21.3q26.2) or t(3;3)(q21.3;q26.2)] is the presence of platelet counts greater than 100×10^9/L, sometimes greater than 1000×10^9/L, and an increase in marrow megakaryocytes, especially micromegakaryocytes.[1] Most of the recurring translocations described above occur in younger patients with a median age in the 30s, whereas other abnormalities, such as del(5q), or −7/del(7q), occur in patients with a median age greater than 50 years. Moreover, many of the latter patients have occupational exposure to mutagenic agents, such as solvents, petroleum, and pesticides.

Mutations

The prognosis of patients with AML is also determined by mutations, most commonly of the *FLT3, NPM1, CEBPA,* or *KIT* genes (Table 13–3).[38] Mutations of the *FLT3* gene, including both point mutations within the tyrosine kinase domain and ITDs, are among the most common genetic changes seen in AML, occurring in 15 to 35 percent of cases. *FLT3*-ITD mutations may occur in any subtype of AML, but are most common in APL and AML with a normal karyotype, and are associated with a poor prognosis, particularly in those cases with loss of the remaining wild type *FLT3* allele.[39] Mutations of the FLT3 tyrosine kinase domain (codons 835 or 836 of the second tyrosine kinase domain) are noted in 5 to 8 percent of AML.[39] Mutations of *NPM1* also occur frequently in AML (35 percent of adult cases, and 80 to 90 percent of acute monocytic leukemia), but are less frequent in patients with recurring cytogenetic abnormalities. In the absence of *FLT3* mutations, *NPM1* mutations are associated with a favorable prognosis.[40] *NPM1* mutations, most commonly involve exon 12, resulting in alterations at the C-terminus, that is, replacement of tryptophan(s) at position 288 and 290, and aberrant localization of the protein to the cytoplasm. *CEBPA* mutations (6 to 15 percent of all AMLs), are often biallelic, and are usually associated with intermediate risk cytogenetics, but are generally associated with a favorable prognosis.[38] Mutations of *KIT* are noted in 2 percent of AMLs, and have prognostic significance among AMLs with t(8;21) and inv(16)/t(16;16) (20 to 25 percent), in which they are associated

TABLE 13–3. Gene Mutations in MDS and AML

Mutated Gene	Disease		
	MDS	AML	t-MDS/t-AML
FLT3 (ITD)	2.4%	15–35%	0%
FLT3 (TKD)	1%	5–8%	<1%
NRAS	10–15%	10%	10%
KIT[D816]	~1%	2%	NA
KMT2A (ITD)	3%	7%	2–3%
RUNX1	10–15%	12%	15–30%
TP53	5–10%	5–10%	25–30%
PTPN11	~1%	~1%	3%
NPM1	Rare	35%	4–5%
CEBPA	1–8%	6–18%	Rare
JAK2[V617F]	2–5%	2–5%	2–5%
DNMT3A	8%	10%	16%

with a poor prognosis.[33] With respect to epigenetic changes, transcriptional silencing via DNA methylation of the *CDKN2B* (*p15*[INK4B]) gene is observed in a high percentage of patients with AML or therapy-related myeloid neoplasm, and is associated with −7/del(7q), and a poor prognosis.[41]

Whole-genome and exome sequencing studies implicated a number of additional genes in pathogenesis of AML, including *DNMT3A, TET2, ASXL1, IDH1, IDH2, PHF6, WT1, TP53, RUNX1,* and *EZH2*. Still, AML genomes have a relatively few mutations compared to other adult cancers (average of 13 mutations), and only approximately 20 genes appear to be mutated in AML with a significant frequency.[42] Several of the newly identified genetic abnormalities have prognostic importance in AML, including *DNMT3A, TET2, ASXL1,* and *PHF6* mutations, and *KMT2A-PTD*, which are all associated with a poor outcome.[43] As more data accumulate regarding the clinical relevance of the specific mutation in homogeneously treated clinical cohorts it will become important to develop and implement assays that allow for cost-effective, rapid molecular profiling in the clinical setting.

In addition, the emerging molecular analysis of tumor tissue presents an opportunity to identify individuals with germline predisposition to cancer.[44–46] Depending on the type of bioinformatic analysis that is performed on tumor tissue, it is possible to identify germline mutations when analyzing an individual's primary tumor, as every cell in that person's body will contain the germline mutation. For example, the current standard for molecular analysis in the case of a patient presenting with a new AML is to perform mutational analysis of *CEBPA*. *CEBPA* is mutated sporadically in AML, but the familial form is associated with biallelic *CEBPA* mutations, most commonly with the germline mutation found within the 5′ end of the gene, accompanied by the acquisition of a second 3′ mutation in the leukemia. Germline 3′ *CEBPA* mutations have also been identified.[47,48] In approximately 10 percent of AML patients found to have biallelic *CEBPA* mutations within their leukemia cells, one of these mutated alleles is actually a germline mutation and, therefore, any AML patient found to have biallelic *CEBPA* mutations should undergo genetic counseling and molecular testing of germline tissue.[44,49–51] This type of scenario may become more common as next-generation sequencing of tumor tissue is performed more frequently. The American College of Medical Genetics and Genomics (ACMG) has published a series of commentaries and recommendations regarding disclosure of genetic information when clinical genetic sequencing is performed.[52,53] The ACMG recommends disclosure of genetic information regarding 24 genes that confer germline cancer predisposition.[53] Figure 13–4 shows the frequency of common cytogenetic abnormalities in AML occurring *de novo*.

THERAPY-RELATED MYELOID NEOPLASMS

Therapy-related myeloid neoplasms (t-MNs), comprised of therapy-related MDS (t-MDS) and therapy-related AML (t-AML), are a late complication of cytotoxic therapy used in the treatment of both malignant and nonmalignant diseases.[54] In patients who received alkylating agents, the characteristic recurring chromosome abnormalities observed are loss of part or all of chromosomes 5 [del(5q)] and/or part or all of chromosome 7 [−7/del(7q)] (see Fig. 13–4). Clinically, these patients have a long latency period (5 years), present with MDS, which often progresses rapidly to AML with multilineage dysplasia and a poor prognosis. In our experience, 92 percent of t-MN patients had an abnormal karyotype and 70 percent had an abnormality of one or both chromosomes 5 and 7,[55] and these observations have been confirmed in other series.[56] In contrast, only approximately 20 percent of patients with AML *de novo* have a similar abnormality of chromosomes 5 or 7 or both.[1]

By cytogenetic and molecular analysis, investigators have defined a 970-kb commonly deleted segment (CDS) containing 19 genes on the long arm of chromosome 5 (5q31.2) predicted to contain a myeloid tumor suppressor gene.[57] A second, nonoverlapping CDS in 5q32 is implicated in MDS with an isolated del(5q).[58] Parallel studies revealed a 2.5-Mb CDS within 7q22 containing 16 genes. Molecular analysis of the genes within these regions did not reveal inactivating mutations in the remaining alleles, nor was there evidence of transcriptional silencing.[57] These observations are compatible with a haploinsufficiency model (gene dosage effect resulting from the loss of one allele), and several candidate haploinsufficient genes (*EGR1, APC, CSNK1A1, RPS14*) have been identified on 5q. The EGR1 transcription factor is downstream of cytokine signaling pathways. In a mouse model, loss of a single allele of *Egr1* cooperates with mutations induced by an alkylating agent in the development of myeloid diseases.[59] *RPS14* encodes an essential component of the 40S subunit of ribosomes, and haploinsufficiency of this gene appears to be responsible for the defect in erythropoiesis in MDS with an isolated del(5q).[60] Other studies show that haploinsufficiency of two micro-RNAs, miR-145 and miR-146a, encoded by sequences near the

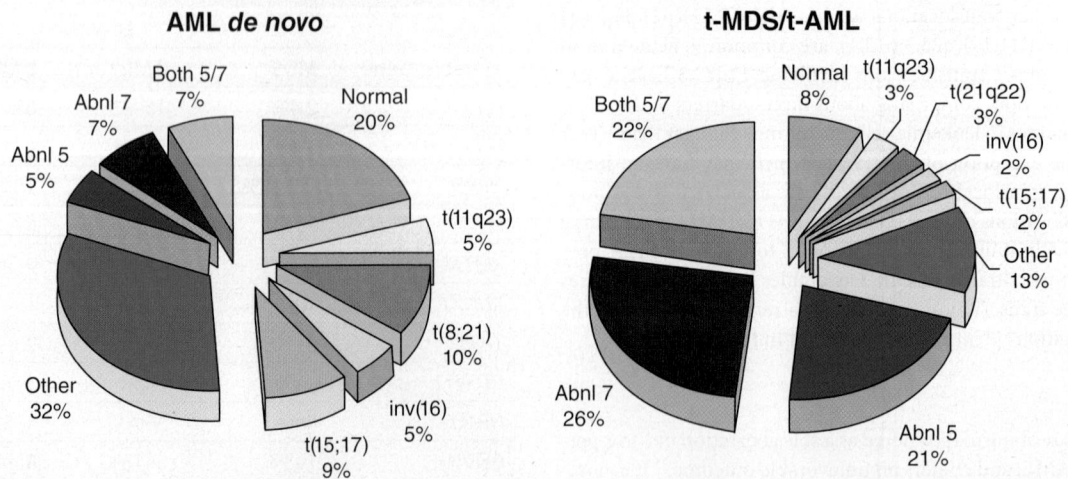

Figure 13–4. Frequency of recurring abnormalities in myeloid leukemias.

RPS14 gene, cooperate with loss of RPS14 and mediate the megakary-ocytic dysplasia seen in this disease.[61] These studies raise the possibility that haploinsufficiency for one or more of these genes in hematopoietic stem cells (HSCs) may contribute to the pathogenesis of MDS or AML with a del(5q), and a study demonstrated that haploinsufficiency for two del(5q) genes, *EGR1* and *APC*, together with loss of *TP53* leads to AML in a mouse model.[62]

A second subtype of t-AML has been identified that is distinctly different from the more common leukemia that follows alkylating agents or irradiation. This type of t-AML is seen in patients receiving drugs known to inhibit topoisomerase II, for example, etoposide, teni-poside, and doxorubicin. Clinically, these patients have a shorter latency period (1 to 2 years), present with overt leukemia, often with monocytic features, without a preceding myelodysplastic phase, and have a more favorable response to intensive induction therapy. Balanced transloca-tions involving the *KMT2A* gene at 11q23.3, or the *RUNX1/AML1* gene at 21q22.3 are common in this subgroup.[54]

ACUTE LYMPHOBLASTIC LEUKEMIA

ALL is the most frequent leukemia in children (Chap. 91). In both childhood and adult ALL, the identification of prognostic subgroups based on recurring cytogenetic abnormalities (Table 13–4) and molec-ular markers has resulted in the application of risk-adapted therapies.[63] The most useful prognostic indicators are karyotype (including ploidy), age, white blood cell count, and response to initial therapy (day 14 mar-row response and end-induction minimal residual disease). Based on these parameters, the Children's Oncology Group has defined four risk groups: lower risk (5-year event-free survival [EFS], at least 85 percent), with either the *ETV6/RUNX1* fusion, or simultaneous trisomies of chro-mosomes 4, 10, and 17; standard and high risk (those remaining in the respective National Cancer Institute risk groups); and very high risk (5-year EFS, 45 percent or below), with extreme hypodiploidy (fewer than 44 chromosomes), or the *BCR-ABL1* fusion, and induction fail-ure.[64] Genome-wide profiling studies using CMA revealed a high fre-quency of submicroscopic copy-number abnormalities in pediatric ALL, including deletions of *PAX5* (32 percent), *IKZF1* (*IKAROS*, 29 percent), *CDKN2A/B* (50 percent), *BTG1*, and *EBF1* (8 percent). Many of these abnormalities disrupt genes and pathways controlling B-cell develop-ment and differentiation, and the most clinically significant among them appears to be genetic alterations of *IKZF1*, which are invariably associated with a very poor outcome in B-cell progenitor ALL.[9]

Translocation 9;22
The incidence of the t(9;22) in ALL is 30 percent in adults (the inci-dence may approach 50 percent in adults older than 60 years of age) and 5 percent in children. Thus, the Ph chromosome is the most frequent rearrangement in adult ALL. Approximately 70 percent of the patients show additional abnormalities, a frequency that is substantially higher than that observed in CML with +der(22)t(9;22),+21, abnormalities of 9p, +8, −7, and +X (noted in descending frequency). Monosomy 7 is associated with a poorer outcome.[65] A chromosomally normal cell line is frequently noted in the marrow of Ph chromosome-positive ALL patients (70 percent), but is rare in untreated CML. Most cases have a B-lineage phenotype (CD10+, CD19+, and TdT+), but there is frequent expression of myeloid-associated antigens (CD13 and CD33). The dis-ease in both adults and children is characterized by high white blood cell counts, a high percentage of circulating blasts, and a poor prognosis. As in CML, the t(9;22) in ALL results in a *BCR-ABL1* fusion gene. How-ever, in more than half of the patients, the break in *BCR* is more prox-imal, resulting in a smaller fusion protein with even greater tyrosine

kinase activity (BCR-ABL1[p190]). Genetic alterations of the *IKZF1* gene are detectable in up to 80 percent of patients with Ph chromosome–pos-itive ALL, and are associated with an unfavorable outcome even with the use of TKIs.[66]

Translocations Involving 11q
Translocations involving the *KMT2A* gene at 11q23.3 are observed in 5 percent of ALL patients.[67] Of these, the most common is the t(4;11) (q21.3;q23.3) (Fig. 13–5). The t(11;19)(q23.3;p13.3) is second in fre-quency. However, this rearrangement is not limited to ALL in that approximately 50 percent of these cases have AML, usually monoblas-tic. Of note is the high frequency of translocations involving 11q23.3 in infant ALL (60 to 80 percent). Patients with the t(4;11) have a pro B-cell phenotype (CD10−, CD19+), with coexpression of monocytic (CD15+), or, less commonly, T-cell markers. Clinically, both children and adults have aggressive features with hyperleukocytosis, extramed-ullary disease, and a poor response to conventional chemotherapy.[67] Adults with the t(4;11) have a remission rate of 75 percent, but a median EFS of only 7 months. Rearrangements affecting *KMT2A* represent a major class of mutations in acute leukemia and identify patients with a poor outcome.

Translocation 12;21
The t(12;21)(p13.2;q22.3) has been identified in a high proportion (approximately 25 percent) of childhood precursor B-cell leukemia, but is uncommon in adults (approximately 5 percent of ALL cases) (Fig. 13–6).[68] The translocation is not easily detected by cytogenetic anal-ysis because of the similarity in size and banding pattern of 12p and 21q. However, the rearrangement can be detected reliably using reverse transcriptase polymerase chain reaction (RT-PCR) or FISH analysis. The t(12;21) defines a distinct subgroup of patients characterized by an age between 1 and 10 years, B-cell lineage immunophenotype (CD10+, CD19+, HLA-DR+), and a favorable outcome, particularly when other favorable risk factors are present. In one study, patients with the t(12;21) had a 5-year EFS of 91 percent as compared to 65 percent for patients without this rearrangement. However, the t(12;21) may be associated with late disease recurrences. The t(12;21) results in a fusion protein containing the N-terminus of ETV6/TEL, a transcriptional repres-sor of the ETS family, and most of the RUNX1/AML1 transcription factor.

Hyperdiploidy
The leukemia cells of some patients with ALL are characterized by a gain of many chromosomes (see Fig. 13–6). Two distinct subgroups are recognized: a group with 1 to 4 extra chromosomes (47 to 50), and the more common group with more than 50 chromosomes. Chromosome numbers usually range from 51 to 60, and a few patients may have up to 65 chromosomes. Hyperdiploidy (>50 and usually <66 chromosomes) is common in children (approximately 30 percent), but is rarely observed in adults (<5 percent). Certain additional chromosomes are com-mon (X chromosome, and chromosomes 4, 6, 10, 14, 17, 18, and 21). Chromosome 21 is gained most frequently (100 percent of cases). Patients who have hyperdiploidy with more than 50 chromosomes have all of the previously recognized clinical factors that indicate a good prognosis, including age between 1 and 9 years, low white blood cell count (median 6700/μL), and favorable immunophenotype (early pre-B cell or pre-B cell).[69] The favorable prognosis associated with high hyper-diploidy is associated with gains of chromosomes 4, 10, and 17, whereas a gain of chromosomes 5 and i(17q) is associated with a poor outcome.[69]

TABLE 13–4. Cytogenetic-Immunophenotypic Correlations in Malignant Lymphoid Diseases

Disease	Chromosome Abnormality	Frequency*	Involved Genes†		Consequence‡
ACUTE LYMPHOBLASTIC LEUKEMIA					
Precursor B	t(12;21)(p13.2;q22.3)	25%	ETV6/TEL	RUNX1/AML1	Fusion protein–TF
	t(9;22)(q34.1;q11.2)	10%#	ABL1	BCR	Fusion protein–altered cytokine signaling pathways
	t(4;11)(q21.3;q23.3)	5%	AFF4	KMT2A	Fusion protein–TF
	t(17;19)(q22;p13.3)	1%	HLF	TCF3 (E2A)	Fusion protein-TF
	t(11;19)(q23.3;p13.3)	1%	KMT2A	MLLT1/ENL	Fusion protein–TF
Pre-B	t(1;19)(q23;p13.3)	6% (30%)	PBX1	TCF3 (E2A)	Fusion protein-TF
B (SIg+)	t(8;14)(q24.2;q32.3)	5% (95%)	MYC	IGH	Deregulated expression–TF
	t(2;8)(p12;q24.2)	<1% (1%)	IGK	MYC	Deregulated expression–TF
	t(8;22)(q24.2;q11.2)	<1% (4%)	MYC	IGL	Deregulated expression–TF
Other	Hyperdiploidy (50–60)	10%			
	del(12p), t(12p)	10%			
T	t(11;14)(p15.4;q11.2)	1%	LMO1	TRA	Deregulated expression–TF
	t(11;14)(p13;q11.2)	3%	LMO2	TRA	Deregulated expression–TF
	t(8;14)(q24.2;q11.2)	<1%	MYC	TRA	Deregulated expression–TF
	inv(14)(q11.2q32.1)	<1%	TRA	TCL1A	Deregulated expression–TF
	t(10;14)(q24.3;q11.2)	3%	TLX1	TRA	Deregulated expression–TF
	t(1;14)(p33;q11.2)	1%	TALI	TRD	Deregulated expression–TF
	t(7;9)(q34;q34.3)		TRB	NOTCH1	Deregulated expression–TF
	t(7;19)(q34;p13.3)	2%			
	del(9p), t(9p)	<1%	CDKN2A,		Tumor suppressor gene–cell-cycle regulation
		<1% (10%)	CDKN2B		
LYMPHOMA					
B-Cell Lymphoma					
Burkitt	t(8;14)(q24.2;q32.3)	95%	MYC	IGH	Deregulated expression–TF
	t(2;8)(p12;q24.2)	1%	IGK	MYC	Deregulated expression–TF
	t(8;22)(q24.2;q11.2)	4%	MYC	IGL	Deregulated expression–TF
Follicular SNCL	t(14;18)(q32.3;q21.3)	80%	IGH	BCL2	Deregulated expression–antiapoptosis protein
DLBCL	t(14;18)(q32.3;q21.3)	20%	IGH	BCL2	
DLBCL	t(3;22)(q27;q11.2)	45% for all	BCL6	IGL	Deregulated expression–TF
	t(3;14)(q27;q32.3)	t(3q27)	BCL6	IGH	Deregulated expression–TF
MCL	t(11;14)(q13.3;q32.3)	~100%	CCND1	IGH	Deregulated expression–TF
LPL	t(9;14)(p13.2;q32.3)		PAX5	IGH	Deregulated expression–TF
SLL	t(14;19)(q32.3;q13.3)		IGH	BCL3	Deregulated expression–TF
MALT	t(11;18)(q22.2;q21.3)	40–50%	BIRC3/API2	MALT1	Fusion Protein–NFκB activation
	t(1;14)(p22.3;q32.3)	10%	BCL10	IGH	Deregulated expression–increased NFκB activation
	t(14;18)(q32.3;q21.3)	10–20%	IGH	MALT1	Deregulated expression–increased NFκB activation
	t(3;14)(p13;q32.3)	10%	FOXP1	IGH	Deregulated expression–TF
	t(X;14)(p11.4;q32.3)	rare	GPR34	IGH	Deregulated expression–G-protein–coupled receptor
PCMZL	t(14;18)(q32.3;q21.3)	rare	IGH	MALT1	Deregulated expression–increased NFκB activation
PCFCL	t(14;18)(q32.3;q21.3)	40%	IGH	BCL2	Deregulated expression–anti-apoptosis protein

(continued)

TABLE 13–4. Cytogenetic-Immunophenotypic Correlations in Malignant Lymphoid Diseases (Continued)

Disease	Chromosome Abnormality	Frequency*	Involved Genes†		Consequence‡
T-Cell Lymphoma					
ALK+ ALCL	t(2;5)(p23.2;q35.1)	75%	*ALK*	*NPM1*	Deregulated expression–tyrosine kinase
ALK– ALCL	t(6;7)(p25.3;q32.3)	10–15%	*IRF4, DUSP22*		Deregulated expression of TF (IRF4) and phosphatase (DUSP22)
Nasal/NK cell	i(1q), i(7q), i(17q)				
Hepatosplenic	i(7q)	>95%			
Peripheral	t(5;9)(q33.3;q22.2)	15%	*ITK*	*SYK*	Constitutively active tyrosine kinase (SYK)
CHRONIC LYMPHOCYTIC LEUKEMIA					
B	t(11;14)(q13.3;q32.3)	10%	*CCND1*	*IGH*	Deregulated expression–cell-cycle regulation
	t(14;19)(q32.3;q13.2)	5%	*IGH*	*BCL3*	Deregulated expression–increased NFκB activation
	t(2;14)(p13;q32.3)	5%		*IGH*	
	t(14q32.3)	15%	*IGH*		
	del(13q)	30%			
	+12	25%			
T	t(8;14)(q24.2;q11.2)	5%	*MYC*	*TRA*	Deregulated expression–TF
	inv(14)(q11.2q32.3)	5%	*TRA/TRD*	*IGH*	Deregulated expression
	inv(14)(q11.2q32.1)	5%	*TRA/TRD*	*TCL1A*	Deregulated expression–TF
MULTIPLE MYELOMA					
B	–13/del(13q)	40%			
	t(4;14)(p16;q32)	15%	*FGFR3*	*IGH*	Deregulated expression–growth factor receptor
			WHSC1/MMSET	*IGH*	Deregulated chromatin modification and gene expression–histone methyltransferase
	t(14;16)(q32.3;q23)	5%	*IGH*	*MAF*	Deregulated expression–TF
	t(6;14)(p21;q32.3)	4%	*CCND3*	*IGH*	Deregulated expression–cell-cycle regulation
	t(11;14)(q13.3;q32.3)	15%	*CCND1*	*IGH*	Deregulated expression–cell-cycle regulation
	t(14q32.3)	50%	*IGH*		
	del(17p)/t(17p)	30%	*TP53*		Loss of function–DNA damage response
	gain of 1q				
	hyperdiploidy: +3,+5,+7,+9,+11	20%			
ADULT T-CELL LEUKEMIA/LYMPHOMA					
	t(14;14)(q11.2;q32.3)		*TRA*	*IGH*	Deregulated expression
	inv(14)(q11.2q32.3)		*TRA/TRD*	*IGH*	Deregulated expression
	+3				

ALCL, anaplastic large cell lymphoma; DLBCL, diffuse large B-cell lymphoma; LPL, lymphoplasmacytoid lymphoma; MALT, mucosa-associated lymphoid tissue; MCL, mantle cell lymphoma; NFκB, nuclear factor κB; NK, natural killer; PCFCL, primary cutaneous follicular center lymphoma; PCMZL, primary cutaneous marginal zone lymphoma; SIg, surface immunoglobulin; SLL, small lymphocytic lymphoma; SNCL, small noncleaved cell lymphoma; TF, transcription factor.

*The percentage refers to the frequency within the disease overall. The number in the parentheses refers to the frequency within the morphologic or immunologic subtype of the disease.

†Genes are listed in order of citation in the karyotype; e.g., for precursor B ALL, *ETV6* is at 12p13.2 and *RUNX1* is at 21q22.3.

‡By cytogenetic analysis, the frequency in children is approximately 5%, and in adults it is approximately 25%; using molecular probes, this frequency is 30% in adults overall, and 50% in adults older than 60 years of age.

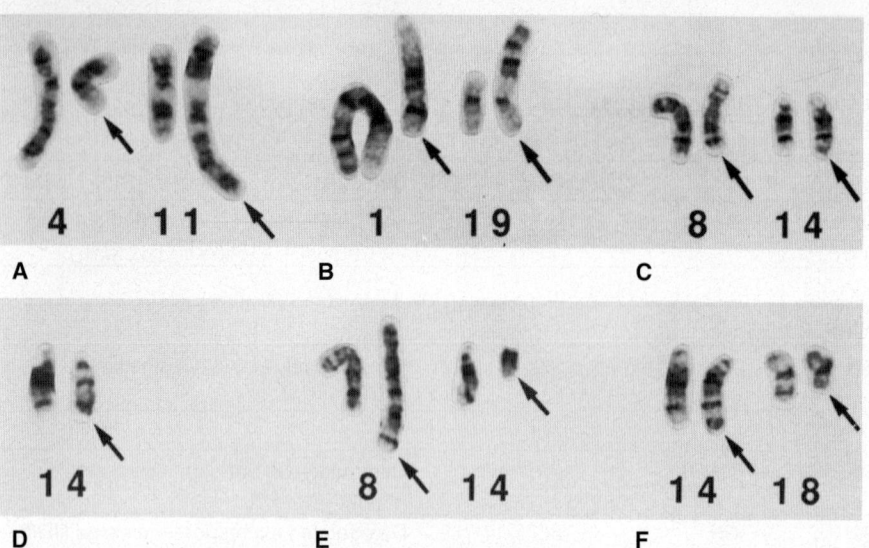

Figure 13–5. Partial karyotypes of trypsin-Giemsa-banded metaphase cells depicting recurring chromosomal rearrangements observed in lymphoid malignant diseases. The rearranged chromosomes are identified with *arrows.* **A.** t(4;11) (q21.3;q23.3) in ALL. **B.** t(1;19)(q23;p13.3) in pre-B cell ALL. **C.** t(8;14)(q24.2;q32) in B-cell ALL and Burkitt lymphoma. **D.** inv(14)(q11.2q32.1) in T-cell leukemia/lymphoma. **E.** t(8;14)(q24.2;q11.2) in T-cell leukemia/lymphoma. **F.** t(14;18)(q32.3;q21.3) in B-cell lymphoma.

Translocation 1;19 and translocation 8;14

The t(1;19)(q23;p13.3) has been identified in approximately 6 percent of children with a B-lineage leukemia (see Fig. 13–5). The leukemia cells have cytoplasmic immunoglobulin and are CD10+, CD19+, CD34–, and CD9+. A reciprocal translocation involving the long arms of chromosomes 8 and 14 [t(8;14)(q24.2;q32.3)] is observed in mature B-cell ALL (see Fig. 13–5).[70] These patients have a high incidence of central nervous system involvement and/or abdominal nodal involvement at diagnosis. Although the outcome for both children and adults with a t(8;14) has been poor, the use of high intensity chemotherapy has markedly improved the outcome (EFS of 80 percent in children).[70]

Philadelphia Chromosome–like Acute Lymphocytic/Lymphoblastic Leukemia

Ph-like ALL is a novel subgroup of high-risk ALL, characterized by increased expression of HSC genes, and a similar gene expression profile to Ph-positive ALL. Like Ph-positive ALL, Ph-like cases are also characterized by a high frequency of *IKZF1* deletions and mutations, which confer a poor prognosis.[9,10] Ph-like ALL comprises up to 15 percent of pediatric ALL and up to 30 percent of adult ALL and is associated with a higher risk of relapse compared to other Ph-negative cases. Genetic alterations responsible for the activated kinase and cytokine receptor signaling signature in Ph-like ALL are starting to be elucidated, and include point mutations and gene fusions affecting *CRLF2, JAK2, ABL1, PDGFRB, EPOR, EBF1, FLT3, IL7R, SH2B3,* and other genes.[71]

T-CELL ACUTE LYMPHOBLASTIC LEUKEMIA

T lymphoblastic leukemia/lymphoma has a distinct pattern of recurring karyotypic abnormalities.[72] Rearrangements involving 14q11.2 (see Fig. 13–5) and two regions of chromosome 7, (7q34) and (7p14), are particularly frequent in T-cell malignancies (see Table 13–4). The most common are the t(10;11)(q24.3;q11.2) (7 percent of childhood and 30 percent of adult cases, *TLX1* gene); the cryptic t(5;14)(q35.1;q32.1) (*TLX3*, 20 percent of childhood and 10 to 15 percent of adult cases), t(11;14) (p13;q11.2) (approximately 3 percent, *LMO2* gene), and t(7;9) (q34;q34.3) (approximately 2 percent, *NOTCH1* gene). Approximately 30 percent of patients have activating mutations of the *NOTCH1* gene. Patients with T-cell ALL are most often young males and often have a mediastinal tumor mass, high white blood cell count, and leukemia

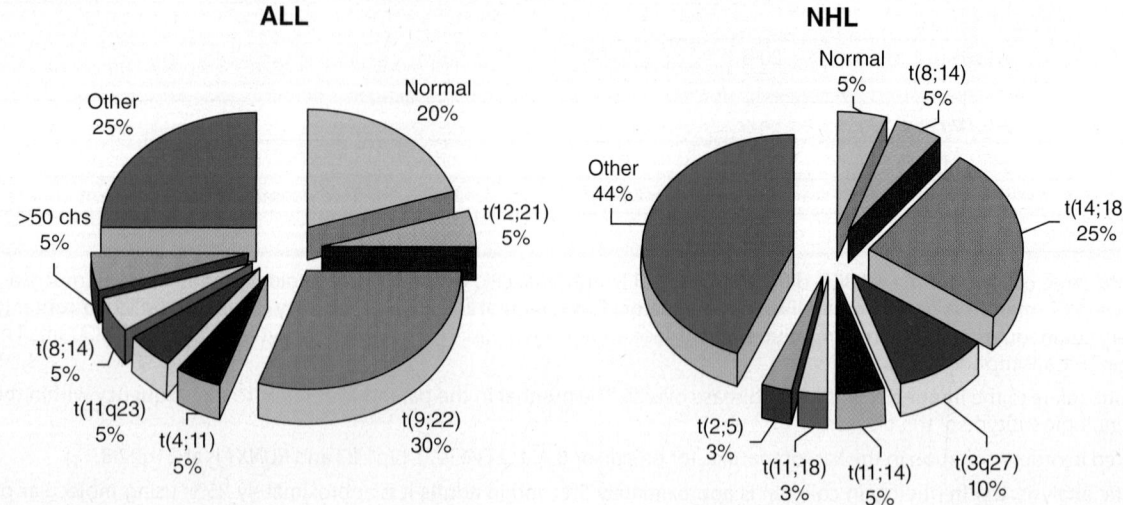

Figure 13–6. Frequency of recurring abnormalities in acute lymphocytic/lymphoblastic leukemias (ALL) and non-Hodgkin lymphomas (NHL).

cells in the cerebrospinal fluid. These same clinical characteristics are associated with lymphoblastic lymphoma, another T-cell malignancy.

CHRONIC LYMPHOCYTIC LEUKEMIA

The chromosomal abnormalities associated with chronic lymphocytic leukemia (CLL) have been delineated through the use of FISH (Chap. 92).[73] When conventional cytogenetic techniques are used, only 50 percent of CLL patients have detectable chromosomal abnormalities. The most common abnormality is trisomy 12 (20 to 60 percent), followed by structural abnormalities of 13q and 14q (see Table 13-4). However, when FISH analysis is used to study specific abnormalities, chromosomal abnormalities can be detected in greater than 80 percent of patients. The most frequent chromosomal changes seen by FISH are: loss or deletion of 13q (55 percent); deletion of 11q, the location of the *ATM* gene (18 percent); trisomy of 12q (16 percent); deletion of 17p, the location of the *TP53* gene; and deletion of 6q (6 percent). The LOH affecting 17p frequently coincides with the *TP53* mutations (7 percent) and can be detected by CMA.[74] Patient survival correlates with cytogenetic subtype, with a shorter median survival observed in patients with 17p (32 months) or 11q (79 months) deletions, than in those with no detectable abnormality (111 months), trisomy of 12q (114 months), or −13/del(13q) (133 months). Two micro-RNA genes (miR-16−1 and miR-15a) are possible target genes in the 13q14.3 region. FISH probes capable of detecting the deletions of 11q, 13q, and 17p, trisomy 12, and immunoglobulin heavy chain *(IGH)* translocations are commercially available, and facilitate the application of risk-adapted treatment strategies.

The prognosis of patients with CLL is also determined by two other molecular abnormalities: the status of the *IGH* variable region and the expression level of CD38 (Chap. 92). Patients whose CLL cells express *IGH* genes containing somatic mutations have a 24-year median survival compared to only 6 to 8 years in those patients who do not have somatic *IGH* gene mutations.[75] This simple grouping of patients based on the mutation status of the *IGH* gene may reflect the fact that CLL cells that have few or no *IGH* mutations also often contain chromosomal aberrations that confer a poor prognosis, for example deletions of 11q or 17p, or trisomy 12, whereas CLL cells with *IGH* mutations often contain deletions of 13q, which confer a more favorable clinical course. Unfortunately, testing for somatic mutations in the *IGH* gene is not currently commercially available. ZAP-70, an enzyme normally expressed in T lymphocytes and critical for T-cell activation, is upregulated in CLL cells that contain unmutated *IGH* genes, conferring a poor prognosis (Chap. 92).[76] Patients whose CLL cells have mutated IGH and lack expression of ZAP-70 and CD38, a membrane protein with signaling activity have the longest treatment-free period after initial diagnosis.[77]

T-cell CLL and large granular lymphocytic leukemia are uncommon disorders in which the malignant lymphocytes have a T-cell immunophenotype. Rearrangements involving band 14q11.2 with or without an accompanying break in 14q32.1 have been reported in T-CLL as well as in T-cell lymphomas (see Table 13-4).[72] The most common is inv(14) (q11.2q32.1).

LYMPHOMA

Cytogenetic analyses of patients with lymphoma have demonstrated that more than 90 percent of cases are characterized by clonal chromosomal abnormalities and, more importantly, many of the recurring abnormalities correlate with histology and immunophenotype (see Table 13-4; Chaps. 95 and 96).[78] For example, the t(14;18) is observed in a high proportion of follicular small cleaved cell lymphomas (70 to 90 percent), most patients with a t(3;22)(q27;q11.2) or t(3;14)(q27;q32.3) have DLBCL, and patients

with a t(8;14)(q24.2;q32.3) have either small noncleaved cell or DLBCL (Chap. 98). Band 14q32.3, the location of *IGH* is frequently involved in translocations in B-cell neoplasms (approximately 70 percent). In contrast, a large proportion of T-cell neoplasms are characterized by rearrangements that involve 14q11.2, 7q34, or 7p14, the locations of the T-cell receptor genes (Chap. 104). Gene expression profiling has proven useful in distinguishing unique genetic subtypes of lymphoma.[79]

The t(8;14) is characteristic of both endemic and nonendemic Burkitt tumors, as well as Epstein-Barr virus (EBV)–negative and EBV-positive tumors (see Fig. 13–5; Chap. 102). Moreover, the t(8;14) has also been observed in other lymphomas, particularly small noncleaved cell (non-Burkitt) and large cell immunoblastic lymphomas, HIV-associated Burkitt lymphoma (100 percent) and HIV-related DLBCL (30 percent).[80] Two other variant translocations also occur in Burkitt lymphoma, t(2;8)(p12;q24.2) and t(8;22)(q24.2;q11.2). All three translocations involve chromosome band 8q24.2. These same translocations have been seen in some patients with B-cell ALL. The t(8;14) involves a break within the *IGH* locus on chromosome 14, and a break either 5′ or within the *MYC* gene on chromosome 8, and relocates the *MYC* coding exons to chromosome 14. MYC is a transcription factor that plays a critical role in a number of cellular processes including DNA replication, proliferation, and apoptosis; its oncogenic properties are a result of its constitutive expression.

Between 70 and 90 percent of follicular lymphomas (Chap. 99) and 20 percent of DLBCL have the t(14;18) (see Fig. 13–6), in which the *BCL2* gene at 18q21.3 is juxtaposed to the *IGH* J segment, leading to the deregulated expression of *BCL2*.[81] Common secondary abnormalities include −7, +18, and del(6q). Other malignancies that overexpress *BCL2*, but do not harbor the t(14;18), include hairy cell leukemia and CLL. The *BCL2* gene encodes a 26-kDa mitochondrial membrane protein that functions to increase cell survival through antiapoptosis and preventing programmed cell death.

The t(11;14) (q13.3;q32.3) is observed in virtually all cases of mantle cell lymphoma (Chap. 100), 3 percent of myeloma (Chap 107), and up to 20 percent of prolymphocytic leukemias (Chap. 92).[82,83] Many cases also have deletions or point mutations of the *ATM* gene (11q22.3). Mantle cell lymphomas are currently regarded as a poor prognostic group with a median survival from diagnosis of 3 years. This translocation results in the activation of the cyclin D1 *(CCND1)* gene by the *IGH* gene (J region).[82] The *CCND1* gene is located 100 to 130 kb away from the breakpoint on 11q13.3. The D-type cyclins act as growth factor sensors, causing cells to go through the restriction start point of the cell cycle at G_1 and committing them to divide via phosphorylation and inactivation of RB1.

The *BCL6* gene was cloned from the recurring breakpoint at 3q27 in cells characterized by a t(3;22)(q27;q11.2), t(3;14)(q27;q32.3) or, rarely, t(2;3)(p12;q27).[78] *BCL6* rearrangements occur in 40 percent of DLBCLs and, in some series, up to 10 percent of follicular lymphomas. The translocations lead to the truncation of the *BCL6* gene within the first exon or the first intron, substitution of its promoter sequences with an *IG* promoter, and deregulated expression. The *BCL6* gene product is a 96-kDa POZ/Zn finger, nuclear protein that acts as a potent transcriptional repressor. It is predominantly expressed in the B-cell lineage, particularly in mature B cells, and may suppress genes involved in lymphocyte activation, differentiation, cell cycle arrest, and apoptosis. Somatic mutations have been identified in the 5′ regulatory regions of *BCL6* in approximately 20 percent of DLBCLs without translocations leading to deregulation of *BCL6*, suggesting that overexpression of *BCL6* is more broadly involved than initially recognized.[84]

Extranodal marginal zone B-cell lymphomas of mucosa-associated lymphoid tissue (MALT lymphoma) are comprised of several genetic subgroups, one characterized by trisomy 3 plus other abnormalities

(60 percent), and another by the t(11;18)(q21.2;q21.3)(25 to 50 percent) and its variants (Chap. 101).[85] Of note is that the t(11;18) is not observed in primary large B-cell gastric lymphoma. The t(11;18) results in the fusion of the apoptosis-inhibitor gene *BIRC3 (API2)*, to a novel gene at 18q21.3, *MALT1*, whose product activates the nuclear factor κB (NFκB) pathway.

A number of recurring chromosomal abnormalities have been recognized in T-cell leukemias and lymphomas (see Table 13–4; Chap. 104). Similar to B-cell neoplasms, in which rearrangements frequently involve the chromosomal bands containing the immunoglobulin gene loci, T-cell neoplasms often have rearrangements involving band 14q11.2, the site of the T-cell receptor α-chain *(TRA)* and δ-chain *(TRD)* genes or, less often, one of two regions of chromosome 7 (7q34 and 7p14) to which the T-cell receptor β-chain *(TRB)* and γ-chain *(TRG)* genes have been localized, respectively.[78] These translocations result from aberrant V-D-J recombination events. With few exceptions, the involved gene on the partner chromosome encodes a transcription factor, whose expression is deregulated or activated as a result of the rearrangement (see Table 13–4). As a consequence of a chromosomal rearrangement that brings an oncogene under the controlling influence of promoters and enhancers that are active in T-cell receptor synthesis, T-cells may gain a proliferative advantage, resulting in malignant clonal expansion.

A distinctive subtype of lymphoma, namely, anaplastic large cell lymphoma (ALCL) is characterized by a young age at presentation, and skin and/or lymph node infiltration by large, often bizarre lymphoma cells, which preferentially involve the paracortical areas and lymph node sinuses (Chap. 98). The majority of such tumors express one or more T-cell antigens, a minority express B-cell antigens, and some express both T- and B-cell antigens (the null phenotype). A reciprocal translocation, t(2;5)(p23.2;q35.1), t(1;2)(q25;p23), or variant rearrangement involving the *ALK* tyrosine kinase gene at 2p23.2 appears to be restricted to ALCL of either T-cell or null phenotype, and is present in a high percentage of these cases.[86] The tumor cells are positive for CD30 on the cell membrane and in the Golgi region, and ALK expression is detectable in 60 to 85 percent of cases, where it confers a more favorable outcome (5-year survival, 80 percent in ALK+ vs. 40 percent in ALK– tumors). The t(2;5) has also been found in CD30+ primary cutaneous lymphomas.

MYELOMA

As in CLL, the application of molecular cytogenetic tools, such as FISH, has led to the discovery of numerous chromosomal abnormalities in myeloma, its precursor essential monoclonal gammopathy (Chaps. 105 and 106), and plasma cell leukemia (Chap. 107).[83,87] Monoclonal gammopathy is characterized by chromosomal aneuploidy, *IGH* translocations (45 percent of patients), and deletions of 13q (15 to 50 percent). Plasma cell myeloma is a malignancy of postfollicular B cells and is characterized by the acquisition of complex chromosomal rearrangements. As in monoclonal gammopathy, the earliest changes involve deletions of 13q14, and translocations of the *IGH* gene, which deregulate the expression of oncogenes located near the translocation breakpoints. Loss of chromosome 13 or a del(13q) is the most frequently observed chromosomal loss in myeloma and confers a poor prognosis.[83] With the use of FISH, deletions of 13q are detected in 40 to 50 percent of patients with myeloma and may be associated with specific 14q translocations.

Among the most frequent chromosomal rearrangements noted in plasma cell malignancies are translocations involving the *IGH* locus on 14q32. *IGH* translocations are detectable by interphase FISH analysis in approximately 10 percent of patients with monoclonal gammopathy, 40 to 50 percent of patients with myeloma, and more than 60 percent of patients with plasma cell leukemia.[83] The t(11;14)(q13.3;q32.2) is found in 15 percent of cases, and results in cyclin D1 overexpression and may deregulate expression of *MYEOV* (myeloma overexpressed

gene). The t(4;14)(p16.3;q32.3) is noted in approximately 15 percent of patients and deregulates the expression of the fibroblast growth factor receptor 3 gene *(FGFR3)* translocated to the der(14), and the *WHSC1/MMSET* domain remaining on the der(4) chromosomes. The t(14;16) (q32.3;q23), noted in 5 percent of cases, results in the overexpression of the *MAF* transcription factor gene. Cyclin D3 overexpression occurs in the context of the t(6;14)(p21.1;q32.3), observed in 4 percent of patients. The translocation partners for the remaining 10 to 15 percent of myeloma cases are currently unknown. The t(4;14) and t(14;16) are both associated with a poor clinical outcome, whereas the t(11;14) confers a favorable prognosis. Translocations involving unknown partners confer an intermediate prognosis.

Chromosome 1 abnormalities are prevalent in multiple myeloma, frequently resulting in both gain of 1q and loss of 1p, and are associated with a shorter survival.[88] Furthermore, gene expression profiling studies that identified a high-risk disease signature noted a significant enrichment of genes located on chromosome 1.[88] For this reason, it is now recommended that a comprehensive FISH testing panel for multiple myeloma include detection of chromosome 1 abnormalities, particularly using probes for 1q.

Additional events occur with disease progression, including mutations of *NRAS* and *KRAS*, *MYC* deregulation, and epigenetic alterations. Activating mutations of *NRAS* or *KRAS* have been identified in monoclonal gammopathy (approximately 5 percent), and at a higher frequency in myeloma (30 to 40 percent); but the frequency may be higher in patients who relapse (80 percent).[89] Several genes are silenced through aberrant promoter hypermethylation in both monoclonal gammopathy and myeloma, including *DAPK1* (67 percent), *SOCS1*, *CDKN2B (p15)*, and *CDKN2A (p16)*.[83]

REFERENCES

1. Carlson KM, Le Beau MM, Cytogenetics/Fluorescent in situ Hybridization in *Clinical Hematology*, edited by N S Young, SL Gerson, KA High, pp 1336–1351. Elsevier, Philadelphia, PA, 2005.
2. Gilliland DG: Molecular genetics of human leukemias: New insights into therapy. *Semin Hematol* 39:6–11, 2002.
3. Shaffer LG, McGowan-Jordan J, Schmid C, editors: *ISCN 2013: An International System for Human Cytogenetic Nomenclature (2013). Recommendations of the International Standing Committee on Human Cytogenetic Nomenclature.* S. Karger, Basel, 2013.
4. Gozzetti A, Le Beau MM: Fluorescence in situ hybridization: Uses and limitations. *Semin Hematol* 37:320–333, 2000.
5. Fonseca R, Bergsagel PL, Drach J, et al: International Myeloma Working Group molecular classification of multiple myeloma: Spotlight review. *Leukemia* 23:2210–2221, 2009.
6. Hartmann L, Biggerstaff JS, Chapman DB, et al: Detection of genomic abnormalities in multiple myeloma: The application of FISH analysis in combination with various plasma cell enrichment techniques. *Am J Clin Pathol* 136:712–720, 2011.
7. Radich JP, Oehler V: Monitoring chronic myelogenous leukemia in the age of tyrosine kinase inhibitors. *J Natl Compr Canc Netw* 5:497–504, 2007.
8. Alizadeh AA, Eisen MB, Davis RE, et al: Distinct types of diffuse large B-cell lymphoma identified by gene expression profiling. *Nature* 403:503–511, 2000.
9. Mullighan CG, Su X, Zhang J, et al: Deletion of IKZF1 and prognosis in acute lymphoblastic leukemia. *N Engl J Med* 360:470–480, 2009.
10. Den Boer ML, van Slegtenhorst M, De Menezes RX, et al: A subtype of childhood acute lymphoblastic leukaemia with poor treatment outcome: A genome-wide classification study. *Lancet Oncol* 10:125–134, 2009.
11. Best T, Li D, Skol AD, et al: Variants at 6q21 implicate PRDM1 in the etiology of therapy-induced second malignancies after Hodgkin's lymphoma. *Nat Med* 17:941–943, 2011.
12. Melo JV, Barnes DJ. Chronic myeloid leukaemia as a model of disease evolution in human cancer. *Nat Rev Cancer* 7:441–453, 2007.
13. O'Hare T, Eide CA, Deininger MW. New Bcr-Abl inhibitors in chronic myeloid leukemia: Keeping resistance in check. *Expert Opin Investig Drugs* 17:865–878, 2008.
14. Hughes T, White D: Which TKI? An embarrassment of riches for chronic myeloid leukemia patients. *Hematology Am Soc Hematol Educ Program* 2013:168–175, 2013.
15. Nowak D, Ogawa S, Muschen M, et al: SNP array analysis of tyrosine kinase inhibitor-resistant chronic myeloid leukemia identifies heterogeneous secondary genomic alterations. *Blood* 115:1049–1053, 2010.
16. Deininger MW, Cortes J, Paquette R, et al: The prognosis for patients with chronic myeloid leukemia who have clonal cytogenetic abnormalities in Philadelphia chromosome–negative cells. *Cancer* 110:1509–1519, 2007.

17. Barnes DJ, Melo JV: Cytogenetic and molecular genetic aspects of chronic myeloid leukaemia. *Acta Haematol* 108:180–202, 2002.

18. Tefferi A: Molecular drug targets in myeloproliferative neoplasms: Mutant ABL1, JAK2, MPL, KIT, PDGFRA, PDGFRB and FGFR1. *J Cell Mol Med* 13:215–237, 2009.

19. Adeyinka A, Dewald GW: Cytogenetics of chronic myeloproliferative disorders and related myelodysplastic syndromes. *Hematol Oncol Clin North Am* 17:1129–1149, 2003.

20. Levine RL, Pardanani A, Tefferi A, et al: Role of JAK2 in the pathogenesis and therapy of myeloproliferative disorders. *Nat Rev Cancer* 7:673–683, 2007.

21. Zipperer E, Wulfert M, Germing U, et al: MPL 515 and JAK2 mutation analysis in MDS presenting with a platelet count of more than 500 x 10(9)/l. *Ann Hematol* 87:413–415, 2008.

22. Nangalia J, Massie CE, Baxter EJ, et al: Somatic CALR mutations in myeloproliferative neoplasms with nonmutated JAK2. *N Engl J Med* 369:2391–2405, 2013.

23. Klampfl T, Gisslinger H, Harutyunyan AS, et al: Somatic mutations of calreticulin in myeloproliferative neoplasms. *N Engl J Med* 369:2379–2390, 2013.

24. Vardiman JW, Thiele J, Arber DA, et al: The 2008 revision of the WHO classification of myeloid neoplasms and acute leukemia: Rationale and important changes. *Blood* 114:937–951, 2009.

25. Olney HJ, Le Beau MM: Evaluation of recurring cytogenetic abnormalities in the treatment of myelodysplastic syndromes. *Leuk Res* 31:427–434, 2007.

26. Greenberg PL, Tuechler H, Schanz J, et al: Revised international prognostic scoring system for myelodysplastic syndromes. *Blood* 120:2454–2465, 2012.

27. Nimer SD: Clinical management of myelodysplastic syndromes with interstitial deletion of chromosome 5q. *J Clin Oncol* 24:2576–2582, 2006.

28. Tiu RV, Gondek LP, O'Keefe CL, et al: Prognostic impact of SNP array karyotyping in myelodysplastic syndromes and related myeloid malignancies. *Blood* 117:4552–4560, 2011.

29. Makishima H, Maciejewski JP: Pathogenesis and consequences of uniparental disomy in cancer. *Clin Cancer Res* 17:3913–3923, 2011.

30. Haase D, Germing U, Schanz J, et al: New insights into the prognostic impact of the karyotype in MDS and correlation with subtypes: Evidence from a core dataset of 2124 patients. *Blood* 110:4385–4395, 2007.

31. Schanz J, Tuchler H, Sole F, et al: New comprehensive cytogenetic scoring system for primary myelodysplastic syndromes (MDS) and oligoblastic acute myeloid leukemia after MDS derived from an international database merge. *J Clin Oncol* 30:820–829, 2012.

32. Mrozek K, Bloomfield CD: Clinical significance of the most common chromosome translocations in adult acute myeloid leukemia. *J Natl Cancer Inst Monogr* (39):52–57, 2008.

33. Mrozek K, Marcucci G, Paschka P, et al: Advances in molecular genetics and treatment of core-binding factor acute myeloid leukemia. *Curr Opin Oncol* 20:711–718, 2008.

34. Mistry AR, Pedersen EW, Solomon E, et al: The molecular pathogenesis of acute promyelocytic leukaemia: Implications for the clinical management of the disease. *Blood Rev* 17:71–97, 2003.

35. Olney HJ, Mitelman F, Johansson B, et al: Unique balanced chromosome abnormalities in treatment-related myelodysplastic syndromes and acute myeloid leukemia: Report from an international workshop. *Genes Chromosomes Cancer* 33:413–423, 2002.

36. Krivtsov AV, Armstrong SA. MLL translocations, histone modifications and leukaemia stem-cell development. *Nat Rev Cancer* 7:823–833, 2007.

37. Farag SS, Archer KJ, Mrozek K, et al: Isolated trisomy of chromosomes 8, 11, 13 and 21 is an adverse prognostic factor in adults with de novo acute myeloid leukemia: Results from Cancer and Leukemia Group B 8461. *Int J Oncol* 21:1041–1051, 2002.

38. Dohner K, Dohner H: Molecular characterization of acute myeloid leukemia. *Haematologica* 93:976–982, 2008.

39. Bacher U, Haferlach T, Kern W, et al: A comparative study of molecular mutations in 381 patients with myelodysplastic syndrome and in 4130 patients with acute myeloid leukemia. *Haematologica* 92:744–752, 2007.

40. Falini B, Mecucci C, Tiacci E, et al: Cytoplasmic nucleophosmin in acute myelogenous leukemia with a normal karyotype. *N Engl J Med* 352:254–266, 2005.

41. Christiansen DH, Andersen MK, Pedersen-Bjergaard J: Methylation of p15INK4B is common, is associated with deletion of genes on chromosome arm 7q and predicts a poor prognosis in therapy-related myelodysplasia and acute myeloid leukemia. *Leukemia* 17:1813–1819, 2003.

42. Cancer Genome Atlas Research Network: Genomic and epigenomic landscapes of adult de novo acute myeloid leukemia. *N Engl J Med* 368:2059–2074, 2013.

43. Patel JP, Gonen M, Figueroa ME, et al: Prognostic relevance of integrated genetic profiling in acute myeloid leukemia. *N Engl J Med* 366:1079–1089, 2012.

44. Churpek JE, Lorenz R, Nedumgottil S, et al: Proposal for the clinical detection and management of patients and their family members with familial myelodysplastic syndrome/acute leukemia predisposition syndromes. *Leuk Lymphoma* 54:28–35, 2013.

45. Nickels EM, Soodalter J, Churpek JE, et al: Recognizing familial myeloid leukemia in adults. *Ther Adv Hematol* 4:254–269, 2013.

46. West AH, Godley LA, Churpek JE. Familial myelodysplastic syndrome/acute leukemia syndromes: A review and utility for translational investigations. *Ann N Y Acad Sci* 1310:111–118, 2014.

47. Taskesen E, Bullinger L, Corbacioglu A, et al: Prognostic impact, concurrent genetic mutations, and gene expression features of AML with CEBPA mutations in a cohort of 1182 cytogenetically normal AML patients: Further evidence for CEBPA double mutant AML as a distinctive disease entity. *Blood* 117:2469–2475, 2011.

48. Udani R, Parlow M, Yin L, et al: *Novel Germline CEBPA Sequence Variations in Familial AML and Cytogenetically Normal AML.* American Society of Hematology Conference 2012, Atlanta, GA, December, 2012.

49. Pabst T, Eyholzer M, Fos J, et al: Heterogeneity within AML with CEBPA mutations; only CEBPA double mutations, but not single CEBPA mutations are associated with favourable prognosis. *Br J Cancer* 100:1343–1346, 2009.

50. Pabst T, Mueller BU: Complexity of CEBPA dysregulation in human acute myeloid leukemia. *Clin Cancer Res* 15:5303–5307, 2009.

51. Renneville A, Mialou V, Philippe N, et al: Another pedigree with familial acute myeloid leukemia and germline CEBPA mutation. *Leukemia* 23:804–806, 2009.

52. ACMG Board of Directors: Points to consider in the clinical application of genomic sequencing. *Genet Med* 14:759–761, 2012.

53. Green RC, Berg JS, Grody WW, et al: ACMG recommendations for reporting of incidental findings in clinical exome and genome sequencing. *Genet Med* 15:565–574, 2013.

54. Godley LA, Larson RA: Therapy-related myeloid leukemia. *Semin Oncol* 35:418–429, 2008.

55. Smith SM, Le Beau MM, Huo D, et al: Clinical-cytogenetic associations in 306 patients with therapy-related myelodysplasia and myeloid leukemia: The University of Chicago series. *Blood* 102:43–52, 2003.

56. Pedersen-Bjergaard J, Andersen MK, Christiansen DH: Therapy-related acute myeloid leukemia and myelodysplasia after high-dose chemotherapy and autologous stem cell transplantation. *Blood* 95:3273–3279, 2000.

57. Lai F, Godley LA, Joslin J, et al: Transcript map and comparative analysis of the 1.5-Mb commonly deleted segment of human 5q31 in malignant myeloid diseases with a del(5q). *Genomics* 71:235–245, 2001.

58. Boultwood J, Fidler C, Strickson AJ, et al: Narrowing and genomic annotation of the commonly deleted region of the 5q-syndrome. *Blood* 99:4638–4641, 2002.

59. Joslin JM, Fernald AA, Tennant TR, et al: Haploinsufficiency of EGR1, a candidate gene in the del(5q), leads to the development of myeloid disorders. *Blood* 110:719–726, 2007.

60. Ebert BL, Pretz J, Bosco J, et al: Identification of RPS14 as a 5q– syndrome gene by RNA interference screen. *Nature* 451:335–339, 2008.

61. Lindsley RC, Ebert BL: Molecular pathophysiology of myelodysplastic syndromes. *Annu Rev Pathol* 8:21–47, 2013.

62. Stoddart A, Fernald AA, Wang J, et al: Haploinsufficiency of del(5q) genes, Egr1 and Apc, cooperate with Tp53 loss to induce acute myeloid leukemia in mice. *Blood* 123:1069–1078, 2014.

63. Harrison CJ. Cytogenetics of paediatric and adolescent acute lymphoblastic leukaemia. *Br J Haematol* 144:147–156, 2009.

64. Schultz KR, Pullen DJ, Sather HN, et al: Risk- and response-based classification of childhood B-precursor acute lymphoblastic leukemia: A combined analysis of prognostic markers from the Pediatric Oncology Group (POG) and Children's Cancer Group (CCG). *Blood* 109:926–935, 2007.

65. Wetzler M, Dodge RK, Mrozek K, et al: Additional cytogenetic abnormalities in adults with Philadelphia chromosome–positive acute lymphoblastic leukaemia: A study of the Cancer and Leukaemia Group B. *Br J Haematol* 124:275–288, 2004.

66. van der Veer A, Zaliova M, Mottadelli F, et al: IKZF1 status as a prognostic feature in BCR-ABL1–positive childhood ALL. *Blood* 123:1691–1698, 2014.

67. Pui CH, Chessells JM, Camitta B, et al: Clinical heterogeneity in childhood acute lymphoblastic leukemia with 11q23 rearrangements. *Leukemia* 17:700–706, 2003.

68. Rubnitz JE, Downing JR, Pui CH, et al: TEL gene rearrangement in acute lymphoblastic leukemia: A new genetic marker with prognostic significance. *J Clin Oncol* 15:1150–1157, 1997.

69. Sutcliffe MJ, Shuster JJ, Sather HN, et al: High concordance from independent studies by the Children's Cancer Group (CCG) and Pediatric Oncology Group (POG) associating favorable prognosis with combined trisomies 4, 10, and 17 in children with NCI Standard-Risk B-precursor Acute Lymphoblastic Leukemia: A Children's Oncology Group (COG) initiative. *Leukemia* 19:734–740, 2005.

70. Faderl S, Jeha S, Kantarjian HM: The biology and therapy of adult acute lymphoblastic leukemia. *Cancer* 98:1337–1354, 2003.

71. Roberts KG, Morin RD, Zhang J, et al: Genetic alterations activating kinase and cytokine receptor signaling in high-risk acute lymphoblastic leukemia. *Cancer Cell* 22:153–166, 2012.

72. Graux C, Cools J, Michaux L, et al: Cytogenetics and molecular genetics of T-cell acute lymphoblastic leukemia: From thymocyte to lymphoblast. *Leukemia* 20:1496–1510, 2006.

73. Caporaso N, Goldin L, Plass C, et al: Chronic lymphocytic leukaemia genetics overview. *Br J Haematol* 139:630–634, 2007.

74. Hagenkord JM, Monzon FA, Kash SF, et al: Array-based karyotyping for prognostic assessment in chronic lymphocytic leukemia: Performance comparison of Affymetrix 10K2.0, 250K Nsp, and SNP6.0 arrays. *J Mol Diagn* 12:184–196, 2010.

75. Zenz T, Mertens D, Dohner H, et al: Molecular diagnostics in chronic lymphocytic leukemia-pathogenetic and clinical implications. *Leuk Lymphoma* 49:864–873, 2008.

76. Crespo M, Bosch F, Villamor N, et al: ZAP-70 expression as a surrogate for immunoglobulin-variable-region mutations in chronic lymphocytic leukemia. *N Engl J Med* 348:1764–1775, 2003.

77. Morilla A, Gonzalez de Castro D, Del Giudice I, et al: Combinations of ZAP-70, CD38 and IGHV mutational status as predictors of time to first treatment in CLL. *Leuk Lymphoma* 49:2108–2115, 2008.

78. Campbell LJ: Cytogenetics of lymphomas. *Pathology* 37:493–507, 2005.

79. Lenz G, Wright GW, Emre NC, et al: Molecular subtypes of diffuse large B-cell lymphoma arise by distinct genetic pathways. *Proc Natl Acad Sci U S A* 105:13520–13525, 2008.

80. Haralambieva E, Boerma EJ, van Imhoff GW, et al: Clinical, immunophenotypic, and genetic analysis of adult lymphomas with morphologic features of Burkitt lymphoma. *Am J Surg Pathol* 29:1086–1094, 2005.

81. Viardot A, Barth TF, Moller P, et al: Cytogenetic evolution of follicular lymphoma. *Semin Cancer Biol* 13:183–190, 2003.

82. Bertoni F, Zucca E, Cotter FE: Molecular basis of mantle cell lymphoma. *Br J Haematol* 124:130–140, 2004.

83. Chng WJ, Glebov O, Bergsagel PL, et al: Genetic events in the pathogenesis of multiple myeloma. *Best Pract Res Clin Haematol* 20:571–596, 2007.

84. Pasqualucci L, Migliazza A, Basso K, et al: Mutations of the BCL6 proto-oncogene disrupt its negative autoregulation in diffuse large B-cell lymphoma. *Blood* 101:2914–2923, 2003.

85. Starostik P, Patzner J, Greiner A, et al: Gastric marginal zone B-cell lymphomas of MALT type develop along 2 distinct pathogenetic pathways. *Blood* 99:3–9, 2002.

86. Chiarle R, Voena C, Ambrogio C, et al: The anaplastic lymphoma kinase in the pathogenesis of cancer. *Nat Rev Cancer* 8:11–23, 2008.

87. Shaughnessy JD Jr, Zhan F, Burington BE, et al: A validated gene expression model of high-risk multiple myeloma is defined by deregulated expression of genes mapping to chromosome 1. *Blood* 109:2276–2284, 2007.

88. Avet-Loiseau H, Li C, Magrangeas F, et al: Prognostic significance of copy-number alterations in multiple myeloma. *J Clin Oncol* 27:4585–4590, 2009.

89. Rasmussen T, Kuehl M, Lodahl M, et al: Possible roles for activating RAS mutations in the MGUS to MM transition and in the intramedullary to extramedullary transition in some plasma cell tumors. *Blood* 105:317–323, 2005.

CHAPTER 14
METABOLISM OF HEMATOLOGIC NEOPLASTIC CELLS

Zandra E. Walton, Annie L. Hsieh, and Chi V. Dang

SUMMARY

The quantum physicist Erwin Schrodinger surmised in his monograph "What is Life?" that the organized matter known as *life* needs to feed on "negative entropy" to avoid decay.[1] He concluded that this feeding on negative entropy is achieved through metabolism, a term derived from Greek that describes an exchange of materials. Because of this centrality to life, metabolism's core pathways—glycolysis and respiration—evolved early in Earth's history and are highly conserved. At every stage of life, metabolism provides the needed nutrients, energy, and building blocks. Embryogenesis, for instance, requires metabolism of maternally derived nutrients to support cellular repair, growth, division, and differentiation. In particular, cell replication requires that the instructions emanating from the DNA sequence, modulated by the epigenome, couple with the import of nutrients and metabolic pathways to produce the components and energy necessary to build two copies of a cell and maintain high replication fidelity of the genome. During growth and development, and especially during adulthood, metabolism also plays the important role of providing bioenergetics for cellular and organismal homeostasis. Metabolism can also feature prominently in disease, and this chapter discusses how the metabolic pathways central to life and normal biology can be subverted in cancer to fuel abnormal growth.

Food, through metabolism, provides the nutrients necessary for homeostasis, repair, and reproduction of many organisms. To align supply and demand, mammalian metabolism is linked to sleep cycles through the central circadian clock that senses light and dark phases of the day via the eye and central nervous system. The central regulation of feeding and sleeping cycles coordinates nutrient availability from food with the circadian oscillation of metabolism of individual cells, which all have a molecular clock comprised of a network of transcription factors that regulates cell metabolism.[2]

Food is digested, absorbed through the gastrointestinal tract, and in part processed or stored in the liver, which is a key metabolic organ.[3] Processed lipids in the form of lipoproteins are synthesized in the liver and disseminated throughout to supply the needs of various organs. Amino acids, with glutamine circulating at the highest level (0.5 mM), supply cells with building blocks for proteins. Some amino acids (nonessential) are synthesized by humans, but essential amino acids must be available from the diet. Complex carbohydrates are broken down and circulate as glucose, a vital nutrient for virtually all mammalian cells. In this regard, an endocrine system (insulin and glucagon) has evolved to control the circulating levels of this precious bioenergetic molecule. When in excess, amino acids and sugars contribute to lipogenesis, and the extra energy is stored as fat depots in adipose tissues. Excess glucose is stored as glycogen, which is deployed to release glucose in starved conditions. It is believed that, during our evolution, periods of gorging and feeding were separated by significant durations of starvation; hence, we have evolved mechanisms to survive starvation.

In contrast to the fed state, when insulin level increases in response to rising glucose to trigger cellular glucose uptake and storage, the starved state triggers glucagon secretion from the pancreas, which mobilizes cellular glycogen stores as nutrient. Prolonged starvation depletes liver and muscle glycogen stores—the only major glycogen stores—and prompts the mobilization of fat stores. The released fatty acids provide glycerol as a substrate for making glucose through gluconeogenic pathways and fatty acids for mitochondrial oxidation. Further prolonged starvation triggers the liver to convert fatty acids to ketone bodies, which can cross the blood–brain barrier to feed

Acronyms and Abbreviations: ABC, activated B-cell type; ALL, acute lymphoid leukemia; AML, acute myeloid leukemia; AMPK, adenosine monophosphate kinase; ASCT2, ASC amino-acid transporter 2; ATRA, all-*trans* retinoic acid; BPTES, a glutaminase inhibitor; CDK, cyclin-dependent kinase; CL, cardiolipin; COO, cell of origin; DFMO, a-difluoromethylornithine; DLBCL, diffuse large B-cell lymphoma; eIF5A, eukaryotic translation initiation factor; ERK, extracellular regulated kinase; ETC, mitochondrial electron transport chain; Ets, E26, E twenty-six; F1,6BP, fructose 1,6 biphosphate; F2,6BP, fructose 2,6 biphosphate; FAO, fatty acid oxidation; FDG-PET, fluorodeoxyglucose positron emission tomography; FH, fumarate hydratase; FOS, a protooncogene; G3P, glycerol 3-phosphate; G6PD, glucose-6-phosphate dehydrogenase; GAP, glyceraldehyde 3-phosphate; GCB, germinal center B-cell type; GDP, guanosine-5'-diphosphate; GLS, glutaminase; GLUT, glucose transporter; GM-CSF, granulocyte-macrophage colony-stimulating factor; GOT, glutamate oxaloacetate transaminase; GPI, glucose phosphate isomerase; GPT, glutamate pyruvate transaminase; GTP, guanosine-5'-triphosphate; 2-HG, 2-hydroxyglutarate; HIF, hypoxia-inducible factor; HSC, hematopoietic stem cell; IDH, isocitrate dehydrogenase; IMPDH, inosine monophosphate dehydrogenase; LDHA, lactate dehydrogenase A; LKB1, Liver kinase B1; LSC, leukemic stem cell; Max, Myc-associated factor X; MDM2, mouse double minute 2 homolog; Miz-1, Myc-interacting zinc finger protein 1; MLL2, mixed-lineage leukemia protein 2; Mlx, Max-like protein X; MondoA, member of the MYC network of transcription factors that upregulates glycolysis (known as MLXIP, MLX interacting protein); mTOR, mammalian target of rapamycin; mTORC1, mTOR complex 1; MYC, a protooncogene that is a major regulator of cell growth and metabolism; NADH, nicotinamide adenine dinucleotide; NADPH, nicotinamide adenine dinucleotide phosphate; NAMPT, nicotinamide phosphoribosyltransferase; NRF2, nuclear respiratory factor-2; NTP, nucleotide triphosphate; ODC, ornithine decarboxylase; OGDH, oxoglutarate dehydrogenase; OXPHOS, oxidative phosphorylation; $_p$53, activates oxidative phosphorylation and inhibits glycolysis; PC, phosphatidyl choline; PDH, pyruvate dehydrogenase; PDK, pyruvate dehydrogenase kinase; PE, phosphatidyl ethanolamine; PEP, phosphoenol pyruvate; PFK, phosphofructokinase; PG, glycerophosphoglycerol; PGC1a, an activator of mitochondrial biogenesis; PI, phosphatidyl inositol; PI3K, phosphoinositol 3'-kinase; PML, promyelocytic leukemia; PRPS, 5-phosphoribosyl-pyrophosphate synthetase; PS, phosphatidyl serine; PTEN, phosphatase and tensin homologue deleted on chromosome 10, an antioncogene; RAS, name given to a family of related proteins belonging to small GTPase involved in signal transduction; ROS, reactive oxygen species; rRNA, ribosomal RNA; SAM, S-adenosylmethionine; SCO_2, cytochrome c oxidase; SDH, succinate dehydrogenase; SLC1A5, ASC amino-acid transporter 2; SOD, superoxide dismutase; TCA, tricarboxylic acid; TET, family of dioxygenases that catalyze conversion of 5-methylcytosine to 5-hydroxymethylcytosine; TFEB, transcription factor EB; THF, tetrahydrofolate; VHL, von Hippel-Lindau protein.

the brain. How whole organisms initiate autophagy (self-eating) during markedly prolonged starvation has not been thoroughly studied. But autophagy is clearly necessary for mammalian development, particularly upon birth when deletion of specific autophagic regulators results in death.[4] Although autophagy plays an important role in mitochondrial and organellar homeostasis and cancer metabolism, it is discussed in Chap. 15; this chapter focuses primarily on intermediary metabolism.

Although most of our cells are differentiated and do not proliferate, stem cell compartments are ubiquitous among tissues, allowing for replacement of used or damaged cells. The hematopoietic stem cell and hematopoiesis constitute probably the best-studied stem cell system.[5] Cytokines, growth factors, and the extracellular matrix provide the cues for stem cells to maintain their quiescent state or to awaken and differentiate to replenish lost cells. In response to growth factors in the presence of nutrient-replete states, stem cells self-renew, proliferate, and then differentiate. In nutrient-deprived states, normal metabolic checkpoints forbid growth factor stimulated cells from proliferating.[6] All of the mechanisms used by normal cells during fed and starved states are potentially exploitable by neoplastic cells for their survival. Genetic mutations drive neoplastic cells to grow and proliferate regardless of the availability of nutrients; in contrast, normal cells sense nutrients and do not proliferate under starved conditions. In this chapter, basic cell metabolism is covered along with discussions about growth signaling and its intersection with metabolism. Alterations in metabolism found in hematologic neoplastic cells are discussed in the context of therapeutic opportunities that are rapidly emerging from the latest basic research and translational efforts.

● CELL GROWTH AND METABOLISM

HOMEOSTASIS

The canonical cell has significant bioenergetic needs for maintenance and homeostasis.[6] Protein synthesis and maintenance of cellular membrane potentials consume most of the ATP produced under homeostatic conditions.[7] In many differentiated or quiescent cells, it is believed that fatty acid oxidation provides the bulk of the energy, followed by the use of glucose. In this regard, mitochondrial respiration is essential for adult tissues and cells. It is notable, however, that specialized cell functions in the various organs could require different metabolic pathways. Glucocorticoid hormone-producing cells, for example, express specialized metabolic pathways. Although cardiac muscle cells depend heavily on fatty acid oxidation, skeletal muscle cells use glucose. The brain depends largely on glucose, but it can feed on ketone bodies under starved states. For differentiated cells, which are the bulk of cells in mammals, homeostasis drives the demand for nutrients, to "the availability of which are determined by feeding and interorgan (liver, muscle, and endocrine tissues) metabolic interplays. For example, lactate produced by exercising muscle circulates back to the liver and is processed via the Cori cycle to produce glucose.[3] Glucose plasma level is tightly controlled by the pancreas, which produces insulin and glucagon, and by the liver (as well as kidney) that can produce glucose through gluconeogenesis.

CELL GROWTH: SIGNALING, NUTRIENTS, AND METABOLISM

Normal cell growth and proliferation are triggered by extracellular cues. Yeast cells, for example, only require the presence of nutrients to initiate cell growth or an increase in cell size.[6] During this growth phase, nutrients are imported and channeled into biomass, which is largely

comprised of ribosomes. It is estimated that ribosomes constitute more than 50 percent of cellular dry mass, and hence ribosome biogenesis is highly regulated and vitally important for cell growth and proliferation. Once a critical cell size (mass) is reached with a balanced nucleotide pool, DNA synthesis begins. Yeast cells sense nutrients, particularly glucose and glutamine, through pathways involving RAS and target of rapamycin complex 1 (TORC1), which silence transcriptional repressors of ribosome biogenesis.[8] With nutrient deprivation, activation of these transcriptional repressors provides a metabolic checkpoint that restrains cells from growing in the absence of adequate bioenergetic support. Hence, the normal feedback loops couple nutrient availability with cell growth: no nutrients, no growth. The normal feedback loops can be artificially disrupted by deletion of transcriptional repressors of ribosomal biogenesis, rendering yeast mutants constitutively activated for growth. These mutants resemble mammalian cancer cells, which have mutations that drive autonomous cell growth with disregard for nutrient availability. The severance of nutrient sensing from growth signaling causes addiction of these yeast mutants to nutrients, such that deprivation of glucose or glutamine results in nonviable mutants. Similarly, cancer cells are addicted to nutrients.[6]

Cell growth in multicellular organisms requires additional cues in addition to the availability of nutrients. Mammalian cells live in a community of cells and are constantly bathed in nutrients derived from the circulation, but they do not proliferate unless there are appropriate cues from growth factors and the extracellular matrix. Mammalian cells can be envisioned as bioreactors that require at least two signals to grow: (1) growth factor and (2) nutrients.[6] Cell growth is arrested in the absence of either growth factor or nutrients. Similar to yeast cells, metabolic checkpoints are critical to the growth of normal mammalian cells.

Growing cells largely depend on glucose, glutamine and other amino acids.[9] Indeed, the core metabolic pathways including glycolysis, glutaminolysis, and the tricarboxylic acid (TCA) cycle link amino acid and glucose metabolism to lipogenesis and nucleotide synthesis (Fig. 14–1). Glycolysis starts with the transport of glucose into cells through several transporters, known as GLUTs, with SLC2A1 (GLUT1) being one that is coupled with cell growth stimulation. Once inside the cell, glucose is phosphorylated in an ATP-consuming step by hexokinases (HK) with HKII being stimulated by many growth signals and directly regulated by the MYC oncogene or the hypoxia inducible factor 1 alpha (HIF-1α). Glucose-6-phosphate (G6P) is used by the pentose phosphate pathway to produce ribose for nucleotide synthesis (Fig. 14–1) or converted to fructose phosphate via an isomerization reaction catalyzed by glucose phosphate isomerase (GPI).[9] Fructose-6-phosphate is further phosphorylated with consumption of a second ATP through a rate-limiting step catalyzed by phosphofructokinase (PFK) to fructose-1,6-bisphosphate (F1,6BP). F1,6BP is converted by aldolase and an isomerase to the three-carbon phosphorylated molecule, glyceraldehyde 3-phosphate (GAP), which is oxidized and phosphorylated using inorganic phosphate by the dehydrogenase, GAPDH, to 1,3-bisphosphoglycerate. The energy gained by nicotinamide adenine dinucleotide (NAD+)-mediated oxidation and phosphorylation is released from 1,3-bisphosphoglycerate by phosphoglycerate kinase, which transfers the high-energy phosphate bond to adenosine diphosphate (ADP) to form ATP. The resulting 3-phosphoglycerate (3-PG) provides a substrate for serine and glycine synthesis, for the production of glycerol, or for the production of phosphoenol pyruvate (PEP) in glycolysis. Pyruvate kinase mediates the transfer of the high-energy phosphate bond from PEP to ADP producing ATP and pyruvate, which is the terminal substrate of glycolysis. Collectively, glycolysis uses ATP to charge up several intermediates for their transformations and uses NAD+ to oxidize intermediates and generate energy through new high-energy phosphate bonds with inorganic phosphate. Each glucose molecule results in the production of a net two ATP molecules from ADP through glycolysis.

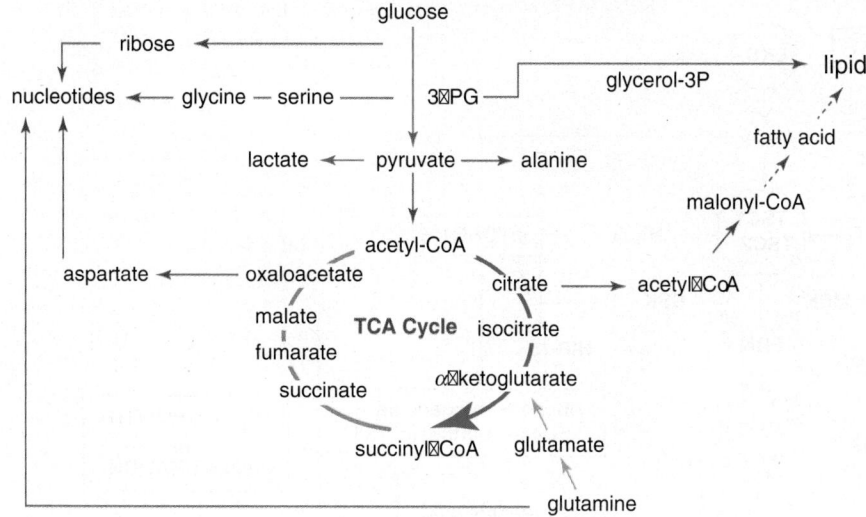

Figure 14–1. Central metabolic pathways involving glycolysis, glutaminolysis, and the tricarboxylic acid *(TCA)* cycle. Glucose is shown metabolized to pyruvate, which can be converted to lactate, alanine, or acetyl-coenzyme A *(acetyl-CoA)*. Upstream of pyruvate, glucose carbons are shunted toward the pentose phosphate pathway for ribose synthesis, glycine, and glycerol synthesis. Acetyl-CoA (2-carbon unit) combines with oxaloacetate (4-carbon) to form citrate (6-carbon), which is subsequently metabolized in the TCA cycle to generate isocitrate, α-ketoglutarate, and other intermediates as depicted. Glutamine is shown to enter the TCA cycle via α-ketoglutarate, after being converted to glutamate. Glucose gives rise to glycerol and citrate, which contributes 2-carbon units for fatty acid synthesis, and contributes to lipid synthesis. Glutamine and glucose are depicted to contribute to nucleotide synthesis.

Pyruvate, derived from glucose through glycolysis, from malate through malic enzyme or from alanine through transamination, could enter the mitochondria through specific transporters and be converted to acetyl-coenzyme A (CoA) by pyruvate dehydrogenase (PDH) (see Fig. 14–1).[10] PDH activity can be attenuated by phosphorylation, mediated by PDH kinase (PDK), which is activated by hypoxia to divert glucose carbons away from the TCA cycle toward lactate production. Under aerobic conditions, acetyl-CoA combines with oxaloacetate coming from a complete turn of the TCA cycle to produce citrate, which can be extruded into the cytoplasm to participate in lipid synthesis or which can be converted to isocitrate in the TCA cycle. Isocitrate is further oxidized to α-ketoglutarate by isocitrate dehydrogenase (IDH) with the production of either nicotinamide adenine dinucleotide (NADH) or nicotinamide adenine dinucleotide phosphate (NADPH) and release of a carbon dioxide molecule. There are three IDH isozymes with IDH1 being located in the cytosol, while IDH2 and IDH3 are in the mitochondrion. NADH in the mitochondrion contributes to the high-energy electrons that drive production of ATP through the electron transport chain. NADPH produced by cytosolic IDH1 or mitochondrial IDH2 could participate in reductive biosynthesis of fatty acids or nucleobases.

In addition to being a key TCA cycle intermediate at the crossroads of several metabolic pathways, a-ketoglutarate (or oxoglutarate) serves as a cofactor for many important oxygenases, such as those involved in the hydroxylation and degradation of the hypoxia inducible factors (HIFs), modification of ribosomes, or those involved in demethylation of DNA and histones.[11,12] Notably, glutamine can enter the TCA cycle at this junction. α-Ketoglutarate is further oxidized by oxoglutarate dehydrogenase (OGDH) to produce succinyl-CoA and carbon dioxide. Succinyl-CoA, which is also used for heme synthesis, is then converted to succinate with the production of a guanosine-5′-triphosphate (GTP) from guanosine-5′-diphosphate (GDP). Succinate is then converted to fumarate by succinate dehydrogenase (SDH), which is mutated in certain familial cancer syndromes. Fumarate hydratase (FH), which is also mutated in cancer syndromes, converts fumarate to malate that is, in turn, converted to oxaloacetate. Oxaloacetate can serve as a substrate for glutamate oxaloacetate transaminase (GOT) for the production of aspartate for nucleotide synthesis, or it can further cycle forward into the TCA cycle by combining with acetyl-CoA to form citrate, thus completing the TCA (citric acid or Krebs) cycle (see Fig. 14–1).

Glutamine also serves as a key metabolic substrate for growing cells (see Fig. 14–1). Glutamine is imported by membrane transporters, such as SLC1A5 or ASCT2.[13,14] Once in the cytosol, glutamine can contribute to protein synthesis or glucosamine or nucleobase biosynthesis by donating its nitrogen. Glutamine is further imported into the mitochondrion and converted to glutamate by glutaminase (GLS) with the release of ammonia. Glutamate is converted to α-ketoglutarate by either glutamate dehydrogenase (primarily in nongrowth states) or aminotransferases (GOT or glutamate pyruvate transaminase [GPT]). In this manner, glutamine serves as a major growth substrate for growing cells. Hence, the TCA cycle is a metabolic roundabout that uses carbons from glucose, glutamine, and fatty acids to generate carbon skeletons for biosynthesis, NADH for the production of ATP, or α-ketoglutarate for catalyzing key oxygenase reactions.

Oxidation of glucose, glutamine, and fatty acids produces energy for growing cells. On the other hand, synthesis of fatty acids and other building blocks require the reductive power of NADPH for bond formation. NADPH is produced from several well-characterized pathways, including the pentose phosphate pathway, malic enzyme, IDH, and the folate pathway.[15] Glucose-6-phosphate dehydrogenase (G6PD) is well-known for its role in oxidation of G6P to 6-phosphogluconolactone and the concurrent reduction of NADP+ to NADPH, which contribute to an antioxidant state through maintaining reduced glutathione. Specifically, loss of G6PD function is associated with severe hemolytic anemia in patients who inherit hypomorphic alleles of G6PD (see Chap. 47). Malic enzyme mediates the oxidation of malate to pyruvate using nicotinamide adenine dinucleotide phosphate (NADP+), which is reduced to NADPH. IDH1 oxidizes isocitrate to α-ketoglutarate with the production of NADPH from NADP+. Lastly, it was recently documented that the folate pathway plays a major role in NADPH production through the oxidation of methylene-tetrahydrofolate (THF) to formyl-THF.[15] The largest consumer of NADPH, on the other hand, involves fatty acid synthesis with reduction of glutathione following closely behind. Thus production of NADPH is critical for both biosynthesis and for redox homeostasis.

● SIGNAL TRANSDUCTION: ONCOGENES, TUMOR SUPPRESSORS AND METABOLISM

Growth factors and nutrients drive the growth and proliferation of cells (Fig. 14–2 and Chap. 17). Growth factor engagement of a (usually dimeric) growth factor receptor triggers allosteric alterations that lead to autophosphorylation, in the case of the receptor tyrosine

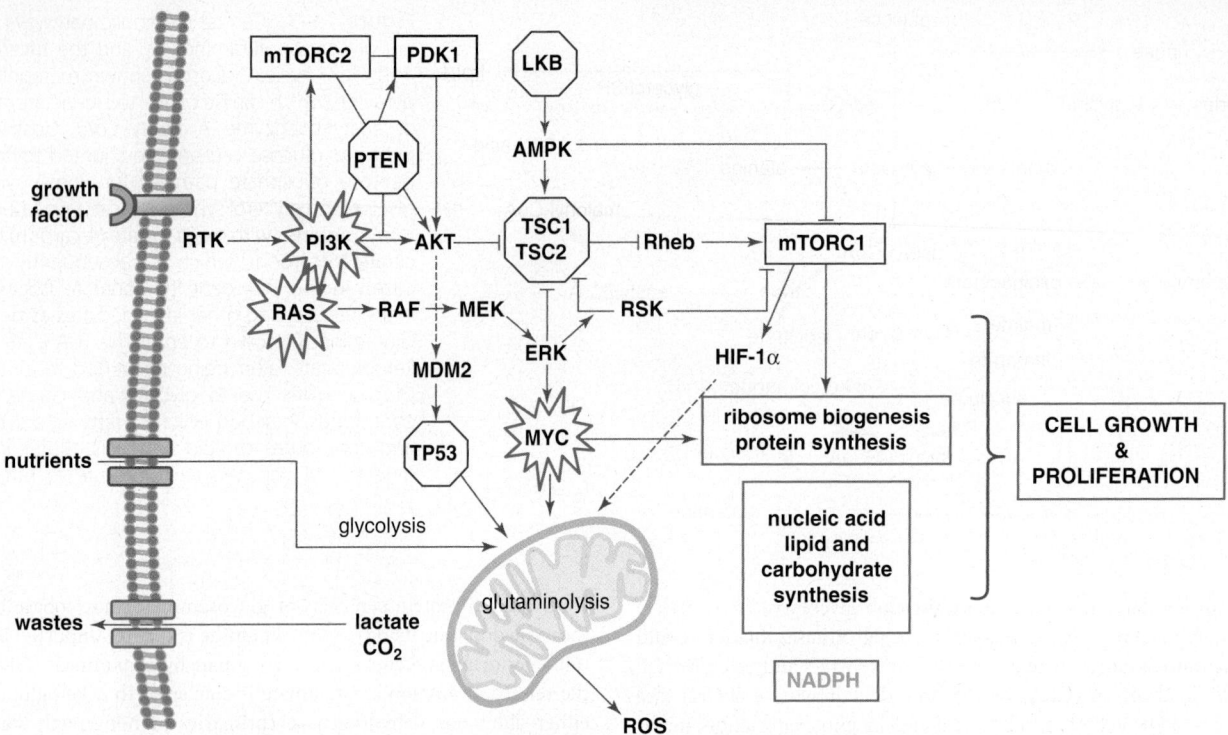

Figure 14–2. Canonical signal transduction pathways emanating from a receptor tyrosine kinase and their connections to metabolism. The phosphoinositol 3'-kinase *(PI3K)-PTEN-Akt* and *Ras-Raf-ERK* (extracellular regulated kinase) pathways are shown with connections to *MYC* and hypoxia-inducible factor 1 *(HIF-1α),* which trigger metabolic transcriptional programs. All of these pathways coordinate a response to growth factors and drive nutrients into the cell to generate ATP and building blocks for lipid, nucleotide, and protein synthesis. The net result is cell growth and generation of waste products, such as reactive oxygen species *(ROS),* lactate and carbon dioxide. Tumor suppressors *(red octagons)* and protooncogenes *(green bursts)* are highlighted.

kinase family, or phosphorylation by Janus kinase in the cases of the hematopoietic cytokine receptor family. The phosphorylated receptor then recruits adaptor molecules that initiate a cascade of phosphorylation events, which culminate in the activation of concurrent pathways through phosphoinositol 3'-kinase (PI3K)/PTEN/AKT and RAS-RAF-ERK (extracellular regulated kinase) (Fig. 14–2). These cascades relay signals to mTOR complex, which is a vital hub for metabolic sensing and short-term post-transcriptional control of cell growth.[16] mTOR, potentially coupled with additional outputs of the RAS-RAF-ERK pathway, also activates a genomic response to the growth signal. In essence, the mTOR pathway provides an immediate response to growth stimulus and nutrients followed thereafter by a transcriptional response that provides an increase in specific mRNAs needed for the production of new building blocks for the growing cell. The initial growth response occurs in cells that have a basal number of ribosomes, which serve to translate delayed early response genes. The cascade down the ERK pathway also activates the expression of early response genes such as FOS and MYC. The activation of MYC is probably mediated through the ERK-activation of Ets transcription factors, whose regulatory motifs are found in the MYC gene.[17] Furthermore, ERK phosphorylates and stabilizes the MYC protein, enhancing ERK's ability to drive a transcriptional response to growth.[18,19]

The immediate sensing of nutrients is mediated through the adenosine monophosphate kinase (AMPK) and mTOR pathways, which, in turn, modulate cellular responses through phosphorylation of regulatory proteins (see Fig. 14–2).[9,16,20] In the presence of nutrients, the import of branched-chain amino acids is sensed through lysosomes to activate mTOR complex 1 (mTORC1). Import of glutamine, which is converted to glutamate, is thought to play an important role in

activating mTOR through the antiporter, SLC7A1, which exports glutamate in exchange for leucine. Leucine is one of the most potent activators of mTORC1, which, in turn, phosphorylates key regulatory proteins to increase protein translation, mitochondrial biogenesis and respiration, glycolysis, and lipogenesis. Many of these effects are also mediated through mTORC1's regulation of transcription factors such as PGC1α (mitochondrial biogenesis), HIF-1α (glycolysis), and SREBP (lipogenesis). mTORC1 also phosphorylates and inactivates the transcription factor TFEB, which is a master positive regulator of lysosome biogenesis.[16] Presumably, inhibition of TFEB would also diminish the machinery involved in autophagy. Although mTORC1 also stimulates ribosome biogenesis, the mechanism by which this occurs is not yet known. Activation of the mTORC2 complex is less well defined, but mTORC2 is responsible for the subsequent activation of AKT that plays a critical role in activating glycolysis. Thus, growth factor signaling stimulates nutrient uptake that in turn activates mTOR to stimulate cell growth.

In nutrient-deprived states, the AMPK pathway regulates cellular responses that optimize energy production and diminish energy utilization pathways (see Fig. 14–2).[20,21] AMPK is allosterically altered by binding to adenosine monophosphate (AMP), which makes AMPK permissive for phosphorylation and activation by the tumor suppressor LKB1. The phosphorylated AMPK in turn phosphorylates and regulates many pathways involved in energy regulation. One of the earliest discoveries was that AMPK phosphorylates and inactivates acetyl-CoA carboxylase, which is involved in fatty acid synthesis. Thus, by diminishing lipogenesis, AMPK is able to inhibit an energy consuming process as well as inhibit cell growth by curbing lipogenesis. AMPK also attenuates protein synthesis through phosphorylation of RNA polymerase I, which is required for ribosome biogenesis. On the other hand, AMPK increases energy yield by stimulating glycolysis through phosphorylation and activation of PFK-2. AMPK stimulates mitochondrial biogenesis through phosphorylation of PGC1α and increases autophagy to recycle energy by phosphorylating ULK-1.[21] Thus, increased AMPK activity conserves energy and maximizes energy production.

Together with posttranscriptional responses to growth signaling and nutrients, the nuclear transcriptional response is necessary to sustain the growth program through production of components of the ribosome and mRNAs that give rise to all other components of the cell. mTOR through its direct activation of specific transcription factors contributes to lipogenesis and mitochondrial biogenesis. Growth signaling also activates the MYC protooncogene, that regulates gene expression broadly to support cell growth and proliferation (see Figs. 14–2 and 14–3).[19] Loss of function of Drosophila dMYC results in decreased cell and body size, a phenotype that underscores MYC's role in cell growth.[22] This phenotype mimics the loss of ribosome protein gene function in a group of mutant flies termed *Minutes*. Hence, *Drosophila* genetics links MYC to cell growth control. Furthermore, MYC is the only transcription factor capable of stimulating the activity of RNA polymerases I, II, and III, all of which are involved in ribosome biogenesis.

MYC dimerizes with its partner Max to bind a specific DNA sequence, termed E-box (CACGTG), and activate transcription.[23] It can also inhibit transcription partly through direct binding to Miz-1 and diminishing the expression of Miz-1 target genes, including the cyclin-dependent kinase (CDK) inhibitor p21 and genes involved in autophagy. Upon MYC activation, it is binding to proximal promoters accounts for most of it is transcriptional function in normal cells. When MYC is experimentally expressed at levels comparable to those found in cancers,[19] excess MYC triggers p53-dependent checkpoints (see Fig. 14–3) that cause cell growth arrest or apoptosis. In multistep tumorigenesis, therefore, p53 is often lost, unleashing MYC's full oncogenic potential. A high, unchecked level of MYC allows it to alter the transcriptome by amplifying selected target genes.[24] MYC was first shown to

directly regulate genes involved in glycolysis, thereby linking an oncogenic transcription factor to metabolism.[6,19] Since these initial observations, high-throughput methods have mapped MYC to a broad swath of metabolic enzyme genes involved in glycolysis, glutaminolysis, and lipogenesis. MYC also directly regulates genes involved in mitochondrial biogenesis and the production of ribosomes. Specifically, genes highly induced by MYC include those involved in nucleolar function and ribosome biogenesis, such as Ncl, NPM1, fibrillarin, and NOP52. Collectively, these studies uncover MYC's role as a central regulator of cell growth through coupling of energy metabolism with cellular biosynthetic processes.

Ribosome biogenesis is a critically important process for cell growth or cell mass accumulation.[25,26] Ribosomes are produced through RNAs that are transcribed by RNA polymerases I (rRNA [ribosomal RNA]), II (mRNA), and III (tRNAs [transfer RNAs] and small RNAs). rRNA is synthesized in the nucleolus from high copy numbers of rDNA, whose chromatin structure and transcription depends on nutrient availability. Under nutrient limitation, rDNA chromatin becomes less accessible, thereby restricting ribosome biogenesis.[26] Ribosomal proteins produced from mRNAs reenter the nucleolus, where components of ribosomes are assembled into mature ribosomal particles, which are exported to the cytosol. The production of rRNAs and proteins also provides an opportunity for bioenergetic sensing of adequate nutrients to support nucleic acid and protein synthesis required for growth. In this regard, specific ribosomal protein subunits (RPL5, RPL11, and others) can bind and inhibit MDM2 (mouse double minute 2 homolog), which binds to and mediates the degradation of p53.[25] Thus, it is surmised that ribosomal proteins in excess of rRNAs would activate p53, triggering checkpoints that block progression through the cell cycle, presumably in response to nutrient limitation sensed as an imbalance in rRNA and ribosomal protein synthesis.

In addition to sensing ribosome biogenesis, p53 also responds to genotoxic stresses by directly regulating metabolism (see Fig. 14–2). P53, in general, activates oxidative phosphorylation and inhibits glycolysis.[27] P53 can activate HK, which phosphorylates glucose in the first step of glycolysis, and stimulate TIGAR that shunts glucose to the pentose phosphate pathway through decreasing the levels of fructose-2,6-bisphosphate (F2,6BP), which allosterically activates PFK. P53 also increases the efficiency of mitochondrial function through induction of cytochrome c oxidase (SCO$_2$).[28] Overall, it appears that the normal function of p53 is to rewire metabolism to mitigate oxidative stress through increased production of NADPH and the antioxidant glutathione. Gain of p53 function through specific mutations, on the other hand, appears to alter metabolism through specific target genes that are involved in cholesterol biosynthesis or phospholipase function.[29,30]

Other tumor suppressors are also involved in metabolism (see Fig. 14–2). PTEN negatively modulates PI3K, and hence its loss stimulates the PI3K pathway that is a potent regulator of cell metabolism through stimulation of glycolysis and activation of mTOR, AKT, MYC, and HIF.[31] The tumor suppressor LKB1, which is lost in some lung cancers, normally activates the AMPK pathway and diminishes lipogenesis.[21] Loss of the von Hippel-Lindau (VHL) tumor suppressor activates HIF, which transcriptionally regulates glucose metabolism.[32] In addition to any direct roles they play in regulating the cell-cycle machinery, tumor suppressors—similar to protooncogenes—also regulate metabolism. By coopting cellular responses to growth factor stimulation in the presence of nutrients, activation of oncogenes and disablement of tumor suppressors achieve coordinated posttranscriptional and transcriptional mobilizations that drive nutrients into ATP production and the building blocks for growing cells.

Growth factor stimulation also results in the production of metabolic wastes and toxins, including carbon dioxide, lactate, and reactive

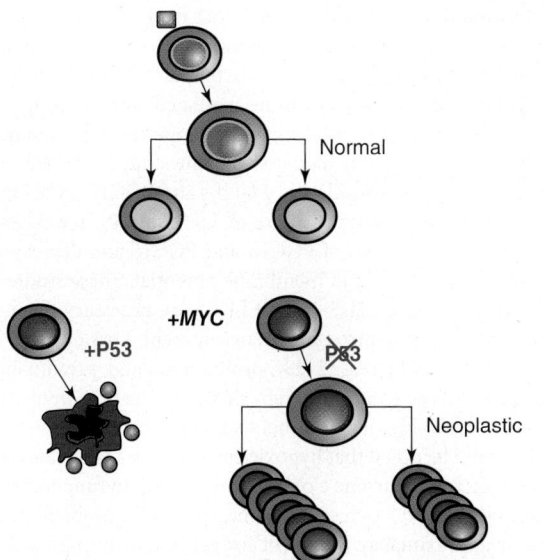

Figure 14–3. Diagram depicting fates of growth factor-stimulated normal cells and MYC transforming cell. Upon engaging a growth factor *(pink square)*, the stimulated cell reacts as a bioreactor, which grows and duplicates itself. MYC overexpression triggers checkpoints via p53, which induces cell death. With loss of p53 MYC's full transforming potential is unleashed through its transcriptional activities.

oxygen species (ROS) (Fig. 14–2). In this regard, various mechanisms have evolved to eliminate these wastes that accumulate as cells discard entropy into the environment after consuming "negative entropy" (macromolecules) to survive and grow. Carbon dioxide and protons are neutralized by carbonic anhydrase. Lactate is exported by monocarboxylate transporters.[33] Reactive oxygen species (ROS) are generated by the mitochondria and other cellular reaction pathways, such as via NADPH oxidases or disulfide bond formation.[34] ROS participates in signaling at ambient levels; however, very high levels of ROS result in oxidative cellular stress.[34,35] In particular, electrons leaking from the mitochondrial electron transport chain (ETC) contribute to a large fraction of cellular ROS.[35] Electrons are donated to the chain by NADH or succinate at mitochondrial complexes I, II, and III, which all generate ROS. Complexes I and II release ROS into the mitochondrial matrix, whereas complex III releases ROS into space on both sides of the inner mitochondrial membrane. Complex I accepts electrons from NADH, which is generated from TCA cycle oxidation, and passes them on to ubiquinone or coenzyme Q that also accepts electrons from succinate via complex II (SDH). Coenzyme Q then passes electrons to complex III, which, in turn, passes them onto cytochrome c. Finally, electrons are passed from cytochrome c to complex IV or cytochrome c oxidase that generates water from electrons, protons, and oxygen, which serves as the final electron acceptor. Upon accepting electrons at complexes I, III, and IV, a proton is pumped into the intermembrane space, creating a proton gradient across the inner mitochondrial membrane. The proton gradient is dissipated through complex V or ATP synthase with the generation of ATP from ADP. During the process of making ATP, leakage of electrons from complexes I, II, and III generates superoxide from oxygen.

Superoxide is highly reactive and could damage membranes and proteins if unattenuated. Hence, superoxide dismutases (SODs) have evolved to convert superoxide to hydrogen peroxide, which is, in turn, neutralized by catalases and converted to water and oxygen. In addition to enzymatic ROS neutralizers, the family of peroxiredoxins also plays an important role in titrating mitochondrial and cytosolic ROS by neutralizing hydrogen peroxide. Because oxidative stress imposed by ROS is a part of normal metabolism, a system of cellular response to this stress has evolved. Immediate response to ROS is mediated by SOD, catalase, peroxiredoxins, and glutathione. A sustained response to ROS is mediated chiefly through NRF2, which is a transcription factor that is negatively regulated by KEAP1, a protein that is directly inhibited by oxidative modification of sensitive cysteine residues.[36] NRF2 activates many genes involved in redox homeostasis, including SODs and catalase. Intriguingly, KEAP1 has been identified as a tumor suppressor in human cancers, illustrating that increased NRF2 activity or antioxidant response is protumorigenic in the setting of heightened metabolic rates and oxidative stress.

METABOLISM AND THE EPIGENOME

Cells have evolved a genome that mediates posttranscriptional and transcriptional mechanisms to import nutrients and harness energy and building blocks for the growing cell. In turn, metabolic intermediates generated from various nutrients can modulate gene expression, seemingly as an adaptive response to the metabolic milieu.[37–39] The epigenome is richly regulated by metabolic intermediates such as acetyl-CoA, S-adenosylmethionine (SAM), α-ketoglutarate, NAD+, and N-acetylglucosamine.[40] Acetyl-CoA mediates histone acetylation and modulates gene expression by rendering the genome accessible to specific transcriptional factors. SAM permits methylation of histones and DNA to prevent access of the transcriptional machinery to certain DNA sequences. α-Ketoglutarate serves as a cofactor for histone and DNA demethylation reactions, thereby countering the modifications

provided by SAM. NAD+ serves as a cofactor for sirtuins that play a key role in histone deacetylation. N-acetylglucosamine, which is produced from glucose and glutamine, serves to modify histones. Other metabolic intermediates such as propionate, butyrate, formate, and crotonate also play a role in modifying histones, which have emerged as the metabolic sensor for gene expression.[40]

The evolution of cancers is not only driven by hard-wired somatic DNA mutations and predisposing germline alleles but also by erasable covalent modifications of DNA and histones. A deregulated epigenetic regulatory system, which randomly silences or makes more accessible portions of the genome, could enhance the adaptability of cancer cells and thus provide a selection advantage that does not require DNA mutations. In this regard, deep sequencing of human cancers, particularly leukemias, has revealed that chromatin-modifying proteins, such as MLL2 (mixed-lineage leukemia protein 2), are frequently mutated at the somatic level.[41,42] Thus, somatic mutations in chromatin modifiers are surmised to increase the degrees of freedom for cancer cell adaptation to the dynamic tumor microenvironment and permit tumor progression.

● HEMATOLOGIC NEOPLASMS AND METABOLISM

Normal hematopoietic stem cells (HSCs) and committed multipotent progenitor cells appear to have different metabolic programs, which may be adopted in the neoplastic state. The HSC resides in a hypoxic environment, and hence low mitochondrial mass and high glycolytic rates appear favored for survival. One of the mechanisms by which the hypoxic HSC niche induces stem cell quiescence is through HIF-1α and inhibits, which transactivates genes involved in glycolysis and inhibits DNA replication.[32] Two studies of HSCs documented that HIF-1α is essential for the quiescent state, such that deletion of HIF-1α resulted in HSC proliferation and depletion of the HSC compartment.[43,44] Conversely, loss of VHL stabilized HIF-1α resulted in an expansion of the HSCs incapable of replenishing hematopoietic cells, resulting in cytopenia. Intriguingly, three studies showed that the LKB1 tumor suppressor also plays a role in HSC quiescence; loss of LKB1 resulted in cell proliferation and loss of the HSC compartment.[45–47] Interestingly, loss of LKB1 in HSCs does not seem to be mediated solely through AMPK, as loss of AMPK in HSCs did not phenocopy the HSC nonquiescent phenotype seen with LKB1 loss. Instead, one study identified the mitochondrial biogenesis coregulators, PGC1α and PGC1β, as being central to the LKB1 loss phenotype.[45] Loss of LKB1 in HSCs was associated with decreased expression of PGC1α and PGC1β and decreased mitochondrial DNA content and membrane potential. These studies collectively suggest that both HIF-1α and LKB1 are necessary for induction of quiescence by the hypoxic microenvironment. Loss of either HIF-1α or LKB1 resulted in increased HSC proliferation and, presumably, commitment toward progenitors, thereby depleting the HSC pool. Although the hypoxic HSC microenvironment suggests that glycolysis predominates, it should be noted that hypoxic cells can still respire and consume oxygen. In fact, cytochrome c oxidase only ceases to function at oxygen tension well below 0.5 percent (as compared to the ambient 21 percent oxygen or approximately 6 percent oxygen found in perfused normal tissues). As such, the observation that loss of LKB1 is associated with a mitochondriopathy in HSCs suggests that mitochondrial function is essential for HSC maintenance, and may resolve the paradox that HSCs seems to rely also on glutamine oxidation (Fig. 14–4).

The HSC uses symmetric commitment to replenish and maintain the stem cell pool and asymmetric division for the generation of committed progenitors (see Fig. 14–4). HIF-1α and LKB1 appear to play a

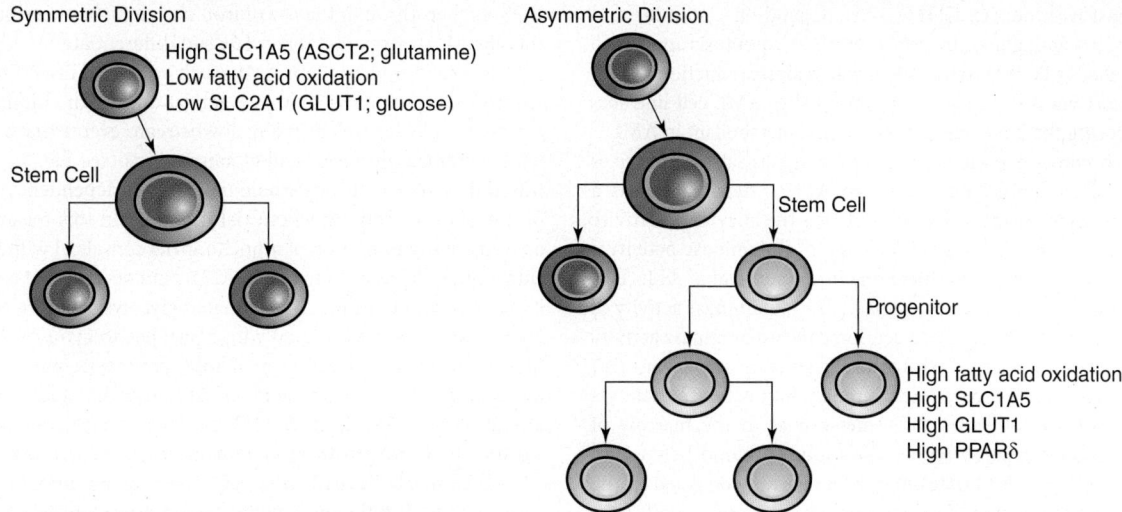

Figure 14–4. Metabolic features of hematopoietic stem cells undergoing symmetric and asymmetric division. Some of these features appear to be preserved in leukemic stem cells.

role in maintaining symmetric commitment. Fatty acid and glutamine oxidation, which requires mitochondrial function, may be required for asymmetric commitment toward progenitors. Surprisingly, despite anticipated HIF-mediated upregulation of glycolysis, the inducible glucose transporter GLUT1 is not highly expressed in HSCs and is only expressed upon differentiation.[48] Instead, the glutamine transporter ASCT2 (SLC1A5) is more highly expressed in HSCs, suggesting that glutamine oxidation via the TCA cycle unexpectedly plays a role in hypoxic stem cell metabolism. Consistent with the notion that hypoxic cells continue to respire, recent studies with human B cells or fibroblasts illustrate this capacity to oxidize glutamine in hypoxia when glucose is largely shunted away from the TCA cycle as lactate.[49,50] Interestingly, glutamine metabolism also appears to influence cell fate. For example, persistent glutamine metabolism in HSCs seems required for erythroid differentiation as glutamine deprivation blunts erythroid nucleotide synthesis and favors differentiation toward the myelomonocytic lineage even in the presence of erythropoietin.[48] Fatty acid oxidation, on the other hand, appears to be necessary for asymmetric division. Activation of peroxisome proliferator-activated receptor (PPAR)-δ, which augments mitochondrial function and fatty acid oxidation through the promyelocytic leukemia (PML)-PPARδ–fatty acid oxidation (FAO) pathway, increases asymmetric stem cell division, whereas inhibition of FAO enhances symmetric stem cell commitment.[51] These findings suggest that mitochondrial oxidation of fatty acids and glutamine may play a role in asymmetric division and lineage commitment, while hypoxia-promoted glycolysis and, surprisingly, glutamine oxidation may be associated with the quiescent HSC pool. How these metabolic cues may affect cellular states through the epigenome is not yet known, however.

LEUKEMIAS

The history of the treatment of acute lymphocytic leukemia (ALL) underscores the importance of metabolism in our understanding of cancer. In fact, the first antimetabolite drug effective against any cancer, 4-aminopteroylglutamic acid (aminopterin), disrupts folate metabolism, which is intimately tied to NADPH production and nucleotide biosynthesis.[52] The dependency of ALL on asparagine also provided a therapeutic opportunity through the use of L-asparaginase, which depletes plasma asparagine from patients.[53] The use of these antimetabolites

led to the current state of therapy in which more than 90 percent of children with ALL achieve complete a substantial improvement from the uniformly lethal disease it presented as 60 years ago. Despite this remarkable clinical progress, our understanding of metabolism in acute leukemias is still rudimentary. However, advances in metabolomics and next-generation DNA sequencing have revealed new insights that provide additional texture to this understanding.

Leukemias have diverse oncogenic drivers, with many chromosomal translocations found in ALLs and some acute myelogenous leukemias (AMLs).[54,55] Whatever the oncogenic driver may be, the leukemic cells share common central metabolic pathways that support growth and replication, particularly glycolysis, glutaminolysis, and FAO (see Fig. 14–1). However, the fluxes through each of these pathways are likely different and dependent on the genomic alterations that are hardwired by mutations. Much of our current understanding comes from *in vitro* studies of leukemic cell lines that have revealed their high glycolytic rates and use of glutamine. Many early studies, including those of Otto Warburg, revealed that leukemic cells have very high rates of conversion of glucose to lactate.[56] Recent studies extend these observations; specifically, high glycolytic rates in primary and relapsed AML correlate with resistance to all *trans*-retinoic acid (ATRA). For these cases better overall survival and attainment of complete remission are achieved with induction chemotherapy.[57] Another study documents that primary childhood ALLs have gene expression profiles that suggest increased glycolysis and decreased oxidative phosphorylation and FAO.[58] Gene expression profiling also catalogued another link between glucose metabolism and leukemia with the discovery that MondoA expression is significantly elevated in ALL.[59] MondoA belongs to a family of transcription factors, including carbohydrate response element binding protein, which senses nutrient states and regulates metabolism.[23] MondoA was discovered as an extended family member of the MYC:Max network of transcription factors. MondoA dimerizes with Mlx (Max-like protein X) to bind target DNA sequences and regulate glucose metabolism. Thus ALL seems to depend on MondoA, with lowered MondoA expression in ALL reducing glycolytic metabolism and enhancing ALL cell differentiation.

Studies of AML cell lines *in vitro* also revealed their dependency on glutamine, which contributes in part to oxidation-reduction (redox) homeostasis through the generation of glutathione.[60,61] Primary AML cells, in contrast with normal CD34+ cells, depend on glutamine and undergo apoptosis with glutamine withdrawal.[62,63] Apoptosis appears to follow diminished mTORC1 activation. Furthermore, reduction of glutamine transport via ASCT2 (SLC1A5) diminishes AML cell line survival, underscoring the importance of glutamine metabolism in AML.[63] Clinical and laboratory experience with L-asparaginase also emphasizes the centrality of glutamine metabolism in ALL. L-Asparaginase is a highly effective agent against ALL, not only via the enzymatic activity embodied in its name, but also via "off-target" glutaminase activity.[63] Because glutamine also plays a critical role in the survival of ALL cells, they are likewise sensitive to L-asparaginase. The glutaminase activity of L-asparaginase additionally serves to reinforce the asparaginase activity of the drug, as glutamine released from the leukemic microenvironment can be used to regenerate asparagine in conjunction with aspartate via asparagine synthetase.[53] In one study, metabolites in the marrow of pediatric ALL were compared with those found in blood before and after standard therapy. Metabolites that were relatively depleted in the marrow prior to therapy include glutamine, glucose, and certain fatty acids.[64] These observations suggest that lymphoblasts or the microenvironment have heightened glycolysis, glutaminolysis, and perhaps fatty acid consumption. Upon therapy, there was severe depletion of asparagine and glutamine, with a more rapid recovery of peripheral glutamine levels after (therapy as also corroborated by another study).[65] Intriguingly, obese children with ALL do not respond well to L-asparaginase therapy, even with a significant reduction in asparagine and glutamine levels.[66] This phenomenon appears to be partly from the induction of glutamine synthetase in the marrow, which releases glutamine from adipocytes.[66] The notion that the tumor microenvironment, particularly mesenchymal cells, might contribute to the production of asparagine appears to be supported by the finding that marrow aspartate levels were higher than in the blood after L-asparaginase treatment while asparagine levels remained low. Thus, metabolism in the tumor microenvironment may affect therapeutic outcome.

Leukemic stem cells (LSCs) appear to adopt the ability of normal HSCs to use oxidative phosphorylation (see Fig. 14-4). Accumulating evidence suggests that FAO and ROS may also play important roles in LSC and HSC survival, self-renewal, and differentiation.[51,67] In one study, AML LSCs with high clonogenicity were isolated from stem cells with low ROS levels.[68] Gene expression analysis comparing these cells with leukemic cells with high ROS levels or with normal CD34+ HSCs revealed elevated expression of Bcl-2, which plays a role in mitochondrial metabolism, in addition to its canonical role in apoptosis.[69] The LSCs with high Bcl-2 expression appear to be metabolically quiescent as compared with normal CD34+ HSCs, demonstrating low oxygen consumption and lactate production. In contrast, ROS high leukemic cells are more metabolically active and have lower colony-forming units. The ROS-low cells are dependent on oxidative phosphorylation and incapable of mounting a glycolytic response, as evidenced by inhibition of Bcl-2 resulting in diminished oxidative metabolism and decreased survival of the LSCs. By contrast, ROS-high leukemic and normal HSCs can mount a glycolytic response in response to Bcl-2 inhibition. In a separate study, inhibition of Bcl-2 with a small molecule in combination with the fatty oxidation inhibitor etomoxir resulted in a decrease in the AML LSC compartment,[68] suggesting that FAO may play a role in the survival of LSCs. If the AML LSCs are similar, at least in part, to normal HSCs, which use FAO for generation of progenitors, then the proliferation of AML cells from LSCs may require fatty acids. Collectively, these results suggest that LSCs may rely on oxidative phosphorylation and may use fatty acids as a source of fuel for survival and generation of more differentiated AML cells from the LSC pool. Use of FAO is expected to increase ROS, which seems to be required for myeloid differentiation from the HSC compartment. In this regard, induction of ROS, such as through the use of iron chelators, has been suggested as a therapeutic strategy that forces LSCs to differentiate.[67]

Frequent mutations in AML, such as FLT3-ITD,[70,71] result in constitutive receptor tyrosine kinase activation, which culminates in activation of PI3K, as well as many downstream events that are associated with increased glycolysis and glutaminolysis (see Fig. 14-2). It is surmised that these pathways would increase the dependency of AML cells on metabolism and mitochondrial function. In this regard, AML cells are sensitive to inhibition of mitochondrial complex I with metformin.[72] Intriguingly, a large study of 400 AML patients revealed a serum metabolic signature pointing to heightened glycolysis and TCA cycle activity in AML that is associated with resistance to cytosine arabinoside.[73] These observations led to a metabolic prognostic score based on the levels of six circulating metabolites. Although this study documents the alteration of metabolism in AML patients, the general applicability of the metabolic prognostic score remains to be determined.

The metabolic pathways (glycolysis, glutaminolysis, and FAO) associated with different leukemic states are surmised to support cellular function, but it could be speculated that these specific pathways are compatible with maintenance of the epigenome of that cellular state. Specifically, the concentrations (and fluxes) of specific metabolic intermediates (e.g., SAM, acetyl-CoA, and α-ketoglutarate) associated with specific metabolic states could modulate the epigenome. The epigenetic influence of metabolism is perhaps best illustrated by the discovery of germline mutations in key metabolic enzymes found in familial cancer syndromes and of somatic mutations of IDH1 and IDH2 in a variety of cancers, including AML and angioimmunoblastic lymphoma.[42]

Somatic mutations of IDH were first discovered in gliomas through deep sequencing.[74] Whole-genome sequencing subsequently revealed the same in a karyotypically normal case of AML.[75] These findings bolstered the notion that hardwired mutations of metabolism could be tumorigenic. A breakthrough in our understanding of IDH mutations in hematologic neoplasm came from a landmark biochemical study of mutant IDH, which revealed a neomorphic activity of the mutant enzymes.[76] Instead of just being inactive, unable to convert isocitrate to α-ketoglutarate (Fig. 14-5), the mutant enzymes reduces α-ketoglutarate to form the oncometabolite 2-hydroxyglutarate (2-HG), which can be detected at high levels in AML.[77] The role of 2-HG in cell growth was illustrated by studies of the leukemic granulocyte-macrophage colony-stimulating factor (GM-CSF)-dependent TF1 cell line, which when deprived of GM-CSF displays diminished growth partially rescuable by exposure to 2-HG.[78,79] Biochemical studies of 2-HG indicate that it could compete with α-ketoglutarate in many oxygenase reactions that depend on α-ketoglutarate as a cofactor, specifically enzymes that are involved in DNA or histone demethylation.

The ability of 2-HG to interfere with epigenetic modifications suggests that IDH mutations promote tumorigenesis through the epigenome.[39] In this regard, genomics of AML reveal the mutual exclusivity of mutations of either IDH1 or IDH2 with mutations in TET2.[42] TET2 produces a DNA demethylating enzyme and hence it appears that high levels of 2-HG production via IDH mutations phenocopies the loss of TET2 in AML. Furthermore, whole-genome methylation analysis uncovers distinct methylomes associated with IDH mutations, underscoring the role of IDH mutations in altering the epigenome in a way that makes myeloid progenitor cells permissive for leukemogenesis.[80] The emergence of specific drugs that inhibit IDH1 or IDH2 reveal that inhibition of mutant IDHs results in differentiation of AML cells. These observations indicate that the epigenome maintained by high levels of 2-HG prevents activation of a myeloid differentiation program, similar to the PML-RAR mutation found in acute PML, which can be induced to differentiate with retinoids. Intriguingly, IDH mutations are also found in other cancers, including angioimmunoblastic lymphomas, but not in other types of lymphomas.[81]

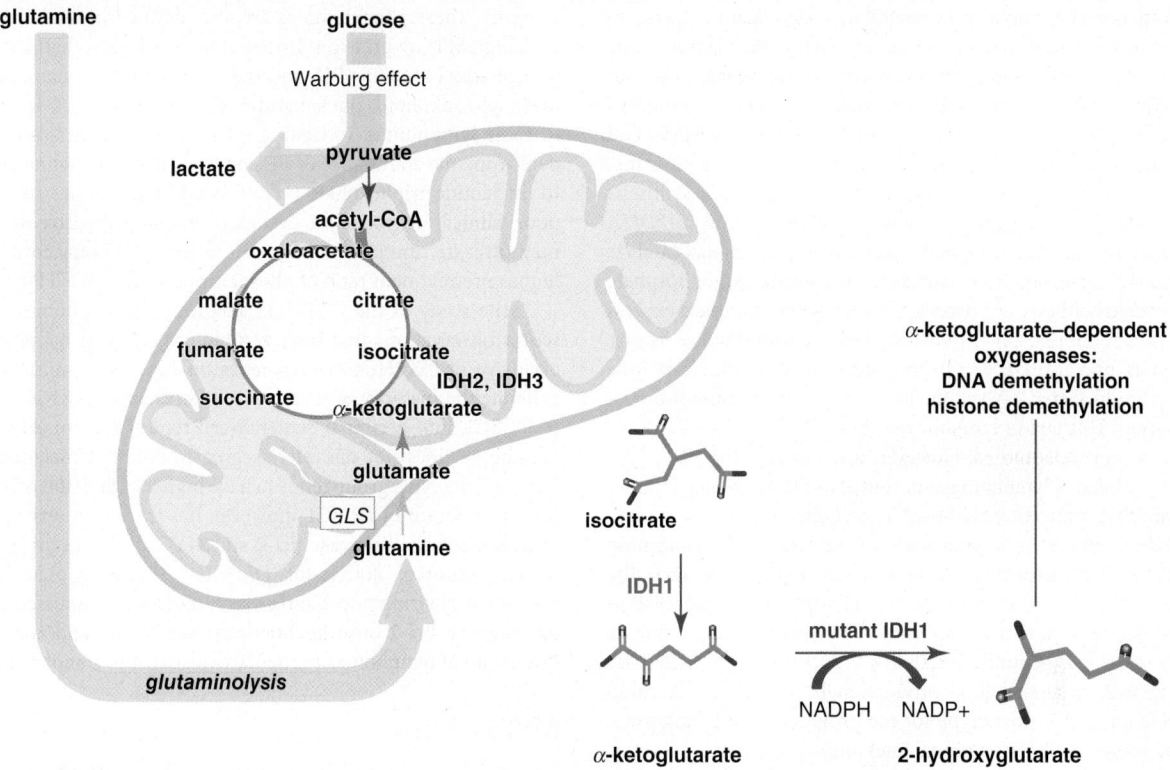

Figure 14–5. Neomorphic enzymatic activity of mutant isocitrate dehydrogenases (IDHs). IDH1 is shown localized in the cytosol, while IDH2 and IDH3 are found participating in the TCA cycle in mitochondria. Isocitrate generated from citrate is oxidized by IDH2 or IDH3 to produce α-ketoglutarate, which is further oxidized in the TCA cycle. IDH1 is depicted to convert isocitrate to α-ketoglutarate in the cytosol. Mutant IDH1 is shown to reduce α-ketoglutarate to 2-hydroxyglutarate (2-HG) with the production of NADP+ from NADPH. Glutamine is the main source of α-ketoglutarate that serves as substrate for mutant IDHs.

LYMPHOMAS

The lymphomas are a broad group of lymphoid malignancies spanning from the more indolent to the most aggressive forms, each with a spectrum of genomic alterations.[82–85] The majority of lymphomas evolve from B-cells at different stages of differentiation in the course of the germinal center reaction (Chap. 78). B-cells activated by T-cell–dependent antigens undergo rapid bursts of growth, forming germinal centers where somatic hypermutation occurs for generation of antibody diversity and plasmacytic differentiation. These phases of B-cell development demand high levels of bioenergetic support and are the stages from which lymphomagenesis is launched. Mantle cell lymphoma arises from the mantle zone. Burkitt lymphoma, emanating from MYC activation, emerges from the pregerminal center compartment. The germinal center type B-cell lymphoma arises from the germinal center compartment, and the activated B-cell (ABC) type of lymphoma develops from the plasmacytic stage. The lymphomas retain the high energetic demands of the precursor cells, and hence the aggressive lymphomas are staged and followed by fluorodeoxyglucose positron emission tomography (FDG-PET), which documents the high levels of glucose uptake and retention in these lymphomas.[86,87] It should be noted that the basis for high FDG-PET is the uptake and retention of 2-deoxyglucose through phosphorylation by HKs. A highly positive FDG-PET does not indicate whether glucose ends up being converted to lactate or being oxidized through the TCA cycle.

Burkitt lymphoma and diffuse large B-cell lymphoma (DLBCL) have high glycolytic flux driving glucose to lactate production. In clinically advanced cases, these lymphomas can present with severe lactic acidosis without any evidence of septicemia.[88,89] The high glycolytic flux is driven by MYC or PI3K activation of glycolysis in these lymphomas and by HIF-1α, which is stabilized in hypoxic regions of the lymphomas (see Fig. 14–2). High glycolytic flux renders models of lymphomas sensitive to glycolytic inhibitors as well as inhibitors of monocarboxylate transporters that export lactate.[90] Inhibition of these transporters and subsequent buildup of lactate result in the inability of lactate dehydrogenase to recycle NADH to NAD+, culminating in inhibition of glycolysis because GAPDH requires NAD+ for its function upstream in the glycolytic pathway. The inhibition of glycolysis causes lymphoma cells to rely further on oxidative phosphorylation, rendering them sensitive to the antidiabetic drug and mitochondrial complex I inhibitor, metformin.

Genetic alterations in lymphomas including B-cell receptor mutations and MYC activation link the genome to alterations in cell metabolism. B-cell receptor activating mutations increase PI3K signaling and render DLBCLs highly glycolytic.[91] High glycolytic rates allow for the synthesis of ribose, glycine, and aspartate, which are building blocks for nucleotide biosynthesis (see Fig. 14–1). Glutamine is also essential for the production of nucleotides and fatty acids. In this regard, glutaminolysis is increased by oncogenic MYC in a model of human Burkitt lymphoma.[49,92–94] Hypoxic lymphoma cells increase glucose flux to lactate but continue to respire in a glutamine dependent fashion, such that inhibition of GLS with the small molecule BPTES diminishes lymphoma progression in preclinical xenograft models.[49]

The rapid proliferation of aggressive lymphomas demands ample nucleotide pools for RNA and DNA synthesis. Many of the key nucleotide metabolic genes are direct targets of the MYC transcription factor, which plays a prominent role in many types of lymphomas.[95,96]

Activation of normal lymphocytes results in a significant increase in 5-phosphoribosyl-pyrophosphate synthetase (PRPS). PRPS2 is not only a target of MYC essential for lymphomagenesis in transgenic mice, but its expression couples the regulation of protein synthesis with nucleotide synthesis.[97] *Prps2* transcription is directly activated by MYC, and the 5′-untranslated region (UTR) of *Prps2* requires the oncogenic translational factor eIF4E for its translation, thereby linking protein synthesis with the regulation of nucleotide metabolism. *IMPDH1* and *IMPDH2*, which encode the inosine monophosphate dehydrogenases that catalyze the oxidation of inosine monophosphate to xanthosine monophosphate in nucleotide biosynthesis, are also MYC target genes. Increased expression of inosine monophosphate dehydrogenases (IMPDHs) is a feature of lymphomas, and IMPDH is also thought to play an additional role as a transcription factor.[98] Mycophenolic acid is an immunosuppressant that targets IMPDH in lymphocytes, but its role in the therapy of lymphomas is not well-studied. However, it is not only the size of the nucleotide pool that is lymphomagenic, but also the imbalanced nature of that pool. DNA replication fidelity relies on balanced pools of nucleotides, with deoxyguanosine triphosphate (dGTP) tending to be limiting amongst the deoxynucleoside triphosphates (dNTPs).[99,100] As such, the relative deficiency of deoxycytidine kinase in lymphomas could result in diminished deoxycytidine triphosphate (dCTP) pools that can induce replication stress and genomic instability.[101] Alterations in nucleotide pools along with increased ROS production by mitochondria could then provide a mutator phenotype for the progression of lymphomas, which have relatively high mutational rates among cancers.

Polyamines play an important role in cell growth by providing polycations involved in DNA replication and dynamics. The synthesis of the polyamines, spermine and spermidine, starts with the synthesis of their precursor, putrescine, from ornithine catalyzed by ornithine decarboxylase (ODC), whose gene is one of the first recognized MYC targets.[102] ODC is essential for transgenic murine lymphomagenesis and its activity could be inhibited by α-difluoromethylornithine (DFMO), which has not had a significant clinical impact despite being studied over the last several decades.[103] Spermidine is also involved as a cofactor in a unique posttranslational alteration of lysine to hypusine. Although this unusual amino acid is found in all eukaryotes, the only known protein containing hypusine is eukaryotic translation initiation factor eIF5A, which is required for lymphocyte activation.[104] Hypusinated eIF5A attenuates the translation of MYC, thereby providing a negative feedback loop, whose disruption accelerates MYC-mediated lymphomagenesis. The tumor-suppressive function of spermidine-dependent hypusinated eIF5A could underlie the reason why DFMO has not made a significant clinical impact.

Intriguingly, gene expression profiling also identified a group of DLBCL that displays high levels of expression of genes involved in oxidative phosphorylation, termed the OXPHOS group of DLBCL.[105] The OXPHOS group depends more on FAO for survival and growth as compared to the B-cell receptor group, which could also be defined by gene expression profiling. FAO requires functional peroxisomes or mitochondria.[106] Fatty acids longer than 12 carbons are conjugated with carnitine and then transported into peroxisomes or mitochondria via carnitine-palmitoyl transferase. Upon entry into the mitochondrial matrix, fatty acids are degraded into acetyl-CoA for further oxidation in the TCA cycle. In this regard, it is notable that MYC induces mitochondrial biogenesis in proliferating cells through activation of genes involve in the genesis and function of mitochondria.[19,107]

In addition to FAO as a signature of a subset of DLBCL, alterations in lipid contents have also been documented. Using MYC-inducible models of lymphoma, glycerophosphoglycerol (PG) and cardiolipin (CL) were found to be elevated in a MYC-dependent manner.[108] Both PG and specifically CL are important for mitochondrial membrane integrity. These phospholipids are also elevated in human lymphomas with high MYC expression. On the other hand, phosphatidyl serine (PS), phosphatidyl inositol (PI), and the most abundant mammalian membrane phospholipid, phosphatidyl ethanolamine (PE), were decreased in these lymphomas. Intriguingly, ^{31}P-MRS imaging has been used to determine the abundance of PE and phosphatidyl choline (PC) relative to nucleotide triphosphate (NTP) in DLBCL and has uncovered that poor clinical response to cyclophosphamide, hydroxydaunorubicin, methotrexate, and prednisone (CHOP)-based therapy correlates with a higher pretreatment ratio of phosphomonoesters to NTP levels.[109]

The study of the OXPHOS subgroup of lymphomas also underscores observations that high aerobic glycolysis in lymphomas is not exclusive of OXPHOS, which relies on functional mitochondria that generate the majority of ATP.[105] The cell-of-origin (COO) classification of DLBCL into germinal center B-cell type (GCB) or ABC groups of lymphoma does not discretely segregate different metabolic features, although the ABC group tends to have higher expression of MYC. A significant fraction of DLBCL, however, has translocations or alterations in expression that increase Bcl-2 and MYC levels, resulting in a highly resistant group of "double-hit" DLBCL.[110] The ability of MYC to induce metabolic rewiring and biomass accumulation (discussed above) and the effect of Bcl-2 on mitochondrial metabolism and apoptosis make this group of lymphomas particularly resistant to standard therapy.

MYELOMAS

Multiple myeloma is characteristically a MYC-driven cancer, particularly since MYC is overexpressed through spurious chromosomal rearrangements and MYC amplification.[111,112] In this regard, it is anticipated that heightened glycolysis and glutaminolysis play vital roles in myeloma development and progression. Although few studies have delineated the metabolic changes in myeloma, clinical FDG-PET scans are used to monitor disease response to therapy,[113] suggesting that myeloma has increased glucose uptake and retention relative to neighboring normal marrow. Moreover, expression of the glucose transporters GLUT4, GLUT8, and GLUT11 are elevated in myeloma.[114] The dependency of myeloma on glycolysis appears to sensitize myeloma cell lines to PDK1 inhibition, which diverts pyruvate away from lactate and into acetyl-CoA.[115] These observations suggest that inhibition of glucose metabolism could potentiate response of myeloma to therapies.

It is notable that several studies showed significant inhibition of myeloma growth and survival with inhibition of NAD+ synthesis through nicotinamide phosphoribosyltransferase (NAMPT).[116] The production of NAD+ is required for multiple metabolic processes, including glycolysis that depends on NAD+ for oxidation of glycolytic intermediates. In this regard, a preclinical model of B cell neoplasia with plasmacytoid features displays sensitivity to a combination of NAMPT and lactate dehydrogenase A (LDHA) inhibition. The expression of NAMPT, which is a direct target of MYC, is elevated in myeloma.[116] The NAMPT inhibitor, FK866, diminishes myeloma tumorigenesis, triggers autophagic cell death, and synergizes with proteasome inhibitors, which have significant clinical activity in multiple myeloma.[117] Collectively, these studies suggest an important role of glucose metabolism in myeloma. However, relatively little is known currently about glutamine or fatty acid metabolism in this disease.

More than ninety years have passed since Otto Warburg first documented metabolic alterations in cancers, including the high rate conversion of glucose to lactate termed the Warburg effect or aerobic glycolysis. Much of our understanding of cancer metabolism has resulted from studies of solid tumors, which share many basic metabolic features with hematologic neoplasms. In particular, the central metabolic pathways of glycolysis and glutaminolysis seem to be similarly exploited by solid and hematologic neoplasm alike for cell growth, proliferation, and survival. Glucose and glutamine flux into cells provides for the production of ATP and building blocks for the growing cell. Furthermore, glutamine and glucose are also substrates for glutathione synthesis, which is vital for redox homeostasis of growing cells that produce ROS as metabolic byproducts. Resting cells, on the other hand, tend to rely on FAO, which provides the most efficient energy production. In this regard, evidence has emerged indicating that neoplastic stem cells also rely on FAO and, hence, could be targeted therapeutically via this route. Glucose, glutamine, and mitochondrial metabolism pathways offer similar inhibition strategies for proliferating hematologic neoplastic cells. One of the most remarkable therapeutic developments, however, is the discovery of IDH mutations in AML and lymphoma and the development of specific drugs targeting the mutant forms of IDH1 and IDH2. Furthermore, alterations of the AML methylome and the ability of mutant IDH inhibitors to induce differentiation of AML cells underscore the link between metabolites and the epigenome. It is through advances in our understanding of cancer metabolism that we have been able to develop therapies like these for mutant IDH, capitalize on the avidity of glucose uptake by hematologic neoplasms for diagnostic and followup FDG-PET scanning, and develop many more metabolic strategies that are hoped to provide new gains against these deadly malignancies.

REFERENCES

1. Schrodinger E: What is Life? Cambridge University Press, Cambridge, UK 1944.
2. Bass J: Circadian topology of metabolism. *Nature* 491:348–356, 2012.
3. Berg J, Tymoczko JL, Stryer L: Biochemistry. WH Freeman, New York, 2002.
4. Rabinowitz JD, White E: Autophagy and metabolism. *Science* 330:1344–1348, 2010.
5. Orkin SH, Zon LI: Hematopoiesis: An evolving paradigm for stem cell biology. *Cell* 132:631–644, 2008.
6. Dang CV: Links between metabolism and cancer. *Genes Dev* 26:877–890, 2012.
7. Rolfe DF, Brown GC: Cellular energy utilization and molecular origin of standard metabolic rate in mammals. *Physiol Rev* 77:731–758, 1997.
8. Lippman SI, Broach JR: Protein kinase A and TORC1 activate genes for ribosomal biogenesis by inactivating repressors encoded by Dot6 and its homolog Tod6. *Proc Natl Acad Sci U S A* 106:19928–19933, 2009.
9. Cantor JR, Sabatini DM: Cancer cell metabolism: One hallmark, many faces. *Cancer Discov* 2:881–898, 2012.
10. Schell JC, Rutter J: The long and winding road to the mitochondrial pyruvate carrier. *Cancer Metab* 1:6, 2013.
11. Chowdhury R, Sekirnik R, Brissett NC, et al: Ribosomal oxygenases are structurally conserved from prokaryotes to humans. *Nature* 510:422–426, 2014.
12. McDonough MA, Loenarz C, Chowdhury R, et al: Structural studies on human 2-oxoglutarate dependent oxygenases. *Curr Opin Struct Biol* 20:659–672, 2010.
13. Hensley CT, Wasti AT, DeBerardinis RJ: Glutamine and cancer: Cell biology, physiology, and clinical opportunities. *J Clin Invest* 123:3678–3684, 2013.
14. DeBerardinis RJ, Cheng T: Q's next: The diverse functions of glutamine in metabolism, cell biology and cancer. *Oncogene* 29:313–324, 2010.
15. Fan J, Ye J, Kamphorst JJ, et al: Quantitative flux analysis reveals folate-dependent NADPH production. *Nature* 510:298–302, 2014.
16. Laplante M, Sabatini DM: Regulation of mTORC1 and its impact on gene expression at a glance. *J Cell Sci* 126:1713–1719, 2013.
17. Roussel MF, Davis JN, Cleveland JL, et al: Dual control of myc expression through a single DNA binding site targeted by ets family proteins and E2F-1. *Oncogene* 9:405–415, 1994.
18. Farrell AS, Sears RC: MYC degradation. *Cold Spring Harb Perspect Med* 4, 2014.
19. Dang CV: MYC on the path to cancer. *Cell* 149:22–35, 2012.
20. Hardie DG: AMP-activated protein kinase: An energy sensor that regulates all aspects of cell function. *Genes Dev* 25:1895–1908, 2011.
21. Mihaylova MM, Shaw RJ: The AMPK signalling pathway coordinates cell growth, autophagy and metabolism. *Nat Cell Biol* 13:1016–1023, 2011.
22. Gallant P: Myc function in *Drosophila. Cold Spring Harb Perspect Med* 3:a014324, 2013.
23. Conacci-Sorrell M, McFerrin L, Eisenman RN: An overview of MYC and its interactome. *Cold Spring Harb Perspect Med* 4:a014357, 2014.
24. Dang CV: Gene regulation: Fine-tuned amplification in cells. *Nature* 511:417–418, 2014.
25. Golomb L, Volarevic S, Oren M: p53 and ribosome biogenesis stress: The essentials. *FEBS Lett* 588:2571–2579, 2014.
26. Mayer C, Grummt I: Ribosome biogenesis and cell growth: MTOR coordinates transcription by all three classes of nuclear RNA polymerases. *Oncogene* 25:6384–6391, 2006.
27. Vousden KH, Ryan KM: p53 and metabolism. *Nat Rev Cancer* 9:691–700, 2009.
28. Matoba S, Kang JG, Patino WD, et al: P53 regulates mitochondrial respiration. *Science* 312:1650–1653, 2006.
29. Freed-Pastor WA, Mizuno H, Zhao X, et al: Mutant p53 disrupts mammary tissue architecture via the mevalonate pathway. *Cell* 148:244–258, 2012.
30. Xiong S, Tu H, Kollareddy M, et al: Pla2g16 phospholipase mediates gain-of-function activities of mutant p53. *Proc Natl Acad Sci U S A* 111:11145–11150, 2014.
31. Ortega-Molina A, Serrano M: PTEN in cancer, metabolism, and aging. *Trends Endocrinol Metab* 24:184–189, 2013.
32. Semenza GL: HIF-1 mediates metabolic responses to intratumoral hypoxia and oncogenic mutations. *J Clin Invest* 123:3664–3671, 2013.
33. Parks SK, Chiche J, Pouyssegur J: Disrupting proton dynamics and energy metabolism for cancer therapy. *Nat Rev Cancer* 13:611–623, 2013.
34. Finkel T: Signal transduction by reactive oxygen species. *J Cell Biol* 194:7–15, 2011.
35. Schieber M, Chandel NS: ROS function in redox signaling and oxidative stress. *Curr Biol* 24:R453–R462, 2014.
36. Leinonen HM, Kansanen E, Polonen P, et al: Role of the Keap1-Nrf2 pathway in cancer. *Adv Cancer Res* 122:281–320, 2014.
37. Dawson MA, Kouzarides T: Cancer epigenetics: From mechanism to therapy. *Cell* 150:12–27, 2012.
38. Bhaumik SR, Smith E, Shilatifard A: Covalent modifications of histones during development and disease pathogenesis. *Nat Struct Mol Biol* 14:1008–1016, 2007.
39. Kaelin WG Jr, McKnight SL: Influence of metabolism on epigenetics and disease. *Cell* 153:56–69, 2013.
40. Choudhary C, Weinert BT, Nishida Y, et al: The growing landscape of lysine acetylation links metabolism and cell signalling. *Nat Rev Mol Cell Biol* 15:536–550, 2014.
41. Neff T, Armstrong SA: Recent progress toward epigenetic therapies: The example of mixed lineage leukemia. *Blood* 121:4847–4853, 2013.
42. Shih AH, Abdel-Wahab O, Patel JP, Levine RL: The role of mutations in epigenetic regulators in myeloid malignancies. *Nat Rev Cancer* 12:599–612, 2012.
43. Simsek T, Kocabas F, Zheng J, et al: The distinct metabolic profile of hematopoietic stem cells reflects their location in a hypoxic niche. *Cell Stem Cell* 7:380–390, 2010.
44. Takubo K, Goda N, Yamada W, et al: Regulation of the HIF-1alpha level is essential for hematopoietic stem cells. *Cell Stem Cell* 7:391–402, 2010.
45. Gan B, Hu J, Jiang S, et al: Lkb1 regulates quiescence and metabolic homeostasis of haematopoietic stem cells. *Nature* 468:701–704, 2010.
46. Gurumurthy S, Xie SZ, Alagesan B, et al: The Lkb1 metabolic sensor maintains haematopoietic stem cell survival. *Nature* 468:659–663, 2010.
47. Nakada D, Saunders TL, Morrison SJ: Lkb1 regulates cell cycle and energy metabolism in haematopoietic stem cells. *Nature* 468:653–658, 2010.
48. Oburoglu L, Tardito S, Fritz V, et al: Glucose and glutamine metabolism regulate human hematopoietic stem cell lineage specification. *Cell Stem Cell* 15:169–184, 2014.
49. Le A, Lane AN, Hamaker M, et al: Glucose-independent glutamine metabolism via TCA cycling for proliferation and survival in B cells. *Cell Metab* 15:110–121, 2012.
50. Fan J, Kamphorst JJ, Mathew R, et al: Glutamine-driven oxidative phosphorylation is a major ATP source in transformed mammalian cells in both normoxia and hypoxia. *Mol Syst Biol* 9:712, 2013.
51. Ito K, Carracedo A, Weiss D, et al: A PML-PPAR-delta pathway for fatty acid oxidation regulates hematopoietic stem cell maintenance. *Nat Med* 18:1350–1358, 2012.
52. Farber S, Diamond LK: Temporary remissions in acute leukemia in children produced by folic acid antagonist, 4-aminopteroyl-glutamic acid. *N Engl J Med* 238:787–793, 1948.
53. Emadi A, Zokaee H, Sausville EA: Asparaginase in the treatment of non-ALL hematologic malignancies. *Cancer Chemother Pharmacol* 73:875–883, 2014.
54. Pui CH, Relling MV, Downing JR: Acute lymphoblastic leukemia. *N Engl J Med* 350:1535–1548, 2004.
55. Meyer SC, Levine RL: Translational implications of somatic genomics in acute myeloid leukaemia. *Lancet Oncol* 15:e382–e394, 2014.
56. Koppenol WH, Bounds PL, Dang CV: Otto Warburg's contributions to current concepts of cancer metabolism. *Nat Rev Cancer* 11:325–337, 2011.
57. Herst PM, Howman RA, Neeson PJ, et al: The level of glycolytic metabolism in acute myeloid leukemia blasts at diagnosis is prognostic for clinical outcome. *J Leukoc Biol* 89:51–55, 2011.
58. Boag JM, Beesley AH, Firth MJ, et al: Altered glucose metabolism in childhood pre-B acute lymphoblastic leukaemia. *Leukemia* 20:1731–1737, 2006.
59. Wernicke CM, Richter GH, Beinvogl BC, et al: MondoA is highly overexpressed in acute lymphoblastic leukemia cells and modulates their metabolism, differentiation and survival. *Leuk Res* 36:1185–1192, 2012.
60. Kitoh T, Kubota M, Takimoto T, et al: Metabolic basis for differential glutamine requirements of human leukemia cell lines. *J Cell Physiol* 143:150–153, 1990.
61. Onuma T, Waligunda J, Holland JF: Amino acid requirements in vitro of human leukemic cells. *Cancer Res* 31:1640–1644, 1971.
62. Goto M, Miwa H, Shikami M, et al: Importance of glutamine metabolism in leukemia cells by energy production through TCA cycle and by redox homeostasis. *Cancer Invest* 32:241–247, 2014.
63. Willems L, Jacque N, Jacquel A, et al: Inhibiting glutamine uptake represents an attractive new strategy for treating acute myeloid leukemia. *Blood* 122:3521–3532, 2013.
64. Tiziani S, Kang Y, Harjanto R, et al: Metabolomics of the tumor microenvironment in pediatric acute lymphoblastic leukemia. *PLoS One* 8:e82859, 2013.

65. Steiner M, Hochreiter D, Kasper DC, et al: Asparagine and aspartic acid concentrations in bone marrow versus peripheral blood during Berlin-Frankfurt-Munster-based induction therapy for childhood acute lymphoblastic leukemia. *Leuk Lymphoma* 53:1682–1687, 2012.

66. Ehsanipour EA, Sheng X, Behan JW, et al: Adipocytes cause leukemia cell resistance to L-asparaginase via release of glutamine. *Cancer Res* 73:2998–3006, 2013.

67. Abdel-Wahab O, Levine RL: Metabolism and the leukemic stem cell. *J Exp Med* 207:677–680, 2010.

68. Samudio I, Harmancey R, Fiegl M, et al: Pharmacologic inhibition of fatty acid oxidation sensitizes human leukemia cells to apoptosis induction. *J Clin Invest* 120:142–156, 2010.

69. Lagadinou ED, Sach A, Callahan K, et al: BCL-2 inhibition targets oxidative phosphorylation and selectively eradicates quiescent human leukemia stem cells. *Cell Stem Cell* 12:329–341, 2013.

70. Small D: Targeting FLT3 for the treatment of leukemia. *Semin Hematol* 45:S17–S21, 2008.

71. Zheng R, Small D: Mutant FLT3 signaling contributes to a block in myeloid differentiation. *Leuk Lymphoma* 46:1679–1687, 2005.

72. Scotland S, Saland E, Skuli N, et al: Mitochondrial energetic and AKT status mediate metabolic effects and apoptosis of metformin in human leukemic cells. *Leukemia* 27:2129–2138, 2013.

73. Chen WL, Wang JH, Zhao AH, et al: A distinct glucose metabolism signature of acute myeloid leukemia with prognostic value. *Blood* 124:1645–1654, 2014.

74. Yan H, Parsons DW, Jin G, et al: IDH1 and IDH2 mutations in gliomas. *N Engl J Med* 360:765–773, 2009.

75. Mardis ER, Ding L, Dooling DJ, et al: Recurring mutations found by sequencing an acute myeloid leukemia genome. *N Engl J Med* 361:1058–1066, 2009.

76. Dang L, White DW, Gross S, et al: Cancer-associated IDH1 mutations produce 2-hydroxyglutarate. *Nature* 465:966, 2010.

77. Gross S, Cairns RA, Minden MD, et al: Cancer-associated metabolite 2-hydroxyglutarate accumulates in acute myelogenous leukemia with isocitrate dehydrogenase 1 and 2 mutations. *J Exp Med* 207:339–344, 2010.

78. Losman JA, Looper RE, Koivunen P, et al: (R)-2-hydroxyglutarate is sufficient to promote leukemogenesis and its effects are reversible. *Science* 339:1621–1625, 2013.

79. Koivunen P, Lee S, Duncan CG, et al: Transformation by the (R)-enantiomer of 2-hydroxyglutarate linked to EGLN activation. *Nature* 483:484–488, 2012.

80. Figueroa ME, Abdel-Wahab O, Lu C, et al: Leukemic IDH1 and IDH2 mutations result in a hypermethylation phenotype, disrupt TET2 function, and impair hematopoietic differentiation. *Cancer Cell* 18:553–567, 2010.

81. Cairns RA, Iqbal J, Lemonnier F, et al: IDH2 mutations are frequent in angioimmunoblastic T-cell lymphoma. *Blood* 119:1901–1903, 2012.

82. Schmitz R, Young RM, Ceribelli M, et al: Burkitt lymphoma pathogenesis and therapeutic targets from structural and functional genomics. *Nature* 490:116–120, 2012.

83. Pasqualucci L, Khiabanian H, Fangazio M, et al: Genetics of follicular lymphoma transformation. *Cell Rep* 6:130–140, 2014.

84. Dominguez-Sola D, Dalla-Favera R: Burkitt lymphoma: Much more than MYC. *Cancer Cell* 22:141–142, 2012.

85. Schneider C, Pasqualucci L, Dalla-Favera R: Molecular pathogenesis of diffuse large B-cell lymphoma. *Semin Diagn Pathol* 28:167–177, 2011.

86. Kostakoglu L, Cheson BD: Current role of FDG PET/CT in lymphoma. *Eur J Nucl Med Mol Imaging* 41:1004–1027, 2014.

87. Alvarez Paez AM, Nogueiras Alonso JM, Serena Puig A: 18F-FDG-PET/CT in lymphoma: Two decades of experience. *Rev Esp Med Nucl Imagen Mol* 31:340–349, 2012.

88. Chan FH, Carl D, Lyckholm LJ: Severe lactic acidosis in a patient with B-cell lymphoma: A case report and review of the literature. *Case Rep Med* 2009:534561, 2009.

89. Friedenberg AS, Brandoff DE, Schiffman FJ: Type B lactic acidosis as a severe metabolic complication in lymphoma and leukemia: A case series from a single institution and literature review. *Medicine (Baltimore)* 86:225–232, 2007.

90. Doherty JR, Yang C, Scott KE, et al: Blocking lactate export by inhibiting the Myc target MCT1 Disables glycolysis and glutathione synthesis. *Cancer Res* 74:908–920, 2014.

91. Bhatt AP, Jacobs SR, Freemerman AJ, et al: Dysregulation of fatty acid synthesis and glycolysis in non-Hodgkin lymphoma. *Proc Natl Acad Sci U S A* 109:11818–11823, 2012.

92. Dutta P, Le A, Vander Jagt DL, et al: Evaluation of LDH-A and glutaminase inhibition in vivo by hyperpolarized 13C-pyruvate magnetic resonance spectroscopy of tumors. *Cancer Res* 73:4190–4195, 2013.

93. Liu W, Le A, Hancock C, et al: Reprogramming of proline and glutamine metabolism contributes to the proliferative and metabolic responses regulated by oncogenic transcription factor c-MYC. *Proc Natl Acad Sci U S A* 109:8983–8988, 2012.

94. Le A, Cooper CR, Gouw AM, et al: Inhibition of lactate dehydrogenase A induces oxidative stress and inhibits tumor progression. *Proc Natl Acad Sci U S A* 107:2037–2042, 2010.

95. Liu YC, Li F, Handler J, et al: Global regulation of nucleotide biosynthetic genes by c-Myc. *PLoS One* 3:e2722, 2008.

96. Mannava S, Grachtchouk V, Wheeler LJ, et al: Direct role of nucleotide metabolism in C-MYC-dependent proliferation of melanoma cells. *Cell Cycle* 7:2392–2400, 2008.

97. Cunningham JT, Moreno MV, Lodi A, et al: Protein and nucleotide biosynthesis are coupled by a single rate-limiting enzyme, PRPS2, to drive cancer. *Cell* 157:1088–1103, 2014.

98. Calvo-Vidal MN, Cerchietti L: The metabolism of lymphomas. *Curr Opin Hematol* 20:345–354, 2013.

99. Mathews CK: DNA precursor metabolism and genomic stability. *FASEB J* 20:1300–1314, 2006.

100. Song S, Pursell ZF, Copeland WC, et al: DNA precursor asymmetries in mammalian tissue mitochondria and possible contribution to mutagenesis through reduced replication fidelity. *Proc Natl Acad Sci U S A* 102:4990–4995, 2005.

101. Austin WR, Armijo AL, Campbell DO, et al: Nucleoside salvage pathway kinases regulate hematopoiesis by linking nucleotide metabolism with replication stress. *J Exp Med* 209:2215–2228, 2012.

102. Bello-Fernandez C, Packham G, Cleveland JL: The ornithine decarboxylase gene is a transcriptional target of c-Myc. *Proc Natl Acad Sci U S A* 90:7804–7808, 1993.

103. Nilsson JA, Keller UB, Baudino TA, et al: Targeting ornithine decarboxylase in Myc-induced lymphomagenesis prevents tumor formation. *Cancer Cell* 7:433–444, 2005.

104. Scuoppo C, Miething C, Lindqvist L, et al: A tumour suppressor network relying on the polyamine-hypusine axis. *Nature* 487:244–248, 2012.

105. Monti S, Savage KJ, Kutok JL, et al: Molecular profiling of diffuse large B-cell lymphoma identifies robust subtypes including one characterized by host inflammatory response. *Blood* 105:1851–1861, 2005.

106. Caro P, Kishan AU, Norberg E, et al: Metabolic signatures uncover distinct targets in molecular subsets of diffuse large B cell lymphoma. *Cancer Cell* 22:547–560, 2012.

107. Zirath H, Frenzel A, Oliynyk G, et al: MYC inhibition induces metabolic changes leading to accumulation of lipid droplets in tumor cells. *Proc Natl Acad Sci U S A* 110:10258–10263, 2013.

108. Eberlin LS, Gabay M, Fan AC, et al: Alteration of the lipid profile in lymphomas induced by MYC overexpression. *Proc Natl Acad Sci U S A* 111:10450–10455, 2014.

109. Arias-Mendoza F, Payne GS, Zakian K, et al: Noninvasive phosphorus magnetic resonance spectroscopic imaging predicts outcome to first-line chemotherapy in newly diagnosed patients with diffuse large B-cell lymphoma. *Acad Radiol* 20:1122–1129, 2013.

110. Lindsley RC, LaCasce AS: Biology of double-hit B-cell lymphomas. *Curr Opin Hematol* 19:299–304, 2012.

111. Affer M, Chesi M, Chen WD, et al: Promiscuous MYC locus rearrangements hijack enhancers but mostly super-enhancers to dysregulate MYC expression in multiple myeloma. *Leukemia* 28:1725–1735, 2014.

112. Kuehl WM, Bergsagel PL: Molecular pathogenesis of multiple myeloma and its premalignant precursor. *J Clin Invest* 122:3456–3463, 2012.

113. Agarwal A, Chirindel A, Shah BA, Subramaniam RM: Evolving role of FDG PET/CT in multiple myeloma imaging and management. *AJR Am J Roentgenol* 200:884–890, 2013.

114. McBrayer SK, Cheng JC, Singhal S, et al: Multiple myeloma exhibits novel dependence on GLUT4, GLUT8, and GLUT11: Implications for glucose transporter-directed therapy. *Blood* 119:4686–4697, 2012.

115. Fujiwara S, Kawano Y, Yuki H, et al: PDK1 inhibition is a novel therapeutic target in multiple myeloma. *Br J Cancer* 108:170–178, 2013.

116. Cea M, Cagnetta A, Fulciniti M, et al: Targeting NAD+ salvage pathway induces autophagy in multiple myeloma cells via mTORC1 and extracellular signal-regulated kinase (ERK1/2) inhibition. *Blood* 120:3519–3529, 2012.

117. Cagnetta A, Cea M, Calimeri T, et al: Intracellular NAD(+) depletion enhances bortezomib-induced anti-myeloma activity. *Blood* 122:1243–1255, 2013.

CHAPTER 15

APOPTOSIS MECHANISMS: RELEVANCE TO THE HEMATOPOIETIC SYSTEM

John C. Reed

SUMMARY

Apoptosis was originally coined to describe the morphologic features of a form of cell death characterized by cell shrinkage, membrane blebbing, and nuclear condensation. This type of cell death occurs in a wide variety of physiologic contexts, and thus is sometimes referred to as programmed cell death. Apoptosis occurs in all animal species as a means to balance cell proliferation with cell loss. The physiologic benefits of apoptosis include eliminating cells that are unneeded, defective, or infected, and maintenance of tissue homeostasis by continuously renewing adult tissues so as to maintain appropriate organ mass. In the hematopoietic system, production of leukocytes is delicately balanced against cell death, until a need arises for rapidly generating immune and inflammatory cells for combating pathogens. The life span of hematopoietic cells is regulated by numerous cytokines and lymphokines, as well as by signals derived from microanatomical niches through cell adhesion molecules and other regulators. Defects in the regulation of hematopoietic cell life span contribute to myriad diseases, including disorders characterized by inappropriate cell accumulation, such as leukemia, lymphoma, and autoimmunity, and diseases where pathologic loss of cells occurs, such as immunodeficiency and various blood dyscrasias.

Acronyms and Abbreviations: ALL, acute lymphocytic leukemia; ALPS, autoimmune lymphoproliferative syndrome; Asp, aspartic acid; B-CLL, B-cell chronic lymphocytic leukemia; BH, Bcl-2 homology domain; CARDs, caspase recruitment domains; caspases, cysteine aspartyl proteases; CLLs, chronic lymphocytic leukemias; CHOP, C/EBP homologous protein; CML, chronic myelogenous leukemias; CTL, cytolytic T lymphocyte; Cyt-c, cytochrome c; DD, death domain; DEDs, death effector domains; DISC, death-inducing signaling complex; DLBCL, diffuse large B-cell lymphoma; DR, death receptor; EBV, Epstein-Barr virus; ER, endoplasmic reticulum; FasL, Fas ligand; FKHD, forkhead transcription factors; IAP, inhibitor of apoptosis; IBD, inflammatory bowel disease; IgH, immunoglobulin heavy chain; IKKs, I-κB kinases; IL, interleukin; KSV, Kaposi sarcoma virus; MALT, mucosa-associated lymphoid tissue; miRNAs, microRNAs; MLKL, mixed-lineage kinase domain-like; MMs, multiple myelomas; MOMP, mitochondrial outer membrane permeabilization; MPT, mitochondrial permeability transition; NHLs, non-Hodgkin lymphomas; NK, natural killer; PARP, poly-ADP ribosyl polymerase; PCD, programmed cell death; PI3K, phosphatidylinositol 3'-kinase; pro/pre–B-cells, B-lymphocyte progenitors; ROS, reactive oxygen species; TNF, tumor necrosis factor; TNFR1, TNF receptor-1; UBCs, ubiquitin conjugating enzymes.

It is now well established that defects in the normal mechanisms that control programmed cell death (PCD) occur commonly in human diseases. Cell numbers in the body are governed not only by cell division, which determines the rate of cell production, but also by cell death, which dictates the rate of cell loss. In the course of a typical day, an average adult human produces, and in parallel eradicates, approximately 50 to 70 billion cells, representing approximately 1 million cells per second. Normally, these two processes of cell division and cell death are tightly coupled so that no net increase in cell numbers occurs, or so that such increases represent only temporary responses to environmental stimuli. However, alternations in the expression or function of the genes that control PCD can upset this delicate balance, contributing to or causing disease.

In most cases, PCD occurs by apoptosis. Apoptosis is defined by its morphologic features. As viewed with the assistance of the light- (or, preferably, electron-) microscope, the characteristics of the apoptotic cell include chromatin condensation and nuclear fragmentation (pyknosis), plasma membrane blebbing, and cell shrinkage. Eventually, the cell breaks into small membrane-surrounded fragments (apoptotic bodies), which are cleared by phagocytosis, without inciting an inflammatory response. The release of apoptotic bodies is what inspired the term "apoptosis" from the Greek, meaning "to fall away from" and conjuring notions of the falling of leaves in the autumn from deciduous trees.[1]

In recent years, the molecular machinery responsible for apoptosis has been elucidated, revealing a family of intracellular proteases, caspases (cysteine aspartyl proteases), which are responsible directly or indirectly for most of the morphologic and biochemical changes that characterize the phenomenon of apoptosis.[2,3] Diverse regulators of the caspases have also been discovered, including activators and inhibitors of these cell death proteases. Inputs from signal transduction pathways into the core of the cell death machinery have also been identified, demonstrating ways of linking environmental stimuli to cell death responses or cell survival maintenance. Knowledge of the molecular mechanisms of apoptosis is providing insights into the pathogenesis of many diseases, revealing strategies for possible novel treatments.

● CASPASES—PROTEASES THAT CAUSE APOPTOSIS

Intracellular proteases called *caspases* are responsible for most of the morphologic changes that we recognize as "apoptosis," as well as many of the biochemical changes often associated with this route of cell demise. Specifically, activation of a family of intracellular cysteine proteases that cleave their substrates at aspartic acid residues, known as "caspases" for *cysteine asp*artyl-specific prote*ases*.[4] These proteases are present as inactive zymogens in essentially all animal cells, but can be triggered to assume active states, generally involving their proteolytic processing at conserved aspartic acid (Asp) residues. During activation, the zymogen proproteins are cleaved to generate the large (~20 kDa) and small (~10 kDa) subunits of the active enzymes, typically liberating an N-terminal prodomain from the processed polypeptide chain. The active enzymes consist of heterotetramers composed of two large and two small subunits, generally with two active sites per molecule.[2,3]

The observation that caspases cleave their substrates at Asp residues and are also activated by proteolytic processing at Asp residues makes evident that these proteases collaborate in proteolytic cascades, where caspases activate themselves and each other. Humans contain 11 caspases. They can be subgrouped according to either their amino-acid sequence similarities or their protease specificities.

From a functional perceptive, it is useful to view the caspases as either upstream "initiator" caspases or downstream "effector" caspases.[5] The zymogen forms of upstream initiator caspases possess large N-terminal prodomains, which function as protein interaction modules, allowing them to interact with various proteins that trigger caspase activation. In contrast, the proforms of downstream effector caspases contain only short N-terminal prodomains, serving no apparent function. Downstream caspases are largely dependent on upstream caspases for their proteolytic processing and activation. The substrates of effector caspases are myriad, as revealed in recent years by unbiased proteomics approaches. Substrates include cytoskeletal and nuclear matrix proteins, chromatin-modifying (e.g., poly-ADP ribosyl polymerase [PARP]) and DNA repair proteins, inhibitory subunits of endonucleases (CIDE-family proteins), protein kinases (often separating the autorepressing regulatory domains from catalytic domains) and other signal transduction proteins.

CASPASE ACTIVATION PATHWAYS

Several pathways for activating caspases have been delineated (Fig. 15–1). The simplest is exploited by cytolytic T lymphocytes (CTLs)

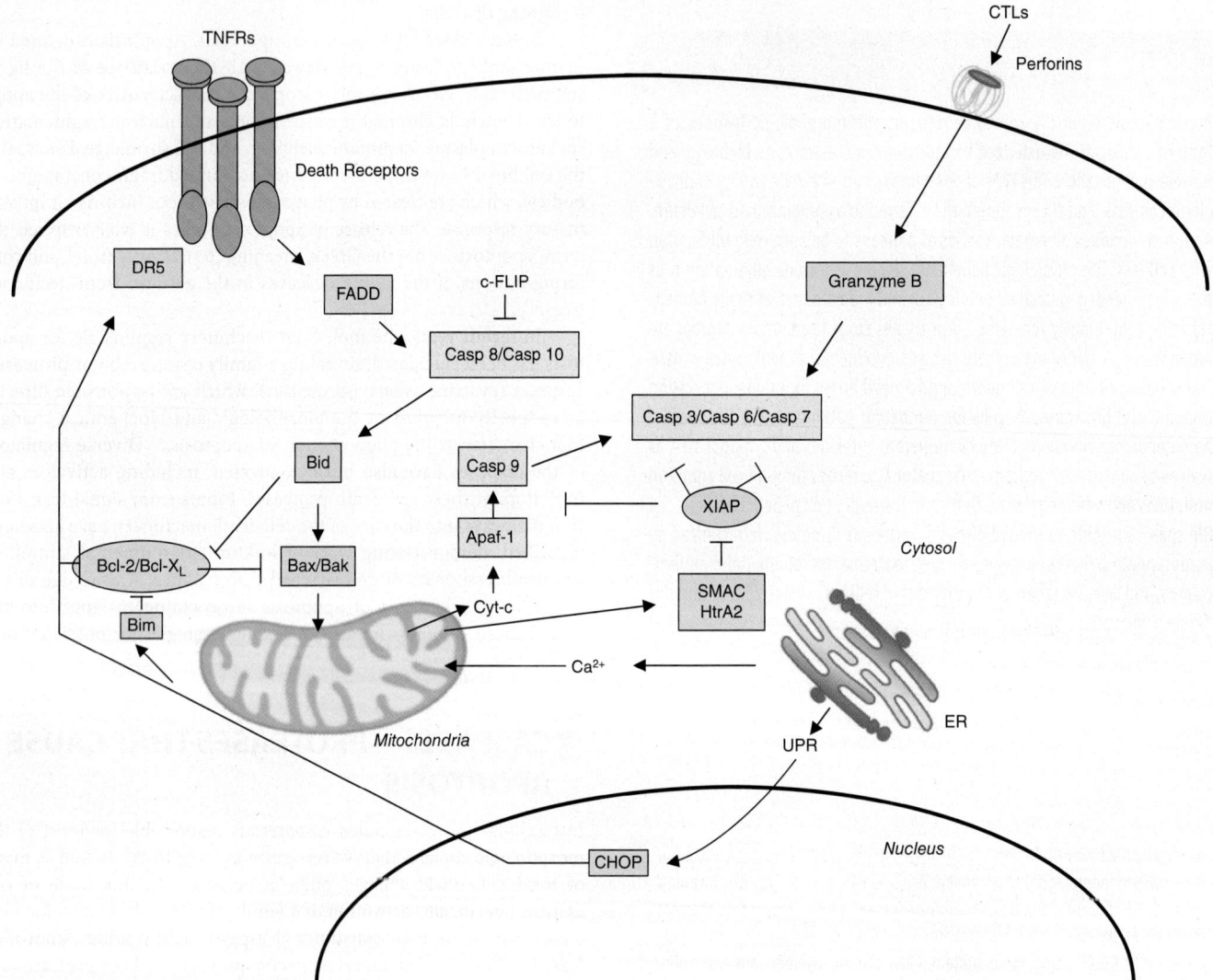

Figure 15–1. Pathways for caspase activation. The major pathways for caspase activation in mammalian cells are presented. The extrinsic (*left, upper*) is induced by members of the tumor necrosis factor (TNF) family of cytokine receptors such as TNF receptor-1 (TNFR1), Fas, and the tumor necrosis factor–related apoptosis-inducing ligand (TRAIL) receptors. These proteins recruit adapter proteins to their cytosolic death domains (DDs), including the Fas-associated death domain (FADD), which then bind the death effector domain (DED)–containing procaspases, particularly procaspase-8, inducing their activation. Cytolytic T lymphocytes (CTLs) and natural killer (NK) cells introduce the protease granzyme B into target cells (*right, upper*). This protease cleaves and activates multiple members of the caspase family. The intrinsic pathway (*left, lower*) is initiated by release of cytochrome c from mitochondria, induced by various stimuli, including elevations in the levels of pore-forming proapoptotic Bcl-2 family proteins, such as Bax and Bak. In the cytosol, cytochrome c binds and activates Apaf-1, allowing it to associate with and activate procaspase-9. Active caspase-9 (intrinsic) and caspase-8 (extrinsic) have been shown to directly cleave and activate the effector protease, caspase-3. Because other caspases also become involved in these pathways (not shown), the schematic represents an oversimplification of the events that occur *in vivo*. Additionally, disturbances in the function of the endoplasmic reticulum (ER) are also linked to the intrinsic and extrinsic apoptosis pathways, through both Ca^{2+} transfer to mitochondria and via transcriptional mechanisms that include induction of CHOP expression, which, in turn, stimulates expression of death receptor 5 (DR5) and Bim (proapoptotic Bcl-2 family member) (*right, lower*). Rectangles indicate proapoptotic proteins whereas ellipses indicate antiapoptotic proteins.

and natural killer (NK) cells, which introduce apoptosis-inducing proteases, particularly granzyme B (a serine protease), into effective intracellular compartments of target cells via perforin-dependent mechanisms.[6] Unlike the caspases, granzyme B is a serine protease. However, similar to the caspases, granzyme B specifically cleaves its substrates at Asp residues. Granzyme B is capable of cleaving and activating multiple caspases and some caspase substrates.[7] Endogenous and viral inhibitors of granzyme B have been identified, accounting for resistance to this apoptotic inducer.[8-10]

Another caspase-activation pathway is represented by tumor necrosis factor (TNF) family receptors. Eight of the approximately 30 known members of the TNF family in humans contain a so-called death domain (DD) in their cytosolic tails.[11] Several of these DD-containing TNF family receptors use caspase activation as a signaling mechanism, including TNF receptor-1 (TNFR1)/CD120a; Fas/APO1/CD95; death receptor (DR)-3 (DR3)/Apo2/Weasle; DR4/ tumor necrosis factor–related apoptosis-inducing ligand receptor 1 (TRAILR1); DR5/TRAILR2; and DR6. Ligation of these receptors at the cell surface results in receptor clustering and recruitment of several intracellular proteins, including certain procaspases, to the cytosolic domains of these receptors, forming a "death-inducing signaling complex" that triggers caspase activation and leads to apoptosis.[12,13]

The specific caspases summoned to the DISC are caspase-8 and, in some cases, caspase-10. These caspases contain so-called death effector domains (DEDs) in their N-terminal prodomains that bind to a corresponding DED in the Fas-associated death domain (FADD), a bipartite adapter protein containing a DD and a DED. FADD functions as a molecular bridge between the DD and DED domain families, and is, in fact, the only protein in the human genome with this dual domain structure. Consequently, cells from mice in which the *fadd* gene has been knocked out are resistant to apoptosis induction by TNF family cytokines and their receptors. Cells derived from *caspase-8* knockout mice also fail to undergo apoptosis in response to ligands or antibodies that activate TNF family DRs, demonstrating an essential role for this caspase in this pathway.[14] However, mice lack the highly homologous protease, caspase-10, which is found in humans, having arisen from an apparent gene duplication on chromosome 2.[15] Thus, caspases 8 and 10 may play redundant roles in human cells.

Mitochondria also play important roles in apoptosis, releasing cytochrome c (Cyt-c) into the cytosol, which then causes assembly of a multiprotein caspase-activating complex, referred to as the "apoptosome."[16,17] The central component of the apoptosome is Apaf1, a caspase-activating protein that oligomerizes upon binding Cyt-c and which specifically binds procaspase-9. Apaf1 and procaspase-9 interact with each other via their caspase recruitment domains (CARDs). Such CARD–CARD interactions play important roles in many steps in apoptosis pathways. In addition to Cyt-c, mitochondria also release several other proteins of relevance to apoptosis, including endonuclease G, AIF (an activator of nuclear endonucleases), and SMAC (Diablo) and Omi (HtrA), antagonists of a family of caspase-inhibitory proteins known as the IAPs (inhibitors of apoptosis) (see section "Inhibitors of Apoptosis" below).

The central importance of the Cyt-c–dependent pathway for apoptosis is underscored by the observation that cells derived from mice in which either the *apaf1* or *procaspase-9* genes have been ablated are incapable of undergoing apoptosis in response to agents that trigger Cyt-c release from mitochondria.[18] Nevertheless, such cells can die by nonapoptotic routes,[19] demonstrating that mitochondria control both caspase-dependent and caspase-independent cell death pathways. Moreover, distinguishing mitochondria-driven apoptotic from nonapoptotic cell death can be challenging in many contexts because of the similar morphologic features caused probably by some of the proteins released from these organelle such as endonuclease G and AIF, which promote chromatin condensation and DNA fragmentation. The mitochondrial mechanisms for apoptotic and nonapoptotic cell death are activated by myriad stimuli, including growth factor deprivation, oxidants, Ca^{2+} overload, DNA-damaging agents, microtubule-modifying drugs, and much more.[17,20] In this sense, mitochondria are sometimes viewed as central integrators of cell stress signals that dictate ultimately cell life and death decisions.

Mitochondria can also participate in cell death pathways induced via TNF family DRs, through crosstalk mechanisms involving proteins such as Bid, BAR, and Bap31.[21-24] However, mitochondrial ("intrinsic") and DR ("extrinsic") pathways for caspase activation are fully capable of independent operation in most types of cells.[25]

Cell death mechanisms are also linked to endoplasmic reticulum (ER). In most cases, however, these ER-initiated signals ultimately seem to impinge on mitochondria as the downstream effectors of the cell death pathway. In this regard, the ER is a central regulator of intracellular Ca^{2+}, and ER membranes form close contacts with mitochondria to create structures where Ca^{2+} effluxes from ER into mitochondria, thereby impacting mitochondrial function in profound ways that can either promote cell life or cause death. Too much Ca^{2+} entry into mitochondria, for instance, triggers a phenomenon called mitochondrial permeability transition (MPT) in which the organelles swell and eventually rupture.

However, in addition to the role of ER Ca^{2+} and mitochondria-driven cell death, another pathway for apoptosis has been linked to accumulation of unfolded proteins in the ER. Specifically, ER stress induces expression of the proapoptotic transcription factor CHOP, which, in turn, stimulates expression of DR5 (TRAILR2), causing caspase-8-dependent apoptosis.[26] Additionally, CHOP has been reported to directly stimulate transcription of the gene encoding Bim, a proapoptotic member of the Bcl-2 family (see section "Suppressors of Apoptosis" below) that stimulates Cyt-c release from mitochondria. Thus, ER stress has multiple potential routes of stimulating cell death pathways, with the predominant pathway probably varying among cell types and pathophysiologic contexts.

Although diverse mechanisms exist for activating initiator Caspases, as outlined above, in most instances, the biochemical mechanisms appear to be remarkably similar. Much of caspase activation and can be explained by the "induced proximity model,"[27] in which forcing dimerization of procaspases results in conformational states that promote protease activation, typically resulting in cleavage events that lock the proteases into their fully active state. This mechanism is clearly operative in the caspase-activation pathways induced by TNF family receptors (extrinsic pathway) and Cyt-c/mitochondria ("intrinsic pathway").

● SUPPRESSORS OF APOPTOSIS

Given the critical importance of making the correct choices about cell life–death decisions in complex multicellular organisms, it is not surprising that the pathways governing caspase activation are under exquisite control by networks of proteins that directly or indirectly communicate with these proteases. A delicate balance between proapoptotic and antiapoptotic regulators of apoptosis pathways is at play on a continual basis, ensuring the survival of long-lived cells and the proper turnover of short-lived cells in a variety of tissues, including the marrow, thymus, and peripheral lymphoid tissues. The antiapoptotic proteins responsible for creating roadblocks to cell death have been mapped to specific caspase-activation pathways.

BCL-2 FAMILY

The Bcl-2 family represents a large group of proteins (number >26 in humans) that control mitochondria-dependent steps in cell-death pathways, including dictating whether Cyt-c is or is not released from these

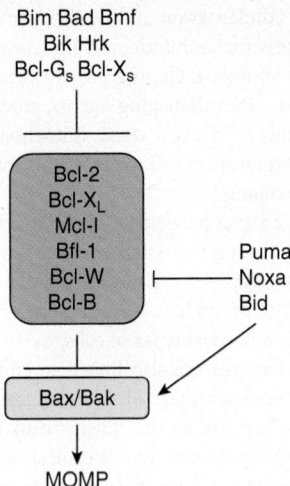

Figure 15–2. Network of interactions among Bcl-2 family proteins. The functional and physical interactions among proapoptotic and antiapoptotic Bcl-2 family proteins are depicted. Illustrative members of the Bcl-2 family are shown.

organelles (Fig. 15–2). Both proapoptotic and antiapoptotic Bcl-2 family proteins have been delineated.[28] These proteins are best known for their roles in controlling the intrinsic (mitochondrial) cell-death pathway,[20] although effects on the ER-pathway for cell death have also been documented.[29] Even though the human genome encodes at least 26 Bcl-2 family proteins, only six of these are antiapoptotic (in humans, Bcl-2, Bcl-X$_L$ [BCL2L1], Bcl-W [BCL2L2], Mcl-1 [BCL2L3], Bfl-1 [BCL2L5], and Bcl-B [BCL2L10]). Several types of animal viruses also harbor Bcl-2 family genes within their genomes, including herpes viruses implicated in cancer such as the Epstein-Barr virus (EBV) and Kaposi sarcoma virus (KSV). The relative ratios of anti- and proapoptotic Bcl-2 family proteins dictate the ultimate sensitivity or resistance of cells to various apoptotic stimuli, including growth factor deprivation, hypoxia, radiation, anticancer drugs, oxidants, and Ca^{2+} overload.

Various Bcl-2 family members play important roles in controlling the life spans of hematopoietic cells, as evidenced by phenotypes generated in genetically engineered mice (gene knockouts and transgenics) and also (in some cases) by human clinical experiences with experimental therapeutics targeting some of these proteins. For example, antiapoptotic protein Bcl-2 is required for survival of mature T cells and B cells, with deficiency of Bcl-2 causing lymphopenia. Conversely, the proapoptotic protein Bim is necessary for limiting expansion of T and B lymphocytes, with deficiency of Bim causing lymphocytosis. Bim also plays important role in eradicating autoreactive T cells in the thymus ("negative selection"), having important implications for mechanisms of autoimmune diseases.[30] Bcl-X$_L$ is required for platelet homeostasis, such that either genetic or pharmacologically induced Bcl-X$_L$ deficiency causes thrombocytopenia. Antiapoptotic protein Mcl-1 is particularly important for survival of the myeloid lineage in mice, as well as contributing to lymphocyte survival. Conversely, antiapoptotic protein Bcl-W is not required for hematopoiesis in mice, despite being widely expressed in myeloid lineage cells. It should be noted that direct comparisons of gene manipulations in mice with the human circumstance are not always possible because of genomic differences in the Bcl-2 family genes of mice versus humans (e.g., human Bfl-1 versus murine A1; human Bcl-B versus murine Boo/Diva).

Many members of the Bcl-2 family have a hydrophobic stretch of amino acids near their carboxyl-terminus that anchors them in the outer mitochondrial membrane.[17] In contrast, other Bcl-2 family members

such as Bid, Bim, and Bad, lack these membrane-anchoring domains, but dynamically target mitochondria in response to specific stimuli. Still others have the membrane-anchoring domain but keep it latched against the body of the protein until stimulated to expose it (e.g., Bax).[31]

Based on their predicted (or experimentally determined) three-dimensional structures, Bcl-2 family proteins can be broadly divided into two groups. One subset of these proteins is probably similar in structure to the pore-forming domains of bacterial toxins, such as the colicins and diphtheria toxin.[32–35] These α-helical pore-like proteins include both antiapoptotic proteins (Bcl-2, Bcl-X$_L$, Mcl-1, Bfl-1, Bcl-W, Bcl-B) and proapoptotic proteins (Bax, Bak, Bok, and Bid). Most of the proteins in this subcategory can be recognized by conserved stretches of amino acid sequence homology, including the presence of Bcl-2 homology (BH) domains, BH1, BH2, BH3, and sometimes BH4. However, this is not uniformly the case, as the Bid protein contains only a BH3 domain but has been determined to share the same overall protein-fold with Bcl-X$_L$, Bcl-2, and Bax.[33,34] Where tested to date, these proteins have all been shown to form ion-conducting channels in synthetic membranes *in vitro*, including Bcl-2, Bcl-X$_L$, Bax, and Bid,[36–40] but the significance of this pore activity remains unclear.

The other subset of Bcl-2 family proteins appears to have in common only the presence of the BH3 domain, including Bad, Bik, Bim, Hrk, Bcl-G$_s$, p193, APR (Noxa), and PUMA. These "BH3-only" proteins are uniformly proapoptotic. Their cell-death–inducing activity depends, in most cases, on their ability to dimerize with antiapoptotic Bcl-2 family members, functioning as *trans*-dominant inhibitors of proteins such as Bcl-2 and Bcl-X$_L$.[41,42] However, some of these proteins (e.g., Bid, PUMA, Bim) can also interact with proapoptotic proteins (e.g., Bax, Bak), functioning as agonists of the killers, in addition to dimerizing with antiapoptotics (e.g., Bcl-2; Bcl-X$_L$) to function as antagonists of these cell-survival proteins (see Fig. 15–2).[28,43] Binding of Bid to Bax or Bak promotes insertion of these proteins into membranes where they oligomerize, apparently forming large pores through which molecules such as Cyt-c, SMAC, and Omi can escape from mitochondria or causing an increase in the permeability of the outer membrane of mitochondria through more complex mechanisms.[44,45] Bax and Bak thus induce mitochondrial outer membrane permeabilization (MOMP), which is a critical event that not only causes release of death-inducing mitochondrial proteins but also secondarily causes necrosis by uncoupling of oxidative phosphorylation (when Cyt-c becomes limiting) and diversion of electrons from the respiratory chain into production of toxic free radicals.[46,47]

The BH3 domain mediates dimerization among Bcl-2 family proteins. This domain consists of an amphipathic α-helix of approximately 16 amino acids that inserts into a hydrophobic crevice on the surface of antiapoptotic proteins such as Bcl-2 and Bcl-X$_L$.[48] The BH3-only proteins link a wide variety of environmental stimuli to the mitochondrial pathway for apoptosis, with some examples outlined below.

In addition to mitochondria, mechanistic links for Bcl-2 family proteins to ER stress and autophagy have also been delineated. For example, Bax and Bak can bind the ER stress signaling protein, IRE-1, thereby stimulating its intrinsic autokinase activity and its endoribonuclease activity.[49] Proapoptotic (Bak/Bax) and antiapoptotic (Bcl-2/Bcl-X$_L$) family members also have opposing effects on basal ER Ca^{2+} levels, probably via effects on Ca^{2+} channel proteins in ER membranes (e.g., IP3Rs, BI-1, and TmBim3). Autophagy protein Beclin contains a BH3-like domain that mediates interactions with antiapoptotic Bcl-2 family proteins, which sequester Beclin and thereby reduce autophagic flux.[50] Autophagy, which is a lysosome-dependent catabolic pathway, can either promote cell survival by providing access to nutrients during times of nutrient insufficiency and hypoxia, or it can cause cell death when stimulated to an extreme.[51]

FLIP

The c-FLIP proteins are another type of apoptosis suppressor that operates via directly binding to certain caspases and their upstream activator, FADD. The *c-FLIP* gene of humans resides in a tandem gene cluster on chromosome 2, which contains the genes encoding procaspases 8 and 10, suggestive of gene duplication events. Two isoforms of c-FLIP are produced from a single gene, including the long form, which is highly similar in overall sequence to procaspases 8 and 10, containing tandem copies of DEDs, followed by a pseudocaspase domain that lacks enzymatic activity. The shorter isoform consists only of the DED domains, thus resembling analogous proteins encoded in the genomes of some mammalian viruses.[52] FLIP-S is exclusively antoptotic whereas FLIP-L can be either pro- or antiapoptotic, depending on its levels of expression relative to procaspases 8 and 10.[53] In general, FLIP proteins form complexes with procaspases 8 and 10, preventing their dimerization and activation, as well as competing for binding to adapter protein FADD, which is required for caspase recruitment to DR complexes.[54,55] Thus, in most circumstances, FLIP proteins create blockades in the extrinsic pathway for apoptosis.

Additionally, a role in suppressing nonapoptotic cell death (necroptosis) has been described for FLIP in partnership with caspase-8.[56] In this regard, TNFR1 signaling has been shown to stimulate caspase-independent cell death in some circumstances (commonly called "necroptosis") via a mechanism that is suppressed by FLIP and caspase-8 but that is dependent on the protein kinase Rip3 (see section "Inhibitors of Apoptosis" below). It is thought that dimers consisting of the longer isoform of c-FLIP plus caspase-8 direct the proteolytic activity of caspase-8 to substrates that promote cell survival rather than cell death.[57] Among the relevant substrates is the kinase Rip1, an upstream activator of Rip3. Thus, FLIP proteins play complex roles in cell death regulation mediated by various members of the TNF Receptor family.

INHIBITORS OF APOPTOSIS

The IAP proteins (n = 8 in humans) suppress apoptosis via a diversity of mechanisms, including directly binding to and inhibiting certain caspases.[58,59] IAPs are characterized by the presence of protein interaction domains called BIRs (baculovirus internal repeats), numbering between 1 and 3 per protein. Most IAPs also carry RING domains that endow them with E3 ligase activity through interactions with ubiquitin conjugating enzymes (UBCs). Some of the apoptogenic proteins released from mitochondria, notably SMAC and HtrA2, bind certain BIRs and thereby compete for protein interactions on the surface of IAPs. Some examples of IAP mechanisms are provided here.

XIAP (so-called because its encoding gene resides on the X-chromosome) contains 3 BIR domains. BIR2 of XIAP binds downstream effector proteases, caspases-3 and -7, to suppress apoptosis at a distal point. BIR3 of XIAP binds upstream initiator protease, caspase-9, to suppress an apical step in the mitochondrial pathway for apoptosis.

The c-IAP1 (BIRC2) and c-IAP2 (BIRC3) proteins are also capable of binding to caspases 3, 7, and 9, although they are less potent by far as direct enzymatic inhibitors and may rely on their E3 ligase activity for controlling caspase degradation. However, these IAP family members also participate in other cell death-relevant mechanisms by impacting signal transduction by TNF family receptors. Binding of TNF to one of its principal cellular receptors expressed widely on cells, TNFR1, is capable of triggering at least three different signaling pathways, each involving overlapping but distinct protein complexes that are assembled at the receptor (Fig. 15–3). One of these TNFR1-initiated pathways causes caspase activation and apoptosis by DISC assembly (described in the section "Caspase Activation Pathways," and Fig. 15-1 above). Another pathway causes activation of the kinase Rip3, usually via the upstream

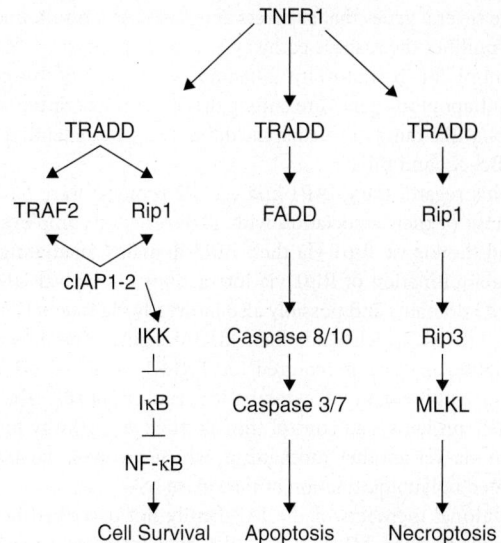

Figure 15–3. Opposing pathways for cell death and cell survival are induced by tumor necrosis factor receptor (TNFR). TNFR1 is the best studied of the death domain (DD)-containing TNF family receptors, which include in humans Fas (CD95), tumor necrosis factor–related apoptosis-inducing ligand (TRAIL) receptor-1 (TRAILR1, DR4), TRAILR2 (DR5), DR3, and DR6. DD-containing adapter protein TRADD (tumor necrosis factor receptor death domain) binds the DD in the cytosolic domain of TNFR1, which then connects to at least one of three different pathways that are outlined here. A cell survival pathway results in nuclear factor (NF)-κB activation, whereby TRADD recruits the DD-containing protein Rip1 and also binds the E3 ligase/adapter protein TRAF2 (tumor receptor-associated factor 2). Rip1 and TRAF2 bind c-IAP1 (inhibitor of apoptosis 1) and c-IAP2. The resulting complex promotes noncanonical ubiquitination of the kinase Rip1, triggering a signal transduction kinase pathway that results in activation of I-κB kinases (IKKs) that cause I-κB ubiquitination and proteasomal degradation, thereby releasing sequestered NF-κB to allow its translocation into the nucleus where it stimulates expression of multiple antiapoptotic genes. In the TNFR1-mediated apoptosis pathway, the DD of TRADD associates with the DD of FADD, which, in turn, binds caspases 8 and 10 via their death effector domains (DEDs), triggering protease activation and thereby stimulating apoptosis. The TNFR1-mediated pathway for necrosis (necroptosis) involves a cascade of events that include recruitment of Rip1, which, in turn, activates Rip3, which activates mixed-lineage kinase domain-like (MLKL) kinase and which causes mitochondrial and probably lysosomal changes that stimulate reactive oxygen species (ROS) generation and lead to necrosis.

kinase Rip1, which associates with TNFR1 complexes.[60] The Rip3-dependent cell death pathway is caspase-independent, leading to nonapoptotic cell death ("necroptosis") through a process involving reactive oxygen species (ROS) generated by mitochondria. Another serine/threonine kinase, mixed-lineage kinase domain-like (MLKL) protein, appears to be a critical downstream mediator of Rip3-induced necroptosis. This Rip3-dependent pathway for necroptosis is suppressed by c-IAP1 and c-IAP2, probably via their roles as E3 ligases and possibly involving ubiquitin/proteasome-mediated reductions in Rip3 protein levels.[61] Finally, TNFR1 stimulates a cell survival pathway in which c-IAP1 and c-IAP2 participate. In this TNFR1-mediated survival pathway, the kinase Rip1 comes together with the E3 ligases c-IAP1, c-IAP2, and tumor receptor-associated factor 2 (TRAF2) to stimulate noncanonical (lysine 63, rather than lysine 48) ubiquitination of Rip1, initiating a signal transduction pathway that causes activation of transcription factor nuclear factor (NF)-κB. NF-κB influences the expression of many target genes involved in host defenses and immune regulation, among which are several genes that suppress apoptosis. As a result, this NF-κB pathway nullifies the caspase pathway, negating apoptosis,[62] in addition to accounting for the untoward inflammatory actions of this cytokine. Several antiapoptotic genes are among the direct transcriptional targets of NF-κB (REL)-family proteins, including the genes encoding c-FLIP, c-IAP2, Bcl-X$_L$, and Bfl-1.

In this regard, the c-IAP1 and c-IAP2 proteins were first identified because of their association with TNF receptor complexes. These IAPs bind the kinase Rip1 via their BIR3 domains, mediating noncanonical ubiquitination of Rip1 via interactions of atypical UBCs with their RING domains and possibly also indirectly via interactions of the E3 ligase TRAF2, which binds their BIR1 domains. The noncanonical ubiquitination of Rip1 is required for TNFR1-mediated NF-κB activation and suppression of cytokine-induced apoptosis. The c-IAP1 and c-IAP2 proteins also control the "alternative" pathway for NF-κB activation via yet another mechanism, which involves classical lysine 48 mediated polyubiquitination of the kinase Nik.

Additional members of the IAP family not described here (Survivin, Apollon/Bruce, ML-IAP, etc.) also have interesting mechanisms of interacting with components of cell-death pathways and they also can have other roles beyond cell-death regulation. For example, XIAP, c-IAP1, and c-IAP2 have other documented cellular activities, which include, for example, their interactions with kinases (e.g., Rip2) or kinase-binding adapter proteins (TAB/Tak) involved in processes such as innate immunity and morphogenesis. In these circumstances, the most relevant activity of IAPs appears to be their noncanonical E3 ligase activity, as well as a protein scaffold role where they serve as platforms for assembling multiprotein complexes. Additional roles for IAP family members include cell division, where, for example, the Survivin protein plays a fundamental role in chromosome segregation and cytokinesis.

Several of the IAPs are opposed by proteins released from mitochondria, SMAC and HtrA2. SMAC and Htra2 bind BIR domains on IAPs, thus displacing caspases and other associated proteins. In many cases, SMAC binding to IAPs induces their polyubiquitination and proteasomal degradation. Thus, factors that cause MOMP take the breaks off the caspases by eliminating various IAP family proteins.

SIGNAL TRANSDUCTION AND APOPTOSIS REGULATION

Various receptor-mediated signal transduction pathways converge on the core components of the cell death machinery outlined above, including receptors for growth factors, lymphokines and cytokines. Some examples illustrating the intimate links between receptor-mediated signal transduction and apoptosis pathways are provided here (Fig. 15–4).

LYMPHOKINES

Many lymphokine receptors signal via Jak/STAT pathways. STAT family transcription factors are known to stimulate transcription of the

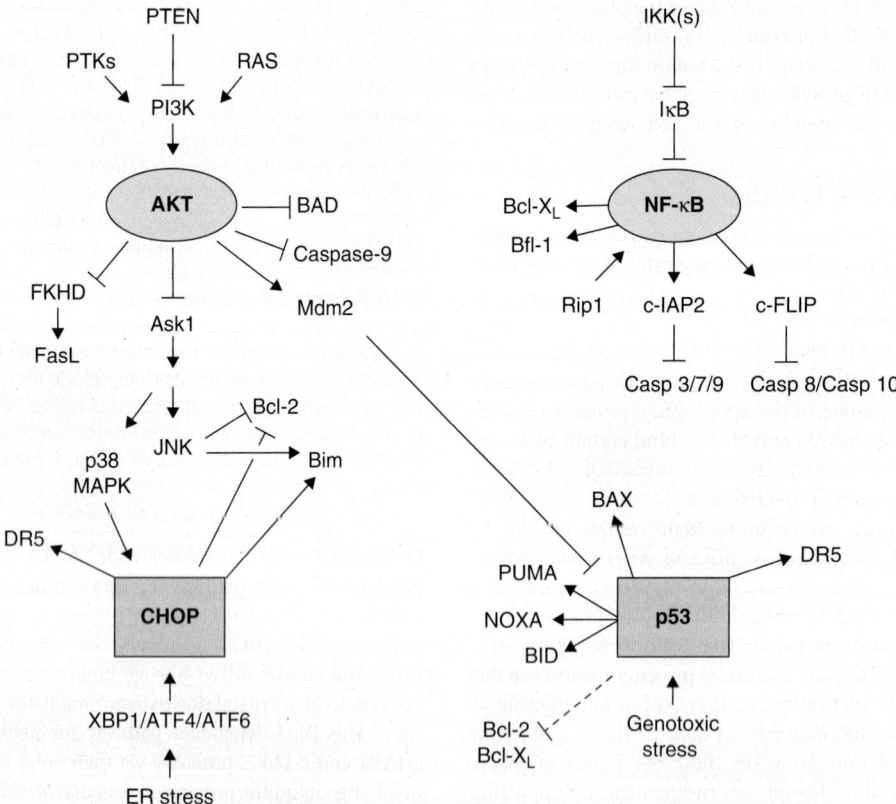

Figure 15–4. Signal transduction and apoptosis regulation. Some of the transcription factors and kinases that play prominent roles in apoptosis regulation are depicted, including kinases Akt (PKB) and the transcription factors p53, NF-κB, and CHOP. Illustrative examples of the connections to apoptosis-regulating proteins and genes are shown, without attempting to be comprehensive. The protein kinase Akt (PKB) is activated in response to second-messengers produced by PI3K, a lipid kinase that is activated by many growth factor receptors and oncoproteins. PTEN is a lipid phosphatase that prevents accumulation of these second messengers, the expression of which is lost in many tumors through gene deletions, gene mutations, and other mechanisms.[89] Akt can phosphorylate and either activate (arrows) or inactivate (⊣) multiple proteins directly or indirectly relevant to apoptosis.[90] Expression of the transcription factor CHOP is stimulated by transcription factors that are elaborated during ER stress, including XBP1, ATF4, and ATF6. See text for additional details.

BCL-X gene as at least one of their mechanisms of suppressing apoptosis. Examples with relevance to hematopoietic system include erythropoietin-mediated stimulation of survival of erythrocyte precursors and interleukin (IL)-3 and IL-7-mediasted stimulation of survival of B-lymphocyte progenitors (pro/pre–B-cells). Additionally, Jak family nonreceptor protein tyrosine kinases are capable of stimulating phosphatidylinositol 3'-kinase (PI3K) activity,[63] which, in turn, causes activation of Akt family kinases. The murine gene encoding Akt was first discovered by virtue of its similarity to the v-akt oncogene found in some murine leukemia viruses and through its activation in thymomas caused by retrovirus insertions near the c-akt gene.[64] Humans contain three AKT genes. Akt can phosphorylate multiple proteins within the core apoptosis machinery. For example, the proapoptotic Bcl-2 family member Bad is a target of Akt, where phosphorylation of Bad causes its sequestration by 14–3–3 family proteins, thus inhibiting Bad from heterodimerizing with Bcl-X$_L$.[65] Akt also can phosphorylate human caspase-9, blocking apoptosis downstream of mitochondria.[66] Another substrate of Akt that is relevant to apoptosis is forkhead transcription factors (FKHD). Some FKHD family members appear to control apoptosis, perhaps by affecting transcription of the gene encoding FasL.[67] Phosphorylation of FKHD by Akt prevents its entry into the nucleus.

CYTOKINES

Several cytokines stimulate the activation of NF-κB (REL) family transcription factors. NF-κB directly binds the promoters and induces expression of several antiapoptotic genes, including the BCL-2 family members BCL-X and BFL-1, the IAP-family member C-IAP2, and C-FLIP.[62] Thus, elevations in NF-κB activity can increase cellular resistance to apoptosis, affecting (1) the Intrinsic (mitochondrial) pathway through elevations in antiapoptotic Bcl-2 family proteins, (2) the extrinsic (TNF family DR) pathway through upregulation of c-Flip, and (3) downstream common pathways involving effector caspases as a result of overexpression of c-IAP2.

The first example of NF-κB involvement in malignancy was provided by studies of the avian Rev-T retrovirus, a transforming retrovirus that causes rapidly fatal lymphomas in young chickens and which carries the v-Rel oncogene. The cellular homologue of this viral oncogene is C-REL, which encodes the p65 subunit of NF-κB. Amplification of the C-REL gene has been reported in non-Hodgkin lymphomas (NHLs), occurring particularly in diffuse large B-cell lymphoma and commonly associated with extranodal presentation.[68] Other genetic alterations associated with dysregulation of NF-κB include chromosomal translocations involving the I-κB family member BCL-3 in B-CLL.[69] I-κB family proteins bind and sequester NF-kB complexes, preventing the transcription factor from entering the nucleus.[70] Typically, I-κB is regulated by ubiquitin-mediated turnover by the 26S proteasome. Mutations in I-κB thus may enhance NF-κB activity, either by producing unstable proteins or reducing the affinity of I-κB for NF-κB. The anticancer activity of drugs that inhibit the proteasome, approved for multiple myeloma, may be attributable in part to suppression of I-κB degradation, thereby inhibiting NF-κB induction.[71]

GENOTOXIC STRESS

Gamma-radiation and many DNA-damaging anticancer drugs potently stimulate apoptosis of hematopoietic cells. The principal mediator of apoptosis induced by genotoxic stress is p53. The p53 protein is a tetrameric transcription factor, whose levels are controlled by the E3 ligase Mdm2. This transcription factor directly induces expression of BH3-only proteins Noxa (APR), Bid, and PUMA,[72–74] thus linking p53 to the death machinery. Additionally, p53 directly binds and transcriptionally activates the human BAX gene promoter. Loss of p53 activity occurs in many human malignancies by a variety of mechanism, including gene deletion, gene mutations that result in mutant p53 proteins lacking transcriptional activity, and MDM2 gene amplification. Small molecule drugs that block Mdm2 protein interaction with p53 have shown promising preclinical activity against hematopoietic malignancies.

Interestingly, in addition to its role as a nuclear transcription factor, evidence has emerged suggesting that p53 may promote apoptosis also via nontranscriptional mechanisms under some circumstances. Specifically, a cytoplasmic pool of p53 reportedly associates with mitochondria, directly inducing activation of the Bax and inhibiting Bcl-2 and Bcl-X$_L$.[75] Importantly, even mutant p53 is capable of activating this cell-death pathway, raising hopes of finding pharmacologic interventions that would entice mutant p53 to attack mitochondria and trigger apoptosis of cancer cells in which this important tumor-suppressor gene product has suffered somatic mutations that inactive its nuclear (transcriptional) functions.

● HEMATOLOGIC DISEASES AND APOPTOSIS

Either insufficient or excessive apoptosis plays important roles in a wide diversity of hematologic diseases. Convincing evidence has gathered to support a major role for insufficient apoptosis in the context of most (if not all) hematologic malignancies, where defects in apoptosis prolong cell life span and thereby promote cell accumulation, as well as complementing the proapoptotic effects of certain oncogenes (e.g., C-MYC; CYCLIN-D1), permitting growth factor independent cell survival, and promoting resistance to chemotherapy, radiation, and immune-mediated cell killing. Defects in apoptosis also seem to underlie some aspects of autoimmunity, where a failure to eradicate autoreactive lymphocytes occurs. Conversely, excessive apoptosis has been implicated in the depletion of CD4+ T-lymphocytes seen in chronic HIV infection, bacteria-mediated killing of macrophages, myelodysplastic disorders where marrow failure occurs resulting in anemia and failed myelopoiesis, and many other conditions. Some examples of the human diseases that have been linked to genomic alterations of apoptosis genes are highlighted here, without an attempt to be comprehensive.

ALTERNATIONS IN APOPTOSIS GENES IN HEMATOLOGIC MALIGNANCIES

Defects in apoptosis (cell death) are recognized as one of the hallmarks of essentially all cancers. Not surprisingly, therefore, myriad examples of alternations in genes regulating the core apoptosis machinery have been delineated in human cancers. Hematologic malignancies have, in fact, revealed many of the first and most striking examples of the critical importance of cell death as a constraint to inappropriate cell expansion and accumulation. Here, some illustrative examples are provided without an attempt to be comprehensive, particularly focusing on the families of apoptosis-regulating genes outlined above with emphasis on genomic alterations. Additionally, myriad epigenetic mechanisms modulate the expression of apoptosis genes in hematologic malignancies, which are not covered here.

BCL-2 FAMILY

The Bcl-2 family derives its name from discovery of the founding member as a result of its involvement in B-cell lymphomas and leukemias. The human BCL-2 gene is involved in t(14;18) chromosomal translocations found commonly in NHLs. In this regard, the BCL-2 gene normally resides on chromosome 18, but it becomes merged with the immunoglobulin heavy-chain (IgH) locus on chromosome 14, probably as a result of aberrant actions of the V-D-J gene recombination machinery responsible for antibody generation in B-cells. In this context, the *BCL-2* gene becomes deregulated in its expression via the powerful *cis*-acting enhancer elements of the IgH locus. Chromosomal translocations activating *BCL-2* occur in most indolent NHLs (especially follicular B-cell lymphomas) as well as a substantial proportion of aggressive NHLs (perhaps commonly arising from progression of a previously undiagnosed low-grade B-lymphoma). Gene amplification provides another mechanism for *BCL-2* gene dysregulation, and is reported in nearly 20 percent of aggressive B-NHLs, particularly diffuse large B-cell lymphomas (DLBCLs). Thus, by studying the cytogenetics of B-cell malignancies, the world's first example of an antiapoptotic gene (*BCL-2*) was discovered.

Additionally, loss of genes encoding microRNAs (miRNAs) that posttranscriptionally suppress *BCL-2* by inducing Bcl-2 mRNA degradation accounts for the widespread dysregulation of *BCL-2* gene in B-cell chronic lymphocytic leukemia (B-CLL). In this context, approximately 90 percent of B-CLLs have homozygous loss of function mutations or deletions involving *miRNA15* and *miRNA16* on chromosome 13q14, thus derepressing *BCL-2* gene expression. This somatic loss of *miRNA15* and *miRNA16* genes in CLL was the first example of miRNA genes operating as tumor suppressors.

Genetic lesions responsible for dysregulation of other members of the Bcl-2 family have also been identified in various types of hematologic and nonhematologic malignancies. Among these somatic genetic mechanisms is the amplification of the *BCL-X (BCL2L2)* or *MCL-1 (BCL2L3)* gene loci, which occurs probably in one in 10 human solid tumors. Conversely, homozygous gene mutations that inactivate the proapoptotic *BAX* gene have also been identified in occasional hematopoietic malignancies and some solid tumors. In this regard, deletions or inactivating mutations in the tumor-suppressor p53 also reduce the expression of several proapoptotic Bcl-2 family genes, including the *BAX*, PUMA, NOXA, and *BID* genes, which are direct transcriptional targets of p53 (see above).[76] The incidence of p53 gene deletions and mutations varies among hematologic malignancies, ranging from rare (<5 percent) in T-cell leukemias and low-grade B-cell lymphomas to frequent (>30 percent) in disorders such as high-grade B-cell lymphomas, Burkitt lymphomas, and relapsed/aggressive acute lymphocytic leukemia (ALL), chronic lymphocytic leukemias (CLLs) that have progressed to Richter syndrome, and chronic myelogenous leukemias (CML) in blast crisis.[77]

INHIBITORS OF APOPTOSIS

Genomic lesions involving the IAP family genes are also associated with hematologic malignancies. For example, in marginal zone mucosa-associated lymphoid tissue (MALT) B-cell lymphoma, the most common of the extranodal NHLs, t(11;18)(q21;q21) chromosomal translocations occur frequently.[78] These translocations fuse the three BIR domains of c-IAP2 with portions of the gene encoding MALT1, a caspase-like protein. The predominant mechanism by which the resulting c-IAP2/MALT1 fusion protein suppresses apoptosis appears to be hyperactivation of NF-κB. In this regard, the BIR1 domain of c-IAP1 binds NF-κB–inducing E3 ligase TRAF2, and this interaction has been shown to be critical for NF-κB induction by c-IAP2/MALT1 fusion proteins. Additionally, the C-terminal region of MALT1 also binds a related NF-κB–inducing E3 ligase, TRAF6, making additional contributions to NF-κB stimulation. Interestingly, *TRAF2* gene amplification has also been described in a significance number of human malignancies.

CASPASES

Inactivating mutations have been described in a variety of cancers. In approximately 15 percent of NHLs, mutations that alter the activity of caspase-10 have been reported. The resulting mutant caspase-10 proteins may operate as dominant-negative inhibitors of DR-mediated apoptosis.[79] Although exhaustive analysis has not been performed to date, overall mutations inactivating caspase-encoding genes appear to be relatively rare in hematopoietic malignancies, though epigenetic silencing may be more common.

TUMOR NECROSIS FACTOR FAMILY DEATH RECEPTORS

Somatic mutations in the *FAS (CD95)* gene have been found in multiple myelomas (MMs) and NHLs.[80] Missense mutations within the DD of Fas (CD95) were associated with retention of the wild-type allele, suggesting a dominant-negative mechanism, whereas missense mutations outside the DD were associated with allelic loss.[80] The observation that tumor-suppressor p53 can induce transcription of the DRs Fas (CD95) and DR5 (TRAILR2) in some types of tumor cells,[81,82] suggests an additional cancer-relevant mechanism by which reductions in the expression TNF family DRs could occur in human malignancies, namely, secondarily to genomic lesions that inactivate p53 or that cause overexpression of endogenous p53 antagonists.[83]

OTHER GENOMICALLY BASED DISEASES INVOLVING APOPTOSIS GENES

Hereditary deficiency of XIAP is a very strong risk factor for early onset inflammatory bowel disease (IBD). This function of XIAP is probably not related to its role in apoptosis, but rather stems from the function of XIAP as a component of NACHT and Leucine rich repeat domain-containing receptor (NLR) family protein complexes involved in innate immunity. Causative mutations have been identified in the *FAS (CD95)* gene of humans in patients with autoimmune lymphoproliferative syndrome (ALPS), also known as Canale-Smith syndrome.[84] Thus, the Fas/Fas ligand (FasL) system plays a critical role in lymphocyte homeostasis *in vivo*. At least some of the mutant Fas proteins found in humans with ALPS have been shown to operate as *trans*-dominant inhibitors of wild-type Fas, probably explaining the dominant inheritance pattern of this disorder. Likewise, germline mutations in Fas and FasL have been discovered as the underlying basis for the lymphoproliferative autoimmune phenotype of *lpr/lpr* and *gdl/gdl* strain mice, respectively.[85,86] In contrast to humans, however, the mutations in the *fas* gene of *lpr*-strain mice produce disease with a recessive inheritance pattern.[85] FasL, like most TNF family members, is a trimer, and the receptor also forms trimers and probably higher-order oligomers, thus explaining why some Fas mutants display dominant-negative effects on wild-type Fas while others do not. Indeed, mutant versions of Fas from some patients with hereditary ALPS have been demonstrated to antagonize wild-type Fas,[87] probably forming mixed oligomers of wild-type and mutant molecules. Additionally, mutations in caspase-10 gene that produce altered proteins that interfere with Fas-induced apoptosis have been identified in patients with ALPS.[88]

These examples of autoimmune disorders associated with hereditary alternations in apoptosis-regulatory genes highlight the intricate linkages between cell death regulation and host–pathogen interactions. Many components of the apoptosis machinery play important roles in aspects of innate and adaptive immunity, possibly reflecting the notion that altruistic cell suicide may be the best defense against pathogens for multicellular organisms. Moreover, a subfamily of the caspases (e.g., caspases 1, 4, and 5 in humans) has as its primary role the proteolytic processing and activation of inflammatory cytokines (pro–IL-1β, pro–IL-18, etc.), with apoptosis representing a secondary function that is observed mostly in the context of excessive stimulation.

CONCLUSIONS

Programmed cell-death mechanisms play critical roles in hematopoietic and immune cell homeostasis. Elaboration of the complex cell-death pathways and the networks of proteins that modulate these pathways have provided insights into the underlying mechanisms of cell life–death decisions, although many mechanistic details remain still to be revealed. In several cases, the available information has already sparked efforts to translate the base of information into therapeutic strategies. Among the experimental therapeutics targeting components of the cell death machinery that have entered clinical testing are small molecule inhibitors of Bcl-2 family and IAP family proteins, as well as large molecule modulators of TNF family DRs. Compounds that modulate upstream inputs into cell death pathways are also advancing through clinical evaluations, such as small molecule inhibitors of Mdm2 (which cause p53 protein accumulation) and small molecule inhibitors of Akt family kinases. Many other targets within the cell-death pathways are the subject of preclinical drug discovery efforts today. The stage is thus set for continued progress in manipulating cell-death pathways for therapeutic benefit of multiple diseases, including disorders of the hematopoietic system.

REFERENCES

1. Kerr JF, Wyllie AH, Currie AR: Apoptosis: A basic biological phenomenon with wide-ranging implications in tissue kinetics. *Br J Cancer* 26(4):239–257, 1972.
2. Thornberry NA, Lazebnik Y: Caspases: Enemies within. *Science* 281:1312–1316, 1998.
3. Cryns V, Yuan Y: Proteases to die for. *Genes Dev* 12:1551–1570, 1999.
4. Alnemri ES, Livingston DJ, Nicholson DW, et al: Human ICE/CED-3 Protease Nomenclature. *Cell* 87:171, 1996.
5. Salvesen GS, Dixit VM: Caspases: Intracellular signaling by proteolysis. *Cell* 91:443–446, 1996, 1997.
6. Motyka B, Korbutt G, Pinkoski MJ, et al: Mannose 6-phosphate/insulin-like growth factor II receptor is a death receptor for granzyme B during cytotoxic T cell-induced apoptosis. *Cell* 103:491–500, 2000.
7. Martin SJ, Amarante-Mendes GP, Shi L, et al: The cytotoxic cell protease granzyme B initiates apoptosis in a cell-free system by proteolytic processing and activation of the ICE/CED-3 family protease, CPP32, via a novel two-step mechanism. *EMBO J* 15(10):2407–2416, 1996.
8. Zhou Q, Krebs J, Snipas S, et al: Interaction of the baculovirus antiapoptotic protein p35 with caspases. Specificity, kinetics, and characterization of the caspase/p35 complex. *Biochemistry* 37:10757–10765, 1998.
9. Quan LT, Caputo A, Bleackley RC, et al: Granzyme B is inhibited by the cowpox virus serpin cytokine response modifier A. *J Biol Chem* 270:10377–10379, 1995.
10. Sun J, Ooms L, Bird CH, et al: A new family of 10 murine ovalbumin serpins includes two homologs of proteinase inhibitor 8 and two homologs of the granzyme B inhibitor (proteinase inhibitor 9). *J Biol Chem* 272:15434–15441, 1997.
11. Locksley RM, Killeen N, Lenardo MJ: The TNF and TNF receptor superfamilies: Integrating mammalian biology. *Cell* 104:487–501, 2001.
12. Wallach D, Varfolomeev EE, Malinin NL, et al: Tumor necrosis factor receptor and Fas signaling mechanisms. *Annu Rev Immunol* 17:331–367, 1999.
13. Yuan J: Transducing signals of life and death. *Curr Opin Cell Biol* 9:247–251, 1997.
14. Varfolomeev EE, Schuchmann M, Luria V, et al: Targeted disruption of the mouse Caspase 8 gene ablates cell death induction by the TNF receptors, Fas/Apo1, and DR3 and is lethal prenatally. *Immunity* 9:267–276, 1998.
15. Reed JC, Doctor KS, Godzik A: The domains of apoptosis: A genomics perspective. *Sci STKE* 2004(239):re9, 2004.
16. Reed JC: Cytochrome C: Can't live with it; Can't live without it. *Cell* 91:559–562, 1997.
17. Green DR, Reed JC: Mitochondria and apoptosis. *Science* 281:1309–1312, 1998.
18. Hakem R, Hakem A, Duncan GS, et al: Differential requirement for caspase 9 in apoptotic pathways *in vivo*. *Cell* 94:339–352, 1998.
19. Haraguchi M, Torii S, Matsuzawa S, et al: Apoptotic protease activating factor (Apaf-1)-independent cell death suppression by Bcl-2. *J Exp Med* 191:1709–1720, 2000.
20. Kroemer G, Reed JC: Mitochondrial control of cell death. *Nat Med* 6:513–519, 2000.
21. Brunger AT, Adams PD, Clore GM, et al: Crystallography & NMR system: A new software suite for macromolecular structure determination. *Acta Crystallogr D Biol Crystallogr* 54(Pt 5):905–921, 1998.
22. Abuamer Y, Ross F, McHugh K, et al: Tumor necrosis factor-a activation of nuclear transcription factor-k-B in marrow macrophages is mediated by C-SRC tyrosine phosphorylation of I-k-B-a. *J Biol Chem* 273(45):29417–29423, 1998.
23. Adams MD, Celniker SE, Holt RA, et al: The genome sequence of *Drosophila melanogaster*. *Science* 287(5461):2185–2195, 2000.
24. Ng FWH, Nguyen M, Kwan T, et al: p28 Bap31, a Bcl-2/Bcl-X$_L$-and procaspase-8-associated protein in the endoplasmic reticulum. *J Cell Biol* 139:327–338, 1997.
25. Vaux DL, Strasser A: The molecular biology of apoptosis. *Proc Natl Acad Sci U S A* 93:2239–2244, 1996.
26. Chen G, Henter ID, Manji HK: Translational research in bipolar disorder: Emerging insights from genetically based models. *Mol Psychiatry* 15(9):883–895, 2010.
27. Salvesen GS, Dixit VM: Caspase activation: The induced-proximity model. *Proc Natl Acad Sci U S A* 96:10964–10967, 1999.
28. Youle RJ, Strasser A: The BCL-2 protein family: Opposing activities that mediate cell death. *Nat Rev Mol Cell Biol* 9(1):47–59, 2008.
29. Demaurex N, Distelhorst C: Apoptosis—The calcium connection. *Science* 300(5616):65–67, 2003.
30. Bouillet P, Purton JF, Godfrey DI, et al: BH3-only Bcl-2 family member Bim is required for apoptosis of autoreactive thymocytes. *Nature* 415(6874):922–926, 2002.
31. Nechushtan A, Smith C, Hsu Y-T, Youle R: Conformation of the Bax C-terminus regulates subcellular location and cell death. *EMBO J* 18:2330–2341, 1999.
32. Muchmore SW, Sattler M, Liang H, et al: X-ray and NMR structure of human Bcl-XL, an inhibitor of programmed cell death. *Nature* 381:335–341, 1996.
33. Chou J, Li H, Salvesen G, et al: Solution structure of BID, an intracellular amplifier of apoptotic signaling. *Cell* 96:615–624, 1999.
34. McDonnell JM, Fushman D, Milliman CL, et al: Solution structure of the proapoptotic molecule BID: A structural basis for apoptotic agonists and antagonists. *Cell* 96:625–634, 1999.
35. Schendel S, Montal M, Reed JC: Bcl-2 family proteins as ion-channels. *Cell Death Differ* 5:372–380, 1998.
36. Minn AJ, Velez P, Schendel SL, et al: Bcl-x$_L$ forms an ion channel in synthetic lipid membranes. *Nature* 385:353–357, 1997.
37. Schendel SL, Xie Z, Montal MO, et al: Channel formation by antiapoptotic protein Bcl-2. *Proc Natl Acad Sci U S A* 94:5113–5118, 1997.
38. Antonsson B, Conti F, Ciavatta A, et al: Inhibition of Bax channel-forming activity by Bcl-2. *Science* 277:370–372, 1997.
39. Schlesinger P, Gross A, Yin X-M, et al: Comparison of the ion channel characteristics of proapoptotic BAX and antiapoptotic BCL-2. *Proc Natl Acad Sci U S A* 94:11357–11362, 1997.
40. Schendel S, Azimov R, Pawlowski K, et al: Ion channel activity of the BH3 only Bcl-2 family member, BID. *J Biol Chem* 274:21932–21936, 1999.
41. Kelekar A, Thompson CB: Bcl-2-family proteins—The role of the BH3 domain in apoptosis. *Trends Cell Biol* 8:324–330, 1998.
42. Huang DC, Strasser A: BH3-only proteins-essential initiators of apoptotic cell death. *Cell* 103:839–842, 2000.
43. Walensky LD, Pitter K, Morash J, et al: A stapled BID BH3 helix directly binds and activates BAX. *Mol Cell* 24(2):199–210, 2006.
44. Kuwana T, Mackey MR, Perkins G, et al: Bid, bax, and lipids cooperate to form supramolecular openings in the outer mitochondrial membrane. *Cell* 111(3):331–342, 2002.
45. Korsmeyer SJ, Wei MC, Saito M, et al: Pro-apoptotic cascade activates BID, which oligomerizes BAK or BAX into pores that result in the release of cytochrome *c*. *Cell Death Differ* 7:1166–1173, 2000.
46. Spierings D, McStay G, Saleh M, et al: Connected to death: The (unexpurgated) mitochondrial pathway of apoptosis. *Science* 310:66–67, 2005.
47. Green DR, Kroemer G: The pathophysiology of mitochondrial cell death. *Science* 305:626–629, 2004.
48. Sattler M, Liang H, Nettesheim D, et al: Structure of Bcl-xL-Bak peptide complex: Recognition between regulators of apoptosis. *Science* 275:983–986, 1997.
49. Hetz C, Bernasconi P, Fisher J, et al: Proapoptotic BAX and BAK modulate the unfolded protein response by a direct interaction with IRE1alpha. *Science* 312:572–576, 2006.
50. Pattingre S, Tassa A, Qu X, et al: Bcl-2 antiapoptotic proteins inhibit Beclin 1-dependent autophagy. *Cell* 122(6):927–939, 2005.
51. Levine B, Kroemer G: Autophagy in the pathogenesis of disease. *Cell* 132(1):27–42, 2008.
52. Tschopp J, Thome M, Hofmann K, Meinl E: The fight of viruses against apoptosis. *Curr Opin Genet Dev* 8(1):82–87, 1998.
53. Chang DW, Xing Z, Pan Y, et al: c-FLIP$_L$ is a dual function regulator for caspase-8 activation and CD95-mediated apoptosis. *EMBO J* 21:3704–3714, 2002.
54. Tschopp J, Irmler M, Thome M: Inhibition of Fas death signals by FLIPs. *Curr Opin Immunol* 10:552–558, 1998.
55. Tschopp J, Martinon F, Hofmann K: Apoptosis: Silencing the death receptors. *Curr Biol* 9:R381-R384.
56. Vanlangenakker N, Bertrand MJ, Bogaert P, et al: TNF-induced necroptosis in L929 cells is tightly regulated by multiple TNFR1 complex I and II members. *Cell Death Dis* 2:e230, 2011.
57. Oberst A, Dillon CP, Weinlich R, et al: Catalytic activity of the caspase-8-FLIP(L) complex inhibits RIPK3-dependent necrosis. *Nature* 471(7338):363–367, 2011.

58. Deveraux QL, Reed JC: IAP family proteins: Suppressors of apoptosis. *Genes Dev* 13:239–252, 1999.

59. Salvesen GS, Duckett CS: IAP proteins: Blocking the road to death's door. *Nat Rev Mol Cell Biol* 3:401–410, 2002.

60. Giampietri C, Starace D, Petrungaro S, et al: Necroptosis: Molecular signalling and translational implications. *Int J Cell Biol* 2014:490275, 2014.

61. McComb S, Cheung HH, Korneluk RG, et al: cIAP1 and cIAP2 limit macrophage necroptosis by inhibiting Rip1 and Rip3 activation. *Cell Death Differ* 19(11):1791–1801, 2012.

62. Karin M, Lin A: NF-kappaB at the crossroads of life and death. *Nat Immunol* 3:221–227, 2002.

63. Rane SG, Reddy EP: Janus kinases: Components of multiple signaling pathways. *Oncogene* 19(49):5662–5679, 2000.

64. Ahmed NN, Franke TF, Bellacosa A, et al: The proteins encoded by c-akt and v-akt differ in post-translational modification, subcellular localization and oncogenic potential. *Oncogene* 8:1957–1963, 1993.

65. Datta S, Brunet A, Greenberg M: Cellular survival: A play in three Akts. *Genes Dev* 13:2905–2927, 1999.

66. Cardone MH, Roy N, Stennicke HR, et al: Regulation of cell death protease caspase-9 by phosphorylation. *Science* 282:1318–1320, 1998.

67. Brunet A, Bonni A, Zigmond MJ, et al: Akt promotes cell survival by phosphorylating and inhibiting a forkhead transcription factor. *Cell* 96:857–868, 1999.

68. Houldsworth J, Mathew S, Rao PH, et al: REL proto-oncogene is frequently amplified in extranodal diffuse large cell lymphoma. *Blood* 87:25–29, 1996.

69. Karnolsky IN: Cytogenetic abnormalities in chronic lymphocytic leukemia. *Folia Medica (Plovdiv)* 42:5–10, 2000.

70. Karin M, Cao Y, Greten FR, Li Z-W: NF-kB in cancer: From innocent bystander to major culprit. *Nat Rev Cancer* 2:301–310, 2002.

71. Hayashi T, Faustman D: Essential role of human leukocyte antigen-encoded proteasome subunits in NF-kappaB activation and prevention of tumor necrosis factor-alpha-induced apoptosis. *J Biol Chem* 275:5238–5247, 2000.

72. Oda E, Ohki R, Murasawa H, et al: Noxa, a BH3-only member of the Bcl-2 family and candidate mediator of p53-induced apoptosis. *Science* 288:1053–1058, 2000.

73. Nakano K, Vousden KH: *PUMA*, a novel proapoptotic gene, is induced by p53. *Mol Cell* 7:683–694, 2001.

74. Yu J, Zhang L, Hwang PM, et al: PUMA induces the rapid apoptosis of colorectal cancer cells. *Mol Cell* 7:673–682, 2001.

75. Chipuk JE, Kuwana T, Bouchier-Hayes L, et al: Direct activation of Bax by p53 mediates mitochondrial membrane permeabilization and apoptosis. *Science* 303:1010–1014, 2004.

76. Miyashita T, Reed JC: Tumor suppressor p53 is a direct transcriptional activator of human Bax gene. *Cell* 80:293–299, 1995.

77. Imamura J, Miyoshi I, Koeffler HP: p53 in hematologic malignancies. *Blood* 84(8):2412–2421, 1994.

78. Remstein ED, James CD, Kurtin PJ: Incidence and subtype specificity of API2-MALT1 fusion translocations in extranodal, nodal, and splenic marginal zone lymphomas. *Am J Pathol* 156(4):1183–1188, 2000.

79. Shin MS, Kim HS, Kang CS, et al: Inactivating mutations of CASP10 gene in non-Hodgkin lymphomas. *Blood* 99(11):4094–4099, 2002.

80. Gronbaek K, Straten PT, Ralfkiaer E, et al: Somatic Fas mutations in non-Hodgkin's lymphoma: Association with extranodal disease and autoimmunity. *Blood* 92:3018–3024, 1998.

81. Wu GS, Burns TF, McDonald ER 3rd, et al: KILLER/DR5 is a DNA damage-inducible p53-regulated death receptor gene. *Nat Genet* 17:141–143, 1997.

82. Owen-Schaub LB, Zhang W, Cusack JC, et al: Wild-type human p53 and a temperature-sensitive mutant induce Fas/APO-1 expression. *Mol Cell Biol* 15(6):3032–3040, 1995.

83. Momand J, Jung D, Wilczynski S, Niland J: The MDM2 gene amplification database. *Nucleic Acids Res* 26(15):3453–3459, 1998.

84. Drappa J, Vaishnaw AK, Sullivan KE, et al: Fas gene mutations in the Canale-Smith syndrome, an inherited lymphoproliferative disorder associated with autoimmunity. *N Engl J Med* 335(22):1643–1649, 1996.

85. Watanabe-Fukunaga R, Brannan CI, Copeland NG, et al: Lymphoproliferation disorder in mice explained by defects in Fas antigen that mediates apoptosis. *Nature* 356:314–317, 1992.

86. Takahashi T, Tanaka M, Brannan CI, et al: Generalized lymphoproliferative disease in mice, caused by a point mutation in the Fas ligand. *Cell* 76:969–976, 1994.

87. Fisher GH, Rosenberg FJ, Straus SE, et al: Dominant interfering fas gene mutations impair apoptosis in a human autoimmune lymphoproliferative syndrome. *Cell* 81:935–946, 1995.

88. Wang J, Zheng L, Lobito A, et al: Inherited human Caspase 10 mutations underlie defective lymphocyte and dendritic cell apoptosis in autoimmune lymphoproliferative syndrome type II. *Cell* 98(1):47–58, 1999.

89. Cantley L, Neel BG: New insights into tumor suppression: PTEN suppresses tumor formation by restraining the phosphoinositide 3-kinase/AKT pathway. *Proc Natl Acad Sci U S A* 96:4240–4245, 1999.

90. Testa JR, Bellacosa A: AKT plays a central role in tumorigenesis. *Proc Natl Acad Sci U S A* 98:10983–10985, 2001.

CHAPTER 16
CELL-CYCLE REGULATION AND HEMATOLOGIC DISORDERS

Yun Dai, Prithviraj Bose, and Steven Grant

SUMMARY

Complex feedback pathways regulate the passage of cells through the G_1, S, G_2, and M phases of the growth cycle. Two key checkpoints control the commitment of cells to replicate DNA synthesis and to mitosis. Many oncogenes and defective tumor-suppressor genes promote malignant change by stimulating cell-cycle entry, or disrupting the checkpoint response to DNA damage. Advances in the understanding of genetic and epigenetic mechanisms of gene regulation provide the basis for novel therapeutic approaches. This chapter presents the pathways and the genetic and epigenetic alterations that regulate cell replication, and highlights the various oncogenes and tumor-suppressor genes that are involved in hematologic malignancies.

Mitosis is the final step of a defined program—the cell cycle—that can be separated into four phases: the G_1, S, G_2, and M phases (Fig. 16–1). A number of surveillance systems (checkpoints) control the cell cycle and interrupt its progression when DNA damage occurs or when cells have failed to complete a necessary event.[1] These checkpoints have been

Acronyms and Abbreviations: ALL, acute lymphoid leukemia; AML, acute myelogenous leukemia; APC, anaphase-promoting complex; APL, acute promyelocytic leukemia; ATM, ataxia-telangiectasia mutated; ATR, ATM and Rad3 related; cdc, cell division cycle; cdk, cyclin-dependent kinase; CDKI, cyclin-dependent kinase inhibitor; Chk, checkpoint kinase; CLL, chronic lymphocytic leukemia; CML, chronic myelogenous leukemia; CTD, carboxy-terminal domain; DDR, DNA damage response; DSIF, DRB-sensitivity–inducing factor; ER, endoplasmic reticulum; FLAM, flavopiridol, cytarabine, mitoxantrone; GADD, growth arrest and DNA damage; HAT, histone acetyltransferase; HDAC, histone deacetylase; HDACI, histone deacetylase inhibitor; HR, homologous recombination; Id1, inhibitor of DNA-binding 1; INK4, inhibitor of kinase 4; JAK, Janus-associated kinase; MAPK, mitogen-activated protein kinase; MCL, mantle cell lymphoma; MDM2, murine double minute protein 2; MLL, mixed-lineage leukemia; MTA, 5'-deoxy-5'-(methylthio)adenosine; MTAP, methylthioadenosine phosphorylase; NELF, negative elongation factor; N-TEF, negative transcription elongation factor; ODC, ornithine decarboxylase; PDGF, platelet derived growth factor; PI3K, phosphatidylinositol 3'-kinase; PLZF, promyelocytic leukemia Kruppel-like zinc finger; PML, promyelocytic leukemia; P-TEFb, positive transcription elongation factor; RAR*a*, retinoic acid receptor *a*; RB, retinoblastoma gene; rPTK, receptor protein-tyrosine kinase; STAT, signal transducer and activator of transcription; TGF-β, transforming growth factor-β; TKI, tyrosine kinase inhibitor; UPR, unfolded protein response.

given an empirical definition: When the occurrence of event B is dependent on the completion of prior event A, the dependence is a result of a checkpoint if a loss-of-function mutation can be found that relieves the dependence.[1] Three major cell-cycle checkpoints have been discovered: the DNA damage checkpoint, the replication checkpoint, and the spindle-pole body duplication checkpoint.[2-4] The functional consequence of failure to "satisfy" the requirements of a cell-cycle checkpoint is usually death by apoptosis. However, small numbers of genetically altered cells may survive. Cells with defective checkpoints have an advantage when selection favors multiple genetic changes. Cancer cells often are missing one or more checkpoints, which facilitates a greater rate of genomic evolution.[5]

A disturbance of cell-cycle regulation is an important pathway in the development of many hematologic malignancies as a result of mutations in tumor-suppressor genes or oncogenes. Until the end of the 20th century, it was believed that the only mechanism by which the "gatekeepers" of the cell cycle could be inactivated was deletion or mutation (gain-of-function or loss-of-function mutations). Progress in the understanding of the regulation of gene expression put emphasis on another mechanism of gene inactivation, called *epigenetic regulation* (Chap. 10). This term summarizes several molecular modifications, including histone deacetylation, CpG-island hypermethylation, ubiquitination, and phosphorylation, etc.

● CYCLINS AND CYCLIN-DEPENDENT KINASES

Table 16–1 lists Cdks, associated partners, and their functions.

Early experiments on the control of mitosis in human cells provided evidence for the existence of factors called *M-phase* and *S-phase promoting factors*.[6] The key element of S-phase promoting factor was thought to be cell division cycle (cdc) 2. Experiments performed in *Xenopus* eggs showed that cdc2 is an M-phase–specific histone H1 kinase,[7] but is just one subunit of a regulatory complex. A second component is cyclin B, which is synthesized in interphase and degraded in midmitosis. More than 10 members of the mammalian cyclin family have been identified. Most of these cyclins interact with a group of cdc2-related kinases called *cyclin-dependent kinases* (cdks),[8,9] while others are involved in alternate splicing processes.[10] Phosphorylation of tyrosine 15 is the key event in regulating human cdc2 activity. Threonine 14 also is phosphorylated in G_2 phase. Dephosphorylation at both phosphorylation sites is required for mitotic initiation. Cdc2 interacts with cyclin B in mitosis, whereas the cdc2/cyclin A complex is formed before mitosis and is required for progression through late G_2 phase.[11] Thus, cyclins A and B are also called the *mitotic* cyclins, because they are upregulated in late G_2 or G_2/M phase and undergo proteolysis in M phase. The exit from mitosis is characterized by the abrupt ubiquitination and subsequent degradation of cyclin B. Cells with a defective cyclin B degradation mechanism or without mitotic cyclin B easily become aneuploid. There is evidence that cyclin A acts at the G_2/M transition and binds cdk2 in S phase. Cyclin A is mandatory for the downregulation of anaphase-promoting complex (APC).[12] Overexpression of cyclin A in G_1 phase leads to an accelerated entry into S phase.[13] Because cdc2 is able to interact with mitotic and G_1 cyclins, it is likely that one protein kinase potentially can fulfill several different functions in the cell cycle at various checkpoints. Notably, there is increasing evidence that cdc2 is directly involved in regulating the DNA damage response (DDR), including DNA damage checkpoint activation and DNA repair (particularly homologous recombination [HR]).[14] There are several cdc2-related protein kinases in humans that interact with the corresponding cyclins. Originally, three cdc2-related proteins were isolated, which

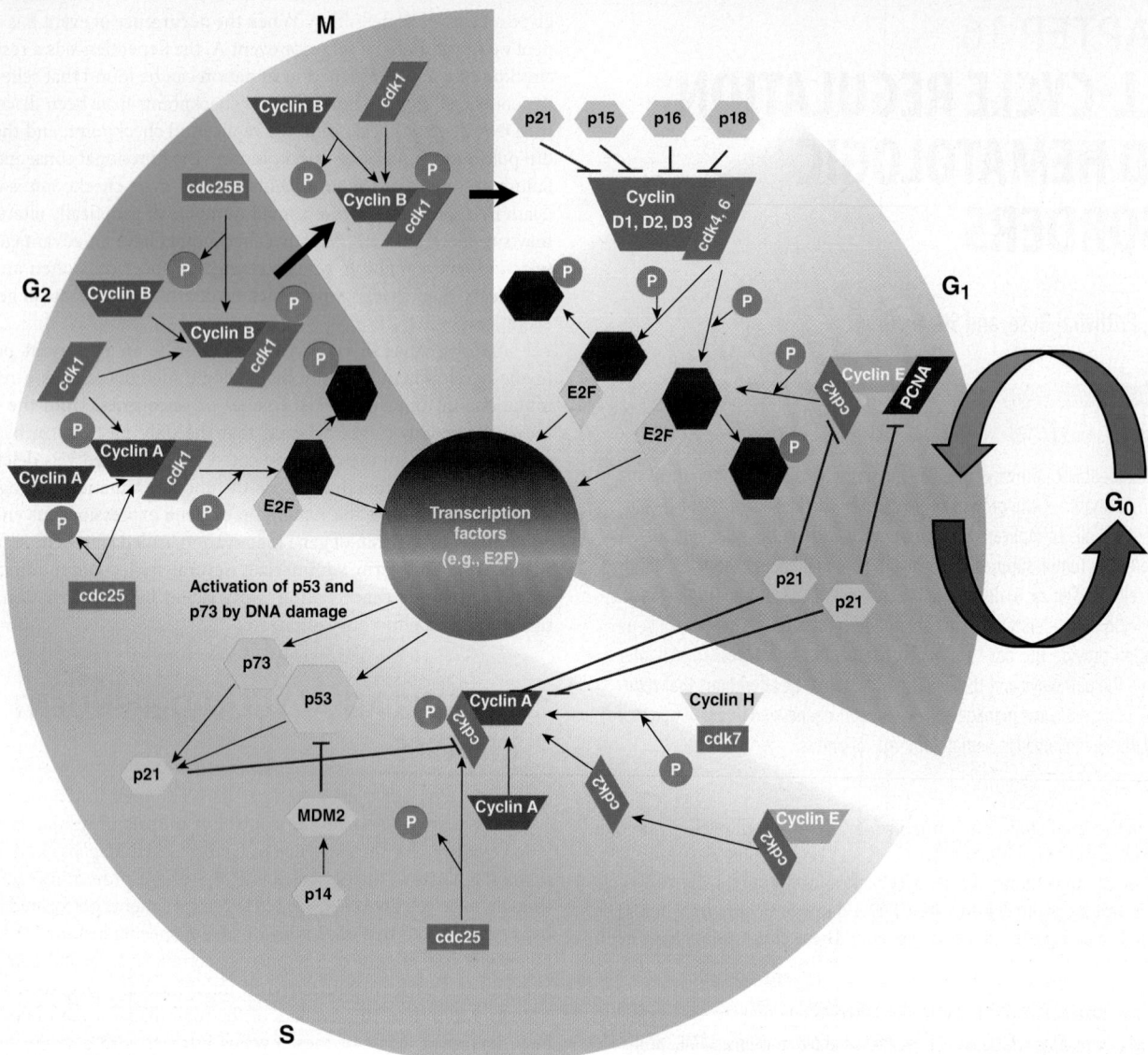

Figure 16–1. Cell-cycle regulation in mammalian cells.

were able to replace deficient cdc28 function in budding yeast: cdk1, cdk2, and cdk3.[15–17] Other cdks are termed cdk4,[18] cdk5,[19] and cdk6.[20] Cdk4/6 has been in the focus of tumor-suppressor gene research for the past several years, because it complexes with cyclin D (a G_1 cyclin). This complex is an important element in the $p16^{INK4A}$-retinoblastoma (RB) gene pathway, which is commonly disrupted in cancer. Interestingly, the neural cdk5 is also expressed at high levels in certain cancer types (e.g., myeloma), potentially representing a therapeutic target in these diseases.[21] Moreover, cdk5 may serve as a prognostic marker and help to identify patients most likely to respond to treatment (e.g., with bortezomib).[22] In addition, inhibition of cdk1 and/or cdk5 may contribute to disruption of the unfolded protein response (UPR) secondary to endoplasmic reticulum (ER) stress inducers.[23] Three transcription-regulatory cdks have been characterized. Cdk7 interacts with cyclin H and is responsible for phosphorylating cdks on threonine residues.[24] Cdk8 interacts with cyclin C, Med12, and Med13, and forms a complex called "cdk8" subcomplex. Several substrates for cdk8, when complexed with the above-mentioned proteins, have been detected, including RNA polymerase II and histone H3.[25] Cdk8 directly antagonizes the repression of β-catenin transcription by the transcription

factor E2F1 in colorectal cancer.[26] The suppression of β-catenin by E2F1 contributes to apoptosis. Therefore, overexpression of cdk8 (and RB) accounts for a reduced rate of apoptosis and increased cell growth.[26] Cdk9 binds cyclin T and displays a tissue-specific expression pattern.[27] That cdk9/cyclin T specifically interacts with the tat element of HIV-1 links this cyclin-dependent kinase directly to the replication pathway of HIV, and circumstantially to HIV-1–related malignancies (e.g., Kaposi sarcoma).[28] Cdk10[29] and cdk11[30] define a novel class of cyclin-dependent kinases; both cdks interact with apoptosis-related factors[30] or transcription factors such as ets.[31] Cdk10 has two isoforms with different functions. A role at the G_2/M transition has been suggested for the first isoform of cdk10, whereas the alternative splicing form interacts with the N-terminus of the Ets2 transcription factor. This interaction affects the G_2/M transition in mice.[32] Two known cyclin-dependent kinases, cdk12 and cdk13, interact with both forms of cyclin L (cyclin L_1 and L_2). This complex seems to be involved in alterative RNA-splicing,[10,33] and thus is involved in the pre–messenger RNA processing machinery. All cyclins share an approximately 150-amino-acid region, called the *cyclin box*, which interacts with the cdks.[34] The G_1 cyclins (C, D, and E) and the mitotic cyclins (A and B)[35] form distinct categories, although cyclin H,

TABLE 16–1. CDKs, Associated Cyclins, and their Functions

Cdk	Associated Partner Cyclin	Function
Cdk1	Cyclin A, B	G_2/M
Cdk2	Cyclin A, D, E; C	G_1/S; S; G_2/M
Cdk3	Cyclin C	$G_{0\,exit}$
Cdk4	Cyclin D	G_1; G_1/S
Cdk5	p35, p39	Neuronal processes (neuron survival/death, migration, cortical layering, synaptic plasticity, etc.)
Cdk6	Cyclin D	G_1; G_1/S
Cdk7	Cyclin H, Mat1	Cdk1, 2, 4/6 activation; transcriptional regulation
Cdk8	Cyclin C, MED12, MED13	Transcriptional regulation
Cdk9	Cyclin T1, T2	Transcriptional regulation
Cdk10	Ets-2	G_2/M
Cdk11	RanBPM, RNPS1, casein kinase, cyclin L	RNA splicing; transcriptional regulation; apoptosis
Cdk12	Cyclin K, L (?)	Transcriptional regulation; alternative splicing
Cdk13	Cyclin K, L (?)	Transcriptional regulation; alternative splicing

cyclins L1 and L2, and the type T cyclins (T_1, T_2a, and T_2b) fall outside these two major groups.

Cyclin A binds and activates cdk2 mainly in S phase. However, microinjection of anti–cyclin A antibodies into cells causes cell cycle arrest just before S phase.[11] This observation, together with the finding that overexpression of cyclin A leads to accelerated S-phase entry, suggests that cyclin A is involved in transformation.[13] Cyclin A is able to compensate for loss of cyclin E function. Cyclin E is important for the duplication of centrosomes. In cyclin E-defective cells, cyclin A can take over the function of cyclin E in S phase, whereas cyclin A is important for centrosome amplification in G_2-arrested cells, irrespective of whether cyclin E is present.[36] The importance of cyclin A in cell division is underlined by other reports.[37] In addition to its role at the G_1/S boundary, cyclin A acts in late G_2 phase, where it complexes with cdk1. Cyclin E, the other cyclin that interacts with cdk2, may control the progression from G_1 to S phase, and the time point when cdk2 "switches" from cyclin E to cyclin A binding is right after prereplication complex assembly terminates while DNA replication initiates. Cells overexpressing cyclin E progress much faster through G_1 into S phase, but the time required for DNA synthesis remains normal.[38] On the other hand, a bifurcation in cdk2 activity determines whether cells immediately commit to the next cell cycle or enter a transient state of quiescence as they exit mitosis.[39] Cyclin E levels are also regulated by environmental factors, including transforming growth factor-β (TGF-β) and irradiation. These effects are, in part, mediated by small proteins, the cyclin-dependent kinase inhibitors. Cyclin E accumulates at the G_1/S boundary of the cell cycle, where it stimulates functions associated with entry into and progression through S phase.[40] In normal cells, cyclin E levels are highly regulated so that peak cyclin E–cdk2 kinase activity occurs only for a short interval near the G_1/S boundary.[40] Cyclin E–cdk2 complexes

become active during S phase and are then rapidly ubiquitinated after phosphorylation.[41] The poor prognostic implications of overexpression of cyclin E has been observed in a variety of human malignancies,[42] leading to a high cyclin E level throughout the cell cycle. The direct linkage between cyclin E overexpression and tumorigenesis is not completely understood. It has been suggested that the cyclin E–cdk2 complex phosphorylates and inactivates the RB protein[43] or leads to genomic instability via generation of aneuploid cells.[44] Cyclin E overexpression delays progression through early phases of mitosis and causes mitosis to be executed aberrantly, thus dysregulating mitotic progression.[45]

The B-type cyclins associate with cdk1 to form the classical mitotic cyclin–cdk complexes.[46] Cyclin B is synthesized in S phase and accumulates, and in the midst of M phase is ubiquitinated and degraded, allowing the cell to exit from mitosis. The G_2/M checkpoint is very often defective in malignant cells, leading to uncontrolled M-phase entry and aneuploidy. The cellular localization of the cdk1–cyclin B complexes is strictly cell-cycle–dependent. Although the complexes accumulate in the cytoplasm during G_2 and S phase, they move to the nucleus in mitosis and bind to the mitotic spindle.[47,48] The cyclin B family has different family members with distinct functions. At mitotic entry, cyclin B_1–cdk1 promotes chromosome condensation, nuclear membrane dissolution, mitotic aster assembly, and Golgi breakdown, whereas cyclin B_2–cdk1 can only induce Golgi disassembly.[49] At prophase, cyclin B_1 accumulates in the nucleus[50] and then localizes to condensed chromatin, spindle microtubules, centrosomes, and chromatin during prometaphase.[51] Distinct sequence elements are responsible for the localization of cyclin B_1 to the chromatin, centrosomes, and kinetochores during mitosis.[52]

The three cyclin D molecules—D_1, D_2, and D_3—function mainly in G_1 phase, where they bind cdk4 and cdk6. These complexes phosphorylate RB, restraining its inhibitory effects on E2F and related transcription factors. Cyclin D_1 is the major D cyclin in most cell types. All three cyclin D molecules act in late G_1 phase, just before entry into S phase. Cyclin D_1 also exhibits a variety of non–cell-cycle regulatory functions. For example, cyclin D_1 regulates microRNA biogenesis by induction of Dicer, a central regulator of microRNA maturation.[53] Many tumors have high cyclin D_1 levels without amplification or mutation of the cyclin D_1 structural gene. Instead, cyclin D levels may be regulated by a feedback loop dependent on RB. Alterations of the *RB* gene in cancer may secondarily cause upregulation of cyclin D transcription. As a result of its central role in cell-cycle control, the cyclin D–cdk4 complex is an important target for anticancer drugs. Mice lacking cyclin D_1 are completely resistant to ErbB-2–driven breast cancer.[54] ErbB-2–induced mammary tumor development is also prohibited by the inactivation of the cyclin D_1 partner cdk4, underlining the role of this complex in human malignancies.[55] As aberrations of the p16–cdk4–cyclin D-RB pathway are common in the majority of cancers, the development of selective cdk4 inhibitors (e.g., palbociclib) launched promising efforts to target tumors displaying either cyclin D_1 overexpression (e.g., breast cancer, mantle cell lymphoma, multiple myeloma) or cdk4 amplification (e.g., liposarcoma).[56] Moreover, cyclin D_1–cdk4 is also involved in regulation of glucose metabolism in postmitotic cells, suggesting a novel cell-cycle–independent function of this complex.[57] However, cdk6, a functional homologue of cdk4, may also play an important role in tumorigenesis under certain circumstances. For example, acute myelogenous leukemia (AML) cells carrying mixed-lineage leukemia (MLL) rearrangements (e.g., MLL-AF9, MLL-AF4, and MLL-AF6) specifically rely on cdk6, rather than cdk4, to proliferate,[58] suggesting that cdk6 might represent a target in MLL-driven leukemia.[59] Interestingly, SUMOylation stabilizes the cdk6 protein, which may contribute to progression of some tumors (e.g., glioblastoma).[60] Notably, cyclin D–dependent cdk4/6 also phosphorylates a variety of substrates (e.g., RB1 and its relatives RBL1 and RBL2, SMAD2, SMAD3, FOXM1, MEP50, etc.), forming a central node in a complex signaling network that governs the overall transcriptional and biologic response of cells to activation or inhibition of the kinases.[61]

Cdk7 plays dual functions in regulation of cell cycle and gene transcription. In the former case, cdk7, together with its partner cyclin H, acts as a cdk-activating kinase, which fully activates various cell-cycle–regulatory cdks (e.g., cdk1, cdk2, cdk4, and cdk6) by phosphorylating their T loop in a context-specific manner.[62] For example, whereas cdk7 is required to determine cyclin specificity and activation order of cdc1 and cdk2 during S and G_2 phases, it is also required to maintain the activity of cdk4 as cells exiting quiescence and G_1 progression through the restriction point.[63] Cdk7, as a component of the general transcription factor TFIIH (cdk7/cyclin H/Mat1 complex), phosphorylates the carboxy-terminal domain (CTD, serines 5 and 7) of RNA polymerase II, which is responsible for transcription initiation and promoter clearance, a critical step in switching initiation to elongation during transcription.[64] As transcription factors that co-opt the general transcriptional machinery to sustain the oncogenic state, pharmacologic inhibition of cdk7 may represent a novel approach to treat tumor types (e.g., T-cell acute lymphoblastic leukemia [T-ALL]) that are particularly dependent on transcription.[65]

Cdk9, as a catalytic subunit, partners with the regulatory subunit cyclin T, an 87-kDa cyclin C–related protein with three isoforms, to form a complex known as positive transcription elongation factor b (P-TEFb).[66] The so-called cdk9-related pathway consists of two cdk9 isoforms (cdk9–42 and cdk9–55), cyclin T_1, cyclin T_{2a}, cyclin T_{2b}, and cyclin K.[27] Cdk9 and its binding partner cyclin T_1 comprise the P-TEFb.[67] P-TEFb hyperphosphorylates the CTD (primarily serine 2) of RNA polymerase II, essential for transcription elongation. P-TEFb also phosphorylates the negative transcription elongation factors (N-TEFs), including DRB-sensitivity inducing factor (DSIF) and the negative elongation factor (NELF), to release the transcription block (a pause immediately after transcription initiation) of both N-TEFs on hypophosphorylated forms of RNA polymerase II. In addition, cdk9 also plays a role in ribosomal RNA processing through activation of RNA polymerase II.[68] In normal cells, the activity of P-TEFb is stringently maintained in a functional equilibrium to accommodate transcriptional demands for different biologic activities.[69] As a rule in oncogenic transformation, upregulated antiapoptotic or prosurvival proteins in transformed cells must be sustained by constitutive RNA polymerase II activity that governs transcription elongation, in which cdk9 is the primary processivity factor.[70] In other words, transformed cells are addicted to transcription because of the requirement for continuous production of antiapoptotic proteins, particularly those with short half-lives. Of note, abnormal activities in the cdk9-related pathway occur in many human malignancies.[71] For example, high levels of cdk9/cyclin T_1 expression are found in several types of hematologic malignancies, including B- and T-cell precursor-derived lymphomas, anaplastic large cell lymphoma, and follicular lymphomas, whereas strong nuclear staining for both proteins are observed in Hodgkin and Reed-Sternberg cells of classical Hodgkin lymphoma. In this context, selective cdk9 inhibitors preferentially target malignant cells in preclinical hematologic tumor models, including leukemia and multiple myeloma.[72,73] Mcl-1, the Bcl-2 family antiapoptotic protein with an estimated half-life of less than 3 hours,[74] represents one of the most common downstream targets for cdk9 inhibition.[75] Moreover, cdk9 inhibition disrupts the process of cytoprotective autophagy, for example, through downregulation of the adaptor protein SQSTM1/p62, resulting in an inefficient form of autophagy from cargo-loading failure, which, in turn, triggers apoptosis via upregulation of the BH3-only protein NBK/Bik.[76] Moreover, cdk inhibitors also induce upregulation of other BH3-only proteins such as Bim and Noxa.[77] Although it remains to be determined whether these events stem from inhibition of

specific cdk(s), it is now clear that in addition to cell cycle-regulatory cdks, transcription-regulatory cdks, such as cdk9, represent another class of therapeutic targets. In addition, P-TEFb forms a complex with the HIV tat protein that binds the transactivation response element. The modification of RNA polymerase II by cdk9/cyclin T facilitates the efficient multiplication of the viral genome.[78] Other binding partners of cdk9 include tumor necrosis factor receptor-associated factor 2,[79] as well as inhibitory MAQ1 (or HEXIM1) and 7SK small nuclear RNA.[80] Furthermore, cdk9 is expressed throughout the cell cycle[81] and is also involved in viral (HIV, herpes) replication.[27]

Other members of the transcription-regulatory cdk subfamily include cdk8 and cdk12. Cdk8 is a subunit of the large Mediator complex (~1.2 MDa) composed of 25 to 30 proteins, which acts as a molecular bridge between DNA-binding transcription factors and RNA polymerase II. Cdk8 binds to cyclin C, MED12, and MED13 in the cyclin C–cdk8 module of the Mediator.[82] The cdk8/cyclin C pair facilitates phosphorylation of both serine 2 and serine 5 at the CTD of RNA polymerase II.[83] Cdk8 can perform both positive and negative functions in transcriptional regulation during different transcription stages (e.g., preinitiation and elongation), which provide a mechanism to respond to different promoter contexts (e.g., transcription factors or cdk8 module binding).[82] Unlike cdk7 and cdk9, which govern global gene expression, cdk8 promotes only gene-specific transcription. Recently, cdk8 expression has been detected in 70 percent colorectal cancers and correlated with β-catenin activation, suggesting that cdk8 may act as a oncogene in certain types of cancer (e.g., colorectal and pancreatic cancer).[84,85] Cdk12 and cdk13 have been identified as CTD kinases, both of which are unusually large proteins that contain a central kinase domain and share the same partner, cyclin K.[86] Cdk12/cyclin K_1 phosphorylates the CTD (preferably serine 2) of RNA polymerase II.[87] Interestingly, cdk12/cyclin K only regulates expression of a small subset of genes, predominantly long genes with high exon numbers and DDR genes, including critical regulators of genomic stability, for example, *BRCA1*, *ATR* (ataxia-telangiectasia mutated [ATM] and Rad3 related), *FANCI*, and *FANCD2*.[88]

The cdk10 gene encodes two different cdk-like putative kinases; it is postulated that they exert their function at the G_2/M transition.[29] These two isoforms predominate in human tissues, except in brain and muscle, and the relative isoform levels do not vary during the cell cycle.[29] Cdk10 interacts with the N-terminus of the Ets2 transcription factor, which contains the highly conserved pointed transactivation domain. The pointed domain is implicated in protein–protein interactions and Ets2 requires an intact pointed domain to bind Cdk10, which inhibits Ets2 transactivation in mammalian cells.[31] This could be an important factor for the development of follicular lymphoma, because cdk10 is overexpressed in this cancer.[89] In addition, cdk10 silencing increases Ets2-driven transcription of c-RAF, resulting in mitogen-activated protein kinase (MAPK) pathway activation and loss of tumor cell reliance upon estrogen signaling.[90] Cdk10 promoters are frequently hypermethylated in malignant tumors, resulting in low expression levels of cdk10 and impaired cell-cycle regulation.[90]

Cdk11 is associated with cyclin L.[91] It is part of the large family of p34(cdc2)-related kinases whose functions appear to be linked with cell-cycle progression, tumorigenesis, and apoptotic signaling. Cdk11 interacts with the p47 subunit of eukaryotic initiation factor 3 during apoptosis and is therefore directly involved in cell death mechanisms.[92] Casein kinase 2 phosphorylates the cdk11 aminoterminal domain, suggesting that cdk11 participates in signaling pathways that include casein kinase 2 and that its function may help to coordinate the regulation of RNA transcription and processing events.[91] So far two isoforms of cdk11 have been identified, a larger p110 and a smaller p46 isoform. During Fas- or tumor necrosis factor-α–induced apoptosis, the caspase-processed p46 isoform is generated from the larger p110 isoform and it promotes apoptosis when it is ectopically expressed in human cells. Cdk11 also stabilizes the microtubule assembly of cells[93]; cdk11 is therefore mandatory for the maintenance of sister chromatid cohesion[94] and its disruption can contribute to the development of cancer.[95]

SUBSTRATES AND INHIBITORS OF CYCLIN-DEPENDENT KINASES

Many cyclin–cdk substrates have been identified by immunoprecipitation or two-hybrid assays, but only a few of them are thought to exert a direct function in cell-cycle control. The regulation of the cell cycle has been studied extensively during the last decade and a consensus paradigm of cell-cycle regulation has been suggested.[50,96] According to this paradigm, the important switch of the cell cycle is the RB family of proteins (Fig. 16–2). In its hypophosphorylated state, RB binds to and inhibits a class of transcription factors, of which the best characterized is the E2F transcription factor. Hyperphosphorylation causes RB to detach from its binding site, permitting transcriptional activation of genes necessary for DNA synthesis and cell division. This phosphorylation of RB is regulated in a cell-cycle–dependent manner.[97] A widely accepted model suggests that RB is phosphorylated by different regulators such as cyclin E/cdk2 at the so-called "R" point, a time point during G_1 when cell cycle progression becomes independent of exogenous stimuli.[98] Interference with RB function impairs G_1 checkpoint regulation and fosters unrestrained cell growth, a nearly universal characteristic of

malignancy. RB controls the activity of several other cell-cycle regulatory elements such as Skp2.[99] The Skp2 regulation follows an autocrine loop where Skp2 triggers degradation of the cdk inhibitor p27^{kip1}, followed by cyclin E/cdk2 activation, consecutive cdk2-induced RB-phosphorylation, and further E2F-dependent Skp2 expression.[100] Causes of reduced RB activity include changes in the structural gene, the sequestration and inactivation of the protein by viral oncogene products, and hyperphosphorylation of RB as a result of increased cdk4 and cyclin D activity or deletion of the gene for the $p16^{INK4A}$ inhibitor of cdk4. Deletions, mutations, and translocations of RB are common in various malignancies, while homozygous deletions of the $p16^{INK4A}$ gene are even more frequent. Many different transforming viruses (papillomavirus, simian virus 40) produce proteins that interact with RB. Both cyclin D_1–cdk4 and cyclin $D_1(D_2, D_3)$–cdk6 complexes are able to phosphorylate RB.[101,102] The time point of RB phosphorylation correlates strongly with the appearance of the cyclin D_1–cdk4 complex.[103] The link between RB and cyclin D is supported by the observation that loss of RB function leads to a decrease in the cellular cyclin D level.[104] However, cyclin D is not the only cyclin that is involved in the RB regulatory pathway.[99,102] Ectopic expression of both cyclin A and cyclin E restores RB hyperphosphorylation and causes cell-cycle arrest in cancer cell lines. Perhaps the cdk2–cyclin A complex contributes to additional phosphorylation of RB, whereas the cdk2–cyclin E complex prolongs the phosphorylation time.[105]

The key regulatory element for the G_1-to-S transition is the RB–E2F complex. After RB is phosphorylated by cdk4 and/or cdk6 complexes during G_1 phase and cdk2 at G_1/S interphase, E2F proteins are released and promote the transcription of genes essential for the transition to S phase.[99,106] As mentioned above, the p16^{INK4A}/cyclin D_1/cdk4/RB/E2F cascade is probably one of the most important cascades in cell-cycle control, and is frequently affected in human cancer. For example, this pathway is defective in nearly 100 percent of AML cell lines and most of the primary AML samples, although the exact mechanism of inactivation is not always clear. Two RB-related pocket proteins, p107 and p130, also form complexes with the transcription factor E2F,[107] bind to the region of the adenovirus E1A protein required for transformation, and are able to induce G_1 arrest when they are overexpressed in human malignant cell lines.[108,109] Unlike RB, the p107 and p130 proteins contain a so-called spacer region that interacts with cdk2/cyclin A and cdk2/cyclin E,[110] although it seems to be unlikely that these two complexes regulate the activity of p107 and p130.[105] Instead, p107 may bind and inactivate the cyclin A and cyclin E complexes. Thus, p107 may regulate the cell cycle by several different mechanisms. Because both p107 and p130 are regulated through phosphorylation, efficient cell-cycle entry is accompanied by phosphorylation of all the RB-related proteins.[111]

In addition to its cell-cycle regulatory properties, RB also influences hematopoietic differentiation.[112] RB interacts with the transcription factor PU.1, which blocks erythroid differentiation in the proerythroblast stage when ectopically overexpressed in marrow cells,[113,114] and represses GATA-1 activity.[115] An important event in this differentiation process is the interaction between hematopoietic stem cells and the microenvironment of the marrow. In addition, hypophosphorylated RB promotes monocytic over neutrophilic differentiation in bipotent progenitor cells, an event that is switched to neutrophilic differentiation if RB expression is inhibited. This finding points to an important property of RB independent of cell-cycle control.[116]

Besides regulation by phosphorylation, specific protein inhibitors of cdk enzymatic activity have been identified.[117] The cyclin-dependent kinase inhibitors (CDKIs) cause cells to arrest in G_1 phase, followed by differentiation and/or senescence. The first CDKI identified was p21^{cip1}.[118] It binds to several cyclin/cdk complexes, including cyclin A/cdk2, cyclin D/cdk4, and cyclin E/cdk2 (see Fig. 16–2).[97,119] Several different cell-cycle

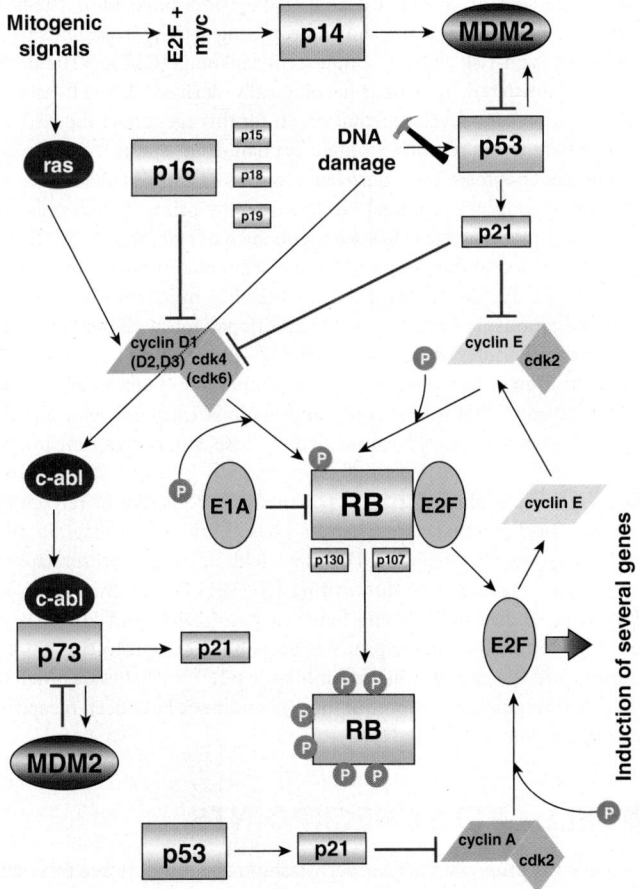

Figure 16–2. Interactions between cyclin-dependent kinase inhibitors (p16, p14, p21), p53, and the retinoblastoma protein (RB).

regulatory pathways are affected by p21[cip1]. In addition, a basal p21[cip1]–cdk2 axis determines quiescent and cycling cell states and thus controls population heterogeneity in both normal cells and tumors, which can make anticancer treatment selectivity challenging.[120] The molecule has a p53 binding site in its promoter, and an increase in p53 levels results in transcriptional activation of p21[cip1], slowing cell-cycle progression. In addition to this p53-dependent pathway, p21[cip1] is also regulated in a p53-independent manner. For example, histone deacetylase inhibitors (HDACIs) are able to induce p21[cip1] expression in p53[null] leukemia cells through an alternative nuclear factor (NF)-κB–dependent mechanism, which may limit the antileukemia activity of these agents.[121,122] Several binding partners of p21[cip1], including Pim-1, have been identified. Pim-1 associates with and phosphorylates p21[cip1] *in vivo*, which influences the subcellular localization of p21[cip1].[123] p21[cip1] is phosphorylated by Pim-1 at two distinct sites, Thr145 and Ser146; phosphorylation on Thr[145] results in a nuclear localization of p21[cip1] and a disruption of the cell cycle, while phosphorylation on Ser[146] leads to a cytoplasmic localization of p21[cip1],[124] suggesting that overexpression of Pim-1 in certain tumors plays a key role in tumorigenesis.[125] Like RB, expression and function of p21[cip1] is also affected by several different mechanisms, including mutation and histone deacetylation (see "The Role of Histone Deacetylases in Cell-Cycle Regulation" below). Other members of the p21[cip1] family of CDKIs include p27[kip1] and p57[kip2].[101,126] As a cdk inhibitor, p27[kip1] has tumor-suppressor activity. Besides cdks, p27[kip1] regulates additional cellular processes, including cell motility, some of which seem to mediate the oncogenic activities of p27[kip1]. For example, the constellation of high p27[kip1] and low Myc expression is characteristic of chronic lymphocytic leukemia (CLL) cells.[127] These activities of p27[kip1] are regulated through multiple phosphorylation sites. The multiple functions of p27[kip1] are dependent on a number of different conditions, and dictate whether the protein displays anti- or protumorigenic properties.[128] High-level expression of p27[kip1] leads to a cell-cycle block in G_1 phase after treatment of cells with TGF-β. One major difference between p21[cip1] and p27[kip1] is that the former binds predominantly to cdk2 whereas the latter binds cdk4.

The cellular levels of a number of cell-cycle regulators, including p21[cip1] and p27[kip1], are regulated by ubiquitination and subsequent proteolysis. Polyubiquitinated proteins are degraded by the 26S proteasome complex. There are two major ubiquitination systems in the cell; they are designated *SCF* and *APC*.[108,110] SCF is named for three of its core components, Skp, Cullin, and an F-box–containing protein. Important examples of SCF substrates are Cln1, Sic1, Wee1, Cdc6/Cdc18, E2F, cyclin D_1, cyclin E, p21[cip1], p27[kip1], and p57[kip2].[129]

A second group of CDKIs belongs to the inhibitor of the kinase 4 (INK4) family and includes *p15[INK4B]*, *p16[INK4A]*, *p18[INK4C]*, and *p19[INK4D]*.[104,107,130,131] They all bind and inhibit the cyclin D_1–cdk4 and/or cyclin D_1–cdk6 complex, which regulate cell-cycle progression via RB.[104,130] TGF-β is also a potent inducer of *p15[INK4B]*,[104] one of the mechanisms by which the cytokine regulates the proliferation of hematopoietic cells (Chap. 16). *p16[INK4A]* is probably the most important CDKI, because the gene is inactivated by several mechanisms (deletion, mutation, hypermethylation) in many different human cancers.[132] Surprisingly, *p16[INK4A]* and *p14[ARF]* are overexpressed in some cases of human hematologic malignancies.[133] This overexpression is probably a result of defects downstream of *p16[INK4A]*, particularly caused by mutations in the RB gene.[134] In hematologic malignancies, the highest frequencies of *p14[ARF]*, *p15[INK4B]*, or *p16[INK4A]* inactivations are found in T-ALL,[135] secondary high-grade lymphomas, and mantle cell lymphoma (MCL).[136,137] The potency of *p14[ARF]* and *p16[INK4A]* in terms of tumorigenicity becomes obvious because the reexpression of both genes by either retroviral transfection or demethylation of the promoter regions results in a complete reversion of the malignant phenotype.[138,139] *p14[ARF]* has multiple

tumor-suppressor functions, some of which are mediated by signaling to p53. On the other hand, it has been shown that *p14[ARF]* is able to drive tumor progression in a p53-independent fashion, especially in myc-driven lymphomas.[140]

● PHARMACOLOGIC INHIBITION OF CYCLIN-DEPENDENT KINASES

Perturbations of the cell cycle, for example, overexpression of cyclins or underexpression of endogenous CDKIs, are nearly universal in human malignancies, and cdks, as critical regulators of cell-cycle progression and RNA transcription, represent attractive targets for anticancer drug development, as their inhibition can lead to both cell-cycle arrest and apoptosis.[141,142] Additionally, pharmacologic inhibition of transcriptional cdks, for example, cdk9, affects proteins with short half-lives, for example, the antiapoptotic proteins Mcl-1 and XIAP (X-linked inhibitor of apoptosis), cell-cycle regulators, p53, and NF-κB–responsive gene products.[142] Hematologic malignancies may be particularly susceptible to cdk inhibition and apoptosis induction. A number of pharmacologic CDKIs have been developed and subjected to various phases of preclinical and clinical testing in hematologic malignancies (for a review, see Ref. 143). The selective cdk4/6 inhibitor palbociclib has been approved by the FDA as a potential treatment for hormone-responsive metastatic breast cancer. In MCL, a disease characterized by cyclin D_1 overexpression, this agent has demonstrated encouraging clinical activity.[144] Whether selective or broad-spectrum inhibition is the superior therapeutic strategy continues to be debated,[143] and may be tumor type-specific. The "pan-CDKI" flavopiridol (alvocidib), the first CDKI to enter the clinic, has shown promising activity in patients with genetically high-risk chronic lymphocytic leukemia (CLL), particularly when administered by a pharmacologically derived "hybrid" schedule,[145,146] but recent developmental efforts for this agent have focused on AML, where it was recently granted "orphan drug" status.[147] Flavopiridol induces apoptosis in primary leukemic blasts and recruits surviving leukemic cells into a proliferative state, thereby priming such cells for killing by S-phase-active cytotoxic agents such as cytarabine.[148,149] These observations led to the design of "timed sequential therapy" regimens, for example, FLAM (flavopiridol, cytarabine, mitoxantrone), which exhibited promising clinical activity in AML patients with nonfavorable cytogenetics.[150] Interestingly, both "bolus" and "hybrid" schedules of administration of flavopiridol produce comparably encouraging results in this setting.[151] Other rational combinations involving pan-CDKIs such as flavopiridol or roscovitine involve those with proteasome inhibitors (PIs),[152,153] HDACIs[154] or BH3-mimetics.[75] The first strategy has been explored in phase I trials in patients with recurrent or refractory indolent B-cell neoplasms,[155,156] and a phase I trial of bortezomib and dexamethasone plus the pan-CDKI dinaciclib in patients with relapsed myeloma is ongoing as of this writing (NCT01711528). Synergism in preclinical studies in leukemia between pan-CDKIs and HDACIs is based predominantly on reciprocal effects on the cytoprotective NF-κB pathway and the endogenous cdk inhibitor p21[WAF1/CIP1], besides Mcl-1/XIAP downregulation.[154] Some of these phenomena have been recapitulated in patients with AML.[157]

● CELL-CYCLE CHECKPOINTS

The cell cycle progresses in an orderly fashion and is monitored by safety mechanisms known as cell-cycle checkpoints, which, upon activation, function to halt cell division.[158] When DNA damage occurs, distinct, albeit overlapping and cooperating, checkpoint pathways are activated, which block S-phase entry (the G₁/S-phase checkpoint), delay S-phase progression (the intra–S- or S-phase checkpoint), or prevent mitotic entry (the G₂/M-phase checkpoint). These events direct phase-specific DNA repair mechanisms through repair-specific gene transcription. If repair fails, checkpoints trigger apoptosis.[159] Checkpoints are thus important quality control measures that ensure the proper sequence of cell-cycle events and allow cells to respond to DNA damage.[160]

The G₁/S checkpoint is the first defense against genomic stress in cycling cells. In response to DNA damage, the G₁/S checkpoint prevents cells from entering the S-phase by inhibiting the initiation of DNA replication. At this checkpoint, the checkpoint kinase Chk2 is activated by the proximal transducer ATM to phosphorylate (and thereby inhibit) the cdc25A phosphatase, thus preventing activation of cyclin E(A)/cdk2 and temporarily halting the cell cycle. G₁ arrest is sustained by ATM/Chk2-mediated phosphorylation of murine double minute protein 2 (MDM2) and p53, resulting in p53 stabilization and accumulation. p53 transcriptionally activates the endogenous cdk inhibitor p21, which, in turn, inhibits cyclin E(A)/cdk2 and preserves the association of Rb with E2F.[160]

The intra-S or S-phase checkpoint is activated in response to structural DNA damage as well as stalled replication forks. Upon activation of this checkpoint, ATR/Chk1 and ATM/Chk2 phosphorylate cdc25A, resulting in enhanced proteolysis of the phosphatase and inhibition of its function through 14-3-3 σ binding. Cyclin E(A)/cdk2 is thereby inhibited, and progression through the S-phase halted.[158]

The G₂/M checkpoint prevents mitotic entry of cells that have either incurred DNA damage during G₂, or that have escaped the G₁/S and intra-S checkpoints despite earlier genomic insults. The key downstream target of the G₂/M checkpoint is the promitotic cyclin B/cdk1 (cdc2) complex. During interphase, this complex is inactivated through phosphorylation by Myt1 and Wee1.[158] Chk1 may phosphorylate Wee1, mediating binding of Wee1 to 14-3-3 proteins, which, in turn, may stimulate the kinase activity of Wee1 against cdk1 (cdc2). Thus, both Chk1 and 14-3-3 proteins may act together as positive regulators of Wee1.[161] Activation of cyclin B/cdk1 (cdc2) requires dephosphorylation by the cdc25 phosphatases (A, B, and C). Notably, phosphorylation/inactivation of cdk1 (cdc2) involves two inhibitory sites, for example, Tyr15 and Thr14, and dephosphorylation of both sites is necessary for full cdk1 (cdc2) activation. Initiation of the G₂/M checkpoint is mediated by ATR/Chk1, which phosphorylates (and thereby inhibits) cdc25A, B, and C, whereas maintenance of this checkpoint requires p53 and its downstream effectors p21, 14-3-3 σ, and growth arrest and DNA damage (GADD) 45.[158]

Checkpoint dysfunction is common in human cancers and is considered a pathologic hallmark of neoplastic transformation.[162] Conversely, agents used for cancer treatment, such as cytotoxic chemotherapy and ionizing radiation, activate cell-cycle checkpoints.[158] Cancer cells are particularly dependent upon the S- and G₂/M-phase checkpoints for repair of DNA damage because of preexisting defects in G₁/S checkpoint mechanisms, such as p53 and RB mutations. Because the S-phase checkpoint facilitates slowing, rather than arrest, of the cell cycle, a cancer cell harboring DNA damage may progress through the S-phase checkpoint, only to halt at the G₂/M checkpoint. The latter is, therefore, a key guardian of the cancer cell genome, and its abrogation can lead to enhanced tumor cell death while sparing normal cells, which maintain an intact G₁/S-phase checkpoint. G₂/M checkpoint abrogation prevents cancer cells from repairing DNA damage, forcing them into a premature and lethal mitosis ("mitotic catastrophe").[160]

Based upon these concepts, synergism between DNA-damaging agents (cytotoxic chemotherapy) and G₂/M checkpoint abrogators have been examined both preclinically and in clinical studies. In human AML cell lines, the Chk1 inhibitor MK-8776 (SCH900776) markedly increased cytarabine-induced apoptosis, with negligible impact on normal myeloid progenitors,[163] leading to a phase I trial of the combination in patients with relapsed and refractory acute leukemias.[164] Chk1 inhibitors increase HDACI lethality in human leukemia cells.[165] This may reflect the ability of HDACIs to induce DNA damage in AML cells,[166] inhibit both homologous recombination and nonhomologous end-joining mechanisms of DNA repair,[167] and downregulate/inactivate Chk1.[168] However, clinical development of MK-8776 has been halted. Based upon the ability of Hsp90 inhibitors to downregulate Chk1, a phase I study of the combination of cytarabine and the Hsp90 inhibitor tanespimycin was conducted in adults with recurrent or refractory acute leukemia; however, the combination exhibited limited clinical activity.[169]

Wee1 is a validated therapeutic target in AML.[170] The combination of cytarabine and the Wee1 inhibitor AZD1775 synergistically induces apoptosis in myeloid cell lines.[171] Similarly, genome-wide short hairpin RNA screens strongly implicate cell-cycle checkpoint proteins, particularly Wee1, as critical mediators of AML cell survival after cytarabine exposure.[172] In AML cell lines, synergistic inhibition of proliferation by the combination of AZD1775 and Ara-C occurred regardless of p53 functionality.[173] Another combinatorial strategy in AML involves coadministration of AZD1775 with HDACIs.[174] Besides inducing DNA damage and inhibiting DNA repair, HDACIs downregulate several proteins critical to checkpoint function, such as ATR, Chk1, and Wee1,[168,175–177] and Wee1 inhibition promotes premature mitotic entry of cells bearing unrepaired DNA damage.[178] Efforts to extend these pre-clinical findings to the clinic are underway.

● ONCOGENES

Table 16–2 lists the common genomic aberrations seen in hematologic malignancies. Tables 16–3 and 16–4 list common somatic mutations encountered in the major myeloid and lymphoid malignancies, respectively.

The complicated cell-cycle network has its parallel in the several different oncogenes and tumor-suppressor genes that influence carcinogenesis and tumor progression. The products of oncogenes, the oncoproteins, lead to or facilitate the transformation of a normal into a malignant cell. Oncogenes can be carried into the cell by viruses or they can arise from mutations in normal cellular genes. In addition, they can also arise from leukemia- or lymphoma-associated translocations where two usually separated genes are fused together and form a novel fusion protein. The familiar concept of this kind of protooncogene activation can be blurred by the fusion proteins because they possess unique capabilities not shared by either of the individual fusion partners. Oncoproteins can interact directly with cell-cycle regulatory proteins or control their activity through phosphorylation and dephosphorylation. Not all mutations in oncogenes lead to an altered function of the resulting product. The nomenclature in the oncogene and tumor-suppressor gene field is not always clear. As a general guideline, if a mutation causes a functional loss of the gene product (loss of function), and the recessive loss of function leads directly to uncontrolled cell division, the underlying gene can be named a *tumor-suppressor gene*. On the other hand, if the mutation leads to an altered gene product (gain of function) that interacts abnormally with other proteins to influence the cell cycle, this gene is an *oncogene*, acting in a dominant fashion. Translocations are typical of oncogenes, whereas homozygous deletions and hypermethylation of CpG-nucleotide repeats in the promoter regions ("epigenetic silencing") are characteristic features of tumor-suppressor genes.

Numerous oncogenes/oncogene candidates are described in the literature, and most of them are involved in the pathogenesis and development of many different tumors types, especially the

TABLE 16–2. Common genomic aberrations seen in the major hematologic malignancies.

Chromosomal abnormality	Genes/loci affected or fusion gene where applicable	Functional consequence, if known	Approximate incidence (in newly diagnosed patients)	Prognostic/therapeutic implications, if any
ACUTE MYELOID LEUKEMIA				
t(8;21)(q22;q22) – diagnostic of AML regardless of blast count	RUNX1-RUNX1T1 (AML1-ETO)	Fusion protein alters transcriptional regulation of normal RUNX1 target genes and activates new target genes to prevent apoptosis and/or differentiation	7% in adults; most frequent abnormality in children with AML	Favorable prognosis in adults(not children) unless c-kit mutated; respond particularly well to high dose cytarabine-based regimens; generally not allografted in CR1
inv(16)(p13.1q22) or t(16;16) (p13.1;q22) - diagnostic of AML regardless of blast count	CBFB-MYH11	Fusion protein disrupts function of RUNX1/CBFB transcription factor→ repression of transcription; association with M4 FAB subtype and abnormal bone marrow eosinophils	5% in adults	Favorable prognosis unless c-kit mutated; respond particularly well to high dose cytarabine-based regimens; generally not allografted in CR1
t(15;17)(q24.1;q21.1) - diagnostic of AML (APL) regardless of blast count	PML-RARA	Fusion protein causes transcriptional repression, preventing differentiation of promyelocytes	13% (APL, most common form of AML related to therapy with bimolane for psoriasis)	Differentiation block overcome by pharmacologic doses of ATRA; high cure rates; low/intermediate risk patients can be cured without chemotherapy
11q23 rearrangements	KMT2A (MLL) and various partner genes, e.g., AF9 (most common partner) or partial tandem duplication	Complex effects (CDKs important in leukemogenesis); can also result in lymphoid phenotype (e.g., KMT2A-AF4 fusion with t(4;11)(q21;q23)	6% in young adults and up to 12% in children; often seen in AML following therapy with DNA topoisomerase II inhibitors	Poor prognosis unless t(9;11)(p22;q23) leading to KMT2A-AF9 fusion (intermediate prognosis); MLL translocations predict improved outcome with high dose daunorubicin
inv(3)(q21q26.2) or t(3;3)(q21;q26.2) or ins(5;3)(q14;q21q26.2)	MECOM (EV1)	MECOM (EV1) activation can promote or repress transcription depending on binding partners through interaction with transcriptional and epigenetic regulators	1% (3q abnormalities as a whole in 4.4%)	Adverse prognosis; association with thrombocytosis and increased, often abnormal, bone marrow megakaryocytes
t(6;9)(p23;q34)	DEK-NUP214 (DEK-CAN)	Fusion protein is a nucleoporin that acts as a transcription factor and also alters nuclear transport	1%	Poor prognosis; high incidence of FLT3-ITD; association with basophilia, dysplasia and pancytopenia
Trisomy 8			13%	Intermediate prognosis
Loss of chromosome 7 or del7q	CUX1, EZH2	CUX1 encodes a transcription factor and EZH2 a histone methyltransferase; both act as tumor suppressors	-7 seen in 9%	Poor prognosis; strong associations with older age, secondary AML, complex karyotype and prior therapy with alkylating agents or radiation
Loss of chromosome 5 or del5q	RPS14, miR-145/146a, EGR1, NPM1, APC, CTNNA1	Unclear; cooperative loss of multiple genes on 5q likely required for pathogenesis	-5 seen in 6%	Poor prognosis; strong associations with older age, secondary AML, complex karyotype and with prior therapy with alkylating agents or radiation
del17p	TP53	Loss of tumor suppressor "guardian of genome", failure of cell cycle checkpoint mechanisms, disruption of DDR	TP53 mutations seen in only 9% of older patients with de novo AML, but much more common in secondary and t-AML	Very poor prognosis, high risk of treatment failure not overcome even by allogeneic HSCT; strong association with complex karyotype

(continued)

TABLE 16–2. Common genomic aberrations seen in the major hematologic malignancies. (Continued)

Chromosomal abnormality	Genes/loci affected or fusion gene where applicable	Functional consequence, if known	Approximate incidence (in newly diagnosed patients)	Prognostic/therapeutic implications, if any
Complex karyotype (≥3 acquired, unrelated abnormalities in the absence of t(8;21), inv(16)/t(16;16) or t(15;17))	Multiple		10-12%, increases with age; much more common in secondary or t-AML	Very poor prognosis; 5q, 17p and 7q abnormalities most common; TP53 alterations the most important prognostic factor
Monosomal karyotype (≥2 monosomies, or a single monosomy in the presence of structural abnormalities)	Multiple		13%, increases with age	Extremely poor prognosis not overcome even by allogeneic HSCT
CHRONIC MYELOID LEUKEMIA				
t(9;22)(q34;q11)	BCR-ABL1 (vast majority of cases characterized by the p210 "major" fusion protein)	Fusion protein (constitutively active tyrosine kinase) drives all aspects of pathogenesis in chronic phase; other pathways also important in advanced phases	All cases (atypical CML, Bcr-Abl negative, is a separate entity)	High degree of "oncogene addiction" in chronic phase allows successful targeting of the Bcr-Abl kinase by small molecule inhibitors; outcomes dismal in blastic phase with loss of addiction to Bcr-Abl signaling
MYELODYSPLASTIC SYNDROMES				
del5q33.1 or del5q31	RPS14, miR-145/146a, EGR1, APC, CTNNA1	In 5q- syndrome, haploinsufficiency of RPS14 leads to impaired maturation of 40S ribosomal units, causing premature TP53-dependent apoptosis of erythroid precursors	15% overall	Most common chromosomal abnormality in MDS; del5q31 more common with higher risk or t-MDS; del5q33.1 seen in the indolent 5q- syndrome responsive to lenalidomide; del5q considered "good" in IPSS-R
del7q or loss of chromosome 7	EZH2?	Unclear loss of which genes on 7q pathogeneic, since vast majority of patients with EZH2 mutations do not have del7q or -7	10% in de novo MDS; up to 50% in t-MDS	del7q considered "intermediate" in IPSS-R; -7 considered "poor"
Trisomy 8	c-MYC, others?	Higher expression of anti-apoptotic genes, c-MYC overexpression?	<10%	Considered "intermediate" in IPSS-R
del20q	Unknown	Unknown	<5%	Considered "good" in IPSS-R
Loss of Y chromosome	Multiple	Not felt to be pathogenic in MDS	Common normal finding in men	Considered "very good" in IPSS-R
Complex karyotype (≥3 abnormalities)	Multiple		18%	Considered "very poor" in IPSS-R if >3 abnormalities; "poor" if only 3
t(5;12)(q33;p13)	ETV6-PDGFRB (TEL-PDGFRB)	Fuses ETV6 transcription factor gene with PDGFR beta gene	Rare	Seen in the context of MDS/MPN; responds to imatinib
B-CELL ACUTE LYMPHOBLASTIC LEUKEMIA				
t(9;22)(q34;q11)	BCR-ABL1 (most cases characterized by the p190 "minor" fusion protein	Fusion protein leads to constitutively active tyrosine kinase; often associated with IKZF1 splicing abnormalities	25-30% in adults, 2-5% in children	Traditionally "high risk", with allogeneic HSCT in CR1 commonly recommended; cure rates improved in "TKI era"

(continued)

TABLE 16–2. Common genomic aberrations seen in the major hematologic malignancies.(Continued)

Chromosomal abnormality	Genes/loci affected or fusion gene where applicable	Functional consequence, if known	Approximate incidence (in newly diagnosed patients)	Prognostic/therapeutic implications, if any
t(8;14)(q24.2;q32) or t(2;8)(p12;q24.2) or t(8;22)(q24.2;q11.2)	c-MYC, immuno-globulin heavy and light chain genes	Constitutive expression of oncogenic c-MYC	1% (Burkitt's lymphoma/leukemia – FAB L3 morphology; mature B-cell phenotype)	Poor prognosis; high incidence of CNS involvement and TLS; treated with short, intensive regimens
t(12;21)(p12;q22)	ETV6-RUNX1 (TEL-AML1)	Fusion protein inhibits transactivation of gene expression by normal RUNX1	15-25% in children, 3-4% in adults	Favorable prognosis
Intrachromosomal amplification of chromosome 21 (secondary chromosomal abnormalities common)	RUNX1 (AML1)		3-5% of older children	Poor prognosis with standard risk regimens, overcome by intensive therapy (high risk regimens)
11q23 abnormalities	KMT2A (MLL), most commonly KMT2A-AF4(AFF1) caused by t(4;11)(q21;q23); 2nd most common is t(11;19)(q23;p13.3)	KMT2A encodes a histone methyltransferase that regulates transcription of genes such as IKZF1 and HOX genes	5-7% overall; 60-80% in infants	Poor prognosis; frequent co-expression of myeloid antigens; about half the patients with t(11;19)(q23;p13.3) have AML, mostly FAB M5a subtype
t(1;19)(q23;p13.3) or der(19)t(1;19)(q23;p13.3) and its variant t(17;19)(q21;p13.3)	PBX1-TCF3 (PBX-1-E2A) or HLF-E2A	Activation of gene transcription by fusion protein via unclear mechanisms	30% of childhood precursor B-cell ALL (5% of all pediatric ALL)	Studies with conflicting results; probably favorable prognosis
del9p	PAX5, JAK2 (in Down syndrome associated ALL)		5-10%	Poor prognosis
Hyperdiploidy	Multiple		40%	Favorable prognosis in patients with >50 chromosomes
Hypodiploidy	Multiple		5-6%	Poor prognosis
T-CELL ACUTE LYMPHOBLASTIC LEUKEMIA				
Translocations involving 7p14 (TCRγ) or 7q34(TCRβ) or 14q11.2 (TCRα/δ)	TCR genes; multiple partners – usually cell cycle inhibitors or transcription factors		35%	
Cryptic interstitial deletion at 1p32	SIL-TAL1	Fusion gene functions as transcription factor	9-30% of childhood T-ALL; frequency decreases in adults	
11q23 abnormalities	KMT2A (MLL) with various partners		8%	
t(10;11)(p13;q14)	CALM-AF10		10%	
t(9;9)(q34;q34)	NUP214-ABL1	Fusion of nuclear pore complex component with intracellular tyrosine kinase as a result of episomal amplification of in-frame fusion	Up to 6%	Responsive to imatinib?

(continued)

TABLE 16–2. Common genomic aberrations seen in the major hematologic malignancies.(Continued)

Chromosomal abnormality	Genes/loci affected or fusion gene where applicable	Functional consequence, if known	Approximate incidence (in newly diagnosed patients)	Prognostic/therapeutic implications, if any
del9p21	p16 (INK4/ARF)	Loss of endogenous CDK inhibitor function	65% in children; 15% in adults	
del6q			20-30%	
CHRONIC LYMPHOCYTIC LEUKEMIA				
del13q	*MIR15A, MIR16-1, RB1*, associated with *MYD88* mutations	Loss of tumor suppressor function of Rb; loss of miR15a and miR16-1 derepresses Bcl-2 but also increases TP53 mRNA; MYD88 is a critical adaptor molecule of the IL-1 TLR pathway that activates NF-κB and augments BTK signaling	55%	Favorable prognosis when sole cytogenetic abnormality; MYD88 mutations associated with mutated *IGHV*; BTK (BCR pathway) inhibition highly effective in CLL
del11q	*ATM*; associated with *SF3B1* mutations	ATM is a proximal transducer of the DDR network; SF3B1 functions in mRNA splicing	18%	Poor prognosis but overcome by FCR; the most common type of karyotypic evolution over time; associated with bulky lymphadenopathy
Trisomy 12q	Associated with *NOTCH1* and *FBXW7* mutations		16%	Unclear - conflicting study results; NOTCH1 mutations confer unfavorable prognosis and are associated with unmutated IGHV
del17p	*TP53*	Loss of tumor suppressor "guardian of genome", failure of cell cycle checkpoint mechanisms, disruption of DDR	7%	Poor prognosis not overcome by cytotoxic chemotherapy; alemtuzumab and BCR pathway inhibitors effective, as well as allogeneic HSCT
del6q			7%	
T-CELL PROLYMPHOCYTIC LEUKEMIA				
t(14;14)(q11;q32) or inv(14)(q11;q32) or t(X;14)(q28;q11)	*TCR-TCL1* *MTCP1-TCR*	Overexpression of the *TCL-1* oncogene or its homolog *MTCP1*	90%	
Chromosome 8 abnormalities	idic(8p11), t(8;8), trisomy 8q	Up-regulation of oncogenic c-MYC	70-80%	
MULTIPLE MYELOMA				
del13q14 or monosomy 13 or hypodiploidy	Multiple		48%	Intermediate risk with modern therapies only if detected on karyotyping, or by FISH in presence of other abnormalities (otherwise standard risk)
del17p13	*TP53*	Loss of tumor suppressor "guardian of genome", failure of cell cycle checkpoint mechanisms, disruption of DDR	11%	High risk
Gain of 1q21	*CKS1B*	*CKS1B* favors cell cycle progression by promoting degradation of the endogenous CDK inhibitor p27 with release of CDKs and mitotic entry	30-43%	Controversial; conflicting study results
del1p	*FAM46C, CDKN2C*	Loss of endogenous CDK inhibitor function leads to excessive proliferation	30%	High risk

(continued)

TABLE 16–2. Common genomic aberrations seen in the major hematologic malignancies.(Continued)

Chromosomal abnormality	Genes/loci affected or fusion gene where applicable	Functional consequence, if known	Approximate incidence (in newly diagnosed patients)	Prognostic/therapeutic implications, if any
t(11;14)(q13;q32)	CCND1-IgH	Overexpression of cyclin D1	21% (10-31%)	Standard risk; very high prevalence in non-secretory cases; associated with lower levels of monoclonal proteins, CD20 expression, lambda light chains and lymphoplasmacytic morphology
t(6;14)(p25;q32)	CCND3-IgH	Overexpression of cyclin D3		Standard risk
t(8;14)(q24;q32)	c-MYC-IgH	c-MYC overexpression		Standard risk
t(4;14)(p16.3;q32.3)	MMSET-IgH	MMSET is a histone methyltransferase and its deregulation/overexpression is key to pathogenesis; FGFR3 also often overexpressed	14%	Intermediate to high risk; adverse prognosis overcome by bortezomib/HSCT
t(14;16)(q32.3;q23)	IgH-c-MAF	MAF encodes a transcription factor that can activate or repress transcription depending on binding site/partner		High risk
t(14;20)(q32;q11)	IgH-MAFB	MAF encodes a transcription factor that can activate or repress transcription depending on binding site/partner		High risk
Hyperdiploidy (trisomies of odd numbered chromosomes other than 1, 13, 21)	Multiple		39%	Standard risk; in the presence of concurrent trisomies, "high risk" cytogenetics become standard risk

NON-HODGKIN'S LYMPHOMA (selected abnormalities)

Chromosomal abnormality	Fusion gene created, where applicable	Pathogenetic mechanism	Disease association	Therapeutic relevance
t(2;5)(p23;q35) and variants	ALK-NPM and others	Constitutively active tyrosine kinase triggers malignant transformation and activates anti-apoptotic pathways	ALK+ anaplastic large cell lymphoma	ALK targeting with small molecule inhibitors, e.g., crizotinib
t(11;14)(q13;q32)	CCND1-IgH	Overexpression of cyclin D1 drives cellular proliferation	Mantle cell lymphoma (almost all cases)	Efficacy of CDK4/6 inhibitors, e.g., palbociclib
t(14;18)(q32;q21)	IgH-BCL2	Constitutive expression of anti-apoptotic Bcl-2 promotes cellular survival	Follicular lymphoma (80%), diffuse large B-cell lymphoma (30%)	Selective targeting of Bcl-2 with BH3-mimetics, e.g., venetoclax
t(11;18)(q21;q21) t(14;18)(q32;q21) t(1;14)(p22;q32) t(3;14)(p13;q32)	API2 (IAP2)-MALT1 IgH-MALT1 BCL10-IgH FOXP1-IgH	Overexpression of BCL10 results in NF-κB activation through BCL10/MALT1 signaling complex; FOXP1 is a transcription factor of unknown function	MALT lymphoma (extranodal marginal zone lymphoma)	Nuclear expression of BCL10 or NF-κB in gastric MALT lymphoma associated with resistance to antibiotic therapy

(continued)

TABLE 16-2. Common genomic aberrations seen in the major hematologic malignancies.(Continued)

Chromosomal abnormality	Genes/loci affected or fusion gene where applicable	Functional consequence, if known	Approximate incidence (in newly diagnosed patients)	Prognostic/therapeutic implications, if any
9p24 amplification	Contains genes that encode PD-L1, PD-L2, JAK2	PDL-1 commonly over-expressed; MHC class II transactivator rearrangements (38% of PMBL) lead to PD-1 overexpression also	Primary mediastinal B-cell lymphoma	PD-1 immune checkpoint pathway a potential target
3q27 abnormalities (mutations, rearrangements)	Locus for *BCL6* transcriptional repressor	Bcl-6 overexpression results in down-regulation of many target proteins, including p53 tumor suppressor	Diffuse large B-cell lymphoma (almost all cases)	New inhibitors that disrupt Bcl-6 function being developed

hematologic malignancies. Among the chromosomal translocations, some of the most well-studied are found in AML and other myeloid neoplasms. These include t(8;21)(q22;q22), leading to the AML1-ETO or RUNX1-RUNX1T1 rearrangement, del4(q12;q12), t(5;12)(q31-q32;p13), leading to the TEL-platelet derived growth factor receptor (PDGFR) β rearrangement, t(15;17)(q22;12), leading to the promyelocytic leukemia (PML)-retinoic acid receptor (RAR) α rearrangement, inv16(p13;q22) or t(16;16)(p13;q22), leading to the CBFβ-MYH11 rearrangement, t(9;22)(q34;q11), leading to the BCR-ABL rearrangement, t(3;3)(q21;q26), t(8;16)(p11;p13), t(6;9)(p23;q34), t(7;11)(p15;p15), t(9;11)(p22;q23), t(6;11)(q27;q23), t(11;19)(q23;p13.1), and t(11;19)(q23;p13.3), all of which translocate the *MLL* gene located at 11q23, t(16;21)(p11;q22), and t(1;22) (p13;q13).[179,180] Leukemias carrying *MLL* rearrangements are driven by dysregulated epigenetic mechanisms in which fusion proteins containing N-terminal sequences of MLL can cause human leukemia without the requirement for a "second hit."[181] *MLL*-rearranged leukemias provide a paradigm for how epigenetic dysregulation can lead to cancer through inappropriate chromatin structure with subsequent activation of target genes with oncogenic activity. An improved molecular understanding of how MLL fusions upregulate binding targets has led to the identification of a number of potential mechanism-based therapeutic vulnerabilities for this poor-prognosis malignancy. Potential novel therapeutic approaches include inhibition of P-TEFb (cdk9/cyclin T), the histone modifying enzymes DOT1L (methyltransferase) or TIP60 (acetyltransferase), and disruption of the interaction of MLL fusions with other epigenetic systems such as CpG island methylation and polycomb genes, for example, PRC2.[181] In contrast, in secondary myeloid leukemias, recurrent numerical and unbalanced cytogenetic abnormalities predominate such as del(5q), del(7q), 7/del(7q), and del(20q), and are often associated with a poor prognosis.[180,182] Table 16-2 lists some of the fusion partners. Apart from the chromosomal translocations in AML as described above, there also aberrant fusion proteins in acute lymphoid leukemia (ALL), such as t(9;22), which is also found in chronic myelogenous leukemia (CML), t(4;11) in prolymphoblastic leukemia, and t(12;21) in childhood ALL. Some lymphomas are characterized by chromosomal translocations that juxtapose an oncogene to the immunoglobulin heavy-chain gene, which then drives overexpression of the oncogene, for example, t(8;14) in Burkitt lymphoma, t(11;14) in MCL, or t(14;18) in follicular lymphoma; for a review see Ref. 125.[183] The same is true of myeloma, where abnormalities such as t(4;14), t(6;14), t(11;14), t(14;16), and t(14;20) are frequently seen. An excellent overview of chromosomal rearrangements in cancer and the affected genes is available.[180]

The precise mechanism by which the fusion proteins lead to tumorigenesis is not always well understood. Nevertheless, in patients with AML, abnormal expression of the transcription factor RUNX1 (AML1) is able to promote cell-cycle progression by shortening G_1 phase and by repressing p21^{cip1} promoter activity. RUNX1 is absolutely required for the establishment of adult-type hematopoiesis[184]; it regulates genes specific to the lymphoid, myeloid, and megakaryocyte lineages,[185] and mice lacking RUNX1 do not develop definitive hematopoiesis, indicating a role in adult hematopoietic stem cell formation.[186] In contrast, the fusion product AML1/ETO, derived from the t(8;21), slows cell-cycle progression, suggesting that one gene in different "fusion situations" can cause different effects on the cell cycle.[187] Activation of the RUNX1-repression domain or fusing the gene to ETO results in downregulation of cdk4 and Myc, directly linking this fusion protein to cell-cycle checkpoints.[187] Additional evidence for the direct involvement of RUNX1 in cell-cycle control comes from the observation that the transcription factor binds to the p19^{INK4D} promoter and downregulates p19^{INK4D} expression in megakaryocytes.[188] Inhibiting the oligomerization domain of ETO interferes with RUNX1/ETO oncogenic activity and these cells lose their progenitor cell characteristics, arrest cell-cycle progression, and undergo cell death.[189] Another interesting chromosomal translocation fusion product that affects cell-cycle control is found in patients with acute PML (APL) or its variant form (vAPL). The PML-RARα, which results from t(15;17)(q22;12), upregulates cyclin A_1 expression, whereas PML itself seems to be a negative regulator of cell growth because its overexpression leads to growth suppression and G_1 arrest in a variety of different cell types.[190] PML is crucial for the growth-inhibiting activity of retinoic acid and its absence abrogates the retinoic acid-dependent transactivation of p21^{cip1}.[191] Another mechanism by which PML elicits irreversible growth arrest is believed to involve activation of the tumor-suppressor pathway p16^{INK4A}/RB.[192] Recent data point toward a linkage between PML and the nucleoporins, especially Nup98 and Nup214. In some AML specimens, these nucleoporins are expressed as oncogenic fusion proteins and become directed—complexed with PML—to common cytoplasmic compartments during the M-to-G_1 transition of the cell cycle. In APL cells, the loss of function of normal PML causes an increase in cytoplasmic-bound versus nuclear-membrane-bound nucleoporins.[193] Consequently, PML by itself is a tumor-suppressor gene that positively regulates cell-cycle progression. Further evidence for a tumor-suppressor gene function of PML comes from transgenic mice models where PML$^{-/-}$ mouse embryonic fibroblasts are enriched in S phase and the G_0/G_1 phase is minimized.[194] In APL, this regulatory role is disrupted by the fusion to RARα. One mechanism by which

TABLE 16–3. Common somatic mutations encountered in the major myeloid malignancies.

Gene	Functional class of encoded protein	Nature of mutation and functional consequence	Approximate incidence	Prognostic and/or therapeutic implications, if any
ACUTE MYELOID LEUKEMIA (AML)				
FLT3 (most commonly mutated gene in AML)	Tyrosine kinase (signaling molecule)	Internal tandem duplications or tyrosine kinase domain mutations ("class I" mutations that confer survival and proliferation advantages)	Up to 35% (25% ITD, 10% TKD); higher in CN AML (31% ITD; 11% TKD)	*FLT3-ITD* AML characterized by higher WBC counts and blast %, early relapses and poor survival; multiple inhibitors in development; allogeneic HSCT in CR1 usually recommended; prognostic impact of TKD mutations unclear; conflicting studies
NPM1 (most commonly mutated gene in CN AML)	Nucleophosmin	"Class II" mutations that impair differentiation of hematopoietic cells	27% (53% of CN AML)	Mutated *NPM1* with WT *FLT3* confers favorable prognosis in CN AML if *IDH1/2* also mutated; patients generally not allografted in CR1; may predict improved outcome with high dose daunorubicin
MLL-PTD	Histone methyltransferase	Partial tandem duplication; for translocations see Table 2	5-7% of CN AML	Poor prognosis; mutually exclusive of NPM1; DOT1L inhibitors in early clinical trials; CDK9 and HDAC inhibitors appear promising
DNMT3A	DNA methyl transferase	Loss of function mutations causing reduced methylation in mutant genomes	22%	Strongly associated with intermediate risk cytogenetics; independent predictor of poor outcome that may be overcome by high dose daunorubicin; mutually exclusive with *MLL* translocations
IDH1/2	Krebs cycle enzymes	IDH mutants produce 2-hydroxyglutarate from alpha-ketoglutarate, which inhibits TET enzymes, causing DNA hypermethylation	15-30%	Increased frequency in older patients; new small molecule IDH inhibitors promising; *IDH2* R140Q mutations associated with improved survival
TET2	Catalyzes alpha-ketoglutarate-dependent conversion of 5-methylcytosine to 5-hydroxymethylcytosine, leading to DNA demethylation	Loss of function mutations→ increased promoter methylation→increased self-renewal and impaired differentiation	10%	*TET2* mutations mutually exclusive with *IDH1/2* mutations and confer poor prognosis in patients with intermediate risk AML
ASXL1	Member of polycomb family of chromatin binding proteins; epigenetic modifier; functions as ligand-dependent coactivator of retinoid acid receptor	Loss of function mutations	3-5% in younger patients, 16% in older patients	Poor prognosis; may be mutually exclusive of *NPM1* mutations
CEBPA	Myeloid transcription factor	"Class II" mutations that impair differentiation of hematopoietic cells	13% of CN AML	Biallelic *CEBPA* mutations associated with favorable prognosis in patients with intermediate risk AML
RUNX1 (AML1)	Myeloid transcription factor – master regulator of hematopoiesis	Gain of function mutations in proximal Runt homology domain, or loss of function mutations in distal transactivation domain	5%	Mutually exclusive of *FLT3* and *NPM1* mutations

(continued)

TABLE 16–3. Common somatic mutations encountered in the major myeloid malignancies. (Continued)

Gene	Functional class of encoded protein	Nature of mutation and functional consequence	Approximate incidence	Prognostic and/or therapeutic implications, if any
TP53	Master regulator of cell cycle, DNA damage response and apoptosis (tumor suppressor)	17p deletions and inactivating point mutations; MDM2 overexpression; other mechanisms of loss of function	TP53 mutations seen in only 9% of older patients with de novo AML, but much more common in secondary and t-AML	Extremely poor prognosis; MDM2 (negative regulator of TP53) antagonists in clinical trials; mutually exclusive of FLT3 and NPM1 mutations
PHF6	X-linked tumor suppressor	Loss of function mutations	3%	Mutations confer poor prognosis
NRAS	Survival signaling molecule	"Class I" mutations that confer survival and proliferation advantages	13% of CN AML; RAS mutated in 19% of elderly patients with AML	RAS mutations predict for benefit of post remission HiDAC
WT1	Transcription factor that may act both as a tumor suppressor gene and an oncogene	Loss of function mutations	10%; most frequent in CN AML	Unclear effect on prognosis; likely negative impact
KIT	Tyrosine kinase (signaling molecule)	Activating mutations	30-40% of CBF AML	Mutated c-KIT confers adverse prognosis in CBF AML; ?role of TKIs
MYELODYSPLASTIC SYDROMES (MDS)				
SF3B1	RNA splicing protein – core component of U2 snRNP, which recognizes the 3′ splice site at intron-exon junctions	Spliceosome mutations→decreased or increased transcription of normal pre-mRNA, exon skipping, intron retention and cryptic splice sites; SF3B1 mutations lead to abnormal splicing of ABCB7	24%	Extremely strong correlation with ringed sideroblasts; indolent course with prolonged survival (RARS); acquisition of JAK2 V617F causes RARS-T
TET2	Catalyzes alpha-ketoglutarate-dependent conversion of 5-methylcytosine to 5-hydroxymethylcytosine, leading to DNA demethylation	Loss of function mutations→ increased promoter methylation→increased self-renewal and impaired differentiation	20-22%	Predict response to HMAs, but overall confer poor prognosis, even after HSCT
SRSF2	RNA splicing protein	Spliceosome mutations→decreased or increased transcription of normal pre-mRNA, exon skipping, intron retention and cryptic splice sites	14%	Co-occurrence of TET2 and SRSF2 mutations highly specific for CMML; mutually exclusive with SF3B1 mutation; progression from SRSF2- mutated RCMD-RS to RAEB may involve appearance of STAG2 mutations
ASXL1	Member of polycomb family of chromatin binding proteins; epigenetic modifier; functions as ligand-dependent coactivator of retinoic acid receptor	Loss of function mutations in C-terminal generate a dominant-negative protein that inhibits its wild type counterpart and other members of polycomb protein complex	10%; >40% of patients with CMML	Poor prognosis
DNMT3A	DNA methyl transferase	Loss of function mutations causing reduced methylation in mutant genomes	10-15%	Poor prognosis, even after HSCT

(continued)

TABLE 16–3. Common somatic mutations encountered in the major myeloid malignancies. (Continued)

Gene	Functional class of encoded protein	Nature of mutation and functional consequence	Approximate incidence	Prognostic and/or therapeutic implications, if any
RUNX1 (AML1)	Myeloid transcription factor – master regulator of hematopoiesis	Gain of function mutations in proximal Runt homology domain, or loss of function mutations in distal transactivation domain	7-15%; higher in t-MDS	Poor prognosis; RUNX1 mutations often accompanied by activation of Ras pathway
U2AF1	RNA splicing protein	Spliceosome mutations→decreased or increased transcription of normal pre-mRNA, exon skipping, intron retention and cryptic splice sites	5-10%	
TP53	Master regulator of cell cycle, DNA damage response and apoptosis (tumor suppressor)	17p deletions and inactivating point mutations	5-15%; higher in t-MDS	Poor prognosis, even after HSCT
EZH2	Tumor suppressor - histone methyltransferase (catalytic subunit of polycomb repressive complex, PRC2)	Loss of function mutations→loss of PRC2 activity→increase in hematopoietic stem cell number and activity	6%	Poor prognosis, including in lower risk patients
IDH1/2	Krebs cycle enzymes	IDH mutants produce 2-hydroxyglutarate from alpha-ketoglutarate, which inhibits TET enzymes, causing DNA hypermethylation	3.5%	IDH2 more frequently mutated than IDH1 and often co-mutated with SRSF2; IDH mutations cause differentiation block; inhibitors in development
ETV6 (TEL)	Transcription factor		0.2-2.7%	Poor prognosis; ETV6-PDGFRB rearrangement in MDS/MPN responds to imatinib
NRAS	Survival signaling molecule	Ras-Raf-MEK-ERK pathway activation	10-15%	Poor prognosis
CBL	Tyrosine kinase-associated ubiquitin ligase that negatively regulates Ras pathway and JAK-STAT signaling by targeting receptor TKs for degradation	Mutants encode a dominant negative protein that inhibits the ubiquitin ligase activity of the wild type protein and of its homolog, CBLB	<5%; 15% of patients with CMML	Unclear impact on prognosis
JAK2	Tyrosine kinase (JAK-STAT signaling critical to hematopoiesis)	Activating mutations (V617F)	5%; 50% in RARS-T	None; evolution from RARS to RARS-T involves acquiring JAK2 V617F in SF3B1 mutants
PHILADELPHIA CHROMOSOME NEGATIVE MYELOPROLIFERATIVE NEOPLASMS (Ph neg MPNs)				
CSF3R	WBC growth factor receptor	Activating mutations lead to oncogenic signaling through SRC family (TNK2 or JAK) kinases	59% of patients with atypical CML or chronic neutrophilic leukemia	Could help diagnose CML-like disorders without the Philadelphia chromosome or Bcr-Abl
JAK2	Tyrosine kinase (JAK-STAT signaling critical to hematopoiesis)	Activating mutations in exons 14 (V617F) and 12	Present in almost all cases of PV and about half of cases of ET and MF	JAK-STAT pathway overactive with or without mutations in JAK2; small molecule TKI ruxolitinib approved for MF and PV

(continued)

TABLE 16–3. Common somatic mutations encountered in the major myeloid malignancies. (Continued)

Gene	Functional class of encoded protein	Nature of mutation and functional consequence	Approximate incidence	Prognostic and/or therapeutic implications, if any
MPL	Thrombopoietin receptor	Activating mutations, e.g., W515L	5-10% of cases of ET or MF	*MPL* W515L activates JAK-STAT signaling; associated with older age, female sex, lower Hgb level and higher platelet count
CBL	TK-associated ubiquitin ligase that negatively regulates signal transduction by targeting receptor TKs for degradation (tumor suppressor)	Mutants encode a dominant negative protein that inhibits the ubiquitin ligase activity of the wild type protein and of its homolog, CBLB (inactivating mutations)	6% of cases of MF	Enhanced JAK-STAT signaling
LNK	Membrane-bound adaptor protein that inhibits wild type and mutant JAK2 signaling	Inactivating mutations	Rare cases of JAK2 V617F-negative ET or MF; more common in blast phase of MF (13%)	Enhanced JAK-STAT signaling
CALR	Endoplasmic reticulum chaperone (calreticulin)	Frameshift mutations in exon 9 create mutant protein with novel C-terminal→altered subcellular localization and impaired Ca^{2+} binding	Absent in PV; present in most (~73%) patients with ET or MF without JAK2 or MPL mutations (helps distinguish clonal MPNs from reactive causes of thrombocytosis)	Predicts for more indolent clinical course than JAK2 V617F; patients have lower Hgb levels and higher platelet counts; mutant CALR activates JAK-STAT signaling in myeloid cells
TET2	Catalyzes alpha-ketoglutarate-dependent conversion of 5-methylcytosine to 5-hydroxymethylcytosine, leading to DNA demethylation	Loss of function mutations→increased promoter methylation→increased self-renewal and impaired differentiation	16% in PV, 5% in ET, 17% in MF; 14% in post-PV or post-ET MF; incidence increases with age	No effect on survival, leukemic transformation or thrombosis; may correlate with anemia in MF
ASXL1	Member of polycomb family of chromatin binding proteins; epigenetic modifier; functions as ligand-dependent coactivator of retinoic acid receptor	Loss of function mutations in C-terminal generate a dominant-negative protein that inhibits its wild type counterpart and other members of polycombprotein complex	8% of patients with MPNs	
IDH1/2	Krebs cycle enzymes	IDH mutants produce 2-hydroxyglutarate from alpha-ketoglutarate, which inhibits TET enzymes, causing DNA hypermethylation	<5% of cases of MF (much higher (~22%) in blast phase); 1-2% of cases of ET and PV	
EZH2	Tumor suppressor-histone methyltransferase (catalytic subunit of polycomb repressive complex, PRC2)	Loss of function mutations→loss of PRC2 activity→increase in hematopoietic stem cell number and activity	13% in MF; 12% in MDS/MPN overlap syndromes	Independently associated with shorter survival in patients with MF
DNMT3A	DNA methyl transferase	Loss of function mutations causing reduced methylation in mutant genomes	7-10%	
IKZF1	Transcription factor	Generally deletions (del7p) rather than mutations; late events	Rare in chronic phase MPNs, but 19% in blast phase	Important step in leukemic transformation

(continued)

TABLE 16–3. Common somatic mutations encountered in the major myeloid malignancies. (Continued)

Gene	Functional class of encoded protein	Nature of mutation and functional consequence	Approximate incidence	Prognostic and/or therapeutic implications, if any
CHRONIC MYELOID LEUKEMIA (CML)				
BCR-ABL	Constitutively active tyrosine kinase (fusion protein)	Point mutations that confer resistance to one or more small molecule TKIs	40-90% of cases of resistance to imatinib (15% T315I)	"Gatekeeper" T315I mutant inhibited only by ponatinib
c-MYC	Oncoprotein	Overexpression often due to acquired trisomy 8	34% of cases with clonal evolution (trisomy 8)	Genomic instability characteristic of progression to advanced phases
TP53	Master regulator of cell cycle, DNA damage response and apoptosis (tumor suppressor)	Loss of function often associated with isochromosome 17	Mutated in 25-30% of patients in myeloid blast phase	Inactivation of tumor suppressor genes characteristic of progression to blast phase
p16 (INK4A/ARF)	Endogenous CDK inhibitor (tumor suppressor)	Deletions affect exon 2 of locus	Deleted in 50% of cases of lymphoid blast phase	Inactivation of tumor suppressor genes characteristic of progression to blast phase

this fusion protein (and also the PML Kruppel-like zinc finger [PLZF]-RARα fusion derived from the rare t[11;17]) affects cell-cycle control is its strong interaction with SMRT or N-CoR, two corepressor elements that are important for the recruitment of HDACs, as described below in "The Role of Histone Deacetylases in Cell-Cycle Regulation." In accordance with this is the finding that retrovirally transduced PML-RARα induces a maturation arrest in the corresponding cells, implying that these cells are unable to express certain transcription factors as a consequence of the conformational changes caused by the recruitment of HDACs.[195] A variant of this chromosomal translocation results in a fusion protein between RARα and the PLZF protein, which is observed in a subset of patients with APL.[195,196]

The translocation t(9;22), which fuses the BCR gene to the c-ABL gene, is a characteristic feature of CML (Chap. 88). The chromosome 9 breakpoints, where the c-abl gene is located, involve a large region of about 200 kb, but fusion genes invariably include the abl exon 2. The corresponding breakpoints on chromosome 22 are located in a much smaller region, including the BCR gene.[197] The bcr-abl fusion protein localizes to the cytoskeleton and displays enhanced tyrosine kinase activity.[198] It is also found in some cases of ALL and in occasional cases of AML.[199,200] Bcr-abl not only regulates cell proliferation, apoptosis, differentiation, and adhesion, but also induces resistance to cytostatic drugs by modulation of DNA repair mechanisms, cell-cycle checkpoints, and the Bcl-2 family of apoptosis regulators. Upon DNA damage, bcr-abl enhances repair of DNA lesions and prolongs activation of cell-cycle checkpoints (e.g., G$_2$/M), providing more time for repair of otherwise lethal lesions, so that these cells have a significant survival advantage.[199] The bcr-abl fusion product is so far the only oncogenic product that is sufficient to induce malignant growth *in vivo* without the presence of other abnormal molecular changes. Several reports have shown that bcr-abl–positive cells display pronounced G$_2$/M delay in response to various chemotherapeutics and irradiation. The exact mechanism of G$_2$/M delay in bcr-abl–positive cells has not been characterized in detail, but it seems that the cdc2-cyclin B$_1$ regulation is affected. In addition, bcr-abl, through both kinase-dependent and kinase-independent mechanisms, converts p27[kip1] from a nuclear tumor suppressor to a cytoplasmic oncogene, which may contribute to bcr-abl tyrosine kinase inhibitor (TKI)-resistance.[201] The bcr-abl signal transduction process involves adapter molecules such as GRB2 and GAB2, as well as signaling pathways (e.g., phosphatidylinositol 3′-kinase [PI3K],

Janus-associated kinase [JAK]–signal transducer and activator of transcription [STAT]).[198] In addition, although there is no direct evidence that the abnormal bcr-abl product affects the M checkpoint itself, some data suggest that bcr-abl–positive CML cells contain elevated MAD2 and BUB1 levels, proteins that inhibit the APC and therefore cause mitotic spindle arrest.[202] Amplification of the fusion sequence is frequently used to detect minimal residual disease in patients under therapy with interferon-α, TKIs,[203] and after stem cell transplantation.[204] The etv6 gene is the only known non-bcr fusion partner of abl, sometimes observed as etv6-abl in ALL or myeloproliferative syndromes (t[9;12][q34;p13]).[205] The affected cells show only a minor response to imatinib.

Mutant-activated receptor protein-tyrosine kinases (rPTKs) comprise a family of very-well-characterized oncogenes. The constitutive activation of rPTK usually is achieved by mutations that lead to the dimerization and activation of their cytoplasmic catalytic domains.[206] Other possible causes of rPTK dimerization are chromosomal translocations that create chimeric proteins. In the t(2;5) translocation, found in several anaplastic large cell lymphomas, N-terminal nucleophosmin sequences on the long arm of chromosome 5 are fused to the cytoplasmic domain of the ALK protein on chromosome 2.[207,208] The characteristic translocation of chronic myelomonocytic leukemia, t(5;12), fuses sequences from the transcription factor TEL to the cytoplasmic domain of the PDGFRβ (TEL-PDGFβR), resulting in the formation of a TEL-PDGFβR fusion protein and constitutive activation of the receptor tyrosine kinase (RTK),[209] while targeting Id1 (inhibitor of DNA-binding 1) inhibits growth of leukemia cells expressing oncogenic FLT3-ITD and BCR-ABL tyrosine kinases.[210] Patients with the t(5;12) translocation respond to imatinib, as the drug also inhibits the PDGFR. The chromosomal area surrounding the TEL gene is a fragile site, because the TEL gene is involved in several other translocations in human acute leukemias (e.g., t[12;9]). One of the TGF-β receptors also is involved in oncogenesis, and mutations are frequently found in colon cancer. TGF-β receptor signaling acts through the SMAD family of transcription factors.

Two important oncogene families encode the Ras and Rho family proteins. Ras itself is a G protein, and activating mutations in H-Ras, K-Ras, and N-Ras have been found in nearly all kinds of human cancers. Several different Ras mutations are able to transform normal cells in tissue culture.[211,212] Mutations in many different Ras-related pathways have been identified in cancer (e.g., Raf1, p110 PI3K, Rin1, Mekk1),

TABLE 16–4. Common somatic mutations encountered in the major lymphoid malignancies.

Gene	Functional class of encoded protein	Nature of mutation and functional consequence	Approximate incidence	Prognostic and/or therapeutic implications, if any
CHRONIC LYMPHOCYTIC LEUKEMIA (most mutations frequencies higher with time and with treatment)				
TP53	Master regulator of cell cycle, DNA damage response and apoptosis (tumor suppressor); strong correlation with del17p	Deletions and inactivating point mutations	7-12%	Poor prognosis; BCR pathway inhibitors, alemtuzumab and allogeneic HSCT only effective currently approved treatments
NOTCH1	Transmembrane receptors, signaling through which regulates cell death, proliferation and differentiation	Gain of function frameshift mutations lead to a truncated, constitutively active protein that lacks degradation signals	10-12%	Strong correlation with trisomy 12; may predict for lack of benefit of adding rituximab to fludarabine plus cyclophosphamide (CLL8 trial); associated with unmutated IGHV and poor outcome
FBXW7	Ubiquitin ligase known to be a tumor suppressor	Loss of function mutations→impaired degradation of Notch1, c-Myc, c-Jun, cyclin E1, Mcl-1	2.5% (newly diagnosed patients)	Associated with trisomy 12 and with NOTCH1 mutations; nearly exclusive of SF3B1 mutations
SF3B1	RNA splicing protein – core component of U2 snRNP, which recognizes the 3′ splice site at intron-exon junctions	Spliceosome mutations→decreased or increased transcription of normal pre-mRNA, exon skipping, intron retention and cryptic splice sites; associated with aberrant DDR	9-18%	Found primarily in patients with del11q and normal karyotype; confer adverse prognosis; almost mutually exclusive with NOTCH1 and FBXW7 mutations
BIRC3	Negative regulator of non-canonical NF-κB pathway	Inactivating mutations, deletions and insertions that disrupt gene function→non-canonical NF-κB activation	4% (newly diagnosed patients)	Associated with fludarabine refractoriness (24%); mutually exclusive of TP53 abnormalities
MYD88	Critical adaptor molecule of the interleukin-1/toll-like receptor signaling (TLR) pathway	Mutations activate toll-like receptor pathway via IRAK1/4 to engage NF-κB and MAPK pathways	1.5% (newly diagnosed patients)	Younger patients; associated with del13q, mutated IGHV and low CD38/ZAP-70 expression; favorable outcome
XPO1	Exportin; controls localization of cyclin B and members of MAPK pathway		3.4% (newly diagnosed patients)	May be associated with CD38/ZAP-70 positivity, NOTCH1 mutations and unmutated IGHV
SAMHD1	Enzyme that degrades the intracellular pool of dNTPs, limiting DNA synthesis; involved in DDR	Inactivating mutations lead to loss of tumor suppressor function→increased cellular survival and proliferation	3% (up to 11% in relapsed/refractory setting)	May serve as biomarker of chemoresistance, fludarabine in particular
ATM	Proximal transducer of DNA damage signals within DDR network	Mutations disrupt DDR and impair apoptosis	18%	ATM gene inactivation associated with del11q
IGHV	Immunoglobulin heavy chain variable region	"Mutated" indicates sequence >2% different from germline sequence; indicative of antigen exposure of B-cells	62%	Mutated IGHV generally confers favorable prognosis
NFKBIE	Inhibitor of NF-κB activity with specific role in B-cell biology		11% (advanced phase patients)	
EGR2	Transcription factor that participates in control of cellular differentiation	Missense mutations affect transcription of target genes	8% (advanced phase patients)	Associated with shorter time to treatment and poor survival

(continued)

TABLE 16–4. Common somatic mutations encountered in the major lymphoid malignancies. (Continued)

Gene	Functional class of encoded protein	Nature of mutation and functional consequence	Approximate incidence	Prognostic and/or therapeutic implications, if any
Wnt pathway genes	Critical for proliferation and cell fate determination of many cell types, including B-cells	Activating mutations in different genes→greater dependence on Wnt pathway signaling (already hyperactive in CLL)	14% overall	Not associated with any known CLL prognostic factor; multiple Wnt-pathway inhibitors being developed
Ras/Raf/MAPK pathway genes	Major cellular pathway that controls proliferation, differentiation, transcription regulation and development	Activating mutations; some in subclones	<5%	May be amenable to therapeutic targeting by small molecule inhibitors
HAIRY CELL LEUKEMIA (HCL)				
BRAF	Serine-threonine kinase; part of the Ras/Raf/MAPK signaling pathway which regulates cell survival, proliferation and differentiation	Activating V600E mutation	Nearly all cases	Efficacy of small molecule kinase inhibitors, e.g., vemurafenib, dabrafenib; may help distinguish from other B-cell lymphomas and leukemias
B-CELL ACUTE LYMPHOBLASTIC LEUKEMIA (B-ALL)				
RB1	Tumor suppressor involved in cell cycle control	Various abnormalities lead to dysregulated cell cycle progression	51%	
p16 (CDKN2A) p15 (CDKN2B)	Endogenous CDK inhibitors	Various abnormalities (deletion, methylation) lead to unrestrained cell cycle progression	40% 70%	Poor prognosis
TP53	Master regulator of cell cycle, DNA damage response and apoptosis (tumor suppressor)	Deletions and inactivating point mutations	16% (92% in patients with low hypodiploidy, 63% with MYC translocations, 23% with complex karyotype)	Poor prognosis; more common in B-ALL than T-ALL; frequency increases with age; "double hit" of TP53 do worst
IKZF1	Transcription factor	Splicing abnormalities	>80% of patients with Ph+ ALL	Poor prognosis independent of Ph status
"PHILADELPHIA CHROMOSOME LIKE" B-ALL (10-13% of children; 21-27% of adolescents /young adults)				
ABL1, ABL2, CSF1R, PDGFRB	Various rearrangements involving different fusion partners, e.g., EBF1-PDGFRB, NUP214-ABL1	Signaling pathway activation (CRKL phosphorylation seen with fusions involving ABL1/2)	12.6%	Sensitive to Bcr-Abl TKIs, e.g., imatinib, dasatinib
EPOR	Various rearrangements involving different fusion partners, e.g., IGH-EPOR	Activation of JAK-STAT signaling	3.9%	Sensitive to JAK1/2 inhibitor ruxolitinib
JAK2	Various rearrangements involving different fusion partners, e.g., PAX5-JAK2, ATF7IP-JAK2, BCR-JAK2, STRB3-JAK2	Activation of JAK-STAT signaling	7.4%	Sensitive to JAK1/2 inhibitor ruxolitinib
CRLF2	Various rearrangements involving different fusion partners, e.g., P2RY8-CRLF2, IGH-CRLF2	Activation of JAK-STAT signaling	49.7%	55% have concomitant JAK1/2 mutation; sensitive to ruxolitinib even without concomitant JAK mutations
IL7R, FLT3, SH2B3 (LNK), JAK1, JAK3, TYK2, IL2RB	Various alterations	Activation of JAK-STAT signaling	12.6%	Role for therapeutic JAK inhibition?
Ras/Raf/MAPK pathway genes	Major cellular pathway that controls proliferation, differentiation, transcription regulation and development	Activating mutations	4.3%	MEK inhibitors?

(continued)

TABLE 16–4. Common somatic mutations encountered in the major lymphoid malignancies. (Continued)

Gene	Functional class of encoded protein	Nature of mutation and functional consequence	Approximate incidence	Prognostic and/or therapeutic implications, if any
NTRK3, DGKH		Fusion proteins, e.g., ETV6-NTRK3	0.9%	ETV6-NTRK3 sensitive to ALK inhibitor crizotinib
IKZF1	Transcription factor	Deletions or point mutations	68% (vs. 16% in Bcr-Abl negative non-"Ph-like" ALL)	Inferior survival; more common in patients with kinase fusions than those with point mutations
T-CELL ACUTE LYMPHOBLASTIC LEUKEMIA (T-ALL)				
NOTCH1	NOTCH1 signaling necessary for commitment to T-cell lineage and for thymic proliferation of T-cell progenitors	NOTCH1 may interact with PRC2, which influences stem cell renewal through epigenetic silencing of genes	>50%	NOTCH1 and FBXW7 mutant T-ALL may enjoy superior survival; miR223 appears to promote NOTCH1-driven T-ALL; gamma secretase inhibitors under study
JAK1/JAK3/ SH2B3 (LNK) Ras/Raf/ MAPK pathway genes	Tyrosine kinases (JAK-STAT signaling critical to hematopoiesis) Major cellular pathway that controls proliferation, differentiation, transcription regulation and development	Enhanced cellular survival and proliferation	More frequent in early T-cell precursor (ETP) ALL; also FLT3, transcription factors (GATA3, ETV6, RUNX1, IKZF1) and histone modifiers (e.g., EZH2) often mutated in ETP ALL	ETP ALL carries a poor prognosis and has a mutational spectrum similar to myeloid tumors; V658F mutation in JAK1 homologous to V617F in JAK2
PHF6	X-linked tumor suppressor	Deletions or inactivating mutations→aberrant expression of TLX1 (HOX11) transcription factor oncogene	16% in children, 38% in adults	May explain greater incidence of T-ALL in males
MULTIPLE MYELOMA (MM)				
KRAS, NRAS, BRAF	Major cellular pathway that controls proliferation, differentiation, transcription regulation and development	Activating mutations lead to activation of the MAPK pathway	23%, 20% and 6% for KRAS, NRAS and BRAF, respectively	Can coexist, but usually only one clonal; combined MEK/BRAF inhibition worth exploring in clonal, BRAF-mutant multiple myeloma
FGFR3	Fibroblast growth factor receptor	Overexpression rather than mutation	23%	
MAF	Transcription factor	Overexpressed rather than mutation	13%	c-MAF overexpression associated with poor survival
DIS3 and FAM46C	Ribonuclease (DIS3) involved in RNA processing; both genes encode RNA-binding proteins; FAM46C functions in regulation of translation	Point mutations with loss of heterozygosity lead to loss of tumor suppressor function of DIS3	11% each	DIS3 aberrations more common in non-hyperdiploid cases; associated with del13q14 and IGH translocations and may predict for worse survival; these mutations rarely seen in other cancers
LRRK2	Serine threonine kinase that phosphorylates translation initiation factor 4EBP	Mutations lead to disruption of translational control	8%	Protein homeostasis critical in MM because of high rate of immunoglobulin production; explains success of proteasome inhibitors
TP53	Master regulator of cell cycle, DNA damage response and apoptosis (tumor suppressor)	Deletions and inactivating point mutations	8%	Poor prognosis; strong correlation with del17p
TRAF3, BIRC2, BIRC3, CYLD, BTRC, CARD11, IKBIP, IKBKB, MAP3K1, LTB, MAP3K14, RIPK4, TLR4, TNFRSF1A	Genes associated with regulation of the NF-κB signaling pathway	Activation of NF-κB signaling, e.g., through deletions and mutations in CYLD or inactivating mutations in LTB	TRAF3 mutated in 5%; CYLD in 2%; others less frequent	Underlies fundamental role of NF-κB signaling and therapeutic efficacy of proteasome inhibitors

(continued)

TABLE 16–4. Common somatic mutations encountered in the major lymphoid malignancies.(Continued)

Gene	Functional class of encoded protein	Nature of mutation and functional consequence	Approximate incidence	Prognostic and/or therapeutic implications, if any
MLL, MLL2, MLL3, UTX, WHSC1, WHSC1L1	Histone modifying enzymes	Mutations lead to epigenetic derepression of transcription factor HOXA9		Aberrant HOXA9 expression could represent a new therapeutic target
PRDM1	Transcriptional repressor involved in plasmacytic differentiation	Missense and truncating frame shift or splice site mutations→loss of tumor suppressor function	5%	
RB1	Tumor suppressor involved in cell cycle control	Mutations lead to dysregulated cell cycle progression	3%	
ACTG1	Cytoplasmic actin found in nonmuscle cells		2%	
EGR1	Transcription factor	Somatic hypermutation	3%	Not clear if "driver" or "passenger" mutations
IRF4 (MUM1)	Transcription factor whose expression propels B-cells towards plasmacytic differentiation	Missense mutations, e.g., K123R, lead to gain of function		
SP140	Transcription factor (tumor suppressor)	Missense, frame shift and splice site alterations		
CDKN2C, CDKN1B, CCND1	Cell cycle regulatory genes	Overexpression of cyclins and/or deficiency of endogenous CDK inhibitors→enhanced proliferation	Cyclin D1 overexpressed in 36%	Efficacy of pharmacologic CDK inhibition, e.g., with dinaciclib, palbociclib
PTPRD	Tyrosine phosphatase that dephosphorylates STAT3, which promotes IL-6 signaling	Homozygous deletions of tumor suppressor gene		
MAX	Transcription factor that functions as heterodimerization partner for MYC	Loss of heterozygosity of tumor suppressor gene		
WALDENSTROM'S MACROGLOBULINEMIA (WM)/LYMPHOPLASMACYTIC LYMPHOMA (LPL)				
MYD88	Critical adaptor molecule of the interleukin-1/toll-like receptor (TLR) signaling pathway	Mutations, e.g., L265P, activate toll-like receptor pathway via IRAK1/4 to engage NF-κB and MAPK pathways	91% of all patients with LPL	Can help diagnose WM/LPL in cases of uncertainty; explains high efficacy of BTK (ibrutinib) and proteasome (bortezomib) inhibitors in WM
DIFFUSE LARGE B-CELL LYMPHOMA – GERMINAL CENTER B-CELL (GCB) AND ACTIVATED B-CELL (ABC)				
EZH2	Histone methyltransferase (catalytic subunit of polycomb repressive complex, PRC2)	Gain of function mutations, e.g., at Y641, promote lymphomagenesis through transcriptional silencing of key antiproliferative tumor suppressor genes, e.g., CDKN1A	22% of GCB DLBCL, not seen in ABC DLBCL	EZH2 inhibitors in early phase clinical trials
PTEN	Negative regulator of PI3K/Akt/mTOR pathway (tumor suppressor)	PTEN deletion leads to constitutive activation of and addiction to PI3K/Akt/mTOR signaling	11% of GCB DLBCL	Inhibtiors of PI3K (e.g., idelalisib), Akt and mTOR (e.g., everolimus, temsirolimus) being explored
BCL-2	Founding member of Bcl-2 family of mitochondrial apoptosis regulators; anti-apoptotic	Promotes cellular survival and a major determinant of resistance to chemotherapy	The most mutated gene in GCB DLBCL; t(14;18) found in 34% of cases of GCB DLBCL	Selective Bcl-2 antagonist (BH3-mimetic) venetoclax in clinical trials

(continued)

TABLE 16–4. Common somatic mutations encountered in the major lymphoid malignancies.(Continued)

Gene	Functional class of encoded protein	Nature of mutation and functional consequence	Approximate incidence	Prognostic and/or therapeutic implications, if any
BCL-6	Transcription factor; represses many target genes involved in proliferation, survival, cell growth and metabolism	Routinely overexpressed in DLBCL; activation may underlie resistance to treatment	Mutated (70%) or rearranged (40%) in essentially all cases of DLBCL	Small molecule inhibitors that disrupt Bcl-6 function in development
CARD11	Part of signaling complex of adaptor proteins that lead to BCR-dependent NF-κB activation upon antigenic stimulation	BCR signaling and NF-κB activation critical in ABC DLBCL	Up to 10% of cases of ABC DLBCL	CARD11 mutations predict for lack of efficacy of inhibition of upstream BCR pathway targets, e.g., BTK (ibrutinib) or PKC-beta
CD79B	B-cell co-receptor	BCR signaling and NF-κB activation critical in ABC DLBCL	21% of cases of ABC DLBCL	CD79B mutations correlate with sensitivity to selective PKC-beta inhibitor sotrastaurin
MYD88	Critical adaptor molecule of the interleukin-1/toll-like receptor (TLR) signaling pathway	Mutations, e.g., L265P, activate toll-like receptor pathway via IRAK1/4 to engage NF-κB and MAPK pathways→IL-6 /IL-10 production→autocrine JAK activation	30% of cases of ABC DLBCL	
TNFAIP3 (A20)	Negative regulator of NF-κB pathway (tumor suppressor)	Inactivating mutations and deletions	Biallelic inactivation occurs in 30% of cases of ABC DLBCL	Can coexist with mutations in both MYD88 and CD79B
IRF4 (MUM1)	Transcription factor whose expression propels B-cells towards plasmacytic differentiation	A direct target of the NF-κB pathway that can induced by both the BCR and TLR pathways	Constitutive NF-κB activation is a pathogenic hallmark of ABC DLBCL	Lenalidomide selectively kills ABC DLBCL cells by cereblon-dependent IRF4 down-regulation
c-MYC (cases harboring additional oncogenic rearrangements involving BCL2, BCL6 or CCND1 designated "double hit")	Oncoprotein	Suppresses transcription of tumor suppressor tristetraprolin	10% of patients with newly diagnosed DLBCL carry an underlying MYC rearrangement (translocation, amplification)	May be possible to target MYC using BET bromodomain BRD4 inhibitors
BTK/Syk/ Lyn/PKC-β/ MALT1/ JAK-STAT	Kinases involved in BCR signaling (JAK-STAT signaling driven by activating MYD88 mutations)	Therapeutic targets without activating mutations	"Chronic active" BCR signaling and NF-κB activation fundamental in ABC DLBCL	Multiple small molecule inhibitors being studied, e.g., ibrutinib (BTK), enzastaurin (PKC-β), ruxolitinib (JAK1/2)
FOLLICULAR LYMPHOMA (FL)				
MLL2, CRE-BBP, EZH2, MEF2B	Histone modifying enzymes	CREBBP, MLL2, EZH2 alterations early events in lymphomagenesis and progression	Very high frequency overall; EZH2 mutated in 7-27% (gain of function mutations, e.g., at Y641)	Potential role for EZH2 inhibitors as in GCB DLBCL?
HIST1H-1B-E, OCT2 (POU2F2), IRF8, ARID1A	Linker histones – proteins that facilitate folding of higher order chromatin structures and regulate access of histone modifying enzymes and chromatin remodeling complexes to target genes		27% (HIST1H1B-E), 8% (OCT2/POU2F2), 6% (IRF8), 11% (ARID1A)	Mutations in HIST1H1B-E and in EZH2 or ARID1A largely mutually exclusive

(continued)

TABLE 16–4. Common somatic mutations encountered in the major lymphoid malignancies. (Continued)

Gene	Functional class of encoded protein	Nature of mutation and functional consequence	Approximate incidence	Prognostic and/or therapeutic implications, if any
STAT6, SOCS1	JAK-STAT signaling pathway genes	Mutations contribute to constitutive STAT6 activation and promotion of tumor cell survival	STAT6 12%, SOCS1 8%	Eventual role for JAK inhibitors?
CARD11, CD79B, TNFAIP3	NF-κB pathway genes - mutually exclusive mutations	Constitutive activation of NF-κB	CARD11 and TNFAIP3 each 11% (overall one third)	Implications for therapy as for ABC DLBCL
EBF1	Transcription factor important in B-cell development	Loss of function mutations lead to reduction in EBF1 target gene expression	17% overall (genes important in B-cell development)	
BCL2	Founding member of Bcl-2 family of mitochondrial apoptosis regulators; anti-apoptotic	Promotes cellular survival and a major determinant of resistance to chemotherapy; overexpression characteristic of FL	Mutation frequency 12% at diagnosis; 53% at transformation (different from t(14;18) present in 80-90%)	Correlate with risk for transformation and death; Bcl-2 antagonist (BH3-mimetic) venetoclax in clinical trials in FL
NOTCH1/2	Transmembrane receptors, signaling through which regulates cell death, proliferation and differentiation	Gain of function mutations lead to truncated protein that lacks degradation signals	6.3%	Female predominance, greater splenic involvement, lower frequency of t(14;18); gamma secretase inhibitors under study
CDKN2A	p16(INK4a) and p14 (ARF) tumor suppressors	Inactivation of tumor suppressor gene through deletion or methylation	Deletion (8%), methylation (19%)	May predict for inferior survival, particularly in rituximab-treated patients
MANTLE CELL LYMPHOMA (MCL)				
IGHV	Immunoglobulin heavy chain variable region	Mutations support antigen-driven selection in the clonogenicexpansion of MCL tumor cells	15-40%	Correlate with SOX11 negativity, indolent clinical course, non-nodal presentation
SOX11	Transcription factor overexpressed (not mutated) in the vast majority of cases of MCL	Promotes angiogenesis via PDGF, regulates PAX5 expression and blocks terminal B-cell differentiation	>90% of cases of MCL, both cyclin D1 positive and negative (can help diagnose in latter situation)	Expression correlates with unmutated IGHV, aggressive clinical course and karyotypic complexity
ATM	Proximal transducer of DNA damage signals within DDR network	Mutations disrupt DDR and impair apoptosis	55% in SOX11+ MCL; 0% in SOX11- cases; 42% overall	Correlate with del11q
CCND1	Cyclin D1	Activating mutations/overexpression drive cell cycle progression	Mutations more frequent in SOX11- cases (86% vs. 18%), and cases with mutated IGHV (58% vs. 19%); 14% overall	Likely acquired in germinal center microenvironment; CDK4/6 inhibitor palbociclib effective in MCL
TP53	Master regulator of cell cycle, DNA damage response and apoptosis (tumor suppressor)	Deletions and inactivating point mutations	19-28%	Equally distributed regardless of SOX11 or IGHV status; correlate with del17p
WHSC1 (MMSET), MLL2, MEF2B	Histone methyltransferases	WHSC1 mutations increase H3K36 methylation→ genome wide hypomethylation of H3K27→ significant overexpression of proliferation and cell cycle regulation genes	Found virtually only in SOX11+/IGVH unmutated MCL (WHSC1 15%, MLL2 18%, MEF2B 5%); of all cases of MCL, WHSC1 mutated in 10%; MLL2 in 20% and MEF2B in 3.2%	WHSC1-mutant gene expression signature very similar to that seen in multiple myeloma with t(4;14); MLL2 and MEF2B mutations similar to those in DLBCL or FL

(continued)

TABLE 16–4. Common somatic mutations encountered in the major lymphoid malignancies.(Continued)

Gene	Functional class of encoded protein	Nature of mutation and functional consequence	Approximate incidence	Prognostic and/or therapeutic implications, if any
TRAF2, BIRC3	BIRC3 is a negative regulator of non-canonical NF-κB pathway; TRAF2 transduces signals from TNF receptors to NF-κB	Inactivating or splice site mutations (BIRC3) and activating mutations (TRAF2) lead to enhanced NF-κB activation	6% (TRAF2); 10% (BIRC3)	BIRC3 mutations correlate with del11q; both suggest NIK (rather than BCR) signaling and alternative NF-κB pathway activation (resistance to BCR pathway inhibitors, e.g., ibrutinib)
TLR2	Toll-like receptor 2 (TLR pathway mediates innate immunity independent of antigenic stimulation)	Mutations lead to significantly increased production of IL-6, IL-1RA and IL-8	Seen only in SOX-11-/IGHV mutated MCL	
NOTCH1/2	Transmembrane receptors, signaling through which regulates cell death, proliferation and differentiation	Gain of function mutations lead to truncated protein that lacks degradation signals	9.5%	A subset of tumors with adverse biological and clinical features; i.e., blastoid morphology and worse survival
LARGE GRANULAR LYMPHOCYTIC LEUKEMIA (LGL leukemia)				
STAT3	Signal transducer and activator of transcription, e.g., transducing signals from cytokine receptor-associated Janus kinases to the nucleus	Activating mutations	40%	May correlate with greater prevalence of neutropenia and rheumatoid arthritis

and numerous downstream signaling effects of those mutations have also been defined. The Ras and the Rho families of oncoproteins are linked by a small G protein called *Rac*, which is required for transformation by Ras.[213,214] The normal formation of actin filaments is required for G_1/S-phase entry. Recent data have shown the Rho-guanosine triphosphatases play a key role in the Wnt-signaling pathway, where they are involved in cellular polarization processes.[215] Thus, alterations in the Rho pathway may lead to premature entry into M phase by interference with cytoskeletal organization. The Ras/Raf/MEK/ERK cascade couples signals from the surface to the intracellular space and triggers cell proliferation signals that influence the cell cycle. Abnormal activation of this cascade occurs in several leukemias because of activating mutations in the Ras protooncogene.[216] Ectopic overexpression of Raf proteins is associated with cell proliferation, whereas overexpression of activated Raf is associated with cell-cycle arrest in G_1 phase.[217,218] Different *Raf* genes have different functions in cells, although A-Raf and B-Raf share three conserved domains termed CR1, CR2, and CR3.[219] A-Raf is able to upregulate the expression of cyclin D_1, cdk2, cyclin E, and cdk4, whereas B-Raf and Raf-1 induce p21^{cip1}, leading to a G_1 arrest.[216,219] The mode of action of these Raf molecules is not fully understood but one explanation why they act differently may be because they activate different downstream pathways, namely the MAPK (MEK [MAP/ERK (extracellular signal-regulated kinase)]). The three different MAPK cascades are the ERK–, c-Jun N-terminal kinase (JNK)/stress-activated protein kinase (SAPK)–, and p38 pathways. The MAP kinase pathways consist of three types of kinases in a series, MAPKKK, MAPKK, and MAPK (ERK), each sequentially activating the next kinase. The MAPK cascades all transmit responses from several different surface receptors to the nucleus.[220] One explanation for the oncogenic effects of the MAPK pathway is that ERK activates c-Myc via phosphorylation on serine 62.[221] In addition, repression of c-Myc is required for terminal differentiation of many cell types, including hematopoietic cells. Thus, deregulated expression of c-Myc in both M1 AML cells and in normal myeloid cells derived from murine marrow blocks terminal differentiation and its associated growth arrest, and also induces apoptosis, which

is dependent on the extrinsic Fas/CD95 pathway. New data suggest a linkage between c-Myc downregulation, the p16^{INK4A}/cyclinD1/RB, and SMAC/Diablo apoptotic pathways.[222] Several different transcription factors have been implicated in the downregulation of c-Myc expression during differentiation, including CCAAT/enhancer binding protein (C/EBP) α, CTCF, BLIMP-1, and RFX1. Alterations in the expression and/or function of these transcription factors, or of the c-Myc and Max interacting proteins, such as MM-1 and Mxi1, can influence the neoplastic process.[223,224]

Experiments on oncoproteins have focused on apoptosis, the lethal response of a cell to either DNA damage or to signaling through cell surface "death" receptors. Key regulators of apoptosis induced by DNA damage are the multiple members of the Bcl-2 family of proteins, which include Bcl-2, Bcl-x$_L$, Mcl-1, Bax, Bak, Bim, and Bad, among others. Bcl-2 is involved in the t(14;18) chromosomal translocation, which is found classically in follicular lymphoma.[225] The disruption of these loci increases expression of Bcl-2, and results in the uncontrolled accumulation of malignant B cells, because of an impaired balance between growth and apoptosis.[226,227] It also has been shown that Bcl-x$_L$, Bax, and Bad are involved in the regulation of AML cells. For example, the ratio between Bax and Bcl-2 is a prognostic factor in this myeloid neoplasm.[228] Additionally, Mcl-1 may be even more critical to the development and maintenance of AML than Bcl-2 or Bcl-x$_{XL}$.[229] The nuclear HDAC complex, which regulates the structural conformation of DNA and therefore the activation of several genes, is targeted by ETO, the fusion partner of the *RUNX1* gene in some patients with AML. The t(8;21) translocation that occurs in such patients allows the formation of a stable complex between the HDAC complex and ETO, contributing to leukemogenesis.[230,231] PLZF, PLZF-RARα, and BCL-6 are other oncogenes that target the HDAC complex.[232,233]

TUMOR-SUPPRESSOR GENES

Almost every cancer harbors one or more abnormalities of tumor-suppressor genes. These include mutations, translocations, deletions, and epigenetic modifications. In addition, at least two epigenetic mechanisms—the hypermethylation of CpG islands in the promoter region and the aberrant acetylation of histones (especially histone H4)—can silence tumor-suppressor genes in a variety of human cancer cell lines and primary tumors.

The products of three important tumor-suppressor genes (*RB*, *P53*, and *p16^INK4A*) are interconnected biochemically. The *RB* gene maps to chromosome 13q14 and has several downstream effectors, among which the transcription factor E2F is the best characterized.[234] The *RB* gene family consists of three closely related proteins, RB, p107, and p130. All three proteins are able to interact with several E2F family members.

Transcriptional activation and repression are mediated via complexes consisting of RB family members, E2F family members, and so-called DP proteins.[235] Besides its role in cell-cycle control, RB can modulate RNA polymerase activity, thus linking cell-cycle progression to transcriptional regulation. Many cellular proteins have been identified that bind to RB. These proteins can be divided into different groups, including transcription factors, growth factors, protein kinases, protein phosphatases, and nuclear matrix proteins. Mutations of RB are frequent in cancer e.g., leukemias; soft-tissue sarcomas; and breast, esophagus, prostate, and renal carcinomas.[236] Several viral or oncoproteins can bind to and inactivate RB.[112,237]

The p53 gene has been called a "guardian" of the genome because it transmits signals arising from various forms of DNA damage, leading to cell-cycle arrest or apoptosis. p53 protein is also the target of leukemogenic mutations. Damaging factors, such as hypoxic stress, chemicals, or irradiation either can alter the p53 protein itself or can stabilize its cellular inhibitor, MDM2 (in humans the homologue is termed HDM2).[238] The MDM2 protein inhibits p53 transcription and stimulates p53 degradation.[239,240] For the former, MDM2 is able to bind to the transactivation domain of p53 through a p53-interacting domain on the MDM2 amino terminus, which inhibits p53 from binding to its transcriptional coactivators, thereby preventing activation of p53 transcriptional targets. For the latter, MDM2 binds to p53 through a RING-domain and ubiquitinates p53 through the E3 ubiquitin ligase activity of MDM2, causing p53 nuclear export and ultimate degradation.[241] Moreover, MDM2 is able to affect chromosomal stability independently of p53.[242] The MDM2 binding region contains several phosphorylation sites.[243] These residues (e.g., serine 395) are phosphorylated by DNA damage-activated kinases (e.g., ATM and Chk2), which is required for p53 activation.[244] The *p14^ARF* tumor-suppressor gene, which is encoded within the *p16^INK4A* locus by alternate splicing, controls MDM2 activity.[245] In *de novo* AML, although p53 mutations are not common,[246] overexpression of MDM2 is frequently encountered,[247] and there is current interest in exploring MDM2 antagonists, for example, RO5503781, in combination with cytarabine in patients with relapsed or refractory AML. Additionally, the MDM2 antagonist nutlin-3A causes p53-dependent apoptosis in AML cells by disrupting the p53-MDM2 interaction[248] and synergizes with BH3-mimetics,[249] MEK/ERK inhibitors,[250,251] aurora kinase inhibitors,[249] cdk1 inhibitors,[252] XIAP antagonists,[253] FLT3 inhibitors,[254,255] and inhibitors of nuclear export, such as CRM1.[256] The *p14^ARF* gene shares exons 2 and 3 with *p16^INK4A* but has a distinct exon 1. The discovery that two important tumor-suppressor genes are encoded by the same chromosomal locus and share several exons was unexpected and is unique in human biology. The *p16^INK4A* gene function depends on p53, because overexpression of *p16^INK4A* causes cell-cycle arrest in p53 wild-type cells but not in p53-deficient cells.[257] The transcription of *p16^INK4A* is regulated by E2F, which is under the control of RB.[258] This indicates the existence of yet another feedback loop, which links the RB pathway to p53.[259] The Ras protein is another identified *p16^INK4A* factor involved in MDM2-p53-p21-RB regulation.[260,261] Different signaling routes that connect DNA damage with p53 include a cascade of Ser/Thr

kinases, for example, ATM, ATR, Chk1 and Chk2, which phosphorylate p53.[262] Abnormalities of p53 are found in slightly more than 50 percent of all human tumors and, surprisingly, even in some normal cells. It is unclear if these "normal" cells represent a pool of premalignant cells in an otherwise healthy individual or, more likely, p53 changes are just one step in multistage tumorigenesis. Two different p53 homologues, p63 and p73, have been described, which show DNA binding, transactivation, and oligomerization domains similar to p53.[263] This similarity in the DNA binding domain allows p63 and p73 to regulate p53 target genes, induce cell-cycle arrest and apoptosis, and therefore act as tumor suppressors.[264] The p73 gene has been localized to chromosome 1p36, a common region of cytogenetic changes in cancer. p73 protein can also bind p53, inhibiting its transcriptional regulatory activity.[265] Although p53 mutations are found frequently in almost all cancers, p63 and p73 mutations are much more rare.[264,266] However, the p73 gene is inactivated by hypermethylation of CpG islands in its promoter region in both leukemias and lymphomas.[267]

Homozygous deletions of the *p16^INK4A*/*p14^ARF* gene locus on human chromosome 9p21 have been detected in gliomas,[107,268] primary cancers of lung,[107,269] bladder,[270] head and neck,[271] as well as in acute T-cell leukemias[272,273] and mesotheliomas.[274] Because inherited mutations of *p16^INK4A* exon 2 may interfere with its expression and/or function, without causing an amino acid change in *p14^ARF*, it is clear that *p16^INK4A* inactivation alone is an important step in the evolution of malignant disease. However, in established tumor cell lines, nearly all chromosome 9p21 deletions disable the entire *p16^INK4A*/*p14^ARF* locus. Both proteins act as suppressors of the G_1-S transition, even though they function in two different pathways: *p16^INK4A* acts as an inhibitor of cyclin D_1/cdk4/6 complexes whereas *p14^ARF* stabilizes p53 by inhibition of MDM2. Several models provide insight into the different modes of action of *p16^INK4A* and *p14^ARF* on cell-cycle regulation. Interestingly, if the entire p19^ARF/p16^INK4A locus is disrupted in mice (the mouse homologue of p14^ARF is p19^ARF), the mice develop lymphomas, lymphoid leukemias, and sarcomas, suggesting that these tumor-suppressor genes do not act in a lineage-specific manner on cell-cycle regulation but in a more general way. Retroviral expression of p16^INK4A restores the normal phenotype in some cell types underlining the strong tumor-suppressor potency of p16^INK4A. The *p15^INK4B* gene, also located on chromosome 9p21, approximately 20 kb centromeric of *p16^INK4A*, is deleted somewhat less frequently. Analyses of primary tumors, however, show that not all 9p21 deletions encompass these three tumor suppressor genes. One mechanism for disruption of the *p15^INK4B*/*p14^ARF*/*p16^INKA* region in T-cell leukemias may be the action of an illegitimate variable diversity joining (V[D]J) recombinase.[275] Several other binding partners of p16^INK4A have been identified.[276] The RB gene interacts with one of these factors, BRG1, to remodel chromatin structures. BRG1 also acts upstream of RB with p16^INK4A and functions as a tumor suppressor.[276]

The p15^INK4B/p16^INK4A/p14^ARF locus on chromosome 9p21 is a hotspot in the development of human cancer and approximately 50 percent of all human malignancies show abnormalities in at least one of these tumor-suppressor genes. Another gene lies about 100 kb telomeric of p16^INK4A, and this gene, methylthioadenosine phosphorylase (MTAP), encodes an important enzyme in purine metabolism. Some early gliomas show MTAP deletions without deletions of other genes on 9p21, suggesting that MTAP by itself has tumor-suppressor properties. The reexpression of MTAP in breast cancer cells severely inhibits their ability to form colonies in soft agar or collagen, supporting this hypothesis.[277] In addition, MTAP-expressing cells are suppressed for tumor formation when implanted into severe combined immune deficiency (SCID) mice. Recent findings suggest that the enzyme ornithine decarboxylase (ODC) is overexpressed in MTAP-deleted tumors, providing evidence for a new pathway in tumorigenesis. Overexpression of

ODC has been observed in many tumors and is linked to the Ras pathway.[278] Reexpression of MTAP in ODC overexpressing cells decreases ODC levels and inhibits tumor cell growth.[279] In addition, high levels of 5'-deoxy-5'-(methylthio) adenosine (MTA) induce matrix metalloproteinase and growth factor gene expression in melanoma cells, leading to enhanced invasion and vasculogenic mimicry. In addition, MTA induced the secretion of β-fibroblast growth factor and the upregulation of activator protein-1, demonstrating a tumor-supporting role of MTA, which is increased in MTAP-deficient cells.[280]

The mechanisms by which the above-mentioned genes are inactivated are rather different. Especially in permanent cell lines, *p15^{INK4B}/ p14^{ARF}/p16^{INK4A}* and MTAP are homozygously deleted. One allele of MTAP is also deleted in AML lines, but not in primary AML samples. Mutations in *p15^{INK4B}/p14^{ARF}/p16^{INK4A}* genes are rare, and if present, occur in exon 2. Hypermethylation of CpG islands in the promoter areas of p15INK4B/*p14^{ARF}/p16^{INK4A}* are frequently found in hematologic malignancies.[281-283] The availability of demethylating agents such as 5-azacytidine and 5-aza-2'-deoxycytidine (decitabine) makes this phenomenon an interesting target for chemotherapy.[284,285] Decitabine has been used to treat patients suffering from different hematologic malignancies and was reported to have activity in advanced myelodysplastic syndrome (MDS), accompanied by demethylation of the *p16^{INK4A}* promoter.[285] Azacytidine and decitabine are approved for the treatment of MDS[286-288] and also widely used for the treatment of AML, particularly older patients considered unfit for cytotoxic chemotherapy, particularly when blast counts are low.[289-291] However, p16^{INK4A} and p15^{INK4B} are not the only targets of these demethylating agents in hematologic malignancies.[292] Transcriptional regulation by methylation is mediated by a multiprotein complex consisting of a MeCP2, a methylcytosine-binding protein with a transcriptional repressor domain that binds the corepressor mSin3A, which is itself one element of a multiprotein complex that includes HDAC1 and HDAC2.[293,294] Therefore, reexpression of silenced genes can be achieved by demethylating DNA or by destabilizing HDACs, and it could be demonstrated that both mechanisms are tightly linked. HDACIs and demethylating agents act synergistically to induce genes silenced in cancer by hypermethylation.[139] Another new mechanism of gene regulation and inactivation *in vivo* is degradation by microRNAs. This has also been shown for several members of the p16^{INK4A}/ cdk4/cyclin D$_1$/RB pathway.[295]

THE ROLE OF HISTONE DEACETYLASES IN CELL–CYCLE REGULATION

HDACs catalyze the deacetylation of lysine residues in the histone N-terminal tails and are found in large multiprotein complexes with transcriptional corepressors. Human HDACs are grouped into three classes based on their similarity to known yeast factors: class I HDACs are similar to the yeast transcriptional repressor yRPD3; class II HDACs are similar to the yeast transcriptional repressor yHDA1; and class III HDACs are similar to the yeast transcriptional repressor ySIR2 (Table 16–5; Fig. 16–3).[296,297] Eleven different HDACs have been identified so far. The physiologic counterparts of

TABLE 16–5. Different Types and Classes of Histone Deacetylases

Enzyme	Mechanism of Deacetylase Activity	Tissue Expression	Interacting Protein
Class I			
HDAC1	Zn^{2+} dependent	Ubiquitous	HDAC2, Sin3, CoREST, NuRD, RB/E2F1, p53, MYOD, NF-κB, YY1, DNMT1, DNMT3A, MBD2, SP1, SP3, BRCA1, MeCP2, ATM, AML1-ETO, PML, PLZF, BCL6, AR, ER
HDAC2	Zn^{2+} dependent	Ubiquitous	HDAC1, Sin3, CoREST, NuRD, RB, NF-κB, BRCA1, DNMT1, AML1-ETO, PML, PLZF, BCL6
HDAC3	Zn^{2+} dependent	Ubiquitous	HDAC4, HDAC5, HDAC7, RB, NF-κB, STAT1, STAT3, GATA1, GATA2, NCoR/SMRT, AML1-ETO, PML, PLZF, PML-RARα, PLZF-RARα, BCL6,
HDAC8	Zn^{2+} dependent	Ubiquitous	SMC3, EST1B, Hsp70
Class IIa			
HDAC4	Zn^{2+} dependent	Tissue specific	MEF2, HDAC3-NCoR, GATA1
HDAC5	Zn^{2+} dependent	Tissue specific	MEF2, HDAC3-NCoR, GATA1, GATA2
HDAC7	Zn^{2+} dependent	Tissue specific	MEF2, HDAC3-NCoR, ERα
HDAC9	Zn^{2+} dependent	Tissue specific	MEF2
Class IIb			
HDAC6	Zn^{2+} dependent	Tissue specific	α-tubulin, Hsp90, HDAC11
HDAC10	Zn^{2+} dependent	Tissue specific	RB
Class III			
Sirt1–7	NAD$^+$ dependent	?	p53
Class IV			
HDAC11	Zn^{2+} dependent	Tissue specific	Interleukin 10, HDAC6

HDAC, histone deacetylase; NAD, nicotinamide adenine dinucleotide; NF-κB, nuclear factor kappa B; RB, retinoblastoma.

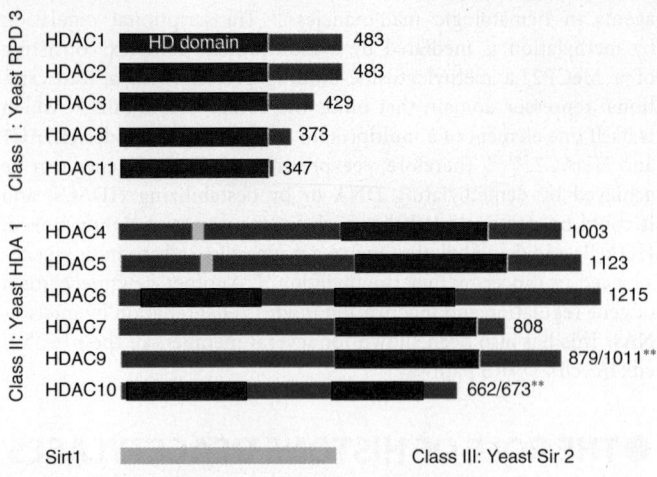

*HD domain, histone deacetylase; **two-splice variants

Figure 16–3. Classes of human histone deacetylases.

the HDACs are histone acetyl transferases (HATs). In the nucleosome, positively charged hypoacetylated histones bind tightly to the phosphate backbone of the DNA and maintain the chromatin in an inactive, silent state. Both HAT and HDAC are recruited to target genes in complexes with sequence-specific transcription factors and their cofactors. Examples of these cofactors include NCoR or SMRT (Fig. 16–4). Several different transcription factors are assembled with these complexes, including Bcl-6, MAD1, PML, and ETO.[296] HDACs are involved in different cellular mechanisms, including proliferation and differentiation. Irregular activation of HDACs leads to the loss of cell-cycle control.[298] Gene silencing by HDAC complexes is an important

mechanism in the development of AML, most notably APL. The PML-RARα fusion protein is an oncoprotein that represses retinoic acid-dependent transcription by recruitment of HDAC to RAR-regulated genes (Fig. 16–4B), halting myeloid maturation because of cell-cycle arrest. In the PML-RARα fusion protein, the RARα is not responsive to physiologic concentrations of retinoic acid and supraphysiologic doses of all-*trans*-retinoic acid are necessary to overcome the tight HDAC-recruitment and the consequent cell-cycle block.[296] The rare translocation t(11;17) fuses the RARα gene to the PLZF gene, which directly interacts with the NCoR–mSin3a–HDAC complex to suppress gene transcription. This block can only be overcome by the addition of a HDACI. Another well-known example of transcriptional silencing by the recruitment of an HDAC repressor is the AML1-ETO fusion protein which results from the t(8;21) translocation. As already described, the addition of an HDACI can relieve ETO-mediated transcriptional repression.[299] Although 11 HDACs have been described, only limited information is available about their redundant biologic and physiologic functions. As shown in Figure 16–4B, inhibitors of HDAC activity lead to the reexpression of silenced genes and to the induction of differentiation. Most of these inhibitors, such as depsipeptide (romidepsin), belinostat or vorinostat,[300] do not exhibit isoenzyme selectivity and may therefore be of limited therapeutic value, at least as single agents. These drugs are currently approved for patients with previously treated peripheral and cutaneous T-cell lymphomas, although they continue to be studied for other indications, for example, vorinostat for AML in combination with chemotherapy (NCT01802333). The pan-HDACI panobinostat, in combination with bortezomib and dexamethasone, has been approved in the treatment of patients with relapsed or refractory myeloma,[301] while the class I–selective HDACI entinostat is currently being studied in phase III clinical trials in advanced hormone-responsive breast cancer in conjunction with aromatase inhibitors (NCT02115282). Finally, pracinostat (pan-HDACI) and mocetinostat (isotype-selective) have been granted "orphan drug" status for AML,[147] and for MDS and diffuse large B-cell lymphoma with specific mutations in HATs (e.g., CREBBP and EP300), respectively. However, the HDACI valproic acid, an established antiepileptic agent, is the first drug within this group that selectively inhibits one HDAC, namely HDAC2.[302] Valproic acid induces proteasomal degradation of HDAC2. Basal and valproic acid-induced HDAC2 turnover strongly depend on the E2 ubiquitin conjugase Ubc8 and the E3 ubiquitin ligase RLIM. Thus, polyubiquitination and proteasomal degradation provide an isoenzyme-selective mechanism for downregulation of HDAC2.[302] This also underlines the importance of another cell-cycle element, the proteasome.

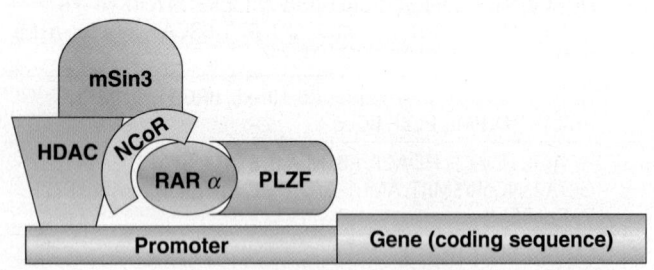

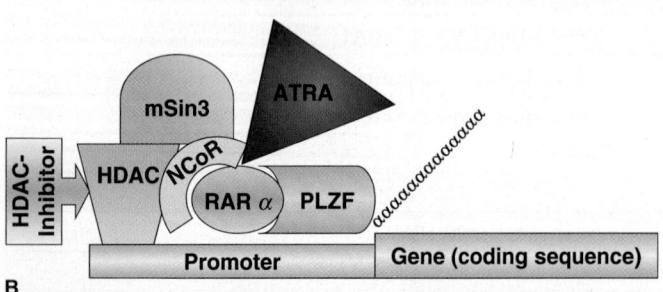

Figure 16–4. A. Transcriptional silencing by the recruitment of histone deacetylases (HDACs) in acute myelogenous leukemia (AML) with t(11;17). See text for further description. **B.** Transcriptional reactivation and induction of differentiation by histone deacetylase inhibitors and all-*trans*-retinoic acid (ATRA) in AML with t(11;17). See text for further description.

● THE PROTEASOME: THE RECYCLING MACHINERY

The proteasome is a 2.4 MDa, multicentric protease complex with an important role in cellular protein regulation. Its structure consists of a cylindrical core, the so-called 20S particle, composed of four stacked rings with a total of seven proteins in each ring. The second part of the proteasome, two copies of a 19S particle, is bound to the 20S core. Only proteins that have been ubiquitinated can be degraded in the proteasome. The ubiquitination of different substrate proteins involves the sequential action of three enzymes: E1 (an ATP-dependent ubiquitin-activating enzyme), E2 (a ubiquitin-conjugating enzyme), and E3 (ubiquitin-protein ligase). The ubiquitin-proteasome pathway plays a critical role in the degradation of intracellular proteins involved in cell-cycle control, transcription activation, apoptosis, and tumor growth through an ATP-dependent mechanism.[303] Proteins such as HDAC2 are tagged with several ubiquitin molecules and then degraded in the machinery.[302] Several tumors depend on rapid cell cycling, which requires expression and degradation of numerous regulatory proteins. Some of the proteins that undergo proteasome-mediated degradation include cyclins (cyclins A, B, D, E), endogenous cdk inhibitors (p27[kip1], p21[cip1]), p53, RB, cdc25 phosphatase, and others.[304] The rapid turnover of these proteins triggers the rapid growth rate of certain human malignancies, thus the proteasome is an excellent new target for the development of new drugs, as attested to by the success of the proteasome inhibitors bortezomib[305,306] and carfilzomib[307] in patients with MCL and myeloma. These agents inhibit the proteolytic activity of the proteasome and so cells accumulate in the G_2-M phase of the cell cycle with a decrease of cells in G_1.[304,308] For example, p27[kip1], p21[cip1] are upregulated in myeloma cells after the treatment with bortezomib, leading to cell-cycle arrest and apoptosis.[309]

The proteasome is also required for activation of the nuclear transcription factor NF-κB, which in response to environmental stress or cytotoxic agents, plays a role in maintaining cell viability through the transcription of inhibitors of apoptosis, and the DDR including DNA-damage checkpoints[310] and DNA repair.[311] Based on these observations, targeting the proteasome has become a successful approach to cancer treatment[312] and with a better understanding of the human cell-cycle machinery, it will be possible in the future to identify new targets for antineoplastic therapies.

REFERENCES

1. Hartwell LH, Weinert TA: Checkpoints: Controls that ensure the order of cell cycle events. *Science* 246(4930):629–634, 1989.
2. Elledge SJ: Cell cycle checkpoints: Preventing an identity crisis. *Science* 274(5293):1664–1672, 1996.
3. Russell P: Checkpoints on the road to mitosis. *Trends Biochem Sci* 23(10):399–402, 1998.
4. Murray AW: The genetics of cell cycle checkpoints. *Curr Opin Genet Dev* 5(1):5–11, 1995.
5. Hartwell LH, Kastan MB: Cell cycle control and cancer. *Science* 266(5192):1821–1828, 1994.
6. Rao PN, Johnson RT: Mammalian cell fusion: Studies on the regulation of DNA synthesis and mitosis. *Nature* 225(5228):159–164, 1970.
7. Lohka MJ, Hayes MK, Maller JL: Purification of maturation-promoting factor, an intracellular regulator of early mitotic events. *Proc Natl Acad Sci U S A* 85(9):3009–3013, 1988.
8. Sherr CJ: Mammalian G1 cyclins. *Cell* 73(6):1059–1065, 1993.
9. Pines J: Cyclins and cyclin-dependent kinases: Take your partners. *Trends Biochem Sci* 18(6):195–197, 1993.
10. Chen HH, Wong YH, Geneviere AM, Fann MJ: CDK13/CDC2L5 interacts with L-type cyclins and regulates alternative splicing. *Biochem Biophys Res Commun* 354(3):735–740, 2007.
11. Pagano M, Pepperkok R, Verde F, et al: Cyclin A is required at two points in the human cell cycle. *EMBO J* 11(3):961–971, 1992.
12. Rape M, Kirschner MW: Autonomous regulation of the anaphase-promoting complex couples mitosis to S-phase entry. *Nature* 432(7017):588–595, 2004.
13. Resnitzky D, Hengst L, Reed SI: Cyclin A-associated kinase activity is rate limiting for entrance into S phase and is negatively regulated in G1 by p27Kip1. *Mol Cell Biol* 15(8):4347–4352, 1995.
14. Trovesi C, Manfrini N, Falcettoni M, Longhese MP: Regulation of the DNA damage response by cyclin-dependent kinases. *J Mol Biol* 425(23):4756–4766, 2013.
15. Meyerson M, Enders GH, Wu CL, et al: A family of human cdc2-related protein kinases. *EMBO J* 11(8):2909–2917, 1992.
16. Solomon MJ: Activation of the various cyclin/cdc2 protein kinases. *Curr Opin Cell Biol* 5(2):180–186, 1993.
17. Lew J, Wang JH: Neuronal cdc2-like kinase. *Trends Biochem Sci* 20(1):33–37, 1995.
18. Matsushime H, Ewen ME, Strom DK, et al: Identification and properties of an atypical catalytic subunit (p34PSK-J3/cdk4) for mammalian D type G1 cyclins. *Cell* 71(2):323–334, 1992.
19. Xiong Y, Zhang H, Beach D: D type cyclins associate with multiple protein kinases and the DNA replication and repair factor PCNA. *Cell* 71(3):505–514, 1992.
20. Meyerson M, Harlow E: Identification of G1 kinase activity for cdk6, a novel cyclin D partner. *Mol Cell Biol* 14(3):2077–2086, 1994.
21. Zhu YX, Tiedemann R, Shi CX, et al: RNAi screen of the druggable genome identifies modulators of proteasome inhibitor sensitivity in myeloma including CDK5. *Blood* 117(14):3847–3857, 2011.
22. Levacque Z, Rosales JL, Lee KY: Level of cdk5 expression predicts the survival of relapsed multiple myeloma patients. *Cell Cycle* 11(21):4093–4095, 2012.
23. Nguyen TK, Grant S: Dinaciclib (SCH727965) inhibits the unfolded protein response through a CDK1- and 5-dependent mechanism. *Mol Cancer Ther* 13(3):662–674, 2014.
24. Fesquet D, Labbe JC, Derancourt J, et al: The MO15 gene encodes the catalytic subunit of a protein kinase that activates cdc2 and other cyclin-dependent kinases (CDKs) through phosphorylation of Thr161 and its homologues. *EMBO J* 12(8):3111–3121, 1993.
25. Knuesel MT, Meyer KD, Donner AJ, et al: The human CDK8 subcomplex is a histone kinase that requires Med12 for activity and can function independently of mediator. *Mol Cell Biol* 29(3):650–661, 2009.
26. Morris EJ, Ji JY, Yang F, et al: E2F1 represses beta-catenin transcription and is antagonized by both pRB and CDK8. *Nature* 455(7212):552–556, 2008.
27. Romano G, Giordano A: Role of the cyclin-dependent kinase 9-related pathway in mammalian gene expression and human diseases. *Cell Cycle* 7(23):3664–3668, 2008.
28. Chen D, Fong Y, Zhou Q: Specific interaction of Tat with the human but not rodent P-TEFb complex mediates the species-specific Tat activation of HIV-1 transcription. *Proc Natl Acad Sci U S A* 96(6):2728–2733, 1999.
29. Sergere JC, Thuret JY, Le Roux G, et al: Human CDK10 gene isoforms. *Biochem Biophys Res Commun* 276(1):271–277, 2000.
30. Hu D, Mayeda A, Trembley JH, et al: CDK11 complexes promote pre-mRNA splicing. *J Biol Chem* 278(10):8623–8629, 2003.
31. Kasten M, Giordano A: Cdk10, a Cdc2-related kinase, associates with the Ets2 transcription factor and modulates its transactivation activity. *Oncogene* 20(15):1832–1838, 2001.
32. Bagella L, Giacinti C, Simone C, Giordano A: Identification of murine cdk10: Association with Ets2 transcription factor and effects on the cell cycle. *J Cell Biochem* 99(3):978–985, 2006.
33. Chen HH, Wang YC, Fann MJ: Identification and characterization of the CDK12/cyclin L1 complex involved in alternative splicing regulation. *Mol Cell Biol* 26(7):2736–2745, 2006.
34. Hunt T: Cyclins and their partners: From a simple idea to complicated reality. *Semin Cell Biol* 2(4):213–222, 1991.
35. Lees EM, Harlow E: Sequences within the conserved cyclin box of human cyclin A are sufficient for binding to and activation of cdc2 kinase. *Mol Cell Biol* 13(2):1194–1201, 1993.
36. Hanashiro K, Kanai M, Geng Y, et al: Roles of cyclins A and E in induction of centrosome amplification in p53-compromised cells. *Oncogene* 27(40):5288–5302, 2008.
37. Krug U, Yasmeen A, Beger C, et al: Cyclin A1 regulates WT1 expression in acute myeloid leukemia cells. *Int J Oncol* 34(1):129–136, 2009.
38. Ohtsubo M, Roberts JM: Cyclin-dependent regulation of G1 in mammalian fibroblasts. *Science* 259(5103):1908–1912, 1993.
39. Spencer SL, Cappell SD, Tsai FC, et al: The proliferation-quiescence decision is controlled by a bifurcation in CDK2 activity at mitotic exit. *Cell* 155(2):369–383, 2013.
40. Ekholm SV, Reed SI: Regulation of G(1) cyclin-dependent kinases in the mammalian cell cycle. *Curr Opin Cell Biol* 12(6):676–684, 2000.
41. Strohmaier H, Spruck CH, Kaiser P, et al: Human F-box protein hCdc4 targets cyclin E for proteolysis and is mutated in a breast cancer cell line. *Nature* 413(6853):316–322, 2001.
42. Ekholm-Reed S, Mendez J, Tedesco D, et al: Deregulation of cyclin E in human cells interferes with prereplication complex assembly. *J Cell Biol* 165(6):789–800, 2004.
43. Zhang HS, Postigo AA, Dean DC: Active transcriptional repression by the Rb-E2F complex mediates G1 arrest triggered by p16INK4a, TGFbeta, and contact inhibition. *Cell* 97(1):53–61, 1999.
44. Rajagopalan H, Jallepalli PV, Rago C, et al: Inactivation of hCDC4 can cause chromosomal instability. *Nature* 428(6978):77–81, 2004.
45. Keck JM, Summers MK, Tedesco D, et al: Cyclin E overexpression impairs progression through mitosis by inhibiting APC(Cdh1). *J Cell Biol* 178(3):371–385, 2007.
46. McGowan CH, Russell P, Reed SI: Periodic biosynthesis of the human M-phase promoting factor catalytic subunit p34 during the cell cycle. *Mol Cell Biol* 10(7):3847–3851, 1990.
47. Buendia B, Draetta G, Karsenti E: Regulation of the microtubule nucleating activity of centrosomes in Xenopus egg extracts: Role of cyclin A-associated protein kinase. *J Cell Biol* 116(6):1431–1442, 1992.
48. Gallant P, Nigg EA: Cyclin B2 undergoes cell cycle-dependent nuclear translocation and, when expressed as a non-destructible mutant, causes mitotic arrest in HeLa cells. *J Cell Biol* 117(1):213–224, 1992.
49. Draviam VM, Orrechia S, Lowe M, et al: The localization of human cyclins B1 and B2 determines CDK1 substrate specificity and neither enzyme requires MEK to disassemble the Golgi apparatus. *J Cell Biol* 152(5):945–958, 2001.
50. Pines J: The cell cycle kinases. *Semin Cancer Biol* 5(4):305–313, 1994.
51. Arnaoutov A, Dasso M: The Ran GTPase regulates kinetochore function. *Dev Cell* 5(1):99–111, 2003.
52. Bentley AM, Normand G, Hoyt J, King RW: Distinct sequence elements of cyclin B1 promote localization to chromatin, centrosomes, and kinetochores during mitosis. *Mol Biol Cell* 18(12):4847–4858, 2007.

53. Yu Z, Wang L, Wang C, et al: Cyclin D1 induction of Dicer governs microRNA processing and expression in breast cancer. *Nat Commun* 4:2812, 2013.

54. Yu Q, Sicinska E, Geng Y, et al: Requirement for CDK4 kinase function in breast cancer. *Cancer Cell* 9(1):23–32, 2006.

55. Landis MW, Pawlyk BS, Li T, et al: Cyclin D1-dependent kinase activity in murine development and mammary tumorigenesis. *Cancer Cell* 9(1):13–22, 2006.

56. Dickson MA: Molecular pathways: CDK4 inhibitors for cancer therapy. *Clin Cancer Res* 20(13):3379–3383, 2014.

57. Lee Y, Dominy JE, Choi YJ, et al: Cyclin D1-Cdk4 controls glucose metabolism independently of cell cycle progression. *Nature* 510(7506):547–551, 2014.

58. Placke T, Faber K, Nonami A, et al: Requirement for CDK6 in MLL-rearranged acute myeloid leukemia. *Blood* 124(1):13–23, 2014.

59. Antony-Debre I, Steidl U: CDK6, a new target in MLL-driven leukemia. *Blood* 124(1):5–6, 2014.

60. Bellail AC, Olson JJ, Hao C: SUMO1 modification stabilizes CDK6 protein and drives the cell cycle and glioblastoma progression. *Nat Commun* 5:4234, 2014.

61. Choi YJ, Anders L: Signaling through cyclin D-dependent kinases. *Oncogene* 33(15):1890–1903, 2014.

62. Schachter MM, Fisher RP: The CDK-activating kinase Cdk7: Taking yes for an answer. *Cell Cycle* 12(20):3239–3240, 2013.

63. Schachter MM, Merrick KA, Larochelle S, et al: A Cdk7-Cdk4 T-loop phosphorylation cascade promotes G1 progression. *Mol Cell* 50(2):250–260, 2013.

64. Fisher RP: Secrets of a double agent: CDK7 in cell-cycle control and transcription. *J Cell Sci* 118(Pt 22):5171–5180, 2005.

65. Kwiatkowski N, Zhang T, Rahl PB, et al: Targeting transcription regulation in cancer with a covalent CDK7 inhibitor. *Nature* 511(7511):616–620, 2014.

66. Wei P, Garber ME, Fang SM, et al: A novel CDK9-associated C-type cyclin interacts directly with HIV-1 Tat and mediates its high-affinity, loop-specific binding to TAR RNA. *Cell* 92(4):451–462, 1998.

67. Peng J, Zhu Y, Milton JT, Price DH: Identification of multiple cyclin subunits of human P-TEFb. *Genes Dev* 12(5):755–762, 1998.

68. Burger K, Muhl B, Rohrmoser M, et al: Cyclin-dependent kinase 9 links RNA polymerase II transcription to processing of ribosomal RNA. *J Biol Chem* 288(29):21173–21183, 2013.

69. Ji X, Lu H, Zhou Q, Luo K: LARP7 suppresses P-TEFb activity to inhibit breast cancer progression and metastasis. *Elife* 3:e02907, 2014.

70. Wang S, Fischer PM: Cyclin-dependent kinase 9: A key transcriptional regulator and potential drug target in oncology, virology and cardiology. *Trends Pharmacol Sci* 29(6):302–313, 2008.

71. Romano G: Deregulations in the cyclin-dependent kinase-9-related pathway in cancer: Implications for drug discovery and development. *ISRN Oncol* 2013:305371, 2013.

72. Walsby E, Pratt G, Shao H, et al: A novel Cdk9 inhibitor preferentially targets tumor cells and synergizes with fludarabine. *Oncotarget* 5(2):375–385, 2014.

73. Yin T, Lallena MJ, Kreklau EL, et al: A novel CDK9 inhibitor shows potent antitumor efficacy in preclinical hematologic tumor models. *Mol Cancer Ther* 13(6):1442–1456, 2014.

74. Stewart DP, Koss B, Bathina M, et al: Ubiquitin-independent degradation of antiapoptotic MCL-1. *Mol Cell Biol* 30(12):3099–3110, 2010.

75. Chen S, Dai Y, Harada H, et al: Mcl-1 down-regulation potentiates ABT-737 lethality by cooperatively inducing Bak activation and Bax translocation. *Cancer Res* 67(2):782–791, 2007.

76. Chen S, Zhou L, Zhang Y, et al: Targeting SQSTM1/p62 induces cargo loading failure and converts autophagy to apoptosis via NBK/Bik. *Mol Cell Biol* 34(18):3435–3449, 2014.

77. Chen S, Dai Y, Pei XY, et al: CDK inhibitors upregulate BH3-only proteins to sensitize human myeloma cells to BH3 mimetic therapies. *Cancer Res* 72(16):4225–4237, 2012.

78. Fujinaga K, Cujec TP, Peng J, et al: The ability of positive transcription elongation factor B to transactivate human immunodeficiency virus transcription depends on a functional kinase domain, cyclin T1, and Tat. *J Virol* 72(9):7154–7159, 1998.

79. MacLachlan TK, Sang N, De Luca A, et al: Binding of CDK9 to TRAF2. *J Cell Biochem* 71(4):467–478, 1998.

80. Michels AA, Nguyen VT, Fraldi A, et al: MAQ1 and 7SK RNA interact with CDK9/cyclin T complexes in a transcription-dependent manner. *Mol Cell Biol* 23(14):4859–4869, 2003.

81. Garriga J, Bhattacharya S, Calbo J, et al: CDK9 is constitutively expressed throughout the cell cycle, and its steady-state expression is independent of SKP2. *Mol Cell Biol* 23(15):5165–5173, 2003.

82. Poss ZC, Ebmeier CC, Taatjes DJ: The Mediator complex and transcription regulation. *Crit Rev Biochem Mol Biol* 48(5):575–608, 2013.

83. Belakavadi M, Fondell JD: Cyclin-dependent kinase 8 positively cooperates with Mediator to promote thyroid hormone receptor-dependent transcriptional activation. *Mol Cell Biol* 30(10):2437–2448, 2010.

84. Firestein R, Shima K, Nosho K, et al: CDK8 expression in 470 colorectal cancers in relation to beta-catenin activation, other molecular alterations and patient survival. *Int J Cancer* 126(12):2863–2873, 2010.

85. Xu W, Wang Z, Zhang W, et al: Mutated K-ras activates CDK8 to stimulate the epithelial-to-mesenchymal transition in pancreatic cancer in part via the Wnt/β-catenin signaling pathway. *Cancer Lett* 356(2 Pt B):613–627, 2015.

86. Bosken CA, Farnung L, Hintermair C, et al: The structure and substrate specificity of human Cdk12/Cyclin K. *Nat Commun* 5:3505, 2014.

87. Cheng SW, Kuzyk MA, Moradian A, et al: Interaction of cyclin-dependent kinase 12/CrkRS with cyclin K1 is required for the phosphorylation of the C-terminal domain of RNA polymerase II. *Mol Cell Biol* 32(22):4691–4704, 2012.

88. Blazek D, Kohoutek J, Bartholomeeusen K, et al: The Cyclin K/Cdk12 complex maintains genomic stability via regulation of expression of DNA damage response genes. *Genes Dev* 25(20):2158–2172, 2011.

89. Husson H, Carideo EG, Neuberg D, et al: Gene expression profiling of follicular lymphoma and normal germinal center B cells using cDNA arrays. *Blood* 99(1):282–289, 2002.

90. Iorns E, Turner NC, Elliott R, et al: Identification of CDK10 as an important determinant of resistance to endocrine therapy for breast cancer. *Cancer Cell* 13(2):91–104, 2008.

91. Trembley JH, Hu D, Slaughter CA, et al: Casein kinase 2 interacts with cyclin-dependent kinase 11 (CDK11) in vivo and phosphorylates both the RNA polymerase II carboxyl-terminal domain and CDK11 in vitro. *J Biol Chem* 278(4):2265–2270, 2003.

92. Shi J, Feng Y, Goulet AC, et al: The p34cdc2-related cyclin-dependent kinase 11 interacts with the p47 subunit of eukaryotic initiation factor 3 during apoptosis. *J Biol Chem* 278(7):5062–5071, 2003.

93. Yokoyama H, Gruss OJ, Rybina S, et al: Cdk11 is a RanGTP-dependent microtubule stabilization factor that regulates spindle assembly rate. *J Cell Biol* 180(5):867–875, 2008.

94. Hu D, Valentine M, Kidd VJ, Lahti JM: CDK11(p58) is required for the maintenance of sister chromatid cohesion. *J Cell Sci* 120(Pt 14):2424–2434, 2007.

95. Chandramouli A, Shi J, Feng Y, et al: Haploinsufficiency of the cdc2l gene contributes to skin cancer development in mice. *Carcinogenesis* 28(9):2028–2035, 2007.

96. Sherr CJ: Cancer cell cycles. *Science* 274(5293):1672–1677, 1996.

97. Gu Y, Turck CW, Morgan DO: Inhibition of CDK2 activity in vivo by an associated 20K regulatory subunit. *Nature* 366(6456):707–710, 1993.

98. Blagosklonny MV, Pardee AB: The restriction point of the cell cycle. *Cell Cycle* 1(2):103–110, 2002.

99. Assoian RK, Yung Y: A reciprocal relationship between Rb and Skp2: Implications for restriction point control, signal transduction to the cell cycle and cancer. *Cell Cycle* 7(1):24–27, 2008.

100. Yung Y, Walker JL, Roberts JM, Assoian RK: A Skp2 autoinduction loop and restriction point control. *J Cell Biol* 178(5):741–747, 2007.

101. Nourse J, Firpo E, Flanagan WM, et al: Interleukin-2-mediated elimination of the p27Kip1 cyclin-dependent kinase inhibitor prevented by rapamycin. *Nature* 372 (6506):570–573, 1994.

102. Santamaria D, Ortega S: Cyclins and CDKS in development and cancer: Lessons from genetically modified mice. *Front Biosci* 11:1164–1188, 2006.

103. Genovese C, Trani D, Caputi M, Claudio PP: Cell cycle control and beyond: Emerging roles for the retinoblastoma gene family. *Oncogene* 25(38):5201–5209, 2006.

104. Serrano M, Hannon GJ, Beach D: A new regulatory motif in cell-cycle control causing specific inhibition of cyclin D/CDK4. *Nature* 366(6456):704–707, 1993.

105. Chan FK, Zhang J, Cheng L, et al: Identification of human and mouse p19, a novel CDK4 and CDK6 inhibitor with homology to p16ink4. *Mol Cell Biol* 15(5):2682–2688, 1995.

106. DeGregori J, Leone G, Ohtani K, et al: E2F-1 accumulation bypasses a G1 arrest resulting from the inhibition of G1 cyclin-dependent kinase activity. *Genes Dev* 9(23):2873–2887, 1995.

107. Nobori T, Miura K, Wu DJ, et al: Deletions of the cyclin-dependent kinase-4 inhibitor gene in multiple human cancers. *Nature* 368(6473):753–756, 1994.

108. Bai C, Sen P, Hofmann K, et al: SKP1 connects cell cycle regulators to the ubiquitin proteolysis machinery through a novel motif, the F-box. *Cell* 86(2):263–274, 1996.

109. Feldman RM, Correll CC, Kaplan KB, Deshaies RJ: A complex of Cdc4p, Skp1p, and Cdc53p/cullin catalyzes ubiquitination of the phosphorylated CDK inhibitor Sic1p. *Cell* 91(2):221–230, 1997.

110. Skowyra D, Koepp DM, Kamura T, et al: Reconstitution of G1 cyclin ubiquitination with complexes containing SCFGrr1 and Rbx1. *Science* 284(5414):662–665, 1999.

111. Sun A, Bagella L, Tutton S, et al: From G0 to S phase: A view of the roles played by the retinoblastoma (Rb) family members in the Rb-E2F pathway. *J Cell Biochem* 102(6):1400–1404, 2007.

112. Krug U, Ganser A, Koeffler HP: Tumor suppressor genes in normal and malignant hematopoiesis. *Oncogene* 21(21):3475–3495, 2002.

113. Hagemeier C, Bannister AJ, Cook A, Kouzarides T: The activation domain of transcription factor PU.1 binds the retinoblastoma (RB) protein and the transcription factor TFIID in vitro: RB shows sequence similarity to TFIID and TFIIB. *Proc Natl Acad Sci U S A* 90(4):1580–1584, 1993.

114. Walkley CR, Sankaran VG, Orkin SH: Rb and hematopoiesis: Stem cells to anemia. *Cell Div* 3:13, 2008.

115. Zhang P, Zhang X, Iwama A, et al: PU.1 inhibits GATA-1 function and erythroid differentiation by blocking GATA-1 DNA binding. *Blood* 96(8):2641–2648, 2000.

116. Bergh G, Ehinger M, Olsson I, et al: Involvement of the retinoblastoma protein in monocytic and neutrophilic lineage commitment of human bone marrow progenitor cells. *Blood* 94(6):1971–1978, 1999.

117. Sherr CJ, Roberts JM: Inhibitors of mammalian G1 cyclin-dependent kinases. *Genes Dev* 9(10):1149–1163, 1995.

118. Zhang H, Xiong Y, Beach D: Proliferating cell nuclear antigen and p21 are components of multiple cell cycle kinase complexes. *Mol Biol Cell* 4(9):897–906, 1993.

119. Li Y, Jenkins CW, Nichols MA, Xiong Y: Cell cycle expression and p53 regulation of the cyclin-dependent kinase inhibitor p21. *Oncogene* 9(8):2261–2268, 1994.

120. Overton KW, Spencer SL, Noderer WL, et al: Basal p21 controls population heterogeneity in cycling and quiescent cell cycle states. *Proc Natl Acad Sci U S A* 111(41): E4386–E4393, 2014.

121. Dai Y, Rahmani M, Grant S: An intact NF-kappaB pathway is required for histone deacetylase inhibitor-induced G1 arrest and maturation in U937 human myeloid leukemia cells. *Cell Cycle* 2(5):467–472, 2003.

122. Dai Y, Rahmani M, Dent P, Grant S: Blockade of histone deacetylase inhibitor-induced RelA/p65 acetylation and NF-kappaB activation potentiates apoptosis in leukemia cells through a process mediated by oxidative damage, XIAP downregulation, and c-Jun N-terminal kinase 1 activation. *Mol Cell Biol* 25(13):5429–5444, 2005.

123. Wang Z, Bhattacharya N, Mixter PF, et al: Phosphorylation of the cell cycle inhibitor p21Cip1/WAF1 by Pim-1 kinase. *Biochim Biophys Acta* 1593(1):45–55, 2002.

124. Zhang Y, Wang Z, Magnuson NS: Pim-1 kinase-dependent phosphorylation of p21Cip1/WAF1 regulates its stability and cellular localization in H1299 cells. *Mol Cancer Res* 5(9):909–922, 2007.

125. Ellwood-Yen K, Graeber TG, Wongvipat J, et al: Myc-driven murine prostate cancer shares molecular features with human prostate tumors. *Cancer Cell* 4(3):223–238, 2003.

126. Kato JY, Matsuoka M, Polyak K, et al: Cyclic AMP-induced G1 phase arrest mediated by an inhibitor (p27Kip1) of cyclin-dependent kinase 4 activation. *Cell* 79(3):487–496, 1994.

127. Caraballo JM, Acosta JC, Cortes MA, et al: High p27 protein levels in chronic lymphocytic leukemia are associated to low Myc and Skp2 expression, confer resistance to apoptosis and antagonize Myc effects on cell cycle. *Oncotarget* 5(13):4694–4708, 2014.

128. Vervoorts J, Luscher B: Post-translational regulation of the tumor suppressor p27(KIP1). *Cell Mol Life Sci* 65(20):3255–3264, 2008.

129. Koepp DM, Harper JW, Elledge SJ: How the cyclin became a cyclin: Regulated proteolysis in the cell cycle. *Cell* 97(4):431–434, 1999.

130. Hirai H, Roussel MF, Kato JY, et al: Novel INK4 proteins, p19 and p18, are specific inhibitors of the cyclin D-dependent kinases CDK4 and CDK6. *Mol Cell Biol* 15(5):2672–2681, 1995.

131. Hannon GJ, Beach D: P15INK4B is a potential effector of TGF-beta-induced cell cycle arrest. *Nature* 371(6494):257–261, 1994.

132. Adams L, Roth MJ, Abnet CC, et al: Promoter methylation in cytology specimens as an early detection marker for esophageal squamous dysplasia and early esophageal squamous cell carcinoma. *Cancer Prev Res (Phila)* 1(5):357–361, 2008.

133. Lee YK, Park JY, Kang HJ, Cho HC: Overexpression of p16INK4A and p14ARF in haematological malignancies. *Clin Lab Haematol* 25(4):233–237, 2003.

134. Drexler HG: Review of alterations of the cyclin-dependent kinase inhibitor INK4 family genes p15, p16, p18 and p19 in human leukemia-lymphoma cells. *Leukemia* 12(6):845–859, 1998.

135. Sulong S, Moorman AV, Irving JA, et al: A comprehensive analysis of the CDKN2A gene in childhood acute lymphoblastic leukemia reveals genomic deletion, copy number neutral loss of heterozygosity, and association with specific cytogenetic subgroups. *Blood* 113(1):100–107, 2009.

136. Diccianni MB, Batova A, Yu J, et al: Shortened survival after relapse in T-cell acute lymphoblastic leukemia patients with p16/p15 deletions. *Leuk Res* 21(6):549–558, 1997.

137. Belaud-Rotureau MA, Marietta V, Vergier B, et al: Inactivation of p16INK4a/CDKN2A gene may be a diagnostic feature of large B cell lymphoma leg type among cutaneous B cell lymphomas. *Virchows Arch* 452(6):607–620, 2008.

138. Bender CM, Pao MM, Jones PA: Inhibition of DNA methylation by 5-aza-2'-deoxycytidine suppresses the growth of human tumor cell lines. *Cancer Res* 58(1):95–101, 1998.

139. Cameron EE, Bachman KE, Myohanen S, et al: Synergy of demethylation and histone deacetylase inhibition in the re-expression of genes silenced in cancer. *Nat Genet* 21(1):103–107, 1999.

140. Humbey O, Pimkina J, Zilfou JT, et al: The ARF tumor suppressor can promote the progression of some tumors. *Cancer Res* 68(23):9608–9613, 2008.

141. Schwartz GK, Shah MA: Targeting the cell cycle: A new approach to cancer therapy. *J Clin Oncol* 23(36):9408–9421, 2005.

142. Shapiro GI: Cyclin-dependent kinase pathways as targets for cancer treatment. *J Clin Oncol* 24(11):1770–1783, 2006.

143. Bose P, Simmons GL, Grant S: Cyclin-dependent kinase inhibitor therapy for hematologic malignancies. *Expert Opin Investig Drugs* 22(6):723–738, 2013.

144. Leonard JP, LaCasce AS, Smith MR, et al: Selective CDK4/6 inhibition with tumor responses by PD0332991 in patients with mantle cell lymphoma. *Blood* 119(20):4597–4607, 2012.

145. Byrd JC, Lin TS, Dalton JT, et al: Flavopiridol administered using a pharmacologically derived schedule is associated with marked clinical efficacy in refractory, genetically high-risk chronic lymphocytic leukemia. *Blood* 109(2):399–404, 2007.

146. Lin TS, Ruppert AS, Johnson AJ, et al: Phase II study of flavopiridol in relapsed chronic lymphocytic leukemia demonstrating high response rates in genetically high-risk disease. *J Clin Oncol* 27(35):6012–6018, 2009.

147. Bose P, Grant S: Orphan drug designation for pracinostat, volasertib and alvocidib in AML. *Leuk Res* 38(8):862–865, 2014.

148. Bible KC, Kaufmann SH: Cytotoxic synergy between flavopiridol (NSC 649890, L86-8275) and various antineoplastic agents: The importance of sequence of administration. *Cancer Res* 57(16):3375–3380, 1997.

149. Karp JE, Ross DD, Yang W, et al: Timed sequential therapy of acute leukemia with flavopiridol: In vitro model for a phase I clinical trial. *Clin Cancer Res* 9(1):307–315, 2003.

150. Zeidner JF, Foster MC, Blackford A, et al: Randomized multicenter phase II trial of timed-sequential therapy with flavopiridol (alvocidib), cytarabine, and mitoxantrone (FLAM) versus "7+3" for adults with newly diagnosed acute myeloid leukemia (AML). *ASCO Meeting Abstracts* 32(15 Suppl):7002, 2014.

151. Karp JE, Garrett-Mayer E, Estey EH, et al: Randomized phase II study of two schedules of flavopiridol given as timed sequential therapy with cytosine arabinoside and mitoxantrone for adults with newly diagnosed, poor-risk acute myelogenous leukemia. *Haematologica* 2012;97(11):1736–1742, 2014.

152. Dai Y, Rahmani M, Grant S: Proteasome inhibitors potentiate leukemic cell apoptosis induced by the cyclin-dependent kinase inhibitor flavopiridol through a SAPK/JNK- and NF-kappaB-dependent process. *Oncogene* 22(46):7108–7122, 2003.

153. Dai Y, Rahmani M, Pei XY, et al: Bortezomib and flavopiridol interact synergistically to induce apoptosis in chronic myeloid leukemia cells resistant to imatinib mesylate through both Bcr/Abl-dependent and -independent mechanisms. *Blood* 104(2):509–518, 2004.

154. Almenara J, Rosato R, Grant S: Synergistic induction of mitochondrial damage and apoptosis in human leukemia cells by flavopiridol and the histone deacetylase inhibitor suberoylanilide hydroxamic acid (SAHA). *Leukemia* 16(7):1331–1343, 2002.

155. Holkova B, Kmieciak M, Perkins EB, et al: Phase I trial of bortezomib (PS-341; NSC 681239) and "nonhybrid" (bolus) infusion schedule of alvocidib (flavopiridol; NSC 649890) in patients with recurrent or refractory indolent B-cell neoplasms. *Clin Cancer Res* 20(22):5652–5662, 2014.

156. Holkova B, Perkins EB, Ramakrishnan V, et al: Phase I trial of bortezomib (PS-341; NSC 681239) and alvocidib (flavopiridol; NSC 649890) in patients with recurrent or refractory B-cell neoplasms. *Clin Cancer Res* 17(10):3388–3397, 2011.

157. Holkova B, Supko JG, Ames MM, et al: A phase I trial of vorinostat and alvocidib in patients with relapsed, refractory, or poor prognosis acute leukemia, or refractory anemia with excess blasts-2. *Clin Cancer Res* 19(7):1873–1883, 2013.

158. Tse AN, Carvajal R, Schwartz GK: Targeting checkpoint kinase 1 in cancer therapeutics. *Clin Cancer Res* 13(7):1955–1960, 2007.

159. Dai Y, Grant S: New insights into checkpoint kinase 1 in the DNA damage response signaling network. *Clin Cancer Res* 16(2):376–383, 2010.

160. Bucher N, Britten CD: G2 checkpoint abrogation and checkpoint kinase-1 targeting in the treatment of cancer. *Br J Cancer* 98(3):523–528, 2008.

161. Lee MH, Yang HY: Negative regulators of cyclin-dependent kinases and their roles in cancers. *Cell Mol Life Sci* 58(12–13):1907–1922, 2001.

162. Kastan MB, Bartek J: Cell-cycle checkpoints and cancer. *Nature* 432(7015):316–323, 2004.

163. Schenk EL, Koh BD, Flatten KS, et al: Effects of selective checkpoint kinase 1 inhibition on cytarabine cytotoxicity in acute myelogenous leukemia cells *in vitro*. *Clin Cancer Res* 18(19):5364–5373, 2012.

164. Karp JE, Thomas BM, Greer JM, et al: Phase I and pharmacologic trial of cytosine arabinoside with the selective checkpoint 1 inhibitor Sch 900776 in refractory acute leukemias. *Clin Cancer Res* 18(24):6723–6731, 2012.

165. Dai Y, Chen S, Kmieciak M, et al: The novel Chk1 inhibitor MK-8776 sensitizes human leukemia cells to HDAC inhibitors by targeting the intra-S checkpoint and DNA replication and repair. *Mol Cancer Ther* 12(6):878–889, 2013.

166. Petruccelli LA, Dupere-Richer D, Pettersson F, et al: Vorinostat induces reactive oxygen species and DNA damage in acute myeloid leukemia cells. *PLoS One* 6(6):e20987, 2011.

167. Koprinarova M, Botev P, Russev G: Histone deacetylase inhibitor sodium butyrate enhances cellular radiosensitivity by inhibiting both DNA nonhomologous end joining and homologous recombination. *DNA Repair (Amst)* 10(9):970–977, 2011.

168. Brazelle W, Kreahling JM, Gemmer J, et al: Histone deacetylase inhibitors downregulate checkpoint kinase 1 expression to induce cell death in non-small cell lung cancer cells. *PLoS One* 5(12):e14335, 2010.

169. Kaufmann SH, Karp JE, Litzow MR, et al: Phase I and pharmacological study of cytarabine and tanespimycin in relapsed and refractory acute leukemia. *Haematologica* 96(11):1619–1626, 2011.

170. Weisberg E, Nonami A, Chen Z, et al: Identification of Wee1 as a novel therapeutic target for mutant RAS-driven acute leukemia and other malignancies. *Leukemia* 29(1):27–37, 2015.

171. Tibes R, Bogenberger JM, Chaudhuri L, et al: RNAi screening of the kinome with cytarabine in leukemias. *Blood* 119(12):2863–2872, 2012.

172. Porter CC, Kim J, Fosmire S, et al: Integrated genomic analyses identify WEE1 as a critical mediator of cell fate and a novel therapeutic target in acute myeloid leukemia. *Leukemia* 26(6):1266–1276, 2012.

173. Van Linden AA, Baturin D, Ford JB, et al: Inhibition of Wee1 sensitizes cancer cells to antimetabolite chemotherapeutics in vitro and in vivo, independent of p53 functionality. *Mol Cancer Ther* 12(12):2675–2684, 2013.

174. Zhou L, Zhang Y, Chen S, et al: A regimen combining the Wee1 inhibitor AZD1775 with HDAC inhibitors targets human acute myeloid leukemia cells harboring various genetic mutations. *Leukemia* 29(4):807–818, 2015.

175. Ha K, Fiskus W, Rao R, et al: Hsp90 inhibitor-mediated disruption of chaperone association of ATR with hsp90 sensitizes cancer cells to DNA damage. *Mol Cancer Ther* 10(7):1194–1206, 2011.

176. Sugimoto K, Sasaki M, Isobe Y, et al: Hsp90-inhibitor geldanamycin abrogates G2 arrest in p53-negative leukemia cell lines through the depletion of Chk1. *Oncogene* 27(22):3091–3101, 2008.

177. Tse AN, Sheikh TN, Alan H, et al: 90-kDa heat shock protein inhibition abrogates the topoisomerase I poison-induced G2/M checkpoint in p53-null tumor cells by depleting Chk1 and Wee1. *Mol Pharmacol* 75(1):124–133, 2009.

178. Aarts M, Sharpe R, Garcia-Murillas I, et al: Forced mitotic entry of S-phase cells as a therapeutic strategy induced by inhibition of WEE1. *Cancer Discov* 2(6):524–539, 2012.

179. Mrozek K, Heinonen K, Bloomfield CD: Clinical importance of cytogenetics in acute myeloid leukaemia. *Best Pract Res Clin Haematol* 14(1):19–47, 2001.

180. Frohling S, Dohner H: Chromosomal abnormalities in cancer. *N Engl J Med* 359(7):722–734, 2008.

181. Neff T, Armstrong SA: Recent progress toward epigenetic therapies: The example of mixed lineage leukemia. *Blood* 121(24):4847–4853, 2013.

182. Dann EJ, Rowe JM: Biology and therapy of secondary leukaemias. *Best Pract Res Clin Haematol* 14(1):119–137, 2001.

183. Vega F, Medeiros LJ: Chromosomal translocations involved in non-Hodgkin lymphomas. *Arch Pathol Lab Med* 127(9):1148–1160, 2003.

184. Ichikawa M, Asai T, Chiba S, et al: Runx1/AML-1 ranks as a master regulator of adult hematopoiesis. *Cell Cycle* 3(6):722–724, 2004.

185. Elagib KE, Racke FK, Mogass M, et al: RUNX1 and GATA-1 coexpression and cooperation in megakaryocytic differentiation. *Blood* 101(11):4333–4341, 2003.

186. Okuda T, van Deursen J, Hiebert SW, et al: AML1, the target of multiple chromosomal translocations in human leukemia, is essential for normal fetal liver hematopoiesis. *Cell* 84(2):321–330, 1996.

187. Scandura JM, Boccuni P, Cammenga J, Nimer SD: Transcription factor fusions in acute leukemia: Variations on a theme. *Oncogene* 21(21):3422–3444, 2002.

188. Gilles L, Guieze R, Bluteau D, et al: P19INK4D links endomitotic arrest and megakaryocyte maturation and is regulated by AML-1. *Blood* 111(8):4081–4091, 2008.

189. Wichmann C, Chen L, Heinrich M, et al: Targeting the oligomerization domain of ETO interferes with RUNX1/ETO oncogenic activity in t(8;21)-positive leukemic cells. *Cancer Res* 67(5):2280–2289, 2007.

190. Lin RJ, Sternsdorf T, Tini M, Evans RM: Transcriptional regulation in acute promyelocytic leukemia. *Oncogene* 20(49):7204–7215, 2001.

191. Le XF, Vallian S, Mu ZM, et al: Recombinant PML adenovirus suppresses growth and tumorigenicity of human breast cancer cells by inducing G1 cell cycle arrest and apoptosis. *Oncogene* 16(14):1839–1849, 1998.

192. Bischof O, Nacerddine K, Dejean A: Human papillomavirus oncoprotein E7 targets the promyelocytic leukemia protein and circumvents cellular senescence via the Rb and p53 tumor suppressor pathways. *Mol Cell Biol* 25(3):1013–1024, 2005.

193. Jul-Larsen A, Grudic A, Bjerkvig R, Boe SO: Cell-cycle regulation and dynamics of cytoplasmic compartments containing the promyelocytic leukemia protein and nucleoporins. *J Cell Sci* 122(Pt 8):1201–1210, 2009.

194. Salomoni P, Pandolfi PP: The role of PML in tumor suppression. *Cell* 108(2):165–170, 2002.

195. Hayakawa F, Abe A, Kitabayashi I, et al: Acetylation of PML is involved in histone deacetylase inhibitor-mediated apoptosis. *J Biol Chem* 283(36):24420–24425, 2008.

196. Chen Z, Brand NJ, Chen A, et al: Fusion between a novel Kruppel-like zinc finger gene and the retinoic acid receptor-alpha locus due to a variant t(11;17) translocation associated with acute promyelocytic leukaemia. *EMBO J* 12(3):1161–1167, 1993.

197. Tefferi A, Gilliland DG: Oncogenes in myeloproliferative disorders. *Cell Cycle* 6(5):550–566, 2007.

198. Ren R: Mechanisms of BCR-ABL in the pathogenesis of chronic myelogenous leukaemia. *Nat Rev Cancer* 5(3):172–183, 2005.

199. Skorski T: BCR/ABL regulates response to DNA damage: The role in resistance to genotoxic treatment and in genomic instability. *Oncogene* 21(56):8591–8604, 2002.

200. Gleissner B, Thiel E: Molecular genetic events in adult acute lymphoblastic leukemia. *Expert Rev Mol Diagn* 3(3):339–355, 2003.

201. Agarwal A, Mackenzie RJ, Besson A, et al: BCR-ABL1 promotes leukemia by converting p27 into a cytoplasmic oncoprotein. *Blood* 124(22):3260–3273, 2014.

202. Chi YH, Ward JM, Cheng LI, et al: Spindle assembly checkpoint and p53 deficiencies cooperate for tumorigenesis in mice. *Int J Cancer* 124(6):1483–1489, 2009.

203. Fabbro D, Ruetz S, Buchdunger E, et al: Protein kinases as targets for anticancer agents: From inhibitors to useful drugs. *Pharmacol Ther* 93(2–3):79–98, 2002.

204. Spinelli O, Peruta B, Tosi M, et al: Clearance of minimal residual disease after allogeneic stem cell transplantation and the prediction of the clinical outcome of adult patients with high-risk acute lymphoblastic leukemia. *Haematologica* 92(5):612–618, 2007.

205. Tirado CA, Sebastian S, Moore JO, et al: Molecular and cytogenetic characterization of a novel rearrangement involving chromosomes 9, 12, and 17 resulting in ETV6 (TEL) and ABL fusion. *Cancer Genet Cytogenet* 157(1):74–77, 2005.

206. Rodrigues GA, Park M: Dimerization mediated through a leucine zipper activates the oncogenic potential of the met receptor tyrosine kinase. *Mol Cell Biol* 13(11):6711–6722, 1993.

207. Fujimoto J, Shiota M, Iwahara T, et al: Characterization of the transforming activity of p80, a hyperphosphorylated protein in a Ki-1 lymphoma cell line with chromosomal translocation t(2;5). *Proc Natl Acad Sci U S A* 93(9):4181–4186, 1996.

208. Amin HM, Lai R: Pathobiology of ALK+ anaplastic large-cell lymphoma. *Blood* 110(7):2259–2267, 2007.

209. Golub TR, Barker GF, Lovett M, Gilliland DG: Fusion of PDGF receptor beta to a novel ets-like gene, tel, in chronic myelomonocytic leukemia with t(5;12) chromosomal translocation. *Cell* 77(2):307–316, 1994.

210. Tam WF, Gu TL, Chen J, et al: Id1 is a common downstream target of oncogenic tyrosine kinases in leukemic cells. *Blood* 112(5):1981–1992, 2008.

211. Graham SM, Cox AD, Drivas G, et al: Aberrant function of the Ras-related protein TC21/R-Ras2 triggers malignant transformation. *Mol Cell Biol* 14(6):4108–4115, 1994.

212. Saxena N, Lahiri SS, Hambarde S, Tripathi RP: RAS: Target for cancer therapy. *Cancer Invest* 26(9):948–955, 2008.

213. Khosravi-Far R, Solski PA, Clark GJ, et al: Activation of Rac1, RhoA, and mitogen-activated protein kinases is required for Ras transformation. *Mol Cell Biol* 15(11):6443–6453, 1995.

214. Yip SC, El-Sibai M, Coniglio SJ, et al: The distinct roles of Ras and Rac in PI 3-kinase-dependent protrusion during EGF-stimulated cell migration. *J Cell Sci* 120(Pt 17):3138–3146, 2007.

215. Schlessinger K, Hall A, Tolwinski N: Wnt signaling pathways meet Rho GTPases. *Genes Dev* 23(3):265–277, 2009.

216. Chang F, Steelman LS, Lee JT, et al: Signal transduction mediated by the Ras/Raf/MEK/ERK pathway from cytokine receptors to transcription factors: Potential targeting for therapeutic intervention. *Leukemia* 17(7):1263–1293, 2003.

217. Crump M: Inhibition of raf kinase in the treatment of acute myeloid leukemia. *Curr Pharm Des* 8(25):2243–2248, 2002.

218. Davis RK, Chellappan S: Disrupting the Rb-Raf-1 interaction: A potential therapeutic target for cancer. *Drug News Perspect* 21(6):331–335, 2008.

219. Thiel G, Ekici M, Rossler OG: Regulation of cellular proliferation, differentiation and cell death by activated Raf. *Cell Commun Signal* 7:8, 2009.

220. Johnson NL, Gardner AM, Diener KM, et al: Signal transduction pathways regulated by mitogen-activated/extracellular response kinase kinase kinase induce cell death. *J Biol Chem* 271(6):3229–3237, 1996.

221. Seth A, Gonzalez FA, Gupta S, et al: Signal transduction within the nucleus by mitogen-activated protein kinase. *J Biol Chem* 267(34):24796–24804, 1992.

222. Amendola D, De Salvo M, Marchese R, et al: Myc down-regulation affects cyclin D1/cdk4 activity and induces apoptosis via Smac/Diablo pathway in an astrocytoma cell line. *Cell Prolif* 42(1):94–109, 2009.

223. Zhang H, Gao P, Fukuda R, et al: HIF-1 inhibits mitochondrial biogenesis and cellular respiration in VHL-deficient renal cell carcinoma by repression of C-MYC activity. *Cancer Cell* 11(5):407–420, 2007.

224. Hoffmann I, Clarke PR, Marcote MJ, et al: Phosphorylation and activation of human cdc25-C by cdc2/Cyclin B and its involvement in the self-amplification of MPF at mitosis. *EMBO J* 12(1):53–63, 1993.

225. Kramer MH, Hermans J, Wijburg E, et al: Clinical relevance of BCL2, BCL6, and MYC rearrangements in diffuse large B-cell lymphoma. *Blood* 92(9):3152–3162, 1998.

226. Bonnotte B, Favre N, Moutet M, et al: Bcl-2-mediated inhibition of apoptosis prevents immunogenicity and restores tumorigenicity of spontaneously regressive tumors. *J Immunol* 161(3):1433–1438, 1998.

227. Yin DX, Schimke RT: Inhibition of apoptosis by overexpressing Bcl-2 enhances gene amplification by a mechanism independent of aphidicolin pretreatment. *Proc Natl Acad Sci U S A* 93(8):3394–3398, 1996.

228. Del Principe MI, Del Poeta G, Venditti A, et al: Apoptosis and immaturity in acute myeloid leukemia. *Hematology* 10(1):25–34, 2005.

229. Glaser SP, Lee EF, Trounson E, et al: Anti-apoptotic Mcl-1 is essential for the development and sustained growth of acute myeloid leukemia. *Genes Dev* 26(2):120–125, 2012.

230. Gelmetti V, Zhang J, Fanelli M, et al: Aberrant recruitment of the nuclear receptor corepressor-histone deacetylase complex by the acute myeloid leukemia fusion partner ETO. *Mol Cell Biol* 18(12):7185–7191, 1998.

231. Wang J, Hoshino T, Redner RL, et al: ETO, fusion partner in t(8;21) acute myeloid leukemia, represses transcription by interaction with the human N-CoR/mSin3/HDAC1 complex. *Proc Natl Acad Sci U S A* 95(18):10860–10865, 1998.

232. Wong CW, Privalsky ML: Components of the SMRT corepressor complex exhibit distinctive interactions with the POZ domain oncoproteins PLZF, PLZF-RARalpha, and BCL-6. *J Biol Chem* 273(42):27695–27702, 1998.

233. David G, Alland L, Hong SH, et al: Histone deacetylase associated with mSin3A mediates repression by the acute promyelocytic leukemia-associated PLZF protein. *Oncogene* 16(19):2549–2556, 1998.

234. Yunis JJ, Ramsay N: Retinoblastoma and subband deletion of chromosome 13. *Am J Dis Child* 132(2):161–163, 1978.

235. Grana X, Garriga J, Mayol X: Role of the retinoblastoma protein family, pRB, p107 and p130 in the negative control of cell growth. *Oncogene* 17(25):3365–3383, 1998.

236. Bookstein R, Lee WH: Molecular genetics of the retinoblastoma suppressor gene. *Crit Rev Oncog* 2(3):211–227, 1991.

237. Chellappan S, Kraus VB, Kroger B, et al: Adenovirus E1A, simian virus 40 tumor antigen, and human papillomavirus E7 protein share the capacity to disrupt the interaction between transcription factor E2F and the retinoblastoma gene product. *Proc Natl Acad Sci U S A* 89(10):4549–4553, 1992.

238. Stommel JM, Wahl GM: Accelerated MDM2 auto-degradation induced by DNA-damage kinases is required for p53 activation. *EMBO J* 23(7):1547–1556, 2004.

239. Kubbutat MH, Jones SN, Vousden KH: Regulation of p53 stability by Mdm2. *Nature* 387(6630):299–303, 1997.

240. Eischen CM, Lozano G: P53 and MDM2: Antagonists or partners in crime? *Cancer Cell* 15(3):161–162, 2009.

241. Shadfan M, Lopez-Pajares V, Yuan ZM: MDM2 and MDMX: Alone and together in regulation of p53. *Transl Cancer Res* 1(2):88–89, 2012.

242. Bouska A, Eischen CM: Mdm2 affects genome stability independent of p53. *Cancer Res* 69(5):1697–1701, 2009.

243. Roth J, Dobbelstein M, Freedman DA, et al: Nucleo-cytoplasmic shuttling of the hdm2 oncoprotein regulates the levels of the p53 protein via a pathway used by the human immunodeficiency virus rev protein. *EMBO J* 17(2):554–564, 1998.

244. Li YC, Wahl GM: What a difference a phosphate makes: Life or death decided by a single amino acid in MDM2. *Cancer Cell* 21(5):595–596, 2012.

245. Quelle DE, Zindy F, Ashmun RA, Sherr CJ: Alternative reading frames of the INK4a tumor suppressor gene encode two unrelated proteins capable of inducing cell cycle arrest. *Cell* 83(6):993–1000, 1995.

246. Stirewalt DL, Kopecky KJ, Meshinchi S, et al: FLT3, RAS, and TP53 mutations in elderly patients with acute myeloid leukemia. *Blood* 97(11):3589–3595, 2001.

247. Faderl S, Kantarjian HM, Estey E, et al: The prognostic significance of p16(INK4a)/p14(ARF) locus deletion and MDM-2 protein expression in adult acute myelogenous leukemia. *Cancer* 89(9):1976–1982, 2000.

248. Kojima K, Konopleva M, Samudio IJ, et al: MDM2 antagonists induce p53-dependent apoptosis in AML: Implications for leukemia therapy. *Blood* 106(9):3150–3159, 2005.

249. Kojima K, Konopleva M, Samudio IJ, et al: Concomitant inhibition of MDM2 and Bcl-2 protein function synergistically induce mitochondrial apoptosis in AML. *Cell Cycle* 5(23):2778–2786, 2006.

250. Zhang W, Konopleva M, Burks JK, et al: Blockade of mitogen-activated protein kinase/extracellular signal-regulated kinase kinase and murine double minute synergistically induces Apoptosis in acute myeloid leukemia via BH3-only proteins Puma and Bim. *Cancer Res* 70(6):2424–2434, 2010.

251. Kojima K, Konopleva M, Samudio IJ, et al: Mitogen-activated protein kinase kinase inhibition enhances nuclear proapoptotic function of p53 in acute myelogenous leukemia cells. *Cancer Res* 67(7):3210–3219, 2007.

252. Kojima K, Shimanuki M, Shikami M, et al: Cyclin-dependent kinase 1 inhibitor RO-3306 enhances p53-mediated Bax activation and mitochondrial apoptosis in AML. *Cancer Sci* 100(6):1128–1136, 2009.

253. Carter BZ, Mak DH, Schober WD, et al: Simultaneous activation of p53 and inhibition of XIAP enhance the activation of apoptosis signaling pathways in AML. *Blood* 115(2):306–314, 2010.

254. Kojima K, McQueen T, Chen Y, et al: p53 activation of mesenchymal stromal cells partially abrogates microenvironment-mediated resistance to FLT3 inhibition in AML through HIF-1alpha-mediated down-regulation of CXCL12. *Blood* 118(16):4431–4439, 2011.

255. Kojima K, Konopleva M, Tsao T, et al: Selective FLT3 inhibitor FI-700 neutralizes Mcl-1 and enhances p53-mediated apoptosis in AML cells with activating mutations of FLT3 through Mcl-1/Noxa axis. *Leukemia* 24(1):33–43, 2010.

256. Kojima K, Kornblau SM, Ruvolo V, et al: Prognostic impact and targeting of CRM1 in acute myeloid leukemia. *Blood* 121(20):4166–4174, 2013.

257. Kamijo T, Zindy F, Roussel MF, et al: Tumor suppression at the mouse INK4a locus mediated by the alternative reading frame product p19ARF. *Cell* 91(5):649–659, 1997.

258. Bates S, Phillips AC, Clark PA, et al: p14ARF links the tumour suppressors RB and p53. *Nature* 395(6698):124–125, 1998.

259. Palmero I, Pantoja C, Serrano M: P19ARF links the tumour suppressor p53 to Ras. *Nature* 395(6698):125–126, 1998.

260. Prives C: Signaling to p53: Breaking the MDM2-p53 circuit. *Cell* 95(1):5–8, 1998.

261. Sherr CJ: Tumor surveillance via the ARF-p53 pathway. *Genes Dev* 12(19):2984–2991, 1998.

262. Kurz EU, Lees-Miller SP: DNA damage-induced activation of ATM and ATM-dependent signaling pathways. *DNA Repair (Amst)* 3(8–9):889–900, 2004.

263. Senoo M, Manis JP, Alt FW, McKeon F: P63 and p73 are not required for the development and p53-dependent apoptosis of T cells. *Cancer Cell* 6(1):85–89, 2004.

264. Deyoung MP, Ellisen LW: P63 and p73 in human cancer: Defining the network. *Oncogene* 26(36):5169–5183, 2007.

265. Di Como CJ, Gaiddon C, Prives C: P73 function is inhibited by tumor-derived p53 mutants in mammalian cells. *Mol Cell Biol* 19(2):1438–1449, 1999.

266. Melino G, Lu X, Gasco M, et al: Functional regulation of p73 and p63: Development and cancer. *Trends Biochem Sci* 28(12):663–670, 2003.

267. Kawano S, Miller CW, Gombart AF, et al: Loss of p73 gene expression in leukemias/lymphomas due to hypermethylation. *Blood* 94(3):1113–1120, 1999.

268. Olopade OI, Jenkins RB, Ransom DT, et al: Molecular analysis of deletions of the short arm of chromosome 9 in human gliomas. *Cancer Res* 52(9):2523–2529, 1992.

269. Schmid M, Malicki D, Nobori T, et al: Homozygous deletions of methylthioadenosine phosphorylase (MTAP) are more frequent than p16INK4A (CDKN2) homozygous deletions in primary non-small cell lung cancers (NSCLC). *Oncogene* 17(20):2669–2675, 1998.

270. Stadler WM, Olopade OI: The 9p21 region in bladder cancer cell lines: Large homozygous deletion inactivate the CDKN2, CDKN2B and MTAP genes. *Urol Res* 24(4):239–244, 1996.

271. Gonzalez MV, Pello MF, Lopez-Larrea C, et al: Deletion and methylation of the tumour suppressor gene p16/CDKN2 in primary head and neck squamous cell carcinoma. *J Clin Pathol* 50(6):509–512, 1997.

272. Yamada Y, Hatta Y, Murata K, et al: Deletions of p15 and/or p16 genes as a poor-prognosis factor in adult T-cell leukemia. *J Clin Oncol* 15(5):1778–1785, 1997.

273. Hori Y, Hori H, Yamada Y, et al: The methylthioadenosine phosphorylase gene is frequently co-deleted with the p16INK4a gene in acute type adult T-cell leukemia. *Int J Cancer* 75(1):51–56, 1998.

274. Kratzke RA, Otterson GA, Lincoln CE, et al: Immunohistochemical analysis of the p16INK4 cyclin-dependent kinase inhibitor in malignant mesothelioma. *J Natl Cancer Inst* 87(24):1870–1875, 1995.

275. Cayuela JM, Gardie B, Sigaux F: Disruption of the multiple tumor suppressor gene MTS1/p16(INK4a)/CDKN2 by illegitimate V(D)J recombinase activity in T-cell acute lymphoblastic leukemias. *Blood* 90(9):3720–3726, 1997.

276. Becker TM, Haferkamp S, Dijkstra MK, et al: The chromatin remodelling factor BRG1 is a novel binding partner of the tumor suppressor p16INK4a. *Mol Cancer* 8:4, 2009.

277. Christopher SA, Diegelman P, Porter CW, Kruger WD: Methylthioadenosine phosphorylase, a gene frequently codeleted with p16(cdkN2a/ARF), acts as a tumor suppressor in a breast cancer cell line. *Cancer Res* 62(22):6639–6644, 2002.

278. Lan L, Trempus C, Gilmour SK: Inhibition of ornithine decarboxylase (ODC) decreases tumor vascularization and reverses spontaneous tumors in ODC/Ras transgenic mice. *Cancer Res* 60(20):5696–5703, 2000.

279. Subhi AL, Diegelman P, Porter CW, et al: Methylthioadenosine phosphorylase regulates ornithine decarboxylase by production of downstream metabolites. *J Biol Chem* 278(50):49868–49873, 2003.

280. Stevens AP, Spangler B, Wallner S, et al: Direct and tumor microenvironment mediated influences of 5′-deoxy-5′-(methylthio)adenosine on tumor progression of malignant melanoma. *J Cell Biochem* 106(2):210–219, 2009.

281. Jaffrain-Rea ML, Ferretti E, Toniato E, et al: p16 (INK4a, MTS-1) gene polymorphism and methylation status in human pituitary tumours. *Clin Endocrinol (Oxf)* 51(3):317–325, 1999.

282. Baylin SB, Herman JG, Graff JR, et al: Alterations in DNA methylation: A fundamental aspect of neoplasia. *Adv Cancer Res* 72:141–196, 1998.

283. Boultwood J, Wainscoat JS: Gene silencing by DNA methylation in haematological malignancies. *Br J Haematol* 138(1):3–11, 2007.

284. Timmermann S, Hinds PW, Munger K: Re-expression of endogenous p16ink4a in oral squamous cell carcinoma lines by 5-aza-2′-deoxycytidine treatment induces a senescence-like state. *Oncogene* 17(26):3445–3453, 1998.

285. Hennessy BT, Garcia-Manero G, Kantarjian HM, Giles FJ: DNA methylation in haematological malignancies: The role of decitabine. *Expert Opin Investig Drugs* 12(12):1985–1993, 2003.

286. Silverman LR, Demakos EP, Peterson BL, et al: Randomized controlled trial of azacitidine in patients with the myelodysplastic syndrome: A study of the cancer and leukemia group B. *J Clin Oncol* 20(10):2429–2440, 2002.

287. Kantarjian H, Issa JP, Rosenfeld CS, et al: Decitabine improves patient outcomes in myelodysplastic syndromes: Results of a phase III randomized study. *Cancer* 106(8):1794–1803, 2006.

288. Fenaux P, Mufti GJ, Hellstrom-Lindberg E, et al: Efficacy of azacitidine compared with that of conventional care regimens in the treatment of higher-risk myelodysplastic syndromes: A randomised, open-label, phase III study. *Lancet Oncol* 10(3):223–232, 2009.

289. Blum W, Garzon R, Klisovic RB, et al: Clinical response and miR-29b predictive significance in older AML patients treated with a 10-day schedule of decitabine. *Proc Natl Acad Sci U S A* 107(16):7473–7478, 2010.

290. Fenaux P, Mufti GJ, Hellstrom-Lindberg E, et al: Azacitidine prolongs overall survival compared with conventional care regimens in elderly patients with low bone marrow blast count acute myeloid leukemia. *J Clin Oncol* 28(4):562–569, 2010.

291. Kantarjian HM, Thomas XG, Dmoszynska A, et al: Multicenter, randomized, open-label, phase III trial of decitabine versus patient choice, with physician advice, of either supportive care or low-dose cytarabine for the treatment of older patients with newly diagnosed acute myeloid leukemia. *J Clin Oncol* 30(21):2670–2677, 2012.

292. Xiong J, Epstein RJ: Growth inhibition of human cancer cells by 5-aza-2′-deoxycytidine does not correlate with its effects on INK4a/ARF expression or initial promoter methylation status. *Mol Cancer Ther* 8(4):779–785, 2009.

293. Razin A: CpG methylation, chromatin structure and gene silencing-a three-way connection. *EMBO J* 17(17):4905–4908, 1998.

294. Jones PL, Veenstra GJ, Wade PA, et al: Methylated DNA and MeCP2 recruit histone deacetylase to repress transcription. *Nat Genet* 19(2):187–191, 1998.

295. Bueno MJ, Perez de Castro I, Malumbres M: Control of cell proliferation pathways by microRNAs. *Cell Cycle* 7(20):3143–3148, 2008.

296. Vigushin DM, Coombes RC: Histone deacetylase inhibitors in cancer treatment. *Anticancer Drugs* 13(1):1–13, 2002.

297. Thiagalingam S, Cheng KH, Lee HJ, et al: Histone deacetylases: Unique players in shaping the epigenetic histone code. *Ann N Y Acad Sci* 983:84–100, 2003.

298. Haberland M, Montgomery RL, Olson EN: The many roles of histone deacetylases in development and physiology: Implications for disease and therapy. *Nat Rev Genet* 10(1):32–42, 2009.

299. Wang J, Saunthararajah Y, Redner RL, Liu JM: Inhibitors of histone deacetylase relieve ETO-mediated repression and induce differentiation of AML1-ETO leukemia cells. *Cancer Res* 59(12):2766–2769, 1999.

300. Zhou W, Zhu WG: The changing face of HDAC inhibitor depsipeptide. *Curr Cancer Drug Targets* 9(1):91–100, 2009.

301. San-Miguel JF, Hungria VT, Yoon SS, et al: Panobinostat plus bortezomib and dexamethasone versus placebo plus bortezomib and dexamethasone in patients with relapsed or relapsed and refractory multiple myeloma: A multicentre, randomised, double-blind phase 3 trial. *Lancet Oncol* 15(11):1195–1206, 2014.

302. Kramer OH, Zhu P, Ostendorff HP, et al: The histone deacetylase inhibitor valproic acid selectively induces proteasomal degradation of HDAC2. *EMBO J* 22(13):3411–3420, 2003.

303. McBride WH, Iwamoto KS, Syljuasen R, et al: The role of the ubiquitin/proteasome system in cellular responses to radiation. *Oncogene* 22(37):5755–5773, 2003.

304. Richardson PG, Mitsiades C, Hideshima T, Anderson KC: Proteasome inhibition in the treatment of cancer. *Cell Cycle* 4(2):290–296, 2005.

305. Kouroukis TC, Baldassarre FG, Haynes AE, et al: Bortezomib in multiple myeloma: Systematic review and clinical considerations. *Curr Oncol* 21(4):e573–e603, 2014.

306. Bose P, Batalo MS, Holkova B, Grant S: Bortezomib for the treatment of non-Hodgkin's lymphoma. *Expert Opin Pharmacother* 15(16):2443–2459, 2014.

307. Kortuem KM, Stewart AK: Carfilzomib. *Blood* 121(6):893–897, 2013.

308. Elliott PJ, Ross JS: The proteasome: A new target for novel drug therapies. *Am J Clin Pathol* 116(5):637–646, 2001.

309. Pei XY, Dai Y, Grant S: Synergistic induction of oxidative injury and apoptosis in human multiple myeloma cells by the proteasome inhibitor bortezomib and histone deacetylase inhibitors. *Clin Cancer Res* 10(11):3839–3852, 2004.

310. Wu ZH, Shi Y, Tibbetts RS, Miyamoto S: Molecular linkage between the kinase ATM and NF-kappaB signaling in response to genotoxic stimuli. *Science* 311(5764):1141–1146, 2006.

311. Volcic M, Karl S, Baumann B, et al: NF-kappaB regulates DNA double-strand break repair in conjunction with BRCA1-CtIP complexes. *Nucleic Acids Res* 40(1):181–195, 2012.

312. Rajkumar SV, Richardson PG, Hideshima T, Anderson KC: Proteasome inhibition as a novel therapeutic target in human cancer. *J Clin Oncol* 23(3):630–639, 2005.

CHAPTER 17
SIGNAL TRANSDUCTION PATHWAYS

Kenneth Kaushansky

SUMMARY

Most external influences upon cells of any organ are mediated by biochemical and molecular mechanisms that are triggered by interactions with membrane, cytoplasmic, or nuclear receptors. Our understanding of the receptors and the intermediate molecules that couple them with cellular pathways that influence the proliferation, activation, differentiation, or survival of hematopoietic cells has expanded significantly. Proteins on the surface of blood cells that transmit vital information from the extracellular environment include single-pass, homodimeric, heterodimeric, and heterotrimeric transmembrane proteins that do, or do not, contain intrinsic kinase activity, but either way signal by inducing the tyrosine phosphorylation of a multitude of cytoplasmic proteins, seven transmembrane domain proteins that signal through G proteins, heterodimeric integrins that recruit large focal adhesions, and large families of heterodimeric proteins that induce serine and threonine phosphorylation. This chapter describes the receptors that influence blood cell production and function, the secondary mediators and the biochemical modifications they undergo to alert the cell to an external influence, the molecular mechanisms that allow for the coordination of multiple signals impacting a cell simultaneously, and the processes upon which they impact.

Acronyms and Abbreviations: AP2, adaptor protein-2; BCR, B-cell antigen receptor; BMP, bone morphogenic protein; CNTF, ciliary neurotrophic factor; CT-1, cardiotrophin-1; DD, death domain; DR, death receptor; EPO, erythropoietin; EPOR, erythropoietin receptor; ERK, extracellular response kinase; FADD, Fas-associated death domain; FAK, focal adhesion kinase; Gab, Grb binding; GH, growth hormone; GM-CSF, granulocyte-macrophage colony-stimulating factor; GPCR, G-protein-coupled receptor; HCR, hematopoietic cytokine receptor; IAP, inhibitors of apoptosis; IKK, I-κB kinase; IL, interleukin; IRS, insulin receptor substrate; ITAM, immunoreceptor tyrosine-based activation motif; ITIM, immunoreceptor tyrosine-based inhibitory motif; JAK, Janus family kinase; JNK, c-Jun N-terminal kinase; LIF, leukemia inhibitory factor; M-CSF, macrophage colony-stimulating factor; MAPK, mitogen-activated protein kinase; NR, nuclear receptor; OSM, oncostatin M; PI3K phosphoinositol 3′-kinase; PIAS, protein inhibitor of activated STATs; PIP, phosphoinositol phosphate; PKC, protein kinase C; PTP, protein tyrosine phosphatase; RACK, receptor for activated C kinase; RTK, receptor tyrosine kinase; SARA, SMAD anchor for receptor activation; SCID, severe combined immunodeficiency; SH2, Src homology 2; SOCS, suppressors of cytokine signaling; STATs, signal transducers and activators of transcription; SUMO, small ubiquitin-like modifier; TGF, transforming growth factor; TM, transmembrane; TNF, tumor necrosis factor; TRADD, TNF receptor death domain; TRAF, TNF receptor-associated factor; TRAIL, tumor necrosis factor-related apoptosis-inducing ligand.

● AN OVERVIEW OF CELL SIGNALING

Blood cells and their marrow-based progenitors are exquisitely responsive to their environment. A wide variety of cues are detected by mature blood cells that impact significantly on their function. For example, leukocytes respond to noxious stimuli by chemokine-induced migration toward inflammatory stimuli, cross endothelial cell barriers and the extracellular matrix by engaging integrins, and then respond to chemotactic gradients to enter inflammatory foci to contact and engulf microorganisms on encountering bacterial products. Likewise, platelets adhere to reactive endothelial surfaces or denuded subendo-thelial cell matrix by engagement of extracellular adhesive proteins. Adherent platelets can also recruit additional platelets and aggregate with them through interactions with platelet integrins, secrete growth factors that will recruit cells that mediate repair of vascular injury and then contract to strengthen the platelet plug by engagement of numerous granule substances. Even the anucleate erythrocyte responds to mechanical deformation and hypoxemia with adenosine triphosphate (ATP) release. Adrenergic receptors also play important roles in the normal erythrocyte response to parasitic infection or in the pathologic red cell's interactions with endothelial cell surfaces (e.g., patients with hemoglobinopathies). Each of these events induces an intracellular signal that leads to further cellular reactivity toward the initiating stimulus, or that prepares the cell for subsequent functional events. Like the functional activation of mature blood cells, the generation of blood cells is under tight regulation, mediated by soluble hematopoietic growth factors, cytokines, and components of the marrow microenvironment. Here again, the erythropoietin (EPO) response to anemia is sensed by erythroid progenitor cell surface receptors; their coordinated reaction involves a myriad of signals that impact on the survival, growth, and differentiation of both undifferentiated and lineage-committed cells. Although anemia induces red cell production and inflammation leads to the production and functional activation of leukocytes, many of the intracellular signals that mediate these two responses overlap substantially. This chapter illuminates a number of principles that mediate the growth and functional responses of blood cells and their progenitors in health and disease. A better understanding of how blood cells respond to their environment can lead to improved strategies to intervene in pathologic processes in which too many or too few blood cells are produced, or in which the functional activation of blood cells is insufficient or overly exuberant and leads to disease. Moreover, a thorough knowledge of how the signaling pathways that mediate growth and cell survival are disrupted in the hematologic malignancies has begun to allow the rational intervention in such diseases.

● TYPES OF RECEPTORS AND THEIR MECHANISMS OF ACTIVATION

THE HEMATOPOIETIC CYTOKINE RECEPTOR FAMILY

The Erythropoietin Receptor

The erythropoietin receptor (EPOR) was cloned in 1989,[1] settling several controversies and setting many important paradigms in receptor biology. Like other hematopoietic cytokines of this class (granulocyte colony-stimulating factor [G-CSF], thrombopoietin [TPO], and growth hormone [GH]), EPO binds to a homodimeric receptor[2,3] with picomolar affinity.[4] Numerous studies in these and multiple other cell-signaling systems demonstrate the importance of phosphorylation of vital cytoplasmic mediators in signal transduction,[5-7] yet one initial conundrum was that the cloned EPOR bears no kinase domain.[1] Rather, subsequent

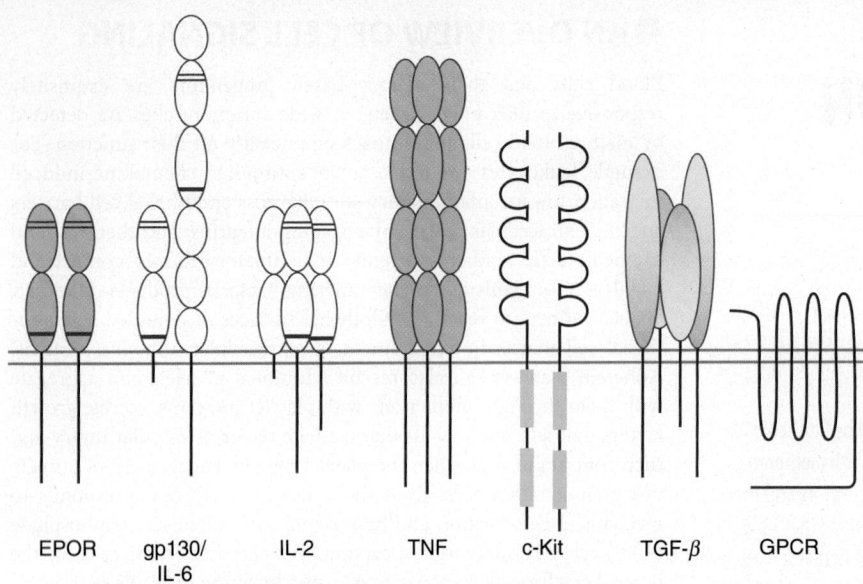

Figure 17–1. An illustration of cell surface receptors. Each member of the cell surface receptors is depicted as an extracellular region of one or multiple domains, with conserved disulfide bonds indicated by *thin cross lines,* and the conserved WS box indicated by a *thick cross line.* The founding member of each receptor class is indicated. EPOR, erythropoietin receptor; GPCR, G-protein–coupled receptor; gp130, glycoprotein 130; IL, interleukin; TGF, transforming growth factor; TNF, tumor necrosis factor. Each receptor subunit illustrated is a single-pass transmembrane protein with the exception of the heptahelical GPCR.

EPOR   gp130/   IL-2   TNF   c-Kit   TGF-*β*   GPCR
            IL-6

studies revealed that the EPOR employs a cytoplasmic kinase of the Janus family (JAK) to initiate signaling.[8] JAK kinases bind to the cytoplasmic domain of hematopoietic receptors through motifs termed *Box1* and *Box2* domains. This information, along with the availability of the tertiary structure of EPOR and of EPO bound to EPOR,[9,10] has provided a key insight into the initiation of signal transduction. EPOR exists as a preformed cell surface dimer (Fig. 17–1), in a conformation that separates the two cytoplasmic domains of the subunits (and hence the two tethered JAK molecules). EPO binds sequentially to the two subunits of the preformed EPOR dimer at two distinct faces of the molecule, first to one subunit with the high-affinity face of the ligand (also termed *site I*), and then to the second subunit of EPOR with a lower-affinity face (termed *site II*), but an interaction that reduces the off-rate of the ligand. Upon engagement of the two EPOR subunits, a conformational change ensues, shifting the distance between the two cytoplasmic domains of the receptor subunits, that is thought to bring the two inactive JAK molecules into sufficiently close juxtaposition to allow cross-phosphorylation and kinase activation. Once the two tethered JAK molecules are active, multiple additional tyrosine residues become phosphorylated, residues of the receptor itself and those on a number of tethered signaling molecules, events that trigger the totality of cellular EPO responses. Although direct proof for this model of signal initiation is not available for other cytokine receptors of this class, it is widely assumed that a variety of growth factors, interleukins, and hormones activate cellular events in the same manner.

The understanding that a single molecule of EPO can bind simultaneously to two EPOR molecules, and the realization that multiple other cytokines employ a similar stoichiometry of activation has allowed for therapeutic engineering of cytokines into peptide and chemical receptor antagonists. Following EPO binding to a first molecule of EPOR through site I, the receptor conformational change becomes dependent on binding of EPO site II to a second EPOR subunit. By altering the residues at site II, it is possible to block binding at site II, and hence block receptor activation. If site I is altered to increase its affinity for binding to a first receptor subunit so that the affinity of the mutant protein rivals that of the intact molecule, a potent rationally designed antagonist is generated. This strategy has been successfully employed to create pegvisomant, a GH antagonist useful for the treatment of acromegaly.

The engagement of two receptor subunits by a cognate ligand is one mechanism of inducing the receptor conformational change necessary for JAK activation, but several other mechanisms exist that have been exploited by man and nature. Small molecules and dimeric antibodies can induce signaling through the EPOR and at least for the former, can serve as EPO mimetics for therapeutic use.[11] Moreover, the 55-kDa glycoprotein (gp55) of the Friend erythroleukemia virus hijacks the EPOR for virus-induced proliferation[12] by directly binding to EPOR and (presumably) by inducing the same receptor conformational changes as induced by the authentic hormone. Thus, there are many ways to activate EPOR, and many subtleties dependent on the actual tertiary structural changes induced.[13]

The Interleukin-6 Receptor Family The interleukin (IL)-6 family of cytokine receptors displays several properties distinct from those of EPOR and its related receptors.[14] Unlike the receptors discussed thus far, the IL-6R family members are composed of a heterodimer. The α subunit of each receptor binds cognate ligand with modest affinity, but plays no role in signaling. Instead, a second receptor subunit, glycoprotein (gp)130 (named for its apparent molecular weight [Mr]), or oncostatin-M (OSM) receptor, molecules that alone have no affinity for ligand, but together with the α *subunit* enhance the binding affinity of the heterodimeric receptor, and are responsible for initiating signal transduction in the presence of ligand.[15] In addition, soluble forms of some of the receptors, such as IL-6R, if loaded with IL-6, can bind to cells bearing only gp130 and activate the latter.[16] Like EPOR and other members of that subfamily, gp130 and OSM-R engage JAKs to initiate signal transduction.[17] Moreover, it is almost certain that the mature IL-6R complex is composed of at least two molecules of IL-6R and two of gp130,[18] the latter required to bring the requisite two JAK molecules to the signaling complex. In addition to serving as signaling subunit for IL-6R, gp130 serves as the signaling receptor subunit for IL-11, OSM, leukemia inhibitory factor (LIF), ciliary neurotrophic factor (CNTF), cardiotrophin-1 and -2 (CT-1, CT-2), cardiotrophin-like cytokine (CLC), and IL-27, and OSM-R serves as a signaling subunit for OSM and IL-31. Similar to its role in the IL-6R, gp130 binds to each of these ligands only in the additional presence of a cytokine-specific receptor subunit (e.g., IL-11R, LIF-R) to form a complete signaling receptor. As a consequence of this shared coreceptor physiology, when two or more of the cytokine-specific receptors are present on a cell, the two corresponding ligands can compete for a limiting amount of gp130, and hence for cytokine-specific signaling. This physiology also allows therapeutically engineered cytokine-receptor complexes to stimulate signaling in all cells that express gp130.[19] Furthermore, the same principles that allow the rationale design of an EPO or GH antagonist can be used to engineer IL-6 antagonists for treatment of pathologic states dependent on interactions with receptors that require gp130 for receptor signaling.[20]

The Interleukin-2 Receptor Family The IL-2 family of receptors is also quite complex, in most cases sharing one, two, or three subunits with receptors for other cytokines of the same class (see Fig. 17–1). IL-2Rβ is shared with the IL-15R, and IL-2Rγ (also termed γ_C [for common]) is shared with the IL-4, IL-7, IL-9, IL-15, and IL-21 receptors.[21] Another feature of the IL-2R not yet discussed for the EPOR or IL-6R families is that of a devoted JAK. While JAK2 is employed by all the EPOR subfamily members along with some of the IL-6R subfamily members, and JAK1 and TYK2 are also shared amongst these latter receptors, the fourth and final JAK family member, JAK3, is engaged almost exclusively by γ_C (one study identified JAK3 activation by IL-8, implying use by the CXCR1 and/or CXCR2 receptors).[22] In addition to providing a more fundamental understanding of the principles of signal transduction, careful investigation of the IL-2 family of receptors also has afforded detailed insights into a number of clinically important immunodeficiency states.[23] The complexity of this family of receptors was illustrated by the progressive investigation into the origins of severe combined immunodeficiency (SCID).[24] As is discussed in Chap. 80, SCID is a severe loss of natural killer (NK) and T lymphocytes, and has been traced to deficiencies of either γ_C or JAK3, a phenotype recapitulated quite well (but not perfectly) by genetic elimination of the same molecules in mice. However, genetic elimination of IL-2 leads to a phenotype quite different than SCID of humans or engineered mice. Instead, of the multiple cytokines for which γ_C and JAK3 support signaling, only elimination of IL-7 or the IL-7R recapitulates the phenotype,[25,26] a finding now consistent with the finding that IL-7 affects common lymphoid progenitors (Chap. 18), while other cytokines in the family affect more differentiated lymphoid cells.

THE TUMOR NECROSIS FACTOR RECEPTOR SUPERFAMILY

At present the tumor necrosis factor (TNF) superfamily of receptors and ligands comprises at least 30 receptors and 20 ligands,[27,28] and illustrates several novel points in signal transduction pathways: trimeric binding (see Fig. 17–1), receptor promiscuity, and decoy receptors. Although many TNF ligand family members (TNF-α, TNF-β, CD40L [CD154], receptor activator of nuclear factor-κB ligand [RANKL; osteoprotegerin ligand (OPGL)], OX40L, etc.) can bind to several receptors, the ligands are, for the most part, subfamily specific. For example, TNF-α only binds to the six TNF-α receptors and TNF-related apoptosis-inducing ligand (TRAIL) binds to the five TRAIL receptors,[29] although it can also bind to the receptor termed *osteoprotegerin* (OPG). Ligands in this family bind as trimers to homotrimeric receptors, leading to recruitment of secondary signaling molecules to the cytoplasmic domain of the receptors. In general, there are two classes of cytoplasmic domains in these receptors, based on whether they contain the death domain (DD), a region capable of binding signaling mediators that initiate apoptosis (Chap. 15). As such, receptors that do not contain a DD or other signaling domain can function as "decoy receptors," diverting ligand from initiating programmed cell death in the target cell. For example, among the TNF-α receptors, TNFRI (death receptor [DR]2) contains a DD, and among the five TRAIL receptors, DR4 and DR5 contain DDs, whereas TNFR2 and DcR1 and DcR2 and OPG act as decoy receptors for TNF and TRAIL, respectively. The biologic consequences of ligand binding to individual TNFR family members depend on the relative affinity of their cytoplasmic domains for multiple adaptor proteins; TNF receptor death domain (TRADD) and Fas-associated death domain (FADD)

engagement trigger apoptosis pathways, whereas recruitment of one of the seven TNF receptor-associated factor (TRAF) family members leads to activation of transcription factors such as nuclear factor-κB (NF-κB) and kinases such as c-Jun N-terminal kinase (JNK) that lead to cell survival, proliferation, and activation of inflammation.

THE RECEPTOR TYROSINE KINASES

The receptor tyrosine kinases (RTKs) comprise another class of receptors that contains members vital for hematopoiesis and mature blood cell function (see Fig. 17–1). The first hematopoietic member of this family to be identified was the eukaryotic version of the *v-fms* oncogene, designated *c-fms*. Further study revealed that the protooncogene is the sole receptor for macrophage colony-stimulating factor (M-CSF),[31] and although somewhat distinct in possessing a split kinase domain, was immediately grouped with other RTKs, such as the receptors for insulin, vascular endothelial cell growth factor and epidermal growth factor, among several others. Subsequently, two additional hematopoietic receptor family members have been identified, c-Kit and Flt-3. These receptors were each cloned based on their homology to the viral oncogene *v-kit* or *c-fms*, respectively.[32,33] Like all other members of the family, upon engagement of their cognate ligand the kinase domains of homodimeric RTKs become activated, leading to the phosphorylation of receptor cytoplasmic domain tyrosine residues and other tethered substrates. In an apparent example of convergent evolution, like members of the hematopoietic cytokine receptor (HCR) family, RTKs were also found to employ JAKs in their signaling pathways[34]; as a result, many of the same secondary signaling pathways are activated by both classes of receptors. But perhaps serving as an even more striking example of convergent evolution, the tertiary structure of the index ligand for a hematopoietic RTK, M-CSF, bears substantial homology to essentially all the ligands of the HCR family, such as granulocyte-macrophage colony-stimulating factor (GM-CSF).[35]

TRANSFORMING GROWTH FACTOR β FAMILY

The transforming growth factor (TGF) receptor family consists of seven type I and five type II receptors that heterodimerize to form receptors for multiple TGF-β family members, including the TGF-β/activin/nodal and bone morphogenic protein (BMP) subfamilies. The precise stoichiometry of binding involves a ligand dimer, stabilized by disulfide and/or hydrophobic bonds, and two type I and two type II subunits (see Fig. 17–1); the tertiary structure of the complex has been carefully investigated.[36] Both type I and type II receptors contain an N-terminal ligand binding, transmembrane, and cytoplasmic ser/thr kinase domains; the type I receptors additionally contain a Gly/Ser (GS)-rich domain.[36] For TGF-β subfamily members, the type II subunit bears a high-affinity ligand binding site, which on TGF-β or activin engagement recruits type I receptors, bringing the two cytoplasmic domains into close juxtaposition, enabling the type II kinase to phosphorylate Ser residues on the type I receptor GS domain, thereby activating the type I kinase. Cell-surface-bound coreceptors also exist and aid in generating the signaling complex for TGF-β, but not activin or BMP ligands. For BMP family members, the type I receptor bears the high-affinity ligand binding site, such that BMP initially binds to type I receptor, with the type II subunit subsequently recruited to form the signaling complex. Once the two receptor kinases are activated, they recruit and phosphorylate the SMAD (Sma- and Mad-related protein) adaptor proteins, allowing their nuclear translocation and transcriptional activation. However, SMAD-independent TGF-β signaling pathways also exist.[37]

G-PROTEIN–COUPLED RECEPTOR FAMILY

Several molecules that play essential roles in blood cell development or function signal by engaging G-protein–coupled receptors (GPCRs), the largest family of cell surface receptors in organisms as diverse as yeast and humans, estimated to comprise approximately 1000 distinct gene products, or approximately 3 percent of the human genome. Also termed *serpentine* or *heptahelical receptors* (for their seven transmembrane domains that form four extracellular and three intracellular loops; see Fig. 17-1), GPCRs are so named because they use three small guanine nucleotide (or G)-binding proteins (Gα, Gβ, and Gγ) for signal transduction. In the unstimulated state, all three G proteins bind to the intracellular loops of the receptor. Individual ligands engage GPCR in one of many different ways. For example, small lipophilic molecules (e.g., epinephrine) bind to transmembrane (TM) domains of the receptor, disrupting the interactions between TM3 and TM6, leading to conformational changes that alter G-protein binding.[38] Other GPCRs use additional extracellular domains (e.g., the "Venus flytrap" domain)[39] to bind and dimerize receptors. Still others, which are engaged by proteases, are activated by protease cleavage of the receptor amino terminus, leading to the "unmasking" of a hexapeptide at the new amino terminus, which then interacts with one of the receptor extracellular or TM domains.[40] By each of these and other mechanisms a conformational change occurs in the GPCR, allowing monomeric Gα and dimeric G$\beta\gamma$ complexes to dissociate from the intracellular loops and each to engage secondary signaling pathways.[41] Examples of critical molecules that employ GPCRs and display hematologic activity are thrombin, adrenergic hormones, and chemokines. The outcomes of such engagement include cellular growth and survival, functional activation, and migration.

INTEGRINS AND OTHER ADHESION MOLECULES

Although adhesion molecules were named for the vital structural role they play in tissue cohesion, physically bridging cells in the marrow with each other and with extracellular matrix macromolecules, and at sites at which mature blood cells interact with the endothelium, engagement of blood and progenitor cell integrins and other adhesion molecules also generates vital cellular signals that affect their survival, proliferation, and functional activation.[42–44] In fibroblasts, cell adhesion is most clearly manifest at contact sites termed focal adhesions, and the signaling complexes that form on cytoplasmic domains of the integrins that support them are termed focal adhesion complexes.[45] Within such complexes are components of the actin cytoskeleton, kinases both specific for focal adhesions and several others found in other cytoplasmic sites,[46–48] and a number of scaffolding molecules upon which adhesion strengthening and signaling take place. Moreover, growth factor receptors functionally interact with integrins, adding to signaling complexity. Thus, adhesion molecules must also be considered as signaling receptors.

NUCLEAR RECEPTORS

Nuclear receptors (NRs) are nascent transcription factors that play a wide variety of roles in cellular physiology by binding small lipophilic hormones. Some NRs, such as glucocorticoid hormone receptors, remain sequestered in the cytoplasm in the absence of their cognate ligand, and upon ligand engagement translocate to the nucleus and bind and activate palindromic, direct repeat, or inverted palindromic sequences that comprise nucleotide hormone response elements.[49] Other NRs, such as receptors for vitamin A metabolites (retinoids), remain bound to nuclear DNA and repress transcription, until engaged by ligand upon which nuclear coactivators are recruited leading to enhancement of gene transcription.[50–52] Although sex, glucocorticoid, and thyroid hormones may play subtle roles in blood cell biology, retinoid receptors, which most commonly bind as heterodimers with the RXR receptor to retinoid response elements of the form PuGTTCA(N)2,5PuGTTCA, play vital developmental roles in a myriad of cell systems, and play similar roles in hematopoiesis. Amongst the hematopoietic targets of retinoid receptors are c-myc, C/EBPε, and p21.[53] However, because this class of receptors represents a nearly direct pathway from stimulus to response, without intervening signaling, they are not discussed further in this chapter.

THE DIVERSITY OF DOWNSTREAM SIGNALS

PROTEIN PHOSPHORYLATION

Protein phosphorylation is the critical first and vital response to engagement of signaling molecules of nearly all classes of cell surface receptors, including those that affect blood cell production and function. Numerous studies reveal that protein tyrosine phosphorylation is detectible within a minute of the addition of a wide variety of hematopoietic cytokines to blood cells and their progenitors. Evidence from nearly all studies employing chemical inhibitors of kinase function or various knockout and knockin strategies shows that JAK activation is critical for hematopoietic cell survival, growth, and differentiation, and mature cell response to a wide range of stimuli (Fig. 17–2).[54,55] Several studies have elucidated an important mechanism of regulation of JAK kinases, one that is altered in the myeloproliferative diseases polycythemia vera, essential thrombocytosis, and idiopathic myelofibrosis (Chaps. 84 to 86).

Based on homologies to a number of other proteins JAK kinases display 7 domains. These include (1) the domains that tether the kinase to the cytoplasmic domain of the cytokine receptor (JH3-JH7), (2) the kinase domain (JH1), and (3) a pseudokinase domain (JH2), so termed because of its homology to other tyrosine kinases but lack of kinase activity. Nevertheless, despite its lack of kinase activity, the pseudokinase domain inhibits the kinase activity of the kinase domain, as shown by single- and double-domain expression studies.[56] Based on the known structures of other kinases, the kinase and pseudokinase domains of JAK2 have been modeled.[57] Both structural and functional studies revealed that unexpectedly, the "pseudokinase" domain is, in fact, a kinase that phosphorylates two negative regulatory tyrosine residues, and suggests that the Val$_{617}$Phe mutation present in virtually all patients with polycythemia vera and approximately half with essential thrombocythemia and idiopathic myelofibrosis (Chaps. 84 to 86)[58–61] acts to stiffen the pseudokinase domain, altering its function.[57]

Among the phosphorylation targets of JAKs and other immediately responsive kinases in both normal and neoplastic hematopoiesis are the signaling receptor itself, adaptor molecules (Shc, Grb2, IRS, Gab, Tensin2) that once modified recruit additional signaling substrates, regulatory subunits of secondary kinases (p85 phosphoinositol 3′-kinase [PI3K]), latent transcription factors (signal transducers and activators of transcription [STATs]), and several phosphatases (SHP2, SHIP). By catalyzing the phosphorylation of Tyr residues present in certain receptor motifs, RTKs and JAK2 modify many signaling proteins to acquire the capacity to bind Src homology (SH)-2 domain-containing proteins. Perhaps equally important are ser/thr phosphorylation sites induced by activated TGF-β receptors. However, most of the downstream signaling components of all of the receptors that use JAK2 and other kinases to transduce growth and differentiation cues have been derived from candidate gene approaches; the availability of antibodies to specific signaling mediators has dictated the molecules that have been studied. An unbiased approach to identifying the entire "signaling space" used by all

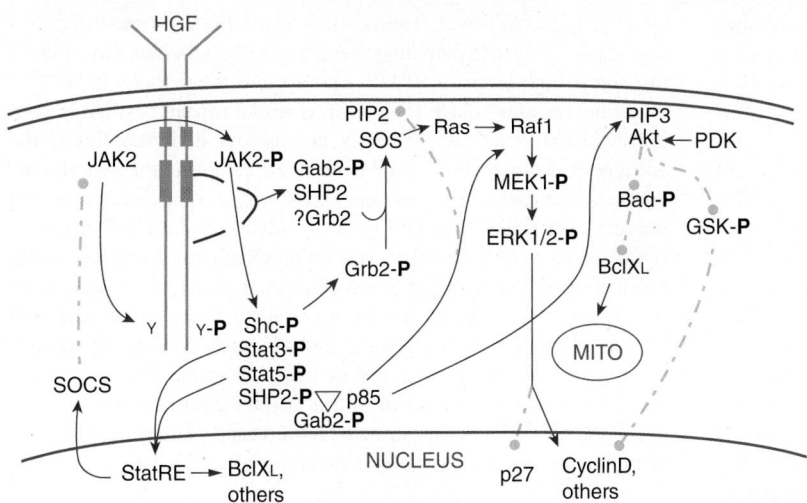

Figure 17–2. An illustration of signal transduction pathways. Signal transduction ensues when a hematopoietic growth factor (HGF) binds to its cognate receptor, resulting in a change in receptor conformation bringing two tethered JAK molecules into close proximity (attachment site to receptor is indicated by two *green boxes*, representing the box1 and box2 motifs). Molecules that become phosphorylated upon activation are indicated by **P**. A multiprotein complex that forms on a scaffolding molecule, such as Gab2, is indicated by the *triangle*. Stimulatory pathways (vis-à-vis cell proliferation) are indicated by *solid lines with arrowheads*. Inhibitory pathways are indicated by *broken lines with ball heads*. The nucleus and the mitochondria (MITO) are indicated.

of the receptors noted above is required if we are to fully understand the influence of the extracellular milieu on hematopoiesis. An example of such an approach has been reported.[63]

MEMBRANE LIPID MODIFICATION

Upon recruitment to a doubly phosphorylated receptor cytoplasmic domain or adapter protein, the p85 regulatory subunit of PI3K undergoes conformational changes enabling the binding of its p110 kinase subunit, resulting in activation of the kinase (see Fig. 17–2).[64] The major target of PI3K is membrane inositols, perhaps most importantly $PI_{4,5}$ phosphate (PIP2), converting the latter into $PI_{3,4,5}P$ (PIP3). Once present in adequate amounts, PIP3 recruits proteins with pleckstrin homology domains to the inner cytoplasmic membrane, which become phosphorylated by their juxtaposition to another PH domain containing kinase, PDK.[65] Among the best known of the recruited proteins are protein kinase B (also termed Akt), a kinase that phosphorylates a broad range of substrates in a wide variety of cells, all with the ultimate effect of enhancing cell survival and/or cell cycling.[66] For example, Akt phosphorylates Bad, a proapoptotic protein that once so modified is targeted for degradation.[67] Akt indirectly activates NF-κB,[67] a transcription factor that influences several cell-cycle and survival proteins,[68] including the antiapoptotic Bcl and IAP (inhibitors of apoptosis) proteins and the cell-cycle activators c-Myc and cyclin D. In addition, forkhead family members, which when present enhance transcription of cell-cycle inhibitors such as p27 and the proapoptotic protein Fas ligand, are phosphorylated and inactivated by Akt.[69] Akt is activated by the bcr-abl oncogene in blood cells of patients with chronic myelogenous leukemia (CML), as it is in patients with polycythemia vera, and blockade of PI3K reduces cell proliferation substantially.[70]

NUCLEAR TRANSLOCATION

In addition to the posttranslational modification of signaling molecules illustrated in the preceding examples, relocalization of signaling molecules is also a vital process that conveys information within the cell. This cellular strategy is well illustrated by the activation of NF-κB,[68] a family of transcription factors activated by growth factor, nuclear, TGF/BMP family, and integrin receptors that affect genes vital for cell survival and growth. In the unstimulated cell, NF-κB subunits reside in the cytoplasm, sequestered from their nuclear targets by virtue of its binding to I-κB. Upon cellular activation of Akt, I-κB kinase (IKK) is activated by phosphorylation, which then phosphorylates I-κB, thereby releasing

NF-κB and targeting I-κB for proteasomal destruction, allowing NF-κB to translocate to the nucleus and bind and activate target genes.

A second example of cytoplasmic sequestration blocking nuclear function involves the SMAD proteins that mediate TGF-β receptor signaling.[36] Once recruited to the phosphorylated type I TGF-β receptor, SMAD2 is phosphorylated, reducing its affinity for the SMAD anchor for receptor activation (SARA), a molecule that helps tether SMAD2 to the receptor. Once free of SARA, a SMAD2/SMAD4 complex forms, which is competent to translocate to the nucleus, either by the generation of a nuclear localization signal or because of the elimination of the SARA blockade of the SMAD2 nuclear pore complex interaction site. In addition to ingress, the formation of a SMAD2/SMAD4 complex also blocks a nuclear export signal present on the latter.[71]

ENGAGEMENT OF ADAPTOR PROTEINS

Another general theme to emerge from numerous studies on signal transduction is that multimolecular complexes of signaling intermediaries often assemble on scaffolding or adaptor proteins, which develop the capacity to assemble signaling complexes upon phosphorylation.[72] Insulin receptor substrates (IRSs) were the first such adaptors identified, and are phosphorylated by the activated insulin receptor.[73] IRS proteins are also modified by several other receptor-activated kinases, including JAKs.[54] Grb-binding (Gab) proteins are a family of at least three adapters, so named because of their ability to bind to the adaptor Grb2, a signaling intermediate necessary for Ras activation.[74] Both IRS and Gab proteins present multiple sites for phosphorylation, and once so modified present numerous SH2-binding and other protein–protein interacting motifs (see Fig. 17–2), which allow assembly of signaling complexes. Additional molecules serve this function in other signaling receptors, such as Tensin2 binding to the thrombopoietin receptor, c-Mpl,[63] which recruits p85 PI3K to the receptor, and paxillin binding on the cytoplasmic tails of α-integrin.[48] Paxillin presents four different types of protein–protein interaction domains (SH3, SH2, LD [Leu-Asp], and LIM [lin-11/Isl-1/Mec-3]) enabling it to bind downstream kinases (focal adhesion kinase [FAK], the related Pyk2 kinase, Src kinase, and paxillin-associated kinase [PAK]), other adaptor molecules (Crk, PIX, PKL), and phosphatases (PTP-PEST). As many cellular kinases can phosphorylate adaptor proteins (e.g., in addition to integrin engagement, GH binding leads to paxillin phosphorylation), such complexes can function as a nexus to coordinate multiple cellular stimuli into a concerted response.

Another example of the capacity of adaptor proteins to translate extracellular signals into intracellular physiologic change is found in the response to TNF ligands. The capacity of receptors that bear DDs to induce apoptosis is dependent on the binding of the adaptor protein FADD to the cytoplasmic domain of TNFR, which then recruits and activates the initiating caspases 8 and 10, leading to activation of the executioner caspases 3, 6, and 7 (Chap. 15).[28,29,75] This extracellular signal-mediated apoptotic pathway stands in contrast to a second, cell-intrinsic apoptosis pathway, in which DNA damage, cell-cycle checkpoint defects, or loss of survival factors leads to enhanced expression of proapoptotic bcl family members (bax, bad, bclXs, bid). Once proapoptotic proteins overcome the level of antiapoptotic family members (bc12, BclXL), mitochondrial TM potential declines, leading to leakage of cytochrome c and SMAC, the former engaging the apoptotic protease-activating factor (APAF) adaptor, thereby activating caspase 9 and, subsequently, the executioner family of caspases, the latter inhibiting members of the IAP family that otherwise attenuate caspase action. It should also be noted that although these two apoptosis pathways can be discussed as distinct entities, merging at the level of caspase 3, they interact. For example, activation of caspase 8 by TNF family members can also cleave bid to cause mitochondrial leakage of cytochrome c, thereby engaging the cell intrinsic pathway, serving to amplify the extracellular signal pathway to programmed cell death.

Binding of TNF family members to their receptors does not always result in apoptosis. Although there are likely many mechanisms for this finding, one is mediated by the binding of adaptors. Different TNF family receptors employ one of six TRAFs to engage and activate IKK, which leads to the release of NF-κB, a transcription factor that induces expression of several prosurvival and proliferation-associated genes.[68]

SIGNALING SPECIFICITY WITHIN EACH RECEPTOR FAMILY

Once a large number of receptor/cytokine systems were identified and tools to study some of their downstream signaling events developed, it became clear that most cytokine receptors stimulate a very similar cadre of signaling events as other members of the same family. For example, EPO, TPO, GH, GM-CSF, IL-6, and leptin all stimulate the phosphorylation of JAK2, yet lead to quite different cellular effects. One theory of hematopoiesis posits that growth factors merely serve to prevent apoptosis; the stochastic induction of one or another set of transcription factors is responsible for the distinct lineage differentiation events of hematopoiesis.[76] If this is true, then overlapping signaling events supported by a diverse range of cytokines might not be surprising as they would subserve the same end point, inhibition of programmed cell death. However, it is also clear that some cytokines and extracellular stimuli induce changes in critical transcription factors, and that the fate of multipotent progenitor cells can be influenced by the cytokines to which they are exposed; if so, each cytokine would need to induce distinct signals. Careful studies of signaling events have supported this hypothesis. For example, JAK3 is engaged only by cytokine receptors that use γ_C,[77] and although EPO activates the same JAK as TPO (JAK2), the former leads to activation of STAT5,[78] whereas the latter leads to STAT1, STAT3, and STAT5 activation,[79] which targets a different set of genes. Moreover, engagement of integrin $\alpha_5\beta_1$ stimulates EPO-induced erythroid development, whereas stimulation of integrin $\alpha_4\beta_1$ mediates signals that inhibit erythropoiesis and enhances TPO-induced megakaryocyte growth.[80,81] Additional examples of relative signaling specificity that separates sets of cytokines are the predominance of STAT5 activation by IL-2, compared with STAT1 and STAT3 by the closely related IL-21,[82] and the almost exclusive engagement of STAT4

by IL-12 and STAT6 by IL-4 and IL-13.[83] This same STAT-mediated "lineage choice" is seen in pathologic hematopoiesis. Individuals more likely to express high levels of STAT1 who acquire the pathologic Jak2^{V617F} mutation are more likely to develop essential thrombocythemia than polycythemia vera.[84] Consequently, because our understanding of the entirety of downstream signals is far from complete, the cytoplasmic domains of cytokine receptors bear almost no homology other than that required to engage JAKs, and there already exists a modest degree of signaling specificity, it is likely that although several cytokines engage overlapping sets of signaling intermediaries, each will result in a unique set of signaling events. It is almost certain that the use of unbiased screens of the entirety of signaling molecules will be required to decipher all the interactions induced by ligand engagement of the multiple receptor families described in this chapter. Such efforts have been described for the epidermal growth factor receptor family,[85] and should be highly informative in studies of hematopoietic signaling.

SIGNALING INSULATION

Many of the kinases and other intermediaries that play important roles in signal transduction are not absolutely substrate specific; nevertheless, they do participate in specific pathways free from interference from other pathways. Perhaps the best example of this is found in the mitogen-activated protein kinase (MAPK) pathway.[86] At least three major MAPK pathways operate in most cells, the p42/p44 ERK (extracellular response kinase), p38, and JNK, each of which is triggered by distinct stimuli (mitogens such as cytokines for ERK, inflammatory mediators and hypoxia for p38, and stress and noxious stimuli for JNK), but all of which eventuate in the activation of a cascade of kinases, a MAPK kinase kinase (also termed MEKK), which phosphorylates and activates a MAPK kinase (also termed a MEK), and finally the MAPK. The MAPKKK (MAP kinase kinase kinase) for ERK1/2 is Raf-1 and the MAPKK for ERK1/2 is MEK1; the MAPKKK for p38 is MEKK1 and the MAPKK is MKK3; and for JNK they are MEKK1 and MKK4 or MKK7, respectively. Because each of these kinases display only limited substrate specificity *in vitro*, it would be difficult to explain how MEKK1 activation does not lead to ERK activation without some mechanism to insulate the signals. Several scaffolding proteins have now been identified that assemble specific MAPKKK, MAPKK, and MAPKs.[87] By forming complexes of the cascade on pathway-specific scaffolding molecules, signaling integrity is preserved. Moreover, once the MAPK is activated, additional scaffolding molecules can link the specific MAPK to its target transcription factors.[88] Additional examples of "insulating" signaling scaffolds include those for NF-κB and the TNF receptor,[89] the B-cell antigen receptor (termed BLNK),[90] and protein kinase C (PKC) and integrins (termed RACKs).[91]

EXTINGUISHING SIGNALS

In addition to initiating signaling by extracellular ligands, the cell must also be able to extinguish the stimulus to prepare for additional events and to guard against continuous cell growth. Several mechanisms have been identified that extinguish the signals initiated by extracellular stimuli.

RECEPTOR DOWN-MODULATION

Shortly after binding to ligand, HCRs and RTKs are rapidly internalized,[92] serving to down-modulate further signaling.[93] Receptor internalization is dependent on membrane clathrin,[93] which represents a major mechanism of endocytosis of cell-surface proteins, and on at least one element of ligand-induced signaling.[94] The sites on hematopoietic receptors responsible for internalization are mapped,[95] potentially allowing intervention in this process. For example, activation of c-Mpl by TPO leads to engagement of the adaptor protein-2 (AP2) complex, which results in clathrin binding and receptor internalization. The kinetics of this process is delayed, taking approximately 30 minutes for near complete internalization, allowing the TPO signal to persist only a short time.[96]

PHOSPHATASES

As discussed earlier in "The Diversity of Downstream Signals," phosphorylation of numerous proteins and membrane lipids plays a vital role in signal transduction within the cell. Thus, elimination of these modifications through the action of phosphatases would be expected to terminate such signals. Moreover, because some of the same signals are activated in malignant transformation, protein tyrosine phosphatases (PTPs) might also be expected to play an important role in malignancy, and possibly in autoimmunity.

Hematopoietic cell phosphatase (also termed SHP1) bears two SH2 domains that interact with cytokine and inhibitory immune coreceptors at ITIM (immunoreceptor tyrosine-based inhibitory motif) sites that have been modified by Tyr phosphorylation. Once so engaged, SHP1 becomes activated and dephosphorylates associated phosphotyrosine activation sites on receptors, adaptor molecules, and their associated kinases.[97] One of the earliest clues that SHP1 plays an important role in hematopoietic signaling came from the discovery that the motheaten mouse phenotype is a result of a genetic loss of function of SHP1.[98] These mice demonstrate a massive expansion and tissue accumulation of monocytes and myeloid cells, resulting in chronic inflammation, massive immune defects, and premature death. Careful analysis of the mice revealed they manifest defective controls over the cellular activation and proliferation response to exogenous stimuli, such as that induced by engagement of the B-cell antigen receptor (BCR) complex. At steady state SHP1 is thought to engage the BCR (through presently unclear mechanisms) and maintains the antigen-binding subunits (immunoglobulin [Ig]α and Igβ) in a dephosphorylated, quiescent state. The phosphatase is displaced from the complex upon antigen engagement, but is later re-recruited to the complex once ITIM containing inhibitory coreceptors such as CD22, PIR-B, CD72, and FcγRIIb are phosphorylated and recruited to the activated complex.[99] Once recruited to the BCR complex, SHP1 removes the activating Tyr phosphate sites on the ITAM (immunoreceptor tyrosine-based activation motif) sites of Igα/β, the coreceptor CD19, the adaptor BLNK and Lyn kinase, and the BCR returns to its quiescent state. Similar roles for SHP1 have been identified in T cells,[100] NK cells,[101] monocytes and macrophages,[102] and erythroid cells.[103] The latter is of particular interest, as mutation of the site on EPOR to which SHP1 binds causes familial erythrocytosis, as a result of prolongation of EPO signaling. Of interest, this mutation was identified in a family containing a two-time Olympic gold medalist.[104]

SOCS Proteins

Another mechanism of growth factor signal termination is mediated by the suppressors of cytokine signaling (SOCS) proteins. The cloning of a STAT-inducible gene, *CIS*,[105] and several additional genes that bear substantial sequence homology,[106,107] yielded a family of proteins that can directly suppress growth factor receptor-induced signals. The engagement of either HCRs or RTKs leads to STAT activation, as discussed earlier in "The Diversity of Downstream Signals." One of the transcriptional targets of STATs are the SOCS and PIAS (protein inhibitor of activated STATs) genes (see Fig. 17–2), which, upon transcription and translation, bind to phosphotyrosine residues and inhibit either JAK kinases, STATs, or the phosphorylated receptors themselves, blocking

recruitment of signaling adaptor molecules.[108] Ubiquitin and SUMO (small ubiquitin-like modifier) also play a vital role in SOCS- and PIAS-mediated repression of cytokine signaling.[108] Like for the hematopoietic phosphatases, dysfunction of SOCS proteins has been implicated in malignancy.[109]

INHIBITORY SIGNALS

Finally, some signals negatively impact signals derived from other receptors. One example is the interaction of the growth inhibitory signals derived from TGF-β and the growth promoting signals triggered by several hematopoietic growth factors. TGF-β is constitutively expressed in the marrow stroma, and acts to reduce hematopoietic stem cell (HSC) cycling by driving the nuclear localization of a SMAD2–SMAD4 complex, which, in turn, is regulated by an inhibitable nuclear export signal present on the complex. Stem cell factor (SCF), FMS-like tyrosine kinase 3 (Flt-3) ligand, and TPO all induce promote HSC survival and growth, in part through activation of the MAPKs: ERK1 and ERK2. In turn, activated ERK1/2 then phosphorylates several sites on the linker region of SMAD2, inhibiting the nuclear localization of the inhibitory SMAD2/SMAD4 complex, reducing the suppressive effects of TGF-β on the cell cycle.[110] Another form of this type of crosstalk between cytokines is illustrated by TPO and interferon (IFN)-α, the latter suppressing megakaryopoiesis driven by the former. By induction of SOCS-1, not usually induced by TPO, IFN-α inhibits TPO-mediated signaling.[111]

● SIGNAL COORDINATION AND CROSSTALK

In the foregoing discussion, several examples of the convergence of signaling pathways and receptor crosstalk were summarized. Over the past decade, two types of cell membrane-based supramolecular organizations have been identified: lipid rafts and tetraspanin webs. In their seminal fluid–mosaic model of the cell membrane, Singer and Nicolson posited that integral membrane proteins float in a random array of membrane lipids.[112] This model was modified to account for local heterogeneity of the lipid bilayer. Lipid rafts, local concentrations of specific membrane lipids and proteins, are defined by the methods to isolate them—the insoluble components of a cold detergent extraction in which raft components "float" to the top of a density gradient.[113] Upon discovery that many of the proteins present in such rafts were involved in signal transduction, it became apparent that these membrane subdomains could represent a structural basis for communication between seemingly disparate components of the signal transduction apparatus.[37,114,115]

A second level of membrane-based structural organization of signaling molecules has been elucidated: the tetraspanin-enriched microdomain or "web." The tetraspanin family of membrane proteins is characterized by four TM domains punctuating two extracellular regions, a CCG motif, and several other conserved cysteine residues in the extracellular domain. The tetraspanins now include more than 30 members,[116] most or all of which interact with other cell surface molecules, and have been functionally linked to cell adhesion, migration, differentiation, and signal transduction. Members of this family are thought to act as molecular facilitators of protein–protein interaction by associating with "partners," the bimolecular complexes then interact with others in a slightly less avid manner, and the complexes loosely associate in microdomains. CD9, CD63, and CD81 are the tetraspanins most closely linked to hematopoietic cell function, are usually found in association with β_1 and β_3 integrins,[117] affect many hematopoietic cell types,[118–120] and act in concert with multiple signaling receptors, kinases, and phosphatases.[121,122]

REFERENCES

1. D'Andrea AD, Lodish HF, Wong GG: Expression cloning of the murine erythropoietin receptor. *Cell* 57:277, 1989.

2. Watowich SS, Hilton DJ, Lodish HF: Activation and inhibition of erythropoietin receptor function: Role of receptor dimerization. *Mol Cell Biol* 14:3535, 1994.

3. Livnah O, Stura EA, Middleton SA, et al: Crystallographic evidence for preformed dimers of erythropoietin receptor before ligand activation. *Science* 283:987, 1999.

4. Broudy VC, Lin N, Egrie J, et al: Identification of the receptor for erythropoietin on human and murine erythroleukemia cells and modulation by phorbol ester and dimethyl sulfoxide. *Proc Natl Acad Sci U S A* 85:6513, 1988.

5. Kanakura Y, Druker B, Cannistra SA, et al: Signal transduction of the human granulocyte-macrophage colony-stimulating factor and interleukin-3 receptors involves tyrosine phosphorylation of a common set of cytoplasmic proteins. *Blood* 76:706, 1990.

6. Spivak JL, Fisher J, Isaacs MA, et al: Protein kinases and phosphatases are involved in erythropoietin-mediated signal transduction. *Exp Hematol* 20:500, 1992.

7. Otani H, Erdos M, Leonard WJ: Tyrosine kinase(s) regulate apoptosis and bcl-2 expression in a growth factor-dependent cell line. *J Biol Chem* 268:22733, 1993.

8. Witthuhn BA, Quelle FW, Silvennoinen O, et al: JAK2 associates with the erythropoietin receptor and is tyrosine phosphorylated and activated following stimulation with erythropoietin. *Cell* 74:227, 1993.

9. Syed RS, Reid SW, Li C, et al: Efficiency of signalling through cytokine receptors depends critically on receptor orientation. *Nature* 395:511, 1998.

10. Cheetham JC, Smith DM, Aoki KH, et al: NMR structure of human erythropoietin and a comparison with its receptor bound conformation. *Nat Struct Biol* 5:861, 1998.

11. Wrighton NC, Farrell FX, Chang R, et al: Small peptides as potent mimetics of the protein hormone erythropoietin. *Science* 273:458, 1996.

12. Li JP, D'Andrea AD, Lodish HF, et al: Activation of cell growth by binding of Friend spleen focus-forming virus gp55 glycoprotein to the erythropoietin receptor. *Nature* 343:762, 1990.

13. Livnah O, Johnson DL, Stura EA, et al: An antagonist peptide-EPO receptor complex suggests that receptor dimerization is not sufficient for activation. *Nat Struct Biol* 5:993, 1998.

14. Taga T, Kishimoto T: Gp130 and the interleukin-6 family of cytokines. *Annu Rev Immunol* 15:797, 1997.

15. Cornelissen C, Juliane Lüscher-Firzlaff J, Malte Baron J, Lüscher B. Signaling by IL-31 and functional consequences. *Eur J Cell Biol* 91:552, 2012.

16. Jones SA, Rose-John S: The role of soluble receptors in cytokine biology: The agonistic properties of the sIL-6R/IL-6 complex. *Biochim Biophys Acta* 1592:251, 2002.

17. Stahl N, Boulton TG, Farruggella T, et al: Association and activation of Jak-Tyk kinases by CNTF-LIF-OSM-IL-6 beta receptor components. *Science* 263:92, 1994.

18. Pflanz S, Kurth I, Grotzinger J, et al: Two different epitopes of the signal transducer gp130 sequentially cooperate on IL-6-induced receptor activation. *J Immunol* 165:7042, 2000.

19. Baiocchi M, Marcucci I, Rose-John S, et al: An IL-6/IL-6 soluble receptor (IL-6R) hybrid protein (H-IL-6) induces EPO-independent erythroid differentiation in human CD34(+) cells. *Cytokine* 12:1395, 2000.

20. Adachi Y, Yoshio-Hoshino N, Nishimoto N. The blockade of IL-6 signaling in rational drug design. *Curr Pharm Des* 14:1217, 2008.

21. Waldmann TA: T-cell receptors for cytokines: Targets for immunotherapy of leukemia/lymphoma. *Ann Oncol* 11(Suppl 1):101, 2000.

22. Henkels KM, Frondorf K, Gonzalez-Mejia ME, et al. IL-8-induced neutrophil chemotaxis is mediated by Janus Kinase 3 (Jak3). *FEBS Lett* 585:159, 2011.

23. Leonard WJ: The molecular basis of X-linked severe combined immunodeficiency: Defective cytokine receptor signaling. *Annu Rev Med* 47:229, 1996.

24. Uribe L, Weinberg KI: X-linked SCID and other defects of cytokine pathways. *Semin Hematol* 35:299, 1998.

25. von Freeden-Jeffry U, Vieira P, Lucian LA, et al: Lymphopenia in interleukin (IL)-7 gene-deleted mice identifies IL-7 as a nonredundant cytokine. *J Exp Med* 181:1519, 1995.

26. Appasamy PM: Biological and clinical implications of interleukin-7 and lymphopoiesis. *Cytokines Cell Mol Ther* 5:25, 1999.

27. Ashkenazi A: Targeting death and decoy receptors of the tumour-necrosis factor superfamily. *Nat Rev Cancer* 2:420, 2002.

28. Aggarwal BB: Signalling pathways of the TNF superfamily: A double-edged sword. *Nat Rev Immunol* 3:745, 2003.

29. Wang S, El-Deiry WS: TRAIL and apoptosis induction by TNF-family death receptors. *Oncogene* 22:8628, 2003.

30. Cabal-Hierro L, Lazo PS: Signal transduction by tumor necrosis factor receptors. *Cell Signal* 24:1297, 2012.

31. Sherr CJ: The role of the CSF-1 receptor gene (C-*fms*) in cell transformation. *Leukemia* 2:132S, 1988.

32. Lyman SD, Jacobsen SE: c-Kit ligand and Flt3 ligand: Stem/progenitor cell factors with overlapping yet distinct activities. *Blood* 91:1101, 1998.

33. Broudy VC: Stem cell factor and hematopoiesis. *Blood* 90:1345, 1997.

34. Linnekin D: Early signaling pathways activated by c-Kit in hematopoietic cells. *Int J Biochem Cell Biol* 31:1053, 1999.

35. Pandit J, Bohm A, Jancarik J, et al: Three-dimensional structure of dimeric human recombinant macrophage colony-stimulating factor. *Science* 258:1358, 1992.

36. Shi Y, Massague J: Mechanisms of TGF-beta signaling from cell membrane to the nucleus. *Cell* 113:685, 2003.

37. Feng XH, Derynck R: Specificity and versatility in tgf-beta signaling through Smads. *Annu Rev Cell Dev Biol* 21:659, 2005.

38. Chen S, Lin F, Xu M, et al: Phe(303) in TMVI of the alpha(1B)-adrenergic receptor is a key residue coupling TM helical movements to G-protein activation. *Biochemistry* 41:588, 2002.

39. Bessis AS, Rondard P, Gaven F, et al: Closure of the Venus flytrap module of mGlu8 receptor and the activation process: Insights from mutations converting antagonists into agonists. *Proc Natl Acad Sci U S A* 99:11097, 2002.

40. Coughlin S: Protease-activated receptors in hemostasis, thrombosis and vascular biology. *J Thromb Haemost* 3:1800, 2005.

41. Slupsky JR, Quitterer U, Weber CK, et al: Binding of Gbetagamma subunits to cRaf1 downregulates G-protein-coupled receptor signalling. *Curr Biol* 9:971, 1999.

42. Levesque JP, Simmons PJ: Cytoskeleton and integrin-mediated adhesion signaling in human CD34+ hemopoietic progenitor cells. *Exp Hematol* 27:579, 1999.

43. Martin KH, Slack JK, Boerner SA, et al: Integrin connections map: To infinity and beyond. *Science* 296:1652, 2002.

44. Rose DM, Alon R, Ginsberg MH: Integrin modulation and signaling in leukocyte adhesion and migration. *Immunol Rev* 218:126, 2007.

45. Mitra SK, Schlaepfer DD: Integrin-regulated FAK-Src signaling in normal and cancer cells. *Curr Opin Cell Biol* 18:516, 2006.

46. Sastry SK, Burridge K: Focal adhesions: A nexus for intracellular signaling and cytoskeletal dynamics. *Exp Cell Res* 261:25, 2000.

47. Schwartz MA, Ginsberg MH: Networks and crosstalk: Integrin signalling spreads. *Nat Cell Biol* 4:E65, 2002.

48. Schaller MD: Paxillin: A focal adhesion-associated adaptor protein. *Oncogene* 20:6459, 2001.

49. Aranda A, Pascual A: Nuclear hormone receptors and gene expression. *Physiol Rev* 81:1269, 2001.

50. Mehta K: Retinoids as regulators of gene transcription. *J Biol Regul Homeost Agents* 17:1, 2003.

51. Ahuja HS, Szanto A, Nagy L, et al: The retinoid X receptor and its ligands: Versatile regulators of metabolic function, cell differentiation and cell death. *J Biol Regul Homeost Agents* 17:29, 2003.

52. Carlberg C: Current understanding of the function of the nuclear vitamin D receptor in response to its natural and synthetic ligands. *Recent Results Cancer Res* 164:29, 2003.

53. Collins SJ: Retinoic acid receptors, hematopoiesis and leukemogenesis. *Curr Opin Hematol* 15:346, 2008.

54. Ihle JN, Kerr IM: Jaks and Stats in signaling by the cytokine receptor superfamily. *Trends Genet* 11:69, 1995.

55. Parganas E, Wang D, Stravopodis D, et al: Jak2 is essential for signaling through a variety of cytokine receptors. *Cell* 93:385, 1998.

56. Saharinen P, Vihinen M, Silvennoinen O: Autoinhibition of Jak2 tyrosine kinase is dependent on specific regions in its pseudokinase domain. *Mol Biol Cell* 14:1448, 2003.

57. Silvennoinen O, Ungureanu D, Niranjan Y, et al: New insights into the structure and function of the pseudokinase domain in JAK2. *Biochem Soc Trans* 41:1002, 2013.

58. James C, Ugo V, LeCouedic JP, et al: A unique clonal JAK2 mutation leading to constitutive signaling causes polycythaemia vera. *Nature* 434:1144, 2005.

59. Baxter EJ, Scott LM, Campbell PJ, et al: Acquired mutation of the tyrosine kinase JAK2 in human myeloproliferative disorders. *Lancet* 365:1054, 2005.

60. Kralovics R, Passamonti F, Buser AS, et al: A gain-of-function mutation of JAK2 in myeloproliferative disorders. *N Engl J Med* 352:1779, 2005.

61. Levine RL, Wadleigh M, Cools J, et al: Activating mutation in the tyrosine kinase JAK2 in polycythemia vera, essential thrombocythemia, and myeloid metaplasia with myelofibrosis. *Cancer Cell* 7:387, 2005.

62. Kaushansky K: On the molecular origins of the chronic myeloproliferative disorders: It all makes sense. *Blood* 105:4187, 2005.

63. Jung AS, Kaushansky A, Macbeath G, Kaushansky K: Tensin 2 is a novel mediator in thrombopoietin (TPO)-induced cellular proliferation by promoting Akt signaling. *Cell Cycle* 10:1838, 2011.

64. Rameh LE, Cantley LC: The role of phosphoinositide 3-kinase lipid products in cell function. *J Biol Chem* 274:8347, 1999.

65. Vanhaesebroeck B, Alessi DR: The PI3K-PDK1 connection: More than just a road to PKB. *Biochem J* 346 Pt 3:561, 2000.

66. Chang F, Lee JT, Navolanic PM, et al: Involvement of PI3K/Akt pathway in cell cycle progression, apoptosis, and neoplastic transformation: A target for cancer chemotherapy. *Leukemia* 17:590, 2003.

67. Datta SR, Brunet A, Greenberg ME: Cellular survival: A play in three Akts. *Genes Dev* 13:2905, 1999.

68. Karin M, Lin A: NF-kappaB at the crossroads of life and death. *Nat Immunol* 3:221, 2002.

69. Tothova Z, Gilliland DG: FoxO transcription factors and stem cell homeostasis: Insights from the hematopoietic system. *Cell Stem Cell* 1:140, 2007.

70. Kawauchi K, Ogasawara T, Yasuyama M, et al: Involvement of Akt kinase in the action of STI571 on chronic myelogenous leukemia cells. *Blood Cells Mol Dis* 31:11, 2003.

71. Inman GJ, Nicolas FJ, Hill CS: Nucleocytoplasmic shuttling of Smads 2, 3, and 4 permits sensing of TGF-beta receptor activity. *Mol Cell* 10:283, 2002.

72. Pawson T, Scott JD: Signaling through scaffold, anchoring, and adaptor proteins. *Science* 278:2075, 1997.

73. White MF: The IRS-1 signaling system. *Curr Opin Genet Dev* 4:47, 1994.
74. Gu H, Neel BG: The "Gab" in signal transduction. *Trends Cell Biol* 13:122, 2003.
75. Micheau O, Tschopp J: Induction of TNF receptor I-mediated apoptosis via two sequential signaling complexes. *Cell* 114:181, 2003.
76. Cantor AB, Orkin SH: Hematopoietic development: A balancing act. *Curr Opin Genet Dev* 11:513, 2001.
77. Liu KD, Gaffen SL, Goldsmith MA, et al: Janus kinases in interleukin-2-mediated signaling: JAK1 and JAK3 are differentially regulated by tyrosine phosphorylation. *Curr Biol* 7:817, 1997.
78. Wakao H, Harada N, Kitamura T, et al: Interleukin 2 and erythropoietin activate STAT5/MGF via distinct pathways. *EMBO J* 14:2527, 1995.
79. Drachman JG, Sabath DF, Fox NE, et al: Thrombopoietin signal transduction in purified murine megakaryocytes. *Blood* 89:483, 1997.
80. Kapur R, Cooper R, Zhang L, et al: Cross-talk between alpha(4)beta(1)/alpha(5)beta(1) and c-Kit results in opposing effect on growth and survival of hematopoietic cells via the activation of focal adhesion kinase, mitogen-activated protein kinase, and Akt signaling pathways. *Blood* 97:1975, 2001.
81. Fox N, Kaushansky K: Engagement of integrin alpha 4 beta 1 but not alpha 5 beta 1 enhances thrombopoietin (TPO)-induced megakaryocyte (MK) growth. *Blood* 98:292a, 2001.
82. Habib T, Nelson A, Kaushansky K: IL-21: A novel IL-2-family lymphokine that modulates B, T, and natural killer cell responses. *J Allergy Clin Immunol* 112:1033, 2003.
83. Bacon CM, Petricoin EF 3rd, Ortaldo JR, et al: Interleukin 12 induces tyrosine phosphorylation and activation of STAT4 in human lymphocytes. *Proc Natl Acad Sci U S A* 92:7307, 1995.
84. Chen E, Beer PA, Godfrey AL, et al: Distinct clinical phenotypes associated with JAK2V617F reflect differential STAT1 signaling. *Cancer Cell* 18:524, 2010.
85. Jones RB, Gordus A, Krall JA, MacBeath G: A quantitative protein interaction network for the ErbB receptors using protein microarrays. *Nature* 439:168, 2006.
86. Cobb MH, Goldsmith EJ: How MAP kinases are regulated. *J Biol Chem* 270:14843, 1995.
87. Whitmarsh AJ, Davis RJ: Structural organization of MAP-kinase signaling modules by scaffold proteins in yeast and mammals. *Trends Biochem Sci* 23:481, 1998.
88. Lee CM, Onesime D, Reddy CD, et al: JLP: A scaffolding protein that tethers JNK/p38MAPK signaling modules and transcription factors. *Proc Natl Acad Sci U S A* 99:14189, 2002.
89. Soond SM, Terry JL, Colbert JD, et al: TRUSS, a novel tumor necrosis factor receptor 1 scaffolding protein that mediates activation of the transcription factor NF-kappaB. *Mol Cell Biol* 23:8334, 2003.
90. Chiu CW, Dalton M, Ishiai M, et al: BLNK: Molecular scaffolding through "cis"-mediated organization of signaling proteins. *EMBO J* 21:6461, 2002.
91. Besson A, Wilson TL, Yong VW: The anchoring protein RACK1 links protein kinase Cepsilon to integrin beta chains. Requirements for adhesion and motility. *J Biol Chem* 277:22073, 2002.
92. Yee NS, Langen H, Besmer P: Mechanism of kit ligand, phorbol ester, and calcium-induced down-regulation of c-kit receptors in mast cells. *J Biol Chem* 268:14189, 1993.
93. Vieira AV, Lamaze C, Schmid SL: Control of EGF receptor signaling by clathrin-mediated endocytosis. *Science* 274:2086, 1996.
94. Broudy VC, Lin NL, Liles WC, et al: Signaling via Src family kinases is required for normal internalization of the receptor c-Kit. *Blood* 94:1979, 1999.
95. Dahlen DD, Broudy VC, Drachman JG: Internalization of the thrombopoietin receptor is regulated by 2 cytoplasmic motifs. *Blood* 102:102, 2003.
96. Hitchcock I, Chen M, Fox NE, Kaushansky K: YRRL motifs in the cytoplasmic domain of the thrombopoietin receptor regulate receptor internalization and degradation. *Blood* 112:2222, 2008
97. Zhang J, Somani AK, Siminovitch KA: Roles of the SHP-1 tyrosine phosphatase in the negative regulation of cell signalling. *Semin Immunol* 12:361, 2000.
98. Tsui HW, Siminovitch KA, De Souza L, et al: Motheaten and viable motheaten mice have mutations in the haematopoietic cell phosphatase gene. *Nat Genet* 4:124, 1993.
99. Otipoby KL, Draves KE, Clark EA: CD22 regulates B cell receptor-mediated signals via two domains that independently recruit Grb2 and SHP-1. *J Biol Chem* 276:44315, 2001.
100. Pani G, Fischer KD, Mlinaric-Rascan I, et al: Signaling capacity of the T cell antigen receptor is negatively regulated by the PTP1C tyrosine phosphatase. *J Exp Med* 184:839, 1996.
101. Binstadt BA, Brumbaugh KM, Dick CJ, et al: Sequential involvement of Lck and SHP-1 with MHC-recognizing receptors on NK cells inhibits FcR-initiated tyrosine kinase activation. *Immunity* 5:629, 1996.
102. Kim CH, Qu CK, Hangoc G, et al: Abnormal chemokine-induced responses of immature and mature hematopoietic cells from motheaten mice implicate the protein tyrosine phosphatase SHP-1 in chemokine responses. *J Exp Med* 190:681, 1999.
103. Sharlow ER, Pacifici R, Crouse J, et al: Hematopoietic cell phosphatase negatively regulates erythropoietin-induced hemoglobinization in erythroleukemic SKT6 cells. *Blood* 90:2175, 1997.
104. Longmore GD: Erythropoietin receptor mutations and Olympic glory. *Nat Genet* 4:108, 1993.
105. Yoshimura A, Ohkubo T, Kiguchi T, et al: A novel cytokine-inducible gene CIS encodes an SH2-containing protein that binds to tyrosine phosphorylated interleukin 3 and erythropoietin receptors. *EMBO J* 14:2816, 1995.
106. Naka T, Narazaki M, Hirata M, et al: Structure and function of a new STAT-induced STAT inhibitor. *Nature* 387:924, 1997.
107. Starr R, Willson TA, Viney EM, et al: A family of cytokine-inducible inhibitors of signalling. *Nature* 387:917, 1997.
108. Wormald S, Hilton DJ: Inhibitors of cytokine signal transduction. *J Biol Chem* 279:821, 2004.
109. Inagaki-Ohara K, Kondo T, Ito M, Yoshimura A. SOCS, inflammation, and cancer. *JAK-STAT* 2:e24053, 2013.
110. Grimm OH, Gurdon JB: Nuclear exclusion of Smad2 is a mechanism leading to loss of competence. *Nat Cell Biol* 4:519, 2002.
111. Wang Q, Miyakawa Y, Fox N, et al: Interferon-alpha directly represses megakaryopoiesis by inhibiting thrombopoietin-induced signaling through induction of SOCS-1. *Blood* 96:2093, 2000.
112. Singer SJ, Nicolson GL: The fluid mosaic model of the structure of cell membranes. *Science* 175:720, 1972.
113. Brown DA, Rose JK: Sorting of GPI-anchored proteins to glycolipid-enriched membrane subdomains during transport to the apical cell surface. *Cell* 68:533, 1992.
114. Viola A, Schroeder S, Sakaikibara Y, et al: T lymphocyte costimulation mediated by reorganization of membrane microdomains. *Science* 283:680, 1999.
115. Sonnino S, Prinetti A: Membrane domains and the "lipid raft" concept. *Curr Med Chem* 20:4, 2013.
116. Hemler ME: Tetraspanin proteins mediate cellular penetration, invasion, and fusion events and define a novel type of membrane microdomain. *Annu Rev Cell Dev Biol* 19:397, 2003.
117. Cook GA, Longhurst CM, Grgurevich S, et al: Identification of CD9 extracellular domains important in regulation of CHO cell adhesion to fibronectin and fibronectin pericellular matrix assembly. *Blood* 100:4502, 2002.
118. Miyazaki T, Muller U, Campbell KS: Normal development but differentially altered proliferative responses of lymphocytes in mice lacking CD81. *EMBO J* 16:4217, 1997.
119. Clay D, Rubinstein E, Mishal Z, et al: CD9 and megakaryocyte differentiation. *Blood* 97:1982, 2001.
120. Anzai N, Lee Y, Youn BS, et al: C-kit associated with the transmembrane 4 superfamily proteins constitutes a functionally distinct subunit in human hematopoietic progenitors. *Blood* 99:4413, 2002.
121. Skubitz KM, Campbell KD, Iida J, et al: CD63 associates with tyrosine kinase activity and CD11/CD18, and transmits an activation signal in neutrophils. *J Immunol* 157:3617, 1996.
122. Kurita-Taniguchi M, Hazeki K, Murabayashi N, et al: Molecular assembly of CD46 with CD9, alpha3-beta1 integrin and protein tyrosine phosphatase SHP-1 in human macrophages through differentiation by GMCSF. *Mol Immunol* 38:689, 2002.

CHAPTER 18
HEMATOPOIETIC STEM CELLS, PROGENITORS, AND CYTOKINES

Kenneth Kaushansky

SUMMARY

Blood cell production is an enormously complex process in which a small number of hematopoietic stem cells expand and differentiate into an excess of 10^{11} cells each day. Based on a number of strategies available to the experimental hematologist a hierarchy of hematopoietic stem, progenitor, and mature blood cells is emerging in which each successive developmental stage loses the potential to differentiate into a specific type or class of cells. The characteristics of the stem and progenitor cells that give rise to the cells of the blood are the subject of this chapter, including the roles played by transcription factors and external signals in lineage fate determination, the cytokines and cell adhesion molecules that support cell survival, self-renewal, expansion, and differentiation, and the cell surface properties that allow for their purification, and biochemical and genetic characterization. A thorough understanding of hematopoietic stem and progenitor cells and their supportive microenvironment can provide critical insights into developmental biology of multiple cell systems, favorably impact blood cell development for therapeutic benefit, impact genetic therapy for a number of blood and other human diseases, and potentially provide the tools necessary to allow the regeneration of multiple organs.

Acronyms and Abbreviations: AGM, aorta-gonad-mesonephros; BFU-E, burst-forming unit–erythroid; BFU-MK, burst-forming unit–megakaryocyte; CAFC, cobblestone area-forming cell; CAR, CXCL12–abundant reticular; CFC, colony-forming cell; CFU-E, colony-forming unit–erythroid; CFU-GM, colony-forming unit–granulocyte-macrophage; CFU-MK, colony-forming unit–megakaryocyte; CLP, common lymphoid progenitor; CMP, common myeloid progenitor; EBF, early B-cell factor; ECM, extracellular matrix; EGF, epidermal growth factor; EPO, erythropoietin; EPOR, erythropoietin receptor; FAK, focal adhesion kinase; FL, Flt-3 ligand; G-CSF, granulocyte colony-stimulating factor; G-CSF-R, granulocyte colony-stimulating factor receptor; GM-CSF, granulocyte-macrophage colony-stimulating factor; GM-CSF-R, granulocyte-monocyte colony-stimulating factor receptor; GMP, granulocyte-macrophage progenitor; HSC, hematopoietic stem cell; Ig, immunoglobulin; IL, interleukin; IRF4, interferon regulatory factor 4; LEF, lymphoid-enhancer binding factor; LR, laminin receptor; LTC, long-term culture; LTC-IC, long-term culture-initiating cell; MAPK, mitogen-activated protein kinase; M-CSF, macrophage colony-stimulating factor; MEP, megakaryocyte-erythroid progenitor; MK, megakaryocyte; MSC, mesenchymal stem cell; PI3K, phosphoinositol 3′-kinase; R, receptor; RAG, recombination activating gene; ROS, reactive oxygen species; SCF, stem cell factor; SCL, stem cell leukemia; SDF-1, stromal-derived factor-1; SLAM, signaling lymphocyte activation molecule; TCF, T-cell factor; TGF, transforming growth factor; TPO, thrombopoietin; VCAM, vascular cell adhesion molecule; VLA, very-late antigen.

AN OVERVIEW OF HEMATOPOIESIS

Blood cell production is an enormous and complex process. Based on the adult blood volume (5 L), the number of each of the blood cell types per microliter of blood, and their circulatory half-life, it can be calculated that each day an adult human produces 2×10^{11} erythrocytes, 1×10^{11} leukocytes, and 1×10^{11} platelets. These numbers can all increase approximately 10-fold in states of blood cell destruction or enhanced need. Over the past four decades experimental hematologists have developed a model of blood cell production in which a hierarchical developmental progression of primitive, multipotential hematopoietic stem cells (HSCs) gradually lose one or more developmental potentials and ultimately become committed to a single cell lineage, which matures into the corresponding blood cell type.[1] Perhaps one of the most compelling arguments supporting this model of hematopoiesis is derived from extensive purification schemes using cell surface markers that yield cells at each predicted developmental stage (Fig. 18–1).[2] Although hematopoietic development is considered by most investigators as an irreversible stepwise and progressive loss of developmental potentials, studies now suggest that cells undergoing apparent differentiation steps might oscillate between different stages depending on their position in the cell cycle.[3] But regardless of the precise relationships between different stages of hematopoietic development, the availability of this model and the data leading to its construction have provided important insights into the biology and clinical uses of hematopoietic stem and progenitor cells. This chapter focuses on our understanding of the molecular basis for blood cell development, beginning with the HSC and its offspring, the lineage-committed progenitor cells.

DEVELOPMENTAL BIOLOGY OF HEMATOPOIESIS

Blood cell production begins in the yolk sac,[4] where extraembryonic mesoderm develops into angioblasts and primitive erythroid precursors at day 7 postcoitum of the mouse; cells of the outer layer of the undifferentiated mesoderm at this time flatten and become endothelial cells, and the inner cells round up to become clusters of erythroid precursors,[5] termed blood islands (Chap. 7). Like in the embryo proper, there is much evidence to suggest that these two cells are derived from a common precursor (the hemangioblast).[6] Once adjacent blood islands begin to coalesce on day 8, the endothelial cells form vascular channels, which by day 8.5 connect with the embryonic vasculature, allowing yolk sac blood cells to exit the blood islands, complete their maturation, and enucleate in the embryonic bloodstream.[7] In both mouse and man there is a stage of embryonic development where both primitive erythrocytes (as characterized by ζ globin phenotype) and definitive red cells are produced in the yolk sac, although the former appears only very transiently. Although not as well characterized, yolk sac myelopoiesis and thrombopoiesis also occur, perhaps as part of the development of multipotent progenitors that appear by day 8.5 postcoitum. Cells capable of differentiating into multiple cell lineages become recognizable early during yolk sac hematopoiesis.[8] However, such cells reproducibly engraft only in the marrow of myeloablated embryonic animals and not in adults,[9] making it unlikely that such cells are true HSCs, although this topic remains controversial. By day 11 postcoitum repopulating HSCs are clearly present in the yolk sac, but the relationship of these cells and the HSCs that are clearly demonstrable a day earlier in a region of the embryonic paraaortic splanchnopleure known as the aorta-gonad-mesonephros (AGM) is not certain. By day 12.5, postcoitum hematopoiesis in the murine yolk sac is eliminated.

Although it was long believed that the developmental origin of the adult mammalian hematopoietic system was the yolk sac, subsequent

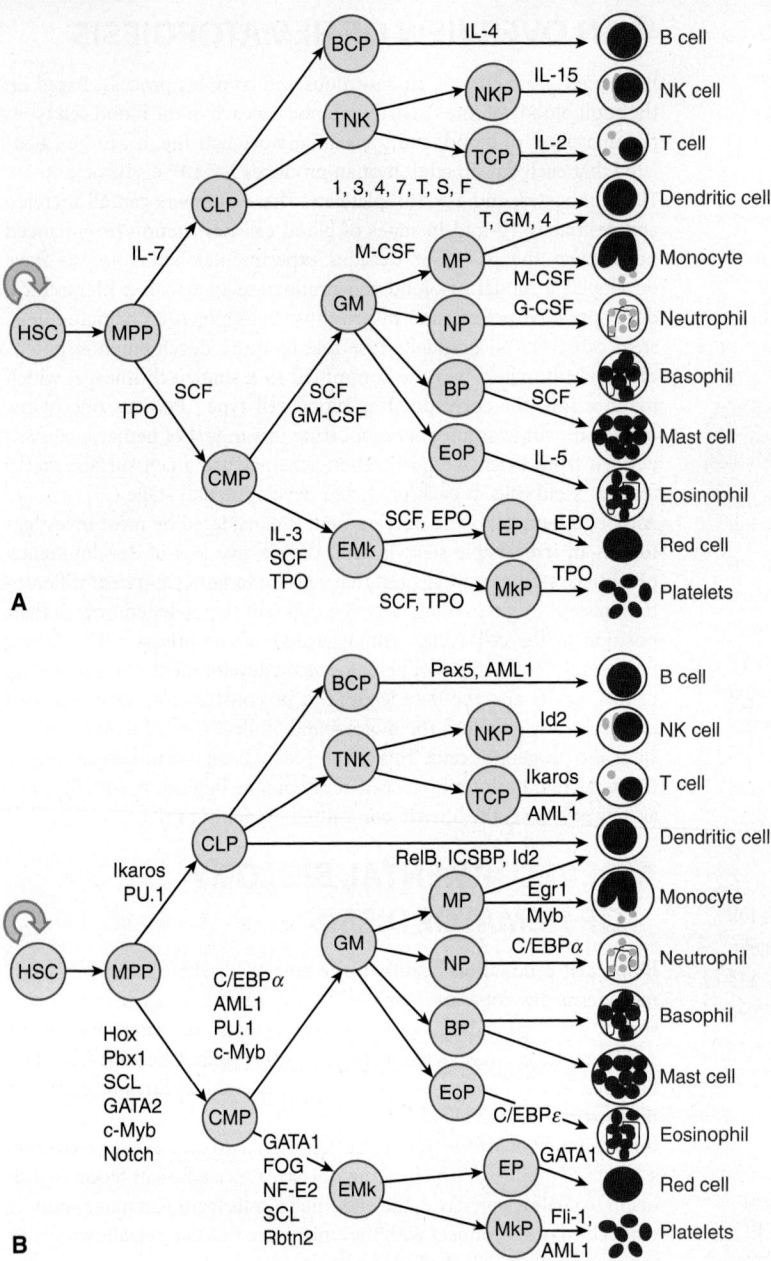

Figure 18–1. The figure displays the hematopoietic progenitors that have been defined by *in vitro* assays or by more complex tissue-based assays. In **(A)** the growth factors responsible for cell survival and proliferation at each corresponding stage of hematopoietic development are shown, and in **(B)** the corresponding transcription factors are illustrated. See text for definitions, except that T,GM,4 represents tumor necrosis factor alpha (TNF-α), GM-CSF and IL-4, and 1,3,4,7,T,S,F represents IL-1, IL-3, IL-4, IL-7, TNF-α, SCF, and Flt3 ligand. Although a single type of macrophage is illustrated, the blood monocyte can differentiate into a plethora of tissue specific macrophage types, including the hepatic Kupffer cell, the brain microglia, and the bone osteoclast (details are provided in Chaps. 67 and 69). Similarly, a single dendritic cell is shown, but of two distinct origins, lymphoid or myeloid (Chap. 20).

research has shown that the first adult-type HSCs are derived from mesodermal cells within the ventral wall of the dorsal aorta of the AGM.[10–12] The AGM remains a source of hematopoiesis between days 9.5 and 11.5 postcoitum in the mouse, and days 30 and 37 in the human.[13,14] Of interest, the development of hematopoietic cells in this region (as well as in the yolk sac) occurs in a "reverse" direction, that is, single lineage-committed progenitors appear prior to multilineage progenitors, which appear prior to stem cells. This region also has cells that express a number of molecules in common with endothelial cells, including CD34, the transcription factors SCL and GATA-2, and the receptors c-KIT and FLK-1.[15] Moreover, cell culture experiments have established that such cells display combined endothelial and hematopoietic potential, establishing them as "hemangioblasts," the postulated combined endothelial cell–hematopoietic precursor.[16]

Approximately 2 days following the appearance of HSCs in the AGM region, hematopoiesis begins in the murine fetal liver. Careful dissection experiments of the 1970s indicate that fetal liver hematopoiesis

is dependent on an exogenous source of hematopoietic cells,[17] which populate the fetal liver in two waves, consisting of erythroid and multilineage progenitors around day 9 of murine gestation and committed progenitors and true HSCs at day 11.[18] Although there is no direct proof, the temporal appearance of these cell types in the AGM approximately 1 to 2 days prior to their appearance in the fetal liver strongly suggests that the former is the source for populating the latter. In humans the fetal liver becomes the major source of blood cells around 5 weeks of gestation, and the marrow begins to populate with hematopoietic cells at 8 weeks of gestation. Unlike the random pattern of cells seen in the yolk sac, hematopoiesis in the fetal liver is well organized; erythroid cells are usually found in clusters surrounding a central macrophage and CD15+ myelopoietic cells localize mainly around portal triad vessels, although lymphoid precursors fail to demonstrate a specific localization pattern and are randomly found amongst hepatocytes.[19] Up to 50 percent of the fetal liver is composed of hematopoietic cells at days 12 to 14 of murine embryonic life, a proportion that begins to decrease as hepatocytes replace hematopoietic cells and the latter shift to the marrow, prior to birth.

The final shift in the site of hematopoiesis occurs before birth; although the marrow begins to populate with liver derived hematopoietic cells at day 16 in the mouse and at 8 weeks gestation in the human, it is mostly myeloid in nature and contributes little to the circulating blood until just before birth.[20] Hematopoietic stem and progenitor cells circulate in large numbers during fetal life, as clinically witnessed by the use of umbilical cord blood as a rich source of HSCs for transplantation. However, shortly after birth neonatal blood has very few primitive hematopoietic cells, as they begin to home to and lodge in the marrow. Genetic studies reveal that marrow localization of HSCs is dependent on the chemokine CXCL12 (previously known as stromal cell-derived factor [SDF]-1)[21] as elimination of the chemokine or its receptor (CXCR4) leads to marrow hypoplasia.[22] The shifts in localization of hematopoiesis during mammalian development are likely the result of changes both in the cell surface adhesion molecules on hematopoietic stem and progenitors that occur during ontogeny, and the characteristics of stromal cells of the yolk sac, AGM, fetal liver, and adult marrow that provide the microenvironmental support of HSC survival, homing and lodgment, self-renewal, proliferative expansion, and differentiation (Chap. 7).

● THE HEMATOPOIETIC STEM CELL

FUNCTIONAL DEFINITION

Although the concept of a common "mother cell" of all blood elements in the adult dates to Maximov in 1909, and its potential for participation in disease as proposed by Danchakoff in 1916,[23] the basic concepts of a hierarchical organization of stem and progenitor cells leading to mature blood cell production were coalesced by Till and McCulloch using a spleen colony-forming assay, experimentally establishing the existence of multipotential hematopoietic cells.[24] The capacity to transplant marrow cells and reconstitute all aspects of hematopoiesis in myeloablated recipients provided an *in vivo* assay for the HSC, but it was not until the development of clonal *in vitro* assays of lineage-committed progenitors that a coherent model of blood cell production began to emerge. The pioneering work of Pluznik and Sachs[25] and of Bradley and Metcalf[26] provided methods to enumerate and characterize marrow cells committed to the hematopoietic lineage. These investigators independently developed culture conditions that allowed colonies of leukocytes to develop from single progenitors. However, as a result of the more fastidious conditions required for erythropoiesis and megakaryopoiesis *in vitro*, the description of methods to culture these progenitors did not occur for another decade or more.[27–31] Work using density fractionation, cell sorting, and fluorescent dye exclusion methods has yielded purified populations of stem cells,[32–36] common myeloid[37] and lymphoid[38] progenitors, and lineage-restricted hematopoietic progenitors,[39,40] methods that have greatly advanced our understanding of the cell and molecular biology of blood cell development. Figure 18–1 depicts a working model of this process.

STEM CELL KINETICS

Based on transplantation data indicating that there are a remarkably similar total-body number of HSCs in mice and cats, it has been estimated that all mammals, including humans, possess 2×10^4 stem cells,[41] and because only a small fraction of these are cycling (and therefore contributing to blood cell production) at any given time, it is also clear that daily blood cell development from the few cycling stem cells to produce the approximately 4×10^{11} mature blood cells represents a massive amplification process. However, the capacity of HSCs to contribute to hematopoiesis changes with age (Chap. 9). The number of HSCs

increases with age in some but not all strains of mice.[42,43] Also, HSC differentiation in aged animals is skewed toward the myeloid rather than lymphoid lineage.[44] The molecular basis for these changes are undergoing intense study.[45–48]

Another measure of stem cell kinetics is the time it takes for transplanted marrow cells to repopulate a lethally irradiated animal. Studies using retroviral markers suggest that HSCs can be divided into short-term and long-term repopulating cells, based on the timing of their appearance in the blood following intravenous transplantation (fewer than or more than 3 months following transplantation in mice).[49] However, a rapidly repopulating stem cell has been identified using a direct marrow injection strategy, a cell capable of generating large numbers of erythroid and myeloid cells within 2 weeks of injection.[50] Moreover, by transplanting luciferase-labeled single stem cells, a strategy that allows the serial tracking of the cells during life, initially detected foci were found to expand locally, seed other sites in the marrow or spleen, and then recede with different kinetics.[51] From these experimental approaches it is clear that HSCs are heterogeneous.

STEM CELL ASSAYS

Transplantation Assays

Assays of Murine Stem Cells Experimental transplantation in animals affords the clearest estimation of HSC properties as the capacity to durably regenerate all of hematopoiesis in an otherwise lethally irradiated animal remains the gold standard for the field; moreover, the technique can be made quantitative. Typically, either 2×10^5 genetically marked, whole murine marrow cells, or reduced numbers of variably purified cells are infused intravenously into recipient animals who had previously received 90 to 110 cGy of whole-body irradiation. Blood cells and marrow are monitored for hematopoietic recovery in the following weeks and months, and the success of the transplant is measured by survival, and long-range contribution to hematopoiesis in the recipient. The contribution of donor cells to recovery is established by analysis of the posttransplant blood or marrow cells; the most common method of distinguishing donor from residual recipient blood and marrow cells is the use of flow cytometry against isoforms of the cell membrane-bound phosphatase CD45, present on virtually all hematopoietic cells. In a more quantitative embodiment of the strategy, limiting numbers of the genetically distinct cells (e.g., CD45.1+) are mixed with a "just adequate" (for full recovery) number of alternately marked cells (e.g., CD45.2+) and the proportion of CD45.1 to total CD45.1+ plus CD45.2+ cells is assessed following transplantation, yielding a calculation of the number of stem cells in the initial inoculum, an approach termed *competitive repopulation*.[52] Because there exist both "short-term" and "long-term" repopulating cells, the degree of donor cell chimerism is tested 3 or more months following transplantation, to be certain that only the latter are evaluated. For example, transplantation of megakaryocyte-erythroid progenitor (MEP) cells allows for survival in a lethally irradiated mouse, as these cells allow sufficient time for endogenous recovery of the small number of relatively radio-resistant HSCs in the recipient mouse.[53] Consequently, survival alone following cell transplantation is not a sufficient measure of the presence of stem cells in a given population. Thus, with the appropriate caveats, this approach allows an assessment of the numbers or "quality" of HSCs in the test population (i.e., some genetically altered stem cell populations repopulate less robustly than wild-type cells as a consequence of defects in cytokine receptors or other genes that affect the self-renewal, survival, or proliferation of stem cells). Based on the use of these experimental tools, we know most about murine HSCs. Obviously, this approach is not available to assess human HSCs. Instead, a number of alternate experimental approaches have been developed.

Assays of Human Hematopoietic Stem Cells Severely immuno-compromised mice can be engrafted by human HSCs, provided their survival can be supported in a strictly controlled animal care environment and that the experiments take place prior to the development of other untoward effects in such animals (e.g., tumor formation). The first assay employing this strategy relies on the combined immuno-deficiency created by the severe combined immunodeficiency (SCID) and nonobese diabetic (NOD) genetic mutations.[54] Subsequently, these mice were found to bear some ability to reject or alter the developmental characteristics of human cell repopulation, leading other investigators to add genetic defects to the NOD-SCID background that improve the engraftment of normal and pathologic human marrow cells, such as NOD-SCID/β_2-microglobulin null,[55] or the most commonly used NOD-SCID/γc null,[56] or by crossing with mice that also express human hematopoietic cytokines.[57] Such animal models have allowed the assessment of (1) stem cell numbers in human CD34+ cells from mobilized blood or umbilical cord blood,[58] (2) assessment of the effects of gene therapy vectors,[59,60] cell-cycle inhibitors,[61] or cytokine cocktails designed to expand stem cell numbers[58–64] on the retention of repopulating capacity, or (3) the study of fundamental biologic properties of human HSCs *in vivo*, such as the cell-cycle restriction of repopulating cells.[65]

Surrogate In Vitro *Stem Cell Assays*

Although *in vivo* assays remain the gold standard, NOD-SCID and more severely immunocompromised mice are difficult to maintain and remain expensive and quite cumbersome methods to assess human HSC quality and quantity. As a result, a number of culture-based methods were developed to more quickly and quantitatively evaluate human HSC function. Generally, each relies on long-term cell growth in culture and other special features to establish their validity as a model of the human HSC.

The ability to grow marrow cells in culture for extended periods of time provided an important tool to explore HSC biology.[66] In long-term cultures human or murine marrow is incubated in serum-containing medium under defined conditions, and after several weeks the stromal layer that has developed is recharged with fresh marrow cells, which then produce mature blood cells and their progenitors for many months. Cell fractionation studies show that the HSC resides adherent to the stromal cell layer in such cultures,[67] and that enzymatic disruption of the stromal layer will allow one to reseed a secondary stromal cell layer with the capacity to produce hematopoietic cells for a period of weeks to months, thereby defining an *in vitro* assayable cell termed the *long-term culture-initiating cell* (LTC-IC).[68] A second assay that was developed based on similar principles is the cobblestone area-forming cell (CAFC), which, when evaluated by phase-contrast microscopy, gives rise to complex colonies of multiple hematopoietic cell types under the stromal cell layer of long-term cultures.[69] Unfortunately, when careful comparisons are made between these assays and transplantation studies, the true HSCs comprise only a fraction of the repopulating cells found in marrow. Thus, conclusions about stem cell behavior from such *in vitro* assays cannot be considered rigorous.

CELL SURFACE PHENOTYPE

Numerous investigators have used monoclonal antibodies to an increasing number of hematopoietic cell surface proteins to negatively and/or positively enrich for stem and primitive hematopoietic progenitor cells. Although the function of only a few of these stem cell markers is known, it has not impeded their use for research and/or therapeutic benefit. Others have taken advantage of the capacity of primitive hematopoietic cells to extrude fluorescent organic chemicals or on their buoyant density to obtain purified populations of these scarce marrow

cells; most successful stem cell purification strategies employ several such techniques.

The antigenic proteins and glycoproteins that exclusively or predominantly present on HSCs include (1) CD34, a 90- to 110-kDa type I glycoprotein that is postulated to mediate cell adhesion and/or cell-cycle arrest[70–72]; (2) CD90 (Thy1),[73] a heavily glycosylated glycophosphoinositol-linked protein that participates in T-cell adhesion to stromal cells[74]; (3) CD117 (the c-Kit receptor),[75] which supports primitive hematopoietic cell survival and proliferation[76,77]; (4) AA4,[34] a murine molecule homologous to the human phagocyte C1q complement receptor[78]; (5) Sca1,[79] a murine surface molecule shown by knockout studies to be necessary for normal stem cell development[80]; (6) CD133,[81] a 115-kDa pentaspan cell-surface glycoprotein expressed on the apical surface of neuroepithelial and HSCs that has been proposed to function in establishing or maintaining plasma membrane protrusions[82]; (7) CD164,[83] a cell-surface sialomucin that is present in several alternately spliced isoforms and that enhances blood cell homing and inhibits CD34+/CD38− cell proliferation,[84] and CD150, a member of the signaling lymphocyte activation molecule (SLAM) family of lymphocyte proliferation receptors[85]; and (8) CD110 (the thrombopoietin [TPO] receptor c-Mpl)[86] present on virtually all repopulating HSCs,[87] and established to be vital for human HSC physiology as genetic elimination of the receptor leads to congenital amegakaryocytic thrombocytopenia at birth and aplastic anemia shortly thereafter (Chap. 117).

Many or most of the surface membrane proteins found on HSCs are also present on cells that have begun to differentiate toward specific lineages, precluding the exclusive use of positive selection alone for stem cell purification. Thus, a number of stem cell purification strategies include negative selection, based on cell surface markers absent on HSCs but present on mature blood cells and their corresponding unilineage-committed progenitors. Typically, cocktails of negatively selecting antibodies include CD38, HLA-DR, CD3, CD4, CD5, or CD8 for T lymphocytes; CD11b, CD14, or Gr-1 to exclude macrophages and granulocytes; CD10, CD19, CD20, or B220 to eliminate B lymphocytes; and glycophorin A or Ter119 to remove erythroid cells. The products that result from the use of such combinations of negative-selecting antibodies are termed *Lin−* cells.

A particularly difficult problem is presented by separating true HSCs from their progeny committed to the lymphoid or myeloid lineage, but not differentiated beyond that stage. Several studies clarify the cell surface profile of the common lymphoid progenitor (CLP) as Lin−/interleukin (IL)-7R(receptor)α+/Thy1−/Sca-110^w/c-kit^{low}[37] and the common myeloid progenitor (CMP) as Lin−/IL-7Rα−/c-Kit+/Sca-1−.[36] The cell surface phenotype of human HSCs includes CD34+/CD38−/KDR(VEGFR2)+/Thy1+/CD133+/Lin−, although most of these markers require careful clinical assessment before their widespread use in patients can be considered. At present, at least for murine cells, that problem has been solved. The most effective cell sorting method for purifying murine HSC is the E-SLAM approach, negatively selecting for CD48 and positively selecting for CD45, CD201, and CD150. It is estimated that such a cell population is at least 50 percent pure HSC based on single-cell transplantation experiments in mice.

STEM CELL INTEGRINS

Integrins are a family of heterodimeric single-pass transmembrane proteins (18 α and 8 β subunits form at least 24 different cell surface adhesion receptors in humans) characterized by multiple immunoglobin (Ig)-like extracellular domains that allow two-way communication between a cell and its environment.[89] A large number of cell types require contact for survival; *in vitro*, this is usually manifest as integrin-dependent cell adhesion, either to extracellular matrix protein(s) or to other cells. In such cultures, disruption of adherence causes programmed cell death; for example, endothelial cells undergo apoptosis upon forced detachment *in vitro*, as a result of disruption of multiple integrins.[90] Integrins also influence the proliferation of cells by affecting the G_1 to S phase transition of the cell cycle.[91] These effects also operate *in vivo*; α_1 integrin (a component of the $\alpha_1\beta_1$ collagen receptor) null mice have a hypoplastic dermis, and the growth of α_1 −/− fibroblasts on collagen is substantially reduced.[92]

Hematopoietic stem and progenitor cells express multiple integrins, including $\alpha_4\beta_1$ (also termed *very-late antigen* [VLA] 4), which binds to either vascular cell adhesion molecule (VCAM) 1 or fibronectin, and $\alpha_5\beta_1$ (VLA5), which binds to a region of fibronectin distinct from the $\beta_1\beta_1$ binding domain. Moreover, primitive hematopoietic cells are thought to express integrin αIIbβ_3, the platelet fibrinogen receptor, based on the death of multiple hematopoietic lineages in mice expressing a suicide transgene under control of the integrin αIIb promoter.[93] However, the physiologic significance of this finding is uncertain at present.

The avidity of progenitor cell–integrin interactions can be altered by external effectors; numerous cytokines and chemokines, including cytokines critical for stem cell function (stem cell factor [SCF], TPO, and CXCL12), enhance integrin-mediated binding.[94–96] Counterreceptors for both integrins, such as VCAM1 and fibronectin (FN), are highly expressed in the marrow matrix and on marrow stromal cells (see "Matrix Proteins" in "The Hematopoietic Microenvironment" later). Integrin-based interactions with the stroma are responsible for homing and retention of stem and primitive progenitor cells in the marrow, as antibodies that interfere with the interaction can mobilize stem and progenitor cells into the blood.[97] However, it is uncertain whether integrins can influence the survival or growth of HSCs, or affect their ultimate developmental fate.

METABOLIC CHARACTERISTICS

One of the hallmarks of HSCs is their resistance to chemotherapy-induced cytotoxicity. A primary reason for this property is high-level expression of drug efflux pumps of the multidrug resistance class of proteins.[98] The presence of these verapamil-sensitive efflux pumps has enabled the separation of HSCs based on their low-level retention of various fluorescent markers such as rhodamine 123 and Hoechst 33342, the "Rh^lo/Ho^lo" population of murine cells and the side population (SP) of cells in human marrow.[99] However, before such maneuvers can be used for clinical stem cell enrichment procedures, the lack of toxicity of the fluorescent dyes must be confirmed. Nevertheless, such experimental strategies continue to shed important insights into HSC biology.

As a consequence of residing physically removed from the marrow vasculature, the stem cell microenvironment is hypoxic (see "Anatomy" in "Hematopoietic Microenvironment"). The metabolic consequence is that HSCs display a low metabolic state, with most of its ATP generation derived from glycolysis. As the HSC rarely undergoes cell division, it can "afford" the low metabolic state of cells dependent on glycolysis. One of the transcription factors critical for HSC physiology, MEIS1,[100] appears responsible for this metabolic profile, by driving expression of hypoxia-inducible factor (HIF)-1α, that upregulates expression of the glycolytic enzyme machinery.[101] In addition, HIF-1α also induces pyruvate dehydrogenase kinases (PDK1-4) that prevent mitochondrial pyruvate oxidation by suppressing pyruvate dehydrogenase complex, the first step that fuels the Krebs cycle. Stem cell down-modulation of mitochondrial oxidative phosphorylation acts to reduce the generation of reactive oxygen species (ROS), which is highly toxic to HSCs. It has been suggested that this property, the avoidance of ROS generation, contributes to the longevity of the stem cell pool in any individual.

As HSCs mature into committed progenitors, they migrate toward the marrow vasculature, and into a higher oxygen tension atmosphere. This would appear to be required to gain the additional metabolic rate afforded by oxidative phosphorylation. As one component of this "metabolic switch," marrow hematopoietic progenitor cells express lower levels of PDKs, reducing PDK-mediated suppression of oxidative phosphorylation seen in HSCs.[102]

CELL-CYCLE CHARACTERISTICS

Adult hematopoietic cells display altered engraftment capacity dependent on their phase in the cell cycle. Using primitive hematopoietic cell populations several investigators have demonstrated that only quiescent G_0/G_1 phase cells engraft into lethally irradiated recipient animals; cells in the S and early G_2 phase display minimal engraftment capacity,[102,103] a situation that can be experimentally manipulated; elimination of p21, a key cell-cycle progression gene, enhances stem cell expansion.[104] This finding correlates well with findings that the profile of expressed genes in a highly selected population of primitive hematopoietic cells shifts when they are induced from $G_{0/1}$ phase into the cell cycle.[105] However, even though this cell-cycle dependence of engraftment of stem cells is true for adult cells, the corresponding cell populations derived from umbilical cord blood or fetal liver is not cell-cycle dependent.[106] A better understanding of these findings is very likely to shed important new insights into the genes that regulate engraftment.

GENE EXPRESSION PROFILE

It can be argued that the most critical feature of the HSC is its ability to quantitatively balance its three fates—apoptosis, self-renewal, and differentiation—into the mature elements of the blood. Moreover, the undifferentiated cell must express (at the least) the initiating genes responsible for all possible developmental lineages. A useful conceptual framework for this process can be constructed by considering the gene expression profiles of stem and committed hematopoietic progenitors that develop into the multiple hematopoietic differentiation pathways. At each developmental step genes associated with the adopted pathway should remain expressed or be upregulated, while the genes that specify the alternate lineage(s) are likely silenced. A thorough understanding of these gene expression profiles should help to explain the circuitry of specific aspects of hematopoiesis, and of developmental biology in general.

Initial studies using immortalized multipotent hematopoietic cell lines reinforced this conceptual framework; pluripotency is characterized by the expression of multiple genes associated with multiple cell fates.[107] Studies of purified HSCs and lineage-committed progenitors have also strengthened this hypothesis, revealing coexpression of several different lineage-affiliated gene sets in single primitive hematopoietic cells.[108] In contrast, the downstream progenitors of HSCs were found to express only lineage-appropriate transcripts, such as for the granulocyte colony-stimulating factor receptor (G-CSF-R) in granulocyte-macrophage progenitors (GMPs), or β-globin and the erythropoietin receptor (EPOR) in committed erythroid progenitors.[36] Similar findings were reported for lymphoid committed cells, although some promiscuity was detected in B-cell progenitors.[109]

With these principles established, more ambitious efforts to catalogue all the genes expressed by each stage of hematopoietic development have been made possible by advances in microarray and whole transcriptome sequencing approaches to gene expression.[110] On an even broader scale, and as might be expected, comparisons of different types of stem cells (e.g., liver, skin, neural) reveals an overlap in the expressed genes, supporting the hypothesis that the mechanisms responsible for critical stem cell properties, such as self-renewal, are shared among the cells derived from multiple organs.[111] This observation also provides a powerful tool to identify such proteins. Such studies have also begun to identify novel genes expressed in HSCs, potentially allowing our better understanding of their role in hematopoiesis.

TRANSCRIPTION FACTOR PROFILE

An important goal of modern cell biology is to provide a molecular explanation for the gene or sets of genes required to orchestrate specific developmental events. Fundamental to this process is an understanding of the proteins present in cells that regulate gene transcription in a lineage-, ontogenic stage-, and developmental level-specific manner. Unlike what is claimed for many organ-specific programs, no single lineage-unique family of master regulators exerts executive control over hematopoiesis. Rather, an assemblage of specific and nonunique factors and signals converge to determine lineage and differentiation patterns. Several transcription factors have been identified in stem cell populations or have been shown to affect stem cell differentiation into the lymphoid and myeloid lineages. In addition to transcription factors that regulate HSC expansion, a number of epigenetic and microRNA changes have been identified that affect gene expression in these cells. The *BMI1* gene encodes a protein that forms part of a polychrome group repressor complex, which represses a number of important target genes including the cell-cycle regulator p16/INK4a, a pathway that regulates HSC function in normal and malignant hematopoiesis.[112] In addition, methylation can affect HSC gene expression, as the DNA methyltransferases DNMT3A and DNMT3B affect HSC self-renewal.[113] And microRNA (miRNA) species are regularly being identified that regulate transcription and translation of critical HSC genes. For example, 9 miRNA were overexpressed and 22 downregulated in CD34+/CD38− HSCs compared with CD34+/CD38+ cells. Among the most upregulated miRNAs in the more primitive cells was miR-520h, predicted to target ATP-binding cassette, subfamily G (ABCG2) gene, known to be involved in stem cell maintenance. Transduction of miR-520h into CD34+ cells increased the numbers of several progenitor cell types (colony-forming unit–erythroid [CFU-E], burst-forming unit–erythroid [BFU-E], and colony-forming unit–granulocyte-macrophage [CFU-GM]) as well as the total number of CD34+ cells (reviewed in Ref. 114).

Hematopoietic Stem Cell Self-Renewal and Expansion

Members of the Hox family of transcription factors are important regulators of hematopoietic cell decisions, at least at the level of self-renewal/expansion, based on (1) a similar role in multiple organ systems[115]; (2) their lineage- and differentiation-stage-specific expression pattern in hematopoietic cells[116]; (3) disruption of their usual level or pattern of expression that leads to hematologic expansion or malignancies[117]; and (4) their elimination,[118] or elimination of the gene(s) that regulate them,[119] which leads to significant defects in hematopoiesis. In addition, members of the extradenticle family of homeodomain-containing proteins serve as cofactors for Hox proteins, altering their cellular localization, DNA-binding affinities, and specificities. Like Hox genes, genetic elimination of some of these cofactor proteins can lead to HSC defects. For example, Pbx1 null mice display greatly reduced numbers of CMPs,[120] and overexpression or altered expression of MEIS1 is associated with hematologic malignancy.[121]

Hematopoietic Stem Cell to Common Lymphoid Progenitor Commitment

The Ikaros gene encodes a family of lymphoid-restricted zinc-finger transcription factors related to the *Drosophila* hunchback gene.[122]

All isoforms of *Ikaros* contain a highly conserved carboxyl-terminal activation domain and two zinc-finger domains that mediate their dimerization. However, only isoforms 1 to 3 of the six known alternately spliced forms contain more than three of the four N-terminal zinc fingers required for DNA binding to the consensus DNA core motif GGGA.[123] The PU.1 gene is 1 of approximately 30 members of the Ets family of transcription factors that bind to the purine-rich sequence 5′-GGAA-3′.[122] Genetic elimination of the Ikaros and PU.1 genes have established their critical role in commitment of HSCs to the lymphoid lineage; fetal stem cells in Ikaros −/− mice fail to generate any definitive T- or B-lymphocyte precursors,[124] and although thymocyte precursors can be identified postnatally, they undergo aberrant differentiation or fail to develop into the CD4, dendritic, and some γδT-cell subsets in adult mice. Consequently, Ikaros is essential for all of lymphopoiesis early during ontogeny, and for several subsets of lymphocytes later in life. In a similar fashion, PU.1-deficient mice also lack any definitive T- and B-cell precursors in their lymphoid organs at birth (and myeloid cells; see "HSC to CMP Commitment" below),[125] and if knockout mice are maintained on antibiotics and survive the first 48 hours of life, they begin to develop normal-appearing T cells 3 to 5 days later. In contrast, mature B cells and macrophages remain undetectable in the older mice, indicating absolute tissue dependence for this lineage.

Hematopoietic Stem Cell to Common Myeloid Progenitor Commitment

The SCL (stem cell leukemia) gene encodes one of the transcription factors responsible for the initial stages of myeloid development, a gene first identified at the site of chromosomal rearrangement in a patient with SCL.[126] SCL belongs to the helix-loop-helix family of transcription factors, which form dimers and bind DNA at consensus E-box motifs (CANNTG).[127] Although initially identified as a gene rearranged in T-cell acute lymphocytic leukemia, an essential role for SCL in hematopoietic development was established by gene ablation studies, which revealed a complete absence of primitive blood cells and lethality in scl−/− embryos at day 9.5 postcoitum.[128] Consistent with this panhematopoietic phenotype, previous studies showed that SCL is downregulated in differentiating granulocytic and monocytic progenitor cells and that forced expression of the gene in hematopoietic cell lines inhibits cytokine-induced granulocytic and monocytic differentiation.[129,130] Consistent with their respective roles in promoting stem cell and mature cell survival and proliferation, SCF sustains SCL expression in primary CD34+ cells, maintaining them in an undifferentiated state, whereas granulocyte-monocyte colony-stimulating factor (GM-CSF) downregulates SCL levels and favors granulocyte and monocyte differentiation.[130,131] Together, these results suggest that SCL expression is required for HSC and CMP maintenance, and that down-modulation of the transcription factor is essential for myeloid differentiation.

The GATA transcription factor family contains six members possessing a highly related DNA-binding domain composed of two conserved zinc-finger motifs.[132] GATA1 and GATA2 are present in hematopoietic cells, GATA2 is found in the same cells as SCL, with GATA1 expression restricted to latter stages of erythroid/megakaryocytic (MEP) differentiation. Because genetic elimination of GATA2 is lethal as a result of numerous nonhematopoietic defects, and because individual hematopoietic lineage-specific knockouts have not yet been engineered, the role of GATA2 in early hematopoiesis is uncertain. However, like SCL, elimination of GATA2 expression is required for hematopoietic cell maturation.[133]

As noted above, numerous lines of evidence indicate that HSCs express the TPO receptor, c-Mpl, as best exemplified by its expression on all AA4+/Sca+ cells that are capable of long-term hematopoietic repopulation.[87]

Several investigators have shown that the 5' flanking region of the c-mpl gene contains a functionally important GATA site and that GATA1 transactivates the gene in hematopoietic cell lines.[134] Because GATA1 does not appear in hematopoietic cells until they have lost their repopulating capacity, it is possible that GATA2 fulfills this role in HSCs, although there is no evidence yet available establishing that this protein can transactivate the c-mpl GATA site.[135]

STEM CELL AGING

While blood cell counts do not change substantially in elderly mammals, a number of alterations are demonstrable in HSCs derived from older individuals. In aged mice, the HSC compartment expands, although each HSC has reduced capacity to expand.[136] Upon transplantation, aged marrow HSCs display a myeloid skewing, generating reduced numbers of T- and B-lymphoid precursors, that along with thymic involution helps to explain the immune depletion seen in older adults. Similar findings were reported when aged human stem cells were transplanted into immunocompromised mice.[137] This topic has been reviewed.[138]

●THE HEMATOPOIETIC MICROENVIRONMENT

It has been estimated that the concentration of cells within the marrow is 10^9/mL; as a result, multiple cell–cell and cell–matrix interactions occur. A major advance in experimental hematology has been the capacity to grow hematopoietic cells in long-term culture. When high concentrations of marrow cells are placed in serum-containing cultures, a stromal cell layer and extracellular proteinaceous matrix form, and when subsequently recharged with fresh marrow cells, these long-term cultures (LTCs) are capable of supporting hematopoiesis for months with simple demidepletion and replacement of culture medium. It is assumed that the cell–cell and cell–matrix interactions that develop in such cultures more closely resemble those found *in vivo*, helping to explain the longevity of such cultures and their capacity to maintain hematopoietic stem and primitive progenitor cells far longer *ex vivo* than do nonstromal cell-containing cultures. The molecular basis for the improved hematopoietic environment of LTCs is thought to rely on stromal cell surface molecules that promote cell–cell contact, prevent programmed cell death, and regulate growth.

The microenvironmental effects on HSCs have far reaching clinical implications as well; our ability to mobilize marrow stem cells for transplantation has greatly changed the way we treat hematologic and other malignancies, and ultimate success in the efforts of experimental hematologists to expand HSCs *ex vivo* with cocktails of cytokines and stromal cells for applications in gene therapy and regenerative medicine will undoubtedly derive only from a thorough understanding of the molecular bases for the interaction of HSCs with their microenvironment (Fig. 18–2).

Marrow stromal cells influence hematopoiesis in a number of ways, by producing several cytokines that positively or negatively affect hematopoietic cell growth,[139–142] including some, like SCF, that are expressed on their cell surfaces, resulting in enhanced biologic activity.[143] Stromal cells are the origin of a number of extracellular matrix proteins that either directly affect hematopoietic cells, or do so indirectly by binding growth factors and presenting them in a functional context.[144] They also bear the Jagged/Delta family ligands that stimulate Notch proteins to undergo cleavage and translocation into the nucleus, events that are critical mediators of cell fate decision making,[145,146] including for hematopoietic cells.[147] Cell–cell interactions mediated by integrins

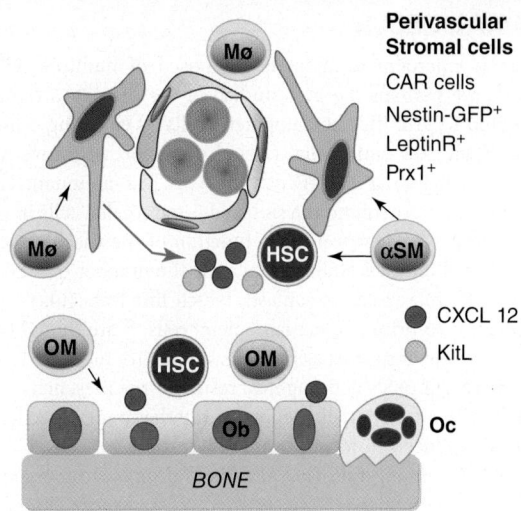

Figure 18-2. The figure depicts multiple elements of the hematopoietic microenvironment. The niche has two major regions in the marrow, supported by osteoblasts or vascular cells. Several cell types provide cytokines that maintain osteoblasts (Ob), which, in turn, support hematopoietic stem cells (HSC) by secreting CXCL12 and other cytokines. Osteoclasts (Oc) are also shown but are of lesser importance in HSC maintenance, and may inhibit HSC survival/proliferation. Macrophages that express *a* smooth muscle actin (αSM) support perivascular cells, including the CXCL12 abundant reticular (CAR) cells, that, in turn, provide CXCL12 and SCF (here termed *c-kit ligand* [KitL]) to HSCs. In addition to paracrine support, direct perivascular cell–stem cell contact, through integrins, also support HSCs. *(Reproduced with permission from Calvi LM, Link DC: Cellular complexity of the bone marrow hematopoietic stem cell niche.* Calcif Tissue Int 94(1):112–124, 2014.)

present on hematopoietic cells and counterreceptors on stromal cells are also very important for hematopoiesis.[65,72] In addition to bringing hematopoietic cells into close proximity to cells producing soluble or cell-bound cytokines, and hence raising the local concentration of these growth promoting proteins, integrin engagement leads to intracellular signaling, usually promoting entry into the cell cycle and preventing programmed cell death.[148] Reflecting the vital and sometimes lineage specific roles of the hematopoietic microenvironment, the extracellular matrix and stromal cells reside in a highly organized structure (Chap. 5).

ANATOMY

Hematopoiesis is highly compartmentalized within areas of red marrow, with erythropoiesis occurring in clusters surrounding a central macrophage,[149] granulocyte development associated with stromal cells,[150] and megakaryopoiesis occurring adjacent to the endothelial sinusoidal cells.[151] In the adult marrow, the specialized niche in which HSCs develop into differentiated progeny has been termed the *hematon* by Peault, a structure that includes Str01+ mesenchymal cells, desmin-positive perivascular lipocytes, Flk1+ endothelial cells, macrophages, and hematopoietic progenitors.[152] From these structures can be derived all lineages of committed colony-forming cells (e.g., CFU-GM and BFU-E) and primitive cells that score positive in CAFC assays, LTC-IC, and high proliferative potential colony-forming cell assays (Chap. 5).

One consequence (or perhaps cause) of this anatomical arrangement is that the stem cell microenvironment is quite hypoxia. It is estimated that the O_2 level of the stem cell niche is approximately 5 percent. The HSC response to hypoxia is discussed in "Metabolic Characteristics" above.

STROMAL CELLS

The marrow microenvironment is composed of multiple cell types. Fibroblasts are perhaps the best-studied of the marrow stromal cells, and can bind to primitive hematopoietic cells by engaging cell-surface integrins.[153] Marrow endothelial cells also support primitive hematopoietic cells, including LTC-IC.[154] The CXCL12–abundant reticular (CAR) cells, which surround the sinusoidal endothelial cells *in vivo*, are also likely to play the critical niche function of the vascular wall.[155,156] However, based on their ability to increase the number of HSCs when experimentally increased, osteoblasts, which line trabecular bone and reside adjacent to primitive hematopoietic cells,[157] are thought to provide a critical role in serving as the HSC supportive niche.[158] The origin of all of these cell types is thought to reside in the mesenchymal stromal cell (MSC), a functionally defined entity that under specific conditions can be induced to form fibroblasts, endothelial cells, CAR cells, and osteoblasts, amongst others,[159] and hold promise to therapeutically manipulate hematopoiesis.[160] MSCs are discussed more extensively in Chap. 30.

Marrow stromal cells affect HSCs in multiple ways. Each of these cells is known to produce a number of cytokines critical for primitive and mature hematopoietic cell development. For example, although a number of organs produce TPO constitutively,[161] marrow stromal cells are induced to produce the hormone in states of thrombocytopenia.[162,163] Stromal cells produce SCF constitutively in both soluble and membrane bound forms,[76] and FLT-3 ligand (FL) is produced both constitutively by stromal cells and lymphocytes and can be induced to high levels in the presence of pancytopenia.[164]

Besides growth factor production, stromal cells are also known to display counterreceptors for the integrins present on hematopoietic cells, including VCAM-1,[165] interactions that promote cell survival and proliferation in several ways.[166] Osteoblast-derived annexin II serves as an adhesion molecule for HSCs.[167] Stromal cells also elaborate extracellular matrix components, including collagen, laminin, FN, heparins, hyaluronan, and tenascin, which display important effects on HSCs (see "Matrix Proteins" later). These substances, in turn, engage a number of HSC integrins and other cell-surface molecules, and form a solid matrix on which hematopoietic cells firmly attach. Of considerable clinical interest, it appears that interference with cell–matrix interactions,[168] or digestion of the extracellular matrix itself,[169] is involved in mobilizing HSCs by some agents such as granulocyte colony-stimulating factor (G-CSF) and IL-8.

It has long been known that the marrow is innervated by the autonomic nervous system,[170] which influences HSCs in several ways, such as directing HSC trafficking by acting on nestin-positive microenvironmental cells.[171] One or more of these functions appear to be critical for HSC homeostasis, as marrow nerve injury impairs hematologic recovery following chemotherapy-induced injury.[172]

Cytokines

The regulation of stem cell survival, proliferation, and differentiation has been difficult to address because of the rarity of stem cells and the requirement that they be assessed using cumbersome transplantation assays. Several cytokines are able to exert effects on HSCs. The pursuit of the cytokines that affect HSCs is of more than pure physiologic interest, as the availability of the right combination of such proteins could allow expansion of the cells for therapeutic use without sacrificing their pluripotent and self-renewal capacities. Three proteins—SCF, FL, and TPO—and their corresponding receptors (c-Kit, Flt3, and c-Mpl, respectively) exert important effects on the number and/or growth of HSCs both *in vitro* and *in vivo* (Table 18–1).

Stem Cell Factor The molecule termed SCF, steel factor, mast cell growth factor, or c-Kit ligand was cloned by several groups based on its

TABLE 18–1. Cytokines and Hormones Active on Stem Cells and Progenitors

Cytokine	Principal Activities
IL-1	Induces production of other cytokines from many cells, works in synergy with other cytokines on primitive hematopoietic cells
IL-2	T-cell growth factor
IL-3	Stimulates the growth of multiple myeloid cell types, involved in delayed type hypersensitivity
IL-4	Stimulates B cell growth and modulates the immune response by affecting immunoglobulin class switching
IL-5*	Eosinophil growth factor and affects mature cell function
IL-6	Stimulates B lymphocyte growth; works in synergy with other cytokines on megakaryocytic progenitors
IL-7*	Principal regulator of early lymphocyte growth
IL-9	Produced by Th2 lymphocytes; costimulates the growth of multiple myeloid cell types
IL-11	Shares activities with IL-11; also affects the gut mucosa
IL-15*	Modulates T lymphocyte activity and stimulates natural killer cell proliferation
IL-21	Affects growth and maturation of B, T, and natural killer cells
SCF*	Affects primitive hematopoietic cells of all lineages and the growth of basophils and mast. Also termed c-Kit Ligand
EPO*	Stimulates the proliferation of erythroid progenitors
M-CSF*	Promotes the proliferation of monocytic progenitors
G-CSF*	Stimulates growth of neutrophilic progenitors, acts in synergy with IL-3 on primitive myeloid cells and activates mature neutrophils
GM-CSF	Affects granulocyte and macrophage progenitors and activates macrophages
TPO*	Affects hematopoietic stem cells and megakaryocytic progenitors
CXCL12	Chemokine that attracts HSCs by binding to the CXC4 receptor

*Primary regulator of the corresponding cell lineage.

binding to a cell surface receptor encoded by the protooncogene c-Kit,[76] previously identified as responsible for the severe defects in hematopoiesis, pigmentation, and gametogenesis in W mice. As the phenotype of mice bearing alleles of W was quite similar to those of steel (Sl), but in transplantation studies one strain displayed a stem cell autonomous defect (W) while the other was not (Sl), it had been hypothesized that the two genes represented the receptor for a growth factor and the cytokine itself, respectively, a tenet proven true with the cloning of SCF.

The extracellular domain of c-Kit is composed of five immunoglobulin-like domains, which leads through a typical transmembrane domain to the intracellular domain that bears a split domain-type tyrosine kinase. A single molecule of SCF binds to the first three immunoglobulin domains $(D_1D_2D_3)$ of two c-Kit receptors. The two D4 domains of a dimeric c-Kit receptor display substantial electrostatic repulsion toward each other, precluding the juxtaposing of the two transmembrane domains, and by extension, the two intracellular kinase domains. Once SCF binds to c-Kit the affinity for dimer formation overcomes the D4 electrostatic repulsion and the two kinase domains are brought together to initiate signaling.[173] The intracellular mediators activated by SCF binding to c-Kit include phosphoinositol 3'-kinase (PI3K), mitogen-activated protein kinases (MAPKs), phospholipase C gamma (PLCγ), and c-Src (Chap. 17; reviewed in Ref. 174).

SCF is synthesized by marrow fibroblasts and other cell types. Soluble SCF is a highly glycosylated 36-kDa protein released from its initial site on the cell membrane by proteolytic processing. An alternatively spliced form of SCF messenger RNA (mRNA), that does not encode the cleavage site, remains on the cell membrane, and is a more potent stimulus of c-Kit-receptor-bearing cells.[140] The ratio of soluble to membrane encoding SCF mRNA varies widely in different tissues, ranging from 10:1 in the brain, to 4:1 in the marrow, to 0.4:1 in the testis.

The importance of SCF to hematopoiesis is easily demonstrated; although nullizygous mice (Sl/Sl) are embryonic lethal because of a number of developmental defects, the presence of a partially functional allele (Sl^d) allows compound heterozygotes (Sl/Sl^d) to survive into adulthood, albeit with severe anemia because of diminished numbers/quality of HSCs. In addition to its critical role in the development of embryonic and fetal hematopoiesis, treatment of adult mice with an antibody that neutralizes the SCF receptor, c-Kit, also results in severe pancytopenia, indicating an important hematopoietic role for the receptor/ligand pair throughout life.

When present in culture SCF alone can maintain the long-term repopulating ability of murine Sca-1+/Rh^{lo}/Lin− hematopoietic cells, suggesting that the cytokine can promote the survival of HSCs *in vitro*.[175] However, alone, SCF is only a weak stimulator of cell proliferation, primarily inducing the development of mast cells both *in vitro* and *in vivo*. Nevertheless, in the additional presence of IL-3, IL-6, IL-11, G-CSF, or TPO, SCF exerts profound effects on the generation of hematopoietic progenitor cells of all lineages,[176–178] pointing to primitive hematopoietic cells as critical targets. The molecular mechanisms of such synergy are beginning to emerge.[179] A physical association of c-Kit and EPOR has been detected following SCF stimulation of cells bearing both receptors, an event that is essential for their functional synergy.[180]

Flt3 Ligand FL was cloned as the binding partner for the then newly identified novel orphan receptor Flt3,[181] a protein most closely related to the receptors for macrophage colony-stimulating factor (M-CSF) (hence the term flt = fms-like tyrosine kinase), and c-Kit. FL is expressed by T lymphocytes and marrow stromal cells.[164,181] The Flt3 receptor is a 160-kDa cell-surface molecule expressed primarily on primitive hematopoietic cells.[182] Like c-Kit, activation of Flt-3 results in activation of several signaling mediators, including the p85 subunit of phosphatidylinositol 3-kinase, SHP, PLCγ, and a guanosine 5'-triphosphatase (GTPase)-activating protein, activating Ras.[183] Normal Flt3 signaling also activates the MAPKs extracellular regulated kinase (ERK)-1 and ERK2 but leads to only weak phosphorylation of signal transducer and activator of transcription (STAT)-5, in contrast to an oncogenic form of the receptor, identified in 25 percent of patients with myelodysplastic syndromes or acute myelogenous leukemia.[184,185] In the leukemic cells of such patients Flt3 bears an internal tandem duplication of the kinase domain, resulting in the constitutive activation of the receptor. Clinically, this is associated with reduced likelihood of patient survival; hence, this observation has led to an attempt to control the growth of such mutant-receptor-bearing cells with specific Flt3 kinase inhibitors,[186] with some success (Chap. 88).

FL was initially cloned using a soluble form of the receptor to identify ligand-bearing cells.[187] As their receptors bear a number of common structural features, it was not surprising to find that FL shares significant structural homology, as well as biologic properties with both M-CSF and SCF. Like the other two cytokines, FL displays a 4α-helix bundle tertiary structure and exists in both membrane-bound and soluble states, the result of alternate splicing of the primary transcript that does or does not include a cleavage site for its release from the cell membrane.[188]

Unlike SCF levels that remain relatively static regardless of blood cell counts,[76] blood concentrations of FL can rise more than 25-fold in response to pancytopenia.[189] Interestingly, only pancytopenia, and not individual lineage deficiencies cause an increase in blood FL concentrations, suggesting that the cytokine is a bona fide regulator of stem or primitive hematopoietic cells. Consistent with this conclusion, transplantation data indicate that HSCs from Flt3-deficient mice do not effectively reconstitute the hematopoietic system,[190] being three- to eightfold less efficient in repopulation as wild-type cells, a conclusion reinforced by its genetic combination with c-Kit mutant mice.[190]

Like SCF, FL appears to act on HSCs only in synergy with other hematopoietic cytokines,[191,192] a finding particularly true for its combination with TPO.[193,194] In addition, FL is a potent stimulus of B lymphopoiesis and granulocyte-macrophage proliferation and development, particularly of the latter toward the dendritic cell lineage.[195,196]

Thrombopoietin TPO is a 45- to 70-kDa hormone that was cloned by both traditional biochemical purification and expression cloning strategies based on the use of a then orphan class I cytokine receptor, first identified as the cellular homologue of the murine-transforming oncogene v-mp1.[197] TPO bears extensive sequence homology to erythropoietin (EPO), sharing 20 percent identity and an additional 25 percent similarity. The hormone is produced in several organs, including the liver, kidney, skeletal muscle, and the marrow stroma. Based on murine liver transplantation studies about half of steady-state TPO production occurs in that organ,[198] but in states of thrombocytopenia the marrow stroma increases production substantially.[160,163] The hormone acts on megakaryocyte (MK) progenitors to enhance their survival and proliferation and on immature MKs to promote their differentiation, but surprisingly not on mature cells during platelet formation.[199] Multiple lines of evidence also indicate that TPO can exert profound effects on the HSC. The hormone also supports the survival of candidate HSC populations, and acts in synergy with IL-3 and SCF to induce these cells into the cell cycle and increase their output of both primitive and committed hematopoietic progenitor cells of all lineages.[200,201] These properties are also seen *in vivo*. For example, administration of the hormone to myelosuppressed animals leads to more rapid recovery of all hematopoietic lineages, including primitive cells,[202–205] and genetic elimination of TPO or its receptor severely reduces the number of marrow stem and progenitor cells of all lineages to 15 to 25 percent of normal values.[87,206,207] In addition, as noted in "Flt3 Ligand" above, TPO acts in synergy with FL to expand primitive hematopoietic cells in suspension culture, and when used to supplement LTC, the hormone maintained HSC numbers for up to 2 months,[207] compared to standard LTCs in which repopulating HSCs are no longer detectable at this time.

The TPO receptor, the product of the cellular protooncogene c-Mpl, is a member of the cytokine receptor family that includes EPO, G-CSF, growth hormone, leptin, and many others. Upon binding TPO, the homodimeric c-Mpl activates its tethered Jak2 kinases, leading to phosphorylation of three of the cytoplasmic domain tyrosine residues. These phosphotyrosine residues then act as docking sites for several secondary signaling molecules, including STATs, MAPKs, and PI3K, ultimately leading to the expression of a number of transcription factors (e.g., homeobox-containing proteins, HIFs) and cell-survival molecules (e.g., BclXL). A more complete discussion of the molecular mechanisms by which TPO affects the HSC is found in Chap. 17.

CXCL12 (Previously Termed Stromal Cell-Derived Factor 1)
CXCL12 is produced by a number of the cells that occupy the

hematopoietic microenvironment, and has profound effects on HSC localization to the stem cell niche.[22] However, this chemokine is also thought to display direct effects on the survival and proliferation of hematopoietic stem and progenitor cells, both alone and in synergy with other hematopoietic cytokines.[208,209]

Notch Ligands The human homologue of *Drosophila* Notch was identified as an altered gene product in T-cell leukemia.[210] The discovery that the hematopoietic microenvironment displays Notch ligands, and that Notch isoforms appear on primitive hematopoietic cells,[211,212] opened the possibility that Notch affects HSCs. This assertion has been directly proven: The Notch ligands Delta1 and Delta4 expand primitive hematopoietic cells.[213,214] It is possible that the favorable effect of marrow osteoblasts on HSCs is a result of their expression of Notch ligands, as inhibition of Notch processing blocks the expansion in HSCs seen in mice in which osteoblasts have been experimentally expanded.[158]

Wnt Proteins A role for Wnt proteins in hematopoiesis was suggested by their localization at sites of fetal blood cell production and their ability to expand hematopoietic progenitor cells.[215] Wnt 3a has been shown to expand long-term repopulating HSCs.[216,217] As Wnt proteins are expressed on primitive hematopoietic cells,[218] it is also possible that in addition to classical paracrine signaling, Wnts could act in an autocrine fashion in HSC biology.

Transforming Growth Factor β The transforming growth factor (TGF) family of ligands (TGF-β, activins, bone morphogenetic proteins [BMP]) bind to members of the TGF-β receptor family and trigger activation of the SMAD (Sma- and Mad-related protein) group of intracellular mediators.[219] Unlike the cytokines discussed above, TGF-β members inhibit HSC cycling,[220,221] and so blunt cell expansion, at least *in vitro*. Nevertheless, the situation *in vivo* is complex; genetic elimination of TGF-β does not alter HSC self-renewal or regeneration *in vivo*,[222] likely because of redundancy in the TGF-β system of ligands.[223] In contrast, genetic elimination of several of the SMAD proteins disrupts normal HSC homeostasis.[224,225] Recent data suggests that BMP4 might be the critical member of the TGF family that affects HSC biology.[226]

The mechanisms by which these cytokines exert their effects on HSCs are only now beginning to be understood at the molecular level, but it is already clear that effects on the transcription factors that govern HSC survival, self-renewal, and expansion likely play critical roles. It has long been understood that Wnt proteins act to stimulate an increase in intracellular levels of β-catenin, a nascent transcription factor. Upon being liberated from proteasomal degradation in the presence of Wnt, β-catenin translocates to the nucleus and alters transcription of genes displaying the T-cell factor (TCF)/lymphoid-enhancer binding factor (LEF) consensus sequence.[227] Moreover, TGF-β–induced alterations in SMAD protein phosphorylation affects their ability to activate transcription directly.[228] However, most of the cytokine receptors that affect HSCs do not directly affect transcription factors; rather, several cytokines affect signaling pathways that alter the expression, activity, or subcellular localization of HSC transcription factors.

As discussed in "Hematopoietic Stem Cell to Common Myeloid Progenitor Commitment" above, SCL is a helix-loop-helix transcription factor critical for hematopoiesis. SCF enhances the survival of primitive hematopoietic cells in culture by maintaining their expression of SCL,[131] which enhances expression of the SCF receptor c-Kit.[229] Two additional transcription factors that play vital roles in HSC expansion, HOXB4 and HOXA9, are both affected by cytokines. Exogenous expression of HOXB4 to levels only twice normal are associated with a marked and rapid expansion of transduced HSCs on their transplantation into lethally irradiated recipients.[116] In both model cell lines and primitive hematopoietic cells TPO doubles the expression of HOXB4, in a p38 MAPK-dependent fashion.[230] Of probably greater significance is the effect of TPO on HOXA9, a gene that also induces rapid expansion of

HSCs on its introduction into these cells, and whose genetic elimination leads to a profound deficit in numbers of HSC *in vivo*.[118] Although the hormone fails to affect total cellular levels of HOXA9 in either model cells or primary primitive murine HSC populations, TPO greatly enhances HOXA9 nuclear translocation by inducing expression of its translocation partner, MEIS1, and leading to ERK1/2 MAPK-induced MEIS1 phosphorylation.[231]

A third mechanism by which cytokines affect HSC expansion is through global inhibitors of signaling. In addition to its direct effects on HSC survival and self-renewal pathways, TPO has been shown to interact with the adaptor protein LNK,[232] which inhibits signaling pathways derived from a broad range of hematopoietic cytokines,[233,234] including TPO.[235] From these data it appears that TPO and LNK alternately regulate HSC expansion and each other.[236]

MATRIX PROTEINS

Fibronectin

FN is a 450-kDa fibril-forming glycoprotein composed of two subunits that is a major component of the hematopoietic microenvironment. FN is produced by both marrow stromal (endothelial cells and fibroblasts) and blood cells,[237] and is implicated in marrow homing of hematopoietic cells.[238] Distinct domains of FN have been identified that interact with different integrins, for example, those for integrin $\alpha_4\beta_1$ and for integrin $\alpha_5\beta_1$.[148] HSCs display multiple integrins and their engagement contributes to cell survival and/or expansion. For example, *ex vivo* culture of human CD34+ cells on FN maintains the repopulating capacity of HSCs, whereas growing the cells in suspension obliterates their ability to repopulate hematopoiesis.[239] FN binding to $\alpha_4\beta_1$ integrins also enhances the generation of large numbers of committed hematopoietic progenitors[240] and LTC-IC[241] from primitive precursors. Multiple molecular mechanisms for the effects of FN on integrin-bearing cells have been identified, and serve as a paradigm for the supportive effects of this entire class of microenvironmental signals.

Integrin engagement by FN triggers a number of intracellular signaling events that affect the cellular cytoskeleton and transcriptional events. Complexes composed of kinases, adaptors, and cytoskeletal components are recruited to sites of integrin engagement, initiated by interactions with integrin cytoplasmic domains.[89] A critical molecule for integrin-based signaling is paxillin, a 68-kDa protein that contains a number of protein–protein binding domains, and which binds to the cytoplasmic domain of the integrin.[242] Additional binding partners also help trigger intracellular signaling, including focal adhesion kinase (FAK) and the closely related Pyk2 kinase. Upon recruitment, FAK and Pyk2 are activated and initiate Tyr phosphorylation of paxillin and other associated molecules, creating additional protein binding sites and activating tethered secondary messenger molecules. One vital signaling pathway downstream of FAK and Pyk2 is PI3K, which is mediated by the association of its regulatory p85 subunit with the adhesion kinases (Chap. 14).[243] FAK also directly activates a pathway that results in upregulation of the cyclin D promoter,[244] affecting cell proliferation. Integrin engagement also leads to Src activation, engagement of Grb2, and activation of Ras,[245] pathways also activated by SCF and TPO, and potentially providing a mechanism by which diverse extrinsic stimuli of HSCs may converge.

Hyaluronan

Another stromal cell matrix glycoprotein is hyaluronan, which binds to two hematopoietic cell-surface receptors, RHAMM and CD44. Although most CD34+ marrow cells express CD44, only a fraction of them adhere to hyaluronan,[246] a process that can be mediated by cytokines, as a result of either increased surface expression of CD44 or an alteration in its conformation. Consistent with the latter notion, certain epitopes on CD44 have been shown to be inducible,[247] and antibodies to CD44 can alter the adherence of CD34+ cells to marrow stroma.[248] Nevertheless, other data suggests that RHAMM is the primary receptor for hyaluronan.[249] It is also of considerable interest that primitive hematopoietic cells also express hyaluronan, and that it plays an important role in their lodgment in the marrow and subsequent proliferation.[250]

Heparan Sulfate

LTCs that support hematopoiesis develop a heparan sulfate proteoglycan layer. Immunochemical analysis has shown that marrow stromal cell lines synthesize and secrete numerous members of the syndecan family of heparan sulfate, including glypican, betaglycan, and perlecan.[18] Evidence is accumulating that heparan sulfate-containing proteoglycans may be vital components of the stem cell niche. For example, the structure of the heparan sulfate secreted from stromal cell lines that support long-term hematopoiesis are significantly larger and more highly sulfated than heparan sulfate from nonsupportive stromal cell lines, and when used alone in LTCs, the former can support LTC-IC, whereas desulfated heparan sulfate cannot.[251]

Tenascin

Tenascins are large, extracellular matrix (ECM) glycoproteins found in several tissues, synthesis of which is upregulated in response to tissue regeneration. Tenascins are multimeric proteins composed of numerous modules. For example, tenascin-C is composed of six subunits linked like spokes in a wheel by their C-terminal fibrinogen-like domains, each subunit being composed of multiple epidermal growth factor (EGF)-like and FN type III modules. Two forms of tenascin of molecular mass (Mr) 280 and 220 kDa are also expressed at high levels by marrow stromal cells.[252] Marrow cells can adhere to tenascin-C within the fibrinogen-like domain and to two sets of the FN type III-like repeats, and when so engaged, they undergo a proliferative response.[253] Genetic elimination of tenascin leads to modest deficiencies in marrow hematopoietic progenitor cells,[254] although as the levels of FN in such mice are also reduced, it is unclear if direct tenascin engagement of hematopoietic cells is responsible, or the defect is a result of the secondary reduction of FN engagement of β_1 integrins.

Laminins

Laminins are heterotrimeric ($\alpha\beta\gamma$) extracellular proteins that regulate cellular function by adhesion to integrin and nonintegrin receptors. At present, 5 α chains, 3 β chains, and 2 γ chains have been characterized, which combine to form at least 12 distinct laminin isoforms.[255] Laminins containing γ_2 and either β_1 and α_5 chains are expressed in marrow, but only the latter (laminin-10/11) binds to $\alpha_6\beta_1$ integrin on primitive hematopoietic cell lines[256] and to primary human CD34+/CD38− stem and progenitor cells.[257] A second, nonintegrin laminin receptor (LR) also binds laminins, as well as other components of the ECM, such as FN, collagen, and elastin, and is composed of an acylated dimer of 32-kDa subunits.[258] Although not an integrin, the LR associates with integrins (e.g., integrin $\alpha_6\beta_4$) to modulate laminin binding.[259] Functionally, aminin-10/11 facilitates SDF-1α–stimulated transmigration of CD34+ cells,[260] and displays mitogenic activity toward human hematopoietic progenitor cells.[255] The nonintegrin LR associates with the GM-CSF receptor (GM-CSF-R) to modulate its signaling properties, down-modulating receptor signaling in the absence of laminin, and releasing the inhibition when bound by its ligand.[261] This arrangement could provide a novel molecular explanation for how laminins affect cell proliferation; whether this physiology extends to other cytokines that affect HSCs is under investigation.

Collagen Types I, III, V, and VI

Collagen types I, III, IV, and VI have been identified in LTC or *in situ* from marrow sections by a number of methods.[35,262] Most of the marrow-derived collagen types are assembled into long fibrils, which form the fine, background reticulin staining seen on marrow biopsies, although type IV collagen is assembled into a meshwork seen most commonly as part of basement membranes. Collagens also interact with laminins in the marrow. Collagen types I and VI are strong adhesive substrates for various hematopoietic cell lines and marrow mononuclear cells, including committed myeloid and erythroid progenitors.[262] Classic collagen receptors on blood cells are of two types, the β_1 integrins ($\alpha_1\beta_1$ and $\alpha_2\beta_1$) and the nonintegrin glycoprotein VI, present predominantly on platelets.

THE AGING MARROW MICROENVIRONMENT

Like the HSC itself (see "Stem Cell Aging" earlier), the HSC niche undergoes several changes with aging. Although the number of osteoblasts decreases, they generate higher levels of ROS, inducing p38 MAPK signaling, potentially accounting for the reduction in self-renewal capacity of HSCs derived from older mammals. The number of adipocytes increases as a result of the skewed differentiation of aged MSCs; increased adiposity and reduced osteogenesis lead to decreased CXCL12 levels in the aged marrow. This finding could be responsible for altered HSC mobilization in elderly individuals. In contrast, increased levels of the CC-chemokine ligand 5 (CCL5; also known as RANTES [regulated upon activation, normal T-cell expressed and secreted]), in the niche could contribute to the altered myeloid/lymphoid skewing seen in HSCs of older individuals.[263] This topic has been reviewed but clearly requires additional study.[138]

● CONTROVERSIES IN HEMATOPOIESIS

LINEAGE FATE DETERMINATION

One of the most contentious issues in hematopoiesis is the origin of stem cell commitment to specific blood cell lineages. Two schools of thought exist: extrinsic and intrinsic control. The former, championed by Metcalf and others,[264] argues that cytokines, ECM, or other stimuli instruct the hematopoietic stem or progenitor cell to differentiate into specific cell types. In contrast, Dexter and others[265] argue that a hierarchy of transcription factors direct a cell toward a specific lineage, mechanistically explained by a stochastic rise in one or more of a mutually antagonistic set of transcription factors, that drive developmental pathways by enhancing expression of the genes that characterize that pathway, and by interfering with the levels or function of the transcription factors that drive the alternate lineage fate choice.

The Case for Transcription Factors

A strong case has been made for intrinsic control of stem cell lineage determination.[265] As Enver and colleagues state: "Simply put, the question is this: Is unilineage commitment the result of a cell-autonomous, internally driven program, or rather is it the consequence of a cell responding to an external, environmentally imposed agenda?" These and several other investigators argue that the stochastic rise in one or another lineage determining transcription factor in the multilineage progenitor leads to its ultimate lineage commitment.

It is abundantly clear that transcription factors can direct lineage commitment in hematopoietic cells. A partial list of transcription factors restricted to specific hematopoietic lineages includes Pax5 (B cells),[266] Ikaros (B/T cells),[267] PU.1 and C/EBPα (myeloid and B cells),[268,269] GATA1 (erythrocytes and MKs),[132,270] Fli1 (MKs),[271] and C/EBPε (granulocytes).[272] A number of loss-of-function studies have revealed the nonredundant role of these proteins in development of the corresponding cell lineage. For example, genetic elimination of Pax5 eliminates B cells[273]; elimination of Ikaros leaves a mouse devoid of fetal T cells, fetal and adult B cells, and their progenitors[124]; and loss of C/EBPα leads to absolute neutropenia.[274] Moreover, the exogenous expression of several transcription factors in lineage committed progenitor cells can redirect cell fate. For example, C/EBPα is expressed in myeloid progenitor cells, and introduction of a regulatable C/EBPα gene into purified erythroid progenitors causes their switch to the myeloid lineage.[275] In further support of this hypothesis, several lines of evidence have been gathered, including the finding that forced expression of the antiapoptotic gene bcl$_2$ in a growth factor-dependent multipotential hematopoietic cell line resulted in growth factor independence and spontaneous differentiation into all of the possible cell lineages that develop when the corresponding growth factor(s) are added to the wild-type cells.[276]

In addition to providing these and other arguments in favor of a transcription factor–based intrinsic regulatory mechanism of stem cell fate, proponents of the intrinsic hypothesis point to feed-forward switch-like molecular mechanisms in which a stochastic increase in one of a binary set of such transcription factors reduces the level or activity of those transcription factors responsible for alternate cell fates. An example of this physiology is illustrated by the mutually antagonistic effects of the erythroid transcription factor GATA1 and the myeloid transcription factor PU.1; GATA1 acts to inhibit the myeloid activation potential of PU.1,[277] and PU.1 blocks the binding of GATA1 to its genetic target sites.[278] Thus, when the level of GATA1 stochastically rises above that of PU.1 in a CMP, the granulocyte-macrophage potential would be extinguished and the MEP potential of the cell would march forward, unfettered. Alternately, CMPs in which PU.1 levels rise above that of GATA1 would develop along the myeloid lineages, both through the direct stimulation of myeloid gene expression by PU.1, and indirectly by the blockade of GATA1-mediated erythroid and megakaryocytic gene expression programs.

The Case for Humoral Mediators

Although much evidence has been garnered in favor of an intrinsic mechanism of stem and progenitor cell fate determination, proponents of an extrinsic instructive hypothesis have also generated a large amount of compelling evidence in favor of the importance of extrinsic signals. One illustrative example of the capacity of certain extrinsic signals to impact specific patterns of differentiation is that the exogenous expression of an IL-2Rβ transgene in CLPs induces their differentiation into myeloid cells.[279] Subsequent studies revealed that the presence of the exogenous receptor leads to upregulation of the GM-CSF-R in the CLP, and that exogenous expression of GM-CSF-R could also lead a CLP toward monocyte/macrophage development.[2] In separate studies, other cytokines were shown to direct myeloid lineage fate determination; compared to the differentiation profile seen when marrow cells were cultured with SCF alone, an antiapoptotic stimulus, the addition of IL-5 greatly enhanced the number of marrow progenitor cells that gave rise to eosinophilic colonies, whereas the addition of TPO induced a predominance of megakaryocytic colonies, without significant changes in the number of apoptotic cells in any of the three culture conditions. These results were interpreted to indicate that while the SCF could keep nearly all progenitor cells alive under the cell culture conditions employed, the second cytokine directed the multilineage progenitors into specific cell fates.[280]

A number of external signaling events have been found to directly impact the transcriptional apparatus of the cell. For example, as previously noted, two transcription factors that lead to the self-renewal and expansion of HSCs, HOXB4, and HOXA9 are induced to higher levels of expression or to translocate into the nucleus of stem cells in response

to TPO.[235,236] Moreover, SCL, a transcription factor that when expressed in maturing hematopoietic cells inhibits cytokine-induced granulocytic and monocytic differentiation, maintaining them in an undifferentiated state, is enhanced by SCF and down-modulated by GM-CSF.[131] And the level of c-Myb, which determines whether a MEP develops an erythroid or MK fate is affected by TPO, mediated by its induction of miR150.[281] Thus, strong evidence supporting both extrinsic and intrinsic control of lineage determination has been presented, and like the case for most conflicts in biology, it is most likely that elements of both mechanisms operate in hematopoiesis.

● STEM CELL SURVIVAL, EXPANSION, SELF-RENEWAL, AND DIFFERENTIATION

Like nearly every other cell type, the HSC is subjected to a number of noxious stimuli, and must possess mechanism to survive such insults. Moreover, the regulation of HSC levels is carefully regulated, such as seen following transplantation, through both cell expansion and programmed cell death. The mechanisms that drive HSC survival are beginning to be determined.

A number of cytokines affect cell survival by regulating inhibitors of apoptosis, such as the Bcl proteins. In addition, in response to sublethal DNA damage, cytokines can also act to trigger DNA repair mechanisms. For example, TPO acts to increase the efficiency of DNA-protein kinase-dependent nonhomologous end-joining in response to irradiation or chemotherapy, helping to repair double-stranded DNA breaks.[282]

The ability to divide symmetrically to generate identical daughters is a feature of most cells, including HSCs. However, the multipotent stem cell possesses an added ability to undergo asymmetric cell divisions, yielding one committed progenitor daughter and one stem cell daughter, or two differentiating progeny; regulating the balance between symmetric and asymmetric stem cell divisions becomes critical in maintaining proper HSC numbers and in meeting the demand for differentiated cells. The beginnings of the molecular origins of asymmetric division in the HSC are under study.[283]

A question related to the previous discussion of whether intrinsic or extrinsic factors determine HSC lineage fate, is whether intrinsic or extrinsic factors determine the possible outcomes for a dividing HSC (two HSC progeny [stem cell expansion], one HSC and one differentiating cell [a self-renewal division], or two differentiating progeny). It is clear that feedback mechanisms exist that govern the size of the stem cell pool, as following myeloablation and transplantation of a limited number of HSCs, the pool expands toward that seen in a normal individual but not beyond, even when subjected to forced overexpression of genes that enhance HSC expansion.[284] HSCs do not appear to have a limit on their capacity for expansion; experiments using serial transplantation of marrow cells revealed that even after four such maneuvers the transplantation of a limiting number of HSCs was associated with a 10-fold expansion in the recipient,[284] a level of expansion remarkably consistent from one serial transplant to the next. Thus, there does not appear to be an intrinsic limit on HSC expansion that sets the size of the stem cell pool. Rather, evidence from quantitative transplants suggests that there exist both intrinsic and extrinsic controls on the size of the stem cell pool.

Following transplantation the degree to which a limiting number of transplanted HSCs expand depends on the source of the cells; fetal liver cells expand to a far greater degree than a similar number of adult marrow-derived HSCs, indicating that an intrinsic mechanism governs stem cell expansion divisions. However, evidence for an extrinsic mechanism that regulates stem cell expansion also exists, as the transplantation of a smaller number of either fetal liver or adult marrow HSCs resulted in slower marrow recovery but ultimately greater levels of HSC expansion than did infusion of larger numbers of cells. These results were interpreted to suggest that the more rapid recovery of marrow function associated with the administration of a larger marrow inoculum, with its increased numbers of stem cells, prematurely shut down HSC expansion, calling attention to an extrinsic regulatory mechanism. Moreover, the differences in expansion capacity amongst fetal and adult stem cells might also reflect the influence of extrinsic factors. When adult human marrow cells are transplanted, they retain their stem cell capacity only if quiescent at the time of transfer. In contrast, fetal liver and cord blood stem cells contribute to long-term hematopoiesis regardless of the phase of the cell cycle in which they reside at the time of harvest.[286] It is postulated that this latter property of fetal stem cells depends on the fetal hematopoietic microenvironment, making it likely that extrinsic factors play the key role in the decision to self-renew or differentiate. Strong experimental evidence has been generated indicating that stem cell numbers in an individual are governed by the number of hematopoietic niches.[287] This data strongly suggests that, at the very least, the availability of stem cell niches places an upper limit upon HSC expansion.

Clues from the developmental biology of lower organisms may also shed important insights into the mechanisms that regulate the decision between symmetric and asymmetric HSC divisions.[288] Within the niche of developing *Drosophila* gonadal tissue exist hierarchies of cells. When female gonadal stem cells divide, the cell directly contacting the niche supportive cells remains a stem cell, the daughter that loses contact differentiates and initiates oogenesis. A similar niche architecture also sets the stage for gonadal stem cell retention in the fly testis and in many tissues of many organisms. The developing principle is that a stem cell in contact with the stem cell determining niche stromal cell, or residing in a region of the niche possessing the highest concentration of a stem cell–determining soluble factor, will remain a stem cell, and those removed from contact or soluble factor will differentiate. In such a niche, the axis of stem cell division then determines cell fate; if the axis of cell division is parallel to the front of stem cell–determining contact or soluble mediator gradient, the proximal cell will remain a stem cell while the distal cell differentiates; if the axis of cell division is perpendicular, both cells will remain under the influence of the "stemness" factor(s), and remain stem cells. Consequently, spindle-polarizing signals could be responsible for the fate of the daughters of stem cell division, a focus of much research, but at present, few established mechanisms.

STEM CELL PLASTICITY

A remarkable observation has been repeatedly made in patients who underwent sex-mismatched (male into female) marrow transplantation, suffered subsequent organ damage, and were carefully studied until the time of their death. In such settings, Y chromosome-bearing cells were identified at the site of repair of previous myocardial infarctions, strokes, and other organ damage. These observations suggest that hematopoietic cells can contribute to the replacement of damaged cells of multiple organs. More direct experimentation has lent additional support to this idea; several investigators have found that marrow cells are capable of giving rise to cells of multiple organs, including nerve,[289,290] liver,[291,292] skeletal muscle,[293] and cardiac muscle,[294] in a process termed *transdifferentiation*. However, direct evidence establishing this conclusion is lacking, as most such studies have assayed only partially purified cell populations that might also contain alternate types of stem cells,[295] and almost none have been performed using single cells, a requirement for robust proof of their multipotency. An alternate explanation for the presence of marked hematopoietic cells at nonhematopoietic sites of organ damage has been termed *cell fusion*. It has long been appreciated

that marrow cells (especially macrophages) can fuse with other cells, and spontaneous *in vitro* fusion of embryonic stem cells with marrow-derived cells yields hybrids that display stem cell function[296,297]; further experimentation is required to prove or disprove the concept of HSC plasticity,[300] a proof that will have far reaching implications for regenerative medicine.

HEMATOPOIETIC PROGENITORS

The loss of one or more developmental potentials of the HSC results in a progenitor committed to any number of specific hematopoietic cell lineages. Besides the loss of pluripotency, committed hematopoietic progenitors display a number of characteristics that differ from their parents, including the lack of capacity for self-renewal, a higher fraction of cells traversing the cell cycle, reduced ability to efflux foreign substances, and a change in their surface protein profile. On the genetic level, the transition of HSCs to committed progenitors is marked by the downregulation of a large number of HSC-associated genes and progressive upregulation of a limited number of lineage-specific genes. This section highlights some of the features of specific lineage-committed progenitors that allow for their purification, characterization, and, potentially, their manipulation for therapeutic benefit. Details of the morphologic, biochemical, and genetic aspects of the differentiation of each of these progenitors is found in the chapters corresponding to their mature blood cell types.

PROGENITOR CELL ASSAYS

Assays for most hematopoietic progenitor cells consist of marrow or (occasionally) blood cells, either unfractionated or purified to varying degrees, a semisolid support (either methylcellulose or agar, which prevents cellular migration), and a source of hematopoietic growth factors. The cultures are incubated in a humidified environment at 37°C for 2 to 7 days for murine cells, or 5 to 14 days for human cells, during which time the vast majority of the cells that began culture as mature blood cells die, allowing the few hematopoietic progenitors present to proliferate and differentiate into mature blood cells. As the cells in such culture systems are immobilized by the semisolid supporting matrix, all of the progeny in the resultant colonies are derived from a single progenitor, allowing one to retrospectively determine the developmental capacity of that cell, termed a *colony-forming cell* (CFC) or *unit* (CFU). The requirement for a source of hematopoietic growth factors was initially fulfilled by using cellular underlayers containing fibroblasts, lymphocytes, or monocytes, or tissue culture medium conditioned by a variety of normal and neoplastic cellular sources, but essentially all the requisite growth factors are now available in purified recombinant form. Despite substantial progress in our understanding of the developmental requirements of committed hematopoietic progenitors, we still do not have an adequate *in vitro* colony-forming assay for some well-characterized hematopoietic progenitor cells (e.g., those committed to the T lymphocytic or natural killer [NK] cell lineages) that still require more complex assays (e.g., fetal thymus explant assay).

CHARACTERISTICS OF SPECIFIC PROGENITOR CELL TYPES

Lymphoid Progenitors

Common Lymphoid Progenitors The existence of a population of cells committed to all lymphoid lineages but devoid of myeloid capacity was theorized to exist based on a number of analyses. For example, patients with adenosine deaminase deficiency, or mice with genetic elimination of the γ_C receptor, the signaling kinase JAK3, or the transcription factor Ikaros, lack T and B lymphocytes and have few, if any, myeloid defects, arguing that the defects in these disorders might affect a CLP; however, this does not prove the existence of a cell common for all. Work using cell sorting for CD10+/CD34+/Thy−/c-Kit−/Lin− human marrow cells revealed the capacity to develop into T, B, NK, and lymphoid dendritic cell progenitors,[298] but the report did not demonstrate a common progenitor capable of giving rise to each lineage on a clonal level.

More recent work, based upon the importance of IL-7 for all single-lineage lymphoid progenitor cells, and on the severe lymphopenia seen when the gene was eliminated in mice,[299] has indicated that the IL-7R marks a CLP that can be used in flow cytometry to isolate a population of IL7R+/Lin−/Thy−/Sca^{lo}/Kit^{lo} cells that engrafts all of lymphopoiesis but no myelopoiesis in congenic mice.[37] For example, the injection of 2000 such CD45.1+ cells plus 1×10^5 whole-marrow CD45.2+ cells into lethally irradiated CD45.2 recipients lead to 3 to 20 percent CD45.1+ B and T lymphocytes, which disappear after approximately 6 months. In contrast, this strategy never results in the appearance of CD45.1+ myeloid cells. When limiting dilution studies were performed, approximately 1 in 20 such cells could give rise to short-term B-lymphopoiesis when injected intravenously, and an equal number could give rise to T-lymphopoiesis when injected into the thymus. In colony-forming assays using IL-7, SCF, and FL, approximately 20 percent of such cells gave rise to pre-B and pro-B cell colonies in vitro. Thus, given the low likelihood of proper homing when injected into mice, it is almost certain that the CLP exists and is IL7R+/Lin−/Thy−/Sca^{lo}/Kit^{lo}. When a genetic expression analysis was performed comparing HSCs to CLPs, the latter demonstrated a down-modulation of many molecules associated with HSCs, such as the cell-surface receptors c-Mpl, β_1-integrin, and Tie2, and the transcription factors HOXA9 and EGR1, and upregulation of the IL-7R and the recombination activating protein recombination activating gene (RAG) 2.[300]

T Lymphocyte/NK Cell, T Lymphocyte, and NK Cell Progenitors
Simple colony-forming assays for mixed T/NK cell progenitors have not been developed, but the existence of the bipotent progenitor can be inferred from studies in which CD44+CD25−FcγRII/III− fetal thymic cells are cultured with genetically marked, deoxyguanosine treated fetal thymic lobes under 70 percent oxygen at 37°C. Without cytokine supplementation, such cultures yield primarily CD3+/Thy1+ T cells, but if IL-2 plus IL-15 are added, the NK cell potential (CD3−/NK1.1+) of these cells is realized, and if IL-7 is also added, the number of single cells that yield cells of both lineages increases significantly.[301] As this type of readout is possible from single day 12 fetal thymus cells, such studies establish that bipotent T/NK cell progenitors exist.

E box–binding proteins consisting of HEB, E2–2, and the E2A gene products E12 and E47 form a distinct subgroup within the large family of basic helix loop helix transcription factors.[302] Heterodimers or homodimers form between family members through their helix-loop-helix (HLH) region, and through their basic regions bind to canonical E-box DNA sequences and thereby affect gene expression, including T-cell targets such as CD4[303] and the pre-Tα,[304] and assist in recombination of the γδ T-cell receptors.[305] It is now clear that E2A is required for the transition from the bipotent T/NK progenitor to committed T-cell progenitors as its genetic elimination leads to preservation of the former but elimination of the latter.[301]

Another important subgroup of HLH proteins is the Id family, which contain an HLH region but lack a DNA binding domain, thereby acting as a sink for functional HLH proteins and thus negatively regulating the function of E proteins.[306] Id proteins appear to be essential for NK cell development, as genetic elimination of Id2 leads to a profound loss of NK cell progenitors[307] and forced overexpression of Id3 leads to a shift of T/NK cells preferentially into the NK cell lineage.[308]

It is also clear that Notch activation plays a vital role in T-cell lineage commitment from the CLP. Overexpression of active Notch1 directs marrow stem cells into immature CD4+/CD8+ T cells and inhibits B-lymphocyte development.[309] Overexpression of Notch1 in RAG-deficient precursors also results in differentiation to the T-cell lineage, although only to the immature CD4−/CD8− stage, indicating that Notch cannot substitute for pre–T-cell-receptor signaling.[310]

B-Lymphocyte Progenitors B-cell progenitors include the pro-B cell, the earliest cell irreversibly committed to the lineage, which are CD34+/CD10+/CD38+/CD19+/CD20+, the pre-B cell, which displays the initial stages of immunoglobulin rearrangement, expresses immunoglobulin heavy chains in their cytoplasm and are CD34−/CD10+/CD19+/CD20+/CD38−, and immature B cells which begin immunoglobulin light-chain production, express cell-surface IgM, and are CD10+/CD19+/CD20+. Pro-B cells can be detected in a simple colony-forming assay.[311] Normally, B-cell precursor development occurs in contact with the hematopoietic microenvironment, mediated by precursor cell integrin $\beta_1\beta_1$ and stromal cell VCAM or matrix FN. A number of cytokines affect B-cell progenitor proliferation,[312] including IL-7,[313] insulin-like growth factor (IGF)-1,[314] SDF-1,[315] and SCF,[316] although based on genetic knockout studies, B cells are absolutely dependent only on IL-7[299] and SDF-1.[22]

A number of cytokines also inhibit B-cell precursor development, including interferon (IFN) α/β,[317] IFN-γ,[318] IL-4,[319] and TGF-β.[320] The role of these and other inhibitory cytokines in B lymphopoiesis is complex, as in some situations a cytokine can inhibit one stage and stimulate another stage of development, and some might act indirectly.

A number of transcription factors are required for mature B cell function, including PU.1, nuclear factor-κB (NF-κB), early B-cell factor (EBF), interferon regulatory factor 4 (IRF4), and Oct2, many of which bind to the promoters and enhancers involved in immunoglobulin gene expression. In contrast to these relatively later stage effects, E2A is required for commitment to the lineage.[321] The marrow of E2A-deficient mice is devoid of CD19 B cells, as well as most B-cell lineage-specific genes, including RAG1/2, Pax5, EBF, and VpreB. Moreover, no immunoglobulin rearrangement is detectable, and there are no IL-7 responsive cells. Reintroduction of E2A into the marrow cells of null mice reconstitutes pre–B-cell development.[322]

E2A sits upon a hierarchy of B-cell lineage-specific genes and transcription factors[323]; E2A directly regulates the expression of RAG1, λ5, D-J$_H$, V-Jκ, and the transcription factor EBF, the latter, in turn, regulating VpreB, mb-1, D-J$_H$, V-Jκ, and the transcription factor Pax5, which, in turn, regulates CD19 and LEF1 and shuts down genes associated with alternate lineages, such as M-CSF-R (monocytic), myeloperoxidase (neutrophilic), GATA1 (MEP), and pTα (T lymphocytic). As noted earlier in the section "Notch Ligands", a critical condition for B-cell commitment is the absence of Notch signaling.

Myeloid Progenitors
Common Myeloid Progenitors Flow cytometry has also been extensively used to purify myeloid progenitors; an IL-7R−/Lin−/c-Kit+/Sca-1− population of murine marrow cells, which by virtue of being Sca1− excludes HSCs, develop into all myeloid lineages.[36] Based on expression of CD34 and the Fcγ RII/III, three distinct subpopulations can be identified by further flow cytometry, IL-7Rα−/Lin−/c-Kit+/Sca-1−/CD34+/FcRγ^{lo}, IL-7Rα−/Lin−/c-Kit+/Sca-1−/CD34−/FcRγ^{lo}, and IL-7Rα−/Lin−/c-Kit+/Sca-1−/CD34+/FcRγ^{hi}. When tested in colony-forming assays in the presence of SCF, FL, IL-11, IL-3, GM-CSF, EPO, and TPO, each cell population yielded distinct mature cell types.[36] IL-7Rα−/Lin−/c-Kit+/Sca-1−/CD34+/FcRγ^{lo} cells give rise to all myeloid colony types, including CFU-Mix, BFU-E, CFU-megakaryocyte (CFU-MK), MEP, CFU-GM, CFU-granulocyte (CFU-G), and CFU-macrophage (CFU-M), consistent with that expected for the CMP. In contrast, IL-7Rα−/Lin−/c-Kit+/Sca-1−/CD34+/FcRγ^{hi} cells form

only CFU-M–, CFU-G–, and CFU-GM–derived colonies in response to any of the growth factors, alone or in combination, and thus represent granulocyte/macrophage lineage-restricted progenitors (GMP). Finally, IL-7Rα–/Lin–/c-Kit+/Sca-1–/CD34–/FcRγ^{lo} cells form only BFU-E–, CFU-MK–, and mixed megakaryocyte-erythroid colonies, leading to their designation as MEP. To demonstrate their capacity to differentiate *in vivo*, limiting numbers of each cell population were transplanted into congenic mice; in such studies, cell fate outcomes correspond strictly with those of the *in vitro* colony assays. For example, 6 days after injection of 5000 CMPs, both donor-derived Gr-1+/Mac-1+ myelomonocytic cells and TER119+ erythroid cells were detectable in recipients. In contrast, when 5000 GMPs were transplanted, only Gr-1+/Mac-1+ cells were recovered, and only for a transient period of time. Likewise, MEPs reconstituted only TER119+ cells in similar experiments, and the genetically marked progeny from each of these progenitor populations disappear within 4 weeks of transplantation, indicating their limited self-renewal capacity.

Erythroid/Megakaryopoietic, Erythroid, and Megakaryopoietic Progenitors Culture conditions necessary for *in vitro* erythropoiesis have been known for nearly 35 years,[324,325] with colony morphologies ranging from small compact clusters of 20 to 50 erythrocytes developing with 2 to 5 days in murine and human marrow plasma clot cultures (CFU-E), to large highly complex colonies containing up to thousands of cells taking from 7 to 14 days to develop in methylcellulose or agar (BFU-E). The cytokine requirement for the former is simple—EPO, whereas a cytokine that stimulates earlier cells, such as IL-3 or SCF, is required for the latter progenitor cell type.

Culture conditions that support the proliferation of MK progenitors have been established for both mouse and humans.[29,31] Using either methylcellulose, agar, or a plasma clot, two colony morphologies that contain exclusively MKs have been described. The CFU-MK is a cell that develops into a simple colony containing from 3 to 50 mature MKs, larger, more complex colonies that include satellite collections of MKs and contain up to several hundred cells are derived from the burst-forming unit–megakaryocyte (BFU-MK). Because of the difference in their proliferative potential and by analogy to erythroid progenitors, BFU-MK and CFU-MK are thought to represent primitive and mature progenitors restricted to the MK lineage. And like their erythroid counterparts, the cytokine requirements for CFU-MK are simple: TPO stimulates the growth of 75 percent of all CFU-MK, with IL-3 being required along with TPO for the remainder,[77] whereas IL-3 or SCF is required alone with TPO for more complex, larger MK colony formation from their more primitive progenitors.

Progenitors for erythrocytes and MKs display many common features: they share a number of transcription factors (SCL, GATA1, GATA2, NF-E2), cell-surface molecules (TER119), and cytokine receptors (for IL-3, SCF, EPO, and TPO), and most erythroid and MK leukemia cell lines display, or can be induced to display, features of the alternate lineage.[326] Moreover, the cytokines most responsible for development of these two lineages—EPO and TPO—are the two most closely related proteins in the hematopoietic cytokine family,[148] and display synergy in stimulating the growth of progenitors of both lineages.[77] For these and other reasons it has been postulated that erythropoiesis and megakaryopoiesis share a common progenitor cell,[327] a hypothesis now established[36] with the identification of IL-7Rα–/Lin–/c-Kit+/Sca-1–/CD34–/FcRγ^{lo} cells.

Like other primitive hematopoietic cells, bipotent MEP progenitors resemble small lymphocytes but can be distinguished by a specific pattern of cell-surface protein display. As noted above, MEPs are IL-7Rα–/Lin–/c-Kit+/Sca-1–/CD34–/FcRγ^{lo}. Cells committed to the MK lineage then begin to express CD41 and CD61 (integrin αIIbβ$_3$), CD42 (glycoprotein Ib), and glycoprotein V. Those that are committed

to the erythroid lineage begin to express CD41 and the transferrin receptor (CD71), and as they mature lose CD41 expression but express the thrombospondin receptor (CD36), glycophorin, and, ultimately, globin.[328] These and other cell-surface markers provide experimental hematologists several strategies to purify committed MK[39,329] and erythroid[330] progenitors. Another useful method to identify megakaryoblasts is histochemical staining for von Willebrand factor, and in rodents, acetylcholinesterase.[331]

The transcription factors expressed by erythroid and MK progenitors that allow for their commitment to the lineage are becoming increasingly well understood. GATA1 is an X-linked gene encoding a 50-kDa polypeptide that contains two zinc fingers required for DNA binding.[270] Genetic elimination of the transcription factor established the critical role of this transcription factor in hematopoiesis; GATA1 –/– mice are embryonic lethal as a consequence of failure of erythropoiesis,[332] and MK-specific elimination of GATA1 leads to severe thrombocytopenia as a consequence of dysmegakaryopoiesis.[333] GATA1 acts in concert with another protein that affects transcription without binding to DNA, friend of GATA (FOG).[334] The importance of this interaction to megakaryopoiesis is clear: several different mutations of the site on GATA1 responsible for FOG binding lead to congenital thrombocytopenia.[335]

The Ets family of transcription factors includes about 30 members that bind to a purine box sequence, proteins that interact in both positive and antagonistic ways. For example, PU.1, initially termed Spi-1 based on its association with spleen focus-forming virus-induced erythroleukemias, blocks erythroid differentiation, although it appears important for MK development.[336] Moreover, the Ets factor Fli-1 is essential for megakaryopoiesis[337] and mutations in the transcription factor are also associated with congenital thrombocytopenia in man.[271]

Granulocyte/Monocytic, Granulocyte, and Monocytic Progenitors As noted above, GMPs (CFU-GM) are IL-7Rα–/Lin–/c-Kit+/Sca-1–/CD34+/FcRγ^{hi}, reflecting their beginning differentiation toward phagocytic cells (i.e., FcRγ-positive). In the human, GMP are CD34+/CD33+/CD13+ markers, which are of clinical significance. For example, CD33 is also termed Siglec-2, a member of a family of sialic-acid-binding surface membrane proteins of the immunoglobulin superfamily that are involved in cell–cell interactions and signaling. Although the role of CD33 is not yet known with certainty, it has become a therapeutic target because of its high-level expression on the blasts of several forms of acute myelogenous leukemia[338]; the use of gemtuzumab ozogamicin, in which a humanized anti-CD33 monoclonal antibody has been fused to *N*-acetyl-gamma calicheamicin 1,2-dimethyl hydrazine dichloride, a potent antitumor antibiotic, has resulted in a complete remission rate of 15 to 20 percent as a single agent in patients with relapsed disease.[339] These initial successes have prompted its testing in earlier stage disease along with other active agents.[340] When marrow grafts are purged of CD33-bearing cells durable engraftment occurs, but is often quite delayed, indicating that CD33 is not present on the HSC, but that the presence of GMPs in a transplantation product is vital for rapid engraftment.

CD13 is also termed *aminopeptidase N*, an ectopeptidase present in many organs other than the marrow, a member of a family of proteases that play an important role in cell growth by virtue of their cleavage of biologically important peptides, in some cases inactivating, and in some cases activating them, and by serving a cell adhesive function as well. CD13 is present on early hematopoietic cells, including myeloid and lymphoid lineage progenitors, but disappears from the latter class of cells and its expression rises as monocytes mature. Although it functions to scavenge peptides in the intestinal brush border and degrade endorphins and enkephalins in the synaptic cleft, its role in hematopoiesis is less clear, although IL-8 is a substrate of its proteolytic activity.

Once bipotent GMPs differentiate, they further restrict their developmental potential. Monocytic progenitors are characterized by a predominance of PU.1, whereas granulocytic cells by members of the C/EBP family—C/EBPα and C/EBPε—are vital for the expression of neutrophil and eosinophil granule proteins.[272,341] A recent study suggests that the developmental decision of a bipotent GMP into each of the two lineages might be mediated by alterations in the relative levels of PU.1 and C/EBP expression[342]; haploinsufficiency of PU.1 (PU.1+/−) results in a reduction in CFU-M frequency in the marrow and an increase in CFU-G levels, even ameliorating the neutropenia seen in G-CSF null mice. Moreover, by increasing expression of C/EBPα, a transcription factor that drives granulocytic differentiation, G-CSF further influences the choice between the granulocytic and monocytic lineages. However, it is also clear that PU.1 plays an important role in both lineages, and it is likely that additional investigation will yield new insights into the molecular mechanisms that establish the ordered process we term *myelopoiesis*.

REFERENCES

1. Ogawa M: Differentiation and proliferation of hematopoietic stem cells. *Blood* 81:2844, 1993.
2. Kondo M, Wagers AJ, Manz MG, et al: Biology of hematopoietic stem cells and progenitors: Implications for clinical application. *Annu Rev Immunol* 21:759, 2003.
3. Colvin GA, Lambert JF, Moore BE, et al: Intrinsic hematopoietic stem cell/progenitor plasticity: Inversions. *J Cell Physiol* 199:20, 2004.
4. Moore MA, Metcalf D: Ontogeny of the haemopoietic system: Yolk sac origin of *in vivo* and *in vitro* colony forming cells in the developing mouse embryo. *Br J Haematol* 18:279, 1970.
5. Flamme I, Frolich T, Risau W: Molecular mechanisms of vasculogenesis and embryonic angiogenesis. *J Cell Physiol* 173:206, 1997.
6. Jaffredo T, Gautier R, Eichmann A, et al: Intraaortic hemopoietic cells are derived from endothelial cells during ontogeny. *Development* 125:4575, 1998.
7. Palis J, Yoder MC: Yolk-sac hematopoiesis: The first blood cells of mouse and man. *Exp Hematol* 29:927, 2001.
8. Huang H, Zettergren LD, Auerbach R: *In vitro* differentiation of B cells and myeloid cells from the early mouse embryo and its extraembryonic yolk sac. *Exp Hematol* 22:19, 1994.
9. Cumano A, Dieterlen-Lievre F, Godin I: Lymphoid potential, probed before circulation in mouse, is restricted to caudal intraembryonic splanchnopleura. *Cell* 86:907, 1996.
10. Peault B, Oberlin E, Tavian M: Emergence of hematopoietic stem cells in the human embryo. *C R Biol* 325:1021, 2002.
11. Robin C, Ottersbach K, de Bruijn M, et al: Developmental origins of hematopoietic stem cells. *Oncol Res* 13:315, 2003.
12. Golub R, Cumano A: Embryonic hematopoiesis. *Blood Cells Mol Dis* 51:226, 2013.
13. Wood HB, May G, Healy L, et al: CD34 expression patterns during early mouse development are related to modes of blood vessel formation and reveal additional sites of hematopoiesis. *Blood* 90:2300, 1997.
14. Tavian M, Coulombel L, Luton D, et al: Aorta-associated CD34+ hematopoietic cells in the early human embryo. *Blood* 87:67, 1996.
15. Marshall CJ, Moore RL, Thorogood P, et al: Detailed characterization of the human aorta-gonad-mesonephros region reveals morphological polarity resembling a hematopoietic stromal layer. *Dev Dyn* 215:139, 1999.
16. Marshall CJ, Kinnon C, Thrasher AJ: Polarized expression of bone morphogenetic protein-4 in the human aorta-gonad-mesonephros region. *Blood* 96:1591, 2000.
17. Johnson GR, Moore MA: Role of stem cell migration in initiation of mouse foetal liver haemopoiesis. *Nature* 258:726, 1975.
18. Dzierzak E, Medvinsky A: Mouse embryonic hematopoiesis. *Trends Genet* 11:359, 1995.
19. Timens W, Kamps WA: Hemopoiesis in human fetal and embryonic liver. *Microsc Res Tech* 39:387, 1997.
20. Clapp DW, Freie B, Lee WH, et al: Molecular evidence that in situ-transduced fetal liver hematopoietic stem/progenitor cells give rise to medullary hematopoiesis in adult rats. *Blood* 86:2113, 1995.
21. Ara T, Tokoyoda K, Sugiyama T, et al: Long-term hematopoietic stem cells require stromal cell-derived factor-1 for colonizing bone marrow during ontogeny. *Immunity* 19:257, 2003.
22. Nagasawa T, Hirota S, Tachibana K, et al: Defects of B-cell lymphopoiesis and bone-marrow myelopoiesis in mice lacking the CXC chemokine PBSF/SDF-1. *Nature* 382:635, 1996.
23. Danchakoff V: Origin of the blood cells. Development of the haematopoietic organs and regeneration of the blood cells from the standpoint of the monophyletic school. *Anat Rec* 10:397, 1916.
24. Till JE, McCulloch CE: A direct measurement of the radiation sensitivity of normal mouse bone marrow cells. *Radiat Res* 14:213, 1961.
25. Pluznik DH, Sachs L: The cloning of normal "mast" cells in tissue culture. *J Cell Physiol* 66:319, 1965.
26. Bradley TR, Metcalf D: The growth of mouse bone marrow cells *in vitro*. *Aust J Exp Biol Med Sci* 44:287, 1966.
27. Silver RK, Erslev AJ: The action of erythropoietin on erythroid cells *in vitro*. *Scand J Haematol* 13:338, 1974.
28. Hara H, Ogawa M: Erythropoietic precursors in mice with phenylhydrazine-induced anemia. *Am J Hematol* 1:453, 1976.
29. Metcalf D, MacDonald HR, Odartchenko N, et al: Growth of mouse megakaryocyte colonies *in vitro*. *Proc Natl Acad Sci U S A* 72:1744, 1975.
30. McLeod DL, Shreve MM, Axelrad AA: Induction of megakaryocyte colonies with platelet formation *in vitro*. *Nature* 261:492, 1976.
31. Vainchenker W, Bouguet J, Guichard J, et al: Megakaryocyte colony formation from human bone marrow precursors. *Blood* 54:940, 1979.
32. Spangrude GJ, Heimfeld S, Weissman IL: Purification and characterization of mouse hematopoietic stem cells. *Science* 241:58, 1988.
33. Civin CI, Strauss LC, Fackler MJ, et al: Positive stem cell selection—Basic science. *Prog Clin Biol Res* 333:387; discussion 402, 1990.
34. Matthews W, Jordan CT, Wiegand GW, et al: A receptor tyrosine kinase specific to hematopoietic stem and progenitor cell-enriched populations. *Cell* 65:1143, 1991.
35. Penn PE, Jiang DZ, Fei RG, et al: Dissecting the hematopoietic microenvironment. IX. Further characterization of murine bone marrow stromal cells. *Blood* 81:1205, 1993.
36. Kiel MJ, Yilmaz OH, Iwashita T, et al: SLAM family receptors distinguish hematopoietic stem and progenitor cells and reveal endothelial niches for stem cells. *Cell* 121:1109, 2005.
37. Akashi K, Traver D, Miyamoto T, et al: A clonogenic common myeloid progenitor that gives rise to all myeloid lineages. *Nature* 404:193, 2000.
38. Kondo M, Weissman IL, Akashi K: Identification of clonogenic common lymphoid progenitors in mouse bone marrow. *Cell* 91:661, 1997.
39. Muta K, Krantz SB, Bondurant MC, et al: Distinct roles of erythropoietin, insulin-like growth factor I, and stem cell factor in the development of erythroid progenitor cells. *J Clin Invest* 94:34, 1994.
40. Nakorn TN, Miyamoto T, Weissman IL: Characterization of mouse clonogenic megakaryocyte progenitors. *Proc Natl Acad Sci U S A* 100:205, 2003.
41. Abkowitz JL, Catlin SN, McCallie MT, et al: Evidence that the number of hematopoietic stem cells per animal is conserved in mammals. *Blood* 100:2665, 2002.
42. Yilmaz OH, Kiel MJ, Morrison SJ: SLAM family markers are conserved among hematopoietic stem cells from old and reconstituted mice and markedly increase their purity, *Blood* 107:924, 2006.
43. Chen J, Astle CM, Harrison DE: Genetic regulation of primitive hematopoietic stem cell senescence. *Exp Hematol* 28:442, 2000.
44. Roobrouck VD, Ulloa-Montoya F, Verfaillie CM: Self-renewal and differentiation capacity of young and aged stem cells. *Exp Cell Res* 314:1937, 2008.
45. Dykstra B, de Haan G: Hematopoietic stem cell aging and self-renewal. *Cell Tissue Res* 331:91, 2008.
46. Chambers SM, Shaw CA, Gatza C, et al: Aging hematopoietic stem cells decline in function and exhibit epigenetic dysregulation. *PLoS Biol* 5:e201, 2007.
47. Rossi DJ, Bryder D, Seita J, et al: Deficiencies in DNA damage repair limit the function of haematopoietic stem cells with age. *Nature* 447:725, 2007.
48. Nijnik A, Woodbine L, Marchetti C, et al: DNA repair is limiting for haematopoietic stem cells during ageing. *Nature* 447:686, 2007.
49. Mazurier F, Gan OI, McKenzie JL, et al: Lentivector-mediated clonal tracking reveals intrinsic heterogeneity in the human hematopoietic stem cell compartment and culture-induced stem cell impairment. *Blood* 103:545, 2004.
50. Mazurier F, Doedens M, Gan OI, et al: Rapid myeloerythroid repopulation after intrafemoral transplantation of NOD-SCID mice reveals a new class of human stem cells. *Nat Med* 9:959, 2003.
51. Cao YA, Wagers AJ, Beilhack A, et al: Shifting foci of hematopoiesis during reconstitution from single stem cells. *Proc Natl Acad Sci U S A* 101:221, 2004.
52. Harrison DE: Competitive repopulation: A new assay for long-term stem cell functional capacity. *Blood* 55:77, 1980.
53. Nakorn TN, Traver D, Weissman IL, Akashi K: Myeloerythroid restricted progenitors are sufficient to confer radioprotection and provide the majority of day 8 CFU-S. *J Clin Invest* 109:1579, 2002.
54. Larochelle A, Vormoor J, Hanenberg H, et al: Identification of primitive human hematopoietic cells capable of repopulating NOD/SCID mouse bone marrow: Implications for gene therapy. *Nat Med* 2:1329, 1996.
55. Thanopoulou E, Cashman J, Kakagianne T, et al: Engraftment of NOD/SCID-beta2 microglobulin null mice with multi-lineage neoplastic cells from patients with myelodysplastic syndrome. *Blood* 103:4285, 2004.
56. Ito M, Hiramatsu H, Kobayashi K, et al: NOD/SCID/gamma(c)(null) mouse: An excellent recipient mouse model for engraftment of human cells. *Blood* 100:3175, 2002.
57. Feuring-Buske M, Gerhard B, Cashman J, et al: Improved engraftment of human acute myeloid leukemia progenitor cells in beta 2-microglobulin-deficient NOD/SCID mice and in NOD/SCID mice transgenic for human growth factors. *Leukemia* 17:760, 2003.
58. Tanavde VM, Malehorn MT, Lumkul R, et al: Human stem-progenitor cells from neonatal cord blood have greater hematopoietic expansion capacity than those from mobilized adult blood. *Exp Hematol* 30:816, 2002.
59. Miyoshi H, Smith KA, Mosier DE, et al: Transduction of human CD34+ cells that mediate long-term engraftment of NOD/SCID mice by HIV vectors. *Science* 283:682, 1999.

60. Scherr M, Battmer K, Blomer U, et al: Lentiviral gene transfer into peripheral blood-derived CD34+ NOD/SCID-repopulating cells. *Blood* 99:709, 2002.

61. Cashman J, Dykstra B, Clark-Lewis I, et al: Changes in the proliferative activity of human hematopoietic stem cells in NOD/SCID mice and enhancement of their transplantability after *in vivo* treatment with cell cycle inhibitors. *J Exp Med* 196:1141, 2002.

62. Guenechea G, Segovia JC, Albella B, et al: Delayed engraftment of nonobese diabetic/severe combined immunodeficient mice transplanted with *ex vivo*-expanded human CD34(+) cord blood cells. *Blood* 93:1097, 1999.

63. Ueda T, Tsuji K, Yoshino H, et al: Expansion of human NOD/SCID-repopulating cells by stem cell factor, Flk2/Flt3 ligand, thrombopoietin, IL-6, and soluble IL-6 receptor. *J Clin Invest* 105:1013, 2000.

64. Zielske SP, Gerson SL: Cytokines, including stem cell factor alone, enhance lentiviral transduction in nondividing human LTCIC and NOD/SCID repopulating cells. *Mol Ther* 7:325, 2003.

65. Glimm H, Oh IH, Eaves CJ: Human hematopoietic stem cells stimulated to proliferate *in vitro* lose engraftment potential during their S/G(2)/M transit and do not reenter G(0). *Blood* 96:4185, 2000.

66. Dexter TM, Allen TD, Lajtha LG: Conditions controlling the proliferation of haemopoietic stem cells *in vitro*. *J Cell Physiol* 91:335, 1977.

67. Coulombel L, Eaves AC, Eaves CJ: Enzymatic treatment of long-term human marrow cultures reveals the preferential location of primitive hemopoietic progenitors in the adherent layer. *Blood* 62:291, 1983.

68. Sutherland HJ, Lansdorp PM, Henkelman DH, et al: Functional characterization of individual human hematopoietic stem cells cultured at limiting dilution on supportive marrow stromal layers. *Proc Natl Acad Sci U S A* 87:3584, 1990.

69. Ploemacher RE, van der Sluijs JP, Voerman JS, et al: An *in vitro* limiting-dilution assay of long-term repopulating hematopoietic stem cells in the mouse. *Blood* 74:2755, 1989.

70. Fackler MJ, Krause DS, Smith OM, et al: Full-length but not truncated CD34 inhibits hematopoietic cell differentiation of M1 cells. *Blood* 85:3040, 1995.

71. Krause DS, Fackler MJ, Civin CI, et al: CD34: Structure, biology, and clinical utility. *Blood* 87:1, 1996.

72. Verfaillie CM: Adhesion receptors as regulators of the hematopoietic process. *Blood* 92:2609, 1998.

73. Baum CM, Weissman IL, Tsukamoto AS, et al: Isolation of a candidate human hematopoietic stem-cell population. *Proc Natl Acad Sci U S A* 89:2804, 1992.

74. Barda-Saad M, Rozenszajn LA, Ashush H, et al: Adhesion molecules involved in the interactions between early T cells and mesenchymal bone marrow stromal cells. *Exp Hematol* 27:834, 1999.

75. Sanchez MJ, Holmes A, Miles C, et al: Characterization of the first definitive hematopoietic stem cells in the AGM and liver of the mouse embryo. *Immunity* 5:513, 1996.

76. Broudy VC: Stem cell factor and hematopoiesis. *Blood* 90:1345, 1997.

77. Broudy VC, Lin NL, Kaushansky K: Thrombopoietin (c-mpl ligand) acts synergistically with erythropoietin, stem cell factor, and interleukin-11 to enhance murine megakaryocyte colony growth and increases megakaryocyte ploidy *in vitro*. *Blood* 85:1719, 1995.

78. Dean YD, McGreal EP, Akatsu H, et al: Molecular and cellular properties of the rat AA4 antigen, a C-type lectin-like receptor with structural homology to thrombomodulin. *J Biol Chem* 275:34382, 2000.

79. Uchida N, Weissman IL: Searching for hematopoietic stem cells: Evidence that Thy-1.110 Lin– Sca-1+ cells are the only stem cells in C57BL/Ka-Thy-1.1 bone marrow. *J Exp Med* 175:175, 1992.

80. Ito CY, Li CY, Bernstein A, et al: Hematopoietic stem cell and progenitor defects in Sca-1/Ly-6A-null mice. *Blood* 101:517, 2003.

81. Miraglia S, Godfrey W, Yin AH, et al: A novel five-transmembrane hematopoietic stem cell antigen: Isolation, characterization, and molecular cloning. *Blood* 90:5013, 1997.

82. Fargeas CA, Florek M, Huttner WB, et al: Characterization of prominin-2, a new member of the prominin family of pentaspan membrane glycoproteins. *J Biol Chem* 278:8586, 2003.

83. Watt SM, Buhring HJ, Rappold I, et al: CD164, a novel sialomucin on CD34(+) and erythroid subsets, is located on human chromosome 6q21. *Blood* 92:849, 1998.

84. Zannettino AC, Buhring HJ, Niutta S, et al: The sialomucin CD164 (MGC-24v) is an adhesive glycoprotein expressed by human hematopoietic progenitors and bone marrow stromal cells that serves as a potent negative regulator of hematopoiesis. *Blood* 92:2613, 1998.

85. Kiel MJ, Yilmaz OH, Iwashita T, et al: SLAM family receptors distinguish hematopoietic stem and progenitor cells and reveal endothelial niches for stem cells. *Cell* 121:1109, 2005.

86. Zeigler FC, de Sauvage F, Widmer HR, et al: *In vitro* megakaryocytopoietic and thrombopoietic activity of c-mpl ligand (TPO) on purified murine hematopoietic stem cells. *Blood* 84:4045, 1994.

87. Solar GP, Kerr WG, Zeigler FC, et al: Role of c-mpl in early hematopoiesis. *Blood* 92:4, 1998.

88. Kent DG, Copley MR, Benz C, et al: Prospective isolation and molecular characterization of hematopoietic stem cells with durable self-renewal potential. *Blood* 113:6342, 2009.

89. Hynes RO: Integrins: Versatility, modulation, and signaling in cell adhesion. *Cell* 69:11, 1992.

90. Fukai F, Mashimo M, Akiyama K, et al: Modulation of apoptotic cell death by extracellular matrix proteins and a fibronectin-derived antiadhesive peptide. *Exp Cell Res* 242:92, 1998.

91. Fang F, Orend G, Watanabe N, et al: Dependence of cyclin E-CDK2 kinase activity on cell anchorage. *Science* 271:499, 1996.

92. Pozzi A, Wary KK, Giancotti FG, et al: Integrin alpha1beta1 mediates a unique collagen-dependent proliferation pathway *in vivo*. *J Cell Biol* 142:587, 1998.

93. Tropel P, Roullot V, Vernet M, et al: A 2.7-kb portion of the 5′ flanking region of the murine glycoprotein alphaIIb gene is transcriptionally active in primitive hematopoietic progenitor cells. *Blood* 90:2995, 1997.

94. Kovach NL, Lin N, Yednock T, et al: Stem cell factor modulates avidity of alpha 4 beta 1 and alpha 5 beta 1 integrins expressed on hematopoietic cell lines. *Blood* 85:159, 1995.

95. Zauli G, Bassini A, Vitale M, et al: Thrombopoietin enhances the alpha IIb beta 3-dependent adhesion of megakaryocytic cells to fibrinogen or fibronectin through PI 3 kinase. *Blood* 89:883, 1997.

96. Peled A, Kollet O, Ponomaryov T, et al: The chemokine SDF-1 activates the integrins LFA-1, VLA-4, and VLA-5 on immature human CD34(+) cells: Role in transendothelial/stromal migration and engraftment of NOD/SCID mice. *Blood* 95:3289, 2000.

97. Papayannopoulou T: Mechanisms of stem-/progenitor-cell mobilization: The anti-VLA-4 paradigm. *Semin Hematol* 37:11, 2000.

98. Chaudhary PM, Roninson IB: Expression and activity of P-glycoprotein, a multidrug efflux pump, in human hematopoietic stem cells. *Cell* 66:85, 1991.

99. Wolf NS, Kone A, Priestley GV, et al: *In vivo* and *in vitro* characterization of long-term repopulating primitive hematopoietic cells isolated by sequential Hoechst 33342-rhodamine 123 FACS selection. *Exp Hematol* 21:614, 1993.

100. Ariki R, Morikawa S, Mabuchi Y, et al: Homeodomain transcription factor meis1 is a critical regulator of adult bone marrow hematopoiesis. *PLoS One* 9:e87646, 2014.

101. Simsek, T, Kocabas, F, Zheng J, et al: The distinct metabolic profile of hematopoietic stem cells reflects their location in a hypoxic niche. *Cell Stem Cell* 7, 380, 2010.

102. Klimmeck D, Hansson J, Raffel S, et al: Proteomic cornerstones of hematopoietic stem cell differentiation: distinct signatures of multipotent progenitors and myeloid committed cells. *Mol Cell Proteomics* 11, 286, 2012.

102. Habibian HK, Peters SO, Hsieh CC, et al: The fluctuating phenotype of the lymphohematopoietic stem cell with cell cycle transit. *J Exp Med* 188:393, 1998.

103. Orschell-Traycoff CM, Hiatt K, Dagher RN, et al: Homing and engraftment potential of Sca-1(+)lin(–) cells fractionated on the basis of adhesion molecule expression and position in cell cycle. *Blood* 96:1380, 2000.

104. Stier S, Cheng T, Forkert R, et al: *Ex vivo* targeting of p21Cip1/Waf1 permits relative expansion of human hematopoietic stem cells. *Blood* 102:1260, 2003.

105. Lambert JF, Liu M, Colvin GA, et al: Marrow stem cells shift gene expression and engraftment phenotype with cell cycle transit. *J Exp Med* 197:1563, 2003.

106. Wilpshaar J, Falkenburg JH, Tong X, et al: Similar repopulating capacity of mitotically active and resting umbilical cord blood CD34(+) cells in NOD/SCID mice. *Blood* 96:2100, 2000.

107. Hu M, Krause D, Greaves M, et al: Multilineage gene expression precedes commitment in the hemopoietic system. *Genes Dev* 11:774, 1997.

108. Miyamoto T, Iwasaki H, Reizis B, et al: Myeloid or lymphoid promiscuity as a critical step in hematopoietic lineage commitment. *Dev Cell* 3:137, 2002.

109. Nutt SL, Heavey B, Rolink AG, et al: Commitment to the B-lymphoid lineage depends on the transcription factor Pax5. *Nature* 401:556, 1999.

110. Phillips RL, Ernst RE, Brunk B, et al: The genetic program of hematopoietic stem cells. *Science* 288:1635, 2000.

111. Terskikh AV, Easterday MC, Li L, et al: From hematopoiesis to neuropoiesis: Evidence of overlapping genetic programs. *Proc Natl Acad Sci U S A* 98:7934, 2001.

112. Lessard J, Sauvageau G: Bmi-1 determines the proliferative capacity of normal and leukaemic stem cells. *Nature* 423:255, 2003.

113. Tadokoro Y, Ema H, Okano M, Li E, Nakauchi H: *De novo* DNA methyltransferase is essential for self-renewal, but not for differentiation, in hematopoietic stem cells. *J Exp Med* 204:715, 2007.

114. Starnes LM, Sorrentino A: Regulatory circuitries coordinated by transcription factors and microRNAs at the cornerstone of hematopoietic stem cell self-renewal and differentiation. *Curr Stem Cell Res Ther* 6:142, 2011.

115. Cillo C, Cantile M, Faiella A, et al: Homeobox genes in normal and malignant cells. *J Cell Physiol* 188:161, 2001.

116. Magli MC, Largman C, Lawrence HJ: Effects of HOX homeobox genes in blood cell differentiation. *J Cell Physiol* 173:168, 1997.

117. Sauvageau G, Thorsteinsdottir U, Eaves CJ, et al: Overexpression of HOXB4 in hematopoietic cells causes the selective expansion of more primitive populations *in vitro* and *in vivo*. *Genes Dev* 9:1753, 1995..

118. Lawrence HJ, Helgason CD, Sauvageau G, et al: Mice bearing a targeted interruption of the homeobox gene HOXA9 have defects in myeloid, erythroid, and lymphoid hematopoiesis. *Blood* 89:1922, 1997.

119. Yagi H, Deguchi K, Aono A, et al: Growth disturbance in fetal liver hematopoiesis of Mll-mutant mice. *Blood* 92:108, 1998.

120. DiMartino JF, Selleri L, Traver D, et al: The Hox cofactor and proto-oncogene Pbx1 is required for maintenance of definitive hematopoiesis in the fetal liver. *Blood* 98:618, 2001.

121. Calvo KR, Knoepfler PS, Sykes DB, et al: Meis1a suppresses differentiation by G-CSF and promotes proliferation by SCF: Potential mechanisms of cooperativity with Hoxa9 in myeloid leukemia. *Proc Natl Acad Sci U S A* 98:13120, 2001.

122. Georgopoulos K: Transcription factors required for lymphoid lineage commitment. *Curr Opin Immunol* 9:222, 1997.

123. Molnar A, Georgopoulos K: The Ikaros gene encodes a family of functionally diverse zinc finger DNA-binding proteins. *Mol Cell Biol* 14:8292, 1994.

124. Wang JH, Nichogiannopoulou A, Wu L, et al: Selective defects in the development of the fetal and adult lymphoid system in mice with an Ikaros null mutation. *Immunity* 5:537, 1996.

125. McKercher SR, Torbett BE, Anderson KL, et al: Targeted disruption of the PU.1 gene results in multiple hematopoietic abnormalities. *EMBO J* 15:5647, 1996.

126. Begley CG, Aplan PD, Denning SM, et al: The gene SCL is expressed during early hematopoiesis and encodes a differentiation-related DNA-binding motif. *Proc Natl Acad Sci U S A* 86:10128, 1989.

127. Lecuyer E, Hoang T: SCL: From the origin of hematopoiesis to stem cells and leukemia. *Exp Hematol* 32:11, 2004.

128. Shivdasani RA, Mayer EL, Orkin SH: Absence of blood formation in mice lacking the T-cell leukaemia oncoprotein tal-1/SCL. *Nature* 373:432, 1995.

129. Brady G, Billia F, Knox J, et al: Analysis of gene expression in a complex differentiation hierarchy by global amplification of cDNA from single cells. *Curr Biol* 5:909, 1995.

130. Hoang T, Paradis E, Brady G, et al: Opposing effects of the basic helix-loop-helix transcription factor SCL on erythroid and monocytic differentiation. *Blood* 87:102, 1996.

131. Caceres-Cortes JR, Krosl G, Tessier N, et al: Steel factor sustains SCL expression and the survival of purified CD34+ bone marrow cells in the absence of detectable cell differentiation. *Stem Cells* 19:59, 2001.

132. Martin DI, Tsai SF, Orkin SH: Increased gamma-globin expression in a nondeletion HPFH mediated by an erythroid-specific DNA-binding factor. *Nature* 338:435, 1989.

133. Persons DA, Allay JA, Allay ER, et al: Enforced expression of the GATA-2 transcription factor blocks normal hematopoiesis. *Blood* 93:488, 1999.

134. Deveaux S, Filipe A, Lemarchandel V, et al: Analysis of the thrombopoietin receptor (MPL) promoter implicates GATA and Ets proteins in the coregulation of megakaryocyte-specific genes. *Blood* 87:4678, 1996.

136. Yamaguchi Y, Ackerman SJ, Minegishi N, et al: Mechanisms of transcription in eosinophils: GATA-1, but not GATA-2, transactivates the promoter of the eosinophil granule major basic protein gene. *Blood* 91:3447, 1998.

136. Dykstra B, Olthof S, Schreuder J, et al: Clonal analysis reveals multiple functional defects of aged murine hematopoietic stem cells. *J Exp Med* 208:2691, 2011.

137. Pang WW, Price EA, Sahoo D, et al: Human bone marrow hematopoietic stem cells are increased in frequency and myeloid-biased with age. *Proc Natl Acad Sci U S A* 108:20012, 2011.

138. Geiger H, de Haan G, Florian MC: The aging hematopoietic stem cell compartment. *Nat Rev Immunol* 13:376, 2013.

139. Kaushansky K, Lin N, Adamson JW: Interleukin 1 stimulates fibroblasts to synthesize granulocyte-macrophage and granulocyte colony-stimulating factors. Mechanism for the hematopoietic response to inflammation. *J Clin Invest* 81:92, 1988.

140. Toksoz D, Zsebo KM, Smith KA, et al: Support of human hematopoiesis in long-term bone marrow cultures by murine stromal cells selectively expressing the membrane-bound and secreted forms of the human homolog of the steel gene product, stem cell factor. *Proc Natl Acad Sci U S A* 89:7350, 1992.

141. Selleri C, Maciejewski JP, Sato T, et al: Interferon-gamma constitutively expressed in the stromal microenvironment of human marrow cultures mediates potent hematopoietic inhibition. *Blood* 87:4149, 1996.

142. Guerriero A, Worford L, Holland HK, et al: Thrombopoietin is synthesized by bone marrow stromal cells. *Blood* 90:3444, 1997.

143. Miyazawa K, Williams DA, Gotoh A, et al: Membrane-bound Steel factor induces more persistent tyrosine kinase activation and longer life span of c-kit gene-encoded protein than its soluble form. *Blood* 85:641, 1995.

144. Gordon MY, Riley GP, Watt SM, et al: Compartmentalization of a haematopoietic growth factor (GM-CSF) by glycosaminoglycans in the bone marrow microenvironment. *Nature* 326:403, 1987.

145. Artavanis-Tsakonas S, Matsuno K, Fortini ME: Notch signaling. *Science* 268:225, 1995.

146. Nye JS, Kopan R: Developmental signaling. Vertebrate ligands for Notch. *Curr Biol* 5:966, 1995.

147. Karanu FN, Murdoch B, Miyabayashi T, et al: Human homologues of Delta-1 and Delta-4 function as mitogenic regulators of primitive human hematopoietic cells. *Blood* 97:1960, 2001.

148. Kapur R, Cooper R, Zhang L, et al: Cross-talk between alpha(4)beta(1)/alpha(5)beta(1) and c-Kit results in opposing effect on growth and survival of hematopoietic cells via the activation of focal adhesion kinase, mitogen-activated protein kinase, and Akt signaling pathways. *Blood* 97:1975, 2001.

149. Shaklai M, Tavassoli M: Cellular relationship in the rat bone marrow studied by freeze fracture and lanthanum impregnation thin-sectioning electron microscopy. *J Ultrastruct Res* 69:343, 1979.

150. Westen H, Bainton DF: Association of alkaline-phosphatase-positive reticulum cells in bone marrow with granulocytic precursors. *J Exp Med* 150:919, 1979.

151. Tavassoli M, Aoki M: Localization of megakaryocytes in the bone marrow. *Blood Cells* 15:3, 1989.

152. Blazsek I, Chagraoui J, Peault B: Ontogenic emergence of the hematon, a morphogenetic stromal unit that supports multipotential hematopoietic progenitors in mouse bone marrow. *Blood* 96:3763, 2000.

153. Simmons PJ, Masinovsky B, Longenecker BM, et al: Vascular cell adhesion molecule-1 expressed by bone marrow stromal cells mediates the binding of hematopoietic progenitor cells. *Blood* 80:388, 1992.

154. Rafii S, Shapiro F, Pettengell R, et al: Human bone marrow microvascular endothelial cells support long-term proliferation and differentiation of myeloid and megakaryocytic progenitors. *Blood* 86:3353, 1995.

155. Sugiyama T, Kohara H, Noda M, Nagasawa T: Maintenance of the hematopoietic stem cell pool by CXCL12-CXCR4 chemokine signaling in bone marrow stromal cell niches. *Immunity* 25:977, 2006.

156. Calvi LM, Link DC: Cellular complexity of the bone marrow hematopoietic stem cell niche. *Calcif Tissue Int* 94:112, 2014.

157. Islam A, Glomski C, Henderson ES: Bone lining (endosteal) cells and hematopoiesis: A light microscopic study of normal and pathologic human bone marrow in plastic-embedded sections. *Anat Rec* 227:300, 1990.

158. Ellis SL, Nilsson SK: The location and cellular composition of the hemopoietic stem cell niche. *Cytotherapy* 14:135, 2012.

159. Keating A: Mesenchymal stromal cells. *Curr Opin Hematol* 13:419, 2006.

160. Dazzi F, Horwood NJ: Potential of mesenchymal stem cell therapy. *Curr Opin Oncol* 19:650, 2007.

161. Lok S, Kaushansky K, Holly RD, et al: Cloning and expression of murine thrombopoietin cDNA and stimulation of platelet production *in vivo*. *Nature* 369:565, 1994.

162. McCarty JM, Sprugel KH, Fox NE, et al: Murine thrombopoietin mRNA levels are modulated by platelet count. *Blood* 86:3668, 1995.

163. Sungaran R, Markovic B, Chong BH: Localization and regulation of thrombopoietin mRNa expression in human kidney, liver, bone marrow, and spleen using *in situ* hybridization. *Blood* 89:101, 1997.

164. Solanilla A, Dechanet J, El Andaloussi A, et al: CD40-ligand stimulates myelopoiesis by regulating flt3-ligand and thrombopoietin production in bone marrow stromal cells. *Blood* 95:3758, 2000.

165. Quirici N, Soligo D, Caneva L, et al: Differentiation and expansion of endothelial cells from human bone marrow CD133(+) cells. *Br J Haematol* 115:186, 2001.

166. Yanai N, Sekine C, Yagita H, et al: Roles for integrin very late activation antigen-4 in stroma-dependent erythropoiesis. *Blood* 83:2844, 1994.

167. Jung Y, Wang J, Song J, et al: Annexin II expressed by osteoblasts and endothelial cells regulates stem cell adhesion, homing, and engraftment following transplantation. *Blood* 110:82, 2007.

168. Scott LM PG, Koni P, Papayannopoulou T: Adult mice with conditional VCAM-1 ablation show altered hemopoietic progenitor biodistribution, homing and regeneration patterns. *Blood* 102, 2003.

169. Carstanjen D, Ulbricht N, Iacone A, et al: Matrix metalloproteinase-9 (gelatinase B) is elevated during mobilization of peripheral blood progenitor cells by G-CSF. *Transfusion* 42:588, 2002.

170. Yamazaki K, Allen TD: Ultrastructural morphometric study of efferent nerve terminals on murine bone marrow stromal cells, and the recognition of a novel anatomical unit: the "neuro-reticular complex" *Am J Anat J Anat* 187:261, 1990.

171. Méndez-Ferrer S, Michurina TV, Ferraro F, et al: Mesenchymal and hematopoietic stem cells form a unique bone marrow niche. *Nature* 466:829, 2010.

172. Lucas D, Scheiermann C, Chow A, et al: Chemotherapy-induced bone marrow nerve injury impairs hematopoietic regeneration. *Nat Med* 19:695, 2013.

173. Yuzawa S, Opatowsky Y, Zhang Z, et al: Structural basis for activation of the receptor tyrosine kinase kit by stem cell factor. *Cell* 130:323, 2007.

174. Liang J, Wu YL, Chen BJ, et al: The c-kit receptor-mediated signal transduction and tumor-related diseases. *Int J Biol Sci* 9:435, 2013.

175. Li CL, Johnson GR: Stem-cell factor enhances the survival but not the self-renewal of murine hematopoietic long-term repopulating cells. *Blood* 84:408, 1994.

176. Bernstein ID, Andrews RG, Zsebo KM: Recombinant human stem-cell factor enhances the formation of colonies by CD34+ and CD34+Lin cells, and the generation of colony-forming cell progeny from CD34+Lin cells cultured with interleukin-3, granulocyte colony-stimulating factor, or granulocyte-macrophage colony-stimulating factor. *Blood* 77:2316, 1991.

177. Brandt J, Briddell RA, Srour EF, et al: Role of c-Kit ligand in the expansion of human hematopoietic progenitor cells. *Blood* 79:634, 1992.

178. Ariyama Y, Misawa S, Sonoda Y: Synergistic effects of stem-cell factor and interleukin-6 or interleukin-11 on the expansion of murine hematopoietic progenitors in liquid suspension-culture. *Stem Cells* 13:404, 1995.

179. Kent D, Copley M, Benz C, et al: Regulation of hematopoietic stem cells by the steel factor/KIT signaling pathway. *Clin Cancer Res* 14:1926, 2008.

180. Wu H, Klingmuller U, Acurio A, et al: Functional interaction of erythropoietin and stem cell factor receptors is essential for erythroid colony formation. *Proc Natl Acad Sci U S A* 94:1806, 1997.

181. Lyman SD, James L, Johnson L, et al: Cloning of the human homolog of the murine Flt3 ligand—A growth factor for early hematopoietic progenitor cells. *Blood* 83:2795, 1994.

182. Rosnet O, Schiff C, Pebusque MJ, et al: Human Flt3/Flk2 gene—CDNA cloning and expression in hematopoietic cells. *Blood* 82:1110, 1993.

183. Parcells BW, Ikeda AK, Simms-Waldrip T, et al: FMS-like tyrosine kinase 3 in normal hematopoiesis and acute myeloid leukemia. *Stem Cells* 24:1174, 2006.

184. Thiede C, Steudel C, Mohr B, et al: Analysis of FLT3-activating mutations in 979 patients with acute myelogenous leukemia: Association with FAB subtypes and identification of subgroups with poor prognosis. *Blood* 99:4326, 2002.

185. Zwaan CM, Meshinchi S, Radich JP, et al: FLT3 internal tandem duplication in 234 children with acute myeloid leukemia: Prognostic significance and relation to cellular drug resistance. *Blood* 102:2387, 2003.

186. O'Farrell AM, Foran JM, Fiedler W, et al: An innovative phase I clinical study demonstrates inhibition of FLT3 phosphorylation by SU11248 in acute myeloid leukemia patients. *Clin Cancer Res* 9:5465, 2003.

187. Lyman SD, James L, Vanden Bos T, et al: Molecular cloning of a ligand for the flt3/flk-2 tyrosine kinase receptor: A proliferative factor for primitive hematopoietic cells. *Cell* 75:1157, 1993.

188. Lyman SD, James L, Escobar S, et al: Identification of soluble and membrane-bound isoforms of the murine flt3 ligand generated by alternative splicing of mRNAs. *Oncogene* 10:149, 1995.

189. Lyman SD, Seaberg M, Hanna R, et al: Plasma/serum levels of flt3 ligand are low in normal individuals and highly elevated in patients with Fanconi anemia and acquired aplastic anemia. *Blood* 86:4091, 1995.

190. Mackarehtschian K, Hardin JD, Moore KA, et al: Targeted disruption of the flk2/flt3 gene leads to deficiencies in primitive hematopoietic progenitors. *Immunity* 3:147, 1995.

191. Rasko JE, Metcalf D, Rossner MT, et al: The flt3/flk-2 ligand: Receptor distribution and action on murine haemopoietic cell survival and proliferation. *Leukemia* 9:2058, 1995.

192. Robinson S, Mosley RL, Parajuli P, et al: Comparison of the hematopoietic activity of flt-3 ligand and granulocyte-macrophage colony-stimulating factor acting alone or in combination. *J Hematother Stem Cell Res* 9:711, 2000.

193. Kobayashi M, Laver JH, Kato T, et al: Thrombopoietin supports proliferation of human primitive hematopoietic cells in synergy with steel factor and/or interleukin-3. *Blood* 88:429, 1996.

194. Piacibello W, Sanavio F, Garetto L, et al: Extensive amplification and self-renewal of human primitive hematopoietic stem cells from cord blood. *Blood* 89:2644, 1997.

195. Namikawa R, Muench MO, de Vries JE, et al: The FLK2/FLT3 ligand synergizes with interleukin-7 in promoting stromal-cell-independent expansion and differentiation of human fetal pro-B cells *in vitro*. *Blood* 87:1881, 1996.

196. Strobl H, Bello-Fernandez C, Riedl E, et al: Flt3 ligand in cooperation with transforming growth factor-beta1 potentiates *in vitro* development of Langerhans-type dendritic cells and allows single-cell dendritic cell cluster formation under serum-free conditions. *Blood* 90:1425, 1997.

197. Kaushansky K: Thrombopoietin: The primary regulator of platelet production. *Blood* 86:419, 1995.

198. Qian S, Fu F, Li W, et al: Primary role of the liver in thrombopoietin production shown by tissue-specific knockout. *Blood* 92:2189, 1998.

199. Kaushansky K: Thrombopoietin. *N Engl J Med* 339:746, 1998.

200. Sitnicka E, Lin N, Priestley GV, et al: The effect of thrombopoietin on the proliferation and differentiation of murine hematopoietic stem cells. *Blood* 87:4998, 1996.

201. Kobayashi M, Laver JH, Kato T, et al: Recombinant human thrombopoietin (Mpl ligand) enhances proliferation of erythroid progenitors. *Blood* 86:2494, 1995.

202. Kaushansky K, Broudy VC, Grossmann A, et al: Thrombopoietin expands erythroid progenitors, increases red cell production, and enhances erythroid recovery after myelosuppressive therapy. *J Clin Invest* 96:1683, 1995.

203. Akahori H, Shibuya K, Obuchi M, et al: Effect of recombinant human thrombopoietin in nonhuman primates with chemotherapy-induced thrombocytopenia. *Br J Haematol* 94:722, 1996.

204. Neelis KJ, Hartong SC, Egeland T, et al: The efficacy of single-dose administration of thrombopoietin with coadministration of either granulocyte/macrophage or granulocyte colony-stimulating factor in myelosuppressed rhesus monkeys. *Blood* 90:2565, 1997.

205. Farese AM, Hunt P, Grab LB, et al: Combined administration of recombinant human megakaryocyte growth and development factor and granulocyte colony-stimulating factor enhances multilineage hematopoietic reconstitution in nonhuman primates after radiation-induced marrow aplasia. *J Clin Invest* 97:2145, 1996.

206. Alexander WS, Roberts AW, Nicola NA, et al: Deficiencies in progenitor cells of multiple hematopoietic lineages and defective megakaryocytopoiesis in mice lacking the thrombopoietic receptor c-Mpl. *Blood* 87:2162, 1996.

207. Yagi M, Ritchie KA, Sitnicka E, et al: Sustained *ex vivo* expansion of hematopoietic stem cells mediated by thrombopoietin. *Proc Natl Acad Sci U S A* 96:8126, 1999.

208. Broxmeyer HE, Kohli L, Kim CH, et al: Stromal cell-derived factor-1/CXCL12 directly enhances survival/antiapoptosis of myeloid progenitor cells through CXCR4 and G(alpha)i proteins and enhances engraftment of competitive, repopulating stem cells. *J Leukoc Biol* 73:630, 2003.

209. Lee Y, Gotoh A, Kwon H-J, et al: Enhancement of intracellular signaling associated with hematopoietic progenitor cell survival in response to SDF-1/CXCL12 in synergy with other cytokines. *Blood* 99:4307, 2002.

210. Ellisen LW, Bird J, West DC, et al: TAN-1, the human homolog of the *Drosophila* notch gene, is broken by chromosomal translocations in T lymphoblastic neoplasms. *Cell* 66(4):649, 1991.

211. Milner LA, Kopan R, Martin DI, Bernstein ID: A human homologue of the *Drosophila* developmental gene, Notch, is expressed in CD34+ hematopoietic precursors. *Blood* 83:2057, 1994.

212. Karanu FN, Murdoch B, Gallacher L, et al: The notch ligand jagged-1 represents a novel growth factor of human hematopoietic stem cells. *J Exp Med* 192:1365, 2000.

213. Karanu FN, Murdoch B, Miyabayashi T, et al: Human homologues of Delta-1 and Delta-4 function as mitogenic regulators of primitive human hematopoietic cells. *Blood* 97:1960, 2001.

214. Varnum-Finney B, Brashem-Stein C, Bernstein ID: Combined effects of Notch signaling and cytokines induce a multiple log increase in precursors with lymphoid and myeloid reconstituting ability. *Blood* 101:1784, 2003.

215. Austin TW, Solar GP, Ziegler FC, et al: A role for the Wnt gene family in hematopoiesis: Expansion of multilineage progenitor cells. *Blood* 89:3624, 1997.

216. Willert K, Brown JD, Danenberg E, et al: Wnt proteins are lipid-modified and can act as stem cell growth factors. *Nature* 423:448, 2003.

217. Reya T, Duncan AW, Ailles L, et al: A role for Wnt signaling in self-renewal of hematopoietic stem cells. *Nature* 423:409, 2003.

218. Van Den Berg DJ, Sharma AK, Bruno E, Hoffman R: Role of members of the Wnt gene family in human hematopoiesis. *Blood* 92:3189, 1998.

219. Shi Y, Massague J: Mechanisms of TGF-beta signaling from cell membrane to the nucleus. *Cell* 113:685, 2003.

220. Sitnicka E, Ruscetti FW, Priestley GV, et al: Transforming growth factor beta 1 directly and reversibly inhibits the initial cell divisions of long-term repopulating hematopoietic stem cells. *Blood* 88:82, 1996.

221. Batard P, Monier MN, Fortunel N, et al: TGF-(beta)1 maintains hematopoietic immaturity by a reversible negative control of cell cycle and induces CD34 antigen up-modulation. *J Cell Sci* 113(Pt 3):383, 2000.

222. Larsson J, Blank U, Helgadottir H, et al: TGF-beta signaling-deficient hematopoietic stem cells have normal self-renewal and regenerative ability *in vivo* despite increased proliferative capacity *in vitro*. *Blood* 102:3129, 2003.

223. Larsson J, Karlsson S: The role of Smad signaling in hematopoiesis. *Oncogene* 29:5676, 2005.

224. Blank U, Karlsson G, Moody JL, et al: Smad7 promotes self-renewal of hematopoietic stem cells *in vivo*. *Blood* 108:4246, 2006.

225. Karlsson G, Blank U, Moody JL, et al: Smad4 is critical for self-renewal of hematopoietic stem cells. *J Exp Med* 204:467, 2007.

226. Lengerke C, Schmitt S, Bowman TV, et al: BMP and Wnt specify hematopoietic fate by activation of the Cdx-Hox pathway. *Cell Stem Cell* 2:72, 2008.

227. Timm A, Grosschedl R: Wnt signaling in lymphopoiesis. *Curr Top Microbiol Immunol* 290:225, 2005.

228. Ross S, Hill CS: How the Smads regulate transcription. *Int J Biochem Cell Biol* 40:383, 2008.

229. Krosl G, He G, Lefrancois M, et al: Transcription factor SCL is required for c-kit expression and c-Kit function in hemopoietic cells. *J Exp Med* 188:439, 1998.

230. Kirito K, Fox N, Kaushansky K: Thrombopoietin stimulates Hoxb4 expression: An explanation for the favorable effects of TPO on hematopoietic stem cells. *Blood* 102:3172, 2003.

231. Kirito K, Fox N, Kaushansky K: Thrombopoietin (TPO) induces the nuclear translocation of HoxA9 in hematopoietic stem cells (HSC): A potential explanation for the favorable effects of TPO on HSCs. *Mol Cell Biol* 24:6751, 2004.

232. Tong W, Lodish HF: Lnk inhibits Tpo-mpl signaling and Tpo-mediated megakaryocytopoiesis. *J Exp Med* 200:569, 2004.

233. Tong W, Zhang J, Lodish HF: Lnk inhibits erythropoiesis and EPO-dependent JAK2 activation and downstream signaling pathways. *Blood* 105:4604, 2005.

234. Takaki S, Sauer K, Iritani BM, et al: Control of B cell production by the adaptor protein lnk: Definition of a conserved family of signal-modulating proteins. *Immunity* 13:599, 2000.

235. Seita J, Ema H, Ooehara J, et al: Lnk negatively regulates self-renewal of hematopoietic stem cells by modifying thrombopoietin-mediated signal transduction. *Proc Natl Acad Sci U S A* 104:2349, 2007.

236. Buza-Vidas N, Antonchuk J, Qian H, et al: Cytokines regulate postnatal hematopoietic stem cell expansion: opposing roles of thrombopoietin and LNK. *Genes Dev* 20:2018, 2006.

237. Schick PK, Wojenski CM, Bennett VD, et al: The synthesis and localization of alternatively spliced fibronectin EIIIB in resting and thrombin-treated megakaryocytes. *Blood* 87:1817, 1996.

238. Prosper F, Stroncek D, McCarthy JB, et al: Mobilization and homing of peripheral blood progenitors is related to reversible downregulation of alpha4 beta1 integrin expression and function. *J Clin Invest* 101:2456, 1998.

239. Dao MA, Hashino K, Kato I, et al: Adhesion to fibronectin maintains regenerative capacity during *ex vivo* culture and transduction of human hematopoietic stem and progenitor cells. *Blood* 92:4612, 1998.

240. Yokota T, Oritani K, Mitsui H, et al: Growth-supporting activities of fibronectin on hematopoietic stem/progenitor cells *in vitro* and *in vivo*: Structural requirement for fibronectin activities of CS1 and cell-binding domains. *Blood* 91:3263, 1998.

241. Bhatia R, Williams AD, Munthe HA: Contact with fibronectin enhances preservation of normal but not chronic myelogenous leukemia primitive hematopoietic progenitors. *Exp Hematol* 30:324, 2002.

242. Liu S, Kiosses WB, Rose DM, et al: A fragment of paxillin binds the alpha 4 integrin cytoplasmic domain (tail) and selectively inhibits alpha 4-mediated cell migration. *J Biol Chem* 277:20887, 2002.

243. Sarkar S, Svoboda M, de Beaumont R, et al: The role of Aktand RAFTK in beta1 integrin mediated survival of precursor B-acute lymphoblastic leukemia cells. *Leuk Lymphoma* 43:1663, 2002.

244. Zhao J, Bian ZC, Yee K, et al: Identification of transcription factor KLF8 as a downstream target of focal adhesion kinase in its regulation of cyclin D1 and cell cycle progression. *Mol Cell* 11:1503, 2003.

245. Schlaepfer DD, Hunter T: Focal adhesion kinase overexpression enhances ras-dependent integrin signaling to ERK2/mitogen-activated protein kinase through interactions with and activation of c-Src. *J Biol Chem* 272:13189, 1997.

246. Legras S, Levesque JP, Charrad R, et al: CD44-mediated adhesiveness of human hematopoietic progenitors to hyaluronan is modulated by cytokines. *Blood* 89:1905, 1997.

247. Bendall LJ, James A, Zannettino A, et al: A novel CD44 antibody identifies an epitope that is aberrantly expressed on acute lymphoblastic leukaemia cells. *Immunol Cell Biol* 81:311, 2003.

248. Bendall LJ, Kirkness J, Hutchinson A, et al: Antibodies to CD44 enhance adhesion of normal CD34+ cells and acute myeloblastic but not lymphoblastic leukaemia cells to bone marrow stroma. *Br J Haematol* 98:828, 1997.

249. Pilarski LM, Pruski E, Wizniak J, et al: Potential role for hyaluronan and the hyaluronan receptor RHAMM in mobilization and trafficking of hematopoietic progenitor cells. *Blood* 93:2918, 1999.

250. Nilsson SK, Haylock DN, Johnston HM, et al: Hyaluronan is synthesized by primitive hemopoietic cells, participates in their lodgment at the endosteum following transplantation, and is involved in the regulation of their proliferation and differentiation *in vitro*. *Blood* 101:856, 2003.

251. Gupta P, Oegema TR Jr, Brazil JJ, et al: Structurally specific heparan sulfates support primitive human hematopoiesis by formation of a multimolecular stem cell niche. *Blood* 92:4641, 1998.

252. Klein G, Beck S, Muller CA: Tenascin is a cytoadhesive extracellular matrix component of the human hematopoietic microenvironment. *J Cell Biol* 123:1027, 1993.

253. Seiffert M, Beck SC, Schermutzki F, et al: Mitogenic and adhesive effects of tenascin-C on human hematopoietic cells are mediated by various functional domains. *Matrix Biol* 17:47, 1998.

254. Ohta M, Sakai T, Saga Y, et al: Suppression of hematopoietic activity in tenascin-C-deficient mice. *Blood* 91:4074, 1998.

255. Siler U, Seiffert M, Puch S, et al: Characterization and functional analysis of laminin isoforms in human bone marrow. *Blood* 96:4194, 2000.

256. Gu Y, Sorokin L, Durbeej M, et al: Characterization of bone marrow laminins and identification of alpha5-containing laminins as adhesive proteins for multipotent hematopoietic FDCP-Mix cells. *Blood* 93:2533, 1999.

257. Siler U, Rousselle P, Muller CA, et al: Laminin gamma2 chain as a stromal cell marker of the human bone marrow microenvironment. *Br J Haematol* 119:212, 2002.

258. Landowski TH, Dratz EA, Starkey JR: Studies of the structure of the metastasis-associated 67 kDa laminin binding protein: Fatty acid acylation and evidence supporting dimerization of the 32 kDa gene product to form the mature protein. *Biochemistry* 34:11276, 1995.

259. Ardini E, Tagliabue E, Magnifico A, et al: Co-regulation and physical association of the 67-kDa monomeric laminin receptor and the alpha6beta4 integrin. *J Biol Chem* 272:2342, 1997.

260. Gu YC, Kortesmaa J, Tryggvason K, et al: Laminin isoform-specific promotion of adhesion and migration of human bone marrow progenitor cells. *Blood* 101:877, 2003.

261. Chen J, Carcamo JM, Borquez-Ojeda O, et al: The laminin receptor modulates granulocyte-macrophage colony-stimulating factor receptor complex formation and modulates its signaling. *Proc Natl Acad Sci U S A* 100:14000, 2003.

262. Klein G, Muller CA, Tillet E, et al: Collagen type VI in the human bone marrow microenvironment: A strong cytoadhesive component. *Blood* 86:1740, 1995.

263. Ergen AV, Boles NC, Goodell MA: Rantes/Ccl5 influences hematopoietic stem cell subtypes and causes myeloid skewing. *Blood* 119:2500, 2012.

264. Metcalf D: Lineage commitment and maturation in hematopoietic cells: The case for extrinsic regulation. *Blood* 92:345; discussion 352, 1998.

265. Enver T, Heyworth CM, Dexter TM: Do stem cells play dice? *Blood* 92:348; discussion 352, 1998.

266. Souabni A, Cobaleda C, Schebesta M, et al: Pax5 promotes B lymphopoiesis and blocks T cell development by repressing Notch1. *Immunity* 17:781, 2002.

267. Georgopoulos K, Moore DD, Derfler B: Ikaros, an early lymphoid-specific transcription factor and a putative mediator for T cell commitment. *Science* 258:808, 1992.

268. Hromas R, Orazi A, Neiman RS, et al: Hematopoietic lineage- and stage-restricted expression of the ETS oncogene family member PU.1. *Blood* 82:2998, 1993.

269. Hohaus S, Petrovick MS, Voso MT, et al: PU.1 (Spi-1) and C/EBP alpha regulate expression of the granulocyte-macrophage colony-stimulating factor receptor alpha gene. *Mol Cell Biol* 15:5830, 1995.

270. Martin DI, Zon LI, Mutter G, et al: Expression of an erythroid transcription factor in megakaryocytic and mast cell lineages. *Nature* 344:444, 1990.

271. Hart A, Melet F, Grossfeld P, et al: Fli-1 is required for murine vascular and megakaryocytic development and is hemizygously deleted in patients with thrombocytopenia. *Immunity* 13:167, 2000.

272. Gombart AF, Kwok SH, Anderson KL, et al: Regulation of neutrophil and eosinophil secondary granule gene expression by transcription factors C/EBP epsilon and PU.1. *Blood* 101:3265, 2003.

273. Enver T: B-cell commitment: Pax5 is the deciding factor. *Curr Biol* 9:R933, 1999.

274. Zhang DE, Zhang P, Wang ND, et al: Absence of granulocyte colony-stimulating factor signaling and neutrophil development in CCAAT enhancer binding protein alpha-deficient mice. *Proc Natl Acad Sci U S A* 94:569, 1997.

275. Cammenga J, Mulloy JC, Berguido FJ, et al: Induction of C/EBPalpha activity alters gene expression and differentiation of human CD34+ cells. *Blood* 101:2206, 2003.

276. Fairbairn LJ, Cowling GJ, Reipert BM, et al: Suppression of apoptosis allows differentiation and development of a multipotent hemopoietic cell line in the absence of added growth factors. *Cell* 74:823, 1993.

277. Nerlov C, Querfurth E, Kulessa H, et al: GATA-1 interacts with the myeloid PU.1 transcription factor and represses PU.1-dependent transcription. *Blood* 95:2543, 2000.

278. Zhang P, Zhang X, Iwama A, et al: PU.1 inhibits GATA-1 function and erythroid differentiation by blocking GATA-1 DNA binding. *Blood* 96:2641, 2000.

279. Kondo M, Scherer DC, Miyamoto T, et al: Cell-fate conversion of lymphoid-committed progenitors by instructive actions of cytokines. *Nature* 407:383, 2000.

280. Metcalf D: Lineage commitment in the progeny of murine hematopoietic prepogenitor cells: Influence of thrombopoietin and interleukin 5. *Proc Natl Acad Sci U S A* 95:6408, 1998.

281. Barroga C, Pham H, Kaushansky K: Thrombopoietin regulates c-myb expression by modulating microRNA (miR)150 expression. *Exp Hematol* 36:1585, 2008.

282. de Laval B, Pawlikowska P, Petit-Cocault L, et al: Thrombopoietin-increased DNA-P-K-dependent DNA repair limits hematopoietic stem and progenitor cell mutagenesis in response to DNA damage. *Cell Stem Cell* 12:37, 2013.

283. Zimdahl B, Ito T, Blevins A, et al: Lis1 regulates asymmetric division in hematopoietic stem cells and in leukemia. *Nat Genet* 46:245, 2014.

284. Thorsteinsdottir U, Sauvageau G, Humphries RK: Enhanced *in vivo* regenerative potential of HOXB4-transduced hematopoietic stem cells with regulation of their pool size. *Blood* 94:2605, 1999.

285. Iscove NN, Nawa K: Hematopoietic stem cells expand during serial transplantation *in vivo* without apparent exhaustion. *Curr Biol* 7:805, 1997.

286. Wilpshaar J, Bhatia M, Kanhai HH, et al: Engraftment potential of human fetal hematopoietic cells in NOD/SCID mice is not restricted to mitotically quiescent cells. *Blood* 100:120, 2002.

287. Czechowicz A, Kraft D, Weissman IL, Bhattacharya D: Efficient transplantation via antibody-based clearance of hematopoietic stem cell niches. *Science* 318:1296, 2007.

288. Fuchs E, Tumbar T, Guasch G: Socializing with the neighbors: Stem cells and their niche. *Cell* 116:769, 2004.

289. Mezey E, Chandross KJ, Harta G, et al: Turning blood into brain: Cells bearing neuronal antigens generated *in vivo* from bone marrow. *Science* 290:1779, 2000.

290. Brazelton TR, Rossi FM, Keshet GI, et al: From marrow to brain: Expression of neuronal phenotypes in adult mice. *Science* 290:1775, 2000.

291. Lagasse E, Connors H, Al-Dhalimy M, et al: Purified hematopoietic stem cells can differentiate into hepatocytes *in vivo*. *Nat Med* 6:1229, 2000.

292. Alison MR, Poulsom R, Jeffery R, et al: Hepatocytes from non-hepatic adult stem cells. *Nature* 406:257, 2000.

293. Ferrari G, Cusella-De Angelis G, Coletta M, et al: Muscle regeneration by bone marrow-derived myogenic progenitors. *Science* 279:1528, 1998.

294. Orlic D, Kajstura J, Chimenti S, et al: Bone marrow cells regenerate infarcted myocardium. *Nature* 410:701, 2001.

295. Jiang Y, Jahagirdar BN, Reinhardt RL, et al: Pluripotency of mesenchymal stem cells derived from adult marrow. *Nature* 418:41, 2002.

296. Ying QL, Nichols J, Evans EP, et al: Changing potency by spontaneous fusion. *Nature* 416:545, 2002.

297. Terada N, Hamazaki T, Oka M, et al: Bone marrow cells adopt the phenotype of other cells by spontaneous cell fusion. *Nature* 416:542, 2002.

298. Galy A, Travis M, Cen D, et al: Human T, B, natural killer, and dendritic cells arise from a common bone marrow progenitor cell subset. *Immunity* 3:459, 1995.

299. von Freeden-Jeffry U, Vieira P, Lucian LA, et al: Lymphopenia in interleukin (IL)-7 gene-deleted mice identifies IL-7 as a nonredundant cytokine. *J Exp Med* 181:1519, 1995.

300. Terskikh AV, Miyamoto T, Chang C, et al: Gene expression analysis of purified hematopoietic stem cells and committed progenitors. *Blood* 102:94, 2003.

301. Ikawa T, Kawamoto H, Fujimoto S, et al: Commitment of common T/natural killer (NK) progenitors to unipotent T and NK progenitors in the murine fetal thymus revealed by a single progenitor assay. *J Exp Med* 190:1617, 1999.

302. Massari ME, Murre C: Helix-loop-helix proteins: Regulators of transcription in eucaryotic organisms. *Mol Cell Biol* 20:429, 2000.

303. Sawada S, Littman DR: A heterodimer of HEB and an E12-related protein interacts with the CD4 enhancer and regulates its activity in T-cell lines. *Mol Cell Biol* 13:5620, 1993.

304. Takeuchi A, Yamasaki S, Takase K, et al: E2A and HEB activate the pre-TCR alpha promoter during immature T cell development. *J Immunol* 167:2157, 2001.

305. Bain G, Romanow WJ, Albers K, et al: Positive and negative regulation of V(D)J recombination by the E2A proteins. *J Exp Med* 189:289, 1999.

306. Norton JD: ID helix-loop-helix proteins in cell growth, differentiation and tumorigenesis. *J Cell Sci* 113 Pt 22:3897, 2000.

307. Yokota Y, Mansouri A, Mori S, et al: Development of peripheral lymphoid organs and natural killer cells depends on the helix-loop-helix inhibitor Id2. *Nature* 397:702, 1999.

308. Heemskerk MH, Blom B, Nolan G, et al: Inhibition of T cell and promotion of natural killer cell development by the dominant negative helix loop helix factor Id3. *J Exp Med* 186:1597, 1997.

309. Pui JC, Allman D, Xu L, et al: Notch1 expression in early lymphopoiesis influences B versus T lineage determination. *Immunity* 11:299, 1999.

310. Allman D, Karnell FG, Punt JA, et al: Separation of Notch1 promoted lineage commitment and expansion/transformation in developing T cells. *J Exp Med* 194:99, 2001.

311. Denis KA, Witte ON: *In vitro* development of B lymphocytes from long-term cultured precursor cells. *Proc Natl Acad Sci U S A* 83:441, 1986.

312. Takatsu K: Cytokines involved in B-cell differentiation and their sites of action. *Proc Soc Exp Biol Med* 215:121, 1997.

313. Namen AE, Lupton S, Hjerrild K, et al: Stimulation of B-cell progenitors by cloned murine interleukin-7. *Nature* 333:571, 1988.

314. Gibson LF, Piktel D, Landreth KS: Insulin-like growth factor-1 potentiates expansion of interleukin-7-dependent pro-B cells. *Blood* 82:3005, 1993.

315. Nagasawa T, Kikutani H, Kishimoto T: Molecular cloning and structure of a pre-B-cell growth-stimulating factor. *Proc Natl Acad Sci U S A* 91:2305, 1994.

316. McNiece IK, Langley KE, Zsebo KM: The role of recombinant stem cell factor in early B cell development. Synergistic interaction with IL-7. *J Immunol* 146:3785, 1991.

317. Gongora R, Stephan RP, Zhang Z, et al: An essential role for Daxx in the inhibition of B lymphopoiesis by type I interferons. *Immunity* 14:727, 2001.

318. Yoshikawa H, Nakajima Y, Tasaka K: IFN-gamma induces the apoptosis of WEHI 279 and normal pre-B cell lines by expressing direct inhibitor of apoptosis protein binding protein with low pI. *J Immunol* 167:2487, 2001.

319. Mitchell PL, Clutterbuck RD, Powles RL, et al: Interleukin-4 enhances the survival of severe combined immunodeficient mice engrafted with human B-cell precursor leukemia. *Blood* 87:4797, 1996.

320. Lee G, Namen AE, Gillis S, et al: Normal B cell precursors responsive to recombinant murine IL-7 and inhibition of IL-7 activity by transforming growth factor-beta. *J Immunol* 142:3875, 1989.

321. Bain G, Maandag EC, Izon DJ, et al: E2A proteins are required for proper B cell development and initiation of immunoglobulin gene rearrangements. *Cell* 79:885, 1994.

322. Bain G, Robanus Maandag EC, te Riele HP, et al: Both E12 and E47 allow commitment to the B cell lineage. *Immunity* 6:145, 1997.

323. Kee BL, Quong MW, Murre C: E2A proteins: Essential regulators at multiple stages of B-cell development. *Immunol Rev* 175:138, 2000.

324. Iscove NN, Sieber F: Erythroid progenitors in mouse bone marrow detected by macroscopic colony formation in culture. *Exp Hematol* 3:32, 1975.

325. Clarke BJ, Housman D: Characterization of an erythroid precursor cell of high proliferative capacity in normal human peripheral blood. *Proc Natl Acad Sci U S A* 74:1105, 1977.

326. Long MW, Heffner CH, Williams JL, et al: Regulation of megakaryocyte phenotype in human erythroleukemia cells. *J Clin Invest* 85:1072, 1990.

327. McDonald TP, Sullivan PS: Megakaryocytic and erythrocytic cell lines share a common precursor cell. *Exp Hematol* 21:1316, 1993.

328. Nakahata T, Okumura N: Cell surface antigen expression in human erythroid progenitors: Erythroid and megakaryocytic markers. *Leuk Lymphoma* 13:401, 1994.

329. Hodohara K, Fujii N, Yamamoto N, et al: Stromal cell-derived factor-1 (SDF-1) acts together with thrombopoietin to enhance the development of megakaryocytic progenitor cells (CFU-MK). *Blood* 95:769, 2000.

330. Sawada K, Krantz SB, Dai CH, et al: Purification of human blood burst-forming units-erythroid and demonstration of the evolution of erythropoietin receptors. *J Cell Physiol* 142:219, 1990.

331. Sporn LA, Chavin SI, Marder VJ, et al: Biosynthesis of von Willebrand protein by human megakaryocytes. *J Clin Invest* 76:1102, 1985.

332. Pevny L, Simon MC, Robertson E, et al: Erythroid differentiation in chimaeric mice blocked by a targeted mutation in the gene for transcription factor GATA-1. *Nature* 349:257, 1991.

333. Shivdasani RA, Fujiwara Y, McDevitt MA, et al: A lineage-selective knockout establishes the critical role of transcription factor GATA-1 in megakaryocyte growth and platelet development. *EMBO J* 16:3965, 1997.

334. Tsang AP, Visvader JE, Turner CA, et al: FOG, a multitype zinc finger protein, acts as a cofactor for transcription factor GATA-1 in erythroid and megakaryocytic differentiation. *Cell* 90:109, 1997.

335. Nichols KE, Crispino JD, Poncz M, et al: Familial dyserythropoietic anaemia and thrombocytopenia due to an inherited mutation in GATA1. *Nat Genet* 24:266, 2000.

336. Doubeikovski A, Uzan G, Doubeikovski Z, et al: Thrombopoietin-induced expression of the glycoprotein IIb gene involves the transcription factor PU.1/Spi-1 in UT7-Mpl cells. *J Biol Chem* 272:24300, 1997.

337. Athanasiou M, Clausen PA, Mavrothalassitis GJ, et al: Increased expression of the ETS-related transcription factor FLI-1/ERGB correlates with and can induce the megakaryocytic phenotype. *Cell Growth Differ* 7:1525, 1996.

338. Giles F, Estey E, O'Brien S: Gemtuzumab ozogamicin in the treatment of acute myeloid leukemia. *Cancer* 98:2095, 2003.

339. Pagano L, Fianchi L, Caira M, Rutella S, Leone G: The role of gemtuzumab ozogamicin in the treatment of acute myeloid leukemia patients. *Oncogene* 26:3679, 2007.

340. Stasi R: Gemtuzumab ozogamicin: an anti-CD33 immunoconjugate for the treatment of acute myeloid leukaemia. *Expert Opin Biol Ther* 8:527, 2008.

341. Khanna-Gupta A, Zibello T, Sun H, et al: C/EBP epsilon mediates myeloid differentiation and is regulated by the CCAAT displacement protein (CDP/cut). *Proc Natl Acad Sci U S A* 98:8000, 2001.

342. Dahl R, Walsh JC, Lancki D, et al: Regulation of macrophage and neutrophil cell fates by the PU.1:C/EBPalpha ratio and granulocyte colony-stimulating factor. *Nat Immunol* 4:1029, 2003.

CHAPTER 19
THE INFLAMMATORY RESPONSE

Jeffrey S. Warren and Peter A. Ward

SUMMARY

The acute inflammatory response is characterized by a rapid but relatively short-lived localized increase in blood flow, an increase in microvascular permeability and the sequential recruitment of different types of leukocytes. Acute inflammation may be followed by "chronic" inflammation and a super-imposed series of reparative processes (e.g., angiogenesis, production of extracellular matrix, parenchymal regeneration and scar formation). The early hemodynamic changes at a site of inflammation establish low shear conditions that enable marginated leukocytes to engage in low-affinity selectin-mediated rolling interactions with activated endothelial cells. In response to locally produced soluble and cell surface mediators, endothelial cells and rolling leukocytes sequentially express several sets of complementary adhesion molecules that include selectins, integrins, and members of the immunoglobulin superfamily. Leukocyte and endothelial cell adhesion molecules mediate the high-affinity adhesive interactions necessary for leukocyte emigration from the vascular space along chemotactic gradients. Analogous, temporally regulated, soluble mediators and cellular adhesion molecules also orchestrate succeeding monocyte- and lymphocyte-rich chronic inflammatory responses. This paradigm is modulated by a vast network of surface-active and soluble inflammatory mediators. Recruited leukocytes and cells indigenous to the anatomic site of inflammation both play critical roles in host defense, resolution of inflammation and tissue repair.

HISTORY

The sentinel clinical features of acute inflammation—rubor, calor, tumor, and dolor—have been recognized for at least 5000 years.[1] Dr. John Hunter, the renowned late 18th-century Scottish surgeon, observed that the inflammatory response is not a disease *per se* but rather a nonspecific and salutary response to a variety of insults. Through his microscopic examinations of transparent vital membrane preparations, German pathologist Julius Cohnheim concluded that the inflammatory response is fundamentally a vascular phenomenon. Phagocytosis was described late in the 19th century by Elie Metchnikoff and his colleagues at the Pasteur Institute. Morphologic studies, using both live animals and fixed histologic preparations, transformed our understanding of inflammation and led to the currently held concepts of inflammation-associated hemodynamic alterations, *acute* inflammation and *chronic* inflammation.[1,2] During the past 5 decades, the modern techniques of biochemistry, tissue culture, monoclonal antibody production, recombinant DNA technology, and the genetic manipulation of isolated cells and whole animals have enabled a more detailed understanding of the cellular and molecular mechanisms which underpin the inflammatory response, the active resolution of inflammation, and the transition to tissue repair and restitution. These studies, in concert with "experiments of nature," such as chronic granulomatous disease (Chap. 66) and the leukocyte adhesion deficiency disorders (Chap. 66), have permitted the formulation of complex, yet elegant, models of acute and chronic inflammation and led to the promise of incisive therapeutic approaches. A large array of human diseases is marked by either defects in the development of the inflammatory response or the deleterious effects of the inflammatory response itself.

GENERAL CHARACTERISTICS OF INFLAMMATION

It is useful to consider inflammation as an acute or chronic (persistent) process. *Acute* inflammation lasts from minutes to several days and is characterized by pronounced local hemodynamic and microvascular changes and leukocyte accumulation.[2,3] The acute inflammatory response is consistently marked by microvascular leakage and the accumulation of neutrophils. The four cardinal signs of acute inflammation, alluded to above, can be accounted for within the physiologic parameters of inflammation. The systemic effects of inflammation, particularly acute inflammation, account for the familiar clinical findings of fever, acute-phase response and altered sensorium. In turn, *sepsis* is a systemic inflammatory response syndrome that occurs in response to infection; *severe sepsis* is sepsis complicated by acute organ dysfunction; and *septic shock* is sepsis complicated by either fluid resuscitation-resistant hypotension or by hyperlactatemia.[4]

The *chronic* inflammatory response, which lasts much longer and is more varied in its effects, is marked by growth of new capillaries and proliferation of resident fibroblasts.[2,3] Cellular infiltrates typically include monocytes and lymphocytes, but there are many variations in the cellular composition, anatomic distribution and tempo of development of chronic inflammatory lesions. Chronic inflammatory processes can be classified according to these variations. For example, granulomatous inflammation is a chronic process marked by nodular aggregates of mononuclear phagocytes that have become "transformed" into epithelioid histiocytes, so-called because of their similar appearance to epithelial cells.[2] Granulomas may be distributed along blood vessels (e.g., angiocentric), along upper airways (e.g., bronchocentric), or randomly throughout the interstitium or parenchyma of an organ. Granulomas may vary morphologically. Tuberculous granulomas often contain areas of caseous necrosis while sarcoidosis-associated granulomas are often cellular and exhibit fibrosis but usually without areas of necrosis.[2] Other chronic inflammatory processes are marked by a preponderance of eosinophils or plasma cells. In contrast to the more stereotyped appearance of an acute inflammatory lesion, the particular appearance of a chronic inflammatory lesion can sometimes provide insight into its cause (e.g.,

Acronyms and Abbreviations: ADAM, a disintegrin and metalloproteinase; BPI, bacterial permeability-increasing protein; CAP37, cationic antimicrobial protein; DARC, Duffy antigen receptor for chemokines; CD, cluster of differentiation; eNOS, endothelial nitric oxide synthase; HEV, high-endothelial venule; HPETE, hydroperoxyeicosatetraenoic acid; ICAM, intercellular adhesion molecule; IFN, interferon; Ig, immunoglobulin; IL, interleukin; iNOS, inducible nitric oxide synthase; LT, leukotriene; $LTB_4/C_4/D_4/E_4$, leukotriene $B_4/C_4/D_4/E_4$; MadCAM, mucosal addressin cell adhesion molecule; MASP, mannan-binding lectin-associated serine protease; MBL, mannan-binding lectin; NADPH, nicotinamide adenine dinucleotide phosphate (reduced); NO, nitric oxide; PAF, platelet-activating factor; PARs, proteinase-activated receptors; PNAd, peripheral node addressin; PSGL-1, P-selectin glycoprotein ligand-1; RGD, arginine-glycine-aspartic acid peptide sequence; TACE, tumor necrosis factor-α converting enzyme; TNF, tumor necrosis factor; VCAM, vascular cell adhesion molecule; VLA, very-late antigen.

caseating granulomas in tuberculosis, eosinophil-rich infiltrates in a parasitic infection and plasma cell-rich infiltrates in viral hepatitis).

Superimposed upon acute and chronic inflammatory responses is *repair*.[2,5] Resolution or termination of the inflammatory response is an important step in the pathway to repair; it occurs through a complex set of regulated processes.[5] Repair, which may entail the regeneration of parenchymal cells damaged as the result of an insult *per se* or as "bystanders" to the inflammatory response, is characterized by the growth of new capillaries (angiogenesis) and the activation of fibroblasts which produce extracellular matrix molecules (e.g., scar tissue). In some circumstances an inflammatory response is self-limited (e.g., sunburn), whereas in other situations the response may persist for many years (e.g., tuberculous granulomas). The elimination or persistence of an insult has a major influence on outcome–whether ongoing chronic inflammation, complete regeneration or scar formation. There is great complexity in terms of the networks of proinflammatory and antiinflammatory soluble mediators (e.g., cytokines) and the phenotypes, as well as the functional and regulatory roles of both indigenous cells and recruited inflammatory cells in inflammation, resolution and repair.[2,3,5-7]

This chapter first addresses acute inflammation, which encompasses localized changes in blood flow, alterations in microvascular permeability and neutrophil exudation.[2,3] In addition to hemodynamic changes, inflammation encompasses endothelial cell activation, low-affinity leukocyte–endothelial adhesion, high-affinity or stationary leukocyte–endothelial adhesive interactions, leukocyte emigration, leukocyte activation, and the subsequent dampening and resolution of the inflammatory response. The highly regulated migration of leukocytes from the vasculature into sites of inflammation and of lymphocytes through secondary lymphoid tissues and, in turn, into sites of microbial invasion, are pivotal to host defense in the contexts of inflammation and immunity.[2,3,6] This extraordinary complexity of regulatory processes that control inflammation is exemplified by, but not limited to, proinflammatory cytokines (e.g., tumor necrosis factor [TNF]-α, interleukin [IL]-1β, IL-6) that drive inflammation, countered by rises in antiinflammatory cytokines (e.g., IL-4, IL-10, IL-11, IL-13, transforming growth factor [TGF]-β, IL-1ra and soluble cytokine receptors) that dampen inflammatory responses (see "Cytokines and Chemolines").[2,7] Both the termination of an inflammatory process and the transition from an active inflammatory milieu to a wound-healing, tissue-remodeling environment are actively regulated processes. The concept of "active" termination of the inflammatory response, including the roles of chemokine depletion, neutrophil apoptosis, resolvins and protectins, and the shift from interferon (IFN)-γ–driven "classical M1" macrophages to IL-4/IL-13–driven "alternative M2" macrophages, is introduced at the end of the first section of this chapter (M1 and M2 Macrophages). The section "Regulators of the Inflammatory Response" of this chapter introduces (and where appropriate, reiterates) the vast array of soluble and surface-active mediators that regulate both acute and chronic inflammatory responses, as well as some aspects of resolution. These mediators include substances that range from short-lived reactive oxygen and nitrogen intermediates to entire regulatory systems (e.g., complement and coagulation). Many mediators of inflammation have become targets for therapeutic interruption strategies. See section "Chronic Inflammation and Repair." This chapter provides a framework for understanding the basic processes of inflammation while promoting an appreciation for the highly complex and integrated nature of the regulated inflammatory response.

● ACUTE INFLAMMATION

HEMODYNAMIC CHANGES

The hemodynamic changes that occur early in acute inflammation include arteriolar vasodilatation and localized increases in microvascular permeability (Fig. 19–1). In many circumstances, arteriolar vasodilation follows a rapid and transient period of vasoconstriction.[2,3] Arteriolar vasodilation results in increased blood flow, thus explaining the familiar redness and warmth that characterize a site of acute inflammation. The increase in blood flow, coupled with increases in microvascular permeability, results in hemoconcentration and increased local viscosity. These hemodynamic changes are critical to subsequent leukocyte emigration because selectin-mediated low-affinity rolling leukocyte–endothelial adhesive interactions occur only under such conditions of low shear force. Experimental studies using *in vitro* flow chambers and transparent vital membrane preparations in live animals indicate that selectin-mediated leukocyte–endothelial rolling adhesive interactions cannot occur in the face of the shear forces that exist under conditions of normal blood flow velocity. Increased microvascular permeability leads initially to protein-poor transudation followed by protein-rich plasma exudation, another characteristic of acute inflammation.[2] Microvascular leakage occurs through a variety of temporally regulated mechanisms, including rapid, reversible, and short-lived venular endothelial cell contraction attended by widening of intercellular junctions; so-called endothelial cell retraction, which is less-well understood but involves long-lived cytokine-mediated cytoskeletal changes; direct endothelial injury and disruption by physical trauma; leukocyte-mediated endothelial cell injury; and leakage via new capillaries that do not yet possess completely "closed" intercellular junctions.[2] Increases in rate of transcytosis by which plasma constituents cross endothelial cells in vesicles or vacuoles (vesiculovacuolar organelles) occur in neoplastic blood vessels and may play a role in inflammation.[2,8] Alterations in local blood flow occur at the level of arterioles, the key to vascular resistance and regulated largely by the autonomic nervous system, nitric oxide (NO) (formerly called endothelium-derived relaxing factor), vasoactive peptides, and eicosanoids. A variety of soluble mediators can induce increases in microvascular permeability through several of the above-mentioned mechanisms.

LEUKOCYTES

The recruitment of leukocytes into a site of inflammation is a fundamental characteristic of the inflammatory response.[2,3,9] The orchestrated recruitment of particular types of leukocytes into specific tissues, whether sites of acute inflammation, in the course of physiologic lymphocyte recirculation through lymph nodes or in the cellular immune response to microbial invasion, is referred to as *homing*.[3] The general mechanisms of leukocyte homing are similar, but the leukocytes and particular mediator molecules vary. For example, neutrophils bind and traverse postcapillary venules in acute inflammation, naïve T lymphocytes bind and traverse lymph node high-endothelial venules (HEVs) in lymphocyte recirculation, and effector and memory T lymphocytes bind and traverse postcapillary endothelial cells in sites of chronic infection.[3] The importance of white blood cells in host defense is highlighted in patients with either numerical leukocyte deficiencies or functional defects. Leukocytes are critical because of their central role in the phagocytosis and killing or containment of microbes and in the digestion of necrotic tissue debris. Leukocyte-derived products, such as proteolytic enzymes and reactive oxygen intermediates, contribute to tissue injury.

Leukocyte Adhesion and Transmigration

Vascular stasis that results from the hemodynamic changes of early acute inflammation leads to displacement of leukocytes from the central axial column of circulating blood cells to positions along the endothelial surface. This process, margination, is enhanced under conditions of slow blood flow.[2,3] Leukocytes adhere transiently and weakly to the endothelial surface. Vital membrane preparations and flow chamber studies using endothelial cell monolayers and suspensions of purified leukocytes have revealed that cells "tumble and roll" along the

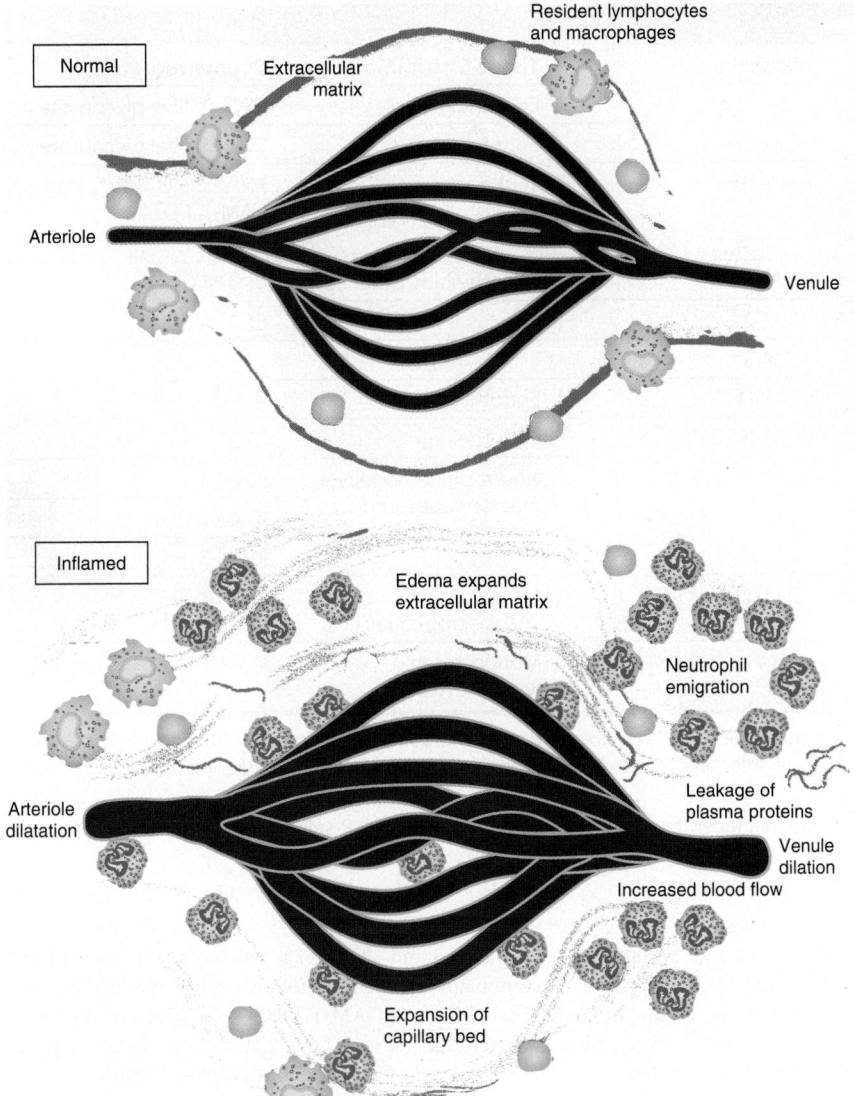

Figure 19–1. Early hemodynamic events in acute inflammation. Vascular dilatation, increased microvascular permeability, fluid transudation, and leukocyte recruitment and emigration occur after a transient period of arteriolar vasoconstriction. *(Modified with permission from Cotran RS, Kumar V, Collins T, Robbins SL (eds): Robbins Pathologic Basis of Disease, 6th ed. Philadelphia, PA: Saunders/Elsevier, 1999.)*

endothelial surface.[10] Transient, weak, rolling neutrophil–endothelial adhesive interactions occur within minutes of initiation of an acute inflammatory response and can, depending upon the time point within the evolution of an inflammatory response, involve neutrophils, lymphocytes, monocytes, basophils, or eosinophils. Leukocyte–endothelial cell-rolling adhesive interaction is a specific and necessary step that precedes high-affinity, or so-called stationary adhesion and emigration.[9–11] Early rolling adhesive interactions are mediated largely by selectins and their carbohydrate-rich counterreceptors.[2,3,9,10] In turn, the cell-surface expression of selectins (and other intercellular adhesion molecules) is regulated by locally produced proinflammatory mediators.[9–11]

Selectins contain an extracellular N-terminal carbohydrate-binding region that is homologous to mammalian lectins, an epidermal growth factor-like domain, a series of complement regulatory domains, and a lipophilic transmembrane domain (Table 19–1).[2,3,9,10] P-selectin is expressed by endothelial cells and platelets, E-selectin by endothelial cells, and L-selectin by most white blood cells. P-selectin is constitutively synthesized and stored in endothelial intracytoplasmic granules (Weibel-Palade bodies).[9] When endothelial cells are exposed to histamine, thrombin, platelet-activating factor (PAF) or tissue factor, preformed P-selectin is rapidly (within minutes) translocated to the

endothelial surface where it engages marginated leukocytes via carbohydrate moieties that contain sialic acid residues (e.g., P-selectin glycoprotein ligand-1 [PSGL-1]).[2,3,10,12] This transient, low-affinity, binding interaction accounts in part for the early rolling interactions (Fig. 19–2). The development of single knockout mice (i.e., lacking individual selectins [P–/–; E–/– or L–/–], double knockout mice (e.g., E–/– and P–/–), and even triple knockout mice, has confirmed that leukocyte rolling can be almost completely accounted for by selectins.[13,14] Exposure of endothelial cells to TNF-α or IL-1β results in new protein synthesis–dependent expression of E-selectin, a response that occurs within 1 to 2 hours and peaks at 4 to 6 hours.[2,3,9] As in the case of P-selectin–mediated leukocyte adhesion, E-selectin–mediated adhesion occurs via a series of sialylated and fucosylated carbohydrate moieties related to the sialyl Lewis X and sialyl Lewis A blood group antigens, but found on leukocytes (Table 19–1).[9,10] Selectin counterreceptors consist of several different mucin-like glycoproteins coated with various sialyl moieties. L-selectin is constitutively expressed by leukocytes, participates in neutrophil and monocyte binding to activated endothelium in inflammatory sites, lymphocyte–endothelial cell homing (e.g., lymphocyte homing to lymph nodes via HEVs), leukocyte–leukocyte adhesive interactions via sulfur-containing mucin-like glycoproteins, and is cleaved from

TABLE 19-1. Adhesion Molecules in Inflammation

Family	Structure	Members	Tissue Distribution	Counterreceptor*
Selectin	N-terminal lectin domain, epidermal growth factor domain, multiple complement regulatory repeats, transmembrane, and short cytoplasmic tail	P-selectin	Endothelium, platelets	PSGL-1, SLe^x glycoprotein
		E-selectin	Endothelium	PSGL-1, SLe^x glycoprotein
		L-selectin	Leukocytes	PNAds: GlyCAM-1, Mad-CAM-1, CD34
Immunoglobulin superfamily	Multiple immunoglobulin domains, transmembrane region and cytoplasmic tail	ICAM-1	Endothelium, other cells	CD11a/CD18
		ICAM-2		CD11b/CD18
		ICAM-3		
		VCAM-1	Endothelium	VLA-4
		CD31 (PECAM)	Endothelium	CD31
Integrin (β_2; leukocyte)	Heterodimers: distinct α subunits with common β subunits	CD11a/CD18 (LFA-1)	Neutrophils, monocytes, macrophages, and lymphocytes	ICAM-1
				ICAM-2
				ICAM-3
		CD11b/CD18 (Mac-1)	Neutrophils, monocytes, and macrophages	ICAM-1, iC3b, LPS, and fibronectin
		VLA-4	Monocytes and lymphocytes	VCAM-1 and fibronectin

CD, cluster of differentiation; ICAM, intercellular adhesion molecule; LFA-1, leukocyte function-associated antigen-1; LPS, lipopolysaccharide; PECAM, platelet endothelial cell adhesion molecule; PSGL-1, P-selectin glycoprotein ligand-1; sLe^x, sialyl Lewis X; VCAM, vascular cell adhesion molecule; VLA, very-late antigen.

*"Counterreceptor" refers to a complementary moiety to which a receptor specifically binds. For example, P-selectin binds to PSGL-1.

cells by means of "sheddase" enzymes such as a disintegrin and metalloproteinase (ADAM)-17 (TNF-α converting enzyme [TACE]) when the leukocyte is activated (see Table 19-1).[3,15] The relevant mucin-like glycoprotein counter-receptors on HEVs are collectively referred to as peripheral node addressins (PNAds) and include mucosal addressin cell adhesion molecule (MadCAM)-1, GlyCAM-1, and CD34.[3,15] L-selectin shedding facilitates leukocyte emigration by allowing the weakly adherent white blood cell to detach from the endothelium. Low-affinity rolling adhesive interactions set the stage for β-integrin– and immunoglobulin superfamily mediated high-affinity adhesive interactions and leukocyte transmigration.[2,3,9]

Weak selectin-mediated rolling and high-affinity stationary adhesive interactions are not temporally or mechanistically completely discrete. For example, TNF-α and IL-1β both induce E-selectin, which is not expressed by quiescent cells, and both increase endothelial expression of intercellular adhesion molecule (ICAM)-1 and vascular cell adhesion molecule (VCAM)-1, which are constitutively expressed in low cell-surface densities.[2,3] ICAM-1 is involved in the recruitment of all types of leukocytes and VCAM-1 is involved in the recruitment of chronic inflammatory leukocytes (lymphocytes, monocytes, eosinophils, and basophils).[2,3,9] ICAM-1 binds to β_2 (leukocyte) integrins, which are heterodimeric structures that contain one species of α chain (e.g., CD11a, CD11b, CD11c, CD11d) and a common β chain (CD18).[16] VCAM-1 binds to β_1 integrins (e.g., very-late antigen [VLA]-4/$\alpha_4\beta_1$) (see Table 19-1).[2,3] Activated endothelial cells secrete PAF and CXCL8 (IL-8), which activate overlying selectin-bound leukocytes.[2,3,9,16] Individual leukocyte CD11a/CD18 (LFA-1) heterodimers undergo a transient conformational change and groups of CD11a/CD18 molecules form multimolecular clusters.[2,3,9] Both the conformational change in CD11a/CD18 and the clustering contribute to increases in binding affinity to endothelial ICAM 1.[3,16] CD11b/CD18 (Mac 1) binds ICAM-1, ICAM-2, and iC3b (see section "Complement"), the latter of which opsonizes complement-coated particulates. CD11c/CD18 also binds to iC3b and initiates phagocytosis, but plays a lesser role in

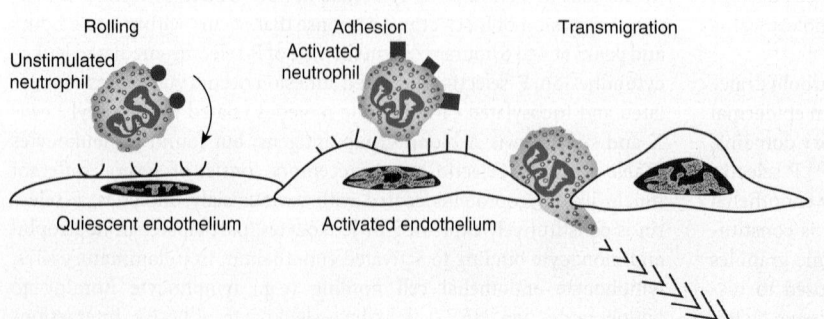

Rolling — Unstimulated neutrophil — Quiescent endothelium

Adhesion — Activated neutrophil — Activated endothelium

Transmigration

Chemotactic gradient

Figure 19-2. Leukocyte–endothelial adhesive interactions. Early in the acute inflammatory response, marginated leukocytes engage in transient, low-affinity, selectin-mediated rolling adhesive interactions with endothelial cells. As the response evolves, activated leukocytes and endothelial cells engage in high-affinity, β_2-integrin– and immunoglobulin superfamily mediated adhesive interactions. A variety of chemotactic factors trigger the motive force for leukocyte emigration.

neutrophil adhesion than do CD11a/CD18 and CD11b/CD18. Intercellular adhesion molecules are found on a variety of cell types other than endothelial cells. The roles of CD11c/CD18, CD11d/CD18, and ICAM-3 in leukocyte–endothelial adhesion are less-well established. β_1-Integrins, notably VLA-4, are found primarily on chronic inflammatory leukocytes (e.g., lymphocytes, monocytes, basophils, and eosinophils) and mediate leukocyte binding via VCAM-1.[2,3,9] β_1-Integrin–mediated adhesive interactions occur via arginine-glycine-aspartic acid peptide sequences (RGDs) displayed by VCAM-1, as well as on exposed surfaces of matrix molecules (e.g., fibronectin). β_2-Integrin–ICAM-1 and β_1-integrin–VCAM-1–mediated adhesive interactions occur later (hours to days) in the inflammatory response than do selectin-mediated interactions.

β_1- and β_2-integrins are clearly important in leukocyte recruitment into sites of acute and chronic inflammation. Eighteen different integrin α subunits, eight integrin β subunits, and 24 in vivo heterodimer combinations have been identified in mammals.[17] In addition to leukocyte–endothelial cell adhesion interactions, integrins function in a variety of other cell–cell and cell–extracellular matrix interactions. A large number of integrin-targeted small molecule, peptide, and designer antibodies have been developed for therapeutic applications.[17] Inflammatory–immunologic diseases treated with integrin antagonists include, among others, multiple sclerosis, Crohn disease, and age-related macular degeneration.

High-affinity stationary adhesive interactions precede leukocyte transmigration across the endothelium into the subjacent interstitium. The functional importance of complementary leukocyte–endothelial adhesive interactions has been clarified by in vitro binding studies and in vivo studies that have employed neutralizing antibodies directed against adhesion molecules, pharmacologic antagonists of adhesion molecules, and knockout mice.[2,3] The functional importance of leukocyte integrins (CD11a/CD18, CD11b/CD18, CD11c/CD18) has also been highlighted by clinical and experimental observations in patients with rare genetic leukocyte adhesion deficiencies (Chap. 66).

β_2-Integrin ICAM-1 and ICAM-2, as well a β_1-integrin (VLA-4) VCAM-1, induce adhesive interactions that lead to cytoskeletal reorganization in leukocytes that flatten and spread out on the endothelial surface, extend pseudopodia between endothelial cells, and migrate along extravascular chemotactic gradients. Most leukocytes exit the vascular space between adjacent endothelial cells (paracellular transmigration). Paracellular transmigration depends not only on integrin-ligand interactions but also on CD31 (PECAM-1 [platelet-endothelial cell adhesion molecule-1]) expressed on both leukocytes and endothelial cells, and transient reversible disassembly of tight interendothelial vascular endothelial (VE)–cadherin junctional complexes.[18] There is evidence that leukocytes can also exit the vascular space via a less-well-characterized transcellular pathway.

Leukocyte Chemotaxis and Activation

Leukocytes bound tightly to endothelium emigrate from the vascular space into the interstitium by extending pseudopods between intercellular junctions (see Fig. 19–2).[18] Secreted neutral proteases such as elastase, cathepsin G, and proteinase 3, play a role in the passage or "invasion" of leukocytes through the subendothelial extracellular matrix. Collagenases are particularly important in leukocyte transmigration through basement membranes. A variety of matrix metalloproteinases, produced by several cell types, participate in leukocyte migration, and also play roles in resolution of inflammation and tissue remodeling. Leukocyte emigration and subsequent movement through the interstitium follow chemical concentration gradients; processes facilitated by binding interactions between leukocyte integrins and complementary sites on extracellular matrix molecules (e.g., fibronectin).[9] A wide variety of

soluble mediators can provide the motive trigger for this process.[2,3,19] Chemotactic factors for neutrophils include peptides derived from bacteria (e.g., N-formyl peptides), complement-derived peptides (e.g., C5a), cell membrane-derived chemotactic lipids (e.g., PAF), and cytokines and chemokines produced by a variety of cell types (e.g., CXCL8 [IL-8] from endothelial cells).[2,3,19] Chemotactic factors vary with respect to their specificity for different types of leukocytes. For example, C5a and N-formyl peptides both induce neutrophil and monocyte chemotaxis, and CXCL8 [IL-8] induces neutrophil chemotaxis, whereas CCL2 (monocyte chemoattractant protein [MCP]-1) induces chemotactic responses in monocytes and a specific subset of memory T lymphocytes.[3] The Th17 subset of CD4 T-helper lymphocytes secretes IL-17 and IL-22 which participate in the recruitment of neutrophils.[3] (There are several species of IL-17, including homodimers IL-17A–IL-17F as well as heterodimeric species.[20]) Each of these chemotactic factors activates "target" cells by engaging specific cell surface receptors, which, in turn, are linked to the contractile cell motility apparatus.[3,19]

In addition to chemotaxis, soluble and cell-surface mediators induce leukocyte activation manifested by a wide array of changes in cellular function (e.g., leukocyte integrin upregulation and increased binding affinity [e.g., CD11b/CD18], selectin shedding [e.g., L-selectin], lysosome degranulation, and initiation of the respiratory burst). There have been great advances in understanding of the biochemical pathways involved in chemotaxis, cell activation, and degranulation.[21] Although there are many nuances in the signal transduction pathways involved in these processes, several themes have emerged. Cell surface receptors are activated by specific ligands (e.g., C5a, leukotriene B$_4$ [LTB$_4$], CXCL8 [IL-8] and receptor activation is transduced via specific G proteins and membrane-associated phospholipases, which leads to mobilization of intracellular calcium, influx of extracellular calcium and phosphorylation of series of cytosolic proteins.[19] Rare genetic diseases linked to receptor and effector defects (e.g., IFN-γ receptor defects and nicotinamide adenine dinucleotide phosphate [reduced form] [NADPH] oxidase defects) have provided insight into leukocyte function and the importance of such specific activities in host defense (Chap. 66).

A principal result of neutrophil and monocyte recruitment is provision of large numbers of activated leukocytes that can release lytic substances and reactive oxygen and nitrogen intermediates needed to destroy foreign invaders, and a vehicle to contain foreign particulates through phagocytosis. Some recruited monocytes differentiate into macrophages and recruited effector and memory lymphocytes play pivotal roles in the adaptive immune response.[3,6] The products and functions of activated inflammatory cells are at once salutary because they contain and destroy invaders and deleterious because they cause tissue damage. The roles of neutrophil apoptosis (programmed cell death) in the termination of acute inflammatory responses and IFN-γ–driven M1 macrophages and IL-4/IL-13–driven M2 macrophages in the transition of an inflammatory milieu to a wound-healing or tissue-remodeling milieu are discussed in "M1 and M2 Macrophages".

Leukocyte activation, especially of neutrophils and mononuclear phagocytes, results in the secretion of microbicidal peptides (e.g., defensins, bactericidal permeability-increasing protein [BPI], cationic antimicrobial protein [e.g., CAP37]) and lytic enzymes (e.g., myeloperoxidase, elastase, cathepsin G).[6,21,22] The release of such granular constituents is accompanied by the generation of reactive oxygen and nitrogen intermediates (e.g., O_2^-, H_2O_2, NO), the generation of arachidonate metabolites (e.g., leukotrienes and prostaglandins) and the production of other proinflammatory mediators (see section "Regulators of the Inflammatory Response").[21,22] In some circumstances these mediators are released into phagolysosomes where they contribute to the destruction of engulfed microbes, while in other circumstances they are secreted into the extracellular milieu where they amplify the inflammatory response and cause tissue damage. The various types of neutrophil granules (primary azurophilic, secondary specific, tertiary gelatinase-containing, and secretory vesicles) are released in a differentially coordinated fashion.[21,22]

An important recently formulated concept is that of the "inflammasome," a cytosolic multiprotein complex that is formed in a variety of leukocytes and leads to the generation of IL-1β via activated caspase-1–mediated cleavage of pro–IL-1β.[23] Inflammasome formation can be induced by a wide variety of microbial products (e.g., lipopolysaccharide) as well as by other proinflammatory molecules (e.g., urate crystals, damage-associated molecular patterns also known as "alarmins").[23] Pathogens can activate immune cells via several classes of pattern-recognition receptors, including C-type lectin receptors, toll-like receptors (TLRs), retinoic acid–inducible gene (RIG) 1-like cytosolic receptor and nucleotide-binding oligomerization domain (NOD)-like receptors.[23,24]

Effective phagocytosis involves three distinct steps: (1) recognition and attachment, (2) engulfment, and (3) degradation (killing in the case of microbes) of the ingested material.[21,22] Phagocytosis is greatly enhanced when particles (e.g., bacteria) are coated with opsonins, which, in turn, function as ligands for leukocyte surface receptors. The major opsonins include the Fc domains of immunoglobulin (Ig) G and IgM and the complement-derived fragments C3b and iC3b, which are generated via activation of the complement cascades and covalently bound to the surfaces of nearby large molecules and particles (e.g., microbes). There are a variety of Fc receptors (FcγRI, FcγRII, FcγRIIIB, etc.) and complement receptors (e.g., CR1, CR3, CR4) that specifically engage their respective opsonins when the latter coat foreign particulates.[6] In addition to facilitating receptor-mediated phagocytosis of opsonized particles, Fc receptors trigger cell activation with the attendant release of granular constituents and the generation of reactive oxygen intermediates.[6] Other important recognition molecules expressed by leukocytes include integrins, the C1q receptor, mannose receptors, scavenger receptors and TLRs.[6,24,25] Mannose receptors bind to mannose and fucose moieties, which are present on some microbes but not mammalian cells; scavenger receptors bind to a variety of microbes, as well as to oxidized and acetylated low-density lipoproteins; and TLRs bind to a variety of microbial moieties including endotoxins (lipopolysaccharide) and prokaryotic nucleic acids (e.g., double-stranded RNA).[6,24,25] Humans express at least nine species of TLR, some of which are expressed on external cell surfaces and others on the inner surfaces of endosomes.[24,25] Some enhanced phagocytic reactions occur independently of opsonins. The engulfment, degranulation, and oxidative burst triggered as the result of engagement of FcR is enhanced by the concurrent engagement of complement receptors. In some circumstances, engulfment is enhanced by the simultaneous binding of the leukocyte to specific extracellular matrix molecules (e.g., fibronectin) or soluble cytokines. Engulfment results in the formation of phagosomes, which fuse with lysosomes to form phagolysosomes in which foreign particles are oxidized and degraded. Numerous mechanisms for killing and/or degradation of microbes have been elucidated (Table 19–2). Although these mechanisms are classified as either oxygen-dependent or oxygen-independent, both types of processes may be involved in the destruction of a given microorganism, and a given microorganism may vary greatly in its susceptibility to various mechanisms of destruction.[6,21,22] Extracellular release of reactive oxygen and nitrogen intermediates, lysosomal enzymes, lipid mediators, and cationic proteins can all contribute to inflammation-related tissue injury.

As noted above, acute inflammation may be followed by chronic inflammation and a superimposed series of reparative processes that can result in resolution or scar formation. Resolution of inflammation was long viewed to be a passive process that included a poorly understood decline in concentrations of proinflammatory mediators

TABLE 19–2. Killing and Degradation of Microorganisms in Phagocytes

Oxygen-Dependent		Oxygen-Independent
Superoxide anion	(O_2^-)	Arachidonate metabolites (prostaglandins, leukotrienes)
Hydrogen peroxide	(H_2O_2)	Platelet-activating factor
Hydroxyl radical	$(HO\cdot)$	Lysosomal proteases
Singlet oxygen	$(^1O_2)$	Lactoferrin
N-chloramines	$(R\text{-}NHC1, R\text{-}NCl_2)$	Lysozyme
Hypohalous acids	$(HO\text{-}X)$	Cationic proteins (e.g., bactericidal permeability-increasing protein, major basic protein, defensins)
Nitric oxide	(NO)	
Peroxynitrite	$(ONOO^-)$	

and cells.[5] It has become clear that the balance between a proinflammatory and an antiinflammatory milieu is regulated by networks of proinflammatory mediators (e.g., proinflammatory cytokines: TNF-α, IL-1β, IL-6) and antiinflammatory mediators (e.g., antiinflammatory cytokines: IL-4, IL-10, IL-11, IL-13, TGFβ, IL-1ra, and soluble cytokine receptors). Clearance of inflammatory cells and mediators is an active process that encompasses leukocyte apoptosis, inactivation and sequestration of proinflammatory chemokines, and egress of leukocytes *from* sites of inflammation.[5] Detailed serial biochemical analyses of inflammatory exudates by liquid chromatography-mass spectroscopy have, along with structure–function analyses and *in vivo* animal studies, elucidated the identities of "resolvins" and "protectins," lipids derived from omega-3 polyunsaturated fatty acids that facilitate resolution of inflammation.[5,26,27] The recognition of functionally distinguishable macrophages as "classical, IFN-γ–driven M1" phenotype and "alternative, IL-4/IL-13–driven M2" phenotype has provided insight into the transition of an active inflammatory milieu to a wound-healing or tissue-remodeling milieu.[5,28,2928] It has become clear that there are several different macrophage phenotypes, a reflection of the great complexity of the transition from active inflammation to resolution and remodeling. Insight into actively regulated termination of inflammation as well as the transition from active inflammation to resolution and remodeling has provided for new therapeutic strategies.

ACUTE-PHASE RESPONSE

The acute-phase response is a stereotyped host response to insults that include trauma, tissue damage, and infection.[3] TNF-α, IL-1β, and IL-6 are consistently produced regardless of trigger. As discussed throughout, these soluble cytokines mediate several proinflammatory processes. (Proinflammatory cytokines TNF-α, IL-1β, IL-6, and antiinflammatory cytokines are further discussed in "Cytokines and Chemokines".) TNF-α, IL-1β and IL-6 act on the hypothalamus to increase the body temperature set point, resulting in fever. Because they are produced endogenously and induce fever in the context of a systemic host response, these mediators have sometimes been referred to as "endogenous pyrogens." Exogenous pyrogens (e.g., endotoxin or lipopolysaccharide) originate from outside the host but induce TNF-α, IL-1β, and IL-6. The downstream effects of these cytokines are responsible for several familiar clinical manifestations of infection, including fever, altered sensorium, and the production of fibrinogen, serum amyloid protein, C3, C4, and C-reactive protein by hepatocytes and other cell types. The biochemical fingerprints of an acute-phase response are revealed through several widely available laboratory tests (C-reactive protein measurement, serum protein electrophoresis). Severe, overwhelming infections attended by high serum concentrations of endotoxin can induce very high concentrations of TNF-α, IL-1β, and IL-6.[4] High concentrations of TNF-α are directly responsible for several of the key manifestations of severe sepsis and septic shock (e.g., cardiac suppression, intravascular thrombosis, capillary leakage and insulin resistance).[3,4]

Interruption of TNF-α has been a therapeutic strategy in localized inflammatory conditions like the joint inflammation (and destruction) of rheumatoid arthritis and bowel wall inflammation in Crohn disease and ulcerative colitis, as well as in severe sepsis and septic shock.[30] Anti-TNF-α therapy (via engineered monoclonal antibodies [infliximab and adalimumab] that neutralize TNF-α as well as inhibitory soluble TNF receptors [etanercept]) has been effective in conditions such as rheumatoid arthritis and inflammatory bowel disease, but not in severe sepsis or septic shock in humans.[4,30] Major adverse events associated with anti–TNF-α therapies include an increased risk of mycobacterial infection, development of autoantibodies (but not autoimmune disease), and injection site inflammation.[30] There have been isolated reports of cytopenias, skin cancer and worsened congestive heart failure.[30]

RESOLUTION OF INFLAMMATION

Since the advent of morphologic examinations of tissue from inflammatory lesions, it has been recognized that resolution of acute inflammation is marked by the disappearance of neutrophils and the engulfment of cellular debris by recruited monocytes and tissue macrophages. It has been relatively recent that resolution of inflammation has been understood to be an active process.[5] Key aspects of resolution include: (1) cessation of neutrophil influx effected by chemokine inactivation and sequestration; (2) neutrophil apoptosis; (3) functional polarization or switching of macrophages from a proinflammatory (M1) to a wound-healing and tissue-remodeling (M2) phenotype; and (4) the rapid, localized generation of proresolution lipid mediators that include lipoxins, resolvins, and protectins.[5]

INACTIVATION AND SEQUESTRATION OF CHEMOKINES

As described in the preceding section, neutrophil influx into an inflammatory site is in part mediated by locally generated chemokines. The actions of proinflammatory chemokines are terminated as a result of their cleavage into inactive fragments and through sequestration or removal from participation by binding to indigenous nonfunctional decoy receptors or to locally generated decoy receptors. Examples include the cleavage of neutrophil-directed CXC-chemokines within a critical ELR motif by macrophage-derived matrix metalloproteinase 12 and matrix metalloproteinase cleavage of the monocyte-directed CC-chemokine, CCL7.[5,31] Cleaved CCL7 can still bind its cognate receptors, CCR1, CCR2, and CCR3, but these cells are not mobilized by the truncated version of CCL7.[5]

Chemokine receptors that lack an intact highly-conserved DRY motif, which normally links the receptor to key signal transduction molecules, function as decoy receptors. The best understood of these are the "Duffy antigen receptor for chemokines" (DARC) and D6.[5] DARC is expressed by endothelial cells at sites of leukocyte egress and binds both CC and CXC chemokines. Functional studies reveal that disruption of DARC leads to increased neutrophil recruitment into sites of inflammation. D6 binds several different CC chemokines, thus rendering them

ineffective. Chemokine decoy receptors can also be derived *in situ* from previously active receptors in sites of inflammation. IL-10 facilitates maintenance of CCR1, CCR2, and CCR5 expression, but induces the functional inactivity of these receptors thus hastening the resolution of inflammation.

NEUTROPHIL APOPTOSIS

Contrary to a long-held belief that extravascular neutrophil life spans are fixed, recent studies suggest that neutrophil life spans can be modulated by local mediators.[5] Low concentrations of macrophage-derived TNF-α and Fas-ligand prolong neutrophil life span, whereas high concentrations of the same ligands lead to shortened life spans.[5] The latter results in neutrophil apoptosis via phosphoinositide 3-kinase–triggered oxygen metabolite generation and Btk-NADPH–modulated pathways. Other local regulators of neutrophil apoptosis include oxygen tension-modulated hypoxia-inducible factor 1α and granulocyte-macrophage colony-stimulating factor (GM-CSF).[5]

In turn, apoptotic neutrophils attenuate inflammation via the secretion of annexin A1, which inhibits the recruitment of additional neutrophils as well enhances neutrophil apoptosis and phagocytosis by macrophages.[5] Lactoferrin, a neutrophil secondary granule protein, also inhibits neutrophil recruitment and induces apoptosis following its release into the inflammatory milieu. (The effect of lactoferrin on neutrophil survival is influenced by its degree of iron saturation.) Macrophage ingestion of apoptotic neutrophils is called "efferocytosis," a process directed by distinct "find me" and "eat me" signals.[5] "Find me" signals include the nucleotides ATP and uridine triphosphate (UTP), fractalkine (CX$_3$CL1), lysophosphatidylcholine and sphingosine-1-phosphate (S-1-P). The corresponding counterreceptors for these "find me" signals include P2Y2 receptors, CX$_3$CR1, G2A, and S-1-P$_{1-5}$ receptors, respectively. This set of "find me/eat me" ligand receptor pairs fits within a larger set of apoptotic cell-efferocyte interactions. In some cases, apoptotic cell "find me" molecules are expressed as a function of apoptosis *per se,* whereas in other cases, existing surface molecules are either modified or linked with mediators that facilitate recognition and ingestion by efferocytes.

M1 AND M2 MACROPHAGES

It was recognized during the 1980s and 1990s that various cytokines can differentially modulate macrophage function.[5] From original specific observations of an IFN-γ–activated macrophage phenotype and an IL-4–activated macrophage phenotype, emerged the concept of "classical, IFN-γ–activated, M1" macrophages and "alternative, IL-4–activated, M2" macrophages.[5] Such macrophages are sometimes described as being "polarized" by IFN-γ, IL-4, or other mediators. Several different activated macrophage "phenotype signatures" have been elucidated, a recognition that has led to a series of designations with "M1" and "M2" representing the most extreme differences.[5] There are several M2 subtypes.[5] IFN-γ–activated macrophages (M1) produce tissue-toxic radicals (e.g., NO) and proinflammatory cytokines (e.g., TNF-α), whereas M2 macrophages produce less NO and more IL-10 and TGF-β, the latter being important mediators of wound healing and/or tissue-remodeling.[5] Insight into the role of tissue macrophages in the resolution of active inflammation and the transition to wound-healing and tissue-remodeling has helped foster the concept of inflammation as an actively regulated response.

LIPID REGULATORS: RESOLVINS AND PROTECTINS

The transition from peak acute inflammation, marked by maximum concentrations of neutrophils, toward resolution, is accompanied by marked changes not only in the local cytokine–chemokine milieu, but also in the lipid milieu. Specifically, there is a shift from high local concentrations of proinflammatory prostaglandins and leukotrienes to antiinflammatory lipoxins, resolvins, and protectins. Basic lipoxin biochemistry is outlined later in the section "Inflammatory Lipids". Resolvins and protectins, derived from omega-3 polyunsaturated fatty acids, each encompass several classes of related molecules.[5,26,27] The synthesis of both resolvins and protectins occurs through enzymatic pathways; the mediators themselves exert their effects through specific receptors on neutrophils, macrophages and dendritic cells.[5,26,27] Antiinflammatory mechanisms exerted by resolvins and protectins are diverse and include enhancement of macrophage-mediated clearance of apoptotic neutrophils, upregulation of cell-surface CCR5 which sequesters proinflammatory chemokines, and the shift of biochemical pathways toward an antiinflammatory phenotype.[3,26,27] The identification and characterization of both resolvins and protectins has laid the groundwork for new therapeutic strategies to modulate inflammation.[5,26] Efficacy of several "proresolving lipids" has been reported in animal models of inflammation.[5] Resolvin E1, a synthetic resolvin analogue (RX-100045), and LXA4-based compounds are under investigation in several human inflammatory diseases.[5]

REGULATORS OF THE INFLAMMATORY RESPONSE

The foregoing sections have provided a conceptual framework for the inflammatory response, specifically, the hemodynamic alterations, mechanisms of specific leukocyte–endothelial adhesive interactions, chemotaxis, leukocyte activation, phagocytosis, intracellular microbial killing mechanisms, active termination/resolution of the acute inflammatory response, and the contributions of M1 and M2 macrophages to inflammation and tissue repair. The many steps that constitute this paradigm are regulated by soluble mediators produced by endothelial cells and leukocytes at a site of inflammation, by other resident cells (e.g., tissue macrophages, fibroblasts, mast cells) and as byproducts of bloodborne proteins (e.g., complement system, coagulation cascade; Table 19–3). There are many examples of "crosstalk" among regulatory systems (e.g., proteinase-activated receptors), complex regulatory networks (e.g., proinflammatory and antiinflammatory cytokine balance), and pleiotropism exhibited by individual mediators (e.g., TNF-α and IL-1β).

REACTIVE OXYGEN INTERMEDIATES

Since the early 1970s it has been recognized that activated phagocytes exhibit a transient but marked increase in oxygen consumption and the mechanistically coupled generation of reduced oxygen metabolites.[32] Although small quantities of reactive oxygen intermediates are produced as byproducts of several metabolic pathways, the chief source is the leukocyte cytosol and membrane-associated NADPH oxidase, an enzyme complex that is defective in most patients with chronic granulomatous disease (Chap. 66). Reactive oxygen intermediates include superoxide anion (O_2^-), hydrogen peroxide (H_2O_2), hydroxyl radical ($HO\bullet$), and singlet oxygen ($^1O_2$).[32] These reduced oxygen products play a major role in intraphagolysosomal killing of microorganisms, and when released extracellularly, are directly or indirectly responsible for a variety of proinflammatory processes, including endothelial cell lysis, extracellular matrix degradation, activation of latent proteolytic enzymes (collagenase, gelatinase), inactivation of antiproteases, interaction with metabolites of L-arginine, and generation of chemotactic factors from arachidonic acid and the complement component, C5.[33] In addition to their role in endothelial cytotoxicity, reactive oxygen intermediates are cytotoxic to fibroblasts, erythrocytes, tumor cells and

TABLE 19–3. Inflammatory Mediator Systems

Mediator System	Source	Major Actions
Reactive oxygen intermediates (O_2^-, H_2O_2, HOX, HO)	Leukocytes, endothelial cells	Tissue damage through cytolysis, matrix degradation, activation of complement, and generation of chemotactic lipids
Reactive nitrogen intermediates (NO, $ONOO^-$, NO_2^-, NO_3^-)	Monocytes, macrophages, lymphocytes, endothelial cells	Cytostasis of cells, inhibition of DNA synthesis, inhibition of mitochondrial respiration, and formation of OH
Lysosomal granule constituents (proteases, lysozyme, lactoferrin, cationic proteins)	Neutrophils, monocytes	Tissue damage through proteolysis, matrix degradation, and catalysis of oxidant-generating reactions
Cytokines and chemokines (TNF, IL-1, IL-8, MCP-1, etc.)	Monocytes, macrophages, and endothelial cells	Cell activation, induction of adhesion, chemotaxis, fever, and acute-phase response
Platelet-activating factor	Leukocytes, endothelial cells	Vascular permeability and cell activation
Arachidonic acid metabolites (prostaglandins, 5-HPETE, leukotrienes)	Cell membranes (endothelial cells, platelets, leukocytes)	Coagulation, vasodilation, vascular permeability, cell activation, and chemotaxis
Kinins (bradykinin, kallikrein)	Plasma	Pain, vascular permeability, and vasodilation
Vasoactive amines (serotonin, histamine)	Platelets, mast cells, and basophils	Vascular permeability, induction of adhesion
Complement	Plasma, macrophages	Chemotaxis, vascular permeability, and cell activation
Coagulation	Plasma	Chemotaxis, vascular permeability, and complement activation

5-HPETE, 5 hydroperoxyeicosatetraenoic acid; IL, interleukin; MCP-1, monocyte chemoattractant protein-1; TNF, tumor necrosis factor.

many types of parenchymal cells.[33] Implicated biochemical mechanisms include lipid peroxidation, formation of carbonyl moieties and nitrosylation products, intracellular enzyme inactivation, protein oxidation, and oxidant-mediated DNA damage. Reactive oxygen intermediates (e.g., O_2^-) can also undergo reactions with reactive nitrogen intermediates (e.g., NO; see "Reactive Nitrogen Intermediates" below) to generate toxic NO derivatives.[33] Within limits, host cells are protected by antioxidant defense systems (e.g., superoxide dismutase, catalase, reduced glutathione).[33]

REACTIVE NITROGEN INTERMEDIATES

Described in 1980 as "endothelium-derived relaxing factor," NO is the soluble, gaseous, short-acting biosynthetic product of L-arginine, O_2, NADPH, and NO synthase (NOS).[34] As suggested by its original name, NO mediates vascular smooth muscle relaxation. NO binds to the heme moiety of guanylyl cyclase to trigger the generation of intracytoplasmic cyclic guanosine monophosphate (cGMP) and, through the activation of a series of kinases, induces smooth-muscle relaxation and vasodilation.[35] Three different forms of NOS have been characterized: endothelial (eNOS), neuronal (nNOS), and inducible (iNOS).[35] Nitric oxide can be produced either constitutively (eNOS, nNOS) or induced (iNOS) in a wide variety of cell types (e.g., endothelial cells, neurons, macrophages, respectively). Nitric oxide produced by eNOS plays a particularly important role in the localized regulation of vascular tone, whereas NO derived from nNOS is important in neuronal signal transduction. NO also plays important roles in the inhibition of smooth-muscle proliferation and in inflammation. The roles of NO in inflammation include inhibition of cell-mediated inflammation, reduction in platelet aggregation and adhesion, and as a regulator of leukocyte recruitment. Specifically, NO produced by cytokine-iNOS reduces leukocyte recruitment into sites of inflammation. NO can react with reactive oxygen intermediates to form both reactive oxygen and nitrogen species (e.g., $NO + O_2^- \rightarrow NO_2^- + HO\bullet$); it can inhibit DNA synthesis; it can directly kill microbes and tumor cells; and it can inactivate cytosolic glutathione and other sulfhydryl enzymes. NO and its generating enzymes, eNOS, nNOS, and iNOS, represent a regulatory system that has varied effects on the inflammatory response depending upon location and setting.

LYSOSOMAL GRANULE CONSTITUENTS

The activation of neutrophils, monocytes and macrophages results in the release, either through exocytosis or as the result of cell death, of a wide variety of proinflammatory mediators that have important roles in the inflammatory response. Neutrophils contain three major types of granules and also secretory vesicles (Chap. 60). Large, primary (azurophilic) granules contain myeloperoxidase, lysozyme, a variety of cationic proteins, defensins, phospholipase, acid hydrolases and neutral proteases (e.g., proteinase 3, collagenases, elastase). Smaller, secondary (specific) granules contain lactoferrin, lysozyme, type IV collagenase, subunits of NADPH oxidase and the β_2-integrin, CD11b/CD18. Tertiary granules contain gelatinase, subunits of NADPH oxidase and CD11b/CD18. Acid proteases function most efficiently within phagolysosomes where the pH is low, whereas neutral proteases can function efficiently within extracellular inflammatory exudates. Lysosomal granule constituents contribute to the inflammatory response and tissue injury through a wide array of mechanisms (e.g., degradation of extracellular matrix, proteolytic generation of chemotactic peptides and catalysis of reactive oxygen metabolite generation).

CYTOKINES AND CHEMOKINES

Cytokines are proteins that exhibit a variety of proinflammatory and antiinflammatory effects. They are produced by many cell types and modulate the function of other cell types. Individual cells may produce many different cytokines, and an individual cytokine may exert a wide variety of effects; they are pleiotropic.[2,3,6] In addition to their important roles in regulating various aspects of the immune response (e.g., lymphocyte activation, proliferation, and differentiation), many cytokines participate in innate immunity (e.g., TNF-α, IL-1β, IL-6, type I interferons), mediate the acute-phase response (TNF-α, IL1β, IL-6), activate inflammatory cells (e.g., IFN-γ) and participate in hematopoiesis (e.g., IL-3, granulocyte-monocyte colony-stimulating factor, granulocyte colony-stimulating factor, macrophage colony-stimulating factor).[2,3] Among the most thoroughly characterized cytokines are TNF-α and IL-1β, which are structurally dissimilar but share many biologic activities and can function as autocrine, paracrine and endocrine mediators of inflammation (Table 19–4).[2,3] TNF-α and IL-1β are produced by various cell types and are pleiotropic. Particularly important functions in inflammation include endothelial, leukocyte and fibroblast activation.

TABLE 19–4. Interleukin-1 and Tumor Necrosis Factor in Inflammation

Acute-phase response
Fever
Shock
Neutrophilia
Somnolence
Anorexia
Endothelial activation
Induction of IL-1, IL-6, IL-8
Procoagulant phenotype
Inhibition of fibrinolysis
Leukocyte adherence
Fibroblast activation
Proliferation
Collagen synthesis
Collagenase and protease induction

Elevated local (and sometimes systemic) concentrations of TNF-α, IL-1β, and IL-6 are consistently observed during the development of an inflammatory response. Based on their roles in the systemic acute-phase response and in the orchestration of important localized mechanistic steps in inflammation (e.g., induction of endothelial leukocyte adhesion molecules, phagocyte activation, procoagulant mediator induction), these mediators are prototypic "proinflammatory" cytokines. Their expression is regulated by nuclear factor κB (NFκB). NFκB is a transcription factor that exists as a heterodimer complexed with IκB (inhibitor κB) in the cytosol of many different cells types.[3,6] When cells are activated by various microbial products, viruses, reactive oxygen intermediates, cytokines, and chemotherapeutic agents, IκB is phosphorylated before it dissociates from NFκB heterodimers. Unbound NFκB translocates into the cell nucleus where it participates in the upregulation of as many as 200 different genes, including TNF-α, IL-1β and IL-6.

The proinflammatory cytokines and their activities are counterbalanced by a wide variety of "antiinflammatory" cytokines, including IL-4, IL-10, IL-11, IL-13, TGFβ, IL-1ra, and several soluble cytokine receptors.[2,3,7] IL-4, a 20-kDa peptide produced by CD4 Th2 cells, inhibits IL-1β synthesis and induces IL-1ra (IL-1 receptor antagonist). Soluble IL-1ra binds IL-1β (and IL-1α), preventing their binding to IL-1 receptors. IL-10 is also secreted by CD4 Th2 cells (and regulatory T cells, monocytes, and macrophages). Acting through its cognate receptor, IL-10 suppresses the expression of proinflammatory cytokines, adhesion molecules, chemokines, and cell-surface activation molecules of neutrophils, monocytes, macrophages, and T lymphocytes.[7] IL-10 also induces the shedding of TNF-α receptors, which then function as soluble TNF-α antagonists. IL-11, IL-13, and TGFβ also each exert a set of activities that counter the proinflammatory actions of TNF-α, IL-1β, and IL-6. Recognition of the many counterbalancing actions between proinflammatory and antiinflammatory cytokines has led to the concept of "proinflammatory–antiinflammatory cytokine balance." This concept is the basis for rational therapeutic strategies to manipulate or "reset" this balance.

TNF-α, IL-1β, and IL-6 are key proximate mediators of the "acute-phase response." Stimuli such as bacterial endotoxin (lipopolysaccharide), exotoxins, immune complexes and physical stimuli (e.g., heat or trauma) can induce macrophages (and other cell types) to secrete TNF-α, IL-1β, and IL-6.[2,3,7] In turn, TNF-α, IL-1β, and IL-6 mediate fever, somnolence, increased production of proteins such as α_1-antitrypsin (α_1-antiprotease) and α_2-macroglobulin, and decreased production of proteins such as albumin and transferrin. As noted, the acute-phase response is a stereotyped host metabolic response to a wide variety of insults. In addition to the systemic acute-phase response, TNF-α and IL-1β induce endothelial activation marked by increases in leukocyte adherence and a procoagulant state, leukocyte activation marked by cytokine secretion, and fibroblast activation marked by proliferation, collagen synthesis, and collagenase production.[2,3,7] These actions are critical components of inflammation and wound healing; they exemplify the linkage between the inflammatory response and the coagulation system.

TNF-α, originally identified as "cachexin or cachectin" because of its role in the systemic wasting that accompanies some chronic infections and cancer, can induce cytokine production in a variety of cells.[2,3] TNF-α can induce neutrophil activation and the expression of adhesion molecules on endothelial cells. In contrast to IL-1β, TNF-α also possesses potent cytotoxic activities for some types of cells. Both IL-1β and TNF-α are produced in response to endotoxemia and both can mediate a systemic shock-like response.

IL-1β, which exhibits a wide variety of biologic activities, was initially termed *endogenous pyrogen* because of its ability to induce temperature elevation and the acute-phase response.[2,3,36] IL-1β is relevant to acute inflammation because of its ability to induce cytokine production in monocytes, macrophages, fibroblasts and endothelial cells. IL-1β can also induce NOS.[36] As noted previously, IL-1β can activate endothelial cells, resulting in the expression of adhesion molecules and a procoagulant phenotype.[2,3,36]

IL-6 participates in the acute-phase response through the induction of proinflammatory mediators production by hepatocytes, via the differentiation of CD4 T lymphocytes that produce IL-17 and through the induction of marrow neutrophil production.[2,3] IL-6 is produced by a variety of cell types following activation by TNF-α, IL-1β, and pathogen-associated molecular patterns (PAMPs) such as lipopolysaccharides (endotoxin), mannans, flagellin, and microbial nucleic acids.[3,6]

Chemokines, or "intercrines," are small proteins, which, in addition to many of the general properties of cytokines, exhibit prominent chemotactic activities.[3,6,37] Chemokines are grouped into four classes based on the amino acid sequence positions of conserved cysteine (C) residues in mature peptides.[6,37] The four classes include CC, CXC, XC, and CX$_3$C chemokines. There are four families of corresponding chemokine receptors: CCR, CXCR, XCR, and CX$_3$CR, respectively. Nomenclature

of chemokines is based on the locations of N-terminal cysteine residues whereby "CC" indicates two adjacent residues, "CXC" indicates two cysteine residues separated by one intervening amino acid, and so on. Individual chemokines contain the letter "L" for ligand, followed by individual numbers (e.g., CCL1, CCL2, CCL3, etc.); more than 40 have been identified. The two most studied subfamilies include the alpha, or "CXC" chemokines, and the beta, or "CC" chemokines. Alpha chemokines, of which IL-8 (CXCL8) is the prototype, consistently exhibit neutrophil chemotactic activity, whereas the beta, or "CC" chemokines, of which MCP-1 (CCL2) is the prototype, exhibit monocyte chemotactic activity (Table 19–5).[37,38] Both *in vitro* and *in vivo* studies have provided insight into the roles of chemokines in inflammation. For example, MCP-1 knockout mice (MCP-1 −/−) exhibit reductions in monocyte influx into sites of experimentally induced peritonitis and delayed-type hypersensitivity.[39] Complementary studies using knockout mice devoid of the MCP-1 receptor CCR2 do not form typical granulomas.[39] These types of studies, as well as many that have employed specific chemokine-neutralizing antibodies or soluble chemokine receptor antagonists, have provided valuable insight into the pathophysiology of inflammation. Seemingly contradictory experimental results suggest that leukocyte recruitment mechanisms are multiple, overlapping or redundant, and not completely understood. Chemokine receptors noted above (CCR, CXCR, etc.) activate leukocytes through membrane receptors (sometimes called "serpentine" receptors) that contain seven transmembrane domains and are linked to cytosolic heterotrimeric G proteins.[3,6]

INFLAMMATORY LIPIDS

Lipid mediators of inflammation, commonly derived from cell membrane precursor molecules, can act either intracellularly or extracellularly, the latter in a short-lived, localized manner.[41] Arachidonic acid, a 20-carbon polyunsaturated fatty acid (5,8,11,14-eicosatetraenoic acid) derived either from dietary sources or by conversion from linoleic acid, is maintained in cell membranes as an esterified phospholipid. Three families of inflammatory mediators derived from arachidonic acid are generated via the cyclooxygenase and lipoxygenase pathways. Arachidonic acid is released from membrane phospholipids via cellular phospholipases such as phospholipase A$_2$. Phospholipase activation is triggered by mechanical/physical or chemical stimuli. Arachidonic acid can be metabolized via the cyclooxygenase pathway to prostaglandins (e.g., PGG$_2$, PGH$_2$, PGD$_2$, PGE$_2$, PGF$_2$), prostacyclin (PGI$_2$) or thromboxane (TXA$_2$).[41] Prostacyclin mediates vasodilation and the inhibition of platelet aggregation; thromboxane has the opposite effects; and PGD$_2$, PGE$_2$, and PGF$_2$ mediate vasodilation and edema. Activation

TABLE 19–5. Chemokines

Family	Members	Abbreviation(s)	Primary Target Cell(s)
α-Chemokines (CXC)	Interleukin-8	IL-8	Neutrophils
	Platelet factor 4	PF4	Neutrophils
	Melanocyte growth-stimulatory activity	MGSA or GROα	Neutrophils
	Neutrophil-activating peptide-2	NAP-2	Neutrophils
	γ-Interferon-inducible protein	γ-IP-10	Neutrophils
β-Chemokines (CC)	Monocyte chemoattractant protein-1	MCP-1/MCAF or JE	Monocytes, basophils
	Regulated on activation, normal T-cell expressed and presumably secreted	RANTES	Monocytes, eosinophils, basophils
	Macrophage inflammatory protein-1α	MIP-1α	Monocytes, eosinophils
	Macrophage inflammatory protein-1β	MIP-1β	Monocytes

of the lipoxygenase pathway results in the synthesis of 5-hydroperoxyeicosatetraenoic acid (5-HPETE), which is a potent chemoattractant of neutrophils and can be enzymatically modified to yield a series of other leukotrienes. LTB$_4$ induces neutrophil chemotaxis, aggregation, degranulation, and adherence, while LTC$_4$, LTD$_4$, and LTE$_4$ trigger smooth-muscle constriction, increases in vascular permeability and bronchoconstriction.[41] Members of both of these families of lipid-derived mediators and their catabolites have been detected in inflammatory exudates. There are two important branches within the lipoxygenase pathway.[41,42] Lipoxins (A$_4$ [LXA$_4$] and B$_4$ [LXB$_4$]) are generated via the 12-lipooxygenase branch of the lipoxygenase pathway in conjunction with a unique transcellular biosynthetic pathway.[42] Neutrophils generate LTA$_4$ via the 5-lipoxygenase pathway branch; in turn, lipoxins (LXA$_4$ and LXB$_4$) are generated through the action of platelet 12-lipooxygense on neutrophil LTA$_4$. Prevention of neutrophil-platelet binding interrupts this pathway. Lipoxins inhibit neutrophil chemotaxis and adhesion to endothelium.[42] As noted above, resolvins and protectins each encompass several molecular species—all derived from omega-3 polyunsaturated fatty acids.[26,27]

PAF is a potent proinflammatory lipid produced by a variety of cell types, including neutrophils, monocytes, endothelial cells and IgE-sensitized basophils.[43] Derived from the cell membrane constituent, choline phosphoglyceride, PAF is an acetyl glycerol ether phosphocholine that is synthesized following the activation of phospholipase A$_2$. PAF triggers platelet aggregation and degranulation, increases vascular permeability, and promotes leukocyte accumulation and activation. *In vivo* studies using specific PAF antagonists have suggested a role for PAF in a variety of acute inflammatory lesions.[43]

KININS

The kinin system is activated by contact activation of clotting factor XII (Hageman factor) (Chaps. 113 and 114).[44] Activation of the kinin system results in the generation of bradykinin, a nine-amino-acid vasoactive peptide. Bradykinin possesses several activities, including the capacity to increase vascular permeability, induce smooth-muscle contraction, trigger vasodilation, and cause pain.[44] Activated Hageman factor (factor XIIa), also known as the prekallikrein activator, converts plasma prekallikrein to kallikrein. In turn, kallikrein cleaves high-molecular-weight kininogen to produce bradykinin. Models of septic shock reveal decreases in plasma kininogen that parallel decreases in peripheral arterial resistance.[44]

VASOACTIVE AMINES

Histamine and serotonin (5-hydroxytryptamine) are low-molecular-weight vasoactive amines. Histamine is contained in mast cell and basophil granules, whereas platelets are a chief source of serotonin.[45] Localized release of histamine results in wheal formation as a consequence of increases in vascular permeability. Histamine induces the formation of reversible openings in endothelial tight junctions, triggers the formation of prostacyclin by endothelial cells and induces NO release from the endothelium. In addition, histamine, like thrombin, can induce the rapid upregulation of endothelial P-selectin.[45] Serotonin, acting through receptors on vascular smooth-muscle cells, is responsible for vasoconstriction, whereas interaction with endothelial receptors results in vasodilation (via release of NO) and increased permeability.[2] Release of histamine and serotonin from mast cells and platelets can be triggered by IgE-mediated type I hypersensitivity reactions, directly by C3a or C5a, and directly by neutrophil granule-derived cationic proteins.

COMPLEMENT

The complement system, including its soluble and cell membrane-associated regulators, consists of nearly two dozen plasma proteins that give rise to mediators of chemotaxis, increased vascular permeability, opsonic activity, phagocyte activation, and cytolysis.[46] In a manner analogous to coagulation, the complement system is activated through a cascade of proteolytic cleavage reactions. There are three convergent pathways (Fig. 19–3). The first of these, the "classical pathway," is initiated primarily (but not exclusively) by complement-fixing immune complexes (IgG subclasses 1 to 3 and IgM), whereas the second, the "alternative pathway," is triggered by a variety of substances that include

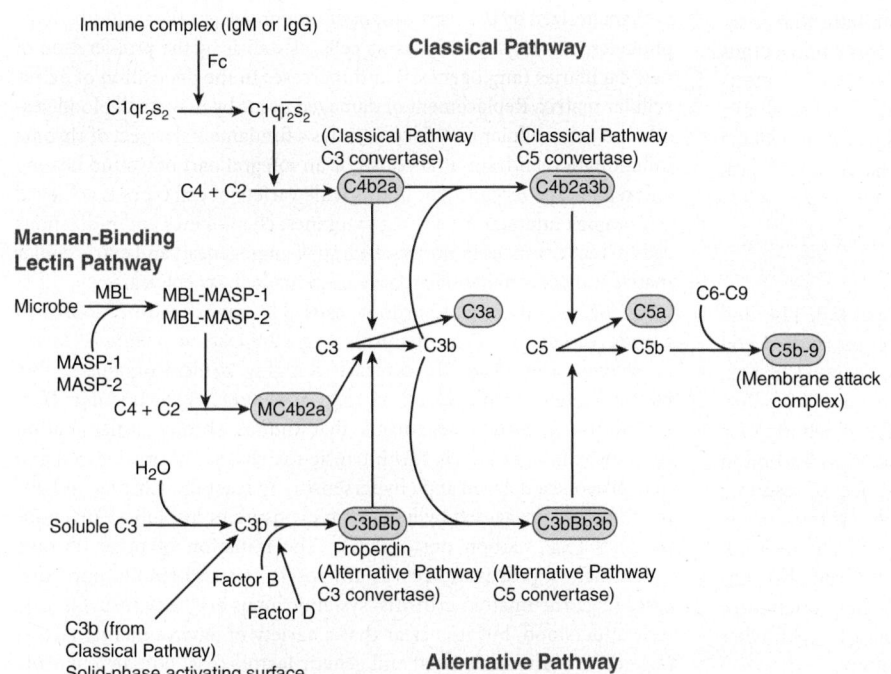

Figure 19–3. The complement system. The complement system consists of a series of soluble and surface-associated mediators that are functionally organized into the classical, alternative, and mannan-binding lectin (MBL) pathways. The three pathways of complement converge and lead to the production of the pore-forming membrane attack complex. The classical pathway is most often activated by IgG- and IgM-containing immune complexes, the alternative pathway can be activated by a variety of carbohydrate-coated particulates, and the MBL pathway also by various carbohydrate-coated surfaces. In all three cases, complex multicomponent enzyme complexes, called C3 and C5 convertases, are formed. A variety of soluble proinflammatory peptide fragments (e.g., C3a, C5a) are generated as a result of complement activation.

IgA aggregates, endotoxin, cobra venom factor, and polysaccharide moieties found on some bacterial and fungal cell walls. The third pathway, the "mannan-binding" lectin (MBL) pathway, is activated when MBL binds to a microorganism coated with certain carbohydrate moieties (e.g., mannans). Upon binding, MBL activates MBL-associated serine proteases (e.g., MASP-1, MASP-2) which function in a manner analogous to C1r and C1s of the classical pathway. MBL recognizes carbohydrate moieties infrequently present in mammalian hosts, thus constituting a system for recognizing foreign particulates. As such, the alternative and MBL pathways are considered to be part of the innate system of host defense.[6] The classical pathway is initiated by the fixation of C1 (C1qr$_2$s$_2$) by the Fc portion of surface-bound IgG or IgM immunoglobulins. Activated C1 (C1qr$_2$s$_2$) cleaves C2 and C4, which leads to the formation of the "classical pathway" C3 convertase, C4b2a. Activation of the alternative pathway results in the formation of an "alternative pathway" C3 convertase following direct cleavage of C3 and subsequent interactions of C3b with factors B and D in the presence of Mg^{2+}. The resulting complex, C3bBb, is stabilized by properdin, leading to the stable C3 convertase, C3bBbP. C3 convertases generated via any of the three pathways efficiently cleave C3 to form C3a and C3b.

These enzymatic reactions exhibit high activity levels, thus serving to dramatically amplify the cascade. C3b can bind to either the classical or alternative pathway C3 convertase to form a C5 convertase, which cleaves C5 into C5a and C5b. C5a is released into the fluid phase, like C3a, whereas C5b combines first with C6 and then C7 to form C5b-7, which, in turn, binds with C8 and multiple C9 molecules to form C5b-9, the membrane attack complex. In addition to the cell-activating and cytolytic activities of C5b-9, individual complement cleavage products and complexes mediate a variety of specific and potent proinflammatory activities.[46] These functions, combined with the rapid amplification in numbers of complement-derived mediators, emphasize the vital role of complement in acute inflammation. The most important activation products of complement appear to be C5a, a major chemotactic factor, and the anaphylatoxins (C3a, C4a, C5a), of which C3a is the most abundant. C5b-9 is a major cytotoxic product, provided that this complex is assembled on the surface of a susceptible cell (e.g., bacterium).

A series of soluble and cell membrane-associated complement proteins play important roles in the regulation of the complement cascade.[46] The pivotal regulator of the proximal arm of classical pathway is C1 esterase inhibitor (C1E-INH), a serine protease inhibitor that covalently bonds to the activated esterase subunits of the C1qrs complex thus preventing activation of the downstream zymogen cascade.[46] Defects in C1E-INH, from genetic defects or those acquired (e.g., neutralizing antibodies against C1E-INH), can result in angioedema. Angioedema can manifest in a variety of ways including as life-threatening laryngeal soft tissue swelling.

COAGULATION SYSTEM

The coagulation system is reviewed in detail in Chaps. 113, 114, and 116. The interrelationships among the coagulation system and several inflammatory mediator systems are important in the context of host defense and the pathophysiology of septic shock.[4] Activation of the clotting cascade results in the generation of fibrinopeptides which increase vascular permeability and are chemotactic for leukocytes. Thrombin and tissue factor induce endothelial expression of P-selectin, resulting in increased neutrophil adhesion.[12] In addition, plasmin is responsible for the activation of Hageman factor, which then can activate the kinin system and can cleave C3 into its active components.[44] It can also generate "fibrin-split" or "fibrin-degradation" products. The induction of tissue factor in endothelial cells exposed to TNF-α and IL-1β further links the coagulation system to the inflammatory response.

PROTEINASE-ACTIVATED RECEPTORS

Proteinase-activated receptors (PARs) define an important general mechanism that links several seemingly disparate regulatory systems involved in inflammation.[47] PARs subsume a G-protein–coupled receptor subfamily defined by a common activation mechanism.[47] Individual PARs include an N-terminal extracellular domain, seven transmembrane helices connected by three intracellular and three extracellular loops, and linkage to cytosolic G-protein–mediated signal transduction pathways.[47] PARs are activated when extracellular proteinases cleave the N-terminal extracellular domain at a specific site which results in the creation of a "tethered ligand." The tethered ligand is the residual, now unmasked N-terminal portion of the PAR; it interacts with the nearby nontruncated extracellular PAR domain and activates the receptor. The PAR family possesses of four members: PAR$_1$, PAR$_2$, PAR$_3$, and PAR$_4$. The extracellular domain of each PAR possesses several potential cleavage sites. For example, the canonical PAR$_1$ tethered ligand sequence created after cleavage by thrombin is the amino acid sequence, SFLLRN.[47] A wide variety of proteinases that are pivotal in inflammation, thrombosis, hemostasis, and wound healing (as well as in development and cancer progression) can activate PARs. PAR$_1$, PAR$_3$, and PAR$_4$ are susceptible to cleavage by thrombin. Other coagulation system-related proteinases, such as factor Xa, activated protein C, plasmin, and kallikreins can also activate PAR$_1$. Likewise, PAR$_1$ can also be activated by matrix metalloproteinase-1, neutrophil elastase, and neutrophil proteinase-3. Various proteinases cleave the N-terminal extracellular domain of PARs at different, yet specific, sites. Examples of PAR activation relevant to inflammation include thrombin-induced CCL2 expression in osteoblasts and PAR$_2$ and PAR$_4$ activation in animal models of arthritis. A goal of rational therapeutic design is to target crosstalk interactions using paired drugs or bifunctional agents. Although no PAR-targeting compounds have yet come into clinical use, this is a promising area.[47]

● CHRONIC INFLAMMATION AND REPAIR

The chronic inflammatory response and repair processes are, like the acute inflammatory response, highly regulated. By definition, "chronic" inflammation connotes a process that lasts at least several days and more often, weeks to months, sometimes years. Chronic inflammation is characterized by the recruitment of mononuclear cells including lymphocytes, monocytes and plasma cells, as well as by the proliferation of new capillaries (angiogenesis) and increases in the deposition of extracellular matrix. Replacement of damaged tissue by new small blood vessels and extracellular matrix constitutes a fundamental aspect of chronic inflammation and, simultaneously, is an integral part of wound healing and repair. The recruitment of this wide variety of cell types is achieved by complex interactions among cytokines, chemokines and indigenous cells. Great advances in understanding of angiogenesis and extracellular matrix molecule metabolism have been made in recent years.

Chronic inflammation can be caused by persistent infections with a wide variety of microorganisms (e.g., *Treponema pallidum*, *Mycobacterium tuberculosis*). In contrast to highly virulent organisms that trigger acute pyogenic infections (e.g., *Streptococcus pneumoniae*, *Haemophilus influenzae*), organisms that induce chronic inflammation typically exhibit relatively low intrinsic toxicity, are poorly cleared and may provoke a delayed-type hypersensitivity reaction. Chronic inflammation is also triggered by long-term exposure to insoluble exogenous particles (e.g., carbon dust, silica).[2] The initiation of other chronic inflammatory processes such as atherosclerosis and autoimmune diseases (e.g., rheumatoid arthritis, systemic lupus erythematosus) is less-well understood, but it is clear that a variety of environmental factors (e.g., diet in atherosclerosis) and genetic factors (e.g., human leukocyte antigen [HLA]-linked susceptibility in rheumatoid arthritis) are important. The characteristics of individual chronic inflammatory responses are dependent on the location of the injury and the type of injurious agent. As noted throughout this chapter, the recruitment of mononuclear cells into an inflammatory lesion is governed by the same general paradigm that orchestrates the recruitment of neutrophils into sites of acute inflammation. Unlike most acute conditions, chronic inflammatory processes are sometimes marked by a relatively specific morphology (e.g., granuloma formation in tuberculosis, eosinophil infiltration in parasitic infections) and by the coexistence of tissue repair (i.e., angiogenesis and extracellular matrix production).

A key cell type in chronic inflammatory processes is the macrophage.[3,5] Tissue macrophages are derived primarily from circulating blood monocytes and can adopt relatively specific functions based on their differentiation in selected body sites (e.g., hepatic Kupffer cells, alveolar macrophages, central nervous system microglia). In the setting of chronic inflammation, tissue macrophages can be activated by immunologic means (IFN-γ secreted by antigen-activated CD4 T lymphocytes) and by nonimmunologic means (microbial endotoxin, extracellular matrix proteins and foreign particulates; Chap. 67). In turn, activated macrophages enlarge, become more metabolically active, exhibit enhanced phagocytosis and secrete a large array of mediators.[3,5] Mediators secreted by activated macrophages include proteases, reactive oxygen and nitrogen intermediates, coagulation factors, arachidonic acid-derived lipids and cytokines. These mediators, as detailed in preceding sections, participate in inflammation. Activated macrophages also secrete collagenases that participate in tissue remodeling, angiogenic factors (e.g., fibroblast growth factor) and profibrogenic growth factors (fibroblast growth factor, TGF-β, platelet-derived growth factor).[3,5] Consequently, activated tissue macrophages participate in inflammation *per se*, tissue remodeling, angiogenesis and fibrosis.

Although macrophages play a central role in all facets of chronic inflammation, other cell types are also important. Lymphocytes (both B and T cells) are recruited into chronic inflammatory lesions via leukocyte–endothelial adhesive interactions and via chemotactic mechanisms analogous to those involved in neutrophil recruitment. Antigen-activated CD4 Th1 lymphocytes produce IFN-γ, which, as discussed above, is an important activator of tissue macrophages.[3] Activated CD4 Th2 lymphocytes produce a variety of proinflammatory mediators that are involved in lymphocyte activation (e.g., IL-2) and in immune regulation (e.g., IL-5 in IgE production).[3]

Eosinophils and mast cells also play important roles in some types of chronic inflammation. Mast cells, which tend to be distributed along small blood vessels, possess high-affinity FcεRI receptors for IgE.[48] Engagement of mast cell-bound IgE triggers degranulation that leads to histamine and arachidonic acid–derived lipid release (Chap. 63). Eosinophils are characteristically formed in IgE-mediated allergic reactions and in parasitic infections (Chap. 62). Eotaxin, a CC chemokine, binds to and activates eosinophils via CCR3.[3,48] Recruited eosinophils secrete various granule proteins that help kill parasites, but which can also cause tissue damage. As inferred above, the histopathologic appearance of many chronic inflammatory lesions can provide insight into their pathogenesis and cause. A variety of poorly degraded, intrinsically low toxicity agents can induce granulomatous inflammation (e.g., *M. tuberculosis*).[49] Many parasites induce an eosinophilic response (e.g., *Toxocara canis*). Finally, the induction of tissue remodeling, angiogenesis and fibrosis can contribute to both tissue damage and repair, and can also suggest underlying etiology (e.g., lung fibrosis associated with asbestos). The tremendous advances in understanding of the inflammatory response hold great promise for the future of both diagnostics and therapeutics.

REFERENCES

1. Weissman G: Inflammation: Historical perspectives, in *Inflammation: Basic Principles and Clinical Correlates*, 2nd ed, edited by JJ Gallin, IM Goldstein, R Snyderman, p 5. Raven Press, New York, 1992.
2. Acute and chronic inflammation, in *Robbins and Cotran Pathologic Basis of Disease*, 8th ed, edited by V Kumar, AK Abbas, N Fausto, p 43. Saunders Elsevier, Philadelphia, 2010.
3. Leukocyte migration into tissues, in *Cellular and Molecular Immunology*, 7th ed, edited by AK Abbas, AH Lichtman, S Pillai, p 37. Elsevier Saunders, Philadelphia, 2012.
4. Angus DC, van der Poll T: Severe sepsis and septic shock. *N Engl J Med* 369:840, 2013.
5. Ortega-Gómez A, Perretti M, Soehnlein O: Resolution of inflammation: An integrated view. *EMBO Mol Med* 5:661, 2013.
6. Innate immunity, in *Cellular and Molecular Immunology*, 7th ed, edited by AK Abbas, AH Lichtman, S Pillai, p 55. Elsevier Saunders, Philadelphia, 2012.
7. Sultani M, Stringen AM, Bowen JM, Gibson RJ: Anti-inflammatory cytokines: Important immunoregulatory factors contributing to chemotherapy-induced gastrointestinal mucositis. *Chemother Res Pract* 10:1, 2012.
8. Dvorak AM, Feng D: The vesiculo-vacuolar organelle (vvo). A new endothelial cell permeability organelle. *J Histochem Cytochem* 49:419, 2001.
9. Ley KO, Laudanna C, Cybulsky MJ, Nourshargh S: Getting to the site of inflammation: The leukocyte adhesion cascade updated. *Nat Rev Immunol* 7:678, 2007.
10. Chen S, Springer TA: Selectin receptor-ligand bonds: Formation limited by shear rate and dissociation governed by the Bell model. *Proc Natl Acad Sci U S A* 98:950, 2001.
11. Kinashi T: Intracellular signaling controlling integrin activation in lymphocytes. *Nat Rev Immunol* 5:546, 2005.
12. Sim D, Flaumenhoft R, Furie B, Furie B: Interactions of platelets, blood-borne tissue factor, and fibrin during arteriolar thrombus formation in vivo. *Microcirculation* 12:301, 2005.
13. Jung U, Key K: Mice lacking two or all three selectins demonstrate overlapping and distinct functions for each selectin. *J Immunol* 162:6755, 1999.
14. Jung U, Ramos CL, Bullard DC, Ley K: Gene-targeted mice reveal importance of L-selectin-dependent rolling for neutrophil adhesion. *Am J Physiol Heart Circ Physiol* 274:H1785, 1998.
15. Bajenoff M, Egen JG, Qi H, et al: Highways, byways and breadcrumbs: Directing lymphocyte traffic in the lymph node. *Trends Immunol* 28:346, 2007.
16. Shimaoka M, Takagi J, Springer TA: Conformational regulation of integrin structure and function. *Annu Rev Biophys Biomol Struct* 31:485, 2002.
17. Millard M, Odde S, Neamati N: Integrin targeted therapeutics. *Theranostics* 1:154, 2011.
18. Luscinskas FW, Ma S, Nusrat A, et al: Leukocyte transendothelial migration: A junctional affair. *Semin Immunol* 14:105, 2002.
19. Ciacchetti G, Allen PG, Glogauer M: Chemotactic signaling pathways in neutrophils: From receptor to actin assembly. *Crit Rev Oral Biol Med* 13:220, 2002.
20. Iwakura Y, Ishigame H, Saijo S, Nakae S: Functional specialization of interleukin-17 family members. *Immunity* 34:149, 2011.
21. Dale DC, Boxer L, Liles WC: The phagocytes: Neutrophils and monocytes. *Blood* 112:935, 2008.
22. Nauseef WM: How human neutrophils kill and degrade microbes: An integrated view. *Immunol Rev* 219:88, 2007.
23. Schroder K, Tschopp J: The inflammasomes. *Cell* 190:821, 2010.
24. Takeuchi O, Akira S: Pattern recognition receptors and inflammation. *Cell* 140:805, 2010.
25. Blasius AL, Beutler B: Intracellular toll-like receptors. *Immunity* 32:305, 2010.
26. Kohli P, Levy BD: Resolvins and protectins: Mediating solutions to inflammation. *Br J Pharmacol* 158:960, 2009.
27. Serhan CN, Chiang N, Van Dyke TE: Resolving inflammation: Dual anti-inflammatory and pro-resolution lipid mediators. *Nat Rev Immunol* 8:349, 2008.
28. Stout RD: Macrophage functional phenotypes: No alternatives in dermal wound healing? *J Leukoc Biol* 87:19, 2010.
29. Martinez FO, Helming L, Gordon S: Alternative activation of macrophages: An immunologic functional perspective. *Annu Rev Immunol* 27:451, 2009.
30. Ding T, Deighton C: Complications of anti-TNF therapies. *Fut Rheumatol* 2:587, 2007.
31. Dean RA, Cox JH, Bellac IL, et al: Macrophage-specific metalloelastase (MMP-12) truncates and inactivates ELR + CXC chemokines and generates CCL2, -7, -8, and -13 antagonists: Potential role of the macrophage in terminating polymorphonuclear leukocyte influx. *Blood* 112: 3455, 2008.
32. Babior BM: Phagocytes and oxidative stress. *Am J Med* 109:33, 2003.
33. Bosmann M, Ward PA: Invited review. The inflammatory response in sepsis. *Trends Immunol* 34:129, 2013.
34. Furchgott RF, Zawadzki JV: The obligatory role of endothelial cells in the relaxation of arterial smooth muscle by acetylcholine. *Nature* 288:373, 1980.
35. Laroux FS, Pavlick KP, Hines IN, et al: Role of nitric oxide in inflammation. *Acta Physiol Scand* 173:113, 2001.
36. Sims JE, Smith DE: The IL-1 family: Regulators of immunity. *Nat Rev Immunol* 10:89, 2010.
37. Bromley SK, Mempel TR, Lyster AD: Orchestrating the orchestrators: Chemokines in control of T cell traffic. *Nat Immunol* 9:970, 2008.
38. Sallusto F, Baggiolini M: Chemokines and leukocytes traffic. *Nat Immunol* 9:949, 2008.
39. Lu B, Rutledge BJ, Gu L, et al: Abnormalities in monocyte recruitment and cytokine expression in monocyte chemoattractant protein 1-deficient mice. *J Exp Med* 187:601, 1998.

40. Kuziel WA, Morgan SJ, Dawson TC, et al: Severe reduction in leukocyte adhesion and monocyte extravasation in mice deficient in CC chemokine receptor 2. *Proc Natl Acad Sci U S A* 94:12053, 1997.

41. Zurier RB: Prostaglandins, leukotrienes, and related compounds, in *Kelley's Textbook of Rheumatology*, 6th ed, edited by ED Harris Jr, RC Budd, GS Firestein, MC Genovese, JS Sargent, S Ruddy, p 356. Saunders Elsevier, Philadelphia, 2005.

42. Levy BD, Serhan CN: Polyisoprenyl phosphates: Natural antiinflammatory lipid signals. *Cell Mol Life Sci* 59:729, 2002.

43. Zimmerman GA, McIntyre TM, Prescott SM, Stafforini DM: The platelet-activating factor signaling system and its regulators in syndromes of inflammation and thrombosis. *Crit Care Med* 30: S294, 2002.

44. Golias CH, Charalabopoulos A, Stagikas D, et al: The kinin system-bradykinin: Biological effects and clinical implications. Multiple role of the kinin system-bradykinin. *Hippokratia* 11:124, 2007.

45. Repka-Ramirez MS, Baraniuk JN: Histamine in health and disease. *Clin Allergy Immunol* 17:1, 2002.

46. Effector mechanisms of humoral immunity, in *Cellular and Molecular Immunology*, 7th ed, edited by AK Abbas, AH Lichtman, S Pillai, p 269. Elsevier Saunders, Philadelphia, 2012.

47. Giesler F, Ungefronen H, Settmacher U, et al: Proteinase-activated receptors (PARs)—Focus on receptor-receptor interactions and their physiological and pathological impact. *Cell Commun Signal* 11:86, 2013.

48. Gould HJ, Sutton BJ, Beavil AJ, et al: The biology of IgE and the basis of allergic disease. *Annu Rev Immunol* 21:579, 2003.

49. Cellular pathology II: Adaptations, intracellular accumulations, and cell aging, in *Robbins Pathologic Basis of Disease*, 8th ed, edited by Kumar V, Abbas AK, Faustos N. Elsevier Saunders, Philadelphia, 2010.

CHAPTER 20
INNATE IMMUNITY

Bruce Beutler

SUMMARY

The innate immune system provides immediate protection against infection and serves an essential antigen-presenting role that allows the adaptive immune response to occur during the days and weeks that follow. The sensory apparatus that allows detection of infectious microbes has been deciphered in large part, and it is now known that Toll-like receptors, NOD-like receptors, RIG-I–like helicases, C-type lectin receptors, and cytosolic sensors of DNA, most notably cyclic guanosine monophosphate/adenosine monophosphate synthetase, permit recognition of specific molecules of microbial origin. Much has also been learned of the biochemical events that follow activation of these sensors. Susceptibility to infection in humans is strongly heritable, and among the many loci that influence it, those that encode proteins vital to the innate immune response are of central importance. Moreover, autoinflammatory and autoimmune diseases are dependent upon the activation of innate immune signaling pathways.

Acronyms and Abbreviations: BIR, baculovirus inhibitor of apoptosis repeat; CARD, caspase activating and recruitment domain; CD, cluster of differentiation; cGAS, cyclic AMP/GMP synthetase; CTLA, cytotoxic T-lymphocyte antigen; DAI, DNA-dependent activator of IRFs; ERK, extracellular signal-regulated kinase; FADD, Fas-associated death domain; G-CSF, granulocyte colony-stimulating factor; GM-CSF, granulocyte-monocyte colony-stimulating factor; IFN, interferon; IκB; inhibitor of κB; IKK, IκB kinase; IL, interleukin; IPAF, ice-protease activating factor; IPS-1, IFN-β promoter stimulator 1; IRAK, interleukin-1 receptor-associated kinase; IRF, interferon response factor; JAK, Janus kinase; JNK, c-Jun N-terminal kinase; LPS, lipopolysaccharide; LRR, leucine-rich repeat; MAL, MyD88 adaptor-like; MDA5, melanoma differentiation-associated gene 5; MDP, muramyl dipeptide; MyD88, myeloid differentiation primary response 88; NACHT, a nucleotide-binding domain present in NAIP, CIITA, HET-E, and TP-1; NADPH, nicotinamide adenine dinucleotide phosphate; NBS, nucleotide binding sequence; NEMO, NF-κB essential modulator; NF-κB, nuclear factor-κB; NK, natural killer; NLR, NOD-like receptor; NOD, nucleotide-binding oligomerization domain; PAR-2, proteinase-activated G-protein–coupled receptor; PRAT4A, protein associated with TLR4; PYD, pyrin domain; RIG-I, retinoic acid inducible gene I; RIP, receptor-interacting protein; RLH, RIG-I–like helicase; ROS, reactive oxygen species; SARM, sterile-α and armadillo motif; SOCS-1, suppressor of cytokine signaling 1; STAT, signal transducer and activator of transcription; STING, stimulator of interferon genes; TAK-1, transforming growth factor-β–activating kinase 1; TBK1, TANK-binding kinase 1; TIR, Toll/interleukin-1 receptor; TLR, Toll-like receptor; TNF, tumor necrosis factor; Tpl2, tumor progression locus 2; TRAF, TNF receptor–associated factor; TRAM, TRIF-related adaptor molecule; TRIF, Toll/interleukin-1 receptor (TIR) domain-containing adaptor inducing IFN-β; UCM, upregulation of costimulatory molecules.

INNATE IMMUNITY VERSUS ADAPTIVE IMMUNITY

In humans, as in all mammals, resistance to microbial infection is based partly upon lymphocytes, which yield highly specific responses to microbial antigens: either the production of antibodies or the expansion of T-cell cell clones that are directly cytotoxic to infected cells (Chaps. 75 and 76). This, the *adaptive* immune response, is a recent fixture in evolution, witnessed only in vertebrates and traceable to the development of a mechanism for recombination of genomic DNA that arose approximately 450 to 500 million years ago, operating on genes encoding proteins with immunoglobulin domains in some lineages and on genes encoding proteins with leucine-rich repeats in other lineages.[1,2] A more fundamental type of immunity, known as *innate* immunity, is represented in one form or another in all multicellular organisms. For this reason, a great deal of progress in the innate immunity field has come from the study of model animals such as *Drosophila melanogaster*, and model plants such as *Arabidopsis thaliana*. Despite the vast evolutionary divergence of these organisms from *Homo sapiens*, these species use defensive proteins and signaling pathways that are ancestrally related to those represented in humans.

Like the adaptive immune system, the innate immune system is endowed with a means of detecting microbes, destroying them, and at the same time, exercising self-tolerance. These mechanisms are far older than the analogous adaptive mechanisms and as a consequence are more refined. Although it is sometimes termed the "primitive" immune system, the innate immune system is both sophisticated and highly effective. Moreover, adaptive immunity is largely dependent upon innate immunity in the sense that antigen presentation and adaptive immune activation depend upon innate immune cells.

Innate immunity, which acts immediately to protect the host in the event of microbial inoculation, fills a temporal gap that would otherwise exist in the global immune response. Days or weeks are required for an effective adaptive immune response to develop when the naïve host encounters a new pathogen. During this time, innate immunity alone protects the host. Indeed, innate immunity is objectively more important than adaptive immunity. In a nonsterile environment, survival would be impossible without it (Table 20–1).

TYPES OF INNATE IMMUNITY

Innate immunity embraces a large number of host resistance mechanisms, which may be divided into cellular and noncellular components, and also into afferent and effector components. Noncellular components of innate immunity include antimicrobial peptides, which selectively disrupt microbial cell membranes, complement, components of which also disrupt cell membranes, and the proteins hemopexin and haptoglobin, which deny iron to invasive microbes. Cellular components include myeloid cells (granulocytes, monocyte/macrophages, mast cells, and dendritic cells) and lymphoid cells (natural killer [NK] cells and NKT cells). As such, it can be seen that despite their recent evolutionary origin, some lymphoid cells have been coopted to serve in the innate immune system rather than the adaptive immune system. Many other cells are also endowed with some degree of innate (often "cell-autonomous") immune function. For example, fibroblasts can sense viral infection and respond with interferon (IFN) production.

Once initiated, the innate immune response runs its course in a preprogrammed fashion, proceeding from microbe sensing all the way through to microbial killing, making division into "afferent" and "effector" functions somewhat arbitrary. Nonetheless, the proteins

TABLE 20–1. Comparisons between Innate and Adaptive Immunity

	Innate Immunity	Adaptive Immunity
Sensing mechanism	TLRs, NK receptors; NLRs, RLHs, fMLP receptor	Immunoglobulins, T-cell receptors
Cellular components	Macrophages, dendritic cells, granulocytes, mast cells, NK cells	T cells, B cells
Efferent mechanisms	Cytokine production, inflammatory response, phagocytosis, pathogen killing	Antibody production, cytokine production, cell killing
Purpose	Alert other innate and adaptive immune cells to pathogen presence; directly kill pathogen; encourage the development of an adaptive immune response	Assist in efficacy of innate immune response, produce highly specific ligands for pathogens
Time scale of response	Quick (maximal in minutes to hours)	Slow (maximal in days to weeks)
Specific memory	No	Yes
Phylogeny	Ancient (all multicellular organisms)	Recent (vertebrates only)

fMLP, N-formyl-methionyl-leucyl-phenylalanine; NK, natural killer; NLR, NOD (nucleotide-binding oligomerization domain)-like receptor; RLH, RIG (retinoic acid inducible gene)-I–like helicase; TLR, Toll-like receptor.

responsible for microbial recognition, signaling, and the development of a transcriptional response within innate immune cells are generally considered "afferent" components; the cytokines that mediate the response and the cellular weaponry that is used to destroy viruses and bacteria may be considered "effector" components.

The remainder of this chapter emphasizes the afferent arm of cellular innate immunity, as the effector mechanisms (neutrophil-mediated killing, complement, and antimicrobial peptides) are covered in other chapters. Our understanding of innate immune responses has improved dramatically as forward and reverse genetic methods have been used to dissect the signaling pathways that permit host recognition of microbes. The initial interactions between molecules of microbes and molecules of the host that trigger an innate immune response have been studied in great detail over the past decade. The afferent pathways are each capable of activating responses that partly overlap with one another.

MICROBE RECOGNITION BY THE TOLL-LIKE RECEPTORS

Discovery of the Mammalian Toll Like Receptors as the Primary Sensors of the Innate Immune System

The Toll-like receptors (TLRs) collectively mediate the recognition of most microbes. Ten TLRs are encoded in the human genome. The molecular specificity of nine of these TLRs has been established, at least in part. Although publications can be found to suggest that some of the TLRs (notably TLRs 2 and 4) detect dozens of molecules, the evidence favoring most of these interactions is slender, and a conservative viewpoint is preferred; hence, Table 20–2 presents only those interactions that are deemed certain.

The microbe-sensing function of the mammalian TLR was discovered as a result of inquiry into the mechanism of endotoxin sensing. Endotoxin (later identified as lipopolysaccharide [LPS]) was first described by Pfeiffer as a toxic component of *Vibrio cholerae* more than 100 years ago.[3] Its chemical structure was established many years later (reviewed in Ref. 4), and a toxic "lipid A" moiety of LPS was synthesized artificially in 1985 and found to have full biologic activity.[5] The identity of the LPS receptor was established in 1998, through the positional cloning of *Lps*, a locus that was known to be required for all cellular responses to endotoxin, and for the effective clearance of Gram-negative bacterial infections[6] in laboratory mice. In LPS-unresponsive mice, the *Tlr4* locus was shown to be mutationally altered or deleted.[7] It had previously been recognized that Toll, a *Drosophila* protein also known for its developmental effects,[8] was required for the innate immune response to fungal infection in flies.[9] Hence, the

TABLE 20–2. Toll-Like Receptors, Microbial Specificities, and Transducers

TLR	Known Macromolecular Associations	Ligand(s)	Adapter Use	Refs.
1	TLR2	Tri-acyl lipopeptides	MyD88, MAL	12, 137–139
2	TLRs 1 or 6, or homodimer	Lipopeptides, lipoteichoic acid, zymosan, protozoal GPI	MyD88, MAL	11
3	–	dsRNA	TRIF	14, 42, 120
4	CD14, MD-2	LPS	MyD88, MAL, TRIF, TRAM	7, 21, 41, 42, 120, 140
5	–	Flagellin	MyD88	13
6	TLR2	Di-acyl lipopeptides, glucans, lipoteichoic acid	MyD88, MAL	141
7	–	ssRNA, imidazoquinolines	MyD88	142
8	–	ssRNA, imidazoquinolines	MyD88	143
9	–	Unmethylated CpG motifs	MyD88	10
10	–	Unknown	Unknown	144

dsRNA, double-stranded RNA; GPI, glycosylphosphatidylinositol; LPS, lipopolysaccharide; MAL, MyD88 adaptor-like; MyD88, myeloid differentiation 88; ssRNA, single-stranded ribonucleic acid; TRAM, TRIF-related adaptor molecule; TRIF, Toll/interleukin-1 receptor (TIR) domain-containing adaptor inducing IFN-β.

discovery of an LPS-sensing function for TLR4, a homologue of Toll, made evolutionary sense.

Other molecules of microbial origin (for example, di- and tri-acylated lipopeptides and lipoproteins, lipoteichoic acid, unmethylated DNA bearing CpG dinucleotides in a particular context, flagellin, and double-stranded RNA [dsRNA]) were known to elicit responses qualitatively similar to those elicited by LPS. The other TLR paralogs seemed excellent candidate receptors for these molecules. Reverse genetic methods established that each of these molecules is indeed recognized by a particular TLR or heteromeric combination of TLRs.[10–14] Moreover, genetic complementation analyses have shown that at least some microbial ligands directly engage the TLRs in order to elicit a signal.[15,16] On the other hand, other molecules enhance the signal, and also participate in ligand recognition. Dectin-1 is a type II transmembrane C-type lectin that recognizes glucans present in the cell walls of fungi, signals via spleen tyrosine kinase (Syk) and the Card9/Bcl-10/MALT1 complex to activate nuclear factor-κB (NF-κB),[17,18] and enhances TLR2/6 signaling.[19] Similarly, proteinase-activated G-protein–coupled receptor (PAR-2) signaling enhances TLR4 responses to LPS.[20] Other examples include the binding of cluster of differentiation (CD) 14 to LPS[21] which augments LPS responses,[22] as well as the enhancement of responses to bacterial diacylglycerides by CD36.[23] It is likely that these accessory molecules form complexes with the TLRs, which are responsible for transducing the signal across the cell membrane. TLR4 exists in a tight complex with MD-2, a small secreted protein that is required for TLR4 to reach the cell surface and required for LPS sensing as well.[24]

Structure of the Toll-Like Receptors

The TLRs are single-spanning transmembrane proteins with leucine-rich repeat (LRR) motifs in their extracellular domains and a characteristic TIR (Toll/interleukin [IL]-1 receptor) motif in their cytoplasmic domains. The TIR domain is based on an ancient protein fold[25] evident in cytosolic plant disease resistance proteins (where it often is represented together with a nucleotide binding sequence [NBS] and/or LRR motifs), in proteins of the IL-1 and IL-18 receptor family, in the adapter proteins that carry signals from TLRs, and in the TLRs themselves.

The structure of the TLR2/1, 2/6, 3, 4, 5, and 8 ectodomains has been determined by x-ray crystallography, which showed a horseshoe-shape characteristic of LRR-containing proteins. TLRs form homodimers or heterodimers induced by the simultaneous binding of ligands to LRRs of distinct receptor chains. The nature of the ligand-receptor interaction has also been determined for several of the above receptors, and appears to be different in each individual case (Fig. 20–1). To activate TLR4, LPS interacts with MD-2, which has a hydrophobic pocket that accommodates the lipid A moiety of LPS.[26,27] TLR2/1 heterodimers are "crosslinked" by the engagement of two acyl chains by TLR1 and a single acyl chain by TLR2.[28] TLR3 molecules bind a linear, negatively charged dsRNA oligonucleotide, which triggers activation.[29]

TLRs 3, 7, 8, and 9 are believed to be intracellular. Little (TLR3) or no (TLRs 7 and 9) surface expression can be detected, and tagged versions of the molecules are found to reside within the interior of transfected cells.[30] The ectodomains of these TLRs project into endocytic vesicles and there detect foreign molecules rather than within the

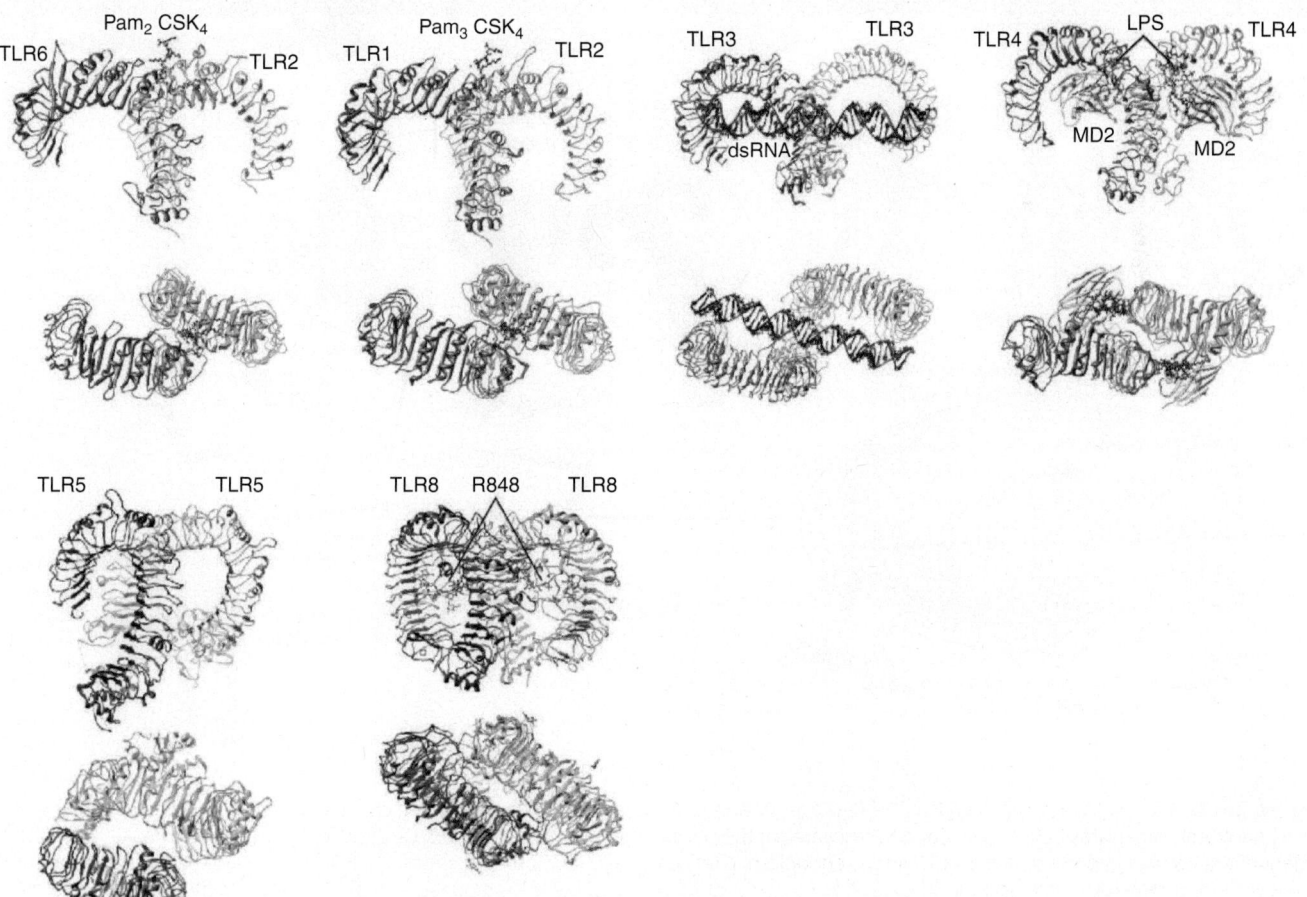

Figure 20–1. Structures of Toll-like receptors (TLRs) and their ligands. TLR2-TLR6-Pam₂CSK₄ lipopeptide (3A79), TLR2-TLR1-Pam₃CSK₄ lipopeptide (2Z7X), TLR3-dsRNA (3CIY), TLR4-MD2-LPS (3FXI), TLR5 (3J0A), and TLR8-R848 (3W3L) are shown. Side view (*upper panels*) and top view (*lower panels*) are shown. Protein Databank ID numbers are indicated in parentheses. Figures were generated with UCSF Chimera. dsRNA, double-stranded RNA.

extracellular space. TLRs 3, 7, 8, and 9 are trafficked from the endoplasmic reticulum (ER) to endosomal compartments via the secretory pathway, and depend on the aid of chaperones to do so. For example, UNC93B1, a 12-transmembrane spanning ER protein, directly binds and is necessary for TLRs 3, 7, and 9 to gain access to the endosomal compartment.[31] UNC93B1 is believed to escort these molecules, and perhaps others, to their destination in the cell.[32] PRAT4A (encoded by *TNRC5*) serves a critical role in chaperoning multiple TLRs to their destination,[33] while the ER chaperone protein, gp96 (also called GRP94 or HSP90B1) is critical for all TLR maturation (Fig. 20–2).[34] Proteolysis of TLR7 and 9 is known to occur in the endolysosome, and at least for TLR9, this cleavage increases ligand binding and is necessary for activating downstream signaling pathways.[35,36] In plasmacytoid dendritic cells, TLR7 and TLR9 are further trafficked from endosomes to lysosome-related organelles; this trafficking is necessary for the abundant production of type I IFN for which these cells are specialized.[37,38] The

adaptor protein complex 3 (AP-3), which directs subcellular trafficking through the secretory pathway, and the peptide/histidine transporter 1 (PHT1) are necessary for TLR7 and TLR9 trafficking to lysosome-related organelles.

Toll/Interleukin-1 Receptor Adapter Signaling

The signaling events initiated by the TLRs are increasingly complex and have been studied in great detail [reviewed in Refs. 39 and 40]. Figure 20-3 illustrates the pathways as they are presently understood. It must be recognized that not all TLRs operate within the same cells, nor are all cells equivalent in their responses to TLR ligation. Notably, macrophages and conventional (myeloid) dendritic cells respond to different stimuli than do lymphoid cells, or plasmacytoid dendritic cells (which are specialized for type I IFN production). Moreover, some cells not usually regarded as "professional" components of the innate immune system are capable of responding to TLR ligands in one way or another.

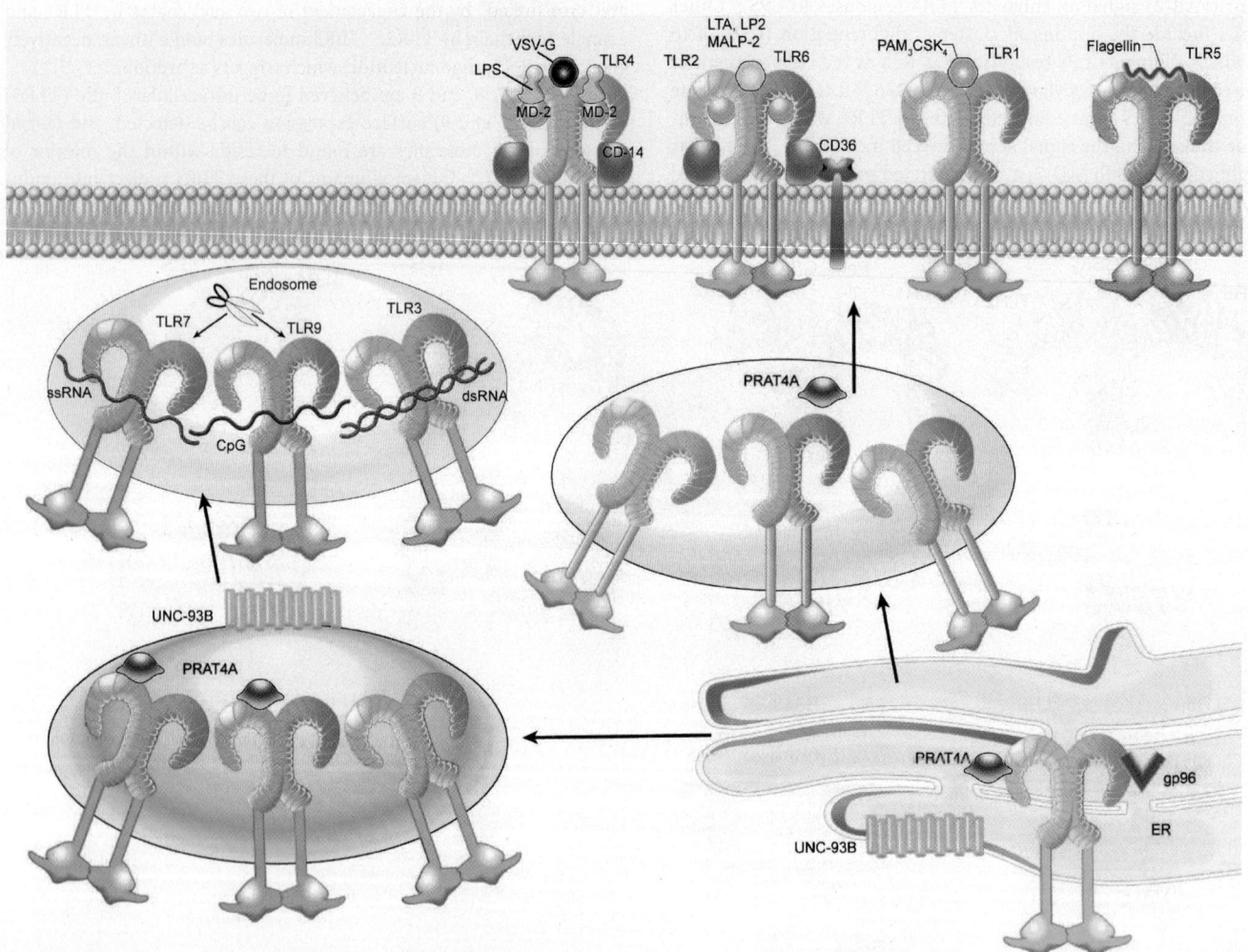

Figure 20–2. The Toll-like receptors (TLRs). The TLRs exist in homo- or heterodimeric form and are capable of sensing diverse molecules derived from pathogenic organisms. TLRs 1, 2, 4, 5, and 6 are located at the cell surface, while TLRs 3, 7, and 9 are located in the endosome. All TLR maturation is dependent on the chaperone protein gp96 in the endoplasmic reticulum (ER). Two other ER proteins, PRAT4A and UNC93B1, play important roles in TLR trafficking. PRAT4A is necessary for TLRs 1, 2, 4, 7, and 9 responses, while UNC93B1 is required for TLRs 3, 7, and 9 trafficking. At the cell surface, a TLR4 complex composed of TLR4, MD2, and CD14 specifically binds to lipopolysaccharide (LPS) and vesicular stomatitis virus glycoprotein G (VSV-G). The TLR2/6 heterodimer, along with CD36 and CD14, recognizes diacylated lipopeptides and lipoteichoic acid (LTA). The TLR1/2 heterodimer senses triacylated lipopeptides (PAM₃CSK₄), and TLR5 recognizes flagellin. TLR7 is able to bind to single-stranded RNA, TLR9 to CpG DNA, and TLR3 to double-stranded RNA. Proteolysis of both TLR7 and TLR9 by lysosomal cysteine proteases including cathepsins and asparagine endopeptidase occurs in the endolysosome, and at least in the case of TLR9, is required for function. Abbreviations are as used in the text.

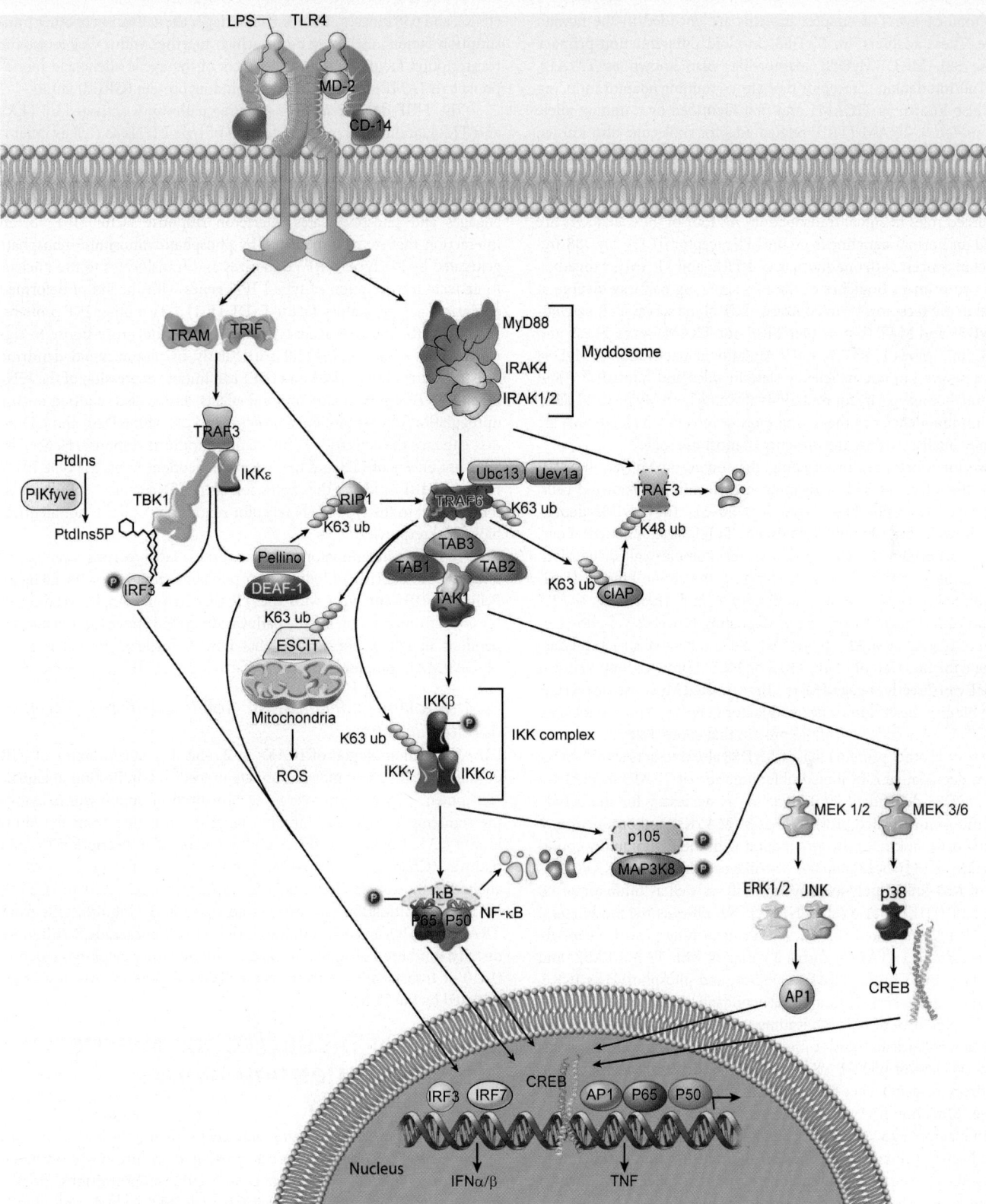

Figure 20–3. Overview of Toll-like receptor (TLR) signaling pathways. Shown are the activating events downstream of TLR activation that ultimately lead to the induction of thousands of genes including those encoding tumor necrosis factor (TNF) and type I interferon (IFN), which are critical in activating innate and adaptive immune responses. TLR4 activation is shown as a prototypical model. Once TLR complexes recognize a specific molecule, they recruit combinations of adaptor proteins (MyD88 [myeloid differentiation primary response 88], TRIF [Toll/interleukin-1 receptor domain-containing adaptor inducing IFN-β], TRAM [TRIF-related adaptor molecule], MAL [MyD88 adaptor-like]) and initiate activation of downstream signaling molecules. See text for details of MyD88-dependent and TRIF-dependent signaling. When bound to vesicular stomatitis virus glycoprotein G (VSV-G), TLR4 can signal through TRAM to induce interferon response factor (IRF) 7 activation, a process that is partially dependent on TRIF (not shown). K63 and K48 ubiquitination are represented by *chained circles*. Proteins that are degraded are shown with a *dotted outline*. LP2, lipopeptide 2; LTA, lipoteichoic acid. PAM$_3$CSK$_4$ is a triacyl lipopeptide. Phosphorylation events are represented by *P*-labeled circles. Abbreviations are as used in the text.

A total of five TIR adapter proteins are encoded in the human genome. These adapters are MyD88 (myeloid differentiation primary response 88), MAL (MyD88 adaptor-like; also known as TIRAP), TRIF (Toll/interleukin-1 receptor domain-containing adaptor inducing IFN-β; also known as TICAM1 and first identified by a mutant allele known as *Lps2*), TRAM (TRIF-related adaptor molecule; also known as TICAM2), and SARM (sterile-α and armadillo motif). The function of SARM remains unknown, and it is the most distantly related paralog among the adaptors. However, the four remaining adapters have well-defined roles in signal transduction. All four of these adapters are required for normal signaling from the LPS receptor, TLR4; MyD88 and MAL act in concert with one another, and TRIF and TRAM act together, so that two primary branches of the LPS signaling pathway diverge at the level of the receptor.[41,42] In contrast, TRIF alone serves TLR3 signaling; MyD88 and MAL (but neither TRIF nor TRAM) serve TLR2; and MyD88 alone serves TLRs 7, 8, and 9. Mutational inactivation of MyD88 creates a severe immunodeficiency state in mice and humans,[43,44] and compound homozygosity for mutations affecting both MyD88 and TRIF causes immunodeficiency that is still more severe, in which animals are essentially unable to sense the presence of most microbes.[42]

Two main branches of signaling, dependent on MyD88 or TRIF, mediate the effects of TLR activation in conventional dendritic cells, macrophages, and fibroblasts (see Fig. 20–3). The MyD88-dependent pathway is used by all TLRs except TLR3, as mentioned above. MyD88 is believed to assemble into a helical complex called the Myddosome upon receptor activation, engaging the serine kinases IRAK (interleukin-1 receptor-associated kinase) 4 and IRAK2 or IRAK1 through death domain interactions.[45] Signaling proceeds via phosphorylation of IRAK2 or IRAK1 by IRAK4. No comparable structural data illuminate the function of MAL, TRIF, or TRAM proteins, but it is clear that TRIF can directly engage TLR3.[46] The activated Myddosome recruits the E3 ubiquitin ligase tumor necrosis factor (TNF) receptor-associated factor (TRAF) 6, a cellular scaffold protein that coordinates the recruitment of several other protein kinases. MyD88 also interacts with TRAF3; however, degradative K48-linked ubiquitination of TRAF3 by cIAP1/2 during MyD88-dependent TLR signaling is necessary for the activation of mitogen-activated protein kinases (MAPKs) and production of inflammatory cytokines.[47] In conjunction with the E2 ubiquitin-conjugating enzyme 13 (Ubc13) and the Ubc-like protein Uev1a, TRAF6 adds chains of K63-linked polyubiquitin to itself, as well as inhibitor of κB (IκB) kinase γ (IKKγ; also called NEMO [NF-κB essential modulator]) and to TRAF2 (reviewed in Ref. 48). Transforming growth factor-β–activating kinase 1 (TAK-1) forms a complex with TAB1, TAB2, and TAB3, is recruited to the TRAF6 complex, and phosphorylates IKKβ, which in complex with IKKα and IKKγ phosphorylates IκB (an inhibitor of the p65 form of NF-κB), leading to its K48-ubiquitin–mediated degradation.[48] Nuclear translocation of homo- or heterodimers composed of p65 and/or p50 NF-κB ensues. NF-κB drives the transcription of hundreds of genes encoding proteins that form the inflammatory response. Mitochondrial reactive oxygen species (ROS) are also produced in macrophages as a result of TLR4, TLR2, and TLR1 activation; this antibacterial response depends on the translocation of TRAF6 to mitochondria to engage and ubiquitinate a protein called ECSIT, which functions in mitochondrial respiratory chain assembly.[49]

At the same time, the IKK complex activated by TAK-1 phosphorylates the p105 form of NF-κB and MAP3K8 (also known as Tpl2), proteins that form a complex in which MAP3K8 is inactive under basal conditions. This leads to the degradation of p105 NF-κB, and to the activation of MAP3K8.[50,51] MAP3K8 phosphorylates and activates MEK1 and MEK2, while independently MEK3 and MEK6 are activated by TAK-1.[40] The MEKs activate MAPK family members, including extracellular signal-regulated kinase (ERK) 1 and ERK2, c-Jun N-terminal kinase (JNK), and p38 kinases. These kinases trigger the activation of other transcription factors, including c-Jun, which together with c-Fos forms the transcription factor AP1, and members of the cyclic adenosine monophosphate (AMP) response element-binding protein (CREB) family.

The TRIF-dependent TLR signaling pathway is activated by TLR3 and TLR4, and results in the induction of type I IFNs as well as inflammatory response genes (see Fig. 20–3). Upon receptor activation, TRIF interacts with TRAF3, which recruits TANK-binding kinase 1 (TBK1) and IKKε (both distantly homologous to the IKKs).[52,53] This complex engages and phosphorylates interferon response factor (IRF) 3, an interaction that may be mediated by phosphatidylinositol-5-phosphate generated by PIKfyve.[54] IRF3 dimerizes and translocates to the nucleus to activate transcription of type I IFN genes with the aid of deformed epidermal autoregulatory factor-1 (DEAF-1).[55] Two other IRF proteins, IRF1 and IRF7, also activate type I IFN genes, but in response to signaling from TLR7 and TLR9 particularly in plasmacytoid dendritic cells.[56,57] Activation of IRF3 and IRF1 can initiate expression of the IFN-β gene.[58,59] IFN-β mediates antiviral effects, and is also required for the upregulation of costimulatory proteins (e.g., CD40, CD80, and CD86) that enhance the activation of an adaptive immune response. Hence, the adjuvant effects of LPS and dsRNA are dependent upon the type I IFN receptor.[60] IRF7 induces the expression of the IFNα genes.[59,61] Both α and β IFNs bind to the type I IFN receptor rendering similar if not identical biological responses.

To induce inflammatory response genes, TRIF recruits receptor-interacting protein (RIP) 1 following its polyubiquitination by the E3 ligase Pellino.[62] RIP1 interacts with the TRAF6/TAK-1 complex leading to NF-κB activation following the pathway described above for MyD88-dependent signaling. For reasons that remain unclear, the heteromeric MyD88/MAL complex is incapable of driving type I IFN gene expression.

Countervailing Influences in Toll/Interleukin-1 Receptor Adapter Signaling

IRAK-M, a homologue of IRAKs 1, 2, and 4, is an inhibitor of TIR domain signaling and may participate in feedback inhibition of signaling known as "endotoxin tolerance."[63] In addition, suppressor of cytokine signaling 1 (SOCS-1) inhibits signal transduction from the Janus kinase (JAK)/signal transducer and activator of transcription (STAT) pathway (Chap. 17) activated by type I IFN, one of the key cytokines elicited in the course of an innate immune response.[64] A20 and CYLD, both deubiquitination enzymes, remove the K63 ubiquitin tails from TRAF6, NEMO, and RIP, inhibiting the activation cascade.[48] Still more distally, inhibition of signaling via antiinflammatory cytokines (such as IL-10 or transforming growth factor [TGF]-β) acts to limit responses initiated by the TLRs.

SENSORS OF THE NUCLEOTIDE-BINDING OLIGOMERIZATION DOMAIN-LIKE RECEPTOR FAMILY

An extensive family of proteins defined by their motif structure has recently been recognized for its participation in innate immune responses to intracellular microbes as well as noninfectious inflammatory stimuli, including, for example, uric acid crystals and aluminum hydroxide particles. Collectively called the nucleotide-binding oligomerization domain (NOD)-like receptors (NLRs), the proteins contain CARD (caspase activating and recruitment domain), Pyrin, or BIR (baculovirus inhibitor of apoptosis repeat) domains followed by nucleotide-binding NACHT domains and LRR domains arranged in tandem, and have been assigned to several subfamilies (Fig. 20–4).[65] Mutations within different representatives of the family produce dominant or semidominant inflammatory diseases. In some cases there is

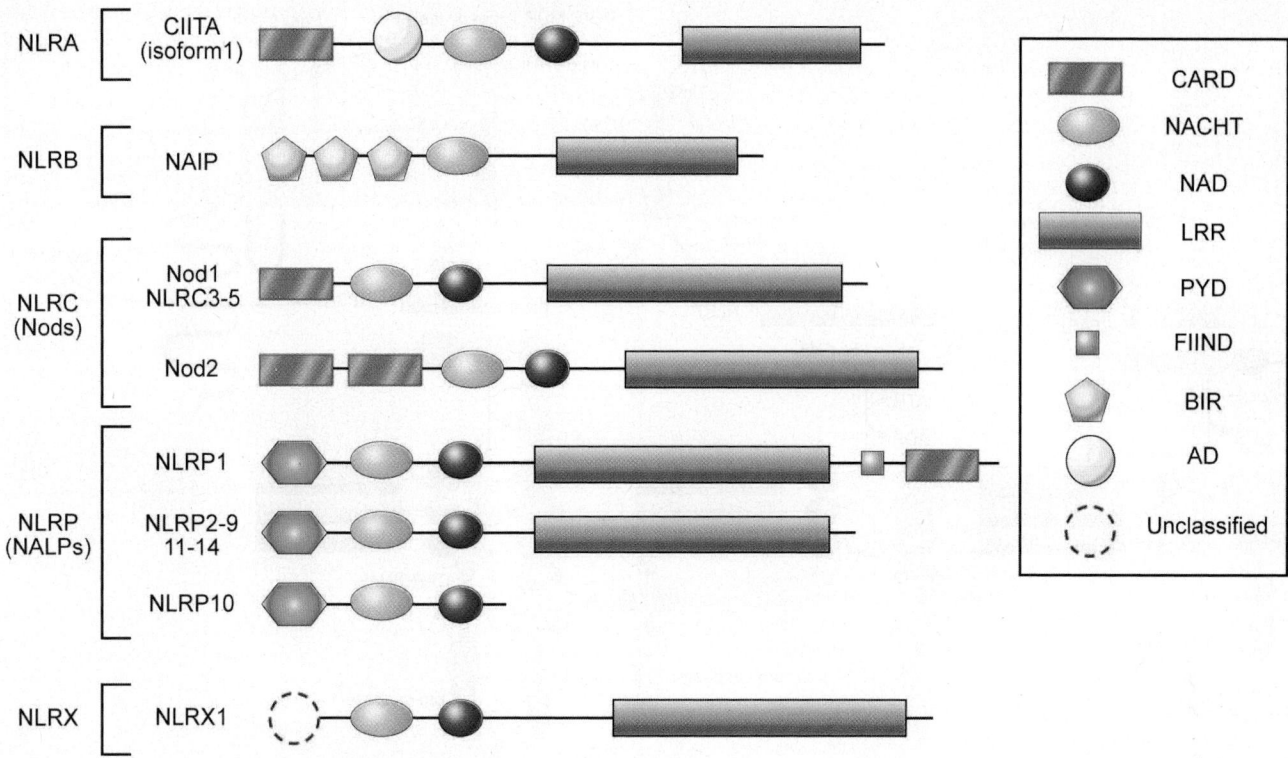

Figure 20–4. Domain structure of nucleotide-binding oligomerization domain (NOD)-like receptors (NLRs). The various members of the NOD-like receptor family are grouped into subfamilies based on domain structure and homology by the Human Genome Gene Nomenclature Committee (HGNC), although sometimes domain classifications and homologies remain unclear. The leucine-rich repeat (LRR) domain contains variable numbers of LRR repeats. Abbreviations are as used in the text.

limited penetrance and strong dependence upon the presence of mutations in other genes. For example, *NOD2* mutations have been clearly shown to enhance the likelihood of Crohn disease[66] and cause Blau syndrome,[67] while distinct *NLPR3* mutations are the proximal cause of cold-induced autoinflammatory syndrome (CIAS1), chronic neurologic cutaneous and articular (CINCA) syndrome, or neonatal onset multisystem inflammatory disease (NOMID).[68-70] Mutations in the structurally related *MEFV* (pyrin-encoding) gene are responsible for familial Mediterranean fever.[71] Pyrin has been shown to interact with the adaptor protein PSTPIP1 (proline serine threonine phosphatase-interacting protein 1). Mutations in the gene encoding this protein also cause an inflammatory disorder, pyogenic arthritis, pyoderma gangrenosum and acne (PAPA) syndrome.[72]

The inflammatory potential of the NLR superfamily is exerted through two signaling pathways: the "inflammasome" pathway and the "NOD1/2" pathway. Each is less fully elucidated at present than the TLR signaling pathways. Moreover, each likely interacts with the TLR signaling pathways and in the case of the inflammasome, is dependent upon the TLR signaling for full expression of activity.

The Inflammasome Pathway

The "inflammasome" pathway (Fig. 20–5) is induced by at least three proteins, and possibly others. Ice-protease activating factor (IPAF/ NLRC4; encoded by *CARD12*), NACHT domain-, LRR-, and pyrin domain (PYD) containing protein 1 (NLRP1, also known as CARD7), and NLRP3 (also known as cryopyrin) each trigger the inflammasome response. Diverse cellular perturbations probably lead to activation of IPAF, NLRP1, and NLRP3. Cytosolic flagellin introduced via type III or type IV bacterial secretion systems activates IPAF.[73] Anthrax lethal factor and muramyl dipeptide (MDP, a product of bacterial cell walls)

introduced via pore-forming toxins activate NLRP1.[74,75] Peptidoglycan (PGN), MDP, lipopeptides, nucleic acids, uric acid crystals, alum, and other foreign substances activate NLRP3.[76-80] Full activation of NLRP3 depends upon a drop in cytosolic potassium concentration, mediated in part by the potassium exporting channel P2X7. Activation of P2X7 recruits the gap junction channel Pannexin-1 (Panx-1), allowing entry of bacterial products and other molecules into the cell.[81] Although it is not clear that the inducers have direct contact with the NLRPs or IPAF, the latter undergo oligomerization (mediated by the NACHT domain). They then signal either directly (in the case of IPAF) or via adapter proteins (ASC in the case of NLRP1, and both ASC and CARDINAL in the case of NLRP3) to activate the cytosolic cysteine proteases caspase-1 and/or caspase-5. Activation occurs through CARD interactions. Homodimeric caspase-1 and caspase-5 act to convert the inflammatory cytokine pro–IL-1β into its active form. Importantly, inflammasome signaling does not initially activate expression of the IL-1β encoding gene. However, TLR signaling, which activates NF-κB, or signaling by IL-1β itself, can do so.[65]

IL-1β signals via its receptor to activate a signaling pathway very similar to those used by the TLRs, dependent upon MyD88 and the downstream signaling cascade components described earlier in this chapter in the section "Toll/Interleukin-1 Receptor Adapter Signaling". As such, IL-1β may be viewed as an endogenous ligand that elicits a response similar to those elicited by microbial ligands. This signal may initially be induced by a focal infection operating in conjunction with a noninfectious inflammatory stimulus.

The Nucleotide-Binding Oligomerization Domain Pathway

NOD1 (CARD4) and NOD2 (CARD15) proteins have been mentioned as sensors of γ-D-glutamyldiaminopimelic acid (DAP) and MDP,

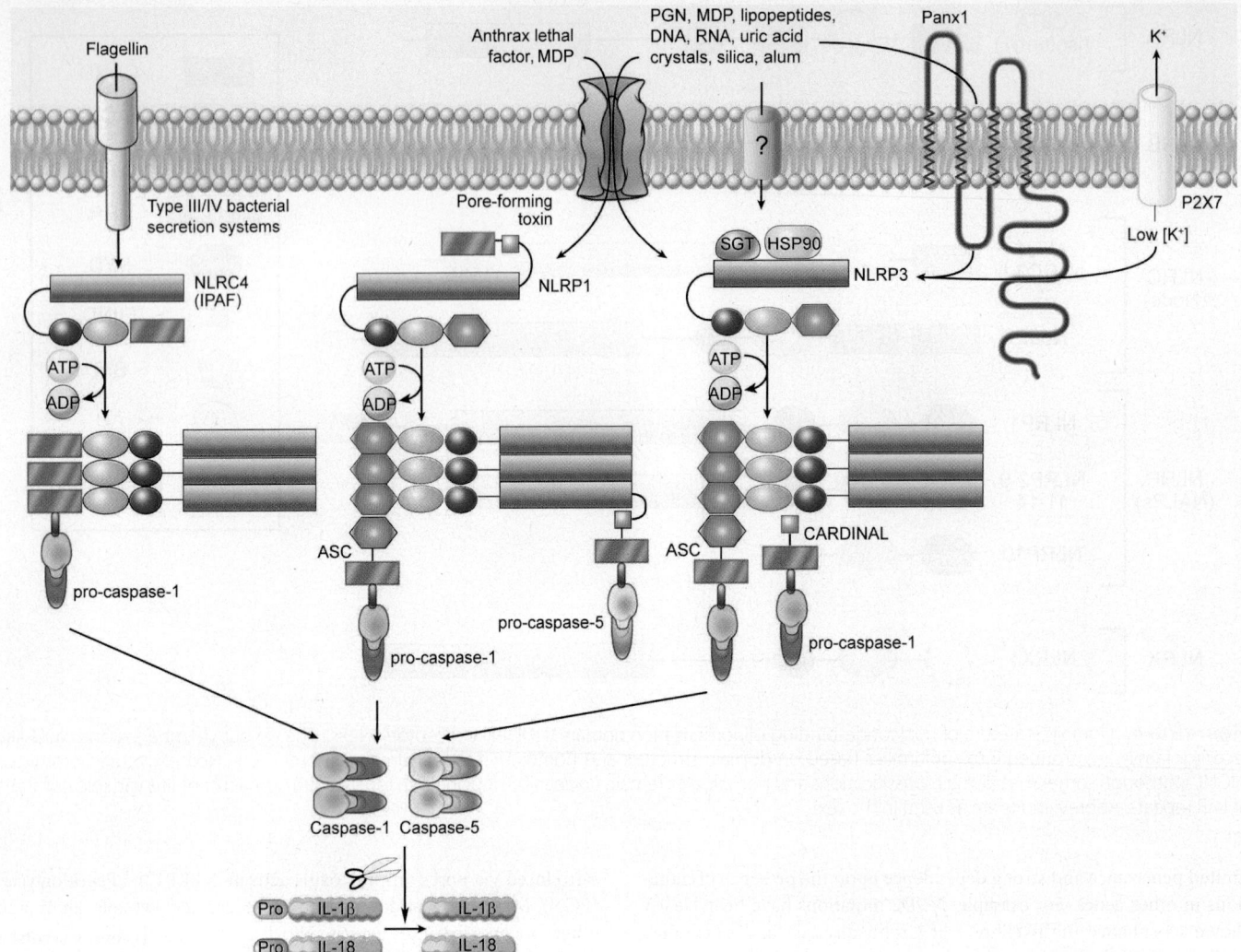

Figure 20–5. Inflammasome complexes formed by NLRP1 (NALP1), NLRP3 (NALP3), and NLRC4 (IPAF [ice-protease activating factor]). In the absence of activating signals, NOD-like receptors (NLRs) are present in the cytosol in inactive conformations. The SGT1/HSP90 chaperone complex associates with and keeps NLRP3 in an activation-ready state. Upon activation, binding and hydrolysis of ATP results in oligomerization and inflammasome formation. NLRP1 and NLRP3 engage procaspase-1 through adaptor proteins (ASC or ASC/CARDINAL for NLRP3), while NLRC4 is able to bind procaspase-1 directly. NLRP1 is also able to engage procaspase-5. This engagement leads to the autoproteolytic maturation of the caspases, which then cleave the pro forms of inflammatory cytokines to their biologically active forms. Protein domains shown are the same as in Fig. 20–4.

respectively, both components of microbial cell walls. They are believed to detect intracellular bacteria or fragments thereof.[82-84] NOD2 has been strongly implicated in the pathogenesis of Crohn disease through linkage disequilibrium mapping and sequence analysis,[66] but mutations of NOD2 cause disease with low penetrance, suggesting the importance of other genetic and environmental factors. No clear disease association has been defined for NOD1. The NOD proteins do not form the core of inflammasomes, although recent data suggests that NOD2 is able to associate with NLRP1 and caspase-1 upon stimulation with MDP.[85] In response to microbial stimuli, the NOD proteins oligomerize and signal via TRAF2, TRAF5, and TRAF6 to cause K63 ubiquitination of RICK2 (also known as RIP2, or CARDIAK), a protein with a domain structure similar to receptor interacting protein (RIP), known for its involvement in TNF signal transduction. RICK2 activates TAK-1, and by way of TAK-1, elicits the activation of both NF-κB and the mitogen-activated protein (MAP) kinase cascade, leading to activation of the transcription factor AP1 (Fig. 20–6).

SENSORS OF THE RIG-I–LIKE HELICASE PATHWAYS

While TLRs are capable of detecting nucleic acids within the endosomal compartment and do make an essential contribution to the detection of some viruses (notably herpesviruses), other viruses are detected chiefly or entirely by cytosolic receptors. Among these, the RIG-I–like helicases (RLHs), including retinoic acid inducible gene I (RIG-I), melanoma differentiation-associated gene 5 (MDA5), and LGP2, are the best known sensors and are believed to undergo direct interaction with nucleic acids to initiate a response. RIG-I and MDA5 sense specific viruses; for example, viruses detected by RIG-I include influenza A, Sendai, and vesicular stomatitis viruses, and MDA5 detects encephalomyocarditis and murine hepatitis viruses.[86] RLH proteins have RNA helicase domains (involved in binding nucleic acids), as well as a regulatory domain (RD) that has been implicated in inhibiting downstream signaling,[87] but is also necessary for RNA sensing.[88,89] Both RIG-I and

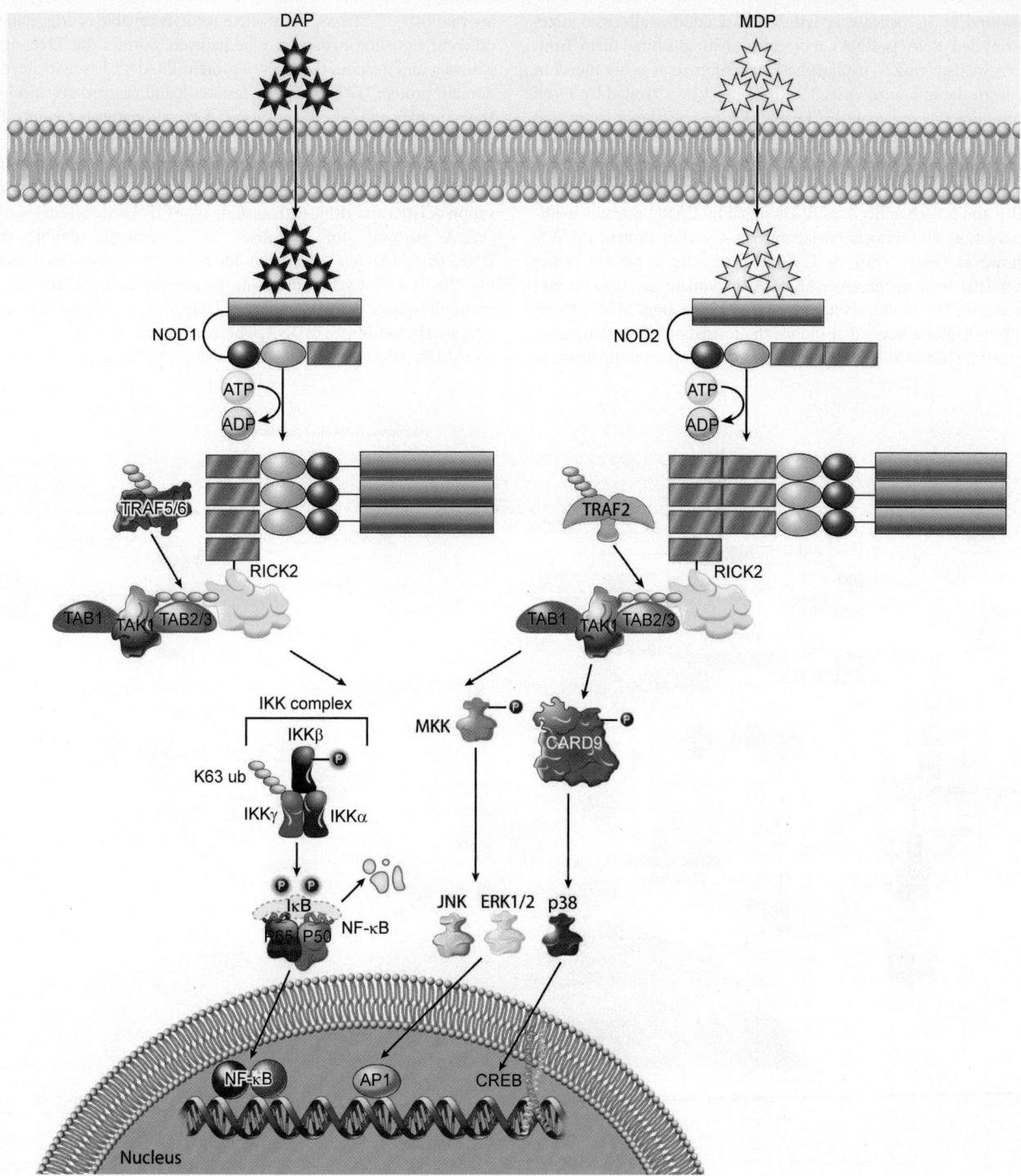

Figure 20–6. The nucleotide-binding oligomerization domain (NOD) 1/2 signaling pathways. Upon sensing PGN-derived motifs in the cytosol (γ-D-glutamyldiaminopimelic acid [DAP] and muramyl dipeptide [MDP]), NOD1 and NOD2 oligomerize and form complexes with the serine/threonine kinase RICK2. Signaling through tumor necrosis factor receptor–associated factors (TRAFs, which are E3 ubiquitin ligases) results in K63 ubiquitination *(chained circles)* of RICK2, and transforming growth factor-β–activating kinase (TAK)-1 recruitment. Activation of the TAK-1 complex leads to IκB kinase (IKK) and MKK activation, resulting in signaling cascades similar to those activated in response to TLR ligands. Caspase activating and recruitment domain (CARD) 9 is important for p38 activation downstream of NOD2. NOD-like receptor (NLR) protein domains shown are the same as in Fig. 20–4. Phosphorylation events are represented by *P*-labeled *circles*. Abbreviations are as used in the text.

MDA5 have more proximal CARD domains involved in signaling, whereas LGP2 does not. On this basis it was initially believed that LGP2 might have an inhibitory function.[90] However, it appears to contribute to sensing in a positive manner, and may augment RIG-I and MDA5 signaling.[89,91,92]

Although TLR3 can detect dsRNA and its synthetic analogue poly I:C, the dominant sensor of poly I:C (long polymers in particular) *in vivo* is MDA5[93]; shorter poly I:C polymers are better detected by RIG-I. RIG-I is able to form stable complexes with dsRNA molecules containing blunt ends or 5′-overhangs, while dsRNA with 3′-overhangs are unwound by its helicase activity.[88] RIG-I additionally recognizes single-stranded RNA (ssRNA) molecules, distinguishing them from host RNA by detecting 5'-triphosphate structures such as are found in ssRNA from the influenza virus.[94,95] RIG-I must be activated by T-cell receptor interacting molecule 25 (TRIM25), a host resistance factor that ubiquitinates RIG-I (K63 linkages).

Upon virus recognition the RLHs initiate signaling, leading to type I IFN and inflammatory cytokine production dependent, respectively, upon IRF and NF-κB activation. RLHs signal by CARD domain-mediated interaction with mitochondrial antiviral signaling protein (MAVS; also known as IPS-1, VISA, or CARDIF), an integral protein of the mitochondrial outer membrane with a CARD domain that projects into the cytoplasm.[96–99] Upon activation by RIG-I interaction, MAVS forms prion-like polymeric fibers that induce the formation of similar aggregates by untouched MAVS molecules, which thereby gain competence to

activate IRF3.[100] MAVS, in its active form, is capable of triggering three different signaling pathways. One pathway mimics the TNF signaling pathway, and includes the adaptor protein TRADD, Fas-associated death domain protein (FADD), RIP1, caspase-8 and caspase-10, and leads to IKK complex and NF-κB activation. A second pathway recruits TRAF6 and MEKK1, leading to activation of the MAP kinases and AP1. These two pathways are responsible for inflammatory cytokine production. The third pathway entails activation of TBK1 and IKKε, and leads to the activation of IRF3 and IRF7, with ensuing type I IFN production (Fig. 20–7).

A pathway for responses to cytoplasmic double-stranded DNA (dsDNA) has also been identified in mammalian cells (see Fig. 20–7).[101,102] Cyclic adenosine monophosphate (AMP)/guanosine monophosphate (GMP) synthetase (cGAS) is an enzyme allosterically activated by binding to dsDNA, whereon it synthesizes cyclic GMP:AMP (cGAMP). cGAMP activates stimulator of IFN genes (STING),[103] a

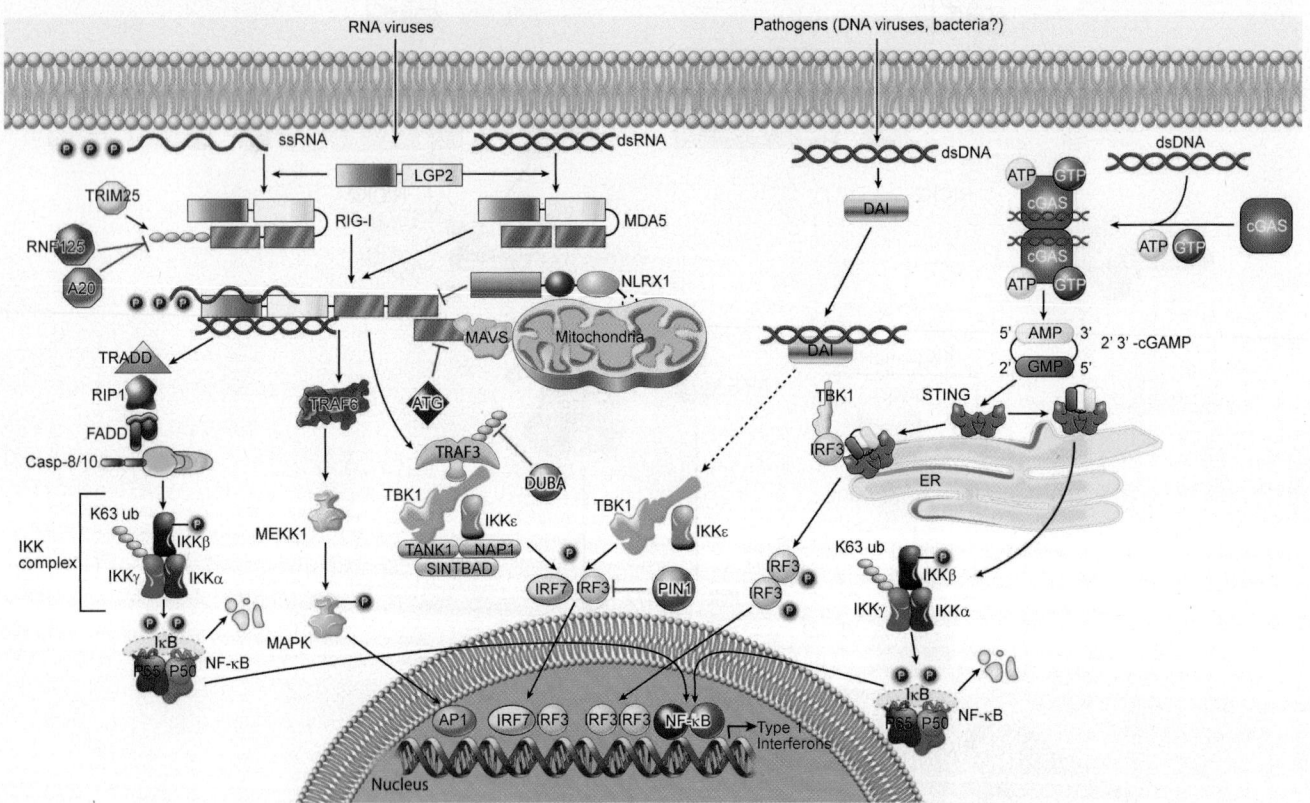

Figure 20–7. Cytosolic sensors and signaling pathways. Retinoic acid inducible gene I (RIG-I) and melanoma differentiation associated gene 5 (MDA5) respond to different viral infections, recognizing single-stranded RNA (ssRNA) and double-stranded RNA (dsRNA), respectively. RIG-I also detects short dsRNA sequences. LGP2 is able to bind to dsRNA, and appears to modulate RIG-I and MDA5 signaling. Full RIG-I activity requires K63 ubiquitination *(chained circles)* by T-cell receptor interacting molecule 25 (TRIM25). RIG-I and MDA5 activate mitochondrial antiviral signaling protein (MAVS), which interacts with a complex containing receptor-interacting protein 1 (RIP1), Fas-associated death domain (FADD), and tumor necrosis factor (TNF) receptor-associated death domain (TRADD), as well as with TNF receptor–associated factor (TRAF) 6, and TRAF3. Association of FADD with procaspase 8 or procaspase 10 results in cleavage to the mature, active caspase 8 or caspase 10, which go on to activate nuclear factor (NF)-κB. Recruitment of TRAF6 leads to activation of the mitogen-activated protein (MAP) kinase pathway and AP1, while K63-ubiquitinated TRAF3 activates interferon response factor (IRF) 3 and IRF7 through the kinases IκB kinase (IKK)ε and TANK-binding kinase (TBK). The latter also associate with TRAF family member-associated NF-κB activator (TANK), NAK-associated protein 1 (NAP1), and similar to NAP1 TBK1 adaptor (SINTBAD). MAVS is negatively regulated by the autophagy conjugate Atg12–Atg5, and potentially by NLRX1, while RIG-I is negatively regulated by the IFN-inducible ubiquitin ligase RNF125 (K48 linkage) and the deubiquitinase A20. The TRAF3-dependent pathway is negatively controlled by the deubiquitinase DUBA. The peptidyl-prolyl-isomerase Pin1 triggers phosphorylated IRF3 ubiquitination and degradation. dsDNA is sensed by cyclic adenosine monophosphate (AMP)/guanosine monophosphate (GMP) synthetase (cGAS), which synthesizes cGAMP from ATP and guanosine triphosphate (GTP). cGAMP binds and activates STING (stimulator of interferon genes), which recruits TBK1 to phosphorylate IRF3. STING also activates the IKK complex. dsDNA can also be sensed by DNA-dependent activator of IRFs (DAI). STING also associates with RIG-I (not shown). The caspase activating and recruitment domains (CARDs) are indicated by *rust-colored rectangles*, helicase domains by *white rectangles*, RD domains by *green rectangles*. NLRX1 domains are the same as in Fig. 20–4 except for the unclassified domain, which is shown inserted into the mitochondrial membrane. Phosphorylation events are represented by *P*-labeled circles. Unknown signaling pathway(s) are represented by a dotted arrow. Abbreviations are as used in the text.

penta-spanning ER membrane protein that undergoes a conformational change leading to the activation of TBK1 to phosphorylate IRF3, which dimerizes and translocates to the nucleus to induce type I IFNs. STING also activates the IKK complex, leading to degradation of IκB and release of NF-κB to enter the nucleus and induce other cytokines. A putative cytosolic DNA sensor DAI (for DNA-dependent activator of IRFs) has also been described. DAI contains DNA binding domains and enhances DNA-mediated induction of type I IFNs *in vitro*.[104] However, the role of DAI as a sensor of cytoplasmic DNA appears to be redundant.[105]

Both the RLH-MAVS pathway and the cGAS-STING pathway become activated in B cells when they are stimulated by type 2 T-cell–independent antigens, such as pneumococcal vaccine (PPSV23).[106] These pathways sense the induction of endogenous retroviruses, leading to sustained B-cell activation and an immunoglobulin (Ig) M response.

KEY EFFECTOR CYTOKINES IN THE INNATE IMMUNE RESPONSE

Cells of the innate immune system exhibit a measure of autonomy (e.g., neutrophils directly engulf and destroy pathogens), but also initiate the adaptive immune response to microbes and summon "reinforcements" to the site of infection. These functions depend upon the production of cytokines, too numerous to describe in this chapter. However, a few of the key mediators are listed here.

Tumor Necrosis Factor-α

A homotrimeric cytokine that is made by many cells, TNF is synthesized in greatest amounts by mononuclear phagocytes that have been exposed to LPS or other TLR-activating stimuli. It was recognized as a key endogenous mediator of endotoxicity,[107] and later, as a mediator of other forms of inflammation (including sterile inflammation, as observed in rheumatoid arthritis and cancer, Crohn disease, ankylosing spondylitis, and psoriasis). The TNF signaling pathway depends upon two receptors, involves NF-κB activation, and is ancestrally related to the *Drosophila Imd* (immunodeficiency) pathway for recognition of Gram-negative bacteria.[108] The ancient phylogenetic origins of TNF signaling, its large representation in distant species, the therapeutic efficacy of TNF neutralization in the diseases just mentioned, and the immunocompromising effects of TNF and TNF receptor mutations in animals all suggest that TNF is one of the most important of the cytokines utilized by the innate immune system for effective containment of infection.

Interleukin-1α and β

Once known as pleiotropic inflammatory cytokines, IL-1α and IL-1β, two distantly related ligands that share the same set of receptors, are produced in response to innate immune stimuli and evoke fever, swelling, and neutrophil adhesion in the region of an infectious nidus. The type I IL-1 receptor, responsible for most or all of the agonist activity of the IL-1 proteins, has two chains, each of which is endowed with a cytoplasmic TIR domain. The receptor complex signals via MyD88 and no other adapters are known to be required. IL-1 signaling may act as an amplification mechanism that augments the primary infectious signal, and transmits awareness of infection to cells that lack the innate immune sensors required for detection of microbes.

Interleukin-6

Signaling via a receptor that uses the JAK/STAT pathway, IL-6 activates many elements of the "acute phase response"; that is, hepatic production of fibrinogen, serum amyloid A protein, and C-reactive protein. It also has thrombopoietic activity, both directly (minor effect) and through its stimulation of thrombopoietin production (major effect) (Chap. 111), which stimulates platelet production, often consumed in the course of a serious infection.

Interleukin-12

A cytokine made in abundance by dendritic and other cells in response to TLR stimulation, IL-12 activates the production of IFN-γ by lymphoid cells, which, in turn, increases the microbicidal activity of mononuclear phagocytes. Unlike most cytokines, IL-12 is a heterodimeric protein, and the IL-12 p40 subunit is subject to induction, whereas the p35 subunit is synthesized constitutively. Mutations of the genes encoding IL-12 or its receptor, or IFN-γ or its receptor, are known to cause relatively severe susceptibility to infection by mycobacteria and other intracellular infections. Hence the IL-12/IFN-γ feedback loop is considered one of the most important innate/adaptive immune interactions.

Chemokines

A family of small proteins, highly redundant in receptor specificity and organized into CC and CXC subfamilies, the chemokines are induced by primary microbial stimuli and by TNF and IL-1. Binding to G-protein–coupled receptors, they exhibit phagocyte chemotactic activity (Chaps. 61 and 68), and are believed to contribute to the egress of neutrophils from blood into infected tissue.

Granulocyte Colony-Stimulating Factor and Granulocyte-Macrophage Colony-Stimulating Factor

The central hematopoietic response is attuned to events in the peripheral tissues, and granulocyte colony-stimulating factor (G-CSF) and granulocyte-macrophage colony-stimulating factor (GM-CSF) promote the production and release of granulocytes and monocytes to cope with an infectious challenge. These cytokines are produced by macrophages, endothelial cells and fibroblasts in direct response to TLR signaling (Chap. 61), and also in response to secondary cytokines such as TNF. They signal via JAK/STAT-coupled receptors.

Interferons

Type I IFNs (IFN-α and IFN-β) are expressed immediately in response to LPS, dsRNA, or unmethylated DNA, and have broad activity in the containment of viral infections. LPS-induced type I IFN production depends upon TLR4 and the adapters TRIF and TRAM. dsRNA-induced type I IFN depends upon TLR3 and TRIF (but not TRAM). Unmethylated CpG motifs in DNA stimulate type I IFN production that depends upon MyD88. Although many cells are induced into an antiviral state as the result of IFN stimulation, NK cells, which are specialized for the elimination of virus-infected targets, are particularly dependent upon type I IFN signaling (Chap. 77),[109] and require it for the elimination of specific pathogens such as cytomegalovirus.[110] The type I IFNs are also involved in protection against bacterial infection,[111] and type I IFN signaling has been shown to be important to the development of endotoxic shock.[112] Plasmacytoid dendritic cells are a particularly important source of type I IFN.[113]

Type II IFN (IFN-γ) has less antiviral activity than type I IFN, is produced by T cells in response to IL-12 receptor stimulation, and is crucial for the elimination of intracellular pathogens such as mycobacteria, which reside within macrophages of the infected host.

● THE ACTIVATION OF ADAPTIVE IMMUNITY

The adjuvant effect of microbes has been known since the classic studies of Lewis and Loomis[114] who coined the term "allergic irritability" to describe the augmented production of antibodies against a protein antigen in guinea pigs infected with *Mycobacterium tuberculosis*. Freund and McDermott[115] demonstrated that heat-killed mycobacteria were capable of eliciting an exaggerated antibody response as well when coadministered with a protein antigen, indicating that molecular components of microbes (rather than infection *per se*) were responsible for adjuvanticity. LPS was shown to be endowed with adjuvant activity in 1955,[116] and by 1975 the *Lps* locus was shown to be required for this effect of LPS (as it is required for all other cellular effects of LPS).[117] By deduction, the positional cloning of *Lps* thus revealed the essential role of TLR4 in LPS-mediated adjuvanticity.[7]

Activation of an adaptive immune response to a specific antigen has long been known to depend upon two signals that occur in the course of antigen presentation. First, the T-cell receptor must be activated. In addition, costimulatory molecules upregulated on the antigen-presenting cell (e.g., CD40, CD69, CD80, and CD86) are known to interact with receptors (or in some cases ligands) on the T cell. An exchange of signals occurs over a period of approximately 12 hours,[118] ultimately leading to autonomous expansion of the T-cell clone and, in turn, activation of specific B cells. Some of these signals are well characterized. For example, CD80 and CD86 both engage CD28 and cytotoxic T-lymphocyte antigen (CTLA) on the T-cell surface, and abrogation of signaling via these costimulatory receptors is known to substantially attenuate the adaptive immune response.[119]

Upregulation of costimulatory molecules (UCM) is therefore essential, although not by itself sufficient, for activation of the adaptive immune response. LPS depends upon TRIF (and specifically, upon TRIF-mediated type I IFN gene expression) to elicit UCM[42,60,120]; absent TRIF, LPS cannot exert an adjuvant effect. TRAM is also required for UCM.[41] Although MyD88 does not elicit UCM, it does contribute to LPS-induced adjuvanticity in an experimental setting.[60] It is likely that IL-12, a cytokine that is largely MyD88-dependent, also contributes to the adjuvant effect, along with other proteins yet to be identified.

Even though several publications initially suggested that TLR signaling is required for adaptive immune responses to occur, it has been observed that mice lacking all TLR signaling are quite capable of mounting adaptive immune responses, including antibody responses and recall responses to defined antigens administered with diverse adjuvants.[121] It is now evident that there is much redundancy in adaptive immune responses, and several innate immune pathways can independently trigger such responses.

DISEASES CAUSED BY INNATE IMMUNE DEFECTS

Premature death from infection is strongly heritable in humans.[122] Defects of the innate immune sensing apparatus are expected to cause hypersusceptibility to infection in humans as they clearly do in mice, and specific examples of such mutations have recently come to light including the NLR disorders discussed above (see "Sensors of the NOD-Like Receptor Family"). Missense mutations of TLR4 that are rare among the normal white population are quite common in patients with systemic meningococcal disease, and have been assigned a role in susceptibility on this basis.[123] A nonsense mutation of TLR5 was found to be overrepresented in patients who developed Legionnaire disease as compared to a comparably exposed population that remained disease-free.[124] Mutations of IRAK4 and MyD88 create susceptibility to suppurative Gram-positive infections.[44,125] In humans, both TLR3[126] and UNC93B1[127] mutations cause susceptibility to recurrent Herpes simplex virus encephalitis, and presumably to other diseases as well.

On the effector side, examples of immunocompromise from innate immune defects are far better known, and include diseases caused by

mutations affecting IFN-γ,[128] IL-12[129] and its receptor,[130,131] defects of granule formation,[132] and defects of nicotinamide adenine dinucleotide phosphate (NADPH) oxidase.[133]

THE GENERAL STRATEGY OF INNATE IMMUNE RESPONSES AND THE CONCEPT OF FORWARD FEEDBACK LOOPS IN AUTOIMMUNITY

Although the term "autoimmunity" is reserved for inappropriate adaptive immune responses that damage tissues of the host, the innate immune system may also cause injury or death, and typically does so when systemic activation occurs in the course of a serious infection. Innate immune responses, which entail cytokine-mediated inflammation and coagulation, evolved to contain small inoculates of microorganisms by encouraging the influx of granulocytes to engulf and destroy these pathogens, and by stimulating the development of an adaptive immune response. The mechanisms that are employed to these ends can be lethal if they are generalized rather than focal. In several examples, the importance of microbes as drivers of inflammation has been cited, and forward-feedback loops may perpetuate inflammation or autoimmunity. It has been reported, for example, that endogenous DNA, signaling via TLR9, is responsible for the generation and perpetuation of antinucleoprotein antibodies in a mouse model of systemic lupus erythematosus.[134] The involvement of TLRs 3 and 7 may also be important.

In hemophagocytic lymphohistiocytosis (HLH), an amplification loop involving a microbial driver, CTL expansion, and IFN-γ driven myeloid expansion has been well described in mice.[135] In SHP1 deficiency in mice, autoimmunity and inflammation also depend upon a microbial driver and activation of TIR domain signaling pathways.[136] NOMID and other mutations capable of activating the NLRP3 inflammasome have been mentioned earlier in this chapter. Beyond this, the innate immune system may also contribute to sterile inflammation (autoinflammatory disease), as witnessed in many human diseases that have so far eluded etiologic decipherment.

REFERENCES

1. Pancer Z, Amemiya CT, Ehrhardt GR, et al: Somatic diversification of variable lymphocyte receptors in the agnathan sea lamprey. *Nature* 430:174, 2004.
2. Cooper MD, Alder MN: The evolution of adaptive immune systems. *Cell* 124:815, 2006.
3. Pfeiffer R: Untersuchungen über das Choleragift. *Z Hyg Infektionskr* 11:393, 1892.
4. Raetz CR, Whitfield C: Lipopolysaccharide endotoxins. *Annu Rev Biochem* 71:635, 2002.
5. Galanos C, Luderitz O, Rietschel ET, et al: Synthetic and natural *Escherichia coli* free lipid A express identical endotoxic activities. *Eur J Biochem* 148:1, 1985.
6. Rosenstreich DL, Weinblatt AC, O'Brien AD: Genetic control of resistance to infection in mice. *CRC Crit Rev Immunol* 3:263, 1982.
7. Poltorak A, He X, Smirnova I, et al: Defective LPS signaling in C3H/HeJ and C57BL/10ScCr mice: Mutations in *Tlr4* gene. *Science* 282:2085, 1998.
8. Anderson KV, Bokla L, Nusslein-Volhard C: Establishment of dorsal-ventral polarity in the *Drosophila* embryo: The induction of polarity by the Toll gene product. *Cell* 42:791, 1985.
9. Lemaitre B, Nicolas E, Michaut L, et al: The dorsoventral regulatory gene cassette spätzle/Toll/cactus controls the potent antifungal response in *Drosophila* adults. *Cell* 86:973, 1996.
10. Hemmi H, Takeuchi O, Kawai T, et al: A Toll-like receptor recognizes bacterial DNA. *Nature* 408:740, 2000.
11. Takeuchi O, Kaufmann A, Grote K, et al: Preferentially the R-stereoisomer of the mycoplasmal lipopeptide macrophage-activating lipopeptide-2 activates immune cells through a Toll-Like receptor 2- and MyD88-dependent signaling pathway. *J Immunol* 164:554, 2000.
12. Takeuchi O, Sato S, Horiuchi T, et al: Cutting edge: Role of Toll-like receptor 1 in mediating immune response to microbial lipoproteins. *J Immunol* 169:10, 2002.

13. Hayashi F, Smith KD, Ozinsky A, et al: The innate immune response to bacterial flagellin is mediated by Toll- like receptor 5. *Nature* 410:1099, 2001.

14. Alexopoulou L, Holt AC, Medzhitov R, Flavell RA: Recognition of double-stranded RNA and activation of NF-kappaB by Toll-like receptor 3. *Nature* 413:732, 2001.

15. Poltorak A, Ricciardi-Castagnoli P, Citterio A, Beutler B: Physical contact between LPS and Tlr4 revealed by genetic complementation. *Proc Natl Acad Sci U S A* 97:2163, 2000.

16. Bauer S, Kirschning CJ, Hacker H, et al: Human TLR9 confers responsiveness to bacterial DNA via species-specific CpG motif recognition. *Proc Natl Acad Sci U S A* 98:9237, 2001.

17. Gross O, Gewies A, Finger K, et al: Card9 controls a non-TLR signalling pathway for innate anti-fungal immunity. *Nature* 442:651, 2006.

18. Rogers NC, Slack EC, Edwards AD, et al: Syk-dependent cytokine induction by Dectin-1 reveals a novel pattern recognition pathway for C type lectins. *Immunity* 22:507, 2005.

19. Gantner BN, Simmons RM, Canavera SJ, et al: Collaborative induction of inflammatory responses by dectin-1 and Toll-like receptor 2. *J Exp Med* 197:1107, 2003.

20. Rallabhandi P, Nhu QM, Toshchakov VY, et al: Analysis of proteinase-activated receptor 2 and TLR4 signal transduction: A novel paradigm for receptor cooperativity. *J Biol Chem* 283:24314, 2008.

21. Wright SD, Ramos RA, Tobias PS, et al: CD14, a receptor for complexes of lipopolysaccharide (LPS) and LPS binding protein. *Science* 249:1431, 1990.

22. Haziot A, Ferrero E, Kontgen F, et al: Resistance to endotoxin shock and reduced dissemination of gram-negative bacteria in CD14-deficient mice. *Immunity* 4:407, 1996.

23. Hoebe K, Georgel P, Rutschmann S, et al: CD36 is a sensor of diacylglycerides. *Nature* 433:523, 2005.

24. Nagai Y, Akashi S, Nagafuku M, et al: Essential role of MD-2 in LPS responsiveness and TLR4 distribution. *Nat Immunol* 3:667, 2002.

25. Xu Y, Tao X, Shen B, et al: Structural basis for signal transduction by the Toll/interleukin-1 receptor domains. *Nature* 408:111, 2000.

26. Kim HM, Park BS, Kim JI, et al: Crystal structure of the TLR4-MD-2 complex with bound endotoxin antagonist Eritoran. *Cell* 130:906, 2007.

27. Ohto U, Fukase K, Miyake K, Satow Y: Crystal structures of human MD-2 and its complex with antiendotoxic lipid IVa. *Science* 316:1632, 2007.

28. Jin MS, Kim SE, Heo JY, et al: Crystal structure of the TLR1-TLR2 heterodimer induced by binding of a tri-acylated lipopeptide. *Cell* 130:1071, 2007.

29. Liu L, Botos I, Wang Y, et al: Structural basis of Toll-like receptor 3 signaling with double-stranded RNA. *Science* 320:379, 2008.

30. Ahmad-Nejad P, Hacker H, Rutz M, et al: Bacterial CpG-DNA and lipopolysaccharides activate Toll-like receptors at distinct cellular compartments. *Eur J Immunol* 32:1958, 2002.

31. Tabeta K, Hoebe K, Janssen EM, et al: The Unc93b1 mutation 3d disrupts exogenous antigen presentation and signaling via Toll-like receptors 3, 7 and 9. *Nat Immunol* 7:156, 2006.

32. Kim YM, Brinkmann MM, Paquet ME, Ploegh HL: UNC93B1 delivers nucleotide-sensing Toll-like receptors to endolysosomes. *Nature* 452:234, 2008.

33. Takahashi K, Shibata T, Akashi-Takamura S, et al: A protein associated with Toll-like receptor (TLR) 4 (PRAT4A) is required for TLR-dependent immune responses. *J Exp Med* 204:2963, 2007.

34. Yang Y, Liu B, Dai J, et al: Heat shock protein gp96 is a master chaperone for Toll-like receptors and is important in the innate function of macrophages. *Immunity* 26:215, 2007.

35. Ewald SE, Lee BL, Lau L, et al: The ectodomain of Toll-like receptor 9 is cleaved to generate a functional receptor. *Nature* 456:658, 2008.

36. Park B, Brinkmann MM, Spooner E, et al: Proteolytic cleavage in an endolysosomal compartment is required for activation of Toll-like receptor 9. *Nat Immunol* 9:1407, 2008.

37. Blasius AL, Arnold CN, Georgel P, et al: Slc15a4, AP-3, and Hermansky-Pudlak syndrome proteins are required for Toll-like receptor signaling in plasmacytoid dendritic cells. *Proc Natl Acad Sci U S A* 107:19973, 2010.

38. Sasai M, Linehan MM, Iwasaki A: Bifurcation of Toll-like receptor 9 signaling by adaptor protein 3. *Science* 329:1530, 2010.

39. Beutler B, Jiang Z, Georgel P, et al: Genetic analysis of host resistance: Toll-Like receptor signaling and immunity at large. *Annu Rev Immunol* 24:353, 2006.

40. Kawai T, Akira S: TLR signaling. *Semin Immunol* 19:24, 2007.

41. Yamamoto M, Sato S, Hemmi H, et al: TRAM is specifically involved in the Toll-like receptor 4-mediated MyD88-independent signaling pathway. *Nat Immunol* 4:1144, 2003.

42. Hoebe K, Du X, Georgel P, et al: Identification of Lps2 as a key transducer of MyD88-independent TIR signaling. *Nature* 424:743, 2003.

43. Takeuchi O, Hoshino K, Akira S: Cutting edge: TLR2-deficient and MyD88-deficient mice are highly susceptible to *Staphylococcus aureus* infection. *J Immunol* 165:5392, 2000.

44. von Bernuth H, Picard C, Jin Z, et al: Pyogenic bacterial infections in humans with MyD88 deficiency. *Science* 321:691, 2008.

45. Lin SC, Lo YC, Wu H: Helical assembly in the MyD88-IRAK4-IRAK2 complex in TLR/IL-1R signalling. *Nature* 465:885, 2010.

46. Oshiumi H, Matsumoto M, Funami K, et al: TICAM-1, an adaptor molecule that participates in Toll-like receptor 3-mediated interferon-beta induction. *Nat Immunol* 4:161, 2003.

47. Tseng PH, Matsuzawa A, Zhang W, et al: Different modes of ubiquitination of the adaptor TRAF3 selectively activate the expression of type I interferons and proinflammatory cytokines. *Nat Immunol* 11:70, 2010.

48. Chen ZJ: Ubiquitin signalling in the NF-kappaB pathway. *Nat Cell Biol* 7:758, 2005.

49. West AP, Brodsky IE, Rahner C, et al: TLR signalling augments macrophage bactericidal activity through mitochondrial ROS. *Nature* 472:476, 2011.

50. Waterfield M, Jin W, Reiley W, et al: IkappaB kinase is an essential component of the Tpl2 signaling pathway. *Mol Cell Biol* 24:6040, 2004.

51. Beinke S, Deka J, Lang V, et al: NF-kappaB1 p105 negatively regulates TPL-2 MEK kinase activity. *Mol Cell Biol* 23:4739, 2003.

52. Fitzgerald KA, McWhirter SM, Faia KL, et al: IKKepsilon and TBK1 are essential components of the IRF3 signaling pathway. *Nat Immunol* 4:491, 2003.

53. Sato S, Sugiyama M, Yamamoto M, et al: Toll/IL-1 receptor domain-containing adaptor inducing IFN-beta (TRIF) associates with TNF receptor-associated factor 6 and TANK-binding kinase 1, and activates two distinct transcription factors, NF-kappa B and IFN-regulatory factor-3, in the Toll-like receptor signaling. *J Immunol* 171:4304, 2003.

54. Kawasaki T, Takemura N, Standley DM, et al: The second messenger phosphatidylinositol-5-phosphate facilitates antiviral innate immune signaling. *Cell Host Microbe* 14:148, 2013.

55. Ordureau A, Enesa K, Nanda S, et al: DEAF1 is a Pellino1-interacting protein required for interferon production by Sendai virus and double-stranded RNA. *J Biol Chem* 288:24569, 2013.

56. Kawai T, Sato S, Ishii KJ, et al: Interferon-alpha induction through Toll-like receptors involves a direct interaction of IRF7 with MyD88 and TRAF6. *Nat Immunol* 5:1061, 2004.

57. Shinohara ML, Lu L, Bu J, et al: Osteopontin expression is essential for interferon-alpha production by plasmacytoid dendritic cells. *Nat Immunol* 7:498, 2006.

58. Negishi H, Fujita Y, Yanai H, et al: Evidence for licensing of IFN-gamma-induced IFN regulatory factor 1 transcription factor by MyD88 in Toll-like receptor-dependent gene induction program. *Proc Natl Acad Sci U S A* 103:15136, 2006.

59. Honda K, Ohba Y, Yanai H, et al: Spatiotemporal regulation of MyD88-IRF-7 signalling for robust type-I interferon induction. *Nature* 434:1035, 2005.

60. Hoebe K, Janssen EM, Kim SO, et al: Upregulation of costimulatory molecules induced by lipopolysaccharide and double-stranded RNA occurs by Trif-dependent and Trif-independent pathways. *Nat Immunol* 4:1223, 2003.

61. Kaisho T: Type I interferon production by nucleic acid-stimulated dendritic cells. *Front Biosci* 13:6034, 2008.

62. Chang M, Jin W, Sun SC: Peli1 facilitates TRIF-dependent Toll-like receptor signaling and proinflammatory cytokine production. *Nat Immunol* 10:1089, 2009.

63. Kobayashi K, Hernandez LD, Galan JE, et al: IRAK-M is a negative regulator of Toll-like receptor signaling. *Cell* 110:191, 2002.

64. Kinjyo I, Hanada T, Inagaki-Ohara K, et al: SOCS1/JAB is a negative regulator of LPS-induced macrophage activation. *Immunity* 17:583, 2002.

65. Ye Z, Ting JP: NLR, the nucleotide-binding domain leucine-rich repeat containing gene family. *Curr Opin Immunol* 20:3, 2008.

66. Hugot JP, Chamaillard M, Zouali H, et al: Association of NOD2 leucine-rich repeat variants with susceptibility to Crohn's disease. *Nature* 411:599, 2001.

67. Miceli-Richard C, Lesage S, Rybojad M, et al: CARD15 mutations in Blau syndrome. *Nat Genet* 29:19, 2001.

68. Hoffman HM, Mueller JL, Broide DH, et al: Mutation of a new gene encoding a putative pyrin-like protein causes familial cold autoinflammatory syndrome and Muckle-Wells syndrome. *Nat Genet* 29:301, 2001.

69. Feldmann J, Prieur AM, Quartier P, et al: Chronic infantile neurological cutaneous and articular syndrome is caused by mutations in CIAS1, a gene highly expressed in polymorphonuclear cells and chondrocytes. *Am J Hum Genet Hum Genet* 71:198, 2002.

70. Neven B, Callebaut I, Prieur AM, et al: Molecular basis of the spectral expression of CIAS1 mutations associated with phagocytic cell-mediated autoinflammatory disorders CINCA/NOMID, MWS, and FCU. *Blood* 103:2809, 2004.

71. The International FMF Consortium: Ancient missense mutations in a new member of the RoRet gene family are likely to cause familial Mediterranean fever. *Cell* 90:797, 1997.

72. Wise CA, Gillum JD, Seidman CE, et al: Mutations in CD2BP1 disrupt binding to PTP PEST and are responsible for PAPA syndrome, an autoinflammatory disorder. *Hum Mol Genet* 11:961, 2002.

73. Miao EA, Andersen-Nissen E, Warren SE, Aderem A: TLR5 and Ipaf: Dual sensors of bacterial flagellin in the innate immune system. *Semin Immunopathol* 29:275, 2007.

74. Boyden ED, Dietrich WF: Nalp1b controls mouse macrophage susceptibility to anthrax lethal toxin. *Nat Genet* 38:240, 2006.

75. Bruey JM, Bruey-Sedano N, Luciano F, et al: Bcl-2 and Bcl-XL regulate proinflammatory caspase-1 activation by interaction with NALP1. *Cell* 129:45, 2007.

76. Martinon F, Agostini L, Meylan E, Tschopp J: Identification of bacterial muramyl dipeptide as activator of the NALP3/cryopyrin inflammasome. *Curr Biol* 14:1929, 2004.

77. Mariathasan S, Newton K, Monack DM, et al: Differential activation of the inflammasome by caspase-1 adaptors ASC and Ipaf. *Nature* 430:213, 2004.

78. Cassel SL, Eisenbarth SC, Iyer SS, et al: The Nalp3 inflammasome is essential for the development of silicosis. *Proc Natl Acad Sci U S A* 105:9035, 2008.

79. Eisenbarth SC, Colegio OR, O'Connor W, et al: Crucial role for the Nalp3 inflammasome in the immunostimulatory properties of aluminium adjuvants. *Nature* 453:1122, 2008.

80. Dostert C, Petrilli V, Van Bruggen R, et al: Innate immune activation through Nalp3 inflammasome sensing of asbestos and silica. *Science* 320:674, 2008.

81. Pelegrin P, Barroso-Gutierrez C, Surprenant A: P2X7 receptor differentially couples to distinct release pathways for IL-1beta in mouse macrophage. *J Immunol* 180:7147, 2008.

82. Girardin SE, Boneca IG, Carneiro LA, et al: Nod1 detects a unique muropeptide from Gram-negative bacterial peptidoglycan. *Science* 300:1584, 2003.

83. Girardin SE, Boneca IG, Viala J, et al: Nod2 is a general sensor of peptidoglycan through muramyl dipeptide (MDP) detection. *J Biol Chem* 278:8869, 2003.

84. Girardin SE, Travassos LH, Herve M, et al: Peptidoglycan molecular requirements allowing detection by Nod1 and Nod2. *J Biol Chem* 278:41702, 2003.

85. Hsu LC, Ali SR, McGillivray S, et al: A NOD2-NALP1 complex mediates caspase-1-dependent IL-1beta secretion in response to Bacillus anthracis infection and muramyl dipeptide. *Proc Natl Acad Sci U S A* 105:7803, 2008.

86. Loo YM, Gale M Jr: Immune signaling by RIG-I-like receptors. *Immunity* 34:680, 2011.

87. Saito T, Hirai R, Loo YM, et al: Regulation of innate antiviral defenses through a shared repressor domain in RIG-I and LGP2. *Proc Natl Acad Sci U S A* 104:582, 2007.

88. Takahasi K, Yoneyama M, Nishihori T, et al: Nonself RNA-sensing mechanism of RIG-I helicase and activation of antiviral immune responses. *Mol Cell* 29:428, 2008.

89. Pippig DA, Hellmuth JC, Cui S, et al: The regulatory domain of the RIG-I family ATPase LGP2 senses double-stranded RNA. *Nucleic Acids Res* 37:2014, 2009.

90. Rothenfusser S, Goutagny N, Diperna G, et al: The RNA helicase Lgp2 inhibits TLR-independent sensing of viral replication by retinoic acid-inducible gene-I. *J Immunol* 175:5260, 2005.

91. Venkataraman T, Valdes M, Elsby R, et al: Loss of DExD/H box RNA helicase LGP2 manifests disparate antiviral responses. *J Immunol* 178:6444, 2007.

92. Satoh T, Kato H, Kumagai Y, et al: LGP2 is a positive regulator of RIG-I- and MDA5-mediated antiviral responses. *Proc Natl Acad Sci U S A* 107:1512, 2010.

93. Gitlin L, Barchet W, Gilfillan S, et al: Essential role of mda-5 in type I IFN responses to polyriboinosinic:polyribocytidylic acid and encephalomyocarditis picornavirus. *Proc Natl Acad Sci U S A* 103:8459, 2006.

94. Hornung V, Ellegast J, Kim S, et al: 5'-Triphosphate RNA is the ligand for RIG-I. *Science* 314:994, 2006.

95. Pichlmair A, Schulz O, Tan CP, et al: RIG-I-mediated antiviral responses to single-stranded RNA bearing 5'-phosphates. *Science* 314:997, 2006.

96. Kawai T, Takahashi K, Sato S, et al: IPS-1, an adaptor triggering RIG-I- and Mda5-mediated type I interferon induction. *Nat Immunol* 6:981, 2005.

97. Seth RB, Sun L, Ea CK, Chen ZJ: Identification and characterization of MAVS, a mitochondrial antiviral signaling protein that activates NF-kappaB and IRF 3. *Cell* 122:669, 2005.

98. Xu LG, Wang YY, Han KJ, et al: VISA is an adapter protein required for virus-triggered IFN-beta signaling. *Mol Cell* 19:727, 2005.

99. Meylan E, Curran J, Hofmann K, et al: Cardif is an adaptor protein in the RIG-I antiviral pathway and is targeted by hepatitis C virus. *Nature* 437:1167, 2005.

100. Hou F, Sun L, Zheng H, et al: MAVS forms functional prion-like aggregates to activate and propagate antiviral innate immune response. *Cell* 146:448, 2011.

101. Sun L, Wu J, Du F, et al: Cyclic GMP-AMP synthase is a cytosolic DNA sensor that activates the type I interferon pathway. *Science* 339:786, 2013.

102. Wu J, Sun L, Chen X, et al: Cyclic GMP-AMP is an endogenous second messenger in innate immune signaling by cytosolic DNA. *Science* 339:826, 2013.

103. Ishikawa H, Barber GN: STING is an endoplasmic reticulum adaptor that facilitates innate immune signalling. *Nature* 455:674, 2008.

104. Takaoka A, Wang Z, Choi MK, et al: DAI (DLM-1/ZBP1) is a cytosolic DNA sensor and an activator of innate immune response. *Nature* 448:501, 2007.

105. Wang Z, Choi MK, Ban T, et al: Regulation of innate immune responses by DAI (DLM-1/ZBP1) and other DNA-sensing molecules. *Proc Natl Acad Sci U S A* 105:5477, 2008.

106. Zeng M, Hu Z, Shi X, et al: MAVS, cGAS, and endogenous retroviruses in T-independent B cell responses. *Science* 346:1486, 2014.

107. Beutler B, Milsark IW, Cerami AC: Passive immunization against cachectin/tumor necrosis factor protects mice from lethal effect of endotoxin. *Science* 229:869, 1985.

108. Georgel P, Naitza S, Kappler C, et al: *Drosophila* immune deficiency (IMD) is a death domain protein that activates antibacterial defense and can promote apoptosis. *Dev Cell* 1:503, 2001.

109. Orange JS, Biron CA: Characterization of early IL-12, IFN-alpha/beta, and TNF effects on antiviral state and NK cell responses during murine cytomegalovirus infection. *J Immunol* 156:4746, 1996.

110. Andrews DM, Scalzo AA, Yokoyama WM, et al: Functional interactions between dendritic cells and NK cells during viral infection. *Nat Immunol* 4:175, 2003.

111. Mancuso G, Midiri A, Biondo C, et al: Type I IFN signaling is crucial for host resistance against different species of pathogenic bacteria. *J Immunol* 178:3126, 2007.

112. Karaghiosoff M, Steinborn R, Kovarik P, et al: Central role for type I interferons and Tyk2 in lipopolysaccharide-induced endotoxin shock. *Nat Immunol* 4:471, 2003.

113. Cella M, Jarrossay D, Facchetti F, et al: Plasmacytoid monocytes migrate to inflamed lymph nodes and produce large amounts of type I interferon. *Nat Med* 5:919, 1999.

114. Lewis PA, Loomis D: The formation of anti-sheep hemolytic amboceptor in the normal and tuberculous guinea pig. *J Exp Med* 40:503, 1924.

115. Freund J, McDermott K: Sensitization to horse serum by means of adjuvants. *Proc Soc Exp Biol Med* 49:548, 1942.

116. Condie RM, Zak SJ, Good RA: Effect of meningococcal endotoxin on the immune response. *Proc Soc Exp Biol Med* 90:355, 1955.

117. Skidmore BJ, Chiller JM, Morrison DC, Weigle WO: Immunologic properties of bacterial lipopolysaccharide (LPS): Correlation between the mitogenic, adjuvant, and immunogenic activities. *J Immunol* 114:770, 1975.

118. Germain RN, Jenkins MK: *In vivo* antigen presentation. *Curr Opin Immunol* 16:120, 2004.

119. Borriello F, Sethna MP, Boyd SD, et al: B7-1 and B7-2 have overlapping, critical roles in immunoglobulin class switching and germinal center formation. *Immunity* 6:303, 1997.

120. Yamamoto M, Sato S, Hemmi H, et al: Role of adaptor TRIF in the MyD88-independent Toll-like receptor signaling pathway. *Science* 301:640, 2003.

121. Gavin AL, Hoebe K, Duong B, et al: Adjuvant-enhanced antibody responses in the absence of Toll-like receptor signaling. *Science* 314:1936, 2006.

122. Sorensen TI, Nielsen GG, Andersen PK, Teasdale TW: Genetic and environmental influences on premature death in adult adoptees. *N Engl J Med* 318:727, 1988.

123. Smirnova I, Mann N, Dols A, et al: Assay of locus-specific genetic load implicates rare Toll-like receptor 4 mutations in meningococcal susceptibility. *Proc Natl Acad Sci U S A* 100:6075, 2003.

124. Hawn TR, Verbon A, Lettinga KD, et al: A common dominant TLR5 stop codon polymorphism abolishes flagellin signaling and is associated with susceptibility to Legionnaires' disease. *J Exp Med* 198:1563, 2003.

125. Picard C, Puel A, Bonnet M, et al: Pyogenic bacterial infections in humans with IRAK-4 deficiency. *Science* 299:2076, 2003.

126. Zhang SY, Jouanguy E, Ugolini S, et al: TLR3 deficiency in patients with herpes simplex encephalitis. *Science* 317:1522, 2007.

127. Casrouge A, Zhang SY, Eidenschenk C, et al: Herpes simplex virus encephalitis in human UNC-93B deficiency. *Science* 314:308, 2006.

128. Jouanguy E, Altare F, Lamhamedi S, et al: Interferon-gamma-receptor deficiency in an infant with fatal bacille Calmette-Guerin infection. *N Engl J Med* 335:1956, 1996.

129. Picard C, Fieschi C, Altare F, et al: Inherited interleukin-12 deficiency: IL12B genotype and clinical phenotype of 13 patients from six kindreds. *Am J Hum Genet Hum Genet* 70:336, 2002.

130. Altare F, Durandy A, Lammas D, et al: Impairment of mycobacterial immunity in human interleukin-12 receptor deficiency. *Science* 280:1432, 1998.

131. De Jong R, Altare F, Haagen IA, et al: Severe mycobacterial and Salmonella infections in interleukin-12 receptor-deficient patients. *Science* 280:1435, 1998.

132. Barbosa MD, Nguyen QA, Tchernev VT, et al: Identification of the homologous beige and Chediak-Higashi syndrome genes. *Nature* 382:262, 1996.

133. Royer-Pokora B, Kunkel LM, Monaco AP, et al: Cloning the gene for an inherited human disorder—chronic granulomatous disease—on the basis of its chromosomal location. *Nature* 322:32, 1986.

134. Leadbetter EA, Rifkin IR, Hohlbaum AM, et al: Chromatin-IgG complexes activate B cells by dual engagement of IgM and Toll-like receptors. *Nature* 416:603, 2002.

135. Crozat K, Hoebe K, Ugolini S, et al: Jinx, an MCMV susceptibility phenotype caused by disruption of Unc13d: A mouse model of type 3 familial hemophagocytic lymphohistiocytosis. *J Exp Med* 204:853, 2007.

136. Croker BA, Lawson BR, Berger M, et al: Inflammation and autoimmunity caused by a SHP1 mutation depend on IL-1, MyD88, and a microbial trigger. *Proc Natl Acad Sci U S A* 105:15028, 2008.

137. Fitzgerald KA, Palsson-McDermott EM, Bowie AG, et al: Mal (MyD88-adapter-like) is required for Toll-like receptor-4 signal transduction. *Nature* 413:78, 2001.

138. Horng T, Barton GM, Medzhitov R: TIRAP: An adapter molecule in the Toll signaling pathway. *Nat Immunol* 2:835, 2001.

139. Yamamoto M, Sato S, Hemmi H, et al: Essential role for TIRAP in activation of the signalling cascade shared by TLR2 and TLR4. *Nature* 420:324, 2002.

140. Poltorak A, Smirnova I, He XL, et al: Genetic and physical mapping of the *Lps* locus-identification of the Toll-4 receptor as a candidate gene in the critical region. *Blood Cells Mol Dis* 24:340, 1998.

141. Takeuchi O, Kawai T, Muhlradt PF, et al: Discrimination of bacterial lipoproteins by Toll-like receptor 6. *Int Immunol* 13:933, 2001.

142. Hemmi H, Kaisho T, Takeuchi O, et al: Small anti-viral compounds activate immune cells via the TLR7 MyD88-dependent signaling pathway. *Nat Immunol* 3:196, 2002.

143. Jurk M, Heil F, Vollmer J, et al: Human TLR7 or TLR8 independently confer responsiveness to the antiviral compound R-848. *Nat Immunol* 3:499, 2002.

144. Chuang T, Ulevitch RJ: Identification of hTLR10: A novel human Toll-like receptor preferentially expressed in immune cells. *Biochim Biophys Acta* 1518:157, 2001.

CHAPTER 21
DENDRITIC CELLS AND ADAPTIVE IMMUNITY

Madhav Dhodapkar, Crystal L. Mackall, and Ralph M. Steinman*

SUMMARY

Dendritic cells are a multifunctional group of cells that serve as sentinels of the immune system and thus regulate many immune functions. Dendritic cells play a central role in initiating adaptive immune responses to pathogens and initiating antitumor immune responses. Dendritic cell receptors sense environmental stimuli and can respond rapidly to both foreign pathogens and danger signals derived from tissue damage or immune complexes. Through their capacity to present antigen to T cells in immune-activating or immune-dampening contexts, dendritic cells can both induce T-cell proliferation (activation) or lack of activation (tolerance). In this way, dendritic cells help regulate immune responses mediated by T cells and B cells of the adaptive immune system. This chapter describes the varied types and functions of this important class of cells.

● FUNCTIONS OF DENDRITIC CELLS

Host defense is mediated by innate and adaptive immune responses, and dendritic cells (DCs) play essential roles in linking together innate and adaptive immunity.[1-3] The innate immune response provides rapid resistance to pathogens, but the potency of innate responses does not increase following initial exposure. Adaptive responses, mediated by B and T lymphocytes, generate immune memory, resulting in more rapid and more potent responses following antigen reexposure (Chaps. 75 and 76).

DENDRITIC CELLS AND INNATE IMMUNITY

DCs provide innate immune resistance through production of cytokines, including interleukin (IL)-12 and type I interferons, and by activating other innate lymphocytes such as natural killer (NK) cells, NKT cells, and $\gamma\delta$ T cells (Chap. 75). Innate responses are most often initiated by "pattern recognition receptors" (Chap. 20), which respond

---

Acronyms and Abbreviations: CD, cluster of differentiation; CMV, cytomegalovirus; DC, dendritic cell; GM-CSF, granulocyte-monocyte colony-stimulating factor; GVHD, graft-versus-host disease; GVL, graft-versus-leukemia; Ig, immunoglobulin; IL, interleukin; M-CSF, monocyte colony-stimulating factor; MHC, major histocompatibility complex; NK, natural killer; Th, T helper; TLR, toll-like receptor; TNF, tumor necrosis factor; Tr, T regulatory.

---

to evolutionarily conserved molecules found in microbes, parasites and viruses.[4,5] Pattern recognition receptors include toll-like receptors (TLRs), nucleotide-binding oligomerization domain-like receptors, retinoic acid-inducible gene 1-like receptors, and numerous C-type lectins. Pattern recognition receptors recognize a wide array of ligands, such as single- or double-stranded RNA, lipopolysaccharides, and other microbial constituents. DCs express pattern recognition receptors and respond to pattern recognition receptor agonists by becoming potent immunostimulatory cells and by presenting captured antigens to T cells in the context of major histocompatibility antigens. Pattern recognition receptors on DCs can also be activated via noninfectious stimuli induced by tissue damage and malignant cells, including uric acid crystals and heat shock and chromatin proteins. Such pathways are likely important for activating DCs toward tumor-associated antigens following transplantation or in disease states such as cancer or allergy.

Activated or matured DCs can prime resting NK cells, which then reciprocally act back on DCs, enhancing DC maturation and initiating adaptive immune responses.[6] NK cells can also negatively regulate DC function by killing immature DCs, a feature that is important in NK mediated graft-versus-leukemia (GVL), without graft-versus-host disease (GVHD), following hematopoietic stem cell transplantation.[7] Such immune crosstalk between NK cells and DCs, is emblematic of the exquisite interdependence and complexity of the immune response.[8-10]

DENDRITIC CELLS AND ADAPTIVE IMMUNITY

Adaptive immunity imparts immune memory to the host, which allows a more rapid and more effective immune response to rechallenge with the same antigen. Adaptive immunity is mediated by B and T lymphocytes, but its induction is largely regulated by DCs. Immune memory increases the frequency and function of antigen-specific lymphocytes, leading to enhanced levels of protective antibodies, cytokines, and killer molecules. Through an elaborate series of gene rearrangements, hypermutation, and selection, antibody on B cells and T-cell receptors on T cells provide remarkable diversity and specificity. This array might be thought of as the largest combinatorial library of specificities in the world!

DCs function as sentinels of the immune system (Table 21–1)[1,3,11] and provide a critical bridge between innate and adaptive immunity. Indeed, the presence of antigen and lymphocyte is rarely sufficient to induce adaptive immune responses. Rather, a third party, the DC system of antigen-presenting cells provides the pivotal immune initiation signal required to induce an adaptive immune response. DCs sense a wide range of environmental stimuli, producing cytokines, such as IL-12 and type I interferons that help stimulate immune responses. DCs express most types of TLRs, with specific subsets of DCs differentially expressing distinct TLRs; for example, plasmacytoid DCs express significant levels of TLR-7 and TLR-9.[12] DCs can also respond to endogenous stimuli, ranging from inflammatory cytokines, including tumor necrosis factor (TNF)-α, IL-1, or interferons, to byproducts of cell death or tissue damage. DCs capture microbes and tumor cells, processing their component antigens for presentation to the adaptive immune system. DC activation, via innate immune receptors, leads to DC maturation and initiation of adaptive immunity. In addition to antigen processing and presentation, sentinel DCs produce chemokines and cytokines. They migrate to lymphoid tissues, where they recruit naïve antigen-specific lymphocytes and instruct their subsequent development.

A variety of DC subsets exist and the biology of DC activation can vary significantly according to the exposure. During immunization, DCs initiate clonal expansion of T cells and can directly and indirectly influence the growth of B cells. In addition, DCs can modulate differentiation of lymphocytes, such that the properties of the lymphocytes are

---

*Deceased. Substantial portions of his contribution have been retained in the current version of this chapter.

TABLE 21–1. Role of Dendritic Cell in Immunity

Sensors: rapid and appropriate differentiation in response to pathogen-associated molecular patterns and other signals

Sentinels: positioned in peripheral tissues to optimize antigen capture and migrate to lymphoid tissues

Tolerance: deletion and anergy of self-reactive lymphocytes and induction of regulatory T cells

Innate resistance: activation of innate lymphocytes, including NK and NKT cells, secretion of protective cytokines

Adaptive immunity: differentiation of quiescent, naïve T cells to form effectors, establishment of memory lymphocytes, antibody responses

TABLE 21–2. Important Components of Dendritic Cell Function

Cell processes or dendrites and motility: numerous and continually probing

Antigen handling: specialized antigen uptake receptors and processing pathways for classic (MHC) and nonclassic (CD1 and others) presenting molecules, including cross-presentation onto MHC class I and CD1

MHC class II products: high and regulated expression

Migration in lymphatics to lymphoid organs and localization to T-cell areas

Environmental sensing: multiple receptors for microbial and non-microbial products and exaggerated responses to the products

Cytokine receptors, including hematopoietins (flt3L and granulocyte-macrophage colony-stimulating factor, but not monocyte colony-stimulating factor, granulocyte colony-stimulating factor)

Chemokine receptors, especially for homing to tissues (CCR6) and lymph nodes (CCR7, CCR2)

Induction of peripheral tolerance via intrinsic and extrinsic pathways

Activation of innate lymphocytes (e.g., natural killer cells)

appropriate to the invading pathogen.[13] For example, under the influence of DCs, T cells can preferentially produce interferon-γ (T-helper [Th] type 1 cells) to activate macrophages to resist infection by intracellular microbes; or IL-4, IL-5, and IL-13 (Th2 cells) to mobilize white cells to resist helminths; or IL-17 (Th17 cells) to mobilize phagocytes at body surfaces to resist extracellular bacteria.

An essential counterpart to adaptive immunity is adaptive tolerance, which is the silencing of cells with receptors reactive to self or harmless environmental antigens. T cells develop tolerance centrally in the thymus and peripherally in lymphoid organs.[14,15] DCs play a role in inducing tolerance, especially with regard to T cells. DCs can silence self-reactive T cells, through either deletion or functional inactivation. DCs can also drive T cells to suppress immunity by expressing IL-10 (T regulatory [Tr]1 cells) or FOXP3.[16]

● DENDRITIC CELL BIOLOGY

DCs are "antigen-presenting cells." An antigen-presenting cell is *any* cell that uses its major histocompatibility complex (MHC) products (or other antigen-presenting molecules, such as the CD1 molecules that present glycolipids and lipoglycans) to bind and display (i.e., "present") fragments of antigen to lymphocytes. DCs are more specialized or professional than other antigen-presenting cells. This is because DCs have efficient and regulated pathways for antigen uptake and processing, and DCs possess dozens of features that allow them to initiate and control immunity (Table 21–2). For example, when DCs mature in response to infection, hundreds, even thousands, of gene transcripts can be upregulated or downregulated.[17,18]

ANTIGEN UPTAKE AND PROCESSING

DCs express a wide array of endocytic receptors, which enhance the efficiency of antigen capture, processing, and presentation. Many endocytic receptors are predicted to be C-type lectins, and in some cases their natural ligands have not been identified. DCs also express Fcγ and Fcε receptors, which recognize immune complexes, as well as scavenger receptors. Recognition of pathogens by DC receptors can have two outcomes. One outcome is immune activation followed by antigen presentation and development of a productive immune responses. Alternatively, pathogens may use DC receptors to evade the host immune response. For example, DC-SIGN (CD209) a lectin expressed on DCs, is used by HIV-1 and cytomegalovirus (CMV) to reach T cells and endothelial cells, respectively[19,20]; by Dengue virus to replicate within DCs[21]; and by *Mycobacterium tuberculosis* to trigger production of the suppressive cytokine IL-10.[22]

Following uptake, efficient processing of antigen yields peptides that bind to MHC class II and class I products. "Exogenous" antigens refer to molecules processed directly following uptake, whereas "endogenous" antigens are processed following biosynthesis in the antigen-presenting cell. Classic pathways of antigen presentation emphasize processing of "exogenous" antigens for presentation on MHC II–peptide complexes to CD4+ T lymphocytes, whereas "endogenous" antigens were targeted for presentation on MHC class I–peptide complexes to CD8+ T cells. However, it is now clear that there is significant overlap in these pathways such that exogenous antigens may also be presented on MHC I products to CD8+ T cells. This pathway is termed *cross-presentation* and is important for initiation of antitumor immune responses. Cross-presentation is well developed in DCs, especially those found in lymphoid tissues, and leads to either tolerance or activation of CD8+ T lymphocytes, depending upon the DC maturation stimulus.[23] For instance, products of dying cells, from transplants, tumors, foci of infection, and self-tissues are endocytosed by DCs then presented on MHC Class I to CD8+ cells.[24,25] Importantly, cross-presentation of antigens onto MHC class I can involve the proteasome and transporters for antigenic peptides, which are used in the presentation of endogenous antigens.

DCs are a major cell type involved in cross-presentation of proteins,[26,27] and probably of lipids.[28,29] Cross-presentation has been documented involving nonreplicating microbes, dying cells, ligands for the DEC205 receptor, and immune complexes, including antibody-coated tumor cells. This pathway allows DCs to induce tolerance or immunity to antigens not synthesized *de novo* in these cells. Fcγ receptors, in addition to mediating presentation, can influence DC maturation, either enhancing maturation through activating forms of the receptor or preventing maturation through inhibitory forms.[30] Such consequences of antibody binding to DC Fc receptors, with regard to DC maturation and cross-presentation, are important features for consideration when trying to understand the use of antibodies as therapeutic agents.

Some DCs subsets also express the CD1 family of antigen-presenting molecules. For example, CD1a typically is found on epidermal Langerhans cells in skin, whereas CD1b and CD1c are expressed on dermal DCs. CD1 molecules present glycolipids, whereas microbial glycolipids are the best studied to date with regard to CD1a, CD1b, and

CD1c. CD1d molecules on DCs also efficiently present the synthetic glycolipid α-galactosylceramide.[31] This process leads to activation of distinct lymphocytes with a restricted T-cell repertoire, the NKT cells.[32] NKT cells have significant potential as effector cells because they can produce large amounts of interferon-γ and lyse tumor targets.

A newer "nonclassical" pathway for antigen presentation involves presentation of "endogenous" proteins on MHC class II.[33] This pathway involves autophagy and is also well developed in DCs.[34] It allows nuclear, mitochondrial and cytoplasmic proteins to be presented from digestive compartments, including as a first example, the Epstein-Barr nuclear antigen 1.[35]

MATURATION OF DENDRITIC CELLS

Immature DCs efficiently take up antigen but do not induce immunity, defined as the production of immune effectors and the establishment of memory. For immune induction to occur, DCs require additional stimuli that lead to an intricate differentiation process called "maturation." Maturation involves changes in endocytic and antigen processing machineries, production of chemokines and cytokines, and expression of many cell-surface molecules, including those of the B7, TNF, and Notch ligand families. DCs have an endocytic system that is tightly regulated and devoted to presentation of captured antigens, rather than clearance and scavenging.

In the case of DCs derived from marrow and monocyte precursors, DC maturation is accompanied by exquisite changes in the endocytic system with attendant consequences for antigen processing and presentation. During maturation, antigen uptake is dampened as a result of inactivation of a rho-guanosine triphosphatase termed *cdc42*.[36] At the same time, machinery associated with antigen processing is augmented. Lysosomal processing is activated by assembly of an active proton pump, which acidifies the lysosome so that processing of antigens and the MHC class II associated invariant chain can proceed. MHC–peptide complexes form within the endocytic system of the maturing DCs,[37,38] then traffic in distinct nonlysosomal compartments to the cell surface. Internalization and degradation of MHC II also occurs via ubiquitination is also inhibited in mature DCs.[39] DC maturation also increases presentation on MHC I via, in part, the formation of an "immunoproteasome," a combinatorial form of proteasome that increases the spectrum of peptides destined to be presented on MHC I.[40]

A hallmark of DC maturation in response to several stimuli is upregulation of costimulatory molecules such as CD80 and CD86, resulting at least in part from production of inflammatory cytokines, particularly TNF-α.[32] Importantly however, CD86 upregulation should not be equated directly with immune activation, which requires other DC functions, such as those triggered by CD40 ligation, including production of cytokines such as IL-12 or type I interferons, and/or engagement of other receptors such as CD70.[32]

DCs enhance antibody formation by several mechanisms. The classical pathway involves induction of antigen-specific CD4+ helper T cells, which then help B-cell growth and antibody secretion. However, DCs can also directly affect B cells to enhance immunoglobulin (Ig) secretion and isotype switching, including production of the IgA class of antibodies, which contribute to mucosal immunity.[41,42] DCs can induce a B-cell class switch in a CD40-independent manner, through production of ligands such as B-lymphocyte stimulator (B-cell activating factor belonging to the TNF family [BAFF]) and a proliferation-induced ligand (APRIL), including T-cell–independent induction of IgA antibodies to commensal organisms.[43] Plasmacytoid DCs stimulate antibody responses to influenza virus in culture.[44] Production of antibodies by any of these mechanisms may lead to interaction with DC FcγR and thereby an adaptive response by T cells.

● DENDRITIC CELL SUBSETS

The primary function of DCs is to survey host tissues and initiate responses upon encountering danger signals. To optimally perform these functions, DCs are present in every tissue of the body, and are enriched in lymphoid tissues. Immature DCs are strategically positioned along body surfaces (skin, airway, gut) and in the interstitial spaces of many organs, such as the heart and kidneys. DCs are able to extend their processes through the tight junctions in epithelia, without altering the epithelial barrier, allowing them to sample antigens from harmless environmental antigens and commensal microorganisms. In the steady state, DCs migrate continuously from tissues into afferent lymphatics and probably blood. By electron microscopy, DCs in lymphoid tissues often are termed *interdigitating cells*, appearing as large stellate cells with a lucent "empty"-appearing cytoplasm.

One method of categorizing DCs is to describe them based upon the tissue in which they reside. Lymphoid tissue–resident DCs have undergone intensive study, especially in murine models. The scarcity of DCs in nonlymphoid tissues, on the other hand, limited understanding of their importance for many years and continues to render study of these cells challenging. Because circulating DCs are the most accessible subset in humans, they have received intense study; however, blood DCs may not reflect accurately the biology of tissue resident cells. Briefly, all DCs subsets are CD45+CD11c+class II+ cells that lack markers associated with T-cell, B-cell, erythroid, granulocytic, and NK lineages. However, such a definition is not complete as some macrophages express this phenotype yet are distinct from the DC lineage. Additional confidence in a DC lineage is provided by expression of Flt-3 (FMS-like tyrosine kinase 3, CD135), which mediates signals important in the differentiation of this lineage, c-kit and/or CCR7.

An alternative method for classifying DC subsets separates the major lineages as classical dendritic cells (cDCs) versus plasmacytoid dendritic cells (pDCs). cDCs are the most plentiful and incorporate lymphoid tissue–resident and nonlymphoid tissue–resident DCs. Although both pDCs and cDCs derive from a common progenitor, pDCs are distinct from cDCs in appearance (they resemble plasma cells) and they reside primarily in blood and lymphoid tissue, but are not found in nonlymphoid tissues. pDCs are important mediators of innate immunity, because of their capacity to rapidly produce high levels of interferon (IFN)−α upon encounter with pathogens that engage the TLR-7 and TLR-9 receptors, which are plentiful in this subset. cDCs are frequently further subdivided into lymphoid-resident cDCs versus nonlymphoid-resident cDCs. In mice, most lymphoid-resident cDCs are CD8α+CD11b− whereas most nonlymphoid-resident cDCs are CD103+CD11b−. CD8α+CD11b− lymphoid tissue–resident cDC have a similar origin, phenotype, and transcriptional profile as CD103+CD11b− nonlymphoid-resident cDC. In contrast, CD11b+ cDCs can be found in both lymphoid and nonlymphoid tissue, and this subset is notable for its ability to derive from monocytes in response to granulocyte-monocyte colony-stimulating factor (GM-CSF), monocyte colony-stimulating factor (M-CSF), and other inflammatory mediators. CD8α+ and CD8α− cDCs show a remarkable division of labor in terms of the nature of induced host response. While CD8α+ DCs efficiently cross-prime CD8+ T-cell immunity through MHC class I antigen presentation,[45] CD8α− DCs stimulate predominantly CD4+ T-cell response through MHC class II presentation.[46] These differences may be explained in part by the fact that CD8α+ DCs have high endosomal pH, low antigen degradation, high antigen export to cytosol, and more presynthesized stores of MHC class I molecules.[47,48]

In humans, essentially all DCs lack lineage markers for T cells, B cells, NK cells, and erythroid and granulocytic lineages, and express CD45 and MHC class II. Human pDCs are described as

Lin−classII+CD303(BDCA2)+CD304(BDCA4)+, whereas human cDC blood subsets generally correlate with lymphoid tissue cDC subsets. Human cDCs are either CD1c(BDCA1)+ or CD141(BDCA3)+, with the CD1c+ subset being significantly more plentiful than the CD141+ subset. In humans, BDCA3+ DCs have been proposed as human equivalents of murine CD8α+ DCs, and may have superior cross-presentation capability compared to other human DC subsets.[49] However, the capacity for cross-presentation is not restricted to this subset of human DCs. The DEC205/CD205 lectin receptor is also a useful marker for DCs in human lymph nodes.[50] Nonlymphoid tissue–resident DCs in humans remain incompletely characterized, with the exception of Langerhans cells. First described more than 100 years ago, Langerhans cells are cDCs found in the epidermis, characterized by a "tennis racket" appearance by light microscopy as a result of internalized Langerin, which localizes in "Birbeck granules."[51] Langerhans cells are characterized by expression of CD1a as well as EpCAM and CD207(Langerin). Uncontrolled proliferation of Langerhans cells is responsible for the clinical disorder known as Langerhans cell histiocytosis (LCH).

Further insights into the functional diversity of DC subsets has come from discovery of distinct transcriptional factors that underlie their development and functional properties.[52] For example, z-DC, was identified as a transcriptional factor regulating the development of classical DCs.[53,54] Functional specialization of DC subsets is likely to impact the next generation of vaccines, as discussed in "Dendritic Cells in Immunotherapy" below.

One of the most important discoveries in DC biology has been identification of a clonogenic DC progenitor within the marrow that is committed to the DC lineage and unable to give rise to other cell types. Such progenitors, described as pro-DCs can generate plasmacytoid and CD8α+ and CD8α− classical DCs, but no other cell subset.[55,56] Subsequent work confirmed that the committed DC progenitor derives from a more primitive cell that is capable of giving rise to monocytes and macrophages.[57] Progenitors can also be identified that specifically gave rise to cDCs but not pDCs.[56] In mice, administration of Flt-3 ligand expands progeny of DC-committed progenitors. This series of discoveries dispelled the notion that DCs in vivo were largely derived from inflammation driven monocyte differentiation and firmly established DCs as a distinct hematopoietic lineage. Still, in states of inflammation, DCs can be induced from mature monocytes in the presence of inflammatory mediators such as GM-CSF and M-CSF.

● DENDRITIC CELLS IN IMMUNOTHERAPY

In view of their central role as antigen-presenting cells, DCs have been targeted to both boost T-cell immunity in the setting of resistance against pathogens/tumors or suppress T cells in the setting of autoimmune disease.[58] Although both are relevant to hematologic diseases, much of the current effort has been in the context of vaccination to boost T-cell immunity against tumors. Immunity to standard subcutaneously injected protein vaccines is also likely impacted by the biology of lymph node–resident and migratory DC subsets.[59] Two broad strategies have been attempted to harness the ability of DCs to boost T-cell immunity. One approach involves adoptive transfer of antigen-loaded DCs.[60] In most of these studies, DCs were generated ex vivo from precursors such as blood monocytes, although some of these studies also utilized more primitive progenitors, such as CD34+ hematopoietic stem cells or circulating DCs.[61] One of the first studies involved the injection of idiotype-pulsed DCs against lymphoma.[62] Most of these studies were small, and while DCs were well tolerated, they led to only modest clinical effects in terms of objective tumor regression. Although these

studies provided important fundamental insights into DC biology, such as the link between DC maturation and their immunogenicity,[63,64] they did not exploit the biology of naturally occurring DCs and their subsets. These studies also emphasized the need to combine vaccine-based approaches with strategies to overcome suppressive elements in the tumor bed, including inhibitory immune checkpoints, and address the vaccine-induced induction of regulatory T cells.[65] Recent promising clinical results with T-cell immune checkpoint blockade such as with antibodies against PD1/PDL1 in human cancer is setting the stage for the next generation of combination therapies with vaccines.[66,67] In addition to T cells, DCs are also being explored to activate other immune cells such as innate NKT cells. Combination of NKT-cell–targeted vaccine with low-dose lenalidomide led to synergistic immune activation and tumor regressions in early myeloma.[68]

Another strategy involves targeting antigens directly to DCs *in situ*. Coupling antigens to antibodies against DEC205, an antigen-uptake receptor on DCs, leads to enhanced activation of T-cell immunity in several models.[58] Even in this setting, DC activation is essential to elicit immunity and targeting antigens to DEC205 in steady state results in the induction of tolerance.[69] Early clinical studies with targeting antigens to DEC205 combined with approaches to activate DCs demonstrate clear induction of humoral and cellular immune responses.[70] Promising but preliminary results in patients who receive T-cell checkpoint blockade following the vaccine supports the investigation of combination approaches.[70] Other emerging approaches to targeting DCs *in situ* include nanoparticles. These technologies hold promise for flexibility and personalization of the vaccine, but the nature of optimal DC subset or adjuvant/DC maturation stimulus remains to be clarified.[71] It is notable that potent human vaccines, such as the yellow fever vaccine, simultaneously engage multiple DC subsets,[72] raising the prospect that to optimize the generation of T-cell immunity a combination of DC subsets will need to targeted *in vivo*.[73]

A setting where the biology of DCs plays a central role in hematology is allogeneic stem cell transplantation. The immunologic activity of donor T cells in allogeneic stem cell transplantation is a critical factor for eradicating residual malignancy, a process termed GVL, but can also lead to detrimental GVHD. There is considerable evidence that the induction of GVHD is dependent on the remaining host antigen-presenting cells of which DCs are the most potent.[74,75] The role of DCs in mediating the GVL effect is less-well understood, although a role for DCs has been implicated.[76] DC subsets, particularly pDCs, have also emerged as critical regulators of autoimmune hematologic disorders such as immune thrombocytopenia in children.[77]

Consequently, targeting DCs may be of benefit in the setting of autoimmunity as well as GVHD.

REFERENCES

1. Steinman RM, Banchereau J: Taking dendritic cells into medicine. *Nature* 449:419–426, 2007.
2. Belkaid Y, Oldenhove G: Tuning microenvironments: Induction of regulatory T cells by dendritic cells. *Immunity* 29:362–371, 2008.
3. Melief CJ: Cancer immunotherapy by dendritic cells. *Immunity* 29:372–383, 2008.
4. Beutler BA: TLRs and innate immunity. *Blood* 113:1399–1407, 2009.
5. Rakoff-Nahoum S, Medzhitov R: Toll-like receptors and cancer. *Nat Rev Cancer* 9: 57–63, 2009.
6. Zitvogel L: Dendritic and natural killer cells cooperate in the control/switch of innate immunity. *J Exp Med* 195:F9-F14, 2002.
7. Ruggeri L, Capanni M, Urbani E, et al: Effectiveness of donor natural killer cell alloreactivity in mismatched hematopoietic transplants. *Science* 295:2097–2100, 2002.
8. Walzer T, Dalod M, Robbins SH, et al: Natural-killer cells and dendritic cells: "l'union fait la force". *Blood* 106:2252–2258, 2005.
9. Munz C, Steinman RM, Fujii S: Dendritic cell maturation by innate lymphocytes: Coordinated stimulation of innate and adaptive immunity. *J Exp Med* 202:203–207, 2005.
10. Fujii S, Shimizu K, Hemmi H, Steinman RM: Innate Valpha14(+) natural killer T cells mature dendritic cells, leading to strong adaptive immunity. *Immunol Rev* 220:183–198, 2007.

11. Pulendran B: Modulating vaccine responses with dendritic cells and Toll-like receptors. *Immunol Rev* 199:227–250, 2004.
12. Gilliet M, Cao W, Liu YJ: Plasmacytoid dendritic cells: Sensing nucleic acids in viral infection and autoimmune diseases. *Nat Rev Immunol* 8:594–606, 2008.
13. Zhu J, Paul WE: CD4 T cells: Fates, functions, and faults. *Blood* 112:1557–1569, 2008.
14. Dhodapkar MV, Steinman RM, Krasovsky J, et al: Antigen-specific inhibition of effector T cell function in humans after injection of immature dendritic cells. *J Exp Med* 193:233–238, 2001.
15. Steinman RM, Hawiger D, Nussenzweig MC: Tolerogenic dendritic cells. *Annu Rev Immunol* 21:685–711, 2003.
16. Yamazaki S, Dudziak D, Heidkamp GF, et al: CD8+ CD205+ splenic dendritic cells are specialized to induce Foxp3+ regulatory T cells. *J Immunol* 181:6923–6933, 2008.
17. Granucci F, Vizzardelli C, Pavelka N, et al: Inducible IL-2 production by dendritic cells revealed by global gene expression analysis. *Nat Immunol* 2:882–888, 2001.
18. Huang Q, Liu D, Majewski P, et al: The plasticity of dendritic cell responses to pathogens and their components. *Science* 294:870–875, 2001.
19. Geijtenbeek TB, Kwon DS, Torensma R, et al: DC-SIGN, a dendritic cell-specific HIV-1-binding protein that enhances trans-infection of T cells. *Cell* 100:587–597, 2000.
20. Halary F, Amara A, Lortat-Jacob H, et al: Human cytomegalovirus binding to DC-SIGN is required for dendritic cell infection and target cell trans-infection. *Immunity* 17:653–664, 2002.
21. Tassaneetrithep B, Burgess TH, Granelli-Piperno A, et al: DC-SIGN (CD209) mediates dengue virus infection of human dendritic cells. *J Exp Med* 197:823–829, 2003.
22. van Kooyk Y, Geijtenbeek TB: DC-SIGN: Escape mechanism for pathogens. *Nat Rev Immunol* 3:697–709, 2003.
23. Bonifaz LC, Bonnyay DP, Charalambous A, et al: In vivo targeting of antigens to maturing dendritic cells via the DEC-205 receptor improves T cell vaccination. *J Exp Med* 199:815–824, 2004.
24. Liu K, Iyoda T, Saternus M, et al: Immune tolerance after delivery of dying cells to dendritic cells in situ. *J Exp Med* 196:1091–1097, 2002.
25. Inaba K, Turley S, Yamaide F, et al: Efficient presentation of phagocytosed cellular fragments on the major histocompatibility complex class II products of dendritic cells. *J Exp Med* 188:2163–2173, 1998.
26. Hildner K, Edelson BT, Purtha WE, et al: Batf3 deficiency reveals a critical role for CD8alpha+ dendritic cells in cytotoxic T cell immunity. *Science* 322:1097–1100, 2008.
27. Jung S, Unutmaz D, Wong P, et al: In vivo depletion of CD11c+ dendritic cells abrogates priming of CD8+ T cells by exogenous cell-associated antigens. *Immunity* 17:211–220, 2002.
28. Shimizu K, Kurosawa Y, Taniguchi M, et al: Cross-presentation of glycolipid from tumor cells loaded with alpha-galactosylceramide leads to potent and long-lived T cell mediated immunity via dendritic cells. *J Exp Med* 204:2641–2653, 2007.
29. Wu DY, Segal NH, Sidobre S, et al: Cross-presentation of disialoganglioside GD3 to natural killer T cells. *J Exp Med* 198:173–181, 2003.
30. Kalergis AM, Ravetch JV: Inducing tumor immunity through the selective engagement of activating Fcgamma receptors on dendritic cells. *J Exp Med* 195:1653–1659, 2002.
31. Vincent MS, Gumperz JE, Brenner MB: Understanding the function of CD1-restricted T cells. *Nat Immunol* 4:517–523, 2003.
32. Fujii S, Liu K, Smith C, et al: The linkage of innate to adaptive immunity via maturing dendritic cells in vivo requires CD40 ligation in addition to antigen presentation and CD80/86 costimulation. *J Exp Med* 199:1607–1618, 2004.
33. Schmid D, Pypaert M, Munz C: Antigen-loading compartments for major histocompatibility complex class II molecules continuously receive input from autophagosomes. *Immunity* 26:79–92, 2007.
34. Schmid D, Munz C: Innate and adaptive immunity through autophagy. *Immunity* 27:11–21, 2007.
35. Paludan C, Schmid D, Landthaler M, et al: Endogenous MHC class II processing of a viral nuclear antigen after autophagy. *Science* 307:593–596, 2005.
36. Garrett WS, Chen LM, Kroschewski R, et al: Developmental control of endocytosis in dendritic cells by Cdc42. *Cell* 102:325–334, 2000.
37. Trombetta ES, Ebersold M, Garrett W, et al: Activation of lysosomal function during dendritic cell maturation. *Science* 299:1400–1403, 2003.
38. Inaba K, Turley S, Iyoda T, et al: The formation of immunogenic major histocompatibility complex class II-peptide ligands in lysosomal compartments of dendritic cells is regulated by inflammatory stimuli. *J Exp Med* 191:927–936, 2000.
39. Chow A, Toomre D, Garrett W, Mellman I: Dendritic cell maturation triggers retrograde MHC class II transport from lysosomes to the plasma membrane. *Nature* 418:988–994, 2002.
40. Shin JS, Ebersold M, Pypaert M, et al: Surface expression of MHC class II in dendritic cells is controlled by regulated ubiquitination. *Nature* 444:115–118, 2006.
41. Tezuka H, Abe Y, Iwata M, et al: Regulation of IgA production by naturally occurring TNF/iNOS-producing dendritic cells. *Nature* 448:929–933, 2007.
42. Fayette J, Dubois B, Vandenabeele S, et al: Human dendritic cells skew isotype switching of CD40-activated naive B cells towards IgA1 and IgA2. *J Exp Med* 185:1909–1918, 1997.
43. Macpherson AJ, Uhr T: Induction of protective IgA by intestinal dendritic cells carrying commensal bacteria. *Science* 303:1662–1665, 2004.
44. Jego G, Palucka AK, Blanck JP, et al: Plasmacytoid dendritic cells induce plasma cell differentiation through type I interferon and interleukin 6. *Immunity* 19:225–234, 2003.
45. Shortman K, Heath WR: The CD8+ dendritic cell subset. *Immunol Rev* 234:18–31, 2010.
46. Dudziak D, Kamphorst AO, Heidkamp GF, et al: Differential antigen processing by dendritic cell subsets in vivo. *Science* 315:107–111, 2007.
47. Savina A, Peres A, Cebrian I, et al: The small GTPase Rac2 controls phagosomal alkalinization and antigen crosspresentation selectively in CD8(+) dendritic cells. *Immunity* 30:544–555, 2009.
48. Segura E, Amigorena S: Cross-presentation by human dendritic cell subsets. *Immunol Lett* 158:73–78, 2014.
49. Bachem A, Guttler S, Hartung E, et al: Superior antigen cross-presentation and XCR1 expression define human CD11c+CD141+ cells as homologues of mouse CD8+ dendritic cells. *J Exp Med* 207:1273–1281, 2010.
50. Granelli-Piperno A, Pritsker A, Pack M, et al: Dendritic cell-specific intercellular adhesion molecule 3-grabbing nonintegrin/CD209 is abundant on macrophages in the normal human lymph node and is not required for dendritic cell stimulation of the mixed leukocyte reaction. *J Immunol* 175:4265–4273, 2005.
51. Merad M, Sathe P, Helft J, et al: The dendritic cell lineage: Ontogeny and function of dendritic cells and their subsets in the steady state and the inflamed setting. *Annu Rev Immunol* 31:563–604, 2013.
52. Murphy KM: Transcriptional control of dendritic cell development. *Adv Immunol* 120:239–267, 2013.
53. Meredith MM, Liu K, Darrasse-Jeze G, et al: Expression of the zinc finger transcription factor zDC (Zbtb46, Btbd4) defines the classical dendritic cell lineage. *J Exp Med* 209:1153–1165, 2012.
54. Meredith MM, Liu K, Kamphorst AO, et al: Zinc finger transcription factor zDC is a negative regulator required to prevent activation of classical dendritic cells in the steady state. *J Exp Med* 209:1583–1593, 2012.
55. Onai N, Obata-Onai A, Schmid MA, et al: Identification of clonogenic common Flt3+M-CSFR+ plasmacytoid and conventional dendritic cell progenitors in mouse bone marrow. *Nat Immunol* 8:1207–1216, 2007.
56. Naik SH, Sathe P, Park HY, et al: Development of plasmacytoid and conventional dendritic cell subtypes from single precursor cells derived in vitro and in vivo. *Nat Immunol* 8:1217–1226, 2007.
57. Liu K, Victora GD, Schwickert TA, et al: In vivo analysis of dendritic cell development and homeostasis. *Science* 324:392–397, 2009.
58. Steinman RM: Decisions about dendritic cells: Past, present, and future. *Annu Rev Immunol* 30:1–22, 2012.
59. Anandasabapathy N, Feder R, Mollah S, et al: Classical Flt3L-dependent dendritic cells control immunity to protein vaccine. *J Exp Med* 211:1875–1891, 2014.
60. Anguille S, Smits EL, Lion E, et al: Clinical use of dendritic cells for cancer therapy. *Lancet Oncol* 15:e257–e267, 2014.
61. Palucka K, Banchereau J: Dendritic-cell-based therapeutic cancer vaccines. *Immunity* 39:38–48, 2013.
62. Hsu FJ, Benike C, Fagnoni F, et al: Vaccination of patients with B-cell lymphoma using autologous antigen-pulsed dendritic cells. *Nat Med* 2:52–58, 1996.
63. Dhodapkar MV, Steinman RM, Krasovsky J, et al: Antigen specific inhibition of effector T cell function in humans after injection of immature dendritic cells. *J Exp Med* 193:233–238, 2001.
64. Dhodapkar MV, Krasovsky J, Steinman RM, Bhardwaj N: Mature dendritic cells boost functionally superior CD8(+) T-cell in humans without foreign helper epitopes. *J Clin Invest* 105:R9–R14, 2000.
65. Banerjee D, Dhodapkar MV, Matayeva E, et al: Expansion of FOXP3high regulatory T cells by human dendritic cells (DCs) in vitro and after DC injection of cytokine matured DCs in myeloma patients. *Blood* 108:2655–2661, 2006.
66. Sznol M, Chen L: Antagonist antibodies to PD-1 and B7-H1 (PD-L1) in the treatment of advanced human cancer. *Clin Cancer Res* 19:1021–1034, 2013.
67. Pardoll DM: The blockade of immune checkpoints in cancer immunotherapy. *Nat Rev Cancer* 12:252–264, 2012.
68. Richter J, Neparidze N, Zhang L, et al: Clinical regressions and broad immune activation following combination therapy targeting human NKT cells in myeloma. *Blood* 121:423–430, 2013.
69. Hawiger D, Inaba K, Dorsett Y, et al: Dendritic cells induce peripheral T cell unresponsiveness under steady state conditions in vivo. *J Exp Med* 194:769–779, 2001.
70. Dhodapkar MV, Sznol M, Zhao B, et al: Induction of antigen-specific immunity with a vaccine targeting NY-ESO-1 to the dendritic cell receptor DEC-205. *Sci Transl Med* 6:232ra51, 2014.
71. Kreutz M, Tacken PJ, Figdor CG: Targeting dendritic cells—Why bother? *Blood* 121:2836–2844, 2013.
72. Pulendran B, Tang H, Denning TL: Division of labor, plasticity, and crosstalk between dendritic cell subsets. *Curr Opin Immunol* 20:61–67, 2008.
73. Sehgal K, Ragheb R, Fahmy TM, et al: Nanoparticle-mediated combinatorial targeting of multiple human dendritic cell (DC) subsets leads to enhanced T cell activation via IL-15-dependent DC crosstalk. *J Immunol* 193:2297–2305, 2014.
74. Hashimoto D, Merad M: Harnessing dendritic cells to improve allogeneic hematopoietic cell transplantation outcome. *Semin Immunol* 23:50–57, 2011.
75. Merad M, Hoffmann P, Ranheim E, et al: Depletion of host Langerhans cells before transplantation of donor alloreactive T cells prevents skin graft-versus-host disease. *Nat Med* 10:510–517, 2004.
76. Toubai T, Mathewson N, Reddy P: The role of dendritic cells in graft-versus-tumor effect. *Front Immunol* 5:66, 2014.
77. Sehgal K, Guo X, Koduru S, et al: Plasmacytoid dendritic cells, interferon signaling, and FcγR contribute to pathogenesis and therapeutic response in childhood immune thrombocytopenia. *Sci Transl Med* 5:193ra89, 2013.

Part V **Therapeutic Principles**

22. Pharmacology and Toxicity of
    Antineoplastic Drugs 315

23. Hematopoietic
    Cell Transplantation. 353

24. Treatment of Infections in the
    Immunocompromised Host 383

25. Antithrombotic Therapy 393

26. Immune Cell Therapy 409

27. Vaccine Therapy 421

28. Therapeutic Apheresis: Indications,
    Efficacy, and Complications 427

29. Gene Therapy for Hematologic
    Diseases. 437

30. Regenerative Medicine:
    Multipotential Cell Therapy for
    Tissue Repair 447

CHAPTER 22
PHARMACOLOGY AND TOXICITY OF ANTINEOPLASTIC DRUGS

Benjamin Izar, Dustin Dzube, James M. Cleary, Constantine S. Mitsiades, Paul G. Richardson, Jeffrey A. Barnes, and Bruce A. Chabner

SUMMARY

The safe and effective use of anticancer drugs in the treatment of hematologic malignancies requires an in-depth knowledge of the pharmacology of these agents. In this field of medicine, the margin of safety is narrow and the potential for serious toxicity is real. At the same time, anticancer drugs cure many hematologic malignancies and provide palliation for others. The discovery and development of treatments for leukemia and lymphoma have provided a paradigm for approaches to the improved treatment of the more common solid tumors.

The intelligent use of these drugs begins with an understanding of their mechanism of action. Cytotoxic anticancer drugs inhibit the synthesis of DNA or directly attack its integrity through the formation of DNA adducts or enzyme-mediated breaks. These DNA-directed actions are recognized by repair processes and by the checkpoints that monitor DNA integrity, including most prominently p53. If DNA damage cannot be repaired, and if the DNA damage reaches thresholds for activating programmed cell death, then DNA damage is translated into tumor regression. Attention has turned to the possibility of identifying molecular targets unique to tumor cells, or dramatically

overexpressed in those cells, including molecules involved in cell signaling and cell-cycle control, but the principles of drug action and resistance to these compounds remain the same. Resistance to drug action can arise from alterations in any one of the critical steps required for drug activity; these steps include drug uptake and distribution through the bloodstream or across the blood–brain barrier; transport across the cell membrane; transformation of the parent drug to its active form within the tumor cell or in the liver; interaction of the drug with its target protein or nucleic acid; enzymatic or chemical inactivation of the agent; drug transport out of the cell; and elimination of the agent from the body through the kidneys or through metabolic transformation. The underlying mutability of tumors leads to the spontaneous generation of cells with alterations in drug uptake, transformation, inactivation, and target binding. In the presence of the selective pressure of drug, resistant tumors replace sensitive cells as the dominant tumor population. Combination chemotherapy overcomes resistance that carries specificity for single agents, but the expression of multidrug resistance genes, as well as loss of the apoptotic response, can result in resistance even to combination drug therapy.

In addition to the molecular determinants of drug action, pharmacokinetics (the disposition of drugs in humans) plays a critical role in determining drug effectiveness and toxicity. Drug regimens are designed to achieve a maximally effective concentration in plasma and tumor cells for an effective duration of exposure. Because of the potential of these agents for toxicity, it is critical for hematologists and oncologists to understand the pathways of drug clearance and to adjust dose in the presence of compromised organ function. Drugs such as methotrexate, hydroxyurea, and the newer purine antagonists (fludarabine and cladribine) are eliminated primarily by renal excretion and should not be used in full doses in patients with renal dysfunction. Similarly, hepatic dysfunction with an elevated serum bilirubin concentration should alert clinicians to decrease doses of the taxanes, vinca alkaloids, and the anthracyclines. In addition, clinicians must be alert to the potential for drug interactions, particularly the ability of drugs that induce or inhibit cytochrome metabolism to alter patterns of drug elimination.

Acronyms and Abbreviations: ABVD, Adriamycin (doxorubicin), bleomycin, vinblastine, and dacarbazine; ADCC, antibody-dependent cellular cytotoxicity; αKG, α-ketoglutarate; ALL, acute lymphocytic leukemia; AML, acute myelogenous leukemia; APL, acute promyelocytic leukemia; ara-C, cytarabine; ara-CTP, cytarabine triphosphate; ara-G, arabinosylguanine; ara-GTP, arabinosylguanine triphosphate; ara-U, arabinosyluracil; ATRA, all-*trans* retinoic acid; BCNU, bischloroethylnitrosourea; BCRP, breast cancer resistance protein transporter; BET, bromodomain and extraterminal; BTK, Bruton tyrosine kinase; CHF, congestive heart failure; CLL, chronic lymphocytic leukemia; CML, chronic myelogenous leukemia; COMFORT, Controlled Myelofibrosis Study with Oral JAK Inhibitor Treatment; CrCl, creatinine clearance; CYP, cytochrome P450; dCK, deoxycytidine kinase; dCTP, deoxycytidine triphosphate; DHFR, dihydrofolate reductase; DNMT, DNA methyltransferase; DTIC, dimethyltriazenoimidazole carboxamide; EPO, erythropoietin; ET, essential thrombocythemia; etoposide, VP-16; EZH2, enhancer of zest homologue 2; FBP, folate-binding protein; GM-CSF, granulocyte-macrophage colony-stimulating factor; HDAC, histone deacetylase; hENT, human equilibrative nucleoside transporter; 2HG, 2-hydroxyglutarate; Hgb, hemoglobin; HGPRT, hypoxanthine guanine phosphoribosyltransferase; IC_{50}, inhibiting growth by concentration 50 percent; IDH, isocitrate dehydrogenase; IL, interleukin; IMiD, immunomodulatory drug; IRF4, interferon regulatory factor 4; IRIS, International Randomized Study of Interferon and STI571; JAK, Janus-type tyrosine kinase; JMJC, Jumonji-C domain; MDR, multidrug resistance; MDS, myelodysplastic syndrome; mesna, sodium 2-mercaptoethane sulfonate; MLL, mixed-lineage leukemia; MOPP, nitrogen mustard, vincristine (Oncovin), procarbazine, and prednisone; 6-MP, 6-mercaptopurine; MPN, myeloproliferative neoplasm; MRI, magnetic resonance imaging; MRP, multidrug resistance-associated protein; MTD, maximum tolerated dose; MUGA, multigated acquisition scan; NK, natural killer; OCT1, organic cation transporter-1; PDGFR, platelet-derived growth factor receptor; PEG, monomethoxypolyethylene glycol; PMF, primary myelofibrosis; PRC2, polycomb repressive complex 2; PRPP, phosphoribosyl pyrophosphate; PV, polycythemia vera; RARα, retinoic acid receptor-α; REMS, risk evaluation and mitigation strategy; RNR, ribonucleotide reductase; SAMe, S-adenosyl-L-methionine; S-phase, synthetic-phase; STAT, signal transducer and activator of transcription; teniposide, VM-26; 6-TG, 6-thioguanine; TKI, tyrosine kinase inhibitor; Topo II, topoisomerase II; TPMT, 5-thiopurine-methyltransferase; TPO, thrombopoietin.

Inherited genetic variations in drug-metabolizing enzymes may lead to an increased risk of drug toxicity and may alter the antitumor response. The most important of these familial syndromes affecting treatment of leukemia is the deficiency of thiopurine methyltransferase, which slows the elimination of 6-mercaptopurine (6-MP) and leads to unanticipated toxicity during maintenance chemotherapy for acute lymphocytic leukemia. Pharmacokinetic monitoring has a standard role in the use of certain therapies, particularly high-dose methotrexate, and in the evaluation of new drugs or new drug combinations. To ensure appropriate dosing, and management of toxicity, there is no substitute for therapy based on standard protocols and peer-reviewed clinical trials. Adherence to protocols ensures that the pharmacologic variables affecting drug disposition can be taken into account early in the course of treatment and that serious untoward events can be avoided while maintaining effective therapy.

The leukemias and lymphomas have been the initial testing ground for cancer chemotherapy. Because of their rapid rates of proliferation, lack of surgical treatment options, ready access to malignant cells, and availability of mouse models of leukemia, the hematologic malignancies drew the attention of early investigators interested in treating cancer with drugs. The first evidence for activity of a chemical antitumor agent came in 1942, from the experimental work and subsequent clinical trials conducted by Goodman, Gilman, and colleagues at Yale, and their observation that nitrogen mustard caused tumor regression in a patient with Hodgkin lymphoma.[1] Six years later, Sidney Farber, a pathologist at Children's Hospital in Boston, made the even more startling discovery of remission induction by aminopterin and then methotrexate in acute lymphocytic leukemia (ALL). His work ushered in the modern era of chemotherapy.[2] Over the next 20 years, clinical trials in these diseases established the basic principles of cyclic combination therapy and dose intensification,[3] developed effective strategies for management of infectious and hemorrhagic complications, and led to the cure of these diseases with chemotherapy. High-dose chemotherapy with marrow reconstitution has further extended the cure rate in leukemias and lymphomas. As our understanding of the biologic and molecular basis for malignancy has advanced, the concept of molecularly targeted therapy achieved its first striking success with the development of imatinib mesylate for chronic myelogenous leukemia (CML).[4] Studies of relapsing patients on imatinib provided the first clear evidence for target mutation as a mechanism of clinical drug resistance.[5] The first effective use of a monoclonal antibody, rituximab, has extended the cure rate for patients with large cell lymphomas, and the first clear demonstration of drug-induced differentiation by all-trans retinoic acid (ATRA) has led to a remarkable improvement in the cure rate of acute promyelocytic leukemia (APL).[6] Other unique noncytotoxic drugs with unusual mechanisms of action, such as L-asparaginase, thalidomide, and bortezomib, have become valuable components of regimens for specific kinds of hematologic malignancies. Molecular studies of the abnormalities in pathways that control proliferation and survival lymphomas and leukemias have revealed distinct subsets of disease have identified new therapeutic targets.

● BASIC PRINCIPLES OF CANCER CHEMOTHERAPY

The safe and effective use of chemotherapy in clinical practice requires a thorough understanding of the basic aspects of drug action as well as knowledge of the important clinical toxicities, pharmacokinetics, and

drug interactions of the various agents. Antineoplastic chemotherapy is a complex undertaking, with the potential for serious or fatal side effects. Patients are best served if their treatment is based on evidence from clinical trials, which define optimal doses, schedules, and drug combinations. The specific protocol chosen for treatment should be appropriate not only for the stage and histology of the tumor but should consider individual patient comorbidities, age, and susceptibility to specific potential toxicities. Thus, bleomycin is not a safe choice for a patient with serious underlying renal or lung disease, nor is doxorubicin an appropriate drug for use in a patient with a history of congestive heart failure; even in patients with normal cardiac or pulmonary function, total dose limits should be respected for these agents. Even though clinical trials define the benefits and risks of a cohort of patients of a defined age range and physiology, these results may not be easily extrapolated to patients at the extreme ends of the spectrum.

Depending on the major route of drug clearance, doses should be modified for renal or hepatic dysfunction (Table 22–1). Changes in the dose and schedule of a drug (dose-dense chemotherapy) offer potentially greater antitumor effects, but often lead to unique toxicities. With the development of techniques for marrow or blood stem cell storage and replacement of marrow after chemotherapy, potentially lethal doses of chemotherapy can be administered in an attempt to cure malignancies

TABLE 22–1. Dose Modification in Patients with Renal or Hepatic Dysfunction

Renal dysfunction (creatinine clearance <60 mL/min)

Reduce dose in proportion to reduction in creatinine clearance.

Drugs
1. Methotrexate
2. Cisplatin
3. Carboplatin
4. Bleomycin
5. Etoposide
6. Hydroxyurea
7. Deoxycoformycin
8. Fludarabine phosphate
9. Cladribine
10. Topotecan
11. imatinib
12. Dasatinib (likely, but no guidelines available)
13. Lenalidomide

Hepatic dysfunction

For bilirubin >1.5 mg/dL reduce initial dose by 50%.

For bilirubin >3.0 mg/dL reduce initial dose by 75%.

Drugs
1. Amsacrine
2. Doxorubicin
3. Daunorubicin
4. Vincristine
5. Vinblastine
6. Paclitaxel and docetaxel
7. Mitoxantrone
8. Gleevec
9. Dasatinib

refractory to standard regimens. In general, these regimens may produce organ toxicities not seen at conventional doses—including pneumonitis, cardiac failure, vascular endothelial damage, and hepatic and renal insufficiency—and are ordinarily reserved for patients of younger age and with normal baseline organ function.

The success of chemotherapy in curing hematologic malignancy is incompletely understood. Although targeted therapies exploit clear differences in biology conferred by mutations or amplification of key genes, an explanation for the differential effects of cytotoxic drugs on tumor versus normal tissues is less obvious. The greater susceptibility of malignant cells to drug toxicity, as reflected in the phenomenon of leukemia remission induction, with restoration of normal marrow function, may result from the relative resistance of normal marrow stem cells to drug injury. These stem cells exist in a nonreplicating phase of the cell cycle, where they are less susceptible to damage by DNA-directed agents, and they express genes that protect against chemical and hypoxic damage. In addition, there is growing evidence that cancer cells lack cell-cycle checkpoints that recognize DNA damage and activate repair of DNA strand breaks, base deletions, or other lesions induced by chemotherapy. This differential in repair capability may allow normal cells to repair damage and promote recovery from chemotherapy-induced injury.

COMBINATION CHEMOTHERAPY

Most leukemias and lymphomas are highly drug sensitive, but, with the exception of the curability of Burkitt lymphoma (treated with cyclophosphamide) and hairy cell leukemia (treated with cladribine), are rarely, if ever, cured with single-agent chemotherapy. Combination chemotherapy forestalls the emergence of drug-resistant cells and thus is curative in settings where individual agents are ineffective. Empiric principles have resulted from the clinical experience of the past 4 decades of combination therapy. In general, drugs selected for combination therapy should have demonstrable antineoplastic activity, or at least biologic effects, against the tumor in question. The lone exception may be targeted drugs that inhibit signal transduction or angiogenesis; antibodies such as trastuzumab or rituximab may exhibit limited antitumor activity on their own, but may significantly augment the action of cytotoxic agents.[7] Individual agents in a combination should be chosen based on their different mechanisms of action and lack of a common mechanism of resistance such as multidrug resistance (MDR). The dose-limiting toxicities of the agents chosen should not overlap; otherwise, they could not be used together at or near full doses. The clinical use of specific combinations should be based on preclinical evidence of synergistic interaction, and single-agent activity in the disease in question. Favorable molecular or biochemical drug interactions may be dependent on specific schedules of administration. Pharmacokinetic interactions should be defined in initial trials of drug combinations so as to avoid under- or overdosing of individual agents.

Another important consideration in designing clinical protocols is dose intensity, the dose administered per unit time, which should be maintained throughout a treatment regimen. Achieving this objective may require the use of hematopoietic growth factors to hasten marrow recovery, prevent repeated episodes of febrile neutropenia, and allow ontime administration of the next treatment cycle.

Interdigitation of chemotherapy with surgery and irradiation makes it possible to take advantage of favorable cytokinetic or radiosensitizing effects of chemotherapy, but drugs may enhance radiation or surgical toxicity to normal organs, an interaction that requires careful consideration in designing a multidisciplinary regimen. Thus, 5-fluorouracil and cisplatin are potent radiosensitizers used with radiation therapy to enhance local tumor control in solid tumors.

In the treatment of lymphomas, the toxicity of radiation therapy to sensitive organs such as skin, lung, heart, and brain may be significantly increased by concurrent administration of anthracyclines, a consideration that has prompted the use of radiation therapy either before or after anthracycline antibiotics, but not concurrently. Likewise, bleomycin sensitizes the lungs to damage by high concentration of inspired O_2 during surgery. Antiangiogenic therapies, rarely used in hematologic malignancies, are associated with an increased risk of bowel perforation in patients who have recently undergone intraabdominal surgery.

CELL KINETICS AND CANCER CHEMOTHERAPY

The cell-killing characteristics of cancer chemotherapeutic agents vary according to their mechanism of action. Many of the most effective agents in antileukemic therapy belong to the antimetabolite class, including cytarabine and methotrexate. These drugs kill cells most effectively during the DNA synthetic phase (S-phase) of the cell cycle. For these agents, a prolonged period of tumor exposure to drug is essential so as to maximize the number of cells exposed during the vulnerable period of the cell cycle. As would be predicted, the antimetabolite drugs are primarily active against rapidly dividing tumors such as acute leukemias and intermediate and high-grade lymphomas. Other anticancer drugs, such as the topoisomerase inhibitors and alkylating agents, do not require cells to be exposed during a specific phase of the cell cycle, although like the antimetabolites, these drugs are generally more effective against actively proliferating cells as compared to resting cells. Still others, most notably the nitrosoureas and busulfan, are equally toxic to dividing and nondividing cells, and at the same time, deplete marrow stem cells. In general, the toxicity of alkylating agents is determined by the total dose of drug, whereas for the cell-cycle-specific drugs (such as methotrexate and cytarabine), both drug concentration and duration of exposure determine cytocidal effect. However, for drugs that act through alternate mechanisms, such as the taxanes, myelosuppression correlates best with the duration of exposure above a threshold plasma concentration, which is approximately 50 to 100 nM for paclitaxel and 200 nM for docetaxel.[8]

High-dose regimens achieve a number of worthwhile objectives for these agents, including an enhancement of cross-membrane transport, saturation of anabolic pathways inside the cell, and prolongation of the period of effective drug concentration. However, achieving these objectives is realized at the cost of increased toxicity to normal proliferating marrow precursor cells and may produce significant and unexpected damage to normal organs, such as hepatic venoocclusive disease (alkylating agents), cerebellar toxicity (certain alkylating agents and cytarabine [ara-C]), or pulmonary toxicity (nitrosoureas and alkylating agents). Because hematopoietic stem cells can be harvested, stored, and reinfused, dose-limiting toxicities of high-dose chemotherapy are generally those affecting nonhematologic organs.

The choice of an appropriate dose and schedule of drug administration depends on a number of factors: (1) the drug's cell-cycle dependence; (2) the often empirically derived relationship between antitumor effects, drug dose, and schedule; (3) pharmacokinetic behavior and the need to maintain a specific drug concentration for a given period of time; (4) potential interactions with other components of the treatment regimen; and (5) patient tolerance. Multiple clinical trials are required to establish safe and effective single-agent regimens and drug combinations. For molecularly targeted drugs, the aim is to maintain inhibition of the target for prolonged periods of time, keeping drug levels above a threshold for toxicity to tumor cells, but balancing these considerations against the potential for toxicity to normal tissues, such as skin, liver, and intestinal epithelium.

DRUG RESISTANCE

Inadequate treatment of a sensitive tumor tends to select for the outgrowth of drug-resistant clones of the original tumor. The reasons for emergence of drug resistance are manifold. Cancer cells often harbor basic defects in DNA repair as one of their hallmark mutations and spontaneously generate drug-resistant mutants, even in the absence of drug exposure. Thus it has been demonstrated in the specific example of imatinib treatment of CML that drug-resistant cells, carrying specific mutations in the *BCR-ABL* gene, can be identified in marrow prior to treatment and become the dominant tumor population under the selective pressure of drug treatment.[5] A similar finding of pretreatment mutations explains drug resistance to inhibitors to the epidermal growth factor receptor in non–small-cell lung cancer.[9] In addition, many cancer drugs, especially alkylating agents, and irradiation are mutagenic and increase the rate of generation of drug-resistant mutants, as demonstrated in the selection of mismatch repair mutants by temozolomide.[10] To discourage the outgrowth of resistant cells, multiple agents with differing mechanisms of resistance should be used simultaneously, because the likelihood of there being a doubly or triply resistant cell is the product of the probabilities of the independent drug-resistant mutations occurring at the same time in a single cell. The probability of a cell division resulting in mutation at any given genetic locus is approximately 10^{-6} for any given episode of cell division in somatic cells; thus the probability of two independent mutations arising in the same cell is 10^{-12}. Mutation rates may be distinctly higher in tumor cells and may be further increased by exposure to alkylating agents and irradiation. Some mutations, such as those affecting apoptosis, may confer resistance to multiple agents of diverse mechanisms of action. Thus, the probability of encountering MDR cells is much higher in reality.

In choosing drugs for combination therapy, one must bear in mind potential mechanisms of resistance. Classical MDR occurs as a consequence of increased expression of drug efflux pumps such as the P-glycoprotein or the MDR-associated proteins (MRPs),[11,12] and confers resistance to a broad spectrum of agents derived from natural products, including taxanes, anthracyclines, vinca alkaloids, and epipodophyllotoxins, and potentially to a number of "targeted" agents. Other mechanisms of resistance that induce amplification of a target gene, such as dihydrofolate reductase (DHFR)[13] or *BCR-ABL* kinase,[14] may be highly specific for a single drug. Table 22–2 lists the common mechanisms of resistance. Although the presence of these biochemical changes is not routinely determined in tumor biopsies prior to therapy, these mechanisms should be considered in developing new protocols and in choosing cytotoxic therapy. In relapse after targeted therapy of CML or certain non–small cell lung cancers, the choice of second-line therapies may rely on studies of tumor cell resistance, as reflected in repeat biopsies of solid tumors or cell sampling in CML.

In addition to drug-specific mechanisms of resistance, mutations that abolish recognition of DNA damage, such as the loss of components of the mismatch repair gene complex (MLH6 or MSH2)[15] seem to block initiation of apoptosis by cisplatin, thiopurines, or alkylating agents. Other mutations that block the induction of apoptosis, such as loss of p53[16] or overexpression of the antiapoptotic factors such as BCL-2,[17] may render tumor cells insensitive to a broad array of drugs and modalities, including ionizing irradiation, alkylating agents, antimetabolites, and anthracyclines. Although the specific contribution of p53 mutation and altered apoptosis to clinical resistance is still uncertain, emerging evidence suggests that these factors are commonly associated with clinical resistance and aggressive tumor growth and may be more relevant causes of drug resistance in the clinic than are the classical drug-specific mechanisms found in experimental tumors.

The contribution of tumor stem cells to treatment resistance and disease recurrence is an intriguing, but as yet undefined, possibility. It is clear that many tissues, including marrow, contain stem cells capable of repopulating organs, even from single cells.[18] Likewise, many tumors contain stem cells, which, on careful evaluation, preserve many of the surface antigens of their normal counterpart, and display resistance to DNA damage, reactive oxygen species generated by drugs or irradiation, and readily export toxic natural products.[19] It is possible, but still to be established, that these drug-resistant stem cells represent the ultimate barrier to successful cancer treatment.

●CELL-CYCLE-SPECIFIC AGENTS

A number of anticancer drugs, particularly those developed during the era of cytotoxic chemotherapy, exert their antitumor effects on DNA synthesis. Cells are thus most vulnerable during periods of active DNA synthesis (S-phase), and least affected during quiescent (G_0) stages of their life cycle. Thus tumors that have a high proliferative rate, such as leukemias and aggressive lymphomas, are most vulnerable to these agents.

METHOTREXATE

Farber and associates showed that the folate antagonist aminopterin induced a complete remission in children with ALL, thereby launching the modern era of chemotherapy. Unfortunately, these remissions were short-lived, and the leukemia invariably became resistant to further treatment. Subsequently, methotrexate, a 4-amino, N-10 methyl analogue of folic acid, supplanted aminopterin because it had more predictable side effects. Methotrexate continues to be a key drug in the induction and maintenance therapy of ALL, in the intrathecal prophylaxis and treatment of CNS leukemia, in the primary treatment of CNS lymphomas, and in combination therapy of high-grade lymphomas.

Mechanisms of Action

Methotrexate enters cells through an active uptake process mediated in most tumor cells by the reduced folate transporter[20] and is actively effluxed from cells by the MRP class of exporters.[21] A second uptake transporter, the membrane folate-binding protein (FBP), has lower affinity for methotrexate, but may contribute to uptake of other antifolates, such as pemetrexed. The FBP is found on many solid malignancies, and is an active target for folate analogue- and antibody-mediated drug development. A third, low pH transporter may also participate in methotrexate influx, particularly in the intestine, but its role in tumor uptake is uncertain.[22] By virtue of its 4-amino substitution, methotrexate potently inhibits the enzyme DHFR, which recycles oxidized dihydrofolate to its active tetrahydrofolate state. Inhibition of DHFR leads to rapid depletion of the intracellular tetrahydrofolate coenzymes required for thymidylate and purine biosynthesis. As a result, DNA synthesis is blocked and cell replication stops. Methotrexate is retained intracellularly as a consequence of an enzymatic process that adds up to six glutamate moieties in an unusual peptide linkage to the γ-carboxyl group of the drug (Fig. 22–1). Polyglutamation is an important determinant of leukemic cell sensitivity to methotrexate. Methotrexate polyglutamates, in addition to their long persistence in cells and their potent inhibition of DHFR, have greatly increased inhibitory effects on other folate-dependent enzymes, including thymidylate synthase and enzymes that synthesize purines (Fig. 22–2). Cells that convert the drug to polyglutamates efficiently, such as leukemic myeloblasts and lymphoblasts, are more susceptible to the drug than are normal myeloid precursors, which have limited capability for polyglutamation.[23] Accumulation of polyglutamates correlates with increased cytotoxicity and treatment response in childhood lymphoblastic leukemia.[24] Hyperdiploid ALLs are particularly efficient in transporting methotrexate and in producing polyglutamated species, factors that may contribute to their favorable

TABLE 22–2. Mechanisms of Resistance to Anticancer Drugs

Mechanisms	Drugs Affected	Clinical Role
1. Decreased drug uptake		
Reduced folate transporter	Methotrexate	ALL
Nucleoside transporter	cytarabine	AML
2. Increased drug efflux		
MDR transporter (P-glycoprotein)	Anthracyclines, vinca alkaloids, taxanes, etoposide	Myeloma, AML, non-Hodgkin lymphoma
MRP transporters, breast cancer- resistant protein	Anthracyclines, vinca alkaloids, taxanes, etoposide	Breast cancer
3. Decreased drug activation in tumor		
Deoxycytidine kinase deletion	cytarabine, fludarabine, cladribine, clofarabine	AML, CLL, hairy cell leukemia
Hypoxanthine phosphoribosyltransferase deletion	6-Mercaptopurine	Uncertain
Folylpolyglutamation	Methotrexate	Acute leukemias
4. Increased drug inactivation defect		
Thiopurine methyltransferase	6-Mercaptopurine	ALL
Bleomycin hydrolase	Bleomycin	Uncertain
Glutathione transferase	Alkylating agents	Uncertain
5. Decreased target enzyme		
Topoisomerase I	Camptothecins	Uncertain
Topoisomerase II	Anthracyclines, etoposide	Uncertain
6. Increased target enzyme		
Dihydrofolate reductase	Methotrexate	Acute leukemia, small cell lung cancer
Thymidylate synthase	5-Fluorouracil	Solid tumors
Adenosine deaminase	Deoxycoformycin	Lymphoid tumors
7. Mutated intracellular target		
BCR-ABL kinase	Imatinib mesylate, dasatinib	CML
Tubulin	Vinca alkaloids, taxanes	Uncertain
Topoisomerase I	Camptothecins	Uncertain
Topoisomerase II	Anthracyclines, etoposide	Uncertain
8. Increase DNA repair		
Guanine-O-6-methyltransferase	Procarbazine, nitrosoureas temozolomide	Brain tumors
Nucleotide excision repair	Platinating drugs	Ovarian cancer
9. Decreased DNA damage recognition		
p53 mutation	Many cancer drugs, radiation	Leukemias, lymphomas
Mismatch DNA repair mutations	Platinating agents, methylating drugs, thiopurines	Colon cancer, glioblastoma, leukemias

ALL, acute lymphocytic leukemia; AML, acute myelogenous leukemia; CLL, chronic lymphocytic leukemia; CML, chronic myelogenous leukemia; MDR, multidrug resistance; MRP, multidrug resistance-associated protein. See text for references and explanation.

prognosis.[25] Polyglutamates are slowly degraded to their readily effluxed monoglutamate form by γ-glutamyl hydrolase, and a polymorphism (T127I) that deceases γ-glutamyl hydrolase activity is associated with enhanced polyglutamate accumulation in leukemic cells.[26] Acquired resistance to methotrexate in patients with leukemia is associated with several different alterations: increased levels of DHFR as a consequence of gene amplification,[13] defective polyglutamation,[27] impaired drug uptake,[28] or increased efflux by the MRP class of transporters.[29]

Clinical Pharmacology

Methotrexate is well absorbed when administered orally at low doses (5 to 10 mg/m^2), but when doses exceed 30 mg/m^2, absorption is variable. Consequently, doses greater than 25 mg/m^2 should be administered parenterally.

The concentration of methotrexate in plasma declines in a polyexponential manner. A very rapid initial disposition phase persists for only a few minutes after intravenous administration. The intermediate disposition phase has a 2- to 4-hour half-life and continues for 12 to 24 hours after dosing. The terminal phase of drug decay is considerably slower, with an 8- to 10-hour half-life, and this phase becomes important in determining drug toxicity and the effectiveness of leucovorin rescue in patients treated with high-dose methotrexate. Methotrexate is primarily excreted unchanged by the kidney, while a minor fraction of the drug (7 to 30 percent) is inactivated by hepatic hydroxylation at

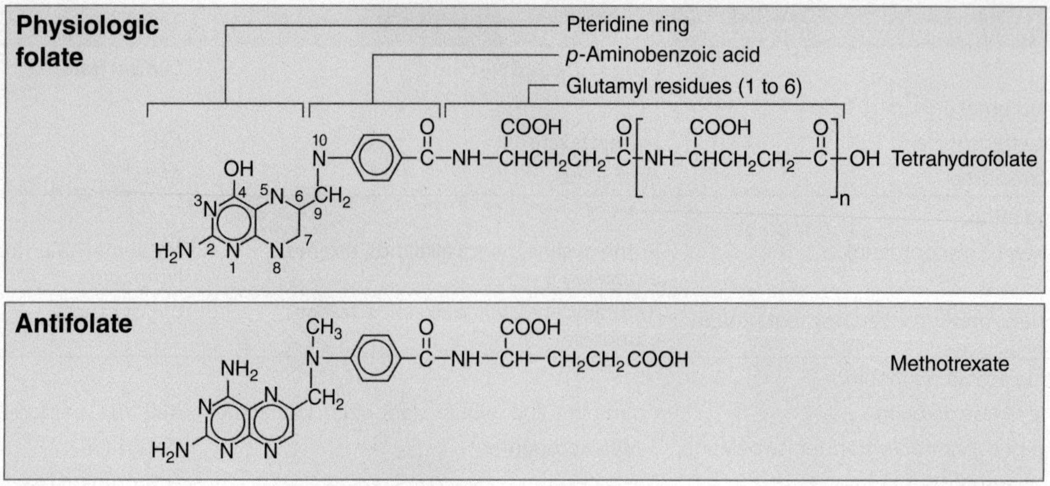

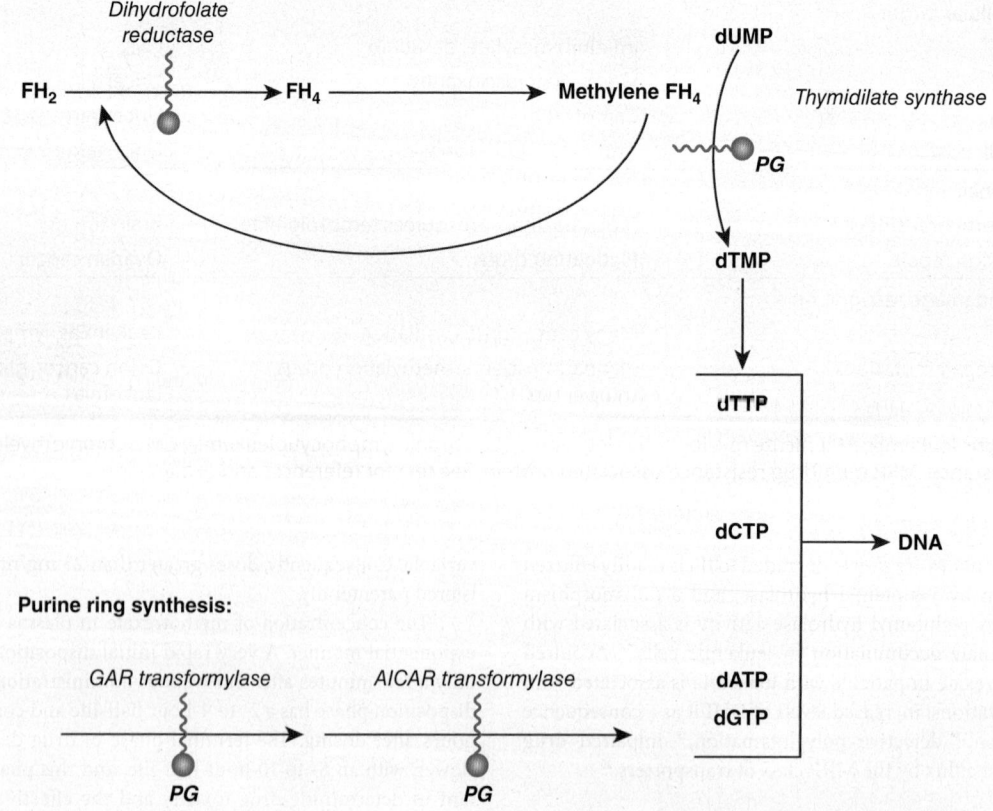

Figure 22–1. Structures of folate, tetrahydrofolate, and its analogue methotrexate. The vitamin is absorbed as a monoglutamate and converted intracellularly to a polyglutamate, in which form it is both physiologically active and is stored in cells. Methotrexate, the 2,4-diamino analogue of folic acid, is shown in the bottom panel and is also converted to a polyglutamate intracellularly. *(Reproduced with permission from Brunton L, Chabner B, and Knollman B: Goodman & Gilman's The Pharmacological Basis of Therapeutics, 12th ed. New York, NY: McGraw-Hill; 2011.)*

the 7 position. Thus, doses should be reduced in proportion to the decrease in creatinine clearance (CrCl) in patients with renal impairment (CrCl <60 mL/min), because the prolonged exposure to high blood levels may result in life-threatening hematologic and gastrointestinal toxicity.[30] High-dose methotrexate (>0.5 g/m²) followed by leucovorin rescue is used to treat patients with high-grade lymphoma, osteosarcoma, and ALL.

In ALL, dose adjustment of methotrexate to maintain a specific area under the concentration × time (C × T) curve improves treatment outcome.[31] Patients receiving high-dose methotrexate can be rescued from drug toxicity by administering small doses of N-10-formyltetrahydrofolate (leucovorin), which replenishes the intracellular pool of reduced folates. Leucovorin is administered intravenously or orally in doses of 10 to 15 mg/m² at 6-hour intervals, starting 6 to 24 hours

Figure 22–2. Mechanism of methotrexate action. Sites of enzyme inhibition by methotrexate and its polyglutamates *(PG)*. AICAR, aminoimidazole-carboxamide ribonucleotide; dUMP, deoxyuridine monophosphate; FH_2, dihydrofolate; FH_4, tetrahydrofolate; GAR, glycine amide ribonucleotide.

after the infusion of methotrexate, and continuing until plasma concentrations of the drug fall below 1 μM. In patients receiving high-dose methotrexate, drug levels are routinely assayed 24 to 48 hours after dosing to determine the rate of drug elimination and the safety of discontinuing leucovorin. Both methotrexate and its hydroxylated metabolite are organic acids, which, like uric acid, are much more soluble in alkaline urine. In patients receiving such therapy, renal toxicity may result from intrarenal precipitation of the parent drug or its 7-OH metabolite, and is generally the primary cause of decreased drug clearance and overwhelming toxicity. Renal dysfunction can be prevented by alkalinizing the urine to pH 7 with intravenous sodium bicarbonate prior to and during therapy. Patients should be given intensive hydration, as well. If drug concentrations in plasma exceed 1 μM at 48 hours after high-dose therapy, leucovorin should be continued at higher doses of 50 to 100 mg/m^2 every 6 hours until methotrexate concentrations fall below 0.1 μM. The higher doses of leucovorin are necessary to compete with methotrexate for transport and polyglutamation. In cases of extreme renal failure, with stable drug levels in the 10 μM range, leucovorin will not be effective. In this setting, continuous flow hemodialysis may provide a sustained reduction in drug levels.[32] An alternative effective measure in this circumstance is the administration of glucarpidase, a commercially available bacterial enzyme that instantly degrades antifolates[33] and prevents further toxicity.

Adverse Effects

The dose-limiting toxicities of methotrexate are myelosuppression and gastrointestinal toxicity. Toxic doses of methotrexate can induce thrombocytopenia and/or leukopenia, although leukopenia is more common. An early indication of methotrexate toxicity to the gastrointestinal tract is oral mucositis, whereas more severe toxicity may be manifested as diarrhea and gastrointestinal bleeding. Less-common toxic effects of methotrexate are skin rash (10 percent), pneumonitis, and chemical hepatitis. Transaminase elevations are frequently seen after high-dose methotrexate but rapidly return to normal in most patients, and without sequelae, but low-dose chronic administration, as employed to treat psoriasis or rheumatoid arthritis, may lead to portal fibrosis and cirrhosis.

Methotrexate, given intrathecally in doses of 12 mg every 4 days for children older than age 3 years and for adults, is used to prevent or treat meningeal leukemia and lymphoma. Dose adjustment is required for children younger than age 3 years, and should be made according to established protocols. Because the drug distributes poorly into the ventricular system after spinal injection, patients with active meningeal leukemia are frequently treated through an indwelling ventricular reservoir. Toxicities caused by intrathecal administration of methotrexate include acute arachnoiditis with nuchal rigidity and headache, as well as more chronic CNS toxicities, such as dementia, motor deficits, seizures, and coma.[34] Rarely, these neurotoxicities develop hours after intrathecal drug administration, but more commonly they occur in the days or weeks after initiation of intrathecal treatment, and are most often seen in patients with active meningeal leukemia. Leucovorin is ineffective in reversing or preventing these toxicities. Patients with such signs should undergo evaluation to rule out progressive CNS tumor, and if malignancy is not found, intrathecal cytarabine should be used for further therapy.

Methotrexate and 6-mercaptopurine (6-MP) are synergistic in their inhibition of purine biosynthesis. L-Asparaginase, an inhibitor of protein synthesis, blocks cells from entering DNA synthesis and antagonizes the effects of methotrexate, when used before the antifolate. The two drugs are not used concurrently.

Nonsteroidal antiinflammatory drugs, which diminish renal blood flow, may reduce methotrexate clearance, as may nephrotoxic antibiotics and platinum derivatives, and these or other renal toxins should be avoided in patients during high-dose methotrexate.

CYTARABINE (CYTOSINE ARABINOSIDE, ARABINOSYL CYTOSINE, ARA-C)

Ara-C is an antimetabolite analogue of cytidine, differing in the configuration at the substituent on C_2' position of the sugar, in which the C_2'-hydroxyl group is *cis*-oriented relative to the C_1'-N-glycosyl bond, in contrast to the *trans* configuration of the ribose nucleoside. Ara-C is a mainstay in the induction of remission in patients with acute myelogenous leukemia (AML).

High doses (1 to 3 g/m^2) of intravenous ara-C given at 12-hour intervals for 6 to 12 doses are more effective alone or in a combination with anthracyclines than conventional doses (100 to 150 mg/m^2 q12h) in consolidation therapy of AML, and they confer particular benefit in patients with cytogenetic abnormalities (t[8:21], inv[16], t[9:16], and del[16]) related to the core binding factor that regulates hematopoiesis.[35] Other subsets of leukemia may have increased sensitivity to ara-C. ALL patients with mixed lineage leukemia (*MLL*) gene translocations have upregulation of the human equilibrative nucleoside transporter (hENT) and have a greater sensitivity to ara-C.[36] AML patients with *K-RAS* gene mutations seem to derive greater benefit from high-dose ara-C than do patients with wild-type K-RAS in their tumors.[37]

Mechanism of Action

Ara-C is converted to the nucleoside triphosphate, cytarabine triphosphate (ara-CTP) intracellularly. The first step is catalyzed by deoxycytidine kinase (dCK); polymorphisms of the *dCK* gene may affect the rate of activation, and ultimately response.[38] Ara-CTP is an inhibitor of DNA polymerase and is also incorporated into DNA, where it terminates strand elongation.[39] If repair is unsuccessful, apoptosis is initiated. Ara-C and its mononucleotide are deaminated and inactivated by two intracellular enzymes, cytidine deaminase and deoxycytidylate deaminase, respectively.

Acquired ara-C resistance in experimental leukemias consistently results from the loss of dCK.[40] Other changes implicated in experimental tumors include decreased drug uptake because of decreased expression of the equilibrative nucleoside transporter, increased deamination, increased pool size of competitive deoxycytidine triphosphate, and inhibition of the apoptotic pathway. Some of these changes, particularly loss of dCK activity, have been reported in studies of human leukemia, but these results have not been confirmed in definitive trials.[41]

Clinical Pharmacology

Ara-C is administered intravenously either as a bolus injection or, more commonly, as a continuous infusion. It is not orally bioavailable because of its degradation by cytidine deaminase, which is present in the gastrointestinal epithelium and liver. Two standard schedules of administration are used: (1) rapid infusion of 100 mg/m^2 every 12 hours for 7 days; or (2) continuous infusion of 100 to 200 mg/m^2 per day for up to 7 days. Ara-C distributes rapidly throughout total-body water and is eliminated from plasma with a biologic half-life of 7 to 20 minutes. Most of the dose is excreted as arabinosyluracil (ara-U), an inactive metabolite, which is formed in plasma, the liver, granulocytes, and other tissues. Inhibition of ara-C deamination by ara-U may be responsible for the prolongation of the biologic half-life of the drug as larger doses are administered.[42] Single-bolus injections and short infusions (30 minutes to 1 hour duration) at doses as high as 5 g/m^2 produce little myelotoxicity because of the drug's rapid clearance, whereas continuous intravenous infusion of only 1 g/m^2 over 48 hours produces severe marrow toxicity. High-dose ara-C (3 g/m^2 q12h for 3 days on days 1, 3, and 5), is routinely used for consolidation therapy of AML, but lower doses of 1 gm/m^2 or less should be used in patients older than 60 years to avoid CNS toxicity. Unlike most drugs, a relatively high concentration of ara-C is achieved in the cerebrospinal fluid after intravenous administration, and may approach 50 percent of the corresponding plasma concentration.

Ara-C is also used intrathecally to treat meningeal leukemia. Doses of 50 to 70 mg in adults are usually employed and afford cerebrospinal fluid levels of the drug near 1 mM, which decline with a half-life of 2 hours. Ara-C (50 mg given every 2 weeks) has been impregnated into a gel matrix, in a formulation called DepoCyt, for sustained release into the cerebrospinal fluid, thus avoiding the need for repeated spinal taps. Initial clinical results in spinal lymphomatous meningitis indicate that it has efficacy equal to that of methotrexate.[43]

Adverse Effects

The dose-limiting toxicity for conventional dosing regimens of intravenous ara-C, 100 to 150 mg/m^2 per day for 5 to 10 days, is myelosuppression. Nausea and vomiting also occur at these doses, the severity of which increases markedly when higher doses are employed, although repeated administration of the drug results in some tolerance. The nadir of the white count and platelet count occurs at about days 7 to 10 after the last dose of drug. Cerebellar, gastrointestinal, and liver toxicity, as well as conjunctivitis have also been observed when high-dose regimens are used. Hepatotoxicity ranges from abnormalities in serum transaminase levels to frank jaundice. The severity of these effects increases as the duration of therapy is prolonged; however, toxic effects rapidly subside upon discontinuation of treatment. Pulmonary infiltrates as a result of noncardiogenic pulmonary edema, and occasionally associated with severe pulmonary dysfunction, occur in leukemic patients receiving ara-C, as do gastrointestinal ulcerations with bleeding and infrequently perforation. Ara-C treatment is also reported to predispose to *Streptococcus viridans* pneumonia.[44]

In patients older than 60 years of age, and in patients with renal dysfunction, intravenous high-dose ara-C (3 g/m^2 every 12 hours, days 1, 3, and 5, for six doses) causes a high incidence of cerebellar toxicity, manifested as ataxia and slurred speech.[45] Confusion and dementia may supervene, leading to a fatal outcome. Cerebellar toxicity is more frequent in patients with abnormal renal function because of slowed elimination of ara-U, with consequent inhibition of ara-C deamination. Intrathecal ara-C is usually well tolerated, but neurologic side effects have been reported (seizures, alterations in mental status).

GEMCITABINE

Although primarily used for solid tumors, gemcitabine, a 2'-2'-difluoro analogue of deoxycytidine, has significant activity against Hodgkin lymphoma. Its mechanism of action is similar to ara-C, in that, as a triphosphate, it competes with deoxycytidine triphosphate for incorporation into the elongating DNA strand, where it terminates DNA synthesis. It is also self-potentiating in that at a second site of action, it inhibits ribonucleotide reductase and thereby reduces competitive pools of deoxycytidine triphosphate (dCTP). It achieves higher nucleotide levels in tumor cells than does ara-CTP, and has a longer intracellular half-life. Its clinical pharmacokinetics are determined primarily by its rapid deamination by cytidine deaminase, yielding a short plasma half-life ($t_{1/2}$) of 15 to 30 minutes. Standard schedules use 1000 mg/m^2 infused over 30 minutes, and produced peak drug concentrations of 20–60 μM in plasma. Longer infusion times may produce higher intracellular triphosphate concentrations, but the benefit is uncertain.[46]

Resistance in solid tumors arises from low expression of hENT, increased expression of ribonucleotide reductase, and low levels of the initial activating enzyme, dCK. Gemcitabine is an extremely potent radiosensitizer and should not be used concurrently with radiation therapy except in clinical trials.

Toxicities are acute myelosuppression, mild hepatic enzyme elevations, uncommonly a reversible pneumonitis, and with prolonged usage, a progressive hemolytic uremic syndrome with capillary leak, leading to pleural effusions, ascites, and renal failure.[47]

5-AZACYTIDINE AND 5-AZA-2'-DEOXYCYTIDINE

Both 5-azacytidine and decitabine (5-aza-2'-deoxycytidine), its closely related deoxy analogue, exhibit cytotoxic activity and also induce differentiation of malignant cells at low doses. The latter action results from their incorporation into DNA and their covalent inactivation of DNA methyltransferase. The resulting inhibition of methylation of cytosine bases in DNA leads to enhanced transcription of otherwise silent genes.[48] The differentiating effects of 5-azacytidine are the basis for the induction of fetal hemoglobin synthesis in patients with sickle cell anemia and thalassemia[53] and its approved use in low-dose therapy of myelodysplastic syndromes (MDS). The usual doses of 5-azacytidine are 75 mg/m^2 subcutaneously or intravenously per day for 7 days, repeated every 28 days, whereas decitabine is used in doses of 20 mg intravenously every day for 5 days every 4 weeks. Responses become apparent in myelodysplasia after two to five courses.

5-Azacytidine and decitabine are rapidly deaminated to chemically unstable uridine metabolites that immediately degrade into inactive products. Pharmacologic activity results from phosphorylation of the parent compound by cytidine kinase (for 5-azacytidine) or dCK (for decitabine), with subsequent conversion to a triphosphate nucleotide that becomes incorporated into DNA. The primary clinical toxicities of both 5-azacytidine and decitabine[49] include reversible myelosuppression, nausea and vomiting with higher doses, hepatic dysfunction, myalgia, and fever and rash. Resistance likely results from defects in drug activation or alternative mechanisms for gene silencing, such as histone methylation or acetylation.

PURINE ANALOGUES

Purine analogues (Fig. 22–3) occupy an important role in maintenance for childhood ALL, and in the past decade newer analogues have shown remarkable activity in chronic leukemias and small cell lymphomas. With methotrexate, 6-MP is a critical component in the maintenance phase of curative therapy of childhood ALL. Other purine analogues include azathioprine, a prodrug of 6-MP and potent immunosuppressive agent; allopurinol, an inhibitor of xanthine oxidase, useful in the prevention of uric acid nephropathy; 2 chlorodeoxyadenosine, effective in the treatment of hairy cell leukemia and other lymphoid malignancies; 6-thioguanine (6-TG), an infrequently used antileukemic agent; and fludarabine phosphate (2-fluoroara-adenosine monophosphate), an effective agent for chronic lymphocytic leukemia (CLL) and follicular lymphomas, and for suppression of graft-versus-host disease in transplantation. A new purine analogue, nelarabine, is an ara-guanine prodrug, with strong activity against T-cell diseases, including lymphoblastic leukemias and lymphomas.[50] The basis for this T-cell sensitivity appears to be the resistance of arabinosylguanine (ara-G) to degradation by the catabolic enzyme, purine nucleoside phosphorylase. High levels of arabinosylguanine triphosphate (ara-GTP) accumulate in T-cell neoplasms, leading to Fas ligand-mediated apoptosis. The most recent addition, clofarabine, also an adenosine analogue, has notable activity against childhood ALL and adult AML. Deoxycoformycin, a potent inhibitor of adenosine deaminase, is also effective in the treatment of T-cell malignancies and hairy cell leukemia.

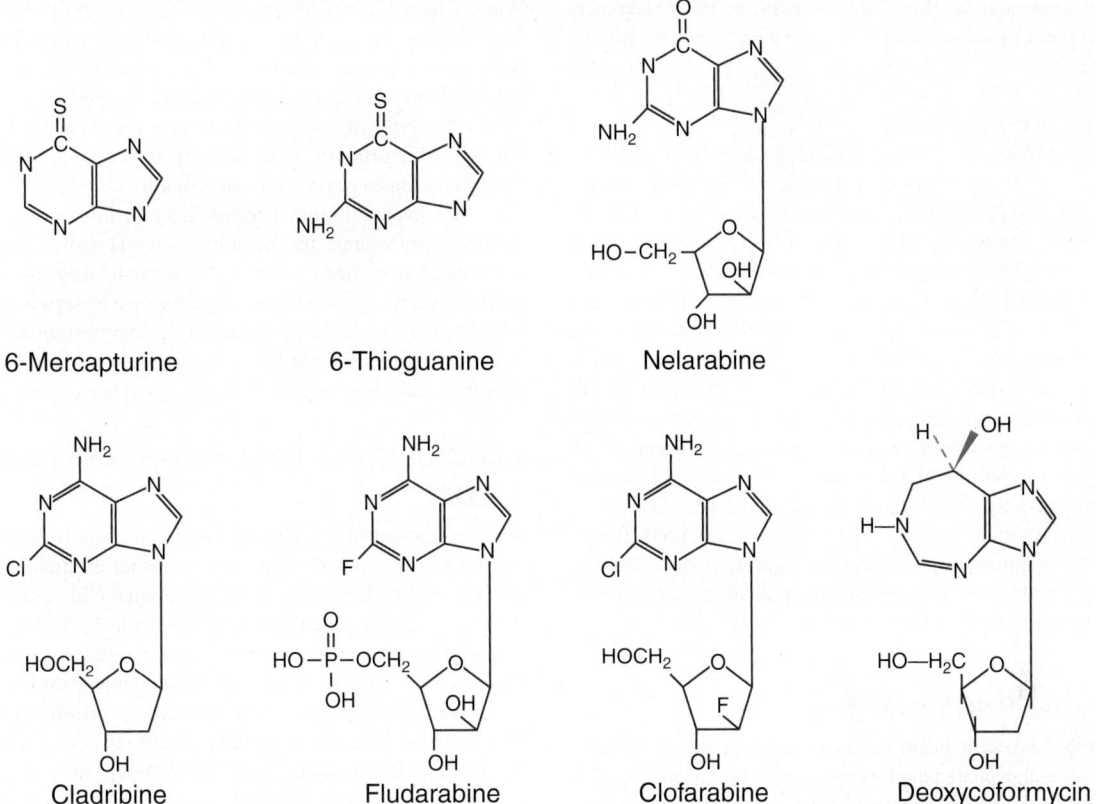

Figure 22–3. Purine analogues.

Mechanism of Action of 6-Thiopurines

Both 6-MP and 6-TG have a thiol group substituted for the 6-hydroxy group of hypoxanthine or guanine, respectively, and are converted to nucleotides by hypoxanthine guanine phosphoribosyltransferase. They block synthesis of purines. The nucleotides of both 6-MP and 6-TG are incorporated into DNA, where they become methylated and are recognized by the mismatch repair system. Attempts to correct miscoding lead to strand breaks and apoptosis.[51] Cell death correlates with the extent of their incorporation into DNA. 6-MP has the added effect of inhibiting de novo purine synthesis through the action of its metabolite, methyl-thioinosine monophosphate.[52]

In experimental tumor cells, resistance to 6-MP is most commonly caused by decreased activity of hypoxanthine guanine phosphoribosyl-transferase (HGPRT), by increased efflux by the transporter MRP-4, and by the absence of an effective mismatch repair process. Resistance in human leukemia is poorly understood, but is linked to HGPRT deficiency. Patients differ in their rates of metabolic clearance of 6-MP and in their ability to efflux 6-thiopurines from cells. Rapid systemic clearance of the drug, as mediated by methylation of the thiol group by 5-thiopurine-methyltransferase (TPMT),[53] is associated with a high leukemia recurrence rate in ALL maintenance therapy. Low levels of red blood cell thiopurine nucleotides correlate with a high level of activity of TPMT (more often found in patients of African descent) and a high risk of clinical relapse in patients with ALL,[54] whereas decreased expression of TPMT, resulting from an inherited polymorphism in the number of tandem repeats in the 5′ promoter region, is associated with increased drug toxicity. A commercial test for enzyme polymorphism, based on red cell enzyme activity or thioguanine nucleotide content, is available. A second polymorphism of significance involves the cellular efflux protein, MRP-4; an inactive variant is associated with high 6-TG nucleotide concentrations in cells, and may be responsible for great sensitivity of Japanese patients to 6-thiopurines, as the variant occurs in 18 percent of the Japanese population.[55] A polymorphism affecting the inosine triphosphate pyrophosphorylase enzyme (rs41320251) responsible for degrading a thiopurine nucleotide intermediate is associated with increased methyl-mercaptopurine nucleotides and a high incidence of febrile neutropenia in children with ALL.[56]

Methotrexate and 6-MP are highly synergistic, possibly because methotrexate blocks the de novo synthesis of purines, elevates phosphoribosyl pyrophosphate (PRPP), and enhances the activation of 6-MP. 6-MP blocks warfarin anticoagulation in some patients, leading to a requirement for higher doses of warfarin in patients receiving chronic 6-MP therapy for immunosuppression.

Clinical Pharmacology of 6-Thiopurines

Both 6-TG and 6-MP are given orally at doses of 50 to 100 mg/m² per day. Oral absorption of 6-MP is erratic, as only 16 to 50 percent of an oral dose is systemically available.[57] Food and antibiotics may decrease absorption. Both 6-MP and 6-TG are inactivated by metabolism, and have half-lives of approximately 1 to 1.5 hour in plasma. Peak plasma levels of 6-MP occur 2 hours after administration and reach 1 to 2 μM. During 6-TG treatment, 6-TG nucleotides accumulate to much higher levels in leukemic cells, as compared to 6-MP. Inactive 6-thiomethyl nucleotides are almost 30-fold higher after 6-MP, than after 6-TG.[58] 6-MP is inactivated by metabolism to 6-thiouric acid, a reaction catalyzed by xanthine oxidase. Allopurinol inhibits the metabolic inactivation of 6-MP, but not of 6-TG. Therefore, it is generally recommended that dosages of orally administered 6-MP be reduced by 75 percent in patients receiving allopurinol. 6-TG is inactivated primarily by S-methylation, followed by oxidation and desulfuration, but a second pathway, mediated by guanase and xanthine oxidase, contributes to clearance. Dose reduction is not necessary when 6-TG and allopurinol are administered together.

Adverse Effects of 6-Thiopurines

Both 6-TG and 6-MP are myelotoxic, producing nadirs of white blood cells and platelets at 7 to 10 days after treatment.[59] Moderate nausea and vomiting may also be observed. Patients may experience mild but rapidly reversible hepatotoxicity after treatment with either compound. Cirrhosis has occurred in some children with leukemia who are receiving long-term therapy with 6-MP. TPMT, which inactivates 6-thiopurines, occurs in several polymorphic forms that fail to metabolize the analogues. Approximately one person in 10 of the white population is heterozygous for ineffective polymorphic forms of the enzyme and will have significantly greater myelosuppression, whereas one patient in 300 is homozygous for the inactive forms, accumulates high concentrations of thioguanine nucleotides in both tumor and normal cells, and is at risk for overwhelming toxicity, even with greatly reduced doses of 6-MP.[60]

Other toxicities may include hypersensitivity reactions (fever, rash), interstitial pneumonitis; pancreatitis; opportunistic infection, and an increased incidence of AML in patients receiving chronic immunosuppressive treatment with 6-MP.

FLUDARABINE PHOSPHATE

Originally synthesized as a deamination-resistant analogue of adenosine, fludarabine phosphate contains two important substitutions: a fluorine attached to the purine ring, which renders the drug resistant to deamination, and an arabinose sugar in place of deoxyribose, which leads to its pharmacologic activity as an inhibitor of DNA synthesis and ribonucleotide reductase. It has outstanding activity in CLL.[61] It is strongly immunosuppressive, like the other purine analogues, and is frequently used for this purpose in nonmyeloablative allogeneic marrow transplantation[62] and in the treatment of autoimmune diseases.

Activation of fludarabine phosphate requires removal of the phosphate group in plasma to allow cellular uptake by nucleoside transporters, and then intracellular rephosphorylation. Fludarabine is activated to the monophosphate level by dCK. The triphosphate inhibits DNA polymerase and becomes incorporated into both DNA and RNA.[63] Its mechanism of cytotoxicity results from DNA chain termination and induction of apoptosis, although it also inhibits ribonucleotide reductase (RNR), a self-potentiating activity that decreases intracellular deoxyadenosine triphosphate (dATP) and increases fludarabine incorporation into DNA.[64] Its triphosphate has a long intracellular half-life of 15 hours in CLL cells. Resistance has been ascribed to decreased active uptake, a deficiency of dCK, increased efflux, or increased RNR.

The drug is available in the United States as an intravenous preparation, and for oral use. It has 60 to 80 percent bioavailability. Because it is resistant to adenosine deaminase, fludarabine is eliminated primarily by renal excretion (60 percent), with a terminal half-life of 10 hours. For patients treated with fludarabine, the standard intravenous dose is 25 mg/m² daily for 5 days, whereas the approved oral dose is 40 mg/m² daily for 5 days. In patients with renal impairment, a 20 percent dose reduction for a CrCl of 17 to 40 mL/min/m², and a 40 percent dose reduction for a CrCl less than 17 mL/min/m² yields an area under the curve approximately equal to that seen in patients with normal renal function receiving full doses of fludarabine.[65,66]

When administered at these doses, fludarabine causes only moderate myelosuppression. In CLL patients, its antileukemic effect will lead to a progressive improvement in marrow function over a period of two to three cycles of treatment, with a median time to disease progression of 31 months. However, the drug also exerts cytotoxic effects against both B and T lymphocytes, lowering CD4 T-cell counts to 150 to 200 cells/μL and predisposing patients to opportunistic infections. In patients with a large tumor burden, rapid tumor lysis may rarely lead to hyperuricemia, renal failure, and hypocalcemia (tumor lysis syndrome).[67] Thus, patients should be well hydrated and their urine alkalinized prior to beginning therapy. The primary acute toxicity is reversible myelosuppression. Peripheral sensory and motor neuropathy may occur during standard-dose therapy; autoimmune phenomena, including prolonged hypothyroidism, neutropenia and hemolytic anemia with both warm and cold antibodies, have been reported.[68] Approximately 10 percent of CLL patients receiving fludarabine may develop a hypersensitivity syndrome of pulmonary infiltrates, hypoxemia, and fever, responsive to glucocorticoids.[69] Myelodysplasia and acute leukemias, with chromosome 7p deletions, have been reported as infrequent late complications.[70]

CLADRIBINE (2-CHLORODEOXYADENOSINE, 2-CDA)

The extreme sensitivity of normal and malignant lymphocytes to deamination-resistant purine analogues is further exemplified by the potent activity of cladribine in hairy cell leukemia, CLL, and low-grade lymphomas.[71] A single course of cladribine, typically 0.09 mg/kg per day for 7 days by continuous intravenous infusion, induces complete response in 80 percent of patients with hairy cell leukemia. Administration by subcutaneous injection or by 2-hour intravenous infusion daily for 5 days to the same total dose achieves similar results. The drug has much the same intracellular fate as fludarabine, undergoing phosphorylation by dCK and further conversion to a triphosphate that becomes incorporated into DNA. The triphosphate of cladribine has a long intracellular half-life of 9.7 hours in CLL cells isolated from patients treated with the drug.[72] The triphosphate has multiple metabolic effects, disrupting oxidative phosphorylation in mitochondria, inhibiting RNR and depleting nicotinamide adenine dinucleotide levels in tumor cells. All of these actions may explain the drug's toxicity to slowly dividing lymphoid malignancies such as hairy cell leukemia and CLL. The actual mechanisms by which cladribine induces DNA strand breaks are not completely understood. However, similar to fludarabine, it inhibits DNA chain extension and daughter strand synthesis.[73] Furthermore, the drug's inhibition of RNR lowers levels of the competitive dATP. The cumulative effects of cladribine induce apoptosis (programmed cell death).

Cladribine is eliminated primarily (>50 percent) by renal excretion, with a terminal plasma half-life of 7 hours. In a patient with renal failure, continuous flow hemodialysis effectively cleared the drug and prevented serious myelosuppression.[74] Cladribine retains effectiveness in at least a fraction of hairy cell leukemia patients resistant to deoxycoformycin or fludarabine, although clinical experience with sequential use of these drugs is limited. Toxicities of cladribine include transient myelosuppression, fever, tumor lysis syndrome, and occasional opportunistic infections possibly related to immunosuppression. The development of cumulative thrombocytopenia during treatment with repeated courses of the drug may limit its use. Resistance develops in experimental tumors through decreased uptake, loss of the activating enzyme dCK, increased RNR activity, increased efflux,[75] or by induction of 5′-nucleotidase activity.

CLOFARABINE (2-CHLORO-2′-FLUORO-ARABINOSYLADENINE)

This analogue has halogen substitutions on both the purine ring and arabinose sugar, resulting in a ready uptake and activation, to a highly stable intracellular triphosphate (half-life of 24 hours), which terminates DNA synthesis, inhibits RNR, and induces apoptosis. The usual adult dose is 52 mg/m^2 given as a 2-hour infusion daily for 5 days. Clofarabine has a plasma half-life of 6.5 hours. The primary route of clearance is through renal excretion, and dose adjustment according to CrCl is recommended for patients with abnormal renal function.

Toxicities are myelosuppression; uncommonly, fever, hypotension, and pulmonary edema, suggestive of capillary leak caused by cytokine release; hepatic transaminitis; hypokalemia; and hypophosphatemia. As a single agent, the drug is well tolerated as second-line treatment for AML patients with remission rates of 30 percent.[76]

NELARABINE (6-METHOXY-ARABINOSYLGUANINE)

A guanine nucleoside analogue, nelarabine has useful activity as a secondary agent for T-cell lymphoblastic lymphoma and acute T-cell leukemias. Its mode of action is similar to the other purine analogues, in that it becomes incorporated into DNA and terminates DNA synthesis. Its selective action for T cells may relate to the ability of T cells to activate purine nucleosides and the lack of susceptibility of this drug to purine nucleoside phosphorylase, a degradative reaction.

Usual doses are an intravenous 2-hour infusion of 1500 mg/m^2 for adults on days 1, 3, and 5, and a lower dose of 650 mg/m^2 per day for 5 days for children. The drug is rapidly demethylated by adenosine deaminase after administration, yielding the ara-G, which is cleared by hydrolysis and has a longer plasma half-life of 3 hours. ara-G is converted intracellularly to its triphosphate[77] which becomes incorporated into DNA. The primary toxicities are myelosuppression and abnormal liver function tests, but the drug may cause a spectrum of neurologic abnormalities, including seizures, delirium, somnolence, and the Guillain-Barré syndrome of ascending paralysis.

PENTOSTATIN (2′-DEOXYCOFORMYCIN)

Pentostatin contains a unique seven-carbon primary ring system that closely resembles the transition-state intermediate of the adenosine deaminase reaction. As such, pentostatin is a potent inhibitor of the enzyme, leading to accumulation of intracellular adenosine and deoxyadenosine nucleotides. In addition, the triphosphate of pentostatin is incorporated into DNA. The imbalance in purine nucleotide pools produced by pentostatin probably accounts for its cytotoxicity.

Although initial trials of pentostatin demonstrated striking renal and neurologic toxicities at doses of 10 mg/m^2 intravenously per day or greater, lower doses (4 mg/m^2 biweekly) are extremely effective in inducing pathologically confirmed complete responses in hairy cell leukemia. At this lower dose, severe depletion of normal T cells occurs and may predispose to opportunistic infection.[78] The optimal dose may be lower than 4 mg/m^2 biweekly. The drug is eliminated entirely by renal excretion, necessitating proportional dose reduction in patients with reduced CrCl.

RIBONUCLEOTIDE REDUCTASE INHIBITOR: HYDROXYUREA

Hydroxyurea inhibits RNR, the enzyme that converts ribonucleotide diphosphates to deoxyribonucleotides. It chelates iron, an essential cofactor in the RNR reaction. In malignant disease, hydroxyurea is most commonly used for treating polycythemia vera, essential thrombocythemia, and the chronic phase of CML and to lower the myeloblast count in patients presenting with AML or blastic crisis of CML. It has also become the standard agent for preventing painful crisis and reducing hospitalization in patients with sickle cell disease and in thalassemia patients with hemoglobin (Hgb) C/SS. Its antisickling activity results from induction of Hgb F through its activation of a specific promoter for the γ-globin gene. It may also exert antisickling activity and decrease occlusion of small vessels through its generation of nitric oxide, a vasodilator, and through decreased expression of adhesion molecules such as L-selectin, on neutrophils.[79] Resistance occurs in experimental tumors as a consequence of amplification of the catalytic subunit of RNR or through mutations in RNR that lower affinity for the enzyme.

Clinical Pharmacology

Hydroxyurea is well absorbed orally, even when large doses such as 50 to 75 mg/kg orally are given for rapid lowering of the white blood cell count. In chronic therapy of myeloproliferative neoplasm, starting doses of 15 mg/kg orally are adjusted upward or downward based on neutrophil counts. In managing patients with sickle cell disease, neutrophils should be maintained above 2000 per mL.[80] Hydroxyurea may also be given intravenously to rapidly lower the white blood cell count in patients with extreme leukemic leukocytosis or thrombocytosis. Peak plasma levels following oral administration are achieved at about 1 hour and decline with a half-life of 3 to 4 hours thereafter. Renal excretion is the major route of drug elimination, and doses should be decreased in proportion to the deficit in CrCl.

Adverse Effects

The major toxicities of hydroxyurea are leukopenia and the induction of megaloblastic changes. Nausea, drug fever, pneumonitis, maculopapular skin rash, and painful leg ulcers have been observed with this drug, although it is generally well tolerated. Hydroxyurea, like ara-C, is an S-phase–specific agent. Accordingly, single large doses cause little toxicity other than myelosuppression. The nadir of the leukocyte count occurs 3 to 5 days after a single dose of drug, and the leukocyte count recovers rapidly. It is a potent teratogen and should not be used in women of childbearing age. Its potential to cause leukemic transformation is uncertain, but small cases series suggest this may occur in patients with a myeloproliferative neoplasm.[81]

⬤ ANTITUBULINS

VINCA ALKALOIDS

Vinblastine and vincristine are commonly used in the treatment of hematologic neoplasms: vinblastine because of its excellent activity in the treatment of Hodgkin lymphoma and vincristine in lymphomas and childhood leukemia. Both drugs have activity in solid-tumor therapy, particularly in treating childhood sarcomas (vincristine), and testicular cancer (vinblastine).

Mechanism of Action

The vinca alkaloids exert their cytotoxic action by their binding to tubulin, a structural protein found in the cytoplasm of cells. Microtubules, assembled through polymerization of tubulin dimers, form the spindle along which the chromosomes migrate during mitosis. Microtubules are an important structural component of neuronal axons. Binding of the vinca alkaloids to tubulin leads to inhibition of formation of the mitotic spindle,[82] arresting cells in metaphase and inducing apoptosis. Resistance to the vinca alkaloids may be acquired through the expression of the MDR efflux pump. Alternatively, resistant cells may contain mutant tubulin with decreased avidity of vinca binding.[83] The clinical importance of these resistance mechanisms, however, is uncertain.

Clinical Pharmacology

Vincristine and vinblastine are both administered by the intravenous route. The average single dose of vincristine is 1.4 mg/m^2 and that of vinblastine 8 to 9 mg/m². Sequential doses of the drugs are usually given at 1- or 2-week intervals. These doses provide peak plasma drug concentrations of approximately 1 μM. The plasma pharmacokinetics of both vinca analogues are characterized by a very rapid initial disposition phase followed by a slow terminal phase of decay, with half-lives of 20 to 85 hours. Almost 70 percent of a dose of vincristine is metabolized by the liver and excreted in the feces. Cytochrome P450 (CYP)-mediated metabolism is also the major route of inactivation of vinblastine, producing a variety of inactive metabolic produced in the liver are excreted in the bile. Inducers of CYP3A4, such as phenylhydantoin, enhance clearance, while inhibitors delay clearance and increase toxicity. The dose of vincristine or vinblastine should be reduced in patients with hepatic impairment. Although specific guidelines for dose reduction have not been developed, a 50 percent decrease in dose is recommended for patients presenting with a bilirubin level of 1.5 to 3 mg/dL and a 75 percent reduction for levels greater than 3 mg/dL. Dose reduction is not necessary for patients with impaired renal function, as very little intact drug is excreted in urine.

Adverse Effects

The dose-limiting side effect of vincristine is neurotoxicity, which usually occurs when the total dose received exceeds 6 mg/m². The initial signs of neurotoxicity are paresthesia of the fingers and lower extremities and loss of deep tendon reflexes. Continued administration may lead to profound loss of motor strength, such as weakness of dorsiflexion of the foot and extension of the wrists. Elderly patients are particularly susceptible to such toxicities. Occasionally, cranial nerve palsies may lead to vocal cord paralysis or diplopia, and severe jaw pain may result from vincristine administration. At high doses of vincristine (>3 mg total single dose), autonomic neuropathy may cause obstipation and paralytic ileus. Sensory changes and reflex abnormalities slowly improve when the drug is discontinued; motor impairment improves less rapidly and may be irreversible. Inappropriate antidiuretic hormone release resulting in symptomatic dilutional hyponatremia has been ascribed to vincristine.

While marrow suppression is not common with vincristine administration, myelosuppression may be noted in patients with impaired marrow function as a consequence of prior treatment with other drugs. Platelet counts are relatively unaffected.

The primary toxicity of vinblastine is leukopenia. The white count reaches a nadir at day 7 and reverses rapidly thereafter. Mucositis may result from higher doses (>8 mg/m²) of vinblastine or when it is used in combination with other cytotoxic drugs. Neurotoxicity is rare, but ileus can occur at high doses.

Both drugs cause severe pain and local toxicity if extravasated. Neither drug should ever be given intrathecally. Vincristine administered inadvertently into the cerebrospinal fluid causes acute neurologic dysfunction, coma, and death. Attempts at replacement of the cerebral spinal fluid with an electrolyte solution, Ringer lactate, supplemented with 15 ml/L of fresh-frozen plasma, have been reported to avert a fatal outcome, but do not prevent severe neurologic sequelae.[84]

TAXANES

The taxanes, paclitaxel, docetaxel, and Abraxane, are a second class of antimitotic compounds that differ in mechanism and toxicity profile from the vinca alkaloids that are primarily used in patients with solid tumors. Paclitaxel was purified from an extract of the bark of *Taxus brevifolia*, whereas docetaxel is a closely related semisynthetic derivative. Abraxane is paclitaxel embedded in an albumin microparticle. The taxanes bind to the β-tubulin subunit of microtubules and promote the polymerization of microtubules, leading to disordered mitotic spindle

formation and a block in the progression through mitosis.[85] They induce apoptosis in tumor cells irrespective of the p53 status of the cells and kill cells at 10 nM concentrations or less in cell culture in a time-dependent manner.[86] In experimental settings, resistance is related to increased drug efflux, mutations in β-tubulin, or increased expression of antiapoptotic proteins such as survivin,[87] or of the mitosis-related aurora kinase.[88]

The taxanes are subject to MDR mediated by the *mdr* and *mrp* genes, as well as to β-tubulin mutations. Because they are highly insoluble in aqueous solution, paclitaxel and docetaxel are formulated in lipid-based solvents that cause occasional hypersensitivity reactions. Thus, paclitaxel is given after pretreatment with antihistamines (cimetidine, diphenhydramine), and dexamethasone. Both drugs are cleared primarily by hepatic CYP metabolism, although by different isoenzymes (paclitaxel predominantly by CYP2B6 and docetaxel by CYP3A4) with terminal plasma half-lives of 10 to 13 hours. Their metabolism is stimulated by phenytoin and other CYP-inducing drugs and inhibited by ketoconazole. Their major toxicities, aside from hypersensitivity, are a sharp but brief leukopenia, milder thrombocytopenia, and mucositis. High-dose or repeated cycles of the taxanes cause a sensory and motor peripheral neuropathy that is reversible with drug discontinuation. Occasional patients have experienced atrial conduction block or atrial or ventricular arrhythmias after paclitaxel administration, and the combination of paclitaxel with doxorubicin may produce a greater incidence of congestive heart failure than seen with doxorubicin alone.[89] A syndrome of progressive fluid retention and peripheral edema occurs in patients receiving multiple cycles of docetaxel and can be at least partially prevented by pretreatment with glucocorticoids.[90]

The taxanes have not found a valuable role in the treatment of hematologic malignancy. However, a number of analogues and new formulations are under development. Abraxane, consisting of paclitaxel bound to albumen microparticles, does not require a lipid solvent, is virtually free of hypersensitivity as a side effect, and enters cells by a separate albumen-mediated transporter. It is approved for treatment of relapsed breast cancer and pancreatic cancer. Cabazitaxel, approved for prostate cancer, is a new analogue with decreased susceptibility to MDR. An entirely new class of natural products, the epothilones, have a similar mechanism of action, are less susceptible to MDR, and have activity against breast cancer.[91]

● TOPOISOMERASE INHIBITORS

CAMPTOTHECINS

This group of compounds includes synthetic derivatives of 20 (S)-camptothecin, a naturally product from the *Camptotheca acuminata* tree. The camptothecins interact with a unique target, topoisomerase I, stabilizing the enzyme's complex with DNA and preventing the resealing of DNA single-strand breaks induced by the enzyme. Resistance arises through mutation, deletion, or decreased expression of the topoisomerase I gene. The primary agents in clinical use are irinotecan, which is approved for treatment of colon cancer, and topotecan, approved for second-line treatment of ovarian cancer and small cell lung cancer. Irinotecan, most commonly administered intravenously at a dose of 125 mg/m² once each week for 4 weeks every 42 days, has shown promise against lymphomas in phase II trials performed in Japan.[92] Response rates of 42 percent in previously treated patients with non-Hodgkin lymphoma, and of 38 percent in patients with refractory or relapsed adult T-cell leukemia-lymphoma, remain to be confirmed. Topotecan has remission-inducing activity in patients with myelodysplasia and chronic myelomonocytic leukemia, both as a single agent (1.5 mg/m² per day for 5 days) and in combination with ara-C.[93,94] Objective responses have also been observed in phase I clinical trials in patients with AML.[95] Irinotecan and topotecan differ substantially in their profile of toxicities and pharmacokinetic behavior. Irinotecan is a water-soluble prodrug that is converted to the active species, SN-38, by carboxyl esterase-mediated cleavage. Irinotecan and SN-38 are both eliminated by glucuronidation and biliary excretion. Therefore, irinotecan must be used with caution and at lower doses in patients with Gilbert disease (and lacking glucuronyl transferase 1A1) or in those with hepatic dysfunction.[96] In contrast to the hepatic extraction and excretion of irinotecan, approximately two-thirds of the dose of topotecan is eliminated by renal excretion, with the remainder being cleared by biliary excretion. Dose adjustment proportional to CrCl is indicated in patients with renal failure.[97] Topotecan toxicity consists mainly of myelosuppression and, to a lesser degree, mucositis, whereas irinotecan causes a profound diarrhea, which is responsive to loperamide, and a more modest myelosuppression. The maximum tolerated dose of topotecan for the 5-day schedule of 30-minute intravenous infusions/day is 4.5 mg/m² per day in patients with leukemia.[98] This is considerably greater than the approved dose for solid tumors, and gastrointestinal side effects, such as mucositis and diarrhea, become dose-limiting at these higher doses.

ANTHRACYCLINE ANTIBIOTICS

The anthracyclines are a unique class of natural products that inhibit topoisomerase II (Topo II), an enzyme important in DNA strand passage allowing the untangling of DNA prior to replication or repair. Doxorubicin, daunorubicin, idarubicin, and epirubicin are closely related in structure, each possessing a rigid planar core to which is linked a daunosamine sugar. The molecules differ in side-chain substitutions attached to the anthracycline ring system, and exhibit different spectra of antitumor activity and toxicity. Mitoxantrone, a closely related, nonglycosidic anthracenedione, has very similar pharmacologic properties to those of the anthracyclines. The anthracyclines are produced by a *Streptomyces* species, whereas mitoxantrone is a synthetic compound. Doxorubicin (Adriamycin) has broad activity against solid and hematologic malignancies. It is an important component of the standard multidrug regimens used to treat Hodgkin lymphoma (doxorubicin, bleomycin, vinblastine, and dacarbazine [ABVD]) and aggressive non-Hodgkin lymphoma (cyclophosphamide, doxorubicin, vincristine, and prednisone). Daunorubicin and idarubicin are used almost exclusively in combination with ara-C for the treatment of AML, whereas epirubicin is primarily effective against solid tumors. Mitoxantrone is employed for the treatment of AML and breast cancer, and as an immunosuppressive for patients with multiple sclerosis. Liposome-encapsulated doxorubicin (Doxil) and daunorubicin derivatives are approved for treatment of solid tumors; they provide a more prolonged, lower peak concentration of drug, and have decreased cardiac toxicity. The daunorubicin liposome is of interest in treating AML.[99] A novel anthracycline, pixantrone, which has lesser cardiotoxicity, has received conditional approval in Europe for refractory non-Hodgkin B-cell lymphoma.[100]

Mechanism of Action

Anthracyclines target the replication and structural integrity of DNA. Their primary mechanism of toxicity stems from their interaction with Topo II, an enzyme that creates DNA strand breaks and promotes strand passage through those breaks. Strand passage is essential in untangling DNA in preparation for replication and repair. Once the strand passage and unwinding is complete, Topo II reseals the broken DNA strands. The anthracyclines inhibit the resealing step by forming a complex with Topo II and the broken DNA strand to which the enzyme is linked. Accumulation of strand breaks activates apoptosis. The planar molecular structure of these drugs promotes their intercalation between opposing strands of the DNA helix and may contribute to the specificity of sites of DNA breakage. In addition to their inhibition of Topo II, anthracyclines generate free radicals by virtue of the oxidation-reduction cycling of their quinone group, an action catalyzed by the binding of Fe²⁺. Free radical generation is thought to be responsible for their cardiac toxicity.

The importance of the presence of Topo II in determining response to anthracyclines is best illustrated by the greater benefit of anthracycline-based breast cancer treatment in patients with amplification of the target enzyme on chromosome 17, near the *HER2* gene with which it coamplifies.[101] Anthracycline-containing regimens are particularly effective in *HER2*-amplified breast cancers.[102]

Anthracyclines enter cells through a passive transport process. Their lipophilic structure allows them to achieve high intracellular concentrations. Anthracyclines are pumped out of the cell by a series of ATP-dependent transporters, including the P-glycoprotein MDR transporter, the breast cancer resistance protein transporter (BCRP) and related efflux pumps.[11] Other mechanisms for anthracycline resistance include decreased Topo II activity or Topo II mutations in the enzyme that inhibit drug binding, as well as defects in apoptosis or impaired checkpoint recognition of DNA strand breaks.

Clinical Pharmacology

Daunorubicin and idarubicin are readily converted to active hydroxyl metabolites, whereas doxorubicin produces limited amounts of alcohol metabolite. The alcohols of daunorubicin and doxorubicin are less active as antitumor agents, but do possess cardiotoxic activity.

All anthracyclines are eliminated by the formation of inactive metabolic products (aglycons, side-chain-modified products, glucuronides, sulphates, and oxidative metabolite) in the liver. Only a minor fraction of the dose of any of the anthracyclines is excreted in the urine as the parent drug or alcohol metabolite. The pharmacokinetics of the clinically useful anthracyclines are predominantly influenced by their terminal disposition phase, which exceeds 24 hours. Although prolongation of the half-life of doxorubicin has been reported in studies of patients with compromised liver function, no clear correlations of liver function with toxicity have been established. However, in patients with elevated serum bilirubin levels, initial doses of doxorubicin and daunorubicin should be reduced by 50 percent, and adjust there after according to tolerance. Idarubicin, the only anthracycline amenable to oral administration, has a bioavailability of 20 percent for the parent drug and 40 percent for parent drug plus idarubicinol, the primary active metabolite. Idarubicinol has a very prolonged biologic half-life, ranging from 50 to 60 hours, and is likely responsible for the antitumor activity of this drug. In contrast to the metabolites of doxorubicin and daunorubicin, idarubicinol is eliminated primarily by renal excretion. No dose adjustment for hepatic dysfunction is indicated.

Mitoxantrone has a long terminal half-life of 23 to 42 hours. Only a minor fraction of unchanged drug is excreted in the urine (<10 percent) or stool (<20 percent). The majority of the drug is metabolized or bound to tissues. Patients with impaired hepatic function may have a more prolonged elimination of mitoxantrone.

The usual dose of doxorubicin when administered as a single agent by bolus intravenous injection is 45 to 75 mg/m² every 3 to 4 weeks, depending on the tumor treated and the drug combination. Less cardiac toxicity may result from schedules that avoid high peak plasma concentrations, such as weekly doses (15 to 25 mg/m²) or continuous intravenous infusion over 48 to 96 hours, as in the EPOCH (etoposide, prednisone, vincristine, cyclophosphamide, and doxorubicin) regimen.[103] When given in combination with other myelotoxic agents such as cyclophosphamide, the dose of doxorubicin is usually decreased because of overlapping marrow toxicity. Daunorubicin has been used as the anthracycline of choice in the treatment of AML. To minimize the cardiotoxic effects of daunorubicin, in standard "3+7" therapy in AML the daunorubicin dosage (45 to 60 mg/m^2 for adults <60 years) is given daily for 3 days to avoid high peak concentrations, although larger doses (90 mg/m^2/day), may produce higher complete remission rates. In the elderly, a lower dose of 30 mg/m^2 daily for 3 days is typically used in combination therapy.

Adverse Effects

Myelosuppression is the primary acute toxicity of this class of drugs, with a nadir occurring 7 to 10 days after single-dose administration and recovery by 2 weeks. Mitoxantrone produces less nausea and vomiting than does either daunorubicin or doxorubicin. Doxorubicin may cause mucositis, especially when used in maximally tolerated divided doses given over 2 to 3 days or when used in combination with other drugs that cause mucositis. Anthracyclines can also cause radiation recall in previously irradiated tissues, especially when the drug is administered just prior to or in the weeks following irradiation. Alopecia often occurs. Extravasation of these drugs can result in tissue necrosis so they should be administered through an indwelling central venous catheter. Dexrazoxane injected subcutaneously, lessens tissue damage after extravasation.[104] Patients receiving doxorubicin should also be warned that their urine may turn red.

Cardiotoxicity is the major late toxic effect of anthracyclines.[105] Cardiotoxicity most likely results from free radical formation catalyzed by the anthracycline's quinone moiety, although cardiac Topo IIb (not the major topoisomerase involved in DNA replication) may play a role in mediating this effect. Iron as a reduction-oxidation (redox) cofactor contributes to toxicity, as it accumulates in mitochondria during treatment.[106] Cardiac proteins, including the cardiac myosin-binding protein C, show evidence of alkylation and degradation after anthracycline treatment.[107]

Clinically, anthracycline-induced cardiotoxicity presents after repeated cycles of treatment. Rarely, acute effects are manifest as arrhythmias, conduction abnormalities, or a "pericarditis–myocarditis syndrome." The more common long-term consequence is congestive heart failure (CHF), which can develop during or several months after treatment. Studies in breast cancer have demonstrated a 0.5 to 1 percent risk of cardiomyopathy in patients treated with adjuvant anthracyclines.[108] The risk is higher in patients receiving trastuzumab or paclitaxel in combination with doxorubicin.

The risk of anthracycline-induced cardiotoxicity increases with total dose, but is difficult to estimate for any individual patient. In patients with normal cardiac function prior to treatment, the subsequent rate of doxorubicin-induced CHF reaches less than 1 percent at total doses of 400 mg/m^2, but climbs steeply thereafter to 7 to 20 percent at total doses of 550 mg/m^2.[109] The threshold for cardiotoxicity varies among the different anthracyclines. For example, the inflection threshold for daunorubicin (600 to 700 mg/m^2) is significantly higher than for doxorubicin (400 mg/m^2). However, it should be remembered that these thresholds are based on population studies, and for any individual patient the risk is impossible to predict. The clinician must pay close attention to symptoms of CHF, such as dyspnea, cough, orthopnea, and weight gain or ankle edema, throughout a course of treatment and irrespective of total dose.

Besides the cumulative dose of anthracycline, other risk factors for anthracycline-induced cardiomyopathy include mediastinal (mantle) radiation, preexisting heart disease, and patient age, the risk being highest in children younger than the age of 4 years. Children who receive greater than 300 mg/m^2 have a significant risk of having decreased myocardial contractility, decreased ventricular dimension, and an increased incidence of cardiac events (such as conduction defects, myocardial

infarction, and CHF) in their adult years. The incidence of may be decreased by coadministering dexrazoxane, an iron chelator, during chemotherapy.[110] It is recommended that the total doxorubicin dose be limited to 300 mg/m^2 in children. In addition, children treated with anthracyclines should have long-term cardiology followup.[110]

Ejection fraction measurements have been helpful in detecting a decline in myocardial function, a sign of impending myocardial failure. Ejection fraction measurements, usually by multigated acquisition scan (MUGA), should be performed to verify normal cardiac function prior to starting anthracycline-based chemotherapy, and should be repeated at the earliest clinical sign of cardiac dysfunction, and before every two cycles of treatment when the total dose of doxorubicin exceeds 300 mg/m^2. Anthracyclines should be discontinued if the ejection fraction falls below 40 percent, or if the ejection fraction drops a total of 20 percent from pretreatment levels.

As cardiotoxicity of anthracyclines results from the generation of free radicals by an anthracycline–iron complex, dexrazoxane, an iron chelator, decreases free radical formation *in vitro* and decreases the risk of cardiotoxicity in children receiving treatment for ALL, and in adults with metastatic breast cancer.[110] Fortunately, dexrazoxane does not cause any apparent diminution of antitumor activity. Adding dexrazoxane to an anthracycline-based regimen represents an alternative to discontinuing anthracyclines in patients who are approaching total-dose thresholds of drug, but who still require treatment. Two trials have shown a higher rate of secondary leukemia and MDS in patients receiving doxorubicin and dexrazoxane.[111,112] In adult patients, dexrazoxane should be added only in patients who have received a total dose of at least 300 mg/m^2 doxorubicin or 540 mg/m^2 epirubicin.

Treatment with Topo II inhibitors, including anthracyclines, mitoxantrone, and the epipodophyllotoxins (see "Epipodophyllotoxins" below), increases the risk of AML. AML typically develops 6 months to 5 years after exposure to the Topo II inhibitor.[107] This heightened risk derives from the increased DNA double-strand breaks generated by the Topo II inhibitor. These double-stranded DNA breaks can give rise to balanced chromosomal translocations involving the *MLL* or *PML* genes.[111] Anthracyclines and mitoxantrone have affinity for specific DNA sequences and cause translocations at specific hot spots in the genome, including a 6-base pair breakpoint region in the *PML* gene causing the 15;17 translocation, the 11q23 translocation involving the *MLL* gene, and the 11;20 translocation involving the *NUP98* gene.[113,114]

EPIPODOPHYLLOTOXINS

Two semisynthetic derivatives of podophyllotoxin, VP-16 (etoposide) and VM-26 (teniposide), inhibit Topo II and have significant clinical activity in hematologic malignancies. Etoposide has been incorporated into combination therapy regimens for Hodgkin lymphoma, large cell non-Hodgkin lymphomas, leukemias, and various solid tumors, and is a frequent component of high-dose chemotherapy regimens. Teniposide has limited value in clinical oncology. Its use is generally restricted to childhood acute leukemia, where it appears to be synergistic with ara-C. These compounds induce double-stranded breaks in DNA through their sequence-specific binding to DNA in complex with Topo II.[115] One mechanism of resistance is increased expression of the MDR drug exporter.[11] A second mechanism results from decreased Topo II activity or mutation of the enzyme, resulting in decreased drug binding.[116,117]

Clinical Pharmacology

Etoposide is administered in doses of 100 to 120 mg/m^2 per day for 3 days, either consecutively or every other day. Approximately 30 to 40 percent of an intravenous dose of etoposide is excreted intact in the urine, while the remainder is cleared by hepatic glucuronidation or demethylation; thus, doses of etoposide require modification for patients with compromised renal or hepatic function.[118] The plasma half-life of etoposide is 15 hours. The clinical activity of etoposide is highly schedule dependent. Single conventional doses are essentially without antitumor effect as compared to consecutive daily doses for 3 to 5 days. The pharmacokinetics of teniposide are very similar to those of etoposide, with a terminal plasma half-life of 20 to 48 hours. However, little parent drug appears intact in the urine, and dose modification for patients with renal dysfunction is unnecessary.

Adverse Effects

When administered intravenously, both etoposide and teniposide should be infused over a 30-minute period to avoid hypotensive episodes. The major toxicity of both drugs is leukopenia, which is rapidly reversible; thrombocytopenia is less common. Nausea and vomiting often follow etoposide administration. Alopecia may occur with both drugs. Other toxicities, such as fever, mild elevation of liver function tests, and peripheral neuropathy, are relatively uncommon. Because the major toxicity of etoposide is limited to the marrow, this drug is a valuable component of high-dose regimens used with marrow transplantation. In high-dose etoposide protocols (1.5 g/m^2 or greater given over 3 to 5 days) oropharyngeal mucositis becomes a prominent toxicity. Less-frequent high-dose toxicities include hepatocellular damage and, rarely, anaphylactic-like symptoms, probably related to the formulation vehicle. Secondary AML associated with translocation at 11q23 or the *PML* gene may follow etoposide treatment in children with ALL[119] and in adults with solid tumors.[120]

AGENTS ACTIVE THROUGHOUT THE CELL CYCLE

THE ALKYLATING DRUGS

These drugs are important in the treatment of hematopoietic malignancies either as single agents or as components of standard- or high-dose regimens. Their role as treatment for both acute and chronic hematologic malignancies results from their unique mechanism of cell killing and their lack of cell-cycle specificity. They may eradicate noncycling cells that escape cycle-active components of the treatment. Although these agents share the common property of forming covalent bonds with electron-rich sites on DNA (oxygen and nitrogen substituents), they exhibit important differences in their intrinsic reactivity, route of cellular uptake, favored sites of alkylation on DNA bases, and the specific mechanism of DNA repair that determines cell survival. These differences are borne out in experimental settings, where cross-resistance to alkylating agents is incomplete. Thus, protocols employing multiple alkylators, particularly in high-dose regimens, have a rational basis.[121] Alkylating agents differ as well in their patterns of toxicity. The majority of these drugs cause myelosuppression and mucositis as their primary acute toxicities, as well as delayed pulmonary fibrosis and late secondary leukemias. These secondary leukemias often arise after a period of myelodysplasia, are usually highly drug resistant AML, and carry defects in chromosomes 5 or 7. Busulfan, bischloroethylnitrosourea (BCNU), or cyclophosphamide are most likely to cause vascular endothelial damage (hepatic venoocclusive disease) when used in high doses. However, these same drugs are often used in high-dose regimens, as they cause less mucositis than other alkylating agents. 4-Hydroperoxycyclophosphamide, an activated analogue of cyclophosphamide, appears to spare marrow stem cells relative to tumor cells and has been used for *in vitro* purging of marrow in autologous transplantation.[122]

Although platinum analogues are not true alkylating agents in that they form metal adducts rather than carbon adducts with DNA, RNA, and protein, their range of toxicities and mechanisms of resistance have much in common with the classical alkylators. They have few indications in hematologic malignancy, aside from carboplatin and its role in high-dose chemotherapy for lymphomas. Their DNA adducts are subject to repair by nucleotide excision repair and double-strand break repair, processes dependent on functional p53 activity.[123] Polymorphisms of the repair pathways, especially the mismatch repair process, may be associated with drug resistance,[124] whereas errors in double-strand break repair (as found in *BRCA1*- and *BRCA2*-solid tumors), may create sensitivity to platinating drugs.

Mechanism of Action

All alkylating agents (Fig. 22–4) have in common the generation of highly reactive carbonium intermediates that attack electron-rich sites on DNA, such as the *N-7*, *O-2*, and *O-6* positions of guanine and the *N-1*, *N-3*, and *N-7* positions of adenine. For many of these agents, the alkylating group must undergo a preliminary activation reaction mediated either by chemical rearrangement of the molecule, as in the case of nitrogen mustard and the nitrosoureas, or by metabolic activation followed by chemical rearrangement, as for cyclophosphamide, ifosfamide, and procarbazine. Most alkylating agents have two reactive sites, usually two chloroethyl groups, enabling them to form intrastrand and, less frequently, interstrand crosslinks.

A second class of alkylating drugs, exemplified by busulfan, dimethyltriazenoimidazole carboxamide (DTIC) and the closely related temozolomide, and procarbazine, produce only single-strand alkylation but may be highly carcinogenic, as, for example, procarbazine. In general, all the commonly used alkylating drugs, including cyclophosphamide, ifosfamide, melphalan, chlorambucil, and the methylating drugs, produce the same spectrum of myelosuppressive, carcinogenic, and genotoxic actions, and depend on an intact mismatch repair system to recognize their adducts and initiate apoptosis.

Experimental systems have elucidated the mechanisms of resistance to alkylating agents.[125] Some mechanisms are specific for certain alkylating agents (e.g., impaired uptake of nitrogen mustard as a consequence of an alteration in the membrane carrier for choline, or deletion of the amino acid carrier used by melphalan), whereas others appear to be less specific (e.g., drug inactivation associated with an increase in intracellular sulfhydryl compounds, and enhanced nucleotide-excision repair of DNA adducts). The primary resistance mechanisms for various alkylating drugs, as documented in experimental tumors, include increased degradation by aldehyde dehydrogenase (specifically for cyclophosphamide)[126]; increased conjugation of the reactive intermediates with glutathione or glutathione transferase (all chloroethylating agents and platinum analogues); increased repair of the O-6 guanine alkyl lesions by a specific alkyl transferase (nitrosoureas, procarbazine, temozolomide, and dacarbazine)[127]; increased nucleotide excision repair (all platinum derivatives and chloroethylating agents, except possibly nitrosoureas); decreased uptake (melphalan, nitrogen mustard); decreased ability to recognize DNA damage because of defective mismatch repair, especially the loss of the MLH6 component[128] (most alkylating agents and platinum derivatives); and defective recognition of DNA alkylation and strand breaks and initiation of apoptosis (p53 loss-of- function mutants), which affects all alkylators. The basis of alkylating agent resistance in the clinic is still incompletely understood.

Clinical Pharmacology

In general, the alkylating agents and their reactive intermediates have short residence times in the systemic circulation and within cells. They are eliminated predominantly by hydrolysis of the reactive site, by

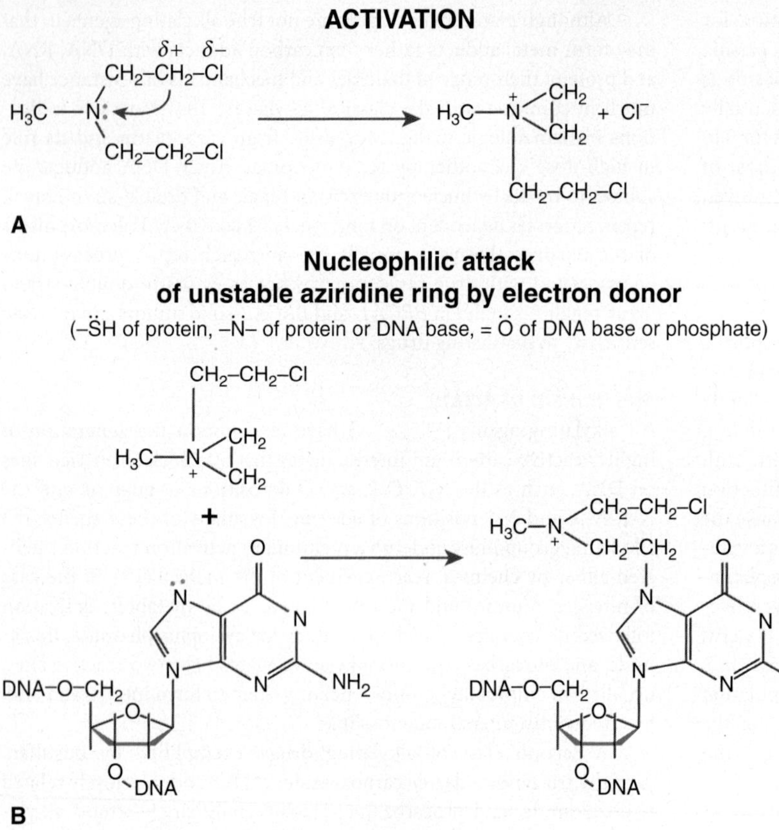

ACTIVATION

A

**Nucleophilic attack
of unstable aziridine ring by electron donor**
(–S̈H of protein, –N̈– of protein or DNA base, = Ö of DNA base or phosphate)

B

Figure 22–4. Mechanism of action of alkylating agents attacking a purine base in DNA. (*Reproduced with permission from Brunton L, Chabner B, and Knollman B:* Goodman & Gilman's The Pharmacological Basis of Therapeutics, *12th ed. New York, NY: McGraw-Hill; 2011.*)

chemical or biochemical conjugation to the sulfhydryl groups of glutathione or proteins, or by oxidative metabolism in the case of ifosfamide and cyclophosphamide. Therefore, dose reduction is not required in patients with diminished renal or hepatic function.

A few of the drugs require enzymatic activation. Cyclophosphamide and ifosfamide are closely related molecules that undergo hepatic CYP-mediated activation. Their active metabolites include a highly labile phosphoramide mustard and a second toxic metabolite, acrolein, which is excreted in the urine.[129] To counteract toxicity of acrolein to kidneys and bladder, mercaptoethane sulfonate (mesna) is administered simultaneously in equivalent doses to the alkylator. Procarbazine and DTIC require metabolic activation by hepatic CYP isoenzymes, whereas temozolomide, a structural congener of DTIC, spontaneously activates to a methylating intermediate, and has become the preferred drug for treating glioblastomas.

Nitrogen mustard is a highly reactive compound in its parent form, and thus can be administered topically for treatment of skin cancers and cutaneous lymphoma. It is a potent vesicant, and care must be taken in the mixing and administering the drug. It is still a preferred component of combination therapy in conjunction with vincristine (Oncovin), procarbazine and prednisone (MOPP) for childhood Hodgkin lymphoma. Extravasation may lead to severe tissue injury. The second-generation alkylating agents, which include cyclophosphamide, melphalan, busulfan, and chlorambucil, are more chemically stable and absorbed reasonably well when given orally.

The newest alkylating drug, bendamustine, is approved for both CLL and relapsed lymphomas, and consists of a purine base with a *bis*-chloroethyl side chain. In experimental systems it is only partially cross-resistant with other alkylators, and produces a bulky DNA adduct that is slowly removed by base excision repair. It strongly induces p53 phosphorylation and apoptosis, as well as cell necrosis, a distinct cell

death response.[130] Bendamustine metabolism produces two minor toxic metabolites: hydroxylation of its 4 position and N-demethylation. The bulk of parent drug is eliminated through its reactivity with sulfhydryls and adduct formation. The drug displays much the same pattern of toxicity of other alkylating drugs, with perhaps less myelosuppression.

Carboplatin, often used in high-dose therapy of lymphomas, is primarily excreted by the kidneys. Its dosing is based on renal function, aiming at a specific area under the curve of 5 to 7, according to the formula:

$$\text{Dose (mg/m}^2) = \text{Area under the curve} \times (\text{glomerular filtration rate} + 25)$$

Adverse Effects of Alkylating Agents

Marrow toxicity, which is cumulative and a function of total dose, is the most important acute toxic effect of alkylators. Nitrosoureas produce a characteristic delayed myelosuppression that reaches a nadir 4 to 6 weeks after administration. Busulfan, like the nitrosoureas, depletes stem cells and can cause profound marrow hypoplasia or permanent aplasia. The dose-limiting toxicity of DTIC is nausea and vomiting rather than marrow suppression. Carboplatin causes an acute thrombocytopenia, as well as a more chronic sensory neuropathy.

Other common toxicities include denudation of the gastrointestinal epithelium, pneumonitis, cardiac, and endothelial damage, which become evident during high-dose therapy. Virtually every organ system may be damaged by alkylating agents. Because alkylating agents react with DNA, mutations and secondary leukemias are major long-term effects of these agents. This hazard appears to be related to the total dose administered. The monofunctional methylating agents (e.g., procarbazine) are especially potent in this regard. All alkylating agents, but particularly busulfan and the nitrosoureas, may produce pulmonary fibrosis. The nitrosoureas also cause nephrotoxicity, particularly after total doses of 1200 mg/m² BCNU, whereas cyclophosphamide and ifosfamide cause chronic bladder toxicity, hemorrhage, and, in rare cases, bladder carcinomas. Urinary toxicity of the latter two agents is prevented by coadministration of mesna, a sulfhydryl that detoxifies acrolein at acid pH.

High-Dose Alkylating Agent Therapy

The development of hematopoietic cell transplantation has made it possible to administer doses of chemotherapy that would otherwise produce life-threatening aplasia. To be of benefit, however, high-dose therapy must employ agents that have a relatively steep dose–response relationship. The drugs used must not have lethal extramedullary toxicity at high doses. Among the classes of cytotoxics, alkylators have a particularly favorable linear relationship between dose and cytotoxicity in experimental tumor systems. Extramedullary organ toxicities are infrequent until doses are increased manyfold, making them ideal candidates for high-dose regimens. Depending on the agent and the toxicity profile, doses may only be escalated by as little as twofold as seen with cisplatin because of renal toxicity, or to as high as 18-fold in the case of thiotepa (Table 22–3).[131-137] However, when agents are combined into a high-dose regimen, overlapping extramedullary toxicities of the agents must be considered so as to avoid serious organ compromise (Table 22–4).[138-142] Overlapping extramedullary toxicities (particularly the risk of pulmonary or hepatic dysfunction or secondary leukemia) cannot be completely avoided, but rational drug selection can minimize the dose reductions of the individual agents, compared to their single-agent maximum tolerated dose (MTD), while at the same time ensuring safety of the combination regimen. This is illustrated in

TABLE 22–3. Dose-Limiting Extramedullary Toxicities of Single-Agent Chemotherapy

Drug	Maximum Tolerated Dose (mg/m²)*	Increase Over Standard Dose†	Major Toxicities‡
Cyclophosphamide	7000	7.0	Cardiac
Ifosfamide	16,000	2.7	Renal, CNS
Thiotepa§	1005	18.0	GI, CNS
Melphalan§	180	5.6	GI
Busulfan§	640	9.0	GI, hepatic
BCNU§	1050	5.3	Lung, hepatic
Cisplatin	200	2.0	Renal, neuropathy
Carboplatin§	2000	5.0	Hepatic, renal
Etoposide	3000	6.0	GI
Cytarabine	3000	10–30	Neurologic, mucositis

BCNU, bischloroethyl nitrosourea; GI, gastrointestinal.

*Independent of hematopoietic toxicity. Dose may be given over multiple days.

†Fold increase. This is an approximation because standard doses may vary.

‡All drugs listed in this table cause vascular endothelial damage and venoocclusive disease, as well as late secondary leukemias.

§With stem cell support.

Table 22–4, which shows the fraction of the single-agent MTD that can be administered in combination with other drugs. As might be expected, this fraction is quite variable depending on the drug combinations, with the average fractional MTD used in combination ranging from 0.5 to 1. Depending on the regimen, significant gastrointestinal, pulmonary, hepatic, and/or renal toxicities are encountered and become dose limiting. For these reasons, high-dose regimens are safest in patients who are younger (<70 years) and who have had minimal prior chemotherapy and radiation therapy.

AGENTS OF DIVERSE MECHANISMS

BLEOMYCIN

Bleomycin is a mixture of cytotoxic peptides produced by the fungus *Streptomyces verticillis*.[143] Because it has antitumor activity with minimal marrow toxicity, it is commonly used as part of combination regimens (such as ABVD) to treat Hodgkin lymphoma and with cisplatin and vinblastine to treat germ cell tumors. Bleomycin acts by causing both single- and double-strand breaks in DNA. These breaks form as a consequence of a bleomycin–Fe (II) complex that binds to DNA and undergoes redox cycling with molecular oxygen. The drug's reactive complex abstracts a proton from deoxyribose, leading to cleavage of the sugar at the 3′-carbon.[144] In experimental tumors, resistance to bleomycin has been attributed to increased tumor cell concentrations of an aminohydrolase that cleaves and inactivates the drug.[145] Some resistant cell lines exhibit enhanced capacity to repair strand breaks, and in others, resistance results from decreased drug accumulation. Additional factors, such as increased free radical detoxification, may also influence toxicity. The tumor specificity of bleomycin, its severe cutaneous and pulmonary toxicity, and its lack of toxicity to marrow and the gastrointestinal tract may be a result of widely differing levels of metal ions and bleomycin hydrolase, the detoxifying enzyme, in these tissues. A polymorphism in the hydrolase gene, identified by SNP A1450G, may confer resistance to the drug as the result of its enhanced hydrolase activity.[146] Cell killing occurs throughout the cell cycle.

Clinical Pharmacology

Bleomycin may be administered intravenously or intramuscularly in doses of 10 to 20 U/m² per week to cumulative doses of 250 U for systemic therapy, as well as intrapleurally or intraperitoneally for control of malignant effusions. The half-life of drug elimination from plasma is estimated to be 2 to 3 hours. After a single intravenous injection, more than half the dose is excreted, unchanged, in the urine within 24 hours.[147] Bleomycin elimination may be markedly impaired in patients with poor renal function; such patients are at risk of overwhelming skin and lung toxicity. Dose reduction by 50 percent should be considered in patients with a CrCl in the range of 30 to 80 mL/min, and drug should be withheld in the present of CrCl less than 30 mL/min.

Adverse Effects

Bleomycin has minimal effects on normal marrow; however, in patients given other myelosuppressive drugs or who are recovering from marrow toxicity from these agents, additional mild myelosuppression may be observed. The primary toxicities that result from bleomycin are pulmonary fibrosis and skin changes. In experimental settings, the drug activates the Hedgehog pathway and induces the secretion of numerous cytokines, including interleukin (IL)-6, tumor necrosis factor-α and transforming growth factor-β, by alveolar macrophages and inflammatory cells, leading to collagen deposition.[148] The risk of pulmonary toxicity is related to the cumulative dose administered, increasing to 10 percent in patients given more than 450 mg. Risk is also greater in

TABLE 22–4. Toxicities and Doses of High-Dose Regimens Administered with Stem Cell Support

Regimen	Dose (mg/m²)	Fraction of MTD*	Major Toxicities	Tumor Targets	Reference
Cyclophosphamide	6000	0.86	GI, cardiac	Breast	135
Thiotepa	500	0.5			
Carboplatin	800	0.4			
Cyclophosphamide	6000	0.86	Lung, GI	Lymphomas	136
BCNU	300	0.29			
Etoposide	750	0.25			
Busulfan	640	1.0	Lung, GI, hepatic	Lymphoma	137
Cyclophosphamide	8000	1.0			
Ifosfamide	16,000	1.0	Renal, hepatic, GI	Lymphomas	138
Carboplatin	1800	0.9			
Etoposide	1500	0.5			
Cyclophosphamide	5625	0.8	Cardiac, hepatic, renal	Breast	139
BCNU	600	0.57			
Cisplatin	164	0.82			

BCNU, bischloroethylnitrosourea; GI, gastrointestinal; MTD, maximum tolerated dose.
*This is the fraction of the single-agent MTD (see Table 22–3, Col. 2).

patients older than age 60 years,[149] in patients with underlying lung disease, in patients receiving bleomycin who are given high oxygen concentrations, and in patients who have had previous radiotherapy to the lungs. Single intravenous doses of 25 mg/m² or more predispose to this toxic effect. Symptoms of pulmonary toxicity include cough and dyspnea. Chest radiographs show nonspecific infiltrates, especially in the lower lobes. Chest computed tomography changes may show extensive infiltrates, fibrosis in later stages of evolution, atelectasis, or cavitation. Positron emission tomography scans are strongly positive. Open-lung biopsy may be required to distinguish bleomycin pulmonary toxicity from infection or malignant disease. Pathologic findings of bleomycin toxicity include an inflammatory alveolar infiltrate with edema, pulmonary hyaline formation, and squamous metaplasia of the alveolar lining cells. These changes progress to intraalveolar and interstitial fibrosis over a period of months. Patients with bleomycin lung toxicity have a measurable decrease in carbon monoxide diffusing capacity, a test of possible value in predicting potential pulmonary toxicity.[150] Because there is no specific therapy for patients with bleomycin lung toxicity, close attention should be paid to early pulmonary symptoms and radiographic changes. In patients with bleomycin pulmonary toxicity, some improvement may be seen on discontinuation of the drug, but the pulmonary fibrosis is usually not reversible. Glucocorticoids may decrease inflammation, but are of no proven benefit once fibrosis has occurred. O₂ supplementation must be avoided, as it promotes the oxidative injury to pulmonary tissue.

The dermatologic toxicity of bleomycin is also dose related. Erythema, hyperpigmentation, hyperkeratosis, and even ulceration may occur when the drug is given in conventional daily doses for longer than 2 to 3 weeks. Areas of skin pressure, especially of the hands, fingers, and joints, are initially affected, and Raynaud phenomenon may become apparent in the distal digits. Nail changes and alopecia may also occur with continued use of the drug. In combination regimens (e.g., ABVD) where bleomycin is used intermittently, skin toxicity is rarely a dose-limiting problem.

Fever and malaise after injection are common symptoms and may be alleviated by acetaminophen. Hypersensitivity reactions have also been observed. Idiosyncratic cardiovascular collapse has been rarely noted. A 1- or 2-mg test dose administered to such susceptible patients may result in hypotension, tachycardia, pulmonary insufficiency, or anaphylactoid reactions within 30 to 60 minutes. Their occurrence precludes further treatment with bleomycin.

L-ASPARAGINASE

The enzyme L-asparaginase is used clinically in the treatment of lymphoid malignancies, particularly in poor-risk B-cell ALL, T-cell ALL, natural killer (NK)-cell leukemia, and in high-grade lymphomas.

Mechanism of Action

The cells causing these lymphoid malignancies require exogenous L-asparagine for growth; they obtain this amino acid from the systemic pool of amino acids generated by the liver. The enzyme L-asparaginase, which catalyzes the hydrolysis of asparagine to aspartic acid and ammonia, rapidly depletes L-asparagine from plasma and induces an asparagine deficiency in lymphoid malignant cells. Resistant tumors are able to respond by induction of asparagine synthetase,[151] thereby restoring intracellular pools of asparagine. For reasons not well understood, hyperdiploid ALL cells are particularly sensitive to L-asparaginase, whereas cells containing the BCR-ABL translocation are more resistant.[152]

Three L-asparaginase preparations are available in the United States.[153] The product purified from *Escherichia coli* is employed as a first-line agent, while a second preparation (pegaspargase), derived by attachment of polyethylene glycol to the *E. coli* enzyme, is used for first-time therapy and for patients hypersensitive to the unmodified enzyme. A third preparation, purified from *Erwinia chrysanthemi*, can be obtained from the National Cancer Institute of the United States for patients hypersensitive to the *E. coli* enzyme or to pegaspargase. The various preparations differ in their pharmacokinetics, immunogenicity, and recommended doses. The *E. coli* enzyme is usually given in doses of 6000 to 10,000 IU intramuscularly every third day for 3 to 4 weeks, although much higher doses (25,000 IU once weekly) may be more effective in ALL treatment. Levels are maintained continuously above 0.2 IU/mL plasma, leading to total abolition of asparagine in the systemic circulation. The *E. coli* enzyme has an elimination half-life of 14 to 24 hours. Monomethoxypolyethylene glycol (PEG) conjugated to the *E. coli* enzyme reduces its immunogenicity and extends its half-life to 6 days. Pegaspargase is used in patients hypersensitive to the unmodified enzyme, in doses of 2500 IU/m² intramuscularly every 2 weeks. Single doses deplete L-asparagine from plasma for 2 to 3 weeks. Some patients develop hypersensitive to both preparations of *E. coli* enzyme, particularly if first exposed to the unmodified enzyme; they may be treated with enzyme from *Erwinia*, which has a low incidence of hypersensitivity and approximately equal catalytic activity to the *E. coli* preparation, but a more rapid clearance.[154] Consequently, the *Erwinia* enzyme must be used in higher doses.

Adverse Effects

Reactions to the first dose are uncommon, but after two or more doses of the unmodified enzyme, hypersensitivity may develop in up to 20 percent of patients, varying from urticarial reactions to hypotension, laryngospasm, and cardiac arrest. Skin testing to predict allergic reactions is helpful in some, but not all, cases, and should be performed to confirm a clinical suspicion of hypersensitivity. Hypersensitive patients may have antibodies to L-asparaginase in their plasma. More than half the patients with such circulating antibodies will not display an overt allergic reaction to the drug, but these patients may have more rapid disappearance of drug from plasma and an inadequate clearance of asparagine from plasma and cells, leading to therapeutic failure. Patients who are treated with L-asparaginase should be observed carefully for several hours after dosing, and epinephrine should be available in case anaphylactic reactions occur. Anaphylaxis is less likely when *E. coli* L-asparaginase is given intramuscularly than when it is administered intravenously. Pegaspargase has much reduced immunogenicity and hypersensitivity reactions are uncommon. However, up to 20 percent of patients previously exposed to unmodified L-asparaginase will develop allergy to subsequent pegaspargase, with undetectable enzyme levels in plasma, and an additional 8 percent will have silent inactivation of the enzyme. The other major toxic effects of L-asparaginase are a consequence of the ability of this drug to inhibit protein synthesis in normal tissues. Inhibition of protein synthesis in the liver will result in hypoalbuminemia, a decrease in clotting factors, a decrease in serum lipoproteins, and a marked increase in plasma triglycerides. Inhibition of insulin production may lead to hyperglycemia. The clotting abnormalities that are regularly observed as a consequence of L-asparaginase treatment include initial decreases in the anticoagulant factors antithrombin III,

protein C, and protein S, leading to either arterial or venous thrombosis in occasional patients, and a predilection to thrombosis of cortical sinus vessels.[155] With more prolonged therapy, bleeding sequelae may result from inhibition of the synthesis of procoagulant proteins such as fibrinogen and factors II, VII, IX, and X. Consequently, monitoring of coagulation factors is recommended. High doses of L-asparaginase may cause cerebral dysfunction that manifests as confusion, stupor, seizures, or coma, and cortical sinus thrombosis has been documented by magnetic resonance imaging scan in such patients.[156] Clinical thromboembolic episodes may occur in up to 35 percent of children with ALL.[157] These events are mostly asymptomatic thrombi associated with central venous catheters; less frequently, cortical sinus and atrial thrombi may occur. Altered mental status may also result from hyperammonemia and diabetic ketoacidosis.[158] Preexisting clotting abnormalities, such as antiphospholipid antibodies or factor V Leiden deficiency, may predispose to thromboembolic complications.[159]

Acute nonhemorrhagic pancreatitis occurs as a complication of L-asparaginase treatment, especially in patients who have extreme elevations of plasma triglycerides (>2 g/dL).[160] Because L-asparaginase manifests little toxicity in marrow or gastrointestinal mucosa, it has been used in combination with other drugs that do have such toxicities.

● IMMUNOMODULATORY DRUGS

THALIDOMIDE, LENALIDOMIDE, AND POMALIDOMIDE

Thalidomide (α-phthalimidoglutarimide; Fig. 22–5), approved in 1953 as a sedative, was withdrawn shortly thereafter because of its teratogenicity. It causes dysmelia (i.e., stunted limb growth) when used during early pregnancy. However, it has since reemerged as an important antibacterial and antitumor agent, with clear effectiveness against leprosy and myeloma, especially when combined with other agents.[161] Its analogues, lenalidomide and pomalidomide (see Fig. 22–5), have proven to be less toxic, and more effective for treating relapsed and refractory patients with myeloma. Lenalidomide is highly active in first-line combination therapy with dexamethasone, and also with bortezomib[162] for myeloma, as well as being approved for the treatment of myelodysplasia in patients with the 5q– variant of this syndrome. The newest immunomodulatory

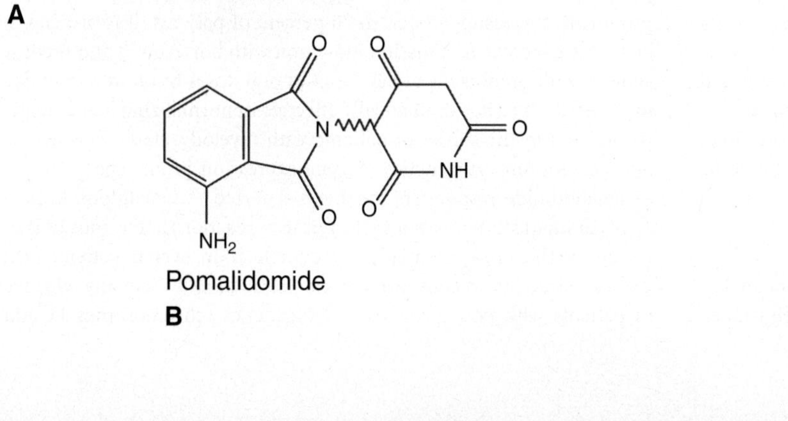

Figure 22–5. Thalidomide, lenalidomide and pomalidomide. *(Reproduced with permission from Brunton L, Chabner B, and Knollman B:* Goodman & Gilman's The Pharmacological Basis of Therapeutics, *12th ed. New York, NY: McGraw-Hill; 2011.)*

Lenalidomide

Thalidomide

A

Pomalidomide

B

drug (IMiD), pomalidomide, is approved for patients refractory to lenalidomide and bortezomib.[163]

The mechanism of action of thalidomide and analogues is incompletely understood, as the compounds have a number of different actions, including a prominent antiangiogenic effect against tumors,[164] immune modulation, and inhibition of cytokine secretion. They inhibit neovascularization in the mouse cornea, block proliferation of endothelial cells in culture,[165] and inhibit secretions of vascular endothelial growth factor and other angiogenic cytokines.[166] Thalidomide potently stimulates phosphorylation of the CD28 costimulatory molecule.[167] This effect can lead to enhancement of T-cell function and activation of signaling pathways. Thalidomide has inhibitory effects on cytokine secretion, lowering levels of tumor necrosis factor-α and γ-interferon in leprosy patients. In addition it enhances NK-cell numbers and function, suppresses T-regulatory cells, and stimulates cytolytic T-cell function. It downregulates interferon regulatory factor 4 (IRF4), a myeloma survival factor. Although lenalidomide and pomalidomide have not been studied as extensively as thalidomide preclinically, they have the same spectrum of biologic actions but with greater potency.

An additional IMiD site of action related to degradation of key proteins has been identified. The IMiDs interact with cereblon, a protein that forms a complex with ubiquitin E3, and thereby promote the degradation of myc protein and other transcription factors. This effect on E3 and cereblon binding partners has been implicated in the teratogenic effects and antitumor activity of the IMiD compounds.[168]

Clinical Pharmacology of Thalidomide and Its Congeners

Thalidomide consists of two enantiomers that rapidly interconvert in solution and biologic fluids. Its two imide bonds are unstable and undergo hydrolysis in solution. The poorly soluble drug undergoes slow and somewhat variable oral absorption with peak levels achieved in 2.9 to 4.3 hours[169,170] after oral doses ranging from 50 to 400 mg. There is no evidence for induction of metabolism on a daily dosing regimen. Drug concentrations in plasma decay with a half-life of 5 to 7 hours, the major pathways for elimination including spontaneous hydrolysis of the imide esters, and further CYP-mediated metabolism by the liver. At high doses of 1200 mg, the rate of clearance of drug from plasma decreases. Less than 1 percent of the drug is excreted unchanged in the urine. No dose adjustment is required for renal dysfunction, although its propensity for causing neuropathy may aggravate any underlying neuropathy secondary to prior exposures, renal failure or amyloidosis, making dose reduction prudent, especially when used in combination with other agents.

Lenalidomide is well absorbed orally in doses up to 400 mg, and usually given in doses up to 25 mg daily; it exhibits a plasma half-life of 3 hours. Approximately 70 percent of administered drug is excreted unchanged by the renal route, the remainder appearing in the feces unchanged. Dose adjustments are therefore recommended for patients in moderate (10 mg/day for CrCl of 30 to 50 mL/min) or severe (10 mg every other day for CrCl <30 mL/min) renal failure. For those on dialysis, the recommended dose is 5 mg once daily, with the same day dose given following dialysis.

Pomalidomide is given orally in doses of up to 4 mg per day. It has a long plasma half-life of 7.5 hours in myeloma patients, and is eliminated by CYP1A2 and CYP3A4 hydroxylation in the liver with minimal renal clearance. Inducers or inhibitors of CYP3A4 metabolism (prominently antibiotics and HIV drugs) and inhibitors of the MDR1 efflux transporter (natural products and targeted cancer therapies) should be used in combination with pomalidomide with caution.[171]

Clinical Use

Thalidomide has been evaluated against a number of human malignancies, with occasional responses in brain tumors, renal cell cancer,

hepatoma, and Kaposi sarcoma. It has established value in treating myeloma refractory to first-line chemotherapy, as well as in newly diagnosed patients.[172,173] In responding patients, all aspects of the disease, including marrow infiltration with tumor cells, anemia, and performance status, improved with therapy. Thalidomide has synergistic myeloma-inhibiting activity with glucocorticoids, interferon-α, bortezomib, and cytotoxic agents. However, lenalidomide, which has less-prominent side effects and probably greater efficacy, has replaced thalidomide in first-line regimens for myeloma. Pomalidomide is reserved for patients refractory to lenalidomide and bortezomib, and retains impressive activity in this setting.

Thalidomide is generally well tolerated in oral doses of 50 to 1200 mg daily, although higher doses are more challenging. In treating myeloma, a 1-month trial is usually sufficient to observe a decline in paraprotein and an improvement in symptoms, with doses typically used ranging from 50 to 200 mg/daily. Doses can be escalated up to 200 mg every 2 weeks until dose-limiting toxicity is reached at 600 to 800 mg/day, but these higher doses are rarely used. Patients older than age 65 years are less tolerant of side effects, particularly sedation, constipation, fatigue, and peripheral sensory neuropathy, and receive a median dose of at most 400 mg/day, with lower doses (e.g., 100 mg/day) being preferable,[174] whereas younger patients may tolerate up to a median of at most 800 mg/day, although again lower doses (e.g., 200 mg/day) are preferable. With extended treatment at doses below 400 mg/day, the peripheral sensory neuropathy may become bothersome, but usually improves with dose reduction or drug discontinuation. To avoid undue sedation, the drug is given either in divided doses, morning and evening, or as a single evening dose. Other side effects include rash, dizziness and orthostatic hypotension, neutropenia, mood changes or depression, and nausea. Hypersensitivity and bradycardia also have been reported. Rarely patients may develop an interstitial pneumonitis or fulminant hepatic failure.

Trials of thalidomide in combination with cytotoxic drugs or biologics originally disclosed some unexpected toxicities.[175] Thalidomide in combination with doxorubicin or with prednisone is associated with an increased incidence of thromboembolism, a complication that can be prevented by concurrent treatment with low-molecular-weight heparin or aspirin.[176] Because of its teratogenicity, patients of childbearing age should take precautions to prevent pregnancy while on therapy. In trials of thalidomide and interferon against renal cell carcinoma, in which high doses of interferon (9 million IU subcutaneously three times per week) were used, four of 13 patients developed complex partial seizures and visual disturbances.[177] Two of 19 patients on thalidomide with low-dose interferon (1.5 to 3 million IU three times weekly) developed complex partial seizures in a trial against melanoma.

In the United States, thalidomide and its analogues are approved for use under a special risk evaluation and mitigation strategy (REMS), with restricted pharmacy access and a special consent form, to assure that pregnant women are not given these agents.

The analogue, lenalidomide, with significant activity against myeloma, causes much less sedation, constipation, and neurotoxicity, but prominent myelosuppression in 20 percent of patients. It is proving to be highly effective in remission induction with bortezomib and prednisone or with prednisone alone. Used in oral doses of up to 25 mg/day for 21 of 28 days, it is dramatically effective in normalizing hematologic parameters in the subset of patients with myelodysplasia who have a 5q– deletion on cytogenetics. A gene expression profile characteristic of lenalidomide responders has been reported.[178] Lenalidomide produces dramatic tumor swelling (tumor flare reaction) and tumor lysis in patients with CLL, a potentially fatal complication, even in patients with disease refractory to conventional agents. In CLL, it is equally effective in patients with poor prognostic cytogenetics (chromosomes 11 and

17 deletions). It must be started in low doses (beginning at 2.5 to 5 mg/day and escalating thereafter) to avoid tumor flare reaction and renal failure.[179] It has rarely been associated with severe hepatic and renal toxicity.

Like thalidomide, lenalidomide in combination with anthracyclines or glucocorticoids causes a 15 percent incidence of thrombotic events, and in these combinations should be administered with low-molecular-weight heparin, although prospective trials of anticoagulation are lacking.[180]

Pomalidomide's prominent toxicity is neutropenia in 50 to 60 percent of patients, and thrombocytopenia in 25 percent. It has little sedating effects and causes neuropathy in 10 percent or fewer subjects. It is highly active in relapsed, refractory myeloma and particularly in combination with various agents, including dexamethasone and proteasome inhibitors, such as bortezomib and carfilzomib. Rare toxicities include thromboembolism (3 percent) and isolated cases of hepatic failure.[163]

● DIFFERENTIATING AGENTS

Certain chemical agents have the ability to cause terminal differentiation (maturation) of malignant cells.[181,182] The most prominent among these are members of the vitamin A family (carotenes and retinoids), vitamin D and its analogues, phenylacetic acid, various cytotoxic agents used in low concentrations (such as hydroxyurea), inhibitors of DNA methylation such as 5-azacytidine and 5-aza-2′-deoxycytidine or decitabine, and inhibitors of histone deacetylase, exemplified by vorinostat, depsipeptide, and various benzamides.[183] In addition, biologic agents such as the interferons and interleukins induce terminal differentiation of both malignant and normal cells, but the role of terminal differentiation in the anticancer action of these drugs in humans is uncertain, as they have multiple biologic effects.

RETINOIDS

As the first effective terminal differentiating agent in cancer therapy, ATRA induces complete responses in a high percentage of patients with APL, and has become a standard member of the combination regimen for treatment and cure of this disease.[184] ATRA acts through binding to a nuclear receptor formed by the heterodimerization of the retinoic acid receptor-α (RARα) and its partner, the retinoid X receptor. In APL, an abnormal fusion protein, composed of portions of the RARα and a unique transcription factor (the *PML* gene product), results from the characteristic 15;17 chromosomal translocation found in this disease.[185] The fusion protein has a lower affinity for retinoids than does the wild-type molecule. High concentrations of retinoids are required to displace a corepressor bound to the protein, and activate key differentiation factors such as CCAAT/enhancer binding protein (C/EBP) and PU.1.[186] The fusion protein forms a variety of homo- and heterodimers that regulate genes and increase leukemic stem cell renewal, and suppress apoptosis and DNA repair, further contributing to progression of leukemia. In experimental settings, resistance to ATRA differentiating activity results from mutation or loss of retinoid binding in the *PML-RARα* fusion gene, indicating that the fusion gene product plays a role in retinoid responsiveness, and sensitivity can be restored by transfection of a functional *RARα* gene.[187]

ATRA is administered to APL patients in oral doses of 25 to 45 mg/m² per day until complete remission is achieved and reaches peak serum levels of 300 ng/mL 1 to 2 hours after administration.[188] It is also used in remission maintenance, with 6-MP, methotrexate, or ara-C. The parent drug disappears from serum with a half-life of less than 1 hour during the initial course of treatment, but its rate of clearance greatly accelerates with continued treatment, a factor that may contribute to resistance

to ATRA therapy. Induction of CYP26A1-mediated metabolism is suspected to underlie this accelerated clearance, and may account for the high rate of disease recurrence if ATRA is used as a single agent.[189] The primary toxicities of ATRA resemble those of other retinoids and vitamin A, specifically dry skin, cheilitis, mild and reversible hepatic dysfunction, bone tenderness and hyperostosis on radiography, hypercalcemia, hyperlipidemia, and occasional cases of pseudotumor cerebri. Imidazole antifungals block the degradation of ATRA and may lead to hypercalcemia and renal failure. In addition, approximately 15 percent of patients with APL, particularly those with an initial leukemic cell count greater than 5000/μL, develop a syndrome of hyperleukocytosis, fever, altered mental status, pleural and pericardial effusions, and respiratory failure (the "retinoic acid syndrome").[190] Hyperleukocytosis and leukocyte adherence to small vessels results from a rapid increase in the number of mature leukemic cells in the blood and from the increased expression of integrins on the leukemic cell surface and secretion of cytokines in response to ATRA. In patients with white blood cell counts above 20×10^3 cells/μL, pleural and pericardial effusions and peripheral edema develop rapidly, and respiratory distress, cardiac failure, and renal insufficiency may lead to death. Anecdotal reports indicate that high-dose glucocorticoids reverse this syndrome, which is mediated by leukocyte adhesion and clogging of small vessels and/or by cytokine release.[191] The early introduction of cytotoxic chemotherapy during remission induction, and the use of dexamethasone sodium phosphate (10 mg twice daily for 3 or more days in patients with initial leukemic counts of greater than 5000 cells/μL), drastically lower the incidence of the syndrome and improve the safety of ATRA therapy.

ARSENIC TRIOXIDE

In the 1930s, arsenic was used to treat CML and other malignancies with little effect. Based on further clinical trials of arsenic trioxide (As_2O_3) in Harbin, China, in 1992, it resurfaced as an impressively effective treatment for relapsed APL, and appears to also be active against myeloma and myelodysplasia.[192] Its mechanism of action probably stems from its ability to promote free radical production.[193] It inhibits the detoxification of free radicals and inactivates glutathione, an important radical scavenger.[194] It promotes degradation of the PML-RARα fusion protein,[195] and upregulates p53 and proapoptotic proteins. The cumulative effect is to induce maturation and promote apoptosis in APL cells. In addition, it has antiangiogenic effects. The sum of these actions is potent antitumor activity in some but not all tumor cells. In APL patients refractory to ATRA and conventional chemotherapy, it produces strikingly durable complete responses, and is therefore under study as a part of primary treatment regimens for this disease.

Patients are treated with a 2-hour intravenous infusion of 0.15 mg/kg day for up to 60 days, or until marrow remission is achieved, with further consolidation therapy beginning 3 weeks after remission. Remissions appear in 2 to 3 months with evidence of leukemic cell differentiation and a progressive blood leukocytosis after 2 weeks of therapy.[196] Side effects of arsenic trioxide in APL may include hyperglycemia, elevated liver enzymes, and hypokalemia, none of which require discontinuation of therapy. Occasional patients complain of fatigue, dysesthesias, and lightheadedness. A pulmonary distress syndrome, similar to that encountered with APL cell maturation after ATRA therapy, occurs in approximately 10 percent of patients, and is managed with glucocorticoids, oxygen, and temporary withholding of arsenic trioxide. Arsenic trioxide prolongs the cardiac QT interval, and uncommonly produces atrial or ventricular arrhythmias; it is important to maintain serum potassium at normal concentrations during arsenic trioxide therapy, and to avoid use of other drugs that prolong the QT interval, such as macrolide antibiotics, methadone, or quinidine.

Torsade de pointes occurs infrequently during arsenic trioxide treatment, but requires immediate treatment with intravenous magnesium sulfate, potassium repletion, and defibrillation if the arrhythmia and hemodynamic instability persist.[197]

A maximum plasma concentration of 5.5 to 7.3 μM was achieved in the initial studies from China, and small amounts of drug and the methylated metabolite are eliminated in the urine, the rest remaining in tissues.[198]

● EPIGENETIC AGENTS

DEMETHYLATING AGENTS

DNA methyltransferases (DNMTs) regulate transcription by methylating CpG promoter regions of DNA and thereby silencing gene expression. Mutations associated with AML, including isocitrate dehydrogenase 1 and 2 (IDH1 and IDH2) mutations, TET2, and mutations that activate DNMT, result in increased DNA methylation. Hypermethylation blocks differentiation and drives cellular proliferation. Two DNA demethylating agents, azacitidine and decitabine, have been approved for treatment of MDS. Both drugs become incorporated into DNA, substituting for cytosine bases, and form a suicide covalent bond with DNMT. The two drugs differ in their activation pathways and in their effects on nucleic acid methylation. Decitabine is phosphorylated by dCK whereas azacitidine is activated by cytidine kinase. Decitabine nucleotide is incorporated only into DNA, while azacitidine is found in both RNA and DNA. The clinical response to these drugs has not been correlated with either global changes in DNA methylation or with methylation of specific genes. Indeed, while traditional thinking has taught that DNA methylation invariably leads to gene silencing, newer studies have demonstrated that many actively transcribed genes have high levels of DNA methylation and that the tissue context and specific patterns of methylated DNA may play an important role in determining transcriptional activity.[199]

Azacitidine received FDA approval for therapy of MDS on the basis of reported improvement in Hgb, white cells, or platelets, delayed progression to AML, improved quality of life, and improved overall survival.[200] In a more recent four-arm phase III trial in higher-risk MDS patients, azacitidine was compared with best supportive care, low-dose ara-C, or induction chemotherapy with anthracycline and ara-C. The median overall survival was 24.5 months in the azacitidine arm compared with 15 months for the other arms.[201]

Decitabine was approved on the basis of a 30 percent overall hematologic response rate in MDS patients.[202] For those with intermediate or high-risk disease, time to AML or death was significantly delayed, but there is no improvement as yet in overall survival with this drug.[203] While the two agents have not been compared head to head in MDS, a meta-analysis showed a significant overall survival benefit versus supportive care only for azacitidine.[204] A retrospective review found no significant difference in efficacy between the two compounds except in patients older than 65 years of age, for whom azacitidine resulted in improved survival and a more favorable toxicity profile.

Both agents increase HgbF levels in sickle cell anemia and thalassemia, and reduce symptomatic episodes, but have been superseded by hydroxyurea for this indication.

Azacitidine is approved for parenteral or subcutaneous administration at 75 mg/m²/day for 7 days every 28 days, a regimen that has been shown to result in maximal DNA hypomethylation. A daily-times-five regimen appears to have similar efficacy.[205] The median number of cycles needed for response is three, but 80 percent of responses occurred before the sixth cycle.[206] An oral formulation is currently being developed and has demonstrated activity in MDS and chronic myelomonocytic leukemia. The decitabine dose resulting in optimal hypomethylation is 20 mg/m² intravenously daily for 5 days every 4 weeks,[205] although alternative schedules employing lower doses have been used. Dose adjustment and delays in repeat cycles may become necessary because of myelosuppression.

The primary clinical toxicities of both drugs include reversible myelosuppression, nausea and vomiting with higher doses, hepatic dysfunction, myalgias, fever, and rash. Both compounds are rapidly deaminated and converted to a chemically unstable azauridine or aza-deoxyuridine metabolite that immediately degrades into inactive products.[202]

A significant portion of patients with MDS does not respond to demethylating agents, and all will ultimately relapse. Azacitidine is initially phosphorylated by a different kinase (uridine-cytidine kinase) and so may benefit patients unresponsive to azacytidine.[205]

Clinical trials of azacytosine nucleosides with histone deacetylase (HDAC) inhibitors have demonstrated promising results in phase I trials in MDS and AML.[205,207] Second-generation hypomethylating agents are currently in clinical trials and hold the promise of more convenient dosing schedules and improved toxicity profiles.[205]

HISTONE DEACETYLASE INHIBITORS

Histone acetylation is an important determinant of gene expression and is regulated by the addition and removal of acetyl groups from lysine amino acid residues on histones. The removal of acetyl groups facilitates chromatin compaction thereby decreasing gene expression and is mediated by HDACs. The four classes of HDACs are differentially expressed. HDACs 1 to 3 are overexpressed in many cancer types. Overexpression of these HDACs is associated with repression of tumor suppressor and DNA repair genes, and confers a poor prognosis.[208,209] HDAC inhibitors reverse these changes. They maintain chromatin acetylation and decompaction and promote expression of tumor-suppressor genes, thereby inducing terminal differentiation and apoptosis of tumor cells. Interestingly, HDACs may paradoxically play a role as tumor suppressors as well, as knockout models in mice exhibit spontaneous tumorigenesis through a p53-mediated mechanism.[208,210,211] HDACs deacetylate multiple nonhistone proteins, including p53 and members of the DNA repair complex, but these actions have uncertain significance.

Three HDAC inhibitors are approved for clinical use: vorinostat and romidepsin. Vorinostat is a hydroxamic acid derivative, whereas romidepsin is a natural product produced by *Chromobacterium violaceum*. Both HDAC inhibitors block the zinc-dependent enzymatic activity of these HDACs and work predominantly against class 1 HDACs (HDACs 1 to 3).[212] In lymphoma cells, romidepsin was able to overcome the prosurvival effects of BCL-2 whereas vorinostat was not.

HDAC inhibitors are active in cutaneous T-cell lymphoma. Pabinostat was recently approved, in combination with bortezomib and dexamethasone, for relapsed multiple myeloma. Romidepsin is useful against peripheral T-cell lymphoma. FDA approval of vorinostat was based upon an overall partial response rate of 30 percent and a median response duration of 168 days in patients with cutaneous T-cell lymphoma who had progressed on at least two prior regimens.[213] Romidepsin was approved for use in cutaneous T-cell lymphoma as well after clinical trials demonstrated an overall response rate of 34 percent, including 7 percent complete responses in previously treated patients.[214]

Romidepsin is approved for use in patients with who have received at least one prior therapy.[212] In these patients it achieved objective response rates of up to 38 percent. The median progression free survival for the 15 percent of patients in complete remission was 29 months.[215,216]

Vorinostat is administered orally at 400 mg/day. It is predominantly cleared by glucuronidation and side change oxidation by cytochrome metabolism, and should be dose reduced to 300 mg/day for mild and moderate hepatic impairment. It is contraindicated in patients with severe hepatic impairment.[217] It has a plasma half-life of 2 hours, although histones remain hyperacetylated for many hours. Renal elimination does not play a major role in the drug's clearance.[218] Romidepsin is administered as a 4-hour intravenous infusion of 14 mg/m² on days 1, 8, and 15 of a 28-day treatment cycle. A dose reduction to 10 mg/m² is possible in patients who experience high-grade toxicities.[219] Romidepsin is metabolized primarily by CYP3A4 and by glucuronidation, and is rapidly cleared with a short half-life of approximately 3.5 hours. Asian patients with the 2B57 genotype of uridine diphosphate (UDP)-glucuronyl transferase may experience delayed clearance and increased toxicity.

Both HDACs are generally well tolerated. The most common adverse events for vorinostat are diarrhea, fatigue, nausea, and anorexia, and laboratory abnormalities including, hyperglycemia, thrombocytopenia, and proteinuria.[213] For romidepsin, nausea, vomiting, infection, fatigue, and myelosuppression were the primary toxicities.[212] Significant QTc prolongation and T-wave flattening but the electrocardiogram (ECG) changes were not associated with clinical cardiotoxicity. Still, it is important to ensure electrolyte levels are normalized prior to and throughout therapy.

Multiple newer HDACs have been extensively tested in clinical trials, although none has proven superior to vorinostat or romidepsin. One new agent, panobinostat, has demonstrated promising results in phase II trials against cutaneous T-cell lymphoma, Hodgkin lymphoma, and Waldenström macroglobulinemia.[208]

FUTURE EPIGENETIC TARGETS

Isocitrate Dehydrogenase 2 Inhibitors

Isocitrate dehydrogenase (IDH) is a metabolic enzyme that converts isocitrate to α-ketoglutarate (αKG) (Fig. 22–6), a cofactor in dioxygenase reaction that precedes demethylation of histones and the DNA.

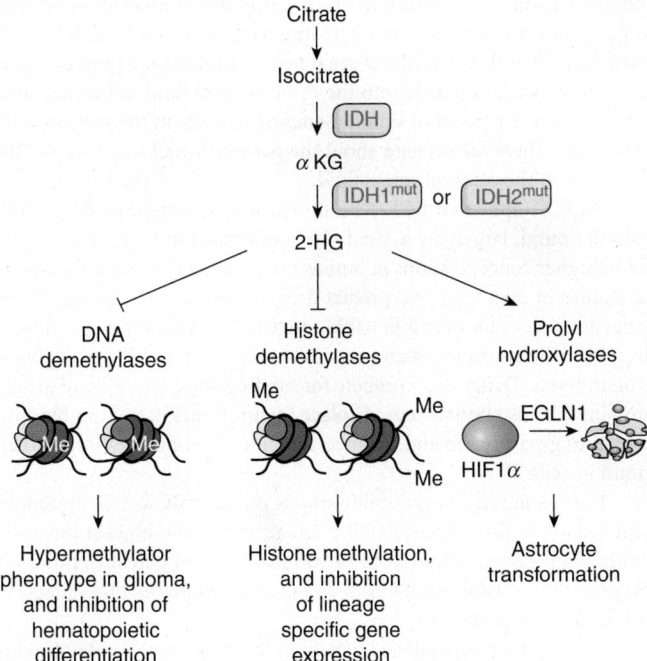

Figure 22–6. Isocitrate dehydrogenase (IDH) mutations produce 2-hydroxyglutarate (2HG), an inhibitor of demethylation reactions. The R-isomer of 2HG activates *EGLN1* gene encoded enzymes, prolyl hydroxylases, which, in turn, activate the ubiquitination and degradation of hypoxia inducible factors (HIFs). (*Reproduced with permission from Schulze A, Harris AL: How cancer metabolism is tuned for proliferation and vulnerable to disruption.* Nature 491(7424):364–373, 2012.)

Certain cancers, including subsets of AML, gliomas, intrahepatic cholangiosarcomas, breast and lung cancers, and central chondrosarcomas harbor IDH1/2 mutations that confer a gain of function. These mutated enzymes (commonly mutated at arginine 132 of IDH1 or arginine 170 of IDH2) convert αKG to the oncometabolite (R)-2-hydroxyglutarate (2HG). High concentrations of 2HG inhibit histone and DNA demethylation by competing with the dioxygenase function of the TET family of enzymes and Jumonji-C domain (JMJC) family of histone lysine demethylases. The result of IDH mutations is hypermethylation of both DNA and histones and a block in differentiation.[220] IDH1 or IDH2 mutations are present in 25 percent of AML where they confer a favorable prognosis. At the same time, IDH mutations in MDS and other myeloproliferative neoplasms may place patients at an increased risk for transformation to AML.[221] High levels of 2HG are measurable in plasma and urine in patients with IDH mutations, and may serve as a sensitive measure of treatment response and may reflect the presence of minimal residual disease.[222] 2HG in IDH mutant solid tumors may also be imaged by magnetic resonance imaging (MRI) spectroscopy.

Small molecule inhibitors of IDH mutant enzymes have been identified. One such inhibitor binds at the dimer interface in an allosteric fashion and exhibits uncompetitive inhibition of mutant IDH2, with great specificity for mutant IDH2 as compared to the wild-type enzyme. Mutant AML cells cultured *ex vivo* in the presence of these inhibitors undergo differentiation.[220]

An oral formulation of the mutant IDH2 inhibitor has shown promising remission-inducing activity in its initial clinical trial.[220A]

DOT1L Inhibitors

Histone methylation also plays a role in transcriptional regulation. Histone methylation leads to exposure of DNA promoter sites, with effects on gene expression. DOT1L, a histone methyltransferase, catalyzes the hypermethylation of specific lysine residues on histone H3 (H3K79), and thereby regulates RNA polymerase II–mediated transcriptional elongation. In leukemias characterized by translocations involving the *MLL* gene, fusion proteins are created that recruit DOT1L to transcription factor (HOXA9 and MEIS1) promoter sites, resulting in leukemogenesis. MLL translocations are seen in 5 to 10 percent of acute leukemias of lymphoid, myeloid, or mixed/indeterminate lineages and are especially common in infant acute leukemias and secondary AML induced by Topo II inhibitors.[221] An aminonucleoside DOT1L inhibitor has entered clinical trials. It occupies the *S*-adenosyl-L-methionine (SAMe) binding pocket of DOT1L and induces conformational changes, thereby contributing to high-affinity binding and specificity of the inhibitor.

Preclinical data demonstrate nanomolar antiproliferative activity specific for MLL-rearranged cell lines, and in a rat xenograft model of MLL-rearranged leukemia, addition of the inhibitor led to complete tumor regression. Based upon these preclinical data, the DOT1L inhibitor has recently entered clinical trials in relapsed/refractory patients with leukemia involving the translocation of the *MLL* gene at 11q23 (NCT01684150).[221]

Enhancer of Zest Homologue 2 Inhibitors

Enhancer of zest homologue 2 (EZH2) is the catalytic subunit of the polycomb repressive complex 2 (PRC2), and methylates lysine K-27 on histone H3 as well as other nonhistone targets. Monoallelic point mutations in EZH2 lead to increased catalytic activity and hyperdimethylation or hypertrimethylation of H3K27 with concomitant transcriptional repression of DNA-damage response pathways in germinal center diffuse large B-cell lymphoma and follicular lymphoma.[223] The Y641 residue is most commonly mutated with up to 22 percent of germinal center diffuse large B-cell lymphoma and 10 percent of follicular lymphoma harboring the mutation.[223] Interestingly, loss-of-function mutations of EZH2 in myeloid malignancies confer a worse prognosis, suggesting that EZH2 may act either as an oncogene or as a tumor suppressor depending on context and site of mutation.

EZH2 inhibitors have been identified through high-throughput biochemical assays using mutant EZH2 with the PRC2 complex and histone substrates. Preclinical data demonstrate increased EZH2 inhibitor selectivity for cell lines carrying activating EZH2 mutations. In mouse models with subcutaneous xenografts of diffuse large B-cell lymphoma cell lines harboring EZH2 activating mutations, marked tumor regression was observed. Based upon these results, EZH2 inhibitors are now in early phase 1 and phase 2 clinical trials in patients with relapsed and refractory diffuse large B-cell lymphoma with EZH2 mutations.[224]

Bromodomain and Extraterminal Inhibitors

The class of bromodomain and extraterminal (BET) family of proteins couple histone acetylation with transcriptional activation by recognizing acetylated lysine residues in histones and recruiting members of the pTEF-b complex to promoters.[225] BET proteins also interact with nonhistone acetylated proteins including p53. BET inhibitors selectively bind to the high conserved bromodomains of the BET proteins thereby inhibiting their ability to bind acetylated lysine residues within histones.

Preclinical data[226] with BET inhibitors demonstrate activity in both myeloma and AML, particularly in cell lines containing MLL fusion proteins or mutant NPM1c+. BET inhibitors induce early cell-cycle arrest and apoptosis via inhibition of c-MYC and other downstream targets.[226] Survival benefits have also been seen in MLL mouse models. HDAC and BET inhibitors act synergistically by maintaining both histone lysine residues and p53 in an acetylated state thereby inducing greater reliance on BET mediated transcription.[227,228] Based upon these results the first BET inhibitors have entered early phase clinical trials.[229]

● SMALL MOLECULES WITH SPECIAL MOLECULAR TARGETS

BCR-ABL TYROSINE KINASE INHIBITORS

The era of targeted cancer therapy was pioneered in the treatment of CML with imatinib mesylate. This carefully designed compound is an inhibitor of ABL tyrosine kinase activity and particularly efficacious against the mutant ABL characteristic of the BCR-ABL fusion protein. This protein is a result of the translocation t(9;22)(q24,q11.2), also known as Philadelphia chromosome, a transforming genetic event, which produces growth factor independent proliferation and sensitizes affected leukemic cells to inhibition with imatinib and other tyrosine kinase inhibitors (TKIs).[230] Imatinib was selected for clinical study by scientists at Ciba-Geigy (later Novartis) based on a high-throughput screen for kinase inhibition and was the first drug of this class approved in 2001 for the treatment of CML based on the large phase III International Randomized Study of Interferon and STI571 (IRIS) trial, which showed induction of durable remissions in a large proportion of patients.[231,232] Since then the three additional second-generation agents dasatinib, nilotinib and bosutinib, as well as the third-generation TKI ponatinib, have been approved for imatinib-refractory or intolerant patients (Table 22–5). Another non-TKI agent, omacetaxine is approved for patients with resistance or intolerance to two or more TKIs.[233]

Mechanism of Action

Imatinib, nilotinib, dasatinib, bosutinib, and ponatinib (Fig. 22–7) are all inhibitors of the BCR-ABL kinase, as well as the c-KIT kinase[234] and the platelet-derived growth factor receptor (PDGFR) kinase. The c-KIT

kinase is the target for imatinib in the treatment of gastrointestinal stromal tumors,[235] while activating mutations of PDGFR are the target of inhibition in the treatment of hypereosinophilia syndrome,[236] chronic myelomonocytic leukemia,[237] MDS with PDGFR rearrangement[237A] and dermatofibrosarcoma protuberans.[238] Dasatinib and ponatinib also inhibit the Src family kinases, an important secondary target in CML.[239] Dasatinib (inhibiting growth by concentration 50 percent [IC_{50}] = <1 nM), nilotinib (IC_{50} = <20 nM),[240] bosutinib (IC_{50} = <1 nM), and ponatinib (IC_{50} = <1 nM and 10 nM for T315I) are more potent inhibitors of BCR-ABL compared to imatinib (IC_{50} = 100 nM). Crystallographic and mutagenesis studies indicate that imatinib and nilotinib bind to a segment of the BCR-ABL tyrosine kinase domain that fixes the enzyme in a closed or inactive state, in which the protein is unable to bind its substrate, ATP.[240-242] The contact points between imatinib and the enzyme become sites of mutations in drug-resistant leukemic cells, preventing tight binding of the drug and locking the enzyme in its active configuration, in which it has access to substrate. Nilotinib has been modified to overcome a number of resistance mutations to imatinib.[239,241,243-245] Dasatinib is unique in that it is able to bind BCR-ABL in both the active and inactive configuration, which may be one of the mechanisms that allows it to overcome resistance.[239] Importantly, ponatinib is the only agent with significant activity against the most common resistance mutation T315I, a gatekeeper mutation that prevents other TKIs from binding to the ATP binding site of BCR-ABL.[246]

Clinical Pharmacology

The BCR-ABL kinase inhibitors are all well absorbed by the oral route and subject to clearance by hepatic CYP3A4 metabolism. The absorption of dasatinib and ponatinib is pH-dependent and may be affected by the use of H_2 blockers and proton pump inhibitors. The absorption of bosutinib may be impaired by concomitant magnesium intake. The bioavailability of nilotinib is increased if taken with meals and therefore should be taken on an empty stomach. Clearance of imatinib is delayed in patients with renal dysfunction, apparently as a result of decreased P450 activity in the presence of renal failure. Limited data indicate that imatinib penetrates poorly into the cerebrospinal fluid, achieving concentrations of 1 percent of simultaneous drug levels in the systemic circulation.[247] There are no data about the penetration of other BCR-ABL inhibitors in the cerebral spinal fluid.

All FDA-approved BCR-ABL inhibitors are more than 94 percent protein bound, largely by α_1-acid glycoprotein, a binding protein present in higher concentrations in humans than in mice.[248] Thus, therapeutic studies in mice may overpredict drug activity. α_1-Acid glycoprotein concentrations vary over a fourfold range in human subjects, and total drug concentrations in plasma appear to be a function of α_1-acid glycoprotein levels. Drugs that compete for binding sites with α_1-acid glycoprotein, such as clindamycin, displace imatinib mesylate from binding to α_1-acid glycoprotein and, in mice, increase the concentration of drug found in cells.

There is significant variability among different BCR-ABL inhibitors with regard to their bioavailability. Imatinib has the highest bioavailability (98 percent), followed by bosutinib (23 to 64 percent), nilotinib (50 percent), and dasatinib (14 to 34 percent), while the bioavailability is unknown for ponatinib.

Despite their unparalleled benefit in the treatment of patients with CML and other malignancies, resistance to TKIs represent a major limitation. Although there are multiple mechanisms of resistance, one can divide resistance to TKIs into two general categories: primary resistance, which refers to a *de novo* lack of response to a drug, and secondary (acquired) resistance, in which resistance to a drug emerges after a period of drug response. The most important and most frequently found resistance mechanisms to TKIs are point mutations in three

TABLE 22–5. Tyrosine Kinase Inhibitors in Treatment of Chronic Myelogenous Leukemia

	Targets	Unique Pharmacokinetics	Mechanism of Clearance	Half-Life	Dosing	Drug Interactions	Toxicity
Imatinib	BCR-ABL, c-Kit, platelet-derived growth factor receptor (PDGFR)	98 percent bioavailability; transport via OCT-1	Hepatic; dose adjustments for severe hepatic and renal impairment	18 hours	Once daily at 400–800 mg	CYP3A4 inducers (dexamethasone, phenytoin, carbamazepine, etc.) CYP3A4 inhibitors (aprepitant, clarithromycin, itraconazole, etc.)	Dose-related fluid retention, heart failure, hepatotoxicity, nausea and vomiting, diarrhea, abdominal pain, skin reactions, myelosuppression
Dasatinib	BCR-ABL, c-Kit, PDGFR, Src family kinases	pH-dependent absorption	Hepatic	3–5 hours	Once daily at 100 mg or twice daily at 70 mg	CYP3A4 inducers (dexamethasone, phenytoin, carbamazepine, etc.) CYP3A4 inhibitors (aprepitant, clarithromycin, itraconazole, etc.) Antacids, H_2 blockers, proton pump inhibitors	Fluid retention (>20%) including pleural and pericardial effusions, heart failure, hepatotoxicity, nausea and vomiting, diarrhea, abdominal pain, skin reactions, myelosuppression, QT prolongation (in vitro), hypocalcemia, hypophosphatemia
Nilotinib	BCR-ABL, c-Kit, PDGFR	Increased bioavailability if taken with food	Hepatic	17 hours	Twice daily at 400 mg	CYP3A4 inducers (dexamethasone, phenytoin, carbamazepine, etc.) CYP3A4 inhibitors (aprepitant, clarithromycin, itraconazole, etc.) Drugs that prolong the QT interval	Fluid retention, heart failure, hepatotoxicity, nausea and vomiting, diarrhea, abdominal pain, skin reactions, myelosuppression, QT prolongation, hypocalcemia, hypophosphatemia, elevated serum lipase and amylase
Bosutinib	BCR-ABL, SRC, LYN, HCK	Absorption may be affected by magnesium intake	Hepatic; dose adjustments for severe hepatic and renal impairment	22 hours	Once daily at 500–600 mg	CYP3A4 inducers (dexamethasone, phenytoin, carbamazepine, etc.) CYP3A4 inhibitors (aprepitant, clarithromycin, itraconazole, etc.) Antacids, H_2 blockers, proton pump inhibitors	Myelosuppression, skin reactions, QT prolongation, Fluid retention, diarrhea, hypophosphatemia, hyper-/hypomagnesemia
Ponatinib	BCR-ABL (including T315I), VEGFR, PDGFR, FGFR, SRC, KIT, RET, TIE-2, FLT-3	pH-dependent absorption	Hepatic	24 hours	Once daily at 30–45 mg	CYP3A4 inducers (dexamethasone, phenytoin, carbamazepine, etc.) CYP3A4 inhibitors (aprepitant, clarithromycin, itraconazole, etc.) Ponatinib is an inhibitor of ABCG2 and P-glycoprotein	Arterial thrombosis, hepatotoxicity, gastrointestinal perforation, wound healing complications, hemorrhage, myelosuppression, cardiac arrhythmias, pancreatitis

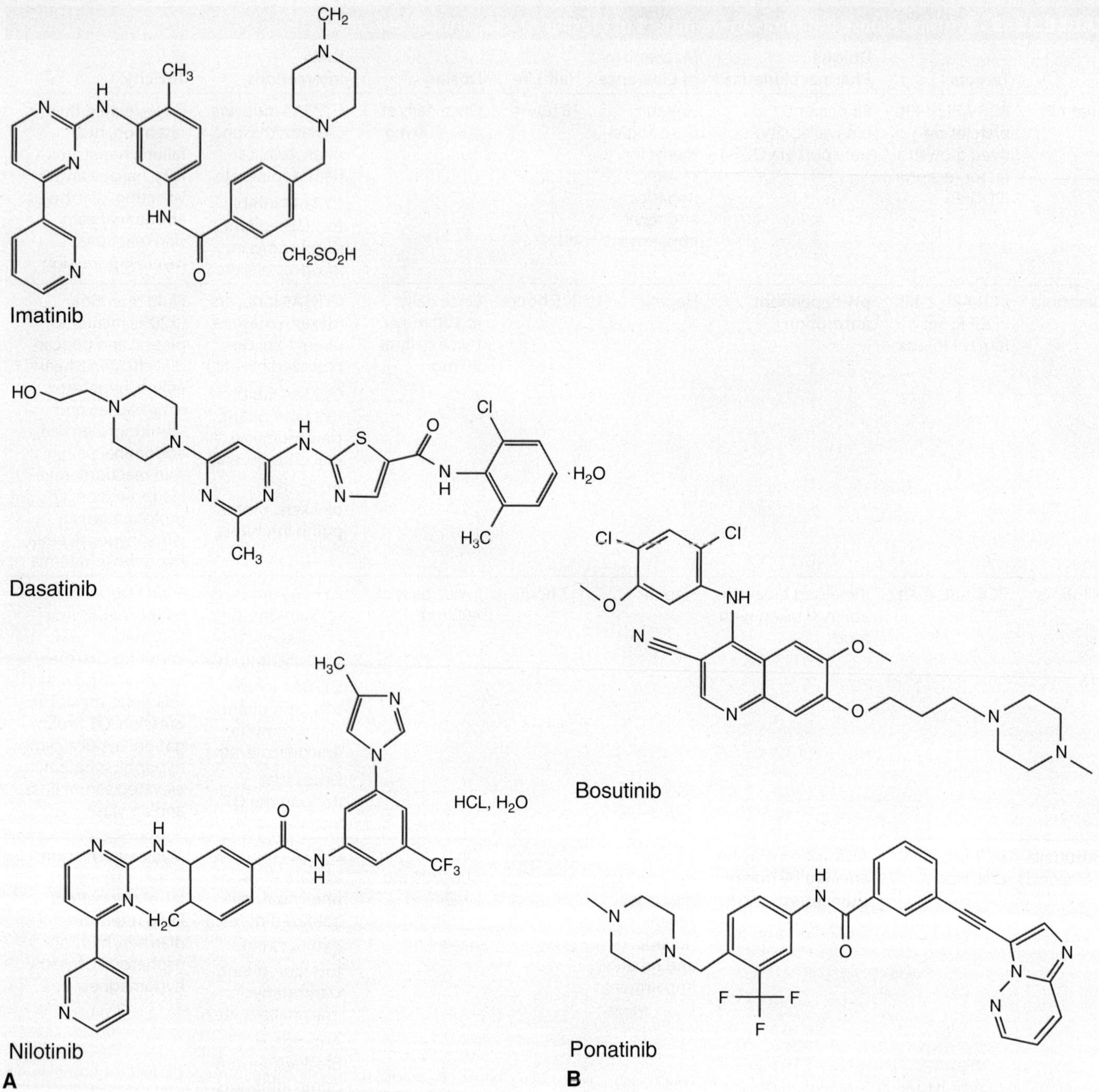

Figure 22–7. BCR-ABL tyrosine kinase inhibitors.

different segments of the kinase domain leading to inability of the drug to effectively inhibit the BCR-ABL kinase activity.[249] The most common mutations associated with clinical resistance affect amino acids 255 and 315, both of which serve as contact points; these mutations confer high-level resistance to imatinib and nilotinib. There is variable efficacy of different BCR-ABL inhibitors to particular resistance mutations. For example, dasatinib can bind to both the active and inactive conformation and can overcome resistance to substitution at 255 but not 315.[241,250] Nilotinib has good activity against most resistance mutations, but lacks activity against substitutions at 255 and 315. Of all approved TKIs, ponatinib is the only agent with activity against the gatekeeper mutation T315I. In a phase II trial of heavily pretreated patients with Philadelphia chromosome positive leukemias, including those who failed dasatinib or nilotinib and with T315I mutations, ponatinib produced major cytogenetic responses in more than half of the patients.[246]

Mutations also affect the phosphate-binding region and the "activation loop" of the domain with varying degrees of associated resistance. Some mutations, such as at amino acids 351 and 355, confer low levels of resistance to imatinib, while these tumor cells remaining sensitive to higher imatinib doses and also sensitive to both nilotinib and dasatinib.[241,251] This may explain the clinical response of some resistant patients to dose escalation of imatinib.

Some kinase mutations known to cause drug resistance may be present at low allelic frequencies prior to initiation of therapy. Malignant cells carrying these mutations may grow out under the pressure of drug and are therefore detected at higher rates after drug exposure.

This observation was made particularly in patients with Philadelphia chromosome–positive ALL or with CML progressing to blastic crisis [252,253] and strongly supports the hypothesis that drug-resistant cells arise through spontaneous mutation, and are further selected by drug exposure.

The site of the resistance mutation has predictive and prognostic implications. Among CML patients, mutations are detectable in some patients receiving imatinib, including one-third of those undergoing treatment in the accelerated phase and in late (longer than 4 years from diagnosis) chronic phase CML.[252] Most patients with mutations demonstrate clinical resistance at the time a mutation is detected, or shortly thereafter. Prior to the development of second generation TKIs, mutations involving the phosphate binding loop were associated with rapid disease progression and death within a median of 4.5 months. The availability of highly active second- and third-generation TKIs that are effective against all known kinase mutations resulted in improved disease control and overall survival in these patients.[246,254-256] As first-line agents, nilotinib and dasatinib are similarly effective, demonstrating high rates of progression free survival and overall survival. The choice of a second-line TKI depends on disease and patient characteristics as well as the side-effect profile of the different agents. For example, currently, there is no alternative to ponatinib for CML with T315I mutation. In patients with targeted CHF or pleural effusions, dasatinib should be avoided given high rate of pleural effusions in up to 35 percent of patients. These patients should be given nilotinib or bosutinib instead. In patients with severe diabetes or a history of pancreatitis, one should avoid nilotinib and choose another second-generation TKI when possible. Patients who fail two or more TKIs, including those with T315I mutation, may also respond to omacetaxine mepesuccinate, a cytotoxic natural product that was FDA approved.[233]

In addition to kinase mutation, amplification of the wild-type kinase gene, leading to overexpression of the enzyme, has been identified in tumor samples from a few patients with resistance to treatment.[257] The *MDR* gene, which codes for a drug efflux protein, confers resistance to imatinib experimentally[258]; thus far this mechanism has not been implicated in clinical resistance. In addition to efflux mechanisms, influx mechanisms may also play an important role. Recent studies indicate that imatinib but not nilotinib or dasatinib is taken into cells via the organic cation transporter-1 (OCT1) and that downregulation of this pathway may confer resistance.[259]

Not all resistance is explained by kinase amplification or mutation, or by pharmacokinetic factors. There is a growing awareness of the appearance of mutant Philadelphia chromosome–negative clones carrying the karyotype of myelodysplastic cells in patients receiving imatinib for CML, and a few cases of progression to MDS and AML have been reported.[260,261] Ongoing research into novel agents for resistant CML includes evaluation of HDAC inhibitors, heat shock protein inhibitors, and targeted therapies of alternative pathways.

Adverse Effects

Imatinib, dasatinib, nilotinib, and bosutinib have modest toxicity. All cause low levels of gastrointestinal distress, including nausea and vomiting. Significant diarrhea occurs more frequently with use of imatinib and bosutinib. All can promote fluid retention resulting in peripheral edema and pleural effusions, with dasatinib causing significantly more edema than the other drugs of this class.[262,263] Although all agents cause rashes, imatinib and bosutinib tend to promote more-severe (grades III/IV) rashes in up to one-third of patients. Mild elevation of transaminases is seen with all BCR-ABL inhibitors, but more-severe elevation with bosutinib. Bilirubinemia is a rather uncommon adverse effect but it is frequently observed with use of nilotinib. Dasatinib and nilotinib cause a prolongation of the QT interval that is not seen in patients

receiving other TKIs. Other nonhematologic adverse effects include hypophosphatemia (primarily dasatinib and nilotinib), muscle pain, pancreatitis, and weight gain (particularly imatinib). All agents can induce neutropenia, anemia and thrombocytopenia that can require transfusion support, dose reduction, or discontinuation. Most nonhematologic adverse reactions are self-limited and respond to dose adjustments. After the adverse events have resolved, many times the drug may be retitrated back to initial dosing. Ponatinib poses a clearly increased risk of arterial thrombosis, and should be used with caution in patients with a history of myocardial infarction, angina, stroke, or peripheral arterial disease.

JANUS KINASE INHIBITORS

Myeloproliferative neoplasms (MPNs) are a group of heterogeneous clonal hematopoietic stem cell disorders that include CML and "BCR-ABL–negative" MPNs polycythemia vera (PV), essential thrombocythemia (ET), and primary myelofibrosis (PMF).[264] A phenotypic characteristic of these disease is the accumulation of mature-appearing myeloid cells. The majority of patients with BCR-ABL–negative MPNs carry a mutation in the Janus-type tyrosine kinase *(JAK)* gene, the most common being JAK^{V617F}.[265-267] Family members of the JAKs include JAK1 to JAK3 and TYK. Physiologically, JAK are necessary for intracellular signal transduction of receptors that have no intrinsic tyrosine kinase activity, such as receptors for erythropoietin (EPO), thrombopoietin (TPO), and granulocyte-macrophage colony-stimulating factor (GM-CSF).[268] Upon ligand binding to the receptor, JAK autophosphorylation leads to binding of signal transducer and activator of transcription (STAT), which dimerizes with another STAT protein, translocates into the nucleus, and promotes transcription of STAT-responsive genes, which are involved in the control of cell proliferation, apoptosis, and cell differentiation.[265] The substitution mutation $JAK2^{V617F}$ is the most common gain-of-function alteration and occurs in 65 to 97 percent of cases in PV, 23 to 57 percent of cases in ET, and 34 to 57 percent of cases in PMF.[261-263] Expression of this mutation results in ligand independent growth or increased sensitivity to the cytokine/growth factor.

In 2011 the FDA approved the first specific JAK inhibitor ruxolitinib (Jakafi) for the treatment of PMF, PV, and ET. This approval was the consequence of two phase III trials: Controlled Myelofibrosis Study with Oral JAK Inhibitor Treatment (COMFORT)-I trial that investigated the activity of ruxolitinib (15 mg or 20 mg orally twice daily) versus placebo in 309 patients with PMF, PV, or ET, and the COMFORT-II trial that assessed ruxolitinib versus best available therapy in 219 patients with PMF, PV, or ET.[266,267] In the COMFORT-I trial, ruxolitinib produced greater than 35 percent spleen volume reduction (primary outcome) in 42 percent of patients at 24 weeks, improved symptom control, and overall survival compared to the placebo group. In the COMFORT-II trial 28 percent versus 0 percent of patients had greater than 35 percent spleen volume reduction, as well as superior reduction of disease-related symptoms, functionality and quality of life with modest toxicities compared to best available treatment (mostly hydroxyurea and glucocorticoids).

Mechanism of Action

Ruxolitinib inhibits all JAK kinases independent of their mutational status and to similar degree independent from the disease subtype. There is variable activity against JAK1 (IC_{50} = 1 nM), JAK2 (IC_{50} = 7.2 nM), TYK2 (IC_{50} = 9.3 nM), and JAK3 (IC_{50} = 98 nM), respectively. Molecular dynamics simulations suggest that ruxolitinib targets the ATP-binding site of the kinase in its active conformation.[268] Administration of ruxolitinib results in decreased expression of STAT responsive genes.

Clinical Pharmacology

Ruxolitinib is orally administered, rapidly absorbed, and with a high bioavailability of at least 95 percent. It undergoes CYP3A4-dependent metabolism and is primarily eliminated in urine. The elimination half-life is approximately 3 hours. High-throughput *in vitro* screens identified mutations that confer primary resistance to ruxolitinib, including the gatekeeper mutation M929I.[269]

Adverse Effects

Most nonhematologic adverse effects are relatively infrequent and mild in nature. These include, but are not limited to, diarrhea, nausea, peripheral edema, nasopharyngitis, pyrexia, arthralgia, cough, and dyspnea. Ruxolitinib can cause anemia and thrombocytopenia that may require transfusions. However, toxicity can be ameliorated with dose reduction or treatment interruptions and only a very small portion of patients had to discontinue the drug. The rate of higher-grade neutropenia was low (~7 percent).[266,267]

IBRUTINIB

CLL is a slowly progressive, indolent hematologic malignancy of mature B lymphocytes.[270] For decades, alkylating agents were the mainstay for treatment of CLL, with modest benefit for survival. The addition of rituximab, an antibody directed against CD20 on B lymphocytes, improves survival in CLL patients.[271] However, subsets of patients with particular deletion, such as 17p13.1, have poor response to this treatment. Furthermore, none of the available therapies are curative.[271] Although no common driver mutation is found in CLL, Bruton tyrosine kinase (BTK), a downstream mediator of the B-cell receptor, appears to be critical for B-cell activation, proliferation, and survival. A selective BTK inhibitor, ibrutinib, was developed and proved highly active in high-risk relapsed CLL. It achieved a high rate of overall (88 percent) and progression-free survival (75 percent) at 26 months of followup.[272] In a subsequent phase III trial including 391 patients with previously treated CLL, ibrutinib was compared to ofatumumab (an anti-CD20 antibody approved for relapsed CLL). Ibrutinib achieved a superior overall response rate, progression-free and overall survival.[273] Based on these findings, ibrutinib was granted accelerated approval by the FDA for this indication. It has also been approved for the treatment of patients with mantle cell lymphoma.

Mechanism of Action

Ibrutinib irreversibly inhibits the BTK active site by forming a covalent bond with a cysteine residue. Inhibition of the BTK results in disruption of activation of multiple downstream pathways important for B-cell activation, proliferation, and adhesion.

Clinical Pharmacology

Ibrutinib is orally administered once daily. The bioavailability has not been established. The half-life is 4 to 6 hours. Ibrutinib is metabolized in the liver primarily by CYP3A4 and only minimally cleared intact in urine (1 percent). No dose adjustments are required for liver or renal dysfunction. Dose adjustment may be necessary for patients who have more than grade 3 hematologic of nonhematologic adverse effect. Using whole exome sequencing, distinct resistance mutations were identified in six patients.[274] In five patients, a cysteine-to-serine mutation (C481S) at the binding site of BTK was found. Interestingly, the resulting protein remains sensitive to ibrutinib; however, inhibition in this case is reversible. Three other mutations (L845F, R665W, and S707Y) found in two patients involving a downstream target of BTK, phospholipase γ2

(PLCγ2). Currently, it is unclear whether dose escalation may overcome these resistance mechanisms.

Adverse Effects

The vast majority of adverse effects to ibrutinib are mild in nature. Almost half of the patients experience diarrhea, and approximately one-third of patients develop upper respiratory infections, cough, or fatigue. Other adverse effects include nausea, vomiting, constipation, pyrexia, rashes, edema, hypertension, and headaches. Approximately 15 percent of patients developed grades 3 to 4 neutropenia, dose reduction allowed continuation of the drug.[272,273]

PROTEAOSOME INHIBITORS

Bortezomib and Carfilzomib

This class of agents targets the ubiquitin-proteasome pathway, the complex regulatory system whereby normal and malignant cells eliminate potentially toxic misfolded proteins and control the intracellular levels of important regulatory proteins.[275] The importance of this pathway and its substrates in diverse aspects of the pathophysiology of human tumors creates opportunities for therapeutic interventions. The multimeric 20S core particle of the proteasome exhibits three distinct proteolytic activities, namely chymotryptic, tryptic, and post–glutamyl peptide hydrolytic-like activities. Both bortezomib (previously known as PS-341) and carfilzomib (Fig. 22-8) inhibit the chymotryptic-like activity by binding to the β5 subunit of the 20S core. Bortezomib, a boronic dipeptide, is a reversible inhibitor of the chymotryptic-like activity, while carfilzomib, an epoxyketone, forms with the β5 subunit an irreversible adduct through two covalent bonds.[276] Bortezomib has potent clinical activity against myeloma[277-279] and other plasma cell dyscrasias, including amyloidosis[280] and Waldenström macroglobulinemia,[281] and is also active in mantle cell lymphoma.[282,283] Bortezomib induces complex molecular sequelae, such as decreased levels of antiapoptotic molecules

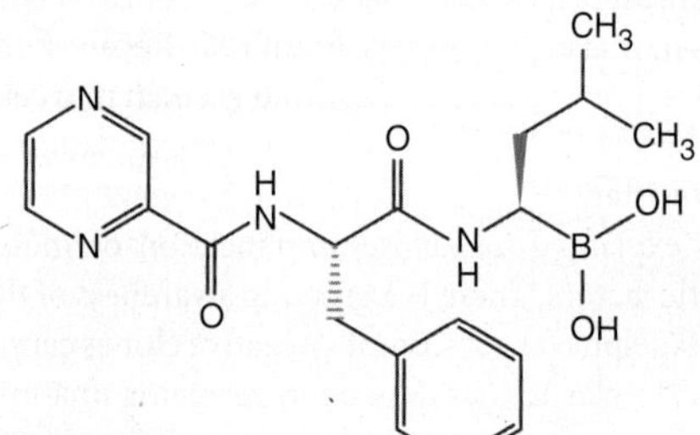

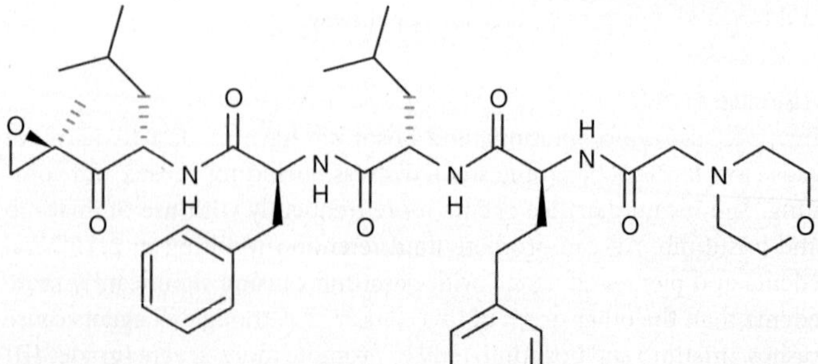

Figure 22–8. Bortezomib and carfilzomib.

(including nuclear factor [NF]-κB, caspase inhibitors, and Bcl-2 family members).[284-287] The composite outcome of these events is an irreversible commitment of myeloma cells to apoptosis,[285] as well as the sensitization of myeloma cells to diverse established agents (e.g., alkylator,[287,288] anthracyclines,[287,289] and thalidomide derivatives) or investigational agents such as HDAC inhibitors[287]. As a result, bortezomib has been a key component of diverse antimyeloma combination regimens.[290] However, patients eventually develop resistance to bortezomib or experience sensory peripheral neuropathy,[291] the main dose-limiting toxicity for this drug. Carfilzomib and other second-generation proteasome inhibitors were thus developed to circumvent these limitations. In 2012, carfilzomib received FDA accelerated approval for the treatment of myeloma patients relapsed and refractory to bortezomib and at least one thalidomide derivative.[292] The observation that carfilzomib can be active in some bortezomib-refractory cases has been attributed to the fact that new proteasomes must be synthesized to fully restore proteasome capacity in cells treated with this irreversible inhibitor. However, the reversible-versus-irreversible nature of a proteasome inhibitor may not be the only determinant of its clinical activity; for example, another second-generation proteasome inhibitor in clinical trials, MLN2238, and its clinically administered prodrug, ixazomib (MLN9708), exhibit preclinical[293] and clinical activity in bortezomib-resistant cells, despite reversible binding to β5.[294]

Despite the important role of the proteasome for normal cells, the administration of bortezomib and carfilzomib is associated with a clinically meaningful therapeutic window, likely because the clinically achievable levels of these agents do not completely shut down the chymotrypsin-like activity[295] of the proteasome and also spare its other proteolytic (trypsin-like and caspase-like)[296] activities. Consequently, there is only modest (<40 percent) decrease in the overall rate of protein degradation in either normal or tumor cells. Although normal cells can recover from this degree of perturbation, malignant plasma cells may not, because their available active proteasome particles ("proteasome capacity") are apparently close to their functional saturation by the increased quantities of unassembled or misfolded proteins ("proteasome load"), such as immunoglobulins.[297] It is not yet determined, if this concept also applies to mantle cell lymphoma.

The safety profile of both bortezomib and carfilzomib includes thrombocytopenia, possibly reflecting a requirement for constitutive proteasome activity in platelets to degrade the apoptosis regulator, Bax, and preserve their normal life span.[298] Unlike bortezomib, carfilzomib does not cause peripheral neuropathy, but cardiopulmonary side effects (e.g., dyspnea, hypoxemia, pulmonary hypertension) and serum creatinine elevations have been reported.[292] These differences may be explained by reports that bortezomib, but not carfilzomib, also inhibits the neuroprotective molecule, Htra2/Omi,[299] and blocks a number of serum proteases, including cathepsin G and cathepsin A, which may contribute to renal injury.[300-302]; inhibition of proteases may contribute to renal injury.[303] The mechanistic basis for cardiopulmonary adverse events with proteasome inhibition remains under investigation.

The clinical activity of bortezomib and carfilzomib, as well as the promising early studies with additional second-generation proteasome inhibitors, has validated the notion that pathways for intracellular regulation of protein homeostasis represent an important therapeutic target for plasma cell dyscrasias, mantle cell lymphoma, and potentially other neoplasias.

●THERAPEUTIC MONOCLONAL ANTIBODIES

Monoclonal antibodies are an important class of agents for the treatment of hematologic malignancies. As a group, lymphoid cells express a variety of antigens that are attractive targets for monoclonal-based therapy, as shown in Table 22–6. Development of monoclonal antibodies against specific targets has been largely accomplished by the empiric method of immunizing mice against human tumor cells and screening the hybridomas for antibodies of interest. Because murine antibodies have a short half-life and induce a human antimouse antibody immune response, they are partially or fully humanized when used as therapeutic

TABLE 22–6. Dose and Toxicity of FDA-Approved Monoclonal Antibody-Based Drugs

Drug	Mechanism	Dose and Schedule	Major Toxicity
Rituximab	Antibody-dependent cytotoxicity, complement activation, induction of apoptosis	375 mg/m² infusion weekly × 4 as single agent, 375 mg/m² infusion in combination with chemotherapy	Infusion related; late-onset neutropenia
Ofatumumab	Antibody-dependent cellular cytotoxicity, complement-dependent cytotoxicity	8 weekly followed by 4 monthly infusions during a 24-week period (dose 1 = 300 mg; doses 2 to 12 = 2000 mg)	Infusion related; late-onset neutropenia
Obinutuzumab	Direct cell death and antibody-dependent cellular cytotoxicity	100 mg infusion on cycle 1 day 1, 900 mg on day 2; 1000 mg on days 8 and 15 of cycle 1 and subsequently 1000 mg on day 1 of cycles 2 through 6 in combination with chlorambucil	Infusion reactions, neutropenia
Alemtuzumab	Complement activation, antibody-dependent cytotoxicity, possible induction of apoptosis	Escalation 3, 10, 30 mg infusion TIW followed by 30 mg TIW for 4 to 12 weeks	Infusion-related toxicity with fever, rash, and dyspnea; T-cell depletion with increased infections
Brentuximab vedotin	Antibody drug conjugate comprising an anti-CD 30 monoclonal antibody linked to mono-methylauristatin E	1.8 mg/kg infusion every 3 weeks	Peripheral neuropathy, neutropenia
⁹⁰Y-ibritumomab tiuxetan	Targeted radiotherapy	0.4 mCi/kg infusion	Hematologic toxicity, myelodysplasia

reagents. Presently, several monoclonal antibodies have received FDA approval for non-Hodgkin lymphoma and CLL, including rituximab and alemtuzumab. Although several mechanism(s) of action have been described for monoclonal antibodies, including direct induction of apoptosis, antibody-dependent cellular cytotoxicity (ADCC), and complement-dependent cytotoxicity, the clinically important mechanisms for most antibodies remain uncertain.[304]

Monoclonal antibodies may also be engineered to combine the antibody with a toxin (immunotoxin) or a radioactive isotope (radioimmunoconjugates), or to contain a second specificity (bispecific antibodies).[305–307] For example, it is possible to conjugate an antibody with specificity to B-cell lymphomas with an antibody against CD3, which binds to and activates normal T cells, so as to enhance T-cell–mediated lysis of the lymphoma cell. One such example of a bispecific antibody blinatumomab contains anti-CD3 and anti-CD19 specificity. Monoclonal antibodies raised against the immunoglobulin idiotype on a B-cell lymphoma represent another therapeutic strategy, which was first reported in 1982 by Miller and associates.[308]

NAKED MONOCLONAL ANTIBODIES

Rituximab

Rituximab, the first monoclonal to receive FDA approval, is a chimeric antibody containing the human immunoglobulin G_1 and κ constant regions with murine variable regions. Rituximab targets the B-cell antigen CD20 expressed on the surface of normal B cells and on more than 90 percent of B-cell neoplasms, and is present from the pre–B-cell stage through terminal differentiation to plasma cells.[309] To date, the biologic functions of CD20 remain uncertain, although incubation of B cells with anti-CD20 antibody has variable effects on cell-cycle progression, depending on the monoclonal antibody type.[310,311] Monoclonal antibody binding to CD20 generates transmembrane signals that produce a number of events including autophosphorylation and activation of serine/tyrosine protein kinases, and induction of c-myc oncogene expression and major histocompatibility complex class II molecules.[312] CD20 promotes transmembrane Ca^{2+} conductance through its possible function as a Ca^{2+} channel.[312] These studies demonstrate the importance of CD20 in B-cell regulation, but do not in themselves indicate how ligation of the receptor produces cell death independent of ADCC or complement-mediated pathways.

Rituximab was initially approved as a single agent for relapsed indolent lymphomas, but it has shown activity in a wide variety of clinical settings. It is approved in combination with chemotherapy for the initial treatment of follicular and diffuse large B cell lymphoma.[313,314] Rituximab has also been shown to be effective in combination with chemotherapy for CLL and indolent B-cell non-Hodgkin lymphomas including mantle cell lymphoma, Waldenström macroglobulinemia, and marginal lymphomas.[313] It is used in combination with salvage chemotherapy for many indolent and aggressive B-cell non-Hodgkin lymphomas even after prior rituximab treatment.[315] The use of maintenance rituximab has gained increased acceptance based the demonstration of delayed time to progression and improved overall survival in the relapse setting.[316–318]

Rituximab is given by intravenous infusion both as a single agent and in combination with chemotherapy at a dose of 375 mg/m^2. As a single agent it is given weekly for 4 weeks with maintenance dosing every 3 to 6 months. It has a half-life of approximately 22 days.[319] Given the risk of infusional reactions, pretreatment with antihistamines, acetaminophen, and glucocorticoids have become standard. During the first administration, the rate must be increased slowly to prevent infusional reactions. Infusions are started at 50 mg/h and in the absence of infusion reactions the rate can be increased in 50 mg/h increments every 30

minutes to a maximum rate of 400 mg/h. On subsequent infusion in the absence of reactions, infusions may start at 100 mg/h and increased in 100 mg/h increments every 30 minutes to a maximum rate of 400 mg/h. Patients with a high degree of circulating tumor cells are at increased risk for tumor lysis syndrome and are given a reduced dose of 50 mg/m^2 on day 1 of treatment in addition to standard tumor lysis prophylaxis. The remainder of the dose can then be given on day 3.

Resistance to rituximab may occur by down regulation of CD20, impaired ADCC, decreased complement activation, limited effects on signaling and induction of apoptosis, and inadequate blood levels.[304,320] Studies in relapsed indolent B-cell non-Hodgkin lymphoma have shown a correlation between higher mean serum rituximab levels and clinical responses,[321] suggesting that dose escalation may be a way to overcome rituximab resistance. Also polymorphisms in two of the receptors for the antibody Fc region responsible for complement activation, FcγRIIIa, and FcγRIIa may predict the clinical response to rituximab monotherapy in patients with follicular lymphoma but not in CLL.[322,323]

Rituximab has a several known toxicities including infusional reactions which can be life-threatening. Most are usually mild and include fever, chills, throat itching, urticaria, and mild hypotension, all of which can respond to decreased infusion rates and antihistamines. There are reports of severe mucocutaneous skin reactions including Stevens-Johnson syndrome.[324] Reactivation of hepatitis B virus also has been reported and it is recommended that patients be screened for hepatitis B prior to initiation of therapy. There also are case reports of progressive multifocal leukoencephalopathy caused by the John Cunningham virus and resulting in death.[325] Hypogammaglobulinemia and delayed neutropenia may occur from 1 to 5 months after administration with resultant serious infections.[326,327]

Ofatumumab

Ofatumumab is a fully human immunoglobulin G_1 kappa (IgG$_1\kappa$), monoclonal antibody which targets a unique epitope on the CD20 antigen found on the surface of normal and malignant pre-B and mature B cells. Ofatumumab offers many potential advantages over rituximab. It has an increased affinity for CD20 compared to rituximab.[328] In vitro experiments have shown it is superior to rituximab in ability to induce cell lysis.[328] Ofatumumab and rituximab both show similar antibody-dependent cellular cytotoxicity, but ofatumumab displays increased complement dependent cytotoxicity.[329] In addition, ofatumumab is a fully human monoclonal antibody with a low incidence of human–antihuman antibody formation.[330]

Ofatumumab has been approved for use in patients with CLL refractory to fludarabine and alemtuzumab. In a phase II trial, 138 patients received eight weekly infusions of ofatumumab followed by four monthly infusions during a 24-week period (dose 1 = 300 mg; doses 2 to 12 = 2000 mg). The overall response rate was 58 percent with median progression-free survival of approximately 14 months.[331] No dose-limiting effects were observed in the phases I/II studies of ofatumumab. Most common adverse reactions (>10 percent) were infusion reactions, neutropenia, pneumonia, pyrexia, cough, diarrhea, anemia, fatigue, dyspnea, rash, nausea, bronchitis, and upper respiratory tract infections. Similar to rituximab above, ofatumumab is being investigated in combination with chemotherapy for both indolent and aggressive B cell non-Hodgkin lymphoma.

Obinutuzumab

Obinutuzumab is a third naked monoclonal antibody that targets the CD20 antigen. It differs from rituximab in that it is a glycoengineered type 2 antibody that, in preclinical studies, showed improved efficacy by inducing direct cell death and by enhanced ADCC.[332] Obinutuzumab was recently approved in combination with chlorambucil of the treatment of patients with previously untreated CLL. This approval was based on a phase III, 781-person trial with three arms comparing single-agent chlorambucil versus chlorambucil plus rituximab versus chlorambucil plus obinutuzumab.[333] A main feature of this trial was that it enrolled mainly older patients (median age: 73 years) with multiple medical comorbidities representative of the majority of patients diagnosed with CLL. The median progression-free survival was greatly improved in obinutuzumab plus chlorambucil arm at 26.7 months versus 11.1 months with chlorambucil alone and 16.3 months with rituximab plus chlorambucil. Obinutuzumab is similar to other monoclonal antibodies associated with infusion reactions. The first dose was split over 2 days with the patient receiving 100 mg intravenously on cycle 1 day 1 and 900 mg on day 2. Patients then received 1000 mg on days 8 and 15 of cycle 1 and subsequently 1000 mg on days 1 of cycles 2 through 6. Patients concurrently received chlorambucil orally at a dose of 0.5 mg/kg on days 1 and 15 of each cycle. This combination was, in general, well tolerated. There was a slightly increased risk of grade 3 neutropenia (33 vs. 28 percent) compared to the rituximab control group, but no increased risk of infection (12 vs. 14 percent). Other common toxicities included infusion reactions, anemia, thrombocytopenia, and leukopenia.

Alemtuzumab

Alemtuzumab is a humanized monoclonal antibody targeted against the CD52 antigen present on the surface of normal neutrophils and lymphocytes as well as most B- and T-cell lymphomas.[334] CD52 is expressed at reasonable levels and does not modulate with antibody binding, making it a good target for unconjugated monoclonal antibodies. Mechanistically, alemtuzumab can induce tumor cell death through ADCC and complement dependent cytotoxicity.[335] Clinical activity has been demonstrated in CLL, including in patients with purine analogue refractory disease.[336,337] In refractory CLL, overall response rates are approximately 38 percent with complete responses of 6 percent in multiple series. Response rates in patients with untreated CLL are higher (overall response rates of 83 percent and complete responses of 24 percent).[336] The most concerning side effects are acute infusion reactions and depletion of normal neutrophils and T cells. Opportunistic infections are a serious consequence, particularly in patients who have received purine analogues.[336,337] Patients should receive antibiotic prophylaxis against *Pneumocystis carinii* and herpes virus during treatment. Serious infections with cytomegalovirus are seen and monitoring is recommended. Alemtuzumab in combination with chemotherapy has been explored in the treatment of T-cell lymphomas but trials were limited by significant infectious complications.[338]

Elotuzumab, Daratumumab, and Others

A number of naked antibodies have been developed for the therapeutic targeting of myeloma. Mechanistically, this approach depends on the recruitment of ADCC, complement-dependent cytotoxicity, and apoptosis, as well as growth arrest via the selected targeting of signaling pathways (Fig. 22–9).[339] Targets include surface molecules as well as signaling molecules (Table 22–7).[339] Of these antibodies, one of the most promising is elotuzumab, which specifically targets CS1 (also known as SLAMF7) through which its mechanism of action includes the enhancement of NK-cell activation directly via SLAMF7 and indirectly by CD16, as well as the targeted killing of SLAMF7-expressing myeloma cells by ADCC.[340,341] Combinatorial strategies for this particular approach have been especially promising, including regimens with lenalidomide and dexamethasone where high qualities of response and impressive progression-free survival have been seen.[341]

Separately, daratumumab as a first-in-class monoclonal antibody that effectively targets CD38 has shown particularly encouraging activity as both a monotherapy and in combination.[342] Similarly, the CD38-targeting monoclonal antibody SAR650984 has shown impressive activity, validating this as an appropriate target as well as further supporting the therapeutic potential of this class of antibodies.[339,340] Combination studies are ongoing and the outlook for the rational development of several monoclonal antibody combinations in myeloma now looks very promising.[341,342]

IMMUNOTOXINS

Immunotoxins combine immune proteins such as antibodies, antibody Fab fragments, or interleukins and toxins such as ricin A chain or *Pseudomonas* exotoxin. These molecules have the advantage of the high specificity of the protein for its receptor or antigen, and its ability to

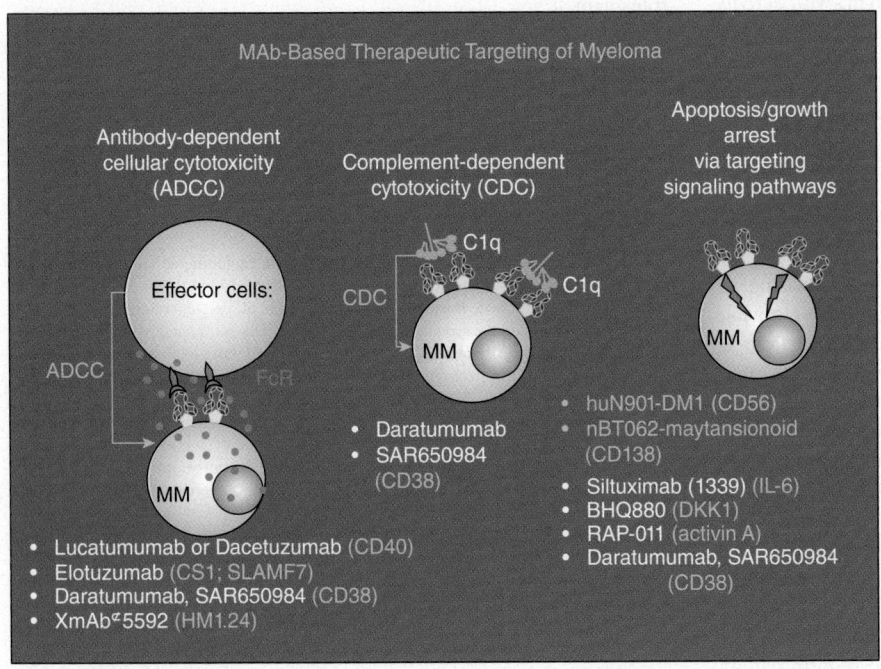

Figure 22–9. Monoclonal-based therapeutic targeting of myeloma. MAb, monoclonal antibody. *(Adapted with permission from Tai YT, Anderson KC: Antibody-based therapies in multiple myeloma, Bone Marrow Res 2011.)*

TABLE 22-7. Monoclonal Antibodies in Myeloma

Target	mAb	Stage of Development
Surface molecules		
CS1/SLAMF7	Elotuzumab	Phase 2/3
CD38	Daratumumab	Phase 1/2/3
	SAR650984	Phase 1/2
	MOR202	Phase 1/2
CD74	Milatuzumab	Phase 1/2
CD40	Dacetuzumab	Phase 1
CD56	Lorvotuzumab mertansine	Phase 1
CD138	BT062	Phase 1
Signaling molecules		
IL-6	Siltuximab	Phase 3
RANKL	Denosumab	Phase 3
B cell activating factor (BAFF)	Tabalumab	Phase 2/3
VEGF	Bevacizumab	Phase 2
DKK1	BHQ880	Phase 2

Data from Richardson et al. et al. IMW 2013 (Abstract P-214), poster presentation.

Plesner et al. ASH 2013 (Abstract 1987), poster presentation.

Martin et al. ASH 2013 (Abstract 284), oral presentation.

http://www.clinicaltrials.gov/ct2/show/NCT00421525

http://www.clinicaltrials.gov/ct2/show/NCT00079716

http://www.clinicaltrials.gov/ct2/show/NCT00346255

http://www.clinicaltrials.gov/ct2/show/NCT01001442

Wong et al. ASH 2013 (Abstract 505), oral presentation.

Hageman et al. *Ann Pharmacother* 2013;47:1069-74.

internalize once bound to its receptor, together with the potency of the toxin molecule. Two agents, denileukin diftitox (which combines IL-2 and the catalytically active fragment of diphtheria toxin) with activity in non-Hodgkin lymphoma and gemtuzumab ozogamicin (composed of an antibody that recognizes CD33 linked to a potent chemical toxin, calicheamicin) with activity in AML, show a proof of principle but have been removed from the market.[343,344] Brentuximab vedotin is currently the only approved antibody drug conjugate for hematologic malignancies but several others are in development.

Brentuximab Vedotin

Brentuximab vedotin is an antibody drug conjugate comprising an anti-CD30 monoclonal antibody conjugated by a protease-cleavable linker to the potent antimicrotubule agent monomethylauristatin E. When brentuximab vedotin binds to CD30-expressing cells, it is internalized with proteolytic cleavage of the linker resulting in release of monomethylauristatin E, disrupting the microtubule network within the cell, and subsequently inducing cell-cycle arrest and apoptotic death of the cells.[345] It is approved for the treatment of Hodgkin lymphoma after the failure of an autologous stem cell transplant or after the failure of at least two prior multiagent chemotherapy regimens in patients who were not candidates for transplantation. It is also approved for the treatment of patients with systemic anaplastic large cell lymphoma after the failure of at least one prior multiagent chemotherapy regimen. In a study of refractory Hodgkin lymphoma, brentuximab vedotin had an impressive overall response rate of 75 percent and a complete remission rate of 34 percent with 96 percent of patients having some improvement in their disease.[346] The median progression-free survival for all patients was 5.6 months but notably the median duration of response for those achieving a complete remission was 20.5 months. In refractory anaplastic large cell lymphoma, a similarly impressive overall response rate of 86 percent was seen with 57 percent of patients achieving a complete remission and 97 percent of patients having a reduction in tumor volume.[307] The overall duration of response was 12.6 months and those in a complete remission experiencing a duration of response of 13.2 months. Dosing is at 1.8 mg/kg as an intravenous infusion every 3 weeks. Dose reductions to 1.2 mg/kg are recommended for patients with hepatic or severe renal impairment. The main toxicity is cumulative peripheral neuropathy reported in up to 54 percent of the patients in the above trials. Patients experiencing new or worsening peripheral neuropathy may require a delay, dose reduction, or discontinuation of brentuximab vedotin. Other common toxicities include neutropenia, thrombocytopenia, fatigue, and nausea.

RADIOIMMUNOCONJUGATES

Radioimmunoconjugates provide monoclonal antibody targeted delivery of radioactive particles to tumor cells.[306,347] Iodine-131 is a commonly used radioisotope because it is readily available, relatively inexpensive, and easily conjugated to a monoclonal antibody. The β-emitter ^{90}Y has emerged as an attractive alternative to ^{131}I, based on its higher energy and longer path length, which may be more effective in tumors with larger diameters. It also has a short half-life and remains conjugated, even after endocytosis, providing a safer profile for outpatient use. Clinically, radioimmunoconjugates were developed with murine monoclonal antibodies against CD20 conjugated with ^{131}I (tositumomab) or ^{90}Y (ibritumomab tiuxetan). Response rates in relapsed lymphoma of 65 to 80 percent were achieved.[306,347,348] Both drugs were well tolerated with most toxicity attributable to marrow suppression; however, there have been worrisome reports of secondary leukemias. Collaboration between treating physicians and nuclear medicine departments is required for administration. ^{131}I tositumomab is no longer available, but ^{90}Y ibritumomab tiuxetan remains in clinical use and is being investigated as a consolidation therapy and as conditioning prior to hematopoietic cell transplant.

REFERENCES

1. Goodman L, Wintrobe M, Dameshek W, et al: Nitrogen mustard therapy: Use of methyl bis (B-chloroethyl) amino hydrochloride for Hodgkin's disease, lymphosarcoma, leukemia and certain allied and miscellaneous disorders. *JAMA* 126:132, 1946.
2. Farber S, Diamond L, Mercer R, et al: Temporary remissions in acute leukemia in children produced by folic acid antagonist, 4-aminopteroyl-glutamic acid (aminopterin). *N Engl J Med* 238:787, 1948.
3. Devita VT, Serpick AA, Carbone PP: Combination chemotherapy in the treatment of advanced Hodgkin's disease. *Ann Intern MedIntern Med* 73:881–895, 1970.
4. Druker BJ, Tamura S, Buchdunger E, et al: Effects of a selective inhibitor of the Abl tyrosine kinase on the growth of Bcr-Abl positive cells. *Nat Med* 2:561–566, 1996.
5. Shah NP, Skaggs BJ, Branford S, et al: Sequential ABL kinase inhibitor therapy selects for compound drug-resistant BCR-ABL mutations with altered oncogenic potency. *J Clin Invest* 117:2562–2569, 2007.
6. Tallman MS: Treatment of relapsed or refractory acute promyelocytic leukemia. *Best Pract Res Clin Haematol* 20:57–65, 2007.
7. Slamon DJ, Leyland-Jones B, Shak S, et al: Use of chemotherapy plus a monoclonal antibody against HER2 for metastatic breast cancer that overexpresses HER2. *N Engl J Med* 344:783–792, 2001.
8. Bruno R, Hille D, Riva A, et al: Population pharmacokinetics/pharmacodynamics of docetaxel in phase II studies in patients with cancer. *J Clin Oncol* 16:187–196, 1998.
9. Maheswaran S, Sequist LV, Nagrath S, et al: Detection of mutations in EGFR in circulating lung-cancer cells. *N Engl J Med* 359:366–377, 2008.
10. Yip S, Miao J, Cahill DP, et al: MSH6 mutations arise in glioblastomas during temozolomide therapy and mediate temozolomide resistance. *Clin Cancer Res* 15:4622–4629, 2009.

11. Borst P, Elferink RO: Mammalian ABC transporters in health and disease. *Annu Rev Biochem* 71:537–592, 2002.
12. Kruh GD, Zeng H, Rea PA, et al: MRP subfamily transporters and resistance to anticancer agents. *J Bioenerg Biomembr* 33:493–501, 2001.
13. Goker E, Waltham M, Kheradpour A, et al: Amplification of the dihydrofolate reductase gene is a mechanism of acquired resistance to methotrexate in patients with acute lymphoblastic leukemia and is correlated with p53 gene mutations. *Blood* 86:677–684, 1995.
14. Nimmanapalli R, Bhalla K: Mechanisms of resistance to imatinib mesylate in Bcr-Abl-positive leukemias. *Curr Opin Oncol* 14:616–620, 2002.
15. Fink D, Aebi S, Howell SB: The role of DNA mismatch repair in drug resistance. *Clin Cancer Res* 4:1–6, 1998.
16. Kirsch DG, Kastan MB: Tumor-suppressor p53: Implications for tumor development and prognosis. *J Clin Oncol* 16:3158–3168, 1998.
17. Holleman A, den Boer ML, Cheok MH, et al: Expression of the outcome predictor in acute leukemia 1 (OPAL1) gene is not an independent prognostic factor in patients treated according to COALL or St Jude protocols. *Blood* 108:1984–1990, 2006.
18. Leong KG, Wang, BE, Johnson L, Gao WQ: Generation of a prostate from a single adult stem cell. *Nature* 456:804–808, 2008.
19. Diehn M, Cho RW, Lobo NA, et al: Association of reactive oxygen species levels and radioresistance in cancer stem cells. *Nature* 458:780–783, 2009.
20. Moscow JA, Connolly T, Myers TG, et al: Reduced folate carrier gene (RFC1) expression and anti-folate resistance in transfected and non-selected cell lines. *Int J Cancer* 72:184–190, 1997.
21. Barrado J, Synold T, Laver J, et al: Co-administration of probenecid, an inhibitor of a cMOAT/MRP-like plasma membrane ATPase, greatly enhanced the efficacy of a new 10-deazaaminopterin against human solid tumors in vivo. *Clin Cancer Res* 6:3705–3712, 2000.
22. Zhao R, Qiu A, Tsai E, et al: The proton-coupled folate transporter: Impact on pemetrexed transport and on antifolates activities compared with the reduced folate carrier. *Mol Pharmacol* 74:854–862, 2008.
23. Galpin AJ, Schuetz JD, Masson E, et al: Differences in folylpolyglutamate synthetase and dihydrofolate reductase expression in human B-lineage versus T-lineage leukemic lymphoblasts: Mechanisms for lineage differences in methotrexate polyglutamylation and cytotoxicity. *Mol Pharmacol* 52:155–163, 1997.
24. Masson E, Relling MV, Synold TW, et al: Accumulation of methotrexate polyglutamates in lymphoblasts is a determinant of antileukemic effects in vivo. A rationale for high-dose methotrexate. *J Clin Invest* 97:73–80, 1996.
25. Synold TW, Relling MV, Boyett JM, et al: Blast cell methotrexate-polyglutamate accumulation in vivo differs by lineage, ploidy, and methotrexate dose in acute lymphoblastic leukemia. *J Clin Invest* 94:1996–2001, 1994.
26. Cheng Q, Wu B, Kager L, et al: A substrate specific functional polymorphism of human gamma-glutamyl hydrolase alters catalytic activity and methotrexate polyglutamate accumulation in acute lymphoblastic leukaemia cells. *Pharmacogenetics* 14:557–567, 2004.
27. Longo GS, Gorlick R, Tong WP, et al: Gamma-Glutamyl hydrolase and folylpolyglutamate synthetase activities predict polyglutamylation of methotrexate in acute leukemias. *Oncol Res* 9:259–263, 1997.
28. Ge Y, Haska CL, LaFiura K, et al: Prognostic role of the reduced folate carrier, the major membrane transporter for methotrexate, in childhood acute lymphoblastic leukemia: A report from the Children's Oncology Group. *Clin Cancer Res* 13:451–457, 2007.
29. Rothem L, Aronheim A, Assaraf YG: Alterations in the expression of transcription factors and the reduced folate carrier as a novel mechanism of antifolate resistance in human leukemia cells. *J Biol Chem* 278:8935–8941, 2003.
30. Stoller RG, Hande KR, Jacobs SA, et al: Use of plasma pharmacokinetics to predict and prevent methotrexate toxicity. *N Engl J Med* 297:630–634, 1977.
31. Evans WE, Crom WR, Abromowitch M, et al: Clinical pharmacodynamics of high-dose methotrexate in acute lymphocytic leukemia. Identification of a relation between concentration and effect. *N Engl J Med* 314:471–477, 1986.
32. Wall SM, Johansen MJ, Molony DA, et al: Effective clearance of methotrexate using high-flux hemodialysis membranes. *Am J Kidney Dis* 28:846–854, 1996.
33. Widemann BC, Schwartz S, Jayaprakash N, et al: Efficacy of glucarpidase (carboxypeptidase g2) in patients with acute kidney injury after high-dose methotrexate therapy. *Pharmacotherapy* 34:427–439, 2014.
34. Shapiro WR, Allen JC, Horten BC: Chronic methotrexate toxicity to the central nervous system. *Clin Bull* 10:49–52, 1980.
35. Bloomfield CD, Lawrence D, Byrd JC, et al: Frequency of prolonged remission duration after high-dose cytarabine intensification in acute myeloid leukemia varies by cytogenetic subtype. *Cancer Res* 58:4173–4179, 1998.
36. Stam RW, den Boer ML, Meijerink JP, et al: Differential mRNA expression of Ara-C-metabolizing enzymes explains Ara-C sensitivity in MLL gene-rearranged infant acute lymphoblastic leukemia. *Blood* 101:1270–1276, 2003.
37. Neubauer A, Maharry K, Mrózek K, et al: Patients with acute myeloid leukemia and RAS mutations benefit most from postremission high-dose cytarabine: A Cancer and Leukemia Group B study. *J Clin Oncol* 26:4603–4609, 2008.
38. Lamba JK, Crews K, Pounds S, et al: Pharmacogenetics of deoxycytidine kinase: Identification and characterization of novel genetic variants. *J Pharmacol Exp Ther* 323:935–945, 2007.
39. Kufe DW, Munroe D, Herrick D, et al: Effects of 1-beta-D-arabinofuranosylcytosine incorporation on eukaryotic DNA template function. *Mol Pharmacol* 26:128–134, 1984.
40. Owens JK, Shewach DS, Ullman B, Mitchell BS: Resistance to 1-beta-D-arabinofuranosylcytosine in human T-lymphoblasts mediated by mutations within the deoxycytidine kinase gene. *Cancer Res* 52:2389–2393, 1992.
41. Flasshove M, Strumberg D, Ayscue L, et al: Structural analysis of the deoxycytidine kinase gene in patients with the acute myeloid leukemia and resistance to cytosine arabinoside. *Leukemia* 8:780–785, 1993.
42. Capizzi R, Powell B: Sequential high-dose ara-C and asparaginase versus high-dose ara-C alone in the treatment of patients with relapsed and refractory acute leukemias. *Semin Oncol* 14(2 Suppl 1):40–50, 1987.
43. Cole BF, Glantz MJ, Jaeckle KA, et al: Quality-of-life-adjusted survival comparison of sustained-release cytosine arabinoside versus intrathecal methotrexate for treatment of solid tumor neoplastic meningitis. *Cancer* 97:3053–3060, 2003.
44. Kern W, Kurrle E, Schmeiser T: Streptococcal bacteremia in adult patients with leukemia undergoing aggressive chemotherapy. A review of 55 cases. *Infection* 18:138–145, 1990.
45. Herzig RH, Hines JD, Herzig GP, et al: Cerebellar toxicity with high-dose cytosine arabinoside. *J Clin Oncol* 5:927–932, 1987.
46. Gandhi V: Questions about gemcitabine dose rate: Answered or unanswered? *J Clin Oncol* 25:5691–5694, 2007.
47. Walter RB, Joerger M, Pestalozzi BC: Gemcitabine-associated hemolytic-uremic syndrome. *Am J Kidney Dis* 40:E16, 2002.
48. Claus R, Lübbert M: Epigenetic targets in hematopoietic malignancies. *Oncogene* 22:6489–6496, 2003.
49. Kantarjian HM, O'Brien S, Cortes J, et al: Results of decitabine (5-aza-2'deoxycytidine) therapy in 130 patients with chronic myelogenous leukemia. *Cancer* 98:522–528, 2003.
50. Rodriguez CO Jr, Stellrecht CM, Gandhi V: Mechanisms for T-cell selective cytotoxicity of arabinosyl guanine. *Blood* 102:1842–1848, 2003.
51. Karran P, Attard N: Thiopurines in current medical practice: Molecular mechanisms and contributions to therapy-related cancer. *Nat Rev Cancer* 8:24–36, 2008.
52. Fotoohi AK, Coulthard SA, Albertioni F: Thiopurines: Factors influencing toxicity and response. *Biochem Pharmacol* 79:1211–1220, 2010.
53. Lennard L, Lilleyman JS: Are children with lymphoblastic leukaemia given enough 6-mercaptopurine? *Lancet* 2:785–787, 1987.
54. Lennard L, Lilleyman JS, Van Loon J, Weinshilboum RM: Genetic variation in response to 6-mercaptopurine for childhood acute lymphoblastic leukaemia. *Lancet* 336:225–229, 1990.
55. Krishnamurthy P, Schwab M, Takenaka K, et al: Transporter-mediated protection against thiopurine-induced hematopoietic toxicity. *Cancer Res* 68:4983–4989, 2008.
56. Stocco G, Cheok MH, Crews KR, et al: Genetic polymorphism of inosine triphosphate pyrophosphatase is a determinant of mercaptopurine metabolism and toxicity during treatment for acute lymphoblastic leukemia. *Clin Pharmacol Ther* 85:164–172, 2009.
57. Zimm S, Collins JM, Riccardi R, et al: Variable bioavailability of oral mercaptopurine. Is maintenance chemotherapy of acute lymphoblastic leukemia being optimally delivered? *N Engl J Med* 308:1005–1009, 1983.
58. Erb N, Harms DO, Janka-Schaub G: Pharmacokinetics and metabolism of thiopurines in children with acute lymphoblastic leukemia receiving 6-thioguanine versus 6-mercaptopurine. *Cancer Chemother Pharmacol* 42:266–272, 1998.
59. Harms DO, Göbel U, Spaar HJ, et al: Thioguanine offers no advantage over mercaptopurine in maintenance treatment of childhood ALL: Results of the randomized trial COALL-92. *Blood* 102:2736–2740, 2003.
60. Jones TS, Yang W, Evans WE, Relling MV: Using HapMap tools in pharmacogenomic discovery: The thiopurine methyltransferase polymorphism. *Clin Pharmacol Ther* 81:729–734, 2007.
61. Keating MJ, O'Brien S, Lerner S, et al: Long-term follow-up of patients with chronic lymphocytic leukemia (CLL) receiving fludarabine regimens as initial therapy. *Blood* 92:1165–1171, 1998.
62. Slavin S, Nagler A, Naparstek E, et al: Nonmyeloablative stem cell transplantation and cell therapy as an alternative to conventional bone marrow transplantation with lethal cytoreduction for the treatment of malignant and nonmalignant hematologic diseases. *Blood* 91:756–763, 1998.
63. Brockman RW, Cheng YC, Schabel FM, Montgomery JA: Metabolism and chemotherapeutic activity of 9-beta-D-arabinofuranosyl-2-fluoroadenine against murine leukemia L1210 and evidence for its phosphorylation by deoxycytidine kinase. *Cancer Res* 40:3610–3615, 1980.
64. Gandhi V, Plunkett W: Cellular and clinical pharmacology of fludarabine. *Clin Pharmacokinet* 41:93–103, 2002.
65. Lichtman SM, Etcubanas E, Budman DR, et al: The pharmacokinetics and pharmacodynamics of fludarabine phosphate in patients with renal impairment: A prospective dose adjustment study. *Cancer Invest* 20:904–913, 2002.
66. Martell RE, Peterson BL, Cohen HJ, et al: Analysis of age, estimated creatinine clearance and pretreatment hematologic parameters as predictors of fludarabine toxicity in patients treated for chronic lymphocytic leukemia: A CALGB (9011) coordinated intergroup study. *Cancer Chemother Pharmacol* 50:37–45, 2002.
67. Cheson BD, Frame JN, Vena D, et al: Tumor lysis syndrome: An uncommon complication of fludarabine therapy of chronic lymphocytic leukemia. *J Clin Oncol* 16:2313–2320, 1998.
68. Cheson BD: Infectious and immunosuppressive complications of purine analog therapy. *J Clin Oncol* 13:2431–2448, 1995.
69. Helman DL Jr, Byrd JC, Ales NC, Shorr AF: Fludarabine-related pulmonary toxicity: A distinct clinical entity in chronic lymphoproliferative syndromes. *Chest* 122:785–790, 2002.
70. Tam CS, O'Brien S, Wierda W, et al: Long-term results of the fludarabine, cyclophosphamide, and rituximab regimen as initial therapy of chronic lymphocytic leukemia. *Blood* 112:975–980, 2008.

71. Estey EH, Kurzrock R, Kantarjian HM, et al: Treatment of hairy cell leukemia with 2-chlorodeoxyadenosine (2-CdA). *Blood* 79:882–887, 1992.

72. Albertoni M, Daub DM, Arden KC, et al: Genetic instability leads to loss of both p53 alleles in a human glioblastoma. *Oncogene* 16:321–326, 1998.

73. Beutler E: Cladribine (2-chlorodeoxyadenosine). *Lancet* 340:952–956, 1992.

74. Crews KR, Wimmer PS, Hudson JQ, et al: Pharmacokinetics of 2-chlorodeoxyadenosine in a child undergoing hemofiltration and hemodialysis for acute renal failure. *J Pediatr Hematol Oncol* 24:677–680, 2002.

75. de Wolf C, Jansen R, Yamaguchi H, et al: Contribution of the drug transporter ABCG2 (breast cancer resistance protein) to resistance against anticancer nucleosides. *Mol Cancer Ther* 7:3092–3102, 2008.

76. Bonate PL, Arthaud L, Cantrell WR Jr, et al: Discovery and development of clofarabine: A nucleoside analogue for treating cancer. *Nat Rev Drug Discov* 5:855–863, 2006.

77. Sanford M, Lyseng-Williamson KA: Nelarabine. *Drugs* 68:439–447, 2008.

78. Steis RG, Urba WJ, Kopp WC, et al: Kinetics of recovery of CD4+ T cells in peripheral blood of deoxycoformycin-treated patients. *J Natl Cancer Inst* 83:1678–1679, 1991.

79. Halsey C, Roberts IA: The role of hydroxyurea in sickle cell disease. *Br J Haematol* 120:177–186, 2003.

80. Platt OS: Hydroxyurea for the treatment of sickle cell anemia. *N Engl J Med* 358:1362–1369, 2008.

81. Sterkers Y, Preudhomme C, Laï JL, et al: Acute myeloid leukemia and myelodysplastic syndromes following essential thrombocythemia treated with hydroxyurea: High proportion of cases with 17p deletion. *Blood* 91:616–622, 1998.

82. Madoc-Jones H, Mauro F: Interphase action of vinblastine and vincristine: Differences in their lethal action through the mitotic cycle of cultured mammalian cells. *J Cell Physiol* 72:185–196, 1968.

83. Cabral FR, Brady RC, Schibler MJ: A mechanism of cellular resistance to drugs that interfere with microtubule assembly. *Ann N Y Acad Sci* 466:745–756, 1986.

84. Dyke RW: Treatment of inadvertent intrathecal injection of vincristine. *N Engl J Med* 321:1270–1271, 1989.

85. Rowinsky EK, Donehower RC: Paclitaxel (taxol). *N Engl J Med* 332:1004–1014, 1995.

86. Lopes NM, Adams EG, Pitts TW, Bhuyan BK: Cell kill kinetics and cell cycle effects of taxol on human and hamster ovarian cell lines. *Cancer Chemother Pharmacol* 32:235–242, 1993.

87. Zaffaroni N, Pennati M, Colella G, et al: Expression of the anti-apoptotic gene survivin correlates with Taxol resistance in human ovarian cancer. *Cell Mol Life Sci* 59:1406–1412, 2002.

88. Anand S, Penrhyn-Lowe S, Venkitaraman AR: AURORA-A amplification overrides the mitotic spindle assembly checkpoint, inducing resistance to Taxol. *Cancer Cell* 3:51–62, 2003.

89. Gianni L, Viganò L, Locatelli A, et al: Human pharmacokinetic characterization and in vitro study of the interaction between doxorubicin and paclitaxel in patients with breast cancer. *J Clin Oncol* 15:1906–1915, 1997.

90. Semb KA, Aamdal S, Oian P: Capillary protein leak syndrome appears to explain fluid retention in cancer patients who receive docetaxel treatment. *J Clin Oncol* 16:3426–3432, 1998.

91. Rivera E, Lee J, Davies A: Clinical development of ixabepilone and other epothilones in patients with advanced solid tumors. *Oncologist* 13:1207–1223, 2008.

92. Ohno R, Okada K, Masaoka T, et al: An early phase II study of CPT-11: A new derivative of camptothecin, for the treatment of leukemia and lymphoma. *J Clin Oncol* 8:1907–1912, 1990.

93. Beran M, Kantarjian H, O'Brien S, et al: Topotecan, a topoisomerase I inhibitor, is active in the treatment of myelodysplastic syndrome and chronic myelomonocytic leukemia. *Blood* 88:2473–2479, 1996.

94. Beran M, Estey E, O'Brien S, et al: Topotecan and cytarabine is an active combination regimen in myelodysplastic syndromes and chronic myelomonocytic leukemia. *J Clin Oncol* 17:2819–2830, 1999.

95. Kantarjian HM, Beran M, Ellis A, et al: Phase I study of Topotecan, a new topoisomerase I inhibitor, in patients with refractory or relapsed acute leukemia. *Blood* 81:1146–1151, 1993.

96. Iyer L, King CD, Whitington PF, et al: Genetic predisposition to the metabolism of irinotecan (CPT-11). Role of uridine diphosphate glucuronosyltransferase isoform 1A1 in the glucuronidation of its active metabolite (SN-38) in human liver microsomes. *J Clin Invest* 101:847–854, 1998.

97. Grochow LB, Rowinsky EK, Johnson R, et al: Pharmacokinetics and pharmacodynamics of topotecan in patients with advanced cancer. *Drug Metab Dispos* 20:706–713, 1992.

98. Rowinsky EK, Kaufmann SH, Baker SD, et al: A phase I and pharmacological study of topotecan infused over 30 minutes for five days in patients with refractory acute leukemia. *Clin Cancer Res* 2:1921–1930, 1996.

99. Creutzig U, Zimmermann M, Bourquin JP, et al: Randomized trial comparing liposomal daunorubicin with idarubicin as induction for pediatric acute myeloid leukemia: Results from Study AML-BFM 2004. *Blood* 122:37–43, 2013.

100. Péan E, Flores B, Hudson I, et al: The European Medicines Agency review of pixantrone for the treatment of adult patients with multiply relapsed or refractory aggressive non-Hodgkin's B-cell lymphomas: Summary of the scientific assessment of the committee for medicinal products for human use. *Oncologist* 18:625–633, 2013.

101. O'Malley FP, Chia S, Tu D, et al: Topoisomerase II alpha and responsiveness of breast cancer to adjuvant chemotherapy. *J Natl Cancer Inst* 101:644–650, 2009.

102. Press MF, Sauter G, Buyse M, et al: Alteration of topoisomerase II-alpha gene in human breast cancer: Association with responsiveness to anthracycline-based chemotherapy. *J Clin Oncol* 29:859–867, 2011.

103. Gutierrez M, Chabner BA, Pearson D, et al: Role of a doxorubicin-containing regimen in relapsed and resistant lymphomas: An 8-year follow-up study of EPOCH. *J Clin Oncol* 18:3633–3642, 2000.

104. Kane RC, McGuinn WD, Dagher R, et al: Dexrazoxane (Totect): FDA review and approval for the treatment of accidental extravasation following intravenous anthracycline chemotherapy. *Oncologist* 13:445–450, 2008.

105. Moreb JS, Oblon DJ: Outcome of clinical congestive heart failure induced by anthracycline chemotherapy. *Cancer* 70:2637–2641, 1992.

106. Ichikawa Y, Ghanefar M, Bayeva M, et al: Cardiotoxicity of doxorubicin is mediated through mitochondrial iron accumulation. *J Clin Invest* 124:617–630, 2014.

107. Aryal B, Jeong J, Rao VA: Doxorubicin-induced carbonylation and degradation of cardiac myosin binding protein C promote cardiotoxicity. *Proc Natl Acad Sci U S A* 111:2011–2016, 2014.

108. Burstein HJ, Winer EP: Primary care for survivors of breast cancer. *N Engl J Med* 343:1086–1094, 2000.

109. Shan K, Lincoff AM, Young JB: Anthracycline-induced cardiotoxicity. *Ann Intern Med* Intern Med 125:47–58, 1996.

110. Lipshultz SE, Alvarez JA, Scully RE: Anthracycline associated cardiotoxicity in survivors of childhood cancer. *Heart* 94:525–533, 2008.

111. Tebbi CK, London WB, Friedman D, et al: Dexrazoxane-associated risk for acute myeloid leukemia/myelodysplastic syndrome and other secondary malignancies in pediatric Hodgkin's disease. *J Clin Oncol* 25:493–500, 2007.

112. Salzer WL, Devidas M, Carroll WL, et al: Long-term results of the pediatric oncology group studies for childhood acute lymphoblastic leukemia 1984–2001: A report from the children's oncology group. *Leukemia* 24:355–370, 2010.

113. Mistry AR, Felix CA, Whitmarsh RJ, et al: DNA topoisomerase II in therapy-related acute promyelocytic leukemia. *N Engl J Med* 352:1529–1538, 2005.

114. Pedersen-Bjergaard J: Insights into leukemogenesis from therapy-related leukemia. *N Engl J Med* 352:1591–1594, 2005.

115. Binaschi M, Zunino F, Capranico G: Mechanism of action of DNA topoisomerase inhibitors. *Stem Cells* 13:369–379, 1995.

116. Bugg BY, Danks MK, Beck WT, Suttle DP: Expression of a mutant topoisomerase II in CCRF-CEM human leukemia cells selected for resistance to teniposide. *Proc Natl Acad Sci U S A* 88:7654–7658, 1991.

117. Zwelling LA, Hinds M, Chan D, et al: Characterization of an amsacrine-resistant line of human leukemia cells. Evidence for a drug-resistant form of topoisomerase II. *J Biol Chem* 264:16411–16420, 1989.

118. Stewart CF, Arbuck SG, Fleming RA, Evans WE: Changes in the clearance of total and unbound etoposide in patients with liver dysfunction. *J Clin Oncol* 8:1874–1879, 1990.

119. Winick NJ, McKenna RW, Shuster JJ, et al: Secondary acute myeloid leukemia in children with acute lymphoblastic leukemia treated with etoposide. *J Clin Oncol* 11:209–217, 1993.

120. Ratain MJ, Kaminer LS, Bitran JD, et al: Acute nonlymphocytic leukemia following etoposide and cisplatin combination chemotherapy for advanced non-small-cell carcinoma of the lung. *Blood* 70:1412–1417, 1987.

121. Peters WP, Shpall EJ, Jones RB, et al: High-dose combination alkylating agents with bone marrow support as initial treatment for metastatic breast cancer. *J Clin Oncol* 6:1368–1376, 1988.

122. Yeager AM, Kaizer H, Santos GW, et al: Autologous bone marrow transplantation in patients with acute nonlymphocytic leukemia, using ex vivo marrow treatment with 4-hydroperoxycyclophosphamide. *N Engl J Med* 315:141–147, 1986.

123. Reed E: Platinum-DNA adduct, nucleotide excision repair and platinum based anticancer chemotherapy. *Cancer Treat Rev* 24:331–344, 1998.

124. Gurubhagavatula S, Liu G, Park S, et al: XPD and XRCC1 genetic polymorphisms are prognostic factors in advanced non-small-cell lung cancer patients treated with platinum chemotherapy. *J Clin Oncol* 22:2594–2601, 2004.

125. Tew K, Colvin M, Jones R, et al: Alkylating agents, in *Cancer Chemotherapy and Biotherapy: Principles and Practice*, 4th ed, edited by p 297. 2006.

126. Hilton J: Role of aldehyde dehydrogenase in cyclophosphamide-resistant L1210 leukemia. *Cancer Res* 44:5156–5160, 1984.

127. Erickson LC: The role of O-6 methylguanine DNA methyltransferase (MGMT) in drug resistance and strategies for its inhibition. *Semin Cancer Biol* 2:257–265, 1991.

128. Hunter C, Smith R, Cahill DP, et al: A hypermutation phenotype and somatic MSH6 mutations in recurrent human malignant gliomas after alkylator chemotherapy. *Cancer Res* 66:3987–3991, 2006.

129. Droller MJ, Saral R, Santos G: Prevention of cyclophosphamide-induced hemorrhagic cystitis. *Urology* 20:256–258, 1982.

130. Leoni LM, Bailey B, Reifert J, et al: Bendamustine (Treanda) displays a distinct pattern of cytotoxicity and unique mechanistic features compared with other alkylating agents. *Clin Cancer Res* 14:309–317, 2008.

131. Elias AD, Eder JP, Shea T, et al: High-dose ifosfamide with mesna uroprotection: A phase I study. *J Clin Oncol* 8:170–178, 1990.

132. Gianni AM, Bregni M, Siena S, et al: Recombinant human granulocyte-macrophage colony-stimulating factor reduces hematologic toxicity and widens clinical applicability of high-dose cyclophosphamide treatment in breast cancer and non-Hodgkin's lymphoma. *J Clin Oncol* 8:768–778, 1990.

133. Lazarus HM, Reed MD, Spitzer TR, et al: High-dose i.v. thiotepa and cryopreserved autologous bone marrow transplantation for therapy of refractory cancer. *Cancer Treat Rep* 71:689–695, 1987.

134. Ozols RF, Corden BJ, Jacob J, et al: High-dose cisplatin in hypertonic saline. *Ann Intern MedIntern Med* 100:19–24, 1984.

135. Peters WP, Henner WD, Grochow LB, et al: Clinical and pharmacologic effects of high dose single agent busulfan with autologous bone marrow support in the treatment of solid tumors. *Cancer Res* 47:6402–6406, 1987.

136. Phillips GL, Wolff SN, Fay JW, et al: Intensive 1,3-bis (2-chloroethyl)-1-nitrosourea (BCNU) monochemotherapy and autologous marrow transplantation for malignant glioma. *J Clin Oncol* 4:639–645, 1986.

137. Shea TC, Flaherty M, Elias A, et al: A phase I clinical and pharmacokinetic study of carboplatin and autologous bone marrow support. *J Clin Oncol* 7:651–661, 1989.

138. Dunphy FR, Spitzer G, Buzdar AU, et al: Treatment of estrogen receptor-negative or hormonally refractory breast cancer with double high-dose chemotherapy intensification and bone marrow support. *J Clin Oncol* 8:1207–1216, 1990.

139. Eder JP, Elias A, Shea TC, et al: A phase I-II study of cyclophosphamide, thiotepa, and carboplatin with autologous bone marrow transplantation in solid tumor patients. *J Clin Oncol* 8:1239–1245, 1990.

140. Jones RJ, Piantadosi S, Mann RB, et al: High-dose cytotoxic therapy and bone marrow transplantation for relapsed Hodgkin's disease. *J Clin Oncol* 8:527–537, 1990.

141. Kessinger A, Armitage JO, Smith DM, et al: High-dose therapy and autologous peripheral blood stem cell transplantation for patients with lymphoma. *Blood* 74:1260–1265, 1989.

142. Wilson WH, Jain V, Bryant G, et al: Phase I and II study of high-dose ifosfamide, carboplatin, and etoposide with autologous bone marrow rescue in lymphomas and solid tumors. *J Clin Oncol* 10:1712–1722, 1992.

143. Umezawa H, Maeda K, Takeuchi T, Okami Y: New antibiotics, bleomycin A and B. *J Antibiot (Tokyo)* 19:200–209, 1966.

144. Burger RM: Cleavage of nucleic acids by bleomycin. *Chem Rev* 98:1153–1170, 1998.

145. Sebti SM, Jani JP, Mistry JS, et al: Metabolic inactivation: A mechanism of human tumor resistance to bleomycin. *Cancer Res* 51:227–232, 1991.

146. De Haas EC, Zwart N, Meijer C, et al: Variation in bleomycin hydrolase gene is associated with reduced survival after chemotherapy for testicular germ cell cancer. *J Clin Oncol* 26:1817–1823, 2008.

147. Alberts DS, Chen HS, Liu R, et al: Bleomycin pharmacokinetics in man. I. Intravenous administration. *Cancer Chemother Pharmacol* 1:177–181, 1978.

148. Karmiol S, Remick DG, Kunkel SL, Phan SH: Regulation of rat pulmonary endothelial cell interleukin-6 production by bleomycin: Effects of cellular fatty acid composition. *Am J Respir Cell Mol Biol* 9:628–636, 1993.

149. Evens AM, Hong F, Gordon LI, et al: The efficacy and tolerability of Adriamycin, bleomycin, vinblastine, dacarbazine and Stanford V in older Hodgkin lymphoma patients: A comprehensive analysis from the North American intergroup trial E2496. *Br J Haematol* 161:76–86, 2013.

150. Comis RL: Detecting bleomycin pulmonary toxicity: A continued conundrum. *J Clin Oncol* 8:765–767, 1990.

151. Hutson RG, Kitoh T, Moraga Amador DA, et al: Amino acid control of asparagine synthetase: Relation to asparaginase resistance in human leukemia cells. *Am J Physiol J Physiol* 272(5 Pt 1):C1691–C1699, 1997.

152. Kaspers GJ, Veerman AJ, Pieters R, et al: *In vitro* cellular drug resistance and prognosis in newly diagnosed childhood acute lymphoblastic leukemia. *Blood* 90:2723–2729, 1997.

153. Holle LM: Pegaspargase: An alternative? *Ann Pharmacother* 31:616–624, 1997.

154. Ettinger LJ, Ettinger AG, Avramis VI, Gaynon PS: Acute lymphoblastic leukaemia: A guide to asparaginase and pegaspargase therapy. *BioDrugs* 7:30–39, 1997.

155. Semeraro N, Montemurro P, Giordano P, et al: Unbalanced coagulation-fibrinolysis potential during L-asparaginase therapy in children with acute lymphoblastic leukaemia. *Thromb Haemost* 64:38–40, 1990.

156. Bushara KO, Rust RS: Reversible MRI lesions due to pegaspargase treatment of non -Hodgkin's lymphoma. *Pediatr Neurol* 17:185–187, 1997.

157. Mitchell LG, Andrew M, Hanna K, et al: A prospective cohort study determining the prevalence of thrombotic events in children with acute lymphoblastic leukemia and a central venous line who are treated with L-asparaginase: results of the Prophylactic Antithrombin Replacement in Kids with Acute Lymphoblastic Leukemia Treated with Asparaginase (PARKAA) Study. *Cancer* 97:508–516, 2003.

158. Heitink-Pollé KM1, Prinsen BH, de Koning TJ, et al: High incidence of symptomatic hyperammonemia in children with acute lymphoblastic leukemia receiving pegylated asparaginase. *JIMD Rep* 7:103–108, 2013.

159. Nowak-Göttl U, Wermes C, Junker R, et al: Prospective evaluation of the thrombotic risk in children with acute lymphoblastic leukemia carrying the MTHFR TT 677 genotype, the prothrombin G20210A variant, and further prothrombotic risk factors. *Blood* 93:1595–1599, 1999.

160. Parsons SK, Skapek SX, Neufeld EJ, et al: Asparaginase-associated lipid abnormalities in children with acute lymphoblastic leukemia. *Blood* 89:1886–1895, 1997.

161. Strobeck M: Multiple myeloma therapies. *Nat Rev Drug Discov* 6:181–182, 2007.

162. Roussel M, Lauwers-Cances V, Robillard N, et al: Front-line transplantation program with lenalidomide, bortezomib, dexamethasone combination as induction and consolidation followed by lenalidomide maintenance in patients with multiple myeloma: A phase II study by the Intergroupe Francophone du Myélome. *J Clin Oncol* 32: 2712–2717, 2014.

163. Richardson PG, Siegel DS, Vij R, et al: Pomalidomide alone or in combination with low-dose dexamethasone in relapsed and refractory multiple myeloma: A randomized phase 2 study. *Blood* 123:1826–1832, 2014.

164. D'Amato RJ, Loughnan MS, Flynn E, Folkman J: Thalidomide is an inhibitor of angiogenesis. *Proc Natl Acad Sci U S A* 91:4082–4085, 1994.

165. Moreira AL, Friedlander DR, Shif B, et al: Thalidomide and a thalidomide analogue inhibit endothelial cell proliferation *in vitro. J Neurooncol* 43:109–114, 1999.

166. Muller GW, Chen R, Huang SY, et al: Amino-substituted thalidomide analogs: Potent inhibitors of TNF-alpha production. *Bioorg Med Chem Lett* 9:1625–1630, 1999.

167. LeBlanc R, Hideshima T, Catley LP, et al: Immunomodulatory drug costimulates T cells via the B7-CD28 pathway. *Blood* 103:1787–1790, 2004.

168. Zhu YX, Braggio E, Shi CX, et al: Identification of cereblon binding proteins and relationship with response and survival following pomalidomide and dexamethasone in multiple myeloma. *Blood* 124:536–545, 2014.

169. Richardson PG, Schlossman RL, Weller E, et al: Immunomodulatory drug CC-5013 overcomes drug resistance and is well tolerated in patients with relapsed multiple myeloma. *Blood* 100:3063–3067, 2002.

170. Teo SK, Scheffler MR, Kook KA, et al: Thalidomide dose proportionality assessment following single doses to healthy subjects. *J Clin Pharmacol* 41:662–667, 2001.

171. Scott LJ: Pomalidomide: A review of its use in patients with recurrent multiple myeloma. *Drugs* 74:549–562, 2014.

172. Piscitelli SC, Figg WD, Hahn B, et al: Single-dose pharmacokinetics of thalidomide in human immunodeficiency virus-infected patients. *Antimicrob Agents Chemother* 41:2797–2799, 1997.

173. Singhal S, Mehta J, Desikan R, et al: Antitumor activity of thalidomide in refractory multiple myeloma. *N Engl J Med* 341:1565–1571, 1999.

174. Mileshkin L, Biagi JJ, Mitchell P, et al: Multicenter phase 2 trial of thalidomide in relapsed/refractory multiple myeloma: Adverse prognostic impact of advanced age. *Blood* 102:69–77, 2003.

175. Rajkumar SV, Hayman S, Gertz MA, et al: Combination therapy with thalidomide plus dexamethasone for newly diagnosed myeloma. *J Clin Oncol* 20:4319–4323, 2002.

176. Musallam KM, Dahdaleh FS, Shamseddine AI, Taher AT: Incidence and prophylaxis of venous thromboembolic events in multiple myeloma patients receiving immunomodulatory therapy. *Thromb Res* 123:679–686, 2009.

177. Nathan PD, Gore ME, Eisen TG: Unexpected toxicity of combination thalidomide and interferon alpha-2a treatment in metastatic renal cell carcinoma. *J Clin Oncol* 20: 1429–1430, 2002.

178. Ebert BL, Galili N, Tamayo P, et al: An erythroid differentiation signature predicts response to lenalidomide in myelodysplastic syndrome. *PLoS Med* 5:e35, 2008.

179. Andritsos LA, Johnson AJ, Lozanski G, et al: Higher doses of lenalidomide are associated with unacceptable toxicity including life-threatening tumor flare in patients with chronic lymphocytic leukemia. *J Clin Oncol* 26:2519–2525, 2008.

180. Weber DM, Chen C, Niesvizky R, et al: Lenalidomide plus dexamethasone for relapsed multiple myeloma in North America. *N Engl J Med* 357:2133–2142, 2007.

181. Kizaki M, Nakazato T, Ito K, et al: A novel therapeutic approach for hematological malignancies based on cellular differentiation and apoptosis. *Int J Hematol* 76 (Suppl 1): 250–252, 2002.

182. Parkinson D, Smith M: Retinoid therapy for acute promyelocytic leukemia: A coming of age for the differentiation therapy of malignancy. *Ann Intern Med* 117:338–340, 1992.

183. Sandor V, Bakke S, Robey RW, et al: Phase I trial of the histone deacetylase inhibitor, depsipeptide (FR901228, NSC 630176), in patients with refractory neoplasms. *Clin Cancer Res* 8:718–728, 2002.

184. Warrell RP Jr, Frankel SR, Miller WH Jr, et al.: Differentiation therapy of acute promyelocytic leukemia with tretinoin (all-trans-retinoic acid). *N Engl J Med* 324:1385–1393, 1991.

185. Kakizuka A, Miller WH Jr, Umesono K, et al: Chromosomal translocation t(15;17) in human acute promyelocytic leukemia fuses RAR alpha with a novel putative transcription factor, PML. *Cell* 66:663–674, 1991.

186. Collins SJ: Retinoic acid receptors, hematopoiesis and leukemogenesis. *Curr Opin Hematol* 15:346–351, 2008.

187. Robertson KA, Emami B, Collins SJ: Retinoic acid-resistant HL-60R cells harbor a point mutation in the retinoic acid receptor ligand-binding domain that confers dominant negative activity. *Blood* 80:1885–1889, 1992.

188. Muindi JR, Frankel SR, Huselton C, et al: Clinical pharmacology of oral all-trans retinoic acid in patients with acute promyelocytic leukemia. *Cancer Res* 52:2138–2142, 1992.

189. Muindi J, Frankel SR, Miller WH Jr, et al: Continuous treatment with all-trans retinoic acid causes a progressive reduction in plasma drug concentrations: Implications for relapse and retinoid "resistance" in patients with acute promyelocytic leukemia. *Blood* 79:299–303, 1992.

190. Frankel SR, Eardley A, Lauwers G, et al: The "retinoic acid syndrome" in acute promyelocytic leukemia. *Ann Intern MedIntern Med* 117:292–296, 1992.

191. De Botton S, Dombret H, Sanz M, et al: Incidence, clinical features, and outcome of all trans-retinoic acid syndrome in 413 cases of newly diagnosed acute promyelocytic leukemia. The European APL Group. *Blood* 92:2712–2718, 1998.

192. Soignet SL, Maslak P, Wang ZG, et al: Complete remission after treatment of acute promyelocytic leukemia with arsenic trioxide. *N Engl J Med* 339:1341–1348, 1998.

193. Miller WH Jr, Schipper HM, Lee JS, et al: Mechanisms of action of arsenic trioxide. *Cancer Res* 62:3893–3903, 2002.

194. Wang ZY, Chen Z: Acute promyelocytic leukemia: From highly fatal to highly curable. *Blood* 111:2505–2515, 2008.

195. Lallemand-Breitenbach V, Jeanne M, Benhenda S, et al: Arsenic degrades PML or PML-RARalpha through a SUMO-triggered RNF4/ubiquitin-mediated pathway. *Nat Cell Biol* 10:547–555, 2008.

196. Chen GQ, Shi XG, Tang W, et al: Use of arsenic trioxide (As2O3) in the treatment of acute promyelocytic leukemia (APL): I. As2O3 exerts dose-dependent dual effects on APL cells. *Blood* 89:3345–3353, 1997.

197. Gupta A, Lawrence AT, Krishnan K, et al: Current concepts in the mechanisms and management of drug-induced QT prolongation and torsade de pointes. *Am Heart J* 153:891–899, 2007.

198. Shen ZX, Chen GQ, Ni JH, et al: Use of arsenic trioxide (As2O3) in the treatment of acute promyelocytic leukemia (APL): II. Clinical efficacy and pharmacokinetics in relapsed patients. *Blood* 89:3354–3360, 1997.

199. Dawson MA, Kouzarides T: Cancer epigenetics: From mechanism to therapy. *Cell* 150:12–27, 2012.

200. Silverman LR, Demakos EP, Peterson BL, et al: Randomized controlled trial of azacitidine in patients with the myelodysplastic syndrome: A study of the cancer and leukemia group B. *J Clin Oncol* 20:2429–2440, 2002.

201. Fenaux P, Mufti GJ, Hellstrom-Lindberg E, et al: Efficacy of azacitidine compared with that of conventional care regimens in the treatment of higher-risk myelodysplastic syndromes: A randomised, open-label, phase III study. *Lancet Oncol* 10:223–232, 2009.

202. Kantarjian H, Issa JP, Rosenfeld CS, et al: Decitabine improves patient outcomes in myelodysplastic syndromes: Results of a phase III randomized study. *Cancer* 106:1794–1803, 2006.

203. Lübbert M, Suciu S, Baila L, et al: Low-dose decitabine versus best supportive care in elderly patients with intermediate- or high-risk myelodysplastic syndrome (MDS) ineligible for intensive chemotherapy: Final results of the randomized phase III study of the European Organisation for Research and Treatment of Cancer Leukemia Group and the German MDS Study Group. *J Clin Oncol* 29:1987–1996, 2011.

204. Lee YG, Kim I, Yoon SS, et al: Comparative analysis between azacitidine and decitabine for the treatment of myelodysplastic syndromes. *Br J Haematol* 161:339–347, 2013.

205. Khan H, Vale C, Bhagat T, Verma A: Role of DNA methylation in the pathogenesis and treatment of myelodysplastic syndromes. *Semin Hematol* 50:16–37, 2013.

206. Campbell RM, Tummino PJ: Cancer epigenetics drug discovery and development: The challenge of hitting the mark. *J Clin Invest* 124:64–69, 2014.

207. Navada SC, Steinmann J, Lübbert M, Silverman LR: Clinical development of demethylating agents in hematology. *J Clin Invest* 124:40–46, 2014.

208. West AC, Johnstone RW: New and emerging HDAC inhibitors for cancer treatment. *J Clin Invest* 124:30–39, 2014.

209. Duan H, Heckman CA, Boxer LM: Histone deacetylase inhibitors down-regulate bcl-2 expression and induce apoptosis in t(14;18) lymphomas. *Mol Cell Biol* 25:1608–1619, 2005.

210. Luo J, Su F, Chen D, et al: Deacetylation of p53 modulates its effect on cell growth and apoptosis. *Nature* 408:377–381, 2000.

211. Heideman MR, Wilting RH, Yanover E, et al: Dosage-dependent tumor suppression by histone deacetylases 1 and 2 through regulation of c-Myc collaborating genes and p53 function. *Blood* 121:2038–2050, 2013.

212. McGraw AL: Romidepsin for the treatment of T-cell lymphomas. *Am J Health Syst Pharm* 70:1115–1122, 2013.

213. Mann BS, Johnson JR, Cohen MH, et al: FDA approval summary: Vorinostat for treatment of advanced primary cutaneous T-cell lymphoma. *Oncologist* 12:1247–1252, 2007.

214. Piekarz RL, Frye R, Turner M, et al: Phase II multi-institutional trial of the histone deacetylase inhibitor romidepsin as monotherapy for patients with cutaneous T-cell lymphoma. *J Clin Oncol* 27:5410–5417, 2009.

215. Piekarz RL, Frye R, Turner M, et al: Phase 2 trial of romidepsin in patients with peripheral T-cell lymphoma. *Blood* 117:5827–5834, 2011.

216. Coiffier B, Pro B, Prince HM, et al: Romidepsin for the treatment of relapsed/refractory peripheral T-cell lymphoma: Pivotal study update demonstrates durable responses. *J Hematol Oncol* 7:11, 2014.

217. Ramalingam SS, Kummar S, Sarantopoulos J, et al: Phase I study of vorinostat in patients with advanced solid tumors and hepatic dysfunction: A National Cancer Institute Organ Dysfunction Working Group study. *J Clin Oncol* 20:4507 4512, 2010.

218. Iwamoto M, Friedman EJ, Sandhu P, et al: Clinical pharmacology profile of vorinostat, a histone deacetylase inhibitor. *Cancer Chemother Pharmacol* 72:493–508, 2013.

219. Wong NS, Seah EZh, Wang LZ, et al: Impact of UDP-glucuronyltransferase 2B17 genotype on vorinostat metabolism and clinical outcomes in Asian women with breast cancer. *Pharmacogenet Genomics* 21:760–768, 2011.

220. Wang F, Travins J, DeLaBarre B, et al: Targeted inhibition of mutant IDH2 in leukemia cells induces cellular differentiation. *Science* 340:622–626, 2013.

220A. Stein E, Tallman M, Pollyea D et al: Clinical safety and activity in a phase I trial of AG-221, a first in class, potent inhibitor of the IDH2-mutant protein, in patients with IDH2 mutant positive advanced hematologic malignancies [abstract]. In: Proceedings of the 105th Annual Meeting of the American Association for Cancer Research; 2014 Apr 5-9; San Diego (CA: AACR; 2014. Abstract nr CT103).

221. Daigle SR, Olhava EJ, Therkelsen CA, et al: Potent inhibition of DOT1L as treatment of MLL-fusion leukemia. *Blood* 122:1017–1025, 2013.

222. Fathi AT, Sadrzadeh H, Borger DR, et al: Prospective serial evaluation of 2-hydroxyglutarate, during treatment of newly diagnosed acute myeloid leukemia, to assess disease activity and therapeutic response. *Blood* 120:4649–4652, 2012.

223. McCabe MT, Ott HM, Ganji G, et al: EZH2 inhibition as a therapeutic strategy for lymphoma with EZH2-activating mutations. *Nature* 492:108–112, 2012.

224. Knutson SK, Kawano S, Minoshima Y, et al: Selective inhibition of EZH2 by EPZ-6438 leads to potent antitumor activity in EZH2-mutant non-Hodgkin lymphoma. *Mol Cancer Ther* 13:842–854, 2014.

225. Wyspiańska BS, Bannister AJ, Barbieri I, et al: BET protein inhibition shows efficacy against JAK2V617F-driven neoplasms. *Leukemia* 28:88–97, 2014.

226. Delmore JE, Issa GC, Lemieux ME, et al: BET bromodomain inhibition as a therapeutic strategy to target c-Myc. *Cell.* 146(6):904–17, 2011. (http://www.ncbi.nlm.nih.gov/pubmed/21889194) Last accessed June 2015.

227. Fiskus W, Sharma S, Qi J, et al: Highly active combination of BRD4 antagonist and histone deacetylase inhibitor against human acute myelogenous leukemia cells. *Mol Cancer Ther* 13:1142–1154, 2014.

228. Stewart HJ, Horne GA, Bastow S, Chevassut TJ: BRD4 associates with p53 in DNMT3A-mutated leukemia cells and is implicated in apoptosis by the bromodomain inhibitor JQ1. *Cancer Med* 2:826–835, 2013.

229. Zhao Y, Yang CY, Wang S: The making of I-BET762, a BET bromodomain inhibitor now in clinical development. *J Med Chem* 56:7498–7500, 2013.

230. Druker BJ: Perspectives on the development of a molecularly targeted agent. *Cancer Cell* 1:31–36, 2002.

231. Druker BJ, Guilhot F, O'Brien SG, et al: Five-year follow-up of patients receiving imatinib for chronic myeloid leukemia. *N Engl J Med* 355:2408–2417, 2006.

232. O'Brien SG, Guilhot F, Larson RA, et al: Imatinib compared with interferon and low-dose cytarabine for newly diagnosed chronic-phase chronic myeloid leukemia. *N Engl J Med* 348:994–1004, 2003.

233. Cortes J, Lipton JH, Rea D, et al: Phase 2 study of subcutaneous omacetaxine mepesuccinate after TKI failure in patients with chronic-phase CML with T315I mutation. *Blood* 120:2573–2580, 2012.

234. Heinrich MC, Griffith DJ, Druker BJ, et al: Inhibition of c-kit receptor tyrosine kinase activity by STI 571, a selective tyrosine kinase inhibitor. *Blood* 96:925–932, 2000.

235. Demetri GD, von Mehren M, Blanke CD, et al: Efficacy and safety of imatinib mesylate in advanced gastrointestinal stromal tumors. *N Engl J Med* 347:472–480, 2002.

236. Cools J, DeAngelo DJ, Gotlib J, et al: A tyrosine kinase created by fusion of the PDGFRA and FIP1L1 genes as a therapeutic target of imatinib in idiopathic hypereosinophilic syndrome. *N Engl J Med* 348:1201–1214, 2003.

237. Magnusson MK, Meade KE, Nakamura R, et al: Activity of STI571 in chronic myelomonocytic leukemia with a platelet-derived growth factor beta receptor fusion oncogene. *Blood* 100:1088–1091, 2002.

237A. Passamonti F: PDGFREB disease: Right diagnosis to prolong survival. *Blood.* 123:3526–8. 2014.

238. Sirvent N, Maire G, Pedeutour F: Genetics of dermatofibrosarcoma protuberans family of tumors: From ring chromosomes to tyrosine kinase inhibitor treatment. *Genes Chromosomes Cancer* 37:1–19, 2003.

239. Shah NP, Tran C, Lee FY, et al: Overriding imatinib resistance with a novel ABL kinase inhibitor. *Science* 305:399–401, 2004.

240. Weisberg E, Manley PW, Breitenstein W, et al: Characterization of AMN107, a selective inhibitor of native and mutant Bcr-Abl. *Cancer Cell* 7:129–141, 2005.

241. O'Hare T, Walters DK, Stoffregen EP, et al: *In vitro* activity of Bcr-Abl inhibitors AMN107 and BMS-354825 against clinically relevant imatinib-resistant Abl kinase domain mutants. *Cancer Res* 65:4500–4505, 2005.

242. Wisniewski D, Lambek CL, Liu C, et al: Characterization of potent inhibitors of the Bcr-Abl and the c-kit receptor tyrosine kinases. *Cancer Res* 62:4244–4255, 2002.

243. Khorashad JS, Kelley TW, Szankasi P, et al: BCR-ABL1 compound mutations in tyrosine kinase inhibitor-resistant CML: Frequency and clonal relationships. *Blood* 121:489–498, 2013.

244. Soverini S, Colarossi S, Gnani A, et al: Contribution of ABL kinase domain mutations to imatinib resistance in different subsets of Philadelphia-positive patients: By the GIMEMA Working Party on Chronic Myeloid Leukemia. *Clin Cancer Res* 12:7374–7379, 2006.

245. Soverini S, Hochhaus A, Nicolini FE, et al: BCR-ABL kinase domain mutation analysis in chronic myeloid leukemia patients treated with tyrosine kinase inhibitors: Recommendations from an expert panel on behalf of European LeukemiaNet. *Blood* 118:1208–1215, 2011.

246. Cortes JE, Kim DW, Pinilla-Ibarz J, et al: A phase 2 trial of ponatinib in Philadelphia chromosome–positive leukemias. *N Engl J Med* 369:1783–1796, 2013.

247. Takayama N, Sato N, O'Brien SG, et al: Imatinib mesylate has limited activity against the central nervous system involvement of Philadelphia chromosome-positive acute lymphoblastic leukaemia due to poor penetration into cerebrospinal fluid. *Br J Haematol* 119:106–108, 2002.

248. Gambacorti-Passerini C, Zucchetti M, Russo D, et al: Alpha1 acid glycoprotein binds to imatinib (STI571) and substantially alters its pharmacokinetics in chronic myeloid leukemia patients. *Clin Cancer Res* 9:625–632, 2003.

249. Shah NP, Nicoll JM, Nagar B, et al: Multiple BCR-ABL kinase domain mutations confer polyclonal resistance to the tyrosine kinase inhibitor imatinib (STI571) in chronic phase and blast crisis chronic myeloid leukemia. *Cancer Cell* 2:117–125, 2002.

250. O'Hare T, Eide CA, Deininger MW: Bcr-Abl kinase domain mutations, drug resistance, and the road to a cure for chronic myeloid leukemia. *Blood* 110:2242–2249, 2007.

251. Corbin AS, La Rosée P, Stoffregen EP, et al: Several Bcr-Abl kinase domain mutants associated with imatinib mesylate resistance remain sensitive to imatinib. *Blood* 101:4611–4614, 2003.

252. Branford S, Rudzki Z, Walsh S, et al: Detection of BCR-ABL mutations in patients with CML treated with imatinib is virtually always accompanied by clinical resistance, and mutations in the ATP phosphate-binding loop (P-loop) are associated with a poor prognosis. *Blood* 102:276–283, 2003.

253. Roche-Lestienne C, Laï, JL, Darré S, et al: A mutation conferring resistance to imatinib at the time of diagnosis of chronic myelogenous leukemia. *N Engl J Med* 348: 2265–2266, 2003.

254. Cortes JE, Kantarjian HM, Brümmendorf TH, et al: Safety and efficacy of bosutinib (SKI-606) in chronic phase Philadelphia chromosome-positive chronic myeloid leukemia patients with resistance or intolerance to imatinib. *Blood* 118:4567–4576, 2011.

255. Kantarjian HM, Giles FJ, Bhalla KN, et al: Nilotinib is effective in patients with chronic myeloid leukemia in chronic phase after imatinib resistance or intolerance: 24-month follow-up results. *Blood* 117:1141–1145, 2011.

256. Shah NP, Kim DW, Kantarjian H, et al: Potent, transient inhibition of BCR-ABL with dasatinib 100 mg daily achieves rapid and durable cytogenetic responses and high transformation-free survival rates in chronic phase chronic myeloid leukemia patients with resistance, suboptimal response or intolerance to imatinib. *Haematologica* 95:232–240, 2010.

257. Morel F, Bris MJ, Herry A, et al: Double minutes containing amplified bcr-abl fusion gene in a case of chronic myeloid leukemia treated by imatinib. *Eur J Haematol* 70:235–239, 2003.

258. Mahon FX, Belloc F, Lagarde V, et al: MDR1 gene overexpression confers resistance to imatinib mesylate in leukemia cell line models. *Blood* 101:2368–2373, 2003.

259. White DL, Saunders VA, Dang P, et al: OCT-1-mediated influx is a key determinant of the intracellular uptake of imatinib but not nilotinib (AMN107): Reduced OCT-1 activity is the cause of low in vitro sensitivity to imatinib. *Blood* 108:697–704, 2006.

260. Andersen MK, Pedersen-Bjergaard J, Kjeldsen L, et al: Clonal Ph-negative hematopoiesis in CML after therapy with imatinib mesylate is frequently characterized by trisomy 8. *Leukemia* 16:1390–1393, 2002.

261. Bumm T, Müller C, Al-Ali HK, et al: Emergence of clonal cytogenetic abnormalities in Ph- cells in some CML patients in cytogenetic remission to imatinib but restoration of polyclonal hematopoiesis in the majority. *Blood* 101:1941–1949, 2003.

262. Kantarjian HM, Giles F, Gattermann N, et al: Nilotinib (formerly AMN107), a highly selective BCR-ABL tyrosine kinase inhibitor, is effective in patients with Philadelphia chromosome-positive chronic myelogenous leukemia in chronic phase following imatinib resistance and intolerance. *Blood* 110:3540–3546, 2007.

263. Talpaz M, Shah NP, Kantarjian H, et al: Dasatinib in imatinib-resistant Philadelphia chromosome-positive leukemias. *N Engl J Med* 354:2531–2541, 2006.

264. Tefferi A, Vardiman JW: Classification and diagnosis of myeloproliferative neoplasms: The 2008 World Health Organization criteria and point-of-care diagnostic algorithms. *Leukemia* 22:14–22, 2008.

265. Baxter EJ, Scott LM, Campbell PJ, et al: Acquired mutation of the tyrosine kinase JAK2 in human myeloproliferative disorders. *Lancet* 365:1054–1061, 2005.

266. James C, Ugo V, Le Couédic JP, et al: A unique clonal JAK2 mutation leading to constitutive signalling causes polycythaemia vera. *Nature* 434:1144–1148, 2005.

267. Levine RL, Wadleigh M, Cools J, et al: Activating mutation in the tyrosine kinase JAK2 in polycythemia vera, essential thrombocythemia, and myeloid metaplasia with myelofibrosis. *Cancer Cell* 7:387–397, 2005.

268. Ihle JN, Witthuhn BA, Quelle FW, et al: Signaling through the hematopoietic cytokine receptors. *Annu Rev Immunol* 13:369–398, 1995.

269. Sonbol MB, Firwana B, Zarzour A, et al: Comprehensive review of JAK inhibitors in myeloproliferative neoplasms. *Ther Adv Hematol* 4:15–35, 2013.

270. Chiorazzi N, Rai KR, Ferrarini M: Chronic Lymphocytic Leukemia. *N Engl J Med* 352:804–815, 2005.

271. Hallek M, Fischer K, Fingerle-Rowson G, et al: Addition of rituximab to fludarabine and cyclophosphamide in patients with chronic lymphocytic leukaemia: A randomised, open-label, phase 3 trial. *Lancet* 376:1164–1174, 2010.

272. Byrd JC, Furman RR, Coutre SE, et al: Targeting BTK with ibrutinib in relapsed chronic lymphocytic leukemia. *N Engl J Med* 369:32–42, 2013.

273. Byrd JC, Brown JR, O'Brien S, et al: Ibrutinib versus ofatumumab in previously treated chronic lymphoid leukemia. *N Engl J Med* 371:213–223, 2014.

274. Woyach JA, Furman RR, Liu TM, et al: Resistance mechanisms for the Bruton's tyrosine kinase inhibitor ibrutinib. *N Engl J Med* 370:2286–2294, 2014.

275. Goldberg AL: Protein degradation and protection against misfolded or damaged proteins. *Nature* 426:895–899, 2003.

276. Demo SD, Kirk CJ, Aujay MA, et al: Antitumor activity of PR-171, a novel irreversible inhibitor of the proteasome. *Cancer Res* 67:6383–6391, 2007.

277. Orlowski RZ, Stinchcombe TE, Mitchell BS, et al: Phase I trial of the proteasome inhibitor PS-341 in patients with refractory hematologic malignancies. *J Clin Oncol* 20: 4420–4427, 2002.

278. Richardson PG, Barlogie B, Berenson J, et al: A phase 2 study of bortezomib in relapsed, refractory myeloma. *N Engl J Med* 348:2609–2617, 2003.

279. Richardson PG, Sonneveld P, Schuster MW, et al: Bortezomib or high-dose dexamethasone for relapsed multiple myeloma. *N Engl J Med* 352:2487–2498, 2005.

280. Sitia R, Palladini G, Merlini G: Bortezomib in the treatment of AL amyloidosis: Targeted therapy? *Haematologica* 92:1302–1307, 2007.

281. Goy A, Younes A, McLaughlin P, et al: Phase II study of proteasome inhibitor bortezomib in relapsed or refractory B-cell non-Hodgkin's lymphoma. *J Clin Oncol* 23:667–675, 2005.

282. Fisher RI, Bernstein SH, Kahl BS, et al: Multicenter phase II study of bortezomib in patients with relapsed or refractory mantle cell lymphoma. *J Clin Oncol* 24:4867–4874, 2006.

283. O'Connor OA, Wright J, Moskowitz C, et al: Phase II clinical experience with the novel proteasome inhibitor bortezomib in patients with indolent non-Hodgkin's lymphoma and mantle cell lymphoma. *J Clin Oncol* 23:676–684, 2005.

284. Mitsiades N, Mitsiades CS, Poulaki V, et al: Molecular sequelae of proteasome inhibition in human multiple myeloma cells. *Proc Natl Acad Sci U S A* 99:14374–14379, 2002.

285. Mitsiades N, Mitsiades CS, Poulaki V, et al: Apoptotic signaling induced by immunomodulatory thalidomide analogs in human multiple myeloma cells: Therapeutic implications. *Blood* 99:4525–4530, 2002.

286. Mitsiades N, Mitsiades CS, Richardson PG, et al: The proteasome inhibitor PS-341 potentiates sensitivity of multiple myeloma cells to conventional chemotherapeutic agents: Therapeutic applications. *Blood* 101:2377–2380, 2003.

287. Mitsiades CS, Mitsiades NS, McMullan CJ, et al: Transcriptional signature of histone deacetylase inhibition in multiple myeloma: Biological and clinical implications. *Proc Natl Acad Sci U S A* 101:540–545, 2004.

288. San Miguel JF, Schlag R, Khuageva NK, et al: Bortezomib plus melphalan and prednisone for initial treatment of multiple myeloma. *N Engl J Med* 359:906–917, 2008.

289. Orlowski RZ, Nagler A, Sonneveld P, et al: Randomized phase III study of pegylated liposomal doxorubicin plus bortezomib compared with bortezomib alone in relapsed or refractory multiple myeloma: Combination therapy improves time to progression. *J Clin Oncol* 25:3892–3901, 2007.

290. Richardson PG, Weller E, Lonial S, et al: Lenalidomide, bortezomib, and dexamethasone combination therapy in patients with newly diagnosed multiple myeloma. *Blood* 116:679–686, 2010.

291. Richardson PG, Briemberg H, Jagannath S, et al: Frequency, characteristics, and reversibility of peripheral neuropathy during treatment of advanced multiple myeloma with bortezomib. *J Clin Oncol* 24:3113–3120, 2006.

292. Herndon TM, Deisseroth A, Kaminskas E, et al: U.S. Food and Drug Administration approval: Carfilzomib for the treatment of multiple myeloma. *Clin Cancer Res* 19: 4559–4563, 2013.

293. Chauhan D, Tian Z, Zhou B, et al: In vitro and in vivo selective antitumor activity of a novel orally bioavailable proteasome inhibitor MLN9708 against multiple myeloma cells. *Clin Cancer Res* 17:5311–5321, 2011.

294. Kupperman E, Lee EC, Cao Y, et al: Evaluation of the proteasome inhibitor MLN9708 in preclinical models of human cancer. *Cancer Res* 71:1970–1980, 2010.

295. Aghajanian C, Soignet S, Dizon DS, et al: A phase I trial of the novel proteasome inhibitor PS341 in advanced solid tumor malignancies. *Clin Cancer Res* 8:2505–2511, 2002.

296. Goldberg AL: Functions of the proteasome: From protein degradation and immune surveillance to cancer therapy. *Biochem Soc Trans* 35:12–17, 2007.

297. Meister S, Schubert U, Neubert K, et al: Extensive immunoglobulin production sensitizes myeloma cells for proteasome inhibition. *Cancer Res* 67:1783–1792, 2007.

298. Nayak MK, Kulkarni PP, Dash D: Regulatory role of proteasome in determination of platelet life span. *J Biol Chem* 288:6826–6834, 2013.

299. Arastu-Kapur S, Anderl JL, Kraus M, et al: Nonproteasomal targets of the proteasome inhibitors bortezomib and carfilzomib: A link to clinical adverse events. *Clin Cancer Res* 17:2734–2743, 2011.

300. Groll M, Berkers CR, Ploegh HL, Ovaa H: Crystal structure of the boronic acid-based proteasome inhibitor bortezomib in complex with the yeast 20S proteasome. *Structure* 14:451–456, 2006.

301. Adams J, Behnke M, Chen S, et al: Potent and selective inhibitors of the proteasome: Dipeptidyl boronic acids. *Bioorg Med Chem Lett* 8:333–338, 1998.

302. Dorsey BD, Iqbal M, Chatterjee S, et al: Discovery of a potent, selective, and orally active proteasome inhibitor for the treatment of cancer. *J Med Chem* 51:1068–1072, 2008.

303. Shimoda N, Fukazawa N, Nonomura K, Fairchild RL: Cathepsin g is required for sustained inflammation and tissue injury after reperfusion of ischemic kidneys. *Am J Pathol* 170:930–940, 2007.

304. Maloney DG, Smith B, Rose A: Rituximab: Mechanism of action and resistance. *Semin Oncol* 29:2–9, 2002.

305. Klinger M, Brandl C, Zugmaier G, et al: Immunopharmacologic response of patients with B-lineage acute lymphoblastic leukemia to continuous infusion of T cell-engaging CD19/CD3-bispecific BiTE antibody blinatumomab. *Blood* 119:6226–6233, 2012.

306. Witzig TE, Gordon LI, Cabanillas F, et al: Randomized controlled trial of yttrium-90-labeled ibritumomab tiuxetan radioimmunotherapy versus rituximab immunotherapy for patients with relapsed or refractory low-grade, follicular, or transformed B-cell non-Hodgkin's lymphoma. *J Clin Oncol* 20:2453–2463, 2002.

307. Pro B, Advani R, Brice P, et al: Brentuximab vedotin (SGN-35) in patients with relapsed or refractory systemic anaplastic large-cell lymphoma: Results of a phase II study. *J Clin Oncol* 30:2190–2196, 2012.

308. Miller RA, Maloney DG, Warnke R, Levy R: Treatment of B-cell lymphoma with monoclonal anti-idiotype antibody. *N Engl J Med* 306:517–522, 1982.

309. Stashenko P, Nadler LM, Hardy R, Schlossman SF: Characterization of a human B lymphocyte-specific antigen. *J Immunol* 125:1678–1685, 1980.

310. Tedder TF, Forsgren A, Boyd AW, et al: Antibodies reactive with the B1 molecule inhibit cell cycle progression but not activation of human B lymphocytes. *Eur J ImmunolJ Immunol* 16:881–887, 1986.

311. Smeland E, Godal T, Ruud E, et al: The specific induction of myc protooncogene expression in normal human B cells is not a sufficient event for acquisition of competence to proliferate. *Proc Natl Acad Sci U S A* 82:6255–6259, 1985.

312. Deans JP, Schieven GL, Shu GL, et al: Association of tyrosine and serine kinases with the B cell surface antigen CD20. Induction via CD20 of tyrosine phosphorylation and activation of phospholipase C-gamma 1 and PLC phospholipase C-gamma 2. *J Immunol* 151:4494–4504, 1993.

313. Marcus R, Imrie K, Belch A, et al: CVP chemotherapy plus rituximab compared with CVP as first-line treatment for advanced follicular lymphoma. *Blood* 105:1417–1423, 2005.

314. Habermann TM, Weller EA, Morrison VA, et al: Rituximab-CHOP versus CHOP alone or with maintenance rituximab in older patients with diffuse large B-cell lymphoma. *J Clin Oncol* 24:3121–3127, 2006.

315. Davis TA, Grillo-López AJ, White CA, et al: Rituximab anti-CD20 monoclonal antibody therapy in non-Hodgkin's lymphoma: Safety and efficacy of re-treatment. *J Clin Oncol* 18:3135–3143, 2000.

316. Salles G, Seymour JF, Offner F, et al: Rituximab maintenance for 2 years in patients with high tumour burden follicular lymphoma responding to rituximab plus chemotherapy (PRIMA): A phase 3, randomised controlled trial. *Lancet* 377:42–51, 2011.

317. van Oers MH, Van Glabbeke M, Giurgea L, et al: Rituximab maintenance treatment of relapsed/resistant follicular non-Hodgkin's lymphoma: Long-term outcome of the EORTC 20981 phase III randomized intergroup study. *J Clin Oncol* 28:2853–2858, 2010.

318. Hainsworth JD, Litchy S, Burris HA 3rd, et al: Rituximab as first-line and maintenance therapy for patients with indolent non-Hodgkin's lymphoma. *J Clin Oncol* 20:4261–4267, 2002.

319. Maloney DG, Grillo-López AJ, Bodkin DJ, et al: IDEC-C2B8: Results of a phase I multiple-dose trial in patients with relapsed non-Hodgkin's lymphoma. *J Clin Oncol* 15:3266–3274, 1997.

320. Cartron G, Watier H, Golay J, Solal-Celigny P: From the bench to the bedside: Ways to improve rituximab efficacy. *Blood* 104:2635–2642, 2004.

321. Berinstein NL, Grillo-López AJ, White CA, et al: Association of serum Rituximab (IDEC-C2B8) concentration and anti-tumor response in the treatment of recurrent low-grade or follicular non-Hodgkin's lymphoma. *Ann Oncol* 9:995–1001, 1998.

322. Cartron G, Dacheux L, Salles G, et al: Therapeutic activity of humanized anti-CD20 monoclonal antibody and polymorphism in IgG Fc receptor FcgammaRIIIa gene. *Blood* 99:754–758, 2002.

323. Farag SS, Flinn IW, Modali R, et al: Fc gamma RIIIa and Fc gamma RIIa polymorphisms do not predict response to rituximab in B-cell chronic lymphocytic leukemia. *Blood* 103:1472–1474, 2004.

324. Lowndes S, Darby A, Mead G, Lister A: Stevens-Johnson syndrome after treatment with rituximab. *Ann Oncol* 13:1948–1950, 2002.

325. Kranick SM, Mowry EM, Rosenfeld MR: Progressive multifocal leukoencephalopathy after rituximab in a case of non-Hodgkin lymphoma. *Neurology* 69:704–706, 2007.

326. Cattaneo C, Spedini P, Casari S, et al: Delayed-onset peripheral blood cytopenia after rituximab: Frequency and risk factor assessment in a consecutive series of 77 treatments. *Leuk Lymphoma* 47:1013–1017, 2006.

327. Cabanillas F, Liboy I, Pavia O, Rivera E: High incidence of non-neutropenic infections induced by rituximab plus fludarabine and associated with hypogammaglobulinemia: A frequently unrecognized and easily treatable complication. *Ann Oncol* 17:1424–1427, 2006.

328. Teeling JL, French RR, Cragg MS, et al: Characterization of new human CD20 monoclonal antibodies with potent cytolytic activity against non-Hodgkin lymphomas. *Blood* 104:1793–1800, 2004.

329. Teeling JL, Mackus WJ, Wiegman LJ, et al: The biological activity of human CD20 monoclonal antibodies is linked to unique epitopes on CD20. *J Immunol* 177:362–371, 2006.

330. Hagenbeek A, Gadeberg O, Johnson P, et al: First clinical use of ofatumumab, a novel fully human anti-CD20 monoclonal antibody in relapsed or refractory follicular lymphoma: Results of a phase 1/2 trial. *Blood* 111:5486–5495, 2008.

331. Wierda WG, Kipps TJ, Mayer J, et al: Ofatumumab as single-agent CD20 immunotherapy in fludarabine-refractory chronic lymphocytic leukemia. *J Clin Oncol* 28:1749–1755, 2010.

332. Patz M, Isaeva P, Forcob N, et al: Comparison of the in vitro effects of the anti-CD20 antibodies rituximab and GA101 on chronic lymphocytic leukaemia cells. *Br J Haematol* 152:295–306, 2011.

333. Goede V, Fischer K, Busch R, et al: Obinutuzumab plus chlorambucil in patients with CLL and coexisting conditions. *N Engl J Med* 370:1101–1110, 2014.

334. Kumar S, Kimlinger TK, Lust JA, et al: Expression of CD52 on plasma cells in plasma cell proliferative disorders. *Blood* 102:1075–1077, 2003.

335. Villamor N, Montserrat E, Colomer D: Mechanism of action and resistance to monoclonal antibody therapy. *Semin Oncol* 30:424–433, 2003.

336. Hillmen P, Skotnicki AB, Robak T, et al: Alemtuzumab compared with chlorambucil as first-line therapy for chronic lymphocytic leukemia. *J Clin Oncol* 25:5616–5623, 2007.

337. Keating MJ, Flinn I, Jain V, et al: Therapeutic role of alemtuzumab (Campath-1H) in patients who have failed fludarabine: Results of a large international study. *Blood* 99:3554–3561, 2002.

338. Gallamini A, Zaja F, Patti C, et al: Alemtuzumab (Campath-1H) and CHOP chemotherapy as first-line treatment of peripheral T-cell lymphoma: Results of a GITIL (Gruppo Italiano Terapie Innovative nei Linfomi) prospective multicenter trial. *Blood* 110:2316–2323, 2007.

339. Varga C, Laubach J, Hideshima T, et al: Novel targeted agents in the treatment of multiple myeloma. *Hematol Oncol Clin North Am* 28:903–925, 2014.

340. Richardson PG, Lonial S, Jakubowiak AJ, et al: Monoclonal antibodies in the treatment of multiple myeloma. *Br J Haematol* 154:745–754, 2011.

341. Lonial S, Kaufman J, Laubach J, Richardson P: Elotuzumab: A novel anti-CS1 monoclonal antibody for the treatment of multiple myeloma. *Expert Opin Biol Ther* 13:1731–1740, 2013.

342. Laubach JP, Tai YT, Richardson PG, Anderson KC: Daratumumab granted breakthrough drug status. *Expert Opin Investig Drugs* 23:445–452, 2014.

343. Dang NH, Pro B, Hagemeister FB, et al: Phase II trial of denileukin diftitox for relapsed/refractory T-cell non-Hodgkin lymphoma. *Br J Haematol* 136:439–447, 2007.

344. Larson RA, Sievers EL, Stadtmauer EA, et al: Final report of the efficacy and safety of gemtuzumab ozogamicin (Mylotarg) in patients with CD33-positive acute myeloid leukemia in first recurrence. *Cancer* 104:1442–1452, 2005.

345. Francisco JA, Cerveny CG, Meyer DL, et al: CAC10-vcMMAE, an anti-CD30-monomethyl auristatin E conjugate with potent and selective antitumor activity. *Blood* 102:1458–1465, 2003.

346. Younes A, Gopal AK, Smith SE, et al: Results of a pivotal phase II study of brentuximab vedotin for patients with relapsed or refractory Hodgkin's lymphoma. *J Clin Oncol* 30:2183–2189, 2012.

347. Horning SJ, Younes A, Jain V, et al: Efficacy and safety of tositumomab and iodine-131 tositumomab (Bexxar) in B-cell lymphoma, progressive after rituximab. *J Clin Oncol* 23:712–719, 2005.

348. Horning SJ, Weller E, Kim K, et al: Chemotherapy with or without radiotherapy in limited-stage diffuse aggressive non-Hodgkin's lymphoma: Eastern Cooperative Oncology Group study 1484. *J Clin Oncol* 22:3032–3038, 2004.

CHAPTER 23
HEMATOPOIETIC CELL TRANSPLANTATION

Andrew R. Rezvani, Robert Lowsky, and Robert S. Negrin

SUMMARY

Over the past 60 years, the field of hematopoietic cell transplantation (HCT) has evolved from experimental animal models of marrow transplantation to curative therapy for tens of thousands of people yearly who are affected by a wide variety of marrow failure states, myeloid and lymphoid malignancies, immune deficiencies, and inborn errors of metabolism. Advances in transplantation immune biology combined with improvements in supportive care have made this evolution possible and have ushered in the modern era of HCT. This chapter discusses the biologic principles and clinical applications of HCT along with its future applications. Selected results demonstrating important principles are highlighted.

Acronyms and Abbreviations: ALL, acute lymphoblastic leukemia; ALK+, anaplastic lymphoma kinase–positive; AML, acute myeloid leukemia; APC, antigen-presenting cells; ASBMT, American Society for Blood & Marrow Transplantation; ATG, antithymocyte globulin; BCNU, 1,3-bis(2-choloroethyl)-1-nitrosurea; BEAM, BCNU, etoposide, cytarabine, and melphalan; BMT-CTN, Blood & Marrow Transplant Clinical Trials Network; BU, busulfan; CIBMTR, Center for International Blood and Marrow Transplant Research; CLL, chronic lymphocytic leukemia; CML, chronic myelogenous leukemia; CMV, cytomegalovirus; CR, complete remission; CR1, first complete remission; CT, computed tomography; CXCL12, extracellular-matrix-bound stromal cell–derived factor-1; CXCR4, chemokine-related receptor 4; CY, cyclophosphamide; DAH, diffuse alveolar hemorrhage; DLI, donor lymphocyte infusion; EBMT, European Society for Blood and Marrow Transplantation; ECP, extracorporeal photopheresis; FDG, 18-fluorodeoxyglucose; FLU, fludarabine; G-CSF, granulocyte colony-stimulating factor; GI, gastrointestinal; GM-CSF, granulocyte-monocyte colony-stimulating factor; GVHD, graft-versus-host disease; GVT, graft-versus-tumor; HCT, hematopoietic cell transplantation; HCT-CI, HCT-specific Comorbidity Index; HL, Hodgkin lymphoma; HLA, human leukocyte antigen; HSC, hematopoietic stem cell; HSV, herpes simplex virus; IFN, interferon; Ig, immunoglobulin; IL, interleukin; IPS, idiopathic pneumonia syndrome; KTLS, c-kit+, Thy-1.1lo, lineage marker−/lo, and Sca-1+; MDS, myelodysplastic syndrome; MHC, major histocompatibility complex; MMF, mycophenolate mofetil; MSC, mesenchymal stromal cell; MTX, methotrexate; NHL, non-Hodgkin lymphoma; NIH, National Institutes of Health; NK, natural killer; NMDP, National Marrow Donor Program; PAM, Pretransplant Assessment of Mortality; PBPC, peripheral blood progenitor cell; PCA, patient-controlled anesthesia; PCR, polymerase chain reaction; PET, positron emission tomography; Ph, Philadelphia chromosome; PSGL-1, P-selectin glycoprotein ligand-1; PTLD, posttransplantation lymphoproliferative disorder; RIC, reduced-intensity conditioning; SCID, severe combined immunodeficiency; SOS, sinusoidal obstruction syndrome; SRL, sirolimus; TAC, tacrolimus; TBI, total-body irradiation; Th, T-cell helper; TKI, tyrosine kinase inhibitor; TLI, total lymphoid irradiation; TNF, tumor necrosis factor; TPN, total parenteral nutrition; T_{reg}, regulatory T cell; TRM, transplant-related mortality; UCB, umbilical cord blood; VCAM, vascular cell adhesion molecule; VOD, venoocclusive disease; VZV, varicella-zoster virus.

●HISTORY

The successful clinical application of hematopoietic cell transplantation (HCT) required a century of key developmental discoveries (Table 23–1). Between 1868 and 1906, European and American investigators established that marrow cells were the source of blood cell production. In 1939, the first documented human marrow transplant was performed in a patient with gold-induced marrow aplasia.[1] The patient was infused intravenously with marrow from a brother with an identical ABO blood type. The transplant was not successful, and the patient died 5 days after the marrow infusion.

In 1922, a Danish investigator modified radiation injury in guinea pigs by shielding their femora against radiation, preventing the typical radiation-induced thrombocytopenia and hemorrhage.[2] This work went essentially unnoticed for more than 2 decades. The period of 1949 to 1954 was marked by a political climate concerned with the threat of continued atomic warfare, which stimulated support for experiments studying the effects of irradiation and led to the development of the field of organ and marrow transplantation. Jacobson and colleagues found that mice could survive an otherwise lethal irradiation exposure if the spleen (a hematopoietic organ in the mouse) was protected by lead foil.[3] Soon afterward, Lorenz and colleagues showed that lethally irradiated mice and guinea pigs were protected by the administration of syngeneic marrow after irradiation, thereby demonstrating the therapeutic efficacy of allogeneic and xenogeneic marrow suspensions.[4] These investigators and others considered that chemicals and/or components from the shielded spleen or infused marrow stimulated endogenous hematopoietic cell recovery after total-body irradiation (TBI).[5-7] In 1954, Barnes and Loutit showed that if mice were immunized against marrow cells from mice of another strain and then lethally irradiated, no protection was observed by the injection of marrow cells from the strain to which they were immunized. However, if nonimmunized mice were lethally irradiated and injected with the same marrow cells, normal protection was seen and all mice survived more than 60 days. This experiment supported the cellular hypothesis of hematopoiesis and was the first to consider that hematopoietic recovery resulted from cellular repopulation and not from humoral factors.[8]

In 1956, Barnes and associates described the treatment of murine leukemia by supralethal irradiation and marrow grafting.[9] Researchers pointed out that irradiation alone would not kill all leukemia cells, but that residual leukemia cells might be eliminated by transplanted cells through immunologic mechanisms, and the term adoptive immune therapy was coined. Their publication stimulated tremendous interest, and the period from 1956 to 1959 was characterized by an increasing appreciation of the potential application of marrow grafting to treat individuals exposed to lethal irradiation and to treat human leukemia. Thomas and colleagues began clinical studies in patients with terminal leukemias, and in 1957 described six patients treated with irradiation and intravenous infusion of marrow from healthy donors.[10] Only two patients developed transient detectable donor hematopoietic engraftment, and none of the six survived beyond 100 days from the cell infusion. In 1959, Thomas and associates described a patient with terminal leukemia who received total body irradiation (TBI) and an intravenous infusion of marrow from an identical twin.[11] The patient showed prompt hematopoietic recovery and disappearance of the leukemia for 4 months, confirming for the first time that lethal irradiation followed by compatible marrow could have an antileukemic effect and restore normal marrow function. In the same year, Mathé and associates reported the infusion of marrow into six patients exposed to potentially lethal irradiation in a reactor accident in Belgrade, Serbia.[12] Five patients survived, yet there was no clear evidence of donor hematopoietic

TABLE 23–1. Key Historical Periods in Hematopoietic Cell Transplantation

Years	Event
1868–1906	Discovery that marrow was the source of the various blood cell types
1896–1900	Discovery of ABO system making blood transfusions possible
1939	First documented clinical marrow transplant
1949–1954	Development of preclinical models of marrow and organ transplantation
1956–1959	Early efforts of marrow grafting to treat human diseases
1960–1965	Development of the hierarchical stem/progenitor cell model of hematopoiesis
1960s	Period of pessimism for the clinical application of marrow grafting for the treatment of human diseases
1968–1969	First successful allogeneic HCT in patients with SCID
1975	First successful series of allogeneic HCT for leukemia
1978	First successful series of autologous HCT for leukemia
1988	Isolation of the murine HSC
1990	Nobel Prize in Physiology or Medicine awarded to Dr. E.D. Thomas
2008	More than 700,000 patients worldwide transplanted, more than 125,000 have survived 5 years or beyond after transplantation

HCT, hematopoietic cell transplantation; HSC, hematopoietic stem cell; SCID, severe combined immunodeficiency.

engraftment and thus no firm agreement over the contribution of marrow transplantation to patient recovery.

The first attempts at autologous marrow transplantation appeared during this time as well. In 1958, Kurnick and colleagues described two patients with metastatic cancer whose marrow was collected and stored by freezing.[13] Following intensive radiation therapy, the marrow was thawed and infused intravenously. One patient died from transplantation complications, while the other showed hematopoietic recovery after a prolonged period of pancytopenia. In Philadelphia, an autologous marrow transplant was carried out after high-dose nitrogen mustard conditioning in a patient with malignant lymphoma who lived for more than 30 years after transplantation, the majority of that time in complete remission.[14]

Despite the many successful preclinical models of marrow transplantation and the predictive value of *in vitro* histocompatibility testing, the period of 1960 to 1967 was marked by increasing pessimism about allogeneic marrow grafting in humans. In a published compendium of 203 human allogeneic marrow grafts carried out throughout the 1950s and 1960s, none were considered successful.[15] The first positive results came from studies of children with severe combined immunodeficiency (SCID). In 1968, Gatti and colleagues performed the first successful allogeneic marrow HCT in a child with SCID.[16] The lymphoid elements of the donor graft corrected the immunodeficiency, and two similar cases were reported shortly thereafter.[17,18] These patients remained alive and well 25 years later.[19]

These successes stimulated a resurgence of enthusiasm for marrow transplantation, and by 1975 strikingly improved results were published by the Seattle team.[20] These investigators reported the outcomes of 37 patients with aplastic anemia and 73 patients with leukemia who had reached an advanced stage of their disease before transplantation. This study stressed the importance of histocompatibility and proper preparation of the patient before transplantation, detailed the technique of marrow transplantation, emphasized the role of posttransplant immunosuppression and supportive care, and raised the possibility of using unrelated donors. This report ushered in the modern era of allogeneic HCT. In 1977 and 1980, the first successful HCT procedures from unrelated marrow donors were reported.[21,22] At the end of 1978, the first series of successful autologous HCT for lymphoma were reported.[23,24] In 1990, the Nobel Prize in Physiology or Medicine was awarded to E. Donnall Thomas in recognition of his pioneering work in the field of marrow transplantation. By 2013, more than 700,000 patients worldwide had undergone transplantation during the previous 3 decades and more than 19,000 transplants were being performed annually.[25]

● STEM CELL MODEL OF HEMATOPOIESIS

At the single-cell level, stem cells self-renew and give rise to progeny that differentiate into functional cells carrying out specific functions (Chap. 18).[26] Progenitor cells can be multipotent, oligopotent, or unipotent, but lack self-renewal capabilities. Hematopoietic stem cells (HSCs) are cells that give rise to more HSCs and form all elements of the blood. HSCs are entirely responsible for the development, maintenance, and regeneration of blood-forming tissues for life, and are the most important, if not the only, cells required for successful engraftment in hematopoietic transplantations.[26] In the adult mouse marrow, all HSC activity is contained in a population marked by the composite phenotype of c-kit$^+$, Thy-1.1^{lo}, lineage marker$^{-/lo}$, and Sca-1$^+$ (designated KTLS).[27,28] When transplanted at the single-cell level into irradiated mice, KTLS HSCs gave rise to lifelong hematopoiesis, including a steady state of thousands of HSCs with more than 10^9 blood cells produced daily in the mouse.[27–29] In humans, the combination of positive selection for CD34, Thy-1, and negative selection for lineage markers identified a homologous HSC population.[30]

Following the success in rodent models, purified populations of human HSCs were tested in three separate clinical trials of patients with myeloma, non-Hodgkin lymphoma (NHL), and metastatic breast cancer.[31–33] The goal of these trials was to purify HSC and thereby reduce the risk of occult malignant cells contaminating the autografts. These trials presented technical challenges primarily because of the rarity of HSC in marrow and granulocyte colony-stimulating factor (G-CSF)–mobilized blood. However, adequate numbers of HSC could be isolated that were tumor-free in the majority of patients. The times to neutrophil and platelet recovery following purified HSC infusion were comparable to those seen with unmanipulated marrow, but T-cell recovery (especially that of CD4+ T cells) was delayed by up to 6 months in almost all patients. A number of patients developed unusual infections (e.g., severe cases of influenza, respiratory syncytial virus, cytomegalovirus [CMV] and *Pneumocystis* pneumonia), thus raising concern over "pure" HSCs as the sole source of hematopoietic reconstitution in clinical transplantation. Although these studies were not powered to detect an impact of purified HSCs on relapse or overall survival, these outcomes appeared favorable compared to historical controls.[34] Cotransplantation of antigen-specific mature T cells is being investigated as an approach to address the T-cell–specific immunodeficiency seen in patients receiving purified HSC autografts.[35]

TRAFFICKING AND HOMING OF HEMATOPOIETIC STEM CELLS

The ability of HSCs to migrate from marrow to blood and back has been conserved throughout evolution. Although the biologic role and physiologic significance of constitutive HSC circulation remains unclear, this capacity to traffic leads to hematopoietic cell reconstitution and is essential for the success of HCT in the treatment of hematologic and nonhematologic diseases.

The restoration of adequate hematopoiesis after transplantation requires a series of balanced interactions between the infused HSCs and the complex supporting marrow microenvironment (Chap. 5). Initially, infused HSCs must adhere to the marrow endothelium with sufficient strength to overcome the shear forces of blood flow.[36] Adhesion and arrest of HSCs are mediated primarily by the selectin ligand P-selectin glycoprotein ligand-1 (PSGL-1) and by the hematopoietic cell L- and E-selectin ligands, which interact principally with endothelial E-selectin.[37,38] Other HSC surface adhesion molecules that mediate adherence to the marrow endothelium include members of the integrin superfamily, principally very late antigen-4, integrin $\alpha 4\beta 7$ and lymphocyte function antigen-1, that interact with endothelial immunoglobulin (Ig) superfamily receptors (e.g., vascular cell adhesion molecule [VCAM]-1), and the hyaluronate receptor CD44.[39,40] HSCs that are null for the β integrins cannot migrate to their marrow niche even though they proliferate and differentiate in the fetal liver.[41] Following firm adherence, the transendothelial movement and intraparenchymal homing to hematopoietic niches within the inner endosteal surface of the bone are predominantly regulated by a gradient of extracellular-matrix-bound stromal cell–derived factor-1 (also known as CXCL12).[12] Mice deficient in CXCR4 develop fetal liver hematopoiesis but die prenatally as a consequence of the lack of marrow hematopoiesis.[42] The requirement for CXCR4 expression on HSCs for homing and engraftment is well-documented,[43] and has led to the development of CXCR4 antagonists such as plerixafor, which help mobilize marrow stem cells for clinical use.[44]

Following successful homing, the initial adhesion of HSC within the hematopoietic niche appears to be regulated at least in part by annexin II.[45] The marrow niche is a complex biologic unit that includes potentially self-renewing mesenchymal stromal cells (MSCs), regulatory T cells (T_{reg}), and cells with the defined phenotype of parathyroid-hormone-receptor-bearing osteoblasts.[46,47] MSCs promote engraftment when cotransplanted with HSCs.[48] Osteoblasts, possibly in conjunction with sinusoidal endothelial cells, also appear to play a pivotal role in the regulation of HSC engraftment by producing a number of molecules, such as annexin II, VCAM-1, intercellular adhesion molecule-1, CD44, CD164, and osteopontin, which promote engraftment.[49,50] Stimulation of osteoblasts with parathyroid hormone results in expansion and mobilization of the HSC pool in animals,[51] although a clinical trial in human cord-blood recipients did not demonstrate a benefit.[52] In addition to the regulators of HSC adhesion and homing, the function of HSCs is further regulated by intrinsic genetic programs for quiescence, self-renewal, proliferation, differentiation, and apoptosis that are dependent on communication with a network of interacting cells in the marrow microenvironment, including various T-cell subpopulations, adipocytes, and fibroblasts. Given the complexity of HSC trafficking and control, it is surprising that clinical HCT has a relatively low rate of graft failure.

SOURCES OF HEMATOPOIETIC CELLS

In humans, HSCs for transplantation can be collected from several sources, including directly from the marrow; from the blood after mobilization; and from umbilical cord blood (UCB) obtained at the time of delivery.

MARROW

Marrow has historically been the traditional source of HSCs for allogeneic and autologous transplantation. Marrow for transplantation is typically aspirated by repeated placement of large-bore needles into both sides of the posterior iliac crest, generally involving 50 to 100 aspirations per side, with the patient under regional or general anesthesia. The lowest cell dose which ensures stable long-term engraftment has not been defined with certainty; typical collections contain at least 2×10^8 total nucleated marrow cells per kg of recipient body weight. Current guidelines indicate that collection of up to 20 mL/kg of donor body weight is considered safe.

Marrow harvesting is considered a very safe procedure, and serious side effects are rare. A review of almost 10,000 healthy adult volunteer unrelated donors by the National Marrow Donor Program (NMDP) found that the risk of serious adverse events was 2.38 percent, most of which were mechanical or anesthesia-related and self-limited. Unexpected, life-threatening, or chronic complications occurred in 0.99 percent of donors.[53] Evaluation of pediatric marrow donor safety is more limited, but a safety review of 453 pediatric donors by the European Group for Blood & Marrow Transplantation (EBMT) found no serious adverse events; pain was the most common complaint but lasted a median of only 1 day after donation.[54] A survey of pediatric transplantation hematologists confirmed that 90 percent of centers were willing to perform a marrow harvest on children, even on those younger than 6 months old.[55]

BLOOD

HSCs are normally present in the blood at very low levels. However, a number of different stimuli, including chemotherapy, hematopoietic growth factors, and inhibitors of certain chemokine receptors, result in the mobilization of HSC from marrow to blood. Once mobilized, HSC can be collected by apheresis; this product has been termed "peripheral blood progenitor cells (PBPCs)" to differentiate it from "blood stem cells," a term that should be reserved for instances where the HSC population itself has been isolated. Agents used to mobilize HSCs include G-CSF, granulocyte-monocyte colony-stimulating factor (GM-CSF), interleukin (IL)-3, thrombopoietin, and the CXCR4 antagonist plerixafor.[44,56,57]

Autologous PBPCs are most commonly mobilized with G-CSF, with or without additional chemotherapy. In contrast, PBPCs for allogeneic HCT are typically mobilized with G-CSF alone, so as to avoid exposing healthy donors to chemotherapy. PBPC mobilization and collection is very safe; a review of nearly 7000 healthy unrelated PBPC donors performed by the NMDP found that the rate of serious adverse events was 0.56 percent, making PBPC donation significantly safer than marrow donation.[53] The most common side effect of PBPC mobilization and collection is bone pain as a result of G-CSF administration. More serious side effects, such as splenic rupture or intracranial hemorrhage, have been described in case reports but are extremely rare.[58,59]

Theoretical concern exists about the potential of short-term growth factor therapy to increase the risk of leukemia in normal donors. However, long-term followup of healthy adult PBPC donors has shown no late effects of G-CSF administration or donation—in particular, no increased risk of cancer, autoimmune disease, or stroke.[53] Detailed white cell subset analysis by fluorescent-activated cell sorting of healthy donors at 1 year after donation shows no changes in B, T, and natural killer (NK) cells or monocytes and neutrophils compared with analysis before G-CSF administration.[60]

The adequacy of PBPC products is generally measured through the absolute number of CD34+ cells per kg of recipient body weight. Most laboratories measure CD34+ cell content by fluorescent-activated cell sorting. A threshold of greater than 2×10^6 CD34+ cells/kg is often considered the minimum acceptable dose for PBPC products, although successful engraftment can occur with lower doses.[61] Platelet recovery appears most impacted by low PBPC CD34+ cell dose. Higher CD34+ cell doses are associated with more rapid engraftment, and thus a dose of equal to or greater than 4×10^6 CD34+ cells/kg is considered optimal.[61] The impact of very high CD34+ cells doses in allogeneic HCT is somewhat unclear; some studies have associated doses greater than 8×10^6 CD34+ cells/kg with a higher risk of extensive chronic graft-versus-host disease (GVHD) in matched-related-donor HCT, although this association was not confirmed in unrelated-donor allogeneic HCT. Because there is no evidence of benefit for CD34+ cell doses greater than 8×10^6/kg in allogeneic HCT, this threshold is sometimes, although not universally, used as a maximum.[61]

Although inadequate mobilization of healthy donors is rare, patients with malignancies undergoing mobilization for autologous HCT often have difficulty collecting adequate numbers of CD34+ cells because of marrow damage from previous chemotherapy or radiation therapy. Approximately 10 to 20 percent of patients preparing for autologous HCT do not mobilize sufficient numbers of CD34+ cells using G-CSF alone or in combination with chemotherapy. Unfortunately, it has proven difficult to identify these individuals prospectively. For patients with NHL, Hodgkin lymphoma (HL), and myeloma who fail mobilization with G-CSF alone, the majority proceed to collect a transplantable dose of CD34+ cells (>2×10^6 cells/kg) when remobilized with plerixafor plus G-CSF.[62] Studies of allogeneic HCT using plerixafor-mobilized grafts have also confirmed prompt and stable donor cell engraftment.[63] Animal models suggest that plerixafor-mobilized PBPCs have a different phenotype and cytokine profile than G-CSF–mobilized PBPCs and may be associated with a higher risk of acute GVHD; however, the relevance of these findings to human allogeneic HCT is unclear.[64] For patients who are thought to be at high risk of poor mobilization, strategies include the upfront use of plerixafor and/or chemotherapy to supplement G-CSF mobilization, as well as large-volume leukapheresis.[61] In 2014, the American Society for Blood & Marrow Transplantation (ASBMT) published guidelines on the mobilization and collection of PBPCs for autologous and allogeneic HCT.[61]

There is some evidence that circadian activity in the hypothalamus regulates the cyclic release of HSCs by altering the expression of CXCL12 in the marrow microenvironment, with the peak time for HSC release in humans in the evening.[65] Preliminary clinical data suggest that CD34+ yield is higher in donors collected in the later afternoon compared to the morning, and more abundant PBPC collections were reported from healthy donors when apheresis was performed at 8:00 PM as opposed to 8:00 AM.[66] Efforts to exploit this circadian rhythm dependence to increase HSC yield in PBPC products have thus far been inconclusive.[67]

Mobilized Peripheral Blood Progenitor Cells versus Marrow
In the setting of autologous HCT, the superiority of PBPCs over marrow as a stem-cell source is clear. Randomized trials have shown that PBPC autografts in this setting are associated with more rapid engraftment, better quality of life, and lower costs compared to marrow autografts.[68–70]

On the basis of these and other results, most transplantation centers use mobilized PBPCs for autologous HCT and have adopted a minimum CD34+ cell of 2×10^6 CD34+ cells/kg.[61]

In the allogeneic setting, the situation is considerably more complex. PBPC grafts contain approximately 10-fold more T cells compared to marrow grafts, leading to concern over a potentially increased incidence and severity of GVHD. At the same time, G-CSF can induce functional immune tolerance in healthy individuals, and T cells from G-CSF–mobilized PBPC grafts show a predominantly immune-tolerant profile with upregulation of genes related to T-cell helper type 2 (Th2) and T_{reg} cells, and downregulation of genes associated with Th1 cells, cytotoxicity, antigen presentation, and GVHD.[71]

A number of randomized clinical trials have compared PBPC and marrow grafts in the setting of allogeneic HCT.[72–75] These studies have consistently reported similar or better overall and disease-free survival with PBPCs compared to marrow allografts. Most, although not all, of these randomized trials found a higher risk of chronic GVHD with PBPCs compared to marrow allografts, and one reported a longer duration of immunosuppression in patients receiving a PBPC graft.[73] PBPC allografts were also associated with faster engraftment and a lower risk of graft failure. Systematic reviews and meta-analyses have similarly reached varying conclusions.[76–78] A 2014 systematic review performed by the Cochrane Library found that overall survival was similar with PBPC and marrow allografts, and that PBPC allografts were associated with faster engraftment but also a higher incidence of chronic GVHD. The effects of stem cell source on relapse and on acute GVHD were unclear.[76]

Currently, the choice between PBPCs and marrow allografts is generally individualized and depends on patient, donor, and institutional considerations. Patients with advanced or high-risk hematologic malignancies may preferentially be given PBPC grafts to reduce their risk of relapse, a strategy with some support in the literature.[79] Conversely, patients with standard-risk malignancies are often given marrow allografts to reduce their risk of chronic GVHD. Likewise, patients transplanted for nonmalignant diseases such as aplastic anemia are typically given marrow allografts to reduce their risk of chronic GVHD, as they derive no benefit from T-cell–mediated graft-versus-malignancy effects. In settings where the risk of GVHD is particularly high—for example, with human leukocyte antigen (HLA)-mismatched unrelated donors—many institutions prefer to use marrow allografts to mitigate this risk. For patients receiving reduced-intensity conditioning (RIC), most centers use PBPC allografts exclusively, as engraftment in this setting is largely dependent on the presence of donor T cells in the allograft. Donor factors also play a role in the choice of allograft product, as some donors may specifically decline either marrow donation or PBPC mobilization and collection. Finally, with the recent predominance of PBPC as a graft source, institutional resources for and expertise in marrow collection have decreased, sometimes limiting the availability of marrow allograft products.

ALTERNATIVE SOURCES OF HEMATOPOIETIC STEM CELLS

One of the most significant advances in allogeneic HCT in the past 10 years is the increasing experience with alternative donors for patients who lack HLA-identical siblings or suitably HLA-matched unrelated donors. Each full sibling has a 25 percent chance of being HLA-identical with another, so the likelihood of finding an HLA-identical sibling donor is proportionate to the number of siblings available. HLA-matched unrelated donors can be identified for approximately 75 percent of patients of northern European ancestry, but the odds of finding a suitable unrelated donor are much lower for patients who belong to ethnic groups that are underrepresented in donor registries, those of mixed ethnicity, and those with uncommon HLA haplotypes.[80] As a result, a substantial fraction of patients who would benefit from allogeneic HCT lack "conventional" related or unrelated donors. For such patients, there are two widely used alternative sources of HSC for allogeneic HCT: UCB and HLA-haploidentical family members.

Umbilical Cord Blood

UCB, collected from the umbilical vessels in the placenta at the time of delivery, is a rich source of HSCs. Because these cells are immunologically naïve, it is feasible to cross major histocompatibility barriers, thus extending the donor pool to individuals for whom finding suitably HLA-matched adult donors can be difficult or impossible.[81] The first successful allogeneic HCT using UCB, in a child with Fanconi anemia, was reported by Gluckman and colleagues in 1989.[82] Since then, hundreds of thousands of UCB units have been collected and stored; searchable registries have been established to facilitate identification of suitable UCB units for transplantation; and more than 20,000 allogeneic HCTs have been performed using UCB.[83] Cord blood units are fully HLA-typed before cryopreservation, and thus suitable units can be rapidly identified (as compared to unrelated-donor searches, which can take 2 to 6 months to complete).

Most UCB units are HLA-typed as HLA-A and HLA-B using low-resolution (serologic) methods, and as HLA-DRB1 using high-resolution (molecular) methods. UCB units matched at equal to or greater than 4/6 HLA loci are generally considered suitable for use, although UCB units matched at 5/6 or 6/6 HLA loci should be used if available because they are associated with lower transplant-related mortality.[84,85] The role of HLA matching between UCB units in double UCB transplantation remains somewhat unclear, and unit-to-unit HLA matching does not appear to impact long-term engraftment rates or GVHD incidence.[85,86]

A major limitation has been the relatively small number of HSC available in cord blood units relative to the size of the average adult recipient.[87] As a result, most UCB transplants in adults use two UCB units rather than one. The minimum acceptable cell doses for single-unit UCB transplantation are generally set at equal to or greater than 2.5×10^7 total nucleated cells or equal to or greater than 2×10^5 CD34+ cells/kg of recipient weight.[84,88] It is difficult to locate units meeting these criteria for average-sized adult recipients, and thus most adult UCB transplants are performed using two UCB units. With double UCB transplantation, transient mixed donor chimerism from the two units is often observed, but ultimately one UCB unit dominates, eradicates the other unit, and is responsible for establishment of long-term hematopoiesis.[86] Despite extensive investigation, the factors determining which unit becomes dominant remain somewhat unclear,[89] although CD8+ T-cell responses against the nonengrafting unit have been implicated.[90] For recipients with a single suitably sized UCB unit, single-unit UCB transplantation is preferable to double UCB transplantation, because of better platelet recovery and a lower risk of GVHD.[88] For the majority of adult recipients, who lack a suitable single UCB unit, double UCB transplantation is typically used and produces equivalent overall survival.[89] For children, a single UCB unit appears superior to double UCB transplantation.[88] A major area of active research in UCB transplantation is the expansion of HSC or other hematopoietic progenitor cells in UCB products, with the goal of improving engraftment rates, shortening the period of preengraftment neutropenia, and reducing the need for double-unit UCB transplantation. Several approaches have been described in the literature, including Notch-mediated or prostaglandin-mediated expansion of progenitor cells and *ex vivo* mesenchymal cell coculture.[91–93]

Recipients of UCB allografts have a higher risk of opportunistic infections—particularly viral infection or reactivation—compared to recipients of PBPC or marrow allografts. Presumably the immunologic naïveté of UCB, which allows its use across HLA barriers, also contributes to impaired antiviral immunity and immune reconstitution after allogeneic HCT.[94] CD8+ T-cell recovery is significantly delayed after UCB compared to marrow allotransplantation (median time to reach $>0.25 \times 10^9$ CD8+ T cells/L, 7.7 months vs. 2.8 months, respectively), whereas CD4+ T cell and NK cell recovery is similar with these two graft sources.[95] A novel syndrome of cord colitis has been described in UCB recipients and tentatively linked to *Bradyrhizobium enterica*, a newly identified bacterium,[96,97] although other groups have questioned the existence of a distinct cord colitis syndrome and instead attributed the findings in question to conventional GVHD.[98,99]

Human Leukocyte Antigen–Haploidentical Donors

Virtually all patients have HLA-haploidentical family members—including any parent, any child, and some siblings—available as donors. Haploidentical related donor HCT has been evaluated for more than 2 decades as an alternative source of HSCs. However, as a result of the substantial HLA disparity involved, early attempts at haploidentical HCT were associated with severe GVHD in T-cell-replete transplants and with graft rejection in T-cell–depleted transplants.[100,101] Extensive *ex vivo* depletion of CD3+ and CD19+ lymphocytes, coupled with megadose CD34+ cells and antithymocyte globulin, can successfully overcome the barriers to engraftment.[102] The extensive T-cell depletion used in these protocols to prevent GVHD would also be expected to result in weak or no graft-versus-malignancy effects. Yet despite the lack of T-cell–mediated alloreactivity and the unfavorable prognostic features at the time of transplantation, relapse rates with this approach remained at 18 to 30 percent in patients with acute leukemia transplanted in first complete remission (CR1).[103] The low rate of relapse was attributed to a strong antitumor effect mediated by donor NK cell alloreactivity. Transplantation from NK-cell-alloreactive donors was associated with a significantly lower leukemia relapse rate and improved overall survival, leading some authorities to recommend selection of haploidentical donors based on NK cell alloreactivity.[104] However, this approach to haploidentical HCT remains hampered by prolonged immune reconstitution and a high risk of serious infection.[105]

More recently, the group at Johns Hopkins has pioneered the use of posttransplantation cyclophosphamide (CY) as GVHD prophylaxis in T-cell-replete haploidentical HCT.[106] In this approach, unmanipulated marrow from an HLA-haploidentical donor is infused after nonmyeloablative conditioning. A period of 48 to 72 hours elapses after infusion, during which alloreactive donor T-cell clones become activated and proliferate. CY is then administered on days +3 and +4 after allogeneic HCT, preferentially eradicating the activated alloreactive donor T-cell clones while leaving other, nonalloreactive clones relatively untouched.[107] This approach has been remarkably well-tolerated and results in very low rates of GVHD and transplant-related mortality (TRM).[108] Additionally, because this approach avoids indiscriminate T-cell depletion, immune reconstitution is relatively robust, and the typical complications of T-cell-depleted allotransplantation (such as posttransplantation lymphoproliferative disorder [PTLD]) are not seen.[109] The major limitation of this approach is a relatively high rate of relapse, perhaps driven by the eradication of the alloreactive donor T-cell clones which would mediate graft-versus-tumor (GVT) effects along with those mediating GVHD.[108]

Retrospective studies have examined the question of selecting the optimal HLA-haploidentical donor when several such donors are available. Early evidence suggested that lower TRM was seen with HLA-haploidentical sibling donors compared to parental donors, while maternal donors were associated with less chronic GVHD and better overall survival than paternal donors.[110,111] In contrast, a 2014 paper reporting outcomes of HLA-haploidentical HCT in China found less GVHD and better overall survival with paternal compared to maternal donors.[112] As with previous studies, haploidentical siblings (particularly those disparate for noninherited maternal antigens) were associated with the best outcomes. There is some preclinical evidence that exposure to noninherited maternal antigens through breastfeeding may reduce the risk of GVHD in maternal-donor haploidentical HCT,[113] and thus the disparate clinical results with maternal donors may be explained in part by variations in demographic patterns of breastfeeding. In view of the conflicting state of the existing literature, there is no universal standard approach to selecting an HLA-haploidentical donor; the decision is often guided by donor availability and health status, although the literature arguably contains weak support to prefer HLA-haploidentical siblings over parents, and mothers over fathers, as donors.

Comparison of Alternative Donor Options

Although both UCB and HLA-haploidentical HCT have been established as feasible and effective options for patients lacking conventional donors, the optimal alternative-donor source remains unclear. Given the lack of robust comparative data, the choice between UCB and haploidentical HCT is often guided by institutional experience, comfort level, and research priorities. To address the relative merits of these approaches, the United States Blood & Marrow Transplant Clinical Trials Network (BMT-CTN) conducted parallel multicenter phase II clinical trials of RIC followed by either UCB or haploidentical HCT (the latter using T-cell-replete marrow as a graft source and posttransplantation CY as GVHD prophylaxis). These trials reported similar overall and disease-free survival at 1 year with the two approaches.[108] UCB transplantation was associated with a higher risk of GVHD and nonrelapse mortality, while haploidentical HCT was associated with a higher risk of relapse. Based on these results, the BMT-CTN is currently conducting a national, multicenter phase III clinical trial randomizing participants between UCB and haploidentical HCT. In addition to clinical outcomes, this trial is designed to measure quality-of-life and cost differences between the two alternative-donor approaches in a comprehensive effort to clarify their relative advantages and disadvantages.

● CONCEPTS OF CURATIVE THERAPY

AUTOLOGOUS HEMATOPOIETIC CELL TRANSPLANTATION

The relationship between the dose of chemoradiotherapy administered and the number of tumor cells killed has been extensively studied *in vitro* and in preclinical animal models, and forms the rationale for myeloablative autologous HCT. For chemosensitive tumors (including most hematologic malignancies), a steeply rising dose–response curve is observed. The curative potential of autologous HCT is, therefore, derived from high-dose chemotherapy or chemoradiotherapy administered as transplant conditioning to enhance tumor cell kill and overcome drug resistance. This level of dose escalation is possible in autologous HCT because dose-limiting toxicities to the hematopoietic system are circumvented by the infusion of autologous HSCs, which rebuild hematopoiesis after high-dose conditioning.

Autologous HCT is associated with relatively low TRM. The use of mobilized PBPCs rather than marrow as a graft source has decreased the duration of neutropenia, and therewith combined with improved supportive care and patient selection has reduced the TRM associated with autologous HCT from approximately 8 to 10 percent in historical studies to 1 to 3 percent at most centers. In addition, the reduced risks and

faster engraftment times seen with PBPC have enabled many centers to pursue outpatient autologous HCT, further easing the logistical burden on patients as well as treatment costs.

Tumor Contamination in the Autograft

A consistent concern in autologous HCT is the possibility that residual tumor cells may contaminate the HSC product and contribute to relapse. The relative contributions of autograft contamination and residual disease in the patient are difficult, if not impossible, to distinguish. Several investigators have approached this question by marking the HSC product at the time of harvest and then assaying for the marker gene in malignant cells at the time of subsequent relapse. Studies using this approach have been performed in patients with leukemia, lymphoma, and myeloma, and have reached conflicting conclusions about the contribution of autograft contamination to relapse.[114,115]

A number of *ex vivo* and *in vivo* purging strategies have been investigated in autologous HCT. These include administration of rituximab before autologous HSC collection in patients with CD20+ malignancies; *ex vivo* positive selection for CD34+ cells; chemotherapy-based purging using CY derivatives; and purging via oncolytic viruses.[116-120] Single-arm or uncontrolled studies have suggested a possible benefit in some of these instances, but there is little or no evidence from randomized clinical trials at present to support the efficacy of autograft purging, and its use remains investigational. One of the few randomized clinical trials in the field concluded that *in vivo* purging with rituximab administered before autologous HSC collection was as effective, and likely safer, than *ex vivo* CD34+ selection.[121] Another randomized clinical trial found that CD34+ selection significantly reduced autograft contamination with myeloma cells, but did not improve clinical outcomes.[122] Purging strategies carry some potential for harm, as they deplete the autograft of mature T cells and increase the risk of infectious complications, particularly CMV or other viral reactivation, after autologous HCT.[123,124] At present, given the lack of convincing evidence of clinical benefit, purging strategies are not widely used and most centers collect and infuse unmanipulated autologous HSC (although these cells are often mobilized with a regimen containing chemoimmunotherapy, which arguably represents a form of *in vivo* purging). Because relapse remains a major concern after autologous HCT, ongoing research is focused on identifying more efficient and clinically effective means of autograft purging.

ALLOGENEIC HEMATOPOIETIC CELL TRANSPLANTATION

Allogeneic HCT is a considerably more complicated procedure than autologous HCT. It involves more pretransplantation preparation, poses a greater risk of complications to the patient, is associated with a significantly higher rate of TRM, and requires at least temporary postgrafting immunosuppression to enable engraftment and prevent GVHD. The decision to pursue allogeneic HCT is based on diagnosis, prognosis, and remission status, as well as the availability of an appropriate donor and the psychosocial resources of the patient to cope with the demands of the process. Decisions about eligibility for allogeneic HCT are typically made on a center-by-center and case-by-case basis, with inherent elements of subjectivity and patient and physician judgment.

A major obstacle to successful allogeneic HCT is the immune competence of the recipient. The potential to reject infused donor cells is mediated predominantly through regimen-resistant host T and NK cells. Strategies to reduce host immunity and promote donor hematopoietic cell engraftment include pretransplantation conditioning (most often chemotherapy and/or radiation) and postgrafting immunosuppressive medications. Donor T cells in the allograft play a key role in hematopoietic engraftment, and depletion of T lymphocytes from the allograft before transplantation is associated with a substantial increase in the occurrence of graft rejection.[125,126] With modern conditioning regimens, rates of allograft rejection are low (typically <5 percent) for patients who have received previous chemotherapy, which weakens their immune response to the allograft. In contrast, graft rejection in seen more often in patients who have not received cytotoxic chemotherapy before allogeneic HCT (for instance, some patients with myeloproliferative neoplasms) or those with nonmalignant diseases such as aplastic anemia, thalassemia, or sickle cell disease, who are often highly sensitized against donor antigens by virtue of being heavily transfused before allogeneic HCT.

Graft-Versus-Tumor Effects

The dominant mechanism of cancer eradication following allogeneic HCT is the immunologic recognition and destruction of residual host tumor cells by donor-derived immune cells. This phenomenon, termed the GVT effect, has been conclusively demonstrated and represents one of the most significant biologic findings of the past half-century, with implications well beyond the transplantation setting. The existence of GVT effects is supported by the following lines of evidence:

- *Tumor relapse is lower after allogeneic than after syngeneic HCT:* The appreciation of alloreactive GVT effects stemmed from the observation that recipients of genotypically identical (syngeneic) grafts had significantly higher rates of disease relapse than did patients who received grafts from HLA-identical siblings.[127,128]
- *Tumor relapse is higher in recipients of T-cell–depleted grafts:* Further support for the allogeneic GVT effect came from studies of T-cell depletion of the graft.[129] T-cell depletion was performed in the expectation that it would reduce the risk of GVHD. However, the later observation that these patients had a much higher risk of disease recurrence as well as graft rejection was unanticipated. These results linked GVHD with GVT effects, and supported the concept that patients who developed some degree of alloreactivity, as manifested by clinically apparent GVHD, had a reduced risk of disease relapse.
- *Donor lymphocyte infusions can induce remission:* Perhaps the most definitive evidence for the existence of GVT effects came from the application of donor lymphocyte infusions (DLIs). In the early 1990s, Kolb and others demonstrated that patients with relapsed malignancies after allogeneic HCT could, in some cases, be returned to complete remission by the simple infusion of donor-derived lymphocytes.[130-132] With increasing experience, it became clear that some diseases (such as chronic myelogenous leukemia [CML]) respond very well to DLI whereas others (for instance, acute lymphoblastic leukemia [ALL]) are much less responsive. Long-term followup of patients successfully treated with DLIs revealed that responders had remarkably durable remissions and excellent outcomes.[132] These observations definitively established the GVT effect as a biologic entity capable of controlling an otherwise lethal condition such as leukemia.

Targets and Effector Cells in Graft-Versus-Tumor Reactions

The biology of the GVT effect remains incompletely understood. A number of immunologic targets recognized by donor immune effector cells have been proposed, including alloantigens (such as major or minor histocompatibility antigens depending upon donor–recipient genetic differences), lineage-specific antigens, and malignancy-specific antigens such as products of chromosomal translocations. Donor T cells clearly play a key role in GVT, and there is emerging evidence that NK cells are also responsible for tumor cell control, especially in the setting of T-cell-depleted HLA-haploidentical HCT.[133] Humoral immunity has also been implicated as playing a role in the GVT effect.[134] Based

on preclinical models, the common effector cells that could potentially mediate a clinical GVT effect include (1) CD8+ cytotoxic T lymphocytes that recognize tumor-associated antigens in context of class I major histocompatibility complex (MHC) antigens; (2) CD4+ T cells that recognize tumor-associated antigens in context of class II MHC antigens and mediate their effects via Th1 cytokines such as interferon (IFN)-γ and IL-2, upregulating expression of class I MHC antigens and promoting expansion and activation of CD8+ cytotoxic T lymphocytes; and (3) NK cells that recognize stress ligands and cells lacking MHC expression.[135-141] The impact of NK cells seems especially pronounced in HLA-haploidentical or mismatched allotransplantation.[104,142]

A major question continues to be whether the subset of T cells that induce GVHD is the same population of T cells responsible for the GVT effect. One of the central aims of research in allogeneic HCT is to separate the beneficial GVT effects from deleterious GVHD. Clinical evidence suggests that, in principle, the two should be separable, as some patients experience an apparent GVT effect in the absence of apparent GVHD.[143] Although numerous approaches have succeeded in separating GVT effects from GVHD in preclinical and animal models, none of these approaches have yet been translated successfully to widespread clinical use. One approach supported by preclinical models involves the use of T_{reg},[144] and recent studies in the HLA-haploidentical setting are supportive of this concept.[145,146]

⬤ TRANSPLANT PREPARATIVE REGIMENS

The transplant preparative regimens used in HCT must accomplish two goals. Because the majority of autologous and allogeneic HCT are performed in individuals with cancer, these regimens were designed, at least initially, to maximize tumor cytoreduction and disease eradication. In the case of allogeneic HCT, the regimen must be sufficiently immunosuppressive to overcome host rejection of the graft. In autologous HCT, where efficacy depends on exploiting the dose–response curve, high-dose conditioning regimens are universally used. In contrast, in allogeneic HCT much or all of the clinical benefit derives from donor alloimmunity, enabling the use of RIC designed to facilitate donor engraftment with minimal toxicity.

TOTAL-BODY IRRADIATION

TBI has been a primary component of many autologous and allogeneic HCT preparative regimens since the inception of the field. TBI has excellent activity against a variety of hematolymphoid malignancies, has pronounced immunosuppressive properties, and is able to treat sanctuary sites like the testicles and the central nervous system. Aside from one very early study of high-dose TBI alone, most preparative regimens combine TBI with cytotoxic agents such as CY. Dose-finding studies suggest that higher TBI doses are associated with a lower risk of relapse with dose escalation as high as 15.75 Gy, but doses above 12 Gy are associated with higher risks of GVHD and TRM, which offset the reduced risk of relapse.[147] Currently, most high-dose TBI-based conditioning regimens use a dose between 12 and 13.2 Gy. Long-term concerns with TBI-based regimens include the development of cataracts and hypothyroidism, impairment of growth and development in children, and secondary malignancies.[148-150]

Hyperfractionated TBI, in which relatively small dose fractions are given two to three times a day over a few days, minimizes leukemia regrowth and reduces lung and gastrointestinal toxicity, allowing higher TBI doses to be administered safely. Several clinical studies confirm decreased overall lung toxicity with fractionation.[151,152] Excellent results are also reported with the combination of fractionated TBI and VP-16 (etoposide), particularly promising results in patients with ALL.[153,154]

An alternate form of irradiation is radioimmunotherapy, which involves the use of antibodies to deliver locally acting radionucleotides to targeted sites. In theory, this strategy could provide excellent targeted antitumor effects without increased systemic toxicity. Clinical trials incorporating anti-CD45 monoclonal antibodies conjugated to radioactive iodine (^{131}I) or yttrium (^{90}Y) show promising early results in both the autologous and the allogeneic setting.[155–158] One approach to further improving the targeting of radiation is the use of α-particle emitters. Alpha particles have a very short effective range but carry immense kinetic energy, making them an attractive option to maximize malignant cell killing while minimizing bystander damage. Preclinical studies using bismuth-213 (^{213}Bi) and astatine-211 (^{211}At) have demonstrated efficacy,[159–162] and this approach is currently being translated into clinical trials.

CHEMOTHERAPY-ONLY REGIMENS

Autologous

Patients with NHL or HL have often received prior intensive local radiotherapy, often to the mediastinum, which results in a high incidence of fatal interstitial pneumonitis following TBI.[163] Therefore, non-TBI-containing conditioning regimens were developed. The choices of drugs include agents that can be significantly dose-escalated and have improved tumor cell killing at higher doses, yet have nonoverlapping toxicities; for example, a common preparative regimen for autologous HCT in lymphoma includes 1,3-bis(2-choloroethyl)-1-nitrosurea (carmustine or bis-chloroethylnitrosourea [BCNU]), VP-16, and CY.[164] The dose-limiting non-hematologic toxicity of BCNU affects the lungs; VP-16 affects the liver; and CY, the heart. Consequently, using these drugs below the maximally tolerated doses results in relatively low regimen-related toxicity but maximizes tumor cell kill to overcome drug resistance. Many other chemotherapy-only regimens have been developed for autologous HCT according to similar principles, including BCNU, etoposide, cytarabine, and melphalan (BEAM) (for lymphomas) and high-dose melphalan (for myeloma).

Allogeneic

A variety of chemotherapy-only conditioning regimens have been developed for allogeneic HCT. The most widely used combines oral busulfan (BU), at a total dose of 16 mg/kg given over 4 days, with CY at a total dose of 120 mg/kg given intravenously over 2 days (referred to as BU/CY).[165,166] A randomized comparison between fractionated TBI plus CY (TBI/CY) and BU/CY in patients transplanted for CML demonstrated that the BU/CY regimen was better tolerated, but there was no significant difference in overall or event-free survival, TRM, or GVHD incidence.[167] The development of intravenous BU further improved the availability and tolerability of this regimen, although steady-state plasma concentrations remain variable after intravenous BU and therapeutic drug monitoring arguably remains necessary.[168,169] Interestingly, pretreatment with BU may deplete hepatic glutathione and thus potentiate the toxicity of CY.[170,171] Reversing the sequence of conditioning agents (from BU/CY to CY/BU) has been studied as a means of reducing regimen-related toxicity, and this alteration to the regimen has been associated with reduced exposure to toxic CY metabolites and a lower risk of hepatotoxicity.[172]

Other high-dose chemotherapy-only conditioning regimens remain in use on an institution-, disease-, and patient-specific basis. The most common modification to BU/CY is the substitution of fludarabine (FLU) for CY (BU/FLU). This regimen has been proposed to avoid the hepatotoxicity of CY and to reduce regimen-related toxicity compared to BU/CY. However, two recent randomized clinical trials comparing BU/CY and BU/FLU have found increased risks of graft rejection and pneumonitis, as well as decreased overall and disease-free survival, with BU/FLU, raising the concern that this regimen is inferior to BU/CY.[173,174]

REDUCED-INTENSITY TRANSPLANTATION

The demonstration that immune-mediated mechanisms are critical in eradicating malignancy after allotransplant challenged the rationale for relatively toxic full-dose conditioning. A number of reduced-intensity regimens have been developed which have lower regimen-related toxicity but are sufficiently immunosuppressive to allow full donor engraftment, shifting the responsibility for tumor eradication largely or entirely to immunologic GVT effects. The development of RIC is one of the most transformative advances in the field of allogeneic HCT in the past several decades, as it has allowed the expansion of eligibility for allogeneic HCT to older and less medically fit patients who would otherwise be ineligible for high-dose conditioning. Additionally, patients with relatively indolent disease may not require the immediate cytoreductive capacity of an aggressive preparative regimen and may be particularly suitable candidates for transplantation using RIC. These regimens are also useful in patients with nonmalignant diseases where the goal is strictly the establishment of donor hematopoiesis; examples include genetic disorders, autoimmune diseases, and the induction of tolerance in combined solid-organ and same-donor marrow transplantation.

A variety of RIC regimens with differing dose intensities have been developed. One significant regimen came from detailed studies in a canine model using a backbone of low-dose 2 Gy TBI followed by postgrafting immunosuppression with mycophenolate mofetil (MMF) and cyclosporine (CSP).[175] This work was translated to patients with a variety of malignancies and resulted in reliable donor engraftment with the addition of intravenous FLU 90 mg/m^2.[176] This reduced-intensity regimen has been used successfully in more than 1000 patients with a wide variety of malignancies, especially in older patients and those with more indolent diseases such as follicular NHL or chronic lymphocytic leukemia (CLL).[177–179] Another commonly used RIC regimen consists of intravenous FLU (between 90 and 150 mg/m^2) and CY (between 900 and 2,000 mg/m^2).[180] This regimen, combined with rituximab or ^{90}Y ibritumomab tiuxetan, has produced excellent long-term disease-free survival in patients with indolent lymphoma.[181] A third common reduced-intensity regimen was developed in a rodent model using fractionated low-dose total lymphoid irradiation (TLI) combined with depletive T-cell antibodies (antithymocyte serum), which showed that recipients were protected from GVHD induction by donor-derived T cells.[182] Rodents conditioned with this approach did not develop lethal acute GVHD despite the infusion of megadoses of donor T lymphocytes. TLI and antithymocyte serum altered residual host T-cell subsets to favor regulatory NK/T cells which suppress GVHD by polarizing the infused donor T cells toward secretion of noninflammatory cytokines such as IL-4, and by promoting expansion of donor CD4+CD25+FoxP3+ T$_{regs}$.[183] This approach was successfully translated to clinical transplantation; patients conditioned with TLI and antithymocyte globulin (ATG) developed sustained donor-derived hematopoiesis with very low incidences of acute GVHD and TRM.[184,185] The relative merits of RIC versus high-dose conditioning continue to be studied; a national multicenter prospective randomized trial comparing high-dose to RIC in patients with acute myeloid leukemia (AML) or myelodysplastic syndrome (MDS) is ongoing under the auspices of the BMT-CTN.

Mixed Chimerism Following Reduced-Intensity Conditioning

A feature common to all RIC protocols is the incomplete eradication, at least initially, of host hematopoietic elements. As a consequence, a significant percentage of patients have mixed donor–recipient chimerism for months after transplantation before fully converting, if ever, to complete donor type. Most reports suggest that persistent mixed chimerism is a significant risk factor for disease relapse.[185,186] Interventions such as withdrawal of immunosuppressive medications, CD34-selected donor cell boost, and DLI have been used to convert mixed chimerism to complete donor type, although these interventions are not without risk and can precipitate GVHD. A significant percentage of patients who received alemtuzumab-containing conditioning regimens required DLI to promote donor engraftment and protect against immune-mediated graft rejection, but the risk of developing post-DLI GVHD was significant.[187] Mixed chimerism is not unique to RIC; prior to the addition of ATG, almost 60 percent of patients who received high-dose conditioning and allogeneic HCT for severe aplastic anemia had mixed chimerism, of whom two-thirds eventually converted to complete donor hematopoiesis while the remainder experienced late graft failure.[188]

Persistent mixed chimerism may have a role in allogeneic transplantation for noncancer patients. In organ transplantation, tolerance, defined as immunosuppressive drug withdrawal without graft rejection, was achieved in kidney transplant recipients who received the same donor marrow when sustained mixed chimerism was established, and not in recipients who experienced donor hematopoietic graft loss.[189]

● EVALUATION AND SELECTION OF CANDIDATES FOR TRANSPLANTATION

Most transplantation candidates are referred by hematologists or oncologists to the tertiary center where HCT will be performed. Patients considered for transplantation require in-depth evaluation and counseling by experienced transplantation physicians, nurses, and social workers. A detailed review of initial diagnostic studies, previous drug and radiation treatments, and responses to these interventions, as well as a psychosocial assessment of the patient and their caregivers, are of the utmost importance. Table 23–2 highlights the issues and topics that should be addressed during counseling meetings with transplantation candidates and their caregivers.[190] Important factors which consistently impact outcomes following HCT include, but are not limited to, disease status at transplantation, type and compatibility of donor, recipient age, and comorbid medical conditions. Early referral for transplantation consultation is critical, particularly if allogeneic HCT is under consideration, because of the time required to identify a suitable donor.

DISEASE STATUS AT THE TIME OF TRANSPLANTATION

Disease status at the time of transplantation is perhaps the most powerful predictor of long-term disease-free survival following allogeneic and autologous HCT. Early studies of allogeneic HCT were performed using predominantly patients with refractory and progressive disease.[191] Although a small percentage of these patients were salvaged, transplantation was unsuccessful in the majority of patients due to progressive malignancy. Patients with acute leukemias transplanted in complete remission (CR) have substantially better outcomes compared to those transplanted with active disease.[192] Even very minimal amounts of residual disease are associated with significantly higher relapse risk in patients undergoing allogeneic HCT for AML, regardless of conditioning intensity,[193–195] underscoring the importance of disease status at transplant as a prognostic factor. Likewise, disease status as determined by positron emission tomography (PET) prior to transplant is an important predictor of progression-free survival for patients with diffuse large B-cell lymphoma and HL undergoing autologous HCT.[196–199] These scenarios highlight a truism: patients who have advanced poorly controlled disease at the start of transplant conditioning have significantly inferior

TABLE 23–2. Topics Addressed During Counseling Meetings with Transplant Candidate and Care Provider

I. Rationale for why transplantation is a therapeutic option
II. How the transplantation is performed
Autologous
Allogeneic—choice for full-dose versus RIC
III. Source of cells
Marrow versus blood versus other source
IV. Risks of procedure
V. Graft failure and graft rejection
VI. Risk of GVHD
Acute and chronic forms, compatibility of graft
Likelihood for long-term immune suppression medication
VII. Nonrelapse mortality at 100 days and 1 year
VIII. Risks of relapse
IX. Timing of transplant
X. Projected result
XI. Requirement for dedicated care provider
XII. Other
Financial implications
Durable power of attorney
Banking of sperm, *in vitro* fertilized eggs
Duration of stay near the transplantation center
Return to home and work
Sexual activity
Quality-of-life issues
Habits such as smoking, alcohol, and drug addiction

GVHD, graft-versus-host disease; RIC, reduced-intensity conditioning.

outcomes compared to patients transplanted earlier in the course of their disease and to those who have achieved good, albeit temporary, control of their disease. On the other hand, attempts to salvage patients with advanced disease who have failed multiple therapies are rarely successful, and transplantation is often best considered early in the course of therapy. These discussions are complex, as earlier transplantation, especially allogeneic, carries significant risks to the patient. A number of other disease-specific considerations are important in determining the appropriate timing for transplantation, including the presence and/or persistence of cytogenetic and molecular abnormalities, the immune phenotype, and evidence of extramedullary or extranodal disease. Advanced genetic characterization of leukemia and lymphoma may provide improved insight into cohorts of patients for which HCT should be performed earlier in the course of disease.

AGE

Historically, older age was a significant barrier to allogeneic HCT, since older patients suffered severe and often prohibitive toxicity after high-dose conditioning regimens.[200] However, the impact of older age is mitigated by the increasing use of RIC for allogeneic HCT.[201] High-dose conditioning and allogeneic HCT is generally reserved for patients 60 years of age or younger, whereas allotransplantation with RIC has been performed successfully in patients into their eighth decade of life. Most centers in the United States do not have a stringent age cutoff for allogeneic HCT, although careful screening for comorbid medical conditions, such as heart, lung, kidney, and liver disease, is particularly important in older patients, and allotransplantation in patients 70 years of age and older remains somewhat controversial. Existing data suggest that allogeneic HCT can be safely performed in selected patients age 60 to 75 years, with a 5-year overall survival of 35 percent.[202,203] Some investigators have proposed that age is a poor and imprecise prognostic marker, and instead advocate the use of comorbidity assessment and scoring to determine eligibility for allogeneic HCT.[204] However, caution is warranted since this approach has not been prospectively validated; retrospective cohort studies necessarily suffer severely from patient selection bias, as they include only those older patients who were deemed appropriate candidates to proceed to allogeneic HCT. Outcomes for this selected group of older patients cannot be generalized to the population of older adults as a whole.

In contrast to allogeneic HCT, autologous HCT relies on high-dose conditioning for its antitumor efficacy. Thus, there is no way to reduce conditioning intensity without sacrificing some degree of efficacy. As a result, age limitations are often stricter for autologous HCT than for allogeneic HCT, as candidates for the former must be able to tolerate intensive, high-dose chemotherapy. It is unusual for autologous HCT to be offered to patients older than 75 years of age.[205,206]

COMORBID MEDICAL CONDITIONS

Comorbid medical conditions have a significant impact on transplantation outcomes. Routine screening of heart and lung function to detect occult abnormalities is of critical importance, especially in older patients. Evaluation of liver and kidney function, as well as exposure to potential pathogens such as CMV, hepatitides B and C, herpes viruses, and HIV are routine and should be performed in all patients. Another major factor is the nutritional status of the patient, as extremes such as cachexia or obesity require special considerations and adversely impact TRM.[207,208]

Several scoring instruments have been devised to allow quantification and comparison of pretransplantation comorbidities. The most widely used of these are the EBMT Risk Score,[209] the Pretransplant Assessment of Mortality (PAM) score,[210] and the HCT-specific Comorbidity Index (HCT-CI; later modified to incorporate age).[204,211] A number of efforts have been made to validate, revise, or combine these scores in diverse populations, with variable success.[212-216] Several caveats are important when considering quantitative scoring of pretransplantation comorbidities. First, because these scoring instruments were derived from retrospective cohorts of patients, they suffer from an inescapable selection bias, as only patients who were deemed fit for transplantation were included in their derivation. This selection bias limits the ability to generalize their use to unselected patient populations. Second, transplantation outcomes have not remained stable over time; instead, TRM has steadily decreased over time with the availability of better supportive care and other refinements.[217,218] Thus, it is conceivable that the relative impacts of specific comorbidities on transplantation outcomes are not fixed, but may vary over time. Efforts are currently underway to prospectively validate these comorbidity scoring instruments.

Every effort should be made to encourage potential patients to maintain good health practices, including discontinuation of alcohol use, tobacco smoking, and illicit drug use (if applicable). Centers vary in their approach to abstinence, but it is common to require that patients cease all tobacco use permanently as a condition of proceeding to autologous or, especially, allogeneic HCT. The risk of pulmonary complications from chemotherapy (e.g., BCNU) or from chronic GVHD involving the lung is potentiated by smoking, as is the risk of secondary cancers of the lung and other organs. A special situation deserving consideration is the use of marijuana, which is increasingly legal,

available, and widely used by cancer patients to combat chemotherapy-related nausea and anorexia. Anecdotally, an increasing number of patients referred for transplantation consultation are actively using marijuana to control these symptoms during their pretransplantation chemotherapy. Cases of severe or fatal pulmonary aspergillosis from inhaled spores have been reported in immunosuppressed patients using marijuana.[219,220] Transplant center policies regarding medical marijuana use and abstinence have lagged behind the rapidly changing legal status of marijuana in the United States, creating a challenge in assessing and counseling patients.

● DISEASES TREATED WITH TRANSPLANTATION

Numerous malignant and nonmalignant hematologic disorders, as well as selected solid tumors, may be treated with HCT. The results obtained with transplantation are reviewed in detail in the disease-specific chapters of this book, and are discussed only briefly here.

In general terms, autologous HCT is recommended for patients whose malignancy exhibits chemosensitivity to conventional dose therapy and does not extensively involve the marrow; included are most lymphomas, germ cell tumors, and other selected pediatric tumors. In these instances, tumor eradication is a result of dose escalation of cytotoxic therapy in the conditioning regimen, and the autograft serves as hematopoietic cell rescue. In contrast, allogeneic transplantation is generally pursued for hematologic malignancies and disorders that primarily originate in the marrow, such as acute and chronic leukemias, aplastic anemia, MDSs, and myeloproliferative neoplasms. For some diseases with extensive marrow involvement, such as the low-grade lymphomas and myeloma, the decision to pursue autologous versus allogeneic HCT is more complex. In these settings, allogeneic transplantation has generally been more successful in controlling disease recurrence and reducing relapse risk. However, the associated risks, including GVHD and prolonged immunosuppression, result in a higher TRM compared to autologous HCT. Thus, the decision to pursue an allogeneic or autologous HCT for patients with these diseases depends on the combination of patient characteristics such as comorbidities and age, availability of a suitable donor, disease-specific characteristics, and often patient preference. For some hematologic conditions, such as MDSs, myeloproliferative neoplasms, and aplastic anemia, only allogeneic transplants are generally appropriate.

In addition, patients with selected solid tumors, such as testicular cancer, neuroblastoma, and other pediatric tumors, have had successful outcomes with autologous HCT.[221-224] Extensive studies in women with breast and ovarian carcinoma, and more limited studies in patients with renal cell carcinoma and small cell lung cancer, have failed to demonstrate a role for HCT.[225,226] Outside of the investigational setting, there are no currently accepted indications for allogeneic HCT to treat nonhematologic solid tumors.

A variety of congenital and acquired nonmalignant disorders can be successfully treated with HCT. The most well-established nonmalignant indication is for allogeneic HCT in patients with severe aplastic anemia, where outstanding results have been achieved, particularly for younger patients with HLA-matched sibling donors, where long-term disease-free survival rates of 88 to 100 percent have been reported.[227,228] Hematopoietic cell transplantation for patients with clinically significant hemoglobin disorders, such as thalassemia major, has been very successful, especially in patients without significant liver disease.[229,230] Likewise, allogeneic HCT is considered a treatment option for young patients with severe forms of sickle cell disease.[231,232] Guidelines for patient selection and management of patients with thalassemia or sickle cell disease were published in 2014 by EBMT.[233] In patients with hemoglobin disorders, transplantation serves as a form of gene therapy, using allogeneic hematopoietic cells as vectors for genes essential for normal hematopoiesis. Eventually the vector may well be autologous stem cells transformed by the insertion of normal genes.[234]

For patients with SCID syndrome and other congenital immunodeficiencies, allogeneic HCT remains the treatment of choice.[235,236] The role of allogeneic HCT for patients with storage diseases, a diverse group of disorders that typically involve a single gene defect in a lysosomal hydrolytic enzyme or peroxisomal function, is evolving and it appears that subsets of mucopolysaccharidoses derive the most benefit.[237]

SELECTED RESULTS OF HEMATOPOIETIC CELL TRANSPLANTATION

A comprehensive discussion of transplantation outcomes is beyond the scope of this chapter; please refer to other disease-focused chapters of this text for more complete information. A brief overview of transplantation-related outcomes in a number of diseases is presented here.

Acute Myeloid Leukemia

Allogeneic HCT has a major role in the management of patients with AML. For patients in CR1, the decision to proceed to allogeneic HCT as opposed to chemotherapy-based consolidation is predicated on prognostic markers and donor availability, as well as patient preference. For patients beyond CR1, allogeneic HCT often offers the only potentially curative treatment option.

First Complete Remission A question of significant practical importance is how best to treat a younger AML patient who achieves a CR1 following induction chemotherapy. Several large prospective trials have been conducted using so-called genetic randomization: that is, patients in CR1 with an HLA-identical sibling received allogeneic HCT, while those without an HLA-identical sibling received chemotherapy-based consolidation or autologous HCT.[238,239] Two meta-analyses have focused on the comparative outcomes of allogeneic HCT versus chemotherapy, both of which found that allogeneic HCT in CR1 yielded better overall and disease-free survival for patients with intermediate- and poor-risk cytogenetics, but not for those with favorable-risk cytogenetics.[240,241] For patients with poor-risk cytogenetics, there is little dispute that allogeneic HCT is the preferred postremission therapy for medically fit patients with available donors. Conversely, patients younger than 60 years of age with favorable-risk cytogenetics who promptly achieve CR1 with induction chemotherapy are generally not considered for allogeneic HCT, and instead should receive chemotherapy-based consolidation. For younger patients with intermediate-risk cytogenetics, allogeneic HCT in CR1 from an HLA-identical sibling donor is the best available postremission therapy, but its advantage over other approaches is not as substantial as in the setting of poor-risk cytogenetics. One caveat is that the studies demonstrating the superiority of allogeneic HCT were performed using genetic randomization, and thus the results are, strictly speaking, only applicable to patients with HLA-identical sibling donors. That said, single-center and registry data suggest that outcomes with HLA-matched unrelated donor allotransplantation for AML in CR1 are similar to those with HLA-identical sibling donors,[242,243] so it is reasonable to extrapolate the results of the genetic-randomization studies to patients with HLA-matched unrelated donors.

Patients older than 60 years of age typically have substantially higher relapse rates with chemotherapy alone (60 to 80+ percent)[244,245] and have poorer outcomes than younger patients with equivalent cytogenetics, suggesting that older adults may benefit from allogeneic HCT

in CR1. There are no prospective, genetically randomized trials in older adults with AML comparing allogeneic HCT to chemotherapy in CR1, but retrospective comparisons suggest that allogeneic HCT can reduce relapse risk and improve outcomes in this demographic.[244,245] The decision to proceed to allogeneic HCT in older adults is often based less on disease risk factors and more on medical comorbidities and the estimated risk of TRM, which may be prohibitive.

In the genomic era of AML risk stratification, patients with intermediate-risk disease are often categorized based on the results of molecular testing for mutations of *FLT3*, *NPM1*, and *CEBPA*. Patients with intermediate-risk cytogenetics and biallelic *CEBPA* mutations or *NPM1* mutations in the absence of *FLT3* mutations have good-risk disease and are often not considered for allogeneic HCT in CR1.[246] In contrast, patients with internal tandem duplications in *FLT3* have poorer prognoses and are often considered for allogeneic HCT in CR1.

Detailed guidelines have been published by the European LeukemiaNet AML Working Party to guide the use of allogeneic HCT in AML patients in CR.[247] Based on existing data, many experts would recommend allogeneic HCT for all medically fit patients younger than 60 years old with AML in CR1 *except* for those with favorable-risk disease (including those with intermediate-risk cytogenetics and favorable molecular markers) who achieve CR1 with their first cycle of induction and have no evidence of minimal residual disease. For all other younger CR1 patients—including those with intermediate-risk cytogenetics and negative molecular markers, and those in any cytogenetic risk group who do not promptly achieve CR with induction or who have minimal residual disease—allogeneic HCT should be strongly considered as the best postremission option.[248] For older adults with AML in CR1, allogeneic HCT should be considered for all medically fit patients except those with favorable-risk disease, although there are fewer data to support this recommendation and medical comorbidities play an increasingly important role in decision making as patients age.

The role of consolidation chemotherapy before allotransplantation in patients in CR1 is unclear. Many transplant physicians recommend at least 1 to 2 cycles of consolidation, especially for patients slated to receive RIC, in order to maximize pretransplantation cytoreduction. However, two recent retrospective studies have questioned the benefit of consolidation chemotherapy, and instead favored moving forward to allogeneic HCT as soon as a suitable donor is available.[249,250] Consolidation chemotherapy is to maintain remission during prolonged donor searches, but its benefit is less clear in patients who have a donor identified.

Aml Beyond First Complete Remission For patients with AML who relapse after attaining a CR1, allogeneic HCT is the treatment of choice. While no prospective randomized trials have compared allogeneic HCT to salvage chemotherapy alone in this setting, retrospective data strongly support the use of allogeneic HCT.[251] Autologous HCT has been used historically in patients who lacked suitable allogeneic donors,[252] but with the advent of improved alternative-donor options the use of autologous HCT for AML has become rare except in developing countries without the capability to perform allogeneic HCT. Patients with AML beyond CR1 who lack suitably HLA-matched donors are candidates for HLA-haploidentical or UCB allotransplantation, as retrospective studies have associated these approaches with equivalent overall and disease-free survival compared to allotransplantation from conventional donor sources.[253,254]

The likelihood of long-term survival is very low in AML patients whose disease fails to achieve CR1 following induction therapy (primary induction failure) and in those whose disease is chemorefractory at relapse. Allogeneic HCT with myeloablative conditioning has been reported to cure approximately 19 to 30 percent of such patients in retrospective analyses.[192,255] These retrospective reports undoubtedly suffer from substantial selection bias; presumably patients with relapsed or refractory AML were not transplanted indiscriminately, but only if their physicians felt they had an above-average chance of responding. These success rates are therefore very unlikely to pertain to the overall population of adults with relapsed or refractory AML. Attempts have been made to construct prognostic tools to identify the subset of patients most likely to benefit from allogeneic HCT,[192] and some authorities have argued that allogeneic HCT is underused in this population.[248] Currently there is no single standard of care for treatment of patients with AML in refractory relapse or primary induction failure; reasonable options include additional salvage chemotherapy to induce remission; enrollment on a clinical trial; allogeneic HCT (in carefully selected patients); and palliative care, and the optimal choice must be individualized based on patient characteristics and donor availability.

Acute Lymphoblastic Leukemia

Allogeneic HCT is widely used in adult patients with ALL, especially those patients with high-risk features (most often defined as white blood cell count at diagnosis >30,000 [or >100,000 in T-cell ALL], adverse cytogenetics, progenitor B-cell immunophenotype, age >60 years, or failure to achieve CR within 4 weeks of induction chemotherapy).[256] Patients with none of these features are considered to have standard-risk disease; there is no clear "favorable-risk" population in adult ALL. While the advisability of allogeneic HCT is uncontroversial as postremission therapy for adults with high-risk ALL, it is also the treatment of choice for eligible adults with standard-risk ALL in CR1. Several large genetically randomized prospective trials have demonstrated a survival benefit for allogeneic HCT in CR1 for adults with standard-risk ALL.[257,258] A 2013 meta-analysis confirmed the benefit of upfront allogeneic HCT for adults 35 years of age or younger; for older adults, the benefit was more difficult to demonstrate owing to increasing TRM.[259] As with all genetically randomized clinical trial data, these findings apply only to patients with HLA-identical sibling donors, strictly speaking, although many authorities extrapolate the observed benefit to HLA-matched unrelated donors and possibly even alternative donors on the basis of generally equivalent outcomes.

On the basis of existing data, we believe that myeloablative allogeneic HCT is the optimal therapy for all eligible adults with ALL in CR1 and available HLA-identical sibling donors—a recommendation supported by a recent Cochrane Library systematic review.[260] Allogeneic HCT is likely also the optimal therapy for those with HLA-matched unrelated donors, although this recommendation relies more on extrapolation from data in the HLA-identical sibling setting. The decision to proceed with alternative-donor allogeneic HCT in a patient with standard-risk ALL in CR1 is less clear-cut and depends on patient preference and institutional comfort level. In any case, we believe that all adults with ALL should be referred for transplantation consultation early in their course to assist in determining the optimal treatment approach.

Conditioning-regimen intensity appears to play a major role in the success of allogeneic HCT for ALL. Results with nonmyeloablative allogeneic HCT for Philadelphia chromosome–negative (Ph–) ALL beyond CR1 have been poor, with virtually no survivors.[261] For older adults with Ph– ALL who are not candidates for intensive conditioning, the optimal approach remains unclear, particularly for those beyond CR1.

Philadelphia Chromosome–Positive Acute Lymphoblastic Leukemia The postremission management of patients with Philadelphia chromosome–positive (Ph+) ALL deserves special attention. Historically, Ph+ ALL carried a very poor prognosis with conventional chemotherapy, and this chromosomal abnormality was considered a high-risk feature. High-dose TBI-based conditioning and allotransplant has historically been the standard of care for postremission therapy of Ph+ ALL in adults, and resulted in 10-year overall survivals of

54 percent and 29 percent for patients transplanted in CR1 and beyond CR1, respectively, in the pre–tyrosine kinase inhibitor (TKI) era.[262]

The development of TKIs targeting *bcr/abl* has markedly improved the prognosis of Ph+ ALL. With the incorporation of TKI therapy into pretransplant induction and posttransplant maintenance, Ph+ ALL now carries one of the best prognoses of all forms of adult ALL, even with nonmyeloablative conditioning.[261,263] Most authorities continue to recommend allogeneic HCT as postremission therapy for adults with ALL in the TKI era. The pediatric literature suggests that it may be safe to forgo allotransplantation in favor of TKI-based chemotherapy alone in Ph+ ALL,[264] but these data cannot be extrapolated to the adult setting because of the very different clinical behavior of adult versus pediatric ALL. For adults with Ph+ ALL who are not candidates for allotransplantation, TKI-containing chemotherapy regimens coupled with close monitoring of minimal residual disease may be an alternative, but this approach has not been tested in clinical trials.

Myeloma

Autologous HCT is not curative in myeloma, but a number of randomized clinical trials have demonstrated prolongation of event-free survival by a median of approximately 1 year when single or double autologous HCT is incorporated into the treatment program.[265–267] Some of these trials also reported improved overall survival with autologous HCT. In addition, early autologous HCT is associated with an improved quality of life in patients with myeloma, likely because it is associated with a shorter period of chemotherapy.[268] However, these studies were performed before the introduction of modern highly active antimyeloma therapies such as thalidomide, lenalidomide, and bortezomib. In 2014, results were published from a randomized trial comparing upfront tandem autologous HCT to lenalidomide-based maintenance therapy after induction with lenalidomide and dexamethasone.[269] Patients randomized to upfront autologous HCT had significantly improved 4-year overall survival compared to those randomized to the nontransplant arm (81.6 percent vs. 65.3 percent, p = 0.02; Fig. 23–1).[269] Patients randomized to the nontransplantation arm remained eligible for autologous HCT at the time of myeloma progression, but only 62.8 percent actually received autologous HCT, suggesting that delayed autologous HCT is not feasible for many patients as a result of rapid clinical deterioration following relapse. These results support the continued role of upfront autologous HCT as the standard of care for medically fit patients with myeloma in the modern era, although several caveats apply. First, the maintenance regimen in the nontransplantation arm consisted of low-dose melphalan in combination with lenalidomide and dexamethasone, and it is unclear whether these findings can be generalized to other, more commonly used maintenance regimens. Second, patients randomized to upfront autologous HCT received planned tandem autologous HCT with intravenous melphalan 200 mg/m² conditioning for each transplant. This approach is relatively uncommon, as tandem autologous HCT has fallen out of favor based on evidence that it does not improve overall survival.[270] In current practice, second autologous HCT is usually reserved for patients who fail to achieve at least a very good partial remission after first autologous HCT,[271] and is often performed using a lower dose of intravenous melphalan (140 mg/m²) as conditioning. As a result, it is unclear whether the benefit observed in this trial extends to the setting of single autologous HCT. Nonetheless, upfront autologous HCT continues to be widely used in myeloma, and the recent trial adds support for this approach, particularly since nearly 40 percent of patients intended to undergo transplantation never received the intervention.

Allogeneic HCT remains the only therapy thought to be potentially curative in myeloma, and has been widely studied, most often as part of a tandem autologous/allogeneic double-transplant approach.

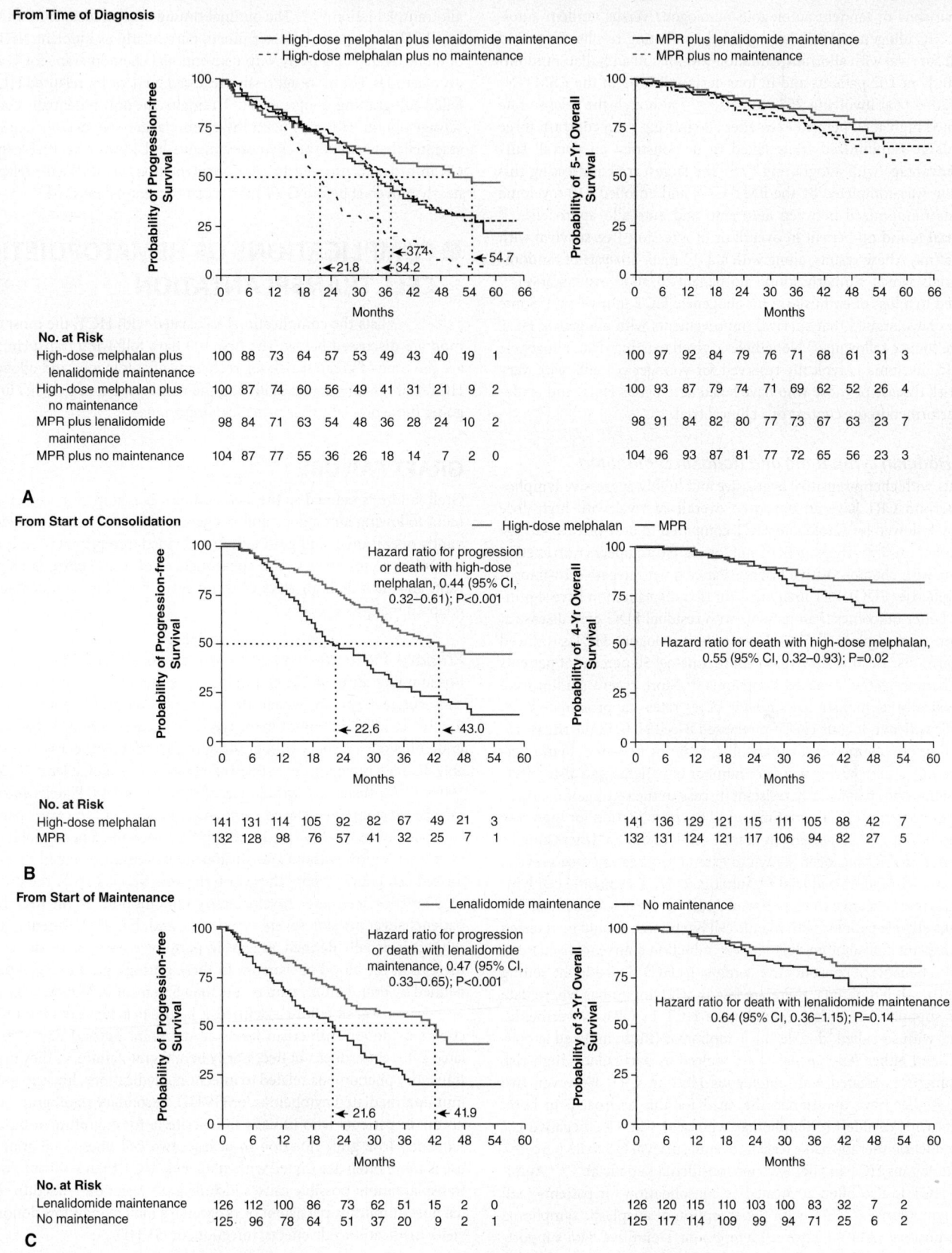

Figure 23–1. Results from a prospective randomized clinical trial comparing upfront autologous hematopoietic cell transplantation to maintenance therapy in myeloma.[269] Panel A shows progression-free survival and 5-year overall survival from the time of diagnosis. Panel B shows progression-free survival and 4-year overall survival from the start of consolidation therapy. Panel C shows progression-free survival and 3-year overall survival from the start of maintenance or no maintenance. CI, confidence interval; MPR, melphalan,prednisone, and lenalidomide. *(Reproduced with permission from Palumbo A, Cavallo F, Gay F, et al: Autologous transplantation and maintenance therapy in multiple myeloma. N Engl J Med 4;371(10):895–905, 2014.)*

Comparisons of tandem autologous/autologous versus tandem autologous/RIC allogeneic HCT have yielded conflicting results. Improved overall survival with allotransplantation was seen in an Italian randomized study of 162 patients and in long-term followup of the EBMT-N-MAM2000 trial involving 257 patients,[272–274] although the relapse rate remained high at 60 percent even after allografting.[273] In contrast, three other large randomized trials failed to demonstrate an overall survival advantage with allografting.[275–277] The largest trial addressing this question was completed by the BMT-CTN and enrolled 710 myeloma patients randomized between auto-auto and auto-allo approaches.[278] This trial found no benefit in overall or progression-free survival with allografting. These results, along with a 2013 meta-analysis of randomized trials which similarly found no benefit to allotransplantation,[279] have led to a loss of enthusiasm for allogeneic HCT in myeloma. Some authors have argued that survival improvements with allogeneic HCT require longer followup.[273] Nonetheless, given existing data, allogeneic HCT in myeloma is typically reserved for younger patients with very high-risk disease or those who have failed autologous HCT, and is ideally performed in the context of a clinical trial.

Non-Hodgkin Lymphoma and Hodgkin Lymphoma

Patients with chemosensitive aggressive and highly aggressive lymphomas beyond CR1 have an improved overall survival with high-dose therapy followed by autologous HCT compared to best-of-care salvage chemotherapy.[280,281] The benefit of autologous HCT appears restricted to patients with chemosensitive disease. Patients with negative 18-fluorodeoxyglucose (FDG)-PET imaging prior to transplantation have significantly better outcomes than patients with residual FDG-avid disease at the time of transplant.[197,282,283] Historically, autologous HCT produced long-term disease-free survival in approximately 50 percent of patients with chemosensitive relapsed lymphoma.[284] More recent studies have paradoxically demonstrated poorer cure rates (approximately 20 percent) with autologous HCT for relapsed B-cell NHL in the rituximab era.[285] One possibility is that rituximab-containing first-line chemotherapy is successful in curing a greater number of patients, but also selects for patients with particularly resistant disease in the setting of relapse.

Autologous HCT is sometimes used as consolidation for high-risk lymphomas in CR1, especially in mantle cell lymphoma, where autologous HCT in CR1 has been shown to extend progression-free survival in a phase III randomized trial.[286] Autologous HCT in mantle cell lymphoma is most effective when performed early in the disease course,[287,288] and thus eligible patients with mantle cell lymphoma should be referred for transplant consultation during their induction course to discuss the risks and benefits of consolidative autologous HCT. Outside the setting of mantle cell lymphoma, there are few B-cell lymphomas where data clearly support consolidative autologous HCT in CR1. Nevertheless, patients with so-called "double-hit" lymphomas (those mutated at both c-MYC and either bcl-2 or bcl-6) are viewed as particularly high-risk and sometimes treated with autologous HCT in CR1. However, two recent studies have questioned the need for this approach; in both, patients with double-hit lymphomas who achieved PET-negative CR with induction therapy had excellent overall survival (75 to 83 percent), and autologous HCT in CR1 was not considered beneficial.[289,290] Autologous HCT is also often advocated as consolidation for patients with T-cell lymphomas in CR1, with the exception of anaplastic lymphoma kinase-positive (ALK+) large cell lymphoma. Definitive data supporting this practice are not available, but this approach appears reasonable in view of the very high relapse rate associated with these lymphomas.

Allogeneic HCT is highly active and potentially curative for NHL, particularly indolent NHL. Excellent disease-free survival has been reported with both early and late allogeneic HCT in indolent NHL, even in heavily pretreated patients and those with active disease at allotransplantation.[179,181] The optimal timing of allogeneic HCT in indolent NHL remains to be determined, particularly as indolent NHL can often be treated effectively with conventional chemotherapy for years or even decades. For more aggressive relapsed NHL or for relapsed HL after failed autografting, allogeneic HCT remains the only potentially curative salvage option. However, with these more aggressive malignancies, it is essential that patients be chemoresponsive and, ideally, in a PET-negative CR in order to proceed to allotransplantation, as otherwise relapse is nearly universal before GVT effects can become established.[291,292]

● COMPLICATIONS OF HEMATOPOIETIC CELL TRANSPLANTATION

Table 23-3 lists the complications associated with HCT; the most common are discussed below. The first 100 days following transplantation are the time of greatest risk for recipients of autologous and allogeneic HCT. Care by physicians skilled in the management of patients undergoing these procedures is of critical importance.

GRAFT FAILURE

Graft failure is defined as the lack of donor hematopoietic cell engraftment following autologous and allogeneic HCT. Criteria are predominantly operational, and graft failure is divided into primary (early) and secondary (late) phases. The consequences of graft failure are significant, and include high risks of death from infection, hemorrhage, or relapsed malignancy.

Primary (Early) and Secondary (Late) Graft Failure

Myeloid engraftment has commonly been defined as the first of three consecutive days on which the absolute neutrophil count exceeds 5×10^8/L. Myeloid engraftment typically occurs within 21 days of the graft infusion, irrespective of graft source. Platelet recovery is more variably defined, often as the first day of a platelet count of at least 20, 50, or 100×10^9/L, sustained without transfusion for 7 days. Platelet recovery may be substantially delayed compared with myeloid recovery, particularly with lower CD34+ cell doses or UCB allografts. A hemoglobin level of at least 8 g/dL without transfusion support is an accepted threshold for red cell engraftment. These criteria were derived from the predictable kinetics seen after myeloablative conditioning. With RIC, many patients never develop severe cytopenias, and thus engraftment in these settings is usually defined, at least in part, by assessment of donor chimerism in the blood or marrow. In these settings, graft loss is typically defined by donor chimerism of less than 5 percent in blood CD3+ cells.

Primary graft failure is defined as failure to achieve these threshold counts or donor chimerism levels at any point beyond day +28. Isolated cytopenias does not necessarily herald graft failure, as they may be transitory phenomena related to infection, medications, lineage-specific immune-mediated cytopenias, or GVHD. Secondary (late) graft failure occurs in patients who initially meet criteria for engraftment but subsequently lose graft function in at least two cell lines. Late graft failure is more often associated with allogeneic HCT than with autologous transplantation; possible causes include graft rejection related to residual host immunity, persistent or progressive malignancy, low donor cell yield, medication side effects, infection, or GVHD.

Graft Rejection and Poor Graft Function

Graft rejection is a subset of primary or secondary graft failure caused by immune-mediated rejection of donor cells by residual host effector cells. A diagnosis of graft rejection requires analysis of blood or marrow for donor hematopoietic chimerism; graft rejection is defined as

TABLE 23–3. Complications of Hematopoietic Cell Transplantation

Vascular access complications

Graft failure

Blood group incompatibilities and hemolytic complications

Acute GVHD

Chronic GVHD

Infectious complications

    Bacterial infections

    Fungal infections

    Cytomegalovirus infection

    Herpes simplex virus infections

    Varicella-zoster virus infections

    Epstein-Barr virus infections

    Adenovirus, respiratory viruses, HHV-6, -7, -8, and other viruses

Gastrointestinal complications

    Mucosal ulceration/bleeding

    Nutritional support

Hepatic complications

    Sinusoidal obstructive syndrome

    Hepatitis: infectious versus noninfectious

Lung injury

    Interstitial pneumonitis: infectious versus noninfectious

    Diffuse alveolar hemorrhage

    Engraftment syndrome

    Bronchiolitis obliterans

Kidney and bladder complications

Endocrine complications

Drug–drug interactions

Growth and development

Late onset nonmalignant complications

    Osteoporosis/osteopenia, avascular necrosis, dental problems, cataracts, chronic fatigue, psychosocial effects, and rehabilitation

Secondary malignancies

Neurologic complications

    Infectious, transplant conditioning and immune suppression medication toxicities

GVHD, graft-versus-host disease; HHV, human herpes virus subtypes.

the inability to detect a meaningful percentage (usually >5 percent) of donor hematopoietic elements. In contrast, *poor graft function* describes the failure to achieve adequate blood counts following allogeneic HCT in the presence of substantive donor hematopoietic cell chimerism.

Graft Failure Following Reduced-Intensity Conditioning

Allogeneic HCT following RIC is associated with incomplete eradication of host hematopoiesis. As a consequence, a significant percentage of patients have mixed donor/host hematopoietic chimerism for several months after transplantation before converting to complete donor type.[186,293] Primary engraftment following reduced-intensity allogeneic HCT is defined by neutrophil, platelet, and hemoglobin count recovery as outlined above as well as stable donor T-cell chimerism. As described above, graft failure is said to have occurred when blood donor T-cell chimerism is less than 5 percent at any point after reduced-intensity allogeneic HCT. Donor T-cell chimerism levels greater than 5 percent but less than 95 percent are generally termed "mixed chimerism," while full donor chimerism is defined by blood donor T-cell chimerism of 95 percent or greater.

Incidence of Graft Failure

The incidence of graft failure varies widely in published reports. To estimate the incidence of graft failure following autologous HCT, consider that in most centers the TRM associated with autologous HCT is less than 5 percent, of which only a small subset can be attributed to graft failure. Another surrogate marker for estimating the incidence of graft failure following autologous HCT is the requirement for hematopoietic cell rescue using a backup autograft product. A study of 300 patients who underwent autologous HCT revealed that 4.7 percent required their backup product.[294] Thus, it is reasonable to estimate that the incidence of graft failure following autologous HCT is somewhere between 1 and 5 percent.

Graft failure following allogeneic HCT is more complex, because of confounding factors such as histocompatibility, ABO matching, graft-versus-host and host-versus-graft reactions, and the use of postgrafting immunosuppression. The overall incidence of graft failure after allogeneic HCT is approximately 5 to 6 percent.[295] In general, graft failure is uncommon after high-dose conditioning and in patients who are heavily pretreated with cytotoxic chemotherapy before coming to allogeneic HCT. Even in the myeloablative setting, though, the incidence of graft failure varies with conditioning regimen, as illustrated in a randomized trial where graft failure occurred in zero of 64 (0 percent) of patients receiving BU/CY but in five of 62 (8 percent) of patients receiving BU/FLU.[174] The risk of graft rejection is highest in patients who are heavily presensitized or who have autoimmunity directed at hematopoietic cells (as in aplastic anemia), those who receive low CD34+ cell doses,[295,296] and those with diseases such as myelofibrosis where the marrow microenvironment is significantly perturbed.

The consequences of graft failure, and its optimal treatment, depend in large part upon the likelihood of autologous hematopoietic recovery. In patients who have received high-dose conditioning, autologous marrow recovery is likely to be severely delayed if not absent, and graft failure is associated with high mortality rates as a consequence of prolonged cytopenias. Second-salvage allogeneic HCT has been used successfully to treat graft failure in this setting; reported outcomes vary from dismal to encouraging,[297,298] and likely depend substantially on patient selection. There is no consensus on whether to use the same or a different donor for salvage allogeneic HCT for graft rejection, and the decision often depends on donor availability. The time needed to identify and collect a second allograft product are often prohibitive for patients with graft rejection and pancytopenia, and thus readily available HSC sources such as UCB and HLA-haploidentical family members have sometimes been used.

For patients with graft failure after RIC, autologous hematopoietic recovery is more likely. For these patients, the optimal strategy often involves withdrawing postgrafting immunosuppression and awaiting autologous count recovery. However, for patients with malignant disease, the risk of relapse is substantially elevated in the setting of graft failure,[295] presumably as a result of a loss of GVT effects.

REGIMEN-RELATED ORGAN TOXICITIES

The severity of organ toxicities associated with HCT is a function of the intensity of conditioning therapy, the amount of prior therapy received, patient comorbidities before transplantation, and posttransplantation factors such as immunosuppressive medication and antimicrobial agents.

Mucositis

Mucositis occurs in more than 90 percent of patients receiving high-dose regimens and is often regarded as the most difficult issue from the patient's perspective.[299] Current management is supportive and includes frequent rinsing with saline solutions and antimicrobials, cryotherapy, pain control (often with continuous intravenous infusions of opioids), and parenteral nutrition when needed. Improvement typically occurs within 10 to 21 days of transplantation, around the time of engraftment. Fully ablative regimens, TBI-based conditioning, and the administration of posttransplantation methotrexate (MTX) for GVHD prevention are associated with more severe mucositis.[300] Severe mucositis may result in significant tissue edema, upper airway obstruction, and/or aspiration pneumonitis, although fortunately these complications are rare. Regimen-related gastroenteritis results in nausea, vomiting, and diarrhea, which may persist for weeks after the transplant. Breaches in the mucosal lining predispose to bacterial translocation from the gastrointestinal tract, with increased risk of bacteremia and sepsis. Palifermin (keratinocyte growth factor) can reduce patient-controlled anesthesia (PCA) and total parenteral nutrition (TPN) usage because of mucositis, predominantly in patients receiving TBI-based conditioning,[301] but at a cost of $5500 to $14,000 per day.[302] Initial hopes that this agent would prevent GVHD after allogeneic HCT have not been realized,[303,304] and the benefits of palifermin appear limited to ameliorating mucositis.

Sinusoidal Obstructive Syndrome

Sinusoidal obstructive syndrome (SOS) is a clinical syndrome of regimen-related hepatotoxicity characterized by tender hepatomegaly, fluid retention, weight gain, and elevated serum bilirubin following autologous or allogeneic HCT. This syndrome was formerly called venoocclusive disease (VOD), but this term is no longer used as it inaccurately describes the underlying pathobiology: the liver injury is initiated by damage to hepatic sinusoidal epithelium, and obstruction of hepatic venules is not essential to the development of the syndrome.[305] The incidence of SOS varies significantly with the intensity of conditioning and with the stringency of diagnostic criteria, from less than 10 percent to as high as 30 to 40 percent. CY is a key culprit in the development of SOS, and large interpatient variability in CY metabolism may account for the syndrome's unpredictability.[306,307] Other contributing factors include the preadministration of BU in the BU/CY regimen, which potentiates CY hepatotoxicity[172]; preexisting hepatic fibrosis, as in patients with cirrhosis or with hepatic extramedullary hematopoiesis as in myelofibrosis[308]; and pretreatment with higher doses of gemtuzumab ozogamicin.[309,310] The incidence of SOS appears to be decreasing over time,[311] likely a result of the prevalence of RIC regimens and the prophylactic use of ursodiol, which prevents SOS and other forms of hepatic injury during allogeneic HCT.[312,313]

SOS is generally is classified as mild (clinically apparent yet resolves without treatment), moderate (requiring diuretics and pain medication for abdominal discomfort yet completely resolves before day +100), or severe (not resolving before day +100 or death).[314] Severe SOS has a tendency to progress to multiorgan failure and is associated with a mortality rate of greater than 80 percent.[315] Therapy for SOS is supportive and includes management of sodium and water balance with diuretics, preservation of renal blood flow, and paracentesis for ascites associated with significant discomfort or pulmonary compromise. Patients with a poor prognosis can be recognized early after SOS onset by steep rises in serum bilirubin, body weight, and other liver enzymes; hepatic venous pressure measurement greater than 20 torr; development of portal vein thrombosis; and multiorgan failure requiring mechanical ventilation or renal dialysis.[316]

There are few satisfactory therapies for severe SOS; the most commonly used is intravenous defibrotide, a mixture of single-stranded porcine oligodeoxyribonucleotides which induces antithrombotic and fibrinolytic effects in preclinical models.[317] Its mechanism of action against SOS remains unknown. A randomized phase II dose-finding trial involving 149 patients with severe SOS reported day +100 survival of 42 percent with few adverse events, and a dose of 25 mg/kg/day was selected for ongoing randomized phase III trials.[318] However, defibrotide is not yet approved by the FDA and remains available only on an investigational or compassionate-use basis in the United States.

Pulmonary Complications

Noncardiogenic and noninfectious diffuse lung injury, also referred to as idiopathic pneumonia syndrome (IPS), remains a significant problem following autologous or allogeneic HCT, occurring in 10 to 15 percent of transplant recipients.[319] Risk factors for idiopathic IPS include high-dose conditioning, TBI, GVHD, older recipient age, prior history of cigarette smoking, prior thoracic/mediastinal irradiation, and abnormal gas exchange as measured by pretransplant pulmonary function testing.[320] Preclinical models suggest that donor T cells play a key role in the development of IPS, indicating that it may be a form of graft-versus-host reaction.[319] In a small subset of patients, diffuse alveolar hemorrhage (DAH) develops, characterized by progressive shortness of breath, cough, and hypoxemia. Classically, DAH is defined by the demonstration of progressively bloodier aliquots in bronchoalveolar lavage fluid. Mortality from this complication is high (often >75 percent) despite aggressive treatment. Another subset of patients with IPS develop periengraftment respiratory distress without a bloody bronchoalveolar lavage. In the autologous setting, the IPS often responds promptly to glucocorticoids, whereas in the allogeneic setting response rates are lower, indicating that perhaps some cases may be complicated by GVHD.

The management of suspected IPS begins with bronchoscopy to rule out infectious etiologies and to evaluate for DAH. Care is supportive and aimed at maximizing respiratory function and preventing volume overload or multiorgan failure. Patients are typically treated with high-dose glucocorticoids (methylprednisolone at 2 mg/kg/day or higher), along with broad-spectrum antimicrobials and intensive supportive care. Retrospective studies have suggested that tumor necrosis factor (TNF) blockade with etanercept may be effective as an adjunct to high-dose glucocorticoids,[321] but a prospective randomized study failed to find an additive benefit,[322] and thus etanercept cannot be routinely recommended at this time. Patients with IPS who progress to require mechanical ventilation have a very poor prognosis, and a frank discussion of the goals of care is indicated in this setting, particularly in the presence of multiorgan failure.[323]

Lung inflammation following the administration of BCNU is a separate form of noninfectious lung injury seen in HCT recipients who receive this agent as part of their conditioning regimens. BCNU-induced pneumonitis is often characterized by a nonproductive cough with increasing dyspnea and bilateral pulmonary infiltrates on chest radiography, with or without fevers, and often occurs 1 to 2 months after transplantation.[324] Pulmonary function tests reveal a restrictive pattern of lung injury and a decrease in diffusing capacity compared to pretransplant values. Prompt treatment with glucocorticoids reduces mortality and morbidity and is crucial to a successful outcome. If untreated or recognized late, significant pulmonary fibrosis may develop.

INFECTIONS

Susceptibility to infection is a significant challenge in the clinical management of transplant recipients. The essential principles are prevention, judicious monitoring, and expeditious treatment of all bacterial, fungal, and viral infections. These basic principles are widely accepted, yet the day-to-day strategy for implementing them varies widely among transplant physicians and centers. Two universally important measures for reducing infections in immunocompromised transplant recipients are effective handwashing policies and a strategy for preventing transmission of respiratory viruses, including metapneumovirus, respiratory syncytial virus, parainfluenza, and influenza.

The duration of neutropenia and severity of oral and gastrointestinal mucosal damage from the conditioning regimen are risk factors for infection before neutrophil recovery has occurred. Following neutrophil recovery, deficiencies of B- and T-cell–mediated immunity persist and increase susceptibility to opportunistic infections. Immune recovery following autologous HCT is relatively rapid compared to after allogeneic transplantation. Most autologous transplant recipients recover T-cell immunity specific for herpes viruses, including CMV, by 3 months after transplantation.[325] The degree and duration of immunodeficiency following allogeneic HCT are influenced, in part, by the type of immunosuppressive therapy and severity of GVHD. Chronic GVHD is associated with chronic B- and T-cell immune deficiencies that may persist for years, and Ig production and reticuloendothelial function may also be impaired.[326–328]

Bacterial Infections

Bacterial infections are common during the period of immediate neutropenia that follows the preparative transplantation regimen, and can be caused by both Gram-positive and Gram-negative organisms.[329] The increased risk of bacterial infections is not only caused by neutropenia, but also from loss of epithelial integrity from regimen-related injury, bacterial translocation, and the presence of indwelling intravenous catheters. Some centers institute preventive measures in addition to rigorous hand washing, such as gowning and masking, although there is little evidence that these actions reduce infection risk. Removal of venous catheters is sometimes required for patients who do not respond promptly to treatment. Chapter 24 reviews specific strategies and regimens for treating bacterial infections in neutropenic patients.

Patients who require ongoing immunosuppressive therapy for the control of chronic GVHD are at risk for recurrent bacteremia with encapsulated bacteria and sinopulmonary infections. Preventive strategies differ from institution to institution, although some form of antibiotic prophylaxis is often used in these patients. Infrequent bacterial pathogens which should also be considered, especially in the presence of pulmonary infiltrates or nodules, are *Legionella*, *Nocardia*, *Mycobacterium tuberculosis*, and atypical mycobacteria.

Fungal Infections

Fungal infections are serious and potentially fatal complications following HCT, and are seen most commonly in allogeneic HCT recipients as a result of the requirement for postgrafting immunosuppressive medication. The incidence of fungal infection varies considerably among transplantation centers because of a variety of factors, including geographic location, nearby construction, and prophylactic regimens. *Candida* and *Aspergillus* are the most common fungal pathogens; however, other organisms can also cause life-threatening infections. Chapter 24 discusses the treatment and prophylaxis of fungal infections.

Fluconazole prophylaxis decreases the incidence of invasive and superficial *Candida albicans* infections and may decrease the 100-day mortality in allogeneic HCT recipients.[330] Fluconazole has limited activity against *Candida krusei*, *Torulopsis glabrata*, and *Aspergillus* species, and some centers reported an increased incidence of resistant *Candida* infections in patients receiving prophylactic fluconazole.[331] More aggressive prophylaxis with mold-active agents such as voriconazole or itraconazole can prevent invasive mold infections, including aspergillosis, but these agents are associated with a higher risk of adverse events and no clear benefit to mortality.[332,333]

Viral Infections

Infection with herpesviruses can cause significant morbidity and mortality in HCT recipients. Most infections are a result of viral reactivation and follow a relatively predictable temporal pattern in the absence of prophylaxis: *Herpes simplex* virus (HSV) causes clinically apparent disease at approximately 2 to 3 weeks after HCT, CMV disease usually occurs during the second to third month, and varicella-zoster virus (VZV) recurrences present at a median of 5 months after HCT.[334]

CMV is an important viral pathogen in HCT recipients. Infection occurs from reactivation of latent virus or is newly acquired from the donor graft or blood transfusions. Reactivation is a common problem in allogeneic HCT, but is relatively rare after autologous HCT except in the setting of CD34+ selection and T-cell depletion.[123] Before effective prevention strategies were introduced, CMV infection developed in 70 percent of CMV-seropositive transplant recipients and 32 percent of CMV-seronegative recipients and was a frequent cause of TRM.[335] Currently, all allogeneic HCT recipients at risk for CMV infection (those who are CMV-seropositive or who have a CMV-seropositive donor) require monitoring with preemptive therapy for CMV reactivation; this approach has markedly reduced the risk of progression to frank CMV disease such as enteritis or pneumonitis.[336] Prophylactic antiviral therapy against CMV is used by some centers, particularly in high-risk situations such as UCB recipients. More commonly, allogeneic HCT recipients are monitored with plasma CMV polymerase chain reaction (PCR) assays at least weekly through at least day +100 after HCT, and are treated preemptively if these studies yield values which exceed institutionally established thresholds.[334] The preemptive approach avoids the toxicity of universal antiviral prophylaxis, reduces the risk of acquired antiviral resistance, and limits overtreatment of CMV while preventing development of tissue disease. However, CMV tissue disease such as enteritis or pneumonitis can, rarely, develop despite negative plasma CMV PCR, and CMV enteritis or pneumonitis cannot be definitively ruled out by blood tests alone.

Prophylaxis with acyclovir or, more potently, valacyclovir can reduce the risk of CMV reactivation after allogeneic HCT, but does not obviate the need for CMV surveillance.[337,338] Intravenous ganciclovir is typically the first-line treatment for CMV reactivation or tissue disease, although oral valganciclovir may be equally effective as preemptive therapy.[339,340] The most common adverse effect of these antiviral drugs is myelosuppression, which often requires growth-factor support. Intravenous foscarnet is as effective as ganciclovir in CMV prevention and treatment,[341] and does not cause myelosuppression. However, foscarnet is nephrotoxic and requires cumbersome pre- and posthydration, and is thus most often used as second-line therapy in patients who cannot tolerate ganciclovir because of myelosuppression. Patients with CMV reactivation are typically treated with an induction dose of anti-CMV therapy (ganciclovir, valganciclovir, or foscarnet) for at least 2 weeks, followed by maintenance antiviral therapy until CMV assays are persistently negative. It is not uncommon for patients to experience additional late reactivations after antiviral therapy is discontinued, and these patients require ongoing monitoring beyond day +100.

Investigational approaches to CMV prevention and treatment include CMX-001, an oral prodrug that is converted to cidofovir intracellularly and lacks renal toxicity. A placebo-controlled randomized trial of CMX-001 as CMV prophylaxis in allogeneic HCT found that this agent reduced the incidence of CMV activation from 37 percent to 10 percent.[342] Diarrhea was the most common adverse effect; myelosuppression and nephrotoxicity were not observed. Letermovir, a novel terminase inhibitor, has also shown efficacy in preventing CMV reactivation in allogeneic HCT in randomized, placebo-controlled clinical trials.[343] Maribavir, another antiviral agent with a novel mechanism of action, was effective in preventing CMV in a randomized dose-finding study,[344] but failed to demonstrate a benefit in a randomized phase III clinical trial.[345] Donor-derived CMV-specific cytotoxic lymphocytes have also been used investigationally with some success.[346]

HSV and VZV are two other members of the herpesvirus family that cause significant morbidity in the posttransplantation setting. These viruses share the characteristics of latency, reactivation, and neurotropism. Virtually all HSV disease occurring after HCT is a result of reactivation, and the serologic status of the transplant recipient determines the risk for disease and the requirement for prophylaxis. Oral mucositis, cutaneous infections, esophagitis, genital herpes, and pneumonia are the most common clinical manifestations. Acyclovir is highly effective for the prevention and treatment of HSV and should be administered to all HSV-seropositive transplant recipients, beginning before or during conditioning. Acyclovir prophylaxis is often continued for at least 1 year after HCT (or longer if patients remain on immunosuppressive therapy), as this approach reduces the risk of late HSV recurrence.[347] Acyclovir is well tolerated immediately after transplantation with no effect on the recovery of neutrophil counts. Valacyclovir is an acceptable alternative. Patients do not require concomitant acyclovir prophylaxis while receiving maribavir, foscarnet, valganciclovir, ganciclovir, or cidofovir for treatment of another virus, because these agents have adequate anti-HSV activity. Acyclovir resistance is rare in HSV and can be treated using foscarnet.[348]

Recurrent VZV disease can occur after both allogeneic and autologous HCT. The initial manifestations of recurrence are localized in approximately half of patients. Treatment with acyclovir within 24 to 48 hours of the onset of herpes zoster prevents dissemination and shortens the course of cutaneous disease. The failure of VZV infections to resolve quickly or their recurrence shortly after acyclovir therapy is discontinued is usually a function of the limited host immune response and is generally not a result of acyclovir resistance. For the rare cases of acyclovir-resistant VZV, foscarnet is the most commonly used alternate therapy.[348] Acyclovir, given for at least 1 year after HCT, is highly effective in preventing VZV recurrence.[349] Pilot studies of vaccination with live attenuated VZV in allogeneic HCT recipients suggest that this approach is safe and effective in selected patients (median of 4 years posttransplantation, off systemic immunosuppression, blood CD4+ cell count >200/μL),[350] but larger studies are required before vaccination can be widely recommended. Heat-inactivated VZV vaccination has also been reported as efficacious in recipients of autologous HCT.[351]

ACUTE GRAFT-VERSUS-HOST DISEASE

Acute GVHD remains one of the most serious and challenging complications of allogeneic HCT. The requirements for the development of acute GVHD were described more than 40 years ago: the graft must contain immunologically competent cells, the recipient must express tissue antigens not found in the donor, and the recipient must be immunologically suppressed such that an effective response against transplanted cells cannot occur.[352] HLA disparities are potent triggers of GVHD, but in the setting of HLA-matched donor/recipient pairs GVHD is mediated by minor histocompatibility antigen disparities which provoke a donor T-cell response.[353,354] There are two primary classes of MHC antigens in humans: HLA class I antigens have a broad distribution and are expressed on nearly all cells, whereas HLA class II antigen expression is restricted to macrophages, dendritic cells, B cells, and activated T cells. Minor histocompatibility antigens are endogenous cellular proteins which are subject to significant genetic polymorphism and are presented to donor T cells as small peptides bound in the grooves of the major histocompatibility antigens.[355] Some minor histocompatibility antigens associated with GVHD include CD31, HA-1, and the male-specific *DBY* gene.[356,357] There are likely hundreds if not thousands

of minor histocompatibility antigens relevant to allogeneic HCT, of which only a handful have been identified to date. Efforts are underway to utilize genome-wide association studies to broaden our knowledge of these determinants of GVT effects and GVHD.[358]

The most important risk factor for the development of acute GVHD is the degree of HLA disparity between donor and recipient. The increased incidence of acute GVHD with fully HLA-matched unrelated donors compared to HLA-identical sibling donors is likely related to increased disparity in minor histocompatibility antigens or unrecognized disparities in the phenotypically matched major histocompatibility loci.[359] Other risk factors for acute GVHD development include conditioning intensity, use of TBI, and possibly graft source (although the effect of graft source on acute GVHD incidence is not consistently observed).[72,359]

Classically, acute GVHD was defined temporally by its occurrence before day +100 after allogeneic HCT. With RIC, acute GVHD can occur beyond day +100, and the distinction between acute and chronic GVHD is now based on organ involvement and histology rather than time of onset.[360] Acute GVHD affects the skin, gastrointestinal (GI) tract, and liver (although liver involvement is increasingly rare, for reasons which are not entirely clear).[218] The overall incidence of acute GVHD after allogeneic HCT is 40 to 60 percent,[359] although the incidence may vary widely in specific settings depending on conditioning regimen, HLA matching, and graft source.

Skin involvement manifests as a rash, which may be localized and maculopapular or diffusely erythematous with bullae and desquamation in very severe cases. Definitive diagnosis requires skin biopsy and interpretation by an experienced pathologist.[361] However, skin biopsies are often inconclusive, and the diagnosis is often made on clinical grounds in patients with a skin rash consistent with acute GVHD arising during the appropriate timeframe after allogeneic HCT. Decision analysis supports the concept that the diagnosis of skin GVHD can be made clinically and does not require skin biopsy in patients with a pretest likelihood of acute GVHD of 30 percent or greater (the majority of allogeneic HCT recipients).[362]

GI manifestations of acute GVHD can affect the upper GI tract (presenting as nausea, emesis, anorexia, and weight loss), the lower GI tract (presenting as diarrhea with or without abdominal cramping and hematochezia), or both. Upper-GI involvement with acute GVHD is likely underdiagnosed, since the symptoms may be mild and posttransplant anorexia and nausea are often nonspecific and multifactorial. Diagnosis requires upper endoscopy and endoscopic biopsy, with interpretation by an experienced pathologist. The diagnosis of upper-GI acute GVHD is clinically important, because this syndrome often responds dramatically to even low-dose treatment and, if left untreated, can cause significant nutritional compromise.

Lower-GI involvement with acute GVHD is a more serious and feared complication of allogeneic HCT. These patients present with substantial diarrhea, often several liters per day, accompanied by pain and bleeding. The diarrhea of acute GVHD is secretory, related to epithelial injury, and typically persists around the clock. Abdominal computed tomography (CT) findings, particularly bowel-wall thickening, are common in acute GVHD,[363] but CT findings alone are insufficient for diagnosis. Patients with suspected lower-GI GVHD should undergo endoscopic evaluation and biopsy as soon as feasible, although in the setting of myeloablative conditioning it is often difficult to differentiate regimen-related GI injury from acute GVHD endoscopically or histologically before day +20. Flexible sigmoidoscopy is viewed as a sufficient diagnostic test in most cases,[364,365] and is far easier to perform than full colonoscopy as it does not require an aggressive preparatory regimen. Visual inspection of the gut mucosa is often sufficient to advance a diagnosis of acute GVHD and initiate treatment,[366] particularly if the endoscopist has experience in evaluating allogeneic HCT recipients, but biopsies remain essential to rule out CMV enteritis and other etiologies.[365] Mucosal denudation is a particularly concerning endoscopic finding,[366] and is associated with a grim prognosis.

Hepatic GVHD presents with abnormal liver function tests, most commonly elevated bilirubin and alkaline phosphatase. Liver biopsy is required for definitive diagnosis, but is rarely performed because of the low pretest likelihood of hepatic GVHD in the modern era and because of procedural risk. When biopsies are performed, the most common finding associated with hepatic GVHD is bile-duct injury and loss resulting in cholestasis.[367] Numerous other etiologies can cause abnormal liver function tests in allogeneic HCT recipients, including SOS, viral hepatitis, regimen-related hepatotoxicity, and medication-related hepatotoxicity (particularly with triazoles and CSP). Hepatic GVHD is relatively uncommon except in the setting of severe multisystem acute GVHD.

Pathophysiology

The current model of acute GVHD requires three steps. In step 1, the transplantation conditioning regimen damages host tissue, leading to increased secretion of inflammatory cytokines such as TNF-α and IL-1. These cytokines enhance alloreactivity of donor T cells by upregulating the expression of major and minor host tissue histocompatibility antigens and also affect other molecules on host antigen-presenting cells (APCs). Regimen-related damage to the GI tract results in leakage of endotoxins such as lipopolysaccharides into the systemic circulation, where they serve as additional inflammatory stimuli.[353] In step 2, resting donor T cells become activated in secondary lymphoid organs by host or donor APCs, which present alloantigens to the T-cell receptor in the context of MHC. Costimulatory signals are required for full T-cell activation. Donor T-cell activation is characterized by cellular proliferation and predominance of Th1 cells and the secretion of IL-2 and IFN-γ. In step 3, cellular effectors mediate tissue injury and destruction in the target organs, resulting in the clinical manifestations of acute GVHD. This step involves the continued release of inflammatory cytokines that direct specific antihost donor-derived T cells to migrate to the target tissues of acute GVHD, namely, skin, liver, and gut. Neutrophils and mononuclear phagocytes contribute to local tissue injury by amplifying the proinflammatory response.

Prevention

Without some form of GVHD prophylaxis, virtually all patients undergoing allogeneic HCT would develop severe or fatal acute GVHD. Immunosuppressive drugs are the mainstay of acute GVHD prevention, and all patients undergoing allogeneic HCT with a T-cell-replete graft require prophylaxis. On the basis of randomized clinical trials published in the 1980s, the most commonly used regimen in myeloablative allogeneic HCT is the combination of a calcineurin inhibitor (CSP or tacrolimus [TAC]) with a short course of MTX, generally given on days +1, +3, +6, and +11 after allotransplantation.[368,369] The addition of prednisone to this backbone paradoxically increased the risk of acute GVHD in a randomized clinical trial, and thus glucocorticoids are rarely used for GVHD prophylaxis.[370] Two randomized studies demonstrated that TAC was superior to CSP in preventing acute GVHD after myeloablative allogeneic HCT,[371,372] and thus TAC has largely supplanted CSP in this setting. A recent randomized clinical trial conducted by the BMT-CTN compared TAC/sirolimus (TAC/SRL) to the standard TAC/MTX regimen as GVHD prophylaxis after myeloablative allogeneic HCT. The primary endpoint (day +114 survival free of acute GVHD grades II to IV) was not significantly different in the two arms, nor were overall or progression-free survival.[300] The toxicity profiles of the two regimens

differed somewhat, but did not impact TRM. Interestingly, there was a strong trend toward a higher incidence of chronic GVHD in the SRL-containing arm (53 percent vs. 45 percent, p = 0.06).

Donor T-cell depletion has been explored as a means of GVHD prevention, using either mechanical *ex vivo* T-cell depletion or *in vivo* T-cell depletion in the form of ATG or alemtuzumab. T-cell-depletion strategies have generally been successful in reducing GVHD, but in many instances the reduction in donor T cells contributes to an increased incidence of graft rejection, infection, and relapse which may negate the advantage of GVHD prevention. A recent randomized clinical trial of ATG versus placebo added to standard CSP/MTX GVHD prophylaxis reported lower rates of acute and chronic GVHD in the ATG arm, although TRM and overall survival were not improved.[373] Longer followup from this study confirmed a significantly lower rate of chronic GVHD in the ATG arm (45 percent vs. 12 percent, p <0.0001).[374] However, ATG was associated with an increased risk of PTLD, a complication that is virtually nonexistent after T-cell-replete allogeneic HCT. In fact, there were 4 deaths from PTLD in the ATG arm (versus none in the placebo arm). Perhaps as a result, the study did not show improvements in TRM or overall survival with ATG. A subsequent randomized clinical trial aimed at replicating and extending these results with ATG has been completed in the United States.

In the setting of reduced-intensity allotransplantation, a number of immunosuppressive regimens have been used, the most common being CSP plus MMF.[177,185] Posttransplant CY has demonstrated impressive efficacy in the setting of HLA-haploidentical HCT, and has been studied in the setting of HLA-matched allotransplantation as well.[375,376] The combination of TLI and ATG is associated with very low rates of acute and chronic GVHD even with standard CSP/MMF postgrafting immunosuppression,[184,185] suggesting that protective conditioning can play a significant role in GVHD prevention.

Several laboratories have reported that naïve (CD62L+) T cells induce experimental acute GVHD, whereas effector memory (CD62L−) T cells do not.[377,378] Based on this insight, depletion of naïve donor T cells has been investigated as a means of preventing acute GVHD in humans.[379] Murine models of marrow transplantation show that simultaneous infusions of T_{reg} limited the proliferation and clonal expansion of activated donor T cells and protected against acute GVHD development in murine models.[144] Pilot studies of T_{reg} infusions in humans have demonstrated safety and some efficacy in preventing GVHD,[145,146,380] although larger trials are required to confirm these preliminary findings. Importantly, relapse rates did not appear to be increased by the addition of T_{reg}, consistent with murine models.[144,146]

Another investigational avenue in GVHD prevention involves inhibition of lymphocyte trafficking through CCR5 blockade. A recent trial combining the CCR5 antagonist maraviroc with standard GVHD prophylaxis demonstrated low rates of acute GVHD, particularly GI GVHD.[381] The BMT-CTN is currently conducting a three-arm randomized clinical trial comparing novel approaches to GVHD prophylaxis: posttransplant CY; maraviroc; and bortezomib-based immunosuppression.

Treatment

The standard first-line therapy for acute GVHD requiring systemic treatment is methylprednisolone or prednisone, at a dose of 1 to 2 mg/kg/day with subsequent tapering once disease activity resolves. Higher doses of methylprednisolone (10 mg/kg per day) do not prevent evolution to grades III to IV acute GVHD or improve survival.[382] Patients with acute GVHD grade II or less can be safely treated with a starting dose of 1 mg/kg/day of methylprednisolone, an approach that reduces overall glucocorticoid exposure and toxicity.[383] Complete resolution of acute GVHD is reported in less than 50 percent of patients after first-line treatment with glucocorticoids, and the likelihood for long-term survival is low among individuals who develop glucocorticoid-refractory acute GVHD.[384] Various approaches, including third-party mesenchymal stem cells, MMF, and TNF blockade, have been combined with glucocorticoids in upfront treatment of acute GVHD, but none has proven superior to glucocorticoids alone.[385,386]

There is no standard second-line therapy for patients with glucocorticoid-refractory acute GVHD. Practices vary widely, although groups such as the ASBMT have published guidelines in an effort to codify and standardize treatment.[387] Even though many agents have been used in this setting, none has proven superior or even reliably effective. Options include enrollment on a clinical trial, treatment with a second-line agent of choice, and palliative care. Agents that have been studied include daclizumab, SRL, MMF, ABX-CBL (a CD147-specific monoclonal antibody), anti-TNF agents, visilizumab, ruxolitinib,[388,389] and ATG, among others. In the absence of comparative clinical trial data, the choice of second-line agent is often guided by institutional experience, physician preference, and side-effect profiles. Outcomes with second-line therapy remain poor, and novel treatments for glucocorticoid-refractory acute GVHD are needed.

CHRONIC GRAFT-VERSUS-HOST DISEASE

Chronic GVHD is the major determinant of quality of life in long-term survivors of allogeneic HCT.[390,391] Despite its impact, however, it remains poorly understood and treatment options remain limited and largely empiric. Historically, any form of GVHD occurring beyond day +100 after allogeneic HCT was defined as chronic GVHD. However, with an increasing appreciation of the biologic differences between acute and chronic GVHD and the recognition that late acute GVHD occurs beyond day +100 with RIC, chronic GVHD was redefined on the basis of pathognomonic clinical and histologic criteria by a National Institutes of Health (NIH) consensus conference in 2005.[360] The NIH consensus criteria include global and organ-specific scoring to evaluate the severity of chronic GVHD, and these staging tools have been validated to correlate with clinical severity and outcomes.[392,393] The Center for International Blood and Marrow Transplant Research (CIBMTR) has also developed a chronic GVHD risk-stratification algorithm that identifies age, donor–recipient gender mismatch, serum bilirubin, platelet count, donor type, and performance status, among other factors, as predictors of outcome in patients with chronic GVHD.[394] The presence of chronic GVHD is consistently associated with more potent GVT effects and a lower risk of posttransplantation relapse,[177,395] although the negative impact of chronic GVHD on TRM may outweigh the benefit against relapse.[177]

In contrast to acute GVHD, which is limited to the skin, gut, and liver, chronic GVHD has diverse manifestations which can affect nearly any organ system and which overlap considerably with those of autoimmune disorders such as scleroderma, lichen planus, Sjögren syndrome, and dermatomyositis. The most common clinical features of chronic GVHD include lichenoid skin lesions that may progress to generalized scleroderma, keratoconjunctivitis sicca, lichenoid oral lesions, esophageal and vaginal strictures, intestinal abnormalities, chronic liver disease, and bronchiolitis obliterans. Comprehensive assessment of chronic GVHD requires a detailed history and physical examination, but can be performed in the clinic in less than 20 minutes.[396] Instructional videos and training tools demonstrating clinical assessment of chronic GVHD are available.[397]

The pathophysiology of chronic GVHD remains poorly understood. In contrast to acute GVHD, where there is a track record of translation from relevant animal models to humans, existing murine models of chronic GVHD suffer from serious shortcomings,[398] limiting the understanding of its pathobiology and restricting the study of novel therapies. Efforts continue to develop more relevant murine models,[399] although translational success remains elusive.

Although chronic GVHD is frequently preceded by acute GVHD, progress in reducing the incidence of acute GVHD has generally not translated into a reduction in the incidence of chronic GVHD. If anything, the incidence of chronic GVHD is likely increasing, as a result of the increasing use of PBPC as a graft source and the increasing at-risk pool of long-term survivors of allogeneic HCT. The only approaches proven to prevent chronic GVHD are the use of marrow as a graft source rather than PBPC,[72] and the use of ex vivo or in vivo T-cell depletion (which carries increased risks of infection, PTLD, and relapse).[373,400] It has been suggested that posttransplant CY may prevent chronic GVHD, as low rates have been reported in single-arm studies,[375,376] but this comparison is confounded by graft source (predominantly marrow in trials of posttransplant CY) and requires confirmation in randomized clinical trials. Recipient statin use has been associated with a significantly reduced risk of chronic GVHD, but a higher risk of relapse, in patients receiving CSP-based GVHD prophylaxis regimens.[401] Rituximab has been studied as a prophylactic agent because of the demonstrated role of B cells in the genesis of chronic GVHD. Results have been mixed; a clinical trial performed at Stanford University demonstrated that rituximab potently abrogated B-cell alloimmunity, but did not lead to a statistically significant reduction in chronic GVHD incidence.[402] A nonrandomized study from the Dana-Farber Cancer Institute reported that rituximab decreased glucocorticoid-requiring chronic GVHD (but not overall chronic GVHD incidence) in comparison with a concurrent control cohort,[403] a finding which requires confirmation in randomized clinical trials.

Despite decades of investigation of novel therapies, the standard of care for initial systemic treatment of chronic GVHD remains prednisone 1 mg/kg/day, with or without a calcineurin inhibitor.[404] Numerous investigational agents have demonstrated promise in uncontrolled phase II clinical trials. However, these agents have uniformly proven disappointing when subjected to randomized phase III studies. At least six large randomized trials conducted over the past 20 years testing various alternate regimens, including azathioprine, thalidomide, MMF, and hydroxychloroquine, have failed to demonstrate the efficacy of any novel regimen for treatment of established chronic GVHD.[405–410]

Patients with chronic GVHD typically require prolonged courses of immunosuppressive therapy. The median time to discontinuation of all systemic immunosuppression in patients with chronic GVHD resolution is approximately 2 years.[411] Approximately half of patients with chronic GVHD will fail to respond to glucocorticoids and require second-line therapy.[412] As with acute GVHD, there is no single standard of care for glucocorticoid-refractory chronic GVHD, and enrollment on a clinical trial should be strongly considered. Treatment choice depends on patient and physician preference, side-effect profile, and institutional priorities, as there are no data to guide a more systematic approach. Typical second-line agents include extracorporeal photopheresis (ECP), SRL, thalidomide, pentostatin, rituximab, and imatinib, among others.[412] ECP is logistically cumbersome but can be effective and causes relatively few adverse effects[413]; this approach is currently being studied in a randomized clinical trial conducted by the BMT-CTN. Low-dose IL-2 has been reported to facilitate T_{reg} expansion and homeostasis in a small single-center study of patients with chronic GVHD,[414,415] although the degree of T_{reg} expansion was not significantly associated with clinical response.[414] Nonetheless, therapies targeting T_{reg}s are under active investigation in the treatment of chronic GVHD, as is the Bruton tyrosine kinase inhibitor ibrutinib.[416] More effective prevention and treatment of chronic GVHD remains a crucial research need in allogeneic HCT.

RELAPSED MALIGNANCY AFTER HCT

Relapse following autologous or allogeneic HCT is an ominous clinical event. Every effort should be made to verify relapse pathologically, as it is common for patients to have residual radiographic abnormalities following transplantation, especially in patients with lymphoma. Patients with myeloma have gradual reductions in biochemical markers of disease which may take several months after autologous HCT to reach maximal response. Following RIC, the allogeneic GVT effect may take weeks to months to result in tumor eradication, and it may be difficult to distinguish persistent yet slowly regressing disease from slowly progressive disease, particularly with indolent NHL or CLL.

Relapse after Autologous Hematopoietic Cell Transplantation

Disease relapse remains the most common cause of treatment failure after autologous HCT. Relapse often occurs at sites of previous disease, suggesting that residual disease within the patient rather than autograft contamination is responsible.[417] Additional cytotoxic chemotherapy alone is highly unlikely to be curative in patients relapsing after autologous HCT, as the disease has already survived supralethal doses of chemotherapy. Treatment options for patients with relapse after autologous HCT include irradiation, immunomodulators, and/or targeted therapies. For selected patients, salvage allogeneic HCT may be feasible using RIC. Strategies to reduce the risk of relapse in high-risk patients undergoing autologous HCT include consolidative involved-field radiotherapy, antitumor vaccination,[418] maintenance therapy with targeted agents,[269,419,420] and planned tandem allogeneic HCT.[421]

Relapse after Allogeneic Hematopoietic Cell Transplantation

Treatment of disease relapse following allogeneic HCT is generally unsuccessful. In particular, patients with high-risk malignancies and early relapse (<100 days after allogeneic HCT) have a dismal prognosis, with 2-year overall survival of less than 5 percent.[422] Salvage chemotherapy can result in disease responses, but they are unlikely to be durable. Performing a second myeloablative transplantation procedure has largely been unsuccessful because of excessive toxicity and TRM of greater than 50 percent. More recently, selected patients have been treated with a second allogeneic HCT using RIC. Treatment-related toxicity with this approach is not prohibitive and successful disease eradication has been reported, although relapse remains the major cause of death.[423] There is no consensus on whether to use the same donor or a different donor for second-salvage allogeneic HCT in the setting of relapse. More importantly, the majority of patients with relapse after allogeneic HCT are ineligible for second allotransplant because their diseases cannot be adequately controlled or cytoreduced. Experimental therapies with chimeric antigen receptor-bearing autologous T cells or other investigational approaches warrant consideration in these cases. In our view, palliative care is a reasonable option, particularly in the setting of early or chemorefractory relapse after allogeneic HCT, and should be presented to patients.

In the setting of retained donor T-cell chimerism, posttransplantation relapse has sometimes been treated by rapidly tapering immunosuppressive medications to stimulate a GVT effect. Although this approach is occasionally successful in patients with indolent malignancies such as low-grade NHL or CLL, it is rarely effective against more aggressive diseases such as acute leukemias, and carries a high risk of precipitating severe GVHD.

In patients who are off immunosuppression without evidence of GVHD at the time of relapse, DLI has been used to augment GVT. The mechanism by which DLI works is unclear; it may normalize the T-cell repertoire or reverse so-called T-cell "exhaustion."[424,425] Historically, the best outcomes for DLI have been reported for CML, although TKIs have

supplanted DLI for the most part in this setting.[426] DLI alone is typically insufficient to control aggressive hematologic malignancies,[427] and thus patients are often treated with reinduction chemotherapy or other cytoreduction before receiving DLI as consolidation.

The major potential adverse effects of DLI are GVHD and marrow aplasia. The risk of GVHD after DLI is at least 20 percent and likely as high as 50 to 70 percent.[428,429] Marrow aplasia typically occurs in the setting of residual host hematopoiesis; when host HSC are eradicated by DLI, there may be too few donor HSC to support hematopoietic recovery and prolonged aplasia (>6 weeks) can ensue.[430] Thus, chimerism should be evaluated before DLI, and DLI should be used with caution in patients with significant residual host hematopoiesis. There are limited data on the optimal cell dose of DLI. In a retrospective analysis, doses greater than 1×10^8 CD3+ cells/kg were associated with a high risk of GVHD (55 percent) without a corresponding benefit in disease control, while doses of 1×10^7 CD3+ cells/kg or less were associated with the lowest rates of GVHD (21 percent).[428] Modifications of DLI, including selection of CD8+ effector lymphocytes or production of cytokine-induced killer cells,[141] are under investigation to improve the safety and efficacy of this approach.

● FUTURE DIRECTIONS

In recent years, research in HCT has helped to establish alternative-donor allotransplantation, improve outcomes through better supportive care,[218] and expand transplant eligibility to previously ineligible populations using RIC,[202] among other advancements. Current research directions in HCT are diverse; two avenues among many are briefly summarized here.

The past several years have seen an explosion of research interest in the microbiome and the role of host/microbiome interaction in regulating immunity. The relevance of this field to allogeneic HCT is immediately obvious, as the gut and skin are key targets of GVHD. Preclinical evidence suggests that gut microbiota play a critical role in the development of GI GVHD.[431,432] In humans, preliminary evidence links changes in the microbiome to respiratory complications,[433] GI GVHD,[432,434] bacteremia,[435] and mortality after allogeneic HCT.[436] While our understanding of these interactions is still in its infancy and the clinical implications of these findings remain unclear, studies are underway revisiting older strategies, such as total gut decontamination, as well as more modern efforts to tailor the microbiome to optimize transplant outcomes.[437]

Allogeneic HCT is also under investigation as a platform to promote tolerance of solid-organ allografts. Solid-organ transplants typically require lifelong immunosuppression to maintain graft function, but investigators in the 1990s noted that renal allotransplantation could be accomplished without immunosuppressive therapy in recipients of allogeneic HCT, provided that the kidney allograft was obtained from the original marrow donor.[438,439] The development of reduced-intensity regimens has spurred research in this field, as these regimens are less toxic and often produce mixed rather than complete donor chimerism—a desirable characteristic in this setting since mixed chimerism reduces the risk of GVHD.

Investigators at Northwestern University described a cohort of 15 HLA-mismatched living-donor kidney transplant recipients given RIC and an infusion of donor marrow enriched with facilitator cells. Six of the 15 patients developed sustained chimerism and were completely withdrawn from immunosuppressive medication without renal allograft rejection.[440,441] Investigators in Boston reported that four of 10 HLA-haplotype matched living-donor kidney transplant recipients were able to discontinue immunosuppression for up to 11.4 years without subsequent graft dysfunction after establishment of transient mixed chimerism.[442]

Stanford investigators used TLI-ATG conditioning in 16 living-donor kidney transplant recipients from HLA-matched siblings treated with infusion of CD34-selected hematopoietic progenitor cells and a defined dose of T cells. Fifteen patients developed multilineage mixed chimerism without GVHD, and eight were withdrawn from antirejection medications without subsequent rejection episodes. Four additional chimeric patients were in the midst of drug withdrawal, and only four patients were not withdrawn because of the return of the underlying disease or rejection episodes.[189,443] Case reports have also described the use of allogeneic HCT as a tolerance-induction platform in lung transplantation.[444]

REFERENCES

1. Osgood EE, Riddle MC, Mathews TJ: Aplastic anemia treated with daily transfusions and intravenous marrow. *Ann Intern Med* 13:357–367, 1939.
2. Fabricius-Moller J: *Experimental Studies on the Hemorrhagic Diathesis of X-Ray Sickness.* Levin and Munksgards Forlag, Copenhagen, 1922.
3. Jacobson LO, Marks EK, Robson MJ: The effect of spleen protection on mortality following X-irradiation. *J Lab Clin Med* 34:1538, 1949.
4. Lorenz E, Uphoff D, Reid TR, et al: Modification of irradiation injury in mice and guinea pigs by bone marrow injections. *J Natl Cancer Inst* 12:197–201, 1951.
5. Cole LJ, Fishler MC, Bond VP: Subcellular fractionation of mouse spleen radiation protection activity. *Proc Natl Acad Sci U S A* 39:759–772, 1953.
6. Hilfinger MF Jr, Ferguson JH, Riemenschneider PA: The effect of homologous bone marrow emulsion on rabbits after total body irradiation. *J Lab Clin Med* 42:581–591, 1953.
7. Lorenz E, Congdon CC: Modification of lethal irradiation injury in mice by injection of homologous or heterologous bone. *J Natl Cancer Inst* 14:955–965, 1954.
8. Barnes DWH, Loutit JF: *Spleen Protection: The Cellular Hypothesis.* Butterworth, London, 1955.
9. Barnes DW, Corp MJ, Loutit JF, et al: Treatment of murine leukaemia with X rays and homologous bone marrow; preliminary communication. *Br Med J* 2:626–627, 1956.
10. Thomas ED, Lochte HL Jr, Lu WC, et al: Intravenous infusion of bone marrow in patients receiving radiation and chemotherapy. *N Engl J Med* 257:491–496, 1957.
11. Thomas ED, Lochte HL Jr, Cannon JH, et al: Supralethal whole body irradiation and isologous marrow transplantation in man. *J Clin Invest* 38:1709–1716, 1959.
12. Mathe G, Jammet H, Pendic B, et al: [Transfusions and grafts of homologous bone marrow in humans after accidental high dosage irradiation] [in French]. *Rev Fr Etud Clin Biol* 4:226–238, 1959.
13. Kurnick NB, Montano A, Gerdes JC, et al: Preliminary observations on the treatment of postirradiation hematopoietic depression in man by the infusion of stored autogenous bone marrow. *Ann Intern Med* 49:973–986, 1958.
14. Haurani FI: Thirty-one-year survival following chemotherapy and autologous bone marrow in malignant lymphoma. *Am J Hematol* 55:35–38, 1997.
15. Bortin MM: A compendium of reported human bone marrow transplants. *Transplantation* 9:571–587, 1970.
16. Gatti RA, Meuwissen HJ, Allen HD, et al: Immunological reconstitution of sex-linked lymphopenic immunological deficiency. *Lancet* 2:1366–1369, 1968.
17. De Koning J, Van Bekkum DW, Dicke KA, et al: Transplantation of bone-marrow cells and fetal thymus in an infant with lymphopenic immunological deficiency. *Lancet* 1:1223–1227, 1969.
18. Bach FH, Albertini RJ, Joo P, et al: Bone-marrow transplantation in a patient with the Wiskott-Aldrich syndrome. *Lancet* 2:1364–1366, 1968.
19. Bortin MM, Bach FH, van Bekkum DW, et al: 25th anniversary of the first successful allogeneic bone marrow transplants. *Bone Marrow Transplant* 14:211–212, 1994.
20. Thomas E, Storb R, Clift RA, et al: Bone-marrow transplantation (first of two parts). *N Engl J Med* 292:832–843, 1975.
21. Hansen JA, Clift RA, Thomas ED, et al: Transplantation of marrow from an unrelated donor to a patient with acute leukemia. *N Engl J Med* 303:565–567, 1980.
22. O'Reilly RJ, Dupont B, Pahwa S, et al: Reconstitution in severe combined immunodeficiency by transplantation of marrow from an unrelated donor. *N Engl J Med* 297:1311–1318, 1977.
23. Appelbaum FR, Herzig GP, Ziegler JL, et al: Successful engraftment of cryopreserved autologous bone marrow in patients with malignant lymphoma. *Blood* 52:85–95, 1978.
24. Appelbaum FR, Deisseroth AB, Graw RG Jr, et al: Prolonged complete remission following high dose chemotherapy of Burkitt's lymphoma in relapse. *Cancer* 41:1059–1063, 1978.
25. Center for International Blood & Marrow Transplant Research: *Progress Report January-December 2013...* Available at: http://www.cibmtr.org/About/ProceduresProgress/Documents/CIBMTR%20Progress%20Report%202013.pdf.
26. Weissman IL: Stem cells: Units of development, units of regeneration, and units in evolution. *Cell* 100:157–168, 2000.
27. Spangrude GJ, Heimfeld S, Weissman IL: Purification and characterization of mouse hematopoietic stem cells. *Science* 241:58–62, 1988.
28. Ikuta K, Weissman IL: Evidence that hematopoietic stem cells express mouse c-kit but do not depend on steel factor for their generation. *Proc Natl Acad Sci U S A* 89:1502–1506, 1992.
29. Osawa M, Hanada K, Hamada H, et al: Long-term lymphohematopoietic reconstitution by a single CD34-low/negative hematopoietic stem cell. *Science* 273:242–245, 1996.
30. Baum CM, Weissman IL, Tsukamoto AS, et al: Isolation of a candidate human hematopoietic stem-cell population. *Proc Natl Acad Sci U S A* 89:2804–2808, 1992.
31. Negrin RS, Atkinson K, Leemhuis T, et al: Transplantation of highly purified CD34+Thy-1+ hematopoietic stem cells in patients with metastatic breast cancer. *Biol Blood Marrow Transplant* 6:262–271, 2000.
32. Vose JM, Bierman PJ, Lynch JC, et al: Transplantation of highly purified CD34+Thy-1+ hematopoietic stem cells in patients with recurrent indolent non-Hodgkin's lymphoma. *Biol Blood Marrow Transplant* 7:680–687, 2001.
33. Michallet M, Philip T, Philip I, et al: Transplantation with selected autologous peripheral blood CD34+Thy1+ hematopoietic stem cells (HSCs) in multiple myeloma: Impact of HSC dose on engraftment, safety, and immune reconstitution. *Exp Hematol* 28:858–870, 2000.
34. Muller AM, Kohrt HE, Cha S, et al: Long-term outcome of patients with metastatic breast cancer treated with high-dose chemotherapy and transplantation of purified autologous hematopoietic stem cells. *Biol Blood Marrow Transplant* 18:125–133, 2012.
35. Muller AM, Shashidhar S, Kupper NJ, et al: Co-transplantation of pure blood stem cells with antigen-specific but not bulk T cells augments functional immunity. *Proc Natl Acad Sci U S A* 109:5820–5825, 2012.
36. Hidalgo A, Robledo MM, Teixido J: CD44-mediated hematopoietic progenitor cell adhesion and its complex role in myelopoiesis. *J Hematother Stem Cell Res* 11:539–547, 2002.
37. Frenette PS, Subbarao S, Mazo IB, et al: Endothelial selectins and vascular cell adhesion molecule-1 promote hematopoietic progenitor homing to bone marrow. *Proc Natl Acad Sci U S A* 95:14423–14428, 1998.
38. Katayama Y, Hidalgo A, Furie BC, et al: PSGL-1 participates in E-selectin-mediated progenitor homing to bone marrow: Evidence for cooperation between E-selectin ligands and alpha4 integrin. *Blood* 102:2060–2067, 2003.
39. Papayannopoulou T, Craddock C, Nakamoto B, et al: The VLA4/VCAM-1 adhesion pathway defines contrasting mechanisms of lodgement of transplanted murine hemopoietic progenitors between bone marrow and spleen. *Proc Natl Acad Sci U S A* 92:9647–9651, 1995.
40. Vermeulen M, Le Pesteur F, Gagnerault MC, et al: Role of adhesion molecules in the homing and mobilization of murine hematopoietic stem and progenitor cells. *Blood* 92:894–900, 1998.
41. Hirsch E, Iglesias A, Potocnik AJ, et al: Impaired migration but not differentiation of haematopoietic stem cells in the absence of beta1 integrins. *Nature* 380:171–175, 1996.
42. Nagasawa T, Hirota S, Tachibana K, et al: Defects of B-cell lymphopoiesis and bone-marrow myelopoiesis in mice lacking the CXC chemokine PBSF/SDF-1. *Nature* 382:635–638, 1996.
43. Lapidot T: Mechanism of human stem cell migration and repopulation of NOD/SCID and B2mnull NOD/SCID mice. The role of SDF-1/CXCR4 interactions. *Ann N Y Acad Sci* 938:83–95, 2001.
44. Liles WC, Broxmeyer HE, Rodger E, et al: Mobilization of hematopoietic progenitor cells in healthy volunteers by AMD3100, a CXCR4 antagonist. *Blood* 102:2728–2730, 2003.
45. Jung Y, Wang J, Song J, et al: Annexin II expressed by osteoblasts and endothelial cells regulates stem cell adhesion, homing, and engraftment following transplantation. *Blood* 110:82–90, 2007.
46. Calvi LM, Adams GB, Weibrecht KW, et al: Osteoblastic cells regulate the haematopoietic stem cell niche. *Nature* 425:841–846, 2003.
47. Mendez-Ferrer S, Michurina TV, Ferraro F, et al: Mesenchymal and haematopoietic stem cells form a unique bone marrow niche. *Nature* 466:829–834, 2010.
48. Masuda S, Ageyama N, Shibata H, et al: Cotransplantation with MSCs improves engraftment of HSCs after autologous intra-bone marrow transplantation in nonhuman primates. *Exp Hematol* 37:1250–1257.e1, 2009.
49. Zannettino AC, Buhring HJ, Niutta S, et al: The sialomucin CD164 (MGC-24v) is an adhesive glycoprotein expressed by human hematopoietic progenitors and bone marrow stromal cells that serves as a potent negative regulator of hematopoiesis. *Blood* 92:2613–2628, 1998.
50. Nilsson SK, Johnston HM, Whitty GA, et al: Osteopontin, a key component of the hematopoietic stem cell niche and regulator of primitive hematopoietic progenitor cells. *Blood* 106:1232–1239, 2005.
51. Brunner S, Zaruba MM, Huber B, et al: Parathyroid hormone effectively induces mobilization of progenitor cells without depletion of bone marrow. *Exp Hematol* 36:1157–1166, 2008.
52. Ballen K, Mendizabal AM, Cutler C, et al: Phase II trial of parathyroid hormone after double umbilical cord blood transplantation. *Biol Blood Marrow Transplant* 18:1851–1858, 2012.
53. Pulsipher MA, Chitphakdithai P, Logan BR, et al: Lower risk for serious adverse events and no increased risk for cancer after PBSC vs BM donation. *Blood* 123:3655–3663, 2014.
54. Styczynski J, Balduzzi A, Gil L, et al: Risk of complications during hematopoietic stem cell collection in pediatric sibling donors: A prospective European Group for Blood and Marrow Transplantation Pediatric Diseases Working Party study. *Blood* 119:2935–2942, 2012.
55. Chan KW, Gajewski JL, Supkis D Jr, et al: Use of minors as bone marrow donors: Current attitude and management. A survey of 56 pediatric transplantation centers. *J Pediatr* 128:644–648, 1996.

56. Siena S, Bregni M, Brando B, et al: Circulation of CD34+ hematopoietic stem cells in the peripheral blood of high-dose cyclophosphamide-treated patients: Enhancement by intravenous recombinant human granulocyte-macrophage colony-stimulating factor. *Blood* 74:1905–1914, 1989.

57. Chao NJ, Schriber JR, Grimes K, et al: Granulocyte colony-stimulating factor "mobilized" peripheral blood progenitor cells accelerate granulocyte and platelet recovery after high-dose chemotherapy. *Blood* 81:2031–2035, 1993.

58. Becker PS, Wagle M, Matous S, et al: Spontaneous splenic rupture following administration of granulocyte colony-stimulating factor (G-CSF): Occurrence in an allogeneic donor of peripheral blood stem cells. *Biol Blood Marrow Transplant* 3:45–49, 1997.

59. Falzetti F, Aversa F, Minelli O, et al: Spontaneous rupture of spleen during peripheral blood stem-cell mobilisation in a healthy donor. *Lancet* 353:555, 1999.

60. Storek J, Dawson MA, Maloney DG: Normal T, B, and NK cell counts in healthy donors at 1 year after blood stem cell harvesting. *Blood* 95:2993–2994, 2000.

61. Duong HK, Savani BN, Copelan E, et al: Peripheral blood progenitor cell mobilization for autologous and allogeneic hematopoietic cell transplantation: Guidelines from the American Society for Blood and Marrow Transplantation. *Biol Blood Marrow Transplant* 20:1262–1273, 2014.

62. Calandra G, McCarty J, McGuirk J, et al: AMD3100 plus G-CSF can successfully mobilize CD34+ cells from non-Hodgkin's lymphoma, Hodgkin's disease and multiple myeloma patients previously failing mobilization with chemotherapy and/or cytokine treatment: Compassionate use data. *Bone Marrow Transplant* 41:331–338, 2008.

63. Devine SM, Vij R, Rettig M, et al: Rapid mobilization of functional donor hematopoietic cells without G-CSF using AMD3100, an antagonist of the CXCR4/SDF-1 interaction. *Blood* 112:990–998, 2008.

64. Lundqvist A, Smith AL, Takahashi Y, et al: Differences in the phenotype, cytokine gene expression profiles, and in vivo alloreactivity of T cells mobilized with plerixafor compared with G-CSF. *J Immunol* 191:6241–6249, 2013.

65. Mendez-Ferrer S, Lucas D, Battista M, et al: Haematopoietic stem cell release is regulated by circadian oscillations. *Nature* 452:442–447, 2008.

66. Lucas D, Battista M, Shi PA, et al: Mobilized hematopoietic stem cell yield depends on species-specific circadian timing. *Cell Stem Cell* 3:364–366, 2008.

67. Shi PA, Isola LM, Gabrilove JL, et al: Prospective cohort study of the circadian rhythm pattern in allogeneic sibling donors undergoing standard granulocyte colony-stimulating factor mobilization. *Stem Cell Res Ther* 4:30, 2013.

68. Schmitz N, Linch DC, Dreger P, et al: Randomised trial of filgrastim-mobilised peripheral blood progenitor cell transplantation versus autologous bone-marrow transplantation in lymphoma patients. *Lancet* 347:353–357, 1996.

69. Vose JM, Sharp G, Chan WC, et al: Autologous transplantation for aggressive non-Hodgkin's lymphoma: Results of a randomized trial evaluating graft source and minimal residual disease. *J Clin Oncol* 20:2344–2352, 2002.

70. Vellenga E, van Agthoven M, Croockewit AJ, et al: Autologous peripheral blood stem cell transplantation in patients with relapsed lymphoma results in accelerated haematopoietic reconstitution, improved quality of life and cost reduction compared with bone marrow transplantation: The Hovon 22 study. *Br J Haematol* 114:319–326, 2001.

71. Toh HC, Sun L, Soe Y, et al: G-CSF induces a potentially tolerant gene and immunophenotype profile in T cells *in vivo*. *Clin Immunol* 132:83–92, 2009.

72. Anasetti C, Logan BR, Lee SJ, et al: Peripheral-blood stem cells versus bone marrow from unrelated donors. *N Engl J Med* 367:1487–1496, 2012.

73. Friedrichs B, Tichelli A, Bacigalupo A, et al: Long-term outcome and late effects in patients transplanted with mobilised blood or bone marrow: A randomised trial. *Lancet Oncol* 11:331–338, 2010.

74. Mielcarek M, Storer B, Martin PJ, et al: Long-term outcomes after transplantation of HLA-identical related G-CSF-mobilized peripheral blood mononuclear cells versus bone marrow. *Blood* 119:2675–2678, 2012.

75. Couban S, Simpson DR, Barnett MJ, et al: A randomized multicenter comparison of bone marrow and peripheral blood in recipients of matched sibling allogeneic transplants for myeloid malignancies. *Blood* 100:1525–1531, 2002.

76. Holtick U, Albrecht M, Chemnitz JM, et al: Bone marrow versus peripheral blood allogeneic haematopoietic stem cell transplantation for haematological malignancies in adults. *Cochrane Database Syst Rev* 4:Cd010189, 2014.

77. Zhang H, Chen J, Que W: Allogeneic peripheral blood stem cell and bone marrow transplantation for hematologic malignancies: Meta-analysis of randomized controlled trials. *Leuk Res* 36:431–437, 2012.

78. Chang YJ, Weng CL, Sun LX, et al: Allogeneic bone marrow transplantation compared to peripheral blood stem cell transplantation for the treatment of hematologic malignancies: A meta-analysis based on time-to-event data from randomized controlled trials. *Ann Hematol* 91:427–437, 2012.

79. Bensinger WI, Martin PJ, Storer B, et al: Transplantation of bone marrow as compared with peripheral-blood cells from HLA-identical relatives in patients with hematologic cancers. *N Engl J Med* 344:175–181, 2001.

80. Gragert L, Eapen M, Williams E, et al: HLA match likelihoods for hematopoietic stem-cell grafts in the U.S. registry. *N Engl J Med* 371:339–348, 2014.

81. Arcese W, Rocha V, Labopin M, et al: Unrelated cord blood transplants in adults with hematologic malignancies. *Haematologica* 91:223–230, 2006.

82. Gluckman E, Broxmeyer HA, Auerbach AD, et al: Hematopoietic reconstitution in a patient with Fanconi's anemia by means of umbilical-cord blood from an HLA-identical sibling. *N Engl J Med* 321:1174–1178, 1989.

83. Gluckman E, Ruggeri A, Volt F, et al: Milestones in umbilical cord blood transplantation. *Br J Haematol* 154:441–447, 2011.

84. Barker JN, Scaradavou A, Stevens CE: Combined effect of total nucleated cell dose and HLA match on transplantation outcome in 1061 cord blood recipients with hematologic malignancies. *Blood* 115:1843–1849, 2010.

85. Ponce DM, Gonzales A, Lubin M, et al: Graft-versus-host disease after double-unit cord blood transplantation has unique features and an association with engrafting unit-to-recipient HLA match. *Biol Blood Marrow Transplant* 19:904–911, 2013.

86. Avery S, Shi W, Lubin M, et al: Influence of infused cell dose and HLA match on engraftment after double-unit cord blood allografts. *Blood* 117:3277–3285; quiz 3478, 2011.

87. Wagner JE, Barker JN, DeFor TE, et al: Transplantation of unrelated donor umbilical cord blood in 102 patients with malignant and nonmalignant diseases: Influence of CD34 cell dose and HLA disparity on treatment-related mortality and survival. *Blood* 100:1611–1618, 2002.

88. Wagner JE Jr, Eapen M, Carter S, et al: One-unit versus two-unit cord-blood transplantation for hematologic cancers. *N Engl J Med* 371:1685–1694, 2014.

89. Sideri A, Neokleous N, Brunet De La Grange P, et al: An overview of the progress on double umbilical cord blood transplantation. *Haematologica* 96:1213–1220, 2011.

90. Gutman JA, Turtle CJ, Manley TJ, et al: Single-unit dominance after double-unit umbilical cord blood transplantation coincides with a specific CD8+ T-cell response against the nonengrafted unit. *Blood* 115:757–765, 2010.

91. Delaney C, Heimfeld S, Brashem-Stein C, et al: Notch-mediated expansion of human cord blood progenitor cells capable of rapid myeloid reconstitution. *Nat Med* 16:232–236, 2010.

92. de Lima M, McNiece I, Robinson SN, et al: Cord-blood engraftment with *ex vivo* mesenchymal-cell coculture. *N Engl J Med* 367:2305–2315, 2012.

93. Cutler C, Multani P, Robbins D, et al: Prostaglandin-modulated umbilical cord blood hematopoietic stem cell transplantation. *Blood* 122:3074–3081, 2013.

94. Risdon G, Gaddy J, Broxmeyer HE: Allogeneic responses of human umbilical cord blood. *Blood Cells* 20:566–570; discussion 571–572, 1994.

95. Renard C, Barlogis V, Mialou V, et al: Lymphocyte subset reconstitution after unrelated cord blood or bone marrow transplantation in children. *Br J Haematol* 152:322–330, 2011.

96. Herrera AF, Soriano G, Bellizzi AM, et al: Cord colitis syndrome in cord-blood stem-cell transplantation. *N Engl J Med* 365:815–824, 2011.

97. Bhatt AS, Freeman SS, Herrera AF, et al: Sequence-based discovery of *Bradyrhizobium enterica* in cord colitis syndrome. *N Engl J Med* 369:517–528, 2013.

98. Milano F, Shulman HM, Guthrie KA, et al: Late-onset colitis after cord blood transplantation is consistent with graft-versus-host disease: Results of a blinded histopathological review. *Biol Blood Marrow Transplant* 20:1008–1013, 2014.

99. Shimoji S, Kato K, Eriguchi Y, et al: Evaluating the association between histological manifestations of cord colitis syndrome with GVHD. *Bone Marrow Transplant* 48:1249–1252, 2013.

100. Ash RC, Horowitz MM, Gale RP, et al: Bone marrow transplantation from related donors other than HLA-identical siblings: Effect of T cell depletion. *Bone Marrow Transplant* 7:443–452, 1991.

101. Aversa F, Velardi A, Tabilio A, et al: Haplo-identical stem cell transplantation in leukemia. *Blood Rev* 15:111–119, 2001.

102. Aversa F, Tabilio A, Velardi A, et al: Treatment of high-risk acute leukemia with T-cell-depleted stem cells from related donors with one fully mismatched HLA haplotype. *N Engl J Med* 339:1186–1193, 1998.

103. Aversa F: Haplo-identical haematopoietic stem cell transplantation for acute leukaemia in adults: Experience in Europe and the United States. *Bone Marrow Transplant* 41:473–481, 2008.

104. Ruggeri L, Capanni M, Urbani E, et al: Effectiveness of donor natural killer cell alloreactivity in mismatched hematopoietic transplants. *Science* 295:2097–2100, 2002.

105. Aversa F, Terenzi A, Tabilio A, et al: Full haplotype-mismatched hematopoietic stem-cell transplantation: A phase II study in patients with acute leukemia at high risk of relapse. *J Clin Oncol* 23:3447–3454, 2005.

106. Luznik L, Jalla S, Engstrom LW, et al: Durable engraftment of major histocompatibility complex-incompatible cells after nonmyeloablative conditioning with fludarabine, low-dose total body irradiation, and posttransplantation cyclophosphamide. *Blood* 98:3456–3464, 2001.

107. O'Donnell PV, Luznik L, Jones RJ, et al: Nonmyeloablative bone marrow transplantation from partially HLA-mismatched related donors using posttransplantation cyclophosphamide. *Biol Blood Marrow Transplant* 8:377–386, 2002.

108. Brunstein CG, Fuchs EJ, Carter SL, et al: Alternative donor transplantation after reduced intensity conditioning: Results of parallel phase 2 trials using partially HLA-mismatched related bone marrow or unrelated double umbilical cord blood grafts. *Blood* 118:282–288, 2011.

109. Kanakry JA, Kasamon YL, Bolanos-Meade J, et al: Absence of post-transplantation lymphoproliferative disorder after allogeneic blood or marrow transplantation using post-transplantation cyclophosphamide as graft-versus-host disease prophylaxis. *Biol Blood Marrow Transplant* 19:1514–1517, 2013.

110. van Rood JJ, Loberiza FR Jr, Zhang MJ, et al: Effect of tolerance to noninherited maternal antigens on the occurrence of graft-versus-host disease after bone marrow transplantation from a parent or an HLA-haplo-identical sibling. *Blood* 99:1572–1577, 2002.

111. Stern M, Ruggeri L, Mancusi A, et al: Survival after T cell-depleted haplo-identical stem cell transplantation is improved using the mother as donor. *Blood* 112:2990–2995, 2008.

112. Wang Y, Chang YJ, Xu LP, et al: Who is the best donor for a related HLA haplotype-mismatched transplant? *Blood* 124:843–850, 2014.

113. Aoyama K, Koyama M, Matsuoka K, et al: Improved outcome of allogeneic bone marrow transplantation due to breastfeeding-induced tolerance to maternal antigens. *Blood* 113:1829–1833, 2009.

114. Alici E, Bjorkstrand B, Treschow A, et al: Long-term follow-up of gene-marked CD34+ cells after autologous stem cell transplantation for multiple myeloma. *Cancer Gene Ther* 14:227–232, 2007.

115. Brenner MK, Rill DR, Moen RC, et al: Gene-marking to trace origin of relapse after autologous bone-marrow transplantation. *Lancet* 341:85–86, 1993.

116. Kasamon YL, Jones RJ, Gocke CD, et al: Extended follow-up of autologous bone marrow transplantation with 4-hydroperoxycyclophosphamide (4-HC) purging for indolent or transformed non-Hodgkin lymphomas. *Biol Blood Marrow Transplant* 17:365–373, 2011.

117. Bartee E, Chan WM, Moreb JS, et al: Selective purging of human multiple myeloma cells from autologous stem cell transplantation grafts using oncolytic myxoma virus. *Biol Blood Marrow Transplant* 18:1540–1551, 2012.

118. Pettengell R, Schmitz N, Gisselbrecht C, et al: Rituximab purging and/or maintenance in patients undergoing autologous transplantation for relapsed follicular lymphoma: A prospective randomized trial from the lymphoma working party of the European group for blood and marrow transplantation. *J Clin Oncol* 31:1624–1630, 2013.

119. Yahng SA, Yoon JH, Shin SH, et al: Influence of ex vivo purging with CliniMACS CD34(+) selection on outcome after autologous stem cell transplantation in non-Hodgkin lymphoma. *Br J Haematol* 164:555–564, 2014.

120. Gribben JG, Freedman AS, Neuberg D, et al: Immunologic purging of marrow assessed by PCR before autologous bone marrow transplantation for B-cell lymphoma. *N Engl J Med* 325:1525–1533, 1991.

121. van Heeckeren WJ, Vollweiler J, Fu P, et al: Randomised comparison of two B-cell purging protocols for patients with B-cell non-Hodgkin lymphoma: In vivo purging with rituximab versus ex vivo purging with CliniMACS CD34 cell enrichment device. *Br J Haematol* 132:42–55, 2006.

122. Stewart AK, Vescio R, Schiller G, et al: Purging of autologous peripheral-blood stem cells using CD34 selection does not improve overall or progression-free survival after high-dose chemotherapy for multiple myeloma: Results of a multicenter randomized controlled trial. *J Clin Oncol* 19:3771–3779, 2001.

123. Holmberg LA, Boeckh M, Hooper H, et al: Increased incidence of cytomegalovirus disease after autologous CD34-selected peripheral blood stem cell transplantation. *Blood* 94:4029–4035, 1999.

124. Crippa F, Holmberg L, Carter RA, et al: Infectious complications after autologous CD34-selected peripheral blood stem cell transplantation. *Biol Blood Marrow Transplant* 8:281–289, 2002.

125. Kernan NA, Flomenberg N, Dupont B, et al: Graft rejection in recipients of T-cell-depleted HLA-nonidentical marrow transplants for leukemia. Identification of host-derived antidonor allocytotoxic T lymphocytes. *Transplantation* 43:842–847, 1987.

126. Kernan NA, Bordignon C, Heller G, et al: Graft failure after T-cell-depleted human leukocyte antigen identical marrow transplants for leukemia: I. Analysis of risk factors and results of secondary transplants. *Blood* 74:2227–2236, 1989.

127. Fefer A, Cheever MA, Thomas ED, et al: Bone marrow transplantation for refractory acute leukemia in 34 patients with identical twins. *Blood* 57:421–430, 1981.

128. Gale RP, Horowitz MM, Ash RC, et al: Identical-twin bone marrow transplants for leukemia. *Ann Intern Med* 120:646–652, 1994.

129. Martin PJ, Clift RA, Fisher LD, et al: HLA-identical marrow transplantation during accelerated-phase chronic myelogenous leukemia: Analysis of survival and remission duration. *Blood* 72:1978–1984, 1988.

130. Kolb HJ, Mittermuller J, Clemm C, et al: Donor leukocyte transfusions for treatment of recurrent chronic myelogenous leukemia in marrow transplant patients. *Blood* 76:2462–2465, 1990.

131. Drobyski WR, Keever CA, Roth MS, et al: Salvage immunotherapy using donor leukocyte infusions as treatment for relapsed chronic myelogenous leukemia after allogeneic bone marrow transplantation: Efficacy and toxicity of a defined T-cell dose. *Blood* 82:2310–2318, 1993.

132. Dazzi F, Szydlo RM, Cross NC, et al: Durability of responses following donor lymphocyte infusions for patients who relapse after allogeneic stem cell transplantation for chronic myeloid leukemia. *Blood* 96:2712–2716, 2000.

133. Ruggeri L, Mancusi A, Capanni M, et al: Donor natural killer cell allorecognition of missing self in haplo-identical hematopoietic transplantation for acute myeloid leukemia: Challenging its predictive value. *Blood* 110:433–440, 2007.

134. Bellucci R, Alyea EP, Chiaretti S, et al: Graft-versus-tumor response in patients with multiple myeloma is associated with antibody response to BCMA, a plasma-cell membrane receptor. *Blood* 105:3945–3950, 2005.

135. Faber LM, van der Hoeven J, Goulmy E, et al: Recognition of clonogenic leukemic cells, remission bone marrow and HLA-identical donor bone marrow by CD8+ or CD4+ minor histocompatibility antigen-specific cytotoxic T lymphocytes. *J Clin Invest* 96:877–883, 1995.

136. Bonnet D, Warren EH, Greenberg PD, et al: CD8(+) minor histocompatibility antigen-specific cytotoxic T lymphocyte clones eliminate human acute myeloid leukemia stem cells. *Proc Natl Acad Sci U S A* 96:8639–8644, 1999.

137. Scheibenbogen C, Letsch A, Thiel E, et al: CD8 T-cell responses to Wilms tumor gene product WT1 and proteinase 3 in patients with acute myeloid leukemia. *Blood* 100:2132–2137, 2002.

138. Delmon L, Ythier A, Moingeon P, et al: Characterization of antileukemia cells' cytotoxic effector function. Implications for monitoring natural killer responses following allogeneic bone marrow transplantation. *Transplantation* 42:252–256, 1986.

139. Higuchi CM, Thompson JA, Cox T, et al: Lymphokine-activated killer function following autologous bone marrow transplantation for refractory hematological malignancies. *Cancer Res* 49:5509–5513, 1989.

140. Linn YC, Niam M, Chu S, et al: The anti-tumour activity of allogeneic cytokine-induced killer cells in patients who relapse after allogeneic transplant for haematological malignancies. *Bone Marrow Transplant* 47:957–966, 2012.

141. Laport GG, Sheehan K, Baker J, et al: Adoptive immunotherapy with cytokine-induced killer cells for patients with relapsed hematologic malignancies after allogeneic hematopoietic cell transplantation. *Biol Blood Marrow Transplant* 17:1679–1687, 2011.

142. Venstrom JM, Pittari G, Gooley TA, et al: HLA-C-dependent prevention of leukemia relapse by donor activating KIR2DS1. *N Engl J Med* 367:805–816, 2012.

143. Ringden O, Labopin M, Gorin NC, et al: Is there a graft-versus-leukaemia effect in the absence of graft-versus-host disease in patients undergoing bone marrow transplantation for acute leukaemia? *Br J Haematol* 111:1130–1137, 2000.

144. Edinger M, Hoffmann P, Ermann J, et al: CD4+CD25+ regulatory T cells preserve graft-versus-tumor activity while inhibiting graft-versus-host disease after bone marrow transplantation. *Nat Med* 9:1144–1150, 2003.

145. Di Ianni M, Falzetti F, Carotti A, et al: Tregs prevent GVHD and promote immune reconstitution in HLA-haplo-identical transplantation. *Blood* 117:3921–3928, 2011.

146. Martelli MF, Di Ianni M, Ruggeri L, et al: HLA-haplo-identical transplantation with regulatory and conventional T-cell adoptive immunotherapy prevents acute leukemia relapse. *Blood* 124:638–644, 2014.

147. Clift RA, Buckner CD, Appelbaum FR, et al: Long-term follow-Up of a randomized trial of two irradiation regimens for patients receiving allogeneic marrow transplants during first remission of acute myeloid leukemia. *Blood* 92:1455–1456, 1998.

148. Faraci M, Barra S, Cohen A, et al: Very late nonfatal consequences of fractionated TBI in children undergoing bone marrow transplant. *Int J Radiat Oncol Biol Phys* 63:1568–1575, 2005.

149. Thomas O, Mahe M, Campion L, et al: Long-term complications of total body irradiation in adults. *Int J Radiat Oncol Biol Phys* 49:125–131, 2001.

150. Kolb HJ, Socie G, Duell T, et al: Malignant neoplasms in long-term survivors of bone marrow transplantation. Late Effects Working Party of the European Cooperative Group for Blood and Marrow Transplantation and the European Late Effect Project Group. *Ann Intern Med* 131:738–744, 1999.

151. Cosset JM, Baume D, Pico JL, et al: Single dose versus hyperfractionated total body irradiation before allogeneic bone marrow transplantation: A non-randomized comparative study of 54 patients at the Institut Gustave-Roussy. *Radiother Oncol* 15:151–160, 1989.

152. Shank B, O'Reilly RJ, Cunningham I, et al: Total body irradiation for bone marrow transplantation: The Memorial Sloan-Kettering Cancer Center experience. *Radiother Oncol* 18 (Suppl 1):68–81, 1990.

153. Marks DI, Forman SJ, Blume KG, et al: A comparison of cyclophosphamide and total body irradiation with etoposide and total body irradiation as conditioning regimens for patients undergoing sibling allografting for acute lymphoblastic leukemia in first or second complete remission. *Biol Blood Marrow Transplant* 12:438–453, 2006.

154. Jamieson CH, Amylon MD, Wong RM, et al: Allogeneic hematopoietic cell transplantation for patients with high-risk acute lymphoblastic leukemia in first or second complete remission using fractionated total-body irradiation and high-dose etoposide: A 15-year experience. *Exp Hematol* 31:981–986, 2003.

155. Pagel JM, Gooley TA, Rajendran J, et al: Allogeneic hematopoietic cell transplantation after conditioning with 131I-anti-CD45 antibody plus fludarabine and low-dose total body irradiation for elderly patients with advanced acute myeloid leukemia or high-risk myelodysplastic syndrome. *Blood* 114:5444–5453, 2009.

156. Gopal AK, Guthrie KA, Rajendran J, et al: (9)(0)Y-Ibritumomab tiuxetan, fludarabine, and TBI-based nonmyeloablative allogeneic transplantation conditioning for patients with persistent high-risk B-cell lymphoma. *Blood* 118:1132–1139, 2011.

157. Gopal AK, Gooley TA, Rajendran JG, et al: Myeloablative I-131-tositumomab with escalating doses of fludarabine and autologous hematopoietic transplantation for adults age ≥ 60 years with B cell lymphoma. *Biol Blood Marrow Transplant* 20:770–775, 2014.

158. Mawad R, Gooley TA, Rajendran JG, et al: Radiolabeled anti-CD45 antibody with reduced-intensity conditioning and allogeneic transplantation for younger patients with advanced acute myeloid leukemia or myelodysplastic syndrome. *Biol Blood Marrow Transplant* 20:1363–1368, 2014.

159. Nakamae H, Wilbur DS, Hamlin DK, et al: Biodistributions, myelosuppression, and toxicities in mice treated with an anti-CD45 antibody labeled with the alpha-emitting radionuclides bismuth-213 or astatine-211. *Cancer Res* 69:2408–2415, 2009.

160. Park SI, Shenoi J, Pagel JM, et al: Conventional and pretargeted radioimmunotherapy using bismuth-213 to target and treat non-Hodgkin lymphomas expressing CD20: A preclinical model toward optimal consolidation therapy to eradicate minimal residual disease. *Blood* 116:4231–4239, 2010.

161. Pagel JM, Kenoyer AL, Back T, et al: Anti-CD45 pretargeted radioimmunotherapy using bismuth-213: High rates of complete remission and long-term survival in a mouse myeloid leukemia xenograft model. *Blood* 118:703–711, 2011.

162. Orozco JJ, Back T, Kenoyer A, et al: Anti-CD45 radioimmunotherapy using (211)At with bone marrow transplantation prolongs survival in a disseminated murine leukemia model. *Blood* 121:3759–3767, 2013.

163. Pecego R, Hill R, Appelbaum FR, et al: Interstitial pneumonitis following autologous bone marrow transplantation. *Transplantation* 42:515–517, 1986.

164. Law LY, Horning SJ, Wong RM, et al: High-dose carmustine, etoposide, and cyclophosphamide followed by allogeneic hematopoietic cell transplantation for non-Hodgkin lymphoma. *Biol Blood Marrow Transplant* 12:703–711, 2006.

165. Santos GW, Tutschka PJ, Brookmeyer R, et al: Marrow transplantation for acute non-lymphocytic leukemia after treatment with busulfan and cyclophosphamide. *N Engl J Med* 309:1347–1353, 1983.

166. Tutschka PJ, Copelan EA, Klein JP: Bone marrow transplantation for leukemia following a new busulfan and cyclophosphamide regimen. *Blood* 70:1382–1388, 1987.

167. Clift RA, Buckner CD, Thomas ED, et al: Marrow transplantation for chronic myeloid leukemia: A randomized study comparing cyclophosphamide and total body irradiation with busulfan and cyclophosphamide. *Blood* 84:2036–2043, 1994.

168. Pidala J, Kim J, Anasetti C, et al: Pharmacokinetic targeting of intravenous busulfan reduces conditioning regimen related toxicity following allogeneic hematopoietic cell transplantation for acute myelogenous leukemia. *J Hematol Oncol* 3:36, 2010.

169. Lee JW, Kang HJ, Lee SH, et al: Highly variable pharmacokinetics of once-daily intravenous busulfan when combined with fludarabine in pediatric patients: Phase I clinical study for determination of optimal once-daily busulfan dose using pharmacokinetic modeling. *Biol Blood Marrow Transplant* 18:944–950, 2012.

170. DeLeve LD: Cellular target of cyclophosphamide toxicity in the murine liver: Role of glutathione and site of metabolic activation. *Hepatology* 24:830–837, 1996.

171. DeLeve LD, Wang X: Role of oxidative stress and glutathione in busulfan toxicity in cultured murine hepatocytes. *Pharmacology* 60:143–154, 2000.

172. Rezvani AR, McCune JS, Storer BE, et al: Cyclophosphamide followed by intravenous targeted busulfan for allogeneic hematopoietic cell transplantation: Pharmacokinetics and clinical outcomes. *Biol Blood Marrow Transplant* 19:1033–1039, 2013.

173. Liu DH, Xu LP, Zhang XH, et al: Substitution of cyclophosphamide in the modified BuCy regimen with fludarabine is associated with increased incidence of severe pneumonia: A prospective, randomized study. *Int J Hematol* 98:708–715, 2013.

174. Lee JH, Joo YD, Kim H, et al: Randomized trial of myeloablative conditioning regimens: Busulfan plus cyclophosphamide versus busulfan plus fludarabine. *J Clin Oncol* 31:701–709, 2013.

175. Storb R, Yu C, Wagner JL, et al: Stable mixed hematopoietic chimerism in DLA-identical littermate dogs given sublethal total body irradiation before and pharmacological immunosuppression after marrow transplantation. *Blood* 89:3048–3054, 1997.

176. McSweeney PA, Niederwieser D, Shizuru JA, et al: Hematopoietic cell transplantation in older patients with hematologic malignancies: Replacing high-dose cytotoxic therapy with graft-versus-tumor effects. *Blood* 97:3390–3400, 2001.

177. Storb R, Gyurkocza B, Storer BE, et al: Graft-versus-host disease and graft-versus-tumor effects after allogeneic hematopoietic cell transplantation. *J Clin Oncol* 31:1530–1538, 2013.

178. Sorror ML, Storer BE, Sandmaier BM, et al: Five-year follow-up of patients with advanced chronic lymphocytic leukemia treated with allogeneic hematopoietic cell transplantation after nonmyeloablative conditioning. *J Clin Oncol* 26:4912–4920, 2008.

179. Rezvani AR, Storer B, Maris M, et al: Nonmyeloablative allogeneic hematopoietic cell transplantation in relapsed, refractory, and transformed indolent non-Hodgkin's lymphoma. *J Clin Oncol* 26:211–217, 2008.

180. Khouri IF, Keating M, Korbling M, et al: Transplant-lite: Induction of graft-versus-malignancy using fludarabine-based nonablative chemotherapy and allogeneic blood progenitor-cell transplantation as treatment for lymphoid malignancies. *J Clin Oncol* 16:2817–2824, 1998.

181. Khouri IF, Saliba RM, Erwin WD, et al: Nonmyeloablative allogeneic transplantation with or without 90yttrium ibritumomab tiuxetan is potentially curative for relapsed follicular lymphoma: 12-year results. *Blood* 119:6373–6378, 2012.

182. Lan F, Zeng D, Higuchi M, et al: Host conditioning with total lymphoid irradiation and antithymocyte globulin prevents graft-versus-host disease: The role of CD1-reactive natural killer T cells. *Biol Blood Marrow Transplant* 9:355–363, 2003.

183. Pillai AB, George TI, Dutt S, et al: Host natural killer T cells induce an interleukin-4-dependent expansion of donor CD4+CD25+Foxp3+ T regulatory cells that protects against graft-versus-host disease. *Blood* 113:4458–4467, 2009.

184. Lowsky R, Takahashi T, Liu YP, et al: Protective conditioning for acute graft-versus-host disease. *N Engl J Med* 353:1321–1331, 2005.

185. Kohrt HE, Turnbull BB, Heydari K, et al: TLI and ATG conditioning with low risk of graft-versus-host disease retains antitumor reactions after allogeneic hematopoietic cell transplantation from related and unrelated donors. *Blood* 114:1099–1109, 2009.

186. Baron F, Baker JE, Storb R, et al: Kinetics of engraftment in patients with hematologic malignancies given allogeneic hematopoietic cell transplantation after nonmyeloablative conditioning. *Blood* 104:2254–2262, 2004.

187. Morris E, Thomson K, Craddock C, et al: Outcomes after alemtuzumab-containing reduced-intensity allogeneic transplantation regimen for relapsed and refractory non-Hodgkin lymphoma. *Blood* 104:3865–3871, 2004.

188. Hill RS, Petersen FB, Storb R, et al: Mixed hematologic chimerism after allogeneic marrow transplantation for severe aplastic anemia is associated with a higher risk of graft rejection and a lessened incidence of acute graft-versus-host disease. *Blood* 67:811–816, 1986.

189. Scandling JD, Busque S, Dejbakhsh-Jones S, et al: Tolerance and withdrawal of immunosuppressive drugs in patients given kidney and hematopoietic cell transplants. *Am J Transplant* 12:1133–1145, 2012.

190. Blume KG, Krance RA: The evaluation and counseling of candidates for hematopoietic cell transplantation, in *Thomas' Hematopoietic Cell Transplantation* ed 4, edited by Appelbaum FR, Forman SJ, Negrin RS, Blume KG, p 445. Wiley-Blackwell, Hoboken, NJ, 2009.

191. Thomas ED, Buckner CD, Banaji M, et al: One hundred patients with acute leukemia treated by chemotherapy, total body irradiation, and allogeneic marrow transplantation. *Blood* 49:511–533, 1977.

192. Duval M, Klein JP, He W, et al: Hematopoietic stem-cell transplantation for acute leukemia in relapse or primary induction failure. *J Clin Oncol* 28:3730–3738, 2010.

193. Walter RB, Gooley TA, Wood BL, et al: Impact of pretransplantation minimal residual disease, as detected by multiparametric flow cytometry, on outcome of myeloablative hematopoietic cell transplantation for acute myeloid leukemia. *J Clin Oncol* 29:1190–1197, 2011.

194. Walter RB, Buckley SA, Pagel JM, et al: Significance of minimal residual disease before myeloablative allogeneic hematopoietic cell transplantation for AML in first and second complete remission. *Blood* 122:1813–1821, 2013.

195. Walter RB, Gyurkocza B, Storer BE, et al: Comparison of minimal residual disease as outcome predictor for AML patients in first complete remission undergoing myeloablative or nonmyeloablative allogeneic hematopoietic cell transplantation. *Leukemia* 29:137–144, 2015.

196. Crocchiolo R, Canevari C, Assanelli A, et al: Pre-transplant 18FDG-PET predicts outcome in lymphoma patients treated with high-dose sequential chemotherapy followed by autologous stem cell transplantation. *Leuk Lymphoma* 49:727–733, 2008.

197. Moskowitz CH, Matasar MJ, Zelenetz AD, et al: Normalization of pre-ASCT, FDG-PET imaging with second-line, non-cross-resistant, chemotherapy programs improves event-free survival in patients with Hodgkin lymphoma. *Blood* 119:1665–1670, 2012.

198. Akhtar S, Al-Sugair AS, Abouzied M, et al: Pre-transplant FDG-PET-based survival model in relapsed and refractory Hodgkin's lymphoma: Outcome after high-dose chemotherapy and auto-SCT. *Bone Marrow Transplant* 48:1530–1536, 2013.

199. Smeltzer JP, Cashen AF, Zhang Q, et al: Prognostic significance of FDG-PET in relapsed or refractory classical Hodgkin lymphoma treated with standard salvage chemotherapy and autologous stem cell transplantation. *Biol Blood Marrow Transplant* 17:1646–1652, 2011.

200. Wallen H, Gooley TA, Deeg HJ, et al: Ablative allogeneic hematopoietic cell transplantation in adults 60 years of age and older. *J Clin Oncol* 23:3439–3446, 2005.

201. Corradini P, Zallio F, Mariotti J, et al: Effect of age and previous autologous transplantation on nonrelapse mortality and survival in patients treated with reduced-intensity conditioning and allografting for advanced hematologic malignancies. *J Clin Oncol* 23:6690–6698, 2005.

202. Sorror ML, Sandmaier BM, Storer BE, et al: Long-term outcomes among older patients following nonmyeloablative conditioning and allogeneic hematopoietic cell transplantation for advanced hematologic malignancies. *JAMA* 306:1874–1883, 2011.

203. Brunner AM, Kim HT, Coughlin E, et al: Outcomes in patients age 70 or older undergoing allogeneic hematopoietic stem cell transplantation for hematologic malignancies. *Biol Blood Marrow Transplant* 19:1374–1380, 2013.

204. Sorror ML, Storb RF, Sandmaier BM, et al: Comorbidity-age index: A clinical measure of biologic age before allogeneic hematopoietic cell transplantation. *J Clin Oncol* 32:3249–3256, 2014.

205. Kumar SK, Dingli D, Lacy MQ, et al: Autologous stem cell transplantation in patients of 70 years and older with multiple myeloma: Results from a matched pair analysis. *Am J Hematol* 83:614–617, 2008.

206. Badros A, Barlogie B, Siegel E, et al: Autologous stem cell transplantation in elderly multiple myeloma patients over the age of 70 years. *Br J Haematol* 114:600–607, 2001.

207. Deeg HJ, Seidel K, Bruemmer B, et al: Impact of patient weight on non-relapse mortality after marrow transplantation. *Bone Marrow Transplant* 15:461–468, 1995.

208. Dickson TM, Kusnierz-Glaz CR, Blume KG, et al: Impact of admission body weight and chemotherapy dose adjustment on the outcome of autologous bone marrow transplantation. *Biol Blood Marrow Transplant* 5:299–305, 1999.

209. Gratwohl A, Hermans J, Goldman JM, et al: Risk assessment for patients with chronic myeloid leukaemia before allogeneic blood or marrow transplantation. Chronic Leukemia Working Party of the European Group for Blood and Marrow Transplantation. *Lancet* 352:1087–1092, 1998.

210. Parimon T, Au DH, Martin PJ, et al: A risk score for mortality after allogeneic hematopoietic cell transplantation. *Ann Intern Med* 144:407–414, 2006.

211. Sorror ML, Maris MB, Storb R, et al: Hematopoietic cell transplantation (HCT)-specific comorbidity index: A new tool for risk assessment before allogeneic HCT. *Blood* 106:2912–2919, 2005.

212. Barba P, Martino R, Perez-Simon JA, et al: Combination of the Hematopoietic Cell Transplantation Comorbidity Index and the European Group for Blood and Marrow Transplantation score allows a better stratification of high-risk patients undergoing reduced-toxicity allogeneic hematopoietic cell transplantation. *Biol Blood Marrow Transplant* 20:66–72, 2014.

213. Barba P, Pinana JL, Martino R, et al: Comparison of two pretransplant predictive models and a flexible HCT-CI using different cut off points to determine low-, intermediate-, and high-risk groups: The flexible HCT-CI Is the best predictor of NRM and OS in a population of patients undergoing allo-RIC. *Biol Blood Marrow Transplant* 16:413–420, 2010.

214. Pollack SM, Steinberg SM, Odom J, et al: Assessment of the hematopoietic cell transplantation comorbidity index in non-Hodgkin lymphoma patients receiving reduced-intensity allogeneic hematopoietic stem cell transplantation. *Biol Blood Marrow Transplant* 15:223–230, 2009.

215. Yamamoto W, Ogusa E, Matsumoto K, et al: Predictive value of risk assessment scores in patients with hematologic malignancies undergoing reduced-intensity conditioning allogeneic stem cell transplantation. *Am J Hematol* 89:E138–E141, 2014.

216. Nakaya A, Mori T, Tanaka M, et al: Does the hematopoietic cell transplantation specific comorbidity index (HCT-CI) predict transplantation outcomes? A prospective multicenter validation study of the Kanto Study Group for Cell Therapy. *Biol Blood Marrow Transplant* 20:1553–1559, 2014.

217. Horan JT, Logan BR, Agovi-Johnson MA, et al: Reducing the risk for transplantation-related mortality after allogeneic hematopoietic cell transplantation: How much progress has been made? *J Clin Oncol* 29:805–813, 2011.

218. Gooley TA, Chien JW, Pergam SA, et al: Reduced mortality after allogeneic hematopoietic-cell transplantation. *N Engl J Med* 363:2091–2101, 2010.

219. Hamadeh R, Ardehali A, Locksley RM, et al: Fatal aspergillosis associated with smoking contaminated marijuana, in a marrow transplant recipient. *Chest* 94:432–433, 1988.

220. Szyper-Kravitz M, Lang R, Manor Y, et al: Early invasive pulmonary aspergillosis in a leukemia patient linked to aspergillus contaminated marijuana smoking. *Leuk Lymphoma* 42:1433–1437, 2001.

221. Ladenstein R, Potschger U, Hartman O, et al: 28 years of high-dose therapy and SCT for neuroblastoma in Europe: Lessons from more than 4000 procedures. *Bone Marrow Transplant* 41 (Suppl 2):S118–S127, 2008.

222. Yalcin B, Kremer LC, Caron HN, et al: High-dose chemotherapy and autologous haematopoietic stem cell rescue for children with high-risk neuroblastoma. *Cochrane Database Syst Rev* 8:Cd006301, 2013.

223. Matthay KK, Reynolds CP, Seeger RC, et al: Long-term results for children with high-risk neuroblastoma treated on a randomized trial of myeloablative therapy followed by 13-cis-retinoic acid: A children's oncology group study. *J Clin Oncol* 27:1007–1013, 2009.

224. Lazarus HM, Stiff PJ, Carreras J, et al: Utility of single versus tandem autotransplants for advanced testes/germ cell cancer: A Center for International Blood and Marrow Transplant Research (CIBMTR) analysis. *Biol Blood Marrow Transplant* 13:778–789, 2007.

225. Howard DH, Kenline C, Lazarus HM, et al: Abandonment of high-dose chemotherapy/hematopoietic cell transplants for breast cancer following negative trial results. *Health Serv Res* 46:1762–1777, 2011.

226. Berry DA, Ueno NT, Johnson MM, et al: High-dose chemotherapy with autologous stem-cell support as adjuvant therapy in breast cancer: Overview of 15 randomized trials. *J Clin Oncol* 29:3214–3223, 2011.

227. Kahl C, Leisenring W, Deeg HJ, et al: Cyclophosphamide and antithymocyte globulin as a conditioning regimen for allogeneic marrow transplantation in patients with aplastic anaemia: A long-term follow-up. *Br J Haematol* 130:747–751, 2005.

228. Burroughs LM, Woolfrey AE, Storer BE, et al: Success of allogeneic marrow transplantation for children with severe aplastic anaemia. *Br J Haematol* 158:120–128, 2012.

229. Gaziev J, Marziali M, Isgro A, et al: Bone marrow transplantation for thalassemia from alternative related donors: Improved outcomes with a new approach. *Blood* 122:2751–2756, 2013.

230. La Nasa G, Caocci G, Efficace F, et al: Long-term health-related quality of life evaluated more than 20 years after hematopoietic stem cell transplantation for thalassemia. *Blood* 122:2262–2270, 2013.

231. Lucarelli G, Isgro A, Sodani P, et al: Hematopoietic SCT for the Black African and non-Black African variants of sickle cell anemia. *Bone Marrow Transplant* 49:1376–1381, 2014.

232. Hsieh MM, Fitzhugh CD, Weitzel RP, et al: Nonmyeloablative HLA-matched sibling allogeneic hematopoietic stem cell transplantation for severe sickle cell phenotype. *JAMA* 312:48–56, 2014.

233. Angelucci E, Matthes-Martin S, Baronciani D, et al: Hematopoietic stem cell transplantation in thalassemia major and sickle cell disease: Indications and management recommendations from an international expert panel. *Haematologica* 99:811–820, 2014.

234. Romero Z, Urbinati F, Geiger S, et al: Beta-globin gene transfer to human bone marrow for sickle cell disease. *J Clin Invest* 2013. [Epub ahead of print]

235. Pai SY, Logan BR, Griffith LM, et al: Transplantation outcomes for severe combined immunodeficiency, 2000–2009. *N Engl J Med* 371:434–446, 2014.

236. Moratto D, Giliani S, Bonfim C, et al: Long-term outcome and lineage-specific chimerism in 194 patients with Wiskott-Aldrich syndrome treated by hematopoietic cell transplantation in the period 1980–2009: An international collaborative study. *Blood* 118:1675–1684, 2011.

237. Boelens JJ, Aldenhoven M, Purtill D, et al: Outcomes of transplantation using various hematopoietic cell sources in children with Hurler syndrome after myeloablative conditioning. *Blood* 121:3981–3987, 2013.

238. Cornelissen JJ, van Putten WL, Verdonck LF, et al: Results of a HOVON/SAKK donor versus no-donor analysis of myeloablative HLA-identical sibling stem cell transplantation in first remission acute myeloid leukemia in young and middle-aged adults: Benefits for whom? *Blood* 109:3658–3666, 2007.

239. Suciu S, Mandelli F, de Witte T, et al: Allogeneic compared with autologous stem cell transplantation in the treatment of patients younger than 46 years with acute myeloid leukemia (AML) in first complete remission (CR1): An intention-to-treat analysis of the EORTC/GIMEMAAML-10 trial. *Blood* 102:1232–1240, 2003.

240. Koreth J, Schlenk R, Kopecky KJ, et al: Allogeneic stem cell transplantation for acute myeloid leukemia in first complete remission: Systematic review and meta-analysis of prospective clinical trials. *JAMA* 301:2349–2361, 2009.

241. Yanada M, Matsuo K, Emi N, et al: Efficacy of allogeneic hematopoietic stem cell transplantation depends on cytogenetic risk for acute myeloid leukemia in first disease remission: A metaanalysis. *Cancer* 103:1652–1658, 2005.

242. Walter RB, Pagel JM, Gooley TA, et al: Comparison of matched unrelated and matched related donor myeloablative hematopoietic cell transplantation for adults with acute myeloid leukemia in first remission. *Leukemia* 24:1276–1282, 2010.

243. Saber W, Opie S, Rizzo JD, et al: Outcomes after matched unrelated donor versus identical sibling hematopoietic cell transplantation in adults with acute myelogenous leukemia. *Blood* 119:3908–3916, 2012.

244. Farag SS, Maharry K, Zhang MJ, et al: Comparison of reduced-intensity hematopoietic cell transplantation with chemotherapy in patients age 60–70 years with acute myelogenous leukemia in first remission. *Biol Blood Marrow Transplant* 17:1796–1803, 2011.

245. Kurosawa S, Yamaguchi T, Uchida N, et al: Comparison of allogeneic hematopoietic cell transplantation and chemotherapy in elderly patients with non-M3 acute myelogenous leukemia in first complete remission. *Biol Blood Marrow Transplant* 17:401–411, 2011.

246. Schlenk RF, Dohner K, Krauter J, et al: Mutations and treatment outcome in cytogenetically normal acute myeloid leukemia. *N Engl J Med* 358:1909–1918, 2008.

247. Cornelissen JJ, Gratwohl A, Schlenk RF, et al: The European LeukemiaNet AML Working Party consensus statement on allogeneic HSCT for patients with AML in remission: An integrated-risk adapted approach. *Nat Rev Clin Oncol* 9:579–590, 2012.

248. Appelbaum FR: Indications for allogeneic hematopoietic cell transplantation for acute myeloid leukemia in the genomic era. *Am Soc Clin Oncol Educ Book* e327–e333, 2014.

249. Yeshurun M, Labopin M, Blaise D, et al: Impact of postremission consolidation chemotherapy on outcome after reduced-intensity conditioning allogeneic stem cell transplantation for patients with acute myeloid leukemia in first complete remission: A report from the Acute Leukemia Working Party of the European Group for Blood and Marrow Transplantation. *Cancer* 120:855–863, 2014.

250. Warlick ED, Paulson K, Brazauskas R, et al: Effect of postremission therapy before reduced-intensity conditioning allogeneic transplantation for acute myeloid leukemia in first complete remission. *Biol Blood Marrow Transplant* 20:202–208, 2014.

251. Armistead PM, de Lima M, Pierce S, et al: Quantifying the survival benefit for allogeneic hematopoietic stem cell transplantation in relapsed acute myelogenous leukemia. *Biol Blood Marrow Transplant* 15:1431–1438, 2009.

252. Kroger N, Brand R, van Biezen A, et al: Autologous stem cell transplantation for therapy-related acute myeloid leukemia and myelodysplastic syndrome. *Bone Marrow Transplant* 37:183–189, 2006.

253. Laughlin MJ, Eapen M, Rubinstein P, et al: Outcomes after transplantation of cord blood or bone marrow from unrelated donors in adults with leukemia. *N Engl J Med* 351:2265–2275, 2004.

254. Rocha V, Labopin M, Sanz G, et al: Transplants of umbilical-cord blood or bone marrow from unrelated donors in adults with acute leukemia. *N Engl J Med* 351:2276–2285, 2004.

255. Fung HC, Stein A, Slovak M, et al: A long-term follow-up report on allogeneic stem cell transplantation for patients with primary refractory acute myelogenous leukemia: Impact of cytogenetic characteristics on transplantation outcome. *Biol Blood Marrow Transplant* 9:766–771, 2003.

256. Pui CH, Evans WE: Treatment of acute lymphoblastic leukemia. *N Engl J Med* 354:166–178, 2006.

257. Cornelissen JJ, van der Holt B, Verhoef GE, et al: Myeloablative allogeneic versus autologous stem cell transplantation in adult patients with acute lymphoblastic leukemia in first remission: A prospective sibling donor versus no-donor comparison. *Blood* 113:1375–1382, 2009.

258. Goldstone AH, Richards SM, Lazarus HM, et al: In adults with standard-risk acute lymphoblastic leukemia, the greatest benefit is achieved from a matched sibling allogeneic transplantation in first complete remission, and an autologous transplantation is less effective than conventional consolidation/maintenance chemotherapy in all patients: Final results of the International ALL Trial (MRC UKALL XII/ECOG E2993). *Blood* 111:1827–1833, 2008.

259. Gupta V, Richards S, Rowe J: Allogeneic, but not autologous, hematopoietic cell transplantation improves survival only among younger adults with acute lymphoblastic leukemia in first remission: An individual patient data meta-analysis. *Blood* 121:339–350, 2013.

260. Pidala J, Djulbegovic B, Anasetti C, et al: Allogeneic hematopoietic cell transplantation for adult acute lymphoblastic leukemia (ALL) in first complete remission. *Cochrane Database Syst Rev* 10:Cd008818, 2011.

261. Ram R, Storb R, Sandmaier BM, et al: Non-myeloablative conditioning with allogeneic hematopoietic cell transplantation for the treatment of high-risk acute lymphoblastic leukemia. *Haematologica* 96:1113–1120, 2011.

262. Laport GG, Alvarnas JC, Palmer JM, et al: Long-term remission of Philadelphia chromosome-positive acute lymphoblastic leukemia after allogeneic hematopoietic cell transplantation from matched sibling donors: A 20-year experience with the fractionated total body irradiation-etoposide regimen. *Blood* 112:903–909, 2008.

263. Mizuta S, Matsuo K, Nishiwaki S, et al: Pretransplant administration of imatinib for allo-HSCT in patients with BCR-ABL-positive acute lymphoblastic leukemia. *Blood* 123:2325–2332, 2014.

264. Schultz KR, Carroll A, Heerema NA, et al: Long-term follow-up of imatinib in pediatric Philadelphia chromosome-positive acute lymphoblastic leukemia: Children's Oncology Group study AALL0031. *Leukemia* 28:1467–1471, 2014.

265. Attal M, Harousseau JL, Stoppa AM, et al: A prospective, randomized trial of autologous bone marrow transplantation and chemotherapy in multiple myeloma. Intergroupe Francais du Myelome. *N Engl J Med* 335:91–97, 1996.

266. Child JA, Morgan GJ, Davies FE, et al: High-dose chemotherapy with hematopoietic stem-cell rescue for multiple myeloma. *N Engl J Med* 348:1875–1883, 2003.

267. Fermand JP, Katsahian S, Divine M, et al: High-dose therapy and autologous blood stem-cell transplantation compared with conventional treatment in myeloma patients aged 55 to 65 years: Long-term results of a randomized control trial from the Group Myelome-Autogreffe. *J Clin Oncol* 23:9227–9233, 2005.

268. Fermand JP, Ravaud P, Chevret S, et al: High-dose therapy and autologous peripheral blood stem cell transplantation in multiple myeloma: Up-front or rescue treatment? Results of a multicenter sequential randomized clinical trial. *Blood* 92:3131–3136, 1998.

269. Palumbo A, Cavallo F, Gay F, et al: Autologous transplantation and maintenance therapy in multiple myeloma. *N Engl J Med* 371:895–905, 2014.

270. Kumar A, Kharfan-Dabaja MA, Glasmacher A, et al: Tandem versus single autologous hematopoietic cell transplantation for the treatment of multiple myeloma: A systematic review and meta-analysis. *J Natl Cancer Inst* 101:100–106, 2009.

271. Attal M, Harousseau JL, Facon T, et al: Single versus double autologous stem-cell transplantation for multiple myeloma. *N Engl J Med* 349:2495–2502, 2003.

272. Bruno B, Rotta M, Patriarca F, et al: A comparison of allografting with autografting for newly diagnosed myeloma. *N Engl J Med* 356:1110–1120, 2007.

273. Gahrton G, Iacobelli S, Bjorkstrand B, et al: Autologous/reduced-intensity allogeneic stem cell transplantation vs autologous transplantation in multiple myeloma: Long-term results of the EBMT-NMAM2000 study. *Blood* 121:5055–5063, 2013.

274. Giaccone L, Storer B, Patriarca F, et al: Long-term follow-up of a comparison of nonmyeloablative allografting with autografting for newly diagnosed myeloma. *Blood* 117:6721–6727, 2011.

275. Rosinol L, Perez-Simon JA, Sureda A, et al: A prospective PETHEMA study of tandem autologous transplantation versus autograft followed by reduced-intensity conditioning allogeneic transplantation in newly diagnosed multiple myeloma. *Blood* 112:3591–3593, 2008.

276. Garban F, Attal M, Michallet M, et al: Prospective comparison of autologous stem cell transplantation followed by dose-reduced allograft (IFM99–03 trial) with tandem autologous stem cell transplantation (IFM99–04 trial) in high-risk *de novo* multiple myeloma. *Blood* 107:3474–3480, 2006.

277. Lokhorst HM, van der Holt B, Cornelissen JJ, et al: Donor versus no-donor comparison of newly diagnosed myeloma patients included in the HOVON-50 multiple myeloma study. *Blood* 119:6219–6225; quiz 6399, 2012.

278. Krishnan A, Pasquini MC, Logan B, et al: Autologous haemopoietic stem-cell transplantation followed by allogeneic or autologous haemopoietic stem-cell transplantation in patients with multiple myeloma (BMT CTN 0102): A phase 3 biological assignment trial. *Lancet Oncol* 12:1195–1203, 2011.

279. Armeson KE, Hill EG, Costa LJ: Tandem autologous vs autologous plus reduced intensity allogeneic transplantation in the upfront management of multiple myeloma: Meta-analysis of trials with biological assignment. *Bone Marrow Transplant* 48:562–567, 2013.

280. Philip T, Armitage JO, Spitzer G, et al: High-dose therapy and autologous bone marrow transplantation after failure of conventional chemotherapy in adults with intermediate-grade or high-grade non-Hodgkin's lymphoma. *N Engl J Med* 316:1493–1498, 1987.

281. Yuen AR, Rosenberg SA, Hoppe RT, et al: Comparison between conventional salvage therapy and high-dose therapy with autografting for recurrent or refractory Hodgkin's disease. *Blood* 89:814–822, 1997.

282. Moskowitz AJ, Yahalom J, Kewalramani T, et al: Pretransplantation functional imaging predicts outcome following autologous stem cell transplantation for relapsed and refractory Hodgkin lymphoma. *Blood* 116:4934–4937, 2010.

283. Terasawa T, Dahabreh IJ, Nihashi T: Fluorine-18-fluorodeoxyglucose positron emission tomography in response assessment before high-dose chemotherapy for lymphoma: A systematic review and meta-analysis. *Oncologist* 15:750–759, 2010.

284. Philip T, Guglielmi C, Hagenbeek A, et al: Autologous bone marrow transplantation as compared with salvage chemotherapy in relapses of chemotherapy-sensitive non-Hodgkin's lymphoma. *N Engl J Med* 333:1540–1545, 1995.

285. Gisselbrecht C, Glass B, Mounier N, et al: Salvage regimens with autologous transplantation for relapsed large B-cell lymphoma in the rituximab era. *J Clin Oncol* 28:4184–4190, 2010.

286. Dreyling M, Lenz G, Hoster E, et al: Early consolidation by myeloablative radiochemotherapy followed by autologous stem cell transplantation in first remission significantly prolongs progression-free survival in mantle-cell lymphoma: Results of a prospective randomized trial of the European MCL Network. *Blood* 105:2677–2684, 2005.

287. LaCasce AS, Vandergrift JL, Rodriguez MA, et al: Comparative outcome of initial therapy for younger patients with mantle cell lymphoma: An analysis from the NCCN NHL Database. *Blood* 119:2093–2099, 2012.

288. Fenske TS, Zhang MJ, Carreras J, et al: Autologous or reduced-intensity conditioning allogeneic hematopoietic cell transplantation for chemotherapy-sensitive mantle-cell lymphoma: Analysis of transplantation timing and modality. *J Clin Oncol* 32:273–281, 2014.

289. Cohen JB, Geyer SM, Lozanski G, et al: Complete response to induction therapy in patients with Myc-positive and double-hit non-Hodgkin lymphoma is associated with prolonged progression-free survival. *Cancer* 120:1677–1685, 2014.

290. Petrich AM, Gandhi M, Jovanovic B, et al: Impact of induction regimen and stem cell transplantation on outcomes in double-hit lymphoma: A multicenter retrospective analysis. *Blood* 124:2354–2361, 2014.

291. Burroughs LM, O'Donnell PV, Sandmaier BM, et al: Comparison of outcomes of HLA-matched related, unrelated, or HLA-haplo-identical related hematopoietic cell transplantation following nonmyeloablative conditioning for relapsed or refractory Hodgkin lymphoma. *Biol Blood Marrow Transplant* 14:1279–1287, 2008.

292. Rezvani AR, Norasetthada L, Gooley T, et al: Non-myeloablative allogeneic haematopoietic cell transplantation for relapsed diffuse large B-cell lymphoma: A multicentre experience. *Br J Haematol* 143:395–403, 2008.

293. Kohrt H, Lowsky R: Nonmyeloablative conditioning with total lymphoid irradiation and antithymocyte globulin: An update. *Curr Opin Hematol* 16:460–465, 2009.

294. Pottinger B, Walker M, Campbell M, et al: The storage and re-infusion of autologous blood and BM as back-up following failed primary hematopoietic stem-cell transplantation: A survey of European practice. *Cytotherapy* 4:127–135, 2002.

295. Olsson R, Remberger M, Schaffer M, et al: Graft failure in the modern era of allogeneic hematopoietic SCT. *Bone Marrow Transplant* 48:537–543, 2013.

296. Baron F, Maris MB, Storer BE, et al: High doses of transplanted CD34+ cells are associated with rapid T-cell engraftment and lessened risk of graft rejection, but not more graft-versus-host disease after nonmyeloablative conditioning and unrelated hematopoietic cell transplantation. *Leukemia* 19:822–828, 2005.

297. Schriber J, Agovi MA, Ho V, et al: Second unrelated donor hematopoietic cell transplantation for primary graft failure. *Biol Blood Marrow Transplant* 16:1099–1106, 2010.

298. Gyurkocza B, Cao TM, Storb RF, et al: Salvage allogeneic hematopoietic cell transplantation with fludarabine and low-dose total body irradiation after rejection of first allografts. *Biol Blood Marrow Transplant* 15:1314–1322, 2009.

299. Vera-Llonch M, Oster G, Ford CM, et al: Oral mucositis and outcomes of allogeneic hematopoietic stem-cell transplantation in patients with hematologic malignancies. *Support Care Cancer* 15:491–496, 2007.

300. Cutler C, Logan B, Nakamura R, et al: Tacrolimus/sirolimus vs tacrolimus/methotrexate as GVHD prophylaxis after matched, related donor allogeneic HCT. *Blood* 124:1372–1377, 2014.

301. Goldberg JD, Zheng J, Castro-Malaspina H, et al: Palifermin is efficacious in recipients of TBI-based but not chemotherapy-based allogeneic hematopoietic stem cell transplants. *Bone Marrow Transplant* 48:99–104, 2013.

302. Nooka AK, Johnson HR, Kaufman JL, et al: Pharmacoeconomic analysis of palifermin to prevent mucositis among patients undergoing autologous hematopoietic stem cell transplantation. *Biol Blood Marrow Transplant* 20:852–857, 2014.

303. Levine JE, Blazar BR, DeFor T, et al: Long-term follow-up of a phase I/II randomized, placebo-controlled trial of palifermin to prevent graft-versus-host disease (GVHD) after related donor allogeneic hematopoietic cell transplantation (HCT). *Biol Blood Marrow Transplant* 14:1017–1021, 2008.

304. Jagasia MH, Abonour R, Long GD, et al: Palifermin for the reduction of acute GVHD: A randomized, double-blind, placebo-controlled trial. *Bone Marrow Transplant* 47:1350–1355, 2012.

305. Shulman HM, Fisher LB, Schoch HG, et al: Veno-occlusive disease of the liver after marrow transplantation: Histological correlates of clinical signs and symptoms. *Hepatology* 19:1171–1181, 1994.

306. McCune JS, Batchelder A, Deeg HJ, et al: Cyclophosphamide following targeted oral busulfan as conditioning for hematopoietic cell transplantation: Pharmacokinetics, liver toxicity, and mortality. *Biol Blood Marrow Transplant* 13:853–862, 2007.

307. McCune JS, Batchelder A, Guthrie KA, et al: Personalized dosing of cyclophosphamide in the total body irradiation-cyclophosphamide conditioning regimen: A phase II trial in patients with hematologic malignancy. *Clin Pharmacol Ther* 85:615–622, 2009.

308. Wong KM, Atenafu EG, Kim D, et al: Incidence and risk factors for early hepatotoxicity and its impact on survival in patients with myelofibrosis undergoing allogeneic hematopoietic cell transplantation. *Biol Blood Marrow Transplant* 18:1589–1599, 2012.

309. McKoy JM, Angelotta C, Bennett CL, et al: Gemtuzumab ozogamicin-associated sinusoidal obstructive syndrome (SOS): An overview from the research on adverse drug events and reports (RADAR) project. *Leuk Res* 31:599–604, 2007.

310. Wadleigh M, Richardson PG, Zahrieh D, et al: Prior gemtuzumab ozogamicin exposure significantly increases the risk of veno-occlusive disease in patients who undergo myeloablative allogeneic stem cell transplantation. *Blood* 102:1578–1582, 2003.

311. Carreras E, Diaz-Beya M, Rosinol L, et al: The incidence of veno-occlusive disease following allogeneic hematopoietic stem cell transplantation has diminished and the outcome improved over the last decade. *Biol Blood Marrow Transplant* 17:1713–1720, 2011.

312. Ohashi K, Tanabe J, Watanabe R, et al: The Japanese multicenter open randomized trial of ursodeoxycholic acid prophylaxis for hepatic veno-occlusive disease after stem cell transplantation. *Am J Hematol* 64:32–38, 2000.

313. Ruutu T, Eriksson B, Remes K, et al: Ursodeoxycholic acid for the prevention of hepatic complications in allogeneic stem cell transplantation. *Blood* 100:1977–1983, 2002.

314. McDonald GB, Hinds MS, Fisher LD, et al: Veno-occlusive disease of the liver and multiorgan failure after bone marrow transplantation: A cohort study of 355 patients. *Ann Intern Med* 118:255–267, 1993.

315. Coppell JA, Richardson PG, Soiffer R, et al: Hepatic veno-occlusive disease following stem cell transplantation: Incidence, clinical course, and outcome. *Biol Blood Marrow Transplant* 16:157–168, 2010.

316. Bearman SI, Anderson GL, Mori M, et al: Venoocclusive disease of the liver: Development of a model for predicting fatal outcome after marrow transplantation. *J Clin Oncol* 11:1729–1736, 1993.

317. Echart CL, Graziadio B, Somaini S, et al: The fibrinolytic mechanism of defibrotide: Effect of defibrotide on plasmin activity. *Blood Coagul Fibrinolysis* 20:627–634, 2009.

318. Richardson PG, Soiffer RJ, Antin JH, et al: Defibrotide for the treatment of severe hepatic veno-occlusive disease and multiorgan failure after stem cell transplantation: A multicenter, randomized, dose-finding trial. *Biol Blood Marrow Transplant* 16:1005–1017, 2010.

319. Panoskaltsis-Mortari A, Griese M, Madtes DK, et al: An official American Thoracic Society research statement: Noninfectious lung injury after hematopoietic stem cell transplantation: Idiopathic pneumonia syndrome. *Am J Respir Crit Care Med* 183:1262–1279, 2011.

320. Weiner RS, Horowitz MM, Gale RP, et al: Risk factors for interstitial pneumonia following bone marrow transplantation for severe aplastic anaemia. *Br J Haematol* 71:535–543, 1989.

321. Tizon R, Frey N, Heitjan DF, et al: High-dose corticosteroids with or without etanercept for the treatment of idiopathic pneumonia syndrome after allo-SCT. *Bone Marrow Transplant* 47:1332–1337, 2012.

322. Yanik GA, Horowitz MM, Weisdorf DJ, et al: Randomized, double-blind, placebo-controlled trial of soluble tumor necrosis factor receptor: Enbrel (etanercept) for the treatment of idiopathic pneumonia syndrome after allogeneic stem cell transplantation: Blood and marrow transplant clinical trials network protocol. *Biol Blood Marrow Transplant* 20:858–864, 2014.

323. Gilbert C, Vasu TS, Baram M: Use of mechanical ventilation and renal replacement therapy in critically ill hematopoietic stem cell transplant recipients. *Biol Blood Marrow Transplant* 19:321–324, 2013.

324. Alessandrino EP, Bernasconi P, Colombo A, et al: Pulmonary toxicity following carmustine-based preparative regimens and autologous peripheral blood progenitor cell transplantation in hematological malignancies. *Bone Marrow Transplant* 25:309–313, 2000.

325. Reusser P, Attenhofer R, Hebart H, et al: Cytomegalovirus-specific T-cell immunity in recipients of autologous peripheral blood stem cell or bone marrow transplants. *Blood* 89:3873–3879, 1997.

326. Dulude G, Roy DC, Perreault C: The effect of graft-versus-host disease on T cell production and homeostasis. *J Exp Med* 189:1329–1342, 1999.

327. Douek DC, Vescio RA, Betts MR, et al: Assessment of thymic output in adults after haematopoietic stem-cell transplantation and prediction of T-cell reconstitution. *Lancet* 355:1875–1881, 2000.

328. Bosch M, Khan FM, Storek J: Immune reconstitution after hematopoietic cell transplantation. *Curr Opin Hematol* 19:324–335, 2012.

329. Collin BA, Leather HL, Wingard JR, et al: Evolution, incidence, and susceptibility of bacterial bloodstream isolates from 519 bone marrow transplant patients. *Clin Infect Dis* 33:947–953, 2001.

330. Robenshtok E, Gafter-Gvili A, Goldberg E, et al: Antifungal prophylaxis in cancer patients after chemotherapy or hematopoietic stem-cell transplantation: Systematic review and meta-analysis. *J Clin Oncol* 25:5471–5489, 2007.

331. van Burik JH, Leisenring W, Myerson D, et al: The effect of prophylactic fluconazole on the clinical spectrum of fungal diseases in bone marrow transplant recipients with special attention to hepatic candidiasis. An autopsy study of 355 patients. *Medicine (Baltimore)* 77:246–254, 1998.

332. Marr KA, Crippa F, Leisenring W, et al: Itraconazole versus fluconazole for prevention of fungal infections in patients receiving allogeneic stem cell transplants. *Blood* 103:1527–1533, 2004.

333. Ethier MC, Science M, Beyene J, et al: Mould-active compared with fluconazole prophylaxis to prevent invasive fungal diseases in cancer patients receiving chemotherapy or haematopoietic stem-cell transplantation: A systematic review and meta-analysis of randomised controlled trials. *Br J Cancer* 106:1626–1637, 2012.

334. Tomblyn M, Chiller T, Einsele H, et al: Guidelines for preventing infectious complications among hematopoietic cell transplantation recipients: A global perspective. *Biol Blood Marrow Transplant* 15:1143–1238, 2009.

335. Neiman P, Wasserman PB, Wentworth BB, et al: Interstitial pneumonia and cytomegalovirus infection as complications of human marrow transplantation. *Transplantation* 15:478–485, 1973.

336. Einsele H, Ehninger G, Hebart H, et al: Polymerase chain reaction monitoring reduces the incidence of cytomegalovirus disease and the duration and side effects of antiviral therapy after bone marrow transplantation. *Blood* 86:2815–2820, 1995.

337. Ljungman P, de La Camara R, Milpied N, et al: Randomized study of valacyclovir as prophylaxis against cytomegalovirus reactivation in recipients of allogeneic bone marrow transplants. *Blood* 99:3050–3056, 2002.

338. Winston DJ, Yeager AM, Chandrasekar PH, et al: Randomized comparison of oral valacyclovir and intravenous ganciclovir for prevention of cytomegalovirus disease after allogeneic bone marrow transplantation. *Clin Infect Dis* 36:749–758, 2003.

339. van der Heiden PL, Kalpoe JS, Barge RM, et al: Oral valganciclovir as pre-emptive therapy has similar efficacy on cytomegalovirus DNA load reduction as intravenous ganciclovir in allogeneic stem cell transplantation recipients. *Bone Marrow Transplant* 37:693–698, 2006.

340. Ruiz-Camps I, Len O, de la Camara R, et al: Valganciclovir as pre-emptive therapy for cytomegalovirus infection in allogeneic haematopoietic stem cell transplant recipients. *Antivir Ther* 16:951–957, 2011.

341. Reusser P, Einsele H, Lee J, et al: Randomized multicenter trial of foscarnet versus ganciclovir for preemptive therapy of cytomegalovirus infection after allogeneic stem cell transplantation. *Blood* 99:1159–1164, 2002.

342. Marty FM, Winston DJ, Rowley SD, et al: CMX001 to prevent cytomegalovirus disease in hematopoietic-cell transplantation. *N Engl J Med* 369:1227–1236, 2013.

343. Chemaly RF, Ullmann AJ, Stoelben S, et al: Letermovir for cytomegalovirus prophylaxis in hematopoietic-cell transplantation. *N Engl J Med* 370:1781–1789, 2014.

344. Winston DJ, Young JA, Pullarkat V, et al: Maribavir prophylaxis for prevention of cytomegalovirus infection in allogeneic stem cell transplant recipients: A multicenter, randomized, double-blind, placebo-controlled, dose-ranging study. *Blood* 111:5403–5410, 2008.

345. Marty FM, Ljungman P, Papanicolaou GA, et al: Maribavir prophylaxis for prevention of cytomegalovirus disease in recipients of allogeneic stem-cell transplants: A phase 3, double-blind, placebo-controlled, randomised trial. *Lancet Infect Dis* 11:284–292, 2011.

346. Blyth E, Clancy L, Simms R, et al: Donor-derived CMV-specific T cells reduce the requirement for CMV-directed pharmacotherapy after allogeneic stem cell transplantation. *Blood* 121:3745–3758, 2013.

347. Erard V, Wald A, Corey L, et al: Use of long-term suppressive acyclovir after hematopoietic stem-cell transplantation: Impact on herpes simplex virus (HSV) disease and drug-resistant HSV disease. *J Infect Dis* 196:266–270, 2007.

348. Hatchette T, Tipples GA, Peters G, et al: Foscarnet salvage therapy for acyclovir-resistant varicella zoster: Report of a novel thymidine kinase mutation and review of the literature. *Pediatr Infect Dis J* 27:75–77, 2008.

349. Erard V, Guthrie KA, Varley C, et al: One-year acyclovir prophylaxis for preventing varicella-zoster virus disease after hematopoietic cell transplantation: No evidence of rebound varicella-zoster virus disease after drug discontinuation. *Blood* 110:3071–3077, 2007.

350. Chou JF, Kernan NA, Prockop S, et al: Safety and immunogenicity of the live attenuated varicella vaccine following T replete or T cell-depleted related and unrelated allogeneic hematopoietic cell transplantation (alloHCT). *Biol Blood Marrow Transplant* 17:1708–1713, 2011.

351. Hata A, Asanuma H, Rinki M, et al: Use of an inactivated varicella vaccine in recipients of hematopoietic-cell transplants. *N Engl J Med* 347:26–34, 2002.

352. Billingham RE: The biology of graft-versus-host reactions. *Harvey Lect* 62:21–78, 1966.

353. Ferrara JL, Levine JE, Reddy P, et al: Graft-versus-host disease. *Lancet* 373:1550–1561, 2009.

354. Spierings E, Kim YH, Hendriks M, et al: Multicenter analyses demonstrate significant clinical effects of minor histocompatibility antigens on GvHD and GvL after HLA-matched related and unrelated hematopoietic stem cell transplantation. *Biol Blood Marrow Transplant* 19:1244–1253, 2013.

355. Spierings E: Minor histocompatibility antigens: Past, present, and future. *Tissue Antigens* 84:374–360, 2014.

356. Behar E, Chao NJ, Hiraki DD, et al: Polymorphism of adhesion molecule CD31 and its role in acute graft-versus-host disease. *N Engl J Med* 334:286–291, 1996.

357. Sahaf B, Yang Y, Arai S, et al: H-Y antigen-binding B cells develop in male recipients of female hematopoietic cells and associate with chronic graft vs. host disease. *Proc Natl Acad Sci U S A* 110:3005–3010, 2013.

358. Oostvogels R, Lokhorst HM, Minnema MC, et al: Identification of minor histocompatibility antigens based on the 1000 Genomes Project. *Haematologica* 99:1854–1859, 2014.

359. Jagasia M, Arora M, Flowers ME, et al: Risk factors for acute GVHD and survival after hematopoietic cell transplantation. *Blood* 119:296–307, 2012.

360. Filipovich AH, Weisdorf D, Pavletic S, et al: National Institutes of Health consensus development project on criteria for clinical trials in chronic graft-versus-host disease: I. Diagnosis and staging working group report. *Biol Blood Marrow Transplant* 11:945–956, 2005.

361. Sale GE, Lerner KG, Barker EA, et al: The skin biopsy in the diagnosis of acute graft-versus-host disease in man. *Am J Pathol* 89:621–636, 1977.

362. Firoz BF, Lee SJ, Nghiem P, et al: Role of skin biopsy to confirm suspected acute graft-vs-host disease: Results of decision analysis. *Arch Dermatol* 142:175–182, 2006.

363. Shimoni A, Rimon U, Hertz M, et al: CT in the clinical and prognostic evaluation of acute graft-vs-host disease of the gastrointestinal tract. *Br J Radiol* 85:e416–e423, 2012.

364. Ross WA, Ghosh S, Dekovich AA, et al: Endoscopic biopsy diagnosis of acute gastrointestinal graft-versus-host disease: Rectosigmoid biopsies are more sensitive than upper gastrointestinal biopsies. *Am J Gastroenterol* 103:982–989, 2008.

365. Liu A, Meyer E, Johnston L, et al: Prevalence of graft versus host disease and cytomegalovirus infection in patients post-haematopoietic cell transplantation presenting with gastrointestinal symptoms. *Aliment Pharmacol Ther* 38:955–966, 2013.

366. Kreisel W, Dahlberg M, Bertz H, et al: Endoscopic diagnosis of acute intestinal GVHD following allogeneic hematopoietic SCT: A retrospective analysis in 175 patients. *Bone Marrow Transplant* 47:430–438, 2012.

367. Shulman HM, Sharma P, Amos D, et al: A coded histologic study of hepatic graft-versus-host disease after human bone marrow transplantation. *Hepatology* 8:463–470, 1988.

368. Storb R, Pepe M, Deeg HJ, et al: Long-term follow-up of a controlled trial comparing a combination of methotrexate plus cyclosporine with cyclosporine alone for prophylaxis of graft-versus-host disease in patients administered HLA-identical marrow grafts for leukemia. *Blood* 80:560–561, 1992.

369. Storb R, Leisenring W, Deeg HJ, et al: Long-term follow-up of a randomized trial of graft-versus-host disease prevention by methotrexate/cyclosporine versus methotrexate alone in patients given marrow grafts for severe aplastic anemia. *Blood* 83:2749–2750, 1994.

370. Storb R, Pepe M, Anasetti C, et al: What role for prednisone in prevention of acute graft-versus-host disease in patients undergoing marrow transplants? *Blood* 76:1037–1045, 1990.

371. Ratanatharathorn V, Nash RA, Przepiorka D, et al: Phase III study comparing methotrexate and tacrolimus (Prograf, FK506) with methotrexate and cyclosporine for graft-versus-host disease prophylaxis after HLA-identical sibling bone marrow transplantation. *Blood* 92:2303–2314, 1998.

372. Nash RA, Antin JH, Karanes C, et al: Phase 3 study comparing methotrexate and tacrolimus with methotrexate and cyclosporine for prophylaxis of acute graft-versus-host disease after marrow transplantation from unrelated donors. *Blood* 96:2062–2068, 2000.

373. Finke J, Bethge WA, Schmoor C, et al: Standard graft-versus-host disease prophylaxis with or without anti-T-cell globulin in haematopoietic cell transplantation from matched unrelated donors: A randomised, open-label, multicentre phase 3 trial. *Lancet Oncol* 10:855–864, 2009.

374. Socie G, Schmoor C, Bethge WA, et al: Chronic graft-versus-host disease: Long-term results from a randomized trial on graft-versus-host disease prophylaxis with or without anti-T-cell globulin ATG-Fresenius. *Blood* 117:6375–6382, 2011.

375. Kanakry CG, Tsai HL, Bolanos-Meade J, et al: Single-agent GVHD prophylaxis with posttransplantation cyclophosphamide after myeloablative, HLA-matched BMT for AML, ALL, and MDS. *Blood* 124:3817–3827, 2014. .

376. Kanakry CG, O'Donnell PV, Furlong T, et al: Multi-institutional study of post-transplantation cyclophosphamide as single-agent graft-versus-host disease prophylaxis after allogeneic bone marrow transplantation using myeloablative busulfan and fludarabine conditioning. *J Clin Oncol* 32:3497–3505, 2014.
377. Anderson BE, Taylor PA, McNiff JM, et al: Effects of donor T-cell trafficking and priming site on graft-versus-host disease induction by naive and memory phenotype CD4 T cells. *Blood* 111:5242–5251, 2008.
378. Chen BJ, Cui X, Sempowski GD, et al: Transfer of allogeneic CD62L– memory T cells without graft-versus-host disease. *Blood* 103:1534–1541, 2004.
379. Bleakley M, Heimfeld S, Jones LA, et al: Engineering human peripheral blood stem cell grafts that are depleted of naive T cells and retain functional pathogen-specific memory T cells. *Biol Blood Marrow Transplant* 20:705–716, 2014.
380. Brunstein CG, Miller JS, Cao Q, et al: Infusion of ex vivo expanded T regulatory cells in adults transplanted with umbilical cord blood: Safety profile and detection kinetics. *Blood* 117:1061–1070, 2011.
381. Reshef R, Luger SM, Hexner EO, et al: Blockade of lymphocyte chemotaxis in visceral graft-versus-host disease. *N Engl J Med* 367:135–145, 2012.
382. Bacigalupo A: Management of acute graft-versus-host disease. *Br J Haematol* 137:87–98, 2007.
383. Mielcarek M, Storer BE, Boeckh M, et al: Initial therapy of acute graft-versus-host disease with low-dose prednisone does not compromise patient outcomes. *Blood* 113:2888–2894, 2009.
384. Castilla-Llorente C, Martin PJ, McDonald GB, et al: Prognostic factors and outcomes of severe gastrointestinal GVHD after allogeneic hematopoietic cell transplantation. *Bone Marrow Transplant* 49:966–971, 2014.
385. Couriel DR, Saliba R, de Lima M, et al: A phase III study of infliximab and corticosteroids for the initial treatment of acute graft-versus-host disease. *Biol Blood Marrow Transplant* 15:1555–1562, 2009.
386. Bolanos-Meade J, Logan BR, Alousi AM, et al: Phase III clinical trial steroids/mycophenolate mofetil vs steroids/placebo as therapy for acute graft-versus-host disease: BMT CTN 0802. *Blood* 124:3221–3227, 2014.
387. Martin PJ, Rizzo JD, Wingard JR, et al: First- and second-line systemic treatment of acute graft-versus-host disease: Recommendations of the American Society of Blood and Marrow Transplantation. *Biol Blood Marrow Transplant* 18:1150–1163, 2012.
388. Choi J, Cooper ML, Alahmari B, et al: Pharmacologic blockade of JAK1/JAK2 reduces GvHD and preserves graft-versus-leukemia effect. *PLoS One* 9:e109799, 2014.
389. Spoerl S, Mathew NR, Bscheider M, et al: Activity of therapeutic JAK 1/2 blockade in graft-versus-host disease. *Blood* 123:3832–3842, 2014.
390. Fraser CJ, Bhatia S, Ness K, et al: Impact of chronic graft-versus-host disease on the health status of hematopoietic cell transplantation survivors: A report from the Bone Marrow Transplant Survivor Study. *Blood* 108:2867–2873, 2006.
391. Pidala J, Kurland B, Chai X, et al: Patient-reported quality of life is associated with severity of chronic graft-versus-host disease as measured by NIH criteria: Report on baseline data from the Chronic GVHD Consortium. *Blood* 117:4651–4657, 2011.
392. Baird K, Steinberg SM, Grkovic L, et al: National Institutes of Health chronic graft-versus-host disease staging in severely affected patients: Organ and global scoring correlate with established indicators of disease severity and prognosis. *Biol Blood Marrow Transplant* 19:632–639, 2013.
393. Moon JH, Sohn SK, Lambie A, et al: Validation of National Institutes of Health global scoring system for chronic graft-versus-host disease (GVHD) according to overall and GVHD-specific survival. *Biol Blood Marrow Transplant* 20:556–563, 2014.
394. Arora M, Klein JP, Weisdorf DJ, et al: Chronic GVHD risk score: A Center for International Blood and Marrow Transplant Research analysis. *Blood* 117:6714–6720, 2011.
395. Lee SJ, Klein JP, Barrett AJ, et al: Severity of chronic graft-versus-host disease: Association with treatment-related mortality and relapse. *Blood* 100:406–414, 2002.
396. Carpenter PA: How I conduct a comprehensive chronic graft-versus-host disease assessment. *Blood* 118:2679–2687, 2011.
397. Carpenter PA: *How to Conduct a Comprehensive Chronic GVHD Assessment. Vol. 2014.* Fred Hutchinson Cancer Research Center, Seattle, WA, 2011.
398. Chu YW, Gress RE: Murine models of chronic graft-versus-host disease: Insights and unresolved issues. *Biol Blood Marrow Transplant* 14:365–378, 2008.
399. Srinivasan M, Flynn R, Price A, et al: Donor B-cell alloantibody deposition and germinal center formation are required for the development of murine chronic GVHD and bronchiolitis obliterans. *Blood* 119:1570–1580, 2012.
400. Wagner JE, Thompson JS, Carter SL, et al: Effect of graft-versus-host disease prophylaxis on 3-year disease-free survival in recipients of unrelated donor bone marrow (T-cell Depletion Trial): A multi-centre, randomised phase II-III trial. *Lancet* 366:733–741, 2005.
401. Rotta M, Storer BE, Storb R, et al: Impact of recipient statin treatment on graft-versus-host disease after allogeneic hematopoietic cell transplantation. *Biol Blood Marrow Transplant* 16:1463–1466, 2010.
402. Arai S, Sahaf B, Narasimhan B, et al: Prophylactic rituximab after allogeneic transplantation decreases B-cell alloimmunity with low chronic GVHD incidence. *Blood* 119:6145–6154, 2012.
403. Cutler C, Kim HT, Bindra B, et al: Rituximab prophylaxis prevents corticosteroid-requiring chronic GVHD after allogeneic peripheral blood stem cell transplantation: Results of a phase 2 trial. *Blood* 122:1510–1517, 2013.
404. Wolff D, Gerbitz A, Ayuk F, et al: Consensus conference on clinical practice in chronic graft-versus-host disease (GVHD): First-line and topical treatment of chronic GVHD. *Biol Blood Marrow Transplant* 16:1611–1628, 2010.
405. Sullivan KM, Witherspoon RP, Storb R, et al: Prednisone and azathioprine compared with prednisone and placebo for treatment of chronic graft-v-host disease: Prognostic influence of prolonged thrombocytopenia after allogeneic marrow transplantation. *Blood* 72:546–554, 1988.
406. Koc S, Leisenring W, Flowers ME, et al: Thalidomide for treatment of patients with chronic graft-versus-host disease. *Blood* 96:3995–3996, 2000.
407. Arora M, Wagner JE, Davies SM, et al: Randomized clinical trial of thalidomide, cyclosporine, and prednisone versus cyclosporine and prednisone as initial therapy for chronic graft-versus-host disease. *Biol Blood Marrow Transplant* 7:265–273, 2001.
408. Koc S, Leisenring W, Flowers ME, et al: Therapy for chronic graft-versus-host disease: A randomized trial comparing cyclosporine plus prednisone versus prednisone alone. *Blood* 100:48–51, 2002.
409. Martin PJ, Storer BE, Rowley SD, et al: Evaluation of mycophenolate mofetil for initial treatment of chronic graft-versus-host disease. *Blood* 113:5074–5082, 2009.
410. Gilman AL, Schultz KR, Goldman FD, et al: Randomized trial of hydroxychloroquine for newly diagnosed chronic graft-versus-host disease in children: A Children's Oncology Group study. *Biol Blood Marrow Transplant* 18:84–91, 2012.
411. Stewart BL, Storer B, Storek J, et al: Duration of immunosuppressive treatment for chronic graft-versus-host disease. *Blood* 104:3501–3506, 2004.
412. Wolff D, Schleuning M, von Harsdorf S, et al: Consensus Conference on Clinical Practice in Chronic GVHD: Second-Line Treatment of Chronic Graft-versus-Host Disease. *Biol Blood Marrow Transplant* 17:1–17, 2011.
413. Abu-Dalle I, Reljic T, Nishihori T, et al: Extracorporeal photopheresis in steroid-refractory acute or chronic graft-versus-host disease: Results of a systematic review of prospective studies. *Biol Blood Marrow Transplant* 20:1677–1686, 2014.
414. Koreth J, Matsuoka K, Kim HT, et al: Interleukin-2 and regulatory T cells in graft-versus-host disease. *N Engl J Med* 365:2055–2066, 2011.
415. Matsuoka K, Koreth J, Kim HT, et al: Low-dose interleukin-2 therapy restores regulatory T cell homeostasis in patients with chronic graft-versus-host disease. *Sci Transl Med* 5:179ra43, 2013.
416. Dubovsky JA, Flynn R, Du J, et al: Ibrutinib treatment ameliorates murine chronic graft-versus-host disease. *J Clin Invest* 124:4867–4876, 2014.
417. Mundt AJ, Sibley G, Williams S, et al: Patterns of failure following high-dose chemotherapy and autologous bone marrow transplantation with involved field radiotherapy for relapsed/refractory Hodgkin's disease. *Int J Radiat Oncol Biol Phys* 33:261–270, 1995.
418. Holman PR, Costello C, deMagalhaes-Silverman M, et al: Idiotype immunization following high-dose therapy and autologous stem cell transplantation for non-Hodgkin lymphoma. *Biol Blood Marrow Transplant* 18:257–264, 2012.
419. Attal M, Lauwers-Cances V, Marit G, et al: Lenalidomide maintenance after stem-cell transplantation for multiple myeloma. *N Engl J Med* 366:1782–1791, 2012.
420. McCarthy PL, Owzar K, Hofmeister CC, et al: Lenalidomide after stem-cell transplantation for multiple myeloma. *N Engl J Med* 366:1770–1781, 2012.
421. Cohen S, Kiss T, Lachance S, et al: Tandem autologous-allogeneic nonmyeloablative sibling transplantation in relapsed follicular lymphoma leads to impressive progression-free survival with minimal toxicity. *Biol Blood Marrow Transplant* 18:951–957, 2012.
422. Mielcarek M, Storer BE, Flowers ME, et al: Outcomes among patients with recurrent high-risk hematologic malignancies after allogeneic hematopoietic cell transplantation. *Biol Blood Marrow Transplant* 13:1160–1168, 2007.
423. Duncan CN, Majhail NS, Brazauskas R, et al: Long-term survival and late effects among 1-year survivors of second allogeneic hematopoietic cell transplantation for relapsed acute leukemia and myelodysplastic syndromes. *Biol Blood Marrow Transplant* 21:151–158, 2015.
424. Claret EJ, Alyea EP, Orsini E, et al: Characterization of T cell repertoire in patients with graft-versus-leukemia after donor lymphocyte infusion. *J Clin Invest* 100:855–866, 1997.
425. Bachireddy P, Hainz U, Rooney M, et al: Reversal of in situ T-cell exhaustion during effective human antileukemia responses to donor lymphocyte infusion. *Blood* 123:1412–1421, 2014.
426. Shanavas M, Messner HA, Kamel-Reid S, et al: A comparison of long-term outcomes of donor lymphocyte infusions and tyrosine kinase inhibitors in patients with relapsed CML after allogeneic hematopoietic cell transplantation. *Clin Lymphoma Myeloma Leuk* 14:87–92, 2014.
427. Collins RH Jr, Shpilberg O, Drobyski WR, et al: Donor leukocyte infusions in 140 patients with relapsed malignancy after allogeneic bone marrow transplantation. *J Clin Oncol* 15:433–444, 1997.
428. Bar M, Sandmaier BM, Inamoto Y, et al: Donor lymphocyte infusion for relapsed hematological malignancies after allogeneic hematopoietic cell transplantation: Prognostic relevance of the initial CD3+ T cell dose. *Biol Blood Marrow Transplant* 19:949–957, 2013.
429. Scarisbrick JJ, Dignan FL, Tulpule S, et al: A multicentre UK study of GVHD following DLI: Rates of GVHD are high but mortality from GVHD is infrequent. *Bone Marrow Transplant* 50:62–67, 2015.
430. Keil F, Haas OA, Fritsch G, et al: Donor leukocyte infusion for leukemic relapse after allogeneic marrow transplantation: Lack of residual donor hematopoiesis predicts aplasia. *Blood* 89:3113–3117, 1997.
431. Heimesaat MM, Nogai A, Bereswill S, et al: MyD88/TLR9 mediated immunopathology and gut microbiota dynamics in a novel murine model of intestinal graft-versus-host disease. *Gut* 59:1079–1087, 2010.

432. Jenq RR, Ubeda C, Taur Y, et al: Regulation of intestinal inflammation by microbiota following allogeneic bone marrow transplantation. *J Exp Med* 209:903–911, 2012.

433. Ames NJ, Sulima P, Ngo T, et al: A characterization of the oral microbiome in allogeneic stem cell transplant patients. *PLoS One* 7:e47628, 2012.

434. Holler E, Butzhammer P, Schmid K, et al: Metagenomic analysis of the stool microbiome in patients receiving allogeneic stem cell transplantation: Loss of diversity is associated with use of systemic antibiotics and more pronounced in gastrointestinal graft-versus-host disease. *Biol Blood Marrow Transplant* 20:640–645, 2014.

435. Taur Y, Xavier JB, Lipuma L, et al: Intestinal domination and the risk of bacteremia in patients undergoing allogeneic hematopoietic stem cell transplantation. *Clin Infect Dis* 55:905–914, 2012.

436. Taur Y, Jenq RR, Perales MA, et al: The effects of intestinal tract bacterial diversity on mortality following allogeneic hematopoietic stem cell transplantation. *Blood* 124:1174–1182, 2014.

437. Vossen JM, Guiot HF, Lankester AC, et al: Complete suppression of the gut microbiome prevents acute graft-versus-host disease following allogeneic bone marrow transplantation. *PLoS One* 9:e105706, 2014.

438. Helg C, Chapuis B, Bolle JF, et al: Renal transplantation without immunosuppression in a host with tolerance induced by allogeneic bone marrow transplantation. *Transplantation* 58:1420–1422, 1994.

439. Sayegh MH, Fine NA, Smith JL, et al: Immunologic tolerance to renal allografts after bone marrow transplants from the same donors. *Ann Intern Med* 114:954–955, 1991.

440. Leventhal J, Abecassis M, Miller J, et al: Chimerism and tolerance without GVHD or engraftment syndrome in HLA-mismatched combined kidney and hematopoietic stem cell transplantation. *Sci Transl Med* 4:124ra28, 2012.

441. Leventhal J, Abecassis M, Miller J, et al: Tolerance induction in HLA disparate living donor kidney transplantation by donor stem cell infusion: Durable chimerism predicts outcome. *Transplantation* 95:169–176, 2013.

442. Kawai T, Sachs DH, Sprangers B, et al: Long-term results in recipients of combined HLA-mismatched kidney and bone marrow transplantation without maintenance immunosuppression. *Am J Transplant* 14:1599–1611, 2014.

443. Scandling JD, Busque S, Dejbakhsh-Jones S, et al: Tolerance and chimerism after renal and hematopoietic-cell transplantation. *N Engl J Med* 358:362–368, 2008.

444. Szabolcs P, Buckley RH, Davis RD, et al: Tolerance and immunity after sequential lung and bone marrow transplantation from an unrelated cadaveric donor. *J Allergy Clin Immunol* 135:567–570.e3, 2015.

CHAPTER 24
TREATMENT OF INFECTIONS IN THE IMMUNOCOMPROMISED HOST

Lisa Beutler and Jennifer Babik

SUMMARY

Infection is a major cause of morbidity and mortality in patients with severe inherited or acquired neutropenia or aplastic anemia, qualitative disorders of neutrophils, and, notably, those persons receiving chemotherapy for treatment of hematologic neoplasms. Severe neutropenia and monocytopenia often result from the combined effects of replacement of marrow with malignant cells and superimposed intense chemotherapy. The severity and duration of the neutropenia determine the risk of infection. Bacterial infections may result in rapid clinical deterioration and even death. Fungal, viral, and parasitic infections also may result in potentially lethal complications during or after chemotherapy. This chapter considers methods of diagnosis of bacterial, fungal, viral, and protozoal infection and describes treatment regimens. Because prevention of infection during periods of neutropenia should reduce morbidity and improve outcome, attention is focused on prophylaxis against bacterial, parasitic, viral, and/or fungal infections.

RISK FACTORS AND INFECTING ORGANISMS

SEVERITY OF NEUTROPENIA

Bacterial, fungal, viral, and parasitic organisms may cause infection in neutropenic patients.[1] Bacterial infections are the most frequent and usually the most serious. The risk for bacterial infection increases when the neutrophil count falls to less than 0.5×10^9/L and becomes especially pronounced at neutrophil counts less than 0.1×10^9/L.[1] The rate of decline and duration of neutropenia are important in determining the risk of bacterial infection. Disruption of mucosal barriers, especially in the oral cavity, esophagus, and bowel, further favors the development of infection by providing portals of entry.

Acronyms and Abbreviations: CMV, cytomegalovirus; CT, computed tomography; ESBL, extended-spectrum β-lactamase; Ig, immunoglobulin; IVIG, intravenous immunoglobulin; LFT, liver function test; MRSA, methicillin-resistant *Staphylococcus aureus*; PCP, *Pneumocystis jiroveci* pneumonia; RSV, respiratory syncytial virus; VRE, vancomycin-resistant *Enterococcus*.

BACTERIAL PATHOGENS

Historically, Gram-negative bacilli have been the most commonly isolated pathogens. These organisms include *Klebsiella*, *Escherichia coli*, *Pseudomonas*, and *Proteus*. These bacteria are responsible for a variety of infections, including pneumonia, soft-tissue infections, perirectal infections, and bacteremia. Urinary tract infections are less frequent unless a urinary catheter is present or urinary tract obstruction has developed. Meningitis is uncommon.

At present, roughly half of all documented infections in neutropenic patients are caused by Gram-positive pathogens. This likely results from the popularity of semipermanent venous catheters and from the use of prophylactic regimens that are active against Gram-negative rods. Staphylococcal species and *Enterococcus* are now the pathogens most frequently isolated from neutropenic patients.[2] Several reports document the increasing frequency of viridans group streptococci as a major pathogen in neutropenic patients, especially in those receiving a hematopoietic stem cell transplant, perhaps because these patients have a higher incidence of mucositis.[3] Among infections caused by both Gram-negative and Gram-positive organisms, antibiotic resistance is a growing problem and is discussed under "Bacterial Infections" below. Anaerobic infections are less common unless periodontal or gastrointestinal pathology coexists.

Patients with Hodgkin lymphoma, other lymphomas, or chronic lymphocytic leukemia primarily suffer from impaired cell-mediated immunity and diminished antibody production.[4] Consequently, the spectrum of infections in these patients differs from that found in neutropenic patients. Bacterial infections, when they occur, tend to result from encapsulated organisms such as *Pneumococcus* or *Haemophilus*. *Listeria* and *Nocardia* infections also are seen more frequently in this group of patients.[5]

FUNGAL PATHOGENS

Fungal infections are common during periods of prolonged neutropenia and in patients with lymphomas or chronic lymphocytic leukemia who have impaired cell-mediated immunity. *Candida* species are most frequently isolated. Historically, *Candida albicans* had been the most common isolate; however, in recent years the number of non-*albicans Candida* infections has increased, partly as a consequence of widespread prophylaxis against *C. albicans*.[6] The gastrointestinal tract serves as a reservoir for *Candida*, and erosive esophagitis may develop. *Candida* may also enter the bloodstream via indwelling catheters.

Aspergillus and fungi that cause mucormycosis also may cause invasive disease. The use of mold-active prophylaxis may be associated with an increased incidence of mucormycosis.[7] These organisms tend to colonize and infect the sinuses and bronchopulmonary tree.

Infections with *Cryptococcus*, *Aspergillus*, *Coccidioides*, *Histoplasma*, and *Candida* are more common in patients with leukemia or lymphoma who require chronic glucocorticoid treatment. *Coccidioides* and *Histoplasma* are endemic mycoses. *Coccidioides* is endemic in the southwestern United States, in particular in Arizona and the San Joaquin Valley in California. *Histoplasma* is endemic in the Ohio and Mississippi River Valleys. Emerging fungal infections with organisms such as *Scedosporium* have become more common with increased use of mold-active prophylaxis.[8]

Pneumocystis jiroveci is a ubiquitous, endogenous fungus that may cause pneumonia in neutropenic patients and in those with defective cell-mediated immunity.

VIRAL PATHOGENS

Viral infections are especially frequent in patients with impaired cell-mediated immunity. Among viruses that cause infections in immunocompromised hosts, herpes simplex, varicella zoster, cytomegalovirus (CMV), and adenoviruses are the most important. Cutaneous lesions and mucositis often are caused by herpes simplex. Herpes zoster infections may be especially severe and have a propensity for dissemination. Left untreated, primary varicella infections are associated with a high mortality rate. CMV may cause febrile illnesses associated with pneumonia, hepatitis, and/or gastrointestinal tract ulcerations. Respiratory syncytial virus (RSV) and influenza virus are important pathogens causing respiratory illness in stem cell transplant recipients in the winter months.[9] Virus-associated hemorrhagic cystitis caused by BK virus and adenovirus is common among hematopoietic stem cell transplant recipients.[10]

MYCOBACTERIAL PATHOGENS

The association between lymphoid malignancies and tuberculosis, particularly among patients born outside the United States, has been recognized for more than a century. It threatens to become a more frequent, serious problem with the resurgence of tuberculosis and the increased prevalence of drug-resistant strains.[11,12] Nontuberculous mycobacterial infections are common in HIV-positive patients, but are less common in patients receiving chemotherapy.[13]

● RECOGNITION AND DIAGNOSIS OF INFECTION

The development of an infection in a neutropenic patient may be accompanied by dramatic clinical manifestations or by none at all. Any fever that develops is very suggestive of infection. However, hypothermia, declining mental status, myalgia, or lethargy also may indicate infection in these patients. The usual local signs of infection, such as pus formation, may be absent or delayed because they are mediated by neutrophils.[14]

A careful physical examination should be performed when such a change in condition is observed. Special attention should be paid to the mouth and teeth for evidence of thrush, ulcerations, or periodontal disease. The skin should be examined in detail. Innocuous-appearing skin lesions may be septic emboli or evidence of disseminated fungal infection. Ordinarily trivial injuries inflicted by venipuncture or intravenous catheters may become infected and result in sepsis. An increased incidence of perianal and perirectal infection is observed in neutropenic patients.[15] Examination of the rectum and perineum may provide a clue to the source of fever in patients without other clinical findings. Although such examinations should not be performed unnecessarily on an immunocompromised patient, rectal or pelvic examination should not be deferred when searching for a cause of fever.

Chest radiographic films should be obtained initially and may need to be repeated, although this practice has been questioned in patients without respiratory complaints.[16] Chest computed tomography (CT) may reveal lesions not detected on routine radiograms.[17] Additional imaging should be guided by clinical presentation.

Blood cultures should be collected prior to initiation of antibiotic therapy, and periodically thereafter if fever persists. If an indwelling venous catheter is present, a blood culture as well as cultures from each lumen of the catheter should be obtained for bacterial and fungal pathogens. Differential time to positivity of central and peripheral cultures may be helpful in diagnosing catheter-associated infections.[18] Sending two or three cultures improves the likelihood of recovering fastidious organisms. If differential time to positivity cannot be performed, potentially infected intravenous lines should be cultured upon removal.

Other cultures should be obtained based on presenting symptoms and risk factors. Urine cultures should be sent in patients with an indwelling urinary catheter, those whose urinalysis is suspicious for infection, and those who have urinary symptoms. Sputum cultures may be helpful in patients with respiratory symptoms or findings on chest radiographs, but must be interpreted with caution, because the results may reflect the flora colonizing the oropharynx rather than the pathogens infecting the lung. Pulmonary fungal and viral infections, which may be difficult to document using conventional culture techniques, may be diagnosed by polymerase chain reaction and antigen detection sent from nasal washes or bronchoalveolar lavage samples.[19,20] Skin lesions of a suspicious nature should be biopsied and cultured. Stool should be cultured as well as examined for ova and parasites, and *Clostridium difficile* in patients with diarrhea. In some patients, testing for rotavirus, norovirus, and adenovirus also may be appropriate.

Patients with findings on chest CT that are consistent with pneumonia who do not respond to initial therapy and in whom initial microbiologic testing is negative may benefit from transbronchial biopsy or CT-guided biopsy of affected tissue.[21]

● TREATMENT AND PREVENTION

INITIAL TREATMENT

Bacterial Infections

Many different regimens have been evaluated and found to be acceptable for empiric therapy in febrile patients with neutropenia. Current recommendations support single-drug therapy with an antipseudomonal β-lactam as initial empiric therapy in febrile neutropenic patients.[22] Piperacillin-tazobactam,[23] imipenem,[24] meropenem,[25] cefepime,[26] and ceftazidime[27] have each been studied as a single agent. These drugs are active against most of the virulent pathogens infecting neutropenic patients. Doripenem, another carbapenem with antipseudomonal activity has not been studied in a prospective randomized control trial in febrile neutropenia. Ertapenem, a carbapenem that is attractive for its daily dosing schedule, lacks activity against pseudomonas and should not be used as empiric therapy.[28] Differences in institutional sensitivity patterns should guide initial antibiotic selection, which should subsequently be tailored to culture results.

Although Gram-negative coverage with a single agent is associated with improved outcomes,[29] among patients who are unstable or in whom antibiotic resistance is suspected, it is reasonable to add a second antibiotic active against Gram-negative organisms. Aminoglycosides may provide synergy against Gram-negative bacilli and further broaden the spectrum of antimicrobial activity, but they increase the risk of nephrotoxicity. No good evidence supports the simultaneous use of two β lactam drugs Fluoroquinolones in conjunction with another antibiotic are effective in patients who have not received quinolone prophylaxis.[30]

Patients with catheters, patients presenting with sepsis, patients with evidence of skin or soft-tissue infection, and other high-risk patients should be treated empirically for Gram-positive infections with vancomycin. Among patients without these risk factors, Gram-positive coverage should be added if fever persists for more than 3 to 5 days after Gram-negative treatment is initiated.[22]

The emergence of multidrug-resistant organisms has influenced the approach to empiric therapy. Approximately 60 percent of the hospital-acquired strains of *Staphylococcus aureus* now are methicillin-resistant *S. aureus* (MRSA), as are a growing number of community-acquired strains.[31] Vancomycin, quinupristin/dalfopristin,[32] linezolid,[33] daptomycin,[34] ceftaroline,[35] and tigecycline[36] are active against MRSA. However, it should be noted that daptomycin should not be used in pneumonia because of inactivation by surfactant. Tigecycline should be avoided in bloodstream infections because of inadequate serum levels, and the drug now carries a black box warning because of increased mortality seen with this agent. Dalbavancin, a second-generation glycopeptide that can be administered once per week, has been approved for treatment of MRSA skin and soft-tissue infections.[37] Ceftobiprole is a broad-spectrum cephalosporin that is also active against MRSA, but is not yet approved in the United States.[38]

The emergence of vancomycin-resistant *S. aureus* strains may limit the use of vancomycin in the treatment of *S. aureus* infections in the future, although, fortunately, these isolates are currently quite rare.[39] Toxicities of anti-MRSA agents as well as a comprehensive list of antibiotics with activity against MRSA still in development are reviewed in Ref. 40. Linezolid is a commonly used alternative to vancomycin, but causes thrombocytopenia and therefore must be used with caution in patients who are receiving chemotherapy.[41] Daptomycin is a good alternative to vancomycin for bloodstream infections.

Vancomycin-resistant *Enterococcus* (VRE) is being isolated with increasing frequency and presents a major challenge, particularly among neutropenic patients.[42,43] Cefepime and ceftazidime lack activity against enterococcus. Linezolid,[44] daptomycin,[45] and quinupristin/dalfopristin,[32] are the best agents currently available for treatment of serious VRE infections. Tigecycline also has activity against VRE,[36] but should not be used in bloodstream infections because of inadequate serum levels. Quinupristin/dalfopristin is not active against *Enterococcus faecalis*. The minimum inhibitory concentration of the organism should be checked before initiating daptomycin because VRE isolates can have daptomycin resistance, even in the absence of prior daptomycin usage.[46]

Drug resistance among Gram-negative pathogens is also of great clinical concern in neutropenic patients. As a result of the rising prevalence of multidrug resistant Gram-negative organisms, older drugs, such as colistin, have been reintroduced into practice.[47] Enteric pathogens, particularly *Klebsiella* and *E. coli* which produce extended-spectrum β-lactamases are a large and growing clinical problem. In up to 25 percent of cases of Gram-negative rod bacteremia in neutropenic patients, cultures ultimately grow extended-spectrum β-lactamase (ESBL)-producing pathogens.[48] These organisms are resistant to all cephalosporins and exhibit varying and unpredictable degrees of sensitivity to aminoglycosides and quinolones. The carbapenems (imipenem, meropenem, doripenem, ertapenem) are active against these pathogens. Carbapenemase-producing organisms, currently relatively rare, may become an important clinical problem in the future. Data regarding treatment of infections caused by carbapenemase-producing organisms are limited to retrospective and noncontrolled, nonrandomized prospective studies but suggest that combination therapy with a carbapenem plus colistin, aminoglycoside, or tigecycline may be more effective than monotherapy.[49,50]

Fungal Infections

Systemic fungal infections are relatively common in neutropenic patients, and empiric antifungal therapy should be considered in febrile patients if empiric antibiotic therapy is not effective within 5 to 7 days.[51] Historically, amphotericin B deoxycholate had been the drug of choice for the majority of fungal infections that develop in neutropenic hosts, although its position has been largely supplanted by the introduction of liposomal formulations of amphotericin in most centers, newer azole drugs, and echinocandins.[52,53]

There are three lipid-associated formulations of amphotericin currently available in the United States. AmBisome (liposomal amphotericin B); Abelcet (amphotericin B lipid complex); and Amphotec/Amphocil (amphotericin B colloidal dispersion). These three agents are not interchangeable. These formulations, particularly AmBisome, are less nephrotoxic, and appear to be at least as efficacious as nonlipid formulations. Infusion-related symptoms are not consistently less common with these preparations, but are generally manageable.[54] Serum creatinine, potassium, and magnesium levels should be monitored closely while giving these medications. Amphotericin products remain the first-line agent in treatment of mucormycosis, although they are frequently used in combination with echinocandins.[55]

Although there are limited data to support its efficacy, it is common practice to give intravenous fluids prior to and sometimes after amphotericin infusion to mitigate nephrotoxicity.[56] Fever and chills associated with administration of amphotericin may be treated or prevented with diphenhydramine hydrochloride, acetaminophen, or hydrocortisone.[57]

Fluconazole, an azole drug that can be administered orally or intravenously, is approved for treatment of *C. albicans*, *Cryptococcus neoformans*, and *Coccidioides immitis*. It is less active against non-*albicans Candida* species and is completely inactive against *Candida krusei*. It also lacks activity against *Aspergillus*.[58]

In contrast to fluconazole, itraconazole has modest activity against *Aspergillus*. It is less active than voriconazole but may have a role in milder infections or when voriconazole is not tolerated.[59]

Voriconazole is another azole drug, which is also available in intravenous and oral formulations. A large study concluded that voriconazole is as effective as liposomal amphotericin B as empiric therapy for neutropenic patients who are febrile, but these results are controversial.[52,60] Oral voriconazole may be a good alternative to the intravenous formulation in neutropenic patients with uncomplicated persistent fever.[61] It is the first-line therapy against *Aspergillus*.[62] Side effects of voriconazole, which may limit its use in some patients, include visual abnormalities, hallucinations, and liver function test (LFT) abnormalities. Recent data suggest that voriconazole use in transplant recipients is associated with an increased rate of nonmelanoma skin cancers. The mechanism by which this occurs is currently unknown.[63] Neurologic side effects may be related to blood levels of the drug, which vary widely depending upon a large number of factors including CYP2C19 genotype. There is mounting evidence that therapeutic drug monitoring improves safety and efficacy of voriconazole in the treatment of invasive fungal infections.[64,65]

Posaconazole is the newest approved azole. It is now available in intravenous and oral formulations. Its primary use has been prophylactic; however, it has shown promise as salvage therapy for invasive aspergillosis.[66] Unlike the older triazoles, posaconazole is active against many species that cause mucormycosis, and it has been used successfully when other therapy has failed; however, there is no clinical trial data available at this time.[67]

Isavuconazole is an investigational broad-spectrum azole available in oral and intravenous formulations. It is currently in phase III trials comparing it to voriconazole for treatment of *Aspergillus*. It also has some activity against species that cause mucormycosis.[68]

The echinocandins, which include caspofungin, micafungin, and anidulafungin, are a class of intravenous drugs that has activity against a wide variety of *Candida* species as well as *Aspergillus*. They are generally well tolerated, and may become especially important as the prevalence of non-*albicans Candida* infections rises.[69] Currently, only caspofungin is approved for first-line empirical use in febrile neutropenia.[70] Caspofungin is also the only echinocandin approved as salvage therapy for aspergillosis; however, mounting evidences suggests that micafungin is also effective in the treatment of invasive *Aspergillus* infections.[71] The echinocandins may have synergy with other antifungal agents against *Aspergillus* species and in treating mucormycosis.[55,72] A randomized controlled trial evaluating echinocandins as part of combination therapy in *Aspergillus* treatment has been performed and results are expected soon. Anidulafungin, the newest approved echinocandin, has shown excellent efficacy in the treatment of candidiasis.[73]

P. jiroveci pneumonia may be treated with trimethoprim-sulfamethoxazole. Pentamidine or primaquine-clindamycin should be used for moderate to severe infections in patients who are allergic to or otherwise intolerant of trimethoprim-sulfamethoxazole, although data for alternative regimens is much more robust in the HIV-positive patient population.[74] Other alternative regimens include dapsone-trimethoprim and atovaquone, although these are best used for mild PCP. Glucocorticoids are commonly given as adjunctive treatment in severe PCP, though the data for this among non–HIV-infected patients are conflicting.[75]

Empiric therapy with antifungal agents is currently the standard of care in high-risk neutropenic patients with persistent fever. However, preemptive antifungal treatment is being evaluated as a possible alternative to empiric therapy in select patients. With preemptive strategies, microbiologic, molecular, and radiologic monitoring is used to detect early evidence of invasive fungal infections and prompt initiation of therapy.[76] Data from studies comparing empiric therapy with preemptive strategies are mixed.[77-79] Surveillance with fungal cell wall components 1,3-β-D-glucan[80] and galactomannan[81] in the blood plays a role in preemptive therapy. Real-time polymerase chain reaction of fungal gene products is another technique that appears to have high sensitivity and specificity for detecting candidemia, although it will require standardization before widespread use is possible.[82]

Although currently not as large a problem as drug-resistant bacteria, the development of drug-resistant fungal organisms is a potential clinical threat. Prophylactic use of antifungals likely contributes to breakthrough infection with innately resistant species.[83] Cross-resistance within and between classes of antifungals is another potentially important problem, which is deserving of clinical study.[84]

Viral Infections

A limited number of options are available for treatment of viral infections. Acyclovir is active against herpes simplex and, at higher doses, against varicella zoster. Other agents, such as famciclovir and valacyclovir, are as effective in treating herpes simplex and zoster infections, and may be administered less frequently, but are not available for intravenous administration.[85]

Ganciclovir, valganciclovir, and foscarnet have efficacy in treatment of CMV disease and are also active against herpes simplex.[86] They are most effective when they are used early in the course of the infection. Hence, frequent screening for CMV and early preemptive treatment in high-risk patients, such as transplant recipients, may allow for improved outcomes.[87] Ganciclovir or valganciclovir is usually the first-line therapy against CMV, but results in marrow suppression in a significant percentage of patients who receive them. Foscarnet, a second-line agent, may be complicated by azotemia and electrolyte abnormalities.

Ribavirin plus an adjunctive immunomodulator such as RSV immunoglobulin (Ig) or intravenous immunoglobulin (IVIG) are used to treat RSV pneumonia in immunocompromised patients. Ribavirin can also be used to treat RSV upper respiratory tract infections, and may prevent spread to the lower respiratory tract as well as decrease mortality; however, prospective studies are needed.[88] The optimal route of ribavirin administration (oral versus inhaled) is not yet known. Oseltamivir or zanamivir should be used if influenza A is suspected.[89]

Mycobacterial Infections

Rates of *Mycobacterium tuberculosis* infection are high among patients with hematologic malignancy worldwide, and tuberculosis should be ruled out in neutropenic patients with lung infiltrates who have tuberculosis risk factors. First-line therapy for tuberculosis includes rifampin, isoniazid, pyrazinamide, and ethambutol.[90]

Infections with multidrug-resistant tuberculosis, defined as microbes resistant to rifampin and isoniazid, are difficult to treat and are associated with poor prognoses. The prevalence of multidrug-resistant tuberculosis varies tremendously by country.[91] Drugs used to treat multidrug-resistant tuberculosis include fluoroquinolones, amikacin, capreomycin, and kanamycin. Extensively drug-resistant *M. tuberculosis*, which is defined as being resistant to rifampin, isoniazid, fluoroquinolones, and at least one injectable second-line agent, is a potentially a huge clinical problem.[92]

Although relatively uncommon, nontuberculous mycobacterial infections also occur in patients with hematologic malignancy. *Mycobacterium avium-intracellulare* complex is treated with clarithromycin, rifabutin, and ethambutol. Treatment of infections with rapidly growing mycobacteria is complicated and should be guided by an infectious disease specialist.[13]

Table 24–1 lists the drugs used as empiric therapy in neutropenic patients.

ADJUSTING THERAPY

Adjustment or modification of the initial antimicrobial regimen may be necessary for several reasons. Results of cultures may suggest another regimen would be more active or less toxic. All cultures may remain negative while the patient fails to respond to the regimen. Fever may recur following an initial response to therapy, raising the possibility of a second infection.

Adjusting therapy based on a culture report usually is straightforward, but the other two situations may pose dilemmas. In these circumstances, resistant organisms or noninfectious causes of fever, such as drug fever or recurrence of malignancy, must be considered. Repeat cultures and careful clinical reappraisal may prove helpful.

DURATION OF THERAPY

Antibiotic therapy for a specific infection is commonly continued for a defined minimum period of time *and* until the granulocyte count reaches 0.5×10^9/L. Although this strategy reduces the number of relapsing infections, it may increase the risk of superinfection and antibiotic toxicity. In low-risk patients whose fever resolves without a documented source of infection, empiric intravenous therapy can usually be stopped and replaced by an oral regimen until counts recover. Alternatively, there is some evidence that returning to a prophylactic regimen in select patients before the absolute neutrophil count reaches 0.5×10^9/L is also a reasonable approach.[93] If antibiotics are discontinued or deescalated, close observation is required, and therapy should be reinstituted at any suggestion of recurrent infection.

FEVER FOLLOWING RECOVERY FROM CHEMOTHERAPY

Fevers occasionally persist or even begin after the granulocyte count has returned to normal levels. Drug fever and engraftment syndrome are considerations in this setting, although a deep-seated infection must be excluded.[94] Hepatosplenic candidiasis is one important consideration in these patients, although its incidence has likely decreased in the setting of widespread antifungal prophylaxis discussed under "Fungal Infections" below.[95] Elevated serum alkaline phosphatase levels and the presence of multiple "punched-out" lesions in the liver on CT are common findings with hepatic involvement. Blood cultures are frequently negative so biopsy may be required to establish a microbiologic diagnosis.[96] Hepatosplenic candidiasis requires prolonged therapy. Several regimens have been proposed, including fluconazole,[97] caspofungin,[98] and liposomal amphotericin B,[99] but there are no randomized trial data. Persistent symptoms despite treatment may be a result of immune reconstitution inflammatory syndrome and may be relieved by adjuvant treatment

TABLE 24–1. Coverage and Side Effects of Drugs Used as Empiric Therapy

Drug Category	Drug	Brand Name	Activity	Toxicity
Antipseudomonal penicillins	Piperacillin-tazobactam	Zosyn	Methicillin-sensitive *Staphylococcus, Streptococcus, Enterococcus faecalis,* anaerobes, *Pseudomonas aeruginosa,* enteric Gram-negative rods	Hypokalemia, antiplatelet effect
Antipseudomonal cephalosporins	Ceftazidime	Fortaz	*P. aeruginosa,* enteric Gram-negative rods, methicillin-sensitive *Staphylococcus**	
	Cefepime	Maxipime	*P. aeruginosa,* enteric Gram-negative rods, methicillin-sensitive *Staphylococcus*	Cefepime-induced neurotoxicity
Aminoglycosides	Amikacin	Amikin	Enteric Gram-negative rods, *P. aeruginosa*	Nephrotoxicity, ototoxicity
	Tobramycin	Nebcin		
	Gentamicin	Garamycin		
Glycopeptide	Vancomycin	Vancocin	*Staphylococcus* (including MRSA), *Streptococcus, E. faecalis, Corynebacterium*	Ototoxicity, red-man syndrome with rapid infusion
Carbapenem	Imipenem	Primaxin	Gram-negative rods, *Pseudomonas aeruginosa* (except for ertapenem), methicillin-sensitive *Staphylococcus,* Streptococci, Enterococcus (imipenem), anaerobes	Nausea, seizures (imipenem)
	Meropenem	Merrem		
	Ertapenem	Invanz		
	Doripenem	Doribax		
Monobactam	Aztreonam	Azactam	Gram-negative rods, *P. aeruginosa*	
Sulfonamides	Trimethoprim-sulfamethoxazole	Bactrim; Septra	*Pneumocystis jiroveci,* some Gram-negative rods, *Staphylococcus, Nocardia*	Sulfa allergy, increased creatinine, nausea, rash
Fluoroquinolones	Ciprofloxacin	Cipro	Gram-negative rods, *P. aeruginosa,* viridans streptococci	Nausea. Rare Achilles tendon rupture
	Levofloxacin	Levaquin	Gram-negative rods, *P. aeruginosa,* viridans streptococci†	
Nucleosides	Acyclovir	Zovirax	HSV, VZV	Crystalluria
	Valacyclovir	Valtrex	HSV, VZV	
	Famciclovir	Famvir	HSV, VZV	
	Ganciclovir	Cytovene	CMV	Marrow suppression
	Valganciclovir	Valcyte	CMV	Marrow suppression
Phosphonoformate	Foscarnet	Foscavir	CMV	Renal failure, electrolyte abnormalities
Polyene antifungals	Amphotericin B	Fungizone	*Candida, Aspergillus,* other fungi including mucormycosis	Fever, chills, nausea, vomiting, renal failure hypokalemia, hypomagnesemia
	Ampho-B lipid complex	Abelcet	*Candida, Aspergillus,* other fungi including mucormycosis	Fever, chills, nausea, vomiting, increased creatinine
	Ampho-B cholesteryl sulfate complex	Amphotec	*Candida, Aspergillus,* other fungi including mucormycosis	Fever, chills, nausea, vomiting, increased creatinine
	Liposomal ampho-B	AmBisome	*Candida, Aspergillus,* other fungi including mucormycosis	Fever, chills, nausea, vomiting, increased creatinine
Azole	Fluconazole	Diflucan	*Candida, Cryptococcus, Coccidioides immitis*	LFT abnormality
	Itraconazole	Sporonox	*Candida, Aspergillus, Histoplasma*	CHF; drug–drug interactions
	Voriconazole	Vfend	*Aspergillus, Coccidioides, Histoplasma*	Loss of vision with intravenous prep
	Posaconazole	Noxafil	*Aspergillus, Coccidioides, Histoplasma,* mucormycosis	Nausea, diarrhea, LFT abnormality

(continued)

TABLE 24–1. Coverage and Side Effects of Drugs Used as Empiric Therapy (Continued)

Drug Category	Drug	Brand Name	Activity	Toxicity
Echinocandin	Caspofungin	Cancidas	*Aspergillus, Candida*, mucormycosis[‡]	
	Micafungin	Mycamine	*Aspergillus, Candida*, mucormycosis[‡]	
	Anidulafungin	Eraxis	*Aspergillus, Candida*, mucormycosis[‡]	
Oxazolidinone	Linezolid	Zyvox	Staphylococci (including MRSA), *Enterococcus* (including VRE), streptococci	Thrombocytopenia, anemia, small risk of serotonin syndrome with concomitant SSRIs, mitochondrial side effects with prolonged use
Lipopeptide	Daptomycin	Cubicin	Staphylococci (including MRSA), *Enterococcus* (including VRE), streptococci	Creatinine kinase elevation

Ampho-B, amphotericin B; CHF, congestive heart failure; CMV, cytomegalovirus; HSV, herpes simplex virus; LFT, liver function test; SSRI, selective serotonin reuptake inhibitor; VRE, vancomycin-resistant *Enterococcus*; VZV, varicella-zoster virus.

*Ceftazidime has less activity than cefepime against methicillin-sensitive *Staphylococcus aureus* and viridans streptococci.

†Levofloxacin has more reliable activity against viridans streptococci than ciprofloxacin.

‡Echinocandins are commonly used in combination with amphotericin in the treatment of mucormycosis, but are not used as monotherapy.

with glucocorticoids.[100] Cure is difficult to achieve regardless of the regimen used and mortality is high.[101]

Indwelling catheter infections are another important consideration in persistent fever after hematologic recovery. Diagnosing catheter infections remains a major challenge, and the use of catheter-sparing diagnostic techniques should be considered, as the need to remove catheters is patient and organism dependent. Coagulase-negative *Staphylococcus* spp. are most commonly isolated and are generally amenable to catheter-sparing treatment. If the catheter is to be retained, a 10- to 14-day course of antibiotics is recommended.[102] If a tunnel infection is present, successful therapy is less likely without catheter removal.

Gram-negative,[103] *S. aureus*,[104] and fungal[105] infections of the catheter usually necessitate its removal. This may be followed, if necessary, by insertion of a new catheter at a different site once blood cultures have cleared. Antibiotic therapy for at least 14 days is recommended. Chlorhexidine and silver-impregnated central venous catheters may prevent bloodstream infections in neutropenic patients.[106] Catheter infections and their management are reviewed in detail elsewhere.[102]

OUTPATIENT THERAPY

Twenty years ago, treatment of the febrile neutropenic patient outside of the hospital would have been unthinkable. Economic pressures, coupled with the widespread availability of home infusion services and more potent oral antibiotics, have made outpatient therapy an option for some of these patients.[107]

Outcomes among patients with neutropenic fever treated as outpatients seem to be comparable to those observed in hospitalized patients, provided the patients are selected properly and appropriate monitoring can be ensured. Suitable candidates for home therapy include patients who are expected to have a short duration of neutropenia and who have few comorbidities.[108,109] Individuals who remain febrile, who require multiple antibiotics, or who are unreliable are not candidates for home therapy. Rigorous family education is crucial for a successful outcome.

PREVENTION OF INFECTIONS

Bacterial Infections

In view of the high mortality rate associated with infections in neutropenic patients, preventive measures remain a priority. Careful attention to sterile technique and personal hygiene is of the utmost importance

in the prevention of bacterial infection during neutropenia. Instrumentation should be avoided whenever possible. Intravenous access sites should be carefully maintained. In addition, systemic antibiotics are currently widely used as prophylaxis against Gram-negative infections in neutropenic patients.

The use of prophylactic antibiotics reduces the number of Gram-negative infections and all-cause mortality in high-risk patients who are expected to have prolonged, severe neutropenia and is recommended in these patients.[110] By contrast, the use of antibiotic prophylaxis in lower-risk patients expected to have a shorter duration of neutropenia is of much less certain benefit, and is not recommended in most cases.[111] Several studies show a reduction in mortality in high-risk patients given prophylactic antibiotics, but the contribution of this practice to the emergence of drug-resistant pathogens must be taken into account when deciding whether to employ it.[112,113] Furthermore, although the agents used for this purpose are generally safe, the risk of drug toxicity must also be taken into consideration. Adverse events associated with antibiotic prophylaxis include drug fever, rash, and worsening of cytopenias. Infection with *C. difficile* is a potentially serious risk of prophylaxis.[114] Incidence of *C. difficile* infection is high in stem cell transplant recipients, and patients who receive high-risk antibiotics including fluoroquinolones more frequently acquire infection with this organism.[115] This potential complication deserves strong consideration, as drug-resistant, hypervirulent strains of this organism have become more prevalent over the last several years.[116]

The fluoroquinolones, particularly ciprofloxacin and levofloxacin, have received considerable attention for their ability to prevent Gram-negative infections in neutropenic patients.[110] Ciprofloxacin has more activity against *Pseudomonas*, whereas levofloxacin is more active against Gram-positive organisms. Unfortunately, indiscriminate use of these agents in the community, as well as prophylactic use, has led to a greatly increased prevalence of quinolone-resistant Gram-negative organisms. Up to 85 percent of Gram-negative isolates from patients with febrile neutropenia are resistant to quinolones,[117] and quinolone prophylaxis has resulted in an increased incidence of quinolone-resistant viridans streptococci.[118] Prophylactic use also eliminates these agents from therapeutic use in the same patient.[119] For these reasons, some centers abandoned the use of prophylactic quinolones in certain patients.[120–122] These studies consistently showed a decrease in fluoroquinolone resistance in isolates from neutropenic patients. While some studies have failed to show an increase in the incidence of bacteremia with discontinuation of prophylaxis,[120] in at least two cases, institutional cessation of quinolone prophylaxis resulted in an increased incidence of bacteremia caused by Gram-negative organisms, which was reversed by reinstitution of fluoroquinolone prophylaxis.[121,122] In summary, there is, at present, a clear role for quinolone prophylaxis in some patients. However, because of increasing resistance to these drugs, it is important to continuously monitor their efficacy and discourage their unnecessary use.

The use of granulocyte-macrophage colony-stimulating factor and granulocyte colony-stimulating factor to raise the absolute neutrophil count has been shown to decrease the incidence of fever in patients on high risk chemotherapy regimens, elderly patients, and patients with certain comorbid conditions.[123,124] However, there is no definitive evidence that prophylaxis with these agents reduces infection-related mortality or overall survival.[125]

Low-bacteria diets are often recommended to patients expected to experience neutropenia, but their effectiveness at preventing infection has not been shown.[126] Similarly, the efficacy of reverse isolation, though often employed as a prophylactic measure, has not been demonstrated.[127]

Viral Infections

Acyclovir and its prodrug valacyclovir are effective at preventing recurrent herpes simplex infections in patients receiving chemotherapy.[128] Long-term treatment with acyclovir also prevents reactivation of varicella-zoster virus in hematopoietic stem cell transplant recipients,[129] as well as in patients undergoing chemotherapy for multiple myeloma.[130] Varicella-zoster immunoglobulin is recommended as postexposure prophylaxis for high-risk, nonimmune patients.[131]

Hematopoietic stem cell transplant recipients have a high risk of CMV infection. Patients at particular risk include those who are seropositive before transplantation, seronegative patients who receive transplants from seropositive donors, and those who receive highly immunosuppressive conditioning regimens prior to transplantation.[132,133] The use of CMV seronegative blood components can markedly decrease the transmission of CMV to seronegative patients; leukocyte reduction similarly prevents transmission.[134] Ganciclovir,[135] oral valganciclovir,[136] and CMV immune globulin infusions have been used to prevent CMV infection in transplant recipients. Ganciclovir and valganciclovir frequently cause myelosuppression, which may complicate the management of neutropenic patients on these medications.[137] In addition, the emergence of CMV antiviral resistance has been reported in association with preventive treatment.[138] CMV prophylaxis among patients receiving conventional chemotherapy has not been as widely studied, but currently there is no evidence supporting its use in this population.[139] Many centers take a preemptive approach, screening patients regularly for CMV viremia and initiating therapy only when CMV is detected. Prophylactic immunotherapy may have benefit in patients unable to tolerate the potential myelotoxicity of antiviral therapy.[140] Recent randomized controlled trials have suggested that novel anti-CMV agents letermovir and brincidofovir may be effective at preventing CMV replication in stem cell transplant recipients.[141,142]

Immunizations with killed vaccines such as influenza are recommended. Live-attenuated vaccines, such as measles and zoster, should be avoided during immunosuppression.[143]

Fungal Infections

The high mortality rate of invasive fungal infections in neutropenic patients makes their prevention extremely important. Antifungal prophylaxis in these patients has been studied for more than 2 decades, yet there is still a great deal of controversy surrounding its efficacy.[144] Studies on prevention of fungal infections in neutropenic patients are difficult to evaluate. Results of the various studies have been conflicting,

partly because different definitions and outcomes were applied, different doses of antifungal agents were administered, and the numbers of study patients have often been small.

As with antibacterial prophylaxis, the clearest benefit of antifungal prophylaxis is seen in patients expected to have severe, prolonged neutropenia, particularly allogeneic transplant recipients. Antifungal prophylaxis is not indicated in patients who are undergoing chemotherapy with low levels of myelotoxicity.[22] When deciding whether to treat prophylactically, drug toxicity must be taken into account. In addition, prophylactic use of antifungal agents may select for more resistant strains of fungus and lead to breakthrough infection with organisms inherently resistant to the agent used for prophylaxis. For example, certain prophylactic regimens active against *Candida* may actually increase the incidence of *Aspergillus* infections.[145] The ability of antifungal agents to prevent systemic infection in high-risk patients has been shown in several studies, but their ability to reduce all-cause mortality has not been definitively established.[146]

Several azole drugs have been studied as prophylactic agents. A number of studies document a statistically significant reduction in superficial and invasive fungal infections when fluconazole is used prophylactically.[147] However, breakthrough infection with *Aspergillus*, *Candida glabrata*, and *Candida krusei* have occurred with fluconazole prophylaxis.[83] Itraconazole and voriconazole[148] have a broader spectrum of activity, are more effective at preventing *Aspergillus* infection, and are generally well tolerated.[149] Prophylaxis with posaconazole is associated with a reduced risk of *Aspergillus* infection, and a trend toward lower mortality.[150]

Echinocandins have become popular antifungal prophylactic agents. Caspofungin has been shown to be as effective as itraconazole in preventing *Aspergillus* and *Candida* infections.[151] Micafungin was shown to be superior to fluconazole at preventing systemic fungal infections in hematopoietic stem cell transplant recipients.[152] Anidulafungin, the newest echinocandin, remains to be studied as a prophylactic agent.

P. jiroveci pneumonia can be prevented with trimethoprim-sulfamethoxazole.[153] Dapsone and atovaquone have each been used as a second-line prophylactic agent in hematopoietic stem cell transplant recipients, and in some cases may be preferred based on the risk of marrow suppression from trimethoprim-sulfamethoxazole.[154,155] Although *P. jiroveci* is a ubiquitous organism, institutional variability in the incidence of infection is observed; therefore, the need for prophylaxis varies.

● INFECTIONS IN HEMATOPOIETIC STEM CELL TRANSPLANTATION RECIPIENTS

Patients receiving hematopoietic stem cell transplants are at risk for the same infections occurring in patients rendered neutropenic by chemotherapy. Graft-versus-host disease and the immunosuppressive agents used to treat it result in a particularly high incidence of infection in this group of patients. CMV and varicella zoster virus, are especially troublesome. Infection in stem cell transplant patients has been reviewed[156] and is discussed in Chap. 23.

REFERENCES

1. Bodey GP, Buckley M, Sathe YS, Freireich EJ: Quantitative relationships between circulating leukocytes and infection in patients with acute leukemia. *Ann Intern MedIntern Med* 64:328, 1966.
2. Ramphal R: Changes in the etiology of bacteremia in febrile neutropenic patients and the susceptibilities of the currently isolated pathogens. *Clin Infect Dis* 39:S25, 2004.
3. Reilly AF, Lange BJ: Infections with viridans group streptococci in children with cancer. *Pediatr Blood Cancer* 49:774, 2007.
4. Wadhwa PD, Morrison VA: Infectious complications of chronic lymphocytic leukemia. *Semin Oncol* 33:240, 2006.

5. Morrison V: Infections in patients with leukemia and lymphoma, in *Infectious Complications in Cancer Patients*, edited by Stosor V, Zembower TR, p 319. Springer International Publishing, Switzerland, 2014.

6. Hachem R, Hanna H, Kontoyiannis D, et al: The changing epidemiology of invasive candidiasis: *Candida glabrata* and *Candida krusei* as the leading causes of candidemia in hematologic malignancy. *Cancer* 112:2493, 2008.

7. Chamilos G, Marom EM, Lewis RE, et al: Predictors of pulmonary zygomycosis versus invasive pulmonary aspergillosis in patients with cancer. *Clin Infect Dis* 41:60, 2005.

8. Walsh TJ, Gamaletsou MN: Treatment of fungal disease in the setting of neutropenia. *Hematology Am Soc Hematol Educ Program* 2013:423, 2013.

9. Mikulska M, Del Bono V, Gandolfo N, et al: Epidemiology of viral respiratory tract infections in an outpatient haematology facility. *Ann Hematol* 93:669, 2014.

10. Mori Y, Miyamoto T, Kato K, et al: Different risk factors related to adenovirus- or BK virus-associated hemorrhagic cystitis following allogeneic stem cell transplantation. *Biol Blood Marrow Transplant* 18:458, 2012.

11. Kamboj M, Sepkowitz KA: The risk of tuberculosis in patients with cancer. *Clin Infect Dis* 42:1592, 2006.

12. De La Rosa GR, Jacobson KL, Rolston KV, et al: *Mycobacterium tuberculosis* at a comprehensive cancer centre: Active disease in patients with underlying malignancy during 1990–2000. *Clin Microbiol Infect* 10:749, 2004.

13. Chen CY, Sheng WH, Lai CC, et al: Mycobacterial infections in adult patients with hematological malignancy. *Eur J Clin Microbiol Infect Dis* 31:1059, 2012.

14. Sickles EA, Greene WH, Wiernik PH: Clinical presentation of infection in granulocytopenic patients. *Arch Intern MedIntern Med* 135:715, 1975.

15. Chen CY, Cheng A, Huang SY, et al: Clinical and microbiological characteristics of perianal infections in adult patients with acute leukemia. *PLoS One* 8:e60624, 2013.

16. Korones DN, Hussong MR, Gullace MA: Routine chest radiography of children with cancer hospitalized for fever and neutropenia: Is it really necessary? *Cancer* 80:1160, 1997.

17. Heussel CP, Kauczor HU, Heussel G, et al: Early detection of pneumonia in febrile neutropenic patients: Use of thin-section CT. *AJR Am J Roentgenol* 169:1347, 1997.

18. Chen WT, Liu TM, Wu SH, et al: Improving diagnosis of central venous catheter-related bloodstream infection by using differential time to positivity as a hospital-wide approach at a cancer hospital. *J Infect* 59:317, 2009.

19. Maschmeyer G, Beinert T, Buchheidt D, et al: Diagnosis and antimicrobial therapy of lung infiltrates in febrile neutropenic patients: Guidelines of the infectious diseases working party of the German Society of Haematology and Oncology. *Eur J Cancer* 45:2462, 2009.

20. Cuenca-Estrella M, Meije Y, Diaz-Pedroche C, et al: Value of serial quantification of fungal DNA by a real-time PCR-based technique for early diagnosis of invasive *Aspergillosis* in patients with febrile neutropenia. *J Clin MicrobiolMicrobiology* 47:379, 2009.

21. Gupta S, Sultenfuss M, Romaguera JE, et al: CT-guided percutaneous lung biopsies in patients with haematologic malignancies and undiagnosed pulmonary lesions. *Hematol Oncol* 28:75, 2010.

22. Freifeld AG, Bow EJ, Sepkowitz KA, et al: Clinical practice guideline for the use of antimicrobial agents in neutropenic patients with cancer: 2010 update by the infectious diseases society of America. *Clin Infect Dis* 52:e56, 2011.

23. Bow EJ, Rotstein C, Noskin GA, et al: A randomized, open-label, multicenter comparative study of the efficacy and safety of piperacillin-tazobactam and cefepime for the empirical treatment of febrile neutropenic episodes in patients with hematologic malignancy. *Clin Infect Dis* 43:447, 2006.

24. Klastersky JA: Use of imipenem as empirical treatment of febrile neutropenia. *Int J Antimicrob Agents* 21:393, 2003.

25. Feld R, DePauw B, Berman S, et al: Meropenem versus ceftazidime in the treatment of cancer patients with febrile neutropenia: A randomized, double-blind trial. *J Clin Oncol* 18:3690, 2000.

26. Raad II, Escalante C, Hachem RY, et al: Treatment of febrile neutropenic patients with cancer who require hospitalization: A prospective randomized study comparing imipenem and cefepime. *Cancer* 98:1039, 2003.

27. Egerer G, Goldschmidt H, Salwender H, et al: Efficacy of continuous infusion of ceftazidime for patients with neutropenic fever after high-dose chemotherapy and peripheral blood stem cell transplantation. *Int J Antimicrob Agents* 15:119, 2000.

28. Zhanel GG, Wiebe R, Dilay L, et al: Comparative review of the carbapenems. *Drugs* 67:1027, 2007.

29. Paul M, Dickstein Y, Schlesinger A, et al: Beta-lactam versus beta-lactam-aminoglycoside combination therapy in cancer patients with neutropenia. *Cochrane Database Syst Rev* 6:CD003038, 2013.

30. Bliziotis IA, Michalopoulos A, Kasiakou SK, et al: Ciprofloxacin vs an aminoglycoside in combination with a beta-lactam for the treatment of febrile neutropenia: A meta-analysis of randomized controlled trials. *Mayo Clin Proc* 80:1146, 2005.

31. Klein EY, Sun L, Smith DL, Laxminarayan R: The changing epidemiology of methicillin-resistant *Staphylococcus aureus* in the United States: A national observational study. *Am J Epidemiol* 177:666, 2013.

32. Klastersky J: Role of quinupristin/dalfopristin in the treatment of Gram-positive nosocomial infections in haematological or oncological patients. *Cancer Treat Rev* 29:431, 2003.

33. Falagas ME, Siempos II, Vardakas KZ: Linezolid versus glycopeptide or beta-lactam for treatment of Gram-positive bacterial infections: Meta-analysis of randomised controlled trials. *Lancet Infect Dis* 8:53, 2008.

34. Rolston KV, Besece D, Lamp KC, et al: Daptomycin use in neutropenic patients with documented gram-positive infections. *Support Care Cancer* 22:7, 2014.

35. Wilcox MH, Corey GR, Talbot GH, et al: CANVAS 2: The second phase III, randomized, double-blind study evaluating ceftaroline fosamil for the treatment of patients with complicated skin and skin structure infections. *J Antimicrob Chemother* 65:iv53, 2010.

36. Florescu I, Beuran M, Dimov R, et al: Efficacy and safety of tigecycline compared with vancomycin or linezolid for treatment of serious infections with methicillin-resistant Staphylococcus aureus or vancomycin-resistant enterococci: A phase 3, multicentre, double-blind, randomized study. *J Antimicrob Chemother* 62 (Suppl 1):i17, 2008.

37. Boucher HW, Wilcox M, Talbot GH, et al: Once-weekly dalbavancin versus daily conventional therapy for skin infection. *N Engl J Med* 370:2169, 2014.

38. Awad SS, Rodriguez AH, Chuang YC, et al: A phase 3 randomized double-blind comparison of ceftobiprole medocaril versus ceftazidime plus linezolid for the treatment of hospital-acquired pneumonia. *Clin Infect Dis* 2014.

39. Appelbaum PC: Reduced glycopeptide susceptibility in methicillin-resistant *Staphylococcus aureus* (MRSA). *Int J Antimicrob Agents* 30:398, 2007.

40. Rodvold KA, McConeghy KW: Methicillin-resistant staphylococcus aureus therapy: Past, present, and future. *Clin Infect Dis* 58:S20, 2014.

41. Beekmann SE, Gilbert DN, Polgreen PM, IDSA Emerging Infections Network: Toxicity of extended courses of linezolid: Results of an Infectious Diseases Society of America Emerging Infections Network survey. *Diagn Microbiol Infect Dis* 62:407, 2008.

42. DiazGranados CA, Jernigan JA: Impact of vancomycin resistance on mortality among patients with neutropenia and enterococcal bloodstream infection. *J Infect Dis* 191:588, 2005.

43. Kang Y, Vicente M, Parsad S, et al: Evaluation of risk factors for vancomycin-resistant Enterococcus bacteremia among previously colonized hematopoietic stem cell transplant patients. *Transpl Infect Dis* 15:466, 2013.

44. Smith PF, Birmingham MC, Noskin GA, et al: Safety, efficacy and pharmacokinetics of linezolid for treatment of resistant Gram-positive infections in cancer patients with neutropenia. *Ann Oncol* 14:795, 2003.

45. Rolston KV, Besece D, Lamp KC, et al: Daptomycin use in neutropenic patients with documented gram-positive infections. *Support Care Cancer* 22:7, 2014.

46. Kelesidis T, Chow AL, Humphries R, et al: Case-control study comparing de novo and daptomycin-exposed daptomycin-nonsusceptible *Enterococcus* infections. *Antimicrob Agents Chemother* 56:2150, 2012.

47. Cassir N, Rolain JM, Brouqui P: A new strategy to fight antimicrobial resistance: The revival of old antibiotics. *Front Microbiol* 5:551, 2014.

48. Kim SH, Kwon JC, Choi SM, et al: *Escherichia coli* and *Klebsiella pneumoniae* bacteremia in patients with neutropenic fever: Factors associated with extended-spectrum beta-lactamase production and its impact on outcome. *Ann Hematol* 92:533, 2013.

49. Rafailidis PI, Falagas ME: Options for treating carbapenem-resistant Enterobacteriaceae. *Curr Opin Infect Dis* 27:479, 2014.

50. Nordmann P, Cuzon G, Naas T: The real threat of Klebsiella pneumoniae carbapenemase-producing bacteria. *Lancet Infect Dis* 9:228, 2009.

51. Schiel X, Link H, Maschmeyer G, et al: A prospective, randomized multicenter trial of the empirical addition of antifungal therapy for febrile neutropenic cancer patients: Results of the Paul Ehrlich Society for Chemotherapy (PEG) Multicenter Trial II. *Infection* 34:118, 2006.

52. Jorgensen KJ, Gotzsche PC, Dalboge CS, Johansen HK: Voriconazole versus amphotericin B or fluconazole in cancer patients with neutropenia. *Cochrane Database Syst Rev* 2:CD004707, 2014.

53. Walsh TJ, Teppler H, Donowitz GR, et al: Caspofungin versus liposomal amphotericin B for empirical antifungal therapy in patients with persistent fever and neutropenia. *N Engl J Med* 351:1391, 2004.

54. Johansen HK, Gotzsche PC: Amphotericin B lipid soluble formulations versus amphotericin B in cancer patients with neutropenia. *Cochrane Database Syst Rev* 9:CD000969, 2014.

55. Spellberg B, Ibrahim AS: Recent advances in the treatment of mucormycosis. *Curr Infect Dis Rep* 12:423, 2010.

56. Girmenia C, Cimino G, Di Cristofano F, et al: Effects of hydration with salt repletion on renal toxicity of conventional amphotericin B empirical therapy: A prospective study in patients with hematological malignancies. *Support Care Cancer* 13:987, 2005.

57. O'Connor N, Borley A: Prospective audit of the effectiveness of hydrocortisone premedication on drug delivery reactions following amphotericin B lipid complex *. *Curr Med Res Opin* 25:749, 2009.

58. Cuenca-Estrella M, Arendrup MC, Chryssanthou E, et al: Multicentre determination of quality control strains and quality control ranges for antifungal susceptibility testing of yeasts and filamentous fungi using the methods of the Antifungal Susceptibility Testing Subcommittee of the European Committee on Antimicrobial Susceptibility Testing (AFST-EUCAST). *Clin Microbiol Infect* 13:1018, 2007.

59. Kim SJ, Cheong JW, Min YH, et al: Success rate and risk factors for failure of empirical antifungal therapy with itraconazole in patients with hematological malignancies: A multicenter, prospective, open-label, observational study in Korea. *J Korean Med Sci* 29:61, 2014.

60. Walsh TJ, Pappas P, Winston DJ, et al: Voriconazole compared with liposomal amphotericin B for empirical antifungal therapy in patients with neutropenia and persistent fever. *N Engl J Med* 346:225, 2002.

61. Przepiorka D, Buadi FK, McClune B: Oral voriconazole for empiric antifungal treatment in patients with uncomplicated febrile neutropenia. *Pharmacotherapy* 28:58, 2008.

62. Walsh TJ, Anaissie EJ, Denning DW, et al: Treatment of aspergillosis: Clinical practice guidelines of the Infectious Diseases Society of America. *Clin Infect Dis* 46:327, 2008.

63. Williams K, Mansh M, Chin-Hong P, et al: Voriconazole-associated cutaneous malignancy: A literature review on photocarcinogenesis in organ transplant recipients. *Clin Infect Dis* 58:997, 2014.

64. Pascual A, Calandra T, Bolay S, et al: Voriconazole therapeutic drug monitoring in patients with invasive mycoses improves efficacy and safety outcomes. *Clin Infect Dis* 46:201, 2008.

65. Park WB, Kim NH, Kim KH, et al: The effect of therapeutic drug monitoring on safety and efficacy of voriconazole in invasive fungal infections: A randomized controlled trial. *Clin Infect Dis* 55:1080, 2012.

66. Raad II, Hanna HA, Boktour M, et al: Novel antifungal agents as salvage therapy for invasive aspergillosis in patients with hematologic malignancies: Posaconazole compared with high-dose lipid formulations of amphotericin B alone or in combination with caspofungin. *Leukemia* 22:496, 2008.

67. Vehreschild JJ, Birtel A, Vehreschild MJ, et al: Mucormycosis treated with posaconazole: Review of 96 case reports. *Crit Rev MicrobiolMicrobiology* 39:310, 2013.

68. Falci DR, Pasqualotto AC: Profile of isavuconazole and its potential in the treatment of severe invasive fungal infections. *Infect Drug Resist* 6:163, 2013.

69. Colombo AL, Ngai AL, Bourque M, et al: Caspofungin use in patients with invasive candidiasis caused by common non-albicans *Candida* species: Review of the caspofungin database. *Antimicrob Agents Chemother* 54:1864, 2010.

70. Mikulska M, Viscoli C: Current role of echinocandins in the management of invasive aspergillosis. *Curr Infect Dis Rep* 13:517, 2011.

71. Enoch DA, Idris SF, Aliyu SH, et al: Micafungin for the treatment of invasive aspergillosis. *J Infect* 68:507, 2014.

72. Zhang M, Sun W, Wu T, et al: Efficacy of combination therapy of triazole and echinocandin in treatment of invasive aspergillosis: A systematic review of animal and human studies. *J Thorac Dis* 6:99, 2014.

73. Reboli AC, Rotstein C, Pappas PG, et al: Anidulafungin versus fluconazole for invasive candidiasis. *N Engl J Med* 356:2472, 2007.

74. Shankar SM, Nania JJ: Management of *Pneumocystis jiroveci* pneumonia in children receiving chemotherapy. *Paediatr Drugs* 9:301, 2007.

75. Lemiale V, Debrumetz A, Delannoy A, et al: Adjunctive steroid in HIV-negative patients with severe Pneumocystis pneumonia. *Respir Res* 14:87, 2013.

76. Almyroudis NG, Segal BH: Prevention and treatment of invasive fungal diseases in neutropenic patients. *Curr Opin Infect Dis* 22:385, 2009.

77. Cordonnier C, Pautas C, Maury S, et al: Empirical versus preemptive antifungal therapy for high-risk, febrile, neutropenic patients: A randomized, controlled trial. *Clin Infect Dis* 48:1042, 2009.

78. Pagano L, Caira M, Nosari A, et al: The use and efficacy of empirical versus pre-emptive therapy in the management of fungal infections: The HEMA e-Chart Project. *Haematologica* 96:1366, 2011.

79. Tan BH, Low JG, Chlebicka NL, et al: Galactomannan-guided preemptive vs. empirical antifungals in the persistently febrile neutropenic patient: A prospective randomized study. *Int J Infect Dis* 15:e350, 2011.

80. Senn L, Robinson JO, Schmidt S, et al: 1,3-Beta-D-glucan antigenemia for early diagnosis of invasive fungal infections in neutropenic patients with acute leukemia. *Clin Infect Dis* 46:878, 2008.

81. Pfeiffer CD, Fine JP, Safdar N: Diagnosis of invasive aspergillosis using a galactomannan assay: A meta-analysis. *Clin Infect Dis* 42:1417, 2006.

82. McMullan R, Metwally L, Coyle PV, et al: A prospective clinical trial of a real-time polymerase chain reaction assay for the diagnosis of candidemia in nonneutropenic, critically ill adults. *Clin Infect Dis* 46:890, 2008.

83. Hachem R, Hanna H, Kontoyiannis D, et al: The changing epidemiology of invasive candidiasis: *Candida glabrata* and *Candida krusei* as the leading causes of candidemia in hematologic malignancy. *Cancer* 112:2493, 2008.

84. Rodriguez-Tudela JL, Alcazar-Fuoli L, Mellado E, et al: Epidemiological cutoffs and cross-resistance to azole drugs in Aspergillus fumigatus. *Antimicrob Agents Chemother* 52:2468, 2008.

85. Glenny AM, Fernandez Mauleffinch LM, Pavitt S, Walsh T: Interventions for the prevention and treatment of herpes simplex virus in patients being treated for cancer. *Cochrane Database Syst Rev* (1):CD006706, 2009.

86. Biron KK: Antiviral drugs for cytomegalovirus diseases. *Antiviral Res* 71:154, 2006.

87. Almyroudis NG, Jakubowski A, Jaffe D, et al: Predictors for persistent cytomegalovirus reactivation after T-cell-depleted allogeneic hematopoietic stem cell transplantation. *Transpl Infect Dis* 9:286, 2007.

88. Chemaly RF, Shah DP, Boeckh MJ: Management of respiratory viral infections in hematopoietic cell transplant recipients and patients with hematologic malignancies. *Clin Infect Dis* 59 (Suppl 5):S344, 2014.

89. Chemaly RF, Torres HA, Aguilera EA, et al: Neuraminidase inhibitors improve outcome of patients with leukemia and influenza: An observational study. *Clin Infect Dis* 44:964, 2007.

90. Al-Anazi KA, Al-Jasser AM, Evans DA: Infections caused by mycobacterium tuberculosis in patients with hematological disorders and in recipients of hematopoietic stem cell transplant, a twelve year retrospective study. *Ann Clin Microbiol Antimicrob* 6:16, 2007.

91. Wright A, Zignol M, Van Deun A, et al: Epidemiology of antituberculosis drug resistance 2002-07: An updated analysis of the Global Project on Anti-Tuberculosis Drug Resistance Surveillance. *Lancet* 373:1861, 2009.

92. Jassal M, Bishai WR: Extensively drug-resistant tuberculosis. *Lancet Infect Dis* 9:19, 2009.

93. Hodgson-Viden H, Grundy PE, Robinson JL: Early discontinuation of intravenous antimicrobial therapy in pediatric oncology patients with febrile neutropenia. *BMC Pediatr* 5:10, 2005.

94. Barton TD, Schuster MG: The cause of fever following resolution of neutropenia in patients with acute leukemia. *Clin Infect Dis* 22:1064, 1996.

95. Rammaert B, Desjardins A, Lortholary O: New insights into hepatosplenic candidosis, a manifestation of chronic disseminated candidosis. *Mycoses* 55:e74, 2012.

96. Anttila VJ, Ruutu P, Bondestam S, et al: Hepatosplenic yeast infection in patients with acute leukemia: A diagnostic problem. *Clin Infect Dis* 18:979, 1994.

97. Torres-Valdivieso MJ, Lopez J, Melero C, et al: Hepatosplenic candidosis in an immunosuppressed patient responding to fluconazole. *Mycoses* 37:443, 1994.

98. Arda B, Soyer N, Sipahi OR, et al: Possible hepatosplenic candidiasis treated with liposomal amphotericin B and caspofungin combination. *J Infect* 52:387, 2006.

99. Walsh TJ, Whitcomb P, Piscitelli S, et al: Safety, tolerance, and pharmacokinetics of amphotericin B lipid complex in children with hepatosplenic candidiasis. *Antimicrob Agents Chemother* 41:1944, 1997.

100. Legrand F, Lecuit M, Dupont B, et al: Adjuvant corticosteroid therapy for chronic disseminated candidiasis. *Clin Infect Dis* 46:696, 2008.

101. Chen CY, Chen YC, Tang JL, et al: Hepatosplenic fungal infection in patients with acute leukemia in Taiwan: Incidence, treatment, and prognosis. *Ann Hematol* 82:93, 2003.

102. Mermel LA, Allon M, Bouza E, et al: Clinical practice guidelines for the diagnosis and management of intravascular catheter-related infection: 2009 Update by the Infectious Diseases Society of America. *Clin Infect Dis* 49:1, 2009.

103. Hanna H, Afif C, Alakech B, et al: Central venous catheter-related bacteremia due to gram-negative bacilli: Significance of catheter removal in preventing relapse. *Infect Control Hosp Epidemiol* 25:646, 2004.

104. Ghanem GA, Boktour M, Warneke C, et al: Catheter-related *Staphylococcus aureus* bacteremia in cancer patients: High rate of complications with therapeutic implications. *Medicine (Baltimore)* 86:54, 2007.

105. Raad I, Hanna H, Boktour M, et al: Management of central venous catheters in patients with cancer and candidemia. *Clin Infect Dis* 38:1119, 2004.

106. Jaeger K, Zenz S, Juttner B, et al: Reduction of catheter-related infections in neutropenic patients: A prospective controlled randomized trial using a chlorhexidine and silver sulfadiazine-impregnated central venous catheter. *Ann Hematol* 84:258, 2005.

107. Flowers CR, Seidenfeld J, Bow EJ, et al: Antimicrobial prophylaxis and outpatient management of fever and neutropenia in adults treated for malignancy: American Society of Clinical Oncology clinical practice guideline. *J Clin Oncol* 31:794, 2013.

108. Freifeld A, Sepkowitz K: The conundrum of fluoroquinolone prophylaxis. *Nat Clin Pract Oncol* 3:524, 2006.

109. Moores KG: Safe and effective outpatient treatment of adults with chemotherapy-induced neutropenic fever. *Am J Health Syst Pharm* 64:717, 2007.

110. Gafter-Gvili A, Fraser A, Paul M, et al: Antibiotic prophylaxis for bacterial infections in afebrile neutropenic patients following chemotherapy. *Cochrane Database Syst Rev* 1:CD004386, 2012.

111. Cullen M, Steven N, Billingham L, et al: Antibacterial prophylaxis after chemotherapy for solid tumors and lymphomas. *N Engl J Med* 353:988, 2005.

112. Macesic N, Morrissey CO, Cheng AC, et al: Changing microbial epidemiology in hematopoietic stem cell transplant recipients: Increasing resistance over a 9-year period. *Transpl Infect Dis* 16:887, 2014.

113. Bow EJ: Fluoroquinolones, antimicrobial resistance and neutropenic cancer patients. *Curr Opin Infect Dis* 24:545, 2011.

114. Leibovici L, Paul M, Cullen M, et al: Antibiotic prophylaxis in neutropenic patients: New evidence, practical decisions. *Cancer* 107:1743, 2006.

115. Alonso CD, Treadway SB, Hanna DB, et al: Epidemiology and outcomes of *Clostridium difficile* infections in hematopoietic stem cell transplant recipients. *Clin Infect Dis* 54:1053, 2012.

116. Cartman ST, Heap JT, Kuehne SA, et al: The emergence of "hypervirulence" in *Clostridium difficile*. *Int J Med Microbiol* 300:387, 2010.

117. Trecarichi EM, Tumbarello M: Antimicrobial-resistant Gram-negative bacteria in febrile neutropenic patients with cancer: Current epidemiology and clinical impact. *Curr Opin Infect Dis* 27:200, 2014.

118. Prabhu RM, Piper KE, Litzow MR, et al: Emergence of quinolone resistance among viridans group streptococci isolated from the oropharynx of neutropenic peripheral blood stem cell transplant patients receiving quinolone antimicrobial prophylaxis. *Eur J Clin Microbiol Infect Dis* 24:832, 2005.

119. Baden LR: Prophylactic antimicrobial agents and the importance of fitness. *N Engl J Med* 353:1052, 2005.

120. Verlinden A, Jansens H, Goossens H, et al: Clinical and microbiological impact of discontinuation of fluoroquinolone prophylaxis in patients with prolonged profound neutropenia. *Eur J Haematol* 93:302, 2014.

121. Kern WV, Klose K, Jellen-Ritter AS, et al: Fluoroquinolone resistance of Escherichia coli at a cancer center: Epidemiologic evolution and effects of discontinuing prophylactic fluoroquinolone use in neutropenic patients with leukemia. *Eur J Clin Microbiol Infect Dis* 24:111, 2005.

122. Reuter S, Kern WV, Sigge A, et al: Impact of fluoroquinolone prophylaxis on reduced infection-related mortality among patients with neutropenia and hematologic malignancies. *Clin Infect Dis* 40:1087, 2005.

123. Aarts MJ, Peters FP, Mandigers CM, et al: Primary granulocyte colony-stimulating factor prophylaxis during the first two cycles only or throughout all chemotherapy cycles in patients with breast cancer at risk for febrile neutropenia. *J Clin Oncol* 31:4290, 2013.

124. Dranitsaris G, Rayson D, Vincent M, et al: Identifying patients at high risk for neutropenic complications during chemotherapy for metastatic breast cancer with doxorubicin or pegylated liposomal doxorubicin: The development of a prediction model. *Am J Clin Oncol*J *Clin Oncol* 31:369, 2008.

125. Aapro MS, Bohlius J, Cameron DA, et al: 2010 Update of EORTC guidelines for the use of granulocyte-colony stimulating factor to reduce the incidence of chemotherapy-induced febrile neutropenia in adult patients with lymphoproliferative disorders and solid tumours. *Eur J Cancer* 47:8, 2011.

126. Gardner A, Mattiuzzi G, Faderl S, et al: Randomized comparison of cooked and non-cooked diets in patients undergoing remission induction therapy for acute myeloid leukemia. *J Clin Oncol* 26:5684, 2008.

127. Russell JA, Poon MC, Jones AR, et al: Allogeneic bone-marrow transplantation without protective isolation in adults with malignant disease. *Lancet* 339:38, 1992.

128. Warkentin DI, Epstein JB, Campbell LM, et al: Valacyclovir versus acyclovir for HSV prophylaxis in neutropenic patients. *Ann Pharmacother* 36:1525, 2002.

129. Boeckh M, Nichols WG: The impact of cytomegalovirus serostatus of donor and recipient before hematopoietic stem cell transplantation in the era of antiviral prophylaxis and preemptive therapy. *Blood* 103:2003, 2004.

130. Vickrey E, Allen S, Mehta J, Singhal S: Acyclovir to prevent reactivation of varicella zoster virus (herpes zoster) in multiple myeloma patients receiving bortezomib therapy. *Cancer* 115:229, 2009.

131. Centers for Disease Control and Prevention (CDC): Updated recommendations for use of VariZIG—United States, 2013. *MMWR Morb Mortal Wkly Rep* 62:574, 2013.

132. Ljungman P: The role of cytomegalovirus serostatus on outcome of hematopoietic stem cell transplantation. *Curr Opin Hematol* 21:466, 2014.

133. Ringden O, Erkers T, Aschan J, et al: A prospective randomized toxicity study to compare reduced-intensity and myeloablative conditioning in patients with myeloid leukaemia undergoing allogeneic haematopoietic stem cell transplantation. *J Intern Med* 274:153, 2013.

134. Kekre N, Tokessy M, Mallick R, et al: Is cytomegalovirus testing of blood products still needed for hematopoietic stem cell transplant recipients in the era of universal leukoreduction? *Biol Blood Marrow Transplant* 19:1719, 2013.

135. van der Heiden PL, Kalpoe JS, Barge RM, et al: Oral valganciclovir as pre-emptive therapy has similar efficacy on cytomegalovirus DNA load reduction as intravenous ganciclovir in allogeneic stem cell transplantation recipients. *Bone Marrow Transplant* 37:693, 2006.

136. Ayala E, Greene J, Sandin R, et al: Valganciclovir is safe and effective as pre-emptive therapy for CMV infection in allogeneic hematopoietic stem cell transplantation. *Bone Marrow Transplant* 37:851, 2006.

137. Ar MC, Ozbalak M, Tuzuner N, et al: Severe bone marrow failure due to valganciclovir overdose after renal transplantation from cadaveric donors: Four consecutive cases. *Transplant Proc* 41:1648, 2009.

138. Allice T, Busca A, Locatelli F, et al: Valganciclovir as pre-emptive therapy for cytomegalovirus infection post-allogenic stem cell transplantation: Implications for the emergence of drug-resistant cytomegalovirus. *J Antimicrob Chemother* 63:600, 2009.

139. Sandherr M, Einsele H, Hebart H, et al: Antiviral prophylaxis in patients with haematological malignancies and solid tumours: Guidelines of the Infectious Diseases Working Party (AGIHO) of the German Society for Hematology and Oncology (DGHO). *Ann Oncol* 17:1051, 2006.

140. Gerdemann U, Katari UL, Papadopoulou A, et al: Safety and clinical efficacy of rapidly-generated trivirus-directed T cells as treatment for adenovirus, EBV, and CMV infections after allogeneic hematopoietic stem cell transplant. *Mol Ther* 21:2113, 2013.

141. Chemaly RF, Ullmann AJ, Stoelben S, et al: Letermovir for cytomegalovirus prophylaxis in hematopoietic-cell transplantation. *N Engl J Med* 370:1781, 2014.

142. Marty FM, Winston DJ, Rowley SD, et al: CMX001 to prevent cytomegalovirus disease in hematopoietic-cell transplantation. *N Engl J Med* 369:1227, 2013.

143. Curtis KK, Connolly MK, Northfelt DW: Live, attenuated varicella zoster vaccination of an immunocompromised patient. *J Gen Intern Med.* 23:648, 2008.

144. Akan H, Antia VP, Kouba M, et al: Preventing invasive fungal disease in patients with haematological malignancies and the recipients of haematopoietic stem cell transplantation: Practical aspects. *J Antimicrob Chemother* 68 (Suppl 3):iii5, 2013.

145. Maschmeyer G: The changing face of febrile neutropenia-from monotherapy to moulds to mucositis. Prevention of mould infections. *J Antimicrob Chemother* 63 (Suppl 1):i27, 2009.

146. Michallet M, Ito JI: Approaches to the management of invasive fungal infections in hematologic malignancy and hematopoietic cell transplantation. *J Clin Oncol* 27:3398, 2009.

147. Goodman JL, Winston DJ, Greenfield RA, et al: A controlled trial of fluconazole to prevent fungal infections in patients undergoing bone marrow transplantation. *N Engl J Med* 326:845, 1992.

148. Vehreschild JJ, Bohme A, Buchheidt D, et al: A double-blind trial on prophylactic voriconazole (VRC) during induction chemotherapy for acute myelogenous leukaemia (AML). *J Infect* 55:445, 2007.

149. Ping B, Zhu Y, Gao Y, et al: Second- versus first-generation azoles for antifungal prophylaxis in hematology patients: A systematic review and meta-analysis. *Ann Hematol* 92:831, 2013.

150. Cornely OA, Maertens J, Winston DJ, et al: Posaconazole vs. fluconazole or itraconazole prophylaxis in patients with neutropenia. *N Engl J Med* 356:348, 2007.

151. Mattiuzzi GN, Alvarado G, Giles FJ, et al: Open-label, randomized comparison of itraconazole versus caspofungin for prophylaxis in patients with hematologic malignancies. *Antimicrob Agents Chemother* 50:143, 2006.

152. van Burik JA, Ratanatharathorn V, Stepan DE, et al: Micafungin versus fluconazole for prophylaxis against invasive fungal infections during neutropenia in patients undergoing hematopoietic stem cell transplantation. *Clin Infect Dis* 39:1407, 2004.

153. Green H, Paul M, Vidal L, Leibovici L: Prophylaxis for Pneumocystis pneumonia (PCP) in non-HIV immunocompromised patients. *Cochrane Database Syst Rev* (3):CD005590, 2007.

154. Colby C, McAfee S, Sackstein R, et al: A prospective randomized trial comparing the toxicity and safety of atovaquone with trimethoprim/sulfamethoxazole as *Pneumocystis carinii* pneumonia prophylaxis following autologous peripheral blood stem cell transplantation. *Bone Marrow Transplant* 24:897, 1999.

155. Sangiolo D, Storer B, Nash R, et al: Toxicity and efficacy of daily dapsone as *Pneumocystis jiroveci* prophylaxis after hematopoietic stem cell transplantation: A case-control study. *Biol Blood Marrow Transplant* 11:521, 2005.

156. Appelbaum FR, Forman SJ, Negrin RS, Blume KG: *Thomas' Hematopoietic Cell Transplantation.* Wiley-Blackwell, New York, 2009.

CHAPTER 25
ANTITHROMBOTIC THERAPY

Gregory C. Connolly and Charles W. Francis

SUMMARY

Antithrombotic drugs are among the most commonly used drugs in medicine and are generally separated into anticoagulants, fibrinolytic agents, and platelet inhibitors based on their primary mechanism of action. For many decades, warfarin, which acts by inhibiting vitamin K action, was the only oral anticoagulant available. Vitamin K antagonists have a prolonged effect, unpredictable pharmacokinetics, and require monitoring, but warfarin was widely used for prevention and treatment. The introduction of novel targeted oral anticoagulants has changed the landscape of anticoagulation. Rivaroxaban, apixaban, and edoxaban are novel oral inhibitors of factor Xa, whereas dabigatran is an orally available inhibitor of thrombin. Unfractionated heparin and the low-molecular-weight heparins are the most commonly used rapidly acting parenteral anticoagulants; they inhibit activated serine proteases through antithrombin. One synthetic agent in this class, fondaparinux, is specific for inhibition of factor Xa, and is effective for prevention and treatment of venous thromboembolism. Several parenteral direct thrombin inhibitors have excellent anticoagulant action and offer an alternative to heparins. A number of fibrinolytic agents are available, all of which convert plasminogen to plasmin to accelerate clot lysis. Differences among them include their degree of fibrin specificity, half-life, and antigenicity. Antiplatelet agents play an important role in prevention and treatment of arterial thrombosis. Aspirin is a cyclooxygenase-1 inhibitor that is effective and widely used in the prevention of stroke and myocardial infarction. Drugs that modulate cyclic adenosine monophosphate levels include dipyridamole, pentoxifylline, and cilostazol, and are primarily used in treatment of peripheral vascular disease. Adenosine diphosphate receptor blockers such as ticlopidine, clopidogrel, and prasugrel are effective in treatment of coronary and peripheral arterial disease. Examples of inhibitors of fibrinogen interaction with $a_{IIb}\beta_3$ are abciximab, tirofiban, and eptifibatide. These drugs are highly effective in treatment of patients with acute coronary syndromes.

Acronyms and Abbreviations: ACT, activated clotting time; ADP, adenosine diphosphate; aPTT, activated partial thromboplastin time; cAMP, cyclic adenosine monophosphate; COX, cyclooxygenase; CYP, cytochrome P450; DVT, deep vein thrombosis; FFP, fresh-frozen plasma; Gla, γ-carboxyglutamic acid; HIT, heparin-induced thrombocytopenia; INR, international normalized ratio; ISI, international sensitivity index; LMWH, low-molecular-weight heparin; MI, myocardial infarction; NSAID, nonsteroidal antiinflammatory drug; PE, pulmonary embolism; PG, prostaglandin; PGI₂, prostacyclin; PRP, platelet-rich plasma; PT, prothrombin time; TNK, tenecteplase; t-PA, tissue-type plasminogen activator; VTE, venous thromboembolism.

Antithrombotic agents are highly effective and are among the most commonly used drugs in medicine because thrombotic diseases are the leading cause of mortality and morbidity in Western countries. Antithrombotic agents are characterized separately as anticoagulants, antiplatelet agents, or fibrinolytic drugs, depending on their primary mechanism, although there is overlap in their activities and clinical indications (Table 25–1). Their greatest use is in prevention of thrombosis in patients at high risk, but they also have important applications for treating acute thrombosis. For many agents, the risk-to-benefit ratio is narrow, with the result that bleeding complications occur, and bleeding is the most common adverse effect. Consequently, the clinician should carefully weigh the risks and benefits for each patient when selecting treatment. Generally, these drugs do not cause bleeding by themselves; instead, they exacerbate preexisting bleeding or predispose to bleeding from pathologic lesions that may be found in the gastrointestinal or genitourinary tracts or central nervous system. A careful review of comorbid conditions that may increase bleeding risk is important when deciding on therapy.

Anticoagulant therapy acts to decrease fibrin formation by inhibiting the formation and action of thrombin, and its most common uses are in preventing systemic embolization in patients with atrial fibrillation and for secondary prevention of venous thromboembolism. Anticoagulant therapy is sometimes monitored using coagulation testing because of marked biologic variation in effect with some agents. Antiplatelet agents act to inhibit platelet function, and their primary uses are in preventing thrombotic complications of cerebrovascular and coronary artery disease. They also have a role in treatment of acute myocardial infarction and some effect in preventing venous thrombosis. Fibrinolytic agents accelerate lysis of thrombi by increasing conversion of plasminogen to plasmin, and are primarily used in the acute management of myocardial infarction, in clearing occluded catheters and also in selected patients with stroke or venous thromboembolism. Fibrinolytic therapy is associated with a higher risk of bleeding complications than treatment with either anticoagulants or antiplatelet agents. Treatment of acute thrombosis often involves combinations of agents with multiple actions for maximum effect.

Antithrombotic therapy has changed considerably with the introduction of several novel target-specific oral anticoagulants. These drugs offer more predictable pharmacokinetics and fewer drug interactions than warfarin, thus eliminating the need for frequent monitoring. These agents have been studied in numerous phase III randomized clinical trials that have compared these agents to standard anticoagulation therapies. In most cases, the new anticoagulants are equivalent to conventional anticoagulation in reducing thrombotic events, while in many cases they are associated with lower rates of major bleeding complications.

VITAMIN K ANTAGONISTS

The development of vitamin K antagonists as oral anticoagulants began in the 1920s with investigation of a hemorrhagic disease in cattle, the cause of which was eventually traced to ingestion of moldy hay leading to hypoprothrombinemia.[1] A coumarin that inhibited vitamin K was purified and eventually introduced into clinical practice in the 1940s. Several coumarin derivatives with differing pharmacologic properties are now available as anticoagulants worldwide, and are collectively referred to as vitamin K antagonists, but warfarin is nearly universally used in North America. These agents are widely used to prevent or treat common thrombotic diseases and represent the most commonly used oral anticoagulant currently available.[2]

TABLE 25–1. Types and Function of Antithrombotic Agents

Anticoagulants—decrease fibrin formation by inhibiting thrombin or thrombin formation

Agents

Oral—warfarin and other vitamin K antagonists, dabigatran (direct thrombin inhibitor) and oral direct X_a inhibitors (rivaroxaban, apixaban, edoxaban)

Parenteral—heparin, low-molecular-weight heparins, fondaparinux, direct thrombin inhibitors (argatroban, desirudin, bivalirudin)

Antiplatelet agents—inhibit platelet function

Agents

Aspirin, clopidogrel, prasugrel, dipyridamole, abciximab, eptifibatide, tirofiban, vorapaxar

Fibrinolytic agents—plasminogen activators and accelerate clot lysis

Agents

Streptokinase, urokinase, alteplase, reteplase, tenecteplase

TABLE 25–2. Effect of Drugs on Warfarin Response

POTENTIATE EFFECT

α-Methyldopa	Indomethacin
Acetaminophen	Isoniazid
Acetohexamide	Mefenamic acid
Allopurinol	Methimazole
Androgenic and anabolic steroids	Methotrexate
Antibiotics that disrupt intestinal flora (tetracyclines, streptomycin, erythromycin, kanamycin, nalidixic acid, neomycin)	Methylphenidate
	Nalidixic acid
	Nortriptyline
	Oxyphenbutazone
Cephaloridine	p-Aminosalicylic acid
Chloral hydrate	Paromomycin
Chloramphenicol	Phenylbutazone
Chlorpromazine	Phenyramidol
Chlorpropamide	Phenytoin
Cimetidine	Propylthiouracil
Clofibrate	Quinidine
Diazoxide	Salicylate
Disulfiram	Sulfinpyrazone
Ethacrynic acid	Sulfonamides
Glucagon	Thyroid hormone
Guanethidine	Tolbutamide

DEPRESS EFFECT

Antipyrine	Glutethimide
Azathioprine	Griseofulvin
Barbiturates	Haloperidol
Carbamazepine	Phenobarbital
Digitalis	Prednisone
Ethanol	Rifampin
Ethchlorvynol	Vitamin K

PHARMACOLOGY

The coumarins are competitive inhibitors of vitamin K. They inhibit γ-carboxylation reactions required for synthesis of several coagulation proteins, including factors II, VII, IX, and X, as well as proteins C and S, which are involved in inhibitory regulation of hemostasis. The synthesis of these proteins requires a posttranslational modification of several glutamic acid residues, converting them to γ-carboxylated glutamic acid (Gla), which is required for proper membrane interaction and biologic activity (Chap. 115).[3,4] The carboxylation reaction requires reduced vitamin K, which is converted to vitamin K epoxide in the reaction. Vitamin K epoxide subsequently undergoes reduction by an enzyme that is inhibited by warfarin.[5–7] Therefore, treatment with warfarin causes reduced γ-carboxylation, leading to synthesis of molecules with impaired activity.[8–10]

Warfarin preparations consist of a racemic mixture of S and R enantiomers in approximately equal proportion in an oral formulation with high bioavailability. Warfarin is water soluble and rapidly absorbed after oral administration, reaching a peak concentration after 60 to 90 minutes. An intravenous preparation is also available for patients who cannot take oral medications or who have malabsorption. It is tightly bound to plasma proteins with a half-life of 35 to 45 hours, with only the free, nonbound form having biologic activity. Warfarin is metabolized through the cytochrome P450 (CYP) system, the activity of which is influenced by environmental factors and also by genetic polymorphisms that alter the structure of common enzymes. Other vitamin K antagonists have similar activities but exhibit differences in absorption and elimination.

Because warfarin is a vitamin K antagonist, its action is influenced by the vitamin K content of the diet. Naturally occurring vitamin K is found in a variety of vegetables, and changes in diet can affect the vitamin K availability and warfarin effect.[11] This may be seen particularly in patients receiving warfarin who are on strict weight-reduction diets or in those with little oral intake because of illness. Also, diarrhea can affect vitamin K availability, as can administration of broad-spectrum antibiotics leading to marked warfarin sensitivity in hospitalized patients. Ingestion of vitamin K in dietary supplements or vitamins also affects sensitivity to warfarin. Liver disease can increase sensitivity to warfarin because of impaired synthesis of coagulation factors, and hyper- or

hypometabolic states may also alter sensitivity. Hereditary resistance to warfarin has been described and related to specific mutations in vitamin K epoxide reductase.[12] Many drug interactions can influence the pharmacodynamics of warfarin by altering synthesis or clearance of vitamin K–dependent coagulation factors or interfering with warfarin metabolism, and patients should be advised to consult their physician or pharmacist about effects on anticoagulation when changing drug therapy or starting new medications (Table 25–2).[11] Other commonly used drugs affecting hemostasis, such as aspirin, nonsteroidal antiinflammatory agents, heparins, and other anticoagulants can add to the antihemostatic effects of warfarin and can lead to bleeding.

ADMINISTRATION AND MONITORING

The anticoagulant effect of warfarin is the result of decreased levels of vitamin K–dependent coagulation factors, and their concentration represents a balance of synthesis and metabolism. Warfarin administration impairs synthesis, and levels of vitamin K–dependent factors fall in relation to their metabolism. This is short for factor VII, with a half-life of approximately 5 hours, but longer for factors X and IX ($t_{1/2}$ = 24 hours) and longest for factor II (prothrombin) with a half-life of approximately 72 hours. The desired anticoagulant effect results from a balanced reduction of all factors and requires several days to achieve. Imbalances in reduction of coagulation factors may occur during initiation of therapy as factor VII level falls rapidly, whereas others, especially factor II, decline more slowly. The initial rapid fall in factor VII level may lead to an early elevation in the prothrombin time (PT) expressed as international normalized ratio (INR) without reflecting the desired anticoagulant effect. Because protein C is a natural inhibitor of coagulation with a short half-life (approximately 8 hours), its level may fall rapidly, theoretically inducing a procoagulant state during initiation of therapy.

As a result of the delayed anticoagulant effect of warfarin, therapy is initiated with a rapidly acting agent, such as heparin or low-molecular-weight heparin (LMWH), if immediate anticoagulation is needed. For example, patients with venous thromboembolism are typically given heparin or an LMWH for rapid effect, and warfarin is also administered within the first 24 hours. After a period of 5 or more days, the necessary anticoagulant effect of warfarin is achieved, and the parenteral anticoagulant can be stopped. Anticoagulation is initiated with a dose close to the expected daily maintenance requirement, which is usually between 5 and 10 mg.[13-15] There is, however, great variability in the doses required, and smaller amounts should be used for frail, elderly, or poorly nourished patients, or those with an increased bleeding risk. In patients with a low level of protein C or protein S as a result of an inherited deficiency, initiation of warfarin therapy without concomitant heparin or other immediately acting anticoagulant can lead to very low levels of these natural anticoagulants with ensuing thrombosis such as skin necrosis.

The anticoagulant effect of the vitamin K antagonists is monitored using the PT, which is sensitive to decreases in vitamin K–dependent factors and is progressively lengthened as the vitamin K–dependent factors reach lower levels. A critical component of the PT is the thromboplastin reagent that is used. Variability in thromboplastin composition leads to variation in results. The widespread introduction of the INR has improved standardization of results.[16] Manufacturers determine the potency of thromboplastins by measuring the international sensitivity index (ISI), and this is used as a correction factor for the responsiveness of the thromboplastin in the PT. The INR represents the ratio of the patient PT to control PT corrected by the ISI. By this method, INR values obtained in different laboratories can be reliably compared for therapeutic monitoring.

During initiation of therapy, the INR is checked every 2 to 3 days for 1 to 2 weeks until a stable therapeutic effect is achieved. The target INR for most indications is 2.5 with a desirable therapeutic range from 2 to 3. A higher INR is recommended for patients with mechanical heart valve replacement and for those who failed anticoagulant therapy despite well-documented INR values in the 2 to 3 range. During chronic therapy, the INR should be monitored regularly, depending on stability of the response, and minor dose adjustments are frequently needed. A recent randomized trial in patients on chronic warfarin therapy with a stable dose for 6 months demonstrated that INR monitoring every 12 weeks was noninferior to monitoring every 4 weeks with regards to time in therapeutic range (74.1 vs. 71.6 percent).[17] Monitoring can also be performed using portable instruments that are suitable for home use, enabling selected patients to learn to modify their warfarin doses in response to their INR value.[18] A nonblinded randomized study compared home monitoring to INR monitoring in a specialized coagulation clinic in a cohort of patients on chronic warfarin and capable of conducting home monitoring.[19] In this trial, rates of the primary composite end point (thrombosis, major bleeding or death) were equivalent, but home monitoring was associated with significant improvement in patient satisfaction, quality of life and time in therapeutic range. Specialized clinics devoted to monitoring warfarin typically achieve better results in maintaining patients within the therapeutic range, resulting in fewer bleeding complications.[20,21] Problems with keeping patients within the therapeutic range often result from failure of compliance, changes in diet, medication or alcohol intake, or intercurrent illnesses.

Warfarin sensitivity is affected by polymorphisms in CYP and vitamin K epoxide reductase complex (VKORC), and pharmacogenomics may become important in dosing. The clearance of warfarin is the result of hepatic metabolism and CYP2C9 is the most important enzyme mediating its clearance.[22] A number of polymorphisms have been identified, but the most important are CYP2C9*2 and CYP2C9*3, which are found in approximately 11 percent and 7 percent of patients and result in reductions of enzymatic activity of approximately 30 percent and 80 percent, respectively.[23-25] This reduced metabolic clearance leads to increased drug levels and an increased anticoagulant effect. VKORC1 converts oxidized vitamin K to the active reduced form as required for posttranslational carboxylation. VKORC1 is the target of warfarin, which functions as a competitive inhibitor. Numerous coding polymorphisms have been identified that can affect the response to warfarin.[26,27] Common haplotypes can be separated into low-dose (A) and high-dose (B) groups with different sensitivities to warfarin.

Evidence is clear that polymorphisms in either CYP2C9 or VKORC1 affect warfarin sensitivity. Retrospective studies have shown that patients with at least one variant allele have an increased risk of INRs over the desired range and the variant groups also require more time to achieve stable dosing compared to patient with wild type allele.[28,29] Additional prospective observational studies indicate that CYP2C9 and VKORC1 genotype affect warfarin sensitivity.[30-32] Several prospective studies have incorporated genotyping for CYP2C9 and VKORC1 into algorithms that typically include clinical variables such as age, gender, and drug interactions in an attempt to use genetic information to improve warfarin dosing. The results of these trials are conflicting possibly as a consequence of different trial design and patient populations. Incorporation of CYP2C9 and VKORC1 polymorphisms into a dosing algorithm in one randomized study more accurately predicted warfarin dose and reduced dose modifications, but did not improve time in therapeutic range.[33] Another randomized study compared dosing based on genotype and clinical variables to clinical variable alone in almost 1000 patients starting warfarin. This showed no difference in time in therapeutic range, bleeding, or thromboembolism.[34] Genotype-based dosing resulted in significantly decreased time in the therapeutic range for black patients in this study suggesting such an approach is detrimental for this subgroup. A third study conducted in Europe reported a significant improvement in time in therapeutic range (67.4 vs. 60.3 percent), episodes of excessive anticoagulation (INR >4), and median time to reach a therapeutic INR (21 vs. 29 days) with genotype-based dosing.[35] A similarly designed study by the same European group in patients starting acenocoumarol or phenprocoumon showed no improvement in these same measures with genotype based dosing.[36] Further research is needed before genetic testing becomes part of standard care for patients receiving warfarin.

COMPLICATIONS

The most serious and common complication of warfarin is bleeding, and its risk is related primarily to patient characteristics, the degree of the anticoagulation, and the duration of therapy. The rate of major bleeding with 3 to 6 months of warfarin treatment in recent clinical trials of patients with venous thromboembolism was 1.2 to 2.2 percent.[37-39]

TABLE 25–3. HAS-BLED Score for Predicting Bleeding Risk on Coumadin

Variable	Points
Hypertension (uncontrolled, systolic >160 torr)	1 point
Abnormal renal or liver function	1 point each, max 2 points
Stroke (prior history)	1 point
Bleeding history of predisposition	1 point
Labile INR (<60% time in therapeutic range)	1 point
Elderly (>65 years old)	1 point
Drugs/alcohol use (nonsteroidal antiinflammatory drugs, aspirin, anti-platelet agents)	1 point for each, max 2 points

INR, international normalized ratio.

Bleeding rate: 0 points = 0.8%, 1 point = 1.3%, 2 points = 2.2%, ≥3 points = 7.8%

Several risk models have been developed to predict bleeding risk in patients on warfarin. The HAS-BLED score was derived and validated in a prospective cohort of more than 6000 patients on warfarin for atrial fibrillation (Table 25–3).[40] Variables in this model include hypertension, abnormal renal or liver function, stroke, prior bleeding complications, labile INR, age older than 65 years, and drug or alcohol abuse. The intensity of anticoagulation as reflected by the INR is the most important predictor of bleeding risk, which is low in the therapeutic range but increases as the INR prolongs further. The cumulative risk of bleeding increases with a longer duration of treatment, whereas the absolute risk is greatest early, possibly caused by pathologic lesions present at the time therapy is started.

A rare complication of warfarin therapy is skin necrosis, which if it occurs usually presents early in the course of anticoagulation.[41] Thrombosis in dermal and subdermal venules is the underlying cause, and this may be caused by disproportionately rapid reduction in proteins C and S. Skin necrosis typically begins with burning and tingling at the affected site, which usually involves a region with a large amount of subcutaneous tissue, such as the breast, buttock, or thigh. Painful hemorrhagic full-thickness skin infarction may develop, and frequently will require skin grafting. Other complications from warfarin are rare. Occasional patients report alopecia; hypersensitivity reactions are rare and are almost uniformly caused by the dye used in the pill rather than by the warfarin itself.

Warfarin use in patients with heparin-induced thrombocytopenia (HIT) may be complicated by limb gangrene caused by occlusive venous thrombosis; this effect is likely a result of a combination of inadequate parenteral anticoagulant effect and reduced levels of protein C, in concert with relatively preserved levels of factors II and X that are seen early after the initiation of warfarin administration.[42] This complication highlights the need for parenteral anticoagulants to be continued in patients with HIT until the coagulopathy has largely resolved, as indicated by a return of the platelet count to normal or near normal levels.

Oral anticoagulation should be avoided in pregnancy because warfarin crosses the placenta, and exposure during organogenesis in the first trimester can lead to fetal embryopathy with significant cranial bone malformations.[43] Anticoagulation during pregnancy increases bleeding complications, especially later in pregnancy. Warfarin may be considered during the second trimester, but heparin or an LMWH is a preferable alternative in most situations. Vitamin K antagonists are safe during lactation.[44]

REVERSAL OF ANTICOAGULATION

Anticoagulation must be reversed for episodes of bleeding, surgery, trauma, or overdosage. Appropriate interventions for patients with excessively prolonged INRs without bleeding include holding warfarin doses, administering low doses of vitamin K (0.5 to 1.0 mg), and increasing the frequency of monitoring (Table 25–4).[45] Serious bleeding and major warfarin overdosage requires factor replacement and larger vitamin K doses that may need to be given intravenously. Four-factor concentrates have been developed and tested for reversal of warfarin. A large, open-label, prospective phase IIIB noninferiority study in nonsurgical patients on warfarin requiring reversal for major bleeding compared fresh-frozen plasma (FFP) to four-factor prothrombin complex concentrate (PCC) (factors II, VII, IX, X, protein C, and protein S).[46] Four-factor PCC was as effective in achieving hemostasis as plasma (72.4 percent with four-factor PCC vs. 65.4 percent with plasma; absolute difference, 7.1 percent [95 percent confidence interval, −5.8 to 19.9]) and superior to FFP with regards to INR correction within 0.5 hours of infusion (62.2 percent receiving four-factor PCC vs. 9.6 percent receiving FFP; absolute difference, 52.6 percent [95 percent confidence interval, 39.4 to 65.9]). The rate of adverse events, such as death and thromboembolism, was similar between groups.

Anticoagulated patients who need invasive procedures represent management problems, and decisions about periprocedural anticoagulation should be based on balancing the risk of thromboembolism with that of bleeding from the procedure. Evidence-based guidelines for bridging therapy are available,[45] and the topic has been reviewed.[47] The goal is to reduce the intensity of anticoagulation during and immediately after surgery, while avoiding thromboembolism caused by the underlying disease. Generally, the risk of recurrence is greatest in the period shortly after an episode of acute thrombosis and declines progressively over time. If possible, elective surgery and other invasive

TABLE 25–4. Reversing Warfarin Therapy

Indication	Action
INR <6	Lower the dose, consider withholding 1 or more doses
	Recheck in 3–7 days
INR 6–10	Lower the dose and withhold 1–3 doses
	Consider administering vitamin K, 1–2 mg orally
	Recheck INR in 24–48 hours
INR >10	Withhold doses until INR in desired range and cause of elevation ascertained
	Give vitamin K, 2–4 mg orally
	Recheck INR in 24 hours
Serious bleeding and major overdose	Administer four-factor prothrombin complex concentrate if available for rapid reversal. If four-factor prothrombin complex concentrate not available administer fresh-frozen plasma. Also give 5–10 mg vitamin K intravenously

INR, international normalized ratio.

procedures associated with a high bleeding risk should be postponed during the first several months following acute thrombosis. The bleeding risk is usually highest during surgery and decreases rapidly to baseline after approximately 7 to 10 days. Most surgery can be done with a minimal bleeding risk in patients receiving warfarin and an INR of 1.5 or less. A recent cohort study of 1496 patients on chronic anticoagulation undergoing periprocedural bridging therapy showed that bleeding occurred in 5.1 percent of patients, and risk factors for bleeding included mitral mechanical valve, active cancer, prior bleeding history, and reinitiation of anticoagulation within 24 hours of procedure.[48] A randomized study of anticoagulated patients undergoing defibrillator placement showed that bridging therapy was associated with a significant increase in device-pocket hematoma (16 percent vs. 3.5 percent) without a reducing thromboembolic complications.[49] Patients at moderate or high risk of thrombotic recurrence should receive heparin or LMWH "bridging therapy" when their INR becomes subtherapeutic. Postprocedural bridging therapy should be undertaken only in patients in whom the risks of this therapy (principally bleeding) are less than the perceived benefits (a reduced risk of thromboembolism).

● HEPARIN

PHARMACOLOGY

Heparin (and the related LMWHs) is the most widely used, rapidly acting, parenteral anticoagulant. Heparin is a heterogeneous mixture of sulfated glycosaminoglycan molecules with varying chain lengths (molecular mass [Mr] 5000 to 30,000 daltons). Heparin has no direct anticoagulant effect, but serves to activate plasma antithrombin (AT), a serine protease inhibitor. Only about one-third of heparin molecules contain the necessary unique pentasaccharide sequence required to interact with AT and thus display anticoagulant activity.[50] AT inhibits thrombin, factor Xa, and other coagulation serine proteases in a reaction that is slow by itself, but is accelerated approximately 1000-fold in the presence of heparin.[51] To inhibit thrombin, heparin binds to both the active enzyme and AT, forming a ternary complex. The inhibition of factor Xa, however, occurs through binding to heparin–AT complex without the requirement for heparin binding directly also to factor Xa. The requirement for a ternary heparin–AT–thrombin complex requires heparin molecules with 19 or more saccharide units, whereas smaller heparin molecules are effective in promoting factor Xa inactivation. Thrombin and factor Xa are relatively protected from inhibition by the heparin–AT complex when they are surface immobilized within thrombi or on cells.[52]

ADMINISTRATION AND MONITORING

Heparin is not absorbed after oral ingestion, so must be given either subcutaneously or intravenously. The pharmacokinetics of unfractionated heparin is complex, a result of extensive protein binding, with a dose-dependent half-life in the range of 1 to 2.5 hours.[53] A common protocol uses an initial intravenous bolus of 5000 units or 75 U/kg, followed by a maintenance infusion of 1250 to 1660 U/h or 18 U/kg per hour. The anticoagulant effect is immediate, but laboratory monitoring is needed because of the variability in response among patients. Monitoring is most convenient with the activated partial thromboplastin time (aPTT), which is sensitive to plasma heparin concentrations of 0.1 U/mL or higher. Because different reagents and measuring systems have differing sensitivities to heparin, it is recommended that the therapeutic range be established for each laboratory by calibrating the aPTT to a plasma heparin concentration of 0.2 to 0.4 units by protamine sulfate titration, or 0.3 to 0.7 U/mL using an anti–factor Xa assay.[54] The usual aPTT range for heparin therapy is between 1.5 and 2.5 times the

mean of the normal range. Clinically useful nomograms are available for adjusting the heparin dose using either fixed- or weight-based dosing.[55] Alternatively, monitoring can be performed using anti-Xa levels, which is a useful approach when the aPTT is unreliable, as in patients with baseline prolongation of the aPTT as a consequence of expressing a lupus anticoagulant. Rapid achievement of a therapeutic level, as assessed by the aPTT or anti-Xa level, is important in ensuring an adequate anticoagulant effect.

Some patients fail to display an adequately prolonged aPTT following treatment with unfractionated heparin, despite apparently adequate or even supratherapeutic doses of the drug. This phenomenon is termed *heparin resistance* and is usually caused by an acute-phase response that results in high levels of procoagulant proteins, including factor VIII. The antithrombotic effect of heparin correlates best with plasma heparin levels, which may be adequate in these circumstances despite a subtherapeutic aPTT.[56] For patients who require heparin doses of greater than 35,000 U/day to increase the aPTT into the therapeutic range, consideration should be given to using heparin levels determined by an anti-Xa assay. Substitution of LMWH for unfractionated heparin is another consideration. Although AT deficiency may cause heparin resistance, most AT-deficient patients can be adequately anticoagulated with heparin in usual doses. No monitoring is recommended when low doses of heparin are used for prophylaxis of venous thromboembolic disease, although minimal prolongation of the aPTT may occur. Care is required in very light weight and frail elderly who may be anticoagulated with usual "prophylactic" doses of unfractionated heparin; aPTT monitoring might be considered in such patients.

A large study demonstrated that patients with acute venous thromboembolism can be safely treated with fixed, weight-adjusted heparin doses without aPTT monitoring.[57] In this study, 708 patients were allocated randomly to receive either unfractionated heparin with a subcutaneous bolus dose of 333 U/kg followed by a twice-daily dose of 250 U/kg, or LMWH over 3 months of follow up. Recurrent venous thromboembolism occurred in 13 patients who were allocated to unfractionated heparin and in 12 who were allocated to LMWH. Major bleeding occurred in four and five patients, respectively. This study calls into question the need for routine aPTT monitoring of therapeutic dose, weight-adjusted unfractionated heparin and warrants validation.

REVERSAL

Heparin has a short half-life, and its anticoagulant effect disappears several hours after discontinuation of an intravenous infusion. Therefore, stopping the infusion and local measures are usually adequate to control bleeding. However, in major or life-threatening bleeding, the anticoagulant effect can be neutralized with protamine sulfate, which is a basic polypeptide that binds tightly to the acidic heparin molecule. The usual dose of protamine required is 1 mg to neutralize 100 units of heparin. The dose to be administered is based on the amount of heparin remaining in the circulation. Protamine is routinely used to neutralize heparin after cardiopulmonary bypass using standard formulas and activated clotting time monitoring.

ADVERSE EFFECTS

The most frequent complication of heparin administration is bleeding, which is related to the dose and intensity of treatment, as well as to patient characteristics. HIT is an immune-mediated platelet consumption caused by an antibody directed against a complex of heparin and platelet factor 4 (Chap. 118). Despite thrombocytopenia, HIT is more commonly associated with thrombotic complications than bleeding, and it occurs in approximately 3 percent of patients, depending on the type of heparin, the dose and route of administration, and the indication for heparin anticoagulation (e.g., more common in "surgical patients" than in "medical patients"). The "4T" score is a clinical prediction tool with good negative predictive value.[58] Platelet counts should be monitored during treatment and heparin discontinued if thrombocytopenia occurs, and an alternative anticoagulant that does not interact with the heparin-platelet factor 4 complexes should be administered. Vitamin K antagonists should be given only after the platelet count has risen to greater than 150,000/μL. Long-term heparin therapy can also cause osteoporosis, and radiographic evidence of bone loss occurs in approximately 15 percent of women who receive prolonged treatment during pregnancy, with symptomatic vertebrae fractures in approximately 2 percent. The bone loss may resolve after heparin is discontinued.

LOW-MOLECULAR-WEIGHT HEPARIN

Limitations of unfractionated heparin led to studies correlating structural and functional relationships of heparin, and this eventually resulted in the development of LMWHs, several of which are available. LMWH preparations are produced by treating heparin chemically or enzymatically to decrease the size of the polysaccharide chains, yielding products with restricted molecular weight distributions with a mean of approximately 4000 to 5000 daltons.[59] Like heparin, LMWHs exert antithrombotic effects through interaction with AT. In the presence of LMWH, AT inactivates factor Xa in the same way as unfractionated heparin, but it is less able to inactivate thrombin because the shorter polysaccharide length does not allow formation of the necessary ternary complex. Consequently, LMWHs have a greater proportion of anti–factor Xa than AT activity.

LMWHs also have different pharmacokinetic properties than unfractionated heparin.[54] Following subcutaneous administration, LMWHs are nearly completely absorbed, a clear benefit over unfractionated heparin, which exhibits variable and dose-dependent absorption. LMWHs also exhibit less binding to plasma proteins and cells than unfractionated heparin, resulting in more predictable blood levels and anticoagulant effects. LMWHs have a longer plasma half-life than unfractionated heparins, allowing once- or twice-daily subcutaneous administration.

LMWHs have significant renal clearance, and high levels can accumulate in patients with renal insufficiency. Care must be taken in dosing LMWHs in patients with reduced renal function as bleeding risks are increased,[60] and monitoring with anti–factor Xa levels may be needed. Similarly, monitoring may be necessary to achieve appropriate levels in very obese patients, although weight-based dosing probably achieves better anticoagulation. Protamine sulfate does not completely reverse the anticoagulant effect of LMWH but is partially effective and can be useful in patients with serious hemorrhage.[61] Several LMWH preparations are available and approved for both prophylaxis and treatment of venous and arterial thrombotic diseases. Each preparation differs slightly and is pharmacologically unique, although the agents are likely similarly effective for the treatment and prevention of venous thrombosis.

Similar to unfractionated heparin, the most common adverse effect is bleeding, which occurs at approximately the same frequency and severity when used in similar patient groups for the same indication. HIT is much less common than with unfractionated heparin,[62] occurring only in 0.3 to 0.45 percent of patients. However, cross-reactivity of the antibody occurs, and LMWH is not an acceptable choice for continued anticoagulation in patients with HIT induced by treatment with unfractionated heparin. Animal studies suggest that osteoporosis may be less common with LMWH, and this is reported by several small clinical trials.[63]

● CHOICE OF HEPARIN OR LOW-MOLECULAR-WEIGHT HEPARIN

The factors governing the choice of heparin or LMWH concern effectiveness, safety, convenience, and cost. For treatment of venous thromboembolic disease, the safety and efficacy of heparin and LMWH are comparable. A meta-analysis of 14 studies comparing unfractionated heparin to LMWH in 4754 patients showed that LMWH-treated patients had less recurrent venous thromboembolic complications (4.3 percent vs. 5.6 percent, odds ratio [OR] 0.76, 95 percent confidence interval 0.57 to 1.01) and fewer major bleeding events (1.3 percent vs. 2.1 percent, OR 0.6, 95 percent confidence interval 0.39 to 0.93).[64] LMWH also offers better convenience because subcutaneous administration permits outpatient treatment. However, LMWHs may be difficult to use in patients with renal insufficiency because of decreased clearance, and intravenous heparin may offer advantages in such patients. LMWHs are incompletely reversed by protamine sulfate, making them more difficult to use for cardiac bypass surgery. Unfractionated heparin may be preferable in patients who require an invasive procedure on an urgent basis because of its shorter half-life. LMWHs may offer some advantages for patients with acute coronary syndromes.

DANAPAROID

Danaparoid is a mixture of glycosaminoglycans and is composed of approximately 84 percent heparan sulfate, 12 percent dermatan sulfate, and 4 percent chondroitin sulfate. It is an AT-dependent anticoagulant with predominant anti–factor Xa activity. The plasma half-life is approximately 24 hours with predominant renal clearance. Danaparoid is not reversed by protamine sulfate. Danaparoid differs structurally from heparin and it has been used successfully to treat patients with HIT. Although there is *in vitro* cross-reactivity of 10 to 20 percent of heparin antibodies with danaparoid, this is of uncertain clinical relevance. Danaparoid is administered subcutaneously, and levels may be monitored with anti–factor Xa assays performed using a danaparoid standard curve. At the time of writing danaparoid has not been approved in the United States, and availability elsewhere was limited.

FONDAPARINUX

Fondaparinux is a unique heparin-like anticoagulant with highly selective AT-dependent anti–factor Xa activity.[54] It is a completely synthetic pentasaccharide whose structure is based on the heparin sequence that interacts with AT. It binds reversibly and with high affinity to AT, resulting in a conformational change that renders it effective in inhibiting factor Xa, but because of its small size, does not inhibit thrombin. Whereas unfractionated heparin and all LMWHs are derived from animal sources, fondaparinux is synthesized in a structurally homogenous form containing no animal products. Consequently, fondaparinux does not induce allergic responses. Because it inhibits factor Xa but has no direct action on thrombin, its mechanism of action depends on reducing thrombin generation.

Pharmacologic studies show that maximum plasma levels are reached approximately 2 hours after subcutaneous administration with an elimination half-life of approximately 17 hours independent of the dose.[65] Bioavailability is nearly complete after subcutaneous or intravenous administration. There is a low intra- and intersubject variability with little accumulation after multiple daily doses. Because elimination is primarily renal and the agent is excreted unchanged in the urine, fondaparinux is contraindicated in patients with severe renal impairment. Fondaparinux plasma levels can be measured with the anti–factor Xa assay, but there is no effect on other coagulation assays including the activated clotting time (ACT), aPTT, or thrombin clotting time.

Clinical studies have evaluated the use of fondaparinux in several conditions, and it is approved by the FDA for prevention of venous thromboembolism (VTE) in patients undergoing major orthopedic surgery or with hip fracture, prophylaxis after abdominal surgery, and treatment of deep venous thrombosis (DVT) or pulmonary embolism (PE). For prophylaxis it is administered subcutaneously in a dose of 2.5 mg once daily, whereas a weight-adjusted dose is used for treatment of VTE. The principal adverse effect is bleeding, and its frequency and severity have been comparable to those observed with LMWH. Elevated levels may occur in patients with renal insufficiency, and caution should be exercised in using fondaparinux in patients with renal compromise. Fondaparinux is a good choice for an anticoagulant in patients with HIT as there is no cross-reactivity.[66]

BIVALIRUDIN

Bivalirudin, a direct thrombin inhibitor, is a recombinant protein based on the structure of hirudin, is composed of a dodecapeptide analogue of the carboxyterminal region of hirudin linked by a four-glycine residue to a structure directed to the active site of thrombin.[67] Pharmacokinetic studies show that plasma clearance is rapid (4.6 mL/min/kg) in patients with normal renal function with a volume of distribution of 0.2 L/kg and elimination half-life of approximately 30 minutes.[54] There is dose-dependent prolongation of the ACT and aPTT that correlates with plasma concentrations. the drug is eliminated by both renal and hepatic clearance, and consequently, dose modification is recommended for patients with moderate-to-severe functional liver or kidney disease.

Bivalirudin is effective when used with aspirin in patients with unstable angina or postinfarction angina undergoing angioplasty, and it is approved for this use.[68] It is also approved for patients with HIT undergoing percutaneous coronary intervention. In some clinical trials, bivalirudin also shows efficacy in preventing restenosis after coronary angioplasty, as an adjunct to streptokinase in acute myocardial infarction, and in preventing venous thrombosis after orthopedic surgery and in patients with HIT. However, these indications have not been approved by the FDA. The most common adverse effect is bleeding, and no specific antidote is available. The infusion should be discontinued in patients with bleeding complications and blood levels monitored with the aPTT or other coagulation parameters. Antibivalirudin antibodies have not been detected following therapy.

ARGATROBAN

Argatroban is a small-molecule arginine derivative that reversibly and directly inhibits thrombin by binding to the active catalytic site of the enzyme with a K_i of 3.9×10^{-8} mol/L.[54] Because of its small size, argatroban is an effective inhibitor of thrombin, both bound to surfaces and in solution.[69] The anticoagulant effect can be assessed with either the aPTT or ACT, and both correlate with plasma concentrations of the drug. Argatroban is approximately 50 percent protein bound and has a volume of distribution of 0.2 L/kg and an elimination half-life of 39 to 51 minutes.[70] Metabolism is primarily hepatic, and the clearance and half-life are prolonged in patients with hepatic functional abnormalities requiring dose reduction. Renal function has less effect on argatroban pharmacokinetics.

Argatroban is approved for treatment and prophylaxis of HIT and for percutaneous interventions in patients with HIT. It also shows some benefit in patients with thrombotic stroke in clinical trials. For treatment of HIT, argatroban is administered at 2 mcg/kg per hour and adjusted to maintain the aPTT at 1.5 to 3 times baseline. For patients with HIT who are undergoing percutaneous coronary interventions, the drug is administered as a bolus of 350 mcg/kg followed by a continuous infusion of 15 to 400 mcg/kg per minute for a target ACT of 300 to 450

seconds. As with other direct thrombin inhibitors, the main side effect is bleeding, and no specific agent is available to reverse its action. The anticoagulant effect may be prolonged in patients with hepatic impairment. If overdosage or excess bleeding occurs, the infusion should be discontinued and the aPTT and other coagulation parameters monitored.

The transition from argatroban to warfarin in patients requiring long-term anticoagulation is complicated because argatroban has a significant effect on both the PT and the aPTT. In patients transitioning to warfarin an INR should be measured; if it is greater than 4.0, the argatroban should be stopped for several hours and the INR remeasured. If the INR is still greater than 2.0, the argatroban can be discontinued; if it is less than 2.0, the argatroban should be reinstituted and the same procedure followed on the next day.

LEPIRUDIN

Lepirudin is closely related to hirudin, a natural anticoagulant found in the salivary glands of the leech. The half-life is 1 to 3 hours in normal volunteers with predominantly renal catabolism, but it may be as long as 2 days in dialysis-dependent patients.[71] Lepirudin prolongs the aPTT in a concentration-dependent manner.[72] The manufacturer discontinued marketing of this product and it is no longer available.

DABIGATRAN ETEXILATE

Dabigatran etexilate, one of the novel oral anticoagulants, is a direct thrombin inhibitor prodrug with a bioavailability of approximately 6 percent after oral administration. The absorbed drug is rapidly converted by esterases to dabigatran. Peak levels occur 1 to 2 hours after an oral dose; the half-life is approximately 12 hours. Dabigatran does not require a cofactor and reversibly inhibits the active site of thrombin. Dabigatran does not interfere with drugs that are metabolized by the CYP enzyme system and it produces a predictable anticoagulant response, which allows therapy without the need for monitoring.[73] Dabigatran prolongs several coagulation assays. The PT, aPTT, and ACT lack sensitivity for therapeutic drug levels, while the dilute thrombin time and ecarin clotting time appear to correlate well across a broad range of drug levels.[74] None of these tests have been shown to predict clinical outcomes such as thrombosis or bleeding.

The major side effect of dabigatran is hemorrhage. No specific antidote is currently available, although such antidotes are in development.[75] Consequently, bleeding complications are managed symptomatically. Although not well studied, there are published case reports showing that dialysis or hemoperfusion likely removes this compound from the circulation.[76] In animal models the administration of various coagulation factor concentrates or recombinant activated factor VII (factor VIIa) improved prolonged bleeding times, although these agents did not cause correlative changes in anticoagulation tests.[77]

Dabigatran etexilate, and the other novel oral anticoagulants, are effective in various clinical settings (Table 25–5). Dabigatran is now FDA approved for management of VTE and prevention of stroke and systemic embolism in nonvalvular atrial fibrillation. In the RE-LY trial, patients with nonvalvular atrial fibrillation and a risk of stroke were randomized to dabigatran etexilate (110 mg BID or 150 mg BID) or dose-adjusted warfarin.[78] In this noninferiority trial, rates of stroke or systemic embolism were 1.69 percent per year with warfarin, 1.53 percent per year with dabigatran etexilate 110 mg (relative risk [RR] 0.91, p<0.001 for noninferiority) and 1.11 percent per year with dabigatran etexilate 150 mg (RR 0.66, p<0.001 for superiority). The rates of major bleeding in the RE-LY trial were similar between higher dose dabigatran and warfarin, but significantly lower for low-dose dabigatran compared to warfarin. The rate of intracranial bleeding was lower for both doses of dabigatran compared to warfarin. The RE-COVER trial was a randomized double-blind

TABLE 25–5. Studies with Novel Targeted Oral Anticoagulants

Anticoagulant	Indication	Study	Efficacy	Safety
Dabigatran	Nonvalvular atrial fibrillation	RE-LY[78]	Dabigatran (150 mg BID dose) superior to warfarin at stroke reduction	Similar rates of major bleeding and lower rates of intracranial bleeding with dabigatran
	VTE	RECOVER[37]	Dabigatran (150 mg BID dose) noninferior to warfarin for prevention of recurrent VTE	Similar rates of major bleeding and decreased rates of total bleeding events with dabigatran
	Mechanical heart valves	RE-ALIGN[80]	Trial stopped early because of increased rates of thrombosis and bleeding in patients receiving dabigatran	
	Hip arthroplasty	RE-NOVATE[140]	Dabigatran (220 mg once daily or 150 mg once daily for 28–35 days) were noninferior to enoxaparin (40 mg once daily for 28–35 days) at prevention of total VTE or death	Major bleeding occurred in 1.4% of the dabigatran group and 0.9% of the enoxaparin group (p = 0.40)
	Hip arthroplasty	RE-NOVATEII[141]	Dabigatran (220 mg once daily for 28–35 days) was noninferior to enoxaparin (40 mg once daily for 28–35 days) at prevention of total VTE or death (7.7% vs. 8.8%). Major VTE plus death was less common in dabigatran group (2.2% vs. 4.2%)	Major bleeding rates were similar (1.4% vs. 0.9%)
	Knee arthroplasty	RE-MODEL[142]	Dabigatran (220 mg once daily or 150 mg once daily for 6–10 days) were noninferior to enoxaparin (40 mg once daily for 6–10 days) at prevention of total VTE or death	The incidence of major bleeding did not differ between the three groups
Rivaroxaban	Nonvalvular atrial fibrillation	ROCKET-AF[83]	Rivaroxaban noninferior to warfarin at stroke reduction	Similar rates of overall bleeding, but significantly fewer intracranial bleeds with rivaroxaban (0.5% vs. 0.7%)
	Acute coronary syndrome	ATLAS ACS[143]	Rivaroxaban (2.5 or 5 mg BID) significantly reduced the combined end point of cardiovascular death, MI or stroke compared to placebo	Rivaroxaban increased the rates of major bleeding (2.1% vs. 0.6%) and intracranial hemorrhage (0.6% vs. 0.2%) without a significant increase in fatal bleeding (0.3% vs. 0.2%)
	PE	EINSTEIN-PE[39]	Rivaroxaban was noninferior to warfarin for treatment of acute PE	Similar overall bleeding rates but significantly fewer major bleeds with rivaroxaban (1.1% vs. 2.1%)
	DVT	EINSTEIN-DVT[38]	Rivaroxaban was noninferior to warfarin for treatment of acute DVT	Similar bleeding rates
	Hip arthroplasty	RECORD1[84]	Extended duration rivaroxaban (10 mg daily 31–39 days) was superior to Lovenox (40 mg daily 31–39 days) for prevention of major VTE (0.2% vs. 2.0%)	Similar rates of major bleeding (0.3% vs. 0.1%)
	Hip arthroplasty	RECORD2[144]	Extended duration rivaroxaban (10 mg daily 31–39 days) was superior to short duration Lovenox (40 mg daily 10–14 days) at prevention of any DVT, nonfatal PE or death (2.0% vs. 9.3%)	Similar rates of bleeding (5.5% vs. 6.6%)
	Knee arthroplasty	RECORD3[85]	Short duration rivaroxaban (10 mg daily 10–14 days) was superior to short duration Lovenox (40 mg daily 10–14 days) at prevention of any DVT, nonfatal PE or death (9.2% vs. 18.9%)	Similar rates of major bleeding (0.5% vs. 0.6%)
	VTE prophylaxis in medically ill patients	MAGELLAN[86]	The rate of any proximal DVT or symptomatic VTE with extended duration rivaroxaban (10 mg daily for 31–39 days) was noninferior at 10 days (2.7% vs. 2.7%) and superior at 35 days (4.4% vs. 5.7%) when compared to standard prophylaxis (Lovenox 40 mg daily for 10–14 days)	The composite of major or clinically relevant nonmajor bleeding occurred more often in patients receiving extended duration rivaroxaban at day 10 (2.8% vs. 1.2%) and at day 35 (4.1% vs. 1.7%)

(Continued)

TABLE 25–5. Studies with Novel Targeted Oral Anticoagulants (Continued)

Anticoagulant	Indication	Study	Efficacy	Safety
Apixaban	Nonvalvular atrial fibrillation	ARISTOTLE[93]	Apixaban was superior to warfarin for stroke prevention (1.3% vs. 1.6%)	Significantly fewer major bleeds with apixaban (2.1% vs. 3.1%)
	Nonvalvular atrial fibrillation not suitable for warfarin	AVERROES[94]	Apixaban superior to aspirin for stroke prevention (1.6% vs. 3.7%)	Similar bleeding rates with apixaban and aspirin
	Acute coronary syndrome	APPRAISE-2[145]	The trial was terminated prematurely because of an increase in major bleeding events without a reduction in cardiovascular ischemic events	
	VTE	AMPLIFY[95]	Apixaban was noninferior to warfarin for treatment of acute VTE	Significantly fewer major bleeding events with apixaban (0.6% vs. 1.8%)
	VTE extended treatment	AMPLIFY-EXT[96]	Apixaban was superior to placebo for prevention of recurrent VTE (1.7% vs. 8.8%)	Apixaban was not associated with increased major bleeding
	Knee arthroplasty	ADVANCE1[98]	Apixaban (2.5 mg BID for 10–14 days) did not meet prespecified criteria for noninferiority in prevention of the composite end point including any DVT, nonfatal PE and death when compared to Lovenox (30 mg BID for 10–14 days)	Apixaban was associated with significantly fewer major and clinically relevant nonmajor bleeding events (2.9% vs. 4.3%)
	Knee arthroplasty	ADVANCE2[99]	Apixaban (2.5 mg BID for 10–14 days) was superior to Lovenox (40 mg once daily 10–14 days) for prevention of the composite endpoint including any DVT, nonfatal PE and death (15% vs. 24%)	Similar rates of major and clinically relevant nonmajor bleeding events (4% vs. 5%)
	Hip arthroplasty	ADVANCE3[97]	Apixaban (2.5 mg BID for 35 days) was superior to Lovenox (40 mg once daily 35 days) for prevention of the composite endpoint including any DVT, nonfatal PE and death (1.4% vs. 3.9%)	Similar rates of major and clinically relevant nonmajor bleeding events (4.8% vs. 5.0%)
	VTE prophylaxis in medically ill patients	ADOPT[146]	The rate of any DVT, symptomatic PE, or death at 60 days with extended duration apixaban (2.5 mg BID for 30 days) was not superior to standard duration Lovenox (40 mg once daily 6–14 days) (2.7% vs. 3.1%)	Major bleeding was significantly more common in patients receiving apixaban (0.5% vs. 0.2%)
Edoxaban	Nonvalvular atrial fibrillation	ENGAGE-AF[101]	Edoxaban was noninferior to warfarin for stroke prevention	Significantly fewer major bleeding events with edoxaban (1.6% vs. 3.4%)
	VTE	HOKUSAI-VTE[102]	Edoxaban noninferior to warfarin for treatment of acute VTE	Significantly fewer overall bleeding events with edoxaban (8.2% vs. 10.3%)

DVT, deep vein thrombosis; MI, myocardial infarction; PE, pulmonary embolism; VTE, venous thromboembolism.

noninferiority trial comparing dabigatran etexilate (150 mg BID) to dose-adjusted warfarin in patients with acute VTE who received initial parenteral anticoagulation for a median of 9 days.[37] The rates of recurrent VTE were similar (2.4 vs. 2.1 percent, P<0.001 for noninferiority). In a meta-analysis of three large randomized trials, dabigatran was as effective as LMWH for prevention of VTE and VTE-related mortality after hip and knee replacement, and had a similar bleeding risk.[79] Dabigatran does not appear to be safe or effective in prevention of thromboembolic complications following heart valve replacement. The RE-ALIGN study randomized patients to dabigatran or warfarin following valve replacement and was terminated early because of excess thrombotic and bleeding complications in dabigatran-treated patients.[80]

RIVAROXABAN

Rivaroxaban is a direct factor Xa inhibitor that is administered orally and produces its anticoagulant effect through reversible binding with factor Xa. Rivaroxaban can inhibit both free and thrombus-associated factor Xa. Like dabigatran, it is dependent on renal excretion, and bioaccumulation may occur in patients with renal insufficiency.

Rivaroxaban produces its peak anticoagulant effect within 4 hours of oral administration and has a terminal elimination half-life of 5.7 to 9.2 hours. PT is more accurate than the aPTT in measuring rivaroxaban effects; however, the sensitivity varies by specific reagent and is not good at lower therapeutic drug levels.[81] A rivaroxaban calibrated anti-Xa assay appears to be the most accurate test as it correlates well with drug level across a broad therapeutic range.[82]

Rivaroxaban is effective in a number of clinical settings. In the EINSTEIN-PE[39] and EINSTEIN-DVT[38] randomized clinical trials treatment with rivaroxaban (15 mg BID for 3 weeks followed by 20 mg once daily) was noninferior to standard anticoagulation (LMWH followed by warfarin) in preventing recurrent thrombosis in patients with acute VTE. In a large randomized trial of patients with nonvalvular atrial fibrillation, rivaroxaban was noninferior to warfarin for prevention of stroke or systemic embolism.[83] Prophylactic rivaroxaban (10 mg once daily) significantly reduced rates of postoperative VTE compared to the LMWH Lovenox (40 mg once daily) following hip arthroplasty (1.1 percent vs, 3.7 percent, p<0.001)[84] and knee arthroplasty (9.6 percent vs. 18.9 percent),[85] and in hospitalized acutely medically ill patients was noninferior to Lovenox for standard 10-day thromboprohylaxis.[86]

The principal side effect of rivaroxaban therapy is bleeding. In a pooled analysis of the EINSTEIN studies, major bleeding was less common in patients receiving rivaroxaban compared to standard anticoagulation (1.0 percent vs. 1.7 percent, p = 0.002), and this includes a significant reduction in intracranial bleeding.[87] In another meta-analysis of phase III trials comparing rivaroxaban to standard anticoagulation, rivaroxaban was associated with a reduced risk of fatal bleeding complications.[88] There is no antidote for the anticoagulant effect of rivaroxaban. Prothrombin complex concentrates partially reverse prolonged coagulation times in healthy volunteers receiving rivaroxaban,[89] and PCC and recombinant activated factor VIIa improved bleeding times after rivaroxaban treatment in animal studies.[90] However, these agents have not been proven effective in managing rivaroxaban treated patients with bleeding complications.

APIXABAN

Apixaban is an orally administered direct inhibitor of factor Xa which is metabolized primarily by the hepatic cytochrome CYP3A4 enzyme. The onset of action and half-life are 3 hours and 12 hours respectively, and approximately 25 percent is excreted by the kidney. Apixaban affects standard anticoagulation assays less than rivaroxaban, and the effect is variable for different reagents within an assay group. In general the PT is more sensitive than aPTT, and chromogenic apixaban specific anti-Xa assays display the most accurate linear correlation across a therapeutic dose range.[91] There is no antidote for reversal of apixaban. In animal studies recombinant activated factor VIIa but not PCCs reduced bleeding times in apixaban-treated animals.[92]

Apixaban, like rivaroxaban and dabigatran, has been studied in several clinical settings. Two large phase III randomized clinical trials with slightly different designs led to the approval of apixaban for management of nonvalvular atrial fibrillation. In the ARISTOTLE trial, patients with nonvalvular atrial fibrillation and a risk for stroke were randomized to apixaban (5 mg BID) or dose-adjusted warfarin. Apixaban was superior to warfarin in reducing the rate of embolic or hemorrhagic stroke and systemic embolism (1.27 percent vs. 1.6 percent per year, p = 0.01), and fewer patients experienced major bleeding complications (2.13 percent vs. 3.09 percent, p<0.001).[93] The AVERROES trial was terminated early because of a clear reduction in stroke and systemic embolism in patients with nonvalvular atrial fibrillation deemed unsuitable or unwilling to take vitamin K antagonists randomized to apixaban versus aspirin (1.6 percent vs. 3.7 percent, p<0.001).[94] Interestingly, there was no difference in major bleeding or intracranial bleeding between apixaban and aspirin. Apixaban (10 mg BID for 7 days then 5 mg BID) has also been shown to be noninferior to standard anticoagulation (LMWH then dose-adjusted warfarin) in initial management of acute VTE,[95] and effective for secondary VTE prevention in patients treated for an extended time following acute VTE.[96] Major bleeding rates were significantly lower with apixaban compared to standard anticoagulation in the initial period after acute VTE (0.6 percent vs. 1.8 percent, p<0.001), and rates of major bleeding were equivalent in patients receiving extended thromboprophylactic dosing of apixaban compared to placebo (0.1 percent in the 5-mg apixaban group, 0.2 percent in the 2.5-mg apixaban group, 0.5 percent in the placebo group). Prophylactic apixaban (2.5 mg BID) is better than Lovenox (40 mg daily) at preventing postoperative VTE following hip replacement.[97]

Following total knee replacement apixaban did not meet prespecified noninferiority criteria in ADVANCE-1, where VTE rates were similar in patients receiving apixaban (2.5 mg BID) and twice daily Lovenox (30 mg BID) (9.0 percent vs. 8.8 percent),[98] however in ADVANCE-2 apixaban was proven to be noninferior to once daily Lovenox in prevention of postoperative VTE following knee replacement.[99]

EDOXABAN

Edoxaban is a direct oral factor Xa inhibitor with peak onset approximately 1 to 2 hours after administration and a half-life of approximately 8 hours.[100] Like other direct Xa inhibitors, edoxaban is renally excreted. Multiple coagulation tests can be affected by edoxaban, but partial thromboplastin time (PTT) and anti-Xa assay show the best correlation with drug levels.

Edoxaban is effective in management of atrial fibrillation and acute venous thromboembolism, and in the prevention of VTE following hip or knee arthroplasty. In the ENGAGE AF-TIMI trial, the annualized rate of stroke or systemic embolism in patients with nonvalvular atrial fibrillation and moderate to high risk of thrombosis was 1.50 percent with warfarin, 1.18 percent with high-dose edoxaban (P<0.001 for noninferiority), and 1.61 percent with low-dose edoxaban (P = 0.005 for noninferiority).[101] Edoxaban-treated patients experienced significantly fewer major bleeding events (3.43 percent with warfarin vs. 2.75 percent with high-dose edoxaban and 1.61 percent with low-dose edoxaban). In the Hokusai-VTE study, edoxaban was noninferior to warfarin in preventing recurrent VTE in patients with acute PE or DVT (3.2 percent vs. 3.4 percent), and bleeding complications were reduced in the edoxaban treated group (8.5 percent vs. 10.3 percent).[102]

● FIBRINOLYTIC THERAPY

Fibrinolytic therapy is administered by infusing high doses of a plasminogen activator to accelerate the conversion of plasminogen to the active fibrinolytic enzyme plasmin, which proteolytically degrades fibrin (Chap. 135). The specific biochemical and pharmacologic properties of different agents are important determinants of the administration regimen, the efficacy of clot lysis, and the nature of adverse effects. For example, some fibrinolytic drugs are bacterial products that are antigenic and can cause allergic responses, whereas others are recombinant human proteins. Some agents activate plasminogen prominently, both in blood and at the clot surface, and induce a systemic fibrinolytic state in addition to accelerating clot lysis. In contrast, the activity of other agents is more specifically limited to the clot surface with fewer systemic effects. Fibrinolytic therapy is used for treatment of both venous and arterial thrombosis and represents standard treatment for many patients presenting with acute myocardial infarction because it accelerates reperfusion, decreases mortality, and reduces morbidity (Chap. 135). Thrombolytic therapy has also become standard for many patients presenting with thrombosis of peripheral arteries, bypass grafts, and catheters.[103] It is used for treatment of selected patients with thrombotic stroke. Fibrinolytic therapy improves outcome in selected patients with large pulmonary emboli (Chap. 135).

STREPTOKINASE

Streptokinase was the first plasminogen activator used clinically. It is derived from β-hemolytic streptococci and has a unique indirect mechanism of action. By itself, streptokinase has no enzymatic activity, but it combines with plasminogen to form an equimolar streptokinase–plasminogen complex that can then convert other plasminogen molecules to plasmin. Additionally, the streptokinase–plasminogen complex can undergo proteolytic cleavage itself, resulting in activation. When administered in therapeutic doses, streptokinase is an effective thrombolytic agent. The streptokinase–plasmin(ogen) complex can bind to fibrin through the "kringle" domains of plasmin and activate clot-bound plasminogen to accelerate clot lysis (Chap. 135), but can also act on plasminogen in the blood to produce plasmin, giving rise to systemic proteolysis termed the *lytic state*. This results in consumption of plasminogen and α_2-antiplasmin, degradation of fibrinogen, factor V, and factor VIII, proteolysis of platelet membrane proteins by plasmin, and platelet activation. Streptokinase has a rapid plasma clearance with a half-life of approximately 20 minutes, but the duration of the proteolytic effect is more prolonged.[104]

Streptokinase can be used to treat either venous or arterial thrombosis. Higher doses given over a shorter time are typically used for arterial disease. For either venous or arterial thrombosis, a sufficient dose must be administered to overcome circulating neutralizing antibodies, which are common because of the frequency of streptococcal infections in the population. Occasionally, individuals have a high titer of antibodies that neutralize this amount of streptokinase, resulting in resistance. Streptokinase is antigenic, and high-titer antibodies develop 1 to 2 weeks after use, precluding retreatment until the titer declines. High titers can also cause febrile or hypotensive reactions. The first large study to demonstrate the utility of coronary reperfusion employed streptokinase.[105] Although not widely used in North America, streptokinase is still extensively used given its low cost, widespread availability, and familiarity.

TISSUE-TYPE PLASMINOGEN ACTIVATOR AND RECOMBINANT TISSUE PLASMINOGEN ACTIVATOR (ALTEPLASE)

Tissue-type plasminogen activator (t-PA) is a naturally occurring plasminogen activator that is structurally and immunologically distinct from urokinase. t-PA is synthesized by endothelial cells as a single-chain polypeptide and was originally produced from cell culture for pharmacologic use, but is now synthesized by recombinant techniques (alteplase). t-PA directly converts plasminogen to plasmin in a reaction that is accelerated several-hundred-fold in the presence of fibrin. In the absence of fibrin, t-PA has much less activity, and this property accounts for the relative "fibrin specificity" of t-PA observed physiologically. However, when administered pharmacologically in a high dose, significant proteolysis of plasma fibrinogen often occurs, but this is typically less prominent than observed with treatment using either streptokinase or urokinase. The half-life of t-PA following intravenous administration is approximately 5 minutes, which requires a constant infusion to maintain therapeutic plasma levels. t-PA is not antigenic because it is a physiologic enzyme.[104]

t-PA has been evaluated in treatment of VTE, myocardial infarction, stroke, catheter thrombosis, and peripheral arterial occlusion. In patients with PE, a regimen of 100 mg intravenously over 2 hours results in a high rate of clot lysis and hemodynamic improvement. t-PA has been evaluated in many large studies for acute myocardial infarction and administration results in improved mortality and morbidity. t-PA has also been evaluated in treatment of stroke and results in significant benefit in highly selected patients who are treated within hours of symptom onset (Chap. 135). In the CaVenT study,[106] use of alteplase in catheter-directed thrombolysis of ileofemoral DVT resulted in an 18 percent reduction in postthrombotic syndrome.

RETEPLASE

Recombinant technology has been used to engineer many t-PA mutants in an attempt to improve pharmacologic properties. The structural

modifications in reteplase include removal of the finger, kringle 1, and EGF (epidermal growth factor) receptor domains. These changes result in enhanced fibrin specificity and a significantly longer half-life of 15 minutes compared to 4 minutes with t-PA, so it can be administered as an intravenous bolus rather than a continuous infusion. Its mode of administration (two 10-U IV boluses given over 2 minutes, 30 minutes apart) make it particularly useful for prehospital administration in remote areas, or areas with limited access to primary percutaneous coronary interventions.[129]

TENECTEPLASE

Tenecteplase (TNK) is another bioengineered variant of t-PA with a longer half-life, increased resistance to inactivation by plasminogen activator inhibitor-1, and improved fibrin specificity. Advantages include a longer half-life, greater fibrin specificity, ease and rapidity of administration, and similar clinical efficacy as t-PA for treatment of acute myocardial infarction. It has a half-life of more than 30 minutes and can be administered as a single IV bolus. Large studies in patients with ST elevation myocardial infarction have shown it to be equivalently effective as other t-PA derivatives.[104] The PEITHO study examined the use of heparin with TNK or placebo in hemodynamically stable patients with large pulmonary emboli associated with right ventricular dysfunction. Thrombolysis resulted in a reduction in the primary end point of death or hemodynamic decompensation at 7 days following randomization (6 percent vs. 3 percent). The administration of thrombolytic agents was associated with increased bleeding complications, which was more prominent in elderly patients.

●ANTIPLATELET DRUGS

Platelets play an important role in hemostasis and thrombosis and inhibitors of platelet function are important therapeutic agents (Chap. 134). Platelets adhere to exposed subendothelium, become activated, release contents of their dense and α granules, and form aggregates. Additional platelets from the circulating blood are then recruited by adenosine diphosphate (ADP), which is released from dense granules, and also by thromboxane A_2 synthesized by activated platelets in the aggregate. Simultaneous with the initial platelet adhesion and aggregation, thrombin generation is initiated. The activated platelet phospholipid membrane is an effective surface for binding of coagulation factors to enhance the rate of thrombin generation. As thrombin is formed it activates additional platelets and also cleaves fibrinopeptides from fibrinogen to form fibrin in and around the platelet plug, consolidating it. The role of platelets in initiating thrombosis is greater in the arterial circulation than in the venous circulation because higher shear forces present in arteries activate platelets. Consequently, antiplatelet drugs are more effective in arterial than in venous thrombosis. Table 25–6 summarizes the types of drug, their use in clinical settings, their mechanism of action, and their dosages.

CYCLOOXYGENASE-1 INHIBITORS

Cyclooxygenase (COX)-1 is an enzyme that is present in most cells. It converts arachidonic acid released from membrane phospholipids by phospholipase A_2 or phospholipase C and diacylglycerol to prostaglandin (PG) G_2 (Chap. 112). A peroxidase converts PGG_2 to PGH_2, which is then converted by thromboxane synthase in platelets to thromboxane A_2. Thromboxane A_2 is a potent activator of platelets. In endothelial cells, PGH_2 is converted to prostacyclin, a potent inhibitor of platelet function, through an increase in intraplatelet cyclic adenosine monophosphate (cAMP).

TABLE 25–6. Antiplatelet Agents by Mechanism of Action and Clinical Use

Agent and Indications		Dosages
Cyclooxygenase inhibitors		
Aspirin	Coronary and cerebrovascular disease	75–650 mg daily
	VTE secondary prevention	
Agents that increase cAMP		
Dipyridamole	Coronary, cerebrovascular, peripheral arterial disease	75–100 mg QID
Pentoxifylline	Peripheral arterial disease	400 mg BID
Cilostazol	Peripheral arterial disease	100 mg BID
ADP receptor blockers		
Ticlopidine	Cerebrovascular disease	250 mg BID
Clopidogrel	Coronary, cerebrovascular disease, PCI	75 mg daily, loading dose 300 mg
Prasugrel	ACS, PCI	10 mg daily, 60-mg loading dose
Ticagrelor	ACS	90 mg BID, 180-mg loading dose
ADP mimetic		
Cangrelor	Not approved in United States at time of this writing	
$\alpha_{IIb}\beta_3$ inhibitors		
Abciximab	ACS, PCI	0.25 mg/kg, then 10 mcg/kg/min
Eptifibatide	ACS, PCI	ACS 180 mcg/kg, then 2 mcg/kg/min
		PCI 180 mcg/kg, then 2 mcg/kg/min with 180 mcg/kg at 10 min
Tirofiban	ACS, PCI	0.4 mcg/kg/min × 30 min, then 0.1 mcg/kg/min
Thrombin receptor blocker		
Vorapaxar	Coronary disease, peripheral arterial disease	2.08 mg daily

ACS, acute coronary syndrome; ADP, adenosine diphosphate; cAMP, cyclic adenosine monophosphate; PCI, percutaneous coronary intervention; VTE, venous thromboembolism.

Aspirin (acetylsalicylic acid) was recognized as an inhibitor of platelet function in the 1960s, although the mechanism of its action was unknown at that time. It prolonged the bleeding time in normal subjects slightly, although usually not out of the normal range, and its effect lasted for several days. It was demonstrated that acetylation of COX is important in platelet inhibition by aspirin. Because platelets cannot synthesize new COX, irreversible enzyme inhibition by aspirin means that inhibition persists for the life span of the platelet. Most cells have two forms of COX, known as COX-1 and COX-2. COX-1 is synthesized constitutively, whereas COX-2 is only synthesized under stress conditions. Both COX-1 and COX-2 are inhibited by aspirin and most nonsteroidal antiinflammatory drugs (NSAIDs), with aspirin acetylating both forms. The nonaspirin COX inhibitors are reversible inhibitors, so they are active only while in the circulation. It was thought initially that only COX-1 is found in platelets, but COX-2 has been detected in platelets and its effect is particularly apparent when there was a rapid platelet turnover. Because COX-1 is the major COX in platelets, COX-2–specific inhibitors have minimal effect on platelet function.

Aspirin and several of the commonly used NSAIDs (e.g., indomethacin, ibuprofen, and naproxen) have similar *in vitro* effects on platelet function. Platelet aggregometry demonstrates that the second wave of aggregation induced by ADP or epinephrine in citrated platelet-rich plasma (PRP) is abolished after aspirin ingestion and that aggregation induced by low concentrations of collagen is markedly decreased. Arachidonic acid–induced aggregation is abolished after aspirin ingestion. Additionally, secretion of dense granule components (ADP, ATP, and serotonin) and of α-granule proteins by ADP, epinephrine, collagen, and arachidonic acid is inhibited in PRP after aspirin ingestion or with addition of indomethacin to PRP. Because of these *in vitro* effects of aspirin, the drug has been used extensively as an inhibitor of platelet function *in vivo*, with beneficial effects in primary and secondary prevention and in treatment of myocardial infarction (Chap. 135). Aspirin is also beneficial in stroke prevention with carotid artery disease and embolic stroke, although anticoagulation with warfarin or its analogues is generally more effective than aspirin in embolic stroke in most patients with a cardiac embolic source.[107] Aspirin is less often used to prevent venous thrombosis, although two recent large randomized studies showed significant benefit for secondary prevention of recurrent VTE compared to placebo.[108,109] Other drugs that inhibit COX-1 are not used to prevent either arterial or venous thrombosis.

A daily dose of 81 to 325 mg is recommended for most indications, as lower-dose aspirin appears as effective and may be associated with a lower risk of gastrointestinal bleeding than higher doses.[110,111] Broadly, aspirin is currently recommended for primary and secondary prevention of a wide variety of atherosclerotic outcomes including stroke, myocardial infarction, and peripheral vascular disease.

DRUGS THAT MODULATE CYCLIC ADENOSINE MONOPHOSPHATE LEVELS

cAMP in platelets is formed from ATP by the action of adenylate cyclase and degraded by cAMP phosphodiesterase, and basal levels of cAMP in platelets are low. Elevated levels of intraplatelet cAMP are induced by inhibition of cAMP phosphodiesterase, or by stimulation of adenylate cyclase activity, resulting in inhibition of platelet activation through several pathways: (1) modulation of phosphorylation of specific proteins; (2) inhibition of several steps in metabolism of phosphoinositol phosphates; and (3) lowering of intracellular Ca^{2+}, and accumulation of Ca^{2+} by platelet microsomes. Agents that inhibit the cAMP phosphodiesterase include theophylline, papaverine, and dipyridamole, as well as pentoxifylline and cilostazol. Several prostaglandins stimulate adenylate cyclase, including PGE_1, PGD_2, and PGI_2 (prostacyclin). Drugs that elevate cAMP levels are dipyridamole, pentoxifylline, and cilostazol. Dipyridamole can be used alone or in combination with aspirin. A very large study of dipyridamole in combination with low-dose aspirin (25 mg) found the combination equivalently effective to clopidogrel for the secondary prevention of noncardioembolic stroke.[112] Recent systematic reviews have also suggested that the combination of dipyridamole and aspirin is superior to aspirin alone for the prevention of cerebrovascular events.[113]

The other two phosphodiesterase inhibitors (pentoxifylline and cilostazol) are used primarily in patients with peripheral vascular disease. In addition to their inhibitory effect on platelets they may exert a beneficial effect on blood rheology and the microcirculation by increasing red cell deformability, thereby reducing blood viscosity. Cilostazol increases vascular endothelial growth factor levels, which may lead to an increase in collateral circulation. It has been shown to reduce risk of stroke in Asian populations,[114,115] and increases walking distance in patients with peripheral vascular disease.[116] Pentoxifylline inhibits vascular smooth-muscle cell proliferation and collagen synthesis, which may enhance vasodilation. Pentoxifylline probably is an effective treatment for ulcers associated with peripheral vascular disease; however, it is only modestly effective for treatment of peripheral vascular disease.[117]

ADENOSINE DIPHOSPHATE RECEPTOR BLOCKERS

The third class of platelet inhibitors is the ADP receptor blockers, which include thienopyridines (ticlopidine, clopidogrel, and prasugrel) and nonthienopyridines (ticagrelor and cangrelor). There are three ADP receptors on platelet membranes (Chap. 112), with the thienopyridines inhibiting one of them, the P2Y12 receptor. The inhibition of binding of ADP to the P2Y12 receptor results in inhibition of adenylate cyclase.

Ticlopidine was available for clinical use before clopidogrel. The Canadian American Ticlopidine Study was a randomized, placebo-controlled, double-blind study showing a 30 percent risk reduction for recurrent cardiovascular events with ticlopidine.[118] A review of four trials of ticlopidine plus aspirin versus oral anticoagulants for coronary stenting showed benefit to the combination in terms of reduced risk of nonfatal myocardial infarction and revascularization at 30 days, combined negative events (mortality, myocardial infarction, revascularization at 30 days), and major bleeding, but increased the risk of thrombocytopenia and neutropenia.[119]

In clinical practice fear of toxicity has largely led ticlopidine to be abandoned in favor of clopidogrel. In a direct comparison of ticlopidine and clopidogrel in patients undergoing coronary stenting (CLASSICS trial), clopidogrel was associated with a significantly lower rate of major adverse events (4.6 percent vs. 9.1 percent).[120] The first clinical trial of clopidogrel was the Clopidogrel Versus Aspirin in Patients at Risk of Ischemic Events (CAPRIE) trial, a large randomized, blinded trial of clopidogrel versus aspirin in 19,000 patients at risk of ischemic events.[121] Patients were enrolled after recent myocardial infarction (MI) or stroke, or if they had symptomatic peripheral arterial disease. The primary outcome was the occurrence of ischemic stroke, MI, or vascular death. With a mean followup of 1.91 years, there was a relative risk reduction of 8.7 percent in the clopidogrel group (p = 0.043). No major differences were noted in terms of safety. Clopidogrel is also used in acute coronary syndromes, based on studies like the Clopidogrel in Unstable Angina to Prevent Recurrent Events (CURE) study, which showed a significant reduction in the combined end point of cardiovascular death, nonfatal MI, or stroke with clopidogrel and aspirin versus aspirin alone.[122] Several studies have demonstrated the effectiveness of clopidogrel in patients undergoing percutaneous coronary intervention, and a recent meta-analysis of several large studies showed that clopidogrel treatment prior to intervention is associated with decreased incidence of major cardiac events (MI, stroke, urgent revascularization) compared to treatment after intervention.[123] The degree of platelet inhibition after clopidogrel therapy varies. Larger loading doses of clopidogrel appear to reduce variability in response; the safety and efficacy of such doses are being compared in ongoing studies.[124]

Prasugrel is a "third-generation" P2Y12 blocking agent. Unlike clopidogrel it can be converted to its active metabolite via esterases present in either the liver or the gut. Like clopidogrel it irreversibly blocks the P2Y12 receptor.[144] Evidence for the use of prasugrel comes predominately from one large study of prasugrel compared with clopidogrel. This study randomized 13,608 patients with moderate-to-high-risk acute coronary syndromes and who were scheduled to undergo percutaneous coronary intervention to receive prasugrel (a 60-mg loading dose and a 10-mg daily maintenance dose) or clopidogrel (a 300-mg loading dose and a 75-mg daily maintenance dose) for up to 15 months.[125] Although prasugrel significantly reduced death from cardiovascular causes, nonfatal MI, and nonfatal stroke, it significantly increased all forms of bleeding, including major and fatal hemorrhage.

Ticagrelor is a member of the cyclopentyltriazolopyrimidines chemical class, a group of agents that reversibly inhibit the P2Y12 platelet receptor. Ticagrelor does not require hepatic activation and has a more rapid onset of action than clopidogrel. The PLATO trial was a large phase III randomized study comparing ticagrelor and aspirin (180 mg loading dose followed by 90 mg twice daily) to clopidogrel (300 to 600 mg dose followed by 75 mg daily) and aspirin for treatment of acute coronary syndrome.[126] Patients receiving ticagrelor experienced the composite primary end point (death from vascular causes, MI, or stroke) less often than patients receiving clopidogrel (9.8 percent vs. 11.7 percent, hazard ratio [HR] 0.84) without a significant difference in the rates of major bleeding (11.6 percent vs. 11.2 percent).

Cangrelor, the first parenteral ADP receptor blocker, is not currently available for clinical use, but has been tested in three large randomized clinical trials of patients undergoing intracoronary stent implantation procedures. Advantages of this agent include parenteral administration, very rapid onset, and short half-life. The CHAMPION studies (PLATFORM,[127] PCI,[128] and PHOENIX[129]) compared cangrelor to clopidogrel or placebo in patients undergoing coronary interventions. Although only the PHOENIX trial showed a significant reduction (4.7 percent vs. 5.9 percent) in the 48-hour composite end point (death, MI, ischemia-driven revascularization, or stent thrombosis), in a pooled analysis of patient level data from the three CHAMPION trials cangrelor use was associated with a significant reduction in the primary efficacy end point compared to control (3.8 percent vs. 4.7 percent, OR 0.81).[130]

$\alpha_{IIb}\beta_3$ BLOCKERS

Fibrinogen binds specifically and saturably to the surface of activated platelets, and the $\alpha_{IIb}\beta_3$ complex is the fibrinogen receptor. This complex mediates platelet aggregation induced by all physiologic agonists. Fibrinogen binds only to the activated conformation of the receptor $\alpha_{IIb}\beta_3$. Monoclonal antibodies have been developed against $\alpha_{IIb}\beta_3$ complex on resting or activated platelets, which prevent aggregation by blocking ligand binding. *Abciximab*, is the Fab$'_2$ fragment of a chimeric mouse–human antibody. Initial human pharmacodynamic studies were performed in patients with unstable angina and in patients undergoing high-risk coronary angioplasty, and dose-related inhibition of platelet function was found. No spontaneous bleeding was observed, despite prolongation of the template bleeding time. Because of the mouse component of abciximab, it may induce antimouse antibodies, preventing repeated use in patients.

The first large clinical trial of abciximab was the Evaluation of c7E3 for the Prevention of Ischemic Complications (EPIC) trial,[131] published in 1994, in which the drug was used in patients with high-risk coronary angioplasty. Abciximab reduced ischemic events after angioplasty when given together with heparin and aspirin, but it also increased the risk of bleeding. Subsequent studies of patients undergoing percutane-ous coronary intervention, the Evaluation in PTCA to Improve Long-term Outcome with Abciximab GP IIb/IIIa ($\alpha_{IIb}\beta_3$) Blockade (EPILOG) study[132] and EPISTENT trial,[133] demonstrated efficacy in both low-risk and high-risk patients without any increase in major bleeding. Abcix-imab has also been tested in patients with acute ischemic stroke, but resulted in significant increase intracranial hemorrhage without any clinical efficacy so it has not been further pursued for this clinical indication.[134]

Other types of inhibitors of fibrinogen binding to platelets have also been developed. Those in clinical use are eptifibatide, a cyclic heptapeptide based on a rattlesnake venom peptide, and tirofiban, a nonpeptide derivative of tyrosine. Pharmacokinetic and pharmacody-namic studies in animals and humans showed a rapid onset of action, short plasma half-life, and rapid reversibility of action. The pharmaco-dynamics of eptifibatide are substantially altered by anticoagulants that chelate calcium, and pharmacokinetic modeling suggests that optimal dosing is obtained by giving a second bolus 10 minutes after the first bolus. Eptifibatide is not immunogenic.

The first major clinical trial of eptifibatide was the Integrilin to Minimize Platelet Aggregation and Coronary Thrombosis (IMPACT) II trial in patients undergoing any kind of coronary intervention.[135] There was a highly significant reduction in the composite end point of death, MI, coronary artery bypass grafting, repeat urgent or emergent coronary intervention, or stent placement for abrupt closure at 24 hours with both eptifibatide dosing arms. There was no increase in major bleeding. The effect was no longer significant at 30 days on intention-to-treat analysis.

Animal studies with tirofiban were performed in dogs. Dose-dependent inhibition of *ex vivo* platelet aggregation was achieved, with rapid reversibility at the end of the infusion. Electrically induced cor-onary artery thrombosis was markedly reduced by tirofiban infusion, without significant extension of the bleeding time. Pharmacokinetic and pharmacodynamic studies in humans showed that tirofiban provided a well-tolerated reversible means of inhibiting platelet function. Bleed-ing time was prolonged, and ADP-induced aggregation was blocked by at least 80 percent in normal volunteers. The plasma half-life was 1.6 hours. ADP- and collagen-induced platelet aggregation in normal vol-unteers returned to 55 percent and 89 percent of baseline, respectively, by 3 hours after the end of infusion. Similar results were found in a dose-ranging study in patients undergoing coronary angioplasty. Based on these results tirofiban has been extensively studied as an adjunct to therapies for patients with, or at risk of, acute coronary syndromes. Clinical results for patients treated with tirofiban have been reviewed.[136]

THROMBIN RECEPTOR BLOCKERS

Platelet activation occurs through a variety of cell surface receptors including the thrombin receptor, a potent platelet activator mediated by its binding to and cleaving the protease-activated receptor (PAR)-1. Vorapaxar is an irreversible PAR-1 thrombin receptor antagonist, which has been studied in two large phase III randomized studies. In the TRACER study 12,944 patients with non–ST elevation acute cor-onary syndromes were randomized to vorapaxar or placebo plus stan-dard care.[137] Vorapaxar use was associated with a significant reduction in death from cardiovascular causes (14.7 percent vs. 16.4 percent), but was also associated with a significant increase in major bleeding events, including intracranial hemorrhage (1.1 percent vs. 0.2 percent). The TRA 2P-TIMI 50 study randomized 26,449 patients with prior MI, stroke, or peripheral artery disease to vorapaxar versus placebo.[138] This phase III study also demonstrated clinical efficacy with a reduction in death from cardiovascular cause (11.2 percent vs. 12.4 percent), but it was at the expense of increased major bleeding complications. Efforts are underway to identify subgroups that may have the greatest net

benefit from vorapaxar. Atopaxar is a low-molecular-weight inhibitor of PAR-1, which has been studied in phase II trials of patients with acute coronary syndrome or high-risk coronary artery disease.[139] These studies showed an increase in minimal bleeding events (16.4 percent vs. 4.5 percent) but no difference in clinically significant bleeding.

REFERENCES

1. Link KP: The discovery of dicumarol and its sequels. *Circulation* 19(1):97–107, 1959.
2. Ageno W, Gallus AS, Wittkowsky A, et al: Oral anticoagulant therapy: Antithrombotic Therapy and Prevention of Thrombosis, 9th ed: American College of Chest Physicians Evidence-Based Clinical Practice Guidelines. *Chest* 141(2 Suppl):e44S–e88S, 2012.
3. Nelsestuen GL, Zytkovicz TH, Howard JB: The mode of action of vitamin K. Identifi-cation of gamma-carboxyglutamic acid as a component of prothrombin. *J Biol Chem* 249(19):6347–6350, 1974.
4. Stenflo J, Fernlund P, Egan W, Roepstorff P: Vitamin K dependent modifications of glutamic acid residues in prothrombin. *Proc Natl Acad Sci U S A* 71(7):2730–2733, 1974.
5. Whitlon DS, Sadowski JA, Suttie JW: Mechanism of coumarin action: Significance of vitamin K epoxide reductase inhibition. *Biochemistry* 17(8):1371–1377, 1978.
6. Morris DP, Soute BA, Vermeer C, Stafford DW: Characterization of the purified vitamin K-dependent gamma-glutamyl carboxylase. *J Biol Chem* 268(12):8735–8742, 1993.
7. Fasco MJ, Hildebrandt EF, Suttie JW: Evidence that warfarin anticoagulant action involves two distinct reductase activities. *J Biol Chem* 257(19):11210–11212, 1982.
8. Paul B, Oxley A, Brigham K, et al: Factor II, VII, IX and X concentrations in patients receiving long term warfarin. *J Clin Pathol* 40(1):94–98, 1987.
9. Malhotra OP: Dicoumarol-induced prothrombins containing 6, 7, and 8 gamma-carboxyglutamic acid residues: Isolation and characterization. *Biochem Cell Biol* 67(8):411–421, 1989.
10. Ratcliffe JV, Furie B, Furie BC: The importance of specific gamma-carboxyglutamic acid residues in prothrombin. Evaluation by site-specific mutagenesis. *J Biol Chem* 268(32):24339–24345, 1993.
11. Holbrook AM, Pereira JA, Labiris R, et al: Systematic overview of warfarin and its drug and food interactions. *Arch Intern Med* 165(10):1095–1106, 2005.
12. Loebstein R, Dvoskin I, Halkin H, et al: A coding VKORC1 Asp36Tyr polymorphism predisposes to warfarin resistance. *Blood* 109(6):2477–2480, 2007.
13. Harrison L, Johnston M, Massicotte MP, et al: Comparison of 5-mg and 10-mg loading doses in initiation of warfarin therapy. *Ann Intern Med* 126(2):133–136, 1997.
14. Crowther MA, Ginsberg JB, Kearon C, et al: A randomized trial comparing 5-mg and 10-mg warfarin loading doses. *Arch Intern Med* 159(1):46–48, 1999.
15. Kovacs MJ, Rodger M, Anderson DR, et al: Comparison of 10-mg and 5-mg warfa-rin initiation nomograms together with low-molecular-weight heparin for outpatient treatment of acute venous thromboembolism. A randomized, double-blind, controlled trial. *Ann Intern Med* 138(9):714–719, 2003.
16. Loeliger EA, van den Besselaar AM, Lewis SM: Reliability and clinical impact of the normalization of the prothrombin times in oral anticoagulant control. *Thromb Haemost* 53(1):148–154, 1985.
17. Schulman S, Parpia S, Stewart C, et al: Warfarin dose assessment every 4 weeks versus every 12 weeks in patients with stable international normalized ratios: A randomized trial. *Ann Intern Med* 155(10):653–659, W201–W203, 2011.
18. Heneghan C, Alonso-Coello P, Garcia-Alamino JM, et al: Self-monitoring of oral anti-coagulation: A systematic review and meta-analysis. *Lancet* 367(9508):404–411, 2006.
19. Matchar DB, Jacobson A, Dolor R, et al: Effect of home testing of international normal-ized ratio on clinical events. *N Engl J Med* 363(17):1608–1620, 2010.
20. Matchar DB, Samsa GP, Cohen SJ, et al: Improving the quality of anticoagulation of patients with atrial fibrillation in managed care organizations: Results of the managing anticoagulation services trial. *Am J Med* 113(1):42–51, 2002.
21. Wilson SJ, Wells PS, Kovacs MJ, et al: Comparing the quality of oral anticoagulant man-agement by anticoagulation clinics and by family physicians: A randomized controlled trial. *CMAJ* 169(4):293–298, 2003.
22. Kaminsky LS, Zhang ZY: Human P450 metabolism of warfarin. *Pharmacol Ther* 73(1):67–74, 1997.
23. Moridani M, Fu L, Selby R, et al: Frequency of CYP2C9 polymorphisms affecting war-farin metabolism in a large anticoagulant clinic cohort. *Clin Biochem* 39(6):606–612, 2006.
24. Crespi CL, Miller VP: The R144C change in the CYP2C9*2 allele alters interaction of the cytochrome P450 with NADPH:cytochrome P450 oxidoreductase. *Pharmacogenet-ics* 7(3):203–210, 1997.
25. Takanashi K, Tainaka H, Kobayashi K, et al: CYP2C9 Ile359 and Leu359 variants: Enzyme kinetic study with seven substrates. *Pharmacogenetics* 10(2):95–104, 2000.
26. D'Andrea G, D'Ambrosio RL, Di Perna P, et al: A polymorphism in the VKORC1 gene is associated with an interindividual variability in the dose-anticoagulant effect of war-farin. *Blood* 105(2):645–649, 2005.
27. Rieder MJ, Reiner AP, Gage BF, et al: Effect of VKORC1 haplotypes on transcriptional regulation and warfarin dose. *N Engl J Med* 352(22):2285–2293, 2005.
28. Higashi MK, Veenstra DL, Kondo LM, et al: Association between CYP2C9 genetic variants and anticoagulation-related outcomes during warfarin therapy. *JAMA* 287(13):1690–1698, 2002.

29. Sconce EA, Khan TI, Wynne HA, et al: The impact of CYP2C9 and VKORC1 genetic polymorphism and patient characteristics upon warfarin dose requirements: Proposal for a new dosing regimen. *Blood* 106(7):2329–2333, 2005.

30. Schwarz UI, Ritchie MD, Bradford Y, et al: Genetic determinants of response to warfarin during initial anticoagulation. *N Engl J Med* 358(10):999–1008, 2008.

31. Wadelius M, Chen LY, Lindh JD, et al: The largest prospective warfarin-treated cohort supports genetic forecasting. *Blood* 113(4):784–792, 2009.

32. International Warfarin Pharmacogenetics Consortium, Klein TE, Altman RB, et al: Estimation of the warfarin dose with clinical and pharmacogenetic data. *N Engl J Med* 360(8):753–764, 2009.

33. Anderson JL, Horne BD, Stevens SM, et al: Randomized trial of genotype-guided versus standard warfarin dosing in patients initiating oral anticoagulation. *Circulation* 116(22):2563–2570, 2007.

34. Kimmel SE, French B, Kasner SE, et al: A pharmacogenetic versus a clinical algorithm for warfarin dosing. *N Engl J Med* 369(24):2283–2293, 2013.

35. Pirmohamed M, Burnside G, Eriksson N, et al: A randomized trial of genotype-guided dosing of warfarin. *N Engl J Med* 369(24):2294–2303, 2013.

36. Verhoef TI, Ragia G, de Boer A, et al: A randomized trial of genotype-guided dosing of acenocoumarol and phenprocoumon. *N Engl J Med* 369(24):2304–2312, 2013.

37. Schulman S, Kearon C, Kakkar A, et al: Dabigatran versus warfarin in the treatment of acute venous thromboembolism. *N Engl J Med* 361(24):2342–2352, 2009.

38. EINSTEIN Investigators, Bauersachs R, Berkowitz SD, et al: Oral rivaroxaban for symptomatic venous thromboembolism. *N Engl J Med* 363(26):2499–2510, 2010.

39. EINSTEIN–PE Investigators, Büller HR, Prins MH, et al: Oral rivaroxaban for the treatment of symptomatic pulmonary embolism. *N Engl J Med* 366(14):1287–1297, 2012.

40. Pisters R, Lane DA, Nieuwlaat R, et al: A novel user-friendly score (HAS-BLED) to assess 1-year risk of major bleeding in patients with atrial fibrillation: The Euro Heart Survey. *Chest* 138(5):1093–1100, 2010.

41. Egred M, Rodrigues E: Purple digit syndrome and warfarin-induced skin necrosis. *Eur J Intern Med* 16(4):294–295, 2005.

42. Warkentin TE, Sikov WM, Lillicrap DP: Multicentric warfarin-induced skin necrosis complicating heparin-induced thrombocytopenia. *Am J Hematol* 62(1):44–48, 1999.

43. Marik PE, Plante LA: Venous thromboembolic disease and pregnancy. *N Engl J Med* 359(19):2025–2033, 2008.

44. Ito S: Drug therapy for breast-feeding women. *N Engl J Med* 343(2):118–126, 2000.

45. Douketis JD, Spyropoulos AC, Spencer FA, et al: Perioperative management of antithrombotic therapy: Antithrombotic Therapy and Prevention of Thrombosis, 9th ed: American College of Chest Physicians Evidence-Based Clinical Practice Guidelines. *Chest* 141(2 Suppl):e326S–e350S.

46. Sarode R, Milling TJ Jr, Refaai MA, et al: Efficacy and safety of a 4-factor prothrombin complex concentrate in patients on vitamin K antagonists presenting with major bleeding: A randomized, plasma-controlled, phase IIIb study. *Circulation* 2013;128(11):1234–1243, 2012.

47. Baron TH, Kamath PS, McBane RD: Management of antithrombotic therapy in patients undergoing invasive procedures. *N Engl J Med* 368(22):2113–2124, 2013.

48. Tafur AJ, McBane R 2nd, Wysokinski WE, et al: Predictors of major bleeding in peri-procedural anticoagulation management. *J Thromb Haemost* 10(2):261–267, 2012.

49. Birnie DH, Healey JS, Wells GA, et al: Pacemaker or defibrillator surgery without interruption of anticoagulation. *N Engl J Med* 368(22):2084–2093, 2013.

50. Casu B, Oreste P, Torri G, et al: The structure of heparin oligosaccharide fragments with high anti-(factor Xa) activity containing the minimal antithrombin III-binding sequence. Chemical and 13C nuclear-magnetic-resonance studies. *Biochem J* 197(3):599–609, 1981.

51. Damus PS, Hicks M, Rosenberg RD: Anticoagulant action of heparin. *Nature* 246(5432):355–357, 1973.

52. Weitz JI, Hudoba M, Massel D, et al: Clot-bound thrombin is protected from inhibition by heparin-antithrombin III but is susceptible to inactivation by antithrombin III-independent inhibitors. *J Clin Invest* 86(2):385–391, 1990.

53. de Swart CA, Nijmeyer B, Roelofs JM, Sixma JJ: Kinetics of intravenously administered heparin in normal humans. *Blood* 60(6):1251–1258, 1982.

54. Garcia DA, Baglin TP, Weitz JI, et al: Parenteral anticoagulants: Antithrombotic Therapy and Prevention of Thrombosis, 9th ed: American College of Chest Physicians Evidence-Based Clinical Practice Guidelines. *Chest* 141(2 Suppl):e24S–e43S.

55. Cruickshank MK, Levine MN, Hirsh J, et al: A standard heparin nomogram for the management of heparin therapy. *Arch Intern Med* 1991;151(2):333–337, 2012.

56. Levine MN, Hirsh J, Gent M, et al: A randomized trial comparing activated thromboplastin time with heparin assay in patients with acute venous thromboembolism requiring large daily doses of heparin. *Arch Intern Med* 154(1):49–56, 1994.

57. Kearon C, Ginsberg JS, Julian JA, et al: Comparison of fixed-dose weight-adjusted unfractionated heparin and low-molecular-weight heparin for acute treatment of venous thromboembolism. *JAMA* 296(8):935–942, 2006.

58. Cuker A, Gimotty PA, Crowther MA, Warkentin TE: Predictive value of the 4Ts scoring system for heparin-induced thrombocytopenia: A systematic review and meta-analysis. *Blood* 120(20):4160–4167, 2012.

59. Weitz JI: Low-molecular-weight heparins. *N Engl J Med* 337(10):688–698, 1997.

60. Lim W, Dentali F, Eikelboom JW, Crowther MA: Meta-analysis: Low-molecular-weight heparin and bleeding in patients with severe renal insufficiency. *Ann Intern Med* 144(9):673–684, 2006.

61. Van Ryn-McKenna J, Cai L, Ofosu FA, et al: Neutralization of enoxaparine-induced bleeding by protamine sulfate. *Thromb Haemost* 63(2):271–274, 1990.

62. Linkins LA, Dans AL, Moores LK, et al: Treatment and prevention of heparin-induced thrombocytopenia: Antithrombotic Therapy and Prevention of Thrombosis, 9th ed: American College of Chest Physicians Evidence-Based Clinical Practice Guidelines. *Chest* 141(2 Suppl):e495S–e530S.

63. Rajgopal R, Bear M, Butcher MK, Shaughnessy SG: The effects of heparin and low molecular weight heparins on bone. *Thromb Res* 2008;122(3):293–298, 2012.

64. van Den Belt AG, Prins MH, Lensing AW, et al: Fixed dose subcutaneous low molecular weight heparins versus adjusted dose unfractionated heparin for venous thromboembolism. *Cochrane Database Syst Rev* (2):CD001100, 2000.

65. Donat F, Duret JP, Santoni A, et al: The pharmacokinetics of fondaparinux sodium in healthy volunteers. *Clin Pharmacokinet* 41(Suppl 2):1–9, 2002.

66. Parody R, Oliver A, Souto JC, Fontcuberta J: Fondaparinux (ARIXTRA) as an alternative anti-thrombotic prophylaxis when there is hypersensitivity to low molecular weight and unfractionated heparins. *Haematologica* 88(11):ECR32, 2003.

67. Maraganore JM, Bourdon P, Jablonski J, et al: Design and characterization of hirulogs: A novel class of bivalent peptide inhibitors of thrombin. *Biochemistry* 1990;29(30):7095–7101, 2003.

68. Warkentin TE, Greinacher A, Koster A: Bivalirudin. *Thromb Haemost* 99(5):830–839, 2008.

69. Berry CN, Girardot C, Lecoffre C, Lunven C: Effects of the synthetic thrombin inhibitor argatroban on fibrin- or clot-incorporated thrombin: Comparison with heparin and recombinant Hirudin. *Thromb Haemost* 72(3):381–386, 1994.

70. Swan SK, Hursting MJ: The pharmacokinetics and pharmacodynamics of argatroban: Effects of age, gender, and hepatic or renal dysfunction. *Pharmacotherapy* 20(3):318–329, 2000.

71. Cardot JM, Lefevre GY, Godbillon JA: Pharmacokinetics of rec-hirudin in healthy volunteers after intravenous administration. *J Pharmacokinet Biopharm* 22(2):147–156, 1994.

72. Tripodi A, Chantarangkul V, Arbini AA, et al: Effects of hirudin on activated partial thromboplastin time determined with ten different reagents. *Thromb Haemost* 70(2):286–288, 1993.

73. Blech S, Ebner T, Ludwig-Schwellinger E, et al: The metabolism and disposition of the oral direct thrombin inhibitor, dabigatran, in humans. *Drug Metab Dispos* 36(2):386–399, 2008.

74. Hawes EM, Deal AM, Funk-Adcock D, et al: Performance of coagulation tests in patients on therapeutic doses of dabigatran: A cross-sectional pharmacodynamic study based on peak and trough plasma levels. *J Thromb Haemost* 11(8):1493–1502, 2013.

75. Schiele F, van Ryn J, Canada K, et al: A specific antidote for dabigatran: Functional and structural characterization. *Blood* 121(18):3554–3562, 2013.

76. Esnault P, Gaillard PE, Cotte J, et al: Haemodialysis before emergency surgery in a patient treated with dabigatran. *Br J Anaesth* 111(5):776–777, 2013.

77. van Ryn J, Schurer J, Kink-Eiband M, Clemens A: Reversal of dabigatran-induced bleeding by coagulation factor concentrates in a rat-tail bleeding model and lack of effect on assays of coagulation. *Anesthesiology* 120(6):1429–1440, 2014.

78. Connolly SJ, Ezekowitz MD, Yusuf S, et al: Dabigatran versus warfarin in patients with atrial fibrillation. *N Engl J Med* 361(12):1139–1151, 2009.

79. Friedman RJ, Dahl OE, Rosencher N, et al: Dabigatran versus enoxaparin for prevention of venous thromboembolism after hip or knee arthroplasty: A pooled analysis of three trials. *Thromb Res* 126(3):175–182, 2010.

80. Eikelboom JW, Connolly SJ, Brueckmann M, et al: Dabigatran versus warfarin in patients with mechanical heart valves. *N Engl J Med* 369(13):1206–1214, 2013.

81. Hillarp A, Baghaei F, Fagerberg Blixter I, et al: Effects of the oral, direct factor Xa inhibitor rivaroxaban on commonly used coagulation assays. *J Thromb Haemost* 9(1):133–139, 2011.

82. Francart SJ, Hawes EM, Deal AM, et al: Performance of coagulation tests in patients on therapeutic doses of rivaroxaban. A cross-sectional pharmacodynamic study based on peak and trough plasma levels. *Thromb Haemost* 111(6):1133–1140, 2014.

83. Patel MR, Mahaffey KW, Garg J, et al: Rivaroxaban versus warfarin in nonvalvular atrial fibrillation. *N Engl J Med* 365(10):883–891, 2011.

84. Eriksson BI, Borris LC, Friedman RJ, et al: Rivaroxaban versus enoxaparin for thromboprophylaxis after hip arthroplasty. *N Engl J Med* 358(26):2765–2775, 2008.

85. Lassen MR, Ageno W, Borris LC, et al: Rivaroxaban versus enoxaparin for thromboprophylaxis after total knee arthroplasty. *N Engl J Med* 358(26):2776–2786, 2008.

86. Cohen AT, Spiro TE, Spyropoulos AC, et al: Rivaroxaban for thromboprophylaxis in acutely ill medical patients. *N Engl J Med* 368(20):1945–1946, 2013.

87. Prins MH, Lensing AW, Bauersachs R, et al: Oral rivaroxaban versus standard therapy for the treatment of symptomatic venous thromboembolism: A pooled analysis of the EINSTEIN-DVT and PE randomized studies. *Thromb J* 11(1):21, 2013.

88. Wasserlauf G, Grandi SM, Filion KB, Eisenberg MJ: Meta-analysis of rivaroxaban and bleeding risk. *Am J Cardiol* 112(3):454–460, 2013.

89. Levi M, Moore KT, Castillejos CF, et al: Comparison of three-factor and four-factor prothrombin complex concentrates regarding reversal of the anticoagulant effects of rivaroxaban in healthy volunteers. *J Thromb Haemost* 12(9):1428–1436, 2014.

90. Perzborn E, Gruber A, Tinel H, et al: Reversal of rivaroxaban anticoagulation by haemostatic agents in rats and primates. *Thromb Haemost* 110(1):162–172, 2013.

91. Hillarp A, Gustafsson KM, Faxälv L, et al: Effects of the oral, direct factor Xa inhibitor apixaban on routine coagulation assays and anti-FXa assays. *J Thromb Haemost* 12(9):1545–1553, 2014.

92. Martin AC, Le Bonniec B, Fischer AM, et al: Evaluation of recombinant activated factor VII, prothrombin complex concentrate, and fibrinogen concentrate to reverse apixaban in a rabbit model of bleeding and thrombosis. *Int J Cardiol* 168(4):4228–4233, 2013.

93. Granger CB, Alexander JH, McMurray JJ, et al: Apixaban versus warfarin in patients with atrial fibrillation. *N Engl J Med* 365(11):981–992, 2011.

94. Connolly SJ, Eikelboom J, Joyner C, et al: Apixaban in patients with atrial fibrillation. *N Engl J Med* 364(9):806–817, 2011.

95. Agnelli G, Buller HR, Cohen A, et al: Oral apixaban for the treatment of acute venous thromboembolism. *N Engl J Med* 369(9):799–808, 2013.

96. Agnelli G, Buller HR, Cohen A, et al: Apixaban for extended treatment of venous thromboembolism. *N Engl J Med* 368(8):699–708, 2013.

97. Lassen MR, Gallus A, Raskob GE, et al: Apixaban versus enoxaparin for thromboprophylaxis after hip replacement. *N Engl J Med* 363(26):2487–2498, 2010.

98. Lassen MR, Raskob GE, Gallus A, et al: Apixaban or enoxaparin for thromboprophylaxis after knee replacement. *N Engl J Med* 361(6):594–604, 2009.

99. Lassen MR, Raskob GE, Gallus A, et al: Apixaban versus enoxaparin for thromboprophylaxis after knee replacement (ADVANCE-2): A randomised double-blind trial. *Lancet* 375(9717):807–815, 2010.

100. Ogata K, Mendell-Harary J, Tachibana M, et al: Clinical safety, tolerability, pharmacokinetics, and pharmacodynamics of the novel factor Xa inhibitor edoxaban in healthy volunteers. *J Clin Pharmacol* 50(7):743–753, 2010.

101. Giugliano RP, Ruff CT, Braunwald E, et al: Edoxaban versus warfarin in patients with atrial fibrillation. *N Engl J Med* 369(22):2093–2104, 2013.

102. Hokusai-VTE Investigators, Büller HR, Décousus H, et al: Edoxaban versus warfarin for the treatment of symptomatic venous thromboembolism. *N Engl J Med* 369(15):1406–1415, 2013.

103. Hilleman DE, Dunlay RW, Packard KA: Reteplase for dysfunctional hemodialysis catheter clearance. *Pharmacotherapy* 23(2):137–141, 2003.

104. Van de Werf FJ, Topol EJ, Sobel BE: The impact of fibrinolytic therapy for ST-segment-elevation acute myocardial infarction. *J Thromb Haemost* 7(1):14–20, 2009.

105. Effectiveness of intravenous thrombolytic treatment in acute myocardial infarction. Gruppo Italiano per lo Studio della Streptochinasi nell'Infarto Miocardico (GISSI). *Lancet* 1(8478):397–402, 1986.

106. Enden T, Haig Y, Kløw NE, et al: Long-term outcome after additional catheter-directed thrombolysis versus standard treatment for acute iliofemoral deep vein thrombosis (the CaVenT study): A randomised controlled trial. *Lancet* 379(9810):31–38, 2012.

107. You JJ, Singer DE, Howard PA, et al: Antithrombotic therapy for atrial fibrillation: Antithrombotic Therapy and Prevention of Thrombosis, 9th ed: American College of Chest Physicians Evidence-Based Clinical Practice Guidelines. *Chest* 141(2 Suppl):e531S–e575S, 2012.

108. Brighton TA, Eikelboom JW, Mann K, et al: Low-dose aspirin for preventing recurrent venous thromboembolism. *N Engl J Med* 367(21):1979–1987, 2012.

109. Becattini C, Agnelli G, Schenone A, et al: Aspirin for preventing the recurrence of venous thromboembolism. *N Engl J Med* 366(21):1959–1967, 2012.

110. Jessup M, Antman E: Reducing the risk of heart attack and stroke: The American Heart Association/American College of Cardiology prevention guidelines. *Circulation* 130(6):e48–e50, 2014.

111. Kernan WN, Ovbiagele B, Black HR, et al: Guidelines for the prevention of stroke in patients with stroke and transient ischemic attack: A guideline for healthcare professionals from the American Heart Association/American Stroke Association. *Stroke* 45(7):2160–2236, 2014.

112. Sacco RL, Diener HC, Yusuf S, et al: Aspirin and extended-release dipyridamole versus clopidogrel for recurrent stroke. *N Engl J Med* 359(12):1238–1251, 2008.

113. Li X, Zhou G, Zhou X, Zhou S: The efficacy and safety of aspirin plus dipyridamole versus aspirin in secondary prevention following TIA or stroke: A meta-analysis of randomized controlled trials. *J Neurol Sci* 332(1–2):92–96, 2013.

114. Huang Y, Cheng Y, Wu J, et al: Cilostazol as an alternative to aspirin after ischaemic stroke: A randomised, double-blind, pilot study. *Lancet Neurol* 7(6):494–499, 2008.

115. Shinohara Y, Katayama Y, Uchiyama S, et al: Cilostazol for prevention of secondary stroke (CSPS 2): An aspirin-controlled, double-blind, randomised non-inferiority trial. *Lancet Neurol* 9(10):959–968, 2010.

116. Thompson PD, Zimet R, Forbes WP, Zhang P: Meta-analysis of results from eight randomized, placebo-controlled trials on the effect of cilostazol on patients with intermittent claudication. *Am J Cardiol* 90(12):1314–1319, 2002.

117. Jull A, Arroll B, Parag V, Waters J: Pentoxifylline for treating venous leg ulcers. *Cochrane Database Syst Rev* (3):CD001733, 2007.

118. Gent M, Blakely JA, Easton JD, et al: The Canadian American Ticlopidine Study (CATS) in thromboembolic stroke. *Lancet* 1(8649):1215–1220, 1989.

119. Cosmi B, Rubboli A, Castelvetri C, Milandri M: Ticlopidine versus oral anticoagulation for coronary stenting. *Cochrane Database Syst Rev* (4):CD002133, 2001.

120. Bertrand ME, Rupprecht HJ, Urban P, et al: Double-blind study of the safety of clopidogrel with and without a loading dose in combination with aspirin compared with ticlopidine in combination with aspirin after coronary stenting: The clopidogrel aspirin stent international cooperative study (CLASSICS). *Circulation* 102(6):624–629, 2000.

121. CAPRIE Steering Committee: A randomised, blinded, trial of clopidogrel versus aspirin in patients at risk of ischaemic events (CAPRIE). CAPRIE Steering Committee. *Lancet* 348(9038):1329–1339, 1996.

122. Yusuf S, Zhao F, Mehta SR, et al: Effects of clopidogrel in addition to aspirin in patients with acute coronary syndromes without ST-segment elevation. *N Engl J Med* 345(7):494–502, 2001.

123. Bellemain-Appaix A, O'Connor SA, Silvain J, et al: Association of clopidogrel pretreatment with mortality, cardiovascular events, and major bleeding among patients undergoing percutaneous coronary intervention: A systematic review and meta-analysis. *JAMA* 308(23):2507–2516, 2012.

124. Sabatine MS: Novel antiplatelet strategies in acute coronary syndromes. *Cleve Clin J Med* 76(Suppl 1):S8–S15, 2009.

125. Wiviott SD, Braunwald E, McCabe CH, et al: Prasugrel versus clopidogrel in patients with acute coronary syndromes. *N Engl J Med* 357(20):2001–2015, 2007.

126. Wallentin L, Becker RC, Budaj A, et al: Ticagrelor versus clopidogrel in patients with acute coronary syndromes. *N Engl J Med* 361(11):1045–1057, 2009.

127. Bhatt DL, Lincoff AM, Gibson CM, et al: Intravenous platelet blockade with cangrelor during PCI. *N Engl J Med* 361(24):2330–2341, 2009.

128. Harrington RA, Stone GW, McNulty S, et al: Platelet inhibition with cangrelor in patients undergoing PCI. *N Engl J Med* 361(24):2318–2329, 2009.

129. Bhatt DL, Stone GW, Mahaffey KW, et al: Effect of platelet inhibition with cangrelor during PCI on ischemic events. *N Engl J Med* 368(14):1303–1313, 2013.

130. Steg PG, Bhatt DL, Hamm CW, et al: Effect of cangrelor on periprocedural outcomes in percutaneous coronary interventions: A pooled analysis of patient-level data. *Lancet* 382(9909):1981–1992, 2013.

131. Use of a monoclonal antibody directed against the platelet glycoprotein IIb/IIIa receptor in high-risk coronary angioplasty. The EPIC Investigation. *N Engl J Med* 330(14):956–961, 1994.

132. EPILOG Investigators: Platelet glycoprotein IIb/IIIa receptor blockade and low-dose heparin during percutaneous coronary revascularization. *N Engl J Med* 336(24):1689–1696, 1997.

133. EPISTENT Investigators: Randomised placebo-controlled and balloon-angioplasty-controlled trial to assess safety of coronary stenting with use of platelet glycoprotein-IIb/IIIa blockade. *Lancet* 352(9122):87–92, 1998.

134. Adams HP Jr, Effron MB, Torner J, et al: Emergency administration of abciximab for treatment of patients with acute ischemic stroke: Results of an international phase III trial: Abciximab in Emergency Treatment of Stroke Trial (AbESTT-II). *Stroke* 39(1):87–99, 2008.

135. Randomised placebo-controlled trial of effect of eptifibatide on complications of percutaneous coronary intervention: IMPACT-II. Integrilin to Minimise Platelet Aggregation and Coronary Thrombosis-II. *Lancet* 349(9063):1422–1428, 1997.

136. Valgimigli M, Biondi-Zoccai G, Tebaldi M, et al: Tirofiban as adjunctive therapy for acute coronary syndromes and percutaneous coronary intervention: A meta-analysis of randomized trials. *Eur Heart J* 31(1):35–49, 2010.

137. Tricoci P, Huang Z, Held C, et al: Thrombin-receptor antagonist vorapaxar in acute coronary syndromes. *N Engl J Med* 366(1):20–33, 2012.

138. Morrow DA, Braunwald E, Bonaca MP, et al: Vorapaxar in the secondary prevention of atherothrombotic events. *N Engl J Med* 366(15):1404–1413, 2012.

139. Goto S, Ogawa H, Takeuchi M, et al: Double-blind, placebo-controlled Phase II studies of the protease-activated receptor 1 antagonist E5555 (atopaxar) in Japanese patients with acute coronary syndrome or high-risk coronary artery disease. *Eur Heart J* 31(21):2601–2613, 2010.

140. Eriksson BI, Dahl OE, Rosencher N, et al: Dabigatran etexilate versus enoxaparin for prevention of venous thromboembolism after total hip replacement: A randomised, double-blind, non-inferiority trial. *Lancet* 370(9591):949–956, 2007.

141. Eriksson BI, Dahl OE, Huo MH, et al: Oral dabigatran versus enoxaparin for thromboprophylaxis after primary total hip arthroplasty (RE-NOVATE II*). A randomised, double-blind, non-inferiority trial. *Thromb Haemost* 105(4):721–729, 2011.

142. Eriksson BI, Dahl OE, Rosencher N, et al: Oral dabigatran etexilate vs. subcutaneous enoxaparin for the prevention of venous thromboembolism after total knee replacement: The RE-MODEL randomized trial. *J Thromb Haemost* 5(11):2178–2185, 2007.

143. Mega JL, Braunwald E, Wiviott SD, et al: Rivaroxaban in patients with a recent acute coronary syndrome. *N Engl J Med* 366(1):9–19, 2012.

144. Kakkar AK, Brenner B, Dahl OE, et al: Extended duration rivaroxaban versus short-term enoxaparin for the prevention of venous thromboembolism after total hip arthroplasty: A double-blind, randomised controlled trial. *Lancet* 372(9632):31–39, 2008.

145. Alexander JH, Lopes RD, James S, et al: Apixaban with antiplatelet therapy after acute coronary syndrome. *N Engl J Med* 365(8):699–708, 2011.

146. Goldhaber SZ, Leizorovicz A, Kakkar AK, et al: Apixaban versus enoxaparin for thromboprophylaxis in medically ill patients. *N Engl J Med* 365(23):2167–2177, 2011.

CHAPTER 26
IMMUNE CELL THERAPY

Carolina Berger and Stanley R. Riddell

SUMMARY

T cells represent an important component of the host response to pathogens and tumors. Adoptive T-cell therapy, in which T cells are isolated or engineered to be specific for molecules expressed on diseased cells and administered to patients, has shown efficacy in infections and malignancy. Clinical applications of T-cell therapy have been facilitated by identification of target antigens expressed by viruses and tumors, improvement in strategies for the isolation and genetic engineering of antigen-specific T cells with intrinsic qualities that enable their persistence *in vivo*, and recognition that transferring T cells into a lymphopenic environment improves the efficiency of cell transfer and treatment efficacy. Insights into the obstacles to routinely achieving an effective antitumor response either by T-cell therapy or vaccination have been derived from careful analysis of clinical trials, and further development of immune cell therapy combined with interventions that target specific regulatory or inhibitory pathways that are present in tumor microenvironments and impede effective immunity represent promising areas for future applications.

Acronyms and Abbreviations: ALL, acute lymphatic leukemia; BCMA, B-cell maturation antigen; CAR, chimeric antigen receptor; cDNA, complementary DNA; CDR3, complementarity determining region 3; CEA, carcinoembryonic antigen; CLL, chronic lymphatic leukemia; CMV, cytomegalovirus; CRS, cytokine release syndrome; CTL, cytotoxic T lymphocyte; DLI, donor lymphocyte infusion; E, early viral protein; EBV, Epstein-Barr virus; EGFR, epidermal growth factor receptor; ERBB2IP, erbb2 interacting protein; GD2, disialoganglioside; GVHD, graft-versus-host disease; GVL, graft-versus-leukemia; HHV-6, human herpes virus-6; HLA, human leukocyte antigen; HSCT, hematopoietic stem cell transplantation; HSV, herpes simplex virus; HSV-TK, herpes simplex virus thymidine kinase; iCasp9, inducible caspase-9; IE, immediate early viral protein; IFN-γ, interferon-γ; IL, interleukin; L1CAM, L1-cell adhesion molecule; LCL, lymphoblastoid cell line; LPD, lymphoproliferative disease; mAbs, monoclonal antibodies; mHAgs, minor histocompatibility antigens; MHC, major histocompatibility complex; PBMC, peripheral blood mononuclear cell; PD-1 receptor, programmed death-1 receptor; PML-RARa, promyelocytic leukemia–retinoic acid receptor a protein; scFV, single-chain variable fragment; SNP, single nucleotide polymorphism; T_{CM}, central memory T cell; TCR, T-cell receptor; T_E, effector T cell; T_{EM}, effector memory T cell; Th, T helper; TIL, tumor-infiltrating lymphocyte; T_{REG}, regulatory T cell; T_{SCM}, T memory stem cell; WT-1, Wilms tumor antigen-1.

● ADOPTIVE CELLULAR THERAPY OF VIRAL DISEASES

Two broad subsets of antigen-specific T cells cooperate to terminate acute viral infections and control reactivation of latent viruses. CD8+ cytotoxic T lymphocytes (CTLs) recognize viral peptides presented by major histocompatibility complex (MHC) class I molecules and lyse infected cells, and produce inflammatory cytokines. CD4+ T-helper (Th) cells recognize viral peptides presented by class II MHC molecules and produce cytokines that amplify T-cell responses and promote B-cell proliferation and antibody production. A deficiency of CD8+ and CD4+ Th cells occurs after allogeneic hematopoietic stem cell transplantation (HSCT) as a consequence of the administration of intensive chemoradiotherapy, anti–T-cell monoclonal antibodies (mAbs), and/or immunosuppressive drugs, and these patients are at risk for life-threatening viral infections.[1-5] Clinical trials have shown that adoptive T-cell therapy has antiviral activity against cytomegalovirus (CMV), Epstein-Barr virus (EBV), and adenovirus infection in immunocompromised allogeneic HSCT recipients.[6,7]

T-CELL THERAPY OF CYTOMEGALOVIRUS INFECTION

The first application of adoptive T-cell therapy with antigen-specific T cells in humans was to treat CMV infection after allogeneic HSCT. CMV is a DNA virus that infects hematopoietic progenitors, monocytes, and endothelial cells.[8] To evade complete elimination by host immunity, CMV encodes proteins that interfere with antigen presentation in cells that contain replicating virus, and establishes latency.[9] Normal CMV+ individuals maintain high levels of CD8+ and CD4+ T cells that are specific for CMV antigens, and these responses are essential to control infection.[10-12] CMV frequently reactivates in individuals with a T-cell immunodeficiency, such as after allogeneic HSCT and solid-organ transplantation, and contributes to morbidity and mortality. Lymphocytopenia and a deficiency of functional CMV-specific T cells persist for several months in many HSCT recipients, including cord blood transplant recipients, and CMV reactivation is frequent.[13-15] Antiviral drugs are used to suppress CMV,[16-18] but often provide only temporary control of reactivation, and restoration of immune function is essential to contain CMV infection.[13,19-21]

Target Antigens for Cytomegalovirus-Specific T Cells

Studies of the specificity of CMV-specific T cells isolated from immunocompetent CMV seropositive individuals identified antigens to target in T-cell therapy.[15,21] A majority of CD8+ CTLs elicited by *in vitro* stimulation with autologous CMV-infected cells recognize virion proteins, including the pp65 and pp150 matrix proteins that are introduced into the cytoplasm of cells immediately following viral entry and processed and presented for T-cell recognition. Although virion proteins are important targets for CD8+ T cells, stimulation of peripheral blood mononuclear cells (PBMCs) from normal CMV+ donors with panels of CMV peptides, or with cells infected with a CMV strain in which the immune evasion genes had been deleted, identified significant CD8+ T-cell responses to intermediate-early (IE) or early (E) viral proteins.[10,11] IE and E are not efficiently presented to T cells *in vitro* by cells replicating wild-type CMV, but evidence from animal models suggests that IE-specific T cells recognize cells that are reactivating CMV from latency.[22] Thus, reconstitution of responses both to virion and IE or E antigens may be necessary to restore control of both the latent and replicating pools of virus in immune-deficient hosts.[23]

CD4+ Th cells are required for optimal CD8+ CTL responses and may eliminate CMV-infected cells that express class II MHC *in vivo*. Studies using recombinant CMV proteins or peptide panels have identified CD4+ T-cell responses to pp65, IE-1, glycoprotein B, and the major capsid protein (UL86) in normal CMV+ individuals.[10,24,25]

Techniques for Adoptive Transfer and Tracking of Cytomegalovirus-Specific T Cells

The application of T-cell therapy for CMV in allogeneic HSCT recipients required the development of approaches to reliably isolate CMV-specific T cells from the stem cell donor, and to remove potentially alloreactive T cells that could cause graft-versus-host disease (GVHD). The first clinical trial of T-cell therapy employed CD8+ CMV-specific T-cell clones that were isolated and expanded by *in vitro* culture of donor lymphocytes with autologous CMV-infected fibroblasts.[26] The donor-derived T-cell clones were screened to exclude alloreactivity with noninfected recipient cells prior to adoptive transfer, to minimize the risk of causing serious GVHD. In a phase I study, 14 allogeneic HSCT recipients received four escalating weekly intravenous doses (3.3×10^7 to 1×10^9/m^2) of CD8+ CMV-specific CTL clones as prophylaxis for CMV disease. The treatment did not cause toxicity or exacerbate GVHD, CMV-specific cytolytic activity was increased after therapy to levels equivalent to those in the donor, and transferred CTLs persisted for more than 12 weeks.[27] None of the 14 patients developed CMV viremia or disease, which in the absence of antiviral drug therapy was expected to occur in approximately 50 percent or 40 percent of these patients, respectively.[27]

The results of the initial trials with CMV-specific T-cell clones suggested this approach can provide an alternative to antiviral drugs for controlling CMV infection after HSCT. However, the isolation and propagation of antigen-specific T-cell clones requires specific expertise and is time-consuming. Culture methods for enrichment of polyclonal CMV-specific T cells circumvent prolonged *ex vivo* manipulation and T-cell expansion and enabled broader application of this approach (Fig. 26–1).[28,29] Clinical trials with polyclonal CD4+ and/or CD8+ T-cell lines generated by short-term culture confirmed the efficacy of adoptive therapy for CMV and suggested that low cell doses (as low as 10^5/kg) of polyclonal T cells can be therapeutically effective.[28,30–32]

A key requirement for T-cell therapy for rapidly progressing and/or life-threatening CMV infections is to further reduce the time needed to generate the CMV-specific T cells for adoptive transfer and to improve the feasibility of this approach (see Fig. 26–1). Techniques have been developed for rapidly isolating antigen-specific T cells directly from the blood using conventional human leukocyte antigen (HLA) multimers or reversible streptamers that are comprised of soluble HLA molecules folded with the viral cognate peptide and bind T cells based on T-cell receptor (TCR) specificity.[33–36] Alternatively, mAbs and immunomagnetic bead-selection strategies have been developed to capture T cells that produce interferon (IFN)-γ or have upregulated activation markers in response to antigen stimulation.[37–39] A pilot study in 18 patients showed that CMV-specific T cells (mean cell dose 2.1×10^4/kg) isolated by IFN-γ capture techniques and transferred after brief *ex vivo* culture had a clinical effect.[40] CMV-specific T cells were also purified from the blood of HSCT donors using HLA-peptide tetramers or reversible streptamers, transferred directly to the patients at low cell doses, and mediated antiviral activity.[35,36]

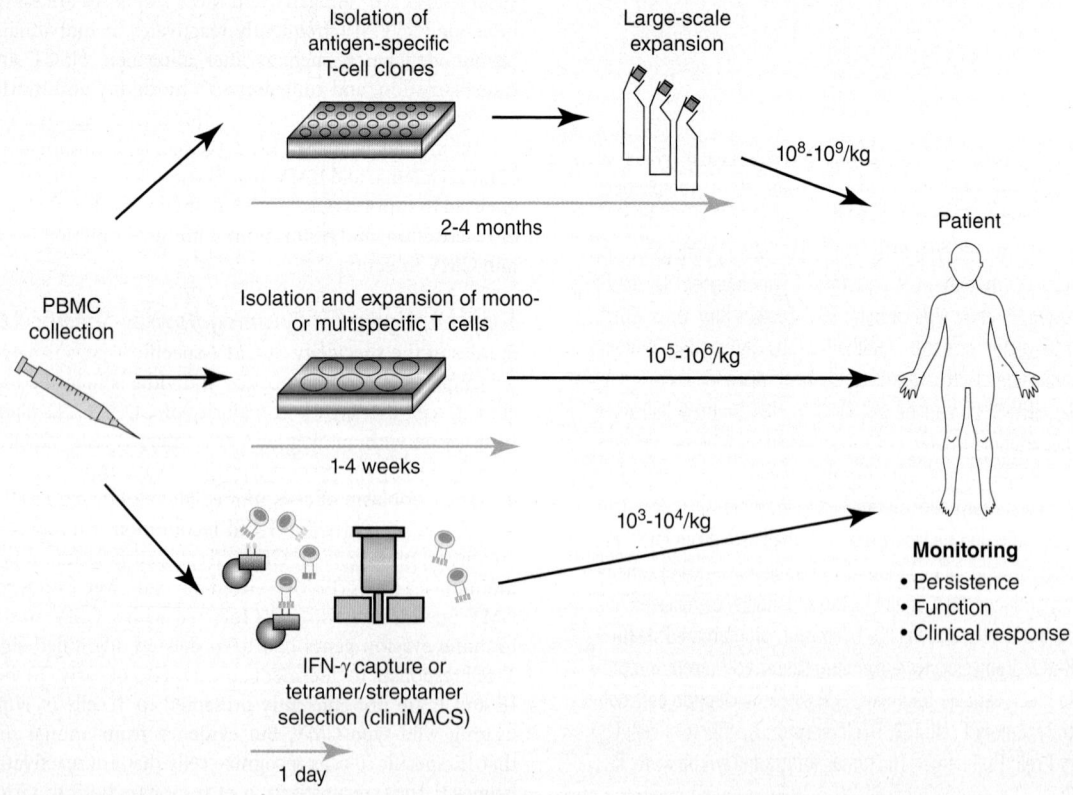

Figure 26–1. Scheme for adoptive T-cell therapy with antigen-specific T cells. Antigen-specific T cells can be isolated by *in vitro* culture, expanded in long- or short-term culture, and then transferred in large numbers to patients. Alternatively, antigen-specific T cells can be isolated using direct methods and transferred immediately to the patient at low numbers. Patients are monitored after each cell infusion for toxicity, T-cell persistence, and efficacy.

Transferred T cells must persist as functional memory T cells and migrate to sites of virus replication to be effective. Therefore, it was essential to verify the presence of the transferred T cells in the blood based on functional or structural properties. In the initial studies of adoptive therapy with CD8+ CMV-specific T-cell clones, assays of cytolytic activity provided an indirect semiquantitative functional measure for the presence of the transferred immune effectors.[27] New approaches that use flow cytometric analysis of blood samples have been developed, such as staining with HLA multimers or intracellular staining, to detect cytokines produced after antigen stimulation. These techniques are being employed to enumerate and analyze the function of cells on a single-cell level.[11,34] The unique DNA sequences of the rearranged TCR Vα or Vβ genes have also been used to evaluate survival of transferred T cells in the first trial of CMV-specific T-cell therapy.[27] Quantitative real-time polymerase chain reaction with TCR-specific primers that flank the unique complementarity determining region 3 (CDR3) sequence can provide precise quantitation of transferred T cells in blood samples. Advances in high-throughput sequencing and computational analysis of the TCR sequences have now enabled much more sensitive analysis and sequencing of the CDR3 and detection of unique sequences in transferred T cells.[36,41,42]

Selection of Defined Subsets of Cytomegalovirus-Specific T cells for Adoptive Therapy

The pool of memory T cells contains both CD45RO+CD62L+ central memory (T_{CM}), and CD62L– effector memory (T_{EM}) subsets that differ in phenotype, function, and migration.[43–45] Studies in animal models have revealed profound differences in the ability of adoptively transferred T cells from distinct subsets to persist *in vivo* and revert to the memory pool. The transfer of effector cells derived from CD8+CD62L+ T_{CM} or a rare subset of CD62L+ cells termed *memory stem cells* (T_{SCM}) that share cell-surface markers of both naïve T cell (T_N) and T_{CM} cells, displayed superior survival *in vivo*, and/or mediated superior antitumor activity compared with more differentiated T_{EM}.[46–49] Studies in mice provide increasing evidence for a progressive differentiation model of T-cell subsets. Fate mapping studies and single-cell transfer experiments show that naïve T cells differentiate into memory and effector subsets (Fig. 26–2), and demonstrated that the stem cell–like properties of self-renewal and differentiation are present in CD62L+ T_{CM} cells.[50–52] It is uncertain whether the intermediate phenotype T_{SCM} has self-renewal capability or represents a cell that is of sufficient frequency to be reliably isolated for immunotherapy. Nevertheless, these findings suggest that selecting less differentiated memory subsets as a starting population for clinical adoptive T-cell therapy can allow very low numbers of T cells to be effective, and this concept has been validated in animal models and patients with CMV infection.[53] Given the considerable potential of this approach, methods are now being developed for clinically applicable serial selection strategies for human T_{CM} subsets.[54]

T-CELL THERAPY OF EPSTEIN-BARR VIRUS INFECTION

EBV is a ubiquitous γ-herpesvirus (Chap. 82) that persists in immunocompetent hosts lifelong without causing disease. Some latently infected B cells express only the EBNA-1 protein, which has glycine-alanine repeats that inhibit its translation and processing for presentation to CD8+ T cells.[55] Infected B cells may activate the latency III program of viral genes that includes EBNA-1, EBNA-2, EBNA-3A, EBNA-3B, EBNA-3C, LMP-1, LMP-2A, and LMP-2B, and induces cell proliferation.[56] In normal hosts, both the CD8+ CTL and CD4+ Th cell response to EBV infection is mainly directed against lytic viral proteins and the EBNA-3A, -3B, and -3C latency proteins.[57,58] The CD4+ Th cell response may also contribute to eliminating class II MHC+ EBV-infected cells *in vivo*[58] and EBV-specific CD8+ and CD4+ T cells cooperate to prevent the outgrowth of EBV+ B cells in immunocompetent hosts.[59,60] Thus, tumors comprised of proliferating EBV+ B cells can arise in individuals with a T-cell deficiency, such as solid-organ or HSCT patients receiving intense immunosuppression, especially if T-cell depletion is used as part of the conditioning regimen.[61,62] Historically, patients with EBV-induced lymphoproliferative disease (EBV-LPD) had a grave prognosis, responding poorly to antiviral drugs or chemotherapy, although early detection of EBV reactivation and treatment with mAbs specific for CD20 have improved outcomes.[63] Ultimately, restoration of EBV-specific T cells is necessary for control of the virus.

Techniques for Isolation and Adoptive Transfer of Epstein-Barr Virus–Specific T Cells

The efficacy of T-cell therapy for EBV-LPD was first demonstrated in a study in which a low dose of unselected donor lymphocytes was administered to five patients with EBV-LPD after T-cell–depleted allogeneic HSCT. Complete resolution of EBV-LPD was achieved in all patients,[64] but this was complicated by GVHD and two patients developed a fatal respiratory failure, demonstrating the importance of selecting EBV-specific T cells for therapy.[64] The adoptive transfer of donor EBV-specific T-cell lines derived by *in vitro* culture with EBV-transformed lymphoblastoid cell lines (LCLs) was effective in 2 of 3 HSCT recipients with established EBV-LPD without causing GVHD.[65] One patient had progressive LPD with a mutation in the EBNA-3B gene that eliminated the region encoding the epitopes targeted by the CTL line.[66] To diminish the probability of escape variants, subsequent studies administered donor EBV-specific T-cell lines prophylactically to a cohort of patients at risk for EBV-LPD after T-cell–depleted allogeneic HSCT.[67] No GVHD was observed, and there were no cases of LPD, although this was expected to occur in 14 percent of the patients.[67] A 9-year followup report summarized the results in a total of 114 HSCT recipients, 101 of which safely received prophylactic infusions of EBV-specific CTLs.[68] None of the 101 patients progressed to EBV-LPD and 11 of 13 patients with LPD achieved sustained complete remissions.[68] Thus, transfer of

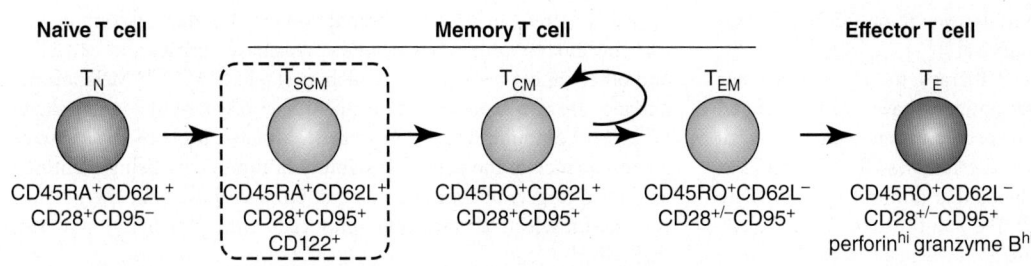

Figure 26–2. Linear differentiation of T-cell subsets. The phenotype of naïve, memory, and effector subsets is shown and the linear pathway of differentiation from a naïve T cell is based on recent data from fate mapping studies in murine models.[50,51]

EBV-specific T cells safely reconstituted immunity, mediated antiviral activity, and protected the majority of patients from EBV-LPD.

MULTISPECIFIC T-CELL THERAPY OF VIRAL INFECTIONS

Severe infections with a broad array of viruses remain a serious problem for immunocompromised patients.[2–5,7,69] In addition to CMV and EBV, infections with adenovirus, BK virus, human herpes virus-6 (HHV-6), herpes simplex virus (HSV), and/or varicella-zoster virus can pose a serious problem. Antiviral drugs may benefit a subset of patients, but the effects are often limited and accompanied by toxicities.[70] There is inferential evidence that restoration of T-cell immunity is also critical for protection against these infections, suggesting that multivirus-specific T-cell products would have greater utility.[71] EBV-LCLs that had been transfected with a recombinant adenovirus that encoded CMVpp65 were used to stimulate donor-derived PBMC and simultaneously expand T cells specific for adenovirus, CMV, and EBV.[31,72,73] The infusion of such multispecific T cells into HSCT recipients augmented T-cell responses to all three viruses and promoted virus clearance. These initial reports of adoptive T-cell therapy with "broad-spectrum" T cells to treat the multiplicity of distinct viral infections that may complicate the clinical outcome of HSCT are encouraging. Studies have further extended this work and demonstrated the feasibility and clinical utility of rapidly generated T-cell lines that recognize 12 immunogenic antigens from five viruses, including CMV, EBV, adenovirus, BK virus, and HHV-6. Adoptive transfer of these T cells to 11 allogeneic transplant recipients produced a greater than 90 percent sustained virologic and clinical response.[74]

⬤ ADOPTIVE CELLULAR THERAPY OF MALIGNANCY

There is evidence from murine models that the host immune system has a dynamic relationship with a developing tumor and can recognize, control, and even eliminate cancer.[75–77] Immunogenic proteins in human tumors have now been identified by screening of tumor complementary DNA (cDNA) libraries with tumor-specific T cells isolated from the blood or tumor environment,[78] or by screening of patient sera for antibody responses to tumor-associated proteins.[79] Distinct categories of tumor antigens have been uncovered, and several are being investigated as targets for T-cell therapy or vaccination (Table 26–1). However, the clinical translation of adoptive T-cell therapy and other immunotherapeutic modalities for human cancers has proven to be more challenging than for opportunistic viral infections. This reflects many issues, including the difficulty isolating highly avid tumor-specific T cells from cancer patients, and evasion mechanisms that tumors employ to avoid immune elimination including the local recruitment of regulatory T cells (T_{REG}) or myeloid-derived suppressor cells, loss of antigen or HLA expression, and expression or secretion of inhibitory molecules or cytokines.[80–83] Additionally, a problem distinct from the results of T-cell therapy for viruses is that transferred tumor-reactive T cells persisted only transiently in most early clinical trials, even if high-dose interleukin (IL)-2 was given to support their survival.[84–88]

The development of immune cell therapy for malignancy has focused on melanoma because target antigens have been identified and this tumor has responded to nonspecific immune therapy with IL-2,[89] and on amplifying the graft-versus-leukemia (GVL) effect after allogeneic HSCT because of the evidence that donor T cells mediate tumor eradication in this setting.[90–92] The ability to engineer T cells to have tumor specificity by introducing TCR genes that recognize

TABLE 26–1. Categories of Tumor Antigens

A. Classes of antigens for MHC-restricted T cells
- Antigens arising from mutations or gene rearrangements (e.g., CDK-4, BCR/ABL)
- Tissue-specific differentiation antigens (e.g., Tyrosinase, gp100)
- Cancer-testes antigens (e.g., MAGE-1, NY-ESO-1)
- Nonmutated overexpressed self-proteins (e.g., Her2/neu, WT-1)
- Oncofetal antigens (e.g., CEA)
- Viral proteins in virus associated malignancies (e.g., HPV E6 and E7, EBV LMP-1)

B. Classes of tumor cell surface molecules for chimeric antigen receptor-modified T cells
- B-cell differentiation molecules (e.g., CD19, CD20, CD22)
- Myeloid differentiation molecules (e.g., CD123)
- Adhesion molecules (e.g., CD44v6, GD2, L1 CAM, mesothelin)
- Oncofetal antigens (e.g., ROR1)
- Signaling molecules (e.g., Her-2)
- Hypoxia induced (e.g., CAIX)

tumor-associated antigens,[93] or chimeric antigen receptor (CAR) genes that encodes a single chain mAb domain linked to the CD3ζ chain of the TCR, and confers recognition of a tumor-associated, cell-surface molecule, is facilitating the broader application of T-cell therapy for both human hematologic malignancies and common epithelial cancers.[94–97]

CELLULAR THERAPY OF MELANOMA

Early studies demonstrated that the adoptive transfer of autologous polyclonal tumor-infiltrating lymphocytes (TILs), isolated and expanded from resected melanoma specimens, combined with the administration of high-dose IL-2 resulted in a 31 percent response rate in patients with advanced melanoma.[98] Most of the responses were transient, but these results validated the potential to eradicate a human solid tumor with immunotherapy. These results also encouraged efforts to define the antigens recognized by TILs in responding patients, and to refine the approaches to augmenting T-cell responses to tumor antigens.

Target Antigens for Melanoma-Specific T Cells

Melanoma has served as a model for the discovery of human tumor antigens because T cells specific for melanoma cells can often be detected in the blood or the tumor microenvironment. A landmark in cancer immunotherapy was the identification by cDNA expression cloning of MAGE-1, which is a member of the cancer-testes antigen class of tumor associated antigens.[78] Several additional shared tumor/self-melanocyte differentiation antigens recognized by CD8+ and/or CD4+ T cells have been discovered, including differentiation proteins that function in normal melanocyte physiology such as tyrosinase, gp100, and MART-1; and other cancer testis antigens such as NY-ESO-1.[78,99,100] Melanosome antigens are also expressed in normal tissues (skin, retina), and toxicity because of autoimmunity is a concern. Mutated proteins that arise as a consequence of the genetic instability of tumors are being identified as critical targets of immune recognition, and these offer the greatest promise for selectively targeting tumor cells without recognition of normal cells.[101]

Techniques for Isolation and Adoptive Transfer of Melanoma-Specific T Cells

The adoptive transfer of tumor-specific T-cell clones or oligoclonal populations of T cells expanded *ex vivo* can, in principle, allow control over the magnitude and function of the tumor-reactive T-cell response in the patient. If the tumor is easily accessible, tumor-reactive T cells can sometimes be isolated directly from the tumor biopsies by culture in high-dose IL-2.[102] Melanoma-reactive T cells can also be isolated using autologous dendritic cells pulsed with synthetic peptide antigen, but this approach can enrich low-avidity T cells that have a limited capacity to persist and function *in vivo*.[103]

Initial clinical trials of T-cell therapy for melanoma employed CD8+ T-cell clones specific for MART-1 or gp100; or clonal or polyclonal melanoma-reactive T cells derived and expanded from TILs.[84,104,105] The transferred T-cell clones given with low-dose IL-2 mediated transient antitumor activity in some patients with advanced disease, but did not persist for long term.[104] The response rate was higher in patients treated with polyclonal TILs and high-dose IL-2.[105] T-cell persistence was highly variable and only rarely sustained despite the infusion of large T-cell numbers (up to 10^{11}).[84,104] The inability of T cells to persist *in vivo* could reflect an inadequate antigen-specific CD4+ Th response, terminal differentiation of T cells during expansion, activation-induced T-cell death at the tumor site, or cell death as a consequence of IL-2 withdrawal.[84,106]

A major advance in the field was the demonstration that the transferred human T-cell persistence and therapeutic efficacy could be improved by pretreatment of the patient with a lymphodepleting regimen containing cyclophosphamide and fludarabine.[107,108] In these studies, high-dose IL-2 was administered daily after TIL transfer until toxicity required it be discontinued. A subset of the patients achieved prolonged high-level engraftment of one or a few tumor-reactive CD8+ T-cell clonotypes present in the infused polyclonal T-cell product.[107–110] In a followup analysis of a large cohort of patients, the overall and complete response rates were approximately 50 percent and 20 percent, respectively.[108,111] The antitumor activity correlated with the persistence of high levels of transferred tumor-reactive CD8+ T cells. Several mechanisms make the lymphopenic environment favorable for T-cell transfer, including less competition for homeostatic cytokines such as IL-15 and IL-7 that promote lymphocyte survival,[112,113] and the elimination of CD4+CD25+ T_{REG} cells.[114] Studies in murine models have confirmed that severe lymphodepletion can be exploited to improve the antitumor efficacy of the transferred T cells.[115] The addition of 2 Gy or 12 Gy of total-body irradiation to the lymphodepleting treatment with cyclophosphamide and fludarabine before TIL transfer increased the response rate to 52 percent and 72 percent, respectively.[116] The results of TIL therapy in a metastatic tumor that is unresponsive to conventional therapy were achieved with moderate toxicity, demonstrating the encouraging potential of this therapy.

Studies of the mechanisms of tumor eradication in melanoma are providing insights for treatment of other cancers with T-cell therapy. Exome sequencing of melanoma has shown that the frequency of mutational events is high,[101,117] and detailed analysis of the specificity of TILs showed that in addition to T cells specific for shared tumor/self-melanocyte differentiation antigens,[118] such mutated gene products encoded neoepitopes that were often targets of immune recognition.[101,108,119] The identification of neoepitope T cells in nonmelanoma cancers is of considerable interest because mutations in other tumors may be similarly targeted. In one example, TIL therapy was used to successfully treat a patient with metastatic cholangiocarcinoma.[120] Whole-exome sequencing of the tumor identified a mutation within the erbb2 interacting protein (ERBB2IP) that was recognized by a subset of CD4+ T cells in the TIL product. Treatment with a greater than 95 percent pure population of mutation-reactive T cells resulted in dramatic and durable tumor regression in this patient.[120] These results illustrate the potential of patient specific T-cell therapy targeting immunogenic mutations present in their tumor and highlight the need to apply advanced genomic technologies to the discovery of targets for immune therapy in cancer.[108,120]

Collectively, significant progress has been made in cellular therapy for melanoma, but additional studies are necessary to define the optimal and safest regimens for adoptive therapy with tumor-reactive T cells. Advances in our understanding of the role of individual cytokines in T-cell survival *in vitro* and *in vivo*, or the regulation of T-cell activation and homeostasis will provide new opportunities for improving the persistence of *in vitro* expanded T cells after transfer, perhaps obviating use of toxic chemoradiotherapy to deplete lymphocytes before T-cell infusions. Most of the initial efforts have focused on the CD8+ T-cell response to tumor antigens, but newer data highlights the potential of tumor-specific CD4+ T cells. Combining T-cell therapy with targeted depletion of T_{REG}, checkpoint inhibitors, and vaccines is also under investigation, and may help overcome mechanisms by which tumors evade elimination by limiting the quantity and quality of the host response.

CELLULAR THERAPY OF LEUKEMIA

Allogeneic donor T cells contained in or derived from the stem cell graft can mount a GVL effect that can contribute to the eradication of hematologic cancers, including leukemia.[90] This is underscored by studies on the antitumor effects of infusions of unselected donor lymphocytes (DLI) given to patients who relapse after allogeneic HSCT. DLI can have potent antitumor effects in patients with relapsed chronic myeloid leukemia, but has been less effective in acute leukemias, and often complicated by the development of acute and chronic GVHD.[91] The identification of leukemia-associated antigens that can be targeted to selectively promote a GVL effect without causing GVHD remains an important goal.[92,121]

Target Antigens for Leukemia-Specific T Cells

GVHD and GVL effects usually coexist, but a GVL effect can be observed after HSCT in the absence of GVHD.[90] Thus, it is presumed there are antigens that are expressed by leukemia cells that can be targeted by allogeneic T cells. Several categories of such antigens have been identified. These include (1) minor histocompatibility antigens (mHAgs) that are selectively expressed in hematopoietic cells including leukemic cells, (2) tumor-specific proteins resulting from chromosome translocations or mutations, and (3) normal proteins that are overexpressed in leukemic cells. Proteins in the latter two classes could be targets both in the transplantation and nontransplantation setting, whereas mHAgs are only relevant after allogeneic HSCT.

Minor Histocompatibility Antigens

The increased potency of the GVL effect after allogeneic HSCT compared with syngeneic HSCT emphasizes the importance of disparity in major HLA and mHAgs for immune-mediated eradication of malignancy.[90,122] Class I and class II molecules on recipient T cells display mHAgs, which are peptides derived from proteins that differ between the donor and recipient as a result of genetic polymorphism.[92,123] In murine models, the adoptive transfer of T cells specific for a single mHAg eradicated leukemia without causing GVHD.[124] In humans, donor T cells reactive with recipient mHAgs can be isolated after transplantation from most allogeneic HSCT recipients.[125] Analysis of the specificity of such T-cell clones shows that many mHAgs are expressed preferentially in hematopoietic cells, including leukemic blasts, and might permit the separation of GVL from GVHD.[125] mHAg-specific CD8+ CTLs prevent engraftment of human leukemia in nonobese diabetic/severe combined immunodeficiency mice, providing evidence that the leukemic stem cell can be recognized by allogeneic T cells.[126]

Most mHAgs result from nonsynonymous single nucleotide polymorphisms (SNPs) in the coding sequence of donor and recipient genes that alter the HLA binding or TCR contact of HLA-bound peptides. There are several million SNPs with an allele frequency of greater than 5 percent in the human genome, including approximately 50,000 SNPs that lead to amino acid changes in proteins.[127] Identification of the polymorphic genes that encode mHAgs is facilitated by the data on genetic variation from the human HapMap project, which has enabled the use of whole-genome association analysis for mHAg discovery in addition to conventional techniques for antigen discovery.[123] Identifying the subset of mHAgs that will be the most useful to target to augment the GVL effect requires consideration of several factors, including the allele frequency of the mHAg encoding gene, the HLA restricting allele that presents the mHAg, and the expression and presentation of the mHAg in leukemia cells and nonhematopoietic tissues.[128] Most mHAg discovery efforts have focused on CD8+ T cells, but CD4+ T cells are likely to play a key role either as direct effector cells in the GVL response, or to support the function and persistence of CD8+ T cells, and efforts to define class II MHC-restricted mHAgs remain an important area of investigation.

Autosome-encoded mHAgs that could be targets for therapy of leukemia after allogeneic HSCT include HA-1 and HA-2, which are encoded by *KIAA0023* and *MYO1G*, respectively, and presented by HLA-A2; peptides encoded by *BCL2A1*, which encodes two mHAgs presented by HLA-A24 and HLA-B44, respectively; LRH-1, encoded by the *P2X5* gene and presented by HLA-B7; SP110, which is derived by a novel peptide-splicing mechanism and presented by HLA-A3; and PANE-1, which is presented by HLA-A3 and selectively expressed on B-lymphoid malignancies.[123,128,129] Additionally, the HLA-A2–restricted and hematopoietic-specific mHAg UTA2–1 has been described.[130] Direct evidence for a role of these mHAgs in the GVL effect is provided by studies using HLA-A/peptide tetramers to detect expansion of mHAg-reactive T cells in patients who responded to treatment with DLI for treatment of relapse following transplantation.[131,132]

There is also evidence for a role of Y-chromosome–encoded mHAgs in the GVL effect. Male recipients of allogeneic HSCT from female donors have a higher risk of GVHD but exhibit a lower risk of leukemia relapse than do other donor/recipient gender combinations, even after controlling for GVHD.[133] Several H-Y antigens are ubiquitously expressed in tissues, providing an explanation for the increased GVHD. Identifying mHAgs encoded by the Y chromosome that are selectively expressed on leukemia cells has been more challenging. A *UTY* epitope presented by HLA-B8 is preferentially presented in hematopoietic cells including acute myeloid leukemia, but the gene is expressed in other tissues and it is not clear if targeting this antigen could avoid GVHD.[134]

Leukemia-Associated Proteins
Leukemia-associated proteins that could be targets for cellular therapy have been identified.[121] These include mutated proteins, such as p21/Ras, or the products of chromosome translocations, such as BCR/ABL, and the promyelocytic leukemia–retinoic acid receptor α protein (PML-RARα), which can provide unique peptides that represent potential tumor-specific targets.[135,136] Nonpolymorphic proteins, such as proteinase 3, Wilms tumor antigen-1 (WT-1), or cyclin A1, which are overexpressed in some leukemias or the leukemic stem cells, also represent potential targets for T-cell therapy.[137–142] T cells specific for WT-1, which is expressed at high levels in myeloid leukemias but at low levels in normal hematopoietic cells, have been isolated from normal donors by *in vitro* stimulation of PBMCs with synthetic peptides.[143] WT-1–specific

CTL selectively lysed leukemic blasts and prevented engraftment of leukemia in immunodeficient mice, suggesting that these T cells may mediate an antileukemic effect without affecting normal hematopoiesis *in vivo*.[140,144] Recent work has identified WT-1–specific T cells after HLA-identical sibling HSCT and correlated these cells with a GVL effect.[145] In a recent pilot trial, 11 high-risk leukemia patients received infusions of WT-1–specific T cells.[146] In four of these patients, the infused T cells were generated in the presence of IL-21, which modulates the differentiation of T cells in culture. The transferred T cells exhibited evidence of leukemic activity, and CTL that were generated with IL-21 had superior antileukemic activity and survived long-term as memory T cells.[146] Additional study in a larger number of patients is needed, but these results offer a potential safe and effective treatment for patients with limited treatment options.

GENETIC RETARGETING OF T CELLS

Extending cellular therapy to patients from whom tumor-reactive T cells cannot be isolated and to other malignancies can be accomplished by using gene transfer approaches to retarget patient T cells to recognize tumor antigens (Fig. 26–3). Two approaches that have already been translated to the clinic are discussed below. The first is the use of retroviral or lentiviral vectors to transfer of TCR α- and β-chain genes isolated from tumor-reactive T cells into T cells obtained from the patient, and the second is the expression of non–MHC-restricted synthetic CARs that target a tumor cell-surface molecule.

Genetic Retargeting of T Cells with T-Cell Receptor Genes
Antigen specificity is conferred by the TCR, therefore the transfer of TCR α- and β-chain genes from a T cell of defined specificity into any T cell, will transfer antigen recognition. This strategy can impart specificity to viral antigens, tumor-associated antigens, or mHAgs,[93,147,148] and can confer potent tumor recognition. However, TCRs are MHC-restricted and a given TCR construct can only be used to treat patients with tumors expressing the target molecule and also express the MHC

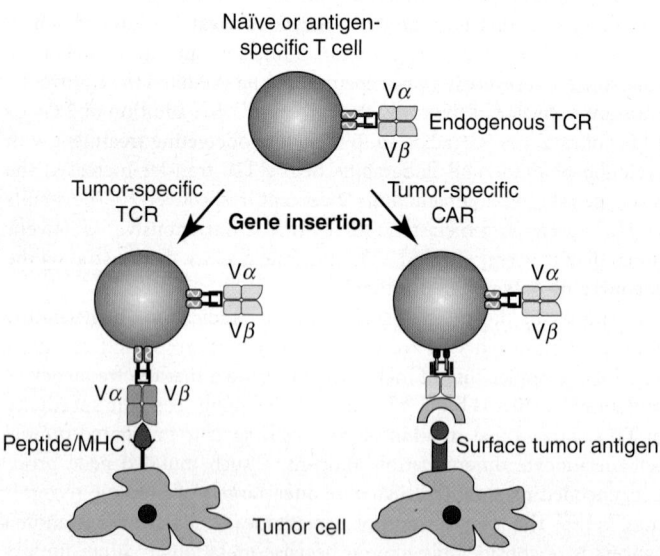

Figure 26–3. Engineering tumor-reactive T cells by insertion of genes that encode tumor-specific T-cell receptors (TCRs) or chimeric antigen receptors (CARs). After isolation of T cells from the desired T-cell subset, the tumor targeting receptor is introduced in the T cells by gene transfer, and the engineered redirected T cells are expanded for reinfusion to the patient.

restricting allele. Moreover, it can be difficult to achieve the same surface level of TCR expression in transduced T cells as observed in the parental T-cell clone from which the TCR genes were isolated. This problem was apparent in the first clinical trial in which MART-1 TCR-engineered T cells were used to treat melanoma and the low TCR expression likely contributed in part to the limited antitumor activity of the TCR-modified T cells.[149] Another problem is that the TCR transfer endows T cells with additional rearranged TCR chains, leading to T cells that could potentially express four different TCR molecules on the cell surface: the natural endogenous TCR, the exogenously introduced TCR, and two mixed heterodimers consisting of endogenous and exogenous TCR chains. Such mismatched TCRs could result in potentially deleterious self-reactive specificities.[150] This problem can be mitigated by the introduction of cysteine residues into the extracellular constant region of the introduced α and β TCR chains to provide for disulfide bond formation[151,152] or by using murine constant domains in place of the human constant regions,[153] both of which promote preferential pairing of the introduced chains. More recently, strategies to knock out or silence the endogenous TCR have been developed.[154,155] These modifications provide for more stable pairing during assembly and export, and better competition for limiting components of the TCR complex.[156]

Strategies to enhance the potency of the TCR, such as by enhancing TCR affinity, may increase the risk of toxicity, particularly if self-antigens are targeted.[157–161] In a clinical trial, autologous T cells were modified to express optimized high-affinity MART-1 or gp100 TCR transgenes and transferred to 36 melanoma patients. Nine of the patients exhibited clinical antitumor responses, but "on-target" toxicities to normal melanocytes in the skin, eye, and ear that required local glucocorticoid treatment were observed in a significant fraction of patients that received the high-avidity TCR.[157] In a separate trial, autologous T cells modified to express a high-affinity TCR specific for the carcinoembryonic antigen (CEA) were transferred to three patients with colorectal cancer. The serum CEA levels decreased in all three patients and there was some regression of metastatic disease. However, the clinical trial was closed early when all three patients developed severe colitis, putatively from recognition of normal epithelial cells that express CEA.[161] Toxicity was also observed in a study in which nine cancer patients were treated with autologous T cells modified to express an anti–MAGE-A3 TCR. Five patients experienced cancer regression, but three patients experienced serious and/or fatal neurologic toxicity. This occurred because of previously unrecognized expression of MAGE-A12, which encodes the identical epitope, in the human brain that resulted in neuronal cell destruction.[160] Additional safety concerns of targeting MAGE-A3 using an affinity-enhanced TCR construct were identified after an unexpected fatal cardiac toxicity. Detailed analysis showed cross-reactivity of the engineered MAGE-A3 TCR-modified T cells with a titin-derived peptide.[158,159]

Such serious "on-target and off-target" toxicities of TCR gene transfer suggested that targeting antigens with restricted expression on tumor cells such as mutant epitopes or cancer testes antigens is preferable. NY-ESO-1 is expressed in many human cancers, but not in normal tissues, except testis. A TCR specific for an HLA-A2-restricted NY-ESO-1 epitope was used for the treatment of melanoma and synovial sarcoma.[162] Toxicity was not observed, and encouraging results showed that the TCR-engineered T cells mediated objective responses in four of six patients with synovial cell carcinoma and five of 11 melanoma patients.

Genetic Retargeting of T Cells with Chimeric Antigen Receptors

A notable advance in T-cell therapy has been the development of CARs that link recognition domains of antibodies to molecules involved in

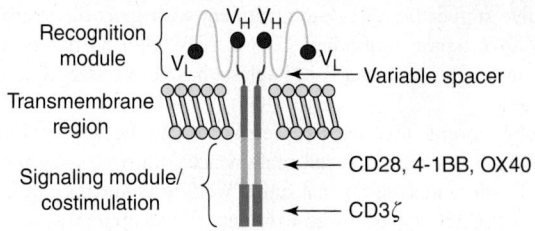

Figure 26–4. Structure of a chimeric antigen receptor (CAR). The CAR is typically composed of a recognition module that is fused in tandem to nonsignaling extracellular and transmembrane domains and intracellular signaling elements. The recognition module, spacer domain, and signaling modules of the CAR can be modified to optimize tumor cell recognition and T-cell function.

signaling T-cell effector function.[94–96,163,164] CARs typically consist of a single-chain variable fragment (scFV) derived from the V_H and V_L sequences of a mAb specific for a tumor cell-surface molecule, fused to a *trans*-membrane domain, as well as the CD3ζ-signaling domain alone, or in combination with one or more costimulatory signaling modules, such as CD28,4–1BB, OX40, or CD27 (Fig. 26–4).[94–96,165,166] CARs can be introduced into T cells by gene transfer to target surface molecules expressed on tumors. Unlike conventional TCRs, CARs are not MHC-restricted and have the advantage that a single construct can be used to treat all patients expressing the tumor antigen.

A large number of CARs targeting a variety of molecules expressed on hematologic malignancies have been developed.[96,167,168] Examples for candidate targets for the treatment of hematologic malignancies include CD19,[96] CD20,[169] and the orphan tyrosine kinase receptor ROR1[170–172] expressed on B-cell lymphomas and leukemias; Lewis Y,[173] CD44v6,[174] CD33 and/or CD123 expressed on acute myeloid leukemia[168,175–177]; and NKG2D ligands[178] or the B-cell maturation antigen (BCMA)[179] expressed on myeloma.

Efficient methods for T-cell activation, gene transfer, and expansion of T cells for therapy have been developed and the results of pilot clinical trials of T cells modified to express CARs specific for CD19, CD20, ERBB2, the disialoganglioside GD2, and mesothelin have been reported and provided evidence of *in vivo* antitumor activity.[180–187] However, serious toxicity has also been observed including a fatal toxicity shortly after infusion of a single high dose of ERBB2-specific CAR-T cells that contained both CD28 and 4–1BB costimulatory domains, and was attributed to cytokine release and recognition of normal lung epithelium that expresses low amounts of ERBB2.[188] Toxicity to normal tissues was also observed in patients receiving CAIX CAR-engineered T cells for the treatment of metastatic renal cell carcinoma.[189,190]

The most encouraging results with CAR-T cells have been obtained targeting the B-cell lineage-restricted CD19 molecule that is expressed on B-cell leukemias and lymphomas. Dramatic and durable remissions in patients with chronic lymphatic leukemia (CLL) and acute lymphatic leukemia (ALL) have been reported after infusion of autologous T cells transduced with CD19-specific CARs that contained either a CD28 or a 4–1BB costimulatory domain.[182,183,191,192] In these studies, infused T cells were shown to expand *in vivo*, induce tumor lysis and a deficiency of normal CD19+ B cells, and persist long-term in some patients. The complete response rate appears to be higher in patients with ALL than those with CLL or lymphoma for reasons that have not been elucidated. Tumor regression is often associated with a cytokine release syndrome (CRS) initiated by activation of CAR-T cells *in vivo*, associated with elevated levels of IFN-γ, IL-6, and tumor necrosis factor, and resulting in high fever, hypotension, and neurologic abnormalities.[183,193] CRS is more severe in patients with high tumor burden and can require intensive supportive care, and treatment with glucocorticoids and/or anti IL-6 receptor antibodies. CAR-T cells often do not persist long term, although prolonged B-cell aplasia has been observed in a subset of patients.

The finding that durable responses can be achieved in some patients with advanced B-cell malignancies illustrates the potency of CAR-T cells, and suggests that future work to define optimal design of the CD19 CAR constructs and to identify the optimal subset(s) of T cells to modify may further improve outcomes, particularly in CLL and lymphoma where response rates and durability are lower. The demonstration of the superior engraftment properties of effector T (T_E) cells derived from T_{CM} would suggest that selection or enrichment of T_{CM} prior to gene insertion may provide a superior T-cell product for adoptive therapy.[48,194] This hypothesis is being examined prospectively in clinical trials of CAR–T-cell therapy. Moreover, integrating T-cell therapy earlier after diagnosis or after autologous HSCT, in which marked tumor cytoreduction can be achieved by intensive conditioning, may further improve outcome and reduce the toxicity resulting from CAR-mediated tumor lysis.

CAR-modified T cells also may have applications in the treatment of solid tumors. Candidate surface molecules on solid tumors that are being actively pursued as targets include GD2,[186] mesothelin,[187] L1-cell adhesion molecule (L1CAM),[85] ROR1,[170,171] prostate stem cell antigen,[195] folate receptor,[196] and the fibroblast activation protein.[197] Significant antitumor activity without toxicity has been reported in patients with neuroblastoma treated with T cells modified with a first-generation GD2 CAR.[186] The persistence of the transferred cells was relatively short in that study, however, perhaps owing to the lack of costimulation in the CAR. GD2 is expressed on normal peripheral nerves, and on-target toxicity from a sustained T-cell response will need to be monitored if more potent CARs are being examined. Suitable animal models for preclinical toxicity studies are urgently needed and are being developed.[197–199] It will also be important to address the multiple evasion mechanisms that tumors employ to avoid immune elimination.[96] For example, the programmed death-1 (PD-1) receptor is a negative regulator of T_E mechanisms that limits immune responses against cancer, and the combination of checkpoint blockade and T-cell therapy is of future interest.[200–202]

Suicide Genes for Conditional Ablation

The results of clinical trials of T-cell therapy have revealed toxicity to normal tissues in some patients. The introduction of a suicide gene into the T cells that could be activated if toxicity occurred has long been the subject of research. The HSV-thymidine kinase (*HSV-TK*) gene has been used in gene therapy trials in the clinic and was effective in reversing GVHD after DLI.[203] However, the viral thymidine kinase is immunogenic and can result in premature elimination of transferred T cells that do not cause toxicity.[204] Novel suicide genes based on inducing conditional cell death through activation of CD95 (Fas) or caspases using a chemical dimerizer such as AP1903 to activate an engineered chimeric human CD95 or caspase transgene product may circumvent the problem of immunogenicity.[205–207] Recently, 10 patients undergoing haploidentical HSCT for relapsed acute leukemia were treated with donor T cells modified to express an inducible *caspase9* gene (iCasp9). The iCasp9 T cells engrafted and conferred protection against infectious diseases. A subset of the patients developed GVHD. A single dose of the dimerizing drug, given to those patients who developed GVHD ablated more than 90 percent of the iCasp9-modified T cells rapidly and eliminated the GVHD without recurrence or adverse events.[208,209] A truncated epidermal growth factor receptor (EGFR) marker/suicide gene that could be targeted *in vivo* using a clinical grade anti-EGFR antibody

(Erbitux) has been developed, but its efficacy for ablating transferred T cells in patients has not been established.

● FUTURE DIRECTIONS IN T-CELL THERAPY

The field of adoptive T-cell therapy is now emerging as a viable and effective therapeutic approach for treating human infections and cancer. Advances in the understanding of cell intrinsic properties of T-cell subsets, discovery of target antigens that distinguish tumor cells from normal cells, and improvements in the methodology for introducing genes into T cells have combined to make it feasible to treat patients with certain malignancies using highly effective T-cell products. Several challenges remain. For most common human tumors, target antigens have not yet been defined, and tumor heterogeneity and other mechanisms that tumors use to evade T-cell recognition represent barriers to effective therapy. Thus, additional research to identify and validate a larger number of target molecules for TCR- and CAR-recognition is essential to broaden therapeutic applications, and improve efficacy. Combination therapies with T cells and checkpoint inhibitors are promising for overcoming local and systemic evasion mechanisms that limit antitumor immunity. Finally, it would be ideal if expression of the tumor targeting receptors or the survival of transferred T cells were under regulatory control by small molecules that could be administered to the patient to reduce toxicity.

REFERENCES

1. Klenerman P, Hill A: T cells and viral persistence: Lessons from diverse infections. *Nat Immunol* 6:873, 2005.
2. Tomblyn M, Chiller T, Einsele H, et al: Guidelines for preventing infectious complications among hematopoietic cell transplantation recipients: A global perspective. *Biol Blood Marrow Transplant* 15:1143, 2009.
3. Pollack M, Heugel J, Xie H, et al: An international comparison of current strategies to prevent herpesvirus and fungal infections in hematopoietic cell transplant recipients. *Biol Blood Marrow Transplant* 17:664, 2011.
4. Wingard JR, Hsu J, Hiemenz JW: Hematopoietic stem cell transplantation: An overview of infection risks and epidemiology. *Hematol Oncol Clin North Am* 25:101, 2011.
5. Hsu JW, Wingard JR: Advances in the management of viral infections. *Cancer Treat Res* 161:157, 2014.
6. Riddell SR, Greenberg PD: T-cell therapy of cytomegalovirus and human immunodeficiency virus infection. *J Antimicrob Chemother* 45 (Suppl T3):35, 2000.
7. Leen AM, Heslop HE, Brenner MK: Antiviral T-cell therapy. *Immunol Rev* 258:12, 2014.
8. Boeckh M, Geballe AP: Cytomegalovirus: Pathogen, paradigm, and puzzle. *J Clin Invest* 121:1673, 2011.
9. Powers C, DeFilippis V, Malouli D, et al: Cytomegalovirus immune evasion. *Curr Top Microbiol Immunol* 325:333, 2008.
10. Sylwester AW, Mitchell BL, Edgar JB, et al: Broadly targeted human cytomegalovirus-specific CD4+ and CD8+ T cells dominate the memory compartments of exposed subjects. *J Exp Med* 202:673, 2005.
11. Manley TJ, Luy L, Jones T, et al: Immune evasion proteins of human cytomegalovirus do not prevent a diverse CD8+ cytotoxic T cell response in natural infection. *Blood* 104:1075, 2004.
12. Li C-R, Greenberg PD, Gilbert MJ, et al: Recovery of HLA-restricted cytomegalovirus (CMV)-specific T-cell responses after allogeneic bone marrow transplant: Correlation with CMV disease and effect of ganciclovir prophylaxis. *Blood* 83:1971, 1994.
13. Boeckh M, Nichols WG, Papanicolaou G, et al: Cytomegalovirus in hematopoietic stem cell transplant recipients: Current status, known challenges, and future strategies. *Biol Blood Marrow Transplant* 9:543, 2003.
14. McGoldrick SMB: Cytomegalovirus-specific T cells are primed early after cord blood transplant but fail to control virus in vivo. *Blood* 121:2796, 2013.
15. Sellar RS, Peggs KS: Therapeutic strategies for cytomegalovirus infection in haematopoietic transplant recipients: A focused update. *Expert Opin Biol Ther* 14:1121, 2014.
16. Reusser P, Einsele H, Lee J, et al: Randomized multicenter trial of foscarnet versus ganciclovir for preemptive therapy of cytomegalovirus infection after allogeneic stem cell transplantation. *Blood* 99:1159, 2002.
17. Marty FM, Winston DJ, Rowley SD, et al: CMX001 to prevent cytomegalovirus disease in hematopoietic-cell transplantation. *N Engl J Med* 369:1227, 2013.
18. Chemaly RF, Ullmann AJ, Stoelben S, et al: Letermovir for cytomegalovirus prophylaxis in hematopoietic-cell transplantation. *N Engl J Med* 370:1781, 2014.

19. Moss P, Rickinson A: Cellular immunotherapy for viral infection after HSC transplantation. *Nat Rev Immunol* 5:9, 2005.

20. Terrazzini N, Kern F: Cell-mediated immunity to human CMV infection: A brief overview. *F1000Prime Rep* 6:28, 2014.

21. Hanley PJ, Bollard CM: Controlling cytomegalovirus: Helping the immune system take the lead. *Viruses* 6:2242, 2014.

22. Simon CO, Holtappels R, Tervo HM, et al: CD8 T cells control cytomegalovirus latency by epitope-specific sensing of transcriptional reactivation. *J Virol* 80:10436, 2006.

23. Sacre K, Nguyen S, Deback C, et al: Expansion of human cytomegalovirus (HCMV) immediate-early 1-specific CD8+ T cells and control of HCMV replication after allogeneic stem cell transplantation. *J Virol* 82:10143, 2008.

24. Fuhrmann S, Streitz M, Reinke P, et al: T cell response to the cytomegalovirus major capsid protein (UL86) is dominated by helper cells with a large polyfunctional component and diverse epitope recognition. *J Infect Dis* 197:1455, 2008.

25. Crompton L, Khan N, Khanna R, et al: CD4+ T cells specific for glycoprotein B from cytomegalovirus exhibit extreme conservation of T-cell receptor usage between different individuals. *Blood* 111:2053, 2008.

26. Riddell SR, Watanabe KS, Goodrich JM, et al: Restoration of viral immunity in immunodeficient humans by the adoptive transfer of T cell clones. *Science* 257:238, 1992.

27. Walter EA, Greenberg PD, Gilbert MJ, et al: Reconstitution of cellular immunity against cytomegalovirus in recipients of allogeneic bone marrow by transfer of T-cell clones from the donor. *N Engl J Med* 333:1038, 1995.

28. Peggs KS, Verfuerth S, Pizzey A, et al: Adoptive cellular therapy for early cytomegalovirus infection after allogeneic stem-cell transplantation with virus-specific T-cell lines. *Lancet* 362:1375, 2003.

29. Kleihauer A, Grigoleit U, Hebart H, et al: Ex vivo generation of human cytomegalovirus-specific cytotoxic T cells by peptide-pulsed dendritic cells. *Br J Haematol* 113:231, 2001.

30. Micklethwaite KP, Clancy L, Sandher U, et al: Prophylactic infusion of cytomegalovirus-specific cytotoxic T lymphocytes stimulated with Ad5f35pp65 gene-modified dendritic cells after allogeneic hemopoietic stem cell transplantation. *Blood* 112:3974, 2008.

31. Leen AM, Myers GD, Sili U, et al: Monoculture-derived T lymphocytes specific for multiple viruses expand and produce clinically relevant effects in immunocompromised individuals. *Nat Med* 12:1160, 2006.

32. Einsele H, Roosnek E, Rufer N, et al: Infusion of cytomegalovirus (CMV)-specific T cells for the treatment of CMV infection not responding to antiviral chemotherapy. *Blood* 99:3916, 2002.

33. Keenan RD, Ainsworth J, Khan N, et al: Purification of cytomegalovirus-specific CD8 T cells from peripheral blood using HLA-peptide tetramers. *Br J Haematol* 115:428, 2001.

34. Knabel M, Franz TJ, Schiemann M, et al: Reversible MHC multimer staining for functional isolation of T-cell populations and effective adoptive transfer. *Nat Med* 8:631, 2002.

35. Cobbold M, Khan N, Pourgheysari B, et al: Adoptive transfer of cytomegalovirus-specific CTL to stem cell transplant patients after selection by HLA-peptide tetramers. *J Exp Med* 202:379, 2005.

36. Schmitt A, Tonn T, Busch DH, et al: Adoptive transfer and selective reconstitution of streptamer-selected cytomegalovirus-specific CD8+ T cells leads to virus clearance in patients after allogeneic peripheral blood stem cell transplantation. *Transfusion* 51:591, 2011.

37. Becker C, Pohla H, Frankenberger B, et al: Adoptive tumor therapy with T lymphocytes enriched through an IFN-γ capture assay. *Nat Med* 7:1159, 2001.

38. Rauser G, Einsele H, Sinzger C, et al: Rapid generation of combined CMV-specific CD4+ and CD8+ T-cell lines for adoptive transfer into allogeneic stem cell transplant recipients. *Blood* 103:3565, 2004.

39. Wolfl M, Kuball J, Ho WY, et al: Activation-induced expression of CD137 permits detection, isolation, and expansion of full repertoire of CD8+ T cells responding to antigen without requiring knowledge of epitope specificities. *Blood* 110:201, 2007.

40. Feuchtinger T, Opherk K, Bethge WA, et al: Adoptive transfer of pp65-specific T cells for the treatment of chemorefractory cytomegalovirus disease or reactivation after haploidentical and matched unrelated stem cell transplantation. *Blood* 116:4360, 2010.

41. Robins HS, Srivastava SK, Campregher PV, et al: Overlap and effective size of the human CD8+ T cell receptor repertoire. *Sci Transl Med* 2:47ra64, 2010.

42. Robins H, Desmarais C, Matthis J, et al: Ultra-sensitive detection of rare T cell clones. *J Immunol Methods* 375:14, 2012.

43. Sallusto F, Geginat J, Lanzavecchia A: Central memory and effector memory T cell subsets: Function, generation, and maintenance. *Annu Rev Immunol* 22:745, 2004.

44. Hertoghs KML, Moerland PD, van Stijn A, et al: Molecular profiling of cytomegalovirus-induced human CD8+ T cell differentiation. *J Clin Invest* 120:4077, 2010.

45. Farber DL, Yudanin NA, Restifo NP: Human memory T cells: Generation, compartmentalization and homeostasis. *Nat Rev Immunol* 14:24, 2014.

46. Berger C, Jensen MC, Lansdorp PM, et al: Adoptive transfer of effector CD8+ T cells derived from central memory cells establishes persistent T cell memory in primates. *J Clin Invest* 118:294, 2008.

47. Gattinoni L, Zhong X-S, Palmer DC, et al: Wnt signaling arrests effector T cell differentiation and generates CD8+ memory stem cells. *Nat Med* 15:808, 2009.

48. Wang X, Berger C, Wong CW, et al: Engraftment of human central memory-derived effector CD8+ T cells in immunodeficient mice. *Blood* 117:1888, 2011.

49. Gattinoni L, Lugli E, Ji Y, et al: A human memory T cell subset with stem cell-like properties. *Nat Med* 17:1290, 2011.

50. Gerlach C, Rohr JC, Perié L, et al: Heterogeneous differentiation patterns of individual CD8+ T cells. *Science* 340:635, 2013.

51. Buchholz VR, Flossdorf M, Hensel I, et al: Disparate individual fates compose robust CD8+ T cell immunity. *Science* 340:630, 2013.

52. Graef P, Buchholz VR, Stemberger C, et al: Serial transfer of single-cell-derived immunocompetence reveals stemness of CD8+ central memory T cells. *Immunity* 41:116, 2014.

53. Stemberger C, Graef P, Odendahl M, et al: Lowest numbers of primary CD8+ T cells can reconstitute protective immunity upon adoptive immunotherapy. *Blood* 124:628, 2014.

54. Stemberger C, Dreher S, Tschulik C, et al: Novel serial positive enrichment technology enables clinical multiparameter cell sorting. *PLoS One* 7:e35798, 2012.

55. Yin Y, Manoury B, Fåhraeus R: Self-inhibition of synthesis and antigen presentation by Epstein-Barr virus-encoded EBNA1. *Science* 301:1371, 2003.

56. Thorley-Lawson DA, Gross A: Persistence of the Epstein-Barr virus and the origins of associated lymphomas. *N Engl J Med* 350:1328, 2004.

57. Annels NE, Callan MFC, Tan L, et al: Changing patterns of dominant TCR usage with maturation of an EBV-specific cytotoxic T cell response. *J Immunol* 165:4831, 2000.

58. Amyes E, Hatton C, Montamat-Sicotte D, et al: Characterization of the CD4+ T cell response to Epstein-Barr virus during primary and persistent infection. *J Exp Med* 198:903, 2003.

59. Rickinson AB, Long HM, Palendira U, et al: Cellular immune controls over Epstein-Barr virus infection: New lessons from the clinic and the laboratory. *Trends Immunol* 35:159, 2014.

60. Adhikary D, Behrends U, Boerschmann H, et al: Immunodominance of lytic cycle antigens in Epstein-Barr virus-specific CD4+ T cell preparations for therapy. *PLoS One* 2:e583, 2007.

61. Curtis RE, Travis LB, Rowlings PA, et al: Risk of lymphoproliferative disorders after bone marrow transplantation: A multi-institutional study. *Blood* 94:2208, 1999.

62. Meij P, van Esser JWJ, Niesters HGM, et al: Impaired recovery of Epstein-Barr virus (EBV)-specific CD8+ T lymphocytes after partially T-depleted allogeneic stem cell transplantation may identify patients at very high risk for progressive EBV reactivation and lymphoproliferative disease. *Blood* 101:4290, 2003.

63. Kuehnle I, Huls MH, Liu Z, et al: CD20 monoclonal antibody (rituximab) for therapy of Epstein-Barr virus lymphoma after hemopoietic stem-cell transplantation. *Blood* 95:1502, 2000.

64. Papadopoulos EB, Ladanyi M, Emanuel D, et al: Infusions of donor leukocytes to treat Epstein-Barr-virus-associated lymphoproliferative disorders after allogeneic bone marrow transplantation. *N Engl J Med* 330:1185, 1994.

65. Rooney CM, Smith CA, Ng CYC, et al: Use of gene-modified virus-specific T lymphocytes to control Epstein-Barr-virus-related lymphoproliferation. *Lancet* 345:9, 1995.

66. Gottschalk S, Edwards OL, Sili U, et al: Generating CTLs against the subdominant Epstein-Barr virus LMP1 antigen for the adoptive immunotherapy of EBV-associated malignancies. *Blood* 101:1905, 2003.

67. Rooney CM, Smith CA, Ng CYC, et al: Infusion of cytotoxic T cells for the prevention and treatment of Epstein-Barr virus-induced lymphoma in allogeneic transplant recipients. *Blood* 92:1549, 1998.

68. Heslop HE, Slobod KS, Pule MA, et al: Long term outcome of EBV specific T-cell infusions to prevent or treat EBV-related lymphoproliferative disease in transplant recipients. *Blood* 115:925, 2010.

69. Styczynski J, Reusser P, Einsele H, et al: Management of HSV, VZV and EBV infections in patients with hematological malignancies and after SCT: Guidelines from the Second European Conference on Infections in Leukemia. *Bone Marrow Transplant* 43:757, 2008.

70. Leen AM, Bollard CM, Myers GD, et al: Adenoviral infections in hematopoietic stem cell transplantation. *Biol Blood Marrow Transplant* 12:243, 2006.

71. Chakrabarti S, Mautner V, Osman H, et al: Adenovirus infections following allogeneic stem cell transplantation: Incidence and outcome in relation to graft manipulation, immunosuppression, and immune recovery. *Blood* 100:1619, 2002.

72. Hanley PJ, Cruz CRY, Savoldo B, et al: Functionally active virus-specific T-cells that target CMV, adenovirus and EBV can be expanded from naïve T-cell populations in cord blood and will target a range of viral epitopes. *Blood* 114:1958, 2009.

73. Gerdemann U, Katari UL, Papadopoulou A, et al: Safety and clinical efficacy of rapidly-generated trivirus-directed T cells as treatment for adenovirus, EBV, and CMV infections after allogeneic hematopoietic stem cell transplant. *Mol Ther* 21:2113, 2013.

74. Papadopoulou A, Gerdemann U, Katari UL, et al: Activity of broad-spectrum T cells as treatment for AdV, EBV, CMV, BKV, and HHV6 infections after HSCT. *Sci Transl Med* 6:242ra83, 2014.

75. Koebel CM, Vermi W, Swann JB, et al: Adaptive immunity maintains occult cancer in an equilibrium state. *Nature* 450:903, 2007.

76. Matsushita H, Vesely MD, Koboldt DC, et al: Cancer exome analysis reveals a T-cell-dependent mechanism of cancer immunoediting. *Nature* 482:400, 2012.

77. Mittal D, Gubin MM, Schreiber RD, et al: New insights into cancer immunoediting and its three component phases—elimination, equilibrium and escape. *Curr Opin Immunol* 27:16, 2014.

78. van der Bruggen P, Traversari C, Chomez P, et al: A gene encoding an antigen recognized by cytolytic T lymphocytes on a human melanoma. *Science* 254:1643, 1991.

79. Chen Y-T, Scanlan MJ, Sahin U, et al: A testicular antigen aberrantly expressed in human cancers detected by autologous antibody screening. *Proc Natl Acad Sci U S A* 94:1914, 1997.

80. Drake CG, Jaffee E, Pardoll DM: Mechanisms of immune evasion by tumors. *Adv Immunol* 90:51, 2006.

81. Ahmadzadeh M, Johnson LA, Heemskerk B, et al: Tumor antigen–specific CD8 T cells infiltrating the tumor express high levels of PD-1 and are functionally impaired. *Blood* 114:1537, 2009.

82. Schietinger A, Greenberg PD: Tolerance and exhaustion: Defining mechanisms of T cell dysfunction. *Trends Immunol* 35:51, 2014.

83. Gros A, Robbins PF, Yao X, et al: PD-1 identifies the patient-specific CD8+ tumor-reactive repertoire infiltrating human tumors. *J Clin Invest* 124:2246, 2014.

84. Dudley ME, Wunderlich J, Nishimura MI, et al: Adoptive transfer of cloned melanoma-reactive T lymphocytes for the treatment of patients with metastatic melanoma. *J Immunother* 24:363, 2001.

85. Park JR, DiGiusto DL, Slovak M, et al: Adoptive transfer of chimeric antigen receptor re-directed cytolytic T lymphocyte clones in patients with neuroblastoma. *Mol Ther* 15:825, 2007.

86. Yee C, Thompson JA, Roche P, et al: Melanocyte destruction after antigen-specific immunotherapy of melanoma: Direct evidence of T cell-mediated vitiligo. *J Exp Med* 192:1637, 2000.

87. Kershaw MH, Westwood JA, Parker LL, et al: A phase I study on adoptive immunotherapy using gene-modified T cells for ovarian cancer. *Clin Cancer Res* 12:6106, 2006.

88. Robbins PF, Dudley ME, Wunderlich J, et al: Cutting edge: Persistence of transferred lymphocyte clonotypes correlates with cancer regression in patients receiving cell transfer therapy. *J Immunol* 173:7125, 2004.

89. Rosenberg SA: Progress in human tumour immunology and immunotherapy. *Nature* 411:380, 2001.

90. Horowitz MM, Gale RP, Sondel PM, et al: Graft-versus-leukemia reactions after bone marrow transplantation. *Blood* 75:555, 1990.

91. Kolb H-J, Schmid C, Barrett AJ, et al: Graft-versus-leukemia reactions in allogeneic chimeras. *Blood* 103:767, 2004.

92. Bleakley M, Turtle CJ, Riddell SR: Augmentation of anti-tumor immunity by adoptive T-cell transfer after allogeneic hematopoietic stem cell transplantation. *Expert Rev Hematol* 5:409, 2012.

93. Schumacher TNM: T-cell-receptor gene therapy. *Nat Rev Immunol* 2:512, 2002.

94. Eshhar Z: Tumor-specific T-bodies: Towards chinical application. *Cancer Immunol Immunother* 45:131, 1997.

95. Jensen MC, Riddell SR: Design and implementation of adoptive therapy with chimeric antigen receptor-modified T cells. *Immunol Rev* 257:127, 2014.

96. Barrett DM, Singh N, Porter DL, et al: Chimeric antigen receptor therapy for cancer. *Annu Rev Med* 65:10. 1-10. 15, 2014.

97. Kershaw MH, Westwood JA, Darcy PK: Gene-engineered T cells for cancer therapy. *Nat Rev Cancer* 13:525, 2013.

98. Rosenberg SA, Yannelli JR, Yang JC, et al: Treatment of patients with metastatic melanoma with autologous tumor-infiltrating lymphocytes and interleukin 2. *J Natl Cancer Inst* 86:1159, 1994.

99. Rosenberg SA: A new era for cancer immunotherapy based on the genes that encode cancer antigens. *Immunity* 10:281, 1999.

100. Engelhard VH, Bullock TNJ, Coletta TA, et al: Antigens derived from melanocyte differentiation proteins: Self-tolerance, autoimmunity, and use for cancer immunotherapy. *Immunol Rev* 188:136, 2002.

101. Robbins PF, Lu YC, El-Gamil M, et al: Mining exomic sequencing data to identify mutated antigens recognized by adoptively transferred tumor-reactive T cells. *Nat Med* 19:747, 2013.

102. Dudley ME, Wunderlich JR, Shelton TE, et al: Generation of tumor-infiltrating lymphocyte cultures for use in adoptive transfer therapy for melanoma patients. *J Immunother* 26:332, 2003.

103. Yee C: The use of endogenous T cells for adoptive transfer. *Immunol Rev* 257:250, 2014.

104. Yee C, Thompson JA, Byrd D, et al: Adoptive T cell therapy using antigen-specific CD8+ T cell clones for the treatment of patients with metastatic melanoma: In vivo persistence, migration, and antitumor effect of transferred cells. *Proc Natl Acad Sci U S A* 99:16168, 2002.

105. Dudley ME, Wunderlich JR, Yang JR, et al: A phase I study of nonmyeloablative chemotherapy and adoptive transfer of autologous tumor antigen-specific T lymphocytes in patients with metastatic melanoma. *J Immunother* 25:243, 2002.

106. Gattinoni L, Klebanoff CA, Palmer DC, et al: Acquisition of full effector function in vitro paradoxically impairs the in vivo antitumor efficacy of adoptively transferred CD8+ T cells. *J Clin Invest* 115:1616, 2005.

107. Dudley ME, Wunderlich JR, Robbins PF, et al: Cancer regression and autoimmunity in patients after clonal repopulation with antitumor lymphocytes. *Science* 298:850, 2002.

108. Hinrichs CS, Rosenberg SA: Exploiting the curative potential of adoptive T-cell therapy for cancer. *Immunol Rev* 257:56, 2014.

109. Dudley ME, Wunderlich JR, Yang JC, et al: Adoptive cell transfer therapy following non-myeloablative but lymphodepleting chemotherapy for the treatment of patients with refractory metastatic melanoma. *J Clin Oncol* 23:2346, 2005.

110. Huang J, Khong HT, Dudley ME, et al: Survival, persistence, and progressive differentiation of adoptively transferred tumor-reactive T cells associated with tumor regression. *J Immunother* 28:258, 2005.

111. Rosenberg SA, Yang JC, Sherry RM, et al: Durable complete responses in heavily pre-treated patients with metastatic melanoma using T-cell transfer immunotherapy. *Clin Cancer Res* 17:4550, 2011.

112. Schluns KS, Lefrançois L: Cytokine control of memory T-cell development and survival. *Nat Rev Immunol* 3:269, 2003.

113. Chapuis AG, Thompson JA, Margolin KA, et al: Transferred melanoma-specific CD8+ T cells persist, mediate tumor regression, and acquire central memory phenotype. *Proc Natl Acad Sci U S A* 109:4592, 2012.

114. Colombo MP, Piconese S: Regulatory T-cell inhibition versus depletion: The right choice in cancer immunotherapy. *Nat Rev Cancer* 7:880, 2007.

115. Wrzesinski C, Paulos CM, Gattinoni L, et al: Hematopoietic stem cells promote the expansion and function of adoptively transferred antitumor CD8+ T cells. *J Clin Invest* 117:492, 2007.

116. Dudley ME, Yang JC, Sherry R, et al: Adoptive cell therapy for patients with metastatic melanoma: Evaluation of intensive myeloablative chemoradiation preparative regimens. *J Clin Oncol* 26:5233, 2008.

117. Prickett TD, Agrawal NS, Wei X, et al: Analysis of the tyrosine kinome in melanoma reveals recurrent mutations in ERBB4. *Nat Genet* 41:1127, 2009.

118. Kvistborg P, Shu CJ, Heemskerk B, et al: TIL therapy broadens the tumor-reactive CD8+ T cell compartment in melanoma patients. *Oncoimmunology* 1:409, 2012.

119. Lu YC, Yao X, Crystal JS, et al: Efficient identification of mutated cancer antigens recognized by T cells associated with durable tumor regressions. *Clin Cancer Res* 20:3401, 2014.

120. Tran E, Turcotte S, Gros A, et al: Cancer immunotherapy based on mutation-specific CD4+ T cells in a patient with epithelial cancer. *Science* 344:641, 2014.

121. Rezvani K, Barrett AJ: Characterizing and optimizing immune responses to leukaemia antigens after allogeneic stem cell transplantation. *Best Pract Res Clin Haematol* 21:437, 2008.

122. Spierings E, Kim YH, Hendriks M, et al: Multicenter analyses demonstrate significant clinical effects of minor histocompatibility antigens on GvHD and GvL after HLA-matched related and unrelated hematopoietic stem cell transplantation. *Biol Blood Marrow Transplant* 19:1244, 2013.

123. Bleakley M, Riddell SR: Molecules and mechanisms of the graft-versus-leukemia effect. *Nat Rev Cancer* 4:371, 2004.

124. Fontaine P, Roy-Proulx G, Knafo L, et al: Adoptive transfer of minor histocompatibility antigen-specific T lymphocytes eradicates leukemia cells without causing graft-versus-host disease. *Nat Med* 7:789, 2001.

125. Warren EH, Greenberg PD, Riddell SR: Cytotoxic T-lymphocyte-defined human minor histocompatibility antigens with a restricted tissue distribution. *Blood* 91:2197, 1998.

126. Bonnet D, Warren EH, Greenberg PD, et al: CD8+ minor histocompatibility antigen-specific cytotoxic T lymphocyte clones eliminate human acute myeloid leukemia stem cells. *Proc Natl Acad Sci U S A* 96:8639, 1999.

127. Carlson CS, Eberle MA, Rieder MJ, et al: Additional SNPs and linkage-disequilibrium analyses are necessary for whole-genome association studies in humans. *Nat Genet* 33:518, 2003.

128. Spierings E, Hendriks M, Absi L, et al: Phenotype frequencies of autosomal minor histocompatibility antigens display significant differences among populations. *PLoS Genet* 3:e103, 2007.

129. Warren EH, Vigneron NJ, Gavin MA, et al: An antigen produced by splicing of noncontiguous peptides in the reverse order. *Science* 313:1444, 2006.

130. Oostvogels R, Minnema MC, van Elk M, et al: Towards effective and safe immunotherapy after allogeneic stem cell transplantation: Identification of hematopoietic-specific minor histocompatibility antigen UTA2-1. *Leukemia* 27:642, 2013.

131. Marijt WAE, Heemskerk MHM, Kloosterboer FM, et al: Hematopoiesis-restricted minor histocompatibility antigens HA-1- or HA-2-specific T cells can induce complete remissions of relapsed leukemia. *Proc Natl Acad Sci U S A* 100:2742, 2003.

132. de Rijke B, van Horssen-Zoetbrood A, Beekman JM, et al: A frameshift polymorphism in P2X5 elicits an allogeneic cytotoxic T lymphocyte response associated with remission of chronic myeloid leukemia. *J Clin Invest* 115:3506, 2005.

133. Randolph SSB, Gooley TA, Warren EH, et al: Female donors contribute to a selective graft-versus-leukemia effect in male recipients of HLA-matched, related hematopoietic cell transplants. *Blood* 103:347, 2004.

134. Warren EH, Gavin MA, Simpson E, et al: The human UTY gene encodes a novel HLA-B8-restricted H-Y antigen. *J Immunol* 164:2807, 2000.

135. Van Elsas A, Nijman HW, Van der Minne CE, et al: Induction and characterization of cytotoxic T-lymphocytes recognizing a mutated p21ras peptide presented by HLA-A*0201. *Int J Cancer* 61:389, 1995.

136. Bocchia M, Korontsvit T, Xu Q, et al: Specific human cellular immunity to bcr-abl oncogene-derived peptides. *Blood* 87:3587, 1996.

137. Molldrem J, Dermime S, Parker K, et al: Targeted T-cell therapy for human leukemia: Cytotoxic T lymphocytes specific for a peptide derived from proteinase 3 preferentially lyse human myeloid leukemia cells. *Blood* 88:2450, 1996.

138. Molldrem JJ, Lee PP, Wang C, et al: Evidence that specific T lymphocytes may participate in the elimination of chronic myelogenous leukemia. *Nat Med* 6:1018, 2000.

139. Sergeeva A, Alatrash G, He H, et al: An anti-PR1/HLA-A2 T-cell receptor-like antibody mediates complement-dependent cytotoxicity against acute myeloid leukemia progenitor cells. *Blood* 117:4262, 2011.

140. Bellantuono I, Gao L, Parry S, et al: Two distinct HLA-A0201-presented epitopes of the Wilms tumor antigen 1 can function as targets for leukemia-reactive CTL. *Blood* 100:3835, 2002.

141. Doubrovina E, Carpenter T, Pankov D, et al: Mapping of novel peptides of WT-1 and presenting HLA alleles that induce epitope-specific HLA-restricted T cells with cytotoxic activity against WT-1(+) leukemias. *Blood* 120:1633, 2012.

142. Ochsenreither S, Majeti R, Schmitt T, et al: Cyclin-A1 represents a new immunogenic targetable antigen expressed in acute myeloid leukemia stem cells with characteristics of a cancer-testis antigen. *Blood* 119:5492, 2012.

143. Menssen HD, Renkl HJ, Entezami M, et al: Wilms' tumor gene expression in human CD34+ hematopoietic progenitors during fetal development and early clonogenic growth. *Blood* 89:3486, 1997.

144. Gao L, Bellantuono I, Elsässer A, et al: Selective elimination of leukemic CD34+ progenitor cells by cytotoxic T lymphocytes specific for WT1. *Blood* 95:2198, 2000.

145. Rezvani K, Yong ASM, Savani BN, et al: Graft-versus-leukemia effects associated with detectable Wilms tumor-1–specific T lymphocytes after allogeneic stem-cell transplantation for acute lymphoblastic leukemia. *Blood* 110:1924, 2007.

146. Chapuis AG, Ragnarsson GB, Nguyen HN, et al: Transferred WT1-reactive CD8+ T cells can mediate antileukemic activity and persist in post-transplant patients. *Sci Transl Med* 5:174ra27, 2013.

147. Cooper LJN, Kalos M, Lewinsohn DA, et al: Transfer of specificity for human immunodeficiency virus type 1 into primary human T lymphocytes by introduction of T-cell receptor genes. *J Virol* 74:8207, 2000.

148. van Loenen MM, de Boer R, Hagedoorn RS, et al: Optimization of the HA-1-specific T-cell receptor for gene therapy of hematologic malignancies. *Haematologica* 96:477, 2011.

149. Morgan RA, Dudley ME, Wunderlich JR, et al: Cancer regression in patients after transfer of genetically engineered lymphocytes. *Science* 314:126, 2006.

150. Bendle GM, Linnemann C, Hooijkaas AI, et al: Lethal graft-versus-host disease in mouse models of T cell receptor gene therapy. *Nat Med* 16:565, 2010.

151. Cohen CJ, Li YF, El-Gamil M, et al: Enhanced antitumor activity of T cells engineered to express T-cell receptors with a second disulfide bond. *Cancer Res* 67:3898, 2007.

152. Kuball J, Dossett ML, Wolfl M, et al: Facilitating matched pairing and expression of TCR-chains introduced into human T-cells. *Blood* 109:2331, 2007.

153. Cohen CJ, Zhao Y, Zheng Z, et al: Enhanced antitumor activity of murine-human hybrid T-cell receptor (TCR) in human lymphocytes is associated with improved pairing and TCR/CD3 stability. *Cancer Res* 66:8878, 2006.

154. Provasi E, Genovese P, Lombardo A, et al: Editing T cell specificity towards leukemia by zinc finger nucleases and lentiviral gene transfer. *Nat Med* 18:807, 2012.

155. Bunse M, Bendle GM, Linnemann C, et al: RNAi-mediated TCR knockdown prevents autoimmunity in mice caused by mixed TCR dimers following TCR gene transfer. *Mol Ther* 22:1983, 2014.

156. Kirchgessner H, Dietrich J, Scherer J, et al: The transmembrane adaptor protein TRIM regulates T cell receptor (TCR) Expression and TCR-mediated signaling via an association with the TCRζ Chain. *J Exp Med* 193:1269, 2001.

157. Johnson LA, Morgan RA, Dudley ME, et al: Gene therapy with human and mouse T cell receptors mediates cancer regression and targets normal tissues expressing cognate antigen. *Blood* 114:535, 2009.

158. Linette GP, Stadtmauer EA, Maus MV, et al: Cardiovascular toxicity and titin cross-reactivity of affinity enhanced T cells in myeloma and melanoma. *Blood* 122:863, 2013.

159. Cameron BJ, Gerry AB, Dukes J, et al: Identification of a titin-derived HLA-A1–presented peptide as a cross-reactive target for engineered MAGE A3–directed T cells. *Sci Transl Med* 5:197ra103, 2013.

160. Morgan RA, Chinnasamy N, Abate-Daga D, et al: Cancer regression and neurological toxicity following anti-MAGE-A3 TCR gene therapy. *J Immunother* 36:133, 2013.

161. Parkhurst MR, Yang JC, Langan RC, et al: T cells targeting carcinoembryonic antigen can mediate regression of metastatic colorectal cancer but induce severe transient colitis. *Mol Ther* 19:620, 2011.

162. Robbins PF, Morgan RA, Feldman SA, et al: Tumor regression in patients with metastatic synovial cell sarcoma and melanoma using genetically engineered lymphocytes reactive with NY-ESO-1. *J Clin Oncol* 29:917, 2011.

163. Turtle CJ, Hudecek M, Jensen MC, et al: Engineered T cells for anti-cancer therapy. *Curr Opin Immunol* 24:633, 2012.

164. Riddell SR, Jensen MC, June CH: Chimeric antigen receptor-modified T cells: Clinical translation in stem cell transplantation and beyond. *Biol Blood Marrow Transplant* 19:52, 2013.

165. Sadelain M, Rivière I, Brentjens RJ: Targeting tumours with genetically enhanced T lymphocytes. *Nat Rev Cancer* 3:35, 2003.

166. Brentjens RJ, Santos E, Nikhamin Y, et al: Genetically targeted T cells eradicate systemic acute lymphoblastic leukemia xenografts. *Clin Cancer Res* 13:5426, 2007.

167. Kalos M, June CH: Adoptive T cell transfer for cancer immunotherapy in the era of synthetic biology. *Immunity* 39:49, 2013.

168. Maus MV, Grupp SA, Porter DL, et al: Antibody modified T cells: CARs take the front seat for hematologic malignancies. *Blood* 123:2625, 2014.

169. Wang J, Jensen M, Lin Y, et al: Optimizing adoptive polyclonal T cell immunotherapy of lymphomas, using a chimeric T cell receptor possessing CD28 and CD137 costimulatory domains. *Hum Gene Ther* 18:712, 2007.

170. Hudecek M, Schmitt TM, Baskar S, et al: The B-cell tumor associated antigen ROR1 can be targeted with T cells modified to express a ROR1-specific chimeric antigen receptor. *Blood* 116:4532, 2010.

171. Hudecek M, Lupo-Stanghellini MT, Kosasih PL, et al: Receptor affinity and extracellular domain modifications affect tumor recognition by ROR1-specific chimeric antigen receptor T cells. *Clin Cancer Res* 19:3153, 2013.

172. Borcherding N, Kusner D, Liu GH, et al: ROR1, an embryonic protein with an emerging role in cancer biology. *Protein Cell* 5:496, 2014.

173. Ritchie DS, Neeson PJ, Khot A, et al: Persistence and efficacy of second generation CAR T cell against the LeY antigen in acute myeloid leukemia. *Mol Ther* 21:2122, 2013.

174. Casucci M, Nicolis di Robilant B, Falcone L, et al: CD44v6-targeted T cells mediate potent antitumor effects against acute myeloid leukemia and multiple myeloma. *Blood* 122:3461, 2013.

175. Dutour A, Martin V, Pizzitola I, et al: In vitro and in vivo antitumor effect of anti-CD33 chimeric receptor-expressing EBV-CTL against CD33 acute myeloid leukemia. *Adv Immunol* 2012:683065, 2012.

176. Pizzitola I, Anjos-Afonso F, Rouault-Pierre K, et al: Chimeric antigen receptors against CD33/CD123 antigens efficiently target primary acute myeloid leukemia cells in vivo. *Leukemia* 28:1596, 2014.

177. Gill S, Tasian SK, Ruella M, et al: Preclinical targeting of human acute myeloid leukemia and myeloablation using chimeric antigen receptor–modified T cells. *Blood* 123:2343, 2014.

178. Sentman CLP, Meehan KRM: NKG2D CARs as cell therapy for cancer. *Cancer J* 20:156, 2014.

179. Carpenter RO, Evbuomwan MO, Pittaluga S, et al: B-cell maturation antigen is a promising target for adoptive T-cell therapy of multiple myeloma. *Clin Cancer Res* 19:2048, 2013.

180. Till BG, Jensen MC, Wang J, et al: Adoptive immunotherapy for indolent non-Hodgkin lymphoma and mantle cell lymphoma using genetically modified autologous CD20-specific T cells. *Blood* 112:2261, 2008.

181. Till BG, Jensen MC, Wang J, et al: CD20-specific adoptive immunotherapy for lymphoma using a chimeric antigen receptor with both CD28 and 4-1BB domains: Pilot clinical trial results. *Blood* 119:3940, 2012.

182. Grupp SA, Kalos M, Barrett D, et al: Chimeric antigen receptor–modified T cells for acute lymphoid leukemia. *N Engl J Med* 368:1509, 2013.

183. Brentjens RJ, Davila ML, Riviere I, et al: CD19-targeted T cells rapidly induce molecular remissions in adults with chemotherapy-refractory acute lymphoblastic leukemia. *Sci Transl Med* 5:177ra38, 2013.

184. Kochenderfer JN, Rosenberg SA: Treating B-cell cancer with T cells expressing anti-CD19 chimeric antigen receptors. *Nat Rev Clin Oncol* 10:267, 2013.

185. Cruz CR, Micklethwaite KP, Savoldo B, et al: Infusion of donor-derived CD19-redirected virus-specific T cells for B-cell malignancies relapsed after allogeneic stem cell transplant: A phase 1 study. *Blood* 122:2965, 2013.

186. Pule MA, Savoldo B, Myers GD, et al: Virus-specific T cells engineered to coexpress tumor-specific receptors: Persistence and antitumor activity in individuals with neuroblastoma. *Nat Med* 14:1264, 2008.

187. Beatty GL, Haas AR, Maus MV, et al: Mesothelin-specific chimeric antigen receptor mRNA-engineered T cells induce antitumor activity in solid malignancies. *Cancer Immunol Res* 2:112, 2014.

188. Morgan RA, Yang JC, Kitano M, et al: Case report of a serious adverse event following the administration of T cells transduced with a chimeric antigen receptor recognizing ERBB2. *Mol Ther* 18:843, 2010.

189. Lamers CHJ, Sleijfer S, Vilto AG, et al: Treatment of metastatic renal cell carcinoma with autologous T-lymphocytes genetically retargeted against carbonic anhydrase IX: First clinical experience. *J Clin Oncol* 24:e20-e22, 2006.

190. Lamers CH, Sleijfer S, van Steenbergen S, et al: Treatment of metastatic renal cell carcinoma with CAIX CAR-engineered T cells: Clinical evaluation and management of on-target toxicity. *Mol Ther* 21:904, 2013.

191. Kalos M, Levine BL, Porter DL, et al: T cells with chimeric antigen receptors have potent antitumor effects and can establish memory in patients with advanced leukemia. *Sci Transl Med* 3:95ra73, 2011.

192. Davila ML, Riviere I, Wang X, et al: Efficacy and toxicity management of 19-28z CAR T cell therapy in B cell acute lymphoblastic leukemia. *Sci Transl Med* 6:224ra25, 2014.

193. Lee DW, Gardner R, Porter DL, et al: Current concepts in the diagnosis and management of cytokine release syndrome. *Blood* 124:188, 2014.

194. Terakura S, Yamamoto TN, Gardner RA, et al: Generation of CD19-chimeric antigen receptor modified CD8+ T cells derived from virus-specific central memory T cells. *Blood* 119:72, 2012.

195. Abate-Daga D, Lagisetty KH, Tran E, et al: A novel chimeric antigen receptor against prostate stem cell antigen mediates tumor destruction in a humanized mouse model of pancreatic cancer. *Hum Gene Ther* 25:1003, 2014.

196. Kandalaft L, Powell D, Coukos G: A phase I clinical trial of adoptive transfer of folate receptor-alpha redirected autologous T cells for recurrent ovarian cancer. *J Transl Med* 10:157, 2012.

197. Tran E, Chinnasamy D, Yu Z, et al: Immune targeting of fibroblast activation protein triggers recognition of multipotent bone marrow stromal cells and cachexia. *J Exp Med* 210:1125, 2013.

198. van der Stegen SJC, Davies DM, Wilkie S, et al: Preclinical in vivo modeling of cytokine release syndrome induced by ErbB-retargeted human T cells: Identifying a window of therapeutic opportunity? *J Immunol* 191:4589, 2013.

199. Berger C, Berger M, Anderson DE, et al: A non-human primate model for analysis of safety, persistence, and function of adoptively transferred T cells. *J Med Primatol* 40:88, 2011.

200. Riley JL: Combination checkpoint blockade—taking melanoma immunotherapy to the next level. *N Engl J Med* 369:187, 2013.

201. Wolchok JD, Kluger H, Callahan MK, et al: Nivolumab plus ipilimumab in advanced melanoma. *N Engl J Med* 369:122, 2013.

202. Hamid O, Robert C, Daud A, et al: Safety and tumor responses with lambrolizumab (anti-PD-1) in melanoma. *N Engl J Med* 369:134, 2013.

203. Bonini C, Ferrari G, Verzeletti S, et al: HSV-TK gene transfer into donor lymphocytes for control of allogeneic graft-versus-leukemia. *Science* 276:1719, 1997.

204. Riddell SR, Elliott M, Lewinsohn DA, et al: T-cell mediated rejection of gene-modified HIV-specific cytotoxic T lymphocytes in HIV-infected patients. *Nat Med* 2:216, 1996.

205. Berger C, Blau CA, Huang ML, et al: Pharmacologically regulated Fas-mediated death of adoptively transferred T cells in a nonhuman primate model. *Blood* 103:1261, 2004.

206. Straathof KC, Pulè MA, Yotnda P, et al: An inducible caspase 9 safety switch for T-cell therapy. *Blood* 105:4247, 2005.

207. Budde LE, Berger C, Lin Y, et al: Combining a CD20 chimeric antigen receptor and an inducible caspase 9 suicide switch to improve the efficacy and safety of T cell adoptive immunotherapy for lymphoma. *PLoS One* 8:e82742, 2013.

208. Di Stasi A, Tey S-K, Dotti G, et al: Inducible apoptosis as a safety switch for adoptive cell therapy. *N Engl J Med* 365:1673, 2011.

209. Zhou X, Di Stasi A, Tey SK, et al: Long-term outcome after haploidentical stem cell transplant and infusion of T cells expressing the inducible caspase 9 safety transgene. *Blood* 123:3895, 2014.

CHAPTER 27
VACCINE THERAPY

Katayoun Rezvani and Jeffrey J. Molldrem*

SUMMARY

Vaccines are biologic substances that are designed to stimulate the host immune system to elicit a neutralizing response against clinically relevant targets, including pathogens and tumors. Active immunotherapy with vaccines has been extremely effective as prevention against infectious pathogens. However, effective vaccine therapy of chronic infectious diseases or cancer, in the therapeutic setting, remains a promising but largely unrealized goal. Hematologic malignancies are an excellent model system for vaccine therapies, in part because of accessibility to the hematopoietic and lymphatic space and susceptibility to immune effector mechanisms and availability of tumor cells for mechanistic studies.

●ADVANTAGES OF CANCER VACCINE THERAPY

Immunity elicited by therapeutic cancer vaccines offers several advantages over passive immunotherapy using monoclonal antibodies. In active immune therapy, all components of the effector immune response are host derived without murine or xenogeneic components that could cause indirect toxicity. The lack of foreign components also allows the host response to be sustained. Also, if the vaccine contains more than a single determinant of the target antigen, the immune response could be broad in scope, recognizing more than a single epitope in the antigen (polyclonal). This feature might be of particular importance for cancer immunotherapy, as mutation of individual peptide epitopes is a possible mechanism of immune evasion by tumors. In addition to inducing antibodies, which can recognize intact proteins on the surface of tumor cells, vaccines activate T cells that can recognize peptide fragments derived from proteins that may be endogenously processed and presented on the surface of tumor cells. Such T cells have various effector mechanisms capable of neutralizing tumor cells, including lysis of the tumor cell by cell-to-cell contact and the local production of cytokines that might directly neutralize tumor cells (e.g., interferon-γ).

*This chapter was written by Sattva S. Neelpu and Larry W. Kwak in the eighth edition and portions of that text have been retained.

●COMPONENTS OF THERAPEUTIC CANCER VACCINES

Most therapeutic cancer vaccines that are being tested in clinical trials have at least three components: antigenic material derived from the tumor, a carrier, and an adjuvant. The antigenic material is usually a protein or peptide derived from the tumor that is either uniquely expressed or is overexpressed in the tumor, compared with normal tissues. A unique tumor antigen or the overexpression of the antigen to prevent the tumor is necessary to prevent the induction of an unwanted autoimmune response against normal tissues following vaccination. The carrier is necessary for delivery of the tumor antigen to antigen-presenting cells, such as dendritic cells, so as to induce the immune response against the tumor antigen. The third component of a cancer vaccine, the adjuvant, is usually a cytokine or other nonspecific immune stimulant to facilitate an enhanced immune response against the tumor antigen.

ANTIGEN DISCOVERY

Both conventional and novel technologies used to define cancer-associated antigens, such as serologic analysis by recombinant expression cloning (SEREX), serial analysis of gene expression (SAGE), screening tumor complementary DNA (cDNA) libraries with tumor-reactive T cells, and characterization of peptides eluted from tumor-derived human leukocyte antigen (HLA) molecules, have resulted in a rapidly growing list of candidate tumor antigens for various hematologic malignancies (Table 27–1). The majority of these candidate antigens have been identified since 1998. Furthermore, the application of genomic and proteomic techniques, combined with the feasibility of isolating sufficient quantities of clonogenic tumor cells from individual patients, should identify additional targets that are differentially expressed in tumors as compared with normal tissues.

Desirable characteristics for candidate target antigens for immune therapy include antigens that are selectively or aberrantly expressed by the tumor or that are required to maintain the malignant cell phenotype or cell survival. Even though the adaptive immune response is comprised of both humoral and cellular components, most efforts at tumor vaccination have focused on eliciting T-cell responses because of their central role in regulating and mediating the overall adaptive response (Chap. 76). Host T-cell recognition of such antigens requires that they are naturally processed and presented by tumor cells into peptides that bind host HLA molecules. Optimally, the candidate antigen should contain both CD4+ and CD8+ T-cell epitopes. Antigens recognized by humoral immune responses must be expressed on the tumor cell surface, and the relevant epitopes must be accessible to antibody molecules. Immunogenic tumor antigens should provoke a strong effector response and not induce tolerance.

Vaccine therapy does not necessarily require a completely defined tumor antigen. Vaccines can consist of whole tumor cells or subcellular components containing putative antigens. For example, autologous tumor cells engineered to overexpress cytokines such as granulocyte-macrophage colony-stimulating factor (GM-CSF),[15,16] or activated ex vivo by CD40 receptor engagement,[17] can be effective at inducing tumor-specific T cells with as yet undefined antigen specificity. Similarly, transfer of the gene encoding CD40-ligand into chronic lymphocytic leukemia cells induced CD4+ and CD8+ T-cell responses in human patients.[18] Vaccination with membrane proteins extracted from tumor cells and incorporated into liposomes along with interleukin (IL)-2 is another strategy that is in clinical testing.[19]

TABLE 27–1. Examples of Candidate Human Tumor Antigens for Hematologic Cancers

Antigen	Reference
Minor histocompatibility antigens (HA-1, HA-2)	1
Proteinase-3	2
Wilms tumor antigen-1	3
B-cell receptor (immunoglobulin idiotype)	4
Anaplastic lymphoma kinase	5
Sperm protein 17	6
Sperm protein associated with the nucleus on X chromosome (SPAN-X)	7
CML-66	8
Survivin	9
HM1.24	10
Immature laminin receptor protein	11
BCR-ABL fusion protein	12
Aurora kinase	13
Fibromodulin	14

VACCINE DELIVERY

Effective delivery of the target antigen to the immune system is critical for the successful induction of immunity. For most tumor antigens, this is a daunting challenge, as most antigens (with the exception of viral antigens associated with cancers) are weakly immunogenic, self, or tissue-differentiation antigens.

Many vaccine-delivery strategies use dendritic cells. These key antigen-presenting cells are principally responsible for initiating a host immune response.[20] The cells, represented in minute quantities, have the powerful capacity to take up antigens, and once activated, to present processed peptides to T cells. Accordingly, optimizing the delivery of tumor antigens to specialized antigen-presenting cells is critical. Such efforts have included isolation of dendritic cells from blood, followed by physical loading with protein or peptide antigens, or introducing the genes for candidate antigens by transfection with cDNA or messenger RNA, or by fusion with whole tumor cells. Loaded dendritic cells have been administered to patients as vaccines.[21]

An alternative strategy is to target the delivery of antigens to dendritic cells *in vivo*. Traditional approaches focused on attempts to make the antigen look foreign to the host immune system; for example, by chemical linkage to larger, highly immunogenic proteins (carriers) or incorporation into liposomes. Rational approaches to increase the efficiency of antigen delivery to dendritic cells have included genetic fusion of the gene encoding the antigen to one encoding biologically active molecules that has the ability to target cell-surface receptors on antigen-presenting cells. Such targeting molecules have included cytokines, chemokines, antibody Fc or Fab fragments, transferrin, CD40, and mannose, which serve as ligands for specific receptors on antigen-presenting cells.[22] Such molecular vaccines can be administered as naked DNA or as fusion proteins. Other promising approaches to target dendritic cells *in vivo* are represented by recombinant viral or bacterial vectors or virus-like particles.[23,24]

IMMUNOSTIMULANTS TO ENHANCE VACCINE EFFICACY

Traditionally, immunologic adjuvants, described by the late Charles Janeway as "immunology's dirty little secret," such as alum and oil-in-water emulsions (e.g., incomplete Freund adjuvant), provide a physical depot for slow release of antigen. Adjuvants also serve as general immune stimulants by providing a danger signal to activate antigen-presenting cells. This feature describes classical adjuvant components, such as bacterial cell wall extracts, as well as unmethylated CpG DNA sequences, which deliver maturation signals to dendritic cells through toll-like receptors (Chap. 20).[25] The incorporation of either recombinant cytokines or their genes into vaccine formulations may increase vaccine potency by broadly enhancing the function of either antigen-presenting cells or T cells. Consequently, cytokines, such as interferon-γ, IL-2, and IL-15, may be useful as components of vaccines.[26] Such cytokines also can help direct the type of immune response elicited. For example, IL-12 elicits primarily T-helper (Th) type 1 cell responses, whereas the inclusion of IL-4 or IL-10 generally induces predominantly Th2 cell responses (Chap. 76). Some cytokines, such as GM-CSF, which can induce dendritic cell differentiation, can also function as an adjuvant by recruiting antigen-presenting cells to local vaccination sites.[27]

● CLINICAL TRIAL DESIGN

Cancer vaccine trials might not fit into the paradigm developed for chemotherapeutic agents, which have direct effects on tumor and normal host cells. For example, studies in heavily pretreated patients with terminal disease might be inappropriate for vaccines, which generally require an intact host immune system. For this reason, even safety cannot be evaluated completely in patients who cannot make an immune response, because any toxicity will likely be indirect, resulting from the immune response elicited. In addition, animal models show that the immune system may be more effective at clearing minimal residual disease than at clearing advanced tumor cell burdens. Accordingly, several late-stage clinical trials of cancer vaccines are testing this approach in the setting of clinical remission, after primary surgery or chemotherapy.

Although conventional clinical trials generally test one experimental agent at a time, vaccine formulations may contain several components. The simultaneous optimization of multiple variables (e.g., vaccine and adjuvant dose and schedule, and routes of administration) in a single clinical study often requires the application of novel, more flexible clinical trial design.[28]

ASSAYS OF VACCINE EFFICACY

The development of surrogate measures of vaccine efficacy has potential value for answering the scientific question of whether it is even possible to vaccinate human patients against a candidate antigen. Traditional assays of immune response, including simple lymphoproliferation and cytotoxicity assays, requiring prolonged periods of prior stimulation, are being replaced by quantitative assays that can measure effector function of T cells directly sampled from blood (e.g., enzyme-linked immunospot assay) and by sensitive tetramer binding assays (Table 27–2).[29] In some cases, tetramer-binding assays have been combined with intracellular cytokine production to provide both quantitative and functional analyses of antigen-specific T cells.[30] An important aim of clinical trials is to determine which, if any, of these measures of immune response are valid surrogates for vaccine efficacy.

TABLE 27–2. Monitoring of Human Immune Responses

Type of Response	Representative Assay
CD4+ T cells	Cytokine induction
	Cytokine ELISPOT (IFN-γ)
	Intracellular cytokine
	Proliferation
CD8+ T cells	Cytotoxicity
	Limiting dilution analysis
	Tetramer
	Cytokine ELISPOT (IFN-γ)
	Intracellular cytokine
Antibody	ELISA
	Flow cytometry
	ELISPOT
Multiple	Microarray
	Cytokine mRNA by RT-PCR
	T-cell spectratyping

ELISA, enzyme-linked immunoabsorbent assay; ELISPOT, enzyme-linked immunospot assay; IFN, interferon; mRNA, messenger RNA; RT-PCR, reverse transcriptase polymerase chain reaction.

CLINICAL TRIALS OF PEPTIDE VACCINATION IN MYELOID LEUKEMIAS

Peptide vaccines derived from primary granule proteins, including proteinase 3, the Wilms tumor 1 protein (WT1), and the fusion sequence of the BCR-ABL protein of chronic myelogenous leukemia, show promising results in early trials of patients with myeloid leukemias.[27–31] Both WT1 and PR1 vaccines (a 9 amino acid peptide derived from proteinase 3) induce peptide-specific cytotoxic CD8+ T cells, which are associated with a fall in WT1 expression, and have induced complete and partial remissions in patients with myeloid leukemia who have relapsed. Other vaccines, such as BCR-ABL peptides and heat-shock protein 70 peptide complexes, have also been administered to patients with chronic myelogenous leukemia on conventional treatment with imatinib or interferon-α. Vaccination was associated with a reduction in BCR-ABL transcripts and cytogenetic or molecular responses in some patients.[31] These preliminary trials show that peptide vaccines that target patients with myeloid malignancies are safe and can induce responses in a subset of patients.

B-CELL ANTIGEN-RECEPTOR VACCINES AS SCIENTIFIC PROOF OF PRINCIPLE

B cells are clonally restricted to express surface immunoglobulin receptors that have unique epitopes present in the antibody variable region termed idiotypes (Chap. 75). Idiotypes expressed by B-cell malignancies are clonally distributed and thus can serve as tumor-specific target antigen for specific immunotherapy. Idiotypes were initially validated as tumor-rejection antigens in mouse models of myeloma and lymphoma,[31,32] and the first clinical trial testing this approach in human patients with lymphoma was reported in 1992.[33,34] Customized idiotype proteins were isolated by heterohybridoma fusion, conjugated chemically to keyhole limpet hemocyanin (KLH), which functioned as a

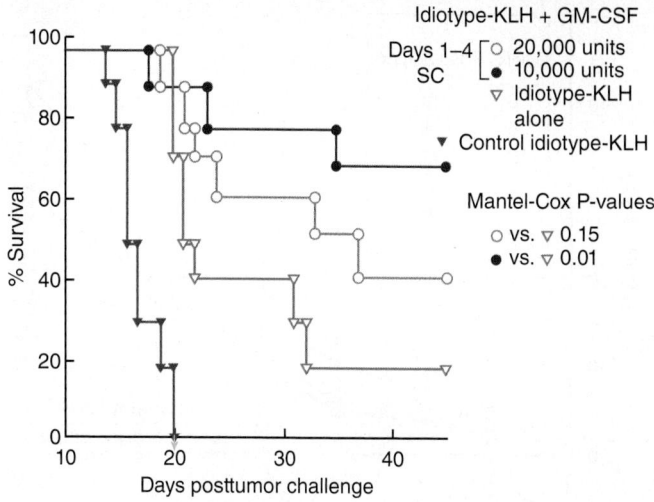

Figure 27–1. Granulocyte-monocyte colony-stimulating factor (GM-CSF) enhances lymphoma vaccine potency. Mice were vaccinated subcutaneously with idiotype keyhole limpet hemocyanin (KLH) protein, together with or without various doses of GM-CSF and challenged with a lethal dose of syngeneic lymphoma cells. The use of 10,000 units of GM-CSF plus idiotype KLH conjugate on days 1 to 4 (*closed dots*) resulted in a significantly longer survival after tumor challenge than did idiotype KLH conjugate vaccination alone.

carrier, and emulsified in a simple oil-in-water emulsion. These vaccines elicited predominantly antibody responses.

Subsequently, guided by additional data from murine lymphoma models (Fig. 27–1), recombinant GM-CSF protein was substituted as the immunologic adjuvant. Soluble GM-CSF, initially mixed with the vaccine and then administered for three additional daily doses subcutaneously as close as possible to the original site of immunization, significantly enhanced vaccine potency, consistent with previous gene therapy studies.[35] The cellular mechanism of this effect required CD8+ and CD4+ T cells.[36]

A phase II study was designed to test these vaccines in the setting of minimal residual disease, defined as first remission after chemotherapy in follicular lymphoma patients.[4] Previously untreated patients first received treatment with uniform chemotherapy to achieve complete remission. After a 6-month break to allow for immune reconstitution, idiotype proteins conjugated with KLH plus GM-CSF vaccines were administered in five monthly doses. Surrogate assays for vaccine efficacy were developed that used autologous lymphoma cells as targets for both B- and T-cell responses. In 19 patients (86 percent), vaccination elicited CD8+ cytotoxic T-lymphocyte cells reactive with the lymphoma cell (Fig. 27–2). More than half of the patients remain in continuous first complete remission, even after a median followup of more than 7 years. A randomized, controlled phase III trial testing this vaccine formulation in follicular lymphoma patients in first remission was reported to improve disease-free survival as compared with controls, suggesting that therapeutic cancer vaccines could induce meaningful clinical benefit in cancer patients.[37]

IMPEDIMENTS TO VACCINE THERAPY

Despite the success of the idiotype vaccine phase III trial in follicular lymphoma, most other phase III trials of cancer vaccines have been disappointing and objective clinical response rates have been low. Potential reasons for the failure despite the high immunogenicity of vaccines[38] may be categorized into factors affecting the afferent or priming phase

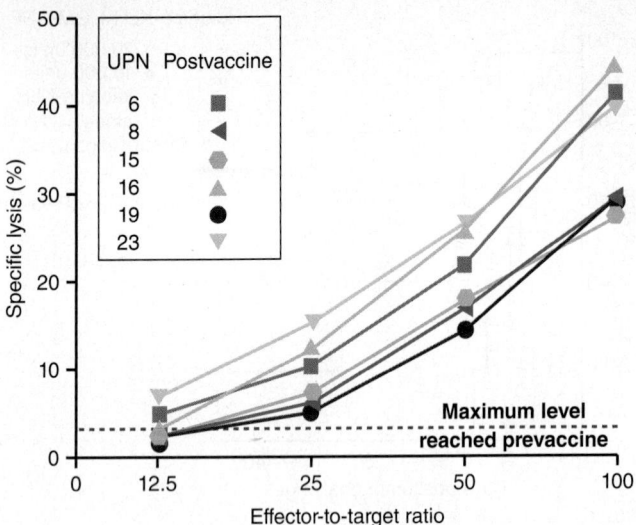

Figure 27–2. T-cell–mediated lysis of human autologous lymphoma cells after vaccination with idiotype keyhole limpet hemocyanin (KLH) protein plus granulocyte-monocyte colony-stimulating factor (GM-CSF). Representative results are shown from six individual patients, designated by unique patient number *(UPN)*. *(Adapted with permission from Bendandi M, Gocke CD, Kobrin CB, et al: Complete molecular remissions induced by patient-specific vaccination plus granulocyte-monocyte colony-stimulating factor against lymphoma. Nat Med 5(10):1171–1177, 1999.)*

of the immune response and factors influencing the efferent or effector phase of the immune response. For instance, during the afferent phase of the immune response, it is possible that the magnitude of the T-cell response or the avidity of the induced T-cells was not high enough following vaccination. During the effector phase of the immune response, it is possible that the antitumor T-cells may not have trafficked to the tumor site or, if they trafficked, they may not have been able to overcome newly recognized immunosuppressive mechanisms present in the tumor microenvironment. Several immunosuppressive mechanisms were shown to impair the function of tumor-specific effector T cells in the tumor microenvironment in several animal models and in some human cancers.[39] Important negative regulatory pathways that inhibit T-cell function include extrinsic suppression by regulatory T-cells; direct inhibition through inhibitory ligands such as cytotoxic T-lymphocyte antigen-4 (CTLA-4); programmed death-ligand (PD L) 1, PD-L2, and B7-H4; soluble factors such as transforming growth factor β and IL-10; and metabolic dysregulation of essential amino acids such as tryptophan.[39] Therapeutic monoclonal antibodies such as ipilimumab and pembrolizumab that block the immune checkpoint pathways mediated by CTLA-4 and programmed cell death protein-1 (PD-1), respectively, prevent downregulation of T-cell responses and enhance anti-tumor immunity[40] and are effective in the treatment of nonhematopoietic tumors. Such immune checkpoint inhibitors offer a novel therapeutic approach that might be highly relevant for hematopoietic tumors.

● FUTURE DIRECTIONS

Advances in understanding of immune tolerance and tumor-induced immunosuppression have now provided several novel agents to augment both the afferent and efferent phases of the immune responses in combination strategies with therapeutic vaccines. It is, therefore, an appropriate time to consider the best way in which leukemia vaccines might be incorporated into the overall treatment strategy for that cancer.

One strategy is to vaccinate patients after chemotherapy, when a state of minimal residual disease has been achieved. Moreover, lymphopenia induced by chemotherapy can also enhance antitumor immunity by promoting expansion of vaccine-induced effector T cells and minimizing tumor-induced immune suppression.[33] In this setting, the profound lymphopenia from chemotherapy results in release of cytokines, such as IL-15, providing a powerful proliferative drive to lymphocytes, which could be exploited to increase specific lymphocyte responses to the vaccine. Moreover, this strategy can eradicate cells that suppress antitumor responses such as regulatory T cells, and may overcome inherent defects in T-cell signaling, processing, or presentation.[33] In addition, the afferent phase of the immune response could be enhanced by using more potent vaccines with novel adjuvants such as toll-like receptor ligands, or by vaccinating donors of transplant recipients who have a healthy immune system as opposed to patients who may be immunocompromised either from the cancer or from therapy.[41] Alternatively, vaccines could be used in combination with agents that inhibit immunosuppressive mechanisms, such as immune checkpoint receptors/ligands[42] and/or deplete regulatory T cells,[43] to augment the afferent and/or effector phase of the immune response. The use of these agents in combination with therapeutic cancer vaccines may lead to enhanced antitumor immunity and improved clinical outcome.

REFERENCES

1. Marijt WA, Heemskerk MH, Kloosterboer FM, et al: Hematopoiesis-restricted minor histocompatibility antigens HA-1- or HA-2-specific T cells can induce complete remissions of relapsed leukemia. *Proc Natl Acad Sci U S A* 100:2742, 2003.
2. Molldrem JJ, Komanduri K, Wieder E: Overexpressed differentiation antigens as targets of graft-versus-leukemia reactions. *Curr Opin Hematol* 9:503, 2002.
3. Bellantuono I, Gao L, Parry S, et al: Two distinct HLA-A0201-presented epitopes of the Wilms tumor antigen 1 can function as targets for leukemia-reactive CTL. *Blood* 100:3835, 2002.
4. Bendandi M, Gocke CD, Kobrin CB, et al: Complete molecular remissions induced by patient-specific vaccination plus granulocyte-monocyte colony-stimulating factor against lymphoma. *Nat Med* 5:1171, 1999.
5. Passoni L, Scardino A, Bertazzoli C, et al: ALK as a novel lymphoma-associated tumor antigen: Identification of 2 HLA-A2.1-restricted CD8+ T-cell epitopes. *Blood* 99:2100, 2002.
6. Lim SH, Wang Z, Chiriva-Internati M, et al: Sperm protein 17 is a novel cancer-testis antigen in multiple myeloma. *Blood* 97:1508, 2001.
7. Wang Z, Zhang Y, Liu H, et al: Gene expression and immunologic consequence of SPAN-Xb in myeloma and other hematologic malignancies. *Blood* 101:955, 2003.
8. Yang XF, Wu CJ, Mclaughlin S, et al: CML66, a broadly immunogenic tumor antigen, elicits a humoral immune response associated with remission of chronic myelogenous leukemia. *Proc Natl Acad Sci U S A* 98:7492, 2001.
9. Zeis M, Siegel S, Wagner A, et al: Generation of cytotoxic responses in mice and human individuals against hematological malignancies using survivin-RNA-transfected dendritic cells. *J Immunol* 170:5391, 2003.
10. Chiriva-Internati M, Liu Y, Weidanz JA, et al: Testing recombinant adeno-associated virus-gene loading of dendritic cells for generating potent cytotoxic T lymphocytes against a prototype self-antigen, multiple myeloma HM1.24. *Blood* 102:3100, 2003.
11. Siegel S, Wagner A, Kabelitz D, et al: Induction of cytotoxic T-cell responses against the oncofetal antigen-immature laminin receptor for the treatment of hematologic malignancies. *Blood* 102:4416, 2003.
12. Pinilla-Ibarz J, Cathcart K, Korontsvit T, et al: Vaccination of patients with chronic myelogenous leukemia with bcr-abl oncogene breakpoint fusion peptides generates specific immune responses. *Blood* 95:1781, 2000.
13. Ochi T, Fujiwara H, Suemori K, et al: Aurora-A kinase: A novel target of cellular immunotherapy for leukemia. *Blood* 113:66, 2009.
14. Mayr C, Bund D, Schlee M, et al: Fibromodulin as a novel tumor-associated antigen (TAA) in chronic lymphocytic leukemia (CLL), which allows expansion of specific CD8+ autologous T lymphocytes. *Blood* 105:1566, 2005.
15. Levitsky HI, Montgomery J, Ahmadzadeh M, et al: Immunization with granulocyte-macrophage colony-stimulating factor-transduced, but not B7-1-transduced, lymphoma cells primes idiotype-specific T cells and generates potent systemic antitumor immunity. *J Immunol* 156:3858, 1996.
16. Dranoff G: Cytokines in cancer pathogenesis and cancer therapy. *Nat Rev Cancer* 4:11, 2004.
17. von Bergwelt-Baildon MS, Vonderheide RH, Maecker B, et al: Human primary and memory cytotoxic T lymphocyte responses are efficiently induced by means of CD40-activated B cells as antigen-presenting cells: Potential for clinical application. *Blood* 99:3319, 2002.

18. Wierda WG, Cantwell MJ, Woods SJ: CD40-ligand (CD154) gene therapy for chronic lymphocytic leukemia. *Blood* 96:2917, 2000.

19. Neelapu SS, Gause BL, Harvey L, et al. A novel proteoliposomal vaccine induces antitumor immunity against follicular lymphoma. *Blood* 109:5160, 2007.

20. Liu YJ: Dendritic cell subsets and lineages, and their functions in innate and adaptive immunity. *Cell* 106:259, 2001.

21. Cerundolo V, Hermans IF, Salio M: Dendritic cells: A journey from laboratory to clinic. *Nat Immunol* 5:7, 2004.

22. Biragyn A, Kwak LW: Designer cancer vaccines are still in fashion. *Nat Med* 6:966, 2000.

23. Tartour E, Benchetrit F, Haicheur N, et al: Synthetic and natural non-live vectors: Rationale for their clinical development in cancer vaccine protocols. *Vaccine* 20 (Suppl 4):A32, 2002.

24. Zhang L, Tang Y, Akbulut H, et al: An adenoviral vector cancer vaccine that delivers a tumor-associated antigen/CD40-ligand fusion protein to dendritic cells. *Proc Natl Acad Sci U S A* 100:15101, 2003.

25. Kreig AM: CpG motifs in bacterial DNA and their immune effects. *Annu Rev Immunol* 20:709, 2002.

26. Waldmann TA, Dubois S, Tagaya Y: Contrasting roles of IL-2 and IL-15 in the life and death of lymphocytes: Implications for immunotherapy. *Immunity* 14:105, 2001.

27. Qazilbash MH, Wieder ED, Thall PF, et al: PR1 peptide vaccine-induced immune response is associated with better event-free survival in patients with myeloid leukemia. *Blood* 110:Abstract 283, 2007.

28. Rezvani K, Yong AS, Tawab A, et al: *Ex vivo* characterization of polyclonal memory CD8+ T-cell responses to PRAME-specific peptides in patients with acute lymphoblastic leukemia and acute and chronic myeloid leukemia. *Blood* 113:2245, 2009.

29. Oka Y, Tsuboi A, Taguchi T, et al: Induction of WT1 (Wilms' tumor gene)-specific cytotoxic T lymphocytes by WT1 peptide vaccine and the resultant cancer regression. *Proc Natl Acad Sci U S A* 101:13885, 2004.

30. Brentjens RJ, Rivière I, Park JH, et al: Safety and persistence of adoptively transferred autologous CD19-targeted T cells in patients with relapsed or chemotherapy refractory B-cell leukemias. *Blood* 118:4817, 2011.

31. Bocchia M, Gentili S, Abruzzese E, et al: Effect of a p210 multipeptide vaccine associated with imatinib or interferon in patients with chronic myeloid leukaemia and persistent residual disease: A multicentre observational trial. *Lancet* 365:657, 2005.

32. Pardoll DM: Spinning molecular immunology into successful immunotherapy. *Nat Rev Immunol* 2:227, 2002.

33. Surh CD, Sprent J: Regulation of mature T cell homeostasis. *Semin Immunol* 17:183, 2005.

34. Simon RM, Steinberg SM, Hamilton M, et al: Clinical trial designs for the early clinical development of therapeutic cancer vaccines. *J Clin Oncol* 19:1848, 2001.

35. Lyerly HK: Quantitating cellular immune responses to cancer vaccines. *Semin Oncol* 30(3 Suppl 8):9, 2003.

36. Lee PP, Yee C, Savage PA, et al: Characterization of circulating T cells specific for tumor-associated antigens in melanoma patients. *Nat Med* 5:677, 1999.

37. Lynch RG, Graff RJ, Sirisinha S, et al: Myeloma proteins as tumor-specific transplantation antigens. *Proc Natl Acad Sci U S A* 69:1540, 1972.

38. Stevenson GT, Elliott EV, Stevenson FK: Idiotypic determinants on the surface of immunoglobulin of neoplastic lymphocytes: A therapeutic target. *Fed Proc* 36:2268, 1977.

39. Kwak LW, Campbell MJ, Czerwinski DK, et al: Induction of immune responses in patients with B-cell lymphoma against the surface-immunoglobulin idiotype expressed by their tumors. *N Engl J Med* 327:1209, 1992.

40. Pardoll DM: The blockade of immune checkpoints in cancer immunotherapy. *Nat Rev Cancer* 12:252, 2012.

41. Hsu FJ, Caspar CB, Czerwinski D, et al: Tumor-specific idiotype vaccines in the treatment of patients with B-cell lymphoma—Long-term results of a clinical trial. *Blood* 89:3129, 1997.

42. Dranoff G, Jaffee E, Lazenby A, et al: Vaccination with irradiated tumor cells engineered to secrete murine granulocyte-macrophage colony-stimulating factor stimulates potent, specific, and long-lasting anti-tumor immunity. *Proc Natl Acad Sci U S A* 90:3539, 1993.

43. Kwak LW, Young HA, Pennington RW, et al: Vaccination with syngeneic lymphoma-derive immunoglobulin idiotype combined with granulocyte/macrophage colony-stimulating factor primes mice for a protective T-cell response. *Proc Natl Acad Sci U S A* 93:10972, 1996.

CHAPTER 28
THERAPEUTIC APHERESIS: INDICATIONS, EFFICACY, AND COMPLICATIONS

Robert Weinstein

SUMMARY

Therapeutic apheresis refers to several blood processing methods that are used in the treatment of diverse clinical conditions. In most cases, the disorders so treated are characterized by a specific qualitative or quantitative abnormality of the blood. In hematologic practice, apheresis procedures are used to mitigate hyperviscosity in monoclonal protein disorders or remove pathologic autoantibodies and replete important plasma proteins. Red cell apheresis is used to improve the ratio of normal to abnormal red cells in hemoglobinopathies and protozoan disease, and to remove excess red cells, red cell-associated toxins, or excess iron from the body. Leukocyte apheresis is used to reduce the circulating blast count in acute leukemias with hyperleukocytosis and platelet apheresis is used to lower a very elevated platelet count in patients with myeloproliferative neoplasms. Photopheresis is used in the treatment of cutaneous T-cell lymphoma and chronic graft-versus-host disease. Adverse effects of apheresis with current technologies are typically mild and, usually, do not prevent completion of therapy.

DEFINITION AND HISTORY

The term *apheresis* emerged in 1914 when John J. Abel, of the Johns Hopkins University Pharmacological Laboratory, demonstrated how large quantities of plasma could be removed from dogs by a process he called "plasmapheresis" (from the Greek *apairesos* or Roman *apaheresis*, meaning take away by force).[1] The treatment, by manual plasmapheresis, of hyperviscosity syndrome in patients with Waldenström macroglobulinemia during the 1950s supported the concept that a disease state causally related to a substance in the plasma can be effectively treated by removal of plasma.[2,3] Today, a number of automated apheresis, or blood processing, techniques are used in the treatment of a growing list of clinical disorders. The American Society for Apheresis

Abbreviations and Acronyms: ADAMTS-13, von Willebrand factor cleaving metalloprotease; ARDS, acute respiratory distress syndrome; ASFA, American Society for Apheresis; CDC, United States Centers for Disease Control and Prevention; ECP, extracorporeal photochemotherapy; FCR, fraction of cells remaining; GRADE, Grading of Recommendations Assessment, Development and Evaluation; HUS, hemolytic uremic syndrome; MHC, major histocompatibility complex; 8-MOP, 8-methoxypsoralen; PUVA, psoralen plus ultraviolet A; TPE, therapeutic plasma exchange; TTP, thrombotic thrombocytopenic purpura; UVA, ultraviolet A light; VR, volume of red blood cells to be removed.

(ASFA) categorizes the indications for apheresis (Table 28–1) according to where apheresis fits into the management strategy for the condition under consideration.[4] In addition, ASFA evaluates the individual indications (clinical entities) and issues recommendations regarding the use of apheresis in their treatment according to the GRADE (Grading of Recommendations Assessment, Development and Evaluation) system.[4,5] Table 28–2 lists the covered indications most relevant to the practice of hematology. This chapter considers the various apheresis approaches to hematologic disorders.

THERAPEUTIC PLASMA EXCHANGE

Therapeutic plasma exchange (TPE) is the most commonly performed therapeutic apheresis procedure in the United States and Medicare claims for TPE have doubled over the past 10 years.[6] The term *plasmapheresis* refers to the removal of plasma from the circulation by manual or automated methods; the term *plasma exchange* refers to a therapeutic procedure in which plasmapheresis is combined with replacement of the removed plasma by a substitute colloid fluid, most commonly a mixture of 5 percent human serum albumin and 0.9 percent saline.[4,7] The efficient extraction of the plasma from whole blood, and its replacement with a substitute colloid fluid, is predicated on the hypothesis that the plasma substance targeted for removal (usually an immunoglobulin or other large molecule) does not escape to the extracellular space during the time it takes to perform the plasma exchange procedure.[7] This hypothesis underlies the "one compartment model" that forms the basis for our understanding of the physiology of plasma exchange and the depletion of plasma constituents (Fig. 28–1).

If the "one compartment model" applies, then the intravascular mass of a substance to be removed is a function of its concentration in the plasma (y) and the patient's plasma volume. Its clearance from the plasma by plasmapheresis depends on the fraction of that plasma volume that is removed per unit of time during the exchange. The fraction of the targeted substance remaining in the intravascular space at any time (t) during the exchange procedure can be expressed as

$$y_t = y_0 e^{-x}$$

where y_t is the concentration of targeted substance remaining in the intravascular space at time t, y_0 is the concentration of targeted substance at the start of the procedure (time zero), e is the natural logarithm base (a constant valued at approximately 2.718282) and x represents multiples of the patient's plasma volume processed by time *t*. Figure 28–2 is a plot based on this formula that generates an asymptotic curve that predicts the disappearance of the intravascular target substance as a function of plasma volumes processed (i.e., multiples of the patient's plasma volume). The curve is initially steep, and the processing of one plasma volume removes approximately two-thirds of the substance of interest. Processing of another half plasma volume lowers the remaining substance of interest to approximately 22 percent of its initial level in the blood. But the curve then rapidly flattens, with much less removal of the substance of interest per volume of plasma processed. Thus the "sweet spot" for plasma exchange procedures is the processing of between 1.0 and 1.5 plasma volumes.[7] The "one compartment model" is particularly relevant to the removal of large molecules, such as immunoglobulins, that have a predictable rate of synthesis and volume of distribution within the intravascular space. Smaller molecules, that are synthesized and/or metabolized in a less-predictable fashion, or are distributed within total body water, are less predictably removed according to the model.[7]

As shown in Table 28–2, most indications for plasma exchange in hematologic disorders are weakly recommended based on low-quality evidence. These indications are reviewed in detail elsewhere.[8,9] The discussion herein is restricted to situations where plasma exchange has an important impact on hematologic practice.

TABLE 28–1. Indication Categories for Therapeutic Apheresis According to the American Society for Apheresis

Category	Definition of Category
I	Apheresis is an accepted first-line therapy for these disorders.
II	Apheresis is an accepted second-line therapy for these disorders.
III	Individualize decision making. The optimal role of apheresis has not been conclusively determined in these disorders.
IV	Published evidence indicates that apheresis is ineffective or harmful in these disorders. Seek institutional review board approval if apheresis is planned.

Adapted with permission from Schwartz J, Winters JL, Padmanabhan A: et al: Guidelines on the use of therapeutic apheresis in clinical practice-evidence-based approach from the Writing Committee of the American Society for Apheresis: the sixth special issue. *J Clin Apher* 28(3):145–284, 2013.

HYPERVISCOSITY IN MONOCLONAL GAMMOPATHIES

Hyperviscosity syndrome in the monoclonal gammopathies (Chaps. 106, 107, and 109) is caused by impaired blood flow from an increase in viscosity of blood as a result of immunoglobulin–red cell interactions.[10–12] It is most common in Waldenström macroglobulinemia because of the highly red-cell-aggregating properties of immunoglobulin (Ig) M and, less often, in IgG or IgA myeloma.[13–15] Symptoms typically emerge when serum viscosity rises above 4.0 relative viscosity units (normal being 1.4 to 1.8).[12,16] Although the relevant variable is blood viscosity, the measurement of serum viscosity is relatively simple and can be used as an indicator of risk of symptomatic hyperviscosity. Specific symptoms may include headache, dizziness, vertigo, nystagmus, hearing loss, visual impairment, somnolence or coma and seizures. In addition, congestive heart failure, impaired respiration, coagulation abnormalities, anemia or peripheral neuropathy may be seen.[13] Plasma exchange rapidly relieves symptoms of hyperviscosity by lowering the plasma content of the responsible paraprotein.[2,3,16,17]

The relationship between monoclonal protein level and serum viscosity is nonlinear, therefore a relatively small (20 percent) decrease in plasma protein can affect a major change in viscosity.[10,17] This is noteworthy in that whereas the removal of plasma proteins during plasma exchange from patients without monoclonal proteinemia closely follows the predictions of the "one compartment model" (i.e., $y_t = y_0 e^{-0.94x}$), removal of plasma proteins from patients with monoclonal proteinemia deviates from the model by as much as 50 percent (i.e., $y_t = y_0 e^{-0.5x}$).[18] The difference likely relates to the underestimated expansion in plasma volume that occurs in monoclonal proteinemias.[7] But despite this compromised removal of plasma protein, the nonlinear relationship between serum monoclonal protein level and serum viscosity results in plasma exchange remaining highly effective in alleviating clinical manifestations of hyperviscosity.[19]

OTHER PLASMA PROTEIN-ASSOCIATED CONDITIONS

Cryoglobulinemia

Cryoglobulins are immunoglobulins or complexes of immunoglobulins that reversibly precipitate when exposed to temperatures below 37°C. They can be isolated monoclonal immunoglobulins (type I), a mixture of immunoglobulins including a monoclonal component that exhibits antibody activity toward polyclonal IgG (type II) or mixed polyclonal immunoglobulins of one or more classes (type III). Whereas type I cryoglobulinemia is largely associated with lymphoproliferative disorders, and type III with chronic infections or autoimmune disorders, type II is almost always associated with infection with hepatitis C. Clinical sequelae may include purpura, arthralgia and arthritis, Raynaud phenomenon, peripheral sensory or sensorimotor neuropathy, nephropathy, skin ulcers, or widespread vasculitis.[20,21] The removal of cryoglobulins by plasma exchange can be effective in treating the renal, vasomotor, vasculitic, and neurologic manifestations of cryoglobulinemia,[22–24] but medical treatment of the underlying disorder with which the cryoglobulinemia is associated is also necessary for a persistent good result.

Myeloma Cast Nephropathy

Myeloma cast nephropathy ("myeloma kidney") results from combination of free light chains with Tamm-Horsfall mucoprotein in the distal nephron and the resultant precipitation of obstructing casts.[25] A number of early case reports and small clinical trials suggested that combining plasma exchange with chemotherapy improved the likelihood of recovering renal function in patients with myeloma and renal failure.[26–30] The largest trial to date (104 participants) was unable to demonstrate a difference in primary outcome based on the composite measure of death, dialysis dependence, or glomerular filtration rate below 30 mL/min/1.73 m² at 6 months.[31] The effectiveness and rapidity of modern chemotherapy may have subsumed a salutary effect of plasma exchange.[32] Plasma exchange is not currently considered to be part of first-line treatment for myeloma with cast nephropathy, but may be a reasonable option when renal function does not rapidly improve with chemotherapy.[4]

THROMBOTIC MICROANGIOPATHIES

Idiopathic Thrombotic Thrombocytopenic Purpura

Idiopathic thrombotic thrombocytopenic purpura (TTP) is a medical emergency that presents with microangiopathic hemolytic anemia and thrombocytopenia (Chap. 132). It is typically characterized by central nervous system, cardiac, renal, or other organ impairment as a result of microvascular obstruction by aggregates of platelets and von Willebrand factor.[33,34] It results from inadequate processing of ultralarge von Willebrand factor multimers by the enzyme ADAMTS-13.[35,36] In acquired, idiopathic TTP, this enzymatic defect is caused by an autoantibody inhibitor of ADAMTS-13 that results in severe deficiency of the enzyme.[35,36] An inherited, relapsing form of TTP results from mutations in the ADAMTS-13 gene.[37] TPE, using human plasma as the colloid exchange fluid, is the only therapy for TTP that has been demonstrated highly effective in a randomized clinical trial.[38,39] It has improved the survival rate of TTP from approximately 20 percent to upward of 90 percent, but with a relapse rate over 30 percent.[8] TPE should be initiated for a patient who presents with unexplained microangiopathic hemolytic anemia and thrombocytopenia while awaiting the result of an assay for ADAMTS-13 level and activity.[40] Of note, hemolytic uremic syndrome (HUS), a thrombotic microangiopathy with acute oliguric or anuric renal failure, is rarely associated with severe deficiency of ADAMTS-13. Shiga toxin-associated HUS does not respond to TPE; atypical HUS (i.e., with defects in regulation of the complement system) has shown only limited responses to TPE and is more appropriately treated with eculizumab.[40]

Drug-Associated Thrombotic Microangiopathy

Several drugs are implicated in thrombotic microangiopathies and a TTP-like syndrome (see Table 28–2). The two most common drugs reported to the FDA as associated with TTP are the antiplatelet

TABLE 28–2. Indications for Apheresis in Hematology: Indication Category Assignments and Recommendation Grades

Clinical Disorder	Apheresis Procedure*	Indication Category†	Grade‡ of Recommendation
Amyloidosis, systemic	TPE	IV	2C
Aplastic anemia or pure red cell aplasia	TPE	III	2C
Autoimmune hemolytic anemia (warm)	TPE	III	2C
Babesiosis, severe	RBC exchange	I	1C
Babesiosis, high-risk population		II	2C
Catastrophic antiphospholipid syndrome	TPE	II	2C
Coagulation factor inhibitor			
Alloantibody	TPE	IV	2C
Alloantibody	IA	III	2B
Autoantibody	TPE	III	2C
Autoantibody	IA	III	1C
Cold agglutinin disease	TPE	II	2C
Cryoglobulinemia	TPE	I	2A
	IA	II	2B
Cutaneous T-cell lymphoma; mycosis fungoides; Sézary syndrome (erythrodermic)	ECP	I	1B
Erythrocytosis	Erythrocytapheresis		
Primary (polycythemia vera)		I	1B
Secondary		III	1C
Graft-versus-host disease, skin	ECP		
Chronic		II	1B
Acute		II	1C
Graft-versus-host disease, nonskin (acute/chronic)		III	2C
Hemopoietic stem cell transplant, ABO incompatible			
Major incompatibility, marrow	TPE	II	1B
Major incompatibility, apheresis	TPE	II	2B
Minor incompatibility, apheresis	RBC exchange	III	2C
Hemolytic uremic syndrome	TPE		
Atypical			
Complement gene mutations		II	2C
Factor H antibodies		I	2C
MCP mutations		IV	1C
Infection-associated			
Shiga toxin associated		IV	1C
Str. pneumonia-associated		III	2C
Heparin-induced thrombocytopenia	TPE		
Precardiopulmonary bypass		III	2C
Thrombosis		III	2C
Hereditary hemochromatosis	Erythrocytapheresis	I	1B
Hyperleukocytosis (acute leukemia)	Leukocytapheresis		
Leukostasis		I	1B
Prophylaxis		III	2C
Hyperviscosity in monoclonal gammopathies	TPE		
Symptomatic		I	1B
Prophylaxis for rituximab		I	1C

(Continued)

TABLE 28–2. Indications for Apheresis in Hematology: Indication Category Assignments and Recommendation Grades (Continued)

Clinical Disorder	Apheresis Procedure*	Indication Category[†]	Grade[‡] of Recommendation
Immune thrombocytopenia (refractory)	TPE	IV	2C
	IA	III	2C
Myeloma cast nephropathy	TPE	II	2B
Posttransfusion purpura	TPE	III	2C
Sickle cell disease	RBC exchange		
Acute stroke		I	1C
Acute chest syndrome		II	1C
Multiorgan failure		III	2C
Preoperative management		III	2A
Priapism		III	2C
Sequestration syndrome (spleen, liver, cholestasis)		III	2C
Stroke prophylaxis		II	1C
Vasoocclusive pain		III	2C
Thrombocytosis	Thrombocytapheresis		
Symptomatic		II	2C
Prophylaxis (or secondary)		III	2C
Thrombotic microangiopathy	TPE		
Hemopoietic stem cell transplant-related		III	2C
Drug associated		I	1B
Ticlopidine		III	2B
Clopidogrel		III	2C
Calcineurin inhibitors		IV	2C
Gemcitabine		IV	2C
Quinine		I	1A
Thrombotic thrombocytopenic purpura			

*Apheresis procedures: ECP, extracorporeal photochemotherapy (photopheresis); IA, immunoadsorption apheresis; MCP, monocyte chemoattractant protein; Str., streptococcal. TPE, therapeutic plasma exchange. NOTE: Leukocytapheresis, erythrocytapheresis, thrombocytapheresis refer to removal of white cells, red cells or platelets respectively by apheresis. RBC (red blood cell) exchange refers to apheresis removal of red blood cells and simultaneous replacement of removed red cells with donor red blood cells.

[†]Indication categories: see Table 28–1 for definitions.

[‡]Grade of recommendation: 1 = strong recommendation (i.e., "we recommend"); 2 = weak recommendation (i.e., "we suggest"). A = recommendation based on high-quality published evidence; B = based on moderate-quality published evidence; C = based on low-quality published evidence.

Adapted with permission from Schwartz J, Winters JL, Padmanabhan A: et al: Guidelines on the use of therapeutic apheresis in clinical practice-evidence-based approach from the Writing Committee of the American Society for Apheresis: the sixth special issue. *J Clin Apher* 28(3): 145–284, 2013.

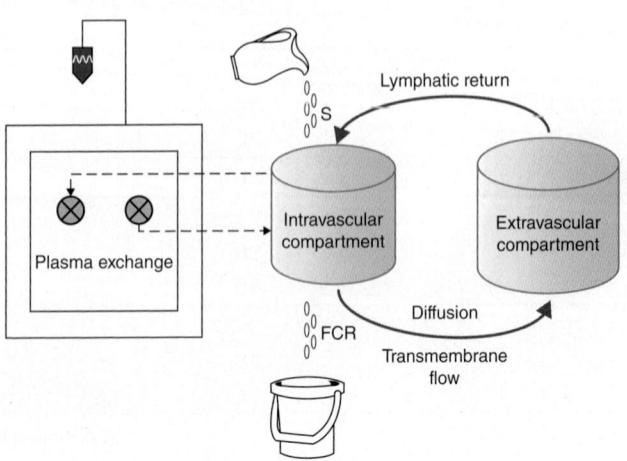

Figure 28–1. Illustration of the "one compartment model" depicting the interaction between intra- and extravascular compartments as relates to plasma exchange. A soluble substance enters the intravascular compartment at synthetic rate *(S)* and is removed at its fraction catabolic rate *(FCR)*. Movement of the substance of interest between the intravascular and (larger) extravascular compartment takes place by the mechanisms shown. The plasma exchange procedure only removes soluble substances directly from the intravascular compartment. *S, FCR,* and the intracompartmental movement of soluble substances are in a balanced steady state and proceed much more slowly than the rate of plasma extraction by the apheresis instrument. Thus, for the purpose of the plasma exchange procedure, the intravascular compartment can be considered to be an isolated system which can be depleted of soluble substances by exchanging the plasma for a replacement fluid.

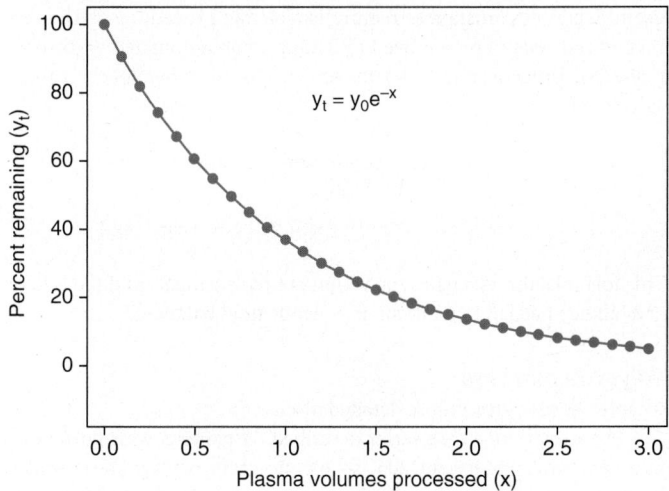

Figure 28–2. Depletion of soluble substances from the intravascular compartment by plasma exchange according to the One Compartment Model. With each incremental volume of plasma removed (and replaced) from the intravascular compartment, a fixed proportion of the remaining intravascular content of a soluble substance of interest is removed. The processing of 1.0 plasma volume depletes the intravascular substance of interest by approximately two thirds. Processing of the next half plasma volume furthers the depletion to almost 80 percent.

thienopyridine derivatives ticlopidine and clopidogrel.[41] Autoantibodies to ADAMTS-13 are seen in ticlopidine-associated TTP, and the contribution of TPE to the survivability of ticlopidine-associated TTP is similar to what is seen in acquired idiopathic TTP.[41,42] Patients with clopidogrel-associated TTP do not appear to benefit from plasma exchange.[41]

ADVERSE EFFECTS OF THERAPEUTIC PLASMA EXCHANGE

Two large studies identified adverse effects in 40 percent of patients but only 12 percent of plasma exchange procedures and in 49 percent of patients but only 17 percent of plasma exchange procedures, respectively.[43,44] This indicates that although a plurality of patients may experience an adverse effect during a course of plasma exchange, they will not necessarily experience them in every procedure during the prescribed course. In both studies, most adverse effects were classified as mild or moderate and did not prevent the successful completion of the procedure. The majority of adverse effects consisted of muscle cramps or paresthesias, transient hypotension, mild nausea, or, in patients receiving plasma as the colloid exchange fluid, fever, chills or urticaria. Muscle cramps, paresthesias, and mild nausea can be attributed to hypocalcemic toxicity that occurs when plasma ionized calcium decreases as a result of the rapid infusion of calcium-free pharmaceutical albumin and, in part, to the use of calcium chelating agents as anticoagulants in plasma exchange procedures.[45,46] A large national survey reported similar findings but with a lower rate of adverse effects during plasma exchange (3.3 percent of procedures without plasma as the colloid replacement fluid, 7.8 percent of procedures with plasma as the colloid replacement fluid) because adverse effects that did not compromise the completion of the procedure were not included.[47] Very few adverse effects are seen as caused by complications of peripheral venous access[47]; however, adverse effects of central venous access placement, although relatively rare, can be severe.[45,47]

● RED CELL APHERESIS

Red cell exchange refers to the removal of a patient's red cells in exchange for donor red cells. When red cells are removed for therapeutic purposes, but not replaced with donor red cells, the process is referred to as *erythrocytapheresis*. Red cell exchange is employed in settings where a clinical disorder is caused by an abnormality (inherited or acquired) of the patient's red blood cells, and erythrocytapheresis may be employed in situations characterized by an untoward elevation in circulating red cell volume or in iron-overload states.[48]

RED CELL EXCHANGE

Therapeutic red cell exchange can be performed manually (i.e., "exchange transfusion") or by apheresis using automated programmable blood-processing equipment.[49-51] This discussion focuses on automated red cell exchange. The programming functions of automated apheresis instruments are used to determine the parameters of red cell exchange procedures. Data that include the patient's gender, height, and weight are used to calculate the patient's total blood volume.[52] Also programmed into the machine are the patient's starting hematocrit, the desired ending hematocrit, the average hematocrit of the replacement red cell units, and the desired fluid balance (typically 100 percent). The desired fraction of the patient's own red cells remaining in the circulation at the end of the procedure (fraction of cells remaining [FCR]) is also programmed into the instrument. The instrument's computer can thus determine how many units of red cells are to be used to obtain the desired hematocrit and FCR. The desired FCR is calculated based on the therapeutic end point targets of the red cell exchange procedure[49,53-55]:

$$FCR\ (as\ \%) = 100$$
$$\times \left(\frac{starting\ hematocrit}{desired\ ending\ hematocrit} \times \frac{desired\ end\ point\ parameter}{starting\ parametre} \right)$$

where the specified starting and end point parameters may be the percent hemoglobin S, the percent parasitized red cells counted on the blood film, etc.

Red Cell Exchange in Sickle Cell Disease

Chapter 49 discusses sickle cell anemia and related abnormalities in greater detail.

In general, clinical studies of the role of transfusion therapy in sickle cell disease have focused mostly on simple transfusion or manual exchange transfusion (reviewed in Ref. 56). Manual versus automated red cell exchange have not been directly compared in a clinical trial, although automated red cell exchange can be completed more efficiently and quickly than manual exchange transfusion.[49] Automated red cell exchange mitigates the accumulation of iron while maintaining a low level of hemoglobin S in patients receiving chronic treatment and, thus, has entered into routine use where available.[57-59] Manual or automated red cell exchange can be initiated using isotonic saline, rather than packed red cells, as the replacement fluid during the early part of the procedure in order to maximize the removal of hemoglobin S–containing red cells and avoid the gratuitous removal of normal red cells.[57,59,60] As shown in Table 28–2, red cell exchange is indicated as first-line therapy in acute vasoocclusive stroke, and may be used in acute chest syndrome refractory to standard management or in prophylaxis (primary or secondary) for vasoocclusive stroke.[56] In the latter two instances, red cell exchange may not be superior to simple transfusion.[56,61] In addition, red cell exchange may not be superior to simple transfusion, as needed, in the management of acute multiorgan failure syndrome, preparation for general anesthesia, complications of pregnancy, or frequent pain episodes.[48,56]

Red Cell Exchange in Protozoan Disease

Chapter 53 discusses infections with microorganisms in greater detail.

Malaria The World Health Organization has suggested that exchange transfusion be considered for nonimmune (i.e., not previously exposed) patients with *falciparum* malaria who have any of the following characteristics: greater than 30 percent parasitemia in the absence of clinical complications, greater than 10 percent parasitemia in the presence of severe[62] disease, greater than 10 percent parasitemia and failure to respond to optimal chemotherapy after 12 to 24 hours, or greater than 10 percent parasitemia and poor prognostic factors (elderly, late-stage parasites [schizonts] in the blood).[63] The Centers for Disease Control and Prevention (CDC) previously recommended strong consideration of exchange transfusion or red cell exchange in severely affected patients.[64] Subsequently, the CDC has rescinded this recommendation based on a literature review and an analysis of the U.S. national malaria surveillance system (patients reported 1985 to 2010) that found no evidence for efficacy of exchange transfusion as adjunctive therapy in severe malaria when rapidly acting antimalarials (specifically artemisinins) were available.[65] It is not certain whether the emergence of artemisinin-resistant *Plasmodium falciparum* will affect their position.[66-68]

Babesiosis Infection with intraerythrocytic protozoan *Babesia microti* is most commonly acquired through the bite of the tick *Ixodes scapularis* and presents with clinical manifestations that range from asymptomatic infection or influenza-like illness to organ failure and death.[69] Complications may include acute respiratory distress syndrome (ARDS), disseminated intravascular coagulopathy, renal failure, or hemolytic anemia. Immunocompromised, elderly, or asplenic individuals are most at risk for severe manifestations.[70,71] Between 2009 and 2013 babesiosis was the most frequent cause of transfusion-transmitted infectious death reported to the FDA.[72] In the United States, the occurrence of babesiosis in Connecticut, Massachusetts, Minnesota, New Jersey, New York, Rhode Island, and Wisconsin accounted for 97 percent of 1124 cases of babesiosis reported to the CDC in 2011.[73] Because the parasite is completely intraerythrocytic, and, despite the lack of clinical trials, observational evidence indicates that the parasite can be efficiently removed using automated red cell exchange.[4,74] Red cell exchange is recommended[4] for patients with severe manifestations, high parasite burdens (>10 percent) or who are at high risk.

Miscellaneous Uses of Red Cell Exchange

Red cell exchange has been successfully used, in conjunction with Rh immunoglobulin, to prevent Rh sensitization of an Rh-negative woman who received emergency transfusion with Rh-positive red blood cells.[75] The macrolide immunosuppressant tacrolimus is highly erythrocyte-bound and overdoses are not responsive to plasma exchange,[76] but can be mitigated using red cell exchange.[77] Red cell exchange can successfully treat refractory methemoglobinemia in patients with glucose-6-phosphate dehydrogenase deficiency or after ingestion of strong oxidants.[78]

RED BLOOD CELL DEPLETION (ERYTHROCYTAPHERESIS)

Although therapeutic phlebotomy is a mainstay of management of polycythemia vera and hereditary hemochromatosis,[79-82] ASFA now considers these clinical entities to be category I (first-line) indications for automated erythrocytapheresis.[4] The role of automated erythrocytapheresis in secondary erythrocytosis is less certain,[83] but it may be useful when circumstances require isovolemic procedures.[84] The volume of red cells to be removed (VR) during an automated erythrocytapheresis procedure in order to achieve a desired hematocrit can be calculated as[85]:

$$VR = \frac{(\text{starting hematocrit-desired hematocrit})}{79} \times [\text{blood volume (ml/kg)}] \times [\text{body weight (kg)}]$$

This formula also estimates the volume of replacement fluid (colloid or crystalloid) needed to maintain isovolemic fluid balance.[83]

Polycythemia Vera

Chapter 84 provides a more detailed discussion.

A retrospective case series described 69 patients with polycythemia vera who underwent 206 isovolemic erythrocytapheresis procedures using 4 percent albumin as replacement fluid.[83,85] Hematocrit was reduced from 56.8 ± 5.6 percent to 41.9 ± 6.6 percent after removal of 1410 ± 418 mL of red blood cells with a hematocrit of 79.7 ± 9.3 percent. Close followup data were provided for a subset of 21 patients whose hematocrits were reduced from 58 ± 5.7 percent to 41.5 ± 4.9 percent by a single erythrocytapheresis procedure and were maintained at less than 50 percent for a median of 6 months.[85] The durability of response to a single procedure was associated with a median 70 percent inhibition of *in vitro* erythropoietin-independent burst-forming unit–erythroid (BFU-E) growth that the authors attributed to iron removal during the apheresis procedure.[86] This claim has not been confirmed. Automated erythrocytapheresis may be useful in polycythemia vera for the rapid induction of hematocrit lowering, followed by maintenance therapeutic phlebotomy, for emergent isovolemic hematocrit lowering in patients with acute thrombotic or microvascular complications, or to avoid perioperative thrombohemorrhagic complications in a patient with an uncontrolled hematocrit who requires urgent surgery.[56,85]

Hereditary Hemochromatosis

Chapter 43 provides a more detailed discussion.

Early observational studies from Europe[87-91] suggested that automated erythrocytapheresis could deplete iron from patients with hereditary hemochromatosis more efficiently and quickly than could conventional therapeutic phlebotomy. A prospective, randomized trial from the Netherlands involving 38 patients with newly diagnosed C282Y-homozygous hemochromatosis compared automated erythrocytapheresis to conventional therapeutic phlebotomy.[92] Study subjects were evenly randomized to either treatment arm. The primary outcome measure was the number of procedures needed to reach a serum ferritin target of 50 mcg/L or less. This was reached in a mean (range) of nine (4 to 20) procedures over 19.6 (7 to 37) weeks in the erythrocytapheresis arm and 27 (11 to 58) procedures over 33.7 (12 to 79) weeks in the phlebotomy arm. Erythrocytapheresis removed 427 (294 to 545) mg of iron with each procedure compared to 205 (136 to 230) mg with each phlebotomy. Secondary outcomes were total duration of treatment, side effects, change in iron status and liver function, quality of life (related to health) and costs. Adverse effects, including hypocalcemia, vasovagal syncope, and mild dizziness, occurred in 3 of 19 patients in the erythrocytapheresis group and in 5 of 19 patients in the phlebotomy group. The 3.5-fold higher cost of performing erythrocytapheresis versus therapeutic phlebotomy was fully counterbalanced by greater time off from work and lost productivity among the phlebotomy group. The investigators were careful to point out that the cost structure of apheresis treatments versus phlebotomy in the Netherlands may not apply to other countries.

ADVERSE EFFECTS OF RED CELL EXCHANGE AND ERYTHROCYTAPHERESIS

Red cell exchange conveys risks related to red cell transfusion including febrile, allergic and hemolytic transfusion reactions, acute lung injury, vasovagal reactions, and transfusion-transmitted disease. Hypocalcemic toxicity resulting from the use of citrate-based anticoagulants in the apheresis circuit and in the red cell replacement units may also occur. Erythrocytapheresis conveys similar risks but not the risks associated with red cell transfusions.[48]

● THERAPEUTIC LEUKOCYTAPHERESIS

ASFA has designated hyperleukocytosis (white blood cell count >100,000/μL in acute myeloid leukemias [Chaps. 83 and 88], white cell count >400,000/μL in acute lymphoblastic leukemia [Chap. 91] with leukostasis as a category I indication for therapeutic leukocytapheresis.[4] Asymptomatic hyperleukocytosis is designated a category III indication, reflecting limited and conflicting published evidence regarding the utility of leukocytapheresis as prophylaxis.[4] Hyperleukocytosis, which occurs in 5 to 13 percent of newly presenting cases of adult acute myelogenous leukemia and 12 to 25 percent of pediatric acute myelogenous leukemia is a risk factor for early mortality, often from leukostasis and pulmonary and/or central nervous system hemorrhage.[93–97] The processing of 1.5 to 2.0 blood volumes, using crystalloid or colloid fluids to maintain fluid balance, with or without a sedimentation agent such as 6 percent hydroxyethyl starch to enhance separation of white cells from red cells, can reduce the circulating white cell count by upward of 60 percent,[4,98] but without a clear effect on the rate of early mortality in patients with acute myeloid leukemia and hyperleukocytosis with or without leukostasis.[99,100] In any case, leukocytapheresis is not undertaken without initiating measures to mitigate the risk of tumor lysis syndrome, including intravenous hydration, lowering of plasma uric acid using allopurinol or urate oxidase, and, if urate oxidase is not used, intravenous sodium bicarbonate to alkalinize the urine.[101] Leukapheresis would ordinarily not be considered primary therapy in patients who present with high blast counts but without symptoms of leukostasis.[4,100]

● THERAPEUTIC THROMBOCYTAPHERESIS

Thrombocytapheresis refers to the selective removal of platelets from a patient, for therapeutic purposes using a blood processing (apheresis) device. ASFA lists symptomatic thrombocytosis in patients with myeloproliferative neoplasms (Chaps. 83 and 85) as a category II indication for thrombocytapheresis.[4] Thrombocytapheresis for prophylaxis in asymptomatic patients or to lower the platelet count in cases of secondary or reactive thrombocytosis[102] is listed as a category III (see Table 28–1) indication because the available data do not firmly establish a role for thrombocytapheresis in these circumstances and decision making should be highly individualized. Secondary thrombocytosis per se does not convey a risk of thromboembolic morbidity absent confounding factors such as malignancy or major surgery.[103–105] Rapid lowering of an elevated platelet count, using apheresis and/or chemotherapy, is indicated for patients with myeloproliferative neoplasms who present with clinical syndromes of thrombocytosis with microvascular thrombosis such as digital or cerebral ischemia.[106] Several case series and case reports have reported successful, rapid lowering of the platelet count in symptomatic patients in whom chemotherapy was either not an immediate option or was judged to have an insufficiently rapid

effect.[107–113] Procedures in which 1.5 to 2.0 blood volumes are processed, and crystalloid replacement fluids are used to manage fluid balance, can lower the platelet count by 30 to 60 percent[108,112,113]; however, thrombocytapheresis without concomitant chemotherapy is ordinarily not a practical means for controlling the platelet count beyond the acute setting. Weekly thrombocytapheresis, beginning in the fifth gestational week, has been used in the management of a high-risk pregnant patient with essential thrombocythemia.[113] Thrombocytapheresis has been reported as effective acute therapy in the case of a patient with immune thrombocytopenic purpura, treated with romiplostim, who developed platelet counts as high as $2 \times 10^6/\mu$L and acute neurologic symptoms in the days following splenectomy,[114] and can be used to prepare acutely symptomatic patients with poorly controlled severe thrombocytosis for cardiovascular surgery.[115]

● EXTRACORPOREAL PHOTOCHEMOTHERAPY (PHOTOPHERESIS)

Extracorporeal photochemotherapy (ECP) is a treatment process in which a patient's mononuclear white blood cells are manipulated outside of the body such that their reinfusion into the patient results in down regulation of cytotoxic T-cell activity.[116] This procedure involves collection of circulating mononuclear cells by centrifugal apheresis, exposing them to 8-methoxypsoralen (8-MOP, a photoactivating agent) and then to ultraviolet A light (UVA), and then reinfusing the treated cells into the patient.[56] ECP was originally approved for Medicare reimbursement in 1998 for palliative treatment of skin manifestations of cutaneous T-cell lymphoma (Chap. 103) unresponsive to other therapy and was further found "reasonable and necessary" for treatment of acute cardiac allograft rejection and chronic graft-versus-host disease (Chap. 23) unresponsive to standard treatments in 2006.[117] It was developed based on an earlier treatment called PUVA (psoralen plus ultraviolet A) in which a patient would take an oral dose of 8-MOP and then stand in a UVA light box thus exposing affected skin to treatment. With ECP, only the white cells collected by apheresis are exposed to 8-MOP and UVA, thus only approximately 0.25 percent of the oral dose equivalent of 8-MOP is used.[116] The precise mechanism of action of ECP is still under investigation, but likely involves a process of immunomodulation.[118] UVA-activated 8-MOP intercalates within nuclear DNA of normal and malignant T lymphocytes and causes the treated T cells, but not treated monocytes, to undergo apoptosis by 24 hours after treatment.[119,120] Immunologic consequences of phagocytosis of reinfused apoptotic cells include induction of major histocompatibility complex (MHC) class I–restricted CD8+ cytotoxic T lymphocytes through the antigen-presenting activity of human dendritic cells and the elaboration by monocytes and macrophages of immunosuppressive cytokines including interleukin (IL)-10 and IL-1 receptor antagonist.[121] Furthermore, ECP results in an increase in CD83+, CD86+ plasmacytoid (DC2) dendritic cells with a concordant diminution in CD80+, CD123+ monocytoid (DC1) dendritic cells. The DC2 cells stimulate T-helper type 2 (Th2) cells to secrete inhibitory cytokines (e.g., IL-4, IL-10, IL-13) while inhibiting stimulation of T-helper type 1 (Th1) cells that secrete proinflammatory cytokines (e.g., IL-2, interferon-γ) and thus inhibiting Th1-mediated alloreactivity.[122] ECP also appears to result in an increase in a population of circulating CD4+, CD25+, CD69– CTLA-4+ regulatory T cells (T_{REG}) that are immunosuppressive and are involved in transplant tolerance.[123] Such induced immunologic responses to ECP are presumed to explain observed clinical benefit in diverse conditions such as cutaneous T-cell lymphoma, chronic graft-versus-host disease, and cardiac transplant rejection.[124–126]

ADVERSE EFFECTS OF EXTRACORPOREAL PHOTOCHEMOTHERAPY

Adverse effects are largely related to volume shifts that result in hypotension, which can be managed by pausing the procedure and/or administering fluids. Transient fevers to 38°C to 39°C have been observed 6 to 8 hours after reinfusion of the treated mononuclear cells.[127]

REFERENCES

1. Abel JJ, Rowntree LG, Turner BB: Plasma removal with return of corpuscles (plasmapheresis). *J Pharmacol Exp Ther* 5:625, 1914.
2. Schwab PJ, Fahey JL: Treatment of Waldenström's macroglobulinemia by plasmapheresis. *N Engl J Med* 263:574, 1960.
3. Solomon A, Fahey JL: Plasmapheresis therapy in macroglobulinemia. *Ann Intern Med* 58:789, 1963.
4. Schwartz J, Winters JL, Padmanabhan A, et al: Guidelines on the use of therapeutic apheresis in clinical practice—Evidence-based approach from the Writing Committee of the American Society for Apheresis: The sixth special issue. *J Clin Apher* 28:145, 2013.
5. Guyatt GH, Oxman AD, Vist GE, et al: GRADE: An emerging consensus on rating quality of evidence and strength of recommendations. *Br Med J (Clin Res Ed)* 336:924, 2008.
6. AMA RUC Database 2014 version 2.
7. Weinstein R: Basic principles of therapeutic blood exchange, in *Apheresis: Principles and Practice*, 3rd ed, edited by BC McLeod, R Weinstein, JL Winters, AM Szczepiorkowski, p 269. AABB Press, Bethesda, MD, 2010.
8. Kiss JE: Therapeutic plasma exchange in hematologic diseases and dysproteinemias, in *Apheresis: Principles and Practice*, 3rd ed, edited by BC McLeod, R Weinstein, JL Winters, AM Szczepiorkowski, p 319. AABB Press, Bethesda, MD, 2010.
9. McLeod BC: Therapeutic plasma exchange, in *Rossi's Principles of Transfusion Medicine*, 4th ed, edited by TL Simon, EL Snyder, BG Solheim, CP Stoell, RG Strauss, M Petrides, p 629. Blackwell Publishing, Chichester, UK, 2009.
10. McGrath MA, Penny R: Paraproteinemia. Blood hyperviscosity and clinical manifestations. *J Clin Invest* 58:1155, 1976.
11. Somer T, Meiselman HJ: Disorders of blood viscosity. *Ann Med* 25:31, 1993.
12. Kwaan HC, Bongu A: The hyperviscosity syndromes. *Semin Thromb Hemost* 25:199, 1999.
13. Weinstein R, Mahmood M: Case records of Massachusetts General Hospital. Weekly clinicopathological exercises. Case 6-2002. A 54-year-old woman with left, then right, central-retinal-vein occlusion. *N Engl J Med* 346:603, 2002.
14. Bloch KJ, Maki DG: Hyperviscosity syndromes associated with immunoglobulin abnormalities. *Semin Hematol* 10:113, 1973.
15. Capra JD, Kunkel HG: Aggregation of gammaG3 proteins: Relevance to the hyperviscosity syndrome. *J Clin Invest* 49:610, 1970.
16. Fahey JL, Barth WF, Solomon A: Serum hyperviscosity syndrome. *JAMA* 192:464, 1965.
17. Beck JR, Quinn BM, Meier FA, Rawnsley HM: Hyperviscosity syndrome in paraproteinemia managed by plasma exchange, monitored by serum tests. *Transfusion* 22:51, 1982.
18. Chopek M, McCullough J: Protein and biochemical changes during plasma exchange, in *Therapeutic Hemapheresis*, edited by EM Berkman, J Umlas, p 13. AABB Press, Washington, DC, 1980.
19. Stone MJ, Bogen SA: Evidence-based focused review of management of hyperviscosity syndrome. *Blood* 119:2205, 2012.
20. Brouet J-C, Clauvel J-P, Danon F, et al: Biologic and clinical significance of cryoglobulins. A report of 86 cases. *Am J Med* 57:775, 1974.
21. Ferri C, Zignego AL, Pileri SA: Cryoglobulins. *J Clin Pathol* 55:4, 2002.
22. Ferri C, Moriconi L, Gremignai G, et al: Treatment of the renal involvement of mixed cryoglobulinemia with prolonged plasma exchange. *Nephron* 43:246, 1986.
23. Berkman EM, Orlin JB: Use of plasmapheresis and partial plasma exchange in the management of patients with cryoglobulinemia. *Transfusion* 20:171, 1980.
24. Shaw M, Van de Pette J, Fenton D, McGibbon DH: Mutilating cryoglobulinemia rapidly improved by plasmapheresis: Diagnostic features on blood film. *J R Soc Med* 78(Suppl 11):37, 1985.
25. Goldschmidt H, Lannert H, Brommer J, Ho AD: Multiple myeloma and renal failure. *Nephrol Dial Transplant* 15:301, 2000.
26. Feest TG, Burge PS, Cohen SL: Successful treatment of myeloma kidney by dieresis and plasmapheresis. *Br Med J* 1:503, 1976.
27. Misiani R, Remuzzi G, Bertani T, Licini R, et al: Plasmapheresis in the treatment of acute renal failure in multiple myeloma. *Am J Med* 66:684, 1979.
28. Zucchelli P, Pasquali S, Cagnoli L, Rovinetti C: Plasma exchange in acute renal failure due to light chain myeloma. *Trans Am Soc Artif Intern Organs* 30:36, 1984.
29. Zucchelli P, Pasquali S, Cagnoli L, Ferrari G: Controlled plasma exchange trial in acute renal failure due to multiple myeloma. *Kidney Int* 33:1175, 1988.
30. Johnson WJ, Kyle RA, Pineda AA, O'Brien PC, et al: Treatment of renal failure associated with multiple myeloma. Plasmapheresis, hemodialysis and chemotherapy. *Arch Intern Med* 150:863, 1990.
31. Clark WF, Stewart AK, Rock GA, et al: Plasma exchange when myeloma presents as acute renal failure. A randomized, controlled trial. *Ann Intern Med* 143:777, 2005.
32. Gertz MA: Managing myeloma kidney. *Ann Intern Med* 143:835, 2005.
33. George JN: Thrombotic thrombocytopenic purpura. *N Engl J Med* 354:1927, 2006.
34. Tsai HM: Current concepts in thrombotic thrombocytopenic purpura. *Annu Rev Med* 57:419, 2006.
35. Furlan M, Robles R, Galbusera M, et al: Von Willebrand factor-cleaving protease in thrombotic thrombocytopenic purpura and the hemolytic uremic syndrome. *N Engl J Med* 339:1578, 1998.
36. Tsai HM, Lian EC: Antibodies to von Willebrand factor-cleaving protease in acute thrombotic thrombocytopenic purpura. *N Engl J Med* 339:1585, 1998.
37. Levy GG, Nichols WC, Lian EC, et al: Mutations in a member of the ADAMTS gene family cause thrombotic thrombocytopenic purpura. *Nature* 413:488, 2001.
38. Rock GA, Shumak KH, Buskard NA, et al: The Canadian apheresis Study Group. Comparison of plasma exchange with plasma infusion in the treatment of thrombotic thrombocytopenic purpura. *N Engl J Med* 325:393, 1991.
39. Henon P: Treatment of thrombotic thrombopenic purpura. Results of a multicenter randomized clinical study. *Presse Med* 20:1761, 1991.
40. Sarode R, Bandarenko N, Brecher ME, et al: Thrombotic thrombocytopenic purpura: 2012 American Society for Apheresis (ASFA) consensus conference on classification, diagnosis, management, and future research. *J Clin Apher* 29:148, 2014.
41. Zakarija A, Kwaan HC, Moake JL, et al: Ticlopidine- and clopidogrel-associated thrombotic thrombocytopenic purpura (TTP): Review of clinical, laboratory, and epidemiological and pharmacovigilance findings (1989–2008). *Kidney Int* 75(Suppl 112):S20, 2009.
42. Tsai H-M, Rice L, Sarode R, et al: Antibody inhibitors to von Willebrand factor metalloproteinase and increased binding of von Willebrand factor to platelets in ticlopidine-associated thrombotic thrombocytopenic purpura. *Ann Intern Med* 132:794, 2000.
43. Sutton DMC, Nair RC, Rock G: Complications of plasma exchange. *Transfusion* 29:124, 1989.
44. Couriel D, Weinstein R: Complications of plasma exchange: A recent assessment. *J Clin Apher* 9:1, 1994.
45. Weinstein R: Hypocalcemic toxicity and atypical reactions in therapeutic plasma exchange. *J Clin Apher* 16:210, 2001.
46. Goss, GA, Weinstein, R: Pentastarch as partial replacement for therapeutic plasma exchange: Effect on plasma proteins, adverse events during treatment, and serum ionized calcium. *J Clin Apher* 14:114, 1999.
47. McLeod BC, Sniecinski I, Ciavarella D, Owen H, et al: Frequency of immediate adverse effects associated with therapeutic apheresis. *Transfusion* 39:282, 1999.
48. Shaz BH: Red cell exchange and other therapeutic alterations of red cell mass, in *Apheresis: Principles and Practice*, 3rd ed, edited by BC McLeod, R Weinstein, JL Winters, AM Szczepiorkowski, p 391. AABB Press, Bethesda, MD, 2010.
49. Swerdlow PS: Red cell exchange in sickle cell disease. *Hematology Am Soc Hematol Educ Program* 48, 2006.
50. Kernoff LM, Botha MC, Jacobs P: Exchange transfusion in sickle cell disease using a continuous-flow blood cell separator. *Transfusion* 17:269, 1977.
51. Klein HG, Garner RJ, Miller DM, et al: Automated partial exchange transfusion in sickle cell anemia. *Transfusion* 20:578, 1980.
52. Nadler SB, Hidalgo JU, Bloch T: Prediction of blood volume in normal human adults. *Surgery* 51:224; 1962.
53. Division of Blood Diseases and Resources: *The Management of Sickle Cell Disease*, 4th ed. NIH Publication No. 02-2117. NHLBI, Bethesda, MD, 2002.
54. Steinberg MH: Management of sickle cell disease. *N Engl J Med* 340:1021, 1999.
55. Platt OS: Prevention and management of stroke in sickle cell anemia. *Hematology Am Soc Hematol Educ Program* 54, 2006.
56. Weinstein R: Specialized therapeutic hemapheresis and phlebotomy, in *Rossi's Principles of Transfusion Medicine*, 4th ed, edited by TL Simon, EL Snyder, BG Solheim, CP Stowell, RG Strauss, M Petrides, p 652. AABB Press, Bethesda, MD, 2009.
57. Kim HC, Dugan NP, Silber JH et al: Erythrocytapheresis therapy to reduce iron overload in chronically transfused patients with sickle cell disease. *Blood* 83:1136, 1994.
58. Hilliard LM, Williams BF, Lounsbury AE: Erythrocytapheresis limits iron accumulation in chronically transfused sickle cell patients. *Am J Hematol* 59:28, 1998.
59. Singer ST, Quirolo, Nishi K: Erythrocytapheresis for chronically transfused children with sickle cell disease: An effective method for maintaining a low hemoglobin S level and reducing iron overload. *J Clin Apher* 14:122, 1999.
60. Sarode R1, Matevosyan K, Rogers ZR: Advantages of isovolemic hemodilution-red cell exchange therapy to prevent recurrent stroke in sickle cell anemia patients. *J Clin Apher* 26:200, 2011.
61. Turner JM, Kaplan JB, Cohen HW, Billett HH: Exchange versus simple transfusion for acute chest syndrome in sickle cell anemia adults. *Transfusion* 49:863, 2009.
62. Trampuz A, Jereb M, Muzlovic I, Prabhu RM: Clinical review: Severe malaria. *Crit Care* 7:315, 2003.
63. Severe falciparum malaria. World Health Organization, Communicable Diseases Cluster. *Trans R Soc Trop Med Hyg* 84(Suppl 1):S1, 2000.
64. Centers for Disease Control and Prevention: *CDC Treatment Guidelines: Treatment of Malaria (Guidelines or Clinicians)*. CDC, Atlanta, GA, 2009.

65. Tan KR, Wiegand RE, Arguin PM: Exchange transfusion for severe malaria: Evidence base and literature review. *Clin Infect Dis* 57:923, 2013.

66. Amaratunga C, Sreng S, Suon S, et al: Artemisinin-resistant Plasmodium falciparum in Pursat province, western Cambodia: A parasite clearance rate study. *Lancet Infect Dis* 12:851, 2012.

67. World Health Organization: Global Plan for Artemisinin Resistance Containment (GPARC). HO Press, Geneva, 2011. Available online at http://www.who.int/malaria/publications/atoz/artemisinin_resistance_containment_2011.pdf (accessed 6 June 2014).

68. Ariey F, Witkowski B, Amaratunga C, et al: A molecular marker of artemisinin-resistant Plasmodium falciparum malaria. *Nature* 505:50, 2014.

69. Vannier E, Krause PJ: Human babesiosis. *N Engl J Med* 366:2397, 2012.

70. Rosner F, Zarrabi MH, Benach JL, et al: Babesiosis in splenectomized adults. Review of 22 reported cases. *Am J Med* 76:696, 1984.

71. Evenson DA, Perry E, Kloster B, et al: Therapeutic apheresis for babesiosis. *J Clin Apher* 13:32, 1998.

72. U.S. Food and Drug Administration: *Fatalities Reported to FDA Following Blood Collection and Transfusion: Annual Summary for Fiscal Year 2013.* Available online at http://www.fda.gov/BiologicsBloodVaccines/SafetyAvailability/ReportaProblem/TransfusionDonationFatalities/ucm391574.htm (accessed 9 June 2014).

73. Centers for Disease Control and Prevention (CDC): Babesiosis surveillance—18 states, 2011. *MMWR Morb Mortal Wkly Rep* 61:505, 2012.

74. Spaete J, Patrozou E, Rich JD, Sweeney JD: Red cell exchange transfusion for babesiosis in Rhode Island. *J Clin Apher* 24:97, 2009.

75. Werch J, Todd C: Resolution by erythrocytapheresis of the exposure of an Rh-negative person to Rh-positive cells: An alternative treatment. *Transfusion* 33:530, 1993.

76. Hale GA, Reece DE, Munn RK, et al: Blood tacrolimus concentrations in bone marrow transplant patients undergoing plasmapheresis. *Bone Marrow Transplant* 25:449, 2000.

77. McCarthy H, Inward C, Marriage S, et al: Red cell exchange transfusion as a rescue therapy for tacrolimus toxicity in a paediatric renal transplant. *Pediatr Nephrol* 26:2245, 2011.

78. Golden PJ, Weinstein R: Treatment of high-risk, refractory acquired methemoglobinemia with automated red blood cell exchange. *J Clin Apher* 13:28, 1998.

79. Streiff, MB, Smith B, Spivak JL: The diagnosis and management of polycythemia vera in the era since the Polycythemia Vera Study Group: A survey of American Society of Hematology members' practice patterns. *Blood* 99:1144, 2002.

80. Tefferi A: Polycythemia vera: A comprehensive review and clinical recommendations. *Mayo Clin Proc* 78:174, 2003.

81. Barton JC, McDonnell SM, Adams PC, et al: Diagnosis and management of hemochromatosis. *Ann Intern Med* 129:932, 1998.

82. Brissot P, de Bels, F: Current approaches to the management of hemochromatosis. *Hematology* 36, 2006.

83. Valbonesi M, Bruni R: Clinical application of therapeutic erythrocytapheresis (TEA). *Transfus Sci* 22:183, 2000.

84. Oechslin E: Hematological management of the cyanotic adult with congenital heart disease. *Int J Cardiol* 97:109, 2004.

85. Kaboth U, Rumpf KW, Lipp T, et al: Treatment of polycythemia vera by isovolemic large-volume erythrocytapheresis. *Klin Wochenschr* 68:18, 1990.

86. Liersch T, Vehmeyer K, Kaboth U: Large volume, isovolemic erythrocytapheresis in treatment of polycythemia vera. Effect of massive iron depletion of proliferation behavior of erythroid precursor cells (BFU-E). *Med Klin (Munich)* 90:390, 1995.

87. Zoller WG, Kellner H, Spengel FA: Erythrocytapheresis. A method for rapid extracorporeal elimination of erythrocytes. Results in 65 patients. *Klin Wochenschr* 66:404, 1988.

88. Conte D, Mandelli C, Cesana M, et al: Effectiveness of erythrocytapheresis in idiopathic hemochromatosis. Report of 14 cases. *Int J Artif Organs* 12:59, 1989.

89. Kellner H, Zoller WG: Repeated isovolemic large-volume erythrocytapheresis in the treatment of idiopathic hemochromatosis. *Z Gastroenterol* 30:779, 1992.

90. Cesana M, Mandelli C, Tiribelli C: Concomitant primary hemochromatosis and beta-thalassemia trait: Iron depletion by erythrocytapheresis and desferrioxamine. *Am J Gastroenterol* 84:150, 1989.

91. Fernández-Mosterín N, Salvador-Osuna C, García-Erce JA, et al: Comparison between phlebotomy and erythrocytapheresis of iron overload in patients with HFE gene mutations. *Med Clin (Barc)* 127:409, 2006.

92. Rombout-Sestrienkova E, Nieman FHM, Essers BAB, et al: Erythrocytapheresis versus phlebotomy in the initial treatment of HFE hemochromatosis patients: Results from a randomized trial. *Transfusion* 52:470, 2012.

93. Bunin NJ, Pui C-H: Differing complications of hyperleukocytosis in children with acute lymphoblastic or acute nonlymphoblastic leukemia. *J Clin Oncol* 3:1590, 1985.

94. Dutcher JP, Schiffer CA, Wiernik PH: Hyperleukocytosis in adult acute nonlymphocytic leukemia: Impact on remission rate and duration, and survival. *J Clin Oncol* 5:1364, 1987.

95. Ventura GJ, Hester JP, Smith TL, et al: Acute myeloblastic leukemia with hyperleukocytosis: Risk factors for early mortality in induction. *Am J Hematol* 27:34, 1988.

96. Porcu P, Cripe LD, Ng EW, et al: Hyperleukocytic leukemias and leukostasis: A review of pathophysiology, clinical presentation and management. *Leuk Lymphoma* 39:1, 2000.

97. Slats AM, Egeler RM, van der Does-van den Berg A, et al: Causes of death–other than progressive leukemia–in childhood acute lymphoblastic (ALL) and myeloid leukemia (AML): The Dutch Childhood Oncology Group experience. *Leukemia* 19:537, 2005.

98. Bruserud Ø, Liseth K, Stamnesfet S, et al: Hyperleukocytosis and leukocytapheresis in acute leukemias: Experience from a single centre and review of the literature of leukocytapheresis in acute myeloid leukaemia. *Transfus Med* 23:397, 2013.

99. Oberoi S, Lehrnbecher T, Phillips B, et al: Leukapheresis and low-dose chemotherapy do not reduce early mortality in acute myeloid leukemia hyperleukocytosis: A systematic review and meta-analysis. *Leuk Res* 38:460, 2014.

100. Pastore F, Pastore A, Wittmann G, et al: The role of therapeutic leukapheresis in hyperleukocytotic AML: *PLoS One* 9(4): E95062, 2014.

101. Lowe EJ, Pui C-H, Hancock ML, et al: Early complications in children with acute lymphoblastic leukemia presenting with hyperleukocytosis. *Pediatr Blood Cancer* 45:10, 2005.

102. Schaefer AI: Thrombocytosis. *N Engl J Med* 350:1211, 2004.

103. Griesshammer M, Bangertner M, Sauer T: Aetiology and clinical significance of thrombocytosis: Analysis of 732 patients with an elevated platelet count. *J Intern Med* 245:295, 1999.

104. Greist A: The role of blood component removal in essential and reactive thrombocytosis. *Ther Apher* 6:36, 2002.

105. Denton A, Davis P: Extreme thrombocytosis in admissions to paediatric intensive care: No requirement for treatment. *Arch Dis Child* 92:515, 2007.

106. Schafer AI: Bleeding and thrombosis in myeloproliferative disorders. *Blood* 64:1, 1984.

107. Baron BW, Mick R, Baron JM: Combined plateletpheresis and cytotoxic chemotherapy for symptomatic thrombocytosis in myeloproliferative disorders. *Cancer* 72:1209, 1993.

108. Taft EG, Babcock RB, Scharfman WB, et al: Plateletpheresis in the management of thrombocytosis. *Blood* 50:927, 1977.

109. Panlilio AL, Reiss RF: Therapeutic plateletpheresis in thrombocythemia. *Transfusion* 19:147, 1979.

110. Goldfinger D, Thompson R, Lowe C: Long-term plateletpheresis in the management of primary thrombocytosis. *Transfusion* 19:336, 1979.

111. Orlin JB, Berkman EM: Improvement of platelet function following plateletpheresis in patients with myeloproliferative diseases. *Transfusion* 20:540, 1980.

112. Janetzko K, Weber K, Klüter H, et al: Efficiency of the cell separator AMICUS for platelet depletion in the treatment of essential thrombocythemia. *J Clin Apher* 16:33, 2001.

113. Yamaguchi K, Hisano M, Sakata M, et al: Periodic plateletpheresis during pregnancy in a high-risk patient with essential thrombocythemia. *J Clin Apher* 21:256, 2006.

114. Raval JS, Redner RL, Kiss JE: Plateletpheresis for postsplenectomy rebound thrombocytosis in a patient with chronic immune thrombocytopenic purpura on romiplostim. *J Clin Apher* 28:321, 2013.

115. Natelson EA: Extreme thrombocytosis and cardiovascular surgery. Risks and management. *Tex Heart Inst J* 39:792, 2012.

116. Ward DM: Extracorporeal photopheresis: How, when and why? *J Clin Apher* 26:276, 2011.

117. Centers for Medicare and Medicaid Services: *Decision Memo for Extracorporeal Photopheresis (CAG-00324R).* (December 19, 2006.), Available online at http://www.cms.gov/medicare-coverage-database/details/nca-decision-memo.aspx?NCAId=255 (accessed 2 January 2015).

118. Babic AM: Extracorporeal photopheresis: Lighting the way to immunomodulation. *Am J Hematol* 83:589, 2008.

119. Yoo EK, Rook AH, Elenitsas R, et al: Apoptosis induction by ultraviolet light A and photochemotherapy in cutaneous T-cell lymphoma: Relevance to mechanism of therapeutic action. *J Invest Dermatol* 107:235, 1996.

120. Tambur AR, Ortegel JW, Morales A, et al: Extracorporeal photopheresis induces lymphocyte but not monocyte apoptosis. *Transplant Proc* 32:747, 2000.

121. Fimiani M, Di Renzo M, Rubegni P: Mechanism of action of extracorporeal photochemotherapy in chronic graft-versus-host disease. *Br J Dermatol* 150:1055, 2004.

122. Gorgun G, Miller KB, Foss FM: Immunologic mechanisms of extracorporeal photochemotherapy in chronic graft-versus-host disease. *Blood* 100:941, 2002.

123. Lamioni A, Parisi F, Isacchi G, et al: The immunological effects of extracorporeal photopheresis unraveled: Induction of tolerogenic dendritic cells in vitro and regulatory T cells in vivo. *Transplantation* 79:846, 2005.

124. McKenna KE, Whittaker S, Rhodes LE, et al: Evidence-based practice of photopheresis 1987-2001: A report of a workshop of the British Photodermatology Group and the UK Skin Lymphoma Group. *Br J Dermatol* 154:7, 2006.

125. Zic JA: The treatment of cutaneous T-cell lymphoma with photopheresis. *Dermatol Ther* 16:337, 2003.

126. Marques MB, Tuncer HH: Photopheresis in solid organ transplant rejection. *J Clin Apher* 21:72, 2006.

127. Choi J, Foss FM: Photopheresis, in *Apheresis: Principles and Practice,* 3rd ed, edited by BC McLeod, R Weinstein, JL Winters, AM Szczepiorkowski, p 615. AABB Press, Bethesda, MD, 2010.

CHAPTER 29
GENE THERAPY FOR HEMATOLOGIC DISEASES

Hua Fung and Stanton Gerson

SUMMARY

The term *gene therapy* describes treatment resulting from expression of a transferred gene (or transgene) in diseased or other cells by engineered vectors. Once within the cell, the transgene can direct synthesis of a therapeutic protein that can complement a genetic deficiency or confer upon the cell a desired phenotype or function. Many clinical trials have involved gene therapy for patients with various gene-deficient hematologic diseases, such as severe combined immunodeficiency, hemophilia, Wiskott-Aldrich syndrome, chronic granulomatous disease, aplastic anemia, hemoglobinopathies, HIV infection, and leukemia. Results from some clinical trials indicate that gene therapy can cure or improve many inherited or acquired hematologic disorders. This chapter reviews the basic principles of gene transfer and the results of selected preclinical and clinical studies.

DEFINITION AND HISTORY

Gene therapy is a promising treatment for several inherited or acquired hematologic disorders. Gene therapy involves the introduction of a functional gene to replace a mutated gene or a therapeutic gene to provide a missing or defective protein to the organism. In some cases, the patient's blood cells are removed and special, targeted cells such as hematopoietic stem cells (HSCs) are selected for engineering. The therapeutic genes are introduced into a vector and delivered into the targeted cells. These targeted, gene-modified cells are reinfused back into the patient. Because this method modifies cells outside the patient's body, it is called *ex vivo* gene therapy (Fig. 29–1A). By contrast *in vivo*

Acronyms and Abbreviations: AAV, adeno-associated virus; ADA-SCID, adenosine deaminase deficiency severe combined immunodeficiency; ARSA, arylsulfatase A; BCNU, 1,3-bis-(2-chloroethyl)-1-nitrosourea; CAR, chimeric antigen receptor; CCR5, chemokine (C-C motif) receptor 5 gene; CGD, chronic granulomatous disease; CLL, chronic lymphocytic leukemia; CRISPR, clustered, regularly interspaced, short palindromic repeats; DSB, double-stranded break; FA, Fanconi anemia; FVIII, factor VIII; FIX, factor IX; GCV, ganciclovir; GVHD, graft-versus-host disease; Hgb, hemoglobin; HR, homologous recombination; HSC, hematopoietic stem cell; HSV, herpes simplex virus; HSV-TK, herpes simplex virus thymidine kinase; iCasp9, inducible caspase 9 protein; IL2RG, interleukin-2 receptor gene; LTRs, the long terminal repeats; MGMT, O^6-methylguanine-DNA methyltransferase; MLD, metachromatic leukodystrophy; SIN, self-inactivating; siRNA, small interfering RNA; TALEN, transcription activator-like effector nuclease; TMZ, temozolomide; WAS, Wiskott-Aldrich syndrome; X-ALD, X-linked adrenoleukodystrophy; X-SCID, X-linked severe combined immunodeficiency; ZFN, zinc-finger nuclease.

gene therapy describes the therapeutic gene-containing vectors being directly injected into the patient (Fig. 29–1B). In the *in vivo* case, the gene is expressed, producing a therapeutic protein for treatment. Theoretically, if the gene-modified cells are long-lived and able to expand inside the body, a single gene therapy can be sufficient to provide a life-long therapeutic effect. Current gene therapy technologies have reached the point that many types of single-gene hematologic deficiency diseases can be permanently corrected, for example, X-linked severe combined immunodeficiency (X-SCID) and adenosine deaminase deficiency severe combined immunodeficiency (ADA-SCID).

Gene therapy has improved significantly in effectiveness since the mid-1980s when the first experiment using stem cell gene transfer was successful. Scientists initially encountered several serious obstacles. First, there was difficulty in delivering a modified gene into HSCs because of their lack of cell-surface receptors and their quiescent state.[1] Second, early X-SCID gene therapy was interrupted because 20 percent of patients developed a T-cell type of leukemia within 3 to 6 years after therapy. This event was caused by gene therapy-related viral vector insertional mutagenesis; the vector contained powerful enhancer elements within its long terminal repeats (LTRs) that inserted close to, and activated the *LMO2* protooncogene.[2] Over 3 decades, these problems have been (for the most part) resolved. With an array of cytokine stimulation cocktails to improve HSC receptivity to engineering, and improved lentiviral vectors, the HSC transduction rate in humans can reach 80 to 100 percent.[3,4] In addition, myeloablative conditioning regimens (e.g., busulfan, melphalan and 1,3-bis-[2-chloroethyl]-1-nitrosourea [BCNU; aka carmustine]) that decrease the number of endogenous stem cells prior to infusion of the engineered HSCs has proven to be an effective method to increase engraftment rates (average: 1 to 2 copies of gene marking/cell).[3,4] High-level stem cell engraftment is a critical factor for the gene therapy of chronic granulomatous disease, X-linked adrenoleukodystrophy (X-ALD) and metachromatic leukodystrophy.[3–6] Moreover, newer, safer self-inactivating (SIN) viral vectors have been developed in which viral LTR enhancers are completely removed. Using these newer vectors, no patient has developed therapy-related malignancy in several clinical trials, some of which have followed patients for as long as 8 years.[3,4] Gene therapy is no longer a hypothetical form of therapy; some trials have achieved clinical correction for as long as 12 years. Gene therapy has, thus, undergone a renaissance. This chapter discusses two critical technical factors in gene therapy: targeted cells and delivered vectors; briefly reviews the gene therapy of several common hematopoietic genetic deficient diseases; and describes new strategies of *in vivo* selection and insertion site-targeted gene therapy.

GENE THERAPY TARGETED CELLS

HEMATOPOIETIC STEM CELLS

HSCs are the cell of choice for many gene therapy applications for several reasons. First, many blood cell disorders originate at the stem cell level and, therefore, gene-corrected HSCs are the best candidate for replacement. Second, HSCs are a long-lived and self-renewing population and may reduce or eliminate the need for repeated administration of gene therapy. HSCs are readily obtained in the blood, marrow, or umbilical cord blood. They are also easily selected and manipulated in the laboratory and can be returned to patients relatively easily. Third, engineered HSCs are able to correct defects in all hematopoietic lineages. Fourth, HSCs migrate to several tissues in the body—primarily the marrow, but also the liver, spleen, and lymph nodes. These may be strategic locations for localized delivery of therapeutic agents for disorders unrelated to the hematopoietic system, such as for patients with liver diseases.

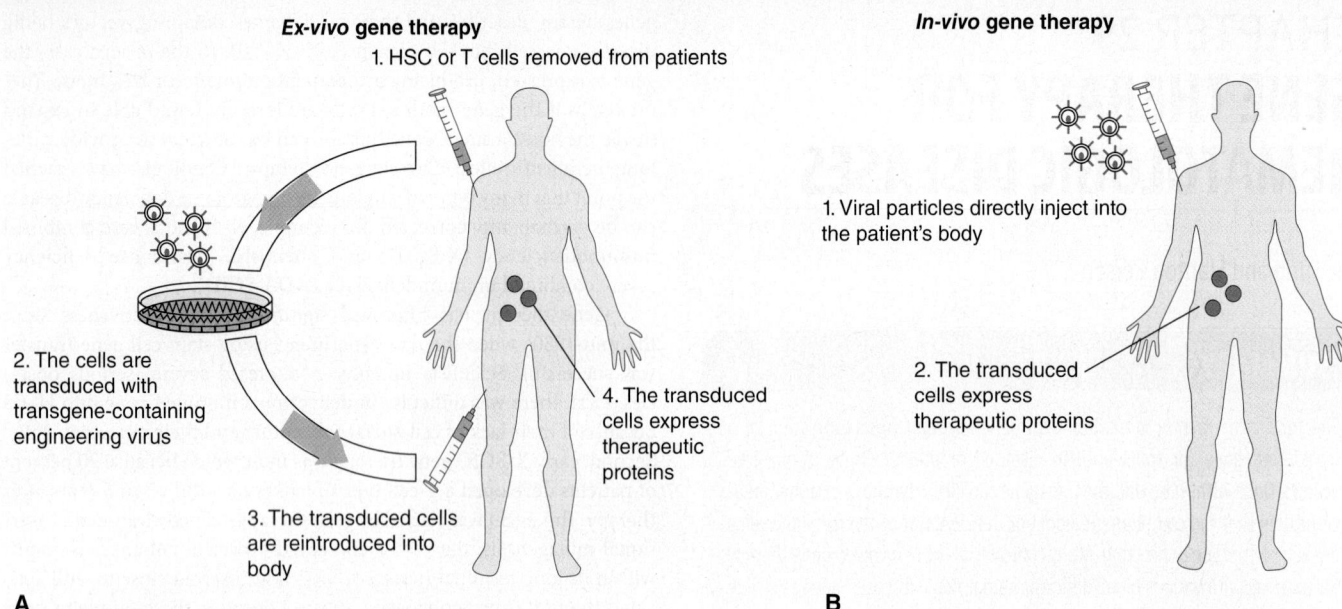

Figure 29–1. A. *Ex vivo* gene therapy involves 4 steps: 1. Obtain patient's blood (HSCs or T cells); 2. transduce the cells in the laboratory by engineering the virus that contains a transgene; 3. infuse the transduced cells into the patient; and 4. the infused transduced cells produce therapeutic proteins. **B.** *In vivo* gene therapy is done by directly injecting viral particles into the patient.

T LYMPHOCYTES

The use of hematopoietic progenitor or precursor cells for gene therapy theoretically would require repeat application. However, for some inherited and acquired diseases involving T cells (e.g., severe combined immunodeficiency [SCID] and AIDS), the use of T-cell precursors is capable of long-term correction of the T-cell deficiency. The underlying mechanism is still not clear, but some types of T cells, such as memory T cells, are long-lived. The memory T-cell compartment has three subsets: T-memory stem cells, central memory T cells, and effector memory T cells.[7] Memory T cells and central memory T cells can expand to large numbers of effector T cells when activated. T-cell gene therapy is effective in some forms of cancer therapy. Long-term effects could be related to memory T stem cells. For example, T effector cells can directly eradicate malignant cells. However, cancer cells are often "invisible" to T cells. For this reason, modified T cells have been created by adding a chimeric antigen receptors (CARs) expressing gene, engineering the T cells to recognize cancer-specific antigens such as CD19 on chronic lymphocytic leukemia (CLL) cells.[8,9] Once the CAR-modified T cells are transfused into the patient, they can attack and eradicate the targeted malignant cells. In clinical trials, anti-CD19 CAR T cells profoundly decreased the level of cancer cells in three patients with end-stage CLL.[8,9]

An advantage of using gene-modified T cells is that the procedure does not disturb the otherwise normal hematopoietic system. However, this is also a limitation of using T cells in gene therapy. For example, when using T cells to correct X-SCID, although T cells recover to near normal levels, the other affected cell types (e.g., B cells, natural killer [NK] cells) are not corrected. In this approach, the patient would require immunoglobulin replacement and the NK cell deficiency would persist. A study compared the outcomes of several clinical trials of HIV therapy comparing CD4+ T-cell treatment to HSC-based treatment. These trials found that overall, the results from HSCs were better than that of CD4+ T cells.[10] One reason offered for this result is that without stimulation, T cells proliferate at a very low rate, estimated at approximately one division every 3.5 years for naïve T cells, and one division every 22 weeks for memory T cells.[11]

● GENE THERAPY VECTORS

The majority of gene therapy studies thus far have employed viral vectors, because of their high efficiency of transgene delivery into the human nucleus. For a long-term effect, genome-integrating retroviral/lentiviral vectors have been employed. However, DNA integration causing critical gene mutagenesis has raised concern about long-term safety. This concern has led to the development of persisting but nonintegrating viral vectors.

NON–GENOME-INTEGRATING VIRAL VECTORS

Adenoviral Vector

Adenoviral vectors do not integrate into the genome, but are highly effective in gene therapy because of their ability to efficiently transduce both dividing and nondividing cells, and to persist relatively well in long-lived targeted cells. Adenoviral vectors also have capacity to hold large segments of DNA (e.g., 7.5 kbp); they are easily manipulated with recombinant DNA techniques and have the ability to produce high titers.[12,13] However, adenoviral vector infection enlists a variety of humoral and cellular immune responses.[14] Therefore, adenoviral vector therapy may result in acute toxicity and autoimmunity, and which clears transgene-expressing cells, reducing the efficacy of therapy.[13] Of interest, this autoimmunity can be targeting to adenovirus-infected cancer cells, and thus used as an oncolytic agent.[15]

ADENO-ASSOCIATED VIRAL VECTORS

The adeno-associated viral vector (AAV) has the abilities to infect both nondividing and dividing cells and to persist without vector integration.[16,17] Upon entering host cells, wild-type AAV DNA becomes episomal or integrates into the genome; in contrast, current, modified AAV vectors are designed to lose their integrating ability.[18] AAV can carry a transgene up to 4.7 kbp. The AAV genome is single-stranded DNA and vector preparations are composed of a mixture of vector particles having one of the two strands of the virus. Upon transduction, the required annealing of the two strands delays gene expression. This limitation can be overcome by using a self-complementary design in which the two strands of the transgene are on a single hairpin genome in an inverted orientation, which allows quick assembly into a transcription unit following transduction.[19]

GENOME-INTEGRATING VIRAL VECTORS

Retroviral Vectors

A feature of retroviral vectors is that they have the ability to stably incorporate their viral DNA into the host genome, which can result in long-term expression of the transgene. Most retroviral vectors are γ-retroviral or lentiviral vectors. Lentiviral vectors are usually HIV-1 based, or may also contain elements of simian immunodeficiency virus, and have at least three advantages over γ-retroviral vectors; first, the lentiviral vector preintegration complex is able to cross the nuclear membrane in host cells even in the absence of mitosis and, therefore, is able to transduce nondividing cells, such as HSCs.[20] Second, the lentiviral vector preintegration complex is more stable and persists longer, which improves the likelihood of integration.[20] Third, γ-retroviral vectors prefer to integrate near gene transcription start sites, such as the CpG islands and conserved noncoding sequences and conserved transcriptional factor binding sites, whereas lentiviral vectors are more evenly distributed, reducing the likelihood of driving the expression of a deleterious gene(s).[22] Lentiviral vectors have thus emerged as an important advance for gene therapy in the hematologic disorders.

● GENE THERAPY FOR HEMATOLOGIC DISEASES

X-LINKED SEVERE COMBINED IMMUNODEFICIENCY

X-SCID is a single-gene-deficient disease caused by mutations in the gene of the interleukin-2 receptor, γIL2RG (Chap. 80).[23] Lack of functional γIL2RG results in a lack of T and NK cells and poorly functional B cells. X-SCID is a fatal disease, and without medical interventions, patients often die within the first 2 years of life.[23] During 1999 to 2006, 20 X-SCID children were treated in two gene therapy trials.[24,25] Because patients lacked an human leukocyte antigen (HLA)-identical donor, precluding stem cell transplantation as a curative therapy, all 20 patients were given a single γ-retroviral vector-mediated gene therapy in which a wild-type γIL2RG gene was delivered into patients' T cells. From 5 to 12 years of observation after the gene transfer procedure, 17 of the 20 treated participants are alive and display nearly full correction of the T-cell deficiency by genetically modified T cells.[24,25]

ADENOSINE DEAMINASE DEFICIENCY SEVERE COMBINED IMMUNODEFICIENCY

Adenosine deaminase (ADA) deficiency is an autosomal-recessive inherited disorder caused by mutation of ADA gene on chromosome 20 (Chap. 80). ADA deficiency leads to inhibition of DNA synthesis, which is particularly toxic to lymphocytes because they are some of the most mitotically active cells. This condition ultimately causes SCID. ADA-SCID is almost always fatal by 2 years of age. Gene therapy with a normal ADA gene expressed in autologous HSC is a potentially curative treatment. However, early attempts at gene therapy did not shown any clinical benefit. In the late 1990s, when improved retroviral vector and preinfusion chemotherapy conditioning were instituted, success occurred. Since 2000, 40 patients have been treated in Italy,

Great Britain, and the United States.[26–28] In these studies HSCs were transduced with a γ-retroviral vector encoding the ADA enzyme. Low-intensity conditioning with either busulfan or melphalan was used to increase engraftment of stem cells. In some patients the corrected ADA gene can be detected in blood mononuclear cells for more than 9 years, and the ADA enzyme remains at a normal level.[27]

WISKOTT-ALDRICH SYNDROME

Wiskott-Aldrich syndrome (WAS) is the result of a mutation in the gene encoding the WAS protein (WASp).[28] The gene is located on the short arm of the X chromosome and WAS is an X-linked recessive genetic disorder. WASP activates actin polymerization in almost all blood cells. Hereditary deficiency in WASP is associated with microthrombocytopenia, recurrent infections, eczema, high incidence of autoimmunity and hematopoietic malignancy (lymphoma or leukemia).[29] In 2010, three patients in Italy were administered a lentiviral vector engineered to express WASp following busulfan conditioning. All three WAS patients showed excellent multilineage engraftment with an average of 0.4 to 0.9 correct gene copy per genome persisting to 30 months. Symptoms of WAS improved substantially. Pretreatment eczema resolved between 6 and 12 months after therapy. The frequency and severity of infections progressively decreased, and cytomegalovirus replication was controlled, allowing withdrawal of antiinfectious prophylaxis in two patients. Improvement of platelet count resulted in discontinuation of platelet transfusions.[3]

LEUKODYSTROPHIES, X-LINKED ADRENOLEUKODYSTROPHY, AND METACHROMATIC LEUKODYSTROPHY

There are two major leukodystrophies, X-ALD and metachromatic leukodystrophy (MLD); both have been successfully treated with gene therapy.[4,6] X-ALD is a severe genetic demyelinating disease caused by mutations in the ABCD1 gene on the X chromosome that encodes the adrenoleukodystrophy (ALD) protein, an adenosine triphosphate binding cassette transporter. ALD deficiency leads to the accumulation of very-long-chain fatty acids and progressive demyelination in the central nervous system. In 2009, two French children were reported to have autologous HSC gene therapy with a lentiviral vector encoding wild-type ABCD1.[6] The patients were given myeloablative regimen conditioning with cyclophosphamide and busulfan. ALD protein was expressed in 23 and 25 percent of blood mononuclear cells in the two patients. Over 3 years of followup, corrected ABCD1 was found in 7 to 14 percent of granulocytes, monocytes, and T and B lymphocytes. Cerebral demyelination was arrested.[6]

MLD is an autosomal recessive disorder caused by mutations in ARSA gene in chromosome 22 that encodes arylsulfatase A (ARSA). Deficiency in ARSA leads to sulfatide accumulation, eventually destroying the myelin sheath of the nervous system. In 2013, three children with the disease received autologous HSC gene therapy with a lentiviral vector encoding wild-type ARSA.[4] After myeloablative conditioning with busulfan, engraftment was excellent with 45 to 80 percent gene marking levels. ARSA activity was restored to above normal values in the hematopoietic lineages and the cerebrospinal fluid.[4] There was a clear therapeutic benefit. In X-ALD and MLD gene therapies, corrected cells did not have an obvious selective advantage. However, in both cases the gene marking levels were high (>10 percent) for as long as 2 years.[4,6] These results indicate that successful gene therapy can be achieved with very high viral transduction rates, even absent a transduced cell selection mechanism.

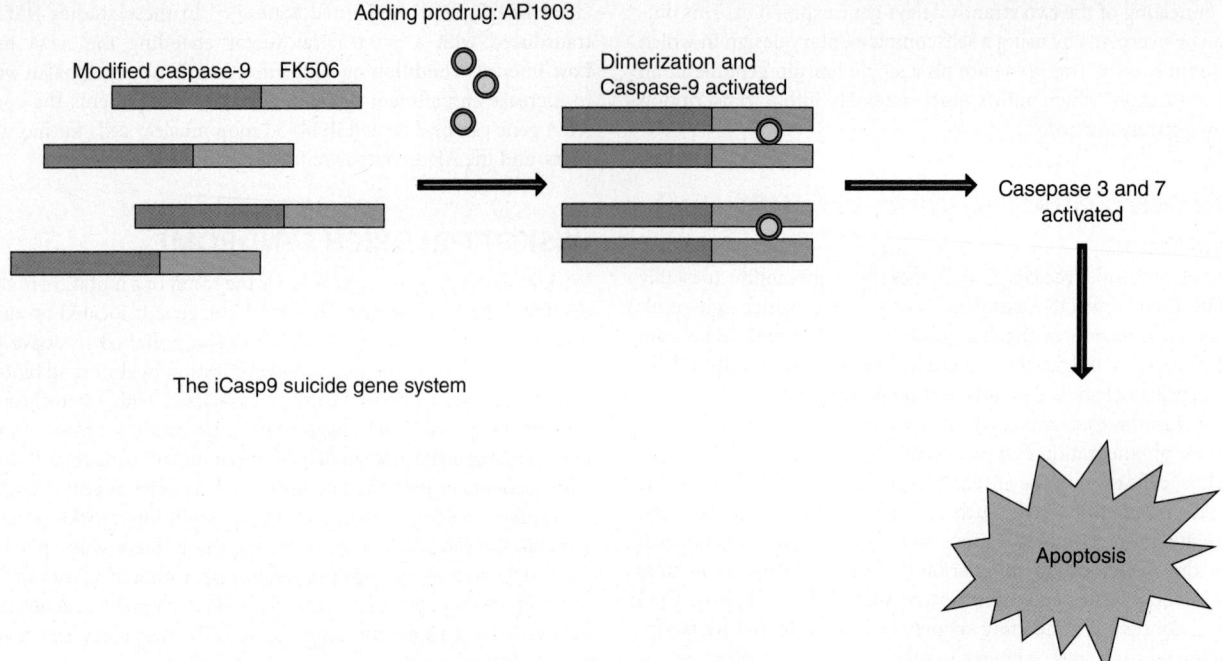

Figure 29–2. Inducible caspase-9 protein (iCasp9) suicide gene therapy system. A fusion protein contains a mutated FK506 protein linked to the modified caspase 9 (deleted for activation and recruitment domains). The prodrug AP1903 interacts with the FK506 domain and triggers the fusion protein dimerization, which activates caspase-9. Activated caspase-9 initiates the cell caspase cascade (caspases 3 and 7) and induces cell death by apoptosis.

Avoiding Graft-versus-Host Disease

Gene therapy can lead to graft-versus-host disease (GVHD), especially after an allogeneic stem cell transplantation. To prevent GVHD, a suicide gene is introduced in the transferred cells; in the event of GVHD, a prodrug is given to activate the suicide gene to kill the transduced cell. This "safety mechanism" can also guard against uncontrolled proliferation of targeted cells. Traditionally, the suicide gene is herpes simplex virus thymidine kinase *(HSV-TK)*, which can be made "suicidal" in the presence of ganciclovir (GCV). Once GCV is phosphorylated by *HSV-TK*, it turns to a nucleotide analogue that inhibits DNA synthesis and kills the cell.[30] Another new suicide gene system was developed by an inducible caspase-9 protein (iCasp9), which activates the mitochondrial apoptotic pathway. Its use is based on caspase-9 dimerization to an active form. The catalytic domain of caspase-9 is fused to a modified FK506-binding domain that can be homodimerized by a chemical inducer, such as AP1903 (Fig. 29–2). In a clinical trial, four patients who had undergone stem cell transplantation for relapsed acute leukemia were treated with the modified T cells. A single dose of AP1903 was given when GVHD developed, which eliminated more than 90 percent of the modified T cells within 30 minutes and eliminated the clinical signs of GVHD.[31] In comparison to HSV-TK, iCasp9 offers several advantages. It induces cell death faster, does not rely on cell proliferation, which makes it ideal for cancer stem cell killing; and, because caspase-9 is downstream of the mitochondria, the sensitivity of cells to its activation should be independent of the antiapoptotic BCL-2 family of proteins, which is often upregulated in hematologic malignancies.

HUMAN IMMUNODEFICIENCY VIRAL INFECTION

The HIV infects helper T cells, such as CD4+ T cells, macrophages, and dendritic cells. The infection kills CD4+ T cells and cripples cell-mediated immunity (Chap. 81). Without treatment, average survival

time after infection with HIV is estimated to be 9 to 11 years. In 2007, a gene therapy trial demonstrated that AIDS can be cured. A patient with an HIV infection and acute myeloid leukemia was given allogenic stem cell transplantation from a selected donor, whose two copies of the chemokine (C-C motif) receptor 5 gene (*CCR5*) were lost because of mutations.[32] CCR5 is the major cellular coreceptor used by HIV to infect CD4+ T cells. The patient has since remained off anti-HIV drugs for 7 years. This case generated enormous interest in gene therapy approaches to cure HIV by blocking CCR5 expression. One of the most promising methods is to create loss of function mutations of *CCR5* with zinc-finger nucleases (ZFNs). ZFNs are artificial restriction enzymes generated by fusing zinc fingers to a nonspecific double-strand DNA cleavage protein, a truncated Fox1.[33] A zinc finger can be engineered to a target 18 to 24 bp sequences in *CCR5* DNA. ZFNs can repeatedly cut the DNA at a targeted site and eventually mutate *CCR5* when repair errors occur. In a 12-patient clinical trial, the patient's CD4+ T cells were infected *ex vivo* with a ZFN-expressing adenoviral vector to disrupt *CCR5*.[34] The modified cells were then reintroduced. CD4 T cells lacking *CCR5* are resistant to HIV infection. Ultimately, the CCR5-mutated cells replace those vulnerable CCR5 wild-type cells. The infusion immediately increased the circulating CD4+ T cell count from a median of 488×10^9/L to 1517×10^9/L in the first week. The modified cells were also found in T-cell–rich gut-associated lymphoid tissues. Patients were off antiviral drugs for 84 days during which time the circulating CD4+ T cells dropped while viral load spiked. Antiviral treatment had to be reinstituted.[34] The CCR5-mutated CD4+ T-cell count remained stable even during the drug-off period, consistent with their resistance to HIV killing. However, CCR5-mutated CD4+ T cells apparently did not expand quickly, which may explain why in this trial the modified cell infusion alone was insufficient to control the HIV infection. Another trial used a lentiviral anti-HIV small interfering RNA (siRNA) expression vector to modify HSCs.[35] Although long-term (18 months) expression of siRNA in multiple blood cell lineages was observed, modified cell levels were less than 0.4 percent. The fact that both modified HSCs and T cells failed to repopulate indicated that the *in vivo* selection of modified HIV-resistant cells may be weak or the modified T cells do not have a proliferative reaction to HIV infection. In both cases, the engraftment rate was very poor (T cell <10 percent and HSC <0.2 percent), which could indicate that the modified cells do not have a sufficient starting number for repopulation. New trials are underway with an improved lentiviral vector, engraftment protocols and a methylguanine DNA methyltransferase (MGMT) *in vivo* selection mechanism.[36] The cure for HIV by gene therapy has shown promise, but some clinical obstacles have to be overcome to achieve success.

DISORDERS OF HEMOGLOBIN

Thalassemia and sickle cell disease represent the most common single-gene defect diseases worldwide (Chaps. 48 and 49). β-Thalassemia is caused by a mutation in the β-globin gene, resulting in reduced adult hemoglobin A (HgbA) and severe anemia.[37] Therefore, gene therapy is used to express a normal β-globin gene. Many efforts have been made to use stem cell gene therapy. However, success has been very limited.[37] Although a weak survival advantage for corrected red cells at an early mature stage was observed, the *in vivo* selection alone appears insufficient to achieve a sustained correction.[38] It is predicated that it would require 20 percent of the primitive hematopoietic cells to be genetically modified, and the gene expressed at near normal levels in those cells, to achieve a definitive therapeutic benefit. Even higher levels of corrected cells (approximately 100 percent) might be required to cure the disease.[38] The first successful clinical trial was reported in 2007.[39] An 18-year-old patient with severe β-thalassemia dependent on monthly red cell transfusion since age 3 years, received HSC lentiviral β-globin gene therapy. The viral transduction rate was approximately 30 percent. The patient continued receiving transfusions for 16 months after the transplantation, at that point the therapeutic HgbA was sufficient and maintained at a sufficient level until 33 months (Fig. 29–3). During the final 21 months, 100 percent of HgbA was from modified cells and the patient was transfusion-free. However, the therapy effect was later found to be from a dominant clone (>60 percent of all viral insertion sites in nucleated blood cells at 24 months), in which the viral insertion causes transcriptional activation of *HMGA2* in erythroid cells.[39] Nevertheless,

the patient remained with a good quality life with a stable Hgb of 9 to 10 g/dL, transfusion-free, and cancer-free for up to 7 years.[40] The dominant clone might indicate a strong *in vivo* selection, however, the level of gene modified cells in this patient has been never greater than 21 percent, and the highest level noted in blood was 10.9 percent and in erythroblasts was 3.3 percent, which is below that predicted. The dominant clone remained stable over time. However, HMGA2 overexpression was detected in erythroid cells, which could enhance *in vivo* selection and proliferation of the corrected cells. Nevertheless, this is but a single case; whether the *in vivo* selection of the dominate clone had a significant role is not clear. More trials are needed.

HEMOPHILIA

Hemophilia is an X-linked single-gene defect, of which 70 percent of affected patients display inheritance and 30 percent develop from *de novo* somatic mutations (Chap. 124). There are two major forms of hemophilia: hemophilia A, caused by loss-of-function mutations of the gene encoding clotting factor VIII (FVIII), and hemophilia B, the result of mutations in the gene encoding clotting factor IX (FIX). Hemophilia A accounts for 80 percent of patients and hemophilia B for 20 percent.[41] The absence of either FVIII or FIX severely impairs the ability to generate thrombin and, subsequently, fibrin, leading to spontaneous bleeding when the factor levels fall below approximately 5 percent of normal. Theoretically, gene therapy using a lentiviral vector that permanently expresses a normal *FVIII* or *FIX* gene in the patient could cure either disease. However, after 2 decades of intense research, gene therapy has been very difficult. FVIII and FIX are produced in hepatocytes, not in derivatives of HSCs.[42] Therefore, hemophilia is not a circumstance for HSC-based gene therapy. The emerging approach to gene therapy for hemophilia is by using *in vivo* gene therapy (see Fig. 29–1). In this approach, viral particles are injected into a patient's vein, muscle, hepatic artery, or omentum.[43] Initially, five clinical trials with retroviral, adenoviral, or AAV vectors failed to achieve long-term expression of the coagulation factor and no measurable clinical benefit was observed.[43] However, a trial by a British-American team reported in 2011 showed exceptional results.[15] This group focused on hemophilia B. The *FIX* gene, unlike the *FVIII* gene, is small and easy to insert into an AAV vector, and 1 to 2 percent of the normal blood levels of FIX

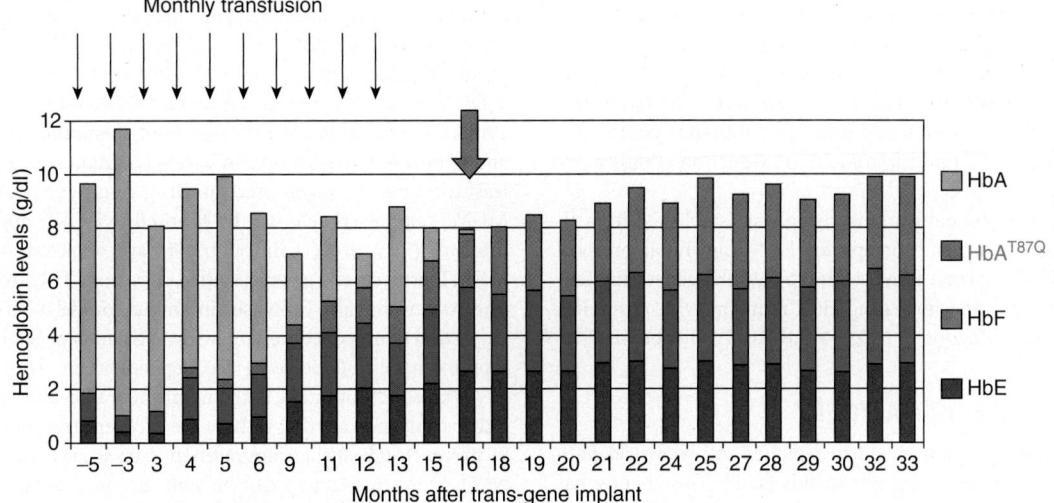

Figure 29–3. A typical successful gene therapy outcome. In this case a β-thalassemia patient was given a lentiviral vector that contains a HgbA^T87Q transgene. After infusion of modified HSCs 16 months *(red arrow)*, HgbA^T87Q *(red)* completely replaced HgbA *(blue)* that was from prior transfusions. At this point, the patient had become transfusion-independent. *(Adapted with permission from Cavazzana-Calvo M, Payen E, Negre O, et al: Transfusion independence and HMGA2 activation after gene therapy of human β-thalassaemia. Nature 16;467(7313):318–322, 2010.)*

is sufficient to markedly reduce the bleeding risk.[43] A new improved AAV vector (AAV8) was used. This vector has a self-complementary genome to improve transduction efficiency, and was designed to produce fivefold higher levels of capsid protein to reduce a potential cytotoxic T-cell response and increase liver tropism. The AAV vector is not genome-integrating and maintains itself as an intracellular episome. Its gene expression in growing cells is transient because episomes may be lost with each cell division. But in quiescent tissues the AAV vector is capable of mediating long-term gene expression as episomal chromatin.[44] A single intravenous infusion of the vector was given to six adult male hemophilia B patients who had been treated with recombinant FIX for many years. No notable acute or chronic toxicities were observed. All six patients displayed stable FIX expression at 2 to 11 percent of normal blood levels for 3 years. Four of these patients discontinued recombinant FIX treatment and remained free of spontaneous hemorrhage.[15,43,45] The same research team is attempting a similar approach for hemophilia A gene therapy; however, *FVIII* gene expression has been inefficient. One reason is gene size. The *FVIII* coding sequence is 7 kb, which far exceeds the normal packaging capacity of AAV vectors. By modifying the B domain, the *FVIII* size was reduced to a 5.2-kb AAV expression cassette, which is more efficiently packaged. Also, a hybrid liver-specific promoter was introduced into the vector. The resulting new AAV vector has shown high (15 percent of normal) FVIII expression for 20 to 45 weeks in four macaques.[46] This AAV vector will be used in a trial of hemophilia A gene therapy in the near future.

FANCONI ANEMIA

Fanconi anemia (FA) is caused by mutations in *Fanconi* genes, which encode the DNA repair proteins that form a function complex (Chap. 35). FA cells are hypersensitive to DNA crosslinking agents.[47] Sixteen *Fanconi* genes have been described. A defect in one of them will lead to FA. The disease is characterized by a high risk of developing marrow failure and later myelodysplasia, acute leukemia, or cancers of other tissues.[47] More than half of patients with FA are the result of *FANCA* gene mutations; therefore current gene therapy has focused on *FANCA* insufficiency. Gene therapy for FA is particularly challenging because of the low numbers of HSCs in the stage of marrow failure, and FA cells are extremely sensitive to DNA damage when exposed to myelosuppressive drugs used to condition the patient for stem cell transplantation. In a rare case, two identical twins had inherited *FANCA* mutations but with normal DNA repair in their blood stem cells. Functional *FANCA* in blood cells was found to be restored by a spontaneous intrauterine self-correcting somatic mutation in a single HSC. The fact that a single HSC was sufficient to restore a fully normal blood system indicates that *FANCA* gene therapy may require transduction of only a few HSCs.[48]

In 2011, an international working group was established to facilitate the development of gene therapy for FA.[49] The initial protocol included delivery of a normal *FANCA* gene by a third-generation lentiviral vector into HSC and increasing HSC number by *in vitro* HSC expansion using a combination of HOXB4 and DELTA-1 proteins.[50]

GENE THERAPY FOR CANCER

Gene therapy for cancer has been widely exploited. A review was published detailing the new developments in this field.[51] This chapter has described a few significant new approaches.

One of the most creative new approaches to cancer-targeted gene therapy is the use of CAR for CLL, in which patient's T cells were modified to target their own cancers (Chap. 92).[7,8] Another strategy is to

enhance conventional chemotherapy by protecting the marrow cells through gene transfer. Chemotherapy has a limited therapeutic window because of its severe toxic effect on marrow cells, and its leukemogenic potential. Because the lethal effect of chemotherapy is mainly DNA damage, especially methylating O^6-guanine, to overcome the side effects, a strong chemoresistant DNA repair gene, a mutant (P140K) of MGMT was introduced into brain tumor patients' autologous HSC by a γ-retroviral vector, thus the patient's transduced marrow progenitor cells could be protected by the modified MGMT, permitting them to tolerate more cycles of chemotherapy. A phase I clinical trial demonstrated that intensification of chemotherapy was feasible, and there was an improvement in therapy outcome and patient survival in these small studies.[52,53] A similar result was also observed in a recent clinical trial with a lentiviral vector (reported at the ASH meeting 2014).

● NEW TECHNOLOGIES USED IN GENE THERAPY

IN VIVO SELECTION AND O^6-METHYLGUANINE-DNA METHYLTRANSFERASE SELECTIVE METHOD

Whether stem cell gene therapy can cure a disease is dependent on the functionality of the gene-corrected cell. In the early successful gene therapy trials for X-SCID and ADA-SCID, a low (0.1 to 1.0 percent) engraftment rate was sufficient for long-term gene correction, and the single most important factor was that the transgene conferred a selective survival advantage on the transgene-bearing cell.[38] In contrast, a main reason for poor responses in other gene therapy trials has been that the gene-corrected cells have no, or only a weak selective advantage, such that the gene-transduced cell levels are insufficient to provide a clinical meaningful benefit. Therefore, *in vivo* selection is a key element in the success of clinical gene therapy.

The gene-corrected cells in the majority of hematologic genetic diseases have no *in vivo* selection advantage.[38] To overcome this problem, a second, selectable gene can be used to be coexpressed with the gene that corrected the defect. The second gene turns the cells into selectable cells.[38] The selectable gene can be cloned into a vector along with correcting gene driven by a single or separate promoter. Experiments have identified several selectable genes including multidrug resistance protein, dihydrofolate reductase, and MGMT.[38] MGMT shows the most promising results in large animal and humans trials. MGMT encodes a DNA repair enzyme O^6-alkylguanine-DNA-alky-transferase, which confers resistance to the cytotoxicity of chemotherapy, such as BCNU and temozolomide (TMZ).[54] A MGMT mutant, P140K-MGMT, has at least a 50-fold stronger effect on drug resistance resistance.[55] P140K-MGMT–expressed cells can be exposed to BCNU and TMZ selection pressure (Fig. 29-4). Clinical trials have demonstrated that P140K-MGMT protects the gene-modified cells from TMZ-induced toxicity.[52] This strategy has also been used in a mouse model of HIV gene therapy.[36]

Successful gene therapy with satisfactory gene marking levels (approximately 30 percent) are dependent on three factors: a high HSC transduction rate, a high engraftment rate, and *in vivo* selection.[38] Other trials indicate that if there are excellent transduction rates (80 to 90 percent) and excellent engraftment rates (gene copy marking/genome >0.5), these two factors can be sufficient to achieve a sustained gene correction, even without an *in vivo* selection mechanism.[4] Nevertheless, if there is a low transduction rate and low engraftment rate, MGMT-mediated *in vivo* selection will be a very valuable tool to improve the likelihood of successful gene therapy.

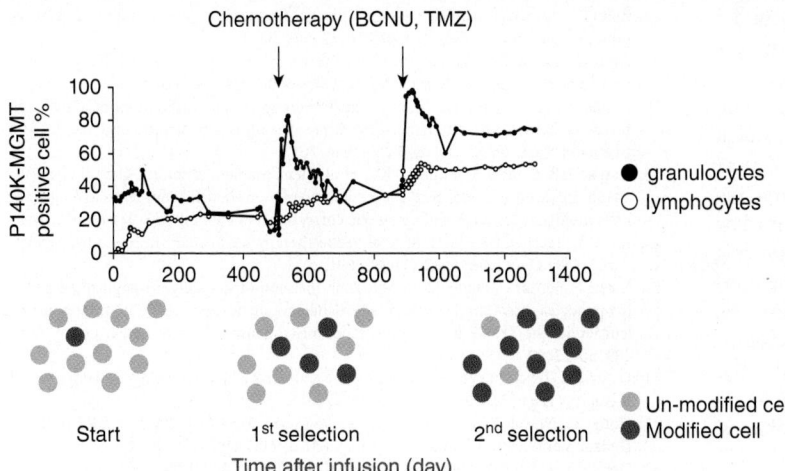

Figure 29–4. An example of P140K-MGMT (O⁶-methyl-guanine-DNA methyltransferase) *in vivo* selection. Studies in a monkey. The P140K-MGMT–modified cells continued to increase after each chemotherapy administration (selective pressures). BCNU, 1,3-bis-(2-chloroethyl)-1-nitrosourea; TMZ, temozolomide. *(Adapted with permission from Beard BC, Trobridge GD, Ironside C, et al: Efficient and stable MGMT-mediated selection of long-term repopulating stem cells in nonhuman primates. J Clin Invest 120(7):2345–2354, 2010.)*

OVERCOMING GENOTOXICITY BY TARGETED-INSERTION GENE THERAPY

To achieve sustained gene correction, some gene therapy approaches have used integrated vectors such as γ-retroviral or lentiviral vectors. Gene therapy for X-SCID,[56] WAS,[57] and chronic granulomatous disease (CGD)[58] has found that γ-retroviral insertion in the vicinity of protooncogenes is associated with the development of lymphoproliferative and myeloproliferative neoplasms. Improved lentiviral vectors have added safety features, such as no preference for integration near promoters, removal of viral promoter-enhancers, and self-inactivation. However, even with these new features, lentiviral vector-induced clonal dominance in human[6] and murine leukemia have been reported.[59] DNA insertion is the most important factor to determine whether a therapy-related cancer will occur, especially as 80 to 90 percent of lentiviral vector insertions are within gene regions.[21] Gene therapy with viral vector insertion, in which the insertion site is uncontrollable, raises the risk of a secondary clonal disease. The FDA has not approved a single-gene therapy in the United States, largely because of the risk of uncontrollable insertional mutagenesis.

One way to reduce this risk is to select preferred sites of DNA insertion. Gene-targeting and gene-editing technologies could make this possible. Gene editing describes insertion of DNA at a desired location.[33] It starts with artificially engineered nucleases, such as ZFNs, which can create a double-stranded break (DSB) at a targeted DNA sequence anywhere in the human genome. The DSBs is repaired by homologous recombination (HR) repair or nonhomologous end-joining repair. The ZFNs can be cotransfected with another plasmid (donor DNA plasmid), in which a desired DNA sequence, such as a transgene has been inserted within a sequence that is homologous to the flanking sequences of the DSB. When this DNA sequence is used as a template by HR, it would result in insertion at a targeted location (Fig. 29–5).

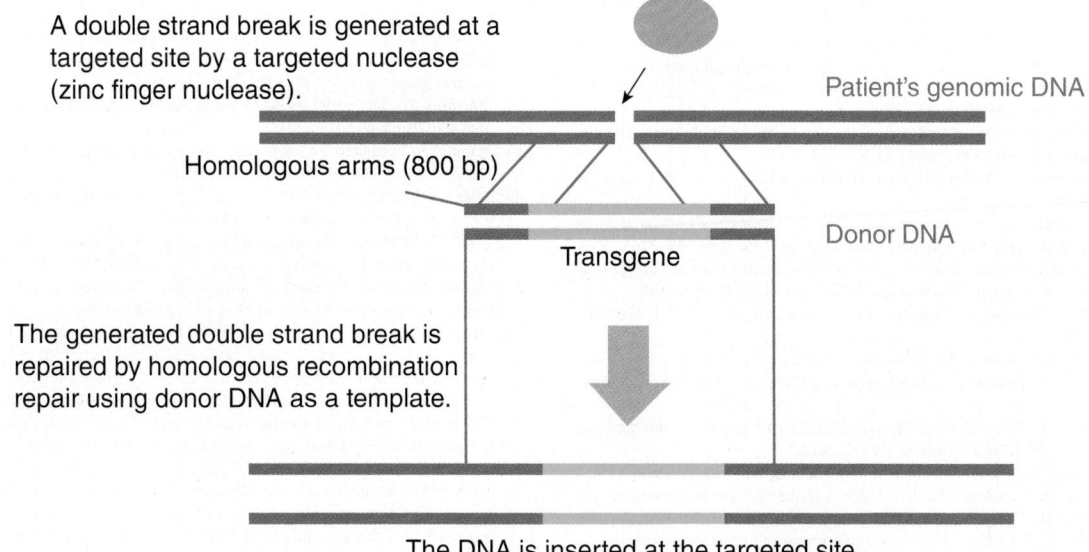

Figure 29–5. Targeted transgene insertion. A targeted nuclease, such as zinc finger nuclease first generates a double-strand break (DSB). Thereafter, the DSB is repaired by homologous recombination repair using donor DNA with a transgene inserted within two homologous arms. When repair is finished, the transgene is inserted at the targeted site.

Using ZFN, a DNA (up to 9.6 kb)[60] can be inserted precisely into a selected location of the human genome. There are several known "safe harbors" in the human genome. For example, the *PPP1R12C* gene on chromosome 19 (*AAVS1* locus) is frequently integrated by an AAV and such an AAV-based integration is not associated with any subsequent pathologic events.[61] Several genes have been inserted into the *AAVS1* site in human cells, including stem cells, using ZFN gene-targeting methods.[60,62] The gene correction rate of gene editing is still very low (approximately 1 percent).[63] Fortunately, gene targeting is a fast-growing field. Many new technologies have developed in recent years. The transcription activator-like effector nuclease (TALEN)[64] and the clustered, regularly interspaced, short palindromic repeats (CRISPR)[65] technology show promise. Both TALEN and CRISPR are much easier and faster to use than the ZFN approach. These new gene-targeted technologies together may solve the retroviral insertion mutagenesis safety problems.

REFERENCES

1. Vollweiler JL, Zielske SP, Reese JS, Gerson SL: Hematopoietic stem cell gene therapy: Progress toward therapeutic targets. *Bone Marrow Transplant* 32(1):1–7, 2003.
2. Howe SJ, Mansour MR, Schwarzwaelder K, et al: Insertional mutagenesis combined with acquired somatic mutations causes leukemogenesis following gene therapy of SCID-X1 patients. *J Clin Invest* 118(9):3143–3150, 2008.
3. Aiuti A, Biasco L, Scaramuzza S, et al: Lentiviral hematopoietic stem cell gene therapy in patients with Wiskott-Aldrich syndrome. *Science* 341(6148):1233151, 2013.
4. Biffi A, Montini E, Lorioli L, et al: Lentiviral hematopoietic stem cell gene therapy benefits metachromatic leukodystrophy. *Science* 341(6148):1233158, 2013.
5. Grez M, Reichenbach J, Schwable J, et al: Gene therapy of chronic granulomatous disease: The engraftment dilemma. *Mol Ther* 19(1):28–35, 2011.
6. Cartier N, Hacein-Bey-Abina S, Bartholomae CC, et al: Hematopoietic stem cell gene therapy with a lentiviral vector in X-linked adrenoleukodystrophy. *Science* 326(5954):818–823, 2009.
7. Gattinoni L, Restifo NP: Moving T memory stem cells to the clinic. *Blood* 121:567–568, 2013.
8. Kalos M, Levine BL, Porter DL, et al: T cells with chimeric antigen receptors have potent antitumor effects and can establish memory in patients with advanced leukemia. *Sci Transl Med* 3(95):95ra73, 2011.
9. Porter DL, Levine BL, Kalos M, et al: Chimeric antigen receptor-modified T cells in chronic lymphoid leukemia. *N Engl J Med* 365(8):725–733, 2011.
10. Savkovic B, Nichols J, Birkett D, et al: A quantitative comparison of anti-HIV gene therapy delivered to hematopoietic stem cells versus CD4+ T cells. *PLoS Comput Biol* 10(6):e1003681, 2014.
11. McLean AR, Michie CA: *In vivo* estimates of division and death rates of human T lymphocytes. *Proc Natl Acad Sci U S A* 92(9):3707–3711, 2014.
12. Kamen A, Henry O: Development and optimization of an adenovirus production process. *J Gene Med* 6 Suppl 1:S184–S192, 2004.
13. Puntel M, A K M GM, Farrokhi C, et al: Safety profile, efficacy, and biodistribution of a bicistronic high-capacity adenovirus vector encoding a combined immunostimulation and cytotoxic gene therapy as a prelude to a phase I clinical trial for glioblastoma. *Toxicol Appl Pharmacol* 268(3):318–330, 2013.
14. Ahi YS, Bangari DS, Mittal SK: Adenoviral vector immunity: Its implications and circumvention strategies. *Curr Gene Ther* 11(4):307–320, 2011.
15. Alemany R: Chapter four—Design of improved oncolytic adenoviruses. *Adv Cancer Res* 115:93–114, 2012.
16. Nathwani AC, Tuddenham EG, Rangarajan S, et al: Adenovirus-associated virus vector-mediated gene transfer in hemophilia B. *N Engl J Med* 365(25):2357–2365, 2011.
17. Xiao PJ, Lentz TB, Samulski RJ: Recombinant adeno-associated virus: Clinical application and development as a gene-therapy vector. *Ther Deliv* 3(7):835–856, 2012.
18. Daya S, Berns KI: Gene therapy using adeno-associated virus vectors. *Clin Microbiol Rev* 21(4):583–593, 2008.
19. Raj D, Davidoff AM, Nathwani AC: Self-complementary adeno-associated viral vectors for gene therapy of hemophilia B: Progress and challenges. *Expert Rev Hematol* 4(5):539–549, 2011.
20. Cooray S, Howe SJ, Thrasher AJ: Retrovirus and lentivirus vector design and methods of cell conditioning. *Methods Enzymol* 507:29–57, 2012.
21. Naldini L, Blomer U, Gage FH, et al: Efficient transfer, integration, and sustained long-term expression of the transgene in adult rat brains injected with a lentiviral vector. *Proc Natl Acad Sci U S A* 93(21):11382–11388, 1996.
22. Cattoglio C, Pellin D, Rizzi E, et al: High-definition mapping of retroviral integration sites identifies active regulatory elements in human multipotent hematopoietic progenitors. *Blood* 116(25):5507–5517, 2010.
23. Cavazzana-Calvo M, Fischer A, Hacein-Bey-Abina S, Aiuti A: Gene therapy for primary immunodeficiencies: Part 1. *Curr Opin Immunol* 24(5):580–584, 2012.
24. Hacein-Bey-Abina S, Hauer J, Lim A, et al: Efficacy of gene therapy for X-linked severe combined immunodeficiency. *N Engl J Med* 363(4):355–364, 2010.
25. Zhang L, Thrasher AJ, Gaspar HB: Current progress on gene therapy for primary immunodeficiencies. *Gene Ther* 20(10):963–969, 2013.
26. Aiuti A, Cattaneo F, Galimberti S, et al: Gene therapy for immunodeficiency due to adenosine deaminase deficiency. *N Engl J Med* 360(5):447–458, 2009.
27. Candotti F, Shaw KL, Muul L, et al: Gene therapy for adenosine deaminase-deficient severe combined immune deficiency: Clinical comparison of retroviral vectors and treatment plans. *Blood* 120(18):3635–3646, 2012.
28. Gaspar HB, Cooray S, Gilmour KC, et al: Hematopoietic stem cell gene therapy for adenosine deaminase-deficient severe combined immunodeficiency leads to long-term immunological recovery and metabolic correction. *Sci Transl Med* 3(97):97ra80, 2011.
29. Aiuti A, Bacchetta R, Seger R, et al: Gene therapy for primary immunodeficiencies: Part 2. *Curr Opin Immunol* 24(5):585–591, 2012.
30. Ciceri F, Bonini C, Stanghellini MT, et al: Infusion of suicide-gene-engineered donor lymphocytes after family haploidentical haemopoietic stem-cell transplantation for leukaemia (the TK007 trial): A non-randomised phase I-II study. *Lancet Oncol* 10(5):489–500, 2009.
31. Di Stasi A, Tey SK, Dotti G, et al: Inducible apoptosis as a safety switch for adoptive cell therapy. *N Engl J Med* 365(18):1673–1683, 2011.
32. Hutter G, Nowak D, Mossner M, et al: Long-term control of HIV by CCR5 Delta32/Delta32 stem-cell transplantation. *N Engl J Med* 360(7):692–698, 2009.
33. Gaj T, Gersbach CA, Barbas CF 3rd: ZFN, TALEN, and CRISPR/Cas-based methods for genome engineering. *Trends Biotechnol* 31(7):397–405, 2013.
34. Tebas P, Stein D, Tang WW, et al: Gene editing of CCR5 in autologous CD4 T cells of persons infected with HIV. *N Engl J Med* 370(10):901–910, 2014.
35. DiGiusto DL, Krishnan A, Li L, et al: RNA-based gene therapy for HIV with lentiviral vector-modified CD34(+) cells in patients undergoing transplantation for AIDS-related lymphoma. *Sci Transl Med* 2(36):36ra43, 2010.
36. Chung J, Scherer LJ, Gu A, et al: Optimized lentiviral vectors for HIV gene therapy: Multiplexed expression of small RNAs and inclusion of MGMT(P140K) drug resistance gene. *Mol Ther* 22(5):952–963, 2014.
37. Drakopoulou E, Papanikolaou E, Anagnou NP: The ongoing challenge of hematopoietic stem cell-based gene therapy for beta-thalassemia. *Stem Cells Int* 2011:987–980, 2011.
38. Neff T, Beard BC, Kiem HP: Survival of the fittest: *In vivo* selection and stem cell gene therapy. *Blood* 107(5):1751–1760, 2006.
39. Cavazzana-Calvo M, Payen E, Negre O, et al: Transfusion independence and HMGA2 activation after gene therapy of human beta-thalassaemia. *Nature* 467(7313):318–322, 2010.
40. Nienhuis AW: Development of gene therapy for blood disorders: An update. *Blood* 122(9):1556–1564, 2013.
41. Pierce GF, Lillicrap D, Pipe SW, Vandendriessche T: Gene therapy, bioengineered clotting factors and novel technologies for hemophilia treatment. *J Thromb Haemost* 5(5):901–906, 2007.
42. Lenting PJ, van Mourik JA, Mertens K: The life cycle of coagulation factor VIII in view of its structure and function. *Blood* 92(11):3983–3996, 1998.
43. Cancio MI, Reiss UM, Nathwani AC, et al: Developments in the treatment of hemophilia B: Focus on emerging gene therapy. *Appl Clin Genet* 6:91–101, 2013.
44. Penaud-Budloo M, Le Guiner C, Nowrouzi A, et al: Adeno-associated virus vector genomes persist as episomal chromatin in primate muscle. *J Virol* 82(16):7875–7885, 2008.
45. Nathwani AC, Reiss UM, Tuddenham EG, et al: Long-term safety and efficacy of factor IX gene therapy in hemophilia B. *N Engl J Med* 371(21):1994–2004, 2014.
46. McIntosh J, Lenting PJ, Rosales C, et al: Therapeutic levels of FVIII following a single peripheral vein administration of rAAV vector encoding a novel human factor VIII variant. *Blood* 121(17):3335–3344, 2013.
47. D'Andrea AD: Susceptibility pathways in Fanconi's anemia and breast cancer. *N Engl J Med* 362(20):1909–1919, 2010.
48. Mankad A, Taniguchi T, Cox B, et al: Natural gene therapy in monozygotic twins with Fanconi anemia. *Blood* 107(8):3084–3090, 2006.
49. Tolar J, Becker PS, Clapp DW, et al: Gene therapy for Fanconi anemia: One step closer to the clinic. *Hum Gene Ther* 23(2):141–144, 2012.
50. Watts KL, Delaney C, Humphries RK, et al: Combination of HOXB4 and Delta-1 ligand improves expansion of cord blood cells. *Blood* 116(26):5859–5866, 2010.
51. Lattime EC, Gerson SL: *Gene Therapy of Cancer: Translational Approaches from Preclinical Studies to Clinical Implementation*, ed 3. Academic Press, San Diego, CA, 2014.
52. Adair JE, Beard BC, Trobridge GD, et al: Extended survival of glioblastoma patients after chemoprotective HSC gene therapy. *Sci Transl Med* 4(133):133ra57, 2012.
53. Adair JE, Johnston SK, Mrugala MM, et al: Gene therapy enhances chemotherapy tolerance and efficacy in glioblastoma patients. *J Clin Invest* 124(9):4082–4092, 2014.
54. Zielske SP, Gerson SL: Lentiviral transduction of P140K MGMT into human CD34(+) hematopoietic progenitors at low multiplicity of infection confers significant resistance to BG/BCNU and allows selection in vitro. *Mol Ther* 5(4):381–387, 2002.
55. Davis BM, Roth JC, Liu L, et al: Characterization of the P140K, PVP(138–140)MLK, and G156A O6-methylguanine-DNA methyltransferase mutants: Implications for drug resistance gene therapy. *Hum Gene Ther* 10(17):2769–2778, 1999.
56. Knight S, Zhang F, Mueller-Kuller U, et al: Safer, silencing-resistant lentiviral vectors: Optimization of the ubiquitous chromatin-opening element through elimination of aberrant splicing. *J Virol* 86(17):9088–9095, 2012.
57. Deichmann A, Brugman MH, Bartholomae CC, et al: Insertion sites in engrafted cells cluster within a limited repertoire of genomic areas after gammaretroviral vector gene therapy. *Mol Ther* 19(11):2031–2039, 2011.

58. Gaussin A, Modlich U, Bauche C, et al: CTF/NF1 transcription factors act as potent genetic insulators for integrating gene transfer vectors. *Gene Ther* 19(1):15–24, 2012.

59. Heckl D, Schwarzer A, Haemmerle R, et al: Lentiviral vector induced insertional haploinsufficiency of Ebf1 causes murine leukemia. *Mol Ther* 20(6):1187–1195, 2012.

60. Fung H, Weinstock DM: Repair at single targeted DNA double-strand breaks in pluripotent and differentiated human cells. *PLoS One* 6(5):e20514, 2011.

61. Smith JR, Maguire S, Davis LA, et al: Robust, persistent transgene expression in human embryonic stem cells is achieved with AAVS1-targeted integration. *Stem Cells* 26(2):496–504, 2011.

62. DeKelver RC, Choi VM, Moehle EA, et al: Functional genomics, proteomics, and regulatory DNA analysis in isogenic settings using zinc finger nuclease-driven transgenesis into a safe harbor locus in the human genome. *Genome Res* 20(8):1133–1142, 2010.

63. Urnov FD, Miller JC, Lee YL, et al: Highly efficient endogenous human gene correction using designed zinc-finger nucleases. *Nature* 435(7042):646–651, 2005.

64. Reyon D, Tsai SQ, Khayter C, et al: FLASH assembly of TALENs for high-throughput genome editing. *Nat Biotechnol* 30(5):460–465, 2012.

65. Sander JD, Joung JK: CRISPR-Cas systems for editing, regulating and targeting genomes. *Nat Biotechnol* 32(4):347–355, 2014.

CHAPTER 30
REGENERATIVE MEDICINE: MULTIPOTENTIAL CELL THERAPY FOR TISSUE REPAIR

Jakub Tolar, Mark J Osborn, Randy Daughters, Anannya Banga, and John Wagner

SUMMARY

Regenerative medicine is a complex and rapidly advancing field that holds tremendous promise in treating, and even curing, many diseases. The understanding and control of tissue repair is one of the most urgent challenges in medicine today. Regenerative medicine seeks to either recruit the patient's reparative cells or to replace the malfunctioning tissue altogether to restore the deficient organ to adequate function. The common link among all types of regenerative therapies is the stem cell, which gives all tissues the capacity to regenerate. The mechanisms underlying the ability of a progenitor cell to differentiate have been challenging to elucidate, with recent experimentation focused on editing the genome itself. It has been even more difficult to determine how a differentiated cell can be instructed to revert to an immature state and undergo a re-specification to another differentiated cellular phenotype or an asymmetrical division to generate more immature cells. Our ability to modify genomes, harness stem cells, and transplant autologous or allogeneic tissues has transformed biomedical inquiry and offers hope to patients with diseases spanning all organ systems, including cardiac, lung, central nervous system, and liver and pancreatic diseases.

Acronyms and Abbreviations: ALS, amyotrophic lateral sclerosis; AMI, acute myocardial infarction; ATI or ATII, alveolar epithelial cells type I or II; BASCs, bronchiolar alveolar stem cells; BDNF, bone-derived neurotrophic factor; BM-derived, marrow-derived; CAR, chimeric antigen receptor; CDCs, cardiac-derived stem cells; COPD, chronic obstructive pulmonary disease; CRISPRs, clustered regularly interspaced short palindromic repeats; dmP-GE$_2$,16,16-dimethyl-prostaglandin E$_2$; DPSCs, dental pulp stem cells; DSB, double-strand break; EC, embryonic carcinoma; ESCs, embryonic stem cells; EPCs, epithelial progenitor cells; FAH, fumarylacetoacetate hydrolase; GVHD, graft-versus-host disease; HCT, hematopoietic cell transplantation; hESC, human embryonic stem cell; HR, homologous recombination; IDLV, integrase-deficient lentiviral; iPSCs, induced pluripotent stem cells; MN, meganuclease; MNCs, mononuclear cells; MSCs, mesenchymal stromal/stem cells; NHEJ, nonhomologous end-joining; NSC, neural stem cell; OPCs, oligodendrocyte progenitor cells; OT, off target; PD, Parkinson disease; SCID-X1, X-linked severe combined immunodeficiency; SCNT, somatic cell nuclear transfer; TALEN, transcription activator-like effector nuclease; TCR, T-cell receptor; TGF-β_1, transforming growth factor-β_1; UBCs, umbilical cord blood cells; VEGF, vascular endothelial growth factor; ZFN, zinc finger nuclease.

● INTRODUCTION

Regenerative medicine is a concept that evolved from knowledge in genome regulation and modification, from understanding of embryonic development and "stemness" of cells, and from 50 years of experience in human transplant biology. Therefore, a narrow view of any of these disciplines is not sufficient for illuminating the mechanisms of action underlying the already accomplished successes and for guiding the potential of novel basic biology discoveries into clinically meaningful regenerative medicine (Fig. 30–1).

Accordingly, this chapter spans major organ systems (marrow, liver, pancreas, brain, and spinal cord) to demonstrate their connectivity and shared biologic responses deployed at the times of acute and chronic injury. Furthermore, the goals of regenerative therapies are different than those of commonly used drugs. Medications are typically aimed at amelioration of symptoms, while regenerative medicine seeks to either recruit the patient's reparative cells or to replace the malfunctioning tissue altogether to restore the deficient organ to adequate function.

Regenerative medicine harnesses the body's own repair mechanisms to replace, restore, or regenerate damaged or malfunctioning cells and tissues in conditions as diverse as diabetes, heart disease, spinal cord injury, and types of blindness. Some regenerative medicine therapies are already in use, for example using unrelated hematopoietic cell transplant to regenerate a patient's immune system after their marrow has been destroyed by chemotherapy or radiation. There are some therapies that are in the early stages of clinical trials, for example using a patient's cells seeded onto a biomesh scaffolding to grow a new trachea, ear, or nose. Some therapies are on the cusp of progressing into clinical trials, such as differentiating human embryonic stem cells into beta cells that could produce insulin in diabetic patients. And some therapies, such as growing new lungs from patient cells and repairing a spinal cord injury with a cellular bridge, remain tantalizingly out of reach.

The zygote has the ability to give rise to a complete organism. Any cellular genome in the organism has the ability to code for any protein in the body. Although we know this, the mechanisms underlying the ability of a progenitor cell to differentiate have been challenging to elucidate. For the earliest critical steps in this long and complex process, we must look at developmental biology. Nuclear transfers in amphibians done by Briggs, King, and Gurdon[1-3] established that bidirectionality of cellular fate determination is possible. It was, established by McGrath and Solter that this process is driven by a multitude of factors of such temporal and spatial complexity that it would make reprogramming of mammalian cells by nuclear transfer impossible.[4,5] Recent experimentation has focused on editing the genome itself, finding success in both mouse and human DNA models. Much work remains to bring this technology into human therapies, but in the foreseeable future, cells and organisms will no longer be seen as being given sealed orders at birth, but rather the instructions contained in their developmental program can be thought of as "software" that can be rewritten and used to reprogram the genomic "hardware" of a cell.

It has been even more difficult to imagine and later define the possibility that a differentiated cell could be instructed to revert to an immature state and undergo a respecification to another differentiated cellular phenotype or an asymmetrical division to generate more immature cells. Yamanaka's experimental proof reduced this perceived complexity to a four-factor recipe sufficient to restore skin fibroblasts to induced pluripotent stem cells (iPSCs).[6,7,8]

This chapter gives a broad overview of the state of regenerative medicine as it stands today, a complex and rapidly advancing field that holds tremendous promise in treating, and even curing, many of the disorders that cause pain and suffering.

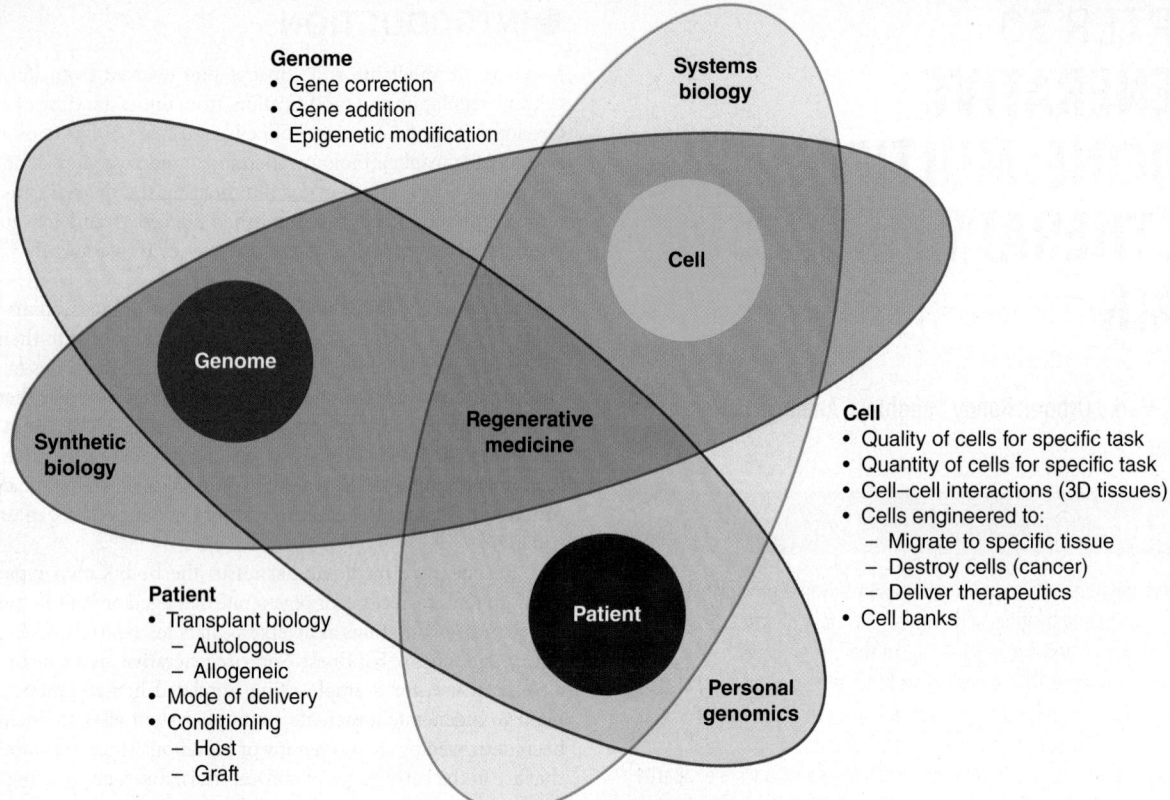

Figure 30–1. The three-body problem of regenerative medicine. The three factors—cell, genome, and patient—influence each other in complex and sometimes unexpected ways. These three separate scientific foci of regenerative medicine must be developed in the context of one another to have meaningful impact.

● MULTIPOTENTIAL CELLS

EMBRYONIC STEM CELLS

Four to 5 days after fertilization, an egg becomes a blastocyst, a ball of approximately 100 to 150 cells. A small group of inner cells within the blastocyst are pluripotent and have the potential to replicate indefinitely and to become any of the differentiated types of tissue in the body. These pluripotent cells are called embryonic stem cells (ESCs). ESCs have the dual ability to self-renew (copy themselves) and differentiate (produce more specialized types of cells of the body)

ESCs were first isolated from mice when embryonic carcinoma (EC) cells[9] were shown to proliferate indefinitely like stem cells and were used to generate a chimeric mouse. Further development of the culture conditions for EC cells that used feeder (supporting) cells, along with discovery of cell-surface antigens, like SSEA-1 and F-9 antigen on EC cells, led to the isolation of the first ESCs from a mouse embryo in 1981.[10] In 1995, Thomson isolated ESC lines from a nonhuman primate,[11] followed by the first successful isolation of human embryonic stem cell (hESC) lines in 1998.[12] The use of human ESCs in research, however, has been severely limited because of the social and religious concerns that the blastocyst is destroyed when the ESC lines are generated.

hESC lines can be cultured on feeder cells where they divide infinitely. They can also be grown without feeder cells, where they develop into clusters known as embryoid bodies. Using cells from a human blastocyst in clinical therapy has been difficult, so the 2006 discovery by Yamanaka and Takahashi that pluripotent stem cells could be created from skin cells[6] revolutionized the stem cell research. Their pioneering work showed that inducing skin cells with four genes (*Oct4*, *SOX2*, *Klf4*, and *c-Myc*) would generate pluripotent embryonic stem-like cells *in vitro*. These cells, known as iPSCs, have the basic properties of hESCs while being derived from somatic cells rather than blastocysts.

An alternative approach for obtaining pluripotent stem cells is somatic cell nuclear transfer (SCNT).[13] In this process, the nucleus of an adult human cell is placed in an egg cell that has had its nucleus removed. As this cell divides it can be a source of pluripotent stem cells. A recent study verified that the SCNT pluripotent stem cells are more similar to ESCs than are iPSCs.[14] Although much research remains to be done, SCNT pluripotent stem cells appear to have potential in regenerative medicine.

There are many disorders and defects that arise from errors in the complex process of embryonic development. Research over the past decade advanced our understanding of the critical steps in the embryonic development of mice; however, information about the embryonic development of humans remains limited. Although there is overlap with what has been learned from studying mouse embryos, human embryonic growth is different and unique. However, by growing hESCs in the laboratory the multitude of regulatory factors that control the different stages of cell, tissue, and organ system development can be studied and can also provide insights into how our adult tissues are maintained and repaired and allows identification of the causes of birth defects by discovering what interferes with the normal path of cell fate acquisition. The hESCs are also used to produce laboratory disease models in specialized cells like nerve, heart, or beta cells and can also be used for development of new drug therapies.

Despite the much-anticipated potential of hESCs to differentiate and replace malfunctioning cells in the body, progress toward clinical use has been hindered by the possibility of teratoma formation or the immune rejection of the allogeneic transplanted cells and production issues.

INDUCED PLURIPOTENT STEM CELLS

Generation of iPSCs has connected several previous observations into a coherent outline. For example, the ability of transcription factor MyoD to change fibroblasts to myoblasts[15] and of transcription factor Antennapedia to change development of antennae into legs in *Drosophilla*,[16] uncovered potential of a differentiated cell to assume an alternative cell fate as a result of defined, externally provided signals.

The understanding of induced pluripotency has become more refined as additional reprogramming factors are identified,[17] the critical role of epigenetic regulation is uncovered,[18] and with the dynamics of iPSC generation (from initially random event to deterministic process) more fully developed.[19]

The reprogramming technology applied to human cells iPSCs allows for modeling various, typically genetic, disorders.[20,21] Furthermore, organoid cultures derived from the patients themselves allow for high throughput drug testing that would be impossible without the supply of differentiated cells from patient-specific iPSCs.

The first preclinical example of iPSC technology conceptually applied to human disease has been amelioration of the sickle cell anemia phenotype in a murine model.[22] At the time of this writing, the first iPSC-based clinical trial opened in Japan for individuals with exudative age-related macular degeneration.[23]

New knowledge derived from the rapidly expanding iPSC field has also reenergized the technology of direct reprogramming, whereby one differentiated cellular phenotype (such as a dermal fibroblast) can be induced to convert into another somatic cell (such as a neuron) without the intermediate iPSC stage. In contrast to the expandable iPSC-based generation of differentiated cells, the process of direct reprogramming makes it more challenging to produce the large numbers of cells needed for therapeutic intervention.

An example of this strategy has been *in vivo trans*-differentiation of exocrine pancreatic cells or biliary epithelial cells into insulin-producing endocrine cells in rodent models.[24,25] A conceptually different concept to solve the same clinical challenge has been blastocyst complementation whereby rat iPSCs were injected into blastocysts that had been derived from mice deficient in pancreatic organogenesis, which resulted in the development of a functional rat pancreas in mice.[26] In addition to reducing the cell numbers needed to create a physiologically meaningful effect, the efficacy of both strategies may be enhanced by targeting them into a permissive cellular niche.

HEMATOPOIETIC STEM CELLS

The earliest advances with clinical potential will most likely arise from understanding reprogramming in hematopoietic stem cells. Not only was hematopoietic cell transplantation the first stem cell therapy, developed close to half a century ago, but reports of using defined factors to turn committed blood progenitor cells into transplantable hematopoietic cells[27,28] suggest that robust generation of clinical-grade, patient-specific autologous grafts for transplantation is possible.

Equally important has been combination of pluripotentiality of ESCs and iPSCs with their commitment to specific lineages, such as hemogenic differentiation program. Derivation of hematopoietic stem cells from murine ESC and their genetic correction has been used in murine severe combined immune deficiency[29]; similarly in a model of sickle cell anemia, hematopoietic stem cells derived from gene-corrected murine iPSCs[22] have established preclinical proof-of-concept for combined gene correction and stem cell engineering. Furthermore, insights from murine embryogenesis were applied to *in vitro* induction of mesoderm and ESC differentiation to blood cells via coculture with feeder cells or generation of embryoid bodies. These seemingly straightforward concepts, however, have proven challenging to mimic in human ESCs and iPSCs. Despite many attempts, current technology appears to lead only to low hematopoietic chimerism after transplantation of hematopoietic stem cells derived from pluripotent human cells.[30,31] An alternative to generation of transplantable human hematopoietic stem cells is direct conversion of fibroblasts to hematopoietic stem cells without the iPSC intermediate. This is done by using forced expression of OCT4[32] and differentiation of human pluripotent progenitor cells by forced expression of GATA-1, ETV2, and TAL-1 into hemoendothelial cells.[33]

The replacement of hematopoiesis by marrow transplantation is the prototype of regenerative medicine. While the initial experimentation with marrow transfers on both sides of the Atlantic was almost immediately recognized as a pioneering effort in hematology, it was only later understood as a turning point in the larger field of regenerative medicine. The critical evidence was the ability of a relatively small number of donor cells to repopulate the host and reconstitute its full lymphohematopoietic system. Although initially applied to leukemia and lymphoma therapy in an effort to replace the malignant lymphohematopoiesis with a healthy wild-type system, it later became clear that the immune elimination of the tumor (graft-versus-leukemia, graft-versus-lymphoma) is the dominant mechanism behind successful therapy in many cases.

This remarkable regenerative capacity of hematopoietic stem cells established marrow, and later cord blood, transplantation as the blueprint for other stem cell therapies.

MESENCHYMAL STROMAL CELLS

Originally defined by how they were identified—they adhered to the surface of a culture dish[34]—marrow-derived mesenchymal stromal/stem cells (MSCs) were then identified as key support cells in the cellular niche. Evidence from different sources (e.g., marrow, umbilical cord blood, and adipose tissue) suggests that MSCs have different functions in various organs (e.g., as pericytes in adventitia of blood vessels, or as supporting cells in marrow periosteal and endovascular hematopoietic niches).[35–37] In addition to this developmental heterogeneity, cultured MSCs display various levels of "stemness," and the cellular products used in therapeutic applications may be more a cell culture artifact than a counterpart to physiologic functionally integrated MSCs. This is not necessarily a disadvantage, as the culture process enables both amplification of cell numbers and defined release criteria for clinical use.

The most striking application of MSCs in medicine to date relies not on the regenerative capacity of MSCs alone but on the immunosuppressive potential of MSC cultures in the setting of severe graft-versus-host disease (GVHD),[38–40] a serious complication of allogeneic hematopoietic cell transplantation (HCT).[41] The treatment options for individuals with glucocorticoid-resistant severe GVHD have been inadequate, and mortality in this subgroup remains high. In a paradigm-changing study, it was demonstrated that culture-expanded MSCs can ameliorate severe GVHD.[38,42] The induction and maintenance of MSC-driven regulation of immune and inflammatory reactions[43] has made it possible to assess their role in autoimmune and inflammatory disorders such as Crohn disease, arthritis, diabetes, organ rejection, and bridge therapy before solid-organ transplantation.[44–46]

The regenerative potential of MSCs has long been sought as a tool to rebuild and replace tissues damaged by acute or chronic injury whereby injected cultured MSCs activate endogenous repair mechanisms and disappear in the process.[47] In this capacity, MSCs in preclinical models have been shown to alleviate ischemic injury in the heart, brain, and kidneys; toxic insults to lung and liver; and degenerative damage to joints; and it is possible that in some settings allogeneic MSCs may be even more effective than autologous MSCs.[48]

Lastly, MSCs are relatively easy to gene-modify and thus can be used as cellular vectors for delivering gene therapeutic agents in both inborn genetic disorders and acquired conditions, such as in anticancer therapy or for trophic factor support after surgery.

● REGENERATIVE MEDICINE

CARDIAC REPAIR

Cardiovascular disease is a leading cause of death in the world, leading to an estimated 17 million deaths per year.[49] As life expectancy in the developed world rises, so too do risk factors associated with chronic heart disease. It is estimated that there are approximately 800,000 new cases of acute myocardial infarction (AMI)[50] annually. Heart failure occurs when there is significant deprivation of oxygen to cardiac tissue, which results in decreased cardiac output and function as a result of loss of cardiomyocytes, scar formation, and tissue remodeling.[50] Identifying ways to regenerate or repair heart tissue will be key to developing effective treatment options for heart failure.

Since the mid-1990s, scientists have been investigating the potential of adult progenitor cells for use in heart regeneration. These early studies were triggered by the discovery that certain adult tissue-specific stem cells could be differentiated *in vitro* to become cardiac-like cells.[51] This discovery led to many preclinical studies that assessed the ability of adult stem cells to repair or enhance cardiac function after various types of injury.

The cells reported to differentiate *in vitro* to cardiac-like cells *in vivo* are satellite cells, which are undifferentiated skeletal muscle myoblasts,[52] which led to studies using autologous skeletal myoblasts surgically implanted into the heart muscle.[53] Although these cells survived for short periods of time, they retained their intrinsic contractile properties and did not fully integrate into the cardiac tissue,[54] which led to arrhythmias and gave little long-term significant benefit in overall heart function.

Some marrow-derived cell populations (lin−; c-kit+) were capable of differentiating to myocytes expressing cardiomyocyte markers such as Nkx2.5, Gata4, and MEF.[55] These marrow-derived cells were shown to survive in infarcted hearts and were capable of differentiating into smooth muscle and endothelial cells but not cardiomyocytes *in vivo*.[56] Additional studies demonstrated that other marrow-derived progenitor cell populations (endothelial progenitors, angioblasts, or CD34+ cells) were able to contribute to angiogenesis and neovascularization of the infarcted myocardium.[57] This differed from more immature marrow progenitor populations, called *side-population cells* (Lin− c-kit+ Sca-1+), that not only contribute to neovascularization but also regenerate myocardium.[58] These marrow-derived side-population cells homed to the border zone of infarction and resulted in improved left ventricular function.[58] The cardiac regeneration capacity of the marrow-derived progenitor cells facilitated large-scale clinical studies using heterogeneous populations of bone mononuclear cells (MNCs), also called *epithelial progenitor cells* (EPCs), for cardiac repair in patients with AMI[59,60] or ischemic cardiomyopathy.[61] These studies showed only moderate improvements, and therefore led to further refinement of the selection criteria for marrow-derived cells (CD34+/CD133+) and changes in the route of administration (intracoronary injection) in the Regeneration by Intracoronary Infusion of Selected Population of Stem Cells in Acute Myocardial Infarction (REGENT) study, which still only showed modest success.[62]

The moderate success of marrow-derived MNCs spurred the investigation of other populations of adult progenitor cells, as well as new routes of administration. The investigations led to the discovery of MSCs, as well as endogenous cardiac-derived stem cells, that could differentiate into cardiomyocytes and endothelial cells in animal models.[63] These findings led to clinical studies comparing marrow-derived MNCs versus the new MSCs used for intracoronary injection into patients with ischemic cardiomyopathy.[64] These tests showed significant improvement in left ventricle ejection fraction in response to MSC treatment.

To date, the clinical success of cell therapy approaches for cardiac regeneration has been mixed. This is in contrast to the promising early preclinical studies that showed significant improvement in many different measures of cardiac function. This difference has been attributed to the differences between rodent cardiac injury models and human clinical pathology, the cell population administration route, the origin of the cell populations, and the limited number of cells injected.

ESCs, because of their pluripotency and unlimited ability to proliferate, have been the subject of extensive preclinical investigation for many tissues, particularly cardiac tissue repair.[65,66] However, there has been less enthusiasm for hESC-derived cardiomyocytes for human cell therapy because their allogeneic nature requires concomitant immunosuppressive therapy and because ethical issues surround their derivation. Despite these challenges, clinical studies have begun to collect ESCs for cardiac differentiation with the intent of being used in a trial for AMI patients. However, as about any somatic cell can be used to generate embryonic stem-like iPSCs,[67] with the capability to differentiate into cardiomyocytes, endothelial cells, and smooth muscle cells.[68] Initial preclinical studies of murine iPSC-derived cardiomyocytes, injected into ischemic myocardium, led to rejection of transplanted cells by immune reaction as well as continuous proliferation that led to teratoma formation.[69] Although iPSCs are attractive for their allogeneic potential they have potential disadvantages for human cell therapy based on their oncogenic nature, epigenetic memory, and maintenance of potency for other cells types.

Growing tissues *in vitro* for use in regenerative therapies has been investigated as another delivery method of cells for heart repair. This tissue engineering approach involves seeding cells onto scaffolds and growing them for later engraftment or for the generation of whole organs.[70] In these systems, cells are transplanted with the scaffolding to the cardiac wall, which provides structural support and a better microenvironment for the migration of cells into the damaged myocardium.[71]

A common theme in most preclinical and clinical cell therapy-based studies is the demonstration of improvements in cardiac function that is not correlated to number of cells injected or their longevity after administration. This observation has led investigators to speculate that transplanted cells improve cardiac function through paracrine rather than structural effects. This model suggests that observed improvements in myocardial regeneration or vasculogenesis are a result of transplanted cells secreting molecules that are known to improve cardiovascular function after injury.[72] The effects of paracrine factors include decreased inflammation, increased angiogenesis, induction of proliferation of cardiomyocytes or protection of existing ones, and activation of endogenous stem cells.[73] Ischemic hearts subjected to secreted factors showed an increase in the expression of genes involved in cardiogenesis and a downregulation of cell-death markers, effects that contribute to survival of ischemic cardiomyocytes.[74] The advantage of the paracrine model is the potential for the commercial development of paracrine factors that have proven potential for cardiac repair.

LUNG REPAIR

The prevalence of lung diseases, like the chronic obstructive pulmonary diseases (COPDs) that include asthma and emphysema, has increased dramatically over the last 50 years. Lung disease is expected to become the third leading cause of disease-related death in the world by 2020. New therapeutic approaches from regenerative medicine are being developed ranging from stem cell therapies to bioengineering of entire tissues of the respiratory system for transplantation. These approaches are based on initial observations that endothelial progenitor cells and mesenchymal stem cells can differentiate *in vitro* to cells expressing lung epithelial markers and contribute to mature functional bioengineered tissues.

Throughout the pulmonary tract there exist many different niche environments containing distinct epithelial cell types that contribute to the complexity of the lung. Identification of a true endogenous stem cell population that is responsible for maintaining lung tissue under steady state and injury has been challenging and has been a source of controversy.[75] Evidence from rodent models and human lungs suggests that the adult endogenous airway, alveolar epithelial cells, lung stroma, and pulmonary vasculature all contain putative stem cell populations that can repair damaged tissue.[76,77] These studies suggest the lung has a regional hierarchy of stem and progenitor cells that are specific for proximal versus distal airways as well as alveoli.

Identifying endogenous lung stem cells is complex because many different subpopulations of basal epithelial cells exhibit restricted patterns or roles in self-renewal for steady-state maintenance or after injury.[78,79] In the distal airway, putative progenitor cells have been identified in the neuroepithelial body,[80] bronchoalveolar duct junction,[81] by specific markers of self-renewing lung epithelial cells,[82,83] and by function as bronchiolar alveolar stem cells (BASCs). This is in contrast to alveolar epithelial repair thought to be regulated by type 2 alveolar epithelial cells (ATII) because they have been shown to be precursors to type 1 (ATI) cells.[84,85] Identification of regionally specific stem cell populations is further complicated by the demonstration that isolated distal airway progenitors (BASCs, CK5+/p63+) can differentiate into ATII and ATI cells.[86,87] Regardless, all of these cells show unique functions in repair after injury, reside in different locations in the distal airway and alveolar epithelium, and play different roles as endogenous lung epithelial progenitors.

Many preclinical studies have shown that EPCs can increase function in pulmonary lung injury models.[88-90] This improvement in function could be because of contributions to structure, paracrine effects, modulation of immune responses, or a combination of these.[90] EPCs have also been demonstrated to preferentially home to sites of injury in the lung after systemic administration[91]; consequently, autologous EPCs have been used clinically in pulmonary hypertension patients and showed improved cardiopulmonary outcomes.[92,93]

Marrow MSCs are known for their immunomodulatory effects in a wide range of diseases.[94,95] The beneficial effect of MSCs results from secretion of soluble mediators and microsomal particles that influence lung progenitor cells directly or indirectly through mediation of inflammatory cells that subsequently promote repair.[96,97] Both preclinical and clinical studies have shown efficacy in either systemic or intratracheal administration of MSCs in acute lung injury models, asthma, COPD, and a host of other inflammation-related lung injuries or diseases.[75,98] Although different studies have shown varying degrees of efficacy, there are still significant gaps in our understanding of the mechanisms of MSC action on ameliorating disease symptoms and of the specific subtype of MSCs used. This is important, as studies have demonstrated that certain MSCs can have negative effects in some lung disease models, such as pulmonary fibrosis.[99,100]

Although there has been significant preclinical investigation into using EPC and MSC therapy approaches to lung repair, clinical studies have been slow to develop. However, there are a growing number of clinical trials in development focused on using MSCs for chronic lung diseases where preclinical data show the most promise. The most recent is the PROCHYMAL phase II trial looking at systemic administration of marrow MSCs for moderate to severe COPD,[101] which showed the safety of using MSCs and also preliminary evidence for decrease in markers of inflammation.

BRAIN AND SPINAL CORD REPAIR

Stem cell-based therapy is rapidly developing as a way to improve outcomes following brain and spinal cord injury or disease. The human CNS is composed of more than 100 billion nerve cells connected in a complex network that must work seamlessly throughout our lives. Conditions affecting the CNS—such as stroke, brain, spinal cord injury, and neurodegenerative diseases—affect millions of people worldwide. Challenges for therapeutic intervention include the complex pathology of these conditions, as well as the specialized anatomical structures of the CNS that prevent easy access from systemic administration of therapies (e.g., the blood–brain barrier).

As with other areas of regenerative medicine, much effort has been spent on the identification of cell types with the best potential for CNS repair. Although it was initially thought that the adult CNS did not contain progenitor cells for repair, it is now recognized that the human CNS does retain an endogenous neural stem cell (NSC) population that retains some capacity for repair, although only in select regions and of a limited nature. Isolated adult and fetal NSCs can be expanded and differentiated into neurons, astrocytes, and oligodendrocytes, the three main CNS cell types. Adult NSCs are retained throughout life, and are found in the striatal subventricular zone and the dentate gyrus of the hippocampus. In preclinical studies, endogenous NSCs have shown to provide the most significant improvement in functional recovery in rodent stroke models.[102] Isolated human fetal NSCs (CD133+),[103] are currently being investigated in a number of clinical studies.[104,105] In addition, multiple NSC-based cell therapy trials are being conducted to determine the safety and efficacy in patients with amyotrophic lateral sclerosis (ALS, sometimes called Lou Gehrig disease).[106,107] Although all trials to date have confirmed the safety of using these cells, any benefit from them has yet to be reported.

Although other adult stem cell types (endothelial progenitor cells, umbilical cord blood cells [UBCs], dental pulp stem cells [DPSCs]) have been investigated preclinically, only MSCs have been shown to have the same level of efficacy as NSCs. Marrow-derived MSCs have been the primary focus of preclinical and clinical studies because of their relative abundance and potential for autologous cell transplantation.[108,109] Administration of MSCs, regardless of route, have been shown to improve outcome measures in rodent models of injury and disease.[106,110] Based on these findings, there have been a number of early phase clinical trials initiated to study the effects of MSC transplantation following CNS injury[111,112] or disease.[113,114] In both cases, MSCs have been shown to be both safe and a feasible approach. Although not designed to test efficacy, many trials have observed improvements in functional outcomes.[115]

From studies of the efficacy of adult stem cells for therapy in preclinical models of CNS injury or disease over the past 20 years, there is strong evidence that transplanted adult stem cells can migrate to the site of injury and promote functional improvement. The mechanism of action, however, remains controversial.[116] There is speculation that the benefits of cell-based therapy arise from multiple factors. From the host of preclinical studies on MSCs for treatment of stroke, improvements in function have been attributed to increased angiogenesis, neurogenesis, prosurvival signals, and mitigation of immune responses.[117,118] These mechanisms are potentially mediated by various soluble factors that act through a paracrine mechanism secreted by transplanted stem cells that benefit the local environment. Many of these secreted factors have begun to be identified and are well-known mediators of neurogenesis (bone-derived neurotrophic factor [BDNF]), angiogenesis (vascular endothelial growth factor [VEGF]), and immune regulation (transforming growth factor-β_1[TGF-β_1]).[117,119]

The use of pluripotent cell types (ESCs, iPSCs) holds significant potential as a therapeutic approach for CNS repair. Clinical application of ESCs/iPSCs is limited because of the inability to isolate pure differentiated populations of neuronal cell types.[120,121] Despite this limitation, considerable progress has been made in preclinical studies for remyelination following spinal cord injury.[122,123] These studies and others have demonstrated that ESCs/iPSCs can be differentiated to oligodendrocyte progenitor cells (OPCs), migrate within the spinal cord, and produce myelin. Again, the efficacy and mechanism of recovery remain controversial.[124-127] In 2010, the Geron Company began recruitment of patients for a phase I clinical trial for treatment of spinal cord injury with ESC-derived OPCs. Despite significant enthusiasm from the patient population, and report of no adverse events on a small cohort of treated patients (n = 4), significant methodologic[128] and economic obstacles forced the early discontinuation of the trial.

LIVER AND PANCREAS REPAIR

The liver is an essential organ that coordinates glycogen storage, drug detoxification, production of various serum proteins, and secretion of bile, which plays a critical role in food digestion and metabolism. It is interspersed with small microscopic canals known as canaliculi through which the bile drains to the gall bladder. The numerous bile canaliculi join together into many larger bile ducts, which join to become a branched structure that forms the common hepatic duct. The part of the common hepatic duct that is outside the liver is called the extra hepatic bile duct, which joins the cystic duct from the gall bladder to form the common bile duct and connect to the exocrine pancreas. This whole branched structure forms the biliary tree.[129] Liver, biliary tree, and pancreas originate from the anterior definitive endoderm and have been found to share stem cell populations during the early stages of development.[130]

The normal liver has extraordinary potential to regenerate following partial removal of the liver or liver injury. The hepatocytes and cholangiocytes (biliary epithelial cells) are normally quiescent, but in response to liver injury, these cells proliferate and contribute to regeneration.[131] Average liver turnover is maintained by differentiation and proliferation of parenchymal or nonparenchymal cells. However, in chronic liver disease, when the liver cannot be repaired by self-duplication of existing hepatocytes, small bipotential progenitor cells are activated that have the ability to differentiate into either hepatocytes or cholangiocytes.[132] Severe injury in alcoholic liver disease has been found to stimulate increased proliferation of hepatic stem/progenitor cells in humans[133] and oval cells in rodents.[134] Some experiments have suggested that stem progenitor cells are not only activated in the injured liver, but that the normal adult human liver contains a large number of liver progenitor cells that may contribute to liver homeostasis.

Liver transplantation is currently the only option in acute liver failure. Two small clinical trials conducted with hepatocyte transplantation resulted in limited restored enzyme function in one patient, but it was not enough for survival and the patient eventually needed a liver transplant.[135] It remains unknown if hepatocytes can contribute to long-term rescue in patients. Additionally, hepatocytes are difficult to produce in clinically sufficient numbers, as they lose their viability and function when cultured *in vitro*.

Transplanted human ESC/iPSC-derived mature hepatocytes can express liver-specific enzymes such as albumin, antitrypsin, and cytochrome P450, which can improve liver function.[136,137] Furthermore, a functional liver organ bud generated from iPSCs was found to be engrafted and integrated within the host organism, even including development of blood vessels.[138] When iPSCs are injected into the blastocysts of fumarylacetoacetate hydrolase (FAH)-deficient mice, iPSC-derived hepatocytes can repopulate the damaged liver efficiently and restore liver function.[139]

The liver and pancreas both harbor a niche of stem cells, collectively known as the hepatic stem/progenitor cells.[140,141] The fetal biliary tree, arising from the ductal plate cells during development and consisting of the intrahepatic and extrahepatic ducts, has been shown to harbor a rich source of stem/progenitor cells.[142] These stem/progenitor cells are quite distinctive from hepatoblasts, which contribute toward the hepatocytes or cholangiocytes during development.[143] These stem/progenitor cells present in the biliary tree differ from hepatoblasts by their ability to self-renew and differentiate into hepatocytes, cholangiocytes, or pancreatic islets, depending on the microenvironment. Sox9 expression is detected throughout the pancreatic ducts, intra- and extrahepatic ducts, and in the intestinal crypt connected through the major duodenal papilla, forming a contiguous Sox9+ zone.[144,145] Remarkably, when an adenovirus contacting three pancreatic transcription factors (Pdx1, Ngn3, and MafA) was delivered into the liver, it was able to reprogram the Sox9+ population of cells within the bile ducts into functional insulin-secreting, beta-like cells.[25] When both *Ad-PNM* and a peroxisome proliferator-activated receptor (PPAR) agonist, WY14643, were given in animals, it resulted in injury to the liver, led to an increase in the cell division rate of Sox9+ cells lining bile ducts, and contributed toward making more insulin-positive beta cells.[146] In an injured liver, the Wnt signaling pathway is activated, which stimulates discreet subsets of progenitor cell populations, which, in turn, engage in liver regeneration.[147] Isolation of stem/progenitor cell populations based on their surface markers like Lgr5 or EpCAM has identified the possibility of differentiating them toward a hepatocyte- or beta-like cell fate.[145,148]

The pancreas plays an important role in digestion, as well as in maintaining blood glucose homeostasis. It is composed of ducts, with the main duct (pancreatic duct) running the length of the pancreas. The pancreatic duct merges with the bile duct to form the major duodenal ampulla, which drains the pancreatic fluid into the first portion of the small intestine, the duodenum. The pancreas is composed of exocrine and endocrine parts. The exocrine component plays an integral part in digestion. The endocrine component contains the islets of Langerhans that produce and secrete hormones into the bloodstream. The pancreatic hormones, insulin and glucagon, work together to maintain proper sugar levels in the blood.

Diabetes mellitus is a metabolic syndrome caused by having an insufficient number of insulin-producing beta cells. In type 1 diabetes, beta cells are destroyed by the body's own immune system. In type 2 diabetes, although the pancreas has functioning beta cells, insulin resistance causes the liver to release too much sugar into the bloodstream, and the beta cells cannot secrete enough insulin to maintain normal glucose homeostasis. The American Diabetes Association estimated in 2012 that approximately 9.3 percent of the United States population is living with diabetes.[149] Beta-cell therapy holds promise for treating type 1 diabetes by replenishing beta cells in the body; however, donor pancreases are in short supply and the demand for transplantable beta cells cannot be met.

In addition, beta-like cells have been successfully generated from hESCs and iPSCs using overexpression of transcription factors, chemicals, or growth factors.[150] Current protocols for differentiation of pluripotent stem cells to beta cells follow a five-stage procedure that recapitulates the embryonic stages of development.[151] Only the first four stages have been carried out successfully *in vitro*. The fifth stage—which involves maturation to glucose-responsive, insulin-secreting beta cells and other islet cells—until recently could only be carried out by implantation *in vivo*.[152] A long-awaited directed differentiation of insulin-producing cells from hESCs has been accomplished; this fully defined *ex vivo* technology is immediately relevant.[153]

Also nonendocrine cells within the pancreas have been found to transdifferentiate or reprogram to a beta cell fate[24] upon their being induced with the three-pancreatic-gene cocktail (Pdx1, Ngn3, and MafA). Another source for adult cell reprogramming to beta cells has been described from glucagon-producing alpha cells. A study showed that overexpression of *Pax4* (a gene responsible for specifying endocrine fate) in the alpha cells was able to force them to become beta-like cells.[154] In another study, it was observed that near-complete ablation of beta cells forced regeneration of beta cells from former alpha cells.[155] However such *in vivo* studies have not been established in humans or other primates.

● GENE EDITED MULTIPOTENTIAL CELLS

The ability to correct defective cells or give them enhanced properties (e.g., antitumor effects) represents a novel approach to transplantation medicine and sets the stage for individualized therapies. Two options exist for this strategy: provision of functional copies of a gene delivered by a viral or nonviral gene transfer system or *in situ* correction of the disease-causing sequence. Several major studies have used clinically employed viral transgenesis of hematopoietic stem cells (HSCs). In 2010, a *γ*-retroviral vector was used to deliver the complementary DNA for the *IL2RG* gene to CD34+ progenitors from patients with X-linked severe combined immunodeficiency (SCID-X1). Normalization of the immune system occurred in most patients; however, four patients developed acute T-cell leukemia from promiscuous LMO2 oncogene activation by the viral vector.[156] To mitigate the potential for viral elements to dysregulate endogenous gene expression, investigators have used self-inactivating lentiviral vectors for the gene therapy of X-linked adrenoleukodystrophy,[157] metachromatic leukodystrophy,[158] and Wiskott-Aldrich syndrome,[159] in gene therapy trials using hematopoietic progenitors.

Despite this, the integrating nature of viral vectors, with a preference for transcriptionally active areas, makes more precise gene targeting a highly desirable goal. Such precision can be achieved with genome editing nucleases that are rationally designed and with engineered proteins that have the unifying characteristic of recognizing and contacting a unique sequence of DNA. Most studies have tethered these proteins to nuclease domains or used their inherent ability to cut DNA. Once the DNA is broken, two predominant repair pathways have been used for therapeutic genome engineering: nonhomologous end-joining (NHEJ) and homologous recombination (HR). NHEJ is an error-prone pathway that, in the absence of a donor template, repairs the DNA break in a way that can cause small insertions or deletions ("indels") that can permanently disrupt coding DNA sequences. Gene repair relies on the error-free HR pathway. In gene repair, the inclusion of an exogenous single- or double-stranded DNA donor template that contains homologous sequences to the target site avoids disruption. In response to a double-strand break (DSB), the donor template acts as the template for repair and allows for the precise and permanent insertion of user-defined sequences at the target locus. Both repair pathways can be used therapeutically. The major candidates employed for DNA cleavage are the meganucleases (MNs), zinc finger nucleases (ZFNs), transcription

activator-like effector nucleases (TALENs), and clustered regularly interspaced short palindromic repeats (CRISPRs)/Cas9 system.

Each class of reagent has been used for stem and progenitor cell genome modification with ZFNS, which is, to date, the first to enter clinical application. Human ESC engineering with ZFNs was first used to target the HUES-3 and HUES-1 cell lines with ZFNs designed for inactivation of the *CCR5* gene, a coreceptor for HIV entry to a cell.[160] ZFNs and a donor sequence containing green fluorescent protein (GFP) were introduced into exon 3 of the *CCR5* gene and approximately 5 percent rates of targeted integration were observed. Importantly, the cells maintained their pluripotency and ability to self-renew.[160] This study established a precedent for inserting genes of interest into a specified spot in the ESC genome via HR. Others extended this to allow for gene addition, a placement of an inducible expression cassette at the so-called safe harbor locus AAVS1. Using ZFNs for the first exon of the *PPP1R12C* gene on chromosome 19, a "standalone" expression cassette was introduced containing a promoter, puromycin gene, and a polyadenylation signal (or gene trap targeting vector) containing a splice acceptor-2A-puromycin gene that relied on proper targeting and splicing with the first exon of the *PPP1R12C* gene.[161] As such, gene targeting at the *AAV* locus allows for placement of a gene with a promoter that drives the desired level of expression or is controlled by the native *PPP1R12C* promoter that is constitutively active.[162] In another study, employing the safe harbor strategy did not appear to alter the pluripotent nature of ESCs.[161–163] The ability to modify genes in pluripotent target cells is important to disease modeling *in vitro*, which has become a new foundation for the acceleration of translational research. Although these studies established the ability to modify ESCs at a site-specific and "safe harbor" locus, widespread use is limited by the relatively small number of approved ESC lines and the even smaller number of disease-specific ones.

As an elegant solution to address the potential paucity of disease-specific stem cells and to remove the potential for variability between stem cell lines, ZFNs have been used to generate isogenic control and Parkinson disease (PD) cell lines.[164] This work centered on engineering the A53T or E46K PD mutations into disease-free ESCs or repairing the mutation in PD patient-derived iPSCs.[164] In this way they mitigated the effects of the numerous genetic differences and modifiers that exist between individuals and ESC and iPSC clones.

Toward realizing the therapeutic potential of stem cells, investigators derived a fibroblast cell line from a humanized mouse model of sickle cell anemia; reprogrammed these cells into iPSCs; performed gene correction using a plasmid donor; differentiated the cells into hematopoietic progenitor cells; and transplanted them into sickle cell mice to reconstitute normal erythropoiesis.[22] Proof of principle for a similar strategy using human cells was demonstrated using ZFNs to correct the sickle cell mutation in iPSCs that were subsequently differentiated into cells of the erythroid lineage.[165] Numerous studies using ZFNs, TALENs, and CRISPR/Cas9 have shown the ability to correct disease-causing mutations in iPSCs or in primary cells that are subsequently differentiated into iPSCs. A major limitation for these strategies for hematologic disorders is the poor and/or absent ability of iPSCs to form from true blood progenitors *ex vivo* that are capable of reconstituting a functional circulatory system. However, the most streamlined path to translational use is likely to be direct modification of a patient's own HSCs. To date only two reports document the ability to mediate HR in HSCs. In 2007, maximal rates of 0.11 percent gene targeting at the *CCR5* locus utilizing ZFNs and a donor containing GFP or a puromycin resistance gene were reached.[160] Subsequently, optimized conditions involving ZFNs delivered as mRNA and the donor construct delivered on an integrase-deficient lentiviral (IDLV) cassette were used to correct the *IL2RG* gene from an individual with SCID-X1 and observed multilineage repopulation in transplanted mice.[166] This specialized delivery methodology in conjunction with the use of the StemRegenin 1 aryl hydrocarbon receptor antagonist[167] and/or 16,16-dimethyl-prostaglandin E$_2$ (dmPGE$_2$)[168,169] allowed for HR in HSCs that normally preferentially employ NHEJ. These data provide a strong platform for first-in-human studies.

The NHEJ arm of DNA repair also holds potential for therapeutic use. A promising avenue of investigation to use NHEJ to permanently disrupt genes has been employed clinically in T cells from HIV patients.[170] However, because of the ability of HIV to infect non–T-cell subsets,[171] studies have also investigated *CCR5* disruption in a preclinical humanized mouse model and showed that the modified cells are resistant to HIV-1 infection.[172,173] These data are especially relevant due to the recent treatment of patients using HCT of grafts with homozygous CCR5Δ32 mutations that disrupt cellular entry of the HIV particles.[174] This treatment protocol was initiated for an individual with HIV/AIDS who developed acute myeloid leukemia (the "Berlin patient") in an attempt to cure both the malignancy and the HIV infection.[174,175] Because of the paucity of CCR5Δ32/CCR5Δ32 donors, ZFN-modified HSCs are thought to be an ideal strategy for widespread implementation of this regimen. However, a 2013 evaluation of this individual showed reinfection, possibly with an HIV strain different from the initial one, indicating that *CCR5* loss alone may not result in full HIV resistance. The CXCR4 receptor is a coreceptor for HIV cellular entry, and a significant number of HIV patients harbor the CXCR4-using HIV strain.[176] A recent combinatorial ZFN approach has been investigated in the laboratory using *CXCR4* and *CCR5* adenoviral-borne ZFNs, with a demonstrated ability to remove both HIV coreceptors simultaneously in human T cells.[177] A potential clinical limitation of this approach is the fact that CXCR4 is a critical homing molecule for HSCs[177] and its disruption may perturb normal HSC homeostasis.

A joint approach using nuclease-induced gene disruption with chimeric antigen receptor (CAR) expression has mitigated the potential for cell-mediated alloreactivity and maximized the antitumor cellular effects. When the T-cell receptor (TCR) α and β chains were disrupted and paired with a Wilms tumor CAR, a potent tumoricidal activity without GVHD resulted.[178] A therapeutic success employing T cells transduced with a CD19-specific CAR have been achieved in patients with chronic lymphoid leukemia.[179] Scientists have extended these findings to include CAR expression with TCR-α disruption via ZFNs.[180] Future improvements to this technology will include more tumor-specific antigen recognition and/or temporizing CAR expression in order to minimize B-cell aplasia and tumor lysis syndrome.[179]

Their blood lineage plasticity and their expansive clinical application makes HSCs a desirable cell type for genome engineering with designer nucleases; however, their limited ability to form extrahematopoietic tissue limits their wide use in comprehensive disease modeling and in regenerative medicine outside the lymphohematopoietic system. ESCs and iPSCs are powerful tools for filling this void and performing nuclease genome modification of multilineage stem cells. Collectively, the convergence of stem cell technology and precision genome engineering holds tremendous potential to increase the therapeutic benefit of cell-based therapies while minimizing allogeneic transplant-associated risks. Crucial to the realization of their clinical potential will be rigorous safety assessments for each platform.

Both nucleases and pluripotent stem cells have potentially deleterious aspects that could limit their effectiveness. For pluripotent stem cells this relates to the presence or accumulation of genetic and epigenetic modifications prior to or during reprogramming. Both ESCs and iPSCs are subject to these modifications *in vitro*, which may manifest in the same line or even within the same culture vessel during propagation.[181] Aneuploidy has been reported in iPSCs, their parental cellular precursors, and ESCs. Studies by the International Stem Cell Initiative

suggest that karyotypic abnormalities may occur in as many as one of every three cell lines.[182] Trisomy 12 is the most common abnormality in human ESCs and iPSCs, and chromosome 17 trisomy occurs frequently in murine ESCs.[182,183]

By definition, engineered nucleases are designed to recognize a specific DNA sequence; however, they may also exhibit off-target (OT) effects due to overlapping or low-complexity sequence recognition between the primary target and the OT site. Unbiased genome-level screens are a powerful way to assess putative OT sites, and ZFN, TALEN, and CRISPR/Cas9 have shown excellent safety profiles to date[184,185]; however, this high-resolution methodology will need to be performed for each gene target candidate. In summary, engineered nucleases allow for unparalleled specificity and flexibility that complement the attributes of progenitor cells. The ability to precisely manipulate the genome will support individualized *ex vivo* therapies and will allow for more uniform disease modeling *in vitro*.

REFERENCES

1. Briggs R, King TJ: Transplantation of living nuclei from blastula cells into enucleated frogs' eggs. *Proc Natl Acad Sci U S A* 38(5):455–463, 1952.
2. Gurdon JB: The developmental capacity of nuclei taken from intestinal epithelium cells of feeding tadpoles. *J Embryol Exp Morphol* 10:622–640, 1962.
3. Gurdon JB, Uehlinger V: "Fertile" intestine nuclei. *Nature* 210(5042):1240–1241, 1966.
4. Solter D, Aronson J, Gilbert SF, McGrath J: Nuclear transfer in mouse embryos: Activation of the embryonic genome. *Cold Spring Harb Symp Quant Biol* 50:45–50, 1985.
5. McGrath J, Solter D: Inability of mouse blastomere nuclei transferred to enucleated zygotes to support development in vitro. *Science* 226(4680):1317–1319, 1984.
6. Takahashi K, Yamanaka S: Induction of pluripotent stem cells from mouse embryonic and adult fibroblast cultures by defined factors. *Cell* 126(4):663–676, 2006.
7. Kuhn TS, Conant J, Haugeland J: *The Road Since Structure: Philosophical essays, 1970–1993, with an autobiographical interview.* University of Chicago Press, Chicago, 2000.
8. Kuhn TS: *The Structure of Scientific Revolutions.* University of Chicago Press, Chicago, 1962.
9. Martin GR, Evans MJ: The morphology and growth of a pluripotent teratocarcinoma cell line and its derivatives in tissue culture. *Cell* 2(3):163–172, 1974.
10. Evans MJ, Kaufman MH: Establishment in culture of pluripotential cells from mouse embryos. *Nature* 292(5819):154–156, 1981.
11. Thomson JA, Kalishman J, Golos TG, et al: Isolation of a primate embryonic stem cell line. *Proc Natl Acad Sci U S A* 92(17):7844–7848, 1995.
12. Thomson JA, Itskovitz-Eldor J, Shapiro SS, et al: Embryonic stem cell lines derived from human blastocysts. *Science* 282(5391):1145–1147, 1998.
13. Hwang WS, Roh SI, Lee BC, et al: Patient-specific embryonic stem cells derived from human SCNT blastocysts. *Science* 308(5729):1777–1783, 2005.
14. Ma H, Morey R, O'Neil RC, et al: Abnormalities in human pluripotent cells due to reprogramming mechanisms. *Nature* 511(7508):177–183, 2014.
15. Davis RL, Weintraub H, Lassar AB: Expression of a single transfected cDNA converts fibroblasts to myoblasts. *Cell* 51(6):987–1000, 1987.
16. Schneuwly S, Klemenz R, Gehring WJ: Redesigning the body plan of Drosophila by ectopic expression of the homoeotic gene Antennapedia. *Nature* 325(6107):816–818, 1987.
17. Yu J, Vodyanik MA, Smuga-Otto K, et al: Induced pluripotent stem cell lines derived from human somatic cells. *Science* 318(5858):1917–1920, 2007.
18. Apostolou E, Hochedlinger K: Chromatin dynamics during cellular reprogramming. *Nature* 502(7472):462–471, 2013.
19. Rais Y, Zviran A, Geula S, et al: Deterministic direct reprogramming of somatic cells to pluripotency. *Nature* 502(7469):65–70, 2013.
20. Park IH, Arora N, Huo H, et al: Disease-specific induced pluripotent stem cells. *Cell* 134(5):877–886, 2008.
21. Dimos JT, Rodolfa KT, Niakan KK, et al: Induced pluripotent stem cells generated from patients with ALS can be differentiated into motor neurons. *Science* 321(5893):1218–1221, 2008.
22. Hanna J, Wernig M, Markoulaki S, et al: Treatment of sickle cell anemia mouse model with iPS cells generated from autologous skin. *Science* 318(5858):1920–1923, 2007.
23. Kamao H, Mandai M, Okamoto S, et al: Characterization of human induced pluripotent stem cell-derived retinal pigment epithelium cell sheets aiming for clinical application. *Stem Cell Reports* 2(2):205–218, 2014.
24. Zhou Q, Brown J, Kanarek A, Rajagopal J, Melton DA: In vivo reprogramming of adult pancreatic exocrine cells to beta-cells. *Nature* 455(7213):627–632, 2008.
25. Banga A, Akinci E, Greder LV, Dutton JR, Slack JM: In vivo reprogramming of Sox9+ cells in the liver to insulin-secreting ducts. *Proc Natl Acad Sci U S A* 109(38):15336–15341, 2012.
26. Kobayashi T, Yamaguchi T, Hamanaka S, et al: Generation of rat pancreas in mouse by interspecific blastocyst injection of pluripotent stem cells. *Cell* 142(5):787–799, 2010.

27. Riddell J, Gazit R, Garrison BS, et al: Reprogramming committed murine blood cells to induced hematopoietic stem cells with defined factors. *Cell* 157(3):549–564, 2014.

28. Doulatov S, Vo LT, Chou SS, et al: Induction of multipotential hematopoietic progenitors from human pluripotent stem cells via respecification of lineage-restricted precursors. *Cell Stem Cell* 13(4):459–470, 2013.

29. Rideout WM 3rd, Hochedlinger K, Kyba M, Daley GQ, Jaenisch R: Correction of a genetic defect by nuclear transplantation and combined cell and gene therapy. *Cell* 109(1):17–27, 2002.

30. Wang L, Menendez P, Cerdan C, Bhatia M: Hematopoietic development from human embryonic stem cell lines. *Exp Hematol* 33(9):987–996, 2005.

31. Ledran MH, Krassowska A, Armstrong L, et al: Efficient hematopoietic differentiation of human embryonic stem cells on stromal cells derived from hematopoietic niches. *Cell Stem Cell* 3(1):85–98, 2008.

32. Szabo E, Rampalli S, Risueno RM, et al: Direct conversion of human fibroblasts to multilineage blood progenitors. *Nature* 468(7323):521–526, 2010.

33. Elcheva I, Brok-Volchanskaya V, Kumar A, et al: Direct induction of haematoendothelial programs in human pluripotent stem cells by transcriptional regulators. *Nat Commun* 5:4372.

34. Friedenstein AJ, Chailakhjan RK, Lalykina KS: The development of fibroblast colonies in monolayer cultures of guinea-pig bone marrow and spleen cells. *Cell Tissue Kinet* 3(4):393–403, 2014.

35. Phinney DG, Prockop DJ: Concise review: Mesenchymal stem/multipotent stromal cells: The state of transdifferentiation and modes of tissue repair—Current views. *Stem Cells* 25(11):2896–2902, 2007.

36. Pittenger MF, Mackay AM, Beck SC, et al: Multilineage potential of adult human mesenchymal stem cells. *Science* 284(5411):143–147, 1999.

37. da Silva Meirelles L, Caplan AI, Nardi NB: In search of the in vivo identity of mesenchymal stem cells. *Stem Cells* 26(9):2287–2299, 2008.

38. Le Blanc K, Rasmusson I, Sundberg B, et al: Treatment of severe acute graft-versus-host disease with third party haploidentical mesenchymal stem cells. *Lancet* 363(9419):1439–1441, 2004.

39. Rasmusson I, Ringden O, Sundberg B, Le Blanc K: Mesenchymal stem cells inhibit lymphocyte proliferation by mitogens and alloantigens by different mechanisms. *Exp Cell Res* 305(1):33–41, 2005.

40. Ringden O, Uzunel M, Rasmusson I, et al: Mesenchymal stem cells for treatment of therapy-resistant graft-versus-host disease. *Transplantation* 81(10):1390–1397, 2006.

41. Holtan SG, Pasquini M, Weisdorf DJ: Acute graft-versus-host disease: A bench-to-bedside update. *Blood* 124(3):363–373, 2014.

42. Ball LM, Bernardo ME, Roelofs H, et al: Multiple infusions of mesenchymal stromal cells induce sustained remission in children with steroid-refractory, grade III-IV acute graft-versus-host disease. *Br J Haematol* 163(4):501–509, 2013.

43. Bernardo ME, Fibbe WE: Mesenchymal stromal cells: Sensors and switchers of inflammation. *Cell Stem Cell* 13(4):392–402, 2013.

44. Dalal J, Gandy K, Domen J: Role of mesenchymal stem cell therapy in Crohn's disease. *Pediatr Res* 71(4 Pt 2):445–451, 2012.

45. Keerthi N, Chimutengwende-Gordon M, Sanghani A, Khan W: The potential of stem cell therapy for osteoarthritis and rheumatoid arthritis. *Curr Stem Cell Res Ther* 8(6):444–450, 2013.

46. Chhabra P, Brayman KL: Stem cell therapy to cure type 1 diabetes: From hype to hope. *Stem Cells Transl Med* 2(5):328–336, 2013.

47. Prockop DJ: Repair of tissues by adult stem/progenitor cells (MSCs): Controversies, myths, and changing paradigms. *Mol Ther* 17(6):939–946, 2009.

48. Tolar J, Wang X, Braunlin E, et al: The host immune response is essential for the beneficial effect of adult stem cells after myocardial ischemia. *Exp Hematol* 35(4):682–690, 2007.

49. Laslett LJ, Alagona P Jr, Clark BA 3rd, et al: The worldwide environment of cardiovascular disease: Prevalence, diagnosis, therapy, and policy issues: A report from the American College of Cardiology. *J Am Coll Cardiol* 60(25 Suppl):S1–S49, 2012.

50. Rosenstrauch D, Poglajen G, Zidar N, Gregoric ID: Stem cell therapy for ischemic heart failure. *Tex Heart Inst J* 32(3):339–347, 2005.

51. Bergmann O, Bhardwaj RD, Bernard S, et al: Evidence for cardiomyocyte renewal in humans. *Science* 324(5923):98–102, 2009.

52. Chiu RC, Zibaitis A, Kao RL: Cellular cardiomyoplasty: Myocardial regeneration with satellite cell implantation. *Ann Thorac Surg* 60(1):12–18, 1995.

53. Pouzet B, Vilquin JT, Hagege AA, et al: Intramyocardial transplantation of autologous myoblasts: Can tissue processing be optimized? *Circulation* 102(19 Suppl 3):III210–III215, 2000.

54. Menasche P: Stem cell therapy for heart failure: Are arrhythmias a real safety concern? *Circulation* 119(20):2735–2740, 2009.

55. Orlic D, Kajstura J, Chimenti S, et al: Bone marrow cells regenerate infarcted myocardium. *Nature* 410(6829):701–705, 2001.

56. Orlic D, Hill JM, Arai AE: Stem cells for myocardial regeneration. *Circ Res* 91(12):1092–1102, 2002.

57. Kocher AA, Schuster MD, Szabolcs MJ, et al: Neovascularization of ischemic myocardium by human bone-marrow-derived angioblasts prevents cardiomyocyte apoptosis, reduces remodeling and improves cardiac function. *Nat Med* 7(4):430–436, 2001.

58. Luth ES, Jun SJ, Wessen MK, et al: Bone marrow side population cells are enriched for progenitors capable of myogenic differentiation. *J Cell Sci* 121(Pt 9):1426–1434, 2008.

59. Strauer BE, Brehm M, Zeus T, et al: Repair of infarcted myocardium by autologous intracoronary mononuclear bone marrow cell transplantation in humans. *Circulation* 106(15):1913–1918, 2002.

60. Assmus B, Schachinger V, Teupe C, et al: Transplantation of progenitor cells and regeneration enhancement in acute myocardial infarction (TOPCARE-AMI). *Circulation* 106(24):3009–3017, 2002.

61. Assmus B, Fischer-Rasokat U, Honold J, et al: Transcoronary transplantation of functionally competent BMCs is associated with a decrease in natriuretic peptide serum levels and improved survival of patients with chronic postinfarction heart failure: Results of the TOPCARE-CHD Registry. *Circ Res* 100(8):1234–1241, 2007.

62. Tendera M, Wojakowski W, Ruzyllo W, et al: Intracoronary infusion of bone marrow-derived selected CD34+CXCR4+ cells and non-selected mononuclear cells in patients with acute STEMI and reduced left ventricular ejection fraction: Results of randomized, multicentre Myocardial Regeneration by Intracoronary Infusion of Selected Population of Stem Cells in Acute Myocardial Infarction (REGENT) Trial. *Eur Heart J* 30(11):1313–1321, 2009.

63. Makino S, Fukuda K, Miyoshi S, et al: Cardiomyocytes can be generated from marrow stromal cells in vitro. *J Clin Invest* 103(5):697–705, 1999.

64. Heldman AW, DiFede DL, Fishman JE, et al: Transendocardial mesenchymal stem cells and mononuclear bone marrow cells for ischemic cardiomyopathy: The TAC-HFT randomized trial. *JAMA* 311(1):62–73, 2014.

65. Boheler KR, Czyz J, Tweedie D, Yang HT, Anisimov SV, Wobus AM: Differentiation of pluripotent embryonic stem cells into cardiomyocytes. *Circ Res* 91(3):189–201, 2002.

66. He JQ, Ma Y, Lee Y, Thomson JA, Kamp TJ: Human embryonic stem cells develop into multiple types of cardiac myocytes: Action potential characterization. *Circ Res* 93(1):32–39, 2003.

67. Yamanaka S, Blau HM: Nuclear reprogramming to a pluripotent state by three approaches. *Nature* 465(7299):704–712, 2010.

68. Wernig M, Meissner A, Foreman R, et al: In vitro reprogramming of fibroblasts into a pluripotent ES-cell-like state. *Nature* 448(7151):318–324, 2007.

69. Liu Z, Wen X, Wang H, et al: Molecular imaging of induced pluripotent stem cell immunogenicity with in vivo development in ischemic myocardium. *PLoS One* 8(6):e66369, 2013.

70. Jawad H, Lyon AR, Harding SE, Ali NN, Boccaccini AR: Myocardial tissue engineering. *Br Med Bull* 87:31–47, 2008.

71. Wendel JS, Ye L, Zhang P, Tranquillo RT, Zhang JJ: Functional consequences of a tissue-engineered myocardial patch for cardiac repair in a rat infarct model. *Tissue Eng Part A* 20(7–8):1325–1335, 2014.

72. Korf-Klingebiel M, Kempf T, Sauer T, et al: Bone marrow cells are a rich source of growth factors and cytokines: Implications for cell therapy trials after myocardial infarction. *Eur Heart J* 29(23):2851–2858, 2008.

73. Thum T, Bauersachs J, Poole-Wilson PA, et al: The dying stem cell hypothesis: Immune modulation as a novel mechanism for progenitor cell therapy in cardiac muscle. *J Am Coll Cardiol* 46(10):1799–1802, 2005.

74. Pavo N, Zimmermann M, Pils D, et al: Long-acting beneficial effect of percutaneously intramyocardially delivered secretome of apoptotic peripheral blood cells on porcine chronic ischemic left ventricular dysfunction. *Biomaterials* 35(11):3541–3550, 2014.

75. Weiss DJ, Bertoncello I, Borok Z, et al: Stem cells and cell therapies in lung biology and lung diseases. *Proc Am Thorac Soc* 8(3):223–272, 2011.

76. Rock JR, Hogan BL: Epithelial progenitor cells in lung development, maintenance, repair, and disease. *Annu Rev Cell Dev Biol* 27:493–512, 2011.

77. McQualter JL, Bertoncello I: Concise review: Deconstructing the lung to reveal its regenerative potential. *Stem Cells* 30(5):811–816, 2012.

78. Perl AK, Wert SE, Loudy DE, et al: Conditional recombination reveals distinct subsets of epithelial cells in trachea, bronchi, and alveoli. *Am J Respir Cell Mol Biol* 33(5):455–462, 2005.

79. Giangreco A, Arwert EN, Rosewell IR, et al: Stem cells are dispensable for lung homeostasis but restore airways after injury. *Proc Natl Acad Sci U S A* 106(23):9286–9291, 2009.

80. Hong KU, Reynolds SD, Giangreco A, et al: Clara cell secretory protein-expressing cells of the airway neuroepithelial body microenvironment include a label-retaining subset and are critical for epithelial renewal after progenitor cell depletion. *Am J Respir Cell Mol Biol* 24(6):671–681, 2001.

81. Giangreco A, Reynolds SD, Stripp BR: Terminal bronchioles harbor a unique airway stem cell population that localizes to the bronchoalveolar duct junction. *Am J Pathol* 161(1):173–182, 2002.

82. Teisanu RM, Chen H, Matsumoto K, et al: Functional analysis of two distinct bronchiolar progenitors during lung injury and repair. *Am J Respir Cell Mol Biol* 44(6):794–803, 2011.

83. Chapman HA, Li X, Alexander JP, et al: Integrin alpha6beta4 identifies an adult distal lung epithelial population with regenerative potential in mice. *J Clin Invest* 121(7):2855–2862, 2011.

84. Dobbs LG, Johnson MD, Vanderbilt J, et al: The great big alveolar TI cell: Evolving concepts and paradigms. *Cell Physiol Biochem* 25(1):55–62, 2010.

85. Buckley S, Shi W, Carraro G, et al: The milieu of damaged alveolar epithelial type 2 cells stimulates alveolar wound repair by endogenous and exogenous progenitors. *Am J Respir Cell Mol Biol* 45(6):1212–1221, 2011.

86. Kim CF, Jackson EL, Woolfenden AE, et al: Identification of bronchioalveolar stem cells in normal lung and lung cancer. *Cell* 121(6):823–835, 2005.

87. Kumar PA, Hu Y, Yamamoto Y, et al: Distal airway stem cells yield alveoli in vitro and during lung regeneration following H1N1 influenza infection. *Cell* 147(3):525–538, 2011.

88. Zhao YD, Courtman DW, Deng Y, et al: Rescue of monocrotaline-induced pulmonary arterial hypertension using bone marrow-derived endothelial-like progenitor cells: Efficacy of combined cell and eNOS gene therapy in established disease. *Circ Res* 96(4):442–450, 2005.

89. Lam CF, Roan JN, Lee CH, et al: Transplantation of endothelial progenitor cells improves pulmonary endothelial function and gas exchange in rabbits with endotoxin-induced acute lung injury. *Anesth Analg* 112(3):620–627, 2011.

90. Balasubramaniam V, Ryan SL, Seedorf GJ, et al: Bone marrow-derived angiogenic cells restore lung alveolar and vascular structure after neonatal hyperoxia in infant mice. *Am J Physiol Lung Cell Mol Physiol* 298(3):L315–323, 2010.

91. Stewart DJ, Mei SH: Cell-based therapies for lung vascular diseases: Lessons for the future. *Proc Am Thorac Soc* 8(6):535–540, 2011.

92. Wang XX, Zhang FR, Shang YP, et al: Transplantation of autologous endothelial progenitor cells may be beneficial in patients with idiopathic pulmonary arterial hypertension: A pilot randomized controlled trial. *J Am Coll Cardiol* 49(14):1566–1571, 2007.

93. Zhu JH, Wang XX, Zhang FR, et al: Safety and efficacy of autologous endothelial progenitor cells transplantation in children with idiopathic pulmonary arterial hypertension: Open-label pilot study. *Pediatr Transplant* 12(6):650–655, 2008.

94. Keating A: Mesenchymal stromal cells: New directions. *Cell Stem Cell* 10(6):709–716, 2012.

95. Prockop DJ, Oh JY: Medical therapies with adult stem/progenitor cells (MSCs): A backward journey from dramatic results in vivo to the cellular and molecular explanations. *J Cell Biochem* 113(5):1460–1469, 2012.

96. Islam MN, Das SR, Emin MT, et al: Mitochondrial transfer from bone-marrow-derived stromal cells to pulmonary alveoli protects against acute lung injury. *Nat Med* 18(5):759–765, 2012.

97. Tropea KA, Leder E, Aslam M, et al: Bronchioalveolar stem cells increase after mesenchymal stromal cell treatment in a mouse model of bronchopulmonary dysplasia. *Am J Physiol Lung Cell Mol Physiol* 302(9):L829–L837, 2012.

98. Matthay MA, Thompson BT, Read EJ, et al: Therapeutic potential of mesenchymal stem cells for severe acute lung injury. *Chest* 138(4):965–972, 2010.

99. Epperly MW, Guo H, Gretton JE, Greenberger JS: Bone marrow origin of myofibroblasts in irradiation pulmonary fibrosis. *Am J Respir Cell Mol Biol* 29(2):213–224, 2003.

100. Yan X, Liu Y, Han Q, et al: Injured microenvironment directly guides the differentiation of engrafted Flk-1(+) mesenchymal stem cell in lung. *Exp Hematol* 35(9):1466–1475, 2007.

101. Weiss DJ, Casaburi R, Flannery R, et al: A placebo-controlled, randomized trial of mesenchymal stem cells in COPD. *Chest* 143(6):1590–1598, 2013.

102. Song M, Kim YJ, Kim YH, et al: Effects of duplicate administration of human neural stem cell after focal cerebral ischemia in the rat. *Int J Neurosci* 121(8):457–461, 2011.

103. Uchida N, Buck DW, He D, et al: Direct isolation of human central nervous system stem cells. *Proc Natl Acad Sci U S A* 97(26):14720–14725, 2000.

104. Goldman SA: Progenitor cell-based treatment of the pediatric myelin disorders. *Arch Neurol Psychiatry* 68(7):848–856, 2011.

105. Sandrock RW, Wheatley W, Levinthal C, et al: Isolation, characterization and preclinical development of human glial-restricted progenitor cells for treatment of neurological disorders. *Regen Men* 5(3):381–394, 2010.

106. Boulis NM, Federici T, Glass JD, et al: Translational stem cell therapy for amyotrophic lateral sclerosis. *Nat Rev Neurol* 8(3):172–176, 2011.

107. Glass JD, Boulis NM, Johe K, et al: Lumbar intraspinal injection of neural stem cells in patients with amyotrophic lateral sclerosis: Results of a phase I trial in 12 patients. *Stem Cells* 30(6):1144–1151, 2012.

108. Minguell JJ, Allers C, Lasala GP: Mesenchymal stem cells and the treatment of conditions and diseases: The less glittering side of a conspicuous stem cell for basic research. *Stem Cells Dev* 22(2):193–203, 2013.

109. Singh SP, Tripathy NK, Nityanand S: Comparison of phenotypic markers and neural differentiation potential of multipotent adult progenitor cells and mesenchymal stem cells. *World J Stem Cells* 5(2):53–60, 2013.

110. Lunn JS, Sakowski SA, Federici T, et al: Stem cell technology for the study and treatment of motor neuron diseases. *Regen Men* 6(2):201–213, 2011.

111. Kondziolka D, Steinberg GK, Wechsler L, et al: Neurotransplantation for patients with subcortical motor stroke: A phase 2 randomized trial. *J Neurosurg* 103(1):38–45, 2005.

112. Bang OY, Lee JS, Lee PH, Lee G: Autologous mesenchymal stem cell transplantation in stroke patients. *Ann Neurol* 57(6):874–882, 2005.

113. Cashman N, Tan LY, Krieger C, et al: Pilot study of granulocyte colony stimulating factor (G-CSF)-mobilized peripheral blood stem cells in amyotrophic lateral sclerosis (ALS). *Muscle Nerve* 37(5):620–625, 2008.

114. Chio A, Mora G, La Bella V, et al: Repeated courses of granulocyte colony-stimulating factor in amyotrophic lateral sclerosis: Clinical and biological results from a prospective multicenter study. *Muscle Nerve* 43(2):189–195, 2011.

115. Deda H, Inci MC, Kurekci AE, et al: Treatment of amyotrophic lateral sclerosis patients by autologous bone marrow-derived hematopoietic stem cell transplantation: A 1-year follow-up. *Cytotherapy* 11(1):18–25, 2009.

116. Lees JS, Sena ES, Egan KJ, et al: Stem cell-based therapy for experimental stroke: A systematic review and meta-analysis. *Int J Stroke* 7(7):582–588, 2012.

117. Zhang ZG, Chopp M: Neurorestorative therapies for stroke: Underlying mechanisms and translation to the clinic. *Lancet Neurol* 8(5):491–500, 2009.

118. Janowski M, Walczak P, Date I: Intravenous route of cell delivery for treatment of neurological disorders: A meta-analysis of preclinical results. *Stem Cells Dev* 19(1):5–16, 2010.

119. Luo Y: Cell-based therapy for stroke. *J Neural Transm* 118(1):61–74, 2011.

120. Keirstead HS, Nistor G, Bernal G, et al: Human embryonic stem cell-derived oligodendrocyte progenitor cell transplants remyelinate and restore locomotion after spinal cord injury. *J Neurosci* 25(19):4694–4705, 2005.

121. Erceg S, Ronaghi M, Stojkovic M: Human embryonic stem cell differentiation toward regional specific neural precursors. *Stem Cells* 27(1):78–87, 2009.

122. Nistor GI, Totoiu MO, Haque N, et al: Human embryonic stem cells differentiate into oligodendrocytes in high purity and myelinate after spinal cord transplantation. *Glia* 49(3):385–396, 2005.

123. Sharp J, Frame J, Siegenthaler M, et al: Human embryonic stem cell-derived oligodendrocyte progenitor cell transplants improve recovery after cervical spinal cord injury. *Stem Cells* 28(1):152–163, 2010.

124. Lu QR, Sun T, Zhu Z, et al: Common developmental requirement for Olig function indicates a motor neuron/oligodendrocyte connection. *Cell* 109(1):75–86, 2002.

125. Zhou Q, Anderson DJ: The bHLH transcription factors OLIG2 and OLIG1 couple neuronal and glial subtype specification. *Cell* 109(1):61–73, 2002.

126. Brustle O, Maskos U, McKay RD: Host-guided migration allows targeted introduction of neurons into the embryonic brain. *Neuron* 15(6):1275–1285, 1995.

127. Pluchino S, Zanotti L, Rossi B, et al: Neurosphere-derived multipotent precursors promote neuroprotection by an immunomodulatory mechanism. *Nature* 436(7048):266–271, 2005.

128. Bretzner F, Gilbert F, Baylis F, Brownstone RM: Target populations for first-in-human embryonic stem cell research in spinal cord injury. *Cell Stem Cell* 8(5):468–475, 2011.

129. Roskams TA, Theise ND, Balabaud C, et al: Nomenclature of the finer branches of the biliary tree: Canals, ductules, and ductular reactions in human livers. *Hepatology* 39(6):1739–1745, 2004.

130. Furuyama K, Kawaguchi Y, Akiyama H, et al: Continuous cell supply from a Sox9-expressing progenitor zone in adult liver, exocrine pancreas and intestine. *Nat Genet* 43(1):34–41, 2011.

131. Duncan AW, Dorrell C, Grompe M: Stem cells and liver regeneration. *Gastroenterology* 137(2):466–481, 2009.

132. Schmelzer E, Zhang L, Bruce A, et al: Human hepatic stem cells from fetal and postnatal donors. *J Exp Med* 204(8):1973–1987, 2007.

133. De Vos R, Desmet V: Ultrastructural characteristics of novel epithelial cell types identified in human pathologic liver specimens with chronic ductular reaction. *Am J Pathol* 140(6):1441–1450, 1992.

134. Wilson JW, Leduc EH: Role of cholangioles in restoration of the liver of the mouse after dietary injury. *J Pathol Bacteriol* 76(2):441–449, 1958.

135. Ito M, Nagata H, Miyakawa S, Fox IJ: Review of hepatocyte transplantation. *J Hepatobiliary Pancreat Surg* 16(2):97–100, 2009.

136. Basma H, Soto-Gutierrez A, Yannam GR, et al: Differentiation and transplantation of human embryonic stem cell-derived hepatocytes. *Gastroenterology* 136(3):990–999, 2009.

137. Asgari S, Moslem M, Bagheri-Lankarani K, et al: Differentiation and transplantation of human induced pluripotent stem cell-derived hepatocyte-like cells. *Stem Cell Rev* 9(4):493–504, 2013.

138. Takebe T, Sekine K, Enomura M, et al: Vascularized and functional human liver from an iPSC-derived organ bud transplant. *Nature* 499(7459):481–484, 2013.

139. Espejel S, Roll GR, McLaughlin KJ, et al: Induced pluripotent stem cell-derived hepatocytes have the functional and proliferative capabilities needed for liver regeneration in mice. *J Clin Invest* 120(9):3120–3126, 2010.

140. Gaudio E, Carpino G, Cardinale V, et al: New insights into liver stem cells. *Dig Liver Dis* 41(7):455–462, 2009.

141. Zhang L, Theise N, Chua M, Reid LM: The stem cell niche of human livers: Symmetry between development and regeneration. *Hepatology* 48(5):1598–1607, 2008.

142. Semeraro R, Carpino G, Cardinale V, et al: Multipotent stem/progenitor cells in the human foetal biliary tree. *J Hepatol* 57(5):987–994, 2012.

143. Carpentier R, Suner RE, van Hul N, et al: Embryonic ductal plate cells give rise to cholangiocytes, periportal hepatocytes, and adult liver progenitor cells. *Gastroenterology* 141(4):1432–1438, 1438.e1431–1434, 2011.

144. Kawaguchi Y: Sox9 and programming of liver and pancreatic progenitors. *J Clin Invest* 123(5):1881–1886, 2013.

145. Cardinale V, Wang Y, Carpino G, et al: Multipotent stem/progenitor cells in human biliary tree give rise to hepatocytes, cholangiocytes, and pancreatic islets. *J Hepatol* 54(6):2159–2172, 2011.

146. Banga A, Greder LV, Dutton JR, Slack JM: Stable insulin-secreting ducts formed by reprogramming of cells in the liver using a three-gene cocktail and a PPAR agonist. *Gene Ther* 21(1):19–27, 2014.

147. Huch M, Dorrell C, Boj SF, et al: In vitro expansion of single Lgr5+ liver stem cells induced by Wnt-driven regeneration. *Nature* 494(7436):247–250, 2013.

148. Huch M, Bonfanti P, Boj SF, et al: Unlimited in vitro expansion of adult bi-potent pancreas progenitors through the Lgr5/R-spondin axis. *EMBO J* 32(20):2708–2721, 2013.

149. American Diabetes Association: *Statistics About Diabetes: Overall Numbers, Diabetes and Prediabetes.* Available online at http://www.diabetes.org/diabetes-basics/statistics/?loc=db-slabnav (accessed 8 August 2014).

150. Zhang D, Jiang W, Liu W, et al: Highly efficient differentiation of human ES cells and iPS cells into mature pancreatic insulin-producing cells. *Cell Res* 19(4):429–438, 2009.

151. Kroon E, Martinson LA, Kadoya K, et al: Pancreatic endoderm derived from human embryonic stem cells generates glucose-responsive insulin-secreting cells in vivo. *Nat Biotechnol* 26(4):443–452, 2008.

152. Rezania A, Bruin JE, Riedel MJ, et al: Maturation of human embryonic stem cell-derived pancreatic progenitors into functional islets capable of treating pre-existing diabetes in mice. *Diabetes* 61(8):2016–2029, 2012.

153. Pagliuca FW, Millman JR, Gurtler M, et al: Generation of functional human pancreatic beta cells in vitro. *Cell* 159(2):428–439, 2014.

154. Collombat P, Xu X, Ravassard P, et al: The ectopic expression of Pax4 in the mouse pancreas converts progenitor cells into alpha and subsequently beta cells. *Cell* 138(3):449–462, 2009.

155. Thorel F, Nepote V, Avril I, et al: Conversion of adult pancreatic alpha-cells to beta-cells after extreme beta-cell loss. *Nature* 464(7292):1149–1154, 2010.

156. Hacein-Bey-Abina S, Garrigue A, Wang GP, et al: Insertional oncogenesis in 4 patients after retrovirus-mediated gene therapy of SCID-X1. *J Clin Invest* 118(9):3132–3142, 2008.

157. Cartier N, Hacein-Bey-Abina S, Bartholomae CC, et al: Hematopoietic stem cell gene therapy with a lentiviral vector in X-linked adrenoleukodystrophy. *Science* 326(5954):818–823, 2009.

158. Biffi A, Montini E, Lorioli L, et al: Lentiviral hematopoietic stem cell gene therapy benefits metachromatic leukodystrophy. *Science* 341(6148):1233158, 2013.

159. Aiuti A, Biasco L, Scaramuzza S, et al: Lentiviral hematopoietic stem cell gene therapy in patients with Wiskott-Aldrich syndrome. *Science* 341(6148):1233151, 2013.

160. Lombardo A, Genovese P, Beausejour CM, et al: Gene editing in human stem cells using zinc finger nucleases and integrase-defective lentiviral vector delivery. *Nat Biotechnol* 25(11):1298–1306, 2007.

161. Hockemeyer D, Soldner F, Beard C, et al: Efficient targeting of expressed and silent genes in human ESCs and iPSCs using zinc-finger nucleases. *Nat Biotechnol* 27(9):851–857, 2009.

162. DeKelver RC, Choi VM, Moehle EA, et al: Functional genomics, proteomics, and regulatory DNA analysis in isogenic settings using zinc finger nuclease-driven transgenesis into a safe harbor locus in the human genome. *Genome Res* 20(8):1133–1142, 2010.

163. Lombardo A, Cesana D, Genovese P, et al: Site-specific integration and tailoring of cassette design for sustainable gene transfer. *Nat Methods* 8(10):861–869, 2011.

164. Soldner F, Laganiere J, Cheng AW, et al: Generation of isogenic pluripotent stem cells differing exclusively at two early onset Parkinson point mutations. *Cell* 146(2):318–331, 2011.

165. Zou J, Mali P, Huang X, Dowey SN, Cheng L: Site-specific gene correction of a point mutation in human iPS cells derived from an adult patient with sickle cell disease. *Blood* 118(17):4599–4608, 2011.

166. Genovese P, Schiroli G, Escobar G, et al: Targeted genome editing in human repopulating haematopoietic stem cells. *Nature* 510(7504):235–240, 2014.

167. Boitano AE, Wang J, Romeo R, et al: Aryl hydrocarbon receptor antagonists promote the expansion of human hematopoietic stem cells. *Science* 329(5997):1345–1348, 2010.

168. North TE, Goessling W, Walkley CR, et al: Prostaglandin E2 regulates vertebrate haematopoietic stem cell homeostasis. *Nature* 447(7147):1007–1011, 2007.

169. Goessling W, Allen RS, Guan X, et al: Prostaglandin E2 enhances human cord blood stem cell xenotransplants and shows long-term safety in preclinical nonhuman primate transplant models. *Cell Stem Cell* 8(4):445–458, 2011.

170. Perez EE, Wang J, Miller JC, et al: Establishment of HIV-1 resistance in CD4+ T cells by genome editing using zinc-finger nucleases. *Nat Biotechnol* 26(7):808–816, 2008.

171. McElrath MJ, Smythe K, Randolph-Habecker J, et al: Comprehensive assessment of HIV target cells in the distal human gut suggests increasing HIV susceptibility toward the anus. *J Acquir Immune Defic Syndr* 63(3):263–271, 2013.

172. Holt N, Wang J, Kim K, et al: Human hematopoietic stem/progenitor cells modified by zinc-finger nucleases targeted to CCR5 control HIV-1 in vivo. *Nat Biotechnol* 28(8):839–847, 2010.

173. Hofer U, Henley JE, Exline CM, et al: Pre-clinical modeling of CCR5 knockout in human hematopoietic stem cells by zinc finger nucleases using humanized mice. *J Infect Dis* 208 Suppl 2:S160–S164, 2013.

174. Allers K, Hutter G, Hofmann J, et al: Evidence for the cure of HIV infection by CCR5Delta32/Delta32 stem cell transplantation. *Blood* 117(10):2791–2799, 2011.

175. Hutter G, Nowak D, Mossner M, et al: Long-term control of HIV by CCR5 Delta32/Delta32 stem-cell transplantation. *N Engl J Med* 360(7):692–698, 2009.

176. de Mendoza C, Rodriguez C, Garcia F, et al: Prevalence of X4 tropic viruses in patients recently infected with HIV-1 and lack of association with transmission of drug resistance. *J Antimicrob Chemother* 59(4):698–704, 2007.

177. Didigu CA, Wilen CB, Wang J, et al: Simultaneous zinc-finger nuclease editing of the HIV coreceptors ccr5 and cxcr4 protects CD4+ T cells from HIV-1 infection. *Blood* 123(1):61–69, 2014.

178. Provasi E, Genovese P, Lombardo A, et al: Editing T cell specificity towards leukemia by zinc finger nucleases and lentiviral gene transfer. *Nat Med* 18(5):807–815, 2012.

179. Porter DL, Levine BL, Kalos M, et al: Chimeric antigen receptor-modified T cells in chronic lymphoid leukemia. *N Engl J Med* 365(8):725–733, 2011.

180. Torikai H, Reik A, Liu PQ, et al: A foundation for universal T-cell based immunotherapy: T cells engineered to express a CD19-specific chimeric-antigen-receptor and eliminate expression of endogenous TCR. *Blood* 119(24):5697–5705, 2012.

181. Liang G, Zhang Y: Genetic and epigenetic variations in iPSCs: Potential causes and implications for application. *Cell Stem Cell* 13(2):149–159, 2013.

182. Amps K, Andrews PW, Anyfantis G, et al: Screening ethnically diverse human embryonic stem cells identifies a chromosome 20 minimal amplicon conferring growth advantage. *Nat Biotechnol* 29(12):1132–1144, 2011.

183. Ben-David U, Benvenisty N: High prevalence of evolutionarily conserved and species-specific genomic aberrations in mouse pluripotent stem cells. *Stem Cells* 30(4):612–622, 2012.

184. Smith C, Gore A, Yan W, et al: Whole-genome sequencing analysis reveals high specificity of CRISPR/Cas9 and TALEN-based genome editing in human iPSCs. *Cell Stem Cell* 15(1):12–13, 2014.

185. Osborn MJ, Starker CG, McElroy AN, et al: TALEN-based gene correction for epidermolysis bullosa. *Mol Ther* 21(6):1151–1159, 2013.

Part VI The Erythrocyte

31. Structure and Composition of the Erythrocyte.........................461

32. Erythropoiesis.........................479

33. Erythrocytes Turnover 495

34. Clinical Manifestations and Classification of Erythrocyte Disorders.........................503

35. Aplastic Anemia: Acquired and Inherited 513

36. Pure Red Cell Aplasia 539

37. Anemia of Chronic Disease.........................549

38. Erythropoietic Effects of Endocrine Disorders 559

39. The Congenital Dyserythropoietic Anemias.........................563

40. Paroxysmal Nocturnal Hemoglobinuria 571

41. Folate, Cobalamin, and Megaloblastic Anemias.........................583

42. Iron Metabolism 617

43. Iron Deficiency and Overload.........................627

44. Anemia Resulting from Other Nutritional Deficiencies 651

45. Anemia Associated with Marrow Infiltration 657

46. Erythrocyte Membrane Disorders.........................661

47. Erythrocyte Enzyme Disorders.........................689

48. The Thalassemias: Disorders of Globin Synthesis 725

49. Disorders of Hemoglobin Structure: Sickle Cell Anemia and Related Abnormalities.........................759

50. Methemoglobinemia and Other Dyshemoglobinemias 789

51. Fragmentation Hemolytic Anemia 801

52. Erythrocyte Disorders as a Result of Chemical and Physical Agents 809

53. Hemolytic Anemia Resulting from Infections with Microorganisms.........................815

54. Hemolytic Anemia Resulting from Immune Injury 823

55. Alloimmune Hemolytic Disease of the Fetus and Newborn 847

56. Hypersplenism and Hyposplenism 863

57. Primary and Secondary Erythrocytoses 871

58. The Porphyrias 889

59. Polyclonal and Hereditary Sideroblastic Anemias 915

CHAPTER 31
STRUCTURE AND COMPOSITION OF THE ERYTHROCYTE

Narla Mohandas*

SUMMARY

Collectively, the erythroid progenitors, terminally differentiating erythroblasts (precursors), and adult red cells are termed the *erythron* to reinforce the idea that they function as an organ. The widely dispersed cells comprising this organ arise from pluripotential hematopoietic stem cells. Following commitment to the erythroid lineage (unipotential progenitor), further maturation gives rise to the erythroid progenitors, burst-forming unit–erythroid and, subsequently, colony-forming unit–erythroid (CFU-E), that can be identified by their development into representative clonal colonies of red cells *in vitro*. The CFU-E then undergoes terminal differentiation, progressing through four to five morphologic stages, each having characteristic light microscopic and ultrastructural features. During terminal erythroid differentiation there is an increasing amount of hemoglobin synthesis accompanied by nuclear chromatin condensation and at the final stage of differentiation there is nuclear extrusion to generate an anucleate polychromatophilic macrocyte (reticulocyte with supravital staining). The human polychromatophilic macrocyte (reticulocyte) matures over 2 to 3 days, first in the marrow and then in circulation into the discoid erythrocyte. During reticulocyte maturation, cytoplasmic inclusions including residual mitochondria and ribosomes are degraded and the reticulocyte loses surface area to achieve the mean cell volume and surface area of a discoidal erythrocyte. Mature erythrocytes are approximately 7 to 8 μm in diameter and undergo extensive deformation to pass through 3-μm diameter capillaries and the 1-μm wide and 0.5-μm thick endothelial slits in the red pulp of the spleen. The ability of the red cell to undergo extensive reversible deformation is essential for both its function and its survival. Red cell deformability is a function of its geometry, the viscosity of the cytoplasm, largely determined by the concentration of hemoglobin. Decreased deformability is a feature of red cells in various pathological states. The erythrocyte is unique among eukaryotic cells in that its principal physical structure is its cell membrane, which encloses a concentrated hemoglobin solution. Thus, all of the structural properties of this cell are in one way or another linked to the cell membrane. In contrast to other cells, the erythrocyte has no cytoplasmic structures or organelles. Only, red cells and platelets do not have a nucleus.

Acronyms and Abbreviations: BFU-E, burst-forming unit–erythroid; CFU-E, colony-forming unit–erythroid; cP, centipoise; DIC, disseminated intravascular coagulation; EMP, erythroblast macrophage protein; ICAM-4, intercellular adhesion molecule-4; IL, interleukin; MCH, mean cell hemoglobin content; MCHC, mean corpuscular hemoglobin concentration; MCV, mean cell volume; MDS, myelodysplastic syndrome; SA:V, surface area-to-volume ratio; TTP, thrombotic thrombocytopenic purpura.

*This chapter contains text written for previous editions of this book by Brian Bull, Paul Herrmann, and Ernest Beutler.

● ERYTHRON

The mass of circulating erythrocytes constitutes an organ responsible for the transport of oxygen to tissues and the removal of carbon dioxide from tissues for exhalation. Collectively, the progenitors, precursors, and adult red cells make up an organ termed the *erythron*, which arises from pluripotent hematopoietic stem cells. Following commitment to the erythroid lineage, unipotential progenitors mature into the erythroid progenitors, the burst-forming unit–erythroid (BFU-E) and, subsequently, the colony-forming unit–erythroid (CFU-E), which then undergoes further maturation to generate anucleate polychromatophilic macrocytes (reticulocytes on supravital staining). The BFU-E and CFU-E are identified by their development into morphologically identifiable clonal colonies of red cells *in vitro*. The reticulocyte further matures, first in the marrow for 2 to 3 days and, subsequently, in the circulation for approximately 1 day, to generate discoid erythrocytes.[1-5] The proerythroblast, the first morphologically recognizable erythroid precursor cell in the marrow undergoes four to five mitoses prior to maturation to an orthochromatic erythroblast, which then undergoes nuclear extrusion. A feature of erythropoiesis is that following each cell division the daughter cells advance in their state of maturation as compared to the parent cell and, ultimately, become functional as mature erythrocytes.[4] In this process, they acquire the human blood group antigens, transport proteins, and all components of the erythrocyte membrane.[4,6]

In the adult stage of development, the total number of circulating erythrocytes is in a steady state, unless perturbed by a pathologic or environmental insult. This effect is not so during growth of the individual *in utero*, particularly in the early stages of embryonic development and also during neonatal development as the total blood volume increases markedly. Consequently, erythrocyte production in the embryo and fetus differs markedly from that in the adult.

THE EARLIEST ERYTHRON

In the very early stages of human growth and development, there are two forms of erythroid differentiation: primitive and definitive.[7-10] Chapters 5 and 7 provide detailed descriptions of embryonic and fetal hematopoiesis. The primitive erythron supplies the embryo with oxygen during the phase of rapid growth before the definitive form of maturation has had a chance to develop and seed an appropriate niche. The hallmark of this primitive erythron is the release of nucleated erythroid precursors containing embryonic hemoglobin. Although primitive in the sense that the cells contain nuclei when released into the circulation, this form of maturation differs from avian and reptilian erythropoiesis in that the nucleus is eventually expelled from the mammalian cells as they circulate. The transient presence of a nucleus in the cells of the circulating primitive erythron can decrease the efficiency of gas exchange in the lungs and microvasculature because the nucleus prevents the red cell from behaving as a fluid droplet.[11] The definitive stage of maturation makes its appearance around week 5 of embryogenesis when multipotential stem cells develop and seed the liver which maintains the erythron for most of fetal life. In later fetal life, skeletal development provides marrow niches to which erythropoiesis relocates being sustained in the form of erythroblastic islands, a central macrophage with circumferential layers of developing erythroid cells.[12] The definitive stage of erythroid maturation predominates during the remainder of fetal development and is the only type of erythroid maturation present through childhood and adult life. All of normal human erythropoiesis occurs in the marrow in the form of erythroblastic islands.[13]

ERYTHROID PROGENITORS

Burst-Forming Unit–Erythroid

The earliest identifiable progenitor committed to the erythroid lineage is the BFU-E (see Chap. 32, Fig. 32–1). A BFU-E is defined *in vitro* by its ability to create a "burst" on semisolid medium—that is, a colony consisting of several hundred to thousands of cells by 10 to 14 days of growth, during which time smaller satellite clusters of cells form around a larger central group of erythroid cells, giving rise to the designation of a "burst." The generation of BFU-E from hematopoietic stem cells requires interleukin (IL)-3, stem cell factor, and erythropoietin for differentiation, proliferation, prevention of apoptosis, and maturation (Chap. 18).[5,13]

Colony-Forming Unit–Erythroid

As erythroid maturation progresses, a later progenitor, the CFU-E, derived from the BFU-E, can be defined *in vitro*. The CFU-E is dependent on erythropoietin for its development and can undergo only a few cell divisions.[5,14] Thus, the CFU-E forms a smaller colony of morphologically recognizable erythroid cells in 5 to 7 days (see Chap. 32, Fig. 32–1). Adhesion between erythroid cells and macrophages occurs at the CFU-E stage of maturation.

Using cell-surface markers, IL-3 receptor, CD34, and CD36, highly purified populations of BFU-E and CFU-E can be isolated from human marrow.[5] Gene expression profiling show distinctive changes in gene expression profiles in hematopoietic stem cells, BFU-E, and CFU-E.[5] Some of the marrow failure syndromes are the result of defects in differentiation of stem cells into erythroid progenitors.

ERYTHROBLASTIC ISLAND

The anatomical unit of erythropoiesis in the normal adult is the erythroblastic island or islet.[13,16,17] The erythroblastic island consists of a centrally located macrophages surrounded by maturing terminally differentiating erythroid cells (Fig. 31–1A). A number of binding proteins are implicated in the cell–cell adhesions important to this process. These include $\alpha_4\beta_1$ integrin, erythroblast macrophage protein (EMP), and intercellular adhesion molecule-4 (ICAM-4) on the erythroblasts and vascular cell adhesion molecule (VCAM-1), EMP, α_v integrin on macrophages.[16] Additional macrophage receptors include CD69 (sialoadhesin) and CD163, but the counterreceptors for these on erythroblasts remains to be defined.[16] Phase-contrast microcinematography reveals that the macrophage is far from passive or immobile. Evidence suggests that either the erythroblastic islands migrate or that erythroid precursors move from island to island, as islands near sinusoids are composed of more mature erythroblasts while islands more distant from the sinusoids are composed of proerythroblasts.[18] The macrophage's pseudopodium-like cytoplasmic extensions move rapidly over cell surfaces of the surrounding wreath of erythroblasts. On phase contrast micrographs, the central macrophage of the erythroblastic island appears sponge-like, with surface invaginations in which the erythroblasts lie (Fig. 31–1B). As the erythroblast matures, it moves along a cytoplasmic extension of the macrophage away from the main body. When the erythroblast is sufficiently mature for nuclear expulsion, the erythroblast makes contact with an endothelial cell, passes through a pore in the cytoplasm of the endothelial cell and enters the circulation as a polychromatophilic macrocyte (reticulocyte).[19–21] The nucleus is ejected prior to egress from the marrow, phagocytized, and degraded by marrow macrophages.[22] In addition to the unique cytologic features described above, the macrophage of the erythroblastic island is also molecularly distinct as demonstrated by a unique immunophenotypic signature.[23] In addition, the macrophage of the erythroblastic island appears to play a stimulatory role in erythropoiesis independent of erythropoietin. The anemia of chronic inflammation and of the myelodysplastic syndrome (MDS) may result, at least in part, from inadequate stimulation of erythropoiesis by these macrophages (Chap. 5).

Despite the central role of erythroid islands in erythropoiesis *in vivo*, morphologically normal development of erythroid cells can be recapitulated *in vitro* without these structures as long as developing cells are provided with supraphysiologic concentrations of appropriate cytokines and growth factors. Such growth, however, occurs at a much slower rate than that observed *in vivo*, when erythroblasts form erythroblastic islands.[24] The erythroblastic island is a fragile structure. It is usually disrupted in the process of obtaining a marrow specimen by needle aspiration but can be seem in marrow biopsies.

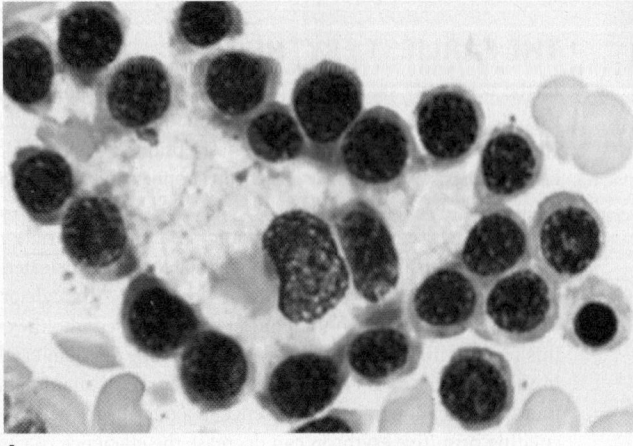
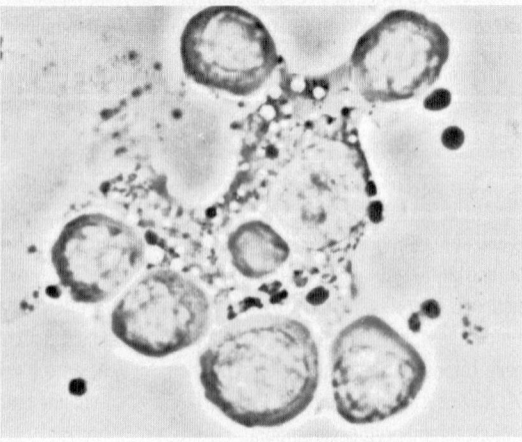

A **B**

Figure 31–1. Erythroblastic island. **A.** Erythroblastic island as seen in Wright-Giemsa–stained marrow. Note central macrophage surrounded by a cohort of attached erythroblasts. **B.** Erythroblastic island in the living state examined by phase-contrast microscopy. The macrophage shows dynamic movement in relation to its surrounding erythroblasts. (*A, reproduced with permission from* Lichtman's Atlas of Hematology, *www.accessmedicine.com.*)

Macrophages in erythroblastic islands not only affect erythroid differentiation and/or proliferation, but also perform other functions, including rapid phagocytosis (<10 min) of extruded nuclei as a result of exposure of phosphatidylserine on the surface of the membrane surrounding the nucleus.[22] This phagocytosis is the reason for the inability to find extruded nuclei in marrow aspirates in spite of the fact that 2 million nuclei are extruded every second during steady-state erythropoiesis. A protective macrophage function linked to efficient phagocytosis has been described. In normal mice, DNase II in macrophages degrades the ingested nuclear DNA but in DNase II knockout mice the inability to degrade DNA results in macrophage toxicity with resultant decrease in number of marrow macrophages and in conjunction with severe anemia.[25] Macrophages can play both positive and negative regulatory roles in human erythropoiesis but the mechanistic basis for these regulatory processes are not completely understood.[16,24] These processes may play a role in the ineffective erythropoiesis in disorders such as MDS, thalassemia, and malarial anemia.

Another potentially important role originally proposed for the central macrophage is direct transfer of iron to developing erythroblasts mediated by ferritin exchange between macrophages and erythroblasts (Chap. 42).[13] Although this is an interesting concept, there is no definitive evidence for this exchange.

ERYTHROID PROGENITORS AND PRECURSORS

Early Progenitors

A "progenitor" in the hematopoietic system is defined as a marrow cell that is a derivative of the pluripotent hematopoietic stem cell through the process of differentiation and is antecedent to a "precursor" cell, the latter being identifiable by light microscopy by its morphologic characteristics (see Chap. 83, Fig. 83–2). In erythropoiesis, the earliest precursor is the proerythroblast. Erythroid progenitor cells are identified as marrow cells capable of forming erythroid colonies in semisolid medium in vitro under conditions in which the appropriate growth factors are present. Progenitor cells also may be identified by characteristic profiles of surface CD antigens using flow cytometry. Numerically, erythroid progenitors, BFU-E and CFU-E represent only a minute proportion of human marrow cells. BFU-E range from 300 to 1700×10^6 mononuclear cells and CFU-E range from 1500 to 5000×10^6 mononuclear cells.[5] In vitro cultures using CD34+ cells from blood, cord blood, and marrow as the starting material have identified the critical cytokines required for erythroid differentiation and maturation and enabled the identification and isolation of pure cohorts of erythroid progenitors and erythroblasts at all stages of terminal erythroid maturation.[4,5]

Precursors

Figure 31–2 shows the sequence of precursors as seen in marrow films. Figure 31–3 shows the marrow precursors as isolated by flow cytometry.

Proerythroblasts On stained films, the proerythroblast appears as a large cell, irregularly rounded or slightly oval.[13] The nucleus occupies approximately 80 percent of the cell area and contains fine chromatin delicately distributed in small clumps. One or several well-defined nucleoli are present. The high concentration of polyribosomes gives the cytoplasm of these cells its characteristic intense basophilia. At very high magnification, ferritin molecules are seen dispersed singly throughout the cytoplasm and lining the clathrin-coated pits on the cell

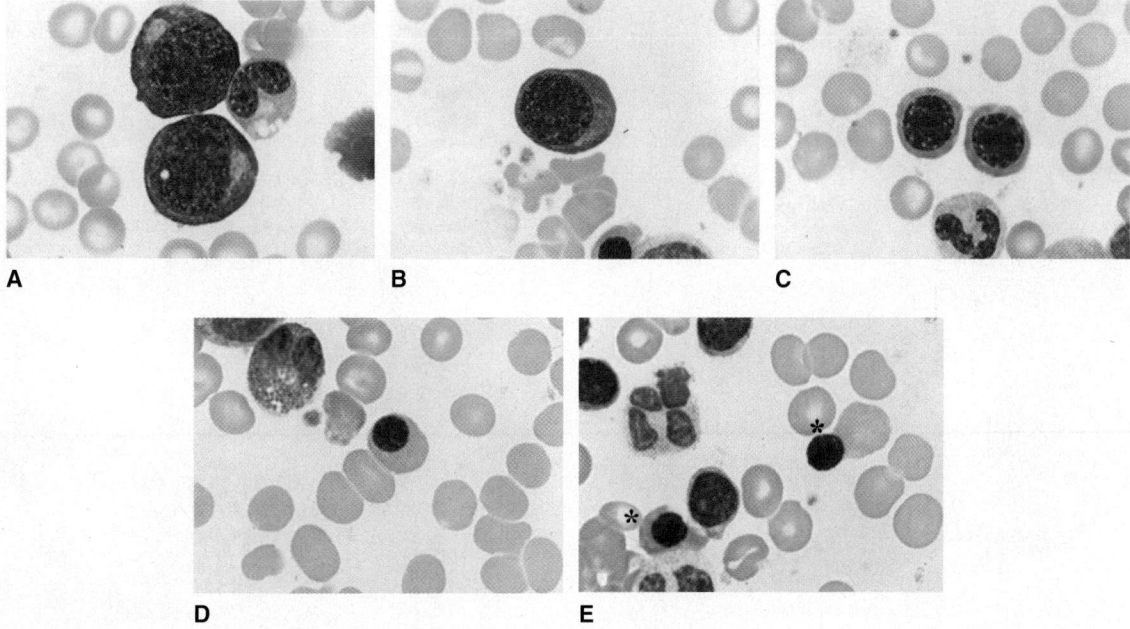

Figure 31–2. Human erythrocyte precursors. Light microscopic appearance. Marrow films stained with Wright stain. There are five stages of erythroblast development recognizable by light microscopy. **A.** Proerythroblasts. Two are present in this field. They are the largest red cell precursor, with a fine nuclear chromatin pattern, nucleoli, basophilic cytoplasm, and often a clear area at the site of the Golgi apparatus. **B.** Basophilic erythroblast. The cell is smaller than the proerythroblast, the nuclear chromatin is slightly more condensed and cytoplasm is basophilic. **C.** Polychromatophilic erythroblasts. The cell is smaller on average than its precursors. The nuclear chromatin is more condensed with a checkerboard pattern developing. Nucleoli are not apparent, usually. The cytoplasm is gray, reflecting the staining modulation induced by hemoglobin synthesis, which adds cytoplasmic content that takes an eosinophilic stain, admixed with the residual basophilia of the fading protein synthetic apparatus. **D.** Orthochromic normoblast. Smaller on average than its precursor, increased condensation of nuclear chromatin, with homogeneous cytoplasmic coloration approaching that of a red cell. **E.** Late orthochromatic erythroblasts (asterisks). The orthochromatic erythroblast to the right is undergoing apparent enucleation. The other three mononuclear cells are lymphocytes. A degenerating four-lobed neutrophil is also present. (Reproduced with permission from Lichtman's Atlas of Hematology, www.accessmedicine.com.)

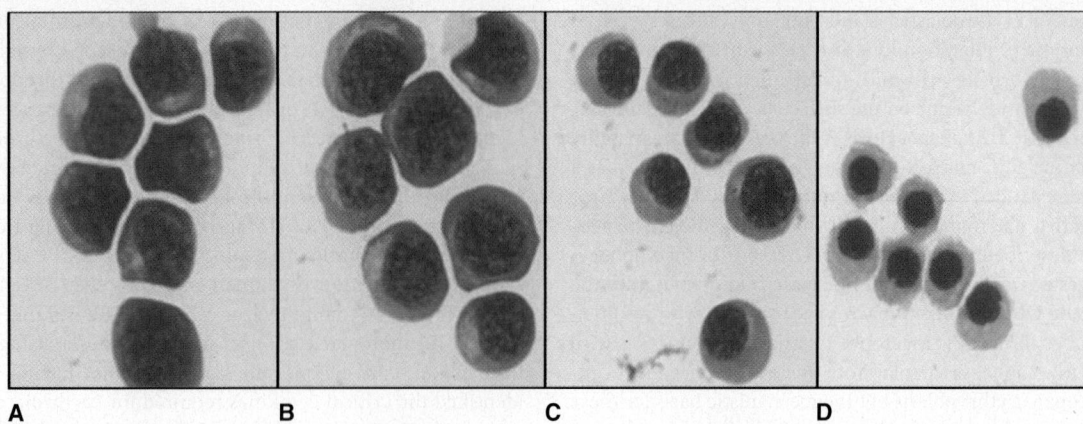

Figure 31–3. Human erythroblast precursors as isolated by cell flow cytometry. Images of populations of human erythroblast precursors at stages of erythroid maturation when sorted from human marrow by flow cytometry. **A** and **B.** Proerythroblasts and early basophilic erythroblasts; **(C)** polychromatic erythroblasts; and **(D)** orthochromatic erythroblasts.

membrane (see Figs. 31–2 and 31–4) Diffuse cytoplasmic density on sections stained for peroxidase indicates hemoglobin is already present. Dispersed glycogen particles are present in the cytoplasm.

Basophilic Erythroblasts Basophilic erythroblasts are smaller than proerythroblasts. The nucleus occupies three-fourths of the cell area and is composed of characteristic dark violet heterochromatin interspersed with pink-staining clumps of euchromatin linked by irregular strands.[13] The whole arrangement often resembles wheel

spokes or a clock face. The cytoplasm stains deep blue, leaving a perinuclear halo that expands into a juxtanuclear clear zone around the Golgi apparatus. Cytoplasmic basophilia at this stage results from the continued presence of polyribosomes (see Figs. 31–2 and 31–5).

Polychromatophilic Erythroblasts Following the mitotic division of the basophilic erythroblast, the cytoplasm changes from deep blue to gray, as hemoglobin dilutes the polyribosome content. Cells at this stage are smaller than basophilic erythroblasts. The nucleus occupies less than half of the cell area. The heterochromatin is located in well-defined clumps spaced regularly about the nucleus, producing a

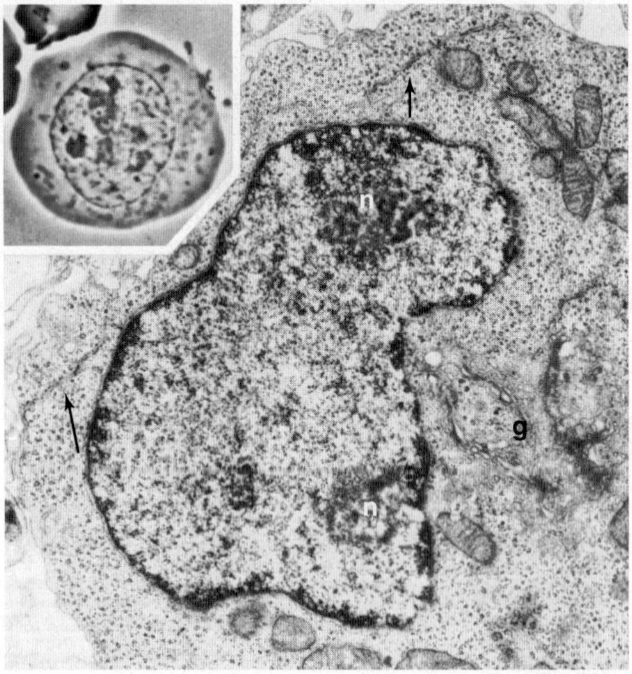

Figure 31–4. Proerythroblast. Phase-contrast micrograph *(inset)* of a proerythroblast showing the immature nucleus with nucleoli and finely dispersed nuclear chromatin. The centrosome (juxtanuclear clear zone) is apparent with its dense accumulation of mitochondria. Electron microscopic section of the proerythroblast shows nucleoli *(n)* in contact with the nuclear membrane. Chromatin is finely dispersed and forms small aggregates in the fixed nuclear membrane. The perinuclear canal is narrow but well defined. Polyribosome groups, many in helical configuration, are dispersed throughout the cytoplasm. The Golgi apparatus *(g)* is well developed, and regions of endoplasmic reticulum *(arrows)* are seen.

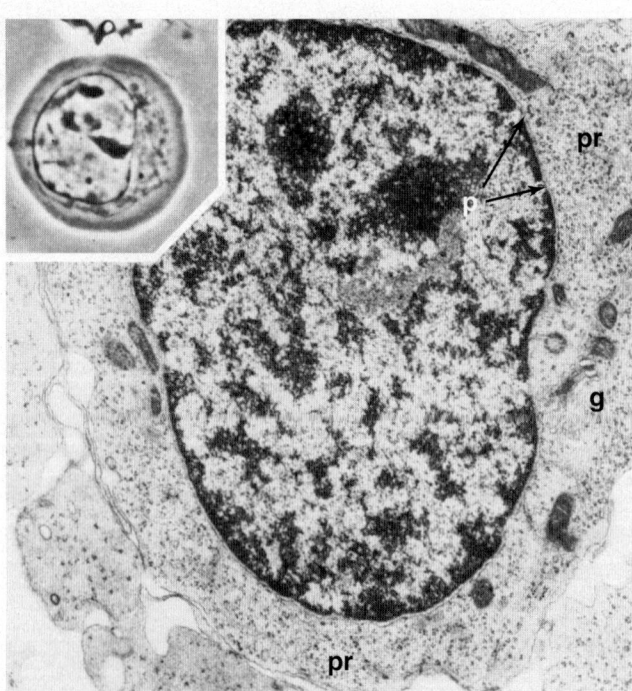

Figure 31–5. Basophilic erythroblast. Phase-contrast photomicrograph *(inset)* shows increased clumping of the nuclear chromatin and further rounding of the cell, with aggregation of the mitochondria and centrosome into the regions of nuclear indentation. Electron microscopic section shows clumping of the nuclear chromatin, nuclear pores *(p)*, organization of the nucleoli, increased density of polyribosomes *(pr)*, well-developed Golgi apparatus *(g)*, and a decrease in smooth endoplasmic reticulum.

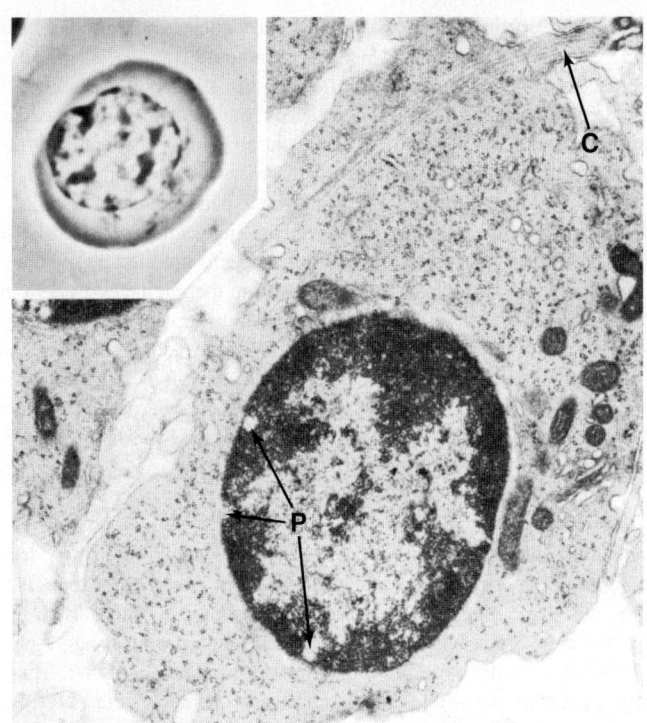

Figure 31–6. Polychromatophilic erythroblast. Phase-contrast micrograph *(inset)* demonstrates diminished size of this cell compared with its precursor. Further clumping of nuclear chromatin gives the nucleus a checkerboard appearance. The centrosome is condensed, and a perinuclear halo has developed. Electron microscopic section demonstrates relative reduction of the density of polyribosomes and dilution by the moderately osmiophilic hemoglobin in the cytoplasm. Nuclear chromatin shows a marked increase in clumping, and nuclear pores *(P)* are enlarged.

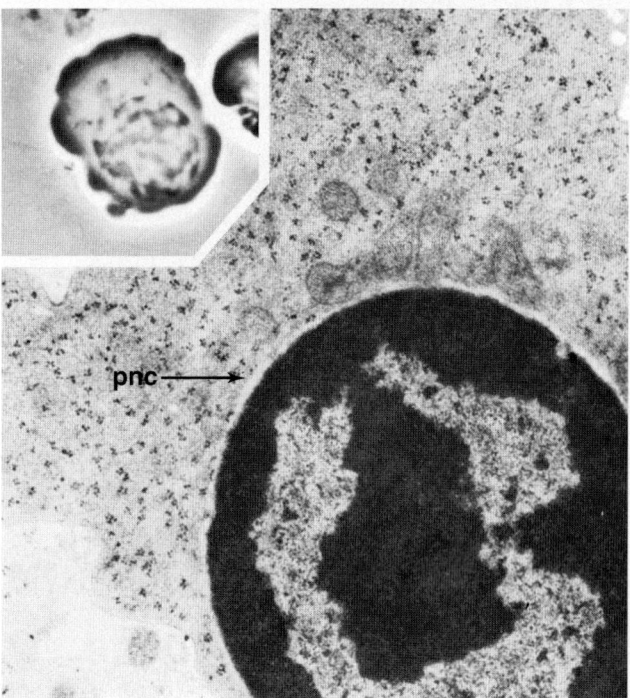

Figure 31–7. Orthochromic erythroblast. Phase-contrast appearance of this cell in the living state *(inset)* shows the irregular borders indicative of its characteristic motility, the eccentric nucleus making contact with the plasmalemma, further pyknosis of the nuclear chromatin, and condensation of the centrosome. Electron microscopic section shows further dilution of polyribosomes, some of which appear to be disintegrating into monoribosomes, by the increasing hemoglobin. The number of mitochondria is decreased, and some mitochondria are degenerating. Nuclear chromatin is clumped into large masses, and a perinuclear canal *(pnc)* is seen.

checkerboard pattern. The nucleolus is lost, but the perinuclear halo persists.[13] It is at this point that erythroblasts lose their mitotic potential. Electron microscopy of the polychromatophilic erythroblast reveals increased aggregation of nuclear heterochromatin.[13] Active ferritin transport across the cell membrane is always evident, and siderosomes along with dispersed ferritin molecules can be identified within the cytoplasm (see Figs. 31–2 and 31–6).

Orthochromic (syn. Orthochromatic) Erythroblasts After the final mitotic division of the erythropoietic series, the concentration of hemoglobin increases within the erythroblast. Under the light microscope, the nucleus appears almost completely dense and featureless. It is measurably decreased in size. This cell is the smallest of the erythroblastic series.[13] The nucleus occupies approximately one-fourth of the cell area and is eccentric. Cell movement can be appreciated under the phase-contrast microscope. Round projections appear suddenly in different parts of the cell periphery and are just as quickly retracted.[13] The movements probably are made in preparation for ejection of the nucleus. The cell ultrastructure is characterized by irregular borders, reflecting its motile state. The heterochromatin forms large masses. Mitochondria are reduced in number and size (see Figs. 31–2, 31–7, and 31–8).

Normal Sideroblasts All normal erythroblasts are sideroblasts in that they contain iron in structures called *siderosomes*, as evident by transmission electron microscopy. These structures are essential for the transfer of iron for heme (hemoglobin) synthesis. By light microscopy, under the usual conditions of Prussian blue staining for iron, a minority of normal erythroblasts (approximately 15 to 20 percent) can be

identified as containing siderosomes and those that can be so identified have very few (one to four) small Prussian blue–positive granules.

Pathologic Sideroblasts A heterogeneous group of erythrocyte disorders is accompanied by ineffective erythropoiesis, abnormal erythroblast morphology and hyperferremia. These disorders include acquired megaloblastic anemia (Chap. 41), congenital dyserythropoietic anemias (Chap. 39), thalassemias (Chap. 48), the inherited and acquired sideroblastic anemias, pyridoxine-responsive anemia, alcohol-induced sideroblastic anemia, and lead intoxication (Chaps. 52 and 59). Some of these conditions are characterized by the presence of pathologic sideroblasts. Pathologic sideroblasts are of two types. One type is an erythroblast that has an increase in number and size of Prussian blue–stained siderotic granules throughout the cytoplasm. Another type is the erythroblast that shows iron-containing granules that are arranged in an arc or a complete ring around the nucleus (Fig. 31–8). These pathologic sideroblasts are referred to as *ring* or *ringed sideroblasts*.[26,27] Electron microscopic studies show that granules in ringed sideroblasts are iron-loaded mitochondria. In cells with iron-loaded mitochondria, many ferritin molecules are deposited between adjacent erythroblast membranes.

RETICULOCYTE

Birth

Prior to enucleation at the late orthochromatic erythroblasts stage, intermediate filaments and the marginal band of microtubules disappear. Enucleation is a highly dynamic process that involves coordinated

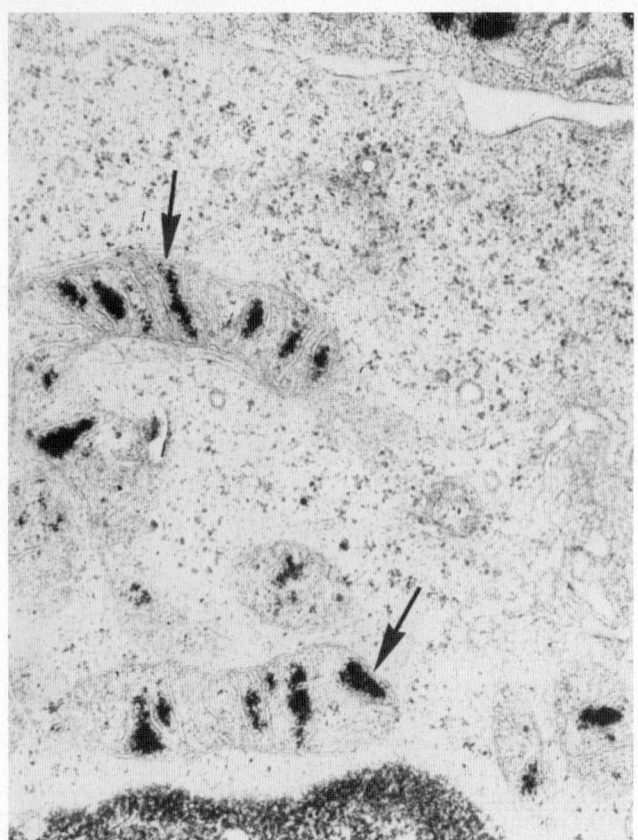

Figure 31–8. Pathologic sideroblast is an erythroblast characterized by the presence of mitochondrial deposits of iron-containing ferruginous micelles *(arrows)* between the cristae.

action of multiple mechanisms.[28–30] Tubulin and actin become concentrated at the point where the nucleus will exit. These changes, accompanied by microtubular rearrangements and actin polymerization, play a role in nuclear expulsion. Expulsion of the nucleus *in vitro* is not an instantaneous phenomenon; it requires a period of 6 to 8 minutes. The process begins with several vigorous contractions around the midportion of the cell, followed by a division of the cell into unequal portions.

The smaller portion consists of the expelled nucleus surrounded by a thin ring of hemoglobin and plasma membrane (Fig. 31–9). *In vivo*, expulsion of the nucleus may occur while the erythroblast is still part of an erythroblastic island or the nucleus may be lost during passage through the wall of a marrow sinus as the nucleus, which cannot traverse the small opening, remains in the marrow. The outer leaflet of the bilaminar membrane surrounding the expelled nucleus is high in phosphatidylserine, a signal for macrophage ingestion (Fig. 31–10).[22] It is not clear what fraction of the expelled nuclei is ingested by the macrophage of the erythroblastic island or by other macrophages resident in marrow. Two hypotheses have been proposed to explain how the reticulocyte exits the marrow.[19–21] The reticulocyte may actively traverse the sinus epithelium to enter the lumen. More likely, however, the reticulocyte may be driven across by a pressure differential because it appears incapable of directed amoeboid motion. The precise mechanism is yet to be defined.

Maturation

Following nuclear extrusion, the reticulocyte retains mitochondria, small numbers of ribosomes, the centriole, and remnants of the Golgi apparatus. It contains no endoplasmic reticulum. Supravital staining with brilliant cresyl blue or new methylene blue produces aggregates of ribosomes, mitochondria, and other cytoplasmic organelles. These aggregates stain deep blue and, arranged in reticular strands, give the reticulocyte its name. Maturation of the reticulocyte requires 48 to 72 hours. During this period, approximately 20 percent of the membrane surface area is lost and cell volume decreases by 10 to 15 percent and the final assembly of the membrane skeleton is completed.[31–33] Living reticulocytes observed by phase-contrast microscopy are irregularly shaped cells with a characteristically puckered exterior and a motile membrane. Examined by electron microscopy, reticulocytes are irregularly shaped and contain many remnant organelles.[13] The organelles, small smooth vesicles, and an occasional centriole are grouped in the region of the cell where the nucleus is expelled. In "young" reticulocytes, the vast majority of ribosomes dispersed throughout the cytoplasm are in the form of polyribosomes. As protein synthesis diminishes during maturation, the polyribosomes gradually transform into monoribosomes. During reticulocyte maturation there is significant remodeling of the membrane, including loss of membrane proteins that include transferrin receptors, Na-K adenosine triphosphatase (ATPase), and adhesion molecules, as well as loss of tubulin and cytoplasmic actin.[33] During the remodeling

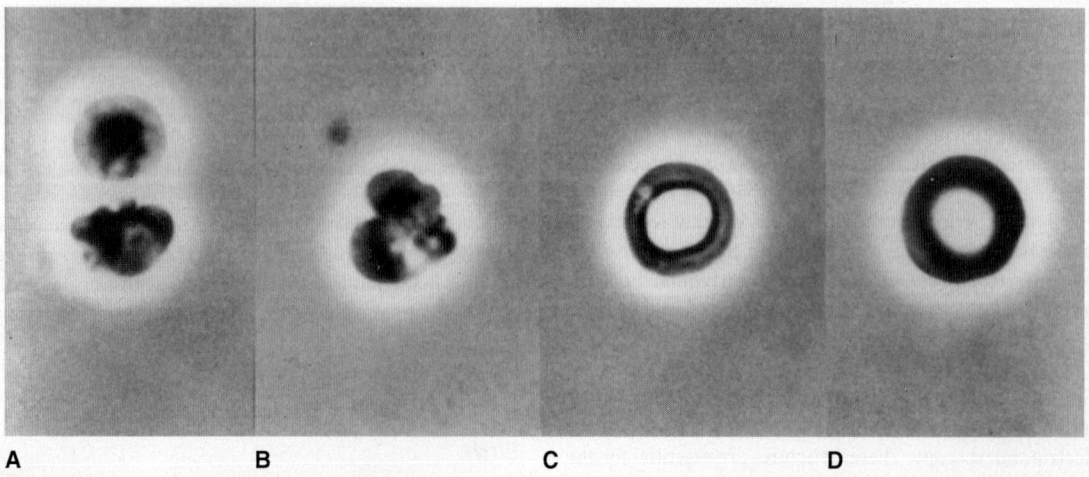

A   B   C   D

Figure 31–9. Morphology of cells during reticulocyte maturation. **A.** Orthochromatic erythroblast extruding its nucleus. **B.** Multilobular, motile reticulocyte generated following nuclear extrusion. **C.** The cup-shaped, nonmotile reticulocyte at a later stage of maturation. **D.** Mature discoid red cell.

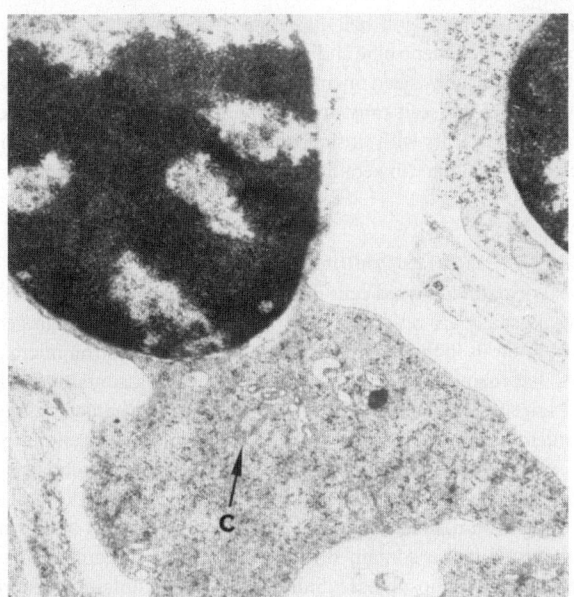

Figure 31–10. Orthochromic erythroblast ejecting its nucleus. A thin rim of cytoplasm surrounds the nucleus. In the cytoplasm, a single centriole *(c)* is partially encircled by some Golgi saccules.

process the membrane becomes more elastic and acquires increased membrane mechanical stability.[32]

Macroreticulocytes

"Stress" reticulocytes are released into the circulation during an intense erythropoietin response to acute anemia or experimentally in response to large doses of exogenously administered erythropoietin.[34] These cells

may be twice the normal volume, with a corresponding increase in mean cell hemoglobin (MCH) content. Whether the increase results from one less mitotic division during maturation or from some other process such as changes in cell cycle is not clear. It is interesting to note that mice do not have the ability to produce stress reticulocytes with increased mean cell volume (MCV) and MCH. In contrast, even under moderate erythropoietic stress, some reticulocytes in the marrow pool shift to the circulating pool. These "shift" reticulocytes with normal MCH contain a higher-than-normal RNA content and now can be quantified. Quantification is commonly performed by applying a fluorescent stain to tag RNA and then dividing reticulocytes into high-, medium-, and low-fluorescence categories using a fluorescence-sensitive flow cytometer. The "stress" reticulocytes of the older literature likely fall in the high- and medium-fluorescence categories. Unfortunately, at present little attention is being paid to discriminate stress and shift reticulocytes.

Pathology of the Reticulocyte

The reticulocyte may show pathologic alterations in size or staining properties. The reticulocyte may contain inclusions visible by light microscopy or identifiable only on ultrastructural analysis. Most pathologic inclusions usually attributed to erythrocytes are actually found within reticulocytes and are nuclear or cytoplasmic remnants derived from late-stage erythroblasts. In splenectomized patients, they may also be found in mature erythrocytes.

RED CELL INCLUSIONS

See Fig. 31–11 for images of red cell inclusions.

Howell-Jolly Bodies

Howell-Jolly bodies are small nuclear remnants that have the color of a pyknotic nucleus on Wright-stained films and give a positive Feulgen reaction for DNA.[35,36] They are spherically shaped, randomly distributed

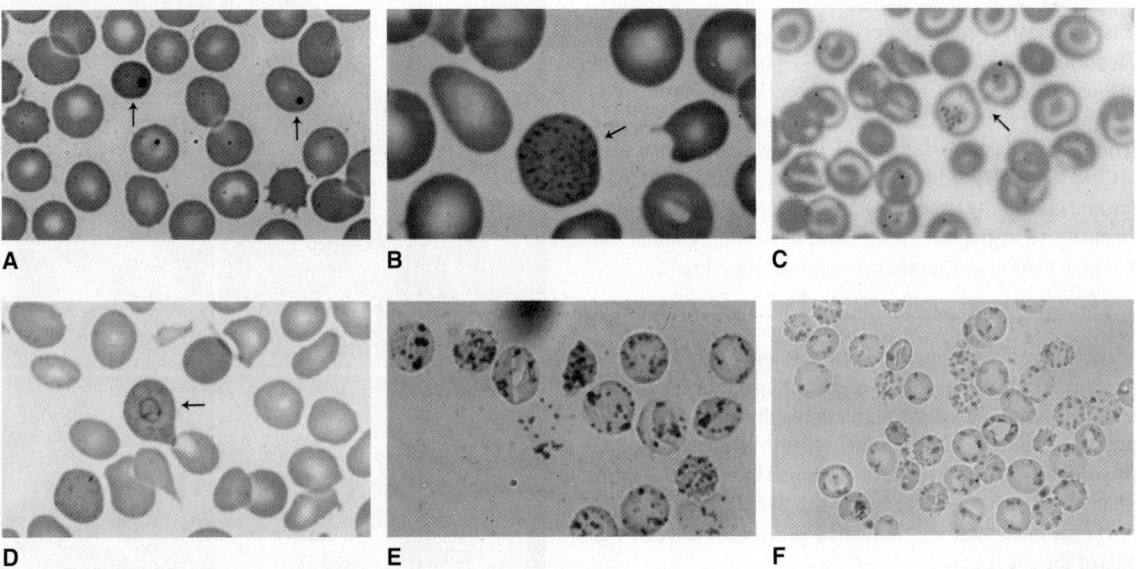

Figure 31–11. Red cell inclusions. Blood films. **A.** Red cells with Howell-Jolly bodies *(arrows)* postsplenectomy. The crisp circular border, dark blue color, and peripheral location are characteristic. **B.** Basophilic stippling. These basophilic inclusions may be fine or coarse. In this case, the cell contains coarse stippling seen in lead poisoning *(arrow)*. **C.** Siderocyte. These cells contain purple granules when stained with Wright stain (Pappenheimer bodies). Compared to basophilic stippling, siderotic granules are usually fewer in number and sometimes clustered. These Prussian blue–stained cells confirm that the granules contain iron (blue reaction product). *Arrow* points to two siderocytes. **D.** Cabot ring. Rare red cell inclusion *(arrow)*. See text for further description. **E.** Heinz bodies. These cells from a patient with glucose-6-phosphate dehydrogenase deficiency were incubated with a supravital dye, which stains the denatured globin precipitates. **F.** Red cells from a patient with hemoglobin H disease (*a*-thalassemia). The hemoglobin precipitates are stained with brilliant cresyl blue. *(Reproduced with permission from Lichtman's Atlas of Hematology, www.accessmedicine.com.)*

in the red cell and usually no larger than 0.5 μm in diameter. Howell-Jolly bodies may be numerous, although generally only one is present. In pathologic situations, they appear to represent chromosomes that have separated from the mitotic spindle during abnormal mitosis, and contain a high proportion of centromeric material along with heterochromatin. More commonly, during normal maturation they arise from nuclear fragmentation or incomplete expulsion of the nucleus. Howell-Jolly bodies are pitted from the reticulocytes during their transit through the interendothelial slits of the splenic sinus. They are characteristically present in the blood of splenectomized persons and in patients suffering from megaloblastic anemia, and hyposplenic states.

Pocked (or Pitted) Red Cells

When viewed by interference-phase microscopy, pocked red cells appear to have surface membrane "pits" or craters.[37–39] The vesicles or indentations characterizing these cells represent autophagic vacuoles adjacent to the cell membrane. The vacuoles appear to be instrumental in disposal of cellular debris as the erythrocyte passes through the microcirculation of the spleen. Within 1 week following splenectomy, pocked red cell counts begin to rise, reaching a plateau at 2 to 3 months. Pocked red blood cell counts sometimes are used as a surrogate test for splenic function.

Cabot Rings

The ring-like or figure-of-eight structures sometimes seen in megaloblastic anemia within reticulocytes and in an occasional, heavily stippled, late-intermediate megaloblast are designated *Cabot rings*.[40,41] Their composition is nuclear. Some investigators have suggested that Cabot rings originate from spindle material that was mishandled during abnormal mitosis. Others have found no indication of DNA or spindle filaments but have shown the rings are associated with adherent granular material containing arginine-rich histone and nonhemoglobin iron.

Basophilic Stippling

Basophilic stippling consists of granulations of variable size and number that stain deep blue with Wright stain. Electron microscopic studies have shown that *punctate basophilia* represents aggregated ribosomes.[42] Clumps form during the course of drying and postvital staining of the cells, much as "reticulum" in reticulocytes precipitates from ribosomes during supravital staining. The clumped ribosomes may include degenerating mitochondria and siderosomes. In conditions such as lead intoxication (Chap. 52), pyrimidine 5′-nucleotidase deficiency (Chap. 47), and thalassemia (Chap. 48), the altered reticulocyte ribosomes have a greater propensity to aggregate. As a result, basophilic granulation appears larger and is referred to as coarse basophilic stippling.

Heinz Bodies

Heinz bodies are composed of denatured proteins, primarily hemoglobin, that form in red cells as a result of chemical insult; in hereditary defects of the hexose monophosphate shunt; in the thalassemias (Chap. 48); and in unstable hemoglobin syndromes (Chap. 49).[43] Heinz bodies are not seen on ordinary Wright- or Giemsa-stained blood films. Heinz bodies are readily visible in red cells stained supravitally with brilliant cresyl blue or crystal violet and are eliminated as red cells traverse the endothelial slits of the splenic sinus.

Hemoglobin H Inclusions

Hemoglobin H is composed of β_4 tetramers, indicating that β chains are present in excess as a result of impaired α-chain production (Chap. 48). Exposure to redox dyes such as brilliant cresyl blue, methylene blue, or new methylene blue, results in denaturation and precipitation of abnormal hemoglobin.[44–46] Brilliant cresyl blue causes the formation of a large number of small membrane-bound inclusions, giving the

cell a characteristic "golf ball–like" appearance when viewed by light microscopy. Methylene blue and new methylene blue generate a smaller number of variably sized membrane-bound and floating inclusions. These changes are seen most frequently in α-thalassemia but also can be found in patients with unstable hemoglobin (Chap. 49) and in rare patients with primary myelofibrosis who develop acquired hemoglobin H disease.

Siderosomes and Pappenheimer Bodies

Normal or pathologic red cells in blood containing siderosomes ("iron bodies") usually are reticulocytes. The iron granulations are larger and more numerous in the pathologic state (Chap. 59). Electron microscopy shows that many of these bodies are mitochondria containing ferruginous micelles rather than the ferritin aggregates characterizing normal siderocytes.[47] Siderosomes usually are found in the cell periphery, whereas basophilic stippling tends to be distributed homogeneously throughout the cell. Pappenheimer bodies are siderosomes that stain with Wright stain. Electron microscopy of Pappenheimer bodies shows that the iron often is contained within a lysosome, as confirmed by the presence of acid phosphatase. Siderosomes may contain degenerating mitochondria, ribosomes, and other cellular remnants.

STRUCTURE AND SHAPE OF ERYTHROCYTES

The normal resting shape of the erythrocyte is a biconcave disc (Fig. 31–12). Variations in the shape and dimensions of the red cell are useful

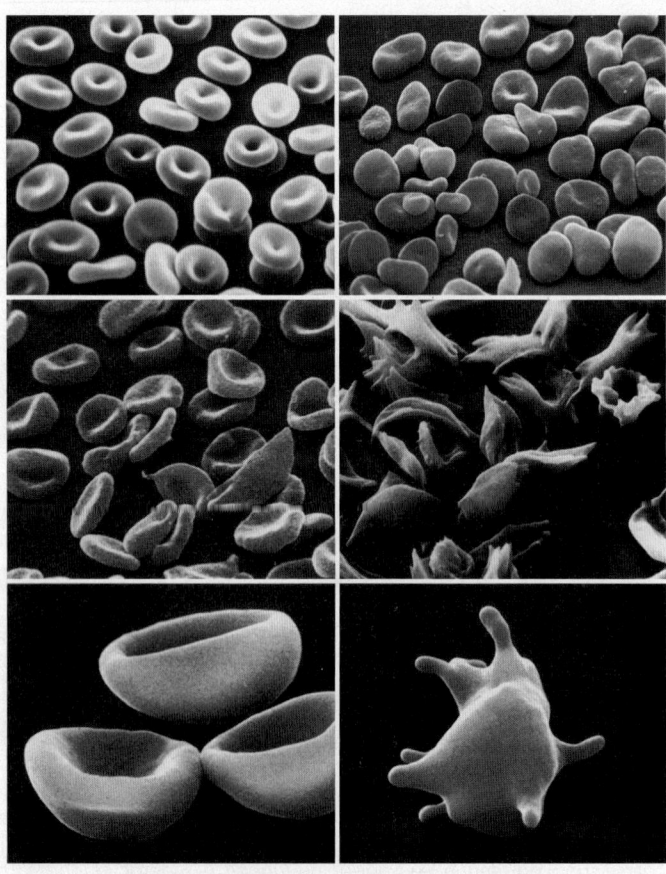

Figure 31–12. Scanning electron micrographs of distinct red cell morphologies. Discoid normal red cells *(top left panel)*. Elliptocytes and fragmented red cells *(top right panel)*. Oxygenated sickle red cells *(middle left panel)* and deoxygenated sickle red cells *(middle right panel)*. Stomatocytic red cells *(bottom left panel)*. Acanthocyte *(bottom right panel)*.

in the differential diagnosis of anemias. Normal human red cells have a diameter of 7 to 8 μm, and the diameter decreases slightly with cell age. The size decrease likely results from loss of membrane surface area during erythrocyte life span by spleen-facilitated vesiculation. The cells have an average volume of approximately 90 fL and a surface area of approximately 140 μm.[2] The membrane is present in sufficient excess to allow the cell to swell to a sphere of approximately 150 fL or to deform so as to enter a capillary with a diameter of 2.8 μm. The normal erythrocyte stains reddish-brown with Wright-stained blood films and pink with Giemsa stain. The central third of the cell appears relatively pale compared with the periphery, reflecting its biconcave shape. Many artifacts can be produced in the preparation of the blood film. They may result from contamination of the glass slide or coverslip with traces of fat, detergent, or other impurities. Friction and surface tension involved in the preparation of the blood film produce fragmentation, "doughnut cells" or anulocytes, and crescent-shaped cells. Observed under the phase-contrast or interference microscope, the red cell shows a characteristic internal scintillation known as red cell flicker.[48] The scintillation results from thermally excited undulations of the red cell membrane. Frequency analysis of the surface undulations has provided an estimate of the membrane curvature elastic constant and of changes in this constant resulting from alcohol, cholesterol loading, and exposure to cross-linking agents.

RED CELL SHAPE AND SURVIVAL IN CIRCULATION

The red cell spends most of its circulatory life within the capillary channels of the microcirculation. During its 100- to 120-day life span, the red cell travels approximately 250 km and loses approximately 15 to 20 percent of its cell surface area. The long survival of the red cell is at least partially a result of the unique capacity of its membrane to "tank tread"—that is, to rotate around the red cell contents and thereby facilitate more efficient oxygen delivery. The physical arrangement of membrane skeletal proteins in a uniform shell of highly folded hexagonal spectrin lattice permits this unusual behavior.[49-51] The arrangement also is responsible for the characteristic biconcave shape of the resting cell. Red cells must also be able to withstand large shear forces and must be able to undergo extensive reversible deformation during transit through the microvasculature and in transiting from the splenic red cell pulp back into circulation. The resiliency and fluidity of the membrane to deformation is regulated by the spectrin-based membrane skeleton.[49] A deficiency in the amount of spectrin or the presence of mutant spectrin in the submembrane skeleton results in abnormally shaped cells in hereditary spherocytosis, elliptocytosis, and pyropoikilocytosis (Chap. 46).[49] In regions of circulatory standstill or very slow flow, red cells travel in aggregates of two to 12 cells, forming rouleaux. Within large vessels, increased shear forces disrupt this aggregation.

RED CELL COMPOSITION

The erythrocyte is a complex cell. The membrane is composed of lipids and proteins, and the interior of the cell contains metabolic machinery designed to sustain the cell through its 120-day life span and maintain the integrity of hemoglobin function. Each component of red blood cells may be expressed as a function of red cell volume, grams of hemoglobin, or square centimeters of cell surface. These expressions are usually interchangeable, but under certain circumstances each may have specific advantages. However, because disease may produce changes in the average red cell size, hemoglobin content, or surface area, the use of any of these measurements individually may, at times, be misleading. For convenience and uniformity, data in the accompanying tables (Tables 31–1 through 31–6) are expressed in terms of cell constituent per milliliter of red cell and per gram of hemoglobin. In many instances, this

process required recalculation of published data. These recalculations assume a hematocrit value of 45 percent and 33 g of hemoglobin per deciliter of red cells. To obtain concentration per gram of hemoglobin, the concentration per milliliter red blood cell can be multiplied by 3.03. The tables list only some of the most commonly referred to constituents of the erythrocyte. The reference on which each value is based is the first number presented in the last column of each table. Where applicable, additional confirmatory references are given. In some instances, only the percentage of the total of the type of constituent present is given. Chapter 46 discusses the detailed protein composition of the red cell membrane and its various protein constituents.

ERYTHROCYTE DEFORMABILITY

During its 120-day life span, the erythrocyte must undergo extensive passive deformation and must be mechanically stable to resist fragmentation and cellular deformability is an important determinant of red cell survival in the circulation. Red cell deformability is influenced by three

TABLE 31–1. Human Erythrocyte Protein and Water Content

Component	mg/mL RBC	Reference(s)
Water	721 ± 17.3	71
Total protein	371	71
Nonhemoglobin protein	9.2	71, 72
Insoluble stroma protein	6.3	72
Enzyme proteins	2.9	72
Extensive study by proteomic methods		73, 74

TABLE 31–2. Human Erythrocyte Phospholipids

Lipid	Amount	Reference
Total phospholipids	2.98 ± 0.20 mg/mL RBC	75
Cephalin	1.17 (0.38–1.91) mg/mL RBC	75
Ethanolamine	29% of total phospholipid	75
	67% of ethanolamine phosphoglyceride	75
Serine phosphoglyceride	10% of total phospholipid	75
Mean plasmalogen content	8% of serine phosphoglyceride	75
Lecithin	0.32 (0.03–0.95) mg/mL	76
Sphingomyelin	0.12–1.13 mg/mL	76
Lysolecithin	1.82% of total phospholipids	77

NOTE: Some results are given as mean ± standard deviation.
RBC, red blood cell.

TABLE 31-3. Human Erythrocyte Coenzyme and Vitamins

Compound	µmol/mL RBC	Reference
Ascorbic acid	0.02892 ± 0.00431	78
Choline free	Trace	79
Cocarboxylase	0.00021	80
Coenzyme A	0.0027	81
Nicotinic acid	0.105	82
Pantothenic acid	0.001 ± 0.00028	83
Pyridoxal phosphate	$20 \infty 10^{-6} \pm 2 \infty 10^{-6}$	84
Pyridoxal	$11 \infty 10^{-6} \pm 3 \infty 10^{-6}$	84
Total vitamin B$_6$ aldehydes	$30 \infty 10^{-6} \pm 8 \infty 10^{-6}$	84
Pyridoxamine phosphate	$8 \infty 10^{-6} \pm 8 \infty 10^{-6}$	84
4-Pyridoxic acid	$4 \infty 10^{-6} \pm 4 \infty 10^{-6}$	84
Riboflavin	0.00059 ± 0.00021	85
Flavin adenine dinucleotide	0.000398 ± 0.000042	86
Thiamine	0.00027	87

NOTE: Some results are given as mean ± standard deviation.
RBC, red blood cell.

TABLE 31-4. Nucleotides

Compound	µmol/mL RBC	Reference(s)
Adenosine monophosphate	0.021 ± 0.003	88–91
Adenosine diphosphate	0.216 ± 0.036	88–91
Adenosine triphosphate	1.35 ± 0.035	90–94
Cyclic adenosine monophosphate	0.015 ± 0.0024	95
Cyclic guanosine monophosphate	0.013 ± 0.0042	95
Guanosine diphosphate	0.018 ± 0.005	90
Guanosine triphosphate	0.052 ± 0.012	89, 90
Inosine monophosphate	0.031 ± 0.005	90–92
Nicotinamide adenine dinucleotide		96, 97
Reduced	0.0018 ± 0.001	96, 97
Oxidized	0.049 ± 0.006	
Nicotinamide adenine dinucleotide phosphate		96, 97
Reduced	0.032 ± 0.002	
Oxidized	0.0014 ± 0.0011	
S-adenosylmethionine	0.005	98
Total nucleotide	1.534 ± 0.033	99
Uridine diphosphoglucose	0.031 ± 0.005	90, 100
Uridine diphosphate N-acetyl glucosamine	0.018	100

NOTE: Some results are given as mean ± standard deviation.
RBC, red blood cell.

distinct cellular components: (1) cell shape or cell geometry, which determines the ratio of cell surface area to cell volume (SA:V); higher values of SA:V facilitate deformation; (2) cytoplasmic viscosity, which is primarily regulated by the mean corpuscular hemoglobin concentration (MCHC) and is therefore influenced by alterations in cell volume; and (3) membrane deformability and mechanical stability, which are regulated by multiple membrane properties, which include elastic shear modulus, bending modulus, and yield stress.[52–55] Either directly or indirectly, membrane components and their organization play an important role in regulating each of the factors that influence cellular deformability.

The biconcave disc shape of the normal red cell creates an advantageous SA:V relationship, allowing the red cell to undergo marked deformation while maintaining a constant surface area. The normal human adult red cell has a volume of 90 fL and a surface area of 140 µm.[2] If the red cell were a sphere of identical volume, it would have a surface area of only 98 µm.[2] Thus, the discoid shape provides approximately 40 µm[2] of excess surface area, or an extra 43 percent, that enables the red cell to undergo extensive deformation. Most deformations occurring *in vivo* and *in vitro* involve no increase in surface area. This is important because the normal red cell can undergo large linear extensions of up to 230 percent of its original dimension while maintaining its surface area, but an increase of even 3 to 4 percent in surface area results in cell lysis. Either membrane loss, leading to a reduction in surface area, or an increase in cell water content, leading to an increase in cell volume, will create a more spherical shape with less redundant surface area. This loss of surface area redundancy results in reduced cellular deformability, compromised red cell function, and diminished survival as a result of splenic sequestration of spherocytic red cells. A 17-percent reduction in surface area results in rapid removal of red cells by the human spleen.[56]

Cytoplasmic viscosity, another regulatory component of red cell deformability, is largely determined by the MCHC, which is determined in large part by cell water content. As the hemoglobin concentration rises from 27 to 35 g/dL (the normal range for red blood cells), the viscosity of hemoglobin solution increases from 5 to 15 centipoise (cP), 5 to 15 times that of water. At these levels, the contribution of cytoplasmic viscosity to cellular deformability is negligible. However, viscosity increases exponentially at hemoglobin concentrations greater than 37 g/dL, reaching 45 cP at 40 g/dL, 170 cP at 45 g/dL, and 650 cP at 50 g/dL. At these levels, cytoplasmic viscosity may become the primary determinant of cellular deformability. Thus, cellular dehydration, usually caused by the failure of normal volume homeostasis mechanisms, can severely impair cellular deformability and thus decrease optimal oxygen delivery by impairing the ability of red cells to undergo rapid deformation necessary for passage through the microvasculature. As examples, cellular dehydration reduces red cell deformability in hereditary xerocytosis, sickle cell anemia, hemoglobin CC, and β-thalassemia.[55,57,58] However, changes in cellular dehydration by itself have little influence on red cell survival.

The property of membrane deformability determines the extent of membrane deformation that can be induced by a defined level of applied force. The more deformable the membrane, the less the force required for the cell to pass through the capillaries and other narrow openings, such as fenestrations in the splenic cords. The property of membrane mechanical stability is defined as the maximum extent of deformation that a membrane can undergo, beyond which it cannot completely

TABLE 31–5. Human Erythrocyte Carbohydrates, Organic Acids, and Metabolites

Compound	µmol/mL RBC	Reference(s)
Dihydroxyacetone phosphate	0.0094 ± 0.0028	88
2,3-Diphosphoglycerate	4.171 ± 0.636	88, 94
Fructose	0.000354 ± 0.0000191	101
Fructose 6-phosphate	0.0093 ± 0.002	88, 91, 94, 102
Fructose 3-phosphate	0.013 ± 0.001	103, 104
Fructose 2,6-diphosphate*	48 ± 13	105
Fructose 1,6-diphosphate	0.0019 ± 0.0006	88, 91, 94, 102
Glucuronic acid	Trace	106
Glucose	In equilibrium with plasma	107, 108
Glucose 6-phosphate	0.0278 ± 0.0075	88, 91, 94, 102
Glucose 1,6-diphosphate	0.18–0.30	91, 109
Glyceraldehyde 3-phosphate	Not detectable	88
Lactic acid	0.932 ± 0.211	72, 88, 110
Mannose 1,6-diphosphate	0.150	109
Octulose 1,8-diphosphate	Trace	111
Pyruvate	0.0533 ± 0.0215	88
3-Phosphoglycerate	0.0449 ± 0.0051	88, 94
2-Phosphoglycerate	0.0073 ± 0.0025	88, 94
Phosphoenol pyruvate	0.0122 ± 0.0022	88
Ribonucleic acid	1.355 mg	112
Ribose 1,5-diphosphate	<0.02	113, 114
Ribulose 5-phosphate	Trace	115
Sedoheptulose 7-phosphate	Trace	115
Sedoheptulose diphosphate	Trace	116
Sialic acid	0.825 ± 0.028	113
Sorbitol	31.1 ± 5.3	101, 103
Sorbitol 3-phosphate	0.013 ± 0.001	104

*Values are given in picomoles.

NOTE: Some results are given as mean ± standard deviation.

RBC, red blood cell.

TABLE 31–6. Human Erythrocyte Electrolytes

Electrolyte	µmol/mL RBC	Reference
Aluminum	0.0026	117
Bromide	0.1225	118, 119
Calcium	0.0089 ± 0.0030	119–121
Chloride	78	119, 122
Chromium	0.0004	123
Cobalt	0.0002	119, 124
Copper	0.018	123, 125, 126
Fluoride	0.0131	127
Iodine, protein-bound	0.0013	128
Lead	0.0082	117, 119, 125, 129
Magnesium	3.06	123, 130–132
Manganese	0.0034	117, 133
Nickel	0.0009	123
Phosphorus (acid soluble):		
Total P	13.2	134
Inorganic P	0.466	134
Lipid P	3.840	135
Unidentified P	0.955	134
Potassium	102.4 ± 3.9	130, 136–140
Rubidium	0.054	119
Silicon	0.036–0.060*	141
Silver	Trace	117
Sodium	6.2 ± 0.8	136–138
Sulfur	0.0044	142
Tin	0.0022	117
Zinc	0.153	123, 143, 144

*Obtained by subtracting plasma concentration from whole-blood concentration.

NOTE: Some results are given as mean ± standard deviation.

RBC, red blood cell.

recover its initial shape. This is the point at which the membrane fails. Normal membrane stability allows human red cells to circulate for 100 to 120 days without fragmenting, while decreased stability leads to cell fragmentation under normal circulating stresses. Both membrane deformability and membrane mechanical stability are regulated by structural organization of membrane proteins.[54] While decreased membrane deformability can reduce effective tissue oxygen delivery it appears to have little effect on red cell survival since Southeast Asian ovalocytes with marked reductions in membrane deformability have near-normal red cell survival. Loss of membrane mechanical stability leading to membrane fragmentation and consequent reduction in SA:V

ratio on the other hand compromises red cell survival as in hemolytic hereditary elliptocytosis.[49]

RED CELL SENESCENCE

The reticulocyte loses membrane as it matures into a discocyte and membrane loss by vesiculation continues throughout the erythrocyte life span. The notion that erythrocyte aging is synonymous with membrane loss, increasing MCHC, and decreasing deformability largely results from studies on density-separated cells and the equating of dense cells with aged cells (Chap. 33). Although it is clear that loss of membrane surface area and decreased cell volume is a feature of normal red cell senescence and that cell density increases with cell age, there is no direct relationship between cell age and cell density since there is a large heterogeneity in cell densities of reticulocytes as they enter circulation. What is clear is that the densest 1 percent of circulating red cells are

TABLE 31–7. Nomenclature of Red Cell Shapes and Associated Disease States

Terminology (Greek Meaning)	Old Terms, Synonyms	Description	Micrograph	Associated Disease States
Discocyte (disc)	Biconcave disc	Biconcave disc form of RBC		
Echinocyte (I–III) (sea urchin)	"Burr cell," crenated cell, "berry cell"	Spiculated RBC with short, equally spaced projections over entire surface; progressing from the "crenated disc" (echinocyte I) to the crenated sphere (echinocyte IV—not shown) with nearly complete loss of spicules		Uremia, liver disease Low-potassium red cells Immediately posttransfusion with aged or metabolically depleted blood Carcinoma of stomach and bleeding peptic ulcers
Acanthocyte (spike)	"Spur cell," acanthoid cell, acanthrocyte	Irregularly spiculated RBC with projections of varying length and position		Abetalipoproteinemia Alcoholic liver disease Postsplenectomy state Malabsorptive states
Stomatocyte (I–III) (mouth)	Mouth cell, cup form, mushroom cap, uniconcave disc, microspherocyte	Bowled-shaped RBC with single concavity; progressing from shallow bowl (I) to near sphere with small dimple (seen as mouth-shaped form in peripheral film)		Hereditary spherocytosis Hereditary stomatocytosis Alcoholism, cirrhosis, obstructive liver disease Erythrocyte sodium-pump defect
Spherostomatocyte (sphere)	Spherocyte, prelytic sphere, microspherocyte	Spherical RBC with dense hemoglobin content; scanning electron microscopy shows a persistent minimal dimple		Hereditary spherocytosis (cells actually spherostomatocytes) Immune hemolytic anemia Posttransfusion Heinz body hemolytic anemia Water-dilution hemolysis Fragmentation hemolysis
Schizocyte (cut)	Schistocyte, helmet cell, fragmented cell	Split RBC, often showing half-disc shape with two or three pointed extremities; may be small, irregular fragment		Microangiopathic hemolytic anemia (TTP, DIC, vasculitis, glomerulonephritis, renal graft rejection) Carcinomatosis Heart-valve hemolysis (prosthetic or pathologic valves) Severe burns March hemoglobinuria
Elliptocyte (oval)	Ovalocyte	Oval to elongated ellipsoid RBC (with polarization of hemoglobin)		Hereditary elliptocytosis Thalassemia Iron deficiency Myelophthisic anemias Megaloblastic anemias

(Continued)

TABLE 31–7. Nomenclature of Red Cell Shapes and Associated Disease States (*Continued*)

Terminology (Greek Meaning)	Old Terms, Synonyms	Description	Micrograph	Associated Disease States
Drepanocyte (sickle)	Sickle cell	RBC containing polymerized hemoglobin S; showing varying shapes from bipolar, spiculated forms to holly-leaf and irregularly spiculated forms		Sickle cell disorders (SS, S trait, SC, SD, S thalassemia, etc.) Hemoglobin C-Harlem Hemoglobin Memphis/S
Codocyte (bell)	Target cell	Bell-shaped RBC that assumes a target shape on dried films of blood		Obstructive liver disease Hemoglobinopathies (S, C) Thalassemia Iron deficiency Postsplenectomy state Lecithin cholesterol acetyltransferase deficiency
Dacryocyte (tear)	Teardrop cell	RBC with a single elongated or pointed extremity		Primary myelofibrosis Myelophthisic anemias Thalassemia
Leptocyte (thin)	Thin cell, wafer cell	Thin, flat RBC with hemoglobin at periphery		Thalassemia Obstructive liver disease (± iron deficiency)
Keratocyte (horn)	Horn cell	RBC with spicules resulting from ruptured vacuole; cell appears half-moon shaped or spindle shaped		DIC or vascular prosthesis

DIC, disseminated intravascular coagulation; RBC, red blood cell; TTP, thrombotic thrombocytopenic purpura.

the most aged—they have the highest levels of glycated hemoglobin (HbA_{1C}), a very good marker of cell age. The loss of membrane surface area of the senescent red cells appears to be a result of membrane oxidation-induced band 3 clustering and consequent membrane vesiculation and the resultant critical decrease in SA:V ratio leads to their removal from circulation[59,60]

PATHOPHYSIOLOGY OF ERYTHROCYTE SHAPES

Chapter 46 discusses erythrocytes in greater detail.

See Table 31–7 and Fig. 31–13 for scanning and blood film appearance of pathologically shaped red cells.

Spherocytes and Stomatocytes

Spherocytes (Chap. 46) represent red cells, with the most decreased SA:V ratio seen in hereditary spherocytosis, immune hemolytic anemia, stored blood, Heinz body hemolytic anemia, and caused by cell fragmentation.[49,61] Stomatocytes are seen in hereditary stomatocytosis, as well as in hereditary spherocytosis, alcoholism, cirrhosis, obstructive liver disease, and erythrocyte sodium pump defects.[49,62,63] Red cells sensitized with antibodies, complement, or immune complexes lose cholesterol and surface area. As a result, they are less deformable and more osmotically fragile. Heinz body formation leads to membrane depletion

by fragmentation, with spherocyte formation. A spherogenic mechanism common to Heinz body hemolytic anemias and immune hemolysis is partial phagocytosis of portions of the cell containing aggregates of denatured hemoglobin and portions of the sensitized membrane, respectively.

Stomatocytosis appear to be an intermediate form in the generation of spherocytosis with varying extents of decreased SA:V ratio as a result of loss of membrane surface area or increased cell volume. Stomatocytosis is a feature of hereditary hydrocytosis caused by increased cell volume and consequent decrease in SA:V ratio. A spectrum of abnormal cells varying from normal discocytes to stomatocytes, spherostomatocytes, and dense microspherocytes is seen in hereditary spherocytosis.

Elliptocytes

Elliptocytes are seen in hereditary elliptocytosis (Chap. 46) as well as in thalassemia (Chap. 48), iron deficiency (Chap. 43), and megaloblastic anemia (Chap. 41).[49] In blood films of normal subjects, elliptical or oval cells usually constitute less than 1 percent of the erythrocytes. In various pathologic situations, with or without anemia (thalassemia trait, folate, and iron deficiency), the number of elliptocytes can increase to 10 percent. Exceptionally, as in dyserythropoiesis, the proportion can be as high as 50 percent. In hereditary elliptocytosis, the number of elliptical

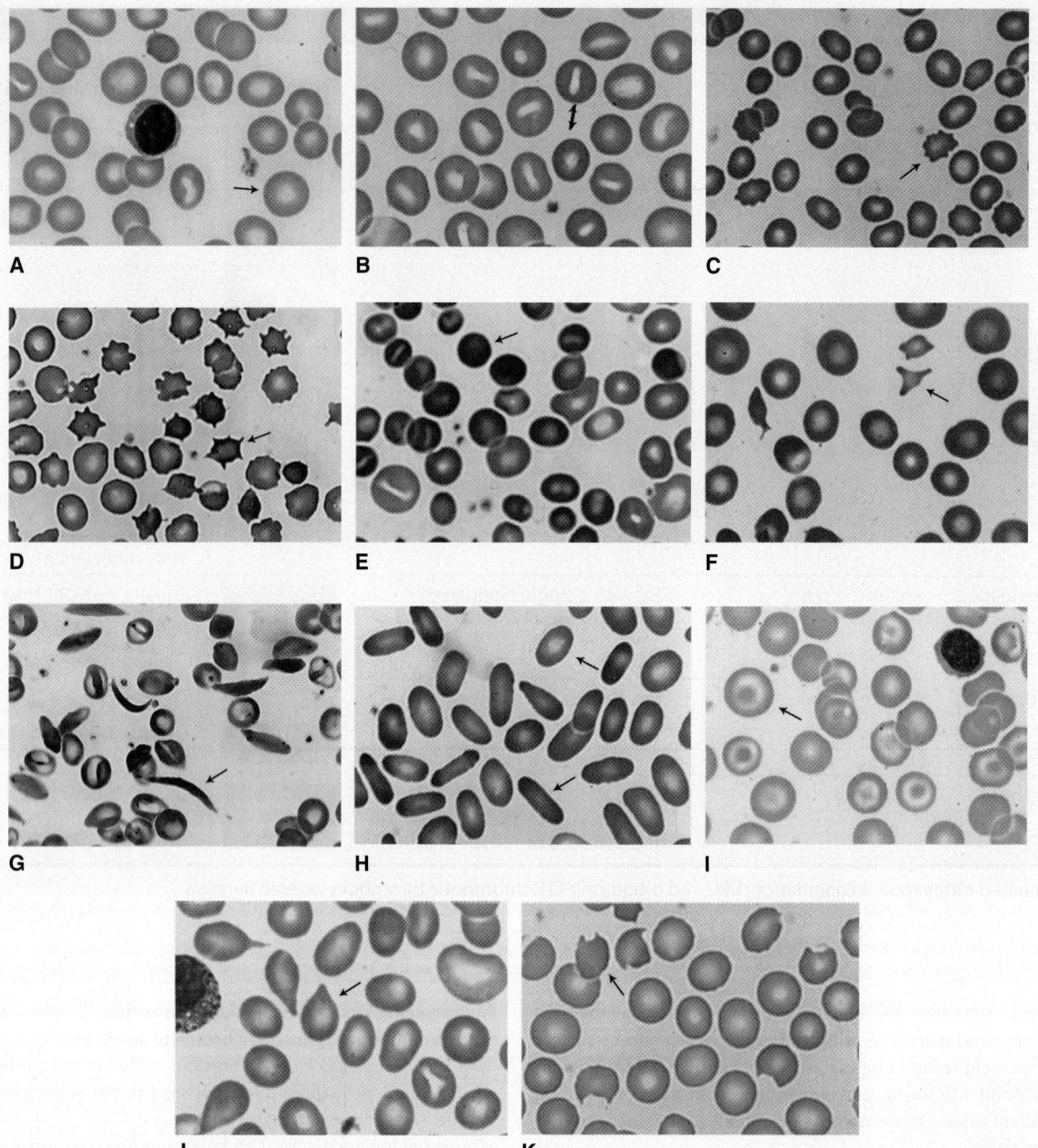

Figure 31–13. A. Normal blood. *Arrow* points to a normochromic-normocytic discocyte. **B.** Stomatocytes. The *double arrow* points to the two morphologic types of stomatocyte: upper cell with a slit-shaped pale area and lower cell with a small central circular pale area. **C.** Echinocytes. The field has several such cells. The *arrow* points to one example with evenly distributed, blunt, short, circumferentially positioned, projections. **D.** Acanthocytes. The *arrow* points to one example with a few spike-shaped projections, unevenly distributed and of varying lengths. **E.** Spherocytes. Small, circular, densely-staining (hyperchromic) cells which, when fully developed, show no central pallor. **F.** Schizocytes (schistocytes, helmet cells, fragmented red cells). These microcytic cell fragments may assume varied shapes. The arrow points to a triangular shape, but two others of different shape are also present in the field. Despite being damaged and very small, they frequently maintain a biconcave appearance as witnessed by their central pallor. **G.** Sickle cells (Drepanocytes). Numerous sickle cells are shown. Two are in the classic shape of the blade on the agricultural sickle *(arrow)*. Many red cells that have undergone the transformation to a "sickle" cell take the slightly less extreme form of elliptical cells with a very narrow diameter with condensed hemoglobin in the center (para-crystallization). About eight such cells are in the field. **H.** Elliptocytes and ovalocytes. The *lower arrow* points to an elliptocyte (cigar-shaped). The *upper arrow* points to an ovalocyte (football-shaped). Because both forms may be seen together in a case of inherited disease (same gene mutation resulting in both shapes), as shown here, it has been proposed that all such shapes be called elliptocytes with a Roman numeral to designate the severity of the shape change toward the elliptical, that is, elliptocytes I, II, and III. **I.** Target cells (Codocytes). The *arrow* points to one characteristic example among several in the field. The hemoglobin concentration corralled by membrane recurvature in the center of the cell gives it the appearance of an archery target. **J.** Tear-drop–shaped cells (Dacryocytes). Three dacryocytes are in this field. One example is indicated by the *arrow*. **K.** Horn cell (Keratocyte). Several examples are in the field. The *arrow* points to a typical such cell with two sharp projections. *(Reproduced with permission from* Lichtman's Atlas of Hematology, *www.accessmedicine.com.)*

erythrocytes varies greatly, from 1 to 98 percent. Qualitative and quantitative anomalies of spectrin and protein 4.1, the major proteins of the membrane skeleton, are associated with hereditary elliptocytosis.[49,64] Severe hemolytic anemia is seen only in the homozygous or compound heterozygotes form of the disease (hereditary pyropoikilocytosis) where extensive cell fragmentation produces *pyropoikilocytes* with marked decreases in SA:V ratio.

Acanthocytes

The acanthocyte (Chap. 46) is irregularly shaped, with two to 10 hemispherically tipped spicules of variable length and diameter. The bases of the spicules on the acanthocyte are of varying girth, unlike the spicules on echinocytes, which have remarkably uniform dimensions. Acanthocytes are seen in neuroacanthocytosis and in abetalipoproteinemia.[65] The lack of anemia in these conditions suggests that these cells have near normal life span in circulation.

Target Cells (Codocytes)

A relative excess of membrane surface area or decreased cell volume leading to increased SA:V ratio results in target cells.[66] Target cells may be seen in obstructive liver disease, hemoglobinopathies (S and C), thalassemia, iron deficiency, postsplenectomy, and lecithin cholesterol acetyltransferase deficiency. In patients with obstructive liver disease, lecithin cholesterol acetyltransferase activity is depressed. This increases the cholesterol-to-phospholipid ratio and produces an absolute increase in the surface area of the red cell membrane. In contrast, membrane excess is only relative in patients with iron-deficiency anemia and thalassemia because of the reduced cell volume. In contrast to spherocytes which exhibit increased osmotic fragility, target red cells are osmotically resistant.

Sickle Cells (Drepanocytes)

The sickle cell (Chap. 49) displays a characteristic variation of form on stained blood films. The fusiform cell in the crescent shape with two pointed extremities is encountered most commonly in deoxygenated blood samples as a result of polymerization of sickle hemoglobin. If sickle cell formation is observed by phase-contrast microscopy, the earliest change with deoxygenation is loss of flicker, followed by slight deformation at the discocyte border with displacement of the hemoglobin to one region of the cell. The cell then elongates and becomes rigid as a result of polymerization of hemoglobin S. Upon reoxygenation, the sickle cell resumes the discocyte form and, in so doing, loses membrane by microspherulation and fragmentation during retraction of long spicules.[67] Evidence suggests that the more typical sickle-shaped cells form under slow deoxygenation. With each sickling–unsickling cycle, membrane damage accumulates resulting in the formation of irreversibly sickled cells (ISCs).[68,69] These cells are incapable of reversion to the biconcave disc shape, even when fully oxygenated. They have an increased hemoglobin concentration, increased cation permeability, decreased potassium, and increased sodium.

Fragmented Cells (Schistocytes)

Schistocytes (Chap. 51) are seen in microangiopathic hemolytic anemias (thrombotic thrombocytopenic purpura [TTP], disseminated intravascular coagulation [DIC], vasculitis, glomerulonephritis, renal graft rejection), carcinomatosis, heart valve hemolysis (prosthetic or pathologic valves), severe burns, and march hemoglobinuria (Chap. 51). Fibrin strands in damaged blood vessels can be arrayed so that they sieve the passing red cells. If a passing red cell folds over or otherwise attaches to the strand, the bloodstream pulls on the arrested cell, stretches it, and eventually fragments it.[70] The spleen rapidly removes the schistocytes with a low relative SA:V ratio; the remainder may circulate for many days.

REFERENCES

1. Malik P, Fischer TC, Barsky LL, et al: An *in vitro* model of human red blood cell production from hematopoietic progenitor cells. *Blood* 91:2664, 1998.
2. Sato T, Maekawa T, Watanabe S, et al: Erythroid progenitors differentiate and mature in response to endogenous erythropoietin. *J Clin Invest* 106:263, 2000.
3. Giarratana MC, Kobari L, Lapillonne HC et al: Ex vivo generation of fully mature human red blood cells from hematopoietic stem cells. *Nat Biotechnol* 23:69, 2005.
4. Hu J, Liu J, Xue F, et al: Isolation and functional characterization of human erythroblasts at distinct stages: Implications for understanding of normal and disordered erythropoiesis in vivo. *Blood* 121:3246, 2013.
5. Li J, Hale J, Bhagia P et al: Isolation and transcriptome analysis of human erythroid progenitors. *Blood* 124:3636, 2014.
6. Southcott MJG, Tanner MJA, Anstee DJ: The expression of human blood group antigens during erythropoiesis in a cell culture system. *Blood* 93:4425, 1999.
7. Palis J: Ontogeny of erythropoiesis. *Curr Opin Hematol* 15:155, 2008.
8. Palis J: Primitive and definitive erythropoiesis in mammals. *Front Physiol* 5:3, 2014.
9. Zambidis ET, Peault B, Park TS, et al: Hematopoietic differentiation of human embryonic stem cells progresses through sequential hematoendothelial, primitive, and definitive stages resembling human yolk sac development. *Blood* 106:860, 2005.
10. Pereda J, Niimi G: Embryonic erythropoiesis in human yolk sac: Two different compartments for two different processes. *Microsc Res Tech* 71:856, 2008.
11. Schmid-Schonbein H, Wells R: Fluid drop-like transition of erythrocytes under shear. *Science* 165:288, 1969.
12. Sadahira Y, Mori M: Role of the macrophage in erythropoiesis. *Pathol Int* 49:841, 1999.
13. Bessis M: *Living Blood Cells and Their Ultrastructure*. Springer-Verlag, Berlin, 1973.
14. Gregory CJ, Eaves AC: Three stages of erythropoietic progenitor cell differentiation distinguished by a number of physical and biologic properties. *Blood* 51:527, 1978.
15. McLeod DL, Shreeve MM, Axelrad AA: Improved plasma culture system for production of erythrocytic colonies in vitro: Quantitative assay method for CFU-E. *Blood* 44:517, 1974.
16. Chasis JA, Mohandas N: Erythroblastic islands: Niches for erythropoiesis. *Blood* 112:470, 2008.
17. Manwani D, Bieker JJ: The erythroblastic island. *Curr Top Dev Biol* 82:23, 2008.
18. Yokoyama T, Etoh T, Kitagawa H, et al: Migration of erythroblastic islands toward the sinusoid as erythroid maturation proceeds in rat bone marrow. *J Vet Med Sci* 65:449, 2003.
19. Lichtman MA, Santillo P: Red cell egress from the marrow—Vis-à-tergo. *Blood Cells* 12:11, 1986.
20. Chamberlain JK, Lichtman MA: Marrow cell egress: Specificity of the site of penetration into the sinus. *Blood* 52:959, 1978.
21. Waugh RE: Reticulocyte rigidity and passage through endothelial-like pores. *Blood* 78:3037, 1991.
22. Yoshida H, Kawane K, Koike M et al: Phosphatidylserine-dependent engulfment by macrophages of nuclei from erythroid precursor cells. *Nature* 437:754, 2005.
23. Jacobsen RN, Forristal CE, Raggatt LJ, et al: Mobilization with granulocyte colony-stimulating factor blocks medullar erythropoiesis by depleting F4/80(+)VCAM1(+)CD169(+)ER-HR3(+)Ly6G(+) erythroid island macrophages in the mouse. *Exp Hematol* 42:547, 2014.
24. Rhodes MM, Kopsombut P, Bondurant MC, et al: Adherence to macrophages in erythroblastic islands enhances erythroblast proliferation and increases erythrocyte production by a different mechanism than erythropoietin. *Blood* 111:1700, 2008.
25. Kawane K, Fukuyama H, Kondoh G, et al: Requirement of DNase II for definitive erythropoiesis in the mouse fetal liver. *Science* 292:1546, 2001.
26. Bowman WD Jr: Abnormal ("ringed") sideroblasts in various hematologic and non-hematologic disorders. *Blood* 18:662, 1961.
27. Hines JD, Grasso JA: The sideroblastic anemias. *Semin Hematol* 7:86, 1970.
28. Konstantinidis DG, Pushkaran S, Johnson JF, et al: Signaling and cytoskeletal requirements in erythroblast enucleation. *Blood* 119:6118, 2012.
29. Ubukawa K, Guo YM, Takahashi M, et al: Enucleation of human erythroblasts involves non-muscle myosin IIB. *Blood* 119:1036, 2012.
30. Keerthivasan G, Small S, Liu H, et al: Vesicle trafficking plays a novel role in erythroblast enucleation. *Blood* 116: 3331, 2010.
31. Pan BT, Johnstone RM: Fate of the transferrin receptor during maturation of sheep reticulocytes *in vitro*: Selective externalization of the receptor. *Cell* 33:967, 1983.
32. Chasis JA, Prenant M, Leung A, et al: Membrane assembly and remodeling during reticulocyte maturation. *Blood* 74:1112, 1989.
33. Liu J, Guo X, Mohandas N, et al: Membrane remodeling during reticulocyte maturation. *Blood* 115: 2021, 2010.
34. Brecher G, Haley JE, et al: Macronormoblasts, macroreticulocytes and macrocytes. *Blood Cells* 1:547, 1975.
35. Jolly JMJ: Recherches sur la formation des globules rouges des mammiféres. *Arch Anat Microsc* 9:133, 1907.
36. Felka T, Lemke J, Lemke C, et al: DNA degradation during maturation of erythrocytes—Molecular cytogenetic characterization of Howell-Jolly bodies. *Cytogenet Genome Res* 119:2, 2007.
37. Holroyde CP, Gardner FH: Acquisition of autophagic vacuoles by human erythrocytes. Physiological role of the spleen. *Blood* 36:566, 1970.
38. O'Grady JG, Harding B, Egan EL, et al: "Pitted" erythrocytes: Impaired formation in splenectomized subjects with congenital spherocytosis. *Br J Haematol* 57:441, 1984.

39. Buchanan GR, Holtkamp CA, Horton JA: Formation and disappearance of pocked erythrocytes: Studies in human subjects and laboratory animals. *Am J Hematol* 25:243, 1987.

40. Kass L: Origin and composition of Cabot rings in pernicious anemia. *Am J Clin Pathol* 64:53, 1975.

41. Kass L, Gray RH: Ultrastructural visualization of Cabot rings in pernicious anemia. *Experientia* 32:507, 1976.

42. Jensen WN, Moreno GD, Bessis MC: An electron microscopic description of basophilic stippling in red cells. *Blood* 25:933, 1965.

43. Heinz R: Uber Blutdegeneration und Regeneration. *Beitr Pathol* 29:299, 1901.

44. Chinprasertsuk S, Piankijagum A, Wasi P: *In vivo* induction of intraerythrocytic inclusion bodies in hemoglobin H disease: An electron microscopic study. *Birth Defects Orig Artic Ser* 23:317, 1987.

45. Sansone G, Sciarratta GV, Ivaldi G, Chiappara G: Hb H-like inclusions in red cells of patients with unstable haemoglobin. *Haematologica* 72:481, 1987.

46. Wickramasinghe SN, Hughes M, Higgs DR et al: Ultrastructure of red cells containing haemoglobin H inclusions induced by redox dyes. *Clin Lab Haematol* 3:51, 1981.

47. Bessis MC, Breton-Gorius J: Iron particles in normal erythroblasts and normal and pathological erythrocytes. *J Biophys Biochem Cytol* 3:503, 1957.

48. Evans J, Gratzer W, Mohandas N, et al: Fluctuations of the red cell membrane: Relation to mechanical properties and lack of ATP-dependence. *Biophys J* 94: 4134, 2008.

49. Mohandas N, Gallagher PG: Red cells: Past, present and future. *Blood* 112:393, 2008.

50. Discher D, Mohandas N, Evans EA: Molecular maps of red cell deformation: Hidden elasticity and in situ connectivity. *Science* 266:1032, 1994.

51. Liu SC, Derick LH, Palek J: Visualization of the hexagonal lattice in the erythrocyte membrane skeleton. *J Cell Biol* 104:527, 1987.

52. Mohandas N, Clark MR, Jacobs MS, Shohet SB: Analysis of factors regulating erythrocyte deformability. *J Clin Invest* 66:563, 1980.

53. Mohandas N, Chasis JA, Shohet SB: The influence of membrane skeleton on red cell deformability, membrane material properties and shape. S*emin Hematol* 20:225, 1983.

54. Chasis JA, Mohandas N: Erythrocyte membrane deformability and stability. Two distinct membrane properties which are independently regulated by skeletal protein associations. *J Cell Biol* 103:343, 1986.

55. Mohandas N, Chasis JA: Red cell deformability, membrane material properties and shape: Regulation by transmembrane, skeletal and cytosolic proteins and lipids. *Semin Hematol* 30:171, 1993.

56. Safeukui I, Buffet P, Delpaine G, et al: Quantitative assessment of sensing and sequestration of spherocytic erythrocytes by human spleen: Implications for understanding clinical variability of membrane disorders. *Blood* 120:424, 2012.

57. Clark MR, Mohandas N, Caggiano V, Shohet SB: Effects of abnormal cation transport on deformability of desiccytes. *J Supramol Struct* 8:521, 1978.

58. Evans E, Mohandas N, Leung A: Static and dynamic rigidities of normal and sickle erythrocytes: Major influence of cell hemoglobin concentration. *J Clin Invest* 73:477, 1984.

59. Pantaleo A, Giribaldi G, Mannu F, et al: Naturally occurring anti-band 3 antibodies and red cell removal under physiological and pathological conditions. *Autoimmun Rev* 7:457, 2008.

60. Arashiki N, Kimata N, Manno S, et al: Membrane peroxidation and methemoglobin formation are both necessary for band 3 clustering: Mechanistic insights into erythrocyte senescence. *Biochemistry* 52:5760, 2013.

61. Cooper RA: Loss of membrane components in pathogenesis of antibody-induced spherocytosis. *J Clin Invest* 51:16, 1972.

62. Lock SP, Smith RS, Hardisty RM: Stomatocytosis: A hereditary red cell anomaly associated with haemolytic anaemia. *Br J Haematol* 7:303, 1961.

63. Delaunay G, Stewart G, Iolascon A: Hereditary dehydrated and overhydrated stomatocytosis: Recent advances. *Curr Opin Hematol* 6:110, 1999.

64. Delaunay J: The molecular basis of hereditary red cell membrane disorders. *Blood Rev* 21:1, 2007.

65. De Franceschi L, Bosman GJ, Mohandas N: Abnormal red cell features associated with hereditary neurodegenerative disorders: The neuroacanthocytosis syndromes. *Curr Opin Hematol* 21:201, 2014.

66. Cooper RA, Jandl JH: Bile salts and cholesterol in the pathogenesis of target cells in obstructive jaundice. *J Clin Invest* 47:809, 1968.

67. Padilla F, Bromberg PA, Jensen WN: Sickle–sickle cycle—Cause of cell fragmentation leading to permanently deformed cells. *Blood* 41:653, 1973.

68. Horiuchi K, Ballas SK, Asakura T: The effect of deoxygenation rate on the formation of irreversibly sickled cells. *Blood* 71:46, 1988.

69. Bertles JF, Milner PF: Irreversibly sickled erythrocytes: A consequence of the heterogeneous distribution of hemoglobin types in sickle-cell anemia. *J Clin Invest* 47:1731, 1968.

70. Bull BS, Kuhn IN: Production of schistocytes by fibrin strands (a scanning electron microscope study). *Blood* 35:104, 1970.

71. Ponder E: *Hemolysis and Related Phenomena.* Grune & Stratton, New York, 1948.

72. Behrendt H: *Chemistry of Erythrocytes.* Charles C Thomas, Springfield, IL, 1957.

73. Tyan YC, Jong SB, Liao JD, et al: Proteomic profiling of erythrocyte proteins by proteolytic digestion chip and identification using two-dimensional electrospray ionization tandem mass spectrometry. *J Proteome Res* 4:748, 2005.

74. Pasini EM, Kirkegaard M, Mortensen P, et al: In-depth analysis of the membrane and cytosolic proteome of red blood cells. *Blood* 108:791, 2006.

75. Farquhar JW: Human erythrocytes phosphoglycerides. I. Quantification of plasmalogens, fatty acids and fatty aldehydes. *Biochim Biophys Acta* 60:80, 1962.

76. Kirk E: The concentration of lecithin, cephalin, ether-insoluble phosphatide, and cerebrosides in plasma and red blood cells of normal adults. *J Biol Chem* 123:637, 1938.

77. Phillips GB, Roome NS: Quantitative chromatographic analysis of the phospholipids of abnormal human red blood cells. *Proc Soc Exp Biol Med* 109:360, 1962.

78. Westerman MP, Zhang Y, McConnell JP, et al: Ascorbate levels in red blood cells and urine in patients with sickle cell anemia. *Am J Hematol* 65:174, 2000.

79. Luecke R, Pearson PB: The microbiological determination of free choline in plasma and urine. *J Biol Chem* 153:259, 1944.

80. Beerstecher E, Spangler S, Granick S, et al: Blood vitamins, hormones, enzymes. Blood coenzymes: Vertebrates, in *Blood and Other Body Fluids*, edited by PL Altman, DS Dittmer, p 108. Federation of American Societies for Experimental Biology, Washington, DC, 1961.

81. Kaplan NO, Lipmann F: The assay of distribution of coenzyme A. *J Biol Chem* 174:37, 1948.

82. Klein JR, Perlzweig WA, Handler P: Determination of nicotinic acid in blood cells and plasma. *J Biol Chem* 145:27, 1942.

83. Pearson PB: The pantothenic acid content of the blood of mammals. *J Biol Chem* 140:423, 1941.

84. Masse PG, Mahuren JD, Tranchant C, Dosy J: B-6, vitamers and 4-pyridoxic acid in the plasma, erythrocytes, and urine of postmenopausal women. *Am J Clin Nutr* 80:946, 2004.

85. Burch HB, Bessey OA, Lowry OH: Fluorometric measurements of riboflavin and its natural derivatives in small quantities of blood serum and cells. *J Biol Chem* 175:457, 1948.

86. Beutler E: Glutathione reductase: Stimulation in normal subjects by riboflavin supplementation. *Science* 165:613, 1969.

87. Burch HB, Bessey OA, Love RH, Lowry OH: The determination of thiamine and thiamine phosphates in small quantities of blood and blood cells. *J Biol Chem* 198:477, 1952.

88. Beutler E: *Red Cell Metabolism: A Manual of Biochemical Methods.* Grune & Stratton, New York, 1984.

89. Bishop C, Rankine D, Talbott JH: The nucleotides in normal human blood. *J Biol Chem* 234:1233, 1959.

90. Mandel P, Chambon P, Karon H, et al: Nucleotides libres des globules rouges et des reticulocytes. *Folia Haematol Int Mag Klin Morphol Blutforsch* 78:525, 1962.

91. Bartlett GR: Human red cell glycolytic intermediates. *J Biol Chem* 234:449, 1959.

92. Yoshikawa H, Nakano M, Miyamoto K, Tatibana M: Phosphorus metabolism in human erythrocyte. II. Separation of acid-soluble phosphorus compounds incorporating p32 by column chromatography with ion exchange resin. *J Biochem* 47:635, 1960.

93. Beutler E, Mathai CK: A comparison of normal red cell ATP levels as measured by the firefly system and the hexokinase system. *Blood* 30:311, 1967.

94. Minakami S, Suzuki C, Saito T, Yoshikawa H: Studies on erythrocyte glycolysis. I. Determination of the glycolytic intermediates in human erythrocytes. *J Biochem* 58:543, 1965.

95. Patterson WD, Hardman JG, Sutherland EW: A comparison of cyclic nucleotide levels in plasma and cells of rat and human blood. *Endocrinology* 95:325, 1974.

96. Canepa L, Ferraris AM, Miglino M, Gaetani GF: Bound and unbound pyridine dinucleotides in normal and glucose-6-phosphate dehydrogenase-deficient erythrocytes. *Biochim Biophys Acta* 1074:101, 1991.

97. Micheli V, Simmonds HA, Bari M, Pompucci G: HPLC determination of oxidized and reduced pyridine coenzymes in human erythrocytes. *Clin Chim Acta* 220:1, 1993.

98. Lagendijk J, Ubbink JB, Vermaak WJH: Quantification of erythrocyte S-adenosyl-L-methionine levels and its application in enzyme studies. *J Chromatogr B Biomed Appl* 576:95, 1992.

99. Overgard-Hansen K, Jorgensen S: Determination and concentration of adenine nucleotides in human blood. *Scand J Clin Lab Invest* 12:10, 1960.

100. Mills GC: Uridine diphosphate glucose and uridine diphosphate N-acetylglucosamine in erythrocytes. *Tex Rep Biol Med* 18:446, 1960.

101. Liang HR, Takagaki T, Foltz RL, Bennett P: Quantitative determination of endogenous sorbitol and fructose in human erythrocytes by atmospheric-pressure chemical ionization LC tandem mass spectrometry. *J Chromatogr B Analyt Technol Biomed Life Sci* 824:36, 2005.

102. Lionetti FJ, McLellan WL, Fortier NL, Foster JM: Phosphate esters produced from inosine in human erythrocyte ghosts. *Arch Biochem* 94:7, 1961.

103. Kawaguchi M, Fujii T, Kamiya Y, et al: Effects of fructose ingestion on sorbitol and fructose 3-phosphate contents of erythrocytes from healthy men. *Acta Diabetol* 33:100, 1996.

104. Petersen A, Szwergold BS, Kappler F, et al: Identification of sorbitol 3-phosphate and fructose 3-phosphate in normal and diabetic human erythrocytes. *J Biol Chem* 265:17424, 1990.

105. Colomer D, Pujades A, Carballo E, Vives Corrons JL: Erythrocyte fructose 2,6-bisphosphate content in congenital hemolytic anemias. *Hemoglobin* 15:517, 1991.

106. Deichmann WB, Dierker M: The spectrophotometric estimation of hexuronates (expressed as glucuronic acid) in plasma or serum. *J Biol Chem* 163:753, 1946.

107. Jung CY: Carrier-mediated glucose transport across human red cell membranes, in *The Red Blood Cell*, edited by DM Surgenor, p 705. Academic Press, New York, 1975.

108. Lacko L, Wittke B, Geck P: The temperature dependence of the exchange transport of glucose in human erythrocytes. *J Cell Physiol* 82:213, 1973.

109. Bartlett GR: Glucose and mannose diphosphates in the red blood cell. *Biochim Biophys Acta* 156:231, 1968.

110. Johnson RE, Edward HT, Dill DB, Wilson JW: Blood as a physicochemical system. XIII. The distribution of lactate. *J Biol Chem* 157:461, 1945.

111. Bartlett GR, Bucolo G: Octulose phosphates from the human red blood cell. *Biochem Biophys Res Commun* 3:474, 1960.

112. Mandel P, Métals P: Les acides nucléiques du plasma sanguin chez l'homme. *C R Seances Soc Biol Fil* 142:241, 1948.

113. Aminoff D, Anderson J, Dabich L, Gathmann WD: Sialic acid content of erythrocytes in normal individuals and patients with certain hematologic disorders. *Am J Hematol* 9:381, 1980.

114. Vanderheiden BS: Ribosediphosphate in the human erythrocyte. *Biochem Biophys Res Commun* 6:117, 1961.

115. Bruns FH, Noltmann E, Vahlhaus E: Über den Stoffwechsel von Ribose-5-phosphat in Hämolysaten. I. Aktivitäts-messung und Eigenschaften der Phosphoribose-isomerase. II. Der Pentosephosphate-Cyclus in roten Blutzellen. *Biochem Z* 330:483, 1958.

116. Bucolo G, Bartlett GR: Sedoheptulose diphosphate formation by the human red blood cell. *Biochem Biophys Res Commun* 3:620, 1960.

117. Kehoe RA, Cholak J, Story RV: A spectrochemical study of the normal ranges of concentration of certain trace metals in biological materials. *J Nutr* 19:579, 1940.

118. Hunter G: Micro-determination of bromide in body fluids. *Biochem J* 60:261, 1955.

119. Ojo JO, Oluwole AF, Durosinmi MA, et al: Baseline levels of elemental concentrations in whole blood, plasma, and erythrocytes of Nigerian subjects. *Biol Trace Elem Res* 43–45:461, 1994.

120. Bernard J-F, Bournier O, Boivin P: Human erythrocytic calcium concentration in hemolytic anemia. *Biomedicine* 23:431, 1975.

121. Shoji S, Komiyama A, Nakamura M, Nomoto S: Calcium content of healthy human erythrocytes. *Clin Chem* 35:1264, 1989.

122. Bernstein RE: Potassium and sodium balance in mammalian red cells. *Science* 120:459, 1954.

123. Herring WB, Leavell BS, Paizao LM, Yoe JH: Trace metals in human plasma and red blood cells: A study of magnesium, chromium, nickel, copper and zinc. I. Observations of normal subjects. *Am J Clin Nutr* 8:846, 1960.

124. Heyrovsky A: The biochemistry of cobalt. III. Amounts of cobalt in plasma, erythrocytes, urine, and feces of normal subjects. *Cas Lek Cesk* 91:680, 1952.

125. Mahalingam TR, Vijayalakshmi S, Prabhu RK, et al: Studies on some trace and minor elements in blood—A survey of the Kalpakkam (India) population. 2. Reference values for plasma and red cells, and correlation with coronary risk index. *Biol Trace Elem Res* 57:207, 1997.

126. Lahey ME, Gubler CJ, Cartwright GE, Wintrobe MM: Studies on copper metabolism. VI. Blood copper in normal human subjects. *J Clin Invest* 32:322, 1953.

127. Largent EJ, Cholak J: Blood electrolytes. Man, in *Blood and Other Body Fluids*, edited by PL Altman, DS Dittmer, p 21. Federation of American Societies for Experimental Biology, Washington, DC, 1961.

128. McClendon JF, Foster WC: Protein-bound iodine in erythrocytes and plasma and elsewhere. *Am J Med Sci* 207:549, 1944.

129. Jensovsky L, Roth Z: Der normale Bleigehalt im menschlichen Blute. *Naturwissenschaften* 48:382, 1961.

130. McCance RA, Widdowson EM: The effect of development, anaemia, and undernutrition on the composition of the erythrocyte. *Clin Sci* 15:409, 1956.

131. Huijgen HJ, Sanders R, van Olden RW, et al: Intracellular and extracellular blood magnesium fractions in hemodialysis patients: Is the ionized fraction a measure of magnesium excess? *Clin Chem* 44:639, 1998.

132. Martin BJ, Lyon TD, Fell GS, McKay P: Erythrocyte magnesium in elderly patients: Not a reliable guide to magnesium status. *J Trace Elem Med Biol* 11:44, 1997.

133. Miller DO, Yoe JH: Spectrophotometric determination of manganese in human plasma and red cells with benzohydroxamic acid. *Anal Chim Acta* 26:224, 1962.

134. Bartlett GR, Savage E, Hughes L, Marlow AA: Carbohydrate intermediates and related cofactors with benzohydroxamic acid. *J Appl Physiol* 6:51, 1953.

135. Ferranti F, Giannetti O: The microdetermination of phosphorus (inorganic, acid-soluble, lipoid and total) in the blood and excretions. *Diagn Tec Lab Napoli Riv Mens* 4:664, 1933.

136. Overman RR, Davis AK: The application of flame photometry to sodium and potassium determinations in biological fluids. *J Biol Chem* 168:641, 1947.

137. Mayer KDF, Starkey BJ: Simpler flame photometric determination of erythrocyte sodium and potassium: The reference range for apparently healthy adults. *Clin Chem* 23:275, 1977.

138. Bernard JF, Bournier O, Renoux M, et al: Unclassified haemolytic anaemia with splenomegaly and erythrocyte cation abnormalities—A disease of the spleen? *Scand J Haematol* 17:231, 1976.

139. Hald PM: Notes on the determination and distribution of sodium and potassium in cells and serum of normal human blood. *J Biol Chem* 163:429, 1946.

140. Streef GM: Sodium and calcium content of erythrocytes. *J Biol Chem* 129:661, 1939.

141. Tamada T: An indirect spectrophotometric method for the determination of silicon in serum, whole blood and erythrocytes. *Anal Sci* 19:1291, 2003.

142. Reed L, Denis W: On the distribution of the non-protein sulfur of the blood between serum and corpuscles. *J Biol Chem* 73:623, 1927.

143. Vallee BL, Gibson JG: The zinc content of normal human whole blood, plasma, leucocytes, and erythrocytes. *J Biol Chem* 176:445, 1948.

144. Zak B, Nalbandian RM, Williams LA, Cohen J: Determination of human erythrocyte zinc: Hemoglobin ratios. *Clin Chim Acta* 7:634, 1962.

CHAPTER 32
ERYTHROPOIESIS

Josef T. Prchal and Perumal Thiagarajan

the transcription factors, hypoxia-inducible factors (HIF), HIF-1 and HIF-2, the principal regulators of the response to hypoxia. HIFs modulate erythropoiesis by regulation of EPO production, by direct EPO-independent mechanism(s) and facilitating iron availability.

SUMMARY

Production of red cells or *erythropoiesis*, is a tightly regulated process by which hematopoietic stem cells differentiate into erythroid progenitors and then mature into red cells. Erythropoiesis generates approximately 2×10^{11} new erythrocytes to replace the 2×10^{11} red cells (approximately 1 percent of the total red cell mass) removed from the circulation each day. Red cell production increases several fold after blood loss or hemolysis. When one of the progeny of the multipotential hematopoietic stem becomes committed to the erythroid lineage, this early erythroid progenitor undergoes a series of divisions and concurrent maturation that eventually result in morphologically recognizable erythroblasts. After expulsion of the nucleus, a macrocyte (polychromatophilic when stained by Wright stain, or a reticulocyte if stained with new methylene blue) leaves the marrow. During the first 24 hours in the circulation, reticulocytes lose their residual organelles (mitochondria and ribosomes) through an autophagic process and undergoes reconditioning of the membrane to become mature red blood cells with a morphology of a biconcave disc. Erythropoiesis is controlled by transcription factors and cytokines, the principal ones being GATA 1 and erythropoietin (EPO), which influence the rate of lineage commitment, proliferation, apoptosis, differentiation, and number of divisions from the earliest progenitor to late erythroblasts. The number of red cells produced varies in response to tissue oxygenation that determines the level of

HISTORY

Erythrocytes evolved largely for the purpose of transporting oxygen to tissues. Thus, the size of the red cell mass and the rate of red cell production must be closely related to supply and demand for oxygen in the tissues. Toward the end of the 19th century, French mountaineers and physiologists established that a low tissue tension of oxygen stimulates red cell production.[1] In 1906, Paul Carnot, a professor at the Sorbonne, and Mademoiselle DeFlandre, his associate, suggested that hypoxia generates a humoral factor capable of stimulating red cell production.[2] Based on questionable experimental data, an influential biochemist Friederich Miescher[3] erroneously proposed that marrow hypoxia directly stimulates red cell production. Finally, in 1950, in an ingenious study on parabiotic rats, Kurt Reissmann[4] provided evidence for the existence of an indirect humoral mechanism. This work, and work of Erslev and colleagues[5,6] who demonstrated that the plasma from anemic rabbits and primates contains an erythrocyte-stimulating factor, provided a strong basis for an existence of the factor appropriately named erythropoietin (EPO). In 1957, Jacobson and coworkers[7] reported that EPO was produced by the kidney, a finding that raised the possibility that EPO isolated in adequate amounts might be of therapeutic benefit to uremic patients. After EPO cloning and production of recombinant EPO in therapeutic quantities, EPO has proved to have not only indications for therapy of anemia, but also has extraerythroid effects that are yet to be fully elucidated, such as its effect on cell growth. Widespread use of EPO for the treatment of anemia has surpassed original expectations.

PHYLOGENY OF RED CELL PRODUCTION

HEMOGLOBIN AND RED CELLS

Hemoglobin is present in the most primitive animal forms, such as *Paramecium* and *Tetrahymena*. Some crustaceans, such as *Daphnia*, are capable of developing an oxygen transport system without circulating red cells.[8] One interesting exception is an Antarctic ice fish (*Chaenocephalus aceratus*) lacking hemoglobin.[9] These ice fish compensate for the absence of hemoglobin by their unusual nitric oxide metabolism.[10–12] They have very large hearts and unusually large diameter capillaries. This permits a large volume of blood to circulate at high flow rate and at low vascular pressure because of decreased peripheral resistance. This permits their survival in the very high oxygen content of Antarctic waters.[12]

An erythroid cell that can synthesize, carry, and protect hemoglobin from oxidation was found only with the development of a circulatory system. Circulating nucleated erythrocytes first appear in the worms of the phylum Nemertina and in the sessile marine creatures of the phylum Phoronida. Erythropoiesis in these primitive invertebrates takes place near or on the peritoneal surface, derived from endothelial cells.[13] Nonnucleated red cells are observed for the first time in the

Acronyms and Abbreviations: BCL11A, a critical switching factor for silencing γ-globin; Bcl-x$_L$, an antiapoptotic factor; BFU-E, burst-forming units—erythroid; CBP, a coactivator of a transcription factor; CFU-E, colony-forming units-erythroid; CFU-Ec-Kit, growth factor receptor also a protooncogene; CIS, a signal transduction protein that downregulates activity of erythropoietin receptor; CPM, counts per minute; EKLF, erythroid Kruppel-like factor; Emp, erythroblast-macrophage protein; EPO, erythropoietin; EPOR, EPO receptor; FOG, "friend of GATA," a GATA-1 interacting protein; Gas6, growth arrest-specific 6; GATA-1, transcription factor; HCP, hematopoietic cell phosphatase; Hct, hematocrit; HIF, hypoxia-inducible transcription factor; ICSH, International Committee on Standardization in Hematology; JAK2, a tyrosine kinase that interacts with erythropoietin receptor; KAP1, KRAB-associated protein-1 is a transcriptional cofactor; KRAB-ZFP, one of the 400 human zinc finger protein-based transcription factors; mDia2, a protein that regulates actin and focal adhesion dynamics; miRNAs, microRNAs are small noncoding RNA molecules; NFE-2, a transcription factor, one of the principal regulator of hematopoiesis; Nix, a protein that is expressed during erythropoiesis and regulates mitochondrial apoptosis (autophagy); OS-9, osteosarcoma protein 9; PU.1, a transcription factor; RACK1, receptor of activated protein kinase C; RCM, red cell mass; SCL/TAL1, stem cell leukemia/T-cell acute lymphoblastic leukemia 1 factor; SOCS3, a signal transduction protein (also known as CIS3) that downregulates activity of erythropoietin receptor; VHL, von Hippel-Lindau protein.

more advanced phylum Annelida. However, the evolutionary advantage derived from enucleation appears to be slight. Nucleated red cells are observed in more advanced animals, such as reptiles and birds.[14] All mammalian erythrocytes are nonnucleated and in most species are disc shaped, but are oval in some species.[15] Enucleation decreases the workload of heart as it reduces one third of the cell weight.

In nonmammalian species, the spleen is the fundamental erythropoietic organ. However, in some fish, the kidneys also are involved in red cell production.[16,17] In vertebrates, an evolutionary shift occurred from the spleen to the liver and from the liver to the bones cavities.[18] The homeostatic regulation of blood or hemoglobin production has been studied in *Daphnia*,[8] where a balance exists between oxygen need and hemoglobin production. In higher animals, this relationship is maintained by adjusting red cell production. Studies of birds,[19] fish,[20] and mammals[21] indicate that red cell production is controlled by EPO, which is capable of adjusting red cell production to the demands for oxygen in the tissues. EPO of mammals has considerable biologic similarity and genetic homology.[22]

ONTOGENY OF RED CELL PRODUCTION

EMBRYONIC AND FETAL ERYTHROPOIESIS

The environment within the bone apparently is optimal for cellular proliferation and maturation. However, bone cavities do not develop until the fifth fetal month. Other, presumably less favorable, sites are responsible for red cell production during early embryonic life (Chap. 7). In the human, large nucleated blood cells are first formed in the yolk sac,[23] and some enucleate.[24] They cluster in blood islands that become enveloped by endothelial cells forming the vascular plexus of the yolk sac.[25] This is referred to as primitive erythropoiesis, and is contrasted with definitive erythropoiesis, which occurs in the fetal liver and in the marrow. During the second gestational month, erythropoiesis moves to fetal liver, wherein smaller, but still macrocytic, nonnucleated cells are produced.[26,27] At birth, the hepatic phase of blood cell production

ceases, and erythropoiesis moves to the marrow (Chaps. 7 and 48 provide details of developmental switching of embryonic, fetal, and adult globin expression).

During the neonatal period, the volume of available marrow space is almost the same as the total volume of hematopoietic cells and marrow vasculature.[28] This process continues for a few years until the growth of bones and bone cavities exceeds the growth of hematopoietic mass. However, whenever the demand on erythropoiesis increases (blood loss, hypoxia, ineffective erythropoiesis, or hemolysis), the lack of reserve space in neonates and small children reactivates extramedullary erythropoiesis in the liver and spleen.[29] In adults, expansion of marrow space continues, and the amount of fatty tissue gradually increases in all bone cavities. Because of the abundant marrow space, compensatory reactivation of extramedullary sites rarely occurs in later life. Extramedullary hematopoiesis during adult years indicates pathologic rather than compensatory blood formation, such as seen in primary myelofibrosis (Chap. 86) wherein the stem cells have abnormal interaction with the extracellular matrix.[30] During fetal life, EPO production is primarily hepatic.[31] At birth, a gradual switch to renal production of EPO occurs. In the adult, the kidney is responsible for approximately 85 percent of total production.[32,33]

CELLULAR COMPONENTS OF ERYTHROPOIESIS

PROGENITOR CELLS

Our ability to evaluate early erythropoiesis rests on functional assays of hematopoietic progenitors. The developmentally earliest progenitor committed to the erythroid lineage is the burst-forming unit–erythroid (BFU-E). It was initially termed a burst because it contains cells still capable of migration. These cells form smaller clusters around a larger central colony, giving the appearance of a sunburst with satellite colonies (Fig. 32–1). However, all the cells in the colony and its satellites are derived from a single BFU-E and, thus, are clonal. BFU-E takes longer

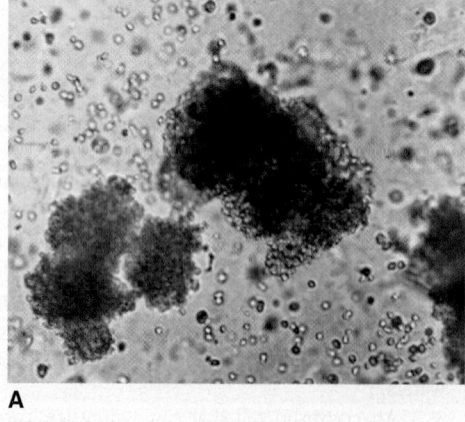 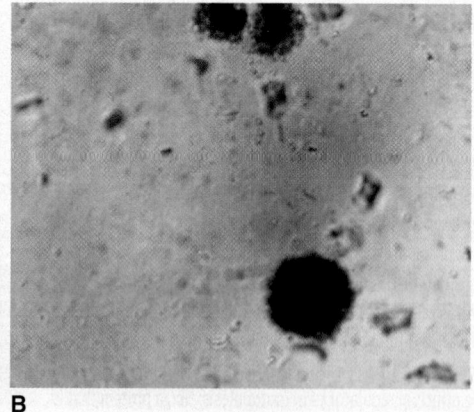

A   B

Figure 32–1. Burst-forming unit–erythroid (BFU-E) and colony-forming unit–erythroid (CFU-E). Erythroid colony growth in methylcellulose medium in presence of erythropoietin. Normal human marrow. The colonies are stained for hemoglobin. **A.** BFU-E. This colony grows from a single marrow erythroid progenitor cell (BFU-E). It was photographed at 14 days in culture. The BFU-E is a differentiated cell, committed to the erythroid lineage. The BFU-E is a more primitive progenitor in the erythroid maturation pathway than the CFU-E. The colony it forms is large, compared to the CFU-E, has spreading margins, and often satellite colonies. **B.** CFU-E. This colony was photographed at day 7 in culture. The CFU-E originates from a more mature single progenitor cell than the BFU-E. The CFU-E is smaller and grows typically in a tight, dense colony, compared to the BFU-E. The sequence established in the erythroid lineage is BFU-E, CFU-E, erythrocyte precursors (proerythroblast, etc). *(Reproduced with permission from Lichtman's Atlas of Hematology, www.accessmedicine.com.)*

than more mature erythroid progenitors to form a colony of erythroblasts (10 to 14 days) and form a large colony approximately 2000 to 3000 cells. BFU-E express low levels of EPO receptors (EPORs). BFU-E mature into colony-forming unit–erythroid (CFU-E), the more mature erythroid progenitor. A CFU-E is identified through more differentiated erythroid progenitor that *in vitro* form smaller colonies (50 to 200 cells) that mature in 3 to 5 days with EPOR density and EPO dependency increase gradually as progenitor cells mature, culminating at the level of the CFU-E.[34,35] BFU-E and CFU-E cannot be identified by microscopy (Chap. 31), but they can be studied *in vitro* by their ability to generate microscopically recognizable hemoglobinized precursors (i.e., erythroblasts) by so-called clonogenic assays on semisolid media.

PRECURSOR CELLS

In contrast, cells that constitute the latter stages of erythropoiesis can be identified by light microscopy (Chap. 31). The earliest morphologically recognizable erythroid precursor in the adult marrow is the pronormoblast. Pronormoblasts are conspicuously large and they have large uncondensed nuclei and deep basophilic cytoplasm as a result of the presence of numerous RNA-containing polyribosomes. Pronormoblast has a volume of 900 fL, 10 times the volume of the mature red blood cell. With each successive division, the precursor cells give rise to daughter cells of half their volume. Furthermore, with each division there is an increase in hemoglobin synthesis and condensation of nucleus. Thus, when the pronormoblasts divide to become basophilic normoblasts, the daughter cells have less blue cytoplasm because of hemoglobin synthesis and also a greater condensation of the nucleus. When the basophilic normoblasts divide further, they give rise to mature cells with more cytoplasmic hemoglobin that is stainable with both acid and basic dyes resulting in muddy-colored cytoplasm. These cells are called polychromatophilic normoblasts. The offspring of polychromatophilic normoblasts are called orthochromic normoblasts. Their nuclear chromatin is completely condensed and cytoplasm is pink from complete hemoglobinization. These cells do not divide further. Following extrusion of the nucleus, the enucleated cells derived from orthochromic orthochromatic erythroblasts are termed *reticulocytes*, named after the cytoplasmic remnants of the endoplasmic reticulum and the persistence of a few mitochondria and strings of ribosomes seen when stained with supravital dyes. Reticulocytes remain in the marrow for 48 to 72 hours before being released to the blood. The reticulocytes have an irregular polylobated shape and various membrane-bound organelles.[36] In the blood, immature erythrocytes (reticulocytes) undergo further maturation with the removal of vestiges of organelles and reconditioning of the membrane to become mature red blood cells with the morphology of a biconcave disk.[37]

The number of erythroid precursor cells determines to a great extent the number of red cells produced. The proerythroblasts also contain EPORs that, in the presence of higher than normal levels of EPO, may accelerate their entry into their first mitotic division. This process may lead to a shortened marrow transit time of erythroblasts[38] and result in release of still immature erythrocytes (polychromatophilic macrocytes), so-called stress reticulocytes (Fig. 32–2).[39] Creation of a normal sized and shaped red cells, devoid of organelles, is the end result of an orderly transformation of a proerythroblast with a large nucleus and a volume of approximately 900 fL to a hemoglobinized anucleate disc-shaped cell with a volume of approximately 90 fL. Although cytoplasmic maturation is continuous, the interposed mitotic divisions cause a stepwise reduction in cytoplasmic and nuclear volumes, enabling recognition of proerythroblasts, erythroblasts, and polychromatophilic macrocytes (reticulocytes) with light microscopy (Chap. 31). Direct measurements of the number of

marrow erythroblasts and reticulocytes have shown approximately 50 erythroblasts and approximately 124 reticulocytes for each proerythroblast (Table 32–1).[40,41] This distribution conforms to the number of cells in a theoretic erythroid pyramid (Table 32–1, Fig. 32–3). In the pyramid, each erythroblast undergoes five mitotic divisions over 5 days before the orthochromatic erythroblast loses its nucleus and as an immature erythrocyte enters a 2- to 3-day period of maturation before its release from the marrow. The size and shape of these erythroid pyramids undoubtedly vary, but such variations play a role in the physiologic control of red cell production. When production is suppressed, as in low EPO as seen in anemia of chronic renal disease, the distribution of erythroblasts appears normal, with no morphologic or ferrokinetic evidence of ineffective erythropoiesis but the number of erythroid progenitors is decreased.[38] When production is increased, as in severe hemolytic anemia, the pyramid of erythroid precursors also appear normal, with no evidence of additional mitotic divisions but the number of erythroid progenitors is increased. Consequently, the rate of red cell production largely depends on the number of erythroid progenitors formed.

As the erythroblast matures, its synthetic activities increase rapidly, producing all proteins characteristic of mature red blood cells, particularly globin. Eventually 95 percent of all protein in the red cell is hemoglobin, almost all hemoglobin A ($\alpha_2\beta_2$) in adults, with only small amounts of hemoglobin F ($\alpha_2\gamma_2$) and hemoglobin A_2 ($\alpha_2\delta_2$). Hemoglobin F is unequally distributed and is present only in some erythrocytes, designated as F cells (Chaps. 48 and 49).

EPOR density declines sharply on early erythroblasts, and EPORs are absent from the more mature erythroblast forms while the number of receptors for transferrin increases, reflecting the increased demands for iron for heme synthesis.

ERYTHROBLAST ENUCLEATION

The microenvironment may be important for proliferation and maturation of erythroblasts. However, *in situ* secreted or circulating growth factors and cytokines appear to be less important for precursor cells than for progenitor cells. Intercellular adhesion molecules secure the structural integrity of the marrow, and fibronectin is of special importance for erythroblasts.[42] Loss of fibronectin receptors heralds the translocation of polychromatophilic macrocytes (reticulocytes) into blood, but some newly emerging erythrocytes remain sticky even after release and are temporarily sequestered by the spleen (Chap. 6). Because erythroid colonies developed *in vitro* consist principally of nucleated red cells, enucleation may primarily be induced by marrow stromal cells (Chaps. 5 and 31).

The extrusion of the spent pyknotic nuclei at terminal erythroid maturation is unique to mammals. This process results in the formation of pliable biconcave disc from rigid spheroidal cells. Enucleation decreases workload of the heart as it reduces one-third of the erythrocyte weight. The retinoblastoma protein and its effector, E2f-2, are critical for erythroid cells to exit the cell cycle for enucleation to take place.[43] During terminal differentiation, the plasma membrane forms an envelope around the nucleus, followed by the formation of the contractile actin ring on the plasma membrane to move the nucleus for disposal.[44] Rac guanosine triphosphatases (GTPases) and their effector mDia2 are required for the contractile actin ring movement in the release of the nucleus.[45] After separation from the cell, the expelled nucleus displays phosphatidylserine and is recognized and engulfed by macrophages.[46] Emp, an erythroblast–macrophage protein initially identified as a mediator of erythroblast–macrophage interactions, also plays a role in the enucleation.[47] Emp associates with F-actin, an interaction important for the normal distribution of F-actin in both

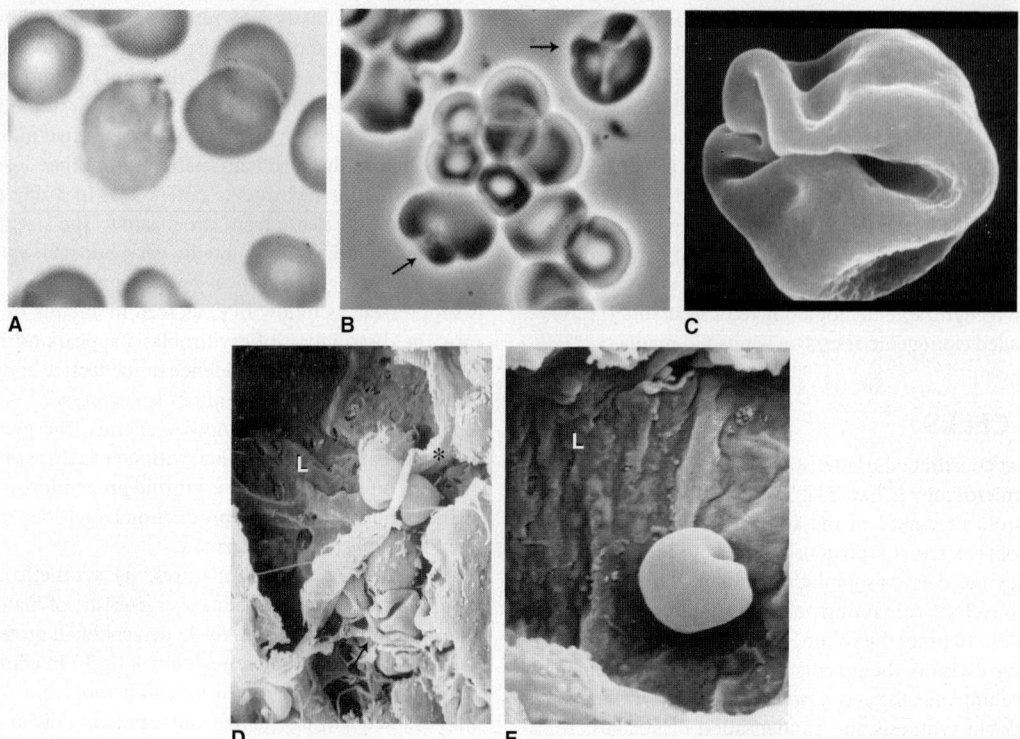

Figure 32–2. Stress reticulocytes. **A.** Blood film. Hemolytic anemia. The polychromatophilic macrocyte with puckering evident by the clover-leaf-shaped clear areas (folds) is a characteristic stress erythrocyte, so named because they are prematurely released from the marrow by high levels of erythropoietin, usually as a result of a hemolytic anemia. They are large, intensely polychromatophilic, and often have evidence of excess surface area as evident by folds. **B.** Phase-contrast microscopy of the blood cells in suspension from a case of hemolytic anemia. The *arrows* point to two macrocytes with puckered (folded) surfaces, characteristic of stress reticulocytes. **C.** A scanning electron micrograph of a stress reticulocyte. Note the markedly increased surface area to volume relationship for a red cell. **D.** Scanning electron micrograph of a marrow sinus of a mouse. *L* denotes the sinus lumen. The *asterisk* is the edge of the endothelial lining of the sinus, torn in preparation for microscopy. The *arrow* points to two anucleate red cells folded amidst the reticular cell extensions that make up the stroma of marrow. Note the severe folding of reticulocytes *in situ*. Note similarity between folds of the cell to the scanning image in **(C)**. Just below the *asterisk* is an enucleated red cell (reticulocyte) half in the hematopoietic space and half in the lumen, presumptively in egress. Note the surface folding required when traversing the narrow pore in endothelium. **E.** A marrow sinus with an anucleate red cell emerging into the lumen. Note the folding required to negotiate the narrow pore through which the cell is exiting. (Chapter 3 provides details of erythrocyte egress.) *(Reproduced with permission from* Lichtman's Atlas of Hematology, *www.accessmedicine.com.)*

erythroblasts and macrophages. Emp null mice do not extrude their nuclei from erythroid cells. Thus, Emp appears to be required for erythroblast enucleation.[48]

Microscopic determination of marrow cellularity and proportion of erythroblasts permits semiquantitative evaluation of erythropoiesis.

TABLE 32–1.	Erythroid Pools	
	Cell Number × 10^8 per kg/Body Weight	
Cell Type	**Observed***	**Theoretic Model (Fig. 31–3)**
Proerythroblasts	1	1
Erythroblasts	49	58
Marrow reticulocytes	82	64
Blood reticulocytes	31	32
Mature red cells	3300	3800

Data from Donohue DM, Reiff RH, Hanson ML, et al.: Quantitative measurement of the erythrocytic and granulocytic cells of the marrow and blood. *J Clin Invest* 37(11):1571-1576, 1958 and Finch CA, Harker LA and Cook JD: Kinetics of the formed elements of human blood. *Blood* 50(4):699–707, 1977.

However, the presence of ineffective erythropoiesis in disease states, such as iron deficiency, anemia of chronic disease, megaloblastic anemias, and thalassemias, makes the morphologic approach misleading (Chaps. 37, 41, 42, and 48). Red cell production can be accurately estimated by ferrokinetic studies using ^{59}Fe. Similarly, the amount of the final product of erythropoiesis, the red cell mass, can also be accurately measured. Unfortunately, the ever-increasing regulation of even minute amounts of radioisotopes used *in vivo* makes these methods available in only a few specialized centers.

Chapters 7, 30, 47, and 48 discuss developmental control of erythropoiesis, differential use of enzyme and globin genes, and the crucial differences between embryonic yolk sac and fetal/adult definite erythropoiesis. This chapter focuses mainly on adult erythropoiesis.

REGULATION OF ERYTHROPOIESIS

Erythropoiesis is a tightly regulated system, but the details are still not fully elucidated. Much remains to be learned from uncovering the molecular basis of many congenital and acquired mutations that disrupt the control of erythropoiesis. Two competing hypothesis have been proposed to explain the differentiation of the hematopoietic progenitors cells toward erythroid lineage.

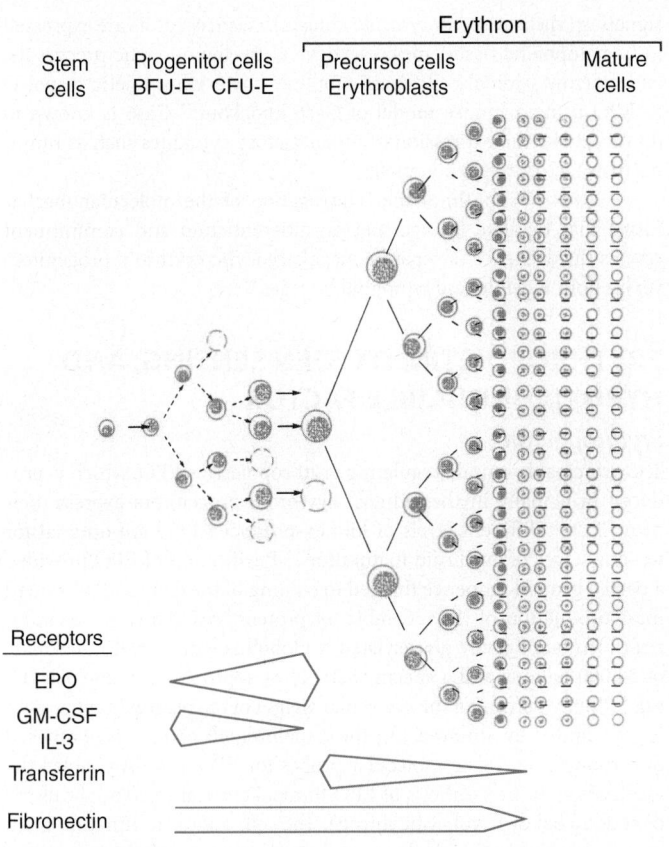

Figure 32–3. Theoretical model of proliferation of erythroid-committed marrow cells, including their most important receptors. BFU-E, burst-forming units–erythroid; CFU-E, colony-forming units–erythroid; EPO, erythropoietin; GM-CSF, granulocyte-macrophage colony-stimulating factor; IL, interleukin.

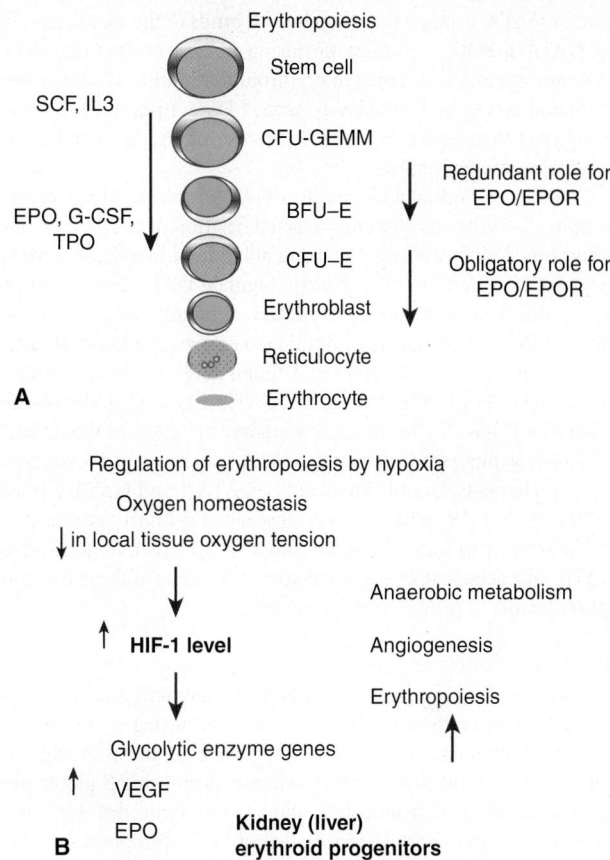

Figure 32–4. A. Cytokine influence on hematopoiesis. CFU-GEMM, colony-forming unit–growing granulocyte, erythrocyte, megakaryocyte, and macrophage precursors; G-CSF, granulocyte colony-stimulating factor; IL3, interleukin-3; SCF, stem cell factor; TPO, thrombopoietin. **B.** Regulation of erythropoiesis by hypoxia. HIF-1 hypoxia inducible factor-1; VEGF, vascular endothelial growth factor 1.

DETERMINISTIC MODEL OF LINEAGE COMMITMENT

According to the deterministic model of lineage commitment, specific extracellular signals, such as cytokines, play an instructive role in lineage specification.

Multipotential progenitors (Chap. 18) and erythroid unipotential progenitors, the BFU-E, require stem cell factor, interleukin-3, granulocyte-macrophage colony-stimulating factor, and/or thrombopoietin for growth and survival (Fig. 32–4).

STOCHASTIC MODEL OF ERYTHROID DIFFERENTIATION

In contrast, the stochastic model proposes that spontaneous formation of a set of transcription factors, independently of extrinsic signals, mediates lineage commitment. These transcription factors activate a unique set of genes for a particular lineage and repress the action of alternative transcription factors and cytokines play only a permissive role. Most of evidence based on gene targeting studies and *in vitro* culture studies support the stochastic model of differentiation. Several transcription factors, such as GATA-1, FOG1, erythroid Kruppel-like factor (EKLF), PU.1, and SCL/TAL1 (stem cell leukemia/T-cell acute lymphoblastic leukemia 1 factor) have been characterized that are involved in erythroid differentiation.

The GATA family of zinc-finger transcription factors was first identified as the nuclear factors that bind to the GATA sequence in the

enhancer region of the globin genes.[49,50] GATA-1 protein is expressed during erythroid differentiation, with highest expression in CFU-Es and pronormoblasts. GATA-1 promotes erythroid differentiation by activating several erythroid-specific genes and represses transcription of Kit receptor and GATA-2. GATA-1 deficient mice die at embryonic day 10.5 with severe anemia from maturation arrest at the stage of pronormoblasts.[51] *In vitro*, GATA-1 null the embryonic stem cells fail to mature beyond pronormoblast and undergo apoptosis. GATA-1 and its cofactor CBP are essential for the formation of an erythroid-specific histone acetylation pattern of histones at the active globin genes and the β-globin locus control region.[52] GATA-1, along with EPO, induces expression of the antiapoptotic protein Bcl-x_L[53] and interacts with multiple proteins, including FOG-1 and PU.1,[54] and FOG-1 acts as a cofactor for GATA-1.[55] GATA-1 interaction with PU.1 appears to counteract erythropoiesis by inducing differentiation of pluripotent stem cell to myeloid and B lymphopoiesis and inhibition of erythropoiesis.[54,56,57] Whereas PU.1 absence appears to be required for completion of terminal erythroid differentiation, low levels of PU.1 expression are essential for fetal erythropoiesis and for proper augmentation of adult erythropoiesis at times of stress.[58]

Friends of GATA

FOG-1, a member of friend of GATA family of zinc finger proteins, act as cofactors for GATA-1. It was first identified in a yeast two-hybrid screen for GATA-1 interacting proteins.[55] It binds to the amino zinc finger of GATA-1. FOG-1−/− mice die during embryonic days 10.5 to 11.5 from severe anemia with arrest in erythroid maturation at a stage similar to that observed in the GATA-1− mice.[59] FOG-1 physically interacts with GATA-1 to augment or inhibit its transcriptional activity depending on the promoter context.

GATA-2 was initially cloned as a GATA motif-binding factor is present in all erythroid cells; and, targeted deletion of GATA-2 resulted in embryonic lethality at day 10.5 from ablation of blood cell development.[60] GATA-1 and GATA-2 directly regulate GATA-2 transcription in a reciprocal fashion during erythroid differentiation.[61,62] GATA-2 autoregulates its transcription by binding to its own regulatory elements in the promoter region. This autoregulation is abolished by the displacement of GATA-2 by GATA-1 (GATA-2/GATA-1 switch), an interaction facilitated by FOG-1.[63] Chromatin immunoprecipitation studies indicate that FOG-1 facilitates occupancy by GATA-1 at selected *cis*-regulatory chromatin elements. Double knockout of GATA-1 and GATA-2 results in embryonic lethality with complete absence of primitive erythropoiesis.[64] The severity of this phenotype compared to either single GATA-1 or GATA-2 knockout suggests overlapping functions of these two transcription factors in primitive erythropoiesis.

Kruppel-like Factor

EKLF is a zinc finger protein identified by subtractive hybridization of the mRNA of erythroid cells with common messages in a myeloid cell line.[65] It interacts with CACCC sequence in the β-globin promoter, where it modifies chromatin structure permitting β-globin gene transcription. EKLF-deficient mice die at embryonic day 14.5 to 15 from severe anemia from defective definitive erythropoiesis.[66] There is a marked decrease in β-globin mRNA and protein levels in EKLF-deficient erythroid cells. Large amounts of iron accumulate in the reticuloendothelial system of EKLF-deficient mice, consistent with an ineffective erythropoiesis.

STEM CELL LEUKEMIA/T-CELL ACUTE LYMPHOBLASTIC LEUKEMIA 1

SCL/TAL1 is a member of basic helix-loop-helix transcription factors essential for maturation of the erythroid and megakaryocytic lineages.[67] Knockout of SCL/TAL1 leads to failure of hematopoiesis.[68] Selective rescue of SCL/TAL1 null embryonic stem cells under the control of stem cell enhancer revealed differentiation blocks in erythroid and megakaryocytic maturation.[69] Conditional knockout studies have revealed that erythroid and megakaryocytic precursors do not develop in the marrow of mice upon deletion of SCL/TAL1.[70] Heterodimerization of SCL with other transcription factors, such as E2A, is a prerequisite for its functions.[71]

BCL11A, a transcription factor initially identified in lymphoid cells, regulates erythroid differentiation, especially in switching from fetal to adult hemoglobin.[71] Fetal hemoglobin (HbF) levels decline after birth and are then replaced by adult hemoglobin A. The molecular mechanisms responsible for this switch are not completely known. Genome-wide association findings have provided a major breakthrough in understanding this phenomenon.[72] There is an inverse correlation between BCL11A and HbF expression in erythroid cells. BCL11A occupies several discrete sites in the β-globin gene cluster and likely plays an important role in hemoglobin switching during erythroid differentiation.

GROWTH ARREST-SPECIFIC 6 PROTEIN

Growth arrest-specific 6 (Gas6) protein is a secreted vitamin K–dependent protein that interacts with cell membranes and leads to intracellular signaling (via its receptor tyrosine kinases). Gas6 receptors are expressed in hematopoietic tissue, megakaryocytes, myelomonocytic precursors, and marrow stromal cells. Gas6 amplifies the erythropoietic response to EPO using a mouse model of Gas6 knockout.[73] Gas6 is known to downregulate the expression of inflammatory cytokines such as tumor necrosis factor-α by macrophages.[74]

Figure 32-5 outlines the interrogation of the molecular mechanisms that regulate lineage-specific differentiation and commitment reveals the existence of separate megakaryocytic/erythroid progenitors versus both myeloid and lymphoid lineages.[75]

ERYTHROPOIETIN, OXYGEN SENSING, AND HYPOXIA-INDUCIBLE FACTOR

Erythropoietin

The principal hormone regulating erythropoiesis is EPO, which is produced principally in the kidney.[7] Erythroid progenitors express their own EPO.[76] Different levels of kidney-produced EPO are optimal for various stages of erythroid maturation.[77] Purification of EPO provided a partial protein sequence that led to cloning of the gene and permitted mass production of the recombinant protein.[78] EPO and its recombinant form are heavily glycosylated α-globulins with a molecular mass of 34,000 daltons and a specific activity of approximately 200,000 IU/mg.[79,80] Sixty percent of the molecular weight of the recombinant protein is contributed by amino acids; the remaining 40 percent is composed of carbohydrate. Using molecular probes for *EPO*, mRNA enabled the localization of the synthesis of EPO to renal cortical interstitial cells[81,82] of endothelial or fibroblastic lineage. The cells appear to function in an all-or-none fashion, with the overall production of mRNA dependent on the number of cells activated.[83]

Certain 5′ sequences located 6000 to 12,000 bp upstream also affect EPO gene transcription.[84] These sequences are not hypoxia sensitive but appear necessary for tissue and cellular specificity.[84] Hepatic production is contributed primarily by hepatocytes but is a much less important source than is the kidney.[85] During fetal life, however, hepatic EPO production is of major importance for red cell production (Chap. 7).[86,87] EPO production is regulated exclusively at the level of its transcription by hypoxia at the transcription level. The transcriptional activation of the EPO gene is controlled by a specific sequence located in the 3′ flanking region termed *hypoxia-responsive element*.[88–90] The core of the enhancer is constituted by the sequence CACGTGCT and mutations in this core sequence abolish hypoxia responsiveness.

EPO is not stored; it is secreted immediately.[81–83] Circulating recombinant EPO and presumably native EPO have a half-life ($T_{1/2}$) of 4 to 12 hours, with a volume of distribution slightly larger than that of the plasma volume.[91] EPO is degraded after it binds to EPOR (see "Erythropoietin Receptor" below).[92]

Erythropoietin Receptor

Interaction of EPO with its receptor EPOR results in (1) stimulation of erythroid cell division, (2) erythroid differentiation by induction of erythroid-specific protein expression, and (3) prevention of erythroid progenitor apoptosis.[93] Earlier models of this interaction were based on the ligand (EPO)-induced homodimerization of EPOR. In reality, EPOR is a preformed homodimer that undergoes a major conformational change upon binding,[94] which initiates the EPO-specific erythroid signal transduction cascade (Fig. 32–6). The cytoplasmic portion of EPOR contains a positive regulatory domain that interacts with Janus kinase 2 (JAK2).[95] Immediately after EPO binding, JAK2 cross-phosphorylates the EPOR itself, and other proteins such as STAT5 (signal transducer and activator of transcription 5), thus initiating a cascade of erythroid-specific signaling.[96] JAK2/STAT5

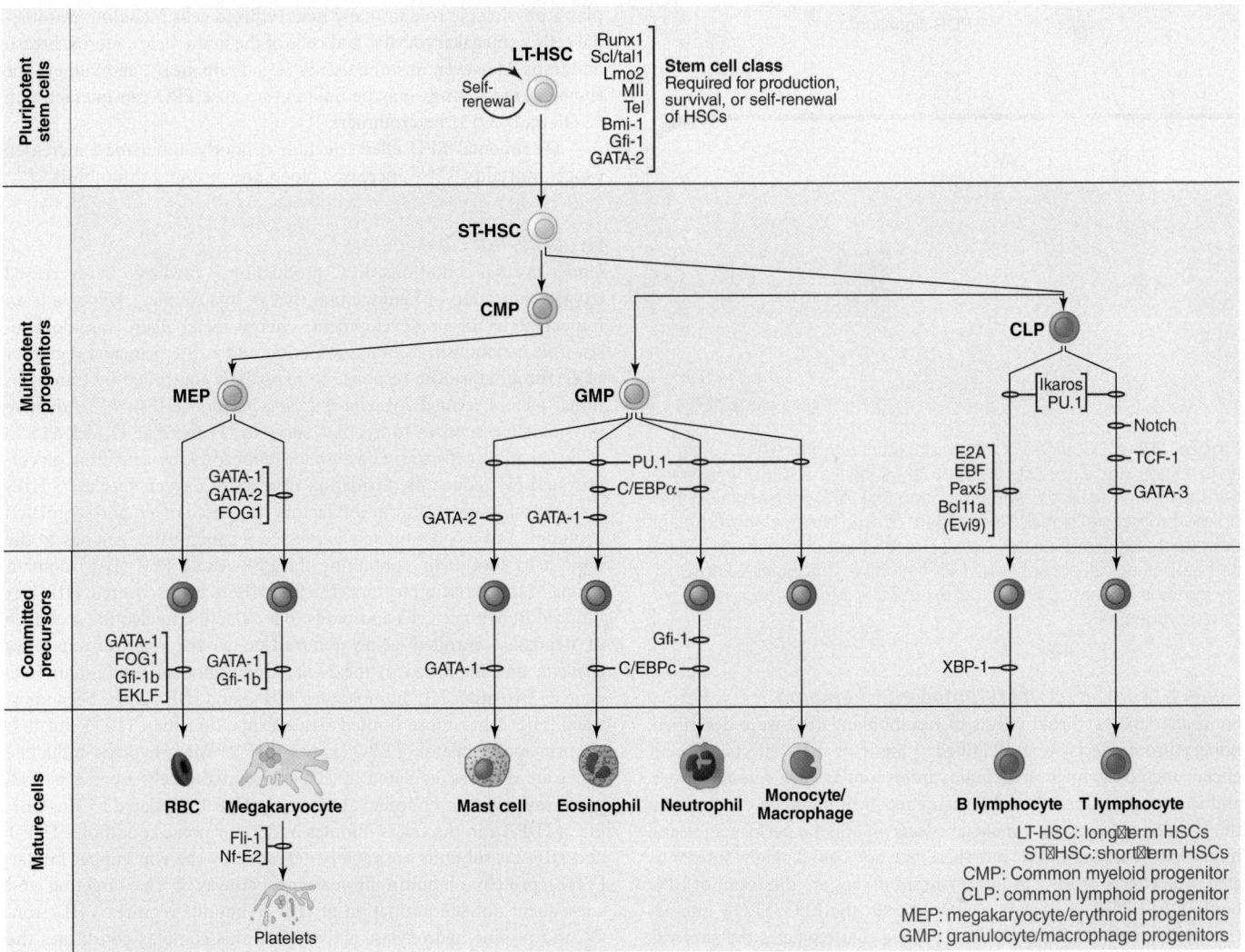

Figure 32–5. Schematic outline of emerging hierarchy of hematopoiesis outlining a separate progenitor for erythroid/megakaryocytic lineage (MEP). RUNX-1, Scl1/Tal1, Lmo1, MllTel, PU-1, GATA-1, GATA-2, gf-1,C/EBPα, FOG1, EKLF, Ikaros, E2A, EBF, PAX-5, BCL 11A, NOTCH, TCF-1 are transcription factors. CLP, common lymphoid progenitor; CMP, common myeloid progenitor; GMP, granulocyte/macrophage progenitor; LT-HSC, long-term hematopoietic stem cell; MEP, megakaryocyte/erythroid progenitor; RBCs, red blood cells; ST-HSC, short-term hematopoietic stem cell. *(Reproduced with permission from Orkin SH1, Zon LI: Hematopoiesis: an evolving paradigm for stem cell biology. Cell 22;132(4):631–644, 2008.)*

signaling plays an essential role in EPO–EPOR–mediated regulation of erythropoiesis (see Fig. 32–6).[97] Deficiency of EPO–EPOR is lethal by abrogating fetal liver erythropoiesis (but not the "primitive" yolk sac erythropoiesis). However, in these *EPO* or *EPOR* knockout mice, differentiation of pluripotential stem cells to BFU-E occurs, but not the subsequent erythroid differentiation. This occurrence demonstrates the crucial role of EPO in terminal erythroid maturation.[35,98,99] The C-terminal cytoplasmic portion of EPOR also possesses a domain essential for prevention of apoptosis (see Fig. 32–6) by inducing expression of Bcl-x$_L$ via phosphoinositide 3′-kinase (PI3K).[53] However, the cytoplasmic portion of EPOR also contains a negative regulatory domain[100] that interacts with hematopoietic cell phosphatase (HCP, also known as SHP1) and down-modulates signal transduction.[101] Once recruited by EPOR tyrosine (Y)429, HCP attaches to the cytoplasmic EPOR domain and dephosphorylates JAK2. Inactivation of the HCP binding site leads to prolonged phosphorylation of JAK2/STAT5.[101,102] CIS3 (also known as SOCS3), another negative regulator of erythropoiesis, binds to the cytoplasmic portion of the EPOR Y401 and suppresses EPO-dependent JAK2/STAT5 signaling.[103,104] Thus, deletion of the distal C-terminal cytoplasmic portion of EPOR results in a truncated EPOR, abolishes

negative regulatory elements, and results in increased proliferation of erythroid progenitor cells. Gain-of-function mutations resulting from deletion of the negative regulatory domain of the *EPOR* gene (Chap. 57) have been demonstrated in a small proportion of individuals with primary familial and congenital polycythemia, but are rarely found in erythroleukemia[105]; however, the rearranged EPOR has also been identified in a subtype of high-risk B-progenitor acute lymphoblastic leukemia.[106]

Because the activation signal after EPO binding to its receptor is rapidly downregulated and EPO briskly disappears after binding to EPOR, EPO–EPOR internalization is one mechanism of downregulation of EPO signaling.[92] After EPO binds to the receptor, EPO–EPOR complexes are ubiquinated, rapidly internalized, and targeted for degradation. This process involves two proteolytic systems, the proteosomes that remove part of the intracellular domain of EPOR at the cell surface and the lysosomes that degrade the EPO–EPOR complex in the cytoplasm.[107]

Another incompletely understood mechanism of erythropoiesis regulation is the presence of several EPOR isoforms, some of which may have an inhibitory function on erythropoiesis.[108–110]

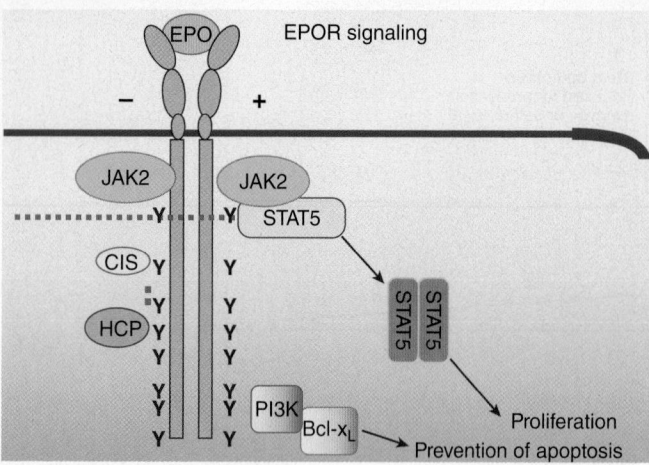

Figure 32–6. Outline of erythropoietin–erythropoietin receptor (EPO–EPOR) signaling. Activation of Janus kinase 2 (JAK2) and signal transducer and activator of transcription 5 (STAT5) represents erythropoiesis-promoting signals. Interaction of CIS, a signal transduction protein that downregulates activity of erythropoietin receptor, and hematopoietic cell phosphatase (HCP) inhibit erythropoiesis. Phosphatidylinositide 3'-kinase (PI3K) activation of Bcl-x$_L$ inhibits apoptosis of erythroid progenitors.

Nonerythroid Effect of Erythropoietin Signaling

Soon after the erythroid effects of recombinant EPO were described, nonerythroid effects were identified.[111] Some of these effects are beneficial, including roles in neural, cardiovascular, and retinal tissues, and in immune function and in tissue repair. It has been claimed that the hormone also exerts beneficial effects on athletic performance and improved neurocognition, but these are not convincingly substantiated. The effects of EPO in nonerythroid tissues are the result of EPO binding to EPOR, and, as in erythroid cells, the EPO–EPOR interaction initiates a signal transduction process that regulates the survival, growth and differentiation of the involved tissue.[112] EPO and EPOR

play a physiologic role in many nonerythroid cells including endothelial cells,[113] megakaryocytes, and cells of the brain, heart, uterus, breast, and testis. However, in some tissues (e.g., brain, heart, and kidney) the signaling mechanism may be different because EPO can interact with EPOR and CD131 heterodimers.[114,115]

Detrimental EPO effects include a poorly understood increased cancer mortality,[95,116,117] increased blood pressure, and thrombosis.[114]

Hypoxia-Inducible Factors

Under normal conditions, EPO production is mediated by decreased oxygen saturation of hemoglobin, that is, hypoxemia.[77] Hypoxia is an important factor in development, energy metabolism, vasculogenesis, iron metabolism, tumor promotion and is the principal regulator of erythropoiesis. The response to hypoxia is controlled by transcriptional factors termed *hypoxia-inducible factors* (HIFs).[118,119] Adaptive physiologic responses to hypoxia serve to (1) increase O$_2$ delivery to cells, (2) allow cells to survive under reduced O$_2$ by activating glycolysis, and (3) reduce the formation of reactive oxygen species.[120] HIFs are heterodimeric transcription factors composed of a highly-regulated α subunit and a constitutively expressed β subunit that belongs to the basic helix-loop-helix containing the PER-ARNT-SIM (PAS)-domain family of transcription factors. The first HIF to be discovered, HIF-1, is induced in hypoxic cells and binds to a *cis*-acting nucleotide sequence of hypoxia-controlled genes referred to as the *hypoxia-responsive element*, first identified in the 3'-flanking region of the human *EPO* gene.[121] Two other HIF homologues, HIF-2 and HIF-3, have been identified. HIF-2 has more limited tissue expression than HIF-1 but it is the principal regulator of EPO expression.[118,119] Many hypoxia-inducible genes are directly regulated by HIF-1. Approximately 3 percent of all genes expressed in endothelial tissue are HIF-1 regulated.[122] The half-life of HIF-1α in the cell is minutes under normoxic conditions. HIF-1 and HIF-2 α subunits are rapidly degraded by the von Hippel-Lindau (VHL) protein–ubiquitin–proteasome pathway.[123] The targeting and subsequent polyubiquitination of HIF α subunits requires VHL, iron, O$_2$, and proline hydroxylase activity, and this complex constitutes the oxygen sensor (Fig. 32-7).[124,125]

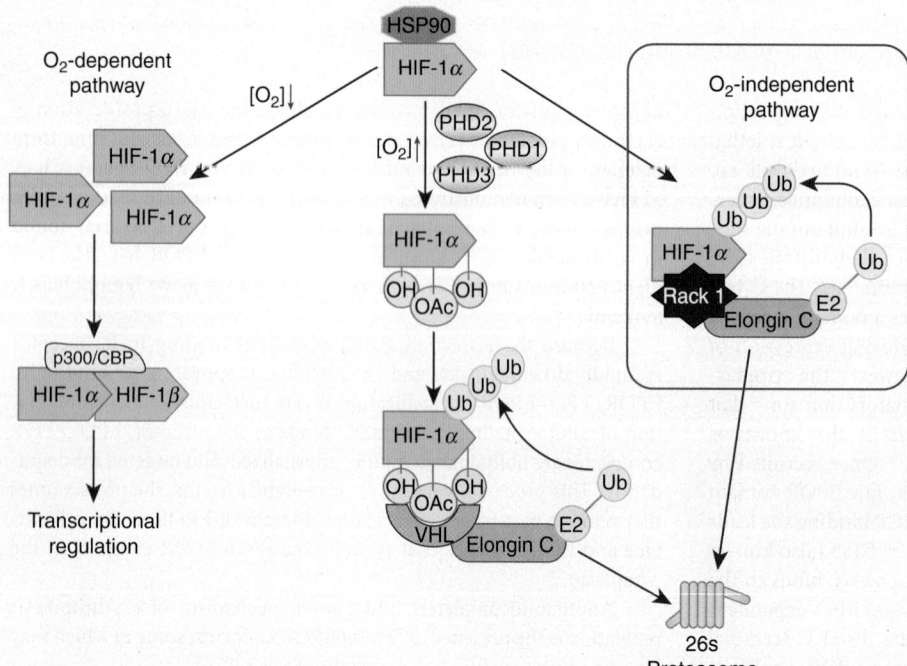

Figure 32–7. Schematic outline of regulation of HIF-2 and HIF-2α subunits by hypoxic and nonhypoxic pathways. HIF, hypoxia-inducible factor; HSP90, heat shock protein 90; PHDs, proline hydroxylases; p300 and CBP, cofactors of hypoxia response transcription with HIF-1; RACK1, receptor of activated protein kinase C; ub, ubiquitin residues; VHL, von Hippel-Lindau protein.

This degradation of HIFs α subunits is initiated by a posttranslational hydroxylation event at residue proline 564 (P564) that is mediated by one of several iron-containing proline hydroxylases (PHDs). The hydroxylation of HIFs α subunits facilitates binding to the VHL protein and subsequent ubiquitination and proteasomal degradation. Osteosarcoma protein 9 (OS-9) binds to both HIF-1α and PHD2 and is required for efficient prolyl hydroxylation.[126] Under hypoxic conditions, HIF-1 and HIF-2 α proteins are not degraded and are translocated to the cell nucleus where they dimerize with HIF-β to form the HIF heterodimer that activates transcription through binding to specific hypoxia-responsive elements on target genes. Another regulatory step involves O_2-dependent asparaginyl-hydroxylation of asparagine (N) 803 in HIF-1α that requires the enzyme HIF-3, also known as FIH-1 (factor inhibiting HIF-1). Hydroxylation of N803 during normoxia blocks the binding of transcription factors p300 and CBP to HIF-1, resulting in inhibition of HIF-1–mediated gene transcription. Under hypoxic conditions, HIF α subunits are not hydroxylated. The unmodified protein escapes VHL-binding, ubiquitination, and degradation (see Fig. 32–7). When N803 of HIF-1α is not asparaginyl-hydroxylated, p300 and CBP can bind to the HIF-1 heterodimer, allowing transcriptional activation of HIF-1 target genes.

HIF-2 Transcription Factor HIF-1α and HIF-2α exhibit a high degree sequence homology but have differing mRNA expression patterns: HIF-1α is expressed ubiquitously, whereas HIF-2α expression is restricted to certain tissues.[118,127] The kidney is the main site of EPO production (i.e., renal interstitial cells), and HIF-2 and, to a lesser degree, HIF-1 are the principal regulator of *EPO* transcription in the kidney.[118,127] In other tissues, such as brain[128] and liver[87] (which generates approximately 15 percent of circulating EPO), *EPO* gene transcription is HIF-2–dependent.[127] The discovery of an iron-responsive element in the 5′ untranslated region of *HIF-2α* reveals a novel regulatory link between iron availability and *HIF-2α* expression[129] that may also influence control of erythropoiesis. The importance of HIF-2α in regulation of *EPO* gene was demonstrated by a gain-of-function *HIF-2α* mutation causing erythrocytosis.[130]

Hypoxia-Independent Regulation of Hypoxia-Inducible Factor While O_2-dependent regulation of the HIF-1α subunit is mediated by prolyl hydroxylases, VHL protein, and the proteasomal complex, hypoxia-independent regulation of HIF-1α has been uncovered. This novel mechanism involves the receptor of activated protein kinase C (RACK1) as a HIF-1α–interacting protein that promotes prolyl hydroxylase/VHL-independent proteasomal degradation of HIF-1α. RACK1 competes with heat shock protein 90 (HSP90) for binding to the PAS-A domain of HIF-1α. HIF-1α degradation is abolished by loss-of-function RACK1. RACK1 binds to the proteasomal subunit, elongin-C, and promotes ubiquitination of HIF-1α (see Fig. 32–7). Therefore, RACK1 and HSP90 are the essential components of an O_2/PHD/VHL-independent mechanism for regulating HIF-1α.[131]

The rapid degradation of HIF is complex and tightly regulated, and mutations affecting the genes that encode the regulatory factors may underlie some of the unexplained congenital polycythemias.

This complex (Chaps. 34 and 57) constitutes the oxygen sensor (see Fig. 32–7).[124,125,132]

INSULIN-LIKE GROWTH FACTOR-1, RENIN–ANGIOTENSIN SYSTEM, AND HEMATOPOIESIS

Although *in vitro* studies of erythropoiesis have provided crucial information about the regulation of erythropoiesis, many experiments were performed in the presence of serum and serum-component proteins capable of stimulating and inhibiting erythropoiesis.[133,134] Using serum-free conditions, insulin-like growth factor-1 (IGF-1) can partially substitute for EPO in BFU-E cultures. Furthermore, anephric, nonanemic patients with no detectable EPO have elevated levels of IGF-1.[135]

● REMOVAL OF ERYTHROCYTE ORGANELLES

NIX-DEPENDENT CLEARANCE OF MITOCHONDRIA BY AUTOPHAGY

During terminal erythroid differentiation, erythroid cells discard all their internal organelles including mitochondria. Autophagy has been suggested to play an important role in this process based on early morphologic studies.[136,137] This is confirmed by studies using chemical inhibitors of autophagy and small interfering ribonucleic acid (siRNA) knockdown of essential autophagy associated genes.[138,139] At the initial stage of autophagy, a double-membrane structure is formed to sequester cytoplasmic components in autophagosomes. Autophagosomes then fuse with lysosomes and become autophagolysosomes to degrade the sequestered components. Mice deficient in a bcl-2 family member, Nix, a protein that is expressed during erythropoiesis and regulates mitochondrial apoptosis (autophagy), display defects in the clearance of mitochondria. Interestingly, the formation of autophagosomes in reticulocytes is normal in the absence of Nix, suggesting that Nix is not required for the initiation of autophagy or the formation of autophagosomes. Instead, mitochondria remain clustered outside of autophagosomes in Nix−/− reticulocytes.[138] This indicates that Nix is required for the sequestration of mitochondria by autophagosomes. Another study using virally transformed Nix−/− erythroid cells also reported defective inclusion of mitochondria by autophagosomes.[140] Therefore, Nix deficiency leads to a specific defect in mitochondrial removal without causing a general block in autophagy or erythroid maturation. Nix−/− reticulocytes are defective in the loss of mitochondrial membrane potential during *in vitro* maturation.[138]

DOWNREGULATION OF CELL SURFACE PROTEINS AND OTHER ORGANELLES

During erythroid maturation, reticulocytes release small vesicles containing cellular proteins. These vehicles are exosomes that are involved in the clearance of cell-surface proteins, such as acetyl cholinesterase, CD71 transferrin receptor and integrin $\alpha_4\beta_1$.[141,142] The enrichment of these surface molecules in exosomes suggests that the exosomal pathway plays a major role in the clearance of these surface molecules. Other cellular components, such as lysosomes, endoplasmic reticulum, Golgi apparatus, ribosomes, and RNA, are also cleared during erythroid maturation. The precise mechanisms for the removal of these components are unclear. In Nix-deficient mice, the loss of CD71 and ribosomes are normal during erythroid maturation, suggesting that exosomal pathways play a major role in the clearance of CD71 or ribosomes.[138]

● MICRORNAS IN ERYTHROPOIESIS

MicroRNAs (miRNAs) are small 18- to 22-nucleotide noncoding RNAs that regulate gene expression by inhibiting protein translation or by destabilizing target mRNAs; they are important regulators of hematopoiesis. The role of miRNAs in regulation of erythropoiesis is being actively defined. Some miRNAs are mainly expressed in early stages of erythropoiesis, others in late stages, and some have biphasic expression during erythroid differentiation. Some appear to have erythroid specific expression.[143] The critical role of miRNAs and their relationship to the essential transcription factors regulating erythropoiesis is outlined by the report that the pivotal transcription factors for erythropoiesis, GATA-1 and NFE-2, directly regulate and control differentiation via miRNA-199b-5p. This miRNA then targets c-Kit, an important receptor on early erythroid cells.[144] Some miRNAs likely play a role in the commitment to erythroid versus megakaryocytic differentiation. Thus, miRNA-18a was reported to be upregulated during erythropoiesis and downregulated during megakaryopoiesis, while miRNA-145 was upregulated in megakaryopoiesis and downregulated in erythropoiesis. Their mRNA targets and their functional significance are being defined.[145] LIN28B and its targeted let-7 have regulated expression during the fetal-to-adult erythroid cell transition.[146] Another important erythroid development and function is regulated by miRNA-351. A complex regulatory transcriptional repressor system controlling heterochromatin formation exists composed of KRAB-ZFP–mediated repression that include cofactor KAP1 (KRAB-associated protein-1). Deletion of KAP1 in mice upregulates miRNA-351 and several other microRNAs, which then downregulate Nix and mitochondrial autophagy (see "Neocytolysis" in Chap. 33), resulting in expansion of mitochondria in erythroid progenitors and severe hypoproliferative anemia phenotype.[147]

MEASUREMENTS OF RED CELL MASS

The red cell mass is maintained and regulated by the kidney and marrow, which, under steady-state conditions, precisely replaces cells lost by senescence. Red cell mass defines pathogenesis of anemia and polycythemia. The kinetics of red cell production and destruction helps establish their pathogenesis. A number of tests have been developed to measure the three main components of red cell kinetics: red cell mass, rate of red cell production, and rate of red cell destruction. Some of these tests are simple but indirect and only semiquantitative, such as hematocrit, reticulocyte count, haptoglobin, lactic dehydrogenase, and unconjugated bilirubin concentration. Examination of the marrow allows assessment of total cellularity and relative erythroid contribution but is limited in that the kinetics of cell production cannot be inferred from a single static image, obtained from a very small fraction of the whole marrow. These tests are very useful in the aggregate but can be supplemented by more complex but direct quantitation; however, most require use of radioisotopes.

HEMATOCRIT

Packed red cell volume is commonly referred as the *hematocrit* (Hct). It is measured as the percentage of the volume of whole blood that is made up by red blood cells. Historically, it was measured by centrifugation but modern counters measure Hct indirectly based on red cell count and the mean red cell volume (MCV). Total-body Hct is the volume of red cells in the body divided by the total blood volume. Blood Hct is the simplest and most widely used test for estimating the size of red cell mass. In most anemic patients, blood Hct gives an excellent approximation of total red cell mass and a functional estimation of the oxygen-carrying capacity and whole-blood viscosity. Its main drawback is that it is an indirect measure that is influenced by changes in plasma volume and may not reflect the size of the red cell mass in dehydrated patients. Dehydration usually is clinically apparent and in most cases can be taken into account when evaluating the significance of a specific Hct determination. Only direct measurement of red cell mass can differentiate between relative and absolute polycythemia. However, when the Hct is greater than 60 percent, almost all patients have an increase in total red cell mass.[148] The extent of the increase cannot be estimated accurately from a Hct measurement alone (Fig. 32–8).

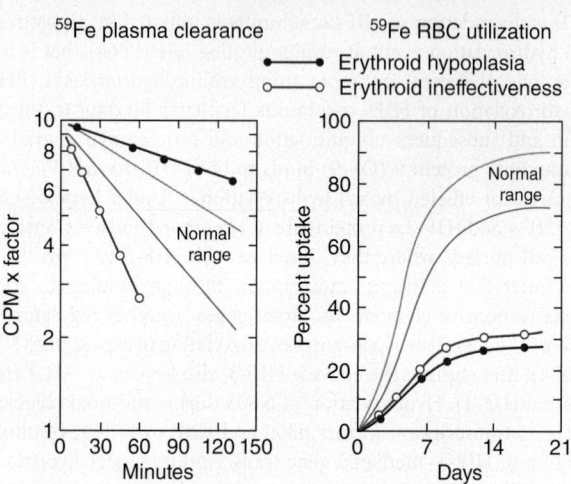

Figure 32–8. Iron clearance and iron utilization in normal subjects, patients with decreased effective red cell production (erythroid hypoplasia), and patients with ineffective red cell production. CPM, counts per minute; RBC, red blood cell.

RED CELL MASS AND PLASMA VOLUME

A more direct and accurate estimate of the size of the red cell mass is obtained from labeling a known volume of red cells and determining the dilution of this label in blood. Radioactive iron is an excellent label of red cells because it is biosynthetically incorporated into hemoglobin *in vivo*. In experimental animals, radioactive iron can be given to a donor animal and the donor's cells transfused into the animal whose red cell volume is being assessed. However, the radiation exposure to the donor and the hazards of transfusing allogeneic cells preclude its use in humans. Thus, almost all current clinical methods use labeling of autologous red cells *in vitro* by any one of a number of isotopes or biotin (Chap. 33). If studies must be performed in radiation-sensitive individuals, such as pregnant women, red cell labeling can be performed by nonradioactive chromium-123 or by biotin, which is detected with streptavidin coupled to a fluorochrome.[149] Among the isotopes available, chromium-51 (^{51}Cr) is the most widely used label, although technetium-99m (^{99m}Tc) is convenient and accurate.[150] Chromium in the form of the chromate ion (CrO_2^-) readily enters the red cell and binds to globin chains. Excess isotope in the incubation mixture can be removed by washing or by using ascorbic acid to reduce the chromate ion to a nonpermeant chromic ion. Approximately 15 minutes after injection of a known amount of labeled cells, a sample of blood is obtained; its volume, Hct, and radioactivity are determined; and the total red cell volume is calculated from the equation:

$$\text{Red cell mass (mL)} = \frac{\text{CPM of isotope injected}}{\text{CPM of red cells in sample}}$$

where CPM = counts per minute. Sampling time is generally 15 minutes. Chromium also labels white cells; thus, one should centrifuge and remove the buffy coat before labeling if the white cell count is elevated ($>25 \times 10^9$/L).

No theoretical objection exists to measuring the red cell mass using labeled cells. It is independent of the Hct of the blood used to measure radioactivity, and replicate determination can be made with a coefficient of variation of approximately 1.5 percent.[126] The principal problem lies in reporting the measured red cell mass. The total red cell mass can be expressed as a volume related to body surface (mL/m^2) or as a volume related to body weight (mL/kg). A committee of the International Committee on Standardization in Hematology (ICSH) has extensively examined existing data and concluded that the most reproducible expressions of red cell mass are related to body surface area estimated from height and weight[151]:

$$RCM_{Males} = (1486 \times S) - 285 \quad RCM_{Females} = (822 \times S) + (1.06 \times Age)$$

where RCM = red cell mass, S = body surface area in square meters, and Age = age in years. The calculated values, ±25 percent, included 98 percent of the measured male values and 99 percent of the measured female values.[13]

Despite the ICSH recommendation, the most common method is to report red cell mass values in terms of milliliters per kilogram. However, this method of expression gives erroneously low values in obese individuals because fat is hypovascular. A better method might be to express the red cell mass in terms of lean weight. In general, lean weight is 20 percent less than actual weight in normal males and 25 percent less in normal females.[150] However, estimation of lean weight in obese individuals is inaccurate. From a practical point of view, RCM probably is best reported in terms of actual weight, with mental adjustments made based on body configuration. In general, the RCM of normal females ranges from 23 to 29 mL/kg of body weight and of normal males ranges from 26 to 32 mL/kg of body weight.[151]

PLASMA LABELS

RCM also can be estimated from plasma volume. Radioactive iodine (^{125}I) is used to label albumin and measure its distribution volume.[152] Other radioactive isotopes of iodine other than ^{99m}Tc have been used, but ^{125}I has virtually supplanted all other plasma labels. Albumin labeled with radioactive iodine is commercially available, and a known amount is injected intravenously. Several blood samples are obtained within the first 15 minutes and centrifuged. CPM per milliliter of plasma is measured, plotted on semilogarithmic paper, and extrapolated to zero time. This procedure is necessary because, in contradistinction to labeled red cells, labeled albumin is removed gradually, beginning immediately after injection. Plasma volume is calculated according to the equation:

$$\text{Plasma volume (mL)} = \frac{\text{CPM of labeled albumin injected}}{\text{CPM mL plasma at 0 hour}}$$

The continuous exchange of intravascular with extravascular albumin is the major problem encountered when plasma volume is measured with labeled albumin. Even with extrapolation to 0 hour, plasma volume is somewhat larger than that measured with a strictly intravascular protein such as fibrinogen.[153] Consequently, if measurement of the plasma volume is used to calculate the size of the total red cell mass, it is a less-reliable measure than determining red cell mass directly with tagged red cells. This inaccuracy is further augmented by the fact that the venous Hct used to calculate red cell mass from measured plasma volume does not reflect accurately the distribution of plasma and red cells in the body. However, from a practical point of view, the results of estimating RCM from plasma volume are surprisingly accurate and have been advocated based on simplicity and low cost.[152]

● TOTAL-BODY HEMATOCRIT

When total RCM is measured with labeled red cells, the value is approximately 10 percent lower than that calculated from plasma volume and the Hct of blood. In fact, the mean Hct of blood in all of the vessels (total-body Hct) clearly is somewhat lower than the Hct measured from blood obtained from large vessels; these differences are a result of varying proportions of plasma in different size vessels.

Generally, the ratio of total-body Hct as estimated by direct measurements of red cell volume and plasma volume to the large-vessel Hct ranges from 0.89 to 0.92.[154] Consequently, when using the determined plasma volume to calculate RCM and total blood volume, a correction factor is necessary, and a value of 0.90 is generally used:

$$\text{Corrected red cell mass} = \frac{\text{Hct} \times \text{plasma volume} \times 0.90}{100 - \text{Hct}}$$

Recommended procedures for determination and evaluation of blood volume are outlined by the ICSH.[155]

● MEASUREMENTS OF RED CELL PRODUCTION

Under normal circumstances, most human red cells produced in the marrow live, or have the potential to live, a normal life span. Under certain conditions, however, a fraction of red cell production is ineffective; with destruction of nonviable red cells either within the marrow or shortly after the cells reach the blood.[38]

EFFECTIVE RED CELL PRODUCTION

Effective erythropoiesis is most simply estimated by determining the reticulocyte count. Most modern automated counters measure reticulocytes by nucleic acid binding dyes such as thiazole orange using flow cytometry. These are fast reliable assays. This count usually is expressed as the percentage of red cells that are reticulocytes, but it also can be expressed as the total number of circulating reticulocytes per unit of blood (absolute reticulocyte count and corrected reticulocyte counts; equation 1 below).

Equation 1

$$\text{Absolute reticulocyte count} = \frac{\% \text{ reticulocytes} \times \text{red cell count}}{100}$$

A simple clinical method to estimate effective erythropoiesis uses the reticulocyte count to calculate the reticulocyte index (see equation 2 below).[156] This measurement depends on several assumptions: (1) the human red cell life span is approximately 100 days (actually approximately 115); (2) the life span is finite and, thus, the oldest 1 of 100 or 1 percent of red cells is removed (and replaced) each day; (3) the reticulocyte is identifiable as such in the blood for 1 day using supravital stain; and (4) the reticulocyte count of 1 percent in a person with a normal Hct represents normal red cell production and thus "1" is the basal reticulocyte index.

In anemic patients, two calculations are needed to measure the reticulocyte index and compare it to the normal of 1 in the basal state. To correct the reticulocyte percentage for the lower red cell count in anemic subjects, the reticulocyte percent is multiplied by the ratio of the patient's Hct over the normal mean Hct, providing a corrected reticulocyte percent.

Conversion of the reticulocyte count (see equation 1 above) to the reticulocyte index (equation 2 below) is achieved by taking into account the estimated life span of reticulocytes. The life span of reticulocytes in blood in a normal individual is approximately 1 day. However, when red cell production is increased under conditions of erythropoietic stress, for example, in severe anemia, reticulocytes are released prematurely and circulate as reticulocytes for 2 to 4 days, except in situations with low EPO levels, as in renal insufficiency. These appear as polychromatophilic erythrocytes on Wright-stained blood film and are called stress or shift reticulocytes.

Equation 2

$$\text{Reticulocyte index} = \frac{\text{corrected reticulocyte \%}}{\text{correction factor (usually 2)}}$$

Accordingly, the corrected reticulocyte percent may give an erroneous impression of the actual rate of daily red cell production. To take this situation into account when estimating the rate of red cell production in anemic patients with high reticulocyte counts, dividing the corrected reticulocyte percent by a factor may provide a more accurate estimate of red cell production.[156] For simplicity, an average factor of 2 often is used; however, the factor depends on the degree of anemia: 1.5 in mild cases, 2.5 in moderate cases, and 3.0 in severe cases.

An example follows: A patient with autoimmune hemolytic anemia has a Hct of 10 and reticulocyte count of 70 percent. The marrow cannot increase production by 70-fold. To measure the approximate true increase, we calculate the reticulocyte index as follows: corrected reticulocyte percent = 70 × 10/45 = 15, and the reticulocyte index = 15/3= 5 × basal. Thus, marrow erythroid production in response to this severe anemia has increased fivefold, a plausible response to this severity of hemolytic anemia.

INEFFECTIVE RED CELL PRODUCTION

Ineffective erythropoiesis is suspected when the reticulocyte count is normal or only slightly increased despite erythroid hyperplasia of the marrow. Ineffective erythropoiesis was first recognized as an entity from the study of isotope incorporation into fecal urobilin following administration of labeled glycine, a precursor of heme.[157] Two peaks were observed: an early peak at 3 to 5 days and a late peak at 100 to 120 days. One of the sources of the early labeled peak was suggested to be the hemoglobin of red cells that had never completed their development, having been destroyed either in the marrow or shortly after reaching the blood. Subsequent studies revealed that in certain disorders, such as pernicious anemia, thalassemia, and sideroblastic anemia, ineffective erythropoiesis is a major component of total erythropoiesis. This component can be quantitated by measuring ^{15}N-labeled glycine incorporation into the early bilirubin peaks[157] or ferrokinetics.[38] Calculated from bilirubin peaks and turnover, ineffective erythropoiesis under normal conditions amounts to approximately 4 to 12 percent of total erythropoiesis. Using ferrokinetic methods, ineffective erythropoiesis is calculated as the difference between total plasma iron turnover and erythrocyte iron turnover plus storage iron turnover (see "Ferrokinetics"). The values estimated from such studies in normal subjects are higher, ranging from 14 to 34 percent.[38] However, the results, both high and low, probably are misleading because none of the methods actually measures cell death, only the turnover of heme and iron. It is possible that little premature death of cells occurs in normal subjects, but much of the early release of bilirubin and iron is derived from the rim of hemoglobin extruded during enucleation of erythroblasts (Chap. 31).

TOTAL ERYTHROPOIESIS

Total erythropoiesis, which is the sum of effective and ineffective red cell production, can be estimated from a marrow examination. Films or sections from marrow aspirates and biopsies are first examined for relative content of fat and hematopoietic tissue. This examination gives an estimate of overall hematopoietic activity within the marrow space. A differential count then is performed, determining the ratio between granulocytic and erythroid precursors (M:E ratio). In a normal adult, the ratio is approximately 3:1 to 5:1. The ratio can be used to estimate whether erythropoiesis is normal, increased, or decreased (Chap. 3).

The ratio is only an approximation of total erythroid activity because the ratio can be altered by changing the myeloid and erythroid components, and an aspirate or biopsy of a small segment of the marrow may not always reflect total marrow activity. These assumptions are valid as long as the marrow reflects the steady-state, if the marrow is recovering from aplasia, or is developing aplasia, it will not accurately reflect output of mature red cells. However, when used in conjunction with determination of red blood cell count and reticulocyte count, under most circumstances the ratio provides qualitative information about the rate and effectiveness of red blood cell production. A more accurate quantitation of total erythropoiesis can be made by measuring the rate of production of red cells (ferrokinetics) or, in steady-state conditions, the rate of destruction of red cells (red cell life span, bilirubin production, carbon monoxide excretion).

FERROKINETICS

In 1950, Huff and associates[158] described a method for measuring the rate of red cell production utilizing a simple model of iron metabolism (Fig. 32–9; Chap. 42). In this method, radioactive iron is complexed to transferrin *in vitro* and injected intravenously. Alternatively, ^{59}Fe can be injected directly intravenously as the gluconate without preincubation with the patient's own plasma, providing enough unbound transferrin is available, because binding is almost instantaneous. The rate of clearance of the transferrin-bound iron from the plasma (^{59}Fe plasma $T_{1/2}$) and the subsequent uptake in the red cells are measured. From these two values and from determinations of plasma iron concentration and plasma volume, the rate of formation of red cells can be calculated.[38]

The initial clearance of iron is exponential, and sampling during this period can be used to calculate $T_{1/2}$. In normal individuals, initial clearance averages approximately 90 minutes. Initial clearance is shorter in patients with hyperplasia of the erythropoietic tissue and longer in patients with marrow hypoplasia (see Fig. 32–9). However, the clearance rate is not a direct measurement of erythropoietic activity because it depends on the size of the pool of unlabeled, circulating iron. Consequently, calculation of the plasma iron turnover rate must include the plasma iron concentration. Clearance is expressed in milligrams of iron. The point of reference can be hemoglobin mass, blood volume,

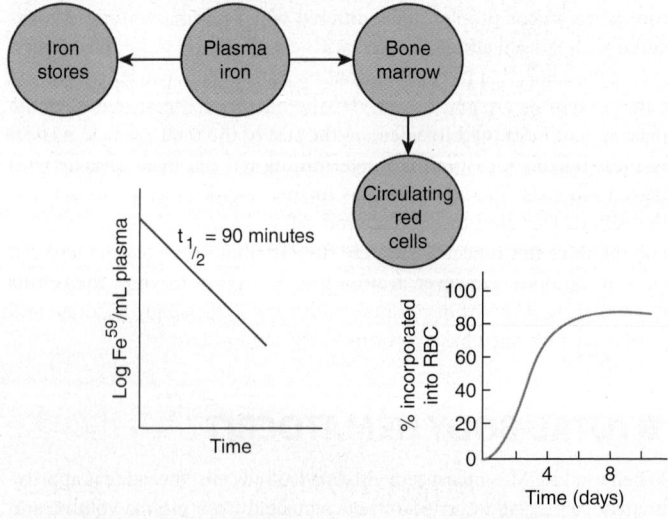

Figure 32–9. Single dynamic pool model of iron metabolism. Radioactive iron injected into the plasma iron pool is cleared from the plasma as a single exponential, and approximately 80 percent is incorporated into circulating blood cells.

or weight, but a commonly used expression is micrograms of iron per deciliters of whole blood per day:

Plasma iron turnover rate (mg iron/dL blood/24 h)

$$= \frac{\text{plasma iron (mg dL)} \times (100 - \text{Hct})}{T_{1/2}(\text{min}) \times 100}$$

Under normal conditions, radioactive iron is incorporated into newly formed red cells after a few days and reaches a maximum approximately 10 to 14 days after injection (see Fig. 32–9). Normal utilization is 70 to 90 percent on day 10 to 14, a value that is so high that further increases have little significance. However, decreased utilization is an important finding and suggests immature red cells are destroyed in the marrow before they are released to the circulation (ineffective erythropoiesis) or that serum iron is diverted to nonerythropoietic tissues (marrow hypoplasia). The shape of the red cell utilization curve also is important. An early and steep rise (rapid marrow transit time) suggests a high EPO level. Finally, an early rise in utilization with a subsequent fall off suggests hemolysis.

When calculating utilization, the blood volume must be known:

Red cell iron utilization (%)

$$= \frac{\text{CPM of l mL blood} \times \text{blood volume} \times 100}{\text{CPM of } ^{59}\text{Fe injected}}$$

Using the plasma iron clearance and utilization of iron, the red cell turnover in milligrams per dL blood for 24-hours is calculated as follows:

Red cell iron turnover (mg iron/dL blood/24 h) = plasma iron turnover × maximal red cell iron utilization

The normal value of red cell iron turnover is 0.30 to 0.70 mg/dL blood per 24 hours.[38] This range fits very well with a crude estimation of the iron used for maintaining the red cell mass in 1 dL of blood or 45 mL of packed red cells. The daily red cell production must equal the daily red cell destruction (45 mL/120 = 0.38 mL), assuming a red cell life span of 120 days. Because 1 mL of packed red cells contains approximately 1 mg of iron, a daily plasma iron turnover of 0.38 mg is needed by 1 dL of blood to maintain homeostasis.

Calculating red cell iron turnover has provided useful information about the total volume and effectiveness of erythroid tissue (Table 32–2). However, an elevated serum iron concentration gives

erroneous impressions of the state of erythropoiesis. Moreover, more prolonged sampling of plasma following an intravenous injection of ^{59}Fe has shown that clearance is not a single exponential, but must be represented by several exponential components.[159] This finding has led to the introduction of more complex models of iron kinetics with a single pool of plasma iron exchanging with a number of extravascular erythroid and nonerythroid pools. Careful analysis of such models has generated computer-supported methods calculating the degree and effectiveness of erythroid activity.[160] Although possibly more accurate than the conventional method of calculating iron turnover, the models appear to be too cumbersome for clinical use. Moreover, even these sophisticated methods may not give an accurate account of the state of erythropoiesis. Despite a constant rate of red cell production, the plasma iron turnover was found to increase with increasing plasma iron and transferrin saturation. This finding was first thought to result from increased nonerythroid iron uptake and led to the introduction of various correction factors in the calculation of red cell iron turnover.[160] However, the iron in plasma is present in two pools, a diferric and a monoferric transferrin pool (Chap. 42), and the erythroid and nonerythroid receptors have a four times greater avidity for diferric transferrin than for monoferric transferrin. Consequently, total plasma iron turnover depends on the degree of saturation and does not necessarily reflect the number of transferrin receptors, presumably a critical measure of erythropoietic capacity.[161] To measure the number of transferrin receptors, adjusting the plasma iron turnover equations for both nonerythroid uptake and degree of transferrin saturation and expressing the plasma turnover in terms of transferrin rather than iron have been proposed.[162] Normal erythroid uptake of transferrin is 60 ± 12 μmol/L of blood per day, a value that has appropriately decreased and increased in patients with hypoplastic and hyperplastic marrow.

REFERENCES

1. Erslev AJ: Blood and mountains, in *Blood, Pure and Eloquent*, edited by MM Wintrobe, p 257. McGraw-Hill, New York, 1980.
2. Carnot P, Deflandre C: Sur l'activité hématopoiétique des serum au cours de la régénération du sang. *Acad Sci Med* 3, 1906.
3. Miescher F: Über die beziehungen zwischen meereshohe und beschaffenheit des blutes. *Koresp Bltt Schweitz Aerzte* 24, 1893.
4. Reissmann KR: Studies on the mechanism of erythropoietic stimulation in parabiotic rats during hypoxia. *Blood* 5(4):372, 1950.
5. Erslev A: Humoral regulation of red cell production. *Blood* 8(4):349, 1953.
6. Erslev A, Lavietes PH, Van Wagenen G: Erythropoietic stimulation induced by anemic serum. *Proc Soc Exp Biol Med* 83(3):548, 1953.
7. Jacobson LO, Goldwasser E, Fried W, et al: Role of the kidney in erythropoiesis. *Nature* 179(4560):633, 1957.
8. Fox H: The hemoglobin of daphnia. *Proc R Soc Lond B Biol Sci* 135, 1948.
9. Hemmingsen EA, Douglas EL: Respiratory characteristics of the hemoglobin-free fish Chaenocephalus aceratus. *Comp Biochem Physiol* 33(4):733, 1970.
10. Garofalo F, Amelio D, Cerra MC, et al: Morphological and physiological study of the cardiac nos/no system in the antarctic (hb-/mb-) icefish Chaenocephalus aceratus and in the red-blooded Trematomus bernacchii. *Nitric Oxide* 20(2):69, 2009.
11. Garofalo F, Pellegrino D, Amelio D, et al: The antarctic hemoglobinless icefish, fifty-five years later: A unique cardiocirculatory interplay of disaptation and phenotypic plasticity. *Comp Biochem Physiol A Mol Integr Physiol* 154(1):10, 2009.
12. Sidell BD, O'Brien KM: When bad things happen to good fish: The loss of hemoglobin and myoglobin expression in antarctic icefishes. *J Exp Biol* 209(Pt 10):1791, 2006.
13. Scott RB: Comparative hematology: The phylogeny of the erythrocyte. *Blut* 12(6):340, 1966.
14. Andrew W: *Comparative Hematology*, Grune & Stratton, New York, 1965.
15. Bolliger A: Observations on the blood of a monotreme Tachyglossus aculeatus. *Aust J Sci* 22, 1959.
16. Iorio RJ: Some morphologic and kinetic studies of the developing erythroid cells of the common gold fish Carassius auratus. *Cell Tissue Kinet* 2, 1969.
17. Jordan HE: Comparative hematology, in *Handbook of Hematology*, edited by H Downey, p 703. Hoeber-Harper, New York, 1938.
18. Robb-Smith AHT: *The Growth of Knowledge of the Functions of the Blood*, Academic Press, New York, 1961.

Condition	Plasma ^{59}FE $T_{1/2}$	Red Blood Cell Uptake (%)
Normal	90 min	80–90
Increased erythropoiesis	Rapid (10–40 min)	80–90
Hemolytic anemia	Rapid	20–90*
Ineffective erythropoiesis	Normal to rapid	10–30
Iron-deficiency anemia	Normal to rapid	100
Decreased erythropoiesis	Slow (≥180 min)	0–20

TABLE 32–2. Plasma Radioactive Iron Clearance and Red Blood Cell Uptake

*Variability a result of variability in intensity of hemolysis and size of iron stores.

19. Rosse WF, Waldmann TA: Factors controlling erythropoiesis in birds. *Blood* 27(5):654, 1966.

20. Zanjani ED, Yu ML, Perlmutter A, et al: Humoral factors influencing erythropoiesis in the fish (blue gourami. Trichogaster trichopterus). *Blood* 33(4):573, 1969.

21. Erslev AJ: Control of red cell production. *Annu Rev Med* 11, 1959.

22. Shoemaker CB, Mitsock LD: Murine erythropoietin gene: Cloning, expression, and human gene homology. *Mol Cell Biol* 6(3):849, 1986.

23. Le Douarin NM: Cell migrations in embryos. *Cell* 38(2):353, 1984.

24. Kingsley PD, Malik J, Emerson RL, et al: "Maturational" globin switching in primary primitive erythroid cells. *Blood* 107(4):1665, 2006.

25. Ferkowicz MJ, Yoder MC: Blood island formation: Longstanding observations and modern interpretations. *Exp Hematol* 33(9):1041, 2005.

26. Hoyes AD, Riches DJ, Martin BG: The fine structure of haemopoiesis in the human fetal liver. I. The haemopoietic precursor cells. *J Anat* 115(Pt 1):99, 1973.

27. Palis J, Robertson S, Kennedy M, et al: Development of erythroid and myeloid progenitors in the yolk sac and embryo proper of the mouse. *Development* 126(22):5073, 1999.

28. Hudson G: Bone-marrow volume in the human foetus and newborn. *Br J Haematol* 11:446, 1965.

29. Brannon D: Extramedullary hematopoiesis in anemia. *Bull Johns Hopkins Hosp* 41, 1927.

30. Erslev AJ: Medullary and extramedullary blood formation. *Clin Orthop Relat Res* 52:25, 1967.

31. Zanjani ED, Poster J, Burlington H, et al: Liver as the primary site of erythropoietin formation in the fetus. *J Lab Clin Med* 89(3):640, 1977.

32. Flake AW, Harrison MR, Adzick NS, et al: Erythropoietin production by the fetal liver in an adult environment. *Blood* 70(2):542, 1987.

33. Zanjani ED, Ascensao JL, McGlave PB, et al: Studies on the liver to kidney switch of erythropoietin production. *J Clin Invest* 67(4):1183, 1981.

34. Sawyer ST, Penta K: Erythropoietin cell biology. *Hematol Oncol Clin North Am* 8(5):895, 1994.

35. Wu H, Liu X, Jaenisch R, et al: Generation of committed erythroid BFU-E and CFU-E progenitors does not require erythropoietin or the erythropoietin receptor. *Cell* 83(1):59, 1995.

36. Bessis M, Breton-Gorius J: [The reticulocyte. Vital staining and electron microscopy] [in French]. *Nouv Rev Fr Hematol* 4:77, 1964.

37. Gronowicz G, Swift H, Steck TL: Maturation of the reticulocyte in vitro. *J Cell Sci* 71:177, 1984.

38. Finch CA, Deubelbeiss K, Cook JD, et al: Ferrokinetics in man. *Medicine (Baltimore)* 49(1):17, 1970.

39. Noble NA, Xu QP, Hoge LL: Reticulocytes II: Reexamination of the in vivo survival of stress reticulocytes. *Blood* 75(9):1877, 1990.

40. Donohue DM, Reiff RH, Hanson ML, et al: Quantitative measurement of the erythrocytic and granulocytic cells of the marrow and blood. *J Clin Invest* 37(11):1571, 1958.

41. Finch CA, Harker LA, Cook JD: Kinetics of the formed elements of human blood. *Blood* 50(4):699, 1977.

42. Goltry KL, Patel VP: Specific domains of fibronectin mediate adhesion and migration of early murine erythroid progenitors. *Blood* 90(1):138, 1997.

43. Dirlam A, Spike BT, Macleod KF: Deregulated e2f-2 underlies cell cycle and maturation defects in retinoblastoma null erythroblasts. *Mol Cell Biol* 27(24):8713, 2007.

44. Repasky EA, Eckert BS: A reevaluation of the process of enucleation in mammalian erythroid cells. *Prog Clin Biol Res* 55:679, 1981.

45. Ji P, Jayapal SR, Lodish HF: Enucleation of cultured mouse fetal erythroblasts requires rac GTPases and mDia2. *Nat Cell Biol* 10(3):314, 2008.

46. Yoshida H, Kawane K, Koike M, et al: Phosphatidylserine-dependent engulfment by macrophages of nuclei from erythroid precursor cells. *Nature* 437(7059):754, 2005.

47. Hanspal M, Hanspal JS: The association of erythroblasts with macrophages promotes erythroid proliferation and maturation: A 30-kd heparin-binding protein is involved in this contact. *Blood* 84(10):3494, 1994.

48. Soni S, Bala S, Gwynn B, et al: Absence of erythroblast macrophage protein (emp) leads to failure of erythroblast nuclear extrusion. *J Biol Chem* 281(29):20181, 2006.

49. Evans T, Felsenfeld G: The erythroid-specific transcription factor eryf1: A new finger protein. *Cell* 58(5):877, 1989.

50. Tsai SF, Martin DI, Zon LI, et al: Cloning of cDNA for the major DNA-binding protein of the erythroid lineage through expression in mammalian cells. *Nature* 339(6224):446, 1989.

51. Pevny L, Lin CS, D'Agati V, et al: Development of hematopoietic cells lacking transcription factor gata-1. *Development* 121(1):163, 1995.

52. Letting DL, Chen YY, Rakowski C, et al: Context-dependent regulation of gata-1 by friend of gata-1. *Proc Natl Acad Sci U S A* 101(2):476, 2004.

53. Gregory T, Yu C, Ma A, et al: Gata-1 and erythropoietin cooperate to promote erythroid cell survival by regulating bcl-xl expression. *Blood* 94(1):87, 1999.

54. Nerlov C, Querfurth E, Kulessa H, et al: Gata-1 interacts with the myeloid pu.1 transcription factor and represses pu.1-dependent transcription. *Blood* 95(8):2543, 2000.

55. Tsang AP, Visvader JE, Turner CA, et al: Fog, a multitype zinc finger protein, acts as a cofactor for transcription factor gata-1 in erythroid and megakaryocytic differentiation. *Cell* 90(1):109, 1997.

56. Cantor AB, Orkin SH: Transcriptional regulation of erythropoiesis: An affair involving multiple partners. *Oncogene* 21(21):3368, 2002.

57. Xie H, Ye M, Feng R, et al: Stepwise reprogramming of b cells into macrophages. *Cell* 117(5):663, 2004.

58. Back J, Dierich A, Bronn C, et al: Pu.1 determines the self-renewal capacity of erythroid progenitor cells. *Blood* 103(10):3615, 2004.

59. Tsang AP, Fujiwara Y, Hom DB, et al: Failure of megakaryopoiesis and arrested erythropoiesis in mice lacking the gata-1 transcriptional cofactor fog. *Genes Dev* 12(8):1176, 1998.

60. Tsai FY, Keller G, Kuo FC, et al: An early haematopoietic defect in mice lacking the transcription factor gata-2. *Nature* 371(6494):221, 1994.

61. Leonard M, Brice M, Engel JD, et al: Dynamics of gata transcription factor expression during erythroid differentiation. *Blood* 82(4):1071, 1993.

62. Mouthon MA, Bernard O, Mitjavila MT, et al: Expression of tal-1 and gata-binding proteins during human hematopoiesis. *Blood* 81(3):647, 1993.

63. Pal S, Cantor AB, Johnson KD, et al: Coregulator-dependent facilitation of chromatin occupancy by gata-1. *Proc Natl Acad Sci U S A* 101(4):980, 2004.

64. Fujiwara Y, Chang AN, Williams AM, et al: Functional overlap of gata-1 and gata-2 in primitive hematopoietic development. *Blood* 103(2):583, 2004.

65. Miller IJ, Bieker JJ: A novel, erythroid cell-specific murine transcription factor that binds to the CACCC element and is related to the Kruppel family of nuclear proteins. *Mol Cell Biol* 13(5):2776, 1993.

66. Nuez B, Michalovich D, Bygrave A, et al: Defective haematopoiesis in fetal liver resulting from inactivation of the eklf gene. *Nature* 375(6529):316, 1995.

67. Aplan PD, Nakahara K, Orkin SH, et al: The scl gene product: A positive regulator of erythroid differentiation. *EMBO J* 11(11):4073, 1992.

68. Robb L, Lyons I, Li R, et al: Absence of yolk sac hematopoiesis from mice with a targeted disruption of the scl gene. *Proc Natl Acad Sci U S A* 92(15):7075, 1995.

69. Sanchez MJ, Bockamp EO, Miller J, et al: Selective rescue of early haematopoietic progenitors in scl(−/−) mice by expressing scl under the control of a stem cell enhancer. *Development* 128(23):4815, 2001.

70. Mikkola HK, Klintman J, Yang H, et al: Haematopoietic stem cells retain long-term repopulating activity and multipotency in the absence of stem-cell leukaemia scl/tal-1 gene. *Nature* 421(6922):547, 2003.

71. Zaitseva MP: [Effect of labor conditions on the development and course of rheumatism] [in Russian]. *Vopr Revm* 10(4):59, 1970.

72. Uda M, Galanello R, Sanna S, et al: Genome-wide association study shows bcl11a associated with persistent fetal hemoglobin and amelioration of the phenotype of beta-thalassemia. *Proc Natl Acad Sci U S A* 105(5):1620, 2008.

73. Angelillo-Scherrer A, Burnier L, Lambrechts D, et al: Role of gas6 in erythropoiesis and anemia in mice. *J Clin Invest* 118(2):583, 2008.

74. Lemke G, Lu Q: Macrophage regulation by tyro 3 family receptors. *Curr Opin Immunol* 15(1):31, 2003.

75. Orkin SH, Zon LI: Hematopoiesis: An evolving paradigm for stem cell biology. *Cell* 132(4):631, 2008.

76. Stopka T, Zivny JH, Stopkova P, et al: Human hematopoietic progenitors express erythropoietin. *Blood* 91(10):3766, 1998.

77. Krantz SB: Erythropoietin. *Blood* 77(3):419, 1991.

78. Lappin TR, Rich IN: Erythropoietin—The first 90 years. *Clin Lab Haematol* 18(3):137, 1996.

79. Jelkmann W: Erythropoietin: Structure, control of production, and function. *Physiol Rev* 72(2):449, 1992.

80. Jelkmann W, Metzen E: Erythropoietin in the control of red cell production. *Ann Anat* 178(5):391, 1996.

81. Koury ST, Bondurant MC, Koury MJ: Localization of erythropoietin synthesizing cells in murine kidneys by in situ hybridization. *Blood* 71(2):524, 1988.

82. Lacombe C, Da Silva JL, Bruneval P, et al: Peritubular cells are the site of erythropoietin synthesis in the murine hypoxic kidney. *J Clin Invest* 81(2):620, 1988.

83. Koury ST, Koury MJ, Bondurant MC, et al: Quantitation of erythropoietin-producing cells in kidneys of mice by in situ hybridization: Correlation with hematocrit, renal erythropoietin mrna, and serum erythropoietin concentration. *Blood* 74(2):645, 1989.

84. Semenza GL, Dureza RC, Traystman MD, et al: Human erythropoietin gene expression in transgenic mice: Multiple transcription initiation sites and cis-acting regulatory elements. *Mol Cell Biol* 10(3):930, 1990.

85. Schuster SJ, Koury ST, Bohrer M, et al: Cellular sites of extrarenal and renal erythropoietin production in anaemic rats. *Br J Haematol* 81(2):153, 1992.

86. Mole DR, Radcliffe PJ: Regulation of endogenous erythropoietin production, in *Erythropoietins and Erythropoiesis*, edited by G Molineux, MA Foote, and SG Elliot, p 19. Birkhäuser-Verlag AG, Basel, 2009.

87. Rankin EB, Biju MP, Liu Q, et al: Hypoxia-inducible factor-2 (hif-2) regulates hepatic erythropoietin in vivo. *J Clin Invest* 117(4):1068, 2007.

88. Semenza GL, Nejfelt MK, Chi SM, et al: Hypoxia-inducible nuclear factors bind to an enhancer element located 3′ to the human erythropoietin gene. *Proc Natl Acad Sci U S A* 88(13):5680, 1991.

89. Regenbogen L, Godel V: Spiral looping of retinal artery. *J Pediatr Ophthalmol* 14(2):117, 1977.

90. Pugh CW, Tan CC, Jones RW, et al: Functional analysis of an oxygen-regulated transcriptional element lying 3′ to the mouse erythropoietin gene. *Proc Natl Acad Sci U S A* 88(23):10553, 1991.

91. Flaharty KK, Caro J, Erslev A, et al: Pharmacokinetics and erythropoietic response to human recombinant erythropoietin in healthy men. *Clin Pharmacol Ther* 47(5):557, 1990.

92. Sawyer ST, Krantz SB, Goldwasser E: Binding and receptor-mediated endocytosis of erythropoietin in friend virus-infected erythroid cells. *J Biol Chem* 262(12):5554, 1987.

93. Ebert BL, Bunn HF: Regulation of the erythropoietin gene. *Blood* 94(6):1864, 1999.

94. Constantinescu SN, Keren T, Socolovsky M, et al: Ligand-independent oligomerization of cell-surface erythropoietin receptor is mediated by the transmembrane domain. *Proc Natl Acad Sci U S A* 98(8):4379, 2001.

95. Witthuhn BA, Quelle FW, Silvennoinen O, et al: Jak2 associates with the erythropoietin receptor and is tyrosine phosphorylated and activated following stimulation with erythropoietin. *Cell* 74(2):227, 1993.

96. Damen JE, Wakao H, Miyajima A, et al: Tyrosine 343 in the erythropoietin receptor positively regulates erythropoietin-induced cell proliferation and stat5 activation. *EMBO J* 14(22):5557, 1995.

97. Parganas E, Wang D, Stravopodis D, et al: Jak2 is essential for signaling through a variety of cytokine receptors. *Cell* 93(3):385, 1998.

98. Divoky V, Prchal JT: Mouse surviving solely on human erythropoietin receptor (EPOR): Model of human EPOR-linked disease. *Blood* 99(10):3873; author reply 3874, 2002.

99. Lin CS, Lim SK, D'Agati V, et al: Differential effects of an erythropoietin receptor gene disruption on primitive and definitive erythropoiesis. *Genes Dev* 10(2):154, 1996.

100. D'Andrea AD, Yoshimura A, Youssoufian H, et al: The cytoplasmic region of the erythropoietin receptor contains nonoverlapping positive and negative growth-regulatory domains. *Mol Cell Biol* 11(4):1980, 1991.

101. Klingmuller U, Lorenz U, Cantley LC, et al: Specific recruitment of sh-ptp1 to the erythropoietin receptor causes inactivation of jak2 and termination of proliferative signals. *Cell* 80(5):729, 1995.

102. Arcasoy MO, Harris KW, Forget BG: A human erythropoietin receptor gene mutant causing familial erythrocytosis is associated with deregulation of the rates of jak2 and stat5 inactivation. *Exp Hematol* 27(1):63, 1999.

103. Marine JC, McKay C, Wang D, et al: Socs3 is essential in the regulation of fetal liver erythropoiesis. *Cell* 98(5):617, 1999.

104. Sasaki A, Yasukawa H, Shouda T, et al: Cis3/socs-3 suppresses erythropoietin (EPO) signaling by binding the EPO receptor and jak2. *J Biol Chem* 275(38):29338, 2000.

105. Prchal JT, Gregg XT: Erythropoiesis. Genetic abnormalities, in *Erythropoietins and Erythropoiesis*, edited by G Molineux, MA Foote, and SG Elliot, p 61. Birkhäuser-Verlag AG, Basel, 2009.

106. Roberts KG, Morin RD, Zhang J, et al: Genetic alterations activating kinase and cytokine receptor signaling in high-risk acute lymphoblastic leukemia. *Cancer Cell* 22(2):153, 2012.

107. Walrafen P, Verdier F, Kadri Z, et al: Both proteasomes and lysosomes degrade the activated erythropoietin receptor. *Blood* 105(2):600, 2005.

108. Arcasoy MO, Jiang X, Haroon ZA: Expression of erythropoietin receptor splice variants in human cancer. *Biochem Biophys Res Commun* 307(4):999, 2003.

109. Barron C, Migliaccio AR, Migliaccio G, et al: Alternatively spliced mRNAs encoding soluble isoforms of the erythropoietin receptor in murine cell lines and bone marrow. *Gene* 147(2):263, 1994.

110. Nakamura Y, Nakauchi H: A truncated erythropoietin receptor and cell death: A reanalysis. *Science* 264(5158):588, 1994.

111. Prchal JT, Semenza GL, Prchal J, et al: Familial polycythemia. *Science* 268(5219):1831, 1995.

112. Noguchi CT, Wang L, Rogers HM, et al: Survival and proliferative roles of erythropoietin beyond the erythroid lineage. *Expert Rev Mol Med* 10:e36, 2008.

113. Anagnostou A, Lee ES, Kessimian N, et al: Erythropoietin has a mitogenic and positive chemotactic effect on endothelial cells. *Proc Natl Acad Sci U S A* 87(15):5978, 1990.

114. Arcasoy MO: The non-haematopoietic biological effects of erythropoietin. *Br J Haematol* 141(1):14, 2008.

115. Brines M, Cerami A: Discovering erythropoietin's extra-hematopoietic functions: Biology and clinical promise. *Kidney Int* 70(2):246, 2006.

116. Agarwal N, Gordeuk VR, Prchal JT: Are erythropoietin receptors expressed in tumors? Facts and fiction—More careful studies are needed. *J Clin Oncol* 25(13):1813; author reply 1815, 2007.

117. Hardee ME, Cao Y, Fu P, et al: Erythropoietin blockade inhibits the induction of tumor angiogenesis and progression. *PLoS One* 2(6):e549, 2007.

118. Hirota K, Semenza GL: Regulation of angiogenesis by hypoxia-inducible factor 1. *Crit Rev Oncol Hematol* 59(1):15, 2006.

119. Yoon D, Pastore YD, Divoky V, et al: Hypoxia-inducible factor-1 deficiency results in dysregulated erythropoiesis signaling and iron homeostasis in mouse development. *J Biol Chem* 281(33):25703, 2006.

120. Fukuda R, Zhang H, Kim JW, et al: Hif-1 regulates cytochrome oxidase subunits to optimize efficiency of respiration in hypoxic cells. *Cell* 129(1):111, 2007.

121. Beck I, Ramirez S, Weinmann R, et al: Enhancer element at the 3′-flanking region controls transcriptional response to hypoxia in the human erythropoietin gene. *J Biol Chem* 266(24):15563, 1991.

122. Manalo DJ, Rowan A, Lavoie T, et al: Transcriptional regulation of vascular endothelial cell responses to hypoxia by Hif-1. *Blood* 105(2):659, 2005.

123. Maxwell PH, Wiesener MS, Chang GW, et al: The tumour suppressor protein VHL targets hypoxia-inducible factors for oxygen-dependent proteolysis. *Nature* 399(6733):271, 1999.

124. Ivan M, Kondo K, Yang H, et al: Hifalpha targeted for VHL-mediated destruction by proline hydroxylation: Implications for O₂ sensing. *Science* 292(5516):464, 2001.

125. Jaakkola P, Mole DR, Tian YM, et al: Targeting of HIF-alpha to the von Hippel-Lindau ubiquitylation complex by O₂-regulated prolyl hydroxylation. *Science* 292(5516):468, 2001.

126. Baek JH, Liu YV, McDonald KR, et al: Spermidine/spermine N(1)-acetyltransferase-1 binds to hypoxia-inducible factor-1alpha (HIF-1alpha) and rack1 and promotes ubiquitination and degradation of HIF-1alpha. *J Biol Chem* 282(46):33358, 2007.

127. Gruber M, Hu CJ, Johnson RS, et al: Acute postnatal ablation of HIF-2alpha results in anemia. *Proc Natl Acad Sci U S A* 104(7):2301, 2007.

128. Chavez JC, Baranova O, Lin J, et al: The transcriptional activator hypoxia inducible factor 2 (HIF-2/EPAS-1) regulates the oxygen-dependent expression of erythropoietin in cortical astrocytes. *J Neurosci* 26(37):9471, 2006.

129. Sanchez M, Galy B, Muckenthaler MU, et al: Iron-regulatory proteins limit hypoxia-inducible factor-2alpha expression in iron deficiency. *Nat Struct Mol Biol* 14(5):420, 2007.

130. Percy MJ, Furlow PW, Lucas GS, et al: A gain-of-function mutation in the HIF2a gene in familial erythrocytosis. *N Engl J Med* 358(2):162, 2008.

131. Liu YV, Baek JH, Zhang H, et al: Rack1 competes with hsp90 for binding to HIF-1alpha and is required for O(2)-independent and hsp90 inhibitor-induced degradation of HIF-1alpha. *Mol Cell* 25(2):207, 2007.

132. Epstein AC, Gleadle JM, McNeill LA, et al: C. Elegans egl-9 and mammalian homologs define a family of dioxygenases that regulate HIF by prolyl hydroxylation. *Cell* 107(1):43, 2001.

133. Correa PN, Eskinazi D, Axelrad AA: Circulating erythroid progenitors in polycythemia vera are hypersensitive to insulin-like growth factor-1 in vitro: Studies in an improved serum-free medium. *Blood* 83(1):99, 1994.

134. Mirza AM, Ezzat S, Axelrad AA: Insulin-like growth factor binding protein-1 is elevated in patients with polycythemia vera and stimulates erythroid burst formation in vitro. *Blood* 89(6):1862, 1997.

135. Brox AG, Congote LF, Fafard J, et al: Identification and characterization of an 8-kd peptide stimulating late erythropoiesis. *Exp Hematol* 17(7):769, 1989.

136. Kent G, Minick OT, Volini FI, et al: Autophagic vacuoles in human red cells. *Am J Pathol* 48(5):831, 1966.

137. Heynen MJ, Tricot G, Verwilghen RL: Autophagy of mitochondria in rat bone marrow erythroid cells. Relation to nuclear extrusion. *Cell Tissue Res* 239(1):235, 1985.

138. Sandoval H, Thiagarajan P, Dasgupta SK, et al: Essential role for nix in autophagic maturation of erythroid cells. *Nature* 454(7201):232, 2008.

139. Kundu M, Lindsten T, Yang CY, et al: Ulk1 plays a critical role in the autophagic clearance of mitochondria and ribosomes during reticulocyte maturation. *Blood* 112(4):1493, 2008.

140. Schweers RL, Zhang J, Randall MS, et al: Nix is required for programmed mitochondrial clearance during reticulocyte maturation. *Proc Natl Acad Sci U S A* 104(49):19500, 2007.

141. Hong CI, De NC, Tritsch GL, et al: Synthesis and biological activities of some N4-substituted 4-aminopyrazolo(3,4-d)pyrimidines. *J Med Chem* 19(4):555, 1976.

142. Eshghi S, Vogelezang MG, Hynes RO, et al: Alpha4beta1 integrin and erythropoietin mediate temporally distinct steps in erythropoiesis: Integrins in red cell development. *J Cell Biol* 177(5):871, 2007.

143. Bruchova H, Yoon D, Agarwal AM, et al: Regulated expression of microRNAs in normal and polycythemia vera erythropoiesis. *Exp Hematol* 35(11):1657, 2007.

144. Li Y, Bai H, Zhang Z, et al: The up-regulation of mir-199b-5p in erythroid differentiation is associated with GATA-1 and NF-E2. *Mol Cells* 37(3):213, 2014.

145. Raghavachari N, Liu P, Barb JJ, et al: Integrated analysis of miRNA and mRNA during differentiation of human cd34+ cells delineates the regulatory roles of microRNA in hematopoiesis. *Exp Hematol* 42(1):14, 2014.

146. Lee YT, de Vasconcellos JF, Yuan J, et al: Lin28b-mediated expression of fetal hemoglobin and production of fetal-like erythrocytes from adult human erythroblasts ex vivo. *Blood* 122(6):1034, 2013.

147. Barde I, Rauwel B, Marin-Florez RM, et al: A KRAB/KAP1-miRNA cascade regulates erythropoiesis through stage-specific control of mitophagy. *Science* 340(6130):350, 2013.

148. Pearson TC, Botterill CA, Glass UH, et al: Interpretation of measured red cell mass and plasma volume in males with elevated venous PCV values. *Scand J Haematol* 33(1):68, 1984.

149. Cavill I, Trevett D, Fisher J, et al: The measurement of the total volume of red cells in man: A non-radioactive approach using biotin. *Br J Haematol* 70(4):491, 1988.

150. Jones J, Mollison PL: A simple and efficient method of labelling red cells with 99mTc for determination of red cell volume. *Br J Haematol* 38(1):141, 1978.

151. Pearson TC, Guthrie DL, Simpson J, et al: Interpretation of measured red cell mass and plasma volume in adults: Expert panel on radionuclides of the international council for standardization in haematology. *Br J Haematol* 89(4):748, 1995.

152. Fairbanks VF, Klee GG, Wiseman GA, et al: Measurement of blood volume and red cell mass: Re-examination of 51cr and 125i methods. *Blood Cells Mol Dis* 22(2):169; discussion 186a, 1996.

153. Larson RA: Studies of the body hematocrit phenomenon: Dynamic hematocrit of large vessel and initial distribution space of albumin and fibrinogen in the whole body. *Scand J Clin Lab Invest* 22(3):189, 1998.

154. Button LN, Gibson JG 2nd, Walter CW: Simultaneous determination of the volume of red cells and plasma for survival studies of stored blood. *Transfusion* 5:143, 1965.

155. Recommended methods for measurement of red-cell and plasma volume: International committee for standardization in haematology. *J Nucl Med* 21(8):793, 1980.

156. Hillman RS, Finch CA: Erythropoiesis: Normal and abnormal. *Semin Hematol* 4(4):327, 1967.

157. Samson D, Halliday D, Nicholson DC, et al: Quantitation of ineffective erythropoiesis from the incorporation of [15N] delta-aminolevulinic acid and [15N] glycine into early labelled bilirubin. I. Normal subjects. *Br J Haematol* 34(1):33, 1976.
158. Huff RL, Hennessy TG, Austin RE, et al: Plasma and red cell iron turnover in normal subjects and in patients having various hematopoietic disorders. *J Clin Invest* 29(8):1041, 1950.
159. Cook JD, Marsaglia G, Eschbach JW, et al: Ferrokinetics: A biologic model for plasma iron exchange in man. *J Clin Invest* 49(2):197, 1970.
160. Ricketts C, Cavill I, Napier JA, et al: Ferrokinetics and erythropoiesis in man: An evaluation of ferrokinetic measurements. *Br J Haematol* 35(1):41, 1977.
161. Bauer W, Stray S, Huebers H, et al: The relationship between plasma iron and plasma iron turnover in the rat. *Blood* 57(2):239, 1981.
162. Beguin Y: The soluble transferrin receptor: Biological aspects and clinical usefulness as quantitative measure of erythropoiesis. *Haematologica* 77(1):1, 1992.

CHAPTER 33
ERYTHROCYTE TURNOVER

Perumal Thiagarajan and Josef Prchal

SUMMARY

The survival of red cells in the circulation can be measured in a variety of ways: (1) by labeling with radioactive isotopes, particularly chromium-51 (^{51}Cr), and assessing the disappearance of the radioactive tag from the circulation over time; (2) by labeling the erythrocytes with biotin or a fluorescent dye and measuring this marker over time; (3) by determining the disappearance of transfused antigen-matched allogeneic erythrocytes using immunologic markers; and (4) by measuring the excretion of carbon monoxide, a product of heme catabolism.

Such studies show that normal human red cells have a finite life span averaging 120 days, with very little random destruction. The mitochondrial and ribosomal removal highlighting maturation of the reticulocyte is accompanied by increasing cell density, but after a few days of intravascular life span there is little further increase in density or other changes in the physical property of the red cells. Thus, cell density is not a good marker for aged red cells. This has made the senescent changes in the red cell that mark it for destruction difficult to study. Candidates for such changes include changes in membrane band 3 and exposure of phosphatidylserine on the membrane, which may be of major importance.

● RED CELL LIFE SPAN

Normal human red blood cells have a life span of approximately 120 days, after which they are engulfed by macrophages. This is an extremely efficient process as macrophages phagocytose approximately 5 million erythrocytes every second without a significant release of hemoglobin into the circulation. The precise molecular mechanism by which macrophages recognize senescent red blood cells for phagocytosis remains largely unknown. As red blood cells age, several physiologic changes occur that may serve as signals for recognition by macrophages.[1,2] These include a decrease in the activity of enzymes,[3] a progressive decrease of ATP content,[4] a loss of lipid asymmetry with exposure of phosphatidylserine,[5] an accumulation of lipid peroxidation products,[6] a desialylation of membrane glycoprotein,[7] an exposure of cryptic senescent antigens,[8] aggregation of band 3 protein (Chap. 46),[9] a decrease in deformability as the result of increased oxidative stress,[10] and an increase

Acronyms and Abbreviations: ADP, adenosine diphosphate; AMP, adenosine monophosphate; BNIP3L, an hypoxic regulated gene that facilitates mitochondrial autophagy; C$_3$, third component of complement; ^{14}C, radioactive carbon; CD44, cell differentiation antigen; CO, carbon monoxide; ^{50}Cr, chromium-50; ^{51}Cr, chromium-51; DFP, diisopropylfluorophosphate; ^{55}Fe or ^{59}Fe, radioactive iron; G6PD, glucose-6-phosphate dehydrogenase; HO, heme oxygenase; Ig, immunoglobulin; ^{111}In, indium-111; ^{15}N, nitrogen; PK, pyruvate kinase; ^{99m}Tc, technetium-99m.

in cell surface-bound immunoglobulins and complement components (Chap. 54).[11,12] All of these changes have been investigated as signals for recognition by the macrophages.

MEASUREMENT OF RED CELL DESTRUCTION

The original method for the measurement of the red cell life span consisted in the transfusion of cells that were compatible but identifiable immunologically—the Ashby technique; type O red cells were infused into individuals with type A or B cells. The differential agglutination technique used anti-A or anti-B antiserum to measure the life span of type O red cells that were transfused to type A or type B recipients and the recipients' own cells were removed using anti-A or anti-B serum.[13] During World War II and shortly after, this method was used extensively, but in recent years, because of the hazards associated with the administration of allogeneic erythrocytes, it has been completely replaced by techniques based on labeling of autologous blood. Furthermore, this method could not be applied to autologous red cells.

In 1946, Shemin and Rittenberg demonstrated that the incorporation of nitrogen (^{15}N)-labeled glycine into heme could be used to measure the life span of the red cells.[14] Since then a number of other isotopic methods have been developed. These can be divided into three groups: (1) those that label a cohort of cells, (2) those that label cells randomly, and (3) those that use indirect measurements such as the rate of production of red cells or the rate of heme breakdown. The first two methodologic approaches yield information about the nature of the shortening of the red cell life span, age-dependent or random. The methodology yields only mean life span.

COHORT METHODS

Cohort methods depend on the biosynthetic incorporation of the label into the developing red cells. In these methods, a group of cells of approximately the same age is labeled. The labels used are glycine-containing labeled ^{15}N,[14] radioactive carbon (^{14}C),[15] or radioactive iron (either ^{55}Fe or ^{59}Fe).[16–18] The main disadvantage of cohort labeling is the need for prolonged periods of sampling, especially if the life span is only moderately reduced (Fig. 33–1). In addition, radioiron from destroyed red cells may be reused, making it difficult to interpret results. Furthermore, the increasing restrictions on use of radiochemicals has drastically decreased availability of these two previously widely used nuclear medicine tests.

A simple double-labeling technique that allows nonradioactive cohort labeling was described using two distinct labeling steps separated by a defined time interval. Cells are subsequently evaluated by the relative proportions of these labels. The initial labeling step uses biotin that binds to all circulating cells (the red blood cells accounting for most of the label) the second administered labeling substance at later time digoxigenin then distinguishes erythrocyte subpopulation of known age.[19]

RANDOM-LABEL METHODS

The random-label methods are the Ashby differential agglutination technique,[13] which uses an immunologic marker, and or the use of various red cell labels such as chromium-50 (^{50}Cr), chromium-51 (^{51}Cr), or chromium-53 (^{53}Cr),[20–22] diisopropylfluorophosphate (DFP) labeled with phosphorus-32 (^{32}P),[23] ^{14}C,[24] or ^{14}C cyanate,[25] a lipophilic dye,[26,27] or biotin.[28,29]

Chromium-51 Method

By far the most commonly used radioactive isotope for the measurement of the red cell life span is ^{51}Cr. As the chromate ion penetrates the red cell membrane it binds to the β and γ chains of globin. Unfortunately, these

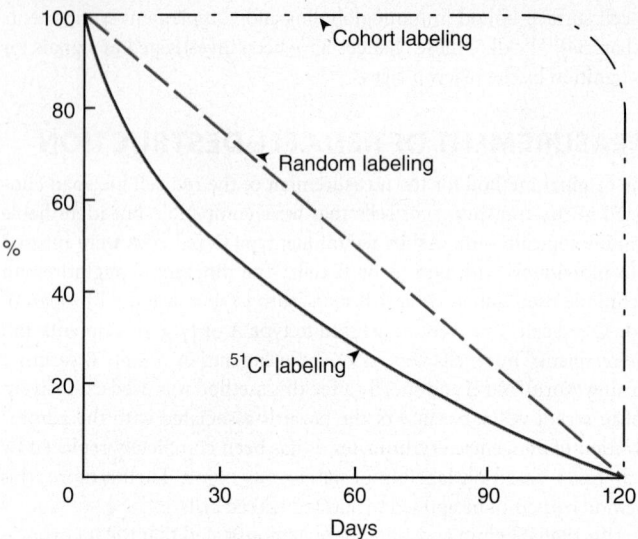

Figure 33–1. Red cell life span measured by cohort labeling or random labeling. When red cells are labeled randomly with chromium-51 (^{51}Cr) there is a daily 1 percent elution that needs to be corrected for in the calculation of total red cell life span.

bonds are not covalent and there is a continuous elution of the isotope, varying from 0.5 to 2.9 percent per day.[30] DFP, on the other hand, is irreversibly bound to red cell cholinesterase. There is some elution of unbound DFP during the first 2 to 3 days of study, but after that, DFP disappearance closely matches red cell destruction.[23,31] Nevertheless, because sample preparation is somewhat complicated, this label is not commonly used.

The life span is estimated by measuring the survival of randomly labeled red cells. Immediately following transfusion, the labeled red cells equilibrate with unlabeled red blood cells (RBCs). This takes normally approximately 5 minutes,[32] but may be longer in patients with splenomegaly. Following equilibration, the cells that have been damaged by the labeling process will be removed from the circulation during the next 24 hours. RBCs that survive this period will usually have their expected long-term survival.[33]

To accurately calculate red cell life span using a random label method requires steady-state conditions or that correction can be made for concurrent blood loss or blood transfusion. Fortunately, it is usually possible to gain an accurate estimate of red cell half-life by sampling three times a week for 1 to 2 weeks.

In the normal human the red cell, life span is finite with an average of approximately 120 days, with very little random destruction, that is, loss irrespective of cell age (0.06 to 0.4 percent per day). In some mammalian species the amount of random destruction is much greater.[34] The survival curve of randomly labeled human red cells should consequently be nearly linear from day 0 to day 120, with a half-life of 60 days. When ^{51}Cr is used as the label, approximately 1 percent of label elutes per day and the survival curve becomes exponential with a half-life of approximately 30 days (see Fig. 33-1). For clinical use, the red cell life span is usually expressed as chromium half-life ($T_{1/2}$) and compared to the normal value for the method of 30 days.

Because merely expressing the red cell life span measured by chromium as chromium $T_{1/2}$ will not give information as to the character of destruction, senescence versus random, it has been recommended that in addition a correction factor for chromium elution be used and the data recorded using linear coordinates.[35] If the data lie on a straight line, the destruction is by senescence and the life span can be calculated

as twice the half-life. If the data indicate exponential disappearance and it is necessary to use a semilogarithmic paper in order to depict the data on a straight line, the destruction is random and the life span is 1.44 times the half-life. One objection to this method is that the degree of chromium elution is not a constant but varies from day to day and is influenced by various disease states.[30] Furthermore, the best fit of data is rarely linear or exponential, but somewhere between. Although computer-assisted methods can resolve ambiguities, the inherent biologic and technical variations in measuring red cell life span are such that it is better to rely on chromium $T_{1/2}$ with intuitive adjustments based on clinical findings.

Biotin Method

A nonradioactive label has also been developed to label the RBCs in humans by covalent attachment of biotin to red cell membrane proteins and enumerating the survival by flow cytometry.[36] Biotin labeling estimates RBC survival comparable to that obtained with a concurrent ^{51}Cr label for both normal volunteers and patients with sickle-cell disease. In addition to being a nonradioactive probe, biotin labeling has other advantages. The transfused cells can be isolated from the patients on avidin substrates for further characterization. Biotin labeling has been used to demonstrate that sickle cells without fetal hemoglobin have a shorter *in vivo* survival compared to those with fetal hemoglobin,[37] and has been also instrumental in showing a role for phosphatidylserine exposure in the clearance of sickle cells.[38]

INDIRECT METHODS

There are two approaches to the calculation of the red cell life span by indirect methods: from a measurement of the rate of production of red cells using radioactive iron and from a measurement of the rate of breakdown of heme to bilirubin,[39] that is, the release of carbon monoxide from catabolized heme.[40] Both of these compounds are derived almost exclusively from catabolized hemoglobin and measurements of their rate of production have provided useful information about the red cell life span. There are too many variables that affect the serum bilirubin level to make it a reliable, quantitative measurement of red cell destruction. The measurement of carbon monoxide (CO) production was formerly very tedious, requiring elaborate rebreathing apparatus. With the development of newer technologies,[41,42] measuring CO levels has become more practical. An advantage of the measurement of blood CO as an indication of the rate of red cell destruction is that it gives the rate of destruction at a single point in time. An instrument by CoSense (Capnia Inc., Palo Alto, CA) obtained FDA 510(k) clearance in December 2013 and provides a substitute for the previous Natus end-tidal breath analyzer (Natus Medical, San Carlos, CA) that had not been available for about a decade. CoSense is compact and portable, and uses a sterile one-time-use single nasal cannula for quantifying end-tidal breath for CO quantification and also samples ambient CO, which is subtracted from the value in exhaled breath and is suitable for use in neonates. This device also counts the breath rate, analyzes CO in individual breaths, and provides CO measurements in parts per million in a matter of minutes.

● IN SITU LOCALIZATION OF RED CELL PRODUCTION AND DESTRUCTION

As part of routine erythrokinetic studies both radioactive iron and radioactive chromium may be used to localize red cell production and red cell destruction. This is accomplished by positioning probes for external counting over the sacrum, liver, spleen, and heart and measuring the distribution of radioactivity in the body.[43]

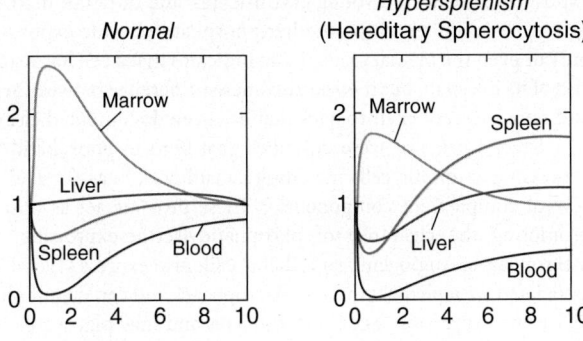

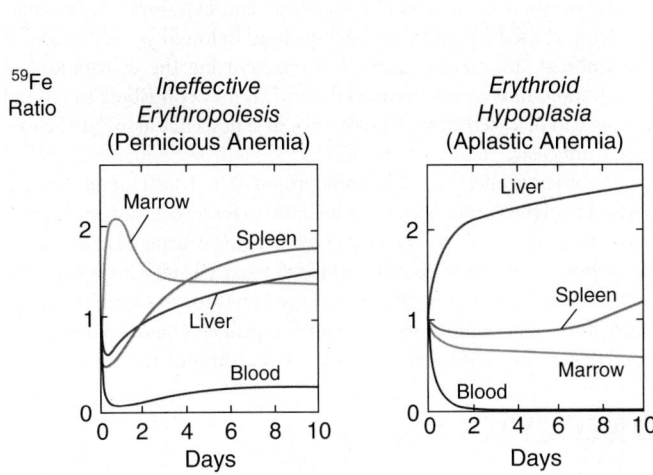

Figure 33–2. Tissue distribution of ^{59}Fe in normal subjects, hypersplenic patients, and anemic patients with ineffective and effective erythropoiesis. The radioactivity is expressed on the ordinate as a ratio relative to the radioactivity measured in the same organ 15 minutes after the intravenous administration of the isotope. (*Redrawn with permission from Hillman RS and Finch CA: Erythropoiesis: Normal and abnormal.* Semin Hematol (4):327–336, 1967.)

In a normal subject, ^{59}Fe injected intravenously is cleared rapidly from the plasma, and within 24 hours approximately 85 percent of the radioactivity can be accounted for in the marrow. The liver and the spleen divide the remaining 15 percent. Over the next 10 days the marrow radioactivity decreases gradually as a result of the release into circulating blood of red cells labeled with radioactive hemoglobin. Patterns showing different uptake and distribution of the radioactive iron have been found for various hematologic disorders.[44] In hypersplenism, the trapping and destruction of iron-labeled cells in the spleen increases splenic radioactivity rapidly, and in patients with erythroid hypoplasia the distribution of radioactive iron between liver and marrow is reversed (Fig. 33–2).

IMAGING MACROPHAGES IN THE MARROW, LIVER, AND SPLEEN

More effective methods demonstrating *in situ* erythropoiesis involve imaging the macrophages in the marrow, liver, and spleen with a technetium-99m (^{99m}Tc) sulfur colloid or indium-111 (^{111}In).[45] Although these isotopes label primarily the monocyte-macrophage system, their uptake is similar to that of ^{59}Fe and they can be used as surrogate markers to estimate the distribution of erythroid tissue.

SURFACE COUNTING FOR CHROMIUM-51

Surface counting for ^{51}Cr-labeled red cells provides a characteristic organ distribution of radioactivity and has been used to demonstrate the degree of red cell sequestration and destruction in an enlarged spleen (see Fig. 33–2).[46] This approach has been used to predict the results of elective splenectomy, but the utility of this method has been challenged.[47] The *in situ* localization of red cell sequestration or destruction can also be determined by following the tissue distribution of ^{59}Fe-labeled red cells, especially if the red cell life span is very short.

SENESCENCE OF NORMAL ERYTHROCYTES

Methodologic Considerations
Labeling a cohort of human erythrocytes with ^{59}Fe and centrifuging the cells in a density gradient demonstrates that reticulocytes and young red cells are less dense than mature red cells.[48,49] However, at the end of the life span of the labeled cohort, radioactivity is fairly evenly distributed throughout red cells of all densities, with only a slight tendency of the radioactivity to be concentrated in the more dense cells. Unfortunately, many studies of the properties of senescent cells in the past have been based upon the characteristics of the most dense fraction of erythrocytes, using various fractionating techniques. In fact, the most dense fraction of red cells is only slightly enriched with old erythrocytes.[50,51] A combination of density separation and elutriation seemed to provide results superior to density separation alone using hemoglobin A$_{1C}$ content as a marker, but the degree of enrichment with older cells has not been documented using actual old red cells as separated by biotinylation or by the mouse hypertransfusion technique.[52]

There are two animal models and one human disease model that provide cells that are truly aged. In mice, *in vivo* aged cells have been produced by serially transfusing mice, maintaining polycythemia to suppress virtually all erythropoiesis.[53] In other species, particularly the rabbit, red cells have been labeled with traces of biotin, which allows them to be recovered from the circulation.[54] The human model is transient erythroblastopenia of childhood (Chaps. 36 and 55), a disorder in which there is cessation of all erythropoiesis for several months; however, the density and deformability of the aged cells in erythroblastopenia of childhood is normal.[50] The use of the latter model has been criticized because this disorder is not fully understood and the red cells in the circulation may not be entirely normal.[55] However, the results that have been obtained are consistent with those obtained in animal models and are probably reliable (see "Properties of Aged Cells" below).

PROPERTIES OF AGED CELLS

Although the activities of a large number of enzymes, including hexokinase, glucose-6-phosphate dehydrogenase (G6PD), and pyruvate kinase (PK), are higher in reticulocytes than in mature erythrocytes, the activities of these enzymes do not normally continue to decline during the aging of the erythrocyte.[54,56] Pyrimidine-5′-nucleotidase[57,58] and adenosine monophosphate (AMP)-deaminase[59–61] appear to be exceptions to this rule in that there is continuing decline of enzyme activity throughout the life span of the red cell. The decrease in the activity of these enzymes is not linear with age but exponential.[3] This stability of many of the red cell enzymes during the aging of normal erythrocytes contrasts to the circumstances that are brought about by mutations in enzymes such as G6PD and PK, where instability of the abnormal enzyme leads to accelerated decay in the amount of enzyme protein, a factor that surely plays an important role in the ultimate demise of the cell (Chap. 47). Fluorescent sorting of blood type NN erythrocytes transfused into humans shows that the most dense fractions are only minimally enriched with old cells,[62] and biotinylated aged cells of rabbits have been found to have only a modestly decreased surface area, volume, cell water, and density, and therefore slightly decreased deformability.[51,63]

As they circulate red cells lose a substantial portion of their membrane and hemoglobin in the form of vesicles (reviewed in Ref. 64). The loss of membrane material in hemoglobin vesicles may play a role in the aging process.[65] In normal blood, a small number of red cell vesicles, approximately 190/μL blood, can be harvested. During storage of RBCs, the aggregates of vesicles are formed and may contribute to acute lung injury by interacting with neutrophils.[66]

MECHANISM OF DESTRUCTION OF NORMAL, AGED CELLS

Several different mechanisms of senescent red cell destruction have been proposed. Determining the actual mechanism(s) is especially difficult because the cells that are marked for removal are bound to be present at very low concentrations or not at all in the circulating blood—they have been removed. Many of the earlier data are predicated upon the isolation of dense cells and the consideration that they are "old"; we now recognize that they are not (see "Methodologic Considerations" above). Moreover, it is likely that there is more than one mechanism that serves to remove effete red cells from the circulation; there is no known mutation that lengthens red cell life span.

Band 3 Clustering Models

It has been proposed that an altered membrane band 3 serves as a receptor for antibodies directed against a neoantigen, designated senescent-cell antigen, and that possibly after-binding complement marks the senescent cell for destruction. It is not known how clustering of band 3 occurs *in vivo* and recent work suggests peroxidation of cytoplasmic aspect of band 3 results in carbonylation. Methemoglobin binds to the cytoplasmic peroxidized domain of band 3 and induces cluster formation.[67] But much, if not all, of the evidence for these models depends upon the assumption that dense cells are old, and the uptake of cells by monocytes as a surrogate for their being marked for destruction.[68] However, immunoglobulin levels on aged, biotinylated rabbit cells are not increased,[69] and the fact that red cell life span has never been demonstrated to be prolonged in agammaglobulinemic patients casts serious doubt upon the concept that immunoglobulins mediate removal of senescent red cells.

Phosphatidylserine Exposure Models

In RBCs, as in most other cells, the anionic phospholipid phosphatidylserine is present exclusively in the inner cytoplasmic leaflet of the membrane bilayer.[70] The exposure of phosphatidylserine on the outer leaflet of the cell membrane is one of the signals that allows macrophages to recognize apoptotic cells. It is likely that this is, indeed, at least one of the signals by which macrophages recognize senescent erythrocytes.[5,71,72] Data from a biotinylated rabbit erythrocyte model suggests that the average time during which phosphatidylserine is exposed is only 0.3 to 0.5 days, so that few cells with increased exposure of the phospholipid are in the circulation at any time.[71] An increase of phosphatidylserine exposure has also been documented in humans descending from high altitudes.[73] The exposure of phosphatidylserine on the outer leaflet of the cell membrane is one of the signals. A proposed model for the destruction of newly formed cells was that endothelial cells might respond to changes in circulating erythropoietin by influencing the interaction of phagocytes with young red cells, targeting the cells by surface adhesion molecules.[74] A study in mice, using somewhat different methods, suggested that phosphatidylserine

exposure is greatest in young erythrocytes, and does not increase with aging.[75] It is not yet clear whether phosphatidylserine exposure is the only or even the primary signal that indicates that a cell has reached the end of its life span, but it is the only major difference between senescent and nonsenescent erythrocytes that has been documented clearly.[72]

Several proteins were described that bind to phosphatidylserine-expressing apoptotic cells including lactadherin,[76] gas-6,[77] Del-1,[78] and several complement components.[79] These proteins act as opsonins in promoting the clearance of phosphatidylserine-expressing cells by macrophages. Angiogenic endothelial cells also express several integrin associated with phagocytosis in macrophages and can engulf phosphatidylserine expressing "aged" erythrocytes and may play a role in clearance of senescent cells.[80]

Eryptosis is defined as cell shrinkage and exposure of phosphatidylserine caused by entry of calcium ions followed by activation of a scramblase, an enzyme capable of randomizing the distribution of phospholipid in both membrane bilayers.[70] It may contribute to red cell clearance in diseased states,[81] but its role in senescence associated clearance is not clear.[82]

Another model that has been proposed is based upon a slight increase in green autofluorescence, believed to represent the result of oxidative damage, which has been observed in aging murine erythrocytes.[83] Interaction of erythrocyte cell surface antigen CD44 with hyaluronic acid may play a role in the clearance of aged erythrocytes from the circulation, but such clearance seems limited to primates, and a patient with CD44 deficiency manifested congenital dyserythropoietic anemia.[84]

● NEOCYTOLYSIS

Hypoxia increases RBCs by enhancing hypoxia-inducible factors (HIFs). Upon return to normoxia, the secondary polycythemia is overcorrected, as the accumulated, newly formed RBCs undergo preferential destruction, a process termed *neocytolysis;* however, its mechanism is unclear.[74] Neocytolysis was originally observed during space travel at zero gravity wherein the mechanism is even less clear. It has been suggested that on return to normoxia, there is excessive generation of reactive oxygen species from increased mitochondrial mass correlating with decreased hypoxia controlled gene BNIP3L transcripts,[85,86] as BNIP3L mediates removal of reticulocyte mitochondria accompanied by reduced catalase activity.[87] Rapid changes in hematocrit in human newborns also suggest that neocytolysis also occurs after birth when a hypoxic fetus is polycythemic at birth, but the neonate rapidly overcorrects its increased red cell mass and becomes anemic in first 2 weeks of life.[88,89]

● MECHANISMS OF DESTRUCTION

"Senescence of Normal Erythrocytes," above, enumerated some mechanisms that may be involved in normally terminating the life of the effete erythrocyte. It has sometimes been assumed that the mechanisms by which red cells are destroyed prematurely in disease states reflect these normal mechanisms. Although there may well be some overlap, the mechanisms of red cell destruction in disease states are likely different. The assumption that the mechanisms that bring around hemolytic anemia represent premature aging of the erythrocyte is no more logical than to suggest that an animal's death through pneumonia, renal failure, or cancer represents premature aging.

INTRAVASCULAR DESTRUCTION

If the red cell membrane is breached in the circulation the red cell is destroyed. This mode of erythrocyte demise occurs at a low frequency, but may be the predominant mode of destruction in some hemolytic disorders, for example, ABO-incompatible transfusions (Chap. 138) and paroxysmal nocturnal hemoglobinuria (Chap. 40), where the surface complement complex creates pores in the red cell membrane, and in cardiac valve hemolysis (Chap. 51) and microangiopathic hemolytic anemia (Chaps. 51 and 132), where the shear stress may be so strong as to break open the membrane.

EXTRAVASCULAR DESTRUCTION

Most commonly, the life of the red cell comes to an end when it is ingested by a macrophage. Clearly, signals that allow the macrophage to distinguish the younger normal red cell from a damaged or senescent cell must exist. Such signals may consist of decreased deformability and/or altered surface properties.

Decreased Deformability

The red cell does not circulate as the biconcave disc customarily observed under the microscope. Instead, it is normally greatly distorted by the shear stresses in the circulation and such distortion is an absolute requirement for the red cell to be able to negotiate the narrow slits that separate the splenic pulp from the sinuses (Chaps. 6 and 56). The deformability of the erythrocyte can be measured clinically using the ektacytometer, an instrument that displays the diffraction pattern of a red cell suspension under shear stress.[90,91] The red cell membrane, a lipid bilayer, bends readily but has very little capacity to stretch. Thus, deformability is largely a function of the excess red cell membrane intrinsic to the biconcave disc shape of the cell, membrane composition, and to some extent, of the viscosity of the hemoglobin solution within the cell. As the red cell loses membrane it assumes a spherical shape and loses its ability to deform. Hereditary spherocytosis and hereditary elliptocytosis are prototypic of hemolytic anemias in which decreased deformability as a result of a decreased surface-to-volume ratio plays a key role in red cell destruction (Chap. 46). However, loss of membrane plays a role in many types of pathologic hemolysis, including autoimmune hemolytic anemia (Chap. 54). In sickle cell disease and hemoglobin C disease (Chap. 49), the internal viscosity of the cell is increased. Loss of water from the red cell, as may occur when the membrane is damaged and leaks potassium as in hereditary xerocytosis (Chap. 46), also markedly impairs the deformability of the cell.

Altered Surface Properties

The surface of the red cell membrane can be altered by binding of antibodies to surface antigens, by binding of complement components, and by chemical alterations, particularly oxidation of membrane components. Immunoglobulin (Ig) G–coated red cells[92] and red cells coated by the third component of complement (C_3)[93,94] are bound by Fc receptors on macrophages and undergo partial phagocytosis. This results in the formation of a spherocyte.

In vitro oxidation of red cells with phenylhydrazine or adenosine diphosphate (ADP) plus iron causes clustering of band 3 protein in the membrane. Although the physiologic significance of this is far from clear, it has been suggested that the clustered protein serves as a recognition site for the binding of IgG.[9,95] Oxidative damage to the membrane may play a role in the removal of sickle cells (Chap. 49) and thalassemic cells from the circulation (Chap. 48).

● FATE OF DESTROYED RED CELLS

INTRAVASCULAR DESTRUCTION

Hemoglobin

When red cells are destroyed in the vascular compartment the hemoglobin escaping into the plasma is bound to haptoglobin. A dimeric glycoprotein, each molecule of haptoglobin can bind two hemoglobin dimers. The binding of hemoglobin not only protects against its potential toxicity, it also triggers the second step of the scavenging process, that is, recognition by macrophage receptor CD163, and subsequent clearance of the entire complex by receptor-mediated endocytosis.[96] CD163 belongs to the scavenger receptor cysteine-rich family of proteins and the haptoglobin–hemoglobin complex is cleared from the plasma with a $T_{1/2}$ of 10 to 30 minutes. The heme of the hemoglobin is converted to iron and biliverdin by heme oxygenase and the biliverdin is further catabolized to bilirubin. CO is released (see "Indirect Methods," above, on measuring red cell life span) in the course of cleavage of heme by heme oxygenase.[97]

Haptoglobin

Free haptoglobin, in contrast to the hemoglobin–haptoglobin complex, has a $T_{1/2}$ of 5 days, and when large amounts of the rapidly turned over haptoglobin–hemoglobin complex are formed, the haptoglobin content of the plasma is depleted. The haptoglobin content of the plasma is diminished not only in the plasma of patients undergoing frank intravascular hemolysis, but also from the plasma of patients who, like those with sickle cell disease, have accelerated red cell destruction occurring primarily within macrophages. Presumably there is either enough intravascular hemolysis in such hemolytic disorders to lower the plasma haptoglobin level or sufficient leakage from the phagocytic cells into the plasma to bind to haptoglobin. Thus the measurement of plasma haptoglobin levels has usefulness in diagnosing the presence of hemolysis, although it cannot, as previously suggested, serve to clearly distinguish extravascular from intravascular hemolysis.

Heme

Free heme that is released into the circulation is bound in a 1:1 ratio to the plasma glycoprotein hemopexin,[98] which is cleared from the plasma with a $T_{1/2}$ of 7 to 8 hours.[99,100] The heme–hemopexin complex is taken up by a low-density lipoprotein-related receptor, CD91.[101] Figure 33–3 illustrates the parallel functions of hemopexin and haptoglobin. When the capacity of hemopexin to bind heme is saturated, excess heme may bind to albumin to form methemalbumin.[102] Excess heme is toxic to cells because of the ability of heme to catalyze the so-called Fenton reaction, generating hydroxyl radicals, a highly reactive oxygen species. To avoid the phenomenon and complement the negative feedback regulation of heme synthesis, the expression of heme oxygenase (HO)-1 is induced in response to an increased level of heme, which subsequently results in the degradation of excess heme not bound to proteins. In contrast to HO-1, HO-2 is constitutively expressed and participates in the regulation of a basal heme level.

EXTRAVASCULAR DESTRUCTION

Red cells that are engulfed by phagocytic cells are degraded within lysosomes into lipids, protein, and heme. The proteins and lipids are reprocessed in their respective catabolic pathways and the heme is cleaved by a microsomal HO.[103] HO catalyzes the oxygen-dependent degradation of heme to biliverdin with the release of CO and "free" iron. Biliverdin is converted into bilirubin by biliverdin reductase α (BVRα), which is expressed ubiquitously in all tissues under basal conditions with high levels in macrophages in the spleen and liver.[104] The overall reduction of biliverdin to bilirubin is very efficient, and under physiologic circumstances, the concentration of serum biliverdin is low.

Bilirubin Excretion

Regardless of the site of destruction of hemoglobin, one of the final products is bilirubin. Bilirubin is very insoluble and transported in

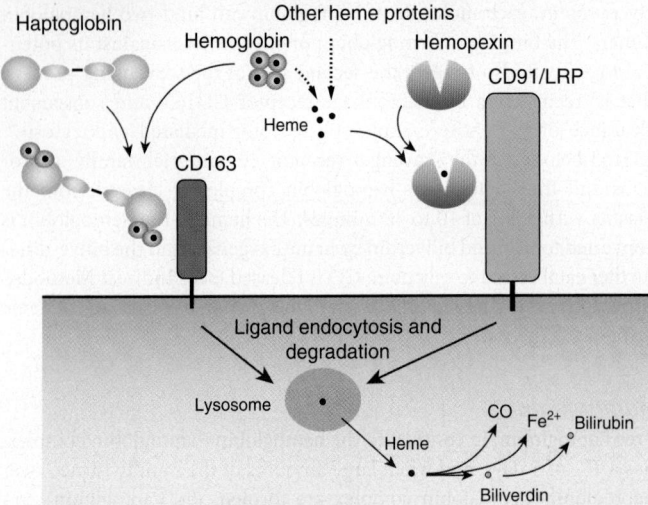

Figure 33–3. Overview of the receptor pathways for endocytosis of extracellular heme and hemoglobin in complex with hemopexin and haptoglobin, respectively. LRP/CD91 and CD163 represent two pathways for uptake of extracellular heme incorporated in hemopexin–heme and haptoglobin–hemoglobin. Both receptors are highly expressed in phagocytic macrophages, which are known to metabolize heme into bilirubin, Fe, and CO. In addition to the expression in macrophages, LRP/CD91 is highly expressed in several other cell types including hepatocytes, neurons, and syncytiotrophoblasts. (*Reproduced with permission from Hvidberg V, Maniecki MB, Jacobsen C, et al.: Identification of the receptor scavenging hemopexin-heme complexes.* Blood *106(7):2572–2579, 2005.*)

plasma bound to albumin. Unconjugated bilirubin is taken up into hepatocytes by transporters of the organic anion-transporting polypeptide (OATP) family, followed by conjugation with glucuronic acid in the microsomes, and ATP-dependent transport into bile. This efflux across the canalicular membrane is mediated by multidrug resistance protein 2, which has high affinity for monoglucuronosyl bilirubin and bisglucuronosyl bilirubin.[105] In the gastrointestinal tract the bilirubin is converted to urobilinogens by bacterial reduction.[106] A small fraction of urobilinogen is reabsorbed and excreted into the urine. Thus, the fecal and urinary urobilinogen excretion have been used as an indicator of the rate of hemolysis, but are only uncommonly used for this purpose in modern practice because the collections are cumbersome and because alternative degradative pathways detract severely from the accuracy of the estimates of the rate of heme catabolism.

REFERENCES

1. Bratosin D, Mazurier J, Tissier JP, et al: Cellular and molecular mechanisms of senescent erythrocyte phagocytosis by macrophages. A review. *Biochimie* 80(2):173, 1998.
2. Lutz HU, Bogdanova A: Mechanisms tagging senescent red blood cells for clearance in healthy humans. *Front Physiol* 4:387, 2013.
3. Clark MR: Senescence of red blood cells: Progress and problems. *Physiol Rev* 68(2):503, 1988.
4. Lichtman MA: Does ATP decrease exponentially during red cell aging? *Nouv Rev Fr Hematol* 17(6):625, 1975.
5. Connor J, Pak CC, Schroit AJ: Exposure of phosphatidylserine in the outer leaflet of human red blood cells. Relationship to cell density, cell age, and clearance by mononuclear cells. *J Biol Chem* 269(4):2399, 1994.
6. Ando K, Beppu M, Kikugawa K: Evidence for accumulation of lipid hydroperoxides during the aging of human red blood cells in the circulation. *Biol Pharm Bull* 18(5):659, 1995.
7. Shinozuka T: Changes in human red blood cells during aging in vivo. *Keio J Med* 43(3):155, 1994.
8. Kay MM: Generation of senescent cell antigen on old cells initiates igg binding to a neoantigen. *Cell Mol Biol (Noisy-le-grand)* 39(2):131, 1993.
9. Low PS, Waugh SM, Zinke K, et al: The role of hemoglobin denaturation and band 3 clustering in red blood cell aging. *Science* 227(4686):531, 1985.
10. Mohanty JG, Nagababu E, Rifkind JM: Red blood cell oxidative stress impairs oxygen delivery and induces red blood cell aging. *Front Physiol* 5:84, 2014.
11. Lutz HU, Gianora O, Nater M, et al: Naturally occurring anti-band 3 antibodies bind to protein rather than to carbohydrate on band 3. *J Biol Chem* 268(31):23562, 1993.
12. Gattegno L, Bladier D, Vaysse J, et al: Inhibition by carbohydrates and monoclonal anti-complement receptor type 1, on interactions between senescent human red blood cells and monocytic macrophagic cells. *Adv Exp Med Biol* 307:329, 1991.
13. Ashby W: The determination of the length of life of transfused blood corpuscles in man. *J Exp Med* 29(3):267, 1919.
14. Shemin D, Rittenberg D: The life span of the human red blood cell. *J Biol Chem* 166(2):627, 1946.
15. Berlin NI, Meyer LM, Lazarus M: Life span of the rat red blood cell as determined by glycine-2-c14. *Am J Physiol* 165(3):465, 1951.
16. Beutler E, Dern RJ, Alving AS: The hemolytic effect of primaquine. Iv. The relationship of cell age to hemolysis. *J Lab Clin Med* 44(3):439, 1954.
17. Birgens HS, Hansen OP, Henriksen JH, et al: Quantitation of erythropoiesis in myelomatosis. *Scand J Haematol* 22(4):357, 1979.
18. Weinstein IM, Beutler E: The use of cr51 and fe59 in a combined procedure to study erythrocyte production and destruction in normal human subjects and in patients with hemolytic or aplastic anemia. *J Lab Clin Med* 45(4):616, 1955.
19. Gifford SC, Yoshida T, Shevkoplyas SS, et al: A high-resolution, double-labeling method for the study of in vivo red blood cell aging. *Transfusion* 46(4):578, 2006.
20. Beutler E, West C: Measurement of the viability of stored red cells by the single-isotope technique using 51cr. Analysis of validity. *Transfusion* 24(2):100, 1984.
21. Lindsell CJ, Franco RS, Smith EP, et al: A method for the continuous calculation of the age of labeled red blood cells. *Am J Hematol* 83(6):454, 2008.
22. Silver HM, Seebeck MA, Cowett RM, et al: Red cell volume determination using a stable isotope of chromium. *J Soc Gynecol Investig* 4(5):254, 1997.
23. Cline MJ, Berlin NI: Measurement of red cell survival with tritiated diisopropylfluorophosphate. *J Lab Clin Med* 60:826, 1962.
24. Milner PF, Charache S: Life span of carbamylated red cells in sickle cell anemia. *J Clin Invest* 52(12):3161, 1973.
25. Eschbach JW, Korn D, Finch CA: 14C cyanate as a tag for red cell survival in normal and uremic man. *J Lab Clin Med* 89(4):823, 1977.
26. Horan PK, Slezak SE: Stable cell membrane labelling. *Nature* 340(6229):167, 1989.
27. Slezak SE, Horan PK: Fluorescent in vivo tracking of hematopoietic cells. Part I. Technical considerations. *Blood* 74(6):2172, 1989.
28. Strauss RG, Mock DM, Widness JA, et al: Posttransfusion 24-hour recovery and subsequent survival of allogeneic red blood cells in the bloodstream of newborn infants. *Transfusion* 44(6):871, 2004.
29. Suzuki T, Dale GL: Biotinylated erythrocytes: In vivo survival and in vitro recovery. *Blood* 70(3):791, 1987.
30. Bentley SA, Glass HI, Lewis SM, et al: Elution correction in 51Cr red cell survival studies. *Br J Haematol* 26(2):179, 1974.
31. McCurdy PR, Sherman AS: Irreversibly sickled cells and red cell survival in sickle cell anemia: A study with both DF32P and 51CR. *Am J Med* 64(2):253, 1978.
32. Franco RS: Measurement of red cell lifespan and aging. *Transfus Med Hemother* 39(5):302, 2012.
33. Mollison P, Engelfriet CP, Contreras M: The transfusion of red cells, in *Blood Transfusion in Clinical Medicine*, edited by Mollison PL. p 95. Blackwell, Oxford, 1987.
34. Eadie GS, Brown IW Jr: Red blood cell survival studies. *Blood* 8(12):1110, 1953.
35. Recommended method for radioisotope red-cell survival studies. International committee for standardization in haematology. *Br J Haematol* 45(4):659, 1980.
36. Cavill I, Trevett D, Fisher J, et al: The measurement of the total volume of red cells in man: A non-radioactive approach using biotin. *Br J Haematol* 70(4):491, 1988.
37. Franco RS, Yasin Z, Palascak MB, et al: The effect of fetal hemoglobin on the survival characteristics of sickle cells. *Blood* 108(3):1073, 2006.
38. Yasin Z, Witting S, Palascak MB, et al: Phosphatidylserine externalization in sickle red blood cells. Associations with cell age, density, and hemoglobin f. *Blood* 102(1):365, 2003.
39. Berlin NI, Berk PD: Quantitative aspects of bilirubin metabolism for hematologists. *Blood* 57(6):983, 1981.
40. Doyle J, Vreman HJ, Stevenson DK, et al: Does vitamin C cause hemolysis in premature newborn infants? Results of a multicenter double-blind, randomized, controlled trial. *J Pediatr* 130(1):103, 1997.
41. Furne JK, Springfield JR, Ho SB, et al: Simplification of the end-alveolar carbon monoxide technique to assess erythrocyte survival. *J Lab Clin Med* 142(1):52, 2003.
42. Vreman HJ, Stevenson DK: Carboxyhemoglobin determined in neonatal blood with a co-oximeter unaffected by fetal oxyhemoglobin. *Clin Chem* 40(8):1522, 1994.
43. Proceedings: Recommended methods for surface counting to determine sites of red-cell destruction. A report by the panel on diagnostic applications of radioisotopes in haematology of the International Committee for Standardization in Haematology (ICSH tentative standard ep8/3: 1975). *Br J Haematol* 30(2):249, 1975.
44. Hillman RS, Finch CA: Erythropoiesis: Normal and abnormal. *Semin Hematol* 4(4):327, 1967.
45. Datz FL, Taylor A Jr: The clinical use of radionuclide bone marrow imaging. *Semin Nucl Med* 15(3):239, 1985.
46. Jandl JH, Greenberg MS, Yonemoto RH, et al: Clinical determination of the sites of red cell sequestration in hemolytic anemias. *J Clin Invest* 35(8):842, 1956.

47. Ferrant A, Cauwe F, Michaux JL, et al: Assessment of the sites of red cell destruction using quantitative measurements of splenic and hepatic red cell destruction. *Br J Haematol* 50(4):591, 1982.

48. Borun ER, Figueroa WG, Perry SM: The distribution of Fe59 tagged human erythrocytes in centrifuged specimens as a function of cell age. *J Clin Invest* 36(5):676, 1957.

49. Luthra MG, Friedman JM, Sears DA: Studies of density fractions of normal human erythrocytes labeled with iron-59 in vivo. *J Lab Clin Med* 94(6):879, 1979.

50. Linderkamp O, Friederichs E, Boehler T, et al: Age dependency of red blood cell deformability and density: Studies in transient erythroblastopenia of childhood. *Br J Haematol* 83(1):125, 1993.

51. Dale GL, Norenberg SL: Density fractionation of erythrocytes by Percoll/Hypaque results in only a slight enrichment for aged cells. *Biochim Biophys Acta* 1036(3):183, 1990.

52. Bosch FH, Werre JM, Roerdinkholder-Stoelwinder B, et al: Characteristics of red blood cell populations fractionated with a combination of counterflow centrifugation and Percoll separation. *Blood* 79(1):254, 1992.

53. Ganzoni AM, Oakes R, Hillman RS: Red cell aging in vivo. *J Clin Invest* 50(7):1373, 1971.

54. Suzuki T, Dale GL: Senescent erythrocytes: Isolation of in vivo aged cells and their biochemical characteristics. *Proc Natl Acad Sci U S A* 85(5):1647, 1988.

55. Haram S, Carriero D, Seaman C, et al: The mechanism of decline of age-dependent enzymes in the red blood cell. *Enzyme* 45(1–2):47, 1991.

56. Zimran A, Forman L, Suzuki T, et al: In vivo aging of red cell enzymes: Study of biotinylated red blood cells in rabbits. *Am J Hematol* 33(4):249, 1990.

57. Beutler E, Hartman G: Age-related red cell enzymes in children with transient erythroblastopenia of childhood and with hemolytic anemia. *Pediatr Res* 19(1):44, 1985.

58. Beutler E: The relationship of red cell enzymes to red cell life-span. *Blood Cells* 14(1):69, 1988.

59. Dale GL, Norenberg SL: Time-dependent loss of adenosine 5′-monophosphate deaminase activity may explain elevated adenosine 5′-triphosphate levels in senescent erythrocytes. *Blood* 74(6):2157, 1989.

60. Paglia DE, Valentine WN, Nakatani M, et al: Amp deaminase as a cell-age marker in transient erythroblastopenia of childhood and its role in the adenylate economy of erythrocytes. *Blood* 74(6):2161, 1989.

61. Dale GL, Norenberg SL, Suzuki T, et al: Altered adenine nucleotide metabolism in senescent erythrocytes from the rabbit. *Prog Clin Biol Res* 319:259; discussion 270, 1989.

62. Clark MR CL, Jensen RH: Density distribution of aging, transfused human red cells. *Blood* 74(Suppl 1):217a, 1989.

63. Waugh RE, Narla M, Jackson CW, et al: Rheologic properties of senescent erythrocytes: Loss of surface area and volume with red blood cell age. *Blood* 79(5):1351, 1992.

64. Tissot JD, Rubin O, Canellini G: Analysis and clinical relevance of microparticles from red blood cells. *Curr Opin Hematol* 17(6):571, 2010.

65. Willekens FL, Werre JM, Groenen-Dopp YA, et al: Erythrocyte vesiculation: A self-protective mechanism? *Br J Haematol* 141(4):549, 2008.

66. Jank H, Salzer U: Vesicles generated during storage of red blood cells enhance the generation of radical oxygen species in activated neutrophils. *ScientificWorldJournal* 11:173, 2011.

67. Arashiki N, Kimata N, Manno S, et al: Membrane peroxidation and methemoglobin formation are both necessary for band 3 clustering: Mechanistic insights into human erythrocyte senescence. *Biochemistry* 52(34):5760, 2013.

68. Arese P, Turrini F, Schwarzer E: Band 3/complement-mediated recognition and removal of normally senescent and pathological human erythrocytes. *Cell Physiol Biochem* 16(4–6):133, 2005.

69. Dale GL, Daniels RB: Quantitation of immunoglobulin associated with senescent erythrocytes from the rabbit. *Blood.* 77(5):1096-9, 1991.

70. Zwaal RF, Comfurius P, Bevers EM: Surface exposure of phosphatidylserine in pathological cells. *Cell Mol Life Sci* 62(9):971, 2005.

71. Boas FE, Forman L, Beutler E: Phosphatidylserine exposure and red cell viability in red cell aging and in hemolytic anemia. *Proc Natl Acad Sci U S A* 95(6):3077, 1998.

72. Kuypers FA, de Jong K: The role of phosphatidylserine in recognition and removal of erythrocytes. *Cell Mol Biol (Noisy-le-grand)* 50(2):147, 2004.

73. Risso A, Turello M, Biffoni F, et al: Red blood cell senescence and neocytolysis in humans after high altitude acclimatization. *Blood Cells Mol Dis* 38(2):83, 2007.

74. Rice L, Alfrey CP: The negative regulation of red cell mass by neocytolysis: Physiologic and pathophysiologic manifestations. *Cell Physiol Biochem* 15(6):245, 2005.

75. Khandelwal S, Saxena RK: A role of phosphatidylserine externalization in clearance of erythrocytes exposed to stress but not in eliminating aging populations of erythrocyte in mice. *Exp Gerontol* 43(8):764, 2008.

76. Dasgupta SK, Abdel-Monem H, Guchhait P, et al: Role of lactadherin in the clearance of phosphatidylserine-expressing red blood cells. *Transfusion* 48(11):2370, 2008.

77. Ishimoto Y, Ohashi K, Mizuno K, et al: Promotion of the uptake of ps liposomes and apoptotic cells by a product of growth arrest-specific gene, gas6. *J Biochem* 127(3):411, 2000.

78. Hanayama R, Tanaka M, Miwa K, et al: Expression of developmental endothelial locus-1 in a subset of macrophages for engulfment of apoptotic cells. *J Immunol* 172(6):3876, 2004.

79. Wang RH, Phillips G Jr, Medof ME, et al: Activation of the alternative complement pathway by exposure of phosphatidylethanolamine and phosphatidylserine on erythrocytes in sickle cell disease patients. *J Clin Invest* 92(3):1326, 1993.

80. Fens MH, Storm G, Pelgrim RC, et al: Erythrophagocytosis by angiogenic endothelial cells is enhanced by loss of erythrocyte deformability. *Exp Hematol* 38(4):282, 2010.

81. Lang F, Gulbins E, Lerche H, et al: Eryptosis, a window to systemic disease. *Cell Physiol Biochem* 22(5–6):373, 2008.

82. Franco RS, Puchulu-Campanella ME, Barber LA, et al: Changes in the properties of normal human red blood cells during in vivo aging. *Am J Hematol* 88(1):44, 2013.

83. Khandelwal S, Saxena RK: Age-dependent increase in green autofluorescence of blood erythrocytes. *J Biosci* 32(6):1139, 2007.

84. Kerfoot SM, McRae K, Lam F, et al: A novel mechanism of erythrocyte capture from circulation in humans. *Exp Hematol* 36(2):111, 2008.

85. Sandoval H, Thiagarajan P, Dasgupta SK, et al: Essential role for nix in autophagic maturation of erythroid cells. *Nature* 454(7201):232, 2008.

86. Fei P, Wang W, Kim SH, et al: Bnip3l is induced by p53 under hypoxia, and its knockdown promotes tumor growth. *Cancer Cell* 6(6):597, 2004.

87. Song J YD, Thiagarajan P, Prchal JT: Molecular basis of neocytolysis, in *54th Annual Meeting American Society of Hematology*, p 2093. ASH Annual Meeting Abstracts, Atlanta, GA, 2012.

88. Javier MC, Krauss A, Nesin M: Corrected end-tidal carbon monoxide closely correlates with the corrected reticulocyte count in Coombs test-positive term neonates. *Pediatrics* 112(6 Pt 1):1333, 2003.

89. Christensen RD, Lambert DK, Henry E, et al: Unexplained extreme hyperbilirubinemia among neonates in a multihospital healthcare system. *Blood Cells Mol Dis* 50(2):105, 2013.

90. Rigal CS: The place of instruments in the scientific work of Marcel Bessis (1917–1994): The electron microscope and the ektacytometer. *Hematol Cell Ther* 42(4):250, 2000.

91. Shin S, Hou JX, Suh JS, et al: Validation and application of a microfluidic ektacytometer (rheoscan-d) in measuring erythrocyte deformability. *Clin Hemorheol Microcirc* 37(4):319, 2007.

92. LoBuglio AF, Cotran RS, Jandl JH: Red cells coated with immunoglobulin g: Binding and sphering by mononuclear cells in man. *Science* 158(3808):1582, 1967.

93. Jandl JH, Tomlinson AS: The destruction of red cells by antibodies in man. II. Pyrogenic, leukocytic and dermal responses to immune hemolysis. *J Clin Invest* 37(8):1202, 1958.

94. Lutz HU SP, Stammler P, Kock D, Taylor RP: Opsonic potential of c3b-anti-band 3 complexes when generated on senescent and oxidatively stressed red cells or in fluid phase, in *Red Blood Cell Aging*, edited by M Magnani. Plenum Press, New York, 1991.

95. Beppu M, Mizukami A, Nagoya M, et al: Binding of anti-band 3 autoantibody to oxidatively damaged erythrocytes. Formation of senescent antigen on erythrocyte surface by an oxidative mechanism. *J Biol Chem* 265(6):3226, 1990.

96. Nielsen MJ, Andersen CB, Moestrup SK: Cd163 binding to haptoglobin-hemoglobin complexes involves a dual-point electrostatic receptor-ligand pairing. *J Biol Chem* 288(26):18834, 2013.

97. Carter K, Worwood M: Haptoglobin: A review of the major allele frequencies worldwide and their association with diseases. *Int J Lab Hematol* 29(2):92, 2007.

98. Piccard H, Van den Steen PE, Opdenakker G: Hemopexin domains as multifunctional liganding modules in matrix metalloproteinases and other proteins. *J Leukoc Biol* 81(4):870, 2007.

99. Sears DA: Disposal of plasma heme in normal man and patients with intravascular hemolysis. *J Clin Invest* 49(1):5, 1970.

100. Wochner RD, Spilberg I, Iio A, et al: Hemopexin metabolism in sickle-cell disease, porphyrias and control subjects—effects of heme injection. *N Engl J Med* 290(15):822, 1974.

101. Hvidberg V, Maniecki MB, Jacobsen C, et al: Identification of the receptor scavenging hemopexin-heme complexes. *Blood* 106(7):2572, 2005.

102. Rosen H, Sears DA, Meisenzahl T: Spectral properties of hemospexin-heme. The Schumm test. *J Lab Clin Med* 74(6):941, 1969.

103. Maines MD: The heme oxygenase system: A regulator of second messenger gases. *Annu Rev Pharmacol Toxicol* 37:517, 1997.

104. Komuro A, Tobe T, Nakano Y, et al: Cloning and characterization of the cdna encoding human biliverdin-ix alpha reductase. *Biochim Biophys Acta* 1309(1–2):89, 1996.

105. Erlinger S, Arias IM, Dhumeaux D: Inherited disorders of bilirubin transport and conjugation: New insights into molecular mechanisms and consequences. *Gastroenterology* 146(7):1625, 2014.

106. Elder G, Gray CH, Nicholson DC: Bile pigment fate in gastrointestinal tract. *Semin Hematol* 9(1):71, 1972.

CHAPTER 34
CLINICAL MANIFESTATIONS AND CLASSIFICATION OF ERYTHROCYTE DISORDERS

Josef T. Prchal

SUMMARY

Anemias are characterized by a decrease and polycythemias by an increase of the red cell mass. In most clinical situations, changes in red cell mass are inferred from the hemoglobin concentration or hematocrit. Some red cell disorders are associated with compensated hemolysis without or with only slight anemia. Their clinical manifestations are evident not by the effects of anemia but by changes associated with catabolism of hemoglobin such as an increase in serum bilirubin and, if sustained, cholelithiasis, decreased haptoglobin, and usually chronic reticulocytosis. Some red cells disorders are only showcased by morphologic abnormalities as exemplified by hereditary elliptocytosis unaccompanied by hemolysis or anemia.

The anemias have their principal effect by decreasing the oxygen-carrying capacity of blood and their severity is best considered in terms of blood hemoglobin concentration. Anemia may cause symptoms because of tissue hypoxia (e.g., fatigue, dyspnea on exertion). Some manifestations are also caused by compensatory attempts to ameliorate hypoxia (e.g., hyperventilation, tachycardia, and increased cardiac output). These manifestations are a function of the severity and rapidity of onset of the anemia. Tissue hypoxia sensing is ubiquitous and is signaled by an increased level of hypoxia-inducible transcription factors (HIFs)-1 and -2. HIFs upregulate transcription of many genes, in addition to the principal erythropoietic factor erythropoietin (EPO), that are involved in erythropoiesis, but also in angiogenesis, energy metabolism, and iron balance. The classification of anemia should take into account new kinetic and molecular findings.

The polycythemias (erythrocytoses) are best expressed in terms of the packed red cell volume (hematocrit), as their clinical manifestations are primarily related to the expanded red cell mass and resulting increased viscosity of blood, and other specific features related to the pathophysiology stemming from a molecular causative defect (e.g., thrombosis in polycythemia vera, cyanosis in congenital methemoglobinemia). The polycythemias may be primary, caused by somatic or germline mutation(s) dysregulating expansion of erythroid progenitors and, thus, red cell production, e.g., clonal expansion of a multipotential hematopoietic cell (polycythemia vera) or gain-of-function mutations of the EPO receptor (EPOR) on red cell progenitors—or secondary, caused by increased levels of circulating erythropoiesis-stimulating factors, usually EPO, as a result of tissue hypoxia (e.g., chronic pulmonary disease, high oxygen-affinity hemoglobin mutants, cobalt poisoning). Some polycythemias have hypersensitive erythroid progenitors, as well as increased levels of EPO, and thus share features of both primary and secondary polycythemia; these include Chuvash polycythemia and some other congenital disorders of hypoxia sensing. Persons with relative (spurious) polycythemia have an increased hematocrit as a result of a decreased plasma volume but a normal red cell mass.

● ANEMIA

PATHOPHYSIOLOGY AND MANIFESTATIONS

Effects on Oxygen Transport

The clinical manifestations of anemia are a function of the degree of tissue hypoxia and the etiology and pathogenesis of the specific anemia (e.g., splenomegaly characteristic of hereditary spherocytosis, neurologic degeneration, or gastric atrophy of pernicious anemia). Decreased oxygen-carrying capacity mobilizes compensatory mechanisms designed to prevent or ameliorate tissue hypoxia. Red cells also transport carbon dioxide from tissues to the lungs and help distribute nitric oxide throughout the body (Chap. 50), but transport of these gases does not appear to be dependent on the concentration of red cells in the blood and is normal in anemic patients. Tissue hypoxia occurs when the pressure of oxygen in the capillaries is too low to provide cells with enough oxygen for cell metabolic needs. In an average person, the red cell mass must provide the total body tissues with approximately 250 mL/min of oxygen to support life. The oxygen-carrying capacity of normal blood is 1.34 mL per gram of hemoglobin (approximately 200 mL/L of normal blood) and cardiac output is approximately 5000 mL/min; thus, 1000 mL/min of oxygen is available at the tissue level. Extraction of one-fourth of this amount reduces the oxygen tension of 100 torr in the arterial end of the capillary to 40 torr in the venous end. This partial extraction ensures the presence of sufficient diffusion pressure throughout the capillaries to provide all cells with enough oxygen for the cell's metabolic needs (Fig. 34–1). In anemia, extraction of the same amount of oxygen leads to greater hemoglobin desaturation and lower oxygen tension at the venous end of the capillary. The resulting hypoxia in the immediate vicinity initiates a number of compensatory, and frequently symptomatic, adjustments in the supply of blood and oxygen.

Hypoxia-Inducible Transcription Factors Hypoxia-inducible transcription factor (HIF)-1 and its homologue with tissue-restricted expression, HIF-2, play a central role in the body's response to hypoxia (Chaps. 32 and 57). HIF-1 was first identified as a factor regulating the transcriptional activity of the erythropoietin (EPO) gene (Chap. 32).[1] The essential role of this transcriptional factor in global regulation of protection against hypoxia soon became clear. Its actions include respiratory control, transcriptional regulation of glycolytic enzyme genes, angiogenesis, and energy metabolism.[2-4] The prediction that degradation of the hypoxia-regulated subunit of HIF-1 (HIF-1α) is controlled by an enzyme sensitive to the presence or absence of oxygen[5] proved to be prescient. Thus, HIF's downregulation is mediated by two principal negative regulators: von Hippel-Lindau tumor suppressor (VHL) and prolyl hydroxylase domain-containing protein 2 (PHD2). Chapter 32

Acronyms and Abbreviations: *EGLN1*, a gene encoding PHD2 protein; *EPAS1*, a gene encoding hypoxia-inducible factor-2α; EPO, erythropoietin; EPOR, erythropoietin receptor; HIF, hypoxia-inducible factor; MCHC, mean corpuscular hemoglobin concentration; MCV, mean corpuscular volume; PFCP, primary familial and congenital polycythemia; PHD2, prolyl hydroxylase domain-containing protein 2; *VHL*, a gene encoding von Hippel-Lindau tumor suppressor.

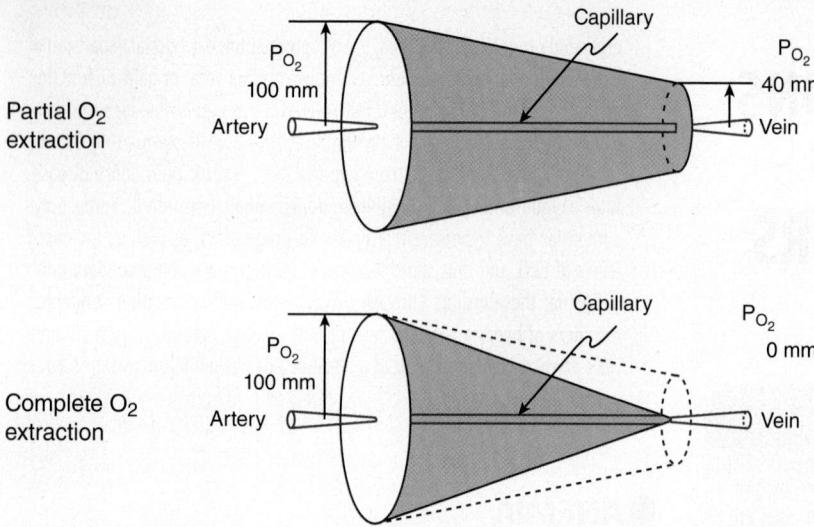

Figure 34–1. Theoretical tissue segment provided with oxygen from one capillary. With an arterial diffusion pressure of oxygen of 100 torr and partial oxygen extraction resulting in a venous oxygen pressure of 40 torr, one capillary can provide oxygen to cells within a truncated cone segment. With complete oxygen extraction, however, oxygen cannot be supplied to cells within a rim of tissue around the apex of the cone.

describes the current knowledge of hypoxia sensing in greater detail; however, it is now clear that HIF-2, not HIF-1, is the major regulator of EPO production (Chap. 32). Tissue-specific factors are responsible for tissue-specific mobilization of the compensatory mechanisms listed below that permit survival under hypoxic conditions. Figure 34–2 outlines the regulation of some physiologic processes by hypoxia.

Decreased Oxygen Consumption Energy metabolism at the optimal oxygen supply is sustained by energy-efficient oxidative phosphorylation. In hypoxia, energy is produced by less-efficient glycolysis accomplished by upregulation of transcription of glycolytic enzyme genes[4] and increased glucose transport, a process known as the *Pasteur effect*. The Pasteur effect and its exception in the metabolism observed in malignant tissue, referred to as the *Warburg effect*, are both explained at the molecular level by changes in HIF-1 levels.[4,6–8]

Decreased Oxygen Affinity Efficient increase in tissue oxygen delivery is accomplished by decreasing the affinity of hemoglobin for oxygen (right-shifted hemoglobin oxygen dissociation curve). This action permits increased oxygen extraction from the same amount of hemoglobin (Chap. 49).[9] Acutely, a very small shift in pH produces a large effect on the dissociation curve because of the Bohr effect (described by Danish physician Christian Bohr in 1904: "hemoglobin's oxygen binding affinity is inversely related both to acidity and to the concentration of carbon dioxide").[10] In chronic anemia, increased oxygen tissue delivery is accomplished by increased amounts of 2,3-bisphosphoglycerate (Chap. 47).[9] The increased synthesis of 2,3-bisphosphoglycerate in anemia is accomplished by increasing the intracellular pH of red cells (Chap. 47) by respiratory alkalosis resulting from increased respiration. This effect is clearly demonstrated in individuals with high-altitude hypoxemia.[11]

Increased Tissue Perfusion The effect of decreased oxygen-carrying capacity on the tissue tension of oxygen can be compensated acutely by increasing tissue perfusion locally via changing vasomotor

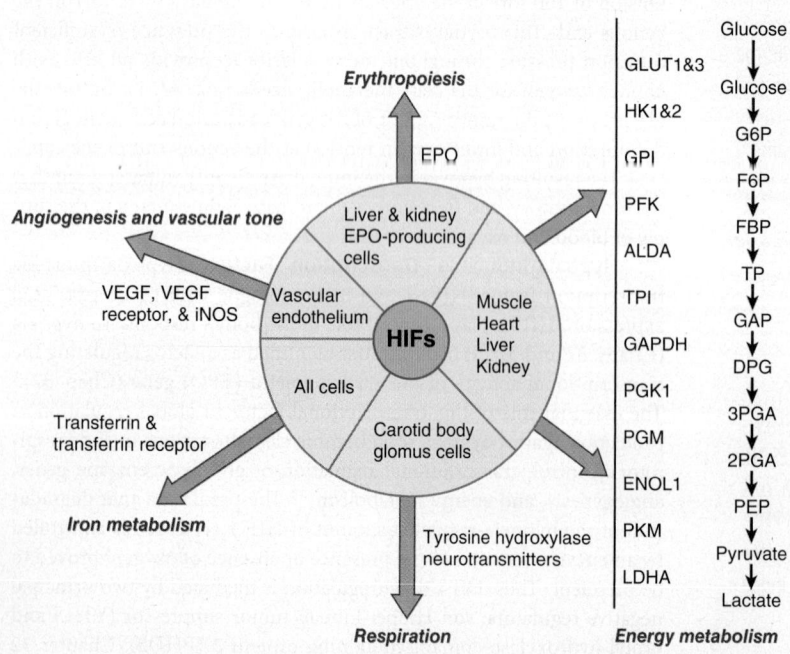

Figure 34–2. Regulation of erythropoiesis, angiogenesis, iron metabolism, respiration, and energy metabolism by hypoxia-inducible factors (HIFs) are examples of physiologic processes regulated by hypoxia. EPO, erythropoietin; iNOS, inducible nitrous oxide synthase; VEGF, vascular endothelial growth factor. *Right panel, left column (in order of listing):* GLUT1&3, glucose transporters 1 and 3; glycolytic enzymes: HK1&2, hexokinase 1 and 2; GPI, glucose phosphate isomerase; PFK, phosphofructokinase; ALDA, aldolase A; TPI, triosephosphate isomerase; GAPDH, glycerol phosphate dehydrogenase; PGK1, phosphoglycerate kinase; PGM, phosphoglycerate mutase; ENOL1, enolase 1; PKM, pyruvate kinase M isoform; LDHA, lactic dehydrogenase A isoform. *Right column:* Metabolic intermediates generated by the depicted enzymes.

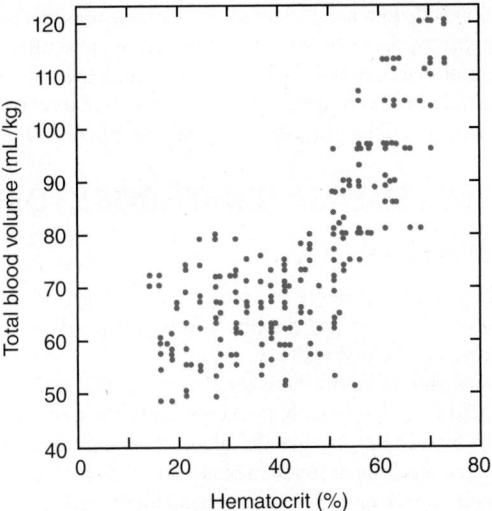

Figure 34–3. Relationship between hematocrit and total blood volume in normal individuals and in patients with anemia and polycythemia. *(Reproduced with permission from Huber H, Lewis SM and Szur L. The Influence of Anaemia, Polycythaemia and Splenomegaly on the Relationship between Venous Haematocrit and Red-Cell Volume. Br J Haematol 10:567–575,1964.)*

activity and, in the long run, by enhanced tissue angiogenesis.[2] Because in chronic anemia the blood volume is not changed (Fig. 34–3),[12] increased tissue perfusion is organ selective, accomplished by shunting the blood from nonvital donor-tissue areas to oxygen-sensitive essential recipient organs. In acute anemia, the major donor areas for redistribution of blood are the mesenteric and iliac beds.[13] In chronic anemia in humans, the donor areas are the cutaneous tissue[14] and the kidneys.[15] Vasoconstriction and oxygen deprivation in the skin cause the characteristic pallor of anemia. In the kidneys, the oxygen supply under normal conditions exceeds oxygen demands. The arteriovenous oxygen difference in the kidney is as low as 1.4 mL/dL (compared with the myocardium, where the difference can be as high as 20 mL/dL), indicating that even a severe reduction in kidney blood perfusion can be tolerated. Nevertheless, enough renal hypoxia must be present to activate HIF-2 and stimulate increased EPO production and erythropoiesis (Chap. 32). The effect on renal excretory mechanisms is slight because the reduction in renal blood flow is offset by a high plasmacrit. Even in severe anemia in which renal blood flow is reduced by almost 50 percent, the total renal plasma flow is only moderately reduced. Thus, organs with the most pressing need for oxygen, such as the myocardium and brain, are largely unimpeded by a moderate reduction in oxygen-carrying capacity, whereas in other tissues severe anemia leads to tissue hypoxia, with some tissue-specific consequences such as retinal hemorrhages.[16]

Increased Cardiac Output
Increased cardiac output is a metabolically expensive compensatory device.[17] It decreases the fraction of oxygen that must be extracted during each circulation, thereby maintaining higher oxygen pressure. Because the viscosity of blood in anemia is decreased and selective vascular dilatation decreases peripheral resistance, high cardiac output can be maintained without any increase in blood pressure.[18] In an otherwise healthy person, a measurable increase in resting cardiac output does not occur until hemoglobin concentration is less than 7 g/dL, and clinical signs of cardiac hyperactivity usually are not present until hemoglobin concentration reaches even lower levels.[19]

Signs of cardiac hyperactivity include tachycardia, increased arterial and capillary pulsation, and hemodynamic "flow" murmurs.[20]

Murmurs usually are heard during systole. Murmurs and bruits have been described in many regions, such as over the jugular vein, the closed eye, and the parietal region of the skull, and may be sensed by the patient as roaring in the ears (tinnitus), especially at night. They disappear promptly after the hemoglobin concentration is restored to normal.[20] The myocardium tolerates a prolonged period of sustained hyperactivity. However, angina pectoris and high-output failure may supervene if anemia is so severe that it exceeds myocardial oxygen demands or if the patient has coronary artery disease. Cardiomegaly, pulmonary congestion, ascites, and edema have been observed, and they require prompt treatment with oxygen and transfusion of packed red cells.

Increased Pulmonary Function
Significant anemia leads to a compensatory increase in respiratory rate that decreases the oxygen gradient from ambient air to alveolar air and increases the amount of oxygen available to oxygenate a greater than normal cardiac output. Consequently, exertional dyspnea and orthopnea are characteristic clinical manifestations of moderate to severe anemia.[19-22]

Increased Red Cell Production
The most appropriate response to anemia is a compensatory increase of red cell production, which may increase about twofold to threefold acutely and fourfold to sixfold chronically, and 10-fold in the most extreme case. The increase is mediated by increased production of EPO. The rate of EPO synthesis is inversely and logarithmically related to hemoglobin concentration (Chap. 32). EPO concentration can increase from approximately 10 mU/mL at normal hemoglobin concentrations to 10,000 mU/mL in severe anemia (Fig. 34–4).[23,24] The change in EPO levels ensures that red cell production increases in response to hemolytic and other anemias or subacute blood loss. If the former is mild, the anemia may be compensated and, if iron is available, the blood loss will be repaired after it ceases. Augmented erythroid activity expands marrow space, which, if intense, can cause sternal tenderness and diffuse bone pains. The proportion and number of reticulocytes increase. Because erythroid transit time through the marrow is shortened, "stress reticulocytes" have increased cell volume and surface area (see Chap. 32, Fig. 32–2). They develop characteristic surface folds as a result of the increased surface-area-to-volume ratio that can be identified in the

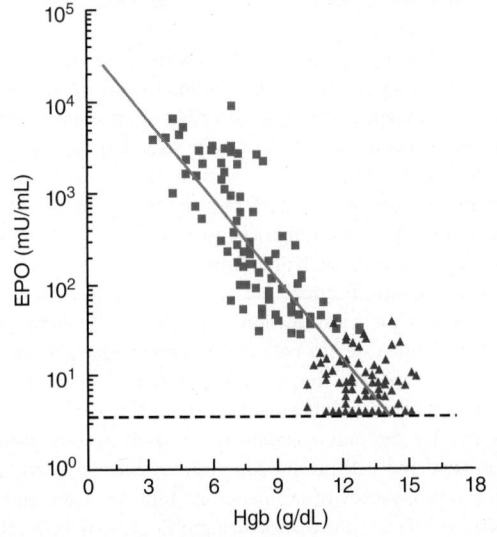

Figure 34–4. Erythropoietin (EPO) levels in plasma of normal individuals and patients with anemia uncomplicated by renal or inflammatory disease. The lower limit of accuracy of the EPO assay is 3 mU/mL and is indicated by the *dashed line*. ■, Anemias; ▲, normals; Hgb, hemoglobin.

blood film. Nucleated red cells may be observed in the blood in severe anemia.[25]

Administration of human recombinant EPO augments or replaces endogenous synthesis. In pharmacologic amounts, the effect on hemoglobin concentration is most noticeable if endogenous production is subnormal as a result of renal failure or systemic illnesses (Chap. 37). In severe anemia where endogenous EPO production (providing production is not impaired) has already increased red cell production maximally, administration of EPO rarely helps, and the patients require transfusion.[24]

Uncorrected Tissue Hypoxia

A certain residual degree of tissue hypoxia remains despite mobilization of compensatory mechanisms. Hypoxia is essential for initiation of adequate cardiovascular and erythropoietic compensation mechanisms, but severe tissue hypoxia can cause the following symptoms: dyspnea on exertion or even at rest; angina; intermittent claudication; muscle cramps, typically at night; headache; light-headedness; and fatigue. A number of diffuse gastrointestinal symptoms are associated with anemia (e.g., abdominal cramps, nausea), but whether the symptoms should be attributed to tissue hypoxia, compensatory redistribution of blood, or the underlying cause of anemia is uncertain.

CLASSIFICATION

Based on determination of the red cell mass, anemia can be classified as either *relative* or *absolute*. Relative anemia is characterized by a normal total red cell mass in an increased plasma volume, resulting in a dilution anemia, a disturbance in plasma volume regulation. However, dilution anemia is of clinical and differential diagnostic importance for the hematologist.

Classification of the *absolute anemias* with decreased red cell mass is difficult because the classification has to consider kinetic, morphologic, and pathophysiologic interacting criteria. Anemia of acute hemorrhage is not a diagnostic problem and is usually a genitourinary or gastrointestinal matter, not a hematologic consideration. Initially, all anemias should be divided into anemias caused by decreased production and anemias caused by increased destruction of red cells. The differentiation is based largely on the reticulocyte count. Subsequent diagnostic breakdown can be based on either morphologic or pathophysiologic criteria.

Morphologic classification subdivides anemia into (1) macrocytic anemia, (2) normocytic anemia, and (3) microcytic hypochromic anemia. The main advantages of this classification are that the classification is simple, is based on readily available red cell indices, for example, mean corpuscular volume (MCV) and mean corpuscular hemoglobin concentration (MCHC), and forces the physician to consider the most important types of curable anemia: vitamin B_{12}, folic acid, and iron-deficiency anemias. Such practical considerations have led to wide acceptance of this classification.

Pathophysiologic classification (Table 34–1) is best suited for relating disease processes to potential treatment. In addition, anemia resulting from vitamin or iron-deficiency states occurs in a significant proportion of patients with normal red cell indices.

This chapter presents a classification based on our present concepts of normal red cell production and red cell destruction. Figure 34–5 outlines the cascade of proliferation, differentiation, and maturation underlying the transformation of a multipotential stem cell, first to erythroid progenitor cells, then to erythroid precursor cells, and finally to mature red cells. Each of these steps can become impaired and cause anemia. Therapeutic intervention depends on identifying the defective step and instituting the specific therapy. The limitation of such a

classification is that, in most anemias, the pathogenesis involves several steps. For example, a decreased rate of production most often results in production of defective red cells with a shortened life span. Thus, the outline provided is a conceptual guide to our present understanding of the processes underlying the production and destruction of red cells.

● POLYCYTHEMIA (ERYTHROCYTOSIS)

PATHOPHYSIOLOGY

The production and presence of an increased number of red cells are associated with general and specific effects generated by changes in blood viscosity and blood volume.

The viscosity of blood increases logarithmically with an increase in hematocrit (Fig. 34–6). At hematocrits above the normal range, the increase in blood viscosity impairs blood flow and increases cardiac workload. The resulting decrease in blood flow reduces the transport of oxygen, with average optimal values at hematocrit readings between 40 and 45 percent.[26,27] In a study of red cells from a number of animal species, the optimal value of oxygen transport corresponded closely to their normal hematocrits,[28] which may explain the evolutionary determination of optimal hematocrit levels.[29] However, before concluding that polycythemia always is a suboptimal condition, consider that it may be inappropriate to correlate viscosity readings, derived from blood tested in a rigid glass viscometer (Ostwald) or even in a cone-plate viscometer, with those in flowing blood through tiny distensible vessels *in vivo*.[30] First, the flow through these narrow channels is rapid (high shear rate), which in a nonnewtonian fluid such as blood causes a marked decrease in viscosity. Second, blood flowing through narrow channels *in vivo* is axial, with a central core of packed red cells sliding over a peripheral layer of lubricating low-viscosity plasma. Finally, and most importantly, absolute polycythemia is not normovolemic but is accompanied by increased blood volume, which, in turn, enlarges the vascular bed and decreases peripheral resistance. Because blood pressure remains stable, the increased blood volume must be associated with increased cardiac output and increased oxygen transport (cardiac output times hemoglobin concentration). Using measurements of cardiac output in dogs[31] and tissue oxygen tension in rats and mice,[30] construction of curves (Fig. 34–7) that relate oxygen transport to hematocrit in normovolemic and hypervolemic states is possible. These curves show that hypervolemia *per se* increases oxygen transport and that the optimum oxygen transport in these conditions occurs at higher hematocrit values than in normovolemic states. Consequently, despite the increased viscosity, a moderate increase in hematocrit is beneficial. The same may not be true of a more pronounced increase in hematocrit. Observations in humans[32] and experimental animals[31] indicate that high viscosity causes reduced blood flow to most tissues and may be responsible for the cerebral and cardiovascular impairment experienced occasionally by high-altitude dwellers,[33] patients with severe polycythemia,[34,35] and athletes self-administering overdoses of EPO (Chap. 57).

MANIFESTATIONS

The rate of red cell production is increased in true polycythemias, but changes in erythroid marrow cellularity can be difficult to assess by microscopy means, although the marrow is hypercellular in a typical patient with polycythemia vera. Under normal conditions, the rate of red cell production is adjusted to maintain the red cell mass at approximately 30 mL per kilogram of body weight. Because the life span of red cells in polycythemia is normal, a doubling of the daily rate of red cell production is adequate to maintain a polycythemic red cell mass of 60 mL/kg. Consequently, the morphology and volume of the marrow are only moderately altered in polycythemia compared with the changes

TABLE 34–1. Classification of Anemia

I. Absolute anemia (decreased red cell volume)

A. Decreased red cell production

1. Acquired

a. Pluripotential hematopoietic stem cell failure

(1) Autoimmune (Aplastic anemia) (Chap. 35)

(a) Radiation-induced

(b) Drugs and chemicals (chloramphenicol, benzene, etc.)

(c) Viruses (non–A-G hepatitis, Epstein-Barr virus, etc.)

(d) Idiopathic

(2) Anemia of leukemia and of myelodysplastic syndromes (Chaps. 87, 88, and 91)

(3) Anemia associated with marrow infiltration (Chap. 45)

(4) Postchemotherapy (Chap. 22)

b. Erythroid progenitor cell failure

(1) Pure red cell aplasia (parvovirus B19 infection, drugs, associated with thymoma, autoantibodies, etc. [Chap. 36])

(2) Endocrine disorders (Chap. 38)

(3) Acquired sideroblastic anemia (drugs, copper deficiency, etc. [Chaps. 59 and 87])

c. Functional impairment of erythroid and other progenitors from nutritional and other causes

(1) Megaloblastic anemias (Chap. 41)

(a) Vitamin B_{12} deficiency

(b) Folate deficiency

(c) Acute megaloblastic anemia because of nitrous oxide (N_2O)

(d) Drug-induced megaloblastic anemia (pemetrexed, methotrexate, phenytoin toxicity, etc.)

(2) Iron-deficiency anemia (Chap. 42)

(3) Anemia resulting from other nutritional deficiencies (Chap. 44)

(4) Anemia of chronic disease and inflammation (Chap. 37)

(5) Anemia of renal failure (Chap. 37)

(6) Anemia caused by chemical agents (lead toxicity [Chap. 52])

(7) Acquired thalassemias (seen in some clonal hematopoietic disorders [Chaps. 48 and 83])

(8) Erythropoietin antibodies (Chap. 36)

2. Hereditary

a. Pluripotential hematopoietic stem cell failure (Chap. 35)

(1) Fanconi anemia

(2) Shwachman syndrome

(3) Dyskeratosis congenita

b. Erythroid progenitor cell failure

(1) Diamond-Blackfan syndrome (Chap. 35)

(2) Congenital dyserythropoietic syndromes (Chap. 39)

c. Functional impairment of erythroid and other progenitors from nutritional and other causes

(1) Megaloblastic anemias (Chap. 41)

(a) Selective malabsorption of vitamin B_{12} (Imerslund-Gräsbeck disease)

(b) Congenital intrinsic factor deficiency

(c) Transcobalamin II deficiency

(d) Inborn errors of cobalamin metabolism (methylmalonic aciduria, homocystinuria, etc.)

(e) Inborn errors of folate metabolism (congenital folate malabsorption, dihydrofolate deficiency, methyltransferase deficiency, etc.)

(2) Inborn purine and pyrimidine metabolism defects (Lesch-Nyhan syndrome, hereditary orotic aciduria, etc.)

(3) Disorders of iron metabolism (Chap. 42)

(a) Hereditary atransferrinemia

(b) Hypochromic anemia caused by divalent metal transporter (DMT)-1 mutation

(4) Hereditary sideroblastic anemia (Chap. 59)

(5) Thalassemias (Chap. 48)

B. Increased red cell destruction

1. Acquired

a. Mechanical

(1) Macroangiopathic (march hemoglobinuria, artificial heart valves [Chap. 51])

(2) Microangiopathic (disseminated intravascular coagulation [DIC]; thrombotic thrombocytopenic purpura [TTP]; vasculitis [Chaps. 51, 122, and 129])

(3) Parasites and microorganisms (malaria, bartonellosis, babesiosis, *Clostridium perfringens*, etc. [Chap. 53])

b. Antibody mediated

(1) Warm-type autoimmune hemolytic anemia (Chap. 54)

(2) Cryopathic syndromes (cold agglutinin disease, paroxysmal cold hemoglobinuria, cryoglobulinemia [Chap. 54])

(3) Transfusion reactions (immediate and delayed [Chaps. 54 and 136])

c. Hypersplenism (Chap. 56)

d. Red cell membrane disorders (Chap. 46)

(1) Spur cell hemolysis

(2) Acquired acanthocytosis and acquired stomatocytosis, etc.

e. Chemical injury and complex chemicals (arsenic, copper, chlorate, spider, scorpion, and snake venoms, etc. [Chap. 52])

f. Physical injury (heat, oxygen, radiation [Chap. 52])

2. Hereditary

a. Hemoglobinopathies (Chap. 49)

(1) Sickle cell disease

(2) Unstable hemoglobins

(Continued)

TABLE 34–1. Classification of Anemia (*Continued*)

b. Red cell membrane disorders (Chap. 46)

   (1) Cytoskeletal membrane disorders (hereditary spherocytosis, elliptocytosis, pyropoikilocytosis)

   (2) Lipid membrane disorders (hereditary abetalipoproteinemia, hereditary stomatocytosis, etc.)

   (3) Membrane disorders associated with abnormalities of erythrocyte antigens (McLeod syndrome, Rh deficiency syndromes, etc.)

   (4) Membrane disorders associated with abnormal transport (hereditary xerocytosis)

c. Red cell enzyme defects (pyruvate kinase, 5′ nucleotidase, glucose-6-phosphate dehydrogenase deficiencies, other red cell enzyme disorders [Chap. 47])

d. Porphyrias (congenital erythropoietic and hepatoerythropoietic porphyrias, rarely congenital erythropoietic protoporphyria [Chap. 58])

C. Blood loss and blood redistribution

  1. Acute blood loss

  2. Splenic sequestration crisis (Chap. 56)

II. Relative (increased plasma volume)

  A. Macroglobulinemia (Chap. 109)

  B. Pregnancy (Chap. 8)

  C. Athletes (Chap. 33)

  D. Postflight astronauts (Chap. 33)

observed in some types of hemolytic anemia, in which the rate of red cell production can be four to six times normal. In erythrocytosis, the number of red cells destroyed daily merely causes a slight increase in bilirubin levels. The presence of secondary gout and splenomegaly are usually signs of a myeloproliferative neoplasm rather than of erythrocytosis alone. Although considerable homology exists between EPO and thrombopoietin,[36] there is no evidence that the two molecules crossreact at the level of their respective receptors.[37] EPO-driven erythrocytosis is generally not associated with increased platelet production.

The increased viscosity and expansion of vascular space are responsible for many of the signs and symptoms of polycythemia. The characteristic *rubor* in patients with polycythemia vera is caused by excessive deoxygenation of blood flowing sluggishly through dilated cutaneous vessels. Nonspecific symptoms such as headaches, dizziness, tinnitus, and a reported feeling of fullness of the face and head probably are caused by a combination of increased viscosity and vascular dilatation. In extreme polycythemia and some specific types of polycythemia (e.g., methemoglobinemia; Chap. 50), cyanosis can result from greater than 4 g/dL of deoxygenated hemoglobin (accomplished more easily at higher hemoglobin concentrations [see "blue bloaters" and "pink puffers" in Chap. 57]) or greater than 1.5 g/dL of methemoglobin.

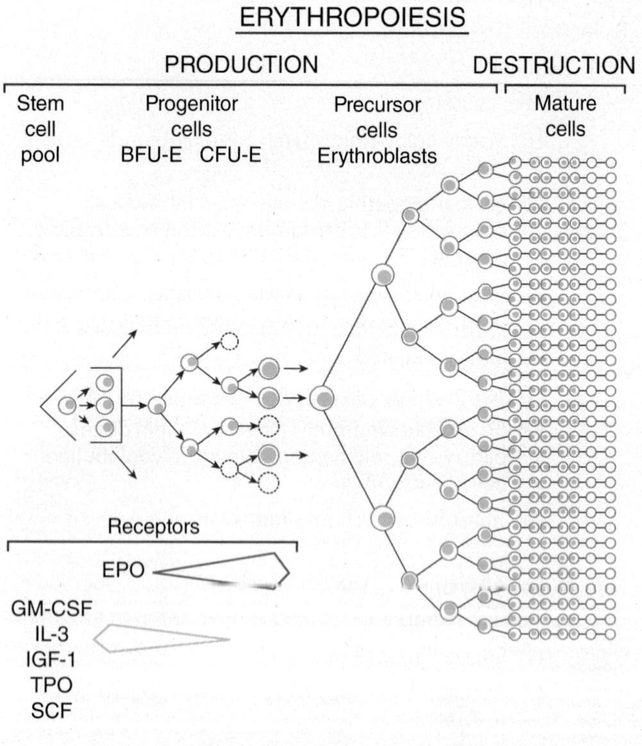

ERYTHROPOIESIS

	PRODUCTION		DESTRUCTION
Stem cell pool	Progenitor cells BFU-E CFU-E	Precursor cells Erythroblasts	Mature cells

Receptors

EPO

GM-CSF
IL-3
IGF-1
TPO
SCF

Figure 34–5. Outline of the process of differentiation, proliferation, and maturation underlying the production and destruction of red blood cells. Multipotential stem cells responding to a number of growth factors, including granulocyte-monocyte colony-stimulating factors (GM-CSF), interleukin 3 (IL-3), insulin growth factor 1 (IGF-1), thrombopoietin (TPO), and stem cell factor (SCF), differentiate to progenitor cells committed to erythroid development. Progenitor cells, burst-forming unit–erythroid (BFU-E), and colony-forming unit–erythroid (CFU-E) proliferate under the control of erythropoietin (EPO) and finally differentiate to precursor cells (erythroblasts). In the presence of adequate amounts of nutrients, such as vitamin B_{12}, folic acid, and iron, precursor cells proliferate and mature into nucleated red cells, reticulocytes, and mature red blood cells. After an average 120-day life span, these cells are destroyed.

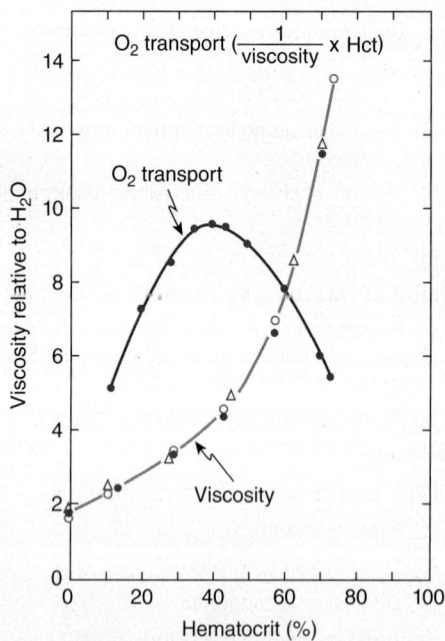

Figure 34–6. Viscosity of heparinized normal human blood related to hematocrit (Hct). Viscosity is measured with an Ostwald viscosimeter at 37°C and expressed in relation to viscosity of saline solution. Oxygen transport is computed from Hct and O_2 flow (1/viscosity) and is recorded in arbitrary units.

TABLE 34-2. Classification of Polycythemia

I. Absolute (true) polycythemia (increased red cell volume) (Chap. 56)

  A. Primary polycythemia

    1. Acquired

      a. Polycythemia vera (Chap. 84)

    2. Hereditary (Chap. 57)

      a. Primary familial and congenital polycythemia (PFCP)

        (1) Erythropoietin receptor mutations

        (2) Unknown gene mutations

  B. Secondary polycythemia

    1. Acquired (Chap. 57)

      a. Hypoxemia

        (1) Chronic lung disease

        (2) Sleep apnea

        (3) Right-to-left cardiac shunts

        (4) High altitude

        (5) Smoking

      b. Carboxyhemoglobinemia (Chap. 50)

        (1) Smoking

        (2) Carbon monoxide poisoning

      c. Autonomous erythropoietin production (Chap. 57)

        (1) Hepatocellular carcinoma

        (2) Renal cell carcinoma

        (3) Cerebellar hemangioblastoma

        (4) Pheochromocytoma

        (5) Parathyroid carcinoma

        (6) Meningioma

        (7) Uterine leiomyoma

        (8) Polycystic kidney disease

      d. Exogenous erythropoietin (EPO) administration ("EPO doping") (Chap. 57)

      e. Complex or uncertain etiology

        (1) Postrenal transplant (probable abnormal angiotensin II signaling) (Chap. 57)

        (2) Androgen/anabolic steroids (Chap. 57)

    2. Hereditary

      a. High-oxygen affinity hemoglobins (Chap. 49)

      b. 2,3-Bisphosphoglycerate deficiency (Chap. 47)

      c. Congenital methemoglobinemias (recessive, i.e., cytochrome b5 reductase deficiency, dominant globin mutations [Chaps. 49 and 57])

  C. Disorders of hypoxia sensing (Chap. 57)

    1. Proven or suspected congenital disorders of hypoxia sensing

      a. Chuvash polycythemia

      b. High erythropoietin polycythemias caused by mutations of von Hippel-Lindau gene other than Chuvash mutation

      c. HIF2a (*EPAS1*) mutations

      d. PHD2 (*EGLN1*) mutations

II. Relative (spurious) polycythemia (normal red cell volume) (Chap. 57)

  A. Dehydration

  B. Diuretics

  C. Smoking

  D. Gaisböck syndrome

Hemorrhage from the nose or stomach in patients with normal platelets and coagulation proteins can be attributed to capillary distention; however, circulatory stagnation causing ischemia and necrosis may contribute. Thrombosis are common in polycythemia vera, but are not seen at similar frequencies in other types of polycythemias (Chaps. 57 and 84). Coronary blood flow is decreased in polycythemia,[34] so the risk of coronary thrombosis in patients with a high hematocrit is assumed to be increased; however, statistical analyses have yielded equivocal evidence of such a relationship.[35,38,39] Polycythemia reportedly does not pose a risk in surgical patients.[40] Although cerebral blood flow is materially reduced in patients with moderately elevated hematocrit,[32,41] such reductions may have little practical significance. In polycythemia vera, however, it has been advocated that normalization of red cell mass should be accomplished before surgery; again, firm data supporting this practice are lacking (Chap. 84).

CLASSIFICATION

Polycythemia, or erythrocytosis, is a condition in which the hematocrit percentage is above the upper limits of normal: greater than 51 percent in men and greater than 48 percent in women. Polycythemia can be classified as: (1) relative, in which the red cell mass is normal but the plasma volume is decreased, or (2) absolute, in which the red cell mass is increased above normal (Chap. 57). Table 34–2 outlines the polycythemic states.

Differentiation of absolute from relative polycythemia can be difficult at hematocrits of less than 60 percent. Designation of a measured red cell mass as normal is imprecise because the red cell mass depends on the patient's age, sex, weight, height, and body frame, and because only increases above the mean of greater than 25 percent are considered abnormal.

Primary Polycythemias

Primary or secondary polycythemias are caused by either acquired (polycythemia vera) or inherited mutations (such as gain-of-function erythropoietin receptor [EPOR] causing primary familial and congenital polycythemia [PFCP]) expressed within hematopoietic progenitors, leading to increased production of red cells.

Secondary Polycythemias

Secondary polycythemias are caused by augmentation of erythropoiesis by circulating stimulatory factors such as EPO (polycythemia of high altitude), cobalt, or insulin-like growth factor 1 (Chap. 57).

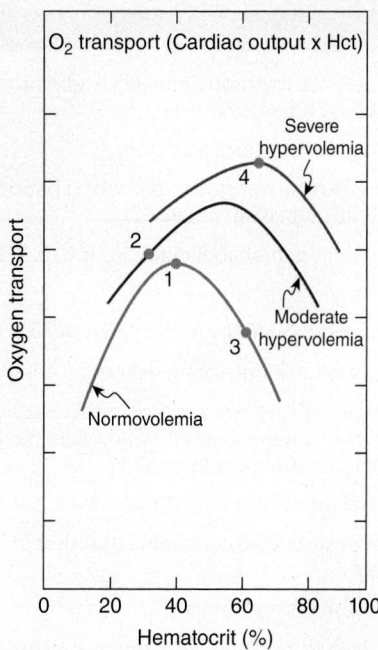

Figure 34–7. Oxygen transport at various hematocrit levels in nor-movolemia, mild hypervolemia, and severe hypervolemia. Oxygen transport is estimated by multiplying hematocrit (Hct) by cardiac output. (1) Optimal oxygen transport for normovolemic subjects is at a hematocrit of approximately 45 percent, with a progressive increase in optimal hematocrit as blood volume increases. (2) Suboptimal hematocrit in a hypervolemic person (anemia of pregnancy) may be associated with higher oxygen transport than in a normovolemic person with normal hematocrit. (3) High hematocrit without an increase in blood volume may be associated with an absolute reduction in oxygen transport and tissue hypoxia. (4) Only high hematocrit coupled with high blood volume enhances oxygen transport to the tissues. *(Data from Murray JF, Gold P and Johnson BL, Jr. The circulatory effects of hematocrit variations in normovolemic and hypervolemic dogs. J Clin Invest. 42:1150-9, 1963 and Thorling EB and Erslev AJ. The "tissue" tension of oxygen and its relation to hematocrit and erythropoiesis. Blood 31(3):332–343, 1968.)*

Disorders of Hypoxia Sensing

Polycythemias from VHL Gene Mutation Chuvash polycythemia and some other disorders of hypoxia sensing, including several recessively inherited mutations of the *VHL* gene, have elevated or inappropriately normal EPO levels in relation to elevated hematocrit. This phenotype is different from other, more common *VHL* mutations encompassing VHL tumor predisposition syndrome, wherein dominantly inherited germline *VHL* mutations precede the acquired somatic mutations that eventually result in tumor genesis (hemangioblastoma, renal cell carcinoma, pheochromocytoma, pancreatic endocrine tumors, and endolymphatic sac tumors). Following the description of Chuvash polycythemia, other homozygous and compound heterozygous inherited *VHL* mutations causing polycythemia, but not tumors, have been described (Chap. 57). Some patients with tumor predisposition VHL syndrome also develop acquired polycythemia as a consequence of EPO production in tumor tissue.[42]

Clinically, Chuvash polycythemia patients are prone to develop thrombosis, they have elevated pulmonary pressure and have increased mortality independent of the increase in hematocrit.[43]

Polycythemias from HIF2α and PHD2 Mutations Dominantly inherited gain-of-function HIF2α (encoded by *EPAS1*) gene mutations have elevated or inappropriately normal EPO levels in relation to elevated hematocrits. All reported polycythemic heterozygotes for loss-of-function PHD2 variants (encoded by *EGLN1* gene) have normal EPO levels.

Because of the rarity of *HIF2a* and *PHD2* mutations, their non-erythroid phenotype is not well defined; however, some *HIF2a* mutations, possibly associated with genetic mosaicism, are associated with congenital polycythemia and later development of pheochromocytoma/paraganglioma and somatistatinoma tumors. In these instances, in most patients, the *HIF2a* mutation is present in the tumors, which frequently recur, but not in leukocytes.[44,45]

REFERENCES

1. Semenza GL, Nejfelt MK, Chi SM, et al: Hypoxia-inducible nuclear factors bind to an enhancer element located 3′ to the human erythropoietin gene. *Proc Natl Acad Sci U S A* 88(13):5680, 1991.
2. Guillemin K, Krasnow MA: The hypoxic response: Huffing and HIFing. *Cell* 89(1):9, 1997.
3. Hochachka PW, Buck LT, Doll CJ, et al: Unifying theory of hypoxia tolerance: Molecular/metabolic defense and rescue mechanisms for surviving oxygen lack. *Proc Natl Acad Sci U S A* 93(18):9493, 1996.
4. Semenza GL: O_2-regulated gene expression: Transcriptional control of cardiorespiratory physiology by HIF-1. *J Appl Physiol (1985)* 96(3):1173; discussion 1170, 2004.
5. Srinivas V, Zhu X, Salceda S, et al: Hypoxia-inducible factor 1alpha (HIF-1alpha) is a non-heme iron protein. Implications for oxygen sensing. *J Biol Chem* 273(29):18019, 1998.
6. Ivan M, Kondo K, Yang H, et al: HIFalpha targeted for VHL-mediated destruction by proline hydroxylation: Implications for O_2 sensing. *Science* 292(5516):464, 2001.
7. Jaakkola P, Mole DR, Tian YM, et al: Targeting of HIF-alpha to the von Hippel-Lindau ubiquitylation complex by O_2-regulated prolyl hydroxylation. *Science* 292(5516):468, 2001.
8. Epstein AC, Gleadle JM, McNeill LA, et al: C. elegans EGL-9 and mammalian homologs define a family of dioxygenases that regulate HIF by prolyl hydroxylation. *Cell* 107(1):43, 2001.
9. Edwards MJ, Novy MJ, Walters CL, et al: Improved oxygen release: An adaptation of mature red cells to hypoxia. *J Clin Invest* 47(8):1851, 1968.
10. Bohr C, Hasselbalch K, Krogh A: [Concerning a biologically important relationship: The influence of the carbon dioxide content of blood on its oxygen binding]. *Skan Arch Physiol* 16:401, 1904.
11. Moore LG, Brewer GJ: Beneficial effect of rightward hemoglobin-oxygen dissociation curve shift for short-term high-altitude adaptation. *J Lab Clin Med* 98(1):145, 1981.
12. Huber H, Lewis SM, Szur L: The influence of anaemia, polycythaemia and splenomegaly on the relationship between venous haematocrit and red-cell volume. *Br J Haematol* 10:567, 1964.
13. Vatner SF: Effects of hemorrhage on regional blood flow distribution in dogs and primates. *J Clin Invest* 54(2):225, 1974.
14. Abramson D, Fierst SM, Flachs K: Resting peripheral blood flow in the anemia state. *Am Heart J* 25, 1954.
15. Bradley SE, Bradley GP: Renal function during chronic anemia in man. *Blood* 2(2):192, 1947.
16. Merin S, Freund M: Retinopathy in severe anemia. *Am J Ophthalmol* 66(6):1102, 1968.
17. Duke M, Abelmann WH: The hemodynamic response to chronic anemia. *Circulation* 39(4):503, 1969.
18. Sharpey-Schafer EP: Cardiac output in severe anemia. *Clin Sci* 5, 1944.
19. Wintrobe MM: The cardiovascular system in anemia; with a note on the particular abnormalities in sickle cell anemia. *Blood* 1:121, 1946.
20. Wales RT, Martin EA: Arterial bruits in anaemia. *Br Med J* 2(5370):1444, 1963.
21. Blumgart HL, Altschule MD: Clinical significance of cardiac and respiratory adjustments in chronic anemia. *Blood* 3(4):329, 1948.
22. Fatemian M, Gamboa A, Leon-Velarde F, et al: Selected contribution: Ventilatory response to CO_2 in high-altitude natives and patients with chronic mountain sickness. *J Appl Physiol (1985)* 94(3):1279; discussion 1253, 2003.
23. Adamson JW: The erythropoietin-hematocrit relationship in normal and polycythemic man: Implications of marrow regulation. *Blood* 32(4):597, 1968.
24. Erslev AJ: Erythropoietin. *N Engl J Med* 324(19):1339, 1991.
25. Ward HP, Holman J: The association of nucleated red cells in the peripheral smear with hypoxemia. *Ann Intern Med* 67(6):1190, 1967.
26. Dintenfass L: A preliminary outline of the blood high viscosity syndromes. *Arch Intern Med* 118(5):427, 1966.
27. Stone HO, Thompson HK Jr, Schmidt-Nielsen K: Influence of erythrocytes on blood viscosity. *Am J Physiol* 214(4):913, 1968.
28. Erslev AJ, Caro J, Schuster SJ: Is there an optimal hemoglobin level? *Transfus Med Rev* 3(4):237, 1989.
29. Murray JF, Gold P, Johnson BL Jr: The circulatory effects of hematocrit variations in normovolemic and hypervolemic dogs. *J Clin Invest* 42:1150, 1963.
30. Thorling EB, Erslev AJ: The "tissue" tension of oxygen and its relation to hematocrit and erythropoiesis. *Blood* 31(3):332, 1968.
31. Fan FC, Chen RY, Schuessler GB, et al: Effects of hematocrit variations on regional hemodynamics and oxygen transport in the dog. *Am J Physiol* 238(4):H545, 1980.

32. Pearson TC, Humphrey PRD, Thomas DJ, et al: Hematocrit, blood viscosity, cerebral blood flow, and vascular occlusion, in *Clinical Aspects of Blood Viscosity and Cell Deformability*, edited by GDO Lowe. Springer-Verlag, New York, 1981.

33. Monge CM, Monge CC: *High-Altitude Diseases: Mechanism and Management*, Charles C Thomas, Springfield, IL, 1966.

34. Kershenovich S, Modiano M, Ewy GA: Markedly decreased coronary blood flow in secondary polycythemia. *Am Heart J* 123(2):521, 1992.

35. Conley CL, Russell RP, Thomas CB, et al: Hematocrit values in coronary artery disease. *Arch Intern Med* 113:170, 1964.

36. Kaushansky K: Thrombopoietin. *N Engl J Med* 339(11):746, 1998.

37. Geddis AE, Kaushansky K: Cross-reactivity between erythropoietin and thrombopoietin at the level of Mpl does not account for the thrombocytosis seen in iron deficiency. *J Pediatr Hematol Oncol* 25(11):919; author reply 920, 2003.

38. Mayer GA: Hematocrit and coronary heart disease. *Can Med Assoc J* 93(22):1151, 1965.

39. Hershberg PI, Wells RE, McGandy RB: Hematocrit and prognosis in patients with acute myocardial infarction. *JAMA* 219(7):855, 1972.

40. Lubarsky DA, Gallagher CJ, Berend JL: Secondary polycythemia does not increase the risk of perioperative hemorrhagic or thrombotic complications. *J Clin Anesth* 3(2):99, 1991.

41. Thomas DJ, du Boulay GH, Marshall J, et al: Cerebral blood-flow in polycythaemia. *Lancet* 2(8030):161, 1977.

42. Friedrich CA: Genotype-phenotype correlation in von Hippel-Lindau syndrome. *Hum Mol Genet* 10(7):763, 2001.

43. Gordeuk VR, Sergueeva AI, Miasnikova GY, et al: Congenital disorder of oxygen sensing: Association of the homozygous Chuvash polycythemia VHL mutation with thrombosis and vascular abnormalities but not tumors. *Blood* 103:3924, 2004.

44. Zhuang Z, Yang C, Lorenzo F, et al: Somatic HIF2A gain-of-function mutations in paraganglioma with polycythemia. *N Engl J Med* 367(10):922, 2012.

45. Lorenzo FR, Yang C, Ng Tang et al: A novel EPAS1/HIF2A germline mutation in a congenital polycythemia with paraganglioma. *J Mol Med (Berl)* 91(4):507, 2013.

CHAPTER 35
APLASTIC ANEMIA: ACQUIRED AND INHERITED

George B. Segel and Marshall A. Lichtman

SUMMARY

Acquired aplastic anemia is a clinical syndrome in which there is a deficiency of red cells, neutrophils, monocytes, and platelets in the blood, and fatty replacement of the marrow with a near absence of hematopoietic precursor cells. Reticulocytopenia is a constant feature. Neutropenia, monocytopenia, and thrombocytopenia, when severe, are life-threatening because of the risk of infection and bleeding, complicated by severe anemia. Most cases occur without an evident precipitating cause and are caused by autoreactive cytotoxic T lymphocytes that suppress or destroy primitive CD34+ multipotential hematopoietic cells. The disorder also can occur after (1) prolonged high-dose exposure to certain toxic chemicals (e.g., benzene), (2) after specific viral infections (e.g., Epstein-Barr virus), (3) as an idiosyncratic response to certain pharmaceuticals (e.g., ticlopidine, chloramphenicol), (4) as a feature of a connective tissue or autoimmune disorder (e.g., lupus erythematosus), or, (5) rarely, in association with pregnancy. The final common pathway may be through cytotoxic T-cell autoreactivity, whether idiopathic or associated with an inciting agent since they all respond in a similar fashion to immunosuppressive therapy. The differential diagnosis of acquired aplastic anemia includes a hypoplastic marrow that can accompany paroxysmal nocturnal hemoglobinuria or hypoplastic oligoblastic (myelodysplastic syndrome) or polyblastic myelogenous leukemia. Allogeneic hematopoietic stem cell transplantation is curative in approximately 80 percent of younger patients with high-resolution human leukocyte antigen–matched sibling donors, although the posttransplant period may be complicated by severe graft-versus-host disease. The disease may be significantly ameliorated or occasionally cured by immunotherapy, especially a regimen coupling antithymocyte globulin with cyclosporine. However, after successful treatment with immunosuppressive agents, the disease may relapse or evolve into a clonal myeloid disorder, such as paroxysmal nocturnal hemoglobinuria, a clonal cytopenia, or oligoblastic

or polyblastic myelogenous leukemia. Several uncommon inherited disorders, including Fanconi anemia, Shwachman-Diamond syndrome, dyskeratosis congenita and others have as a primary manifestation aplastic hematopoiesis.

● ACQUIRED APLASTIC ANEMIA

DEFINITION AND HISTORY

Aplastic anemia is a clinical syndrome that results from a marked diminution of marrow blood cell production. The decrease in hematopoiesis results in reticulocytopenia, anemia, granulocytopenia, monocytopenia, and thrombocytopenia. The diagnosis usually requires the presence of pancytopenia with a neutrophil count fewer than 1500/μL (1.5 × 10^9/L), a platelet count fewer than 50,000/μL (50 × 10^9/L), a hemoglobin concentration less than 10 g/dL (100 g/L), and an absolute reticulocyte count fewer than 40,000/μL (40 × 10^9/L), accompanied by a hypocellular marrow without abnormal or malignant cells or fibrosis.[1] For the purpose of therapeutic decision making, comparative clinical trials, and international sharing of data, the disease has been stratified into moderately severe, severe, and very severe acquired aplastic anemia based on the blood counts (especially the neutrophil count) and the degree of marrow hypocellularity (Table 35–1). Most cases of aplastic anemia are acquired; fewer cases are the result of an inherited disorder, such as Fanconi anemia, Shwachman-Diamond syndrome, and others (see "Hereditary Aplastic Anemia" below).

Aplastic anemia was first recognized by Paul Ehrlich in 1888.[2] He described a young, pregnant woman who died of severe anemia and neutropenia. Thrombocytopenia was difficult to measure and the role of blood dust (platelets) was controversial at that time. Autopsy examination revealed a fatty marrow with essentially no hematopoiesis. The name *aplastic anemia* was subsequently applied to this disease by Chauffard, a French hematologist, in 1904,[3] and although an anachronistic term because the morbidity is the result of pancytopenia, especially neutropenia and thrombocytopenia, the designation is entrenched in medical usage. For the next 40 years, many conditions that caused pancytopenia were confused with aplastic anemia based on incomplete or inadequate histologic study of the patient's marrow.[4] The development of improved instruments for percutaneous marrow biopsy in the last half of the 20th century improved diagnostic precision. In 1972, Thomas and his colleagues established that marrow transplantation from a histocompatible sibling donor could cure the disease.[5] The disease initially was thought to result from an atrophy or chemical injury of primitive marrow hematopoietic cells. The unexpected recovery of marrow recipients who were given immunosuppressive conditioning therapy but who did not engraft with donor stem cells raised the possibility that the disease may not be intrinsic to primitive hematopoietic cells but the result of a suppression of hematopoietic cells by immune cells, notably T lymphocytes.[6] The requirement to treat the recipient of a marrow transplant from an identical twin with immunosuppressive conditioning therapy for optimal results of transplant, buttressed this concept.[7] This supposition was confirmed by a clinical trial that established antilymphocyte globulin (ALG) capable of ameliorating the disease in the majority of patients.[8] Since that time, compelling evidence for a cellular autoimmune mechanism has accumulated (see "Etiology and Pathogenesis" below).

EPIDEMIOLOGY

The International Aplastic Anemia and Agranulocytosis Study and a French study found the incidence of acquired aplastic anemia to be approximately 2 per 1,000,000 persons per year.[1,9] This annual incidence

Acronyms and Abbreviations: A, adenine; ALG, antilymphocyte globulin; ALL, acute lymphocytic leukemia; AML, acute myelogenous leukemia; ATG, antithymocyte globulin; ATR, ataxia-telangiectasia mutated and rad3-related kinase; BFU-E, erythroid burst-forming units; CD, cluster of differentiation; CFU-GM, colony-forming unit–granulocyte-macrophage; CMV, cytomegalovirus; EBV, Epstein-Barr virus; G, guanine; G-CSF, granulocyte colony-stimulating factor; HHV, human herpes virus; HLA, human leukocyte antigen; IL, interleukin; MRI, magnetic resonance imaging; PCP, pentachlorophenol; PNH, paroxysmal nocturnal hemoglobinuria; SCF, stem cell factor; T, thymine; TERC, telomerase RNA component; TERT, telomerase reverse transcriptase; TNF, tumor necrosis factor; TNT, trinitrotoluene; TPO, thrombopoietin.

TABLE 35–1. Degree of Severity of Acquired Aplastic Anemia

Diagnostic Categories	Hemoglobin	Reticulocyte Concentration	Neutrophil Count	Platelet Count	Marrow Biopsy	Comments
Moderately severe	<100 g/L	<40 × 10⁹/L	<1.5 × 10⁹/L	<50 × 10⁹/L	Marked decrease of hematopoietic cells.	At the time of diagnosis at least 2 of 3 blood counts should meet these criteria.
Severe	<90 g/L	<30.0 × 10⁹/L	<0.5 × 10⁹/L	<30.0 × 10⁹/L	Marked decrease or absence of hematopoietic cells.	Search for a histocompatible sibling should be made if age permits.
Very severe	<80 g/L	<20.0 × 10⁹/L	<0.2 × 10⁹/L	<20.0 × 10⁹/L	Marked decrease or absence of hematopoietic cells.	Search for a histocompatible sibling should be made if age permits.

NOTE: These values are approximations and must be considered in the context of an individual patient's situation. (In some clinical trials, the blood count thresholds for moderately severe aplastic anemia are higher, e.g., platelet count <100 × 10⁹/L and absolute reticulocyte count <60,000 × 10⁹/L.) The marrow biopsy may contain the usual number of lymphocytes and plasma cells; "hot spots," focal areas of erythroid cells, may be seen. No fibrosis, abnormal cells, or malignant cells should be evident in the marrow. Dysmorphic features of blood or marrow cells are not features of acquired aplastic anemia. Ethnic differences in the lower limit of the absolute neutrophil count should be considered (Chap. 64).

has been confirmed in studies in Spain (Barcelona),[10] Brazil (State of Parana),[11] and Canada (British Columbia).[12] The highest frequency of aplastic anemia occurs in persons between the ages of 15 and 25 years; a second peak occurs between the ages of 65 and 69.[1] Aplastic anemia is more prevalent in the Far East where the incidence is approximately 7 per 1,000,000 in parts of China,[13] approximately 4 per 1,000,000 in sections of Thailand,[14] approximately 5 per 1,000,000 in areas of Malaysia,[15] and approximately 7 per 1,000,000 among children of Asian descent living in Canada.[12] The explanation for a twofold or greater incidence in the Orient compared to the Occident may be multifactorial,[16] but a predisposition gene or genes is a likely component.[12,17] Studies have not established the use of chloramphenicol in Asia as a cause. Poorly regulated exposure of workers to benzene is a factor,[18] but the attributable risk from benzene and other toxic exposures does not explain the magnitude of the difference in the incidence in Asia compared to that in Europe and South America.[16,17] A relationship to impure water use in Thailand has led to speculation of an infectious etiology, although no agent, including seronegative hepatitis, a known association with the onset of acquired aplastic anemia,[16] has been identified. Seronegative viral hepatitis is a forerunner of approximately 7 percent of cases of acquired aplastic anemia.[17,19] The male-to-female incidence ratio of aplastic anemia in most studies is approximately one.[17]

ETIOLOGY AND PATHOGENESIS

Table 35–2 lists the conditions associated with aplastic anemia.

The final common pathway to the clinical disease is a decrease in blood cell formation in the marrow. The number of marrow CD34+ cells (multipotential hematopoietic progenitors) and their derivative colony-forming unit–granulocyte-macrophage (CFU-GM) and burst-forming unit–erythroid (BFU-E) are reduced markedly in patients with aplastic anemia.[20–23] Long-term culture-initiating cells, an *in vitro* surrogate assay for hematopoietic stem cells, also are reduced to approximately 1 percent of normal values.[23] Potential mechanisms responsible for acquired marrow cell failure include (1) cellular or humoral immune suppression of the marrow multipotential cells, (2) progressive erosion of chromosome telomeres, (3) direct toxicity to hematopoietic multipotential or stem cells, (4) a defect in the stromal microenvironment of the marrow required for hematopoietic cell development, and (5) impaired

TABLE 35–2. Etiologic Classification of Aplastic Anemia

ACQUIRED

Autoimmune

Drugs
  See Table 35–3

Toxins
  Benzene
  Chlorinated hydrocarbons
  Organophosphates

Viruses
  Epstein-Barr virus
  Non-A, -B, -C, -D, -E, or -G hepatitis virus
  Human immunodeficiency virus (HIV)

Paroxysmal nocturnal hemoglobinuria

Autoimmune/connective tissue disorders
  Eosinophilic fasciitis
  Immune thyroid disease (Graves disease, Hashimoto thyroiditis)
  Rheumatoid arthritis
  Systemic lupus erythematosus

Thymoma

Pregnancy

Iatrogenic
  Radiation
  Cytotoxic drug therapy

INHERITED

Fanconi anemia

Dyskeratosis congenita

Shwachman-Diamond syndrome

Other rare syndromes (see Table 35–9)

production or release of essential multilineage hematopoietic growth factors. There is little experimental evidence for a stromal microenvironmental defect or a deficit of critical hematopoietic growth factors or their receptors. Telomerase mutations with consequent telomere shortening may be involved in as many as 40 percent of patients.[25] A susceptibility to the development of aplastic anemia is present in persons with certain human leukocyte antigen (HLA) types, such as HLA-DR15.[25]

Deficiencies in telomere repair could predispose to aplastic anemia by affecting the size of the multipotential hematopoietic cell compartment and by decreasing the multipotential cell's response to marrow injury, and could play a role in the evolution of aplastic anemia to a clonal myeloid disease by contributing to genomic instability.[24] Reduced hematopoiesis in most cases of aplastic anemia results from cytotoxic T-cell–mediated immune suppression of very early CD34+ hematopoietic multipotential progenitor or stem cells.[26] A small fraction of cases is initiated by a toxic exposure, drug exposure, or viral infection, and in these cases the pathogenesis also may relate to autoimmunity as there is evidence of immune dysfunction in seronegative hepatitis, after benzene exposure, and many such patients respond to anti–T-cell therapy.[26]

Autoreactive Cytotoxic T Lymphocytes

In vitro and clinical observations have resulted in the identification of a cytotoxic T-cell–mediated attack on multipotential hematopoietic cells in the CD34+ cellular compartment as the basis for most cases of acquired aplastic anemia.[27] Cellular immune injury to the marrow after drug-, viral-, or toxin-initiated marrow aplasia could result from the induction of neoantigens that provoke a secondary T-cell-mediated attack on hematopoietic cells. This mechanism could explain the response to immunosuppressive treatment in cases that follow exposure to an exogenous agent. Spontaneous or mitogen-induced increases in mononuclear cell production of interferon-γ,[28,29] interleukin (IL)-2,[29] and tumor necrosis factor-α (TNF-α)[30,31] occur. These factors are inhibitory to hematopoietic cell development. Elevated serum levels of interferon-γ are present in 30 percent of patients with aplastic anemia, and interferon-γ expression has been detected in the marrow of most patients with acquired aplastic anemia.[32] Addition of antibodies to interferon-γ enhances *in vitro* colony growth of marrow cells from affected patients.[33] Long-term marrow cultures manipulated to elaborate exaggerated amounts of interferon-γ, markedly reduced the frequency of long-term culture-initiating cells.[26] These observations indicate that acquired aplastic anemia is the result of cellular immune-induced apoptosis of primitive CD34+ multipotential hematopoietic progenitors, mediated by cytotoxic T lymphocytes, in part, through the expression of T-helper type 1 (Th1) inhibitory cytokines, interferon-γ, and TNF-α (Fig. 35–1).[34] The secretion of interferon-γ is a result of the upregulation of the regulatory transcription factor T-bet,[35] and apoptosis of CD34+ cells is, in part, mediated through a FAS-dependent pathway.[26] Because HLA-DR2 is more prevalent in patients with aplastic anemia, antigen recognition may be a factor in those patients. A variety of other potential factors have been found in some patients, including nucleotide polymorphisms in cytokine genes, overexpression of perforin in marrow cells, and decreased expression of SLAM-associated protein (SAP), a modulator protein that inhibits interferon-γ secretion.[26]

A decrease in regulatory T cells (CD4+CD25+FoxP3+) contributes to the expansion of an autoreactive CD8+CD28− T-cell population, which induces apoptosis of autologous hematopoietic multipotential hematopoietic cells.[36–38] T-regulatory cells are a component of the immune system that suppress immune responses of other cells. They provide a "stop" for immune reactions that have achieved their purpose. They also play a role in preventing autoimmune reactions (Chap. 76). One mouse model of immune-related marrow failure, induced by infusion of parental lymph node cells into F1 hybrid recipients, caused a fatal aplastic anemia. The aplasia could be prevented by immunotherapy or with monoclonal antibodies to interferon-γ and TNF-α.[26] Another mouse model of aplastic anemia induced by the infusion of lymph node cells histoincompatible for the minor H antigen, H60, resulted from the expansion of H60-specific CD8 T cells in recipient mice. The result was severe marrow aplasia. The effect of the CD8 T cells could be abrogated by either immunosuppressive agents or administration of CD4+CD25+ regulatory T cells,[39] providing additional experimental evidence for the role of regulatory T cells in the prevention of aplastic anemia.

Several putative target antigens on affected hematopoietic cells have been identified. Autoantibodies to one putative antigen, kinectin, have been found in patients with aplastic anemia. T cells, responsive to kinectin-derived peptides, suppress granulocyte-monocyte colony growth *in vitro*. However, in these studies cytotoxic T lymphocytes with that specificity were not isolated from patients.[40] Thus, the putative antigen(s) that is the target of the autoreactive T cells has not been identified.

Telomere Shortening

A relationship between acquired aplastic anemia and hereditary aplastic anemia (Fanconi anemia or dyskeratosis congenita) in some patients has been suggested because the defects in telomerase and telomere repair, characteristic of Fanconi anemia and dyskeratosis congenita are shared in some adult patients with aplastic anemia, but in these cases there is no family history of such a disorder and no phenotypic abnormalities that characterize the hereditary disorders (see "Fanconi Anemia" and "Dyskeratosis Congenita" below). Telomeres shorten physiologically with age as telomerase becomes less active. T-cell–mediated acquired aplastic anemia is associated with telomere shortening which could reflect an inherited defect in telomerase or a senescent erosion of activity. The telomerase mechanism consists of a telomerase reverse transcriptase (TERT); an RNA template for TERT, the telomerase RNA component (TERC), and other stabilizing proteins.[41,41a] Cells with shortened telomeres normally undergo apoptosis unless DNA repair mechanisms are impaired allowing the development of aneuploidy and neoplastic transformation.

Drugs

Chloramphenicol is the most notorious drug documented to cause aplastic anemia. Although this drug is directly myelosuppressive at very high dose because of its effect on mitochondrial DNA, the occurrence of aplastic anemia appears to be idiosyncratic, perhaps related to an inherited sensitivity to the nitroso-containing toxic intermediates.[42] This sensitivity may produce immunologic marrow suppression, as a substantial proportion of affected patients respond to treatment with immunosuppressive therapy.[43] The risk of developing aplastic anemia in patients treated with chloramphenicol is approximately 1 in 20,000, or 25 times that of the general population.[44] Although its use as an antibiotic has been largely abandoned in industrialized countries, global reports of fatal aplastic anemia continue to appear with topical or systemic use of the drug.

Epidemiologic evidence established that quinacrine (Atabrine) increased the risk of aplastic anemia.[45] This drug was administered to all U.S. troops in the South Pacific and Asiatic theaters of operations as prophylaxis for malaria during 1943 and 1944. The incidence of aplastic anemia was 7 to 28 cases per 1,000,000 personnel per year in the prophylaxis zones, whereas untreated soldiers had 1 to 2 cases per 1,000,000 personnel per year. The aplasia occurred during administration of the offending agent and was preceded by a characteristic rash in nearly half the cases. Many other drugs have been reported to increase the risk of aplastic anemia, but owing to incomplete reporting of information and

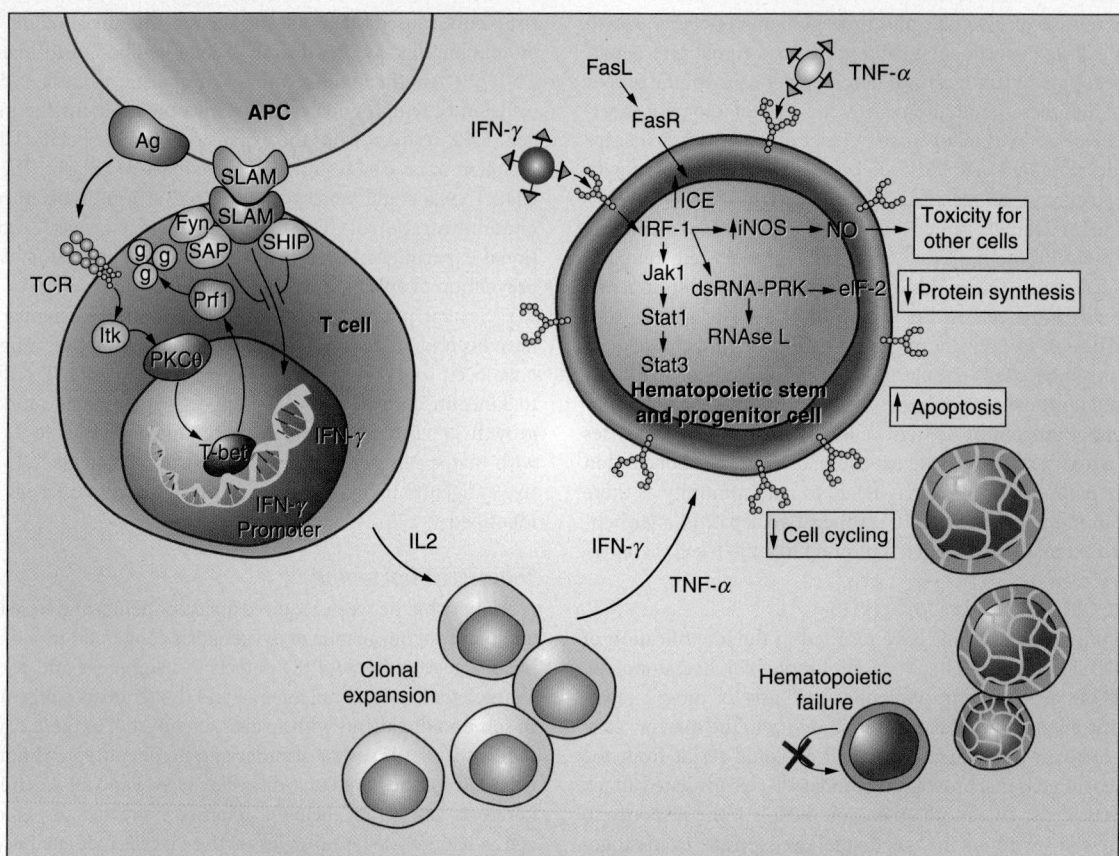

Figure 35–1. Immune pathogenesis of apoptosis of CD34 multipotential hematopoietic cells in acquired aplastic anemia. Antigens are presented to T lymphocytes by antigen-presenting cells (APCs). This triggers T cells to activate and proliferate. T-bet, a transcription factor, binds to the interferon-*γ* (IFN-*γ*) promoter region and induces gene expression. SLAM-associated protein (SAP) binds to Fyn and modulates the signaling lymphocyte activation molecule (SLAM) activity on IFN-*γ* expression, diminishing gene transcription. Patients with aplastic anemia show constitutive T-bet expression and low SAP levels. IFN-*γ* and tumor necrosis factor-*α* (TNF-*α*) upregulate both the T cell's cellular receptors and the Fas receptor. Increased production of interleukin-2 leads to polyclonal expansion of T cells. Activation of the Fas receptor by the Fas ligand leads to apoptosis of target cells. Some effects of IFN-*γ* are mediated through interferon regulatory factor 1 (IRF-1), which inhibits the transcription of cellular genes and entry into the cell cycle. IFN-*γ* is a potent inducer of many cellular genes, including inducible nitric oxide synthase (NOS), and production of the toxic gas, nitric oxide (NO), may further diffuse the toxic effects. These events ultimately lead to reduced cell cycling and cell death by apoptosis. *(Reproduced with permission from Young NS, Calado RT, Scheinberg P: Current concepts in the pathophysiology and treatment of aplastic anemia. Blood 108(8):2509–2519, 2006.)*

the infrequency of the association, the spectrum of drug-induced aplastic anemia may not be fully appreciated. Table 35–3 is a partial list of drugs that have been implicated.[46-54]

Many of these drugs are known to also induce selective cytopenias, such as agranulocytosis, which usually are reversible after discontinuation of the offending agent. These reversible reactions are not correlated with the risk of aplastic anemia, casting doubt on the effectiveness of routine monitoring of blood counts as a strategy to avoid aplastic anemia.

Because aplastic anemia is a rare event with drug use, it may occur because of an underlying metabolic or immunologic predisposition (gene polymorphism) in susceptible individuals. In the case of phenylbutazone-associated marrow aplasia, there is delayed oxidation and clearance of a related compound, acetanilide, as compared to either normal controls or those with aplastic anemia from other causes. This finding suggests excess accumulation of the drug as a potential mechanism for the aplasia. In some cases, drug interactions or synergy may be required to induce marrow aplasia. Cimetidine, a histamine H_2-receptor antagonist, is occasionally implicated in the onset of cytopenias and aplastic anemia, perhaps owing to a direct effect on early hematopoietic progenitor cells.[55] This drug accentuates the marrow-suppressive

effects of the chemotherapy drug carmustine.[56] In several instances, it has been reported as a possible cause of marrow aplasia when given with chloramphenicol.

There appears to be little difference in the age distribution, gender, response to immunotherapy, marrow transplantation, or survival, whether or not a drug exposure preceded the onset of the marrow aplasia.

Toxic Chemicals

Benzene was the first chemical linked to aplastic anemia, based on studies in factory workers before the 20th century.[57-59] Benzene is used as a solvent and is employed in the manufacture of chemicals, drugs, dyes, and explosives. It has been a vital chemical in the manufacture of rubber and leather goods and has been used widely in the shoe industry, leading to an increased risk for aplastic anemia (and acute myelogenous leukemia) in workers exposed to a poorly regulated environment.[59] In studies in China, aplastic anemia among workers was sixfold higher than in the general population.[18]

The U.S. Occupational Safety and Health Administration has lowered the permissible atmospheric exposure limit of benzene to 1 part per million (ppm) (8-hour time-weighted average) and short-term

TABLE 35–3. Drugs Associated with Aplastic Anemia

Category	High Risk	Intermediate Risk	Low Risk
Analgesic			Phenacetin, aspirin, salicylamide
Antiarrhythmic			Quinidine, tocainide
Antiarthritic		Gold salts	Colchicine
Anticonvulsant		Carbamazepine, hydantoins, felbamate	Ethosuximide, phenacemide, primidone, trimethadione, sodium valproate
Antihistamine			Chlorpheniramine, pyrilamine, tripelennamine
Antihypertensive			Captopril, methyldopa
Antiinflammatory		Penicillamine, phenylbutazone, oxyphenbutazone	Diclofenac, ibuprofen, indomethacin, naproxen, sulindac
Antimicrobial			
Antibacterial		Chloramphenicol	Dapsone, methicillin, penicillin, streptomycin, β-lactam antibiotics
Antifungal			Amphotericin, flucytosine
Antiprotozoal		Quinacrine	Chloroquine, mepacrine, pyrimethamine
Antineoplastic drugs			
Alkylating agent	Busulfan, cyclophosphamide, melphalan, nitrogen mustard		
Antimetabolite	Fluorouracil, mercaptopurine, methotrexate		
Cytotoxic antibiotic	Daunorubicin, doxorubicin, mitoxantrone		
Antiplatelet			Ticlopidine
Antithyroid			Carbimazole, methimazole, methylthiouracil, potassium perchlorate, propylthiouracil, sodium thiocyanate
Sedative and tranquilizer			Chlordiazepoxide, chlorpromazine (and other phenothiazines), lithium, meprobamate, methyprylon
Sulfa derivative		Sulfonamides	
Antibacterial			Numerous sulfonamides
Diuretic		Acetazolamide	Chlorothiazide, furosemide
Hypoglycemic			Chlorpropamide, tolbutamide
Miscellaneous			Allopurinol, interferon, pentoxifylline, penicillamine

NOTE: Drugs that invariably cause marrow aplasia with high doses are termed *high risk;* drugs with 30 or more reported cases are listed as moderate risk; others are less often associated with aplastic anemia (low risk).

SOURCE: This list was compiled from the AMA Registry,[46] publications of the International Agranulocytosis and Aplastic Anemia Study,[47–51] and other reviews and studies.[26,52–54] An additional comprehensive source for potentially offending drugs can be found in *The Drug Etiology of Agranulocytosis and Aplastic Anemia*, Oxford, UK: Oxford University Press, 1991.

exposure to 5 ppm (15-minute time-weighted average). The National Institute for Occupational Safety and Health recommends limits of exposure of 0.1 ppm as the 8-hour weighted average and 1 ppm for 15-minute short-term exposure. Previous to that regulatory change, the frequency of aplastic anemia in workers exposed to greater than 100 ppm benzene was approximately 1 in 100 workers, which decreased to 1 in 1000 workers at 10 to 20 ppm exposure.[58]

Organochlorine and organophosphate pesticide compounds have been suspected in the onset of aplastic anemia[60,61] and several studies have indicated an increased relative risk, especially for agricultural exposures[11,16,62,63] and household[11,63] exposures. These relationships are suspect because dose–disease relationships and other important factors have not been delineated, and several studies have not found an association with environmental exposures.[12,64] DDT (dichlorodiphenyltrichloroethane), lindane, and chlordane are insecticides that also have been associated with cases of aplastic anemia.[16,61] Occasional cases still occur following heavy exposure at industrial plants or after its use as a pesticide.[65] Lindane is metabolized in part to pentachlorophenol (PCP), another potentially toxic chlorinated hydrocarbon that is manufactured for use as a wood preservative. Cases of aplastic anemia and related blood disorders have been attributed to PCP over the past 25 years.[61,66] Prolonged exposures to petroleum distillates in the form of Stoddard solvent[67] and acute exposure to toluene through the practice of glue sniffing[68,69] also have been reported to cause marrow aplasia.

Trinitrotoluene (TNT), an explosive used extensively during World Wars I and II, is absorbed readily by inhalation and through the skin.[70] Fatal cases of aplastic anemia were observed in munitions workers exposed to TNT in Great Britain[71] from 1940 to 1946. In most cases, these conclusions have not been derived from specific studies but from accumulation of case reports or from patient histories, making conclusions provisional, although the argument for minimizing exposures to potential toxins is logical in any case.

Viruses

Non-A, -B, -C, -D, -E, -G Hepatitis Virus A relationship between hepatitis and the subsequent development of aplastic anemia has been the subject of a number of case reports, and this association was emphasized by two major reviews in the 1970s.[72,73] In the aggregate, these reports summarized findings in more than 200 cases. In many instances, the hepatitis was improving or had resolved when the aplastic anemia was noted 4 to 12 weeks later. Approximately 10 percent of cases occurred more than 1 year after the initial diagnosis of hepatitis. Most patients were young (ages 18 to 20 years); two-thirds were male, and their survival was short (10 weeks). Although hepatitides A and B have been implicated in aplastic anemia in a small number of cases, most cases are related to non-A, non-B, non-C hepatitis.[74–76] Severe aplastic anemia developed in 9 of 31 patients who underwent liver transplantation for non-A, non-B, non-C hepatitis, but in none of 1463 patients transplanted for other indications.[77] Several lines of evidence indicate there is no causal association with hepatitis C virus, suggesting that an unknown viral agent is involved.[16,78,79] Hepatitis virus B or C can be a secondary infection, if carefully screened blood products are not used for transfusion. In 15 patients with posthepatitic aplastic anemia, no evidence was found for hepatitis A, B, C, D, E, or G, transfusion-transmitted virus, or parvovirus B19.[80] Several reports suggest a relationship of parvovirus B19 to aplastic anemia,[81,82] whereas others have not.[79] This relationship has not been established (Chap. 36). The effect of seronegative hepatitis may be mediated through an autoimmune T-cell effect because of evidence of T-cell activation and cytokine elaboration.[26] These patients also have a similar response to combined immunotherapy as do those with idiopathic aplastic anemia[83,84] (see "Treatment: Combination Immunotherapy" below).

Epstein-Barr Virus Epstein-Barr virus (EBV) has been implicated in the pathogenesis of aplastic anemia.[85,86] The onset usually occurs within 4 to 6 weeks of infection. In some cases, infectious mononucleosis is subclinical, with a finding of reactive lymphocytes in the blood film and serologic results consistent with a recent infection (Chap. 82). EBV has been detected in marrow cells,[86] but it is uncertain whether marrow aplasia results from a direct effect or an immunologic response by the host. Patients have recovered following therapy with antithymocyte globulin.[86]

Other Viruses HIV infection frequently is associated with varying degrees of cytopenia. The marrow is often cellular, but occasional cases of aplastic anemia have been noted.[87–89] Marrow hypoplasia may result from viral suppression and from the drugs used to control viral replication in this disorder. Human herpes virus (HHV)-6 has caused severe marrow aplasia subsequent to marrow transplantation for other disorders.[90]

Autoimmune Diseases

The incidence of severe aplastic anemia was sevenfold greater than expected in patients with rheumatoid arthritis.[52] It is uncertain whether the aplastic anemia is related directly to rheumatoid arthritis or to the various drugs used to treat the condition (gold salts, D-penicillamine, and nonsteroidal antiinflammatory agents). Occasional cases of aplastic anemia are seen in conjunction with systemic lupus erythematosus.[91] *In vitro* studies found either the presence of an antibody[92] or suppressor cell[93,94] directed against hematopoietic progenitor cells. Patients have recovered after plasmapheresis,[92] glucocorticoids,[94] or cyclophosphamide therapy,[93,95] which is compatible with an immune etiology.

Eosinophilic fasciitis, an uncommon connective tissue disorder with painful swelling and induration of the skin and subcutaneous tissue, has been associated with aplastic anemia.[96,97] Although it may be antibody-mediated in some cases, it has been largely unresponsive to therapy.[96] Nevertheless, (1) stem cell transplantation, (2) immunosuppressive therapy using cyclosporine, (3) immunosuppressive therapy using antithymocyte globulin (ATG), or (4) immunosuppressive therapy with ATG and cyclosporine has cured or significantly ameliorated the disease in a few patients.[96,97]

Severe aplastic anemia also has been reported coincident with immune thyroid disease (Graves disease)[98–102] and the aplasia has been reversed with treatment of the hyperthyroidism. Aplastic anemia has occurred in association with thymoma.[102–108] Autoimmune renal disease and aplastic anemia have occurred concurrently. The underlying relationship may be the role of cytotoxic T lymphocytes in the pathogenesis of several autoimmune diseases and in aplastic anemia.[109]

Pregnancy

There are a number of reports of pregnancy-associated aplastic anemia, but the relationship between the two conditions is not always clear.[110–115] In some patients, preexisting aplastic anemia is exacerbated with pregnancy, only to improve following termination of the pregnancy.[110,111] In other cases, the aplasia develops during pregnancy with recurrences during subsequent pregnancies.[111,112] Termination of pregnancy or delivery may improve the marrow function, but the disease may progress to a fatal outcome even after delivery.[110–112] Therapy may include elective termination of early pregnancy, supportive care, immunosuppressive therapy, or marrow transplantation after delivery. Pregnancy in women previously treated with immunosuppression for aplastic anemia can result in the birth of a normal newborn.[115] In this latter study of 36 pregnancies, 22 were uncomplicated, 7 were complicated by a relapse of the marrow aplasia, and 5 without marrow aplasia required red cell transfusion during delivery.[115] One death occurred from cerebral thrombosis in a patient with paroxysmal nocturnal hemoglobinuria (PNH) and marrow aplasia.

Iatrogenic Causes

Although marrow toxicity from cytotoxic chemotherapy or radiation produces direct damage to stem cells and more mature cells, resulting in marrow aplasia, most patients with acquired aplastic anemia cannot relate an exposure that would be responsible for marrow damage.

Chronic exposure to low doses of radiation or use of spinal radiation for ankylosing spondylitis is associated with an increased, but delayed, risk of developing aplastic anemia and acute leukemia.[116,117] Patients who were given thorium dioxide (Thorotrast) as an intravenous contrast medium suffered numerous late complications, including malignant liver tumors, acute leukemia, and aplastic anemia.[118] Chronic radium poisoning with osteitis of the jaw, osteogenic sarcoma, and aplastic anemia was seen in workers who painted watch dials with luminous paint when they moistened the brushes orally.[119]

Acute exposures to large doses of radiation are associated with the development of marrow aplasia and a gastrointestinal syndrome.[120,121] Total-body exposure to between 1 and 2.5 Gy leads to gastrointestinal symptoms and depression of leukocyte counts, but most patients recover. A dose of 4.5 Gy leads to death in half the individuals (LD_{50}) owing to marrow failure. Higher doses in the range of 10 Gy are universally fatal unless the patient receives extensive supportive care followed by marrow transplantation. Aplastic anemia associated with nuclear accidents was seen after the disaster that occurred at the Chernobyl nuclear power station in the Ukraine in 1986.[122]

Antineoplastic drugs such as alkylating agents, antimetabolites, and certain cytotoxic antibiotics have the potential for producing marrow aplasia. In general, this is transient, is an extension of their pharmacologic action, and resolves within several weeks of completing chemotherapy. Although unusual, severe marrow aplasia can follow use of the alkylating agent, busulfan, and may persist indefinitely. Patients may develop marrow aplasia 2 to 5 years after discontinuation of alkylating agent therapy. These cases often evolve into hypoplastic myelodysplastic syndromes.

Stromal Microenvironment and Growth Factors

Short-term clonal assays for marrow stromal cells have shown variable defects in stromal cell function in patients with aplastic anemia. Serum levels of stem cell factor (SCF) have been either moderately low or normal in several studies of aplastic anemia.[123,124] Although SCF augments the growth of hematopoietic colonies from aplastic anemia patient's marrows, its use in patients has not led to clinical remissions. Another early acting growth factor, FLT-3 ligand, is 30- to 100-fold elevated in the serum of patients with aplastic anemia, although the pathobiologic effect of this change is unclear.[125] Fibroblasts grown from patients with severe aplastic anemia have subnormal cytokine production. However, serum levels of granulocyte colony-stimulating factor,[126] erythropoietin,[127] and thrombopoietin (TPO)[128] are usually high. Synthesis of IL-1, an early stimulator of hematopoiesis, is decreased in mononuclear cells from patients with aplastic anemia.[129] Studies of the microenvironment have shown relatively normal stromal cell proliferation and growth factor production.[130] These findings, coupled with the limited response of patients with aplastic anemia to growth factors, suggest that cytokine deficiency is not the etiologic problem in most cases. The most compelling argument is that most patients transplanted for aplastic anemia are cured with allogeneic donor stem cells and autologous stroma.[131]

A rare exception to the negligible pathogenetic role of hematopoietic growth factors in the etiology of aplastic anemia is the homozygous or mixed heterozygous mutation of the TPO receptor gene, *MPL*, which can cause amegakaryocytic thrombocytopenia that evolves, later, into aplastic anemia (Chap. 117). Furthermore, eltrombopag, a TPO receptor agonist, can stimulate mono, or in some patients, bilineage or trilineage recovery of blood counts that may be sustained off therapy (see "Treatment: Cytokines" below).

CLINICAL FEATURES

The onset of symptoms of aplastic anemia may be gradual with pallor, weakness, dyspnea, and fatigue as a result of the anemia. Dependent petechiae, bruising, epistaxis, vaginal bleeding, and unexpected bleeding at other sites secondary to thrombocytopenia are frequent presenting signs of the underlying marrow disorder. Rarely, it may be more dramatic with fever, chills, and pharyngitis or other sites of infection resulting from severe neutropenia and monocytopenia. Physical examination generally is unrevealing except for evidence of anemia (e.g., conjunctival and cutaneous pallor, resting tachycardia) or cutaneous bleeding (e.g., ecchymoses and petechiae), gingival bleeding and intraoral purpura. Lymphadenopathy and splenomegaly are not features of aplastic anemia; such findings suggest an alternative diagnosis such as a clonal myeloid or lymphoid disease.

LABORATORY FEATURES

Blood Findings

Patients with aplastic anemia have varying degrees of pancytopenia. Anemia is associated with a low reticulocyte index. The reticulocyte count is usually less than 1 percent and may be zero despite the high levels of erythropoietin. Absolute reticulocyte counts are usually fewer than 40,000/μL (40 × 10^9/L). Macrocytes may be present in the blood film and the mean cell volume (MCV) increased. The absolute neutrophil and monocyte count are low. An absolute neutrophil count fewer than 500/μL (0.5 × 10^9/L) along with a platelet count fewer than 30,000/μL (30 × 10^9/L) is indicative of severe disease, and a neutrophil count below 200/μL (0.2 × 10^9/L) denotes very severe disease (see Table 35–1). Lymphocyte production is thought to be normal, but patients may have mild lymphopenia. Platelets function normally. Significant qualitative changes of red cell, leukocyte, or platelet morphology on the blood film are not features of classical acquired aplastic anemia. On occasion, only one cell line is depressed initially, which may lead to an early diagnosis of pure red cell aplasia or amegakaryocytic thrombocytopenia. In such patients, other cell lines will fail shortly thereafter (days to weeks) and permit a definitive diagnosis. Table 35–4 is a plan for the initial laboratory investigation.

Plasma Findings

The plasma contains high levels of hematopoietic growth factors, including erythropoietin, TPO, and myeloid colony-stimulating factors. Growth factor levels need not be measured, however, for clinical care. Plasma iron values are usually high, and ^{59}Fe clearance is prolonged, with decreased incorporation into red cells.

Marrow Findings

Morphology The marrow aspirate typically contains numerous spicules with empty, fat-filled spaces, and relatively few hematopoietic cells. Lymphocytes, plasma cells, macrophages, and mast cells may be present. On occasion, occasional spicules are cellular or even hypercellular ("hot spots"), but megakaryocytes usually are reduced. These focal areas of residual hematopoiesis do not appear to be of prognostic significance. Residual granulocytic cells generally appear normal, but it is not unusual to see mild macronormoblastic erythropoiesis, presumably as a result of the high levels of erythropoietin. Marrow biopsy is essential to confirm the overall hypocellularity (Fig. 35–2), as a poor

---

TABLE 35–4. Approach to Diagnosis

History and Physical Examination

- Complete blood counts, reticulocyte count, and examination of the blood film
- Marrow aspiration and biopsy
- Marrow cell cytogenetics to evaluate clonal myeloid disease
- DNA stability test as a marker of Fanconi anemia
- Immunophenotyping of red and white cells, especially for CD55, CD59 to exclude PNH
- Direct and indirect antiglobulin (Coombs) test to rule out immune cytopenia
- Serum lactate dehydrogenase (LDH) and uric acid, which if increased may reflect neoplastic cell turnover
- Liver function tests to assess evidence of any recent viral hepatitis
- Screening tests for hepatitis viruses A, B, and C
- Screening tests for EBV, cytomegalovirus (CMV), and HIV
- Serum B$_{12}$ and red cell folic acid levels to rule out cryptic megaloblastic pancytopenia
- Serum iron, iron-binding capacity, and ferritin as a baseline prior to chronic transfusion therapy

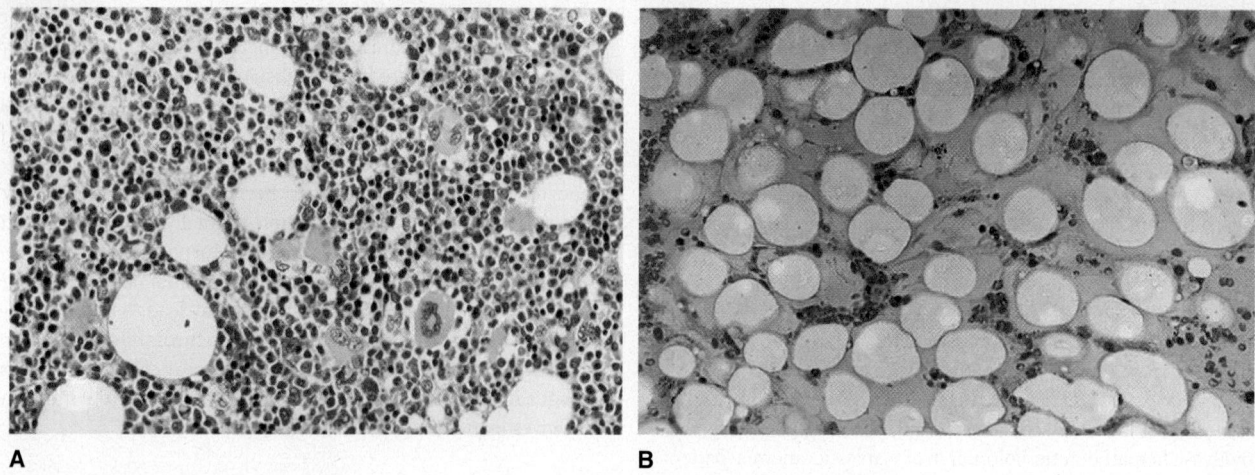

A   **B**

Figure 35–2. Marrow biopsy in aplastic anemia. **A.** A normal marrow biopsy section of a young adult. **B.** The marrow biopsy section of a young adult with very severe aplastic anemia. The specimen is devoid of hematopoietic cells and contains only scattered lymphocytes and stromal cells. The hematopoietic space is replaced by reticular cells (pre-adipocytic fibroblasts) converted to adipocytes.

yield of spicules and cells occurs in marrow aspirates in other disorders, especially if fibrosis is present.

In severe aplastic anemia, as defined by the International Aplastic Anemia Study Group, less than 25 percent cellularity or less than 50 percent cellularity with less than 30 percent hematopoietic cells is seen in the marrow.

Progenitor Cell Growth *In vitro* CFU-GM and BFU-E colony assays reveal a marked reduction in progenitor cells.[19–22]

Cytogenetic and Genetic Studies Cytogenetic analysis may be difficult to perform owing to low cellularity; thus, multiple aspirates may be required to provide sufficient cells for study. The results are normal in aplastic anemia. Clonal cytogenetic abnormalities in otherwise apparent aplastic anemia is indicative of an underlying hypoplastic clonal myeloid disease.[132] The move to newer techniques such as microarray-based comparative genomic hybridization (CGH) permits detection of aneuploidies, deletions, duplications, and/or amplifications of any locus represented on an array. In addition, microarray-based CGH is an effective tool for the detection of submicroscopic chromosomal abnormalities. This approach would increase the sensitivity to detect chromosome abnormalities in very hypocellular marrow samples, compared to standard G-banding, despite dilution of scant hematopoietic cells with nonhematopoietic stromal cells (e.g., fibroblasts). Next-generation sequencing of targeted exons has uncovered 32 mutations associated with myeloid malignancies. These mutations occurred in nearly 20 percent (29 of 150 patients) of cases of aplastic anemia. These mutations include the genes *ASXL1*, *DNMT3A*, and *BCOR*, which are considered driver mutations in myelodysplastic syndrome and acute myelogenous leukemia. Seventeen of the 29 patients with one of these three mutations evolved to overt myelodysplasia.[132a]

Imaging Studies Magnetic resonance imaging (MRI) can be used to distinguish between marrow fat and hematopoietic cells.[133] This approach may be a more useful overall estimate of marrow hematopoietic cell density than morphologic techniques and may help differentiate hypoplastic myelogenous leukemia from aplastic anemia.[128]

DIFFERENTIAL DIAGNOSIS

Any disease that can present with pancytopenia may mimic aplastic anemia if only the blood counts are considered. Measurement of the reticulocyte count and an examination of the blood film and marrow biopsy are essential early steps to arrive at a diagnosis. A reticulocyte

percentage of 0.5 percent to zero is strongly indicative of aplastic erythropoiesis, and when coupled with leukopenia and thrombocytopenia, points to aplastic anemia. Absence of qualitative abnormalities of cells on the blood film and a markedly hypocellular marrow are characteristic of acquired aplastic anemia. The disorders most commonly confused with severe aplastic anemia include the approximately 5 to 10 percent of patients with myelodysplastic syndromes who present with a hypoplastic rather than a hypercellular marrow. Myelodysplasia should be considered if there is abnormal blood film morphology consistent with myelodysplasia (e.g., poikilocytosis, basophilic stippling, neutrophils with hypogranulation or the pseudo–Pelger-Hüet anomaly). Marrow erythroid precursors in myelodysplasia may have dysmorphic features. Pathologic sideroblasts are inconsistent with aplastic anemia and a frequent feature of myelodysplasia. Granulocyte precursors may have reduced or abnormal granulation. Megakaryocytes may have abnormal nuclear lobulation (e.g., unilobular micromegakaryocytes; Chap. 87). If clonal cytogenetic abnormalities are found, a clonal myeloid disorder, especially myelodysplastic syndrome or hypocellular myelogenous leukemia is likely. MRI studies of bone may be useful in differentiating severe aplastic anemia from clonal myeloid syndromes. The former gives a fatty signal and the latter a diffuse cellular pattern.

A hypocellular marrow frequently is associated with PNH. PNH is characterized by an acquired mutation in the *PIG-A* gene that encodes an enzyme that is required to synthesize mannolipids. The gene mutation prevents the synthesis of the glycosylphosphatidylinositol anchor precursor. This moiety anchors several proteins, including inhibitors of the complement pathway to blood cell membranes, and its absence accounts for the complement-mediated hemolysis in PNH. As many as 50 percent of patients with otherwise typical aplastic anemia have evidence of glycosylphosphatidylinositol molecule defects and diminished phosphatidylinositol-anchored protein on leukocytes and red cells as judged by flow cytometry, analogous to that seen in PNH.[134] The decrease or absence of these membrane proteins may make the PNH clone of cells resistant to the acquired immune attack on normal marrow components, or the phosphatidylinositol-anchored protein(s) on normal cells provides an epitope that initiates an aberrant T-cell attack, leaving the PNH clone relatively resistant (Chap. 40).[26]

Occasionally, apparent aplastic anemia may be the prodrome to childhood[135] or, less commonly, adult[136] acute lymphoblastic leukemia. Sometimes, careful examination of marrow cells by light microscopy or flow cytometry will uncover a population of leukemic lymphoblasts. In other cases, the acute leukemia may appear later. Hairy-cell leukemia, Hodgkin disease, or another lymphoma subtype, rarely, may be preceded by a period of marrow hypoplasia. Immunophenotyping of marrow and blood cells by flow cytometry for CD25 may uncover the presence of hairy cells. Other clinical features may be distinctive (Chap. 93). Organomegaly such as lymphadenopathy, hepatomegaly, or splenomegaly are inconsistent with the atrophic (hypoproliferative) features of aplastic anemia. Large granular lymphocytic leukemia has also been associated with aplastic anemia. Rare cases of typical acquired aplastic anemia have been followed by t(9;22)-positive acute lymphocytic leukemia (ALL) or chronic myelogenous leukemia (CML).[136]

RELATIONSHIP AMONG APLASTIC ANEMIA, PAROXYSMAL NOCTURNAL HEMOGLOBINURIA, AND CLONAL MYELOID DISEASES

In addition to the diagnostic difficulties occasionally presented by patients with hypoplastic myelodysplastic syndromes, hypoplastic acute myelogenous leukemia (AML), or PNH with hypocellular marrows, there may be a more fundamental relationship among these three diseases and aplastic anemia. The development of clonal cytogenetic abnormalities such as monosomy 7 or trisomy 8 in a patient with aplastic anemia portends the evolution of a myelodysplastic syndrome or acute leukemia. Occasionally, these cytogenetic markers have been transient, and in cases with disappearance of monosomy 7, hematologic improvement has occurred as well.[137] Persistent monosomy 7 carries a poor prognosis as compared to trisomy 8.[138,139]

As many as 20 percent of patients with aplastic anemia have a 5-year probability of developing myelodysplasia.[137] If one excludes any transformation to a clonal myeloid disorder that occurs up to 6 months after treatment to avoid misdiagnosis among the hypoplastic clonal myeloid diseases, the frequency of a clonal disorder was nearly 15 times greater in patients treated with immunosuppression as compared to those treated with marrow transplantation after 39 months of observation.[140] This finding suggests either that immune suppression by anti–T-cell therapy enhances the evolution of a neoplastic clone or that it does not suppress the intrinsic tendency of aplastic anemia to evolve to a clonal disease, but provides the increased longevity of the patient required to express that potential. The latter interpretation is more likely as patients successfully treated solely with androgens develop clonal disease as frequently as those treated with immunosuppression.[141] Transplantation may reduce the potential to clonal evolution in patients with aplastic anemia by reestablishing robust lymphohematopoiesis.

Telomere shortening also may play a pathogenetic role in the evolution of aplastic anemia into myelodysplasia. Patients with aplastic anemia have shorter telomere lengths than matched controls, and patients with aplastic anemia with persistent cytopenias had greater telomere shortening over time than matched controls. Three of five patients with telomere lengths less than 5 kb developed clonal cytogenetic changes, whereas patients with longer telomeres did not develop such diseases.[23,142]

The findings of mutated genes considered driver mutations in myelodysplastic syndrome or AML (see "Marrow Findings: Cytogenetic and Genetic Studies" earlier) in nearly 20 percent of a population of patients with clinical aplastic anemia indicates that clonal hematopoiesis may develop or be present surreptitiously. The precise relationships to the aplastic anemia lesion is uncertain but could be caused the outgrowth of a clone of cells in the background of severally suppressed polyclonal hematopoietic stem cells. These findings were more common in patients with a long duration of disease and with shorter telomeres.[132a]

The relationship of PNH to aplastic anemia remains enigmatic. Because hematopoietic stem cells lacking the phosphatidylinositol-anchored proteins are present in many or all normal persons in very small numbers,[143] it is not surprising that more than 50 percent of patients with aplastic anemia may have a PNH cell population as detected by immunophenotyping.[134] The probability of patients with aplastic anemia developing a clinical syndrome consistent with PNH is 10 to 20 percent, and this is not a consequence of immunosuppressive treatment.[137] Patients also may present with the hemolytic anemia of PNH and later develop progressive marrow failure so that any pathogenetic explanation should consider both types of development of aplastic marrows in PNH. The *PIG-A* mutation may confer either a proliferative or survival advantage to PNH cells.[144,145] A survival advantage could result if the anchor protein or one of its ligands served as an epitope for the T-lymphocyte cytotoxicity, which induces the marrow aplasia. In this case, the presenting event could either reflect cytopenias or the sensitivity of red cells to complement lysis and hemolysis, depending on the intrinsic proliferative potential of the PNH clone.

Within our current state of knowledge, aplastic anemia is an autoimmune process, and any residual hematopoiesis is presumably polyclonal. This is a critical distinction from hypoplastic leukemia and PNH, which are clonal (neoplastic) diseases. The environment of the aplastic marrow, however, may favor the eventual evolution of a mutant (malignant) clone, especially if immunotherapy is used, whereas hematopoietic stem cell transplantation may either ablate threatening minor clones or establish more robust hematopoiesis, an environment less conducive to clonal evolution.

TREATMENT

Approach to Therapy

Severe anemia, bleeding from thrombocytopenia, and, uncommonly at the time of diagnosis, infection secondary to granulocytopenia and monocytopenia require prompt attention to remove potential life-threatening conditions and improve patient comfort (Table 35–5). More specific treatment of the marrow aplasia involves two principal options: (1) syngeneic or allogeneic hematopoietic stem cell transplantation or (2) combination immunosuppressive therapy with ATG and cyclosporine. The selection of the specific mode of treatment depends

TABLE 35–5. Initial Management of Aplastic Anemia

- Discontinue any potential offending drug and use an alternative class of agents if essential.
- Anemia: transfusion of leukocyte-depleted, irradiated red cells as required for very severe anemia.
- Very severe thrombocytopenia or thrombocytopenic bleeding: consider ε-aminocaproic acid; transfusion of platelets as required.
- Severe neutropenia; use infection precautions.
- Fever (suspected infection): microbial cultures; broad-spectrum antibiotics if specific organism not identified, granulocyte colony-stimulating factor (G-CSF) in dire cases. If child or small adult with profound infection (e.g., Gram-negative bacteria, fungus, persistent positive blood cultures) can consider neutrophil transfusion from a G-CSF pretreated donor.
- Immediate assessment for allogeneic stem cell transplantation: Histocompatibility testing of patient, parents, and siblings. Search databases for unrelated donor, if appropriate.

on several factors, including the patient's age and condition and the availability of a suitable allele-level HLA-matched hematopoietic stem cell donor. In general, transplantation is the preferred treatment for children and most otherwise healthy younger adults. Early histocompatibility testing of siblings is of particular importance because it establishes whether there is an optimal donor available to the patient for transplantation. The preferred stem cell source is a histocompatible sibling matched at the HLA-A, -B, -C, and -DR loci.

Supportive Care

The Use of Blood Products Although it has been recommended that red cell and platelet transfusions be used sparingly in potential transplant recipients to minimize sensitization to histocompatibility antigens, this has become less important since ATG and cyclophosphamide have been used as the preparative regimen for transplantation in aplastic anemia, as their use has markedly reduced the problem of graft rejection.[146]

Cytomegalovirus (CMV)-reduced risk red cells and platelets should be given to a potential transplant recipient to minimize problems with CMV infections after transplantation. Once a patient is shown to be CMV-positive, this restriction is no longer necessary. Leukocyte-depletion filters or CMV serotesting are equivalent methods of decreasing the risk of transmitting CMV.

Red Cell Transfusion Packed red cells to alleviate symptoms of anemia usually are indicated at hemoglobin values below 8 g/dL (80 g/L), unless comorbid medical conditions require a higher hemoglobin concentration. These products should be leukocyte-depleted to lessen leukocyte and platelet sensitization and to reduce subsequent transfusion reactions and radiated to reduce the potential for a transfusion-related graft-versus-host reaction. It is important not to transfuse patients with red cells (or platelets) from family members if transplantation within the family is remotely possible, as this approach may sensitize patients to minor histocompatibility antigens, increasing the risk of graft rejection after marrow transplantation. Following a marrow transplant, or in those individuals in whom transplantation is not a consideration, family members may be ideal donors for platelet products. Because each unit of red cells adds approximately 200 mg of iron to the total body iron, over the long-term transfusion-induced iron overload may occur. This is not a major problem in patients who respond to transplantation or immunosuppressive therapy, but it is an issue in nonresponders who require continued transfusion support. In the latter case, consideration should be given to iron-chelation therapy. Newer oral agents make this procedure easier to effect (Chap. 48).[147]

Platelet Transfusion It is important to assess the risk of bleeding in each patient. Most patients tolerate platelet counts of 10,000/μL (10 × 10⁹/L) without undue bruising or bleeding, unless a systemic infection is present or vascular integrity is impaired.[148,149] A traumatic injury or surgery requires transfusion to greater than 50,000/μL or greater than 100,000/μL, respectively. Administration of ε-aminocaproic acid, 50 mg/kg per dose every 4 hours orally or intravenously, may reduce the bleeding tendency.[150] Pooled random-donor platelets may be used until sensitization ensues, although it is preferable to use single-donor platelets from the onset to minimize sensitization to HLA or platelet antigens. Subsequently, single-donor apheresis products or HLA-matched platelets may be required.

Platelet refractoriness is a major problem with long-term transfusion support.[151] This may occur transiently, with fever or infection, or as a chronic problem secondary to HLA sensitization. In the past, this occurred in approximately 50 percent of patients after 8 to 10 weeks of transfusion support. Filtration of blood and platelet concentrates to remove leukocytes reduces this problem to approximately 15 percent of patients receiving chronic transfusions.[151,152] Patient's should also get ABO-identical platelets because this enhances platelet survival and further decreases refractoriness to platelet transfusion. Single-donor HLA-matched apheresis-harvested platelets may be necessary in previously pregnant or transfused patients who are already allosensitized or who so become after treatment with leukoreduced platelets. The frequency of either of these events is less than 10 percent. Chapter 139 discusses approaches to chronic platelet transfusion.

Management of Neutropenia Neutropenic precautions should be applied to hospitalized patients with a severe depression of the neutrophil count. The level of neutrophils requiring precautions is fewer than 500/μL (0.5 × 10⁹/L). One approach is to use private rooms, with requirements for face masks and handwashing with antiseptic soap. Unwashed fresh fruits and vegetables should be avoided as they are sources of bacterial contamination. It is uncommon for patients with aplastic anemia to present with a significant infection. When patients with aplastic anemia become febrile, cultures should be obtained from the throat, sputum (if any), blood, urine, stool, and any suspicious lesions. Broad-spectrum bactericidal antibiotics should be initiated promptly, without awaiting culture results. The choice of antibiotics depends on the prevalence of organisms and their antibiotic sensitivity in the local setting. Organisms of concern usually include *Staphylococcus aureus* (notably methicillin-and oxacillin-resistant strains), *Staphylococcus epidermidis* (in patients with venous access devices), and Gram-negative organisms. Patients with persistent culture-negative fevers should be considered for antifungal treatment (Chap. 24).

In the past, leukocyte transfusions were used on a daily basis to reduce the short-term mortality from infections. It was unusual to detect more than 100 to 200 neutrophils per microliter for more than a few hours after transfusion. The yield of neutrophils can be increased by administering granulocyte colony-stimulating factor (G-CSF) to the donor,[153] but most physicians avoid using white cell products because present-day antibiotics are usually sufficient to treat a patient for an episode of sepsis. Notable exceptions include documented invasive aspergillosis unresponsive to amphotericin (particularly in the posttransplant setting), infections with organisms resistant to all known antibiotics, and when blood cultures remain positive in spite of antibiotic treatment. Leukocyte transfusion is more effective in children and adults with smaller body size, as transfused leukocytes have a smaller distribution space, which results in higher blood and tissue concentrations.

Specific Treatment

Hematopoietic Stem Cell Transplantation Prompt therapy usually is indicated for patients with severe aplastic anemia. The major curative approach is hematopoietic stem cell transplantation from a histocompatible sibling.[154–156] Chapter 23 describes this treatment modality. Only 20 to 30 percent of patients in the United States have compatible sibling donors (related to average family size). In the unusual case of an identical twin donor, conditioning is required to obliterate the immune disease in the recipient, but it can be limited to cyclophosphamide. In this setting, an 80 to 90 percent survival is expected. Marrow stem cells seem to perform better than blood stem cells when used as a source for patients with aplastic anemia, although this is under continued study. The results of transplantation are best in patients younger than age 20 years (80 to 90 percent long-term survival) but decrease every decade of increasing age thereafter. Posttransplant mortality is increased and survival decreased with increasing age (Fig. 35–3). In patients older than age 40 years, survival in matched sibling transplant is reduced to approximately 50 percent.[157] There are still uncertainties about the optimal conditioning program in younger and older patients. ATG, cyclophosphamide, total-body radiation, fludarabine, and alemtuzumab are among the agents being studied.[154,156–158] Alemtuzumab (Campath)-containing regimens appear to improve outcome by decreasing the

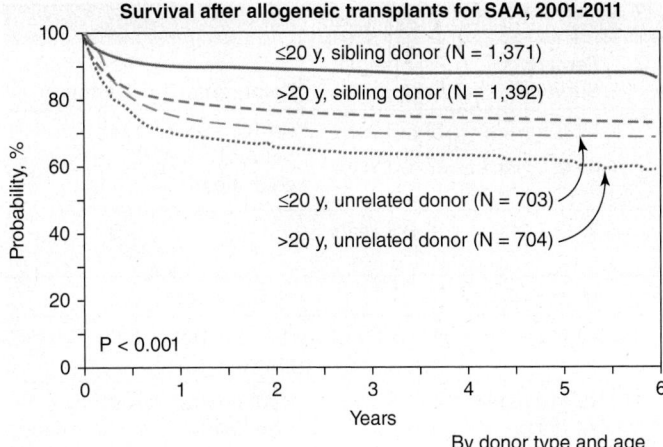

Survival after allogeneic transplants for SAA, 2001-2011

≤20 y, sibling donor (N = 1,371)
>20 y, sibling donor (N = 1,392)
≤20 y, unrelated donor (N = 703)
>20 y, unrelated donor (N = 704)
P < 0.001
By donor type and age

Figure 35–3. Allogeneic hematopoietic stem cell transplantation is the principal treatment for young patients with severe aplastic anemia and available HLA-matched sibling donor. Among the 2763 patients receiving HLA-matched sibling donor hematopoietic stem cell transplantation for severe aplastic anemia (SAA) between 2001 and 2011, the 3-year probabilities of survival were 88% ± 1% for those younger than 20 years and 76% ± 1% for those 20 years of age or older. Among the 1407 recipients of unrelated donor hematopoietic stem cell transplantation, the corresponding probabilities of survival were 70% ± 2% and 63% ± 2%. (*Reproduced with permission from MC Pasquini, Z Wang: Current use and outcome of hematopoietic stem cell transplantation: CIBMTR Summary Slides, 2013. Available at: http://www.cibmtr.org.*)

frequency of chronic graft-versus-host disease, which could make it useful in older patients.[158]

The longer the delay between diagnosis and transplantation, the less likely is a salutary outcome, probably as a result of a greater number of transfusions and a higher likelihood of pretransplantation infection. Acute and chronic graft-versus-host disease are serious complications, and therapy to prevent or ameliorate them is a standard part of post-transplantation treatment.[154,157] Transplantations have been performed using stem cells from partially matched siblings or unrelated, histocompatible donors recruited through the National Marrow Donor Program or similar organizations in other countries.[159] Umbilical cord blood is an alternative source of stem cells from unrelated donors (or, rarely, siblings) for transplantation in children, but the results are optimal with matched sibling transplantation. Alternatively, the use of high-resolution, HLA typing of a matched, unrelated donor markedly improves the prognosis for transplantation.[160] High-resolution DNA matching at HLA-A, -B, -C, and -DRB1 (8 of 8 alleles) is considered the lowest level of matching consistent with the highest level of survival. If there is an HLA mismatch at one or more loci, especially HLA-A or -DRB1, the outcome is compromised,[160] and immunosuppression with combined therapy may be preferred initially, depending on patient age, CMV status, and disease severity. Older patients have a much lower favorable response with alternative, non–matched-sibling, donor transplantations. The use of hematopoietic stem cell transplantation can be considered for patients who do not respond or who no longer respond to immunotherapy.[157] If the patient in question is a candidate for stem cell transplantation based on all relevant factors, transplantation could be considered at any age for a patient with a syngeneic donor; transplantation could be considered as a first-choice therapy up to age 50 years for a patient with an HLA allele-level matched sibling donor; and transplantation could be considered a first-choice therapy if an allele-level HLA-matched unrelated donor is available for patients younger than

age 20 years.[157] These guidelines are subject to the unique or special circumstances of an individual case. For example, if patients with aplastic anemia undergo gene sequencing and a mutation known to be a driver mutation for myelodysplasia or AML is found, allogeneic hematopoietic stem cell transplantation may prove to be a preferred approach.

Components of Anti–T-Lymphocyte (Immunosuppressive) Therapy

Antilymphocyte Serum and Antithymocyte Globulin ATG and ALG act principally by reducing cytotoxic T cells. This involves ATG-induced apoptosis through both FAS and TNF pathways.[161] Cathepsin B also plays a role in T-cell cytotoxicity at clinical concentrations of ATG, but may involve an independent apoptosis pathway.[162] ATG and ALG also release hematopoietic growth factors from T cells.[163,164] Horse and rabbit ATG are licensed in the United States. Skin tests against horse serum should be performed prior to administration.[165] If positive, the patient may be desensitized. ATG therapy is given daily for 4 to 10 days with doses of 15 to 40 mg/kg. Fever and chills are common during the first day of treatment. Concomitant treatment with glucocorticoids, such as methylprednisolone or dexamethasone lessens the reaction to ATG. Several studies have compared equine to rabbit ATG in the immunotherapy of aplastic anemia, contemporaneously or using historical comparisons. The consensus is that equine ATG is superior to rabbit and, if available, is recommended as the first line of therapy (Table 35–6).[166–174] Nevertheless, rabbit ATG is effective and should be considered if equine ATG does not result in a satisfactory outcome (Fig. 35–4).

ATG treatment may accelerate platelet destruction, reduce the absolute neutrophil count, and cause a positive direct antiglobulin (Coombs) test. This effect may lead to an increase in transfusion requirements during the 4- to 10-day treatment interval. Serum sickness, characterized by spiking fevers, skin rashes, and arthralgias, occurs commonly 7 to 10 days from the first dose. The clinical manifestations of serum sickness can be diminished by increasing the glucocorticoid dose from day 10 to day 17 after treatment. Approximately one-third of patients no longer require transfusion support after treatment with ATG alone.[175–177]

Of 358 patients responding to immunosuppressive therapy, principally ATG alone, 74 (21 percent) relapsed after a mean of 2.1 years. The actuarial incidence of relapse was 35 percent at 10 years.[178] Similar results were observed when 227 patients were treated with immunosuppression, primarily ATG alone.[179] The actuarial survival at 15 years was 38 percent following immunosuppression.[178] However, a combination of immunosuppressive agents provides more effective therapy than ATG alone (see "Combination Immunotherapy" below).

Twenty-eight (22 percent) of 129 patients treated with ALG developed myelodysplasia, leukemia, PNH, or combined disorders.[180] This tendency to relapse and to develop clonal hematologic disorders was reviewed by the European Cooperative Group for Bone Marrow Transplantation in 468 patients, most of whom received ATG.[181] The risk of a hematologic complication increased continuously and reached 57 percent at 8 years after immunosuppressive therapy. A further survey found 42 (5 percent) malignancies in 860 patients treated with immunosuppression, whereas only 9 (1 percent) malignancies were seen in 748 patients who received marrow transplants.[182]

There are no predictors that augur the risk of clonal evolution in an individual patient, although shorter telomere length at diagnosis and poorer prognosis are associated.[183]

Cyclosporine Administration of cyclosporine, a cyclic polypeptide that inhibits IL-2 production by T lymphocytes and prevents expansion of cytotoxic T cells in response to IL-2, is another approach to immunotherapy. After the initial report of its ability to induce remission in 1984,[184] several groups have used cyclosporine as

TABLE 35–6. Immunosuppressive Therapy of Aplastic Anemia: Source of Antithymocyte Globulin

Year of Report	Agents Used	No. Pts	Age Range (years)	Percent Response	Percent Survival	Percent Relapse	Comments	Citation
2013	H-ATG + CYA +GM-CSF	46	14–75	48 @ (NR)	84 @ 5 years	23 @ 3 years	H-ATG & R-ATG equivalent	174
	R-ATG +CYA	53	15–66	51 @ (NR)	83 @ 5 years	27 @ 3 years		
2012	R-ATG + CYA + G-CSF + glucoc	24	19–81	64 @ 3 months	70 @ 5 years	28 @ 5 years		170
2012	R-ATG + CYA	46	2-15	85 @ 1 year	??	??	Pediatric age	172
2012	R-ATG + CYA	35	17–75	60 @ 6 months	68 @ 27	NR	H-ATG better than R-ATG*	173
2011	H-ATG + CYA	60	37±3	68 @ 6 months	96 @ 3 years	NR	H-ATG better than R-ATG	169
	R-ATG + CYA	60	31±3	37 @ 6 months	76 @ 3 years			
2011	R-ATG + CYA + glucoc	20	19–80	50 @ 1 years	65 @ 3 years	NR	?R-ATG similar to H-ATG*	171
2010	H-ATG	42	1–66	59 @ 6 months	78 @ 2 years	NR	H-ATG better than R-ATG	167
	R-ATG	29	4–63	34 @ 6 months	55 @ 2 years			
2009	R-ATG + CYA + G-CSF	13	20–83	92 @ 1y	NR	30 @ 18 months	?R-ATG better than H-ATG*	168
2006	H-ATG +CYA +GM-CSF +EPO	30	2–71	73 @ (NR)	80 @ 5 years	NR	H-ATG better than R-ATG	166
	R-ATG +CYA +GM-CSF +EPO	32	2–71	53 @ (NR)	66 @ 5 years	NR		

CYA, cyclosporine; EPO, erythropoietin; Glucoc, glucocorticoids; G-CSF, granulocyte colony-stimulating factor; GM-CSF, granulocyte-monocyte, colony-stimulating factor; H-ATG, horse antithymocyte globulin; No., number; NR, not reported; Pts, patients; R-ATG, rabbit antithymocyte globulin.

*Based on prior studies of H-ATG.

either (1) primary treatment,[185-188] (2) in patients refractory to ATG or glucocorticoids,[186-191] (3) in combination with G-CSFs,[192,193] or (4) in varying combinations with other modes of therapy.[194] Cyclosporine is administered orally at 10 to 12 mg/kg per day for at least 4 to 6 months. Dosage adjustments may be required to maintain trough blood levels of 200 to 400 ng/mL. Renal impairment is common and may require increased hydration or dose adjustments to keep creatinine values below 2 mg/dL. Cyclosporine also may cause moderate hypertension, a variety of neurologic manifestations, and other side effects. Several drug classes interact with cyclosporine to either increase (e.g., some antibiotics and antifungals) or decrease (e.g., some anticonvulsants) blood levels. Responses usually are seen by 3 months and may range from achieving transfusion independence to complete remission. Approximately 25 percent of patients respond to this agent when used alone, but the response rate has ranged from 0 to 80 percent in various reports.[194]

Although immunosuppression with ALG or ATG has been used the longest and has a seemingly better response rate, there are certain advantages to cyclosporine. This drug does not require hospitalization or use of a central venous catheter. Fewer platelet transfusions are required during the first few weeks of therapy compared to treatment with ALG or ATG. A French cooperative trial showed equal effectiveness of cyclosporine compared to ATG plus prednisone.[195] In this crossover study of newly diagnosed patients, survival of approximately 65 percent was observed 12 months after diagnosis.

Combination Immunotherapy Combination treatment of severe aplastic anemia usually includes, for example, ATG, 40 mg/kg per day, for 4 days; cyclosporine, 10 to 12 mg/kg per day, for 6 months and methylprednisolone, 1 mg/kg per day, for 2 weeks.[196] The dose of cyclosporine is adjusted to maintain a trough level of 200 to 400 ng/mL. Prophylaxis for *Pneumocystis carinii* with daily trimethoprim-sulfamethoxazole or with monthly pentamidine inhalations should be considered for these patients as they receive immunosuppressive therapy.

The addition of cyclosporine to the combination of ALG and glucocorticoids improves response rates to approximately 70 percent of patients (Table 35–7).[197,198] G-CSF added to the combined immunosuppressive therapy does not increase response rate or survival.[199] Response is usually defined as a significant improvement in red cells, white cells, and platelets to eliminate risk of infection and bleeding and the requirement for red cell transfusions.

The 5-year survival after completion of combination immunosuppressive therapy may approximate that after stem cell transplantation.[200] Forty-eight children treated between 1983 and 1992 had a 10-year survival of approximately 75 percent for marrow transplantation and approximately 75 percent for combined immunosuppressive

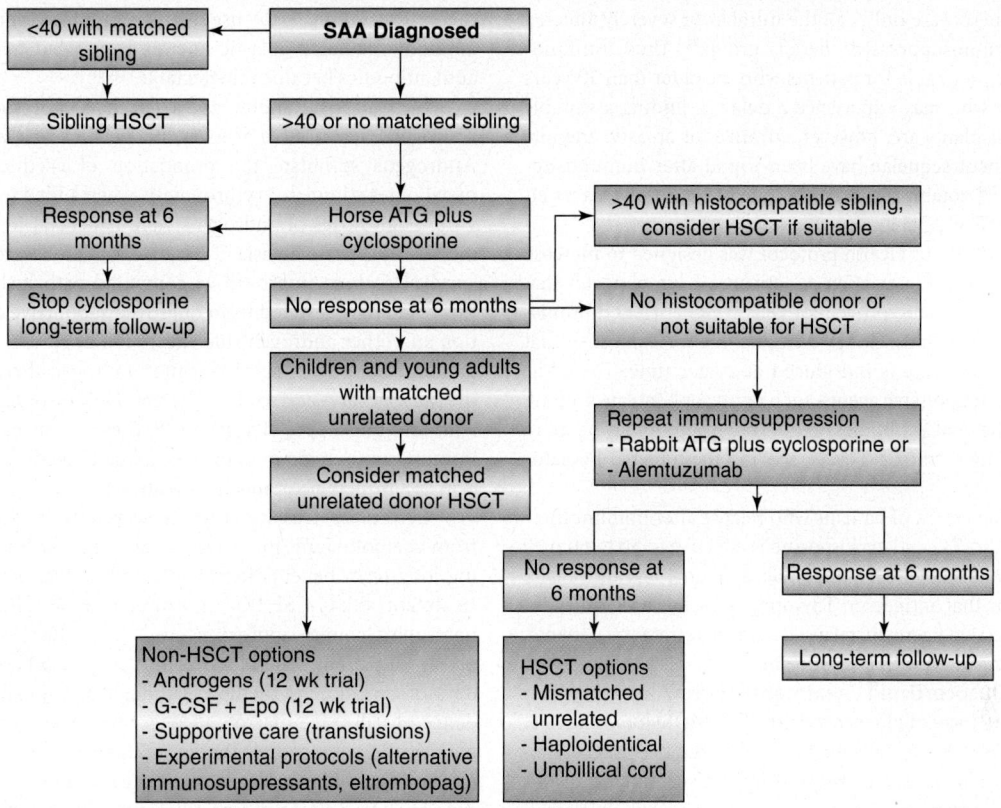

Figure 35–4. Flow chart with general guidelines for treatment. Response to horse ATG plus cyclosporine is followed for 6 months before deciding the patient has not responded adequately unless the patient is doing poorly and the neutrophil count remains less than 200 × 10⁹/L. In that case, one can proceed to next suitable option. In general, transplantation options are reassessed at 6 months after immunotherapy and are dependent on donor availability and quality of match, patient age, comorbid conditions that would increase transplantation risk, and the severity of the depression in neutrophil count. In younger patients, a matched unrelated donor may be appropriate. In older patients, retreating with immunotherapy would be favored unless the neutrophil count persists in the very-severe-risk category. After two unsuccessful attempts at immunotherapy, therapy is individualized and a high-risk transplantation procedure (slight mismatched-related, haploidentical, umbilical cord blood) may be considered, using the relevant variables (e.g., age, comorbidities, performance status, neutrophil count). The age of 40 years is an approximate guideline for considering an initial allogeneic hematopoietic stem cell transplant and may be modified upwards somewhat (e.g., 41 to 50 years) based on the clinical status and other features of the patient. (*Reproduced with permission from Scheinberg P and Young NS: How I treat aplastic anemia. Blood 120(6):1185–1196, 2012.*)

TABLE 35–7. Response to Immunotherapy in Patients with Severe Aplastic Anemia

Year of Publication	Principal Drugs Used	No. Pts (Age-range, years)	Significant Response No. (%)	Survival at 5/10 Years (%)	Relapse at 5 Years (Cum%)	Comments	Reference
2011	ATG+CYA	95(7–80)	63(66)	76*/NR	33*	Fewer early infections with G-CSF; no difference in response or survival	223
	ATG+CYA+G-CSF	97(2–81)	71(73)	78*/NR	32*		
2008	ATG + CYA	77 (<18)	57 (74)	83/80	25	8.5% evolved to clonal myeloid disease	197
2007	ATG + CYA	44 (NR)	31 (70)	NR/88	NR	All cases were associated with hepatitis	198
2007	ATG + CYA	47 (19–75)	31 (66)	80/NR	45	No late clonal diseases at 5 years	199
2007	ATG + CYA + G-CSF	48 (19–74)	37 (77)	90/NR	15	No late clonal diseases at 5 years	199
2006	ATG + CYA	47 (8–71)	37 (79)	80/75	NR	No late clonal diseases at 10 years	166
2006	ATG + CYA + G-CSF + rhuEPO	30 (5–68)	22 (73)	80/75	NR	One patient developed clonal myeloid disease	166

ATG, antithymocyte globulin; Cum%, cumulative percent; CYA, cyclosporine; G-CSF, granulocyte colony-stimulating factor; No. Pts, number of patients; NR, not reported; rhuEPO, recombinant human erythropoietin.

*At 6 years posttreatment.

therapy, although there were only half the number of severely affected patients in the immunosuppressive therapy group.[201] Thus, immunosuppression may be preferable for patients who are older than 30 years of age and in those who may experience a delay in finding a suitable donor. Marrow transplants are, however, curative for aplastic anemia, whereas more frequent sequelae have been found after immunosuppressive therapy,[202–204] notably a substantial rate of evolution to a myelodysplastic syndrome or AML.

A National Institutes of Health protocol was designed to increase immune tolerance by specific deletion of activated T lymphocytes that target primitive hematopoietic progenitor cells.[26] Concurrent administration of cyclosporine with ATG may diminish the ATG effect so that in this program cyclosporine is introduced at a later time. The addition of new immunosuppressive agents, such as mycophenolate mofetil, rapamycin, or monoclonal antibodies, to the IL-2 receptor may be more effective in decreasing cytotoxic T cells, sparing the targeted hematopoietic stem cells.[26]

For the 30 to 40 percent of patients who relapse after immunotherapy, retreatment with ATG and cyclosporine is effective in 50 to 60 percent of them.[205,206] Alternatively, alemtuzumab, a monoclonal anti-CD52 antibody that targets that antigen on T lymphocytes, has been an effective immunosuppressive agent in relapsed and in refractory patients, and it may be administered with cyclosporine.[207–209]

High-Dose Glucocorticoid Treatment Marrow recovery can occur after very high doses of glucocorticoids.[210,211] Methylprednisolone in the range of 500 to 1000 mg daily for 3 to 14 days has been successful, but the side effects, which include marked hyperglycemia and glycosuria, electrolyte disturbances, gastric irritation, psychosis, increased infections, and aseptic necrosis of the hips, can be severe. Glucocorticoids at lower doses commonly are used only as a component of combination therapy for aplastic anemia to ameliorate the toxic effects of ATG and in providing additional lymphocyte suppression.

High-Dose Cyclophosphamide Therapy High-dose cyclophosphamide has been used as a form of immunosuppression.[212] Although it would seem inappropriate to administer high doses of chemotherapy to patients with severe marrow aplasia, this approach was based on observations of autologous recovery after preparative therapy for allogeneic transplants not followed by a transplantation.[6] In an early study, 10 patients who received cyclophosphamide at 45 mg/kg per day intravenously for 4 days with or without cyclosporine for an additional 100 days had gradual neutrophil and platelet recovery over 3 months. Seven patients responded completely and remained in remission 11 years after treatment. High-dose cyclophosphamide treatment may spare hematopoietic stem cells, which have high levels of aldehyde dehydrogenase and are relatively resistant to cyclophosphamide.[213,214] Thus, cyclophosphamide in this situation may be more immunosuppressive than myelotoxic. The most extensive trial of high-dose cyclophosphamide resulted in 65 percent of patients responding completely at 50 months.[215] However, the role of this regimen as initial therapy is not clear because of early toxicity that may exceed that of the ATG and cyclosporine combination.[216] The probability of a durable remission may be superior, but there are insufficient data (comparative clinical trials) to conclude whether high-dose cyclophosphamide provides better long-term results than ATG and cyclosporine. The latter approach is favored at this time.

Rituximab A case report of the successful use of the anti-CD20 humanized mouse antibody rituximab has provided preliminary evidence for its potential effectiveness in treating aplastic anemia.[217] Clinical trials have not examined its efficacy compared to standard immunotherapy (ATG and cyclosporine), in patients refractory to standard therapy, or as a third drug in an immunotherapy regimen. Whether B lymphocytes play a role in the pathogenesis of T-cell–mediated aplastic anemia has not been defined, so rituximab does not appear to have a theoretical rationale for use at this time. However, a singular case of antibody-mediated aplastic anemia responded to rituximab, and the autoantibodies became undetectable.[218,219]

Androgens Randomized trials have not shown efficacy when androgens were used as primary therapy for severe aplastic anemia.[220,221] Androgens stimulate the production of erythropoietin, and their metabolites stimulate erythropoiesis when added to marrow cultures *in vitro*. High doses of androgens were beneficial in some patients with moderately severe aplasia.[220] Series of patients were reported in which survival seemed improved as compared with historical controls, but this could have resulted from improved supportive care.[141] Masculinization and other androgen side effects can be severe, especially in female patients. Long-term survivors after androgen therapy have essentially the same progression to clonal hematologic disorders as patients treated with immunosuppressive agents.[141] These agents have been replaced by immunosuppression or allogeneic hematopoietic stem cell transplantation as a principal approach to treatment.

Cytokines Despite their effectiveness in accelerating recovery from chemotherapy, these agents have been far less effective in achieving long-term benefits in patients with severe aplastic anemia. Daily treatment with G-CSF[222] has improved marrow cellularity and increased neutrophil counts approximately 1.5- to 10-fold. Unfortunately, in nearly all patients, the blood counts return to baseline within several days of cessation of therapy. Although occasional patients show evidence of trilineage marrow recovery with long-term therapy, the vast majority do not respond. Therapy with myeloid growth factors is probably best reserved for episodes of severe infection or as a preventive measure prior to dental work or other procedures that would compromise mucosal barriers in patients who have not responded to stem cell transplant or immunotherapy. G-CSF in a dose of 5 mcg/kg by subcutaneous injection is easiest to administer and seems to be associated with the fewest side effects. The drug can be given daily or fewer times per week depending on the response. Newer pegylated preparations have a longer effect and usually are administered at less frequent, every-other-week intervals. The SAA Working Party of the European Group for Blood and Marrow Transplant reported that G-CSF added to ATG and cyclosporine reduces infection early in treatment, but does not affect survival or length of remission.[223] Generally, prophylactic use of growth factors is not warranted.

IL-1, a potent stimulator of marrow stromal cell production of other cytokines, and IL-3 have been ineffective in small numbers of patients so treated with severe aplastic anemia.[224,225] These disappointing results with cytokines are not unexpected, as previous work has found high serum levels of growth factors in patients with aplastic anemia. Moreover, the majority of patients have suppression of very primitive progenitors, which may be unresponsive to individual factors that act on more mature progenitor cells.

An exception to the poor response to cytokines is the use of eltrombopag, a TPO receptor agonist that binds to the transmembrane region of the TPO receptor and stimulates the Janus kinase (JAK)-signal transducer and activator of transcription (STAT) and mitogen-activated protein (MAP) kinase pathways. TPO may expand stem cell numbers and promote DNA repair.[226–229] Use of this agent in 43 patients with acquired aplastic anemia who did not respond to immunotherapy resulted in improved hematopoiesis and cell counts in 17 (40 percent) with several having improved bi- or trilineage hematopoiesis and cell counts. Five patients had near normalization of all blood counts and had therapy stopped after 9 to 37 months with maintenance of their blood counts for 1 to 13 months of observation.[230] Although many did not normalize their counts, several became red cell and platelet transfusion independent. Eight patients developed new cytogenetic abnormalities (5 of 8 patients developed −7 or del[7]), but none had progressed to AML.

Splenectomy Removal of the spleen does not increase hematopoiesis but may increase neutrophil and platelet counts two- to threefold and improve survival of transfused red cells or platelets in highly sensitized individuals.[231] The surgical morbidity and mortality in patients with few platelets and white cells makes this a questionable therapeutic procedure. Because there are more successful methods of therapy that attack the fundamental problem, this approach is not recommended.

Other Therapy High doses of intravenous γ-globulin have been given to small numbers of patients with severe aplastic anemia[232,233] because of its success in treating certain cases of antibody-mediated pure red cell aplasia. Some improvement was noted in 4 of 6 patients treated. Another treatment that is occasionally successful is lymphocytapheresis to deplete T cells.[234,235] Agents that target other T-cell functions, such as alefacept, a CD2-directed leukocyte function antigen-3 (LFA-3)/Fc fusion protein that consists of the extracellular CD2-binding portion of the human LFA-3 linked to the Fc (hinge, CH2 and CH3 domains) portion of human immunoglobulin (Ig) G_1 are being tested as immunosuppressive drugs in acquired aplastic anemia.[236]

Course and Prognosis

At diagnosis, the prognosis is largely related to the absolute neutrophil and platelet count. The absolute neutrophil count is the most important prognostic feature, with a count of fewer than $500/\mu$L (0.5×10^9/L) considered severe aplastic anemia and a count of fewer than $200/\mu$L (0.2×10^9/L) very severe aplastic anemia, the latter associated with a poor response to immunotherapy and usually a dire prognosis, if early successful allogeneic transplant is not available. In the past, the prognosis appeared worse when the disease followed hepatitis.[72,73] But, more comprehensive results with immunosuppression[210] or hematopoietic stem cell transplantation[237] show an equivalent response to that seen with idiopathic or drug-induced cases.

Before marrow transplantation and immunosuppressive therapy, more than 25 percent of the patients with severe aplastic anemia died within 4 months of diagnosis; half succumbed within 1 year.[235,239] Marrow transplantation is curative for approximately 80 to 90 percent of patients younger than 20 years of age, approximately 70 percent if between the ages of 20 and 40 years, and approximately 50 percent if older than age 40 years.[157,240] Unfortunately, as many as 40 percent of transplant survivors suffer the deleterious consequences of chronic graft-versus-host disease,[157] and the risk of subsequent cancer can be as high as 10 percent in older patients or after immunotherapy prior to hematopoietic stem cell transplantation.[241,242] The best outcomes occur in those patients who have an allele-based HLA-matched sibling; have not been exposed to immunosuppressive therapy prior to transplantation; have not been exposed and sensitized to blood cell products; have had a marrow rather than a blood stem cell donor product; and have not been subjected to high-dose radiation in the conditioning regimen for transplantation.[157,241,243,244]

Combination immunosuppressive therapy with ATG and cyclosporine leads to a marked improvement in approximately 70 percent of the patients; a higher initial absolute reticulocyte and lymphocyte counts are predictive of the response to therapy.[245] Although some patients regain normal blood counts, many continue with moderate anemia or thrombocytopenia. In as many as 40 percent of patients initially responding to immunosuppressive therapy, their disease may relapse or progress to PNH, a myelodysplastic syndrome, or AML over 10 years of observation.[178–186,214–216] Moreover, the beneficial effects of immunotherapy are often lost 10 years after treatment. In 168 transplanted patients the actuarial survival at 15 years was 69 percent, and in 227 patients receiving immunosuppressive therapy it was 38 percent.[178] The long-term survival in pediatric patients younger than age 18 years appears better, with approximately one-third relapsing at 10 years.[246]

Treatment with high-dose cyclophosphamide produces early results similar to that seen with the combination of ATG and cyclosporine.[247,248] However, cyclophosphamide has greater early toxicity and slower hematologic recovery, but may generate more durable remissions. Its use has been too limited to reach a firm conclusion on its relative merits and it is rarely used as the first choice of immunotherapy.

● HEREDITARY APLASTIC ANEMIA

FANCONI ANEMIA

Definition and History

Fanconi anemia is the most common form of constitutional aplastic anemia and was initially described in three brothers by Fanconi in 1927.[249] It is inherited as an autosomal recessive condition that results from defects in genes that modulate the stability of DNA.

Epidemiology

Fanconi anemia is an uncommon disorder and is estimated to be present in 1 in 1 million individuals. It is far more frequent in Afrikaners of European descent.[250] This unusually high frequency has been attributed to a founder effect.

Etiology and Pathogenesis

Sixteen complementation groups, defined by somatic cell hybridization, are associated with the development of Fanconi anemia (FA).[251,252] A complementation group is a genetic subgroup. Identifying a complementation group requires adding a gene to the genome of a cell to correct (complement) the genetic defect. This procedure can be done by cell fusion studies. After fusing two cells together, thereby joining their genetic material, one can test the cells for the genetic defect. In the case of Fanconi anemia, this would be with the diepoxybutane test. In this test, diepoxybutane results in chromosome fragmentation in the cells of patients with Fanconi anemia. Hybrids in which the hypersensitivity to diepoxybutane is corrected (complemented) can be assumed to result from the fusion of cells from different genetic subgroups (complementation groups), whereas hybrids that still show the sensitivity are the result of fusion of cells from the same subgroup. Because one can determine the complementation group without knowing the gene involved, this approach is the first step in understanding the genetic basis of a disease. Once the genes are known, one does not need to use cell fusion studies; rather, retroviral vectors can be used to insert corrected genes into the cells.

The complementation groups have been designated *FANCA, B, C, D1, D2, E, F, G, I, J, L, M, N, O, P,* and *Q.* Table 35–8 lists the gene mutations corresponding to these complementation groups, and Fig. 35–5 summarizes the functions of the known Fanconi anemia proteins.[252] The great majority of patients have mutations of *FANCA, FANCC,* or *FANCG.*[253] It has been proposed that the A and C gene products, which are cytoplasmic proteins, form an "FA core complex" with the products of genes B, E, F, G, L, and M, which are adaptors or phosphorylators.[253,254] The complex translocates to the nucleus, where it is required for the ubiquitination of FANCD2 and protects the cell from DNA crosslinking and participates in DNA repair (Fig. 35–6). DNA damage initiates activation of the FA/BRCA pathway and ubiquitination of FANCD2, which is targeted to the altered DNA and facilitates repair by interacting with DNA repair proteins, BRCA1, FANCD1/BRCA2, FANCN/PALB2, and RAD51. In the presence of a mutant gene product, the normal protective and repair functions are disturbed leading to damaging effects in sensitive tissues, including hematopoietic cells. The genetic damage appears related to the adverse effects of reactive oxygen radicals, such as superoxide and hydrogen peroxide as well as

TABLE 35–8. Gene Mutations Found in Fanconi Anemia

Gene	Chromosome Location	% of Patients	Inheritance	Protein Function
FANCA	16q24.3	~65*	AR	FA core complex
FANCB	Xp22.31	rare	XLR	FA core complex
FANCC	9q22.3	~10	AR	FA core complex
FANCDI (BRCA2)	13q12.3	rare	AR	RAD51 recruitment
FANCD2	3p25.3	rare	AR	Monoubiquitinated protein
FANCE	6p21.3	~10	AR	FA core complex
FANCF	11p15	rare	AR	FA core complex
FANCG (XRCC9)	9p13	~10	AR	FA core complex
FANCI (KIAA1794)	15q25–26	rare	AR	Monoubiquitination of FANCD2
FANCJ (BACH1/BRIP1)	17q22.3	rare	AR	5′ to 3′ DNA helicase/ATPase
FANCL (PHF9/POG)	2q16.1	rare	AR	FA core complex, E3 ubiquitin ligase
FANCM (Hef)	14q21.3	rare	AR	FA core complex, ATPase/translocase, DNA helicase motifs
FANCN (PALB2)	16q12.1	rare	AR	Regulation of BRCA2 localization
FANCO(RAD51C/RAD51L2)	17q25.1	Rare	AR	Homologous combination In DNA repair
FANCP (SLX4/BTBD12/KIAA)	16p13.3	Rare	AR	SLX4 endonuclease subunit
FANCQ (XPF/ERCC4)	16p13.12	Rare	AR	DNA-repair endonuclease XPF

AR, autosomal recessive; ATPase, adenosine triphosphatase; FA, Fanconi anemia; XLR, X-linked recessive.

*There are more than 100 mutant FANCA alleles, approximately 40 percent of which are large intragenic deletions. This table was made using material from references 251 to 256.

aldehydes produced by normal cellular metabolism.[255–257] In addition to the genetic defects leading to DNA instability and an inability to repair DNA, TNF-α and -γ are overexpressed in the marrow of Fanconi anemia patients.[258] The excess TNF-α may play a role in the suppression of erythropoiesis in these patients.

The generation of reactive oxygen radicals and aldehydes, the defective mechanisms of DNA repair, the hypersensitivity to cytokines such as TNF-α, and the age-related shortening of DNA-protective telomeres produce a marked predisposition to clonal evolution and neoplasia in Fanconi anemia patients (see "Therapy and Course" below).

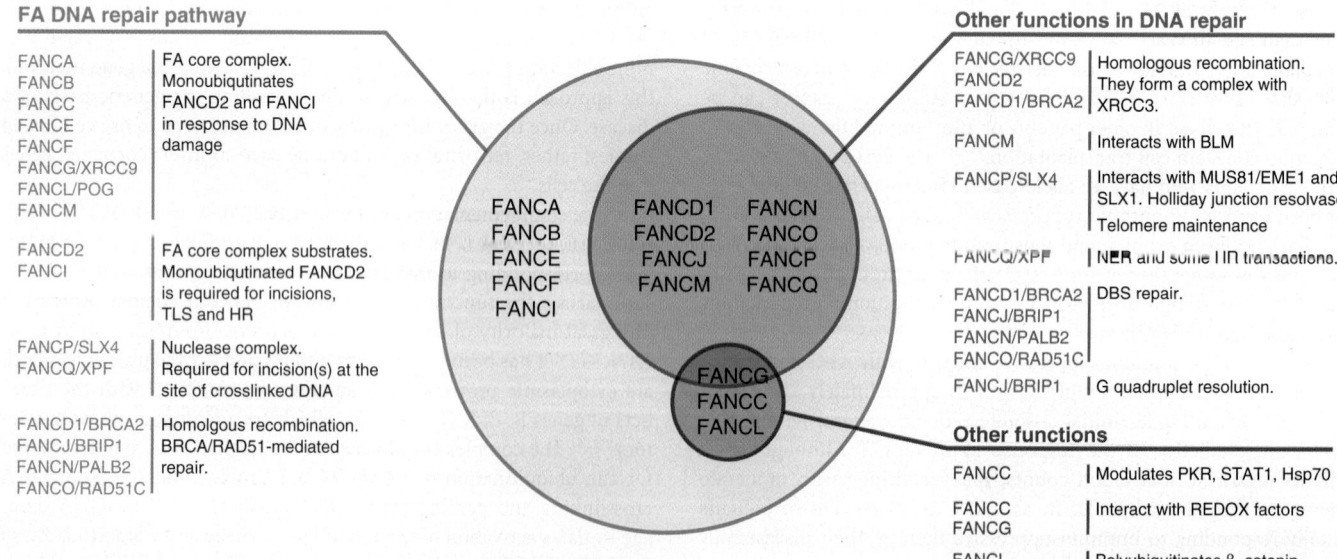

Figure 35–5. Summary of the interactions of the Fanconi Anemia proteins. The primary function of this group of proteins is the repair of crosslinked DNA and to maintain genomic stability (as shown on the *left* side of the figure). The Fanconi anemia DNA repair pathway includes a core complex for monoubiquitination of other components (substrates, FANCD2 and FANCI), as well as a nuclease complex and a complex for homologous recombination DNA repair. A number of these Fanconi anemia proteins also participate in other DNA repair functions such as telomere maintenance and interaction with redox proteins as shown in the *right* side of the figure. (*Reproduced with permission from Garaycoechea JI and Patel KJ Why does the bone marrow fail in Fanconi Anemia? Blood 123(1):26–34, 2014.*)

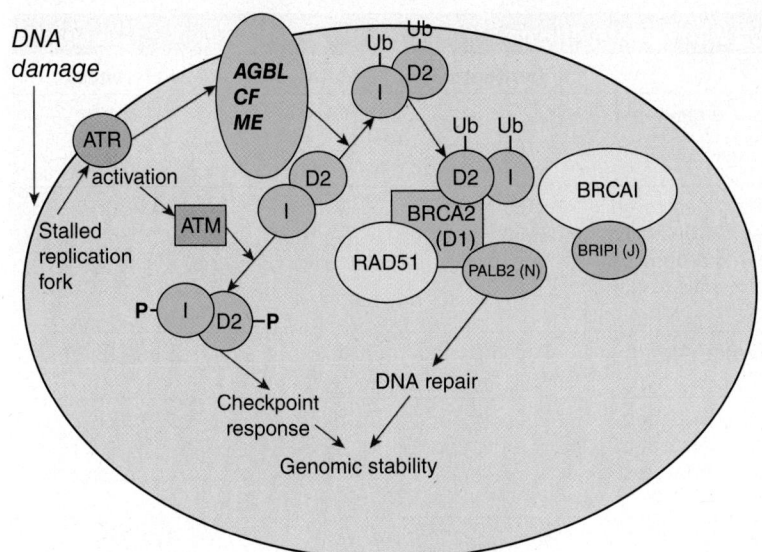

Figure 35–6. Representation of the "FA/BRCA pathway." Following DNA damage when a replication fork encounters a DNA crosslink, ATR (ataxia telangiectasia and rad3-related protein) is activated. This leads to the activation of the Fanconi anemia (FA) pathway, as well as cell-cycle checkpoint activation via the ATM (ataxia telangiectasia mutated) protein. Activation of the FA pathway leads to the formation of the "FA core complex" (consisting of the FA proteins A, B, C, E, F, G, L, and M). This activated FA core complex leads to the monoubiquitination of FANCD2 (FANCD2-Ub) and FANCI (I-Ub). The I-Ub/FANCD2-Ub complex is then targeted to the chromatin containing the crosslink where it interacts with BRCA2 and possibly other DNA repair proteins (e.g., RAD51, J, N) leading to the repair of the DNA damage. Proteins mutated in the different FA subtypes are shown in *yellow. (Reproduced with permission from Dokal I, Vulliamy T: Inherited aplastic anaemias/bone marrow failure syndromes. Blood Rev 22(3):141–153, 2008.)*

Clinical Features

Growth retardation, resulting in short stature, and skeletal anomalies are common. Absent, misshapen, or supernumerary thumbs and dysplastic radii occur in half the patients. Hip and vertebral abnormalities also may occur. Septal heart defects, eye abnormalities, and absent, misshapen, or fused kidneys may be present. Females may have aplasia of the uterus and vagina, absent ovaries, infertility and late menarche and early menopause and males may have hypospermia. Thus, hypogonadism may be evident. Learning disability is frequent, and microcephaly and mental retardation may be a feature. The skin may be generally hyperpigmented or may have areas of abnormal skin pigmentation referred to as *café-au-lait* spots, which are flat, light brown, and from 1 to 12 centimeters in diameter. Hepatosplenomegaly is not a feature of the disease. Some patients have no or minor phenotypic abnormalities and may be diagnosed as a result of the onset of marrow failure or a cancer involving any of many sites as late as the fifth decade of life.

The onset of marrow failure is gradual and usually is evident during the last half of the first decade of life. The manifestations of anemia, including weakness, fatigue, and dyspnea on exertion, and of thrombocytopenia with epistaxis, purpura, or other unexpected bleeding, are the principal findings. Hematologic and visceral manifestations are combined eventually in more than a third of patients, but some may have cytopenias and inconspicuous somatic changes, whereas others may have somatic anomalies with no or a nominal disorder of blood cell formation for months or years. Some who carry the gene may be virtually unaffected.[259–261] In a review of the more than 1300 patients in the literature, 100 patients, or fewer than 7 percent, without anomalies were identified by chromosome breakage studies (see "Laboratory Features" below) because of affected siblings.[227] In the past, children in Fanconi families with an onset of aplastic anemia without congenital somatic abnormalities were thought to have a different disorder termed *Estren-Dameshek syndrome*.[262] However, these children, whose lymphocytes show sensitivity to diepoxybutane, are considered to have Fanconi anemia without skeletal abnormalities.

Laboratory Features

Blood counts and marrow cellularity are often normal until 5 to 10 years of age, when pancytopenia develops over an extended interval. Macrocytosis with anisocytosis and poikilocytosis may be present before any cytopenia occurs. Thrombocytopenia may precede the development of granulocytopenia and anemia. The marrow becomes hypocellular, and *in vitro* colony assays reveal a decrease in CFU-GM and BFU-E.[261]

Random chromatid breaks are present in myeloid cells, lymphocytes, and chorionic villus biopsy samples. This chromosome damage is intensified after exposure to DNA crosslinking agents such as mitomycin C or diepoxybutane. The hypersensitivity of the chromosomes of marrow cells or lymphocytes to the latter agent is used as a diagnostic test for this condition. Cell-cycle progression is prolonged at the G2-to-M transition, and the cells are more susceptible to oxygen toxicity when cultured *in vitro*. It is important to test the lymphocytes from pediatric patients with aplastic anemia for sensitivity to diepoxybutane, because therapy for Fanconi anemia differs from that used for acquired aplastic anemia.

In the near future, clinical laboratories will be able to genotype suspected patients. Determining the specific gene mutation responsible in a patient (see Table 35–8) is important because it confirms the diagnosis, identifies the genotype linked to BRCA2 that may predispose to a cancer (e.g., breast, ovary), and permits carrier detection.[263]

Differential Diagnosis

The differential diagnosis of Fanconi anemia includes other causes of aplastic anemia, particularly those familial syndromes associated with skeletal anomalies and other dysmorphic features. Other familial types of aplastic anemia have been reported with or without associated anomalies. In those instances in which no sensitivity to DNA damaging agents is observed, the syndrome does not represent Fanconi anemia. Several uncommon syndromes of this type are described below and are tabulated in Table 35–9.

Therapy and Course

Most patients with Fanconi anemia do not respond to ATG or cyclosporine but do improve with androgen preparations, often for as long as several years. Cytokines may provide some improvement in blood counts, but their effect may wane. Studies in a mouse model also suggest that cytokine effects may not be sustained.[264] The cumulative median survival is approximately 20 years from progressive marrow failure, conversion to myelodysplastic syndrome, AML (approximately 10 percent of patients), or the development of a variety of other cancers, such as those involving the genitourinary system, digestive system (especially liver), or head and neck.[265] Multiple cancers in an individual patient

TABLE 35–9. Other Rare Inherited Syndromes Associated with Aplastic Anemia

Disorder	Findings	Inheritance	Mutated Gene	References
Ataxia-pancytopenia (myelocerebellar disorder)	Cerebellar atrophy and ataxia; aplastic pancytopenia; ± monosomy 7; increased risk of AML	AD	Unknown	315–317
Congenital amegakaryocytic thrombocytopenia	Thrombocytopenia; absent or markedly decreased marrow megakaryocytes; hemorrhagic propensity; elevated thrombopoietin; propensity to progress to aplastic pancytopenia; propensity to evolve to clonal myeloid disease	AR (compound heterozygotes)	MPL	305–307
DNA ligase IV deficiency	Pre- and postnatal growth delay; dysmorphic facies; aplastic pancytopenia	AR (compound heterozygotes)	LIG4	314, 318, 319
Dubowitz syndrome	Intrauterine and postpartum growth failure; short stature; microcephaly; mental retardation; distinct dysmorphic facies; aplastic pancytopenia; increased risk of AML and ALL	AR	Unknown	320, 321
Nijmegen breakage syndrome	Microcephaly; dystrophic facies; short stature; immunodeficiency; radiation sensitivity; aplastic pancytopenia; predisposition to lymphoid malignancy	AR	NBS1	322, 323
Reticular dysgenesis (type of severe immunodeficiency syndrome)	Lymphopenia; anemia and neutropenia; corrected by hematopoietic stem cell transplantation	XLR	Unknown	308, 309
Seckel syndrome	Intrauterine and post-partum growth failure; microcephaly; characteristic dysmorphic facies (bird-headed profile); aplastic pancytopenia; ? increased risk of AML	AR	ATR (and RAD3-related gene); PCNT	310–314
WT syndrome	Radial/ulnar abnormalities; aplastic pancytopenia; increased risk of AML	AD	Unknown	324

AD, autosomal dominant; ALL, acute lymphocytic leukemia; AML, acute myelogenous leukemia; AR, autosomal recessive; XLR, X-linked recessive.

NOTE: The listed clinical findings in each syndrome are not comprehensive. The designated clinical findings may not be present in all cases of the syndrome. Isolated cases of familial aplastic anemia with or without associated anomalies that are not consistent with Fanconi anemia or other defined syndromes have been reported.[227]

also occur. Cancers may occur as late as the fifth decade of life and precede the diagnosis of Fanconi anemia in 25 percent of patients.[265] The presence of a clonal cytogenetic abnormality or marrow morphology consistent with myelodysplasia markedly reduces the 5-year survival.[232] Allogeneic hematopoietic stem cell transplantation is curative for the marrow manifestations of Fanconi anemia.[266–269] A marked reduction in dosage of the marrow-conditioning regimen of cyclophosphamide and radiation is necessary owing to the undue sensitivity of the tissues to DNA-damaging exposures. The risk of cancer is so high that, where practical, surveillance should be used; for example, frequent pelvic exams in females, hepatic ultrasonography to detect adenomas, and careful oropharyngeal examinations. Therapy of cancer in patients with Fanconi anemia needs to consider the marked sensitivity of their cells to DNA cross-linking agents and radiotherapy.

Normal complementary DNA has been transferred into cells from patients with restoration of resistance to DNA damaging agents.[270,271] Difficulties in this approach include the paucity of stem cells in these patients, as well as the potential toxicity of the gene transfer methodology.

DYSKERATOSIS CONGENITA

Definition

This inherited disorder is characterized by cutaneous and mucous membrane abnormalities, progressive marrow insufficiency, and a predisposition to malignant transformation. It is much more common in

males than in females, and occurs in approximately 1 per 1,000,000 population.[251,272]

Pathogenesis

Dyskeratosis usually is inherited as a recessive X-chromosome–linked disorder although rare cases can have autosomal dominant or autosomal recessive inheritance (Table 35–10). The disease is a reflection of telomere complex dysfunction,[273–276] and it results from defective telomerase activity resulting from mutations in the telomerase-related genes (Fig. 35–7).[274,278,279] The telomerase complex maintains the length of telomeres, which are nucleotide tandem repeat structures residing at the termini of eukaryotic chromosomes (e.g., 5'-TTAGGG-3'). Telomerase restores the guanine (G)-rich telomere repeats that are lost as a result of end-processing during normal cell division. Combined with protein, located at the ends of chromosomes, they maintain chromosome integrity by preventing end-to-end chromosome fusion, preventing chromosome degradation, and preventing chromosome instability. In dyskeratosis congenita, the telomeres are markedly shortened resulting in genomic instability and cell (including marrow cell) apoptosis, and the underlying gene defects may alter Box H/ACA small nucleolar RNAs, such as the telomerase RNA component, TERC, that is central to telomere maintenance.[279a] Rapidly proliferating cells are at highest risk for dysfunction. Mutations of the DKC1 gene are responsible for the X-linked recessive form. DKC1 encodes dyskerin, which is a conserved multifunctional protein component of the telomerase complex. Mutations of the TERT, TERC, and TINF2 genes are the

TABLE 35–10. Gene Mutations in Dyskeratosis Congenita

Gene	Chromosome Location	% of Patients	Inheritance	Protein Function
DKC1	Xq28	30	XLR	Essential part of snoRNPs and telomerase
TERC	3q26	5–10	AD	RNA 3′ end processing and stability
TERT	5p15.33	5–10	AD, AR	Reverse transcriptase component of telomerase
NOP10 (NOLA3)	15q14-q15	<1	AR	RNA binding
TINF2	14q11.2	15	AD	? Binds to TRF1 to regulate telomere length
CTC1	17p13.1	Rare	AR	Telomere maintenance component
NHP2 (NOLA2)	5q35.3	<1	AR	RNA binding protein; associates with NOP10 and *DKC1*
WRAP53 (TCAB1, WDR79)	17p13.1	Rare	AR	Trafficking of telomerase
RTEL1 (NHL)	20q13.33	Rare	AD, AR	Regulator of telomere elongation helicase 1
C16orF57 (USB1)	16q21	2	AR	Unknown; Patient telomeres were normal length
hTR	3q	5–10	AD	hTR is the RNA component of telomerase

AD, autosomal dominant; AR, autosomal recessive; XLR, X-linked recessive.

NOTE: Table prepared from data in references 251, 254, 273, 276 to 279 and OMIM (Online Mendelian Inheritance in Man). Percent of patients is approximate because of continuing identification of mutations.

principal abnormalities in the autosomal dominant form. TERC is the RNA component of the telomerase reverse transcriptase that TERT, the reverse transcriptase, uses to synthesize the 6-bp repeats on the 3′ end of telomeric DNA. Mutations of *TINF2* have been described in patients with dyskeratosis congenital.[280] *TINF2* is a component of the shelterin complex, which prevents end-to-end telomere fusion.[280] It also permits the distinction of telomeres from sites of DNA damage, preventing their inappropriate processing. Recessive mutations in *NHP2* and in *NOP10*, which encode parts of small ribonucleoprotein components associated with the telomerase complex, also have been described in association with dyskeratosis.[281,282] Homozygous recessive mutations in the *TERT* gene produce a severe variant of dyskeratosis, referred to as the Hoyeraal-Hreidarsson syndrome.[272]

Clinical Findings

The cutaneous findings usually appear after 5 years of age and include reticulated, tan to gray, hyperpigmented and hypopigmented cutaneous macules; alopecia of scalp, eyelashes, and eyebrows; adermatoglyphia

(loss of dermal ridges on fingers and toes); hyperkeratosis of palms and soles; mucosal leukoplakia in 75 percent of patients; and dystrophic nails in more than 85 percent of patients.[251,272,273] Other mucosal sites, such as conjunctiva, lacrimal duct, esophagus, urethra, vagina, and anus, can be involved, sometimes with stenosis leading to dysphagia or dysuria. Pulmonary vascular involvement occurs in a significant minority of affected children. Aplastic anemia usually develops in late childhood or early adulthood and is evident in the classical blood and marrow findings described under acquired aplastic anemia. Female carriers of X-linked dyskeratosis congenital may have slight abnormalities such as a dystrophic nail, a single area of hypopigmentation, or slight leukoplakia.[272] The clinical manifestations exhibit disease anticipation, occurring earlier in subsequent generations, and this appears related to earlier shortening of the telomeres.[283]

Diagnosis

The diagnosis results from the combination of phenotypic findings and blood cell deficiencies. Genetic analysis for telomerase complex gene

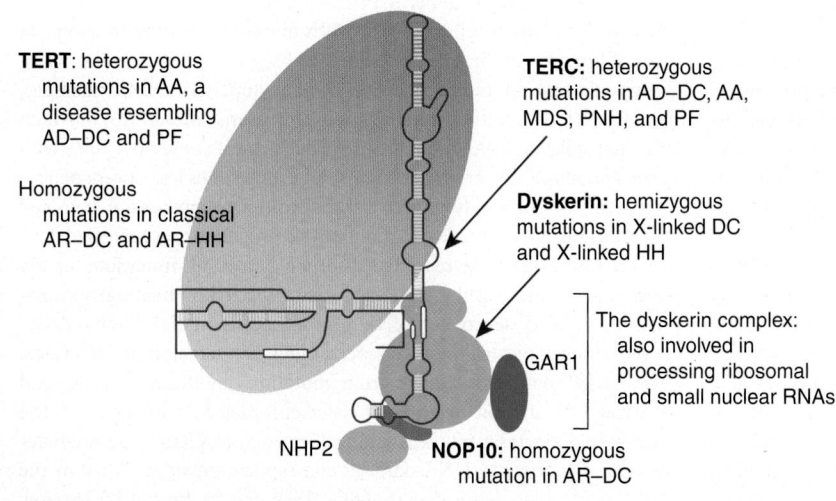

TERT: heterozygous mutations in AA, a disease resembling AD–DC and PF

Homozygous mutations in classical AR–DC and AR–HH

TERC: heterozygous mutations in AD–DC, AA, MDS, PNH, and PF

Dyskerin: hemizygous mutations in X-linked DC and X-linked HH

The dyskerin complex: also involved in processing ribosomal and small nuclear RNAs

GAR1

NHP2 **NOP10:** homozygous mutation in AR–DC

Figure 35–7. Representation of the interaction between dyskerin and the other molecules (GAR1, NHP2, NOP10, TERC, and TERT) of the telomerase complex (and their association with different disease categories). Telomerase is an RNA-protein complex because TERC is an RNA molecule that is never translated. The other molecules (dyskerin, GAR1, NHP2, NOP10, and TERT) are proteins. The minimal active telomerase enzyme is composed of two molecules each of TERT, TERC, and dyskerin. Dyskerin, GAR1, NHP2, and NOP10 are important for the stability of the telomerase complex. AA, aplastic anemia; AD–DC, autosomal dominant dyskeratosis congenita; AR–DC, autosomal recessive dyskeratosis congenita; AR–HH, autosomal recessive Hoyeraal-Hreidarsson syndrome; MDS, myelodysplasia; PF, pulmonary fibrosis; PNH, paroxysmal nocturnal hemoglobinuria; X-linked DC, X-linked dyskeratosis congenita; X-linked HH, X-linked Hoyeraal-Hreidarsson syndrome. *(Reproduced with permission from Dokal I, Vulliamy T: Inherited aplastic anaemias/bone marrow failure syndromes. Blood Rev 22(3):141–153, 2008.)*

mutations should be used to confirm the clinical conclusion. Shortened telomere length in leukocytes also can be assessed by flow cytometric fluorescence in situ hybridization studies.[284]

Management

Stem cell hematopoietic transplantation has had inconsistent results because of frequent and severe posttransplantation complications.[285] Nonmyeloablative transplantation might improve results.[286–288] Transplantation might improve the cytopenias, but not the abnormalities of other organs or the frequency of secondary nonhematopoietic cancer.

Course and Prognosis

The incidence of squamous cell carcinoma of mucosal sites is increased and the squamous cell carcinoma often originates in sites of leukoplakia in the skin, gastrointestinal, or genitourinary tracts.[289] These carcinomas usually develop between the ages of 20 and 30 years. Mortality from neutropenic infection or thrombocytopenic hemorrhage occurs in about two-thirds of patients with aplastic anemia. Median survival is approximately 30 years.

SHWACHMAN-DIAMOND SYNDROME

Definition

This disease is an uncommon inherited disorder that is estimated to occur once in every 75,000 births,[290] manifesting exocrine pancreatic insufficiency with secondary steatorrhea, blood cell deficiencies, and skeletal abnormalities. It was first described in 1964.[291,292]

Pathogenesis

Shwachman-Diamond syndrome results from mutations in the *SBDS* gene on chromosome 7q11, which induces accelerated cellular apoptosis via the FAS pathway.[293] The resulting hyperproliferation may account for the abnormal telomere shortening that has been documented in the leukocytes in this condition.[294] The pathogenetic mechanism that (1) prevents development of pancreatic acinar cells, (2) results in abnormal bone morphogenesis, and (3) causes marrow impairment of blood cell production is not understood. *SBDS* knockdown in experimental animals affects expression of genes involved in brain, bone, and marrow development, and may be the result of the gene's role in RNA processing.[295,296] The *SBDS* gene promotes the release of eukaryotic initiation factor 6 from the pre-60s ribosome.[279a] This action is necessary for the formation of a mature 80s functional ribosome and production of appropriate ribosome joining. The mutations in *SBDS* also result in abnormalities in neutrophil motility and chemotaxis, but pus formation *in vivo* seems adequate.

Clinical Findings

Pancreatic insufficiency, steatorrhea, and neutropenia are present in most patients at the time of diagnosis.[291,292,297] Pallor may reflect anemia and easy bruising; epistaxis or bleeding from other sites reflect thrombocytopenia. Neutropenia occurs in approximately 95 percent, anemia in approximately 50 percent, and thrombocytopenia in approximately 35 percent of patients.[293] Thus, a substantial plurality of patients has bicytopenia or tricytopenia with an hypoplastic marrow. Fetal hemoglobin levels are elevated in approximately 75 percent of the patients, perhaps secondary to erythroid hypoplasia. Cytogenetic abnormalities involving chromosomes 7 and 20 have been described in marrow cells. Nutritional inadequacies related to intestinal malabsorption result in a failure to thrive. Short stature is characteristic. Skeletal abnormalities are present in most patients, notably osteopenia, but also syndactyly, supernumerary metatarsals, coax vera deformity, and dental enamel defects and caries. Hepatic dysfunction as evidenced by elevated serum aminotransaminase is seen in most young patients and appears to resolve with age.[298] Delayed puberty is common. The neutropenia and chemotactic abnormality may result in recurrent infections, including sinusitis, otitis, pneumonia, osteomyelitis, and others. Pancreatic cell lipase production improves with age, and as many as half the patients may have improvement in lipid absorption in the small bowel with time.

Diagnosis

The diagnosis is based on the clinical findings of failure to thrive, steatorrhea, and neutropenia. Pancreatic insufficiency can be established by low serum trypsinogen in patients younger than 3 years of age. The marrow may be initially normal, but develops evidence of marrow failure and sometimes cytogenetic abnormalities, particularly of chromosome 7, as the child ages. The age of expression of clonal hematopoiesis (e.g., myelodysplastic syndrome or AML) is variable.[299] The *SBDS* gene mutation is present in 90 percent of patients with Shwachman-Diamond syndrome.[300] The remaining 10 percent have the clinical features of the syndrome, but the gene defects have not been defined.

Management

Supportive care, particularly with supplemental pancreatic enzymes, to provide proper nutrition, and appropriate and prompt treatment of bacterial infections with antibiotics is important. Many agents, including G-CSF, glucocorticoids, pancreatic extract, vitamins, have been tried to improve the neutropenia with unpredictable results. Some agents have potential risks, such as G-CSF fostering clonal evolution and glucocorticoids fostering immunodeficiency. Severe hematopoietic dysfunction and cytopenias can be corrected with allogeneic hematopoietic stem cell transplantation.[301]

Course and Prognosis

Death from overwhelming sepsis is common. These patients, especially males, have a significant risk of progression to a myelodysplastic syndrome or AML.[292,302,303] Cytogenetic abnormalities are common, and telomeres are shortened,[304] as in other marrow failure syndromes. Survival is a function of the severity of the cytopenias. If the cytopenias are mild, survival is not uncommon into the fourth or fifth decade of life. It is not clear whether Shwachman-Diamond syndrome is associated with an increased incidence of solid tumors.

OTHER INHERITED APLASTIC ANEMIAS

Several other rare syndromes are associated with aplastic pancytopenia, and these are described in Table 35–9. Congenital (hereditary) amegakaryocytic thrombocytopenia (CAMT) results from mutations in the TPO receptor gene, *MPL*,[305–307] The affected children can be divided into two groups: CAMT I with mutations leading to complete loss of function of the TPO receptor, resulting in more severe thrombocytopenia and a rapid progression to pancytopenia (aplastic anemia), and CAMT II, resulting from a variety of missense mutations, in which affected children have an increase in platelet count above 50×10^9/L with time and much slower progression to and sometimes less-severe pancytopenia.[306] Reticular dysgenesis results from a pluripotential stem cell defect as both lymphoid and granulocytic progenitors are affected.[308,309] It is a rare autosomal recessive disorder caused by mutations in the adenylate kinase 2 gene (*AK2*) and characterized by bilateral sensorineural deafness, severe combined immunodeficiency, and agranulocytosis, which subjects infants to severe, often, life-threatening infections. The Seckel syndrome results from mutations in the *ATR* gene, and marrow cells exhibit heightened sister chromatid exchange.[310–314] The ataxia-telangiectasia mutated and rad3-related (ATR) kinase mediates cellular responses to DNA damage and replication stress. Most of the eight syndromes delineated in Table 35–9 can be treated by marrow transplantation, but this step, if successful, does not correct somatic abnormalities, only the hematopoietic and immunologic defect. The restoration of robust lymphohematopoiesis by transplantation may decrease their propensity to undergo clonal evolution to a clonal myeloid or, in some cases, lymphoid disorder.

REFERENCES

1. Incidence of aplastic anemia: The relevance of diagnostic criteria. By the International Agranulocytosis and Aplastic Anemia Study. *Blood* 70:1718, 1987.
2. Ehrlich P: Über einen Fall von Anamie mit Bemerkungen über regenerative Veranderungen des Knochenmarks. *Charite Ann* 13:300, 1888.
3. Chauffard M: Un cas d'anémie pernicieuse aplastique. *Bull Soc Med Hop Paris* 21:313, 1904.
4. Scott JL, Cartwright GE, Wintrobe MM: Acquired aplastic anemia: An analysis of thirty-nine cases and review of the pertinent literature. *Medicine (Baltimore)* 38:119, 1959.
5. Thomas ED, Storb R, Fefer A, et al: Aplastic anemia treated by bone marrow transplantation. *Lancet* 1: 284, 1972.
6. Thomas ED, Storb R, Giblett B, et al: Recovery from aplastic anemia following attempted marrow transplantation. *Exp Hematol* 4:97, 1976.
7. Champlin RE, Feig SA, Sparkes RS, Gale RP: Bone marrow transplantation from identical twins in the treatment of aplastic anaemia: Implication for the pathogenesis of the disease. *Br J Haematol* 56:455, 1984.
8. Speck B, Gluckman E: Treatment of aplastic anemia by antilymphocyte globulin with and without allogeneic bone marrow infusions. *Lancet* 2:1145, 1977.
9. Mary JY, Baumelou E, Guiguet M: Epidemiology of aplastic anemia in France: A prospective multicenter study. *Blood* 75:1646, 1990.
10. Montané E, Ibáñez L, Vidal X, et al: Epidemiology of aplastic anemia: A prospective multicenter study. *Haematologica* 93:518, 2008.
11. Maluf EM, Pasquini R, Eluf JN, et al: Aplastic anemia in Brazil: Incidence and risk factors. *Am J Hematol* 71:268, 2002.
12. McCahon E, Tang K, Rogers PC, et al: The impact of Asian descent on the incidence of acquired severe aplastic anaemia in children. *Br J Haematol* 121:170, 2003.
13. Chongli Y, Ziaobo Z: Incidence survey of aplastic anemia in China. *Chin Med Sci J* 6:203, 1991.
14. Issaragrisil S: Epidemiology of aplastic anemia in Thailand. Thai Aplastic Anemia Study Group. *Int J Hematol* 70:137, 1999.
15. Yong AS, Goh AS, Rahman M, et al: Epidemiology of aplastic anemia in the state of Sabah, Malaysia. *Med J Malaysia* 53:59, 1998.
16. Issaragrisil S, Kaufman DW, Anderson T, et al: The epidemiology of aplastic anemia in Thailand. *Blood* 107:1299, 2006.
17. Young NS, Kaufman DW: The epidemiology of acquired aplastic anemia. *Haematologica* 93:489, 2008.
18. Yin SN, Hayes RB, Linet MS, et al: A cohort study of cancer among benzene-exposed workers in China: Overall results. *Am J Ind Med* 29:227, 1996.
19. Locasciulli A, Bacigalupo A, Bruno B, et al: Hepatitis-associated aplastic anaemia: Epidemiology and treatment results obtained in Europe. A report of The EBMT aplastic anaemia working party. Br J Haematol 149:890, 2010.
20. Kagan WA, Ascensao J, Pahwa R, et al: Aplastic anemia: Presence in human bone marrow of cells that suppress myelopoiesis. *Proc Natl Acad Sci U S A* 73:2890, 1976.
21. Maciejewski JP, Anderson S, Katevas P, Young NS: Phenotypic and functional analysis of bone marrow progenitor cell compartment in bone marrow failure. *Br J Haematol* 87:227, 1994.
22. Scopes J, Bagnara M, Gordon-Smith EC, et al: Haemopoietic progenitor cells are reduced in aplastic anaemia. *Br J Haematol* 86:427, 1994.
23. Maciejewski JP, Selleri C, Sato T, et al: A severe and consistent deficit in marrow and circulating primitive hematopoietic cells (long-term culture-initiating cells) in acquired aplastic anemia. *Blood* 88:1983, 1996.
24. Young NS, Scheinberg P, Calado RT: Aplastic anemia. *Curr Opin Hematol* 15:162, 2008.
25. Sugimori C, Yamazaki H, Feng X, et al: Roles of DRB1 *1501 and DRB1 *1502 in the pathogenesis of aplastic anemia. *Exp Hematol* 35:13, 2007.
26. Young NS, Calado RT, Scheinberg P: Why does the bone marrow fail in Fanconi anemia? *Blood* 108:2509, 2006.
27. Young NS, Maciejewski J: Mechanisms of disease: The pathophysiology of acquired aplastic anemia. *N Engl J Med* 336:1365, 1997.
28. Laver J, Castro-Malaspina H, Kernan NA, et al: In vitro interferon-gamma production by cultured T-cells in severe aplastic anaemia: Correlation with granulomonopoietic inhibition in patients who respond to anti-thymocyte globulin. *Br J Haematol* 69:545, 1988.
29. Gascon P, Zoumbos NC, Scala G, et al: Lymphokine abnormalities in aplastic anemia: Implications for the mechanism of action of antithymocyte globulin. *Blood* 65:407, 1985.
30. Hinterberger W, Adolf G, Bettelheim P, et al: Lymphokine overproduction in severe aplastic anemia is not related to blood transfusions. *Blood* 74:2713, 1989.
31. Shinohara K, Ayame H, Tanaka M, et al: Increased production of tumor necrosis factor alpha by peripheral blood mononuclear cells in the patients with aplastic anemia. *Am J Hematol* 37:75, 1991.
32. Nistico, A, Young, NS: Gamma-interferon gene expression in the bone marrow of patients with aplastic anemia. *Ann Intern Med* 120:463, 1994.
33. Zoumbos N, Gascon P, Djeu J, Young NS: Interferon is a mediator of hematopoietic suppression in aplastic anemia in vitro and possibly in vivo. *Proc Natl Acad Sci U S A* 82:188, 1985.
34. Sloand E, Kim S, Maciejewski JP, et al: Intracellular interferon-gamma in circulating and marrow T cells detected by flow cytometry and the response to immunosuppressive therapy in patients with aplastic anemia. *Blood* 100:1185, 2002.
35. Solomou EE, Keyvanfar K, Young NS: T-bet, a Th1 transcription factor, is up-regulated in T cells from patients with aplastic anemia. *Blood* 107:3983, 2006.
36. Risitano AM, Maciejewski JP, Green S, et al: In vivo dominant immune responses in aplastic anaemia: Molecular tracking of putatively pathogenetic T-cell clones by TCR beta-CDR3 sequencing. *Lancet* 364:355, 2004.
37. Solomou EE, Rezvani K, Mielke S, et al: Deficient CD4+ CD25+ FOXP3+ T regulatory cells in acquired aplastic anemia. *Blood* 110:1603, 2007.
38. Fujisaki J, Wu J, Carlson AL, et al: In vivo imaging of Treg cells providing immune privilege to the haematopoietic stem-cell niche. *Nature* 474:216, 2011.
39. Chen J, Ellison FM, Eckhaus MA, et al: Minor antigen h60-mediated aplastic anemia is ameliorated by immunosuppression and the infusion of regulatory T cells. *J Immunol* 178:4159, 2007.
40. Hirano N, Butler MO, Von Bergwelt-Baildon MS, et al: Autoantibodies frequently detected in patients with aplastic anemia. *Blood* 102:4567, 2003.
41. Young, NS: Current concepts in the pathophysiology and treatment of aplastic anemia. *Hematology Am Soc Hematol Educ Program* 2013:76, 2013.
41a. Townsley DM, Dumitriu B, Young NS. Bone marrow failure and the telomeropathies. *Blood* 124:2775, 2014.
42. Smick K, Condit PK, Proctor RL, Sutcher V: Fatal aplastic anemia: An epidemiological study of its relationship to the drug chloramphenicol. *J Chronic Dis* 17:899, 1964.
43. Modan B, Segal S, Shani M, Sheba C: Aplastic anemia in Israel: Evaluation of the etiological role of chloramphenicol on a community-wide basis. *Am J Med Sci* 270:441, 1975.
44. Yunis AA Chloramphenicol toxicity: 25 years of research. *Am J Med* 87:44N, 1989.
45. Custer RP: Aplastic anemia in soldiers treated with Atabrine (quinacrine). *Am J Med Sci* 212:211, 1946.
46. Best WR: Drug-associated blood dyscrasias. *JAMA* 185:286, 1963.
47. Risks of agranulocytosis and aplastic anemia. A first report of their relation to drug use with special reference to analgesics. The International Agranulocytosis and Aplastic Anemia Study. *JAMA* 256:1749, 1986.
48. Retsagi G, Kelly JP, Kaufman DW: Risk of agranulocytosis and aplastic anaemia in relation to use of antithyroid drugs. International Agranulocytosis and Aplastic Anaemia Study. *BMJ* 297:262, 1988.
49. Anti-infective drug use in relation to the risk of agranulocytosis and aplastic anemia. A report from the International Agranulocytosis and Aplastic Anemia Study. *Arch Intern Med* 149:1036, 1989.
50. Kelly JP, Kaufman DW, Shapiro S: Risks of agranulocytosis and aplastic anemia in relation to the use of cardiovascular drugs: The International Agranulocytosis and Aplastic Anemia Study. *Clin Pharmacol Ther* 49:330, 1991.
51. Kaufmann DW, Kelly JP, Jurgelon JM, et al: Drugs in the aetiology of agranulocytosis and aplastic anaemia. *Eur J Haematol* 57(Suppl):23, 1996.
52. Baumelou E, Guiguet M, Mary JY, et al: Epidemiology of aplastic anemia in France: A case control study. I. Medical history and medication use. *Blood* 81:1471, 1993.
53. Bithell TC, Wintrobe MM: Drug-induced aplastic anemia. *Semin Hematol* 4:194, 1967.
54. Williams DM, Lynch RE, Cartwright GE: Drug-induced aplastic anemia. *Semin Hematol* 10:195, 1973.
55. Tonkonow B, Hoffman R: Aplastic anemia and cimetidine. *Arch Intern Med* 140:1123, 1980.
56. Volkin RL, Shadduck RK, Winkelstein A, et al: Potentiation of carmustine-cranial-irradiation-induced myelosuppression by cimetidine. *Arch Intern Med* 142:243, 1982.
57. Khan HA: Benzene toxicity: A consolidated short review of human and animal studies. *Hum Exp Toxicol* 26:677, 2007.
58. Smith MT: Overview of benzene-induced aplastic anemia. *Eur J Haematol* 60:107, 1996.
59. Snyder R: Benzene and leukemia. *Crit Rev Toxicol* 32:155, 2002.
60. Fleming LE, Timmeny MA: Aplastic anemia and pesticides. An etiologic association? *J Occup Med* 35:1106, 1993.
61. Rugman FP, Cosstick R: Aplastic anaemia associated with organochlorine pesticide: Case reports and review of evidence. *J Clin Pathol* 43:98, 1990.
62. Muir KR, Chilvers CE, Harriss C, et al: The role of occupational and environmental exposures in the aetiology of acquired severe aplastic anaemia: A case control investigation. *Br J Haematol* 123:906, 2003.
63. Valdez Salas B, Garcia Duran EI, Wiener MS: Impact of pesticides use on human health in Mexico: A review. *Rev Environ Health* 15:399, 2000.
64. Ahamed M, Anand M, Kumar A, Siddiqui MK: Childhood aplastic anaemia in Lucknow, India: Incidence, organochlorines in the blood and review of case reports following exposure to pesticides. *Clin Biochem* 39:762, 2006.
65. Rauch AE, Kowalsky SF, Lesar TS, et al: Lindane (Kwell)-induced aplastic anemia. *Arch Intern Med* 150:2393, 1990.
66. Roberts HJ: Pentachlorophenol-associated aplastic anemia, red cell aplasia, leukemia and other blood disorders. *J Fla Med Assoc* 77:86, 1990.
67. Prager D, Peters C: Development of aplastic anemia and the exposure to Stoddard solvent. *Blood* 35:286, 1970.

68. Powers D: Aplastic anemia secondary to glue sniffing. *N Engl J Med* 273:700, 1965.

69. Kirtadze I, Zurabashvili D: Study of chemical composition of glue "RAZI" used by solvent abusers in Tbilisi. *Georgian Med News* 133:65, 2006.

70. Sabbioni G, Sepai O, Norppa H, et al: Comparison of biomarkers in workers exposed to 2,4,6-trinitrotoluene. *Biomarkers* 12:21, 2007.

71. Crawford MAD: Aplastic anaemia due to trinitrotoluene intoxication. *Br Med J* 2:430, 1954.

72. Ajlouni K, Doeblin TD: The syndrome of hepatitis and aplastic anaemia. *Br J Haematol* 27:345, 1974.

73. Hagler L, Pastore RA, Bergin JJ: Aplastic anemia following viral hepatitis: Report of 2 fatal cases and literature review. *Medicine (Baltimore)* 54:139, 1975.

74. Pol S, Driss F, Devergie A, et al: Is hepatitis C virus involved in hepatitis-associated aplastic anemia? *Ann Intern Med* 113:435, 1990.

75. Hibbs JR, Frickhofen N, Rosenfeld SJ, et al: Aplastic anemia and viral hepatitis: Non-A, non-B, non-C? *JAMA* 267:2051, 1992.

76. Honkaniemi E, Gustafsson B, Fischler B, et al: Acquired aplastic anaemia in seven children with severe hepatitis with or without liver failure. *Acta Paediatr* 96:1660, 2007.

77. Tzakis AG, Arditi M, Whitington PF, et al: Aplastic anemia complicating orthotopic liver transplantation for non-A, non-B hepatitis. *N Engl J Med* 319:393, 1988.

78. Brown KE, Tisdale J, Barrett AJ, Dunbar CE, Young NS: Hepatitis-associated aplastic anemia. *N Engl J Med* 336:1059, 1997.

79. Safadi R, Or R, Ilan Y, et al: Lack of known hepatitis virus in hepatitis-associated aplastic anemia and outcome after bone marrow transplantation. *Bone Marrow Transplant* 27:183, 2001.

80. Mishra B, Malhotra P, Ratho RK, et al: Human parvovirus B19 in patients with aplastic anemia. *Am J Hematol* 79:166, 2005.

81. Yetgin S, Cetin M, Ozyürek E, et al: Parvovirus B19 infection associated with severe aplastic anemia in an immunocompetent patient. *Pediatr Hematol Oncol* 21:223, 2004.

82. Wong S, Young NS, Brown KE: Prevalence of parvovirus B19 in liver tissue: No association with fulminant hepatitis or hepatitis-associated aplastic anemia. *J Infect Dis* 187:1581, 2003.

83. Locasciulli A, Bacigalupo A, Bruno B, et al: Hepatitis-associated aplastic anaemia: Epidemiology and treatment results obtained in Europe. A report of The EBMT aplastic anaemia working party. *Br J Haematol* 149:890, 2010.

84. Rauff B, Idrees M, Shah SAR, et al: Hepatitis associated aplastic anemia: A review. *Virol J* 8: 87, 2011.

85. Lazarus KH, Baehner RL: Aplastic anemia complicating infectious mononucleosis: A case report and review of the literature. *Pediatrics* 67:907, 1981.

86. Baranski B, Armstrong G, Truman JT, et al: Epstein-Barr virus in the bone marrow of patients with aplastic anemia. *Ann Intern Med* 109:695, 1988.

87. Vinters HV, Mah V, Mohrmann R, Wiley CA: Evidence for human immunodeficiency virus (HIV) infection of the brain in a patient with aplastic anemia. *Acta Neuropathol* 76:311, 1988.

88. Samuel D, Castaing D, Adam R, et al: Fatal acute HIV infection with aplastic anaemia, transmitted by liver graft. *Lancet* 1:1221, 1988.

89. Morales CE, Sriram I, Baumann MA: Myelodysplastic syndrome occurring as possible first manifestation of human immunodeficiency virus infection with subsequent progression to aplastic anaemia. *Int J STD AIDS* 1:55, 1990.

90. Rosenfeld CS, Rybka WB, Weinbaum D, et al: Late graft failure due to dual bone marrow infection with variants A and B of human Herpesvirus-6. *Exp Hematol* 23:626, 1995.

91. Pavithran K, Raji NL, Thomas M: Aplastic anemia complicating lupus erythematosus—Report of a case and review of the literature. *Rheumatol Int* 22:253, 2002.

92. Bailey FA, Lilly M, Bertoli LF, Ball GV: An antibody that inhibits in vitro bone marrow proliferation in a patient with systemic lupus erythematosus and aplastic anemia. *Arthritis Rheum* 31:901, 1989.

93. Roffe C, Cahill MR, Samanta A, et al: Aplastic anaemia in systemic lupus erythematosus: A cellular immune mechanism? *Br J Rheumatol* 30:301, 1991.

94. Sumimoto S, Kawai M, Kasajima Y, Hamamoto T: Aplastic anemia associated with systemic lupus erythematosus. *Am J Hematol* 38:329, 1991.

95. Winkler A, Jackson RW, Kay DS, et al: High-dose intravenous cyclophosphamide treatment of systemic lupus erythematosus-associated aplastic anemia [letter]. *Arthritis Rheum* 31:693, 1988.

96. Kim SW, Rice L, Champlin R, Udden MM: Aplastic Anemia in eosinophilic fasciitis: Responses to immunosuppression and marrow transplantation. *Haematologica* 28:131, 1997.

97. Debusscher L, Bitar N, DeMaubeuge J, et al: Eosinophilic fasciitis and severe aplastic anemia: Favorable response to either antithymocyte globulin or cyclosporin A in blood and skin disorders. *Transplant Proc* 20:310, 1988.

98. Kumar M, Goldman J: Severe aplastic anemia and Grave's disease in a paediatric patient. *Br J Haematol* 118:327, 2002.

99. Tomonari A, Tojo A, Iseki T, et al: Severe aplastic anemia with autoimmune thyroiditis showing no hematological response to intensive immunosuppressive therapy. *Acta Haematol* 109:90, 2003.

100. Aydin Y, Berker D, Üstün I, et al: A very rare cause of aplastic anemia: Graves disease. *South Med J* 101:666, 2008.

101. Lima CS, Zantut Wittmann DE, Castro V, et al: Pancytopenia in untreated patients with Graves' disease. *Thyroid* 16:403, 2006.

102. Das PK, Wherrett D, Dror Y: Remission of aplastic anemia induced by treatment for Graves disease in a pediatric patient. *Pediatr Blood Cancer* 49:210, 2007.

103. Dincol G, Saka B, Aktan M, et al: Very severe aplastic anemia following resection of lymphocytic thymoma: Effectiveness of antilymphocyte globulin, cyclosporine A and granulocyte-colony stimulating factor. *Am J Hematol* 64:78, 2000.

104. Ritchie DS, Underhill C, Grigg AP. Aplastic anemia as a late complication of thymoma in remission. *Eur J Haematol* 68:389, 2002.

105. Gaglia A, Bobota A, Pectasides E, et al: Successful treatment with cyclosporine of thymoma-related aplastic anemia. *Anticancer Res* 27:3025, 2007.

106. Trisal V, Nademanee A, Lau SK, Grannis FW Jr: Thymoma-associated severe aplastic anemia treated with surgical resection followed by allogeneic stem-cell transplantation. *J Clin Oncol* 25:3374, 2007.

107. Arcasoy MO, Gockerman JP: Aplastic anaemia as an autoimmune complication of thymoma. *Br J Haematol* 137:272, 2007.

108. Park CY, Kim HJ, Kim YJ, et al: Very severe aplastic anemia appearing after thymectomy. *Korean J Intern Med* 18:61, 2003.

109. Abrams EM, Gibson IW, Blydt-Hansen TD: The concurrent presentation of minimal change nephrotic syndrome and aplastic anemia. *Pediatr Nephrol* 24:407, 2009.

110. Aitchison RGM, Marsh JCW, Hows JM, et al: Pregnancy associated aplastic anaemia: A report of 5 cases and review of current management. *Br J Haematol* 73:541, 1989.

111. Pajor A, Kelemen E, Szak'acs Z, Lehoczky D: Pregnancy in idiopathic aplastic anemia (report of 10 patients). *Eur J Obstet Gynecol Reprod Biol* 45:19, 1992.

112. Bourantas K, Makrydimas G, Georgiou I, et al: Aplastic anemia: Report of a case with recurrent episodes in consecutive pregnancies. *J Reprod Med* 42:672, 1997.

113. Kwon JY, Lee Y, Shin JC, et al: Supportive management of pregnancy-associated aplastic anemia. *Int J Gynaecol Obstet* 95:115, 2006.

114. Thakral B, Saluja K, Sharma RR, et al: Successful management of pregnancy-associated severe aplastic anemia. *Eur J Obstet Gynecol Reprod Biol* 131:244, 2007.

115. Tichelli A, Socie G, Marsh J, et al: Outcome of pregnancy and disease course among women with aplastic anemia treated with immunosuppression. *Ann Intern Med* 137:164, 2002.

116. Court-Brown WM, Doll R: Leukaemia and aplastic anaemia in patients irradiated for ankylosing spondylitis. 1957. *J Radiol Prot* 27:B15-B154, 2007.

117. Darby SC, Doll R, Gill SK, Smith PG: Long term mortality after a single treatment course with x-rays in patients treated with ankylosing spondylitis. *Br J Cancer* 55:179, 1987.

118. Johnson SAN, Bateman CJT, Beard MEJ, et al: Long-term haematological complications of Thorotrast. *Q J Med* 182:259, 1977.

119. Martland HS: The occurrence of malignancy in radioactive persons: A general review of data gathered in the study of the radium dial painters, with special reference to the occurrence of osteogeneic sarcoma and the inter-relationship of certain blood diseases. *Am J Cancer* 15:2435, 1931.

120. Cronkite EP, Haley TJ: Clinical aspects of acute radiation injury, in *Manual on Radiation Haematology*, pp 169–173. International Atomic Energy Agency, Vienna, 1971.

121. Mettler FA Jr, Moseley RD Jr: *Medical Effects of Ionizing Irradiation*, pp 1–185. Grune and Stratton, New York, 1985.

122. Gale RP: USSR: Follow-up after Chernobyl. *Lancet* 1:401, 1990.

123. Nimer SD, Leung DHY, Wolin MJ, Golde DW: Serum stem cell factor levels in patients with aplastic anemia. *Int J Hematol* 60:185, 1994.

124. Kojima S, Matsuyama T, Kodera Y: Plasma levels and production of soluble stem cell factor by marrow stromal cells in patients with aplastic anaemia. *Br J Haematol* 99:440, 1997.

125. Lyman SD, Seaberg M, Hanna R, et al: Plasma/serum levels of flt3 ligand are low in normal individuals and highly elevated in patients with Fanconi anemia and acquired aplastic anemia. *Blood* 86:4091, 1995.

126. Kojima S, Matsuyama T, Kodera Y, et al: Measurement of endogenous plasma granulocyte colony-stimulating factor in patients with acquired aplastic anemia by a sensitive chemiluminescent immunoassay. *Blood* 87:1303, 1996.

127. Kojima S, Matsuyama T, Kodera Y: Circulating erythropoietin in patients with acquired aplastic anaemia. *Acta Haematol* 94:117, 1995.

128. Emmons RVD, Reid DM, Cohen RL, et al. Human thrombopoietin levels are high when thrombocytopenia is due to megakaryocyte deficiency and low when due to increased platelet destruction. *Blood* 87:4068, 1996.

129. Nakao S, Matsushima K, Young N: Deficient interleukin I production by aplastic anaemia monocytes. *Br J Haematol* 71:431, 1989.

130. Holmberg LA, Seidel K, Leisenring W, Torok-Storb B: Aplastic anemia: Analysis of stromal cell function in long-term marrow cultures. *Blood* 84:3685, 1994.

131. Stute N, Fehse B, Schroder J, et al: Human mesenchymal stem cells are not of donor origin in patients with severe aplastic anemia who underwent sex-mismatched allogeneic bone marrow transplant. *J Hematother Stem Cell Res* 11:977, 2002.

132. Applebaum FR, Barrall J, Storb R, et al: Clonal cytogenetic abnormalities in patients with otherwise typical aplastic anemia. *Exp Hematol* 15:1134, 1987.

132a. Kulasekararaj AG, Jiang J, Smith AE, et al: Somatic mutations identify a subgroup of aplastic anemia patients who progress to myelodysplastic syndrome. *Blood* 124:2698, 2014.

133. Negendank W, Weissman D, Bey TM, et al: Evidence for clonal disease by magnetic resonance imaging in patients with hypoplastic marrow disorders. *Blood* 78:2872, 1991.

134. Schrezenmeier H, Hertenstein B, Wagner B, et al: A pathogenetic link between aplastic anemia and paroxysmal nocturnal hemoglobinuria is suggested by a high frequency of aplastic anemia patients with a deficiency of phosphatidylinositol glycan anchored proteins. *Exp Hematol* 23:81, 1995.

135. Horsley SW, Colman S, McKinley M, et al: Genetic lesions in a preleukemic aplasia phase in a child with acute lymphoblastic leukemia. *Genes Chromosomes Cancer* 47:333, 2008.

136. Suzan F, Terré C, Garcia I, et al: Three cases of typical aplastic anaemia associated with a Philadelphia chromosome. *Br J Haematol* 112:385, 2001.

137. Socie G, Rosenfeld S, Frickhofen N, et al: Late clonal diseases of aplastic anemia. *Semin Hematol* 37:91–101 2000.

138. Gordon-Smith EC, Marsh JC, Gibson FM: Views on the pathophysiology of aplastic anemia. *Int J Hematol* 76(Suppl 2):163, 2002.

139. Maciejewski JP, Risitano A, Sloand EM, et al: Distinct clinical outcomes for cytogenetic abnormalities evolving from aplastic anemia. *Blood* 99:3129, 2002.

140. Socie G, Henryamar M, Bacigalupo A, et al: Malignant tumors occurring after treatment of aplastic anemia. *N Engl J Med* 329:1152, 1993.

141. Najean Y, Haguenauer O: Long-term (5–20 years) evolution of non-grafted aplastic anemias. *Blood* 76:2222, 1990.

142. Ball SE, Gibson FM, Rizzo S: Progressive telomere shortening in aplastic anemia. *Blood* 91:3582, 1998.

143. Rosse WF: New insights into paroxysmal nocturnal hemoglobinuria. *Curr Opin Hematol* 8:61, 2001.

144. Nakakuma H, Kawaguchi T: Pathogenesis of selective expansion of PNH clones. *Int J Hematol* 77:121, 2003.

145. Scheinberg P, Marte M, Nunez O, Young NS: Paroxysmal nocturnal hemoglobinuria clones in severe aplastic anemia patients treated with horse anti-thymocyte globulin plus cyclosporine. *Haematologica* 95:1075, 2010.

146. Storb R, Blume KG, O'Donnell MR, et al: Cyclophosphamide and antithymocyte globulin to condition patients with aplastic anemia for allogeneic marrow transplantation: The experience in four centers. *Biol Blood Marrow Transplant* 7:39, 2001.

147. Metzgeroth G, Dinter D, Schultheis B, et al: Deferasirox in MDS patients with transfusion-caused iron overload-a phase-II study. *Ann Hematol* 88:301, 2009.

148. Sagmeister M, Oec L, Gmur J: A restrictive platelet transfusion policy allowing long-term support of outpatients with severe aplastic anemia. *Blood* 93:3124, 1999.

149. Lawrence JB, Yomtovian RA, Hammons T, et al: Lowering the prophylactic platelet transfusion threshold: A prospective analysis. *Leuk Lymphoma* 41:67, 2001.

150. Zeigler ZR: Effects of epsilon aminocaproic acid on primary haemostasis. *Haemostasis* 21:313, 1991.

151. Hod E, Schwartz J: Platelet transfusion refractoriness. *Br J Haematol* 142:348, 2008.

152. Slichter SJ, Davis K, Enright H, et al: Factors affecting posttransfusion platelet increments, platelet refractoriness, and platelet transfusion intervals in thrombocytopenic patients. *Blood* 105:4106, 2005.

153. Drewniak A, Boelens JJ, Vrielink H, et al: Granulocyte concentrates: Prolonged functional capacity during storage in the presence of phenotypic changes. *Haematologica* 93:1058, 2008.

154. Armand P, Antin JH: Allogeneic stem cell transplantation for aplastic anemia. *Biol Blood Marrow Transplant* 13:505, 2007.

155. Georges GE, Storb R: Stem cell transplantation for aplastic anemia. *Int J Hematol* 75:141, 2002.

156. Champlin RE, Perez WS, Passweg JR, et al: Bone marrow transplantation for severe aplastic anemia: A randomized controlled study of conditioning regimens. *Blood* 109:4582, 2007.

157. Locasciulli A, Oneto R, Bacigalupo A, et al: Outcome of patients with acquired aplastic anemia given first line bone marrow transplantation or immunosuppressive treatment in the last decade: A report from the European Group for Blood and Marrow Transplantation (EBMT). *Haematologica* 92:11, 2007.

158. Gandhi S, Kulasekararaj AG, Mufti GJ, Marsh JC: Allogeneic stem cell transplantation using alemtuzumab-containing regimens in severe aplastic anemia. *Int J Hematol* 97:573, 2013.

159. Viollier R, Socié G, Tichelli A, et al: Recent improvement in outcome of unrelated donor transplantation for aplastic anemia. *Bone Marrow Transplant* 41:45, 2008.

160. Lee SJ, Klein J, Haagenson M, Baxter-Lowe LA, et al: High-resolution donor-recipient HLA matching contributes to the success of unrelated donor marrow transplantation. *Blood* 110:4576, 2007.

161. Dubey S, Nityanand S: Involvement of Fas and TNF pathways in the induction of apoptosis of T cells by antithymocyte globulin. *Ann Hematol* 82:496, 2003.

162. Michallet M-C, Saltel F, Preville X, et al: Cathepsin-B-dependent apoptosis triggered by antithymocyte globulins: A novel mechanism of T-cell depletion. *Blood* 102:3719, 2003.

163. Mangan KF, D'Alessandro L, Mullaney MT: Action of antithymocyte globulin on normal human erythroid progenitor cell proliferation in vitro: Erythropoietic growth-enhancing factors are released from marrow accessory cells. *J Lab Clin Med* 107:353, 1986.

164. Kawano Y, Nissen C, Gratwohl A, Speck B: Immunostimulatory effects of different antilymphocyte globulin preparations: A possible clue to their clinical effect. *Br J Haematol* 68:115, 1988.

165. Bielory L, Wright R, Nienhuis AW, et al: Antithymocyte globulin hypersensitivity in bone marrow failure patients. *JAMA* 260:3164, 1988.

166. Zheng Y, Liu Y, Chu Y: Immunosuppressive therapy for acquired severe aplastic anemia (SAA): A prospective comparison of four different regimens. *Exp Hematol* 34:826, 2006.

167. Atta EH, Dias DS, Marra VL, de Azevedo AM: Comparison between horse and rabbit antithymocyte globulin as first-line treatment for patients with severe aplastic anemia: A single-center retrospective study. *Ann Hematol* 89:851, 2010.

168. Garg R, Faderl S, Garcia-Manero G, et al: Phase II study of rabbit anti-thymocyte globulin, cyclosporine and granulocyte colony-stimulating factor in patients with aplastic anemia and myelodysplastic syndrome. *Leukemia* 23:1297, 2009.

169. Scheinberg P, Nunez O, Weinstein B, et al: Horse versus rabbit antithymocyte globulin in acquired aplastic anemia. *N Engl J Med* 365:430, 2011.

170. Kadia TM, Borthakur G, Garcia-Manero G, et al: Final results of the phase II study of rabbit anti-thymocyte globulin, ciclosporin, methylprednisone, and granulocyte colony-stimulating factor in patients with aplastic anaemia and myelodysplastic syndrome. *Br J Haematol* 157:312, 2012.

171. Afable MG 2nd, Shaik M, Sugimoto Y, et al: Efficacy of rabbit anti-thymocyte globulin in severe aplastic anemia. *Haematologica* 96: 2069, 2011.

172. Chen, C, Xue HM, Li Y, et al: Rabbit-antithymocyte globulin combined with cyclosporine A as a first-line therapy: Improved, effective and safe for children with acquired severe aplastic anemia. *J Cancer Res Clin Oncol* 138:1105, 2012.

173. Marsh JC, Bacigalupo A, Schrezenmeier H, et al: Prospective study of rabbit antithymocyte globulin and cyclosporine for aplastic anemia from the EBMT Severe Aplastic Anaemia Working Party. *Blood* 119:5391, 2012.

174. Shin SH, Yoon JH, Yahng SA, et al: The efficacy of rabbit antithymocyte globulin with cyclosporine in comparison to horse antithymocyte globulin as a first-line treatment in adult patients with severe aplastic anemia: A single-center retrospective study. *Ann Hematol* 92:817, 2013.

175. Camitta B, O'Reilly RJ, Sensenbrenner L: Antithoracic duct lymphocyte globulin therapy of severe aplastic anemia. *Blood* 62:883, 1983.

176. Champlin R, Ho W, Gale RP: Antithymocyte globulin treatment in patients with aplastic anemia: A prospective randomized trial. *N Engl J Med* 308:113, 1983.

177. Young N, Griffin P, Brittain E, et al: A multicenter trial of antithymocyte globulin in aplastic anemia and related diseases. *Blood* 72:1861, 1988.

178. Schrezenmeier H, Marin P, Raghavachar A, et al: Relapse of aplastic anaemia after immunosuppressive treatment: A report from the European Bone Marrow Transplantation Group SAA Working Party. *Br J Haematol* 85:371, 1993.

179. Doney K, Leisenring W, Storb R, Appelbaum FR: Primary treatment of acquired aplastic anemia: Outcomes with bone marrow transplantation and immunosuppressive therapy. *Ann Intern Med* 126:107, 1997.

180. Tichelli A, Gratwohl A, Nissen C, Speck B: Late clonal complications in severe aplastic anemia. *Leuk Lymphoma* 12:167, 1994.

181. De Planque MM, Bacigalupo A, Würsch A, et al: Long-term follow-up of severe aplastic anaemia patients treated with antithymocyte globulin. *Br J Haematol* 73:121, 1989.

182. Socié G, Henry-Amar M, Bacigalupo A, et al: Malignant tumors occurring after treatment of aplastic anemia. *N Engl J Med* 319:1152, 1993.

183. Calado RT, Cooper JN, Padilla-Nash HM, et al: Short telomeres result in chromosomal instability in hematopoietic cells and precede malignant evolution in human aplastic anemia. *Leukemia* 26:700, 2012.

184. Stryckmans PA, Dumont JP, Velu T, Debusscher L: Cyclosporine in refractory severe aplastic anemia [letter]. *N Engl J Med* 310:655, 1984.

185. Lazzarino M, Morra E, Canevari A, et al: Cyclosporine in the treatment of aplastic anemia and pure red-cell aplasia. *Bone Marrow Transplant* 4(Suppl 4):165, 1989.

186. Hinterberger-Fischer M, Höcker P, Lechner K, et al: Oral cyclosporin-A is effective treatment for untreated and also for previously immunosuppressed patients with severe bone marrow failure. *Eur J Haematol* 43:136, 1989.

187. Tötterman TH, Höglund M, Bengtsson M, et al: Treatment of pure red-cell aplasia and aplastic anaemia with cyclosporin: Long-term clinical effects. *Eur J Haematol* 42:126, 1989.

188. Leeksma OC, Thomas LLM, van der Lelie J, et al: Effectiveness of low dose cyclosporine in acquired aplastic anaemia with severe neutropenia. *Neth J Med* 41:143, 1992.

189. Leonard EM, Raefsky E, Griffith P, et al: Cyclosporine therapy of aplastic anaemia, congenital and acquired red-cell aplasia. *Br J Haematol* 72:278, 1989.

190. Tong J, Bacigalupo A, Piaggio G, et al: Severe aplastic anemia (SAA): Response to cyclosporin A (CyA) in vivo and in vitro. *Eur J Haematol* 46:212, 1991.

191. Nakao S, Yamaguchi M, Shiobara S, et al: Interferon-g gene expression in unstimulated bone marrow mononuclear cells predicts a good response to cyclosporine therapy in aplastic anemia. *Blood* 79:2531, 1992.

192. Kojima S, Fukada M, Miyajima Y, Matsuyama T: Cyclosporine and recombinant granulocyte colony-stimulating factor in severe aplastic anemia [letter]. *N Engl J Med* 313:920, 1990.

193. Bertrand Y, Amri F, Capdeville R, et al: The successful treatment of two cases of severe aplastic anaemia with granulocyte colony-stimulating factor and cyclosporine A [case report]. *Br J Haematol* 79:648, 1991.

194. Schrezenmeier H, Schlander M, Raghavachar A: Cyclosporin A in aplastic anemia—Report of a workshop. *Ann Hematol* 65:33, 1992.

195. Gluckman E, Esperou-Bourdeau H, Baruchel A, et al: Multicenter randomized study comparing cyclosporine-A alone and antithymocyte globulin with prednisone for treatment of severe aplastic anemia. *Blood* 79:2540, 1992.

196. Rosenfeld S, Follmann D, Nunez O, et al: Antithymocyte globulin and cyclosporine for severe aplastic anemia: Association between hematologic response and long-term outcome. *JAMA* 289:1130, 2003.

197. Scheinberg P, Wu CO, Nunez O, et al: Long-term outcome of pediatric patients with severe aplastic anemia treated with antithymocyte globulin and cyclosporine. *J Pediatr* 153:814, 2008.

198. Osugi Y, Yagasaki H, Sako M, et al: Antithymocyte globulin and cyclosporine for treatment of 44 children with hepatitis associated aplastic anemia. *Haematologica* 92:1687, 2007.

199. Teramura M, Kimura A, Iwase S, et al: Treatment of severe aplastic anemia with anti-thymocyte globulin and cyclosporin A with or without G-CSF in adults: A multicenter randomized study in Japan. *Blood* 110:1756, 2007.

200. Bacigalupo A, Brand R, Oneto R, et al: Treatment of acquired severe aplastic anemia: Bone marrow transplantation compared with immunosuppressive therapy—The European Group for Blood and Marrow Transplantation experience. *Semin Hematol* 37:69, 2000.

201. Gillio AP, Boulad F, Small TN, et al: Comparison of long-term outcome of children with severe aplastic anemia treated with immunosuppression versus bone marrow transplantation. *Biol Blood Marrow Transplant* 3:18, 1997.

202. De Planque MM, Kluin-Nelemans HC, Van Krieken HJM, et al: Evolution of acquired severe aplastic anaemia to myelodysplasia and subsequent leukaemia in adults. *Br J Haematol* 70:55, 1988.

203. Tichelli A, Gratwohl A, Würsch A, et al: Late haematological complications in severe aplastic anaemia. *Br J Haematol* 69:413, 1988.

204. Moore MAS, Castro-Malaspina H: Immunosuppression in aplastic anemia—Postponing the inevitable? *N Engl J Med* 314:1358, 1991.

205. Tichelli A, Passweg J, Nissen C, et al: Repeated treatment with horse antilymphocyte globulin for severe aplastic anaemia. *Br J Haematol* 100:393, 1998.

206. Scheinberg P, Nunez O, Young NS: Retreatment with rabbit anti-thymocyte globulin and ciclosporin for patients with relapsed or refractory severe aplastic anaemia. *Br J Haematol* 133:622, 2006.

207. Scheinberg P, Nunez O, Weinstein B, et al: Activity of alemtuzumab monotherapy in treatment-naive, relapsed, and refractory severe acquired aplastic anemia. *Blood* 119:345, 2011.

208. Marsh JC, Kulasekararaj AG: Management of the refractory aplastic anemia patient: What are the options? *Hematology Am Soc Hematol Educ Program* 2013:87, 2013.

209. Risitano AM, Schrezenmeier H: Alternative immunosuppression in patients failing immunosuppression with ATG who are not transplant candidates: Campath (Alemtuzumab). *Bone Marrow Transplant* 48:186, 2013.

210. Bacigalupo A, Van Lint MT, Cerri R, et al: Treatment of severe aplastic anemia with bolus 6-methylprednisolone and antilymphocyte globulin. *Blut* 41:168, 1980.

211. Issaragrisil S, Tangnai-Trisorana Y, Siriseriwan T, et al: Methylprednisolone therapy in aplastic anaemia: Correlation of in vitro tests and lymphocyte subsets with clinical response. *Eur J Haematol* 40:343, 1988.

212. Brodsky RA, Sensenbrenner LL, Jones RJ: Complete remission in severe aplastic anemia after high-dose cyclophosphamide without bone marrow transplantation. *Blood* 87:491, 1996.

213. Jones RJ, Barber JP, Vala MS, et al: Assessment of aldehyde dehydrogenase in viable cells. *Blood* 85:2742, 1995.

214. Kastan MB, Schlaffer I, Russo JE, et al: Direct demonstration of aldehyde dehydrogenase in human hematopoietic progenitor cells. *Blood* 75:1947, 1990.

215. Brodsky RA, Sensenbrenner LL, Smith BD, et al: Durable treatment-free remission following high-dose cyclophosphamide for previously untreated severe aplastic anemia. *Ann Intern Med* 135:477, 2001.

216. Brodsky RA: High-dose cyclophosphamide for aplastic anemia and autoimmunity. *Curr Opin Oncol* 14:143, 2002.

217. Hansen PB, Lauritzen AM: Aplastic anemia successfully treated with rituximab. *Am J Hematol* 80:292, 2005.

218. Hansen PB, Lauritzen AM. Aplastic anemia successfully treated with rituximab. *Am J Hematol* 80:292, 2005.

219. Takamatsu H, Yagasaki H, Takahashi Y, et al: Aplastic anemia successfully treated with rituximab: The possible role of aplastic anemia-associated autoantibodies as a marker for response. *Eur J Haematol* 86:541, 2011.

220. Androgen therapy in aplastic anemia: A comparative study of high and low doses of 4 different androgens. French Cooperative Group for the Study of Aplastic and Refractory Anemias. *Scand J Haematol* 36:346, 1986.

221. Champlin RE, Ho WG, Feig SA, et al: Do androgens enhance the response to antithymocyte globulin in patients with aplastic anemia? A prospective randomized trial. *Blood* 66:184, 1985.

222. Socie G, Mary JY, Schrezenmeier H, et al: Granulocyte-stimulating factor and severe aplastic anemia: A survey by the European Group for Blood and Marrow Transplantation (EBMT). *Blood* 109:2794, 2007.

223. Tichelli A, Schrezenmeier H, Socié G, et al: A randomized controlled study in patients with newly diagnosed severe aplastic anemia receiving antithymocyte globulin (ATG), cyclosporine, with or without G-CSF: A study of the SAA Working Party of the European Group for Blood and Marrow Transplantation. *Blood* 117:4434, 2011.

224. Ganser A, Lindemann A, Siepelt G, et al: Effects of recombinant human interleukin-3 in aplastic anemia. *Blood* 76:1287, 1990.

225. Walsh CE, Liu JM, Anderson SM, et al: A trial of recombinant human interleukin-1 in patients with severe refractory aplastic anaemia. *Br J Haematol* 80:106, 1992.

226. Hirao A: TPO signal for stem cell genomic integrity. *Blood* 123:459, 2014.

227. de Lavel B, Pawlikowska P, Barbieri D, et al: Thrombopoietin promotes NHEJ DNA repair in hematopoietic stem cells through specific activation of Erk and NF-κB pathways and their target, IEX-1. *Blood* 123:509, 2014.

228. Desmond R, Townsley DM, Dumitriu B, et al: Eltrombopag restores tri-lineage hematopoiesis in refractory severe aplastic anemia which can be sustained on discontinuation of drug. *Blood* 123:1818, 2014.

229. Olnes MJ, Scheinberg P, Calvo KR, et al: Eltrombopag and improved hematopoiesis in refractory aplastic anemia. *N Engl J Med* 367:11, 2012; erratum in *N Engl J Med* 367:284, 2012.

230. Desmond R, Townsley DM, Dunbar C, Young NS. Eltrombopag in aplastic anemia. *Semin Hematol* 52:31, 2015.

231. Speck B, Tichelli A, Widmer E, et al: Splenectomy as an adjuvant measure in the treatment of severe aplastic anaemia. *Br J Haematol* 92:818, 1996.

232. Sadowitz PD, Dubowy RL: Intravenous immunoglobulin in the treatment of aplastic anemia. *Am J Pediatr Hematol Oncol* 12:198, 1990.

233. Bodenstein H: Successful treatment of aplastic anemia with high-dose immunoglobulin [letter]. *N Engl J Med* 314:1368, 1991.

234. Ito T, Haraiwa M, Ishikawa Y, et al: Lymphocytapheresis in a patient with severe aplastic anaemia. *Acta Haematol* 80:167, 1988.

235. Morales-Polanco MR, Sanchez-Valle E, Guerrero-Rivera S, et al: Treatment results of 23 cases of severe aplastic anemia with lymphocytapheresis. *Arch Med Res* 28:85, 1997.

236. Tiu RV, Visconte V, Elson P, et al: LFA-3/CD2 pathway, potential target for immunosuppressive therapy in aplastic anemia: A phase I/II clinical trail of alefacept in patients with relapsed/ refractory aplastic anemia. *Blood* 122: abstract 3711, 2013.

237. Kiem HP, McDonald GB, Myerson D, et al: Marrow transplantation for hepatitis-associated aplastic anemia: A follow-up of long-term survivors. *Biol Blood Marrow Transplant* 2:93, 1996.

238. Lewis SM: Course and prognosis in aplastic anemia. *Br Med J* 1:1027, 1965.

239. Lynch RE, Williams DM, Reading JC, Cartwright GE: The prognosis in aplastic anemia. *Blood* 45:517, 1975.

240. Horowitz MM: Current status of allogeneic bone marrow transplantation in acquired aplastic anemia. *Semin Hematol* 37:30, 2000.

241. Ades L, Mary J-Y, Robin M, et al: Long-term outcome after bone marrow transplantation for severe aplastic anemia. *Blood* 103:2490, 2004.

242. Sangiolo D, Storb R, Deeg HJ, et al: Outcome of allogeneic hematopoietic cell transplantation from HLA-identical siblings for severe aplastic anemia in patients over 40 years of age. *Biol Blood Marrow Transplant* 16:1411, 2010.

243. Schrezenmeier H, Passweg JR, Marsh JC, et al: Worse outcome and more chronic GVHD with peripheral blood progenitor cells than bone marrow in HLA-matched sibling donor transplants for young patients with severe acquired aplastic anemia. *Blood* 110:1397, 2007.

244. Locasciulli A: Acquired aplastic anemia in children: Incidence, prognosis and treatment options. *Paediatr Drugs* 4:761, 2002.

245. Scheinberg P, Wu CO, Nunez O, Young NS: Predicting response to immunosuppressive therapy and survival in severe aplastic anaemia. *Br J Haematol* 144:206, 2009.

246. Scheinberg P, Wu CO, Nunez O, Young NS: Long-term outcome of pediatric patients with severe aplastic anemia treated with antithymocyte globulin and cyclosporine. *J Pediatr* 153:814, 2008.

247. Tisdale JF, Dunn DE, Maciejewski J: Cyclophosphamide and other new agents for the treatment of severe aplastic anemia. *Semin Hematol* 37:102, 2000.

248. Brodsky RA, Chen AR, Dorr D, et al: High-dose cyclophosphamide for severe aplastic anemia: Long-term follow-up. *Blood* 115:2136, 2010.

249. Fanconi G: Familiäre infantile perniziosaartige anämie (perniziöses blutbild und konstitution). *Jahrbuch Kinderheil* 117:257, 1927.

250. Rosendorff J, Bernstein R, Macdougall L, Jenkins T: Fanconi anemia: Another disease of unusually high prevalence in the Afrikaans population of South Africa. *Am J Med Genet* 27:793, 1987.

251. Dokal I, Vulliamy T: Inherited aplastic anaemias/bone marrow failure syndromes. *Blood Rev* 22:141, 2008.

252. Garaycoechea JI, Patel KJ: Why does the bone marrow fail in Fanconi anemia? *Blood* 123:26, 2014.

253. Jacquemont C, Taniguchi T: The Fanconi anemia pathway and ubiquitin. *BMC Biochem* 22(8 Suppl 1):S10, 2007.

254. Alter BP, Giri N, Savage SA, et al: Update on inherited bone marrow failure syndromes (IBMFS). *IBMFS Newsletter of the Clinical Genetics Branch*, National Cancer Institute. P.1, Summer 2008.

255. HGNC: HUGO Gene Nomenclature Committee of the National Human Genome Research Institute: Fanconi Anemia, complementation groups. Available at: http://www.genenames.org/genefamilies/fanc (last accessed 16 February 2015).

256. Somyajit K, Subramanya S, Nagaraju G: Distinct roles of FANCO/RAD51C protein in DNA damage signaling and repair. *J Biol Chem* 287:3366, 2012.

257. Kashiyama K, Nakazawa Y, Pliz DT, et al: Malfunction of Nuclease ERCC1-XPF results in diverse clinical manifestations and causes Cockayne syndrome, xeroderma pigmentosa, and Fanconi anemia. *Am J Hum Genet* 92:807, 2013.

258. Dufour C, Corcione A, Svahn J, et al: TNF-α and TNF-γ are overexpressed in the bone marrow of Fanconi anemia patients and TNF-α suppresses erythropoiesis in vitro. *Blood* 102:2053, 2003.

259. D'Apolito M, Zelante L, Savoia A: Molecular basis of Fanconi anemia. *Haematologica* 83:533, 1998.

260. Garcia-Higuera I, Kuang Y, D'Andrea AD: The molecular and cellular biology of Fanconi anemia. *Curr Opin Hematol* 6:83, 1999.

261. Young NA, Alter BP: *Aplastic Anemia: Acquired and Inherited.* WB Saunders, Philadelphia, 1994.

262. Estren S, Damshek W: Familial hypoplastic anemia of childhood: Report of 8 cases in 2 families with beneficial effects of splenectomy in 1 case. *Am J Dis Child* 73:671, 1947.

263. Swhimamura A, D'Andrea AD: Subtyping of Fanconi anemia patients: Implications for clinical management. *Blood* 102:3459, 2003.

264. Carreau M, Liu L, Gan OI, et al: Short-term granulocyte colony-stimulating factor and erythropoietin treatment enhances hematopoiesis and survival in the mitomycin

C-conditioned Fancc(−/−) mouse model, while long-term treatment is ineffective. *Blood* 100:1499, 2002.

265. Alter BP: Cancer in Fanconi anemia. *Cancer* 97:425, 2003.
266. Alter BP, Caruso JP, Drachtman RA, et al: Fanconi anemia: Myelodysplasia as a predictor of outcome. *Cancer Genet Cytogenet* 117:125, 2000.
267. Gluckman E, Wagner JE: Hematopoietic stem cell transplantation in childhood inherited bone marrow failure syndrome. *Bone Marrow Transplant* 41:127, 2008.
268. Huck K, Hanenberg H, Nürnberger W, et al: Favourable long-term outcome after matched sibling transplantation for Fanconi-anemia (FA) and in vivo T-cell depletion. *Klin Padiatr* 220:147, 2008.
269. Ayas M, Al-Jefri A, Al-Seraihi A, et al: Second stem cell transplantation in patients with Fanconi anemia using antithymocyte globulin alone for conditioning. *Biol Blood Marrow Transplant* 14:445, 2008.
270. Kelly PF, Radtke S, von Kalle C, et al: Stem cell collection and gene transfer in Fanconi anemia. *Mol Ther* 15:211, 2007.
271. Dufour C, Svahn J: Fanconi anaemia: New strategies. *Bone Marrow Transplant* 41(Suppl 2):S90, 2008.
272. Dokal I: Dyskeratosis congenita in all its forms. *Br J Haematol* 110:768, 2000.
273. Nelson ND, Bertuch AA: Dyskeratosis congenita as a disorder of telomere maintenance. *Mutat Res* 730:43, 2012.
274. Savage SA, Alter BP: The role of telomere biology in bone marrow failure and other disorders. *Mech Ageing Dev* 129(1–2):35, 2008.
275. Keller RB, Gagne KE, Usmani GN, et al: Mutations in a patient with dyskeratosis congenita. *Pediatr Blood Cancer* 59:311, 2012.
276. Ballew B, Yeager M, Jacobs K, et al: Germline mutations of regulator of telomere elongation helicase 1, RTEL1, in dyskeratosis congenital. *Hum Genet* 132:473, 2013.
277. Vulliamy A, Marrone F, Goldman A, et al: The RNA component of telomerase is mutated in autosomal dominant dyskeratosis congenita. *Nature* 413:432, 2001.
278. Dokal I, Vulliamy T, Mason P, Bessler M: Clinical utility gene card for: Dyskeratosis congenital. *Eur J Hum Genet* Sep 3, 2014. doi: 10.1038/ejhg.2014.170. [Epub ahead of print].
279. Walne A, Bhagat T, Kirwan M, et al: Mutations in the telomere capping complex in bone marrow failure and related syndromes. *Haematologica* 98:334, 2013.
279a. Ruggero D, Shimamura A. Marrow failure: A window into ribosome biology. *Blood* 124:2784, 2014.
280. Savage SA, Giri N, Baerlocher GM, et al: TINF2, a component of the shelterin telomere protection complex, is mutated in dyskeratosis congenita. *Am J Hum Genet* 82:501, 2008.
281. Walne AJ, Vulliamy T, Marrone A, et al: Genetic heterogeneity in autosomal recessive dyskeratosis congenita with one subtype due to mutations in the telomerase-associated protein NOP10. *Hum Mol Genet* 16:1619, 2007.
282. Vulliamy T, Beswick R, Kirwan M, et al: Mutations in the telomerase component of NHP2 cause the premature aging syndrome, dyskeratosis congenital. *Proc Natl Acad Sci U S A* 105:8073, 2008.
283. Vulliamy T, Marrone A, Szydlo R, et al: Disease anticipation is associated with progressive telomere shortening in families with dyskeratosis congenita due to mutations in TERC. *Nat Genet* 36:447, 2004.
284. Alter BP, Baerlocher GM, Savage SA, et al: Very short telomere length by flow fluorescence in situ hybridization identifies patients with dyskeratosis congenita. *Blood* 110:1439, 2007.
285. Ghavamzadeh A, Alimoghadam K, Nasseri P, et al: Correction of bone marrow failure in dyskeratosis congenita by bone marrow transplantation. *Bone Marrow Transplant* 23:299, 1999.
286. Cesaro S, Oneto R, Messina C, et al: Haematopoietic stem cell transplantation for Shwachman-Diamond disease: A study from the European Group for Blood and Marrow Transplantation. *Br J Haematol* 131:231, 2005.
287. Güngör T, Corbacioglu S, Storb R, Seger RA: Nonmyeloablative allogeneic hematopoietic stem cell transplantation for treatment of dyskeratosis congenita. *Bone Marrow Transplant* 31:407, 2003.
288. Dror Y, Freedman MH, Leaker M, et al: Low-intensity hematopoietic stem-cell transplantation across human leucocyte antigen barriers in dyskeratosis congenita. *Bone Marrow Transplant* 31:847, 2003.
289. Alter BP, Neelam G, Savage SA, et al: Cancer in dyskeratosis congenital. *Blood* 113:6549, 2009.
290. Goobie S, Popovic M, Morrison J, et al: Shwachman Diamond syndrome with exocrine pancreatic dysfunction and bone marrow failure maps to the centromeric region of chromosome 7. *Am J Hum Genet* 68:1048, 2001.
291. Ginzberg H, Shin J, Ellis L, et al: Shwachman syndrome: Phenotypic manifestations of sibling sets and isolated cases in a large patient cohort are similar. *J Pediatr* 135:81, 1999.
292. Shimamura A: Shwachman-Diamond syndrome. *Semin Hematol* 43:178, 2006.
293. Rujkijyanont P, Watanabe K, Ambekar C, et al: SBDS-Deficient cells undergo accelerated apoptosis through the FAS pathway. *Haematologica* 93:363, 2008.
294. Thornley I, Dror Y, Sung L, et al: Abnormal telomere shortening in leucocytes of children with Shwachman-Diamond syndrome. *Br J Haematol* 117:189, 2002.
295. Ganapathi KA, Shimamura A: Ribosomal dysfunction and inherited marrow failure. *Br J Haematol* 141:376, 2008.
296. Ganapathi KA, Austin KM, Lee CS, et al: The human Shwachman-Diamond syndrome protein, SBDS, associates with ribosomal RNA. *Blood* 110:1458, 2007.
297. Myers KC, Davies SM, Shimamura A: Clinical and molecular pathophysiology of Shwachman-Diamond syndrome: An update. *Hematol Oncol Clin North Am* 27:117, 2013.
298. Toiviainen-Salo S, Durie PR, Numminen K, et al: The natural history of Shwachman Diamond syndrome associated liver disease from childhood to adulthood. *J Pediatr* 155:807, 2009.
299. Dror Y, Durie P, Ginzberg H, et al: Clonal evolution in marrows of patients with Shwachman-Diamond syndrome: A prospective 5-year follow-up study. *Exp Hematol* 30:659, 2002.
300. Woloszynek JR, Rothbaum RJ, Rawis AS, et al: Mutations of the SBDS gene are present in most patients with Shwachman-Diamond syndrome. *Blood* 104:3588, 2004.
301. Bhatla D, Davies SM, Shenoy S, et al: Reduced-intensity conditioning is effective and safe for transplantation of patients with Shwachman-Diamond syndrome. *Bone Marrow Transplant* 42:159, 2008.
302. Dokal I, Rule S, Chen F, et al: Adult onset of acute myeloid leukaemia (M6) in patients with Shwachman-Diamond syndrome. *Br J Haematol* 99:171, 1997.
303. Dror Y, Squire J, Durie P, Freedman MH: Malignant myeloid transformation with isochromosome 7q in Shwachman-Diamond syndrome. *Leukemia* 12:1591, 1998.
304. Thornely I, Dror Y, Sung L, et al: Abnormal telomere shortening in leukocytes of children with Shwachman-Diamond syndrome. *Br J Haematol* 117:189, 2002.
305. Geddis AE: Inherited thrombocytopenia: Congenital amegakaryocytic thrombocytopenia and thrombocytopenia with absent radii. *Semin Hematol* 43:196, 2006.
306. Germeshausen M, Ballmaier M, Welte K: MPL mutations in 23 patients suffering from congenital amegakaryocytic thrombocytopenia: The type of mutation predicts the course of the disease. *Hum Mutat* 27:296, 2006.
307. King S, Germeshausen M, Strauss G, et al: Congenital amegakaryocytic thrombocytopenia: A retrospective clinical analysis of 20 patients. *Br J Haematol* 131:636, 2005.
308. Stephan JL, Vlekova V, Le Deist F, et al: Severe combined immunodeficiency: A retrospective single-center study of clinical presentation and outcome in 117 patients. *J Pediatr* 123:564, 1993.
309. Bertrand Y, Muller SM, Casanova JL, et al: Reticular dysgenesis: HLA non-identical bone marrow transplants in a series of 10 patients. *Bone Marrow Transplant* 29:759, 2002.
310. Esperou-Bourdeau H, Leblanc T, Schaison G, et al: Aplastic anemia associated with "bird-headed" dwarfism (Seckel syndrome). *Nouv Rev Fr Hematol* 35:99, 1993.
311. O'Driscoll M, Ruiz-Perez VL, Woods CG, et al: A splicing mutation affecting expression of ataxia-telangiectasia and RAD3-related protein (ATR) results in Seckel syndrome. *Nat Genet* 33:497, 2003.
312. Griffith E, Walker S, Martin CA, et al: Mutations in pericentrin cause Seckel syndrome with defective ATR-dependent DNA damage signaling. *Nat Genet* 40:232, 2008.
313. Hayani A, Suarez CR, Molnar Z, et al: Acute myeloid leukemia in a patient with Seckel syndrome. *J Med Genet* 31:148, 1994.
314. O'Driscoll M, Gennery AR, Seidel J, et al: An overview of three new disorders associated with genetic instability: LIG4 syndrome, RS-SCID and ATR-Seckel syndrome. *DNA Repair (Amst)* 3:1227, 2004.
315. Li FP, Hecht F, Kaiser-McCaw B, et al: Ataxia-pancytopenia: Syndrome of cerebellar ataxia, hypoplastic anemia, monosomy 7 and acute myelogenous leukemia. *Cancer Genet Cytogenet* 4:189, 1981.
316. Mahmood F, King MD, Smyth OO, et al: Familial cerebellar hypoplasia and pancytopenia without chromosomal breakages. *Neuropediatrie* 29:302, 1998.
317. González-del AA, Cervera M, Gomez L, et al: Ataxia-pancytopenia syndrome. *Am J Med Genet* 90:252, 2000.
318. Pierce AJ, Jasin M: NHEJ deficiency and disease. *Mol Cell* 8:1160, 2001.
319. O'Driscoll M, Jeggo PA: CSA can induce DNA double-strand breaks: Implications for BMT regimens particularly for individuals with defective DNA repair. *Bone Marrow Transplant* 41:983, 2008.
320. Walters TR, Desposito F: Aplastic anemia in Dubowitz syndrome. *J Pediatr* 106:622, 1985.
321. Berthold F, Fuhrmann W, Lampert F: Fatal aplastic anemia in a patient with Dubowitz syndrome. *Eur J Pediatr* 146:605, 1987.
322. Gennery AR, Slatter MA, Bhattacharya A, et al: The clinical and biological overlap between Nijmegen breakage syndrome and Fanconi anemia. *Clin Immunol* 113:214, 2004.
323. Gadkowska-Dura M, Dzieranowska-Fangrat K, Dura W, et al: Unique morphological spectrum of lymphomas in Nijmegen breakage syndrome (NBS) patients with high frequency of consecutive lymphoma formation. *J Pathol* 216:337, 2008.
324. Gonzalez CH, Durkin-Stamm MV, Geimer NF, et al: The WT syndrome—A "new" autosomal dominant pleiotropic trait of radial/ulnar hypoplasia with high risk of bone marrow failure and/or leukemia. *Birth Defects Orig Artic Ser* 13:31, 1977.

CHAPTER 36
PURE RED CELL APLASIA

Neal S. Young

SUMMARY

Pure red cell aplasia is the diagnosis applied to isolated anemia secondary to failure of erythropoiesis. Cardinal findings are a low hemoglobin level combined with reticulocytopenia and absent or extremely infrequent marrow erythroid precursor. Historical names for pure red cell aplasia include *erythroblast hypoplasia, erythroblastopenia, red cell agenesis, hypoplastic anemia,* and *aregenerative anemia. Aplastic anemia* confers the same meaning, of course, but is applied to pancytopenia and an empty marrow (Chap. 35). Pure red cell aplasia was first separated from aplastic anemia by Kaznelson in 1922. The association of red cell aplasia and thymoma interested physicians in the 1930s and ultimately led to laboratory studies linking pure red cell aplasia to immune mechanisms, including the early identification of antierythroid precursor cell antibodies by Krantz and later characterization of T cells that inhibited erythropoiesis. Red cell aplasia as an acute and life-threatening complication of sickle cell disease and other hemolytic anemias was recognized in the 1940s, presaging the role of a specific virus in the etiology of both acute and chronic erythropoietic failure. Despite its infrequency, pure red cell aplasia has been a subject of much laboratory research because of its link to an immune mechanism of erythropoietic failure and as a manifestation of parvovirus B19 infection and viral destruction of red cell progenitors. However, because of its infrequency, pure red cell aplasia has not been the subject of large or controlled clinical trials; as a result, therapeutic recommendations are based on single cases or small series. Table 36–1 lists a practical classification of pure red cell aplasia.

● INHERITED PURE RED CELL APLASIA (DIAMOND-BLACKFAN ANEMIA)

DEFINITION AND HISTORY

Anemia in infancy and early childhood associated with absent reticulocytes in the blood and erythroid precursor cells in the marrow was described by Joseph[1] in 1936 as a "failure of erythropoiesis" and by Diamond and Blackfan[2] in 1938 as "congenital hypoplastic anemia."

Acronyms and Abbreviations: B19, primate erythroparvovirus 1; BFU-E, burst-forming unit–erythroid; CD20, a cluster of differentiation molecule expressed on the surface of all mature B cells; CFU-E, colony-forming unit–erythroid; CLL, chronic lymphocytic leukemia; FA, Fanconi anemia; *GATA1* gene, globin transcription factor 1; HLA, human leukocyte antigen; Ig, immunoglobulin; IL, interleukin; LGL, large granular lymphocytic leukemia; *RPS14* and *RPS19* genes, ribosomal protein S14 and S19 genes; *STAT3* gene, signal transducer and activator of transcription 3 gene; T cell, thymus-derived lymphocyte.

Gasser[3] first reported a response of a patient to glucocorticoids in 1951, and Diamond and associates[4] presented a series of treated patients. Genetic linkage studies have identified etiologic mutations in ribosomal protein genes.[5–9] Hundreds of cases have been reported, and many excellent reviews have been published.[10] Although Joseph was the first to describe the disorder, the anemia invariably is referred to as either *Blackfan-Diamond* or *Diamond-Blackfan anemia.*

ETIOLOGY AND PATHOGENESIS

An annual incidence of 5 cases per 1 million livebirths has been estimated from registry data.[11] Well-characterized pedigrees are consistent with an autosomal dominant or, less often, recessive inheritance pattern. Sporadic cases are seen most frequently. Retrospective studies may reveal subtle hematologic or biochemical lesions, or an abnormal gene, in an affected parent or another relative without clinical anemia.[12]

Recent genetic studies have led to the characterization of Diamond-Blackfan anemia as a disease of ribosomal biogenesis.[5–7,13,14] Linkage analyses of several dozen European families mapped to a site on chromosome 19q13[15] and the finding of a translocation in one individual allowed cloning of the ribosomal protein S19 *(RPS19)* gene, which encodes a protein involved in ribosome assembly.[5–9] Most mutations are whole gene deletions, translocations or truncations; this pattern suggests a mechanism of haploinsufficiency, and *RPS19* behaves as a dominant gene.[16] (Disruption of both copies of the gene in the mouse prevents implantation.[17]) *RPS19* mutations occur in approximately 25 percent of patients with inherited red cell aplasia[16,18]; and mutations subsequently have been identified in multiple other ribosomal biogenesis genes *(RPS10, RPS26* particularly) in other cases.[16,19,20] More recently, a globin transcription factor 1 *(GATA1)* gene mutation was identified in a Diamond-Blackfan kindred, implicating a signal transduction pathway of erythroid differentiation as also causative of the syndrome.[21] Experiments have implicated *RPS14* in one of the myelodysplastic syndromes characterized by loss of 5q.[22]

Precisely how defects in ribosomal protein genes cause constitutional red cell aplasia is uncertain. Historically, Diamond-Blackfan anemia has been characterized by diminished erythroid progenitor cell numbers (colony forming unit–erythroid [CFU-E] and burst-forming unit–erythroid [BFU-E]).[23,24] In cell culture, early, erythropoietin-independent erythropoiesis is relatively normal; the major defect is in the late stage of erythropoietin-dependent erythroid cell expansion and maturation.[25] A defect in late erythroid differentiation is compatible with the classic findings of macrocytosis and increased hemoglobin F expression in inherited red cell aplasia. Granulopoiesis in the colony-forming unit–granulocyte-macrophage assay and the earlier hematopoietic progenitors as measured *in vitro* by long-term culture-initiating cell assay (an assay for an early multipotential hematopoietic progenitor) frequently are abnormal, but to a lesser degree than are CFU-E and BFU-E.[26] In a zebrafish model, deficiency of *rps19* in early embryogenesis caused a decrease in erythrocytes and also physical anomalies.[27] In tissue culture experiments, silencing of *RPS19* profoundly affects erythropoietic differentiation and, to lesser degrees, myelopoiesis.[28,29] Both *in vivo* and *in vitro* models have implicated accumulation in the cell of free ribosomal proteins, which modulates the inhibitory activity of regulators of tumor protein p53, leading to p53 stabilization and apoptosis.[30] The specificity of this molecular defect for the erythroid pathway may be a result of the extreme requirement of red cell progenitors and precursors for ribosome biogenesis.

Despite responsiveness of patients to glucocorticoids, there is little evidence of an immune mechanism, cellular or humoral, underlying inherited red cell aplasia.

CLINICAL FEATURES

Approximately one-third of patients are diagnosed at birth or within a few weeks of delivery, and almost all are identified within the first year of life.[31] Considerable variations are noted with regard to severity of phenotype, ranging from hydrops fetalis[32,33] to presentation in adulthood, when diagnosis is inferred from associated physical anomalies.[5,34] No sex predominance exists. Increased rates of prematurity in patients and of miscarriages in families have been inferred from collected cases.[35] Symptoms of anemia in early childhood include pallor, apathy, poor appetite, and "failure to thrive." Physical anomalies occur in about a third of cases; most frequent is craniofacial dysmorphism, the classic appearance described by Cathie[36] is "tow-colored hair, snub nose, wide set eyes, thick upper lips, and an intelligent expression." Malformations of the thumbs and short stature are frequent, followed by abnormalities of the urogenital system, web neck, and skeletal and cardiac defects.[11,31,37] These physical anomalies are less prevalent than the abnormalities seen in Fanconi anemia (FA).

LABORATORY FEATURES

The degree of anemia is highly variable at diagnosis. Erythrocytes may be macrocytic or normocytic. Reticulocytopenia is profound. The marrow, which usually is devoid of red blood cell precursors, may show small numbers of megaloblastoid early erythroid cells with apparent "maturation arrest." Platelets are normal or elevated. Leukocytes may be normal or slightly decreased at presentation. Neutrophils often decline with age, and in adult survivors neutropenia occasionally is severe enough to predispose to fatal infection.[38]

Erythrocyte adenosine deaminase level is elevated in approximately 75 percent of patients but also may be increased in other aregenerative anemias of childhood.[39] Serum erythropoietin level, serum iron level, and total iron-binding capacity are high. Ferritin level increases as patients receive multiple transfusions and develop iron overload if they are not treated with chelation therapy.

DIFFERENTIAL DIAGNOSIS

The characteristic triad consists of the clinical diagnostic features of anemia, reticulocytopenia, and a paucity or absence of erythroid precursors in the marrow. These findings may be supplemented by increased activity of red cell adenosine deaminase and ribosomal gene mutation analysis. FA can be excluded by cytogenetic analyses under clastogenic stress and determination of FA gene mutations (Chap. 35). Transient erythroblastopenia of childhood, which unusually occurs in the first year of life, is established by spontaneous recovery. When presentation occurs at older ages, the distinction between inherited and acquired aplastic anemia can be difficult[40]: family history, physical anomalies, and characteristic cytogenetic enzymatic, or genetic findings implicate and indicate an inherited disorder.

THERAPY, COURSE, AND PROGNOSIS

Untreated inherited pure red cell aplasia is fatal; death results from severe anemia and congestive heart failure. Transfusions, glucocorticoids, and allogeneic stem cell transplantation are of proven efficacy.[9,41] Predictors of glucocorticoid administration in glucocorticoid responsive patients include older age at presentation, a family history, and a normal platelet count. Younger age at presentation and premature birth correlate with continued red cell transfusion dependence.[42] Supportive care consists of red cell transfusions. To avoid transfusional hemosiderosis, chelation with desferrioxamine should be initiated early (Chap. 43). Injury to visceral organs from iron overload has been a major cause of death in the past.

Red cell transfusions should be leukocyte depleted to avoid alloimmunization (see Chap. 138). Erythrocytes are administered with the goal of eliminating symptoms and permitting normal growth and sexual development, usually achieved by maintaining hemoglobin levels between 7 and 9 g/dL (70 to 90 g/L).

Glucocorticoids are effective in many patients.[43] Although the mechanism of action of glucocorticoids in this disease is not understood, their toxicities are substantial, and a response is not predictable. Once the diagnosis is established, prednisone is administered orally at 2 mg/kg daily in three or four divided doses.[35,44,45] A reticulocyte response is seen in the majority of patients 1 to 4 weeks later, followed by a rise in hemoglobin level. Once the hemoglobin level reaches 9 to 10 g/dL (90 to 100 g/L), very slow reduction of the glucocorticoid dose is undertaken by decreasing the number of daily doses. When a single daily dose is achieved, an alternate-day schedule is adopted. In general, severe anemia can be avoided with continued glucocorticoid administration. The maintenance dose may be low (1 to 2 mg/day). Some patients may tolerate complete withdrawal of prednisone, but relapse is frequent and most responders become glucocorticoid dependent. A variety of patterns of response have been described, ranging from prompt recovery and apparent cure to refractoriness after a long period of responsiveness.[35] Conversely, a second trial of glucocorticoids years after an apparent therapeutic failure may be successful. In a series of 76 patients followed for many years, 59 were treated with prednisone; 31 initially responded, and two of the 25 who initially failed later responded.[44] Glucocorticoid responsiveness is strongly associated with better survival, and patients who require low doses of prednisone, or those few who spontaneously remit, may have normal life expectancies. Long-term use of high-dose prednisone results in significant toxicity, including some combination of growth retardation, cushingoid facies, buffalo hump, osteoporosis, aseptic necrosis of the hip and fractures, diabetes, hypertension, and cataracts. Red cell transfusions with iron chelation may be preferable to such an outcome.

Allogeneic stem cell marrow transplantation, when successful, is curative (Chap. 23), but the procedure has not been widely applied to children responding to medical measures. The median life expectancy of patients requiring transfusions and iron chelation is 30 to 40 years. A less-favorable outcome is related to poor compliance and cardiac and hepatic disease from iron overload.[46] Because of the morbidity and mortality associated with allogeneic stem cell transplant, most patients have been transplanted late in their disease course, after large numbers of transfusions, accumulation of heavy iron loads, and alloimmunization. Despite the poor predictive factors, 15 of 19 patients of the first published series of cases survived 5 months to many years posttransplant.[37] Comparable survival rates have been reported from European[47] and Japanese registries.[48] Stem cell transplantation from unrelated stem cell donors or use of cord blood stem cells[47,49] has been less successful. Recurrent red cell aplasia despite full engraftment was reported in one child after transplantation.[50]

Other therapies have not gained wide acceptance despite promising pilot studies, including interleukin-3 (IL-3),[51] high-dose methylprednisolone,[52] cyclosporine and other immunosuppressive agents,[53,54] and prolactin induction by metoclopropamide.[55] Leucine, which is effective in animal models,[56] is in clinical trials.

With better survival, the risk of late development of leukemia has become apparent.[14,43] Four of 76 patients followed at Children's Hospital in Boston died of acute myelogenous leukemia, with a calculated relative risk of greater than 200 times expected.[44]

Gene transfer *in vitro* has functionally corrected cells defective in *RSP19*,[57] and in animal models corrected cells show improved erythropoiesis and a survival advantage *in vivo*[58] offering the possibility of gene therapy.

⬤TRANSIENT APLASTIC CRISIS AND TRANSIENT ERYTHROBLASTOPENIA OF CHILDHOOD

DEFINITION AND HISTORY

Temporary failure of erythropoiesis is clinically identical to pure red cell aplasia except for spontaneous resolution of symptoms and of the laboratory findings of normocytic and normochromic anemia and marrow erythroid hypoplasia, usually over the course of a few weeks. Erythrocyte production is halted: (1) by acute primate erythroparvovirus 1 (B19 parvovirus) infection, typically in the context of underlying hemolytic disease (called transient aplastic crisis); (2) in normal children, usually after an infection by another [unknown] childhood virus (transient erythroblastopenia of childhood); or (3) as a transient reaction to a drug.

An anemic crisis was described in the 1940s first by Lyngar[59] and then by Owren,[60] Gasser,[3] and Dameshek and Bloom[61] in kindreds with hereditary spherocytosis. Several children within a family suffered anemic crises and exhibited low, rather than the usually high, reticulocyte numbers. Transient aplastic crisis also was noted as a complication of sickle cell disease.[62,63] Marrow examination showed decrease or absence of erythroid precursor cells, and often giant erythroblasts.[60,61] An infectious etiology was suspected from the history of a preceding febrile illness in families and its simultaneous occurrence in siblings. After the serendipitous discovery of B19 parvovirus in a normal blood donor, Pattison and colleagues screened large numbers of stored sera for evidence of recent infection. Immunoglobulin (Ig) M antibody or viral antigen was found in the blood of Jamaican children in London, all of whom had transient aplastic crisis of sickle cell disease.[64] B19 parvovirus later was established as the agent also responsible for fifth disease.[65] In the large cohort of sickle cell patients in Jamaica reported by Serjeant and colleagues,[66,67] virtually all episodes of transient aplastic crisis could be linked to B19 parvovirus. In retrospect, red cell aplasias blamed on kwashiorkor, vitamin deficiency, bacterial infections, and chemical exposures likely represented parvovirus infection.

Gasser[3] described erythroblastopenia in normal children who ultimately recovered[60]; the disease was recognized as an entity by Wranne[68] in the 1970s. Transient erythroblastopenia of childhood has an unclear etiology but may represent a postviral immune-mediated syndrome. The syndrome is rare and may be declining in incidence.[69]

ETIOLOGY AND PATHOGENESIS

B19 parvovirus, a small DNA virus, commonly infects humans. Most of the adult population has IgG antibodies specific to B19.[65] The virus is tropic for erythroid progenitor cells,[70] mainly because of their P antigen or globoside, the receptor for entry of B19 into the cell[71,72] (Fig. 36–1). Infection lyses the target cell and abrogates erythropoiesis *in vitro* and *in vivo*. Reticulocytopenia probably accompanies B19 parvovirus infection in all infected persons.[73] Anemia only manifests if red cell survival is decreased. Infection ordinarily is terminated by production of neutralizing antibodies to the virus (when such antibodies are absent, persistence of the virus produces chronic pure red cell aplasia). B19 parvovirus may appear in epidemics of fifth disease in the normal population and of transient aplastic crisis, for example, in hematology clinics specializing in sickle cell disease.[74,75] In fifth disease, IgM antibody is present in the blood, and virus levels are either low or are not detectable. Symptoms and signs of a typical "slapped cheek" cutaneous eruption and arthralgia or arthritis are secondary to antibody–virus immune complex deposition.

In contrast, in transient aplastic crisis, high concentrations of virus are present in the circulation, and patients do not develop fifth disease. In children with sickle cell disease, the incidence of B19 parvovirus infection was estimated at approximately 11 percent, and 75 percent of patients were infected by age 20 years.[76] In this setting, parvovirus infection was associated with transient aplastic crisis, a higher frequency of fever, pain, acute chest syndrome, and acute splenic sequestration syndrome.[76] As in normal individuals, parvovirus infection can be asymptomatic in sickle cell disease.[77]

The origins of transient erythroblastopenia of childhood are poorly understood. An apparent viral prodrome is typical,[78] and temporal and seasonal clustering of cases may occur.[79–81] With rare exception,[82] B19 parvovirus is not the etiology,[83,84] and no other virus has been consistently implicated.[78] Erythroid colony numbers (Chap. 32) usually are low.[85] An immune pathophysiology has been inferred from *in vitro* experiments in which IgG from sera of patients inhibited erythropoiesis[86] in the majority of cases.[87] Cell-mediated mechanisms also may play a causal role. In one report, T-cell depletion led to a dramatic increase in CFU-E formation.[88] A possible relationship between transient erythroblastopenia of childhood and inherited red cell aplasia has been suggested by the clustering of polymorphic alleles in familial transient erythroblastopenia.[89]

The same drugs implicated in chronic pure red cell aplasia apply to transient erythropoietic failure.[90] Laboratory investigations of red cell aplasia secondary to diphenylhydantoin[91] and rifampicin[92] are consistent with a hapten mechanism, in which serum antibody affects erythroid progenitor cells only in the presence of drug.

CLINICAL FEATURES

Transient aplastic crisis typically occurs in younger patients who are chronically anemic as a result of hereditary spherocytosis, sickle cell

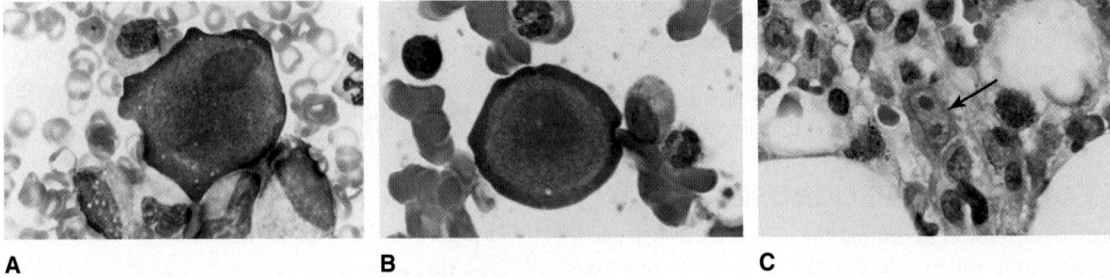

Figure 36–1. A and **B.** Giant early erythroblast precursors in the marrow aspirate of a patient with chronic pure red cell aplasia secondary to persistent B19 parvovirus infection. Note the nuclear inclusions (darker nuclear shading) representing parvovirus infection. **C.** Marrow biopsy section. The arrows point to binucleate erythroid precursor cell with nuclear inclusions representing parvovirus infection. *(Reproduced with permission from Lichtman's Atlas of Hematology, www.accessmedicine.com.)*

disease, or another hemolytic anemia. The decrease in erythropoiesis results in more evident pallor, fatigue on exertion or at rest, lassitude, and dyspnea on exertion. Gastrointestinal complaints or headache may be associated.[93] Parvovirus infection can unmask previously undiagnosed underlying hemolytic anemia. Physical examination may reveal signs of anemia, such as pallor, tachycardia, and a flow murmur. No rash or joint swelling is seen. Elevated serum bilirubin or overt icterus may be a clue to underlying hemolysis.

Transient erythroblastopenia of childhood presents as an acute anemia in a previously well child. The syndrome has an estimated incidence rate of 4 to 5 cases per 1 million children.[94–96] Transient erythroblastopenia is a frequent diagnosis in children with severe anemia,[95,97] and is the most common cause of acquired red cell aplasia in pediatric patients.[94,98] Most patients are 1 to 3 years old,[97,98] but transient erythroblastopenia of childhood can occur in the first year of life and through adolescence. Rare complications include seizures and transient neurologic abnormalities.[99–101]

LABORATORY EVALUATION

In both syndromes, anemia is the hallmark, and hemoglobin levels may be markedly depressed. Reticulocytes usually are absent from the blood, and erythroid precursor cells are not present or markedly decreased in the marrow. Red cell indices are normal. White blood cell and platelet counts are normal or elevated. Occasionally, neutropenia and thrombocytopenia of mild or moderate degree are present (especially if splenic function is intact, as in hereditary spherocytosis and in transient erythroblastopenia of childhood).[97] If the episode is brief and diagnosed during marrow recovery, patients may present with reticulocytosis, and nucleated red blood cells may be seen on the blood film.

DIFFERENTIAL DIAGNOSIS

The reticulocyte count readily distinguishes the cause of increasing anemia in a patient with hemolytic disease as transient aplastic crisis. The most important differential diagnosis for transient erythroblastopenia of childhood is inherited pure red cell aplasia. For the former, the age at presentation is older, the patient usually has no family history (but transient erythroblastopenia of childhood may be familial and can occur simultaneously in siblings),[102] physical anomalies are absent, and the syndrome resolves spontaneously.

In transient erythroblastopenia of childhood (in contrast to inherited red cell aplasia), erythrocyte adenosine deaminase levels are normal, and red cells do not show "stress" patterns of fetal hemoglobin and i antigen (red cell antigen expressed primarily on feral erythrocytes) expression. The patient's medical history, the red cell indices, and appropriate serum assays should allow prompt exclusion of more common causes of anemia in children, such as iron deficiency or other nutritional deficiencies. When transient erythroblastopenia is associated with neutropenia, acute lymphoblastic leukemia and aplastic anemia may be suspected: marrow examination clarifies the diagnosis.[103] A record of current medications, more important in adults, may provide the basis for a tentative diagnosis of drug-induced rather than idiopathic disease.

THERAPY, COURSE, AND PROGNOSIS

Transient aplastic crisis resolves as neutralizing antibodies to B19 parvovirus are made, usually within 1 to 2 weeks of infection. Ensuing reticulocytosis may be brisk, and the hemoglobin may transiently rise to higher-than-normal values. White cell and platelet numbers may "rebound," and some bone pain from marrow expansion may be present. Severe anemia may require transfusion of red blood cells (Chap. 138). No established role for administration of immunoglobulin exists.

Transient erythroblastopenia of childhood typically terminates after a few weeks, but anemia may persist occasionally for months.[98] Transfusions may be required during that interval. Overtreatment of a self-limited illness and misdiagnosis of a more serious disease are to be avoided.

For drug-associated transient failure of erythropoiesis, the suspected offending drug is discontinued and the diagnosis established from subsequent clinical improvement.

●ACQUIRED PURE RED CELL APLASIA

DEFINITION AND HISTORY

Acquired pure red cell aplasia is an uncommon cause of anemia that occurs principally in older adults. The blood counts and marrow appearance are indistinguishable from the picture of Diamond-Blackfan anemia, that is, anemia, severe reticulocytopenia, and absent marrow erythroid precursor cells. The nosologic origins of acquired pure red cell aplasia are obscure. Early descriptions are intermixed with those of aplastic anemia (in retrospect, a poor term for generalized marrow failure). Kaznelson[104] is credited with the first case report in 1922. Early distinction of the two syndromes was stimulated by the relationship of red cell aplasia to thymoma. Although red cell aplasia shares with aplastic anemia an immune pathophysiology and responsiveness to immunosuppressive therapies, the absence of involvement of neutrophils, monocytes, and platelets makes the diagnostic distinction evident. Many of the diverse clinical associations (Table 36–1) are consistent with an immune-mediated pathophysiology. The mechanism

TABLE 36–1. Classification of Pure Red Cell Aplasia

Fetal red cell aplasia (nonimmune hydrops fetalis)

Parvovirus B19 *in utero*

Inherited (Diamond-Blackfan anemia)

RPS19 and other RPS mutations

Acquired

Transient pure red cell aplasia

Acute B19 parvovirus infection in hemolytic disease (transient aplastic crisis; ~100% of cases)

Transient erythroblastopenia of childhood

Chronic pure red cell aplasia

Idiopathic

Large granular lymphocytic leukemia

Chronic lymphocytic leukemia

Clonal myeloid diseases (especially 5q-syndrome)

Persistent B19 parvovirus infection in immunodeficient host (~15% of cases)

Thymoma

Collagen vascular diseases

Post–stem cell transplantation

Anti-ABO antibodies

Drug induced

Antierythropoietin antibodies

Pregnancy

of red cell failure is best understood for T cell–mediated autoimmune destruction and persistent B19 parvovirus infection.

ETIOLOGY AND PATHOGENESIS

Immune-Mediated Erythropoietic Failure

Clinical and laboratory evidence supports both antibody and cellular mechanisms of inhibition of erythropoiesis. Red cell aplasia is associated with autoimmune diseases, such as rheumatoid arthritis, systemic lupus erythematosus, myasthenia gravis, autoimmune hemolytic anemia, acquired hypoimmunoglobulinemia, autoimmune polyglandular syndrome, and especially thymoma, and with lymphoproliferative processes, such as chronic lymphocytic leukemia (CLL) and Hodgkin disease, in which immune dysregulation is common. Serum inhibitors can be detected in the laboratory. Krantz and colleagues showed that immunoglobulin fractions from the patient's blood inhibited heme synthesis and red cell progenitor assays *in vitro*.[87] Antibodies that inhibit BFU-E and CFU-E colony formation are present frequently in patients with red cell aplasia. A pathophysiologic role can be inferred, first from the response of patients to specific treatments directed at antibodies, such as plasmapheresis and a monoclonal antibody to a cluster of differentiation molecule expressed on the surface of all mature B cells, CD20, and second from decreased or absent plasma antibody in recovered patients. Antibodies may be involved in the red cell aplasia of pregnancy.[105]

Autoantibodies to erythropoietin rarely have caused this disease.[106,107] More frequently, red cell aplasia secondary to antibodies is elicited by administration of recombinant erythropoietin to patients undergoing renal dialysis.[108–113] Anemia can be profound, and some patients remain transfusion dependent despite discontinuation of hormone therapy. Glycosylation of recombinant erythropoietin is different from the native molecule, but antibodies are directed against conformational epitopes of the protein and not to the sugar moieties. Erythropoietin immunogenicity associates with human leukocyte antigen (HLA) specificities.[114] The second example of antibodies of known specificity causing red cell aplasia occurs after hematopoietic stem cell transplantation using donors mismatched at a major ABO locus, which can lead to delayed donor erythroid engraftment or late erythropoietic failure.[115–118] In most instances, however, the target antigen(s) responsible for this outcome is(are) not known.

Suppression of erythropoiesis by T cells may be more common than antibody inhibition as a mechanism of erythropoietic failure.[119] Suggestive clinical observations include the frequent association of red cell aplasia with CLL (Chap. 92) in approximately 6 percent of cases[120]; CLL is also associated with autoimmune hemolytic anemia and idiopathic thrombocytopenic purpura[121] and with large granular lymphocytic leukemia (LGL; Chap. 94) in approximately 7 percent of cases.[122] In a series of 47 red cell aplasia patients, four had CLL and nine had LGL.[123] More sensitive flow cytometric and molecular methods may detect clonal T-cell expansion in patients with normal numbers of circulating lymphocytes.[124,125] An attractive molecular mechanism underlying CD8 cell expansion is signal transducer and activator of transcription 3 gene mutations (*STAT3*), leading to constitutive activation of a clone of cytotoxic T cells, which is relatively frequent in patients with large granular lymphocytosis[126] and has been described in patients with pure red cell aplasia.[127–129] Functionally, lymphocytes from patients with idiopathic pure red cell aplasia[130–132] or red cell aplasia associated with CLL,[133,134] LGL,[135–137] thymoma,[138] other lymphoid malignancies,[139,140] Epstein-Barr virus infection,[141] and human T-cell leukemia virus 1 infection[142] suppressed erythropoiesis in colony assays. Several mechanisms of cell killing have been suggested.[122,143] When effector cells show histocompatibility locus A class I–restricted killing, recognition of a specific antigen peptide is implied by a T cell with an $\alpha\beta$ T-cell receptor.[144]

In one man with red cell aplasia and LGL, erythropoiesis was inhibited by non–MHC (major histocompatibility) antigen-restricted $\gamma\delta$ T cells that lysed CFU-E. T cells downregulated class I histocompatibility antigens and thus were unable to engage the natural killer cell's inhibitory receptors.[137]

Persistent B19 Parvovirus Infection

B19 parvovirus specifically infects and is toxic to erythroid progenitor cells. Parvovirus infection normally is terminated within 1 to 2 weeks of infection by the humoral immune response. Linear neutralizing epitopes are localized to a relatively small region of the capsid protein.[145] In the absence of an effective antibody response, infection persists and causes pure red cell aplasia.[65,145] Erythropoietic failure may be the only evidence of parvoviral infection. Persistence of B19 parvovirus infection may occur in the setting of immunodeficiency (Chap. 80), most commonly caused by chemotherapeutic and immunosuppressive drugs,[146] human immunodeficiency virus 1 infection,[147] and occasionally with Nezelof syndrome's subtle immunologic abnormalities.[148] Parvovirus at one time may have accounted for approximately 15 percent of severe anemia in patients with AIDS,[149] but highly effective antiretroviral drug regimens have reduced its role.[150,151] Persistent B19 parvovirus infection can occur in the fetus exposed during the midtrimester of pregnancy (Chap. 55). The infection can cause hydrops fetalis as a result of viral cytotoxicity for erythroid progenitors in the fetal liver and death of the newborn as a result of severe anemia and congestive heart failure.[65] In rare instances, parvovirus-infected or hydropic infants rescued by red cell transfusion show congenital red cell aplasia or dyserythropoietic anemia.[33]

Intrinsic Cellular Defects Leading to Failed Red Blood Cell Production

Red cell aplasia can be the first or the major manifestation of myelodysplasia.[152] Discrete genetic defects can lead to failure of erythropoiesis. Activating point mutations in *N-RAS*, an oncogene in the RAS family occur in some cases of myelodysplastic syndrome.[153,154] Mutant *N-RAS in vitro* can induce a proliferative defect in erythroid progenitor cells.[155] Loss of the *RPS14* gene in 5q– deletions leads to red cell aplasia in this myelodysplastic syndrome.[22,156] *In vitro* colony formation may distinguish such intrinsic cellular defects from immune mediated marrow failure, with higher BFU-E numbers predicting response to immunosuppressive therapies.[157]

Medications

Idiosyncratic drug reactions account for a far smaller proportion of red cell aplasia than of agranulocytosis (Chap. 65). Case reports have implicated various agents, such as diphenylhydantoin, sulfa and sulfonamide drugs, azathioprine, allopurinol, isoniazid, procainamide, ticlopidine, ribavirin, and penicillamine. Causality is impossible to assign from case reports; with nonsteroidal antiinflammatory drugs, gold, and colchicine, the underlying rheumatic syndrome may be the etiologic link.

CLINICAL FEATURES

Symptomatic anemia in the older patient may manifest as pallor, fatigue, lassitude, pulsatile tinnitus, and anginal chest pain (Chap. 34). Iatrogenic Cushing syndrome and the physical stigmata of secondary hemochromatosis are seen in patients after prolonged glucocorticoid administration and long-term red cell transfusion therapy. Concomitant diseases include CLL and lymphomas, collagen vascular disorders, myasthenia gravis, especially in the setting of thymoma, and some cancers. Red cell aplasia also occurs with pregnancy. Persistent B19 parvovirus infection should be suspected in the anemic cancer patient after stem cell transplantation, in patients treated with immunosuppressive drugs, in patients with AIDS, and in patients with a family or personal history suggestive of inherited immune disorder. Other viral infections have been implicated in pure red cell aplasia, including infectious mononucleosis and an unknown agent in seronegative hepatitis.

LABORATORY FEATURES

Anemia is either normocytic or macrocytic, reticulocytopenia is profound, and white cell and platelet counts are generally normal. The marrow shows absent or very few erythroid precursor cells, but normal granulopoiesis and megakaryocytopoiesis. Iron saturation and ferritin level frequently are elevated and rise further after repeated red cell transfusions. Erythroid colony assays may predict responsiveness to immunosuppressive treatment. The presence of marrow or blood BFU-E and CFU-E correlates with hematologic improvement,[130,158,159] but these tests may not be generally available.

Thymomas are frequently associated with autoimmune disease, myasthenia gravis most prominently and occasionally with marrow failure syndromes.[160] In pure red cell aplasia, a thymoma should be sought by chest imaging, including computed tomographic scan. The association of thymoma and pure red cell aplasia has been emphasized but is uncommon: thymoma in only two of 37 red cell aplasia patients,[161] and only two instances of red cell aplasia in a series of 29 thymoma patients.[162] The thymomas usually are encapsulated and have a spindle cell histology. In one series, 10 of 56 cases were considered malignant because of their locally infiltrating character[163]; therefore, the tumors should be surgically excised, if feasible.

CLL should be evident based on elevated lymphocyte count and immunophenotyping for monoclonality. LGL (Chap. 94), which frequently underlies red cell aplasia, may be more subtle. It's diagnosis requires careful examination of the blood film for typical lymphocytic forms, flow cytometry for cell surface markers characteristic of natural killer and cytotoxic lymphocytes, and demonstration of monoclonal T-cell proliferation by molecular studies.

Persistent parvovirus infection can be difficult to diagnose. Giant pronormoblasts scattered on the marrow film are the most characteristic of the condition (see Fig. 36–1), but such typical cells may not be observed. Marrow morphologies that are dysplastic or suggestive of leukemia also have been described. Serum antibodies specific to the virus are absent or only IgM is positive. Parvovirus DNA should be present in high concentrations in the blood and readily detected by molecular techniques.

DIFFERENTIAL DIAGNOSIS

Distinction between inherited and acquired red cell aplasia may be impossible in the younger patient. Rarely, pure red cell aplasia is difficult to distinguish from more generalized marrow failure if other blood counts are borderline. A dysmorphic marrow smear and abnormal chromosomes point to myelodysplasia as responsible for isolated anemia and reticulocytopenia. B19 parvovirus infection should always be suspected and searched for in any immunosuppressed individual who is anemic because the infection can be treated.

THERAPY, COURSE, AND PROGNOSIS

Treatment

Transfusion Therapy As with inherited red cell aplasia, transfusions and iron chelation are basic to management.[164] In an adult, 1 unit of packed erythrocytes per week can replace marrow erythropoiesis, which

for convenience usually is transfused as 2 units every 2 weeks. The goal of preventing symptoms of anemia is achievable in most patients if the nadir hemoglobin is greater than 7 g/dL (70 g/L). A goal greater than 9 g/dL (90 g/L) may be preferable in patients with cardiac or pulmonary disease and in older patients. Even refractory pure red cell aplasia is consistent with a prolonged and perhaps even normal life expectancy, and iron-chelation therapy can be initiated based on the ferritin level (Chap. 43).

Immunosuppression Immunosuppressive agents are used to treat disease of suspected immune origin. Response is likely in the majority of patients, but sequential treatment with a variety of agents often is required. Some patients, however, remain refractory to treatment.[119,164-166] Typically, oral prednisone 1 to 2 mg/kg/day is given first, and about half of patients improve. A 1- to 2-month trial can be associated with significant toxicity and evidence of Cushing syndrome. Higher response rates have been cited for cyclosporine, and some investigators advocate using this drug first.[53,167-171] Cytotoxic agents, especially azathioprine and cyclophosphamide,[172] can be beneficial but are not first-choice because of their mutagenic and leukemogenic properties. These drugs may be preferred for red cell aplasia associated with LGL, in which cytoreduction is required.[124,173,174] Acquired pure red cell aplasia often responds to antithymocyte globulin.[130,159,175] More specific monoclonal antibodies have less toxicity than does antilymphocyte globulin, and can be administered without hospitalization.[176] Daclizumab, a monoclonal antibody directed against the IL-2 receptor, is effective in approximately 40 percent of patients.[177] Success has been reported also using rituximab (anti-CD20 monoclonal antibody)[178-180] and alemtuzumab (anti-CD52).[181-183] Some patients with resistant disease respond to fludarabine and cladribine.[184,185] Plasmapheresis[186,187] has produced long-lasting improvement in a few patients, presumably by removing pathogenic antibodies.[186] The absence of randomized trials and even case series of adequate sample size makes the extrapolation of case reports to quantitative estimates of response problematic for many of these therapies.[164]

A thymoma should be excised to prevent local spread of a malignant tumor, but thymectomy does not necessarily improve marrow function.[163] Red cell aplasia can follow thymectomy. Cyclosporine appears the most effective drug to treat pure red cell aplasia associated with thymoma.[188] Red cell aplasia is rarely an indication for stem cell transplantation because the anemia usually can be managed with less drastic approaches. Unresponsive patients have been cured by infusion of allogeneic stem cells after cyclophosphamide conditioning.[189,190]

Other Therapies Despite early favorable case reports, androgens, erythropoietin, and splenectomy are not routinely used to treat pure red cell aplasia.

Immunoglobulin for Persistent B19 Parvovirus Infection Persistent parvovirus infection results from the inability of the host to mount an effective humoral immune response. It can be effectively treated in almost all cases by administration of commercial immunoglobulin,[191,192] an excellent source of neutralizing antibodies present in a large proportion of the normal population. Infusion of immunoglobulin at 0.4 g/kg/day for 5 to 10 days should produce brisk reticulocytosis and restore a hemoglobin level appropriate for the patient. A single course may be adequate to cure longstanding red cell aplasia resulting from an underlying inherited immunodeficiency syndrome,[193] but patients with AIDS may not show complete clearance of parvovirus from the circulation and may relapse, requiring retreatment[147] or maintenance immunoglobulin injections (Fig. 36–2).[147,194] Patients suffering from persistent B19 parvovirus infection do not have typical manifestations of a viral infection, such as fever. In these patients, immunoglobulin infusions can induce fifth disease symptoms of variable severity, including cutaneous eruptions and arthritis. Older case reports of red cell aplasia

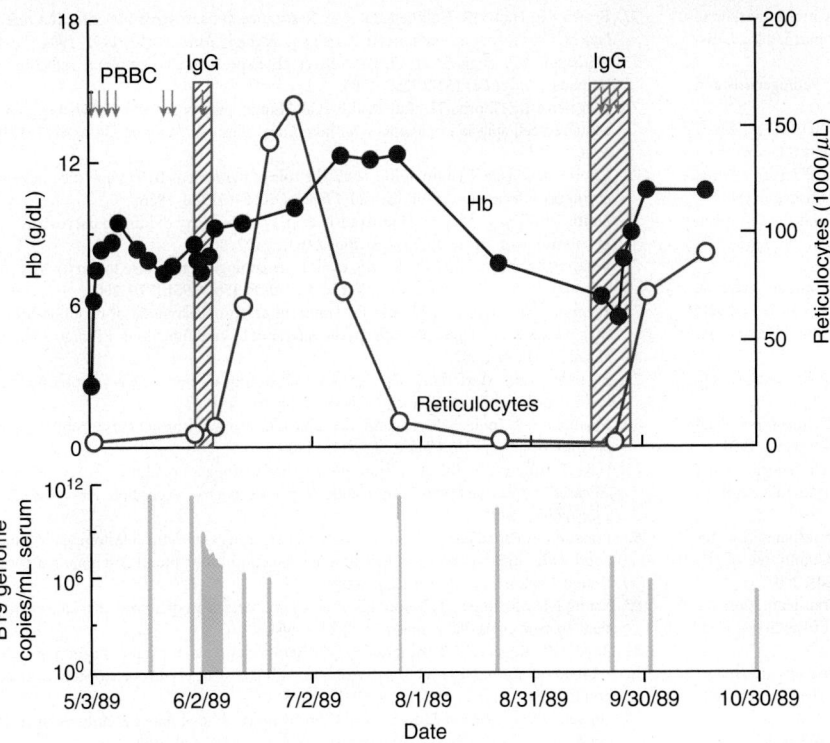

Figure 36–2. Diagram of the clinical course of a HIV-1–infected patient with red cell aplasia caused by B19 persistent parvovirus.[123] Note the increase of the reticulocyte count (open circles) to the first infusion of immunoglobulin (Ig) G (hatched bar) and the subsequent decline in parvovirus titers. Thereafter, the reticulocyte count and the hemoglobin (Hgb) concentration (closed circles) decrease, reflecting the return of the anemia. A second IgG treatment increases the reticulocyte count and Hgb concentration and decreases the parvovirus titers. PRBC, packed red blood cells.

responsive to immunoglobulin infusions likely represent treatment of patients with previously unrecognized parvovirus infection.

REFERENCES

1. Joseph WH: Anemia of infancy and early childhood. *Medicine (Baltimore)* 15:307, 1936.
2. Diamond LK, Blackfan KD: Hypoplastic anemia. *Am J Dis Child* 56:464, 1938.
3. Gasser C: Aplasia of erythropoiesis; acute and chronic erythroblastopenias or pure (red cell) aplastic anaemias in childhood. *Pediatr Clin North Am* 445, 1957.
4. Diamond LK, Wang WC, Alter BP: Congenital hypoplastic anemia. *Adv Pediatr* 22:349, 1976.
5. Farrar JE, Dahl N: Untangling the phenotypic heterogeneity of Diamond Blackfan anemia. *Semin Hematol* 48(2):124, 2011.
6. Ellis SR, Lipton JM: Diamond Blackfan anemia: A disorder of red blood cell development. *Curr Top Dev Biol* 82:217, 2008.
7. Khincha PP, Savage SA: Genomic characterization of the inherited bone marrow failure syndromes. *Semin Hematol* 50(4):333, 2013.
8. Vlachos A, Blanc L, Lipton JM: Diamond Blackfan anemia: A model for the translational approach to understanding human disease. *Expert Rev Hematol* 7(3):359, 2014.
9. Narla A, Vlachos A, Nathan DG: Diamond Blackfan anemia treatment: Past, present, and future. *Semin Hematol* 48(2):117, 2011.
10. Rodon P, Breton P, Courouble G: Treatment of pure red cell aplasia and autoimmune haemolytic anaemia in chronic lymphocytic leukaemia with Campath-1H. *Eur J Haematol* 70(5):319, 2003.
11. Ball SE, McGuckin CP, Jenkins G, et al: Diamond-Blackfan anaemia in the U.K.: Analysis of 80 cases from a 20-year birth cohort. *Br J Haematol* 94(4):645, 1996.
12. Orfali KA, Ohene-Abuakwa Y, Ball SE: Diamond Blackfan anaemia in the UK: Clinical and genetic heterogeneity. *Br J Haematol* 125(2):243–52, 2005.
13. Dianzani I, Loreni F: Diamond-Blackfan anemia: A ribosomal puzzle. *Haematologica* 93(11):1601, 2008.
14. Lipton JM: Diamond blackfan anemia: New paradigms for a "not so pure" inherited red cell aplasia. *Semin Hematol* 43(3):167, 2006.
15. Gustavsson P, Willing TN, van Haeringen A, et al: Diamond-Blackfan anaemia: Genetic homogeneity for a gene on chromosome 19q13 restricted to 1.8 Mb. *Nat Genet* 16(4):368, 1997.
16. Campagnoli MF, Ramenghi U, Armiraglio M, et al: RPS19 mutations in patients with Diamond-Blackfan anemia. *Hum Mutat* 29(7):911, 2008.
17. Matsson H, Davey EJ, Draptchinskaia N, et al: Targeted disruption of the ribosomal protein S19 gene is lethal prior to implantation. *Mol Cell Biol* 24(9):4032, 2004.
18. Willig TN, Draptchinskaia N, Dianzani I, et al: Mutations in ribosomal protein S19 gene and diamond blackfan anemia: Wide variations in phenotypic expression. *Blood* 94(12):4294, 1999.
19. Boria I, Quarello P, Avondo F, et al: A new database for ribosomal protein genes which are mutated in Diamond-Blackfan Anemia. *Hum Mutat* 29(11):E263, 2008.
20. Doherty L, Sheen MR, Vlachos A, et al: Ribosomal protein genes RPS10 and RPS26 are commonly mutated in Diamond-Blackfan anemia. *Am J Hum Genet* 86(2):222, 2010.
21. Sankaran VG, Ghazvinian R, Do R, et al: Exome sequencing identifies GATA1 mutations resulting in Diamond-Blackfan anemia. *J Clin Invest* 122(7):2439, 2012.
22. Ebert BL, Pretz J, Bosco J, et al: Identification of RPS14 as a 5q− syndrome gene by RNA interference screen. *Nature* 451(7176):335, 2008.
23. Perdahl EB, Naprstek BL, Wallace WC, et al: Erythroid failure in Diamond-Blackfan anemia is characterized by apoptosis. *Blood* 83(3):645, 1994.
24. Casadevall N, Croisille L, Auffray I, et al: Age-related alterations in erythroid and granulopoietic progenitors in Diamond-Blackfan anaemia. *Br J Haematol* 87(2):369, 1994.
25. Ohene-Abuakwa Y, Orfali KA, Marius C, et al: Two-phase culture in Diamond Blackfan anemia: Localization of erythroid defect. *Blood* 105(2):838, 2005.
26. Giri N, Kang E, Tisdale JF, et al: Clinical and laboratory evidence for a trilineage haematopoietic defect in patients with refractory Diamond-Blackfan anaemia. *Br J Haematol* 108(1):167, 2000.
27. Uechi T, Nakajima Y, Chakraborty A, et al: Deficiency of ribosomal protein S19 during early embryogenesis leads to reduction of erythrocytes in a zebrafish model of Diamond-Blackfan anemia. *Hum Mol Genet* 17(20):3204, 2008.
28. Flygare J, Olsson K, Richter J, Karlsson S: Gene therapy of Diamond Blackfan anemia CD34(+) cells leads to improved erythroid development and engraftment following transplantation. *Exp Hematol* 36(11):1428–35, 2008.
29. Miyake K, Flygare J, Keifer T, et al: Deficiency of ribosomal protein S19 in CD34+ cells generated by siRNA blocks erythroid development and mimics defects seen in Diamond-Blackfan anemia. *Blood* 105(12):4627–34, 2005.
30. Raiser DM, Narla A, Ebert BL: The emerging importance of ribosomal dysfunction in the pathogenesis of hematologic disorders. *Leuk Lymphoma* 55(3):491, 2014.
31. Halperin DS, Freedman MH: Diamond-Blackfan anemia: Etiology, pathophysiology, and treatment. *Am J Pediatr Hematol Oncol* 11(4):380, 1989.
32. Scimeca PG, Weinblatt ME, Slepowitz G, et al: Diamond-Blackfan syndrome: An unusual cause of hydrops fetalis. *Am J Pediatr Hematol Oncol* 10(3):241, 1988.
33. Brown KE, Green SW, Antunez de Mayolo J, et al: Congenital anaemia after transplacental B19 parvovirus infection. *Lancet* 343(8902):895, 1994.
34. Balaban EP, Buchanan GR, Graham M, et al: Diamond-Blackfan syndrome in adult patients. *Am J Med* 78(3):533, 1985.
35. Alter BP: Diamond-Blackfan anemia, in *Aplastic Anemia, Acquired and Inherited*, edited by NS Young, BP Alter, p 361. WB Saunders, Philadelphia, 1994.
36. Cathie IA: Erythrogenesis imperfecta. *Arch Dis Child* 25(124):313, 1950.
37. Tisdale J, Dunbar CE: Pure red cell aplasia, in *The Bone Marrow Failure Syndromes*, edited by NS Young, p 135. WB Saunders, Philadelphia, 2000.
38. Schofield KP, Evans DI: Diamond-Blackfan syndrome and neutropenia. *J Clin Pathol* 44(9):742, 1991.

39. Glader BE, Backer K: Elevated red cell adenosine deaminase activity: A marker of disordered erythropoiesis in Diamond-Blackfan anaemia and other haematologic diseases. *Br J Haematol* 68(2):165, 1988.

40. Freedman MH: Pure red cell aplasia in childhood and adolescence: Pathogenesis and approaches to diagnosis. *Br J Haematol* 85(2):246, 1993.

41. Vlachos A, Muir E: How I treat Diamond-Blackfan anemia. *Blood* 116(19):3715, 2010.

42. Willig TN, Niemeyer CM, Leblanc T, et al: Identification of new prognosis factors from the clinical and epidemiologic analysis of a registry of 229 Diamond-Blackfan anemia patients. DBA group of Société d'Hématologie et d'Immunologie Pédiatrique (SHIP), Gesellshaft für Pädiatrische Onkologie und Hamatologie (GPOH), and the European Society for Pediatric Hematology and Immunology (ESPHI). *Pediatr Res* 46(5):553, 1999.

43. Vlachos A BS, Dahl N, et al: Diagnosing and treating Diamond Blackfan anaemia: Results of an international clinical consensus conference. *Br J Haematol* 142:849, 2008.

44. Janov AJ, Leong T, Nathan DG, et al: Diamond-Blackfan anemia. Natural history and sequelae of treatment. *Medicine (Baltimore)* 75(2):77, 1996.

45. Willig TN, Gazda H, Sieff CA: Diamond-Blackfan anemia. *Curr Opin Hematol* 7(2):85, 2000.

46. Navenot JM, Muller JY, Blanchard D: Expression of blood group I antigen and fetal hemoglobin in paroxysmal nocturnal hemoglobinuria. *Transfusion* 37(3):291, 1997.

47. Vlachos A, Federman N, Reyes-Haley C, et al: Hematopoietic stem cell transplantation for Diamond Blackfan anemia: A report from the Diamond Blackfan Anemia Registry. *Bone Marrow Transplant* 27(4):381, 2001.

48. Mugishima H, Ohga S, Ohara A, et al: Hematopoietic stem cell transplantation for Diamond-Blackfan anemia: A report from the Aplastic Anemia Committee of the Japanese Society of Pediatric Hematology. *Pediatr Transplant* 11(6):601, 2007.

49. Fagioli F, Quarello P, Zecca M, et al: Haematopoietic stem cell transplantation for Diamond Blackfan anaemia: A report from the Italian Association of Paediatric Haematology and Oncology Registry. *Br J Haematol* 165(5):673, 2014.

50. Wynn RF, Grainger JD, Carr TF, et al: Failure of allogeneic bone marrow transplantation to correct Diamond-Blackfan anaemia despite haemopoietic stem cell engraftment. *Bone Marrow Transplant* 24(7):803, 1999.

51. Ball SE, Tchernia G, Wranne L, et al: Is there a role for interleukin-3 in Diamond-Blackfan anaemia? Results of a European multicentre study. *Br J Haematol* 91(2):313, 1995.

52. Ozsoylu S: High-dose intravenous corticosteroid treatment for patients with Diamond-Blackfan syndrome resistant or refractory to conventional treatment. *Am J Pediatr Hematol Oncol* 10(3):217, 1988.

53. Leonard EM, Raefsky E, Griffith P, et al: Cyclosporine therapy of aplastic anaemia, congenital and acquired red cell aplasia. *Br J Haematol* 72(2):278, 1989.

54. Marmont AM: Congenital hypoplastic anaemia refractory to corticosteroids but responding to cyclophosphamide and antilymphocytic globulin. Report of a case having responded with a transitory wave of dyserythropoiesis. *Acta Haematol* 60(2):90, 1978.

55. Rutella S, Pierelli L, Bonanno G, et al: Role for granulocyte colony-stimulating factor in the generation of human T regulatory type 1 cells. *Blood* 100(7):2562, 2002.

56. Narla A, Payne EM, Abayasekara N, et al: L-Leucine improves the anaemia in models of Diamond Blackfan anaemia and the 5q– syndrome in a TP53-independent way. *Br J Haematol* 167(4):524, 2014.

57. Hamaguchi I, Ooka A, Brun A, et al: Gene transfer improves erythroid development in ribosomal protein S19-deficient Diamond-Blackfan anemia. *Blood* 100(8):2724, 2002.

58. Flygare J, Olsson K, Richter J, et al: Gene therapy of Diamond Blackfan anemia CD34(+) cells leads to improved erythroid development and engraftment following transplantation. *Exp Hematol* 36(11):1428, 2008.

59. Lyngar E: Samtidig optreden av anemisk kriser hos 3 barn i en familie med hymolytisk ikterus. *Nord Med* 14:1246, 1942.

60. Owren PA: Congenital hemolytic jaundice; the pathogenesis of the hemolytic crisis. *Blood* 3(3):231, 1948.

61. Dameshek W, Bloom ML: The events in the hemolytic crisis of hereditary spherocytosis, with particular reference to the reticulocytopenia, pancytopenia and an abnormal splenic mechanism. *Blood* 3(12):1381, 1948.

62. Chernoff AI, Josephson AM: Acute erythroblastopenia in sickle-cell anemia and infectious mononucleosis. *AMA Am J Dis Child* 82(3):310, 1951.

63. Singer K, Motulsky AG, Wile SA: Aplastic crisis in sickle cell anemia; a study of its mechanism and its relationship to other types of hemolytic crises. *J Lab Clin Med* 35(5):721, 1950.

64. Pattison JR, Jones SE, Hodgson J, et al: Parvovirus infections and hypoplastic crisis in sickle-cell anaemia. *Lancet* 1(8221):664, 1981.

65. Young NS, Brown KE: Parvovirus B19. *N Engl J Med* 350(6):586, 2004.

66. Serjeant GR, Serjeant BE, Thomas PW, et al: Human parvovirus infection in homozygous sickle cell disease. *Lancet* 341(8855):1237, 1993.

67. Serjeant GR, Topley JM, Mason K, et al: Outbreak of aplastic crises in sickle cell anaemia associated with parvovirus-like agent. *Lancet* 2(8247):595, 1981.

68. Wranne L: Transient erythroblastopenia in infancy and childhood. *Scand J Haematol* 7(2):76, 1970.

69. van den Akker M, Dror Y, Odame I: Transient erythroblastopenia of childhood is an underdiagnosed and self-limiting disease. *Acta Paediatr* 103(7):e288, 2014.

70. Young N, Harrison M, Moore J, et al: Direct demonstration of the human parvovirus in erythroid progenitor cells infected in vitro. *J Clin Invest* 74(6):2024, 1984.

71. Brown KE, Anderson SM, Young NS: Erythrocyte P antigen: Cellular receptor for B19 parvovirus. *Science* 262(5130):114, 1993.

72. Brown KE, Hibbs JR, Gallinella G, et al: Resistance to parvovirus B19 infection due to lack of virus receptor (erythrocyte P antigen). *N Engl J Med* 330(17):1192, 1994.

73. Anderson MJ, Higgins PG, Davis LR, et al: Experimental parvoviral infection in humans. *J Infect Dis* 152(2):257, 1985.

74. Saarinen UM, Chorba TL, Tattersall P, et al: Human parvovirus B19-induced epidemic acute red cell aplasia in patients with hereditary hemolytic anemia. *Blood* 67(5):1411, 1986.

75. Chorba T, Coccia P, Holman RC, et al: The role of parvovirus B19 in aplastic crisis and erythema infectiosum (fifth disease). *J Infect Dis* 154(3):383, 1986.

76. Smith-Whitley K, Zhao H, Hodinka RL, et al: Epidemiology of human parvovirus B19 in children with sickle cell disease. *Blood* 103(2):422, 2004.

77. Serjeant BE, Hambleton IR, Kerr S, et al: Haematological response to parvovirus B19 infection in homozygous sickle-cell disease. *Lancet* 358(9295):1779, 2001.

78. Skeppner G, Kreuger A, Elinder G: Transient erythroblastopenia of childhood: Prospective study of 10 patients with special reference to viral infections. *J Pediatr Hematol Oncol* 24(4):294, 2002.

79. Beresford CH, Macfarlane SD: Temporal clustering of transient erythroblastopenia (cytopenia) of childhood. *Aust Paediatr J* 23(6):351, 1987.

80. Bhambhani K, Inoue S, Sarnaik SA: Seasonal clustering of transient erythroblastopenia of childhood. *Am J Dis Child* 142(2):175, 1988.

81. Hays T, Lane PA Jr, Shafer F: Transient erythroblastopenia of childhood. A review of 26 cases and reassessment of indications for bone marrow aspiration. *Am J Dis Child* 143(5):605, 1989.

82. Prassouli A, Papadakis V, Tsakris A, et al: Classic transient erythroblastopenia of childhood with human parvovirus B19 genome detection in the blood and bone marrow. *J Pediatr Hematol Oncol* 27(6):333, 2005.

83. Young NS, Mortimer PP, Moore JG, et al: Characterization of a virus that causes transient aplastic crisis. *J Clin Invest* 73(1):224, 1984.

84. Rogers BB, Rogers ZR, Timmons CF: Polymerase chain reaction amplification of archival material for parvovirus B19 in children with transient erythroblastopenia of childhood. *Pediatr Pathol Lab Med* 16(3):471, 1996.

85. Gussetis ES, Peristeri J, Kitra V, et al: Clinical value of bone marrow cultures in childhood pure red cell aplasia. *J Pediatr Hematol Oncol* 20(2):120, 1998.

86. Koenig HM, Lightsey AL, Nelson DP, et al: Immune suppression of erythropoiesis in transient erythroblastopenia of childhood. *Blood* 54(3):742, 1979.

87. Dessypris EN, Krantz SB, Roloff JS, et al: Mode of action of the IgG inhibitor of erythropoiesis in transient erythroblastopenia of children. *Blood* 59(1):114, 1982.

88. Tamary H, Kaplinsky C, Shvartzmayer S, et al: Transient erythroblastopenia of childhood. Evidence for cell-mediated suppression of erythropoiesis. *Am J Pediatr Hematol Oncol* 15(4):386, 1993.

89. Gustavsson P, Klar J, Matsson H, et al: Familial transient erythroblastopenia of childhood is associated with the chromosome 19q13.2 region but not caused by mutations in coding sequences of the ribosomal protein S19 (RPS19) gene. *Br J Haematol* 119(1):261, 2002.

90. Thompson DF, Gales MA: Drug-induced pure red cell aplasia. *Pharmacotherapy* 16(6):1002, 1996.

91. Dessypris EN, Redline S, Harris JW, et al: Diphenylhydantoin-induced pure red cell aplasia. *Blood* 65(4):789, 1985.

92. Mariette X, Mitjavila MT, Moulinie JP, et al: Rifampicin-induced pure red cell aplasia. *Am J Med* 87(4):459, 1989.

93. Smith JC, Megason GC, Iyer RV, et al: Clinical characteristics of children with hereditary hemolytic anemias and aplastic crisis: A 7-year review. *South Med J* 87(7):702, 1994.

94. Kynaston JA, West NC, Reid MM: A regional experience of red cell aplasia. *Eur J Pediatr* 152(4):306, 1993.

95. Farhi DC, Luebbers EL, Rosenthal NS: Bone marrow biopsy findings in childhood anemia: Prevalence of transient erythroblastopenia of childhood. *Arch Pathol Lab Med* 122(7):638, 1998.

96. Skeppner G, Wranne L: Transient erythroblastopenia of childhood in Sweden. Incidence and findings at the time of diagnosis. *Acta Paediatr* 82(6-7):574, 1993.

97. Cherrick I, Karayalcin G, Lanzkowsky P: Transient erythroblastopenia of childhood. Prospective study of fifty patients. *Am J Pediatr Hematol Oncol* 16(4):320, 1994.

98. Glader BE: Diagnosis and management of red cell aplasia in children. *Hematol Oncol Clin North Am* 1(3):431, 1987.

99. Michelson AD, Marshall PC: Transient neurological disorder associated with transient erythroblastopenia of childhood. *Am J Pediatr Hematol Oncol* 9(2):161, 1987.

100. Young RS, Rannels DE, Hilmo A, et al: Severe anemia in childhood presenting as transient ischemic attacks. *Stroke* 14(4):622, 1983.

101. Chan GC, Kanwar VS, Wilimas J: Transient erythroblastopenia of childhood associated with transient neurologic deficit: Report of a case and review of the literature. *J Paediatr Child Health* 34(3):299, 1998.

102. Skeppner G, Forestier E, Henter JI, et al: Transient red cell aplasia in siblings: A common environmental or a common hereditary factor? *Acta Paediatr* 87(1):43, 1998.

103. Leuschner S, Bodewaldt-Radzun S, Rister M: Increase of CALLA-positive stimulated lymphoid cells in transient erythroblastopenia of childhood. *Eur J Pediatr* 149(8):551, 1990.

104. Kaznelson P: Zur Enstehung der Blut Plattchen. *Verh Dtsch Ges Inn Med* 34:557, 1922.

105. Baker RI, Manoharan A, de Luca E, et al: Pure red cell aplasia of pregnancy: A distinct clinical entity. *Br J Haematol* 85(3):619, 1993.

106. Peschle C, Marmont AM, Marone G, et al: Pure red cell aplasia: Studies on an IgG serum inhibitor neutralizing erythropoietin. *Br J Haematol* 30(4):411, 1975.

107. Casadevall N, Dupuy E, Molho-Sabatier P, et al: Autoantibodies against erythropoietin in a patient with pure red-cell aplasia. *N Engl J Med* 334(10):630, 1996.

108. Prabhakar SS, Muhlfelder T: Antibodies to recombinant human erythropoietin causing pure red cell aplasia. *Clin Nephrol* 47(5):331, 1997.

109. Casadevall N, Nataf J, Viron B, et al: Pure red-cell aplasia and antierythropoietin antibodies in patients treated with recombinant erythropoietin. *N Engl J Med* 346(7):469, 2002.

110. Locatelli F and Del Vecchio L. Pure red cell aplasia secondary to treatment with erythropoietin. *J Nephrol* 16(4):461, 2003.

111. Pollock C, Johnson DW, Horl WH, et al: Pure red cell aplasia induced by erythropoiesis-stimulating agents. *Clin J Am Soc Nephrol* 3(1):193, 2008.

112. McKoy JM, Stonecash RE, Cournoyer D, et al: Epoetin-associated pure red cell aplasia: Past, present, and future considerations. *Transfusion* 48(8):1754, 2008.

113. Barger TE, Wrona D, Goletz TJ, et al: A detailed examination of the antibody prevalence and characteristics of anti-ESA antibodies. *Nephrol Dial Transplant* 27(10):3892, 2012.

114. Fijal B, Ricci D, Vercammen E, et al: Case-control study of the association between select HLA genes and anti-erythropoietin antibody-positive pure red-cell aplasia. *Pharmacogenomics* 9(2):157, 2008.

115. Bolan CD, Leitman SF, Griffith LM, et al: Delayed donor red cell chimerism and pure red cell aplasia following major ABO-incompatible nonmyeloablative hematopoietic stem cell transplantation. *Blood* 98(6):1687, 2001.

116. Grigg AP, Juneja SK: Pure red cell aplasia with the onset of graft versus host disease. *Bone Marrow Transplant* 32(11):1099, 2003.

117. Hayden PJ, Gardiner N, Molloy K, et al: Pure red cell aplasia after a major ABO-mismatched bone marrow transplant for chronic myeloid leukaemia: Response to re-introduction of cyclosporin. *Bone Marrow Transplant* 33(4):459, 2004.

118. Helbig G, Stella-Holowiecka B, Wojnar J, et al: Pure red-cell aplasia following major and bi-directional ABO-incompatible allogeneic stem-cell transplantation: Recovery of donor-derived erythropoiesis after long-term treatment using different therapeutic strategies. *Ann Hematol* 86(9):677, 2007.

119. Charles RJ, Sabo KM, Kidd PG, et al: The pathophysiology of pure red cell aplasia: Implications for therapy. *Blood* 87(11):4831, 1996.

120. Chikkappa G, Zarrabi MH, Tsan MF: Pure red-cell aplasia in patients with chronic lymphocytic leukaemia. *Medicine (Baltimore)* 65(5):339, 1986.

121. Visco C, Barcellini W, Maura F, et al: Autoimmune cytopenias in chronic lymphocytic leukaemia. *Am J Hematol* 2014.

122. Go RS, Lust JA, Phyliky RL: Aplastic anemia and pure red cell aplasia associated with large granular lymphocyte leukemia. *Semin Hematol* 40(3):196, 2003.

123. Lacy MQ, Kurtin PJ, Tefferi A: Pure red cell aplasia: Association with large granular lymphocyte leukemia and the prognostic value of cytogenetic abnormalities. *Blood* 87(7):3000, 1996.

124. Yamada O: Clonal T cell proliferation in patients with pure red cell aplasia. *Leuk Lymphoma* 35(1-2):69, 1999.

125. Fujishima N, Hirokawa M, Fujishima M, et al: Oligoclonal T cell expansion in blood but not in the thymus from a patient with thymoma-associated pure red cell aplasia. *Haematologica* 91(12 Suppl):ECR47, 2006.

126. Koskela HL, Eldfors S, Ellonen P, et al: Somatic STAT3 mutations in large granular lymphocyte leukemia. *N Engl J Med* 366(20):1905, 2012.

127. Qiu ZY, Fan L, Wang L, et al: STAT3 mutations are frequent in T-cell large granular lymphocytic leukemia with pure red cell aplasia. *J Hematol Oncol* 6:82, 2013.

128. Ghrenassia E, Roulin L, Aline-Fardin A, et al: The spectrum of chronic CD8+ T-cell expansions: Clinical features in 14 patients. *PLoS One* 9(3):e91505, 2014.

129. Ishida F, Matsuda K, Sekiguchi N, et al: STAT3 gene mutations and their association with pure red cell aplasia in large granular lymphocyte leukemia. *Cancer Sci* 105(3):342, 2014.

130. Abkowitz JL, Powell JS, Nakamura JM, et al: Pure red cell aplasia: Response to therapy with anti-thymocyte globulin. *Am J Hematol* 23(4):363, 1986.

131. Abkowitz JL, Kadin ME, Powell JS, et al: Pure red cell aplasia: Lymphocyte inhibition of erythropoiesis. *Br J Haematol* 63(1):59, 1986.

132. Hanada T, Abe T, Nakamura H, et al: Pure red cell aplasia: Relationship between inhibitory activity of T cells to CFU-E and erythropoiesis. *Br J Haematol* 58(1):107, 1984.

133. Mangan KF, D'Alessandro L: Hypoplastic anemia in B cell chronic lymphocytic leukemia: Evolution of T cell-mediated suppression of erythropoiesis in early-stage and late-stage disease. *Blood* 66(3):533, 1985.

134. Mangan KF, Chikkappa G, Farley PC: T gamma (T gamma) cells suppress growth of erythroid colony-forming units in vitro in the pure red cell aplasia of B-cell chronic lymphocytic leukemia. *J Clin Invest* 70(6):1148, 1982.

135. Hoffman R, Kopel S, Hsu SD, et al: T cell chronic lymphocytic leukemia: Presence in bone marrow and peripheral blood of cells that suppress erythropoiesis in vitro. *Blood* 52(1):255, 1978.

136. Nagasawa T, Abe T, Nakagawa T: Pure red cell aplasia and hypogammaglobulinemia associated with Tr-cell chronic lymphocytic leukemia. *Blood* 57(6):1025, 1981.

137. Handgretinger R, Geiselhart A, Moris A, et al: Pure red-cell aplasia associated with clonal expansion of granular lymphocytes expressing killer-cell inhibitory receptors. *N Engl J Med* 340(4):278, 1999.

138. Mangan KF, Volkin R, Winkelstein A: Autoreactive erythroid progenitor-T suppressor cells in the pure red cell aplasia associated with thymoma and panhypogammaglobulinemia. *Am J Hematol* 23(2):167, 1986.

139. Akard LP, Brandt J, Lu L, et al: Chronic T cell lymphoproliferative disorder and pure red cell aplasia. Further characterization of cell-mediated inhibition of erythropoiesis and clinical response to cytotoxic chemotherapy. *Am J Med* 83(6):1069, 1987.

140. Reid TJ 3rd, Mullaney M, Burrell LM, et al: Pure red cell aplasia after chemotherapy for Hodgkin's lymphoma: In vitro evidence for T cell mediated suppression of erythropoiesis and response to sequential cyclosporin and erythropoietin. *Am J Hematol* 46(1):48, 1994.

141. Socinski MA, Ershler WB, Tosato G, et al: Pure red blood cell aplasia associated with chronic Epstein-Barr virus infection: Evidence for T cell-mediated suppression of erythroid colony forming units. *J Lab Clin Med* 104(6):995, 1984.

142. Levitt LJ, Reyes GR, Moonka DK, et al: Human T cell leukemia virus-I-associated T-suppressor cell inhibition of erythropoiesis in a patient with pure red cell aplasia and chronic T gamma-lymphoproliferative disease. *J Clin Invest* 81(2):538, 1988.

143. Fisch P, Handgretinger R, Schaefer HE: Pure red cell aplasia. *Br J Haematol* 111(4):1010, 2000.

144. Lipton JM, Nadler LM, Canellos GP, et al: Evidence for genetic restriction in the suppression of erythropoiesis by a unique subset of T lymphocytes in man. *J Clin Invest* 72(2):694, 1983.

145. Kurtzman GJ, Cohen BJ, Field AM, et al: Immune response to B19 parvovirus and an antibody defect in persistent viral infection. *J Clin Invest* 84(4):1114, 1989.

146. Geetha D, Zachary JB, Baldado HM, et al: Pure red cell aplasia caused by Parvovirus B19 infection in solid organ transplant recipients: A case report and review of literature. *Clin Transplant* 14(6):586, 2000.

147. Frickhofen N, Abkowitz JL, Safford M, et al: Persistent B19 parvovirus infection in patients infected with human immunodeficiency virus type 1 (HIV-1): A treatable cause of anemia in AIDS. *Ann Intern Med* 113(12):926, 1990.

148. Wiktor-Jedrzejczak W, Szczylik C, Gonas P, et al: Different marrow cell number requirements for the haemopoietic colony formation and the curve of the W/Wv anemia. *Experientia* 35(4):546, 1979.

149. Abkowitz JL, Brown KE, Wood RW, et al: Clinical relevance of parvovirus B19 as a cause of anemia in patients with human immunodeficiency virus infection. *J Infect Dis* 176(1):269, 1997.

150. Mylonakis E, Dickinson BP, Mileno MD, et al: Persistent parvovirus B19 related anemia of seven years' duration in an HIV-infected patient: Complete remission associated with highly active antiretroviral therapy. *Am J Hematol* 60(2):164, 1999.

151. Morelli P, Bestetti G, Longhi E, et al: Persistent parvovirus B19-induced anemia in an HIV-infected patient under HAART. Case report and review of literature. *Eur J Clin Microbiol Infect Dis* 26(11):833, 2007.

152. Garcia-Suarez J, Pascual T, Munoz MA, et al: Myelodysplastic syndrome with erythroid hypoplasia/aplasia: A case report and review of the literature. *Am J Hematol* 58(4):319, 1998.

153. Hirai H: Molecular pathogenesis of MDS. *Int J Hematol* 76(Suppl 2):213, 2002.

154. Pellagatti A, Esoof N, Watkins F, et al: Gene expression profiling in the myelodysplastic syndromes using cDNA microarray technology. *Br J Haematol* 125(5):576, 2004.

155. Darley RL, Hoy TG, Baines P, et al: Mutant N-RAS induces erythroid lineage dysplasia in human CD34+ cells. *J Exp Med* 185(7):1337, 1997.

156. Vlachos A, Farrar JE, Atsidaftos E, et al: Diminutive somatic deletions in the 5q region lead to a phenotype atypical of classical 5q− syndrome. *Blood* 122(14):2487, 2013.

157. DeZern AE, Pu J, McDevitt MA, et al: Burst-forming unit–erythroid assays to distinguish cellular bone marrow failure disorders. *Exp Hematol* 41(9):808, 2013.

158. Lacombe C, Casadevall N, Muller O, et al: Erythroid progenitors in adult chronic pure red cell aplasia: Relationship of in vitro erythroid colonies to therapeutic response. *Blood* 64(1):71, 1984.

159. Mangan KF, Shadduck RK: Successful treatment of chronic refractory pure red cell aplasia with antithymocyte globulin: Correlation with in vitro erythroid culture studies. *Am J Hematol* 17(4):417, 1984.

160. Shelly S, Agmon-Levin N, Altman A, et al: Thymoma and autoimmunity. *Cell Mol Immunol* 8(3):199, 2011.

161. Oski FA: Hematologic consequences of chloramphenicol therapy. *J Pediatr* 94(3):515, 1979.

162. Holbro A, Jauch A, Lardinois D, et al: High prevalence of infections and autoimmunity in patients with thymoma. *Hum Immunol* 73(3):287, 2012.

163. Hirst E, Robertson TI: The syndrome of thymoma and erythroblastopenic anemia. A review of 56 cases including 3 case reports. *Medicine (Baltimore)* 46(3):225, 1967.

164. Sawada K, Fujishima N, Hirokawa M: Acquired pure red cell aplasia: Updated review of treatment. *Br J Haematol* 142(4):505, 2008.

165. Firkin FC, Maher D: Cytotoxic immunosuppressive drug treatment strategy in pure red cell aplasia. *Eur J Haematol* 41(3):212, 1988.

166. Kwong YL, Wong KF, Liang RH, et al: Pure red cell aplasia: Clinical features and treatment results in 16 cases. *Ann Hematol* 72(3):137, 1996.

167. Mamiya S, Itoh T, Miura AB: Acquired pure red cell aplasia in Japan. *Eur J Haematol* 59(4):199, 1997.

168. Yamada O, Motoji T, Mizoguchi H: Selective effect of cyclosporine monotherapy for pure red cell aplasia not associated with granular lymphocyte-proliferative disorders. *Br J Haematol* 106(2):371, 1999.

169. Raghavachar A: Pure red cell aplasia: Review of treatment and proposal for a treatment strategy. *Blut* 61(2-3):47, 1990.

170. Totterman TH, Hoglund M, Bengtsson M, et al: Treatment of pure red-cell aplasia and aplastic anaemia with ciclosporin: Long-term clinical effects. *Eur J Haematol* 42(2):126, 1989.

171. Sawada K, Hirokawa M, Fujishima N, et al: Long-term outcome of patients with acquired primary idiopathic pure red cell aplasia receiving cyclosporine A. A nationwide cohort study in Japan for the PRCA Collaborative Study Group. *Haematologica* 92(8):1021, 2007.

172. Yamada O, Mizoguchi H, Oshimi K: Cyclophosphamide therapy for pure red cell aplasia associated with granular lymphocyte-proliferative disorders. *Br J Haematol* 97(2):392, 1997.

173. Go RS, Li CY, Tefferi A, et al: Acquired pure red cell aplasia associated with lymphoproliferative disease of granular T lymphocytes. *Blood* 98(2):483, 2001.

174. Fujishima N, Sawada K, Hirokawa M, et al: Long-term responses and outcomes following immunosuppressive therapy in large granular lymphocyte leukemia-associated pure red cell aplasia: A Nationwide Cohort Study in Japan for the PRCA Collaborative Study Group. *Haematologica* 93(10):1555, 2008.

175. Harris SI, Weinberg JB: Treatment of red cell aplasia with antithymocyte globulin: Repeated inductions of complete remissions in two patients. *Am J Hematol* 20(2):183, 1985.

176. Robak T: Monoclonal antibodies in the treatment of autoimmune cytopenias. *Eur J Haematol* 72(2):79, 2004.

177. Sloand EM, Scheinberg P, Maciejewski J, et al: Brief communication: Successful treatment of pure red-cell aplasia with an anti-interleukin-2 receptor antibody (daclizumab). *Ann Intern Med* 144(3):181, 2006.

178. Ghazal H: Successful treatment of pure red cell aplasia with rituximab in patients with chronic lymphocytic leukemia. *Blood* 99(3):1092, 2002.

179. Auner HW, Wolfler A, Beham-Schmid C, et al: Restoration of erythropoiesis by rituximab in an adult patient with primary acquired pure red cell aplasia refractory to conventional treatment. *Br J Haematol* 116(3):727, 2002.

180. Scaramucci L, Niscola P, Ales M, et al: Pure red cell aplasia associated with hemolytic anemia refractory to standard measures and resolved by rituximab in an elderly patient. *Int J Hematol* 88(3):343, 2008.

181. Willis F, Marsh JC, Bevan DH, et al: The effect of treatment with Campath-1H in patients with autoimmune cytopenias. *Br J Haematol* 114(4):891, 2001.

182. Ru X, Liebman HA: Successful treatment of refractory pure red cell aplasia associated with lymphoproliferative disorders with the anti-CD52 monoclonal antibody alemtuzumab (Campath-1H). *Br J Haematol* 123(2):278, 2003.

183. Chow JK, Chan TK: Low-dose subcutaneous alemtuzumab is a safe and effective treatment for chronic acquired pure red cell aplasia. *Hong Kong Med J* 19(6):549, 2013.

184. Ahn J, Lee K, Lee J, et al: A case of refractory idiopathic pure red cell aplasia responsive to fludarabine treatment. *Br J Haematol* 112(2):527, 2001.

185. Robak T, Kasznicki M, Blonski JZ, et al: Pure red cell aplasia in patients with chronic lymphocytic leukaemia treated with cladribine. *Br J Haematol* 112(4):1083, 2001.

186. Messner HA, Fauser AA, Curtis JE, et al: Control of antibody-mediated pure red-cell aplasia by plasmapheresis. *N Engl J Med* 304(22):1334, 1981.

187. Freund LG, Hippe E, Strandgaard S, et al: Complete remission in pure red cell aplasia after plasmapheresis. *Scand J Haematol* 35(3):315, 1985.

188. Hirokawa M, Sawada K, Fujishima N, et al: Long-term response and outcome following immunosuppressive therapy in thymoma-associated pure red cell aplasia: A nationwide cohort study in Japan by the PRCA collaborative study group. *Haematologica* 93(1):27, 2008.

189. Muller BU, Tichelli A, Passweg JR, et al: Successful treatment of refractory acquired pure red cell aplasia (PRCA) by allogeneic bone marrow transplantation. *Bone Marrow Transplant* 23(11):1205, 1999.

190. Tseng SB, Lin SF, Chang CS, et al: Successful treatment of acquired pure red cell aplasia (PRCA) by allogeneic peripheral blood stem cell transplantation. *Am J Hematol* 74(4):273, 2003.

191. Kurtzman G, Frickhofen N, Kimball J, et al: Pure red-cell aplasia of 10 years' duration due to persistent parvovirus B19 infection and its cure with immunoglobulin therapy. *N Engl J Med* 321(8):519, 1989.

192. Crabol Y, Terrier B, Rozenberg F, et al: Intravenous immunoglobulin therapy for pure red cell aplasia related to human parvovirus b19 infection: A retrospective study of 10 patients and review of the literature. *Clin Infect Dis* 56(7):968, 2013.

193. Kurtzman GJ, Ozawa K, Cohen B, et al: Chronic bone marrow failure due to persistent B19 parvovirus infection. *N Engl J Med* 317(5):287, 1987.

194. Ramratnam B, Gollerkeri A, Schiffman FJ, et al: Management of persistent B19 parvovirus infection in AIDS. *Br J Haematol* 91(1):90, 1995.

CHAPTER 37
ANEMIA OF CHRONIC DISEASE

Tomas Ganz

SUMMARY

Most patients suffering from chronic infection, chronic inflammation, or some with various malignancies develop a mild to moderate anemia. This anemia, designated *anemia of chronic disease* or *anemia of chronic inflammation*, is characterized by a low serum iron level, a low to normal transferrin level, and a high to normal ferritin level. The anemia is caused by the direct and indirect inhibitory effects of inflammatory cytokines on erythrocyte production. Among the cytokines, interleukin-6 has a central role, acting by increasing hepatocyte production of the iron-regulatory hormone hepcidin. Hepcidin then blocks the release of iron from macrophages and hepatocytes, causing the characteristic hypoferremia associated with this anemia, and limiting the availability of iron to the developing erythrocytes. Effective treatment of the underlying disease restores normal erythropoiesis. When this is not possible, and treatment is necessary, therapeutic trials have revealed that the anemia is often responsive to pharmacologic doses of erythropoietin.

Anemia of chronic kidney disease presents similarly to anemia of inflammation but because the kidneys are the predominant site of erythropoietin production, the pathogenesis of this anemia is frequently dominated by relative erythropoietin deficiency, where erythropoietin concentrations in serum are lower than expected for the severity of anemia. Systemic inflammation from underlying renal disease, or induced by dialysis treatments and their complications, contributes to pathogenesis in a manner similar to anemia of inflammation. Circulating hepcidin concentrations may also rise because of its decreased renal clearance. Suppressive effects of uremia on erythropoiesis and blood losses from hemodialysis may contribute to anemia in end-stage renal disease. A combination of erythropoiesis–stimulating agents and intravenous iron is usually effective in reversing anemia but overtreatment may worsen overall outcomes.

● DEFINITION AND HISTORY

The term *anemia of chronic disease* (ACD) or *anemia of chronic disorders* refers to mild to moderately severe anemia (hemoglobin [Hgb] 7 to 12 g/dL) associated with chronic infections and inflammatory disorders and some malignancies.[1] The newer name, *anemia of inflammation*

Acronyms and Abbreviations: ACD, anemia of chronic disease; AI, anemia of inflammation; CKD, chronic kidney disease; CPG, clinical practice guideline; CRP, C-reactive protein; EPO, erythropoietin; ESA, erythropoiesis-stimulating agent; IDA, iron-deficiency anemia; IL, Interleukin; KDIGO, The Kidney Disease Improving Global Outcomes; sTfR, soluble transferrin receptor; TfR, transferring receptor; TNF, tumor necrosis factor.

(AI), is not only more reflective of the pathophysiology of ACD but also includes *anemia of critical illness*,[2] a condition that presents similarly to ACD but develops within days of the onset of illness. An anemia similar to AI is seen in some older individuals in the absence of an identifiable chronic disease; this condition is sometimes referred to as *unexplained anemia of elderlies* or *anemia of aging* (Chap. 9).[3]

AI is characterized by inadequate erythrocyte production in the setting of low serum iron and low iron-binding capacity (i.e., low transferrin) despite preserved or even increased macrophage iron stores in the marrow. The erythrocytes are usually normocytic and normochromic but can be mildly hypochromic and microcytic. Anemia of critical illness[2] can develop acutely (within days) in intensive care settings where the effects of infection or inflammation are exacerbated by disease-related or iatrogenic blood loss or red cell destruction, which by themselves are not sufficiently severe to cause anemia. Anemia of aging[3] is diagnosed in the older when a normocytic normochromic anemia with low serum iron and preserved iron stores develops without an identified underlying disease. Older patients in this defined subset typically have an elevated sedimentation rate and/or elevated C-reactive protein (CRP), a high plasma interleukin (IL)-6 concentration, and frailty.

Anemia of chronic kidney disease (CKD) usually develops as chronic renal disease progresses and generally becomes more severe with decreasing creatinine clearance (Fig. 37–1). The anemia presents similarly to AI but because the kidney is the main site of erythropoietin (EPO) production in adults, the progressive destruction and fibrosis of the kidneys causes relative EPO deficiency, which frequently dominates the pathogenesis of this anemia. Patients with polycystic kidney disease are often at least partially spared of the anemia, whereas patients with bilateral nephrectomy are particularly severely affected by EPO deficiency. Systemic inflammation, true iron deficiency and decreased clearance of hepcidin are common consequences of the underlying disease and dialysis treatments, and one or more of these factors frequently worsen anemia or diminish the response to EPO therapy.

Physicians have known about the pale appearance of patients with chronic infections for hundreds of years. In 19th-century Europe, tuberculosis was the major killer and the pallor associated with this disease was romanticized in the art literature of the time. The first measurements of red cell mass revealed the association between inflammation and anemia. Discussing "the alterations in the condition of the Blood in Inflammation" in Section 372 of the 1859 edition of the *Principles of Human Physiology*, William B. Carpenter[4] described this connection between inflammation and anemia (author's parentheses): "With this increase in the proportion of fibrin and colorless corpuscles (leukocytes), separately or in combination, there is a diminution of the proportion of the red corpuscles, albumen and the salts of the blood." In 1961, 100 years later, Maxwell Wintrobe, in the fifth edition of *Clinical Hematology*,[5] used the term "simple chronic anemia" for the normocytic anemia associated with the majority of infections and chronic systemic diseases. He described anemia associated with inflammation as a common subtype. Wintrobe proposed "profound alterations in iron and porphyrin metabolism" as the likely cause, and referred to his own experiments that showed a decrease in erythrocyte survival of only 27 percent, which "could easily be met by increased erythropoiesis if the bone marrow functional capacity were not impaired." Despite advances in our understanding of the pathophysiology of this very common form of anemia, our knowledge is incomplete.

Anemia of CKD became a common problem in the 1960s when hemodialysis became widely available and allowed prolonged survival of patients with end-stage renal failure. Anemia of CKD was usually severe enough to limit activities of daily living and was treated by blood transfusions until the late 1980s when recombinant EPO became widely available, and alleviated the most severe forms of this anemia.

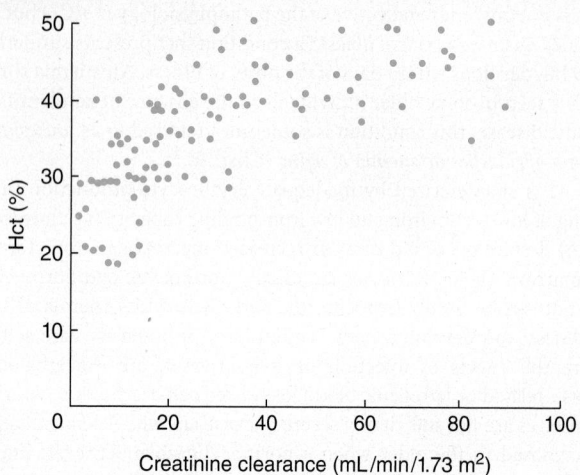

Figure 37–1. Relationship between hematocrit (Hct) and creatinine clearance in patients with CKD. Anemia worsens with decreasing creatinine clearance. *(Reproduced with permission from Radtke HW, Claussner A, Erbes PM, et al: Serum erythropoietin concentration in chronic renal failure: relationship to degree of anemia and excretory renal function. Blood 54(4):877–884, 1979.)*

EPIDEMIOLOGY

The high prevalence of infectious diseases worldwide and the high prevalence of inflammatory and malignant disorders in industrialized countries would suggest that AI is the second or third most common form of anemia after iron-deficiency anemia (IDA) and possibly thalassemia.[6] Although the prevalence of iron deficiency in the industrialized countries is now rapidly decreasing,[6,7] AI is expected to increase as the population ages. Table 37–1 lists the most common diseases associated with AI.

Although anemia can develop early in the progression of CKD, it generally worsens as the kidneys fail.[8–10] Accordingly, the prevalence of patients with anemia of CKD worldwide is influenced by the availability of life-sustaining dialysis therapies. It is estimated that there are currently approximately 600,000 patients with end-stage renal disease in the United States, and approximately 100,000 new patients each year,[11] the majority of whom are anemic or receive treatment for anemia.[9] Additional patients with milder anemia of CKD are found among the estimated 6.7 percent of the U.S. population (or approximately 20 million) identified as having likely CKD (estimated glomerular filtration rate [eGFR] <60 mL/min/1.73 m²) in the 2007–2010 National Health and Nutritional Examination Surveys (NHANES) study.[11]

TABLE 37–1. Common Conditions Associated with Anemia of Inflammation

Category	Diseases Associated with Anemia of Inflammation
Infection	AIDS/HIV, tuberculosis, malaria (contributory), osteomyelitis, chronic abscesses, sepsis
Inflammation	Rheumatoid arthritis, other rheumatologic disorders, inflammatory bowel diseases, systemic inflammatory response syndrome
Malignancy	Carcinomas, multiple myeloma, lymphomas
Cytokine dysregulation	Anemia of aging

ETIOLOGY AND PATHOGENESIS

In the chronic setting, AI predominantly results from the body's inability to increase erythrocyte production to compensate for relatively small decrements in erythrocyte survival (reviewed in Ref. 1). In the steady state, erythrocyte production is sufficiently high so that the resulting anemia is mild to moderate. The anemia associated with acute critical illness has the same pathogenesis as other forms of AI but it develops more rapidly perhaps because of the more extensive erythrocyte destruction and intensive diagnostic phlebotomy common in this setting. The key questions about the pathogenesis of AI, still only partially answered, are: (1) What accounts for the inability of the AI marrow to increase erythropoiesis? and (2) How is this deficit connected to the characteristic hypoferremia and sequestration of iron in macrophages and hepatocytes? Anemia of CKD is similar to AI but the underlying renal pathology also impairs the ability of the kidneys to produce enough EPO leading to insufficient compensatory erythropoiesis.

RED CELL DESTRUCTION

Human studies indicate that transfused AI erythrocytes have a normal life span in normal recipients but transfused normal erythrocytes have a decreased life span in AI recipients.[1] This finding suggests that increased erythrocyte destruction is caused by the activation of hosts factors such as macrophages that prematurely remove aging erythrocytes from the bloodstream. The explanation is consistent with the predominance of young erythrocytes in AI. Whether extrinsic factors, such as bacterial toxins and medications, or host-derived antibodies or complement contribute to this process is unknown.

SUPPRESSIVE EFFECTS OF INFLAMMATION ON ERYTHROPOIETIC PRECURSORS

Some cytokines, chiefly tumor necrosis factor (TNF)-α, IL-1, and the interferons, exert a suppressive effect on erythroid colony formation.[12] Interferon-γ overproduction suppresses erythropoiesis in a mouse model[13] by reducing erythrocyte life span and decreasing erythropoiesis without any evidence of iron restriction. It is not known to what extent and under what conditions these mechanisms contribute to human AI.

INADEQUATE ERYTHROPOIETIN SECRETION AND RESISTANCE TO ERYTHROPOIETIN

The normal response to increased destruction of erythrocytes is transient anemia followed by an increase in EPO production and subsequent compensatory increase in erythropoiesis. One proposed explanation for the inadequate marrow response in AI is less EPO production than expected based on other types of anemia. Studies of patients with rheumatoid arthritis and AI indicated that EPO levels are increased but less so than in IDA.[14–19] The findings were similar in patients with anemias associated with solid tumors or hematologic malignancies.[20,21] However, these comparisons did not take into account the potentiating effect of iron deficiency on hypoxia sensing (Chaps. 32 and 42).[22] This effect could increase EPO production in IDA above that in other types of anemia, and make EPO production in AI appear low in comparison. In support of the EPO suppression hypothesis are experiments with EPO-producing cell lines indicate that production of the hormone is inhibited by inflammatory cytokines including TNF-α and IL-1. The inhibition is mediated by the effects of the transcription factor GATA-1 on the *EPO* gene promoter, and the suppression of EPO production can be reversed by a GATA inhibitor.[23] Moreover, both baseline and hypoxia-induced *EPO* gene expression is suppressed in rats treated with bacterial lipopolysaccharide or IL-1β to mimic a septic state.[24] However, suppression of EPO production is not the major mechanism of AI. If it were, administration of relatively small amounts of EPO should be sufficient to reverse the AI.

In contrast, relative EPO deficiency is often a major contributor to anemia of CKD. Most destructive diseases affecting the kidneys also decrease the release of EPO.[25,26] In the kidney, interstitial fibroblasts of neural crest origin[26,27] are probably the main source of EPO, but the identity of EPO-producing cells in the kidney remains controversial, mostly because the basal production of EPO is very low and ultrasensitive methods are required to detect the source of the hormone. In response to anemia or hypoxia, the number of renal cells producing EPO increases. In advanced CKD, the kidneys undergo end-stage fibrosis, during which these fibroblasts may transdifferentiate into myofibroblasts and lose their ability to produce appropriate amounts of EPO in response to hypoxia.[26,27] However, these or other renal cells can be activated to increase their EPO output by the administration of therapeutic prolyl-hydroxylase inhibitors[28] (Chap. 32), as indicated by the lower stimulated EPO production by anephric patients compared to those with end-stage renal disease and retained kidneys. Studies in animal models indicate that the impairment of EPO production in end-stage kidneys may be reversible and could be therapeutically restored.[26,27]

Inflammation is also a strong contributor to the pathogenesis of anemia of CKD. Patients who had renal disease with inflammation, as measured by increased serum CRP greater than 20 mg/L, required on the average 80 percent higher doses of EPO than patients with simple primary EPO deficiency from renal disease.[29] In another study, patients with CRP greater than 50 mg/L reached lower concentrations of Hgb than patients with CRP less than 50 mg/L, despite higher doses of erythropoiesis-stimulating agents.[30] Inflammation thus induces a state of relative resistance to EPO, contributing to the pathogenesis of anemia of CKD.

ERYTHROPOIESIS RESTRICTION AS A RESULT OF IRON UNAVAILABILITY

Interleukin-6, Hepcidin, and Hypoferremia

Hypoferremia, one of the defining features of AI, develops within hours of the onset of inflammation.[1] Although previous studies of cytokine mediators of hypoferremia of inflammation were inconclusive, subsequent work[31] indicates that the response is dependent on IL-6 which induces the iron-regulatory hormone, hepcidin.[32] Unlike wild-type mice, mice deficient in either hepcidin[33] or IL-6[34] do not become hypoferremic during turpentine-induced inflammation. In human hepatocyte cell cultures, IL-6 is a potent and direct inducer of hepcidin and neither IL-1 nor TNF-α share this activity. The central role of IL-6 is further indicated by the observation that IL-6-deficient mice do not acutely induce hepcidin in response to turpentine inflammation. Infusion of IL-6 into human volunteers induces hepcidin release within hours and causes concomitant hypoferremia.[35] The IL-6–hepcidin axis now appears to be responsible for the induction of hypoferremia during inflammation. However, these studies do not exclude the potential contribution of other cytokines, including activin B and interferon-γ,[13,36] to AI in human diseases or more complex mouse models. In support of multiple pathways of AI in a mouse model of inflammation, either the ablation of hepcidin or the ablation of IL-6 ameliorated the anemia, but neither restored normal Hgb concentration.[37,38]

Serum Iron Concentration Is Dependent on Iron Released from Macrophages and Hepatocytes

In the steady state, almost all of the approximately 20 to 25 mg of iron that daily enters the plasma iron/transferrin pool comes from macrophage recycling of senescent erythrocytes and from hepatocyte iron stores; only approximately 1 to 2 mg come from dietary iron. Only approximately 2 to 4 mg of iron is bound to transferrin but the entire daily iron flow transits through this compartment; thus, the iron in this pool turns over every few hours. During inflammation the release of iron from macrophages and probably also from liver stores is markedly inhibited.[39-45] Studies in transgenic mice lacking hepcidin and mice overexpressing hepcidin indicate that the peptide is a negative regulator of iron release from macrophages and of intestinal iron uptake.[46,47] During inflammation, IL-6 induces hepcidin production, which in turn inhibits iron release from macrophages (and probably from hepatocytes), leading to hypoferremia (Fig. 37–2). Hepcidin acts by binding to cell membrane-associated ferroportin molecules that are the only conduits for iron export, and inducing ferroportin internalization and degradation.[48] As hepcidin concentrations increase, less and less ferroportin is available for iron export and the iron release into plasma from macrophages, hepatocytes, and enterocytes decreases.

Erythropoiesis in Anemia of Inflammation Is Limited by Iron

As an intermediate step during the synthesis of heme, iron becomes incorporated into protoporphyrin IX. Zinc is an alternative protoporphyrin ligand. In iron deficiency, increased amounts of zinc are incorporated into protoporphyrin. In AI, zinc protoporphyrin is also increased.[49]

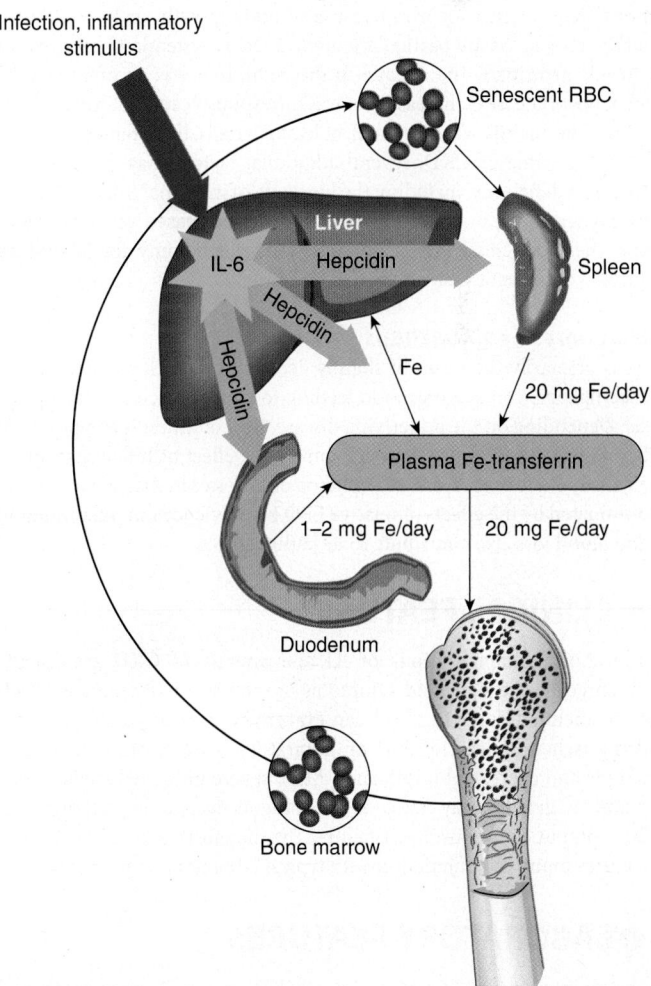

Figure 37–2. Diagram of the effect of inflammation on iron concentrations in plasma. Arrows labeled "Hepcidin" indicate control points where hepcidin inhibits iron flow into the plasma transferrin compartment.

Insufficient iron reaches the sites of heme synthesis in developing erythrocytes, leading to the substitution of zinc. Moreover, the number of sideroblasts, nucleated erythrocyte precursors that stain for iron with Prussian blue, is decreased in AI.[1] A further indication of the limiting role of iron in patients with AI but no evidence of iron deficiency is that coadministration of parenteral iron can resolve the resistance of AI to EPO.[50,51] Attempts to treat AI with iron alone generally have been less successful, as iron became rapidly trapped in the macrophage compartment.[1,52,53]

In the context of anemia of CKD, increased zinc protoporphyrin and decreased reticulocyte Hgb is also characteristic of functional iron deficiency during intense bursts of erythropoiesis stimulated by pharmacologic doses of EPO derivatives.[54]

Inhibition of Intestinal Absorption of Iron and Other Factors Leading to Systemic Iron Deficiency

In longstanding AI, erythrocytes can become hypochromic and microcytic, partly because progressive depletion of iron stores worsens the iron restriction. Intestinal absorption of iron is inhibited[55–57] during inflammation by an IL-6 and hepcidin-mediated mechanism.[58–62] Only 1 to 2 mg of the daily iron needed for erythropoiesis comes from the diet and most adults have 400 to 2000 mg of iron stores (Chap. 42); therefore, a considerable amount of time is needed to deplete the stored iron. True iron deficiency can eventually develop in chronic inflammatory diseases, especially in children who have smaller iron stores and an additional requirement for iron because of body growth, or in conditions where IL-6 levels are particularly high, such as systemic-onset juvenile chronic arthritis.[63] The anemia in these children was accompanied by an appropriate EPO increase, but was unresponsive to oral iron replacement. The anemia was corrected, at least partially, by parenteral iron.

In anemia of CKD, several additional factors may contribute to true iron deficiency, including the blockade of intestinal iron absorption by higher hepcidin concentrations from its decreased renal clearance and the blood losses from hemodialysis, phlebotomy for laboratory studies, and occult gastrointestinal bleeding.

Summary of Pathogenesis

AI is primarily the result of slightly decreased red cell survival and of macrophage iron sequestration leading to iron-restricted erythropoiesis. Depending on the underlying disease, the condition is compounded by inadequate EPO production, suppressive effect of inflammation on erythropoietic precursors, or depletion of iron stores. Anemia of CKD is dominated by the effects of relative EPO insufficiency but inflammation and blood loss also contribute to its pathogenesis.

● CLINICAL FEATURES

The clinical manifestations of AI and anemia of CKD are usually obscured by the signs and symptoms of the underlying disease. Moderate anemia (Hgb <10 g/dL) can exacerbate the symptoms of preexisting ischemic heart disease or respiratory disease, or contribute to fatigue and exertional intolerance. More severe untreated anemia seen mainly with CKD may cause extreme fatigue, dyspnea on exertion, and high-output congestive heart failure. The diagnosis is based on clinical features found in conjunction with typical laboratory abnormalities.

● LABORATORY FEATURES

The erythrocytes in AI and anemia of CKD are usually normocytic and normochromic but, with increasing severity or duration, can sometimes become hypochromic and eventually microcytic.[1] The absolute reticulocyte count is normal or slightly elevated.

HYPOFERREMIA AND INCREASED SERUM TRANSFERRIN

Hypoferremia, a decrease in serum iron concentration, is a defining feature of AI and, in the absence of iron therapy, is also commonly seen in anemia of CKD. It develops within hours of the onset of infection or severe inflammation. The concentration of the iron-binding protein, transferrin (measured as total iron binding capacity), is moderately decreased in AI, unlike in IDA in which transferrin concentration is increased. The decrease in transferrin concentrations develops more slowly than the decrease in serum iron levels because of the longer half-life of transferrin (8 to 12 days)[64] compared to the turnover of plasma iron (approximately 90 minutes).

INCREASED SERUM FERRITIN

Serum ferritin concentrations, which reflect iron stores and inflammation, are increased in AI but decreased in iron deficiency. Thus, serum ferritin is useful in differential diagnosis in patients with low serum iron concentrations.[65] Depleted iron stores in patients with coexisting inflammation may result in intermediate ferritin levels (Table 37–2 and Fig. 37–3) because ferritin is an acute-phase protein and inflammatory cytokines increase ferritin synthesis. In this situation, iron deficiency should be suspected if ferritin concentrations are less than 60 mcg/L. Soluble transferrin receptor (sTfR) levels (Table 37–2) increase with increased demand of the erythroid marrow for iron but inflammation may have a direct suppressive effect on sTfR. As a result, sTfR is increased in iron deficiency but, unlike ferritin, it is unchanged or decreased during infection or inflammation.[66] Although these properties should make sTfR a useful diagnostic parameter alone or in combination with ferritin,[67] the use of sTfR in practice has been hampered by inadequate standardization and inconsistent reports of its clinical utility. Another promising marker that may differentiate AI from systemic iron deficiency is serum hepcidin, as very low serum hepcidin levels in the setting of hypoferremia are diagnostic of systemic iron deficiency. However, the assays have not yet been standardized and the clinical utility of hepcidin measurements in differential diagnosis of anemia has not yet been tested in large heterogeneous patient populations.[68]

Low serum ferritin concentrations are indicative of iron deficiency in anemia of CKD but normal or even high ferritin concentrations do not preclude a clinical response (increased Hgb) after parenteral iron therapy. In these settings, high ferritin levels may largely reflect inflammation, and augmented iron supply may be needed to overcome "functional iron deficiency,"[54] that is, to provide sufficient iron supply for pulsatile erythropoiesis stimulated by intermittently administered pharmacologic doses of EPO or its derivatives.[69]

MARROW IRON STAIN

Marrow aspiration or biopsy is rarely required for the diagnosis of AI. In general, the marrow is normal, unless the underlying disease alters the picture. The most important information obtained from marrow examination is the content and distribution of iron. Iron in a marrow preparation can be found as storage iron in the cytoplasm of macrophages or as functional iron in nucleated red cells. In normal individuals, a few Prussian blue–staining particles can be found inside or adjacent to many macrophages. Approximately one-third of nucleated red cells contain one to four blue inclusion bodies and such cells are called *sideroblasts*. Both sideroblasts and macrophage iron are absent in iron deficiency. In contrast, sideroblasts are decreased or absent but macrophage iron is increased in AI. The increase in storage iron in association with a decreased level of circulating iron and a decreased

TABLE 37–2. Laboratory Studies of Iron Metabolism in Iron-Deficiency Anemia and Anemia of Inflammation

	IDA (n = 48)	AI (n = 58)	COMBI (n = 17)
Hemoglobin, g/L	93 ± 16 (96)	102 ± 12 (103)	88 ± 20 (90)
MCV, fL	75 ± 9 (75)	90 ± 7 (91)	78 ± 9 (79)
Iron, μmol/L (10–40)	8 ± 11 (4)	10 ± 6 (9)	6 ± 3 (6)
Transferrin, g/L (2.1–3.4 m, 2.0–3.1 f)	3.3 ± 0.4 (3.3)	1.9 ± 0.5 (1.8)	2.6 ± 0.6 (2.4)
Transferrin saturation, %	12 ± 17 (5.7)	23 ± 13 (21)	12 ± 7 (8)
Ferritin, μg/L (15–306 m, 5–103 f)	21 ± 55 (11)	342 ± 385 (195)	87 ± 167 (23)
TfR, mg/L (0.85–3.05)	6.2 ± 3.5 (5.0)	1.8 ± 0.6 (1.8)	5.1 ± 2.0 (4.7)
TfR/log ferritin	6.8 ± 6.5 (5.4)	0.8 ± 0.3 (0.8)	3.8 ± 1.9 (3.2)

f, Females; m, males; TfR, transferrin receptor.

Diagnosis was defined by marrow iron stain and appropriate coexisting disease. Patients with a combination of no stainable marrow iron and either coexisting disease or elevated CRP were classified as "COMBI." Normal ranges for this laboratory for males (m) and females (f) are indicated. Measurements are presented as mean ± SD (median).

Modified with permission from Punnonen K, Irjala K, Rajamaki A: Serum transferrin receptor and its ratio to serum ferritin in the diagnosis of iron deficiency. *Blood* 89(3):1052–1057, 1997.

number of sideroblasts is characteristic of AI. Although marrow stain could be considered the gold standard for differential diagnosis of AI and iron deficiency, the discomfort to the patient associated this procedure, reports of variability in interpretation[70] and the wide availability of the serum ferritin assay have decreased the use of marrow stain in this setting.

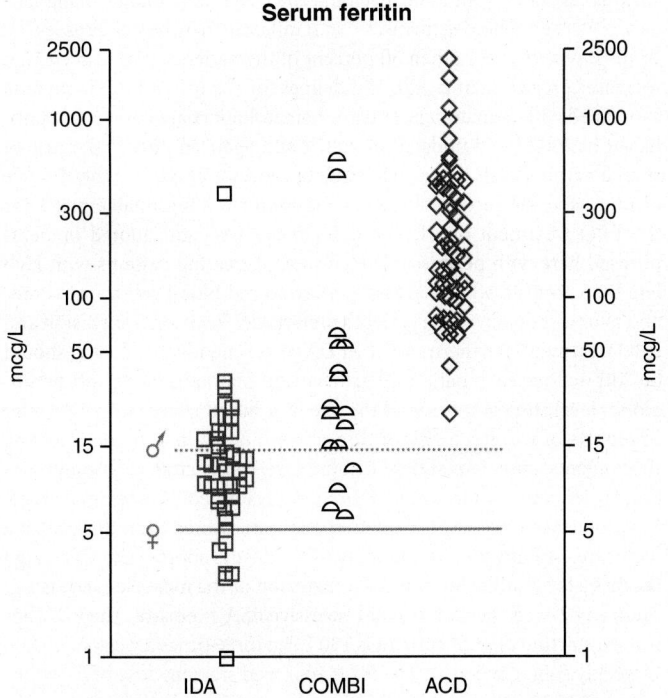

Figure 37–3. Distribution of serum ferritin measurements in patients with iron-deficiency anemia (IDA), anemia of chronic disease (ACD = anemia of inflammation [AI]) and combined IDA and ACD (COMBI). The *horizontal lines* indicate lower normal values for healthy men and women. *(Reproduced with permission from Punnonen K, Irjala K, Rajamaki A: Serum Transferrin Receptor and Its Ratio to Serum Ferritin in the Diagnosis of Iron Deficiency.* Blood *89(3):1052–1057, 1997.)*

DIFFERENTIAL DIAGNOSIS

Most patients with chronic infections, inflammatory diseases, or neoplastic disorders are anemic. The diagnosis of AI should only be made if the anemia is mild to moderate, the serum iron and iron-binding capacity are low, and the serum ferritin is elevated. Anemia of CKD is rare in mild renal disease but common and often severe in end-stage renal disease. Underlying diseases, comorbidities, and their treatments can cause many types of anemia, so other potential causes should be considered.

1. *Drug-induced marrow suppression or drug-induced hemolysis* can complicate infections, inflammatory disorders, CKDs, and cancer. When the marrow is suppressed by cytotoxic drugs or idiopathic toxic reaction, serum iron tends to be high and reticulocyte count low. In hemolysis, reticulocyte counts, haptoglobin, bilirubin, and lactate dehydrogenase often are elevated.

2. *Chronic blood loss* depletes iron stores and decreases serum iron and serum ferritin but increases transferrin (Chap. 43). When AI and chronic blood loss coexist, serum ferritin usually indicates the predominant disorder, although the level can increase as a result of inflammation itself. Chronic blood loss from hemodialysis or occult gastrointestinal bleeding is common in anemia of CKD and its lowering effect on ferritin may be masked by coexisting inflammation. Testing stool for occult blood and looking for other sources of overlooked blood loss, including phlebotomy, urinary loss and menorrhagia, often identify the source of bleeding. Once this issue is addressed, a successful trial of iron repletion confirms the diagnosis of iron deficiency complicating AI or anemia of CKD.

3. *Endocrine disorders*, including hypothyroidism and hyperthyroidism, testicular failure, and diabetes mellitus, can be associated with a chronic normocytic, normochromic anemia (Chap. 38). Unless inflammation or associated iron deficiency is present, serum iron should be normal in these disorders.

4. *Anemia resulting from metastatic invasion of the marrow* by tumors can be the presenting symptom of malignancy. The anemia can develop in the setting of a previous diagnosis of carcinoma or lymphoma and by itself is accompanied by normal or increased serum iron (Chap. 45). It often develops in the setting of preexisting malignancy-related AI. The blood film often is abnormal, with poikilocytes, teardrop-shaped red cells, normoblasts, or immature

TABLE 37–3. Treatments of Anemia of Inflammation and Anemia of Chronic Kidney Disease

Modality	Indications	Typical Setting	Risks and Side Effects	Specific Benefits
Transfusion	• Cardiac ischemia • Lack of response to other modalities	• Hgb <10 g/dL • Chest pain and electro-cardiogram changes	• Infections • Volume overload • Transfusion reaction	• Rapid correction of anemia
Erythropoietin	• Fatigue, exertional intolerance	• Hgb <10 g/dL • Anemia symptoms • Balance against side effects in Hgb 10–12 g/dL	• Response takes several weeks • Rare red cell aplasia with some forms of erythropoietin[107] • May worsen outcome in some cancers[108] • Increased thromboembolic events[79–82,96,109] • Expensive	• Usually well tolerated, relatively safe
Iron (oral or parenteral)[51]	• Coexisting iron deficiency • Resistance to erythro-poietin (investigational)	• Suspected or documented iron deficiency	• Gastrointestinal side effects (oral) • Systemic and local reactions (parenteral) • May decrease resistance to infections?[83,103–105]	• Inexpensive, relatively safe

myeloid cells. Direct marrow examination is necessary to establish the diagnosis.

5. *Thalassemia minor* is a common cause of mild anemia in many parts of the world. It can be confused with AI (Chap. 48). Microcytosis is a life-long condition and usually is more severe in this group of disorders than in AI.

6. *Dilutional anemia* is seen in pregnancy and in patients with severely increased plasma protein levels as a result of multiple myeloma or macroglobulinemia (Chap. 109).

● THERAPY, COURSE, AND PROGNOSIS

Anemia that presents in the setting of infection, inflammation, or malignancy requires sufficient diagnostic studies to rule out reversible and potentially more threatening causes, such as occult hemorrhage; iron, vitamin B$_{12}$, and folate deficiencies; hemolysis; and drug reaction. If the anemia can be designated as AI after such studies, effective treatment of the underlying disease resolves the anemia. If treatment of the underlying disease is not effective and the patient has symptoms or medical complications attributable to anemia, one or more of the available anemia-specific treatment modalities should be considered (Table 37–3). These recommendations are also applicable to anemia of CKD where, for most patients, only renal transplantation can reverse the underlying pathology. However, although anemia generally resolves or improves after renal transplantation, 30 to 40 percent patients continue to be anemic, mainly because of pathologic changes in the transplanted kidney and adverse effects of immunosuppressive drugs.[71-78]

Specific therapy for AI and anemia of CKD employs erythrocyte transfusions, erythropoiesis-stimulating agents (ESAs) and intravenous iron (see Table 37–3). Transfusion of erythrocytes is used to correct AI or anemia of CKD when anemia is moderate to severe and the patient is acutely symptomatic. Because treatment with ESAs often effectively treats chronic anemia but may increase the risk of thromboembolic events,[79–82] guidelines have been proposed for appropriate use of these agents. The widespread adjunctive use of intravenous iron with ESAs may increase their effectiveness and reduce the required doses but

evidence to date has not resulted in a consensus on specific indications for intravenous iron or its optimal dosing.[83]

THERAPY FOR ANEMIA OF INFLAMMATION

EPO therapy for the treatment of AI has been tested in the setting of various cancers,[84,85] multiple myeloma and other hematologic malignancies,[21,86,87] rheumatoid arthritis,[88–91] and inflammatory bowel diseases.[92,93] In most reports, more than 50 percent of the patients experienced Hgb increases greater than 2 g/dL. Guidelines for the use of EPO in anemia associated with hematologic and nonhematologic malignancy were published in 2002[94] and updated in 2007[95] and again in 2010.[96] Because of shared pathogenesis between anemia of cancer and AI, and the absence of more specific recommendations, these form a reasonable guide for the EPO treatment of AI. The guidelines (used and quoted or paraphrased here with permission) recommend treating patients with Hgb less than 10 g/dL when necessary to avoid red blood cell transfusions, and after discussion of the patient's preferences between transfusion and EPO treatment. Furthermore, the FDA recommends that dosing should be "titrated for each patient to achieve and maintain the lowest hemoglobin level sufficient to avoid the need for blood transfusion." Because of reports of increased risk of thromboembolism in patients receiving these agents, clinicians should carefully weigh the risks of thromboembolism in patients for whom ESAs are prescribed. An optimal target Hgb concentration cannot be definitively determined from the available literature. Modification to reduce the ESA dose is appropriate when Hgb reaches a level sufficient to avoid transfusion or the increase exceeds 1 g/dL in any 2-week period to avoid excessive ESA exposure. The FDA-approved starting dose of epoetin is 150 U/kg three times a week or 40,000 U weekly subcutaneously. The FDA-approved starting dose of darbepoetin is 2.25 mcg/kg weekly or 500 mcg every 3 weeks subcutaneously. Alternative starting doses or dosing schedules have shown no consistent difference in effectiveness on outcomes, including transfusion and Hgb response, although they may be considered to improve convenience. Dose escalation should follow FDA-approved labeling; no convincing evidence exists to suggest differences in dose escalation schedules are associated with different effectiveness. Continuing the ESA treatment beyond 6 to 8 weeks in the absence of response (e.g., <1 to 2 g/dL rise in Hgb), does not appear to be beneficial and EPO therapy should be discontinued. The most recent specific guidelines for dose reduction are contained in the FDA-approved package insert. Baseline and periodic monitoring of iron, total iron-binding capacity, transferrin saturation, or ferritin levels and instituting iron repletion when indicated may be valuable in limiting the need for EPO, maximizing symptomatic improvement for patients, and determining the reason for failure to respond adequately to EPO.

THERAPY FOR ANEMIA OF CHRONIC KIDNEY DISEASE

The most current recommendations are The Kidney Disease Improving Global Outcomes (KDIGO) clinical practice guideline (CPG) for anemia in CKD,[97] based upon systematic literature searches last conducted in October 2010 and supplemented with additional evidence through March 2012. For adult patients, these guidelines recommend that a newly anemic patient with CKD should have laboratory studies to rule out vitamin B_{12} and folate deficiencies (Chap. 41), and a therapeutic trial of IV iron if their transferrin saturation is equal to or less than 30 percent and ferritin is equal to or less than 500 ng/mL. After the guidelines were published, the recommendation for a trial of IV iron received some support from a randomized trial showing that IV iron therapy delays or reduces the need for other anemia management including ESAs.[98] However, the entry criteria for this trial were more restrictive than those in the guidelines. The guidelines go on to recommend that individualized therapy with ESAs may be started when Hgb concentrations fall below 10 g/dL and are adjusted to maintain Hgb not exceeding 11.5 g/dL unless the patient perceives an increased quality of life at higher Hgb levels (not exceeding 13 g/dL) and is willing to accept increased risks.

ADJUNCTIVE USE OF INTRAVENOUS IRON WITH ERYTHROPOIETIN

This use of IV iron is an empiric therapeutic strategy based on the idea that iron becomes limiting when marrow production of erythrocytes is pharmacologically stimulated. In some cases occult iron deficiency coexists with AI.[66,93] In other situations, limited iron stores may become depleted when EPO is initiated.[91] In hemodialysis patients with high ferritin, low transferrin saturation (less than 25 percent), and above average EPO requirements, iron supplementation of EPO treatment with a 1-g loading course of intravenous ferric gluconate was shown to lead to a small increase in Hgb and decreased dosage of EPO.[99,100] It is not yet certain whether this strategy is applicable to other AI settings. Pending additional studies, the coadministration of iron with EPO in AI in the absence of demonstrated iron deficiency remains investigational.[51] Because of its ability to decrease the use of ESAs, the use of IV iron is now common practice in CKD patients on hemodialysis, without a clear consensus about the indications and potential risks of this strategy.[83] Concerns exist that iron supplementation in AI or CKD may increase susceptibility to infections,[101,102] but epidemiologic studies have not come to consistent conclusions on this risk.[83,103,104] The use of high bolus doses of iron in patients with intravenous catheters[105] may be associated with increased infections.

REFERENCES

1. Cartwright GE: The anemia of chronic disorders. *Semin Hematol* 3:351, 1966.
2. Corwin HL, Krantz SB: Anemia of the critically ill: "Acute" anemia of chronic disease. *Crit Care Med* 28:3098, 2000.
3. Ershler WB: Biological interactions of aging and anemia: A focus on cytokines. *J Am Geriatr Soc* 51:S18, 2003.
4. Carpenter WB: *Principles of Human Physiology*, edited by FG Smith. Blanchard and Lea, Philadelphia, 1859.
5. Wintrobe MM: *Clinical Hematology*, 5th ed. Lea & Febiger, Philadelphia, 1961.
6. Dallman PR, Yip R, Johnson C: Prevalence and causes of anemia in the United States, 1976 to 1980. *Am J Clin Nutr* 39:437, 1984.
7. Ramakrishnan U, Yip R: Experiences and challenges in industrialized countries: Control of iron deficiency in industrialized countries. *J Nutr* 132:820S, 2002.
8. Hsu CY, McCulloch CE, Curhan GC: Epidemiology of anemia associated with chronic renal insufficiency among adults in the United States: Results from the Third National Health and Nutrition Examination Survey. *J Am Soc Nephrol* 13:504, 2002.
9. Stauffer ME, Fan T: Prevalence of anemia in chronic kidney disease in the United States. *PLoS One* 9:e84943, 2014.
10. McClellan W, Aronoff SL, Bolton WK, et al: The prevalence of anemia in patients with chronic kidney disease. *Curr Med Res Opin* 20:1501, 2004.
11. U.S. Renal Data System: *USRDS 2013 Annual Data Report: Atlas of Chronic Kidney Disease and End-Stage Renal Disease in the United States*. National Institutes of Health, National Institute of Diabetes and Digestive and Kidney Diseases, Bethesda, MD, 2013.
12. Means RT Jr, Krantz SB: Inhibition of human erythroid colony-forming units by gamma interferon can be corrected by recombinant human erythropoietin. *Blood* 78:2564, 1991.
13. Libregts SF, Gutierrez L, de Bruin AM, et al: Chronic IFN-gamma production in mice induces anemia by reducing erythrocyte life span and inhibiting erythropoiesis through an IRF-1/PU.1 axis. *Blood* 118:2578, 2011.
14. Baer AN, Dessypris EN, Goldwasser E, et al: Blunted erythropoietin response to anaemia in rheumatoid arthritis. *Br J Haematol* 66:559, 1987.
15. Hochberg MC, Arnold CM, Hogans BB, et al: Serum immunoreactive erythropoietin in rheumatoid arthritis: Impaired response to anemia. *Arthritis Rheum* 31:1318, 1988.
16. Vreugdenhil G, Wognum AW, van Eijk HG, et al: Anaemia in rheumatoid arthritis: The role of iron, vitamin B12, and folic acid deficiency, and erythropoietin responsiveness. *Ann Rheum Dis* 49:93, 1990.
17. Kendall R, Wasti A, Harvey A, et al: The relationship of haemoglobin to serum erythropoietin concentrations in the anaemia of rheumatoid arthritis: The effect of oral prednisolone. *Br J Rheumatol* 32:204, 1993.
18. Noe G, Augustin J, Hausdorf S, et al: Serum erythropoietin and transferrin receptor levels in patients with rheumatoid arthritis. *Clin Exp Rheumatol* 13:445, 1995.
19. Remacha AF, Rodriguez-de la Serna A, Garcia-Die F, et al: Erythroid abnormalities in rheumatoid arthritis: The role of erythropoietin. *J Rheumatol* 19:1687, 1992.
20. Miller CB, Jones RJ, Piantadosi S, et al: Decreased erythropoietin response in patients with the anemia of cancer. *N Engl J Med* 322:1689, 1990.
21. Cazzola M, Messinger D, Battistel V, et al: Recombinant human erythropoietin in the anemia associated with multiple myeloma or non-Hodgkin's lymphoma: Dose finding and identification of predictors of response. *Blood* 86:4446, 1995.
22. Safran M, Kaelin WG Jr: HIF hydroxylation and the mammalian oxygen-sensing pathway. *J Clin Invest* 111:779, 2003.
23. Imagawa S, Nakano Y, Obara N, et al: A GATA-specific inhibitor (K-7174) rescues anemia induced by IL-1beta, TNF-alpha, or L-NMMA. *FASEB J* 17:1742, 2003.
24. Frede S, Fandrey J, Pagel H, et al: Erythropoietin gene expression is suppressed after lipopolysaccharide or interleukin-1 beta injections in rats. *Am J Physiol* 273:R1067, 1997.
25. Adamson JW, Eschbach J, Finch CA: The kidney and erythropoiesis. *Am J Med* 44:725, 1968.
26. Sato Y, Yanagita M: Renal anemia: From incurable to curable. *Am J Physiol Renal Physiol* 305:F1239, 2013.
27. Asada N, Takase M, Nakamura J, et al: Dysfunction of fibroblasts of extrarenal origin underlies renal fibrosis and renal anemia in mice. *J Clin Invest* 121:3981, 2011.
28. Bernhardt WM, Wiesener MS, Scigalla P, et al: Inhibition of prolyl hydroxylases increases erythropoietin production in ESRD. *J Am Soc Nephrol* 21:2151, 2010.
29. Barany P: Inflammation, serum C-reactive protein, and erythropoietin resistance. *Nephrol Dial Transplant* 16:224, 2001.
30. Macdougall IC, Cooper AC: Erythropoietin resistance: The role of inflammation and pro-inflammatory cytokines. *Nephrol Dial Transplant* 17:39, 2002.
31. Nemeth E, Rivera S, Gabayan V, et al: IL-6 mediates hypoferremia of inflammation by inducing the synthesis of the iron regulatory hormone hepcidin. *J Clin Invest* 113:1271, 2004.
32. Ganz T: Hepcidin, a key regulator of iron metabolism and mediator of anemia of inflammation. *Blood* 102:783, 2003.
33. Nicolas G, Chauvet C, Viatte L, et al: The gene encoding the iron regulatory peptide hepcidin is regulated by anemia, hypoxia, and inflammation. *J Clin Invest* 110:1037, 2002.
34. Nemeth E, Rivera S, Gabayan V, et al: IL-6 mediates hypoferremia of inflammation by inducing the synthesis of the iron regulatory hormone hepcidin. *J Clin Invest* 113:1271, 2004.
35. Nemeth E, Rivera S, Gabayan V, et al: IL-6 mediates hypoferremia of inflammation by inducing the synthesis of the iron regulatory hormone hepcidin. *J Clin Invest* 113:1271, 2004.
36. Besson-Fournier C, Latour C, Kautz L, et al: Induction of activin B by inflammatory stimuli upregulates the iron-regulatory peptide hepcidin through Smad1/5/8 signaling. *Blood* 120:431, 2012.
37. Gardenghi S, Renaud TM, Meloni A, et al: Distinct roles for hepcidin and interleukin-6 in the recovery from anemia in mice injected with heat-killed Brucella abortus. *Blood* 123:1137, 2014.

38. Kim A, Fung E, Parikh SG, et al: A mouse model of anemia of inflammation: Complex pathogenesis with partial dependence on hepcidin. *Blood* 123:1129, 2014.
39. Freireich EM, Miller A, Emerson CP, et al: The effect of inflammation on the utilization of erythrocyte and transferrin-bound radio-iron for red cell production. *Blood* 12:972, 1957.
40. Haurani FI, Burke W, Martinez EJ: Defective reutilization of iron in the anemia of inflammation. *J Lab Clin Med* 65:560, 1965.
41. O'Shea MJ, Kershenobich D, Tavill AS: Effects of inflammation on iron and transferrin metabolism. *Br J Haematol* 25:707, 1973.
42. Hershko C, Cook JD, Finch CA: Storage iron kinetics. VI. The effect of inflammation on iron exchange in the rat. *Br J Haematol* 28:67, 1974.
43. Zarrabi MH, Lysik R, DiStefano J, et al: The anaemia of chronic disorders: Studies of iron reutilization in the anaemia of experimental malignancy and chronic inflammation. *Br J Haematol* 35:647, 1977.
44. Feldman BF, Kaneko JJ, Farver TB: Anemia of inflammatory disease in the dog: Ferrokinetics of adjuvant-induced anemia. *Am J Vet Res* 42:583, 1981.
45. Fillet G, Beguin Y, Baldelli L: Model of reticuloendothelial iron metabolism in humans: Abnormal behavior in idiopathic hemochromatosis and in inflammation. *Blood* 74:844, 1989.
46. Nicolas G, Bennoun M, Devaux I, et al: Lack of hepcidin gene expression and severe tissue iron overload in upstream stimulatory factor 2 (USF2) knockout mice. *Proc Natl Acad Sci U S A* 98:8780, 2001.
47. Nicolas G, Bennoun M, Porteu A, et al: Severe iron deficiency anemia in transgenic mice expressing liver hepcidin. *Proc Natl Acad Sci U S A* 99:4596, 2002.
48. Nemeth E, Tuttle MS, Powelson J, et al: Hepcidin regulates cellular iron efflux by binding to ferroportin and inducing its internalization. *Science* 306:2090, 2004.
49. Hastka J, Lasserre JJ, Schwarzbeck A, et al: Zinc protoporphyrin in anemia of chronic disorders. *Blood* 81:1200, 1993.
50. Taylor JE, Peat N, Porter C, et al: Regular low-dose intravenous iron therapy improves response to erythropoietin in haemodialysis patients. *Nephrol Dial Transplant* 11:1079, 1996.
51. Goodnough LT, Skikne B, Brugnara C: Erythropoietin, iron, and erythropoiesis. *Blood* 96:823, 2000.
52. Hume R, Currie WJ, Tennant M: Anaemia of rheumatoid arthritis and iron therapy. *Ann Rheum Dis* 24:451, 1965.
53. Beamish MR, Davies AG, Eakins JD, et al: The measurement of reticuloendothelial iron release using iron-dextran. *Br J Haematol* 21:617, 1971.
54. Brugnara C, Chambers LA, Malynn E, et al: Red blood cell regeneration induced by subcutaneous recombinant erythropoietin: Iron-deficient erythropoiesis in iron-replete subjects [see comments]. *Blood* 81:956, 1993.
55. Gubler CJ, Cartwright GE, Wintrobe MM: The anemia of infection. X. The effect of infection on the absorption and storage of iron by the rat. *J Biol Chem* 184:563, 1950.
56. Weber J, Werre JM, Julius HW, et al: Decreased iron absorption in patients with active rheumatoid arthritis, with and without iron deficiency. *Ann Rheum Dis* 47:404, 1988.
57. Weber J, Julius HW, Verhoef CW, et al: Absorption and retention of iron in rheumatoid arthritis. *Ann Rheum Dis* 32:83, 1973.
58. Nicolas G, Bennoun M, Porteu A, et al: Severe iron deficiency anemia in transgenic mice expressing liver hepcidin. *Proc Natl Acad Sci U S A* 99:4596, 2002.
59. Nicolas G, Chauvet C, Viatte L, et al: The gene encoding the iron regulatory peptide hepcidin is regulated by anemia, hypoxia, and inflammation. *J Clin Invest* 110:1037, 2002.
60. Anderson GJ, Frazer DM, Wilkins SJ, et al: Relationship between intestinal iron-transporter expression, hepatic hepcidin levels and the control of iron absorption. *Biochem Soc Trans* 30:724, 2002.
61. Roe MA, Collings R, Dainty JR, et al: Plasma hepcidin concentrations significantly predict interindividual variation in iron absorption in healthy men. *Am J Clin Nutr* 89:1088, 2009.
62. Young MF, Glahn RP, Riza-Nieto M, et al: Serum hepcidin is significantly associated with iron absorption from food and supplemental sources in healthy young women. *Am J Clin Nutr* 89:533, 2009.
63. Cazzola M, Ponchio L, de Benedetti F, et al: Defective iron supply for erythropoiesis and adequate endogenous erythropoietin production in the anemia associated with systemic-onset juvenile chronic arthritis. *Blood* 87:4824, 1996.
64. Awai M, Brown EB: Studies of the metabolism of I-131-labeled human transferrin. *J Lab Clin Med* 61:363, 1963.
65. Jacobs A, Worwood M: Ferritin in serum. Clinical and biochemical implications. *N Engl J Med* 292:951, 1975.
66. Punnonen K, Irjala K, Rajamaki A: Serum transferrin receptor and its ratio to serum ferritin in the diagnosis of iron deficiency. *Blood* 89:1052, 1997.
67. Skikne BS: Serum transferrin receptor. *Am J Hematol* 83:872, 2008.
68. Konz T, Montes-Bayon M, Vaulont S: Hepcidin quantification: Methods and utility in diagnosis. *Metallomics* 6:1583, 2014.
69. Goodnough LT, Nemeth E, Ganz T: Detection, evaluation, and management of iron-restricted erythropoiesis. *Blood* 116:4754, 2010.
70. Barron BA, Hoyer JD, Tefferi A: A bone marrow report of absent stainable iron is not diagnostic of iron deficiency. *Ann Hematol* 80:166, 2001.
71. Iwamoto H, Nakamura Y, Konno O, et al: Correlation between post kidney transplant anemia and kidney graft function. *Transplant Proc* 46:496, 2014.

72. Pascual J, Jimenez C, Franco A, et al: Early-onset anemia after kidney transplantation is an independent factor for graft loss: A multicenter, observational cohort study. *Transplantation* 96:717, 2013.
73. Jones H, Talwar M, Nogueira JM, et al: Anemia after kidney transplantation; its prevalence, risk factors, and independent association with graft and patient survival: A time-varying analysis. *Transplantation* 93:923, 2012.
74. Kamar N, Rostaing L, Ignace S, et al: Impact of post-transplant anemia on patient and graft survival rates after kidney transplantation: A meta-analysis. *Clin Transplant* 26:461, 2012.
75. Yabu JM, Winkelmayer WC: Posttransplantation anemia: Mechanisms and management. *Clin J Am Soc Nephrol* 6:1794, 2011.
76. Vanrenterghem Y: Anemia after kidney transplantation. *Transplantation* 87:1265, 2009.
77. Ott U, Busch M, Steiner T, et al: Anemia after renal transplantation: An underestimated problem. *Transplant Proc* 40:3481, 2008.
78. Ghafari A, Noori-Majelan N: Anemia among long-term renal transplant recipients. *Transplant Proc* 40:186, 2008.
79. Bennett CL, Silver SM, Djulbegovic B, et al: Venous thromboembolism and mortality associated with recombinant erythropoietin and darbepoetin administration for the treatment of cancer-associated anemia. *JAMA* 299:914, 2008.
80. Singh AK, Szczech L, Tang KL, et al: Correction of anemia with epoetin alfa in chronic kidney disease. *N Engl J Med* 355:2085, 2006.
81. Pfeffer MA, Burdmann EA, Chen CY, et al: A trial of darbepoetin alfa in type 2 diabetes and chronic kidney disease. *N Engl J Med* 361:2019, 2009.
82. Solomon SD, Uno H, Lewis EF, et al: Erythropoietic response and outcomes in kidney disease and type 2 diabetes. *N Engl J Med* 363:1146, 2010.
83. Gaweda AE, Ginzburg YZ, Chait Y, et al: Iron dosing in kidney disease: Inconsistency of evidence and clinical practice. *Nephrol Dial Transplant* 2014 [Epub ahead of print].
84. Ludwig H, Fritz E, Leitgeb C, et al: Prediction of response to erythropoietin treatment in chronic anemia of cancer [see comments]. *Blood* 84:1056, 1994.
85. Smith RE, Tchekmedyian NS, Chan D, et al: A dose- and schedule-finding study of darbepoetin alpha for the treatment of chronic anaemia of cancer. *Br J Cancer* 88:1851, 2003.
86. Dammacco F, Castoldi G, Rodjer S: Efficacy of epoetin alfa in the treatment of anaemia of multiple myeloma. *Br J Haematol* 113:172, 2001.
87. Hedenus M, Adriansson M, San Miguel J, et al: Efficacy and safety of darbepoetin alfa in anaemic patients with lymphoproliferative malignancies: A randomized, double-blind, placebo-controlled study. *Br J Haematol* 122:394, 2003.
88. Peeters HR, Jongen-Lavrencic M, Bakker CH, et al: Recombinant human erythropoietin improves health-related quality of life in patients with rheumatoid arthritis and anaemia of chronic disease; utility measures correlate strongly with disease activity measures. *Rheumatol Int* 18:201, 1999.
89. Peeters HR, Jongen-Lavrencic M, Vreugdenhil G, et al: Effect of recombinant human erythropoietin on anaemia and disease activity in patients with rheumatoid arthritis and anaemia of chronic disease: A randomised placebo controlled double blind 52 weeks clinical trial. *Ann Rheum Dis* 55:739, 1996.
90. Goodnough LT, Marcus RE: The erythropoietic response to erythropoietin in patients with rheumatoid arthritis. *J Lab Clin Med* 130:381, 1997.
91. Kaltwasser JP, Kessler U, Gottschalk R, et al: Effect of recombinant human erythropoietin and intravenous iron on anemia and disease activity in rheumatoid arthritis. *J Rheumatol* 28:2430, 2001.
92. Schreiber S, Howaldt S, Schnoor M, et al: Recombinant erythropoietin for the treatment of anemia in inflammatory bowel disease. *N Engl J Med* 334:619, 1996.
93. Gasche C, Dejaco C, Reinisch W, et al: Sequential treatment of anemia in ulcerative colitis with intravenous iron and erythropoietin. *Digestion* 60:262, 1999.
94. Rizzo JD, Lichtin AE, Woolf SH, et al: Use of epoetin in patients with cancer: evidence-based clinical practice guidelines of the American Society of Clinical Oncology and the American Society of Hematology. *J Clin Oncol* 20:4083, 2002.
95. Rizzo JD, Somerfield MR, Hagerty KL, et al: Use of epoetin and darbepoetin in patients with cancer: 2007 American Society of Hematology/American Society of Clinical Oncology clinical practice guideline update. *Blood* 111:25, 2008.
96. Rizzo JD, Brouwers M, Hurley P, et al: American Society of Hematology/American Society of Clinical Oncology clinical practice guideline update on the use of epoetin and darbepoetin in adult patients with cancer. *Blood* 116:4045, 2010.
97. Drueke TB, Parfrey PS: Summary of the KDIGO guideline on anemia and comment: Reading between the (guide)line(s). *Kidney Int* 82:952, 2012.
98. Macdougall IC, Bock AH, Carrera F, et al: FIND-CKD: A randomized trial of intravenous ferric carboxymaltose versus oral iron in patients with chronic kidney disease and iron deficiency anaemia. *Nephrol Dial Transplant* 2014.
99. Kapoian T, O'Mara NB, Singh AK, et al: Ferric gluconate reduces epoetin requirements in hemodialysis patients with elevated ferritin. *J Am Soc Nephrol* 19:372, 2008.
100. Coyne DW, Kapoian T, Suki W, et al: Ferric gluconate is highly efficacious in anemic hemodialysis patients with high serum ferritin and low transferrin saturation: Results of the Dialysis Patients' Response to IV Iron with Elevated Ferritin (DRIVE) Study. *J Am Soc Nephrol* 18:975, 2007.
101. Jurado RL: Iron, infections, and anemia of inflammation. *Clin Infect Dis* 25:888, 1997.
102. Oppenheimer SJ: Iron and its relation to immunity and infectious disease. *J Nutr* 131:616S, 2001.

103. Susantitaphong P, Alqahtani F, Jaber BL: Efficacy and safety of intravenous iron therapy for functional iron deficiency anemia in hemodialysis patients: A meta-analysis. *Am J Nephrol* 39:130, 2014.

104. Litton E, Xiao J, Ho KM: Safety and efficacy of intravenous iron therapy in reducing requirement for allogeneic blood transfusion: Systematic review and meta-analysis of randomised clinical trials. *BMJ* 347:f4822, 2013.

105. Brookhart MA, Freburger JK, Ellis AR, et al: Infection risk with bolus versus maintenance iron supplementation in hemodialysis patients. *J Am Soc Nephrol* 24:1151, 2013.

106. Radtke HW, Claussner A, Erbes PM, et al: Serum erythropoietin concentration in chronic renal failure: Relationship to degree of anemia and excretory renal function. *Blood* 54:877, 1979.

107. Rossert J, Casadevall N, Eckardt KU: Anti-erythropoietin antibodies and pure red cell aplasia. *J Am Soc Nephrol* 15:398, 2004.

108. Epoetin: For better or for worse? *Lancet Oncol* 5:1, 2004.

109. Bohlius J, Weingart O, Trelle S, et al: Cancer-related anemia and recombinant human erythropoietin—an updated overview. *Nat Clin Pract Oncol* 3:152, 2006.

CHAPTER 38
ERYTHROPOIETIC EFFECTS OF ENDOCRINE DISORDERS

Xylina T. Gregg

SUMMARY

Anemia is the most common hematopoietic abnormality in endocrine disorders and may be the first manifestation of an endocrine disorder. Polycythemia/erythrocytosis is less common, but occurs in certain endocrine disorders. The pathophysiologic basis of the anemia is often multifactorial, but a direct influence of hormones on erythropoiesis in some instances may contribute to anemia. A decreased plasma volume in some of these disorders may mask the severity of anemia. It has been proposed that anemia in endocrine-deficiency states may be physiologic to adjust for decreased oxygen requirements. Some endocrine disorders are associated with an impaired response to the therapeutic use of erythropoietin.

●THYROID DYSFUNCTION

HYPOTHYROIDISM

Anemia is a well-recognized complication of thyroidectomy and other causes of hypothyroidism and may also occur in subclinical hypothyroidism.[1] In a retrospective review, anemia defined as a hemoglobin less than 13 g/dL in men and less than 12 g/dL in women was present in 57 percent of patients with hypothyroidism.[2] The anemia in hypothyroidism has been described variably as normocytic, macrocytic, or microcytic[3] coexisting deficiencies of iron, vitamin B_{12}, and folate may explain some of this heterogeneity. In a study of approximately 60 anemic patients with untreated primary hypothyroidism, 10 percent had a macrocytic anemia, all of whom had vitamin B_{12} deficiency, 43 percent had a microcytic anemia and iron deficiency, and the remainder had a normocytic anemia.[4] However, even when these deficiencies have been excluded, some hypothyroid patients have a macrocytic anemia.[5] In addition, although most hypothyroid patients have a significant reduction in their red cell mass, anemia is not always evident from hemoglobin and hematocrit values owing to a concomitant reduction of plasma volume.[6,7]

Hypothyroidism may contribute to the development of iron deficiency (Chap. 43) due to associated menorrhagia, although this association is less common than previously thought.[8] Because thyroid hormone may augment iron absorption,[9,10] iron deficiency in hypothyroidism may also be caused by impaired iron absorption, either directly from a lack of thyroid hormone or an associated achlorhydria.[11,12] Conversely, iron deficiency impairs thyroid hormone synthesis by reducing the activity of heme-dependent thyroid peroxidase.[13] In patients with coexisting iron-deficiency anemia and subclinical hypothyroidism, the anemia often does not adequately respond to oral iron therapy. Combined treatment with oral iron and levothyroxine results in superior improvement in hemoglobin and ferritin levels compared with levothyroxine alone in these patients.[14,15]

Although the macrocytosis seen in hypothyroid patients may be due to deficiencies of vitamin B_{12}[4,5] or folate[16] (Chap. 41), hypothyroidism

also causes macrocytosis that resolves with thyroxine treatment.[5] The mean corpuscular volume of hypothyroid patients with low vitamin B_{12} levels is similar to those with uncomplicated hypothyroidism, so this is not a sensitive means of identifying patients with hypothyroidism complicated by B_{12} deficiency.[5] Although there is an established association of hypothyroidism and pernicious anemia,[17,18] the underlying mechanism is unclear. In one analysis of 116 hypothyroid patients, 40 percent had low serum vitamin B_{12} levels.[19] Although the mean hemoglobin was slightly lower in the vitamin B_{12}–deficient group (11.9 g/L vs. 12.4 g/L), the mean corpuscular volume and prevalence of antithyroid antibodies did not differ between the two groups.[19]

However, even when iron deficiency, vitamin B_{12} deficiency, and other confounding causes of anemia have been excluded, anemia can be a direct consequence of thyroid hormone deficiency.[5,16] Dogs subjected to thyroidectomy have a normocytic, normochromic anemia that is associated with reticulocytopenia and marrow erythroid hypoplasia.[20] In hypothyroid humans and thyroidectomized animals, the red cell life span is normal, and results of ferrokinetic studies are compatible with hypoproliferative erythropoiesis.[20,21] Administration of thyroid hormones increases the rate of red cell production in experimental animals,[22] whereas thyroidectomy decreases red cell production.[23] Because thyroid hormones affect the cellular needs for oxygen, these responses are compatible with an appropriate physiologic adjustment. Evidence of a direct effect of thyroid hormones on erythropoiesis exists. Some *in vitro* studies show that triiodothyronine, thyroxine, and noncalorigenic resin triiodothyronine all potentiate the effect of erythropoietin on erythroid colony formation.[24] Thyroid hormones also increase hypoxia-induced production of erythropoietin in the rat kidney and a human hepatoma cell line.[25] However, other *in vitro* studies show an inhibitory effect of triiodothyronine on erythroid colony formation, particularly in combination with all-*trans* retinoic acid.[26]

Hypothyroidism may also affect the response to erythropoietin therapy. After adjusting for other variables, the mean monthly erythropoietin dose required to maintain a target hemoglobin level in hemodialysis patients was significantly higher in hypothyroid compared with euthyroid patients.[27]

Improvement in the hemoglobin concentration in response to thyroid hormone therapy is seen over a several-month period.[5] White blood cell and platelet counts usually are unaffected in hypothyroidism. However, pancytopenia in association with marrow hypoplasia has been reported in a patient with myxedema coma; the hematologic abnormalities in this patient resolved with thyroid hormone replacement.[28]

HYPERTHYROIDISM

Although thyroid hormone administration increases red cell production in animals,[29] humans with hyperthyroidism generally do not have erythrocytosis. Anemia is present in 10 to 25 percent of these patients.[30–32] This finding may be the result of increased plasma volume[7]; however, decreased red cell survival[33] and ineffective erythropoiesis[34] also have been described. Antithyroid treatment ameliorates the anemia.[31,32] A patient with autoimmune hemolytic anemia and hyperthyroidism has been described; the hemolysis in this patient abated with treatment of the hyperthyroidism.[35] Pancytopenia rarely occurs but also may respond to treatment of hyperthyroidism.[36,37]

●ADRENAL GLAND DISORDERS

ADRENOCORTICAL INSUFFICIENCY

A normocytic normochromic anemia may be seen in primary adrenal insufficiency (Addison disease),[12,38] but the anemia may also be masked by the concomitant reduction in plasma volume that is common in this disease.[38] In a series of patients with Addison disease, some patients with normal hemoglobin levels developed transient anemia after initiation of hormone replacement therapy, presumably secondary to an increased plasma volume.[38]

In experimental animals, adrenalectomy causes a mild anemia that responds to glucocorticoids.[39] However, the pathophysiologic basis of the anemia and any influence of adrenal cortical hormones on erythropoiesis are not well defined.

Pernicious anemia occurs in patients with autoimmune adrenal insufficiency, but is seen primarily in patients with type I polyglandular autoimmune syndrome, whose other manifestations include mucocutaneous candidiasis and hypoparathyroidism.[40] Anemia as a result of primary erythropoietin deficiency was reported in one patient with this syndrome.[41]

CUSHING DISEASE AND ALDOSTERONISM

Glucocorticoids interact with erythropoietin *in vitro* to enhance erythroid colony proliferation.[42] Glucocorticoid receptors, activated by their cognate ligand, initiate Janus kinase 2 phosphorylation-mediated cytoplasmic signal transduction, which may stimulate erythropoiesis by a mechanism shared with erythropoietin (Chaps. 32 and 57). Erythrocytosis has been reported in Cushing syndrome,[43] primary aldosteronism,[44] and Bartter syndrome.[45]

However, a study of 63 women and 17 men with Cushing disease found that although the hemoglobin levels in the females were evenly distributed over the normal range, the hemoglobin levels were in the lowest quartile in 14 of the 17 men, and 3 of these 14 were anemic.[46] The reduced hemoglobin levels in the male patients correlated with a low testosterone level and slowly improved after treatment of Cushing disease.

CONGENITAL ADRENAL HYPERPLASIA

The most common cause of congenital adrenal hyperplasia is 21-hydroxylase deficiency, which impairs conversion of 17-hydroxyprogesterone to 11-deoxycortisol.[47] Patients with the "classic form" present during the neonatal period with adrenal insufficiency, but others have a late onset presentation with findings of androgen excess. Erythrocytosis, likely a consequence of increased androgen levels, has been reported in patients with congenital adrenal hyperplasia resulting from 21-hydroxylase deficiency,[48] and erythrocytosis has also been described as the presenting manifestation of this disease.[49]

PHEOCHROMOCYTOMA

Pheochromocytomas and the closely related tumor, paraganglioma, are rarely associated with erythrocytosis. This finding is believed to be a result of autonomous erythropoietin production by the tumor,[50] often mediated by von Hippel-Lindau mutations that cause or contribute to pheochromocytoma development (Chaps. 32 and 57).

However, several individuals with congenital polycythemia have developed recurrent pheochromocytomas, paragangliomas, and sometimes somatostatinomas.[51,52] Their tumors are heterozygous for a heterogeneous gain-of-function mutation of hypoxia-inducible factor-2α gene and erythropoietin transcript is present in tumor tissues (Chaps. 32 and 57). However, these mutations are generally not found in nontumor tissues, so the etiology of the association of these tumors with polycythemia is unknown.[51,52]

A syndrome of congenital polycythemia associated with a mutation in the proline hydroxylase type 2 gene and recurrent paragangliomas has also been described in a single family.[53]

● GONADAL HORMONES

ANDROGENS

Sexually mature males have higher hemoglobin levels than prepubertal males, older males, and females.[54] This difference is attributed to androgen production. Testosterone levels directly correlated with hemoglobin levels in a community population of males 30 to 94 years of age.[55] Another study of males 70 to 81 years of age also found a correlation between hemoglobin and testosterone levels, but when individuals with hemoglobin less than 13 g/dL and/or a testosterone level less than 8 nmol/L were excluded, the association was no longer significant.[56] Orchiectomy results in a median decrease in hemoglobin concentration of 1.2 g/dL.[57] "Medical" castration with combined androgen blockade by gonadotropin-releasing agonists and antiandrogens also causes anemia.[58]

The erythropoietic effects of androgens have been widely exploited for the treatment of various anemias, especially before the development of recombinant erythropoietin. Testosterone therapy in hypogonadal men increased the mean hematocrit from 38.0 percent to 43.1 percent within 3 months.[59] Two meta-analyses found that erythrocytosis (defined as a hematocrit greater than 50 or 52 percent) was greater than three times more likely to occur in a testosterone-treated group compared to placebo.[60,61] Erythrocytosis was reported in a woman treated for breast cancer with an aromatase inhibitor, which prevents the conversion of androstenedione and testosterone to estrogen.[62]

The mechanism of androgen action appears to be complex, with evidence for stimulation of erythropoietin secretion[63] and a direct effect on the marrow.[64] Androgen receptors have been identified in the marrow cells of human males and females. However, the cells expressing the receptors included stromal cells, endothelial cells, macrophages, and myeloid precursors, but not erythroid cells,[65] thus the pathophysiologic significance of this association is unclear. Testosterone administration is associated with an increase in erythropoietin levels and a decrease in hepcidin levels.[63] Although erythropoietin levels declined with continued testosterone administration, they remained inappropriately high despite improved hemoglobin levels, suggesting a new setpoint.[63]

ESTROGENS

Data regarding the role of estrogens is conflicting. Administration of large doses of estrogen led to a moderately severe anemia in rats.[66,67] However, hematopoietic stem cells express estrogen receptor-α and estrogen signaling via this receptor promotes hematopoietic stem cell self-renewal and stimulates erythropoiesis.[68]

● PITUITARY GLAND DISORDERS

PITUITARY INSUFFICIENCY

The most common cause of pituitary insufficiency is pituitary tumors or consequences of their therapy.[69] Other etiologies include hypothalamic tumors or dysfunction, sarcoidosis or other infiltrative diseases, pituitary hemorrhage or infarct, genetic causes, and idiopathic pituitary failure. Regardless of the cause, hypopituitarism results in a moderately severe normochromic normocytic anemia, with an average hemoglobin level of 10 g/dL.[12,70] Anemia and erythroid hypoplasia have also been described in hypophysectomized animals.[71,72]

In rats, removal of the posterior lobe of the pituitary, which secretes vasopressin and oxytocin, does not result in anemia.[73] Thus, the anemia of hypopituitarism presumably results from the absence of the anterior lobe hormones, adrenocorticotropic hormone, thyroid-stimulating hormone, follicle-stimulating hormone, luteinizing hormone, growth hormone, and prolactin, although the exact role of each of these hormones in the pathogenesis of anemia is unknown. The resulting deficiencies of thyroid hormones, adrenal hormones, and androgens are likely the major contributors to anemia. Combined adrenalectomy and thyroidectomy in animals results in an anemia that is similar but not identical to that seen after hypophysectomy.[74] A correlation between low testosterone levels and anemia has been observed in human males with hypopituitarism resulting from nonfunctioning pituitary adenomas.[75]

Red cell survival is normal in hypopituitarism, but the marrow is hypoplastic. The results of ferrokinetic studies are consistent with decreased erythropoiesis.[12] In addition to anemia, leukopenia and even pancytopenia can occur.[76] Replacement therapy with a combination of thyroid, adrenal, and gonadal hormones usually effectively corrects anemia and other cytopenias.[76,77] Erythropoietin therapy also was effective in one case of postoperative hypopituitarism refractory to hormone replacement therapy.[78]

OTHER PITUITARY HORMONES

Growth Hormone

Growth hormone stimulates erythropoietin-induced erythropoiesis *in vitro*,[79,80] and children with isolated growth hormone deficiency become anemic.[81] Growth hormone replacement therapy in both children and adults with growth hormone deficiency increases hemoglobin levels.[82–84]

Prolactin

There is limited information about the influence of prolactin. Prolactin administration in mice increased the number of erythroid and myeloid progenitor cells and partially corrected anemia induced by azidothymidine.[85] Metoclopramide, which stimulates prolactin secretion, improved hemoglobin levels or reduced transfusions in three of nine patients with Diamond-Blackfan anemia.[86] The prolactin receptor can substitute for the erythropoietin receptor in *in vitro* studies of erythroid differentiation.[87,88]

However, macroprolactinomas have not been associated with erythrocytosis, but with anemia, likely the result of a concomitant decrease in testosterone levels.[89] In a retrospective review of 26 males with prolactinomas, a mild anemia was present in one-third, all of whom had a macroprolactinoma.[90] Hemoglobin levels did not correlate with serum prolactin levels, but did correlate with the presence of hypogonadism.[90]

Gonadotropins

Pituitary adenomas that secrete gonadotropins are rare, but have been associated with erythrocytosis, likely due to testosterone excess.[91]

●HYPERPARATHYROIDISM

Anemia not attributable to other causes is present in 3 to 5 percent of patients with primary hyperparathyroidism; these patients usually have severe hyperparathyroidism.[92,93] The anemia is normochromic and normocytic and resolves or improves after parathyroidectomy.[92,93] The cause of the anemia is unknown; marrow fibrosis is present in some but not all patients.[92,94] Although there is no correlation with marrow fibrosis and the duration of hyperparathyroidism, the presence of marrow fibrosis may positively correlate with improvement in anemia after parathyroidectomy.[94]

Although anemia in patients with renal failure is multifactorial, secondary hyperparathyroidism may contribute to refractoriness to erythropoietin therapy. Parathyroidectomy or medical treatment of hyperparathyroidism may improve anemia and decrease requirements for exogenous erythropoietin therapy.[95–98]

REFERENCES

1. Bashir H, Bhat MH, Farooq R, et al: Comparison of hematological parameters in untreated and treated subclinical hypothyroidism and primary hypothyroidism patients. *Med J Islam Repub Iran* 26(4):172–178, 2012.
2. Omar S, Hadj Taeib S, Kanoun F, et al: [Erythrocyte abnormalities in thyroid dysfunction] [in French]. *Tunis Med* 88(11):783–788, 2010.
3. Fein HG, Rivlin RS: Anemia in thyroid diseases. *Med Clin North Am* 59(5):1133–1145, 1975.
4. Das C, Sahana PK, Sengupta N, et al: Etiology of anemia in primary hypothyroid subjects in a tertiary care center in eastern India. *Indian J Endocrinol Metab* 16(Suppl 2): S361–S363, 2012.
5. Horton L, Coburn RJ, England JM, et al: The haematology of hypothyroidism. *Q J Med* 45(177):101–123, 1976.
6. Das KC, Mukherjee M, Sarkar TK, et al: Erythropoiesis and erythropoietin in hypo- and hyperthyroidism. *J Clin Endocrinol Metab* 40(2):211–220, 1975.
7. Muldowney FP, Crooks J, Wayne EJ: The total red cell mass in thyrotoxicosis and myxoedema. *Clin Sci (Lond)* 16(2):309–314, 1957.
8. Kakuno Y, Amino N, Kanoh M, et al: Menstrual disturbances in various thyroid diseases. *Endocr J* 57(12):1017–1022, 2010.
9. Pirzio-Biroli G, Bothwell TH, Finch CA: Iron absorption. II. The absorption of radioiron administered with a standard meal in man. *J Lab Clin Med* 51(1):37–48, 1958.
10. Donati RM, Fletcher JW, Warnecke MA, et al: Erythropoiesis in hypothyroidism. *Proc Soc Exp Biol Med* 144(1):78–82, 1973.
11. Lerman J, Means JH: The gastric secretion in exophthalmic goitre and myxedema. *J Clin Invest* 11(1):167–182, 1932.
12. Daughaday WH, Williams RH, Daland GA: The effect of endocrinopathies on the blood. *Blood* 3(12):1342–1366, 1948.
13. Zimmermann MB, Köhrle J: The impact of iron and selenium deficiencies on iodine and thyroid metabolism: Biochemistry and relevance to public health. *Thyroid* 12(10):867–878, 2002.
14. Cinemre H, Bilir C, Gokosmanoglu F, et al: Hematologic effects of levothyroxine in iron-deficient subclinical hypothyroid patients: A randomized, double-blind, controlled study. *J Clin Endocrinol Metab* 94(1):151–156, 2009.
15. Ravanbod M, Asadipooya K, Kalantarhormozi M, et al: Treatment of iron-deficiency anemia in patients with subclinical hypothyroidism. *Am J Med* 126(5):420–424, 2013.
16. Hines JD, Halsted CH, Griggs RC, et al: Megaloblastic anemia secondary to folate deficiency associated with hypothyroidism. *Ann Intern Med* 68(4):792–805, 1968.
17. Carmel R, Spencer CA: Clinical and subclinical thyroid disorders associated with pernicious anemia. Observations on abnormal thyroid-stimulating hormone levels and on a possible association of blood group O with hyperthyroidism. *Arch Intern Med* 142(8):1465–1469, 1982.
18. Green ST, Ng JP, Chan-Lam D: Insulin-dependent diabetes mellitus, myasthenia gravis, pernicious anaemia, autoimmune thyroiditis and autoimmune adrenalitis in a single patient. *Scott Med J* 33(1):213–214, 1988.
19. Jabbar A, Yawar A, Waseem S, et al: Vitamin B₁₂ deficiency common in primary hypothyroidism. *J Pak Med Assoc* 58(5):258–261, 2008.
20. Cline MJ, Berlin NI: Erythropoiesis and red cell survival in the hypothyroid dog. *Am J Physiol* 204:415–418, 1963.
21. Kiely JM, Purnell DC, Owen CA: Erythrokinetics in myxedema. *Ann Intern Med* 67(3):533–538, 1967.
22. Shalet M, Coe D, Reissmann KR: Mechanism of erythropoietic action of thyroid hormone. *Proc Soc Exp Biol Med* 123(2):443–446, 1966.
23. Gordon AS, Kadow PC: The thyroid and blood regeneration in the rat. *Am J Med Sci* 212(4):385–394, 1946.
24. Golde DW, Bersch N, Chopra IJ, et al: Thyroid hormones stimulate erythropoiesis in vitro. *Br J Haematol* 37(2):173–177, 1977.
25. Fandrey J, Pagel H, Frede S, et al: Thyroid hormones enhance hypoxia-induced erythropoietin production in vitro. *Exp Hematol* 22(3):272–277, 1994.
26. Perrin MC, Blanchet JP, Mouchiroud G: Modulation of human and mouse erythropoiesis by thyroid hormone and retinoic acid: Evidence for specific effects at different steps of the erythroid pathway. *Hematol Cell Ther* 39(1):19–26, 1997.
27. Ng YY, Lin HD, Wu SC, et al: Impact of thyroid dysfunction on erythropoietin dosage in hemodialysis patients. *Thyroid* 23(5):552–561, 2013.
28. Song SH, McCallum CJ, Campbell IW: Hypoplastic anaemia complicating myxoedema coma. *Scott Med J* 43(5):149–150, 1998.
29. Sullivan PS, McDonald TP: Thyroxine suppresses thrombocytopoiesis and stimulates erythropoiesis in mice. *Proc Soc Exp Biol Med* 201(3):271–277, 1992.
30. Nightingale S, Vitek PJ, Himsworth RL: The haematology of hyperthyroidism. *Q J Med* 47(185):35–47, 1978.
31. Perlman JA, Sternthal PM: Effect of 131i on the anemia of hyperthyroidism. *J Chronic Dis* 36(5):405–412, 1983.
32. Gianoukakis AG, Leigh MJ, Richards P, et al: Characterization of the anaemia associated with Graves' disease. *Clin Endocrinol (Oxf)* 70(5):781–787, 2009.
33. McClellan JE, Donegan C, Thorup OA, et al: Survival time of the erythrocyte in myxedema and hyperthyroidism. *J Lab Clin Med* 51(1):91–96, 1958.
34. Donati RM, Warnecke MA, Gallagher NI: Ferrokinetics in hyperthyroidism. *Ann Intern Med* 63(6):945–950, 1965.

35. Ogihara T, Katoh H, Yoshitake H, et al: Hyperthyroidism associated with autoimmune hemolytic anemia and periodic paralysis: A report of a case in which antihyperthyroid therapy alone was effective against hemolysis. *Jpn J Med* 26(3):401–403, 1987.

36. Lima CSP, Zantut Wittmann DE, Castro V, et al: Pancytopenia in untreated patients with graves' disease. *Thyroid* 16(4):403–409, 2006.

37. Akoum R, Michel S, Wafic T, et al: Myelodysplastic syndrome and pancytopenia responding to treatment of hyperthyroidism: Peripheral blood and bone marrow analysis before and after antihormonal treatment. *J Cancer Res Ther* 3(1):43–46, 2007.

38. Baez-Villasenor J, Rath CE, Finch CA: The blood picture in Addison's disease. *Blood* 3(7):769–773, 1948.

39. Bozzini CE, Barrio Rendo ME, Kofoed JA, et al: Effect of hydrocortisone administration on erythropoiesis in the adrenalectomized dog. *Experientia* 24(8):800–801, 1968.

40. Eisenbarth GS, Gottlieb PA: Autoimmune polyendocrine syndromes. *N Engl J Med* 350(20):2068–2079, 2004.

41. Toonkel R, Levine M, Gardner L: Erythropoietin-deficient anemia associated with autoimmune polyglandular syndrome type I. *Am J Hematol* 75(2):84–88, 2004.

42. von Lindern M, Zauner W, Mellitzer G, et al: The glucocorticoid receptor cooperates with the erythropoietin receptor and c-kit to enhance and sustain proliferation of erythroid progenitors in vitro. *Blood* 94(2):550–559, 1999.

43. Plotz CM, Knowlton AI, Ragan C: The natural history of Cushing's syndrome. *Am J Med* 13(5):597–614, 1952.

44. Mann DL, Gallagher NI, Donati RM: Erythrocytosis and primary aldosteronism. *Ann Intern Med* 66(2):335–340, 1967.

45. Erkelens DW, Statius van Eps LW: Bartter's syndrome and erythrocytosis. *Am J Med* 55(5):711–719, 1973.

46. Ambrogio AG, De Martin M, Ascoli P, et al: Gender-dependent changes in haematological parameters in patients with Cushing's disease before and after remission. *Eur J Endocrinol* 170(3):393–400, 2014.

47. White PC, Speiser PW: Congenital adrenal hyperplasia due to 21-hydroxylase deficiency. *Endocr Rev* 21(3):245–291, 2000.

48. Albareda MM, Rodríguez-Espinosa J, Remacha A, et al: Polycythemia in a patient with 21-hydroxylase deficiency. *Haematologica* 85 (E-letters):E08, 2000.

49. Ramos J, Regadera A, Román P, et al: [Congenital adrenal hyperplasia owing to 21-hydroxylase deficiency presenting with erythrocytosis] [in Spanish]. *Med Clin (Barc)* 131(16):638–639, 2008.

50. Drénou B, Le Tulzo Y, Caulet-Maugendre S, et al: Pheochromocytoma and secondary erythrocytosis: Role of tumour erythropoietin secretion. *Nouv Rev Fr Hematol Invest* 37(3):197–199, 1995.

51. Zhuang Z, Yang C, Lorenzo F, et al: Somatic HIF2A gain-of-function mutations in paraganglioma with polycythemia. *N Engl J Med* 367(10):922–930, 2012.

52. Yang C, Sun MG, Matro J, et al: Novel HIF2A mutations disrupt oxygen sensing, leading to polycythemia, paragangliomas, and somatostatinomas. *Blood* 121(13):2563–2566, 2013.

53. Ladroue C, Carcenac R, Leporrier M, et al: PHD2 mutation and congenital erythrocytosis with paraganglioma. *N Engl J Med* 359(25):2685–2692, 2008.

54. Hawkins WW, Speck E, Leonard VG: Variation of the hemoglobin level with age and sex. *Blood* 9(10):999–1007, 1954.

55. Yeap BB, Beilin J, Shi Z, et al: Serum testosterone levels correlate with haemoglobin in middle-aged and older men. *Intern Med J* 39(8):532–538, 2009.

56. Lewerin C, Nilsson-Ehle H, Jacobsson S, et al: Serum estradiol associates with blood hemoglobin in elderly men: The MROS Sweden study. *J Clin Endocrinol Metab* 99(7):2549–2556, 2014.

57. Fonseca R, Rajkumar SV, White WL, et al: Anemia after orchiectomy. *Am J Hematol* 59(3):230–233, 1998.

58. Bogdanos J, Karamanolakis D, Milathianakis C, et al: Combined androgen blockade-induced anemia in prostate cancer patients without bone involvement. *Anticancer Res* 23(2C):1757–1762, 2003.

59. Snyder PJ, Peachey H, Berlin JA, et al: Effects of testosterone replacement in hypogonadal men. *J Clin Endocrinol Metab* 85(8):2670–2677, 2000.

60. Calof OM, Singh AB, Lee ML, et al: Adverse events associated with testosterone replacement in middle-aged and older men: A meta-analysis of randomized, placebo-controlled trials. *J Gerontol A Biol Sci Med Sci* 60(11):1451–1457, 2005.

61. Fernández-Balsells MM, Murad MH, Lane M, et al: Clinical review 1: Adverse effects of testosterone therapy in adult men: A systematic review and meta-analysis. *J Clin Endocrinol Metab* 95(6):2560–2575, 2010.

62. Iyengar A, Sheppard D: A case of erythrocytosis in a patient treated with an aromatase inhibitor for breast cancer. *Case Rep Hematol* 2013:615189, 2013.

63. Bachman E, Travison TG, Basaria S, et al: Testosterone induces erythrocytosis via increased erythropoietin and suppressed hepcidin: Evidence for a new erythropoietin/hemoglobin set point. *J Gerontol A Biol Sci Med Sci* 69(6):725–735, 2014.

64. Beran M, Spitzer G, Verma DS: Testosterone and synthetic and androgens improve the in vitro survival of human marrow progenitor cells in serum-free suspension cultures. *J Lab Clin Med* 99(2):247–253, 1982.

65. Mantalaris A, Panoskaltsis N, Sakai Y, et al: Localization of androgen receptor expression in human bone marrow. *J Pathol* 193(3):361–366, 2001.

66. Dukes PP, Goldwasser E: Inhibition of erythropoiesis by estrogens. *Endocrinology* 69:21–29, 1961.

67. Piliero SJ, Medici PT, Haber C: The interrelationships of the endocrine and erythropoietic systems in the rat with special reference to the mechanism of action of estradiol and testosterone. *Ann N Y Acad Sci* 149(1):336–355, 1968.

68. Nakada D, Oguro H, Levi BP, et al: Oestrogen increases haematopoietic stem-cell self-renewal in females and during pregnancy. *Nature* 505(7484):555–558, 2014.

69. Bates AS, Van't Hoff W, Jones PJ, et al: The effect of hypopituitarism on life expectancy. *J Clin Endocrinol Metab* 81(3):1169–1172, 1996.

70. Greig HB, Metz J, Sunn L: Anaemia in hypopituitarism; treatment with testosterone and cortisone. *S Afr J Lab Clin Med* 2(1):52–61, 1956.

71. Berlin NI, Van Dyke DC, Siri WE, et al: The effect of hypophysectomy on the total circulating red cell volume of the rat. *Endocrinology* 47(6):429–435, 1950.

72. Crafts RC, Meineke HA: The anemia of hypophysectomized animals. *Ann N Y Acad Sci* 77:501–517, 1959.

73. Van Dyke DC, Garcia JF, Simpson ME, et al: Maintenance of circulating red cell volume in rats after removal of the posterior and intermediate lobes of the pituitary. *Blood* 7(10):1005–1016, 1952.

74. Crafts RC: The similarity between anemia induced by hypophysectomy and that induced by a combined thyroidectomy and adrenalectomy in adult female rats. *Endocrinology* 53(5):465–473, 1953.

75. Ellegala DB, Alden TD, Couture DE, et al: Anemia, testosterone, and pituitary adenoma in men. *J Neurosurg* 98(5):974–977, 2003.

76. Kim D-Y, Kim JH, Park YJ, et al: Case of complete recovery of pancytopenia after treatment of hypopituitarism. *Ann Hematol* 83(5):309–312, 2004.

77. Ferrari E, Ascari E, Bossolo PA, et al: Sheehan's syndrome with complete bone marrow aplasia: Long-term results of substitution therapy with hormones. *Br J Haematol* 33(4):575–582, 1976.

78. Nomiyama J, Shinohara K, Inoue H: Improvement of anemia by recombinant erythropoietin in a patient with postoperative hypopituitarism. *Am J Hematol* 47(3):249–250, 1994.

79. Golde DW, Bersch N, Li CH: Growth hormone: Species-specific stimulation of erythropoiesis in vitro. *Science* 196(4294):1112–1113, 1977.

80. Merchav S, Tatarsky I, Hochberg Z: Enhancement of erythropoiesis in vitro by human growth hormone is mediated by insulin-like growth factor I. *Br J Haematol* 70(3):267–271, 1988.

81. Eugster EA, Fisch M, Walvoord EC, et al: Low hemoglobin levels in children with in idiopathic growth hormone deficiency. *Endocrine* 18(2):135–136, 2002.

82. Ten Have SM, van der Lely AJ, Lamberts SW: Increase in haemoglobin concentrations in growth hormone deficient adults during human recombinant growth hormone replacement therapy. *Clin Endocrinol (Oxf)* 47(5):565–570, 1997.

83. Bergamaschi S, Giavoli C, Ferrante E, et al: Growth hormone replacement therapy in growth hormone deficient children and adults: Effects on hemochrome. *J Endocrinol Invest* 29(5):399–404, 2006.

84. Miniero R, Altomare F, Rubino M, et al: Effect of recombinant human growth hormone (rhgh) on hemoglobin concentration in children with idiopathic growth hormone deficiency-related anemia. *J Pediatr Hematol Oncol* 34(6):407–411, 2012.

85. Woody MA, Welniak LA, Sun R, et al: Prolactin exerts hematopoietic growth-promoting effects in vivo and partially counteracts myelosuppression by azidothymidine. *Exp Hematol* 27(5):811–816, 1999.

86. Abkowitz JL, Schaison G, Boulad F, et al: Response of Diamond-Blackfan anemia to metoclopramide: Evidence for a role for prolactin in erythropoiesis. *Blood* 100(8):2687–2691, 2002.

87. Socolovsky M, Dusanter-Fourt I, Lodish HF: The prolactin receptor and severely truncated erythropoietin receptors support differentiation of erythroid progenitors. *J Biol Chem* 272(22):14009–14012, 1997.

88. Socolovsky M, Fallon AE, Lodish HF: The prolactin receptor rescues EPOR-/- erythroid progenitors and replaces EPOR in a synergistic interaction with c-kit. *Blood* 92(5):1491–1496, 1998.

89. Shimon I, Benbassat C, Tzvetov G, et al: Anemia in a cohort of men with macroprolactinomas: Increase in hemoglobin levels follows prolactin suppression. *Pituitary* 14(1):11–15, 2011.

90. Iglesias P, Castro JC, Díez JJ: Clinical significance of anaemia associated with prolactin-secreting pituitary tumours in men. *Int J Clin Pract* 65(6):669–673, 2011.

91. Ceccato F, Occhi G, Regazzo D, et al: Gonadotropin secreting pituitary adenoma associated with erythrocytosis: Case report and literature review. *Hormones (Athens)* 13(1):131–139, 2014.

92. Boxer M, Ellman L, Geller R, et al: Anemia in primary hyperparathyroidism. *Arch Intern Med* 137(5):588–593, 1977.

93. Abarca J, Trigonis C, Hamberger B, et al: Anaemia in primary hyperparathyroidism—fantasy or reality. *Ann Chir Gynaecol* 74(2):74–76, 1985.

94. Bhadada SK, Bhansali A, Ahluwalia J, et al: Anaemia and marrow fibrosis in patients with primary hyperparathyroidism before and after curative parathyroidectomy. *Clin Endocrinol (Oxf)* 70(4):527–532, 2009.

95. Argilés A, Mourad G, Lorho R, et al: Medical treatment of severe hyperparathyroidism and its influence on anaemia in end-stage renal failure. *Nephrol Dial Transplant* 9(12):1809–1812, 1994.

96. Trunzo JA, McHenry CR, Schulak JA, et al: Effect of parathyroidectomy on anemia and erythropoietin dosing in end-stage renal disease patients with hyperparathyroidism. *Surgery* 144(6):915–918; discussion 919, 2008.

97. Battistella M, Richardson RMA, Bargman JM, et al: Improved parathyroid hormone control by cinacalcet is associated with reduction in darbepoetin requirement in patients with end-stage renal disease. *Clin Nephrol* 76(2):99–103, 2011.

98. Oshiro Y, Tanaka H, Okimoto N: A patient undergoing chronic dialysis whose renal anemia was successfully corrected by treatment with cinacalcet. *Clin Exp Nephrol* 15(4):607–610, 2011.

CHAPTER 39
THE CONGENITAL DYSERYTHROPOIETIC ANEMIAS

Achille Iolascon*

SUMMARY

The congenital dyserythropoietic anemias (CDAs) are a heterogeneous group of rare disorders characterized by anemia, the presence of erythroid hyperplasia with multinuclear erythroid precursors in the marrow, ineffective erythropoiesis and secondary iron overload. Only the erythroid series shows significant abnormalities, with rare exceptions. Patients have been classified as types I, II, and III, but several patients appearing with these general characteristics do not fit into any of the three groups. CDA types I and II are inherited as autosomal recessive disorders, and type III disease is inherited as an autosomal dominant disorder. Type I disease is caused by mutations of the *CDAN1* gene. Codanin-1, the gene product, is a cell-cycle-regulated protein of currently unknown function. In codanin-negative cases, *C15ORF41* mutations can cause type I CDA. Type II CDA is also known as hereditary erythroblastic multinuclearity with a positive acidified serum test, or by its acronym HEMPAS. The vast majority of CDA type II cases are caused by mutations of the *SEC23B* gene. This gene encodes the cytoplasmic COPII (coat protein) component

SEC23B, which is involved in the secretory pathway of eukaryotic cells. CDA type III disease is rarer than the other two forms and its erythroid production failure is accompanied by a tendency for the development of retinal angioid streaks and of myeloma in the long term. It is caused by *KIF23* mutations, a gene encoding mitotic kinesin-like protein 1, which plays a critical role in cytokinesis. There is no specific treatment for these disorders. Management includes red cell transfusion, removal of excess body iron by chelation therapy or judicious phlebotomy, splenectomy, and allogeneic hematopoietic stem cell transplantation. Only in severe forms of type I CDA does interferon-*a* decrease transfusion needs.

DEFINITION AND HISTORY

The term *congenital dyserythropoietic anemia* (CDA), coined by Heimpel and Wendt,[1] applies to a group of rare hereditary refractory anemias characterized by ineffective erythropoiesis, erythroid hyperplasia, abnormal morphology of erythroid precursors, and secondary accumulation of tissue iron.

Dyserythropoiesis is a result of derangement of the multistep process of normal erythroid maturation caused by a maturation arrest at early and late polychromatic erythroblasts and a consequent reduction of daily red cell production (Fig. 39–1A). Depending on the degree of the cellular defect, variable degrees of anemia can result.

Dyserythropoiesis can be considered a subtype of marrow failure syndromes characterized by monolineage involvement and abnormalities in erythroid precursor cells (see Fig. 39–1B). Microscopic morphologic characterization defines the heterogeneity of these syndromes (Fig. 39–2). Indeed, the appearance of abnormal morphology of erythroid progenitors can be from other hereditary defects (such as thalassemias) and acquired causes (rapid regeneration of marrow, myelodysplasia, etc.), but these are usually readily apparent from the history, blood examination, and laboratory tests in the former and multilineage involvement and the absence of prevalent multinuclearity in the latter. Furthermore, the term *congenital* could be confusing, as the clinical appearance of hereditary dyserythropoietic anemias can be present during different ages. In addition, it is an archaic residual of older nomenclature and should be replaced by "hereditary" as it has been in diseases such as congenital spherocytosis (now hereditary spherocytosis).

Anemia is usually first noted in infancy or childhood. The life span of circulating erythrocytes is moderately reduced, and the dominant factor in pathogenesis is a large component of ineffective erythropoiesis (intramedullary cell death as a result of precursor cell apoptosis) resulting in anemia of variable severity, normal or slightly elevated reticulocytes, moderate increase in indirect bilirubin, low haptoglobin, and, typically, a gradual increase in ferritin levels. Splenomegaly is common. Congenital dyserythropoietic anemias have been classified into three types—types I, II, and III. In addition, a number of cases that do not fit clearly into any of these three categories have been described.[2]

EPIDEMIOLOGY

The prevalence of CDAs is likely higher than reported as a result of their clinical heterogeneity and diagnostic difficulties, as demonstrated by the fact that the correct diagnosis is often delayed into adulthood.

Merging of information from European registries suggests that the prevalence of CDA I and CDA II in Europe is approximately

Acronyms and Abbreviations: AE1, band 3 anion transport protein; Arf6, adenosine diphosphate (ADP)-ribosylation factor 6; Asf1a, a protein that is a member of the H3/H4 family of histone chaperones; *C15ORF41*, gene encoding a protein with two predicted helix-turn-helix domains of unknown function; CDA, congenital dyserythropoietic anemia; *CDAN1* gene, codanin-1; COP, cytoplasmic coat protein; *COX4I2*, gene encoding cytochrome c oxidase subunit IV isoform; E2F1, transcription factor 1; ER, endoplasmic reticulum; G6PD, glucose-6-phosphate dehydrogenase; GATA1, hematopoietic transcription factor; GDF15, growth differentiation factor 15; HEMPAS, hereditary erythroblastic multinuclearity associated with a positive acidified serum test; HJV, hemojuvelin gene; HLA, human leukocyte antigens; HS, hereditary spherocytosis; KIF23, mitotic kinesin-like protein 1; *LPIN2* (18p11.31), encoding lipin 2; KLF1, a hematopoietic transcription factor; MCV, mean cell volume; MKD, mevalonate kinase deficiency; *MKLP1*, gene encoding mitotic kinesin-like protein 1; *SAR1B*, a gene encoding a small guanosine triphosphatase (GTPase) protein; SDS-PAGE, sodium dodecylsulfate polyacrylamide gel electrophoresis; *UGT1A1*, bilirubin uridine diphosphate (UDP)-glucuronosyltransferase 1A1 gene.

*Dr. Jean Delaunay wrote this chapter in the 8th edition of this textbook. Some of the material from the 8th edition has been retained. Dr. Roberta Russo collaborated in the preparation of this manuscript.

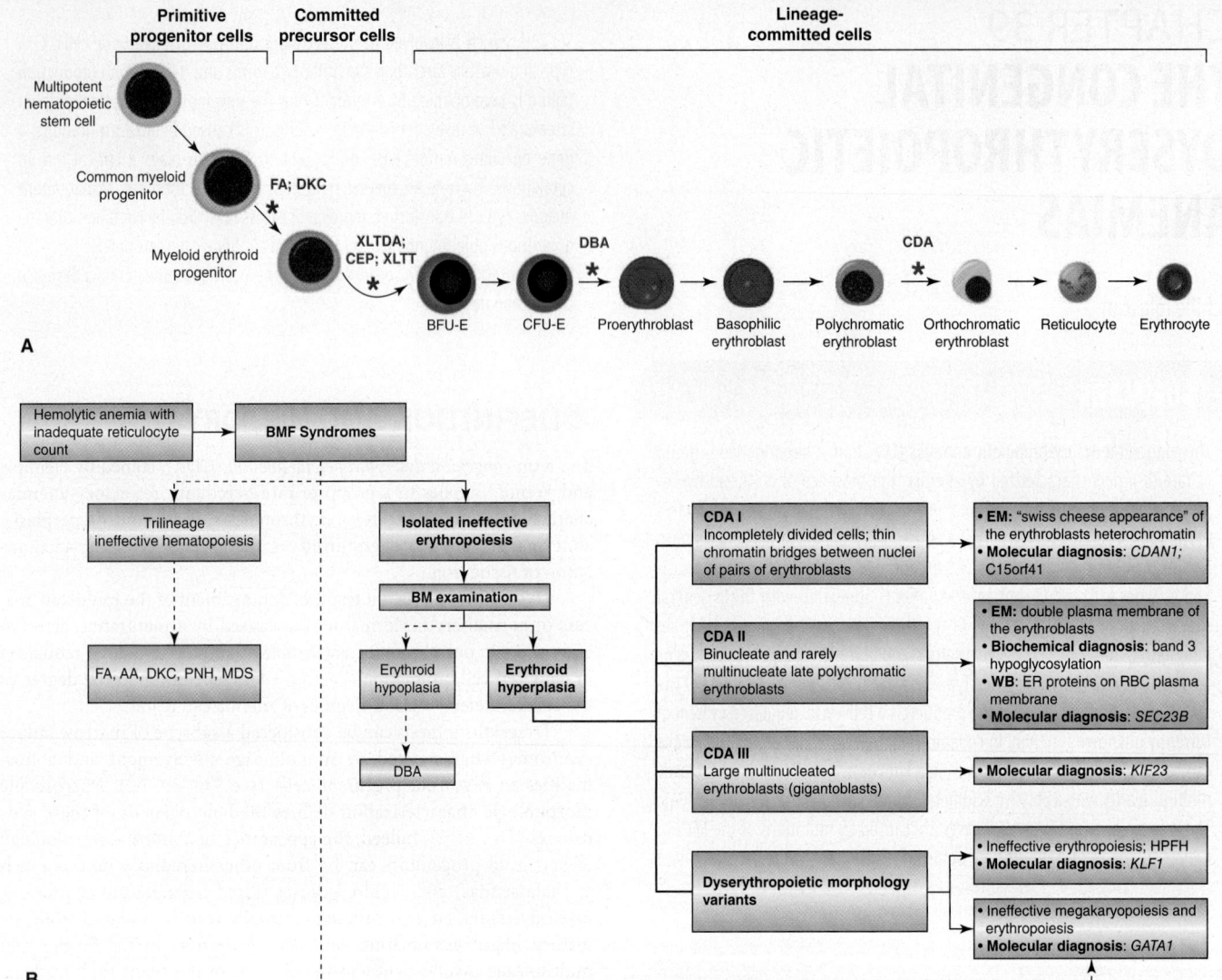

Figure 39–1. Differential diagnosis of congenital dyserythropoietic anemias (CDAs) among marrow failure syndromes. **A.** Erythroid maturation arrest can occur at several stages and can result in different marrow failure syndromes. CDA marrow is characterized by erythroid hyperplasia because the maturation arrest occurs later in these patients. **B.** Flow diagram for differential diagnosis of CDA subtypes based on clinical, morphologic, biochemical, and molecular findings. AA, aplastic anemia; BFU-E, burst-forming unit–erythroid; BM, marrow; BMF, marrow failure; CEP, congenital erythropoietic porphyria; CFU-E, colony-forming unit–erythroid; DBA, Diamond-Blackfan anemia; DKC, dyskeratosis congenita; EM, electron microscopy; ER, endoplasmic reticulum; FA, Fanconi anemia; HPFH, hereditary persistence of fetal hemoglobin; MDS, myelodysplastic syndromes; PNH, paroxysmal nocturnal hemoglobinuria; RBC, red blood cell; WB, western blotting; XLTDA, X-linked thrombocytopenia with dyserythropoietic anemia; XLTT, X linked thrombocytopenia with β-thalassemia.

0.24 and 0.71 cases/million, respectively, whereas CDA III is even less common.[3,4] In 2011, 712 cases from 614 families were included in the German CDA Registry, whereas in the Italian CDA registry 206 cases from 183 families were enrolled. In the literature, 169 cases from 143 families with CDA I and 454 cases from 356 families with CDA II worldwide have been recorded. Hence, CDA I is approximately one-third as frequent as CDA II. Most reported families were from Western European and Middle Eastern countries, but single cases have been also reported in the United States, India, Japan, and China.

The wide variation of incidence of CDA in Europe could be owing to genetic factors and also to the existence of reference centers for the diagnosis of CDA. However, molecular studies have established, at least for CDA type II, the presence of a founder effect in Europeans for the two most common mutations of the *SEC23B* gene.[5,6]

● CONGENITAL DYSERYTHROPOIETIC ANEMIA, TYPE I

CLINICAL FEATURES

CDA I is inherited as an autosomal recessive disorder. It can manifest in any year of pediatric age, but may not be diagnosed until adulthood. There is a continuous spectrum between moderate and severe forms; more severe presentations are predictably diagnosed at earlier ages.[7]

Anemia, usually macrocytic, is typically moderate and associated with intermittent jaundice, splenomegaly, and, sometimes, hepatomegaly. Hemoglobin values fluctuate around 9 to 10 g/dL. The patient usually does not require transfusion.[7–9]

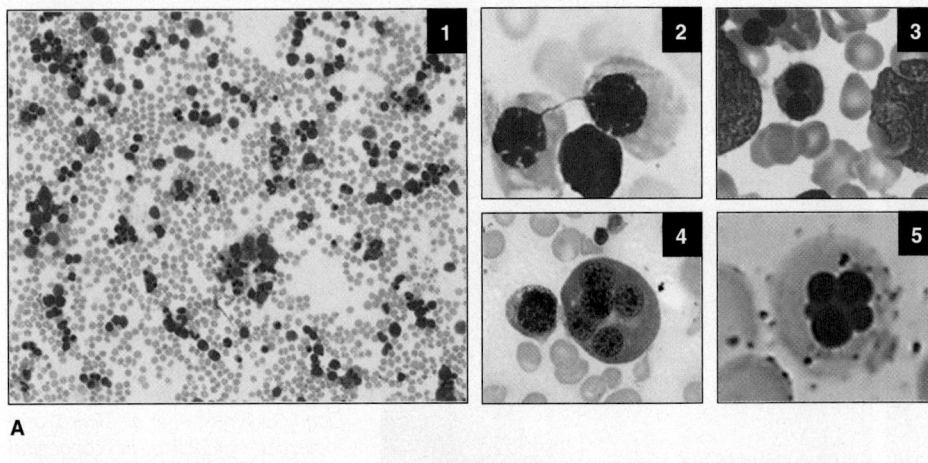

A

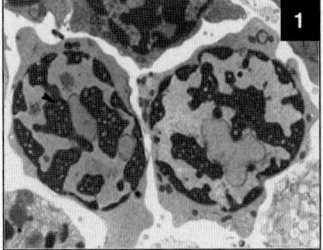

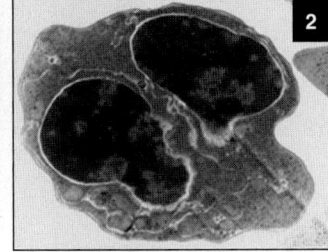

B

Figure 39–2. Marrow morphologic features of congenital dyserythropoietic anemia (CDA) erythroblasts. **A.** Marrow light microscopy of CDA patients almost always shows erythroid hyperplasia (*inset 1*). However, specific morphologic abnormalities in erythroid precursor cells are used as hallmarks for discerning different types of CDAs. The presence of internuclear chromatin bridging is a mark of CDA type I (*inset 2*), whereas the presence of bi- or multinucleated late erythroid precursors is the discriminating feature of CDA type II (*inset 3*). Giant multinucleated erythroblasts (*Inset 4*) and multinucleate erythroblasts (*Inset 5*) are typical features of CDA types III and IV, respectively. **B.** Marrow electron microscopy of CDA I erythroblasts show a typical Swiss cheese-heterochromatin pattern in the nucleus (*inset 1*), whereas CDA type II erythroid precursors display the characteristic double plasma membrane (*inset 2*). CDA type IV has nonspecific features, shared among different CDA types, such as marked heterochromatin, invagination of nuclear membrane, intranuclear precipitated material, and nuclear blebbing (*inset 3*).

Patients diagnosed in the neonatal period often have hepatomegaly and jaundice, and may have exhibited intrauterine growth retardation. Spleen size increases with age. Cholelithiasis is a common complication, and jaundice may be aggravated by the coinheritance of A[TA]$_7$TAA polymorphism in the promoter of the *UGT1A1* gene, the main cause of Gilbert syndrome.[10]

The disease is occasionally associated with a variety of dysmorphologic features (4 to 14 percent of affected individuals), the most common of which involves the bones of the hand and the foot (syndactyly, hypoplasia of one or several phalanges, presence of supplementary metatarsal bones, and clubfoot) (Fig. 39–3).[11] Small stature, almond-shaped blue eyes, hypertelorism, micrognathism, and other abnormalities may also be present.

LABORATORY FEATURES

Anemia is a common finding, usually in the range of 8 to 10 g/dL of hemoglobin. The blood film usually exhibits macrocytosis (mean cell volume [MCV] of approximately 90 to 100 fL), marked poikilocytosis, and occasional nucleated erythrocytes, elliptocytes, and basophilic stippling. The reticulocyte count is inappropriately low for the degree of anemia.[7-9] The marrow has intense erythroid hyperplasia. Binucleate polychromatic erythroblasts are evident at a frequency of approximately 3 to 7 percent. A highly specific feature is the presence of chromatin bridges linking two nuclei in more or less incompletely separated polychromatic erythroblasts with 0.6 to 2.8 strands per 100 erythroblasts (see Fig. 39–2A).[12] Ultrastructural abnormalities consist of a spongy ("Swiss cheese") appearance in the nucleus of up to 60 percent of early and late polychromatic erythroblasts. Nuclei exhibit areas of electrolucency within electron-dense heterochromatin and contain nuclear membrane-lined cytoplasmic intrusions, occasionally with retained cytoplasmic organelles (see Fig. 39–2B).[9,11]

GENETICS

The most frequent mutated gene in CDA I patients, *CDAN1* (chromosome 15q15.1–15.3), spans 15 kb and is composed of 28 exons.[13,14] The encoded protein, codanin-1, contains 1227 amino acids and it is ubiquitously expressed. Codanin-1 is a cell-cycle-regulated protein. The proximal *CDAN1* gene-promoter region appears to be a direct target of transcription factor E2F1, and high levels of codanin-1 are observed in the DNA synthesis (S) phase of the cell mitotic cycle.[15] At mitosis, codanin-1 undergoes phosphorylation and it is excluded from condensed chromosomes. Moreover, codanin-1 binds to Asf1a, a protein involved in chromatin structure dynamics by its role in nucleosome assembly and disassembly.[16]

More than 30 unique mutations have been found in the *CDAN1* gene, and affected subjects are either homozygotes or compound heterozygotes for the mutation(s) they carry. A genotype–phenotype correlation has not been established. A homozygous patient for null-type mutations has not been described, suggesting that an absence of codanin-1 is lethal. Indeed, CDA I knockout mice embryos die *in utero* at 6.5 days before erythropoiesis onset, presumably as a result of the critical role of this protein in developmental processes other than erythropoiesis.[17] In approximately 20 percent of families with the CDA I phenotype, *CDAN1* mutations were not found.[18] One founder mutation, R1042W, was observed in Bedouins.[2,8,19]

A new CDA I causative gene, *C15ORF41*, has been identified in three unrelated pedigrees of Middle Eastern and Southeast Asian origin by whole-genome sequencing.[20] The cellular role of the restriction endonuclease encoded by the *C15ORF41* gene is unknown. This protein interacts with Asf1b, the paralogue of Asf1a, which may support the hypothesis that the primary defect in CDA I is confined to DNA replication and chromatin assembly.

In the erythroid lineage during normal maturation, cell division ceases at the polychromatophilic erythroblast stage and cell size

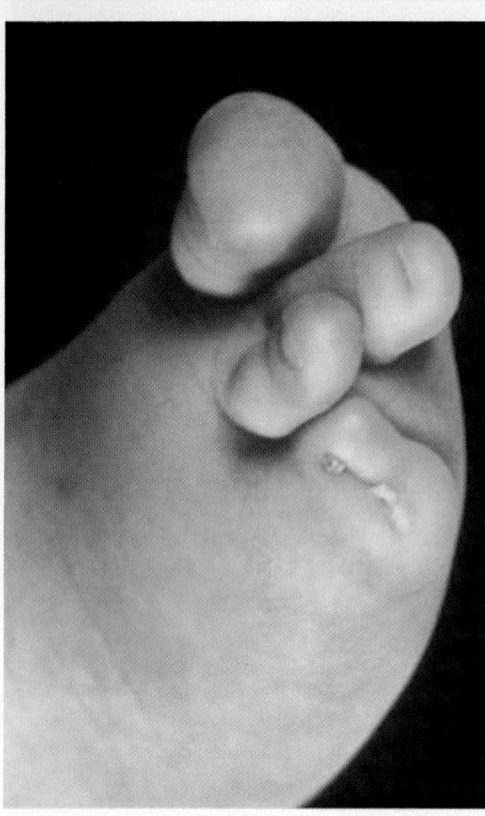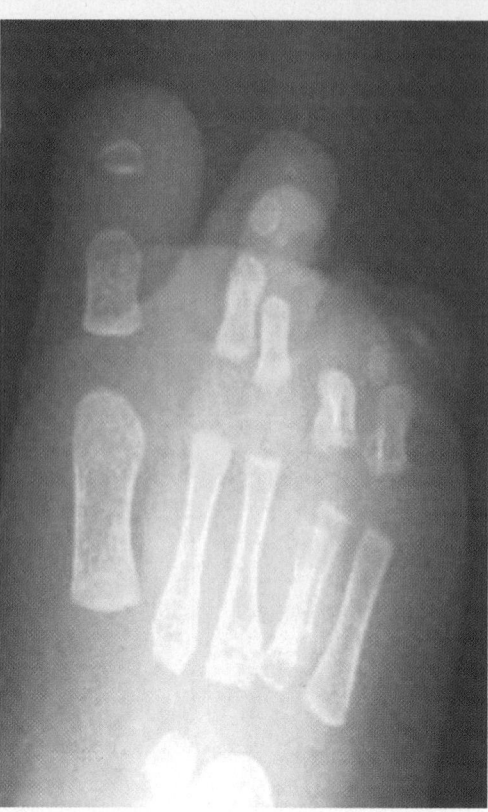

Figure 39–3. Foot dysmorphology in congenital dyserythropoietic anemia (CDA) type I. *Left:* Photograph showing hypoplastic nails, a broad first toe, hypoplastic third toe, and brachysyndactyly of the fourth and the fifth toes. *Right:* Radiograph showing a duplication of the fourth metatarsal bone (both bones being hypoplastic), a duplication of the fourth proximal phalanx, a single middle phalanx for the fourth and fifth toe, and the absence of the fourth distal phalanx. *(Reproduced with permission from Tamary H, Dgany O, Proust A, et al: Clinical and molecular variability in congenital dyserythropoietic anemia type I. Br J Haematol 130(4):628–634, 2005.)*

is progressively reduced.[21] Cell mitotic cycle defects in mice result in S-phase arrest, ineffective erythropoiesis, and macrocytosis.[22] Based on the probable involvement of CDA I mutated genes in DNA replication and chromatin assembly, it can be speculated that CDA I pathogenesis may involve disruption of the intrinsic connection between cell cycle dynamics and erythroid maturation.

Knowledge of the molecular defects in CDA patients permits detection of carriers for prenatal diagnosis.

TREATMENT, COURSE, AND PROGNOSIS

Severe forms of CDA I may present with hydrops fetalis.[23] Pulmonary hypertension was reported in three Bedouin newborns with CDA I.[24] Iron overload as a result of transfusion, hemosiderosis, and/or enhanced iron absorption characteristic of inefficient erythropoiesis is the main concern as patients age. Monitoring for iron overload is required; the following assessments are recommended: (1) annual measurement of serum ferritin concentration, and (2) myocardial T2* magnetic resonance imaging (MRI) and hepatic R2* MRI starting in adolescence (Chap. 43). Inappropriately low serum hepcidin levels could account for iron overload. High levels of *s-hemojuvelin (HJV)* in patients affected with CDA I, compared with controls, have been documented.[25] Hepcidin-to-ferritin ratio was negatively correlated with s-HJV, suggesting that s-HJV may suppress hepcidin.[26] Rare patients develop retinal angioid streaks.[27]

Fertility in patients is not affected. However, fetal anemia during pregnancy in affected women is associated with some morbidity. In some cases, intrauterine transfusions are warranted by the severity of anemia as judged by fetal blood sampling.[23]

Transfusions should be avoided whenever possible because of the risk of iron overload. When anemia is mild and does not require transfusion, small-volume regular phlebotomies may be used to decrease

body iron. Iron chelation or phlebotomies should be instituted when ferritin levels exceed 500 to 1000 mg/L. Iron chelation may be required for iron overload in those patients who cannot tolerate iron depletion by phlebotomies. Splenectomy is usually not beneficial.[2,9] Cholecystectomy for cholelithiasis is commonly performed.

Interferon-α was once used in a child with hepatitis C and CDA I; it was associated with an increase in hemoglobin level. A 9-year followup showed that the treatment remained effective and, on repeated liver biopsies, iron overload was normalized. In this case, the effective dose of interferon-α was 2 million units twice a week. Pegylated interferon could be used as well, at a dose of 30 mcg/wk.[28] The mechanism behind this response is unknown. Allogeneic hematopoietic stem cell transplantation was successful in several transfusion-dependent children.[29]

● CONGENITAL DYSERYTHROPOIETIC ANEMIA, TYPE II

CLINICAL AND LABORATORY FEATURES

CDA II is an autosomal, recessively inherited condition in which the severity of anemia varies from mild to severe and in which approximately 7 percent of cases are transfusion-dependent.[2,8,30,31] This disorder becomes variably manifest in infancy, childhood, or adolescence. Very few cases are characterized by clinical manifestations during intrauterine life, but hydrops fetalis caused by severe anemia has been reported.[32,33] More commonly, anemia is mild and, in several cases, diagnosis has been based on the appearance of complications (mainly iron overload) during adulthood.[2,8]

Erythrocytes of CDA II patients lyse in acidified serum (Ham test; Chap. 40) because of a naturally occurring immunoglobulin M class antibody that recognizes an antigen present on CDA II red cells but which is absent on normal cells. Thus, the acronym HEMPAS (hemolytic anemia with a positive acidified serum test) is commonly used as a synonym for CDA II. The technical difficulty of this test, and the fact that cross-testing of more than 30 normal sera is needed to obtain a reliable result, has undermined its usefulness.[34]

The clinical picture of CDA II includes hemolytic anemia with marrow erythroid expansion, commonly with splenomegaly, hepatomegaly, intermittent jaundice, and cholelithiasis.[30,31] The blood film exhibits moderate to marked anisocytosis and anisochromia and a number of spherocytes. This, along with the patient's clinical appearance, may lead to confusion of CDA II with hereditary spherocytosis (HS; Chap. 46). However, typically in HS, the reticulocyte count in comparison to hemoglobin level is higher and the serum transferrin receptor level is lower. Moreover, the majority of HS cases are inherited as autosomal dominant and, thus, a parent is likely to have findings of spherocytosis on blood examination, whereas CDA II is invariably an autosomal recessive condition. Despite these differentiating features, CDA II is at times only diagnosed after the failure of splenectomy to normalize anemia when performed for suspected HS. In the marrow, 10 to 30 percent of intermediate and late erythroblasts have two or more nuclei or lobulated nuclei (see Fig. 39–2A). Karyorrhexis (fragmentation of the nucleus) is common. Gaucher-like cells may develop as a result of phagocytosis of erythroblasts by macrophages. Ringed sideroblasts are present in severe forms.[12] Electron microscopy shows structures that have been misnamed as "double membrane" (see Fig. 39–2B). These are cisternae of the endoplasmic reticulum (ER) that run along the red cell plasma membrane inner surface, and which contain ER-specific proteins, as shown by immunochemistry labeling.[35] Sodium dodecylsulfate polyacrylamide gel electrophoresis (SDS-PAGE), followed by immunoblots, reveals the presence of calreticulin, glucose-regulated protein 78, and disulfide isomerase; these are specific for the ER and are not detected in normal individuals.[35]

The diagnostic hallmark of CDA II is analysis of erythrocyte membrane proteins by SDS-PAGE identifying narrower band size and faster migration of erythrocyte anion transporters (AE1 or band 3) and band 4.5 proteins.[36,37] Increased destruction of red blood cells in CDA II is associated with hypoglycosylation of AE1, which causes clustering of this protein on the red cell surface and contributes to erythrocyte destruction in the spleen.[38] Rare patients have been reported without this characteristic SDS-PAGE pattern; it is recommended that these should be classified as CDA II–like conditions.

GENETICS

Pathognomonic hypoglycosylation of AE1 protein is the outcome of the expression of the mutated gene *SEC23B*.[39]

Sequencing analysis in 33 patients from 28 unrelated families showed heterogeneous mutations in the *SEC23B* gene, either in compound heterozygous or homozygous states.[2,8,39] An *in vitro* model of gene silencing demonstrated that suppression of SEC23B expression recapitulates the cellular defects in SEC23B-silenced cells.[39] Knockdown of zebrafish SEC23B also leads to aberrant erythrocyte development.[39]

SEC23B is a cytoplasmic coat protein (COP) II component involved in the secretory pathway of eukaryotic cells. COPII is a multisubunit complex essential for transport of correctly folded proteins from the ER toward the Golgi apparatus.[40] This pathway is critical for membrane homeostasis, localization of proteins within cells and secretion of extracellular factors.[40,41]

CDA II belongs to COPII-related human genetic disorders.[42] Alterations in *SAR1B*, a paralogue of SEC23B, are identified as the cause of chylomicron retention disease (Anderson disease),[43] while a specific mutation in the *SEC23A* gene causes craniolenticulosutural dysplasia (Boyadjiev-Jabs syndrome).[44] The specificity of the CDA II phenotype seems to be determined by tissue-specific expression of SEC23B versus SEC23A during erythroid differentiation.[39] Alternatively, this specificity could be explained by the presence of tissue-specific proteins (such as band 3 in red blood cells) which might require high levels and full function of a specific COPII component to be correctly transported.[42,45]

So far, more than 60 different causative mutations have been described worldwide.[2,8] A genotype–phenotype correlation seems to exist. Particularly, compound heterozygosity for missense and nonsense mutations tends to produce more severe clinical presentations than homozygosity or compound heterozygosity for two missense mutations. Homozygosity or compound heterozygosity for two nonsense mutations has not been reported, suggesting it may be lethal.[46] *Sec23b*-deficient mice (*Sec23b gt/gt*) have been generated and are born without anemia but die shortly after birth, with degeneration of secretory organs, including the pancreas and salivary glands.[47]

The disparate phenotypes in mouse and human could result from residual SEC23B function associated with the hypomorphic mutations observed in humans, or, alternatively, might be explained by species-specific functional differences.[48]

TREATMENT, COURSE, AND PROGNOSIS

The clinical course of this condition is quite heterogeneous. Treatment approaches depend on age, severity of phenotype and comorbidity. Most patients have only mild or moderate anemia and do not require medical intervention. Approximately 10 percent of neonates need at least one erythrocyte transfusion, and some remain transfusion-dependent.[8,31] In most adolescents and adults, transfusional needs are limited to aplastic crises, pregnancy, coexistent infections, or major operations.

The more common, moderate forms may only be diagnosed in adult life because of iron overload (Chap. 43) that is consistently observed even in the absence of transfusions.[2,8,49] Patients with severe forms of CDA II may be transfusion-dependent. In some cases, severe phenotypes could be the result of additional genetic abnormalities, such as coinheritance of glucose-6-phosphate dehydrogenase (G6PD) deficiency or thalassemic trait.[50]

The iron overload is associated with high levels of growth differentiation factor 15 (GDF15).[51] However, GDF15 concentrations are significantly lower in CDA II compared to CDA I patients, despite a similar degree of iron overload in both patient groups. It can be speculated that additional signals may determine hepatic hepcidin expression and the degree of iron overload in CDA II.[51]

Ferritin levels should be controlled at least annually, even in patients with only mild anemia. Achievement of normal ferritin concentrations is desirable.[52] Iron chelation should be instituted when ferritin level exceeds 500 to 1000 cg/L (Chap. 43). If phlebotomies are tolerated, this is the preferred treatment. In instances where the patient cannot tolerate phlebotomy, chelating agents may be used.

Cholelithiasis and splenomegaly are common complications. Coinheritance of the UGT1A (TA)7/(TA)7 genotype could account for the increased rate of gallstones.[53] Cholelithiasis, which is frequent in all types of CDA, may require cholecystectomy; decision making should follow therapy guidelines for cholelithiasis.[54] Splenectomy is not universally recommended for CDA II or CDA I; individual decisions should be influenced by transfusion dependency and the presence of a massively enlarged spleen. Generally accepted criteria for splenectomy have not been defined. Splenectomy leads to a moderate, sustained increase in hemoglobin concentrations and decrease of serum bilirubin levels, but it does not prevent iron overload, and hemoglobin levels postsplenectomy generally do not reach normal values.[5,6] In non–transfusion-dependent patients, it is advisable to follow the guidelines for mild cases of HS.[54]

Allogeneic marrow transplantation from an human leukocyte antigen (HLA)-identical sibling has been successful in transfusion-dependent children with very severe CDA II and in one adult with CDA II and β-thalassemia trait.[32,33,55,56]

CONGENITAL DYSERYTHROPOIETIC ANEMIA, TYPE III

CLINICAL AND LABORATORY FINDINGS

Type III is the least-common form of CDA. This condition, which is dominantly inherited, was initially coined "hereditary benign erythrocytosis." One dominantly inherited form was reported as early as 1951 in a woman and her three children, in whom 16.0 to 22.7 percent of hematopoietic stem cell erythroblasts were multinucleated. Giant-size erythrocytes were present in the blood.

Most of our knowledge about CDA III stems from a large family from the province of Västerbotten in northern Sweden.[57] The diagnosis was made in the adults and older children. The spleen was not palpable, nor was iron overload recorded. The large size of this family made it possible to map the responsible gene to 15q22–25.[58] In addition, a number of sporadic cases of CDA III have been reported.[59]

In another case, a number of stillbirths, including at least one stillborn with hydrops fetalis, were noted in an Indian family in which the mother, who initially required transfusions, became transfusion-independent after splenectomy.[60]

Blood films from these patients show macrocytes, occasional extremely large forms (gigantocytes), and poikilocytes. Patients are generally asymptomatic, with no or moderate anemia, mild jaundice, and, commonly, cholelithiasis. The reticulocyte count is typically less than 3 percent.[57,61] Marrow shows marked erythroid hyperplasia, with large multinucleate erythroblasts with large, lobulated nuclei, and giant multinucleate erythroblasts with up to 12 nuclei (see Fig. 39–2A). On electron microscopy, clefts within heterochromatin, autophagic vacuoles, iron-laden mitochondria, and myelin figures in the cytoplasm have been reported.[62]

GENETICS

The causative mutation was found to be 2747C>G (P916R) in the *KIF23* gene.[63] The same mutation was also found in CDA III patients from an American family without any known relation to the Swedish kindred.[63] *KIF23* encodes a kinesin-superfamily molecule, mitotic kinesin-like protein 1 (MKLP1), a mitotic protein essential for cytokinesis.[64,65] MKLP1 interacts with Arf6 (adenosine diphosphate (ADP)-ribosylation factor 6), ultimately forming an extended β-sheet that interacts with the membrane surface at the cleavage furrow. The Arf6–MKLP1 complex plays a crucial role in cytokinesis by connecting the microtubule bundle and membranes at the cleavage plane.[64] Knockdown of Arf6 results in binucleated and multinucleated cells, a hallmark of CDA III erythroblasts.[66] In knockdown and rescue experiments with *in vitro* cell lines, cytokinesis failure and binucleated cells were seen more frequently with the P916R mutant than wild-type GFP-MKLP1, indicating that the P916R mutation impairs the function of MKLP1 in cytokinesis.[63]

COURSE AND PROGNOSIS

In spite of an apparently benign course, CDA III is prone to various long-term complications, including intravascular hemolysis, increased risk of myeloma and other monoclonal gammapathies,[67] and development of angioid streaks.[68]

OTHER CONGENITAL DYSERYTHROPOIETIC ANEMIAS

A number of cases of CDA that do not have specific features of types I, II, or, to some extent, III disease have been reported.[69-74] Classification has been proposed based largely on cell morphology.[75] In addition, several genes have been associated with CDA variants, including mutations in the *GATA1* and *KLF1* genes, which are critical for development of specific blood cell lineages (outlined in Table 39–1).[69-74,76]

Alterations in the erythroid hematopoietic transcription factor *KLF1* gene are associated with CDA type IV,[77] characterized by severe hemolytic anemia, elevated fetal hemoglobin, and deficiency of erythroid proteins CD44 and aquaporin 1 (see Table 39–1).[78]

Additionally, syndromes have been described in which CDA accounts only for one feature of a syndrome phenotype (see Table 39–1). For instance, Majeed syndrome, is comprised of chronic recurrent multifocal osteomyelitis, inflammatory dermatosis, and CDA. The responsible gene is *LPIN2* (18p11.31), encoding lipin 2, an ER-phosphatidate phosphatase.[79] Additionally, dyserythropoiesis associated with exocrine pancreatic insufficiency and calvarial hyperostosis resulting from *COX4I2* gene mutations has been described in two Arab families.[80] Mevalonate kinase deficiency (MKD) resulting from a missense mutation in the *MVK* gene and showing morphologic marrow cell abnormalities similar to CDA II has also been reported.[81]

DIFFERENTIAL DIAGNOSIS

Congenital dyserythropoietic anemias may be confused with thalassemias and other hemolytic anemias. Marked anisocytosis, including a

TABLE 39–1. A Classification Frame for Atypical Congenital Dyserythropoietic Anemias

Group	Main Features
IV	Transfusion-dependent anemia
	Pronounced normoblastic erythroid hyperplasia with a slight to moderate increase in the nonspecific dyserythropoietic erythroblasts with irregular or karyorrhectic nuclei
	No precipitated protein within erythroblasts
V	Near-normal hemoglobin with normal or slightly increased mean corpuscular volume
	Predominantly unconjugated hyperbilirubinemia
	Marked normoblastic/slightly megaloblastic hyperplasia
	Little or no erythroid dysplasia
VI	Normal or near-normal hemoglobin with marked macrocytosis
	Erythroid hyperplasia with cobalamin- and folate-independent florid megaloblastic erythropoiesis
VII	Severe transfusion-dependent anemia
	Severe normoblastic erythroid hyperplasia with irregular nuclear shapes in many erythroblasts
	Intraerythroblastic inclusions that resemble precipitated globin but do not contain globin

Data from Wickramasinghe SN and Wood WG: Advances in the understanding of the congenital dyserythropoietic anaemias. *Br J Haematol* 131(4):431–446, 2005.

normomacrocytic component, and low or moderate reticulocyte count out of keeping with the degree of anemia will point to a diagnosis of CDA. Indeed, CDAs are a subtype of marrow failure syndromes characterized by ineffective erythropoiesis and heterogeneous, type-specific morphologic abnormalities in erythroid precursor cells (see Fig. 39–1). Thus, marrow examination is essential if family history is unrevealing. The marrow, if needed, is quite different than in other types of hemolytic anemia or the thalassemias as multinuclearity of erythroblasts is not a feature of the latter two types of anemia.

REFERENCES

1. Heimpel H, Wendt F: Congenital dyserythropoietic anemia with karyorrhexis and multinuclearity of erythroblasts. *Helv Med Acta* 34(2):103–115, 1968.
2. Iolascon A, Heimpel H, Wahlin A, et al: Congenital dyserythropoietic anemias: Molecular insights and diagnostic approach. *Blood* 122(13):2162–2166, 2013.
3. Gulbis B, Eleftheriou A, Angastiniotis M, et al: Epidemiology of rare anaemias in Europe. *Adv Exp Med Biol* 686:375–396, 2010.
4. Heimpel H, Matuschek A, Ahmed M, et al: Frequency of congenital dyserythropoietic anemias in Europe. *Eur J Haematol* 85(1):20–25, 2010.
5. Iolascon A, Servedio V, Carbone R, et al: Geographic distribution of cda-ii: Did a founder effect operate in southern Italy? *Haematologica* 85(5):470–474, 2000.
6. Russo R, Gambale A, Esposito MR, et al: Two founder mutations in the sec23b gene account for the relatively high frequency of CDA II in the Italian population. *Am J Hematol* 86(9):727–732, 2011.
7. Tamary H, Shalev H, Luria D, et al: Clinical features and studies of erythropoiesis in Israeli Bedouins with congenital dyserythropoietic anemia type I. *Blood* 87(5):1763–1770, 1996.
8. Iolascon A, Esposito MR, Russo R: Clinical aspects and pathogenesis of congenital dyserythropoietic anemias: From morphology to molecular approach. *Haematologica* 97(12):1786–1794, 2012.
9. Heimpel H, Schwarz K, Ebnother M, et al: Congenital dyserythropoietic anemia type I (CDA I): Molecular genetics, clinical appearance, and prognosis based on long-term observation. *Blood* 107(1):334–340, 2006.
10. Wickramasinghe SN, Thein SL, Srichairatanakool S, et al: Determinants of iron status and bilirubin levels in congenital dyserythropoietic anaemia type I. *Br J Haematol* 107(3):522–525, 1999.
11. Wickramasinghe SN: Congenital dyserythropoietic anaemias: Clinical features, haematological morphology and new biochemical data. *Blood Rev* 12(3):178–200, 1998.
12. Heimpel H, Kellermann K, Neuschwander N, et al: The morphological diagnosis of congenital dyserythropoietic anemia: Results of a quantitative analysis of peripheral blood and bone marrow cells. *Haematologica* 95(6):1034–1036, 2010.
13. Tamary H, Shalmon L, Shalev H, et al: Localization of the gene for congenital dyserythropoietic anemia type I to a <1-cm interval on chromosome 15q15.1–15.3. *Am J Hum Genet* 62(5):1062–1069, 1998.
14. Dgany O, Avidan N, Delaunay J, et al: Congenital dyserythropoietic anemia type I is caused by mutations in codanin-1. *Am J Hum Genet* 71(6):1467–1474, 2002.
15. Noy-Lotan S, Dgany O, Lahmi R, et al: Codanin-1, the protein encoded by the gene mutated in congenital dyserythropoietic anemia type I (cdan1), is cell cycle-regulated. *Haematologica* 94(5):629–637, 2009.
16. Ask K, Jasencakova Z, Menard P, et al: Codanin-1, mutated in the anaemic disease CDAI, regulates Asf1 function in S-phase histone supply. *EMBO J* 31(8):2013–2023, 2012.
17. Renella R, Roberts NA, Brown JM, et al: Codanin-1 mutations in congenital dyserythropoietic anemia type 1 affect HP1{alpha} localization in erythroblasts. *Blood* 117(25):6928–6938, 2011.
18. Ahmed MR, Chehal A, Zahed L, et al: Linkage and mutational analysis of the CDAN1 gene reveals genetic heterogeneity in congenital dyserythropoietic anemia type I. *Blood* 107(12):4968–4969, 2006.
19. Tamary H, Dgany O, Proust A, et al: Clinical and molecular variability in congenital dyserythropoietic anaemia type I. *Br J Haematol* 130(4):628–634, 2005.
20. Babbs C, Roberts NA, Sanchez-Pulido L, et al: Homozygous mutations in a predicted endonuclease are a novel cause of congenital dyserythropoietic anemia type I. *Haematologica* 98(9):1383–1387, 2013.
21. Sankaran VG, Ludwig LS, Sicinska E, et al: Cyclin D3 coordinates the cell cycle during differentiation to regulate erythrocyte size and number. *Genes Dev* 26(18):2075–2087, 2012.
22. Li FX, Zhu JW, Hogan CJ, et al: Defective gene expression, S phase progression, and maturation during hematopoiesis in e2f1/e2f2 mutant mice. *Mol Cell Biol* 23(10):3607–3622, 2003.
23. Parez N, Dommergues M, Zupan V, et al: Severe congenital dyserythropoietic anaemia type I: Prenatal management, transfusion support and alpha-interferon therapy. *Br J Haematol* 110(2):420–423, 2000.
24. Shalev H, Moser A, Kapelushnik J, et al: Congenital dyserythropoietic anemia type I presenting as persistent pulmonary hypertension of the newborn. *J Pediatr* 136(4):553–555, 2000.
25. Tamary H, Shalev H, Perez-Avraham G, et al: Elevated growth differentiation factor 15 expression in patients with congenital dyserythropoietic anemia type I. *Blood* 112(13):5241–5244, 2008.
26. Shalev H, Perez-Avraham G, Kapelushnik J, et al: High levels of soluble serum hemojuvelin in patients with congenital dyserythropoietic anemia type I. *Eur J Haematol* 90(1):31–36, 2013.
27. Tamary H, Offret H, Dgany O, et al: Congenital dyserythropoietic anaemia, type I, in a Caucasian patient with retinal angioid streaks (homozygous arg1042trp mutation in codanin-1). *Eur J Haematol* 80(3):271–274, 2008.
28. Lavabre-Bertrand T, Ramos J, Delfour C, et al: Long-term alpha interferon treatment is effective on anaemia and significantly reduces iron overload in congenital dyserythropoiesis type I. *Eur J Haematol* 73(5):380–383, 2004.
29. Ayas M, al-Jefri A, Baothman A, et al: Transfusion-dependent congenital dyserythropoietic anemia type I successfully treated with allogeneic stem cell transplantation. *Bone Marrow Transplant* 29(8):681–682, 2002.
30. Heimpel H, Anselstetter V, Chrobak L, et al: Congenital dyserythropoietic anemia type II: Epidemiology, clinical appearance, and prognosis based on long-term observation. *Blood* 102(13):4576–4581, 2003.
31. Iolascon A, Delaunay J, Wickramasinghe SN, et al: Natural history of congenital dyserythropoietic anemia type II. *Blood* 98(4):1258–1260, 2001.
32. Remacha AF, Badell I, Pujol-Moix N, et al: Hydrops fetalis-associated congenital dyserythropoietic anemia treated with intrauterine transfusions and bone marrow transplantation. *Blood* 100(1):356–358, 2002.
33. Braun M, Wolfl M, Wiegering V, et al: Successful treatment of an infant with CDA type II by intrauterine transfusions and postnatal stem cell transplantation. *Pediatr Blood Cancer* 61(4):743–745, 2014.
34. Crookston JH, Crookston MC, Burnie KL, et al: Hereditary erythroblastic multinuclearity associated with a positive acidified-serum test: A type of congenital dyserythropoietic anaemia. *Br J Haematol* 17(1):11–26, 1969.
35. Alloisio N, Texier P, Denoroy L, et al: The cisternae decorating the red blood cell membrane in congenital dyserythropoietic anemia (type II) originate from the endoplasmic reticulum. *Blood* 87(10):4433–4439, 1996.
36. Scartezzini P, Forni GL, Baldi M, et al: Decreased glycosylation of band 3 and band 4.5 glycoproteins of erythrocyte membrane in congenital dyserythropoietic anaemia type II. *Br J Haematol* 51(4):569–576, 1982.
37. Fukuda MN, Gaetani GF, Izzo P, et al: Incompletely processed N-glycans of serum glycoproteins in congenital dyserythropoietic anaemia type II (HEMPAS). *Br J Haematol* 82(4):745–752, 1992.
38. De Franceschi L, Turrini F, del Giudice EM, et al: Decreased band 3 anion transport activity and band 3 clusterization in congenital dyserythropoietic anemia type II. *Exp Hematol* 26(9):869–873, 1998.
39. Schwarz K, Iolascon A, Verissimo F, et al: Mutations affecting the secretory COPII coat component SEC23B cause congenital dyserythropoietic anemia type II. *Nat Genet* 41(8):936–940, 2009.
40. Fromme JC, Orci L, Schekman R: Coordination of COPII vesicle trafficking by SEC23. *Trends Cell Biol* 18(7):330–336, 2008.
41. Lee MC, Miller EA, Goldberg J, et al: Bi-directional protein transport between the ER and GOLGI. *Annu Rev Cell Dev Biol* 20:87–123, 2004.
42. Russo R, Esposito MR, Iolascon A: Inherited hematological disorders due to defects in coat protein (COP)II complex. *Am J Hematol* 88(2):135–140, 2013.
43. Jones B, Jones EL, Bonney SA, et al: Mutations in a Sar1 GTPase of COPII vesicles are associated with lipid absorption disorders. *Nat Genet* 34(1):29–31, 2003.
44. Boyadjiev SA, Fromme JC, Ben J, et al: Cranio-lenticulo-sutural dysplasia is caused by a SEC23A mutation leading to abnormal endoplasmic-reticulum-to-Golgi trafficking. *Nat Genet* 38(10):1192–1197, 2006.
45. De Matteis MA, Luini A: Mendelian disorders of membrane trafficking. *N Engl J Med* 365(10):927–938, 2011.
46. Iolascon A, Russo R, Esposito MR, et al: Molecular analysis of 42 patients with congenital dyserythropoietic anemia type II: New mutations in the SEC23B gene and a search for a genotype–phenotype relationship. *Haematologica* 95(5):708–715, 2010.
47. Tao J, Zhu M, Wang H, et al: SEC23B is required for the maintenance of murine professional secretory tissues. *Proc Natl Acad Sci U S A* 109(29):E2001–E2009, 2012.
48. Russo R, Langella C, Esposito MR, et al: Hypomorphic mutations of SEC23B gene account for mild phenotypes of congenital dyserythropoietic anemia type II. *Blood Cells Mol Dis* 51(1):17–21, 2013.
49. Fargion S, Valenti L, Fracanzani AL, et al: Hereditary hemochromatosis in a patient with congenital dyserythropoietic anemia. *Blood* 96(10):3653–3655, 2000.
50. Gangarossa S, Romano V, Miraglia del Giudice E, et al: Congenital dyserythropoietic anemia type II associated with G6PD Seattle in a Sicilian child. *Acta Haematol* 93(1):36–39, 1995.
51. Casanovas G, Swinkels DW, Altamura S, et al: Growth differentiation factor 15 in patients with congenital dyserythropoietic anaemia (CDA) type II. *J Mol Med (Berl)* 89(8):811–816, 2011.
52. Hofmann WK, Kaltwasser JP, Hoelzer D, et al: Successful treatment of iron overload by phlebotomies in a patient with severe congenital dyserythropoietic anemia type II. *Blood* 89(8):3068–3069, 1997.
53. Perrotta S, del Giudice EM, Carbone R, et al: Gilbert's syndrome accounts for the phenotypic variability of congenital dyserythropoietic anemia type II (CDA-II). *J Pediatr* 136(4):556–559, 2000.

54. Bolton-Maggs PH, Langer JC, Iolascon A, et al: Guidelines for the diagnosis and management of hereditary spherocytosis—2011 update. *Br J Haematol* 156(1):37–49, 2012.

55. Iolascon A, Sabato V, de Mattia D, et al: Bone marrow transplantation in a case of severe, type II congenital dyserythropoietic anemia (CDA II). *Bone Marrow Transplant* 27(2):213–215, 2001.

56. Unal S, Russo R, Gumruk F, et al: Successful hematopoietic stem cell transplantation in a patient with congenital dyserythropoietic anemia type II. *Pediatr Transplant* 18(4):E130–E133, 2014.

57. Bergstrom I, Jacobsson L: Hereditary benign erythroreticulosis. *Blood* 19:296–303, 1962.

58. Lind L, Sandstrom H, Wahlin A, et al: Localization of the gene for congenital dyserythropoietic anemia type III, CDAN3, to chromosome 15q21-q25. *Hum Mol Genet* 4(1):109–112, 1995.

59. Accame EA, de Tezanos Pinto M: [Congenital dyserythropoiesis with erythroblastic polyploidy. Report of a variety found in Argentinian Mesopotamia (author's transl)] [in Spanish]. *Sangre (Barc)* 26(5-A):545–555, 1981.

60. Jijina F, Ghosh K, Yavagal D, et al: A patient with congenital dyserythropoietic anaemia type III presenting with stillbirths. *Acta Haematol* 99(1):31–33, 1998.

61. Wolff JA, Von Hofe FH: Familial erythroid multinuclearity. *Blood* 6(12):1274–1283, 1951.

62. Sandstrom H, Wahlin A: Congenital dyserythropoietic anemia type III. *Haematologica* 85(7):753–757, 2000.

63. Liljeholm M, Irvine AF, Vikberg AL, et al: Congenital dyserythropoietic anemia type III (CDA III) is caused by a mutation in kinesin family member, KIF23. *Blood* 121(23):4791–4799, 2013.

64. Boman AL, Kuai J, Zhu X, et al: ARF proteins bind to mitotic kinesin-like protein 1 (MKLP1) in a GTP-dependent fashion. *Cell Motil Cytoskeleton* 44(2):119–132, 1999.

65. Joseph N, Hutterer A, Poser I, et al: ARF6 GTPase protects the post-mitotic midbody from 14-3-3-mediated disintegration. *EMBO J* 31(11):2604–2614, 2012.

66. Makyio H, Ohgi M, Takei T, et al: Structural basis for ARF6-MKLP1 complex formation on the Flemming body responsible for cytokinesis. *EMBO J* 31(11):2590–2603, 2012.

67. Sandstrom H, Wahlin A, Eriksson M, et al: Intravascular haemolysis and increased prevalence of myeloma and monoclonal gammopathy in congenital dyserythropoietic anaemia, type III. *Eur J Haematol* 52(1):42–46, 1994.

68. Sandstrom H, Wahlin A, Eriksson M, et al: Angioid streaks are part of a familial syndrome of dyserythropoietic anaemia (CDA III). *Br J Haematol* 98(4):845–849, 1997.

69. David G , VanDorpe A, Lewis SM, Verwilghen RL: Aberrant congenital dyserythropoietic anaemias, in *Dyserythropoiesis*, edited by SM Lewis RV. Academic Press, London, 1977.

70. Bethlenfalvay NC, Hadnagy C, Heimpel H: Unclassified type of congenital dyserythropoietic anaemia (CDA) with prominent peripheral erythroblastosis. *Br J Haematol* 60(3):541–550, 1985.

71. Brien WF, Mant MJ, Etches WS: Variant congenital dyserythropoietic anaemia with ringed sideroblasts. *Clin Lab Haematol* 7(3):231–237, 1985.

72. Pothier B, Morle L, Alloisio N, et al: Aberrant pattern of red cell membrane and cytosolic proteins in a case of congenital dyserythropoietic anaemia. *Br J Haematol* 66(3):393–400, 1987.

73. Ohisalo JJ, Viitala J, Lintula R, et al: A new congenital dyserythropoietic anaemia. *Br J Haematol* 68(1):111–114, 1988.

74. Woessner S, Trujillo M, Florensa L, et al: Congenital dyserythropoietic anaemia other than type I to III with a peculiar erythroblastic morphology. *Eur J Haematol* 71(3):211–214, 2003.

75. Wickramasinghe SN, Wood WG: Advances in the understanding of the congenital dyserythropoietic anaemias. *Br J Haematol* 131(4):431–446, 2005.

76. Ciovacco WA, Raskind WH, Kacena MA: Human phenotypes associated with GATA-1 mutations. *Gene* 427(1–2):1–6, 2008.

77. Arnaud L, Saison C, Helias V, et al: A dominant mutation in the gene encoding the erythroid transcription factor KLF1 causes a congenital dyserythropoietic anemia. *Am J Hum Genet* 87(5):721–727, 2010.

78. Jaffray JA, Mitchell WB, Gnanapragasam MN, et al: Erythroid transcription factor EKLF/KLF1 mutation causing congenital dyserythropoietic anemia type IV in a patient of Taiwanese origin: Review of all reported cases and development of a clinical diagnostic paradigm. *Blood Cells Mol Dis* 51(2):71–75, 2013.

79. Ferguson PJ, Chen S, Tayeh MK, et al: Homozygous mutations in LPIN2 are responsible for the syndrome of chronic recurrent multifocal osteomyelitis and congenital dyserythropoietic anaemia (Majeed syndrome). *J Med Genet* 42(7):551–557, 2005.

80. Shteyer E, Saada A, Shaag A, et al: Exocrine pancreatic insufficiency, dyserythropoietic anemia, and calvarial hyperostosis are caused by a mutation in the COX4I2 gene. *Am J Hum Genet* 84(3):412–417, 2009.

81. Samkari A, Borzutzky A, Fermo E, et al: A novel missense mutation in MVK associated with MK deficiency and dyserythropoietic anemia. *Pediatrics* 125(4):e964–e968, 2010.

CHAPTER 40
PAROXYSMAL NOCTURNAL HEMOGLOBINURIA

Charles J. Parker

SUMMARY

In contrast to all other intrinsic abnormalities of the erythrocyte, paroxysmal nocturnal hemoglobinuria (PNH) is an acquired, not an inherited, disorder. PNH arises as a consequence of somatic mutation, involving one or more hematopoietic stem cells, of *PIGA*, a gene located on the X chromosome that is required for synthesis of the glycosylphosphatidylinositol (GPI) moiety that anchors some proteins to the cell surface. Consequently, all GPI-anchored proteins (GPI-APs) that are normally expressed are deficient on the mutant hematopoietic stem cells and their progeny. The complement-mediated intravascular hemolytic anemia and the resulting hemoglobinuria that are the clinical hallmarks of PNH are a consequence of deficiency of the GPI-anchored complement regulatory proteins, CD55 and CD59. Although PNH is a neoplastic (clonal) disease, it is not a malignant disease in that there is no exaggerated proliferation of neoplastic cells and replacement of marrow or spread to other tissues, and the extent to which the mutant clones expand varies greatly among patients. Thus, the blood cells of patients with PNH are a mosaic of phenotypically normal and abnormal cells. The size of the mutant clone is an important determinant of the clinical manifestations of the disease, which include hemolysis, thrombophilia, and, in many patients, pancytopenia as a result of marrow failure. The diagnosis of PNH is confirmed using flow cytometry to detect and quantify the percentage of blood erythrocytes and leukocytes (i. e., neutrophils and monocytes) that lack GPI-APs measured as intensity of CD55 and CD59 on the cell surface. The intravascular hemolysis of PNH can be controlled with eculizumab, a humanized monoclonal antibody that blocks formation of the cytolytic membrane attack complex of complement.

Acronyms and Abbreviations: APC, alternative pathway of complement; CD55, an antigen encoding DAF; CD59, an antigen encoding MAC-inhibitory protein; DAF, decay-accelerating factor; GPI, glycosylphosphatidylinositol; GPI-APs, glycosylphosphatidylinositol-anchored proteins; GVHD, graft-versus-host disease; HLA, human leukocyte antigen; INR, international normalized ratio of prothrombin assay data; LDH, lactate dehydrogenase; MAC, membrane attack complex of complement; MDS, myelodysplastic syndrome; MIRL, membrane inhibitor of reactive lysis; *PIGA*, phosphatidylinositol glycan class A; PMN, polymorphonuclear cell; PNH, paroxysmal nocturnal hemoglobinuria; PNH-sc, subclinical PNH; RA, refractory anemia; RAEB, refractory anemia with excess of blasts; RAEB-t, refractory anemia with excess of blasts in transformation; RA-PNH+, RA with a population of PNH cells; RA-PNH−, RA without a population of PNH cells; RARS, refractory anemia with ringed sideroblasts; RBCs, red blood cells; RCMD, refractory cytopenias with multilineage dysplasia; WHO, World Health Organization.

Although treatment with eculizumab favorably modifies the natural history of PNH, it has no effect on the underlying disease process (i.e., the *PIGA*-mutant hematopoietic stem cell clone). The *PIGA*-mutant mutant clone can be eradicated and normal hematopoiesis restored by allogeneic hematopoietic stem cell transplantation, but the relatively benign natural history of PNH in patients treated with eculizumab has tempered enthusiasm for transplantation because of concerns about subjecting patients to the risk of treatment-related morbidity.

● DEFINITION AND HISTORY

Although commonly regarded as a type of hemolytic anemia, paroxysmal nocturnal hemoglobinuria (PNH) is properly categorized as a hematopoietic stem cell disorder. PNH arises as a result of clonal expansion of *one or several* hematopoietic stem cells that have acquired a *somatic mutation* of the X-chromosome gene *PIGA* (phosphatidylinositol glycan class A). As a consequence of mutant PIGA, any progeny of affected stem cells (erythrocytes, granulocytes, monocytes, platelets, and lymphocytes) are deficient in all glycosylphosphatidylinositol-anchored proteins (GPI-APs) that are normally expressed on hematopoietic cells. The clinical manifestations of PNH are hemolytic anemia, thrombophilia, and marrow failure, but only the hemolytic anemia is unequivocally a consequence of somatic mutation of *PIGA*. It is not a malignant neoplasm in the classical sense of uncontrolled proliferation of cells, spread to tissues other than marrow, or spatial replacement of hematopoiesis. Its effects can be lethal and it can uncommonly undergo clonal evolution to acute myelogenous leukemia.

Comprehensive, scholarly reviews of the history of PNH have been published.[1-4] The first published clinical description of PNH is attributed to William Gull in 1866, but he failed to distinguish definitively PNH from paroxysmal cold hemoglobinuria. Paul Strübing, in 1882, clearly recognized PNH as a distinct entity and undertook prescient experiments designed to test his hypothesis that the nocturnal hemoglobinuria was a consequence of acidification of plasma that occurred when carbon dioxide and lactic acid accumulated because of slowing of respiration during sleep. In 1911, A.A. Hijmans van den Berg demonstrated that the hemolysis of PNH is caused by a defect in the red cell rather than by the presence of an abnormal plasma factor (as is the case with paroxysmal cold hemoglobinuria; Chap. 54). Thomas Hale Ham is credited with discovering, in the late 1930s, that complement mediates the hemolysis of PNH erythrocytes, although it was not until the alternative pathway of complement was identified and characterized in the mid-1950s by Louis Pillemer that the basis of Ham's original observations became apparent. Ham developed the acidified serum lysis test (Ham test) that, along with the sucrose lysis test (*sugar water test*) of Robert Hartmann and David Jenkins, was used as the standard diagnostic test for PNH until being supplanted in the early 1990s by flow cytometry. Both Hartmann and William Crosby brought attention to the important role that thrombosis (particularly the Budd-Chiari syndrome) plays in the natural history of PNH, and John Dacie and his student and colleague S.M. Lewis were the first to systematically characterize the relationship between PNH and marrow failure.

● EPIDEMIOLOGY

The prevalence of PNH is not known with certainty. Prevalence estimates are influenced by bias in study design and results differ considerably, in large part, because of the heterogeneous nature of the disease. The blood of patients with PNH is a mosaic of normal and abnormal cells, and the extent of the mosaicism varies widely among patients (see "Phenotypic Mosaicism is Characteristic of Paroxysmal Nocturnal Hemoglobinuria" below). Patients with small PNH clones have few or no symptoms related to hemolysis. Thus an argument can be made that asymptomatic patients with small clones do not have clinically significant PNH and should be excluded from prevalence estimates. Others, however, may argue that any patient with flow cytometric evidence of a population of GPI-AP–deficient cells, regardless of clone size, has PNH and should be included in prevalence estimates. Well-designed, rigorous studies of prevalence that address the issue of disease heterogeneity are needed, but, by any definition, PNH is a rare disease. The prevalence of clinically significant PNH (i.e., classic PNH) plus patients with relatively large clones that arise in the setting of another marrow failure syndrome, (see "Clinical Features" and Table 40–2 below) is likely in the order of less than 1 case per 200,000 population, easily fulfilling criteria (<1 case per 50,000 population) for classification as an ultraorphan disease.[5] There is a close association between PNH and aplastic anemia, and environmental factors, drugs, and toxins, that cause aplastic anemia, concordantly increase the risk of developing PNH. Although PNH is reported in all age groups, the peak incidence is in the third and fourth decades of life, similar to that of aplastic anemia (Chap. 35). PNH is an acquired disorder, and there is no known inherited risk for developing the disease. A number of cases have been reported in which only one of a pair of identical twins was affected.

ETIOLOGY AND PATHOGENESIS

COMPLEMENT AND PAROXYSMAL NOCTURNAL HEMOGLOBINURIA

The chronic intravascular hemolysis that is the hallmark clinical manifestation of PNH is mediated by the alternative pathway of complement (APC) (Fig. 40–1).[6] The APC is a component of innate immunity (Chap. 20).[7] This ancient system evolved to protect the host against invasion by pathogenic microorganisms. Unlike the classical pathway of complement that is part of the system of acquired immunity and requires antibody for initiation of activation, the APC is in a state of continuous activation, armed at all times to protect the host (Chap. 19 provides a detailed review of the complement system). The APC cascade can be divided into two functional components: the amplification C3 and C5 convertases and the membrane attack complex (MAC). The C3 and C5 convertases (Fig. 40–1, *top panel*) are enzymatic complexes that initiate and amplify the activity of the APC. Generation of C5b by enzymatic cleavage of C5 by the APC C5 convertase activates the terminal pathway of complement that results ultimately in assembly of the cytolytic MAC.

Because the APC is primed for attack at all times, elaborate mechanisms for self-recognition and for protection of the host against APC-mediated injury have evolved. Both fluid-phase and membrane-bound proteins are involved in these processes. Normal human erythrocytes are protected against APC-mediated cytolysis primarily by decay-accelerating factor (DAF, CD55)[8-10] and membrane inhibitor of reactive lysis (MIRL, CD59).[11] These proteins act at different steps in the complement cascade (see Fig. 40–1, *top panel*). CD55 regulates the formation and stability of the C3 and C5 convertases, whereas CD59 blocks the formation of the MAC. Deficiency of CD55 and CD59 on the erythrocytes of PNH is the pathophysiologic basis of the Coombs-negative, intravascular hemolysis that is the clinical hallmark of the disease (see Fig. 40–1, *bottom panel*). But why are PNH erythrocytes deficient in the two complement regulatory proteins?

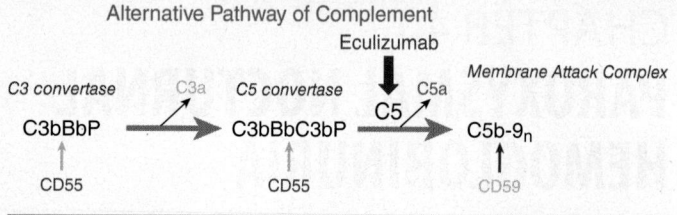

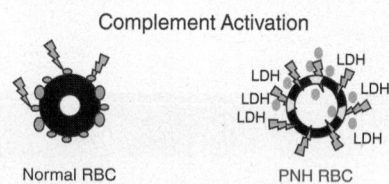

Figure 40–1. Complement-mediated lysis of paroxysmal nocturnal hemoglobinuria (PNH) erythrocytes. *Upper panel.* The hemolytic anemia of PNH is Coombs test–negative because the process is mediated by the antibody-independent alternative pathway of complement (APC). The C3 convertase of the APC consists of activated C3 (C3b), activated factor B (Bb, the enzymatic subunit of the complex), and factor P (a protein that stabilizes the complex, formally called properdin). The C5 convertase has the same components as the C3 convertase except that two C3b molecules are required to bind and position C5 for cleavage by activated factor B (Bb). C3a and C5a are bioactive peptides that are generated by cleavage of C3 and C5, respectively, by their specific activation convertases. The C3 and C5 convertases greatly amplify complement activation by cleaving multiple substrate molecules. The membrane attack complex (MAC) consists of activated C5 (C5b), C6, C7, C8, and multiple molecules of C9 ($C9_n$). The MAC is the cytolytic unit of the complement system. The glycosylphosphatidylinositol (GPI)-anchored complement regulatory protein CD55 restricts formation and stability of both the C3 and the C5 amplification convertases by destabilizing the interaction between activated factor B (Bb) and C3b (indicated by the *blue arrow*), whereas GPI-anchored CD59 blocks formation of the MAC by inhibiting the binding of C9 to the C5b-8 complex (indicated by the *brown arrow*). Inhibition of MAC formation by the humanized monoclonal anti-C5 antibody eculizumab (indicated by the *red arrow*) ameliorates the intravascular hemolysis of PNH. *Lower panel.* Normal erythrocytes *(left)* are protected against complement-mediated lysis primarily by CD55 *(blue circles)* and CD59 *(green circles)*. Deficiency of these GPI-anchored complement regulatory proteins results in APC activation on PNH erythrocytes *(right)*. Because of deficiency of CD55 and CD59, the complement cascade activates on the cell surface. Consequently, MACs form pores in the red cell membrane resulting in colloid osmotic lysis and release of hemoglobin *(red circles)* and other contents of the red cell including lactate dehydrogenase (LDH) into the intravascular space. RBC, red blood cell. *(Modified with permission from Parker CJ: The pathophysiology of paroxysmal nocturnal hemoglobinuria. Exp Hematol 35(4):523–533, 2007.)*

THE MOLECULAR PATHOGENESIS AND GENETIC BASIS OF PAROXYSMAL NOCTURNAL HEMOGLOBINURIA

PNH is a consequence of clonal expansion of one or more hematopoietic stem cells with mutant *PIGA* (located on Xp22.1).[12] The protein product of *PIGA* is a glycosyl transferase[12-16] that is an obligate constituent of a complex biochemical pathway required for synthesis of the glycosylphosphatidylinositol (GPI) moiety that anchors individual proteins belonging to diverse functional groups to the cell surface (Fig. 40–2). As a result of mutant *PIGA*, progeny of the affected stem cells are deficient in all GPI-APs. Although more than 20 GPI-APs are expressed by hematopoietic cells, it is deficiency on red blood cells

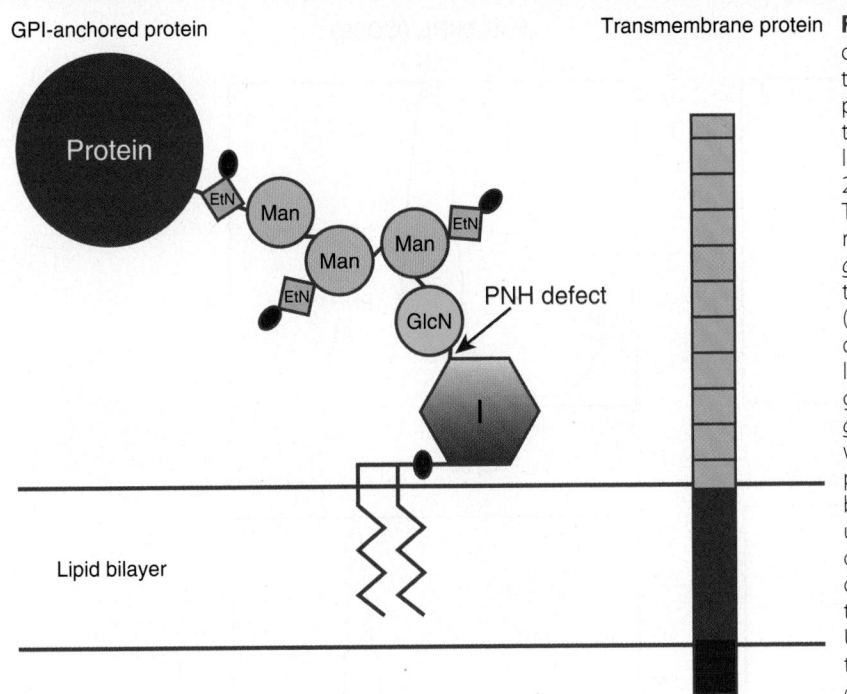

GPI-anchored protein

Transmembrane protein

Figure 40–2. The molecular and genetic basis of paroxysmal nocturnal hemoglobinuria (PNH). There are two types of anchoring mechanisms for plasma membrane proteins: transmembrane and glycosylphosphatidylinositol (GPI). Transmembrane proteins are anchored into the lipid bilayer of the cell by a short series (approximately 25 amino acids) of hydrophobic residues (*blue rectangle*). Transmembrane proteins typically have a short cytoplasmic tail that usually has signaling properties (*red rectangle*). The ectoplasmic portion of the protein is illustrated by the series of *gray-blue squares*. The GPI-anchored protein (AP) consists of the following components: phosphatidylinositol (inositol is represented by the *blue hexagon* labeled I and phosphate is represented by the *red oval*); glucosamine (GLcN, *yellow circle*); three mannose (Man, *green circles*); ethanolamine phosphate (EtN, *blue square* with attached phosphate represented by the *red oval*); the protein entity (*blue circle*). The lipid component (indicated by the series of *diagonal lines* within the lipid bilayer) is usually 1-alkyl,2-acylglycerol for mammalian GPI-APs. PNH cells are deficient in all GPI-APs because somatic mutation of the X-chromosome gene *PIGA* disrupts the first step in the biosynthetic pathway (transfer of the nucleotide sugar UDP-GlcNAc [uridine diphosphate–*N*-acetylglucosamine] to GlcNAc-PI [phosphatidylinositol]) indicated by the arrow.

(RBCs) of the two GPI-anchored complement regulatory proteins, CD55 and CD59, that underlies the hemolytic anemia of PNH.[17] RBCs lacking CD55 and CD59 undergo spontaneous intravascular hemolysis as a consequence of unregulated activation of the APC (see Fig. 40–1, *bottom panel*). Thus, the hallmark clinical manifestation of PNH (intravascular hemolysis and the resultant hemoglobinuria) occurs because the two proteins that regulate complement on erythrocytes happen to be GPI-anchored.

Hypothetically, the PNH phenotype would result from inactivation of any of the more than 25 genes involved in synthesis of the GPI-anchor (see Fig. 40–2), but, with one exception,[18] somatic mutation of no gene involved in GPI-AP synthesis other than *PIGA* has been reported in patients with PNH. This phenomenon is accounted for by the fact that, of the genes involved in the GPI-anchor synthesis pathway, only *PIGA* is located on the X-chromosome. Therefore, somatic mutation of only one allele is required for expression of the phenotype as males have one X-chromosome and, as a consequence of X-inactivation during embryogenesis, females have only one functional X-chromosome in somatic tissues (Chap. 10). On the other hand, mutation of two alleles would be required for inactivation of any of the autosomal genes involved in the GPI-anchor synthesis pathway.[18]

Cells with *PIGA* mutations do not appear to have a proliferative advantage *in vitro* or in hybrid animal models made with *PIGA* knockouts.[19] They have been found to be relatively resistant to apoptosis in some studies,[20–23] but not in others.[24,25] Thus, the basis of clonal selection and clonal expansion of *PIGA* mutant stem cells in patients with PNH remains largely enigmatic[26] although a number of hypotheses have been proposed (reviewed in Ref. 17).

PHENOTYPIC MOSAICISM IS CHARACTERISTIC OF PAROXYSMAL NOCTURNAL HEMOGLOBINURIA

The blood of patients with PNH is a mosaic of normal and abnormal cells (Fig. 40–3). Although PNH is a clonal disease, the extent to which the *PIGA*-mutant clone expands varies widely among patients.[17] As an example, in some cases, greater than 90 percent of the blood cells may

be derived from the *PIGA*-mutant clone, whereas in others, less than 10 percent of the blood cells may be GPI-AP deficient. This unique feature (variability in extent of mosaicism) is clinically relevant because patients with relatively small PNH clones have minimal or no symptoms and require no PNH-specific treatment, whereas those with large clones are often debilitated by the consequences of chronic complement-mediated intravascular hemolysis and respond dramatically to complement inhibitory therapy.

Another remarkable feature of PNH is phenotypic mosaicism (see Fig. 40–3A) based on *PIGA* genotype[27] (see Fig. 40–3B) that determines the degree of GPI-AP deficiency.[17] PNH III cells are completely deficient in GPI-APs, PNH II cells are partially (approximately 90 percent) deficient and PNH I cells express GPI-APs at normal density (putatively, these cells are progeny of residual normal stem cells; see Fig. 40–3A). Phenotype varies among patients (Fig. 40–4). Some patients have only type I and type III cells (the most common phenotype), some have type I, type II, and type III (the second most common phenotype), and some patients have only type I and type II cells (the least-common phenotype). Furthermore, the contribution of each phenotype to the composition of the blood varies. Phenotypic mosaicism is clinically important because PNH II cells are relatively resistant to spontaneous hemolysis, and patients with a high percentage of type II cells have a relatively benign clinical course with respect to hemolysis (Fig. 40–4).

The anemia of PNH is multifactorial as an element of marrow failure is present in all patients, although the degree of marrow dysfunction is variable.[28] In some patients, PNH arises in the setting of aplastic anemia. In this case, marrow failure is the dominant cause of anemia. In other patients with PNH, evidence of marrow dysfunction may be subtle (e.g., an inappropriately low reticulocyte count) with the degree of anemia being determined primarily by the rate of hemolysis that is, in turn, determined by PNH clone size.

● CLINICAL FEATURES

The primary clinical manifestations of PNH are hemolysis, thrombosis, and marrow failure.[28] Constitutional symptoms (fatigue, lethargy, malaise, asthenia) dominate the history, with nocturnal hemoglobinuria

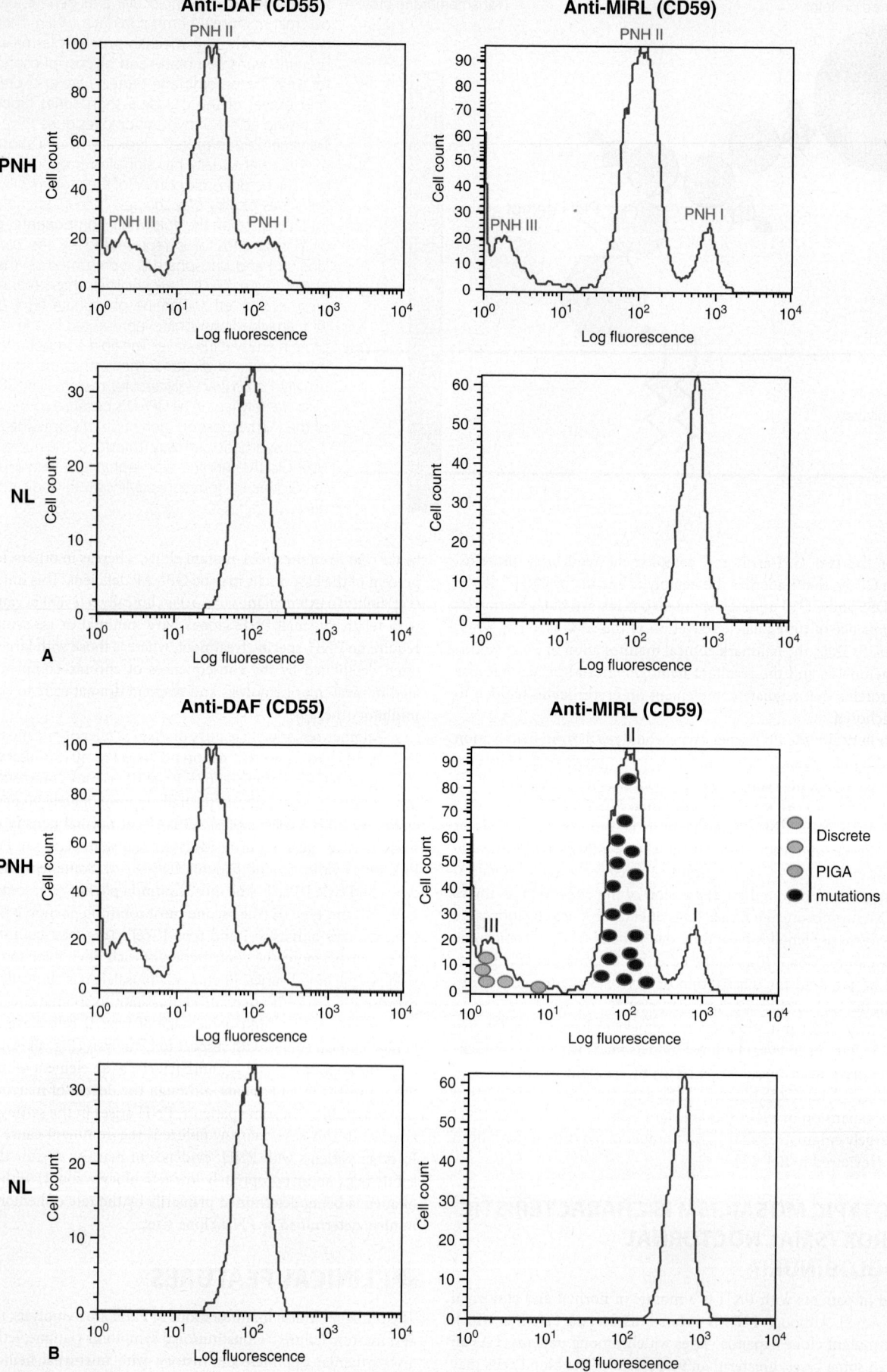

TABLE 40-1. Recommendation for Screening Patients for Paroxysmal Nocturnal Hemoglobinuria*

History of episodic hemoglobinuria

Evidence of nonspherocytic, Coombs-negative intravascular hemolysis (must have high serum lactate dehydrogenase)

Patients with aplastic anemia (screen at diagnosis and once yearly even in the absence of intravascular hemolysis)

Patients with refractory anemia or refractory cytopenias with multilineage dysplasia variants of myelodysplastic syndrome†

Patients with venous thrombosis involving unusual sites (usually have evidence of intravascular hemolysis)

- Budd-Chiari syndrome
- Other intraabdominal sites
- Cerebral veins
- Dermal veins

*Screening by flow cytometric analysis of glycosylphosphatidylinositol-anchored proteins on red blood cells and polymorphonuclear cells.

†There is no indication for screening patients with other myelodysplastic syndrome classifications.

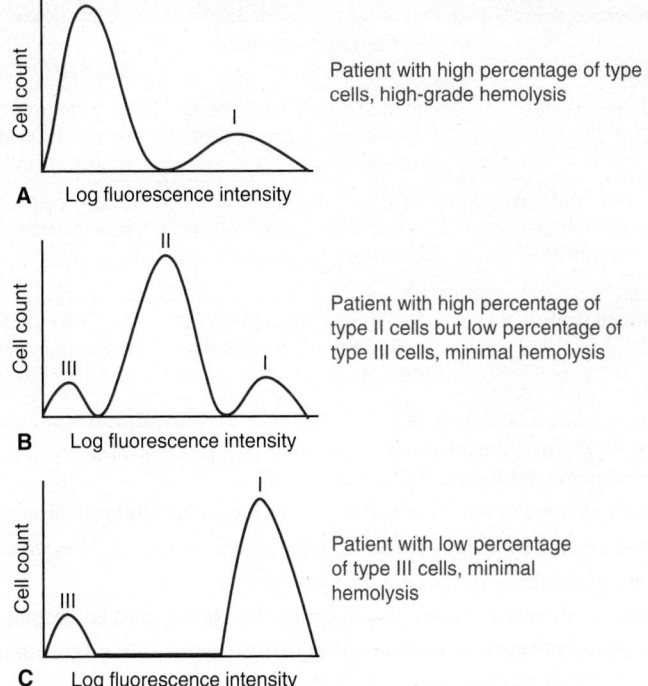

Figure 40–4. Clinical manifestations of paroxysmal nocturnal hemoglobinuria (PNH) are determined by clone size and erythrocyte phenotype. Mock flow cytometry histograms of erythrocytes from hypothetical patients with PNH stained with anti-CD59 are illustrated. Both the proportion and type of abnormal erythrocytes vary greatly among patients with PNH and these characteristics are important determinants of clinical manifestations. In general, patients with a high percentage of type III erythrocytes have clinically apparent hemolysis **(A)**. If the erythrocytes are partially deficient in glycosylphosphatidylinositol-anchored protein (PNH II cells), hemolysis may be modest even if the percentage of the affected cells is high **(B)**. A patient may have a diagnosis of PNH, but if the proportion of type III cells is low, only biochemical evidence of hemolysis may be observed **(C)**. *(Modified with permission from Parker C, Omine M, Richards S, et al: Diagnosis and management of paroxysmal nocturnal hemoglobinuria. Blood 106(12):3699–3709, 2005.)*

being a presenting symptom in only approximately 25 percent of patients.[29] Direct questioning frequently elicits a history of episodic dysphagia and odynophagia, abdominal pain, and male impotence. Venous thrombosis, often occurring at unusual sites (Budd-Chiari syndrome, mesenteric, dermal, or cerebral veins), may complicate PNH. Arterial thrombosis is less common.

●LABORATORY FEATURES

PNH should be suspected in all patients with nonspherocytic, Coombs-negative intravascular hemolysis (Table 40–1).

Although the clinical manifestations of PNH depend in large part on the size of the *PIGA*-mutant clone, the extent of the associate marrow failure also contributes significantly to disease manifestations. Thus, PNH is not a binary process and based on clinical features, marrow characteristics, and the size of the mutant clone as determined by the percentage of GPI-AP–deficient polymorphonuclear cells (PMNs), the International PNH Interest Group recognizes three disease subcategories (Table 40–2).[28]

Reticulocytosis reflects the response to hemolysis, although the reticulocyte count may be lower than expected for the degree of anemia because of underlying marrow failure (see Table 40–1). Serum lactate

dehydrogenase (LDH) concentration is always abnormally high in patients with clinically significant hemolysis and serves as an important surrogate marker for estimating and following the rate of intravascular hemolysis. A close association exists between PNH and aplastic anemia, and to a lesser extent between PNH and low-risk myelodysplastic syndromes (MDSs) (Chaps. 35 and 87 and see "Paroxysmal Nocturnal Hemoglobinuria and Marrow Failure" below). By using high-sensitivity flow cytometry, approximately 50 percent of patients with aplastic

Figure 40–3. Phenotypic mosaicism is a characteristic feature of paroxysmal nocturnal hemoglobinuria (PNH). **A.** The blood of patients with PNH is a mosaic of phenotypically normal and abnormal cells. In some patients, erythrocytes that are partially deficient in glycosylphosphatidylinositol-anchored proteins (GPI-APs) (called PNH II) are present in the blood along with cells that are completely deficient (PNH III) and cells that are phenotypically normal (PNH I). In the case illustrated, erythrocytes from a patient with PNH (PNH, *upper panels*) and from a healthy volunteer (NL, *lower panels*) were stained with fluorescently labeled antibodies (anti-CD55, *left panels*; CD59, *right panels*) and analyzed by flow cytometry. **B.** *PIGA* genotype determines PNH phenotype. The PNH II phenotype is a consequence of *PIGA* mutation that partially inactivates enzyme function (*red circles*), whereas any *PIGA* mutation that causes complete loss of enzyme function generates the PNH III phenotype (*green, yellow,* and *blue circles*). PNH I cells, have wild-type *PIGA* and are the progeny of normal residual hematopoietic stem cells. In a single individual, multiple discrete *PIGA* mutations can be identified, accounting for the phenotypic mosaicism based on GPI-AP expression. DAF, decay-accelerating factor; MIRL, membrane inhibitor of reactive lysis.

TABLE 40–2. Classification of Paroxysmal Nocturnal Hemoglobinuria[*]

Category	Rate of Intravascular Hemolysis[†]	Marrow	Flow Cytometry	Benefit from Eculizumab
Classic	Florid (macroscopic hemoglobinuria is frequent or persistent)	Cellular marrow with erythroid hyperplasia and normal or near-normal morphology[‡]	Large population (>50%) of GPI-AP–deficient PMNs[¶]	Yes
PNH in the setting of another marrow failure syndrome[§]	Mild to moderate (macroscopic hemoglobinuria is intermittent or absent)	Evidence of a concomitant marrow failure syndrome[§]	Although variable, the percentage of GPI-AP deficient PMNs[¶] is usually relatively small (<30%)	Dependent on the size of the PNH clone
Subclinical	No clinical or biochemical evidence of intravascular hemolysis	Evidence of a concomitant marrow failure syndrome[§]	Small (<1%) population of GPI-AP–deficient PMNs detected by high-resolution flow cytometry	No

GPI-AP, glycosylphosphatidylinositol-anchored protein; MDS, myelodysplastic syndrome; PMN, polymorphonuclear cell; PNH, paroxysmal nocturnal hemoglobinuria; RBC, red blood cell.

[*]Based on recommendations of the International PNH Interest Group.[28]

[†]Based on macroscopic hemoglobinuria, serum lactate dehydrogenase concentration, and reticulocyte count.

[‡]Karyotypic abnormalities are uncommon.

[§]Aplastic anemia and refractory anemia/MDS are the most commonly associated marrow failure syndromes.

[¶]Analysis of PMNs is more informative than analysis of RBCs because of selective destruction GPI-AP–deficient RBCs.

anemia and 15 percent of patients with low-risk MDS have been found to have a detectable population of GPI-AP–deficient erythrocytes and granulocytes.[30-33] In approximately 80 percent of these cases, the proportion of GPI-AP deficient cells is <1.0 percent of the total. These patients with very small populations of GPI-AP–deficient erythrocytes have no clinical or biochemical evidence of hemolysis and are designated as subclinical PNH (PNH-sc; see Table 40-2). Varying degrees of leukopenia, thrombocytopenia, and relative reticulocytopenia reflect the extent of marrow insufficiency (see "Paroxysmal Nocturnal Hemoglobinuria and Marrow Failure" below).

Once suspected, diagnosing PNH is straightforward as deficiency of GPI-APs on blood cells is readily demonstrated by flow cytometry (Fig. 40–5).[34,35] Although they have much biologic and historic importance, the acidified serum lysis test (Ham test) and the sucrose lysis test (sugar water test) have largely been abandoned as diagnostic assays because they are both less sensitive and less quantitative than flow cytometry. Flow cytometric analysis of both RBCs and PMNs is warranted, as clone size will be underestimated if only RBCs are examined because GPI-AP–deficient red cells are selectively destroyed by complement. Recent transfusion will also affect the estimate of clone size, if only RBCs are analyzed, but delineation of PNH phenotypes (i.e., the percentage of types I, II, and III cells) requires flow cytometric analysis of the erythrocyte population.

In addition to flow cytometric analysis, the basic initial evaluation of a patient with PNH should include complete blood count to assess the effects of the disease on production of leukocytes and platelets, as well as on erythrocytes (Table 40-3). In patients with classic PNH, the leukocyte and platelet counts are usually normal or nearly normal, whereas leukopenia, thrombocytopenia, or both invariably accompany PNH/aplastic anemia and PNH/MDS. The reticulocyte count is needed to assess the ongoing capacity of the marrow to respond to the anemia. Although the reticulocyte count is elevated in patients with classic PNH, as noted above, it may be inappropriately low for the degree of anemia, reflecting underlying relative insufficiency of hematopoiesis that is characteristic of the disease. The reticulocyte count is decreased in patients with PNH with concomitant aplastic anemia or low-risk MDS.

Serum LDH is always markedly elevated in classic PNH. The degree of serum LDH elevation is variable in patients with PNH/aplastic anemia and PNH/MDS, depending on the size of the PNH clone (see Table 40-2). By definition, patients with PNH-sc have neither clinical nor biochemical evidence of hemolysis (see Table 40-2). Patients with classic PNH are often iron deficient as a result of chronic iron loss in the form of hemoglobinuria and hemosiderinuria (Chap. 43). Marrow aspirate and biopsy are needed to distinguish classic PNH from PNH in the setting of another marrow abnormality. Nonrandom cytogenetic abnormalities are rare in PNH.[26]

● DIFFERENTIAL DIAGNOSIS

PAROXYSMAL NOCTURNAL HEMOGLOBINURIA AND MARROW FAILURE

Although the marrow of patients with classic PNH appears relatively normal morphologically (see Table 40-2), numerous *in vitro* studies have shown that the growth characteristics of marrow-derived stem cells are aberrant.[21,36,37] Moreover, when stem cells are sorted into GPI-AP– and GPI-AP+ populations, compared to the GPI-AP+ population, the growth characteristics of the GPI-AP– population more closely approach those of normal control cells.[21,36] One plausible explanation for this observation is that the GPI-AP– cells are relatively protected from the pathophysiologic process that mediates the marrow injury, thereby providing a basis for natural selection of the *PIGA* mutant clone. In this view of PNH, outgrowth of the *PIGA* mutant clone is seen as an example of Darwinian evolution occurring within the microenvironment of the marrow. Although appealing, definitive experimental support for this hypothesis is lacking.

A close association exists between PNH and aplastic anemia and to a lesser extent between PNH and low-risk MDSs. By using high-resolution flow cytometry,[34] approximately 50 to 60 percent of patients with aplastic anemia and 15 to 20 percent of patients with low-risk MDS have been found to have a detectable population of GPI-AP–deficient erythrocytes and granulocytes.[30,31,33,38,39] In approximately 90 percent of

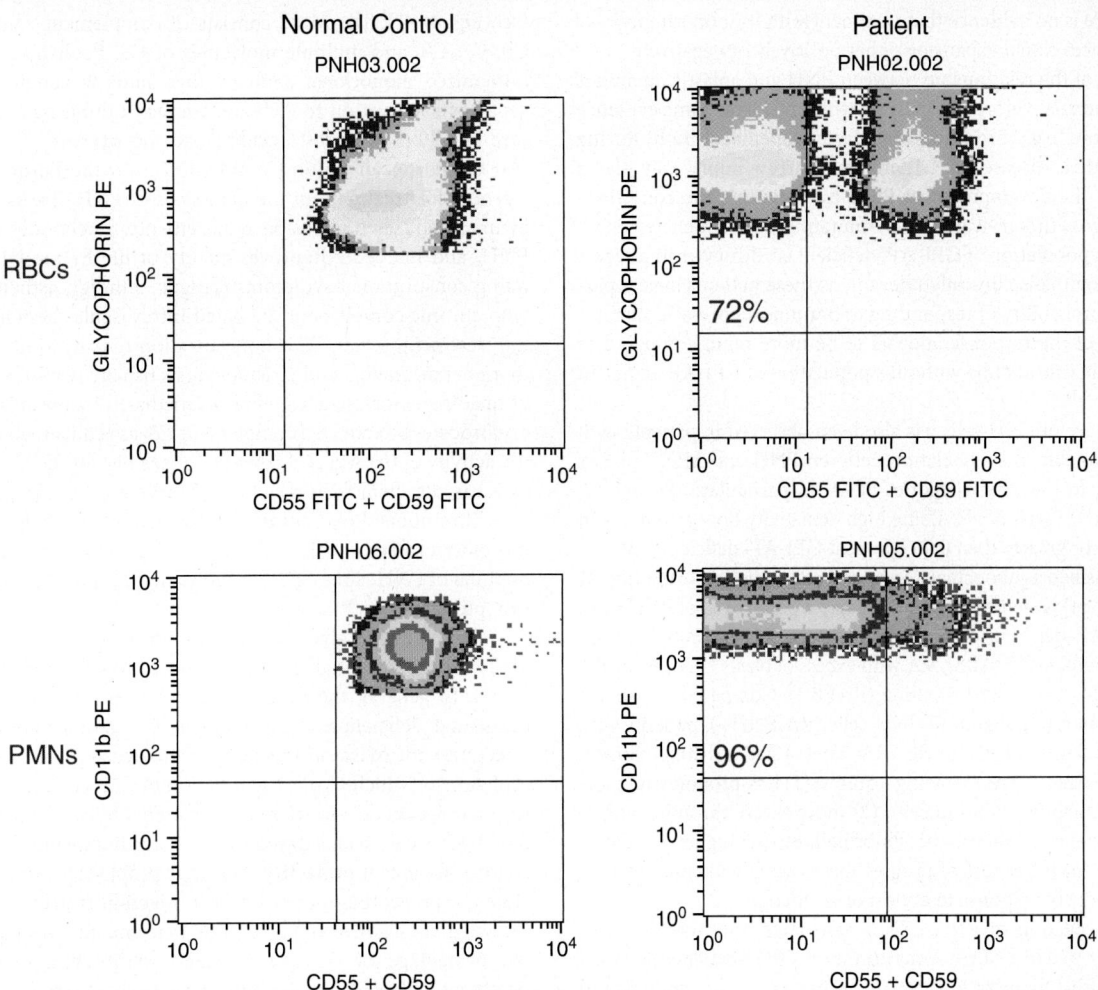

Figure 40–5. Diagnosis of paroxysmal nocturnal hemoglobinuria (PNH) by flow cytometry. Erythrocytes (RBCs) and neutrophils (PMNs) from a healthy volunteer and a patient with PNH were analyzed by flow cytometry using anti–glycophorin A *(top row, vertical axis)* to identify RBCs and anti-CD11b *(bottom row, vertical axis)* to identify PMNs. Glycosylphosphatidylinositol-anchored protein (GPI-AP) expression was detected using a combination of anti-CD55 and anti-CD59 *(top and bottom rows, horizontal axis)*. PNH cells are deficient in both CD55 and CD59 *(upper left quadrant of each histogram)*. The percentage of GPI-AP–deficient (PNH) cells is shown for each sample.

TABLE 40–3. Basic Evaluation for Paroxysmal Nocturnal Hemoglobinuria

Flow cytometric evidence of a population of erythrocytes and granulocytes partially or completely deficient in multiple glycosylphosphatidylinositol-anchored proteins (GPI-APs)*

Complete blood count, reticulocyte count, serum concentration of lactate dehydrogenase,† bilirubin (fractionated) and haptoglobin, determination of iron stores

Marrow aspirate, biopsy, and cytogenetics‡

*Paroxysmal nocturnal hemoglobinuria (PNH) clone size is determined by the percentage of GPI-AP–deficient polymorphonuclear cells.

†The most important surrogate marker for intravascular hemolysis.

‡Marrow aspirate and biopsy are used to distinguish classic PNH from PNH in the setting of another marrow failure syndrome. Nonrandom karyotypic abnormalities are rare in PNH.

these cases, the proportion of GPI-AP–deficient blood neutrophils is less than 25 percent of the total.[38] Those patients with very small populations of GPI-AP–deficient erythrocytes (designated PNH-sc) have no clinical or biochemical evidence of hemolysis and require no specific treatment for PNH (see Table 40–2).

Studies have investigated the natural history of PNH clones in the setting of marrow failure.[38,40,41] The threshold that separates PNH-sc from clinical PNH is reached when the neutrophil clone size is in the range of 20 to 25 percent with a corresponding GPI-AP–deficient erythrocyte population of 3 to 5 percent.[40] Longitudinal studies indicate that clonal expansion occurs in 15 to 50 percent of cases.[38,40,41] In 10 to 25 percent of cases the clone disappears, and in 25 to 60 percent of cases the clone size persists unchanged.[38,40,41] Available evidence indicates that patients who present with PNH-sc do not progress to clinical PNH.[38,40,41] Among patients who present with clinical PNH in the setting of marrow failure, treatment for complications of PNH (eculizumab for hemolysis or anticoagulation for thrombosis) is required in approximately 50 percent of cases.[41] There is no evidence that treatment with immunosuppressive therapy influences clonal expansion either positively or negatively.

The basis of the relationship between PNH and aplastic anemia is speculative. The vast majority of patients with PNH have some evidence of marrow failure (e.g., thrombocytopenia, leukopenia, or both) during the course of their disease.[26,42,43] Therefore, marrow injury may play a central role in the development of PNH by providing the conditions that favor the growth/survival of *PIGA*-mutant, GPI-AP–deficient stem cells. Finding a population of GPI-AP–deficient erythrocytes in patients with aplastic anemia is clinically relevant, as these patients have a particularly high probability of responding to immunosuppressive therapy, and the onset of the response appears to be more rapid compared to patients with aplastic anemia without a population of GPI-AP–deficient erythrocytes.[31,33,44]

The presence of PNH cells has also been observed in patients with MDS.[30,33,39,45] Notably, the association between PNH and MDS appears to be confined to low-risk categories of MDS, particularly the refractory anemia (RA) variant.[30,33,39] Using high-sensitivity flow cytometry in which equal to or greater than 0.003 percent GPI-AP–deficient RBCs or PMNs was classified as abnormal, Wang and colleagues reported that 21 of 119 (18 percent) patients with RA MDS had a population of PNH cells, whereas GPI-AP–deficient cells were not detected in patients with RA with ringed sideroblast (RARS), RA with excess of blasts (RAEB), or RA with excess of blasts in transformation (RAEB-t). Compared to patients with RA without a population of PNH cells (RA-PNH−), patients with RA with a population of PNH cells (RA-PNH+) had a distinct clinical profile characterized by the following features: (1) less-pronounced morphologic abnormalities of blood cells; (2) more severe thrombocytopenia; (3) lower rates of karyotypic abnormalities; (4) higher incidence of HLA-DR15; (5) lower rate of progression to acute leukemia; and (6) higher probability of response to cyclosporine therapy.

That a population of PNH cells is associated only with low-risk MDS was confirmed in a North American study of 137 patients classified by World Health Organization (WHO) criteria.[39,46] The study found a population of PNH cells in 1 of 5 (20 percent) patients with 5q−syndrome, in 6 of 17 (35 percent) patients with RA, and in 2 of 37 (5 percent) patients with refractory cytopenias with multilineage dysplasia (RCMD), whereas no patient with RARS (0 of 9), RCMD-ringed sideroblasts (0 of 6), RAEB (0 of 26), MDS unspecified (0 of 10), myelodysplastic/myeloproliferative disease (0 of 10), primary myelofibrosis (0 of 5), chronic myelomonocytic leukemia (0 of 5), or acute myeloid leukemia (0 of 6) had a detectable population of GPI-AP–deficient blood cells.[39]

When combined with evidence of polyclonal hematopoiesis (based on the pattern of X-chromosome inactivation in female patients), the presence of a population of PNH cells in patients with MDS predicts a relatively benign clinical course and a high probability of response to immunosuppressive therapy in patients.[30] A relatively good response to immunosuppressive therapy for patients with MDS and aplastic anemia was also predicted by expression of HLA-DR15 in studies of both North American and Japanese patients.[47,48] Together, these observations provide compelling indirect evidence that aplastic anemia and a subgroup of low-risk MDS are immune-mediated diseases and that the immune pathophysiologic process provides the selection pressure that favors the outgrowth of *PIGA* mutant, GPI-AP–deficient stem cells.

⬤THERAPY

ECULIZUMAB

The complement-mediated intravascular hemolysis of PNH can be inhibited by blocking formation of the terminal complement pathway generated MAC, the cytolytic component of the complement system

(see Fig. 40–1). The MAC consists of complement components C5b, C6, C7, C8, and multiple molecules of C9. Eculizumab (Soliris) is a humanized monoclonal antibody that binds to complement C5, preventing its activation to C5b and thereby inhibiting MAC formation (see Fig. 40–1).[49] In 2007, eculizumab was approved by both the FDA and the European Union Commission (now the European Medicines Agency) for treatment of the hemolysis of PNH. Treatment with eculizumab reduces transfusion requirements, ameliorates the anemia of PNH, and markedly improves quality of life by resolving the debilitating constitutional symptoms (fatigue, lethargy, asthenia) associated with chronic complement-mediated intravascular hemolysis.[50] Following treatment, serum LDH concentration returns to normal, but mild to moderate anemia and reticulocytosis usually persist, likely the result of ongoing extravascular hemolysis mediated by opsonization of PNH erythrocytes by activated complement C3, as eculizumab does not block the activity of the APC C3 convertase (see Fig. 40–1).[51,52] In some cases, extravascular hemolysis is sufficiently severe so as to require therapy.[53]

Thromboembolic events are the major cause of morbidity and mortality in PNH,[28] and eculizumab appears to ameliorate the thrombophilia of PNH, although the studies that support that conclusion had suboptimal design.[54]

Eculizumab is given by intravenous infusion on a biweekly schedule following an initial loading period consisting of five weekly treatments. In general, the drug is well tolerated; however, patients with congenital deficiency of complement C5 have an increased risk of infection with *Neisseria* species. For this reason, patients treated with eculizumab (which blocks the function of C5; see Fig. 40–1) are at risk for meningococcal septicemia. All patients must be inoculated with a meningococcal vaccine 2 weeks before starting therapy, but the vaccine is not 100 percent protective. Whether prophylactic antibiotic therapy aimed at preventing meningococcal infection is justified for a patient receiving eculizumab remains to be determined. Despite the fact that the percentage of GPI-AP–deficient erythrocytes increases during treatment with eculizumab,[55] there have been no reports of catastrophic hemolytic crises in the relatively few PNH patients who have discontinued treatment with eculizumab.[54,56]

Eculizumab is expensive (approximately $400,000/year in the United States), and it has no effect on either the underlying stem cell abnormality or the associated marrow failure. Consequently, treatment must continue indefinitely and leukopenia, thrombocytopenia, and reticulocytopenia, if present, persist.

OTHER TREATMENT FOR PAROXYSMAL NOCTURNAL HEMOGLOBINURIA

Other than eculizumab, there is no specific treatment for PNH, and for patients who are not being treated with eculizumab, management is largely supportive (reviewed in Ref. 28). Although hemolysis is ameliorated in some patients by treatment with glucocorticoids or androgens, the use of steroids in the management of patients with PNH is controversial.[28] The main value of glucocorticoids may be in attenuating acute hemolytic exacerbations. Under these circumstances, brief pulses of prednisone may reduce the severity and duration of the crisis. The value of glucocorticoids in treating chronic hemolysis is limited by toxicity, and the harm that can accrue from long-term use cannot be overemphasized. An every-other-day schedule may attenuate some of the adverse effects of chronic glucocorticoid use,[57] but patients may note worsening of symptoms on the off day.

Androgen therapy, either alone or in combination with glucocorticoids, has been used successfully to treat the anemia of PNH.[57,58] As with glucocorticoids, the mechanism by which androgenic steroids ameliorate the anemia of PNH is not fully understood, although the rapid onset of action is consistent with complement inhibition.[58] Potential complications of androgen therapy include liver toxicity, prostatic hypertrophy, and virilizing effects. The toxicity profile is more favorable for attenuated synthetic androgens such as danazol, making long-term use of this drug a reasonable management option in responding patients. A starting dose of 400 mg twice a day is recommended, but a lower dose (100 to 400 mg/day) may be adequate to control chronic hemolysis.[28]

Patients with PNH frequently become iron deficient as a result of both hemoglobinuria and hemosiderinuria.[57,58] Clinically important iron loss from hemosiderinuria can occur (Chap. 43), even in the absence of gross hemoglobinuria. Replacement is often associated with exacerbation of hemolysis, regardless of the route of administration.[57,58] Compared with parenteral replacement, oral administration of iron may be accompanied by less-severe hemolytic exacerbations, but urinary iron loss may be so great that repletion may not be achieved.[57] Concern for inducing a hemolytic exacerbation should not deter iron repletion.[57] If a hemolytic exacerbation occurs in the setting of iron repletion, the episode can be controlled by treatment with glucocorticoids or androgens or by suppression of erythropoiesis by transfusion. There is no concern about iron-replacement therapy inducing a hemolytic exacerbation in patients being treated with eculizumab as hemolysis is inhibited by the drug.

Because the hemolysis is a consequence of a defect intrinsic to patient's erythrocytes, the anemia of PNH responds to red cell transfusion. Concerns about inducing a hemolytic exacerbation as a consequence of infusion of small amounts of donor plasma that may be included in red cell preparations appear unwarranted.[59] However, hemofiltration is recommended to prevent transfusion reaction arising from the interaction between donor leukocytes and recipient antibodies. Iatrogenic hemochromatosis from chronic transfusion may be delayed in patients with PNH as a result of iron loss from hemoglobinuria/hemosiderinuria,[57] but iron overload remains a concern in patients who require chronic transfusion when the anemia is primarily a consequence of marrow failure rather than intravascular hemolysis.

Supplemental folate (1 mg/day) is recommended to compensate for increased use (Chap. 41) associated with heightened erythropoiesis that is a consequence of ongoing hemolysis.[28]

The role of splenectomy in the management of patients with PNH has not been investigated systematically. Reports of amelioration of hemolysis and improvement in cytopenias following splenectomy are anecdotal. Concerns about lack of proven efficacy and the potential for postoperative complications, particularly thrombosis, have led some to argue that splenectomy has no role in the management of PNH.[28]

ALLOGENEIC HEMATOPOIETIC STEM CELL TRANSPLANTATION

Prior to the availability of eculizumab, the primary indications for transplantation were marrow failure, recurrent, life-threatening thrombosis, and uncontrollable hemolysis (Table 40-4).[28] The latter process can be eliminated by treatment with eculizumab and the thrombophilia of PNH may also respond to inhibition of intravascular hemolysis by eculizumab.[54,60] Nonetheless, transplantation is the only curative therapy for PNH, and the availability of molecularly defined, matched, unrelated donors, less-toxic conditioning regimens, reduction in transplantation-related morbidity and mortality, and improvements in posttransplantation supportive care make this option a viable alternative to medical management. Studies (see "Course and Prognosis" below) indicate a normal survival for patients with PNH treated with eculizumab, making the decision of whether to recommend medical management or hematopoietic stem cell transplant particularly complex.[60]

TABLE 40–4. Hematopoietic Stem Cell Transplantation for Paroxysmal Nocturnal Hemoglobinuria

Indications for transplantation
- Marrow failure—approach to management depends primarily on the underlying marrow abnormality (e.g., aplastic anemia) but the treatment regimen must be sufficient to eradicate the paroxysmal nocturnal hemoglobinuria (PNH) clone
- Major complications of PNH
- Refractory, transfusion-dependent hemolytic anemia*
- Recurrent, life-threatening, thromboembolic complications†

Conditioning regimens and donors
- Ablative and reduced intensity conditioning regimens have been successful
- For transplantations involving syngeneic twins, an ablative regimen is recommended‡
- Matched unrelated donor transplantations have been successful but experience is limited

Outcomes
- There are no PNH-specific adverse events. Severe, acute graft-versus-host disease occurs in approximately 33% of patients and the incidence of chronic graft-versus-host disease is roughly 35%
- Overall survival for unselected PNH patients who undergo transplantation using an human leukocyte antigen (HLA)-matched sibling donor is in the range of 50–60%

*Treatment with eculizumab controls the intravascular hemolysis of PNH. Mild to moderate extravascular hemolytic anemia persists in most patients with PNH treated with eculizumab, likely as a consequence of opsonization of erythrocytes by activation and degradation products of complement C3.

†Eculizumab may ameliorate the thrombophilia of PNH.

‡Absence of graft-versus-host effect may render nonablative approaches inadequate.

An understanding of the unique pathobiology of PNH and the input of physicians experienced in transplantation and medical management of PNH are essential to develop an appropriate management plan for transplantation-eligible patients.[61]

For patients who are receiving transplantation for marrow failure, the focus of management is on the etiology of the marrow failure (see Table 40-4). For patients with aplastic anemia and a small PNH clone who undergo matched sibling donor allotransplantation, the conditioning regimen of antithymocyte globulin and cyclophosphamide coupled with graft-versus-host effects appear sufficient to eradicate the PNH clone.[28] However, in the unusual situation in which the patient has a syngeneic twin, a more intense conditioning regimen is required, as graft-versus-PNH effect does not contribute to clonal eradication in this circumstance.[62] In the event that a patient with low-risk MDS with a PNH clone requires allotransplantation, the conditioning regimen (marrow ablative or reduced intensity) in combination with graft-versus-tumor effects usually is sufficient to eradicate the PNH clone.

Transplantation for classic PNH is aimed at eradicating the PNH clone, and both marrow ablative[63-65] and reduced-intensity[66,67] conditioning regimens are effective, although experience with the latter is more limited. Successful outcomes have been reported using matched, unrelated donors, as well as matched, sibling donors.[66,68] There are no PNH-specific adverse events associated with transplantation; severe, acute graft-versus-host disease (GVHD) occurs in more than one-third of the patients and the incidence of chronic GVHD is approximately 35 percent. Overall survival for unselected PNH patients who undergo transplantation using an human leukocyte antigen (HLA)-matched sibling donor is in the range of 50 to 60 percent.[28]

MANAGEMENT OF THE THROMBOPHILIA OF PAROXYSMAL NOCTURNAL HEMOGLOBINURIA

Thromboembolic complications are the leading cause of morbidity and mortality in PNH.[69] Prophylaxis against thromboembolic events in patients with PNH is an issue of active debate.[69] Current estimates of risk are based on retrospective analysis,[54,70–73] but risk appears to correlate with size of the PNH clone (based on flow cytometric determination of the percentage of GPI-AP–deficient PMNs), leading to the recommendation that patients with greater than 50 to 60 percent GPI-AP–deficient PMNs be offered prophylactic anticoagulation.[70,71] Treatment with warfarin with a goal international normalized ratio (INR) of between 2.0 and 3.0 is recommended for patients with PNH who require chronic anticoagulation either for treatment of a thromboembolic event or for prophylaxis. There are no empiric data to guide the use of low-molecular-weight heparin or novel oral anticoagulants in these settings, but their use can be considered in patients with adequate renal function who fail warfarin or in patients have difficulty maintaining a consistent therapeutic INR.

Although arterial thrombosis may be observed,[54] thromboembolic events in patients with PNH usually involve the venous system. Acute thrombotic events require anticoagulation with heparin. Systemic thrombolytic therapy,[74,75] or thrombolytic therapy delivered via canalization directly to the affected site,[76] should be strongly considered in patients with acute onset of Budd-Chiari syndrome.

Thrombocytopenia often complicates PNH, and this issue should be addressed when formulating an anticoagulation management plan. Thrombocytopenia is a relative contraindication to anticoagulation, and transfusions should be given to maintain the platelet count in a safe range rather than withholding therapy.[77] Patients with PNH who experience a thromboembolic event should be anticoagulated indefinitely. Recurrent, life-threatening thrombosis merits consideration of marrow transplantation, but such patients are at high-risk for transplantation-related adverse events (see Table 40–4).[61]

Eculizumab reduces the risk of thromboembolic complications.[54] For patients being treated with eculizumab who have no prior history of thromboembolic complications, prophylactic anticoagulation may not be necessary.

PREGNANCY AND PAROXYSMAL NOCTURNAL HEMOGLOBINURIA

Women with PNH can have serious morbidity and increased mortality during pregnancy.[77,78] Because of concerns about fetal/maternal risks from exposure to potentially toxic therapy, anticoagulation and transfusion have been the mainstay of management. Eculizumab has been assigned to pregnancy category C (risk cannot be ruled out) by the FDA. There are no controlled studies of the use of eculizumab in human pregnancy; however, anecdotal reports and small series have identified no significant adverse effects when eculizumab is used during pregnancy, including early in gestation and, in one case, from the time of conception.[51,79,80] Nonetheless, until more is known about the safety of eculizumab in pregnancy, it seems prudent to restricted use of the drug to the third trimester and then only for patients who are at high-risk for thrombosis and who have no acceptable erytherapeutic alternatives.

Moderate to severe thrombocytopenia may complicate the pregnancy, and clinically significant bleeding in this setting necessitates platelet transfusion. The incidence of clinically apparent venous thromboembolism during pregnancy in women with PNH is approximately 10 percent,[77] and these events are associated with a high risk of mortality.[77,78] Similar to nonpregnant patients with PNH, cerebral and hepatic veins are commonly involved sites of thrombosis. Thrombolytic therapy should be considered for those with Budd-Chiari syndrome.

The role of prophylactic anticoagulation for pregnant women with PNH has not been studied prospectively; however, because of the significant morbidity and mortality associated with thromboembolism in this setting, prophylaxis is recommended. Coumadin is contraindicated because of teratogenic potential in the first trimester and hemorrhagic risks later in gestation (Chap. 8). Anticoagulation with heparin should begin immediately once the pregnancy is documented. Low-molecular-weight heparin has a hypothetical advantage over unfractionated heparin because of a lower incidence of drug-induced thrombocytopenia and less osteopenia (Chap. 118). Careful monitoring of the platelet count is required because thrombocytopenia may worsen during the period of anticoagulation. Anticoagulation can be discontinued briefly around the time of delivery. However, it should be restarted as soon as is feasible and continued for at least 6 weeks into the postpartum period, as thrombosis during the puerperium is a major concern.[77,78] Most deliveries can be accomplished vaginally, although premature delivery may be necessary. Despite the many concerns surrounding PNH and pregnancy, successful outcomes appear to be the rule rather than the exception[72,77]; however, management is complicated and should involve the combined efforts of a knowledgeable hematologist and an obstetrician experienced in dealing with high-risk pregnancies.[27]

PEDIATRIC PAROXYSMAL NOCTURNAL HEMOGLOBINURIA

PNH can occur in the young (approximately 10 percent of patients are younger than age 21 years at the time of diagnosis).[28] A retrospective analysis of 26 cases, underscored the many similarities between childhood and adult PNH.[81] Signs and symptoms of hemolysis, marrow failure, and thrombosis dominate the clinical picture, although gross hemoglobinuria as a presenting symptom may be less common in young patients. A generally good response to immunosuppressive therapy was observed,[81] but based on poor long-term survival, hematopoietic cell transplantation is the recommended treatment for childhood PNH. One study[82] confirmed the common presentation of marrow failure in 11 children with PNH, and reported that five patients eventually underwent hematopoietic cell transplant (three matched unrelated donors and two matched family donors), of whom four were long-term survivors. In another study of 12 young patients over an 18-year period, 10 presented with evidence of marrow failure and only one with hemoglobinuria.[40] There were six children with thrombosis and five with myelodysplastic features, indicating that the clinical presentation may be more similar to adult PNH than previously recognized. The safety and effectiveness of eculizumab in pediatric patients below the age of 18 years has not been established, however, there are anecdotal reports of its use in pediatric patients with PNH.[83] Although eculizumab is not approved for PNH patients younger than age 18 years, approval will likely be sought once pharmacodynamic and pharmacokinetic characteristics of the drug are defined for the pediatric/adolescent population.[84] The availability of eculizumab for pediatric PNH may be particularly advantageous as a bridge prior to implementation of more definitive therapy.

● COURSE AND PROGNOSIS

The clinical course of PNH is enormously variable. In rare instances, the patient may succumb to this disease within a few months of the first onset of symptoms. Most patients experience a chronic course in which the severity of the disease waxes and wanes as the normal cells and the PNH clone alternately appear to gain ascendancy. Rarely, the abnormal clone disappears altogether, and the patient appears to be cured. Transformation to acute leukemia is uncommon (in the range of 1 percent). In some instances, but not in others, leukemic blasts are GPI-AP–deficient.[46]

As with so many other diseases, initial reports on PNH tended to emphasize the more severely affected patients, so the prognosis was generally deemed to be very grave. As physicians developed a higher index of suspicion concerning this disorder, and as simplified methods for diagnosis became available, milder cases were diagnosed with a better long-term outlook. Nonetheless, even today, the disease must be considered a very serious one. The most common lethal event is a thrombotic episode such as the Budd-Chiari syndrome,[69,73,85] but the various complications of pancytopenia also may lead to death,[29,43] and in a few patients, the terminal process is development of acute leukemia.[46] In a study of 220 patients with PNH followed for up to 46 years in the preeculizumab era, the Kaplan-Meier survival estimate was 65 percent at 10 years and 48 percent at 15 years after diagnosis.[85] In another preeculizumab era study of 80 consecutive patients the outlook was similar: the median survival after diagnosis was 10 years, with 28 percent of patients surviving for 25 years.[43] Eight-year cumulative incidence rates of the main complications of pancytopenia, thrombosis, and MDS were 15 percent, 28 percent, and 5 percent, respectively. Poor survival was associated with age older than 55 years at the time of diagnosis, the occurrence of thrombosis as a complication, evolution to pancytopenia, MDS or acute leukemia, and thrombocytopenia at diagnosis. The prognosis of patients in whom aplastic anemia antedated PNH was better than in those in whom it did not.[85]

In addition to symptomatic benefit, treatment with eculizumab appears to influence the natural history of PNH. In a retrospective study of the clinical history of 79 patients with classic PNH or PNH/marrow failure treated with eculizumab, the median age at diagnosis was 37 years (range: 12 to 79 years) and the median age at the time of initiation of treatment with eculizumab was 46 years (range: 14 to 84 years).[60] The mean duration of treatment with eculizumab was 39 months (range: 1 to 98 months). Based on flow cytometric analysis of blood neutrophils, the average clone size among the treated patients was 96.4 percent (range: 41.8 to 100 percent). Twenty-four patients (30 percent) had a history of a marrow failure syndrome at the time of diagnosis (23 with aplastic anemia and one with MDS). Thrombotic episodes were reported in 27 percent of patients prior to starting eculizumab (including 12 cases of Budd-Chiari syndrome, four cases of mesenteric vein thrombosis, three cases of cerebral vein thrombosis). The investigators found that treatment with eculizumab reduced the mean yearly transfusion requirement from 19.3 units to 5.0 units. Of 61 patients who had been on eculizumab for more than 1 year, 40 (66 percent) became transfusion-independent. Thrombosis was observed in two patients while on eculizumab. No thrombotic events were reported in 21 patients who discontinue prophylactic anticoagulation after starting treatment with eculizumab.

Survival of the 79 patients treated with eculizumab was the same as that of a group of age- and sex-matched controls from the general population. Two eculizumab patients developed documented meningococcal infection with *Neisseria meningitidis* serogroup B, and thereafter, a program of antibiotic prophylaxis was instituted by the investigators.

A multicenter study involving 195 patients followed for 66 months largely confirmed these findings.[86]

Together, these results demonstrate that treatment with eculizumab alters the natural history of PNH both by reducing or eliminating transfusion requirements through inhibition of intravascular hemolysis and by virtually eradicating thromboembolic complications. Eculizumab treatment may also reduce disease related mortality although the extent to which the drug enhances survival cannot be accurately determined from these studies as the experimental design did not include a randomized control group of patients. Eculizumab does not appear to affect either the marrow failure component of the disease or the clonal hematopoiesis that underlies disease pathophysiology. Although PNH is a clonal disease, it is not a malignant disease, as previously discussed, and it is this characteristic of PNH that allows for successful long-term symptomatic management in the absence of a treatment strategy aimed at eradicating the *PIGA* mutant hematopoietic stem cells.

REFERENCES

1. Crosby WH: Paroxysmal nocturnal hemoglobinuria; a classic description by Paul Strubling in 1882, and a bibliography of the disease. *Blood* 6:270, 1951.
2. Parker CJ: Historical aspects of paroxysmal nocturnal haemoglobinuria: "defining the disease." *Br J Haematol* 117:3, 2002.
3. Parker CJ: Paroxysmal nocturnal hemoglobinuria: An historical overview. *Hematology Am Soc Hematol Educ Program* 2008:93, 2008.
4. Rosse W: A brief history of PNH, in *PNH and the GPI-Linked Proteins*, edited by NS Young, J Moss, p 1. Academic Press, San Diego, 2000.
5. Hughes DA, Tunnage B, Yeo ST: Drugs for exceptionally rare diseases: Do they deserve special status for funding? *QJM* 98:829, 2005.
6. Parker CJ: Hemolysis in PNH, in *PNH and the GPI-Linked Proteins*, edited by NS Young, J Moss, p 49. Academic Press, San Diego, 2000.
7. Thurman JM, Holers VM: The central role of the alternative complement pathway in human disease. *J Immunol* 176:1305, 2006.
8. Nicholson-Weller A, Burge J, Fearon DT, et al: Isolation of a human erythrocyte membrane glycoprotein with decay-accelerating activity for C3 convertases of the complement system. *J Immunol* 129:184, 1982.
9. Nicholson-Weller A, March JP, Rosenfeld SI, Austen KF: Affected erythrocytes of patients with paroxysmal nocturnal hemoglobinuria are deficient in the complement regulatory protein, decay accelerating factor. *Proc Natl Acad Sci U S A* 80:5066, 1983.
10. Pangburn MK, Schreiber RD, Muller-Eberhard HJ: Deficiency of an erythrocyte membrane protein with complement regulatory activity in paroxysmal nocturnal hemoglobinuria. *Proc Natl Acad Sci U S A* 80:5430, 1983.
11. Holguin MH, Fredrick LR, Bernshaw NJ, et al: Isolation and characterization of a membrane protein from normal human erythrocytes that inhibits reactive lysis of the erythrocytes of paroxysmal nocturnal hemoglobinuria. *J Clin Invest* 84:7, 1989.
12. Kinoshita T, Inoue N, Takeda J: Defective glycosyl phosphatidylinositol anchor synthesis and paroxysmal nocturnal hemoglobinuria. *Adv Immunol* 60:57, 1995.
13. Miyata T, Takeda J, Iida Y, et al: The cloning of PIG-A, a component in the early step of GPI-anchor biosynthesis. *Science* 259:1318, 1993.
14. Miyata T, Yamada N, Iida Y, et al: Abnormalities of PIG-A transcripts in granulocytes from patients with paroxysmal nocturnal hemoglobinuria. *N Engl J Med* 330:249, 1994.
15. Takahashi M, Takeda J, Hirose S, et al: Deficient biosynthesis of N-acetylglucosaminyl-phosphatidylinositol, the first intermediate of glycosyl phosphatidylinositol anchor biosynthesis, in cell lines established from patients with paroxysmal nocturnal hemoglobinuria. *J Exp Med* 177:517, 1993.
16. Takeda J, Miyata T, Kawagoe K, et al: Deficiency of the GPI anchor caused by a somatic mutation of the PIG-A gene in paroxysmal nocturnal hemoglobinuria. *Cell* 73:703, 1993.
17. Parker CJ: The pathophysiology of paroxysmal nocturnal hemoglobinuria. *Exp Hematol* 35:523, 2007.
18. Krawitz PM, Hochsmann B, Murakami Y, et al: A case of paroxysmal nocturnal hemoglobinuria caused by a germline mutation and a somatic mutation in PIGT. *Blood* 122:1312, 2013.
19. Rosti V, Tremml G, Soares V, et al: Murine embryonic stem cells without pig-a gene activity are competent for hematopoiesis with the PNH phenotype but not for clonal expansion. *J Clin Invest* 100:1028, 1997.
20. Brodsky RA, Vala MS, Barber JP, Medof ME, Jones RJ: Resistance to apoptosis caused by PIG-A gene mutations in paroxysmal nocturnal hemoglobinuria. *Proc Natl Acad Sci U S A* 94:8756, 1997.
21. Chen R, Nagarajan S, Prince GM, et al: Impaired growth and elevated fas receptor expression in PIGA(+) stem cells in primary paroxysmal nocturnal hemoglobinuria. *J Clin Invest* 106:689, 2000.
22. Heeney MM, Ormsbee SM, Moody MA, et al: Increased expression of anti-apoptosis genes in peripheral blood cells from patients with paroxysmal nocturnal hemoglobinuria. *Mol Genet Metab* 78:291, 2003.
23. Horikawa K, Nakakuma H, Kawaguchi T, et al: Apoptosis resistance of blood cells from patients with paroxysmal nocturnal hemoglobinuria, aplastic anemia, and myelodysplastic syndrome. *Blood* 90:2716, 1997.
24. Ware RE, Nishimura J, Moody MA, et al: The PIG-A mutation and absence of glycosyl-phosphatidylinositol-linked proteins do not confer resistance to apoptosis in paroxysmal nocturnal hemoglobinuria. *Blood* 92:2541, 1998.
25. Yamamoto T, Shichishima T, Shikama Y, et al: Granulocytes from patients with paroxysmal nocturnal hemoglobinuria and normal individuals have the same sensitivity to spontaneous apoptosis. *Exp Hematol* 30:187, 2002.

26. Inoue N, Izui-Sarumaru T, Murakami Y, et al: Molecular basis of clonal expansion of hematopoiesis in 2 patients with paroxysmal nocturnal hemoglobinuria (PNH). *Blood* 108:4232, 2006.
27. Endo M, Ware RE, Vreeke TM, et al: Molecular basis of the heterogeneity of expression of glycosyl phosphatidylinositol anchored proteins in paroxysmal nocturnal hemoglobinuria. *Blood* 87:2546, 1996.
28. Parker C, Omine M, Richards S, et al: Diagnosis and management of paroxysmal nocturnal hemoglobinuria. *Blood* 106:3699, 2005.
29. Dacie JV, Lewis SM: Paroxysmal nocturnal haemoglobinuria: Clinical manifestations, haematology, and nature of the disease. *Ser Haematol* 5:3, 1972.
30. Ishiyama K, Chuhjo T, Wang H, et al: Polyclonal hematopoiesis maintained in patients with bone marrow failure harboring a minor population of paroxysmal nocturnal hemoglobinuria-type cells. *Blood* 102:1211, 2003.
31. Sugimori C, Chuhjo T, Feng X, et al: Minor population of CD55-CD59- blood cells predicts response to immunosuppressive therapy and prognosis in patients with aplastic anemia. *Blood* 107:1308, 2006.
32. Timeus F, Crescenzio N, Longoni D, et al: Paroxysmal nocturnal hemoglobinuria clones in children with acquired aplastic anemia: A multicentre study. *PLoS One* 9:e101948, 2014.
33. Wang H, Chuhjo T, Yasue S, et al: Clinical significance of a minor population of paroxysmal nocturnal hemoglobinuria-type cells in bone marrow failure syndrome. *Blood* 100:3897, 2002.
34. Borowitz MJ, Craig FE, Digiuseppe JA, et al: Guidelines for the diagnosis and monitoring of paroxysmal nocturnal hemoglobinuria and related disorders by flow cytometry. *Cytometry B Clin Cytom* 78:211, 2010.
35. Richards SJ, Rawstron AC, Hillmen P: Application of flow cytometry to the diagnosis of paroxysmal nocturnal hemoglobinuria. *Cytometry* 42:223, 2000.
36. Chen G, Kirby M, Zeng W, et al: Superior growth of glycophosphatidy linositol-anchored protein-deficient progenitor cells in vitro is due to the higher apoptotic rate of progenitors with normal phenotype in vivo. *Exp Hematol* 30:774, 2002.
37. Dunn DE, Liu JM, Young NS: Bone marrow failure in PNH, in *PNH and the GPI-Linked Proteins*, edited by NS Young, J Moss p 113. Academic Press, San Diego, 2000.
38. Sugimori C, Mochizuki K, Qi Z, et al: Origin and fate of blood cells deficient in glycosylphosphatidyl-anchored protein among patients with bone marrow failure. *Br J Haematol* 147:102, 2009.
39. Wang SA, Pozdnyakova O, Jorgensen JL, et al: Detection of paroxysmal nocturnal hemoglobinuria clones in patients with myelodysplastic syndromes and related bone marrow diseases, with emphasis on diagnostic pitfalls and caveats. *Haematologica* 94:29, 2009.
40. Curran KJ, Kernan NA, Prockop SE, et al: Paroxysmal nocturnal hemoglobinuria in pediatric patients. *Pediatr Blood Cancer* 59:525, 2012.
41. Scheinberg P, Marte M, Nunez O, Young NS: Paroxysmal nocturnal hemoglobinuria clones in severe aplastic anemia patients treated with horse anti-thymocyte globulin plus cyclosporine. *Haematologica* 95:1075, 2010.
42. de Latour RP, Mary JY, Salanoubat C, et al: Paroxysmal nocturnal hemoglobinuria: Natural history of disease subcategories. *Blood* 112:3099, 2008.
43. Hillmen P, Lewis SM, Bessler M, et al: Natural history of paroxysmal nocturnal hemoglobinuria. *N Engl J Med* 333:1253, 1995.
44. Kulagin A, Lisukov I, Ivanova M, et al: Prognostic value of paroxysmal nocturnal haemoglobinuria clone presence in aplastic anaemia patients treated with combined immunosuppression: Results of two-centre prospective study. *Br J Haematol* 164:546, 2014.
45. Dunn DE, Tanawattanacharoen P, Boccuni P, et al: Paroxysmal nocturnal hemoglobinuria cells in patients with bone marrow failure syndromes. *Ann Intern Med* 131:401, 1999.
46. Harris JW, Koscick R, Lazarus HM, et al: Leukemia arising out of paroxysmal nocturnal hemoglobinuria. *Leuk Lymphoma* 32:401, 1999.
47. Saunthararajah Y, Nakamura R, Nam JM, et al: HLA-DR15 (DR2) is overrepresented in myelodysplastic syndrome and aplastic anemia and predicts a response to immunosuppression in myelodysplastic syndrome. *Blood* 100:1570, 2002.
48. Sugimori C, Yamazaki H, Feng X, et al: Roles of DRB1 *1501 and DRB1 *1502 in the pathogenesis of aplastic anemia. *Exp Hematol* 35:13, 2007.
49. Parker C: Eculizumab for paroxysmal nocturnal haemoglobinuria. *Lancet* 373:759, 2009.
50. Hillmen P, Young NS, Schubert J, et al: The complement inhibitor eculizumab in paroxysmal nocturnal hemoglobinuria. *N Engl J Med* 355:1233, 2006.
51. Marasca R, Coluccio V, Santachiara R, et al: Pregnancy in PNH: Another eculizumab baby. *Br J Haematol* 150:707, 2010.
52. Parker CJ: Thanks for the complement (inhibitor). *Blood* 118:4503, 2011.
53. Risitano AM, Marando L, Seneca E, Rotoli B: Hemoglobin normalization after splenectomy in a paroxysmal nocturnal hemoglobinuria patient treated by eculizumab. *Blood* 112:449, 2008.
54. Hillmen P, Muus P, Duhrsen U, et al: Effect of the complement inhibitor eculizumab on thromboembolism in patients with paroxysmal nocturnal hemoglobinuria. *Blood* 110:4123, 2007.
55. Hillmen P, Hall C, Marsh JC, et al: Effect of eculizumab on hemolysis and transfusion requirements in patients with paroxysmal nocturnal hemoglobinuria. *N Engl J Med* 350:552, 2004.
56. Ferreira VP, Pangburn MK: Factor H mediated cell surface protection from complement is critical for the survival of PNH erythrocytes. *Blood* 110:2190, 2007.
57. Rosse WF: Treatment of paroxysmal nocturnal hemoglobinuria. *Blood* 60:20, 1982.
58. Hartmann RC, Jenkins DE Jr, McKee LC, Heyssel RM: Paroxysmal nocturnal hemoglobinuria: Clinical and laboratory studies relating to iron metabolism and therapy with androgen and iron. *Medicine (Baltimore)* 45:331, 1966.
59. Brecher ME, Taswell HF: Paroxysmal nocturnal hemoglobinuria and the transfusion of washed red cells: A myth revisited. *Transfusion* 29:681, 1989.
60. Kelly RJ, Hill A, Arnold LM, et al: Long-term treatment with eculizumab in paroxysmal nocturnal hemoglobinuria: Sustained efficacy and improved survival. *Blood* 117:6786, 2011.
61. Peffault de Latour R, Schrezenmeier H, Bacigalupo A, et al: Allogeneic stem cell transplantation in paroxysmal nocturnal hemoglobinuria. *Haematologica* 97:1666, 2012.
62. Endo M, Beatty PG, Vreeke TM, et al: Syngeneic bone marrow transplantation without conditioning in a patient with paroxysmal nocturnal hemoglobinuria: In vivo evidence that the mutant stem cells have a survival advantage. *Blood* 88:742, 1996.
63. Bemba M, Guardiola P, Garderet L, et al: Bone marrow transplantation for paroxysmal nocturnal haemoglobinuria. *Br J Haematol* 105:366, 1999.
64. Hegenbart U, Niederwieser D, Forman S, et al: Hematopoietic cell transplantation from related and unrelated donors after minimal conditioning as a curative treatment modality for severe paroxysmal nocturnal hemoglobinuria. *Biol Blood Marrow Transplant* 9:689, 2003.
65. Raiola AM, Van Lint MT, Lamparelli T, et al: Bone marrow transplantation for paroxysmal nocturnal hemoglobinuria. *Haematologica* 85:59, 2000.
66. Saso R, Marsh J, Cevreska L, et al: Bone marrow transplants for paroxysmal nocturnal haemoglobinuria. *Br J Haematol* 104:392, 1999.
67. Takahashi Y, McCoy JP Jr, Carvallo C, et al: In vitro and in vivo evidence of PNH cell sensitivity to immune attack after nonmyeloablative allogeneic hematopoietic cell transplantation. *Blood* 103:1383, 2004.
68. Woodard P, Wang W, Pitts N, et al: Successful unrelated donor bone marrow transplantation for paroxysmal nocturnal hemoglobinuria. *Bone Marrow Transplant* 27:589, 2001.
69. Hill A, Kelly RJ, Hillmen P: Thrombosis in paroxysmal nocturnal hemoglobinuria. *Blood* 121:4985, 2013.
70. Hall C, Richards S, Hillmen P: Primary prophylaxis with warfarin prevents thrombosis in paroxysmal nocturnal hemoglobinuria (PNH). *Blood* 102:3587, 2003.
71. Moyo VM, Mukina GL, Barrett ES, Brodsky RA: Natural history of paroxysmal nocturnal haemoglobinuria using modern diagnostic assays. *Br J Haematol* 126:133, 2004.
72. Nishimura JI, Kanakura Y, Ware RE, et al: Clinical course and flow cytometric analysis of paroxysmal nocturnal hemoglobinuria in the United States and Japan. *Medicine (Baltimore)* 83:193, 2004.
73. Sloand EM, Young NS: Thrombotic complications in PNH, in *PNH and the GPI-Linked Proteins*, edited by NS Young, J Moss, p 101. Academic Press, San Diego, 2000.
74. Griffith JF, Mahmoud AE, Cooper S, et al: Radiological intervention in Budd-Chiari syndrome: Techniques and outcome in 18 patients. *Clin Radiol* 51:775, 1996.
75. McMullin MF, Hillmen P, Jackson J, et al: Tissue plasminogen activator for hepatic vein thrombosis in paroxysmal nocturnal haemoglobinuria. *J Intern Med* 235:85, 1994.
76. Sholar PW, Bell WR: Thrombolytic therapy for inferior vena cava thrombosis in paroxysmal nocturnal hemoglobinuria. *Ann Intern Med* 103:539, 1985.
77. Ray JG, Burows RF, Ginsberg JS, Burrows EA: Paroxysmal nocturnal hemoglobinuria and the risk of venous thrombosis: Review and recommendations for management of the pregnant and nonpregnant patient. *Haemostasis* 30:103, 2000.
78. Tichelli A, Socie G, Marsh J, et al: Outcome of pregnancy and disease course among women with aplastic anemia treated with immunosuppression. *Ann Intern Med* 137:164, 2002.
79. Danilov AV, Brodsky RA, Craigo S, et al: Managing a pregnant patient with paroxysmal nocturnal hemoglobinuria in the era of eculizumab. *Leuk Res* 34:566, 2010.
80. Kelly R, Arnold L, Richards S, et al: The management of pregnancy in paroxysmal nocturnal haemoglobinuria on long term eculizumab. *Br J Haematol* 149:446, 2010.
81. Ware RE, Hall SE, Rosse WF: Paroxysmal nocturnal hemoglobinuria with onset in childhood and adolescence. *N Engl J Med* 325:991, 1991.
82. van den Heuvel-Eibrink MM, Bredius RG, te Winkel ML, et al: Childhood paroxysmal nocturnal haemoglobinuria (PNH), a report of 11 cases in the Netherlands. *Br J Haematol* 128:571, 2005.
83. Bauters T, Bordon V, Robays H, et al: Successful use of eculizumab in a pediatric patient treated for paroxysmal nocturnal hemoglobinuria. *J Pediatr Hematol Oncol* 34:e346, 2012.
84. Reiss UM, Schwartz J, Sakamoto KM, et al: Efficacy and safety of eculizumab in children and adolescents with paroxysmal nocturnal hemoglobinuria. *Pediatr Blood Cancer* 2014.
85. Socie G, Mary JY, de Gramont A, et al: Paroxysmal nocturnal haemoglobinuria: Long-term follow-up and prognostic factors. French Society of Haematology. *Lancet* 348:573, 1996.
86. Hillmen P, Muus P, Roth A, et al: Long-term safety and efficacy of sustained eculizumab treatment in patients with paroxysmal nocturnal haemoglobinuria. *Br J Haematol* 162:62, 2013.

CHAPTER 41
FOLATE, COBALAMIN, AND MEGALOBLASTIC ANEMIAS

Ralph Green

SUMMARY

Deficiency of either folate or cobalamin (vitamin B_{12}) leads to macrocytic anemia with or without other cytopenias as a result of megaloblastic hematopoiesis, a manifestation of defective DNA synthesis. Folate in its tetrahydro form is a transporter of one-carbon fragments, which it can carry at any of three oxidation levels: methanol, formaldehyde, or formic acid. The oxidation levels of the folate-bound one-carbon fragments can be altered by oxidation and reduction reactions that require nicotinamide adenine dinucleotide phosphate in its oxidized (NADP) or reduced (NADPH) form. The primary source of the folate-bound one-carbon fragments is serine, which is converted to glycine as its terminal carbon is transferred to folate. The one-carbon fragments are used for biosynthesis of purines, thymidine, and methionine. During biosynthesis of purines and methionine, free folate is released in its tetrahydro form. During biosynthesis of thymidine, tetrahydrofolate is oxidized to the dihydro form and must again be fully reduced by dihydrofolate reductase to continue functioning in one-carbon metabolism. Methotrexate acts as an anticancer agent because it is an exceedingly powerful inhibitor of dihydrofolate reductase, thereby interdicting the generation of reduced folate.

In the cell, folates are conjugated by the addition of a chain of seven or eight glutamic acid residues. These residues enable the retention of folates in the cell. When folates are absorbed from the intestine, a process that occurs chiefly in the duodenum and proximal jejunum, all but one of the glutamates is removed by the enzyme glutamate carboxypeptidase II (folate hydrolase). Resulting monoglutamate forms are then taken up by one of two folate-specific transporters located on the apical brush border small bowel epithelium, the reduced folate carrier or the proton-coupled folate transporter. Blood folates are taken up by cells, mainly in the form of methyltetrahydrofolate monoglutamate. The newly absorbed folates are rapidly reglutamylated in the cell by the enzyme folyl-polyglutamyl synthase (FPGS). If glutamylation is prevented, the folates cannot be retained in the cell, resulting in an intracellular folate deficiency.

Cobalamin is required for two reactions: intramitochondrial conversion of methylmalonyl coenzyme A (CoA), a product of catabolism of branched-chain amino acids, and ketogenic amino acids to succinyl CoA, a Krebs cycle intermediate and cytosolic conversion of homocysteine to methionine, a reaction in which the methyl group of methyltetrahydrofolate is donated to the sulfur atom of homocysteine. In cobalamin deficiency, methyltetrahydrofolate accumulates because, for practical purposes, donation of the methyl group to homocysteine is the only method of generating free tetrahydrofolate from methyltetrahydrofolate. Free tetrahydrofolate is an excellent substrate for FPGS; methyltetrahydrofolate is a poor substrate. Consequently, much of the methyltetrahydrofolate taken up by a cobalamin-deficient cell leaks out of the cell before it can be polyglutamylated. The megaloblastic anemia of cobalamin deficiency results from an intracellular folate deficiency that arises because of the cell's limited ability to polyglutamylate methyltetrahydrofolate.

Absorption of cobalamin is a highly complex process. Upon arriving in the stomach, cobalamin is taken up by haptocorrin (HC) binder (also called *R binder* or *cobalophilin*), a glycoprotein found in virtually all secretions. When the cobalamin HC complex enters the duodenum, the HC is digested and the cobalamin is released into the intestinal lumen, where it is taken up by intrinsic factor, a glycoprotein secreted by the gastric parietal cells. The cobalamin-intrinsic factor complex is absorbed by cells in the ileum through receptor-mediated endocytosis, involving cubilin and other proteins. The cobalamin is released within lysosomes and transported to the blood where it circulates bound to transcobalamin (TC), which delivers its cargo of cobalamin to cells throughout the body. Folate (vitamin B_9) and cobalamin (vitamin B_{12}) play key roles in the metabolic machinery of proliferating cells.

Megaloblastic anemia most commonly results from folate or cobalamin (vitamin B_{12}) deficiency. Folate deficiency often was nutritional in origin. It may be seen in alcoholics, the elderly, the poor, but also is seen in patients on hyperalimentation, with hemolytic anemia, or hemodialysis. In the many countries that now practice folic acid fortification of the diet, such as the United States and Canada, the prevalence of folate deficiency has been dramatically reduced and nutritional folate deficiency has been virtually eliminated. In pregnancy, even a mild folate deficiency may be associated with defects in neural tube closure in the fetus, so pregnant women should always receive folate supplements. The incidence of neural tube defects has fallen considerably in North America since the introduction of folic acid fortification. Diagnosis of folate deficiency is based on measurements of folate in serum, which furnishes information about the current level of folate, and in red cells, which provide data on aggregate folate status over the preceding period during which those red cells were produced. Nutritional folate deficiency is treated with folic acid by mouth.

Folate deficiency as a result of malabsorption occurs in tropical and nontropical sprue. Folate deficiency as a result of tropical sprue is treated with folate supplements and antibiotics. In nontropical sprue, the treatment is folate plus a gluten-free diet.

The most common cause of clinically apparent cobalamin deficiency is pernicious anemia (PA), a condition in which the portion of gastric mucosa that contains the parietal cells is destroyed through an autoimmune mechanism. The parietal cells secrete intrinsic factor, which is essential for physiologic cobalamin absorption. Without intrinsic factor, a state of cobalamin deficiency develops over the course of years. Cobalamin deficiency leads not only to megaloblastic anemia but also to a demyelinating disease that manifests itself

Acronyms and Abbreviations: AdoCbl, adenosylcobalamin; AICAR, 5-amino-4-imidazole carboxamide ribotide; ATPase, adenosine triphosphatase; AZT, azidothymidine; CnCbl, cyanocobalamin; CoA, coenzyme A; CUB, cubilin; CUBAM, the binary ileal cubilin receptor complex consisting of cubilin and amnionless; dTMP, deoxythymidine monophosphate; dU, deoxyuridine; dUMP, deoxyuridine monophosphate; FH_4, tetrahydrofolate; FPGS, folylpoly-γ-glutamyl synthase; [^{3}H]Thd, [^{3}H]thymidine; HC, haptocorrin; HCl, hydrochloric acid; IM, intramuscular; LDH, lactate dehydrogenase; MCV, mean corpuscular volume; MeCbl, methylcobalamin; MRI, magnetic resonance imaging; MTHFR, methylenetetrahydrofolate reductase; NADP, nicotinamide adenine dinucleotide phosphate; NADPH, nicotinamide adenine dinucleotide phosphate (reduced form); N_2O, nitrous oxide; OHCbl, hydroxocobalamin; PA, pernicious anemia; PteGlu, pteroylglutamic acid (folic acid); SAH, *S*-adenosylhomocysteine; SAMe, *S*-adenosylmethionine; TC, transcobalamin.

as peripheral neuropathy, spastic paralysis with ataxia (so-called combined system disease of the spinal cord), dementia, psychosis, or some combination of these features. "Subtle" cobalamin deficiency, which may manifest as neurologic symptoms without anemia, appears to be relatively widespread among the elderly. The incidence of gastric cancer is increased by a factor of two to three in patients with PA. Other causes of cobalamin deficiency are gastric resection; stasis of the small intestinal contents as a result of blind loops, strictures, or hypomotility; and disease or resection of the terminal ileum, the site of vitamin B_{12}–intrinsic factor complex absorption. Individuals on a vegan diet can become cobalamin deficient. Cobalamin deficiency is diagnosed by measuring the level of either total or TC-bound vitamin in the blood or by measuring serum methylmalonic acid, which accumulates in the bloodstream in patients with cobalamin deficiency. The cause of cobalamin deficiency was determined by the Schilling test, a measure of cobalamin absorption, but the test is obsolete and no replacement is currently available. In patients with nutritional megaloblastic anemia, folate or cobalamin deficiency as the cause of the anemia must be determined. If a patient with cobalamin deficiency is treated with folic acid, the anemia may be corrected but the neurologic abnormalities persist, progress or may be aggravated. Patients with cobalamin deficiency usually are treated with parenteral cobalamin but large doses of oral cobalamin may be used.

Megaloblastic anemia can develop as an acute disorder with rapid development of leukopenia and/or thrombocytopenia. Nitrous oxide anesthesia or abuse is responsible for some cases of acute megaloblastic anemia. The anemia is rarely also seen in patients with a marginal folate status in intensive care units or severe hemolytic anemia through increased folate demand for augmented erythropoiesis. The condition resembles an immune cytopenia but can be ruled out by examining the marrow, which exhibits a floridly megaloblastic picture.

Other causes of megaloblastic anemia include drugs (e.g., hydroxyurea, nucleoside analogues) and certain inborn errors of metabolism. Of the inherited conditions, TC deficiency is singled out because it causes a severe megaloblastic anemia in infants who respond completely to high-dose cobalamin. Irreversible neurologic complications supervene if the deficiency is not detected in time. Megaloblastic-like morphologic features of varying degree are seen in the myelodysplastic syndromes, and in acute leukemia of the erythroleukemia type. Megaloblastic anemia seen in association with refractory anemia with excess sideroblasts occasionally responds to very high doses of pyridoxine.

●FOLATE

Folate and cobalamin (vitamin B_{12}) play key roles in the metabolism of all cells, particularly proliferating cells.

CHEMISTRY

The group of compounds referred to as folates consists of folic acid and its various derivatives. *Folic acid* (pteroylglutamic acid) is composed of a pteridine moiety, a *p*-aminobenzoate residue, and an L-glutamic acid residue (Fig. 41–1A). The first two together are called *pteroic acid*.[1] In nature, folates occur largely as conjugates in which multiple glutamic acids are linked by peptide bonds involving their γ-carboxyl groups (Fig. 41–1B). Additionally, the naturally occurring polyglutamated folates are reduced in the 5, 6, 7, and 8 positions of the pteridine ring (as described below, Fig. 41–1B). Conjugates are named according to the length of the glutamate chain (e.g., pteroylmonoglutamate,

pteroyldiglutamate, pteroylhexaglutamate). Therapeutic folic acid (pteroylglutamic acid, abbreviated PteGlu, or F) has one glutamic acid and the pteridine ring is not reduced.

To form a functional compound, folate must be reduced to tetrahydrofolate (FH_4; see Fig. 41–1B). In this reduction, dihydrofolate (FH_2) is an intermediate. A single enzyme, FH_2 *reductase*, catalyzes both F→FH_2 and FH_2→FH_4.

The folate family consists largely of FH_4 derivatives bearing a one-carbon substituent (symbolized as FH_4-C). The varieties of FH_4-C differ with regard to the identity of the one-carbon unit and the site of its attachment to FH_4. Figure 41–2 shows one-carbon substituents of biochemical significance and their major interconversions.

These substituents are attached to FH_4 through N^5,N^{10}, or both (see Fig. 41–2). Specific enzymes interconvert these various FH_4 derivatives through oxidations that require nicotinamide adenine dinucleotide phosphate (NADP) and reductions that utilize the reduced form of NADP, NADPH.[2]

Reduced derivatives of folic acid usually are sensitive to air oxidation. An important exception is N^5-formyl FH_4, also called *citrovorum factor*, *leucovorin*, or *folinic acid*, which, because of its stability, is the form preferred for clinical use.

NUTRITION

Sources

Folic acid comes from many sources. The richest vegetable sources are asparagus, broccoli, endive, spinach, lettuce, and lima beans. Each vegetable contains more than 1 mg of folate per 100 g dry weight. The best fruit sources are oranges, lemons, bananas, strawberries, and melons. Folates also are abundant in liver, kidney, yeast, mushrooms, and peanuts. Since the advent of folic acid fortification of the food supply, the median daily intake of folate from an average American diet is estimated to be 350 mcg.[3] Foods are readily depleted of folate by excessive cooking, especially with large amounts of water, discarded before ingestion.

Daily Requirements

In the normal adult, the minimum daily requirement for folic acid is approximately 50 mcg. The average diet contains many times this amount, but some of the folate may be unavailable. Accordingly, the officially recommended dietary allowance of *food* folate for an adult is 0.4 mg.[3] This figure is derived through considerations of the nutrient requirements to satisfy the needs of 97 to 98 percent of healthy individuals and the relative differences in absorption and bioavailability between dietary folate and the more bioavailable synthetic folic acid. One microgram of food folate is the dietary equivalent of 0.6 mcg folic acid added to food. The body is thought to contain approximately 5 mg of folate.[4] When folate intake is reduced to 5 mcg/day, megaloblastic anemia develops in approximately 4 months.[5]

Folic acid requirements increase in hemolytic anemia, leukemia, and other malignant diseases, in alcoholism[6] and during growth; in pregnancy and during lactation requirements increase threefold to sixfold.[7] Adequate folate supplies are particularly important in pregnant and lactating women, in whom the recommended daily allowance is increased to 600 and 500 mcg/day, respectively, to meet requirements.[8]

METABOLISM

Folate-Dependent Enzymes

FH_4 is an intermediate in reactions involving the transfer of one-carbon units from a donor to an acceptor. Table 41–1 summarizes the metabolic systems of animal tissues known to require folic acid coenzymes.

One-carbon units enter the folate pool principally via the serine hydroxymethyltransferase (SHMT) reaction which requires pyridoxal

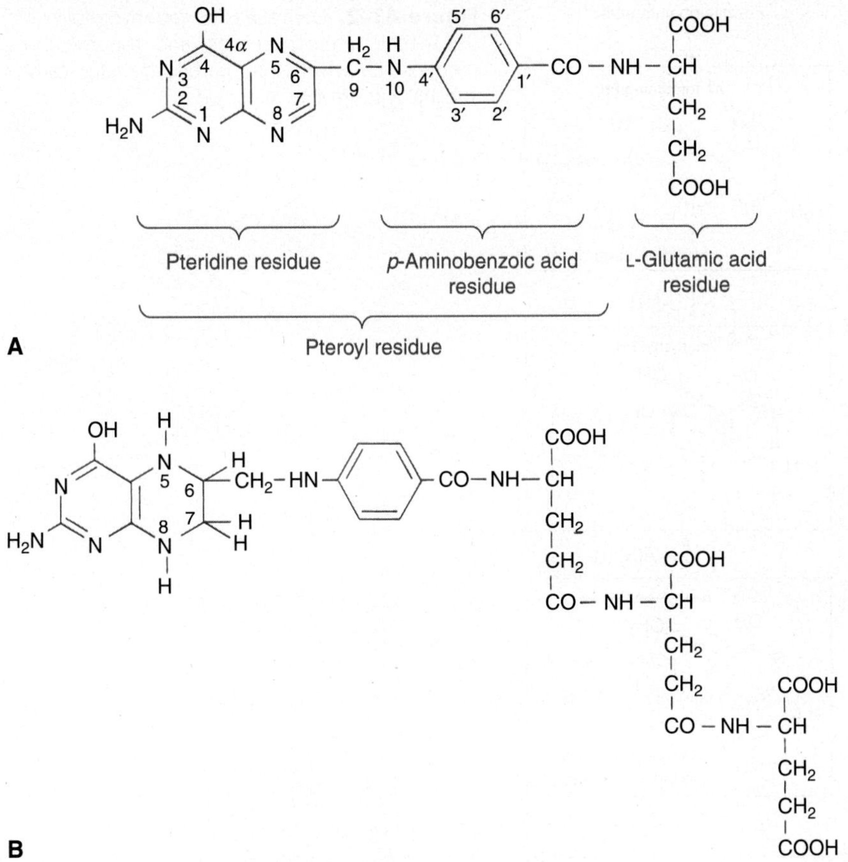

Figure 41-1. Folic acid. **A.** Folic acid (pteroylglutamic acid) and its components. **B.** Tetrahydrofolate triglutamate.

phosphate as a cofactor.[9] There are both cytoplasmic (SHMT1) and mitochondrial (SHMT2) isoforms of SHMT which impart a state of functional redundancy for this important enzyme, which is the primary source of one-carbon units for purine and pyrimidine biosynthesis. The cytoplasmic form can undergo sumoylation during S-phase, allowing nuclear localization.[10]

$$\text{Serine} + FH_4 \rightarrow \text{glycine} + N^5,N^{10}\text{-methylene } FH^4 + H_2O$$

Among the several one-carbon transfers mediated by folic acid, the transfer that appears to be the most important clinically is the methylation of deoxyuridylate to thymidylate, catalyzed by the enzyme thymidylate synthase.[2,10,11] This reaction is an essential step in the synthesis of DNA (Fig. 41-3). In carrying out this reaction, N^5,N^{10}-methylene FH_4 simultaneously transfers and reduces a one-carbon group, itself serving as the hydrogen donor for the reduction.[12] The reaction generates FH_2, which must be reduced again to FH_4 by FH_2 reductase and NADPH before it can again be utilized as a coenzyme:

$$dUMP + N^5,N^{10}\text{-methylene } FH_4 \rightarrow$$
$$FH_2 + dTMP \ FH_2 + NADPH + H^+ \rightarrow FH_4 + NADP^+$$

where dUMP = deoxyuridine monophosphate; dTMP = deoxythymidine monophosphate; and NADP = nicotinamide adenine dinucleotide phosphate. Limitation of thymidylate synthesis in folic acid deficiency causes incorporation of uracil instead of thymine into DNA.[13]

A key enzyme, methylenetetrahydrofolate reductase (MTHFR) regulates the distribution of reduced folates by controlling the rate of NADPH-mediated conversion of N^5,N^{10}-methylene FH_4 to N-methyltetrahydrofolate. Because N^5,N^{10}-methylene FH_4 is the obligate one-carbon donor for thymidylate synthesis, its conversion to N-methyltetrahydrofolate serves as a brake on DNA synthesis and repair, while diverting more folate to the methionine synthase reaction (see

Fig. 41-2). The activity of MTHFR therefore serves as a checkpoint for intracellular folate trafficking and distribution, and thus becomes more critical in states of folate depletion.

A polymorphic form of MTHFR, MTHFR 677C→T, is of some clinical importance. The mutation results in a thermolabile form of the enzyme with a higher K_m (Michaelis-Menten dissociation constant) for its methylene-FH_4 substrate. Retardation of the folate methylation cycle makes more methylene-FH_4 available for thymidylate synthesis (Fig. 41-4), and also affects the levels of homocysteine, an amino acid whose rate of production depends on both folate and cobalamin.

Folate deficiency diminishes purine biosynthesis by slowing (1) the folate-dependent formylation of glycinamide ribotide to N-formylglycinamide ribotide, the reaction that places the C-8 in the purine ring, and (2) the folate-dependent conversion of 5-amino-4-imidazole carboxamide ribotide (AICAR) to 5-formamido-4-imidazole carboxy-amide ribotide, the reaction that places the C-2 in the purine ring.[14] Additional reactions dependent on biopterin, a nonfolate pteridine derivative, that are of potential metabolic importance are hydroxylation of phenylalanine to tyrosine, oxidation of long-chain alkyl ethers of glycerol to fatty acid, hydroxylation of tryptophan to 6-hydroxytryptophan (a precursor of serotonin), 17α-hydroxylation of progesterone,[15] and production of nitric oxide.[16] Tetrahydrofolic acid is weakly active in some of these systems *in vitro*[17]; whether it plays any such role *in vivo* is unknown.

Significance of Folylpolyglutamates

Intracellular folates exist primarily as polyglutamate conjugates.[18] Approximately 75 percent of the folate in human erythrocytes and leukocytes is polyglutamylated.[19] Plasma folate consists largely of the monoglutamate N^5-methyltetrahydrofolate and is transported into the cells in this form.[20] Inside the cells, the polyglutamate chain is sequentially built up by an ATP-dependent *folylpoly-γ-glutamyl synthase* (FPGS).[21]

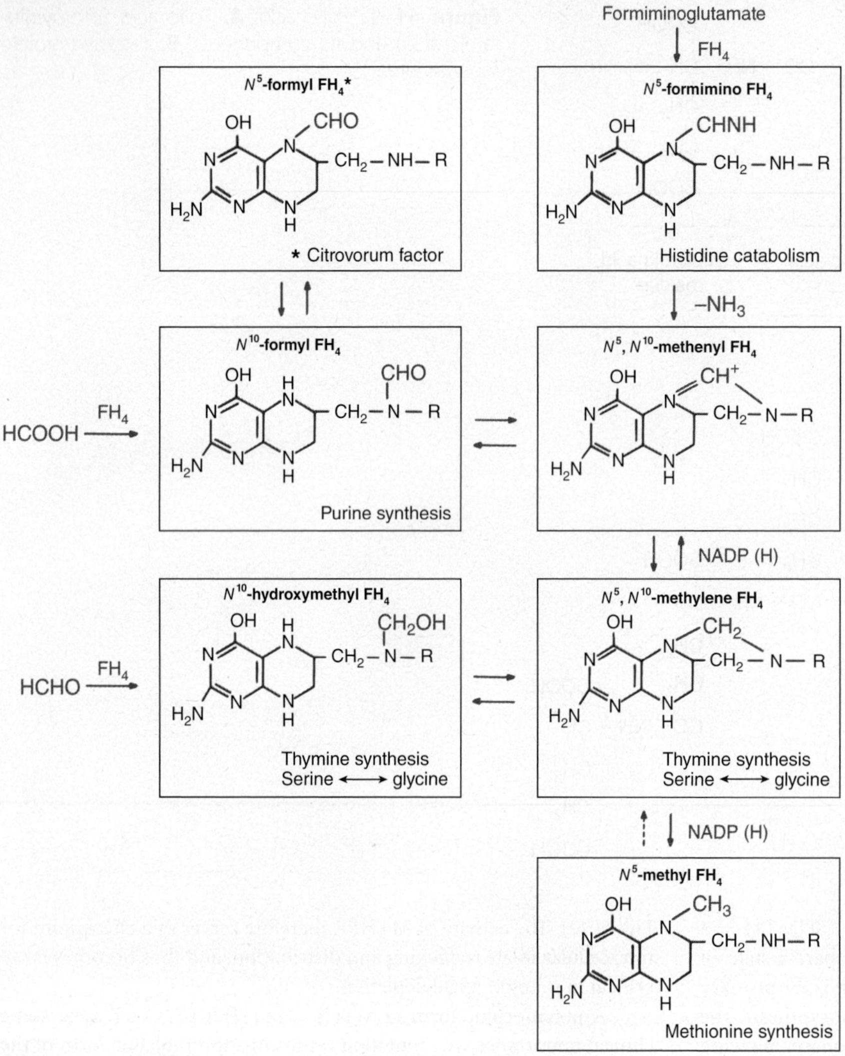

Figure 41–2. Derivatives of tetrahydrofolic acid (FH$_4$), their interconversions, and the metabolic pathways in which they participate. One-carbon substituents are shown in *blue*.

TABLE 41–1. Metabolic Systems Requiring Folic Acid Coenzymes in Animal Cells

System	Related Transformations of Folic Acid Coenzymes
Serine → glycine	Serine + tetrahydrofolate (FH$_4$) → N^5,N^{10}-methylene FH$_4$ + glycine
Thymidylate synthesis	Deoxyuridylate (dUMP) + N^5,N^{10}-methylene FH$_4$ → FH$_2$ + thymidylate (dTMP)
Histidine catabolism	Formiminoglutamate + FH$_4$ → N^5-formimino FH$_4$ + glutamate
Methionine synthesis	Homocysteine + N^5-methyltetrahydrofolate → FH$_4$ + methionine
Purine synthesis	Glycinamide ribotide + N^{10}-formyl FH$_4$ → FH$_4$ + formylglycinamide ribotide
Purine synthesis	5-Amino-4-imidazole carboxamide ribotide + N^{10}-formyl FH$_4$ → FH$_4$ + 5-formamido-4-imidazolecarboxamide ribotide

The activity of human FPGS depends strongly on the form of the folate substrate, declining in the order FH$_4$ > N^{10}-formyl FH$_4$ > N^5-methyltetrahydrofolate, toward which the enzyme is almost inert.[22] In humans, conjugated folates carry on average seven to eight glutamyl residues.[23] Intracellular folylmonoglutamates leak out of the cells at a fairly rapid rate whereas polyglutamates do not, presumably because of the highly charged polyglutamate tail.[24] Therefore, attachment of the polyglutamate chain is essential for retaining folates within cells. Folylpolyglutamates are superior to monoglutamates as substrates for folate-dependent enzyme reactions.[19]

PHYSIOLOGY

Intestinal Absorption

The duodenum and proximal jejunum is the principal site of folate absorption. Absorption of a dose of either monoglutamate or polyglutamate forms of folate begins within minutes. Peak plasma levels are reached in 1 to 2 hours. Because only folylmonoglutamate appears in plasma, all folylpolyglutamates must first be hydrolyzed by the enzyme glutamate carboxypeptidase II (folate hydrolase)[25] during absorption across the intestine.[26] This enzyme (previously referred to as "conjugase") is located on the brush-border membrane and plays an important role in the intestinal absorption of folate.[27] Folylpolyglutamate is hydrolyzed at the brush-border of the intestinal cell (Fig. 41–5). Folate

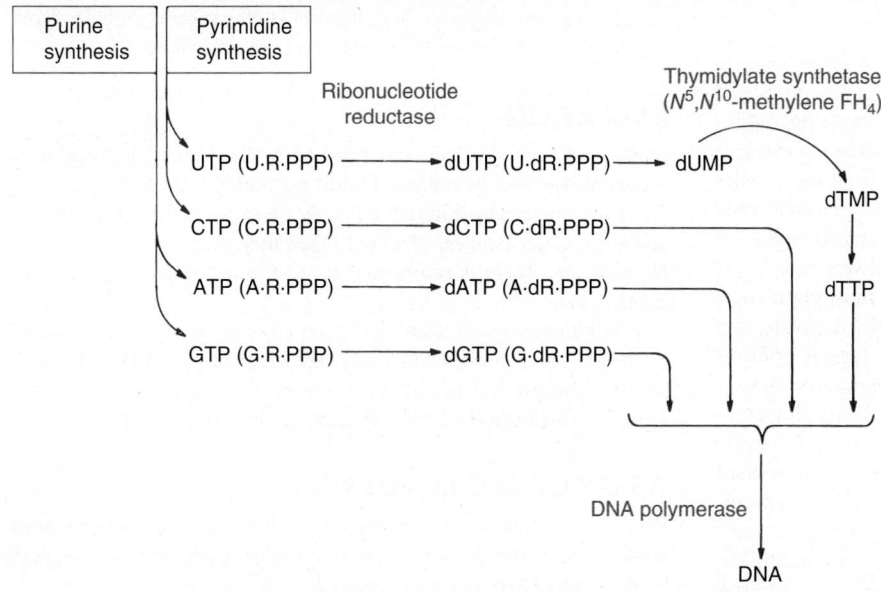

Figure 41–3. Pathways of deoxynucleotide and DNA synthesis.

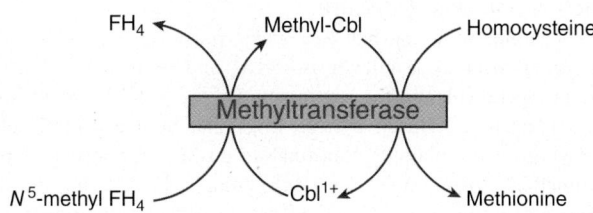

Figure 41–4. N^5-methyltetrahydrofolate–homocysteine methyltransferase reaction.

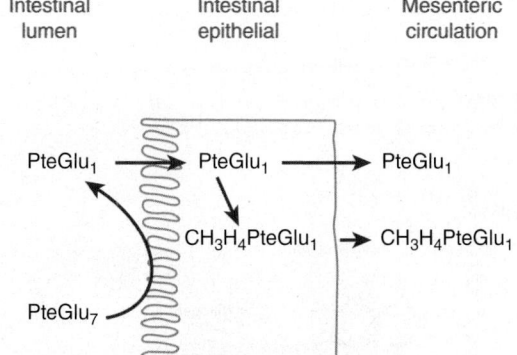

Figure 41–5. Digestion and absorption of folate polyglutamate by the intestine. The polyglutamate (in this case, PteGlu$_7$) is hydrolyzed in the intestinal lumen or at the brush-border. The resulting pteroylglutamate (PteGlu) is transported into the intestinal cell, where it is reduced and methylated, appearing in the circulation chiefly as N^5-methyltetrahydrofolate.

hydrolase purified from human jejunum catalyzes the Zn^{2+}-dependent deconjugation of folate polyglutamates ranging from PteGlu$_2$ to at least PteGlu$_7$.[28] It is an exopeptidase that successively removes single glutamate residues from the end of the polyglutamate chain, ultimately yielding the folylmonoglutamate. The monoglutamate forms are then taken up by one of two folate-specific transporters located on the apical brush-border, the reduced folate carrier (RFC) or the proton-coupled folate transporter (PCFT).[25] Although RFC has a pH optimum of 7.4, PCFT is a high-affinity folate transporter that uses a proton-coupled system to facilitate folate absorption and shows maximum transport activity at a low pH.[25,29] This property is consistent with the observation that cancer cells retain a high affinity for the new-generation antifolate pemetrexed. Defects in the PCFT are the underlying cause of hereditary folate malabsorption.[30]

Folate hydrolases also are found outside the intestine. For example, human plasma contains sufficient hydrolase activity to convert polyglutamates containing more than three glutamyl residues to monoglutamates. Other γ-glutamyl hydrolases appear to be lysosomal carboxypeptidases[31] that are not involved in absorption of folates from the intestine but that play a role in the release of folate from storage sites in the liver and kidney.[25]

Folate monoglutamates are actively transported across the intestinal epithelium by PCFT-mediated transport ($K_m = 1$ to $2~\mu M$) that is independent of Na$^+$, K$^+$, and transmembrane potential.[32] The mechanism uses the pH gradient between the jejunal lumen (pH ~6) and the interior of the epithelial cell to drive folate into the cell against a concentration gradient.[33] Passive transport also may occur.[34] In the intestinal cell, the absorbed folate monoglutamates are reduced if necessary, and then converted to N^5-methyltetrahydrofolate (some N^{10}-formyl FH$_4$ also is made) and transported into the bloodstream without further change.[35]

Folate undergoes an enterohepatic cycle in which it is first secreted against a concentration gradient into the bile, appearing there chiefly as N^5-methyltetrahydrofolate monoglutamate, and then is reabsorbed from the small intestine.[36] Bile contains approximately two to 10 times the folate concentration of normal serum, with biliary excretion accounting for up to 0.1 mg of folate per day. This quantity is sufficiently large that interruption of the enterohepatic cycle by biliary diversion causes serum folate levels to fall by more than 50 percent in less than 1 day.[37] The enterohepatic cycle has been proposed to redistribute folate between hepatic stores and peripheral tissues according to the state of the exogenous folate supplies.[38]

METABOLISM

Tritiated folylmonoglutamate (^{3}H-F) administered intravenously is almost completely removed from the bloodstream in a few minutes.[39] Uptake involves two classes of folate-binding proteins[40]: *high-affinity folate receptors*[41] that concentrate folate in intracellular vesicles and a *membrane folate transporter* that transports folate from the vesicles into the cytosol. The high-affinity receptors, which are attached to the outer surface of the cell membrane by glycosyl-phosphatidylinositol linkages and lack an intracytoplasmic portion,[42] bind very tightly (K_d [distribution coefficient] in the nanomolar range) to most physiologic folate monoglutamates,[43] particularly N^5-methyltetrahydrofolate, the major circulating folate.[44] The folate receptors exist in various isoforms (of which α and β are the most important). Folate receptor-α, despite its missing cytoplasmic extension, is effective in mediating endocytosis.[45] Their very high affinity enables the receptors to take up N^5-methyltetrahydrofolate from the plasma, even at its ambient concentration of approximately 10 nM. The membrane folate transporter is a probenecid-inhibitable organic anion carrier that, among other functions, carries reduced folates and methotrexate in and out of the cytoplasm.[40] Its K_m for folate is in the micromolar range. Once internalized, the folates are retained by the cells partly through polyglutamylation[46] as well as through tight association with a set of intracellular folate-binding proteins.[47] Three of these proteins are enzymes involved in methyl group metabolism: sarcosine dehydrogenase and dimethylglycine dehydrogenase (mitochondrial)[48] and glycine N-methyl transferase (cytosolic).[49] Why these enzymes bind folate so avidly or whether this binding affects overall methyl group metabolism is unknown, although glycine N-methyl transferase is speculated to regulate methyl group metabolism by controlling the tissue concentration of S-adenosylhomocysteine (SAH), one of its reaction products and a potent inhibitor of most methyltransferases.

Folates have been found in all body tissues that have been analyzed. The principal form of the vitamin in tissues and in blood appears to be the N^5-methyl form.[50] The total folate pool turns over very slowly.[51] Degradation accounts for a portion of this turnover. *p*-Aminobenzoylglutamate has been identified as a breakdown product. The fate of the pteridine moiety is unknown.

FOLATE-BINDING PROTEINS OF SERUM AND MILK

The soluble folate-binding proteins of serum and milk are high-affinity folate receptors that are released from cell membranes by proteolysis.[52] These proteins can be detected in approximately 15 percent of normal individuals[53] and are found at increased levels in some pregnant women, women taking oral contraceptives, folate-deficient alcoholics (but not patients with cobalamin deficiency),[54] and patients with uremia, hepatic cirrhosis, and chronic myelogenous leukemia.[55] In normal subjects, the proteins are approximately two-thirds saturated and have a total folate-binding capacity of approximately 175 pg/mL of serum.[56] The proteins may not be detected in some subjects because of complete saturation of the proteins with endogenous unlabeled folate.[57] Serum folate-binding protein has an Mr of 40,000 and prefers oxidized to reduced folates.[55]

Folate-binding proteins have been found in milk and in normal granulocytes.[58] Folate bound to the milk folate binder in suckling animals is absorbed chiefly in the ileum[59] rather than the jejunum, the principal site of absorption of free folate. The milk folate binder, a glycoprotein, also promotes folate transport into the liver via the asialoglycoprotein receptor.[60] The milk folate binder is speculated to protect an infant's folate supply by preventing bacteria from sequestering the vitamin away from the intestinal absorptive surface. The folate-binding

protein in granulocytes has been localized to the specific granules, from which it is released when the granulocytes are stimulated.

EXCRETION

Folates are both resorbed and secreted by the kidney. Resorption is accomplished by a membrane-bound high-affinity folate receptor (K_m for N^5-methyltetrahydrofolate = 0.4 nM) located in the brush-borders of the proximal tubules.[61] Filtered folate may thus be returned to the bloodstream. There is resorption of most, but not all, of the filtered folate.

In humans, intact folates and their cleavage products are excreted by the kidney at a rate of 2 to 5 mcg/day.[62] A small percentage of parenterally administered labeled folate is recoverable in the feces and mainly represents unreabsorbed folate from the enterohepatic cycle.[63]

ASSAY OF SERUM FOLATE

Folates are measured by chemiluminescent methods using various folate binders. These assays are identical in principle to the radioligand binding assays that they have replaced.

● COBALAMIN

CHEMISTRY

Structure and Nomenclature

The cobalamin molecule has two major portions: a porphyrin-like near-planar macrocycle known as corrin, and a nucleotide that lies almost perpendicular to the corrin ring (Fig. 41–6). The corrin moiety contains four reduced pyrrole rings that bind a central cobalt atom whose two remaining coordination positions are occupied by a 5,6-dimethylbenzimidazolyl (5,6-DMB) group, below the ring and various ligands (in this case, —N in the form of CN) above the ring.[64]

Compounds containing the corrin ring are known as *corrinoids*. The cobalamins are corrinoids whose nucleotide contains 5,6-DMB. Two connections exist between the corrin and the nucleotide: (1) a bond between the nucleotide phosphate and a side chain in ring D, and (2) a bond between cobalt and a nitrogen atom of benzimidazole. Figure 41–7 summarizes the numbering and ring designations of the corrin system.

The term *vitamin* B_{12} is sometimes used as a generic term for the cobalamins. The term probably is best reserved, however, as an alternative name for cyanocobalamin, the usual therapeutic form of cobalamin.

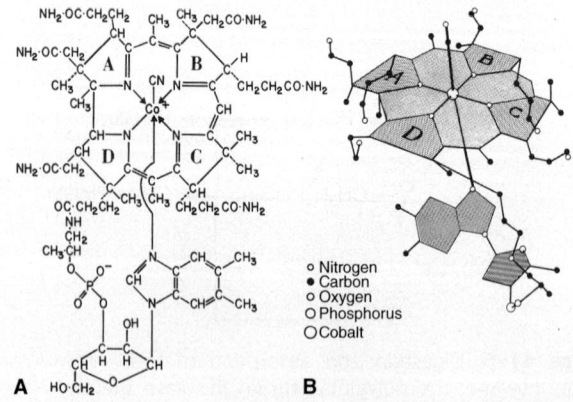

Figure 41–6. A. Structure of cyanocobalamin (CnCbl; vitamin B_{12}). **B.** Partial structure of CnCbl showing the relationship between the corrin ring and the nucleotide.

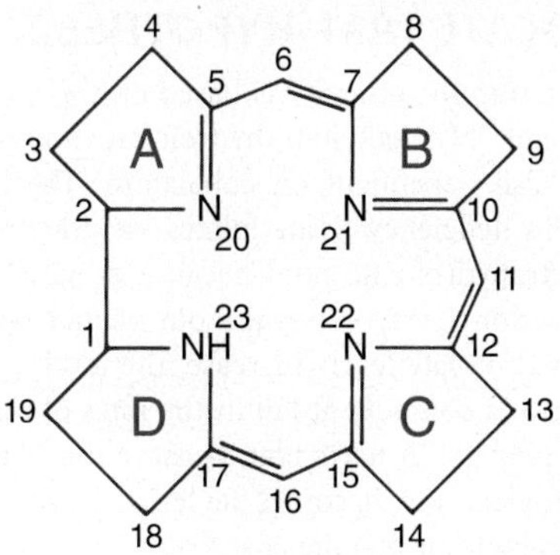

Figure 41–7. Corrin ring showing ring designations and standard numbering of the atoms.

Four cobalamins are important in animal cell metabolism. Two are *cyanocobalamin* (CnCbl; vitamin B$_{12}$) and *hydroxocobalamin* (OHCbl) or *aquocobalamin* (HOH Cbl). The other two cobalamins are alkyl derivatives that are synthesized from OHCbl and serve as coenzymes. In one, *adenosylcobalamin* (AdoCbl), a 5′-deoxyadenosyl replaces OH as the cobalt ligand above the ring (Fig. 41–8).[65] In the second, *methylcobalamin* (MeCbl), the upper ligand is a methyl group. MeCbl is the major form of cobalamin in human blood plasma.[66]

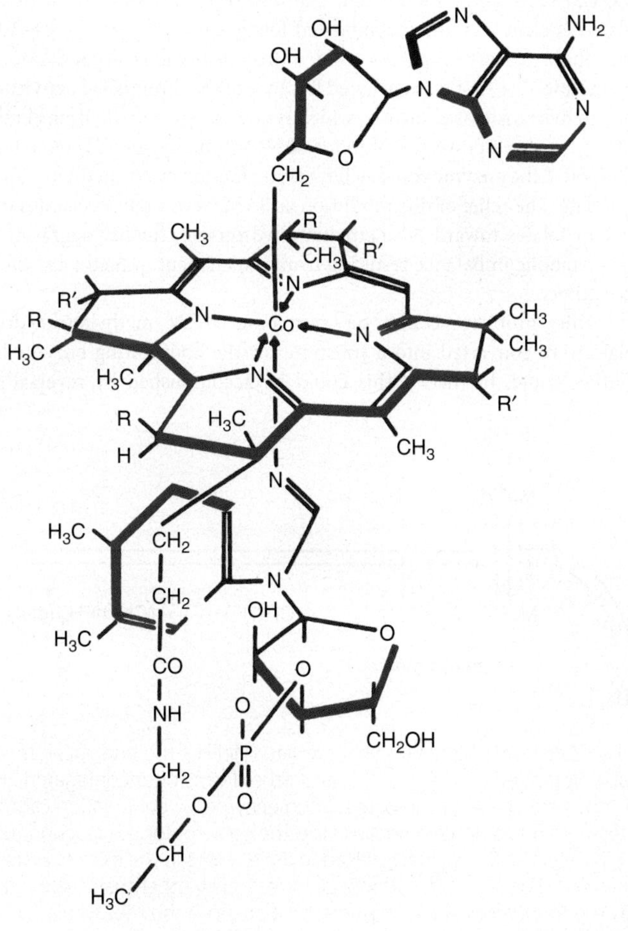

Figure 41–8. Adenosylcobalamin (AdoCbl). R = CH$_2$CONH$_2$; R′ = CH$_2$CH$_2$CONH$_2$.

NUTRITION

Sources

Cobalamin is synthesized only by certain microorganisms; animals ultimately depend on microbial synthesis for their cobalamin supply. Foods that contain cobalamin are of animal origin: meat, liver, seafood, and dairy products. Cobalamin has not been found in plants.

Daily Requirements

The average daily diet in Western countries contains 5 to 30 mcg of cobalamin, of which 1 to 5 mcg is absorbed.[67] Less than 250 ng appears in the urine; the unabsorbed remainder appears in the feces. Total body content is 2 to 5 mg in an adult,[68] with approximately 1 mg in the liver. The kidneys also are rich in cobalamin.[69] Relative to the daily requirement, body reserves of cobalamin are much larger than those of folate.

Cobalamin has a daily rate of obligatory loss of approximately 0.1 percent of the total-body pool, irrespective of the pool size. For this reason, a deficiency state does not develop for several years after cessation of cobalamin intake. The officially recommended dietary allowance (RDA) for adults is 2.4 mcg[2]; growth, hypermetabolic states, and pregnancy increase daily requirements. The RDA for children ages 1 to 13 years is 0.9 to 1.8 mcg. Because of insufficient data, no RDA has been established for infants. Instead, adequate intakes of 0.4 mcg for age 0 to 6 months and 0.5 mcg for age 7 to 12 months have been estimated.

ROLE IN METABOLISM

The only two recognized cobalamin-dependent enzymes in human cells are AdoCbl-dependent *methylmalonyl CoA (coenzyme A) mutase* and MeCbl-dependent *methyltetrahydrofolate-homocysteine methyltransferase*.

Methylmalonyl Coenzyme A Mutase

Methylmalonyl CoA mutase is a mitochondrial enzyme that participates in the disposal of the propionate formed during breakdown of valine, isoleucine, and odd-carbon fatty acids. The enzyme is a homodimer of a 78-kDa subunit that is encoded by a gene on chromosome 6.[70] In the reaction catalyzed by methylmalonyl CoA mutase, methylmalonyl CoA, which is produced during catabolism of propionate,[71] is converted to succinyl CoA, a Krebs cycle intermediate. In the course of this reaction, a hydrogen on the methyl carbon of the substrate exchanges places with the —COSCoA group (Fig. 41–9).

The coenzyme serves as an intermediate hydrogen carrier, accepting the hydrogen from the substrate in the initial phase of the reaction and returning it to the product after migration of —COSCoA.

N^5-Methyltetrahydrofolate-Homocysteine Methyltransferase

MeCbl participates in cobalamin-dependent synthesis of methionine from homocysteine by the enzyme N^5-methyltetrahydrofolate–homocysteine methyltransferase. S-adenosylmethionine (SAMe) and a second enzyme, methionine synthase reductase are required for methyltransferase activity.[72] The reductase converts the oxidized cobalt to

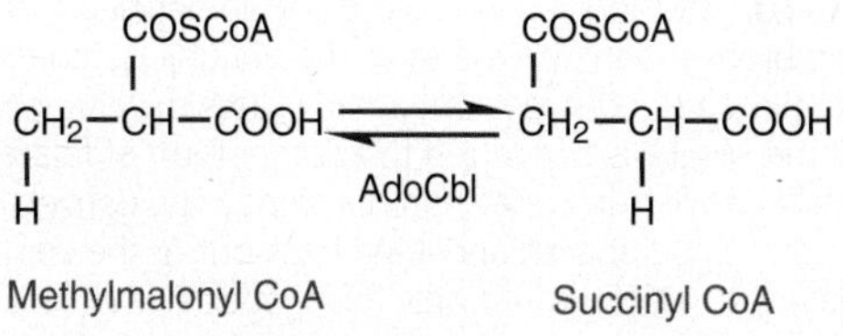

Figure 41–9. Methylmalonyl coenzyme A (CoA) mutase reaction. AdoCbl, adenosylcobalamin.

the readily alkalizable Co^+, which then accepts a methyl group from SAMe, a powerful biologic methylating agent, thereby restoring activity of the methyltransferase. In humans, this pathway also serves as a mechanism critical for converting N^5-methyltetrahydrofolate to FH_4 required for synthesis of polyglutamates as well as other important one-carbon adducts of folate. The demethylation of N^5-methyltetrahydrofolate is a prerequisite for attachment of the polyglutamate chain to newly acquired folate, which is largely taken up by the cell in the form of N^5-methyltetrahydrofolate monoglutamate.[24] Nitrous oxide (N_2O) impairs the methyltransferase by oxidizing cob(I)alamin (a catalytic intermediate in the methyltransferase reaction) to cob(II)alamin. This reaction depletes MeCbl and produces a cobalamin deficiency-like state.

Nonenzymatic Metabolism

Because cobalamin has the capacity to bind cyanide, it may participate in detoxification of cyanide. Tobacco and certain foods (fruits, beans, tubers, and nuts) contain cyanide in the form of thiocyanate. Although the evidence is inconclusive, cobalamin is believed to play a role in neutralizing cyanide taken in via these substances.[64]

FOLATE–COBALAMIN RELATIONSHIP

In both folate deficiency and cobalamin deficiency, the megaloblastic anemias are fully corrected by treatment with the appropriate vitamin. The megaloblastic anemia of cobalamin deficiency also is variably corrected by folic acid supplementation even if no cobalamin is given, although the remission may be partial and only temporary. Conversely, the anemia of folate deficiency is generally not helped at all by cobalamin although partial responses to high doses of cobalamin have been reported in some patients with folate deficiency.[73] These clinical observations indicate that the megaloblastic anemia in cobalamin deficiency actually results from an abnormality in folate metabolism.[24] The observation that urinary excretion of formiminoglutamic acid (FIGlu) and AICAR, normally regarded as a sign of folate deficiency, is seen occasionally in pure cobalamin deficiency[74] provides further evidence that folate metabolism is deranged by cobalamin deficiency. Two explanations have been proposed to account for the folate responsiveness of cobalamin-deficient megaloblastic anemia: (1) the *methylfolate trap* hypothesis, which is accepted by the majority of authorities, and (2) the *formate starvation* hypothesis (Fig. 41–10).

METHYLFOLATE TRAP HYPOTHESIS

The methylfolate trap hypothesis[75] is based on the fact that the folate-requiring enzyme N^5-methyltetrahydrofolate–homocysteine methyltransferase is also dependent on cobalamin. The hypothesis states that in cobalamin deficiency tissue folates are gradually diverted into the N^5-methyltetrahydrofolate pool because of slowing of the methyltransferase reaction,[76] the only route out of that pool for folate. As N^5-methyltetrahydrofolate levels increase, the levels of other forms of folate decline, with a consequent fall in the rates of reactions in which those forms participate. In particular, because the MTHFR reaction is irreversible, methylene-FH_4 becomes depleted, the synthesis of dTMP is slowed, and megaloblastic anemia ensues.

In its simplest form, the hypothesis predicts that in cobalamin deficiency tissue levels of N^5-methyltetrahydrofolate are abnormally high and those of other forms of folate are abnormally low. Although serum N^5-methyltetrahydrofolate levels are frequently elevated in cobalamin deficiency,[77] tissue folate levels, predominantly polyglutamates, decline.[78] The decreased level appears to be related to the substrate specificity of the folate-conjugating enzyme. This enzyme works very poorly with N^5-methyltetrahydrofolate; therefore, it is unable to carry out normal γ-glutamylation of newly internalized N^5-methyltetrahydrofolate monoglutamate in cobalamin-deficient cells because the freshly acquired folate cannot be converted into a suitable substrate (i.e., free FH_4 or formyl FH_4). Thus, although sequestration of tissue folates in an expanded N^5-methyltetrahydrofolate pool may account for some of the effects of the blockade in methyltransferase activity, the major problem seems to be a failure to convert newly acquired folate into a form that can be retained by the cell. The upshot is development of tissue folate deficiency as the unconjugated folate leaks out (see Fig. 41–10). The whole process is aggravated by a drop in tissue levels of SAMe as the methionine supply is curtailed because of the diminished activity of the methyltransferase.[79] SAMe, which is necessary for methyltransferase activity, is also a powerful inhibitor of N^5,N^{10}-methylene FH_4 reductase MTHFR,[80] the enzyme responsible for production of N^5-methyltetrahydrofolate. The relief of this inhibition as SAMe levels fall accelerates the flow of folates toward N^5-methyltetrahydrofolate, further aggravating the metabolic imbalance resulting from impairment in methyltransferase activity.

This problem could be overcome if N^5-methyltetrahydrofolate were converted into a substrate for the conjugating enzyme by another route. In theory, this could be accomplished by reversal of

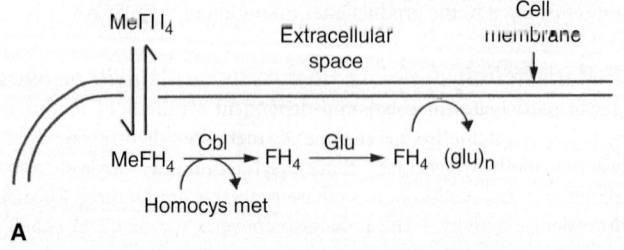

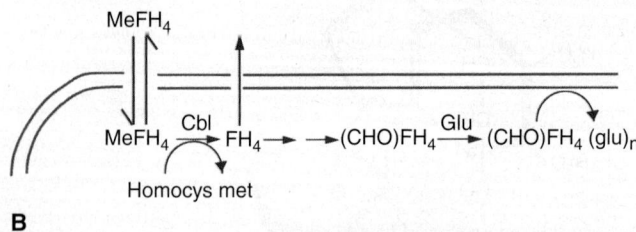

A   **B**

Figure 41–10. Methods by which cobalamin deficiency decreases intracellular folate levels. Methyltetrahydrofolate (MeFH$_4$), the principal form of folate in the bloodstream, circulates in the unconjugated form (i.e., it has no polyglutamate side chain). This and other forms of unconjugated FH$_4$ can be taken into cells but leak out again unless they are conjugated. MeFH$_4$ is not a substrate for the conjugating enzyme, so conjugation cannot occur until the MeFH$_4$ is converted to another form of folate. Cobalamin is necessary for this process because it is the cofactor for the reaction that converts MeFH$_4$ to FH$_4$. In cobalamin deficiency, the conversion of MeFH$_4$ to FH$_4$ is defective. Newly transported folate remains in the form of MeFH$_4$, which cannot be conjugated and leaks back out of the cell. **A.** According to the *methylfolate trap hypothesis*, all forms of FH$_4$ other than MeFH$_4$ can be conjugated, so MeFH$_4$ is the only folate species that leaks out of the cell. **B.** The *formate starvation hypothesis* differs from the methylfolate trap hypothesis solely in assuming that only the formylated folates (N^{10}-formyl FH$_4$ and/or N^5,N^{10}-methenyl FH$_4$) can be conjugated, so newly transported MeFH$_4$, N^5,N^{10}-methylene FH$_4$, and free FH$_4$ leak out of the cell. (CHO) FH$_4$ = N^{10}-formyl FH$_4$. Homocys met, homocysteine methyltransferase.

the N^5,N^{10}-methylene FH_4 reductase reaction. For practical purposes, however, the N^5,N^{10}-methylene FH_4 reductase reaction is irreversible *in vivo*.[81]

FORMATE STARVATION HYPOTHESIS

This hypothesis holds that formate starvation is the basis for folate-responsive megaloblastic anemia of cobalamin deficiency.[82] This theory is based on the diminished capacity of cobalamin-deficient lymphoblasts to incorporate formaldehyde into purine and methionine[79] and on experiments showing that N^5-formyl FH_4 is more effective than FH_4 at correcting some of the abnormalities in folate metabolism seen in cobalamin deficiency.[83] The hypothesis states that with the decrease in methionine production in cobalamin-deficient conditions, the generation of formate is depressed (because normally the methyl group of excess methionine is rapidly oxidized to formate),[84] leading to a decline in the production of N^5-formyl FH_4.

INTESTINAL ABSORPTION

Intrinsic Factor

Intrinsic factor is one of a number of binding proteins in which cobalamin is ensconced as it makes its way through the body (Table 41–2). Intrinsic factor is needed for the absorption of cobalamins taken orally at physiologic dosage levels. Human intrinsic factor is a glycoprotein (Mr approximately 44,000) encoded by a gene on chromosome 11.[85] It has binding sites for cobalamin and a specific ileal receptor, the former situated near the carboxy-terminus and the latter near the aminoterminus of the intrinsic factor molecule.[86] Binding to cobalamin is very tight, and involves the 5,6-DMB lower axial ligand of the molecule. This specificity allows for the exclusion of other noncobalamin corrinoids during the tightly regulated absorptive process.[64] The entrapment of the vitamin alters the conformation of intrinsic factor, producing a more compact form that is resistant to proteolytic digestion.

In humans, intrinsic factor is synthesized and secreted by the parietal cells of the cardiac and fundic mucosa.[87] Secretion of intrinsic factor usually parallels that of hydrochloric acid (HCl). It is enhanced by the presence of food in the stomach, vagal stimulation, histamine, and gastrin. Gastric juice also contains other cobalamin-binding glycoproteins.[88] These proteins were known as the *R proteins* because of their rapid electrophoretic mobility compared with intrinsic factor. Elucidation of the primary protein structure of the R proteins reveals that they belong to the same family of isoproteins as the plasma haptocorrin (HC) binder (previously known as transcobalamins I and III). These HC-like proteins are produced mainly by the salivary glands.

Absorption of Cobalamin: Cubilin

Cobalamins in foods are liberated in the stomach by peptic digestion.[89] They are then bound not to intrinsic factor but to the HC-like protein

because cobalamin binds much more tightly to HC than to intrinsic factor at the acid pH of the stomach.[90] Upon entering the duodenum, cobalamin is released from the cobalamin–HC protein complex through digestion by pancreatic proteases, which in normal subjects act by selectively degrading HC and the cobalamin–HC complex while sparing intrinsic factor.[90] Only at this point can cobalamin bind to intrinsic factor to form the intrinsic factor–cobalamin complex.

The intrinsic factor–cobalamin complex, which is very resistant to digestion,[91] traverses the intestine until it reaches the intrinsic factor receptor, *cubilin*,[92] a 460-kDa peripheral membrane glycoprotein located in the microvillus pits of the ileal mucosa brush-border. Cubilin forms part of a multifunctional epithelial receptor complex also found in the yolk sac and renal proximal tubule cells.[93] In the kidney, it appears to serve a role in the overall body economy through tubular reabsorption of cobalamin,[94] but the function of the cubilin receptor complex in the kidney and other polarized epithelial surfaces extends beyond cobalamin. The ileal cubilin receptor complex consists of two proteins, cubilin (CUB) and amnionless (AMN), the product of two distinct genes, *CUB* and *AMN*. Both proteins, which together have been designated the "CUBAM complex," colocalize in the endocytic compartment and are required for the process of assimilation of cobalamin,[95] AMN serving as a chaperon for endosomal targeting. Mutations affecting either of the two proteins disrupt the normal process of the intestinal phase of cobalamin absorption. In addition to the tightly embracing components of the CUBAM complex, a distinct large multifunctional protein, megalin, which belongs to the low-density lipoprotein family,[96] also participates in the conformational changes that accompany internalization. The concentration of the CUBAM complex rises progressively to a maximum near the terminal ileum.[97] A specific site on the intrinsic factor molecule avidly attaches to the receptor in a binding reaction that requires a pH of 5.4 or greater and Ca^{2+} (or other divalent cations) but no energy.[98]

The intrinsic factor–cobalamin receptor complex is taken into the ileal mucosal cells over 30 to 60 minutes by endocytosis,[99] where the vitamin is processed and released into the portal blood over many hours. The receptors recycle to the microvillus surface to shuttle another load of intrinsic factor–cobalamin complex.[99] That this process has a limited capacity is evident from estimates of the maximum amount of cobalamin that can be absorbed from a single dose via this physiologic pathway.[64,100] Defects in the genes that regulate the complex mechanism of ileal absorption are implicated in autosomal recessive megaloblastic anemia (MGA1), caused by intestinal malabsorption of cobalamin (see "Selective Malabsorption of Cobalamin, Autosomal Recessive Megaloblastic Anemia, Imerslund-Gräsbeck Disease" below).

During its sojourn in the ileal enterocyte, the vitamin first appears in the lysosomes, but by 4 hours most of the vitamin is located in the cytosol.[101] During absorption, the entire intrinsic factor–cobalamin complex appears to be taken into the cell, where the cobalamin is released while the intrinsic factor is degraded.[102]

Cobalamin from a small oral dose (10 to 20 mcg) starts to appear in the blood after 3 to 4 hours, and the vitamin reaches a peak level in 6 to 12 hours. In the portal blood, the cobalamin is complexed with a cobalamin-transporting protein known as *transcobalamin* (TC) previously known as TC II.[103] There is evidence that cobalamin leaves the enterocyte through a portal that is part of the ABC drug transport system, ABCC1 (also known as the multidrug resistance protein1 [MRP1]) located on the basolateral surface of the intestinal epithelium, as well as other polar cells and nonpolar cells (macrophages).[104] The cobalamin–TC complex is now believed to be formed as it exits the ileal enterocyte, one of a variety of cells that synthesize TC, including the neighboring vascular endothelial cells in the submucosa.[105] Large oral doses (1 mg) of cobalamin are absorbed inefficiently (1 to 2 percent of an oral dose)

TABLE 41–2. Cobalamin-Binding Proteins		
Protein	**Source**	**Function**
Intrinsic factor	Gastric parietal cells	Promotes absorption uptake of cobalamin by ileum
Transcobalamin	Probably all cells	Promotes uptake of cobalamin by cells
Haptocorrin	Exocrine glands, phagocytes	Helps dispose of cobalamin analogues (?)

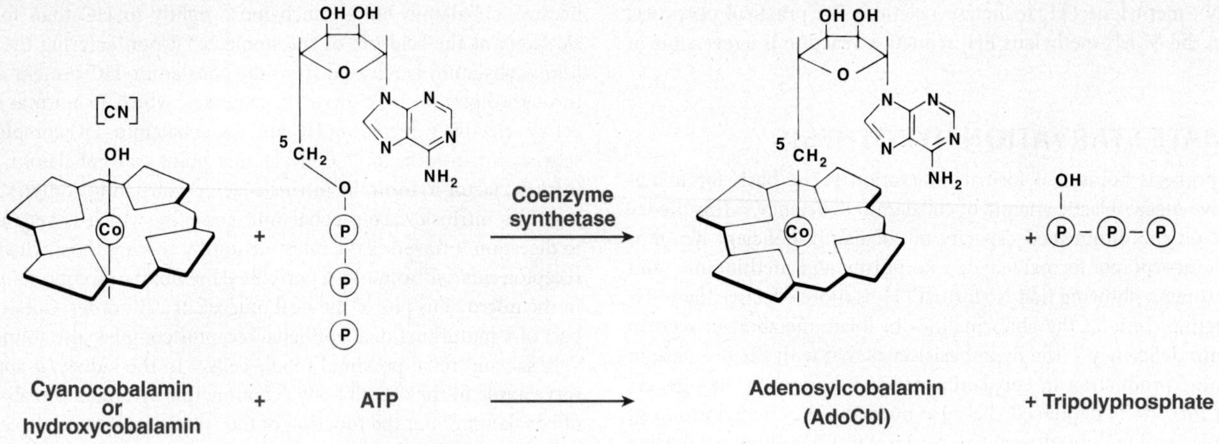

Figure 41–11. Biosynthesis of adenosylcobalamin (AdoCbl).

by simple diffusion that is not mediated by intrinsic factor.[100] In these instances, the vitamin appears in blood within minutes, again as the cobalamin–TC complex.

Like the folates, the cobalamins undergo appreciable enterohepatic recycling.[106] In humans, between 0.5 and 9 mcg/day of cobalamin is secreted into the bile, where it is bound to HC.[107] After entering the intestine, the cobalamin–HC complexes of biliary origin are treated exactly like those delivered from the stomach. The cobalamin is released by digestion of the HC by pancreatic proteases, and then is taken up by intrinsic factor and reabsorbed. From 65 to 75 percent of biliary cobalamin is estimated to be reabsorbed by this mechanism.[108] Because of the size of the cobalamin storage pool and the existence of this enterohepatic circulation, a very long time—as long as 20 years—is required for a clinically significant cobalamin deficiency to develop from a diet providing insufficient cobalamin (e.g., a strictly vegetarian diet).[109] Patients who are unable to absorb the vitamin, however, become clinically deficient in only 3 to 6 years because the absorption of both biliary and dietary cobalamin are interdicted.[110]

COBALAMIN IN THE CELL: TRANSCOBALAMIN

Uptake of Cobalamin By Cells

TC is the plasma protein that mediates the transport of cobalamin into the tissues.[111] A β-globulin protein with a calculated molecular weight of 45,538 from the deduced amino acid sequence,[112,113] TC binds cobalamin with exceedingly high affinity ($K_a \sim 10^{-11}\,M$).[114] Unlike intrinsic factor, whose binding is highly specific for cobalamins, TC shows some promiscuity and also can bind certain corrins that are chemically related to the cobalamins but have no function in mammalian systems and are known as cobalamin "analogues."[115] TC is synthesized by many types of cells, including enterocytes, hepatocytes, endothelial cells, mononuclear phagocytes, fibroblasts, and hematopoietic precursors in the marrow.[64] Although circulating TC carries only a minor fraction of the cobalamin in the plasma, it is the protein on which cobalamin absorbed through the intestine and is transported into the portal blood as the preformed cobalamin–TC complex. It also is the protein with which cobalamin given parenterally associates almost immediately.[116] These cobalamin–TC complexes are transported into the tissues within minutes of appearing in the bloodstream.[117] The transport process begins with binding of the cobalamin–TC complex to a specific membrane receptor that is present on a wide variety of cells.[118] The protein and gene encoding the TC receptor has been purified from placental membranes and characterized.[119] Designated as CD320, the receptor belongs to the low-density

lipoprotein receptor family and its internalization involves megalin. The receptor-bound complex is internalized by receptor-mediated endocytosis and delivered to a lysosome, where the TC is digested and the cobalamin is freed.[120,121]

Formation of Adenosylcobalamin and Methylcobalamin

To become metabolically active, CnCbl and OHCbl must first be converted to AdoCbl and MeCbl, the coenzymatically active cobalamins. The conversion is accomplished by reduction and alkylation. CnCbl and OHCbl are first reduced to the Co++ form [cob(II)alamin] by NADPH- and NADH (nicotinamide adenine dinucleotide phosphate)-dependent reductases that are present in mitochondria and microsomes.[122] CN– and OH– are displaced from the metal during reduction. Some of the cob(II)alamin is reduced further in the mitochondria to the intensely nucleophilic Co+ form [cob(I)alamin]. This is then alkylated by ATP to form AdoCbl in a reaction in which the 5′-deoxyadenosyl moiety of ATP is transferred to the cobalamin and the three phosphates of ATP are released as inorganic triphosphate (Fig. 41–11). The rest of the cobalamin binds to cytosolic N^5-methyltetrahydrofolate–homocysteine methyltransferase, where it is converted to MeCbl. The several steps involved in the conversion of cobalamin to its coenzymatically active forms are regulated by genes that play a critical role in the processing of the vitamin. There are a number of inherited metabolic errors that correspond to one or more of these specific steps and that result in characteristic syndromes affecting aspects of cobalamin metabolism that are discussed later in this chapter.

PLASMA HAPTOCORRIN (TRANSCOBALAMINS I AND III; "R" PROTEINS)

The HCs (previously known as R proteins) are a group of immunologically related proteins of apparent Mr approximately 60,000, consisting of a single polypeptide species variably substituted with oligosaccharides that terminate with different quantities of sialic acid.[123] They are found in milk, plasma, saliva, gastric juice, and numerous other body fluids. They appear to be synthesized by mucosal cells of the organs that secrete them[124] and by phagocytes.[125] Although the HCs bind cobalamin, they lack intrinsic factor activity, that is, they are unable to promote the intestinal absorption of the vitamin.

Plasma HC carries most (70 to 90 percent) of the circulating cobalamin. It contains nine potential glycosylation sites[126] and is encoded by a gene on chromosome 11, the same chromosome that carries the intrinsic factor gene.[127] In contrast to TC, HC clearance from the plasma is very slow (half-life [$T_{1/2}$]: 9 to 10 days).[128] The asialoglycoprotein receptor carries the cobalamin–HC complexes into the hepatocytes, where they are chiefly eliminated. The complexes are degraded, and their load of cobalamins is excreted in the bile.[106,129] HC binds its ligands more tightly than does either intrinsic factor or TC. Furthermore, HC is less restrictive than either intrinsic factor or TC with respect to ligand specificity; it avidly takes up corrinoids of widely varying structure.[130] The ligand-binding properties of HC and its mode of clearance by the liver suggest that HC helps clear the system of nonphysiologic cobalamin analogues that may have been acquired or may have arisen through degradation of cobalamin.[131,132] As the liver metabolizes analogue–HC complexes, it secretes the analogues into the bile. Because these analogues are bound poorly by intrinsic factor,[130] they are poorly reabsorbed from the intestine and are eliminated in the feces. The precise role of HC is unknown, although it may play a role in the body economy of cobalamin by facilitating excretion of cobalamin analogues while conserving cobalamin through enterohepatic recycling. Additionally, it has been proposed that HC may serve an antimicrobial role.[64]

ASSAY OF SERUM COBALAMIN AND THE TRANSCOBALAMINS

As with folate, cobalamin is usually measured with automated competitive displacement assays using intrinsic factor as a cobalamin-binding protein. The misleading results previously provided by competitive ligand displacement assays were explained by the discovery in serum and tissue of a class of cobalamin analogues that are detected by the radioisotope assay when HC-type proteins and not intrinsic factor were used as the binding protein.[133] Current assays use intrinsic factor as the binder and give more reliable values for serum cobalamin. The chemical nature and biologic significance of the analogues are unknown,[134] but recent evidence suggests that they may arise in the gastrointestinal tract.[131,132]

TC and HC are present in plasma in trace quantities (approximately 7 and 20 mcg/L, respectively). In fasting plasma, at least 70 percent of the circulating cobalamin is bound to HC.[135] TC binds only 10 to 25 percent of the total plasma cobalamin,[136] but provides the majority (approximately 75 percent) of the total unsaturated cobalamin-binding capacity of plasma.[135] Table 41–3 lists alterations in unsaturated cobalamin-binding capacity and in HC and TC levels in various disease states. In recent years, assays have been developed that measure the fraction of the plasma cobalamin that is bound to TC. This component, known as holotranscobalamin (holoTC), shows improved specificity compared with the standard cobalamin assay for identifying true cobalamin deficiency, although the assays appear to be generally comparable with respect to sensitivity.[137–143]

⬤ MEGALOBLASTIC ANEMIAS

DEFINITION

Megaloblastic anemias are disorders caused by impaired DNA synthesis. The presence of megaloblastic cells is the morphologic hallmark of this group of anemias. Megaloblastic red cell precursors are larger than normal and have more cytoplasm relative to the size of the nucleus. Promegaloblasts show a blue granule-free cytoplasm and a fine "salt and pepper" granular chromatin that contrasts with the ground-glass texture of its normal counterpart. As the cell differentiates, the chromatin condenses more slowly than normal into darker aggregates that coalesce, but do not fuse homogeneously, giving the nucleus a characteristic fenestrated appearance. Continuing maturation of the cytoplasm as it acquires hemoglobin contrasts with the immature-looking nucleus—a feature termed *nuclear-cytoplasmic asynchrony.*

TABLE 41–3. Levels and Binding Capacity of Cobalamin-Binding Proteins in Disease

Binder	Disease
Increased HC (TCI, R protein)	Myeloproliferative disorders
	Polycythemia vera
	Myelofibrosis
	Benign neutrophilia
	Chronic myelocytic leukemia
	Hepatoma (occasionally)
	Metastatic cancer
Increased TC	Myeloproliferative disorders
	Liver disease
	Inflammatory disorders
	Gaucher disease
	Anti-TC antibodies
Unsaturated cobalamin binders	
Increased	Transient neutropenia
	Elevated HC
Decreased	Liver disease
	Elevated serum cobalamin

Data from Lawler S, Roberts P, Hoffbrand A: Chromosome studies in megaloblastic anaemia before and after treatment. *Scand J Haematol* 8(4):309–320, 1971.

Megaloblastic granulocyte precursors are also larger than normal and show nuclear-cytoplasmic asynchrony. A characteristic cell is the *giant metamyelocyte,* which has a large horseshoe-shaped nucleus, sometimes irregularly shaped, containing ragged open chromatin.

Megaloblastic megakaryocytes may be abnormally large and polylobated, with deficient granulation of the cytoplasm. In severe megaloblastosis, the nucleus may show detached lobes. Further details are provided in "Laboratory Features" below and in Figs. 41–12 and 41–13.

ETIOLOGY AND PATHOGENESIS

Table 41–4 lists the causes of megaloblastic anemia. By far the most common causes worldwide are folate deficiency and cobalamin deficiency. There has, however, been a marked reduction in the prevalence of folate deficiency in North America and a growing number of other countries that have implemented folic acid fortification of the food supply.

Megaloblastic cells have much more cytoplasm and RNA than do their normal counterparts, but they have a relatively normal amount of DNA,[144] suggesting that cytoplasmic constituents (RNA and protein) are synthesized faster than is DNA. Evidence that maturation is retarded in megaloblastic precursors supports this conclusion.[145] DNA synthesis is impaired,[146] and migration of the DNA replication fork and the joining of DNA fragments synthesized from the lagging strand (Okazaki fragments) are delayed,[147] and the S-phase is prolonged.[146]

Slowing of DNA replication in the megaloblastic anemias of folate and cobalamin deficiency appears to arise from failure of the folate-dependent conversion of dUMP to dTMP. Because of this failure, deoxyuridine triphosphate (dUTP) levels become abundant and because DNA polymerase is promiscuous with respect to its substrate specificity, allows dUTP to become incorporated into the DNA of folate-deficient cells in place of deoxythymidine triphosphate (dTTP).[148] DNA excision–repair mechanisms to repair the DNA by replacing uridine with

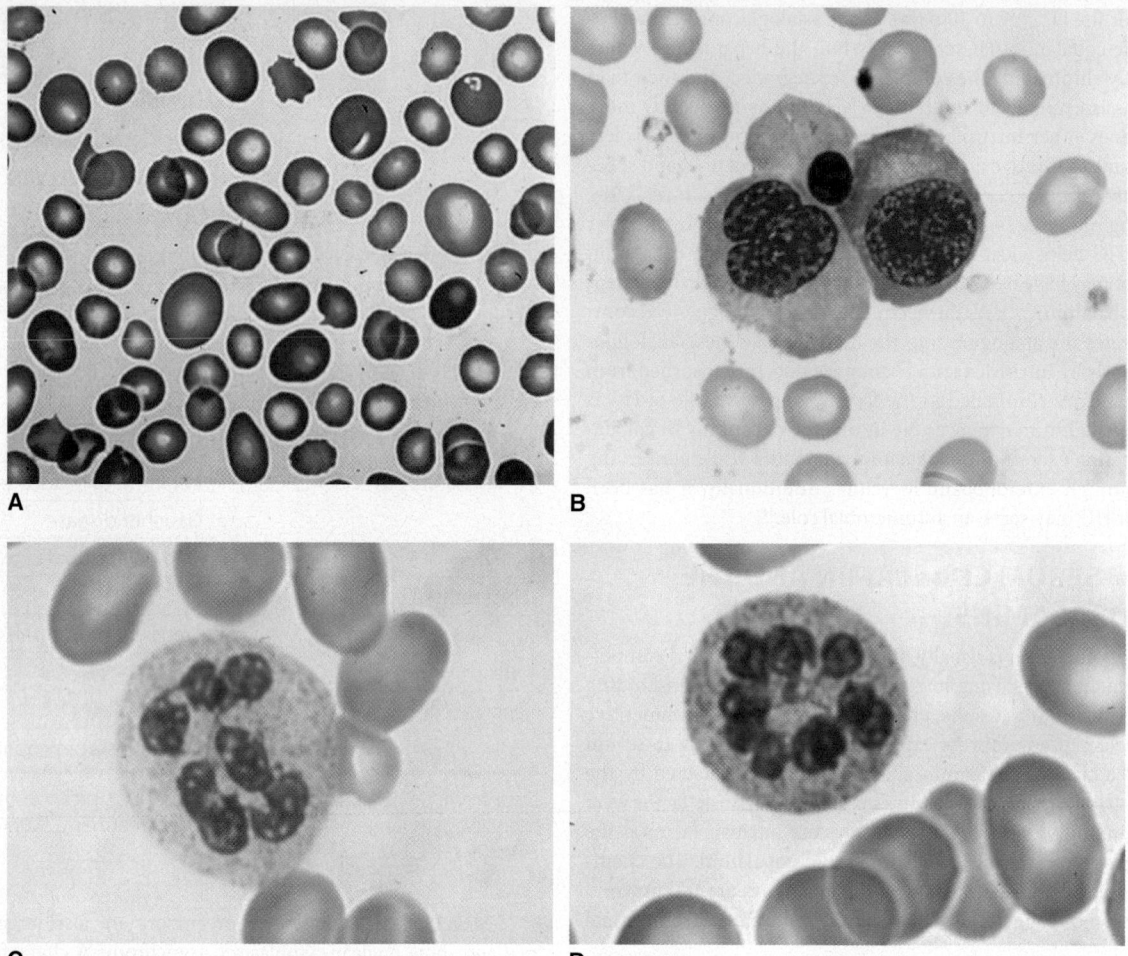

Figure 41–12. **A.** Pernicious anemia. Blood film. Note the striking oval macrocytes, wide variation in red cell size, and poikilocytes. Despite the anisocytosis and microcytes, the mean red cell volume is usually elevated, as in this case (mean corpuscular volume [MCV] = 121 fL). **B.** Marrow precursors in pernicious anemia. Note very large size of erythroblasts (megaloblasts) and asynchronous maturation. Cell on *right* is a polychromatophilic megaloblast with an immature nucleus for that stage of maturation. Cell on *left* is an orthochromatic megaloblast with a lobulated immature nucleus. An orthochromatic megaloblast with a condensed nucleus is between and above those two cells. **C** and **D.** Two examples of hypersegmented neutrophils characteristic of megaloblastic anemia. The morphology of blood and marrow cells in folate-deficient and vitamin B$_{12}$-deficient patients is identical. The extent of the morphologic changes in each case is related to the severity of the vitamin deficiency. *(Reproduced with permission from Lichtman's Atlas of Hematology, www.accessmedicine.com.)*

thymidine fail for the same reason that uridine triphosphate was incorporated into the DNA in the first place. The result is a repetitive iteration of flawed DNA repair that ultimately leads to DNA strand breaks, fragmentation, and apoptotic cell death.[149]

Addition of deoxyuridine (dU) to marrow cells in culture normally decreases the incorporation of tritiated thymidine into DNA, because the dU is converted via dUMP→dTMP to unlabeled dTTP, which competes with the tritiated thymidine. In megaloblastic cells, this effect of added dU is greatly diminished. This finding is consistent with impairment in the dUMP→dTMP reaction in the megaloblastic cells and was the basis for the now defunct *dU suppression test*.[150] The failed excision–repair model following dUTP misincorporation into DNA also explains the chromosome breaks and other abnormalities that occur in megaloblastic cells.[151]

CLINICAL FEATURES

All megaloblastic anemias share certain general clinical features. Because the anemia develops slowly, with opportunity for cardiopulmonary and intraerythrocytic compensatory changes,[152] it produces few symptoms until the hematocrit is severely depressed. Symptoms, when they appear, are those of anemia: weakness, palpitation, fatigue, lightheadedness, and shortness of breath. The blending of severe pallor and slight jaundice caused by a combination of intramedullary and extravascular hemolysis produce a characteristic lemon-yellow skin. Leukocyte and platelet counts may be low, but rarely cause clinical problems. Details of the clinical manifestations are given in the sections on the specific forms of megaloblastic anemia later in this chapter.

LABORATORY FEATURES

Blood Cells

All cell lines are affected. Erythrocytes vary markedly in size and shape, often are large and oval, and in severe cases can show basophilic stippling and nuclear remnants (Cabot rings and Howell-Jolly bodies). Erythroid activity in the marrow is enhanced, although the megaloblastic cells usually die before they are released, accounting for the reduced reticulocyte count. The more severe the anemia, the more pronounced

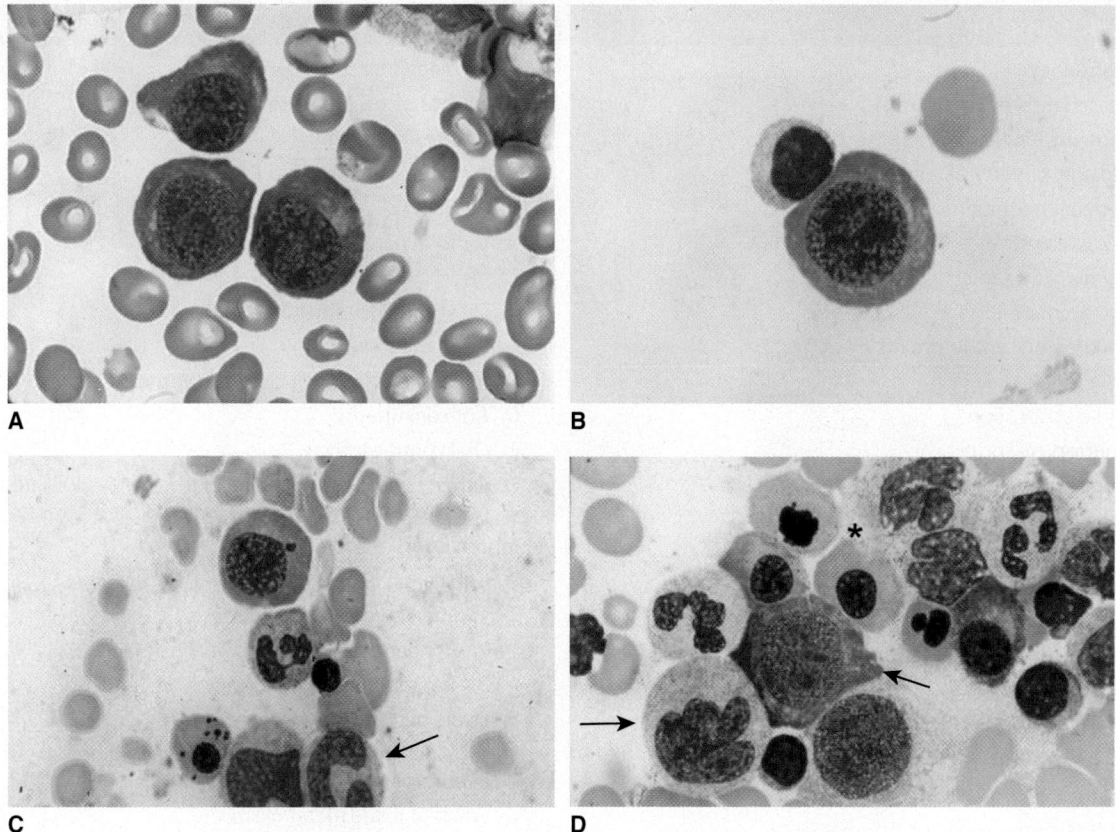

Figure 41–13. Marrow films. Megaloblastic anemia. Patient with pernicious anemia (vitamin B_{12} deficiency). **A.** Basophilic megaloblasts. Large cell size, very characteristic nuclear chromatin pattern with exaggerated proportion of euchromatin. **B.** Polychromatophilic megaloblast. Very large cell size for maturational stage. Large nuclear size and abnormally large proportion of euchromatin without appropriate nuclear condensation at this stage of maturation. Adjacent lymphocyte. **C.** Polychromatophilic megaloblast with small nuclear fragment. *Arrow* indicates giant band neutrophil. At lower left is orthochromatic megaloblast with multiple nuclear fragments. **D.** *Oblique arrow* indicates promegaloblast. *Horizontal arrow* indicates giant band neutrophil. To the left of and below the *asterisk* are four orthochromatic megaloblasts—large cell size for maturational stage: two with delayed nuclear condensation and two with condensed nuclei with abnormal nuclear margins showing small or large budding nuclei. To the right of the asterisk are two giant band neutrophils. On the right at midfield is a plasma cell below which is a lymphocyte. *(Reproduced with permission from Lichtman's Atlas of Hematology, www.accessmedicine.com.)*

the morphologic changes in the red cells. When the hematocrit is less than 20 percent, erythroblasts with megaloblastic nuclei, including an occasional promegaloblast, may appear in the blood. The anemia is macrocytic (mean corpuscular volume [MCV] is 100 to 150 fL or more), although coexisting iron deficiency, thalassemia trait,[153] or inflammation can prevent macrocytosis.[154] Slight macrocytosis may be the earliest sign of megaloblastic anemia. Because of the progressive nature of gradual replacement of normocytic red cells with the macrocytic progeny of a megaloblastic marrow, the earliest observable change in red cell indices is an increase in the red cell distribution width (RDW), reflecting an increase in anisocytosis.

Neutrophil nuclei often have more than the usual three to five lobes (see Fig. 41–12).[155] Typically, more than 5 percent of the neutrophils have five lobes. Cells may contain six or more lobes, a morphology rarely seen in normal neutrophils but not pathognomonic of megaloblastic hematopoiesis. In nutritional megaloblastic anemias caused by folate deficiency, hypersegmented neutrophils are an early sign of megaloblastosis[5] and persist in the blood for many days after treatment.[155] Neutrophil hypersegmentation was not found to be a sensitive test for mild cobalamin deficiency.[156] Cytogenetic studies are nonspecific and show chromosomes that are elongated and broken. Specific therapy corrects these abnormalities, usually within 2 days, although some abnormalities do not disappear for months.[151,157] Platelets are often

reduced in number and slightly smaller than normal with a wider variation in size (increased platelet distribution width [PDW]).[158] The morphologic features of megaloblastic anemia may be grossly exaggerated in patients who have been splenectomized or lack a functional spleen as occurs in celiac disease or sickle cell anemia. Numerous circulating megaloblasts and bizarre red cell morphology may be present.[159]

Marrow

Aspirated marrow is cellular and shows striking megaloblastic changes, especially in the erythroid series with well-hemoglobinized erythroblasts containing nuclei that possess less-mature, more-open nuclear chromatin than their normal counterparts. There is a preponderance of earlier basophilic erythroblasts over more mature forms which gives the overall impression of a maturation arrest (see Fig. 41–13). Sideroblasts are increased in number and contain increased numbers of iron granules. The ratio of myeloid to erythroid precursors falls to 1:1 or lower, and granulocyte reserves may be decreased. In severe cases, promegaloblasts containing an unusually large number of mitotic figures are plentiful. Macrophage iron content often is increased. Megaloblastic features in the granulocytic series is also usually present with giant forms and large horseshoe-shaped nuclei. Occasionally megakaryocytes with hyperlobated nuclei are present.

TABLE 41–4. Causes of Megaloblastic Anemias

I. Folate Deficiency
   A. Decreased intake
      1. Poor nutrition
      2. Old age, poverty, alcoholism
      3. Hyperalimentation
      4. Hemodialysis
      5. Premature infants
      6. Spinal cord injury
      7. Children on synthetic diets
      8. Goat's milk anemia
   B. Impaired absorption
      1. Nontropical sprue
      2. Tropical sprue
      3. Other disease of the small intestine
   C. Increased requirements
      1. Pregnancy
      2. Increased cell turnover
      3. Chronic hemolytic anemia
      4. Exfoliative dermatitis
II. Cobalamin Deficiency
   A. Impaired absorption
      1. Gastric causes
         a. Pernicious anemia
         b. Gastrectomy
         c. Zollinger-Ellison syndrome
      2. Intestinal causes
         a. Ileal resection or disease
         b. Blind loop syndrome
         c. Fish tapeworm
      3. Pancreatic insufficiency
   B. Decreased intake
      1. Vegans

III. Acute Megaloblastic Anemia
   A. Nitrous oxide exposure
   B. Severe illness with
      1. Extensive transfusion
      2. Dialysis
      3. Total parenteral nutrition
IV. Drugs
   A. Dihydrofolate reductase inhibitors
   B. Antimetabolites
   C. Inhibitors of deoxynucleotide synthesis
   D. Anticonvulsants
   E. Oral contraceptives
   F. Others, such as long-term exposure to weak folate antagonists (e.g., trimethoprim or low-dose methotrexate)
V. Inborn Errors
   A. Cobalamin deficiency
      1. Imerslund-Gräsbeck disease
      2. Congenital deficiency of intrinsic factor
      3. Transcobalamin deficiency
   B. Errors of cobalamin metabolism
      1. "Cobalamin mutant" syndromes with homocystinuria and/or methylmalonic acidemia
   C. Errors of folate metabolism
      1. Congenital folate malabsorption
      2. Dihydrofolate reductase deficiency
      3. N^5-methyltetrahydrofolate homocysteine-methyltransferase deficiency
   D. Other errors
      1. Hereditary orotic aciduria
      2. Lesch-Nyhan syndrome
      3. Thiamine-responsive megaloblastic anemia
VI. Unexplained
   A. Congenital dyserythropoietic anemia
   B. Refractory megaloblastic anemia
   C. Erythroleukemia

Coexisting Microcytic Anemia

Many features of megaloblastic anemia may be masked when megaloblastic anemia is combined with a microcytic anemia.[154] The anemia can be normocytic or even microcytic, whereas the blood film may show both microcytes and macroovalocytes (a "dimorphic anemia"). The marrow may contain "intermediate" megaloblasts[160] that are smaller and look less "megaloblastic" than usual. In this kind of mixed anemia, the microcytic component usually is iron-deficiency anemia,[154] but it may be thalassemia minor[153] or the anemia of chronic disease. Even megaloblastic anemia masked by a severe microcytic anemia usually shows hypersegmented neutrophils in the blood and giant metamyelocytes and bands in the marrow. Neutrophil myeloperoxidase levels are high.[161]

Less commonly, the megaloblastic component of a mixed iron-deficiency anemia can be overlooked, and the patient may be treated only with iron. In this situation, the anemia may respond only partly to therapy, and megaloblastic features become more conspicuous as iron stores fill. The masking of macrocytosis in these situations may be responsible for delay or difficulty in diagnosis of pernicious anemia, particularly in certain geographic areas and ethnic groups where there is a high incidence of thalassemia and microcytic hemoglobinopathies.[153,162,163] There are several situations that favor the coexistence of a megaloblastic state with iron deficiency. Both folate and iron deficiency occur in celiac disease,[164] and cobalamin and iron deficiency both complicate gastric reduction surgery for morbid obesity.[165] Furthermore, *Helicobacter pylori* infection is associated with gastric atrophy that can result first in iron deficiency and later lead to cobalamin malabsorption and perhaps even predispose to pernicious anemia.[166,167]

Incomplete Megaloblastic Anemia

If a patient with a full-blown megaloblastic anemia receives cobalamin or folate before marrow aspiration, the anemia persists but the megaloblastic changes may be obscured. Attenuated megaloblastic changes also are seen in patients with early megaloblastic anemia, in patients with coexisting infection,[154] or in patients after transfusion.

Megaloblastic Anemia Misdiagnosed as Acute Leukemia

Occasionally, very severe megaloblastic anemia produces marrow morphology so bizarre as to be mistaken for acute leukemia. In some cases, the erythroid series does not mature, and the megaloblastic pronormoblast dominates the marrow with prominent mitotic figures and dysmorphic forms, raising the possibility of erythroid leukemia.

Megaloblastic Changes in Other Cells

In most forms of megaloblastic anemia, cytologic abnormalities resembling megaloblastosis may appear in other proliferating cells. Epithelial cells from the mouth, stomach, small intestine, and cervix uteri may look megaloblastic, appearing larger than their normal counterparts and containing atypical immature-looking nuclei. Distinguishing these "megaloblastic" changes from the changes of malignancy may be difficult.[168]

Chemical Changes in Body Fluids

Plasma bilirubin, iron, and ferritin levels are increased.[169] Serum lactate dehydrogenase-1 (LDH-1) and LDH-2, both found in red cells, are markedly elevated as a result of rapid intramedullary erythroblast turnover and increase with the severity of the anemia.[170] In megaloblastic anemia LDH-1 is greater than LDH-2, whereas in other anemias LDH-2 is greater than LDH-1.[171] Serum muramidase (lysozyme) levels are high,[172] whereas serum glutamic oxaloacetic transaminase (aspartate transaminase [AST]) is normal.[173] Erythropoietin levels rise, but less than in other anemias of similar severity.[174] Surprisingly, the elevated erythropoietin levels fall sharply within 1 day of beginning treatment, an interval too short either to have been mediated by the hematocrit or to affect it.

Cytokinetics

Megaloblastic anemia is associated with two pathophysiologic abnormalities: *ineffective erythropoiesis* and *hemolysis*. Ineffective erythropoiesis increases the red cell precursor to reticulocyte ratio, plasma iron turnover,[175] LDH-1 and LDH-2 levels,[171] and "early labeled" bilirubin.[176] Both intramedullary and extramedullary hemolysis occurs in megaloblastic anemia, with red cell life span decreased by 30 to 50 percent.[177]

Increased serum muramidase in megaloblastic anemia can be caused by increased granulocyte turnover,[172] possibly induced by disintegration of granulocyte precursors in the marrow (ineffective granulopoiesis). In cobalamin deficiency, platelet production is only 10 percent of that expected from the megakaryocyte mass,[178] perhaps reflecting ineffective thrombopoiesis. Platelets in severe cobalamin deficiency are functionally abnormal.[179]

FOLIC ACID DEFICIENCY

Etiology and Pathogenesis

Folate deficiency is caused by (1) dietary deficiency, (2) impaired absorption, and (3) increased requirements or losses (see Table 41–4).

Decreased Intake Caused by Poor Nutrition Prior to the mid-1990s, inadequate dietary intake was the major cause of folate deficiency. However, in the era of folic acid fortification, the prevalence of folate deficiency has fallen dramatically. In the United States, the prevalence of low plasma folate has dropped from 22 to 1.7 percent of the population.[180] Because folate reserves are limited, deficiency develops rapidly in malnourished persons, typically the old, the poor, and the alcoholic. Folate deficiency can also occur during hyperalimentation[181] and subclinical folate deficiency has been reported in subtotal gastrectomy.[182] Folate deficiency can occur in premature infants, especially with infection, diarrhea, or hemolytic anemia[183]; in children on a synthetic diet because of inborn errors[184]; and in infants raised on goat's milk, which is poor in available folate.[185] Destruction of folate through excessive cooking can aggravate folate deficiency.

In alcoholic cirrhosis, megaloblastic anemia usually is caused by folate deficiency.[186] Alcohol may acutely depress serum folate, even if folate stores are replete,[187] and accelerates the development of megaloblastic anemia in persons with early folate deficiency.[188] Alcohol causes acute marrow suppression, decreases in reticulocyte, platelet, and granulocyte levels[189]; reversible vacuolation of erythroid and myeloid precursors; and dysfunction of granulocytes.[190] These changes occur even if large doses of folate are given with the alcohol.[191]

Decreased Intake Caused by Impaired Absorption Nontropical Sprue Nontropical sprue (*celiac disease* in children) is related to ingestion of wheat gluten.[192] Pathologically, nontropical sprue shows atrophy and chronic inflammation of the small intestinal mucosa that is most severe proximally. Findings include weight loss; glossitis (typical of folate deficiency); other signs of a generalized vitamin deficiency; diarrhea; and passage of light-colored, bulky stools with a particularly foul odor caused by steatorrhea. Iron deficiency, hypocalcemia, osteoporosis, and osteomalacia may occur.

Folate malabsorption occurs in most patients with this disorder.[193] Serum folate levels are low,[194] and megaloblastic anemia occurs frequently.

Tropical Sprue Tropical sprue is endemic in the West Indies, southern India, parts of Southern Africa, and Southeast Asia. It can be acquired by travelers to those regions and persists for many years after the travelers return.[195] Tropical sprue is rapidly corrected by folate therapy, even though folate deficiency does not cause the disease. The precise etiology of tropical sprue is unknown, although the response of the disease to antibiotics suggests infection.[196]

Clinically and pathologically, tropical sprue is like nontropical sprue, except that tropical sprue is more severe in the distal small intestine.[197] Therefore, tropical sprue eventually also leads to cobalamin deficiency[198] and should be strongly considered as a cause of cobalamin deficiency in former residents of the tropics, even though they have been away from the tropics for 20 years or more. Folate malabsorption may occur,[199] possibly because the diseased intestine fails to deconjugate folate polyglutamates.[200] Consequently, megaloblastic anemia is very common in patients with this disease,[201] and may result from both folate and cobalamin deficiency.

Other Intestinal Disorders Malabsorption of folic acid commonly occurs in regional enteritis,[201] after extensive resections of the small intestine,[202] and in conditions such as lymphomatous or leukemic infiltration of the small intestine,[203] Whipple disease,[203] scleroderma and amyloidosis,[204] and diabetes mellitus.[205] Systemic bacterial infections impair folate absorption.[206]

Increased Folate Requirements in Pregnancy During pregnancy (Chap. 8),[207] folate requirements increase five- to 10-fold because of transfer of folate to the growing fetus,[208] which draws down maternal folate stores even in the face of severe maternal folate deficiency.[209] Further increases in requirements may result from the presence of multiple fetuses, a poor diet, infection, coexisting hemolytic anemia, or anticonvulsant medication. Lactation aggravates folate deficiency.[210] Consequently, folate deficiency is very common in pregnancy and is the major cause of the megaloblastic anemia of pregnancy,[211] particularly in developing countries.[212]

Folate deficiency is difficult to diagnose in pregnancy because the signs of deficiency are obscured by the normal hematologic changes of pregnancy. During pregnancy, a physiologic "anemia" develops because of increased plasma volume that is only partly offset by an accompanying increase in red cell mass. Hemoglobin levels may fall to 10 g/dL. The anemia is associated with a physiologic macrocytosis; MCV may increase to 120 fL, although the average at term is 104 fL.[213] Serum and red cell folate levels fall steadily during pregnancy, even in well-nourished women who are not taking a folic acid supplement.[214] Conversely, hypersegmented neutrophils, usually a reliable clue to early megaloblastic anemia, are inconspicuous in early megaloblastic anemia of pregnancy.[215]

Increased Cell Turnover Because of increased marrow cell turnover, the folate requirement rises sharply in chronic *hemolytic anemia*.[216] During bouts of acute hemolysis that can occur in these anemias, the marrow may become megaloblastic within days.

Folic acid deficiency may arise in chronic *exfoliative dermatitis*, in which folate losses of 5 to 20 mcg/day may occur.[217] Patients with psoriasis who are treated with methotrexate have an added reason for developing signs of folate deficiency. Pretreating such patients with folate may prevent these signs without impairing the therapeutic effect of methotrexate.[217] During hemodialysis, folate is lost in the dialysis fluid.[218]

Clinical Features

The clinical picture of folate deficiency includes all the general manifestations of megaloblastic anemia *plus* the following specific features: (1) a history and laboratory studies indicating folate deficiency, (2) absence of the neurologic signs of cobalamin deficiency (see "Cobalamin Deficiency" below), and (3) a full response to *physiologic* doses of folate.

Laboratory Features

The earliest specific indicator of folate deficiency is a low serum or plasma folate. Raised plasma levels of homocysteine may precede the lowering of plasma folate. However, elevated homocysteine has poor specificity as there are several causes of a raised plasma homocysteine.[219] Plasma folate follows folate intake closely, so an isolated low serum folate (less than approximately 3 ng/mL) may simply indicate a drop in folate intake over the preceding few days.[5] Similarly, a low plasma folate, except in malabsorption, rises quickly on refeeding.

A better indicator of the tissue folate status is the red cell folate,[220] which remains relatively unchanged while a red cell is circulating and thus reflects folate status over the preceding 2 to 3 months. Red cell folate usually is quite low in folate-deficient megaloblastic anemia. However, red cell folate also is low in more than 50 percent of patients with cobalamin-deficient megaloblastic anemia[100] owing to the poor retention of methyltetrahydrofolate monoglutamate within the cells; consequently, red cell folate cannot be used to distinguish between folate and cobalamin deficiencies. Conversely, red cell folate may be normal in the megaloblastic state that occurs, often with little accompanying anemia, in rapidly developing folate deficiency (see "Acute Megaloblastic Anemia" below).[221]

The dU suppression test has been used in research on pathogenetic mechanisms in megaloblastic states. It adds little to the clinical evaluation of a megaloblastic anemia. The test is further discussed in "Deoxyuridine Suppression" below.

Differential Diagnosis

Macrocytosis without megaloblastic anemia occurs in alcoholism, liver disease, hypothyroidism, aplastic anemia, certain forms of myelodysplasia, pregnancy, and any condition associated with reticulocytosis (e.g., autoimmune hemolytic anemia). Macrocytosis has also been reported among smokers.[222] However, MCV rarely exceeds 110 fL in these conditions, whereas in folate deficiency, uncomplicated by causes of microcytosis, the MCV is usually over 110 fL.

A full hematologic response to physiologic doses of folate (i.e., 200 mcg daily) distinguishes folate deficiency from cobalamin deficiency, in which a response occurs only at pharmacologic doses of folate (e.g., 5 mg daily). This is not recommended as a diagnostic test because

neurologic problems may develop in cobalamin-deficient patients treated with folate alone. High doses of cobalamin may produce a partial response in folate deficiency.[73]

The diagnosis of nontropical sprue rests on (1) the demonstration of malabsorption, (2) noninvasive serologic testing including detection of antibodies to gliadin, endomysium, tissue transglutaminase, and deamidated gliadin,[223] (3) a jejunal biopsy showing villus atrophy, and (4) the response to a gluten-free diet. In 80 percent of patients, a gluten-free diet gradually reverses the functional disorder by correcting folate malabsorption.[224]

Nonhematologic Effects of Folate Deficiency

The hematologic problems associated with folate deficiency have been recognized for decades. However, folate deficiency has been associated with a number of serious disorders not involving the hematopoietic system. Moreover, these disorders occur at folate levels usually regarded as low normal. They include developmental, neurologic, cardiovascular, and neoplasic diseases.[225]

Abnormalities of Neural Tube Closure

A close association exists between mild folate deficiency and congenital anomalies of the fetus, most notably defects in neural tube closure, but also abnormalities involving the heart, urinary tract, limbs, and other sites.[226] A portion of the neural tube closure defects appear to be associated with antibodies against folate receptors that may be overcome by higher folate intake.[227] Mutations and polymorphisms affecting enzymes of folate metabolism, especially the common 677C→T polymorphism of the *MTHFR* gene (also designated as *MTHFR* 677C→T),[228] also predispose to congenital anomalies. As noted above, this polymorphism results in diminished conversion of its substrate methylene FH_4 to methyltetrahydrofolate, supporting the view that it is the role of folate in methylation through methionine synthesis (see Table 41–1) that is critical in embryonic development. Folic acid fortification programs, which were mandated in the United States and Canada in the mid-1990s, have been highly successful as a public health measure in reducing the incidence of neural tube defect births by between 20 and 50 percent.[229,230]

Cobalamin also plays a significant role as a risk factor for neural tube defects. Levels of TC in normal pregnant women correlate with their likelihood of bearing an infant with a defect in neural tube closure. Patients in the lowest quintile of TC concentration are five times more likely to give birth to a defective infant as patients in the highest quintile.[231] Evidence indicates that in populations exposed to folic acid fortification, there is an approximately threefold increase in the risk of neural tube defects in offspring of mothers in the lowest quartile of TC.[232]

Several poorly defined neuropsychiatric abnormalities that respond to folate therapy have been reported in patients with folate deficiency. The most convincing associations are with depressive illness.[225,233]

Vascular Disease

Even a mildly elevated homocysteine level is a major independent risk factor for atherosclerosis and venous thrombosis, possibly because of an effect on the vascular endothelium.[234] In folate deficiency, homocysteine levels may rise considerably, resulting in varying degrees of hyperhomocysteinemia. This is true also in cobalamin and pyridoxine deficiencies; consequently, the notion of seeking to ameliorate hyperhomocysteinemia and thus diminish the risk of cardiovascular disease has seemed appealing. However, the effect of lowering homocysteine levels by the use of folate, cobalamin, and pyridoxine supplements, on the risk of recurrent vascular disease is unclear. Although there is some evidence that such supplements reduce risk,[235] contradictory evidence suggests that supplement use may actually increase the risk of in-stent coronary restenosis[236] or other adverse cardiovascular outcome.[237] On the other hand, an accelerated rate of decrease in stroke mortality has been observed in the United States and Canada that coincided with the introduction of folic acid fortification in these countries.[238] The disparate designs of these studies makes it difficult to draw firm conclusions regarding the question of whether lowering of plasma homocysteine in subjects at risk for cardiovascular disease has any ameliorative or deleterious effect on outcome. In a meta-analysis of eight randomized trials involving over 37,000 individuals, the authors concluded that supplementation with folic acid in various combinations with vitamin B$_{12}$ and vitamin B$_6$ for periods of up to 7.3 years, despite an overall reduction of plasma homocysteine of 22 percent and 25 percent in folic acid fortified and non-fortified populations, respectively, there were no significant effects on cardiovascular events, overall cancer, or mortality.[239] Critical factors might relate to several considerations including the preexisting degree of vascular damage in relation to the time of the intervention and the form and dosage of administered vitamins.

Another potential link between folate deficiency and morbidity risk that relates to hyperhomocysteinemia is the association between elevated homocysteine levels and incident dementia or cognitive impairment without dementia, independent of the vascular complications of hyperhomocysteinemia.[240,241] The *MTHFR* polymorphism *MTHFR* 677C→T leads to increased homocysteine levels in subjects with low folate or cobalamin levels,[242] although controversy exists as to whether *MTHFR* 677C→T contributes to an increased incidence of vascular disease. Like folate, cobalamin seems to be important in decreasing the risk of vascular disease.[243] A 1561C→T polymorphism in the gene for glutamate carboxypeptidase-II increases serum folate and decreases serum homocysteine in the homozygote, possibly protecting against vascular disease.[244]

HELLP Syndrome

Severe folate deficiency reportedly mimics the hemolysis, elevated liver enzymes, low platelets (HELLP) syndrome (preeclampsia with liver swelling and abnormal liver function studies in pregnant women; Chap. 8).[245] In these patients, the diagnosis of severe folate deficiency can be made based on the presence of anemia and a megaloblastic blood film and marrow. Serum and red cell folate, serum cobalamin, homocysteine, and methylmalonic acid levels all should be assayed before treatment is started.[246] The patient should immediately be given high doses of folate plus cobalamin, the latter in case the megaloblastic anemia actually results from cobalamin deficiency, a possibility rendered more likely in folic acid-fortified populations. A major goal of treatment is preventing preterm delivery of the fetus.

Colon Cancer

A large study of nurses in the United States indicated that supplementation with more than 400 mcg of folic acid per day reduces the incidence of colon cancer by 31 percent.[247] Furthermore, individuals who are homozygous for the 677C→T *MTHFR* mutation also have a decreased incidence for colon cancer compared with 677C→T heterozygotes and normal controls.[248] Other evidence points to possible deleterious effect of folic acid on colon cancer incidence. Although only circumstantial, a recent epidemiologic study reported that after several successive years of a declining incidence of colorectal cancer in the United States and Canada, there was a significant increase in the rate in both countries that coincided with and followed the introduction of folic acid fortification.[249] These apparently contradictory observations may be reconcilable because of the several roles of folate on cellular proliferation and repair as well as on the stage of tumorigenesis.[250] Because folate is critical for *de novo* thymidine synthesis, it plays an important part in DNA repair, thus correcting mutations and DNA strand breaks that could

potentially initiate cancer. On the other hand, the growth of established neoplastic clones might be accelerated by additional folate, allowing more rapid tumor progression. The situation is rendered even more complex if the potential role of folate in epigenetic regulation of gene expression is considered. Folate is necessary for synthesis of the universal methyl donor, SAMe, which is required for both cytosine and histone methylation. In this pathway, too, the role of folate theoretically may be cancer promoting or cancer protective, depending on whether oncogenes or tumor-suppressor genes are silenced by methylation of CpG islands in DNA or by conformational changes in chromatin resulting from histone methylation. The question of a possible effect of increased folate intake through the use of folic acid supplements on overall and site-specific cancer incidence was recently examined in a meta-analysis of 50,000 individuals. The authors concluded that there was no substantial increase or decrease in incidence over a 5-year period of folic acid supplement use.[251]

Therapy, Course, and Prognosis

Folate, usually in the form of folic acid, 1 to 5 mg/day, is given orally, although 1 mg usually is sufficient. At this dose, anemia usually is corrected even in patients with malabsorption. A parenteral preparation containing 5 mg/mL of folate also is available.

Treatment for *tropical sprue* consists of the usual doses of folate, plus cobalamin if indicated. To prevent relapse, treatment should be maintained for at least 2 years. Broad-spectrum antibiotics are helpful adjuncts, although antibiotics alone fail to correct the condition.

Pregnant women must be given at least 400 mcg of folate per day.[252] As to the possibility of overlooking cobalamin deficiency resulting from folate administration, although pernicious anemia (PA) in women of childbearing age is rare in whites, this is not the case among persons of African and Hispanic descent.[253,254] In pregnant women at risk for cobalamin deficiency (e.g., vegans or patients with malabsorption), the risk of an associated cobalamin deficiency is easily prevented with vitamin B$_{12}$, 1 mg given parenterally every 3 months during the pregnancy.

Therapeutic doses of folate partially and temporarily correct the hematologic abnormalities in cobalamin deficiency, but the neurologic manifestations can progress, with disastrous results.[255] Therefore, both folate status and cobalamin status must be evaluated early in the workup of a megaloblastic anemia. If treatment is urgent and the nature of the deficiency is unclear, both folate and cobalamin can be given after suitable specimens have been obtained for assay.

Patients who receive low-dose methotrexate therapy as an immunosuppressant may develop side effects, the worst of which is hepatotoxicity. The incidence of side effects, including hepatotoxicity, has been correlated with reduced folate levels.[256] Administration of folic or folinic acid can prevent or greatly diminish the major side effects without reducing the therapeutic effect of low-dose methotrexate. Coadministration of folic acid together with vitamin B$_{12}$ also reduces side-effects without adversely affecting the therapeutic efficacy of the newer multitargeted antifolate drug, pemetrexed.[257]

COBALAMIN DEFICIENCY
Etiology and Pathogenesis

There are several causes and varying degrees of severity of cobalamin depletion and deficiency. From the hematologic standpoint, it is convenient to divide the causes of B$_{12}$ deficiency into those that frequently lead to megaloblastic anemia and those that usually do not.[64,258]

Table 41–4 lists disorders that lead to cobalamin deficiency.

Decreased Uptake Caused by Impaired Absorption Cobalamin deficiency most often results from defective absorption, most commonly PA, a condition characterized by failure of gastric intrinsic factor production. Many other causes of defective cobalamin absorption involve mainly the stomach, or small intestine and to lesser extent, the pancreas.

Gastric Disorders in Pernicious Anemia PA is a disease of insidious onset that generally begins in middle age or later (usually after age 40 years).[259] In this condition, intrinsic factor secretion fails because of gastric mucosal atrophy. PA is an autoimmune disease. The gastric atrophy of PA probably results from immune destruction of the acid- and pepsin-secreting portion of the gastric mucosa. The term *pernicious anemia* sometimes is used as a synonym for cobalamin deficiency, but it should be reserved for the condition resulting from defective secretion of intrinsic factor by an atrophic gastric mucosa caused by an autoimmune process primarily directed against the parietal cells and their products.

In patients with PA, antibodies occur that recognize the H+/K+-adenosine triphosphatase (ATPase), which resides in the secretory membrane of the parietal cell and is responsible for acidifying the stomach contents. These antiparietal cell antibodies occur in approximately 60 percent of patients with simple atrophic gastritis and in 90 percent of patients with PA, but in only 5 percent of a random 30- to 60-year-old population.[260] Antiparietal cell antibodies also occur in a significant percentage of patients with thyroid disease.[261] Conversely, patients with PA have a higher than expected incidence of antibodies against thyroid epithelium, lymphocytes, and renal collecting duct cells.[262]

Antiparietal cell antibodies are not thought to be responsible for the pathogenesis of PA. Rather, studies in mice suggest the gastric atrophy in PA is caused by CD4+ T cells whose receptors recognize the H+/K+-ATPase. Thus, thymectomized BALB/c mice develop an autoimmune atrophic gastritis similar to that seen in PA patients. CD4+ T cells from these mice produce atrophic gastritis when injected into nude mice.[263]

Antibodies to intrinsic factor ("type I," or "blocking," antibodies) or the intrinsic factor–cobalamin (Cbl) complex ("type II," or "binding," antibodies) are highly specific to PA patients.[264] Blocking antibodies, which prevent formation of the intrinsic factor–Cbl complex, are found in up to 70 percent of PA sera.[264] Binding antibodies, which prevent the intrinsic factor–Cbl complex from binding to its ileal receptors, are found in about half the sera that contain blocking antibody. Some findings in humans support the idea that T cells are responsible for the gastric atrophy in PA. First, lymphocytes from patients with PA are hyperresponsive to gastric antigens.[265] Second, the incidence of PA is higher than expected in patients with agammaglobulinemia, even though their sera contain none of the antibodies typical of PA.[266]

Other Autoimmune Diseases The coexistence of several other autoimmune diseases and PA is further evidence that PA is an autoimmune disease. Antiparietal cell antibodies and PA are unexpectedly frequent in patients with other autoimmune diseases,[267] including autoimmune thyroid disorders (thyrotoxicosis, hypothyroidism, and Hashimoto thyroiditis),[268] type I diabetes mellitus, hypoparathyroidism,[269] Addison disease, postpartum hypophysitis,[270] vitiligo,[271] acquired agammaglobulinemia,[266] infertile female patients younger than age 40 years,[272] and hypospermia and infertility in males.[273,274] Infertility may, however, relate to impairment of DNA synthesis in gonadal cells rather than to an autoimmune mechanism.

Inherited Predisposition to Pernicious Anemia Predisposition to PA can be inherited. The disease is associated with human leukocyte antigen types A2, A3, B7, and B12,[275] and with blood group A.[276] PA and antiparietal cell antibodies occur more frequently than expected in the families of PA patients.[277] In one study, gastric atrophy was found in more than 30 percent of the relatives of patients with PA; of these relatives, 65 percent had antiparietal cell antibodies and 22 percent had antiintrinsic factor antibodies.[278] PA occurs relatively frequently

in northern Europeans (especially Scandinavians)[279] as well as Africans,[163,280] but is uncommon in Asians. In Americans of African descent, the disease tends to begin early, occurs with high frequency in women, and often is severe.[163,254]

Stomach and Intestine in Pernicious Anemia Gastric manifestations of PA include achlorhydria, acquired intrinsic factor deficiency previously demonstrable by the Schilling test, and an increased incidence of certain malignancies. There is an approximately twofold increase in the incidence of gastric cancer, similar increases in the incidence of certain hematologic malignancies, and an increase in the incidence of gastric carcinoid.[279] Achlorhydria may precede by many years the loss of intrinsic factor secretion and the development of PA.[281] The absence of achlorhydria excludes the diagnosis of PA. *H. pylori*, a microorganism that infects the gastric mucosa, is a major cause of gastritis and peptic ulcers. Evidence is conflicting regarding the role of *H. pylori* in PA. In two studies, cultures of gastric biopsies showed a very low incidence of *H. pylori* infection in PA patients.[282] One study reported that anti–*H. pylori* antibodies were found in only a small fraction of the sera from these patients. The other study reported that these antibodies were present in most of the PA sera, indicating that most of the patients described in the study had been infected previously. Whether *H. pylori* participates in the pathogenesis of PA is an open question. An intriguing hypothesis has been advanced that chronic infection with *H. pylori* may be responsible for triggering an autoimmune reaction directed against the host H+/K+-ATPase protein as a result of molecular mimicry.[167,283]

Fasting plasma gastrin levels are high in most patients with PA, whereas somatostatin levels are low.[284] In biopsies from PA stomachs, however, fundal gastrin and somatostatin levels were high, correlating with increases in argyrophilic cells in the basal crypts; antral gastrin and somatostatin were normal. Gastrin levels are high in simple achlorhydria without PA.[285]

The stomach shows characteristic histologic abnormalities in PA (Fig. 41–14). The mucosa of the cardia and fundus is atrophic, containing few chief (i.e., pepsin-secreting) or parietal cells. The withered mucosa is infiltrated with lymphocytes[286] and plasma cells. In contrast, the antral and pyloric mucosa are normal. Gastric atrophy is partly reversible by glucocorticoid treatment, with some regeneration and return of intrinsic factor secretion, further evidence for the autoimmune nature of PA.[287] Clinical response to administration of glucocorticoids or adrenocorticotropic hormone in patients with neurologic disease may reflect temporary amelioration of underlying and undiagnosed PA.[288]

Megaloblastic changes reversible by cobalamin are seen in the gastrointestinal epithelium. Cells recovered by lavage are large[168] and show atypical nuclei resembling early malignant change.[289] Small intestinal biopsy shows decreased mitoses in crypts, shortening of villi, megaloblastic changes in epithelial cells, and infiltration in the lamina propria.[290] These changes may account for the malabsorption of D-xylose and carotene observed in PA.[291]

Recognizing PA may be difficult. PA combines the general features of megaloblastic anemia and features specific for cobalamin deficiency with unique clinical features related to its (probable) autoimmune etiology and gastric pathology. The disease is easily missed because of its (1) insidious onset, (2) tendency to be masked by the use of multivitamin preparations containing folic acid,[292] and (3) many atypical presentations,[293] including its presentation as a neurologic disease without hematologic findings,[77,294] and its tendency to be overlooked in patients with another autoimmune disease.

Antiparietal cell and antiintrinsic factor antibodies are rarely measured, even though antiintrinsic factor antibodies in particular could be of considerable diagnostic value.[221] In the absence of a reliable method to assess vitamin B_{12} absorption, following the Schilling test becoming obsolete, measurement of antiintrinsic factor antibodies in serum

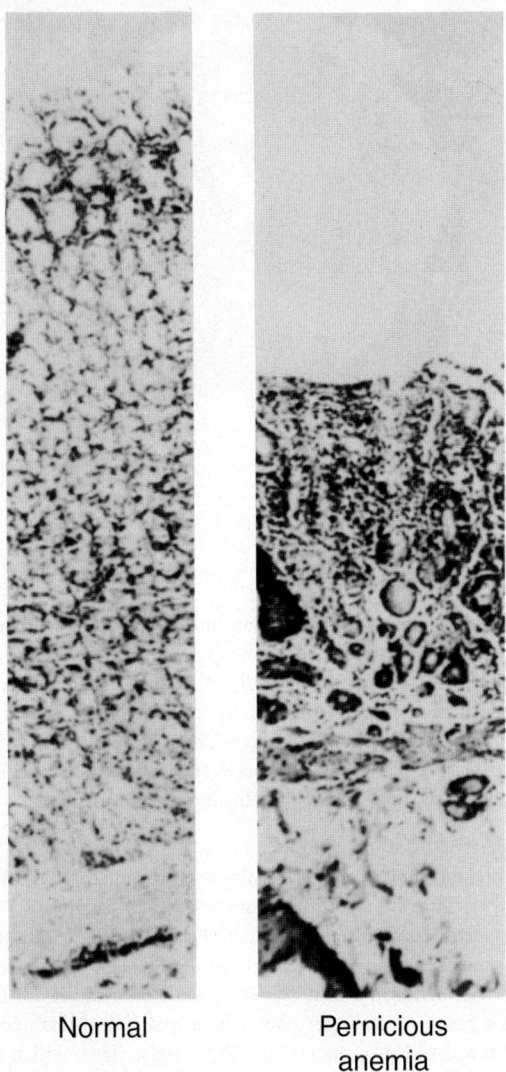

Normal   Pernicious
                    anemia

Figure 41–14. Gastric histology in pernicious anemia. *(Left)* Normal fundus. The thick mucosa is packed with gastric glands composed mostly of chief cells and parietal cells. The mucus-secreting cells are concentrated in the necks of the glands. *(Right)* Fundus in pernicious anemia. Gastric glands in the atrophic mucosa are sparse and consist mainly of mucus-secreting cells. The mucosa is densely infiltrated by lymphocytes.

represents the only available method to confirm a diagnosis of PA. Anti-intrinsic factor antibody is highly specific for PA (although its sensitivity is only modest); its presence in a megaloblastic anemia makes the diagnosis of PA almost certain.

Gastrectomy Syndromes Gastric surgery often leads to anemia. Iron-deficiency anemia is most common, but cobalamin deficiency with megaloblastic anemia can occur. After *total gastrectomy*, cobalamin deficiency develops within 5 or 6 years because the operation removes the source of intrinsic factor.[295] The delay between surgery and the onset of cobalamin deficiency reflects the time needed to exhaust cobalamin stores after cobalamin absorption ceases. This may occur more rapidly because of abrogation of the enterohepatic reabsorption of biliary cobalamin.

After *partial gastrectomy*, few patients show frank cobalamin deficiency, but approximately 5 percent have intermediate megaloblastosis, approximately 25 to 50 percent have low serum cobalamin levels, and

many have varying degrees of decreased cobalamin absorption.[296] Achlorhydria not present before surgery often develops some years after gastrectomy. Postgastrectomy patients with low serum cobalamin levels usually have low serum iron levels,[297] in contrast to the high iron levels otherwise typical of cobalamin deficiency.

Cobalamin deficiency after partial gastrectomy can be caused by mucosal atrophy in the unresected remnant of the stomach[298] or, if a gastrojejunostomy was performed, by bacterial overgrowth in the afferent loop (see "Competing Intestinal Flora and Fauna: 'Blind Loop Syndrome'" below). A surgical procedure that has gained popularity for the treatment of morbid obesity is gastric reduction surgery. This procedure results in multiple deficiencies of micronutrients including cobalamin.[299]

Of the various causes of cobalamin malabsorption described, those that most often lead to megaloblastic anemia include PA, total or partial gastrectomy, intestinal blind loop syndrome, fish tapeworm, ileal resection, regional enteritis (Crohn disease) and tropical sprue.[64] In addition, several of the inherited disorders affecting cobalamin absorption and metabolism, such as congenital intrinsic factor deficiency, selective cobalamin malabsorption and congenital TC deficiency can also result in megaloblastic anemia.

Zollinger-Ellison Syndrome In Zollinger-Ellison syndrome, a gastrin-producing tumor, usually in the pancreas, stimulates the gastric mucosa to secrete immense amounts of HCl. The major clinical problem is a severe ulcer diathesis. Malabsorption of cobalamin occurs when the vast quantities of HCl secreted by the overactive gastric mucosa cannot be completely neutralized by the pancreatic secretions. The resulting acidification of the duodenal contents prevents transfer of Cbl from HC binder to intrinsic factor and also inactivates pancreatic proteases.[300]

Intestinal Diseases Because the terminal ileum is the site for physiologic cobalamin absorption, a number of intestinal disorders can lead to cobalamin deficiency, including (1) extensive resection of the ileum[301]; (2) inflammatory bowel disease or regional ileitis or other disease affecting the ileum (e.g., lymphoma, radiation damage[302]); (3) cobalamin malabsorption associated with hypothyroidism,[303] or certain drugs[304]; (4) the effects of cobalamin deficiency itself[305]; and (5) sprue, either tropical or, less often, nontropical.[198] In each of these disorders, administration of exogenous intrinsic factor, as was carried out in the Schilling test, would fail to correct subnormal cobalamin absorption.

Competing Intestinal Flora and Fauna: "Blind Loop Syndrome" The *blind loop syndrome* is a state of cobalamin malabsorption with megaloblastic anemia caused by intestinal stasis from anatomic lesions (strictures, diverticula, anastomoses, surgical blind loops) or impaired motility (scleroderma, amyloid).[306] Serum cobalamin is low, but intrinsic factor secretion is normal. Cobalamin malabsorption is not corrected by exogenous intrinsic factor but may be corrected by antibiotic treatment. The defect in cobalamin absorption is caused by colonization of the diseased small intestine by bacteria that take up ingested cobalamin before it can be absorbed from the intestine.[307] Steatorrhea is also seen in the blind loop syndrome.

Another cause of cobalamin deficiency is infestation with the fish tapeworm *Diphyllobothrium latum*. Prevalence is highest near the Baltic Sea, Canada, and Alaska, where raw or undercooked fish is consumed. Cobalamin deficiency results from competition between the worm and the host for ingested cobalamin.[308] The clinical picture of *D. latum* infestation ranges from no symptoms to a full-blown megaloblastic anemia with neurologic changes. The infestation is diagnosed by finding tapeworm ova in the feces.

Acquired Immunodeficiency Syndrome A substantial number of patients with AIDS have low serum cobalamin levels with associated evidence of cobalamin malabsorption.[309] In addition, individuals testing seropositive for HIV infection may also have low serum cobalamin and evidence of cobalamin malabsorption.[309] The cause of the malabsorption may be intestinal or gastric or a combination of both.[310, 311]

Pancreatic Disease Some degree of cobalamin malabsorption has been demonstrated in 50 to 70 percent of patients with exocrine pancreatic insufficiency.[312] Cobalamin malabsorption in pancreatic insufficiency is caused by a deficiency in pancreatic proteases, resulting in a partial failure to destroy HC–Cbl complexes whose destruction is a prerequisite for the transfer of cobalamin to intrinsic factor.[313] Pancreatic insufficiency rarely causes clinically significant cobalamin deficiency.[314]

Dietary Cobalamin Deficiency Dietary cobalamin deficiency was previously considered very unusual and restricted largely to complete vegetarians who also do not consume dairy products and eggs (vegans).[315] Low serum cobalamin levels occur in 50 to 60 percent of individuals in this group. The onset of cobalamin deficiency in vegans is slower than in conditions associated with cobalamin malabsorption. Thus it may take 10 to 20 years for an individual consuming a vegan diet to manifest features of cobalamin deficiency.[316] This is because the enterohepatic pathway for biliary cobalamin absorption remains intact, thus conserving body cobalamin stores.[64] Breastfed infants of vegan mothers also may develop cobalamin deficiency.[317] Cobalamin deficiency in vegans presents with mild megaloblastic anemia, glossitis, and neurologic disturbances. In addition to vegans, however, there is mounting evidence of cobalamin inadequacy in children and young adults in developing countries that cannot be explained on the basis of cobalamin malabsorption, and has therefore been attributed to inadequate dietary intake.[318]

Cobalamin deficiency may occur in severe general malnutrition. A megaloblastic anemia not related to cobalamin deficiency may accompany kwashiorkor or marasmus.[319]

Neurologic Effects of Cobalamin Deficiency

Previously, the neurologic abnormalities of cobalamin deficiency were attributed to disordered metabolism of myelin lipids caused by an impaired methylmalonyl CoA mutase reaction.[320] Similar neurologic abnormalities do not, however, occur in patients with inherited methylmalonyl CoA mutase deficiency.[260,321] Authentic combined system disease has occurred in a patient with nutritional folate deficiency[322] and in a patient with MTHFR deficiency.[323] The latter reports suggest the neurologic lesions of cobalamin deficiency result from deranged methyl group metabolism. Animal studies support this hypothesis. Neurologic disorders closely resembling combined system disease develop in cobalamin-deficient fruit bats,[324] pigs, and monkeys.[325] The development of these disorders is prevented by methionine, which is produced in a cobalamin-dependent reaction and is the precursor of the biologic methylating reagent SAMe. A finding that further supports a methylation defect is that brains from cobalamin-deficient pigs contain increased levels of SAH,[326] a powerful methylation inhibitor produced in SAMe-dependent methylation reactions:

$$SAMe + RH \rightarrow SAH + RCH_3$$

where RH is any unmethylated compound and RCH_3 is its methylated form. Against the methylation defect hypothesis is the finding that cobalamin deficiency had no effect on SAMe, SAH, or methylation of phospholipids or myelin basic protein[327] in the brains of fruit bats.

CLINICAL FEATURES

The more typical clinical picture of cobalamin deficiency includes the nonspecific manifestations of megaloblastosis, such as anemia, thrombocytopenia, neutropenia, smooth tongue, cardiomyopathy, pale yellow skin and/or weight loss, plus specific features caused by the lack of cobalamin, chiefly neurologic abnormalities. Disturbances in either or both cellular and hormonal immune functions have been reported

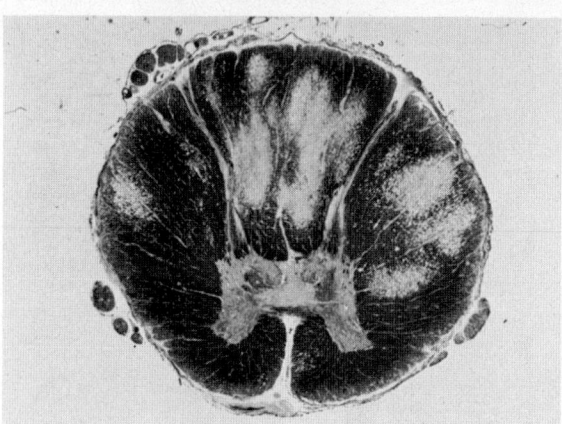

Figure 41–15. Degeneration of spinal cord in combined system disease. *(Reproduced with permission from JW Harris, RW Kellermeyer: The Red Cell: Production, Metabolism, Destruction: Normal and Abnormal, rev ed. Harvard University Press, Cambridge, 1970.)*

in cobalamin deficiency.[328,329] Cobalamin deficiency may also contribute to the risk of vascular disease through elevation of homocysteine levels. Other disease associations with cobalamin deficiency have been described. These include a possible increase in breast cancer risk in premenopausal women[330] and in osteoporosis.[331,332] Because cobalamin reserves are large, years may pass between the cessation of cobalamin absorption and the appearance of deficiency symptoms.

Neurologic Abnormalities

Cobalamin deficiency causes a neurologic syndrome that is particularly dangerous because the syndrome can develop in isolation,[333] with no megaloblastic anemia to suggest a lack of cobalamin,[294,334] and because the syndrome cannot be reversed by treatment when it is sufficiently far advanced. The syndrome usually begins with paresthesias in feet and fingers as a result of early peripheral neuropathy and disturbances of vibratory sense and proprioception. The earliest signs, which precede other neurologic findings by months, are loss of position sense in the second toe and loss of vibration sense for a 256-Hz but not a 128-Hz tuning fork.[335] Left untreated, the neurologic disorder progresses to spastic ataxia resulting from demyelination of the dorsal and lateral columns of the spinal cord, so-called *combined system disease* (Fig. 41–15).[336]

The peripheral nerves, the spinal cord, and the brain are affected by cobalamin deficiency. Somnolence and perversion of taste, smell, and vision with occasional optic atrophy are accompanied by slow waves on the electroencephalogram. A dementia mimicking Alzheimer disease can develop.[337] There is recent evidence linking low cobalamin status with brain volume loss and cerebral white matter lesions.[338,339] Psychological derangements, including psychotic depression and paranoid schizophrenia, can occur.[340] Frank psychosis in cobalamin deficiency has been given the sobriquet *megaloblastic madness*.[341]

The neurologic lesions of cobalamin deficiency can be detected by magnetic resonance imaging (MRI). Demyelination appears as T2-weighted hyperintensity of the white matter.[342] MRI is particularly useful for confirming the diagnosis of a neurologic disorder resulting from cobalamin deficiency. MRI also has been used to follow the progress of neurologic abnormalities during treatment of cobalamin-deficient patients.[342]

Subtle Cobalamin Deficiency

Some observations suggest the existence of a large group of patients who are hematologically normal, with a normal hematocrit and MCV, but who have cobalamin-responsive neuropsychiatric disease.[294]

Neuropsychiatric findings include peripheral neuropathy, gait disturbance, memory loss, and psychiatric symptoms, often with abnormal evoked potentials. Serum cobalamin may be normal, borderline, or low, but tissue cobalamin deficiency is suggested by consistently high levels of serum methylmalonic acid and/or homocysteine. Most of the neuropsychiatric abnormalities appear to respond to cobalamin therapy.

LABORATORY FEATURES

Plasma or Serum Cobalamin Levels

Plasma or serum cobalamin is low in most but not all patients with cobalamin deficiency.[219] Cobalamin levels are usually normal in cobalamin deficiency resulting from exposure to nitrous oxide, TC deficiency, and inborn errors of cobalamin metabolism. Levels also may be normal in cobalamin-deficient patients with high HC levels resulting from myeloproliferative diseases. Conversely, plasma cobalamin levels may be low in the presence of normal tissue cobalamins in vegetarians, in subjects taking megadoses of ascorbic acid,[343] in pregnancy (25 percent), in the presence of HC deficiency,[344,345] and in megaloblastic anemia resulting from folate deficiency (30 percent).[219] Plasma folate may be high in cobalamin deficiency because of retardation in conversion of methyltetrahydrofolate, which is the predominant form in plasma. Patients deficient in both cobalamin and folate may show normal serum folate levels.

Plasma or Serum Holotranscobalamin

The fraction of the cobalamin in plasma that is bound to TC constitutes only 10 to 30 percent of the total plasma cobalamin. Even so, it is this fraction that is functionally important and also better reflects the integrity of the cobalamin absorptive status of an individual.[142,346,347] The major fraction of plasma cobalamin bound to HC is considered functionally inert and is therefore less relevant for the consideration of cobalamin status. Consequently, and with the development of assays to measure the TC-bound fraction of the plasma cobalamin, an increasing body of evidence has accumulated to support the usefulness of TC-associated cobalamin (holoTC).[64,137,140,346]

Methylmalonic Acid

Except when caused by an inborn error, methylmalonic aciduria is a reliable indicator of cobalamin deficiency.[348] Normal subjects excrete only traces of methylmalonate (0 to 3.4 mg/day). In cobalamin deficiency, urine methylmalonate usually is elevated.[349] Cobalamin therapy restores excretion to normal in a few days. Another possible advantage of measurement of urine rather than plasma methylmalonic acid is that in conditions of impaired renal function, when plasma methylmalonic acid may give misleadingly elevated levels, measurement of the metabolite in urine when correlated with creatinine obviates this problem.[350]

Serum or Plasma Methylmalonic Acid and Homocysteine

Elevated plasma or serum methylmalonic acid and homocysteine levels are indicators of *tissue* cobalamin deficiency. Their levels are high in more than 90 percent of cobalamin-deficient patients and rise before plasma cobalamin falls to subnormal levels.[219,351] Elevated plasma methylmalonic acid and/or elevated homocysteine are both indicators of cobalamin deficiency in patients without a congenital disorder in their metabolism. Of the two, methylmalonic acid measurement is both more sensitive and more specific, and elevated methylmalonic acid will persist for several days, even after cobalamin treatment is instituted. Unlike homocysteine levels that rise in folate and pyridoxine deficiencies, as well as in hypothyroidism, methylmalonic acid elevation is seen only in cobalamin deficiency.[219] In renal diseases however, both homocysteine and methylmalonate, acid levels are frequently elevated. Additionally,

intestinal bacteria synthesize propionate, a precursor of methylmalonate, and in conditions of bacterial overgrowth, microbially derived methylmalonic acid may contribute to elevations in plasma methylmalonic acid.[351,352] Although measurement of these metabolites may be used for population screening for evidence of cobalamin deficiency, the finding of an isolated elevation of plasma methylmalonate cannot be taken as *a priori* evidence of clinically attributable cobalamin deficiency, absent any demonstration of a therapeutic response to the administration of cobalamin.[352,353]

Spinal fluid methylmalonic acid levels are markedly elevated in cobalamin deficiency.[354]

Assays of Cobalamin Absorption and Intrinsic Factor

Despite its numerous shortcomings the previous "gold standard" for assessment of cobalamin absorption was the Schilling test. The Schilling test assessed cobalamin absorption by measuring urinary radioactivity after an oral dose of radioactive cobalamin. The test could be performed even after cobalamin deficiency had been corrected. The test consisted of administering a physiologic dose of radiolabeled Co-CnCbl by mouth followed 2 hours later by injection of a large "flushing" dose of unlabeled CnCbl and determination and radioactivity in a 24-hour collection of urine. Subjects with normal absorption excreted 7 percent or more of the radioactivity in the urine. Subjects with subnormal urinary excretion would have the test repeated with addition of an animal-derived intrinsic factor to determine whether the malabsorption could be corrected.[355] The use of the Schilling test has dropped to a point of obsolescence as a consequence of reduced availability of the test components, cost, radioactive waste disposal, and concern about the use of animal-derived tissues for human use, which were required for the intrinsic factor administered in the second part of the test.[64] Replacements for the Schilling test are currently under development. One approach uses measurement of the change in holoTC following oral administration of non–radiolabeled cobalamin.[346,347,356] A different approach involves the use of accelerator mass spectrometry and microbially produced ^{14}C at attomolar concentrations.[357] In this approach, ^{14}C is measured in blood at the time of peak appearance 6 to 8 hours following the dose. Both methods show promise but have not been approved or validated for routine clinical use.

Deoxyuridine Suppression Test

The dU suppression test is based on the finding that unlabeled dU can suppress the uptake of [^{3}H]thymidine ([^{3}H]Thd) into the DNA of cultured lymphocytes or marrow cells through dilution of the label in the thymidine pool.[358] This occurs when the thymidylate synthase reaction is functionally intact, which requires adequate quantities of both folate and cobalamin.

The dU suppression test is chiefly a research tool. It can help diagnose certain special clinical problems,[358] but these problems also can be diagnosed using other laboratory tests, therapeutic trials with vitamins or iron, or watchful waiting. Furthermore, in more than 40 years of use, the test has not moved from the research laboratory into the clinic. The dU suppression test seems unlikely to enjoy more widespread clinical use in the future.

THERAPY, COURSE, AND PROGNOSIS

Treatment of cobalamin deficiency consists of parenteral CnCbl (vitamin B_{12}) or OHCbl to replace daily losses and refill storage pools, which normally contain 2 to 5 mg of cobalamin.[359] Toxicity is highly unusual, and there is no defined upper limit.[2] Doses exceeding 100 mcg saturate the cobalamin-binding proteins (TC and HC), and the excess is lost in the urine. A typical treatment schedule consists of 1000 mcg cobalamin intramuscular (IM) daily for 2 weeks, then weekly until the hematocrit is normal, and then monthly for life. For neurologic manifestations, 1000 mcg every 2 weeks for 6 months is recommended. Higher doses are given for certain inherited disorders (e.g., TC deficiency). *Transfusion* occasionally is required when the hematocrit is less than 15 percent or the patient is debilitated, infected, or in heart failure. In such instances, packed cells should be given slowly to avoid pulmonary edema. Infections can impair the response to cobalamin and must be treated vigorously.

Response to Treatment and Therapeutic Trial

Following parenteral administration of cobalamin to deficient patients, elevated plasma bilirubin, iron, and LDH levels fall rapidly (Fig. 41–16).[360] Decreasing plasma iron turnover and fecal urobilinogen reflect cessation of ineffective erythropoiesis. Within 12 hours, the marrow begins to change from megaloblastic to normoblastic, a process that is complete in 2 to 3 days. Consequently, morphologic diagnosis may be difficult after treatment is initiated. Reticulocytosis begins on days 3 to 5 and peaks on days 4 to 10.[361] The new red cells come from new normoblasts, not from the old megaloblasts, most of which die before leaving the marrow.[149] Blood hemoglobin concentration becomes normal within 1 to 2 months. If normal values are not achieved by 2 months, another cause of anemia should be sought.

Other changes include the following: (1) prompt and dramatic improvement in the sense of well-being; (2) normalization of leukocyte and platelet counts, although neutrophil hypersegmentation may

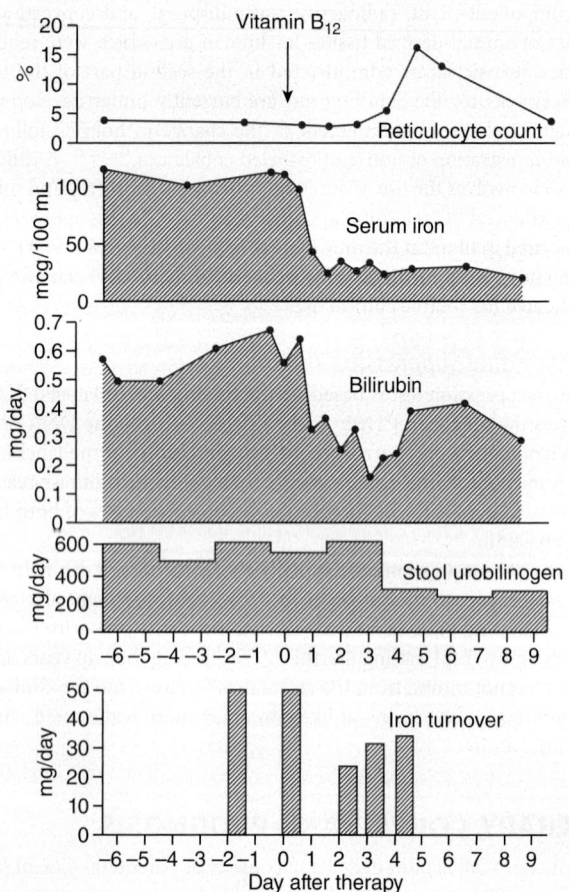

Figure 41–16. Effect of cyanocobalamin on reticulocyte count, serum iron, serum bilirubin, stool urobilinogen, and plasma iron turnover. *(Adapted with permission from Coleman D, Donohue D, Finch C, et al: Erythrokinetics in pernicious anemia. Blood 11(9):807–820, 1956.)*

persist for 10 to 14 days; (3) rise in serum cobalamin and folate. Cobalamin deficiency does not respond to a physiologic dose of folate (100 to 400 mcg/day), although this dose produces a maximal response in folate deficiency. Larger doses of folate (5 to 15 mg/day) can produce a reticulocytosis and partially or temporarily correct the anemia in cobalamin deficiency. To avoid the risk of masking an underlying cobalamin deficiency by inducing a hematologic remission in response to folate, doses in excess of 1 mg folic acid daily should be shunned until an underlying cobalamin deficiency has been ruled out.[3]

Special Circumstances
After Gastrectomy Cobalamin should always be given after total gastrectomy. Cobalamin administration is not necessary after partial gastrectomy, but patients need to be watched for megaloblastic anemia, bearing in mind that this anemia can be masked by postgastrectomy iron deficiency.[352,362]

Blind Loop Syndrome The anemia of the blind loop syndrome can be treated by parenteral cobalamin therapy. It also responds after approximately 1 week to oral broad-spectrum antibiotics (cephalexin monohydrate [Keflex] 250 mg QID plus metronidazole 250 mg TID for 10 days),[363] and cobalamin absorption is restored. Successful surgical correction of an anatomic lesion also cures the syndrome.

Fish Tapeworm Treatment consists of a single oral dose of a 50 mg/kg of niclosamide or a dose of 5 to 10 mg/kg of praziquantel.

Rekindled Use of Oral Cobalamin

Much interest has been kindled[364] regarding the possibility of treating cobalamin deficiency with oral cobalamin as had been proposed previously.[365] Oral cobalamin can be used not only for treatment of dietary cobalamin deficiency that occurs in vegans and in patients with very severe general malnutrition, but also for patients with food cobalamin malabsorption[366] and for patients with PA, provided the patients are followed carefully.[367] In patients lacking intrinsic factor, approximately 1 percent of an oral dose of the vitamin crosses the intestinal epithelium by mass action. Therefore, 1000 to 2000 mcg/day of oral cobalamin supplies most PA patients with their daily cobalamin requirement without the need for injections and their accompanying pain and expense. Cobalamin should be given by mouth to patients with dietary cobalamin deficiency and patients (e.g., hemophiliacs, the frail elderly) who cannot take IM injections.

ACUTE MEGALOBLASTIC ANEMIA

Megaloblastic anemia usually is a chronic condition that requires weeks or months to develop, but a potentially fatal megaloblastic state resulting from acute tissue folate or cobalamin deficiency can arise over the course of only a few days. Patients with acute megaloblastic anemia present with rapidly developing thrombocytopenia and/or leukopenia and counts that sometimes fall to very low levels, but little change in red cell levels unless another cause of anemia is present. The discrepancy between platelet and leukocyte counts on the one hand and red cells on the other hand is a reflection of the much longer red cell life span. The clinical picture can suggest an immune cytopenia. The diagnosis is made from the marrow aspirate, which is floridly megaloblastic, and confirmed by the rapid response to appropriate replacement therapy.

The most common cause of acute megaloblastic anemia is nitrous oxide (N_2O) anesthesia.[368] N_2O rapidly destroys MeCbl,[369] leading to a megaloblastic state. AdoCbl eventually is lost, SAMe and total folate levels decline, and the proportion of folate in the form of N^5-methyltetrahydrofolate increases.[370] Clinical findings develop quickly. Grossly megaloblastic changes are seen in the marrow after 12 to 24 hours.[371] Hypersegmented neutrophils do not appear until 5 days after exposure but then persist for several days.[372] The effects of N_2O disappear spontaneously after a few days; disappearance can be hastened by folinic acid or cobalamin.[373] Fatalities resulting from N₂O-induced megaloblastosis have occurred in tetanus patients given N₂O for weeks.[368] Long-term recreational use of N₂O has led to a neurologic disorder similar to combined system disease.[374]

Acute megaloblastic anemia occurs in other clinical settings. A rapidly developing megaloblastic state with acute thrombocytopenia has occurred in seriously ill patients, often in intensive care units.[375] Especially at risk are patients who are transfused extensively at surgery,[376] those on dialysis or total parenteral nutrition, and those receiving weak folate antagonists such as trimethoprim. Morphologic clues to the diagnosis (e.g., hypersegmented neutrophils) often are absent from the blood film. Both red cell folate and serum cobalamin levels may be normal, but the marrow is always megaloblastic. A rapid response to therapeutic doses of parenteral folate (5 mg/day) and cobalamin (1 mg) is the rule.

MEGALOBLASTIC ANEMIA CAUSED BY DRUGS

Table 41–5 lists the drugs that cause megaloblastic anemia. *Aminopterin* and *methotrexate* are almost structurally identical to folic acid. After they enter cells via the folate carrier[377] and acquire a polyglutamate chain,[378] they act as very powerful inhibitors of FH₂ reductase.[379] By blocking the FH₂→FH₄ reaction and perhaps inhibiting other enzymes of folate metabolism, they effect the rapid withdrawal of folates from the one-carbon fragment carrier pool, causing a fall in nucleotide (especially thymidine) biosynthesis that leads to a major derangement in DNA replication (Chaps. 10 and 22).[380]

Toxic effects include necrotic mouth lesions; ulcerations of the esophagus, small intestine, and colon, with abdominal pain, vomiting, and diarrhea; megaloblastic anemia; alopecia; and hyperpigmentation. The drug is excreted by the kidney, so effects and toxicity are prolonged and enhanced if renal function is impaired. Toxicity caused by these folate antagonists is treated with folinic acid (N⁵-formyl FH₄). Folic acid itself is useless in this setting because the blocked reductase cannot convert folate to the active tetrahydro form. Folinic acid is already in the tetrahydro form, so folinic acid is effective despite reductase blockade. The usual dose of folinic acid is 3 to 6 mg/day IM. Larger doses are given in chemotherapy protocols that use folinic acid to rescue patients deliberately treated with otherwise fatal doses of methotrexate. Folinic acid was used intrathecally in a patient in whom a large overdose of methotrexate was accidentally delivered into the subarachnoid space.[381]

Zidovudine (azidothymidine [AZT]) is used for HIV infections (AIDS; Chap. 81).[382] Its principal toxic effect is severe megaloblastic anemia. Anemia or neutropenia produced by zidovudine limits use of this drug.[383]

HIV infection itself suppresses hematopoiesis, leading to pancytopenia with myelodysplastic features (Chaps. 81 and 87). The blood film shows vacuolated monocytes. Megaloblastosis in HIV infection may result from folate or cobalamin deficiency[384] or AZT or trimethoprim toxicity.

Hydroxyurea is used at high doses to treat chronic myelogenous leukemia, polycythemia vera, and essential thrombocythemia, and at lower doses to treat psoriasis, rheumatoid arthritis, and sickle cell disease (Chap. 22). It inhibits conversion of ribonucleotides to deoxyribonucleotides.[385] Marked megaloblastic changes are routinely found in the marrow 1 to 2 days after initiating hydroxyurea therapy. These changes are rapidly reversed after the drug is withdrawn. Megaloblastosis as a result of N₂O is discussed in "Acute Megaloblastic Anemia" above.

Long-term use of omeprazole and presumably other H⁺/K⁺-ATPase inhibitors is associated with reduced serum cobalamin levels, presumably because of the ability of these drugs to inhibit parietal cell

function.[386] Reduced serum cobalamin levels are not a problem when these drugs are used for short intervals.[387]

Pemetrexed is an antifolate approved for use in mesothelioma. It also has been used for treatment of non–small cell lung cancer. Like other antifolate agents, pemetrexed can result in a megaloblastic anemia that is treated with cobalamin and folate. Coadministration of the drug with cobalamin and folate also reduces toxicity. Trimethoprim is a FH₂ reductase inhibitor that is designed to act on microbial rather than the mammalian enzyme. Still, in patients with borderline folate status, trimethoprim can precipitate a state of folate deficiency.

MEGALOBLASTIC ANEMIA IN CHILDHOOD

Megaloblastic anemia in childhood is usually the result of genetic disorders affecting either the cobalamin binding proteins or the enzymes concerned with intracellular trafficking of cobalamin or its conversion to coenzymatically active forms. Several recent reviews have dealt comprehensively with this topic.[321,388,389]

Defects Involving Cobalamin-Binding Proteins

Several genetic mutations and polymorphisms exist that affect the key binding proteins for cobalamin. Their effects range from being clinically benign to causing severe cobalamin deficiency with megaloblastic anemia and neurologic complications usually manifesting in infancy or early childhood, occasionally in adolescence or early adulthood. In general, the mutations and deletions affecting the encoded proteins cause serious health consequences whereas the polymorphic variants may be totally inconspicuous or result only in a modified likelihood of disease risk.

Cobalamin malabsorption occurs in four childhood conditions associated with a genetic component: (1) cobalamin malabsorption in the presence of normal intrinsic factor secretion, (2) congenital abnormality of intrinsic factor, (3) TC deficiency, and (4) true PA of childhood. The management of cobalamin deficiency in childhood has been comprehensively reviewed.[389]

Selective Malabsorption of Cobalamin, Autosomal Recessive Megaloblastic Anemia, Imerslund-Gräsbeck Disease Imerslund-Gräsbeck disease[390] is an inherited failure of transport of the intrinsic factor–Cbl complex by the ileum, usually accompanied by proteinuria, mostly of albumin.[389] It may be the most common cause of cobalamin deficiency in infancy in some populations.[391] Cobalamin deficiency usually is seen before age 2 years, but may appear earlier or later. Cobalamin malabsorption is not corrected by addition of intrinsic factor. Endogenous intrinsic factor and HCl secretion, TC and HC levels, and gastric and intestinal histology are all normal. Intrinsic factor antibodies are absent. Intrinsic factor–Cbl receptors are present in some but not all patients. The molecular defect responsible for this disease has been elucidated. For the ileal phase of cobalamin absorption, two genes code distinct proteins that form part of the cobalamin–IF receptor (cobalamin-intrinsic factor receptor) complex. The first, which codes for the protein CUBN, is affected by several mutations described in Finnish patients with MGA1.[95,392] The second, affecting the protein AMN results in a milder MGA1 phenotype and is found in Norwegian patients.[95,393] Again, several mutations in the gene coding for the AMN protein have been described.[95] Patients are treated with IM cobalamin. The anemia is corrected, but proteinuria persists.

Congenital Intrinsic Factor Deficiency Congenital intrinsic factor deficiency is an autosomal recessive disease in which parietal cells fail to produce functionally normal intrinsic factor.[394] Patients present with irritability and megaloblastic anemia when cobalamin stores (<25 mcg at birth) are exhausted. The disease usually presents at age 6 to 24 months. HCl secretion and gastric histology are normal, proteinuria is not present, and antiintrinsic factor antibodies are absent.[395] Abnormal cobalamin absorption is corrected by oral intrinsic factor.[396] Treatment consists of standard doses of IM cobalamin.

TABLE 41–5. Drugs That Cause Megaloblastic Anemia

Agents	Comments	Reference
ANTIFOLATES		
Methotrexate	Very potent inhibitor of dihydrofolate reductase	425
Aminopterin	Treat overdose with folinic acid	380
Pyrimethamine	Much weaker than methotrexate and aminopterin	
Trimethoprim	Treat with folinic acid or by withdrawing the drug	426, 427
Sulfasalazine	Can cause acute megaloblastic anemia in susceptible patients, especially those with low folate stores	428
Chlorguanide (Proguanil)		429
Triamterene	Use of folate and cobalamin during pemetrexed treatment reduces toxicity	
Pemetrexed (Alimta)		430
PURINE ANALOGUES		
6-Mercaptopurine	Megaloblastosis precedes hypoplasia, usually mild	431
6-Thioguanine	Responds to folinic acid but not folate	432
Azathioprine		433
Acyclovir	Megaloblastosis at high doses	434
PYRIMIDINE ANALOGUES		
5-Fluorouracil	Mild megaloblastosis	435
Floxuridine (5-fluorodeoxyuridine)		435
6-Azauridine	Blocks uridine monophosphate production by inhibiting orotidylic decarboxylase; occasional megaloblastosis with orotic acid and orotidine in urine	436
Zidovudine (AZT)	Severe megaloblastic anemia is the major side effect	383
RIBONUCLEOTIDE REDUCTASE INHIBITORS		
Hydroxyurea	Marked megaloblastosis within 1–2 days of starting therapy; quickly reversed by withdrawing drug	437
Cytarabine (cytosine arabinoside)	Early megaloblastosis is routine	438
ANTICONVULSANTS		
Phenytoin (diphenylhydantoin)	Occasional megaloblastosis, associated with low folate levels; responds to high-dose folate (1–5 mg/day); how anticonvulsants cause low folate is not understood, but may be related to a drug-induced rise in cytochrome P450	439–441
Phenobarbital		439
Primidone		439
Carbamazepine		442
OTHER DRUGS THAT DEPRESS FOLATES		
Oral contraceptives	Occasional megaloblastosis; sometimes dysplasia of uterine cervix, corrected with folate	443
Glutethimide		
Cycloserine		
H^+/K^+-ATPASE INHIBITORS		
Omeprazole	Long-term use causes decreased serum cobalamin levels	386
Lansoprazole		
MISCELLANEOUS		
N_2O	See "Acute Megaloblastic Anemia" in text	368
p-Aminosalicylic acid	Causes cobalamin malabsorption with occasional mild megaloblastic anemia	444
Metformin		445
Phenformin	Causes cobalamin malabsorption but not anemia	
Colchicine		446
Neomycin		447
Arsenic	Causes myelodysplastic hematopoiesis, sometimes with megaloblastic changes	448

Transcobalamin Deficiency TC deficiency is an autosomal recessive disorder causing a flagrant megaloblastic anemia that generally presents in early infancy.[395] The disease is dangerously deceptive because it results from a very severe deficiency of tissue cobalamin, usually with serum cobalamin levels in the normal range because most of the plasma cobalamin is bound to HC resulting in a misleading test result if reliance is placed simply on serum cobalamin measurement. Undiagnosed TC deficiency causes irreversible CNS damage.[397] Patients are healthy at birth but over the next few weeks develop signs and symptoms of cobalamin deficiency, such as rapidly progressive pancytopenia, mouth ulcers, vomiting, and diarrhea. Recurrent bacterial infections may occur.[395] Neurologic findings are not prominent in the early stages of the disease.[397]

Serum folate and cobalamin are normal (the latter because most cobalamin is carried by HC). Homocysteine and/or methylmalonic acid levels are elevated in the plasma.[398] The marrow is megaloblastic and the cobalamin absorption is usually but not always abnormal and is not corrected by intrinsic factor.[399] The diagnosis is made by measuring plasma TC.[389] Prenatal diagnosis is possible.[400] Serum should be obtained prior to treatment because TC levels in normal individuals drop sharply after cobalamin is given. TC deficiency is treated with cobalamin doses sufficiently large to force enough vitamin into the cells to allow normal function. Initial therapy can consist of oral CnCbl or OHCbl 500 to 1000 mcg twice a week, or IM OHCbl 1000 mcg/week. Blood counts and symptoms should be monitored and doses adjusted upward if necessary.

Several single nucleotide polymorphisms in the TC gene have been described and the allele frequency of the most common form (776 C>G) is high in certain populations.[401,402] HoloTC levels are lower and methylmalonate levels are higher in individuals homozygous for the G allele,[401,402] suggesting that this genotype may be associated with less-favorable cobalamin status.[64]

Haptocorrin Deficiency Congenital deficiency is not associated with clinically manifested cobalamin deficiency, although the plasma or serum cobalamin levels are well below normal,[345] and this is how the condition is recognized. The absence of morbidity in these patients indicates that HCs are not essential for health.

True Juvenile Pernicious Anemia True PA, with gastric atrophy and a defect in intrinsic factor secretion, is exceedingly rare in childhood.[403] Patients usually present in their teens with cobalamin deficiency. Serum antiintrinsic factor antibodies usually are present.[265] The diagnosis and treatment are the same as for PA in adults.

INBORN ERRORS OF COBALAMIN METABOLISM

Cobalamin is converted to AdoCbl and MeCbl by a complex series of transformations involving several steps.[388,398,404] Eight disorders affecting this cobalamin transformation pathway have been described, one for each of the steps. Because the molecular causes of these disorders have not yet been fully characterized, the disorders themselves are not named for a defective protein but instead are designated by sequential capital letters preceded by a *cbl* prefix. The disorders can be grouped into three broad clinical syndromes based on the abnormal metabolites in the patient's urine (Table 41–6). These disorders are usually discovered during investigation of infants with unexplained developmental delay, acidosis, anemia, or unexplained neurologic difficulties. Typically they have normal plasma cobalamin levels.

Methylmalonic Aciduria Only (cblA, cblB, and cblH)

In cblA and cblB, AdoCbl production is impaired but MeCbl production is normal. This may result either from an abnormal methylmalonyl CoA mutase (designated *mut⁰* or *mut–*) or from a defect in activation

TABLE 41–6. Cobalamin Mutant Class Syndromes

Syndrome	Methylmalonic Aciduria	Homocystinuria	Megaloblastic Anemia
cblA, cblB, cblH	+	–	–
cblE, cblC	–	+	+
cblC, cblD, cblF	+	+	±

or production of its cofactor, AdoCbl. The cblH variant appears to represent an interallelic variant of cblA.[405] Patients present in infancy with acidosis because they cannot catabolize methylmalonic acid. Symptoms include lethargy and failure to thrive, vomiting, and neurologic problems. Mental retardation is not prominent, and megaloblastic anemia is absent. Most patients respond to 1000 mcg/day of OHCbl or CnCbl, although mut⁰ and mut– patients are unresponsive.

Homocystinuria Only (CblE and CblG)

In these disorders, N^5-methyltetrahydrofolate-homocysteine methyltransferase is defective and lacks the capacity to produce MeCbl.[406] In patients with cblG, methionine synthase is missing or defective.[407] cblE results from failure to reactivate methionine synthase that was inactivated by oxidation of its bound cobalamin.[408] Patients present in infancy with vomiting, mental retardation, and megaloblastic anemia. They have marked homocystinuria and hyperhomocysteinemia without methylmalonic aciduria or methylmalonic acidemia. They respond well to CnCbl 1000 mcg/day or 1000 mcg/week. Infants diagnosed prenatally and treated from birth usually show normal development. On rare occasions, this disorder may first become apparent in adult life.

Methylmalonic Aciduria and Homocystinuria (Cblc, Cbld, and Cblf)

In these disorders, the defect in Cbl transformation affects AdoCbl and MeCbl, probably because reduction of cobalt from Co⁺⁺ to Co⁺ is defective. These patients have both hyperhomocysteinemia and methylmalonic acidemia. The age at initial presentation ranges from early infancy to adolescence. In addition to lethargy and failure to thrive, affected infants present with serious neurologic difficulties. Older patients present with psychological problems, progressive dementia, and motor signs and symptoms. cblC disease is the most common of the cobalamin inborn errors. In cblF the defect lies in an inability to release cobalamin from lysosomes.[409] Megaloblastic anemia occurs in about half the cases. Patients respond partially to 1000 mcg/day of OHCbl or CnCbl.

A tentative diagnosis of a cobalamin mutation can be made by demonstrating methylmalonic aciduria and/or homocystinuria in a patient with the clinical findings described above in "Methylmalonic Aciduria Only" or "Homocystinuria Only," respectively. Establishing a diagnosis requires a specialized laboratory equipped to do cultured fibroblast complementation studies.[388] In a patient suspected of having a cobalamin mutation, treatment should be started pending the test results because early high-dose cobalamin treatment is risk-free and may reduce the chance of damage to the CNS. Fetuses with these diseases have been successfully treated *in utero* with very large doses of CnCbl given parenterally to the mother.[410]

INBORN ERRORS OF FOLATE METABOLISM

Megaloblastic anemia in infancy has been described in three inherited disorders of folate metabolism.[30,389,411]

Hereditary Folate Malabsorption

Hereditary folate malabsorption is a rare inherited disorder in which patients cannot absorb folate from the gastrointestinal tract or transport it across the choroid plexus and into the cerebrospinal fluid.[29,30] The molecular basis for this disorder is caused by abnormalities in the PCFT.[29] Patients present with severe megaloblastic anemia, seizures, mental retardation, and other CNS findings.[412] Folate levels are low in the serum and nil in the cerebrospinal fluid. Folate given parenterally has corrected the anemia and seizures in some patients but has had no effect on other CNS symptoms or on the cerebrospinal fluid folate level. Treatment with daily folinic acid by injection maintains the spinal fluid level and can lead to normal development.[389]

Dihydrofolate Reductase Deficiency

Dihydrofolate reductase deficiency may present isolated megaloblastic anemia within days or weeks after birth. The anemia responds to folinic acid but not to folic acid.[413]

N^5-Methyltetrahydrofolate–Homocysteine Methyltransferase Deficiency

Decreased methyltransferase activity was described in a liver biopsy from a child with megaloblastic anemia and mental retardation. The anemia failed to respond to folate, cobalamin, or pyridoxal phosphate.[414] The phenotype of this disorder resembles the inborn errors of cobalamin metabolism affecting the methionine synthesis reaction and has not been well characterized as a distinct entity at the molecular level.

Methylene Tetrahydrofolate Reductase Deficiency

In this rare autosomal recessive disorder there is a severe hyperhomocysteinemia and homocystinuria with low plasma methionine. Patients have neurologic and vascular complications but no megaloblastic anemia or methylmalonic aciduria.[389] The polymorphic variations in MTHFR have been discussed earlier as well as their influence on disease susceptibility and the influence of the enzyme on the distribution of major folate species toward either methylation or DNA synthetic pathways.

OTHER INBORN ERRORS

Hereditary Orotic Aciduria

Hereditary orotic aciduria is an autosomal recessive disorder of pyrimidine metabolism[415] characterized by megaloblastic anemia, growth impairment, and excretion of orotic acid in the urine. Cobalamin and folate levels are normal.

Lesch-Nyhan Syndrome

The Lesch-Nyhan syndrome is an X-linked disorder of purine metabolism characterized by hyperuricemia, hyperuricosuria, and a neurologic disease with self-mutilation. It is caused by a hypoxanthine–guanine phosphoribosyltransferase deficiency. One patient described had megaloblastic anemia.[416]

Thiamine-Responsive Megaloblastic Anemia

Seven children with severe megaloblastic anemia, sensorineural deafness, and diabetes mellitus, all beginning in infancy, have been reported. The anemia responded to thiamine (25 to 100 mg/day). The marrow was reported as myelodysplastic in two patients with the disorder.[417] The gene for this puzzling disorder has been mapped to the long arm of chromosome 1, and the underlying biochemical defect is caused by reduced nucleic acid production through impairment of the thiamine dependent pentose cycle enzyme transketolase that results in cell-cycle arrest and the megaloblastic phenotype.[418] This condition is also discussed in Chap. 44.

OTHER CAUSES OF MEGALOBLASTIC ANEMIA

Congenital Dyserythropoietic Anemia

The congenital dyserythropoietic anemias are lifelong anemias. They often are mild, showing dysplastic changes affecting the red cell line only, most typically multinuclearity of the normoblasts. They appear to result from defects in glycosylation of polylactosaminoglycans linked to membrane proteins and ceramides.[419] Of the three types, two (type I usually[420] and type III occasionally[421]) show megaloblastic red cell precursors (Chap. 39).

Refractory Megaloblastic Anemia

Refractory megaloblastic anemia is regarded as a manifestation of some sideroblastic anemias (Chap. 59) and myelodysplastic disorders (Chap. 87).[422] The megaloblastic changes are atypical. Dysplastic features are confined to the erythroid series. Giant metamyelocytes and bands are absent from the marrow. A few patients with refractory megaloblastic anemia respond to pharmacologic doses of pyridoxine (200 mg/day),[423] perhaps because of an effect on serine transformylase, which requires both pyridoxine and folate.

Acute Erythroid Leukemia

In acute erythroid leukemia, a variety of acute myelogenous leukemia (Chap. 89)[424] nucleated red cells appear on the blood film, there is usually marked anisocytosis and anisochromia, and macrocytes are usually present. The marrow shows pronounced erythroid hyperplasia involving very bizarre looking megaloblast-like red cell precursors, often containing multiple nuclei or nuclear fragments (see Chap. 88, Fig. 88–1) together with increased numbers of blasts. The megaloblastoid erythroid precursors frequently appear vacuolated.

Consideration of the rarer causes of megaloblastic anemia is important when the common and correctable causes resulting from folate or cobalamin deficiencies have been excluded. This is particularly important in the pediatric age group, but also in patients who are refractory to treatment with either folate or cobalamin.

REFERENCES

1. Butterworth CJ, Santini RJ, Frommeyer WJ: The pteroylglutamate components of American diets as determined by chromatographic fractionation. *J Clin Invest* 42:1929–1939, 1963.
2. Stover PJ, Field MS: Trafficking of intracellular folates. *Adv Nutr* 2(4):325–331, 2011.
3. Institute of Medicine: *Dietary Reference Intakes for Thiamin, Riboflavin, Niacin, Vitamin B6, Folate, Vitamin B12, Pantothenic Acid, Biotin, and Choline.* The National Academies Press, Washington, DC, 2000.
4. von der Porten AE, Gregory JF 3rd, Toth JP, et al: *In vivo* folate kinetics during chronic supplementation of human subjects with deuterium-labeled folic acid. *J Nutr* 122(6):1293–1299, 1992.
5. Herbert V: Experimental nutritional folate deficiency in man. *Trans Assoc Am Physicians* 75:307–320, 1962.
6. Halsted C: Folate deficiency in alcoholism. *Am J Clin Nutr* 33(12):2736–2740, 1980.
7. Alperin J, Hutchinson H, Levin W: Studies of folic acid requirements in megaloblastic anemia of pregnancy. *Arch Intern Med* 117(5):681–688, 1966.
8. Schwarz R, Johnston RJ: Folic acid supplementation—When and how. *Obstet Gynecol* 88(5):886–887, 1996.
9. Ulevitch R, Kallen R: Purification and characterization of pyridoxal 5′-phosphate dependent serine hydroxymethylase from lamb liver and its action upon beta-phenylserines. *Biochemistry* 16(24):5342–5350, 1977.
10. Anderson DD, Stover PJ: SHMT1 and SHMT2 are functionally redundant in nuclear de novo thymidylate biosynthesis. *PLoS One* 4(6): E5839, 2009.
11. Deacon R, Chanarin I, Perry J, Lumb M: Marrow cells from patients with untreated pernicious anaemia cannot use tetrahydrofolate normally. *Br J Haematol* 46(4):523–528, 2009.
12. Wahba A, Friedkin M: The enzymatic synthesis of thymidylate. I. Early steps in the purification of thymidylate synthetase of *Escherichia coli*. *J Biol Chem* 237:3794–3801, 1962.
13. Fenech M: The role of folic acid and vitamin B12 in genomic stability of human cells. *Mutat Res* 475(1–2):57–67, 2001.
14. Huennekens F: Folic acid coenzymes in the biosynthesis of purines and pyrimidines. *Vitam Horm* 26:375–394, 1968.

15. Kaufman S: The phenylalanine hydroxylating system from mammalian liver. *Adv Enzymol Relat Areas Mol Biol* 35:245–319, 1971.

16. Kwon N, Nathan C, Stuehr D: Reduced biopterin as a cofactor in the generation of nitrogen oxides by murine macrophages. *J Biol Chem* 264(34):20496–20501, 1989.

17. Banerjee S, Snyder S: Methyltetrahydrofolic acid mediates N- and O-methylation of biogenic amines. *Science* 182(107):74–75, 1973.

18. Bird O, McGlohon V, Vaitkus J: Naturally occurring folates in the blood and liver of the rat. *Anal Biochem* 12(1):18–35, 1965.

19. Shane B: Folylpolyglutamate synthesis and role in the regulation of one-carbon metabolism. *Vitam Horm* 45:263–335, 1989.

20. Pratt R, Cooper B: Folates in plasma and bile of man after feeding folic acid—3H and 5-formyltetrahydrofolate (folinic acid). *J Clin Invest* 50(2):455–462, 1971.

21. Kisliuk R: Pteroylpolyglutamates. *Mol Cell Biochem* 39:331–345, 1981.

22. Atkinson I, Garrow T, Brenner A, Shane B: Human cytosolic folylpoly-gamma-glutamate synthase. *Methods Enzymol* 281:134–140, 1997.

23. Sussman D, Milman G, Shane B: Characterization of human folylpolyglutamate synthetase expressed in Chinese hamster ovary cells. *Somat Cell Mol Genet* 12(6):531–540, 1986.

24. Shane B, Stokstad E: Vitamin B12-folate interrelationships. *Annu Rev Nutr* 5:115–141, 1985.

25. Visentin M, Diop-Bove N, Zhao R, Goldman ID: The intestinal absorption of folates. *Annu Rev Physiol* 76:251–274, 2014.

26. Butterworth CJ, Baugh C, Krumdieck C: A study of folate absorption and metabolism in man utilizing carbon-14–labeled polyglutamates synthesized by the solid phase method. *J Clin Invest* 48(6):1131–1142, 1969.

27. Rosenberg I, Godwin H: The digestion and absorption of dietary folate. *Gastroenterology* 60(3):445–463, 1971.

28. Chandler C, Wang T, Halsted C: Pteroylpolyglutamate hydrolase from human jejunal brush borders. Purification and characterization. *J Biol Chem* 261(2):928–933, 1986.

29. Qiu A, Jansen M, Sakaris A, et al: Identification of an intestinal folate transporter and the molecular basis for hereditary folate malabsorption. *Cell* 127(5):917–928, 2006.

30. Zhao R, Matherly L, Goldman I: Membrane transporters and folate homeostasis: Intestinal absorption and transport into systemic compartments and tissues. *Expert Rev Mol Med* 11:e4, 2009.

31. Elsenhans B, Ahmad O, Rosenberg I: Isolation and characterization of pteroylpolyglutamate hydrolase from rat intestinal mucosa. *J Biol Chem* 259(10):6364–6368, 1984.

32. Schron C: PH modulation of the kinetics of rabbit jejunal, brush-border folate transport. *J Membr Biol* 120(2):192–200, 1991.

33. Schron C, Washington CJ, Blitzer B: The transmembrane pH gradient drives uphill folate transport in rabbit jejunum. Direct evidence for folate/hydroxyl exchange in brush border membrane vesicles. *J Clin Invest* 76(5):2030–2033, 1985.

34. Zimmerman J, Selhub J, Rosenberg I: Role of sodium ion in transport of folic acid in the small intestine. *Am J Physiol* 251(2 Pt 1):G218–G222, 1986.

35. Perry J, Chanarin I: Intestinal absorption of reduced folate compounds in man. *Br J Haematol* 18(3):329–339, 1970.

36. Kanazawa S, Herbert V: Mechanism of enterohepatic circulation of vitamin B12: Movement of vitamin B12 from bile R-binder to intrinsic factor due to the action of pancreatic trypsin. *Trans Assoc Am Physicians* 96:336–344, 1983.

37. Steinberg S, Campbell C, Hillman R: Kinetics of the normal folate enterohepatic cycle. *J Clin Invest* 64(1):83–88, 1979.

38. Steinberg S: Mechanisms of folate homeostasis. *Am J Physiol* 246(4 Pt 1):G319–G324, 1984.

39. Johns D, Sperti S, Burgen A: The metabolism of tritiated folic acid in man. *J Clin Invest* 40:1684–1695, 1961.

40. Antony A: The biological chemistry of folate receptors. *Blood* 79(11):2807–2820, 1992.

41. Weitman S, Weinberg A, Coney L, et al: Cellular localization of the folate receptor: Potential role in drug toxicity and folate homeostasis. *Cancer Res* 52(23):6708–6711, 1992.

42. Luhrs C, Slomiany B: A human membrane-associated folate binding protein is anchored by a glycosyl-phosphatidylinositol tail. *J Biol Chem* 264(36):21446–21449, 1989.

43. Green T, Ford HC: Human placental microvilli contain high-affinity binding sites for folate. *Biochem J* 218(1):75–80, 1984.

44. Rothberg K, Ying Y, Kolhouse J, et al: The glycophospholipid-linked folate receptor internalizes folate without entering the clathrin-coated pit endocytic pathway. *J Cell Biol* 110(3):637–649, 1990.

45. Moestrup SK: New insights into carrier binding and epithelial uptake of the erythropoietic nutrients cobalamin and folate. *Curr Opin Hematol* 13(3):119–123, 2006.

46. Hilton J, Cooper B, Rosenblatt D: Folate polyglutamate synthesis and turnover in cultured human fibroblasts. *J Biol Chem* 254(17):8398–8403, 1979.

47. Zamierowski M, Wagner C: High molecular weight complexes of folic acid in mammalian tissues. *Biochem Biophys Res Commun* 60(1):81–87, 1974.

48. Duch D, Bowers S, Nichol C: Analysis of folate cofactor levels in tissues using high-performance liquid chromatography. *Anal Biochem* 130(2):385–392, 1983.

49. Cook R, Wagner C: Glycine N-methyltransferase is a folate binding protein of rat liver cytosol. *Proc Natl Acad Sci U S A* 81(12):3631–3634, 1984.

50. Rosenblatt D, Cooper B, Lue-Shing S, et al: Folate distribution in cultured human cells. Studies on 5,10-CH2-H4PteGlu reductase deficiency. *J Clin Invest* 63(5):1019–1025, 1979.

51. Stites T, Bailey L, Scott K, et al: Kinetic modeling of folate metabolism through use of chronic administration of deuterium-labeled folic acid in men. *Am J Clin Nutr* 65(1):53–60, 1997.

52. Elwood P, Deutsch J, Kolhouse J: The conversion of the human membrane-associated folate binding protein (folate receptor) to the soluble folate binding protein by a membrane-associated metalloprotease. *J Biol Chem* 266(4):2346–2353, 1991.

53. Colman N, Herbert V: Total folate binding capacity of normal human plasma, and variations in uremia, cirrhosis, and pregnancy. *Blood* 48(6):911–921, 1976.

54. Waxman S: Folate binding proteins. *Br J Haematol* 29(1):23–29, 1975.

55. Waxman S, Schreiber C: Measurement of serum folate levels and serum folic acid-binding protein by 3H-PGA radioassay. *Blood* 42(2):281–290, 1973.

56. Colman N, Herbert V: Folate-binding proteins. *Annu Rev Med* 31:433–439, 1980.

57. Waxman S, Schreiber C: Characteristics of folic acid-binding protein in folate-deficient serum. *Blood* 42(2):291–301, 1973.

58. Rothenberg S: A macromolecular factor in some leukemic cells which binds folic acid. *Proc Soc Exp Biol Med* 133(2):428–432, 1970.

59. Mason J, Selhub J: Folate-binding protein and the absorption of folic acid in the small intestine of the suckling rat. *Am J Clin Nutr* 48(3):620–625, 1988.

60. Rubinoff M, Abramson R, Schreiber C, Waxman S: Effect of a folate-binding protein on the plasma transport and tissue distribution of folic acid. *Acta Haematol* 65(3):145–152, 1981.

61. Selhub J, Nakamura S, Carone F: Renal folate absorption and the kidney folate binding protein. II. Microinfusion studies. *Am J Physiol* 252(4 Pt 2):F757–F760, 1987.

62. O'Brien J: Urinary excretion of folic and folinic acids in normal adults. *Proc Soc Exp Biol Med* 104:354–355, 1960.

63. Clifford A, Arjomand A, Dueker S, et al: The dynamics of folic acid metabolism in an adult given a small tracer dose of 14C-folic acid. *Adv Exp Med Biol* 445:239–251, 1998.

64. Green R, Miller JW: Vitamin B12, in *Handbook of Vitamins*, ed 5. Taylor & Francis, Boca Raton, FL, 2014.

65. Lenhert P, Hodgkin D: Structure of the 5,6-dimethyl-benzimidazolylcobamide coenzyme. *Nature* 192:937–938, 1961.

66. Lindstrand K: Isolation of methylcobalamin from natural source material. *Nature* 204:188–189, 1964.

67. Heyssel R, Bozian R, Darby W, Bell M: Vitamin B12 turnover in man. The assimilation of vitamin B12 from natural foodstuff by man and estimates of minimal daily dietary requirements. *Am J Clin Nutr* 18(3):176–184, 1966.

68. Grasbeck R: Calculations on vitamin B12 turnover in man. With a note on the maintenance treatment in pernicious anemia and the radiation dose received by patients ingesting radiovitamin B12. *Scand J Clin Lab Invest* 11:250–258, 1959.

69. JM H: Vitamin B12 concentrations in human tissues. In: MPMJA Kawin B, editor.: Nature; 1966. p. 1264.

70. Nham S, Wilkemeyer M, Ledley F: Structure of the human methylmalonyl-CoA mutase (MUT) locus. *Genomics* 8(4):710–716, 1990.

71. Beck W, Flavin M, Ochoa S: Metabolism of propionic acid in animal tissues. III. Formation of succinate. *J Biol Chem* 229(2):997–1010, 1957.

72. Taylor R, Weissbach H: Enzymic synthesis of methionine: Formation of a radioactive cobamide enzyme with N5-methyl-14C-tetrahydrofolate. *Arch Biochem Biophys* 119(1):572–579, 1967.

73. Zalusky R, Herbert V, Castle W: Cyanocobalamin therapy effect in folic acid deficiency. *Arch Intern Med* 109:545–554, 1962.

74. Knowles J, Prankerd T: Abnormal folic acid metabolism in vitamin B12 deficiency. *Clin Sci* 22:233–238, 1962.

75. Herbert V, Zalusky R: Interrelations of vitamin B12 and folic acid metabolism: Folic acid clearance studies. *J Clin Invest* 41:1263–1276, 1962.

76. Kano Y, Sakamoto S, Hida K, et al: 5-Methyltetrahydrofolate related enzymes and DNA polymerase alpha activities in bone marrow cells from patients with vitamin B12 deficient megaloblastic anemia. *Blood* 59(4):832–837, 1982.

77. Waters A, Mollin D: Observations on the metabolism of folic acid in pernicious anaemia. *Br J Haematol* 9:319–327, 1963.

78. Jeejeebhoy K, Pathare S, Noronha J: Observations on conjugated and unconjugated blood folate levels in megaloblastic anemia and the effects of vitamin B12. *Blood* 26:354–359, 1965.

79. Boss G: Cobalamin inactivation decreases purine and methionine synthesis in cultured lymphoblasts. *J Clin Invest* 76(1):213–218, 1985.

80. Finkelstein JD, Martin JJ: Methionine metabolism in mammals. Adaptation to methionine excess. *J Biol Chem* 261(4):1582–1587, 1986.

81. Katzen H, Buchanan J: Enzymatic synthesis of the methyl group of methionine. 8. Repression-derepression, purification, and properties of 5,10-methylenetetrahydrofolate reductase from *Escherichia coli*. *J Biol Chem* 240:825–835, 1965.

82. Chanarin I, Deacon R, Lumb M, Perry J: Vitamin B12 regulates folate metabolism by the supply of formate. *Lancet* 2(8193):505–507, 1980.

83. Taheri M, Wickremasinghe R, Jackson B, Hoffbrand A: The effect of folate analogues and vitamin B12 on provision of thymine nucleotides for DNA synthesis in megaloblastic anemia. *Blood* 59(3):634–640, 1982.

84. Chanarin I, Deacon R, Lumb M, Perry J: Cobalamin and folate: Recent developments. *J Clin Pathol* 45(4):277–283, 1992.

85. Hewitt J, Gordon M, Taggart R, et al: Human gastric intrinsic factor: Characterization of cDNA and genomic clones and localization to human chromosome 11. *Genomics* 10(2):432–440, 1991.

86. Tang L, Chokshi H, Hu C, et al: The intrinsic factor (IF)-cobalamin receptor binding site is located in the amino-terminal portion of IF. *J Biol Chem* 267(32):22982–22986, 1992.

87. Levine JS, Nakane PK, Allen RH: Immunocytochemical localization of human intrinsic factor: The nonstimulated stomach. *Gastroenterology* 79(3):493–502, 1980.

88. Stenman U: Vitamin B12-binding proteins of r-type, cobalophilin. *Scand J Haematol* 14(2):91–107, 1975.

89. Cooper B, Castle W: Sequential mechanisms in the enhanced absorption of vitamin B12 by intrinsic factor in the rat. *J Clin Invest* 39:199–214, 1960.

90. Allen R, Seetharam B, Podell E, Alpers D: Effect of proteolytic enzymes on the binding of cobalamin to R protein and intrinsic factor. *In vitro* evidence that a failure to partially degrade R protein is responsible for cobalamin malabsorption in pancreatic insufficiency. *J Clin Invest* 61(1):47–54, 1978.

91. Abels J, Schilling R: Protection of intrinsic factor by vitamin B12. *J Lab Clin Med* 64:375–384, 1964.

92. Moestrup S, Kozyraki R, Kristiansen M, et al: The intrinsic factor-vitamin B12 receptor and target of teratogenic antibodies is a megalin-binding peripheral membrane protein with homology to developmental proteins. *J Biol Chem* 273(9):5235–5242, 1998.

93. Barth JL, Argraves WS: Cubilin and megalin: Partners in lipoprotein and vitamin metabolism. *Trends Cardiovasc Med* 11(1):26–31, 2001.

94. Birn H, Willnow T, Nielsen R, et al: Megalin is essential for renal proximal tubule reabsorption and accumulation of transcobalamin-B(12). *Am J Physiol Renal Physiol* 282(3):F408–F416, 2002.

95. Fyfe J, Madsen M, Højrup P, et al: The functional cobalamin (vitamin B12)-intrinsic factor receptor is a novel complex of cubilin and amnionless. *Blood* 103(5):1573–1579, 2004.

96. Christensen E, Birn H: Megalin and cubilin: Multifunctional endocytic receptors. *Nat Rev Mol Cell Biol* 3(4):256–266, 2002.

97. Hagedorn C, Alpers D: Distribution of intrinsic factor-vitamin B12 receptors in human intestine. *Gastroenterology* 73(5):1019–1022, 1977.

98. Kapadia C, Serfilippi D, Voloshin K, Donaldson RJ: Intrinsic factor-mediated absorption of cobalamin in guinea pig ileal cells. *J Clin Invest* 71(3):440–448, 1983.

99. Robertson J, Gallagher N: *In vivo* evidence that cobalamin is absorbed by receptor-mediated endocytosis in the mouse. *Gastroenterology* 88(4):908–912, 1985.

100. Chanarin I: *The Megaloblastic Anaemias*. Blackwell Scientific, Oxford, 1969.

101. Horadagoda N, Batt R: Lysosomal localisation of cobalamin during absorption by the ileum of the dog. *Biochim Biophys Acta* 838(2):206–210, 1985.

102. Rothenberg S, Weisberg H, Ficarra A: Evidence for the absorption of immunoreactive intrinsic factor into the intestinal epithelial cell during vitamin B12 absorption. *J Lab Clin Med* 79(4):587–597, 1972.

103. Hall C: Transcobalamins I and II as natural transport proteins of vitamin B12. *J Clin Invest* 56(5):1125–1131, 1975.

104. Beedholm-Ebsen R, van de Wetering K, Hardlei T, et al: Identification of multidrug resistance protein 1 (MRP1/ABCC1) as a molecular gate for cellular export of cobalamin. *Blood* 115(8):1632–1639, 2010.

105. Quadros E, Regec A, Khan K, et al: Transcobalamin II synthesized in the intestinal villi facilitates transfer of cobalamin to the portal blood. *Am J Physiol* 277(1 Pt 1):G161–G166, 1999.

106. Green R, Jacobsen D, van Tonder S, et al: Enterohepatic circulation of cobalamin in the nonhuman primate. *Gastroenterology* 81(4):773–776, 1981.

107. Grasbeck R, Nyberg W, Reizenstein P: Biliary and fecal vit. B12 excretion in man: An isotope study. *Proc Soc Exp Biol Med* 97(4):780–784, 1958.

108. Green R, Jacobsen D, Van Tonder S, et al: Absorption of biliary cobalamin in baboons following total gastrectomy. *J Lab Clin Med* 100(5):771–777, 1982.

109. Antony A: Vegetarianism and vitamin B-12 (cobalamin) deficiency. *Am J Clin Nutr* 78(1):3–6, 2003.

110. Doscherholmen A, Hagen P: A dual mechanism of vitamin B12 plasma absorption. *J Clin Invest* 36(11):1551–1557, 1957.

111. Seetharam B, Alpers D: Cellular uptake of cobalamin. *Nutr Rev* 43(4):97–102, 1985.

112. Quadros EV, Rothenberg SP, Pan YC, Stein S: Purification and molecular characterization of human transcobalamin II. *J Biol Chem* 261(33):15455–15460, 1986.

113. Platica O, Janeczko R, Quadros E, et al: The cDNA sequence and the deduced amino acid sequence of human transcobalamin II show homology with rat intrinsic factor and human transcobalamin I. *J Biol Chem* 266(12):7860–7863, 1991.

114. Hippe E, Olesen H: Nature of vitamin B12 binding. 3. Thermodynamics of binding to human intrinsic factor and transcobalamins. *Biochim Biophys Acta* 243(1):83–88, 1971.

115. Kolhouse J, Allen R: Absorption, plasma transport, and cellular retention of cobalamin analogues in the rabbit. Evidence for the existence of multiple mechanisms that prevent the absorption and tissue dissemination of naturally occurring cobalamin analogues. *J Clin Invest* 60(6):1381–1392, 1977.

116. Donaldson RJ, Brand M, Serfilippi D: Changes in circulating transcobalamin II after injection of cyanocobalamin. *N Engl J Med* 296(25):1427–1430, 1977.

117. Schneider R, Burger R, Mehlman C, Allen R: The role and fate of rabbit and human transcobalamin II in the plasma transport of vitamin B12 in the rabbit. *J Clin Invest* 57(1):27–38, 1976.

118. Youngdahl-Turner P, Rosenberg L, Allen R: Binding and uptake of transcobalamin II by human fibroblasts. *J Clin Invest* 61(1):133–141, 1978.

119. Quadros E, Nakayama Y, Sequeira J: The protein and the gene encoding the receptor for the cellular uptake of transcobalamin-bound cobalamin. *Blood* 113(1):186–192, 2009.

120. Peters TJ, Quinlan A, Hoffbrand AV: Subcellular localization of radioactive vitamin B12 during absorption by guinea-pig ileum. *Clin Sci* 37(2):568–569, 1969.

121. Pletsch Q, Coffey J: Properties of the proteins that bind vitamin B12 in subcellular fractions of rat liver. *Arch Biochem Biophys* 151(1):157–167, 1972.

122. Watanabe F, Nakano Y: Comparative biochemistry of vitamin B12 (cobalamin) metabolism: Biochemical diversity in the systems for intracellular cobalamin transfer and synthesis of the coenzymes. *Int J Biochem* 23(12):1353–1359, 1991.

123. Burger R, Allen R: Characterization of vitamin B12-binding proteins isolated from human milk and saliva by affinity chromatography. *J Biol Chem* 249(22):7220–7227, 1974.

124. Hurlimann J, Zuber C: Vitamin B12-binders in human body fluids. II. Synthesis *in vitro*. *Clin Exp Immunol* 4(1):141–148, 1969.

125. Simons K, Weber T: The vitamin B12-binding protein in human leukocytes. *Biochim Biophys Acta* 117(1):201–208, 1966.

126. Johnston J, Bollekens J, Allen R, Berliner N: Structure of the cDNA encoding transcobalamin I, a neutrophil granule protein. *J Biol Chem* 264(27):15754–15757, 1989.

127. Johnston J, Yang-Feng T, Berliner N: Genomic structure and mapping of the chromosomal gene for transcobalamin I (TCN1): Comparison to human intrinsic factor. *Genomics* 12(3):459–464, 1992.

128. Burger R, Schneider R, Mehlman C, Allen R: Human plasma R-type vitamin B12-binding proteins. II. The role of transcobalamin I, transcobalamin III, and the normal granulocyte vitamin B12-binding protein in the plasma transport of vitamin B12. *J Biol Chem* 250(19):7707–7713, 1975.

129. Guéant J, Monin B, Boissel P, et al: Biliary excretion of cobalamin and cobalamin analogues in man. *Digestion* 30(3):151–157, 1984.

130. Gottlieb C, Retief F, Herbert V: Blockade of vitamin B12-binding sites in gastric juice, serum and saliva by analogues and derivatives of vitamin B12 and by antibody to intrinsic factor. *Biochim Biophys Acta* 141(3):560–572, 1967.

131. Allen R, Stabler S: Identification and quantitation of cobalamin and cobalamin analogues in human feces. *Am J Clin Nutr* 87(5):1324–1335, 2008.

132. Green R LK-S, Sutter S, Allen LH, Buchholz B, Dueker SR, Miller JW: Evidence that physiological doses of vitamin B12 are metabolized or degraded in the gastrointestinal tract: Implications for vitamin B12 bioavailability and fortification. *FASEB J* 2009:335.

133. Kolhouse J, Kondo H, Allen N, et al: Cobalamin analogues are present in human plasma and can mask cobalamin deficiency because current radioisotope dilution assays are not specific for true cobalamin. *N Engl J Med* 299(15):785–792, 1978.

134. Kondo H, Kolhouse J, Allen R: Presence of cobalamin analogues in animal tissues. *Proc Natl Acad Sci U S A* 77(2):817–821, 1980.

135. Hom B: Plasma turnover of 57cobalt-vitamin B12 bound to transcobalamin I and II. *Scand J Haematol* 4(5):321–332, 1967.

136. Carmel R: The distribution of endogenous cobalamin among cobalamin-binding proteins in the blood in normal and abnormal states. *Am J Clin Nutr* 41(4):713–719, 1985.

137. Nexo E, Hvas AM, Bleie Ø, et al: Holo-transcobalamin is an early marker of changes in cobalamin homeostasis. A randomized placebo-controlled study. *Clin Chem* 48(10):1768–1771, 2002.

138. Hvas A, Nexo E: Holotranscobalamin as a predictor of vitamin B12 status. *Clin Chem Lab Med* 41(11):1489–1492, 2003.

139. Lloyd-Wright Z, Hvas A, Møller J, et al: Holotranscobalamin as an indicator of dietary vitamin B12 deficiency. *Clin Chem* 49(12):2076–2078, 2003.

140. Obeid R, Herrmann W: Holotranscobalamin in laboratory diagnosis of cobalamin deficiency compared to total cobalamin and methylmalonic acid. *Clin Chem Lab Med* 45(12):1746–1750, 2007.

141. Herzlich B, Herbert V: Depletion of serum holotranscobalamin II. An early sign of negative vitamin B12 balance. *Lab Invest* 58(3):332–337, 1988.

142. Lindgren A, Kilander A, Bagge E, Nexø E: Holotranscobalamin-a sensitive marker of cobalamin malabsorption. *Eur J Clin Invest* 29(4):321–329, 1999.

143. Miller JW, Garrod MG, Rockwood AL, et al: Measurement of total vitamin B12 and holotranscobalamin, singly and in combination, in screening for metabolic vitamin B12 deficiency. *Clin Chem* 52(2):278–285, 2006.

144. Bertaux O, Mederic C, Valencia R: Amplification of ribosomal DNA in the nucleolus of vitamin B12-deficient Euglena cells. *Exp Cell Res* 195(1):119–128, 1991.

145. Rondanelli E, Gorini P, Magliulo E, Fiori G: Differences in proliferative activity between normoblasts and pernicious anemia megaloblasts. *Blood* 24:542–552, 1964.

146. Steinberg S, Fonda S, Campbell C, Hillman R: Cellular abnormalities of folate deficiency. *Br J Haematol* 54(4):605–612, 1983.

147. Wickremasinghe R, Hoffbrand A: Reduced rate of DNA replication fork movement in megaloblastic anemia. *J Clin Invest* 65(1):26–36, 1980.

148. Duthie S, McMillan P: Uracil misincorporation in human DNA detected using single cell gel electrophoresis. *Carcinogenesis* 18(9):1709–1714, 1997.

149. Koury M, Horne D, Brown Z, et al: Apoptosis of late-stage erythroblasts in megaloblastic anemia: Association with DNA damage and macrocyte production. *Blood* 89(12):4617–4623, 1997.

150. Metz J, Kelly A, Swett V, et al: Deranged DNA synthesis by bone marrow from vitamin B-12-deficient humans. *Br J Haematol* 14(6):575–592, 1968.

151. Das K, Mohanty D, Garewal G: Cytogenetics in nutritional megaloblastic anaemia: Prolonged persistence of chromosomal abnormalities in lymphocytes after remission. *Acta Haematol* 76(2–3):146–154, 1986.

152. Fernandes-Costa F, Green R, Torrance J: Increased erythrocytic diphosphoglycerate in megaloblastic anaemia. A compensatory mechanism? *S Afr Med J* 53(18):709–712, 1978.

153. Green R, Kuhl W, Jacobson R, et al: Masking of macrocytosis by alpha-thalassemia in blacks with pernicious anemia. *N Engl J Med* 307(21):1322–1325, 1982.

154. Spivak J: Masked megaloblastic anemia. *Arch Intern Med* 142(12):2111–2114, 1982.

155. Lindenbaum J, Nath BJ: Megaloblastic anaemia and neutrophil hypersegmentation. *Br J Haematol* 44(3):511–513, 1980.

156. Carmel R, Green R, Jacobsen DW, Qian GD: Neutrophil nuclear segmentation in mild cobalamin deficiency: Relation to metabolic tests of cobalamin status and observations on ethnic differences in neutrophil segmentation. *Am J Clin Pathol* 106(1):57–63, 1996.

157. Lawler S, Roberts P, Hoffbrand A: Chromosome studies in megaloblastic anaemia before and after treatment. *Scand J Haematol* 8(4):309–320, 1971.

158. Bessman J, Williams L, Gilmer PJ: Platelet size in health and hematologic disease. *Am J Clin Pathol* 78(2):150–153, 1982.

159. Marsh GW, Stewart JS: Splenic function in adult coeliac disease. *Br J Haematol* 19(4):445–457, 1970.

160. Fudenberg H, Estren S: Non-addisonian megaloblastic anemia; the intermediate megaloblast in the differential diagnosis of pernicious and related anemias. *Am J Med* 25(2):198–209, 1958.

161. Gulley M, Bentley S, Ross D: Neutrophil myeloperoxidase measurement uncovers masked megaloblastic anemia. *Blood* 76(5):1004–1007, 1990.

162. Solanki DL, Jacobson RJ, McKibbon J, Green R: Racial patterns in pernicious anemia. *N Engl J Med* 298(24):1365.

163. Solanki D, Jacobson R, Green R, et al: Pernicious anemia in blacks. A study of 64 patients from Washington, D.C., and Johannesburg, South Africa. *Am J Clin Pathol* 1981;75(1):96–99, 1978.

164. Harper J, Holleran SF, Ramakrishnan R, et al: Anemia in celiac disease is multifactorial in etiology. *Am J Hematol* 82(11):996–1000, 2007.

165. Green R: Anemias beyond B12 and iron deficiency: The buzz about other B's, elementary, and nonelementary problems. *Hematology Am Soc Hematol Educ Program* 2012:492–498, 2012.

166. Bunn HF: Vitamin B12 and pernicious anemia—The dawn of molecular medicine. *N Engl J Med* 370(8):773–776, 2014.

167. Hershko C, Ronson A, Souroujon M, et al: Variable hematologic presentation of autoimmune gastritis: Age-related progression from iron deficiency to cobalamin depletion. *Blood* 107(4):1673–1679, 2006.

168. Boddington M, Spriggs A: The epithelial cells in megaloblastic anaemias. *J Clin Pathol* 12(3):228–234, 1959.

169. Hussein S, Laulicht M, Hoffbrand A: Serum ferritin in megaloblastic anaemia. *Scand J Haematol* 20(3):241–245, 1978.

170. Emerson P, Wilkinson J: Lactate dehydrogenase in the diagnosis and assessment of response to treatment of megaloblastic anaemia. *Br J Haematol* 12(6):678–688, 1966.

171. Winston R, Warburton F, Stott A: Enzymatic diagnosis of megaloblastic anaemia. *Br J Haematol* 19(5):587–592, 1970.

172. Hansen N, Karle H: Blood and bone-marrow lysozyme in neutropenia: An attempt towards pathogenetic classification. *Br J Haematol* 21(3):261–270, 1971.

173. Heller P, Weinstein H, West M, Zimmerman H: Enzymes in anemia: A study of abnormalities of several enzymes of carbohydrate metabolism in the plasma and erythrocytes in patients with anemia, with preliminary observations of bone marrow enzymes. *Ann Intern Med* 53:898–913, 1960.

174. de Klerk G, Rosengarten P, Vet R, Goudsmit R: Serum erythropoietin (ESF) titers in polycythemia. *Blood* 58(6):1171–1174, 1981.

175. Myhre E: Studies on the erythrokinetics in pernicious anemia. *Scand J Clin Lab Invest* 16:391–402, 1964.

176. Lindahl J: Quantification of ineffective erythropoiesis in megaloblastic anaemia by determination of endogenous production of 14CO after administration of glycine-2-14C. *Scand J Haematol* 24(4):281–291, 1980.

177. Hamililton H, Sheets R, DeGowin E: Studies with inagglutinable erythrocyte counts. VII. Further investigation of the hemolytic mechanism in untreated pernicious anemia and the demonstration of a hemolytic property in the plasma. *J Lab Clin Med* 51(6):942–955, 1958.

178. Harker L, Finch C: Thrombokinetics in man. *J Clin Invest* 48(6):963–974, 1969.

179. Obeid R, Geisel J, Schorr H, et al: The impact of vegetarianism on some haematological parameters. *Eur J Haematol* 69(5–6):275–279, 2002.

180. Jacques P, Selhub J, Bostom A, et al: The effect of folic acid fortification on plasma folate and total homocysteine concentrations. *N Engl J Med* 340(19):1449–1454, 1999.

181. Ballard H, Lindenbaum J: Megaloblastic anemia complicating hyperalimentation therapy. *Am J Med* 56(5):740–742, 1974.

182. Mollin D, Hines J: Late post-gastrectomy syndromes. observations on the nature and pathogenesis of anaemia following partial gastrectomy. *Proc R Soc Med* 57:575–580, 1964.

183. Hoffbrand A: Folate deficiency in premature infants. *Arch Dis Child* 45(242):441–444, 1970.

184. Royston NJ, Parry TE: Megaloblastic anaemia complicating dietary treatment of phenylketonuria in infancy. *Arch Dis Child* 37(194):430–435, 1962.

185. Ford JD, Scott KJ: The folic acid activity of some milk foods for babies. *J Dairy Res* 35:85, 1968.

186. Savage D, Lindenbaum J: Anemia in alcoholics. *Medicine (Baltimore)* 65(5):322–338, 1986.

187. Eichner E, Hillman R: Effect of alcohol on serum folate level. *J Clin Invest* 52(3):584–591, 1973.

188. Lieber C: Metabolism and metabolic effects of alcohol. *Semin Hematol* 17(2):85–99, 1980.

189. Post R, Desforges J: Thrombocytopenia and alcoholism. *Ann Intern Med* 68(6):1230–1236, 1968.

190. Liu Y: Effects of alcohol on granulocytes and lymphocytes. *Semin Hematol* 17(2):130–136, 1980.

191. Lindenbaum J, Lieber C: Hematologic effects of alcohol in man in the absence of nutritional deficiency. *N Engl J Med* 281(7):333–338, 1969.

192. Trier J: Celiac sprue. *N Engl J Med* 325(24):1709–1719, 1991.

193. Halsted C, Reisenauer A, Romero J, et al: Jejunal perfusion of simple and conjugated folates in celiac sprue. *J Clin Invest* 59(5):933–940, 1977.

194. Hjelt K, Krasilnikoff P: The impact of gluten on haematological status, dietary intakes of haemopoietic nutrients and vitamin B12 and folic acid absorption in children with coeliac disease. *Acta Paediatr Scand* 79(10):911–919, 1990.

195. Klipstein F: Tropical sprue in New York City. *Gastroenterology* 47:457–470, 1964.

196. Klipstein F, Schenk E, Samloff I: Folate repletion associated with oral tetracycline therapy in tropical sprue. *Gastroenterology* 51(3):317–332, 1966.

197. Klipstein F: Progress in gastroenterology: Tropical sprue. *Gastroenterology* 275, 1968.

198. Sheehy T, Perez-Santiago E, Rubini M: Tropical sprue and vitamin B12. *N Engl J Med* 265:1232–1236, 1961.

199. Klipstein F: Folate in tropical sprue. *Br J Haematol* 23: Suppl:119–133, 1972.

200. Corcino J, Coll G, Klipstein F: Pteroylglutamic acid malabsorption in tropical sprue. *Blood* 45(4):577–580, 1975.

201. Chanarin I, Bennett M: Absorption of folic acid and D-xylose as tests of small-intestinal function. *Br Med J* 1(5283):985–989, 1962.

202. Booth C: The metabolic effects of intestinal resection in man. *Postgrad Med J* 37:725–739, 1961.

203. Pitney W, Joske R, Mackinnon N: Folic acid and other absorption tests in lymphosarcoma, chronic lymphocytic leukaemia, and some related conditions. *J Clin Pathol* 13:440–447, 1960.

204. Hoskins L, Norris H, Gottlieb L, Zamcheck N: Functional and morphologic alterations of the gastrointestinal tract in progressive systemic sclerosis (scleroderma). *Am J Med* 33:459–470, 1962.

205. Vinnik I, Kern FJ, Struthers JJ: Malabsorption and the diarrhea of diabetes mellitus. *Gastroenterology* 43:507–520, 1962.

206. Cook G, Morgan J, Hoffbrand A: Impairment of folate absorption by systemic bacterial infections. *Lancet* 2(7894):1416–1417, 1974.

207. Shojania AM: Folic acid and vitamin B12 deficiency in pregnancy and in the neonatal period. *Clin Perinatol* 11(2):433–459, 1984.

208. Landon M, Eyre D, Hytten F: Transfer of folate to the fetus. *Br J Obstet Gynaecol* 82(1):12–19, 1975.

209. Pritchard J, Scott D, Whalley P, Haling RJ: Infants of mothers with megaloblastic anemia due to folate deficiency. *JAMA* 211(12):1982–1984, 1970.

210. Shapiro J, Alberts H, Welch P, Metz J: Folate and vitamin B-12 deficiency associated with lactation. *Br J Haematol* 11:498–504, 1965.

211. Streiff R, Little A: Folic acid deficiency in pregnancy. *N Engl J Med* 276(14):776–779, 1967.

212. de Benoist B. Conclusions of a WHO Technical Consultation on folate and vitamin B12 deficiencies. *Food Nutr Bull* 29(2 Suppl):S238–S244, 2008.

213. Chanarin I, McFadyen I, Kyle R: The physiological macrocytosis of pregnancy. *Br J Obstet Gynaecol* 84(7):504–508, 1977.

214. Avery B, Ledger W: Folic acid metabolism in well-nourished pregnant women. *Obstet Gynecol* 35(4):616–624, 1970.

215. Giles C: An account of 335 cases of megaloblastic anaemia of pregnancy and the puerperium. *J Clin Pathol* 19(1):1–11, 1966.

216. Lindenbaum J, Klipstein F: Folic acid deficiency in sickle-cell anemia. *N Engl J Med* 269:875–882, 1963.

217. Hild D: Folate losses from the skin in exfoliative dermatitis. *Arch Intern Med* 123(1):51–57, 1969.

218. Whitehead V, Comty C, Posen G, Kaye M: Homeostasis of folic acid in patients undergoing maintenance hemodialysis. *N Engl J Med* 279(18):970–974, 1968.

219. Green R: Metabolite assays in cobalamin and folate deficiency. *Baillieres Clin Haematol* 8(3):533–566, 1995.

220. Hoffbrand A, Newcombe F, Mollin D: Method of assay of red cell folate activity and the value of the assay as a test for folate deficiency. *J Clin Pathol* 19(1):17–28, 1966.

221. Lindenbaum J: Status of laboratory testing in the diagnosis of megaloblastic anemia. *Blood* 61(4):624–627, 1983.

222. McNamee T, Hyland T, Harrington J, et al: Haematinic deficiency and macrocytosis in middle-aged and older adults. *PLoS One* 8(11):E77743, 2013.

223. Leffler DA, Schuppan D: Update on serologic testing in celiac disease. *Am J Gastroenterol* 2010;105(12):2520–2524, 2013.

224. Kinnear D, Macintosh P, Cameron D, et al: Intestinal absorption of tritium-labelled folic acid in idiopathic steatorrhea: Effect of a gluten-free diet. *Can Med Assoc J* 89:975–979, 1963.

225. Green R, Miller JW: Folate deficiency beyond megaloblastic anemia: Hyperhomocysteinemia and other manifestations of dysfunctional folate status. *Semin Hematol* 36(1):47–64, 1999.

226. Prevention of neural tube defects: Results of the Medical Research Council Vitamin Study. MRC Vitamin Study Research Group. *Lancet* 338(8760):131–137, 1991.

227. Rothenberg S, da Costa M, Sequeira J, et al: Autoantibodies against folate receptors in women with a pregnancy complicated by a neural-tube defect. *N Engl J Med* 350(2):134–142, 2004.

228. van der Put N, Gabreëls F, Stevens E, et al: A second common mutation in the methylenetetrahydrofolate reductase gene: An additional risk factor for neural-tube defects? *Am J Hum Genet* 62(5):1044–1051, 1998.

229. Honein M, Paulozzi L, Mathews T, et al: Impact of folic acid fortification of the US food supply on the occurrence of neural tube defects. *JAMA* 285(23):2981–2986, 2001.

230. De Wals P, Tairou F, Van Allen M, et al: Reduction in neural-tube defects after folic acid fortification in Canada. *N Engl J Med* 357(2):135–142, 2007.

231. Afman L, Van Der Put N, Thomas C, et al: Reduced vitamin B12 binding by transcobalamin II increases the risk of neural tube defects. *QJM* 94(3):159–166, 2001.

232. Thompson M, Cole D, Ray J: Vitamin B-12 and neural tube defects: The Canadian experience. *Am J Clin Nutr* 89(2):697S–701S, 2009.

233. Ramos MI, Allen LH, Haan MN, et al: Plasma folate concentrations are associated with depressive symptoms in elderly Latina women despite folic acid fortification. *Am J Clin Nutr* 80(4):1024–1028, 2004.

234. D'Angelo A, Selhub J: Homocysteine and thrombotic disease. *Blood* 90(1):1–11, 1997.

235. Schnyder G, Roffi M, Pin R, et al: Decreased rate of coronary restenosis after lowering of plasma homocysteine levels. *N Engl J Med* 345(22):1593–1600, 2001.

236. Lange H, Suryapranata H, De Luca G, et al: Folate therapy and in-stent restenosis after coronary stenting. *N Engl J Med* 350(26):2673–2681, 2004.

237. Bonaa KH, Njolstad I, Ueland PM, et al: Homocysteine lowering and cardiovascular events after acute myocardial infarction. *N Engl J Med* 354(15):1578–1588, 2006.

238. Yang Q, Botto LD, Erickson JD, et al: Improvement in stroke mortality in Canada and the United States, 1990 to 2002. *Circulation* 113(10):1335–1343, 2006.

239. Clarke R, Halsey J, Lewington S, et al: Effects of lowering homocysteine levels with B vitamins on cardiovascular disease, cancer, and cause-specific mortality: Meta-analysis of 8 randomized trials involving 37 485 individuals. *Arch Intern Med* 170(18):1622–1631, 2010.

240. Seshadri S, Beiser A, Selhub J, et al: Plasma homocysteine as a risk factor for dementia and Alzheimer's disease. *N Engl J Med* 346(7):476–483, 2002.

241. Haan MN, Miller JW, Aiello AE, et al: Homocysteine, B vitamins, and the incidence of dementia and cognitive impairment: Results from the Sacramento Area Latino Study on Aging. *Am J Clin Nutr* 85(2):511–517, 2007.

242. Kluijtmans L, Young I, Boreham C, et al: Genetic and nutritional factors contributing to hyperhomocysteinemia in young adults. *Blood* 101(7):2483–2488, 2003.

243. Quinlivan E, McPartlin J, McNulty H, et al: Importance of both folic acid and vitamin B12 in reduction of risk of vascular disease. *Lancet* 359(9302):227–228, 2002.

244. Lievers K, Kluijtmans L, Boers G, et al: Influence of a glutamate carboxypeptidase II (GCPII) polymorphism (1561C—>T) on plasma homocysteine, folate and vitamin B(12) levels and its relationship to cardiovascular disease risk. *Atherosclerosis* 164(2):269–273, 2002.

245. Walker S, Wein P, Ihle B: Severe folate deficiency masquerading as the syndrome of hemolysis, elevated liver enzymes, and low platelets. *Obstet Gynecol* 90(4 Pt 2):655–657, 1997.

246. Hartong SC, Steegers EA, Visser W: Hemolysis, elevated liver enzymes and low platelets during pregnancy due to Vitamin B12 and folate deficiencies. *Eur J Obstet Gynecol Reprod Biol* 131(2):241–242, 2007.

247. Giovannucci E, Stampfer M, Colditz G, et al: Multivitamin use, folate, and colon cancer in women in the Nurses' Health Study. *Ann Intern Med* 129(7):517–524, 1998.

248. Ma J, Stampfer M, Giovannucci E, et al: Methylenetetrahydrofolate reductase polymorphism, dietary interactions, and risk of colorectal cancer. *Cancer Res* 57(6):1098–1102, 1997.

249. Mason JB, Dickstein A, Jacques PF, et al: A temporal association between folic acid fortification and an increase in colorectal cancer rates may be illuminating important biological principles: A hypothesis. *Cancer Epidemiol Biomarkers Prev* 16(7):1325–1329, 2007.

250. Kim Y: Will mandatory folic acid fortification prevent or promote cancer? *Am J Clin Nutr* 80(5):1123–1128, 2004.

251. Vollset SE, Clarke R, Lewington S, et al: Effects of folic acid supplementation on overall and site-specific cancer incidence during the randomised trials: Meta-analyses of data on 50,000 individuals. *Lancet* 381(9871):1029–1036, 2013.

252. Rosenberg I: Folic acid and neural-tube defects—Time for action? *N Engl J Med* 327(26):1875–1877, 1992.

253. Hibbard E, Spencer W: Low serum B12 levels and latent Addisonian anaemia in pregnancy. *J Obstet Gynaecol Br Commonw* 77(1):52–57, 1970.

254. Carmel R, Johnson C: Racial patterns in pernicious anemia. Early age at onset and increased frequency of intrinsic-factor antibody in black women. *N Engl J Med* 298(12):647–650, 1978.

255. Vilter CF, Vilter RW, Spies TD: The treatment of pernicious and related anemias with synthetic folic acid: I. Observations on the maintenance of a normal hematologic status and on the occurrence of combined system disease at the end of one year. *J Lab Clin Med* 32(3):262–273, 1947.

256. Andersen L, Hansen E, Knudsen J, et al: Prospectively measured red cell folate levels in methotrexate treated patients with rheumatoid arthritis: Relation to withdrawal and side effects. *J Rheumatol* 24(5):830–837, 1997.

257. Kim YS, Sun JM, Ahn JS, et al: The optimal duration of vitamin supplementation prior to the first dose of pemetrexed in patients with non-small-cell lung cancer. *Lung Cancer* 81(2):231–235, 2013.

258. Stabler SP: Clinical practice. Vitamin B12 deficiency. *N Engl J Med* 368(2):149–160, 2013.

259. Toh B, van Driel I, Gleeson P: Pernicious anemia. *N Engl J Med* 337(20):1441–1448, 1997.

260. Kano Y, Sakamoto S, Miura Y, Takaku F: Disorders of cobalamin metabolism. *Crit Rev Oncol Hematol* 3(1):1–34, 1985.

261. Irvine W, Davies S, Teitelbaum S, et al: The clinical and pathological significance of gastric parietal cell antibody. *Ann N Y Acad Sci* 124(2):657–691, 1965.

262. Gaarder P, Heier H: A human autoantibody to renal collecting duct cells associated with thyroid and gastric autoimmunity and possibly renal tubular acidosis. *Clin Exp Immunol* 51(1):29–37, 1983.

263. Suri-Payer E, Kehn P, Cheever A, Shevach E: Pathogenesis of post-thymectomy autoimmune gastritis. Identification of anti-H/K adenosine triphosphatase-reactive T cells. *J Immunol* 157(4):1799–1805, 1996.

264. Kapadia C, Donaldson RJ: Disorders of cobalamin (vitamin B12) absorption and transport. *Annu Rev Med* 36:93–110, 1985.

265. Chanarin I, James D: Humoral and cell-mediated intrinsic-factor antibody in pernicious anaemia. *Lancet* 1(7866):1078–1080, 1974.

266. Conn H, Binder H, Burns B: Pernicious anemia and immunologic deficiency. *Ann Intern Med* 68(3):603–612, 1968.

267. Conn HO, Binder H, Burns B: Pernicious anemia and immunologic deficiency. *Ann Intern Med* 68(3):603–612, 1968.

268. Ardeman S, Chanarin I, Krafchik B, Singer W: Addisonian pernicious anaemia and intrinsic factor antibodies in thyroid disorders. *Q J Med* 35(139):421–431, 1966.

269. Comin D, Hines J, Wieland R: Coexistent pernicious anemia and idiopathic hypoparathyroidism in a women. *JAMA* 207(6):1147–1149, 1969.

270. Mazzone T, Kelly W, Ensinck J: Lymphocytic hypophysitis. Associated with antiparietal cell antibodies and vitamin B12 deficiency. *Arch Intern Med* 143(9):1794–1795, 1983.

271. Howitz J, Schwartz M: Vitiligo, achlorhydria, and pernicious anaemia. *Lancet* 1(7713):1331–1334, 1971.

272. Jackson I, Doig W, McDonald G: Pernicious anaemia as a cause of infertility. *Lancet* 2(7527):1159–1160, 1967.

273. Watson A: Seminal vitamin B12 and sterility. *Lancet* 2(7257):644, 1962.

274. Pront R, Margalioth EJ, Green R, et al: Prevalence of low serum cobalamin in infertile couples. *Andrologia* 2009;41(1):46–50, 1962.

275. Ungar B, Mathews J, Tait B, Cowling D: HLA-DR patterns in pernicious anaemia. *Br Med J (Clin Res Ed)* 282(6266):768–770, 1981.

276. Hoskins L, Loux H, Britten A, Zamcheck N: Distribution of ABO blood groups in patients with pernicious anemia, gastric carcinoma and gastric carcinoma associated with pernicious anemia. *N Engl J Med* 273(12):633–637, 1965.

277. Wangel A, Callender S, Spray G, Wright R: A family study of pernicious anaemia. I. Autoantibodies, achlorhydria, serum pepsinogen and vitamin B12. *Br J Haematol* 14(2):161–181, 1968.

278. Varis K, Ihamäki T, Härkönen M, et al: Gastric morphology, function, and immunology in first-degree relatives of probands with pernicious anemia and controls. *Scand J Gastroenterol* 14(2):129–139, 1979.

279. Eriksson S, Clase L, Moquist-Olsson I: Pernicious anemia as a risk factor in gastric cancer. The extent of the problem. *Acta Med Scand* 210(6):481–484, 1981.

280. Savage D, Gangaidzo I, Lindenbaum J, et al: Vitamin B12 deficiency is the primary cause of megaloblastic anaemia in Zimbabwe. *Br J Haematol* 86(4):844–850, 1994.

281. Wilkinson JF: The gastric secretions in pernicious anemia. *Q J Med* 1(3)361, 1932.

282. Karnes WJ, Samloff I, Siurala M, et al: Positive serum antibody and negative tissue staining for Helicobacter pylori in subjects with atrophic body gastritis. *Gastroenterology* 101(1):167–174, 1991.

283. Green R: Protean *H. pylori*: Perhaps "pernicious" too? (Editorial) *Blood* 107(4):1247, 2006.

284. Slingerland D, Cardarelli J, Burrows B, Miller A: The utility of serum gastrin levels in assessing the significance of low serum B12 levels. *Arch Intern Med* 144(6):1167–1168, 1984.

285. Ganguli P, Cullen D, Irvine W: Radioimmunoassay of plasma gastrin in pernicious anaemia, achlorhydria without pernicious anaemia, hypochlorhydria, and in controls. *Lancet* 1(7691):155–158, 1971.

286. Kaye M, Whorwell P, Wright R: Gastric mucosal lymphocyte subpopulations in pernicious anemia and in normal stomach. *Clin Immunol Immunopathol* 28(3):431–440, 1983.

287. Rodbro P, Dige-Petersen H, Schwartz M, Dalgaard O: Effect of steroids on gastric mucosal structure and function in pernicious anemia. *Acta Med Scand* 181(4):445–452, 1967.

288. Ransohoff R, Jacobsen D, Green R: Vitamin B12 deficiency and multiple sclerosis. *Lancet* 335(8700):1285–1286, 1990.

289. Nieburgs H, Glass G: Gastric-cell maturation disorders in atrophic gastritis, pernicious anemia, and carcinoma. Histologic site of origin and diagnostic significance of abnormal cells. *Am J Dig Dis* 8:135–159, 1963.

290. Foroozan P, Trier J: Mucosa of the small intestine in pernicious anemia. *N Engl J Med* 277(11):553–559, 1967.

291. Bezman A, Kinnear D, Zamcheck N: D-Xylose and potassium iodide absorption and serum carotene in pernicious anemia. *J Lab Clin Med* 53(2):226–232, 1959.

292. Ellison A: Pernicious anemia masked by multivitamins containing folic acid. *JAMA* 173:240–243, 1960.

293. Carmel R: Subtle and atypical cobalamin deficiency states. *Am J Hematol* 34(2):108–114, 1990.

294. Lindenbaum J, Healton E, Savage D, et al: Neuropsychiatric disorders caused by cobalamin deficiency in the absence of anemia or macrocytosis. *N Engl J Med* 318(26):1720–1728, 1988.

295. MacLean L, Sundberg R: Incidence of megaloblastic anemia after total gastrectomy. *N Engl J Med* 254(19):885–893, 1956.

296. Gozzard D, Dawson D, Lewis M: Experiences with dual protein bound aqueous vitamin B12 absorption test in subjects with low serum vitamin B12 concentrations. *J Clin Pathol* 40(6):633–637, 1987.

297. Van der Weyden M, Rother M, Firkin B: Megaloblastic maturation masked by iron deficiency: A biochemical basis. *Br J Haematol* 22(3):299–307, 1972.

298. Lees F, Grandjean L: The gastric and jejunal mucosae in healthy patients with partial gastrectomy. *AMA Arch Intern Med* 101(5):943–951, 1958.

299. Chen M, Krishnamurthy A, Mohamed AR, Green R: Hematological disorders following gastric bypass surgery: Emerging concepts of the interplay between nutritional deficiency and inflammation. *Biomed Res Int* 2013:205467, 2013.

300. Shimoda S, Rubin C: The Zollinger-Ellison syndrome with steatorrhea. I. Anticholinergic treatment followed by total gastrectomy and colonic interposition. *Gastroenterology* 1968;55(6):695–704, 2013.

301. Kennedy H, Callender S, Truelove S, Warner G: Haematological aspects of life with an ileostomy. *Br J Haematol* 52(3):445–454, 1982.

302. Anderson C, Walton K, Chanarin I: Megaloblastic anaemia after pelvic radiotherapy for carcinoma of the cervix. *J Clin Pathol* 34(2):151–152, 1981.

303. Tudhope G, Wilson G: Deficiency of vitamin B12 in hypothyroidism. *Lancet* 1(7232):703–706, 1962.

304. Waxman S, Corcino J, Herbert V: Drugs, toxins and dietary amino acids affecting vitamin B12 or folic acid absorption or utilization. *Am J Med* 48(5):599–608, 1970.

305. Lindenbaum J, Pezzimenti JF, Shea N: Small-intestinal function in vitamin B12 deficiency. *Ann Intern Med* 80(3):326–331, 1974.

306. Cameron D, Watson G, Witts L: The clinical association of macrocytic anemia with intestinal stricture and anastomosis. *Blood* 4(7):793–802, 1949.

307. Murphy M, Sourial N, Burman J, et al: Megaloblastic anaemia due to vitamin B12 deficiency caused by small intestinal bacterial overgrowth: Possible role of vitamin B12 analogues. *Br J Haematol* 62(1):7–12, 1986.

308. Nyberg W: The influence of *Diphyllobothrium latum* on the vitamin B12-intrinsic factor complex. I. In vivo studies with Schilling test technique. *Acta Med Scand* 167:185–187, 1960.

309. Harriman G, Smith P, Horne M, et al: Vitamin B12 malabsorption in patients with acquired immunodeficiency syndrome. *Arch Intern Med* 149(9):2039–2041, 1989.

310. Herzlich B, Schiano T, Moussa Z, et al: Decreased intrinsic factor secretion in AIDS: Relation to parietal cell acid secretory capacity and vitamin B12 malabsorption. *Am J Gastroenterol* 87(12):1781–1788, 1992.

311. Remacha A, Cadafalch J: Cobalamin deficiency in patients infected with the human immunodeficiency virus. *Semin Hematol* 36(1):75–87, 1999.

312. Guéant J, Champigneulle B, Gaucher P, Nicolas J: Malabsorption of vitamin B12 in pancreatic insufficiency of the adult and of the child. *Pancreas* 5(5):559–567, 1990.

313. Toskes P, Deren J, Conrad M: Trypsin-like nature of the pancreatic factor that corrects vitamin B12 malabsorption associated with pancreatic dysfunction. *J Clin Invest* 52(7):1660–1664, 1973.

314. Henderson J, Simpson J, Warwick R, Shearman D: Does malabsorption of vitamin B 12 occur in chronic pancreatitis? *Lancet* 2(7771):241–243, 1972.

315. Gilois C, Wierzbicki A, Hirani N, et al: The hematological and electrophysiological effects of cobalamin. Deficiency secondary to vegetarian diets. *Ann N Y Acad Sci* 669:345–348, 1992.

316. Ford M: Megaloblastic anaemia in a vegetarian. *Br J Clin Pract* 34(7):222, 1980.

317. Michaud J, Lemieux B, Ogier H, Lambert M: Nutritional vitamin B12 deficiency: Two cases detected by routine newborn urinary screening. *Eur J Pediatr* 151(3):218–220, 1992.

318. Allen LH: How common is vitamin B-12 deficiency? *Am J Clin Nutr* 89(2):693S–696S, 2009.

319. Wickramasinghe S, Akinyanju O, Grange A, Litwinczuk R: Folate levels and deoxyuridine suppression tests in protein-energy malnutrition. *Br J Haematol* 53(1):135–143, 1983.

320. Frenkel E: Abnormal fatty acid metabolism in peripheral nerves of patients with pernicious anemia. *J Clin Invest* 52(5):1237–1245, 1973.

321. Watkins D, Rosenblatt DS: Inborn errors of cobalamin absorption and metabolism. *Am J Med Genet C Semin Med Genet* 157C(1):33–44, 2011.

322. Lever E, Elwes R, Williams A, Reynolds E: Subacute combined degeneration of the cord due to folate deficiency: Response to methyl folate treatment. *J Neurol Neurosurg Psychiatry* 49(10):1203–1207, 1986.

323. Clayton P, Smith I, Harding B, et al: Subacute combined degeneration of the cord, dementia and parkinsonism due to an inborn error of folate metabolism. *J Neurol Neurosurg Psychiatry* 49(8):920–927, 1986.

324. Green R, Van Tonder S, Oettle G, et al: Neurological changes in fruit bats deficient in vitamin B12. *Nature* 254(5496):148–150, 1975.

325. Weir D, Keating S, Molloy A, et al: Methylation deficiency causes vitamin B12-associated neuropathy in the pig. *J Neurochem* 51(6):1949–1952, 1988.

326. Molloy A, Orsi B, Kennedy D, et al: The relationship between the activity of methionine synthase and the ratio of S-adenosylmethionine to S-adenosylhomocysteine in the brain and other tissues of the pig. *Biochem Pharmacol* 44(7):1349–1355, 1992.

327. Deacon R, Purkiss P, Green R: Vitamin B12 neuropathy is not due to failure to methylate myelin basic protein. *J Neurol Sci* 72(1):113–117, 1986.

328. Kätkä K: Immune functions in pernicious anaemia before and during treatment with vitamin B12. *Scand J Haematol* 32(1):76–82, 1984.

329. Kätkä K, Eskola J, Granfors K, et al: Serum IgA deficiency and anti-IgA antibodies in pernicious anemia. *Clin Immunol Immunopathol* 46(1):55–60, 1988.

330. Zhang S, Willett W, Selhub J, et al: Plasma folate, vitamin B6, vitamin B12, homocysteine, and risk of breast cancer. *J Natl Cancer Inst* 95(5):373–380, 2003.

331. Dhonukshe-Rutten R, Lips M, de Jong N, et al: Vitamin B-12 status is associated with bone mineral content and bone mineral density in frail elderly women but not in men. *J Nutr* 133(3):801–807, 2003.

332. Stone K, Bauer D, Sellmeyer D, Cummings S: Low serum vitamin B-12 levels are associated with increased hip bone loss in older women: A prospective study. *J Clin Endocrinol Metab* 89(3):1217–1221, 2004.

333. Beck W: Neuropsychiatric consequences of cobalamin deficiency. *Adv Intern Med* 36:33–56, 1991.

334. Victor M, Lear A: Subacute combined degeneration of the spinal cord; current concepts of the disease process; value of serum vitamin B12; determinations in clarifying some of the common clinical problems. *Am J Med* 20(6):896–911, 1956.

335. Herbert V: Megaloblastic anemias. *Lab Invest* 52(1):3–19, 1985.

336. Di Lazzaro V, Restuccia D, Fogli D, et al: Central sensory and motor conduction in vitamin B12 deficiency. *Electroencephalogr Clin Neurophysiol* 84(5):433–439, 1992.

337. Fraser T: Cerebral manifestations of Addisonian pernicious anaemia. *Lancet* 2(7148):458–459, 1960.

338. Vogiatzoglou A, Refsum H, Johnston C, et al: Vitamin B12 status and rate of brain volume loss in community-dwelling elderly. *Neurology* 71(11):826–832, 2008.

339. de Lau L, Smith A, Refsum H, et al: Plasma vitamin B12 status and cerebral white-matter lesions. *J Neurol Neurosurg Psychiatry* 80(2):149–157, 2009.

340. Shulman R: Psychiatric aspects of pernicious anaemia: A prospective controlled investigation. *Br Med J* 3(5560):266–270, 1967.

341. Smith AD: Megaloblastic madness. *Br Med J* 2(5216):1840–1845, 1960.

342. Stojsavljević N, Lević Z, Drulović J, Dragutinović G: A 44-month clinical-brain MRI follow-up in a patient with B12 deficiency. *Neurology* 49(3):878–881, 1997.

343. Herbert V, Jacob E, Wong KT, et al: Low serum vitamin B12 levels in patients receiving ascorbic acid in megadoses: Studies concerning the effect of ascorbate on radioisotope vitamin B12 assay. *Am J Clin Nutr* 31(2):253–258, 1978.

344. Carmel R: R-binder deficiency. A clinically benign cause of cobalamin pseudodeficiency. *JAMA* 250(14):1886–1890, 1983.

345. Carmel R: Mild transcobalamin I (haptocorrin) deficiency and low serum cobalamin concentrations. *Clin Chem* 49(8):1367–1374, 2003.

346. Bor M, Nexø E, Hvas A: Holo-transcobalamin concentration and transcobalamin saturation reflect recent vitamin B12 absorption better than does serum vitamin B12. *Clin Chem* 50(6):1043–1049, 2004.

347. von Castel-Roberts K, Morkbak A, Nexo E, et al: Holo-transcobalamin is an indicator of vitamin B-12 absorption in healthy adults with adequate vitamin B-12 status. *Am J Clin Nutr* 85(4):1057–1061, 2007.

348. Barness LA: Vitamin B12 deficiency with emphasis on methylmalonic acid as a diagnostic aid. *Am J Clin Nutr* 20(6):573–582, 1967.

349. Norman E, Morrison J: Screening elderly populations for cobalamin (vitamin B12) deficiency using the urinary methylmalonic acid assay by gas chromatography mass spectrometry. *Am J Med* 94(6):589–594, 1993.

350. Norman E, Martelo O, Denton M: Cobalamin (vitamin B12) deficiency detection by urinary methylmalonic acid quantitation. *Blood* 59(6):1128–1131, 1982.

351. Lindenbaum J, Savage D, Stabler S, Allen R: Diagnosis of cobalamin deficiency: II. Relative sensitivities of serum cobalamin, methylmalonic acid, and total homocysteine concentrations. *Am J Hematol* 34(2):99–107, 1990.

352. Green R: Screening for vitamin B12 deficiency: Caveat emptor. *Ann Intern Med* 124(5):509–511, 1996.

353. Solomon LR: Cobalamin-responsive disorders in the ambulatory care setting: Unreliability of cobalamin, methylmalonic acid, and homocysteine testing. *Blood* 105(3):978–985; author reply 1137, 2005.

354. Stabler S, Allen R, Barrett R, et al: Cerebrospinal fluid methylmalonic acid levels in normal subjects and patients with cobalamin deficiency. *Neurology* 41(10):1627–1632, 1991.

355. Fairbanks V, Wahner H, Phyliky R: Tests for pernicious anemia: The "Schilling test." *Mayo Clin Proc* 58(8):541–544, 1983.

356. Bor M, Cetin M, Aytaç S, et al: Nonradioactive vitamin B12 absorption test evaluated in controls and in patients with inherited malabsorption of vitamin B12. *Clin Chem* 51(11):2151–2155, 2005.

357. Carkeet C, Dueker S, Lango J, et al: Human vitamin B12 absorption measurement by accelerator mass spectrometry using specifically labeled (14)C-cobalamin. *Proc Natl Acad Sci U S A* 103(15):5694–5699, 2006.

358. Metz J: The deoxyuridine suppression test. *Crit Rev Clin Lab Sci* 20(3):205–241, 1984.

359. Boddy K, King P, Mervyn L, et al: Retention of cyanocobalamin, hydroxocobalamin, and coenzyme B12 after parenteral administration. *Lancet* 2(7570):710–712, 1968.

360. Coleman D, Donohue D, Finch C, et al: Erythrokinetics in pernicious anemia. *Blood* 11(9):807–820, 1956.

361. Hillman R, Adamson J, Burka E: Characteristics of vitamin B12 correction of the abnormal erythropoiesis of pernicious anemia. *Blood* 31(4):419–432, 1968.

362. Sumner A, Chin M, Abrahm J, et al: Elevated methylmalonic acid and total homocysteine levels show high prevalence of vitamin B12 deficiency after gastric surgery. *Ann Intern Med* 124(5):469–476, 1996.

363. Paulk EJ, Farrar WJ: Diverticulosis of the small intestine and megaloblastic anemia: Intestinal microflora and absorption before and after tetracycline administration. *Am J Med* 37:473–480, 1964.

364. Kuzminski A, Del Giacco E, Allen R, et al: Effective treatment of cobalamin deficiency with oral cobalamin. *Blood* 92(4):1191–1198, 1998.

365. Crosby W: Improvisation revisited. Oral cyanocobalamin without intrinsic factor for pernicious anemia. *Arch Intern Med* 140(12):1582.

366. Andrès E, Kurtz J, Perrin A, et al: Oral cobalamin therapy for the treatment of patients with food-cobalamin malabsorption. *Am J Med* 2001;111(2):126–129, 1980.

367. Lederle F: Oral cobalamin for pernicious anemia: Back from the verge of extinction. *J Am Geriatr Soc* 46(9):1125–1127, 1998.

368. Amess J, Burman J, Rees G, et al: Megaloblastic haemopoiesis in patients receiving nitrous oxide. *Lancet* 2(8085):339–342, 1978.

369. Kondo H, Osborne M, Kolhouse J, et al: Nitrous oxide has multiple deleterious effects on cobalamin metabolism and causes decreases in activities of both mammalian cobalamin-dependent enzymes in rats. *J Clin Invest* 67(5):1270–1283, 1981.

370. Lumb M, Sharer N, Deacon R, et al: Effects of nitrous oxide-induced inactivation of cobalamin on methionine and S-adenosylmethionine metabolism in the rat. *Biochim Biophys Acta* 756(3):354–359, 1983.

371. O'Sullivan H, Jennings F, Ward K, et al: Human bone marrow biochemical function and megaloblastic hematopoiesis after nitrous oxide anesthesia. *Anesthesiology* 55(6):645–649, 1981.

372. Skacel P, Hewlett A, Lewis J, et al: Studies on the haemopoietic toxicity of nitrous oxide in man. *Br J Haematol* 53(2):189–200, 1983.

373. Kano Y, Sakamoto S, Sakuraya K, et al: Effects of leucovorin and methylcobalamin with N2O anesthesia. *J Lab Clin Med* 104(5):711–717, 1984.

374. Layzer R, Fishman R, Schafer J: Neuropathy following abuse of nitrous oxide. *Neurology* 28(5):504–506, 1978.

375. Easton D: Severe thrombocytopenia associated with acute folic acid deficiency and severe hemorrhage in two patients. *Can Med Assoc J* 130(4):418–420, 422, 1984.

376. Beard M, Hatipov C, Hamer J: Acute onset of folate deficiency in patients under intensive care. *Crit Care Med* 8(9):500–503, 1980.

377. Henderson G, Suresh M, Vitols K, Huennekens F: Transport of folate compounds in L1210 cells: Kinetic evidence that folate influx proceeds via the high-affinity transport system for 5-methyltetrahydrofolate and methotrexate. *Cancer Res* 46(4 Pt 1):1639–1643, 1986.

378. Schoo M, Pristupa Z, Vickers P, Scrimgeour K: Folate analogues as substrates of mammalian folylpolyglutamate synthetase. *Cancer Res* 45(7):3034–3041, 1985.

379. Huennekens FM, Duffy TH, Pope LE: Biochemistry of methotrexate: Teaching an old drug new tricks, in *Cancer Biology and Therapeutics* edited by Corry JG, Szentivanyi A, p 45. *Plenum*, New York, 1987.

380. Kesavan V, Sur P, Doig M, et al: Effects of methotrexate on folates in Krebs ascites and L1210 murine leukemia cells. *Cancer Lett* 30(1):55–59, 1986.

381. Spiegel R, Cooper P, Blum R, et al: Treatment of massive intrathecal methotrexate overdose by ventriculolumbar perfusion. *N Engl J Med* 311(6):386–388, 1984.

382. Yarchoan R, Broder S: Development of antiretroviral therapy for the acquired immunodeficiency syndrome and related disorders. A progress report. *N Engl J Med* 316(9):557–564, 1987.

383. Richman D, Fischl M, Grieco M, et al: The toxicity of azidothymidine (AZT) in the treatment of patients with AIDS and AIDS-related complex. A double-blind, placebo-controlled trial. *N Engl J Med* 317(4):192–197, 1987.

384. Boudes P, Zittoun J, Sobel A: Folate, vitamin B12, and HIV infection. *Lancet* 335(8702):1401–1402, 1990.

385. Krakoff I, Brown N, Reichard P: Inhibition of ribonucleoside diphosphate reductase by hydroxyurea. *Cancer Res* 28(8):1559–1565, 1968.

386. Termanini B, Gibril F, Sutliff VE, et al: Effect of long-term gastric acid suppressive therapy on serum vitamin B12 levels in patients with Zollinger-Ellison syndrome. *Am J Med* 104(5):422–430, 1998.

387. Koop H, Bachem M: Serum iron, ferritin, and vitamin B12 during prolonged omeprazole therapy. *J Clin Gastroenterol* 14(4):288–292, 1992.

388. Rosenblatt DS: Inherited disorders of folate and cobalamin transport and metabolism in *The Metabolic and Molecular bases of Inherited Metabolic Disease*, 8th ed, edited by Fenton WA, p 3897. McGraw-Hill, New York, 2001.

389. Whitehead V: Acquired and inherited disorders of cobalamin and folate in children. *Br J Haematol* 134(2):125–136, 2006.

390. Grasbeck R, Gordin R, Kantero I, Kuhlback B: Selective vitamin B12 malabsorption and proteinuria in young people. A syndrome. *Acta Med Scand* 167;289–296, 1960.

391. Zimran A, Hershko C: The changing pattern of megaloblastic anemia: Megaloblastic anemia in Israel. *Am J Clin Nutr* 37(5):855–861, 1983.

392. Aminoff M, Carter J, Chadwick R, et al: Mutations in CUBN, encoding the intrinsic factor-vitamin B12 receptor, cubilin, cause hereditary megaloblastic anaemia 1. *Nat Genet* 21(3):309–313, 1999.

393. He Q, Madsen M, Kilkenney A, et al: Amnionless function is required for cubilin brush-border expression and intrinsic factor-cobalamin (vitamin B12) absorption *in vivo*. *Blood* 106(4):1447–1453, 2005.

394. Carmel R: Gastric juice in congenital pernicious anemia contains no immunoreactive intrinsic factor molecule: Study of three kindreds with variable ages at presentation, including a patient first diagnosed in adulthood. *Am J Hum Genet* 35(1):67–77, 1983.

395. Cooper B, Rosenblatt D: Inherited defects of vitamin B12 metabolism. *Annu Rev Nutr* 7:291–320, 1987.

396. Miller D, Bloom G, Streiff R, et al: Juvenile "congenital" pernicious anemia. Clinical and immunologic studies. *N Engl J Med* 275(18):978–983, 1966.

397. Thomas P, Hoffbrand A, Smith I: Neurological involvement in hereditary transcobalamin II deficiency. *J Neurol Neurosurg Psychiatry* 45(1):74–77, 1982.

398. Carmel R, Green R, Rosenblatt D, Watkins D: Update on cobalamin, folate, and homocysteine. *Hematology Am Soc Hematol Educ Program* 62–81, 2003.

399. Barshop B, Wolff J, Nyhan W, et al: Transcobalamin II deficiency presenting with methylmalonic aciduria and homocystinuria and abnormal absorption of cobalamin. *Am J Med Genet* 35(2):222–228, 1990.

400. Rosenblatt D, Hosack A, Matiaszuk N: Expression of transcobalamin II by amniocytes. *Prenat Diagn* 7(1):35–39, 1987.

401. Namour F, Olivier J, Abdelmouttaleb I, et al: Transcobalamin codon 259 polymorphism in HT-29 and Caco-2 cells and in Caucasians: Relation to transcobalamin and homocysteine concentration in blood. *Blood* 97(4):1092–1098, 2001.

402. Miller JW, Ramos MI, Garrod MG, et al: Transcobalamin II 775G>C polymorphism and indices of vitamin B12 status in healthy older adults. *Blood* 100(2):718–720, 2002.

403. McIntyre O, Sullivan L, Jeffries G, Silver R: Pernicious anemia in childhood. *N Engl J Med* 272:981–986, 1965.

404. Fowler B: Genetic defects of folate and cobalamin metabolism. *Eur J Pediatr* 157 Suppl 2:S60–S66, 1998.

405. Watkins D, Matiaszuk N, Rosenblatt D: Complementation studies in the cblA class of inborn error of cobalamin metabolism: Evidence for interallelic complementation and for a new complementation class (cblH). *J Med Genet* 37(7):510–513, 2000.

406. Rosenblatt D, Cooper B, Pottier A, et al: Altered vitamin B12 metabolism in fibroblasts from a patient with megaloblastic anemia and homocystinuria due to a new defect in methionine biosynthesis. *J Clin Invest* 74(6):2149–2156, 1984.

407. Leclerc D, Campeau E, Goyette P, et al: Human methionine synthase: CDNA cloning and identification of mutations in patients of the cblG complementation group of folate/cobalamin disorders. *Hum Mol Genet* 5(12):1867–1874, 1996.

408. Gulati S, Chen Z, Brody L, et al: Defects in auxiliary redox proteins lead to functional methionine synthase deficiency. *J Biol Chem* 272(31):19171–19175, 1997.

409. Watkins D, Rosenblatt DS: Failure of lysosomal release of vitamin B12: A new complementation group causing methylmalonic aciduria (cblF). *Am J Hum Genet* 39(3):404–408, 1986.

410. van der Meer S, Spaapen L, Fowler B, et al: Prenatal treatment of a patient with vitamin B12-responsive methylmalonic acidemia. *J Pediatr* 117(6):923–926, 1990.

411. Erbe R: Inborn errors of folate metabolism (second of two parts). *N Engl J Med* 293(16):807–812, 1975.

412. Min S, Oh S, Karp G, et al: The clinical course and genetic defect in the PCFT gene in a 27-year-old woman with hereditary folate malabsorption. *J Pediatr* 153(3):435–437, 2008.

413. Zittoun J: Congenital errors of folate metabolism. *Baillieres Clin Haematol* 8(3):603–616, 1995.

414. Arakawa T, Narisawa K, Tanno K, et al: Megaloblastic anemia and mental retardation associated with hyperfolic-acidemia: Probably due to N5 methyltetrahydrofolate transferase deficiency. *Tohoku J Exp Med* 93(1):1–22, 1967.

415. Fox R, Wood M, Royse-Smith D, O'Sullivan W: Hereditary orotic aciduria: Types I and II. *Am J Med* 55(6):791–798, 1973.

416. van der Zee S, Schretlen E, Monnens L: Megaloblastic anaemia in the Lesch-Nyhan syndrome. *Lancet* 1(7557):1427, 1968.

417. Bazarbachi A, Muakkit S, Ayas M, et al: Thiamine-responsive myelodysplasia. *Br J Haematol* 102(4):1098–1100, 1998.

418. Boros L, Steinkamp M, Fleming J, et al: Defective RNA ribose synthesis in fibroblasts from patients with thiamine-responsive megaloblastic anemia (TRMA). *Blood* 102(10):3556–3561, 2003.

419. Zdebska E, Mendek-Czajkowska E, Ploski R, et al: Heterozygosity of CDAN II (HEMPAS) gene may be detected by the analysis of erythrocyte membrane glycoconjugates from healthy carriers. *Haematologica* 87(2):126–130, 2002.

420. Maeda K, Saeed S, Rebuck J, Monto R: Type I dyserythropoietic anemia. A 30-year follow-up. *Am J Clin Pathol* 73(3):433–438, 1980.

421. Wickramasinghe S, Parry T, Williams C, et al: A new case of congenital dyserythropoietic anaemia, type III: Studies of the cell cycle distribution and ultrastructure of erythroblasts and of nucleic acid synthesis in marrow cells. *J Clin Pathol* 35(10):1103–1109, 1982.

422. Najfeld V, McArthur J, Shashaty G: Monosomy 7 in a patient with pancytopenia and abnormal erythropoiesis. *Acta Haematol* 66(1):12–18, 1981.

423. Camaschella C: Recent advances in the understanding of inherited sideroblastic anaemia. *Br J Haematol* 143(1):27–38, 2008.

424. Roggli V, Saleem A: Erythroleukemia: A study of 15 cases and literature review. *Cancer* 49(1):101–108, 1982.

425. Matherly LH, Barlowe CK, Phillips VM, Goldman ID: The Effects on 4-aminoantifolates on 5-formyltetrahydrofolate metabolism in L1210 cells—A biochemical basis of the selectivity of leucovorin rescue. *J Biol Chem* 262(2):710–717, 1987.

426. Magee F, O'Sullivan H, McCann SR: Megaloblastosis and low-dose trimethoprimsulfamethoxazole. *Ann Intern Med* 95(5):657, 1981.

427. Spector I, Green R, Bowes D, et al: Trimethoprim-sulphamethoxazole therapy and folate nutrition. *S Afr Med J* 1973;47(28):1230–1232, 1981.

428. Swinson CM, Perry J, Lumb M, Levi AJ: Role of Sulphasalazine in the etiology of folate-deficiency in ulcerative-colitis. *Gut* 22(6):456–461, 1981.

429. Boots M, Phillips M, Curtis JR: Megaloblastic anemia and pancytopenia due to proguanil in patients with chronic renal failure. *Clin Nephrol* 18(2):106–108, 1982.

430. Fossella FV: Pemetrexed for treatment of advanced non-small cell lung cancer. *Semin Oncol* 31(1 Suppl 1):100–105, 2004.

431. Bethell FH, Thompson DS: Treatment of leukemia and related disorders with 6-mercaptopurine. *Ann N Y Acad Sci* 60(2):436–438, 1954.

432. Christoph R, Pirnay D, Hartl W: [Megaloblastic anemia following treatment of rheumatoid arthritis with azathioprine] [in German]. *Med Welt* 46:1824–1827, 1971.

433. Klippel JH, Decker JL: Relative macrocytosis in cyclophosphamide and azathioprine therapy. *JAMA* 229(2):180–181, 1974.

434. Amos RJ, Amess JAL: Megaloblastic hematopoiesis due to acyclovir. *Lancet* 1(8318):242–243, 1983.

435. Reyes P, Heidelberger C: Fluorinated pyrimidines. XXV. The inhibition of thymidylate synthetase from ehrlich ascites carcinoma cells by pyrimidine analogs. *Biochim Biophys Acta* 103:177–179, 1965.

436. Cornell RC, Milstein HG, Fox RM, Stoughton RB: Anemia of azaribine in the treatment of psoriasis. *Arch Dermatol* 112(12):1717–1723, 1976.

437. Frenkel EP, Arthur C: Induced ribotide reductive conversion defect by hydroxyurea and its relationship to megaloblastosis. *Cancer Res* 27(6):1016–1019, 1967.

438. Papac RJ: Clinical and hematologic studies with 1-beta-D-arabinosylcytosine. *J Natl Cancer Inst* 40(5):997, 1968.

439. Druskin MS, Bohagura L, Wallen MH: Anticonvulsant-associated megaloblastic anemia. Response to 25 microgm. of folic acid administered by mouth daily. *N Engl J Med* 267(10):483–485, 1962.

440. Gerson CD, Brown N, Herbert V, et al: Inhibition by diphenylhydantoin of folic-acid absorption in man. *Gastroenterology* 63(2):246, 1972.

441. Carl GF, Smith ML, Furman GM, et al: Phenytoin-treatment and folate supplementation affect folate concentrations and methylation capacity in rats. *J Nutr* 121(8):1214–1221, 1991.

442. Isojarvi JIT, Pakarinen AJ, Myllyla VV: Basic haematological parameters, serum gamm-maglutamyl-transferase activity, and erythrocyte folate and serum vitamin B-12 levels during carbamazepine and oxcarbazepine therapy. *Seizure* 6(3):207–211, 1997.

443. Lindenbaum J, Whitehead N, Reyner F: Oral-contraceptive hormones, folate metabolism, and cervical epithelium. *Am J Clin Nutr* 28(4):346–353, 1975.

444. Heinivaa O, Palva IP: Malabsorption and deficiency of vitamin B12 caused by treatment with para-aminosalicylic acid. *Acta Med Scand* 177(3):337–341, 1965.

445. Callaghan TS, Hadden DR: Megaloblastic-anemia due to vitamin-B12 malabsorption associated with long-term metformin treatment. *BMJ* 280(6225):1214–1215, 1980.

446. Webb DI, Chodos RB, Mahar CQ, Faloon WW: Mechanism of vitamin B12 malabsorption in patients receiving colchicine. *N Engl J Med* 279(16):845–850, 1968.

447. Dobbins WO, Herrero BA, Mansbach CM: Morphologic alterations associated with neomycin induced malabsorption. *Am J Med Sci* 255: 63–77, 1968.

448. Lerman BB, Ali N, Green D: Megaloblastic, dyserythropoietic anemia following arsenic ingestion. *Ann Clin Lab Sci* 1980;10(6):515–517, 1968.

CHAPTER 42
IRON METABOLISM

Tomas Ganz

SUMMARY

Iron is a component of nearly all living organisms. It plays an important metabolic role, particularly in electron transfer reactions. Most of the iron in the human body is incorporated into the hemoglobin of circulating red cells, which contain approximately 1 mg of iron per 1 mL of packed cells. Smaller amounts of iron are present in myoglobin and in many enzymes. Iron is stored within cells inside ferritin and circulates in plasma bound to transferrin. Because little iron is lost from the body under normal circumstances, the iron content of the body is controlled by modulating dietary iron absorption. Iron absorption increases in the presence of iron deficiency and it decreases when there is iron overload. The absorption of inorganic iron involves a ferrireductase and a divalent iron transporter, DMT-1, on the gastrointestinal luminal apical membranes of enterocytes, and ferroportin and hephaestin, located on the basolateral enterocyte membranes, in contact with blood. In contrast to elemental iron, heme iron is absorbed by a distinct pathway, which is still not well understood.

Systemic iron homeostasis is orchestrated by the hepatic peptide hormone hepcidin, which regulates plasma iron concentrations, the absorption of dietary iron, and the release of iron from macrophages involved in iron recycling and storage and from hepatocytes that store iron. The cellular iron exporter ferroportin serves as the receptor for hepcidin and is destroyed when the complex is formed. This impairs transport from intestinal mucosal cells, from macrophages and from hepatocytes into the plasma, and lowers iron absorption and release from stores. Hepcidin decreases plasma iron levels by causing iron to be sequestered within cells, predominantly in macrophages or enterocytes, the latter of which are then shed along with their absorbed iron. Once ferric iron enters the plasma, it is bound by transferrin, which, after forming a complex with the transferrin receptor, transports the metal into cells. The transferrin receptor is internalized together with bound transferrin and iron, and the iron is released inside the cell into an acidified vacuole. The transferrin receptor then recycles to the cell surface.

Cellular iron homeostasis is largely achieved through posttranscriptional regulation of key proteins involved in iron transport, storage and utilization. The synthesis of these proteins is regulated by binding of one of the iron-regulatory proteins (IRPs) to iron-responsive elements (IREs) located within stem loop structures of the corresponding messenger ribonucleic acids (mRNAs). IRP-1 is cytoplasmic aconitase that binds to the IRE when it is not complexed with iron and does not bind when iron is present; IRP-2, a closely related protein, is destabilized by the presence of iron. When IRPs bind to IREs at the 5′ end of the mRNA, they prevent translation; when they bind at the 3′ end, they stabilize the mRNA.

Iron is a key element in the metabolism of nearly all living organisms. Iron is a component of heme, which is the active site of electron transport in cytochromes and cytochrome oxidase involved in mitochondrial energy generation. The heme moiety of hemoglobin and myoglobin binds O_2, providing the means to transfer O_2 from the lungs to tissues and to store it. Heme is also the active site of peroxidases that protect cells from oxidative injury by reducing peroxides to water or generate microbicidal hypochlorite in granulocytes. DNA synthesis requires the enzyme ribonucleotide reductase to convert ribonucleotides to deoxyribonucleotides. Neither bacteria nor nucleated cells proliferate when the supply of iron is insufficient.

Acronyms and Abbreviations: ABCB10, ATP-binding cassette (ABC) transporter in the inner membrane of mitochondria; ALA synthase, aminolevulinic acid synthase; BMP, bone morphogenetic protein; dcytb, duodenal cytochrome b; DMT, divalent metal transporter; GDF15, growth differentiation factor 15; HFE, human hemochromatosis protein; HRG1, heme transporter; IL, interleukin; IRE, iron-responsive element; IRP, iron-regulatory protein; NADPH, nicotinamide adenine dinucleotide phosphate; Nramp1, natural resistance-associated macrophage protein one; STEAP3, six-transmembrane epithelial antigen of prostate 3; TfR, transferrin receptor.

In the previous edition, this chapter was written by Ernest Beutler and portions of that chapter have been retained.

● DISTRIBUTION OF IRON IN THE AVERAGE PERSON

Table 42–1 summarizes the most important iron compartments.

HEMOGLOBIN

Hemoglobin, which is 0.34 percent iron by weight, contains approximately 2 g of body iron in men and 1.5 g in women. One mL of packed erythrocytes contains approximately 1 mg of iron. Because the life span of human erythrocytes is approximately 120 days, every day 1/120 of the iron in hemoglobin is recycled by macrophages and returned to the plasma, from where it is largely delivered to marrow erythroblasts for incorporation into newly synthesized hemoglobin.

STORAGE COMPARTMENT

Iron is stored either as ferritin or as hemosiderin. The former is water-soluble; the latter is water-insoluble. The protein ferritin is composed of 24 similar or identical subunits arranged as 12 dimers forming a dodecahedron that approximates a hollow sphere with a cavity capable of storing up to 4500 Fe atoms as hydrous ferric oxide polymers.[1,2] The ferritin subunits are of H (heavy) or L (light) type. H subunits have ferroxidase activity, thereby enabling ferritin to take up or release iron quite rapidly. Ferritin that is rich in H subunits takes up iron more readily, but retains it less avidly than does ferritin composed predominantly of L subunits. Much of the storage iron in liver and spleen is in ferritin containing mostly L subunits.

Ferritin is found in virtually all cells of the body and also in tissue fluids. In plasma ferritin is present in minute concentrations. It is glycosylated and largely composed of L subunits. Except under conditions of inflammation, the plasma (serum) ferritin concentration usually correlates with total-body iron stores, making measurement

TABLE 42–1. Iron Compartments in the Average Person*

Compartment	Iron Content (mg)	Total Body Iron (%)
Hemoglobin iron	2000	67
Storage iron (ferritin, hemosiderin)	1000	27
Myoglobin iron	130	3.5
Labile pool	80	2.2
Other tissue iron	8	0.2
Transport iron	3	0.08

*These values represent estimates for an "average" person, that is, 70 kg (154 lb) in weight and 177 cm (70 inches) in height. The values are derived from data in several sources.

of serum ferritin levels important in the diagnosis of disorders of iron metabolism.

The size of the iron storage compartment is quite variable. Normally, in adult men, it amounts to 800 to 2000 mg; in adult women, it is a few hundred milligrams. The mobilization of storage iron from ferritin involves the reduction of Fe^{3+} to Fe^{2+}, its release from the core crystal and its diffusion out of the apoferritin shell. As it passes from cytosol to plasma, it must be reoxidized to Fe^{3+}, either by hephaestin or ceruloplasmin in the cell membrane or by ceruloplasmin in plasma, before it binds to transferrin. Alternatively, iron may be released from ferritin by autophagy followed by lysosomal degradation.[3]

Hemosiderin is found predominantly in macrophages. Microscopically, in unstained tissue sections or marrow films it appears as clumps or granules of golden refractile pigment. Under pathologic conditions, it may accumulate in large quantities in almost every tissue of the body. Hemosiderin is chemically similar to the iron core of ferritin and may be derived from ferritins whose protein shells have been digested in lysosomes.

MYOGLOBIN

Myoglobin is structurally similar to hemoglobin, but it is monomeric rather than tetrameric: Each myoglobin molecule consists of a heme group nearly surrounded by polypeptide loops of the 154 amino acid protein. It is present in small amounts in all skeletal and cardiac muscle cells, where it may serve as an oxygen reservoir to protect against cellular injury during periods of oxygen deprivation and may scavenge nitric oxide and reactive oxygen species.[4]

LABILE IRON POOL

The existence of a cellular labile iron pool was postulated from studies of the rate of clearance of injected ^{59}Fe from plasma.[5] Iron leaves the plasma and enters the interstitial and intracellular fluid compartments for a brief time before it is incorporated into heme or storage compounds. Some of the iron reenters plasma, causing a biphasic curve of ^{59}Fe clearance 1 to 2 days after injection. The change in slope defines the size of the labile pool, normally 80 to 90 mg of iron. It is now sometimes considered to be equivalent to the chelatable iron pool.[6]

TISSUE IRON COMPARTMENT

Tissue iron (exclusive of hemoglobin, ferritin, hemosiderin, myoglobin, and the labile compartment) normally amounts to 6 to 8 mg. This includes cytochromes and other iron-containing enzymes. Although a small compartment, it is an extremely vital one and is sensitive to iron deficiency.[7,8]

TRANSPORT COMPARTMENT

From the standpoint of its total iron content, normally about 3 mg, the transport compartment of plasma is the smallest but the most active of the iron compartments: Its iron, almost entirely carried by transferrin, normally turns over at least 10 times each day. This is the common pathway for interchange of iron between compartments.

Transferrin

Transferrin is a dumbbell-shaped glycoprotein with a Mr of approximately 80 kDa where each of the two globular domains contains a binding cleft for Fe^{3+}.[9–11] Normally, approximately one-third of the transferrin iron-binding sites are occupied by iron. Human plasma normally contains approximately 25 to 45 μM (200 to 360 mg/dL) transferrin, capable of binding 50 to 90 μM iron but carrying only 10 to 30 μM (50 to 180 mcg/dL) iron. Apotransferrin (transferrin devoid of iron) is synthesized by hepatocytes and by cells of the monocyte–macrophage system.[12,13]

● DIETARY IRON

CONTENT

Average American adult men and women ingest 9 to 10 mg and 12 to 14 mg of iron daily, respectively.[14] The amount of iron absorbed by a normal adult male need only balance the small amount that is excreted, mostly in the stool, approximately 1 mg/day.[15] More iron is needed during growth periods or after blood loss. In women, iron absorbed must be sufficient to replace that lost through menstruation or diverted to the fetus or milk during and after pregnancy. Table 42–2 shows the age- and gender-specific recommended dietary allowances for iron.[16]

BIOAVAILABILITY

In meat-eaters in Western countries, heme from hemoglobin and myoglobin normally comprises approximately 15 percent of dietary iron but is much more efficiently absorbed than nonheme iron, and promotes the absorption of nonheme iron.[17] The absorption of nonheme dietary iron is strongly affected by iron-binding components of food. Oxalates, phytates, and phosphates complex with iron and retard its absorption, whereas simple reducing substances, such as hydroquinone, ascorbate, lactate, pyruvate, succinate, fructose, cysteine, and sorbitol, increase iron absorption.[18] Iron-fortified cereals are major sources of iron in countries where fortification is practiced, but cooking in iron pots may also provide important exogenous iron.[17] Gastric acid secretion,

TABLE 42–2. Recommended Dietary Allowances (RDAs) for Iron[16]

Age	Male	Female	Pregnancy	Lactation
Birth to 6 months	0.27 mg*	0.27 mg*		
7–12 months	11 mg	11 mg		
1–3 years	7 mg	7 mg		
4–8 years	10 mg	10 mg		
9–13 years	8 mg	8 mg		
14–18 years	11 mg	15 mg	27 mg	10 mg
19–50 years	8 mg	18 mg	27 mg	9 mg
51+ years	8 mg	8 mg		

*Adequate intake (AI).

the transit time, and mucus secretion all play roles in iron absorption. Red wine, contrary to popular belief, inhibits iron absorption, probably because of the presence of polyphenols.[19] In mice, alcohol suppresses the response of hepcidin to iron,[20] and this may contribute to iron loading that is seen in some alcoholic subjects.

IRON ABSORPTION

Iron normally enters the body through the gastrointestinal tract, mostly through the enterocytes of the duodenum. The amount of iron absorbed is normally tightly regulated according to body needs. Active erythropoiesis and/or iron deficiency increase absorption; iron overload and systemic inflammation decrease absorption. Nevertheless, the amount of iron absorbed increases with the administered dose even though the percentage absorbed decreases (Fig. 42-1). Accidental or deliberate ingestion of large doses of medicinal iron can therefore cause iron intoxication.

MECHANISM OF TRANSPORT ACROSS THE INTESTINAL MUCOSA

Heme Iron

Understanding the mechanism of iron absorption has been made more difficult by the fact that the pathways for the uptake of inorganic iron and of heme by enterocytes are different but seem to merge within the intestinal cell where heme is converted to inorganic iron. How much heme (if any) is exported intact by enterocytes and bound by plasma heme-binding protein hemopexin is not clear, but hemopexin knockout mice show minor retention of iron in duodenal enterocytes without any effect on systemic iron homeostasis,[21] arguing against a major contribution from this mechanism, at least in mice. Efforts to identify the apical heme import mechanism in enterocytes have not yet been definitive.[22]

Ferric Iron

Following the reduction of ferric iron to ferrous iron, in part by duodenal cytochrome b (dcytb) reductase,[23] ferrous iron is transported into

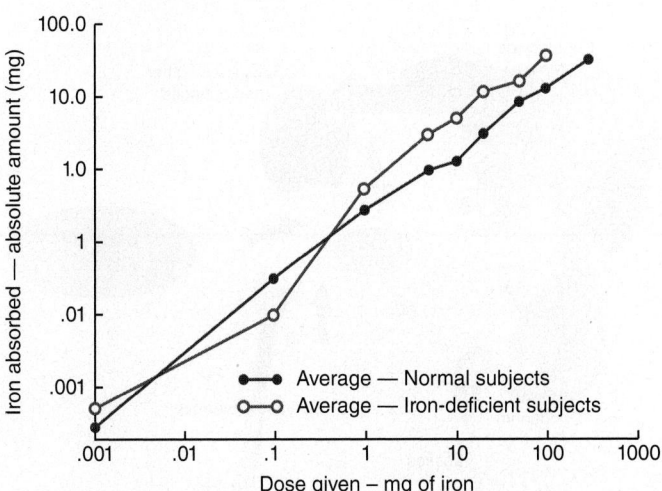

Figure 42-1. The relationship between oral iron dosage and amount of iron absorbed in humans. When the logarithm of the dose is plotted against the logarithm of the amount of iron absorbed, a rectilinear relationship is observed. Thus, at all levels, the greater the dose of iron, the more is absorbed, although the percent of the dose that is absorbed progressively declines. *(Reproduced with permission from Mackenzie B, Garrick MD: Iron Imports. II. Iron uptake at the apical membrane in the intestine. Am J Physiol Gastrointest Liver Physiol 289(6):G981–G986, 2005.)*

the intestinal villus cell by the divalent metal transporter (DMT)-1.[24,25] How iron transits within the enterocytes is not yet known. Basolateral export of ferrous iron is mediated by ferroportin[26-28] in association with hephaestin[29] and plasma ceruloplasmin[30] to oxidize iron to the ferric state. Ferric iron is taken up by plasma apotransferrin. Figure 42-2 illustrates some of the steps that are thought to regulate iron transport across the mucosal cell.

IRON RECYCLING

Role of the Monocyte–Macrophage System

In humans, the destruction and production of erythrocytes generates most of the iron flux in and out of plasma (20 to 25 mg/day recycled in adults compared to 1 to 2 mg/day absorbed). Iron from other cell types is likely also recycled, but this source contributes little to iron flux and has not been studied. Destruction of aged erythrocytes and hemoglobin degradation occur within macrophages (Chap. 32). This proceeds at a rate sufficient to release approximately 20 percent of the hemoglobin iron from the cell to the plasma compartment within a few hours. Approximately 80 percent of this iron is rapidly reincorporated into hemoglobin. Thus, 20 to 70 percent of the hemoglobin iron of nonviable erythrocytes reappears in circulating red cells in 12 days. The remainder of the iron enters the storage pool as ferritin or hemosiderin and then turns over very slowly. In normal subjects, approximately 40 percent of this iron remains in storage after 140 days. When there is an increased iron demand for hemoglobin synthesis, however, storage iron may be mobilized more rapidly.[31] Conversely, in the presence of infection or another inflammatory process (e.g., ulcerative colitis or malignancy), iron is more slowly reused in hemoglobin synthesis and is associated with anemia (Chap. 37).[32,33]

Erythrophagocytosis

As human erythrocytes age during their average 120-day life span, they shrink, stiffen, and their membranes accumulate markers of senescence.[34] These changes eventually trigger phagocytosis by splenic or hepatic sinusoidal macrophages. Macrophages also take up the products of intravascular hemolysis, including hemoglobin (bound by haptoglobin) and heme (bound by hemopexin), using specific endocytic receptors for the complexes.[35] The vesicles involved in phagocytosis and endocytosis must fuse with lysosomes to digest cellular materials or protein complexes and to free heme from hemoglobin. The membrane complex of nicotinamide adenine dinucleotide phosphate (NADPH) cytochrome c reductase, heme oxygenase 1, and biliverdin reductase releases ferrous iron from heme and simultaneously protects erythrophagocytosing macrophages from heme-induced toxicity.[36] The subcellular location of the conversion of heme to iron is not known with certainty. Heme oxygenase 1 is mostly located in the endoplasmic reticulum in erythrophagocytic macrophages[37] with the catalytic face in the cytosol, and little, if any, heme oxygenase in the phagosomal membrane. Moreover, the phagosomal membrane is enriched in the heme transporter HRG1,[38] and macrophage heme has a signaling role in inducing various proteins involved in macrophage iron metabolism, indicating that it may leave the phagosome, and the heme oxygenase-1–mediated release of iron may occur in the cytoplasm. However, the ferrous iron transporter Nramp1, and perhaps DMT-1, may also participate in subcellular iron transport.[39] Ultimately, depending on systemic iron requirements, the released ferrous iron is either exported to plasma via ferroportin[40] or trapped in macrophage cytoplasmic ferritin. By a mechanism potentially important at the low oxygen tensions found in some tissues, plasma ceruloplasmin[41-43] catalyzes the conversion of ferrous to ferric iron, the form of iron loaded to plasma transferrin for systemic distribution.

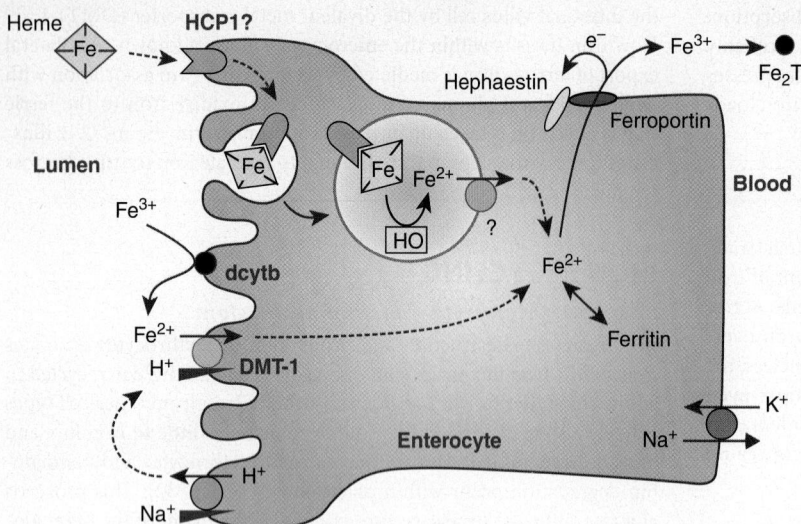

Figure 42–2. Schematic of iron uptake from the intestine and transfer to the plasma by an intestinal villus cell. Nonheme dietary iron includes Fe(II) and Fe(III) salts and organic complexes. Fe^{3+} is reduced to Fe^{2+} by ascorbic acid and apical membrane ferrireductases that include duodenal cytochrome b (dcytb). The acid microclimate at the brush-border provides an H^+ electrochemical potential gradient to drive transport of Fe^{2+} via the divalent metal-ion transporter (DMT-1) into the enterocyte. DMT-1 may also contribute to the absorption of other nutritionally important metal ions (e.g., Mn^{2+}). Heme can be taken up by endocytosis, and Fe^{2+} is liberated within the endosome/lysosome, but the molecular identity of proteins involved, including heme carrier protein 1 (HCP1), is yet to be elucidated. Basolateral export of Fe^2 may be mediated by ferroportin in association with hephaestin. Fe_2Tf, diferric transferrin; HO, heme oxygenase. *(Data from Smith MD, Pannacciulli IM: Absorption of inorganic iron from graded doses: its significance in relation to iron absorption tests and mucosal block theory. Br J Haematol 4(4):428–434, 1958.)*

SYSTEMIC IRON HOMEOSTASIS

The mechanism by which body iron content is regulated by the modulation of iron absorption has been a subject of intense interest for the past 65 years. It has now become clear that intestinal iron absorption, plasma iron concentrations, and tissue distribution of iron are subject to endocrine regulation similar to that of other simple nutrients, for example, glucose or calcium, albeit in a somewhat more complex fashion.

Hepcidin and Ferroportin

Hepcidin, a 25-amino-acid peptide hormone with 4 disulfide bonds,[44-47] is produced predominantly by hepatocytes and plays a central role in systemic iron homeostasis. Hepcidin regulates plasma iron concentrations by controlling the absorption of iron by the intestinal epithelial enterocytes and its release from iron-recycling macrophages and hepatocytes involved in iron storage. The structural similarity of hepcidin and a class of antimicrobial peptides termed *defensins* suggests that the hormone evolved from the latter to modulate iron homeostasis as a mechanism of body defense against microorganisms. Overexpression of hepcidin results in marked iron-deficiency anemia in mice[48] and a refractory anemia resembling the anemia of chronic inflammation in humans,[49] and injection of synthetic hepcidin rapidly lowers plasma iron concentrations.[50] As many microorganisms are dependent on plasma iron for survival in the circulation, hepcidin can exert host defense. In fact, patients with iron overload and high plasma iron levels are susceptible to such infections, such as with *Yersinia enterocolitica* (Chap. 43).

Hepcidin exerts its iron-regulatory effect by binding to ferroportin, a transmembrane iron-export protein expressed on enterocytes, macrophages, and hepatocytes. Once hepcidin has bound to ferroportin, the ferroportin is internalized and undergoes proteolysis.[40,51] With membrane ferroportin depleted, iron cannot be exported from the enterocyte, the macrophage or the hepatocyte into the plasma (Fig. 42–3). This results in decreased iron absorption from the gastrointestinal tract and a fall in the plasma iron concentration. Hepcidin production is stimulated by inflammatory cytokines such as interleukin (IL)-6,[52,53] and the overproduction of hepcidin is one of the factors in the pathogenesis of the anemia of chronic inflammation (Chap. 37).

The regulation of hepcidin production seems to be entirely transcriptional. In humans and laboratory rodents, hepcidin mRNA and plasma hepcidin levels increase in parallel with iron-loading and inflammatory stimuli,[44,54,55] and are decreased by erythropoietic activity[56] and iron deficiency.[57]

Regulation of Hepcidin by Iron

Both elevated plasma iron concentrations and increased liver stores are sensed in the intact organism and regulate hepcidin transcription,[58,59] but the relevant mechanisms are only partially understood. For reasons that are not understood, involving perhaps the complex interactions of hepatocytes with other liver cells, isolated hepatocytes do not show consistently increased hepcidin synthesis after iron treatment, although small effects were observed when the cells were freshly harvested from mice.[60] Important clues are provided by hereditary disorders in which hepcidin transcription is dysregulated. As indicated in Table 42–3, impairment of the function of several genes is associated with iron overload in humans and in experimental animals. In addition to genes that encode the hormone hepcidin itself and its receptor, ferroportin, or encode proteins primarily involved in iron transport, there are a number of genes whose products are likely to function in

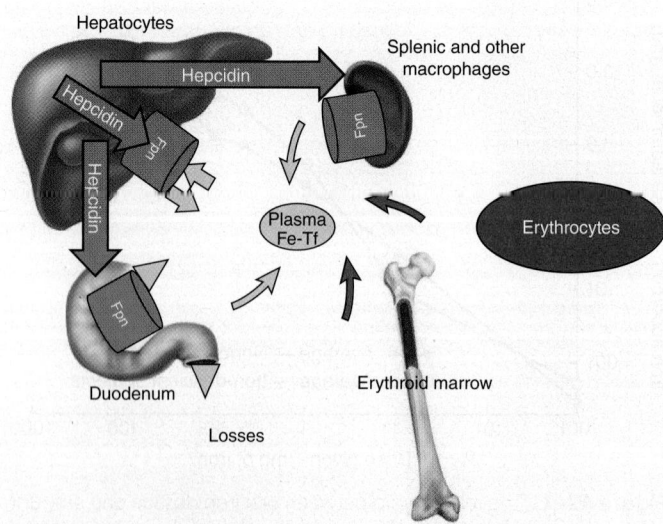

Figure 42–3. Regulation of iron flows into plasma by hepcidin. Ferroportin is the only known transporter that exports iron from cells to plasma (and extracellular fluid). Hepcidin induces ferroportin endocytosis and proteolysis and thereby controls the transfer of iron to plasma from all its major sources: iron-absorbing duodenal enterocytes, iron-storing hepatocytes, and iron-recycling macrophages.

TABLE 42–3. Proteins That Play a Role in Iron Homeostasis in Humans or in Animal Models

Proteins That Affect Iron Homeostasis	Effect of Deficiency or Mutation	References to Human Data	References to Murine Data	Comments
HFE	Parenchymal Fe increased	94	95, 96	Most patients with hereditary hemochromatosis are homozygous for the 845 A→G (C282Y) mutation of this gene. In signaling pathway to hepcidin
Ferroportin (SLC40A1, SLC11A3)	Macrophage Fe increased (loss of function)	97	98	Autosomal dominant, hepcidin receptor, cellular iron exporter
	Parenchymal Fe increased (resistance to hepcidin)	99, 100	101	Autosomal dominant
β_2-Microglobulin	Parenchymal Fe increased	Unknown	102, 103	Facilitates transport of *HFE* to membrane
Transferrin	Parenchymal Fe increased	104–106	107, 108	Plasma iron transporter, holotransferrin concentrations regulate hepcidin
Transferrin receptor-1	Lethal; increased CNS Fe	Unknown	109	Mediates cellular iron uptake, essential for erythropoiesis, may be involved in signaling for hepcidin regulation
Transferrin receptor-2	Parenchymal Fe increased	84, 110	111	Signaling for hepcidin regulation
Hephaestin	Fe deficiency	Unknown	29	Sex-linked gene; deletion of exons is cause of *sla* mouse
Ceruloplasmin	Fe increased	112	42	Brain iron accumulation and neurologic disease
Ferritin H chain	Fe increased	113	Unknown	Dominant IRE mutation
Duodenal cytochrome b (dcytb)	Unknown	Unknown	23	Mild iron restriction under erythropoietic stress
Nramp1 (SLC11A1)	Alters iron distribution in macrophages	Unknown	39	Deficiency increases susceptibility to infection in mice
Nramp2 (DMT-1)	Hypochromic microcytic anemia and hepatic siderosis in people; Fe deficiency in rodents	114, 115	116, 117	Anemia is ameliorated by erythropoietin therapy in humans; same naturally occurring mutations found in the *mk* mouse and the Belgrade rat
Hepcidin	Parenchymal Fe Increased	118	46, 119	The hormone-regulating iron absorption, plasma iron concentration, and systemic distribution
Hemojuvelin	Parenchymal Fe increased	65	120, 121	Signaling for hepcidin regulation
Tmprss6	Fe deficiency	49	70, 72	Signaling for hepcidin regulation, membrane protease, cleaves hemojuvelin
BMP6	Parenchymal Fe increased	Unknown	122, 123	Necessary for iron regulation in mice
BMP receptor subunit	Parenchymal Fe increased	Unknown	124	Necessary for iron regulation in mice
SMAD4 in the liver	Parenchymal Fe increased	Unknown	125	In signaling pathway for hepcidin regulation
Neogenin	Parenchymal Fe increased	Unknown	126, 127	Necessary for hepcidin regulation

BMP, bone morphogenetic protein; HFE, human hemochromatosis protein; IRE, iron-responsive element.

iron sensing, signal transduction and transcriptional regulation. These include human hemochromatosis protein (HFE), transferrin receptor-2, bone morphogenetic proteins (BMPs), BMP receptor and its signaling pathway, and hemojuvelin, all of which encode proteins that normally stimulate hepcidin transcription to prevent iron overload. In the best-supported model, hepcidin transcription is regulated in an iron-dependent manner by the BMP pathway. Complexes of HFE, transferrin receptor-1, and transferrin receptor-2 may be involved in sensing the concentration of iron-transferrin and interact in as yet unknown manner with the BMP receptor to stimulate the transcription of hepcidin.[61-64] Hemojuvelin, whose autosomal recessive mutations cause a very severe form of hereditary hemochromatosis, serves as a coreceptor for the BMPs.[65,66] A soluble fragment of hemojuvelin acts as an inhibitor of the interaction of BMP with the receptor, but it is not clear whether it has a physiologic regulatory role.[67,68] Regulation of hepcidin transcription itself is complex, involving the formation of a complex of liver-specific and response-specific transcription factors bound to a distal BMP-RE2/bZIP/HNF4α/COUP region and to the proximal BMP-RE1/STAT region of the hepcidin promoter, possibly by physical association of the two regions.[69] A pathway that inhibits the transcription of hepcidin exists as well. Tmprss6 (also called matriptase 2) is a membrane serine protease that inhibits hepcidin transcription, likely by proteolysis of hemojuvelin.[70,71] This function was discovered when random mutagenesis in mice produced an iron-deficient animal with mutagenized Tmprss6.[72] Subsequently, humans with mutations of the Tmprss6 orthologue were shown to manifest iron-refractory iron-deficiency anemia that does not respond to oral iron and only partially to parenteral iron therapy.[49]

Regulation of Hepcidin by Erythropoiesis

Intestinal iron absorption is increased severalfold after hemorrhage or erythropoietin administration, and is chronically increased in patients with ineffective erythropoiesis but not in aplastic anemia.[73] These observations led to the hypothesis that the marrow generates an "erythroid regulator"[73] that modulates intestinal iron absorption. Later studies in mouse models[56] provided evidence that the erythroid regulator is a marrow-derived suppressor of hepcidin. Erythroferrone is an erythropoietin-induced erythroblast-secreted glycoprotein that acts on hepatocytes to suppress their hepcidin production and is required for rapid suppression of hepcidin after hemorrhage or erythropoietin administration.[74] It also contributes to hepcidin suppression and iron overload in murine models of β-thalassemia intermedia. Growth differentiation factor 15 (GDF15), a member of the BMP family, may also contribute to pathologic hepcidin suppression in anemias with ineffective erythropoiesis.[75]

Regulation of Hepcidin by Inflammation

Within hours after the onset of systemic infection, plasma iron concentration decreases. The response is thought to contribute to host defense, particularly against microbes with high dependence on environmental iron.[76] This response, hypoferremia of inflammation, is also triggered by noninfectious causes of acute and chronic inflammation. Hypoferremia of inflammation is mediated by cytokine-induced increase in plasma hepcidin concentrations[54] causing hepcidin-induced sequestration of iron in macrophages. The main human cytokine responsible for hepcidin induction is IL-6[52,53] acting via the JAK2-STAT3 pathway,[77–79]

but other cytokines including activin B may also contribute.[80] Chronic inflammation impairs iron supply to erythropoiesis and combines with other effects of inflammation to cause anemia of inflammation (anemia of chronic disease, see Chap. 37).

●TRANSPORT OF IRON

Once an atom of iron enters the blood plasma from dietary iron absorption, it is virtually trapped in the body (Fig. 42–4) and cycles almost endlessly from the plasma to the developing erythroblast (where it is used in hemoglobin synthesis), thence into the circulating blood for approximately 4 months, and then to macrophages. Here it is removed from heme by heme oxygenase and released back into the plasma to repeat the cycle.

The major function of the transport protein transferrin is to move iron from wherever it enters the plasma (intestinal villi, splenic and hepatic sinusoids) to the erythroblasts of the marrow and to other sites of use.

ENDOCYTOSIS OF TRANSFERRIN

Diferric (holo)transferrin binds to the transferrin receptor (TfR)-1 on the cell surface and the holotransferrin–TfR1 complex forms clusters in pits on the cell membrane.[81] The complex is then internalized by endocytosis (Fig. 42–5). Within the cytosol the holotransferrin-TfR1 complex is in a clathrin-coated vesicle. The vesicles fuse with endosomes and become acidified to pH 5 which releases iron from transferrin.

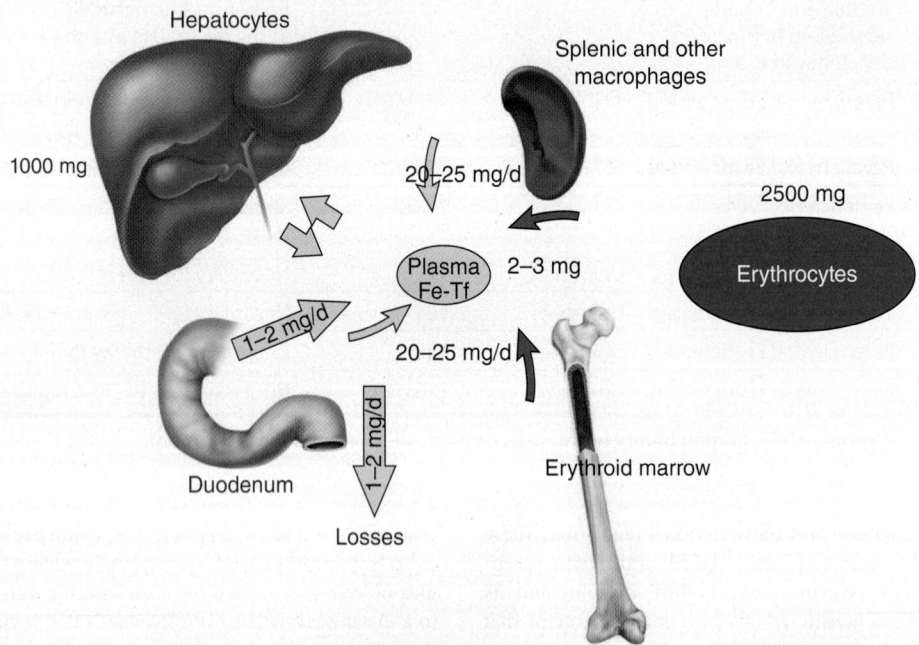

Figure 42–4. The iron cycle in humans. Iron is tightly conserved in a nearly closed system in which each iron atom cycles repeatedly from plasma and extracellular fluid ("plasma") to the marrow, where it is incorporated into hemoglobin. Then it moves into the blood within erythrocytes and circulates for 4 months. It then travels to phagocytes of the mononuclear phagocyte system ("splenic and other macrophages"), where senescent erythrocytes are engulfed and destroyed, hemoglobin is digested, and iron is released to plasma, where the cycle continues. With each cycle, a small proportion of iron is transferred to storage sites, where it is incorporated into ferritin or hemosiderin, a small proportion of storage iron is released to plasma, a small proportion is lost in urine, sweat, feces, or blood, and an equivalent small amount of iron is absorbed from the intestinal tract. In addition, a small proportion (approximately 10 percent) of newly formed erythrocytes normally is destroyed within the marrow and its iron released, bypassing the circulating blood part of the cycle (ineffective erythropoiesis). The numbers indicate the approximate amount of iron (in mg) in various compartments and fluxes of iron (mg/day) that enter and leave each of these iron compartments in healthy adults who do not have bleeding or other blood disorders.

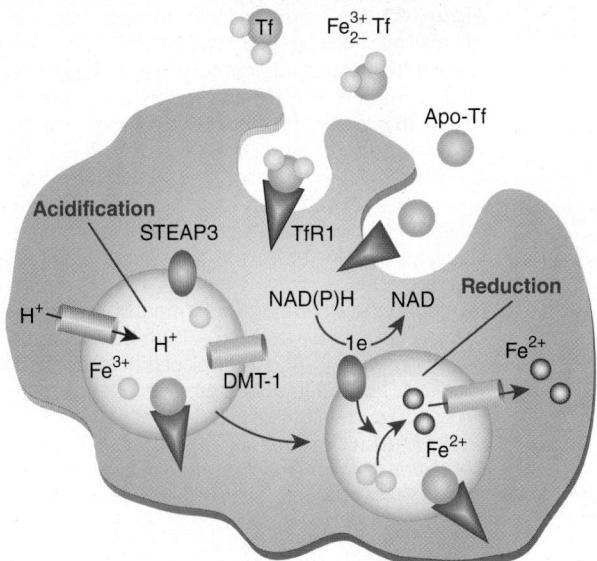

Figure 42–5. The transferrin cycle. Holotransferrin (Fe³⁺₂-Tf) binds to transferrin receptors (TfR1) on the cell surface. The complexes localize to clathrin-coated pits, which invaginate to initiate endocytosis. Specialized endosomes form, and become acidified through the action of a proton pump. Acidification leads to protein conformational changes that release iron from transferrin. STEAP3 (six-transmembrane epithelial antigen of prostate 3) reduces ferric iron to ferrous iron, enabling iron transport out of the endosomes through the activity of the divalent metal transporter-1 protein (DMT-1). Subsequently, apotransferrin (Apo-Tf) and the transferrin receptor both return to the cell surface, where they dissociate at neutral pH. Both proteins participate in further rounds of iron delivery. In nonerythroid cells, iron is stored as ferritin and hemosiderin. *(Reproduced with permission from McKie AT: A ferrireductase fills the gap in the transferrin cycle. Nat Genet 37(11):1159–1160, 2005.)*

Iron-depleted (apo)transferrin and TfR1 remain complexed as they return to the cell membrane, where at neutral pH, apotransferrin separates from its receptor and is released to the interstitial fluid to reenter plasma and take up more iron.

The TfR is a protein consisting of two subunits that are linked by disulfide bonds.[9] Its aminoterminus is on the cytoplasmic side of the membrane, and its carboxyl-terminus is on the outer surface. Because of the role of TfR1 in the binding and endocytosis of diferric transferrin, control of TfR1 biosynthesis is a major mechanism for regulation of iron metabolism. Synthesis of TfR1 is induced by iron deficiency. Iron inhibits TfR1 synthesis by destabilizing TfR1 mRNA by a mechanism that involves the iron-responsive element (IRE)/iron-regulatory protein (IRP) regulatory system (Fig. 42–6).[82,83] TfR1 binds to HFE,[61] using a binding site that overlaps that of holotransferrin. According to a current model of iron sensing, high concentrations of holotransferrin would therefore displace HFE from its complex with TfR1, leaving HFE to signal to the BMP receptor complex to increase hepcidin transcription. This model is supported by studies in which the expression of HFE or its binding site on TfR1 are manipulated.[61]

A second TfR, TfR2, also endocytic for holotransferrin, is not thought to be involved in delivering iron to cells but its hepatic expression is necessary for normal hepcidin expression and regulation.[84] TfR2 influences the BMP complex and its signaling pathway to regulate hepcidin transcription but the molecular mechanism of this effect is not yet understood. TfR2 is also expressed in erythroid precursors where it interacts with the erythropoietin receptor and negatively modulates erythropoiesis, perhaps putting a brake on erythrocyte production during iron deficiency.[85]

INTRACELLULAR IRON HOMEOSTASIS

Each cell must regulate its iron uptake and subcellular distribution, both to assure adequate iron for a multitude of cellular enzymes and to prevent excessive iron accumulation that could be injurious or deny adequate iron to other cells. Accordingly, the synthesis of key cellular proteins involved in iron transport, storage, and use is regulated post-transcriptionally by cellular iron concentrations.[82,83] The mRNA for each of these proteins contains one or several IREs. If the IRE is located at the 5′ end of the mRNA, it serves to regulate translation; 3′ IREs regulate the stability of the mRNA. Each IRE consists of a stem and loop structure, in which the loop is the nucleotide sequence CAGUG (Fig. 42–7). IRE/IRP–regulated mRNAs include those encoding ferritin, TfR1, aminolevulinic acid (ALA) synthase, transferrin, aconitase, DMT-1, and ferroportin. The ferritin mRNA has, as its IRE, a single stem–loop structure in the 5′ (upstream) region. In contrast to the ferritin IRE, there are as many as five stems–loops in the 3′ untranslated portion of TfR mRNA. The IREs are targeted by specific RNA-binding proteins, IRPs. IRP-1 is cytoplasmic aconitase with four iron-sulfur clusters and the ability to bind iron, which is required for its aconitase activity; IRP-2 is highly homologous to IRP-1 but differs by the presence of a 73-amino-acid insertion in the *N*-terminus and a lack of aconitase activity. In the absence of iron, IRP-1 binds to IREs, but in its presence becomes a cytoplasmic aconitase and does not bind IREs. IRP-2 (as well as, to some extent, IRP-1) undergoes ubiquitination and proteasomal degradation in the presence of iron.[86,87] The effect of binding of IRPs to 5′ IREs is to inhibit protein translation; the effect of binding of IRPs to 3′ IREs is to increase the stability of the mRNA and thus to enhance the synthesis of the gene product. Figure 42–6 illustrates these relationships for the regulation of synthesis of ferritin and TfR. The net effect of the IRE/IRP system is to balance cellular iron uptake with storage, use, and in some cell types, export of iron.

IRON IN THE ERYTHROBLAST

Once within the developing erythroblast, iron must be transported to mitochondria to be incorporated into heme, or taken up by ferritin within siderosomes. Within the vesicle, STEAP3 (six-transmembrane epithelial antigen of prostate 3) effects the reduction of ferric (Fe³⁺) to ferrous (Fe²⁺) iron, and another protein, DMT-1 (the same transporter as in intestinal iron absorption), transports Fe²⁺ into the cytosol, where it is taken up by mitochondria by a complex of mitoferrin-1, ABCB10 (ATP-binding cassette [ABC] transporter in the inner membrane of mitochondria) and ferrochelatase for heme synthesis.[88] Physical interaction between mitochondria and endosomes ("kiss and run") may also be required.[89]

Mitochondrial Iron

Mitochondria, working together with cellular cytoplasm, supply each cell with heme. Although heme synthesis is important for all cells, erythroblasts synthesize much more heme than any other cell type. The final steps of heme synthesis take place in mitochondria, where iron is inserted into protoporphyrin by the enzyme ferrochelatase. When heme synthesis is impaired, as in lead poisoning or in the sideroblastic anemias (Chap. 59), the mitochondria accumulates excessive amounts of amorphous iron aggregates. The mitochondria can then be stained by the Prussian blue reaction and are seen by light microscopy as a ring of large blue siderotic granules encircling the erythroblast nucleus (ringed sideroblast). In normal, iron-replete marrow, (much smaller) siderotic granules are also demonstrable, scattered in the cytoplasm of about one-third of erythroblasts. These normal siderotic granules are ferritin aggregates located in lysosomal organelles designated siderosomes.[90] Erythroblasts containing these siderotic granules,

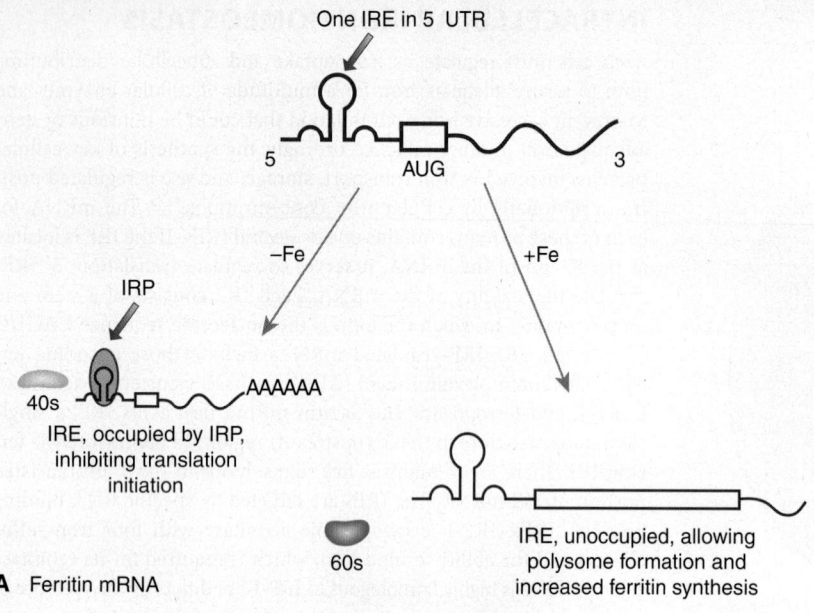

One IRE in 5′ UTR

5′   AUG   3′

−Fe   +Fe

IRP

40s

IRE, occupied by IRP,
inhibiting translation
initiation

60s

IRE, unoccupied, allowing
polysome formation and
increased ferritin synthesis

A   Ferritin mRNA

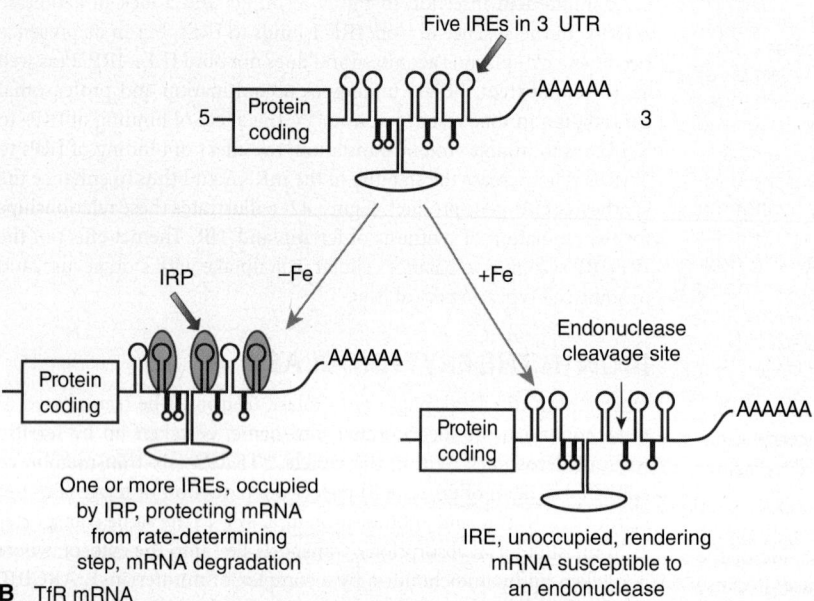

Five IREs in 3′ UTR

5′   Protein coding   AAAAAA   3′

IRP   −Fe   +Fe

Protein coding   AAAAAA

Endonuclease
cleavage site

Protein coding   AAAAAA

One or more IREs, occupied
by IRP, protecting mRNA
from rate-determining
step, mRNA degradation

IRE, unoccupied, rendering
mRNA susceptible to
an endonuclease

B   TfR mRNA

Figure 42–6. The regulation of iron metabolism at the cytoplasmic mRNA level by interaction of iron-regulatory protein (IRP)-1 and the iron-responsive elements (IREs) to apoferritin mRNA **(A)** and transferrin receptor (TfR) mRNA **(B).** When the cytoplasmic iron concentration is low (*left side of illustration*), IRP-1 binds to the IREs of both mRNAs. This represses the translation of apoferritin mRNA, where the IRE is at the 5′ end of the mRNA, thereby reducing the amount of apoferritin formed. It stabilizes and increases the translation of TfR mRNA where the IRE is at the 3′ end of the mRNA, thereby increasing the amount of TfR formed. Conversely, when there is an abundance of iron in the cytoplasm (*right side of illustration*), IRP-1 is displaced from both species of mRNA. This results in derepression of apoferritin synthesis and destabilization and degradation of TfR mRNA. (*Reproduced with permission from Rouault T, Klausner R: Regulation of iron metabolism in eukaryotes.* Curr Top Cell Regul 35:1–19, 1997.)

sideroblasts, normally represent 20 to 50 percent of the erythrocyte precursors of the marrow and as visualized by light microscopy. In iron deficiency and in the anemia that accompanies chronic disorders, sideroblasts almost disappear from the marrow. Conversely, in some states of iron overload, they may become more numerous and contain excessive numbers of granules, some of which may be considerably larger than normal.

Mitochondrial Ferritin

Ring sideroblasts contain a ferritin isoform, mitochondrial ferritin (Chap. 59), which is a product of an intronless, IRE-lacking, ferritin gene on chromosome 5q23.1 that is specifically targeted to mitochondria by a 60-amino-acid-leader sequence.[1,91] Mitochondrial ferritin lacks IRE and, thus, is not subject to iron-dependent translational control. Its function appears to be to reduce the labile iron pool and decrease the level of reactive oxygen species. Mitochondrial ferritin has limited tissue expression and is found in high concentrations in the mitochondria

of normal testes and in the sideroblasts of patients with sideroblastic anemia (Chap. 59).[92]

● IRON EXCRETION

The body conserves iron with remarkable efficiency. Most iron loss occurs by way of desquamated intestinal cells in the feces and it normally amounts to approximately 1 mg/day,[15,93] less than one-thousandth of total-body iron. Exfoliation of skin and dermal appendages and perspiration result in much smaller losses. Even in tropical climates, the loss of iron in sweat is minimal.[90] Very small amounts of iron are lost in the urine. Lactation may cause excretion of approximately 1 mg iron daily, thus doubling the overall rate of iron loss. Blood loss by normal menstruation contributes to negative iron balance.

Although total daily iron loss is normally approximately 1 mg for males,[15] it averages approximately 2 mg for menstruating women.

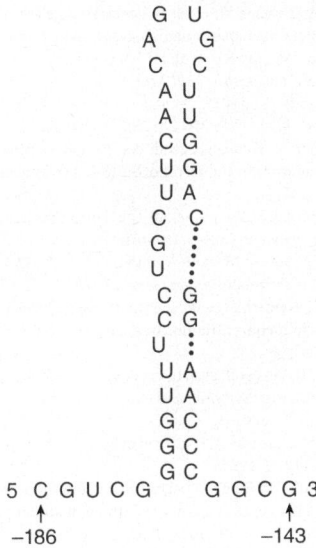

Figure 42–7. The stem–loop structure that is the iron-responsive element of apoferritin mRNA. *(Reproduced with permission from Hentze MW, Caughman SW, Casey JL, et al: A model for the structure and functions of iron-responsive elements.* Gene *72(1–2):201–208, 1988.)*

Persons with marked iron overload, as in hemochromatosis, may lose as much as 4 mg of iron daily, probably because of the shedding of iron-laden cells, principally macrophages.

REFERENCES

1. Arosio P, Levi S: Cytosolic and mitochondrial ferritins in the regulation of cellular iron homeostasis and oxidative damage. *Biochim Biophys Acta* 1800:783, 2010.
2. Koorts AM, Viljoen M: Ferritin and ferritin isoforms I: Structure–function relationships, synthesis, degradation and secretion. *Arch Physiol Biochem* 113:30, 2007.
3. Mancias JD, Wang X, Gygi SP, et al: Quantitative proteomics identifies NCOA4 as the cargo receptor mediating ferritinophagy. *Nature* 509:105, 2014.
4. Ordway GA, Garry DJ: Myoglobin: An essential hemoprotein in striated muscle. *J Exp Biol* 207:3441, 2004.
5. Hosain F, Marsaglia G, Finch CA: Blood ferrokinetics in normal man. *J Clin Invest* 46:1, 1967.
6. Breuer W, Shvartsman M, Cabantchik ZI: Intracellular labile iron. *Int J Biochem Cell Biol* 40:350, 2008.
7. Dallman PR, Beutler E, Finch CA: Effects of iron deficiency exclusive of anaemia. *Br J Haematol* 40:179, 1978.
8. Radlowski EC, Johnson RW: Perinatal iron deficiency and neurocognitive development. *Front Hum Neurosci* 7:1, 2013.
9. Cheng Y, Zak O, Aisen P, et al: Structure of the human transferrin receptor-transferrin complex. *Cell* 116:565, 2004.
10. Bailey S, Evans RW, Garratt RC, et al: Molecular structure of serum transferrin at 3.3-A resolution. *Biochemistry* 27:5804, 1988.
11. Aisen P, Brown EB: Structure and function of transferrin. *Prog Hematol* 9:25, 1975.
12. Thorbecke GJ, Liem HH, Knight S, et al: Sites of formation of the serum proteins transferrin and hemopexin. *J Clin Invest* 52:725, 1973.
13. Haurani FI, Meyer A, O'Brien R: Production of transferrin by the macrophage. *J Reticuloendothel Soc* 14:309, 1973.
14. Egan SK, Tao SS, Pennington JA, et al: US Food and Drug Administration's Total Diet Study: Intake of nutritional and toxic elements, 1991-96. *Food Addit Contam* 19:103, 2002.
15. Dubach R, Moore CV, Callender S: Studies in iron transportation and metabolism. IX. The excretion of iron as measured by the isotope technique. *J Lab Clin Med* 45:599, 1955.
16. Trumbo P, Yates AA, Schlicker S, Poos M: Dietary reference intakes: Vitamin A, vitamin K, arsenic, boron, chromium, copper, iodine, iron, manganese, molybdenum, nickel, silicon, vanadium, and zinc. *J Am Diet Assoc* 101:294, 2001.
17. Heath AL, Fairweather T: Clinical implications of changes in the modern diet: Iron intake, absorption and status. *Best Pract Res Clin Haematol* 15:225, 2002.
18. Hurrell R, Egli I: Iron bioavailability and dietary reference values. *Am J Clin Nutr* 91:1461S, 2010.
19. Cook JD, Reddy MB, Hurrell RF: The effect of red and white wines on nonheme-iron absorption in humans. *Am J Clin Nutr* 61:800, 1995.
20. Anderson ER, Taylor M, Xue X, et al: The hypoxia-inducible factor-C/EBPalpha axis controls ethanol-mediated hepcidin repression. *Mol Cell Biol* 32:4068, 2012.
21. Fiorito V, Geninatti CS, Silengo L, et al: Lack of plasma protein hemopexin results in increased duodenal iron uptake. *PLoS One* 8:e68146, 2013.
22. Korolnek T, Hamza I: Like iron in the blood of the people: The requirement for heme trafficking in iron metabolism. *Front Pharmacol* 5:126, 2014.
23. Choi J, Masaratana P, Latunde-Dada GO, et al: Duodenal reductase activity and spleen iron stores are reduced and erythropoiesis is abnormal in Dcytb knockout mice exposed to hypoxic conditions. *J Nutr* 142:1929, 2012.
24. Gunshin H, Mackenzie B, Berger UV, et al: Cloning and characterization of a mammalian proton-coupled metalion transporter. *Nature* 388:482, 1997.
25. Shawki A, Knight PB, Maliken BD, et al: H(+)-coupled divalent metal-ion transporter-1: Functional properties, physiological roles and therapeutics. *Curr Top Membr* 70:169, 2012.
26. Donovan A, Brownlie A, Zhou Y, et al: Positional cloning of zebrafish ferroportin1 identifies a conserved vertebrate iron exporter. *Nature* 403:776, 2000.
27. McKie AT, Marciani P, Rolfs A, et al: A novel duodenal iron-regulated transporter, IREG1, implicated in the basolateral transfer of iron to the circulation. *Mol Cell* 5:299, 2000.
28. Abboud S, Haile DJ: A novel mammalian iron-regulated protein involved in intracellular iron metabolism. *J Biol Chem* 275:19906, 2000.
29. Vulpe CD, Kuo YM, Murphy TL, et al: Hephaestin, a ceruloplasmin homologue implicated in intestinal iron transport, is defective in the sla mouse. *Nat Genet* 21:195, 1999.
30. Cherukuri S, Potla R, Sarkar J, et al: Unexpected role of ceruloplasmin in intestinal iron absorption. *Cell Metab* 2:309, 2005.
31. Noyes WD, Bothwell TH, Finch CA: The role of the reticulo-endothelial cell in iron metabolism. *Br J Haematol* 6:43, 1960.
32. Haurani FI, Burke W, Martinez EJ: Defective reutilization of iron in the anemia of inflammation. *J Lab Clin Med* 65:560, 1965.
33. O'Shea MJ, Kershenobich D, Tavill AS: Effects of inflammation on iron and transferrin metabolism. *Br J Haematol* 25:707, 1973.
34. Bosman GJCG, Werre JM, Willekens FLA, et al: Erythrocyte ageing in vivo and in vitro: Structural aspects and implications for transfusion. *Transfus Med* 18:335, 2008.
35. Beaumont C, Delaby C: Recycling iron in normal and pathological states. *Semin Hematol* 46:328, 2009.
36. Kovtunovych G, Eckhaus MA, Ghosh MC, et al: Dysfunction of the heme recycling system in heme oxygenase-1 deficient mice: Effects on macrophage viability and tissue iron distribution. *Blood* 116:6054, 2010.
37. Delaby C, Rondeau C, Pouzet C, et al: Subcellular localization of iron and heme metabolism related proteins at early stages of erythrophagocytosis. *PLoS One* 7:e42199, 2012.
38. White C, Yuan X, Schmidt PJ, et al: HRG1 is essential for heme transport from the phagolysosome of macrophages during erythrophagocytosis. *Cell Metab* 17:261, 2013.
39. Soe-Lin S, Apte SS, Andriopoulos B Jr, et al: Nramp1 promotes efficient macrophage recycling of iron following erythrophagocytosis in vivo. *Proc Natl Acad Sci U S A* 106:5960, 2009.
40. Knutson MD, Oukka M, Koss LM, et al: Iron release from macrophages after erythrophagocytosis is up-regulated by ferroportin 1 overexpression and down-regulated by hepcidin. *Proc Natl Acad Sci U S A* 102:1324, 2005.
41. Cherukuri S, Tripoulas NA, Nurko S, et al: Anemia and impaired stress-induced erythropoiesis in aceruloplasminemic mice. *Blood Cells Mol Dis* 33:346, 2004.
42. Harris ZL, Durley AP, Man TK, et al: Targeted gene disruption reveals an essential role for ceruloplasmin in cellular iron efflux. *Proc Natl Acad Sci U S A* 96:10812, 1999.
43. Sarkar J, Seshadri V, Tripoulas NA, et al: Role of ceruloplasmin in macrophage iron efflux during hypoxia. *J Biol Chem* 278:44018, 2003.
44. Pigeon C, Ilyin G, Courselaud B, et al: A new mouse liver-specific gene, encoding a protein homologous to human antimicrobial peptide hepcidin, is overexpressed during iron overload. *J Biol Chem* 276:7811, 2001.
45. Park CH, Valore EV, Waring AJ, et al: Hepcidin, a urinary antimicrobial peptide synthesized in the liver. *J Biol Chem* 276:7806, 2001.
46. Nicolas G, Bennoun M, Devaux I, et al: Lack of hepcidin gene expression and severe tissue iron overload in upstream stimulatory factor 2 (USF2) knockout mice. *Proc Natl Acad Sci U S A* 98:8780, 2001.
47. Ganz T: Hepcidin and iron regulation, 10 years later. *Blood* 117:4425, 2011.
48. Nicolas G, Bennoun M, Porteu A, et al: Severe iron deficiency anemia in transgenic mice expressing liver hepcidin. *Proc Natl Acad Sci U S A* 99:4596, 2002.
49. Finberg KE, Heeney MM, Campagna DR, et al: Mutations in TMPRSS6 cause iron-refractory iron deficiency anemia (IRIDA). *Nat Genet* 40:569, 2008.
50. Rivera S, Nemeth E, Gabayan V, et al: Synthetic hepcidin causes rapid dose-dependent hypoferremia and is concentrated in ferroportin-containing organs. *Blood* 106:2196, 2005.
51. Nemeth E, Tuttle MS, Powelson J, et al: Hepcidin regulates cellular iron efflux by binding to ferroportin and inducing its internalization. *Science* 306:2090, 2004.
52. Nemeth E, Rivera S, Gabayan V, et al: IL-6 mediates hypoferremia of inflammation by inducing the synthesis of the iron regulatory hormone hepcidin. *J Clin Invest* 113:1271, 2004.
53. Rodriguez R, Jung CL, Gabayan V, et al: Hepcidin induction by pathogens and pathogen-derived molecules is strongly dependent on interleukin-6. *Infect Immun* 82:745, 2014.
54. Nicolas G, Chauvet C, Viatte L, et al: The gene encoding the iron regulatory peptide hepcidin is regulated by anemia, hypoxia, and inflammation. *J Clin Invest* 110:1037, 2002.
55. Nemeth E, Valore EV, Territo M, et al: Hepcidin, a putative mediator of anemia of inflammation, is a type II acute-phase protein. *Blood* 101:2461, 2003.

56. Pak M, Lopez MA, Gabayan V, et al: Suppression of hepcidin during anemia requires erythropoietic activity. *Blood* 108:3730, 2006.
57. Ganz T, Olbina G, Girelli D, et al: Immunoassay for human serum hepcidin. *Blood* 112:4292, 2008.
58. Ramos E, Kautz L, Rodriguez R, et al: Evidence for distinct pathways of hepcidin regulation by acute and chronic iron loading in mice. *Hepatology* 53:1333, 2011.
59. Corradini E, Meynard D, Wu Q, et al: Serum and liver iron differently regulate the bone morphogenetic protein 6 (BMP6)-SMAD signaling pathway in mice. *Hepatology* 54:273, 2011.
60. Lin L, Valore EV, Nemeth E, et al: Iron transferrin regulates hepcidin synthesis in primary hepatocyte culture through hemojuvelin and BMP2/4. *Blood* 110:2182, 2007.
61. Schmidt PJ, Toran PT, Giannetti AM, et al: The transferrin receptor modulates Hfe-dependent regulation of hepcidin expression. *Cell Metab* 7:205, 2008.
62. Schmidt PJ, Huang FW, Wrighting DM, et al: Hepcidin expression is regulated by a complex of hemochromatosis-associated proteins. *ASH Annu Meet Abstr* 108:267, 2006.
63. D'Alessio F, Hentze MW, Muckenthaler MU: The hemochromatosis proteins HFE, TfR2, and HJV form a membrane-associated protein complex for hepcidin regulation. *J Hepatol* 57:1052, 2012.
64. Rishi G, Crampton EM, Wallace DF, et al: In situ proximity ligation assays indicate that hemochromatosis proteins Hfe and transferrin receptor 2 (Tfr2) do not interact. *PLoS One* 8:e77267, 2013.
65. Papanikolaou G, Samuels ME, Ludwig EH, et al: Mutations in HFE2 cause iron overload in chromosome 1q-linked juvenile hemochromatosis. *Nat Genet* 36:77, 2004.
66. Babitt JL, Huang FW, Wrighting DM, et al: Bone morphogenetic protein signaling by hemojuvelin regulates hepcidin expression. *Nat Genet* 38:531, 2006.
67. Lin L, Nemeth E, Goodnough JB, et al: Soluble hemojuvelin is released by proprotein convertase-mediated cleavage at a conserved polybasic RNRR site. *Blood Cells Mol Dis* 40:122, 2008.
68. Lin L, Goldberg YP, Ganz T: Competitive regulation of hepcidin mRNA by soluble and cell-associated hemojuvelin. *Blood* 106:2884, 2005.
69. Truksa J, Lee P, Beutler E: Two BMP responsive elements, STAT, and bZIP/HNF4/COUP motifs of the hepcidin promoter are critical for BMP, SMAD1, and HJV responsiveness. *Blood* 113:688, 2009.
70. Silvestri L, Pagani A, Nai A, et al: The serine protease matriptase-2 (TMPRSS6) inhibits hepcidin activation by cleaving membrane hemojuvelin. *Cell Metab* 8:502, 2008.
71. Truksa J, Gelbart T, Peng H, et al: Suppression of the hepcidin-encoding gene Hamp permits iron overload in mice lacking both hemojuvelin and matriptase-2/TMPRSS6. *Br J Haematol* 147:571, 2009.
72. Du X, She E, Gelbart T, et al: The serine protease TMPRSS6 is required to sense iron deficiency. *Science* 320:1088, 2008.
73. Finch C: Regulators of iron balance in humans. *Blood* 84:1697, 1994.
74. Kautz L, Jung G, Valore EV, et al: Identification of erythroferrone as an erythroid regulator of iron metabolism. *Nat Genet* 2014.
75. Tanno T, Bhanu NV, Oneal PA, et al: High levels of GDF15 in thalassemia suppress expression of the iron regulatory protein hepcidin. *Nat Med* 13:1096, 2007.
76. Drakesmith H, Prentice AM: Hepcidin and the iron-infection axis. *Science* 338:768, 2012.
77. Wrighting DM, Andrews NC: Interleukin-6 induces hepcidin expression through STAT3. *Blood* 108:3204, 2006.
78. Pietrangelo A, Dierssen U, Valli L, et al: STAT3 is required for IL-6-gp130-dependent activation of hepcidin in vivo. *Gastroenterology* 132:294, 2007.
79. Verga Falzacappa MV, Vujic SM, Kessler R, et al: STAT3 mediates hepatic hepcidin expression and its inflammatory stimulation. *Blood* 109:353, 2007.
80. Besson-Fournier C, Latour C, Kautz L, et al: Induction of activin B by inflammatory stimuli up-regulates expression of the iron-regulatory peptide hepcidin through Smad1/5/8 signaling. *Blood* 120:431, 2012.
81. Aisen P: Transferrin receptor 1. *Int J Biochem Cell Biol* 36:2137, 2004.
82. Muckenthaler MU, Galy B, Hentze MW: Systemic iron homeostasis and the iron-responsive element/iron-regulatory protein (IRE/IRP) regulatory network. *Annu Rev Nutr* 28:197, 2008.
83. Rouault TA: The role of iron regulatory proteins in mammalian iron homeostasis and disease. *Nat Chem Biol* 2:406, 2006.
84. Nemeth E, Roetto A, Garozzo G, et al: Hepcidin is decreased in TFR2 hemochromatosis. *Blood* 105:1803, 2005.
85. Silvestri L, Nai A, Pagani A, et al: The extrahepatic role of TFR2 in iron homeostasis. *Front Pharmacol* 5:93, 2014.
86. Vashisht AA, Zumbrennen KB, Huang X, et al: Control of iron homeostasis by an iron-regulated ubiquitin ligase. *Science* 326:718, 2009.
87. Salahudeen AA, Thompson JW, Ruiz JC, et al: An E3 ligase possessing an iron-responsive hemerythrin domain is a regulator of iron homeostasis. *Science* 326:722, 2009.
88. Chen W, Dailey HA, Paw BH: Ferrochelatase forms an oligomeric complex with mitoferrin-1 and Abcb10 for erythroid heme biosynthesis. *Blood* 116:628, 2010.
89. Sheftel AD, Zhang AS, Brown C, et al: Direct interorganellar transfer of iron from endosome to mitochondrion. *Blood* 110:125, 2007.
90. Cartwright GE, Deiss A: Sideroblasts, siderocytes, and sideroblastic anemia. *N Engl J Med* 292:185, 1975.
91. Levi S, Arosio P: Mitochondrial ferritin. *Int J Biochem Cell Biol* 36:1887, 2004.
92. Cazzola M, Invernizzi R, Bergamaschi G, et al: Mitochondrial ferritin expression in erythroid cells from patients with sideroblastic anemia. *Blood* 101:1996, 2003.
93. Green R, Charlton R, Seftel H, et al: Body iron excretion in man: A collaborative study. *Am J Med* 45:336, 1968.
94. Feder JN, Gnirke A, Thomas W, et al: A novel MHC class I-like gene is mutated in patients with hereditary haemochromatosis. *Nat Genet* 13:399, 1996.
95. Zhou XY, Tomatsu S, Fleming RE, et al: HFE gene knockout produces mouse model of hereditary hemochromatosis. *Proc Natl Acad Sci U S A* 95:2492, 1998.
96. Ahmad KA, Ahmann JR, Migas MC, et al: Decreased Liver Hepcidin Expression in the Hfe Knockout Mouse. *Blood Cells Mol Dis* 29:361, 2002.
97. Montosi G, Donovan A, Totaro A, et al: Autosomal-dominant hemochromatosis is associated with a mutation in the ferroportin (SLC11A3) gene. *J Clin Invest* 108:619, 2001.
98. Zohn IE, De Domenico I, Pollock A, et al: The flatiron mutation in mouse ferroportin acts as a dominant negative to cause ferroportin disease. *Blood* 109:4174, 2007.
99. Njajou OT, Vaessen N, Joosse M, et al: A mutation in SLC11A3 is associated with autosomal dominant hemochromatosis. *Nat Genet* 28:213, 2001.
100. Sham RL, Phatak PD, Nemeth E, et al: Hereditary hemochromatosis due to resistance to hepcidin: High hepcidin concentrations in a family with C326S ferroportin mutation. *Blood* 114:493, 2009.
101. Altamura S, Groene HJ, Kessler R, et al: In vivo disruption of the hepcidin-ferroportin regulatory circuitry causes fatal systemic and exocrine pancreatic iron overload [abstract]. *ASH Annu Meet Abstr* 175, 2013.
102. De Sousa M, Reimao R, Lacerda R, et al: Iron overload in beta 2-microglobulin-deficient mice. *Immunol Lett* 39:105, 1994.
103. Rothenberg BE, Voland JR: Beta2 knockout mice develop parenchymal iron overload: A putative role for class I genes of the major histocompatibility complex in iron metabolism. *Proc Natl Acad Sci U S A* 93:1529, 1996.
104. Goya N, Miyazaki S, Kodate S, et al: A family of congenital atransferrinemia. *Blood* 40:239, 1972.
105. Bernstein SE: Hereditary hypotransferrinemia with hemosiderosis, a murine disorder resembling human atransferrinemia. *J Lab Clin Med* 110:690, 1987.
106. Hamill RL, Woods JC, Cook BA: Congenital atransferrinemia. A case report and review of the literature. *Am J Clin Pathol* 96:215, 1991.
107. Trenor CC, III, Campagna DR, Sellers VM, et al: The molecular defect in hypotransferrinemic mice. *Blood* 96:1113, 2000.
108. Bartnikas TB, Andrews NC, Fleming MD: Transferrin is a major determinant of hepcidin expression in hypotransferrinemic mice. *Blood* 117:630, 2011.
109. Levy JE, Jin O, Fujiwara Y, et al: Transferrin receptor is necessary for development of erythrocytes and the nervous system. *Nat Genet* 21:396, 1999.
110. Camaschella C, Roetto A, Cali A, et al: The gene TFR2 is mutated in a new type of haemochromatosis mapping to 7q22. *Nat Genet* 25:14, 2000.
111. Fleming RE, Ahmann JR, Migas MC, et al: Targeted mutagenesis of the murine transferrin receptor-2 gene produces hemochromatosis. *Proc Natl Acad Sci U S A* 99:10653, 2002.
112. Harris ZL, Takahashi Y, Miyajima H, et al: Aceruloplasminemia: Molecular characterization of this disorder of iron metabolism. *Proc Natl Acad Sci U S A* 92:2539, 1995.
113. Kato J, Fujikawa K, Kanda M, et al: A mutation, in the iron-responsive element of H ferritin mRNA, causing autosomal dominant iron overload. *Am J Hum Genet* 69:191, 2001.
114. Iolascon A, De FL: Mutations in the gene encoding DMT1: Clinical presentation and treatment. *Semin Hematol* 46:358, 2009.
115. Blanco E, Kannengiesser C, Grandchamp B, et al: Not all DMT1 mutations lead to iron overload. *Blood Cells Mol Dis* 43:199, 2009.
116. Fleming MD, Trenor CC, III, Su MA, et al: Microcytic anaemia mice have a mutation in Nramp2, a candidate iron transporter gene. *Nat Genet* 16:383, 1997.
117. Fleming MD, Romano MA, Su MA, et al: Nramp2 is mutated in the anemic Belgrade (b) rat: Evidence of a role for Nramp2 in endosomal iron transport. *Proc Natl Acad Sci U S A* 95:1148, 1998.
118. Roetto A, Papanikolaou G, Politou M, et al: Mutant antimicrobial peptide hepcidin is associated with severe juvenile hemochromatosis. *Nat Genet* 33:21, 2003.
119. Lesbordes-Brion JC, Viatte L, Bennoun M, et al: Targeted disruption of the hepcidin 1 gene results in severe hemochromatosis. *Blood* 108:1402, 2006.
120. Niederkofler V, Salie R, Arber S: Hemojuvelin is essential for dietary iron sensing, and its mutation leads to severe iron overload. *J Clin Invest* 115:2180, 2005.
121. Huang FW, Pinkus JL, Pinkus GS, et al: A mouse model of juvenile hemochromatosis. *J Clin Invest* 115:2187, 2005.
122. Meynard D, Kautz L, Darnaud V, et al: Lack of the bone morphogenetic protein BMP6 induces massive iron overload. *Nat Genet* 41:478, 2009.
123. Andriopoulos B Jr, Corradini E, Xia Y, et al: BMP6 is a key endogenous regulator of hepcidin expression and iron metabolism. *Nat Genet* 41:482, 2009.
124. Steinbicker AU, Bartnikas TB, Lohmeyer LK, et al: Perturbation of hepcidin expression by BMP type I receptor deletion induces iron overload in mice. *Blood* 118:4224, 2011.
125. Wang RH, Li C, Xu X, et al: A role of SMAD4 in iron metabolism through the positive regulation of hepcidin expression. *Cell Metab* 2:399, 2005.
126. Lee DH, Zhou LJ, Zhou Z, et al: Neogenin inhibits HJV secretion and regulates BMP-induced hepcidin expression and iron homeostasis. *Blood* 115:3136, 2010.
127. Enns CA, Ahmed R, Zhang AS: Neogenin interacts with matriptase-2 to facilitate hemojuvelin cleavage. *J Biol Chem* 287:35104, 2012.
128. Mackenzie B, Garrick MD: Iron Imports. II. Iron uptake at the apical membrane in the intestine. *Am J Physiol Gastrointest Liver Physiol* 289:G981, 2005.
129. Smith MD, Pannacciulli IM: Absorption of inorganic iron from graded doses: Its significance in relation to iron absorption tests and mucosal block theory. *Br J Haematol* 4:428, 1958.
130. McKie AT: A ferrireductase fills the gap in the transferrin cycle. *Nat Genet* 37:1159, 2005.

CHAPTER 43
IRON DEFICIENCY AND OVERLOAD

Tomas Ganz

SUMMARY

Iron deficiency and iron-deficiency anemia are common nutritional and hematologic disorders. In infants and young children, iron deficiency is most commonly caused by insufficient dietary iron. Rarely, it can result from mutations in *TMPRSS6*, a gene encoding a membrane protease that serves normally as a transcriptional suppressor of the primary negative regulator of iron absorption, hepcidin. In young women, iron deficiency is most often the result of blood loss in menstruation or as a result of blood loss during pregnancy, childbirth, and lactation. In older adults, bleeding is often the cause of iron deficiency, and may originate from the gastrointestinal tract, as from hemorrhoids, peptic ulcer, hiatus hernia, colon cancer, or angiodysplasia; from the genitourinary tract; from uterine leiomyomas or carcinoma, or a renal tumor; or from the pulmonary tree, through chronic hemoptysis caused by infection or malignancy, or as a result of idiopathic pulmonary hemosiderosis. Iron deficiency in infants can result in impairment of growth and intellectual development. The hematologic features of iron deficiency are nonspecific and too often confused with other causes of microcytic anemia such as thalassemias, chronic inflammation, and renal neoplasms. A low serum ferritin concentration is a good indicator of iron deficiency, but ferritin levels are increased by inflammation and can be particularly high in cancer, macrophage activation syndromes, hepatitis, or chronic kidney disease, which may mask the detection of iron deficiency coexisting with the anemia of chronic inflammation. The plasma iron is decreased and the iron-binding capacity increased in severe iron deficiency, but these alterations are not uniformly present in mild iron deficiency, and low plasma iron levels are also characteristic of the anemia of inflammation. Other laboratory tests that are useful include assays for serum transferrin receptor, reticulocyte hemoglobin content, percent hypochromic erythrocytes and erythrocyte zinc protoporphyrin. Diagnosis of iron deficiency, particularly in an adult, obliges the clinician to determine the site and cause of blood loss, and to rectify it whenever possible. Ferrous salts, in doses of 100 to 200 mg of elemental iron daily, are the initial treatment in most patients with iron deficiency. Enteric-coated and prolonged-release preparations should be avoided. Complete correction of anemia is expected in 8 to 12 weeks, depending on patient's age. If this response is not achieved, the patient and the diagnosis require reevaluation. Administration of iron should be continued for 12 months after correction of anemia, or for as long as bleeding continues. Parenteral iron is used in patients who need more iron than can be delivered by the oral route, patients who do not tolerate oral iron salts, patients with gastrointestinal disease or following certain forms of bariatric surgery, noncompliant patients, and patients undergoing renal dialysis. All current parenteral iron preparations are much less likely to cause serious adverse events than was the case for high-molecular-weight iron dextran used in the past.

At the opposite end of the iron disorder spectrum, iron storage disease (hemochromatosis) can be the result of mutations of genes that are involved in regulation of iron homeostasis or transport, including the genes encoding HFE, transferrin receptor 2, ferroportin, hemojuvelin, and hepcidin. Because iron is not substantially excreted, iron overload commonly results from chronic erythrocyte transfusions for those anemias that are not caused by blood loss or iron deficiency.

Alternatively, iron overload resembling hereditary hemochromatosis can be the result of hyperabsorption of iron induced by ineffective erythropoiesis, including in β-thalassemias, dyserythropoietic anemias, pyruvate kinase deficiency, congenital dyserythropoietic anemias and some sideroblastic anemias. Here iron overload can develop even in the absence of erythrocyte transfusions or the (ill-advised) administration of medicinal iron, but is further aggravated by these events.

The diagnosis of systemic iron overload depends, in large part, upon increased serum ferritin levels accompanied by increased transferrin saturation, which tend to reflect increased iron stores. However, ferritin levels are also increased in patients with chronic inflammation or neoplasia or with the hyperferritinemia cataract syndrome, a disorder caused by mutations in the iron-responsive element of the ferritin light chain. The transferrin saturation is usually increased in patients with hereditary hemochromatosis even when the ferritin level is normal.

Many subjects with genetic hemochromatosis never develop organ dysfunction, those who do, their clinically significant hemochromatosis is characterized by cirrhosis of the liver, darkening of the skin, diabetes, cardiomyopathies, and possibly by arthropathies. Iron deposition is primarily in hepatocytes, with macrophages and intestinal mucosal cells being relatively iron poor. The most common causes of genetic hemochromatosis are mutations of the *HFE* gene. Two common mutations are involved: the c.854G→A (C282Y) and c.187C→G (H63D) substitutions. Increased transferrin saturation values, serum ferritin levels, and iron stores were found in a majority of homozygotes for the C282Y mutation and in many compound heterozygotes for C282Y/H63D or rarely in homozygotes for H63D. However, clinical manifestations even among homozygotes for the C282Y mutation are rare, in contrast to biochemical and/or histologic manifestations of the increased iron levels, which are common. Only a few percent of C282Y homozygous patients develop clinically significant disease, and cofactors including male gender and alcohol intake potentiate disease development. Juvenile hemochromatosis, an earlier onset and more severe type of hemochromatosis with high penetrance is the result of mutations of the hemojuvelin or the hepcidin gene. Ferroportin mutations produced two types of autosomal dominant iron overload. In one of these, the iron is deposited chiefly in macrophages; the other is similar to classical hereditary hemochromatosis with iron deposition in hepatocytes and other parenchymal cells.

Iron can be removed from patients with hereditary hemochromatosis by serial phlebotomy, but in patients with iron-loading anemias iron chelation therapy with either parenteral desferrioxamine infusions or the oral chelators deferiprone or deferasirox is required.

Acronyms and Abbreviations: BMP, bone morphogenetic protein; cDNA, complementary DNA; DMT, divalent metal transporter; HFE, high iron (*high Fe*)—a mutated protein associated with common hereditary hemochromatosis; HLA, human leukocyte antigen; IL, interleukin; IRE, iron-responsive element; IRP, iron-regulatory protein; MCV, mean corpuscular volume; MRI, magnetic resonance imaging; RDA, recommended daily allowance; RDW, red cell distribution width; TfR, transferrin receptor; TIBC, total iron-binding capacity; UIBC, unsaturated iron-binding capacity.

●IRON DEFICIENCY

DEFINITION AND HISTORY

Iron deficiency is the state in which the content of iron in the body is less than normal. Iron depletion is the earliest stage of iron deficiency, in which storage iron is decreased or absent but serum iron concentration, transferrin saturation, and blood hemoglobin levels are normal. Iron deficiency without anemia is a somewhat more advanced stage of iron deficiency, characterized by absent storage iron, usually low serum iron concentration and transferrin saturation, but without frank anemia. Iron-deficiency anemia, the most advanced stage of iron deficiency, is characterized by absent iron stores, low serum iron concentration, low transferrin saturation, and low blood hemoglobin concentration.

Chlorosis, or "green sickness," was well known to European physicians after the middle of the 16th century. In France, by the middle of the 17th century, iron salts and other remedies (including, oddly enough, phlebotomy) were used in its treatment. Not long thereafter, iron was recommended by Sydenham as a specific remedy for chlorosis. For the 100 years preceding 1930, iron was used in the treatment of chlorosis, often in ineffective doses, although the mechanism of action of iron and the appropriateness of its use were highly controversial. By the beginning of the 20th century, it had been established that chlorosis was characterized by a decrease in the iron content of the blood and by the presence of hypochromic erythrocytes, but it was not until the classic 1932 studies by Heath, Strauss, and Castle[1] that it was shown that the response of anemia to iron was stoichiometrically related to the amount of iron given and that chlorosis was, indeed, iron deficiency. The history of iron deficiency has been reviewed in greater detail elsewhere.[2,3]

EPIDEMIOLOGY

Iron-deficiency anemia is the most common anemia worldwide, and is especially prevalent in women and children in regions where meat intake is low, food is not fortified with iron, and malaria, intestinal infections, and parasitic worms are common.[4–6] Women with frequent pregnancies may be particularly susceptible. In the United States, iron deficiency is most common in children 1 to 4 years old and in adolescent, reproductive age, or pregnant women.[7–9]

ETIOLOGY AND PATHOGENESIS

Etiology

Iron deficiency may occur as a result of chronic blood loss, diversion of iron to fetal and infant erythropoiesis during pregnancy and lactation, inadequate dietary iron intake, malabsorption of iron, intravascular hemolysis with hemoglobinuria, diversion of iron to nonhematopoietic tissues like the lung, genetic factors, or a combination of these factors. Of these, gastrointestinal or menstrual blood loss are the most common. As discussed in Chap. 42, the average adult male has approximately 1000 mg of iron in stores, but on average, women have less than half of this amount. The average daily dietary intake of iron is 10 to 12 mg, but much of this is not absorbed, even when absorption is maximal. Blood loss of each milliliter of packed erythrocytes represents 1 mg of iron. Thus chronic daily blood loss greater than 5 mL of erythrocytes will deplete iron reserves over weeks to months, and even if bleeding stops completely, the repletion of lost iron, including the restoration of iron stores (around 1000 mg in the average adult man), will take many months.

Blood Loss

Gastrointestinal Blood Loss In men and in postmenopausal women, iron deficiency is most commonly caused by chronic bleeding from the gastrointestinal tract. Table 43–1 lists the causes of such blood loss.

TABLE 43–1. Sources of Blood Loss

ALIMENTARY TRACT
Esophagus
Varices
Stomach and duodenum
Ulcer
Hiatus hernia
Gastritis
Carcinoma
Varices
Angiodysplasia
Hemangioma
Leiomyoma (Ménétrier disease)
Mucosal hypertrophy
Hypergastrinemia
Antral vascular ectasia
"Watermelon stomach"
Small intestine
Vascular ectasia
Tumors
Ulceration
Meckel's diverticulum
Colon and anorectal
Hemorrhoids
Carcinoma
Polyp
Diverticulum
Ulcerative colitis
Angiodysplasia
Hemangioma
Telangiectasia
Amebiasis
BILIARY TRACT
Intrahepatic bleeding
Carcinoma
Cholelithiasis
Trauma
Ruptured aneurysm
Aberrant pancreas
GENITOURINARY TRACT
Menorrhagia
Uterine fibroids
Endometriosis
Carcinoma
Vascular abnormalities
RESPIRATORY TRACT
Epistaxis
Carcinoma
Infections
Telangiectases
Idiopathic pulmonary hemosiderosis

After history and physical examination rule out an obvious bleeding source in the genitourinary or respiratory tracts, evaluation of the gastrointestinal tract[10] is necessary because of the potential that the pathologic process causing the blood loss is life-threatening. In the adult, the most common causes are peptic ulcer, erosion in a hiatal hernia, gastritis (including that caused by alcohol or aspirin ingestion), hemorrhoids, vascular anomalies (such as angiodysplasia), and neoplasms.

Gastritis, Varices, Ulcers, and Inflammation Gastritis as a result of drug ingestion is a common cause of bleeding. Aspirin, indomethacin, ibuprofen, and other nonsteroidal antiinflammatory drugs cause gastritis, but may also cause bleeding by inducing gastric or duodenal ulcers, or lesions in the small intestine[11] and even the colon. Gastritis caused by alcohol ingestion[12] can also cause significant blood loss. Chronic blood loss is often the cause of anemia in rheumatoid arthritis (perhaps because of the use of nonsteroidal antiinflammatory medications) and in inflammatory bowel disease.

Chronic blood loss from esophageal or gastric varices can lead to iron-deficiency anemia. Hemorrhoidal bleeding may lead to severe iron-deficiency anemia. Chronic blood loss may result from diffuse gastric mucosal hypertrophy (Ménétrier disease).[13] Peptic ulcers of the stomach or duodenum are common causes of iron deficiency, and an association between infection with *Helicobacter pylori* and iron-deficiency anemia has been documented in numerous studies.[14] Some of these iron-deficient patients who are infected with *H. pylori* do not respond to oral iron alone, but do respond to eradication of *H. pylori*.[15]

Gastric ulceration and bleeding can also occur in disorders of hypergastrinemia, as in Zollinger-Ellison syndrome and pseudo–Zollinger-Ellison syndrome. Although concerns were raised that long-term medical therapy of these disorders with proton pump inhibitors would also cause iron deficiency by raising gastric pH and making iron less soluble, this does not seem to be the case.[16] Anemia that follows subtotal gastrectomy is usually attributed to reduced absorption of dietary iron (see "Malabsorption of Iron" below), but occult intermittent gastrointestinal bleeding from gastrointestinal lesions may also be a contributory factor, and requires endoscopic evaluation.[17]

Diaphragmatic Hernia Diaphragmatic (hiatal) hernia is often associated with gastrointestinal bleeding.[18–20] The frequency of anemia ranges from 8 to 38 percent. Bleeding is much more likely to occur in patients with paraesophageal or large hernias than in those with sliding or small hernias. Mucosal changes cannot always be demonstrated by esophagoscopy or gastroscopy in patients who have had blood loss from hiatus hernia. However, a linear gastric erosion, also called a "Cameron ulcer," commonly occurs on the crests of mucosal folds at the level of the diaphragm, and appears to be the site of bleeding.[21]

Intestinal Parasitism Hookworms are a major cause of gastrointestinal blood loss in many parts of the world.[22]

Vascular Anomalies The lesions of angiodysplasia may occur in any part of the gastrointestinal tract.[23] These tiny vascular anomalies may be the cause of significant blood loss. Endoscopy is usually required for diagnosis, and often needs to be repeated as bleeding can be intermittent. Gastric antral vascular ectasia[24] exhibits a characteristic endoscopic appearance ("watermelon stomach"), and is another cause of blood loss. Hemorrhage into the biliary tract is a rare cause of chronic iron-deficiency anemia.[25]

Tortuous, dilated sublingual venous structures, the cherry hemangiomas commonly seen in the elderly, and the spider telangiectases of chronic liver disease are usually easily distinguished from the lesions of hereditary hemorrhagic telangiectasia. Bleeding from intestinal telangiectases has also been observed in scleroderma[26] and in Turner syndrome,[27] as a manifestation of bleeding from abnormal blood vessels. Cutaneous hemangiomas (blue rubber bleb nevus) may be associated with hemorrhage from intestinal hemangiomas.[28]

In hereditary hemorrhagic telangiectasia (Chap. 122), characteristic lesions commonly occur on fingertips, nasal septum, tongue, lips, margins (helices) of ears, oral and pharyngeal mucosa, palms and soles, and other epithelial and cutaneous surfaces throughout the body. Those lesions that occur in the gastrointestinal tract are particularly likely to bleed and to cause iron deficiency.

Meckel Diverticulum Meckel diverticulum is a very common abnormality representing a vestigial remnant of the omphalomesenteric duct. In children, bleeding from this structure accounts for a small proportion of cases of iron-deficiency anemia.[29]

Genitourinary Tract Heavy menstrual bleeding[30] is a very common cause of iron deficiency. The amount of blood lost with menstruation[31] varies markedly from one woman to another and is often difficult to evaluate by questioning the patient. The average menstrual blood loss is approximately 40 mL per cycle. Blood loss exceeds 80 mL (equivalent to approximately 30 mg of iron) per cycle in only 10 percent of women. The volume of blood lost in the course of one menstrual cycle may be as high as 495 mL in apparently healthy, nonanemic women who do not regard their menstrual flow to be excessive. The amount of menstrual blood lost does not seem to vary markedly from one cycle to another for any given individual. Oral contraceptives reduce menstrual blood loss, but the use of an intrauterine coil for contraception increases menstrual blood loss, especially during the first year of use. Because the daily dietary intake is usually between 10 and 12 mg of iron and only a few milligrams of this can be absorbed, iron balance in many menstruating women is precarious.

Excessive bleeding may be caused by uterine fibroids and malignant neoplasms. Neoplasms, stones, or inflammatory disease of the kidney, ureter, or bladder may cause enough chronic blood loss to produce iron deficiency.

In the absence of hematuria, urinary iron losses as high as 1 mg/day have been reported in rare patients with nephrotic syndrome, some of whom had hypoferremia and hypochromic anemia.[32] We found only one report of a patient in whom abnormally high urinary iron loss may have caused anemia without proteinuria or hematuria.[33]

Bleeding Disorders Hemostatic defects, particularly those related to abnormal platelet function or number may lead to gastrointestinal bleeding, although unless the thrombocytopenia or platelet dysfunction is severe, gastrointestinal bleeding usually signifies an abnormality in the gastrointestinal tract. Gastrointestinal bleeding is common in von Willebrand disease (Chap. 126), but often because of coexistent peptic ulcer disease. Polycythemia vera is typically associated with iron deficiency as a result either of spontaneous gastrointestinal hemorrhage that commonly occurs in this disorder, or phlebotomy therapy, or both (Chap. 84).

When a patient with a disorder of hemostasis suffers from gastrointestinal bleeding, one must consider the possibility that the bleeding may not be caused by a hemostatic defect alone, but that an anatomic lesion of the gastrointestinal tract may also be present.

Nosocomial (Iatrogenic) Anemia Iatrogenic anemia is particularly prevalent in intensive care units[34] where repetitive blood sampling may result in removal of 40 to 70 mL of blood daily, and this iatrogenic phlebotomy can result in iron-deficiency anemia.

The use of extracorporeal dialysis for treatment of chronic renal disease may cause iron deficiency,[35,36] often superimposed upon the anemia of chronic renal disease (Chap. 37). Patients treated with chronic hemodialysis experience multiple sources of blood loss with the dialysis equipment is a major cause, along with gastrointestinal bleeding, blood sampling and bleeding related to vascular access.

Anemia Incident to Blood Donation Each whole-blood donation removes approximately 200 mg of iron from the body. Lesser amounts of iron are removed in the course of donating platelets or leukocytes. Potential donors are screened in blood banks, so that those with frank anemia are not phlebotomized. Yet, by the time they are excluded from donation, some blood donors are iron depleted[37–39] and may readily develop iron-deficiency anemia with relatively small additional blood loss.

Factitious Anemia Factitious anemia as a result of self-inflicted bleeding may present a formidable diagnostic and therapeutic problem. This rare condition has also been called, in literary allusion to a fictitious character, "Lasthénie de Ferjol syndrome" (in Barbey d'Aurevilly's gloomy novel, *Une Histoire Sans Nom*), or part of Munchausen syndrome (based on the Rudolf Raspe book, *The Surprising Adventures of Baron Münchausen*).[40,41] Most patients are women, and are often employed in a medical setting. There is often a history of numerous blood transfusions. The anemia is chronic and may be severe. The site of induced blood loss is obscure. Hence, patients are subjected to numerous radiographic and endoscopic examinations, usually to no avail. The patients are usually refractory to medical advice and therapy. The patients may be depressed and suicidal; some also suffer anorexia nervosa. Psychiatric care is needed, but often is unsuccessful. Rarely, the outcome of self-bleeding may be fatal.[42]

Cow's Milk Anemia Ingestion of whole cow's milk may induce protein-losing enteropathy and gastrointestinal bleeding in infants,[43,44] probably on the basis of hypersensitivity or allergy. In four such cases observed endoscopically, erosive gastritis or gastroduodenitis was demonstrated as the probable source of bleeding. At least during the first year of life, children should not be given whole bovine milk, either raw or pasteurized. More protracted heating, as in preparation of infant formulas, eliminates this problem. Intrinsic lesions of the gastrointestinal tract, such as those listed above, may cause bleeding in infants, as well as in older children.

Respiratory Tract Persistent recurrent hemoptysis may lead to iron-deficiency anemia. It may be a result of congenital anomalies of the respiratory tract, endobronchial vascular anomalies, chronic infections, neoplasms, or valvular heart disease. Severe iron-deficiency anemia is a manifestation of idiopathic pulmonary hemosiderosis[45] and of Goodpasture syndrome (progressive glomerulonephritis with intrapulmonary hemorrhage). In some of these disorders, hemoptysis may not be observed, but sufficient amounts of blood-laden sputum may be swallowed to result in positive tests for occult blood in the stools. Iron deficiency occurs in a large proportion of patients with cystic fibrosis,[46,47] and occurs even in the absence of hemoptysis, suggesting that inflammatory inhibition of dietary iron absorption and iron loss in purulent sputum could contribute to the deficiency.

Pregnancy and Parturition

Although physiologic decrease in hemoglobin concentration is an expected consequence of hemodilution associated with pregnancy, true iron deficiency frequently results in more severe anemia. In pregnancy, the average iron loss resulting from diversion of iron to the fetus, blood loss at delivery (equivalent to an average of 150 to 200 mg of iron), and lactation is altogether approximately 900 mg; in terms of iron content, this is equivalent to the loss of more than 2 L of blood. Approximately 30 mg of iron may be expended monthly in lactation. Because most women begin pregnancy with low iron reserves, these additional demands frequently result in iron-deficiency anemia. Iron depletion has been reported in some 85 to 100 percent of pregnant women. Iron-deficient mothers are likely to have smaller babies. The incidence of anemia and iron deficiency is lower in women who take oral iron supplementation, daily or intermittently.[48–51] In regions with endemic malaria, iron supplementation may increase the risk of malaria and some recommend that it be combined with malarial prophylaxis.[52] Most experts agree that oral iron supplementation during pregnancy is desirable despite side effects. Increasing safety and convenience of parenteral iron therapy may lead to reevaluation of its role in the prevention and treatment of iron-deficiency anemia of pregnancy.[53]

Dietary Iron Deficiency

In infants, iron deficiency is most often a result of the use of unsupplemented milk diets, which contain an inadequate amount of iron. During the first year of life, the full-term infant requires approximately 160 mg and the premature infant approximately 240 mg of iron to meet the needs of an expanding red cell mass. Approximately 50 mg of this need is fulfilled by the destruction of erythrocytes that occurs physiologically during the first week of life (Chaps. 7 and 33); the rest must come from the diet. Milk products are very poor sources of iron, and prolonged breast- or bottle-feeding of infants frequently leads to iron-deficiency anemia unless iron supplementation is implemented. This is especially true of premature infants. The European Society for Pediatric Gastroenterology, Hepatology, and Nutrition (ESPGHAN) Committee on Nutrition urges that all infant formulas be iron-fortified[54]; in North America, the use of iron-fortified formula is now generally accepted, but there is controversy about the appropriate level of fortification.[55] In older children, an iron-poor diet may also contribute to the development of iron-deficiency anemia, particularly during rapid growth periods.

Infants and young women are usually in precarious iron balance, their iron intake being less than 80 percent of the recommended daily allowance (RDA).[56] Fortification of bread and cereals with ferrous sulfate or metallic iron is commonplace. This practice was suspended in Sweden because of concern for the possibility of increasing iron storage in patients with the hemochromatosis genotype, resulting in increased incidence of iron-deficiency anemia.[57]

The scant iron supply of the American diet places young women and children at particular risk of negative iron balance. Because the adult male needs to absorb only approximately 1 mg iron daily from his diet to maintain normal iron balance, iron deficiency in older men is very rarely caused by insufficient dietary intake alone.

Malabsorption of Iron

Gastric secretion of hydrochloric acid is often reduced in iron deficiency.[58] Histamine-fast achlorhydria has been found in as many as 43 percent of patients with iron deficiency. Gastric function may improve after correction of the iron deficiency, so that iron deficiency may be both a cause and a result of impairment of gastric iron secretion. However, in persons older than the age of 30 years, the achlorhydria is usually irreversible. Furthermore, when atrophic gastritis coexists with iron deficiency, no improvement in gastric secretory function has followed iron therapy. Autoimmune gastritis, which is often associated with *H. pylori* infection,[14,15] may play an important role in both iron-deficiency anemia and, in later life, in the development of pernicious anemia.

Intestinal malabsorption of iron is quite an uncommon cause of iron deficiency except after gastrointestinal surgery and in malabsorption syndromes. Ten to 34 percent of patients who have undergone subtotal gastric resection develop iron-deficiency anemia years later. Many such patients have impaired absorption of food iron, caused in part by more rapid gastrojejunal transit and in part by partially digested food bypassing some of the duodenum as a result of the location of the anastomosis. Fortunately, medicinal iron is well absorbed in post–partial gastrectomy patients. Moreover, gastrointestinal blood loss may also play an important role in anemia following gastric resection (see "Gastrointestinal Blood Loss" earlier). In malabsorption syndromes, absorption of iron may be so limited that iron-deficiency anemia develops over a period of years. Celiac disease, whether overt or occult, may be associated with iron-deficiency anemia.[14,15,59,60]

Intravascular Hemolysis and Hemoglobinuria

Iron-deficiency anemia may occur in paroxysmal nocturnal hemoglobinuria (Chap. 40) and in hemolysis resulting from mechanical erythrocyte trauma from intracardiac myxomas, valvular prostheses (particularly if malfunctioning), or patches (Chaps. 33 and 51). In these disorders, up to 10 mg/day of iron is lost in the urine as hemosiderin and ferritin in desquamated tubular cells and as hemoglobin dimers, an amount sufficient to cause systemic iron deficiency.[61,62]

Iron deficiency occurs frequently in athletes engaged in a variety of sports (Chaps. 33 and 51), especially female athletes.[63] There may be mild anemia. Increased intravascular hemolysis, presumably with some renal loss of iron, may play a role, but gastrointestinal blood loss has also been demonstrated in persons engaged in strenuous athletic pursuits. Hemoglobinuria and hemosiderinuria are also seen in competitive and recreational runners, that is, *march hemoglobinuria* (Chaps. 33 and 51). Strenuous exercise also elicits a rise in serum interleukin (IL)-6 and hepcidin, and this could decrease dietary iron absorption.[63]

Women soldiers undergoing basic training experience iron depletion as determined by serum ferritin measurements, and this can be partially reversed by iron supplementation.[64] The etiology may be similar to the iron deficiency seen in athletes.

Genetic Factors

Based on twin studies,[65] genetic factors play a role in iron deficiency. Mutations in multiple genes, including *HFE* and transferrin, show weak associations with iron stores but only mutations of the membrane serine protease Tmprss6[66] have been identified in genome-wide association studies as genetic factors that cause or predispose to iron deficiency. The genetic syndrome of iron-refractory iron deficiency anemia is mediated by inappropriately increased hepcidin as a result of homozygous or compound heterozygous mutations in Tmprss6.[67–69] Increased hepcidin diminishes iron absorption and causes inappropriate retention of available iron in splenic macrophages and Kupffer cells.

PATHOGENESIS

As iron deficiency develops, different compartments are depleted in iron in an overlapping sequence, as illustrated schematically in Fig. 43–1.

Iron-Containing Proteins

As the body becomes depleted of iron, changes occur in many tissues. Hemosiderin and ferritin virtually disappear from marrow and other storage sites. Hemoglobin synthesis in the marrow decreases, first as a result of fewer erythroblasts,[70] but eventually also per erythroblast if iron deficiency becomes more severe, resulting in hemoglobin-deficient erythrocytes. The concentration of many other iron-containing proteins is affected, often in an organ-specific manner.[71] Studies in laboratory animals on defined iron-deficient diets are most informative about this process, because human iron deficiency is often confounded by other forms of malnutrition. In such models of severe (pure) iron deficiency, skeletal muscle myoglobin is mildly depleted but cardiac myoglobin is not. Cytochromes and other mitochondrial ferroproteins are depleted but selectively so. Since these classical studies were performed, it has become apparent that the synthesis of many ferroproteins is regulated in an iron-dependent manner, mainly via the iron-responsive element (IRE)/iron-regulatory protein (IRP) system (Chap. 42). The changes in iron-containing proteins may thus be adaptive,[72] to allow the survival of the organism until more iron becomes available.

Muscular Function and Exercise Tolerance

Decrements in high-intensity exercise performance can be detected even during nonanemic iron deficiency,[63] and worsen with increasing

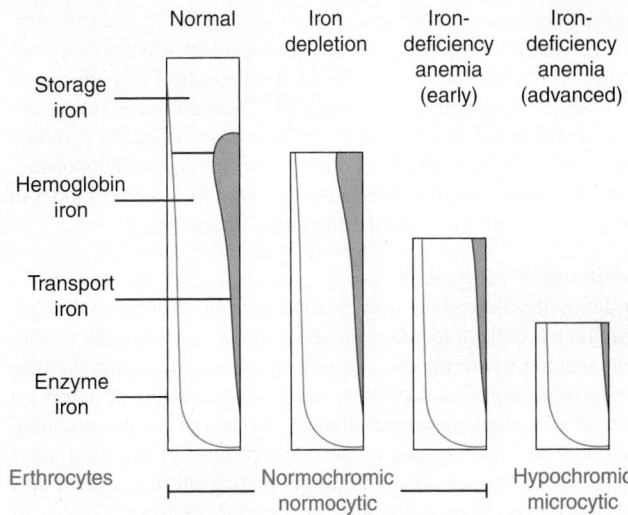

Figure 43–1. Stages in the development of iron deficiency. Early iron deficiency (iron depletion) is usually not accompanied by any abnormalities in blood; at this stage, serum iron concentration is occasionally below normal values and storage iron is markedly depleted. As iron deficiency progresses, development of anemia precedes appearance of morphologic changes in blood, although some cells may be smaller and paler than normal; serum iron concentration is usually low at this time, but it may be normal. With advanced iron depletion, classic changes of hypochromic, microcytic, hypoferremic anemia become manifest. (*Reproduced with permission from* Lichtman's Atlas of Hematology, *www.accessmedicine.com.*)

anemia.[73] The limitation of high-level exercise by oxygen delivery, and, therefore, hemoglobin content of blood, is well known, and has given rise to surreptitious blood doping and erythropoietin abuse by some athletes. The impairment of performance during nonanemic iron deficiency consists of decreased spontaneous activity (seen in humans and in animal models) and decreased ventilatory threshold, that is, the point at which ventilation starts increasing more rapidly than oxygen consumption.[74] Other deficits that have been reported include decreased endurance and increased muscle fatigue. The biochemical basis of the deficits associated with nonanemic iron deficiency is not well understood but is attributed to the depletion of iron-containing mitochondrial proteins that are involved in energy metabolism.[63] The condition is reversible with iron supplementation.

Neurologic Changes

Iron deficiency is associated with both developmental abnormalities in children and with restless leg syndrome in adults, but in neither case has iron deficiency been established as the primary cause.[75,76] The substantia nigra is a particularly iron-rich region of the brain and contains dopaminergic neurons that are suspected of involvement in restless leg syndrome. In mouse models of iron deficiency, iron depletion of the substantia nigra is highly strain-dependent,[77] suggesting that iron deficiency and as yet incompletely characterized genetic variations may cooperate in the pathogenesis of restless leg syndrome by allowing the depletion of iron from susceptible brain regions involved in dopaminergic signaling.[78]

Host Defense and Inflammation

In multiple publications, iron deficiency has been reported to impair various immune functions, but the effects appear minor and inconsistent.[79] Perhaps surprisingly, the evidence for a narrowly protective and proinflammatory effect of iron deficiency appears stronger. Iron deficiency decreases the risk and severity of malaria,[80,81] and iron supplementation may have the opposite effect, especially when not targeted to patients with iron deficiency.[52,82] The mechanism of this effect is of great interest but not yet well understood.[83] There are some indications that iron deficiency may have a proinflammatory effect. In a mouse model, iron deficiency potentiated the systemic effect of lipopolysaccharide in a hepcidin-dependent manner,[84] and in a mouse model of asthma, iron deficiency promoted allergic inflammation.[85]

Growth and Metabolism

Iron-deficient children have been reported to suffer from growth retardation but it is difficult to isolate the effect of iron deficiency from other nutritional and environmental causes of stunting. Two comprehensive analyses of randomized controlled trials did not detect an effect on growth of iron supplementation alone.[86,87] Decreased thermoregulation in response to cold exposure is seen in both humans and laboratory models.[88] It has been attributed to the conflicting effects on blood flow of decreased oxygen content of blood and need to minimize heat loss, as well as the effect of iron deficiency on thyroid function.

Histologic Findings

Severe iron deficiency may lead to histologic changes in various organs. The rapidly proliferating cells of the upper part of the alimentary tract seem particularly susceptible to the effect of iron deficiency. There may be atrophy of the mucosa of the tongue and esophagus,[89] stomach,[90] and small intestine.[91] The epithelium of the lateral margins of the tongue is reduced in thickness despite increase in the progenitor compartment. This thinning presumably reflects accelerated exfoliation of epithelial cells.[92] Buccal mucosa has shown thinning and keratinization of epithelium and increased mitotic activity.[93,94] However, light microscopic and electron microscopic examination of exfoliated oral mucosal cells showed no aberrations in morphology of nuclei or cytoplasm of the cells of patients with iron-deficiency anemia.[95] In iron-deficiency anemia resulting from idiopathic pulmonary hemosiderosis, characteristic pathologic changes are found in the lungs, including intense deposition of iron in the littoral cells of the alveoli and interstitial fibrosis.[45]

Widening of diploic spaces of bones, particularly those of the skull and hands,[96-98] may be a consequence of chronic iron deficiency beginning in infancy. In the skull, this is of the same character as in thalassemia, except that in β-thalassemia major there is maxillary hypertrophy, whereas in severe iron-deficiency anemia maxillary growth and pneumatization are normal.

CLINICAL FEATURES

Clinical Manifestations of Anemia

The anemia in iron-deficient patients can be very severe, with blood hemoglobin levels as low as less than 4 g/dL being encountered in some patients. Severe iron-deficiency anemia is associated with all of the various symptoms of anemia, resulting from hypoxia and the body's response to hypoxia, as described in Chap. 32. Thus, tachycardia with palpitations and pounding in the ears, headache, light-headedness, and even angina pectoris, may all occur in patients who are severely anemic.

Clinical Manifestations That May Be Unrelated to Anemia

The clinical features of iron deficiency encompass nonhematologic effects and symptoms caused by the anemia itself. A number of controlled studies show that various manifestations of iron deficiency can occur in individuals whose hemoglobin is within the accepted normal range.

Decreased Work Performance Objective measurements of work performance and studies using O_2 consumption as an index of work performance have given contradictory results, but a comprehensive review led to the conclusion that severe iron-deficiency anemia (hemoglobin

<8 g/dL) and mild iron deficiency anemia (hemoglobin between 8 and 12 g/dL) led to decreased work performance, primarily as estimated by peak oxygen consumption (VO_2max) measurements, but the evidence that nonanemic iron deficiency had such an effect was less convincing.[99] However, in athletes with low ferritin levels but normal hemoglobin levels, iron-supplemented subjects showed an increased VO_2max without a change in their red cell mass, and in other studies nonanemic subjects treated with iron showed improved performance and/or VO_2max.[63]

Infant and Childhood Development It has been proposed that iron deficiency in infants and children is associated with poor attention span, poor response to sensory stimuli, and retarded behavioral and developmental achievement even in the absence of anemia. The causality of these associations is confounded by other coexisting nutritional deficits and socioeconomic deprivation, so reversibility by iron supplementation would be important in establishing causality. However, in systematic meta-analyses, iron supplementation had weak or no effects on these deficits.[86,100-102]

Hyperactivity Syndromes It has been speculated that there is a relationship between restless legs syndrome, Tourette syndrome, and attention deficit hyperactivity disorder and that iron deficiency contributes to their pathophysiology. Restless legs syndrome, a common nocturnal problem, especially in the elderly, is associated with iron deficiency and is reported to improve on iron therapy, but the beneficial effects are inconsistent and not well predicted by blood ferritin or transferrin saturation.[75,103,104] In children there may be a relationship between iron deficiency and attention deficit hyperactivity disorder, but the association is inconsistent.[105]

Other Neurologic Symptoms Breath holding in children, headaches, and paresthesias have been attributed to iron deficiency but there are no controlled studies to support these impressions. Anecdotal reports of intracranial hypertension with papilledema are buttressed by apparent response to iron therapy.[106-109] Stroke in children and in adults, possibly triggered by thrombocytosis, is associated with iron-deficiency anemia.[110-114]

Oral and Nasopharyngeal Symptoms Burning of the tongue has also been described anecdotally in many accounts of iron deficiency, and although this symptom has been observed to diminish with treatment, no controlled studies have been performed. The tongue symptoms could be a result of concurrent pyridoxine deficiency. Although iron deficiency has been proposed as a cause of atrophic rhinitis, the evidence for this is weak.

Dysphagia In the laryngopharynx, mucosal atrophy may lead to web formation in the postcricoid region, thereby giving rise to dysphagia (Paterson-Kelly also known as Plummer-Vinson syndrome).[115] If these alterations are of long duration, they may lead to pharyngeal carcinoma. Although it has been generally thought that these changes are secondary to longstanding iron deficiency, this mechanism is not universally accepted. The frequency of the condition is considered to have decreased considerably, and it is remarkably rare in many parts of the world where iron deficiency is common.

Pica The craving to eat unusual substances, for example, dirt, clay, ice, laundry starch, salt, cardboard, and hair, is a well-documented manifestation of iron deficiency and is usually cured promptly by iron therapy.[116-119]

Hair Loss Although the association of hair loss with iron deficiency is controversial,[120] low ferritin levels were a risk factor for hair loss in a large multivariate analysis.[121] Remarkably, hair loss sparing the face ("mask mouse") is a sign of iron deficiency in mice.[122]

Physical Findings

The physical findings in iron-deficiency anemia include pallor, glossitis (smooth, red tongue), stomatitis, and angular cheilitis. Koilonychia (spoon nails), once a common finding, is now encountered rarely. Retinal hemorrhages and exudates may be seen in severely anemic patients (e.g., hemoglobin concentration of <5 g/dL). Splenomegaly has occasionally been attributed to iron-deficiency anemia, but when it occurs, it is probably from other causes.

LABORATORY FEATURES

In severe, uncomplicated iron-deficiency anemia, the erythrocytes are hypochromic and microcytic; the plasma iron concentration is diminished; the iron-binding capacity is increased; the serum ferritin concentration is low; the serum transferrin receptor (TfR) and erythrocyte zinc protoporphyrin concentrations are increased; and the marrow is depleted of stainable iron. However, the classic combination of laboratory findings occurs consistently only when iron-deficiency anemia is far advanced, when there are no complicating factors such as infection or malignant neoplasms, and when there has not been previous therapy with transfusions or parenteral iron.

Blood Cells

Erythrocytes Anisocytosis is the earliest recognizable morphologic change of erythrocytes in iron-deficiency anemia (Fig. 43–2).[123] The anisocytosis is typically accompanied by mild ovalocytosis. As the iron deficiency worsens, a mild normochromic, normocytic anemia often develops. With further progression, hemoglobin concentration, erythrocyte count, mean corpuscular volume (MCV), and mean erythrocyte hemoglobin content all decline together.[124,125] As the indices change the erythrocytes appear microcytic and hypochromic on stained blood films. Target cells may sometimes be present. Elongated hypochromic elliptocytes may be seen, in which the long sides are nearly parallel. Such cells have been called "pencil cells," although they more nearly resemble cigars in shape. The red cell indices are consistently abnormal in adults only when iron-deficiency anemia is moderate or severe (e.g., in males with hemoglobin concentrations <12 g/dL or in women with hemoglobin concentrations <10 g/dL) (Fig. 43–3). The distribution of erythrocyte volume (e.g., red cell distribution width [RDW]) is usually increased in established iron-deficiency anemia. The RDW is reported often as the coefficient of variation (in percent) of erythrocyte volume (see "Differential Diagnosis" below).

Leukocytes Leukopenia has been found in some patients with iron-deficiency anemia, but the overall distribution of leukocyte counts in iron-deficient patients seems to be approximately normal.

Platelets Both thrombocytopenia[126] and, more commonly, thrombocytosis[127] have been associated with iron deficiency. Platelet abnormalities correct with iron therapy. Thrombotic complications of iron deficiency have been reported but are very rare.[128] The etiology of either abnormality is not known. Low-iron-diet-induced iron-deficiency anemia developed in a rat model within 2 weeks, and this was accompanied by sustained 50 percent increase in platelet count with increased platelet size but without significant changes in known megakaryocyte growth factors (thrombopoietin, IL-6 or IL-11). It has been suggested that high erythropoietin levels may stimulate thrombopoietin receptors because the two hematopoietic factors are structurally related, but this does not seem to be the case.[129]

Reticulocytes Reticulocyte count is often mildly increased,[130] a finding consistent with the increased erythroid activity of the marrow (see "Marrow" below).

Marrow

Because most of the iron in the body is normally in erythrocytes, and iron is not excreted, decrease in erythrocyte mass generally results in increased storage iron. Iron-deficiency anemia is the exception, as iron stores are depleted before the red cell mass is compromised. Thus, evaluation of iron stores should be a sensitive and usually reliable means for the differentiation between iron-deficiency anemia and all other anemias. Decreased or absent hemosiderin in the marrow is characteristic of iron deficiency, and is readily evaluated after staining by the simple Prussian blue method. Stored iron in the macrophages of the marrow can be seen in marrow spicules in marrow sections, or in marrow aspirate films. Iron granules, normally found in the cytoplasm of approximately 30 percent of erythroblasts, become rare but may not be entirely absent.

Evaluation of the amount of iron in marrow macrophages has long been considered the "gold standard" for the diagnosis of iron deficiency. There are, however, technical barriers to the accurate histochemical determination of marrow iron. First, an invasive procedure, marrow aspiration, is required. Second, the differentiation of iron within macrophages from artifacts takes experience and skill. In one study only 74 of 108 cases had been accurately reported.[131] Moreover, misleading results may be obtained in patients who have been transfused or who have been treated with parenteral iron.[132] The marrow of such patients may contain normal, or even increased, quantities of stainable iron in the face of typical iron-responsive iron-deficiency anemia. In such patients, iron that is seen on marrow examination is not readily available for erythropoiesis. As serum markers of iron deficiency became widely available, the reasons for the primacy of marrow iron estimation have been questioned.[133]

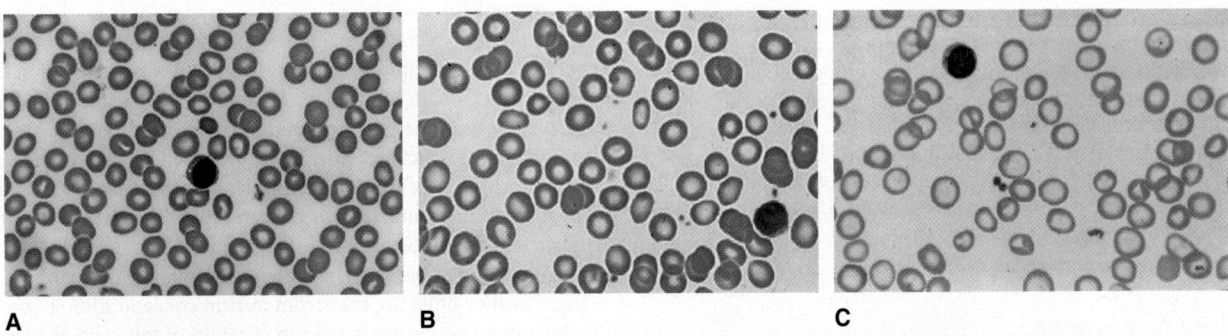

Figure 43–2. Variability in morphologic diagnosis of iron-deficiency anemia from blood film. As in all deficiency states leading to anemia, the blood film morphology and blood cell changes are a function of the severity of the deficiency. **A.** Normal blood film. Normocytic-normochromic red cells with normal shape. **B.** Mild iron deficiency. Serum iron, ferritin, and transferring saturation were consistent with mild iron deficiency. Cannot discern if mean red cell size has decreased. There may be a few red cells that have larger central pallor, but that is arguable. A few cells have oval or elliptical shape. **C.** Severe iron deficiency. Serum iron, ferritin, and transferring saturation were consistent with severe iron deficiency. Note obvious increase in overtly hypochromic cells and higher frequency of microcytes. *(Reproduced with permission from Lichtman's Atlas of Hematology, www.accessmedicine.com.)*

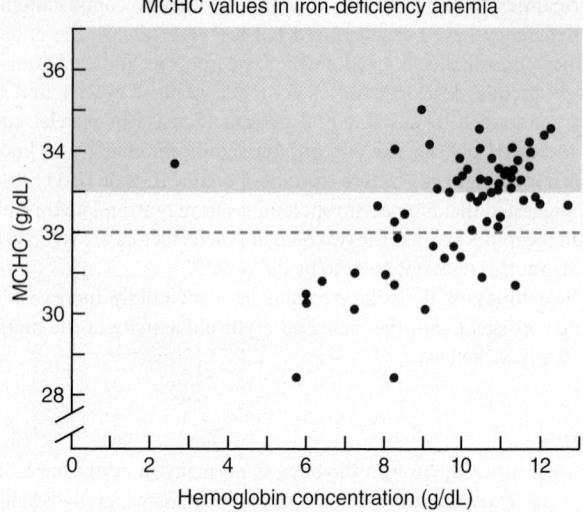

MCHC values in iron-deficiency anemia

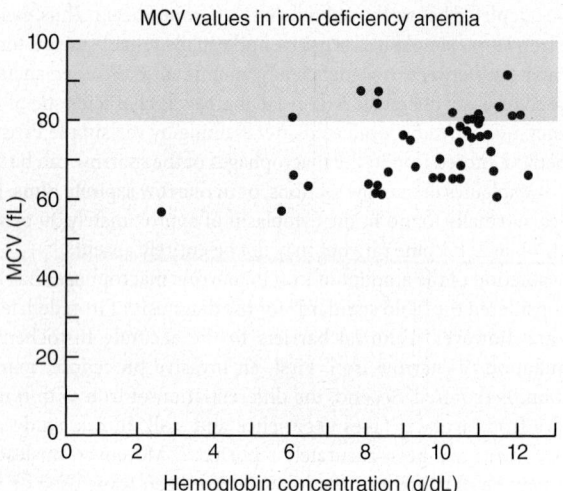

MCV values in iron-deficiency anemia

Figure 43–3. Erythrocyte indices in iron-deficiency anemia of adults; data obtained with Coulter Counter, Model S. Normal ranges of indices observed in approximately 500 healthy adults using the same instrument are indicated by shading. The *dashed line* in the *top panel* indicates the more widely accepted lower normal limit of mean corpuscular hemoglobin concentrations (MCHCs) stated in this text. *(Top)* Correlation between venous blood hemoglobin concentration and MCHC. More than half of 62 patients with iron-deficiency anemia had MCHC values clearly in the normal range. *(Bottom)* Correlation between venous blood hemoglobin concentrations and mean corpuscular volume (MCV). Nearly 70 percent of cases exhibited distinct microcytosis. Thus when indices are determined by automated cell-counting methods, the MCV is much more sensitive than is the MCHC in detecting changes of iron deficiency. However, at least 30 percent of cases of iron-deficiency anemia will be misdiagnosed if physicians rely on the erythrocyte indices. *(Data from Klee GG:* Decision Rules for Accelerated Hematology Laboratory Investigation: *Thesis, University of Minnesota.)*

Serum Iron Concentration

The serum iron concentration is usually low in untreated iron-deficiency anemia, but may rarely be normal.[125,134,135] Iron in blood plasma turns over every few hours and constitutes less than 0.1 percent of total body iron in adults, so iron concentrations are readily perturbed by transient changes in iron supply or demand. Physiologically, the serum iron concentration has a diurnal rhythm; it decreases in late afternoon and evening, reaching a nadir near 9 PM and increases to its maximum between 7 and 10 AM. This effect is rarely of sufficient magnitude to influence diagnosis.[136] Serum iron levels decrease at about the time of menstrual bleeding[137,138] regardless of whether the bleeding is physiologic or induced by withdrawal of contraceptive hormonal preparations.

Importantly, the serum iron concentration is reduced in the presence of either acute or chronic inflammatory processes[139] or malignancy[140] and following acute myocardial infarction.[141,142] The serum iron concentration under these circumstances may be decreased sufficiently to suggest iron deficiency. Conversely, during chemotherapy of malignancy, the serum iron concentration may be quite elevated, as cytotoxic effects of the drugs on erythroblasts inhibit erythropoiesis and related iron uptake by erythroblasts. This effect is observed from the third to the seventh day after inception of chemotherapy of a variety of tumors.[143]

Normal or high concentrations of serum iron are commonly observed even in patients with iron-deficiency anemia if such patients receive iron medication before blood is drawn for these measurements. Even multivitamin preparations, which commonly contain approximately 18 mg of elemental iron per tablet, can result in this effect. Oral iron medication should be withheld for 24 hours before blood samples are obtained. Parenteral injection of iron dextran may result in a very high serum iron concentration (e.g., 500 to 1000 mcg/dL), at least with some methods,[144] for several weeks. The elevation of serum iron levels after infusion of sodium ferric gluconate or iron sucrose is of much shorter duration.[145]

Iron-Binding Capacity and Transferrin Saturation

The iron-binding capacity is a measure of the amount of transferrin in circulating blood. Normally, there is enough transferrin present in 100 mL serum to bind 4.4 to 8.0 μmol (250 to 450 mcg) of iron; because the normal serum iron concentration is approximately 1.8 μmol/dL (100 mcg/dL), transferrin may be found to be approximately one-third saturated with iron. The unsaturated or latent iron-binding capacity (UIBC) is easily measured with radioactive iron or by spectrophotometric techniques. The sum of the UIBC and the plasma iron represents total iron-binding capacity (TIBC). TIBC can also be measured directly. In iron-deficiency anemia, UIBC and TIBC are often increased and serum iron concentrations are decreased so that transferrin saturation of 15 percent or less is usually found. Because transferrin concentration and TIBC are decreased during inflammation, a normal value for transferrin saturation often accompanies a low serum iron concentration in the anemia of chronic inflammation.

Serum Ferritin

Serum ferritin, secreted mainly by macrophages[146] and hepatocytes, contains relatively little iron, yet serum ferritin concentration empirically correlates with total-body iron stores,[147] for reasons that are still obscure. Serum ferritin concentrations of 10 mcg/L or less are characteristic of iron-deficiency anemia. In iron deficiency without anemia, serum ferritin concentration is typically in the range of 10 to 20 mcg/L. An increase in serum ferritin concentration occurs in inflammatory disorders, such as rheumatoid arthritis, in chronic renal disease, and in malignancies.[148] When one of these conditions coexists with iron deficiency, as they often do, the serum ferritin concentration is commonly in the normal range; interpretation of results of this assay then becomes difficult. In patients with rheumatoid arthritis who are anemic, some suggest that concomitant iron deficiency may be suspected when the serum ferritin concentration is less than 60 mcg/L,[149] but such empiric guidelines are unlikely to apply to the full spectrum of severity of inflammation. Increased serum ferritin concentrations are also characteristic of some malignancies, as well as of acute and chronic liver disease and chronic renal failure.[150-153] In Gaucher disease, juvenile rheumatoid arthritis, and various macrophage activation syndromes, and in ferroportin disease characterized by massive iron loading of macrophages, the serum ferritin concentration is commonly in the range of thousands of mcg/L and may mask iron deficiency.[154-158]

Erythrocyte Zinc Protoporphyrin

Erythrocyte protoporphyrin, principally zinc protoporphyrin, is increased in disorders of heme synthesis, including iron deficiency, lead poisoning, and sideroblastic anemias, as well as other conditions.[159-161] This assay analyzes the fluorescence of erythrocytes and uses small blood samples. It is quite sensitive in the diagnosis of iron deficiency and practical for large-scale screening programs designed to identify children with either iron deficiency or lead poisoning.[58,159] It does not differentiate between iron deficiency and anemia that accompanies inflammatory or malignant processes.[162]

Serum Transferrin Receptor

The role of TfR in transporting transferrin iron into cells is described in Chap. 42 section "Transport of Iron". The circulating receptor is a truncated form of the cellular receptor, lacking the transmembrane and cytoplasmic domains of the cellular receptor. It circulates bound to transferrin. Sensitive immunologic methods can detect approximately 5 mg/L of receptor in serum. The levels of circulating TfR mirror the amount of cellular receptor, and therefore are proportional to the number of erythroblasts expressing the receptor. Because receptor synthesis is greatly increased when cells lack iron, the amount of the circulating receptor increases in iron deficiency.[163,164] In anemia of inflammation, the synthesis of the TfR is suppressed by cytokines and this negates the opposing stimulatory effect of iron restriction, resulting in a lower serum TfR concentration than in pure iron deficiency.[165] This test for iron deficiency has gradually come into clinical use, but the methodology has not yet been standardized, making laboratory-to-laboratory comparisons difficult. A method for performing reproducible assays for the soluble TfR has been standardized.[166] Like the serum ferritin and serum iron, serum TfR assay results may be confounded by poorly understood variations in patients with malignancies; in patients in whom the serum TfR concentration is reduced; and in patients with asymptomatic malaria or thalassemia trait,[167,168] in whom, in the absence of iron deficiency, it is increased. The ratio of serum TfR to serum ferritin seems to be a useful but not infallible reflection of body iron stores.[169] Moreover, several studies show that the soluble transferrin index calculated as a ratio of the serum TfR/log ferritin (TfR-F Index) may be superior to other means for detection of iron deficiency.[170-172]

Reticulocyte Hemoglobin Content and Other Novel Erythrocyte Indices

Some automated hematology instruments offer a method for diagnosis of iron deficiency using an assay of hemoglobin content within reticulocytes. This parameter is an indicator of iron restriction of hemoglobin synthesis during 3 to 4 days prior to the test.[173,174] Percent hypochromic erythrocytes offers a longer term assessment of iron restriction during the preceding few months.[173,175]

DIFFERENTIAL DIAGNOSIS

Iron-deficiency anemia is characterized by many abnormal laboratory features. Because none of these are unique, a small deviation from normal will detect most cases of iron deficiency (high sensitivity), but

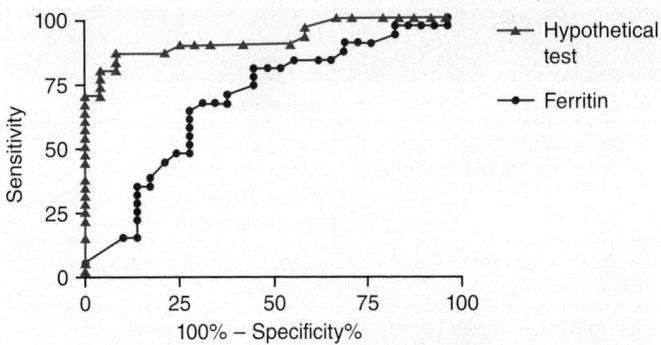

Figure 43–4. Two receiver operator curves. As the specificity increases the sensitivity decreases. The receiver-operator properties of serum ferritin are far from ideal. When the specificity is high (to the *left on the abscissa*) the sensitivity is low; only when the specificity is low is the sensitivity adequate. The curve that would be obtained with a nearly ideal test for iron deficiency gives high specificity and high sensitivity. In the curve shown, a cutoff value could be found that allows one to identify 75 percent of patients with iron deficiency with a specificity of greater than 90 percent. Unfortunately, no such test exists.

also falsely identify non–iron-deficient subjects as being iron deficient (low specificity). On the other hand, a large deviation from normal will exclude most nondeficient patients (high specificity), but miss many iron-deficient subjects (low sensitivity). This tradeoff is shown graphically in so-called *receiver operator characteristic curves.* These curves are constructed by plotting the sensitivity against the false-positive rate (1 – specificity) at various values of the analyte. Figure 43–4 shows receiver operator characteristic curve for some tests for iron deficiency. The situation is complicated in the case of iron deficiency by the fact that the diagnostic problem faced by the physician is not one of differentiating a patient with iron-deficiency anemia from a normal person, but rather from a patient who has an anemia with a different etiology. It is partly for this reason that a simple algorithm for the diagnosis of iron deficiency does not exist. In a severely anemic patient, microcytosis would have very high specificity and high sensitivity compared to normal, but compared to a patient with thalassemia the specificity would be very low. Similarly, a low serum ferritin level is an excellent test in the general population, but it has relatively little value in patients with chronic renal disease. Another problem that is inherent in evaluating diagnostic tests for iron deficiency is the standard that is applied to decide who is iron deficient and who is not. Marrow iron has served as one "gold standard" but has limitations, as discussed earlier (see "Marrow" earlier). Alternatively, the response to iron therapy serves as a powerful indicator of whose anemia is actually a result of a deficiency of iron. Here, too, there are limitations, in that some iron-deficient patients may fail to respond adequately because of factors such as infection. Lacking an absolute test for iron deficiency, the ability of the physician to use judgment relevant to the particular patient's circumstances is of paramount importance.

The forms of anemia that must be distinguished from iron-deficiency anemia most frequently include those of thalassemia minor, chronic inflammatory disease, malignancy, chronic liver disease, and chronic renal disease. It is the microcytic anemias that are most likely to be confused with iron deficiency. These include other conditions in which hemoglobin synthesis is impaired,[176] including thalassemias and thalassemia traits, drug- or toxin-induced impairments of heme synthesis, sideroblastic anemias (Chap. 59), and very rare defects in the delivery of iron to erythrocytes or erythrocyte iron uptake and utilization (Table 43–2).

TABLE 43–2. Microcytic Disorders Other Than Iron Deficiency

Mechanisms	Diseases
Impaired globin chain synthesis or highly unstable hemoglobin	β-Thalassemia or trait, α-thalassemia minima or minor, hemoglobin H, hemoglobin E or trait, combinations of above
Drugs or toxins that inhibit heme synthesis	Lead, isoniazid, pyrazinamide, sirolimus
Disorders that impair heme synthesis directly or by decreased iron delivery to erythroblasts, or decreased uptake or utilization of iron by erythroblasts	sideroblastic anemias, erythropoietic porphyrias, atransferrinemia,[203] aceruloplasminemia,[284] DMT-1 mutations,[207] STEAP3 deficiency[285]

DMT, divalent metal transporter; STEAP3, six-transmembrane epithelial antigen of prostate 3.

Thalassemia Minor

In many parts of the world, and in many communities of North America, the frequency of β-thalassemia minor is second only to that of iron deficiency as a cause of hypochromic microcytic anemia (Chap. 48). In African Americans, homozygosity for α-thalassemia-2, that is the state in which only single α-globin gene is present on each chromosome, is a common cause of microcytosis. Approximately 3 percent of African Americans are homozygous for α-thalassemia-2. The condition is associated with only a very modest lowering of the blood hemoglobin level.[177] Heterozygotes may also have microcytosis, although usually they are hematologically normal. Among persons of Mediterranean ancestry both α- and β-thalassemia are very prevalent, particularly the latter. Among Asians, particularly in those from Southeast Asia, β-thalassemia minor, α-thalassemia minor, and hemoglobin E trait, all occur frequently. All are characterized by microcytosis, and none can be distinguished reliably from the others on the basis of erythrocyte morphology or erythrocyte indices alone. In each of these conditions there may be only mild to moderate microcytosis without any other distinctive changes. However, in the majority of patients with α- or β-thalassemia minor, hemoglobin Lepore trait, and hemoglobin E trait, the erythrocyte count is greater than 5×10^{12}/L (5,000,000/μL), despite low hemoglobin concentration.[178,179] Homozygous hemoglobin E is also characterized by marked hypochromia, microcytosis, abundant target cells, and elevated erythrocyte count, but usually not by more than minimal anemia (Chap. 49).[178]

In contrast to the findings in these hemoglobinopathies, erythrocyte counts of 5×10^{12}/L (5,000,000/μL) or higher are relatively uncommon among adults with iron-deficiency anemia.[180] However, erythrocytosis may be seen in children with iron-deficiency anemia or in polycythemia vera patients who have become iron deficient following hemorrhage or therapeutic phlebotomy. Consequently, while the mean MCV is almost always reduced in α- or β-thalassemia minor and in homozygous hemoglobin E, with values of 60 to 70 fL being the rule, values this low are seen only in severe iron-deficiency anemia. In hemoglobin Lepore trait and hemoglobin E trait, only minimal microcytosis is observed.[178,179,181] Algorithmic rules based on red cell counts, MCV or RDW are not sufficiently reliable for distinguishing iron deficiency from thalassemia in populations with high prevalence of iron deficiency compared to thalassemias.

Mild reticulocytosis, polychromatophilia, and basophilic stippling are more likely to be encountered in β-thalassemia minor, δβ-thalassemia minor, and hemoglobin Lepore trait than in iron-deficiency anemia, but may be absent in these disorders. The serum iron concentration is usually normal or increased in thalassemic syndromes and is usually low in iron-deficiency anemia. Similarly, examination of marrow iron stores helps to differentiate these disorders. The presence of β-thalassemia trait is substantiated by the demonstration of increased proportions of hemoglobin A_2 and F, or by the presence on electrophoresis of hemoglobin H or Lepore (Chap. 48). At present, the diagnosis of α-thalassemia minor is usually made on the basis of exclusion of other causes of microcytosis, but it can be confirmed by direct demonstration of mutations in α-globin genes by DNA-based techniques.

Iron deficiency may mask concurrent thalassemia. The amounts of both hemoglobin A_2 and hemoglobin H are diminished disproportionately to the reduction in hemoglobin A in the presence of iron deficiency[182] (Chap. 46); however, usually the hemoglobin A_2 level remains above the normal range.

Anemia of Inflammation (Anemia of Chronic Disease)

The anemia of inflammation (Chap. 37) is usually normochromic and normocytic, but hypochromic microcytic anemia occurs in 20 to 30 percent of patients with chronic infections or malignancies.[139] Thus these disorders cannot be distinguished from iron-deficiency anemia by examination of the blood film. Furthermore, the serum iron concentration is usually decreased in these disorders,[139] sometimes severely. In uncomplicated iron deficiency, the TIBC is usually increased, whereas in inflammatory and neoplastic diseases it is commonly decreased, but there is considerable overlap among TIBC values of normal subjects, those with iron-deficiency anemia, and those with chronic inflammatory diseases.

Transferrin saturation may be normal in iron-deficiency anemia, and, conversely, low saturation is sometimes observed in chronic inflammation. However, circulating soluble TfRs increase in iron deficiency but not in the anemia of inflammation.[170] The serum ferritin level is usually diminished in iron deficiency, but it is generally increased in chronic inflammatory and neoplastic disorders.[147] Measurement of the ratio of soluble TfR to ferritin has been found to be useful in distinguishing the anemia of chronic inflammation from that of iron deficiency,[170] but meta-analysis of the relevant clinical studies suggested that the ratio may not be better than soluble TfR assay alone at discriminating between iron deficiency anemia and anemia of inflammation.[183] Examination of the marrow for stainable iron is invasive and requires skilled reading but may be helpful in an occasional patient. Iron staining of marrow macrophages is greatly decreased in amount or absent in iron deficiency anemia and normal or increased in the other disorders. Low serum hepcidin concentrations are characteristic of iron deficiency and high serum hepcidin indicates anemia of inflammation, but this assay is not yet clinically available and its clinical value is unknown. As would be expected from the inhibitory effect of hepcidin on the absorption of iron, high hepcidin levels predict a poor response to oral iron therapy[184] and low incorporation of dietary iron into erythrocytes.[185]

Anemia of Chronic Liver Disease

The erythrocytes in the blood film from patients with chronic liver disease may be normochromic and normocytic, macrocytic, or hypochromic. Target cells are frequently present in large numbers. Because the blood film in iron-deficiency anemia may also display these features, differential diagnosis must be based on other observations. Low serum ferritin levels are useful in detecting iron deficiency in the setting of cirrhosis,[186] but normal or even increased serum ferritin does not exclude iron deficiency, especially in the presence of active liver injury.[186,187]

Anemia of Chronic Renal Disease

Iron deficiency is frequent in patients with chronic renal disease (Chap. 37). Iron-deficiency anemia is particularly difficult to diagnose in patients with chronic renal disease (Chap. 37) where iron delivery to the marrow is inadequate because of coexisting inflammation and because of increased demands from pulsatile erythropoiesis as a result of erythropoiesis-stimulating agents. Because the problem is fairly common, and perhaps because of interest in identifying those patients who can benefit from iron therapy and decreasing their use of erythropoiesis-stimulating agents, a large number of studies have been done to determine the best way to diagnose iron deficiency in patients undergoing extracorporeal dialysis. The diagnostic problem is further complicated by the common occurrence of "functional iron deficiency,"[188] that is, a state in which iron stores are adequate but iron delivery to the marrow is insufficient to meet the increased kinetic requirements of erythropoiesis stimulated by intermittent use of erythropoietin and related agents. If response to intravenous iron therapy is used to diagnose iron deficiency, even many patients with abnormally high ferritins will be iron deficient.[150,189] High serum ferritins do not preclude a response to IV iron, not even in patients with chronic kidney disease who are not on hemodialysis.[190] Although measurements of reticulocyte hemoglobin and percent of hypochromic erythrocytes show promise as markers of response to iron therapy, there is insufficient evidence that any individual biomarker or combination of biomarkers can reliably predict the response to iron treatment in chronic kidney disease.[191]

Anemia of Hemolytic Disease

Hemolytic disease can usually be distinguished from iron-deficiency anemia on the basis of the blood film. The marked polychromatophilia, spherocytosis, schistocytes, Heinz bodies, basophilic stippling, and other morphologic features characteristic of various types of hemolysis usually are not seen in iron-deficiency anemia. Furthermore, reticulocytosis is usually marked in hemolytic disorders but minimal or absent in iron-deficiency anemia. However, there are some outstanding exceptions to these generally valid principles.

In unstable hemoglobin disorders, such as hemoglobin H disease or hemoglobin Köln disease, erythrocytic hypochromia may be pronounced. In these disorders, there is moderate reticulocytosis, which helps to differentiate them from iron-deficiency anemia. The serum iron concentration is normal or increased. Chapter 49 discusses the detection of unstable hemoglobins.

When there is chronic intravascular hemolysis, erythrocytes in the blood film may display marked morphologic abnormalities, such as burr cells and schizocytes. Yet because of loss of iron in the urine, iron deficiency may be the dominant cause of the resulting anemia. Evaluation of iron content in marrow aspirates or measurement of serum iron concentration and TIBC may clarify the diagnosis in this form of anemia.

Hypoplastic and Aplastic Anemia

In their early phases, these disorders cannot reliably be differentiated from mild iron-deficiency anemia on the basis of erythrocyte morphology alone (Chap. 35). The reticulocyte count is generally less than 0.5 percent in hypoplastic or aplastic anemia. The presence of neutropenia and thrombocytopenia suggests a diagnosis of aplastic anemia, but mild neutropenia may also occur in iron-deficiency anemia. The serum iron concentration is usually increased in aplastic anemia; and the percentage transferrin saturation is then elevated. Marrow aspiration may produce scant material for cytologic study, and marrow biopsy may be necessary. An iron stain usually reveals increased amounts of hemosiderin in aplastic or hypoplastic anemia. However, if chronic bleeding has occurred, for example, as a consequence of thrombocytopenia, iron stores may be depleted.

Sideroblastic Anemia

In this heterogeneous group of disorders (Chap. 59), the blood findings often simulate those of iron-deficiency anemia. Reticulocytosis is usually absent, and the serum iron concentration and serum ferritin is generally normal or increased. Marrow examination shows characteristic ring sideroblasts and increased amounts of stainable iron.

Congenital Dyserythropoietic Anemia

In the rare congenital dyserythropoietic anemias (Chap. 39), erythrocyte morphologic abnormalities may resemble those of iron deficiency or thalassemia (Chap. 48). In general, in congenital dyserythropoietic anemias, poikilocytosis is very striking and occurs with less reduction in MCV than in iron deficiency or thalassemias. Often, however, such cases are believed to be thalassemic until the marrow is examined.

Megaloblastic Anemia

In pernicious anemia and other types of megaloblastic anemia (Chap. 41), the blood film usually shows changes sufficiently distinctive that there is little difficulty in differential diagnosis. One potential source of error is the change in serum iron concentration that occurs after therapy. In the patient with pernicious anemia or folic acid deficiency, early after starting treatment, the serum iron concentration decreases markedly as iron is used rapidly for hemoglobin synthesis.[192] Thus the finding of a low serum iron concentration in such circumstances should not be taken as evidence of iron deficiency. Iron-deficiency anemia and anemia as a consequence of folic acid or vitamin B_{12} deficiency may coexist. During the course of treatment, with the rapid increase in the number of red cells, the typical manifestations of severe iron deficiency may develop. The mixture of microcytic-hypochromic and normocytic-normochromic cells has been called *dimorphic anemia* (see "Coexisting Microcytic Anemia" in Chap. 41).

Anemia of Hypothyroidism

The anemia of severe hypothyroidism (myxedema; Chap. 38) is usually normochromic and normocytic and may be accompanied by mild-to-moderate depression of serum iron concentration. Marrow examination may be required to determine whether iron deficiency is present, especially as iron deficiency often complicates myxedema because of menorrhagia, which is common in this disorder.

Therapeutic Trial

In the final analysis, the response to iron therapy is the proof of correctness of diagnosis of iron-deficiency anemia. Furthermore, some physicians or patients may not have access to all the techniques described for diagnosis of iron-deficiency anemia. In this event, the patient's response to therapy may become a primary diagnostic measure. Iron administration in such a therapeutic trial is usually by the oral route, but intravenous iron can be used if there is evidence or strong suspicion of coexisting inflammation, iron malabsorption, or intolerance of oral iron preparations. A therapeutic trial under any circumstances should be followed carefully. If the cause of anemia is iron deficiency, adequate iron therapy should result in reticulocytosis with a peak occurring after 1 to 2 weeks of therapy, although if anemia is mild, the reticulocyte response may be minimal. A significant increase in the hemoglobin concentration of the blood should be evident 3 to 4 weeks later, and the hemoglobin concentration should attain a normal value within 2 to 4 months. Unless there is evidence of continued substantial blood loss, the absence of response to oral or, when appropriate, parenteral iron must be taken as evidence that iron deficiency is not the cause of anemia. Iron therapy should be discontinued and another cause for the anemia sought.

Special Studies to Delineate the Cause of Iron Deficiency

The physician who establishes a diagnosis of iron deficiency resulting from blood loss has the obligation to determine the site and cause of hemorrhage. Examination for fecal occult blood is particularly helpful in determining what additional studies should be carried out. Specimens should be examined on at least 3 days, because bleeding may be intermittent. Occasionally, it is helpful to label the patient's erythrocytes with chromium-51 (^{51}Cr) sodium chromate and to determine quantitatively the amount of blood lost daily. When there is reason to believe that bleeding is from the gastrointestinal tract, roentgenographic and other imaging studies and endoscopic investigation are indicated. The other imaging studies often include gastroscopy, esophagoscopy, colonoscopy, and capsule endoscopy, and, rarely, angiography or scintigraphic studies. Numerous clinical studies indicate that intensive investigation of patients, particularly men and postmenopausal women, reveals unexpected bleeding lesions, many of which are curable or treatable.[10,193] *H. pylori* infection should be sought, particularly in patients who are iron deficient but who do not seem to respond to therapy.[14,15] An iron stain of sputum may reveal hemosiderin-laden macrophages when there is intrapulmonary bleeding.

THERAPY

Once it has been established that a patient is deficient in iron, replacement therapy should be instituted. Iron may be administered orally, as simple iron salts; parenterally, as an iron-carbohydrate complex; or, very rarely, as a blood transfusion. In general, the oral route is preferred, but the intravenous route is increasingly used because of the improved safety and convenience of new parenteral iron preparations. In most patients, iron-deficiency anemia is a disorder of long duration and slow progression, and restoration of normal hemoglobin is not urgent unless the patient suffers from acute cardiac problems, in which case blood transfusion is appropriate. There is usually time to wait for normal mechanisms of erythropoiesis to respond to the body's needs and for gradual adjustment of the cardiovascular system to reexpansion of the total circulating erythrocyte volume.

Oral Iron Therapy

Dietary Therapy The patient should be encouraged to eat a diversified diet supplying all nutritional requirements. Nonetheless, it must be emphasized that neither meat nor any other dietary article contains enough iron to be useful therapeutically. Meat contains small amounts of myoglobin and hemoglobin and insignificant amounts of iron in other proteins. Although heme iron is better absorbed than inorganic iron, the quantity of heme iron in meat is actually quite small. In fact, an average (3-ounce) serving of steak provides only about 3 mg of iron, that is, the equivalent of only 3 mL of packed erythrocytes. Provision of sufficient dietary iron to permit a maximal rate or recovery from iron-deficiency anemia might require a daily intake of at least 10 pounds of steak. For these and other reasons, medicinal iron is much superior to dietary iron in the therapy of iron deficiency.

Iron Preparations The pharmaceutical market is glutted with iron preparations in nearly every conceivable form; each promoted to appeal to physician or patient for one reason or another. The following simple principles may help the physician to find a way through this chaos.

1. Each dose of an inorganic iron preparation for an adult should contain between 30 and 100 mg of elemental iron. Doses of this magnitude cause unpleasant side effects relatively infrequently.[194] Smaller doses have been popular in the past, but these may result in a slower recovery of the patient or no recovery at all.
2. The iron should be readily released in acidic or neutral gastric juice or duodenal juice (usually pH 5 to 6), because maximal absorption occurs when iron is presented to the duodenal mucosa. Enteric-coated and prolonged-release preparations dissolve slowly in any of these fluids. Thus with such preparations the iron that eventually is released may be presented to a portion of the intestinal mucosa in which absorption is least efficient. Some patients who have been treated unsuccessfully with enteric-coated or prolonged-release iron preparations respond promptly to the administration of non–enteric-coated ferrous salts.
3. The iron, once released, should be readily absorbed. Iron is absorbed in the ferrous form; consequently, only ferrous salts should be used.
4. Side effects should be infrequent. This seems not to be a particular problem for any of the common commercially available iron compounds. Despite the claims of pharmaceutical companies, there is no convincing evidence that any one effective preparation is superior in this respect to any other.
5. Inexpensive iron preparations can be as effective as the more costly ones. The use of preparations containing several therapeutic agents is unnecessary and may increase side effects. Physicians should be aware that if ferrous sulfate is prescribed generically, the choice of preparation is left to the pharmacist who may dispense enteric-coated tablets. It is advisable to specify "nonenteric" or to prescribe by brand name a product that is not enteric-coated. Although substances such as ascorbic acid, succinate, and fructose enhance iron absorption, the gain is offset to a large extent by the increase in frequency of side effects, cost of therapy, or both. There is no convincing evidence to support the use of chelated forms of iron or of iron in combination with wetting agents.

Dosage For therapy of iron deficiency in adults, the dosage should be sufficient to provide between 150 and 200 mg elemental iron daily. The iron may be taken orally in three or four doses 1 hour before meals. Infants may be given 6 mg/kg[195] daily in divided doses for therapy, or a daily dose of 12.5 mg daily for prophylaxis of iron deficiency

Side Effects Mild gastrointestinal side effects occur occasionally in the form of nausea, heartburn, constipation, or changes in the stool consistency. A metallic taste may be experienced. The majority of patients tolerate the usual therapeutic doses of iron without the least side effect. However, there is no doubt that some patients, perhaps 10 to 20 percent, experience symptoms that may be ascribed to the iron preparation and may be dose-dependent. In such cases, reduction of the frequency of administration to 1 tablet a day for a few days may alleviate the symptoms; later, the patient may be able to tolerate treatment in full dosage. It might also be useful to change to another iron preparation, especially one with a different external appearance.

Carbonyl iron has been proposed as an alternative to iron salts, on the assertion that it can be given in large doses with minimal side effects. This substance is actually metallic iron powder, with a particle size less than 5 μm. Because it is insoluble, it is not absorbed until converted to the ionic form. The bioavailability of carbonyl iron has been estimated to be approximately 70 percent of that of an equivalent amount of ferrous sulfate.[196] Oral doses as high as 600 mg three times daily did not produce toxic effects.[196]

Widespread iron supplementation in regions where malaria and gastrointestinal infections are highly endemic is associated with increased malaria transmission and childhood mortality, presumably from increased infections.[197] Although there is not yet a consensus on optimal strategy in such settings, it seems reasonable to target iron supplementation to children who are iron-deficient.

Acute Iron Poisoning Acute iron poisoning is usually a consequence of the accidental ingestion by infants or small children of iron-containing medications intended for use by adults. Any potent oral preparation may cause acute iron poisoning, and this serious disorder remains a problem, despite public awareness campaigns and safer packaging of medications.[198] In the United States, there were nearly 30,000 reported incidents in 2008. The earliest manifestation of iron poisoning is vomiting, usually within 1 hour of the ingestion. There may be hematemesis or melena. Restlessness, hypotension, tachypnea, and cyanosis may develop soon thereafter, and may be followed within a few hours by coma and death but fatal outcomes are now extremely rare. Usually, medical aid is sought early and, with proper treatment, most iron-poisoned children survive. The initial treatment is prompt evacuation of the stomach. In the home, this may be induced by digital stimulation of the pharyngeal gag reflex. If the patient arrives in the emergency room within minutes of ingestion, gastric intubation and lavage should be performed promptly. Whole-bowel irrigation[198] is currently recommended to for all heavy metal intoxications. Supportive measures should be used as needed for shock or for metabolic acidosis should these develop. IV desferrioxamine is the agent of choice for specific therapy of hyperferremia, at a maximum rate of 15 mg/kg per hour for 1 hour, then lowered to 125 mg/hour. Improvement often appears several hours to a few days after onset of iron poisoning. Children who survive for 3 or 4 days usually recover without sequelae. However, gastric strictures and fibrosis or intestinal stenosis may occur as late complications.

Parenteral Iron Therapy

Indications As parenteral iron preparations have become safer and easier to administer, the use of parenteral iron is increasing. Established indications for the use of parenteral rather than oral iron include malabsorption, either because of systemic inflammation or gastrointestinal pathology, intolerance to iron taken orally, iron need in excess of an amount that can be absorbed in the intestine, and noncompliance. Parenteral iron administration has an erythropoietin-sparing effect in anemic patients on long-term hemodialysis for chronic renal disease.[35,199,200] Because of systemic inflammation and possibly other factors, these patients do not appear to respond adequately to oral iron therapy.

Calculating Dosage The amount of iron that needs to be given is readily estimated by noting that 1 mL of red cells contains approximately 1 mg of iron. However, various formulas have been used for estimating total dose required for treatment. Because total blood volume is approximately 65 mL/kg and the iron content of hemoglobin is 0.34 percent by weight, the simplest formula for estimating the total dose required for correction of anemia only is as follows:

$$\text{The dose of iron (mg)} = \text{Whole-blood hemoglobin deficit (g/dL)} \times \text{Body weight (lb)}$$

Assuming normal mean hemoglobin concentration of 16 g/dL, a male weighing 170 pounds, whose hemoglobin concentration is 7 g/dL, would require $170 \times (16 - 7) = 1530$ mg iron to correct this anemia. To this should be added a sufficient quantity of iron to replete iron stores, approximately 1000 mg for men and approximately 600 mg for women. Thus a 170-pound male with a hemoglobin concentration of 7 g/dL should receive 2530 mg iron.

Parenteral Iron Preparations Because iron salts are highly toxic when given parenterally, all iron preparations consist of colloidal (nanoparticulate) complex of iron with carbohydrates. To make the iron bioavailable for erythropoiesis and other biologic processes, the iron complexes must be ingested by macrophages and digested so that the administered iron can be gradually delivered to plasma transferrin. Currently available preparations include iron sucrose, low-molecular-weight iron dextran, ferric gluconate, ferumoxytol, ferric carboxymaltose, and iron isomaltoside. High-molecular-weight dextran was associated with anaphylactoid adverse events compared to the other preparations and should therefore be avoided.[201] The remaining preparations are safe and serious adverse events are extremely rare.[202] Although the recommended methods of administration, including the use of test

dosing, the amount of iron per infusion, and infusion rates differ among the preparations, these are not based on comparative studies. Currently available data indicate that the preparations do not significantly differ in safety or efficacy. Premedication to prevent allergic responses was commonly used with the older preparations but it is neither needed nor known to be effective with the newer formulations, and may introduce side effects of its own.

COURSE AND PROGNOSIS

Course

If therapy is adequate, the correction of iron-deficiency anemia is usually gratifying. Symptoms such as headache, fatigue, pica, paresthesia, and burning sensation of the oropharyngeal mucosa may abate within a few days. In the blood, the reticulocyte count begins to increase after a few days, usually reaches a maximum at approximately 7 to 12 days, and thereafter decreases. When anemia is mild, little or no reticulocytosis may be observed. Little change in hemoglobin concentration or hematocrit value is to be expected for the first 2 weeks, but then the anemia is corrected rapidly. The hemoglobin concentration in the blood may be halfway back to normal after 4 to 5 weeks of therapy. By the end of 2 months of therapy, and often much sooner, the hemoglobin concentration should have reached a normal level.

When iron-deficiency anemia does not resolve with oral iron treatment, careful inquiry into the nature, duration, and regularity of iron therapy may reveal a reason for the failure of therapy and permit a gratifying response to be elicited with adequate therapy. Other questions that should be asked in evaluation of such a case are these: (1) Has bleeding been controlled? (2) Has the patient been on iron therapy long enough to show a response? (3) Has the dose of iron been adequate? (4) Are there other factors—inflammatory disease, neoplastic disease, hepatic or renal disease, prior gastrointestinal surgery, concomitant deficiencies (vitamin B_{12}, folic acid, thyroid)—that might retard response? Prominent among these are *H. pylori* infection, autoimmune gastritis, and celiac disease.[15] (5) Is the diagnosis of iron deficiency correct?

Intravenous iron should be effective in patients with established iron deficiency who fail to respond to oral iron after several weeks. Continued loss of blood or, rarely, the genetic disorder iron-refractory iron-deficiency anemia,[15] may account for incomplete response to IV iron.

Prognosis

When the cause of the iron deficiency is a benign disorder, the prognosis is excellent, provided bleeding is controlled or can be compensated for by continual iron therapy. If there is a benign cause of recurrent bleeding that is corrected, such as hiatal hernia, menorrhagia, or hereditary hemorrhagic telangiectasia, oral iron therapy may be continued indefinitely; if the bleeding is especially brisk, supplementation with parenterally administered iron or, rarely, with transfusion may be needed. Continuous iron administration may also be required in patients with iron deficiency secondary to intravascular hemolysis with hemoglobinuria.

● IRON STORAGE DISEASE

DEFINITION AND HISTORY

The terms *iron storage disease* and *hemochromatosis* are used to designate an increase of tissue iron resulting in a disease state; *hemosiderosis* denotes an increase of tissue iron stores with or without tissue damage. Classically hemochromatosis has been characterized by bronzing of the skin, cirrhosis, and diabetes, and was once called *bronzed diabetes*. Since the 1970s, usage of the term *hemochromatosis* has expanded well beyond its original meaning. This diagnosis is now commonly applied to persons who have increased body iron as suggested by increased serum

TABLE 43–3. Classification of Hemochromatosis

I. Hereditary Hemochromatosis

A. Classical hemochromatosis (HFE hemochromatosis) (type 1)

B. Juvenile hemochromatosis (type 2)

   1. Abnormality in hemojuvelin

   2. Abnormality of hepcidin

C. Transferrin receptor-2 deficiency (type 3)

D. Ferroportin abnormalities (type 4)

   1. Gain of function (systemic iron overload)

   2. Loss of function (macrophage iron overload)

E. Ferritin H-chain iron-responsive element mutation

F. African iron overload

II. Secondary Hemochromatosis

ferritin levels, and even to those who merely have the hemochromatosis *HFE* genotype, regardless of the level of their iron stores.

Hemochromatosis may be divided into genetic forms and acquired forms. The former have sometimes been designated as *primary* and the latter as *secondary* forms. The disorder once designated *idiopathic hemochromatosis* and now as *hereditary hemochromatosis* usually is applied to the common genetic form of the disorder, found principally in those of northern European ancestry, and as a result of mutations in the *HFE* gene (type I hemochromatosis). In the United States, this is by far the most common form of the disease. *Juvenile hemochromatosis* from hemojuvelin and hepcidin mutations (type 2), hemochromatosis as a result of TfR-2 mutations (type 3), hemochromatosis caused by ferroportin mutations (type 4), and *African iron overload* are much less common. Table 43–3 classifies hereditary hemochromatosis. *Secondary hemochromatosis* occurs in patients who receive multiple blood transfusions, and in patients with ineffective erythropoiesis, even when they do not receive transfusions.

Systemic iron overload and hepatic iron accumulation similar to hemochromatosis are also characteristic of atransferrinemia[203–206] and of human divalent metal transporter (DMT)-1 mutations.[207,208] A fetal and neonatal disorder termed *neonatal hemochromatosis* is characterized by hepatic and extrahepatic iron deposition and fulminant hepatitis caused by maternal immune response to fetal antigens.[209]

Iron accumulation in localized sites, particularly the brain, occurs in disorders other than hemochromatosis. Increased quantities of brain iron are characteristic of aceruloplasminemia, and are found in Alzheimer disease, parkinsonism, Friedreich ataxia, Hallervorden-Spatz syndrome, and multiple system atrophy. Because none of these are primarily hematologic disorders, and because the role of iron deposition in the pathology of the disorders is uncertain, they are not discussed further here.

Hemochromatosis was first described by Trousseau in 1865. The massive accumulation of iron that occurred in this disease was recognized as its hallmark. The ingenious development of serial phlebotomy as treatment for the disease suggested by Finch in 1949, and implemented on a larger scale in 1952,[210] made it clear that iron accumulation was the most important pathogenetic factor. Alcohol consumption and other environmental factors were also commonly found in patients with hemochromatosis.[211] The existence of a long-suspected hereditary factor was firmly established when the disease was shown tightly linked to the human leukocyte antigen (HLA locus). Surprisingly, the gene proved to be *HFE* (initially named *HLA-H*), one of the many HLA-like genes on chromosome 6.[212]

The identification of the *HFE* gene made it possible, for the first time, to assess accurately the gene frequency and penetrance of the *HFE* mutations. This brought about a fusion of the apparently contrasting views of genetic and environmental causes. The penetrance of the homozygous state is so low that it could be considered an essential risk factor that required other genetic or environmental factors for disease development.[213]

EPIDEMIOLOGY

The prevalence of mutations of the *HFE* gene is very high. The most significant of these is the c.845 A→G (C282Y) mutation, and with a gene frequency of approximately 0.07 in the northern European population, approximately 5 in 1000 northern Europeans are homozygous for the mutation. The C282Y and S65C mutations are almost entirely confined to individuals with European ancestry. The H63D mutation is more widespread geographically, but is also most common in Europeans. Within Europe the highest gene frequencies of the C282Y mutation are encountered in the southern British Isles and in northern France but other northern Europeans, including Scandinavians, also have high gene frequencies, consistent with Celtic or possibly Viking origin of the mutation.[214]

Although earlier studies attributed nonspecific symptoms in patients to hemochromatosis, large controlled series have shown that most such symptoms are not present in homozygotes for the C282Y mutation at a higher frequency than in controls,[215–217] or a borderline increase, at most, invariably in groups of patients who were aware of their diagnosis when answering questions about symptoms. These findings are consistent with the very low prevalence of hemochromatosis reported in autopsy series and in hospital surveys. The prevalence of symptomatic clinical hemochromatosis in northern European populations is probably only approximately 5 in 100,000 individuals. If patients with abnormal liver function tests and/or fibrosis on liver biopsy are included, the number of affected may be severalfold higher.[218–221] The factors that determine whether a patient with the C282Y homozygous genotype develops disease are not well understood. The patient's sex is clearly a modifying factor, with more severe manifestations observed in males, as pregnancy and menstrual losses tend to ameliorate the disease in women. Other genetic factors that might interact with the C282Y homozygous genotype in producing clinically significant iron storage disease have been sought, but not found, except rare instances in which coinheritance of mutations of the hepcidin gene may be responsible. An increased proportion of severely affected patients have a large alcohol intake.[222,223]

The widespread perception that classical hereditary hemochromatosis frequently led to clinical disease resulted in enthusiasm for population-based screening. However, the cost-to-benefit analysis used was based upon the assumptions that life-threatening disease manifestations will occur in 43 percent of males and in 28 percent of females, estimates that were based upon the prevalence of disease in patients, most of whom had been diagnosed clinically with hemochromatosis. With the realization that the clinical penetrance is much lower, interest in screening the general population for hemochromatosis has largely disappeared.

The prevalence of other forms of hemochromatosis, including juvenile hemochromatosis, hemochromatosis as a result of ferroportin deficiency, and atransferrinemia, is much lower than that the prevalence of classical hereditary hemochromatosis. These forms of hemochromatosis are very rare.

ETIOLOGY AND PATHOGENESIS

Toxicity of Iron

In living organisms, iron associates with proteins to function in oxygen storage and transport and in various metabolic reactions as an electron donor or electron acceptor. The capacity to catalyze oxidation-reduction reactions appears to cause iron-mediated cellular and tissue injury. One of the pathways that is considered to be of greatest importance is the Haber-Weiss reaction:

$$Fe^{2+} + H_2O_2 \rightarrow Fe^{3+} + OH- + HO\cdot O_2^- + Fe^{3+} \rightarrow O_2 + Fe^{2+}$$

The sum of these two reactions is the Fenton reaction:

$$O_2^- + H_2O_2 \rightarrow O_2 + OH^- + HO\cdot$$

The hydroxyl radical (HO·) has been implicated in producing damage to polysaccharides, DNA, and enzymes, and in causing lipid peroxidation.[224] Although there is no direct evidence that hydroxyl radical generation is the main pathway of tissue damage in hemochromatosis, this common conjecture seems reasonable. Demonstrating a damaging effect of iron alone on experimental animals has been difficult. Although in mouse models of genetic, parenteral, or dietary iron overload subtle biochemical defects have been documented, frank cirrhotic changes have not been found. In gerbils, parenteral iron overload causes hepatic necrosis, fibrosis, and nodular regeneration, as well as cardiac damage.[225] In rats, iron alone does not cause fibrosis, and alcohol alone causes only minor liver abnormalities. However, administration of both excess iron and alcohol results in fibrosis.[226] These findings in rats are quite consistent with the strong association that has been demonstrated to exist between alcohol ingestion and cirrhosis in patients with the hemochromatosis genotype. In a number of species, including birds, rhinoceros, tapir, fruit bats, and others, iron overload has been observed in zoos or other restricted settings, particularly after a diet other than the animal's native diet is fed.

Iron is stored in ferritin in the cytoplasm of all cells. The multiple isoferritins found in human tissues are composed of variable proportions of two subunits: L-ferritin (light) and H-ferritin (heavy).[227] Because free iron is potentially harmful to the cell, it is sequestered and detoxified to the less-soluble ferric form by ferroxidase activity; H-ferritin exerts most of its ferroxidase activity in the cytosol. The mitochondrial ferritin, expressed in the mitochondrial matrix, also has potent ferroxidase activity and is markedly upregulated in sideroblastic anemias.

Causes of Iron Overload

Because body iron content is maintained by regulating absorption, excess body iron can accumulate only when absorption is increased above iron requirements, or when iron is injected into the body, either in the form of medicinal iron or as transfused erythrocytes.

Excessive Iron Absorption A variety of mutations are known to cause increased iron absorption in experimental animals and in man (see Table 43–3 for a summary). Mutations in the genes encoding HFE, hemojuvelin, TfR-2, ferroportin, and hepcidin are all associated with iron overload. The common pathway that causes hyperabsorption of iron is deficiency of hepcidin which allows excessive activity of the iron exporter ferroportin in the duodenum and in macrophages of the reticuloendothelial system. Normally, hepcidin is upregulated when body iron increases. However, this response is blunted or absent in either *Hfe-, TfR-2-,* or *Hjv-*deficient mice,[228] or in the human disease,[229–231] all of which exhibit disproportionately low hepcidin levels for the degree of iron overload. Although the biochemistry of their interactions is not known, there is increasing evidence that HFE, TfR-2, and hemojuvelin are part of the signaling pathway that regulates hepcidin expression. In autosomal dominant hereditary hemochromatosis (class 4), ferroportin mutations interfere with binding of hepcidin to ferroportin[232,233] or with the resulting ferroportin endocytosis.

Ineffective Erythropoiesis Anemias with ineffective erythropoiesis commonly cause systemic iron overload with damage to the liver, heart and the endocrine system. Iron storage disease is particularly common in disorders such as β-thalassemia, hereditary dyserythropoietic anemia, and pyruvate kinase deficiency. The amount of body iron may greatly exceed the quantity that can be accounted for through blood transfusion, and iron overload is common even in patients who are rarely or never transfused.

The iron overload commonly observed in β-thalassemia intermedia and major patients likely results, at least in part, from suppression of the iron-regulatory hormone hepcidin by erythroid factors secreted by massively proliferating erythropoietin-stimulated erythroblasts. Candidate erythroid suppressors of hepcidin include growth differentiation factor 15 (GDF15)[234] and erythroferrone.[235] GDF15 overexpression was also observed in congenital dyserythropoietic anemia.[236,237]

Transfusion or Iron Therapy Iron overload can be iatrogenic in origin. Because erythrocytes contain 1 mg of iron per milliliter, transfusion of 450 mL of whole blood or of 200 mL of red cells adds 200 mg of total iron to the body, iron that will not be excreted. Thus, a patient who receives 2 units of blood monthly for an anemia that is not a result of blood loss will accumulate 4.8 g of iron per year. If the need for transfusion is occasioned by a disorder in which ineffective erythropoiesis plays a prominent role, the accumulation of iron is even greater. Thalassemia is such a circumstance, and iron overload is the most important cause of death in patients with this disorder (Chap. 48).

The homeostatic mechanisms of the body are such that the inappropriate administration of iron by the oral route is very unlikely to produce clinically significant iron overload. Of the few cases that have been described, all but one were documented before the cloning of the *HFE* gene, raising the possibility that the patients had genetic hemochromatosis that was accelerated by excess iron intake. Documented iron overload after iron injection is even less common and has not been accompanied by demonstrable tissue damage.

Pathology

Affected tissues and organs exhibit a deep brown color. Histologic examination reveals prominent hemosiderin deposition in many tissues and organs.

Liver The liver is often enlarged. After cirrhosis has developed, the organ becomes granular or coarsely nodular. In the liver of patients with classical hemochromatosis, TfR-2 mutations, and in juvenile hemochromatosis, hemosiderin is found primarily in hepatocytes. Kupffer cells are relatively spared. Prior to the development of cirrhosis, the hemosiderin accumulates primarily in periportal hepatocytes and is less toward the central veins. The iron of cirrhotic livers is mostly in the periphery of regenerative nodules. Fibrosis begins periportally, then fibrous septa traverse the lobules. Usually, the distortion of the architecture is not as severe or as uniform as in alcoholic cirrhosis. The cirrhosis of hemochromatosis usually has a micronodular appearance. Iron in bile duct epithelium has sometimes been considered a specific marker for hemochromatosis, but is not reliable. The amount of iron in the liver is always greatly increased. This is apparent on inspection of sections stained for iron with the Prussian blue reaction, and can be quantitated on liver biopsy specimens. An iron concentration of more than 300 μmol/g dry weight (or about 50 μmol/g wet weight) is considered strong evidence for hemochromatosis when factors such as transfusions are eliminated as the cause.

In the original description of African iron overload, the liver pathology was deemed to be indistinguishable from that of classical hemochromatosis, but in newer studies[238] it seems that only some of the affected patients manifest iron storage, primarily in the hepatocytes; some have storage primarily in Kupffer cells. In the case of patients with ferroportin mutations that prevent transport of iron, storage of iron takes place mostly in the Kupffer cells, and fibrosis seems to be absent; ferroportin mutations that prevent interaction with hepcidin, on the other hand, are associated with hepatocytes iron overload, as is seen in classical hemochromatosis.[233,239]

Heart Iron accumulates more slowly in the myocardium than in the liver, but the heart is more sensitive to its toxic effects. Myocardial damage is seen when iron loading is rapid, for example, in β-thalassemic patients dying of transfusional iron overload in their 20s and 30s[240] prior to effective chelation therapy, and in juvenile hemochromatosis patients who usually present with iron-induced cardiomyopathy and endocrinopathy rather than liver failure.[241] The myocardium is thickened and the heart is often enlarged; arrhythmias and myocardial failure follows. Accumulation of cardiac iron is the leading cause of death in transfused patients with β-thalassemia major. Patients with transfusion-dependent anemias, such as congenital dyserythropoietic anemia and Diamond-Blackfan syndrome, also develop iron overload-induced cardiomyopathy. In transfused patients with myelodysplastic syndromes, transfusion threshold guidelines of 75 units of blood was suggested as a risk factor of cardiac iron overload but this is not based on firm data. Direct cardiac iron measurement using magnetic resonance imaging predicts cardiac complications and can stratify the risk of subsequent cardiac dysfunction.[242] This technique measures the half-life, T2*, of cardiac muscle darkening (with respect to echo time) produced by magnetically active stored cardiac iron.

Marrow The quantity of iron in the marrow of patients with classical hereditary hemochromatosis is only modestly increased, if increased at all. The iron is characteristically distributed into small, equal-size granules, and these are located in endothelial lining cells rather than in macrophages. Indeed, in classical hereditary hemochromatosis, both macrophages[243] and intestinal mucosal cells are iron-poor relative to the overall iron burden.

Genetics

Genetic factors play an important role in the etiology of iron storage disease. This is true not only in the primary forms of the disorder, but also in secondary hemochromatosis, where genetic disorders of erythropoiesis are the most common causes. The genetics of these disorders, including the thalassemias, dyserythropoietic anemias, and red cell enzymopathies, are described in Chaps. 39, 47, and 48. Mutations of several genes that play an important role in iron homeostasis have been found to lead to iron storage disease.[244]

HFE **Mutations** The most common cause of hereditary hemochromatosis is a mutation of the *HFE* gene. This HLA-like gene resides on chromosome 6. Three polymorphic mutations have been identified. These are located at nucleotides 187,193, and 845 of the cDNA (complementary DNA) and at the protein level encode the H63D, S65C, and C282Y mutations, respectively. The phenotypic severity of these mutations on iron homeostasis is manifested in the following order: C282Y > H63D > S65C. Hereditary hemochromatosis is essentially an autosomal recessive disorder. Approximately two-thirds of homozygotes for the C282Y and a slightly lower percentage of compound heterozygotes for the C282Y and H63D mutations manifest increased serum transferrin saturations and serum ferritin levels. Individuals heterozygous for either the C282Y or the H63D mutation have, on the average, significantly higher transferrin saturations and serum ferritin levels than do wild-type homozygotes. However, the magnitude of this increase is very low.[245] For example, the average transferrin saturation of men with the wild-type genotype is 26.69 percent and heterozygotes for the C282Y mutation have a transferrin saturation averaging 30.63 percent. The effect of the H63D mutation is even less, and that of the S65C mutation barely perceptible.

In spite of the minimal effect of the heterozygous state for *HFE* mutations on iron homeostasis, a number of investigators have proposed that heterozygotes are at increased risk for a variety of disorders.

What has not been taken into account in the studies is that the *HFE* gene is in close proximity to (and therefore likely to be coinherited with) many immune-response genes on chromosome 6; consequently, it is not possible to distinguish the minor effects that *HFE* mutations may have on iron homeostasis from variation in the immune response.

HAMP **(Hepcidin) Mutations** Mutations of hepcidin are rare, and are associated with severe juvenile hemochromatosis.[246]

SCL40A1 **(Ferroportin) Mutations** Mutations of the gene encoding ferroportin cause an autosomal dominant iron storage disease of two types. Gain-of-function mutations, for example the C326S mutation, interfere with hepcidin binding to ferroportin or with the resulting ferroportin endocytosis, so that mutant ferroportin molecules continue exporting iron from enterocytes and macrophages to plasma even in the face of high hepcidin levels[232] that normally cause ferroportin endocytosis and proteolysis. A mouse model of this condition shows that a heterozygous mutation is sufficient to cause severe iron overload but that homozygosity for this mutation is even more severe.[247] Loss-of-function mutations are more common and include ferroportin mutations that do not allow ferroportin protein to localize to the cell surface, or prevent transport of iron. Here storage of iron takes place mostly in the Kupffer cells and splenic macrophages, and cirrhosis does not occur. It is not clear why these act in a dominant manner, nor why all of the reported mutations encode amino acid substitutions and none are completely destructive (frameshift or stop codons).[158,248] An attractive explanation is that these mutations act in a dominant-negative manner, but this mechanism has not yet been supported by convincing biochemical data. A common polymorphism c.744G→T (Gln284His) shows an association with African iron overload,[238,249,250] but is clearly not present in all patients who manifest this syndrome.

TfR-2 **Mutations** Mutations of *TfR-2* cause an autosomal recessive disorder that is indistinguishable clinically from the common HFE-related form of hereditary hemochromatosis.[230,251–253]

Hemojuvelin Mutations Several different mutations of a gene designated as *HFE2* and as *HJV* cause juvenile hemochromatosis.[231,254–258] Hemojuvelin belongs to the class of glycosylphosphatidylinositol-anchored repulsive-guidance molecules, and may act as a coreceptor for bone morphogenetic proteins (BMPs). BMP receptor is now known to be a key regulator of hepcidin transcription.[259]

DMT-1 Human Mutations DMT-1 human mutations are all associated with hepatic hemosiderosis[207,208,260] and most are associated with abnormal liver function tests in addition to microcytic hypochromic anemia. This is in contrast to mice and rats with DMT-1 mutations, as these DMT-1–deficient rodents are iron deficient. This is likely because humans, unlike rodents, can also absorb heme-containing iron, at least to a small degree in a DMT-1 independent manner while the DMT-1 dependent iron utilization by erythroblasts is severely impaired in both humans and rodents.

Animal Models
Naturally Occurring Models
When kept in zoos or other nonnative habitats, a number of animal species, such as myna birds, the toco toucan, Salers cattle, lemurs, and the browsing rhinoceros, are iron-loaded. Rhinoceroses may represent an interesting paradigm for iron storage in captive species. Although the browsing rhinoceros species are iron loaded, grazing species are not, even when kept under similar conditions. It seems likely that because iron is not readily available in the leaves and twigs eaten by the browsing species, these species have evolved to more efficiently take up iron from their diet—more efficiently than needed when fed a zoo diet. Molecular comparisons of iron-regulatory genes in browser versus grazer rhinoceroses identified some promising candidates, but the ultimate cause of the differences in iron handling has not yet been established.[261]

Models Produced by Iron Loading Numerous efforts have been made to create models of hemochromatosis by loading laboratory animals with iron, either by the oral or parenteral route. A few of these appear to simulate the human disease in one respect or another. For example, the iron-loaded gerbil[262–265] develops heart disease, features of which resemble the human disease. Such models have been used for the study of potential chelating agents.

Targeted Disruption Models Targeted disruption of most of the genes associated with human iron disorders has been achieved. Included are *HFE*,[266] TfR-2,[252] ferroportin,[267] hemojuvelin,[255,256] and hepcidin.[268] The targeted disruption of several genes, including those encoding BMP-6,[269,270] or the components of the BMP receptor,[259] caused iron overload in mice, but the equivalent human diseases have not yet been found.

CLINICAL FEATURES

HFE-Related (Type 1) Hereditary Hemochromatosis

Onset The clinical features of the most common form of hereditary hemochromatosis are cirrhosis of the liver, darkening of the skin, cardiomyopathies, and diabetes. These features are only seen in the fully penetrant form of the disease and may depend on additional cofactors such as alcohol consumption. In contrast to the juvenile form of the disease, in which onset is usually in the second or third decade of life, classical hereditary hemochromatosis associated with mutations of the *HFE* gene generally is diagnosed in the fifth or six decade of life.

General Symptomatology Many symptoms are attributed to hereditary hemochromatosis, including abdominal pain, weakness, lethargy, fatigue, loss of libido, impotence, and arthropathies. However, all of these symptoms are common in an aging population, and epidemiologic studies show that none of them are more common in patients with the HFE hemochromatosis, even those with the biochemical phenotype, than they are in the general population.

Arthropathies The arthropathy of patients with hemochromatosis has characteristic features.[218,271,272] It is said to tend to begin at the small joints of the hands, especially the second and third metacarpal joints, and that in some cases episodes of acute synovitis may occur, as in calcium pyrophosphate dehydrate deposition arthropathy (pseudogout; chondrocalcinosis). Radiologically, the arthropathy resembles that of osteoarthritis with joint space loss, subchondral cysts, sclerosis, and osteophytosis. The features that have been considered distinctive include the joint distribution, the presence of shape osteophytes emerging from the radial sides of the metacarpal distal epiphysis, and the presence of radiolucent zones in the subchondral area of the femoral head. It is generally recognized that arthritis does not respond to phlebotomy therapy. The possibility that this type of arthritis depends on linkage of HFE to other HLA genes is made less likely by the occurrence of similar arthritis in juvenile hemochromatosis,[273] which is genetically independent of the HLA locus. Hip arthritis at an early age was also noted in a family with hepcidin-resistant ferroportin mutation and iron overload.[239]

Liver Patients with hepatic iron overload are at a greatly increased risk of developing a hepatocellular carcinoma, especially when cirrhosis is present.[274] Occasional patients with hereditary hemochromatosis have been reported to develop hepatocellular carcinoma even in the absence of cirrhosis suggesting that iron overload could be directly carcinogenic.

Porphyria Cutanea Tarda

Porphyria cutanea tarda is a disease that is well known to be associated with mild iron overload and that responds to phlebotomy treatment (Chap. 58). Numerous studies document that the prevalence of patients with this disorder who also have mutations of the *HFE* gene is considerably increased.[275]

Juvenile Hemochromatosis

The penetrance of the rare juvenile form of the disease seems to be high and cardiomyopathies and endocrine deficiencies are the major clinical features.[276] Joint manifestations were found to be relatively common in patients with juvenile hemochromatosis.[273]

African Iron Overload

It is not clear to what extent African iron overload is symptomatic. Among the Bantu, where the disorder was originally described, there are many complicating factors, including malnutrition and high alcohol intake. Among African Americans various associated disorders have been noted, but a cause-and-effect relationship is not clear.

Secondary Hemochromatosis

The clinical findings in patients with hemochromatosis secondary to blood transfusion and/or disorders of erythropoiesis are, in general, indistinguishable from those found in patients with the primary hemochromatosis.[277]

LABORATORY FEATURES

The main laboratory features of hereditary hemochromatosis are an abnormally high transferrin saturation, and increased serum ferritin level. Five to 10 percent of patients with classical HFE hemochromatosis manifest increased liver enzyme levels in the serum. In secondary hemochromatosis, anemia and other manifestations of the underlying disorder are found. Macrocytosis of the erythrocytes is a common feature; this finding seems unrelated to liver disease and its cause is unknown.

Differential Diagnosis

A large number of methods have been introduced that allow the amount of storage iron to be estimated.[278] The suspicion that a patient may have primary hemochromatosis is generally raised by an increased serum transferrin saturation, particularly when it is found together with an elevated serum ferritin level. Increased transferrin saturation commonly occurs in patients with chronic liver disease who have no mutations in the *HFE* gene.[279] Ferritin is an acute phase protein and levels are elevated in a variety of disorders. Particularly high levels are encountered in patients with macrophage activation syndromes, loss-of-function ferroportin mutations, acute hepatitis, Gaucher disease, in some malignancies, and in patients with the hyperferritinemia-cataract syndrome.[280] The latter disorder is an uncommon autosomal dominant defect in which a mutation in the 5′ IRE of the ferritin light chain prevents binding of the IRPs, resulting in unrestrained constitutive production of the ferritin chains.

Many clinicians have considered a liver biopsy the "gold standard" for the diagnosis of iron overload. The material obtained at biopsy not only provides the opportunity to assess the histopathology of the liver of the patient, but also to quantitate the amount of nonheme iron in the specimen. Dividing the iron content by the patient's age provides an iron index; a value greater than 2 implies the presence of hemochromatosis. Although in some situations liver biopsy may provide useful information, it is an invasive procedure that, although low-risk, is no longer required for the diagnosis of hemochromatosis. Enthusiasm for subjecting every patient with potential hemochromatosis to liver biopsy has diminished with the ready availability of genetic analysis. Moreover, a simple way to determine whether a patient is iron overloaded is to institute a program of phlebotomies. This is an essentially harmless way to determine how much storage iron the body contains. Magnetic resonance imaging (MRI) is also capable of detecting and reliably quantifying the amount of iron in the liver.[281] For detection of cardiac iron overload, T2* MRI[242] is a superior diagnostic approach.

THERAPY

The treatment of hemochromatosis consists of removing the accumulated iron. In the case of patients who are able to mount an erythropoietic response to phlebotomy, removal of blood is generally the treatment of choice. When the patient has marked impairment of erythropoiesis, as in thalassemia and dyserythropoietic anemia, it is necessary to employ chelating agents to remove iron, although occasionally serial phlebotomy will stimulate sufficient erythropoiesis to make it a viable therapy.

Phlebotomy

Each milliliter of packed red cells contains approximately 1 mg of iron. Thus, the removal of 500 mL of blood with a hematocrit of 40 percent removes approximately 200 mg of iron. As the red cell mass is restored to its prephlebotomy size, iron is mobilized from the stores. When the stores have been exhausted the signs of iron deficiency develop, and this is the end point of the initial part of the phlebotomy program. The patient is then followed and a schedule of maintenance phlebotomies is established with the frequency of phlebotomies tailored to maintain the serum ferritin level, the best indicator of body stores, below 100 ng/mL.

The actual volume of blood removed at each phlebotomy depends on the patient's size. Most average-size patients tolerate removal of 500 mL, but patients who weigh 50 kg or less are better treated by the removal of correspondingly smaller volumes of blood. Many patients may complain of symptoms following the first few phlebotomies. Better compliance is achieved if such symptoms are minimized by performing phlebotomies only every 14 days initially, increasing the frequency to weekly phlebotomies once the patient has become accustomed to the procedure and the activity of the marrow has been stimulated so as to replace the lost erythrocytes rapidly. The hematocrit or hemoglobin and the MCV of the red cells should be measured before each phlebotomy is undertaken. If there has been a substantial decrease in the hematocrit or hemoglobin, the phlebotomy should be deferred. The MCV may rise early in the treatment program, but as iron deficiency develops it will fall, signaling that the end point has been reached or is near. The transferrin saturation and serum ferritin level should be measured every 2 or 3 months. When the transferrin saturation is less than 10 percent and the serum ferritin less than 10 ng/mL, phlebotomy should be discontinued and the patient monitored every 4 to 8 weeks. When the serum ferritin is in the 50 to 100 ng/mL range, the maintenance phase should be initiated. Some patients may require phlebotomies monthly to maintain a normal ferritin value, whereas others may only require two or three phlebotomies per year.

Chelation Therapy

Chelation therapy instituted in a timely manner can decrease the potential morbidity caused by iron overload and prolong the life of patients with hereditary chronic iron-loading disorders such as β-thalassemia major or intermedia. It also has a place in the management of some patients with acquired marrow dysplasias provided that the prognosis of the underlying disorder, and the patient's psychological state, justifies the somewhat cumbersome implementation of parenteral chelation. As oral chelating agents become more readily available, the application of chelation therapy to myelodysplastic states may broaden.

Desferrioxamine

Desferrioxamine is a naturally occurring iron-chelating compound elaborated by the microorganism *Streptomyces pilosus,* having evolved to enable the microbe to obtain iron from its environment. One molecule of this chelator binds one atom of iron. Its molecular weight is 560 daltons. The iron complex is excreted into the urine and feces. Urine iron is derived primarily from red cells broken down by macrophages, whereas fecal iron is believed to be from iron chelated in the liver.[282]

Desferrioxamine is poorly absorbed from the gastrointestinal tract and must therefore be given parenterally, either by the subcutaneous or intravenous route. Rapid intravenous or intramuscular injection results in the relatively little iron mobilization; instead, it is necessary to administer desferrioxamine by slow intravenous or subcutaneous infusion over a period of 8 to 10 hours. Increasing doses of desferrioxamine result in increased iron excretion, and the usual recommended dose is 30 to 50 mL/kg.[282,283] Vitamin C (up to 200 mg daily) may be given to enhance iron excretion. The amount of iron excreted will vary from patient to patient and depends to a large extent on the iron burden. Because the treatment is cumbersome and costly, one should be reasonably certain that sufficient good is being accomplished to justify the effort. This can be achieved by measuring urine output of iron after a test desferrioxamine infusion, bearing in mind that urinary excretion may account for only one-third of the iron excreted, fecal excretion accounting for the rest.

Desferrioxamine is usually well tolerated. Minor local reactions, such as local pruritus, induration, or pain at the site of infusion, are not uncommon. Large doses are associated with hearing loss, night blindness and other visual abnormalities, growth retardation, and skeletal changes. At very high doses occasional cases of kidney and lung abnormalities have been reported.[282] Approximately 20 percent of patients on desferrioxamine alone will continue to have cardiac iron overload.

Oral Chelating Agents

The inconvenience and high cost of administration with desferrioxamine has stimulated an intensive search for safe, orally active chelating agents. Deferiprone (L-1) is an orally effective bidentate chelating agent; three molecules of deferiprone bind one iron atom. Its molecular weight is only 139 daltons and it is excreted almost entirely in the urine. The usual dose is 75 mg/kg per day divided into three doses. Deferiprone administration is associated with a number of toxic effects, including gastrointestinal disturbances, arthropathy, transient increases in the serum levels of liver enzymes, and zinc deficiency. The main concern has centered on the propensity of the drug to produce neutropenia and agranulocytosis. The latter complication occurs in approximately 1 percent of patients. It appears to be idiosyncratic, is more common in females, and appears to be reversible. Neutropenia with a granulocyte level between 0.5 and 1.5×10^9/L (500 and 1500/μL) occurs in an additional 5 percent of patients. Treatment should be stopped at the first sign of a fall in the leukocyte count.[282] It has been suggested that deferiprone may be more effective in removing iron from the heart and desferrioxamine more effective with respect to liver iron accumulations.[283] Preliminary investigations suggest that a combination of desferrioxamine and deferiprone may be more effective than either alone. It has been proposed that deferiprone enters cells and removes their iron and then passes the iron to desferrioxamine.[283] The combination may be particularly useful in patients with heart failure from iron overload where it may decrease mortality, and in patients with endocrinopathies.[283]

Deferasirox (ICL670 or Exjade), a tridented triazole component, is a newer oral iron-chelating agent with a long plasma half-life.[283] At a dose of 30 mg/kg per day, it was found as efficient as desferrioxamine and is generally well tolerated. It has been recommended for patients who are noncompliant with desferrioxamine, and like deferiprone, may be effective at removing cardiac iron. Its main toxicity is renal and hepatic, but it may also cause gastrointestinal hemorrhage.[283] Combination therapy with the two oral chelators is still experimental.

COURSE AND PROGNOSIS

The outlook in this disease has changed to one in which the life span of patients with hemochromatosis is normal or nearly so. This is largely a result of the change in the definition of the disorder. In the early

20th century, the diagnosis was reserved for the rare patient with full-blown bronzed diabetes. Today, the diagnosis is applied to any person found to be homozygous for the C282Y mutation, or, indeed, anyone with an increased transferrin saturation and elevated serum ferritin level. In reality, patients with a diagnosis of hemochromatosis based on genetic and/or biochemical criteria have a normal life span. This is not to suggest that patients do not die of hereditary hemochromatosis; it is simply that the penetrance of the disorder as detected on genetic or biochemical bases is so low that the few deaths that do occur cannot be detected even in very sizable series.

For those patients with classical hereditary hemochromatosis who are clinically affected, it is likely that removal of iron by phlebotomy prevents further complications and prolongs life span. Although controlled studies of the effect of phlebotomy are not ethically feasible, serial observations in patients undergoing phlebotomy suggest that cirrhosis is either stabilized or may, at least in some patients, improve. The course of untreated juvenile hemochromatosis seems much less benign. Cardiac deaths seem to be particularly common,[276] and in a few cases cardiac transplantation has been performed successfully, but there are insufficient data concerning this rare disorder to allow one to provide more precise information about the outlook.

Institution of iron chelation has greatly improved outcomes in β-thalassemia major and similar disorders, but the prognosis is grim when iron chelation is not performed (Chap. 48). Death is most frequently a result of cardiac failure but this complication is preventable with modern chelation regimens.

REFERENCES

1. Heath CW, Strauss MB, Castle WB: Quantitative aspects of iron deficiency in hypochromic anemia (the parenteral administration of iron). *J Clin Invest* 11(6):1293–1312, 1932.
2. Beutler E: History of iron in medicine. *Blood Cells Mol Dis* 29(3):297–308, 2002.
3. Poskitt EM: Early history of iron deficiency. *Br J Haematol* 122(4):554–562, 2003.
4. Stoltzfus RJ: Iron interventions for women and children in low-income countries. *J Nutr* 141(4):756S–762S, 2011.
5. McLean E, Cogswell M, Egli I, et al: Worldwide prevalence of anaemia, WHO Vitamin and Mineral Nutrition Information System, 1993–2005. *Public Health Nutr* 12(4):444–454, 2009.
6. Pasricha SR, Drakesmith H, Black J, et al: Control of iron deficiency anemia in low- and middle-income countries. *Blood* 121(14):2607–2617, 2013.
7. Cogswell ME, Looker AC, Pfeiffer CM, et al: Assessment of iron deficiency in US preschool children and nonpregnant females of childbearing age: National Health and Nutrition Examination Survey 2003–2006. *Am J Clin Nutr* 89(5):1334–1342, 2009.
8. Looker AC, Dallman PR, Carroll MD, et al: Prevalence of iron deficiency in the United States. *JAMA* 277(12):973–976, 1997.
9. Mei Z, Cogswell ME, Looker AC, et al: Assessment of iron status in US pregnant women from the National Health and Nutrition Examination Survey (NHANES), 1999–2006. *Am J Clin Nutr* 93(6):1312–1320, 2011.
10. Rockey DC: Occult and obscure gastrointestinal bleeding: Causes and clinical management. *Nat Rev Gastroenterol Hepatol* 7(5):265–279, 2010.
11. Blackler RW, Gemici B, Manko A, et al: NSAID-gastroenteropathy: New aspects of pathogenesis and prevention. *Curr Opin Pharmacol* 19C:11–16, 2014.
12. Bode C, Christian Bode J: Effect of alcohol consumption on the gut. *Best Pract Res Clin Gastroenterol* 17(4):575–592, 2003.
13. Coffey RJ, Washington MK, Corless CL, et al: Menetrier disease and gastrointestinal stromal tumors: Hyperproliferative disorders of the stomach. *J Clin Invest* 117(1):70–80, 2007.
14. Hershko C, Skikne B: Pathogenesis and management of iron deficiency anemia: Emerging role of celiac disease, *Helicobacter pylori*, and autoimmune gastritis. *Semin Hematol* 46(4):339–350, 2009.
15. Hershko CC: How I treat unexplained refractory iron deficiency anemia. *Blood* 123(3):326–333, 2013.
16. Stewart, Termanini, Sutliff, et al: Iron absorption in patients with Zollinger-Ellison syndrome treated with long-term gastric acid antisecretory therapy. *Aliment Pharmacol Ther* 12(1):83–98, 1998.
17. Bini EJ, Unger JS, Weinshel EH: Outcomes of endoscopy in patients with iron deficiency anemia after Billroth II partial gastrectomy. *J Clin Gastroenterol* 34(4):421–426, 2002.
18. Ruhl CE, Everhart JE: Relationship of iron-deficiency anemia with esophagitis and hiatal hernia: Hospital findings from a prospective, population-based study. *Am J Gastroenterol* 96(2):322–326, 2001.
19. Panzuto F, Di Giulio E, Capurso G, et al: Large hiatal hernia in patients with iron deficiency anaemia: A prospective study on prevalence and treatment. *Aliment Pharmacol Ther* 19(6):663–670, 2004.
20. Haurani C, Carlin A, Hammoud Z, et al: Prevalence and resolution of anemia with paraesophageal hernia repair. *J Gastrointest Surg* 16(10):1817–1820, 2012.
21. Camus M, Jensen DM, Ohning GV, et al: Severe upper gastrointestinal hemorrhage from linear gastric ulcers in large hiatal hernias: A large prospective case series of Cameron ulcers. *Endoscopy* 45(05):397–400, 2013.
22. Crompton DWT, Nesheim MC: Nutritional impact of intestinal helminthiasis during the human life cycle. *Annu Rev Nutr* 22(1):35–59, 2002.
23. Hemingway AP: Angiodysplasia as a cause of iron deficiency anaemia. *Blood Rev* 3(3):147–151, 1989.
24. Kar P, Mitra S, Resnick JM, et al: Gastric antral vascular ectasia: Case report and review of the literature. *Clin Med Res* 11(2):80–85, 2013.
25. Chin MW, Enns R: Hemobilia. *Curr Gastroenterol Rep* 12(2):121–129, 2010.
26. Duchini A, Sessoms S: Gastrointestinal hemorrhage in patients with systemic sclerosis and CREST syndrome. *Am J Gastroenterol* 93(9):1453–1456, 1998.
27. Bang JY, Peter S: Obscure gastrointestinal bleeding and Turner syndrome. *Dig Endosc* 25(4):462–464, 2013.
28. Wong CH, Tan YM, Chow WC, et al: Blue rubber bleb nevus syndrome: A clinical spectrum with correlation between cutaneous and gastrointestinal manifestations. *J Gastroenterol Hepatol* 18(8):1000–1002, 2003.
29. Sparberg M: Chronic iron deficiency anemia due to Meckel's diverticulum. *Am J Dis Child* 113(2):286–287, 1967.
30. Pai M, Chan A, Barr R: How I manage heavy menstrual bleeding. *Br J Haematol* 162(6):721–729, 2013.
31. Hallberg L, Rossander-Hulten L: Iron requirements in menstruating women. *Am J Clin Nutr* 54(6):1047–1058, 1991.
32. Brown EA, Sampson B, Muller BR, et al: Urinary iron loss in the nephrotic syndrome—an unusual cause of iron deficiency with a note on urinary copper losses. *Postgrad Med J* 60(700):125–128, 1984.
33. Kildahl-Andersen O, Dahl IM, Thorstensen K, et al: Iron deficiency anemia in a patient with excessive urinary iron loss. *Eur J Haematol* 64(3):204–205, 2000.
34. Hayden SJ, Albert TJ, Watkins TR, et al: Anemia in critical illness: Insights into etiology, consequences, and management. *Am J Respir Crit Care Med* 185(10):1049–1057, 2012.
35. Fishbane S, Frei GL, Maesaka J: Reduction in recombinant human erythropoietin doses by the use of chronic intravenous iron supplementation. *Am J Kidney Dis* 26(1):41–46, 1995.
36. Eschbach JW, Cook JD, Scribner BH, et al: Iron balance in hemodialysis patients. *Ann Intern Med* 87(6):710–713, 1977.
37. Salvin HE, Pasricha SR, Marks DC, et al: Iron deficiency in blood donors: A national cross-sectional study. *Transfusion* 54(10):2434–2444, 2014.
38. Baart AM, van Noord PAH, Vergouwe Y, et al: High prevalence of subclinical iron deficiency in whole blood donors not deferred for low hemoglobin. *Transfusion* 53(8):1670–1677, 2013.
39. Brittenham GM: Iron deficiency in whole blood donors. *Transfusion* 51(3):458–461, 2011.
40. Bernard J: [Lasthénie de Ferjol, Marie de Saint-Vallier, Emilie de Tourville or the novelist and anemia] [in French]. *Nouv Rev Fr Hematol* 24(1):43–44, 1982.
41. Karamanou M, Androutsos G: Lasthenie de Ferjol syndrome: A rare disease with fascinating history. *Intern Med J* 40(5):381–382, 2010.
42. Hirayama Y, Sakamaki S, Tsuji Y, et al: Fatality caused by self-bloodletting in a patient with factitious anemia. *Int J Hematol* 78(2):146–148, 2003.
43. Coello-Ramirez P, Larrosa-Haro A: Gastrointestinal occult hemorrhage and gastroduodenitis in cow's milk protein intolerance. *J Pediatr Gastroenterol Nutr* 3(2):215–218, 1984.
44. Kokkonen J, Simila S: Cow's milk intolerance with melena. *Eur J Pediatr* 135(2):189–194, 1980.
45. Milman N, Pedersen FM: Idiopathic pulmonary haemosiderosis. Epidemiology, pathogenic aspects and diagnosis. *Respir Med* 92(7):902–907, 1998.
46. Reid DW, Withers NJ, Francis L, et al: Iron deficiency in cystic fibrosis: Relationship to lung disease severity and chronic pseudomonas aeruginosa infection. *Chest* 121(1):48–54, 2002.
47. von Drygalski A, Biller J: Anemia in Cystic fibrosis: Incidence, mechanisms, and association with pulmonary function and vitamin deficiency. *Nutr Clin Pract* 23(5):557–563, 2008.
48. Pena-Rosas JP, De-Regil LM, Dowswell T, et al: Daily oral iron supplementation during pregnancy. *Cochrane Database Syst Rev* 12:CD004736, 2012.
49. Pena-Rosas JP, De-Regil LM, Dowswell T, et al: Intermittent oral iron supplementation during pregnancy. *Cochrane Database Syst Rev* 7:CD009997, 2012.
50. Reveiz L, Gyte GM, Cuervo LG, et al: Treatments for iron-deficiency anaemia in pregnancy. *Cochrane Database Syst Rev* (10):CD003094, 2011.
51. Pena-Rosas JP, Viteri FE: Effects and safety of preventive oral iron or iron+folic acid supplementation for women during pregnancy. *Cochrane Database Syst Rev* (4):CD004736, 2009.
52. Sangare L, van Eijk AM, Ter Kuile FO, et al: The association between malaria and iron status or supplementation in pregnancy: A systematic review and meta-analysis. *PLoS One* 9(2):e87743, 2014.
53. Auerbach M: IV Iron in pregnancy: An unmet clinical need. *Am J Hematol* 89(7):789–789, 2014.

54. Domellof M, Braegger C, Campoy C, et al: Iron requirements of infants and toddlers. *J Pediatr Gastroenterol Nutr* 58(1):119–129, 2014.

55. Baker RD, Greer FR; Committee on Nutrition American Academy of Pediatrics: Diagnosis and prevention of iron deficiency and iron-deficiency anemia in infants and young children (0–3 years of age). *Pediatrics* 126(5):1040–1050, 2010.

56. Egan SK, Tao SS, Pennington JA, et al: US Food and Drug Administration's Total Diet Study: Intake of nutritional and toxic elements, 1991–96. *Food Addit Contam* 19(2):103–125, 2002.

57. Hallberg L, Hulthqn L: Perspectives on iron absorption. *Blood Cells Mol Dis* 29(3):562–573, 2002.

58. Jacobs A, Lawrie JH, Entwistle CC, et al: Gastric acid secretion in chronic iron-deficiency anaemia. *Lancet* 2(7456):190–192, 1966.

59. Schmitz U, Ko Y, Seewald S, et al: Iron-deficiency anemia as the sole manifestation of celiac disease. *Clin Investig* 72(7):519–521, 1994.

60. Kilpatrick ZM, Katz J: Occult celiac disease as a cause of iron deficiency anemia. *JAMA* 208(6):999–1001, 1969.

61. Sears DA, Anderson PR, Foy AL, et al: Urinary iron excretion and renal metabolism of hemoglobin in hemolytic diseases. *Blood* 28(5):708–725, 1966.

62. Roeser HP, Powell LW: Urinary iron excretion in valvular heart disease and after heart valve replacement. *Blood* 36(6):785–792, 1970.

63. McClung JP: Iron status and the female athlete. *J Trace Elem Med Biol* 26(2–3):124–126, 2012.

64. Karl JP, Lieberman HR, Cable SJ, et al: Randomized, double-blind, placebo-controlled trial of an iron-fortified food product in female soldiers during military training: Relations between iron status, serum hepcidin, and inflammation. *Am J Clin Nutr* 92(1):93–100, 2010.

65. Whitfield JB, Treloar S, Zhu G, et al: Relative importance of female-specific and non-female-specific effects on variation in iron stores between women. *Br J Haematol* 120(5):860–866, 2003.

66. An P, Wu Q, Wang H, et al: TMPRSS6, but not TF, TFR2 or BMP2 variants are associated with increased risk of iron-deficiency anemia. *Hum Mol Genet* 21(9):2124–2131, 2012.

67. Finberg KE, Heeney MM, Campagna DR, et al: Mutations in TMPRSS6 cause iron-refractory iron deficiency anemia (IRIDA). *Nat Genet* 40(5):569–571, 2008.

68. Guillem F, Lawson S, Kannengiesser C, et al: Two nonsense mutations in the TMPRSS6 gene in a patient with microcytic anemia and iron deficiency. *Blood* 112(5):2089–2091, 2008.

69. Du X, She E, Gelbart T, et al: The serine protease TMPRSS6 is required to sense iron deficiency. *Science* 320(5879):1088–1092, 2008.

70. Kimura H, Finch CA, Adamson JW: Hematopoiesis in the rat: Quantitation of hematopoietic progenitors and the response to iron deficiency anemia. *J Cell Physiol* 126(2):298–306, 1986.

71. Dallman PR: Biochemical basis for the manifestations of iron deficiency. *Ann. Rev Nutr* 6:13–40, 1986.

72. Eisenstein RS, Ross KL: Novel roles for iron regulatory proteins in the adaptive response to iron deficiency. *J Nutr* 133(5):1510S–1516S, 2003.

73. Woodson RD, Wills RE, Lenfant C: Effect of acute and established anemia on O_2 transport at rest, submaximal and maximal work. *J Appl Physiol Respir Environ Exerc Physiol* 44(1):36–43, 1978.

74. Crouter SE, DellaValle DM, Haas JD: Relationship between physical activity, physical performance, and iron status in adult women. *Appl Physiol Nutr Metab* 37(4):697–705, 2012.

75. Allen RP, Auerbach S, Bahrain H, et al: The prevalence and impact of restless legs syndrome on patients with iron deficiency anemia. *Am J Hematol* 88(4):261–264, 2013.

76. McCann JC, Ames BN: An overview of evidence for a causal relation between iron deficiency during development and deficits in cognitive or behavioral function. *Am J Clin Nutr* 85(4):931–945, 2007.

77. Jellen LC, Lu L, Wang X, et al: Iron deficiency alters expression of dopamine-related genes in the ventral midbrain in mice. *Neuroscience* 252(0):13–23, 2013.

78. Earley CJ, Allen RP, Beard JL, et al: Insight into the pathophysiology of restless legs syndrome. *J Neurosci Res* 62(5):623–628, 2000.

79. Oppenheimer SJ: Iron and Its Relation to Immunity and Infectious Disease. *J Nutr* 131(2):616S–6635, 2001.

80. Gwamaka M, Kurtis JD, Sorensen BE, et al: Iron deficiency protects against severe *Plasmodium falciparum* malaria and death in young children. *Clin Infect Dis* 54(8):1137–1144, 2012.

81. Kabyemela ER, Fried M, Kurtis JD, et al: Decreased susceptibility to *Plasmodium falciparum* infection in pregnant women with iron deficiency. *J Infect Dis* 198(2):163–166, 2008.

82. Stoltzfus RJ, Heidkamp R, Kenkel D, et al: Iron supplementation of young children: Learning from the new evidence. *Food Nutr Bull* 28(4 Suppl):S572–S584, 2007.

83. Spottiswoode N, Duffy P, Drakesmith H: Iron, anemia and hepcidin in malaria. *Front Pharmacol* 5, 2014.

84. Pagani A, Nai A, Corna G, et al: Low hepcidin accounts for the proinflammatory status associated with iron deficiency. *Blood* 118(3):736–746, 2011.

85. Hale LP, Kant EP, Greer PK, et al: Iron supplementation decreases severity of allergic inflammation in murine lung. *PLoS One* 7(9):e45667, 2012.

86. Thompson J, Biggs BA, Pasricha SR: Effects of daily iron supplementation in 2- to 5-year-old children: Systematic review and meta-analysis. *Pediatrics* 131(4):739–753, 2013.

87. Sachdev H, Gera T, Nestel P: Effect of iron supplementation on physical growth in children: Systematic review of randomised controlled trials. *Public Health Nutr* 9(7):904–920, 2006.

88. Beard JL, Borel MJ, Derr J: Impaired thermoregulation and thyroid function in iron-deficiency anemia. *Am J Clin Nutr* 52(5):813–819, 1990.

89. Baird IM, Dodge OG, Palmer FJ, et al: The tongue and oesophagus in iron-deficiency anaemia and the effect of iron therapy. *J Clin Pathol* 14:603–609, 1961.

90. Lees F, Rosenthal FD: Gastric mucosal lesions before and after treatment in iron deficiency anaemia. *Q J Med* 27(105):19–26, 1958.

91. Naiman JL, Oski FA, Diamond LK, et al: The gastrointestinal effects of iron-deficiency anemia. *Pediatrics* 33:83–99, 1964.

92. Scott J, Valentine JA, St Hill CA, et al: A quantitative histological analysis of the effects of age and sex on human lingual epithelium. *J Biol Buccale* 11(4):303–315, 1983.

93. Jacobs A: The buccal mucosa in anaemia. *J Clin Pathol* 13:463–468, 1960.

94. Boddington MM: Changes in buccal cells in the anaemias. *J Clin Pathol* 12(3):222–227, 1959.

95. Macleod RI, Hamilton PJ, Soames JV: Quantitative exfoliative oral cytology in iron-deficiency and megaloblastic anemia. *Anal Quant Cytol Histol* 10(3):176–180, 1988.

96. Burko H, Mellins HZ, Watson J: Skull changes in iron deficiency anemia simulating congenital hemolytic anemia. *Am J Roentgenol Radium Ther Nucl Med* 86:447–452, 1961.

97. Moseley JE: Skull changes in chronic iron deficiency anemia. *Am J Roentgenol Radium Ther Nucl Med* 85:649–652, 1961.

98. Shahidi NT, Diamond LK: Skull changes in infants with chronic iron-deficiency anemia. *N Engl J Med* 262:137–139, 1960.

99. Haas JD, Brownlie T: Iron deficiency and reduced work capacity: A critical review of the research to determine a causal relationship. *J Nutr* 131(2):676S–690S, 2001.

100. Wang B, Zhan S, Gong T, et al: Iron therapy for improving psychomotor development and cognitive function in children under the age of three with iron deficiency anaemia. *Cochrane Database Syst Rev* 6:CD001444, 2013.

101. Abdullah K, Kendzerska T, Shah P, et al: Efficacy of oral iron therapy in improving the developmental outcome of pre-school children with non-anaemic iron deficiency: A systematic review. *Public Health Nutr* 16(8):1497–1506, 2013.

102. Hermoso M, Vucic V, Vollhardt C, et al: The effect of iron on cognitive development and function in infants, children and adolescents: A systematic review. *Ann Nutr Metab* 59(2–4):154–165, 2011.

103. Hornyak M, Scholz H, Kohnen R, et al: What treatment works best for restless legs syndrome? Meta-analyses of dopaminergic and non-dopaminergic medications. *Sleep Med Rev* 18(2):153–164, 2014.

104. Trotti LM, Bhadriraju S, Becker LA: Iron for restless legs syndrome. *Cochrane Database Syst Rev* 5:CD007834, 2012.

105. Cortese S, Angriman M, Lecendreux M, et al: Iron and attention deficit/hyperactivity disorder: What is the empirical evidence so far? A systematic review of the literature. *Expert Rev Neurother* 12(10):1227–1240, 2012.

106. Trujillo MH, Desenne JJ, Pinto HB: Reversible papilledema in iron deficiency anemia. Two cases with normal spinal fluid pressure. *Ann Ophthalmol* 4(5):378–380, 1972.

107. Knizley H Jr, Noyes WD: Iron deficiency anemia, papilledema, thrombocytosis, and transient hemiparesis. *Arch Intern MedIntern Med* 129(3):483–486, 1972.

108. Stoebner R, Kiser R, Alperin JB: Iron deficiency anemia and papilledema. Rapid resolution with oral iron therapy. *Am J Dig Dis* 15(10):919–922, 1970.

109. Lubeck MJ: Papilledema caused by iron-deficiency anemia. *Trans Am Acad Ophthalmol Otolaryngol* 63(3):306–310, 1959.

110. Kim LJ, Coelho FM, Tufik S, et al: New perspectives of iron deficiency as a risk factor for ischemic stroke. *Ann Hematol* 93(7):1243–1244, 2014.

111. Chang YL, Hung SH, Ling W, et al: Association between ischemic stroke and iron-deficiency anemia: A population-based study. *PLoS One* 8(12):e82952, 2013.

112. Munot P, De VC, Hemingway C, et al: Severe iron deficiency anaemia and ischaemic stroke in children. *Arch Dis Child* 96(3):276–279, 2011.

113. Maguire JL, deVeber G, Parkin PC: Association between iron-deficiency anemia and stroke in young children. *Pediatrics* 120(5):1053–1057, 2007.

114. Yager JY, Hartfield DS: Neurologic manifestations of iron deficiency in childhood. *Pediatr Neurol* 27(2):85–92, 2002.

115. Novacek G: Plummer-Vinson syndrome. *Orphanet J Rare Dis* 1:36, 2006.

116. Lumish RA, Young SL, Lee S, et al: Gestational iron deficiency is associated with pica behaviors in adolescents. *J Nutr* 144(10):1533–1539, 2014.

117. Uchida T, Kawati Y: Pagophagia in iron deficiency anemia. *Rinsho Ketsueki* 55(4):436–439, 2014.

118. Spencer BR, Kleinman S, Wright DJ, et al: Restless legs syndrome, pica, and iron status in blood donors. *Transfusion* 53(8):1645–1652, 2013.

119. Barton J, Barton JC, Bertoli L: Pica associated with iron deficiency or depletion: Clinical and laboratory correlates in 262 non-pregnant adult outpatients. *BMC Blood Disord* 10(1):9, 2010.

120. Olsen EA, Reed KB, Cacchio PB, et al: Iron deficiency in female pattern hair loss, chronic telogen effluvium, and control groups. *J Am Acad Dermatol* 63(6):991–999, 2010.

121. Deloche C, Bastien P, Chadoutaud S, et al: Low iron stores: A risk factor for excessive hair loss in non-menopausal women. *Eur J Dermatol* 17(6):507–512, 2007.

122. Beutler E, Lee P, Gelbart T, et al: The mask mutation identifies TMPRSS6 as an essential suppressor of hepcidin gene expression, required for normal uptake of dietary iron. *ASH Annu Meet Abstr* 110(11):3, 2007.

123. Bessman JD, Feinstein DI: Quantitative anisocytosis as a discriminant between iron deficiency and thalassemia minor. *Blood* 53(2):288–293, 1979.

124. England JM, Ward SM, Down MC: Microcytosis, anisocytosis and the red cell indices in iron deficiency. *Br J Haematol* 34(4):589–597, 1976.

125. Beutler E: The red cell indices in the diagnosis of iron-deficiency anemia. *Ann Intern Med* 50(2):313–322, 1959.

126. Verma V, Ayalew G, Sidhu G, et al: An analysis of the relationship between severe iron deficiency anemia and thrombocytopenia. *Ann Hematol* 1–3, 2014.

127. Dan K: Thrombocytosis in iron deficiency anemia. *Intern Med* 44(10):1025–1026, 2005.

128. Keung YK, Owen J: Iron deficiency and thrombosis: Literature review. *Clin Appl Thromb Hemost* 10(4):387–391, 2004.

129. Geddis AE, Kaushansky K: Cross-reactivity between erythropoietin and thrombopoietin at the level of Mpl does not account for the thrombocytosis seen in iron deficiency. *J Pediatr Hematol Oncol* 25(11):919–920, 2003.

130. Kasper CK, Whissell DY, Wallerstein RO: Clinical aspects of iron deficiency. *JAMA* 191:359–363, 1965.

131. Barron BA, Hoyer JD, Tefferi A: A bone marrow report of absent stainable iron is not diagnostic of iron deficiency. *Ann Hematol* 80(3):166–169, 2001.

132. Thomason RW, Lavelle J, Nelson D, et al: Parenteral iron therapy is associated with a characteristic pattern of iron staining on bone marrow aspirate smears. *Am J Clin Pathol* 128(4):590–593, 2007.

133. Cavill IA: Iron status indicators: Hello new, goodbye old? *Blood* 101(1):372–373, 2003.

134. Ellis LD, Jensen WN, Westerman MP: Marrow iron. An evaluation of depleted stores in a series of 1,332 needle biopsies. *Ann Intern Med* 61:44–49, 1964.

135. Garby L, Irnell L, Werner I: Iron deficiency in women of fertile age in a Swedish community. II. Efficiency of several laboratory tests to predict the response to iron supplementation. *Acta Med Scand* 185(1–2):107–111, 1969.

136. Dale JC, Burritt MF, Zinsmeister AR: Diurnal variation of serum iron, iron-binding capacity, transferrin saturation, and ferritin levels. *Am J Clin Pathol* 117(5):802–808, 2002.

137. Mardell M, Zilva JF: Effect of oral contraceptives on the variations in serum-iron during the menstrual cycle. *Lancet* 2(7530):1323–1325, 1967.

138. Zilva JF, Patston VJ: Variations in serum-iron in healthy women. *Lancet* 1(7435):459–462, 1966.

139. Cartwright GE: The anemia of chronic disorders. *Semin Hematol* 3(4):351–375, 1966.

140. Adamson JW: The anemia of inflammation/malignancy: Mechanisms and management. *Hematology Am Soc Hematol Educ Program* 159–165, 2008.

141. Huang CH, Chang CC, Kuo CL, et al: Serum iron concentration, but not hemoglobin, correlates with TIMI risk score and 6-month left ventricular performance after primary angioplasty for acute myocardial infarction. *PLoS One* 9(8):e104495, 2014.

142. Syrkis I, Machtey I: Hypoferremia in acute myocardial infarction. *J Am Geriatr Soc* 21(1):28–30, 1973.

143. Follezou JY, Bizon M: Cancer chemotherapy induces a transient increase of serum-iron level. *Neoplasma* 33(2):225–231, 1986.

144. Seligman PA, Schleicher RB: Comparison of methods used to measure serum iron in the presence of iron gluconate or iron dextran. *Clin Chem* 45(6 Pt 1):898–901, 1999.

145. Geisser P, Burckhardt S: The pharmacokinetics and pharmacodynamics of iron preparations. *Pharmaceutics* 3(1):12–33, 2011.

146. Cohen LA, Gutierrez L, Weiss A, et al: Serum ferritin is derived primarily from macrophages through a nonclassical secretory pathway. *Blood* 116(9):1574–1584, 2010.

147. Lipschitz DA, Cook JD, Finch CA: A clinical evaluation of serum ferritin as an index of iron stores. *N Engl J Med* 290(22):1213–1216, 1974.

148. Sears DA: Anemia of chronic disease. *Med Clin North Am* 76(3):567–579, 1992.

149. Hansen TM, Hansen NE: Serum ferritin as indicator of iron responsive anaemia in patients with rheumatoid arthritis. *Ann Rheum Dis* 45(7):596–602, 1986.

150. Fishbane S, Kalantar-Zadeh K, Nissenson AR: Serum ferritin in chronic kidney disease: Reconsidering the upper limit for iron treatment. *Semin Dial* 17(5):336–341, 2004.

151. Milman N, Graudal N, Hegnhøj J, et al: Relationships among serum iron status markers, chemical and histochemical liver iron content in 117 patients with alcoholic and non-alcoholic hepatic disease. *Hepatogastroenterology* 41(1):20–24, 1994.

152. Milman N, Graudal N: Serum ferritin in acute viral hepatitis. *Scand J Gastroenterol* 19(1):38–40, 1984.

153. Matzner Y, Konijn AM, Hershko C: Serum ferritin in hematologic malignancies. *Am J Hematol* 9(1):13–22, 1980.

154. Medrano-Engay B, Irun P, Gervas-Arruga J, et al: Iron homeostasis and inflammatory biomarker analysis in patients with type 1 Gaucher disease. *Blood Cells Mol Dis* 53(4):171–175, 2014.

155. Mekinian A, Stirnemann J, Belmatoug N, et al: Ferritinemia during type 1 Gaucher disease: Mechanisms and progression under treatment. *Blood Cells Mol Dis* 49(1):53–57, 2012.

156. Moore C Jr, Ormseth M, Fuchs H: Causes and significance of markedly elevated serum ferritin levels in an academic medical center. *J Clin Rheumatol* 19(6):324–328, 2013.

157. Lehmberg K, McClain KL, Janka GE, Allen CE: Determination of an appropriate cut-off value for ferritin in the diagnosis of hemophagocytic lymphohistiocytosis. *Pediatr Blood Cancer* 61(11):2101–2103, 2014.

158. Mayr R, Janecke AR, Schranz M, et al: Ferroportin disease: A systematic meta-analysis of clinical and molecular findings. *J Hepatol* 53(5):941–949, 2010.

159. Magge H, Sprinz P, Adams WG, et al: Zinc protoporphyrin and iron deficiency screening: Trends and therapeutic response in an urban pediatric center. *JAMA Pediatr* 167(4):361–367, 2013.

160. Mei Z, Parvanta I, Cogswell ME, et al: Erythrocyte protoporphyrin or hemoglobin: Which is a better screening test for iron deficiency in children and women? *Am J Clin Nutr* 77(5):1229–1233, 2003.

161. Braun J: Erythrocyte zinc protoporphyrin. *Kidney Int Suppl* 69:S57–S60, 1999.

162. Hastka J, Lasserre JJ, Schwarzbeck A, et al: Zinc protoporphyrin in anemia of chronic disorders. *Blood* 81(5):1200–1204, 1993.

163. Skikne BS, Flowers CH, Cook JD: Serum transferrin receptor: A quantitative measure of tissue iron deficiency. *Blood* 75(9):1870–1876, 1990.

164. Skikne BS: Serum transferrin receptor. *Am J Hematol* 83(11):872–875, 2008.

165. Pettersson T, Kivivuori SM, Siimes MA: Is serum transferrin receptor useful for detecting iron-deficiency in anaemic patients with chronic inflammatory diseases? *Br J Rheumatol* 33(8):740–744, 1994.

166. Thorpe SJ, Heath A, Sharp G, et al: A WHO reference reagent for the Serum Transferrin Receptor (sTfR): International collaborative study to evaluate a recombinant soluble transferrin receptor preparation. *Clin Chem Lab Med* 48(6):815–820, 2010.

167. Uaprasert N, Rojnuckarin P, Bhokaisawan N, et al: Elevated serum transferrin receptor levels in common types of thalassemia heterozygotes in Southeast Asia: A correlation with genotypes and red cell indices. *Clin Chim Acta* 403(1–2):110–113, 2009.

168. Mockenhaupt FP, May J, Stark K, et al: Serum transferrin receptor levels are increased in asymptomatic and mild *Plasmodium falciparum*-infection. *Haematologica* 84(10):869–873, 1999.

169. Cook JD, Flowers CH, Skikne BS: The quantitative assessment of body iron. *Blood* 101(9):3359–3363, 2003.

170. Skikne BS, Punnonen K, Caldron PH, et al: Improved differential diagnosis of anemia of chronic disease and iron deficiency anemia: A prospective multicenter evaluation of soluble transferrin receptor and the sTfR/log ferritin index. *Am J Hematol* 86(11):923–927, 2011.

171. Suominen P, Punnonen K, Rajamaki A, et al: Serum transferrin receptor and transferrin receptor-ferritin index identify healthy subjects with subclinical iron deficits. *Blood* 92(8):2934–2939, 1998.

172. Punnonen K, Irjala K, Rajamaki A: Serum transferrin receptor and its ratio to serum ferritin in the diagnosis of iron deficiency. *Blood* 89(3):1052–1057, 1997.

173. Brugnara C, Mohandas N: Red cell indices in classification and treatment of anemias: From M. M. Wintrobe's original 1934 classification to the third millennium. *Curr Opin Hematol* 20(3):222–230, 2013.

174. Brugnara C, Schiller B, Moran J: Reticulocyte hemoglobin equivalent (Ret He) and assessment of iron-deficient states. *Clin Lab Haematol* 28(5):303–308, 2006.

175. Bovy C, Gothot A, Krzesinski JM, et al: Mature erythrocyte indices: New markers of iron availability. *Haematologica* 90(4):549–551, 2005.

176. Iolascon A, De FL, Beaumont C: Molecular basis of inherited microcytic anemia due to defects in iron acquisition or heme synthesis. *Haematologica* 94(3):395–408, 2009.

177. Beutler E, West C: Hematologic differences between African-Americans and whites: The roles of iron deficiency and alpha-thalassemia on hemoglobin levels and mean corpuscular volume. *Blood* 106(2):740–745, 2005.

178. Fairbanks VF, Oliveros R, Brandabur JH, et al: Homozygous hemoglobin E mimics beta-thalassemia minor without anemia or hemolysis: Hematologic, functional, and biosynthetic studies of first North American cases. *Am J Hematol* 8(1):109–121, 1980.

179. Fairbanks VF, Gilchrist GS, Brimhall B, et al: Hemoglobin E trait reexamined: A cause of microcytosis and erythrocytosis. *Blood* 53(1):109–115, 1979.

180. Johnson CS, Tegos C, Beutler E: Thalassemia minor: Routine erythrocyte measurements and differentiation from iron deficiency. *Am J Clin Pathol* 80(1):31–36, 1983.

181. Duma H, Efremov G, Sadikario A, et al: Study of nine families with haemoglobin-Lepore. *Br J Haematol* 15(2):161–172, 1968.

182. Cartei G, Chisesi T, Cazzavillan M, et al: Relationship between Hb and HbA2 concentrations in beta-thalassemia trait and effect of iron deficiency anaemia. *Biomedicine (Taipei)* 25(8):282–284, 1976.

183. Infusino I, Braga F, Dolci A, et al: Soluble transferrin receptor (sTfR) and sTfR/log ferritin index for the diagnosis of iron-deficiency anemia. A meta-analysis. *Am J Clin Pathol* 138(5):642–649, 2012.

184. Bregman DB, Morris D, Koch TA, et al: Hepcidin levels predict nonresponsiveness to oral iron therapy in patients with iron deficiency anemia. *Am J Hematol* 88(2):97–101, 2013.

185. Prentice AM, Doherty CP, Abrams SA, et al: Hepcidin is the major predictor of erythrocyte iron incorporation in anemic African children. *Blood* 119(8):1922–1928, 2012.

186. Intragumtornchai T, Rojnukkarin P, Swasdikul D, et al: The role of serum ferritin in the diagnosis of iron deficiency anaemia in patients with liver cirrhosis. *J Intern Med* 243(3):233–241, 1998.

187. Prieto J, Barry M, Sherlock S: Serum ferritin in patients with iron overload and with acute and chronic liver diseases. *Gastroenterology* 68(3):525–533, 1975.

188. Macdougall IC, Hutton RD, Cavill I, et al: Poor response to treatment of renal anaemia with erythropoietin corrected by iron given intravenously. *BMJ* 299(6692):157–158, 1989.

189. Dukkipati R and Kalantar-Zadeh K. Should we limit the ferritin upper threshold to 500 ng/mL in CKD patients? *Nephrol News Issues* 21(1):34–38, 2007.

190. Macdougall IC, Bock AH, Carrera F, et al: FIND-CKD: A randomized trial of intravenous ferric carboxymaltose versus oral iron in patients with chronic kidney disease and iron deficiency anaemia. *Nephrol Dial Transplant* 29(11):2075–2084, 2014.

191. Chung M, Chan JA, Moorthy D, et al: *Biomarkers for Assessing and Managing Iron Deficiency Anemia in Late-Stage Chronic Kidney Disease: Future Research Needs: Identification of Future Research Needs from Comparative Effectiveness Reviews, No. 83 [Internet].*

Agency for Healthcare Research and Quality, Rockville, MD, 2013. Available at: http://www.ncbi.nlm.nih.gov/books/NBK242350/ (last accessed 14 January 2015).

192. Hilal H, McCurdy PR: A pitfall in the interpretation of serum iron values. *Ann Intern MedIntern Med* 66(5):983–988, 1967.

193. Rockey DC: Occult gastrointestinal bleeding. *Gastroenterol Clin North Am* 34(4):699–718, 2005.

194. Hallberg L, Ryttinger L, Solvell L: Side-effects of oral iron therapy. A double-blind study of different iron compounds in tablet form. *Acta Med Scand Suppl* 459:3–10, 1966.

195. Leung AK, Chan KW: Iron deficiency anemia. *Adv Pediatr* 48:385–408, 2001.

196. Gordeuk VR, Brittenham GM, Hughes M, et al: High-dose carbonyl iron for iron deficiency anemia: A randomized double-blind trial. *Am J Clin Nutr* 46(6):1029–1034, 1987.

197. Harding KB, Neufeld LM: Iron deficiency and anemia control for infants and young children in malaria-endemic areas: A call to action and consensus among the research community. *Adv Nutr* 3(4):551–554, 2012.

198. Chang TP, Rangan C: Iron poisoning: A literature-based review of epidemiology, diagnosis, and management. *Pediatr Emerg Care* 27(10):978–985, 2011.

199. Susantitaphong P, Alqahtani F, Jaber BL: Efficacy and safety of intravenous iron therapy for functional iron deficiency anemia in hemodialysis patients: A meta-analysis. *Am J Nephrol* 39(2):130–141, 2014.

200. Taylor JE, Peat N, Porter C, et al: Regular low-dose intravenous iron therapy improves response to erythropoietin in haemodialysis patients. *Nephrol Dial Transplant* 11(6):1079–1083, 1996.

201. Rodgers GM, Auerbach M, Cella D, et al: High-molecular weight iron dextran: A wolf in sheep's clothing. *J Am Soc Nephrol* 19(5):833–834, 2008.

202. Bircher AJ, Auerbach M: Hypersensitivity from intravenous iron products. *Immunol Allergy Clin North Am* 34(3):707–723, 2014.

203. Aslan D, Crain K, Beutler E: A new case of human atransferrinemia with a previously undescribed mutation in the transferrin gene. *Acta Haematol* 118(4):244–247, 2007.

204. Chen C, Wen S, Tan X: Molecular analysis of a novel case of congenital atransferrinemia. *Acta Haematol* 122(1):27–28, 2009.

205. Knisely AS, Gelbart T, Beutler E: Molecular characterization of a third case of human atransferrinemia. *Blood* 104(8):2607, 2004.

206. Shamsian BS, Rezaei N, Arzanian MT, et al: Severe hypochromic microcytic anemia in a patient with congenital atransferrinemia. *Pediatr Hematol Oncol* 26(5):356–362, 2009.

207. Iolascon A, De Falco L: Mutations in the gene encoding DMT1: Clinical presentation and treatment. *Semin Hematol* 46(4):358–370, 2009.

208. Mims MP, Guan Y, Pospisilova D, et al: Identification of a human mutation of DMT1 in a patient with microcytic anemia and iron overload. *Blood* 105(3):1337–1342, 2005.

209. Whitington PF: Gestational alloimmune liver disease and neonatal hemochromatosis. *Semin Liver Dis* 32(4):325–332, 2012.

210. Davis WD Jr, Arrowsmith WR: The treatment of hemochromatosis by massive venesection. *Ann Intern Med* 39(4):723–734, 1953.

211. MacDonald RA: Hemochromatosis: A perlustration. *Am J Clin Nutr* 23(5):592–603, 1970.

212. Feder JN, Gnirke A, Thomas W, et al: A novel MHC class I-like gene is mutated in patients with hereditary haemochromatosis. *Nat Genet* 13(4):399–408, 1996.

213. Beutler E: Iron storage disease: Facts, fiction and progress. *Blood Cells Mol Dis* 39(2):140–147, 2007.

214. Lucotte G, Dieterlen F: A European allele map of the C282Y mutation of hemochromatosis: Celtic versus Viking origin of the mutation? *Blood Cells Mol Dis* 31(2):262–267, 2003.

215. Adams PC, Deugnier Y, Moirand R, et al: The relationship between iron overload, clinical symptoms, and age in 410 patients with genetic hemochromatosis. *Hepatology* 25(1):162–166, 1997.

216. McDonnell SM, Preston BL, Jewell SA, et al: A survey of 2,851 patients with hemochromatosis: Symptoms and response to treatment. *Am J Med* 106(6):619–624, 1999.

217. Waalen J, Felitti V, Gelbart T, et al: Prevalence of hemochromatosis-related symptoms among individuals with mutations in the HFE gene. *Mayo Clin Proc* 77(6):522–530, 2002.

218. Allen KJ, Gurrin LC, Constantine CC, et al: Iron-overload-related disease in HFE hereditary hemochromatosis. *N Engl J Med* 358(3):221–230, 2008.

219. Beutler E: The HFE Cys282Tyr mutation as a necessary but not sufficient cause of clinical hereditary hemochromatosis. *Blood* 101(9):3347–3350, 2003.

220. Rossi E, Olynyk JK, Jeffrey GP: Clinical penetrance of C282Y homozygous HFE hemochromatosis. *Expert Rev Hematol* 1(2):205–216, 2008.

221. Bacon BR, Britton RS: Clinical penetrance of hereditary hemochromatosis. *N Engl J Med* 358(3):291–292, 2008.

222. Fletcher LM, Powell LW: Hemochromatosis and alcoholic liver disease. *Alcohol* 30(2):131–136, 2003.

223. Fletcher LM, Dixon JL, Purdie DM, et al: Excess alcohol greatly increases the prevalence of cirrhosis in hereditary hemochromatosis. *Gastroenterology* 122(2):281–289, 2002.

224. McCord JM: Iron, free radicals, and oxidative injury. *Semin Hematol* 35(1):5–12, 1998.

225. Carthew P, Dorman BM, Edwards RE, et al: A unique rodent model for both the cardiotoxic and hepatotoxic effects of prolonged iron overload. *Lab Invest* 69(2):217–222, 1993.

226. Tsukamoto H, Horne W, Kamimura S, et al: Experimental liver cirrhosis induced by alcohol and iron. *J Clin Invest* 96(1):620–630, 1995.

227. Arosio P, Ingrassia R, Cavadini P: Ferritins: A family of molecules for iron storage, antioxidation and more. *Biochim Biophys Acta* 1790(7):589–599, 2009.

228. Ramos E, Kautz L, Rodriguez R, et al: Evidence for distinct pathways of hepcidin regulation by acute and chronic iron loading in mice. *Hepatology* 53(4):1333–1341, 2011.

229. Bridle KR, Frazer DM, Wilkins SJ, et al: Disrupted hepcidin regulation in HFE-associated haemochromatosis and the liver as a regulator of body iron homoeostasis. *Lancet* 361:669–673, 2003.

230. Nemeth E, Roetto A, Garozzo G, et al: Hepcidin is decreased in TFR2 hemochromatosis. *Blood* 105(4):1803–1806, 2005.

231. Papanikolaou G, Samuels ME, Ludwig EH, et al: Mutations in HFE2 cause iron overload in chromosome 1q-linked juvenile hemochromatosis. *Nat Genet* 36(1):77–82, 2004.

232. Sham RL, Phatak PD, Nemeth E, et al: Hereditary hemochromatosis due to resistance to hepcidin: High hepcidin concentrations in a family with C326S ferroportin mutation. *Blood* 114(2):493–494, 2009.

233. Fernandes A, Preza GC, Phung Y, et al: The molecular basis of hepcidin-resistant hereditary hemochromatosis. *Blood* 114(2):437–443, 2009.

234. Tanno T, Bhanu NV, Oneal PA, et al: High levels of GDF15 in thalassemia suppress expression of the iron regulatory protein hepcidin. *Nat Med* 13(9):1096–1101, 2007.

235. Kautz L, Jung G, Valore EV, et al: Identification of erythroferrone as an erythroid regulator of iron metabolism. *Nat Genet* 46(7):678–684, 2014.

236. Tamary H, Shalev H, Perez-Avraham G, et al: Elevated growth differentiation factor 15 expression in patients with congenital dyserythropoietic anemia type I. *Blood* 112(13):5241–5244, 2008.

237. Casanovas G, Swinkels DW, Altamura S, et al: Growth differentiation factor 15 in patients with congenital dyserythropoietic anaemia (CDA) type II. *J Mol Med (Berl)* 89(8):811–816, 2011.

238. Barton JC, Acton RT, Rivers CA, et al: Genotypic and phenotypic heterogeneity of African Americans with primary iron overload. *Blood Cells Mol Dis* 31(3):310–319, 2003.

239. Sham RL, Phatak PD, West C, et al: Autosomal dominant hereditary hemochromatosis associated with a novel ferroportin mutation and unique clinical features. *Blood Cells Mol Dis* 34(2):157–161, 2005.

240. Porter JB, Garbowski M: The pathophysiology of transfusional iron overload. *Hematol Oncol Clin North Am* 28(4):683–701, vi, 2014.

241. Pietrangelo A: Juvenile hemochromatosis. *J Hepatol* 45(6):892–894, 2006.

242. Anderson LJ: Assessment of iron overload with T2* magnetic resonance imaging. *Prog Cardiovasc Dis* 54(3):287–294, 2011.

243. Herring WB, Gay RM: Absence of stainable bone marrow iron in hemochromatosis. *South Med J* 74(9):1088–1089, 1094, 1981.

244. Camaschella C, Poggiali E: Inherited disorders of iron metabolism. *Curr Opin Pediatr Pediatrics* 23(1):14–20, 2011.

245. Beutler E, Felitti VJ, Ho NJ, et al: Commentary on HFE S65C variant is not associated with increased transferrin saturation in voluntary blood donors by Naveen Arya, Subrata Chakrabrati, Robert A. Hegele, Paul C. Adams. *Blood Cells Mol Dis* 25(6):358–360, 1999.

246. Roetto A, Papanikolaou G, Politou M, et al: Mutant antimicrobial peptide hepcidin is associated with severe juvenile hemochromatosis. *Nat Genet* 33(1):21–22, 2003.

247. Altamura S, Kessler R, Gr+¦ne HJ, et al: Resistance of ferroportin to hepcidin binding causes exocrine pancreatic failure and fatal iron overload. *Cell Metab* 20(2):359–367, 2014.

248. Wallace DF, Harris JM, Subramaniam VN: Functional analysis and theoretical modeling of ferroportin reveals clustering of mutations according to phenotype. *Am J Physiol Cell Physiol* 298(1):C75–C84, 2010.

249. Barton JC, Acton RT, Lee PL, et al: SLC40A1 Q248H allele frequencies and Q248H-associated risk of non-HFE iron overload in persons of sub-Saharan African descent. *Blood Cells Mol Dis* 39(2):206–211, 2007.

250. Rivers CA, Barton JC, Gordeuk VR, et al: Association of ferroportin Q248H polymorphism with elevated levels of serum ferritin in African Americans in the Hemochromatosis and Iron Overload Screening (HEIRS) Study. *Blood Cells Mol Dis* 38(3):247–252, 2007.

251. Girelli D, Trombini P, Busti F, et al: A time course of hepcidin response to iron challenge in patients with HFE and TFR2 hemochromatosis. *Haematologica* 96(4):500–506, 2011.

252. Kawabata H, Fleming RE, Gui D, et al: Expression of hepcidin is down-regulated in TfR2 mutant mice manifesting a phenotype of hereditary hemochromatosis. *Blood* 105(1):376–381, 2005.

253. Camaschella C, Roetto A, Cali A, et al: The gene TFR2 is mutated in a new type of haemochromatosis mapping to 7q22. *Nat Genet* 25(1):14–15, 2000.

254. Huang FW, Babitt JL, Wrighting DM, et al: Hemojuvelin acts as a bone morphogenetic protein co-receptor to regulate hepcidin expression. *ASH Annu Meet Abstr.* 106(11):511, 2005.

255. Niederkofler V, Salie R, Arber S: Hemojuvelin is essential for dietary iron sensing, and its mutation leads to severe iron overload. *J Clin Invest* 115(8):2180–2186, 2005.

256. Huang FW, Pinkus JL, Pinkus GS, et al: A mouse model of juvenile hemochromatosis. *J Clin Invest* 115(8):2187–2191, 2005.

257. Lee PL, Beutler E, Rao SV, et al: Genetic abnormalities and juvenile hemochromatosis: Mutations of the HJV gene encoding hemojuvelin. *Blood* 103(12):4669–4671, 2004.

258. Lanzara C, Roetto A, Daraio F, et al: Spectrum of hemojuvelin gene mutations in 1q-linked juvenile hemochromatosis. *Blood* 103(11):4317–4321, 2004.

259. Steinbicker AU, Bartnikas TB, Lohmeyer LK, et al: Perturbation of hepcidin expression by BMP type I receptor deletion induces iron overload in mice. *Blood* 118(15):4224–4230, 2011.

260. Blanco E, Kannengiesser C, Grandchamp B, et al: Not all DMT1 mutations lead to iron overload. *Blood Cells Mol Dis* 43(2):199–201, 2009.

261. Ganz T, Goff J, Klasing K, et al: IOD in rhinos—immunity group report: Report from the Immunity, Genetics and Toxicology Working Group of the International Workshop on Iron Overload Disorder in Browsing Rhinoceros (February 2011). *J Zoo Wildl Med* 43(3 Suppl):S117–S119, 2012.

262. Yang T, Brittenham GM, Dong WQ, et al: Deferoxamine prevents cardiac hypertrophy and failure in the gerbil model of iron-induced cardiomyopathy. *J Lab Clin Med* 142(5):332–340, 2003.

263. Brittenham GM, Kuryshev YA, Obejero-Paz CA, et al: Yang et al response. *J Lab Clin Med* 141(6):420–422, 2003.

264. Wood JC, Otto-Duessel M, Gonzalez I, et al: Deferasirox and deferiprone remove cardiac iron in the iron-overloaded gerbil. *Transl Res* 148(5):272–280, 2006.

265. Hershko C, Link G, Konijn AM, et al: The iron-loaded gerbil model revisited: Effects of deferoxamine and deferiprone treatment. *J Lab Clin Med* 139(1):50–58, 2002.

266. Zhou XY, Tomatsu S, Fleming RE, et al: HFE gene knockout produces mouse model of hereditary hemochromatosis. *Proc Natl Acad Sci U S A* 95(5):2492–2497, 1998.

267. Donovan A, Lima CA, Pinkus JL, et al: The iron exporter ferroportin/Slc40a1 is essential for iron homeostasis. *Cell Metab* 1(3):191–200, 2005.

268. Lesbordes-Brion JC, Viatte L, Bennoun M, et al: Targeted disruption of the hepcidin 1 gene results in severe hemochromatosis. *Blood* 108(4):1402–1405, 2006.

269. Meynard D, Kautz L, Darnaud V, et al: Lack of the bone morphogenetic protein BMP6 induces massive iron overload. *Nat Genet* 41(4):478–481, 2009.

270. Andriopoulos B, Jr, Corradini E, Xia Y, et al: BMP6 is a key endogenous regulator of hepcidin expression and iron metabolism. *Nat Genet* 41(4):482–487, 2009.

271. Carroll GJ, Breidahl WH, Bulsara MK, et al: Hereditary hemochromatosis is characterized by a clinically definable arthropathy that correlates with iron load. *Arthritis Rheum* 63(1):286–294, 2011.

272. Elmberg M, Hultcrantz R, Simard JF, et al: Increased risk of arthropathies and joint replacement surgery in patients with genetic hemochromatosis: A study of 3,531 patients and their 11,794 first-degree relatives. *Arthritis Care Res (Hoboken)* 65(5):678–685, 2013.

273. Vaiopoulos G, Papanikolaou G, Politou M, et al: Arthropathy in juvenile hemochromatosis. *Arthritis Rheum* 48(1):227–230, 2003.

274. Ko C, Siddaiah N, Berger J, et al: Prevalence of hepatic iron overload and association with hepatocellular cancer in end-stage liver disease: Results from the National Hemochromatosis Transplant Registry. *Liver Int* 27(10):1394–1401, 2007.

275. Ryan CF, Sendi H, Bonkovsky HL: Hepatitis C, porphyria cutanea tarda and liver iron: An update. *Liver Int* 32(6):880–893, 2012.

276. Camaschella C, Roetto A, De GM: Juvenile hemochromatosis. *Semin Hematol* 39(4):242–248, 2002.

277. Bottomley SS: Secondary iron overload disorders. *Semin Hematol* 35(1):77–86, 1998.

278. Jensen PD: Evaluation of iron overload. *Br J Haematol* 124(6):697–711, 2004.

279. Poullis A, Moodie SJ, Ang L, et al: Routine transferrin saturation measurement in liver clinic patients increases detection of hereditary haemochromatosis. *Ann Clin Biochem* 40(Pt 5):521–527, 2003.

280. Yin D, Kulhalli V, Walker AP: Raised serum ferritin concentration in hereditary hyperferritinemia cataract syndrome is not a marker for iron overload. *Hepatology* 59(3):1204–1206, 2014.

281. Brissot P, Bardou-Jacquet E, Jouanolle AM, et al: Iron disorders of genetic origin: A changing world. *Trends Mol Med* 17(12):707–713, 2011.

282. Porter JB: Practical management of iron overload. *Br J Haematol* 115(2):239–252, 2001.

283. Hoffbrand AV, Taher A, Cappellini MD: How I treat transfusional iron overload. *Blood* 120(18):3657–3669, 2012.

284. Ogimoto M, Anzai K, Takenoshita H, et al: Criteria for early identification of aceruloplasminemia. *Intern Med* 50(13):1415–1418, 2011.

285. Grandchamp B, Hetet G, Kannengiesser C, et al: A novel type of congenital hypochromic anemia associated with a nonsense mutation in the STEAP3/TSAP6 gene. *Blood* 118(25):6660–6666, 2011.

CHAPTER 44
ANEMIA RESULTING FROM OTHER NUTRITIONAL DEFICIENCIES

Ralph Green

SUMMARY

The anemia that results from deficiencies of vitamin B_{12}, folic acid (Chap. 41) or iron (Chap. 43) are, in general, clearly defined and are relatively common. In contrast, characteristics of anemia that may occur with deficiencies of the other vitamins and minerals are poorly defined and relatively rare in humans. When present, they usually exist not as isolated deficiencies of one vitamin or one mineral, but rather, as a combination of deficiencies resulting from malnutrition or malabsorption. In this context, it is difficult to deduce which abnormalities are the result of which deficiency. Studies in experimental animals may not accurately reflect the role of micronutrients in humans. Accordingly, our knowledge of the effects of many micronutrients on hematopoiesis is fragmentary and based on clinical observations and interpretations that may be flawed. Inborn metabolic errors that affect single micronutrient pathways may shed light on specific effects of those micronutrients on hematopoiesis. Daily requirements of some micronutrients are available at: http://www.nal.usda.gov/fnic/dga/rda.pdf, and levels normally found in serum, red cells, and leukocytes are shown in Table 44–1.

● VITAMIN-DEFICIENCY ANEMIAS

VITAMIN A DEFICIENCY

Chronic deprivation of vitamin A results in anemia similar to that observed in iron deficiency.[1–4] Mean corpuscular volume (MCV) and mean corpuscular hemoglobin concentration (MCHC) are reduced. Anisocytosis and poikilocytosis may be present, and serum iron levels are low. Unlike iron-deficiency anemia, but similar to anemia of chronic disease, iron stores in the liver and marrow are increased, serum transferrin concentration usually is normal or decreased, and administration of medicinal iron does not correct the anemia. However, there is some evidence to suggest that vitamin A deficiency may result in impaired iron absorption or utilization[5] and this may be mediated through effects on the expression of genes involved in the regulation of intestinal iron absorption.[6] The suggestion that vitamin A may facilitate iron absorption[7] was not confirmed.[8] Supplementation with vitamin A alone may ameliorate the anemia, although coadministration of vitamin A and iron resulted in a better response than with either nutrient alone.[9]

Surveys conducted in developing countries suggest that vitamin A deficiency represents a public health problem among infants, schoolchildren and women of childbearing age.[10,11] The prevalence of vitamin A deficiency closely coincides with the prevalence of iron deficiency in this demographic setting. However, there is no known causal relationship between the two nutrients beyond both occurring in a setting of generalized malnutrition. Although vitamin A deficiency is recognized to occur in the United States, the relationship between it and anemia is not known.

DEFICIENCIES OF MEMBERS OF THE VITAMIN B GROUP

Isolated nutritional deficiencies of members of the vitamin B group, with the exception of folic acid and vitamin B_{12}, are very uncommon in humans. Evidence linking isolated nutritional deficiencies of pyridoxine, riboflavin, pantothenic acid, and niacin to anemia in patients is inconclusive. In animals, experimentally induced deficiency states are more commonly associated with hematologic abnormalities.

Vitamin B_6 Deficiency

Vitamin B_6 includes pyridoxal, pyridoxine, and pyridoxamine. These components are converted to pyridoxal 5-phosphate, which acts as a coenzyme in decarboxylation and transamination of amino acids and synthesis of aminolevulinic acid, the porphyrin precursor (Chap. 58). Vitamin B_6 deficiency induced in infants is associated with a hypochromic microcytic anemia.[12] A malnourished patient with a hypochromic anemia who failed to respond to iron therapy but subsequently responded to administration of vitamin B_6 has been described.[13] In some anemic pregnant women who did not respond to iron supplementation alone, vitamin B_6 administration resulted in subsequent improvement in hemoglobin level.[14] Occasionally, patients receiving therapy with antituberculosis agents, such as isoniazid, which interfere with vitamin B_6 metabolism, develop a microcytic anemia that can be corrected with large doses of pyridoxine.[15] Pyridoxine is usually prescribed with isoniazid to prevent such an effect. Some patients with sideroblastic anemias (Chap. 59) respond to administration of large doses of pyridoxine, but these patients are not deficient in this vitamin. A review of more than 200 patients with acquired sideroblastic anemia reported that fewer than 7 percent showed greater than 1.5 g/dL improvement in hemoglobin concentration with pyridoxine treatment.[16] Pyridoxine is involved in many metabolic processes. Derangements in these pathways, sometimes involving anemia, are usually the result of inborn errors affecting the pathways of vitamin B_6 metabolism and specific pyridoxal phosphate-dependent enzymes or inborn errors that lead to accumulation of small molecules that react with pyridoxal phosphate and inactivate it.[17] Other acquired conditions that may influence pyridoxine metabolism include drugs that react with pyridoxal phosphate or affect metabolism, malabsorptive states such as celiac disease, and renal dialysis which leads to increased loss of vitamin B_6 vitamers from the circulation as these vitamers are bound to plasma albumin.[18]

Riboflavin Deficiency

Riboflavin deficiency results in a decrease in red cell glutathione reductase activity because this enzyme requires flavin adenine dinucleotide for activation. Glutathione reductase deficiency, induced by riboflavin deficiency, is not associated with hemolytic anemia or increased susceptibility to oxidant-induced injury (Chap. 47).[19] Human volunteers maintained on a semisynthetic riboflavin-deficient diet and fed the riboflavin antagonist, galactoflavin, developed pure red cell aplasia.[20] Vacuolated erythroid precursors are evident prior to the development of aplasia. This anemia is reversed specifically by administration of riboflavin. It

TABLE 44–1. Blood Vitamin and Mineral Levels (Adult Values)

Vitamin or Mineral	Serum Level	Plasma Level	Red Cell Level	White Cell Level
Copper	11–24 μmol/L		14–24 μmol/L	
Folate	7–45 nmol/L		>320 nmol/L	
Riboflavin (B$_2$)	110–640 nmol/L		265–1350 nmol/L	
Vitamin A	1–3 μmol/L			
Vitamin B$_6$		20–122 nmol/L		
Vitamin C		25–85 μmol/L		11–30 attomol/cell
Vitamin E	12–40 μmol/L			
Selenium	1200–2000 nmol/L			
Zinc	11–18 μmol/L			

Data from Burtis CA and Ashwood EF: *Tietz Textbook of Clinical Chemistry*, 3rd ed. Philadelphia, PA: WB Saunders,1999.

has been suggested that riboflavin deficiency causes anemia,[21] possibly by interfering with iron release from ferritin.[20] Although the relationship between dietary riboflavin deficiency and anemia is not clear, inadequate riboflavin intake increased the risk of anemia in Chinese adults and was associated with a high probability of anemia when iron intake was low.[16] Thus, poor riboflavin status may interfere with iron handling and contribute to the etiology of anemia when iron intake is low. There is also some evidence to suggest that riboflavin may exert its effects secondarily on other nutrients, such as folate and cobalamin.[22]

Pantothenic Acid Deficiency

Pantothenic acid deficiency, when artificially induced in humans, is not associated with anemia.[23]

Niacin Deficiency

Pellagra (niacin deficiency) is associated with anemia, which responds to treatment with niacin.[24] However, it is not clear whether the anemia is a direct or indirect effect of niacin deficiency.

Thiamine Deficiency

Megaloblastic anemia, responsive to thiamine, occurs in a childhood syndrome in association with diabetes and sensorineural deafness. There is usually profound anemia, megaloblastic changes with or without ringed sideroblasts in the marrow, and occasionally thrombocytopenia.[25] Most cases have been reported in patients of Middle and Far Eastern descent. The underlying defect in this condition is in the high-affinity thiamine transporter, which primarily affects synthesis of nucleic acid ribose via the nonoxidative branch of the pentose cycle.[26] This decrease in ribose synthesis is a consequence of the thiamine-dependent pentose-cycle enzyme transketolase. Reduced nucleic acid production through impaired transketolase catalysis appears to be the underlying biochemical disturbance that likely induces cell-cycle arrest or apoptosis in marrow cells and leads to thiamine-responsive megaloblastic anemia syndrome in these patients, which responds to lifelong administration of oral thiamine (25 to 100 mg/day). The *SLC19A2* gene on chromosome 1q23.3 is implicated in all cases of thiamine-responsive megaloblastic anemia.[27] The folate carriers and thiamine transporters evolved from the same family of solute carriers.[28]

VITAMIN C (ASCORBIC ACID) DEFICIENCY

Although approximately 80 percent of patients with scurvy[29] are anemic, attempts to induce anemia in human volunteers by severely restricting

dietary ascorbic acid have been unsuccessful.[30] Anemia observed in subjects with scurvy is not simply the result of a deficiency of ascorbic acid, but rather a result of bleeding or deficiency of folic acid.[29] Human subjects with scurvy and megaloblastic anemia fail to correct their anemia with vitamin C administration if they are maintained on a folic acid–deficient diet. When folic acid is given to these patients in a dose of 50 mcg/day orally, a prompt hematologic response is observed.[31]

Ascorbic acid, in common with other compounds that contribute to cellular reducing potential, participates in maintenance of dihydrofolate reductase in its reduced, or active, form. Impaired dihydrofolate reductase activity results in an inability to form tetrahydrofolic acid, the metabolically active form of folic acid (Chap. 41). Patients with scurvy and megaloblastic anemia excrete 10-formylfolic acid as the major urinary folate metabolite. Following ascorbic acid therapy, 5-methyltetrahydrofolic acid becomes the major urinary folate metabolite. This observation has led to the suggestion that ascorbic acid prevents the irreversible oxidation of methyltetrahydrofolic acid to formylfolic acid.[32] Failure to synthesize tetrahydrofolic acid or protect it from oxidation ultimately results in megaloblastic anemia. Under these circumstances, ascorbic acid therapy produces a hematologic response only if enough folic acid is present to interact with the ascorbic acid.[33] Dietary iron deficiency in children often occurs in association with dietary ascorbic acid deficiency. Iron balance may be compromised by ascorbic acid deficiency because this vitamin serves to facilitate intestinal iron absorption by maintaining iron in a more soluble reduced or ferrous (Fe^{2+}) state. Patients with scurvy, particularly children, may require both iron and vitamin C to correct hypochromic microcytic anemia.[34] Vitamin C affects the oxidoreduction involved in compartmental iron release and may stimulate iron mobilization from endosomes, as well as transferrin-dependent iron uptake. Scurvy itself may cause iron deficiency as a consequence of external bleeding. In patients with iron overload from repeated blood transfusions, the level of vitamin C in leukocytes is often decreased because of rapid conversion of ascorbate to oxalate.[35] Deferoxamine (desferrioxamine)-induced iron excretion is diminished when stores of vitamin C are reduced, but excretion returns to expected values with vitamin C supplementation.[36,37] Large doses of ascorbic acid may be harmful in patients with iron overload and should be given only after an infusion of deferoxamine mesylate (Desferal) has been initiated (Chap. 43). The presence of scurvy in patients with iron overload may protect them from tissue damage.[38] In scorbutic guinea pigs and Bantu subjects with nutritional vitamin C deficiency and dietary hemosiderosis, iron accumulates in the monocyte-macrophage system rather than in the parenchymal cells of the liver.[39,40]

VITAMIN E DEFICIENCY

Vitamin E, α-tocopherol, is a fat-soluble vitamin that appears to be an antioxidant in humans. It is not an essential cofactor in any recognized reactions. Nutritional deficiency of vitamin E in humans is extremely uncommon because of the widespread occurrence of α-tocopherol in food. The daily requirement of d-α-tocopherol for adults ranges from 5 to 7 mg, but this requirement varies with the polyunsaturated fatty acid content of the diet and the content of peroxidizable lipids in tissues. Hematologic manifestations of vitamin E deficiency in humans are limited to the neonatal period and to pathologic states associated with chronic fat malabsorption.

Low-birthweight infants are born with low serum and tissue concentrations of vitamin E. When these infants are fed a diet unusually rich in polyunsaturated fatty acids and inadequate in vitamin E, hemolytic anemia frequently develops by 4 to 6 weeks of age, particularly if iron is also present in the diet.[41] This anemia often is associated with morphologic alterations of the erythrocytes,[42] thrombocytosis, and edema of the dorsum of the feet and pretibial area.[43] Treatment with vitamin E produces a prompt increase in hemoglobin level, a decrease in the elevated reticulocyte count, normalization of red cell life span, and disappearance of thrombocytosis and edema. Modifications of infant formulas have all but eliminated vitamin E deficiency in preterm infants.[44]

Vitamin E deficiency is common in patients with cystic fibrosis who are not receiving daily supplements of a water-soluble form of the vitamin.[45] Red cell life span in such patients is shortened to an average chromium-51 (^{51}Cr) half-life of 19 days (normal: approximately 30 days). Severe anemia may be present.[45] After vitamin E therapy, red cell half-life increases to 27.5 days.[46]

Pharmacologic doses of vitamin E have been employed with apparent success in the absence of vitamin deficiency to compensate for genetic defects that limit erythrocyte defense against oxidant injury. Chronic administration of oral vitamin E 400 to 800 U/day lengthened red cell life span in some,[47,48] but not all,[49] studies of patients with hereditary hemolytic anemias associated with glutathione synthetase deficiency or glucose-6-phosphate dehydrogenase deficiency.

Administration of vitamin E (450 U/day for 6 to 36 weeks) to patients with sickle cell anemia significantly reduced the number of irreversibly sickled erythrocytes.[50] Adult patients with sickle cell anemia have been reported to have significantly lower serum tocopherol values compared with normal controls,[51,52] and in children with sickle cell anemia, those with vitamin E deficiency have significantly more irreversibly sickled cells than did children without vitamin E deficiency.[53]

● TRACE METAL DEFICIENCY

COPPER DEFICIENCY

Copper is present in a number of metalloproteins. Cytochrome c oxidase, dopamine β-hydroxylase, urate oxidase, tyrosine and lysyl oxidase, ascorbic acid oxidase, and superoxide dismutase (erythrocuprein) are cuproenzymes. More than 90 percent of copper in the blood is carried bound to ceruloplasmin, an α_2-globulin with ferroxidase activity. Copper is required for absorption and utilization of iron. Copper, in the form of hephaestin,[54] converts iron to the ferric (Fe^{3+}) state for its transport by transferrin.

Copper deficiency has been described in malnourished children,[55] and in both infants and adults receiving parenteral alimentation.[56-58] There is increasing recognition of copper deficiency associated with anemia occurring as a complication following gastric resection or bariatric gastric reduction surgery.[59] Copper deficiency is characterized by anemia, often macrocytic, that is unresponsive to iron therapy; hypoferremia; neutropenia; and, usually, the presence of vacuolated erythroid and granulocytic precursors in marrow.[57-60] The mechanism of neutropenia remains unknown, but there is some evidence that copper deficiency results in inhibition of differentiation and self-renewal of CD34(+) hematopoietic progenitor cells.[61,62] Iron-containing plasma cells, a decrease in granulocyte precursors and ring sideroblasts have also been reported.[59,60] Consequently, copper deficiency should enter the differential diagnosis in patients with features of myelodysplastic syndrome, particularly if there is a history of previous gastric surgery (Chap. 87).[60]

Copper deficiency should be considered in the differential diagnosis of a patient with anemia and associated myeloneuropathy suspected of having cobalamin deficiency with subacute combined degeneration of the spinal cord; neurologic findings, most commonly the result of myeloneuropathy, are frequently present.[63,64]

Radiologic abnormalities generally are present in infants and young children with copper deficiency. These abnormalities include osteoporosis, flaring of the anterior ribs with spontaneous rib fractures, cupping and flaring of long-bone metaphyses with spur formation and submetaphyseal fractures, and epiphyseal separation. These changes are frequently misinterpreted as signs of scurvy.

Copper deficiency with resultant microcytic anemia can be produced by chronic ingestion of massive quantities of zinc. This has been reported in patients using excessive quantities of zinc-containing dental fixatives.[65,66] Dietary zinc in large doses leads to copper deficiency by impairing copper absorption.[67,68]

The diagnosis of copper deficiency can be established by demonstrating a low serum ceruloplasmin or serum copper level, but the copper level is thought to be more reliable because ceruloplasmin behaves as an acute-phase protein.[59] Adequate normal values for the first 2 to 3 months of life are not well defined and normally are lower than the levels observed later in life. Despite these limitations, a serum copper level less than 70 mcg/dL (11 μmol/L) or ceruloplasmin level less than 15 mg/dL after age 1 or 2 months can be regarded as evidence of copper deficiency. In later infancy, childhood, and adulthood, serum copper values should normally exceed 70 mcg/dL. Low serum copper values may be observed in hypoproteinemic states, such as exudative enteropathies and nephrosis, and Wilson disease. In these circumstances, a diagnosis of copper deficiency cannot be established by serum measurements alone but requires analysis of liver copper content or clinical response after a therapeutic trial of copper supplementation.

Copper-deficiency anemia and neutropenia are quickly corrected by administration of copper. Treatment of copper-deficient infants consists of administration of approximately 2.5 mg of copper (approximately 80 mcg/kg per day) oral supplementation as a copper sulfate solution.[69] Intravenous bolus injection of copper chloride also has been used.[60]

ZINC DEFICIENCY

Zinc is required for a large number of zinc metalloenzymes, zinc-activated enzymes, and "zinc finger" transcription factors. Zinc deficiency occurs in a variety of pathologic states in humans, including hemolytic anemias such as thalassemia[70] and sickle cell anemia.[71] Zinc deficiency with or without an associated copper deficiency has been described in a patient receiving intensive desferrioxamine therapy[72] and in patients with decreased renal reabsorption of trace minerals.[73]

Although human zinc deficiency may produce growth retardation, impaired wound healing, impaired taste perception, immunologic abnormalities, and acrodermatitis enteropathica, at present there is no evidence that isolated zinc deficiency produces anemia.

SELENIUM DEFICIENCY

Selenium deficiency occurs in patients who live in areas where the selenium content of the soil is very low[74] and has been observed in patients receiving total parenteral nutrition.[75,76] Although this results in a striking decrease in the level of red cell glutathione peroxidase, there do not appear to be any adverse hematologic consequences.

An examination of the relationship between serum selenium and hematologic indices found that low serum selenium was independently associated with anemia among older men and women in the United States.[77] A similar association has been reported in adolescent girls living in rural Vietnam.[78]

● ANEMIA OF STARVATION

Studies conducted during World War II among prisoners of war and conscientious objectors demonstrated that semistarvation for 24 weeks can result in a mild to moderate normocytic normochromic anemia.[79] Marrow cellularity is usually reduced and is accompanied by a decreased erythroid-to-myeloid ratio. Measurements of red cell volume and plasma volume suggest that dilution is a major factor responsible for a reduction in hemoglobin concentration.

In persons subjected to complete starvation, either for experimental purposes or treatment of severe obesity, anemia was not observed during the first 2 to 9 weeks of fasting.[80] Starvation for 9 to 17 weeks produced a decrease in hemoglobin and marrow hypocellularity.[81] Resumption of a normal diet was accompanied by reticulocytosis and the disappearance of anemia. It has been suggested that the anemia of starvation is a response to a hypometabolic state with its attendant decrease in oxygen requirements.[82]

● ANEMIA OF PROTEIN DEFICIENCY (KWASHIORKOR)

Even strict vegetarians do not seem to develop hematologic problems related to the absence of animal proteins.[83] Vegans may, however, develop vitamin B_{12} deficiency.[84] The anemia in this situation is caused by cobalamin insufficiency rather than animal protein insufficiency, and results from the natural occurrence of cobalamin exclusively in foods of animal origin. Kwashiorkor is largely a disease of the underdeveloped world, but occasionally is seen even among the children of educated and well-to-do parents when the children are fed an inappropriate diet.[85,86]

In infants and children with protein-calorie malnutrition, hemoglobin concentration may fall to 8 g/dL of blood,[86,87] but some children with kwashiorkor have normal hemoglobin levels, probably because of a decreased plasma volume. The anemia is normocytic and normochromic, but the size and shape of red cells on blood film vary considerably. White blood cells and platelets are usually normal. Marrow is cellular or slightly hypocellular, with a reduced erythroid-to-myeloid ratio. Erythroblastopenia, reticulocytopenia, and marrow containing a few giant pronormoblasts may be found, particularly if the child has an infection. With treatment of the infection, erythroid precursors may appear in the marrow, and reticulocyte count may rise. When nutrition is improved by giving high-protein diets (powdered milk or essential amino acids), reticulocytosis, a slight fall in hematocrit because of hemodilution, and then rises in hemoglobin level occurs. Improvement is very slow, however, and during the third or fourth week, when patients are clinically improved and serum protein levels are approaching normal, another episode of erythroid marrow aplasia may develop. This relapse is not associated with infection, does not respond to antibiotics, and does not remit spontaneously. It may respond to either riboflavin or prednisone.

An abrupt fall in hemoglobin following protein feeding may be an ominous harbinger of an adverse and even fatal outcome and prompt transfusion to restore hemoglobin may be life-saving.[87] It has been suggested that erythroblastic aplasia may be a manifestation of riboflavin deficiency.[88]

Although plasma volume is reduced to a variable degree in children with kwashiorkor, total circulating red cell volume decreases in proportion to a decrease in lean body mass as protein deprivation reduces metabolic demands. During repletion, an increase in plasma volume may occur before an increase in red cell volume, and anemia may seem to become more severe despite reticulocytosis. In a report from Turkey of patients with protein-energy malnutrition, the major cause of anemia was identified as associated with either iron deficiency or defective utilization of iron.[89]

From study of anemia of protein deficiency in rats, it was deduced that oxygen consumption and, therefore, erythropoietin production are reduced.[90] Other studies confirmed this observation but related the reduction to calorie deprivation with associated decrease in blood levels of triiodothyronine (T_3) and thyroxine (T_4). As a result, erythropoiesis decreases and reticulocyte count falls. Plasma iron turnover and red cell uptake of radioactive iron are markedly reduced, and red cell volume gradually declines.[90] Protein deficiency also produces a maturation block at the erythroblast level and slight decrease in the erythropoietin-sensitive progenitor cell pool.[91] If exogenous erythropoietin is provided, normal erythropoiesis is restored despite protein depletion,[92] an observation that explains the successful use of starved rats in a bioassay for erythropoietin.

Anemia seen in anorexia nervosa shows some features that resemble protein energy malnutrition. Anemia and leukopenia are found in approximately one-third of patients, and 50 percent of these show marrow atrophy with gelatinous transformation of the marrow stroma.[93]

● ALCOHOLISM

Chronic alcohol ingestion is often associated with anemia. This anemia may result from nutritional deficiencies, chronic gastrointestinal bleeding, hepatic dysfunction, or direct toxic effects of alcohol on erythropoiesis. Quite commonly, all these factors work in concert to produce anemia. Pyridoxal phosphate and folate deficiency are common in alcoholics.[94] Alcohol affects not only red cells, as described here, but also platelet production (Chap. 113).[95,96]

Macrocytosis is common in chronic alcoholics[97] and is often associated with megaloblastic anemia. Among hospitalized malnourished alcoholics, it is the most common type of anemia, occurring alone or in combination with ringed sideroblasts in approximately 40 percent of patients.[98,99] In contrast, megaloblastic anemia is rarely observed in nonhospitalized chronic alcoholics or relatively well-nourished subjects admitted to the hospital for alcohol withdrawal.[100] Anemia, when associated with megaloblastic marrow changes in alcoholics, almost always results from folate deficiency. Iron deficiency often is associated with folate deficiency in alcoholics.[100] In patients with both nutritional deficiencies, the blood film is "dimorphic," with macrocytes, hypersegmented neutrophils, and hypochromic microcytes. This is also the case when folate deficiency coexists with a sideroblastic process.[98,99] Consequently, the MCV may be normal but, because of marked anisopoikilocytosis, the red cell distribution width (RDW) is elevated.[64] Although liver disease is frequently present in alcoholics with megaloblastic anemia, it is not responsible for the folate deficiency. Megaloblastic anemia occurs almost exclusively in alcoholics who have been eating poorly. It is seen more commonly in heavy drinkers of wine and whiskey, which contain little or no folate, than in drinkers of beer, which is a rich source of the vitamin.

In addition to folate deficiency, chronic alcoholics frequently demonstrate multiple other micronutrient deficiencies, including thiamine, pyridoxine, and vitamin A, which aggravate the risk of anemia.[101] Although decreased dietary folate intake appears to be a necessary factor in the etiology of the megaloblastic anemia, ethanol itself interferes with folate metabolism (Chap. 41).[102,103]

Macrocytosis, however, does not always indicate the presence of megaloblastic anemia,[97] reticulocytosis secondary to hemolysis or bleeding, or liver disease. So-called macrocytosis of alcoholism is found in as many as 96 percent of alcoholics.[104] In these patients, the macrocytosis usually is mild, with MCV in the range of 100 to 110 fL, and anemia is usually absent. In the blood film, macrocytes are typically round rather than oval and neutrophil hypersegmentation is not present. The macrocytosis persists until the patient abstains from alcohol. Even then, MCV does not become completely normal for a period of 2 to 4 months in view of the life span of erythrocytes.[103]

Alcohol ingestion for 5 to 7 days produces vacuolization of early red cell precursors, and formation of vacuoles can be observed in *in vitro* marrow cell cultures.[99,105] These changes disappear promptly when alcohol ingestion is discontinued. Vacuolization with a similar appearance occurs in subjects who are fed a phenylalanine-deficient diet, patients treated with chloramphenicol or pyrazinamide, patients in hyperosmolar coma, and individuals deficient in copper or riboflavin.[104]

Two relatively uncommon hematologic complications of alcoholism are Zieve syndrome,[106,107] consisting of alcohol-induced liver disease, often hyperlipidemia, jaundice, and transient spherocytic hemolytic anemia; and spur cell hemolytic anemia, associated with severe alcohol-induced liver disease often requiring hepatic transplantation for resolution.[108,109] Chapter 45 discusses these syndromes.

REFERENCES

1. Blackfan KD, Wolbach SB: Vitamin A deficiency in infants, a clinical and pathological study. *J Pediatr* 3:679–706, 1933.
2. Vitamin A and iron deficiency. *Nutr Rev* 47(4):119–121, 1989.
3. Majia LA, Hodges RE, Arroyave G, et al: Vitamin A deficiency and anemia in Central American children. *Am J Clin Nutr* 30(7):1175–1184, 1977.
4. Hodges RE, Sauberlich HE, Canham JE, et al: Hematopoietic studies in vitamin A deficiency. *Am J Clin Nutr* 31(5):876–885, 1978.
5. Lynch S: Influence of infection/inflammation, thalassemia and nutritional status on iron absorption. *Int J Vitam Nutr Res* 77(3):217–223, 2007.
6. Citelli M, Bittencourt LL, da Silva SV, et al: Vitamin A modulates the expression of genes involved in iron bioavailability. *Biol Trace Elem Res* 149(1):64–70, 2012.
7. Kolsteren P, Rahman SR, Hilderbrand K, et al: Treatment for iron deficiency anaemia with a combined supplementation of iron, vitamin A and zinc in women of Dinajpur, Bangladesh. *Eur J Clin Nutr* 53(2):102–106, 1999.
8. Walczyk T, Davidsson L, Rossander-Hulthen L, et al: No enhancing effect of vitamin A on iron absorption in humans. *Am J Clin Nutr* 77(1):144–149, 2003.
9. Mejia LA, Chew F: Hematological effect of supplementing anemic children with vitamin A alone and in combination with iron. *Am J Clin Nutr* 48(3):595–600, 1988.
10. Calis JC, Phiri KS, Faragher EB, et al: Severe anemia in Malawian children. *N Engl J Med* 358(9):888–899, 2008.
11. Tatala SR, Kihamia CM, Kyungu LH, et al: Risk factors for anaemia in schoolchildren in Tanga Region, Tanzania. *Tanzan J Health Res* 10(4):189–202, 2008.
12. Snyderman SE, Holt LE Jr, Carretero R, et al: Pyridoxine deficiency in the human infant. *J Clin Nutr* 1(3):200–207, 1953.
13. Foy H, Kondi A: Hypochromic anemias of the tropics associated with pyridoxine and nicotinic acid deficiency. *Blood* 13(11):1054–1062, 1958.
14. Hisano M, Suzuki R, Sago H, et al: Vitamin B6 deficiency and anemia in pregnancy. *Eur J Clin Nutr* 64(2):221–223, 2010.
15. McCurdy PR, Donohoe RF, Magovern M: Reversible sideroblastic anemia caused by pyrazinoic acid (Pyrazinamide). *Ann Intern Med* 64(6):1280–1284, 1966.
16. Baumann Kreuziger LM, Wolanskyj AP, Hanson CA, et al: Lack of efficacy of pyridoxine (vitamin B6) treatment in acquired idiopathic sideroblastic anaemia, including refractory anaemia with ring sideroblasts. *Eur J Haematol* 86(6):512–516, 2011.
17. Clayton PT: B6-responsive disorders: A model of vitamin dependency. *J Inherit Metab Dis* 29(2–3):317–326, 2006.
18. Anderson BB, Newmark PA, Rawlins M, et al: Plasma binding of vitamin B6 compounds. *Nature* 250(5466):502–504, 1974.
19. Beutler E, Srivastava SK: Relationship between glutathione reductase activity and drug-induced haemolytic anaemia. *Nature* 226(5247):759–760, 1970.
20. Lane M, Alfrey CP Jr: The anemia of human riboflavin deficiency. *Blood* 25:432–442, 1965.
21. Foy H, Kondi A: A case of true red cell aplastic anaemia successfully treated with riboflavin. *J Pathol Bacteriol* 65(2):559–564, 1953.
22. Powers HJ: Riboflavin (vitamin B-2) and health. *Am J Clin Nutr* 77(6):1352–1360, 2003.
23. Hodges RE, Bean WB, Ohlson MA, et al: Human pantothenic acid deficiency produced by omega-methyl pantothenic acid. *J Clin Invest* 38(8):1421–1425, 1959.
24. Spivak JL, Jackson DL: Pellagra: An analysis of 18 patients and a review of the literature. *Johns Hopkins Med J* 140(6):295–309, 1977.
25. Bay A, Keskin M, Hizli S, et al: Thiamine-responsive megaloblastic anemia syndrome. *Int J Hematol* 92(3):524–526, 2010.
26. Boros LG, Steinkamp MP, Fleming JC, et al: Defective RNA ribose synthesis in fibroblasts from patients with thiamine-responsive megaloblastic anemia (TRMA). *Blood* 102(10):3556–3561, 2003.
27. Beshlawi I, Al Zadjali S, Bashir W, et al: Thiamine responsive megaloblastic anemia: The puzzling phenotype. *Pediatr Blood Cancer* 61(3):528–531, 2014.
28. Zhao R, Goldman ID: Folate and thiamine transporters mediated by facilitative carriers (SLC19A1-3 and SLC46A1) and folate receptors. *Mol Aspects Med* 34(2–3):373–385, 2013.
29. Reuler JB, Broudy VC, Cooney TG: Adult scurvy. *JAMA* 253(6):805–807, 1985.
30. Hodges RE, Baker EM, Hood J, et al: Experimental scurvy in man. *Am J Clin Nutr* 22(5):535–548, 1969.
31. Zalusky R, Herbert V: Megaloblastic anemia in scurvy with response to 50 microgm. of folic acid daily. *N Engl J Med* 265:1033–1038, 1961.
32. Stokes PL, Melikian V, Leeming RL, et al: Folate metabolism in scurvy. *Am J Clin Nutr* 28(2):126–129, 1975.
33. Cox EV, Meynell MJ, Northam BE, et al: The anaemia of scurvy. *Am J Med* 42(2):220–227, 1967.
34. Clark NG, Sheard NF, Kelleher JF: Treatment of iron-deficiency anemia complicated by scurvy and folic acid deficiency. *Nutr Rev* 50(5):134–137, 1992.
35. Wapnick AA, Lynch SR, Krawitz P, et al: Effects of iron overload on ascorbic acid metabolism. *Br Med J* 3(5620):704–707, 1968.
36. Wapnick AA, Lynch SR, Charlton RW, et al: The effect of ascorbic acid deficiency on desferrioxamine-induced urinary iron excretion. *Br J Haematol* 17(6):563–568, 1969.
37. Chapman RW, Hussain MA, Gorman A, et al: Effect of ascorbic acid deficiency on serum ferritin concentration in patients with beta-thalassaemia major and iron overload. *J Clin Pathol* 35(5):487–491, 1982.
38. Cohen A, Cohen IJ, Schwartz E: Scurvy and altered iron stores in thalassemia major. *N Engl J Med* 304(3):158–160, 1981.
39. Lipschitz DA, Bothwell TH, Seftel HC, et al: The role of ascorbic acid in the metabolism of storage iron. *Br J Haematol* 20(2):155–163, 1971.
40. Bothwell TH, Abrahams C, Bradlow BA, et al: Idiopathic and Bantu Hemochromatosis. Comparative Histological Study. *Arch Pathol* 79:163–168, 1965.
41. Williams ML, Shoot RJ, O'Neal PL, et al: Role of dietary iron and fat on vitamin E deficiency anemia of infancy. *N Engl J Med* 292(17):887–890, 1975.
42. Oski FA, Barness LA: Hemolytic anemia in vitamin E deficiency. *Am J Clin Nutr* 21(1):45–50, 1968.
43. Ritchie JH, Fish MB, McMasters V, et al: Edema and hemolytic anemia in premature infants. A vitamin E deficiency syndrome. *N Engl J Med* 279(22):1185–1190, 1968.
44. Zipursky A: Vitamin E deficiency anemia in newborn infants. *Clin Perinatol* 11(2):393–402, 1984.
45. Wilfond BS, Farrell PM, Laxova A, et al: Severe hemolytic anemia associated with vitamin E deficiency in infants with cystic fibrosis. Implications for neonatal screening. *Clin Pediatr (Phila)* 33(1):2–7, 1994.
46. Farrell PM, Bieri JG, Fratantoni JF, et al: The occurrence and effects of human vitamin E deficiency. A study in patients with cystic fibrosis. *J Clin Invest* 60(1):233–241, 1977.
47. Corash L, Spielberg S, Bartsocas C, et al: Reduced chronic hemolysis during high-dose vitamin E administration in Mediterranean-type glucose-6-phosphate dehydrogenase deficiency. *N Engl J Med* 303(8):416–420, 1980.
48. Eldamhougy S, Elhelw Z, Yamamah G, et al: The vitamin E status among glucose-6 phosphate dehydrogenase deficient patients and effectiveness of oral vitamin E. *Int J Vitam Nutr Res* 58(2):184–188, 1988.
49. Johnson GJ, Vatassery GT, Finkel B, et al: High-dose vitamin E does not decrease the rate of chronic hemolysis in glucose-6-phosphate dehydrogenase deficiency. *N Engl J Med* 308(17):1014–1017, 1983.
50. Natta CL, Machlin LJ, Brin M: A decrease in irreversibly sickled erythrocytes in sickle cell anemia patients given vitamin E. *Am J Clin Nutr* 33(5):968–971, 1980.
51. Tangney CC, Phillips G, Bell RA, et al: Selected indices of micronutrient status in adult patients with sickle cell anemia (SCA). *Am J Hematol* 32(3):161–166, 1989.
52. Ren H, Ghebremeskel K, Okpala I, et al: Patients with sickle cell disease have reduced blood antioxidant protection. *Int J Vitam Nutr Res* 78(3):139–147, 2008.
53. Ndombi IO, Kinoti SN: Serum vitamin E and the sickling status in children with sickle cell anaemia. *East Afr Med J* 67(10):720–725, 1990.
54. Anderson GJ, Frazer DM, McKie AT, et al: The ceruloplasmin homolog hephaestin and the control of intestinal iron absorption. *Blood Cells Mol Dis* 29(3):367–375, 2002.
55. Graham GG, Cordano A: Copper depletion and deficiency in the malnourished infant. *Johns Hopkins Med J* 124(3):139–150, 1969.
56. Spiegel JE, Willenbucher RF: Rapid development of severe copper deficiency in a patient with Crohn's disease receiving parenteral nutrition. *JPEN J Parenter Enteral Nutr* 23(3):169–172, 1999.

57. Hirase N, Abe Y, Sadamura S, et al: Anemia and neutropenia in a case of copper deficiency: Role of copper in normal hematopoiesis. *Acta Haematol* 87(4):195–197, 1992.
58. Fuhrman MP, Herrmann V, Masidonski P, et al: Pancytopenia after removal of copper from total parenteral nutrition. *JPEN J Parenter Enteral Nutr* 24(6):361–366, 2000.
59. Halfdanarson TR, Kumar N, Li CY, et al: Hematological manifestations of copper deficiency: A retrospective review. *Eur J Haematol* 80(6):523–531, 2008.
60. Gregg XT, Reddy V, Prchal JT: Copper deficiency masquerading as myelodysplastic syndrome. *Blood* 100(4):1493–1495, 2002.
61. Lazarchick J: Update on anemia and neutropenia in copper deficiency. *Curr Opin Hematol* 19(1):58–60, 2012.
62. Prus E, Peled T, Fibach E: The effect of tetraethylenepentamine, a synthetic copper chelating polyamine, on expression of CD34 and CD38 antigens on normal and leukemic hematopoietic cells. *Leuk Lymphoma* 45(3):583–589, 2004.
63. Kumar N, Gross JB Jr, Ahlskog JE: Copper deficiency myelopathy produces a clinical picture like subacute combined degeneration. *Neurology* 63(1):33–39, 2004.
64. Green R: Anemias beyond B12 and iron deficiency: The buzz about other B's, elementary, and nonelementary problems. *Hematology Am Soc Hematol Educ Program* 2012:492–498, 2012.
65. Gabreyes AA, Abbasi HN, Forbes KP, et al: Hypocupremia associated cytopenia and myelopathy: A national retrospective review. *Eur J Haematol* 90(1):1–9, 2013.
66. Chen M, Krishnamurthy A, Mohamed AR, et al: Hematological disorders following gastric bypass surgery: Emerging concepts of the interplay between nutritional deficiency and inflammation. *Biomed Res Int* 2013:205467, 2013.
67. Hein MS: Copper deficiency anemia and nephrosis in zinc-toxicity: A case report. *S D J Med* 56(4):143–147, 2003.
68. Igic PG, Lee E, Harper W, et al: Toxic effects associated with consumption of zinc. *Mayo Clin Proc* 77(7):713–716, 2002.
69. Cordano A: Clinical manifestations of nutritional copper deficiency in infants and children. *Am J Clin Nutr* 67(5 Suppl):1012S–1016S, 1998.
70. Fuchs GJ, Tienboon P, Linpisarn S, et al: Nutritional factors and thalassaemia major. *Arch Dis Child* 74(3):224–227, 1996.
71. Prasad AS: Zinc deficiency in patients with sickle cell disease. *Am J Clin Nutr* 75(2):181–182, 2002.
72. Yuzbasiyan-Gurkan VA, Brewer GJ, Vander AJ, et al: Net renal tubular reabsorption of zinc in healthy man and impaired handling in sickle cell anemia. *Am J Hematol* 31(2):87–90, 1989.
73. De Virgiliis S, Congia M, Turco MP, et al: Depletion of trace elements and acute ocular toxicity induced by desferrioxamine in patients with thalassaemia. *Arch Dis Child* 63(3):250–255, 1988.
74. Thomson CD, Rea HM, Doesburg VM, et al: Selenium concentrations and glutathione peroxidase activities in whole blood of New Zealand residents. *Br J Nutr* 37(3):457–460, 1977.
75. Kien CL, Ganther HE: Manifestations of chronic selenium deficiency in a child receiving total parenteral nutrition. *Am J Clin Nutr* 37(2):319–328, 1983.
76. Cohen HJ, Brown MR, Hamilton D, et al: Glutathione peroxidase and selenium deficiency in patients receiving home parenteral nutrition: Time course for development of deficiency and repletion of enzyme activity in plasma and blood cells. *Am J Clin Nutr* 49(1):132–139, 1989.
77. Semba RD, Ricks MO, Ferrucci L, et al: Low serum selenium is associated with anemia among older adults in the United States. *Eur J Clin Nutr* 63(1):93–99, 2009.
78. Van Nhien N, Yabutani T, Khan NC, et al: Association of low serum selenium with anemia among adolescent girls living in rural Vietnam. *Nutrition* 25(1):6–10, 2009.
79. Keys A, Brozek J, Henschel A, et al: *The Biology of Semistarvation.* Minnesota Press, Minneapolis, MN, 1950.
80. Thomson TJ, Runcie J, Miller V: Treatment of obesity by total fasting for up to 249 days. *Lancet* 2(7471):992–996, 1966.
81. Drenick EJ, Swendseid ME, Blahd WH, et al: Prolonged starvation as treatment for severe obesity. *JAMA* 187:100–105, 1964.
82. Caro J, Silver R, Erslev AJ, et al: Erythropoietin production in fasted rats. Effects of thyroid hormones and glucose supplementation. *J Lab Clin Med* 98(6):860–868, 1981.
83. Lowik MR, Schrijver J, Odink J, et al: Long-term effects of a vegetarian diet on the nutritional status of elderly people (Dutch Nutrition Surveillance System). *J Am Coll Nutr* 9(6):600–609, 1990.
84. Chanarin I, Malkowska V, O'Hea AM, et al: Megaloblastic anaemia in a vegetarian Hindu community. *Lancet* 2(8465):1168–1172, 1985.
85. Carvalho NF, Kenney RD, Carrington PH, et al: Severe nutritional deficiencies in toddlers resulting from health food milk alternatives. *Pediatrics* 107(4):E46, 2001.
86. Lunn PG, Morley CJ, Neale G: A case of kwashiorkor in the UK. *Clin Nutr* 17(3):131–133, 1998.
87. Adams EB, Scragg JN, Naidoo BT, et al: Observations on the aetiology and treatment of anaemia in kwashiorkor. *Br Med J* 3(5563):451–454, 1967.
88. Foy H, Kondi A: Comparison between erythroid aplasia in marasmus and kwashiorkor and the experimentally induced erythroid aplasia in baboons by riboflavin deficiency. *Vitam Horm* 26:653–684, 1968.
89. Ozkale M, Sipahi T: Hematologic and bone marrow changes in children with protein-energy malnutrition. *Pediatr Hematol Oncol* 31(4):349–358, 2014.
90. Delmonte L, Aschkenasy A, Eyquem A: Studies on the hemolytic nature of protein-deficiency anemia in the rat. *Blood* 24:49–68, 1964.
91. Naets JP, Wittek M: Effect of starvation on the response to erythropoietin in the rat. *Acta Haematol* 52(3):141–150, 1974.
92. Ito K, Reissmann KR: Quantitative and qualitative aspects of steady state erythropoiesis induced in protein-starved rats by long-term erythropoietin injection. *Blood* 27(3):343–351, 1966.
93. Hutter G, Ganepola S, Hofmann WK: The hematology of anorexia nervosa. *Int J Eat Disord* 42(4):293–300, 2009.
94. Gloria L, Cravo M, Camilo ME, et al: Nutritional deficiencies in chronic alcoholics: Relation to dietary intake and alcohol consumption. *Am J Gastroenterol* 92(3):485–489, 1997.
95. Savage D, Lindenbaum J: Anemia in alcoholics. *Medicine (Baltimore)* 65(5):322–338, 1986.
96. Girard DE, Kumar KL, McAfee JH: Hematologic effects of acute and chronic alcohol abuse. *Hematol Oncol Clin North Am* 1(2):321–334, 1987.
97. Fernando OV, Grimsley EW: Prevalence of folate deficiency and macrocytosis in patients with and without alcohol-related illness. *South Med J* 91(8):721–725, 1998.
98. Colman N, Herbert V: Hematologic complications of alcoholism: Overview. *Semin Hematol* 17(3):164–176, 1980.
99. Sullivan LW, Herbert V: Suppression hematopoiesis by ethanol. *J Clin Invest* 43:2048–2062, 1964.
100. Eichner ER, Hillman RS: Effect of alcohol on serum folate level. *J Clin Invest* 52(3):584–591, 1973.
101. Halsted CH: Nutrition and alcoholic liver disease. *Semin Liver Dis* 24(3):289–304, 2004.
102. Lindenbaum J: Folate and vitamin B12 deficiencies in alcoholism. *Semin Hematol* 17(2):119–129, 1980.
103. Seppa K, Laippala P, Saarni M: Macrocytosis as a consequence of alcohol abuse among patients in general practice. *Alcohol Clin Exp Res* 15(5):871–876, 1991.
104. McCurdy PR, Rath CE: Vacuolated nucleated bone marrow cells in alcoholism. *Semin Hematol* 17(2):100–102, 1980.
105. Yeung KY, Klug PP, Lessin LS: Alcohol-induced vacuolization in bone marrow cells: Ultrastructure and mechanism of formation. *Blood Cells* 13(3):487–502, 1988.
106. Zieve L: Jaundice, hyperlipemia and hemolytic anemia: A heretofore unrecognized syndrome associated with alcoholic fatty liver and cirrhosis. *Ann Intern Med* 48(3):471–496, 1958.
107. Melrose WD, Bell PA, Jupe DM, et al: Alcohol-associated haemolysis in Zieve's syndrome: A clinical and laboratory study of five cases. *Clin Lab Haematol* 12(2):159–167, 1990.
108. Chitale AA, Sterling RK, Post AB, et al: Resolution of spur cell anemia with liver transplantation: A case report and review of the literature. *Transplantation* 65(7):993–995, 1998.
109. Malik P, Bogetti D, Sileri P, et al: Spur cell anemia in alcoholic cirrhosis: Cure by orthotopic liver transplantation and recurrence after liver graft failure. *Int Surg* 87(4):201–204, 2002.

CHAPTER 45
ANEMIA ASSOCIATED WITH MARROW INFILTRATION

Vishnu VB Reddy and Josef T. Prchal

SUMMARY

Myelophthisic anemia is caused by marrow infiltration, typically by metastatic cancer, and by any nonhematopoietic conditions, for example, granulomatous inflammation or fibrosis. It can present with an overt leukoerythroblastic picture or with only a few teardrop-shaped red cells on a blood film. These changes may represent an early spread of the tumor (or other nonhematopoietic tissue) to the marrow or may indicate massive replacement of the marrow space. The diagnosis can be made by standard marrow biopsy. Radioisotope scanning and magnetic resonance imaging, although not very sensitive, can be helpful in locating the biopsy site and can also help in estimating the percentage of involvement of the marrow space.

● DEFINITION AND HISTORY

Myelophthisic anemia is the term that has been used to describe diverse pathologic processes, including Fanconi anemia,[1] but currently refers to anemia resulting from the presence of spotty to massive marrow infiltration with abnormal cells or tissue components. Strictly speaking, the blasts of acute leukemia, plasma cells of myeloma, and cells of lymphoma, chronic leukemia, and myeloproliferative neoplasms fit this definition. However, the term *myelophthisic anemia*[2] is best reserved for marrow replacement by nonhematologic tumors and nonhematopoietic tissue. Minimal to moderate involvement usually does not cause symptoms or hematologic changes. Such infiltration is clinically significant, however, because in patients with an established diagnosis of cancer, it indicates metastatic dissemination of the tumor and usually an advanced stage. Although extensive infiltration may lead to anemia or even pancytopenia, anemia can be frequently accompanied by an elevated leukocyte count, often with immature myeloid cells in the blood. Platelets can be increased, decreased, or normal (megakaryocytic fragments are seen occasionally in the blood film). The findings accompanied by teardrop-shaped red cells (dacrocytes), prematurely released nucleated red cells, and immature myeloid cells is referred to as *leukoerythroblastic reaction* (Chaps. 2, 31, and 86), which generally reflects marrow replacement by tumor or extramedullary hematopoiesis.

● ETIOLOGY AND PATHOGENESIS

Tumor metastasis results from the complex interactions between the tumor cells and the surrounding microenvironment. Invasion is the

Acronyms and Abbreviations: MRI, magnetic resonance imaging; ^{99m}Tc, a radioisotope of technetium; ^{99m}Tc sestamibi, a radioisotope of technetium attached to the sestamibi molecule.

primary process of metastasis and occurs often as a result of loss of E-cadherin. E-cadherin is a calcium-dependent cell adhesion molecule that likely plays a role in intercellular adhesion and inhibition of invasion by neoplastic cells. The loss of E-cadherin can be caused by many mechanisms, including mutations and gene silencing.[3] Dysregulation of calcium influx pathways through stromal interaction molecule (STIM) and calcium-permeable transient receptor potential (TRP) also plays a role in tumor invasive and metastatic behavior.[4] Many members of the family of matrix metalloproteinases can also participate in the process of tumor cell invasion. Stromal cells, such as tumor-associated macrophages, and growth factors secreted by them, such as fibroblast growth factor, are also known to promote tumor spread.[5]

Table 45–1 lists the most common causes of extensive cellular infiltration of marrow. In myelofibrotic disorders of both primary and secondary origin, the fibrosis/osteosclerosis restricts the available marrow space and disrupts marrow architecture (Chap. 86). The disruption may cause cytopenias with production of deformed red cells, especially poikilocytes and teardrop-shaped cells, and premature release of erythroblasts, myelocytes, and giant platelets. The leukocyte count also may be elevated. Similar abnormalities following marrow replacement by calcium oxalate crystals have been reported.[6] Anemia seen in metastatic cancer most frequently results from cytokine release leading to anemia of chronic inflammation (Chap. 37), iron deficiency as a result of gastrointestinal or uterine bleeding (Chap. 42), or other nutritional deficiencies (Chaps. 41 and 44). However, marrow replacement causing a myelophthisic anemia as the sole cause of anemia also occurs. The marrow microenvironment is susceptible to implantation of bloodborne malignant cells. Almost all cancers can metastasize to the marrow,[7–11] but the most common are cancers of the lung, breast, and prostate. Metastatic foci in the marrow can be found in 20 to 30 percent of patients with small cell carcinoma of the lung at the time of diagnosis, and in more than 50 percent of patients at autopsy.[12,13] Overt leukoerythroblastic blood picture is less common, and its absence is not a reliable indicator that the marrow is not involved.

The characteristic abnormalities observed in patients with myelophthisic anemia may result partly from an attempt for compensatory extramedullary blood formation that generally reflects extramedullary hematopoiesis predominantly from the spleen. A similar picture can be seen when the marrow is replaced by numerous granulomas,[14,15] for example, sarcoidosis, disseminated tuberculosis, fungal infections, or by macrophages containing indigestible lipids, as in Gaucher and Niemann-Pick diseases (Chap. 72)[16] and in macrophage activation syndrome (MAS).

Marrow necrosis can be an underlying cause of myelophthisic anemia. The morphologic picture, best observed in hematoxylin-and-eosin–stained biopsy of marrow, consists of cell debris and occasional necrotic cells in an eosinophilic amorphus background (Fig. 45–1).[17] Marrow necrosis is generally considered to be very uncommon, accounting for less than 1 percent of marrow biopsies. Metastatic tumors, acute lymphoblastic leukemia (children), and septicemia are generally the underlying cause,[17,18] but sickle cell disease[19–21] and arsenic therapy in acute promyelocytic leukemia are other causes.[22] Necrotic foci range from small to very extensive (<5 to 90 percent of the biopsy volume). Extensive necrosis often results in inability to perform flow cytometry/molecular analysis satisfactorily. A repeat biopsy at a different site may be needed.[17,23,24]

Because myelophthisic anemia is so uncommon, only a few rigorous studies of the pathogenesis of anemia in this entity have been conducted. *In vitro* study of hematopoietic progenitors reveals only a moderate decrease of their proportion and proliferative capacity.[25] Similar reports of erythropoiesis quantitation by ferrokinetic studies reveal only a moderate defect (Chap. 32).[26] The following confounding factors

TABLE 45–1. Causes of Marrow Infiltration

I. Fibroblasts and collagen

  A. Primary myelofibrosis (PMF)

  B. Fibrosis associated with other myeloproliferative neoplasms (MPNs)

  C. Fibrosis of hairy cell leukemia

  D. Metastatic tumors (e.g., breast carcinoma)

  E. Sarcoidosis[14,15]

  F. Secondary myelofibrosis with pulmonary hypertension

II. Other noncellular material

  A. Oxalosis[6]

III. Tumor cells

  A. Carcinomas (breast, lung, prostate, kidney, thyroid and neuroblastoma)[7,8,11]

  B. Sarcoma[10]

IV. Granulomas[14]

  A. Sarcoidosis

  B. Fungal infections

  C. Miliary tuberculosis

V. Macrophages

  A. Gaucher disease

  B. Niemann-Pick disease[16]

  C. Macrophage activation syndrome (MAS)[34,35]

VI. Marrow necrosis

  A. Sickle cell anemia[19]

  B. Solid tumor metastasis[18]

  C. Septicemia[18]

  D. Acute lymphoblastic leukemia

  E. Arsenic therapy[22]

VII. Failure of osteoclast development

  A. Osteopetrosis[36]

contribute to anemia: elevated hepcidin (Chap. 37) and other factors, including hematopoiesis-inhibiting cytokines released from tumor cells (Chap. 37) and iron (Chap. 42) and folate and cobalamin (Chap. 41) deficiencies. When they are excluded, the finding discussed above suggests that only massive marrow replacement leads to anemia.

CLINICAL FEATURES

Symptoms and signs associated with infiltrative marrow disorders usually are related to the underlying disease. Other symptoms, such as fatigue, often from upregulated cytokines, may also contribute to anemia itself. Some patients are asymptomatic, and the incidental discovery of cytopenias and leukoerythroblastic blood morphology leads to diagnosis of an underlying disorder

LABORATORY FEATURES

BLOOD

The anemia usually is mild to moderate, but it can be severe. White cell and platelet counts may vary, but the most characteristic feature is the morphologic appearance of red cells on the blood film. These cells may show anisocytosis and poikilocytosis, but the presence of teardrop forms and nucleated red cells is particularly suggestive of marrow infiltration (Chap. 31; Fig. 45–2). The combination of nucleated red cells and immature myeloid precursors constitutes the leukoerythroblastic picture that is characteristic of marrow infiltration and extramedullary hematopoiesis. The presence of cancer cells on the blood film occurs occasionally and always indicates marrow invasion (Fig. 45–3).[27]

MARROW

Marrow biopsy is the most reliable procedure used to diagnose marrow-infiltrative disease and should be performed in all patients with suspected metastatic carcinoma or hematologic features of myelophthisic anemia. Marrow aspiration[24,28] does not provide a reliable yield of tumor cells and is particularly difficult in primary or secondary myelofibrosis. The inability to aspirate marrow (dry tap) leads to a high degree of suspicion of marrow replacement and accompanying myelofibrosis. Because the diagnostic marrow yield from biopsies depends on the amount of tissue examined, bilateral posterior iliac crest marrow biopsies may be necessary. In patients with metastatic cancer

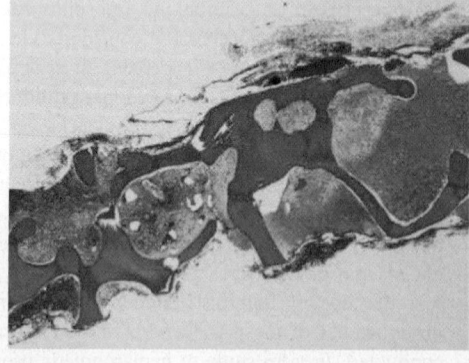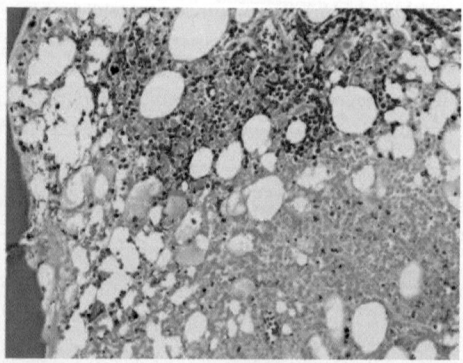

A   **B**

Figure 45–1. Marrow necrosis. **A.** Low-magnification view of the biopsy showing mostly necrosis (*pink area*) and focally preserved tumor to the left (*blue area*). **B.** Higher-magnification view of necrosis with loss of cellular details, granular eosinophilic/pink cell debris.

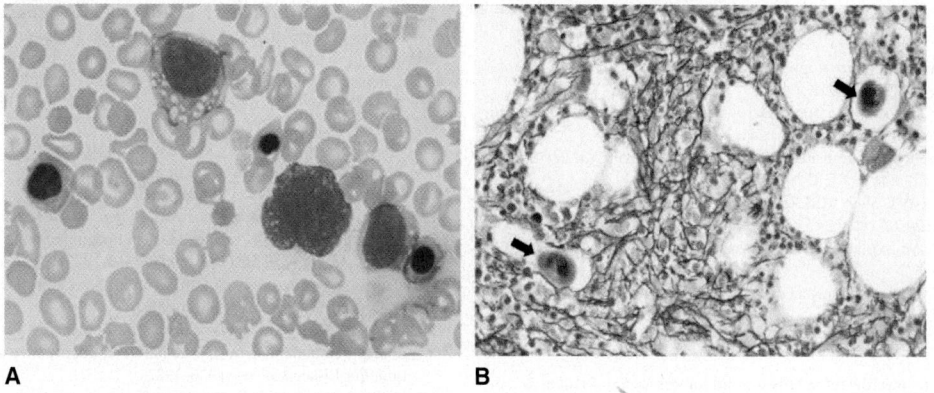

Figure 45–2. Leukoerythroblastosis. **A.** Blood film containing several nucleated red blood cells (RBCs), few circulating blasts, and RBCs showing severe anisopoikilocytosis. **B.** Corresponding marrow biopsy with reticulin fibrosis (3+) and intrasinusoidal megakaryocytes *(black arrows)*.

involving the marrow, the blood CD34-positive cell count can be up to 50 times higher than in patients with metastatic cancer without marrow involvement.[29]

ISOTOPE AND IMAGING PROCEDURES

Technetium-99m (^{99m}Tc) sestamibi uptake reliably identifies marrow infiltration by Gaucher cells. Sestamibi is a pharmaceutical agent used in nuclear medicine imaging. Magnetic resonance imaging (MRI) is also helpful for defining the severity of marrow replacement and is being used with increasing frequency. This imaging approach is especially useful for following resolution of marrow infiltration in patients with type 1 Gaucher disease who are treated with enzyme-replacement therapy.[20,30,31] An isotopic bone scan or MRI study showing focal accumulation of radioactive tracers can be helpful in locating a suitable site for biopsy,[20,32] but a negative study of the area does not exclude the possibility of marrow involvement. On MRI, marrow necrosis characteristically has an extensive, diffuse, geographic pattern of signal abnormality consisting of a central area of variable signal intensity surrounded by a distinct peripheral enhancing rim.[21]

DIFFERENTIAL DIAGNOSIS

The cause of a leukoerythroblastic blood picture is known to occur in a patient with metastatic cancer or overt hematologic malignancy. In the absence of a likely cause after clinical evaluation, the initial approach to diagnosis is the marrow biopsy. Although it is not a very sensitive technique, with the help of immunocytochemistry and flow cytometry for tumor-specific antigens, its diagnostic sensitivity and specificity increases. MRI or isotopic scanning before the marrow may aid in locating the site of the biopsy. Hematologic disorders causing marrow fibrosis, notably primary myelofibrosis, may mimic a myelophthisic disorder, but the distinctions are usually evident. For example, the patient with primary myelofibrosis invariably has splenic enlargement and the patient with metastatic cancer nearly always does not (Chap. 91). If the myelophthisis is the result of a storage disease or other infiltrative cause, the appropriate chemical tests, as well as marrow biopsy, are helpful in diagnosis. Nucleated red cells and leukocytosis can be seen in acute conditions, including overwhelming sepsis, acute severe hypoxia, postcardiac arrest, and chronic conditions such as thalassemia major, congestive heart failure, and severe hemolytic anemia.

THERAPY, COURSE, AND PROGNOSIS

The goal of treatment is managing the underlying disease. Patients with marrow infiltration caused by cancer should be treated appropriately; however, in some instances the presence of marrow infiltration may not adversely affect the outcome. If treatment is successful, not only the malignant cells but also the reactive fibrosis surrounding metastatic foci may completely disappear. In hormone-refractory prostate cancer, the presence of a leukoerythroblastic picture does not seem to influence survival.[33] However, in most patients with cancers metastatic to the marrow, only short-term survival is a rule.

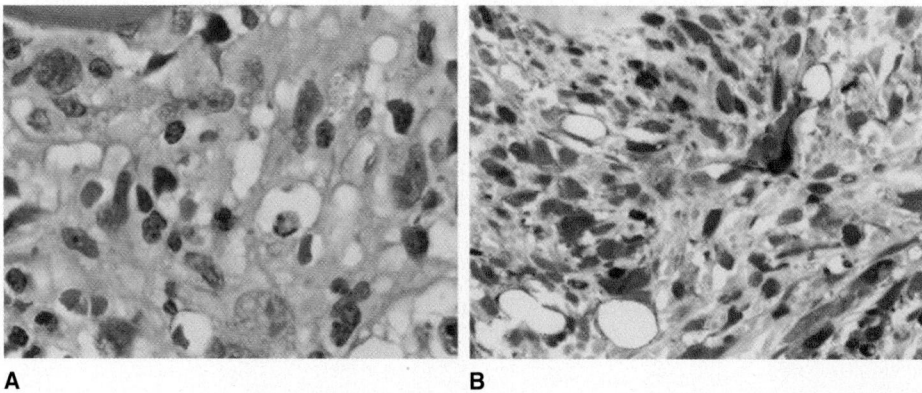

Figure 45–3. Metastatic tumor in the marrow. **A.** Marrow packed with melanoma cells and displacing normal marrow elements. Tumor cells have characteristic large nuclei with prominent pink nucleoli. **B.** S100 immunohistochemical stain highlights melanoma infiltrates in the marrow.

REFERENCES

1. Baumann T: Constitutional general myelophthisis with multiple degeneration (Fanconi syndrome). *Ann Paediatr* 177(2):65, 1951.
2. Rundles RW, Jonsson U: Metastases in bone marrow and myelophthisic anemia from carcinoma of the prostate. *Am J Med Sci* 218(3):241, 1949.
3. Thiery JP: Epithelial-mesenchymal transitions in tumour progression. *Nat Rev Cancer* 2(6):442, 2002.
4. Chen YF, Chen YT, Chiu WT, Shen MR: Remodeling of calcium signaling in tumor progression. *J Biomed Sci* 20:23, 2013.
5. Chiang AC. Massague J: Molecular basis of metastasis. *N Engl J Med* 359(26):2814, 2008.
6. Halil O, Farringdon K: Oxalosis: An unusual cause of leucoerythroblastic anaemia. *Br J Haematol* 122(1):2, 2003.
7. Makoni SN, Laber DA: Clinical spectrum of myelophthisis in cancer patients. *Am J Hematol* 76(1):92, 2004.
8. Mohanty SK, Dash S: Bone marrow metastasis in solid tumors. *Indian J Pathol Microbiol* 46(4):613, 2003.
9. Pham CM, Syed AA, Siddiqui HA, et al: Case of metastatic basal cell carcinoma to bone marrow, resulting in myelophthisic anemia. *Am J Dermatopathol* 35(2):e34, 2013.
10. Shinkoda Y, Nagatoshi Y, Fukano R, et al: Rhabdomyosarcoma masquerading as acute leukemia. *Pediatr Blood Cancer* 52(2):286, 2009.
11. Velasco-Rodriguez D, Castellanos-González M, Alonso-Domínguez JM, et al: Metastatic malignant melanoma detected on bone marrow aspiration. *Br J Haematol* 162(4):432, 2013.
12. Hirsch FR, Hansen HH: Bone marrow involvement in small cell anaplastic carcinoma of the lung: Prognostic and therapeutic aspects. *Cancer* 46(1):206, 1980.
13. Hirsch FR, Osterlind K, Kristjansen PE, Hansen HH: Bone marrow examination in small cell lung cancer. *Ann Intern Med* 106(6):913, 1987.
14. Eid A, Carion W, Nystrom JS: Differential diagnoses of bone marrow granuloma. *West J Med* 164(6):510, 1996.
15. Saliba WR, Elias MS: Recurrent severe hypercalcemia caused by bone marrow sarcoidosis. *Am J Med Sci* 330(3):147, 2005.
16. Hsu YS, Hwu WL, Huang SF, et al: Niemann-Pick disease type C (a cellular cholesterol lipidosis) treated by bone marrow transplantation. *Bone Marrow Transplant* 24(1):103, 1999.
17. Khoshnaw NS, Muhealdeen DN: Bone marrow necrosis in an adult patient with precursor B-cell acute lymphoblastic leukaemia at the time of presentation. *BMJ Case Rep* Apr 4:2014, 2014.
18. Paydas S, Ergin M, Baslamisli F, et al: Bone marrow necrosis: Clinicopathologic analysis of 20 cases and review of the literature. *Am J Hematol* 70(4):300, 2002.
19. Conrad ME, Studdard H, Anderson LJ: Aplastic crisis in sickle cell disorders: Bone marrow necrosis and human parvovirus infection. *Am J Med Sci* 295(3):212, 1988.
20. Howe BM, Johnson GB, Wenger DE: Current concepts in MRI of focal and diffuse malignancy of bone marrow. *Semin Musculoskelet Radiol* 17(2):137, 2013.
21. Tang YM, Jeavons S, Stuckey S, et al: MRI features of bone marrow necrosis. *AJR Am J Roentgenol* 188(2):509, 2007.
22. Chim CS, Lam CC, Wong KF, et al: Atypical blasts and bone marrow necrosis associated with near-triploid relapse of acute promyelocytic leukemia after arsenic trioxide treatment. *Hum Pathol* 33(8):849, 2002.
23. Conrad ME: Bone marrow necrosis. *J Intensive Care Med* 10(4):171, 1995.
24. Langsteger W, Haim S, Knauer M, et al: Imaging of bone metastases in prostate cancer: An update. *Q J Nucl Med Mol Imaging* 56(5):447, 2012.
25. Dainiak N, Kulkarni V, Howard D, et al: Mechanisms of abnormal erythropoiesis in malignancy. *Cancer* 51(6):1101, 1983.
26. Cazzola M, Bergamaschi G, Huebers HA, Finch CA: Pathophysiological classification of acquired bone marrow failure based on quantitative assessment of erythroid function. *Eur J Haematol* 38(5):426, 1987.
27. Gallivan MV, Lokich JJ: Carcinocythemia (carcinoma cell leukemia). Report of two cases with English literature review. *Cancer* 53(5):1100, 1984.
28. Garrett TJ, Gee TS, Lieberman PH, et al: The role of bone marrow aspiration and biopsy in detecting marrow involvement by nonhematologic malignancies. *Cancer* 38(6):2401, 1976.
29. Ciancia R, Martinelli V, Cosentini E, et al: High number of circulating CD34+ cells in patients with myelophthisis. *Haematologica* 90(7):976, 2005.
30. Erba PA, Minichilli F, Giona F, et al: 99mTc-sestamibi scintigraphy to monitor the long-term efficacy of enzyme replacement therapy on bone marrow infiltration in patients with Gaucher disease. *J Nucl Med* 54(10):1717, 2013.
31. Mariani G, Filocamo M, Giona F, et al: Severity of bone marrow involvement in patients with Gaucher's disease evaluated by scintigraphy with 99mTc-sestamibi. *J Nucl Med* 44(8):1253, 2003.
32. Terk MR, Dardashti S, Liebman HA: Bone marrow response in treated patients with Gaucher disease: Evaluation by T1-weighted magnetic resonance images and correlation with reduction in liver and spleen volume. *Skeletal Radiol* 29(10):563, 2000.
33. Shamdas GJ, Ahmann FR, Matzner MB, Ritchie JM: Leukoerythroblastic anemia in metastatic prostate cancer. Clinical and prognostic significance in patients with hormone-refractory disease. *Cancer* 71(11):3594, 1993.
34. George MR: Hemophagocytic lymphohistiocytosis: Review of etiologies and management. *J Blood Med* 5:69, 2014.
35. Ravelli A, Grom AA, Behrens EM, Cron RQ: Macrophage activation syndrome as part of systemic juvenile idiopathic arthritis: Diagnosis, genetics, pathophysiology and treatment. *Genes Immun* 13(4):289, 2012.
36. Stark Z, Savarirayan R: Osteopetrosis. *Orphanet J Rare Dis* 4:5, 2009.

CHAPTER 46
ERYTHROCYTE MEMBRANE DISORDERS

Theresa L. Coetzer

SUMMARY

The human erythrocyte membrane consists of a lipid bilayer containing transmembrane proteins and an underlying membrane skeleton, which is attached to the bilayer by linker protein complexes. The membrane is critical in maintaining the unique biconcave disk shape of the erythrocyte and enabling it to withstand the circulatory shear stress. The integrity of the membrane is ensured by vertical interactions between the skeleton and the transmembrane proteins, as well as by horizontal interactions between skeletal proteins. Inherited defects of membrane proteins compromise these interactions and alter the shape and deformability of the cells, which ultimately results in their premature destruction and hemolytic anemia. The disorders are typically autosomal dominant and exhibit significant clinical, laboratory, biochemical, and genetic heterogeneity.

Hereditary spherocytosis is a common condition characterized by spherically shaped erythrocytes on the blood film, reticulocytosis, and splenomegaly. The underlying defect is a deficiency of one of the membrane proteins, including ankyrin, band 3, *a*-spectrin, *β*-spectrin, or protein 4.2. This weakens the vertical membrane interactions, resulting in loss of membrane and surface area. Spherocytes have diminished deformability, which predisposes them to entrapment and destruction in the spleen. *Hereditary elliptocytosis* is characterized by the presence of elliptical erythrocytes on the blood film. The principal abnormality affects horizontal membrane protein interactions and typically involves *a*-spectrin, *β*-spectrin, protein 4.1R, or glycophorin C. The membrane skeleton is destabilized and unable to maintain the biconcave disk shape, which manifests as an elliptical distortion of the cells in the circulation.

Hereditary pyropoikilocytosis is a rare, severe hemolytic anemia characterized by markedly abnormal erythrocyte morphology caused by defective spectrin. *Southeast Asian ovalocytosis* is largely asymptomatic and is caused by a defect in band 3. The blood film shows large oval red cells with a transverse ridge across the central area. *Acanthocytosis* is typified by contracted, dense erythrocytes with irregular projections, which may be seen in patients with severe liver disease, abetalipoproteinemia, various neurologic disorders, certain aberrant red cell antigens, and postsplenectomy. *Stomatocytosis* is a rare group of inherited disorders associated with abnormal membrane permeability and red cell cation content, which either cause overhydration or dehydration of the cells.

The erythrocyte membrane plays a critical role in the function and structure of the red cell. It is a key determinant of the unique biconcave disk shape and provides the cell with a finely tuned combination of flexibility and durability. These properties enable the erythrocyte to withstand the circulatory shear pressure and allow it to undergo extensive and repeated distortion while negotiating the microvasculature and the spleen, thus ensuring survival during its average 120-day life span. The red cell membrane maintains a nonreactive surface so that erythrocytes do not adhere to the endothelium or aggregate and occlude capillaries. It provides a barrier with selective permeability, which retains vital components inside the cell and permits the efflux of metabolic waste. To facilitate the transfer of carbon dioxide and to maintain pH homeostasis, the membrane exchanges chloride and bicarbonate anions, and it also actively controls the cation and water content of the erythrocyte. The membrane sequesters reducing agents required to prevent oxidative damage to hemoglobin and other cellular components, and it plays a role in regulating metabolism by reversibly binding and inactivating selected glycolytic enzymes.

Abnormalities of the erythrocyte membrane alter the shape of the cell and compromise its integrity and ability to survive the rigors of circulation, which leads to premature destruction and hemolysis. Erythrocyte membrane disorders comprise an important group of hereditary hemolytic anemias, which are classified according to the altered red cell morphology and include hereditary spherocytosis (HS), hereditary elliptocytosis (HE) and related disorders, and the hereditary stomatocytosis (HSt) syndromes. This chapter summarizes our current understanding of the erythrocyte membrane in normal cells followed by a discussion of the underlying molecular defects and their role in the pathophysiology and clinical manifestations of these disorders. The main emphasis is on spherocytosis and elliptocytosis, the two most common and best characterized diseases.

● OVERVIEW OF THE ERYTHROCYTE MEMBRANE

The erythrocyte membrane is the most studied plasma membrane and serves as a paradigm for all cellular membranes. Mature erythrocytes are readily accessible; they contain no intracellular organelles, which facilitates the isolation of pure erythrocyte membranes; and "experiments of nature" resulting in abnormal erythrocyte morphology have provided unique opportunities to investigate the function of membrane components. These studies have revealed the primary structure and several important functions of the red cell membrane. Ongoing research, using the latest molecular technologies, continues to yield important insights into our understanding of membrane structure–function relationships, as well as genotype–phenotype correlations.

Acronyms and Abbreviations: AE1, anion exchanger-1; α^{LELY}, *a*-spectrin low-expression Lyon; α^{LEPRA}, *a*-spectrin low-expression Prague; AGLT, acidified glycerol lysis test; ANK, ankyrin; AQP1, aquaporin-1; BCSH, British Committee for Standards in Haematology; BPG, 2,3-bisphosphoglycerate; CDAII, congenital dyserythropoietic anemia type II; EMA, eosin 5′-maleimide; 4.1R, erythrocyte isoform of protein 4.1; GLT, glycerol lysis test; GLUT-1, glucose transporter-1; GP, glycophorin; GP-A, -B, -C, -D, -E, various members of glycophorin family; GSSG, oxidized glutathione; HARP, hypobetalipoproteinemia, acanthocytosis, retinitis pigmentosa, and pallidal degeneration syndrome; HE, hereditary elliptocytosis; HPP, hereditary pyropoikilocytosis; HS, hereditary spherocytosis; HSt, hereditary stomatocytosis; MAGUK, membrane-associated guanylate kinase; MARCKS, myristoylated alanine-rich C kinase substrate; MCHC, mean corpuscular hemoglobin concentration; MCV, mean corpuscular volume; OF, osmotic fragility; PKAN, pantothenate kinase-associated neurodegeneration; RhAG, Rh-associated glycoprotein; SAO, southeast Asian ovalocytosis; SDS-PAGE, sodium dodecylsulfate polyacrylamide gel electrophoresis; UGT1, uridine diphosphate glucuronosyltransferase 1.

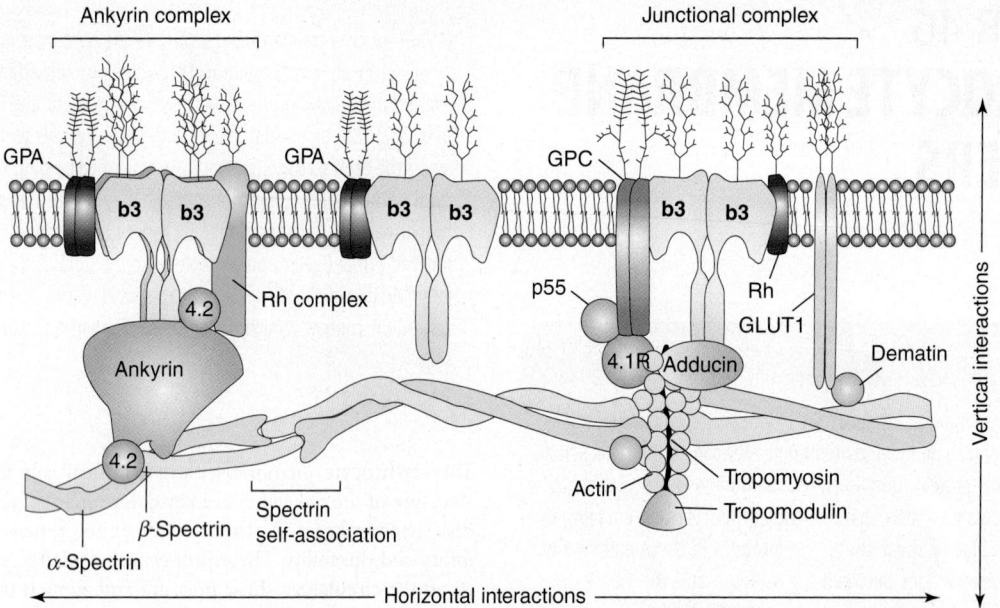

Figure 46–1. Schematic model of the human erythrocyte membrane. The molecular assembly of the major proteins is indicated. *Vertical* interactions are perpendicular to the plane of the membrane and are represented by the ankyrin and junctional protein complexes that connect the membrane spectrin skeleton to the integral proteins embedded in the lipid bilayer. *Horizontal* interactions occur parallel to the plane of the membrane and involve spectrin tetramers and protein 4.1R. The proteins and lipids are not drawn to scale. b3, Band 3; GPA/GPC, glycophorin A/C; GLUT-1, glucose transporter-1.

The erythrocyte membrane is a complex structure consisting of a relatively fluid lipid bilayer stabilized by an underlying two-dimensional membrane skeleton, which maintains the integrity of the biconcave disk shape of the erythrocyte (Fig. 46–1). The skeleton provides the cell with the strength and flexibility to deform rapidly and repeatedly and thus endure the shear stress encountered in the tiny capillaries of the microcirculation and in the spleen. The lipid bilayer separates the erythrocyte cytoplasm from the external plasma environment and contains phospholipids and cholesterol, as well as integral transmembrane proteins, which are tethered to the skeleton by interactions with linker proteins.

● COMPONENTS OF THE ERYTHROCYTE MEMBRANE

MEMBRANE LIPIDS

The lipid bilayer comprises approximately 50 percent of the membrane mass and contains unesterified cholesterol and phospholipids in approximately equal amounts, with small amounts of glycolipids and phosphoinositides (Chap. 31).[1,2] Mature erythrocytes are unable to synthesize fatty acids, phospholipids, or cholesterol *de novo*, and they depend on lipid exchange and limited phospholipid repair.[3]

Cholesterol regulates the fluidity of the membrane and is present in both leaflets, whereas the phospholipids are asymmetrically distributed. The choline phospholipids, phosphatidylcholine and sphingomyelin, are predominantly located in the outer leaflet and play a role in plasma lipid exchange and renewal of membrane phospholipids. Glycolipids carry several important red cell antigens, including A, B, H, and P, and are only found in the external leaflet with their carbohydrate moieties extending into the plasma. The aminophospholipids, phosphatidylserine and phosphatidylethanolamine, as well as phosphatidylinositol are located in the inner leaflet of the lipid bilayer.

This asymmetric distribution of phospholipids is maintained by a dynamic process involving flippase and floppase enzymes, which translocate the aminophospholipids to the inner and outer leaflets, respectively.[4,5] A scramblase mediates bidirectional movement of phospholipids down their concentration gradient.[6] Asymmetry of the phospholipids is important for the survival of the erythrocyte since exposure of phosphatidylserine on the outside surface of the cell, as found in sickle cell disease and thalassemia, has several deleterious consequences. It activates the coagulation cascade and may contribute to thromboses[4]; it facilitates adhesion to the vascular endothelium; it provides a recognition signal for macrophages to phagocytose these cells; and it decreases the interaction of skeletal proteins with the bilayer, which destabilizes the membrane.

Lipid rafts have been identified in erythrocytes.[7] They form detergent-resistant membrane microdomains, enriched in cholesterol and sphingolipids, and are associated with several proteins, including stomatin and flotillin-1 and -2. These rafts play a role in signaling and invasion of malaria parasites.[8]

MEMBRANE PROTEINS

Pioneering studies resolved the major proteins of the red cell membrane by sodium dodecylsulfate polyacrylamide gel electrophoresis (SDS-PAGE) and numbers from 1 to 8 were assigned to each protein starting with the largest protein, which migrated the slowest (Chap. 31).[9] Subsequent research revealed minor bands between the major proteins and these were designated with decimals. Analysis of the individual proteins led to the renaming of some of them, such as band 1 and 2, which are now known as α- and β-spectrin, respectively. Technologic advances have enabled an in-depth analysis of the erythrocyte proteome by mass spectrometry, revealing a total of 340 membrane proteins.[10] Table 46–1 summarizes the properties of the major components.

TABLE 46-1. Major Red Cell Membrane Proteins

Band	Protein	Mr (gel)	Mr (calc)	Copies per Cell (×10³)	Percent-age of Total[a]	Gene Symbol	Chromosomal Localization	Amino Acids	Gene Size (kb)	No. of Exons	Involvement in Hemolytic Anemias
1	α-Spectrin	240	280	240	16	SPTA1	1q22–q23	2429	80	52	HE, HS, HPP
2	β-Spectrin	220	246	240	14	SPTB	14q23–q24.2	2137	>100	32	HE, HS, HPP
2.1	Ankyrin[b]	210	206	120	4.5	ANK1	8p11.2	1881	>100	40	HS
2.9	α-Adducin[c]	103	81	30	2	ADDA	4p16.3	737	85	16	N
2.9	β-Adducin[c]	97	80	30	2	ADDB	2p13–2p14	726	~100	17	N
3	Anion exchanger-1	90–100	102	1200	27	EPB3	17q21–qter	911	17	20	HS, SAO, HAc
4.1	Protein 4.1	80	66	200	5	EL11	1p33–p34.2	588[d]	>100	23	HE
4.2	Protein 4.2	72	77	200	5	EB42	15q15–q21	691	20	13	HS
4.9	Dematin[e]	48 + 52	43	40[f]	1	EPB49	8p21.1	383	–	–	N
4.9	p55[e]	55	53	80	–	MPP1	Xq28	466	–	–	N
5	β-Actin	43	42	400–500	5.5	ACTB	7pter–q22	375	>4	6	N
5	Tropomodulin	43	41	30	–	TMOD	9q22	359	–	–	N
6	G3PD[g]	35	37	500	3.5[g]	GAPD	12p13.31–p13.1	335	5	9	N
7	Stomatin	31	32	–	2.5	EPB72	9q33–q34	288	12	7	HSt
7	Tropomyosin	27 + 29	28	80	1	TPM3	1q31	239	–	–	N
PAS-1	Glycophorin A[h]	36	–	500–1000	85	GYPA	4q28–q31	131	>40	7	HE
PAS-2	Glycophorin C[h]	32	14	50–100	4	GYPC	2q14–q21	128	14	4	HE
PAS-3	Glycophorin B[h]	20	–	100–300	10	GYPB	4q28–q31	72	>30	5	N
	Glycophorin D[h]	23	–	20	1	GYPD	2q14–q21	107	14	4	N
	Glycophorin E	–	–	–	–	GYPE	4q28–q31	59	>30	4	N

—, Information not available; G3PD, glyceraldehyde 3-phosphate dehydrogenase; HAc, hereditary acanthocytosis; HE, hereditary elliptocytosis; HPP, hereditary pyropoikilocytosis; HS, hereditary spherocytosis; HSt, hereditary stomatocytosis; N, no hematologic abnormalities reported; SAO, southeast Asian ovalocytosis.

[a]Quantitation based on scanning of sodium dodecylsulfate polyacrylamide gel electrophoresis of red cell membranes prepared from healthy blood donors. For glycophorins, values indicate the fraction of periodic acid-Schiff–positive material.

[b]Bands 2.1, 2.2, 2.3, and 2.6 are protein isoforms of erythroid ankyrin, at least some of which are produced by alternative splicing of ankyrin messenger RNA.

[c]Because adducin comigrates with band 3, no numerical band designation is available.

[d]Numerous erythroid and nonerythroid isoforms of protein 4.1 produced by alternative splicing have been described. Values correspond to the major erythroid protein 4.1 isoform.

[e]Both dematin and p55 migrate within the 4.9 band.

[f]Forty thousand dematin trimers are present in one red cell.

[g]Variable amounts of band 6 are detected in red cell membranes.

[h]Detectable on periodic acid-Schiff–stained gels only.

The membrane proteins are classified as either integral or peripheral based on the ease with which they can be removed from whole red cell membrane preparations in the laboratory. Integral or transmembrane proteins are embedded in the lipid bilayer by hydrophobic interactions and require detergents to extract them. They often protrude from the bilayer and extend into the plasma and/or the interior of the erythrocyte and these structural features correlate with their functions as transport proteins, receptors, signaling molecules, and carriers of red cell antigens.

Peripheral proteins constitute the membrane skeleton and are loosely attached to the cytoplasmic face of the lipid bilayer and can be extracted by high or low salt concentrations or by high pH. Attachment is mediated indirectly by covalent or noncovalent interactions with the cytoplasmic domains of the transmembrane proteins, as well as by direct interactions with the inner leaflet of the lipid bilayer. These associations are dynamic and the affinity of binding is regulated by post-translational modifications of the proteins, including phosphorylation, methylation, glycosylation, or lipid modification (myristoylation, palmitoylation, or farnesylation). Peripheral proteins typically function either as structural proteins and form part of the membrane skeleton or they serve as linker proteins attaching the skeleton to the bilayer.

Many erythrocyte proteins belong to superfamilies and have homologues in nonerythroid cells that are structurally related but are encoded by different genes. This genetic diversity explains why the clinical expression of most (but not all) red cell membrane protein mutations is confined to the erythroid lineage. Several proteins exist in different isoforms, created by tissue- and developmental stage-specific alternative splicing or by the use of alternative initiation codons or promoters. Many of the membrane proteins are large, multifunctional proteins and therefore the position of a mutation determines the functional abnormality and clinical phenotype.

Integral Membrane Proteins

The most abundant and important transmembrane proteins are band 3, which is the anion exchanger (AE1) of the erythrocyte, and the glycophorins (GPs).

Band 3 The red cell contains approximately 1.2 million copies of AE1, a multifunctional and major integral membrane protein (see Table 46–1). It has a molecular mass of 102 kDa, but migrates as a diffuse band on sodium dodecylsulfate (SDS) gels as a result of heterogeneous N-glycosylation. The 911-amino-acid protein consists of two functional domains; an N-terminal 43-kDa cytoplasmic domain and a 52-kDa transmembrane channel, including a short 33-amino-acid C-terminal cytoplasmic tail[11] (Fig. 46–2). The anion exchange domain encompasses 13 α helical transmembrane segments and one nonhelical segment all connected by hydrophilic loops.[12,13] The short cytoplasmic tail binds carbonic anhydrase II to form a metabolon with the transmembrane domain, enabling the exchange of HCO_3^- and Cl^- anions, which is a critical function of the red cell.[14] The extracellular surface of the transmembrane domain of band 3 carries several antigens, including Diego, I/i, and Wright blood groups.

The N-terminal phosphorylated cytoplasmic domain serves as a major hub for protein-protein interactions, which perform key functions (see Figs. 46–1 and 46–2).[15] It regulates metabolic pathways by sequestering key glycolytic enzymes such as glyceraldehyde-3-phosphate dehydrogenase, phosphoglycerate kinase and aldolase, which are inactive when bound. Phosphorylation at tyrosine 8 prevents binding, which liberates the active enzymes.[16] The cytoplasmic domain interacts with hemoglobin and hemichromes and plays a role in red cell aging[17]; it associates with several peripheral membrane proteins, including the erythrocyte isoform of protein (4.1R),[18,19] protein 4.2,[20] and adducin,[21] as well as phosphatases and kinases. This domain also serves as the major attachment

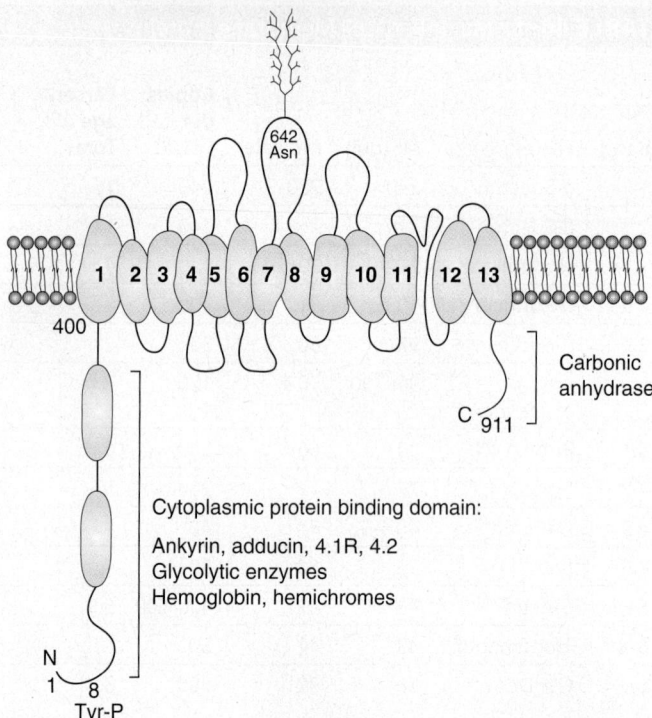

Figure 46–2. Schematic model of human erythrocyte band 3. The N and C terminal regions of the protein extend into the cytoplasm and provide binding sites for several red cell proteins and enzymes. The transmembrane domain forms an anion exchange channel and consists of 13 α helical segments embedded in the lipid bilayer and one nonhelical segment. Asparagine 642 is linked to complex carbohydrates, which protrude on the exterior of the red cell. Tyrosine 8 is phosphorylated. The domains are not drawn to scale.

site of the membrane to the underlying skeleton through its interaction with ankyrin, which binds to spectrin (see Figs. 46–1 and 46–2).[22,23]

Band 3 associates with other transmembrane proteins to form macromolecular complexes (see Fig. 46–1).[24] This includes the major GP, GPA,[25] and the Rh protein complex, consisting of Rh-associated glycoprotein (RhAG), Rh, CD47, LW, and GPB (Chap. 136).[24] In addition, band 3 participates in the protein 4.1-based junctional complex of proteins.[19]

Band 3 is encoded by the *SLC4A1* gene, which produces different tissue-specific isoforms.[11,26] The erythroid isoform is controlled by a promoter upstream of exon 1, whereas transcription of the kidney isoform is initiated from a promoter in intron 3, resulting in a protein lacking the first N-terminal 65 amino acids.

Glycophorins GPs are integral membrane glycoproteins composed of an extracellular hydrophilic N-terminal domain, a single α-helical membrane-spanning domain, and a C-terminal cytoplasmic tail. GPA, GPB, and GPE are homologous and are encoded by closely linked genes that arose by duplication of the ancestral GPA gene.[27] GPC and GPD are encoded by the same gene but make use of alternate initiation codons.[28]

GPs have very high sialic acid content and are responsible for most of the external negative charge of red cells, which prevents the adherence of cells to each other and the vascular endothelium. The GPs carry a large number of blood group antigens, including MN, SsU, Miltenberger, En(a–), M^K, and Gerbich (Chap. 136). They also function as receptors for *Plasmodium falciparum*, the most virulent malaria parasite. Within the lipid bilayer of the membrane, GPA interacts with band

3 as part of a macromolecular complex, and may serve as a chaperone for band 3 targeting to the membrane.[25] GPC associates with protein 4.1R and p55, thereby providing an additional contact site between the membrane and the skeleton (see Fig. 46–1).[19] These interactions play a role in stabilizing the membrane.

Other Integral Membrane Proteins The Rh-RhAG group of proteins is part of a macromolecular band 3 complex, which stabilizes the membrane. RhAG belongs to the ammonium transporter family of proteins, but its function is controversial. Numerous other proteins are embedded in the lipid bilayer, many of which are implicated in clinical immunohematology and membrane disorders, such as the XK, Kell, Kidd, Duffy, and Lutheran glycoproteins (see Fig. 46–1).[11,19] Additional integral membrane proteins include ion pumps and channels, such as stomatin, aquaporin, glucose transporter (GLUT-1), and various cation and anion transporters.

Peripheral Membrane Proteins

Underlying the lipid bilayer is the peripheral membrane skeleton, an interlocking network of structural proteins, which plays a critical role in maintaining the shape and integrity of the red cell. The major proteins of the erythrocyte membrane skeleton are spectrin, actin, proteins 4.1R, 4.2, 4.9, p55, and the adducins, which interact in a horizontal plane.

Linker proteins mediate the vertical attachment of the skeleton to integral membrane proteins in the lipid bilayer (see Fig. 46–1). The primary connecting protein is ankyrin, which links spectrin to the cytoplasmic domain of band 3, as well as to the Rh–RhAG complex. Protein 4.1R provides an additional link with GPC and band 3.

Spectrin Spectrin is the major constituent of the erythrocyte membrane skeleton and is present at approximately 240,000 molecules per cell.[29] It is a multifunctional protein composed of two homologous but structurally distinct subunits, α and β, encoded by separate genes, which may have evolved from duplication of a single ancestral gene[30] (see Table 46–1 and Fig. 46–3). Both α- and β-spectrin contain tandem homologous spectrin repeats that are approximately 106 amino acids long and are folded into three antiparallel helices, A, B, and C. Each repeat is connected to the adjacent repeat by short ordered α-helical linkers (Fig. 46–3).[31,32] Erythrocyte α-spectrin is a 280-kDa protein comprising 20 complete repeats, an N-terminal partial repeat, a central SH3 domain, and a C-terminal calcium-binding EF hand. The β-spectrin subunit is a 246-kDa polypeptide consisting of 16 complete repeats, an N-terminal actin binding domain, a partial repeat near the C-terminus, and a nonhomologous phosphorylated C-terminus. Mild trypsin treatment of spectrin cleaves the two subunits into distinct structural domains: αI-V and βI-IV. The triple helical structure of the spectrin

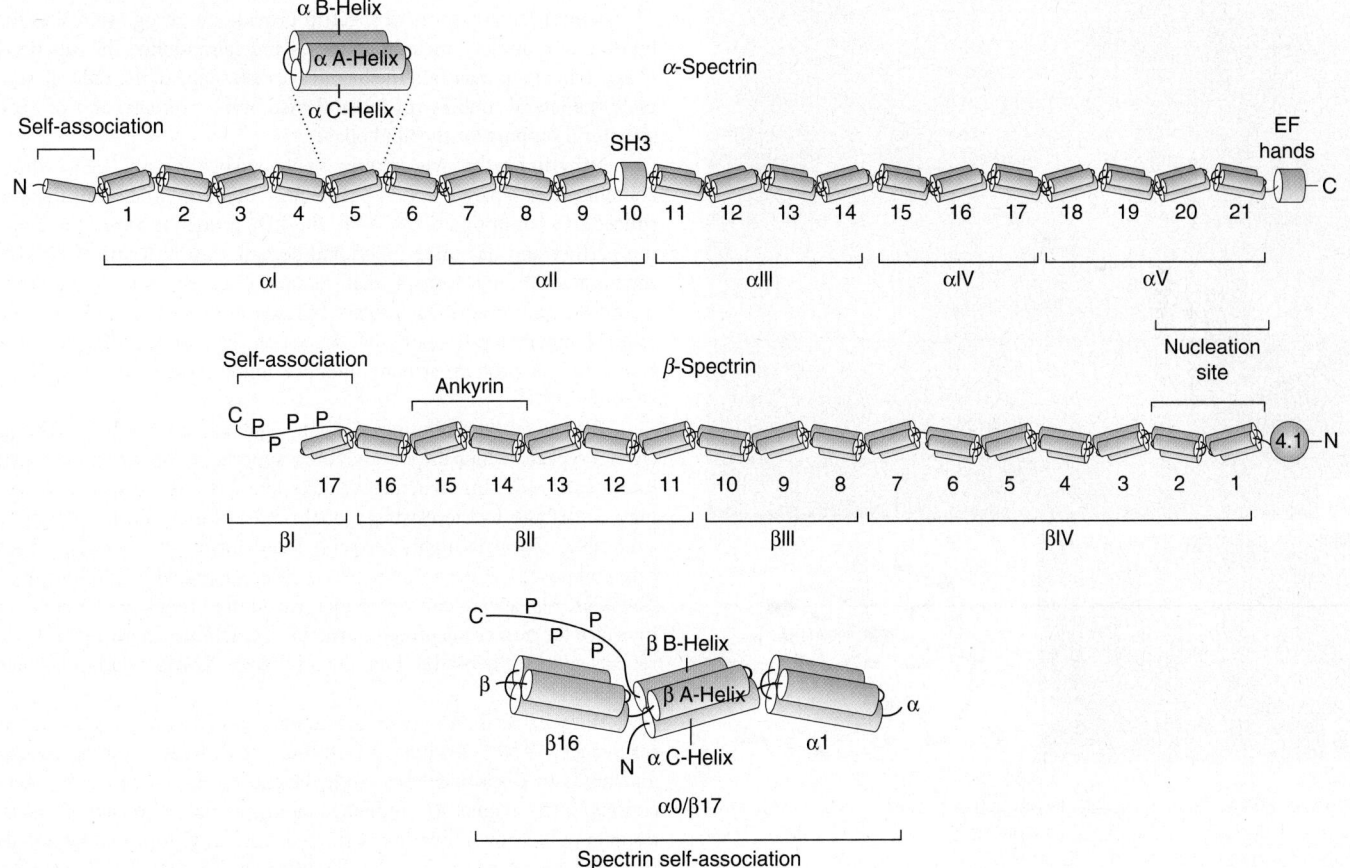

Figure 46–3. Schematic model of human erythrocyte α- and β-spectrin. The proteins consist of multiple homologous spectrin repeats of approximately 106 amino acids numbered from the N-terminal. Each repeat is composed of three α helices. Nonhomologous regions include an SH3 domain and calcium-binding EF hands in α-spectrin, a protein 4.1R binding domain, and a C-terminal phosphorylated tail in β-spectrin. The nucleation site indicates the initial region of interaction between α and β monomers to form an antiparallel heterodimer. Spectrin heterodimer self association into tetramers involves helix C of the α0 partial repeat of α-spectrin and helices A and B of the partial β17 repeat of β-spectrin to form a complete triple helical repeat. Ankyrin binds to repeats 14 and 15 of β-spectrin. Limited tryptic digestion of spectrin cleaves the proteins into discrete αI-V and βI-IV domains.

repeats renders the molecule highly flexible and enables it to extend and condense reversibly, which provides the red cell with elasticity and durability to withstand the shear stress encountered in the circulation.

The core structure of the erythrocyte skeleton consists of spectrin heterotetramers, which are strong but flexible filaments. Tetramers are assembled from the monomers in a series of events. For initial heterodimer formation, the α- and β-spectrin chains align in an antiparallel fashion and interact with high affinity through long-range electrostatic interactions at a nucleation site, comprising repeats α20–21 and β1–2.[33] This triggers the association of the remaining repeats in the two subunits in a zipper-like fashion. Repeats at the N-terminus of α-spectrin (αI domain) and the C-terminus of β-spectrin (βI domain) are the regions involved in heterodimer self-association to form tetramers. Partial repeat β17 consists of two helices (A and B) which interact with the single helix C of partial repeat α0 to form a complete triple helical repeat (see Fig. 46–3). The interface of this tetramerization site is dominated by hydrophobic contacts supplemented by electrostatic interactions.[34] Phosphorylation of the C-terminal region of β-spectrin beyond the self-association site decreases the mechanical stability of the membrane.

At the opposite tail end of the spectrin tetramers, the N terminus of β-spectrin binds to short F-actin filaments, which is potentiated by 4.1R, to form the core of a junctional complex,[35] which links six tetramers together into a hexagonal skeletal network (Fig. 46–4).[36] The C-terminal

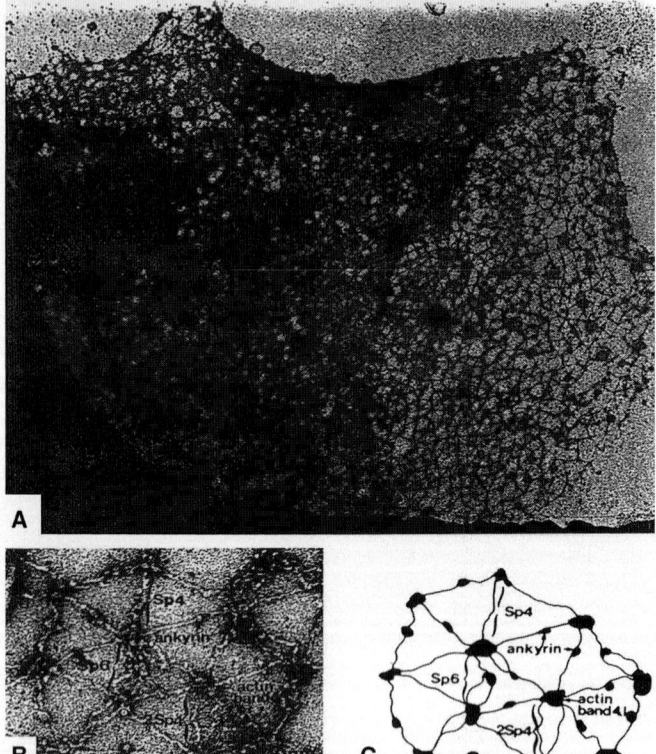

Figure 46–4. Electron micrograph of the human erythrocyte membrane skeleton. Membrane lipids and transmembrane proteins have been removed and the skeletons were extended during preparation and negative staining to reveal the structure. **A.** Low-magnification image reveals an ordered network of proteins. **B** and **C.** High-magnification image and schematic of the hexagonal lattice showing spectrin tetramers (Sp4) and hexamers (Sp6) or double tetramers (2Sp4). Junctional complexes contain actin filaments and protein 4.1R. Globular ankyrin molecules are bound to spectrin tetramers. *(Reproduced with permission from Liu SC et al: Visualisation of the hexagonal lattice in the erythrocyte membrane skeleton.* J Cell Biol *104(3):527–536, 1987.)*

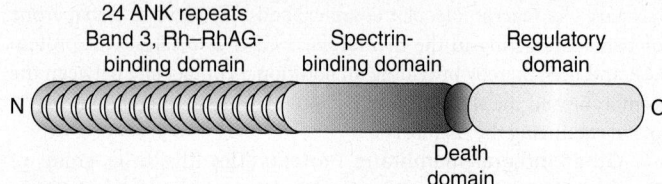

Figure 46–5. Schematic of human erythrocyte ankyrin. The N-terminal domain consists of 24 ANK repeats, which bind to band 3 and the Rh–RhAg complex. The central domain attaches to spectrin. The C-terminal domain varies in different isoforms of ankyrin, which are produced by alternative splicing of the gene. This domain also contains a conserved death domain of unknown function.

EF hand of α-spectrin enhances this spectrin-actin-4.1R interaction.[37] Numerous other proteins participate in the junctional complex, including adducin, protein 4.9, p55, tropomodulin and tropomyosin (see Fig. 46–1).[19] Protein 4.1R binds to GPC and band 3, which serves as a secondary attachment site of the skeleton to integral membrane proteins. The main interaction tethering the skeleton to the lipid bilayer is accomplished by ankyrin, which links β-spectrin to band 3 (see Fig. 46–1). The ankyrin binding site is a flexible pocket formed by repeats 14 and 15 of β-spectrin near the C-terminal end of the molecule.[38,39] Spectrin also interacts with phosphatidylserine on the inner leaflet of the lipid bilayer.

Nonrepeat sequences in spectrin provide the recognition sites for binding to modifiers, including kinases and calmodulin. The functions of spectrin are to maintain the biconcave disk shape of the red cell, regulate the lateral mobility of integral membrane proteins, and provide structural support for the lipid bilayer.

Ankyrin Erythrocyte ankyrin is encoded by the *ANK1* gene, which contains three separate tissue-specific promoters and first exons that are spliced to a common exon 2.[40] The 206-kDa protein is a versatile binding partner and has three functional domains: an N-terminal 89-kDa membrane-binding domain, that contains sites for band 3 and other ligands; a central 62-kDa spectrin-binding domain, and a C-terminal 55-kDa regulatory domain that is responsible for the different isoforms of the protein, which influence ankyrin–protein interactions (Fig. 46–5).[29]

The membrane-binding domain contains 24 tandem ankyrin (ANK) repeats, which are stacked into a superhelical array that is coiled into a solenoid. This structure behaves like a reversible spring, which may contribute to the elasticity of the membrane.[22] Each 33-amino-acid ANK repeat is highly conserved and forms an L-shaped structure composed of two antiparallel α helices separated by a β hairpin.[41] The ANK repeats are connected by unstructured loops and provide an interface for numerous protein–protein interactions. Erythrocyte ANK repeats specifically bind to band 3 and the Rh–RhAg macromolecular complex.[19,29]

The spectrin-binding domain contains a small unique subdomain termed *ZU5-ANK*, which has a β-strand core with several surface loops and binds to β-spectrin through hydrophobic and electrostatic interactions.[42] The regulatory domain contains a highly conserved death domain of unknown function in the red cell. The C-terminal section of the regulatory domain varies in the different isoforms of ankyrin, proteins 2.1 to 2.6, which are created by alternative splicing[43] and which exhibit different binding affinities for band 3 and spectrin. Phosphorylation of ankyrin reduces binding to band 3 and spectrin tetramers.

Protein 4.1R The gene encoding protein 4.1 produces diverse isoforms in different tissues and different developmental stages. This diversity is accomplished by the use of alternate first exons under the control of different promoters, and alternate initiation codons. This

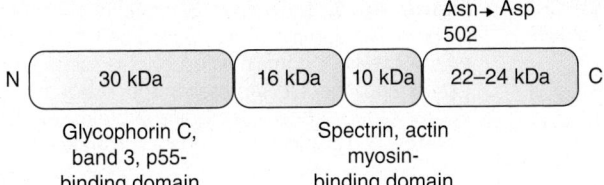

Figure 46–6. Schematic of human erythrocyte protein 4.1R. The protein consists of four domains, with the 30-kDa and the 10-kDa domains involved in binding to other red cell membrane proteins. The C-terminal domain has an asparagine residue at position 502 in isoform 4.1a, which is deamidated in older red cells to form aspartic acid and isoform 4.1b.

transcriptional regulation is coupled to complex pre-mRNA splicing events.[44,45] The erythrocyte isoform, 4.1R, is produced from the downstream initiation codon and contains exon 16, which encodes an essential part of the spectrin-actin binding domain.

Protein 4.1R is a globular phosphoprotein that contains four structural and functional domains of 30 kDa, 16 kDa, 10 kDa, and 22 to 24 kDa (Fig. 46–6). The N-terminal 30-kDa domain is responsible for binding to the cytoplasmic domains of band 3 and GPC, as well as to p55, thereby linking the skeleton to the lipid bilayer.[19] The 10-kDa domain enhances the interaction between spectrin and actin in the junctional complex, which connects spectrin tetramers to each other. The functions of the other two domains are not characterized. Phosphorylation of 4.1R inhibits spectrin–actin–4.1R complex formation and also decreases binding to band 3. Protein 4.1R binds weakly to phosphatidylserine in the lipid bilayer.

Two forms of 4.1R, a and b, are present in red cells, with protein 4.1b predominating in young erythrocytes. The difference between the two isoforms relates to the gradual deamidation of asparagine 502 to aspartic acid in a nonenzymatic, age-dependent manner, which influences the mobility of the protein on SDS gels.[46]

Protein 4.2 Protein 4.2 is a member of the transglutaminase family of proteins,[47] but it has no enzyme activity as it lacks the critical triad of residues that form the active transglutaminase site. The exact role of protein 4.2 has not been elucidated, but it stabilizes the link between the skeleton and the lipid bilayer. Protein 4.2 interacts with several proteins, including the cytoplasmic domain of band 3, and this binding site has been identified as a hairpin region toward the center of the protein 4.2 molecule.[11,47] Interactions with the ANK repeats in the membrane-binding domain of ankyrin[47] and CD47, a component of the Rh complex, have been documented.[19,47] *In vitro* binding studies have revealed an association of protein 4.2 with 4.1R and spectrin. Protein 4.2 binds calcium adjacent to the spectrin-binding loop suggesting that calcium may regulate this interaction. The protein undergoes posttranslational palmitoylation and myristoylation, which suggests an interaction with the lipid bilayer.[47]

p55 This molecule is a phosphoprotein member of the membrane-associated guanylate kinase (MAGUK) family of proteins.[48] In the red cell it is found as part of a ternary complex with GPC and 4.1R and it strengthens the link between the skeleton and the bilayer.[19] p55

contains five domains, including an N-terminal PDZ domain, which binds to GPC; an SH3 domain; a central HOOK domain interacting with the 30-kDa domain of 4.1R; a region with tyrosine phosphorylation sites; and a C-terminal guanylate kinase domain (Fig. 46–7).[48] The protein is extensively palmitoylated, reflecting an interaction with the membrane bilayer.

Adducin Adducin, a calcium/calmodulin-binding phosphoprotein located at the spectrin–actin junctional complex, is composed of $\alpha\beta$ adducin heterodimers, which are structurally similar proteins encoded by separate genes. Adducins contain a 39-kDa globular head region, a small neck region of 9 kDa implicated in oligomerization to form $\alpha_2\beta_2$ heterotetramers, and a 30-kDa cytoplasmic tail with a myristoylated alanine-rich C kinase substrate (MARCKS) phosphorylation domain at the C terminus (Fig. 46–8). The adducin tails cap actin filaments and promote interaction of spectrin and actin.[49] They also bind band 3 and the GLUT-1, and thus form part of the macromolecular junctional complex linking the spectrin skeleton to the lipid bilayer (see Fig. 46–1).[21,50] The function of adducin is regulated by calcium-dependent calmodulin binding and differential phosphorylation. A primary deficiency of adducin in human disease has not been described; however, mice with targeted inactivation of α- or β-adducin suffer from compensated spherocytic anemia, suggesting that the adducin mutations may be candidates for recessively inherited hemolytic anemia.[51]

Actin and Actin-Binding Proteins The erythrocyte contains β-type actin assembled into short F-actin protofilaments of 14 to 16 monomers. The length of the filaments is regulated by a "molecular ruler" of two rod-shaped tropomyosin molecules, which are bound along the filament, as well as by two tropomodulin molecules, which cap the filaments at the pointed ends.[52] At the barbed end actin is capped by an adducin heterodimer. Dematin or protein 4.9 is a trimeric phosphoprotein, which bundles the actin filaments,[53] but also acts as a linker molecule by binding to the transmembrane GLUT-1.[21,50]

● MEMBRANE ORGANIZATION

The structure of the erythrocyte membrane is determined by multiple protein–protein interactions between (1) integral membrane proteins within the lipid bilayer, (2) peripheral proteins in the skeleton, and (3) linker proteins, which tether the skeleton to the transmembrane proteins (see Fig. 46–1). Protein–lipid interactions within the bilayer or between the anionic phospholipids and the underlying membrane skeleton also play a role in cohesion of the membrane components. By using the cytoplasmic domains of embedded proteins as attachment points, the membrane skeleton not only affixes itself to the lipid bilayer but also influences the topology of the transmembrane proteins and constrains their lateral and rotational mobility.

The membrane skeleton resembles a lattice-like network, with approximately 60 percent of the lipid bilayer directly laminated to the underlying skeleton.[36] Electron microscopy of stretched membrane skeletons indicate that the individual proteins can be visualized as a highly ordered meshwork of hexagons (see Fig. 46–4).[36] The corners of each hexagon consist of a globular macromolecular junctional complex of proteins, including 4.1R and actin, which interact with spectrin

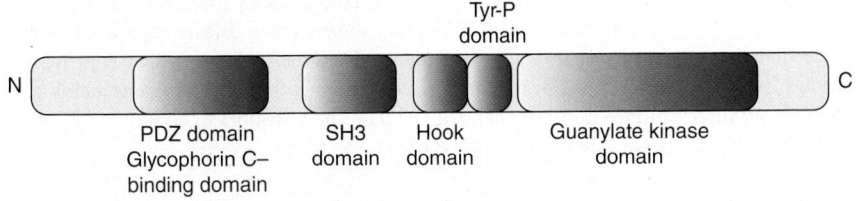

Figure 46–7. Schematic of human erythrocyte p55. The protein is part of the membrane-associated guanylate kinase family and the kinase domain is close to the C terminus. Adjacent is a tyrosine phosphorylation zone. The central HOOK domain binds protein 4.1R.

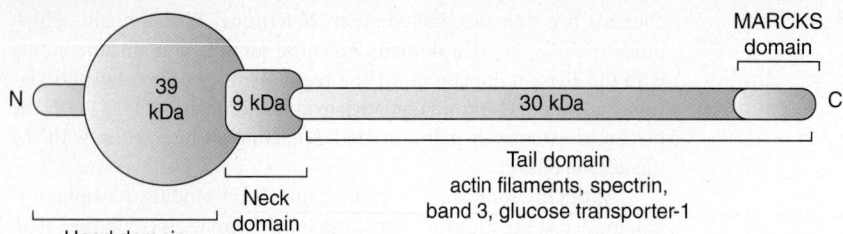

Figure 46–8. Schematic of human erythrocyte adducin. The domain structure for α and β adducin is similar. The neck domain is responsible for oligomerization and the tail represents the major binding site for other red cell membrane proteins. MARCKS, myristoylated alanine-rich C kinase substrate.

tetramers, as well as tropomyosin, tropomodulin, adducin, dematin, and p55.[19,21,50] Spectrin tetramers form the arms of the hexagons, cross-bridging individual junctional complexes. These *horizontal* protein interactions are important in the maintenance of the structural integrity of the cell, accounting for the high tensile strength of the erythrocyte (see Fig. 46–1).

The spectrin/actin skeleton is anchored to the phospholipid bilayer by two major membrane protein complexes: (1) an ankyrin complex that contains transmembrane proteins, band 3, GPA, Rh, and RhAG complex proteins, as well as peripheral proteins ankyrin, protein 4.2, and several glycolytic enzymes, and (2) a distal junctional complex that contains the membrane-spanning proteins band 3, GPC, GLUT-1, Rh, Kell, and XK proteins, in addition to peripheral proteins 4.1R, actin, tropomyosin, tropomodulin, adducin, dematin, and p55. These *vertical* protein–protein interactions are critical in the stabilization of the lipid bilayer, preventing loss of microvesicles from the cells (see Fig. 46–1).

The avidity of these horizontal and vertical interactions is modulated by posttranslational modifications of the participating proteins, especially phosphorylation. The erythrocyte contains multiple protein kinases and phosphatases that constantly phosphorylate and dephosphorylate specific serine, threonine, and tyrosine residues on band 3, β-spectrin, ankyrin, 4.1R, adducin, and dematin, in a dynamic manner, thereby tightly regulating the structural properties of the membrane. Additionally, membrane protein associations are also influenced by a variety of intracellular factors, including calcium, calmodulin, phosphoinositides, and polyanions such as 2,3-bisphosphoglycerate (BPG). Red cell membrane proteins are also subject to a variety of other posttranslational modifications, including myristoylation, palmitoylation, glycosylation, methylation, deamidation, oxidation, and limited proteolytic cleavage, but the functional effects of these alterations are generally not known.

CELLULAR DEFORMABILITY AND MEMBRANE STABILITY

In performing its primary function of oxygen delivery to the tissues, the erythrocyte has to repeatedly negotiate tiny capillaries in the microvasculature, as well as narrow slits in the spleen, which are much smaller than the diameter of the cell. Consequently, it has to undergo extensive distortion and deformation without fragmentation or loss of integrity, and this property of deformability is critical for survival during its average 120-day life span. The structure of the red cell membrane endows the cell with unique material properties, which makes it highly flexible, yet incredibly resilient, and enables a very rapid response to circulatory shear stress.

Elegant biophysical studies have identified three features that regulate the deformability of the cell: (1) the biconcave disk shape, which reflects the cell surface-area-to-volume ratio; (2) the viscoelastic properties of the membrane, which depend on the structural and functional integrity of the membrane skeleton; and (3) the cytoplasmic viscosity, which is determined primarily by intracellular haemoglobin.[54]

The unique biconcave disk shape of the erythrocyte provides a high ratio of surface area to cellular volume and this excess of membrane is critical for survival of the cell. It enables the red cell to stretch and distort when it passes through the microcirculation and protects it from destruction. To maintain the shape of the cell and to prevent loss of membrane microvesicles, the lipid bilayer and the skeleton have to be in direct contact with each other. The cohesion between the two sections of the membrane depends on protein–protein interactions between transmembrane proteins and peripheral proteins in the vertical plane of the membrane. These contacts are represented by the two macromolecular complexes (ankyrin–band 3 complex and the junctional complex) anchoring the skeleton to the integral proteins. To prevent fragmentation of the membrane and loss of the biconcave disk shape, the structural integrity of the membrane skeleton is critical. In this regard, the horizontal interactions of the peripheral proteins of the junctional complex, mainly 4.1R and actin, which link the tail ends of the spectrin tetramers together, is a major determinant of membrane stability. Spectrin heterodimer self-association, which links the head regions of the spectrin tetramers, is also of paramount importance.

The viscoelastic properties of the membrane are intrinsic features of the spectrin skeleton. The enormous distortion imposed on the cell during passage through the microvasculature is accommodated by the dynamic dissociation of spectrin tetramers into dimers, and subsequent reassociation to restore the original shape once the shear stress is removed.[55] The lattice structure of the skeleton facilitates this flexibility, as the individual hexagons are either in a compact configuration, with the junctional complexes close to each other and the spectrin tetramers coiled between them, or in an extended configuration, which allows large unidirectional deformation without disruption of the skeleton (see Fig. 46–4). The structure of the spectrin repeats also play a major role in the elasticity of the skeleton. Each triple helical repeat behaves partly as an independently folding unit and has a different thermal stability.[56] Cysteine labeling studies indicated that shear stress forced the unfolding of the least stable repeats.[57] These studies highlight the flexibility of the spectrin repeats and support the concept that their unfolding and refolding contributes to the deformability of the membrane. In addition, the elasticity of the ANK repeats may also facilitate the dynamic changes in the membrane during circulatory shear stress.[22]

Red cell viscosity is largely determined by the concentration of intracellular hemoglobin, which is tightly regulated to minimize cytoplasmic viscous dissipation during cellular deformation. As the mean cell hemoglobin concentration rises above 37 g/dL, the viscosity increases exponentially, and this compromises the deformability of the cell under increased circulatory shear stress.[54] The hemoglobin concentration is critically dependent on red cell volume, which is primarily determined by the total cation content of the cell. Numerous membrane pumps and ion channels regulate the transport of sodium and potassium across the membrane (Fig. 46–9).

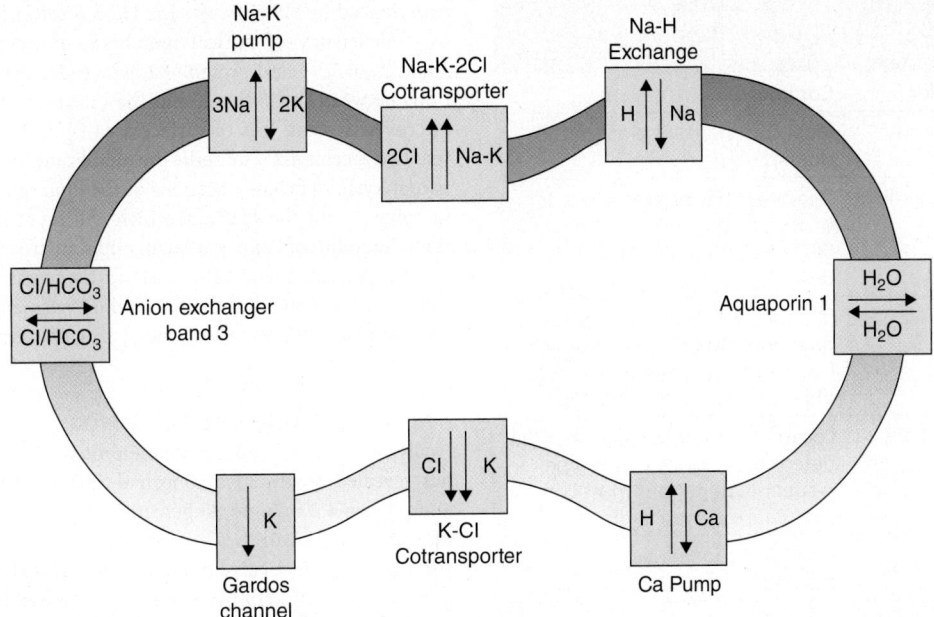

Figure 46–9. Principal ion transport and ion exchange channels and passive permeability pathways of the human erythrocyte.

● MEMBRANE PERMEABILITY

The red cell membrane displays selective permeability to cations and anions and it maintains a high potassium, low sodium, and very low calcium content within the cell.[58] Ion transport pathways in the red cell membrane (see Fig. 46–9) include energy-driven membrane pumps, gradient-driven systems, and various channels. Several transport mechanisms exist for cations, including two energy-driven pumps.[58] The sodium pump is a Na^+K^+ adenosine triphosphatase (ATPase) that extrudes three sodium ions in exchange for two potassium ions entering the red cell. Calcium is pumped out of the cell by a calmodulin-activated Ca^{2+} ATPase, which protects the cell from deleterious effects of calcium, such as echinocytosis (Chap. 31), membrane vesiculation, calpain activation, membrane proteolysis, and cellular dehydration.[58] The Ca^{2+}-activated K^+ channel, also called the Gardos channel, causes selective loss of K^+ in response to increased intracellular Ca^{2+}. The Na^+K^+ gradient established by the sodium pump is used by several passive, gradient-driven systems to move ions across the red cell membrane.[58] The systems include the K^+Cl^- cotransporter, the $Na^+K^+2Cl^-$ cotransporter, and the Na^+H^+ exchanger.

Chloride and bicarbonate anions are readily exchanged through band 3. The red cell is highly permeable to water, which is transported by aquaporin-1 (AQP1),[59] and glucose is taken up by the glucose transporter.[60] The membrane also contains an ATP-driven oxidized glutathione (GSSG) transporter and amino acid transport systems.[58] Larger charged molecules, such as ATP, do not cross the membrane.

● RED CELL MEMBRANE DISORDERS

Hemolytic anemias resulting from defects in the erythrocyte membrane comprise an important group of hereditary anemias. The disorders are characterized by altered red cell morphology, which is reflected in the nomenclature of HS, HE, hereditary pyropoikilocytosis (HPP) and southeast Asian ovalocytosis (SAO), which are the most common disorders in this group. Protein studies have identified the underlying membrane abnormalities and advances in molecular biology have

enabled further characterization of these disorders and, in many cases, identification of the causative mutations. These molecular analyses have provided additional information on the pathogenesis of these disorders and important insights into the structure–function relationships of erythrocyte membrane proteins.

As predicted in 1984 by Jiri Palek[61] and confirmed by subsequent studies, protein defects that compromise *vertical* interactions between the membrane skeleton and the lipid bilayer result in destabilization of the bilayer, loss of membrane microvesicles and spherocyte formation; whereas mutations affecting *horizontal* protein interactions within the membrane skeletal network disrupt the skeleton resulting in defective shape recovery and elliptocytes (Table 46–2). Red cell membrane disorders exhibit significant heterogeneity in their clinical, morphologic, laboratory and molecular characteristics.

HEREDITARY SPHEROCYTOSIS

Definition and History

Hereditary spherocytosis is characterized by the presence of osmotically fragile spherical red blood cells on the blood film (Fig. 46–10B). The disorder was first described in 1871 as microcythemia in a case history by two Belgian physicians.[62]

Epidemiology

HS occurs in all racial and ethnic groups. It is the most common inherited hemolytic anemia in individuals of northern European ancestry, affecting approximately 1 in 2000 individuals in North America and Europe.[63] It is also common in Japan and in Africans from southern Africa. Males and females are affected equally.

Etiology and Pathogenesis

The hallmark of HS erythrocytes is loss of membrane surface area relative to intracellular volume, which accounts for the spherical shape and loss of central pallor of the cell (Figs 46–10B and 46–11C). Spherocytes exhibit decreased deformability and are thus selectively retained, damaged and ultimately destroyed in the spleen, which causes the hemolysis

TABLE 46–2. Erythrocyte Membrane Protein Defects in Inherited Disorders of Red Cell Shape

Protein	Disorder	Comment
Ankyrin	HS	Most common cause of typical dominant HS
Band 3	HS, SAO, NIHF, HAc	"Pincered" HS spherocytes seen on blood film presplenectomy; SAO results from 9-amino-acid deletion
β-Spectrin	HS, HE, HPP, NIHF	"Acanthocytic" spherocytes seen on blood film presplenectomy; location of mutation in β-spectrin determines clinical phenotype
α-Spectrin	HS, HE, HPP, NIHF	Location of mutation in α-spectrin determines clinical phenotype; α-spectrin mutations most common cause of typical HE
Protein 4.2	HS	Primarily found in Japanese patients
Protein 4.1	HE	Found in certain European and Arab populations
GPC	HE	Concomitant protein 4.1 deficiency is basis of HE in GPC defects

GPC, glycophorin C; HAc, hereditary acanthocytosis; HE, hereditary elliptocytosis; HPP, hereditary pyropoikilocytosis; HS, hereditary spherocytosis; NIHF, nonimmune hydrops fetalis; SAO, southeast Asian ovalocytosis.

experienced by HS patients. The HS red cell membrane is destabilized by a deficiency of critical membrane proteins, including spectrin, ankyrin, band 3 and protein 4.2, which decreases the vertical interactions between the skeleton and the bilayer, resulting in the release of microvesicles and loss of surface area (Fig. 46–12). It is hypothesized that two mechanisms underlie the membrane loss: (1) in cells with spectrin/ankyrin deficiency, sections of the lipid bilayer and band 3 are not in contact with the skeleton, which will increase the lateral and rotational mobility of band 3, allowing lipid microvesicles containing band 3 to be generated, and (2) in cells with decreased amounts of band 3/protein 4.2, the stabilizing effect of the transmembrane section of band 3 on the lipid bilayer is lost, facilitating the formation of band 3-free microvesicles.[13]

Red Cell Membrane Protein Defects

Analysis of HS red cell membrane proteins by several research groups has revealed quantitative abnormalities of spectrin, ankyrin, band 3, and protein 4.2 in 70 to 90 percent of the cases.[13,63,64] This spectrum of defects is found worldwide in all the HS cohorts that have been studied; however, the relative frequency of each defect varies with the geographical area and ethnic group. In the United States, parts of Europe, and in Korea, the most common defect is ankyrin deficiency (30 to 60 percent),[63,65,66] whereas it is relatively uncommon elsewhere in the world (<15 percent). In other parts of Europe[64,67] and in South Africa (unpublished), band 3 deficiency is the main defect. In Japan, almost half of the HS cases are caused by a decreased amount of protein 4.2, and in Korea and South Africa, this defect is the second most common, but in other populations it is rare (<6 percent).[63–65] The underlying gene mutations have not been investigated in all HS subjects, but the limited research that has been conducted on the defective genes has identified more than 140 different mutations, which are often unique to a family.

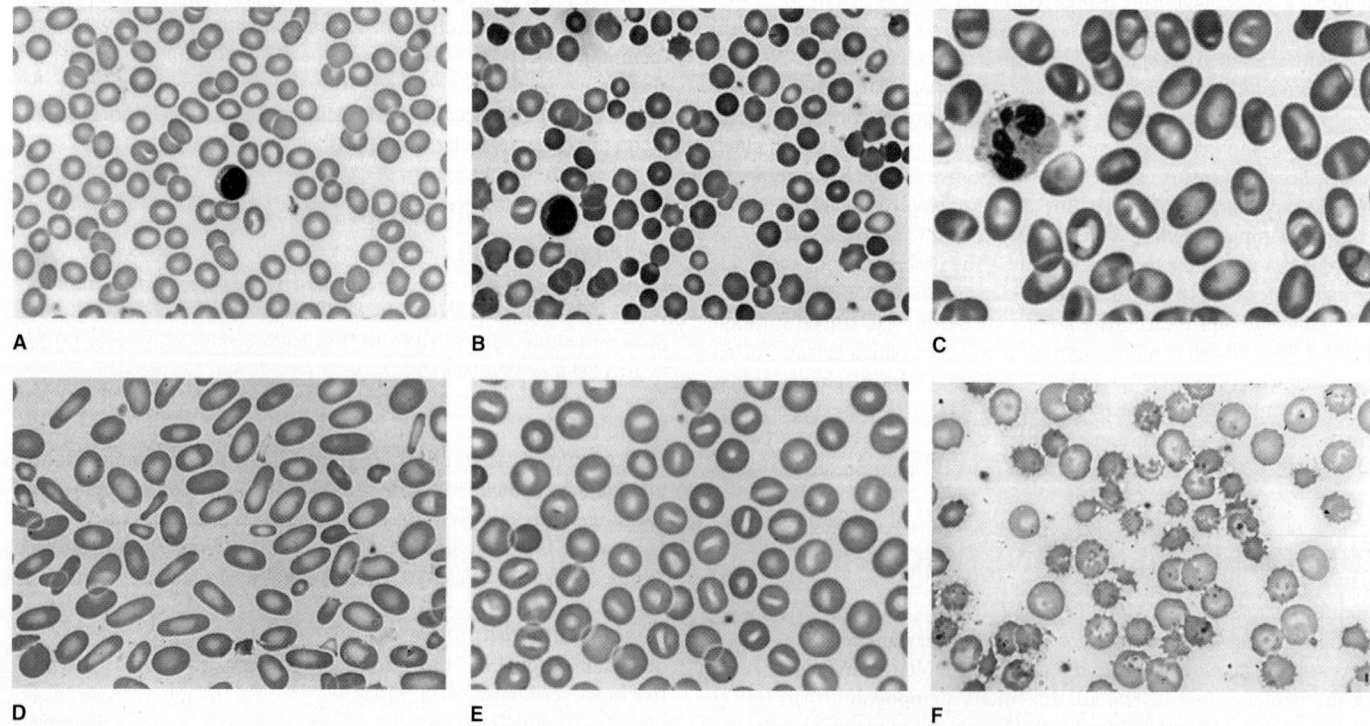

Figure 46–10. Blood films from patients with erythrocyte membrane disorders. **A.** Normal blood film. **B.** HS with dense spherocytes. **C.** SAO with large ovalocytes exhibiting a transverse ridge. **D.** HE with elongated elliptocytes and some poikilocytes. **E.** HSt with cup-shaped stomatocytes. **F.** Hereditary abetalipoproteinemia with acanthocytes. *(Reproduced with permission from Lichtman's Atlas of Hematology, www.accessmedicine.com.)*

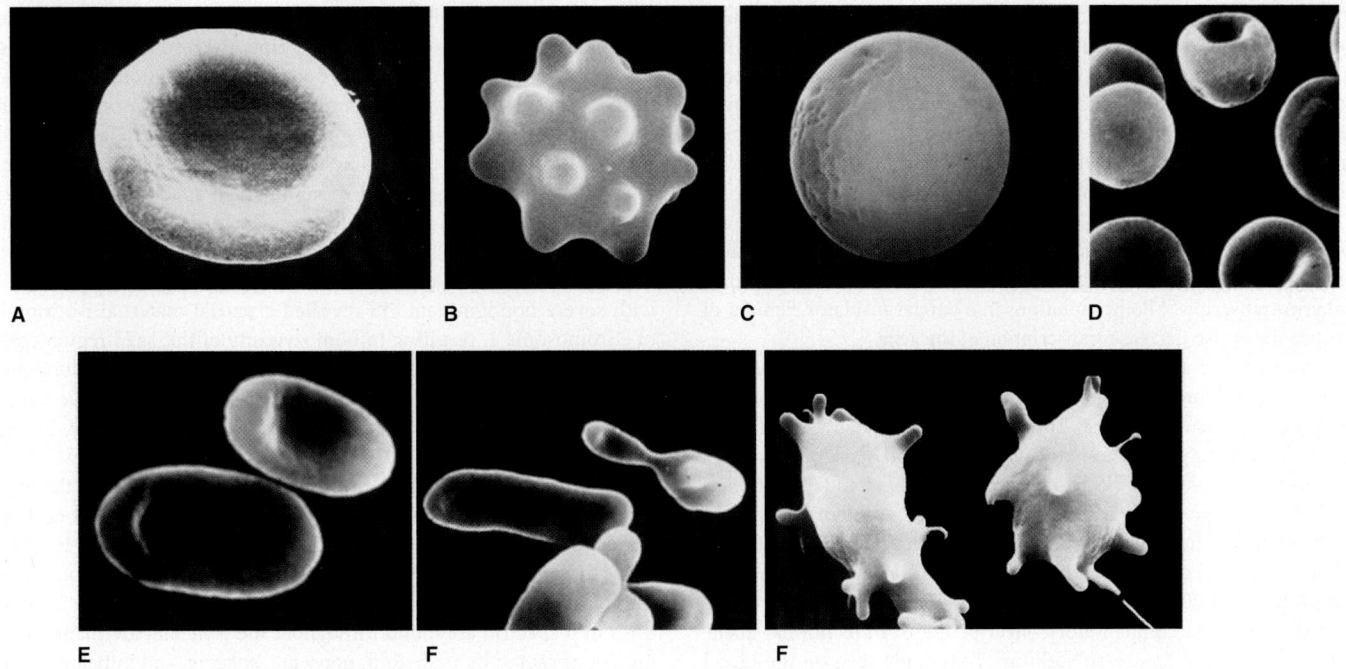

Figure 46–11. Scanning electron micrographs of erythrocytes with abnormal morphology due to membrane defects. **A.** Normal discocyte. **B.** Echinocyte. **C.** Spherocyte. **D.** Stomatocytes. **E.** Ovalocytes. **F.** Elliptocytes. **G.** Acanthocytes. *(Reproduced with permission from Lichtman's Atlas of Hematology, www.accessmedicine.com.)*

Ankyrin Concomitant ankyrin and spectrin deficiency was first described in two patients with severe atypical HS and the primary defect was identified as an ankyrin abnormality.[68] Subsequent DNA analysis of the *ANK1* gene in patients with typical HS identified several mutations,[69] and numerous other studies have shown that ankyrin/spectrin deficiency is a common cause of HS. Ankyrin binds to spectrin with high affinity and attaches it to the membrane, which stabilizes the molecule. Because ankyrin is present in limiting amounts, a deficiency of ankyrin causes an equivalent loss of spectrin.

Different types of ankyrin mutations have been identified throughout the gene, indicating that there are several mechanisms that ultimately result in a decreased amount of ankyrin in the membrane. Interestingly, the majority of these mutations are frameshift and nonsense mutations that either result in unstable transcripts that are destroyed by nonsense-mediated mRNA decay or else produce a truncated defective ankyrin molecule.[66] More than 50 mutations have been documented and they are typically family-specific, although a few recurrent mutations have been described[69,70] and 15 to 20 percent of mutations are *de novo*.[63]

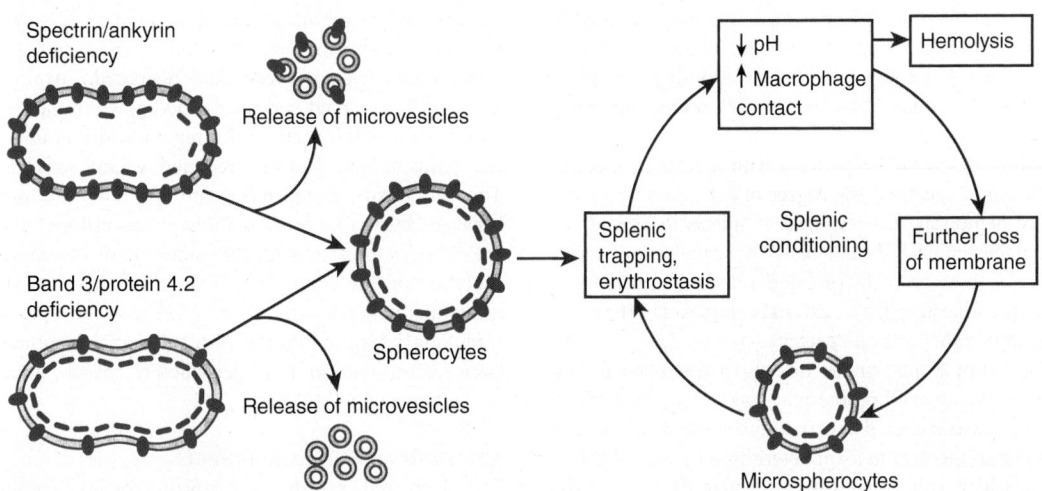

Figure 46–12. Pathobiology of hereditary spherocytosis (HS). The primary defect in HS is a deficiency of one of the membrane proteins, which destabilizes the lipid bilayer and leads to a loss of membrane in the form of microvesicles. This reduces the surface area of the cell and leads to spherocyte formation. Red cells with a deficiency of spectrin or ankyrin produce microvesicles containing band 3, whereas a reduced amount of band 3 or protein 4.1R gives rise to band 3–free microvesicles. Spherocytes have decreased deformability and are trapped in the spleen where the membrane is further damaged by splenic conditioning, which ultimately results in hemolysis.

Missense mutations have been documented in all the ankyrin domains and are thought to disrupt normal ankyrin–protein interactions. A few splicing mutations have been identified, including a mutation in intron 16, which created a new splice acceptor site and a complex pattern of aberrant splicing.[71] Both parents were heterozygous for this mutation and the proband was homozygous, indicating that homozygosity for an ankyrin mutation is compatible with life.

Mutations in the erythroid-specific promoter of the *ANK1* gene are common in recessive HS. A dinucleotide deletion impairs the binding of a transcription factor complex, which leads to a reduced number of ankyrin transcripts.[72] Point mutations in a barrier insulator element of the promoter also decrease transcription of the gene.[73]

Cytogenetic studies have identified a few ankyrin-deficient HS patients with a contiguous gene syndrome that includes deletion of the ankyrin gene locus at 8p11.2. These patients additionally suffer from dysmorphic features, psychomotor retardation, and hypogonadism.[74]

Band 3 A subset of HS patients present with a band 3 deficiency, typically accompanied by a secondary decrease in protein 4.2, a result of the reduction in protein 4.2 binding sites in the cytoplasmic domain of band 3. The extent of band 3 deficiency in heterozygous patients ranges between 20 and 50 percent, depending on the severity of the mutation, and the compensatory effect of the *in trans* normal allele. Mushroom-shaped "pincered" cells are commonly seen on the blood film of HS patients with a band 3 abnormality.

More than 55 underlying mutations have been described; they are variable and occur throughout the band 3 gene.[13,66] Null mutations are typically family-specific and are caused by frameshift or nonsense mutations, or, in a few cases, by abnormal splicing, all of which result in truncated nonfunctional proteins or unstable transcripts that are not translated into protein. Missense mutations are common and often occur in several kindred. Highly conserved arginine residues at the internal boundaries of the transmembrane segments of the protein (see Fig. 46–2) are frequently mutated, including residues 490, 518, 760, 808, and 870.[66,75] The mutations probably interfere with the cotranslational insertion of band 3 into the endoplasmic reticulum and ultimately into the red cell membrane. Short in-frame insertions or deletions have been documented and presumably also impair insertion of the mutant protein into the lipid bilayer.

Mutations in the cytoplasmic domain of band 3 impact on the interaction of band 3 with proteins in the membrane skeleton, or may alter the conformation of the protein rendering it unstable and prone to degradation prior to insertion into the membrane. Some cytoplasmic mutations, such as band 3 Cape Town and band 3 Mondega, are silent in the heterozygous state, but exacerbate the clinical presentation when inherited *in trans* to another mutation.[76,77]

Spectrin Erythrocytes from HS patients with defects in spectrin or ankyrin are deficient in spectrin. The degree of deficiency correlates with the severity of hemolysis, the response to splenectomy and the ability to withstand mechanical shear stress.[78,79] Visualization of the membrane skeleton of these red cells revealed a decreased density of the spectrin filaments connecting the junctional complexes.[80] The causative mutations occur in either α- or β-spectrin genes.

α-Spectrin Defects in α-spectrin are rare and are associated with severe recessive HS. During erythropoiesis α-spectrin is synthesized in a two- to fourfold excess over β-spectrin and heterozygotes thus still produce sufficient α-spectrin to form heterodimers with all the β-spectrin molecules, which will not result in spectrin deficiency. The defect will only be manifested in individuals who are homozygous or doubly heterozygous for mutations in α-spectrin. The mechanism underlying spectrin deficiency has not been fully elucidated, but a low-expression allele or a polymorphism inherited *in trans* to a causative null mutation plays a role. An example of a low-expression allele is α^{LEPRA} (low-expression Prague), which produces less than 20 percent of the normal amount of α-spectrin transcripts as a result of a splicing and mRNA processing defect, but does not cause any symptoms even in the homozygous state. However, in combination with another mutation on the other α-spectrin allele, which produces a nonfunctional truncated protein, it causes severe spectrin deficiency and anemia.[81] A polymorphic missense mutation in the αII domain in spectrin Bug Hill has been identified in several patients with spectrin-deficient, recessive HS who carry another uncharacterized α-spectrin gene defect that causes the disease.[82] Extensive analysis of the α-spectrin gene in a proband with severe nondominant HS revealed a partial maternal isodisomy of chromosome 1, resulting in homozygosity of the 1q23 region containing the maternal *SPTA1* gene, which carried an R891X nonsense mutation.[83] Uniparental disomy therefore unmasked a recessive mutation in the mother, which caused severe clinical symptoms in the child.

β-Spectrin The production of β-spectrin polypeptides is the limiting factor in spectrin heterodimer formation and one mutant allele is sufficient to cause spectrin deficiency in autosomal dominant HS. The blood films of these patients typically show a subpopulation of spiculated cells (acanthocytes and echinocytes) in addition to spherocytes.[63] Mutations in β-spectrin are found throughout the gene and are mainly null mutations caused by frameshift, nonsense, splicing, and initiator codon defects, which silence the mutant allele.[84] With a few exceptions the mutations are all kindred-specific. Truncated β-spectrin chains have also been described and are caused by frameshift mutations, in-frame deletions, or exon skipping. These mutations lead to, for example, reduced synthesis of an unstable protein,[85] or they impair the interaction with ankyrin and thereby the insertion of spectrin into the membrane.[86] A few missense mutations have been identified, including β-spectrin[Kissimmee], which is caused by a mutation in the 4.1R/actin–binding domain of the protein.[87] The mutant protein is unstable and does not bind to 4.1R, and thus it only interacts weakly with actin, which may explain why these red cells are deficient in spectrin.[87]

Protein 4.2 Protein 4.2 deficiency is common in Japanese patients with recessively inherited HS who exhibit almost a complete absence of the protein.[63] Defects in this protein also occur in whites and other population groups, and 13 mutations have been described in the 4.2 gene of individual kindred, including missense mutations and in-frame deletion and insertion of nucleotides. Nonsense, frameshift, and splicing defects result in premature termination of translation and these mutant truncated proteins are not detected on the membrane, indicating that they are unstable and presumably degraded.[47] Amino acids 306 to 320 are highly conserved and five of the known mutations (three missense and two nonsense) occur in this region, which is adjacent to the hairpin that binds to band 3 in the predicted tertiary structure of protein 4.2.[88] The only recurrent and most common mutation, protein 4.2 Nippon, is caused by a point mutation that affects mRNA processing.[89] Patients are either homozygous for this mutation or heterozygous for a second mutation on the other allele.[47] Mutations have also been identified in individual patients with recessive HS from Europe, Tunisia, and Pakistan. South African kindred with autosomal dominant HS from a deficiency of protein 4.2 have been noted, but the underlying mutations have not been investigated.

Secondary Membrane Defects

The decreased membrane surface area in hereditary spherocytes involves a symmetrical loss of each species of membrane lipid. The relative proportions of cholesterol and phospholipids are therefore normal and the asymmetrical distribution of phospholipids is maintained.

HS red cells exhibit increased cation permeability, presumably secondary to the underlying membrane defect.[90] The excessive sodium influx activates the Na$^+$-K$^+$ ATPase cation pump, which increases ATP turnover and glycolysis. Spherocytes are dehydrated, especially cells obtained from the splenic pulp, but the underlying mechanism has not been clearly defined. The acidic environment of the spleen and oxidative damage by splenic macrophages increase the activity of the K$^+$Cl$^-$ cotransporter, which may play a role in dehydration. The hyperactive Na$^+$-K$^+$ ATPase pump may also contribute as three sodium ions are extruded in exchange for two potassium ions, and this loss of monovalent cations is accompanied by the loss of water. Dehydration may also be related to loss of surface area.

Molecular Determinants of Clinical Severity

Affected individuals of the same kindred typically experience similar degrees of hemolysis. However, in some families the clinical expression is variable and this may be influenced by several factors. Low-expression alleles decrease transcription of the gene or influence the expression or incorporation of the protein into the membrane, but there is no phenotypic effect in the heterozygous state because the normal allele compensates for the deleterious effect. However, when inherited with a mutant allele that causes HS, it exacerbates the clinical expression of the disease. Examples of low-expression alleles that influence HS include band 3 Genas, band 3 Mondego, and two α-spectrin alleles, α^{LELY} and α^{LEPRA}.[77,81,91–94]

Variable penetrance of the defective gene, a *de novo* mutation or a mild form of recessively inherited HS may also influence the clinical severity. Double heterozygosity for two mild band 3 mutations can have an additive effect[76] and rare cases caused by homozygous defects in band 3 result in severe transfusion-dependent hemolytic anemia or fetal death.[91,95,96] Coinheritance of other hematologic disorders or Gilbert syndrome, caused by homozygosity for a polymorphism in the promoter of the uridine diphosphate-glucuronosyltransferase (UGT1) gene, can also alter the clinical symptoms.[63,97,98]

Role of the Spleen

The spleen plays a secondary but important role in the pathophysiology of HS. Spherocytes are retained and ultimately destroyed in the spleen and this is the primary cause of the chronic hemolysis experienced by HS patients (see Fig. 46–12). The reduced deformability of spherocytes impedes their passage through the interendothelial slits separating the splenic cords of the red pulp from the splenic sinuses. The decrease in red cell deformability is primarily related to a loss of surface area and, to a lesser extent, to an increase in internal viscosity as a result of mild cellular dehydration. *Ex vivo* experiments using perfused human spleens and red cells treated with lysophosphatidylcholine to induce spherocytosis revealed that the degree of splenic retention correlated with the reduction in the surface-area-to-volume ratio.[99]

The spleen is a metabolically hostile environment with a decreased pH, low concentrations of glucose and ATP, and increased oxidants, all of which are detrimental to the red cell. Spherocytes are "conditioned" during erythrostasis in the spleen and become more osmotically fragile and increasingly spherocytic.[100] Exposure to macrophages in the spleen eventually leads to erythrophagocytosis and destruction.

Inheritance

In approximately 75 percent of HS patients, inheritance is autosomal dominant. In the remaining patients, the disorder may be autosomal recessive or result from *de novo* mutations, which is relatively common.[101,102] Mutations in α-spectrin or protein 4.2 are often associated with recessive HS.

Clinical Features

The clinical manifestations of HS vary widely. The typical clinical picture combines evidence of hemolysis (anemia, jaundice, reticulocytosis, gallstones, splenomegaly) with spherocytosis (spherocytes on the blood film and increased osmotic fragility) and a positive family history. Mild, moderate, and severe forms of HS have been defined according to differences in hemoglobin, bilirubin, and reticulocyte counts (Table 46–3), which can be correlated with the degree of compensation for hemolysis. Initial assessment of a patient with suspected HS should include a family history and questions about history of anemia, jaundice, gallstones, and splenectomy. Physical examination should seek signs such as scleral icterus, jaundice, and splenomegaly.

TABLE 46–3. Classification of Hereditary Spherocytosis

Laboratory Findings	HS Trait or Carrier	Mild Spherocytosis	Moderate Spherocytosis	Moderately Severe Spherocytosis*	Severe Spherocytosis†
Hemoglobin (g/dL)	Normal	11–15	8–12	6–8	<6
Reticulocytes (%)	1–2	3–8	± 8	≥10	≥10
Bilirubin (mg/dL)	0–1	1–2	± 2	2–3	≥3
Spectrin content (% of normal)‡	100	80–100	50–80	40–80§	20–50
Blood film	Normal	Mild spherocytosis	Spherocytosis	Spherocytosis	Spherocytosis and poikilocytosis
Osmotic fragility					
Fresh blood	Normal	Normal or slightly increased	Distinctly increased	Distinctly increased	Distinctly increased
Incubated blood	Slightly increased	Distinctly increased	Distinctly increased	Distinctly increased	Markedly increased

*Values in untransfused patients.

†By definition, patients with severe spherocytosis are transfusion-dependent. Values were obtained immediately prior to transfusion.

‡Normal: 245 ± 27 × 10³ spectrin dimers per erythrocyte.

§Spectrin content is variable in this group of patients, presumably reflecting heterogeneity of the underlying pathophysiology.

Adapted with permission from Eber SW, Armbrust R, Schröter W: Variable clinical severity of hereditary spherocytosis: Relation to erythrocytic spectrin concentration, osmotic fragility, and autohemolysis. *J Pediatr* 1990 Sep;117(3):409–416.

Typical Hereditary Spherocytosis Approximately 60 to 70 percent of HS patients have moderate disease, which typically presents in infancy or childhood but may present at any age. In children, anemia is the most frequent finding (50 percent of cases), followed by splenomegaly, jaundice, or a positive family history.[13,63] No comparable data exist for adults. Hemolysis may be incompletely compensated with mild to moderate anemia (see Table 46–3). The moderate anemia may often be asymptomatic; however, fatigue and mild pallor or both may be present. Jaundice may be intermittent and is seen in about half of patients, usually in association with viral infections. When present, jaundice is acholuric, characterized by unconjugated hyperbilirubinemia without detectable bilirubinuria. Palpable splenomegaly is evident in most (>75 percent) older children and adults. Typically the spleen is modestly enlarged (2 to 6 cm below the costal margin), but it may be massive. No proven correlation exists between the spleen size and the severity of HS. However, given the pathophysiology and response of the disease to splenectomy, such a correlation probably exists.

Mild Hereditary Spherocytosis Approximately 20 to 30 percent of HS patients have mild disease with "compensated hemolysis," that is, red blood cell production and destruction are balanced, and the hemoglobin concentration of the blood is normal (see Table 46–3).[63,103] The life span of spherocytes is decreased, but patients adequately compensate for hemolysis with increased marrow erythropoiesis. These patients are usually asymptomatic. Splenomegaly is mild, reticulocyte counts are generally less than 6 percent, and spherocytes on the blood film may be minimal, which complicates the diagnosis. Many of these individuals escape detection until adulthood when they are being evaluated for unrelated disorders or when complications related to anemia or chronic hemolysis occur. Hemolysis may become severe with illnesses that further increase splenomegaly, such as infectious mononucleosis, or may be exacerbated by other factors, such as pregnancy or sustained, vigorous exercise. Because of the asymptomatic course of HS in these patients, diagnosis of HS should be considered during evaluation of incidentally noted splenomegaly, gallstones at a young age, or anemia resulting from parvovirus B19 infection or other viral infections.

Moderately Severe and Severe Hereditary Spherocytosis Approximately 5 to 10 percent of HS patients have moderately severe disease, as evidenced by indicators of anemia that are more pronounced than in typical moderate HS, and an intermittent requirement for transfusions (see Table 46–3). This category includes patients with dominant and recessive HS. A small number (<5 percent) of patients have severe disease with life-threatening anemia and are transfusion-dependent. They almost always have recessive HS. Most have severe spectrin deficiency, which is thought to result from a defect in α-spectrin,[78,79] but defects in ankyrin or band 3 have also been identified.[91,96] Patients with severe HS often have irregularly contoured or budding spherocytes or bizarre poikilocytes in addition to typical spherocytes and microspherocytes on the blood film. Added to the risks of recurrent transfusions, patients often suffer from hemolytic and aplastic crises and may develop complications of severe uncompensated anemia, including growth retardation, delayed sexual maturation, and aspects of thalassemic facies.

Asymptomatic Carriers Parents of patients with recessive HS are clinically asymptomatic and do not have anemia, splenomegaly, hyperbilirubinemia, or spherocytosis on the blood films. However, most have subtle laboratory signs of HS (see Table 46–3), including slight reticulocytosis, diminished haptoglobin levels, and slightly elevated incubated osmotic fragility, particularly the 100 percent red cell lysis point, which occurs at a higher sodium chloride concentration in carriers compared to normal subjects.[103] The acidified glycerol lysis test may also be useful to detect carriers. In North America and parts of Europe, approximately 1 percent of the population is estimated to be silent carriers.[63]

Pregnancy and Hereditary Spherocytosis
Most patients do well during pregnancy[104] although anemia may be exacerbated by plasma volume expansion and increased hemolysis. A few patients are symptomatic only during pregnancy. Transfusions are rarely required.

Hereditary Spherocytosis in the Neonate
Jaundice is the most common finding in neonates with HS, present in approximately 90 percent of cases. It may be accentuated by coinheritance of Gilbert syndrome, caused by homozygosity for a polymorphism in the promoter of the *UGT1* gene (Chaps. 33 and 47).[63,97,98] Less than half of infants are anemic and severe anemia is rare. A few cases of hydrops fetalis from homozygosity or compound heterozygosity for band 3 or spectrin defects have been reported.[91,105,106]

Complications
Gallbladder Disease Chronic hemolysis leads to formation of bilirubinate gallstones, the most frequently reported complication in up to half of HS patients. Coinheritance of Gilbert syndrome markedly increases the risk of gallstone formation. Although gallstones have been detected in children, they mainly occur in adolescents and young adults.[13,63] Routine management should include interval ultrasonography to detect gallstones because many patients with cholelithiasis and HS are asymptomatic. Interval ultrasonography allows prompt diagnosis and treatment and prevents complications of symptomatic biliary tract disease, including biliary obstruction, cholecystitis, and cholangitis.

Hemolytic, Aplastic and Megaloblastic Crises Hemolytic crises are the most common and are usually associated with viral illnesses and typically occur in childhood.[13,63] They are generally mild and characterized by jaundice, splenomegaly, anemia and reticulocytosis. Medical intervention is seldom necessary. During rare severe hemolytic crises, red cell transfusion may be required.

Aplastic crises following virally induced marrow suppression are uncommon but may result in severe anemia requiring hospitalization and transfusion with serious complications, including congestive heart failure or even death.[13,63] The most common etiologic agent in these cases is parvovirus B19 (Chap. 36). The virus selectively infects erythropoietic progenitor cells and inhibits their growth leading to the characteristic finding of a low number of reticulocytes despite severe anemia. Aplastic crises usually last for 10 to 14 days and may bring asymptomatic, undiagnosed HS patients with compensated hemolysis to medical attention.[63]

Megaloblastic crises may occur in HS patients with increased folate demands, such as pregnant patients, growing children, or patients recovering from an aplastic crisis. This complication can be prevented with appropriate folate supplementation.

Other Complications Leg ulcers, chronic dermatitis on the legs and gout are rare manifestations of HS, which usually heal rapidly after splenectomy. In severe cases, skeletal abnormalities resulting from expansion of the marrow can occur. Extramedullary hematopoiesis can lead to tumors, particularly along the thoracic and lumbar spine or in the kidney hila, in nonsplenectomized patients with mild to moderate HS.[13,63] Postsplenectomy, the masses involute and undergo fatty metamorphosis.

HS has been suggested to predispose patients to hematologic malignancies, including myeloproliferative disorders, particularly myeloma, but cause and effect have not been proven. Thrombosis has been reported in several HS patients, usually postsplenectomy. Untreated HS may aggravate other underlying diseases, such as congestive heart disease and hemochromatosis.[13,63]

Nonerythroid Manifestations

Clinical manifestations are confined to the erythroid lineage in the majority of patients with HS, but a few exceptions have been observed. Several HS kindred have been reported with cosegregating nonerythroid manifestations, particularly neuromuscular abnormalities including cardiomyopathy, slowly progressive spinocerebellar degenerative disease, spinal cord dysfunction, and movement disorders. Erythrocyte ankyrin and β-spectrin are also expressed in muscle, brain, and spinal cord, which raises the possibility that these HS patients suffer from defects of one of these proteins.[13]

An isoform of band 3 is expressed in the kidney and heterozygous defects of band 3 have been described in patients with inherited distal renal tubular acidosis and normal erythrocytes. This finding is in contrast to most patients with heterozygous mutations of band 3, who have normal renal acidification and abnormal erythrocytes. Kindred with HS *and* renal acidification defects resulting from band 3 mRNA processing mutations, band 3[Pribram] and band 3[Campinas], have been described.[107,108] Homozygosity for band 3[Coimbra], a V488M missense mutation, resulted in the absence of band 3 and renal tubular acidosis in a severely affected HS infant.[91]

Laboratory Features

Laboratory findings in HS are variable, which correlate with the heterogeneous clinical presentation.

Blood Film Erythrocyte morphology in HS is not uniform. Typical HS patients have blood films with easily identifiable spherocytes lacking central pallor (see Fig. 46–10B and 46–11C). Patients with mild HS may present with only a few spherocytes, and at the other end of the spectrum, severely affected patients exhibit numerous dense microspherocytes and bizarre erythrocyte morphology with anisocytosis and poikilocytosis. Blood films from patients with band 3 defects often exhibit "pincered" or mushroom-shaped red cells, whereas spherocytic acanthocytes are associated with β-spectrin mutations. When examining blood from a patient with suspected spherocytosis, a high-quality film with the erythrocytes properly separated and some cells with central pallor in the field of examination are important because spherocytes can be an artifact.

Erythrocyte Indices Most patients have mild to moderate anemia with hemoglobin in the 9 to 12 g/dL range (see Table 46–3). Mean corpuscular hemoglobin concentration (MCHC) is increased (>36 g/dL) because of relative cellular dehydration in approximately half of patients, but all HS patients have some dehydrated cells. Some automated hematology analyzers measure the hemoglobin concentration of individual red cells and a demonstration of a population of hyperdense erythrocytes can be useful as a screening test for HS, especially when combined with an increased red cell distribution width. Mean corpuscular volume (MCV) is usually normal except in cases of severe HS, when MCV is slightly decreased.

Markers of Hemolysis Other laboratory features of HS are markers of ongoing hemolysis. Reticulocytosis, variably increased lactate dehydrogenase, increased urinary and fecal urobilinogen, unconjugated hyperbilirubinemia, and decreased serum haptoglobin reflect hemolysis and increased erythropoiesis (Chaps. 32 and 33). The reticulocyte count may appear to be elevated disproportionately relative to the degree of anemia.

Erythrocyte Fragility Tests Spherocytes have a decreased surface area relative to cell volume and this renders them osmotically fragile. Several laboratory tests exploit this characteristic and are used to diagnose HS. The most common osmotic fragility (OF) test measures lysis

of red cells, either from freshly drawn blood or after incubation of the sample at 37°C for 24 hours, in a range of hypotonic concentrations of sodium chloride. Spherocytes typically swell and burst much more readily than normal biconcave disk-shaped red cells. Other tests based on the same principle measure the rate and extent of cell lysis in buffered glycerol solutions and include the glycerol lysis test (GLT) and the acidified glycerol lysis test (AGLT). These tests, however, have relatively poor sensitivity and do not detect all cases of mild HS or those with small numbers of spherocytes, including patients who had recent blood transfusions.[63,67,109] These tests may also be unreliable and give normal results in the presence of iron deficiency, obstructive jaundice, or during the recovery phase of an aplastic crisis.[63] In addition, these tests do not differentiate HS from other disorders with secondary spherocytosis, such as the autoimmune hemolytic anemias (Chap. 54).

Other fragility tests include the cryohemolysis test, based on the sensitivity of HS red cells to cooling at 0°C in hypertonic conditions, and the autohemolysis test, but these tests also do not detect all cases of HS.[13] The reduced surface area of spherocytes can be measured by osmotic gradient ektacytometry, but the highly specialized equipment required for this procedure is only available in a few research-oriented laboratories.

Eosin 5′-Maleimide Flow Cytometry Test Eosin 5′-maleimide (EMA) is a fluorescent dye that binds to the transmembrane proteins, band 3, Rh protein, Rh glycoprotein, and CD47.[110] Patients with HS exhibit decreased fluorescence compared to controls, irrespective of the underlying defective membrane protein, although not all patients with HS are detected. In addition, lower fluorescence values are also observed in patients with HE, HPP, some red cell enzymopathies, and other abnormalities of band 3, such as congenital dyserythropoietic anemia type II (CDAII; Chap. 39). The sensitivity and specificity of the test vary, depending on the cutoff value of the fluorescence, which differs between laboratories.[109,111–113]

Molecular Diagnostics Because HS can be caused by mutations in several different genes and because there are very few common mutations, a simple DNA test to diagnose HS is not feasible. Initial analysis of the red cell membrane proteins by quantitative SDS-PAGE is required to identify the underlying defective protein. The sensitivity of this test varies between laboratories and different patient populations, but typically an abnormality is defined in 75 to 93 percent of cases.[63,64,67] Patients with clinically identified HS and normal SDS-PAGE results may have a slight decrease of 10 to 15 percent in one of the membrane proteins, which may be missed by the densitometric analysis, or they may have an abnormality in a protein that is currently not quantified and not linked to HS, for example, adducin.

Knowledge of the defective protein facilitates subsequent DNA/RNA investigations to characterize the gene defect, although this approach is challenging as the genes causing HS are large and contain many exons. Polymorphisms may be used to identify reduced expression from one allele or loss of heterozygosity because of a null mutation. In families with variable clinical expression of HS, a molecular investigation into low-expression alleles and other modifying genes is useful. A molecular diagnosis is informative in patients with atypical features; severe disease; unclear or recessive inheritance; *de novo* mutations; or undiagnosed hemolytic anemia. Identification of silent carriers and prenatal diagnosis also require molecular testing.

Differential Diagnosis

Clinical features and family history should accompany an initial laboratory investigation comprising a complete blood count with a blood film, reticulocyte count, direct antiglobulin test (Coombs test), and serum bilirubin. Other causes of anemia should be excluded, particularly autoimmune hemolytic anemia, CDAII and HSt. Further diagnostic tests (discussed in "Laboratory Features" earlier), are not standardized as reflected by a European survey of 25 centers.[114] A consistent finding was that all the laboratories used at least two tests to make a final diagnosis, as none of the currently available methods have 100 percent sensitivity. The EMA test was most commonly used. Recent guidelines from the British Committee for Standards in Haematology (BCSH)[115] advocate the use of the EMA test or cryohemolysis, but OF is not recommended for routine use.

In neonates, ABO incompatibility should be considered, but its differentiation from HS becomes clear several months after birth. Other causes of spherocytic hemolytic anemia, such as autoimmune hemolysis, clostridial sepsis, transfusion reactions, severe burns, and bites from snakes, spiders, bees, and wasps (Chaps. 52 to 54), should be viewed in the appropriate clinical context. Occasional spherocytes are seen in patients with a large spleen (e.g., in cirrhosis or myelofibrosis) or in patients with microangiopathic anemias (Chap. 51), but differentiation of these conditions from HS does not usually present diagnostic difficulties.

HS may be obscured in disorders that increase the surface-to-volume ratio of erythrocytes, such as obstructive jaundice, iron deficiency (Chap. 43), β-thalassemia trait, or hemoglobin SC disease (Chaps. 48 and 49), and vitamin B_{12} or folate deficiency (Chap. 41).

Therapy and Prognosis

Splenectomy Splenic sequestration is the primary determinant of erythrocyte survival in HS patients. Thus, splenectomy cures or alleviates the anemia in the overwhelming majority of patients, reducing or eliminating the need for red cell transfusions, which has obvious implications for future iron overload and hemochromatosis-related end-organ damage. The incidence of cholelithiasis is decreased. Postsplenectomy, spherocytosis, and altered OF persist, but the "tail" of the OF curve, created by conditioning of a subpopulation of spherocytes by the spleen, disappears. Erythrocyte life span nearly normalizes, and reticulocyte counts fall to normal or near-normal levels. Changes typical of the postsplenectomy state, including Howell-Jolly bodies, target cells, Pappenheimer bodies (siderocytes), and acanthocytes (Chaps. 2 and 31), become evident on the blood film. Postsplenectomy, patients with the most severe forms of HS still suffer from shortened erythrocyte survival and hemolysis, but their clinical improvement is striking.[79]

Complications of Splenectomy Early complications of splenectomy include local infection, thrombotic complications and in particular hepatic and mesenteric thrombosis, bleeding, and pancreatitis, presumably resulting from injury to the tail of the pancreas incurred during spleen removal. In general, the morbidity of splenectomy for HS is lower than the morbidity of other hematologic disorders. Chapters 5 and 6 discuss the complications of splenectomy.

Indications for Splenectomy In the past, splenectomy, which has a low operative mortality, was considered routine in HS patients. However, the risk of overwhelming postsplenectomy infection and the emergence of penicillin-resistant pneumococci have led to reevaluation of the role of splenectomy in the treatment of HS.[116] Considering the risks and benefits, a reasonable approach is to splenectomize all patients with transfusion-dependent severe spherocytosis and all patients suffering from significant signs or symptoms of anemia, including growth failure, skeletal changes, leg ulcers, and extramedullary hematopoietic tumors. Other candidates for splenectomy are older HS patients suffering from vascular compromise of vital organs.

Whether patients with moderate HS and compensated, asymptomatic anemia should undergo splenectomy is controversial. Patients with mild HS and compensated hemolysis can be followed and referred for splenectomy if clinically indicated. Treatment of patients with mild

to moderate HS and gallstones is debatable, particularly because new treatments for cholelithiasis, including laparoscopic cholecystectomy, and endoscopic sphincterotomy, lower the risk of this complication. If such patients have symptomatic gallstones, a combined cholecystectomy and splenectomy can be performed, particularly if acute cholecystitis or biliary obstruction has occurred. No evidence indicates any benefit to performing cholecystectomy and splenectomy separately, as performed in the past.

Because the risk of postsplenectomy sepsis is very high during infancy and early childhood, splenectomy should be delayed until age 5 to 9 years if possible and to at least 3 years if feasible, even if chronic transfusions are required in the interim. No evidence indicates further delay is useful. In fact, further delay may be harmful because the risk of cholelithiasis increases dramatically in children older than 10 years.

When splenectomy is warranted, laparoscopic splenectomy has become the method of choice in centers with surgeons experienced in the technique.[117] If desired, the procedure can be combined with laparoscopic cholecystectomy. Laparoscopic splenectomy results in less postoperative discomfort, a quicker return to preoperative diet and activities, shorter hospitalization, decreased costs, and smaller scars. The risk of bleeding increases during the operation and approximately 10 percent of laparoscopic operations (for all causes) must be converted to standard splenectomies. Even very large spleens (>600 g) can be removed laparoscopically because the spleen is placed in a large bag, diced, and eliminated via suction catheters.

Partial splenectomy via laparotomy has been advocated for infants and young children with significant anemia associated with erythrocyte membrane disorders.[118] The goal of this procedure is to allow for palliation of hemolysis and anemia while maintaining some residual splenic immune function. Long-term followup data for this procedure have been variable.

Prior to splenectomy, patients should be immunized with vaccines against pneumococcus, *Haemophilus influenzae* type B, and meningococcus, preferably several weeks preoperatively. Use of prophylactic antibiotics postsplenectomy for prevention of pneumococcal sepsis is controversial. Prophylactic antibiotics (penicillin V 125 mg orally twice daily for patients younger than 7 years or 250 mg orally twice daily for those older than 7 years, including adults) have been recommended for at least 5 years postsplenectomy by some and for life by others. The optimal duration of prophylactic antibiotic therapy postsplenectomy is unknown. Presplenectomy and, in severe cases, postsplenectomy, HS patients should take folic acid (1 mg/day orally) to prevent folate deficiency.

Splenectomy Failure Splenectomy failure is uncommon. Failure may result from an accessory spleen missed during splenectomy, from development of splenunculi as a consequence of autotransplantation of splenic tissue during surgery, or from another intrinsic red cell defect, such as pyruvate kinase deficiency (Chap. 47). Accessory spleens occur in 15 to 40 percent of patients and must always be sought. Recurrence of hemolytic anemia years or even decades following splenectomy should raise suspicion of an accessory spleen particularly if Howell-Jolly bodies are no longer found on blood film (Chaps. 2 and 31). Definitive confirmation of ectopic splenic tissue can be achieved by a radiocolloid liver–spleen scan or a scan using ^{51}Cr-labeled, heat-damaged red cells.

Genetic Counseling

After a patient is diagnosed with HS, family members should be examined for the presence of HS. A history, physical examination for splenomegaly, complete blood count, examination of the blood film for spherocytes, and a reticulocyte count should be obtained for parents, children, and siblings, if available.

HEREDITARY ELLIPTOCYTOSIS AND PYROPOIKILOCYTOSIS

Definition and History

HE is characterized by the presence of elliptical or oval erythrocytes on the blood films of affected individuals (Figs. 46–10D and 46–11F.). In 1904, Dresbach, a physiologist at Ohio State University in Columbus, Ohio, published the first description of elliptical red blood cells in one of his students, noticed during a laboratory exercise in which the students were examining their own blood.[119] The report elicited controversy because the student died soon thereafter, leading to speculation that he had actually suffered from pernicious anemia. The demonstration of elliptocytosis in three generations of one family established the hereditary nature of this disorder.[120] A related disorder, HPP is a rare disease first described in 1975 in children with severe neonatal anemia with abnormal poikilocytic red cell morphology reminiscent of that seen in patients suffering from severe burns (Fig. 46–13).[121] The erythrocytes from these patients exhibited increased thermal sensitivity.

Epidemiology and Inheritance

HE has a worldwide distribution but the true incidence is unknown because the disease is heterogeneous and many patients are asymptomatic. In the United States, the incidence is estimated to be 1 in 2000 to 4000 individuals.[13,122] HE occurs in all racial groups but is more prevalent in individuals of West African descent, possibly because elliptocytes may confer some resistance to malaria.[123,124] HPP is typically found in patients of African origin, but it has also been diagnosed in subjects of European and Arabic descent.[122,125,126]

Etiology and Pathogenesis

The primary abnormality in HE and HPP erythrocytes is defective horizontal interactions between components of the membrane skeleton, which weakens the skeleton and compromises its ability to maintain the biconcave disk shape of the red cell during circulatory shear stress. Investigations of erythrocyte membrane proteins in these disorders have identified abnormalities in α- and β-spectrin, protein 4.1, and GPC.[122] The most common defects occur in spectrin, the main structural protein of the erythrocyte membrane skeleton, and they impair the ability of spectrin dimers to self-associate into tetramers and oligomers, thereby disrupting the skeletal lattice.[55] Abnormalities in 4.1R diminish the interaction between the tail ends of spectrin tetramers in the junctional complex and thus destabilize the skeleton. Deficiency of GPC/GPD is associated with reduced levels of 4.1R, which presumably is responsible for the elliptocytosis.

When the integrity of the skeleton is compromised, the capacity of the erythrocyte to undergo flow-induced deformation and

rearrangement of the skeleton is reduced. Disruption of the dynamic dissociation and reassociation of spectrin tetramers causes mechanical instability of the membrane, which precludes the recovery of the normal biconcave disk shape of the cell after prolonged and repeated unidirectional axial distortion in the microcirculation.[127] HE reticulocytes have a normal shape when released into the circulation but the mature red cells become progressively more elliptical as they age and ultimately the abnormal shape becomes permanent.[13,122] As the severity of the defect increases, poikilocytes are formed and the cells become prone to fragmentation. HPP patients exhibit a combination of horizontal (impaired spectrin tetramer formation) and vertical (spectrin deficiency) defects, with the latter causing microspherocytes and exacerbating the hemolytic anemia.[128,129]

Red Cell Membrane Protein Defects

Spectrin Mutations that affect spectrin heterodimer self-association are found in the majority of HE patients and in all patients with HPP. This functional defect results in an increased percentage of spectrin dimers relative to tetramers,[130] which is reflected on a structural level by an abnormal tryptic digest pattern of the protein, whereby the normal peptide is decreased with a concomitant increase in an abnormal peptide of lower molecular weight. Most of the defects affect the 80-kDa αI domain of α-spectrin and of the nine structural variants the most common are Spα$^{I/74}$, Spα$^{I/65}$, and Spα$^{I/46 \text{ or } 50a}$.[128]

More than 50 mutations have been identified in either α- or β-spectrin genes. The majority of the mutations are missense mutations that substitute highly conserved amino acids or those in close proximity. The abnormal amino acids typically have a different charge, or in the case of glycine or proline substitutions, they disrupt the helical structure of the spectrin repeats, which alter the interactions between α and β subunits. Interestingly, mutations in α-spectrin primarily occur in helix C of the repeats, which highlights the importance of this helix in the triple helical bundle (see Fig. 46–3). Several mechanisms have been identified by which the mutations impair spectrin tetramer formation.

Spα$^{I/74}$ mutations are mostly missense mutations found at the self-association site, which consists of helix C of the α0 partial spectrin repeat that interacts with helices B and C of β-spectrin partial repeat 17 to form a complete triple helical bundle.[34] In vitro studies on missense mutations in α0 revealed that the mutant peptides were stable folded structures, similar to wild type, but their binding affinities to β-spectrin peptides were variable. This suggested that their effect on tetramer formation was exerted through defective molecular recognition and disruption of protein-protein interactions at the contact site, rather than an altered structure.[131] These findings contrasted with mutations in the β17 repeat of β-spectrin, which perturbed the structural conformation of this partial repeat and the adjacent β16 repeat.[132] Codon 28

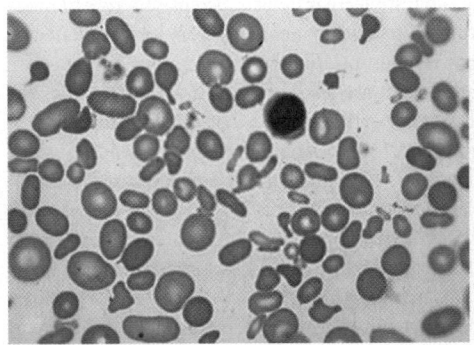
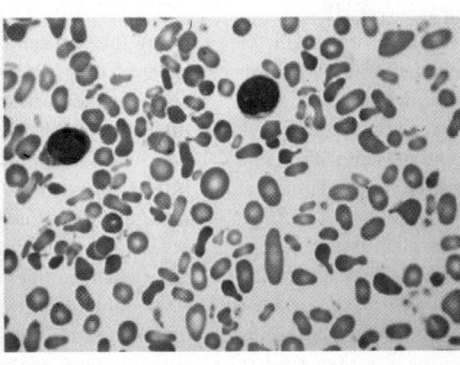

A   B

Figure 46–13. Blood films from a patient with HPP. **A.** Pre-splenectomy. **B.** Post-splenectomy. Note the prominent micro-poikilocytosis, microspherocytosis, and fragmentation especially after splenectomy. (*Reproduced with permission from* Lichtman's Atlas of Hematology, *www.accessmedicine. com.*)

in helix C of $\alpha 0$ has been identified as a mutation "hotspot" since four different point mutations occur in this position, resulting in different amino acid substitutions, and the mutations have also been found in several unrelated kindred.[133] Arginine 28 is a highly conserved amino acid and any changes in this position are typically associated with severe HE or HPP.[133,134] An interesting case of HE Sp$\alpha^{I/74}$ involving an intragenic crossover in the α-spectrin gene and uniparental disomy, together with an underlying R34P mutation, was recently described in a Utah family.[126]

Sp$\alpha^{I/74}$ defects are also caused by mutations in β-spectrin, which presumably expose the αI domain of spectrin to increased tryptic digestion. These abnormalities are all located in partial repeat 17. Missense mutations are found in both helices A and B of the β17 repeat, but some in helix A are particularly severe, including spectrin^{Providence}, spectrin^{Cagliari}, and spectrin^{Buffalo}, which cause severe fetal or neonatal anemia and non-immune hydrops fetalis when inherited in the homozygous state.[105,106,135] Frame-shift mutations and splicing defects predominate in helix B, resulting in truncated spectrin molecules lacking the self-association site.[13,122,136]

Sp$\alpha^{I/65}$ is a mild defect, even in the homozygous state, because of a duplication of leucine 154 in helix C of the $\alpha 1$ repeat.[137] It is very common in blacks from West and Central Africa, as well as Arabs in North Africa, suggesting genetic selection, possibly by protecting carriers against *P. falciparum* malaria.[13,122,123]

Sp$\alpha^{I/46 \text{ or } 50a}$ mutations are distal from the self-association site and usually occur close to the helical linker regions between individual repeats and often involve the substitution of an amino acid with a proline residue, which is a helix breaker.[13,122] *In vitro* studies on Q471P between repeats 4 and 5 of α-spectrin showed that the mutation uncoupled the repeats and caused cooperative unfolding, which abolished the stabilizing influence of the helical linker on adjacent repeats.[138] Because β-spectrin has fewer repeats than α-spectrin, the alignment of the heterodimers places $\alpha 4$ and $\alpha 5$ in contact with $\beta 16$ and $\beta 17$, suggesting that unfolding of the mutant spectrin repeats interferes with the self-association site and prevents tetramer formation.[139] The L260P mutation is in a similar position to Q471P, but is between repeats $\alpha 2$ and $\alpha 3$ of spectrin. When heterodimers are aligned, repeats $\alpha 03$ are not in contact with β-spectrin and they represent an open dimer configuration, which facilitates tetramer formation. Open dimers are in equilibrium with closed dimers whereby $\alpha 0$ to $\alpha 3$ are folded onto $\beta 16$ and $\beta 17$ of the same dimer, thus preventing bivalent tetramer formation.[139] *In vitro* experiments on the L260P mutation revealed a conformational change, which stabilized the mutant spectrin in the closed dimer configuration and reduced tetramer assembly.[140]

Mutations in the αII domain of spectrin implicated in HE are rare. Spectrin$^{St Claude}$ is caused by a single point mutation in intron 19 of α-spectrin,[141,142] which creates complex splicing events that ultimately impair the function of both α- and β-spectrin, resulting in decreased binding to ankyrin, defective spectrin self-association and spectrin deficiency.[141] These membrane abnormalities have profound effects on red blood cell morphology and survival, manifesting as severe HE.

Protein 4.1R Defects in the erythrocyte isoform of protein 4.1 associated with HE are relatively common in some Arab and European populations.[13] Heterozygotes exhibit partial deficiency of 4.1R, manifesting as mild or asymptomatic HE, whereas homozygotes lack 4.1R and p55, have a reduced content of GPC, and present with severe HE. These red blood cells are mechanically unstable and fragment at moderate shear stress, but the stability can be restored by reconstituting the deficient red cells with 4.1R or the 4.1R spectrin–actin binding domain.[143] The 4.1R null erythrocytes demonstrate decreased invasion and growth of *P. falciparum* parasites *in vitro*.[144]

Mutations in the 4.1R gene often affect the erythroid-specific initiation codon, which abolishes transcription, or else they tend to cluster in the spectrin-actin binding domain where exon deletions or duplications result in mutant proteins that are smaller or larger than normal.[122]

Glycophorin C GPC and GPD carry the Gerbich antigens and rare patients with the Leach phenotype are Gerbich-negative and lack both GPs. The underlying mutations are either a 7-kb deletion of genomic DNA or a frameshift mutation.[145] Heterozygous carriers are asymptomatic, with normal red blood cell morphology, whereas homozygous subjects exhibit elliptocytes on the blood film and present with mild HE, presumably as a result of the concomitant partial deficiency of 4.1R.[13,145]

Molecular Determinants of Clinical Severity

HE patients exhibit marked clinical heterogeneity ranging from asymptomatic carrier to severe, transfusion-dependent anemia. In patients with spectrin heterodimer self-association defects, the resultant increase in spectrin dimers and concomitant decrease in spectrin tetramers, weakens the membrane skeleton and facilitates the formation of elliptocytes under circulatory shear stress. The most important determinants of the severity of hemolysis in these patients are the percentage of spectrin dimers and the spectrin content of the membrane skeleton. These parameters are influenced by the degree of dysfunction of the mutant spectrin, and the gene dose (heterozygote versus homozygote or compound heterozygote).[128] Genotype–phenotype correlations indicate that the order of clinical severity of αI domain defects is Sp$\alpha^{I/74}$ > Sp$\alpha^{I/46-50a}$ > Sp$\alpha^{I/65}$ and it depends on the position of the mutations within the proteins, as well as the type of mutation. Defects in the spectrin dimer self-association contact site leading to Sp$\alpha^{I/74}$ mutants are the most severe[128] and, for example, codon 28 mutations, which affect a highly conserved and critical arginine residue, are generally associated with phenotypically severe HE or HPP.[133] A more distal mutation such as the duplication of leucine 154, which causes Sp$\alpha^{I/65}$, is phenotypically very mild, even in the homozygous state.[137] Proline or glycine helix-breaking mutations resulting in Sp$\alpha^{I/46 \text{ or } 50a}$ are more severe even though they are further away from the self-association site.[138]

The clinical expression of HE often varies within the same kindred, despite all the affected individuals carrying the same causative mutation. This heterogeneity is a result of the inheritance of modifier alleles or additional defects. The low-expression α^{LELY} is the most common polymorphism affecting spectrin content and clinical severity. The allele is characterized by an L1857V amino acid substitution, and partial skipping of exon 46 in 50 percent of the α-spectrin mRNA.[94] The six amino acids encoded by exon 46 are essential for spectrin heterodimer assembly and therefore Spα^{LELY} results in a reduced amount of spectrin, as monomers are rapidly degraded.[146] The Spα^{LELY} allele is clinically silent, even when homozygous, because α-spectrin is normally synthesized in three- to fourfold excess.[147] Inheritance of Spα^{LELY} *in cis* to an elliptocytogenic α-spectrin mutation ameliorates symptoms,[148] whereas inheritance *in trans* causes a relative increase in the mutant spectrin and therefore exacerbates the disease.[94]

Coinheritance of other molecular defects also plays a role in modifying the clinical expression. HPP patients are very severely affected because they are homozygous or doubly heterozygous for spectrin self-association mutations and are also deficient in spectrin.[129] Several molecular mechanisms have been identified that underlie the spectrin deficiency, including an RNA processing defect[149]; reduced α-spectrin mRNA and protein synthesis[150]; abnormal splicing resulting in a premature stop codon[151]; and degradation of α-spectrin.[150] A recent study revealed the complexity of genotype–phenotype interactions in two large Utah families of northern European descent in whom a novel R34P mutation in α-spectrin was associated with three morphologic phenotypes.[126] This heterogeneity was caused by an intricate interplay and coinheritance of other factors, including Spα^{LELY} *in trans*, reduced transcription from the α-spectrin gene and intragenic crossover.[126]

In neonates the clinical severity of HE can be affected by the weak binding of BPG to fetal hemoglobin leading to an increase in free BPG, which, in turn, destabilizes the spectrin–actin–protein 4.1 interaction.[152] Finally, hemolytic anemia can be exacerbated by several acquired conditions, including those that alter microcirculatory stress to the cells.

Inheritance

HE is typically inherited as an autosomal dominant disorder. *De novo* mutations are rare.[134] The severity of clinical symptoms is highly variable reflecting heterogeneous molecular abnormalities, as well as the coinheritance of other genetic defects or polymorphisms that modify disease expression. A strong genetic relationship exists between HE and HPP, and parents or siblings of patients with HPP often have typical HE.

Clinical Features

The clinical presentation of HE is heterogeneous, ranging from asymptomatic carriers to patients with severe, life-threatening anemia. The overwhelming majority of patients with HE are asymptomatic and are diagnosed incidentally during testing for unrelated conditions. HPP patients present in infancy or early childhood with a very severe hemolytic anemia.

Asymptomatic carriers who possess the same molecular defect as an affected HE relative but who have normal or near-normal blood films have been identified. The erythrocyte life span is normal, and the patients are not anemic. Asymptomatic HE patients may experience hemolysis in association with infections, hypersplenism, vitamin B_{12} deficiency, or microangiopathic hemolysis, such as disseminated intravascular coagulation or thrombotic thrombocytopenic purpura. In the latter two conditions, increased hemolysis may result from microcirculatory damage superimposed on the underlying mechanical instability of red cells.

HE patients with chronic hemolysis experience moderate to severe hemolytic anemia with elliptocytes and poikilocytes on the blood film. Red cell life span is decreased and patients may develop complications of chronic hemolysis, such as gallbladder disease. In some kindreds, the hemolytic HE has been transmitted through several generations. In other kindreds, not all HE subjects have chronic hemolysis; some have only mild hemolysis, presumably because another genetic factor modifies disease expression. The blood films of the most severe HE patients with chronic hemolysis exhibit elliptocytes, poikilocytes, fragments and small microspherocytes, reminiscent of HPP.

HPP represents a subtype of common HE, as evidenced by the coexistence of HE and HPP in the same family and the presence of the same molecular defects of spectrin.[130] HE relatives are heterozygous for an elliptocytogenic spectrin mutation, whereas HPP patients are homozygous or doubly heterozygous and are also partially deficient in spectrin.[128,129]

Hereditary Elliptocytosis and Pyropoikilocytosis in Infancy

Clinical symptoms of elliptocytosis are uncommon in the neonatal period. Typically, elliptocytes do not appear on the blood film until the patient is 4 to 6 months old. Occasionally, severe forms of HE present in the neonatal period with severe, hemolytic anemia with marked poikilocytosis and jaundice. These patients may require red cell transfusion, phototherapy, or exchange transfusion. Usually, even in severely affected patients, the hemolysis abates between 9 and 12 months of age, and the patient progresses to typical HE with mild anemia. Infrequently, patients remain transfusion dependent beyond the first year of life and require early splenectomy. In cases of suspected neonatal HE or HPP, review of family history and analysis of blood films from the parents usually are of greater diagnostic benefit than other available studies.

A few cases of hydrops fetalis accompanied by fetal or early neonatal death as a result of unusually severe forms of HE have been described.[105] A severely affected hydropic infant salvaged by intrauterine transfusions (Chap. 55) and early exchange transfusion has remained transfusion dependent for more than 2 years.

Laboratory Features

The hallmark of HE is the presence of cigar-shaped elliptocytes on blood films (Figs. 46–10D and 46–11F). These normochromic, normocytic elliptocytes may number from a few to 100 percent. The degree of hemolysis does not correlate with the number of elliptocytes present. Spherocytes, stomatocytes, and fragmented cells may be seen. Osmotic fragility is abnormal in severe HE and in HPP. The reticulocyte count generally is less than 5 percent but may be higher when hemolysis is severe. Other laboratory findings in HE are similar to those of other hemolytic anemias and are nonspecific markers of increased erythrocyte production and destruction. For example, increased serum bilirubin, increased urinary urobilinogen, and decreased serum haptoglobin reflect increased erythrocyte destruction.

HPP blood films exhibit similar features to severe HE, but in addition, they reveal extreme poikilocytosis, some bizarre-shaped cells with fragmentation or budding and often only very few or no elliptocytes (Fig. 46–13). Microspherocytosis is common and MCV is usually low, ranging between 50 to 70 fL. Pyknocytes are prominent on blood films of neonates with HPP. The thermal instability of erythrocytes, originally reported as diagnostic of HPP, is not unique to this disorder because it is also commonly found in HE erythrocytes.

Specialized testing has been used in difficult cases or cases requiring a molecular diagnosis. Tests on isolated membrane proteins include analysis and quantitation of the proteins by SDS-PAGE; extraction of spectrin from the membranes to evaluate the spectrin-dimer-to-tetramer ratio on nondenaturing gels, as well as limited tryptic digestion of spectrin followed by SDS-PAGE or two-dimensional gel electrophoresis to identify the defective domain. Ektacytometry may be used to measure membrane stability and deformability. Genomic DNA and/or complementary DNA analyses are used to determine the underlying mutation.

Differential Diagnosis

Elliptocytes may be seen in association with several disorders, including megaloblastic anemias, hypochromic microcytic anemias (iron-deficiency anemia and thalassemia), myelodysplastic syndromes, and myelofibrosis. In these conditions, elliptocytosis is acquired and generally represents less than one-quarter of red cells seen on the blood film. History and additional laboratory testing usually clarify the diagnosis of these disorders. Pseudoelliptocytosis is an artifact of blood film preparation and these cells are found only in certain areas of the film, usually near its tail. The long axes of pseudoelliptocytes are parallel, whereas the axes of true elliptocytes are distributed randomly.

Therapy and Prognosis

Therapy is rarely needed in patients with HE. In rare cases, occasional red blood cell transfusions may be required. In cases of severe HE and HPP, splenectomy has been palliative, as the spleen is the site of erythrocyte sequestration and destruction. The same indications for splenectomy in HS can be applied to patients with symptomatic HE or HPP. Postsplenectomy, patients with HE or HPP exhibit increased hematocrit, decreased reticulocyte counts, and improved clinical symptoms.

Patients should be followed for signs of decompensation during acute illnesses, characterized by acute decrease of hematocrit from nonspecific suppression of erythropoiesis by a concurrent acute event. HE and particularly HPP patients are at increased risk for parvovirus infection generally requiring short-lasting transfusion support (Chap. 36).[153] Interval ultrasonography to detect gallstones should be performed. Patients with significant hemolysis should receive daily folate supplementation.

SOUTHEAST ASIAN OVALOCYTOSIS

SAO, also known as Melanesian elliptocytosis or stomatocytic elliptocytosis, is widespread in certain ethnic groups of Malaysia, Papua New Guinea, the Philippines, and Indonesia,[123] but is also common in the Cape Coloured population in South Africa.[154] It is characterized by the presence of large oval red cells, many of which contain one or two transverse ridges or a longitudinal slit (Figs. 46–10C and 46–11E).

SAO erythrocytes are rigid and hyperstable because of a structurally and functionally abnormal band 3. SAO band 3 binds tightly to ankyrin, forms oligomers, exhibits restricted lateral and rotational mobility[155,156] and is unable to transport anions.[157] The underlying molecular abnormality is an in-frame deletion of 27 bp in the band 3 gene resulting in the loss of amino acids 400 to 408 located at the boundary of the cytoplasmic and membrane domains of band 3.[158] The defective SLC4A1 allele also carries a linked band 3[Memphis] polymorphism, L56E.

SAO is a dominantly inherited trait and homozygosity is postulated to be lethal during embryonic development.[159] A recent case of homozygous SAO has been described where the fetus was kept alive by two intrauterine transfusions and since birth he has been on a monthly transfusion program.[160] Distal renal tubular acidosis was diagnosed at 3 months as a result of the inability of the SAO band 3 to transport anions.

A remarkable feature of SAO erythrocytes is their resistance to infection by several species of malaria parasites. This has been demonstrated by numerous *in vitro* studies, as well as *in vivo* evidence indicating that SAO provides protection against severe malaria and cerebral malaria.[123,161] Epidemiologic data and the increased prevalence of SAO in populations challenged by malaria suggest a selective advantage of the gene.[123] Numerous factors have been implicated in the protective effect, but the precise mechanism of malaria resistance of SAO red cells has not been fully elucidated.

Clinically, the presence on the blood film of at least 20 percent ovalocytic red cells, some containing a central slit or a transverse ridge, and the notable absence of clinical and laboratory evidence of hemolysis are highly suggestive of SAO. Rapid genetic diagnosis can be made by amplifying the defective region of the band 3 gene and demonstrating heterozygosity for the SAO allele containing the 27 bp deletion.

ACANTHOCYTOSIS

Spiculated red cells are classified into two types: acanthocytes and echinocytes. *Acanthocytes* are contracted, dense cells with irregular projections from the red cell surface that vary in width and length (Figs. 46–10F and 46–11G). *Echinocytes* have small, uniform projections spread evenly over the circumference of the red cell (Fig. 46–11B). Diagnostically, the distinction is not critical, and disorders of spiculated red cells are generally classified together. Normal adults may have up to 3 percent spiculated erythrocytes, but care should be taken when preparing and examining the blood film, because spiculated cells, particularly echinocytes, are common artifacts of blood film preparation and blood storage.

Acanthocytes/echinocytes are found in various inherited disorders and acquired conditions. Spiculated cells can occur transiently in several instances, such as after transfusion with stored blood, ingestion of alcohol and certain drugs, exposure to ionizing radiation or certain venoms, and during hemodialysis.[13] Spiculated cells are commonly seen on the blood films of patients with functional or actual splenectomy, severe liver disease, severe uremia, abetalipoproteinemia, certain inherited neurologic disorders and abnormalities of the Kell blood group. Occasionally acanthocytes and/or echinocytes may be present in patients with glycolytic enzyme defects, myelodysplasia, hypothyroidism, anorexia nervosa, vitamin E deficiency, and in premature infants.[13] Individuals with suppressed expression of Lu[a] and Lu[b], the major antigens of the Lutheran blood group system, may also exhibit acanthocytes.[13]

The molecular mechanisms whereby acanthocytes are generated have not been fully elucidated. However, alterations in band 3 have emerged as a pivotal causative factor. The abnormal red cell membrane lipid composition and altered lipid distribution between the inner and outer leaflets of the bilayer are only found in some, but not all, of these disorders, implying that they may play a secondary role.[162]

ACANTHOCYTOSIS IN SEVERE LIVER DISEASE

Definition

The anemia in patients with liver disease is often called "spur cell anemia" because of the projections on the red cells. Although only a small number of patients with end-stage liver disease acquire spur cell anemia, these individuals typically account for the majority of cases of acanthocytosis seen in clinical practice.

Etiology and Pathogenesis

The anemia in patients with liver disease is of complex etiology. Common causes include blood loss, iron or folate deficiency, hypersplenism, and marrow suppression from alcohol, malnutrition, hepatitis infection, or other factors. Acquired abnormalities of the red cell membrane may contribute to the anemia in some patients.[163]

In vivo acanthocyte formation in spur cell anemia is a two-step process involving accumulation of free (nonesterified) cholesterol in the red cell membrane and remodeling of abnormally shaped red cells by the spleen.[13,163] The diseased liver of the patient produces abnormal lipoproteins with excess cholesterol, which is acquired by circulating erythrocytes, increasing their cholesterol content. The cholesterol preferentially partitions into the outer leaflet, increasing the surface area to volume ratio and forming scalloped edges. In the spleen, membrane fragments are lost and the cells develop the characteristic projections of acanthocytes. Cholesterol interacts with band 3 and changes its conformation, which may affect the membrane skeleton and reduce the deformability of the cell,[162] causing it to be trapped and eventually destroyed in the narrow sinusoids of the spleen.

Clinical Features

Spur cell anemia is characterized by rapidly progressive hemolytic anemia with large numbers of acanthocytes on the blood film. Splenomegaly and jaundice become more prominent and are accompanied by severe ascites, bleeding diatheses, and hepatic encephalopathy. Spur cell anemia is most common in patients with alcoholic liver disease, but similar clinical syndromes have been described in association with advanced metastatic liver disease, cardiac cirrhosis, Wilson disease, fulminant hepatitis, and infantile cholestatic liver disease.[13]

Laboratory Features

Most patients have moderate anemia with a hematocrit of 20 to 30 percent, marked indirect hyperbilirubinemia, and laboratory evidence of severe hepatocellular disease. Blood films reveal significant acanthocytosis and in some patients, echinocytes, target cells and microspherocytes, many with very fine spicules, are visible (see Fig. 46–13).

Differential Diagnosis

Spur cell hemolytic anemia should be distinguished from other hemolytic syndromes associated with liver disease, including congestive splenomegaly, in which patients exhibit chronic, mild hemolysis and occasional spherocytes, and patients with transient hemolytic episodes.

Therapy, Course, and Prognosis

The anemia of spur cell anemia usually is not a significant clinical problem, but it can aggravate pre-existing anemia resulting from, for example, gastrointestinal bleeding, to the point that erythrocyte transfusion is required. The life span of spur cells is markedly decreased because of splenic sequestration, and, as expected, hemolysis abates after splenectomy. However, splenectomy is a dangerous and potentially fatal procedure in these critically ill patients and is generally not recommended.

NEUROACANTHOCYTOSIS

The term *neuroacanthocytosis* describes a heterogeneous group of rare disorders with variable clinical phenotypes and inheritance. The common features are a degeneration of neurons and abnormal acanthocytic erythrocyte morphology. These syndromes may be divided into: (1) lipoprotein abnormalities, which cause peripheral neuropathy, such as abetalipoproteinemia and hypobetalipoproteinemia, (2) neural degeneration of the basal ganglia resulting in movement disorders with normal lipoproteins, such as chorea-acanthocytosis and McLeod syndrome, and (3) movement abnormalities in which acanthocytes are occasionally seen, such as Huntington disease-like 2 (HDL2) and pantothenate kinase-associated neurodegeneration (PKAN).

Abetalipoproteinemia

Definition Abetalipoproteinemia or Bassen-Kornzweig syndrome is a rare autosomal recessive disorder characterized by progressive ataxic neurologic disease, dietary fat malabsorption, retinitis pigmentosa, and acanthocytosis found in people of diverse ethnic backgrounds.[164]

Etiology and Pathogenesis This disorder is caused by a failure to synthesize or secrete lipoproteins containing products of the apolipoprotein B (apoB) gene and this leads to changes in the plasma lipid profile.[164] The primary molecular defect is a lack of the microsomal triglyceride transfer protein, which performs an essential step in apoB-containing lipoprotein synthesis.[165] The relative distribution of erythrocyte membrane phospholipids is altered and the phosphatidylcholine content is decreased with a corresponding increase in sphingomyelin. The excess sphingomyelin is preferentially confined to the outer leaflet of the membrane bilayer, where it presumably causes an expansion of this layer and modifies the conformation of band 3, which contributes to the irregularities in cell surface contour.[162] Red cell precursors and reticulocytes have a normal shape and acanthocytosis only becomes apparent as the red cells mature in the circulation, worsening with increasing red cell age.[166]

Clinical Features The disorder manifests in the first month of life by steatorrhea. Atypical retinitis pigmentosa, which often results in blindness, and progressive neurologic abnormalities characterized by ataxia and intention tremors develop between 5 and 10 years of age and progress to death in the second or third decade.[166]

Laboratory Features Patients usually have mild anemia with normal red cell indices and normal or slightly increased reticulocyte counts.[166] Acanthocytosis is prominent, ranging from approximately 50 to 90 percent of red cells. Despite the red cell lipid abnormalities, the hemolysis is mild and the spleen is normal in patients with abetalipoproteinemia, in contrast to spur cell anemia. There is marked vitamin E deficiency (Chap. 44), which is thought to be a primary stimulus for the neuropathy. Coagulopathy may be observed.[164]

Differential Diagnosis The related disorders hypobetalipoproteinemia, normotriglyceridemic abetalipoproteinemia, and chylomicron retention disease are associated with partial production of apoB-containing lipoproteins or with secretion of lipoproteins containing truncated forms of apoB. Patients with these disorders may experience neurologic disease and acanthocytosis, depending on the severity of the underlying defect.

Therapy, Course, and Prognosis Treatment includes dietary restriction of triglycerides and supplementation with high doses of vitamins A, K, D, and E.[166] Chronic administration of vitamin E can delay or prevent the neurologic symptoms.

Chorea-Acanthocytosis Syndrome

Chorea-acanthocytosis is a rare autosomal recessive movement disorder characterized by atrophy of the basal ganglia and progressive neurodegenerative disease with onset in adolescence or adult life.[167] In some patients, acanthocytosis may precede the onset of neurologic symptoms. The lipoproteins are normal.

Molecular studies have identified approximately 100 mutations in the *VPS13A* gene, which codes for chorein, a protein ubiquitously expressed in the brain and also found in mature red cells.[168–170] It is a member of a conserved protein family involved in trafficking of membrane proteins between cellular compartments, but its role in red cells and the pathogenesis of the disorder and acanthocytes is unknown. The mutations result in the absence or markedly reduced levels of chorein and founder mutations have been identified in Japanese and French-Canadian families.[167]

Patients are not anemic, and red cell survival is only slightly decreased. Plasma and erythrocyte membrane lipids, as well as membrane protein composition and content, are normal, but electron microscopy studies revealed structural abnormalities in the skeleton and an uneven distribution of intra-membrane particles. Red cell membrane fluidity is decreased. Increased serine-threonine and tyrosine phosphorylation of band 3, β-spectrin, and β-adducin has been documented.[171] In particular, abnormal activation of Lyn kinase results in increased tyrosine phosphorylation of band 3, which alters the association of band 3 with β-adducin and the junctional complex of the skeleton.[171] This may lead to localized disruption of the skeleton–membrane interaction, facilitating the formation of protrusions. In one chorea-acanthocytosis kindred a point mutation near the C terminus of band 3 has been identified, which may influence the interaction of band 3 with the skeleton.[172]

McLeod Syndrome

The McLeod phenotype is a rare X-linked defect of the Kell blood group system, whereby cells react poorly with Kell antisera. The XK protein is an integral membrane transport channel protein that is covalently linked to the Kell antigen by disulphide bonds, and mutations in the XK gene cause a deficiency of the XK protein.[167,170] Male hemizygotes who lack XK have up to 85 percent acanthocytes on the blood film with mild, compensated hemolysis and develop late-onset multisystem myopathy or chorea known as the McLeod syndrome. Female heterozygous carriers may have occasional acanthocytes as a result of mosaicism in X chromosome inactivation. Large deletions involving not only the XK locus at Xp21.1, but also contiguous genes, result in the McLeod syndrome being associated with other diseases, such as chronic granulomatous disease of childhood, retinitis pigmentosa, Duchenne muscular dystrophy, and ornithine transcarbamylase deficiency.

Red cell membrane protein and lipid composition are normal, but the distribution of intramembrane particles is altered and increased phosphorylation of membrane proteins, notably band 3, has been noted, which again implicates band 3 as a key player in the generation of acanthocytes.

Other Neuroacanthocytosis Syndromes

The HDL2 disorder is caused by expanded CGT/CAG trinucleotide repeat mutations in the *junctophilin-3* gene, which encodes a protein involved in junctional membrane structures and calcium regulation.[167] The disease is autosomal dominant and presents with late-onset chorea, parkinsonism, and progressive cognitive defects. Acanthocytes are present in some patients. In one unusual kindred autosomal dominant inheritance of chorea-acanthocytosis with polyglutamine neuronal inclusions was described in association with HDL2. Proteolysis of band 3 was also noted, which could contribute to the altered red cell morphology.[170,173]

Acanthocytes have been noted in some patients with PKAN (formerly known as Hallervorden-Spatz syndrome) with features of dystonia, dysarthria, and rigidity in childhood, and in HARP syndrome (hypobetalipoproteinemia, acanthocytosis, retinitis pigmentosa and pallidal degeneration). Both conditions are caused by mutations in pantothenate kinase 2, which is involved in synthesis of coenzyme A and phospholipids.[167,170,174]

Differential Diagnosis of Neuroacanthocytosis with Normal Lipoproteins

Chorea-acanthocytosis, McLeod syndrome, HDL2, and pantothenate kinase disorders present with overlapping neurologic symptoms and clinical phenotypes and also resemble Huntington disease, which renders the clinical diagnosis difficult. Identification of the underlying gene defects and the availability of molecular tests have markedly improved the diagnostic accuracy. This also provides insight into the underlying pathogenesis and suggests that the affected proteins, which are all linked to membrane structure, may participate in a common pathway that ultimately causes degeneration of the basal ganglia.

HEREDITARY STOMATOCYTOSIS SYNDROMES

The intracellular concentration of the monovalent cations, Na^+ and K^+, contribute to erythrocyte volume homeostasis. A net increase in these cations causes water to enter the cells resulting in overhydrated cells or stomatocytes, whereas a net loss dehydrates the cells and forms xerocytes. Disorders of red cell cation permeability are very rare conditions that are inherited in an autosomal dominant fashion with marked clinical and biochemical heterogeneity (Table 46–4).[175]

Stomatocytes are cup-shaped red cells characterized by a central hemoglobin-free area (Figs. 46–10E and 46–11D). The molecular mechanism of stomatocyte formation has not been elucidated, but several theories have been postulated. The lipid bilayer hypothesis predicts that agents or abnormalities that expand the inner leaflet will tend to form stomatocytes.[176] Other theories relegate lipids to a secondary role

TABLE 46–4. Heterogeneity of the Hereditary Stomatocytosis Syndromes

	Stomatocytosis (Hydrocytosis)		Intermediate Syndromes			
	Severe Hemolysis	Mild Hemolysis	Cryohydrocytosis	Stomatocytic Xerocytosis	Xerocytosis with High Phosphatidylcholine	Xerocytosis
Hemolysis	Severe	Mild–moderate	Moderate	Mild	Moderate	Moderate
Anemia	Severe	Mild–moderate	Mild–moderate	None	Mild	Moderate
Blood film	Stomatocytes	Stomatocytes	Stomatocytes	Stomatocytes	Targets	Targets, echinocytes
MCV (80–100 fL)*	110–150	95–130	90–105	91–98	84–92	100–110
MCHC (32–36%)	24–30	26–29	34–40	33–39	34–38	34–38
Unincubated osmotic fragility	Markedly increased	Increased	Normal	Decreased	Markedly decreased	Markedly decreased
RBC Na$^{+5-12†}$	60–100	30–60	40–50	10–20	10–15	10–20
RBC K$^{+90-103}$	20–55	40–85	55–65	75–85	75–90	60–80
RBC Na$^+$+K$^{+95-110}$	110–140	115–145	100–105	87–103	93–99	75–90
Phosphatidylcholine content	Normal	± Increased	Normal	Normal	Increased	Normal
Cold autohemolysis	No	No	Yes	No	No	?
Effect of splenectomy‡	Good	Good	Fair	?	?	? Poor
Inheritance	Autosomal dominant?, autosomal recessive	Autosomal dominant	Autosomal dominant	Autosomal dominant	Autosomal dominant	Autosomal dominant

MCHC, mean corpuscular hemoglobin concentration; MCV, mean corpuscular volume; RBC, red blood cell.

*Values in parentheses are the normal range.

†Values for sodium, potassium, and sodium + potassium are mEq/L RBC.

‡Splenectomy may be contraindicated in these syndromes; see text for details.

Reproduced with permission from Nathan DG, Orkin SH, Oski FA: *Hematology of Infancy and Childhood,* 5th edition. Philadelphia, PA: Saunders/Elsevier; 1998.

and propose that membrane proteins, specifically band 3, play a major role in regulating the structure of the red cell.[162] Band 3 tetramers are attached to the spectrin skeleton and different configurations of band 3 that either face inward or outward can influence the topography of the skeleton and the shape of the cell.

HEREDITARY XEROCYTOSIS

Definition

Hereditary xerocytosis, also known as dehydrated HSt, is the most common form of the cation permeability defects. It is an autosomal dominant hemolytic anemia characterized by an efflux of K^+ and red cell dehydration. Hereditary xerocytosis is part of a pleiotropic syndrome and patients may also exhibit pseudohyperkalemia and perinatal edema.[177]

Etiology and Pathogenesis

The underlying membrane permeability defect is complex and involves a net loss of potassium from the red cells that is not accompanied by a proportional gain of sodium. Consequently, the net intracellular cation content and cell water content are decreased. In some cases, erythrocytes exhibit an increase in phosphatidylcholine and reduced BPG content.[13]

The genetic locus for this disorder was mapped to 16q23–q24.[177] Subsequent refinement of the locus and exome sequencing of several large unrelated multigenerational kindred identified numerous missense mutations in the gene encoding the PIEZO1 protein.[178,179] Cosegregation of some of the mutations in families with multiple disease phenotypes suggested a correlation between PIEZO and perinatal edema.[178] PIEZO proteins were recently identified as mechanosensory molecules that form part of stretch-activated cation channels. The PIEZO1 protein is present in red cell membranes and two PIEZO1 mutations, R2456H and R2488Q, were demonstrated to regulate a mechanosensitive transduction channel, leading to increased cation transport in erythrocytes.[178,179]

Clinical Features

Patients may present with symptoms of compensated hemolytic anemia, including jaundice, splenomegaly, and gallstones. Some patients may also exhibit pseudohyperkalemia and perinatal edema and even hydrops fetalis.[13,177] Variable penetrance is present in this disorder, with significant disparity in clinical symptoms between affected individuals in the same kindred. Patients display a strong tendency to iron overload (Chap. 43).[175]

Laboratory Features

The hematologic picture is that of mild to moderate compensated hemolytic anemia (see Table 46–4) with an elevated reticulocyte count. The K^+ content is decreased and the Na^+ content is increased, but the total monovalent cation content is reduced. The MCHC is increased reflecting cellular dehydration and the MCV is frequently mildly increased.[175] Erythrocytes are resistant to osmotic lysis and the bell-shaped curve obtained by osmotic gradient ektacytometry is shifted to the left. Stomatocytes are not a prominent feature on blood films, but some target cells and spiculated cells are seen. In some of the cells, hemoglobin is concentrated ("puddled") in discrete areas on the cell periphery.

Therapy, Course, and Prognosis

Most patients experience only mild anemia and therapy is not required. The patients should receive folate supplementation and be monitored for complications of hemolysis. Splenectomy does not significantly improve the anemia, which suggests that xerocytes are detected and eliminated in other areas of the reticuloendothelial system. Because of

a markedly high risk of hypercoagulability and life-threatening thrombotic episodes after splenectomy, the procedure is contraindicated.[13]

HEREDITARY STOMATOCYTOSIS/ HYDROCYTOSIS

Definition and History

Hereditary stomatocytosis, also known as hereditary hydrocytosis or overhydrated stomatocytosis, is characterized by a marked passive sodium leak, which causes red cell overhydration and macrocytosis. It is an autosomal dominantly inherited hemolytic anemia. The syndrome was first described in a girl with dominantly inherited hemolytic anemia whose blood film contained stomatocytes.[180] The hallmarks of abnormal cation transport and overhydration of the red cells were discovered subsequently.[181]

Etiology and Pathogenesis

The red cell membrane of stomatocytes has enhanced permeability toward monovalent cations, especially sodium ions. This marked passive sodium leak into the cell represents the principal lesion in this disorder. The Na^+-K^+-ATPase pump, which normally maintains low intracellular sodium and high potassium concentrations, is stimulated but this increase in active transport, coupled to enhanced glycolysis to provide ATP, is insufficient to overcome the leak.[175,182]

The overhydrated red cells of some patients lack stomatin, a 31-kDa integral membrane protein, but no gene mutations have been found implying that the absence of the protein is a secondary phenomenon.[13,175] Stomatin interacts with GLUT-1 and converts it to a dehydroascorbic acid transporter, suggesting that it might be beneficial to inhibit this interaction in stomatocytes, because they require additional glucose for their increased ATP needs.[175]

In some stomatocytosis patients, missense mutations causing amino acid substitutions of conserved residues in the transmembrane domain of the RhAG protein, a component of the band 3–Rh–RhAG multiprotein complex in the membrane, have been described.[183] RhAG is a transport protein that may function as a gas and/or ammonium channel through pore-like structures. The mutations are thought to widen the pores allowing cations to leak through the membrane. A *de novo* missense mutation in the transmembrane domain of band 3 has been described in one patient with stomatocytosis associated with dyserythropoiesis.[184] This changed the transport function of band 3 from an anion exchanger to a cation channel. The tyrosine phosphorylation profile of the stomatocyte membranes revealed increased phosphorylation of band 3 and stomatin, as a result of enhanced activity of the Syk and Lyn tyrosine kinases, suggesting that phospho-signaling pathways involved in cell volume regulation may be perturbed.[184]

Clinical Features

Moderate to severe anemia is present. Jaundice and splenomegaly are common, as are complications of chronic hemolysis, such as cholelithiasis. Patients exhibit a tendency for iron overload, independent of transfusion status or splenectomy. No other organ system abnormalities have been noted.[13,175] A dyserythropoietic phenotype was noted in one patient with mild anemia.[184]

Laboratory Features

The blood film reveals striking stomatocytosis and up to 50 percent of red cells may have abnormal morphology (Figs. 46–10E and 46–11D). In addition to the anemia, red cell indices show decreased MCHC and marked macrocytosis, as reflected by an elevated MCV, which can reach 150 fL in some severely affected patients (see Table 46–4). The K^+ content is decreased and the Na^+ content is markedly increased, leading to elevated total monovalent cation content. The OF of stomatocytes is markedly increased because many of the swollen red cells approach their critical hemolytic volume, which causes a shift of the osmotic gradient ektacytometer curve to the right. Red cell deformability is decreased.

Therapy, Course, and Prognosis

The majority of hydrocytosis patients suffer from significant lifelong anemia. They should be monitored for complications of hemolysis, such as cholelithiasis and parvovirus infection, and should receive folate supplementation. The outcome of splenectomy has been variable, but typically it has been beneficial and improved the hemolytic anemia in severely affected patients.[13] This is expected because stomatocytes expend large amounts of ATP to pump cations in an attempt to avoid osmotic lysis and are, therefore, vulnerable in the metabolically challenging environment of the spleen. However, splenectomy should be carefully considered in patients with this disorder, since they are at high risk of developing hypercoagulability after splenectomy, leading to catastrophic thrombotic episodes.[13]

CRYOHYDROCYTOSIS

The clinical phenotype and biochemical features of some patients with stomatocytes are intermediate between the extremes of hereditary hydrocytosis and hereditary xerocytosis. One of these disorders is cryohydrocytosis in which the mild cation leak is markedly enhanced at low temperatures. It is a very rare condition associated with mild to moderate hemolytic anemia and splenectomy appears to be beneficial.[175] Missense mutations have been found in the transmembrane section of band 3 that cluster between membrane span eight and the last two membrane-spanning domains.[184-186] In vitro studies indicated that the mutant proteins have lost their anion exchange capability and are converted to a nonselective cation channel.[175,186,187]

Two cases of cryohydrocytosis and stomatin deficiency have been described with mutations in GLUT-1, which abolish the glucose transport function of the protein and create a cation leak.[188]

OTHER STOMATOCYTIC DISORDERS

Rh-deficiency syndrome designates rare individuals who either lack all Rh antigens (Rh_null) or exhibit markedly reduced (Rh_mod) Rh antigen expression. Rh antigens are carried on RhCE and RhD proteins that associate with RhAG and enable the formation of the Rh multiprotein complex in the red cell membrane. The Rh complex is either absent or markedly reduced in patients with Rh deficiency syndrome and they present with mild to moderate hemolytic anemia. Stomatocytes and occasional spherocytes are seen on the blood film and the cells have cation transport abnormalities, which cause dehydration. Hemolytic anemia is improved by splenectomy.[13,175] Chapter 136 reviews the structure, localization, and functions of the Rh antigens.

Familial deficiency of high-density lipoproteins is a rare condition that leads to accumulation of cholesteryl esters in many tissues, resulting in clinical findings of large orange tonsils and hepatosplenomegaly. Hematologic manifestations include moderately severe hemolytic anemia with stomatocytosis. Red cell membrane lipid analyses revealed a low cholesterol content and a relative increase in phosphatidylcholine at the expense of sphingomyelin.[13]

ACQUIRED STOMATOCYTOSIS

Normal individuals have up to 3 percent stomatocytes on blood films. Acquired stomatocytosis is common in alcoholics particularly those with acute alcoholism. Vinca alkaloids, such as vincristine and vinblastine, may induce hemolysis with increased sodium permeability and

stomatocytosis at the doses used for chemotherapy of leukemias and lymphomas.[189] Transient stomatocytosis has been observed in long distance runners immediately after a race. The molecular basis of acquired stomatocytosis is unknown.[13]

REFERENCES

1. Jakobik V, Burus I, Decsi T: Fatty acid composition of erythrocyte membrane lipids in healthy subjects from birth to young adulthood. *Eur J Pediatr* 168:141, 2009.
2. Ways P, Hanahan DJ: Characterization and quantification of red cell lipids in normal man. *J Lipid Res* 5:318, 1964.
3. Mulder E, Van Deenen LLM: Incorporation in vitro of fatty acids into phospholipids from mature erythrocytes. *Biochim Biophys Acta* 106:106, 1965.
4. Daleke DL: Regulation of phospholipid asymmetry in the erythrocyte membrane. *Curr Opin Hematol* 15(3):191, 2008.
5. Devaux PF, Herrmann A, Ohlwein N, et al: How lipid flippases can modulate membrane structure. *Biochim Biophys Acta* 1778(7–8):1591, 2008.
6. Sahu SK, Gummadi SN, Manoj N, et al: Phospholipid scramblases: An overview. *Arch Biochem Biophys* 462:103, 2007.
7. Salzer U, Prohaska R: Stomatin, flotillin-1, and flotillin-2 are major integral proteins of erythrocyte lipid rafts. *Blood* 97(4):1141, 2001.
8. Murphy SC, Samuel BU, Harrison T, et al: Erythrocyte detergent-resistant membrane proteins: their characterization and selective uptake during malarial infection. *Blood* 103(5):1920, 2004.
9. Fairbanks G, Steck TL, Wallach DFH: Electrophoretic analysis of the major polypeptides of the human erythrocyte membrane. *Biochemistry* 10(13):2606, 1971.
10. Pasini EM, Kirkegaard M, Mortensen P, et al: In-depth analysis of the membrane and cytosolic proteome of red blood cells. *Blood* 108(3):791, 2006.
11. Van den Akker E, Satchwell TJ, Williamson RC, et al: Band 3 multiprotein complexes in the red cell membrane; of mice and men. *Blood Cells Mol Dis* 45(1):1, 2010.
12. Fujinaga J, Tang X-B, Casey JR: Topology of the membrane domain of human erythrocyte anion exchange protein, AE1. *J Biol Chem* 274(10):6626, 1999.
13. Walensky Loren D, Narla Mohandas Lux SE: Disorders of the red blood cell membrane, in *Blood: Principles and Practice of Hematology*, 2nd ed., edited by Handin RI, Lux SE, Stossel TP, p 1709. Lippincott Williams & Wilkins, New York, 2003.
14. Sterling D, Reithmeier RAF, Casey JR: A transport metabolon: Functional interaction of carbonic anhydrase II and chloride/bicarbonate exchangers. *J Biol Chem* 276(51):47886, 2001.
15. Zhang D, Kiyatkin A, Bolin JT, et al: Crystallographic structure and functional interpretation of the cytoplasmic domain of erythrocyte membrane band 3. *Blood* 96(9):2925, 2000.
16. Chu H, Low PS: Mapping of glycolytic enzyme-binding sites on human erythrocyte band 3. *Biochem J* 400(1):143, 2006.
17. Low PS, Waugh SM, Zinke K, et al: The Role of hemoglobin denaturation and band 3 clustering in red blood cell aging. *Science* 227(4686):531, 1985.
18. Pasternack GR, Anderson RA, Leto TL, et al: Interactions between protein 4.1 and band 3. An alternative binding site for an element of the membrane skeleton. *J Biol Chem* 260(6):3676, 1985.
19. Salomao M, Zhang X, Yang Y, et al: Protein 4.1R-dependent multiprotein complex: New insights into the structural organization of the red blood cell membrane. *Proc Natl Acad Sci U S A* 105(23):8026, 2008.
20. Rybicki AC, Musto S, Schwartz RS: Identification of a band-3 binding site near the N-terminus of erythrocyte membrane protein 4.2. *Biochem J* 309:677, 1995.
21. Anong WA, Franco T, Chu H, et al: Adducin forms a bridge between the erythrocyte membrane and its cytoskeleton and regulates membrane cohesion. *Blood* 114(9):1904, 2009.
22. Lee G, Abdi K, Jiang Y, et al: Nanospring behaviour of ankyrin repeats. *Nature* 440(7081):3, 2006.
23. Michaely P, Bennett V: The ANK repeats of erythrocyte ankyrin form two distinct but cooperative binding sites for the erythrocyte anion exchanger. *J Biol Chem* 270(37):22050, 1995.
24. Bruce LJ, Beckmann R, Ribeiro ML, et al: A band 3-based macro complex of integral and peripheral proteins in the RBC membrane. *Blood* 101(10):4180, 2003.
25. Williamson RC, Toye AM: Glycophorin A: Band 3 aid. *Blood Cells Mol Dis* 41(1):35, 2008.
26. Schofield AE, Martin PG, Spillett D, et al: The structure of the human red blood cell anion exchanger (EPB3, AE1, band 3) gene. *Blood* 84(6):2000, 1994.
27. Rearden A, Magnet A, Kudo S, et al: Glycophorin B and glycophorin E genes arose from the glycophorin A ancestral gene via two duplications during primate evolution. *J Biol Chem* 268(3):2260, 1993.
28. Cartron JP, Le Van Kim C, Colin Y: Glycophorin C and related glycoproteins: structure, function and regulation. *Semin Hematol* 30:152, 1993.
29. Bennett V, Healy J: Organizing the fluid membrane bilayer: diseases linked to spectrin and ankyrin. *Trends Mol Med* 14(1):28, 2008.
30. Thomas GH, Newbern EC, Korte CC, et al: Intragenic duplication and divergence in the spectrin superfamily of proteins. *Mol Biol Evol* 14(12):1285, 1997.
31. Grum VL, Li D, MacDonald RI, et al: Structures of two repeats of spectrin suggest models of flexibility. *Cell* 98(4):523, 1999.
32. Speicher DW, Marchesi VT: Erythrocyte spectrin is comprised of many homologous triple helical segments. *Nature* 311(5982):177, 1984.

33. Li D, Tang H-Y, Speicher DW: A structural model of the erythrocyte spectrin heterodimer initiation site determined using homology modeling and chemical cross-linking. *J Biol Chem* 283(3):1553, 2008.

34. Ipsaro JJ, Harper SL, Messick TE, et al: Crystal structure and functional interpretation of the erythrocyte spectrin tetramerization domain complex. *Blood* 115(23):4843, 2010.

35. Becker PS, Schwartz MA, Morrow JS, et al: Radiolabel-transfer cross-linking demonstrates that protein 4.1 binds to the N-terminal region of β spectrin and to actin in binary interactions. *Eur J Biochem* 193:827, 1990.

36. Liu SC, Derick LH, Palek J: Visualization of the hexagonal lattice in the erythrocyte membrane skeleton. *J Cell Biol* 104:527, 1987.

37. Korsgren C, Lux SE: The carboxyterminal EF domain of erythroid alpha-spectrin is necessary for optimal spectrin-actin binding. *Blood* 116(14):2600, 2010.

38. Ipsaro JJ, Huang L, Mondragón A: Structures of the spectrin-ankyrin interaction binding domains. *Blood* 113(22):5385, 2009.

39. Stabach PR, Simonović I, Ranieri MA, et al: The structure of the ankyrin-binding site of β-spectrin reveals how tandem spectrin-repeats generate unique ligand-binding properties. *Blood* 113(22):5377, 2009.

40. Yocum AO, Steiner LA, Seidel NE, et al: A tissue-specific chromatin loop activates the erythroid ankyrin-1 promoter. *Blood* 120(17):3586, 2012.

41. Michaely P, Tomchick DR, Machius M, Anderson RG: Crystal structure of a 12 ANK repeat stack from human ankyrinR. *EMBO J* 21(23):6387, 2002.

42. Ipsaro JJ, Mondragón A: Structural basis for spectrin recognition by ankyrin. *Blood* 115(20):4093, 2010.

43. Gallagher PG, Tse WT, Scarpa L, et al: Structure and organization of the human ankyrin-1 gene: Basis for complexity of pre-mRNA processing. *J Biol Chem* 272(31):19220, 1997.

44. Hou VC, Conboy JG: Regulation of alternative pre-mRNA splicing during erythroid differentiation. *Curr Opin Hematol* 8(2):74, 2001.

45. Parra MK, Gee SL, Koury MJ, et al: Alternative 5′ exons and differential splicing regulate expression of protein 4.1R isoforms with distinct N-termini. *Blood* 101(10):4164, 2003.

46. Inaba M, Kuwabara M, Takahashi T, et al: Deamidation of human erythrocyte protein 4.1: Possible role in aging. *Blood* 79:3355, 1992.

47. Satchwell TJ, Shoemark DK, Sessions RB, et al: Protein 4.2: A complex linker. *Blood Cells Mol Dis* 42(3):201, 2009.

48. Chishti AH: Function of p55 and its nonerythroid homologues. *Curr Opin Hematol* 5(2):116, 1998.

49. Li X, Matsuoka Y, Bennett V: Adducin preferentially recruits spectrin to the fast growing ends of actin filaments in a complex requiring the MARCKS-related domain and a newly defined oligomerization domain. *J Biol Chem* 273(30):19329, 1998.

50. Khan AA, Hanada T, Mohseni M, et al: Dematin and adducin provide a novel link between the erythrocyte cytoskeleton and erythrocyte membrane by directly interacting with glucose transporter-1. *J Biol Chem* 283(21):14600, 2008.

51. Robledo RF, Ciciotte SL, Gwynn B, et al: Targeted deletion of α-adducin results in absent β- and γ-adducin, compensated hemolytic anemia, and lethal hydrocephalus in mice. *Blood* 112(10):4298, 2008.

52. Fowler VM: Regulation of actin filament length in erythrocytes and striated muscle. *Curr Opin Cell Biol* 8(1):86, 1996.

53. Azim AC, Knoll JHM, Beggs AH, Chishti AH: Isoform cloning, actin binding, and chromosomal localization of human erythroid dematin, a member of the villin superfamily. *J Biol Chem* 270(29):17407, 1995.

54. Mohandas N, Gallagher PG: Red cell membrane: past, present, and future. *Blood* 112(10):3939, 2008.

55. An X, Lecomte MC, Chasis JA, et al: Shear-response of the spectrin dimer-tetramer equilibrium in the red blood cell membrane. *J Biol Chem* 277(35):31796, 2002.

56. An X, Guo X, Zhang X, et al: Conformational stabilities of the structural repeats of erythroid spectrin and their functional implications. *J Biol Chem* 281(15):10527, 2006.

57. Johnson CP, Tang H-Y, Carag C, et al: Forced unfolding of proteins within cells. *Science* 317(5838):663, 2007.

58. Brugnara C: Erythrocyte membrane transport physiology. *Curr Opin Hematol* 4(2):122, 1997.

59. Moon C, Preston GM, Griffin CA, et al: The human aquaporin-CHIP gene. Structure, organization, and chromosomal localization. *J Biol Chem* 268(21):15772, 1993.

60. Mueckler M, Caruso C, Baldwin SA, et al: Sequence and structure of a human glucose transporter. *Science* 229(4717):941, 1985.

61. Palek J: Disorders of the red cell membrane skeleton, in *Erythrocyte Membranes 3: Recent Clinical and Experimental Advances*, edited by Kruckeberg WL, Eaton JW, Brewer GJ, p 177. Alan R. Liss, New York, 1984.

62. Vanlair CF MJ: De la microcythemie. *Bull Acad R Med Belg* 5:515, 1871.

63. Perrotta S, Gallagher PG, Mohandas N: Hereditary spherocytosis. *Lancet* 372(9647):1411, 2008.

64. Iolascon A, Avvisati RA: Genotype/phenotype correlation in hereditary spherocytosis. *Haematologica* 93(9):1283, 2008.

65. An X, Mohandas N: Disorders of red cell membrane. *Br J Haematol* 141(3):367, 2008.

66. Eber S, Lux SE: Hereditary spherocytosis—Defects in proteins that connect the membrane skeleton to the lipid bilayer. *Semin Hematol* 41(2):118, 2004.

67. Mariani M, Barcellini W, Vercellati C, et al: Clinical and hematologic features of 300 patients affected by hereditary spherocytosis grouped according to the type of the membrane protein defect. *Haematologica* 93(9):1310, 2008.

68. Coetzer TL, Lawler J, Liu S-C, et al: Partial ankyrin and spectrin deficiency in severe, atypical hereditary spherocytosis. *N Engl J Med* 318(4):230, 1988.

69. Eber SW, Gonzalez JM, Lux ML, et al: Ankyrin-1 mutations are a major cause of dominant and recessive hereditary spherocytosis. *Nat Genet* 13:214, 1996.

70. Gallagher PG, Ferreira JDS, Costa FF, et al: A recurrent frameshift mutation of the ankyrin gene associated with severe hereditary spherocytosis. *Br J Haematol* 111:1190, 2000.

71. Edelman EJ, Maksimova Y, Duru F, et al: A complex splicing defect associated with homozygous ankyrin-deficient hereditary spherocytosis. *Blood* 109(12):5491, 2007.

72. Gallagher PG, Nilson DG, Wong C, et al: A dinucleotide deletion in the ankyrin promoter alters gene expression, transcription initiation and TFIID complex formation in hereditary spherocytosis. *Hum Mol Genet* 14(17):2501, 2005.

73. Gallagher PG, Steiner LA, Liem RI, et al: Mutation of a barrier insulator in the human ankyrin-1 gene is associated with hereditary spherocytosis. *J Clin Invest* 120(12):4453, 2010.

74. Lux SE, Tse WT, Menninger JC, et al: Hereditary spherocytosis associated with deletion of human erythrocyte ankyrin gene on chromosome 8. *Nature* 345(6277):736, 1990.

75. Jarolim P, Rubin HL, Brabec V, et al: Mutations of conserved arginines in the membrane domain of erythroid band 3 lead to a decrease in membrane-associated band 3 and to the phenotype of hereditary spherocytosis. *Blood* 85(3):634, 1995.

76. Bracher NA, Lyons CA, Wessels G, et al: Band 3 Cape Town (E90K) causes severe hereditary spherocytosis in combination with band 3 Prague III. *Br J Haematol* 113(3):689, 2001.

77. Alloisio N, Texier P, Ribeiro ML, et al: Modulation of clinical expression and band 3 deficiency in hereditary spherocytosis. *Blood* 90(1):414, 1997.

78. Agre P, Casella JF, Zinkham WH, et al: Partial deficiency of erythrocyte spectrin in hereditary spherocytosis. *Nature* 314(6009):380, 1985.

79. Agre P, Asimos A, Casella JF, et al: Inheritance pattern and clinical response to splenectomy as a reflection of erythrocyte spectrin deficiency in hereditary spherocytosis. *N Engl J Med* 315(25):1579, 1986.

80. Liu SC, Derick LH, Agre P PJ: Alteration of the erythrocyte membrane skeletal ultrastructure in hereditary spherocytosis, hereditary elliptocytosis, and pyropoikilocytosis. *Blood* 76:198, 1990.

81. Wichterle H, Hanspal M, Palek J, et al: Combination of two mutant alpha spectrin alleles underlies a severe spherocytic hemolytic anemia. *J Clin Invest* 98(10):2300, 1996.

82. Tse WT, Gallagher PG, Jenkins PB, et al: Amino-acid substitution in α-spectrin commonly coinherited with nondominant hereditary spherocytosis. *Am J Hematol* 54:233, 1997.

83. Bogardus H, Schulz VP, Maksimova Y, et al: Severe nondominant hereditary spherocytosis due to uniparental isodisomy at the SPTA1 locus. *Haematologica* 99(9):e168, 2014.

84. Hassoun H, Vassiliadis JN, Murray J, et al: Characterization of the underlying molecular defect in hereditary spherocytosis associated with spectrin deficiency. *Blood* 90(1):398, 1997.

85. Hassoun H, Vassiliades J, Murray J, et al: Hereditary spherocytosis with spectrin deficiency due to an unstable truncated beta spectrin. *Blood* 87(6):2538, 1996.

86. Hassoun H, Vassiliadis JN, Murray J, et al: Molecular basis of spectrin deficiency in beta spectrin Durham. A deletion within spectrin adjacent to the ankyrin-binding site precludes spectrin attachment to the membrane in hereditary spherocytosis. *J Clin Invest* 96:2623, 1995.

87. Becker PS, Tse WT, Lux SE, et al: β Spectrin Kissimmee: A spectrin variant associated with autosomal dominant hereditary spherocytosis and defective binding to protein 4.1. *J Clin Invest* 92(2):612, 1993.

88. Hammill AM, Risinger MA, Joiner CH, et al: Compound heterozygosity for two novel mutations in the erythrocyte protein 4.2 gene causing spherocytosis in a Caucasian patient. *Br J Haematol* 152:777, 2011.

89. Bouhassira EE, Schwartz RS, Yawata Y, et al: An alanine-to-threonine substitution in protein 4.2 cDNA is associated with a Japanese form of hereditary hemolytic anemia (protein 4.2NIPPON). *Blood* 79(7):1846, 1992.

90. De Franceschi L, Olivieri O, Miraglia del Giudice E, et al: Membrane cation and anion transport activities in erythrocytes of hereditary spherocytosis: Effects of different membrane protein defects. *Am J Hematol* 55(3):121, 1997.

91. Ribeiro LM, Alloisio N, Almeida H, et al: Severe hereditary spherocytosis and distal renal tubular acidosis associated with the total absence of band 3. *Blood* 96(4):1602, 2000.

92. Delaunay J, Nouyrigat V, Proust A, et al: Different impacts of alleles αLEPRA and αLELY as assessed versus a novel, virtually null allele of the SPTA1 gene in trans. *Br J Haematol* 127(1):118, 2004.

93. Alloisio N, Maillet P, Carre G, et al: Hereditary spherocytosis with band 3 deficiency. Association with a nonsense mutation of the band 3 gene (allele Lyon), and aggravation by a low-expression allele occurring in trans (allele Genas). *Blood* 88(3):1062, 1996.

94. Wilmotte R, Maréchal J, Morlé L, et al: Low expression allele αLELY of red cell spectrin is associated with mutations in exon 40 (αV/41 polymorphism) and intron 45 and with partial skipping of exon 46. *J Clin Invest* 91(5):2091, 1993.

95. Toye AM, Williamson RC, Khanfar M, et al: Band 3 Courcouronnes (Ser667Phe): A trafficking mutant differentially rescued by wild-type band 3 and glycophorin A. *Blood* 111(11):5380, 2008.

96. Perrotta S, Borriello A, Scaloni A, et al: The N-terminal 11 amino acids of human erythrocyte band 3 are critical for aldolase binding and protein phosphorylation: implications for band 3 function. *Blood* 106(13):4359, 2005.

97. Delhommeau F, Cynober T, Schischmanoff PO, et al: Natural history of hereditary spherocytosis during the first year of life. *Blood* 95(2):393, 2000.

98. Iolascon A, Faienza MF, Moretti A, et al: UGT1 promoter polymorphism accounts for increased neonatal appearance of hereditary spherocytosis. *Blood* 91(3):1093, 1998.

99. Safeukui I, Buffet PA, Deplaine G, et al: Quantitative assessment of sensing and seques-tration of spherocytic erythrocytes by the human spleen. *Blood* 120(2):424, 2012.

100. Emerson CP Jr, Chu SS, Ham TH, et al: Studies on the destruction of red blood cells. IX. *AMA Arch Intern Med* 97(1):1, 1956.

101. Miraglia del Giudice E, Lombardi C, Francese M, et al: Frequent de novo monoallelic expression of β-spectrin gene (SPTB) in children with hereditary spherocytosis and isolated spectrin deficiency. *Br J Haematol* 101:251, 1998.

102. Miraglia del Giudice E, Francese M, Nobili B, et al: High frequency of de novo muta-tions in ankyrin gene (ANK1) in children with hereditary spherocytosis. *J Pediatr* 132(1):117, 1998.

103. Eber SW, Armbrust R, Schröter W: Variable clinical severity of hereditary spherocyto-sis: relation to erythrocytic spectrin concentration, osmotic fragility, and autohemoly-sis. *J Pediatr* 117(3):409, 1990.

104. Pajor A, Lehoczky D, Szakács Z: Pregnancy and hereditary spherocytosis. Report of 8 patients and a review. *Arch Gynecol Obstet* 253:37, 1993.

105. Gallagher PG, Weed SA, Tse WT, et al: Recurrent fatal hydrops fetalis associated with a nucleotide substitution in the erythrocyte β-spectrin gene. *J Clin Invest* 95:1174, 1995.

106. Gallagher PG, Petruzzi MJ, Weed SA, et al: Mutation of a highly conserved residue of βI spectrin associated with fatal and near-fatal neonatal hemolytic anemia. *J Clin Invest* 99(2):267, 1997.

107. Lima PRM, Gontijo JAR, Lopes de Faria JB, et al: Band 3 Campinas: A novel splicing mutation in the Band 3 gene (AE1) associated with hereditary spherocytosis, hyperac-tivity of Na+/Li+ countertransport and an abnormal renal bicarbonate handling. *Blood* 90(7):2810, 1997.

108. Ryšavá R, Tesař V, Jirsa M Jr, et al: Incomplete distal renal tubular acidosis coinherited with a mutation in the band 3 (AE1) gene. *Nephrol Dial Transplant* 12:1869, 1997.

109. Bianchi P, Fermo E, Vercellati C, et al: Diagnostic power of laboratory tests for heredi-tary spherocytosis: A comparison study in 150 patients grouped according to molecular and clinical characteristics. *Haematologica* 97(4):516, 2012.

110. King M-J, Smythe JS, Mushens R: Eosin-5-maleimide binding to band 3 and Rh-related proteins forms the basis of a screening test for hereditary spherocytosis. *Br J Haematol* 124:106, 2004.

111. Bianchi P, Fermo E, Zanella A: Reply to "Flow cytometry test for hereditary spherocy-tosis." Haematologica. 2012;97(12):e47. *Haematologica* 97(12):e50, 2012.

112. Mackiewicz G, Bailly F, Favre B, et al: Flow cytometry test for hereditary spherocytosis. *Haematologica* 97(12):e47, 2012.

113. Mayeur-Rousse C, Gentil M, Botton J, et al: Testing for hereditary spherocytosis: A French experience. *Haematologica* 97(12):e48, 2012.

114. Bianchi P: Current diagnostic approach and screening methods for hereditary sphero-cytosis. *Thalassemia Reports* 3(s1)(e32):78, 2013.

115. Bolton-Maggs PHB, Langer JC, Iolascon A, et al: Guidelines for the diagnosis and man-agement of hereditary spherocytosis—2011 update. *Br J Haematol* 156(1):37, 2012.

116. Schilling RF: Risks and benefits of splenectomy versus no splenectomy for hereditary spherocytosis—A personal view. *Br J Haematol* 145(6):728, 2009.

117. Rescorla FJ, West KW, Engum SA, et al: Laparoscopic splenic procedures in children: Experience in 231 children. *Ann Surg* 246(4):683, 2007.

118. Tracy ET, Rice HE: Partial splenectomy for hereditary spherocytosis. *Pediatr Clin North Am* 55(2):503, 2008.

119. Dresbach M: Elliptical human red corpuscles. *Science* 19:469, 1904.

120. Hunter WC, Adams RB: Hematologic study of three generations of a white family showing elliptical erythrocytes. *Ann Intern Med* 2(11):1162, 1929.

121. Zarkowsky HS, Mohandas N, Speaker CB, et al: A congenital haemolytic anaemia with thermal sensitivity of the erythrocyte membrane. *Br J Haematol* 29(4):537, 1975.

122. Gallagher PG: Hereditary elliptocytosis: spectrin and protein 4.1R. *Semin Hematol* 41(2):142, 2004.

123. Nurse GT, Coetzer TL, Palek J: The elliptocytoses, ovalocytosis and related disorders. *Baillieres Clin Haematol* 5(1):187, 1992.

124. Glele-Kakai C, Garbarz M, Lecomte M-C, et al: Epidemiological studies of spectrin mutations related to hereditary elliptocytosis and spectrin polymorphisms in Benin. *Br J Haematol* 95(1):57, 1996.

125. Garbarz BM, Lecomte M, Feo C, et al: Hereditary pyropoikilocytosis and elliptocytosis in a white French family with the spectrin alpha I/74 variant related to a CGT to CAT codon change (Arg to His) at position 22 of the spectrin alpha I domain. *Blood* 75:1691, 1990.

126. Swierczek S, Agarwal AM, Naidoo K, et al: Novel exon 2 α spectrin mutation and intragenic crossover: Three morphological phenotypes associated with four distinct α spectrin defects. *Haematologica* 98(12):1972, 2013.

127. Mohandas N, Chasis JA: Red blood cell deformability, membrane material properties and shape: regulation by transmembrane, skeletal and cytosolic proteins and lipids. *Semin Hematol* 30(3):171, 1993.

128. Coetzer T, Palek J, Lawler J, et al: Structural and functional heterogeneity of α spec-trin mutations involving the spectrin heterodimer self-association site: relationships to hematologic expression of homozygous hereditary elliptocytosis and hereditary pyro-poikilocytosis. *Blood* 75(11):2235, 1990.

129. Coetzer TL, Palek J: Partial spectrin deficiency in hereditary pyropoikilocytosis. *Blood* 67:919, 1986.

130. Coetzer T, Lawler J, Prchal JT, et al: Molecular determinants of clinical expression of hereditary elliptocytosis and pyropoikilocytosis. *Blood* 70(3):766, 1987.

131. Gaetani M, Mootien S, Harper S, et al: Structural and functional effects of hereditary hemolytic anemia-associated point mutations in the alpha spectrin tetramer site. *Blood* 111(12):5712, 2008.

132. Lecomte MC, Nicolas G, Dhermy D, et al: Properties of normal and mutant polypeptide fragments from the dimer self-association sites of human red cell spectrin. *Eur Biophys J* 28:208, 1999.

133. Coetzer TL, Sahr K, Prchal J, et al: Four different mutations in codon 28 of α spectrin are associated with structurally and functionally abnormal spectrin αI/74 in hereditary elliptocytosis. *J Clin Invest* 88:743, 1991.

134. Lorenzo F, Miraglia del Giudice E, Alloisio N, et al: Severe poikilocytosis associated with a de novo α28 Arg>Cys mutation in spectrin. *Br J Haematol* 83:152, 1993.

135. Sahr KE, Coetzer TL, Moy LS, et al: Spectrin Cagliari: An Ala>Gly substitution in helix 1 of β spectrin repeat 17 that severely disrupts the structure and self-association of the erythrocyte spectrin heterodimer. *J Biol Chem* 268(30):22656, 1993.

136. Yoon S, Yu H, Eber S, et al: Molecular defect of truncated β-spectrin associated with hereditary elliptocytosis. β-spectrin Göttingen. *J Biol Chem* 266(13):8490, 1991.

137. Roux A-F, Morlé F, Guertarni D, et al: Molecular basis of Sp αI/65 hereditary ellipto-cytosis in North Africa: Insertion of a TTG triplet between codons 147 and 149 in the α-spectrin gene from five unrelated families. *Blood* 73(8):2196, 1989.

138. Johnson CP, Gaetani M, Ortiz V, et al: Pathogenic proline mutation in the linker between spectrin repeats: disease caused by spectrin unfolding. *Blood* 109(8):3538, 2007.

139. Harper SL, Li D, Maksimova Y, et al: A fused α-β "mini-spectrin" mimics the intact erythrocyte spectrin head-to-head tetramer. *J Biol Chem* 285(14):11003, 2010.

140. Harper SL, Sriswasdi S, Tang H-Y, et al: The common hereditary elliptocytosis-associ-ated α-spectrin L260P mutation perturbs erythrocyte membranes by stabilizing spec-trin in the closed dimer conformation. *Blood* 122(17):3045, 2013.

141. Burke JP, Van Zyl D, Zail SS, Coetzer TL: Reduced spectrin-ankyrin binding in a South African hereditary elliptocytosis kindred homozygous for spectrin St Claude. *Blood* 92:2591, 1998.

142. Fournier CM, Gaël N, Gallagher PG, et al: Spectrin St Claude, a splicing mutation of the human α-spectrin gene associated with severe poikilocytic anemia. *Blood* 89(12):4584, 1997.

143. Takakuwa Y, Tchernia G, Rossi M, et al: Restoration of normal membrane stability to unstable protein 4.1-deficient erythrocyte membranes by incorporation of purified pro-tein 4.1. *J Clin Invest* 78:80, 1986.

144. Chishti AH, Palek J, Fisher D, et al: Reduced invasion and growth of Plasmodium fal-ciparum into elliptocytic red blood cells with a combined deficiency of protein 4.1, glycophorin C, and p55. *Blood* 87(8):3462, 1996.

145. Winardi R, Reid M, Conboy J, et al: Molecular analysis of glycophorin C deficiency in human erythrocytes. *Blood* 81(10):2799, 1993.

146. Wilmotte R, Harper SL, Ursitti JA, et al: The exon 46-encoded sequence is essential for stability of human erythroid α-spectrin and heterodimer formation. *Blood* 90(10):4188, 1997.

147. Hanspal M, Palek J: Biogenesis of normal and abnormal red blood cell membrane skel-eton. *Semin Hematol* 29(4):305, 1992.

148. Randon J, Boulanger L, Garbarz M, et al: A variant of spectrin low-expression allele αLELY carrying a hereditary elliptocytosis mutation in codon 28. *Br J Haematol* 88:534, 1994.

149. Gallagher PG, Tse WT, Marchesi SL, et al: A defect in alpha spectrin mRNA accumula-tion in hereditary pyropoikilocytosis. *Trans Assoc Am Physicians* 104:32, 1991.

150. Hanspal M, Fibach E, Nachman J, et al: Molecular basis of spectrin deficiency in hered-itary pyropoikilocytosis. *Blood* 82:1652, 1993.

151. Costa DB, Lozovatsky L, Gallagher PG, et al: A novel splicing mutation of the α-spec-trin gene in the original hereditary pyropoikilocytosis kindred. *Blood* 106(13):4367, 2005.

152. Mentzer WC Jr, Iarocci TA, Mohandas N, et al: Modulation of erythrocyte membrane mechanical stability by 2,3-diphosphoglycerate in the neonatal poikilocytosis/ellipto-cytosis syndrome. *J Clin Invest* 79(3):943, 1987.

153. Lowenthal EA, Prchal JT: Parvovirus B19 induced red blood cell aplasia in a patient with hereditary pyropoikilocytosis. *Blood* 86:411, 1995.

154. Coetzer TL, Beeton L, van Zyl D, et al: Southeast Asian ovalocytosis in a South African kindred with hemolytic anemia. *Blood* 87:1656, 1996.

155. Liu SC, Zhai S, Palek J, et al: Molecular defect of the band 3 protein in southeast Asian ovalocytosis. *N Engl J Med* 323(22):1530, 1990.

156. Mohandas N, Winardi R, Knowles D, et al: Molecular basis for membrane rigidity of hereditary ovalocytosis. *J Clin Invest* 89:686, 1992.

157. Schofield AE, Reardon DM, Tanner MJA: Defective anion transport activity of the abnormal band 3 in hereditary ovalocytic red blood cells. *Nature* 355(6363):836, 1992.

158. Jarolim P, Palek J, Amato D, et al: Deletion in erythrocyte band 3 gene in malaria-resis-tant Southeast Asian ovalocytosis. *Proc Natl Acad Sci U S A* 88:11022, 1991.

159. Liu S-C, Jarolim P, Rubin HL, et al: The homozygous state for the band 3 protein muta-tion in Southeast Asian ovalocytosis may be lethal. *Blood* 84(10):3590, 1994.

160. Picard V, Proust A, Eveillard M, et al: Homozygous Southeast Asian ovalocytosis is a severe dyserythropoietic anemia associated with distal renal tubular acidosis. *Blood* 123(12):1963, 2014.

161. Genton B, AI-Yaman F, Mgone CS, et al: Ovalocytosis and cerebral malaria. *Nature* 378(6557):564, 1995.

162. Wong P: A basis of echinocytosis and stomatocytosis in the disc-sphere transforma-tions of the erythrocyte. *J Theor Biol* 196(3):343, 1999.

163. Cooper RA: Hemolytic syndromes and red cell membrane abnormalities in liver dis-ease. *Semin Hematol* 17(2):103, 1980.

164. Zamel R, Khan R, Pollex RL, Hegele RA: Abetalipoproteinemia: Two case reports and literature review. *Orphanet J Rare Dis* 3:19, 2008.

165. Wetterau JR, Aggerbeck LP, Bouma M, et al: Absence of microsomal triglyceride transfer protein in individuals with abetalipoproteinemia. *Science* 258:999, 1992.

166. Kane J, Havel R: Disorders of the biogenesis and secretion of lipoproteins containing the B apolipoproteins, in *The Metabolic and Molecular Bases of Inherited Disease*, edited by Scriver C, Beaudet A, Sly W, Valle DL, p 1853. McGraw-Hill, New York, 1995.

167. Danek A, Walker RH: Neuroacanthocytosis. *Curr Opin Neurol* 18:386, 2005.

168. Rampoldi L, Dobson-Stone C, Rubio JP, et al: A conserved sorting-associated protein is mutant in chorea-acanthocytosis. *Nat Genet* 28:119, 2001.

169. Ueno S, Maruki Y, Nakamura M, et al: The gene encoding a newly discovered protein, chorein, is mutated in chorea-acanthocytosis. *Nat Genet* 28:121, 2001.

170. Walker RH, Jung HH, Dobson-Stone C, et al: Neurologic phenotypes associated with acanthocytosis. *Neurology* 68(2):92, 2007.

171. De Franceschi L, Tomelleri C, Matte A, et al: Erythrocyte membrane changes of chorea-acanthocytosis are the result of altered Lyn kinase activity. *Blood* 118(20):5652, 2011.

172. Bruce LJ, Kay MM, Lawrence C, Tanner MJ: Band 3 HT, a human red-cell variant associated with acanthocytosis and increased anion transport, carries the mutation Pro-868Leu in the membrane domain of band 3. *Biochem J* 293:317, 1993.

173. Walker RH, Rasmussen A, Rudnicki D, et al: Huntington's disease–like 2 can present as chorea-acanthocytosis. *Neurology* 61(7):1002, 2003.

174. Walker RH, Jung HH, Danek A: Neuroacanthocytosis. *Handb Clin Neurol* 100(89):141, 2011.

175. Bruce LJ: Hereditary stomatocytosis and cation-leaky red cells-Recent developments. *Blood Cells Mol Dis* 42(3):216, 2009.

176. Lim GHW, Wortis M, Mukhopadhyay R: Stomatocyte-discocyte-echinocyte sequence of the human red blood cell: Evidence for the bilayer-couple hypothesis from membrane mechanics. *Proc Natl Acad Sci U S A* 99(26):16766, 2002.

177. Grootenboer S, Schischmanoff PO, Laurendeau I, et al: Pleiotropic syndrome of dehydrated hereditary stomatocytosis, pseudohyperkalemia, and perinatal edema maps to 16q23-q24. *Blood* 96(7):2599, 2000.

178. Andolfo I, Alper SL, De Franceschi L, et al: Multiple clinical forms of dehydrated hereditary stomatocytosis arise from mutations in PIEZO1. *Blood* 121(19):3925, 2013.

179. Zarychanski R, Schulz VP, Houston BL, et al: Mutations in the mechanotransduction protein PIEZO1 are associated with hereditary xerocytosis. *Blood* 120(9):1908, 2012.

180. Lock SP, Smith RS, Hardisty RM: Stomatocytosis: A hereditary red cell anomaly associated with haemolytic anaemia. *Br J Haematol* 7(3):303, 1961.

181. Zarkowsky HS, Oski FA, Sha'afi R, et al: Congenital hemolytic anemia with high sodium, low potassium and red cells. *N Engl J Med* 278(11):573, 1968.

182. Flatt JF, Bruce LJ: The hereditary stomatocytoses. *Haematologica* 94(8):1039, 2009.

183. Bruce LJ, Burton NM, Gabillat N, et al: The monovalent cation leak in overhydrated stomatocytic red blood cells results from amino acid substitutions in the Rh-associated glycoprotein. *Blood* 113(6):1350, 2009.

184. Iolascon A, De Falco L, Borgese F, et al: A novel erythroid anion exchange variant (Gly796Arg) of hereditary stomatocytosis associated with dyserythropoiesis. *Haematologica* 94(8):1049, 2009.

185. Bruce LJ, Robinson HC, Guizouarn H, et al: Monovalent cation leaks in human red cells caused by single amino-acid substitutions in the transport domain of the band 3 chloride-bicarbonate exchanger, AE1. *Nat Genet* 37(11):1258, 2005.

186. Guizouarn H, Martial S, Gabillat N, et al: Point mutations involved in red cell stomatocytosis convert the electroneutral anion exchanger 1 to a nonselective cation conductance. *Blood* 110(6):2158, 2007.

187. Bogdanova A, Goede JS, Weiss E, et al: Cryohydrocytosis: Increased activity of cation carriers in red cells from a patient with a band 3 mutation. *Haematologica* 95(2):189, 2010.

188. Flatt JF, Guizouarn H, Burton NM, et al: Stomatin-deficient cryohydrocytosis results from mutations in SLC2A1: A novel form of GLUT1 deficiency syndrome. *Blood* 118(19):5267, 2011.

189. Neville AJ, Rand CA, Barr RD, et al: Drug-induced stomatocytosis and anemia during consolidation chemotherapy of childhood acute leukemia. *Am J Med Sci* 287(1):3, 1984.

CHAPTER 47
ERYTHROCYTE ENZYME DISORDERS

Wouter W. van Solinge and Richard van Wijk

SUMMARY

Red cells possess active metabolic machinery that provides energy to pump ions against electrochemical gradients, to maintain red cell shape, to keep hemoglobin iron in the reduced form, and to maintain enzyme and hemoglobin sulfhydryl groups. The main source of metabolic energy comes from glucose. Glucose is metabolized through the glycolytic pathway and through the hexose monophosphate shunt. Glycolysis catabolizes glucose to pyruvate and lactate, which represent the end products of glucose metabolism in the erythrocyte, because it lacks the mitochondria required for further oxidation of pyruvate. Adenosine diphosphate (ADP) is phosphorylated to ATP, and nicotinamide adenine dinucleotide (NAD)$^+$ is reduced to NADH in glycolysis. 2,3-Bisphosphoglycerate, an important regulator of the oxygen affinity of hemoglobin, is generated during glycolysis. The hexose monophosphate shunt oxidizes glucose-6-phosphate, reducing NADP$^+$ to reduced nicotinamide adenine dinucleotide phosphate (NADPH). In addition to glucose, the red cell has the capacity to utilize some other sugars and nucleosides as a source of energy. The red cell lacks the capacity for *de novo* purine synthesis, but has a salvage pathway that permits synthesis of purine nucleotides from purine bases. The red cell contains high concentrations of glutathione, which is maintained almost entirely in the reduced state by NADPH through the catalytic activity of glutathione reductase. Glutathione is synthesized from glycine, cysteine, and glutamic acid in a two-step process that requires ATP as a source of energy. Catalase and glutathione peroxidase serve to protect the red cell from oxidative damage. The maturation of reticulocytes into erythrocytes is associated with a rapid decrease in the activity of several enzymes. However, the decrease in activities of other enzymes occurs much more slowly or not at all with aging.

Erythrocyte enzyme deficiencies may lead to hemolytic anemia; expression of the defect in other cell lines may lead to pathologic changes such as neuromuscular abnormalities. Glucose-6-phosphate dehydrogenase (G6PD) deficiency is the most common erythrocyte enzyme defect. In some populations, more than 20 percent of people may be affected by this enzyme deficiency. In the common polymorphic forms, such as G6PD A−, G6PD Mediterranean, or G6PD Canton, hemolysis occurs only during the stress imposed by infection or administration of "oxidative" drugs, and in some individuals upon ingestion of fava beans. Neonatal icterus, which appears largely with the interaction with an independent defect in bilirubin conjugation, is the clinically most serious complication of G6PD deficiency. Patients with uncommon, functionally very severe, genetic variants of G6PD experience chronic hemolysis, a disorder designated hereditary nonspherocytic hemolytic anemia.

Hereditary nonspherocytic hemolytic anemia (HNSHA) also occurs as a consequence of other enzyme deficiencies, the most common of which is pyruvate kinase (PK) deficiency. Glucose phosphate isomerase (GPI), triosephosphate isomerase (TPI), and pyrimidine 5′-nucleotidase (P5′N) deficiency are included among the relatively rare causes of hereditary nonspherocytic hemolytic anemia. In the case of some deficiencies, notably those of glutathione synthetase (GS), TPI, and phosphoglycerate kinase (PGK), the defect is expressed throughout the body, and neurologic and other defects may be a prominent part of the clinical syndrome.

Diagnosis is best achieved by determining red cell enzyme activity either with a quantitative assay or a screening test. Except for the basophilic stippling of erythrocytes that is characteristic, but not specific, of pyrimidine 5′-nucleotidase deficiency, red cell morphology is of little or no help in differentiating one red cell enzyme deficiency from another. A variety of molecular lesions have been defined in most of these enzyme deficiencies. Confirmation of the diagnosis by DNA analysis is recommended: it is necessary for genetic counseling and is helpful in recommendations for treatment, as patients with some enzyme deficiencies (e.g., GPI deficiency) tend to respond favorably to splenectomy whereas others do not (e.g., G6PD deficiency). Some of the defects, such as PK and GPI deficiencies, are transmitted as autosomal recessive disorders, whereas G6PD and PGK deficiencies are X linked.

Acronyms and Abbreviations: ADA, adenosine deaminase; ADP, adenosine diphosphate; AK, adenylate kinase; AP-1, a transcription factor; 2,3-BPG, 2,3-bisphosphoglycerate; BPGM, bisphosphoglycerate mutase enzyme; CDP, cytidine diphosphate; 2,3-DPG, 2,3-diphosphoglycerate; EMP, Embden-Meyerhof direct glycolytic pathway; FAD, flavin adenine dinucleotide; G6PD, glucose-6-phosphate dehydrogenase; GAPDH, glyceraldehyde phosphate dehydrogenase; GCL, glutamate cysteine ligase; GLUT1, glucose transporter 1; GPI, glucose phosphate isomerase; GR, glutathione reductase; GS, glutathione synthetase; GSH, reduced glutathione; GSSG, oxidized glutathione; *HFE,* the gene associated with hereditary hemochromatosis; HK, hexokinase; KLF1, key erythroid transcription factor; LDH, lactate dehydrogenase; miRNA, microRNA; MRP1, multidrug resistance protein 1; NAD, nicotinamide adenine dinucleotide; NADPH, nicotinamide adenine dinucleotide phosphate (reduced form); nt, nucleotide; P5′N1, pyrimidine-5′-nucleotidase-1; PFK, phosphofructose kinase; *PFKM,* gene encoding muscle subunit of PFK; PGK, phosphoglycerate kinase; PK, pyruvate kinase; *PKLR,* gene encoding PK enzyme activity in red cells and liver; SNP, single nucleotide polymorphism; SOD1, superoxide dismutase type 1; TPI, triosephosphate isomerase; WHO, World Health Organization.

● DEFINITION AND HISTORY

Deficiencies in the activities of a number of erythrocyte enzymes may lead to shortening of the red cell life span. Glucose-6-phosphate dehydrogenase (G6PD) deficiency was the first of these to be recognized and is the most common.

The recognition of G6PD deficiency was the result of investigations of the hemolytic effect of the antimalarial drug primaquine, carried out in the 1950s and described in detail elsewhere.[1-3] These early studies defined G6PD deficiency as a hereditary sex-linked enzyme deficiency that affected primarily the erythrocytes, older cells being more severely affected than newly formed ones because of age-dependent decline of mutant enzyme activity. They showed that this enzyme deficiency was very prevalent in individuals of African, Mediterranean, and Asian ethnic origins, but that it could be found in virtually any population. The common (polymorphic) forms of G6PD deficiency were found to be associated with anemia only under conditions of stress, such as the administration of oxidative drugs, infection, and the neonatal period.

Chronic hemolysis in the absence of a stress occurs in uncommon, functionally severe forms of G6PD deficiency and in patients with a variety of other red cell enzyme deficiencies. Such patients suffer from *hereditary nonspherocytic hemolytic anemia*. Although patients fitting the description of hereditary nonspherocytic hemolytic anemia had been documented earlier, the designation was first introduced by Crosby in 1950.[4] Dacie and colleagues[5] subsequently reported several families in which affected members manifested hemolytic anemia from an early age and in whom the osmotic fragility of the red cells was normal. The latter finding was the main feature that distinguished this disorder from hereditary spherocytosis. Thus, defined essentially by exclusion as a hereditary hemolytic anemia that is not hereditary spherocytosis (or without any other major aberration of red cell morphology), it is not at all surprising that hereditary nonspherocytic hemolytic anemia has proven to be extremely heterogeneous both in etiology and in clinical manifestations. Sometimes this disorder is also designated *congenital nonspherocytic hemolytic anemia*, but the name *hereditary hemolytic anemia* is more accurate and is therefore preferable. Although hereditary ovalocytosis, pyropoikilocytosis, and stomatocytosis (Chap. 46), and even thalassemia major and sickle cell disease (Chaps. 48 and 49), are hereditary hemolytic anemias that are also nonspherocytic, they are not included in this category.

Although a deficiency of G6PD was found to be responsible for hemolysis in a few patients with hereditary nonspherocytic hemolytic anemia, in the overwhelming majority of cases the cause remained obscure. In 1954, Selwyn and Dacie[6] studied autohemolysis (spontaneous lysis of red cells after sterile incubation for 24 to 48 hours at 37°C) in four patients with hereditary nonspherocytic hemolytic anemia and found that in two of them lysis was only slightly increased and was prevented by glucose; these patients were designated as type 1, whereas the others, in whom glucose failed to correct autohemolysis, were classified as type 2. Autohemolysis of the erythrocytes of type 2 patients was modified by the addition of ATP. However, ATP does not penetrate the red cell membrane and instead, its modifying influence was nonspecific exerted chiefly by virtue of its effect on the osmolarity and pH of the suspending solution. These findings suggested to DeGruchy and associates[7] that patients with type 2 autohemolysis suffered from a defect in ATP generation. This proposal, born of a misunderstanding of red cell biochemistry, turned out to be correct, as one of the major causes of hereditary nonspherocytic hemolytic anemia proved to be a deficiency of the ATP-generating enzyme pyruvate kinase (PK).[8] PK deficiency was the first of a large number of enzyme defects that have been shown to account for this heterogeneous syndrome.

● EPIDEMIOLOGY

The most common red cell enzyme abnormality is deficiency of G6PD. Its prevalence among white populations ranges from less than 1 in 1000 among northern European populations to 50 percent of the males among Kurdish Jews. The lowest frequencies of G6PD deficiency are found in both North and South America (≤1 percent), and highest rates are predicted across the tropical belt of sub-Saharan Africa (15 to 30 percent; Fig. 47–1). The distribution across Asia and Asia Pacific is generally heterogeneous, ranging from virtually absent to relatively high.[9,10] Although many of the highest frequencies are predicted from sub-Saharan African countries, the very high population densities across Asia infers that the overall population burden is largely focused here. The overall allele frequency of G6PD deficiency across all malaria

endemic countries is predicted to be 8 percent. This corresponds to 220 million affected males and an even greater number of females, although some heterozygous females for this X-chromosome–encoded gene do not have enough deficient erythrocytes to become prone to significant hemolysis.[9] Details on the distribution of G6PD deficiency among various population groups is presented elsewhere. [9–12]

The high frequency of G6PD-deficient genes in many populations implies that G6PD deficiency confers a selective advantage. The suggestion that resistance to malaria accounts for the high frequency of G6PD deficiency paralleling the worldwide distribution of malaria is supported by the sheer diversity of variants in the *G6PD* gene. Many of these are found at polymorphic frequencies in genetically isolated populations, suggesting independent selection of each variant.[11–13] Important supporting evidence was obtained from studies in heterozygotes for G6PD A– that showed a higher degree of infestation of G6PD-sufficient cells than of G6PD-deficient cells.[14] Deficient cells infested with malaria parasites may be phagocytosed more efficiently than normal cells.[15] Which G6PD genotypes confer protection from malarial infection is the subject of debate.[16–18] The majority of studies conclude that G6PD deficiency in hemizygous males, and probably also homozygous females, confers significant protection against malarial infection. The nature of protection from the mosaic state of G6PD deficiency in heterozygous females remains to be established.[18,19]

It has been suggested that a higher prevalence of G6PD deficiency in individuals with sickle cell disease than in the general African population reflects a favorable effect of the enzyme deficiency on the clinical course of the sickling disorders.[20] However, studies aimed at investigating the effects of G6PD deficiency on the clinical manifestations of sickle cell disease have produced conflicting results. Some studies found no evidence for any such effect,[21,22] whereas others reported on lower hemoglobin levels in patients with both disorders, either accompanied[23] or not[24] by signs of increased hemolysis.

PK deficiency is the most common cause of hereditary nonspherocytic hemolytic anemia. Based on large-scale mutation analysis, it has been estimated that the population prevalence of PK deficiency among whites is approximately 50 cases per 1 million population.[25] Estimates of frequencies of other deficiency alleles, such as those for adenylate kinase, diphosphoglycerate mutase, enolase, triosephosphate isomerase (TPI), and phosphoglycerate kinase (PGK), have been made on large numbers of cord bloods.[26] A particularly high incidence of heterozygous TPI deficiency (>4 percent) in Americans of African descent is supported by family studies.[27] Because this is not reflected in a correspondingly high birth incidence, the allele might be lethal in the homozygous state.

In addition to the common G6PD mutations, there are mutations in other enzymes that are repeatedly encountered in the population. In PK, the c.1529G>A, p.(Arg510Gln) mutation is the most common mutation in the United States,[28] and in northern and central Europe[29]; the c.1456C>T, p.(Arg486Trp) mutation is prevalent in southern Europe,[30] and the c.1468C>T, (p.Arg490Trp) mutation in Asia.[31] Similarly, the c.315G>C, p.(Glu104Asp) mutation is recurrently encountered in TPI.[32] In phosphofructose kinase (PFK) deficiency, one-third of the reported patients are of Jewish origin, and in this population, an intronic splice site mutation, c.237+1G>A, and a single base-pair deletion, c.2003delC, are among the most frequently encountered mutations.[33] In a number of these instances, the existence of each mutation in the context of the same haplotype implies that there has been a *founder effect*, that is, the mutation occurred only once, and all individuals now carrying it are descendants of the person who sustained the original mutation. The expansion of the mutation could represent a selective advantage for heterozygotes, but also may result from random factors or from a selective advantage provided by one or more tightly linked genes.

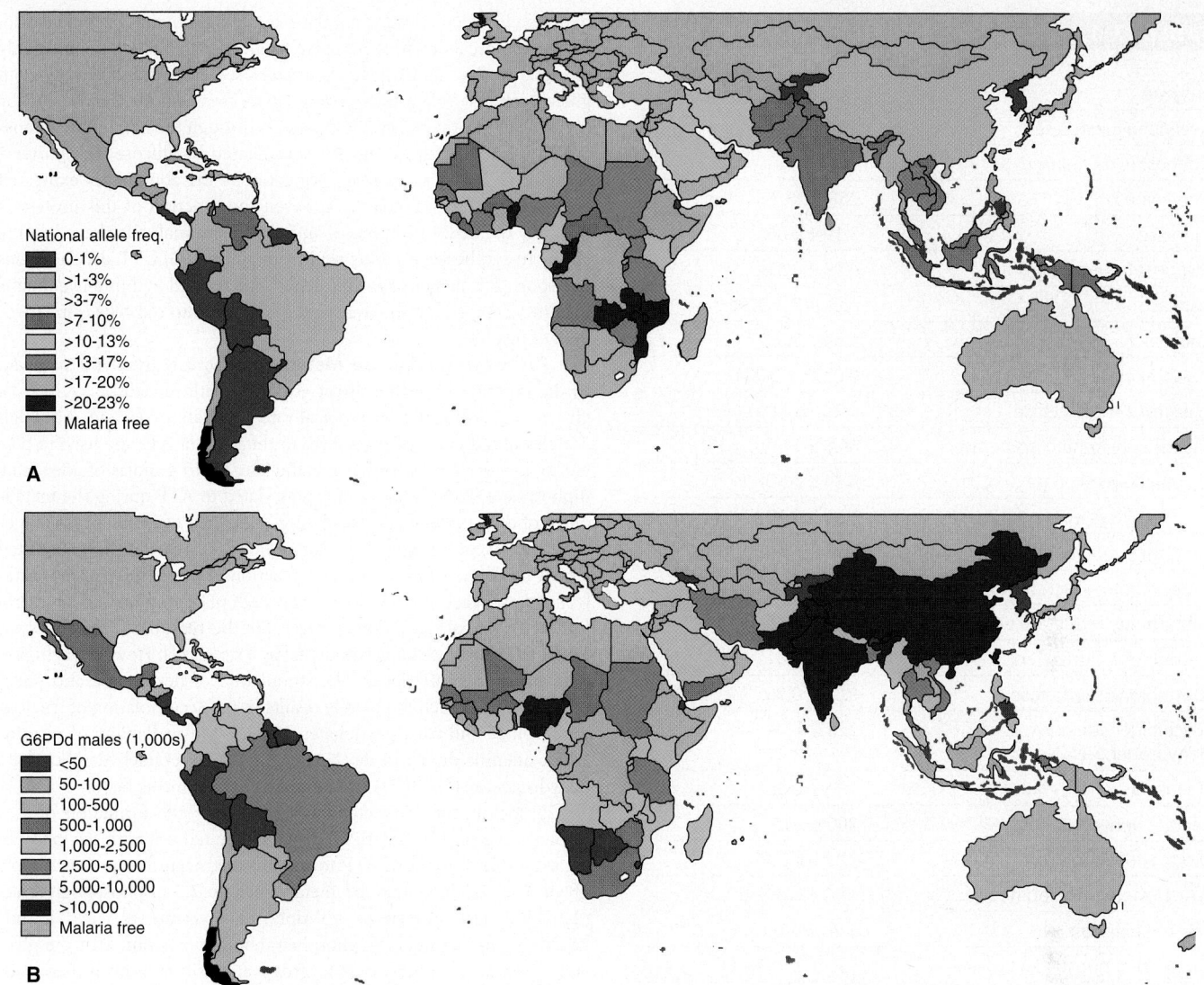

Figure 47–1. Estimated prevalence of glucose-6-phosphate dehydrogenase (G6PD) deficiency. **A.** National-level allele frequencies. **B.** National-level population estimates of G6PD-deficient (G6PDd) males. *(Reproduced with permission from Howes RE, Piel FB, Patil AP, et al: G6PD deficiency prevalence and estimates of affected populations in malaria endemic countries: a geostatistical model-based map. PLoS Med 2012;9(11):e1001339.)*

● ETIOLOGY AND PATHOGENESIS

RED CELL METABOLISM

Although the binding, transport, and delivery of oxygen do not require the expenditure of metabolic energy by the red cell, a source of energy is required if the red cell is to perform its function efficiently and to survive in the circulation for its full life span of approximately 120 days. This energy is needed to maintain (1) the iron of hemoglobin in the divalent form; (2) the high potassium and low calcium and sodium levels within the cell against a gradient imposed by the high plasma calcium and sodium and low plasma potassium levels; (3) the sulfhydryl groups of red cell enzymes, hemoglobin, and membranes in the active, reduced form; and (4) the biconcave shape of the cell. If the red cell is deprived of a source of energy, it becomes sodium and calcium logged and potassium depleted, and the red cell shape changes from a flexible biconcave disk. Such a cell is quickly removed from the circulation by the filtering action of the spleen and the monocyte–macrophage system. Even if it survived, such an energy-deprived cell would gradually turn brown as hemoglobin is oxidized to methemoglobin by the very high concentrations of oxygen within the erythrocyte and would then be unable to perform its function of transporting oxygen and carbon dioxide.

The process of extracting energy from a substrate, such as glucose, and of utilizing this energy is carried out by a large number of enzymes (Table 47–1). Because the red cell loses its nucleus before it enters the circulation and most of its RNA within 1 or 2 days of its release into the circulation, it does not have the capacity to synthesize new proteins to replace those that may become degraded during its life span. The enzymes present in the red cells were formed largely by the nucleated cell in the marrow and, to a lesser extent, the reticulocyte.

Glucose Metabolism

Glucose is the normal energy source of the red cell. It is metabolized by the erythrocyte along two major routes: the glycolytic pathway and the hexose monophosphate shunt. The steps in these pathways are essentially the same as those found in other tissues and in other organisms, including even relatively simple ones such as *Escherichia coli* and yeast. Unlike most other cells, however, the red cell lacks mitochondria and

TABLE 47–1. Activities of Some Red Cell Enzymes

Enzyme	Activity at 37°C IU/g Hgb (mean ± SD)
Acetylcholinesterase	36.93 ± 3.83
Adenosine deaminase	1.11 ± 0.23
Adenylate kinase	258 ± 29.3
Aldolase	3.19 ± 0.86
Bisphosphoglyceromutase	4.78 ± 0.65
Catalase	153,117 ± 2390
Enolase	5.39 ± 0.83
Galactokinase	0.0291 ± 0.004
Galactose-4-epimerase	0.231 ± 0.061
Glucose phosphate isomerase	60.8 ± 11.0
Glucose-6-phosphate dehydrogenase	8.34 ± 1.59
γ-Glutamylcysteine synthetase	1.05 ± 0.19
Glutathione peroxidase*	30.82 ± 4.65
Glutathione reductase without FAD	7.18 ± 1.09
Glutathione reductase with FAD	10.4 ± 1.50
Glutathione-S-transferase	6.66 ± 1.81
Glutathione synthetase	0.34 ± 0.06
Glyceraldehyde phosphate dehydrogenase	226 ± 41.9
Hexokinase	1.78 ± 0.38
Lactate dehydrogenase	200 ± 26.5
Monophosphoglyceromutase	37.71 ± 5.56
NADH-methemoglobin reductase	19.2 ± 3.85(30°)
NADPH diaphorase	2.26 ± 0.16
Nucleoside phosphorylase	359 ± 32
Phosphofructokinase	11.01 ± 2.33
Phosphoglucomutase	5.50 ± 0.62
Phosphoglycerate kinase	320 ± 36.1
Phosphoglycolate phosphatase	1.23 ± 0.10
Phosphomannose isomerase	0.054 ± 0.026
Pyrimidine 5′-nucleotidase	0.138 ± 0.018
Pyruvate kinase	15.0 ± 1.99
6-Phosphogluconate dehydrogenase	8.78 ± 0.78
6-Phosphogluconolactonase	50.6 ± 5.9
Ribosephosphate isomerase	200
Superoxide dismutase	2225 ± 303
Transaldolase	1.21 ± 0.24
Transketolase	0.725 ± 0.17
Triose phosphate isomerase	2111 ± 397

FAD, flavin adenine dinucleotide; NADH, reduced form of nicotinamide adenine dinucleotide; NADPH, nicotinamide adenine dinucleotide phosphate.

*For United States and European subjects.

hence a citric acid cycle. Only the reticulocytes maintain some capacity for the breakdown of pyruvate to CO_2, with the attendant highly efficient production of ATP. The mature red cell extracts energy from glucose almost solely by anaerobic glycolysis. Before glucose can be metabolized by the red cell, it must pass through the membrane. Transport into the interior of the cell is facilitated by glucose transporter 1 receptor GLUT1, and perhaps regulated by the abundantly expressed membrane protein stomatin; however, the function of this protein is not fully defined.[34] In humans, and other mammals that have lost the ability to synthesize ascorbic acid from glucose, GLUT1 also facilitates transport of L-dehydroascorbic acid.[34] The red cell membrane contains insulin receptors, but the transport of glucose into red cells is independent of insulin.

Pathways of Glucose Metabolism Direct glycolytic pathway. In the Embden-Meyerhof direct glycolytic pathway (EMP; Fig. 47–2), glucose is catabolized anaerobically to pyruvate or lactate. Although 2 moles of high-energy phosphate in the form of ATP are used in preparing glucose for its further metabolism, up to 4 moles of adenosine diphosphate (ADP) may be phosphorylated to ATP during the metabolism of each mole of glucose, giving a net yield of 2 moles of ATP per mole of glucose metabolized. The rate of glucose utilization is limited largely by the hexokinase and PFK reactions. Both of the enzymes catalyzing these reactions have a relatively high pH optimum and have very little activity at pH levels lower than 7. For this reason, red cell glycolysis is very pH sensitive, being stimulated by a rise in pH. However, at higher than physiologic pH levels, the stimulation of hexokinase and phosphofructokinase activity merely results in the accumulation of fructose diphosphate and triosephosphates, because the availability of nicotinamide adenine dinucleotide (NAD)+ for the glyceraldehyde phosphate dehydrogenase (GAPDH) reaction becomes a limiting factor.

Branching of the metabolic stream after the formation of 1,3-bisphosphoglycerate (1,3-BPG) provides the red cell with flexibility in regard to the amount of ATP formed in the metabolism of each mole of glucose. 1,3-BPG may be metabolized to 2,3-bisphosphoglycerate (2,3-BPG), also known as 2,3-diphosphoglycerate (2,3-DPG), thus "wasting" the high-energy phosphate bond in position 1 of the glycerate. Removing the phosphate group at position 2 by bisphosphoglycerate phosphatase results in the formation of 3-phosphoglycerate. Both reactions in this unique glycolytic bypass, known as the *Rapoport-Luebering shunt*, are catalyzed by the erythroid-specific multifunctional enzyme bisphosphoglycerate mutase.[35] In mammalian erythrocytes, a separate 2,3-BPG phosphatase activity has been ascribed to multiple inositol polyphosphate phosphatase.[36] In contrast to bisphosphoglycerate mutase, multiple inositol polyphosphate phosphatase-1 is able to remove the phosphate at position 3, thereby bypassing the formation of 3-phosphoglycerate. The precise functional significance of multiple inositol polyphosphate phosphatase-1 for human red cell physiology and regulation of 2,3-BPG levels remains to be established.

3-Phosphoglycerate may also be formed directly from 1,3-BPG through the PGK step, resulting in phosphorylation of 1 mole of ADP to ATP. Although metabolism of glucose through the 2,3-BPG step occurs without any net gain of high-energy phosphate bonds in the form of ATP, metabolism through the PGK step results in the formation of two such bonds per mole of glucose metabolized. This portion of the direct glycolytic pathway has been called the *energy clutch*. Regulation of metabolism at this branch point determines not only the rate of ADP phosphorylation to ATP but also the concentration of 2,3-BPG, an important regulator of the oxygen affinity of hemoglobin (Chaps. 49 and 57). The concentration of 2,3-BPG depends on the balance between its rate of formation and degradation by bisphosphoglycerate mutase. Hydrogen ions inhibit the bisphosphoglycerate mutase reaction and stimulate the phosphatase reaction. Thus, red cell 2,3-BPG levels are

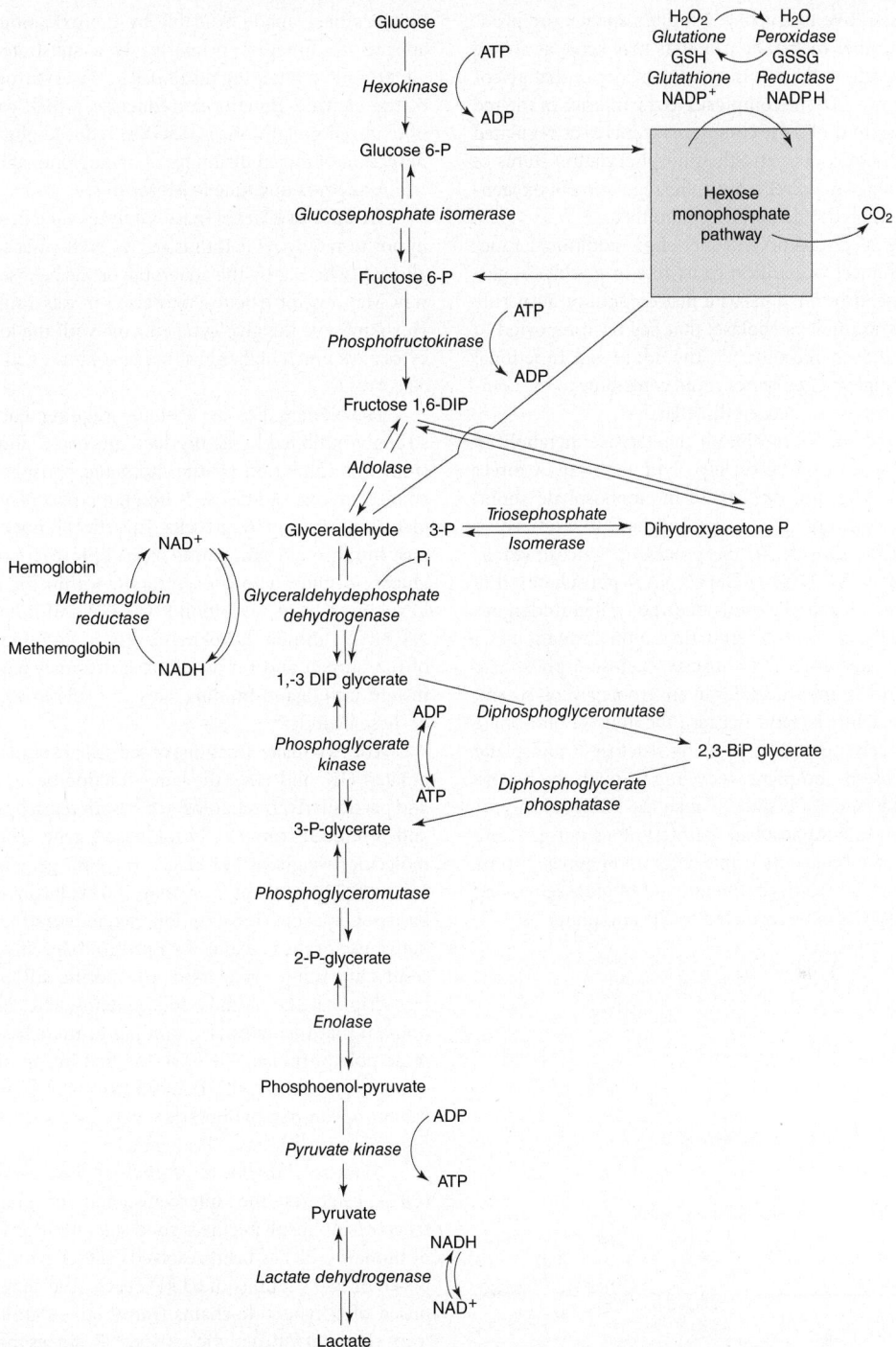

Figure 47–2. Glucose metabolism of the erythrocyte. The details of the hexose monophosphate pathway are shown in Fig. 47–3.

exquisitely sensitive to pH: a rise in pH causes a rise in 2,3-BPG levels, whereas acidosis results in 2,3-BPG depletion. It may be that the ratio of oxyhemoglobin to deoxyhemoglobin also influences 2,3-BPG synthesis by virtue of the fact that only deoxyhemoglobin binds this compound, thus affecting the concentration of free 2,3-BPG that is available for feedback inhibition of the enzymes that lead to its formation. However, the available evidence suggests that the pH is the primary controlling factor.

Metabolism of glucose by way of the EMP may also yield reducing energy in the form of the reduced form of NAD (NADH). The reduction of NAD⁺ to NADH occurs in the GAPDH step. If NADH is reoxidized

in reducing methemoglobin to hemoglobin, the end product of glucose metabolism is pyruvate. If NADH is not reoxidized by methemoglobin, however, pyruvate is reduced in the lactate dehydrogenase (LDH) step, forming lactate as the final end product of glucose metabolism. The lactate or pyruvate formed is transported from the red cell and is metabolized elsewhere in the body. Thus, the erythrocyte has a flexible EMP that can adjust the amount of ADP phosphorylated per mole of glucose according to the requirement of the cell.

The regulation of red cell glycolytic metabolism is very complex. Products of some reactions may stimulate others. For example, the PK reaction is exquisitely sensitive to fructose 1,6-diphosphate, the product of PFK. Conversely, other metabolic products may serve as strong enzyme inhibitors. In addition, there is increasing evidence that glycolytic enzymes assemble into enzyme complexes to the interior of the red cell membrane.[37] The assembly of these complexes seems to be regulated by the oxygen status of hemoglobin and the phosphorylation status of band 3,[37,38] suggesting they play a direct role in the regulation of oxygen-dependent changes in glycolytic and pentose shunt fluxes.[39]

Notably, a number of glycolytic enzymes show additional functional activities. For instance, in addition to its role in glycolysis, glucosephosphate isomerase also functions as a neuroleukin or autocrine motility factor. Another example is enolase, that has been reported to also function as plasminogen receptor.[40,41] The additional functional activities of these "moonlighting" enzymes could contribute to the complexity of the phenotype of the associated disorder.

Hexose Monophosphate Shunt Not all the glucose metabolized by the red cell passes through the direct glycolytic pathway. A direct oxidative pathway of metabolism, the hexose monophosphate shunt, also functions. In this pathway, glucose-6-phosphate is oxidized at position 1, yielding carbon dioxide. In the process of glucose oxidation, $NADP^+$ is reduced to NADPH (reduced NAD phosphate). The pentose phosphate formed when glucose is decarboxylated undergoes a series of molecular rearrangements, eventuating in the formation of a triose, glyceraldehyde-3-phosphate, and a hexose, fructose-6-phosphate (Fig. 47–3). These are normal intermediates in anaerobic glycolysis and thus can rejoin that metabolic stream. Because the glucose phosphate isomerase reaction is freely reversible, allowing fructose-6-phosphate to be converted to glucose-6-phosphate, recycling through the hexose monophosphate pathway is also possible. Unlike the anaerobic glycolytic pathway, the hexose monophosphate pathway does not generate any high-energy phosphate bonds. Its primary function appears to be the formation of NADPH, and, indeed, the amount of glucose passing through this pathway appears to be regulated by the amount of $NADP^+$

that has been made available by the oxidation of NADPH. NADPH appears to function primarily as a substrate for the reduction of glutathione-containing disulfides in the erythrocyte through mediation of the enzyme glutathione reductase, which catalyzes the conversion of oxidized glutathione (GSSG) to reduced glutathione (GSH) and the reduction of mixed disulfides of hemoglobin and GSH.[42]

Enzymes of Glucose Metabolism

Hexokinase Hexokinase catalyzes the phosphorylation of glucose in position 6 by ATP. It thus serves as the first step in the utilization of glucose, whether by the anaerobic or the hexose monophosphate pathway. Mannose or fructose may also serve as a substrate for this enzyme. Hexokinase is the glycolytic enzyme with the lowest activity. Reticulocytes have much higher levels of hexokinase activity than do mature red cells.[43,44]

Hexokinase has an absolute requirement for magnesium. It is strongly inhibited by its product, glucose-6-phosphate, and is released from this inhibition by the inorganic phosphate ion[45,46] and by high concentrations of glucose.[47] Inorganic phosphate enhances the rate of glucose utilization by red cells. This effect is not exerted through hexokinase but through stimulation of the PFK reaction, resulting in a lowered glucose-6-phosphate concentration within the cell and thus releasing hexokinase from inhibition.[48] GSSG[49] and other disulfides, as well as 2,3-BPG,[50] inhibit hexokinase. The determination of the structures of the human and rat hexokinase isozymes have provided substantial insight into ligand-binding sites and subsequent modes of interaction of these ligands.[51,52]

The two major fractions of red cell hexokinase (HK) have been designated HK_I and HK_R; the latter fraction being unique to erythrocytes and particularly to reticulocytes.[53] Both red cell isozymes are monomers and produced from the hexokinase I gene (*HK1*),[54] with an apparent molecular weight of 112 kDa.[55] The *HK1* gene is localized on chromosome 10q22 and spans more than 100 kb. It contains 29 exons,[56,57] which, by tissue-specific transcription, generate multiple transcripts by alternative use of the 5′ exons.[57,58] Erythroid-specific transcriptional control results in a unique red blood cell–specific mRNA that differs from HK_I transcripts at the 5′ end. Consequently, HK_R lacks the porin-binding domain that mediates HK_I binding to mitochondria.[59] A single nucleotide polymorphism (SNP) in the first intron of HK_R was found to be strongly associated with reduced hemoglobin and hematocrit levels in the European population.[60] HK deficiency is a rare cause of hereditary nonspherocytic hemolytic anemia.

Glucose Phosphate Isomerase Glucose phosphate isomerase (GPI) catalyzes the interconversion of glucose-6-phosphate and fructose-6-phosphate, the second step of the EMP. The crystal structure of human GPI has been resolved. The enzyme is a homodimer, composed of two subunits of 63 kDa each. The enzyme's active site is composed of polypeptide chains from both subunits, making the dimeric form essential for catalytic activity.[61] Residues that are not in direct contact with the reacting substrate molecule have also been implicated as important for catalytic function of GPI.[62] The gene encoding GPI (*GPI*) is located on chromosome 19q13.1 and consists of 18 exons, spanning at least 50 kb, with a complementary DNA (cDNA) of 1.9 kb in length.[63] GPI deficiency is one of the relatively more common causes of hereditary nonspherocytic hemolytic anemia.

Phosphofructokinase PFK catalyzes the rate-limiting phosphorylation of fructose-6-phosphate by ATP to fructose-1,6-diphosphate. Under intracellular conditions this reaction is nearly irreversible. Therefore PFK is an important regulator of glycolytic flux. The enzyme has a molecular mass of around 340 kDa. Red cell phosphofructokinase exists as five different homo- or heterotetramers comprised of muscle (M) and liver (L) subunits. Each tetramer displays unique properties with respect to catalytic function and regulation. The enzyme requires magnesium

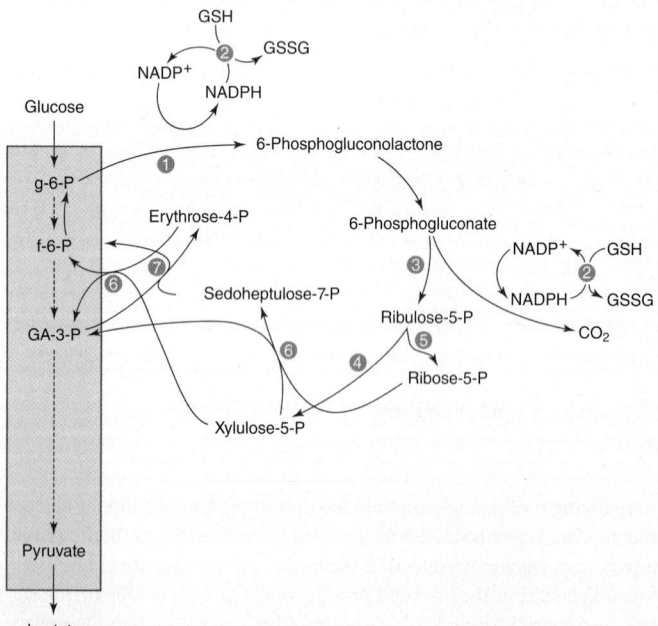

Figure 47–3. Hexose monophosphate pathway of the erythrocyte: (1) glucose-6-phosphate dehydrogenase, (2) glutathione reductase, (3) phosphogluconate dehydrogenase, (4) ribulose-phosphate epimerase, (5) ribosephosphate isomerase, (6) transketolase, and (7) transaldolase.

for activity. PFK activity is tightly controlled and subject to regulation by many metabolic effectors. Among the most important activators are ADP, cyclic adenosine monophosphate (cAMP), and fructose-2,6-diphosphate, whereas PFK is inhibited by its substrate ATP, citrate, and lactate.[64,65] These metabolic effectors exert their effects probably by stabilizing either the minimally active dimeric and fully active tetrameric form of PFK.[66] PFK activity is also regulated by its binding to calmodulin,[67] and association of the enzyme with the red cell membrane[68]; in particular, binding to band 3[69,70] and actin[71] appears to inhibit and stimulate PFK activity, respectively.

A preliminary crystallographic analysis of dimeric wild-type human muscle PFK has been presented.[72] The gene encoding the 85-kDa M subunit *(PFKM)* is located on chromosome 12q13.3 and spans 30 kb. It contains 27 exons and at least three promoter regions.[73] The 80-kDa L-subunit encoding gene *(PFKL)* is located on chromosome 21q22.3; it contains 22 exons and spans more than 28 kb.[74] Deficiency of PFK is associated with mild hemolytic anemia and with type VII glycogen storage disease (Tarui disease).[75]

Aldolase Aldolase reversibly cleaves fructose-1,6-diphosphate into two trioses. The "upper" half of the fructose-1,6-diphosphate molecule becomes dihydroxyacetone phosphate and the "lower" half becomes glyceraldehyde-3-phosphate. Aldolase is a 159-kDa homotetrameric enzyme comprised of subunits of 40 kDa each.[76] Three distinct isoenzymes have been identified: aldolase A, B, and C. The 364-amino-acids-long aldolase A subunits are primarily expressed in erythrocytes and muscle cells.[77] The structure of human aldolase A is known.[78] Red cell aldolase binds to F-actin[79] and the N-terminal part of band 3,[80] which inhibits its activity.[70] The gene for aldolase A *(ALDOA)* is located on chromosome 16q22–24. It spans 7.5 kb and consists of 12 exons. Several transcription-initiation sites were identified and *ALDOA* pre-mRNA is spliced in a tissue-specific manner.[81] Aldolase deficiency is a very rare cause of hereditary nonspherocytic hemolytic anemia.

Triosephosphate Isomerase TPI is the enzyme of the anaerobic glycolytic pathway that has the highest activity. Its metabolic role is to catalyze interconversion of the two trioses formed by the action of aldolase: dihydroxyacetone phosphate and glyceraldehyde-3-phosphate.[82] Although equilibrium is in favor of dihydroxyacetone phosphate, glyceraldehyde-3-phosphate undergoes continued oxidation through the action of GAPDH and is thus removed from the equilibrium. TPI is a dimer consisting of two identical 27-kDa subunits of 248 amino acids.[83] Several crystal structures have been resolved.[84,85] These show that the active site is at the dimer interface and a number of critical residues have been identified. Several water molecules, some of which are highly conserved, are an integral part of the dimer interface. There are no isoenzymes known, but three distinct electrophoretic forms can be distinguished as a result of posttranslational modifications.[86] Red blood cell TPI activity is not red-cell-age dependent. TPI is transcribed from a single gene *(TPI1)*, located on chromosome 12p13. The gene spans 3.5 kb and contains 7 exons. Three processed pseudogenes have been identified.[87] A deficiency of TPI causes hereditary nonspherocytic hemolytic anemia and a severe neuromuscular disorder.

Glyceraldehyde Phosphate Dehydrogenase GAPDH performs the dual functions of oxidizing and phosphorylating glyceraldehyde-3-phosphate, producing 1,3-BPG. In the process, NAD$^+$ is reduced to NADH. This enzyme is closely associated with the red cell membrane[88] where it binds to the N-terminal part of band 3.[70] Membrane binding influences the activity of GAPDH[89] thereby possibly regulating glycolytic flux.[90] Human red blood cell GAPDH has been purified. It is a homotetramer of approximately 150 kDa, composed of 36-kDa subunits, and shows an absolute specificity for NAD$^+$.[91] One of the many nonglycolytic functions of GAPDH[40,41] may include its function as a transferrin receptor.[92] The crystal structure of human liver GAPDH

reveals a homotetramer, each subunit of which is bound to a NAD$^+$ molecule.[93] Deficiency of GAPDH seems a rare occurrence without functional consequences.[94]

Phosphoglycerate Kinase PGK effects the transfer to ADP of the high-energy phosphate from the 1-carbon of 1,3-diphosphoglycerate (1,3-DPG) to form ATP. The reaction is readily reversible and can be bypassed by the Rapoport-Luebering shunt. The isoenzyme PGK-1 is ubiquitously expressed in all somatic cells and is a 48-kDa monomeric enzyme of 417 amino acids.[95] Expression of isozyme PGK-2 has been found in testis.[96] PGK is composed of two domains. The N-terminal domain binds 3-phosphoglycerate and 1,3-DPG, whereas ADP and ATP bind to the C-terminal domain. For catalysis to occur, the protein needs to undergo a large conformational change ("hinge bending").[97-99] The gene encoding PGK *(PGK-1)* is located on the long arm of the X-chromosome (Xq13), spans 23 kb, and is composed of 11 exons. Nonfunctional pseudogenes have been located on chromosome 19 and the X-chromosome.[96] Deficiency of PGK is a rare cause of nonspherocytic hemolytic anemia, often associated with neuromuscular abnormalities.

Bisphosphoglycerate Mutase The same protein molecule is responsible for both bisphosphoglycerate mutase and bisphosphoglycerate phosphatase activities in the erythrocyte.[35,100] This enzyme is particularly important because it regulates the concentration of 2,3-BPG of erythrocytes. In its role as a bisphosphoglyceromutase, the enzyme competes with PGK for 1,3-BPG as a substrate. It changes 1,3-BPG to 2,3-BPG, thereby dissipating the energy of the high-energy acylphosphate bond.[101] It is inhibited by its product 2,3-BPG and by inorganic phosphate, and it is activated by 2-phosphoglycerate and by increased pH levels. It requires 3-phosphoglycerate for activity. In its role as bisphosphoglycerate phosphatase it catalyzes the removal of the phosphate group from carbon 2 of 2,3-BPG.[101] It is inhibited by its product 3-phosphoglycerate and by sulfhydryl reagents. It is most active at a slightly acid pH and is strongly stimulated by bisulfite and phosphoglycolate. Phosphoglycolate, the most potent activator of phosphatase activity, is present in erythrocytes at very low concentrations,[102] but the source of this substance in red cells is unknown.[103,104] Phosphoglycolate phosphatase, the enzyme that hydrolyzes phosphoglycolate, has also been identified in erythrocytes.[105]

Bisphosphoglycerate mutase is a homodimer, with 30-kDa subunits consisting of 258 amino acids. The crystal structure of human bisphosphoglycerate mutase has been determined, providing a rationale for the specific residues that are crucial for synthase, mutase, and phosphatase activity.[106,107] The gene for bisphosphoglycerate mutase *(BPGM)* has been mapped to chromosome 7q31–34 and it consists of 3 exons, spanning more than 22 kb.

A deficiency of bisphosphoglycerate mutase results in a marked decrease in red cell 2,3-BPG levels. The consequent left shift of the oxygen dissociation curve leads to erythrocytosis/polycythemia (Chap. 57).

Phosphoglycerate Mutase An equilibrium is established between 3-phosphoglycerate and 2-phosphoglycerate by phosphoglycerate mutase.[108] 2,3-BPG acts as an essential cofactor for the transformation. Red blood cell phosphoglycerate mutase is a heterodimer consisting of M and B subunits, encoded by separate genes.[109] Only one well-characterized patient with partial red blood cell monophosphoglycerate mutase deficiency has been described who was homozygous for a p.Met230Ile amino acid change in the B subunit.[110] The mutant enzyme was unstable and thus had a short half-life.[111] Unexpectedly, all glycolytic intermediates were decreased, possibly because of lactate accumulation.[112] The exact clinical consequences of this red blood cell enzymopathy remain to be established.

Enolase Enolase is a homodimeric enzyme that establishes an equilibrium between 2-phosphoglycerate and phosphoenolpyruvate.

The reaction is facilitated by the presence of metal ions.[113] Aside from its enzymatic function in the glycolytic pathway, α-enolase (ENO1) has been implicated in numerous diseases, including metastatic cancer, autoimmune disorders, ischemia, and bacterial infection.[114] The gene for enolase (*ENO1*) is located on chromosome 1p36.23. Enolase deficiency is extremely rare. Although it has been reported in association with hereditary nonspherocytic hemolytic anemia,[115,116] a clear cause-and-effect relationship has not yet been firmly established.

Pyruvate Kinase The transfer of phosphate from phosphoenolpyruvate to ADP, forming ATP and pyruvate, is catalyzed by the allosteric enzyme PK. This is the second energy-yielding step of glycolysis. Four PK isoenzymes are present in mammalian tissues: PK-M1 (in skeletal muscle), PK-M2 (in leukocytes, kidney, adipose tissue, and lungs), PK-L (in liver), and PK-R (in red blood cells). The four PK isoenzymes are products of only two genes (*PKLR* and *PKM2*). The PK-M1 and PK-M2 enzymes are formed from the *PKM2* gene by alternative splicing.[117] PK-L (the liver enzyme) and PK-R (the erythrocyte enzyme) are products of the *PKLR* gene, transcribed from two different, tissue-specific promoters.[118,119] There is evidence that other, yet unknown, regulatory elements are involved in *PKLR* gene expression.[120] *PKLR* consists of 12 exons and spans more than 10 kb. Exon 2, but not exon 1, is present in the processed liver transcript; in the red cell enzyme exon 1, but not exon 2, is represented.[119] The red blood cell–specific mRNA is 2 kb in length and codes for a full-length 63-kDa PK-R subunit of 574 amino acids.[121] Red blood cell PK is a heterotetramer comprised of two 62- to 63-kDa and two 57- to 58-kDa subunits, the latter resulting from limited proteolytic cleavage of the full-length subunit.[122,123] Each subunit of PK-R contains an N domain, A domain, B domain, and C domain (Fig. 47–4).[124] Domain A is the most highly conserved, whereas the B and C domains are more variable.[125] The functional role of the N domain is unknown, but it may play a role in enzyme regulation.[126,127] The active site of PK lies in a cleft between the A domain and the flexible B domain. The C domain contains the binding site for fructose-1,6-diphosphate.

Both intra- and intersubunit interactions are considered to be key determinants of the allosteric response, which involves switching of the PK tetramer from the low-affinity T state to the high-affinity R state.[128–132] Red cell PK manifests sigmoid kinetics with respect to phosphoenolpyruvate in the absence of fructose-1,6-diphosphate. Hyperbolic kinetics are observed in the presence of even minute amounts of fructose-1,6-diphosphate,[122,133] so that at low concentrations of phosphoenolpyruvate the enzyme activity is greatly increased by fructose diphosphate. PK deficiency is the most common cause of hereditary nonspherocytic hemolytic anemia.

Lactate Dehydrogenase LDH catalyzes the reversible reduction of pyruvate to lactate by NADH, the last step in the EMP. The enzyme is composed of H (heart) and M (muscle) subunits. In red cells, the predominant subunit is H. Hereditary absence of the H subunit seems to be a benign condition, usually without clinical manifestations,[134,135] although one case with hemolysis has been reported.[136] Absence of the M subunit has been reported as well,[137] and was unaccompanied by hematologic manifestations. Judging from the origin of the reports, LDH deficiency appears to be most common in Japan, where population surveys show a gene frequency of approximately 0.05 for each deficiency, and several mutations have been identified.[138]

Glucose-6-Phosphate Dehydrogenase G6PD is the most extensively studied erythrocyte enzyme. It catalyzes the oxidation of glucose-6-phosphate to 6-phosphogluconolactone, which is rapidly hydrolyzed to 6-phosphogluconic acid, in the first step of the hexose monophosphate pathway. NADP$^+$ is reduced to NADPH in this reaction, generating 1 mole of NADPH. In the erythrocyte, the hexose monophosphate pathway is the only source of NADPH, which is crucial in maintaining high cellular levels of GSH to protect the cell from oxidative stress-induced damage.

The G6PD monomer is composed of 515 amino acids with a calculated molecular weight of approximately 59 kDa.[139] Aggregation of these inactive monomers into catalytically active dimers and higher forms

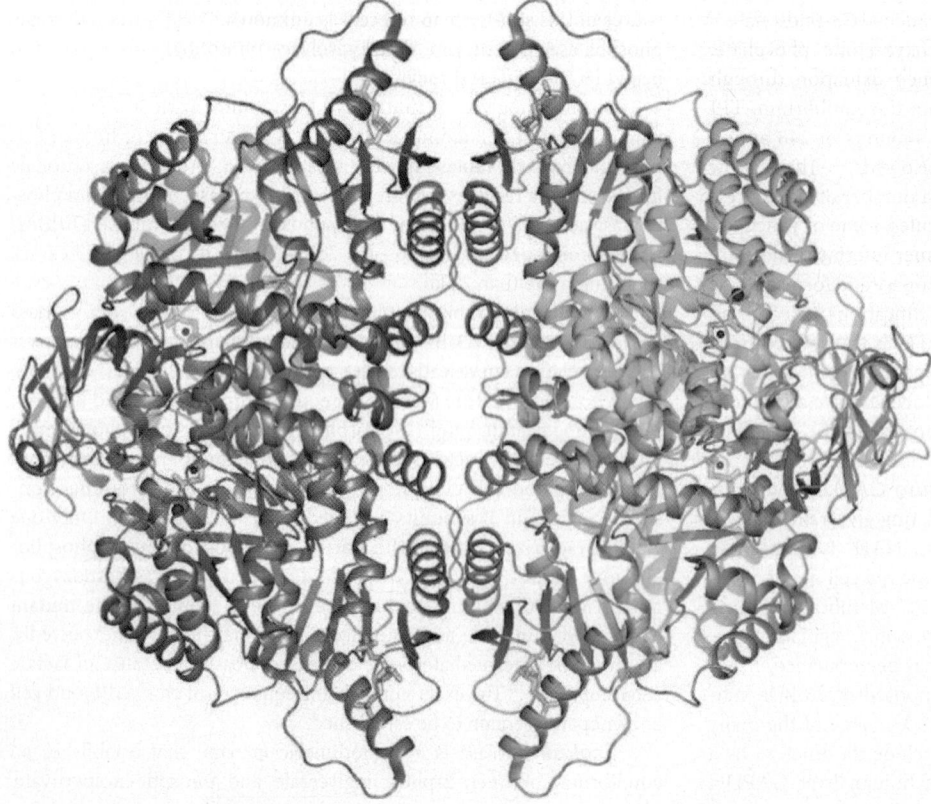

Figure 47–4. Ribbon representation of the human erythrocyte pyruvate kinase tetramer. The substrate phosphoglycolate and fructose-1,6-diphosphate are shown in ball-and-stick representation, and colored *yellow* and *gray*, respectively. Metal ions in the active site are shown as *blue* (potassium) and *pink* (manganese) spheres. Individual subunits are colored lime, cyan, violet, and orange.

requires the presence of NADP$^+$ (Fig. 47–5).[140] Hence, NADP$^+$ is bound to the enzyme both as a structural component, in the subunit interface, and as one of the substrates of the reaction.[141-143] Under physiologic conditions, the active human enzyme exists in a dimer–tetramer equilibrium. Lowering the pH causes a shift toward the tetrameric form.[141,144,145]

G6PD is strongly inhibited by physiologic amounts of NADPH[146] and, to a lesser extent, by physiologic concentrations of ATP.[147] It has much higher enzyme-activity in reticulocytes than in mature red cells, especially for the mutant forms of the enzyme.[43,148] This may complicate diagnosing G6PD deficiency in patients with high reticulocyte counts following a hemolytic episode (see "Laboratory Features" below).

The three-dimensional model of the crystal structure of human G6PD shows that the G6PD monomer is built up by two domains, a N-terminal domain and a large $\beta + \alpha$ domain with an antiparallel nine-stranded sheet. The extensive interface between the two monomers is of crucial importance for enzymatic stability and activity.[143] The fully conserved amino acids 198 to 205 (Arg-Ile-Asp-His-Tyr-Leu-Gly-Lys) are essential for substrate binding and catalysis.[143,149-151]

The *G6PD* gene is located on the X-chromosome (Xq28). It spans 18 kb, and consists of 13 exons of which exon 1 is noncoding. Methylation of certain cytidines at the 3′ end is believed to have a regulatory function.[152,153] The 3′-UTR (untranslated region) also harbors putative microRNA (miRNA) target sites, which potentially could have a functional effect on the downregulation of *G6PD* mRNA, thereby affecting the stability of *G6PD* mRNA and translation, or the miRNA regulation process.[154] G6PD deficiency is one of the world's most common hereditary disorders. Many mutations and variants have been reported and studied.[1,2,155-160]

Phosphogluconolactonase Although 6-phosphogluconolactone is the direct product of the oxidation of glucose-6-phosphate by G6PD and hydrolyzes spontaneously at a physiologic pH, enzymatic hydrolysis is much more rapid and is required for normal metabolic flow through the stimulated hexose monophosphate pathway.[161,162] Partial deficiency of the enzyme has been observed[163] and is probably benign.[164]

Phosphogluconate Dehydrogenase Phosphogluconate dehydrogenase catalyzes the oxidation of phosphogluconate to ribulose-5-phosphate and CO_2 and the reduction of NADP$^+$ to NADPH. Variability of electrophoretic mobility of the enzyme is common in humans and in several animal species.[165] Deficiency of the enzyme has been observed only rarely and appears to be essentially innocuous or possibly associated with mild hemolysis.[166-168]

Ribosephosphate Isomerase Ribosephosphate isomerase catalyzes the interconversion of ribulose-5-phosphate and ribose-5-phosphate.

Deficiency of the enzyme has been described as one of the rarest human disorders.[169] It manifests with progressive leukoencephalopathy and neuropathy. No dysfunction of red cells was reported.[170]

Ribulose-Phosphate Epimerase Ribulose-phosphate epimerase converts ribulose-5-phosphate to xylulose-5-phosphate. The exact activity of this enzyme in human hemolysates has not been reported but seems to be less than that of ribosephosphate isomerase.

Transketolase Transketolase effects the transfer of two carbon atoms from xylulose-5-phosphate to ribose-5-phosphate, resulting in the formation of the 7-carbon sugar sedoheptulose-7-phosphate and the 3-carbon sugar glyceraldehyde-3-phosphate.[171-173] It can also catalyze the reaction between xylulose-5-phosphate and erythrose-4-phosphate, producing fructose-6-phosphate and glyceraldehyde-3-phosphate. Thiamine pyrophosphate is a coenzyme for transketolase, and the activity of erythrocyte transketolase is used as an index of the adequacy of thiamine nutrition.[174]

Transaldolase The conversion of seduhepulose-7-phosphate and glyceraldehyde-3-phosphate into erythrose-4-phosphate and fructose-6-phosphate is catalyzed by transaldolase.[175] This is another one in the series of molecular rearrangements that leads in the conversion of the 5-carbon sugar formed in the phosphogluconate dehydrogenase step to metabolic intermediates of the EMP. Transaldolase deficiency was first reported in 2001 as a new inborn error of the pentose phosphate pathway.[176] To date, 23 patients from 13 families have been described.[177,178] It is a pleiotropic metabolic disorder, and patients present in the neonatal or antenatal period with dysmorphic features, hepatosplenomegaly, abnormal liver function, cardiac defects, thrombocytopenia, bleeding tendencies, and anemia. The latter appears to be hemolytic in nature, possibly because of decreased levels of NADPH.[179,180]

L-Hexonate Dehydrogenase Red cells contain L-hexonate dehydrogenase, an enzyme that has the capacity to reduce aldoses such as glucose, galactose, or glyceraldehyde to their corresponding polyol (i.e., glucose to sorbitol, galactose to dulcitol, and glyceraldehyde to glycerol). NADPH serves as a hydrogen donor for this reaction.[181] Aldose reductase is another enzyme that can catalyze this reaction. It is present in red cells,[182] and increased levels have been implicated in diabetic complications, such as retinopathy[183] and autonomic neuropathy.[184]

Utilization of Substrates Other Than Glucose as Energy Sources

The red cell has the capacity to use several other substrates in addition to glucose as a source of energy. Among these are adenosine, inosine, fructose, mannose, galactose, dihydroxyacetone, and lactate.[185] Although in

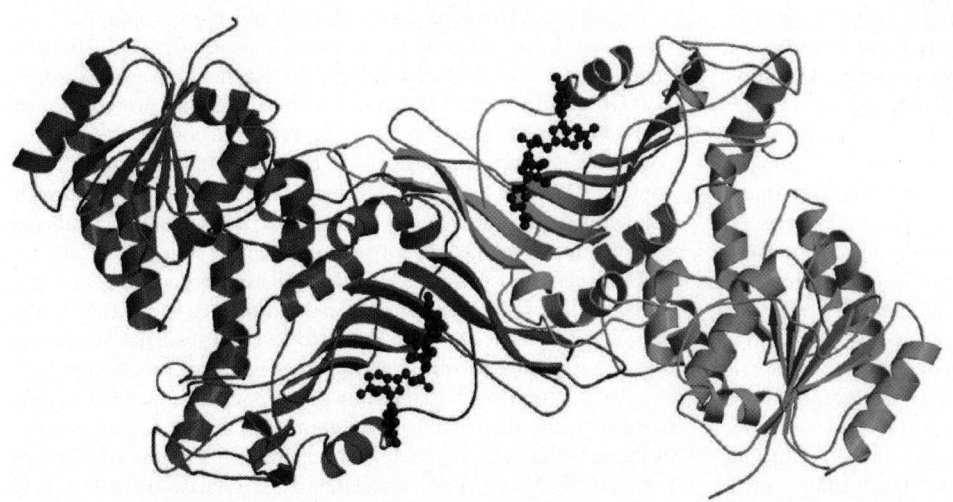

Figure 47–5. A dimer of human glucose-6-phosphate dehydrogenase. Subunits A and B are colored *red* and *blue*. Structural nicotinamide adenine dinucleotide phosphate (NADP$^+$) molecules are drawn in ball-and-stick mode and colored *dark blue*.

the circulation red cells normally rely on glucose as their energy source, the use of other substrates, particularly during blood storage (Chap. 138) and in certain experimental situations, is of interest.

Glutathione Metabolism of the Erythrocyte The red cell contains a high concentration of the sulfhydryl-containing tripeptide GSH. It serves a major role in antioxidant defense, detoxification, and maintenance of thiol status. Reported concentrations range between 0.4 and 3.0 mM, with a terminal half-life ($T_{1/2}$) of approximately 4 days.[187] The wide interindividual range suggests that GSH levels are, at least in part, genetically determined.[188] In its role of defense against oxidative stress GSH is oxidized to glutathione disulfide (GSSG), which can be reverted back to GSH by mediation of glutathione reductase. In addition GSSG can be transported out of the cell.

Glutathione biosynthesis occurs in two ATP-dependent steps:

$$Glutamate + Cysteine + ATP \rightarrow \gamma\text{-}Glutamylcysteine + ADP + Pi$$
$$\gamma\text{-}Glutamylcysteine + Glycine + ATP \rightarrow GSH + ADP + Pi$$

The first step is rate limiting and catalyzed by glutamate cysteine ligase (GCL) (γ-glutamylcysteine synthetase). Feedback inhibition of GCL by GSH is commonly considered a key regulatory step in GSH homeostasis, but other pathways are likely to play a role in maintaining GSH levels.[189] GCL is a heterodimer composed of a catalytic 73-kDa catalytic subunit (GCLC) and a 31-kDa modifier subunit (GCLM).[190,191] An intersubunit disulfide bond has been implicated in stabilization and catalytic efficiency of the heterodimer, acting as a cellular redox switch to couple enzyme activity, and consequently GSH levels, with the reduction-oxidation (redox) state of the cell.[192,193] An alternative model suggests that increased levels of oxidative stress induce the formation of high activity heterodimer complexes from low activity monomeric and holoenzyme forms of the enzyme.[194] GCL subunits are encoded by separate genes, located on chromosome 6p12 (*GCLC*) and 1p22.1 (*GCLM*), respectively. *GCLC* contains 16 exons, encoding for the 637-amino-acids catalytic subunit, whereas *GCLM* contains 7 exons that encode the 274 amino acids of the modifier subunit. A trinucleotide repeat polymorphism in the 5'-UTR affects *GCLC* gene expression and is associated with alterations in GCL activity and GSH levels.[195] GCL deficiency is a very rare cause of hemolytic anemia.

The second step in GSH synthesis is irreversible and mediated by glutathione synthetase (GS). This enzyme is a homodimer composed of 52-kDa subunits,[196] and the crystal structure of human GS has been resolved.[197] There is one gene coding for GS. This 23-kb gene (*GSS*) is located on chromosome 20q11.2 and contains 13 exons, of which the first is noncoding, that code for the 474-amino-acids-long protein. Deficiency of GS is the most common disorder of GSH synthesis and is associated with hemolytic anemia.

One important function of GSH in the erythrocyte is the detoxification of low levels of hydrogen peroxide that may form spontaneously or as a result of drug administration. Hydrogen peroxide is reduced to water through mediation of the enzyme glutathione peroxidase,[198] thereby oxidizing GSH to GSSG (see Fig. 47–7). Several glutathione peroxidases exist but only type 1 appears to be expressed in red blood cells.[199] Glutathione peroxidase is a selenium-containing[200] tetrameric enzyme consisting of 21-kDa subunits. A polymorphism affecting the activity of this enzyme, which is most common in persons of Mediterranean descent,[201] has been described. The consequent decreases in enzyme activity are without clinical effect.[202] In agreement with this, complete loss of glutathione peroxidase activity in mice was found to be without any consequences, even at high levels of oxidative stress, thus suggesting that glutathione peroxidase is of minor significance for red cell function.[199]

GSH also functions in maintaining integrity of the erythrocyte by reducing sulfhydryl groups of membrane proteins,[203] and glycolytic

enzymes,[204] for example, PK.[205] In the process of reducing peroxides or oxidized protein sulfhydryl groups, GSH is converted to GSSG, or may form mixed disulfides. Thus, for instance, GSSG has the capacity to inhibit red cell HK,[49,206] although greater than physiologic levels may be needed for this effect. It may also complex with hemoglobin A to form hemoglobin A$_3$.[207]

Glutathione reductase (GR) provides an efficient mechanism for the reduction of GSSG to regenerate GSH, and thus maintaining high intracellular levels of GSH. A mitochondrial and a cytoplasmic isozyme are both produced from the same mRNA, most likely by alternative initiation of translation.[208] GR is a homodimer, linked by a disulfide bridge. Each 56-kDa subunit contains four domains, of which domains 1 and 2 bind FAD (flavin adenine dinucleotide) and NADPH, respectively, with domain 4 constituting the interface.[209] The protein is encoded by the *GR* gene, located on chromosome 8p21.1. *GR* spans 50 kb, contains 13 exons, and encodes a 522-amino-acids-long protein. GR is a flavin enzyme, and either NADPH or NADH may serve as a hydrogen donor.[210] In the intact cell, only the NADPH system appears to function.[211] The same enzyme system appears to have the capacity to reduce mixed disulfides of GSH and proteins.[42] The activity of red cell GR is strongly influenced by the riboflavin content of the diet,[212] and its activity is used as a biomarker for riboflavin status.[213] Correction of partial GR deficiency by riboflavin administration has been reported to ameliorate hemolysis in a case of unstable hemoglobin.[214] Hereditary deficiency of GR is a very rare disorder and associated with hemolytic anemia.

Red cells also contain thioltransferase that can catalyze GSH-dependent reduction of some disulfides.[215,216]

Oxidized glutathione is actively extruded from the erythrocyte.[217,218] GSSG efflux is likely an important regulator of GSH turnover in red blood cells.[219] The system consists of at least two GSSG-activated adenosine triphosphatases (ATPases) that serve as an enzymatic basis for this transport process.[220] In addition to transporting GSSG, the system appears to have the capacity to transport thioether conjugates of GSH and electrophiles formed by the action of glutathione-S-transferase.[221,222] Preliminary evidence indicates that multidrug resistance protein 1 (MRP1) may be the exporter protein of both glutathione-S conjugates and GSSG.[189,223] Erythrocytes contain glutathione-S-transferases rho, sigma, and theta.[224–226] Glutathione-S-transferase catalyzes the formation of a thioether bond between GSH and a variety of xenobiotics. The role of glutathione-S-transferase in the erythrocyte has not been established. It may be that it serves to cleanse the blood of xenobiotics to which the red cell membrane is permeable. Glutathione-S-transferase could conjugate such substances to glutathione, and the detoxified product of conjugation would be transported out of the red cell for subsequent disposal. The enzyme has the capacity to reversibly bind heme, and a possible role in heme transport has been postulated.[227] Deficiency of this enzyme is associated with hemolytic anemia, but a cause-and-effect relationship has not been established.[228]

Other Antioxidant Enzymes Superoxide radicals that are formed are converted to hydrogen peroxide by the action of the copper-containing enzyme superoxide dismutase (SOD).[229] Red blood cells contain SOD type 1 (*SOD1*). Mutations in *SOD1* are associated with the dominant disorder familial amyotrophic lateral sclerosis.[230] Patients display no hematologic phenotype. In agreement with this, studies on SOD1-deficient mice have shown that a 50 percent reduced SOD activity in red cells is probably sufficient to exert its protective effects.[231] SOD1 null mice are viable, but show elevated levels of oxidative stress that causes regenerative anemia and triggers autoantibody production.[232]

Hydrogen peroxide can be also decomposed to water and oxygen by catalase and peroxiredoxin. Both enzymes are abundantly present in the red blood cell, suggesting an important role in the cell's oxidative defense. Nevertheless, acatalasemia, or catalase deficiency, is a rare benign condition without hematologic consequences. It has been suggested, though, that it may act as a complicating factor in age and diseases such as diabetes[233] and oxidative stress-related conditions.[234] Deficiencies of peroxiredoxin 2, the major red cell peroxiredoxin,[235] have not been reported in humans. Peroxiredoxin 2 null mice, however, develop severe hemolytic anemia with Heinz body formation,[236] and show signs of abnormal erythropoiesis.[237] Based on mouse models, it has been postulated that glutathione peroxidase, catalase, and peroxiredoxin each have distinct roles in the scavenging of hydrogen peroxide and antioxidative defense.[238–240]

Nucleotide Metabolism of the Erythrocyte

Approximately 97 percent of the total nucleotide content of the mature red blood cell consists of interconvertible adenosine phosphates (Chap. 31). Less than 3 percent of total nucleotides are guanosine phosphates. ATP is the most abundant adenosine phosphate (comprising roughly 84 percent of total adenosine ribonucleotides), whereas ADP (14 percent) and adenosine monophosphate (AMP, 1 percent) are present in considerably lower amounts. The interconversion of adenine nucleotides is modulated by adenylate kinase (AK):

$$Mg^{2+} + ATP + AMP \rightarrow Mg^{2+} + ADP + ADP$$

By catalyzing the reversible phosphoryl transfer among ATP, ADP, and AMP, AK contributes to cellular adenine nucleotide homeostasis. Red cells contain the AK1 isozyme, which is present in the cytosol as a monomeric enzyme composed of 194 amino acids. The recombinant purified enzyme has a molecular mass of approximately 22 kDa.[241] The *AK1* gene is localized on chromosome 9q34.1, and consists of 7 exons of which exon 1 is noncoding. AK activity depends on the presence of Mg^2.

ATP serves as a cofactor in a number of reactions, such as the phosphorylation steps mediated by HK and PFK in glycolysis, the synthesis of GSH, and ATPase-dependent function of membrane pumps. Therefore, ATP is crucial in maintenance of the red cell's structure and function. Because the mature red cell is unable to synthesize adenosine phosphates from precursor molecules, it relies on salvage pathways to preserve adenosine ribonucleotides. This is of particular importance for AMP because this adenosine ribonucleotide is at risk of being lost from the adenine pool by dephosphorylation to adenosine and, subsequent, irreversible deamination to inosine by the enzyme adenosine deaminase (ADA). ADA thus plays a regulatory role in the concentration of adenosine ribonucleotides in the red cell. The gene encoding ADA *(ADA)* is located on chromosome 20q13.12. It comprises 12 exons that encode a 363-amino-acid protein.

Deficiency of AK and hyperactivity of ADA are both very rare causes of hereditary nonspherocytic hemolytic anemia.

Additional enzymes of purine metabolism are also present in the red cell. Although disorders of these enzymes are associated with a number of metabolic diseases, their function does not appear to be relevant for the red blood cell as these disorders are without hematologic consequences.[242]

Pyrimidine-5′-Nucleotidase-1 Pyrimidine ribonucleotides are found only in trace amounts in the mature red blood cell. They are lost from the cell together with the degradation of ribosomes and RNA during reticulocyte maturation. Pyrimidine-5′-nucleotidase-1 (P5′N1) mediates this loss by catalyzing the dephosphorylation of pyrimidine nucleoside monophosphates into the corresponding nucleosides (cytidine and uridine), which are freely diffusible across the membrane.[243] P5′N1 is specific for pyrimidine nucleotides and does not use purine nucleotides as substrate.[244] The enzyme requires Mg^{2+} for it activity, and is inhibited by a number of heavy metals, including Pb^{2+}.[245] Like other red blood cell enzymes, P5′N1 activity is much higher in reticulocytes. The enzyme declines in activity during red cell aging.[246] P5′N1 also has

phosphotransferase properties, suggesting an additional role of this enzyme in nucleotide metabolism.[247] The crystal structure of mouse P5′N1 has been published, providing a framework for understanding the kinetics of both nucleotidase and phosphotransferase activities of human P5′N1.[248]

P5′N1 is encoded by the *NT5C3A* gene on chromosome 7p14.3. It comprises 11 exons, and produces three distinct mRNAs by alternative splicing. Red cell P5′N1 is translated from the mRNA lacking exons 2 and R.[249,250] It is a 286-amino-acids-long monomeric protein with an apparent molecular weight of 34 kDa.[249]

A second P5′N is present in red blood cells, the activity of which is generally measured together with that of P5′N1. This enzyme (P5′N2) is encoded by a separate gene, shows little homology to P5′N1, and is not strictly pyrimidine-specific. It is unable to compensate for deficient function of P5′N1.[247,251] P5′N1 deficiency is one of the most common causes of hereditary nonspherocytic hemolytic anemia.

Human red blood cells have been found to express low NAD synthesis activity, mediated by nicotinamide mononucleotide adenylyltransferase.[252] It appears that the predominant isozyme in red blood cells is nicotinamide mononucleotide adenylyltransferase-3.[253] Human dysfunction of this enzyme has not been reported but the deficiency in mice blocks glycolysis at the GAPDH step and is associated with hemolytic anemia.[254]

● GENETICS

The great majority of red cell enzyme deficiencies that cause hemolytic anemia are hereditary. Most are inherited as autosomal recessive disorders, but G6PD deficiency and PGK deficiency are X-chromosome-linked. The vast majority of the genes encoding for the red cell enzymes have been identified, making the molecular diagnosis of hereditary red cell enzyme deficiency possible. Occasionally, acquired forms of enzyme deficiencies, particularly PK deficiency, have been encountered, usually in patients with hematologic neoplasia.[255–259]

ENZYME DEFICIENCIES—BIOCHEMICAL GENETICS AND MOLECULAR BIOLOGY

Table 47–2 lists the erythrocyte enzyme deficiencies shown to cause hemolytic disease. Other red cell enzyme deficiencies (Table 47–3) do not appear to cause hemolysis or other functional abnormality of the erythrocyte.[202] For example, acatalasemia, the state in which there is a virtually total absence of red cell catalase, is devoid of hematologic manifestations.[233] Similarly, red cells without acetylcholinesterase survive normally in most cases.[260]

The lack of clinical manifestations is not always clearcut. In some instances, hemolytic anemia is reported in some individuals with a given deficiency but not in others. For example, most subjects with LDH deficiency have no anemia, but cases with hemolysis have been reported.[136] Such ambiguity could result from differences in environmental and genetic factors or from bias of ascertainment. Erythrocyte enzyme assays are usually performed on patients with hemolytic anemia. Thus, a benign enzyme defect may be thought, mistakenly, to cause hemolysis because it is found in a patient with hemolytic anemia caused by an unrelated and undetected defect. Deficiencies of PGK, GS, or AK are usually associated with hereditary nonspherocytic hemolytic anemia, but cases have been reported in which these deficiencies were unassociated with any hematologic manifestations.[261–263] At times it has been suggested that moderate decreases in the activity of glutathione peroxidase causes hemolytic anemia, but the best available evidence indicates that this enzyme is not ordinarily rate limiting in erythrocyte metabolism and not associated with hemolytic anemia.[264]

TABLE 47–2. Red Cell Enzyme Abnormalities Leading to Hemolytic Disease

Enzyme	Clinical Features	Inheritance	Red Cell Morphology	Diagnosis (Reference)		Response to Splenectomy*	Approximate Frequency†
				Screening Test	Assay		
Hexokinase	HNSHA	AR	Unremarkable	—	580	+ +	Rare
Glucose phosphate isomerase	HNSHA; neurologic abnormalities	AR	Unremarkable	580	580	+ + +	Unusual
Phosphofruc-tokinase	HNSHA and/or muscle glycogen storage disease	AR	Unremarkable	—	580	0	Rare
Aldolase	HNSHA and mild liver glycogen storage; myopathy, mental retardation	AR	Unremarkable	—	580	?	Very rare
Triose-phosphate isomerase	HNSHA and severe neuromuscular disease	AR	Unremarkable	580	580	?	Rare
Phosphoglyc-erate kinase	HNSHA; myoglobi-nuria neuromuscu-lar disorder	SL	Unremarkable	—	580	+ +	Rare
Pyruvate kinase	HNSHA	AR	Usually unre-markable; occasionally contracted echinocytes	580	580	+ +	Unusual
Glucose-6-phosphate dehydrogenase	HNSHA; drug- or infection-induced hemolysis; favism	SL	Usually unre-markable; rarely "bite cells"	580	580	±	Very common
Glutathione reductase	Drug-sensitive hemolytic anemia and favism	AR	Unremarkable	580	580	?	Very rare
Glutamate cysteine synthetase	HNSHA; drug- or infection-induced hemolysis; neuro-logic abnormalities	AR	Unremarkable	644	645	?	Very rare
Glutathione synthetase	HNSHA; drug- or infection-induced hemolysis; neuro-logic defect and 5-oxoprolinuria in some cases	AR	Usually unremarkable	644	645	0	Rare
Pyrimidine 5′-nucleotidase	HNSHA; mental retardation in some cases	AR	Prominent stippling	646	647	0	Unusual
Adenylate kinase	HNSHA	AR	Unremarkable	—	580	?	Rare
Adenosine deaminase (increased activity)	HNSHA	AD	Unremarkable	—	580	?	Very rare

AD, autosomal dominant; AR, autosomal recessive; HNSHA, hereditary nonspherocytic hemolytic anemia; SL, sex-linked; —, not applicable.

*On a scale of 0 to 4+, where 4+ is a complete response. In many cases, data are meager.

†Very common if incidence is >5 percent. Unusual if >100 cases reported. Rare if 10 to 100 cases reported. Very rare if <10 cases reported.

‡Recent reports.

TABLE 47–3. Red Cell Enzyme Abnormalities Not Leading to Hemolytic Disease

Enzyme	Clinical Features	Inheritance	Diagnosis Reference Assay	Estimated Frequency*	Reference
6-Phosphogluconate dehydrogenase (complete deficiency)	None	AR	580	Unusual	166–168
6-Phosphogluconolactonase (partial defect)	Probably none	AD	648	Unusual	163
δ-ALA dehydrase	None	AD	649		
Acetylcholinesterase	None	AR	580	Very rare	260
Adenine phosphoribosyl transferase	Kidney stones	AR	650	Rare	651
Adenosine deaminase (decreased activity)	Immunodeficiency	AR	580	Rare	652
AMP deaminase	None	AR	653	Unusual	654
Bisphosphoglycerate mutase	Erythrocytosis	AR	580	Very rare	377, 380
Carbonic anhydrase I	None	AR	655	Rare	656
Carbonic anhydrase II	Osteoporosis	AR		Rare	657
Catalase	Oral ulcers in some types	AR	580	Rare	658
Cytochrome-b_5-reductase	Methemoglobinemia; mental retardation	AR	580	Unusual	659
Enolase	HNSHA?	AD?	580	Rare	115, 116
Galactokinase	Cataracts	AR	580	Rare	660
Galactose-1-P-uridyltransferase	Cataracts; mental retardation; liver disease	AR	580	Rare	661
Glutathione peroxidase (partial deficiency)	None	AR and AD[662]	580	Very common	580, 662
Glutathione reductase (partial deficiency)	None	Usually not inherited[662]	580	Very common	662, 663
Glutathione-S-transferase	HNSHA	?	580	Very rare	228
Glyceraldehyde-3-phosphate dehydrogenase (partial defect)	None	AD	580	Unusual	94
Glyoxalase I	None	AR		Rare	664
Hypoxanthine-guanine phosphoribosyl transferase (HGPRT)	Lesch-Nyhan syndrome (neurologic symptoms and gout)	SL	665	Rare	666
Inosine triphosphatase	None	AR	656	Rare	667
Lactate dehydrogenase	None	AR	580	Rare	135
NADPH diaphorase	None	AR	580	Rare	668
Phosphoglucomutase	None	AR	580	Rare	669
Transaldolase	Liver disease, thrombocytopenia, HNSHA?	AR	670	Rare	175
Uroporphyrinogen 1 synthase	Porphyria	AD	671	Unusual (common in selected populations)	672

AD, autosomal dominant; ALA, aminolevulinic acid; AMP, adenosine monophosphate; AR, autosomal recessive; HNSHA, hereditary nonspherocytic hemolytic anemia; NADPH, nicotinamide adenine dinucleotide phosphate (reduced form); SL, sex-linked.

*Very common if incidence is >5 percent, common if 1 to 5 percent, unusual if 0.01 to 1 percent, rare if <0.01 percent.

Table 47–3 includes deficiencies that may cause hemolytic anemia but for which a cause-and-effect relationship has not been clearly established, such as those of phosphogluconolactonase,[163] enolase,[115,116] and glutathione-S-transferase.[228]

Patients with unstable hemoglobins (Chap. 49) may present with the clinical picture of hereditary nonspherocytic hemolytic anemia. Hemolytic anemia resulting from abnormalities in the lipid composition of the red cell membrane, particularly increased phosphatidyl choline, occurs rarely (Chap. 46).

Glucose-6-Phosphate Dehydrogenase

The "normal" or wild-type enzyme is designated as G6PD B. Many variants of G6PD have been detected all over the world, associated with a wide range of biochemical characteristics and phenotypes. Accordingly, five classes of G6PD variants can be distinguished based on enzymatic activity and clinical manifestations (Table 47–4).[265] Before it became possible to characterize G6PD variants at the DNA level, they were distinguished from each other on the basis of biochemical characteristics, such as electrophoretic mobility, K_m for NADP and glucose-6-P, ability to use substrate analogues, pH activity profile, and thermal stability. To facilitate comparison of variants characterized in different laboratories, international standards for the methodology were established.[266] In the case of the common G6PD A– and G6PD Mediterranean mutations, the abnormal enzyme may be synthesized at normal or near-normal rates but has decreased stability *in vivo*.[267] The amount of enzyme antigen in the red cells declines concurrently with enzyme activity.[268] This suggests that the mutant protein in these variants is rendered unusually sensitive to proteolysis in the environment of the erythrocyte.[269] Other mutations also result in the formation of enzyme molecules with decreased enzyme activity[268] and with altered kinetic properties,[270] some of which may render them functionally inadequate.[158] By far the majority of mutations (85 percent) are missense mutations causing the substitution of a single amino acid.[158] More severe mutations such as frameshift and nonsense mutations have not been found, indicating that some residual activity is required for survival. In agreement with this, targeted deletion of G6PD in the mouse causes embryonic lethality.[271]

Detailed biochemical and genetic characteristics of some 400 putatively distinct G6PD variants and more than 200 different mutations have been tabulated.[155,160] Table 47–4 lists common G6PD variants that have reached polymorphic frequencies in certain populations.

African Variants Among persons of African descent, a mutant enzyme G6PD A+, with normal activity is polymorphic. It migrates electrophoretically more rapidly than the normal B enzyme, has substitution of Asn to Asp at codon 126, resulting from nucleotide change c.376A>G.[272] G6PD A– is the principal deficient variant found among people of African origin. The red cells contain only 5 to 15 percent of the normal amount of enzyme activity; however because of the instability of the enzyme, the age-dependent decline of the activity renders old red cells severely deficient and susceptible to hemolysis. These two electrophoretically rapid variants are common in African populations have in common a nucleotide substitution at cDNA nucleotide 376 that produces the amino acid substitution responsible for the rapid electrophoretic mobility. Most samples with G6PD A– manifest an additional *in cis* G>A mutation at cDNA nucleotide 202 (c.202G>A; p.Val68Met), which accounts for its *in vivo* instability.[273] Less commonly, the additional mutation is at a different site (c.680G>T or c.968T>C).[273] Thus G6PD A– arose in an individual who already had the G6PD A+ mutation. However, the ancestral human sequence has been deduced to be that of G6PD B, both by showing that this is the sequence of the chimpanzee,[274] our nearest relative, and by analysis of linkage dysequilibrium.[275] Although it has been suggested that only the interaction of p.Val68Met and p.Asn126Asp invariably results in G6PD A– deficiency,[276] the

c.202G>A mutation has been found in a patient to cause deficiency without the presence of the mutation at cDNA nucleotide (nt) 376.[274]

Variants in the Mediterranean Region Among white populations, G6PD deficiency is most common in Mediterranean countries. The most common enzyme variant in this region is G6PD Mediterranean.[270,277] The enzyme activity of the red cells of individuals who have inherited this abnormal gene is barely detectable. Other variants are also prevalent in the Mediterranean region, including G6PD A– and G6PD Seattle (see Table 47–4).

Variants in Asia A great many different variants have been described in Asian populations. Some of these proved to be identical at a molecular level (e.g., G6PD Gifu-like, Canton, Agrigento-like, and Taiwan-Hakka all have the same mutation at cDNA nt 1376 [see Table 47–4]). DNA analysis shows that more than 100 different mutations are found in various Asian populations.[160,278]

Variants Producing Hereditary Nonspherocytic Hemolytic Anemia Some mutations of G6PD result in chronic hemolysis without, but exacerbated by, precipitating causes. These variants are class I mutants (World Health Organization [WHO] class 1).[265] From a functional point of view, these mutations are more severe than the more commonly occurring polymorphic forms of the enzyme, such as G6PD Mediterranean and G6PD A–. On a molecular level, such variants are often caused by mutations located in exons 10 and 11, encoding the subunit interface, or affect residues that bind the structural NADP molecule.[143,158] There are, however, exceptions to this rule.[28,279–281] The clinical severity of these variants can be quite variable.[282]

G6PD deficiency has also been encountered in the rat, dog,[283] mouse,[284] and horse.[285] G6PD deficiency in mice has been rescued by stable *in vivo* expression of the human *G6PD* gene in hematopoietic tissues by a gene transfer approach.[271,286]

Pyruvate Kinase

PK deficiency is the second most common enzyme disorder in glycolysis and the most common cause of nonspherocytic hemolytic anemia.[287] Like G6PD deficiency, the disease is genetically heterogeneous, with different mutations causing different kinetic changes in the enzyme that is formed. There are even cases in which the activity of PK as measured *in vitro* is higher than normal, but a kinetically abnormal enzyme is responsible for the occurrence of hemolytic anemia.[288] Kinetic characterization and analysis of PK mutants is considerably more complex than analysis of G6PD mutants. Most PK-deficient patients are compound heterozygous for two different (missense) mutations, rather than homozygous for one. Assuming that stable mutant monomers are synthesized, up to seven different tetrameric forms of PK may be present in compound heterozygous individuals, each with distinct structural and kinetic properties. This complicates genotype-to-phenotype correlations in these individuals as it is difficult to infer which mutation is primarily responsible for deficient enzyme function and the clinical phenotype.[289,290] More than 230 mutations in the *PKLR* gene encoding the red cell PK have been identified. Seventy percent of these mutations are missense mutations affecting conserved residues in structurally and functionally important domains of PK. There appears to be no direct relationship between the nature and location of the substituted amino acid and the type of molecular perturbation.[124] Hence, the nature of the mutation has relatively little predictive value with respect to the severity of the clinical course and the phenotypic expression of identical mutations can be strikingly different in patients.[29,289–291]

Apart from decreased red blood cell survival ineffective erythropoiesis because of increased numbers of apoptotic cells is implicated as one of the pathophysiologic features of PK deficiency.[292,293] In particular, glycolytic inhibition by mutation of *PKLR* has been suggested to augment oxidative stress, leading to proapoptotic gene expression.[293]

TABLE 47–4. Major Polymorphic G6PD Variants

Variant	Nucleotide Substitution	Amino Acid Substitution	WHO Class[†]	Distribution	Reference
Gaohe	c.95A>G	p.(His32Arg)	III	Chinese	673
Honiara	c.99A>G	p.(Ile33Met)	I	Solomon Islands	674
	c.1360C>T	p.(Arg454Cys)			
Orissa	c.131C>G	p.(Ala44Gly)	III	India, Italy	675, 676
Aures	c.143T>C	p.(Ile48Thr)	III	Algeria, Tunisia	677, 678
Metaponto	c.172G>A	p.(Asp58Asn)	III	Italy	679
A–	c.202G>A	p.(Val68Met)	III	Africa	277
	c.376A>G	p.(Asn126Asp)			
Namoru	c.208T>C	p.(Tyr70His)	II	Vanuatu Archipelago	680
Ube-Konan	c.241C>T	p.(Arg81Cys)	III	Japan, Italy	676, 681
A+	c.376A>G	p.(Asn126Asp)	III-IV	Africa, Mediterranean	272
Vanua Lava	c.383T>C	p.(Leu128Pro)	II	Southwestern Pacific	680
Quing Yan	c.392G>T	p.(Gly131Val)	III	China	682
Mahidol	c.487G>A	p.(Gly163Ser)	III	Southeast Asia	683
Santamaria	c.542A>T	p.(Asp181Val)	II	Costa Rica, Italy	684, 685
	c.376A>G	p.(Asn126Asp)			
Mediterranean, Dallas, Panama, Sassari	c.563C>T	p.(Ser188Phe)	II	Mediterranean	277, 686
Coimbra	c.592C>T	p.(Arg198Cys)	II	India, Portugal	687
A–	c.680G>T	p.(Arg227Leu)	III	Africa	274
	c.376A>G	p.(Asn126Asp)			
Seattle, Lodi, Modena, Ferrara II, Athens-like		p.(Asp282His)	III	United States, Italy	688–690
Montalbano	c.854G>A	p.(Arg285His)	III	Italy	691
Viangchan, Jammu	c.871G>A	p.(Val291Met)	II	China	692, 693
Kalyan, Kerala, Jamnaga, Rohini	c.949G>A	p.(Glu317Lys)	III	India	694, 695
A–, Betica, Selma, Guantanamo	c.968T>C	p.(Leu323Pro)	III	Africa, Spain	274
	c.376A>G	p.(Asn126Asp)			
Chatham	c.1003G>A	p.(Ala335Thr)	II	Italy, Asia, Africa	277
Chinese-5	c.1024C>T	p.(Leu342Phe)	III	China	682
Ierapetra	c.1057C>T	p.(Pro353Ser)	II	Greece	696
Cassano	c.1347G>C	p.(Gln449His)	II	Italy, Greece	697, 698
Union, Maewo, Chinese-2, Kalo	c.1360C>T	p.(Arg454Cys)	II	Italy, Spain, China, Japan	697, 699, 700
Canton, Taiwan-Hakka, Gifu-like, Agrigento-like	c.1376G>T	p.(Arg459Leu)	II	Japan, Italy	701, 702
Cosenza	c.1376G>C	p.(Arg459Pro)	II	Italy	697
Kaiping, Anant, Dhon, Sapporo-like, Wosera	c.1388G>A	p.(Arg463His)	II	China	700, 702

[†]Class 1, severely deficient, associated with nonspherocytic hemolytic anemia; class 2, severe deficiency (1 to 10 percent residual activity), associated with acute hemolytic anemia; class 3, moderate deficiency (10 to 60 percent residual activity); class 4, not deficient (60 to 150 percent activity); class 5, increased activity (>150 percent).

Adapted from PJ Mason, JM Bautista, F Gilsanz[158] and A Minucci, K Moradkhani, MJ Hwang, et al.[160]

Data from Mason, P. J., Bautista, J. M., and Gilsanz, F. G6PD deficiency: The genotype-phenotype association. *Blood reviews.* 21: 267–283, 2007 and Minucci, A., Moradkhani, K., Hwang, M. J., et al. Glucose-6-phosphate dehydrogenase (G6PD) mutations database: Review of the "old" and update of the new mutations. *Blood cells, molecules & diseases* 48: 154–165, 2012.

PK deficiency may be also caused by mutations not directly involving the *PKLR* gene as demonstrated by a deficiency of PK being one of the key features of severe congenital hemolytic anemia caused by mutations in the key erythroid transcription factor KLF1.[294]

There is evidence that PK deficiency provides protection against infection and replication of *Plasmodium falciparum* in human erythrocytes,[295,296] an effect possibly mediated by reduced ATP levels in PK-deficient red blood cells.[297] This suggests that PK deficiency may confer a protective advantage against malaria in human populations in areas where this disease is endemic. In agreement with this, population studies on sub-Saharan African populations indicate that malaria is acting as a selective force in the *PKLR* genomic region.[298–300]

PK deficiency has also been recognized in mice, dogs, and multiple breeds of domestic cats.[301] In all these animals, the deficiency causes severe anemia and marked reticulocytosis, closely resembling human PK deficiency. Basenji dogs with PK deficiency completely lack PKLR enzymatic activity and, instead, only the PK-M2 isozyme is expressed in their red blood cells.[302] A unique feature of PK deficiency in dogs is the progressive development of myelofibrosis and osteosclerosis. Marrow fibrosis may occur in response to damage caused by iron overload,[303] although factors associated with marked erythropoiesis have also been proposed to play a role.[304] Gene therapy approaches have been employed to cure PK deficiency in dogs.[305] PK-deficient mice show delayed switching from PK-M2 to PK-R, resulting in delayed onset of the hemolytic anemia.[306] PK deficiency in mice has been rescued by expression of the human PK-R isozyme in murine hematopoietic stem cells.[307,308]

Other Enzyme Deficiencies

Hexokinase Deficiency Nineteen families with HK deficiency have been described as of the time of this writing[309–311] and only four patients have been characterized at the molecular level.[310–313] Two of these patients were homozygous, either for a highly conserved substitution in the enzyme's active site[313] or a lethal out-of-frame deletion of exons 5 to 8 of *HK1*.[310] In one patient a regulatory mutation was identified in the putative erythroid-specific promoter. *In vitro*, this mutation disrupted binding of the AP-1 transcription factor complex, leading to strongly decreased gene expression.[311]

In mice, a mutation designated *downeast anemia* causes severe hemolytic anemia with extensive tissue iron deposition and marked reticulocytosis, representing a mouse model of generalized HK deficiency.[314]

Glucosephosphate Isomerase Deficiency Glucosephosphate isomerase deficiency is second to PK deficiency in frequency, with respect to glycolytic enzymopathies. To date, approximately 55 families with glucosephosphate isomerase deficiency have been described worldwide.[315–320] Most of these patients are compound heterozygous for mutations that partially inactivate the enzyme. Most of the 31 *GPI* mutations reported to date are missense mutations. Mapping of these mutations to the crystal structure of the human enzyme and recombinant expression of genetic variants has provided considerable insight in the molecular mechanisms causing hemolytic anemia in this disorder.[321,322] The majority of the mutations disrupt key interactions that contribute directly or indirectly to the architecture of the enzyme's active site.[321] In rare cases, GPI deficiency also affects nonerythroid tissues, causing severe neuromuscular symptoms and granulocyte dysfunction.[323–328] The finding that GPI also functions as a neuroleukin,[329] an autocrine motility factor,[330] a nerve growth factor,[331] and a differentiation and maturation mediator[332] has led to the hypothesis that the mutation-dependent loss of cytokine function of GPI could account for the neuromuscular symptoms.[333] An alternative explanation involves disturbed glycerolipid biosynthesis in GPI deficiency, which could have significant effects on membrane formation, membrane function, and axonal migration.[334,335]

Homozygous GPI-deficient mice exhibit hematologic features resembling that of the human enzymopathies. In addition, other tissues are also affected, indicating a reduced glycolytic capability of the whole organism.[336] Complete loss of GPI in mice is embryonically lethal.[337]

Phosphofructokinase Deficiency Because red cells contain both PFK M and L subunits, mutations affecting either gene (*PFKM* or *PFKL*) will lead to a partially reduced red cell enzyme activity in PFK deficiency. Mutations in the *PFKM* gene cause PFKM deficiency or glycogen storage disease VII (Tarui disease).[338] The disease is characterized predominantly by mild to severe myopathy, in particular exercise intolerance, cramps, and myoglobinuria. The associated hemolysis is usually mild but may be absent. As of this writing, there has been only one reported case in which an unstable L subunit was identified. This patient exhibited no signs of myopathy or hemolysis.[75] Approximately 100 cases of PFK deficiency have been reported as of this writing, and 23 mutant *PFKM* alleles are reported. Approximately half of the reported mutations are missense mutations, the remaining mutations mostly affect splicing. Intriguingly, PFK-deficient Ashkenazi Jews share two common mutations: a G>A base change affecting the donor splice site of intron 5 (c.237+1G>A) and a single base deletion in exon 2 (c.2003delC).[33,339] The mode of action by which missense mutations cause disease is largely unknown.[33,340–347]

PFK deficiency in dogs[301] is characterized by the association of hemolytic crises with strenuous exercise.[348] *Pfkm* null mice show exercise intolerance, reduced life span, and progressive cardiac hypertrophy, suggesting that Tarui disease should be considered as a complex systemic disorder rather than a muscle glycogenosis.[349,350]

Aldolase Deficiency At the time of this writing, only six patients with red cell aldolase deficiency had been described, four of whom were characterized at the DNA level. All displayed moderate chronic hemolytic anemia, either by itself[351] or accompanied by myopathy,[352,353] rhabdomyolysis,[354] psychomotor retardation,[352] or mental retardation.[77,352]

Triosephosphate Isomerase Deficiency TPI deficiency is characterized by hemolytic anemia, often accompanied by neonatal hyperbilirubinemia requiring exchange transfusion. In addition, patients display progressive neurologic dysfunction, increased susceptibility to infection, and cardiomyopathy.[355] Most affected individuals die before the age of 6 years, but there are remarkable exceptions.[356] TPI deficiency is the most severe disorder of glycolysis. Key in the pathophysiology of the severe neuromuscular disease is the formation of toxic protein aggregates: accumulation of the substrate dihydroxyacetone phosphate results in elevated levels of the toxic methylglyoxal, leading to the formation of terminal glycation of proteins, whereas mutation-induced changes in the quaternary structure of TPI lead to the formation of an aggregation-prone protein.[357,358] Therefore, it has been suggested that TPI deficiency represents a conformational rather than a metabolic disease.[357]

Approximately 40 patients and 19 different mutations have been reported in TPI deficiency.[355,358–363] The most common mutation is the p.(Glu104Asp) amino acid change which is detected in approximately 80 percent of patients, all descendants from a common ancestor.[364] Studies on recombinant mutant TPI show that the p.(Glu104Asp) does not affect catalysis. Instead, the mutation disrupts a conserved network of buried water molecules, which prevents efficient formation of the active TPI dimer, causing its dissociation in inactive monomers.[85]

TPI-null mice die at an early stage of development.[365] Hemolytic anemia characterizes the only viable mouse model of TPI deficiency.[366] Studies on a *Drosophila* model recapitulating the neurologic phenotype of TPI deficiency[367] suggests that loss of an isomerase-independent function of TPI underlies the neuropathogenesis in TPI deficiency.[368]

Phosphoglycerate Kinase Deficiency PGK deficiency is one of the relatively uncommon causes of hereditary nonspherocytic hemolytic anemia. Mutations in the X chromosome-linked gene may cause mild to severe chronic hemolysis, neurologic dysfunction, and myopathy.[369] Approximately 40 patients with PGK deficiency have been reported.[369,370] Most patients manifest either hemolytic anemia in combination with neurologic symptoms, including mental retardation, seizures, progressive decline of motor function, and developmental delay, or isolated myopathy.[370–372] The combination of all clinical manifestations is a rare event, described in only 2 families.[373,374] Splenectomy has been reported to be beneficial but does not correct the hemolytic process.[341,369] Marrow transplantation has been performed to prevent the manifestation of severe neurologic symptoms.[375]

Twenty-two unique mutations have been identified.[370,371] Most of these mutations (80 percent) are missense mutations. Most of the encoded amino acid changes heavily affect the protein's thermal stability and to a different extent catalytic efficiency.[371,376] In an attempt to correlate the genotype to the phenotype, it was found that amino acid changes grossly impairing protein stability but moderately affecting kinetic properties were associated mostly with hemolytic anemia and neurological symptoms. Mutations perturbing both catalysis and heat stability were associated with myopathy alone, whereas mutations faintly affecting molecular properties of PGK correlated with a wide range of clinical symptoms.[376] Yet, the precise reason for the different clinical manifestations of mutations of the same gene remains unknown, suggesting the involvement of yet unknown alternate function of this enzyme, environmental, metabolic, genetic and/or epigenetic factors.[372,376]

Bisphosphoglycerate Mutase Deficiency Bisphosphoglycerate mutase deficiency is a very rare disorder. Only three affected families have been characterized. Bisphosphoglycerate mutase deficiency appears to be inherited as an autosomal recessive disorder. However, some heterozygous relatives have had a borderline high hemoglobin concentration,[377,378] and in one single affected patient only one mutation was identified.[379] Erythrocytosis was the predominant feature of the clinically normal probands, likely resulting from reduced 2,3-BPG levels[380] and, consequently, the increased oxygen affinity of hemoglobin (Chap. 57).

Glutamate Cysteine Ligase Deficiency GCL deficiency is associated with mild hereditary nonspherocytic hemolytic anemia that may be fully compensated. Drug- and infection-induced hemolytic crises may occur as a consequence of strongly reduced GSH levels. As of this writing, eight cases of GCL deficiency had been described, belonging to six unrelated families.[381–388] In approximately half of the patients with GCL deficiency, the hemolytic anemia was accompanied by impaired neurological function.[388] Six patients have been characterized at the molecular level and five different mutations have been reported.[385–388] In all these cases, the causative mutation affected the catalytic subunit of GCL. The clinically observed mutations have been mapped to a homology model of the human enzyme, based on the crystal structure of GCL of *Saccharomyces cerevisiae*, thus explaining the molecular basis of GSH depletion as a result of GCL deficiency.[192] Complementary expression studies in mice showed that these GCL mutations impair glutathione production by reducing the activity of the catalytic subunit of GCL. Addition of the modifier subunit was able to largely restore enzymatic activity, thereby underscoring the critical role of GCLM.[389] Complete deficiency of GCLC has shown to be lethal in mice,[390,391] whereas GCLM-null mice are viable and show no overt phenotype despite strongly reduced GSH levels, including a reduction of more than 90 percent in red blood cells.[392] Upon exposure to oxidative stress, however, red blood cells from such mice undergo massive hemolysis with fatal outcome.[393]

Glutathione Synthetase Deficiency GS deficiency[394] is the most common abnormality of red cell glutathione metabolism. Three distinct clinical forms of GS deficiency can be distinguished,[395] most likely reflecting different mutations or epigenetic modifications in the *GS*

gene.[396] Patients with mild GS deficiency display mild hemolytic anemia as their only symptom. In contrast, patients with a moderate deficiency usually present in the neonatal period with metabolic acidosis, 5-oxoprolinuria, and mild to moderate hemolytic anemia. In addition to these symptoms, patients with the third and most severe type develop progressive neurologic symptoms such as psychomotor retardation, mental retardation, seizures, ataxia, and spasticity. 5-Oxoprolinuria results from accumulation of γ-glutamylcysteine because of decreased feedback inhibition of GCL by the decreased levels of GSH.[397] Importantly, 5-oxoprolinuria may have other causes.[398,399] Experiments in rats show that acute administration of 5-oxoproline induces oxidative damage in the brain, a mechanism that may be involved in the neurologic symptoms of severe GS deficiency.[400]

The diagnosis of GS deficiency has been established in more than 70 patients from 50 families,[396,397,401,402] of whom approximately 25 percent died in childhood.[401] Thirty-two mutations are identified as being associated with GS deficiency. Based on the nature of the mutation, and taking into account GS activity and GSH levels it seems possible to predict a mild versus a more severe phenotype.[396] The structural effects of a number of missense mutations have been determined.[197]

A long-term followup study showed that early diagnosis, correction of acidosis, and early supplementation with antioxidants vitamins C and E improve survival and long-term outcome.[395] For these reasons it has been argued that GS deficiency should be included in the newborn screening program.[401]

Complete deficiency of GS has shown to be lethal in mice, whereas heterozygous animals survive with no distinct phenotype.[403]

Glutathione Reductase Deficiency Only two families with hereditary GR deficiency have been described and characterized.[404,405] The complete absence of GR in the red cells of members of one family was associated with only rare episodes of hemolysis, possibly caused by fava beans. GR deficiency was caused by homozygosity for a large genomic deletion. GR deficiency in the other family was caused by compound heterozygosity for a nonsense mutation, and a missense mutation affecting a highly conserved residue. GR in red cells was undetectable, but some residual activity was found in the patient's leucocytes.[404]

In vitro studies on members of one of the GR deficiency families has provided experimental evidence that GR deficiency may protect from malarial infection by enhancing phagocytosis of ring-infected red blood cells.[406]

Adenylate Kinase Deficiency AK deficiency has been reported in 12 unrelated families and 7 different mutations have been identified.[263,407–412] In all but one case,[263,413] the deficiency was associated with moderate to severe hemolytic anemia. In some of the patients, mental retardation and psychomotor impairment was also observed.[410,414] Studies on a number of recombinant proteins revealed strongly altered catalytic properties or protein stability resulting from mutation.[241] In contrast, patient's cells sometimes displayed considerable residual enzymatic activity. The activation of expression of other isozymes, that is, AK2 and AK3, has been proposed as one of the factors contributing to this apparent discrepancy.[412]

Adenosine Deaminase Hyperactivity An increased activity of ADA is associated with hereditary nonspherocytic hemolytic anemia. It is the only red cell enzyme disorder that is inherited in an autosomal dominant disorder.[415] Adenosine deaminase hyperactivity results in depletion of red cell ATP.[415,416] Few cases with a 30- to 70-fold increase in activity have been described. The molecular mechanism of this disorder has not been identified but the markedly increased amounts of ADA mRNA in affected individuals indicate that the red blood cell–specific overexpression occurs at the mRNA level,[417] causing an overproduction of a structurally normal enzyme.[418] ADA hyperactivity probably results from a *cis*-acting mutation in the vicinity of the *ADA* gene.[419]

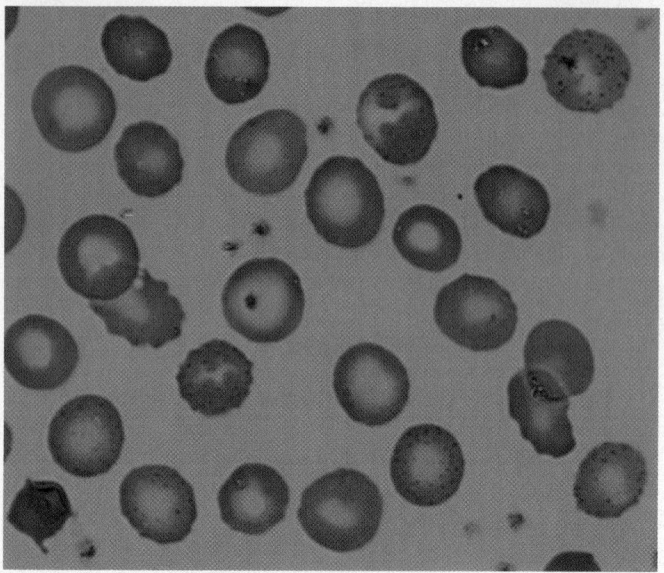

Figure 47–6. Prominent basophilic stippling in pyrimidine-5′-nucleotidase-1 (P5′N1) deficiency.

For reasons that are not understood, milder elevations of red cell ADA activity (two- to sixfold) are also increased in most, but not all, patients with Diamond-Blackfan anemia.[186] Deficiency of ADA is associated with severe combined immunodeficiency (Chap. 80). In this disorder, large quantities of deoxyadenine nucleotides, not normally present in erythrocytes, accumulate.

Pyrimidine 5′-Nucleotidase Deficiency Pyrimidine 5′-nucleotidase deficiency is the most frequent disorder of red cell nucleotide metabolism and a relatively common cause of mild-to-moderate hemolytic anemia.[420–422] More than 100 patients have been reported, but because of the relatively mild phenotype many patients may remain undetected. Deficient enzyme function leads to the accumulation of pyrimidine nucleotides. This results in prominent stippling on the blood film, the hallmark of this disorder (Fig. 47–6).[244] Hence, P5′N1 deficiency is the only red cell enzyme deficiency in which red cell morphology is helpful in establishing the diagnosis. The precise mechanism leading to premature destruction of P5′N1-deficient red cells is unknown. Some proposed pathophysiologic mechanisms have related the accumulation of pyrimidine nucleotide to alterations of the red cell membrane due to increased levels of cytidine diphosphate (CDP)-choline and CDP-ethanolamide,[423] decreased pentose phosphate shunt activity,[424–426] chelation of Mg^{2+} ions that serves as a cofactor for a number of enzymes,[427] decreased phosphoribosyl pyrophosphate synthetase activity,[428,429] increased activity of pyrimidine nucleoside monophosphate kinase,[430] increased levels of GSH,[431] and competition with reactions that require ADP or ATP.[432] However, clear cause-and-effect relationships have not been established.

As of this writing, 27 different mutations have been reported in *NT5C3A* in association with P5′N1 deficiency.[420,433,434] Most patients were found to be homozygous for a specific mutation. The majority of mutations concern frameshift or nonsense mutations, deletions, or mutations that affect splicing. Functional analysis of reported missense mutations was studied using recombinant mutant proteins. These rendered contrasting results between the substantial changes in kinetic behavior and thermostability and the actual residual enzymatic activity in patient's red cells, probably due to compensation by upregulation of other nucleotidases.[435] Of interest is the observation that none of the

reported missense mutations affect residues of the catalytic site, suggesting that the reduced catalytic efficiency and/or instability result from secondary effects related to conformational changes.[248]

Acquired deficiency of P5′N1 may result from lead poisoning. Structural studies have shown that Pb^{2+} specifically binds within the active site, in a different position than Mg^{2+} but with much higher affinity.[248] Because simultaneous binding of Mg^{2+} and Pb^{2+} is not possible, Pb^{2+} outcompetes Mg^{2+}, thereby preventing this essential cofactor from binding, thus abolishing catalytic activity. P5′N1 activity is also inhibited in β-thalassemia and related disorders that result in excess α-globin chains, such as hemoglobin E, probably from oxidative damage induced by excess α-globin chains.[436,437]

MECHANISM OF HEMOLYSIS

G6PD Deficiency

The life span of G6PD-deficient red cells is shortened under many circumstances, particularly during drug administration and infection. The exact reason for this is not known.

Drug-Induced Hemolysis

Drug-induced hemolysis in G6PD-deficient cells is generally accompanied by the formation of Heinz bodies, particles of denatured hemoglobin, and stromal protein (Chap. 49), formed only in the presence of oxygen.[438] Together with the inability to protect their GSH against drug challenge, this suggests that a major component of the hemolytic process is the inability of G6PD-deficient cells to protect sulfhydryl groups against oxidative damage.[2] The mechanism by which Heinz bodies are formed and become attached to red cell stroma has been the subject of considerable investigation and speculation. Exposure of red cells to certain drugs results in the formation of low levels of hydrogen peroxide as the drug interacts with hemoglobin.[439] In addition, some drugs may form free radicals that oxidize GSH without the formation of peroxide as an intermediate.[440] The formation of free radicals of GSH through the action of peroxide or by the direct action of drugs may be followed either by oxidation of GSH to the disulfide form (GSSG) or complexing of the glutathione with hemoglobin to form a mixed disulfide. Such mixed disulfides are believed to form initially with the sulfhydryl group of the β-93 position of β-globin.[441] The mixed disulfide of GSH and hemoglobin is probably unstable and undergoes conformational changes exposing interior sulfhydryl groups to oxidation and mixed disulfide formation. Globin chain separation into free α and β chains also occurs.[442] Once such oxidation has occurred, hemoglobin is denatured irreversibly and will precipitate as Heinz bodies. Normal red cells can defend themselves to a considerable extent against such changes by reducing GSSG to GSH and by reducing the mixed disulfides of GSH and hemoglobin through the GR reaction.[42] However, the reduction of these disulfide bonds requires a source of NADPH. Because G6PD-deficient red cells are unable to reduce $NADP^+$ to NADPH at a normal rate, they are unable to reduce hydrogen peroxide or the mixed disulfides of hemoglobin and GSH. Moreover, because catalase contains tightly bound NADPH[443] that is required for activity, the lack of freely available NADPH generation may, in addition, impede disposal of hydrogen peroxide by the catalase-dependent pathway.[444] When such cells are challenged by drugs, they form Heinz bodies more readily than do normal cells. Cells containing Heinz bodies encounter difficulty in traversing the splenic pulp[445] and are eliminated relatively rapidly from the circulation. Figure 47–7 summarizes a plausible scenario of the metabolic events that leads to red cell damage and eventually destruction. However, it has been shown that in mice, targeted disruption of the gene encoding glutathione peroxidase has little effect on oxidation of hemoglobin of murine red cells challenged with peroxides.[199] In addition,

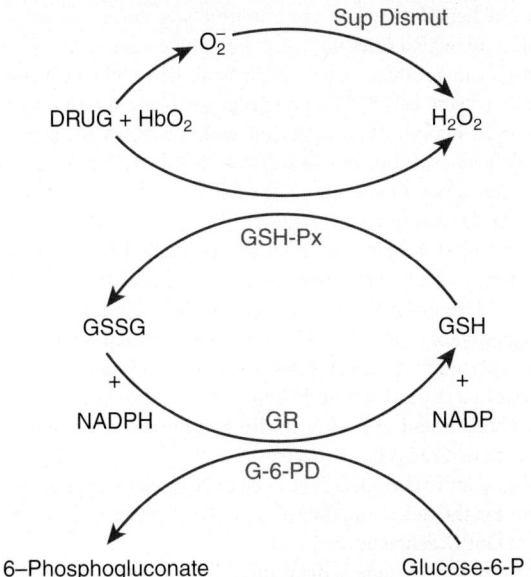

Figure 47–7. Reactions through which hydrogen peroxide is generated and detoxified in the erythrocyte. In glucose-6-phosphate dehydrogenase (G6PD) deficiency and related disorders, inadequate generation of nicotinamide adenine dinucleotide phosphate (reduced form) (NADPH) results in accumulation of GSSG and probably of hydrogen peroxide (H_2O_2). The accumulation of these substances leads to hemoglobin denaturation, Heinz body formation, and, consequently, to decreased red cell survival. GR, glutathione reductase; GSH, reduced glutathione; GSH-Px, glutathione peroxidase; GSSG, glutathione disulfide (oxidized glutathione); HbO_2, oxyhemoglobin; NADP, nicotinamide adenine dinucleotide phosphate; Sup Dismut, superoxide dismutase.

catalase-null mice show negligible antioxidant function of catalase in oxidant injury.[446] If such murine models reflect the situation in man, then different pathways requiring GSH, such as the thioredoxin, and/or peroxiredoxin reactions, may be important.[446,447]

The formation of methemoglobin frequently accompanies the administration of drugs that have the capacity to produce hemolysis of G6PD-deficient cells.[448] The heme groups of methemoglobin become detached from the globin more readily than do the heme groups of oxyhemoglobin.[449] It is not clear whether methemoglobin formation plays an important role in the oxidative degradation of hemoglobin to Heinz bodies or whether formation of methemoglobin is merely an incidental side effect of oxidative drugs.[450,451]

Infection-Induced Hemolysis

The mechanism of hemolysis induced by infection or occurring spontaneously in G6PD-deficient subjects is not well understood. The generation of hydrogen peroxide by phagocytizing leukocytes may play a role in this type of hemolytic reaction.[451]

Favism

Substances capable of destroying red cell GSH have been isolated from fava beans,[452] but scientific evidence that these components (i.e., divicine and isouramil) are indeed responsible for hemolysis is lacking. Favism occurs only in G6PD-deficient subjects, but not all individuals in a particular family may be sensitive to the hemolytic effect of the beans. Nonetheless, some tendency toward familial occurrence has suggested that an additional genetic factor may be important.[453] The observation of increased excretion of glucaric acid[454] led to the suggestion that a defect in glucuronide formation might be present. Specific genotypes

of the acid phosphatase gene have been attributed to a decrease in the *f* isoforms of this tyrosine phosphatase and, consequently, low GSH levels.[455] Immunologic factors do not seem to play a role in favism.[456] Increased levels of red cell calcium[457,458] and consequent "cross-bonding" of membranes may occur. Other membrane alterations that have been described are oxidation and clustering of membrane proteins, hemichrome binding to the internal face of the membrane, destabilization of the membrane, and the release of microvesicles.[459-462]

Icterus Neonatorum

G6PD-deficient neonates are at increased risk of developing severe icterus neonatorum. The icterus is frequently unaccompanied by changes in hematologic indices reflective of a hemolytic process.[463-465] The reason for this discrepancy is unclear. Icterus probably results principally from inadequate processing of bilirubin by the immature liver of G6PD-deficient infants. The demonstrated increase in carboxyhemoglobin levels, indicative of increased heme catabolism, suggests, however, that shortening of red cell life span also plays a role.[466] A predisposing factor for severe jaundice in G6PD deficiency is mutation of the uridine diphosphoglucuronate glucuronosyltransferase-1 gene (*UGT1A1*) promoter,[467] or, in Asia, the c.211G>A coding mutation.[468] In adults, these mutations are associated with Gilbert syndrome. The limited data available on liver G6PD in deficient adults[469] suggest that a considerable degree of deficiency may be present. If such a deficiency also is present in infants, it may play a role in impairing the borderline ability of infant livers with the *UGT1A1* promoter defect to catabolize bilirubin, in particular when a hemolytic process is set off because of contact with environmental factors, for example, neocytolysis (Chap. 33) certain drugs, naphthalene containing mothballs, etc. However, it is becoming apparent that modulation of bilirubin metabolism and serum bilirubin levels is under complex genetic control,[470] and coexpressing of mutations in other genes, for example, *SLCO1B3*,[471] may contribute further to the bilirubin production-conjugation imbalance in G6PD-deficient individuals.[472]

Deficiencies of Other Enzymes of the Hexose Monophosphate Shunt and of Glutathione Metabolism

Deficiencies of glutamate cysteine synthetase, GS, and GR are associated with a decrease in red cell GSH levels. The generally mild hemolysis that occurs in these disorders probably has a pathogenesis similar to the hemolysis that occurs in G6PD deficiency. Other defects of the hexose monophosphate shunt and associated metabolic pathways are not associated with hemolysis (see Table 47–3).

Other Enzyme Deficiencies

How deficiencies of enzymes other than those of the hexose monophosphate pathway result in shortening of red cell life-span remains unknown, although it has been the object of much experimental work and of speculation. It is often believed that ATP depletion is a common pathway in producing damage to the cell leading to its destruction,[473] but the evidence that this is the case is not always compelling.[474] Nevertheless, it seems reasonable to assume that a red cell, deprived of a source of energy becomes sodium and calcium logged and potassium depleted, and the red cell shape changes from a flexible biconcave disk. Such a cell is quickly removed from the circulation by the filtering action of the spleen and the monocyte-macrophage system. Even if it survived, such an energy-deprived cell would gradually turn brown as hemoglobin is oxidized to methemoglobin by the very high concentrations of oxygen within the erythrocyte. Calcium has been proposed to play a central role. In particular, malfunction of ATP-dependent calcium transporters could lead to increased intracellular calcium levels that could affect red cell membrane proteins (i.e., protein 4.1), the lipid bilayer, volume regulation, metabolism, and redox state preservation, consequently leading to proteolysis, oxidation, irreversible cellular shrinkage, phosphatidyl exposure and premature clearance.[475] In agreement with this, PFK deficiency has been shown to result in increased calcium levels, accompanied by volume loss and metabolic dysregulation.[476,477]

It is possible that, at least in some cases, alteration of the levels of red cell intermediate metabolites interferes with synthesis of cell components in early stages of development of the cell. In agreement with this, the lack of pyruvate has been implicated in the ineffective maturation of erythroid progenitors in PK-deficient mice.[478]

CLINICAL FEATURES

COMMON FORMS OF GLUCOSE-6-PHOSPHATE DEHYDROGENASE DEFICIENCY

Individuals who inherit the common (polymorphic) forms of G6PD deficiency, such as G6PD A– or G6PD Mediterranean, usually have no clinical manifestations. The major clinical consequence of G6PD deficiency is hemolytic anemia in adults and neonatal icterus in infants. Usually the anemia is episodic, but some of the unusual variants of G6PD may cause nonspherocytic congenital hemolytic disease (see "Variants Producing Hereditary Nonspherocytic Hemolytic Anemia" above). In general, hemolysis is associated with stress, most notably drug administration, infection, and, in certain individuals, exposure to fava beans.

Drug-Induced Hemolytic Anemia

Table 47–5 is an evidence-based[3,479] list of drugs and other chemicals that are predicted to precipitate hemolytic reactions in G6PD-deficient individuals, and drugs that are innocuous when given in normal doses,

TABLE 47–5. Drugs That Can Trigger Hemolysis in G6PD-Deficient Individuals

Category of Drug	Predictable Hemolysis	Possible Hemolysis
Antimalarials	Dapsone	Chloroquine
	Primaquine	Quinine
	Methylene blue	
Analgesics/ Antipyretic	Phenazopyridine	Aspirin (high doses)
		Paracetamol (Acetaminophen)
Antibacterials	Cotrimoxazole	Sulfasalazine
	Sulfadiazine	
	Quinolones (including nalidixic acid, ciprofloxacin, ofloxacin)	
	Nitrofurantoin	
Other	Rasburicase	Chloramphenicol
	Toluidine blue	Isoniazid
		Ascorbic acid
		Glibenclamide
		Vitamin K
		Isosorbide dinitrate

Reproduced with permission from Luzzatto L, Seneca E: G6PD deficiency: A classic example of pharmacogenetics with on-going clinical implications. *Br J Haematol* 164(4):469–480, 2014.

but may be hemolytic when given in excessive doses. A case in point is ascorbic acid, which does not cause hemolytic anemia in normal doses but which can produce severe, even fatal, hemolysis at doses of 80 g or more intravenously.[480–482] Some drugs, such as chloramphenicol, may induce mild hemolysis in a person with severe, Mediterranean-type G6PD deficiency,[484] but not in those with the milder A– or Canton[485] types of deficiency. Furthermore, there appears, to be a difference in the severity of the reaction to the same drug of different individuals with the same G6PD variant. For example, red cells from a single G6PD-deficient individual were hemolyzed in the circulation of some recipients who were given thiazolsulfone, but their survival was normal in the circulation of others.[438] Sulfamethoxazole, which was clearly hemolytic in experimental studies, does not appear to be a common cause of hemolysis in a clinical setting.[486] Undoubtedly, individual differences in the metabolism and excretion of drugs influence the extent to which G6PD-deficient red cells are destroyed.[487,488]

Several animal models have been developed to serve as a screening platform for the determination of hemolytic toxicity of pharmacologic agents in G6PD deficiency.[489,490–492]

Typically, an episode of drug-induced hemolysis in G6PD-deficient individuals begins 1 to 3 days after drug administration is initiated.[493] Heinz bodies appear in the red cells, and the hemoglobin concentration begins to decline rapidly.[494] As hemolysis progresses, Heinz bodies disappear from the circulation, presumably as they or the erythrocytes that contain them are removed by the spleen. In severe cases, abdominal or back pain may occur. The urine may turn dark or even black. Within 4 to 6 days, there is generally an increase in the reticulocyte count, except in instances in which the patient has received the offending drug for treatment of an active infection as infection depresses erythropoiesis (Chap. 37). Because of the tendency of infections and certain other stressful situations to precipitate hemolysis in G6PD-deficient individuals, many drugs have been incorrectly implicated as a cause. Other drugs, such as aspirin, have appeared on many lists of proscribed medications because very large doses could slightly reduce the red cell life span. It is important to recognize that such drugs do not produce clinically significant hemolytic anemia. Advising patients not to ingest these drugs may not only deprive patients of potentially helpful medications, but will also weaken their confidence in the advice that they have received. Most G6PD-deficient patients, after all, have taken aspirin without untoward effect and are likely to distrust an advisor who counsels them that the ingestion of aspirin will have catastrophic effects.

In the A– type of G6PD deficiency, the hemolytic anemia is self-limited[493] because the young red cells produced in response to hemolysis have nearly normal G6PD levels and are relatively resistant to hemolysis.[495] The hemoglobin level may return to normal even while the same dose of drug that initially precipitated hemolysis is administered. In contrast, hemolysis is not self-limited in the more severe types such as Mediterranean deficiency.[496]

Hemolytic Anemia Occurring During Infection

Anemia often develops rather suddenly in G6PD-deficient individuals within a few days of onset of a febrile illness. The anemia is usually relatively mild, with a decline in the hemoglobin concentration of 3 or 4 g/dL. Hemolysis has been noted particularly in patients suffering from hepatitides A and B, cytomegalovirus, and pneumonia, and in those with typhoid fever.[497–499] The fulminating form of the disease occurs particularly frequently among G6PD-deficient patients who are infected with Rocky Mountain spotted fever.[500] Jaundice is not a prominent part of the clinical picture, except where hemolysis occurs in association with infectious hepatitis.[501,502] In that case, it can be quite intense. Presumably because of the effect of the infection, reticulocytosis is usually absent, and recovery from the anemia is generally delayed until after the active infection has abated. In rare cases, G6PD deficiency may present as transient aplastic crisis caused by viral infection.[503,504]

Favism

Favism is potentially one of the gravest clinical consequences of G6PD deficiency. It occurs much more commonly in children than in adults, and occurs almost exclusively in persons who have inherited variants of G6PD that cause severe deficiency (most frequently associated with the Mediterranean variant), but rarely has the disorder been noted in patients with G6PD A–.[505] The onset of hemolysis may be quite sudden, having been reported to occur within the first hours after exposure to fava beans. More commonly, the onset is gradual, hemolysis being noticed 1 to 2 days after ingestion of the beans.[506] The urine becomes red or quite dark, and in severe cases shock may develop within a short time. Care should be taken to avoid acute renal failure. The oxidative stress causes membrane changes in erythrocytes, leading to extravascular hemolysis (in addition to the intravascular destruction).[3] Sometimes the patient or parent does not realize that fava beans have been ingested, as they may be incorporated into foods such as Yew Dow, eaten by the Chinese,[507] or falafel, eaten in the Middle East. Occasionally ingestion of other foodstuffs, such as unripe peaches[508] or a spiced Nigerian barbecued meat known as red suya,[509] has been reported to precipitate hemolysis. The toxic constituents of the fava beans are transmitted into the milk of breastfeeding mothers, putting affected babies at risk.[510]

Neonatal Icterus

Although serious, the clinical consequences of drug-induced hemolysis, favism, or chronic hemolytic anemia are usually not devastating, and death from favism is a very rare event. The most serious consequence of G6PD deficiency is icterus neonatorum.[463] G6PD-deficient neonates are an estimated three to four times more at risk for hyperbilirubinemia and phototherapy than G6PD-adequate neonates,[511] depending on population groups and geographic area.[512] Jaundice commences in the immediate perinatal period, and is usually evident by 1 to 4 days of age, similar to physiologic jaundice, but is seen at a later time than in blood group alloimmunization.[513] The jaundice may be quite severe and, if untreated, may result in kernicterus. Reports indicate an overrepresentation of G6PD deficiency among cases of kernicterus relative to the frequency of in the background population, also in countries with a low overall frequency of G6PD deficiency.[472] Thus, G6PD deficiency is a preventable cause of mental retardation,[514–516] and this aspect of the disorder has considerable public health significance. Neonatal screening for G6PD deficiency has been associated with a decrease in the number of cases of kernicterus.[472]

Nonspherocytic Hemolytic Anemia

As described, the anemia in G6PD deficiency is usually episodic and acute, but some sporadic variants of G6PD may cause nonspherocytic congenital hemolytic disease, exacerbated by oxidative stress. Affected individuals have a history of severe neonatal jaundice, and features of chronic hemolysis (see "Variants Producing Hereditary Nonspherocytic Hemolytic Anemia" above). The hemolysis is mainly extravascular.

Effects on Other Tissues

In the common variants of G6PD, such as G6PD A– and Mediterranean, and even in most of the severely deficient variants, there is usually no demonstrated defect in leukocyte number or function.[517] However, there have been reports of isolated instances of leukocyte dysfunction associated with rare, severely deficient variants of G6PD.[280,281,518–522] Patients with G6PD deficiency do not have a bleeding tendency, and studies of platelet function have yielded conflicting results.[523,524] Occasionally, cataracts have been observed in patients with variants of G6PD

that produce nonspherocytic hemolytic anemia,[525–527] or in neonatal patients.[528] The incidence of senile cataracts may be increased in G6PD deficiency,[529,530] but this remains controversial.[531,532] Small studies from the Middle East are suggestive that decreased G6PD activity may predispose to the development of diabetes.[533–535]

A number of studies reported on acute rhabdomyolysis in patients with G6PD deficiency, suggesting that this condition could predispose to muscle damage,[535–540] probably through the depletion of NADPH.[541] Others however, have demonstrated that G6PD-deficient individuals can participate in various physical activities, even high-intensity muscle damaging activities[542] without a negative impact on muscle function and redox status.[543,544]

Although claims have been made that an association exists between various kinds of G6PD deficiency and cancer,[545,546] the relationship between G6PD status and cancer is not clear as epidemiologic studies have not demonstrated any difference in risk for cancers between G6PD-deficient and normal patients.[547–549] Some role for G6PD in carcinogenesis may be conceivable, though, given the finding that mutation of p53 abolishes the direct binding of this major tumor-suppressor gene to G6PD, thereby enhancing hexose monophosphate shunt flux and tumor cell biosynthesis.[550]

Population studies are needed to better elucidate the postulated effects of G6PD deficiency on the development of cardiovascular disease.[278,551]

ENZYME DEFICIENCIES OTHER THAN GLUCOSE-6-PHOSPHATE DEHYDROGENASE

Most patients with hereditary nonspherocytic hemolytic anemia manifest only the usual clinical signs and symptoms of chronic hemolysis. The degree of anemia in this group of disorders varies widely. In some cases of very severe PK deficiency, scarcely any deficient cells survive in the circulation, and only transfused cells are found or steady-state hemoglobin levels as low as 5 g/dL are encountered. Other patients with hereditary nonspherocytic hemolytic anemia may manifest compensated hemolysis with a normal steady-state hemoglobin concentration. Chronic jaundice is a common finding, and splenomegaly is often present. Gallstones are common. As in other forms of chronic hemolytic anemia, ankle ulcers may be present.[552,553] Pregnancy has been thought to precipitate hemolysis in patients with PK deficiency, perhaps even in heterozygotes.[554–556] In PK deficiency, the increased 2,3-BPG levels may ameliorate the anemia by lowering the oxygen-affinity of hemoglobin. Some PK-deficient patients present with hydrops fetalis.[557]

In the case of some enzyme defects, characteristic nonhematologic systemic manifestations may be present, and these may be the only sign of the enzyme deficiency. For example, patients with PFK deficiency may have type VII muscle glycogen storage disease. In some patients with this defect, hemolysis is present without muscle manifestations, but in others both muscle abnormalities and hemolysis occur.[558] Glutathione synthetase deficiency may be associated with 5-oxoprolinuria and neuromuscular disturbances, and such abnormalities may occur either with[559] or without hematologic abnormalities.[262] On the other hand, some patients with GS deficiency manifest only the hematologic abnormalities.[382] Spinocerebellar degeneration was documented in the first case of glutamate cysteine synthetase described,[381,384] but was not present in subsequently investigated patients.[382,383] Patients with TPI deficiency nearly always manifest serious neuromuscular disease, and most of the patients who inherit this abnormality die in the first decade of life,[560,561] but there are exceptions, as only one of two brothers with the same genotype manifested neurologic disease (see "Genetic Modifiers of the Phenotypes" below).[562,563] Neurologic symptoms have also been noted in patients with deficiencies of glucosephosphate isomerase and PGK.[333,564] Myoglobinuria has been encountered in patients with PGK,[261,565] aldolase,[352] and G6PD deficiency.[539] Table 47–2 summarizes the clinical features of enzyme deficiencies causing nonspherocytic hemolytic anemia.

GENETIC MODIFIERS OF THE PHENOTYPES

The clinical phenotype of both acute and chronic hemolysis can be modified by coinherited (although unrelated) other defects of the red cells. Combined deficiencies of, for example, GPI and G6PD,[316] of PK and band 3,[566–568] of PK and α-thalassemia,[569] and of PK and G6PD[570] have been documented.

The inheritance of polymorphic *UGT1A1* promoter alleles exacerbates the icterus both in neonates and in adults with G6PD deficiency (see also "Mechanism of Hemolysis" above).[472] Overt iron overload and iron-related morbidity in PK deficiency has been attributed to coinheritance of mutations in *HFE*, the gene associated with hereditary hemochromatosis.[571]

A striking example of complex interplay defining the differences between the genotype and the phenotype was described in a Hungarian family with TPI deficiency. Two adult germline-identical compound heterozygous brothers displayed strikingly different phenotypes. Both had the same severe decrease in TPI activity and congenital hemolytic anemia, but only one suffered from severe neurologic disorder. Studies aimed at the pathogenesis of this differing phenotype indicated functional differences between the two brothers in lipid environment of the red cell membrane proteins influencing the enzyme activities,[562] as well as differences in *TPI1* mRNA expression, and protein expression levels of prolyl oligopeptidase, the activity decrease of which has been reported in well-characterized neurodegenerative diseases.[572]

The variety of clinical features associated with the various enzymopathies, regardless of the underlying molecular mechanism, do unequivocally demonstrate that the phenotype of hereditary red blood cell enzymopathies, is not solely dependent on the molecular properties of mutant proteins but rather reflects a complex interplay between physiologic, environmental, and other (genetic) factors. Putative phenotypic modifiers include differences in genetic background, concomitant functional polymorphisms of other glycolytic enzymes (many enzymes are regulated by their product or other metabolites), posttranslational modification, ineffective erythropoiesis, and different splenic function. As an example, persistent expression of the PK-M2 isozyme has been reported in the red blood cells of patients (and animals) with severe PK deficiency.[29,573] The survival of these patients, though not in all cases may be enabled by this compensatory increase in PK activity.[574]

● LABORATORY FEATURES

Varying degrees of anemia and reticulocytosis are the main hematologic laboratory features of patients with hereditary nonspherocytic hemolytic anemia. Heinz bodies often are found in the erythrocytes of G6PD-deficient patients undergoing drug-induced hemolysis. In the absence of hemolysis, the light-microscopic morphology of G6PD-deficient red cells appears to be normal. Differences in the texture of the membrane of the cells have, however, been observed under electron microscopy.[575] When a hemolytic drug is administered to a G6PD-deficient patient, Heinz bodies (Chap. 31) develop in the erythrocytes immediately preceding and in the early phases of the hemolytic episode. If the hemolytic anemia is very severe, spherocytosis and red cell fragmentation may be seen in the stained film. Despite the fact that "bite cells" may be noted in the blood of a G6PD-deficient patient undergoing drug-induced hemolysis, the association with G6PD deficiency is doubtful because such cells are usually lacking in acute hemolytic

states of patients with common G6PD variants or in G6PD-deficient patients with chronic hemolysis. Moreover, "bite cells" have been noted in G6PD-replete patients.[576,577]

The presence of small, densely staining cells has often been noted in the blood films of patients with hereditary nonspherocytic hemolytic anemia with defects other than G6PD deficiency. Particularly when manifesting an echinocytic appearance, such cells have been thought to be common in PK deficiency. In one reported case,[578] spectacular numbers of such cells were observed. However, cells of this type are seen in many blood films both from patients with other glycolytic enzyme deficiencies and from those with other disorders and it is hazardous to attempt to make an enzymatic diagnosis on the basis of such findings. Basophilic stippling of the erythrocytes is prominent in most patients with pyrimidine 5'-nucleotidase deficiency but is on itself an unspecific finding, and may not be apparent in blood that has been collected in ethylenediaminetetraacetic acid anticoagulant. Leukopenia occasionally is observed in patients with hereditary nonspherocytic hemolytic anemia, possibly secondary to splenic enlargement. Other laboratory stigmata of increased hemolysis may include increased levels of serum bilirubin, decreased haptoglobin levels, and increased serum LDH activity (Chap. 33). Reticulocytosis is frequently observed, which may result in increased mean corpuscular volume of erythrocytes. In PK deficiency, splenectomy increases reticulocyte counts even further because in particular the younger PK-deficient red blood cells are preferentially sequestered by the spleen.[579] Also in P5'N1 deficiency reticulocytes tend to be higher in splenectomized patients compared to non-splenectomized patients.[420]

Diagnosis of red cell enzyme deficiencies usually depends on the demonstration of decreased enzyme activity either through a quantitative assay or a screening test.[580–583] Assay of most of the enzymes generally is carried out by measuring the rate of reduction or oxidation of nicotinamide adenine nucleotides in an ultraviolet spectrophotometer, and a number of screening tests that depend upon the development or loss of fluorescence have been devised.[584]

However, difficulties arise when the patient has been transfused so that the blood drawn represents a mixture of the patient's own cells and those obtained from the blood bank. Under the circumstances, DNA analysis may prove invaluable, because the DNA is extracted from blood leukocytes and transfused leukocytes do not persist in the circulation. Alternatively, density fractionation has been applied to isolate fractions of patient's red cells, in which an enzyme deficiency can be detected.[585]

Although detection of G6PD deficiency in the healthy, fully affected (hemizygous) male can be achieved readily through either assay or screening tests, difficulties arise when a patient with G6PD deficiency of the A– type has undergone a hemolytic episode. As the older, more enzyme-deficient cells are removed from the circulation and are replaced by young cells, the level of the enzyme begins to increase toward normal. Under such circumstances, suspicion that the patient may be G6PD deficient should be raised by the fact that enzyme activity is not increased, even though the reticulocytes count is elevated.[586,587] It is helpful to perform DNA mutational analyses, carry out family studies, or to wait until the circulating red cells have aged sufficiently to betray their lack of enzyme.

Even greater difficulties are encountered in attempting to diagnose heterozygotes for G6PD deficiency.[588] Because the gene is X linked, a population of normal red cells coexists with the deficient cells. This may mask the enzyme deficiency when screening tests are used. Even enzyme assays carried out on erythrocytes of heterozygous females frequently may be in the normal range. Here DNA mutational analyses and histochemical methods that depend upon individual red cell enzyme activity may be useful.[589,590] In addition, the ascorbate cyanide test,[591] in which screening is carried out on a whole-cell population rather than on a lysate, may be more sensitive than the other screening procedures. Prenatal diagnosis of G6PD deficiency is also possible using DNA mutational analyses approach.

Testing for red cells enzyme deficiencies is best done in specialized laboratories. Specimens can be shipped by mail to reference laboratories. As a rule, whole-blood specimens are suitable and can best be sent at 4°C as some enzymes, notably PFK, are relatively unstable.[580] Blood from a healthy volunteer should be shipped with the patient sample to serve as a shipping control. Exceptions are assays for phosphorylated sugar intermediates, 2,3-BPG, and nucleotide intermediates, which are unstable in freshly drawn blood and require immediate deproteinization in perchloric acid.

Several aspects should be kept in mind when interpreting test results. First, care must be taken to remove leukocytes and platelets in assays such as for PK, as these cells contain PK activity, obscuring a deficiency in the red cells. Second, one should be aware of the already mentioned red cell age dependency of, for example, PK, HK, and G6PD. The measurement of these enzymes simultaneously can give an idea about red cell age and relative deficiencies. If patients received blood transfusions, interpreting results from red cell enzyme assays is generally not possible because the presence of donor erythrocytes will obscure any deficiencies. Some mutant enzymes also display a normal activity *in vitro*, whereas *in vivo* severe hemolysis can occur, reflecting the differences between optimal circumstances *in vitro* and the *in vivo* cellular environment. More sophisticated assays to measure, for example, heat instability and kinetics, have to be used in those cases. Interpretation can be particularly challenging in newborn patients given the differences in red cell energy metabolism and enzymatic activities between adults and newborn infants.[592-596] Molecular diagnosis is now available for all red cell enzyme deficiencies.

DIFFERENTIAL DIAGNOSIS

Drug-induced hemolytic anemia resulting from G6PD deficiency is similar in its clinical features and in certain laboratory features, to drug-induced hemolytic anemia associated with unstable hemoglobins (Chap. 49). Other enzyme defects affecting the pentose-phosphate shunt, such as a deficiency of GS, also may mimic G6PD deficiency. The diagnosis of hemoglobinopathies can be excluded by performing a stability test,[597] hemoglobin electrophoresis or DNA sequence analysis. These are normal in G6PD deficiency. Some of the screening tests, particularly the ascorbate cyanide test,[591] may give positive results in the above-named disorders, but a G6PD assay or the fluorescent screening test will be positive only in G6PD deficiency. In addition, defects of the erythrocyte membrane should be excluded (Chap. 46), but these cytoskeletal and other membrane defects are generally associated with characteristic morphologic abnormalities, that makes them easy to differentiate from hemolysis because of enzyme defects.

Physicians often attempt to establish the cause of hereditary nonspherocytic hemolytic anemia on the basis of the appearance of red cells on a blood film. In reality, red cell morphology is helpful only in the diagnosis of pyrimidine 5'-nucleotidase deficiency because of the characteristic stippling of the red cells that is observed in that disorder. The appearance of Heinz bodies suggests the possible presence of an unstable hemoglobin, or defective GSH metabolism. They are more likely to be present after splenectomy.

Because the laboratory diagnosis of these disorders may entail considerable expenditure of time and effort, it is prudent to perform the simplest tests for the most common causes of hereditary nonspherocytic hemolytic anemia first. Accordingly, it is useful to carry out screening tests[580,582] for G6PD and PK activity and an isopropanol stability test to detect an unstable hemoglobin (Chap. 49). If prominent

stippling of erythrocytes is present, examination of the ultraviolet spectrum of a perchloric acid extract of the erythrocytes, reflecting the ratio between pyrimidine and purine nucleotide content, may help to establish the diagnosis of pyrimidine 5'-nucleotidase deficiency.[598] Beyond these relatively simple procedures it is probably rarely useful to pick and choose individual enzyme assays on the basis of family history or clinical manifestations. Rather, it is usually appropriate to submit a blood sample to a reference laboratory that has the capability of performing all the enzyme assays listed in Table 47–3. Preferably, the suspicion of a specific enzyme disorder causing hereditary nonspherocytic hemolytic anemia is confirmed by DNA sequence analysis. This also enables prenatal diagnosis which has already been achieved for some of enzymatic defects.[599-607]

Notably, in an estimated 70 percent of cases of suspected hereditary nonspherocytic hemolytic anemia no enzymatic abnormality is found.[608,609] Current promising approaches such as red cell proteome analysis[610-612] and/or the use of next-generation sequencing technologies[613] may aid in a better and more comprehensive understanding of the etiology of this disorder.

THERAPY

GLUCOSE-6-PHOSPHATE DEHYDROGENASE DEFICIENCY

G6PD-deficient individuals should avoid drugs that are predicted to induce hemolytic episodes (see Table 47–5). However, it is important to realize that such patients are able to tolerate most drugs. Unfortunately, in the past, a number of case reports incorrectly suggested that some drugs had hemolytic potential that subsequently were shown to be safe (see Table 47–5, possible hemolysis). Although it is possible that some of these may be hemolytic in some patients or under some circumstances, this is unlikely, and G6PD-deficient patients should not be deprived of the possible benefit of these drugs.

If hemolysis occurs as a result of drug ingestion or infection, particularly in the milder A– type of deficiency, transfusion usually is not required. If, however, the rate of hemolysis is very rapid, as may occur, for example, in favism, transfusions of packed cells may be useful. Good urine flow should be maintained in patients with hemoglobinuria to avert renal damage. Infants with neonatal jaundice resulting from G6PD deficiency may require phototherapy or exchange transfusion; in areas in which G6PD deficiency is prevalent, care must be taken not to give G6PD-deficient blood to such newborns.[614] A single dose of Sn-mesoporphyrin, a potent inhibitor of heme oxygenase, has been advocated to eliminate the need for phototherapy.[615] Patients with hereditary nonspherocytic hemolytic anemia resulting from G6PD deficiency usually do not require any therapy. Splenectomy is often ineffective, although some improvement has been reported in a number of cases following removal of the spleen.[264,616] In most cases, the anemia is not very severe, but in some instances frequent transfusions have been necessary.[617,618] The antioxidant properties of vitamin E have been tested in G6PD-deficient subjects, and a slight but statistically significant reduction in hemolysis was observed.[619,620] These results could not be confirmed in other studies.[621,622] It has been suggested that desferrioxamine decreases hemolysis.[623,624] Inhibition of histone acetylation by histone deacetylase inhibitors has been shown to increase *G6PD* gene transcription in erythroid progenitor cells and restore G6PD deficiency.[625]

OTHER ENZYME DEFICIENCIES

Most patients with hereditary nonspherocytic hemolytic anemia secondary to red cell enzymopathies do not require therapy, other than blood transfusion during hemolytic periods, if the anemia needs clinically to be corrected. There are patients with PK deficiency who need to be transfused continually. Chronic transfusion therapy usually requires iron chelation if of sufficient iron load. Patients with TPI deficiency generally die as children, not because of the severity of the anemia but because of the severe neuromuscular effects of the enzyme deficiency. It has been proposed that the exogenous replacement of TPI might be useful for the treatment of this deficiency,[626] but no clinical trials have been carried out. PK deficiency[627] and PGK deficiency[375] have been treated successfully by stem cell transplantation, but this is still only very rarely done. Studies are underway to improve gene therapy in PK deficiency.[305,307,308] In PK deficiency, erythroid cells have been treated *ex vivo* with glycolytic intermediates to correct for metabolic dysfunction.[628] Preliminary evidence indicates that small molecule activation of mutant PK may be able to restore glycolytic pathway activity and normalize red cell metabolism in PK deficiency.[629] The jaundice of glucose-phosphate isomerase deficiency has been treated by the administration of phenobarbital.[630]

The principal decision that the physician must make regarding patients with hereditary nonspherocytic hemolytic anemia is whether or not they require a splenectomy. This decision is not made easily as the response is unpredictable, and some patients who fail to respond may develop serious thrombotic complications, resulting thrombocytosis is often exaggerated when splenectomy does not ameliorate the hemolysis. The recommendation that is made should be based upon the following considerations: (1) severity of the disease, (2) family history of response to splenectomy, (3) the underlying defect, and (4) perhaps the need for cholecystectomy. Because it is unusual to obtain more than a partial response to splenectomy, this procedure should probably be reserved for patients whose quality of life is impaired by their anemia. The operation needs to be particularly considered for patients who need frequent transfusion and for those who require gallbladder surgery, in which splenectomy might be carried out as part of the same procedure. The best guide to the likely efficacy of splenectomy is probably the response to splenectomy of other affected family members. Unfortunately, such information is only occasionally available. The physician must therefore rely upon the experience of other patients with hereditary nonspherocytic hemolytic anemia of similar etiology to serve as a guide. However, even as the large group of patients with hereditary nonspherocytic hemolytic anemia represents a heterogeneous population, so individuals with a single enzymatic lesion, such as PK deficiency, are heterogeneous. Each family is likely to be afflicted with a distinct mutant enzyme, and the various mutants may differ both with respect to clinical manifestations and with respect to response to splenectomy. Some of the available information regarding response to splenectomy of patients with hereditary nonspherocytic hemolytic anemia has been reviewed[264] and is summarized in Table 47-2.

Glucocorticoids are of no known value in this group of disorders. Folic acid is often given, as in other patients with increased marrow activity, but without proven hematologic benefit. In the absence of iron deficiency, iron is contraindicated. Iron overload is a complication in this group of disorders, particularly in connection with PK deficiency,[289,571,631,632] even in nontransfused patients.[633] The iron overload is probably multifactorial (Chap. 43), involving chronic hemolysis, ineffective erythropoiesis, splenectomy, coinheritance of hereditary hemochromatosis gene *(HFE)* mutations, growth differentiation factor-15, and hepcidin levels.[571,634,635]

● COURSE AND PROGNOSIS

Hemolytic episodes in the A– type of deficiency are usually self-limited, even if drug administration is continued. This is not the case in the more severe Mediterranean type of deficiency.[636] In patients with hereditary nonspherocytic hemolytic anemia resulting from G6PD deficiency, gallstones may occur.[637] During periods of infections or drug administration, anemia may increase in severity. Otherwise, the hemoglobin level of affected subjects remains relatively stable.

Nearly all patients with drug- or infection-induced hemolysis recover uneventfully. Favism must be considered, by comparison, a relatively dangerous disease. The most serious complication of G6PD deficiency is neonatal icterus. If not recognized early and properly treated, it can lead to kernicterus (see "Clinical Features" above).

In one large population study, a decreasing incidence of G6PD deficiency was noted with increasing age of the population,[638] but no such change was observed in another.[22] Although age stratification might represent evidence of a shorter life span for individuals with the A– deficiency, other factors are more likely explanations. Examination of the health records of more than 65,000 U.S. Veterans Administration males failed to reveal any higher frequency of any illness in G6PD-deficient compared to nondeficient subjects.[639] Furthermore, it appears that there are no indications that G6PD-deficient individuals should systematically be excluded from serving as blood donors,[640] or hematopoietic stem cell donor.[641] In view of the benign nature of the common types of G6PD deficiency, community-based population screening is not recommended. However, screening for G6PD deficiency of all patients admitted to the hospital may be useful in anticipating hemolytic reactions and in understanding them if they occur; however, this recommendation has not been submitted to rigorous analysis and is controversial because of low likelihood of any preventable hemolysis. This is particularly prudent if a drug such as dapsone or rasburicase, known to cause hemolysis in G6PD-deficient individuals, is to be given.[483,642] Study of family members of patients with this X chromosome-linked enzyme deficiency can be helpful in providing appropriate counseling to affected individuals.

The diagnosis of hereditary nonspherocytic hemolytic anemia has been made as late as the seventh decade,[202] and the disease can be fatal in the first few years of life. TPI deficiency appears to have the worst prognosis of all of the known defects that cause this disorder. With few exceptions, patients with this deficiency have died by the fifth or sixth year of life, usually of cardiopulmonary failure. PK deficiency, too, can be fatal in early childhood; the PK mutation prevalent among the Amish of Pennsylvania produces particularly severe disease.[643] Unless the affected homozygous children have their spleens removed, the disorder is commonly lethal. In PK deficiency, compound heterozygotes and homozygotes can suffer of major side effects as a result of the chronic hemolysis and the burden of repeated transfusions and iron chelation. In general, however, hereditary nonspherocytic hemolytic anemia is a relatively mild disease and most affected individuals lead a relatively normal life, apparently without much compromise of life span.

REFERENCES

1. Beutler E: G6PD deficiency. *Blood* 84:3613–3636, 1994.
2. Beutler E: Glucose-6-phosphate dehydrogenase deficiency: A historical perspective. *Blood* 111:16–24, 2008.
3. Luzzatto L, Seneca E: G6PD deficiency: A classic example of pharmacogenetics with on-going clinical implications. *Br J Haematol* 164:469–480, 2014.
4. Crosby WH: Hereditary nonspherocytic hemolytic anemia. *Blood* 5:233–253, 1950.
5. Dacie JV: The congenital anaemias, in *The Haemolytic Anaemias*, p 171. Grune & Stratton, New York, 1960.
6. Selwyn JG, Dacie JV: Autohemolysis and other changes resulting from the incubation in vitro of red cells from patients with congenital hemolytic anemia. *Blood* 9:414–438, 1954.
7. Robinson MA, Loder PB, DeGruchy GC: Red-cell metabolism in non-spherocytic congenital haemolytic anaemia. *Br J Haematol* 7:327–339, 1961.
8. Valentine WN, Tanaka KR, Miwa S: A specific erythrocyte glycolytic enzyme defect (pyruvate kinase) in three subjects with congenital non-spherocytic hemolytic anemia. *Trans Assoc Am Physicians* 74:100–110, 1961.
9. Howes RE, Piel FB, Patil AP, et al: G6PD deficiency prevalence and estimates of affected populations in malaria endemic countries: A geostatistical model-based map. *PLoS Med* 9:e1001339, 2012.

10. Howes RE, Dewi M, Piel FB, et al: Spatial distribution of G6PD deficiency variants across malaria-endemic regions. *Malar J* 12:418, 2013.

11. Howes RE, Battle KE, Satyagraha AW, et al: G6PD deficiency: Global distribution, genetic variants and primaquine therapy. *Adv Parasitol* 81:133–201, 2013.

12. Nkhoma ET, Poole C, Vannappagari V, et al: The global prevalence of glucose-6-phosphate dehydrogenase deficiency: A systematic review and meta-analysis. *Blood Cells Mol Dis* 42:267–278, 2009.

13. Tishkoff SA, Varkonyi R, Cahinhinan N, et al: Haplotype diversity and linkage disequilibrium at human G6PD: Recent origin of alleles that confer malarial resistance. *Science* 293:455–462, 2001.

14. Luzzatto L, Usanga EA, Reddy S: Glucose 6-phosphate dehydrogenase deficient red cells: Resistance to infection by malarial parasites. *Science* 164:839–842, 1969.

15. Cappadoro M, Giribaldi G, O'Brien E, et al: Early phagocytosis of glucose-6-phosphate dehydrogenase (G6PD)-deficient erythrocytes parasitized by plasmodium falciparum may explain malaria protection in G6PD deficiency. *Blood* 92:2527–2534, 1998.

16. Luzzatto L: G6PD deficiency and malaria selection. *Heredity (Edinb)* 108: 456, 2012.

17. Clark TG, Fry AE, Auburn S, et al: Allelic heterogeneity of G6PD deficiency in West Africa and severe malaria susceptibility. *Eur J Hum Genet* 17:1080–1085, 2009.

18. Guindo A, Fairhurst RM, Doumbo OK, et al: X-linked G6PD deficiency protects hemizygous males but not heterozygous females against severe malaria. *PLoS Med* 4:e66, 2007.

19. Bienzle U, Ayeni O, Lucas AO, et al: Glucose-6-phosphate dehydrogenase and malaria. Greater resistance of females heterozygous for enzyme deficiency and of males with non-deficient variant. *Lancet* 1:107–110, 1972.

20. Piomelli S, Reindorf CA, Arzanian MT, et al: Clinical and biochemical interactions of glucose-6-phosphate dehydrogenase deficiency and sickle-cell anemia. *N Engl J Med* 287:213–217, 1972.

21. Gibbs WN, Wardle J, Serjeant GR: Glucose-6-phosphate dehydrogenase deficiency and homozygous sickle cell disease in Jamaica. *Br J Haematol* 45:73–80, 1980.

22. Steinberg MH, West MS, Gallagher D, et al: Effects of glucose-6-phosphate dehydrogenase deficiency upon sickle cell anemia. *Blood* 71:748–752, 1988.

23. Benkerrou M, Alberti C, Couque N, et al: Impact of glucose-6-phosphate dehydrogenase deficiency on sickle cell anaemia expression in infancy and early childhood: A prospective study. *Br J Haematol* 163:646–654, 2013.

24. Nouraie M, Reading NS, Campbell A, et al: Association of G6PD with lower haemoglobin concentration but not increased haemolysis in patients with sickle cell anaemia. *Br J Haematol* 150:218–225, 2010.

25. Beutler E, Gelbart T: Estimating the prevalence of pyruvate kinase deficiency from the gene frequency in the general white population. *Blood* 95:3585–3588, 2000.

26. Mohrenweiser HW: Functional hemizygosity in the human genome: Direct estimate from twelve erythrocyte enzyme loci. *Hum Genet* 77:241–245, 1987.

27. Watanabe M, Zingg BC, Mohrenweiser HW: Molecular analysis of a series of alleles in humans with reduced activity at the triosephosphate isomerase locus. *Am J Hum Genet* 58:308–316, 1996.

28. Baronciani L, Beutler E: Analysis of pyruvate kinase-deficiency mutations that produce nonspherocytic hemolytic anemia. *Proc Natl Acad Sci U S A* 90:4324–4327, 1993.

29. Lenzner C, Nurnberg P, Jacobasch G, et al: Molecular analysis of 29 pyruvate kinase-deficient patients from central Europe with hereditary hemolytic anemia. *Blood* 89:1793–1799, 1997.

30. Manco L, Abade A: Pyruvate kinase deficiency: Prevalence of the 1456C→T mutation in the Portuguese population. *Clin Genet* 60:472–473, 2001.

31. Zanella A, Bianchi P: Red cell pyruvate kinase deficiency: From genetics to clinical manifestations. *Baillieres Best Pract Res Clin Haematol* 13:57–81, 2000.

32. Schneider A, Westwood B, Yim C, et al: The 1591C mutation in triosephosphate isomerase (TPI) deficiency. Tightly linked polymorphisms and a common haplotype in all known families. *Blood Cells Mol Dis* 22:115–125, 1996.

33. Sherman JB, Raben N, Nicastri C, et al: Common mutations in the phosphofructokinase-M gene in Ashkenazi Jewish patients with glycogenesis VII—and their population frequency. *Am J Hum Genet* 55:305–313, 1994.

34. Montel-Hagen A, Kinet S, Manel N, et al: Erythrocyte Glut1 triggers dehydroascorbic acid uptake in mammals unable to synthesize vitamin C. *Cell* 132:1039–1048, 2008.

35. Rosa R, Gaillardon J, Rosa J: Diphosphoglycerate mutase and 2,3-diphosphoglycerate phosphatase activities of red cells: Comparative electrophoretic study. *Biochem Biophys Res Commun* 51:536–542, 1973.

36. Cho J, King JS, Qian X, et al: Dephosphorylation of 2,3-bisphosphoglycerate by MIPP expands the regulatory capacity of the Rapoport-Luebering glycolytic shunt. *Proc Natl Acad Sci U S A* 105:5998–6003, 2008.

37. Puchulu-Campanella E, Chu H, Anstee DJ, et al: Identification of the components of a glycolytic enzyme metabolon on the human red blood cell membrane. *J Biol Chem* 288:848–858, 2013.

38. Campanella ME, Chu H, Low PS: Assembly and regulation of a glycolytic enzyme complex on the human erythrocyte membrane. *Proc Natl Acad Sci U S A* 102:2402–2407, 2005.

39. Lewis IA, Campanella ME, Markley JL, et al: Role of band 3 in regulating metabolic flux of red blood cells. *Proc Natl Acad Sci U S A* 106:18515–18520, 2009.

40. Sriram G, Martinez JA, McCabe ER, et al: Single-gene disorders: What role could moonlighting enzymes play? *Am J Hum Genet* 76:911–924, 2005.

41. Kim J-W, Dang CV: Multifaceted roles of glycolytic enzymes. *Trends Biochem Sci* 30:142–150, 2005.

42. Srivastava SK, Beutler E: Glutathione metabolism of the erythrocyte. The enzymic cleavage of glutathione-haemoglobin preparations by glutathione reductase. *Biochem J* 119:353–357, 1970.

43. Jansen G, Koenderman L, Rijksen G, et al: Age dependent behaviour of red cell glycolytic enzymes in haematological disorders. *Br J Haematol* 61:51–59, 1985.

44. Lakomek M, Schröter W, De Maeyer G, et al: On the diagnosis of erythrocyte enzyme defects in the presence of high reticulocyte counts. *Br J Haematol* 72:445–451, 1989.

45. Wilson JE: Isozymes of mammalian hexokinase: Structure, subcellular localization and metabolic function. *J Exp Biol* 206:2049–2057, 2003.

46. Cárdenas ML, Cornish-Bowden A, Ureta T: Evolution and regulatory role of the hexokinases. *Biochim Biophys Acta* 1401:242–264, 1998.

47. Fujii S, Beutler E: High glucose concentrations partially release hexokinase from inhibition by glucose-6-phosphate. *Proc Natl Acad Sci U S A* 82:1552–1554, 1985.

48. Gerber G, Kloppick E, Rapoport S: Öber den Einfluss des Anorganischen Phosphats auf die Glykolyse; seine Unwirksamkeit auf die Hexokinase des Menschenerythrozyten. *Acta Biol Med Ger* 18:305–312, 1967.

49. Beutler E, Teeple L: The effect of oxidized glutathione (GSSG) on human erythrocyte hexokinase activity. *Acta Biol Med Ger* 22:707–711, 1969.

50. Beutler E: 2,3-Diphosphoglycerate affects enzymes of glucose metabolism in red blood cells. *Nat New Biol* 232:20–21, 1971.

51. Mulichak AM, Wilson JE, Padmanabhan K, et al: The structure of mammalian hexokinase-1. *Nat Struct Biol* 5:555–560, 1998.

52. Aleshin AE, Kirby C, Liu X, et al: Crystal structures of mutant monomeric hexokinase I reveal multiple ADP binding sites and conformational changes relevant to allosteric regulation. *J Mol Biol* 296:1001–1015, 2000.

53. Murakami K, Blei F, Tilton W, et al: An isozyme of hexokinase specific for the human red blood cell (HK$_R$). *Blood* 75:770–775, 1990.

54. Ruzzo A, Andreoni F, Magnani M: Structure of the human hexokinase type I gene and nucleotide sequence of the 5′ flanking region. *Biochem J* 331:607–613, 1998.

55. Magnani M, Serafini G, Stocchi V: Hexokinase type I multiplicity in human erythrocytes. *Biochem J* 254:617–620, 1988.

56. Andreoni F, Ruzzo A, Magnani M: Structure of the 5′ region of the human hexokinase type I (HKI) gene and identification of an additional testis-specific HKI mRNA. *Biochim Biophys Acta* 1493:19–26, 2000.

57. Hantke J, Chandler D, King R, et al: A mutation in an alternative untranslated exon of hexokinase 1 associated with hereditary motor and sensory neuropathy–Russe (HMSNR). *Eur J Hum Genet* 17:1606–1614, 2009.

58. Murakami K, Kanno H, Miwa S, et al: Human HK$_R$ isozyme: Organization of the hexokinase I gene, the erythroid-specific promoter, and transcription initiation site. *Mol Genet Metab* 67:118–130, 1999.

59. Murakami K, Piomelli S: Identification of the cDNA for human red blood cell-specific hexokinase isozyme. *Blood* 89:762–766, 1997.

60. Bonnefond A, Vaxillaire M, Labrune Y, et al: Genetic variant in HK1 is associated with a proanemic state and A1C but not other glycemic control-related traits. *Diabetes* 58:2687–2697, 2009.

61. Read J, Pearce J, Li X, et al: The crystal structure of human phosphoglucose isomerase at 1.6 resolution: Implications for catalytic mechanism, cytokine activity and haemolytic anaemia. *J Mol Biol* 309:447–463, 2001.

62. Somarowthu S, Brodkin HR, D'Aquino JA, et al: A tale of two isomerases: Compact versus extended active sites in ketosteroid isomerase and phosphoglucose isomerase. *Biochemistry* 50:9283–9295, 2011.

63. Xu W, Lee P, Beutler E: Human glucose phosphate isomerase: Exon mapping and gene structure. *Genomics* 29:732–739, 1995.

64. Sola-Penna M, Da Silva D, Coelho WS, et al: Regulation of mammalian muscle type 6-phosphofructo-1-kinase and its implication for the control of the metabolism. *IUBMB Life* 62:791–796, 2010.

65. Schöneberg T, Kloos M, Brüser A, et al: Structure and allosteric regulation of eukaryotic 6-phosphofructokinases. *Biol Chem* 394:977–993, 2013.

66. Costa Leite T, Da Silva D, Guimaraes Coelho R, et al: Lactate favours the dissociation of skeletal muscle 6-phosphofructo-1-kinase tetramers down-regulating the enzyme and muscle glycolysis. *Biochem J* 408:123–130, 2007.

67. Marinho-Carvalho MM, Costa-Mattos PV, Spitz GA, et al: Calmodulin upregulates skeletal muscle 6-phosphofructo-1-kinase reversing the inhibitory effects of allosteric modulators. *Biochim Biophys Acta* 1794:1175–1180, 2009.

68. Higashi T, Richards CS, Uyeda K: The interaction of phosphofructokinase with erythrocyte membrane. *J Biol Chem* 254:9542–9550, 1979.

69. Jenkins JD, Kezdy FJ, Steck TL: Mode of interaction of phosphofructokinase with the erythrocyte membrane. *J Biol Chem* 260:10426–10433, 1985.

70. Chu H, Low PS: Mapping of glycolytic enzyme binding sites on human erythrocyte band 3. *Biochem J* 400:143–151, 2006.

71. Real-Hohn A, Zancan P, Da Silva D, et al: Filamentous actin and its associated binding proteins are the stimulatory site for 6-phosphofructo-1-kinase association within the membrane of human erythrocytes. *Biochimie* 92:538–544, 2010.

72. Kloos M, Bruser A, Kirchberger J, et al: Crystallization and preliminary crystallographic analysis of human muscle phosphofructokinase, the main regulator of glycolysis. *Acta Crystallogr F Struct Biol Commun* 70:578–582, 2014.

73. Yamada S, Nakajima H, Kuehn MR: Novel testis- and embryo-specific isoforms of the phosphofructokinase-1 muscle type gene. *Biochem Biophys Res Commun* 316:580–587, 2004.

74. Elson A, Levanon D, Brandeis M, et al: The structure of the human liver-type phosphofructokinase gene. *Genomics* 7:47–56, 1990.

75. Vora S, Davidson M, Seaman C, et al: Heterogeneity of the molecular lesions in inherited phosphofructokinase deficiency. *J Clin Invest* 72:1995–2006, 1983.

76. Yeltman DR, Harris BG: Fructose-bisphosphate aldolase from human erythrocytes. *Methods Enzymol* 90 Pt E:251–254, 1982.

77. Beutler E, Scott S, Bishop A, et al: Red cell aldolase deficiency and hemolytic anemia: A new syndrome. *Trans Assoc Am Physicians* 86:154–166, 1973.

78. Dalby A, Dauter Z, Littlechild JA: Crystal structure of human muscle aldolase complexed with fructose 1,6-bisphosphate: Mechanistic implications. *Protein Sci* 8:291–297, 1999.

79. Yeltman DR, Harris BG: Localization and membrane association of aldolase in human erythrocytes. *Arch Biochem Biophys* 199:186–196, 1980.

80. Perrotta S, Borriello A, Scaloni A, et al: The N-terminal 11 amino acids of human erythrocyte band 3 are critical for aldolase binding and protein phosphorylation: Implications for band 3 function. *Blood* 106:4359–4366, 2005.

81. Izzo P, Costanzo P, Lupo A, et al: Human aldolase A gene. Structural organization and tissue-specific expression by multiple promoters and alternate mRNA processing. *Eur J Biochem* 174:569–578, 1988.

82. Wierenga RK, Kapetaniou EG, Venkatesan R: Triosephosphate isomerase: A highly evolved biocatalyst. *Cell Mol Life Sci* 67:3961–3982, 2010.

83. Lu HS, Yuan PM, Gracy RW: Primary structure of human triosephosphate isomerase. *J Biol Chem* 259:11958–11968, 1984.

84. Mande SC, Mainfroid V, Kalk KH, et al: Crystal structure of recombinant human triosephosphate isomerase at 2.8 A resolution. Triosephosphate isomerase-related human genetic disorders and comparison with the trypanosomal enzyme. *Protein Sci* 3:810–821, 1994.

85. Rodríguez-Almazán C, Arreola R, Rodríguez-Larrea D, et al: Structural basis of human triosephosphate isomerase deficiency: Mutation E104D is related to alterations of a conserved water network at the dimer interface. *J Biol Chem* 283:23254–23263, 2008.

86. Peters J, Hopkinson DA, Harris H: Genetic and non-genetic variation of triose phosphate isomerase isozymes in human tissues. *Ann Hum Genet* 36:297–312, 1973.

87. Brown JR, Daar IO, Krug JR, et al: Characterization of the functional gene and several processed pseudogenes in the human triosephosphate isomerase gene family. *Mol Cell Biol* 5:1694–1706, 1985.

88. Rogalski AA, Steck TL, Waseem A: Association of glyceraldehyde-3-phosphate dehydrogenase with the plasma membrane of the intact human red blood cell. *J Biol Chem* 264:6438–6446, 1989.

89. Tsai IH, Murthy SN, Steck TL: Effect of red cell membrane binding on the catalytic activity of glyceraldehyde-3-phosphate dehydrogenase. *J Biol Chem* 257:1438–1442, 1982.

90. Low PS, Rathinavelu P, Harrison ML: Regulation of glycolysis via reversible enzyme binding to the membrane protein, band 3. *J Biol Chem* 268:14627–14631, 1993.

91. Mountassif D, Baibai T, Fourrat L, et al: Immunoaffinity purification and characterization of glyceraldehyde-3-phosphate dehydrogenase from human erythrocytes. *Acta Biochim Biophys Sin (Shanghai)* 41:399–406, 2009.

92. Raje CI, Kumar S, Harle A, et al: The macrophage cell surface glyceraldehyde-3-phosphate dehydrogenase is a novel transferrin receptor. *J Biol Chem* 282:3252–3261, 2007.

93. Ismail SA, Park HW: Structural analysis of human liver glyceraldehyde-3-phosphate dehydrogenase. *Acta Crystallogr D Biol Crystallogr* 61:1508–1513, 2005.

94. McCann SR, Finkel B, Cadman S, et al: Study of a kindred with hereditary spherocytosis and glyceraldehyde-3-phosphate dehydrogenase deficiency. *Blood* 47:171–181, 1976.

95. Huang IY, Welch CD, Yoshida A: Complete amino acid sequence of human phosphoglycerate kinase. Cyanogen bromide peptides and complete amino acid sequence. *J Biol Chem* 255:6412–6420, 1980.

96. McCarrey JR, Thomas K: Human testis-specific PGK gene lacks introns and possesses characteristics of a processed gene. *Nature* 326:501–505, 1987.

97. Banks RD, Blake CC, Evans PR, et al: Sequence, structure and activity of phosphoglycerate kinase: A possible hinge-bending enzyme. *Nature* 279:773–777, 1979.

98. Szabo J, Varga A, Flachner B, et al: Communication between the nucleotide site and the main molecular hinge of 3-phosphoglycerate kinase. *Biochemistry* 47:6735–6744, 2008.

99. Palmai Z, Chaloin L, Lionne C, et al: Substrate binding modifies the hinge bending characteristics of human 3-phosphoglycerate kinase: A molecular dynamics study. *Proteins* 77:319–329, 2009.

100. Ikura K, Sasaki R, Narita H, et al: Multifunctional enzyme, bisphosphoglyceromutase/2,3-bisphosphoglycerate phosphatase/phosphoglyceromutase from human erythrocytes. *Eur J Biochem* 66:515–522, 1976.

101. Rose ZB: The enzymology of 2,3-bisphosphoglycerate. *Adv Enzymol Relat Areas Mol Biol* 51:211–253, 1980.

102. Vora S, Spear D: Demonstration and quantitation of phosphoglycolate in human red cells. *Clin Res* 34:664A, 1986.

103. Fujii S, Beutler E: Where does phosphoglycolate come from in red cells? *Acta Haematol* 73:26–30, 1985.

104. Sasaki H, Fujii S, Yoshizaki Y, et al: Phosphoglycolate synthesis by human erythrocyte pyruvate kinase. *Acta Haematol* 77:83–86, 1987.

105. Beutler E, West C: An improved assay and some properties of phosphoglycolate phosphatase. *Anal Biochem* 106:163–168, 1980.

106. Wang Y, Wei Z, Bian Q, et al: Crystal structure of human bisphosphoglycerate mutase. *J Biol Chem* 279:39132–39138, 2004.

107. Patterson A, Price NC, Nairn J: Unliganded structure of human bisphosphoglycerate mutase reveals side-chain movements induced by ligand binding. *Acta Crystallogr Sect F Struct Biol Cryst Commun* 66(Pt 11):1415–1420, 2010.

108. Hass LF, Kappel WK, Muller KB, et al: Evidence for structural homology between human red cell phosphoglycerate mutase and 2,3-bisphosphoglycerate synthase. *J Biol Chem* 253:77–81, 1978.

109. Climent F, Roset F, Repiso A, et al: Red cell glycolytic enzyme disorders caused by mutations: An update. *Cardiovasc Hematol Disord Drug Targets* 9:95–106, 2009.

110. Repiso A, Perez de la Ossa P, Aviles X, et al: Red blood cell phosphoglycerate mutase. Description of the first human BB isoenzyme mutation. *Haematologica* 88:eCR07, 2003.

111. de Atauri P, Repiso A, Oliva B, et al: Characterization of the first described mutation of human red blood cell phosphoglycerate mutase. *Biochim Biophys Acta* 1740:403–410, 2005.

112. Repiso A, Ramirez Bajo MJ, Corrons JL, et al: Phosphoglycerate mutase BB isoenzyme deficiency in a patient with non-spherocytic anemia: Familial and metabolic studies. *Haematologica* 90:257–259, 2005.

113. Hoorn RK: J:, Filkweert JP, Staal GE: J. Purification and properties of enolase of human erythrocytes. *Int J Biochem* 5:845–852, 1974.

114. Kang HJ, Jung SK, Kim SJ, et al: Structure of human alpha-enolase (hENO1), a multifunctional glycolytic enzyme. *Acta Crystallogr D Biol Crystallogr* 64:651–657, 2008.

115. Stefanini M: Chronic hemolytic anemia associated with erythrocyte enolase deficiency exacerbated by ingestion of nitrofurantoin. *Am J Clin Pathol* 58:408–414, 1972.

116. Boulard-Heitzmann P, Boulard M, Tallineau C, et al: Decreased red cell enolase activity in a 40-year-old woman with compensated haemolysis. *Scand J Haematol* 33:401–404, 1984.

117. Noguchi T, Inoue H, Tanaka T: The M_1- and M_2-type isozymes of rat pyruvate kinase are produced from the same gene by alternative RNA splicing. *J Biol Chem* 261:13807–13812, 1986.

118. Kanno H, Fujii H, Miwa S: Structural analysis of human pyruvate kinase L-gene and identification of the promoter activity in erythroid cells. *Biochem Biophys Res Commun* 188:516–523, 1992.

119. Noguchi T, Yamada K, Inoue H, et al: The L- and R-type isozymes of rat pyruvate kinase are produced from a single gene by use of different promoters. *J Biol Chem* 262:14366–14371, 1987.

120. van Oirschot BA, Francois JJ, van Solinge WW, et al: Novel type of red blood cell pyruvate kinase hyperactivity predicts a remote regulatory locus involved in *PKLR* gene expression. *Am J Hematol* 89:380–384, 2014.

121. Kanno H, Fujii H, Hirono A, et al: CDNA cloning of human R-type pyruvate kinase and identification of a single amino acid substitution (Thr[384]→Met) affecting enzymatic stability in a pyruvate kinase variant (PK Tokyo) associated with hereditary hemolytic anemia. *Proc Natl Acad Sci U S A* 88:8218–8221, 1991.

122. Kahn A, Marie J, Garreau H, et al: The genetic system of the L-type pyruvate kinase forms in man. Subunit structure, interrelation and kinetic characteristics of the pyruvate kinase enzymes from erythrocytes and liver. *Biochim Biophys Acta* 523:59–74, 1978.

123. Kahn A, Marie J: Pyruvate kinases from human erythrocytes and liver. *Methods Enzymol* 90:131–140, 1982.

124. Valentini G, Chiarelli LR, Fortin R, et al: Structure and function of human erythrocyte pyruvate kinase. Molecular basis of nonspherocytic hemolytic anemia. *J Biol Chem* 277:23807–23814, 2002.

125. Enriqueta Muñoz M, Ponce E: Pyruvate kinase: Current status of regulatory and functional properties. *Comp Biochem Physiol B Biochem Mol Biol* 135:197–218, 2003.

126. Wang C, Chiarelli LR, Bianchi P, et al: Human erythrocyte pyruvate kinase: Characterization of the recombinant enzyme and a mutant form (R510Q) causing nonspherocytic hemolytic anemia. *Blood* 98:3113–3120, 2001.

127. Fenton AW, Tang Q: An activating interaction between the unphosphorylated n-terminus of human liver pyruvate kinase and the main body of the protein is interrupted by phosphorylation. *Biochemistry* 48:3816–3818, 2009.

128. Jurica MS, Mesecar A, Heath PJ, et al: The allosteric regulation of pyruvate kinase by fructose-1,6-bisphosphate. *Structure* 6:195–210, 1998.

129. Rigden DJ, Phillips SE, Michels PA, et al: The structure of pyruvate kinase from *Leishmania mexicana* reveals details of the allosteric transition and unusual effector specificity. *J Mol Biol* 291:615–635, 1999.

130. Valentini G, Chiarelli L, Fortin R, et al: The allosteric regulation of pyruvate kinase. *J Biol Chem* 275:18145–18152, 2000.

131. Wooll JO, Friesen RH, White MA, et al: Structural and functional linkages between subunit interfaces in mammalian pyruvate kinase. *J Mol Biol* 312:525–540, 2001.

132. Fenton AW, Blair JB: Kinetic and allosteric consequences of mutations in the subunit and domain interfaces and the allosteric site of yeast pyruvate kinase. *Arch Biochem Biophys* 397:28–39, 2002.

133. Blume KG, Hoffbauer RW, Busch D, et al: Purification and properties of pyruvate kinase in normal and in pyruvate kinase deficient human red blood cells. *Biochim Biophys Acta* 227:364–372, 1971.

134. Kitamura M, Iijima N, Hashimoto F, et al: Hereditary deficiency of subunit H of lactate dehydrogenase. *Clin Chim Acta* 34:419–423, 1971.

135. Joukyuu R, Mizuno S, Amakawa T, et al: Hereditary complete deficiency of lactate dehydrogenase H-subunit. *Clin Chem* 35:687–690, 1989.

136. Wakabayashi H, Tsuchiya M, Yoshino K, et al: Hereditary deficiency of lactate dehydrogenase H-subunit. *Intern Med* 35:550–554, 1996.

137. Kanno T, Maekawa M: Lactate dehydrogenase M-subunit deficiencies: Clinical features, metabolic background, and genetic heterogeneities. *Muscle Nerve Suppl* 3:S54–S60, 1995.

138. Maekawa M, Sudo K, Nagura K, et al: Population screening of lactate dehydrogenase deficiencies in Fukuoka Prefecture in Japan and molecular characterization of three independent mutations in the lactate dehydrogenase-B(H) gene. *Hum Genet* 93:74–76, 1994.

139. Persico MG, Viglietto G, Martini G, et al: Isolation of human glucose-6-phosphate dehydrogenase (G6PD) cDNA clones: Primary structure of the protein and unusual 5′ non-coding region. *Nucleic Acids Res* 14:2511–2522, 1986.

140. Kirkman HN, Hendrickson EM: Glucose 6-phosphate dehydrogenase from human erythrocytes. II. Subactive states of the enzyme from normal persons. *J Biol Chem* 237:2371–2376, 1962.

141. Bonsignore A, Cancedda R, Nicolini A, et al: Metabolism of human erythrocyte glucose-6-phosphate dehydrogenase. VI. Interconversion of multiple molecular forms. *Arch Biochem Biophys* 147:493–501, 1971.

142. Canepa L, Ferraris AM, Miglino M, et al: Bound and unbound pyridine dinucleotides in normal and glucose- 6-phosphate dehydrogenase-deficient erythrocytes. *Biochim Biophys Acta* 1074:101–104, 1991.

143. Au SW, Gover S, Lam VM, Adams MJ: Human glucose-6-phosphate dehydrogenase: The crystal structure reveals a structural NADP⁺ molecule and provides insights into enzyme deficiency. *Structure* 8:293–303, 2000.

144. Cohen P, Rosemeyer MA: Subunit interactions of glucose-6-phosphate dehydrogenase from human erythrocytes. *Eur J Biochem* 8:8–15, 1969.

145. Wrigley NG, Heather JV, Bonsignore A, et al: Human erythrocyte glucose 6-phosphate dehydrogenase: Electron microscope studies on structure and interconversion of tetramers, dimers and monomers. *J Mol Biol* 68:483–499, 1972.

146. Yoshida A: Hemolytic anemia and G6PD deficiency. *Science* 179:532–537, 1973.

147. Ben-Bassat I, Beutler E: Inhibition by ATP of erythrocyte glucose-6-phosphate dehydrogenase variants. *Proc Soc Exp Biol Med* 142:410–411, 1973.

148. Zimran A, Torem S, Beutler E: The in vivo ageing of red cell enzymes: Direct evidence of biphasic decay from polycythaemic rabbits with reticulocytosis. *Br J Haematol* 69:67–70, 1988.

149. Cosgrove MS, Naylor C, Paludan S, et al: On the mechanism of the reaction catalyzed by glucose 6-phosphate dehydrogenase. *Biochemistry* 37:2759–2767, 1998.

150. Lee WT, Levy HR: Lysine-21 of Leuconostoc mesenteroides glucose 6-phosphate dehydrogenase participates in substrate binding through charge-charge interaction. *Protein Sci* 1:329–334, 1992.

151. Bautista JM, Mason PJ, Luzzatto L: Human glucose-6-phosphate dehydrogenase. Lysine 205 is dispensable for substrate binding but essential for catalysis. *FEBS Lett* 366:61–64, 1995.

152. Battistuzzi G, D'Urso M, Toniolo D, et al: Tissue-specific levels of human glucose-6-phosphate dehydrogenase correlate with methylation of specific sites at the 3′ end of the gene. *Proc Natl Acad Sci U S A* 82:1465–1469, 1985.

153. Toniolo D, D'Urso M, Martini G, et al: Specific methylation pattern at the 3′ end of the human housekeeping gene for glucose 6-phosphate dehydrogenase. *EMBO J* 3:1987–1995, 1984.

154. Amini F, Ismail EA: R. 3′-UTR variations and G6PD deficiency. *J Hum Genet* 58:189–194, 2013.

155. Beutler E: Genetics of glucose-6-phosphate dehydrogenase deficiency. *Semin Hematol* 27:137–164, 1990.

156. Luzzatto L, Mehta A: Glucose 6-phosphate dehydrogenase deficiency, in *The Metabolic and Molecular Basis of Inherited Disease*, 7th ed, edited by Scriver C, Beaudet AL, Sly WS, Valle D, pp 3367–3398. McGraw Hill, New York, 1995.

157. Mason PJ: New insights into G6PD deficiency. *Br J Haematol* 94:585–591, 1996.

158. Mason PJ, Bautista JM, Gilsanz F: G6PD deficiency: The genotype-phenotype association. *Blood Rev* 21:267–283, 2007.

159. Cappellini MD, Fiorelli G: Glucose-6-phosphate dehydrogenase deficiency. *Lancet* 371:64–74, 2008.

160. Minucci A, Moradkhani K, Hwang MJ, et al: Glucose-6-phosphate dehydrogenase (G6PD) mutations database: Review of the "old" and update of the new mutations. *Blood Cells Mol Dis* 48:154–165, 2012.

161. Beutler E, Kuhl W: Limiting role of 6-phosphogluconolactonase in erythrocyte hexose monophosphate pathway metabolism. *J Lab Clin Med* 106:573–577, 1985.

162. Rakitzis ET, Papandreou P: Kinetic analysis of 6-phosphogluconolactone hydrolysis in hemolysates. *Biochem Mol Biol Int* 37:747–755, 1995.

163. Beutler E, Kuhl W, Gelbart T: 6-Phosphogluconolactonase deficiency, a hereditary erythrocyte enzyme deficiency: Possible interaction with glucose-6-phosphate dehydrogenase deficiency. *Proc Natl Acad Sci U S A* 82:3876–3878, 1985.

164. Thorburn DR, Kuchel PW: Computer simulation of the metabolic consequences of the combined deficiency of 6-phosphogluconolactonase and glucose-6-phosphate dehydrogenase in human erythrocytes. *J Lab Clin Med* 110:70–74, 1987.

165. Shih L, Justice P, Hsia DY: Purification and characterization of genetic variants of 6-phosphogluconate dehydrogenase. *Biochem Genet* 1:359–371, 1968.

166. Parr CW, Fitch LI: Inherited quantitative variations of human phosphogluconate dehydrogenase. *Ann Hum Genet.* 30:339–353, 1967.

167. Caprari P, Caforio MP, Cianciulli P, et al: 6-Phosphogluconate dehydrogenase deficiency in an Italian family. *Ann Hematol* 80:41–44, 2001.

168. Vives Corrons JL, Colomer D, Pujades A, et al: Congenital 6-phosphogluconate dehydrogenase (6PGD) deficiency associated with chronic hemolytic anemia in a Spanish family. *Am J Hematol* 53:221–227, 1996.

169. Wamelink MM, Gruning NM, Jansen EE, et al: The difference between rare and exceptionally rare: Molecular characterization of ribose 5-phosphate isomerase deficiency. *J Mol Med (Berl)* 88:931–939, 2010.

170. Huck JH, Verhoeven NM, Struys EA, et al: Ribose-5-phosphate isomerase deficiency: New inborn error in the pentose phosphate pathway associated with a slowly progressive leukoencephalopathy. *Am J Hum Genet* 74:745–751, 2004.

171. Dische Z, Bishop C, Surgenor DM: The pentose phosphate metabolism in red cells, in *The Red Blood Cell*, pp 189–209. Academic Press, New York, 1964.

172. Brownstone YS, Denstedt OF: The pentose phosphate metabolic pathway in the human erythrocyte. II. The transketolase and transaldolase activity of the human erythrocyte. *Can J Biochem* 39:533–545, 1961.

173. Kochetov GA, Solovjeva ON: Structure and functioning mechanism of transketolase. *Biochim Biophys Acta* 1844:1608–1618, 2014.

174. Soukaloun D, Lee SJ, Chamberlain K, et al: Erythrocyte transketolase activity, markers of cardiac dysfunction and the diagnosis of infantile beriberi. *PLoS Negl Trop Dis* 5:e971, 2011.

175. Wamelink MM, Struys EA, Jakobs C: The biochemistry, metabolism and inherited defects of the pentose phosphate pathway: A review. *J Inherit Metab Dis* 31:703–717, 2008.

176. Verhoeven NM, Huck JH, Roos B, et al: Transaldolase deficiency: Liver cirrhosis associated with a new inborn error in the pentose phosphate pathway. *Am J Hum Genet* 68:1086–1092, 2001.

177. Eyaid W, Al Harbi T, Anazi S, et al: Transaldolase deficiency: Report of 12 new cases and further delineation of the phenotype. *J Inherit Metab Dis* 36:997–1004, 2013.

178. Tylki-Szymanska A, Wamelink MM, Stradomska TJ, et al: Clinical and molecular characteristics of two transaldolase-deficient patients. *Eur J Pediatr* 173:1679–1682, 2014.

179. Valayannopoulos V, Verhoeven NM, Mention K, et al: Transaldolase deficiency: A new cause of hydrops fetalis and neonatal multi-organ disease. *J Pediatr* 149:713–717, 2006.

180. Wamelink MM, Struys EA, Salomons GS, et al: Transaldolase deficiency in a two-year-old boy with cirrhosis. *Mol Genet Metab* 94:255–258, 2008.

181. Beutler E, Guinto E: The reduction of glyceraldehyde by human erythrocytes. L-hexonate dehydrogenase activity. *J Clin Invest* 53:1258–1264, 1974.

182. Das B, Srivastava SK: Purification and properties of aldose reductase and aldehyde reductase II from human erythrocyte. *Arch Biochem Biophys.* 238:670–679, 1985.

183. Reddy GB, Satyanarayana A, Balakrishna N, et al: Erythrocyte aldose reductase activity and sorbitol levels in diabetic retinopathy. *Mol Vis* 14:593–601, 2008.

184. Gupta P, Verma N, Bhattacharya S, et al: Association of diabetic autonomic neuropathy with red blood cell aldose reductase activity. *Can J Diabetes* 38:22–25, 2014.

185. van Solinge WW, van Wijk R: Disorders of red cells resulting from enzyme abnormalities, in *Williams Hematology*, 8th ed, pp 647–674, edited by Kaushansky KJ, Lichtman MA, Beutler E, Kipps TJ, Selighsohn U, Prchal JT. McGraw-Hill, New York, 2010.

186. Fargo JH, Kratz CP, Giri N, et al: Erythrocyte adenosine deaminase: Diagnostic value for Diamond-Blackfan anaemia. *Br J Haematol* 160:547–554, 2013.

187. Dimant E, Landberg E, London IM: The metabolic behavior of reduced glutathione in human and avian erythrocytes. *J Biol Chem* 213:769–776, 1955.

188. van't Erve TJ, Wagner BA, Ryckman KK, et al: The concentration of glutathione in human erythrocytes is a heritable trait. *Free Radic Biol Med* 65:742–749, 2013.

189. Ellison I, Richie JP Jr: Mechanisms of glutathione disulfide efflux from erythrocytes. *Biochem Pharmacol* 83:164–169, 2012.

190. Gipp JJ, Chang C, Mulcahy RT: Cloning and nucleotide sequence of a full-length cDNA for human liver gamma-glutamylcysteine synthetase. *Biochem Biophys Res Commun* 185:29–35, 1992.

191. Gipp JJ, Bailey HH, Mulcahy RT: Cloning and sequencing of the cDNA for the light subunit of human liver gamma-glutamylcysteine synthetase and relative mRNA levels for heavy and light subunits in human normal tissues. *Biochem Biophys Res Commun* 206:584–589, 1995.

192. Biterova EI, Barycki JJ: Mechanistic details of glutathione biosynthesis revealed by crystal structures of *Saccharomyces cerevisiae* glutamate cysteine ligase. *J Biol Chem* 284:32700–32708, 2009.

193. Kumar S, Kasturia N, Sharma A, et al: Redox-dependent stability of the gamma-glutamylcysteine synthetase enzyme of *Escherichia coli*: A novel means of redox regulation. *Biochem J* 449:783–794, 2013.

194. Krejsa CM, Franklin CC, White CC, et al: Rapid activation of glutamate cysteine ligase following oxidative stress. *J Biol Chem* 285:16116–16124, 2010.

195. Nichenametla SN, Lazarus P, Richie JP Jr: A GAG trinucleotide-repeat polymorphism in the gene for glutathione biosynthetic enzyme, GCLC, affects gene expression through translation. *FASEB J* 25:2180–2187, 2011.

196. Gali RR, Board PG: Sequencing and expression of a cDNA for human glutathione synthetase. *Biochem J* 310(Pt 1):353–358, 1995.

197. Polekhina G, Board PG, Gali RR, et al: Molecular basis of glutathione synthetase deficiency and a rare gene permutation event. *EMBO J* 18:3204–3213, 1999.

198. Cohen G, Hochstein P: Glutathione peroxidase: The primary agent for the elimination of hydrogen peroxide in erythrocytes. *Biochemistry* 2:1420–1428, 1963.

199. Johnson RM, Goyette G, Jr, Ravindranath Y, et al: Red cells from glutathione peroxidase-1-deficient mice have nearly normal defenses against exogenous peroxides. *Blood* 96:1985–1988, 2000.

200. Rotruck JT, Pope AL, Ganther HE, et al: Selenium: Biochemical role as a component of glutathione peroxidase. *Science* 179:588–590, 1973.

201. Beutler E, Matsumoto F: Ethnic variation in red cell glutathione peroxidase activity. *Blood* 46:103–110, 1975.

202. Beutler E: Red cell enzyme defects as nondiseases and as diseases. *Blood* 54:1–7, 1979.

203. Jacob HS, Jandl JH: Effects of sulfhydryl inhibition on red blood cells. I. Mechanism of hemolysis. *J Clin Invest* 41:779–792, 1962.

204. Valentine WN, Toohey JI, Paglia DE, et al: Modification of erythrocyte enzyme activities by persulfides and methanethiol: Possible regulatory role. *Proc Natl Acad Sci U S A* 84:1394–1398, 1987.

205. Ogasawara Y, Funakoshi M, Ishii K: Pyruvate kinase is protected by glutathione-dependent redox balance in human red blood cells exposed to reactive oxygen species. *Biol Pharm Bull* 31:1875–1881, 2008.

206. Magnani M, Stocchi V, Ninfali P, et al: Action of oxidized and reduced glutathione on rabbit red blood cell hexokinase. *Biochim Biophys Acta* 615:113–120, 1980.

207. Huisman TH, Dozy AM: Studies on the heterogeneity of hemoglobin. V. Binding of hemoglobin with oxidized glutathione. *J Lab Clin Med* 60:302–319, 1962.

208. Kelner MJ, Montoya MA: Structural organization of the human glutathione reductase gene: Determination of correct cDNA sequence and identification of a mitochondrial leader sequence. *Biochem Biophys Res Commun* 269:366–368, 2000.

209. Karplus PA, Schulz GE: Refined structure of glutathione reductase at 1.54 A resolution. *J Mol Biol* 195:701–729, 1987.

210. Wong KK, Blanchard JS: Human erythrocyte glutathione reductase: PH dependence of kinetic parameters. *Biochemistry* 28:3586–3590, 1989.

211. Beutler E, Yeh MK: Y. Erythrocyte glutathione reductase. *Blood* 21:573–585, 1963.

212. Beutler E: Glutathione reductase: Stimulation in normal subjects by riboflavin supplementation. *Science* 165:613–615, 1969.

213. Hoey L, McNulty H, Strain JJ: Studies of biomarker responses to intervention with riboflavin: A systematic review. *Am J Clin Nutr* 89:1960S–1980S, 2009.

214. Mojzikova R, Dolezel P, Pavlicek J, et al: Partial glutathione reductase deficiency as a cause of diverse clinical manifestations in a family with unstable hemoglobin (Hemoglobin Hana, beta63(E7) His-Asn). *Blood Cells Mol Dis* 45:219–222, 2010.

215. Mieyal JJ, Starke DW, Gravina SA, et al: Thioltransferase in human red blood cells: Kinetics and equilibrium. *Biochemistry* 30:8883–8891, 1991.

216. Mieyal JJ, Starke DW, Gravina SA, et al: Thioltransferase in human red blood cells: Purification and properties. *Biochemistry* 30:6088–6097, 1991.

217. Srivastava SK, Beutler E: The transport of oxidized glutathione from human erythrocytes. *J Biol Chem* 244:9–16, 1969.

218. Prchal J, Srivastava SK, Beutler E: Active transport of GSSG from reconstituted erythrocyte ghosts. *Blood* 46:111–117, 1975.

219. Lunn G, Dale GL, Beutler E: Transport accounts for glutathione turnover in human erythrocytes. *Blood* 54:238–244, 1979.

220. Kondo T, Kawakami Y, Taniguchi N, et al: Glutathione disulfide-stimulated Mg2+-ATPase of human erythrocyte membranes. *Proc Natl Acad Sci U S A* 84:7373–7377, 1987.

221. Board PG: Transport of glutathione S-conjugate from human erythrocytes. *FEBS Lett* 124:163–165, 1981.

222. Kondo T, Murao M, Taniguchi N: Glutathione S-conjugate transport using inside-out vesicles from human erythrocytes. *Eur J Biochem* 125:551–554, 1982.

223. Pulaski L, Jedlitschky G, Leier I, et al: Identification of the multidrug-resistance protein (MRP) as the glutathione-S-conjugate export pump of erythrocytes. *Eur J Biochem* 241:644–648, 1996.

224. Marcus CJ, Habig WH, Jakoby WB: Glutathione transferase from human erythrocytes. Nonidentity with the enzymes from liver. *Arch Biochem Biophys* 188:287–293, 1978.

225. Awasthi YC, Singh SV: Purification and characterization of a new form of glutathione S-transferase from human erythrocytes. *Biochim Biophys Res Commun* 125:1053–1060, 1984.

226. Schroder KR, Hallier E, Meyer DJ, et al: Purification and characterization of a new glutathione S-transferase, class theta, from human erythrocytes. *Arch Toxicol.* 70:559–566, 1996.

227. Harvey JW, Beutler E: Binding of heme by glutathione S-transferase: A possible role of the erythrocyte enzyme. *Blood* 60:1227–1230, 1982.

228. Beutler E, Dunning D, Dabe IB, et al: Erythrocyte glutathione S-transferase deficiency and hemolytic anemia. *Blood* 72:73–77, 1988.

229. Winterbourn CC, Hawkins RE, Brian M, et al: The estimation of red cell superoxide dismutase activity. *J Lab Clin Med* 85:337–341, 1975.

230. Rosen DR, Siddique T, Patterson D, et al: Mutations in Cu/Zn superoxide dismutase gene are associated with familial amyotrophic lateral sclerosis. *Nature* 362:59–62, 1993.

231. Grzelak A, Kruszewski M, Macierzyńska E, et al: The effects of superoxide dismutase knockout on the oxidative stress parameters and survival of mouse erythrocytes. *Cell Mol Biol Lett* 14:23–34, 2009.

232. Iuchi Y, Okada F, Takamiya R, et al: Rescue of anaemia and autoimmune responses in SOD1-deficient mice by transgenic expression of human SOD1 in erythrocytes. *Biochem J* 422:313–320, 2009.

233. Goth L, Nagy T: Inherited catalase deficiency: Is it benign or a factor in various age related disorders? *Mutat Res* 753:147–154, 2013.

234. Takahara S: Progressive oral gangrene probably due to lack of catalase in the blood (acatalasaemia); report of nine cases. *Lancet* 2:1101–1104, 1952.

235. Low FM, Hampton MB, Peskin AV, et al: Peroxiredoxin 2 functions as a noncatalytic scavenger of low-level hydrogen peroxide in the erythrocyte. *Blood* 109:2611–2617, 2007.

236. Lee T-H, Kim S-U, Yu S-L, et al: Peroxiredoxin II is essential for sustaining life span of erythrocytes in mice. *Blood* 101:5033–5038, 2003.

237. Kwon TH, Han YH, Hong SG, et al: Reactive oxygen species mediated DNA damage is essential for abnormal erythropoiesis in peroxiredoxin II(−/−) mice. *Biochem Biophys Res Commun* 424:189–195, 2012.

238. Johnson RM, Ho Y-S, Yu D-Y, et al: The effects of disruption of genes for peroxiredoxin-2, glutathione peroxidase-1, and catalase on erythrocyte oxidative metabolism. *Free Radic Biol Med* 48:519–525, 2010.

239. Nagababu E, Mohanty JG, Friedman JS, et al: Role of peroxiredoxin-2 in protecting RBCs from hydrogen peroxide-induced oxidative stress. *Free Radic Res* 47:164–171, 2013.

240. van Zwieten R, Verhoeven AJ, Roos D: Inborn defects in the antioxidant systems of human red blood cells. *Free Radic Biol Med.* 67:377–386, 2014.

241. Abrusci P, Chiarelli LR, Galizzi A, et al: Erythrocyte adenylate kinase deficiency: Characterization of recombinant mutant forms and relationship with nonspherocytic hemolytic anemia. *Exp Hematol* 35:1182–1189, 2007.

242. Balasubramaniam S, Duley JA, Christodoulou J: Inborn errors of purine metabolism: Clinical update and therapies. *J Inherit Metab Dis* 37:669–686, 2014.

243. Valentine WN, Paglia DE: Erythrocyte disorders of purine and pyrimidine metabolism. *Hemoglobin* 4:669–681, 1980.

244. Valentine WN, Fink K, Paglia DE, et al: Hereditary hemolytic anemia with human erythrocyte pyrimidine 5'-nucleotidase deficiency. *J Clin Invest* 54:866–879, 1974.

245. Paglia DE, Valentine WN: Characteristics of a pyrimidine-specific 5'-nucleotidase in human erythrocytes. *J Biol Chem* 250:7973–7979, 1975.

246. Beutler E, Hartman G: Age-related red cell enzymes in children with transient erythroblastopenia of childhood and with hemolytic anemia. *Pediatr Res* 19:44–47, 1985.

247. Amici A, Emanuelli M, Magni G, et al: Pyrimidine nucleotidases from human erythrocyte possess phosphotransferase activities specific for pyrimidine nucleotides. *FEBS Lett* 419:263–267, 1997.

248. Bitto E, Bingman CA, Wesenberg GE, et al: Structure of pyrimidine 5'-nucleotidase type 1. Insight into mechanism of action and inhibition during lead poisoning. *J Biol Chem* 281:20521–20529, 2006.

249. Marinaki AM, Escuredo E, Duley JA, et al: Genetic basis of hemolytic anemia caused by pyrimidine 5' nucleotidase deficiency. *Blood* 97:3327–3332, 2001.

250. Kanno H, Takizawa T, Miwa S, et al: Molecular basis of Japanese variants of pyrimidine 5'-nucleotidase deficiency. *Br J Haematol* 126:265–271, 2004.

251. Hirono A, Fujii H, Natori H, et al: Chromatographic analysis of human erythrocyte pyrimidine 5'-nucleotidase from five patients with pyrimidine 5'-nucleotidase deficiency. *Br J Haematol* 65:35–41, 1987.

252. Sestini S, Ricci C, Micheli V, et al: Nicotinamide mononucleotide adenylyltransferase activity in human erythrocytes. *Arch Biochem Biophys* 302:206–211, 1993.

253. Di Stefano M, Galassi L, Magni G: Unique expression pattern of human nicotinamide mononucleotide adenylyltransferase isozymes in red blood cells. *Blood Cells Mol Dis* 45:33–39, 2010.

254. Hikosaka K, Ikutani M, Shito M, et al: Deficiency of nicotinamide mononucleotide adenylyltransferase 3 (Nmnat3) causes hemolytic anemia by altering the glycolytic flow in mature erythrocytes. *J Biol Chem* 289:14796–14811, 2014.

255. Arnold H, Blume KG, Lohr GW, et al: "Acquired" red cell enzyme defects in hematological diseases. *Clin Chim Acta* 57:187–189, 1974.

256. Boivin P, Galand C, Hakim J, et al: Acquired erythroenzymopathies in blood disorders: Study of 200 cases. *Br J Haematol* 31:531–543, 1975.

257. Kahn A, Marie J, Bernard J-F, et al: Mechanisms of the acquired erythrocyte enzyme deficiencies in blood diseases. *Clin Chim Acta* 71:379–387, 1976.

258. Kahn A: Abnormalities of erythrocyte enzymes in dyserythropoiesis and malignancies. *Clin Haematol* 10:123–138, 1981.

259. Kornberg A, Goldfarb A: Preleukemia manifested by hemolytic anemia with pyruvate-kinase deficiency. *Arch Intern Med* 146:785–786, 1986.

260. Shinohara K, Tanaka KR: Hereditary deficiency of erythrocyte acetylcholinesterase. *Am J Hematol* 7:313–321, 1979.

261. Rosa R, George C, Fardeau M, et al: A new case of phosphoglycerate kinase deficiency: PGK Creteil associated with rhabdomyolysis and lacking hemolytic anemia. *Blood* 60:84–91, 1982.

262. Marstein S, Jellum E, Halpern B, et al: Biochemical studies of erythrocytes in a patient with pyroglutamic acidemia (5-oxoprolinemia). *N Engl J Med* 295:406–412, 1976.

263. Beutler E, Carson D, Dannawi H, et al: Metabolic compensation for profound erythrocyte adenylate kinase deficiency. *J Clin Invest* 72:648–655, 1983.

264. Beutler E: *Hemolytic Anemia in Disorders of Red Cell Metabolism*. Plenum Press, New York, 1978.

265. Glucose-6-phosphate dehydrogenase deficiency. WHO Working Group. *Bull World Health Organ* 67:601–611, 1989.

266. Betke K, Beutler E, Brewer GJ, et al: Standardization of procedures for the study of glucose-6-phosphate dehydrogenase. Report of a WHO scientific group. *World Health Organ Tech Rep Ser* 366:1–53, 1967.

267. Piomelli S, Corash LM, Davenport DD, et al: In vivo lability of glucose-6-phosphate dehydrogenase in GdA- and Gd Mediterranean deficiency. *J Clin Invest* 47:940–948, 1968.

268. Kahn A, Cottreau D, Boivin P: Molecular mechanism of glucose-6-phosphate dehydrogenase deficiency. *Humangenetik* 25:101–109, 1974.

269. Beutler E: Selectivity of proteases as a basis for tissue distribution of enzymes in hereditary deficiencies. *Proc Natl Acad Sci U S A* 80:3767–3768, 1983.

270. Kirkman HN, Schettini F, Pickard BM: Mediterranean variant of glucose-6-phosphate dehydrogenase. *J Lab Clin Med* 63:726–735, 1964.

271. Longo L, Vanegas OC, Patel M, et al: Maternally transmitted severe glucose 6-phosphate dehydrogenase deficiency is an embryonic lethal. *EMBO J* 21:4229–4239, 2002.

272. Takizawa T, Yoneyama Y, Miwa S, et al: A single nucleotide base transition is the basis of the common human glucose-6-phosphate dehydrogenase variant A(+). *Genomics* 1:228–231, 1987.

273. Hirono A, Beutler E: Molecular cloning and nucleotide sequence of cDNA for human glucose-6-phosphate dehydrogenase variant A(−). *Proc Natl Acad Sci U S A* 85:3951–3954, 1988.

274. Beutler E, Kuhl W, Vives-Corrons JL, et al: Molecular heterogeneity of glucose-6-phosphate dehydrogenase A−. *Blood* 74:2550–2555, 1989.

275. Vulliamy TJ, Othman A, Town M, et al: Polymorphic sites in the African population detected by sequence analysis of the glucose-6-phosphate dehydrogenase gene outline the evolution of the variants A and A−. *Proc Natl Acad Sci U S A* 88:8568–8571, 1991.

276. Town M, Bautista JM, Mason PJ, et al: Both mutations in G6PD A− are necessary to produce the G6PD deficient phenotype. *Hum Mol Genet.* 1:171–174, 1992.

277. Vulliamy TJ, D'Urso M, Battistuzzi G, et al: Diverse point mutations in the human glucose 6-phosphate dehydrogenase gene cause enzyme deficiency and mild or severe hemolytic anemia. *Proc Natl Acad Sci U S A* 85:5171–5175, 1988.

278. Ho HY, Cheng ML, Chiu DT: Glucose-6-phosphate dehydrogenase-beyond the realm of red cell biology. *Free Radic Res* 48:1028–1048, 2014.

279. MacDonald D, Town M, Mason P, et al: Deficiency in red blood cells. *Nature* 350:115–115, 1991.

280. Roos D, van Zwieten R, Wijnen JT, et al: Molecular basis and enzymatic properties of glucose 6-phosphate dehydrogenase volendam, leading to chronic nonspherocytic anemia, granulocyte dysfunction, and increased susceptibility to infections. *Blood* 94:2955–2962, 1999.

281. van Bruggen R, Bautista JM, Petropoulou T, et al: Deletion of leucine 61 in glucose-6-phosphate dehydrogenase leads to chronic nonspherocytic anemia, granulocyte dysfunction, and increased susceptibility to infections. *Blood* 100:1026–1030, 2002.

282. van Wijk R, Huizinga EG, Prins I, et al: Distinct phenotypic expression of two de novo missense mutations affecting the dimer interface of glucose-6-phosphate dehydrogenase. *Blood Cells Mol Dis* 32:112–117, 2004.

283. Smith JE, Ryer K, Wallace L: Glucose-6-phosphate dehydrogenase deficiency in a dog. *Enzyme* 21:379–382, 1976.

284. Sanders S, Smith DP, Thomas GA, et al: A glucose-6-phosphate dehydrogenase (G6PD) splice site consensus sequence mutation associated with G6PD enzyme deficiency. *Mutat Res* 374:79–87, 1997.

285. Stockham SL, Harvey JW, Kinden DA: Equine glucose-6-phosphate dehydrogenase deficiency. *Vet Pathol* 31:518–527, 1994.

286. Rovira A, De Angioletti M, Camacho-Vanegas O, et al: Stable in vivo expression of glucose-6-phosphate dehydrogenase (G6PD) and rescue of G6PD deficiency in stem cells by gene transfer. *Blood* 96:4111–4117, 2000.

287. van Wijk R, van Solinge WW: The energy-less red blood cell is lost: Erythrocyte enzyme abnormalities of glycolysis. *Blood* 106:4034–4042, 2005.

288. Beutler E, Forman L, Rios-Larrain E: Elevated pyruvate kinase activity in patients with hemolytic anemia due to red cell pyruvate kinase "deficiency." *Am J Med* 83:899–904, 1987.

289. Zanella A, Fermo E, Bianchi P, et al: Pyruvate kinase deficiency: The genotype-phenotype association. *Blood Rev* 21:217–231, 2007.

290. Van Wijk R, Huizinga EG, Van Wesel AC: W., et al: Fifteen novel mutations in *PKLR* associated with pyruvate kinase (PK) deficiency: Structural implications of amino acid substitutions in PK. *Hum Mutat* 30:446–453, 2009.

291. Demina A, Varughese KI, Barbot J, et al: Six previously undescribed pyruvate kinase mutations causing enzyme deficiency. *Blood* 92:647–652, 1998.

292. Aizawa S, Kohdera U, Hiramoto M, et al: Ineffective erythropoiesis in the spleen of a patient with pyruvate kinase deficiency. *Am J Hematol* 74:68–72, 2003.

293. Aizawa S, Harada T, Kanbe E, et al: Ineffective erythropoiesis in mutant mice with deficient pyruvate kinase activity. *Exp Hematol* 33:1292–1298, 2005.

294. Viprakasit V, Ekwattanakit S, Riolueang S, et al: Mutations in Krüppel-like factor 1 cause transfusion-dependent hemolytic anemia and persistence of embryonic globin gene expression. *Blood* 123:1586–1595, 2014.

295. Durand PM, Coetzer TL: Pyruvate kinase deficiency protects against malaria in humans. *Haematologica* 93:939–940, 2008.

296. Ayi K, Min-OoG, Serghides L, et al: Pyruvate kinase deficiency and malaria. *N Engl J Med* 358:1805–1810, 2008.

297. Ayi K, Liles WC, Gros P, et al: Adenosine triphosphate depletion of erythrocytes simulates the phenotype associated with pyruvate kinase deficiency and confers protection against *Plasmodium falciparum* in vitro. *J Infect Dis* 200:1289–1299, 2009.

298. Machado P, Pereira R, Rocha AM, et al: Malaria: Looking for selection signatures in the human PKLR gene region. *Br J Haematol* 149:775–784, 2010.

299. Berghout J, Higgins S, Loucoubar C, et al: Genetic diversity in human erythrocyte pyruvate kinase. *Genes Immun* 13:98–102, 2011.

300. Machado P, Manco L, Gomes C, et al: Pyruvate kinase deficiency in sub-Saharan Africa: Identification of a highly frequent missense mutation (G829A;Glu277Lys) and association with malaria. *PLoS One* 7:e47071, 2012.

301. Owen JL, Harvey JW: Hemolytic anemia in dogs and cats due to erythrocyte enzyme deficiencies. *Vet Clin North Am Small Anim Pract* 42:73–84, 2011.

302. Whitney KM, Goodman SA, Bailey EM, et al: The molecular basis of canine pyruvate kinase deficiency. *Exp Hematol* 22:866–874, 1994.

303. Zaucha JA, Yu C, Lothrop CD, Jr, et al: Severe canine hereditary hemolytic anemia treated by nonmyeloablative marrow transplantation. *Biol Blood Marrow Transplant* 7:14–24, 2001.

304. Bader R, Bode G, Rebel W, et al: Stimulation of bone marrow by administration of excessive doses of recombinant human erythropoietin. *Pathol Res Pract* 188:676–679, 1992.

305. Trobridge GD, Beard BC, Wu RA, et al: Stem cell selection in vivo using foamy vectors cures canine pyruvate kinase deficiency. *PLoS One* 7:e45173, 2012.

306. Tsujino K, Kanno H, Hashimoto K, et al: Delayed onset of hemolytic anemia in CBA-*Pk-1^slc^/Pk-1^slc^* mice with a point mutation of the gene encoding red blood cell type pyruvate kinase. *Blood* 91:2169–2174, 1998.

307. Kanno H, Utsugisawa T, Aizawa S, et al: Transgenic rescue of hemolytic anemia due to red blood cell pyruvate kinase deficiency. *Haematologica* 92:731–737, 2007.

308. Meza NW, Alonso-Ferrero ME, Navarro S, et al: Rescue of pyruvate kinase deficiency in mice by gene therapy using the human isoenzyme. *Mol Ther* 17:2000–2009, 2009.

309. Kanno H: Hexokinase: Gene structure and mutations. *Baillieres Best Pract Res Clin Haematol* 13:83–88, 2000.

310. Kanno H, Murakami K, Hariyama Y, et al: Homozygous intragenic deletion of type I hexokinase gene causes lethal hemolytic anemia of the affected fetus. *Blood* 100:1930, 2002.

311. de Vooght KM: K., van Solinge WW, van Wesel AC, et al: First mutation in the red blood cell-specific promoter of hexokinase combined with a novel missense mutation causes hexokinase deficiency and mild chronic hemolysis. *Haematologica* 94:1203–1210, 2009.

312. Bianchi M, Magnani M: Hexokinase mutations that produce nonspherocytic hemolytic anemia. *Blood Cells Mol Dis* 21:2–8, 1995.

313. Van Wijk R, Rijksen G, Huizinga EG, et al: HK Utrecht: Missense mutation in the active site of human hexokinase associated with hexokinase deficiency and severe nonspherocytic hemolytic anemia. *Blood* 101:345–347, 2003.

314. Peters LL, Lane PW, Andersen SG, et al: Downeast anemia (*dea*), a new mouse model of severe nonspherocytic hemolytic anemia caused by hexokinase (HK_I) deficiency. *Blood Cells Mol Dis* 27:850–860, 2001.

315. Kugler W, Lakomek M: Glucose-6-phosphate isomerase deficiency. *Baillieres Best Pract Res Clin Haematol* 13:89–101, 2000.

316. Clarke JL, Vulliamy TJ, Roper D, et al: Combined glucose-6-phosphate dehydrogenase and glucosephosphate isomerase deficiency can alter clinical outcome. *Blood Cells Mol Dis* 30:258–263, 2003.

317. Repiso A, Oliva B, Vives Corrons JL, et al: Glucose phosphate isomerase deficiency: Enzymatic and familial characterization of Arg346His mutation. *Biochim Biophys Acta* 1740:467–471, 2005.

318. Repiso A, Oliva B, Vives-Corrons JL, et al: Red cell glucose phosphate isomerase (GPI): A molecular study of three novel mutations associated with hereditary nonspherocytic hemolytic anemia. *Hum Mutat* 27: 1159, 2006.

319. Rossi F, Ruggiero S, Gallo M, et al: Amoxicillin-induced hemolytic anemia in a child with glucose 6-phosphate isomerase deficiency. *Ann Pharmacother* 44:1327–1329, 2010.

320. Warang P, Kedar P, Ghosh K, et al: Hereditary non-spherocytic hemolytic anemia and severe glucose phosphate isomerase deficiency in an Indian patient homozygous for the L487F mutation in the human GPI gene. *Int J Hematol* 96:263–267, 2012.

321. Read J, Pearce J, Li X, et al: The crystal structure of human phosphoglucose isomerase at 1.6 A resolution: Implications for catalytic mechanism, cytokine activity and haemolytic anaemia. *J Mol Biol* 309:447–463, 2001.

322. Lin HY, Kao YH, Chen ST, et al: Effects of inherited mutations on catalytic activity and structural stability of human glucose-6-phosphate isomerase expressed in Escherichia coli. *Biochim Biophys Acta* 1794:315–323, 2009.

323. Helleman PW, Van Biervliet JP: Haematological studies in a new variant of glucose-phosphate isomerase deficiency (GPI Utrecht). *Helv Paediatr Acta* 30:525–536, 1976.

324. Kahn A, Buc HA, Girot R, et al: Molecular and functional anomalies in two new mutant glucose-phosphate-isomerase variants with enzyme deficiency and chronic hemolysis. *Hum Genet* 40:293–304, 1978.

325. Schroter W, Eber SW, Bardosi A, et al: Generalised glucosephosphate isomerase (GPI) deficiency causing haemolytic anaemia, neuromuscular symptoms and impairment of granulocytic function: A new syndrome due to a new stable GPI variant with diminished specific activity (GPI Homburg). *Eur J Pediatr* 144:301–305, 1985.

326. Beutler E, West C, Britton HA, et al: Glucosephosphate isomerase (GPI) deficiency mutations associated with hereditary nonspherocytic hemolytic anemia (HNSHA). *Blood Cells Mol Dis* 23:402–409, 1997.

327. Zanella A, Izzo C, Rebulla P, et al: The first stable variant of erythrocyte glucose-phosphate isomerase associated with severe hemolytic anemia. *Am J Hematol* 9:1–11, 1980.

328. Shalev O, Shalev RS, Forman L, et al: GPI Mount Scopus—a variant of glucosephosphate isomerase deficiency. *Ann Hematol* 67:197–200, 1993.

329. Chaput M, Claes V, Portetelle D, et al: The neurotrophic factor neuroleukin is 90% homologous with phosphohexose isomerase. *Nature* 332:454–455, 1988.

330. Watanabe H, Takehana K, Date M, et al: Tumor cell autocrine motility factor is the neuroleukin/phosphohexose isomerase polypeptide. *Cancer Res* 56:2960–2963, 1996.

331. Gurney ME, Heinrich SP, Lee MR, et al: Molecular cloning and expression of neuroleukin, a neurotrophic factor for spinal and sensory neurons. *Science* 234:566–574, 1986.

332. Xu W, Seiter K, Feldman E, et al: The differentiation and maturation mediator for human myeloid leukemia cells shares homology with neuroleukin or phosphoglucose isomerase. *Blood* 87:4502–4506, 1996.

333. Kugler W, Breme K, Laspe P, et al: Molecular basis of neurological dysfunction coupled with haemolytic anaemia in human glucose-6-phosphate isomerase (GPI) deficiency. *Hum Genet* 103:450–454, 1998.

334. Haller JF, Smith C, Liu D, et al: Isolation of novel animal cell lines defective in glycerolipid biosynthesis reveals mutations in glucose-6-phosphate isomerase. *J Biol Chem* 285:866–877, 2010.

335. Haller JF, Krawczyk SA, Gostilovitch L, et al: Glucose-6-phosphate isomerase deficiency results in mTOR activation, failed translocation of lipin 1alpha to the nucleus and hypersensitivity to glucose: Implications for the inherited glycolytic disease. *Biochim Biophys Acta* 1812:1393–1402, 2011.

336. Merkle S, Pretsch W: Glucose-6-phosphate isomerase deficiency associated with non-spherocytic hemolytic anemia in the mouse: An animal model for the human disease. *Blood* 81:206–213, 1993.

337. West JD: A genetically defined animal model of anembryonic pregnancy. *Hum Reprod* 8:1316–1323, 1993.

338. Nakajima H, Raben N, Hamaguchi T, et al: Phosphofructokinase deficiency; past, present and future. *Curr Mol Med* 2:197–212, 2002.

339. Raben N, Sherman J, Miller F, et al: A 5′ splice junction mutation leading to exon deletion in an Ashkenazic Jewish family with phosphofructokinase deficiency (Tarui disease). *J Biol Chem* 268:4963–4967, 1993.

340. Tsujino S, Servidei S, Tonin P, et al: Identification of three novel mutations in non-Ashkenazi Italian patients with muscle phosphofructokinase deficiency. *Am J Hum Genet* 54:812–819, 1994.

341. Fujii H, Miwa S: Other erythrocyte enzyme deficiencies associated with non-haematological symptoms: Phosphoglycerate kinase and phosphofructokinase deficiency. *Baillieres Best Pract Res Clin Haematol* 13:141–148, 2000.

342. Raben N, Exelbert R, Spiegel R, et al: Functional expression of human mutant phosphofructokinase in yeast: Genetic defects in French Canadian and Swiss patients with phosphofructokinase deficiency. *Am J Hum Genet* 56:131–141, 1995.

343. Musumeci O, Bruno C, Mongini T, et al: Clinical features and new molecular findings in muscle phosphofructokinase deficiency (GSD type VII). *Neuromuscul Disord* 22:325–330, 2012.

344. Vives Corrons J-L, Koralkova P, Grau JM, et al: First identification of phosphofructokinase deficiency in Spain: Identification of a novel homozygous missense mutation in the PFKM gene. *Front Physiol* 4: 393, 2013.

345. Brüser A, Kirchberger J, Schöneberg T: Altered allosteric regulation of muscle 6-phosphofructokinase causes Tarui disease. *Biochem Biophys Res Commun* 427(1):133–137, 2012.

346. Nichols RC, Rudolphi O, Ek B, et al: Glycogenosis type VII (Tarui disease) in a Swedish family: Two novel mutations in muscle phosphofructokinase gene (PFK-M) resulting in intron retentions. *Am J Hum Genet* 59:59–65, 1996.

347. Hamaguchi T, Nakajima H, Noguchi T, et al: Novel missense mutation (W686C) of the phosphofructokinase-M gene in a Japanese patient with a mild form of glycogenosis VII. *Hum Mutat* 8:273–275, 1996.

348. Inal Gultekin G, Raj K, Lehman S, et al: Missense mutation in *PFKM* associated with muscle-type phosphofructokinase deficiency in the Wachtelhund dog. *Mol Cell Probes* 26:243–247, 2012.

349. Garcia M, Pujol A, Ruzo A, et al: Phosphofructo-1-kinase deficiency leads to a severe cardiac and hematological disorder in addition to skeletal muscle glycogenosis. *PLoS Genet* 5:e1000615, 2009.

350. Gerber K, Harvey JW, D'Agorne S, et al: Hemolysis, myopathy, and cardiac disease associated with hereditary phosphofructokinase deficiency in two Whippets. *Vet Clin Pathol* 38:46–51, 2009.

351. Miwa S, Fujii H, Tani K, et al: Two cases of red cell aldolase deficiency associated with hereditary hemolytic anemia in a Japanese family. *Am J Hematol* 11:425–437, 1981.

352. Kreuder J, Borkhardt A, Repp R, et al: Brief report: Inherited metabolic myopathy and hemolysis due to a mutation in aldolase A. *N Engl J Med* 334:1100–1104, 1996.

353. Esposito G, Vitagliano L, Costanzo P, et al: Human aldolase A natural mutants: Relationship between flexibility of the C-terminal region and enzyme function. *Biochem J* 380:51–56, 2004.

354. Yao DC, Tolan DR, Murray MF, et al: Hemolytic anemia and severe rhabdomyolysis caused by compound heterozygous mutations of the gene for erythrocyte/muscle isozyme of aldolase, ALDOA(Arg303X/Cys338Tyr). *Blood* 103:2401–2403, 2004.

355. Schneider AS: Triosephosphate isomerase deficiency: Historical perspectives and molecular aspects. *Baillieres Best Pract Res Clin Haematol* 13:119–140, 2000.

356. Orosz F, Olah J, Alvarez M, et al: Distinct behavior of mutant triosephosphate isomerase in hemolysate and in isolated form: Molecular basis of enzyme deficiency. *Blood* 98:3106–3112, 2001.

357. Orosz F, Oláh J, Ovádi J: Triosephosphate isomerase deficiency: New insights into an enigmatic disease. *Biochim Biophys Acta* 1792:1168–1174, 2009.

358. Orosz F, Olah J, Ovadi J: Triosephosphate isomerase deficiency: Facts and doubts. *IUBMB Life* 58:703–715, 2006.

359. Serdaroglu G, Aydinok Y, Yilmaz S, et al: Triosephosphate isomerase deficiency: A patient with Val231Met mutation [in process citation]. *Pediatr Neurol* 44:139–142, 2011.

360. Fermo E, Bianchi P, Vercellati C, et al: Triose phosphate isomerase deficiency associated with two novel mutations in TPI gene. *Eur J Haematol* 85:170–173, 2010.

361. Aissa K, Kamoun F, Sfaihi L, et al: Hemolytic anemia and progressive neurologic impairment: Think about triosephosphate isomerase deficiency. *Fetal Pediatr Pathol* 33:234–238, 2014.

362. Manco L, Ribeiro ML: Novel human pathological mutations. Gene symbol: TPI1. Disease: Triosephosphate isomerase deficiency. *Hum Genet* 121: 650, 2007.

363. Sarper N, Zengin E, Jakobs C, et al: Mild hemolytic anemia, progressive neuromotor retardation and fatal outcome: A disorder of glycolysis, triose- phosphate isomerase deficiency. *Turk J Pediatr* 55:198–202, 2013.

364. Schneider A, Westwood B, Yim C, et al: The 1591C mutation in triosephosphate isomerase (TPI) deficiency. Tightly linked polymorphisms and a common haplotype in all known families. *Blood Cells Mol Dis* 22:115–125, 1996.

365. Zingg BC, Pretsch W, Mohrenweiser HW: Molecular analysis of four ENU induced triosephosphate isomerase null mutants in Mus musculus. *Mut Res* 328:163–173, 1995.

366. Pretsch W: Triosephosphate isomerase activity-deficient mice show haemolytic anaemia in homozygous condition. *Genet Res (Camb)* 91:1–4, 2009.

367. Celotto AM, Frank AC, Seigle JL, et al: Drosophila model of human inherited triosephosphate isomerase deficiency glycolytic enzymopathy. *Genetics* 174:1237–1246, 2006.

368. Roland BP, Stuchul KA, Larsen SB, et al: Evidence of a triosephosphate isomerase non-catalytic function crucial to behavior and longevity. *J Cell Sci* 126:3151–3158, 2013.

369. Beutler E: PGK deficiency. *Br J Haematol* 136:3–11, 2007.

370. Tamai M, Kawano T, Saito R, et al: Phosphoglycerate kinase deficiency due to a novel mutation (c. 1180A>G) manifesting as chronic hemolytic anemia in a Japanese boy. *Int J Hematol* 2014.

371. Valentini G, Maggi M, Pey AL: Protein stability, folding and misfolding in human PGK1 deficiency. *Biomolecules* 3:1030–1052, 2013.

372. Spiegel R, Gomez EA, Akman HO, et al: Myopathic form of phosphoglycerate kinase (PGK) deficiency: A new case and pathogenic considerations. *Neuromuscul Disord* 19:207–211, 2009.

373. Morimoto A, Ueda I, Hirashima Y, et al: A novel missense mutation (1060G -> C) in the phosphoglycerate kinase gene in a Japanese boy with chronic haemolytic anaemia, developmental delay and rhabdomyolysis. *Br J Haematol* 122:1009–1013, 2003.

374. Fermo E, Bianchi P, Chiarelli LR, et al: A new variant of phosphoglycerate kinase deficiency (p.I371K) with multiple tissue involvement: Molecular and functional characterization. *Mol Genet Metab* 106:455–461, 2012.

375. Rhodes M, Ashford L, Manes B, et al: Bone marrow transplantation in phosphoglycerate kinase (PGK) deficiency. *Br J Haematol* 152:500–502, 2011.

376. Chiarelli LR, Morera SM, Bianchi P, et al: Molecular insights on pathogenic effects of mutations causing phosphoglycerate kinase deficiency. *PLoS One* 7:e32065, 2012.

377. Lemarchandel V, Joulin V, Valentin C, et al: Compound heterozygosity in a complete erythrocyte bisphosphoglycerate mutase deficiency. *Blood* 80:2643–2649, 1992.

378. Hoyer JD, Allen SL, Beutler E, et al: Erythrocytosis due to bisphosphoglycerate mutase deficiency with concurrent glucose-6-phosphate dehydrogenase (G6PD) deficiency. *Am J Hematol* 75:205–208, 2004.

379. Petousi N, Copley RR, Lappin TR, et al: Erythrocytosis associated with a novel missense mutation in the *BPGM* gene. *Haematologica* 99:e201–e204, 2014.

380. Rosa R, Prehu M-O, Beuzard Y, et al: The first case of a complete deficiency of diphosphoglycerate mutase in human erythrocytes. *J Clin Invest* 62:907–915, 1978.

381. Konrad PN, Richards F II, Valentine WN, et al: γ-Glutamyl-cysteine synthetase deficiency. A cause of hereditary hemolytic anemia. *N Engl J Med* 286:557–561, 1972.

382. Hirono A, Iyori H, Sekine I, et al: Three cases of hereditary nonspherocytic hemolytic anemia associated with red blood cell glutathione deficiency. *Blood* 87:2071–2074, 1996.

383. Beutler E, Moroose R, Kramer L, et al: Gamma-glutamylcysteine synthetase deficiency and hemolytic anemia. *Blood* 75:271–273, 1990.

384. Richards F 2nd, Cooper MR, Pearce LA, et al: Familial spinocerebellar degeneration, hemolytic anemia, and glutathione deficiency. *Arch Intern Med* 134:534–537, 1974.

385. Beutler E, Gelbart T, Kondo T, et al: The molecular basis of a case of γ-glutamylcysteine synthetase deficiency. *Blood* 94:2890–2894, 1999.

386. Ristoff E, Augustson C, Geissler J, et al: A missense mutation in the heavy subunit of γ-glutamylcysteine synthetase gene causes hemolytic anemia. *Blood* 95:1896–1897, 2000.

387. Hamilton D, Wu JH, Alaoui-Jamali M, et al: A novel missense mutation in the γ-glutamylcysteine synthetase catalytic subunit gene causes both decreased enzymatic activity and glutathione production. *Blood* 102:725–730, 2003.

388. Manu Pereira M, Gelbart T, Ristoff E, et al: Chronic non-spherocytic hemolytic anemia associated with severe neurological disease due to γ-glutamylcysteine synthetase deficiency in a patient of Moroccan origin. *Haematologica* 92:e102–E105, 2007.

389. Willis MN, Liu Y, Biterova EI, et al: Enzymatic defects underlying hereditary glutamate cysteine ligase deficiency are mitigated by association of the catalytic and regulatory subunits. *Biochemistry* 50:6508–6517, 2011.

390. Shi ZZ, Osei-Frimpong J, Kala G, et al: Glutathione synthesis is essential for mouse development but not for cell growth in culture. *Proc Natl Acad Sci U S A* 97:5101–5106, 2000.

391. Dalton TP, Dieter MZ, Yang Y, et al: Knockout of the mouse glutamate cysteine ligase catalytic subunit (Gclc) gene: Embryonic lethal when homozygous, and proposed model for moderate glutathione deficiency when heterozygous. *Biochem Biophys Res Commun* 279:324–329, 2000.

392. Yang Y, Dieter MZ, Chen Y, et al: Initial characterization of the glutamate-cysteine ligase modifier subunit Gclm(−/−) knockout mouse. Novel model system for a severely compromised oxidative stress response. *J Biol Chem* 277:49446–49452, 2002.

393. Foller M, Harris IS, Elia A, et al: Functional significance of glutamate-cysteine ligase modifier for erythrocyte survival in vitro and in vivo. *Cell Death Differ* 20:1350–1358, 2013.

394. Shi Z-Z, Habib GM, Rhead WJ, et al: Mutations in the glutathione synthetase gene cause 5-oxoprolinuria. *Nat Genet* 14:361–365, 1996.

395. Ristoff E, Mayatepek E, Larsson A: Long-term clinical outcome in patients with gluta-thione synthetase deficiency. *J Pediatr* 139:79–84, 2001.

396. Njalsson R, Ristoff E, Carlsson K, et al: Genotype, enzyme activity, glutathione level, and clinical phenotype in patients with glutathione synthetase deficiency. *Hum Genet* 116:384–389, 2005.

397. Ristoff E: Inborn errors of GSH metabolism, in *Glutathione and Sulfur Amino Acids in Human Health and Disease*, edited by Masella R, Mazza G, pp 343–362. John Wiley & Sons, New York, 2009.

398. Riudor E, Arranz JA, Alvarez R, et al: Massive 5-oxoprolinuria with normal 5-oxoprolinase and glutathione synthetase activities. *J Inherit Metab Dis* 24:404–406, 2001.

399. Mayatepek E: 5-Oxoprolinuria in patients with and without defects in the gamma-glu-tamyl cycle. *Eur J Pediatr* 158:221–225, 1999.

400. Pederzolli CD, Mescka CP, Zandona BR, et al: Acute administration of 5-oxoproline induces oxidative damage to lipids and proteins and impairs antioxidant defenses in cerebral cortex and cerebellum of young rats. *Metab Brain Dis* 25:145–154, 2010.

401. Simon E, Vogel M, Fingerhut R, et al: Diagnosis of glutathione synthetase deficiency in newborn screening. *J Inherit Metab Dis* 32 Suppl 1:S269–S272, 2009.

402. Burstedt MS, Ristoff E, Larsson A, et al: Rod-cone dystrophy with maculopathy in genetic glutathione synthetase deficiency: A morphologic and electrophysiologic study. *Ophthalmology* 116:324–331, 2009.

403. Winkler A, Njalsson R, Carlsson K, et al: Glutathione is essential for early embryo-genesis—analysis of a glutathione synthetase knockout mouse. *Biochem Biophys Res Commun* 412:121–126, 2011.

404. Kamerbeek NM, van Zwieten R, de Boer M, et al: Molecular basis of glutathione reduc-tase deficiency in human blood cells. *Blood* 109:3560–3566, 2007.

405. Loos H, Roos D, Weening R, et al: Familial deficiency of glutathione reductase in human blood cells. *Blood* 48:53–62, 1976.

406. Gallo V, Schwarzer E, Rahlfs S, et al: Inherited glutathione reductase deficiency and *Plasmodium falciparum* malaria–a case study. *PLoS One* 4:e7303, 2009.

407. Miwa S, Fujii H, Tani K, et al: Red cell adenylate kinase deficiency associated with hereditary nonspherocytic hemolytic anemia: Clinical and biochemical studies. *Am J Hematol* 14:325–333, 1983.

408. Matsuura S, Igarashi M, Tanizawa Y, et al: Human adenylate kinase deficiency associ-ated with hemolytic anemia. A single base substitution affecting solubility and catalytic activity of the cytosolic adenylate kinase. *J Biol Chem* 264:10148–10155, 1989.

409. Qualtieri A, Pedace V, Bisconte MG, et al: Severe erythrocyte adenylate kinase defi-ciency due to homozygous A—>G substitution at codon 164 of human AK1 gene asso-ciated with chronic haemolytic anaemia. *Br J Haematol* 99:770–776, 1997.

410. Bianchi P, Zappa M, Bredi E, et al: A case of complete adenylate kinase deficiency due to a nonsense mutation in AK-1 gene (Arg 107 —> Stop, CGA —> TGA) associated with chronic haemolytic anaemia. *Br J Haematol* 105:75–79, 1999.

411. Corrons JL, Garcia E, Tusell JJ, et al: Red cell adenylate kinase deficiency: Molecu-lar study of 3 new mutations (118G>A, 190G>A, and GAC deletion) associated with hereditary nonspherocytic hemolytic anemia. *Blood* 102:353–356, 2003.

412. Fermo E, Bianchi P, Vercellati C, et al: A new variant of adenylate kinase (delG138) associated with severe hemolytic anemia. *Blood Cells Mol Dis* 33:146–149, 2004.

413. Lachant NA, Zerez CR, Barredo J, et al: Hereditary erythrocyte adenylate kinase defi-ciency: A defect of multiple phosphotransferases? *Blood* 77:2774–2784, 1991.

414. Toren A, Brok-Simoni F, Ben-Bassat I, et al: Congenital haemolytic anaemia associated with adenylate kinase deficiency. *Br J Haematol* 87:376–380, 1994.

415. Valentine WN, Paglia DE, Tartaglia AP, et al: Hereditary hemolytic anemia with increased red cell adenosine deaminase (45- to 70-fold) and decreased adenosine tri-phosphate. *Science* 195:783–785, 1977.

416. Perignon JL, Hamet M, Buc HA, et al: Biochemical study of a case of hemolytic anemia with increased (85 fold) red cell adenosine deaminase. *Clin Chim Acta* 124:205–212, 1982.

417. Chottiner EG, Ginsburg D, Tartaglia AP, et al: Erythrocyte adenosine deaminase over-production in hereditary hemolytic anemia. *Blood* 74:448–453, 1989.

418. Fujii H, Miwa S, Suzuki K: Purification and properties of adenosine deaminase in normal and hereditary hemolytic anemia with increased red cell activity. *Hemoglobin* 4:693–705, 1980.

419. Chen EH, Tartaglia AP, Mitchell BS: Hereditary overexpression of adenosine deaminase in erythrocytes: Evidence for a *cis*-acting mutation. *Am J Hum Genet* 53:889–893, 1993.

420. Zanella A, Bianchi P, Fermo E, et al: Hereditary pyrimidine 5′-nucleotidase deficiency: From genetics to clinical manifestations. *Br J Haematol* 133:113–123, 2006.

421. Rees DC, Duley JA, Marinaki AM: Pyrimidine 5′ nucleotidase deficiency. *Br J Haematol* 120:375–383, 2003.

422. Vives i Corrons JL: Chronic non-spherocytic haemolytic anaemia due to congenital pyrimidine 5′ nucleotidase deficiency: 25 years later. *Baillieres Best Pract Res Clin Hae-matol* 13:103–118, 2000.

423. Swanson MS, Markin RS, Stohs SJ, et al: Identification of cytidine diphosphodiesters in erythrocytes from a patient with pyrimidine nucleotidase deficiency. *Blood* 63:665–670, 1984.

424. Tomoda A, Noble NA, Lachant NA, et al: Hemolytic anemia in hereditary pyrimidine 5′-nucleotidase deficiency: Nucleotide inhibition of G6PD and the pentose phosphate shunt. *Blood* 60:1212–1218, 1982.

425. David O, Ramenghi U, Camaschella C, et al: Inhibition of hexose monophosphate shunt in young erythrocytes by pyrimidine nucleotides in hereditary pyrimidine 5′ nucleotidase deficiency. *Eur J Haematol* 47:48–54, 1991.

426. Rees DC, Duley J, Simmonds HA, et al: Interaction of hemoglobin E and pyrimidine 5′ nucleotidase deficiency. *Blood* 88:2761–2767, 1996.

427. Lachant NA, Tanaka KR: Red cell metabolism in hereditary pyrimidine 5′-nucleotidase deficiency: Effect of magnesium. *Br J Haematol* 63:615–623, 1986.

428. Lachant NA, Zerez CR, Tanaka KR: Pyrimidine nucleotides impair phosphoribosylpy-rophosphate (PRPP) synthetase subunit aggregation by sequestering magnesium. A mechanism for the decreased PRPP synthetase activity in hereditary erythrocyte pyrimidine 5′-nucleotidase deficiency. *Biochim Biophys Acta* 994:81–88, 1989.

429. Zerez CR, Lachant NA, Tanaka KR: Decrease in subunit aggregation of phosphori-bosylpyrophosphate synthetase: A mechanism for decreased nucleotide concentrations in pyruvate kinase-deficient human erythrocytes. *Blood* 68:1024–1029, 1986.

430. Lachant NA, Zerez CR, Tanaka KR: Pyrimidine nucleoside monophosphate kinase hyperactivity in hereditary erythrocyte pyrimidine 5′-nucleotidase deficiency. *Br J Haematol* 66:91–96, 1987.

431. Valentine WN, Anderson HM, Paglia DE, et al: Studies on human erythrocyte nucleo-tide metabolism. II. Nonspherocytic hemolytic anemia, high red cell ATP, and ribose-phosphate pyrophosphokinase (RPK, E.C.2.7.6.1) deficiency. *Blood* 39:674–684, 1972.

432. Oda E, Oda S, Tomoda A, et al: Hemolytic anemia in hereditary pyrimidine 5′-nucleotidase deficiency. II. Effect of pyrimidine nucleotides and their derivatives on gly-colytic and pentose phosphate shunt enzyme activity. *Clin Chim Acta* 141:93–100, 1984.

433. Chiarelli LR, Morera SM, Galizzi A, et al: Molecular basis of pyrimidine 5′-nucleotidase deficiency caused by 3 newly identified missense mutations (c.187T>C, c.469G>C and c.740T>C) and a tabulation of known mutations. *Blood Cells Mol Dis* 40:295–301, 2008.

434. Warang P, Kedar P, Kar R, et al: New missense homozygous mutation (Q270Ter) in the pyrimidine 5′ nucleotidase type I-related gene in two Indian families with hereditary non-spherocytic hemolytic anemia. *Ann Hematol* 92:715–717, 2013.

435. Chiarelli LR, Bianchi P, Fermo E, et al: Functional analysis of pyrimidine 5′-nucleotidase mutants causing nonspherocytic hemolytic anemia. *Blood* 105:3340–3345, 2005.

436. David O, Vota MG, Piga A, et al: Pyrimidine 5′-nucleotidase acquired deficiency in beta-thalassemia: Involvement of enzyme-SH groups in the inactivation process. *Acta Haematol* 82:69–74, 1989.

437. Vives Corrons JL, Pujades MA, Aguilari Bascompte JL, et al: Pyrimidine 5′nucleotidase and several other red cell enzyme activities in beta-thalassaemia trait. *Br J Haematol* 56:483–494, 1984.

438. Dern RJ, Beutler E, Alving AS: The hemolytic effect of primaquine. V. Primaquine sen-sitivity as a manifestation of a multiple drug sensitivity. *J Lab Clin Med* 45:30–39, 1955.

439. Cohen G, Hochstein P: Generation of hydrogen peroxide in erythrocytes by hemolytic agents. *Biochemistry* 3:895–900, 1964.

440. Kosower NS, Song KR, Kosower EM, et al: Glutathione. II. Chemical aspects of azoester procedure for oxidation to disulfide. *Biochim Biophys Acta* 192:8–14, 1969.

441. Birchmeier W, Tuchschmid PE, Winterhalter H: Comparison of human hemoglobin A carrying glutathione as a mixed disulfide with the naturally occurring human hemoglo-bin A3. *Biochemistry* 12:3667–3672, 1973.

442. Rachmilewitz EA, Harari E, Winterhalter KH: Separation of alpha- and beta-chains of hemoglobin A by acetylphenylhydrazine. *Biochim Biophys Acta* 371:402–407, 1974.

443. Kirkman HN, Gaetani GF: Catalase: A tetrameric enzyme with four tightly bound mol-ecules of NADPH. *Proc Natl Acad Sci U S A* 81:4343–4347, 1984.

444. Gaetani GF, Rolfo M, Arena S, et al: Active involvement of catalase during hemolytic crises of favism. *Blood* 88:1084–1088, 1996.

445. Rifkind RA: Heinz body anemia: An ultrastructural study. II. Red cell sequestration and destruction. *Blood* 26:433–448, 1965.

446. Ho YS, Xiong Y, Ma W, et al: Mice lacking catalase develop normally but show differen-tial sensitivity to oxidant tissue injury. *J Biol Chem* 279:32804–32812, 2004.

447. Cheah FC, Peskin AV, Wong FL, et al: Increased basal oxidation of peroxiredoxin 2 and limited peroxiredoxin recycling in glucose-6-phosphate dehydrogenase-deficient erythrocytes from newborn infants. *FASEB J* 28:3205–3210, 2014.

448. Bunn HE: F., Jandl JH: Exchange of heme among hemoglobin molecules. *Proc Natl Acad Sci U S A* 56:974–978, 1966.

449. Jandl JH: The Heinz body hemolytic anemias. *Ann Intern Med* 58:702–709, 1963.

450. Beutler E: Abnormalities of glycolysis (HMP shunt). *Bibl Haematol* 29:146–157, 1968.

451. Baehner RL, Nathan DG, Castle WB: Oxidant injury of Caucasian glucose-6-phosphate dehydrogenase-deficient red blood cells by phagocytosing leukocytes during infection. *J Clin Invest* 50:2466–2473, 1971.

452. Arese P, De Flora A: Denaturation of normal and abnormal erythrocytes II. Pathophysi-ology of hemolysis in glucose-6-phosphate dehydrogenase deficiency. *Semin Hematol* 27:1–40, 1990.

453. Stamatoyannopoulos G, Fraser GR, Motulsky AG, et al: On the familial predisposition to favism. *Am J Hum Genet* 18:253–263, 1966.

454. Cassimos CH: R., Malaka-Zafiriu K, Tsiures J: Urinary d-glucaric acid excretion in nor-mal and G6PD-deficient children with favism. *J. Pediatrics* 84:871–872, 1974.

455. Bottini E, Bottini FG, Borgiani P, et al: Association between ACP1 and favism: A possi-ble biochemical mechanism. *Blood* 89:2613–2615, 1997.

456. Fiorelli G, Podda M, Corrias A, et al: The relevance of immune reactions in acute favism. *Acta Haematol.* 51:211–218, 1974.

457. Turrini F, Naitana A, Mannuzzu L, et al: Increased red cell calcium, decreased calcium adenosine triphosphatase, and altered membrane proteins during fava bean hemolysis in glucose-6-phosphate dehydrogenase-deficient (Mediterranean variant) individuals. *Blood* 66:302–305, 1985.

458. De Flora A, Benatti U, Guida L, et al: Favism: Disordered erythrocyte calcium homeo-stasis. *Blood* 66:294–297, 1985.

459. Fischer TM, Meloni T, Pescarmona GP, et al: Membrane cross bonding in red cells in favic crisis: A missing link in the mechanism of extravascular haemolysis. *Br J Haematol.* 59:159–169, 1985.

460. Caprari P, Bozzi A, Ferroni L, et al: Membrane alterations in G6PD- and PK-deficient erythrocytes exposed to oxidizing agents. *Biochem Med Metab Biol* 45:16–27, 1991.

461. Johnson RM, Ravindranath Y, ElAlfy MS, et al: Oxidant damage to erythrocyte membrane in glucose-6-phosphate dehydrogenase deficiency: Correlation with in vivo reduced glutathione concentration and membrane protein oxidation. *Blood* 83:1117–1123, 1994.

462. Pantaleo A, Ferru E, Carta F, et al: Irreversible AE1 tyrosine phosphorylation leads to membrane vesiculation in G6PD deficient red cells. *PLoS One* 6:e15847, 2011.

463. Kaplan M, Hammerman C: Severe neonatal hyperbilirubinemia. A potential complication of glucose-6-phosphate dehydrogenase deficiency. *Clin Perinatol* 25:575–590, 1998.

464. Kaplan M, Hammerman C: Glucose-6-phosphate dehydrogenase deficiency: A potential source of severe neonatal hyperbilirubinaemia and kernicterus. *Semin Neonatol* 7:121–128, 2002.

465. Kaplan M, Hammerman C: Glucose-6-phosphate dehydrogenase deficiency: A hidden risk for kernicterus. *Semin Perinatol* 28:356–364, 2004.

466. Kaplan M, Hammerman C, Vreman HJ, et al: Severe hemolysis with normal blood count in a glucose-6-phosphate dehydrogenase deficient neonate. *J Perinatol* 28:306–309, 2008.

467. Kaplan M, Renbaum P, Levy-Lahad E, et al: Gilbert syndrome and glucose-6-phosphate dehydrogenase deficiency: A dose-dependent genetic interaction crucial to neonatal hyperbilirubinemia. *Proc Natl Acad Sci U S A* 94:12128–12132, 1997.

468. Huang CS, Chang PF, Huang MJ, et al: Glucose-6-phosphate dehydrogenase deficiency, the UDP-glucuronosyl transferase 1A1 gene, and neonatal hyperbilirubinemia. *Gastroenterology* 123:127–133, 2002.

469. Oluboyede OA, Esan GJ: F., Francis TI, et al: Genetically determined deficiency of glucose 6-phosphate dehydrogenase (type A–) is expressed in the liver. *J Lab Clin Med* 93:783–789, 1979.

470. Kaplan M, Hammerman C, Maisels MJ: Bilirubin genetics for the nongeneticist: Hereditary defects of neonatal bilirubin conjugation. *Pediatrics* 111:886–893, 2003.

471. Sanna S, Busonero F, Maschio A, et al: Common variants in the SLCO1B3 locus are associated with bilirubin levels and unconjugated hyperbilirubinemia. *Hum Mol Genet* 18:2711–2718, 2009.

472. Kaplan M, Hammerman C: Glucose-6-phosphate dehydrogenase deficiency and severe neonatal hyperbilirubinemia: A complexity of interactions between genes and environment. *Semin Fetal Neonatal Med* 15:148–156, 2010.

473. Valentine WN, Paglia DE: The primary cause of hemolysis in enzymopathies of anaerobic glycolysis: A viewpoint. *Blood Cells* 6:819–829, 1980.

474. Beutler E: "The primary cause of hemolysis in enzymopathies of anaerobic glycolysis: A viewpoint." A commentary. *Blood Cells* 6:827–829, 1980.

475. Bogdanova A, Makhro A, Wang J, et al: Calcium in red blood cells-a perilous balance. *Int J Mol Sci* 14:9848–9872, 2013.

476. Ronquist G, Rudolphi O, Engström I, et al: Familial phosphofructokinase deficiency is associated with a disturbed calcium homeostasis in erythrocytes. *J Intern Med* 249:85–95, 2001.

477. Sabina RL, Waldenström A, Ronquist G: The contribution of Ca+ calmodulin activation of human erythrocyte AMP deaminase (isoform E) to the erythrocyte metabolic dysregulation of familial phosphofructokinase deficiency. *Haematologica* 91:652–655, 2006.

478. Aisaki K, Aizawa S, Fujii H, et al: Glycolytic inhibition by mutation of pyruvate kinase gene increases oxidative stress and causes apoptosis of a pyruvate kinase deficient cell line. *Exp Hematol* 35:1190–1200, 2007.

479. Youngster I, Arcavi L, Schechmaster R, et al: Medications and glucose-6-phosphate dehydrogenase deficiency: An evidence-based review. *Drug Saf* 33:713–726, 2010.

480. Campbell GD Jr, Steinberg MH, Bower JD: Ascorbic acid-induced hemolysis in G6PD deficiency. *Ann Intern Med* 82: 810, 1975.

481. Rees DC, Kelsey H, Richards JD: Acute haemolysis induced by high dose ascorbic acid in glucose-6-phosphate dehydrogenase deficiency. *BMJ* 306:841–842, 1993.

482. Mehta JB, Singhal SB, Mehta BC: Ascorbic-acid-induced haemolysis in G6PD deficiency. *Lancet* 336:944–944, 1990.

483. Relling MV, McDonagh EM, Chang T, et al: Clinical Pharmacogenetics Implementation Consortium (CPIC) guidelines for rasburicase therapy in the context of G6PD deficiency genotype. *Clin Pharmacol Ther* 96:169–174, 2014.

484. McCaffrey RP, Halsted CH, Wahab MF, Robertson RP: Chloramphenicol-induced hemolysis in Caucasian glucose-6-phosphate dehydrogenase deficiency. *Ann Intern Med* 74:722–726, 1971.

485. Chan TK, Chesterman CN, McFadzean AJ, Todd D: The survival of glucose-6-phosphate dehydrogenase-deficient erythrocytes in patients with typhoid fever on chloramphenicol therapy. *J Lab Clin Med* 77:177–184, 1971.

486. Markowitz N, Saravolatz LD: Use of trimethoprim-sulfamethoxazole in a glucose-6-phosphate dehydrogenase-deficient population. *Rev Infect Dis* 9 Suppl 2:S218–S229, 1987.

487. Magon AM, Leipzig RM, Zannoni VG, et al: Interactions of glucose-6-phosphate dehydrogenase deficiency with drug acetylation and hydroxylation reactions. *J Lab Clin Med* 97:764–770, 1981.

488. Woolhouse NM, Atu-Taylor LC: Influence of double genetic polymorphism on response to sulfamethazine. *Clin Pharmacol Ther* 31:377–383, 1982.

489. Rochford R, Ohrt C, Baresel PC, et al: Humanized mouse model of glucose 6-phosphate dehydrogenase deficiency for in vivo assessment of hemolytic toxicity. *Proc Natl Acad Sci U S A* 110:17486–17491, 2013.

490. Ko CH, Li K, Li CL, et al: Development of a novel mouse model of severe glucose-6-phosphate dehydrogenase (G6PD)-deficiency for in vitro and in vivo assessment of hemolytic toxicity to red blood cells. *Blood Cells Mol Dis* 47:176–181, 2011.

491. Patrinostro X, Carter ML, Kramer AC, et al: A model of glucose-6-phosphate dehydrogenase deficiency in the zebrafish. *Exp Hematol* 41:697–710 e692, 2013.

492. Zhang P, Gao X, Ishida H, et al: An in vivo drug screening model using glucose-6-phosphate dehydrogenase deficient mice to predict the hemolytic toxicity of 8-amino-quinolines. *Am J Trop Med Hyg* 88:1138–1145, 2013.

493. Dern RJ, Beutler E, Alving AS: The hemolytic effect of primaquine. II. The natural course of the hemolytic anemia and the mechanism of its self-limited character. *J Lab Clin Med* 44:171–175, 1954.

494. Beutler E, Dern RJ, Alving AS: The hemolytic effect of primaquine. III. A study of primaquine-sensitive erythrocytes. *J Lab Clin Med* 44:177–184, 1954.

495. Beutler E, Dern RJ, Alving AS: The hemolytic effect of primaquine. IV. The relationship of cell age to hemolysis. *J Lab Clin Med* 44:439–442, 1954.

496. George JN, Sears DA, McCurdy P, et al: Primaquine sensitivity in caucasians: Hemolytic reactions induced by primaquine in G6PD deficient subjects. *J Lab Clin Med* 70:80–93, 1967.

497. Siddiqui T, Khan AH: Hepatitis A and cytomegalovirus infection precipitating acute hemolysis in glucose-6-phosphate dehydrogenase deficiency. *Mil Med* 163:434–435, 1998.

498. Tugwell P: Glucose-6-phosphate-dehydrogenase deficiency in Nigerians with jaundice associated with lobar pneumonia. *Lancet* 1:968–969, 1973.

499. Choremis C, Kattamis CA, Kyriazakou M, et al: Viral hepatitis in G-6-PD deficiency. *Lancet* 1:269–270, 1966.

500. Walker DH, Hawkins HK, Hudson P: Fulminant Rocky Mountain spotted fever. *Arch Pathol Lab Med* 107:121–125, 1983.

501. Huo TI, Wu JC, Chiu CF, et al: Severe hyperbilirubinemia due to acute hepatitis a superimposed on a chronic hepatitis B carrier with glucose-6-phosphate dehydrogenase deficiency. *Am J Gastroenterol* 91:158–159, 1996.

502. Chau TN, Lai ST, Lai JY, et al: Haemolysis complicating acute viral hepatitis in patients with normal or deficient glucose-6-phosphate dehydrogenase activity. *Scand J Infect Dis* 29:551–553, 1997.

503. Green L, De Lord C, Clark B, et al: Transient aplastic crisis as presentation of a previously unknown G6PD deficiency with iron overload. *Br J Haematol* 154:288, 2011.

504. Garcia S, Linares M, Colomina P, et al: Cytomegalovirus infection and aplastic crisis in glucose-6-phosphate dehydrogenase deficiency. *Lancet* 2:105, 1987.

505. Pietrapertosa A, Palma A, Campanale D, et al: Genotype and phenotype correlation in glucose-6-phosphate dehydrogenase deficiency. *Haematologica* 86:30–35, 2001.

506. Kattamis CA, Kyriazakou M, Chaidas S: Favism. Clinical and biochemical data. *J Med Genet* 6:34–41, 1969.

507. Wong WY, Powars D, Williams WD: "Yewdow"-induced anemia. *West J Med* 151:459–460, 1989.

508. Globerman H, Novak T, Chevion M: Haemolysis in a G6PD-deficient child induced by eating unripe peaches. *Scand J Haematol* 33:337–341, 1984.

509. Williams CK, Osotimehin BO, Ogunmola GB, Awotedu AA: Haemolytic anaemia associated with Nigerian barbecued meat (red suya). *Afr J Med Med Sci* 17:71–75, 1988.

510. Schiliro G, Russo A, Curreri R, et al: Glucose-6-phosphate dehydrogenase deficiency in Sicily. Incidence, biochemical characteristics and clinical implications. *Clin Genet* 15:183–188, 1979.

511. Liu H, Liu W, Tang X, et al: Association between G6PD deficiency and hyperbilirubinemia in neonates: A meta-analysis. *Pediatr Hematol Oncol* 32:92–98, 2015.

512. Valaes T: Severe neonatal jaundice associated with glucose-6-phosphate dehydrogenase deficiency: Pathogenesis and global epidemiology. *Acta Paediatr* 394:58–76, 1994.

513. Kaplan M, Hammerman C, Vreman HJ, et al: Acute hemolysis and severe neonatal hyperbilirubinemia in glucose-6-phosphate dehydrogenase-deficient heterozygotes. *J Pediatr* 139:137–140, 2001.

514. Fok TF, Lau SP: Glucose-6-phosphate dehydrogenase deficiency: A preventable cause of mental retardation. *BMJ* 292: 829, 1986.

515. Singh H: Glucose-6-phosphate dehydrogenase deficiency: A preventable cause of mental retardation. *BMJ* 292:397–398, 1986.

516. Olusanya B, Emokpae A, Zamora T, et al: Addressing the burden of neonatal hyperbilirubinaemia in countries with significant glucose-6-phosphate dehydrogenase deficiency. *Acta Paediatr* 103:1102–1109, 2014.

517. Ardati KO, Bajakian KM, Tabbara KS: Effect of glucose-6-phosphate dehydrogenase deficiency on neutrophil function. *Acta Haematol* 97:211–215, 1997.

518. Cooper MR, DeChatelet LR, McCall CE, et al: Complete deficiency of leukocyte glucose-6-phosphate dehydrogenase with defective bactericidal activity. *J Clin Invest* 51:769–778, 1972.

519. Gray GR, Klebanoff SJ, Stamatoyannopoulos G, et al: Neutrophil dysfunction, chronic granulomatous disease, and nonspherocytic haemolytic anaemia caused by complete deficiency of glucose-6-phosphate dehydrogenase. *Lancet* 2:530–534, 1973.

520. Vives-Corrons JL, Feliu E, Pujades MA, et al: Severe glucose-6-phosphate dehydrogenase (G 6 PD) deficiency associated with chronic hemolytic anemia, granulocyte dysfunction and increased susceptibility to infections. Description of a new molecular variant (G 6 PD Barcelona). *Blood* 59:428–434, 1982.

521. Rosa-Borges A, Sampaio MG, Condino-Neto A, et al: Glucose-6-phosphate dehydrogenase deficiency with recurrent infections: Case report. *J Pediatr (Rio J)* 77:331–336, 2001.
522. Chao YC, Huang CS, Lee CN, et al: Higher infection of dengue virus serotype 2 in human monocytes of patients with G6PD deficiency. *PLoS One* 3:e1557, 2008.
523. Gray GR, Naiman SC, Robinson GC: Platelet function and G6PD deficiency. *Lancet* 1:997, 1974.
524. Schwartz JP, Cooperberg AA, Rosenberg A: Platelet-function studies in patients with glucose-6-phosphate dehydrogenase deficiency. *Br J Haematol* 27:273–280, 1974.
525. Westring DW, Pisciotta AV: Anemia, cataracts, and seizures in patient with glucose-6-phosphate dehydrogenase deficiency. *Arch Intern Med* 118:385–390, 1966.
526. Harley JD, Agar NS, Gruca MA, et al: Cataracts with a glucose-6-phosphate dehydrogenase variant. *BMJ* 2:86, 1975.
527. Harley JD, Agar NS, Yoshida A: Glucose-6-phosphate dehydrogenase variants: Gd (+) Alexandra associated with neonatal jaundice and Gd (–) Camperdown in a young man with lamellar cataracts. *J Lab Clin Med* 91:295–300, 1978.
528. Nair V, Hasan SU, Romanchuk K, et al: Bilateral cataracts associated with glucose-6-phosphate dehydrogenase deficiency. *J Perinatol* 33:574–575, 2013.
529. Panich V, Na-Nakorn S: G 6 PD deficiency in senile cataracts. *Hum Genet* 55:123–124, 1980.
530. Orzalesi N, Sorcinelli R, Guiso G: Increased incidence of cataract in male subjects deficient in glucose-6-phosphate dehydrogenase. *Arch Ophthalmol* 99:69–70, 1981.
531. Bhatia RP, Patel R, Dubey B: Senile cataract and glucose-6-phosphate dehydrogenase deficiency in Indians. *Trop Geogr Med* 42:349–351, 1990.
532. Assaf AA, Tabbara KF, el-Hazmi MA: Cataracts in glucose-6-phosphate dehydrogenase deficiency. *Ophthalmic Paediatr Genet* 14:81–86, 1993.
533. Niazi GA: Glucose-6-phosphate dehydrogenase deficiency and diabetes mellitus. *Int J Hematol* 54:295–298, 1991.
534. Saeed TK, Hamamy HA, Alwan AA: Association of glucose-6-phosphate dehydrogenase deficiency with diabetes mellitus. *Diabet Med* 2:110–112, 1985.
535. Heymann AD, Cohen Y, Chodick G: Glucose-6-phosphate dehydrogenase deficiency and type 2 diabetes. *Diabetes Care* 35:e58, 2012.
536. Ninfali P, Bresolin N, Baronciani L, et al: Glucose-6-phosphate dehydrogenase Lodi[844C]: A study on its expression in blood cells and muscle. *Enzyme* 45:180–187, 1991.
537. Ninfali P, Baronciani L, Bardoni A, et al: Muscle expression of glucose-6-phosphate dehydrogenase deficiency in different variants. *Clin Genet* 48:232–237, 1995.
538. Bresolin N, Bet L, Moggio M, et al: Muscle G6PD deficiency. *Lancet* 2:212–213, 1987.
539. Bresolin N, Bet L, Moggio M, et al: Muscle glucose-6-phosphate dehydrogenase deficiency. *J Neurol* 236:193–198, 1989.
540. Liguori R, Giannoccaro MP, Pasini E, et al: Acute rhabdomyolysis induced by tonic-clonic epileptic seizures in a patient with glucose-6-phosphate dehydrogenase deficiency. *J Neurol* 260:2669–2671, 2013.
541. Mailloux RJ, Harper ME: Glucose regulates enzymatic sources of mitochondrial NADPH in skeletal muscle cells; a novel role for glucose-6-phosphate dehydrogenase. *FASEB J* 24:2495–2506, 2010.
542. Demir AY, van Solinge WW, van Oirschot B, et al: Glucose 6-phosphate dehydrogenase deficiency in an elite long-distance runner. *Blood* 113:2118–2119, 2009.
543. Theodorou AA, Nikolaidis MG, Paschalis V, et al: Comparison between glucose-6-phosphate dehydrogenase-deficient and normal individuals after eccentric exercise. *Med Sci Sports Exerc* 42:1113–1121, 2010.
544. Jamurtas AZ, Fatouros IG, Koukosias N, et al: Effect of exercise on oxidative stress in individuals with glucose-6-phosphate dehydrogenase deficiency. *In Vivo* 20:875–880, 2006.
545. Sulis E: G6PD deficiency and cancer. *Lancet* 1:1185, 1972.
546. Zampella EJ, Bradley EL, Pretlow TG: Glucose-6-phosphate dehydrogenase: A possible clinical indicator for prostatic carcinoma. *Cancer* 49:384–387, 1982.
547. Ferraris AM, Broccia G, Meloni T, et al: Glucose-6-phosphate dehydrogenase deficiency and incidence of hematologic malignancy. *Am J Hum Genet* 42:516–520, 1988.
548. Forteleoni G, Argiolas L, Farris A, et al: G6PD deficiency and breast cancer. *Tumori* 74:665–667, 1988.
549. Pisano M, Cocco P, Cherchi R, et al: Glucose-6-phosphate dehydrogenase deficiency and lung cancer: A hospital based case-control study. *Tumori* 77:12–15, 1991.
550. Jiang P, Du W, Wang X, et al: p53 regulates biosynthesis through direct inactivation of glucose-6-phosphate dehydrogenase. *Nat Cell Biol* 13:310–316, 2011.
551. Hecker PA, Leopold JA, Gupte SA, et al: Impact of glucose-6-phosphate dehydrogenase deficiency on the pathophysiology of cardiovascular disease. *Am J Physiol Heart Circ Physiol* 304:H491–H500, 2013.
552. Müller-Soyano A, Tovar de Roura E, Duke PR, et al: Pyruvate kinase deficiency and leg ulcers. *Blood* 47:807–813, 1976.
553. Curiel CD, Velasquez GA, Papa R: Hemolytic anemia and leg ulcers due to pyruvate kinase deficiency. Report of the second Venezuelan family. *Sangre (Barc)* 22:64–77, 1977.
554. Dolan LM, Ryan M, Moohan J: Pyruvate kinase deficiency in pregnancy complicated by iron overload. *BJOG* 109:844–846, 2002.
555. Wax JR, Pinette MG, Cartin A, et al: Pyruvate kinase deficiency complicating pregnancy. *Obstet Gynecol* 109:553–555, 2007.
556. Fanning J, Hinkle RS: Pyruvate kinase deficiency hemolytic anemia: Two successful pregnancy outcomes. *Am J Obstet Gynecol* 153:313–314, 1985.
557. Ferreira P, Morais L, Costa R, et al: Hydrops fetalis associated with erythrocyte pyruvate kinase deficiency. *Eur J Pediatr* 159:481–482, 2000.
558. Vora S, Rattazzi MC, Scandalios JG, et al: Isozymes of human phosphofructokinase: Biochemical and genetic aspects, in *Isozymes: Current Topics in Biological and Medical Research*, pp 3–23. Alan R. Liss, New York, 1983.
559. Wellner VP, Sekura R, Meister A, et al: Glutathione synthetase deficiency, an inborn error of metabolism involving the gamma-glutamyl cycle in patients with 5-oxoprolinuria (pyroglutamic aciduria). *Proc Natl Acad Sci U S A* 71:2505–2509, 1974.
560. Skala H, Dreyfus JC, Vives-Corrons JL, et al: Triose phosphate isomerase deficiency. *Biochem Med* 18:226–234, 1977.
561. Valentine WN, Schneider AS, Baughan MA, et al: Hereditary hemolytic anemia with triosephosphate isomerase deficiency. *Am J Med* 41:27–41, 1966.
562. Hollán S, Magócsi M, Fodor E, et al: Search for the pathogenesis of the differing phenotype in two compound heterozygote Hungarian brothers with the same genotypic triosephosphate isomerase deficiency. *Proc Natl Acad Sci U S A* 94:10362–10366, 1997.
563. Hollán S, Fujii H, Hirono A, et al: Hereditary triosephosphate isomerase (TPI) deficiency: Two severely affected brothers one with and one without neurological symptoms. *Hum Genet* 92:486–490, 1993.
564. Noel N, Flanagan JM, Ramirez Bajo MJ, et al: Two new phosphoglycerate kinase mutations associated with chronic haemolytic anaemia and neurological dysfunction in two patients from Spain. *Br J Haematol* 132:523–529, 2006.
565. DiMauro S, Dalakas M, Miranda AF: Phosphoglycerate kinase deficiency: Another cause of recurrent myoglobinuria. *Ann Neurol* 13:11–19, 1983.
566. Branca A, Costa E, Rocha S, et al: Coexistence of congenital red cell pyruvate kinase and band 3 deficiency. *Clin Lab Haematol* 26:297–300, 2004.
567. Zarza R, Moscardó M, Alvarez R, et al: Co-existence of hereditary spherocytosis and a new red cell pyruvate kinase variant: PK Mallorca. *Haematologica* 85:227–232, 2000.
568. Vercellati C, Marcello AP, Fermo E, et al: A case of hereditary spherocytosis misdiagnosed as pyruvate kinase deficient hemolytic anemia. *Clin Lab* 59:421–424, 2013.
569. Beutler E, Forman L: Coexistence of α-thalassemia and a new pyruvate kinase variant: PK Fukien. *Acta Haematol* 69:3–8, 1983.
570. Vives Corrons JL, García AM, Sosa AM, et al: Heterozygous pyruvate kinase deficiency and severe hemolytic anemia in a pregnant woman with concomitant, glucose-6-phosphate dehydrogenase deficiency. *Ann Hematol* 62:190–193, 1991.
571. Zanella A, Bianchi P, Iurlo A, et al: Iron status and *HFE* genotype in erythrocyte pyruvate kinase deficiency: Study of Italian cases. *Blood Cells Mol Dis* 27:653–661, 2001.
572. Olah J, Orosz F, Puskas LG, et al: Triosephosphate isomerase deficiency: Consequences of an inherited mutation at mRNA, protein and metabolic levels. *Biochem J* 392:675–683, 2005.
573. Kanno H, Wei DC, Chan LC, et al: Hereditary hemolytic anemia caused by diverse point mutations of pyruvate kinase gene found in Japan and Hong Kong. *Blood* 84:3505–3509, 1994.
574. Diez A, Gilsanz F, Martinez J, et al: Life-threatening nonspherocytic hemolytic anemia in a patient with a null mutation in the PKLR gene and no compensatory PKM gene expression. *Blood* 106:1851–1856, 2005.
575. Danon D, Sheba C, Ramot B: The morphology of glucose 6 phosphate dehydrogenase deficient erythrocytes: Electron-microscopic studies. *Blood* 17:229–234, 1961.
576. Greenberg MS: Heinz body hemolytic anemia. *Arch Intern Med* 136:153–155, 1976.
577. Nathan DM, Siegel AJ, Bunn HF: Acute methemoglobinemia and hemolytic anemia with phenazopyridine. *Arch Intern Med* 137:1636–1638, 1977.
578. Oski FA, Nathan DG, Sidel VW, et al: Extreme hemolysis and red-cell distortion in erythrocyte pyruvate kinase deficiency. *N Engl J Med* 270:1023–1030, 1964.
579. Mentzer WC Jr, Baehner RL, Schmidt-Schonbein H, et al: Selective reticulocyte destruction in erythrocyte pyruvate kinase deficiency. *J Clin Invest* 50:688–699, 1971.
580. Beutler E: *Red Cell Metabolism. A Manual of Biochemical Methods*, 3rd ed., Grune & Stratton, Orlando, FL, 1984.
581. Recommended methods for the characterization of red cell pyruvate kinase variants. International Committee for Standardization in Haematology. *Br J Haematol* 43:275–286, 1979.
582. Beutler E, Blume KG, Kaplan JC, et al: International Committee for Standardization in Haematology: Recommended methods for red-cell enzyme analysis. *Br J Haematol* 35:331–340, 1977.
583. Beutler E, Blume KG, Kaplan JC, et al: International Committee for Standardization in Haematology: Recommended screening test for glucose-6-phosphate dehydrogenase (G6PD) deficiency. *Br J Haematol* 43:465–467, 1979.
584. Beutler E, Mitchell M: Special modifications of the fluorescent screening method for glucose-6-phosphate dehydrogenase deficiency. *Blood* 32:816–818, 1968.
585. Rijksen G, Veerman AJ, Schipper-Kester GP, et al: Diagnosis of pyruvate kinase deficiency in a transfusion-dependent patient with severe hemolytic anemia. *Am J Hematol* 35:187–193, 1990.
586. Herz F, Kaplan E, Scheye ES: Diagnosis of erythrocyte glucose-6-phosphate dehydrogenase deficiency in the negro male despite hemolytic crisis. *Blood* 35:90–93, 1970.
587. Ringelhahn B: A simple laboratory procedure for the recognition of A- (African type) G6PD deficiency in acute haemolytic crisis. *Clin Chim Acta* 36:272–274, 1972.
588. Beutler E, Yoshida A: X-inactivation in heterozygous G6PD variant females, in *Glucose-6-Phosphate Dehydrogenase*, pp 405–415. Academic Press, Orlando, FL, 1986.
589. Beutler E, Yunis JJ: G6PD activity of individual erythrocytes and X-chromosomal inactivation, in *Biochemical Methods in Red Cell Genetics*, pp 95–113. Academic Press, New York, 1969.
590. Vogels IM, van Noorden CJ, Wolf BH, et al: Cytochemical determination of heterozygous glucose-6-phosphate dehydrogenase deficiency in erythrocytes. *Br J Haematol* 63:402–405, 1986.

591. Jacob H, Jandl JH: A simple visual screening test for G6PD deficiency employing ascorbate and cyanide. *N Engl J Med* 274:1162–1167, 1966.

592. Oski FA: Red cell metabolism in the newborn infant. V. Glycolytic intermediates and glycolytic enzymes. *Pediatrics* 44:84–91, 1969.

593. Travis SF, Kumar SP, Paez PC, et al: Red cell metabolic alterations in postnatal life in term infants: Glycolytic enzymes and glucose-6-phosphate dehydrogenase. *Pediatr Res* 14:1349–1352, 1980.

594. Gross RT, Schroeder EA, Brounstein SA: Energy metabolism in the erythrocytes of premature infants compared to full term newborn infants and adults. *Blood* 21:755–763, 1963.

595. Lestas AN, Rodeck CH, White JM: Normal activities of glycolytic enzymes in the fetal erythrocytes. *Br J Haematol* 50:439–444, 1982.

596. Konrad PN, Valentine WN, Paglia DE: Enzymatic activities and glutathione content of erythrocytes in the newborn: Comparison with red cells of older normal subjects and those with comparable reticulocytosis. *Acta Haematol* 48:193–201, 1972.

597. Carrell RW, Kay R: A simple method for the detection of unstable haemoglobins. *Br J Haematol*. 23:615–619, 1972.

598. Valentine WN, Paglia DE, Fink K, et al: Lead poisoning. Association with hemolytic anemia, basophilic stippling, erythrocyte pyrimidine 5′-nucleotidase deficiency, and intraerythrocytic accumulation of pyrimidines. *J Clin Invest* 58:926–932, 1976.

599. Beutler E, Kuhl W, Fox M, et al: Prenatal diagnosis of glucose-6-P dehydrogenase (G6PD) deficiency. *Acta Haematol* 87:103–104, 1992.

600. Baronciani L, Beutler E: Prenatal diagnosis of pyruvate kinase deficiency. *Blood* 84:2354–2356, 1994.

601. Rouger H, Girodon E, Goossens M, et al: PK Mondor: Prenatal diagnosis of a frameshift mutation in the LR pyruvate kinase gene associated with severe hereditary non-spherocytic haemolytic anaemia. *Prenat Diagn* 16:97–104, 1996.

602. Gupta N, Bianchi P, Fermo E, et al: Prenatal diagnosis for a novel homozygous mutation in *PKLR* gene in an Indian family. *Prenat Diagn* 27:117–118, 2007.

603. Kedar PS, Nampoothiri S, Sreedhar S, et al: First-trimester prenatal diagnosis of pyruvate kinase deficiency in an Indian family with the pyruvate kinase-Amish mutation. *Genet Mol Res* 6:470–475, 2007.

604. So C-C, Tang M, Li C-H, et al: First reported case of prenatal diagnosis for pyruvate kinase deficiency in a Chinese family. *Hematology* 16:377–379, 2011.

605. Pekrun A, Neubauer BA, Eber SW, et al: Triosephosphate isomerase deficiency: Biochemical and molecular genetic analysis for prenatal diagnosis. *Clin Genet* 47:175–179, 1995.

606. Repiso A, Corrons JL, Vulliamy T, et al: New haplotype for the Glu104Asp mutation in triose-phosphate isomerase deficiency and prenatal diagnosis in a Spanish family. *J Inherit Metab Dis* 28:807–809, 2005.

607. Arya R, Lalloz MR, Nicolaides KH, et al: Prenatal diagnosis of triosephosphate isomerase deficiency. *Blood* 87:4507–4509, 1996.

608. Hirono A, Forman L, Beutler E: Enzymatic diagnosis in non-spherocytic hemolytic anemia. *Medicine (Baltimore)* 67:110–117, 1988.

609. Beutler E, Luzzatto L: Hemolytic anemia. *Semin Hematol* 36:38–47, 1999.

610. von Löhneysen K, Scott TM, Soldau K, et al: Assessment of the red cell proteome of young patients with unexplained hemolytic anemia by two-dimensional differential in-gel electrophoresis (DIGE). *PLoS One* 7:e34237, 2012.

611. Barasa B, Slijper M: Challenges for red blood cell biomarker discovery through proteomics. *Biochim Biophys Acta* 1844:1003–1010, 2014.

612. Bordbar A, Jamshidi N, Palsson BO: iAB-RBC-283: A proteomically derived knowledge-base of erythrocyte metabolism that can be used to simulate its physiological and patho-physiological states. *BMC Syst Biol* 5:110, 2011.

613. Lyon GJ, Jiang T, Van Wijk R, et al: Exome sequencing and unrelated findings in the context of complex disease research: Ethical and clinical implications. *Discov Med* 12:41–55, 2011.

614. Mimouni F, Shohat S, Reisner SH: G6PD-deficiency donor blood as a cause of hemolysis in two preterm infants. *Isr J Med Sci* 22:120–122, 1986.

615. Kappas A, Drummond GS, Valaes T: A single dose of Sn-mesoporphyrin prevents development of severe hyperbilirubinemia in glucose-6-phosphate dehydrogenase-deficient newborns. *Pediatrics* 108:25–30, 2001.

616. Hamilton JW, Jones FG, McMullin MF: Glucose-6-phosphate dehydrogenase Guadalajara—a case of chronic non-spherocytic haemolytic anaemia responding to splenectomy and the role of splenectomy in this disorder. *Hematology* 9:307–309, 2004.

617. Baronciani L, Tricta F, Beutler E: G6PD "campinas:" A deficient enzyme with a mutation at the far 3′ end of the gene. *Hum Mutat* 2:77–78, 1993.

618. Beutler E, Mathai CK, Smith JE: Biochemical variants of glucose-6-phosphate dehydrogenase giving rise to congenital nonspherocytic hemolytic disease. *Blood* 31:131–150, 1968.

619. Corash L, Spielberg S, Bartsocas C, et al: Reduced chronic hemolysis during high-dose vitamin E administration in Mediterranean-type glucose-6-phosphate dehydrogenase deficiency. *N Engl J Med* 303:416–420, 1980.

620. Spielberg SP, Boxer LA, Corash LM, et al: Improved erythrocyte survival with high dose vitamin E in chronic hemolyzing G6PD and glutathione synthetase deficiencies. *Ann Intern Med* 90:53–54, 1978.

621. Johnson GJ, Vatassery GT, Finkel B, et al: High-dose vitamin E does not decrease the rate of chronic hemolysis in glucose-6-phosphate dehydrogenase deficiency. *N Engl J Med* 308:1014–1017, 1983.

622. Newman JG, Newman TB, Bowie LJ, et al: An examination of the role of vitamin E in glucose-6-phosphate dehydrogenase deficiency. *Clin Biochem* 12:149–151, 1979.

623. Al Rimawi HS, Al Sheyyab M, Batieha A, et al: Effect of desferrioxamine in acute haemolytic anaemia of glucose-6-phosphate dehydrogenase deficiency. *Acta Haematol.* 101:145–148, 1999.

624. Ekert H, Rawlinson I: Deferoxamine and favism. *N Engl J Med* 312:1260, 1985.

625. Makarona K, Caputo VS, Costa JR, et al: Transcriptional and epigenetic basis for restoration of G6PD enzymatic activity in human G6PD-deficient cells. *Blood* 124:134–141, 2014.

626. Ationu A, Humphries A, Lalloz MR, et al: Reversal of metabolic block in glycolysis by enzyme replacement in triosephosphate isomerase-deficient cells. *Blood* 94:3193–3198, 1999.

627. Tanphaichitr VS, Suvatte V, Issaragrisil S, et al: Successful bone marrow transplantation in a child with red blood cell pyruvate kinase deficiency. *Bone Marrow Transplant* 26:689–690, 2000.

628. Kanno H, Aisaki, K.-I., Hamada T, et al: Ex vivo treatment of erythroid cells with glycolytic intermediates for metabolic correction of pyruvate kinase deficiency [abstract]. *Blood* 104: P3689, 2004.

629. Kung C, Hixon J, Kosinski P, et al: Small molecule activation of pyruvate kinase normalizes metabolic activity in red cells from patients with pyruvate kinase deficiency-associated hemolytic anemia, in *American Society of Hematology (ASH) 55th Annual meeting*, New Orleans, LA, 2013.

630. Schroter W: Successful long-term phenobarbital therapy of hyperbilirubinemia in congenital hemolytic anemia due to glucose phosphate isomerase deficiency. *Eur J Pediatr* 135:41–43, 1980.

631. Andersen FD, d'Amore F, Nielsen FC, et al: Unexpectedly high but still asymptomatic iron overload in a patient with pyruvate kinase deficiency. *Hematol J* 5:543–545, 2004.

632. Rider NL, Strauss KA, Brown K, et al: Erythrocyte pyruvate kinase deficiency in an old-order Amish cohort: Longitudinal risk and disease management. *Am J Hematol* 86:827–834, 2011.

633. Zanella A, Berzuini A, Colombo MB, et al: Iron status in red cell pyruvate kinase deficiency: Study of Italian cases. *Br J Haematol* 83:485–490, 1993.

634. Finkenstedt A, Bianchi P, Theurl I, et al: Regulation of iron metabolism through GDF15 and hepcidin in pyruvate kinase deficiency. *Br J Haematol* 144:789–793, 2009.

635. Mojzikova R, Koralkova P, Holub D, et al: Iron status in patients with pyruvate kinase deficiency: Neonatal hyperferritinaemia associated with a novel frameshift deletion in the *PKLR* gene (p.Arg518fs), and low hepcidin to ferritin ratios. *Br J Haematol* 165:556–563, 2014.

636. Pannacciulli I, Tizianello A, Ajmar F, et al: The course of experimentally-induced hemolytic anemia in a primaquine- sensitive Caucasian. A case study. *Blood* 25:92–95, 1965.

637. Meloni T, Forteleoni G, Noja G, et al: Increased prevalence of glucose-6-phosphate dehydrogenase deficiency in patients with cholelithiasis. *Acta Haematol* 85:76–78, 1991.

638. Petrakis NL, Wiesenfeld SL, Sams BJ, et al: Prevalence of sickle-cell trait and glucose-6-phosphate dehydrogenase deficiency. *N Engl J Med* 282:767–770, 1970.

639. Heller P, Best WR, Nelson RB, et al: Clinical implications of sickle-cell trait and glucose-6-phosphate dehydrogenase deficiency in hospitalized black male patients. *N Engl J Med* 300:1001–1005, 1979.

640. Renzaho AM, Husser E, Polonsky M: Should blood donors be routinely screened for glucose-6-phosphate dehydrogenase deficiency? A systematic review of clinical studies focusing on patients transfused with glucose-6-phosphate dehydrogenase-deficient red cells. *Transfus Med Rev* 28:7–17, 2014.

641. Pilo F, Baronciani D, Depau C, et al: Safety of hematopoietic stem cell donation in glucose 6 phosphate dehydrogenase-deficient donors. *Bone Marrow Transplant* 48:36–39, 2013.

642. Pamba A, Richardson ND, Carter N, et al: Clinical spectrum and severity of hemolytic anemia in glucose 6 phosphate dehydrogenase-deficient children receiving dapsone [in process citation]. *Blood* 120:4123–4133, 2012.

643. Bowman HS, McKusick VA, Dronamraju KR: Pyruvate kinase deficient hemolytic anemia in an Amish Isolate. *Hum GenotAm J Hum Genet* 17:1–8, 1965.

644. Beutler E, Duron O, Kelly BM: Improved method for the determination of blood glutathione. *J Lab Clin Med* 61:882–890, 1963.

645. Beutler E, Gelbart T: Improved assay of the enzymes of glutathione synthesis: Gamma-glutamylcysteine synthetase and glutathione synthetase. *Clin Chim Acta* 158:115–123, 1986.

646. Valentine WN, Fink K, Paglia DE, et al: Hereditary hemolytic anemia with human erythrocyte pyrimidine 5′-nucleotidase deficiency. *J Clin Invest* 54:866–879, 1974.

647. Torrance J, West C, Beutler E: A simple rapid radiometric assay for pyrimidine-5′-nucleotidase. *J Lab Clin Med* 90:563–568, 1977.

648. Beutler E, Kuhl W, Gelbart T: Blood cell phosphogluconolactonase: Assay and properties. *Br J Haematol.* 62:577–586, 1986.

649. Bird TD, Hamernyik P, Nutter JY, et al: Inherited deficiency of delta-aminolevulinic acid dehydratase. *Am J Hum Genet* 31:662–668, 1979.

650. Kamatani N, Hakoda M, Otsuka S, et al: Only three mutations account for almost all defective alleles causing adenine phosphoribosyltransferase deficiency in Japanese patients. *J Clin Invest* 90:130–135, 1992.

651. Hidaka Y, Palella TD, O'Toole TE, et al: Human adenine phosphoribosyltransferase. Identification of allelic mutations at the nucleotide level as a cause of complete deficiency of the enzyme. *J Clin Invest* 80:1409–1415, 1987.

652. Resta R, Thompson LF: SCID: The role of adenosine deaminase deficiency. *Immunol Today* 18:371–374, 1997.

653. Ogasawara N, Goto H, Yamada Y, et al: Distribution of AMP-deaminase isozymes in rat tissues. *Eur J Biochem* 87:297–304, 1978.
654. Yamada Y, Goto H, Wakamatsu N, et al: A rare case of complete human erythrocyte AMP deaminase deficiency due to two novel missense mutations in AMPD3. *Hum Mutat* 17:78, 2001.
655. Armstrong JM, Myers DV, Verpoorte JA, et al: Purification and properties of human erythrocyte carbonic anhydrases. *J Biol Chem* 241:5137–5149, 1966.
656. Kendall AG, Tashian RE: Erythrocyte carbonic anhydrase I: Inherited deficiency in humans. *Science* 197:471–472, 1977.
657. Roth DE, Venta PJ, Tashian RE, et al: Molecular basis of human carbonic anhydrase II deficiency. *Proc Natl Acad Sci U S A* 89:1804–1808, 1992.
658. Goth L, Rass P, Pay A: Catalase enzyme mutations and their association with diseases. *Mol Diagn* 8:141–149, 2004.
659. Percy MJ, Lappin TR: Recessive congenital methaemoglobinaemia: Cytochrome b(5) reductase deficiency. *Br J Haematol* 141:298–308, 2008.
660. Simonelli F, Giovane A, Frunzio S, et al: Galactokinase activity in patients with idiopathic presenile and senile cataract. *Metab Pediatr Syst Ophthalmol* 15:53–56, 1992.
661. Karas N, Gobec L, Pfeifer V, et al: Mutations in galactose-1-phosphate uridyltransferase gene in patients with idiopathic presenile cataract. *J Inherit Metab Dis* 26:699–704, 2003.
662. Beutler E: Red cell enzyme defects as non-diseases and as diseases. *Blood* 54:1–7, 1979.
663. Beutler E: Effect of flavin compounds on glutathione reductase activity: In vivo and in vitro studies. *J Clin Invest* 48:1957–1966, 1969.
664. Valentine WN, Paglia DE, Neerhout RC, et al: Erythrocyte glyoxalase II deficiency with coincidental hereditary elliptocytosis. *Blood* 36:797–808, 1970.
665. Johnson LA, Gordon RB, Emmerson BT: Hypoxanthine-guanine phosphoribosyltransferase: A simple spectrophotometric assay. *Clin Chim Acta* 80:203–207, 1977.
666. Larovere LE, Romero N, Fairbanks LD, et al: A novel missense mutation, c.584A > C (Y195S), in two unrelated Argentine patients with hypoxanthine-guanine phosphoribosyl-transferase deficiency, neurological variant. *Mol Genet Metab* 81:352–354, 2004.
667. Sumi S, Marinaki AM, Arenas M, et al: Genetic basis of inosine triphosphate pyrophosphohydrolase deficiency. *Hum Genet* 111:360–367, 2002.
668. Sass MD, Caruso CJ, Farhangi M: TPNH-methemoglobin reductase deficiency: A new red-cell enzyme defect. *J Lab Clin Med* 70:760–767, 1967.
669. Ferrell RE, Escallon M, Aguilar L, et al: Erythrocyte phosphoglucomutase: A family study of a PGM1 deficient allele. *Hum Genet* 67:306–308, 1984.
670. Banki K, Hutter E, Colombo E, et al: Glutathione levels and sensitivity to apoptosis are regulated by changes in transaldolase expression. *J Biol Chem* 271:32994–33001, 1996.
671. Chamberlain BR, Buttery JE: Reappraisal of the uroporphyrinogen I synthase assay, and a proposed modified method. *Clin Chem* 26:1346–1347, 1980.
672. Strand LJ, Meyer UA, Felsher BF, et al: Decreased red cell uroporphyrinogen I synthetase activity in intermittent acute porphyria. *J Clin Invest* 51:2530–2536, 1972.
673. Chao LT, Du CS, Louie E, et al: A to G substitution identified in exon 2 of the G6PD gene among G6PD deficient Chinese. *Nucleic Acids Res* 19:6056, 1991.
674. Hirono A, Ishii A, Kere N, et al: Molecular analysis of glucose-6-phosphate dehydrogenase variants in the Solomon Islands. *Am J Hum Genet* 56:1243–1245, 1995.
675. Kaeda JS, Chhotray GP, Ranjit MR, et al: A new glucose-6-phosphate dehydrogenase variant, G6PD Orissa (44 Ala—>Gly), is the major polymorphic variant in tribal populations in India. *Am J Hum Genet* 57:1335–1341, 1995.
676. Minucci A, Antenucci M, Giardina B, et al: G6PD Murcia, G6PD Ube and G6PD Orissa: Report of three G6PD mutations unusual for Italian population. *Clin Biochem* 43:1180–1181, 2010.
677. Nafa K, Reghis A, Osmani N, et al: G6PD Aures: A new mutation (48 Ile—>Thr) causing mild G6PD deficiency is associated with favism. *Hum Mol Genet.* 2:81–82, 1993.
678. Daoud BB, Mosbehi I, Prehu C, et al: Molecular characterization of erythrocyte glucose-6-phosphate dehydrogenase deficiency in Tunisia. *Pathol Biol (Paris)* 56:260–267, 2008.
679. Calabro V, Giacobbe A, Vallone D, et al: Genetic heterogeneity at the glucose-6-phosphate dehydrogenase locus in southern Italy: A study on a population from the Matera district. *Hum Genet* 86:49–53, 1990.
680. Ganczakowski M, Town M, Bowden DK, et al: Multiple glucose 6-phosphate dehydrogenase-deficient variants correlate with malaria endemicity in the Vanuatu archipelago (southwestern Pacific). *Am J Hum Genet* 56:294–301, 1995.
681. Nakatsuji T, Miwa S: Incidence and characteristics of glucose-6-phosphate dehydrogenase variants in Japan. *Hum Genet* 51:297–305, 1979.
682. Chiu DT, Zuo L, Chao L, et al: Molecular characterization of glucose-6-phosphate dehydrogenase (G6PD) deficiency in patients of Chinese descent and identification of new base substitutions in the human G6PD gene. *Blood* 81:2150–2154, 1993.
683. Vulliamy TJ, Wanachiwanawin W, Mason PJ, et al: G6PD Mahidol, a common deficient variant in South East Asia is caused by a (163)glycine—serine mutation. *Nucleic Acids Res* 17: 5868, 1989.
684. Beutler E, Kuhl W, Saenz GF, et al: Mutation analysis of glucose-6-phosphate dehydrogenase (G6PD) variants in Costa Rica. *Hum Genet* 87:462–464, 1991.
685. Cittadella R, Civitelli D, Manna I, et al: Genetic heterogeneity of glucose-6-phosphate dehydrogenase deficiency in south-east Sicily. *Ann Hum Genet* 61:229–234, 1997.
686. De Vita G, Alcalay M, Sampietro M, et al: Two point mutations are responsible for G6PD polymorphism in Sardinia. *Am J Hum Genet* 44:233–240, 1989.
687. Corcoran CM, Calabro V, Tamagnini G, et al: Molecular heterogeneity underlying the G6PD Mediterranean phenotype. *Hum Genet* 88:688–690, 1992.
688. Kirkman HN, Simon ER, Pickard BM: Seattle variant of glucose-6-phosphate dehydrogenase. *J Lab Clin Med* 66:834–840, 1965.
689. Cappellini MD, Sampietro M, Toniolo D, et al: Biochemical and molecular characterization of a new sporadic glucose-6-phosphate dehydrogenase variant described in Italy: G6PD Modena. *Br J Haematol* 87:209–211, 1994.
690. Cappellini MD, Martinez di Montemuros F, Dotti C, et al: Molecular characterisation of the glucose-6-phosphate dehydrogenase (G6PD) Ferrara II variant. *Hum Genet* 95:440–442, 1995.
691. Viglietto G, Montanaro V, Calabro V, et al: Common glucose-6-phosphate dehydrogenase (G6PD) variants from the Italian population: Biochemical and molecular characterization. *Ann Hum Genet* 54:1–15, 1990.
692. Beutler E, Westwood B, Kuhl W: Definition of the mutations of G6PD Wayne, G6PD Viangchan, G6PD Jammu, and G6PD "LeJeune". *Acta Haematol* 86:179–182, 1991.
693. Poon MC, Hall K, Scott CW, et al: G6PD Viangchan: A new glucose 6-phosphate dehydrogenase variant from Laos. *Hum Genet* 78:98–99, 1988.
694. Ahluwalia A, Corcoran CM, Vulliamy TJ, et al: G6PD Kalyan and G6PD Kerala; two deficient variants in India caused by the same 317 Glu—>Lys mutation. *Hum Mol Genet* 1:209–210, 1992.
695. Sukumar S, Mukherjee MB, Colah RB, et al: Two distinct Indian G6PD variants G6PD Jamnagar and G6PD Rohini caused by the same 949 G—>A mutation. *Blood Cells Mol Dis* 35:193–195, 2005.
696. Beutler E, Westwood B, Prchal JT, et al: New glucose-6-phosphate dehydrogenase mutations from various ethnic groups. *Blood* 80:255–256, 1992.
697. Calabro V, Mason PJ, Filosa S, et al: Genetic heterogeneity of glucose-6-phosphate dehydrogenase deficiency revealed by single-strand conformation and sequence analysis. *Am J Hum Genet* 52:527–536, 1993.
698. Menounos P, Zervas C, Garinis G, et al: Molecular heterogeneity of the glucose-6-phosphate dehydrogenase deficiency in the Hellenic population. *Hum Hered* 50:237–241, 2000.
699. Perng LI, Chiou SS, Liu TC, et al: A novel C to T substitution at nucleotide 1360 of cDNA which abolishes a natural Hha I site accounts for a new G6PD deficiency gene in Chinese. *Hum Mol Genet* 1:205, 1992.
700. Wagner G, Bhatia K, Board P: Glucose-6-phosphate dehydrogenase deficiency mutations in Papua New Guinea. *Hum Biol* 68:383–394, 1996.
701. Stevens DJ, Wanachiwanawin W, Mason PJ, et al: G6PD Canton a common deficient variant in South East Asia caused by a 459 Arg—Leu mutation. *Nucleic Acids Res* 18:7190, 1990.
702. Chiu DT, Zuo L, Chen E, et al: Two commonly occurring nucleotide base substitutions in Chinese G6PD variants. *Biochem Biophys Res Commun* 180:988–993, 1991.

CHAPTER 48

THE THALASSEMIAS: DISORDERS OF GLOBIN SYNTHESIS

David J. Weatherall

SUMMARY

The thalassemias are the commonest monogenic diseases in man. They occur at a high gene frequency throughout the Mediterranean populations, the Middle East, the Indian subcontinent, and Myanmar, and in a line stretching from southern China through Thailand and the Malay peninsula into the island populations of the Pacific. They are also seen commonly in countries in which there has been immigration from these high-frequency populations.

There are two main classes of thalassemias, α and β, in which the α- and β-globin genes are involved, and rarer forms caused by abnormalities of other globin genes. Some extremely rare congenital and acquired thalassemia that have intact globin genes are caused by either mutations of nonglobin genes or factors yet to be elucidated. All thalassemias have in common an imbalanced rate of production of the globin chains of adult hemoglobin, excess α chains in β-thalassemia and excess β chains in α-thalassemia. Several hundred different mutations at the α- and β-globin loci have been defined as the cause of the reduced or absent output of α or β chains. The high frequency and genetic diversity of the thalassemias is related to past or present heterozygote resistance to malaria.

The pathophysiology of the thalassemias can be traced to the deleterious effects of the globin-chain subunits that are produced in excess. In β-thalassemia, excess α chains cause damage to the red cell precursors and red cells and lead to profound anemia. This causes expansion of the ineffective marrow, with severe effects on development, bone formation, and growth. The major cause of morbidity and mortality is the effect of iron deposition in the endocrine organs, liver, and heart, which results from increased intestinal absorption and the effects of blood transfusion. The pathophysiology of the α-thalassemias is different because the excess β chains that result from defective α-chain production form β_4 molecules, or hemoglobin H, which is soluble and does not precipitate in the marrow. However, it is unstable and precipitates in older red cells. Hence, the anemia of α-thalassemia is hemolytic rather than dyserythropoietic.

The clinical pictures of α- and β-thalassemia vary widely, and knowledge is gradually being amassed about some of the genetic and environmental factors that modify these phenotypes.

Because the carrier states for the thalassemias can be identified and affected fetuses can be diagnosed by DNA analysis after the ninth to tenth week of gestation, these conditions are widely amenable to prenatal diagnosis. Currently, marrow transplantation is the only way in which they can be cured. Symptomatic management is based on regular blood transfusion, iron chelation therapy, and the judicious use of splenectomy. Experimental approaches to their management include the stimulation of fetal hemoglobin synthesis and attempts at somatic cell gene therapy.

Acronyms and Abbreviations: AATAAA, the polyadenylation signal site; ATR-16, α-thalassemia chromosome 16-linked mental retardation syndrome; ATR-X, α-thalassemia X-linked mental retardation syndrome; *BCL11A*, B-cell lymphoma/leukemia oncogene important for γ- to β-globin switching; CAP site, a DNA site located in or near a promoter; DNase I, an enzyme used to detect DNA-protein interaction; GATA-1, a transcription factor essential for productive erythropoiesis; HPFH, hereditary persistence of fetal hemoglobin; HS, hypersensitive site to DNase I treatment; IVS, intervening sequence of a gene (i.e., an intron); KLF1, erythroid Kruppel-like factor; LCR, locus control region; MCS, multispecies conserved sequences; NFE-2, "nuclear factor, erythroid 2" is a transcription factor essential for productive erythropoiesis; PHD region, known as plant homeodomain is a DNA region with zinc finger motif commonly deleted in ATR-X α-thalassemia; RFLP, restriction fragment length polymorphism; TATA box, a DNA sequence (*cis*-regulatory element) found in the promoter region of genes.

● DEFINITIONS AND HISTORY

In 1925, Cooley and Lee[1] first described a form of severe anemia that occurred early in life and was associated with splenomegaly and bone changes. In 1932, George H. Whipple and William L. Bradford[2] published a comprehensive account of the pathologic findings in this disease. Whipple coined the phrase *thalassic anemia*[3,4] and condensed it to *thalassemia*, from $\theta\alpha\lambda\alpha\sigma\sigma\alpha$ ("the sea"), because early patients were all of Mediterranean background. The true genetic character of the disorder became fully appreciated after 1940. The disease described by Cooley and Lee is the homozygous state of an autosomal gene for which the heterozygous state is associated with much milder hematologic changes. The severe homozygous condition became known as *thalassemia major*. The heterozygous states, thalassemia trait, were designated according to their severity as *thalassemia minor* or *minima*.[3,5-7] Later, the term *thalassemia intermedia* was used to describe disorders that were milder than the major form but more severe than the traits.

Thalassemia is not a single disease but a group of disorders, each resulting from an inherited abnormality of globin production.[7] The conditions form part of the spectrum of diseases known collectively as the *hemoglobinopathies*, which can be classified broadly into two types. The first subdivision consists of conditions, such as sickle cell anemia, that result from an inherited structural alteration in one of the globin chains. Although such abnormal hemoglobins may be synthesized less efficiently or broken down more rapidly than normal adult hemoglobin, the associated clinical abnormalities result from the physical properties of the abnormal hemoglobin (Chap. 49). The second major subdivision of the hemoglobinopathies, the thalassemias, consists of inherited defects in the rate of synthesis of one or more of the globin chains. The result is imbalanced globin chain production, ineffective erythropoiesis, hemolysis, and a variable degree of anemia.

Several monographs describe the historical aspects of thalassemia in greater detail.[5,7]

TABLE 48–1. Thalassemias and Related Disorders

α-Thalassemia

  α^0

  α^+

  Deletion ($-\alpha$)

  Nondeletion (α^T)

β-Thalassemia

  β^0

  β^+

  Normal hemoglobin A_2

  Dominant

  Unlinked to β-globin genes

$\delta\beta$-Thalassemia

  $(\delta\beta)^+$

  $(\delta\beta)^0$

  $(^A\gamma\,\delta\beta)^0$

γ-Thalassemia

δ-Thalassemia

  δ^0

  δ^+

$\varepsilon\gamma\delta\beta$-Thalassemia

Hereditary Persistence of Fetal Hemoglobin

  Deletion

  $(\delta\beta)^0$, $(^A\gamma\,\delta\beta)^0$

  Nondeletion

  Linked to β-globin genes

  $^G\gamma\,\beta^+$, $^A\gamma\,\beta^+$

  Unlinked to β-globin genes

DIFFERENT FORMS OF THALASSEMIA

Thalassemia can be defined as a condition in which a reduced rate of synthesis of one or more of the globin chains leads to imbalanced globin chain synthesis, defective hemoglobin production, and damage to the red cells or their precursors from the effects of the globin subunits that are produced in relative excess.[7,8] Table 48–1 summarizes the main varieties of thalassemia that have been defined with certainty.

The β-thalassemias are divided into two main varieties. In one form, β^0-thalassemia, there is no β-chain production. In the other form, β^+-thalassemia, there is a partial deficiency of β-chain production. The hallmark of the common forms of β-thalassemia is an elevated level of hemoglobin A_2 in heterozygotes. In a less-common class of β-thalassemias, heterozygotes have normal hemoglobin A_2 levels. Other rare forms include varieties of β-thalassemia intermedia that are inherited in a dominant fashion, that is, heterozygotes are severely affected, and there is a variety in which the genetic determinants are not linked to the β-globin gene cluster.[7,9,10]

The $\delta\beta$-thalassemias are heterogeneous. In some cases, no δ or β chains are synthesized. Originally, these disorders were classified according to the structure of the hemoglobin F produced, that is, $^G\gamma^A\gamma(\delta\beta)^0$- and $^G\gamma(\delta\beta)^0$-thalassemia. This classification is illogical. The conditions are best described by the globin chains that are defectively synthesized, that is, simply $(\delta\beta)^+$-, $(\delta\beta)^0$-, and $(^A\gamma\delta\beta)^0$-thalassemia.[7,10] In the $(\delta\beta)^+$-thalassemias, an abnormal hemoglobin is produced that has normal α chains combined with non-α chains consisting of the N-terminal residues of the δ chain fused to the C-terminal residues of the β chain. These fusion variants, called the *Lepore hemoglobins*, show structural heterogeneity.

The δ-thalassemias[7,10] are characterized by reduced output of δ chains and hence reduced hemoglobin A_2 levels in heterozygotes and an absence of hemoglobin A_2 in homozygotes. They are of no clinical significance except that, when inherited with β-thalassemia trait, the level of hemoglobin A_2 is reduced to the normal range.

A disorder characterized by defective ε-, γ-, δ-, and β-chain synthesis has been defined at the clinical and molecular level.[7,10] The homozygous state for this condition, $\varepsilon\gamma\delta\beta$-thalassemia, presumably is not compatible with fetal survival. It has been observed only in heterozygotes.

Hereditary persistence of fetal hemoglobin (HPFH) is a heterogeneous condition characterized by persistent fetal hemoglobin.[7,9,10] It is classified into deletion and nondeletion forms. The deletion forms of HPFH can be classified, like $\delta\beta$-thalassemia, as $(\delta\beta)^0$ HPFH and then subdivided according to the particular population in which this occurs and its associated molecular defect. In effect, the deletion forms of HPFH are very similar to β-thalassemia except for more efficient γ-chain synthesis and, therefore, less chain imbalance and a milder phenotype. The homozygous state is associated with mild thalassemic changes. In fact, the β-thalassemias and deletion forms of HPFH form a clinical continuum. The nondeletion forms of HPFH also are heterogeneous. In some cases, they are associated with mutations that involve the β-globin gene cluster and in which there is β-chain synthesis *cis* to the HPFH determinant. These conditions are subdivided into $^G\gamma\beta^+$ HPFH and $^A\gamma\beta^+$ HPFH. Again, they often are subclassified according to the population in which they occur, for example, Greek HPFH, British HPFH, and so on. Finally, a heterogeneous group of HPFH determinants is associated with very low levels of persistent fetal hemoglobin, the genetic loci of which, at least in some cases, are not linked to the β-globin gene cluster.

Because α chains are present in both fetal and adult hemoglobins, a deficiency of α-chain production affects hemoglobin synthesis in fetal and in adult life. A reduced rate of α-chain synthesis in fetal life results in an excess of γ chains, which form γ_4 tetramers, or hemoglobin Bart's. In adult life, a deficiency of α chains results in an excess of β chains, which form β_4 tetramers, or hemoglobin H. Because there are two α-globin genes per haploid genome, the genetics of α-thalassemia is more complicated than that of β-thalassemia. There are two main groups of α-thalassemia determinants.[7,10] First, in the α^0-thalassemias (formerly called α-thalassemia 1), no α chains are produced from an affected chromosome; that is, both linked α-globin genes are inactivated. Second, in the α^+-thalassemias (formerly called α-thalassemia 2), the output of one of the linked pair of α-globin genes is defective. The α^+-thalassemias are subdivided into deletion and nondeletion types. Both the α^0-thalassemias and deletion and nondeletion forms of α^+-thalassemia are extremely heterogeneous at the molecular level. There are two major clinical phenotypes of α-thalassemia: the hemoglobin Bart's hydrops syndrome, which usually reflects the homozygous state for α^0-thalassemia, and hemoglobin H disease, which usually results from the compound heterozygous state for α^0- and α^+-thalassemia.

Because the structural hemoglobin variants and the thalassemias occur at a high frequency in some populations, the two types of genetic defect can be found in the same individual. The different genetic varieties of thalassemia and their combinations with the genes for abnormal hemoglobins produce a series of disorders known collectively as the *thalassemia syndromes*.[7]

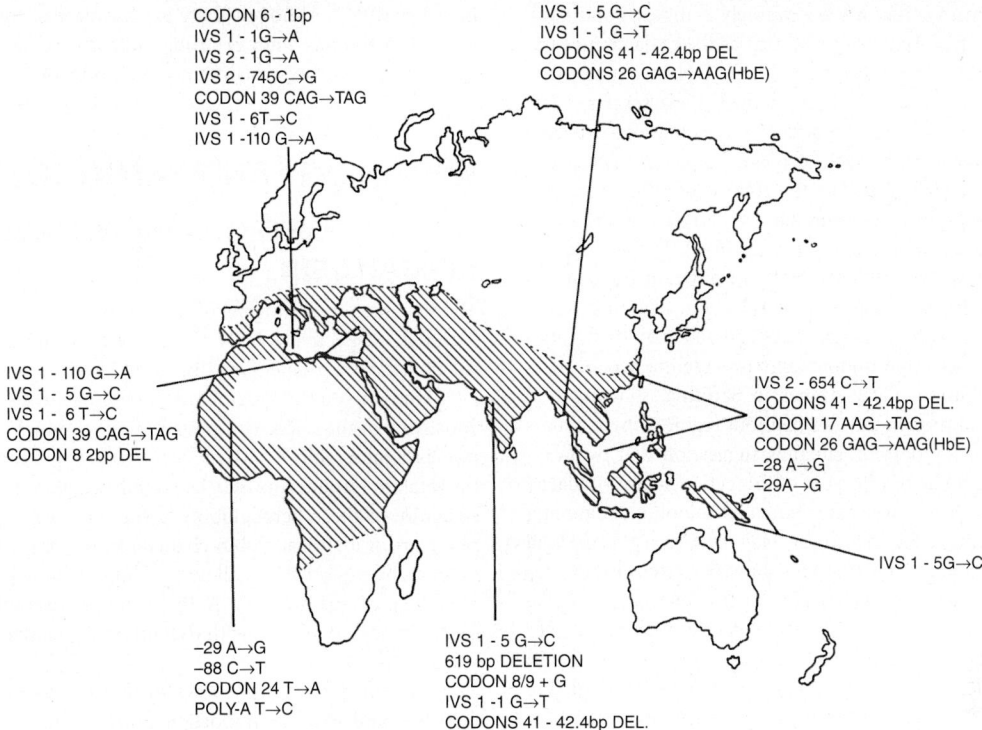

CODON 6 - 1bp
IVS 1 - 1G→A
IVS 2 - 1G→A
IVS 2 - 745C→G
CODON 39 CAG→TAG
IVS 1 - 6T→C
IVS 1 -110 G→A

IVS 1 - 5 G→C
IVS 1 - 1 G→T
CODONS 41 - 42.4bp DEL
CODONS 26 GAG→AAG(HbE)

IVS 1 - 110 G→A
IVS 1 - 5 G→C
IVS 1 - 6 T→C
CODON 39 CAG→TAG
CODON 8 2bp DEL

IVS 2 - 654 C→T
CODONS 41 - 42.4bp DEL.
CODON 17 AAG→TAG
CODON 26 GAG→AAG(HbE)
−28 A→G
−29A→G

IVS 1 - 5G→C

−29 A→G
−88 C→T
CODON 24 T→A
POLY-A T→C

IVS 1 - 5 G→C
619 bp DELETION
CODON 8/9 + G
IVS 1 -1 G→T
CODONS 41 - 42.4bp DEL.

Figure 48–1. World distribution of β-thalassemia.

EPIDEMIOLOGY AND POPULATION GENETICS

The β-thalassemias are distributed widely in Mediterranean populations, the Middle East, parts of India and Pakistan, and throughout Southeast Asia (Fig. 48–1).[7,11,12] The disease is common in Tajikistan, Turkmenistan, Kyrgyzstan, and the People's Republic of China. Because of the extensive migration from areas of high gene frequency such as the Mediterranean region (e.g., Italy, Greece), Africa, and Asia to the Americas, the α- and β-thalassemia genes and clinical disease are relatively common, especially in North, but also South, America. The β-thalassemias are rare in Africa, except for isolated pockets in West Africa, notably Liberia, and in parts of North Africa. However, β-thalassemia occurs sporadically in all racial groups and has been observed in the homozygous state in persons of pure Anglo-Saxon heritage. Thus, a patient's racial background does not preclude the diagnosis.

The δβ-thalassemias have been observed sporadically in many racial groups, although no high-frequency populations have been defined. Similarly, the hemoglobin Lepore syndromes have been found in many populations, but, with the possible exceptions of central Italy, Western Europe, and parts of Spain and Portugal, these disorders have not been found to occur at a high frequency in any particular region.

The α-thalassemias occur widely throughout Africa, the Mediterranean countries, the Middle East, and Southeast Asia (Fig. 48–2).[7,11,12] The α⁰-thalassemias are found most commonly in Mediterranean and Oriental populations, but are extremely rare in African and Middle Eastern populations. However, the deletion forms of α⁺-thalassemia occur at a high frequency throughout West Africa, the Mediterranean, the Middle East, and Southeast Asia. In United States, approximately 30 percent of Americans of African descent carry the gene α⁺-thalassemia. Up to 80 percent of the population of some parts of Papua New Guinea are carriers for the deletion form of α⁺-thalassemia. How common the nondeletion forms of α⁺-thalassemia are in any particular populations

is uncertain, but they have been reported quite frequently in some of the Mediterranean island populations and in the Middle Eastern and Southeast Asian populations. Because the hemoglobin Bart's hydrops syndrome and hemoglobin H disease require the action of an α⁰-thalassemia determinant, these disorders are found at a high frequency only in Southeast Asia and in parts of the Mediterranean region. The α-chain termination mutants, such as hemoglobin Constant Spring, seem to be particularly common in Southeast Asia. Approximately 4 percent of the population in Thailand are carriers.

In 1949, J.B.S. Haldane[13] suggested that thalassemia had reached its high frequency in tropical regions because heterozygotes are protected against malaria.[13] Although many population studies have tested this

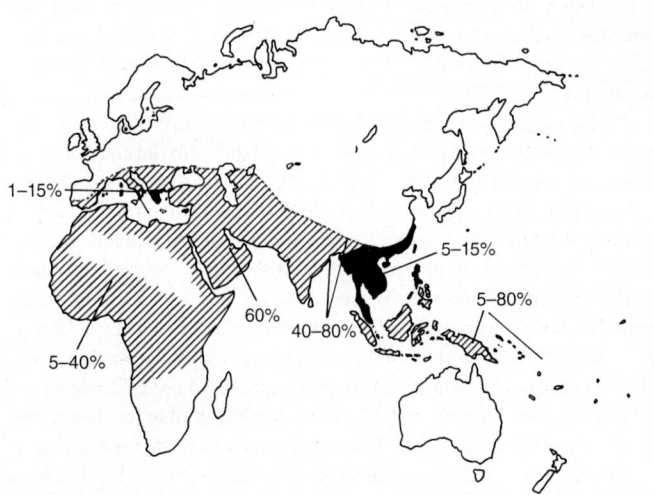

1–15%
5–15%
5–80%
60%
40–80%
5–40%

Figure 48–2. World distribution of α⁺- (hatched areas) and α⁰- thalassemia (shaded areas).

hypothesis, elucidation of some of the extremely complex population genetics underlying polymorphic systems such as the thalassemias has been possible only with the advent of recombinant DNA technology.

In each of the high-frequency areas for the β-thalassemias, a few common mutations and varying numbers of rare mutations are seen (see Fig. 48–1). Furthermore, in each of these regions the pattern of mutations is different, usually found in the context of different haplotypes in the associated β-globin gene cluster.[11,14,15] Similar observations have been made in the α-thalassemias (see Fig. 48–2).[7,11] These studies suggest the thalassemias arose independently in different populations and then achieved their high frequency by selection. Although some movement of the thalassemia genes may have resulted from drift, independent mutation and selection undoubtedly provide the overall basis for their world distribution. Early studies in Sardinia, showing that β-thalassemia is less common in the mountainous regions where malarial transmission is low, supported Haldane's suggestion that β-thalassemia reached its high frequency because of protection against malarial infections.[16] For many years these data remained the only convincing evidence for a protective effect. However, later studies using malaria endemicity data and globin-gene mapping showed a clear altitude-related effect on the frequency of α-thalassemia in Papua New Guinea. In addition, a sharp cline (a gradual change of species phenotype over a geographical area) in the frequency of α-thalassemia has been found in the region stretching south from Papua New Guinea through the island populations of Melanesia to New Caledonia. This is mirrored by a similar gradient in the distribution of malaria.[17] The effect of drift and founder effect in these island populations has been largely excluded by showing that other DNA polymorphisms have a random distribution through the region, with no evidence of a cline similar to that characterizing the distribution of α-thalassemia and malaria.

Firm evidence for protection of individuals with mild forms of α^+-thalassemia against *Plasmodium falciparum* malaria has been provided. In a case-control study performed in Papua New Guinea, the homozygous state for α^+-thalassemia offered approximately 60 percent protection against hospital admittance because of serious complications of malaria, notably coma or profound anemia.[18] Similar levels of protection by α-thalassemia against *P. falciparum* malaria have been found in several different African populations.[19] However, it is becoming clear that there are complex genetic epistatic interactions between protective polymorphisms of this kind. For example, although α-thalassemia and the sickle cell trait both offer strong protection against *P. falciparum* malaria, in those who inherit both traits, the protection is canceled out and they are fully susceptible to the disease.[20] Interactions of this type will have an important effect on the gene frequency of protective polymorphisms in countries in which more than one exists in the same population.

There is growing evidence that both immune and cellular mechanisms may underlie these protective effects of different red cell polymorphisms against malarial infection. Followup studies of cohorts of babies with α-thalassemia suggest that, in the first year of life, they are more prone to *Plasmodium vivax* and *P. falciparum* malaria. Because there is evidence for cross-immunization between these two species, it is possible that this effect induces early immunization that may result in babies with α-thalassemia being more resistant to *P. falciparum* malaria later in life.[21] At the cellular level there is no evidence that α-thalassemia has any effect on the rates of parasite invasion and growth in red cells. However, parasitized α-thalassemic red cells are more susceptible to phagocytosis *in vitro*, and are less able than normal cells to form rosettes, an *in vitro* phenomena whereby uninfected cells bind to infected cells that is strongly associated with severity of infection, and express low levels of complement receptor 1, which is required for rosette formation.[22] These highly complex immune and cellular interactions are discussed in detail

in reviews.[19,23,24] Although there are less data of this kind available for the β-thalassemias, there is strong indirect evidence that their high frequency has also been maintained by protection against *P. falciparum* malaria.

● ETIOLOGY AND PATHOGENESIS

GENETIC CONTROL AND SYNTHESIS OF HEMOGLOBIN

The structure and ontogeny of the hemoglobins are reviewed in Chaps. 7 and 49, respectively. Only those aspects with particular relevance to the thalassemia problem are discussed here.

Human adult hemoglobin is a heterogeneous mixture of proteins consisting of the major component hemoglobin A and the minor component hemoglobin A_2, which constitutes approximately 2.5 percent of the total. In intrauterine life, the main hemoglobin is hemoglobin F. The structure of these hemoglobins is similar. Each consists of two separate pairs of identical globin chains. Except for some of the embryonic hemoglobins (see below), all normal human hemoglobins have one pair of α chains. In hemoglobin A, the α chains are combined with β chains ($\alpha_2\beta_2$), in hemoglobin A_2 with δ chains ($\alpha_2\delta_2$), and in hemoglobin F with γ chains ($\alpha_2\gamma_2$).

Human hemoglobin shows further heterogeneity, particularly in fetal life, and this has important implications for understanding the thalassemias and for approaches to their prenatal diagnosis. Hemoglobin F is a mixture of molecular species with the formulas $\alpha_2\gamma_2^{136Gly}$ and $\alpha_2\gamma_2^{136Ala}$. The γ chains containing glycine at position 136 are designated $^G\gamma$ chains. The γ chains containing alanine are called $^A\gamma$ chains. At birth, the ratio of molecules containing $^G\gamma$ chains to those containing $^A\gamma$ chains is approximately 3:1. The ratio varies widely in the trace amounts of hemoglobin F present in normal adults.

Before week 8 of intrauterine life, three embryonic hemoglobins—Gower 1 ($\xi_2\varepsilon_2$), Gower 2 ($\alpha_2\varepsilon_2$), and Portland ($\xi_2\gamma_2$)—are present. The ξ and ε chains are the embryonic counterparts of the adult α and β and γ and δ chains, respectively. ξ-Chain synthesis persists beyond the embryonic stage of development in some of the α-thalassemias. Persistent ε-chain production has not been found in any of the thalassemia syndromes. During fetal development, an orderly switch from ξ- to α-chain and from ε- to γ-chain production occurs, followed by β- and δ-chain production after birth.

Figure 48–3 shows the different human hemoglobins and the arrangements of the α-gene cluster on chromosome 16 and the β-gene cluster on chromosome 11.

Globin Gene Clusters

Although some individual variability exists, the α-gene cluster usually contains one functional ξ gene and two α genes, designated α_2 and α_1. It also contains four pseudogenes: $\psi\xi_1$, $\psi\alpha_1$, $\psi\alpha_2$, and θ_1.[9,10] These four pseudogenes are remarkably conserved among different species. Although it appears to be expressed early in fetal life, its function is unknown. It likely does not produce a viable globin chain. Each α gene is located in a region of homology approximately 4 kb long, interrupted by two small nonhomologous regions.[25–27] The homologous regions are believed to result from gene duplication, and the nonhomologous segments are believed to arise subsequently by insertion of DNA into the noncoding regions around one of the two genes. The exons of the two α-globin genes have identical sequences. The first intron in each gene is identical. The second intron of α_1 is nine bases longer and differs by three bases from that in the α_2 gene.[27–29] Despite their high degree of homology, the sequences of the two α-globin genes diverge in their 3' untranslated regions 13 bases beyond the TAA stop codon. These differences provide

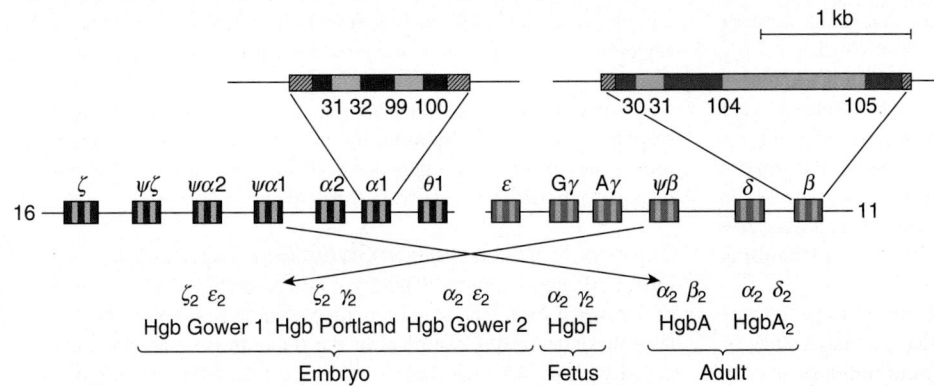

Figure 48–3. Genetic control of human hemoglobin (Hgb). The main globin gene clusters are located on chromosomes 11 and 16. At each stage of development, different genes in these clusters are activated or repressed. The different globin chains directed by individual genes are synthesized independently and combine in random fashion as indicated by the *arrows.*

an opportunity to assess the relative output of the genes, an important part of the analysis of the α-thalassemias.[30,31] Production of α_2 messenger RNA appears to exceed that of α_1 by a factor of 1.5 to 3. $\psi\xi_1$ and ξ_2 genes also are highly homologous. The introns are much larger than those of α-globin genes. In contrast to the latter, IVS-1 is larger than IVS-2. In each ξ gene, IVS-1 contains several copies of a simple repeated 14-bp sequence that is similar to sequences located between the two ξ genes and near the human insulin gene. The coding sequence of the first exon of $\psi\xi_1$ contains three base changes, one of which gives rise to a premature stop codon, thus making $\psi\xi_1$ an inactive pseudogene.

The regions separating and surrounding the α-like structural genes have been analyzed in detail. Of particular relevance to thalassemia is the polymorphic nature of this gene cluster.[32] The cluster contains five hypervariable regions: one downstream from the α_1 gene, one between the ξ and $\psi\xi$ genes, one in the first intron of both the ξ and $\psi\xi$ genes, and one 5' to the cluster. These regions consist of varying numbers of tandem repeats of nucleotide sequences. Taken together with single-base restriction fragment length polymorphisms (RFLPs), the variability of the α-globin gene cluster reaches a heterozygosity level of approximately 0.95. Thus, each parental α-globin gene cluster can be identified in the majority of persons. This heterogeneity has important implications for tracing the history of the thalassemia mutations.

Figure 48–3 shows the arrangement of the β-globin gene cluster on the short arm of chromosome 11. Each of the individual genes and their flanking regions have been sequenced.[33–36] Like the α_1 and α_2 gene pairs, the $^G\gamma$ and $^A\gamma$ genes share a similar sequence. In fact, the $^G\gamma$ and $^A\gamma$ genes on one chromosome are identical in the region 5' to the center of the large intron yet show some divergence 3' to that position. At the boundary between the conserved and divergent regions, a block of simple sequence may be a "hot spot" for initiation of recombination events that lead to unidirectional gene conversion.

Like the α-globin genes, the β-gene cluster contains a series of single-point RFLPs, although in this case no hypervariable regions have been identified.[37,38] The arrangement of RFLPs, or haplotypes, in the β-globin gene cluster falls into two domains. The 5' side of the β gene, spanning approximately 32 kb from the ε gene to the 3' end of the $\psi\beta$ gene, contains three common patterns of RFLPs. The region encompassing about 18 kb to the 3' side of the β-globin gene also contains three common patterns in different populations. Between these regions is a sequence of about 11 kb in which there is randomization of the 5' and 3' domains; hence, a relatively higher frequency of recombination can occur.[38] The β-globin gene haplotypes are similar in most populations but differ markedly in individuals of African origin. These findings suggest the haplotype arrangements were laid down very early during evolution. The findings are consistent with data obtained from mitochondrial DNA polymorphisms pointing to the early emergence of a relatively small population from Africa with subsequent divergence into

other racial groups.[39] Again, they are extremely useful for analyzing the population genetics and history of the thalassemia mutations.

The regions flanking the coding regions of the globin genes contain a number of conserved sequences essential for their expression.[28,33] The first conserved sequence is the TATA box, which serves accurately to locate the site of transcription initiation at the CAP site, usually about 30 bases downstream. It also appears to influence the rate of transcription. In addition, two so-called upstream promoter elements are present. A second conserved sequence, the CCAAT box, is located 70 or 80 bp upstream. The third conserved sequence, the CACCC homology box, is located further 5', approximately 80 to 100 bp from the CAP site. It can be either inverted or duplicated. These promoter sequences also are required for optimal transcription. Mutations in this region of the β-globin gene cause its defective expression and these findings provide the foundation for understating regulation of other human genes. The globin genes also have conserved sequences in their 3' flanking regions, notably AATAAA, which is the polyadenylation signal site.

Regulation of Globin Gene Clusters Figure 48–4 summarizes the mechanism of globin gene expression. The primary transcript is a mRNA precursor containing both intron and exon sequences. During its stay in

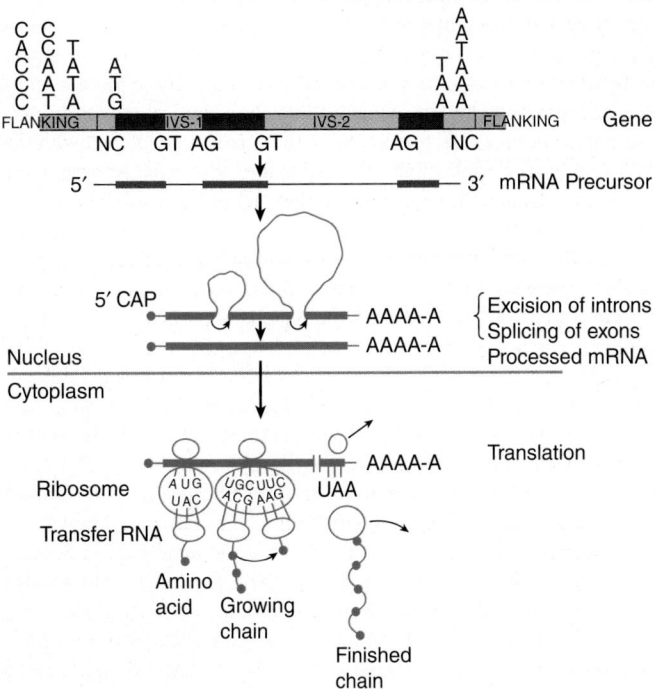

Figure 48–4. Expression of a human globin gene.

the nucleus, it undergoes a good deal of processing that entails capping the 5′ end and polyadenylation of the 3′ end, both of which probably serve to stabilize the transcript (Chap. 10). The intervening sequences are removed from the mRNA precursor in a complex two-stage process that relies on certain critical sequences at the intron–exon junctions.

The method by which globin gene clusters are regulated is important to understanding the pathogenesis of the thalassemias. Many details remain to be determined, but studies performed over the last few years have provided at least an outline of some of the major mechanisms of globin gene regulation.[7,9,40–42]

Most of the DNA within cells that is not involved in gene transcription is packaged into a compact form that is inaccessible to transcription factors and RNA polymerase. Transcriptional activity is characterized by a major change in the structure of the chromatin surrounding a particular gene. These alterations in chromatin structure can be identified by enhanced sensitivity to exogenous nucleases. Erythroid lineage-specific nuclease-hypersensitive sites are found at several locations in the β-globin gene cluster, which vary during different stages of development. In fetal life, these sites are associated with the promoter regions of all four globin genes. In adult erythroid cells, the sites associated with the γ genes are absent. The methylation state of the genes plays an important role in their ability to be expressed. In human and other animal tissues, the globin genes are extensively methylated in nonerythroid organs and are relatively undermethylated in hematopoietic tissues. Changes in chromatin configuration around the globin genes at different stages of development are reflected by alterations in their methylation state.

In addition to the promoter elements, several other important regulatory sequences have been identified in the globin gene clusters. For example, several enhancer sequences thought to be involved with tissue-specific expression have been identified. Their sequences are similar to the upstream activating sequences of the promoter elements. Both consist of a number of "modules," or motifs, that contain binding sites for transcriptional activators or repressors. The enhancer sequences are thought to act by coming into spatial apposition with the promoter sequences to increase the efficiency of transcription of particular genes. It now is clear that transcriptional regulatory proteins may bind to both the promoter region of a gene and to the enhancer. Some of these transcriptional proteins, GATA-1 and NFE-2, for example, appear to be largely restricted to hematopoietic tissues.[40] These proteins may bring the promoter and the enhancer into close physical proximity, permitting transcription factors bound to the enhancer to interact with the transcriptional complex that forms near the TATA box. At least some of these hematopoietic gene transcription factors likely will be developmental-stage specific.

Another set of erythroid-specific nuclease-hypersensitive sites is located upstream from the embryonic globin genes in both the α- and β-gene clusters. These sites mark the regions of particularly important control elements. In the case of the β-globin gene cluster, the region is marked by five hypersensitive sites to DNase I treatment (HS) (an enzyme used to detect DNA-protein interaction).[40] The most 5′ site (HS5) does not show tissue specificity. HS1 through HS4, which together form the locus control region (LCR), are largely erythroid-specific. Each of the regions of the LCR contains a variety of binding sites for erythroid transcription factors. The precise function of the LCR is not known, but it is undoubtedly required to establish a transcriptionally active domain spanning the entire globin gene cluster. The α-globin gene cluster also has a major regulatory element of this kind, in this case HS40.[41] This forms part of four highly conserved noncoding sequences, or multispecies conserved sequences (MCSs), called MSC-R1-R4; of these elements only MSC-R2, that is HS40, is essential for α-globin gene expression. Although deletions of this region inactivate the entire α-globin gene

cluster, its action must be fundamentally different from that of the β-globin LCR because the chromatin structure of the α-gene cluster is in an open conformation in all tissues.

Some forms of thalassemia result from deletions involving these regulatory regions. In addition, the phenotypic effects of deletions of these gene clusters are strongly positional, which may reflect the relative distance of particular genes from the LCR and HS40.

Developmental Changes in Globin Gene Expression

One particularly important aspect of human globin genes is regulation of the switch from fetal to adult hemoglobin. Because many of the thalassemias and related disorders of the β-globin gene cluster are associated with persistent γ-chain synthesis, a full understanding of their pathophysiology must include an explanation for this important phenomenon, which plays a considerable role in modifying their phenotypic expression.

The complex topic of hemoglobin switching has been the subject of several extensive reviews.[7,42] β-Globin synthesis commences early during fetal life, at approximately 8 to 10 weeks' gestation. β-Globin synthesis continues at a low level, approximately 10 percent of the total non–α-globin chain production, up to approximately 36 weeks' gestation, after which it is considerably augmented. At the same time, γ-globin chain synthesis starts to decline so that, at birth, approximately equal amounts of γ- and β-globin chains are produced. Over the first year of life, γ-chain synthesis gradually declines. By the end of the first year, γ-chain synthesis amounts to less than 1 percent of the total non–α-globin chain output. In adults the small amount of hemoglobin F is confined to an erythrocyte population called *F cells*.

How this series of developmental switches is regulated is not clear. The process is not organ specific but is synchronized throughout the developing hematopoietic tissues. Although environmental factors may be involved, the bulk of experimental evidence suggests some form of "time clock" is built into the hematopoietic stem cell. At the chromosomal level, regulation appears to occur in a complex manner involving both developmental stage-specific *trans*-activating factors and the relative proximity of the different genes of the β-globin gene cluster to LCR. Some of the elements involved in the stage-specific regulation of human globin genes have been identified. KLF1 (erythroid Kruppel-like factor), a developmental stage–enriched protein, activates human β-globin gene expression and is involved in human γ- to β-globin gene switching.[43] More recently BCL11A and MYB have also been identified as being involved in this process.[42]

Fetal hemoglobin synthesis can be reactivated at low levels in states of hematopoietic stress and at higher levels in certain hematologic malignancies, notably juvenile myeloid leukemia. However, high levels of hemoglobin F production are seen consistently in adult life only in the hemoglobinopathies.

● MOLECULAR BASIS OF THE THALASSEMIAS

Once cloning and sequencing of globin genes from patients with many different forms of thalassemia were possible, the wide spectrum of mutations underlying these conditions became clear. A picture of remarkable heterogeneity has emerged. For more extensive coverage of this topic, the reader is referred to several monographs and reviews.[7,9,10,44–46]

β-THALASSEMIA

β-thalassemia is extremely heterogeneous at the molecular level.[7] More than 200 different mutations have been found in association with the β-thalassemia phenotype.[7] Broadly, they fall into deletions

TABLE 48-2. Molecular Pathology of the β-Thalassemias

β^0- or β^+-Thalassemia

   Transcription

   Deletions

   Insertions

   Promoter

   5′-UTR

Processing of mRNA

   Junctional

   Consensus splicing sequences

   Cryptic splice sites in introns

   Cryptic splice sites in exons

   Poly (A) addition site

Translation

   Initiation

   Nonsense

   Frameshift

Posttranslational stability

   Unstable β-chain variants

Normal hemoglobin A$_2$ β-thalassemia

   β-Thalassemia and δ-thalassemia, *cis* or *trans*

   "Silent" β-thalassemia

   Some promoter mutations

   CAP +1, CAP +3, etc.

   5′ UTR

   Some splice mutations

Dominant β-thalassemia

   Mainly point mutations or rearrangements in exon 3

   Other unstable variants

UTR, untranslated region.

NOTE: A full list of mutations is given in Refs. 7 and 45.

of the β-globin gene and nondeletional mutations that may affect the transcription, processing, or translation of β-globin messenger (Table 48–2 and Fig. 48–5). Each major population group has a different set of β-thalassemia mutations, usually consisting of two or three mutations forming the bulk and large numbers of rare mutations. Because of this distribution pattern, only approximately 20 alleles account for the majority of all β-thalassemia determinants (see Fig. 48–1).

Gene Deletions

At least 17 different deletions affecting only the β genes have been described. With one exception, the deletions are rare and appear to be isolated, single events. The 619-bp deletion at the 3′ end of the β gene is more common,[48] but even that is restricted to the Sind and Gujarati populations of Pakistan and India, where it accounts for approximately 50 percent of β-thalassemia alleles.[48] The Indian 619-bp deletion removes the 3′ end of the β gene but leaves the 5′ end intact. Many of the other deletions remove the 5′ end of the gene and leave the δ gene intact.[49–53] Homozygotes for these deletions have β^0-thalassemia. Heterozygotes for the Indian deletion have increased hemoglobin A$_2$ and F levels identical to those seen in heterozygotes for the other common forms of β-thalassemia. Heterozygotes for the other deletions all have unusually high hemoglobin A$_2$ levels.[7] Increased δ-chain production results from increased δ-gene transcription in *cis* to the deletion, possibly as a result of reduced competition from the deleted 5′ β gene for transcription factors.

Other Transcriptional Mutations

Several different base substitutions involve the conserved sequences upstream from the β-globin gene.[7] In every case, the phenotype is β^+-thalassemia, although considerable variability exists in the clinical severity associated with different mutations of this type. Several mutations, at positions −88 and −87 relative to the mRNA CAP site, for example,[54,55] are close to the CCAAT box, whereas others lie within the TATA box homology.[56–59]

Some mutations upstream from the β-globin gene are associated with even more subtle alterations in phenotype. For example, a C→T substitution at position −101, which involves one of the upstream promoter elements, is associated with "silent" β-thalassemia, that is, a completely normal ("silent") phenotype that can be identified only by its interaction with more severe forms of β-thalassemia in compound heterozygotes.[60] A single example of an A→C substitution at the CAP site (+1) was described in an Asian Indian who, despite being homozygous for the mutation, appeared to have the phenotype of the β-thalassemia trait.[61]

Upstream regulatory mutations confirm the importance of the role of conserved sequences in this region as regulators of the transcription of the β-globin genes and provide the basis for some of the mildest forms of β-thalassemia, particularly those in African populations, and for some varieties of "silent" β-thalassemia.

RNA-Processing Mutations

One surprise about β-thalassemia has been the remarkable diversity of the single-base mutations that can interfere with the intranuclear processing of mRNA.

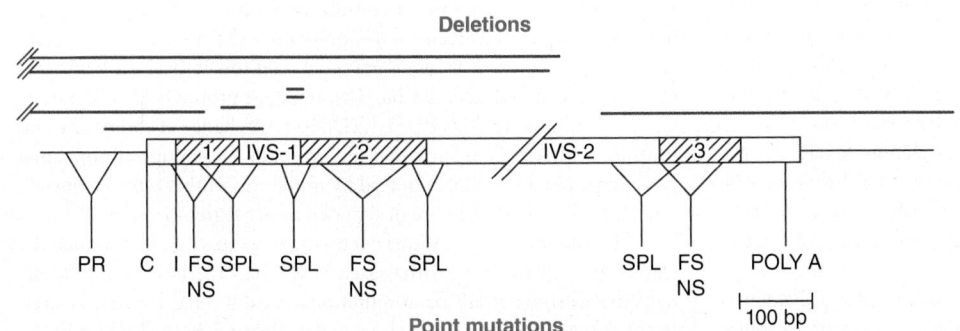

Deletions

Point mutations

PR C I FS SPL SPL FS SPL   SPL FS POLY A
      NS   NS   NS

100 bp

Figure 48–5. Classes of mutations that underlie β-thalassemia. C, CAP site; FS, frameshift; I, initiation site; NS, nonsense mutation; POLY A, polyA addition site mutation; PR, promoter; SPL, splicing mutation. For a complete list see ref. 304.

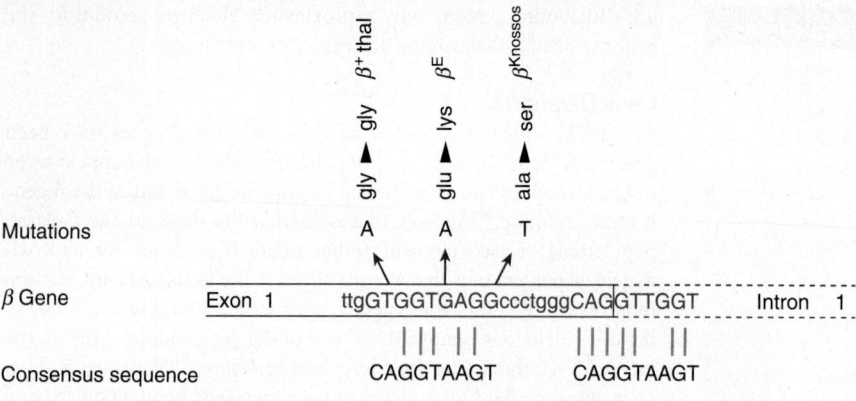

Figure 48–6. Activation of cryptic splice sites in exon 1 as the cause of β^+-thalassemia, hemoglobin E, and hemoglobin Knossos. The similarities between the 5′ splice region of intron 1 and the cryptic splice region in exon 1 are shown in *capitals*.

The boundaries of exons and introns are marked by invariant dinucleotides, GT at the 5′ (donor) and AG at the 3′ (receptor) sites. Single-base changes that involve either of these splice junctions totally abolish normal RNA splicing and result in the β^0-thalassemia phenotype.[7,62–66]

Highly conserved sequences involved in mRNA processing surround the invariant dinucleotides at the splice junctions. Different varieties of β-thalassemia involve single-base substitutions within the consensus sequence of the IVS-1 donor site.[55,58,63–69] These mutations are particularly interesting because of the remarkable variability in their associated phenotypes. For example, substitution of the G in position 5 of IVS-1 by C or T results in severe β^+-thalassemia.[55] On the other hand, a T→C change at position 6, found commonly in the Mediterranean region,[70] results in a very mild form of β^+-thalassemia. The G→C change at position 5 has also been found in Melanesia and appears to be the most common cause of β-thalassemia in Papua New Guinea.[71]

RNA processing is affected by mutations that create new splice sites within either introns or exons. Again, these lesions are remarkably variable in their phenotypic effect, depending on the degree to which the new site is utilized compared with the normal splice site. For example, the G→A substitution at position 110 of IVS-1, which is one of the most common forms of β-thalassemia in the Mediterranean region, leads to only approximately 10 percent splicing at the normal site and hence results in a severe β^+-thalassemia phenotype.[72,73] Similarly, a mutation that produces a new acceptor site at position 116 in IVS-1 results in little or no β-globin mRNA production and the β^0-thalassemia phenotype.[74] Several mutations that generate new donor sites within IVS-2 of the β-globin gene have been described.[55,68]

Another mechanism for abnormal splicing is activation of donor sites within exons (Fig. 48–6). For example, within exon 1 is a cryptic donor site in the region of codons 24 through 27. This site contains a GT dinucleotide. An adjacent substitution that alters the site so that it more closely resembles the consensus donor splice site results in its activation, even though the normal site is active. Several mutations in this region can activate this site so that it is utilized during RNA processing, with the production of abnormal mRNAs.[75–78] Three of the substitutions—A→G in codon 19, G→A in codon 26, and G→T in codon 27—result in reduced production of β-globin mRNA and an amino acid substitution so that the mRNA that is spliced normally is translated into protein. The abnormal hemoglobins produced are hemoglobins Malay, E, and Knossos, respectively, all of which are associated with a β-thalassemia phenotype, presumably as a result of reduced overall output of normal mRNA (Fig. 48–6). A variety of other cryptic splice mutations within introns and exons have been described.[44]

Another class of processing mutations involves the polyadenylation signal site AAUAAA in the 3′ untranslated region of β-globin

mRNA.[79–81] For example, a T→C substitution in this sequence leads to only one-tenth the normal amount of β-globin mRNA and hence the severe β^+-thalassemia phenotype.[79]

Mutations Causing Abnormal Translation of Messenger RNA

Base substitutions that change an amino acid codon into a chain termination codon, that is, nonsense mutations, prevent translation of the mRNA and result in β^0-thalassemia. Many substitutions of this type have been described.[7,44] For example, a codon 17 mutation is common in Southeast Asia,[82,83] and a codon 39 mutation occurs at a high frequency in the Mediterranean region.[84,85]

The insertion or deletion of one, two, or four nucleotides in the coding region of the β-globin gene disrupts the normal reading frame and results, upon translation of the mRNA, in the addition of anomalous amino acids until a termination codon is reached in the new reading frame. Several frameshift mutations of this type have been described.[7,44] Two mutations—the insertion of one nucleotide between codons 8 and 9 and a deletion of four nucleotides in codons 41 and 42—are common in Asian Indians.[63] The latter deletions are found frequently in different populations in Southeast Asia.[83]

An unusual β^+-thalassemia was described in a patient from the Czech Republic in whom a full-length L1 transposon was inserted into the second intron of β-globin, creating a β^+-thalassemia phenotype by an undefined molecular mechanism.[86]

Dominantly Inherited β-Thalassemia

Families in which a picture indistinguishable from moderately severe β-thalassemia has segregated in mendelian dominant fashion have been reported sporadically.[87,88] Because this condition often is characterized by the presence of inclusion bodies in the red cell precursors, it has been called *inclusion body β-thalassemia*. However, because all severe forms of β-thalassemia have inclusions in the red cell precursors, the term *dominantly inherited β-thalassemia* is preferred.[7,89] Sequence analysis has shown that these conditions are heterogeneous at the molecular level, but that many involve mutations of exon 3 of the β-globin gene. The mutations include frameshifts, premature chain termination mutations, and complex rearrangements that lead to synthesis of truncated or elongated and highly unstable β-globin gene products.[7,89–93] The most common mutation of this type is a GAA→TAA change at codon 121 that leads to synthesis of a truncated β-globin chain.[94] Although an abnormal β-chain product from loci affected by mutations of this type is unusual, many of these conditions are designated as hemoglobin variants.

The reason why mutations occurring in exons 1 and 2 produce the classic form of recessive β-thalassemia whereas the bulk of the dominant thalassemias result from mutations in exon 3 has become clearer. In the former case, very little abnormal β-globin mRNA is found in the cytoplasm of the red cell precursors, whereas exon 3 mutations are associated with full-length but abnormal mRNA accumulation. The different phenotypes of these premature termination codons have been suggested to reflect a phenomenon called *nonsense-mediated RNA decay*, a surveillance system to prevent transport of mRNA coding for truncated peptides. Presumably this process is active in the case of exon 1 or 2 mutations, in which affected mRNAs are degraded, but is not active in the case of exon 3 mutations.[95-97] A complete list of the mutations that underlie the dominant β-thalassemias is given in reference 44.

Unstable β-Globin Variants

Some β-globin chain variants are highly unstable but are capable of forming a viable tetramer. The resulting unstable hemoglobins may precipitate in the red cell precursors or in the blood, giving rise to a spectrum of conditions ranging from dominantly inherited β-thalassemia to a hemolytic anemia similar to the anemia associated with other unstable hemoglobins. The first unstable hemoglobin to be described was hemoglobin Indianapolis.[98] Its structure was characterized by DNA analysis performed on stored autopsy material; however, the original description proved to be incorrect.[99]

Silent β-Thalassemia

A number of extremely mild β-thalassemia alleles are either silent or almost unidentifiable in heterozygotes (see Table 48–2). Some alleles are in the region of the promoter boxes of the β-globin gene, but others involve the CAP sites or the 5′ or 3′ untranslated regions.[7,44] These alleles usually are identified by finding a form of β-thalassemia intermedia in which one parent has a typical thalassemia trait and the other parent appears to be normal but, in fact, is a carrier of one of the mild β-thalassemia alleles.

β-Thalassemia Mutations Unlinked to the B-Globin Gene Cluster

Several family studies suggest the existence of mutations that result in the β-thalassemia phenotype but do not segregate with the β-globin genes[100]; however, their molecular basis has not been determined. Further evidence for the existence of novel mutations of this type can be found in reference 7.

Variant Forms of β-Thalassemia

In several forms of β-thalassemia, the hemoglobin A_2 level is normal in heterozygotes. Some cases result from "silent" β-thalassemia alleles, whereas others reflect the coinheritance of β- and δ-thalassemia.[7]

δβ-THALASSEMIA

The δβ-thalassemias are classified into the (δβ)⁺- and (δβ)⁰-thalassemias (Table 48–3). The (δβ)⁰-thalassemias are further divided into (δβ)⁰-thalassemia, in which both the δ- and β-globin genes are deleted, and (ᴬγδβ)⁰-thalassemia, in which the ᴳγ, δ, and β genes are deleted. Because many different deletion forms of δβ-thalassemia have been described, they are further classified according to the country in which they were first identified (Table 48–3).

(δβ)⁰- and (ᴬγδβ)⁰-Thalassemia

Nearly all these conditions result from deletions involving varying lengths of the β-globin gene cluster. Many different varieties have been described in different populations (see Table 48–3), although their heterozygous and homozygous phenotypes are very similar.[7] Rare forms of these conditions result from more complex gene rearrangements. For example, one form of (ᴬγδβ)⁰-thalassemia, found in Indian populations, does not result from a simple linear deletion but rather from a complex

TABLE 48–3. δβ-Thalassemias

(δβ)⁺-Thalassemia
Hgb Lepore thalassemia
Hgb Lepore Washington-Boston
Hgb Lepore Hollandia
Hgb Lepore Baltimore
Phenocopies of (δβ)⁺-thalassemia
Sardinian δβ-thalassemia
Corfu δβ-thalassemia
Chinese δβ-thalassemia
β-Thalassemia with δ-thalassemia
(δβ)⁰-Thalassemia
Sicilian
Indian
Japanese
Spanish
Black
Eastern European
Macedonian
Turkish
Laotian
Thai
(ᴬγδβ)⁰-Thalassemia
Indian
German
Cantonese
Turkish
Malay 2
Belgian
Black
Chinese
Yunnanese
Thai
Italian

Hgb, hemoglobin.

NOTE: Details of the molecular pathology of these conditions are given in Refs. 7 and 45.

rearrangement with two deletions, one affecting the ᴬγ gene and the other the δ and β genes. The intervening region is intact but inverted.[101] Figure 48–7 illustrates some of these conditions.

(δβ)⁺-Thalassemia

The (δβ)⁺-thalassemias usually are associated with the production of structural hemoglobin variants called Lepore.[102] Hemoglobin Lepore contains normal α chains and non-α chains that consist of the first 50 to 80 amino acid residues of the δ chains and the last 60 to 90 residues of the normal C-terminal amino acid sequence of the β chains. Thus,

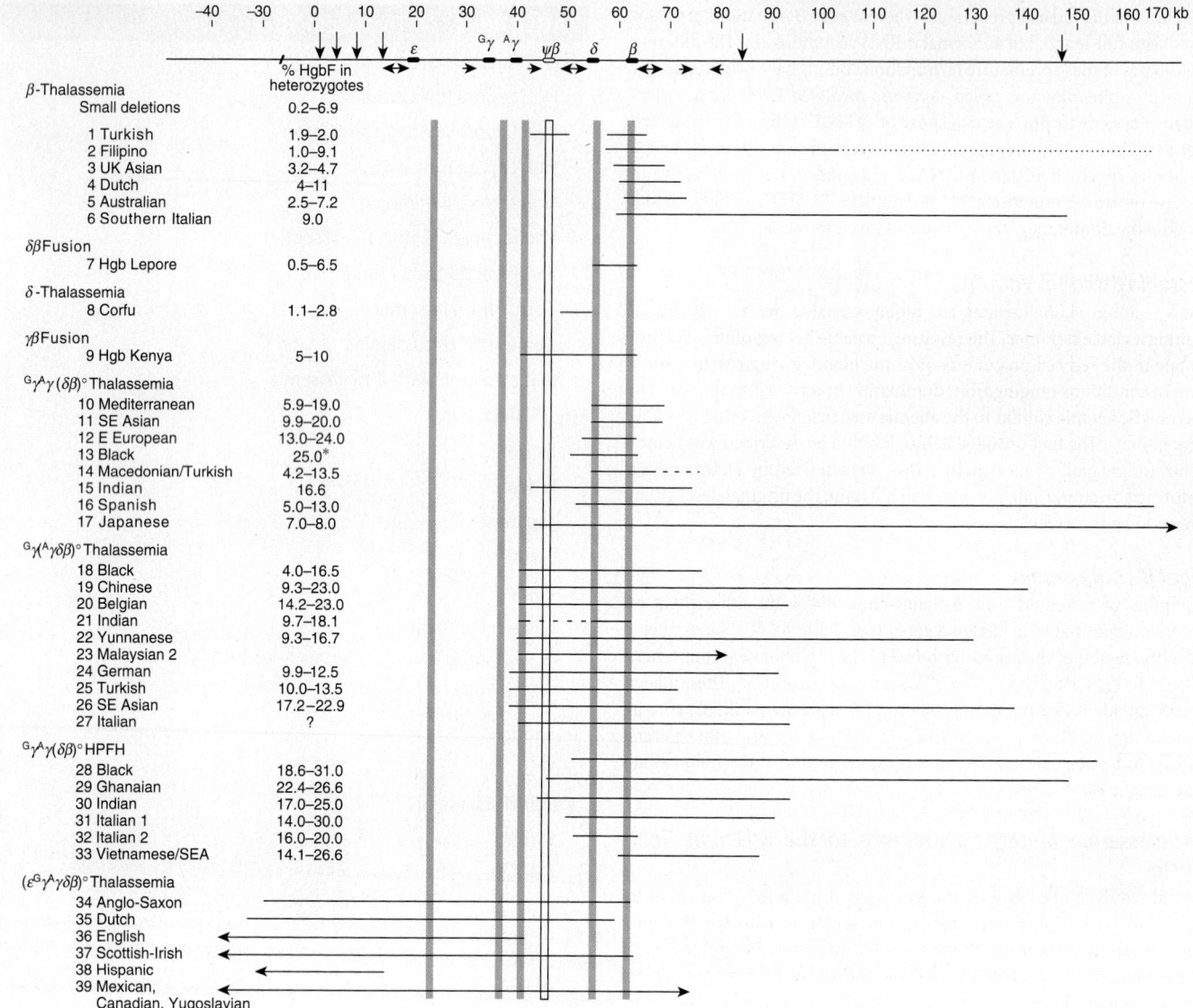

Figure 48–7. Some deletions responsible for the β- and δβ-thalassemias and hereditary persistence of fetal hemoglobin. For a complete list see reference 304.

the Lepore non-α chain is a β-fusion chain. Several different varieties of hemoglobin Lepore have been described—Washington-Boston, Baltimore, and Hollandia—in which the transition from δ to β sequences occurs at different points.[7] The fusion chains probably arose by nonhomologous crossing over between part of the δ locus on one chromosome and part of the β locus on the complementary chromosome (Fig. 48–8). This event results from misalignment of chromosome pairing during meiosis so that a δ-chain gene pairs with a β-chain gene instead of with its homologous partner.[103] Figure 48–8 shows such a mechanism should give rise to two abnormal chromosomes: the first, the Lepore chromosome, will have no normal δ or β loci but simply a δβ fusion gene. Opposite the homologous pairs of chromosomes should be an anti-Lepore (βδ) fusion gene and normal δ and β loci. A variety of anti–Lepore-like hemoglobins have been discovered, including hemoglobins Miyada, P-Congo, Lincoln Park, and P-Nilotic.[7] All the hemoglobin Lepore disorders are characterized by a severe form of δβ-thalassemia. The output of the γ-globin genes on the chromosome with the δβ fusion gene is not increased sufficiently to compensate for the low output of the δβ fusion product. The reduced rate of production of the δβ fusion chains

of hemoglobin Lepore presumably reflects the fact that its genetic determinant has the δ gene promoter region, which is structurally different from the β-globin gene promoter and is associated with a reduced rate of transcription of its gene product.

δβ-Thalassemia-Like Disorders Resulting from Two Mutations in the β-Globin Gene Cluster

A heterogeneous group of nondeletion δβ-thalassemias has been described, most resulting from two mutations in the εγδβ-globin gene cluster (see Table 48–3). Strictly speaking, they are not all δβ-thalassemias, but they often appear in the literature under this title because their phenotypes resemble the deletion forms of (δβ)⁰-thalassemia. In the Sardinian form of δβ-thalassemia, the β-globin gene has the common Mediterranean codon 39 nonsense mutation that leads to an absence of β-globin synthesis. The relatively high expression of the ᴬγ gene in *cis* gives this condition the δβ-thalassemia phenotype because of a point mutation at position –196 upstream from the ᴬγ gene (see "Hereditary Persistence of Fetal Hemoglobin" below). The phenotypic picture, in which heterozygotes have 15 to 20 percent hemoglobin F and

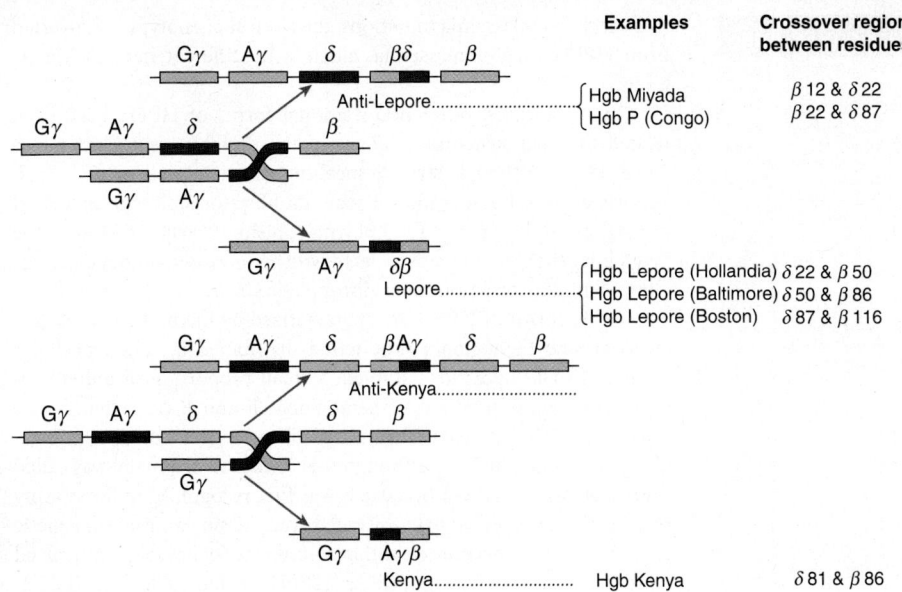

	Examples	Crossover region between residues
Anti-Lepore	Hgb Miyada	β 12 & δ 22
	Hgb P (Congo)	β 22 & δ 87
Lepore	Hgb Lepore (Hollandia)	δ 22 & β 50
	Hgb Lepore (Baltimore)	δ 50 & β 86
	Hgb Lepore (Boston)	δ 87 & β 116
Anti-Kenya		
Kenya	Hgb Kenya	δ 81 & β 86

Figure 48–8. Mechanisms for the production of the Lepore and anti-Lepore hemoglobins. Hgb, hemoglobin.

normal hemoglobin A$_2$ levels, is identical to that of δβ-thalassemia.[103] Another condition having the β-thalassemia phenotype, with greater than 20 percent hemoglobin F in heterozygotes, has been described in a Chinese patient in whom defective β-globin chain synthesis appears to result from an A→G change in the ATA sequence in the promoter region of the β-globin gene.[104] The increased γ-chain synthesis, which appears to involve both $^Gγ$ and $^Aγ$ *cis* to this mutation, remains unexplained. A disorder originally called δβ-thalassemia has been described in the Corfu population.[105,106] The condition results from two mutations in the β-globin gene cluster: first, a 7201-bp deletion that starts in the δ-globin gene, IVS-2, position 818 to 822, and extends upstream to a 5′ breakpoint located 1719 to 1722 bp 3′ to the ψβ-gene termination codon; and second, a G→A mutation at position 5 in the donor site consensus region of IVS-1 of the β-globin gene. The output from this chromosome consists of relatively high levels of γ chains with very low levels of β chains. The condition resembles δβ-thalassemia in the homozygous state, with almost 100 percent hemoglobin F, traces of hemoglobin A, but no hemoglobin A$_2$. Heterozygotes have only slightly elevated hemoglobin F levels, with a phenotype similar to "normal A$_2$β-thalassemia."

εγδβ-THALASSEMIA

These rare conditions[107-113] result from long deletions that begin upstream from the β-gene complex 55 kb or more 5′ to the ε gene and terminate within the cluster (see Fig. 48–7). In two cases, designated Dutch[110,111] and English,[112] the deletions leave the β-globin gene intact, but no β-chain production occurs even though the gene is expressed in heterologous systems.

The molecular basis for inactivation of the β-globin gene *cis* to these deletions was clarified by the discovery of the LCR approximately 50 kb upstream from the εγδβ-globin gene cluster (see "Genetic Control and Synthesis of Hemoglobin" above). Removal of this critical regulatory region seems to completely inactivate the downstream globin gene complex. The Hispanic form of εγδβ-thalassemia[113] results from a deletion that includes most of the LCR, including four of the five DNase-1-hypersensitive sites. These lesions appear to close down the chromatin domain that usually is open in erythroid tissues and delay replication of the β-globin genes in the cell cycle. Thus, although they are rare, the lesions have been of considerable importance because analysis of the

Dutch deletion first pointed to the possibility of a major control region upstream from the β-like-globin gene cluster and ultimately led to the discovery of the β-globin LCR.

HEREDITARY PERSISTENCE OF FETAL HEMOGLOBIN

This heterogeneous group of conditions produces phenotypes very similar to those of the δβ-thalassemias, except that defective β-chain production appears to be almost, but in some forms not completely, compensated by persistent γ-chain production. These conditions are best classified into deletion and nondeletion forms (Table 48–4). In the past, the conditions were classified into pancellular and heterocellular varieties, depending on the intercellular distribution of fetal hemoglobin. However, this subdivision now appears to bear little relevance to their molecular basis and probably relates more to the particular level of fetal hemoglobin and how its cellular distribution is determined.[7]

The deletion forms of HPFH are heterogeneous (see Fig. 48–7). The two African varieties result from extensive deletions of similar length (<70 kb) but with staggered ends, differing phenotypically only in the proportions of $^Gγ$ and $^Aγ$ chains produced.[114] Another type of HPFH results from misalignment during crossing over between the $^Aγ$- and β-globin genes, resulting in production of $^Aγβ$ fusion genes (see Fig. 48–8) that combine with α chains to form the hemoglobin variant called hemoglobin Kenya.[115,116] Hemoglobin Kenya is associated with an increased output of hemoglobin F, although at a lower level than in the deletion forms of HPFH. A theory that adequately explains the phenotypic differences between δβ-thalassemia and the deletion forms of HPFH has not been developed.[7]

The nondeletion determinants of HPFH can be classified into those that map within the β-globin gene cluster and those that segregate independently. The former are subdivided into $^Gγ^+$ and $^Aγ^+$ varieties, indicating persistent $^Gγ$- or $^Aγ$-chain synthesis in association with β-globin production directed by the β gene *cis* (on the same chromosome) to the HPFH determinant. Analysis of the overexpressed γ genes revealed in each case a single-base substitution in the region immediately upstream from the transcription start site.[7,117-120] Clustering of these substitutions and lack of similar changes in normal γ genes suggest they are responsible for persistent hemoglobin F production (Fig. 48–9). This region

TABLE 48–4. Hereditary Persistence of Fetal Hemoglobin

Deletion (Pancellular*)

$(\delta\beta)^0$

Black (HPFH 1)

Ghanaian (HPFH 2)

Indian (HPFH 3)

Italian (HPFH 4 and 5)

Vietnamese (HPFH 6)

$^G\gamma \,(^A\gamma\,\beta)^+$ (Hgb Kenya)

Nondeletion

Linked to β-globin gene cluster (pancellular*)

$^G\gamma\,\beta^+$

Black $^G\gamma$-202 C→G

Tunisian $^G\gamma$-200+C

Black/Sardinian $^G\gamma$-175 T→C

Japanese $^G\gamma$-114 C→T

Australian $^G\gamma$-114 C→G

$^A\gamma\,\beta^+$

Greek/Sardinian/Black $^A\gamma$-117 G→A

British $^A\gamma$-198 T→C

Black $^A\gamma$-202 C→T

Italian/Chinese $^A\gamma$-196 C→T

Brazilian $^A\gamma$-195 C→G

Black $^A\gamma$-175 T→C

Black $^A\gamma$-114 to −102 (del)

Georgia $^A\gamma$-114 C→T

$^G\gamma\,^A\gamma\,\beta^+$

Linked to β-globin gene cluster (heterocellular*)

Atlanta

Czech

Seattle

Others (including some cases of $^G\gamma$-158 T→C)

Unlinked to β-globin gene cluster (heterocellular*)

Chromosome 6

Others

Hgb, hemoglobin; HPFH, hereditary persistence of fetal hemoglobin.

*The intercellular distribution of Hgb F is not always reported, and some inconsistencies are present within groups. Complete details are given in Ref. 7.

of DNA likely is involved in binding of *trans*-acting proteins involved in the normal developmental repression of γ-gene expression, either by decreasing the affinity for an inhibitory factor normally present in adult life or by increasing the affinity for a factor promoting gene expression. The most common of these conditions are Greek $^A\gamma\beta^+$ HPFH and a form of $^G\gamma\beta^+$ HPFH, which has been found in several different African populations. If the upstream point mutations associated with persistent γ-chain production occur on the same chromosome as β-globin genes

that carry β^0-thalassemia mutations, the clinical phenotype is converted from HPFH to $\delta\beta$-thalassemia, albeit with different hemoglobin A_2 levels.

In some cases, other nondeletional forms of HPFH have been related to small structural changes in the β-globin gene cluster (see Table 48–4). Although strictly speaking not a true form of HPFH, because even in homozygotes it may not be associated with increased hemoglobin F levels, the T→C polymorphism at position −158 to the $^G\gamma$-globin gene[121] might be associated with an increased output of hemoglobin F under conditions of erythropoietic stress.

Other forms of HPFH are characterized by the persistence of low levels of fetal hemoglobin production distributed in a heterocellular manner. In all populations studied, a small proportion of individuals have an increased amount of hemoglobin F and F cells, that is, red cells that can be detected when blood films are treated with antibodies against hemoglobin F. Although this condition originally was called the Swiss form of HPFH because it was first recognized in Swiss army recruits,[122] it is observed in every racial group. Using a variety of genetic approaches, it has become clear that a number of genes may be involved in the generation of heterocellular HPFH, including loci at Xp22.2-p22.3,6q23,8q, and 2p15[123–128]; the latter linkage has been identified as the oncogene *BCL11A*. The mechanism whereby these different loci affect the level of F cells in normal individuals and increase their levels in conditions like thalassemia and sickle cell anemia remain to be determined, but their coinheritance with these conditions may have an extremely beneficial effect of their associated phenotypes.[129]

δ-THALASSEMIA

Several point mutations and deletions that reduce δ-globin synthesis have been described. They are summarized in reference 7.

α-THALASSEMIA

Table 48–5 summarizes the different classes of α-thalassemia mutations. The α-globin gene haplotype can be written $\alpha\alpha$, indicating the α_1 and α_2 genes, respectively. A normal individual has the genotype $\alpha\alpha/\alpha\alpha$. A deletion involving one (−α) or both (− −) α genes can be further classified based on its size, written as a superscript; thus, $-\alpha^{3.7}$ indicates a deletion of 3.7 kb including one α gene. When the sizes of the deletions are not established, a superscript describing their geographic or family origin is useful; thus, $- -^{MED}$ describes a deletion of both α genes first identified in individuals of Mediterranean origin. In thalassemia haplotypes in which both genes are intact, that is, nondeletion lesions, the nomenclature $\alpha^{ND}\alpha$ is given, with the superscript ND indicating the gene is thalassemic. However, when the precise molecular defect is known, as in hemoglobin Constant Spring, for example, $\alpha^{ND}\alpha$ can be replaced by the more informative $\alpha^{CS}\alpha$. The molecular pathology and population genetics of the α-thalassemias have been the subject of several extensive reviews.[7,41,45,130,131]

α⁰-Thalassemia

Many deletions that involve both α genes, and therefore abolish α-chain production from the affected chromosome, have been described (Fig. 48–10).[7] Several of the 3′ breakpoints fall within a 6- to 8-kb region at the 3′ end of the α-globin complex, suggesting this represents a breakpoint cluster region with a high level of recombination.[132] In at least five of the deletions, the 5′ breakpoints also appear to cluster. This gives rise to a situation in which the 5′ breakpoints are located approximately the same distance apart and in the same order along a chromosome as their respective 3′ breakpoints. It is possible that such staggered deletions arise from illegitimate recombination events that delete an integral number of chromatin loops as they pass through their nuclear attachment

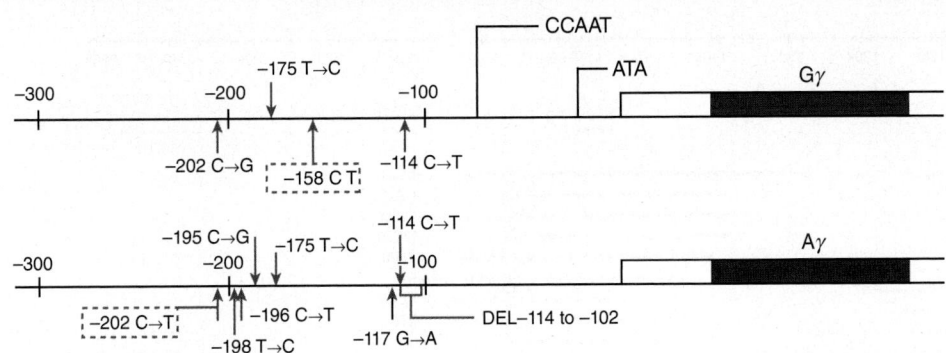

Figure 48–9. Some upstream point mutations associated with hereditary persistence of fetal hemoglobin.

points during replication. This mechanism has also been suggested to underlie some of the deletion forms of HPFH. One of these deletions ($--^{MED}$) involves a more complex rearrangement that introduces a new piece of DNA bridging the two breakpoints in the α-gene cluster. This new sequence originates upstream from the α cluster and appears to

have been replicated into the junction in a manner suggesting that the upstream segment of DNA also lies at the base of a replication loop. At least some of these deletions seem to have arisen by recombination events between Alu repeat sequences.

Several other mechanisms for the generation of α^0-thalassemia have been identified. In one case of unusual genetic interest, a long (>18 kb) deletion that removes the α_1 gene and the region downstream was identified in which the α_2 gene remains intact but is completely inactivated, giving the α^0-thalassemia phenotype. Although the inactive α_2 gene retains all its local and remote *cis*-regulatory elements, its expression is completely silenced and its CpG island is completely methylated as a result of transcription of antisense RNA expressed from a locus that had been juxtaposed to the α_2 gene because of the large deletion.[133,134] In some cases, this condition results from a terminal truncation of the short arm of chromosome 16 to a site 50 kb distal to the α-globin genes.[135] It is interesting that the telomeric consensus sequence (TTAGGGG)n has been added directly to the site of the break. Because this mutation is stably inherited, telomeric DNA alone appears sufficient to stabilize the broken chromosome end. This observation raises the possibility that other genetic diseases result from chromosomal truncations.

Several deletions have been identified that appear to downregulate α-globin genes by removing the α-globin LCR (HS40).[7,136,137] In each case, the α-globin genes are left intact, although in one the 3' breakpoint is found between the ξ and $\psi\xi$ genes, thus removing the ξ gene. These deletions appear to completely inactivate the α-globin gene complex, just as deletions of the β-globin LCR inactivate the entire β-gene complex. Such deletions have not been observed in the homozygous state, presumably because they would be lethal.

α^+-Thalassemia Gene Deletions

The most common forms of α^+-thalassemia ($-\alpha^{3.7}$ and $-\alpha^{4.2}$) involve deletion of one or the other of the duplicated α-globin genes (see Figs. 48–10 and 48–11).

Each α gene is located within a region of homology approximately 4 kb long, interrupted by two nonhomologous regions. The homologous regions are believed to have resulted from an ancient duplication event and to have subsequently subdivided, presumably by insertions and deletions, to give three homologous subsegments referred to as X, Y, and Z (see Fig. 48–11). The duplicated Z boxes are 3.7 kb apart, and the X boxes are 4.2 kb apart. Misalignment and reciprocal crossover between these segments at meiosis can give rise to chromosomes with either single ($-\alpha$) or triplicated ($\alpha\alpha\alpha$) α-globin genes. Such an occurrence between homologous Z boxes deletes 3.7 kb of DNA (rightward deletion). A similar crossover between the two X blocks deletes 4.2 kb of DNA (leftward deletion $-\alpha^{4.2}$).[138] The corresponding triplicated α-gene arrangements are referred to as $\alpha\alpha\alpha^{anti-3.7}$ and $\alpha^{anti-4.2}$.[139–141] More detailed analysis of these crossover events indicates they occur more commonly in the Z box. At least three different $-\alpha^{3.7}$ deletions have been found,

TABLE 48–5. Classes of Mutations That Cause α-Thalassemia

α^0-Thalassemia

    Deletions involving both α-globin genes

    Deletions downstream from α_2 gene

    Truncations of telomeric region of 16p

    Deletions of HS40 region

α^+-Thalassemia

    Deletions involving α_2 or α_1 genes

    Point mutations involving α_2 or α_1 genes

    mRNA processing

        Splice site

        Poly(A) signal

    mRNA translation

        Initiation

        Nonsense, frameshift

        Termination

    Posttranslational

        Unstable α-globin variants

α-Thalassemia Mental Retardation

    ATR-16

    Deletions or telomeric truncations of 16p

    Translocations

    ATR-X

    Mutations of *ATR-X*

    Deletions

    Splice site

    Missense

    Nonsense

NOTE: Complete lists of individual mutations are found in Refs. 7, 10, and 51.

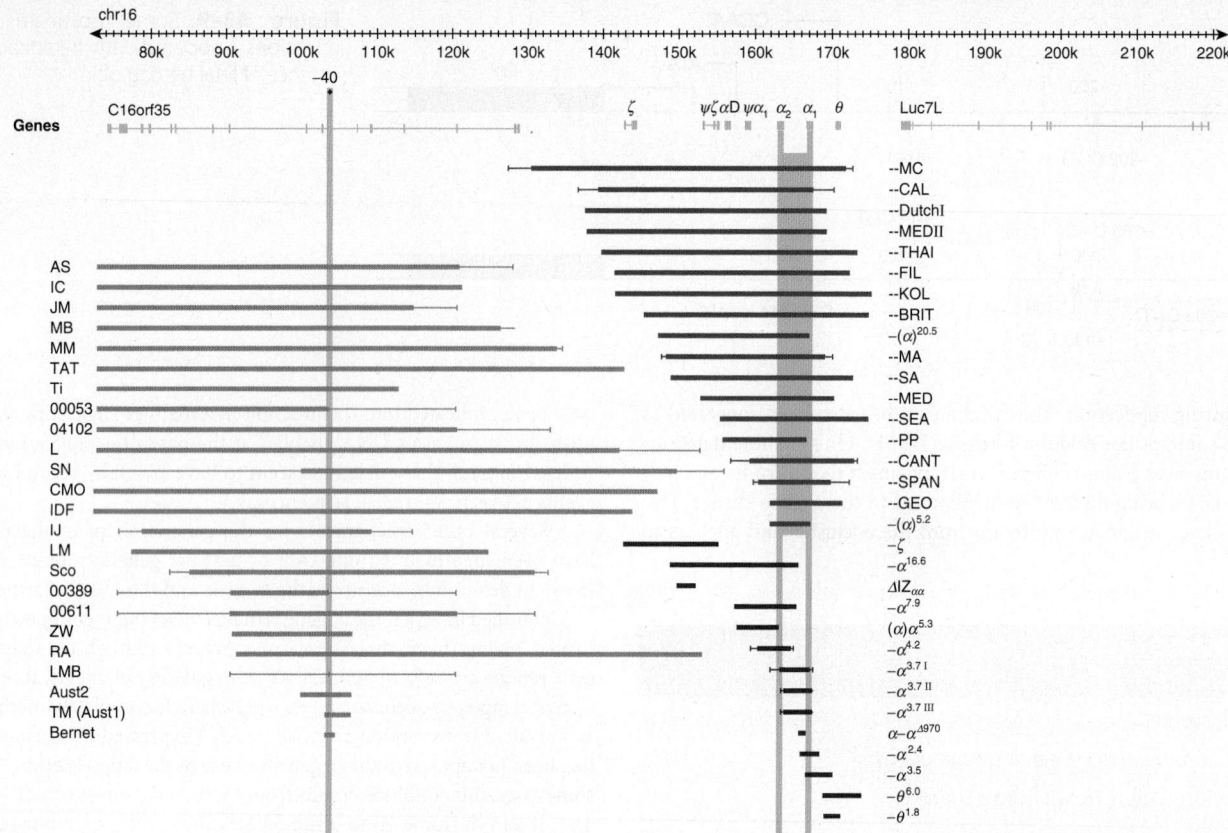

Figure 48–10. Some deletions of the α-globin gene cluster responsible for α⁰-thalassemia. Deletions: MC, initials of patient; CAL, initials of patient; THAI, Thai; FIL, Filipino; CI, Conway Islands; BRIT, United Kingdom; SA, South Africa; MED, Mediterranean; SEA, Southeast Asian; SPAN, Spanish. The top line indicates the size of the region in kilobases (K). The second line shows the different genes that constitute the α-globin gene cluster, HS40, the major regulatory region of the cluster, and the position of other genes in the region. The lines in blue represent the size of the deletions that have been described in α⁰-thalassemia, while those in red below them on the right-hand side of the figure show some of the deletions that have now been reported in different forms of α⁺-thalassemia. The lines in yellow on the left side of the figure represent some of the deletions that have been reported upstream from the α-globin gene cluster, which, because they remove the major regulatory region, result in the phenotype of α⁰-thalassemia. For a more detailed list of these deletions and references to those marked in this diagram, see references 45 and 304.

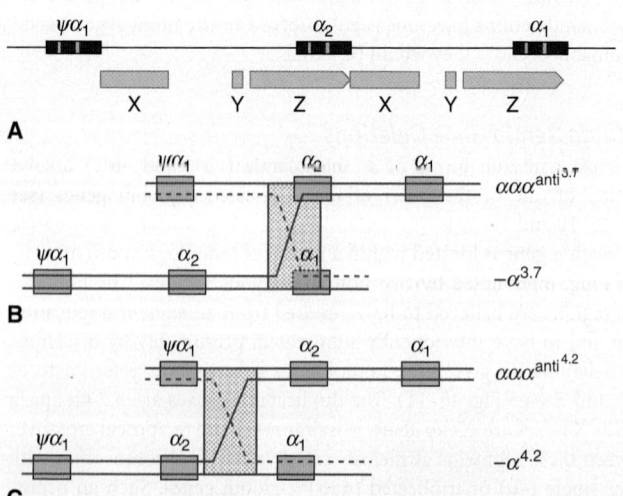

Figure 48–11. Mechanisms for production of the common deletion forms of α⁺-thalassemia. **A.** Normal α-globin gene cluster showing the homology boxes X, Y, and Z. **B.** Rightward crossover through the Z bones, giving rise to the 3.7-kb deletion and a chromosome with three α-globin genes. **C.** Leftward crossover through the Z boxes, giving rise to a 4.2-kb deletion and a chromosome containing three α genes.

depending on exactly where the crossover occurred.[142] These deletions are designated $-\alpha^{3.7I}$, $-\alpha^{3.7II}$, and $-\alpha^{3.7III}$, respectively. Other, rarer deletions of a single α gene have been observed.[7]

Nondeletion α-Thalassemia

Because expression of the α_2 gene is two to three times greater than expression of the α_1 gene, the finding that most of the nondeletion mutants discovered to date affect predominantly α_2 gene expression is not surprising. Presumably this is ascertainment bias because of the greater phenotypic effect of these lesions. It also is possible that defective expression of the α_2 gene has come under greater selective pressure.

Like the β-thalassemia mutations, α-thalassemia mutations[7] can be classified according to the level of gene expression they affect (see Table 48–5). Several processing mutations have been identified. For example, a pentanucleotide deletion includes the 5′ splice site of IVS-1 of the α_2-globin gene. This mutation involves the invariant GT donor splicing sequence and thus completely inactivates the α_2 gene.[143] A second mutant of this type, found commonly in the Middle East, involves the poly-A addition signal site (AATAAA→AATAAG) and downregulates the α_2 gene by interfering with 3′ end processing.[144,145]

A second group of nondeletion α-thalassemias results from mutations that interfere with translation of mRNA.[7] Several mutations involve the initiation codon.[146–149] In one case, for example, the initiation codon

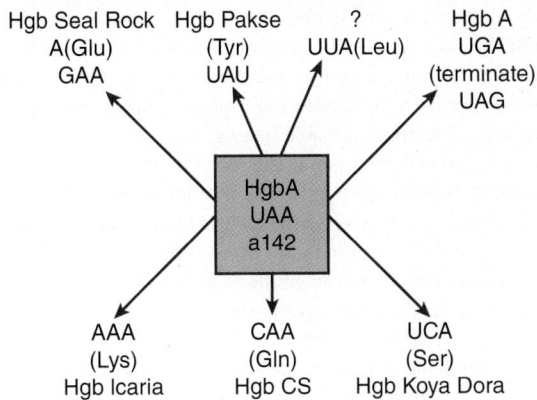

Figure 48–12. Point mutations in the α-globin gene termination codon. Hgb, hemoglobin; Hgb CS, hemoglobin Constant Spring;

is inactivated by a T→C transition.[146] In another case, efficiency of initiation is reduced by a dinucleotide deletion in the consensus sequence around the start signal.[149] Five mutations that affect termination of translation and give rise to elongated α chains have been identified: hemoglobins Constant Spring, Icaria, Koya Dora, Seal Rock, and Pakse.[7] Each mutation specifically changes the termination codon TAA so that an amino acid is inserted instead of the chain terminating (Fig. 48–12). This process is followed by read-through of mRNA that is not normally translated until another "in-phase" stop codon is reached. Thus, each of these variants has an elongated α chain. The "read-through" of α-globin mRNA that usually is not utilized likely reduces its stability.[150] Several nonsense mutations occur, for example, one in exon 3 of the α_2-globin gene.[151] Finally, several mutations occur that cause α-thalassemia by producing highly unstable α-globin chains, including hemoglobins Quong Sze,[152] Suan Doc,[153] Petah Tikvah,[154] and Evanston.[155] A complete list of nondeletion α-thalassemia alleles is given in reference 45.

Interactions of α-Thalassemia Haplotypes

Many α-thalassemia haplotypes have been described, and potentially more than 500 interactions are possible![7] These phenotypes result in four broad categories: (1) normal, (2) conditions characterized by mild hematologic changes but no clinical abnormality, (3) hemoglobin H disease, and (4) hemoglobin Bart's hydrops fetalis syndrome. The heterozygous states for deletion or nondeletion forms of α^+-thalassemia either cause extremely mild hematologic abnormalities or are completely silent. In populations where α-thalassemia is common, the homozygous state for α^+-thalassemia ($-\alpha/-\alpha$) can produce a hematologic phenotype identical to that of the heterozygous state for α^0-thalassemia ($--/\alpha\alpha$), that is, mild anemia with reduced mean cell hemoglobin and mean cell volume values.

Hemoglobin H disease usually results from the compound heterozygous state for α^0-thalassemia and either deletion or non-deletion α^+-thalassemia. It occurs most frequently in Southeast Asia ($--^{SEA}/-\alpha^{3.7}$) and the Mediterranean region (usually $--^{MED}/-\alpha^{3.7}$).

The hemoglobin Bart's hydrops fetalis syndrome usually results from the homozygous state for α^0-thalassemia, most commonly $--^{SEA}/--^{SEA}$ or $--^{MED}/--^{MED}$. A few infants with this syndrome who synthesized very low levels of α chains at birth have been reported. Gene-mapping studies suggest these cases result from interaction of α^0-thalassemia with nondeletion mutations ($\alpha\alpha^{ND}$).

Unusual Forms of α-Thalassemia

Some unusual forms of α-thalassemia are completely unrelated to the common forms of the disease that occur in tropical populations. These

conditions, which can occur in any racial groups, include α-thalassemia associated with mental retardation or leukemia. Their importance lies with the diagnostic problems they may present and, more importantly, the light that elucidation of the α-thalassemia pathology may shed on broader disease mechanisms.

Molecular Pathology of the α-Thalassemia Mental Retardation Syndrome

The first descriptions of noninherited forms of α-thalassemia associated with mental retardation suggested the lesions involving the α-globin gene locus were acquired in the paternal germ cells and that their molecular pathology might help elucidate the associated developmental changes.[156] Two separate syndromes of this type now are evident. In one group of patients, long deletions involve the α-globin gene cluster and remove at least 1 Mb.[157] This condition can arise in several ways, including unbalanced translocation involving chromosome 16, truncation of the tip of chromosome 16, and loss of the α-globin gene cluster and parts of its flanking regions by other mechanisms. These findings localize a region of approximately 1.7 Mb in band 16p13.3 proximal to the α-globin genes as being causative of mental handicap.[41]

The second group is characterized by defective α-globin synthesis associated with severe mental retardation and a relatively homogeneous pattern of dysmorphology.[158] Extensive structural studies have shown no abnormalities of the α-globin genes. These chromosomes direct the synthesis of normal amounts of α-globin in mouse erythroleukemia cells, suggesting that α-thalassemia results from deficiency of a *trans*-activating factor involved in regulation of the α-globin genes. This condition is encoded by a locus on the short arm of the X chromosome.[159] *ATR-X*, the gene involved, is a DNA helicase with many features of a DNA-binding protein. Many different mutations of this gene have been identified in different families with the ATR-X (α-thalassemia X-linked mental retardation) syndrome.[131,160] Studies have identified a plant homeodomain (PHD) region and an adenosine triphosphatase (ATPase)/helicase domain.[161] Because patients with ATR-X syndrome show defective methylation of recombinant DNA arrays and related defects, this condition likely is one of a growing list of disorders that result from disordered chromatin remodeling.[162,163]

α-Thalassemia and Myelodysplasia

The hematologic findings of hemoglobin H disease or mild α-thalassemia occasionally are observed in elderly patients with myeloid leukemia or the myelodysplastic syndrome. Earlier studies suggested this finding resulted from an acquired defect of α-globin synthesis in which the α-globin genes were completely inactivated in the neoplastic hemopoietic cell line.[164] The molecular basis for this observation now is known to reside in a variety of different mutations involving *ATR-X*.[41,165] The relationship of these somatic mutations of *ATR-X* to the neoplastic transformation remains to be determined. The molecular defect of other cases of acquired α-thalassemia, such as that seen in variable combined immunodeficiency,[166] also remains to be defined.

● PATHOPHYSIOLOGY

Almost all the pathophysiologic features of the thalassemias can be related to a primary imbalance of globin-chain synthesis. This phenomenon makes the thalassemias fundamentally different from all the other genetic and acquired disorders of hemoglobin production and, to a large extent, explains their extreme severity in the homozygous and compound heterozygous states (Fig. 48–13).

The anemia of β-thalassemia has three major components. First, and most important, is ineffective erythropoiesis with intramedullary destruction of a variable proportion of the developing red cell

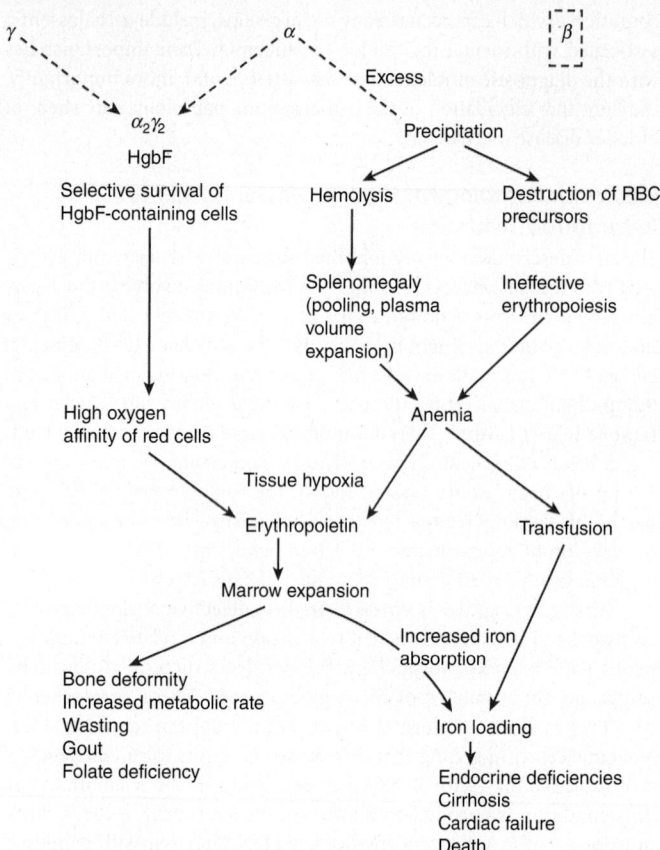

Figure 48–13. Pathophysiology of β-thalassemia. HgbF, hemoglobin F; RBC, red blood cell.

precursors. Second is hemolysis resulting from destruction of mature red cells containing α-chain inclusions. Third are the hypochromic and microcytic red cells that result from the overall reduction in hemoglobin synthesis.

Because the primary defect in β-thalassemia involves β-chain production, synthesis of hemoglobins F and A₂ should be unaffected. Fetal hemoglobin production *in utero* is normal. The clinical manifestations of thalassemia appear only when the neonatal switch from γ- to β-chain production occurs. However, fetal hemoglobin synthesis persists beyond the neonatal period in nearly all forms of β-thalassemia (see "Persistent Fetal Hemoglobin Production and Cellular Heterogeneity" below). β-Thalassemia heterozygotes have an elevated level of hemoglobin A₂. The elevated level appears to reflect not only a relative decrease in hemoglobin A as a result of defective β-chain synthesis but also an absolute increase in the output of δ chains both *cis* and *trans* to the mutant β-globin gene.[7]

Because α chains are shared by hemoglobins F, A, and A₂, there is no increase in hemoglobin F in the α-thalassemias. The excess γ and β chains formed as a result of defective α-chain production produce soluble homotetramers (see "Mechanisms and Consequences of Erythroid Precursor Damage and Red Cell Damage" below). Hence there is less ineffective erythropoiesis than in β-thalassemia and the major cause of anemia is hemolysis and poorly hemoglobinized red cells.

IMBALANCED GLOBIN-CHAIN SYNTHESIS

Measurements of *in vitro* globin-chain synthesis in the blood or marrow of patients with different types of thalassemia[167,168] and family studies that allow examination of the action of thalassemia genes in patients

who also inherited α- or β-globin structural variants[7,9] provide a clear picture of the action of the thalassemia determinants. In homozygous β-thalassemia, β-globin synthesis is either absent or markedly reduced. The result is excessive production of α-globin chains. α-Globin chains are incapable of forming a viable hemoglobin tetramer, so the chains precipitate in red cell precursors. The resulting inclusion bodies can be demonstrated by both light and electron microscopy.[169,170] In the marrow, precipitation can be seen in the earliest hemoglobinized precursors and throughout the erythroid maturation pathway.[171] These large inclusions are responsible for intramedullary destruction of red cell precursors and hence for the ineffective erythropoiesis characterizing all the β-thalassemias. A large proportion of the developing erythroblasts are destroyed within the marrow in severe cases.[172] Any red cells that are released are prematurely destroyed by mechanisms that are considered below in "Mechanisms and Consequences of Erythroid Precursor and Red Cell Damage." β-Thalassemia heterozygotes also have imbalanced globin-chain synthesis, but the magnitude of α-chain excess is much less and presumably can be resolved by the proteolytic enzymes of the red cell precursors.[173] Notwithstanding, a mild degree of ineffective erythropoiesis occurs.

Although there is marked globin-chain imbalance in the severe α-thalassemias,[7,167] the excess γ and β chains form homotetramers that do not precipitate in the red cell precursors to the same extent as excess α chains in β-thalassemia. Hence the pathophysiology of anemia is fundamentally different between the two conditions.

MECHANISMS AND CONSEQUENCES OF ERYTHROID PRECURSOR AND RED CELL DAMAGE

Damage to the red cell membrane by the globin-chain precipitation process occurs by two major routes: generation of hemichromes (Chap. 49) from excess α chains with subsequent structural damage to the red cell membrane, and similar damage mediated through the degradation products of excess α chains.[7,174–176] The degradation products of free α chains—globin, heme, hemin (oxidized heme), and free iron—also play a role in damaging red cell membranes. Excess globin chains bind to different membrane proteins and alter their structure and function. Excess iron, by generating oxygen free radicals, damages several red cell membrane components (including lipids and protein) and intracellular organelles. Heme and its products can catalyze the formation of a variety of reactive oxygen species that can damage the red cell membrane. These changes are reflected in an increased rate of apoptosis of red cell precursors.[177] The red cells are rigid and underhydrated, leak potassium, and have increased levels of calcium and low, unstable levels of ATP. Damage to the red cells can also be mediated by the presence of rigid inclusion bodies during passage of the red cells through the spleen.

The consequences of excess non–α-chain production in the α-thalassemias are quite different. Because α chains are shared by both fetal and adult hemoglobin (Chaps. 6 and 48), defective α-chain production is manifest in both fetal and adult life. In the fetus, it leads to excess γ-chain production; in the adult, it leads to an excess of β chains. Excess γ chains form γ₄ homotetramers or hemoglobin Bart's[178]; excess β chains form β₄ homotetramers or hemoglobin H.[179] The fact that γ and β chains form homotetramers is the reason for the fundamental difference in the pathophysiology of α- and β-thalassemia. Because γ₄ and β₄ tetramers are soluble, they do not precipitate to any significant degree in the marrow, and therefore the α-thalassemias are not characterized by severe ineffective erythropoiesis. However, β₄ tetramers precipitate as red cells age, with the formation of inclusion bodies. Thus, the anemia of the more severe forms of α-thalassemia in the adult results from a shortened survival of red cells consequent to their damage in the microvasculature of the spleen as a result of the presence of the inclusions. In addition, because of the defect in hemoglobin synthesis, the cells are hypochromic and microcytic. Hemoglobin Bart's is more stable than hemoglobin H and does not form large inclusions.

Although, as is the case in β-thalassemia, excess globin chains cause damage to the red cell membrane, the mechanisms are different in the two forms of the disease. As described in "Etiology and Pathogenesis" above, in β-thalassemia, excess α chains result in mechanical instability and oxidative damage to a variety of membrane proteins, notably protein 4.1. However, in α-thalassemia, the membranes are hyperstable, and no evidence of oxidation or dysfunction of this protein is present. Furthermore, the state of red cell hydration is different in α-thalassemia. Accumulation of excess β chains results in increased hydration. These differences in the pathophysiology of membrane damage between α- and β-thalassemia are discussed in detail in references 7 and 174 to 176.

Another factor exacerbates the tissue hypoxia of the anemia of the α-thalassemias. Both hemoglobin Bart's and hemoglobin H show no heme–heme interaction and have almost hyperbolic oxygen dissociation curves with very high oxygen affinities. Thus, they are not able to liberate oxygen at physiologic tissue tensions; in effect, they are useless as oxygen carriers.[7]

As a consequence, infants with high levels of hemoglobin Bart's have severe intrauterine hypoxia. This is the major basis for the clinical picture of homozygous α^0-thalassemia, which results in the stillbirth of hydropic infants late in pregnancy or at term. Oxygen deprivation is reflected by the grossly hydropic state of the infant, presumably as a result of increased capillary permeability, and by severe erythroblastosis. Deficient fetal oxygenation probably is responsible for the enormously hypertrophied placentas and possibly for the associated developmental abnormalities that occur with the severe forms of intrauterine α-thalassemia.[7]

PERSISTENT FETAL HEMOGLOBIN PRODUCTION AND CELLULAR HETEROGENEITY

Children with severe thalassemia have an increased level of hemoglobin F that persists into childhood and later.[7,10] In the β^0-thalassemias, hemoglobin F is the only hemoglobin produced, except for small amounts of hemoglobin A$_2$. Examination of the blood using staining methods specific for hemoglobin F shows that it is heterogeneously distributed among the red cells.[7] Persistent hemoglobin F production is not a major feature of the more severe forms of α-thalassemia.

The mechanism of persistent γ-chain synthesis in the thalassemias is incompletely understood. Normal adults have small quantities of hemoglobin F that are heterogeneously distributed among the red cells. Cells with demonstrable hemoglobin F are called *F cells*. One important mechanism for high hemoglobin F levels in the blood of patients with β-thalassemia is cell selection.[7,180–183] The major cause of ineffective erythropoiesis and shortened red cell survival in β-thalassemia is the deleterious effect of excess α chains on erythroid maturation in the marrow and on the survival of red cells in the blood. Therefore, red cell precursors that produce γ chains are at a selective advantage. Excess α chains combine with γ chains to produce hemoglobin F; therefore, the magnitude of α-chain precipitation is less. Differential centrifugation experiments[181–183] and *in vivo* labeling studies[180] have shown that populations of red cells with relatively large amounts of hemoglobin F are more efficiently produced and survive longer in the blood. The blood of patients with homozygous β-thalassemia shows remarkable cellular heterogeneity with respect to red cell survival, such as populations of cells containing predominantly hemoglobin A that are destroyed very

rapidly in the spleen and elsewhere, cells with a much longer survival that contain relatively more hemoglobin F, and populations of intermediate age and hemoglobin constitution.[7,182]

Although cell selection is probably the main reason for the increased levels of hemoglobin F in the red cells in β-thalassemia, other mechanisms may also be involved. In any form of "stress erythropoiesis," that is, rapid erythroid proliferation, there is a tendency for a relative increase in γ-chain production. Furthermore, as discussed in "Hereditary Persistence of Fetal Hemoglobin" above, several genes or chromosomal locations have been defined in which polymorphisms are involved in the increased basal production of γ chains and a relative increase in the number of F cells in the blood. The interaction of these different loci appear to be responsible for high levels of hemoglobin F production in β-thalassemia and sickle cell anemia with the production of milder phenotypes.[125–128,184] However, biosynthesis studies indicate that marrow expansion and the selective survival of F-cell precursors and their progeny are the major factors in hemoglobin F production in hemoglobin E/β-thalassemia.[183]

Because a reciprocal relation exists between γ- and δ-chain synthesis, the red cells of β-thalassemia homozygotes containing large amounts of hemoglobin F have relatively low hemoglobin A$_2$ levels.[7] Thus, the measured percent hemoglobin A$_2$ in these individuals is the average of a very heterogeneous cell population. This finding probably accounts for the extreme variability in hemoglobin A$_2$ levels found in homozygotes for this disorder. A further consequence of the persistence of hemoglobin F in β-thalassemia is the high oxygen affinity of the red cells.

CONSEQUENCES OF COMPENSATORY MECHANISMS FOR THE ANEMIA OF THALASSEMIA

The profound anemia of homozygous β-thalassemia and the relatively high oxygen affinity of hemoglobin F combine to cause severe tissue hypoxia. Because of the high oxygen affinity of hemoglobins Bart's and H, a similar defect in tissue oxygenation occurs in the more severe forms of α-thalassemia. The major adaptive response to hypoxia is increased erythropoietin production. It has been found that in severely anemic children with hemoglobin E β-thalassemia, age and hemoglobin levels are independent variables in erythropoietin response and that for a given hemoglobin level there is a relatively high erythropoietin in very young children.[185] These observations provide an explanation for the rather unstable phenotype of many intermediate forms of β-thalassemia during early childhood. The major effect of these very high levels of erythropoietin production is expansion of the dyserythropoietic marrow. The results are deformities of the skull and face and porosity of the long bones.[7] Extramedullary hematopoietic tumors may develop in extreme cases. Apart from the production of severe skeletal deformities, marrow expansion may cause pathologic fractures and sinus and middle ear infection as a result of ineffective drainage.

Another important effect of the enormous expansion of the marrow mass is the diversion of calories required for normal development to the ineffective red cell precursors. Thus, patients severely affected by thalassemia show poor development and wasting. The massive turnover of erythroid precursors may result in secondary hyperuricemia and gout and severe folate deficiency.

The effects of gross intrauterine hypoxia in homozygous α^0-thalassemia have been described. In the symptomatic forms of α-thalassemia (e.g., hemoglobin H disease) that are compatible with survival into adult life, bone changes and other consequences of erythroid expansion are seen, although less commonly than in β-thalassemia.

SPLENOMEGALY: DILUTIONAL ANEMIA

Constant exposure of the spleen to red cells with inclusions consisting of precipitated globin chains gives rise to the phenomenon of "work hypertrophy." Progressive splenomegaly occurs in both α- and β-thalassemia and may worsen the anemia.[7,10] A large spleen acts as a sump for red cells, sequestering a considerable proportion of the red cell mass. Furthermore, splenomegaly may cause plasma volume expansion, a complication that can be exacerbated by massive expansion of the erythroid marrow. The combination of pooling of the red cells in the spleen and plasma volume expansion can exacerbate the anemia in both α- and β-thalassemia.

ABNORMAL IRON METABOLISM

β-Thalassemia homozygotes that are anemic manifest increased intestinal iron absorption that is related to the degree of expansion of the red cell precursor population. Iron absorption is decreased by blood transfusion.[7,10] Increased absorption causes a steady accumulation of iron, first in the Kupffer cells of the liver and the macrophages of the spleen and later in the parenchymal cells of the liver. Most patients homozygous for β-thalassemia require regular blood transfusion; thus, transfusional siderosis adds to the iron accumulation. Iron accumulates in the endocrine glands,[7,186] particularly in the parathyroids, pituitary, pancreas, skin leading to increased pigmentation, liver, and, most important, in the myocardium.[7,187] Iron accumulation in the myocardium leads to death by involving the conducting tissues or by causing intractable cardiac failure. Other consequences of iron loading include diabetes, hypoparathyroidism, hypothyroidism, and abnormalities of hypothalamic–pituitary function leading to growth retardation and hypogonadism.[7,186] Recent work on the mechanisms of hepcidin downregulation in association with marrow hypertrophy provides a much better understanding of the mechanisms of iron loading in diseases like thalassemia and may provide new therapeutic options for the future (Chap. 43 and Ref. 188).

Accurate information is available regarding the levels of body iron, as reflected by hepatic iron, at which patients are at risk for serious complications of iron overload.[7,189] These studies, which extrapolate data obtained from patients with genetic hemochromatosis, suggest that patients with hepatic iron levels of approximately 80 μmol of iron per gram of liver, wet weight (~15 mg of iron per gram of liver, dry weight), are at increased risk for hepatic disease and endocrine organ damage. Patients with higher body iron burdens are at particular risk for cardiac disease and early death (Chap. 43).

Disordered iron metabolism is less common in the adult forms of α-thalassemia. The milder degree of anemia, fewer transfusions, and the less marked erythroid expansion of the marrow are likely explanations.

The mechanisms whereby iron, and in particular non–transferrin-bound iron mediate tissue damage, and recent evidence about the central role of hepcidin in the abnormal regulation of iron absorption in disorders like thalassemia are discussed in Chap. 42.

INFECTION

All forms of severe thalassemia appear to be associated with an increased susceptibility to bacterial infection.[7] The reason is not known. The relatively high serum iron levels may favor bacterial growth. Another possible mechanism is blockade of the monocyte–macrophage system as a result of the increased rate of destruction of red cells. No consistent defects in white cell or immune function have been reported, and high serum iron levels as an important factor remain to be unequivocally demonstrated. The one exception is infection with *Yersinia enterocolitica*, a normally nonvirulent pathogen that can produce its own siderophore and hence can thrive in iron excess. Transfusion-dependent patients with thalassemia are at particular risk for blood-borne infections including hepatitis B, hepatitis C, HIV/AIDS, and, in some parts of the world, malaria.

COAGULATION DEFECTS

The increasing knowledge about the potential hypercoagulable state in some forms of thalassemia has been reviewed in detail.[174–176,190] Evidence indicates that patients, particularly after splenectomy and with high platelet counts, may develop progressive pulmonary arterial disease as a result of platelet aggregation in the pulmonary circulation. Furthermore, using thalassemic red cells as a source of phospholipids, enhanced thrombin generation has been demonstrated in a prothrombinase assay. The procoagulant effect of thalassemia cells appears to result from increased expression of anionic phospholipids on the red cell surface (Chap. 33). Normally, neutral or negatively charged phospholipids are confined to the inner leaflet of the red cell membrane, an effect that is mediated by the action of aminophospholipid translocase, an enzyme sometimes known as flippase. In effect, this enzyme flips aminophospholipids that are diffused to the outer leaflet back to the inner leaflet (Chaps. 31 and 46). The current belief is that these aminophospholipids in thalassemic red cells are moved to the outer leaflet, thus providing a surface on which coagulation can be activated. Other nonspecific changes in the coagulation pathway and its antagonists have been observed in patients with different forms of thalassemia.

There is increasing evidence that, as in the case of sickle cell anemia (Chap. 49), the hemolytic component of the anemia of β-thalassemia is associated with the release of hemoglobin and arginase resulting in impaired nitric oxide availability and endothelial dysfunction with progressive pulmonary hypertension.[191] There may be other contributions to this complication including increased coagulability and local structural damage to the lungs relating to excess iron deposition.

CLINICAL HETEROGENEITY

The pathophysiologic mechanisms described above provide the basis for the remarkably diverse clinical findings in the thalassemia syndromes.[7,192] All the manifestations of β-thalassemia can be related to excess α-chain production. Thus, any mechanism that reduces the excess of α chains should reduce the clinical severity of the disease. Several elegant "experiments of nature" have shown that this reasoning is true and, incidentally, have confirmed that globin-chain imbalance is the major factor determining the severity of the thalassemias.

Coinheritance of α-thalassemia can reduce the severity of the more severe forms of β-thalassemia.[193,194] The effect is much more marked in individuals who are homozygotes or compound heterozygotes for different forms of β^+-thalassemia. β^0-Thalassemia homozygotes who have inherited α-thalassemia seem to be protected little, if at all.

Severe β-thalassemia can be modified by the coinheritance of genetic determinants for enhanced production of γ chains. Several determinants may be involved. For example, inheritance of a particular RFLP haplotype in the region 5' to the β-globin gene may be an important factor.[195,196] This particular β-globin gene haplotype is associated with a single base change, C→T, at position –158 relative to the $^G\gamma$-globin gene, an alteration that creates a cleavage site for the restriction enzyme XmnI.[121] An excess of individuals homozygous for T (XmnI+ +) with the phenotype of thalassemia intermedia exist compared with thalassemia major in different populations.[196–198] Whether this polymorphism is the only factor that increases hemoglobin F production in these cases is not absolutely clear. As discussed under "Hereditary Persistence of Fetal Hemoglobin" above, it is now clear that there are loci on chromosomes 2, 6, and 8, and possibly the X chromosome, at which polymorphisms are involved in the elevation of fetal hemoglobin synthesis and that their coinheritance may significantly modify the phenotype of different forms of β-thalassemia.

Some mutations that cause β-thalassemia are associated with a mild phenotype because they result in only modest reduction of β-chain production.[7] For example, mutations at positions –29 and –88 are associated with mild β+-thalassemia in Africans. Similarly, particularly mild phenotypes are commonly found with a base substitution at position 6 in IVS-1 and at position –87 in the 5′-flanking region of the β-globin gene in Mediterranean populations. The homozygous state for the IVS-1 position 6 mutation usually produces an extremely mild form of β-thalassemia. When these "mild" mutations are coinherited with more-severe β-thalassemia determinants, the compound heterozygous states are characterized by a more severe form of thalassemia intermedia. Other forms of thalassemia intermedia are associated with the homozygous state for δβ-thalassemia, the various interactions of β-thalassemia with δβ-thalassemia, and heterozygous β-thalassemia of the severe variety or in association with triplicated α-gene loci.[7,10,198] These complex interactions are the subject of several extensive reviews.[198–200]

These mechanisms for the phenotypic variability of the β-thalassemias represent only the beginning of our understanding of the genetic diversity of these conditions. Hence, defining a series of genetic modifiers that act at different levels is useful.[192] Primary modifiers represent the diversity of mutations at the β-globin gene locus. Secondary modifiers are those, such as α-thalassemia and increased hemoglobin F production, that directly modify the relative degree of the imbalanced globin chain output. However, an increasing number of tertiary modifiers, that is, genetic diversity, have an important effect on the complications of the disease. These include loci involved in iron, bone, and bilirubin metabolism and in determining resistance of susceptibility to infection. Furthermore, phenotypic diversity may reflect different degrees of adaptation to anemia and the effect of the environment. These complex issues have been reviewed[192] and are illustrated in Fig. 48–14. Several extensive reviews of the pathophysiology of the intermediate forms of β-thalassemia in different populations are available.[199,200]

The α-thalassemias, particularly hemoglobin H disease, show considerable clinical diversity. Some of this variability can be related to particular genotypes,[7,41] but the reasons for the heterogeneity of these disorders is not clear.

CLINICAL FEATURES

β- AND δβ-THALASSEMIAS

The most clinically severe form of β-thalassemia is thalassemia major. A milder clinical picture, characterized by a later onset and either no transfusion requirement or at least fewer transfusions than are required to treat the major form of the illnesses, is designated *β-thalassemia intermedia*. *β-Thalassemia minor* is the term used to describe the heterozygous carrier state for β-thalassemia. More extensive accounts of the clinical features of these conditions are given in two monographs.[7,9]

β-THALASSEMIA MAJOR

The homozygous or compound heterozygous state for β-thalassemia, thalassemia major, produces the clinical picture first described by Cooley and Lee[1] in 1925. Affected infants are well at birth. Anemia usually develops during the first few months of life and becomes progressively more severe. The infants fail to thrive and may have feeding problems, bouts of fever, diarrhea, and other gastrointestinal symptoms. The majority of infants who develop transfusion-dependent homozygous β-thalassemia present with these symptoms within the first year of life.

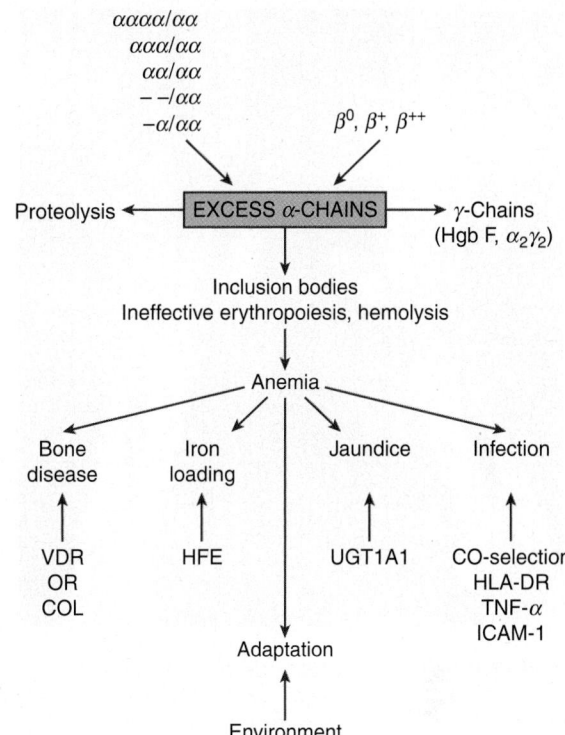

Figure 48–14. Different levels of modification of the β-thalassemia phenotype. COL, various genes involved in collagen metabolism; CO-selection, indicates variable selection of genes involved in susceptibility to infection along with different thalassemia genes; HFE, gene for hereditary hemochromatosis; Hgb F, hemoglobin F; ICAM, intercellular adhesion molecule; OR, estrogen receptor; TNF, tumor necrosis factor; UGT1A1, uridine diphosphate-glucuronyltransferase; VDR, vitamin D receptor. *(Adapted with permission from Weatherall DJ: Phenotype-genotype relationships in monogenic disease: lessons from the thalassaemias.* Nat Rev Genet 2(4):245–255, 2001.)

A later onset suggests the condition will develop into one of the intermediate forms of β-thalassemia (see "Pathophysiology" above).

The course of the disease in childhood depends almost entirely on whether the child is maintained on an adequate transfusion program.[7,9] The classic textbook picture of Cooley anemia describes the disease as it was seen before these children could be maintained with relatively normal hemoglobin levels by regular blood transfusions. If adequate transfusion is possible, children grow and develop normally and have no abnormal physical signs. Few of the complications of the disorder occur during childhood. The disease presents a problem only when the effects of iron loading resulting from ineffective erythropoiesis and from repeated blood transfusions become apparent at the end of the first decade. Children who are treated with an adequate iron chelation regimen develop normally, although some of them remain short in height.

An inadequately transfused child develops the typical features of Cooley anemia. Growth is stunted. With bossing of the skull and overgrowth of the maxillary region, the face gradually assumes a "mongoloid" appearance. These changes are associated with a characteristic radiologic appearance of the skull, long bones, and hands (Fig. 48–15). The diploe widens, with a "hair on end" or "sun ray" appearance and a lacy trabeculation of the long bones and phalanges. Gross skeletal deformities can occur. The liver and spleen are enlarged, and the pigmentation of the skin increases. Many features of a hypermetabolic state, as evidence by fever, wasting, and hyperuricemia, may develop.

The clinical course is characterized by severe anemia with frequent complications. These children are particularly prone to infection, which

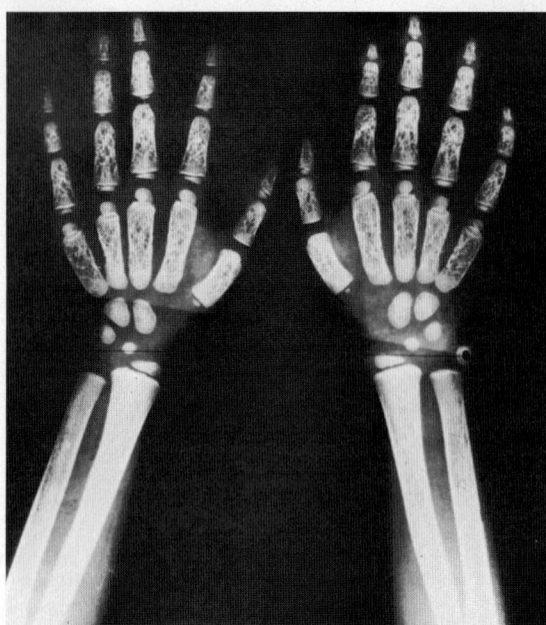

Figure 48–15. Radiologic appearances of the hands in homozygous β-thalassemia. The scattered lucent areas in the bones of the fingers reflect the marked expansion of marrow in distal areas.

is a common cause of death. Spontaneous fractures occur commonly as a result of the expansion of the marrow cavities with thinning of the long bones and skull. Maxillary deformities often lead to dental problems from malocclusion. Formation of massive deposits of extramedullary hematopoietic tissue may cause neurologic complications. With the gross splenomegaly that may occur, secondary thrombocytopenia and leukopenia frequently develop, leading to a further tendency to infection and bleeding. Splenectomy is frequently performed to reduce transfusion frequency and severe thrombocytopenia; however, postsplenectomy infections are particularly common.[7] Bleeding tendency may be seen in the absence of thrombocytopenia. Epistaxis is particularly common. These hemostatic problems are associated with poor liver function in some cases. Chronic leg ulceration may occur but is more common in thalassemia intermedia.

Children who have grown and developed normally throughout the first 10 years of life as a result of regular blood transfusion begin to develop the symptoms of iron loading as they enter puberty, particularly if they have not received adequate iron chelation.[7,9] The first indication of iron loading usually is the absence of the pubertal growth spurt and failure of the menarche. Over the succeeding years, a variety of endocrine disturbances may develop, particularly diabetes mellitus, hypogonadotrophic hypogonadism, and growth hormone deficiency. Hypothyroidism and adrenal insufficiency also occur but are less common.[7,186] Toward the end of the second decade, cardiac complications arise, and death usually occurs in the second or third decade as a result of cardiac siderosis.[187–189] Cardiac siderosis may cause an acute cardiac death with arrhythmia, or intractable cardiac failure. Both of these complications can be precipitated by intercurrent infection.

Even the adequately transfused child who has received chelation therapy may suffer a number of complications. Bloodborne infection, notably with hepatitis B or C,[201] HIV,[202] or malaria,[203] is extremely common in some populations, although the frequency is decreasing with the use of widespread blood-donor screening programs. Delayed puberty and growth retardation are common and probably reflect hypogonadotrophic hypogonadism and damage to the pituitary gland.[201,204]

Osteoporosis is being recognized increasingly and may, at least in part, be a reflection of hypogonadism.[201]

β-THALASSEMIA INTERMEDIA

The clinical phenotype of patients designated as having thalassemia intermedia is more severe than the usual asymptomatic thalassemia trait but milder than transfusion-dependent thalassemia major.[7,199,200] The syndrome encompasses disorders with a wide spectrum of disability. At the severe end, patients present with anemia later than patients with the transfusion-dependent forms of homozygous β-thalassemia and are just able to maintain a hemoglobin level of approximately 6 g/dL without transfusion. However, their growth and development are retarded. The patients become seriously disabled, with marked skeletal deformities, arthritis, and bone pain; progressive splenomegaly; growth retardation; and chronic ulcerations above the ankles. At the other end of the spectrum, patients remain completely asymptomatic until adult life and are transfusion independent, with hemoglobin levels as high as 10 to 12 g/dL. All varieties of intermediate severity are observed. Some patients become disabled simply from the effects of hypersplenism. Intensive studies of the molecular pathology of this condition have provided some guidelines about genotype–phenotype relationships that are useful for genetic counseling (Table 48–6).

Overall, the clinical features of the intermediate forms of β-thalassemia are similar to the features of β-thalassemia major. At the severe end of the spectrum, particularly in cases of growth retardation, patients should be treated with regular transfusion. However, a number of important complications, including progressive hypersplenism, occur in patients with milder forms. Clinically significant iron loading

TABLE 48–6. Genotypes of Patients with β-Thalassemia Intermedia

Mild forms of β-thalassemia

   Homozygosity for mild β⁺-thalassemia alleles

   Compound heterozygosity for two mild β⁺-thalassemia alleles

   Compound heterozygosity for a "silent" or mild and more-severe β-thalassemia allele

Inheritance of α- and β-thalassemia

   β⁺-Thalassemia with α⁰-thalassemia (– –/αα) or α⁺-thalassemia (–α/αα or –α/–α)

   β⁺-Thalassemia with genotype of Hgb H disease (– –/–α)

β-Thalassemia with elevated γ-chain synthesis

   Homozygous β-thalassemia with heterocellular HPFH

   Homozygous β-thalassemia with homozygous $^Gγ$ 158 T→C change (some cases)

   Compound heterozygosity for β-thalassemia and deletion forms of HPFH

Compound heterozygosity for β-thalassemia and β-chain variants

   Hgb E/β-thalassemia

   Other interactions with rare β-chain variants

Heterozygous β-thalassemia with triplicated or quadruplicated α-chain genes (ααα or αααα)

   Dominant forms of β-thalassemia

   Interactions of β- and (δβ)⁺- or (δβ)⁰-thalassemia

Hgb, hemoglobin; HPFH, hereditary persistence of fetal hemoglobin.

as a result of increased absorption is seen even in patients with infrequent transfusions (Chap. 43). Iron overload results in frequent diabetes and endocrine disturbances, typically by fourth decade of life. A high incidence of pigment gallstones, skeletal deformities, bone and joint disease, leg ulcers, and thrombotic tendency, particularly after splenectomy, is observed.[7]

Hematologists should be aware that in patients heterozygous for rare forms of β-thalassemia, a phenotype of thalassemia intermedia that results in the clinical constellation of autosomal dominant thalassemia (discussed in "Pathophysiology" above) is encountered on rare occasions.

β-THALASSEMIA MINOR

The heterozygous state for β-thalassemia is usually identified during family studies of patients with more severe forms of β-thalassemia, population surveys, or, most frequently, by the chance finding of the characteristic hematologic changes during a routine study. There is an extensive literature on this condition,[7] some of which suggests that affected individuals may have symptoms of anemia and, not infrequently, splenomegaly, while other studies suggest that the condition is completely symptomless and palpable splenomegaly does not occur. Surprisingly, none of these studies have been controlled. A controlled study reported that individuals with the β-thalassemia trait suffer from fatigue and other symptoms indistinguishable from those with mild anemias from other causes. There was no difference in the frequency of palpable splenomegaly between the thalassemic and control groups.[205] The trait not infrequently causes a moderately severe anemia of pregnancy, in some cases requiring transfusion. Some β-thalassemia carriers have increased iron stores, although this is most often a result of inappropriate iron therapy based on a misdiagnosis. In countries where there is a relatively high frequency of genetic determinants for hemochromatosis, the possibility of their coinheritance should be borne in mind if a patient with β-thalassemia trait with an unusually high plasma iron or serum ferritin level is encountered.

α-THALASSEMIAS

Hemoglobin Bart's Hydrops Fetalis Syndrome

This disorder is a frequent cause of stillbirth in Southeast Asia. Infants either are stillborn between 34 and 40 weeks' gestation or are born alive but die within the first few hours.[7,206] Pallor, edema, and hepatosplenomegaly are seen. The clinical picture resembles hydrops fetalis as a result of Rh blood group incompatibility. Massive extramedullary hemopoiesis and enlargement of the placenta are noted at autopsy. A variety of congenital anomalies have been observed.

The rescue of a few infants with this syndrome by prenatal detection and exchange transfusion has been reported. These babies have grown and developed normally, although they are blood transfusion–dependent.[207,208]

This condition is associated with a high incidence of maternal toxemia of pregnancy and difficulties at the time of delivery because of the massive placenta.[206] The reason for placental hypertrophy is unknown, although severe intrauterine hypoxia is suspected because a similar phenomenon is observed in hydrops infants with Rh incompatibility.

Hemoglobin H Disease

Hemoglobin H disease was described independently in the United States and in Greece in 1956.[209,210] The clinical findings are variable. A few patients are affected almost as severely as patients with β-thalassemia major, but most patients have a much milder course.[7,211] Lifelong anemia with variable splenomegaly occurs; bone changes are unusual.

As discussed earlier in "Etiology and Pathogenesis," a few attempts have been made to correlate the genotype with the phenotype of hemoglobin H disease. In general, as expected, patients with a nondeletion form of α-thalassemia affecting the predominant α_2 gene interacting with an α^0-thalassemia determinant $\alpha^{ND}\alpha/--$, or $\alpha^{ConstantSpring}\alpha/--$, for example, have higher hemoglobin H levels, a greater degree of anemia, and a more severe clinical course than patients with the $--/-\alpha$ genotype.[212-215]

Milder Forms of α-Thalassemia

Because two α-globin genes exist per haploid genome, a wide spectrum of different conditions with overlapping phenotypes result from their various interactions.[7] The carrier states for the deletion and nondeletion forms of α-thalassemia, $-\alpha/\alpha\alpha$ and $\alpha^{ND}\alpha/\alpha\alpha$, are symptomless. Similarly, the homozygous states for the deletion forms of α^+-thalassemia, $-\alpha/-\alpha$, and the heterozygous state for α^0-thalassemia, $--/\alpha\alpha$, are symptomless, although they are associated with mild anemia and red cell changes. On the other hand, the homozygous states for the nondeletion forms of α-thalassemia, $\alpha^{ND}\alpha/\alpha^{ND}\alpha$, are associated with an extremely diverse series of phenotypes. As mentioned in "Interactions of α-Thalassemia Haplotypes" above in "Etiology and Pathogenesis," they sometimes result in the clinical picture of hemoglobin H disease. In other patients, they are associated with only mild hypochromic anemia.[7] The homozygous states for the chain termination mutants, notably hemoglobin Constant Spring, constitute a special case because they produce a particularly characteristic phenotype. In this case, moderate hemolytic anemia with splenomegaly are seen.[7,216,217]

α-Thalassemia and Mental Retardation

The clinical phenotype of these conditions is heterogeneous. In cases associated with chromosomal deletion (tip of chromosome 16; ATR-16 [α-thalassemia chromosome 16-linked mental retardation syndrome]), the clinical defects vary with the extent of chromosomal defect; only α-thalassemia and mental retardation are constant.[157] To some extent this clinical variation is related to the length of the associated deletions; those which extend for 2000 kb involve the genes that are involved in tuberous sclerosis and polycystic kidney disease. In these cases the latter dominate the clinical picture, but there mental retardation and α-thalassemia are also associated.

The clinical phenotype in the second group of these disorders, which are caused by mutations of ATR-X, includes skeletal abnormalities, dysmorphic face, neonatal hypotonus, genital abnormalities, and a variety of less-constant features, in addition to mental retardation and α-thalassemia.[158]

εγδβ-Thalassemia

The clinical picture varies with the stage of development.[7] Neonates may be significantly anemic and require transfusions. In contrast, children and adults with this condition are asymptomatic. They have the clinical and laboratory picture of heterozygous β-thalassemia, with the exception of a normal hemoglobin A₂ level. The reason for this discrepancy of developmental differences of the clinical phenotype has not been identified. The homozygous state is assumed to be lethal.

● LABORATORY FEATURES

β-THALASSEMIA MAJOR

Hemoglobin levels at presentation may range from 2 to 3 g/dL or even lower.[7] The red cells show marked anisopoikilocytosis, with hypochromia, target cell formation, and a variable degree of basophilic stippling (Fig. 48–16). The appearance of the blood film varies, depending on whether the spleen is intact. In nonsplenectomized patients, large

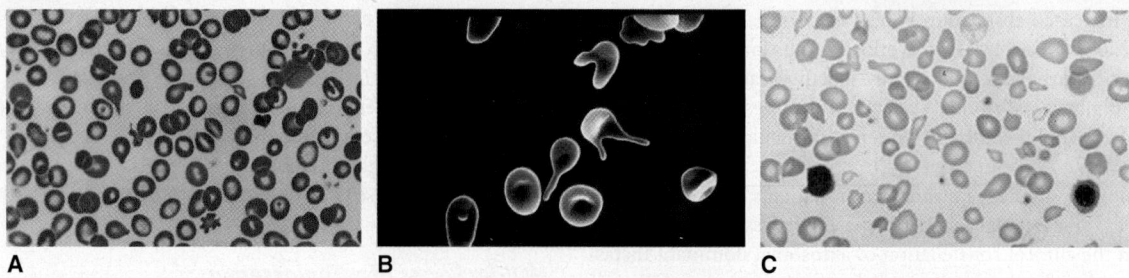

Figure 48–16. Blood films in β-thalassemia. **A.** β-Thalassemia minor. Anisocytosis, poikilocytosis, hypochromia. Occasional spherocytes and stomatocytes. **B.** Scanning electron micrograph of cells in **(A)** showing more detail of the poikilocytes. Note the knizocyte (pinch-bottle cell) at the lower right. **C.** β-Thalassemia major. Marked anisocytosis with many microcytes. Marked poikilocytosis. Anisochromia. Nucleated red cell on the right. Small lymphocyte on the left. *(Reproduced with permission from Lichtman's Atlas of Hematology, www.accessmedicine.com.)*

poikilocytes are common. After splenectomy, large, flat macrocytes and small, deformed microcytes are frequently seen. The reticulocyte count is moderately elevated, and nucleated red cells nearly always are present in the blood. These red cell forms may reach very high levels after splenectomy. The white cell and platelet counts are slightly elevated unless secondary hypersplenism occurs. Staining of the blood with methyl violet, particularly in splenectomized subjects, reveals stippling or ragged inclusion bodies in the red cells.[169] These inclusions can nearly always be found in the red cell precursors in the marrow. The marrow usually shows erythroid hyperplasia with morphologic abnormalities of the erythroblasts, such as striking basophilic stippling and increased iron deposition. Iron kinetic studies indicate markedly ineffective erythropoiesis, and red cell survival usually is shortened. Populations of cells with very short survival and longer-lived populations of cells are seen. The latter contain relatively more fetal hemoglobin. An increased level of fetal hemoglobin, ranging from less than 10 percent to greater than 90 percent, is characteristic of homozygous β-thalassemia. No hemoglobin A is produced in β^0-thalassemia. The fetal hemoglobin is heterogeneously distributed among the red cells. Hemoglobin A_2 levels in homozygous β-thalassemia may be low, normal, or high. However, expressed as a proportion of hemoglobin A, the hemoglobin A_2 level almost invariably is elevated. Differential centrifugation studies indicate some heterogeneity of hemoglobin F and A_2 distribution among thalassemic red cells, but their level in whole blood gives little indication of their total rates of synthesis.

In vitro hemoglobin synthesis studies using marrow or blood show a marked degree of globin-chain imbalance. Marked excess of α-chain over β- and γ-chain production is always observed. Other aspects of the laboratory findings in this condition, including red cell survival, iron absorption, ferrokinetics, erythrokinetics, and the consequences of iron loading, were discussed earlier (see "Etiology and Pathogenesis" above).

The examination of siblings, parents, and children can be very important in confirming the diagnosis by finding the abnormalities in other family members, and the examining physician should make every effort to obtain a complete blood count in family members. With the exception of higher hemoglobin levels, the hematological changes in β-thalassemia intermedia are similar to those in β-thalassemia major (Fig. 48–17).

β-THALASSEMIA MINOR

Hemoglobin values of patients with β-thalassemia minor usually range from 9 to 11 g/dL. The most consistent finding is small, poorly hemoglobinized red cells (see Fig. 48–16), resulting in mean cell hemoglobin (MCH) values of 20 to 22 pg and mean corpuscular volume (MCV) values of 50 to 70 fL. The red cell count is usually normal or elevated and the hemoglobin and hematocrit is usually slightly below normal; however, the red cell indices are particularly useful in screening for heterozygous carriers of thalassemia in population surveys. The marrow in heterozygous β-thalassemia shows slight erythroid hyperplasia with rare red cell inclusions. Megaloblastic transformation as a result of folic acid deficiency occurs occasionally, particularly during pregnancy. A mild degree of ineffective erythropoiesis is noted, but red cell survival is normal or nearly normal. The hemoglobin A_2 level is increased to

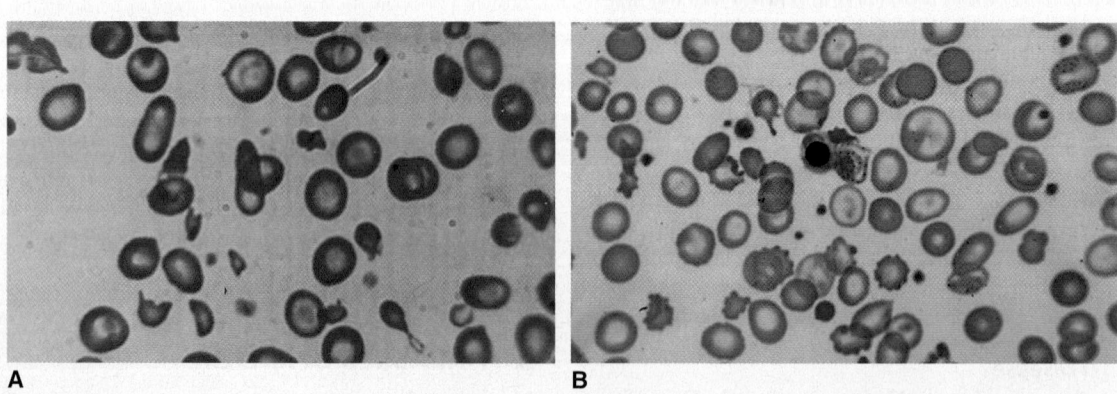

Figure 48–17. A. Thalassemia intermedia. Blood films. Marked anisocytosis, poikilocytosis with elliptical, oval, tear-drop-shaped, and fragmented red cells. Target cells. **B.** Postsplenectomy. Morphology similar to that in **(A)** but with a nucleated red cell, coarsely stippled cell in center of field, and large and numerous platelets, indicative of the changes superimposed by splenectomy. *(Reproduced with permission from Lichtman's Atlas of Hematology, www.accessmedicine.com.)*

3.5 to 7.0 percent. The level of fetal hemoglobin is elevated in approximately 50 percent of cases, usually to 1 to 3 percent and rarely to greater than 5 percent.

α-THALASSEMIAS

Hemoglobin Bart's Hydrops Fetalis Syndrome

In infants with the hydrops fetalis syndrome, the blood film shows severe thalassemic changes with many nucleated red cells. The hemoglobin consists mainly of hemoglobin Bart's, with approximately 10 to 20 percent hemoglobin Portland. Usually no hemoglobin A or F is present, although rare cases that seem to result from interaction of α⁰-thalassemia with a severe nondeletion form of α⁺-thalassemia show small amounts of hemoglobin A.

Hemoglobin H Disease

The blood film shows hypochromia and anisopoikilocytosis. The reticulocyte count usually is approximately 5 percent. Incubation of the red cells with brilliant cresyl blue results in ragged inclusion bodies in almost all cells. These bodies form because of precipitation of hemoglobin H *in vitro* as a result of redox action of the dye. After splenectomy, large, single Heinz bodies are observed in some cells (Fig. 48–18). These bodies are formed by *in vitro* precipitation of the unstable hemoglobin H molecule and are seen only after splenectomy. Hemoglobin H constitutes between 5 and 40 percent of the total hemoglobin. Traces of hemoglobin Bart's may be present, and the hemoglobin A₂ level usually is slightly subnormal.

α⁰-Thalassemia and α⁺-Thalassemia Traits

The α⁰-thalassemia trait is characterized by the presence of 5 to 15 percent hemoglobin Bart's at birth.[7] This hemoglobin disappears during maturation and is not replaced by a similar amount of hemoglobin H. An occasional cell with hemoglobin H inclusion bodies may appear after incubation with brilliant cresyl blue. This phenomenon is often used as a diagnostic test for the α-thalassemia trait. However, the test is difficult to standardize and requires much experience to be useful. In adult life, the red cells of heterozygotes have morphologic changes of heterozygous thalassemia with low MCH and MCV values. The electrophoretic pattern is normal. Globin-synthesis studies show a deficit of α-chain production, with an α-chain–to–β-chain production ratio of approximately 0.7.

The α⁺-thalassemia trait (–α/αα) is characterized by a mild reduction in MCH and MCV values although in some cases there are normal values, 1 to 2 percent of hemoglobin Bart's at birth in some but not all cases, and a slightly reduced α-chain–to–β-chain production ratio of approximately 0.8; thus, this genotype often is referred to as *silent carrier*. Extensive studies comparing the level of hemoglobin Bart's at birth with a DNA analyses demonstrated that there is no detectable hemoglobin Bart's in a significant number of newborns who are heterozygous for α⁺-thalassemia.[218,219] Globin gene synthetic ratios can be distinguished from normal only by studying relatively large numbers of samples and comparing the mean α–to–β ratio with that of normal control subjects. This approach is not reliable for diagnosing individual cases of the α⁺-thalassemia trait, and, unfortunately, no reliable method of diagnosis is available except for DNA analysis.

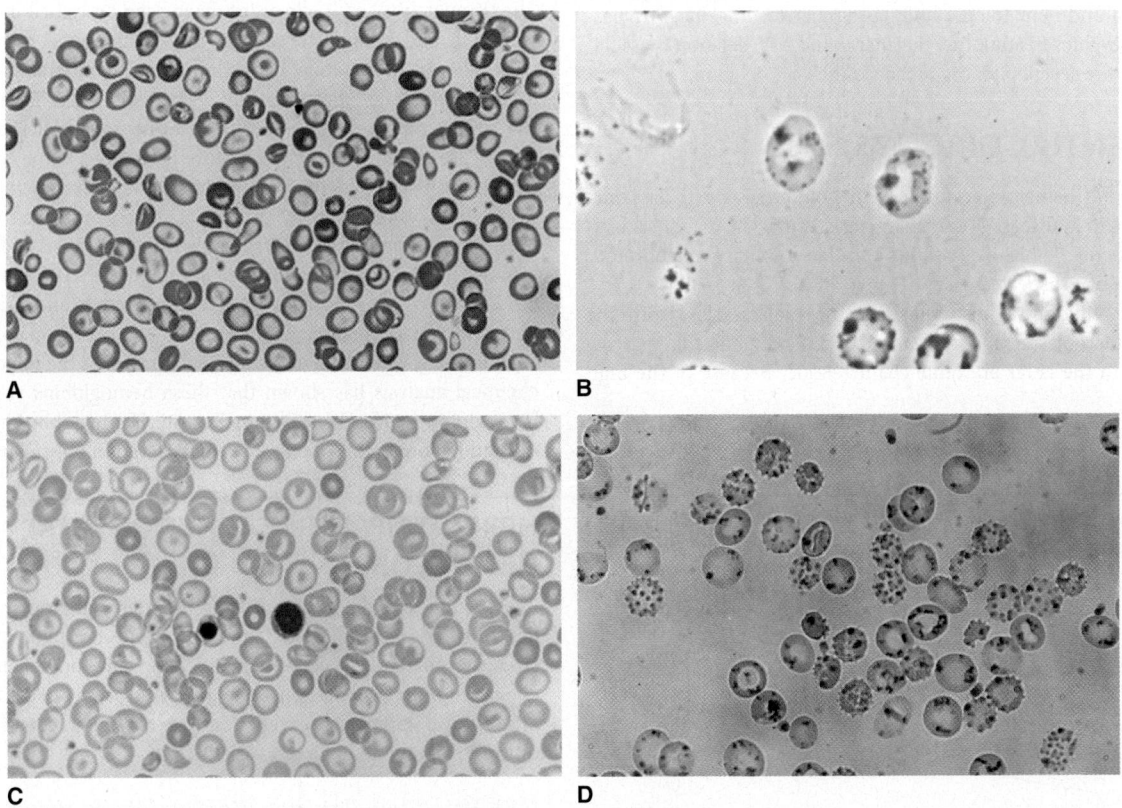

Figure 48–18. Hemoglobin H disease (α-thalassemia). Blood films. **A.** Note hypochromic red cells, anisocytosis, target cells, poikilocytes, including tear-drop-shaped red cells. **B.** Wet preparation stained with crystal violet. Inclusions in red cells (Heinz bodies) usually attached to membrane. **C.** Postsplenectomy. Note reduction in poikilocytes and frequency of target cells, a change consistent with hemoglobin H disease and enhanced by postsplenectomy effects. A nucleated red cell is in this field, reflecting an increase in their prevalence in the blood after splenectomy. **D.** Blood incubated for 90 minutes with brilliant cresyl blue. Numerous hemoglobin H intracellular precipitates (precipitates of excess β-globin chains). The frequent crenation is an artifact of the incubation conditions. (*Reproduced with permission from* Lichtman's Atlas of Hematology, *www.accessmedicine.com.*)

Homozygous State for Nondeletion Types of α-Thalassemia

The homozygous state for nondeletion forms of α-thalassemia involving the dominant (α_2) globin gene causes a more severe deficit of α chains than do the deletion forms of α^+-thalassemia. In some cases, the homozygous state produces hemoglobin H disease.

The homozygous state for hemoglobin Constant Spring or other chain-termination mutations is associated with moderately severe hemolytic anemia in which, for reasons not explained, no hemoglobin H is present but small amounts of hemoglobin Bart's persist into adult life. The homozygous states for the other nondeletion forms of α^+-thalassemia are associated with hemoglobin H disease. In the homozygous state for hemoglobin Constant Spring, the blood picture shows mild thalassemic changes with normal-size red cells.[216,217] The hemoglobin consists of approximately 5 to 6 percent hemoglobin Constant Spring, normal hemoglobin A_2 levels, and trace amounts of hemoglobin Bart's. The remainder is hemoglobin A.

The heterozygous state for hemoglobin Constant Spring shows no hematologic abnormality. The hemoglobin pattern is normal except for the presence of approximately 0.5 percent hemoglobin Constant Spring. The latter can be observed on alkaline starch-gel electrophoresis as a faint band migrating between hemoglobin A_2 and the origin. It is best seen on heavily loaded starch gels and is easily missed if other electrophoretic techniques are used (Fig. 48–19). In the newborn, usually 1 to 3 percent hemoglobin Bart's is present in the cord blood.

Homozygous State for Deletion Forms of α⁺-Thalassemia

The homozygous state for deletion forms of α^+-thalassemia is characterized by a thalassemic blood picture with 5 to 10 percent hemoglobin Bart's at birth and hematologic findings similar to those in α^0-thalassemia heterozygotes in adult life. In general, the $-\alpha^{4.2}$ deletion is associated with a more severe phenotype than is the $-\alpha^{3.7}$ deletion.[7]

DIFFERENTIAL DIAGNOSIS

The clinical and hematologic findings in homozygous β-thalassemia and hemoglobin H disease are so characteristic that the diagnosis usually is not difficult. Figure 48–20 shows a simple flowchart for laboratory investigations of a suspected case.

In early childhood, distinguishing the thalassemias from the congenital sideroblastic anemias may be difficult, but the marrow appearances in the latter are quite characteristic. Because of the high hemoglobin F levels encountered in juvenile chronic myelogenous leukemia, this disorder may superficially resemble β-thalassemia. However, the finding of primitive cells in the marrow, the absence of elevated hemoglobin A_2 levels on hemoglobin electrophoresis, the decrease in carbonic anhydrase in juvenile chronic myelogenous leukemia, and characteristic *in vitro* responses of myeloid progenitors *in vitro* to granulocyte-monocyte colony-stimulating factor (Chap. 87) readily differentiate this disorder from β-thalassemia.

LESS-COMMON FORMS OF THALASSEMIA

(δβ)⁰-Thalassemia

The homozygous state for δβ-thalassemia is clinically milder than Cooley anemia and is one form of thalassemia intermedia.[220–222] Only hemoglobin F is present; hemoglobins A and A_2 are not produced. Heterozygous δβ-thalassemia is hematologically similar to β-thalassemia minor.[7] The fetal hemoglobin level is higher (range: 5 to 20 percent), and the hemoglobin A_2 value is normal or slightly reduced. As in β-thalassemia, the fetal hemoglobin is heterogeneously distributed among the red cells, thus distinguishing this disorder from HPFH (Fig. 48–21).

Heterozygosity for both β-thalassemia and δβ-thalassemia results is a condition clinically similar to but milder than Cooley anemia. The hemoglobin consists largely of hemoglobin F, with a small amount of hemoglobin A_2. This finding is seen because the associated β-thalassemia gene has usually been the β^0 variety. δβ-Thalassemia has also been observed in individuals heterozygous for hemoglobin S or C.[7]

(δβ)⁺-Thalassemia and Hemoglobin Lepore Disorders

The hemoglobin Lepore disorders have been described in the homozygous state and in the heterozygous state, either alone or in association with β- or δβ-thalassemia, hemoglobin S, or hemoglobin C.[7,9,223] In the homozygous state, approximately 20 percent of the hemoglobin is of the Lepore type and 80 percent is fetal hemoglobin. Hemoglobins A and A_2 are absent. The clinical picture is variable. Some cases are identical to transfusion-dependent homozygous β-thalassemia; others are associated with the clinical picture of thalassemia intermedia. In the heterozygous state, the findings are similar to those of β-thalassemia minor. The hemoglobin consists of approximately 10 percent hemoglobin Lepore, with a reduced level of hemoglobin A_2 and a slight but consistent increase in fetal hemoglobin level. The Lepore hemoglobins have been found sporadically in most racial groups. In the majority of cases, chemical analysis has shown that these hemoglobins are identical to hemoglobin Lepore Washington-Boston. Hemoglobin Lepore Hollandia and Lepore Baltimore have been observed in only a few patients.[7,223]

HEREDITARY PERSISTENCE OF FETAL HEMOGLOBIN

The current knowledge about the molecular pathology of HPFH was described earlier in "Etiology and Pathogenesis." Table 48–4 summarizes the currently accepted classification and nomenclature of this complex group of conditions. The different forms of HPFH are of very little clinical importance except that they may interact with thalassemia or the structural hemoglobin variants.

(δβ)⁰ Hereditary Persistence of Fetal Hemoglobin

Homozygotes for $(\delta\beta)^0$ HPFH have 100 percent hemoglobin F. Their blood shows mild thalassemic changes, with reduced MCH and MCV values very similar to those observed in heterozygous β-thalassemia. Similarly, they have imbalanced globin chain production, with ratios in the range of those observed in β-thalassemia heterozygotes.[224] Heterozygotes have approximately 20 to 30 percent hemoglobin F, slightly

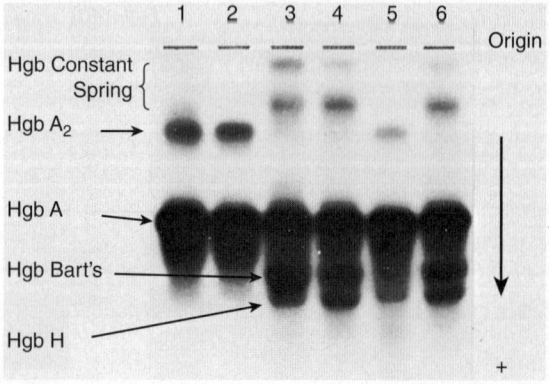

Figure 48–19. Hemoglobin (Hgb) Constant Spring. Starch gel electrophoresis of *1,2,* normal adult; *3,4,* compund heterozygotes for hemoglobin Constant Spring and a^0-thalassemia with hemoglobin H disease; *5,* normal adult; and *6,* compound heterozygote for a^0-thalassemia and hemoglobin Constant Spring.

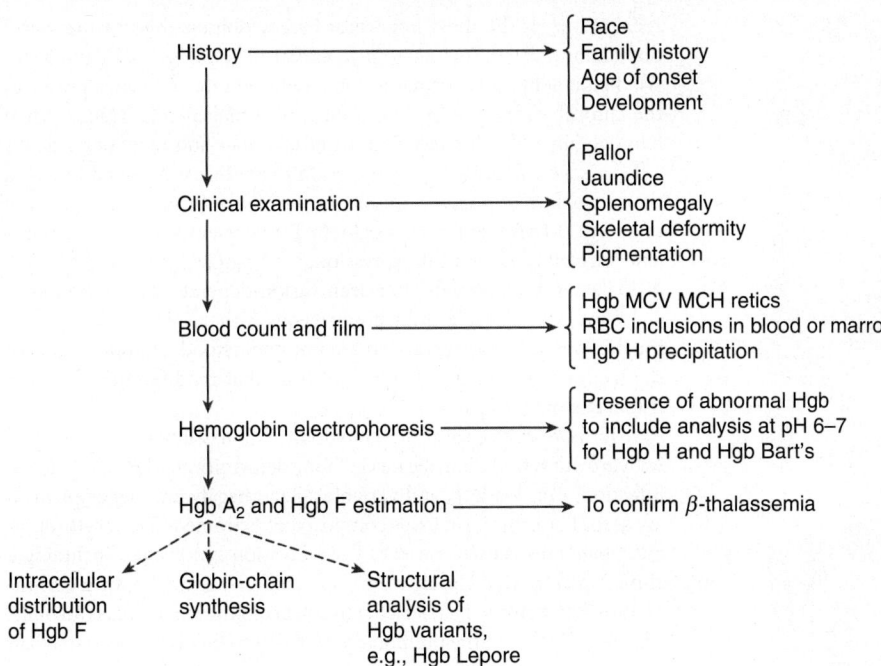

Figure 48-20. Flowchart showing an approach to diagnosis of the thalassemia syndromes. Hgb, hemoglobin; MCH, mean cell hemoglobin; MCV, mean corpuscular volume; RBC, red blood cell count.

reduced hemoglobin A_2 values, and completely normal blood pictures. Thus, this condition appears to be an extremely well-compensated form of $\delta\beta$-thalassemia in which the output of γ chains almost but not entirely compensates for the complete absence of β and δ chains. The different molecular forms of this condition show no difference in phenotype except in the proportion of $^G\gamma$ chains. The African forms of $(\delta\beta)^0$ HPFH have been found in association with hemoglobins S and C or with β-thalassemia (Chap. 49). These compound heterozygous states are associated with little clinical disability.[7]

Nondeletion Types of Hereditary Persistence of Fetal Hemoglobin

Many nondeletion forms of HPFH associated with point mutations upstream from the γ-globin genes have been described (see Table 48-4). $^G\gamma\,\beta^+$ HPFH has been found in the heterozygous and compound heterozygous states with β-globin chain variants in African populations. No associated clinical or hematologic findings have been reported. Compound heterozygotes for $^G\gamma\,\beta^+$ HPFH and hemoglobins S or C produce 45 percent of the abnormal hemoglobin, approximately 30 percent hemoglobin A, and approximately 20 percent hemoglobin F containing only $^G\gamma$ chains.[225,226]

The most common form of nondeletion HPFH is $^A\gamma\,\beta^+$ HPFH, which is found in Greeks.[227-229] In the homozygous state, no clinical or hematologic abnormalities are noted. The hemoglobin findings are characterized by approximately 25 percent fetal hemoglobin and reduced hemoglobin A_2 levels of approximately 0.8 percent.[230] Heterozygotes, who also are hematologically normal, have 10 to 15 percent hemoglobin F, almost all of the $^A\gamma$ variety. Compound heterozygotes with β-thalassemia have high hemoglobin F levels and a clinical picture that is only slightly more severe than the β-thalassemia trait.

In the British form of $^A\gamma\,\beta^+$ HPFH[231] heterozygotes have approximately 5 to 12 percent hemoglobin F, whereas homozygotes have approximately 20 percent. No associated hematologic abnormalities are seen, although surprisingly in this form of nondeletion HPFH the hemoglobin F seems to be unevenly distributed among the red cells.

A heterogeneous group of conditions is associated with persistent production of small amounts of hemoglobin F in adult life. They are categorized under the general heading of *heterocellular HPFH*. Their clinical importance is that, when they are coinherited with different forms of β-thalassemia, they may lead to greater output of hemoglobin F and, hence, to a milder phenotype. This type of interaction should be suspected when one parent of a patient with β-thalassemia intermedia has an unusually high level of hemoglobin F for the β-thalassemia trait. Similarly, unaffected lateral relatives or other family members with slightly elevated hemoglobin F levels may be found.

β-THALASSEMIA ASSOCIATED WITH β-CHAIN STRUCTURAL HEMOGLOBIN VARIANTS

The most clinically important associations of β-thalassemia with β structural hemoglobin variants are sickle cell thalassemia, hemoglobin C thalassemia, and hemoglobin E thalassemia (Chap. 49). In addition, many interactions of β-thalassemia with rare structural variants have been reported.[7,9,10]

Sickle cell thalassemia[7,232,233] occurs in parts of Africa and in the Mediterranean, particularly Greece and Italy. It also has been observed in the Middle East and parts of India. The clinical consequences of carrying one gene for hemoglobin S and one gene for β-thalassemia depend entirely on the type of β-thalassemia mutation. The interaction between the sickle cell gene and β^0-thalassemia is characterized by a clinical disorder that is very similar to sickle cell anemia. Similarly, the interaction of the sickle cell gene with the more severe forms of β^+-thalassemia associated with marked reduction in β-globin synthesis yields a similar clinical phenotype. On the other hand, the interaction of the sickle cell gene with very mild forms of β^+-thalassemia may be quite innocuous.[233] The latter disorder is characterized by mild anemia associated with splenomegaly and a hemoglobin composition of approximately 60 to 70 percent hemoglobin S, 25 percent hemoglobin A, and an elevated level of hemoglobin A_2. In all these interactions, one parent shows the sickle cell trait, and the other parent shows the β-thalassemia trait.

Hemoglobin C thalassemia is a mild hemolytic disorder associated with splenomegaly.[7,9,10] Again, the hemoglobin pattern varies depending on whether the thalassemia gene is the β^+ or β^0 type. This relatively innocuous condition has been recorded mainly in North Africa, but

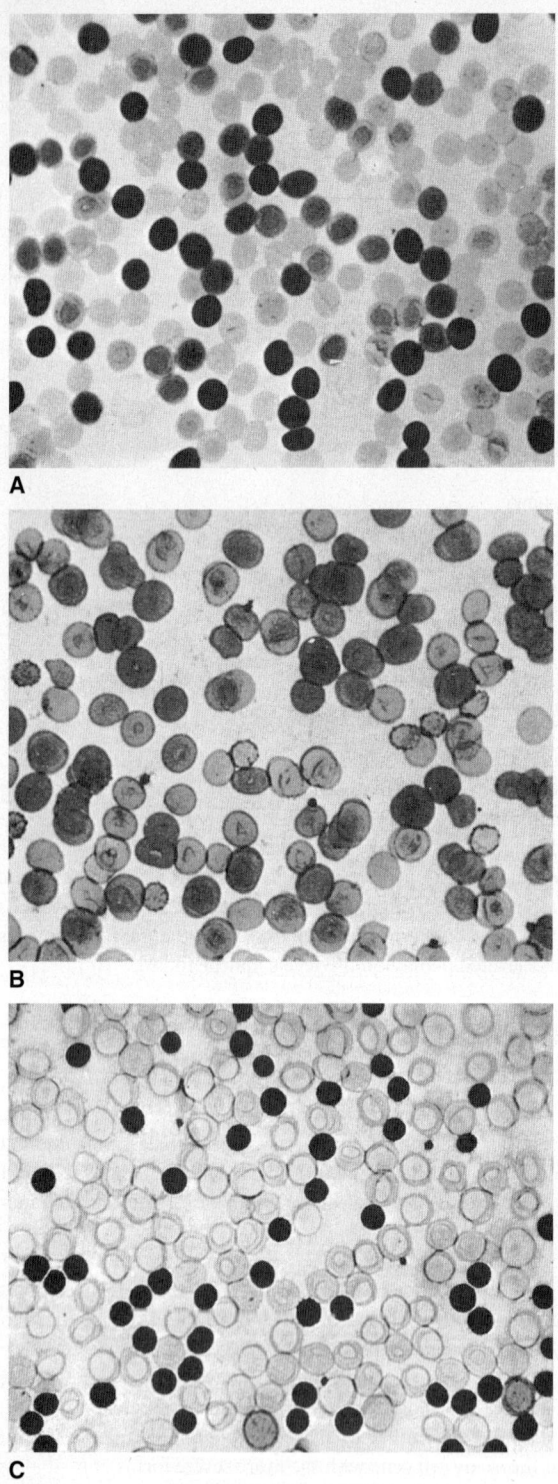

Figure 48–21. Acid elution preparations of blood films from **(A)** $\delta\beta$-thalassemia, **(B)** hereditary persistence of fetal hemoglobin, and **(C)** artificial mixture of fetal and adult red cells. The dark cells contain hemoglobin F. Hemoglobin F is resistant to acid elution.

it also is found in West Africa. It is characterized by a mild hemolytic anemia and splenomegaly with a blood picture showing the numerous target cells characteristic of all the hemoglobin C disorders.

Hemoglobin E thalassemia, which occurs at a high frequency in the eastern half of the Indian subcontinent and throughout Southeast Asia, is one of the most important hemoglobinopathies in the world population.[7,9,10,234–240] As mentioned earlier in "Etiology and Pathogenesis," hemoglobin E is synthesized at a reduced rate and hence produces the clinical phenotype of a mild form of β-thalassemia. Hence, when hemoglobin E is inherited with β-thalassemia—and most often this is a β^0- or severe β^+-thalassemia mutation in Southeast Asia and India—a marked deficit of β-chain production results, with the clinical picture of severe β-thalassemia. Hemoglobin E thalassemia shows a remarkable variability in clinical expression,[234–238] ranging from a mild form of thalassemia intermedia to a transfusion-dependent condition clinically indistinguishable from homozygous β-thalassemia. The reasons for this variability of expression are not understood, although some of the factors involved are identical to those that modify other forms of β-thalassemia.[239,240]

In more-severe cases of hemoglobin E thalassemia, severe anemia with growth retardation, leg ulcers, bone deformity, marked tendency to infection, iron loading, and variable splenomegaly and hypersplenism are seen. Large tumor masses composed of extramedullary erythropoietic tissue may cause a variety of compression syndromes, including a clinical picture that closely mimics a cerebral tumor. Another curious picture that seems to be restricted to splenectomized patients is an obliterative occlusion of the pulmonary vasculature that is believed to result from an extremely high platelet count.[241]

The clinical course and complications in transfusion-dependent patients are similar to those observed in homozygous β-thalassemia. In the milder forms, the main complications are progressive hypersplenism, organ damage as a result of progressive iron loading from an increased rate of absorption, extramedullary erythropoietic tumor masses, bone disease, and infection. The blood picture shows a typical thalassemic pattern. The hemoglobin consists of E, F, and A_2. Usually no hemoglobin A is present because the β^0-thalassemias are particularly common in the parts of the world where hemoglobin E is found.

Newer studies emphasize the complex interactions between genetic factors,[239,240] differences in adaptation to anemia, particularly in early life (see "Pathophysiology" above), and the environment, notably proneness to malarial infection, that underlie the widely differing and unstable phenotypes of patients with hemoglobin E β-thalassemia.[238,239]

β-THALASSEMIA WITH NORMAL HEMOGLOBIN A_2 LEVEL

Rare forms of β-thalassemia are seen in which heterozygotes have normal hemoglobin A_2 levels. Their main clinical importance is that they can be confused with the more severe forms of α-thalassemia in the heterozygous state and therefore may cause difficulties in genetic counseling and prenatal diagnosis. Based on hematologic studies, two main classes of "normal hemoglobin A_2 β-thalassemia"—sometimes called types 1 and 2—are seen.[242] Type 1 is the "silent" form of β-thalassemia. Type 2 is heterogeneous, with many cases representing the compound heterozygous state for β-thalassemia and δ-thalassemia.

"Silent" β-thalassemia[7,243] is characterized by no hematologic changes in heterozygotes. Several mild forms of β-thalassemia that underlie this phenotype are described (see Refs. 44 and 45). Although this condition can be partly identified by demonstrating a mild degree of globin-chain imbalance, with α-to-β synthesis ratios of approximately 1.5:1, it can only be diagnosed with certainty by DNA analysis. Compound heterozygotes for this condition and β^0-thalassemia have a mild form of β-thalassemia intermedia.

Normal hemoglobin A_2 β-thalassemia type 2 in heterozygotes is indistinguishable from typical β-thalassemia with elevated hemoglobin A_2 levels.[242] The homozygous state has not been described. The compound heterozygous state for this gene and for β-thalassemia with raised hemoglobin A$_2$ levels is characterized by a clinical picture of severe transfusion-dependent β-thalassemia. Family data obtained in Italy and Sardinia suggest this condition represents the compound heterozygous state for both β-thalassemia and δ-thalassemia.[244,245] Most of the δ-thalassemias have been observed *trans* to β-thalassemia. However, the form of δ-thalassemia resulting from loss of an A in codon 59 occurs on the same chromosome as the hemoglobin Knossos mutation, which is associated with a mild form of β-thalassemia.[246] This finding explains the normal level of hemoglobin A$_2$ associated with this condition, which is the most common form of normal hemoglobin A$_2$ β-thalassemia in the Mediterranean region.

Several other conditions, mentioned earlier in this chapter in "Etiology and Pathogenesis," are associated with a phenotype that is indistinguishable from normal A$_2$ β-thalassemia. These conditions include the heterozygous states for the Corfu form of δβ-thalassemia and εγδβ-thalassemia.

OTHER UNUSUAL FORMS OF β-THALASSEMIA

The clinical features of the dominant β-thalassemias resemble the features of thalassemia intermedia.[7] Moderate anemia and splenomegaly are seen, with a blood picture showing thalassemic red cell changes. The marrow shows erythroid hyperplasia with well-marked inclusion bodies in the red cell precursors. The latter may be seen in the blood after splenectomy. Hemoglobin analysis shows hemoglobins A and A$_2$ are present, and the hemoglobin F level is not usually elevated much higher than that seen in β-thalassemia trait. Hemoglobin A$_2$ levels are always raised.

Other unusual varieties of β-thalassemia include those categorized by unusually high hemoglobin F or A$_2$ levels. Most of these conditions result from deletions involving the β-globin gene and its promoter region. For example, the so-called Dutch[247] form of β-thalassemia is associated with unusually high hemoglobin F levels in heterozygotes and high hemoglobin A$_2$ levels. Several other conditions of this type, which result from different-size deletions, have been reported (see Ref. 7).

δ⁰-THALASSEMIA

δ⁰-Thalassemia causes a complete absence of hemoglobin A$_2$ in homozygotes and a reduced hemoglobin A$_2$ level in heterozygotes.[248] It is of no clinical significance except for its effect of reducing hemoglobin A$_2$ levels in β-thalassemia heterozygotes.

εγδβ-THALASSEMIA

This heterogeneous condition has been observed only in the heterozygous state in a few families.[7,108,109] It is characterized by neonatal hemolysis and, in adult life, by the hematologic picture of heterozygous β-thalassemia with normal hemoglobin A$_2$ levels.

α-THALASSEMIA IN ASSOCIATION WITH α- AND β-CHAIN HEMOGLOBIN VARIANTS

Several α-globin structural variants are caused by single amino acid substitutions at α-chain loci on chromosomes that carry only a single α-chain gene. Individuals who inherit variants of this type and an α⁰-thalassemia determinant have a form of hemoglobin H disease in which the hemoglobin consists of the α-chain variant hemoglobin and hemoglobin H. Well-documented examples include hemoglobin QH disease (− −/−α^Q),[249,250] hemoglobin G Philadelphia H disease (− −/−α^G),[251,252] and hemoglobin Hasharon H disease (− −/−α^{Hash}).[253] Many examples of the coexistence of the homozygous or heterozygous states for β-chain hemoglobin variants and different α-thalassemia determinants have

been reported.[7,9,10] Particularly well-characterized disorders include the various interactions of α⁰- and α⁺-thalassemia with hemoglobin E[7,234] and hemoglobin S (Chap. 49).[254,255] Carriers for these hemoglobin variants who also have the α⁰- or α⁺-thalassemia traits have thalassemic red cell indices and unusually low levels of the abnormal hemoglobin. Individuals with sickle cell anemia who have α-thalassemia show thalassemic red cell changes, more persistent splenomegaly, and lower hemoglobin F values than do patients without the thalassemia genes.

● THERAPY, COURSE, AND PROGNOSIS

The only forms of treatment available for thalassemic children are regular blood transfusions, iron chelation therapy in an attempt to prevent iron overload, judicious use of splenectomy in cases complicated by hypersplenism, and a good standard of general pediatric care.[7,9,256] Marrow transplantation has an important role in selected cases (Chap. 23).

TRANSFUSION

Children with β-thalassemia who are maintained at a hemoglobin level of 9.5 to 14.0 g/dL grow and develop normally. They do not develop the distressing skeletal complications of thalassemia.[7,256] Maintaining a lower hemoglobin level than this range without any deleterious effects on development and with the added advantage of reducing the level of iron loading may be possible. This regimen maintains a mean pretransfusion level that does not exceed 9.5 g/dL.[257] A transfusion program should not be started too early, and it should be initiated only when the hemoglobin level is too low to be compatible with normal development. If transfusion is started too soon, thalassemia intermedia may be missed, and the child may be transfused unnecessarily. Usually blood transfusions are given every 4 weeks on an outpatient basis. To avoid transfusion reactions, washed, filtered, or frozen red cells should be used so that the majority of the white cells and plasma-protein components are removed (Chap. 138).

IRON CHELATION

Every child who is maintained on a high-transfusion regimen ultimately develops iron overload and dies of siderosis of the myocardium. Therefore, such children must be started on a program of iron chelation within the first 2 to 3 years of life.[256] Deferoxamine (desferrioxamine) was the first chelating agent of proven long-term value for treatment of thalassemia. It is best administered by an 8- to 12-hour overnight pump-driven infusion in the subcutaneous tissues of the anterior abdominal wall.[258,259] Chelation therapy should commence by the time the serum ferritin level reaches approximately 1000 mcg/dL. In practice, this level usually is seen after the 12th to 15th transfusion. To prevent toxicity, infants must not be overchelated when the iron burden is still low. The initial dose usually is 20 mg/kg 5 nights per week, with 100 mg of oral vitamin C (200 mg in older children and adults) on the day of infusion, after the infusion has been initiated.[259] Some evidence and widespread opinion indicate ascorbate precipitates myocardiopathy in these patients if it is given before deferoxamine infusion is started.[260,261] In patients who are heavily iron loaded, particularly those patients with cardiac or endocrine complications, the body iron stores can be effectively lowered by continuous intravenous infusion of deferoxamine at a dose of up to 50 mg/kg body weight. The procedure usually entails insertion of an intravenous delivery system.

Extensive experience with the use of deferoxamine and its toxic effects has been reported.[189] No serious complications occur other than local erythema and painful subcutaneous nodules at the site of infusions and extremely rare severe allergic reactions. These reactions can be controlled, at least in part, by including 5 to 10 mg hydrocortisone in the infusion. Probably of greatest concern is neurosensory toxicity, which has been documented in up to 30 percent of cases. Toxicity causes high-frequency hearing loss that may become symptomatic.[262,263] In a few cases, the toxicity did not respond to discontinuation of the drug, and permanent hearing loss resulted. Ocular toxicity has been reported.[262] Symptoms include visual failure, night and color blindness, and field loss. Reversal of symptoms after discontinuation of the drug has been reported. Deferoxamine may cause bone changes and growth retardation, sometimes associated with bone pain. Body measurements characteristically show a reduced crown-pubis–to–pubis-heel ratio.[264] These changes may be associated with radiologic abnormalities of the vertebral column. These complications can be prevented by exercising extreme care in monitoring patients receiving long-term deferoxamine therapy. Young children or individuals from whom most of the iron has been removed by chelation are at particularly high risk. Formal audiometry and ophthalmologic examinations at 6-month intervals are recommended.

Because of the practical difficulties of a nightly subcutaneous infusion of deferoxamine there has been an intensive search for effective oral chelating drugs. Two of these agents are currently available, deferiprone (Ferriprox, L1) and deferasirox. The extensive literature on these agents has been reviewed.[265-267] Deferiprone is administered at a dosage of 75 mg/kg in three daily doses. Unfortunately there have been limited numbers of long-term trials comparing its efficacy with deferoxamine, but overall it appears to be less effective than deferoxamine at maintaining safe body iron levels. Its administration is accompanied by a number of complications, the most important of which is neutropenia and, in some cases, agranulocytosis with some fatalities. Hence it is recommended that patients receiving this agent have a weekly white cell count. It also causes arthritis which varies in severity and between different ethnic groups. However, by virtue of its membrane-crossing capacity it has been suggested that it may be more effective in removing cardiac iron (Chap. 43). Unfortunately, to date, all the studies that suggest that it may reduce the frequency of cardiac complications in transfusion-dependent thalassemics have been retrospective and there are no long-term controlled data available. It is currently suggested that it should be used in combination with desferrioxamine, particularly for its cardiac-iron sparing effect; again, long-term prospective data are required.

The initial studies of deferasirox were promising[266] and suggested that this agent in doses of 5 or 10 mg/kg per day, or higher in those who are heavily iron-loaded, was as effective as desferrioxamine in containing adequate hepatic iron levels. Preliminary clinical studies also showed that this agent may be effective for removing excess cardiac iron. Recent followup data have confirmed these early observations.[267] The most frequent adverse reactions to deferasirox included gastrointestinal disturbances, transient rashes, and a nonprogressive increase in serum creatinine. It is still too early to be sure about the overall effectiveness of this agent, however, or to assess its long-term safety.

Because of the extremely well-documented data showing long-term survival of patients adequately treated with deferoxamine,[268-270] this agent is still recommended as a first-line choice for management of transfusion-dependent thalassemia. However, particularly in view of problems of compliance and the promising trial results of deferasirox, this drug is also being used increasingly as a first line form of treatment. Further long-term follow up data regarding its efficacy are still required however.

Careful monitoring of the degree of iron accumulation during chelation therapy is absolutely vital. The simplest approach, particularly in countries where most sophisticated technology is not available, is a regular estimation of the serum ferritin level, which should be maintained at less than 1500 mcg/L. The value of hepatic iron concentration assessment was discussed earlier in "Abnormal Iron Metabolism." Newer noninvasive approaches to assessing body iron burden have been developed. There is now strong evidence that, with adequate calibration, the measurement and mapping of liver iron concentrations using magnetic resonance imaging (MRI) is an extremely effective approach for the regular assessment of the effectiveness of chelation therapy.[271] Similarly, there have been advances in the noninvasive estimation of myocardial iron using T2* MRI. Evidence obtained using this approach suggests that there may be a variable correlation between hepatic and cardiac iron concentrations.[272] Clearly functional cardiologic studies should be combined with assessment of cardiac iron levels, particularly the ejection fraction, pulmonary artery pressure, and other parameters of cardiac activity. The true value of these new approaches to assessing myocardial iron levels and function still require further study by prospective controlled trials.

Increasing evidence indicates children maintained at a high hemoglobin level do not develop hypersplenism.[7] However, enlargement of the spleen with increased transfusion requirements occurs commonly in patients maintained at a lower hemoglobin level. Splenectomy should be performed if transfusion requirements increase dramatically or pain develops because of the size of the spleen. Because of the risk of overwhelming pneumococcal infections, splenectomy should not be performed in children younger than age 5 years. Patients should receive a pneumococcal vaccine prior to the procedure. They then should be placed on prophylactic oral penicillin after the operation. *Haemophilus influenzae* type B and meningococcal vaccines also are recommended.

Children with severe thalassemia are still prone to other infections. Presentation with abdominal pain, diarrhea, and vomiting should always suggest an infection with a member of the *Yersinia* class of bacteria. Empirical treatment should start immediately with either an aminoglycoside or a cotrimoxazole. Transfusion-transmitted virus infection is common in some populations. All chronically transfused patients should be tested annually for hepatitis C, hepatitis B, and HIV. Patients with serologic evidence of chronic active hepatitis should be considered for treatment.

As mentioned earlier in "Abnormal Iron Metabolism," subtle endocrine deficiencies are increasingly recognized, particularly those associated with growth retardation and hypogonadism. These patients require expert endocrinologic assessment and replacement therapy when appropriate.

STEM CELL TRANSPLANTATION

By 1997, more than 1000 marrow transplants had been performed at three centers in Italy.[273-276] Based on this experience and on later data,[7] the prognosis evidently depended on the adequacy of iron chelation up to the time of transplantation. Hence, patients were divided into three classes: class I patients had a history of adequate iron chelation and neither liver fibrosis nor hepatomegaly; class II patients had one or two of these characteristics; and class III patients had all three characteristics. Among children in class I who had undergone transplantation early in the course of the disease, disease-free survival was assessed at 90 to 93 percent at 5 years, with a 4 percent risk of mortality related to the procedure. For class II patients, the intermediate-risk group, the survival and disease-free survival rates were 86 percent and 82 percent, respectively. For class III, the high-risk group, the survival and disease-free survival rates were 62 percent and 51 percent, respectively. Apart from the immediate complications of severe infection in the posttransplantation period, most of the problems were related to development of acute or chronic graft-versus-host disease. The overall frequency of mild to severe grades ranges from 27 to 30 percent.[277] Modification of preparative drug regimens has reduced the frequency of drug toxicity. The occurrence of mixed chimerism may be a risk factor for graft-versus-host disease. No case of hematologic malignancy has been observed in the longest followup of patients between 15 and 20 years after transplantation. Recent experience has fully confirmed these pioneering studies[278] and suggests that patients without matched donors could benefit from haploidentical mother-to-child transplantation. The current status of blood stem cell therapy is discussed further in Chap. 23.

GENERAL CARE

Management of thalassemia requires a high standard of general pediatric care. Infection should be treated early. If the diet is deficient in folate, supplements should be given. Supplementation probably is unnecessary in children maintained on a high-transfusion regimen. Particular attention should be paid to the ear, nose, and throat because of chronic sinus infection and middle-ear diseases resulting from bone deformity of the skull. Similarly, regular dental surveillance is essential because poorly transfused thalassemic children have a variety of deformities of the maxilla and poorly developed teeth. In the later stages of the illness, when iron loading becomes the major feature, endocrine replacement therapy may be necessary. Symptomatic treatment for metabolic bone disease and cardiac failure also may be needed.

THERAPIES OF SPECIAL TYPES OF THALASSEMIA

Hemoglobin H disease usually requires no specific therapy, although splenectomy may be of value in cases associated with severe anemia and splenomegaly.[7,9,10] Because splenectomy may be followed by a higher incidence of thromboembolic disease than occurs in splenectomized children with β-thalassemia,[7] the spleen should be removed only in cases of extreme anemia and splenomegaly. Oxidant drugs should not be given to patients with hemoglobin H disease. The management of symptomatic sickle cell thalassemia follows the lines described for sickle cell anemia (Chap. 49).

Thalassemia intermedia presents a particularly complex therapeutic problem. Whether a child with a steady-state hemoglobin level of 6 to 7 g/dL should be transfused is difficult to determine with certainty. Probably the best compromise is to watch such children very closely during the first years of life. If they grow and develop normally and no signs of bone changes are evident, they should be maintained without transfusion. If, however, their early growth pattern is retarded or their activity is limited because of their anemia, they should be placed on a regular transfusion regimen. If hypersplenism plays a role in their anemia as the children grow older, splenectomy should be performed. Because many of these patients have significant iron loading from the gastrointestinal tract, regular estimations of serum iron and ferritin should be obtained and chelation therapy instituted when appropriate.

EXPERIMENTAL APPROACHES TO TREATMENT

Two main experimental approaches are being pursued in the search for more effective therapy of the thalassemias: (1) reactivation or augmentation of fetal hemoglobin production and (2) somatic gene therapy.

The main rationale for employing agents that have been used in attempts to increase hemoglobin F production is based on the observation that patients recovering from cytotoxic drug therapy or during other periods of erythroid expansion may reactivate hemoglobin F synthesis. In addition, the observation that butyrate analogues might have a stimulating effect on hemoglobin F production has led to a number of studies of their potential for management of thalassemia. A number of clinical trials have been performed.[279–282] Agents that have been used

include various cytotoxic drugs, erythropoietin, and several different butyrate analogues. Overall, these agents, used alone or in combination, have produced some small effects on fetal hemoglobin production, but the results of these trials have been disappointing. Some notable exceptions were seen, however, particularly several cases of homozygosity or compound heterozygosity for hemoglobin Lepore in which use of either a combination of sodium phenylbutyrate and hydroxyurea or hydroxyurea alone produced a spectacular rise in hemoglobin F production. In the case of two homozygotes for hemoglobin Lepore, the necessity for further transfusion was eliminated.[283] This finding raises the intriguing possibility that certain mutations, possibly deletions of the β-globin gene cluster, are more susceptible to this type of approach. Recent progress in searching for genetic targets for modifying fetal hemoglobin synthesis has been reviewed recently.[42]

The other experimental approach involves somatic gene therapy. Currently, the therapy is mainly directed at gene transfer into potential hematopoietic stem cells using retroviral vectors.[284] Other approaches also are being taken, including attempts at the restoration of normal splicing in cases of splicing mutations[285] and use of *trans*-splicing ribozymes to correct β-globin gene transcripts.[286] However, studies using murine models with recombinant lentiviral vectors suggest that sustained, high-level globin gene expression may be possible, at least in this experimental system.[287,288] There continues to be slow progress toward somatic-cell gene therapy as applied to the hemoglobin disorders,[289] with at least one apparent success and future plans for several clinical trials.

PROGNOSIS

The prognosis for patients with severe forms of β-thalassemia who are adequately treated by transfusion and chelation has improved dramatically over the years. Three large studies investigated the influence of effective long-term desferrioxamine use on the development of cardiac disease.[268–270] In one study, patients who had maintained sustained reduction of body iron, as estimated by a serum ferritin level less than 2500 mcg/L over 12 years of followup, had an estimated cardiac disease-free survival rate of 91 percent. This finding is in contrast to patients in whom most determinations of serum ferritin level exceeded this value, in whom the estimated cardiac disease-free survival rate was less than 20 percent. In a second study, the relationship between survival and total-body iron burden was measured directly using hepatic storage iron values. Patients who had maintained hepatic iron concentrations of at least 15 mg of iron per gram of liver, dry weight, had a 32 percent probability of survival to age 25 years. No cardiac disease developed in patients who maintained hepatic iron levels below this threshold. These and other studies provide unequivocal evidence that adequate transfusion and chelation are associated with longevity and good quality of life. On the other hand, poor compliance or unavailability of chelating agents still are associated with a poor prospect of survival much beyond the second decade.

PREVENTION

In parts of the world where the incidence of thalassemia is high, the disease places an immense economic burden on society. For example, if all the thalassemic children born in Cyprus were treated by regular blood transfusions and iron-chelating therapy, it was estimated that within 15 years the total medical budget of the island would be required to treat this single disease.[290] Clearly, this approach was not feasible, so considerable effort was directed toward developing programs for prevention of the different forms of thalassemia.

The goal of prevention can be achieved in two ways. The first is prospective genetic counseling, that is, screening total populations while the children still are at school and warning carriers about the potential risks of marriage to another carrier. Few data are available about the value of programs of this type; a pilot study in Greece was unsuccessful.[291] Because it is believed this approach will not be successful in many populations, considerable effort has been directed toward developing prenatal diagnosis programs.

Prenatal diagnosis for prevention of thalassemia entails screening mothers at the first prenatal visit, screening the father in cases in which the mother is a thalassemia carrier, and offering the couple the possibility of prenatal diagnosis and termination of pregnancy if both mother and father are carriers of a gene for a severe form of thalassemia. Currently, these programs are devoted mainly to prenatal diagnosis of the severe transfusion-dependent forms of homozygous β^+ or β^0-thalassemia. Considerable experience has also been gained in prenatal diagnosis of mothers at risk for having a fetus with the hemoglobin Bart hydrops syndrome, considering the distress caused by a long and difficult pregnancy and the obstetric problems resulting from the birth of a hydropic infant with a massive placenta.

The first efforts at prenatal detection of β-thalassemia used fetal blood sampling and globin-chain synthesis analysis carried out at approximately week 18 of pregnancy. Despite the technical difficulties involved, the method was applied successfully in many countries and resulted in a reduced birth rate of infants with β-thalassemia.[292] The technique is associated with a low maternal morbidity rate, a fetal mortality rate of approximately 3 to 4 percent, and an error rate of 1 to 2 percent. Its main disadvantage is that it must be carried out relatively late in pregnancy. For this reason, efforts turned to first trimester prenatal diagnosis.

DNA technology has enabled diagnosis of important hemoglobin disorders *in utero* by fetal DNA analysis. Although analysis can be carried out on DNA derived from amniotic fluid, the approach has drawbacks because, again, it must be done relatively late in pregnancy, and often amniotic fluid cells must be grown in culture to obtain a sufficient amount of DNA.[293] However, DNA can be obtained as early as week 9 of pregnancy by chorionic villus sampling. Although the safety of this technique remains to be fully evaluated and limb reduction deformities may occur when the procedure is carried out very early in pregnancy (9 or 10 weeks), chorionic villus sampling has become the major method for prenatal diagnosis of the thalassemias based on subsequent experience with the technique.[7,293-297]

Remarkable advances in DNA technology have provided a variety of methods for the direct identification of mutations in fetal DNA[77] Even in families with extremely rare mutations, rapid DNA sequencing technology allows a diagnosis to be made very rapidly. The error rate using these different approaches varies, mainly depending on the experience of the particular laboratory; low rates, less than 1 percent, are reported from most centers. Potential sources of error include maternal contamination of fetal DNA and nonpaternity.

The application of this new technology has caused a major reduction in the birth rate of infants with thalassemia throughout the Mediterranean region and the Middle East, and in parts of the Indian subcontinent and Southeast Asia. Several approaches continue to be explored in an attempt to avoid the use of invasive procedures like chorion villous sampling. A variety of methods are being used to harvest fetal DNA from fetal cells in maternal blood or from maternal plasma[298,299] and there are increasing numbers of attempts at preimplantation diagnosis of thalassemias.[300,301] There is every expectation that some of these approaches will reach the clinic in the near future.[302]

THALASSEMIA AS A GLOBAL HEALTH PROBLEM

The remarkable advances in the diagnosis, prevention, and treatment of the thalassemias described in this chapter are only relevant to the richer countries of the world. In many developing countries in which there is a very high frequency of thalassemia, there are very limited facilities for their diagnosis and management. Because many of these countries are going through the epidemiologic transition, which involves improvements in nutrition, cleaner water supplies, and better public health services, babies with serious forms of thalassemia who previously would have died of infection or profound anemia are now surviving to present for treatment.

Approaches to the better control and management of the thalassemias in developing countries have been reviewed.[303,304] They include the development of partnerships between centers in the developed and developing countries for training workers in this field, and, once these partnerships are developed, for the further evolution of partnerships between those developing countries where there is knowledge and expertise of the field with those where no knowledge or facilities exist. Without organizations along these lines, the thalassemias will continue to cause the premature death of hundreds of thousands of infants worldwide.

REFERENCES

1. Cooley TB, Lee P: A series of cases of splenomegaly in children with anemia and peculiar bone changes. *Trans Am Pediatr Soc* 37:29, 1925.
2. Whipple GH, Bradford WL: Racial or familial anemia of children associated with fundamental disturbances of bone and pigment metabolism (Cooley von Jaksch). *Am J Dis Child* 44:336, 1932.
3. Whipple CH, Bradford WL: Mediterranean disease—Thalassemia (erythroblastic anemia of Cooley): Associated pigment abnormalities simulating hemochromatosis. *J Pediatr* 9:279, 1936.
4. Weatherall DJ: Toward an understanding of the molecular biology of some common inherited anemias: The story of thalassemia, in *Blood, Pure and Eloquent*, edited by Wintrobe MM, p 373. McGraw-Hill, New York, 1980.
5. Weatherall DJ: *Thalassaemia: The Biography*. Oxford University Press, Oxford, 2010.
6. Chernoff AI: The distribution of the thalassemia gene: A historical review. *Blood* 14:899, 1959.
7. Weatherall DJ, Clegg JB: *The Thalassaemia Syndromes*, 4th ed. Blackwell, Oxford, 2001.
8. Ingram VM, Stretton AOW: Genetic basis of the thalassemia diseases. *Nature* 184:1903, 1959.
9. Steinberg MH, Forget BG, Higgs DR, Weatherall DJ: *Disorders of Hemoglobin*, 2nd ed. Cambridge University Press, Cambridge, UK, 2009.
10. Weatherall DJ, Clegg JB, Higgs DR, Wood WG: The hemoglobinopathies, in *The Metabolic and Molecular Bases of Inherited Disease*, 8th ed, edited by Scriver CR, Beauder AL, Sly WS, Valle D, p 4571. McGraw-Hill, New York, 2001.
11. Weatherall DJ, Clegg JB: Inherited haemoglobin disorders: An increasing global health problem. *Bull World Health Organ* 79:704, 2001.
12. Christianson A, Howson CP, Modell B: *March of Dimes Global Report on Birth Defects*. March of Dimes Birth Defects Foundation, New York, 2006.
13. Haldane JBS: The rate of mutation of human genes. *Hereditas* 35(Suppl):267, 1949.
14. Orkin SH, Kazazian HH: The mutation and polymorphism of the human β-globin gene and its surrounding DNA. *Annu Rev Genet* 18:131, 1984.
15. Orkin SH, Antonarakis SE, Kazazian HH: Polymorphisms and molecular pathology of the human β-globin gene. *Prog Hematol* 13:49, 1983.
16. Siniscalco M, Bernini L, Filippi G, et al: Population genetics of haemoglobin variants, thalassaemia and glucose-6-phosphate dehydrogenase deficiency, with particular reference to malaria hypothesis. *Bull World Health Organ* 34:379, 1966.
17. Flint J, Hill AVS, Bowden DK, et al: High frequencies of α thalassemia are the result of natural selection by malaria. *Nature* 321:744, 1986.
18. Allen SJ, O'Donnell A, Alexander NDE, et al: α^+-Thalassemia protects children against disease due to malaria and other infections. *Proc Natl Acad Sci U S A* 94:14836, 1997.
19. Williams TN: Red blood cell defects and malaria. *Mol Biochem Parasitol* 149:121, 2006.
20. Williams TN, Mwangi TW, Wambua S, et al: Negative epistasis between the malaria-protective effects of alpha$^+$-thalassemia and the sickle cell trait. *Nat Genet* 37:1253, 2005.
21. Williams TN, Maitland K, Bennett S, et al: High incidence of malaria in α-thalassemic children. *Nature* 383:522, 1996.
22. Cockburn IA, Mackinnon MJ, O'Donnell A, et al: A human complement receptor 1 polymorphism that reduces *Plasmodium falciparum* rosetting confers protection against severe malaria. *Proc Natl Acad Sci U S A* 101:272, 2004.
23. Weatherall DJ: Genetic variation and susceptibility to infection: The red cell and malaria. *Br J Haematol* 141:276, 2008.
24. Williams TN, Weatherall DJ: World distribution, population genetics, and health burden of the hemoglobinopathies. *Cold Spring Harb Perspect Med* 2:a011692, 2012.
25. Orkin SH: The duplicated human α globin genes lie close together in cellular DNA. *Proc Natl Acad Sci U S A* 75:5950, 1978.

26. Lauer J, Shen C-KJ, Maniatis T: The chromosomal arrangement of human α-like globin genes: Sequence homology and α-globin gene deletions. *Cell* 20:119, 1980.

27. Liebhaber SA, Goossens N, Kan YW: Homology and concerted evolution at the α₁ and α₂ loci of human α-globin. *Nature* 290:26, 1981.

28. Liebhaber SA, Goossens MJ, Kan YW: Cloning and complete nucleotide sequence of human 5′-α-globin gene. *Proc Natl Acad Sci U S A* 77:7054, 1980.

29. Proudfoot NJ, Maniatis T: The structure of a human α-globin pseudo-gene and its relationship to α-globin duplication. *Cell* 21:537, 1980.

30. Liebhaber SA, Kan YW: Differentiation of the mRNA transcripts originating from the α₁- and α₂-globin loci in normals and α-thalassemics. *J Clin Invest* 68:439, 1981.

31. Orkin SH, Goff SC: The duplicated human α-globin genes: Their relative expression as measured by RNA analysis. *Cell* 24:345, 1981.

32. Higgs DR, Wainscoat JS, Flint J, et al: Analysis of the human α globin gene cluster reveals a highly informative genetic locus. *Proc Natl Acad Sci U S A* 83:5156, 1986.

33. Fritsch EF, Lawn RM, Maniatis T: Molecular cloning and characterization of the human β-like globin gene cluster. *Cell* 19:959, 1980.

34. Spritz RA, DeRiel JK, Forget BG, Weissman SM: Complete nucleotide sequence of the human δ-globin gene. *Cell* 21:639, 1980.

35. Baralle FE, Shoulders CC, Proudfoot NJ: The primary structure of the human ε globin gene. *Cell* 21:621, 1980.

36. Slightom JL, Blechl AE, Smithies O: Human G gamma- and A gamma-globin genes: Complete nucleotide sequences suggest that DNA can be exchanged between these duplicated genes. *Cell* 21:627, 1980.

37. Jeffrey AJ: DNA sequences in the G gamma-, A gamma-, delta- and beta-globin genes of man. *Cell* 18:1, 1979.

38. Antonarakis SE, Boehm CD, Giardina PVJ, Kazazian HH: Nonrandom association of polymorphic restriction sites in the β-globin gene complex. *Proc Natl Acad Sci U S A* 79:137, 1982.

39. Wainscoat JS, Hill AVV, Boyce A, et al: Evolutionary relationships of human populations from an analysis of nuclear DNA polymorphisms. *Nature* 319:491, 1982.

40. Katsumura KR, DeVilbiss AW, Pope NJ, et al: Transcriptional mechanisms underlying hemoglobin synthesis. *Cold Spring Harb Perspect Med* 3:a015412, 2013.

41. Higgs DR, Weatherall DJ: The alpha thalassaemias. *Cell Mol Life Sci* 66:1154, 2008.

42. Sankaran VG, Orkin SH: The switch from fetal to adult hemoglobin. *Cold Spring Harb Perspect Med* 3:a011643, 2013.

43. Donze D, Townes TM, Bieker JJ: Role of erythroid Kruppel-like factor in human gamma- to beta-globin gene switching. *J Biol Chem* 270:1955, 1995.

44. Thein SL, Wood WG: The molecular basis of β thalassaemia, δβ thalassaemia, and hereditary persistence of fetal hemoglobin, in *Disorders of Hemoglobin*, 2nd ed, edited by Steinberg MH, Forget BG, Higgs DR, Weatherall DJ, p 323. Cambridge University Press, Cambridge, UK, 2009.

45. Higgs DR: The alpha thalassemias. *Cold Spring Harb Perspect Med* 2:a011718, 2012.

46. Giardine B, van Baal S, Kaimakis P, et al: HbVar database of human hemoglobin variants and thalassemia mutations: 2007 Update. *Hum Mutat* 28:206, 2007.

48. Orkin SH, Old JM, Weatherall DJ, Nathan DG: Partial deletion of beta-globin gene DNA in certain patients with beta 0-thalassemia. *Proc Natl Acad Sci U S A* 76:2400, 1979.

48. Thein SL, Old JM, Wainscoat JS, Weatherall DJ: Population and genetic studies suggest a single origin for the Indian deletion beta thalassaemia. *Br J Haematol* 57:271, 1984.

49. Anand R, Boehm CD, Kazazian HH, Vanin EF: Molecular characterization of a beta zero-thalassemia resulting from a 1.4 kilobase deletion. *Blood* 72:636, 1988.

50. Padanilam BJ, Felice AE, Huisman THJ: Partial deletion of the 5′ beta-globin gene region causes beta zero-thalassemia in members of an American black family. *Blood* 64:941, 1984.

51. Popovich BW, Rosenblatt DS, Kendall AG, Nishioka Y: Molecular characterization of an atypical beta-thalassemia caused by a large deletion in the 5′ beta-globin gene region. *Am J Hum Genet* 39:797, 1986.

52. Diaz-Chico JC, Yang KG, Kutlar A, et al: An approximately 300 bp deletion involving part of the 5′ beta-globin gene region is observed in members of a Turkish family with beta-thalassemia. *Blood* 70:583, 1987.

53. Aulehla-Scholz C, Spiegelberg R, Horst J: A beta-thalassemia mutant caused by a 300-bp deletion in the human beta-globin gene. *Hum Genet* 81:298, 1989.

54. Orkin SH, Antonarakis SE, Kazazian HH: Base substitution at position −88 in a beta-thalassemic globin gene. Further evidence for the role of the distal promoter element ACACCC. *J Biol Chem* 259:8679, 1984.

55. Orkin SH, Kazazian HH, Antonarakis SE, et al: Linkage of beta-thalassemia mutations and beta-globin gene polymorphisms with DNA polymorphisms in human globin gene cluster. *Nature* 296:267, 1982.

56. Poncz M, Ballantine M, Solowiejczyk D, et al: beta-Thalassemia in a Kurdish Jew. *J Biol Chem* 257:5994, 1983.

57. Orkin SH, Sexton JP, Cheng TC, et al: TATA box transcription mutation in beta-thalassemia. *Nucleic Acids Res* 11:4827, 1983.

58. Antonarakis SE, Irkin SH, Cheng TC, et al: beta-Thalassemia in American Blacks: Novel mutations in the "TATA" box and an acceptor splice site. *Proc Natl Acad Sci U S A* 81:1154, 1984.

59. Surrey S, Delgrosso K, Malladi P, Schwartz E: Functional analysis of a beta-globin gene containing a TATA box mutation from a Kurdish Jew with beta-thalassemia. *J Biol Chem* 260:6507, 1985.

60. Gonzalez-Redondo JH, Stoming TA, Kutlar A, et al: A C→T substitution at nt −101 in a conserved DNA sequence of the promoter region of the beta-globin gene is associated with "silent" beta-thalassemia. *Blood* 73:1705, 1989.

61. Wong C, Dowling CE, Saiki RK, et al: Characterization of beta-thalassemia mutations using direct genomic sequencing of amplified single copy DNA. *Nature* 330:384, 1987.

62. Treisman R, Orkin SH, Maniatis T: Specific transcription and RNA splicing defects in five cloned beta-thalassemia genes. *Nature* 302:591, 1983.

63. Kazazian HH, Orkin SH, Antonarakis SE: Molecular characterization of seven beta-thalassaemia mutations in Asian Indians. *EMBO J* 3:593, 1984.

64. Padanilam BJ, Huisman THJ: The beta zero-thalassemia in an American Black family is due to a single nucleotide substitution in the acceptor splice junction of the second intervening sequence. *Am J Hematol* 22:259, 1986.

65. Atweh GF, Anagnou NP, Shearin J, et al: beta-Thalassemia resulting from a single nucleotide substitution in an acceptor splice site. *Nucleic Acids Res* 13:777, 1985.

66. Orkin SH, Sexton JP, Goff SC, Kazazian HH: Inactivation of an acceptor splice site by a short deletion in beta-thalassemia. *J Biol Chem* 258:7249, 1983.

67. Atweh GF, Wong C, Reed R, et al: A new mutation in IVS-1 of the human beta globin gene causing beta thalassemia due to abnormal splicing. *Blood* 70:148, 1987.

68. Cheng T, Orkin SH, Antonarakis SE, et al: beta-Thalassemia in Chinese: Use of *in vivo* RNA analysis and oligonucleotide hybridization in systematic characterization of molecular defects. *Proc Natl Acad Sci U S A* 81:2821, 1984.

69. Gonzalez-Redondo JH, Stoming TA, Lanclos KD, et al: Clinical and genetic heterogeneity in Black patients with homozygous beta-thalassemia from the southeastern United States. *Blood* 72:1007, 1988.

70. Tamagnini GP, Lopes MC, Castanheira ME, et al: Beta + thalassaemia—Portuguese type: Clinical, haematological and molecular studies of a newly defined form of beta thalassaemia. *Br J Haematol* 54:189, 1983.

71. Hill AVS, Bowden DK, O'Shaughnessy DF, et al: beta-Thalassemia in Melanesia: Association with malaria and characterization of a common variant. *Blood* 72:9, 1988.

72. Spritz RA, Jagadeeswaran P, Choudary PV, et al: Base substitution in an intervening sequence of a beta+-thalassemic human globin gene. *Proc Natl Acad Sci U S A* 78:2455, 1981.

73. Busslinger M, Moschonas N, Flavell RA: Beta + thalassemia: Aberrant splicing results from a single point mutation in an intron. *Cell* 27:289, 1981.

74. Metherall JE, Collins RS, Pan J, et al: Beta zero thalassaemia caused by a base substitution that creates an alternative splice acceptor site in an intron. *EMBO J* 5:2551, 1986.

75. Orkin SH, Kazazian HH Jr, Antonarakis SE,, et al: Abnormal RNA processing due to the exon mutation of beta E-globin gene. *Nature* 300:768, 1982.

76. Goldsmith ME, Humphries RK, Ley T, et al: "Silent" nucleotide substitution in beta+-thalassemia globin gene activates splice site in coding sequence RNA. *Proc Natl Acad Sci U S A* 88:2318, 1983.

77. Orkin SH, Antonarakis SE, Loukopoulos D: Abnormal processing of beta Knossos RNA. *Blood* 64:311, 1984.

78. Yang KG, Kutlar F, George E, et al: Molecular characterization of beta-globin gene mutations in Malay patients with Hb E-beta-thalassaemia major. *Br J Haematol* 72:73, 1989.

79. Orkin SH, Cheng TC, Antonarakis SE, Kazazian HH Jr: Thalassaemia due to a mutation in the cleavage-polyadenylation signal of the human beta-globin gene. *EMBO J* 4:453, 1985.

80. Jankovic L, Efremov GD, Petkov G, et al: Three novel mutations leading to beta thalassemia. *Blood* 74:226, 1989.

81. Rund D, Filon D, Rachmilewitz EA, et al: Molecular analysis of beta-thalassemia in Kurdish Jews: Novel mutations and expression studies. *Blood* 74:821, 1989.

82. Chang JC, Kan YW: beta-Thalassemia: A nonsense mutation in man. *Proc Natl Acad Sci U S A* 76:2886, 1979.

83. Kazazian HH, Dowling CE, Waber PG, et al: The spectrum of beta-thalassemia genes in China and Southeast Asia. *Blood* 68:964, 1986.

84. Trecartin RF, Liebhaber SA, Chang JC, et al: Beta zero thalassemia in Sardinia is caused by a nonsense mutation. *J Clin Invest* 68:1012, 1981.

85. Rosatelli C, Leoni GB, Tuveri T, et al: Beta thalassaemia mutations in Sardinians: Implications for prenatal diagnosis. *J Med Genet* 24:97, 1987.

86. Kimberland ML, Divoky V, Prchal J, et al: Full-length human L1 insertions retain the capacity for high frequency retrotransposition in cultured cells. *Hum Mol Genet* 8:1557, 1999.

87. Weatherall DJ, Clegg JB, Knox-Macaulay HHM, et al: A genetically determined disorder with features both of thalassaemia and congenital dyserythropoietic anaemia. *Br J Haematol* 24:681, 1973.

88. Stamatoyannopoulos G, Woodson R, Papayannopoulou T, et al: Inclusion-body beta-thalassemia trait: A form of beta thalassemia producing clinical manifestations in simple heterozygotes. *N Engl J Med* 290:939, 1974.

89. Thein SL: Dominant beta thalassaemia: Molecular basis and pathophysiology. *Br J Haematol* 80:273,1992.

90. Thein SL, Hesketh C, Taylor P, et al: Molecular basis for dominantly inherited inclusion body beta thalassaemia. *Proc Natl Acad Sci U S A* 87:3924, 1990.

91. Beris RP, Miescher PA, Diaz-Chico JC, et al: Inclusion body beta-thalassaemia trait in a Swiss family is caused by an abnormal hemoglobin (Geneva) with an altered and extended beta chain carboxy-terminus due to a modification in codon 114. *Blood* 72:801, 1988.

92. Kazazian HH, Dowling CE, Hurwitz RL, et al: Thalassemia mutations in exon 3 of the beta-globin gene often cause a dominant form of thalassemia and show no predilection for malarial-endemic regions of the world. *Am J Hum Genet* 45:A242, 1989.

93. Fei YJ, Stoming TA, Kutlar A, et al: One form of inclusion body beta thalassemia is due to a GAA—TAA mutation at codon 121 of the beta chain. *Blood* 73:1075, 1989.

94. Kazazian HH, Orkin SH, Boehm CD, et al: Characterization of a spontaneous mutation to a beta-thalassemia allele. *Am J Hum Genet* 38:860, 1986.

95. Sachs AB: Messenger RNA degradation in eukaryotes. *Cell* 74:413, 1993.

96. Thermann R, Neu-Yilik J, Deters A, et al: Binary specification of nonsense codons by splicing and cytoplasmic translation. *EMBO J* 17:3484, 1998.

97. Thein SL: Is it dominantly inherited beta thalassaemia or just a beta-chain variant that is highly unstable? *Br J Haematol* 107:12, 1999.

98. Adams JG, Steinberg MH, Boxer LA, et al: The structure of hemoglobin Indianapolis [(beta112(G14) arginine]: An unstable variant detectable only by isotopic labeling. *J Biol Chem* 254:3489, 1979.

99. Coleman MB, Steinberg MH, Adams JG 3rd: Hemoglobin Terre Haute arginine beta 106. A posthumous correction to the original structure of hemoglobin Indianapolis. *Blood* 76:57, 1990.

100. Thein SL, Wood WG, Wickramasinghe SN, Galvin MC: Beta-thalassemia unlinked to the beta-globin gene in an English family. *Blood* 82:961, 1993.

101. Jones RW, Old JM, Trent RJ, et al: Major rearrangement in the human beta-globin cluster. *Nature* 291:39, 1981.

102. Baglioni C: The fusion of two peptide chains in hemoglobin Lepore and its interpretation as a genetic deletion. *Proc Natl Acad Sci U S A* 48:1880, 1962.

103. Ottolenghi S, Giglioni B, Pulazzini A, et al: Sardinian delta beta zero-thalassemia: a further example of a C to T substitution at position −196 of the A gamma globin gene promoter. *Blood* 69:1058, 1987.

104. Atweh GF, Zhu XX, Brickner HE, et al: The beta-globin gene on the Chinese delta beta-thalassemia chromosome carries a promoter mutation. *Blood* 70:1480, 1987.

105. Wainscoat JS, Thein SL, Wood WG, et al: A novel deletion in the beta globin gene complex. *Ann N Y Acad Sci* 445:20, 1985.

106. Kulozik A, Yarwood N, Jones RW: The Corfu delta beta zero thalassemia: A small deletion acts at a distance to selectively abolish beta globin gene expression. *Blood* 71:457, 1988.

107. Fritsch EF, Lawn RM, Maniatis T: Characterization of deletions which affect the expression of fetal globin genes in man. *Nature* 279:598, 1979.

108. Orkin SH, Goff SC, Nathan DG: Heterogeneity of DNA deletion in gamma delta beta-thalassemia. *J Clin Invest* 67:878, 1981.

109. Pirastu M, Kan YW, Lin CC, et al: Hemolytic disease of the newborn caused by a new deletion of the entire beta-globin cluster. *J Clin Invest* 72:602, 1983.

110. Fearon ER, Kazazian HH Jr, Waber PG, et al: The entire beta-globin gene cluster is deleted in a form of gamma delta beta-thalassemia. *Blood* 61:1269, 1983.

111. Van der Ploeg LH, Konings A, Oort M, et al: gamma-beta-Thalassaemia studies showing that deletion of the gamma- and delta-genes influences beta-globin gene expression in man. *Nature* 283:637, 1980.

112. Curtin P, Pirastu M, Kan YW, et al: A distant gene deletion affects beta-globin gene function in an gamma delta beta-thalassemia. *J Clin Invest* 76:1554, 1985.

113. Driscoll MC, Dobkin CS, Alter BP: Gamma delta beta-thalassemia due to a de novo mutation deleting the 5′ beta-globin gene activation-region hypersensitive sites. *Proc Natl Acad Sci U S A* 86:7480, 1989.

114. Tuan D, Feingold E, Newman M, et al: Different 3′ end points of deletions causing delta beta-thalassemia and hereditary persistence of fetal hemoglobin: Implications for the control of gamma-globin gene expression in man. *Proc Natl Acad Sci U S A* 80:6937, 1983.

115. Kendall AG, Ojwang PJ, Schroeder WA, Huisman TH: Hemoglobin Kenya, the product of a gamma-beta fusion gene: Studies of the family. *Am J Hum Genet* 25:548, 1973.

116. Smith DH, Clegg JB, Weatherall DJ, Gilles HM: Hereditary persistence of foetal haemoglobin associated with a gamma beta fusion variant, haemoglobin Kenya. *Nat New Biol* 246:184, 1973.

117. Collins FS, Stoeckert CJ, Serjeant GR, et al: G gamma beta+ hereditary persistence of fetal hemoglobin: Cosmid cloning and identification of a specific mutation 5′ to the G gamma gene. *Proc Natl Acad Sci U S A* 81:4894, 1984.

118. Giglioni B, Casini C, Mantovani R, et al: A molecular study of a family with Greek hereditary persistence of fetal hemoglobin and beta-thalassemia. *EMBO J* 3:2641, 1984.

119. Gelinas R, Endlich B, Pfeiffer C, et al: G to A substitution in the distal CCAAT box of the A gamma-globin gene in Greek hereditary persistence of fetal haemoglobin. *Nature* 313:323, 1985.

120. Tate VE, Wood WG, Weatherall DJ: The British form of hereditary persistence of fetal hemoglobin results from a single base mutation adjacent to an S1 hypersensitive site 5′ to the A gamma globin gene. *Blood* 68:1389, 1986.

121. Gilman JG, Huisman TH: DNA sequence variation associated with elevated fetal G gamma globin production. *Blood* 66:783, 1985.

122. Marti HR: *Normale und Abnormale Menschliche Haemoglobin*. Springer-Verlag, Berlin, 1963.

123. Dover GJ, Smith KD, Chang YC, et al: Fetal hemoglobin levels in sickle cell disease and normal individuals are partially controlled by an X-linked gene located at Xp22.2. *Blood* 80:816, 1992.

124. Craig JE, Rochette J, Fisher CA, et al: Dissecting the loci controlling fetal haemoglobin production on chromosomes 11p and 6q by the regressive approach. *Nat Genet* 12:58, 1996.

125. Garner C, Silver N, Best S, et al: Quantitative trait loci on chromosome 8q influences the switch from fetal to adult hemoglobin. *Blood* 104:2184, 2004.

126. Menzel S, Garner C, Gut I, et al: A QTL influencing F cell production maps to a gene encoding a zinc-finger protein on chromosome 2p15. *Nat Genet* 39:1197, 2007.

127. Uda M, Galanello R, Sanna S, et al: Genome-wide association study shows *BCL11A* associated with persistent fetal hemoglobin and amelioration of the phenotype of beta-thalassemia. *Proc Natl Acad Sci U S A* 105:1620, 2008.

128. Menzel S, Thein SL: Genetic architecture of hemoglobin F control. *Curr Opin Hematol* 16:179, 2009.

129. Wood WG, Weatherall DJ, Clegg JB: Interaction of heterocellular hereditary persistence of foetal haemoglobin with beta thalassaemia and sickle cell anaemia. *Nature* 264:248, 1976.

130. Gibbons RJ, Wada T: ATRX and X-linked (alpha)-thalassemia mental retardation syndrome, in *Inborn Errors of Development*, edited by Epstein CJ, Erickson RP, Wynshaw-Boris A, p 748. Oxford University Press, Oxford, 2004.

131. Gibbons RJ, Wada T, Fisher CA, et al: Mutations in the chromatin-associated protein ATRX. *Hum Mutat* 29:796, 2008.

132. Nicholls RD, Fischel-Ghodsian N, Higgs DR: Recombination at the human alpha-globin gene cluster: Sequence features and topological constraints. *Cell* 49:369, 1987.

133. Barbour VM, Tufarelli C, Sharpe JA, et al: Alpha-thalassemia resulting from a negative chromosomal position effect. *Blood* 96:800, 2000.

134. Tufarelli C, Stanley JA, Garrick D, et al: Transcription of antisense RNA leading to gene silencing and methylation as a novel cause of human genetic disease. *Nat Genet* 34:157, 2003.

135. Wilkie AOM, Lamb J, Harris PC, et al: A truncated human chromosome 16 associated with alpha thalassaemia is stabilized by addition of telomeric repeat (TTAGGG). *Nature* 346:868, 1990.

136. Hatton CS, Wilkie AO, Drysdale HC, et al: Alpha-thalassemia caused by a large (62 kb) deletion upstream of the human alpha globin gene cluster. *Blood* 76:221, 1990.

137. Liebhaber SA, Griese E-U, Cash FE, et al: Inactivation of human alpha-globin gene expression by a de novo deletion located upstream of the alpha-globin gene cluster. *Proc Natl Acad Sci U S A* 81:9431, 1990.

138. Embury SH, Miller JA, Dozy AM, et al: Two different molecular organizations account for the single alpha-globin gene of the alpha-thalassemia-2 genotype. *J Clin Invest* 66:1319, 1980.

139. Higgs DR, Old JM, Pressley L, et al: A novel alpha-globin gene arrangement in man. *Nature* 284:632, 1980.

140. Goossens M, Dozy AM, Embury SH, et al: Triplicated alpha-globin loci in humans. *Proc Natl Acad Sci U S A* 77:518, 1980.

141. Trent RJ, Higgs DR, Clegg JB, Weatherall DJ: A new triplicated alpha-globin gene arrangement in man. *Br J Haematol* 49:149, 1981.

142. Higgs DR, Hill AVS, Bowden DK, Weatherall DJ: Independent recombination events between duplicated human alpha globin genes: Implications for their concerted evolution. *Nucleic Acids Res* 12:6965, 1984.

143. Orkin SH, Goff SC, Hechtman RL: Mutation in an intervening sequence splice junction in man. *Proc Natl Acad Sci U S A* 78:5041, 1981.

144. Higgs DR, Goodbourn SE, Lamb J, et al: Alpha-thalassaemia caused by a polyadenylation signal mutation. *Nature* 306:398, 1983.

145. Thein SL, Wallace RB, Pressley L, et al: The polyadenylation site mutation in the alpha-globin gene cluster. *Blood* 71:313, 1988.

146. Pirastu M, Saglio G, Chang JC, et al: Initiation codon mutation as a cause of alpha thalassemia. *J Biol Chem* 259:12315, 1984.

148. Olivieri NF, Chang LS, Poon AO, et al: An alpha-globin gene initiation codon mutation in a black family with HbH disease. *Blood* 70:729, 1987.

148. Paglietti E, Galanello R, Moi P, et al: Molecular pathology of haemoglobin H disease in Sardinians. *Br J Haematol* 63:485, 1986.

149. Morlé F, Lopez B, Henni T, Godet J: alpha-Thalassaemia associated with the deletion of two nucleotides at position −2 and −3 preceding the AUG codon. *EMBO J* 4:1245, 1985.

150. Weatherall DJ, Clegg JB: The alpha-chain-termination mutants and their relationship to the alpha-thalassaemias. *Philos Trans R Soc London B Biol Sci* 271:411, 1975.

151. Liebhaber SA, Coleman MB, Adams JG 3rd, et al: Molecular basis for nondeletion alpha-thalassemia in American blacks. Alpha 2(116GAG—UAG). *J Clin Invest* 80:154, 1987.

152. Liebhaber SA, Kan YW: A Thalassemia caused by an unstable alpha-globin mutant. *J Clin Invest* 71:461, 1983.

153. Sanguansermsri T, Matragoon S, Changloah L, Flatz G: Hemoglobin Suan-Dok (alpha 2 109 (G16) Leu replaced by Arg beta 2): An unstable variant associated with alpha-thalassemia. *Hemoglobin* 3:161, 1979.

154. Honig GR, Shamsuddin M, Zaizov R, et al: Hemoglobin Petah Tikva (alpha 110 ala replaced by asp): A new unstable variant with alpha-thalassemia-like expression. *Blood* 57:705, 1981.

155. Honig GR, Shamsuddin M, Vida LN, et al: Hemoglobin Evanston (alpha 14 Trp—Arg). An unstable alpha-chain variant expressed as alpha-thalassemia. *J Clin Invest* 73:1740, 1984.

156. Weatherall DJ, Higgs DR, Bunch C, et al: Hemoglobin H disease and mental retardation: A new syndrome or a remarkable coincidence? *N Engl J Med* 305:607, 1981.

157. Wilkie AO, Buckle VJ, Harris PC, et al: Clinical features and molecular analysis of the alpha thalassaemia/mental retardation syndromes: I. Cases due to deletions involving chromosome band 16p13.3. *Am J Hum Genet* 46:1112, 1990.

158. Wilkie AO, Zeitlin HC, Lindenbaum RH, et al: Clinical features and molecular analysis of the alpha-thalassemia/mental retardation syndromes: II. Cases without detectable abnormality of the alpha globin complex. *Am J Hum Genet* 46:1127, 1990.

159. Gibbons RJ, Suthers GK, Wilkie AO, et al: X-linked alpha-thalassemia/mental retardation (ATR-X) syndrome: Localization to Xq12–21.31 by X-inactivation and linkage analysis. *Am J Hum Genet* 51:1136, 1992.

160. Gibbons RJ, Picketts DJ, Villard L, Higgs DR: Mutations in a putative global transcriptional regulator cause X-linked mental retardation with alpha-thalassemia (ATR-X syndrome). *Cell* 80:837, 1995.

161. Gibbons RJ, Bachoo S, Picketts DJ, et al: Mutations in transcriptional regulator *ATRX* establish the functional significance of a PHD-like domain. *Nat Genet* 17:146, 1997.

162. Ausió J, Levin DB, De Amorim GV, et al: Syndromes of disordered chromatin remodeling. *Clin Genet* 64:83, 2003.

163. Gibbons RJ, McDowell TL, Raman S, et al: Mutations in ATRX, encoding a SWI/SNF-like protein, cause diverse changes in the pattern of DNA methylation. *Nat Genet* 24:368, 2000.

164. Weatherall DJ, Old J, Longley J, et al: Acquired haemoglobin H disease in leukaemia: Pathophysiology and molecular basis. *Br J Haematol* 38:305, 1978.

165. Gibbons RJ: alpha-Thalassemia, mental retardation, and myelodysplastic syndrome. *Cold Spring Harb Perspect Med* 2:a011759, 2012.

166. Belickova M, Schroeder HW, Guan YL, et al: Clonal hematopoiesis and acquired thalassemia in common variable immunodeficiency. *Mol Med* 1:56, 1995.

167. Weatherall DJ, Clegg JB, Naughton MA: Globin synthesis in thalassemia: An in vitro study. *Nature* 208:1061, 1965.

168. Weatherall DJ, Clegg JB, Na-Nakorn S, Wasi P: The pattern of disordered haemoglobin synthesis in homozygous and heterozygous beta-thalassaemia. *Br J Haematol* 16:251, 1969.

169. Fessas P: Inclusions of hemoglobin in erythroblasts and erythrocytes of thalassemia. *Blood* 21:21, 1963.

170. Wickramasinghe SN, Hughes M: Some features of bone marrow macrophages in patients with beta-thalassaemia. *Br J Haematol* 38:23, 1978.

171. Yataganas X, Fessas P: The pattern of hemoglobin precipitation in thalassemia and its significance. *Ann N Y Acad Sci* 165:270, 1969.

172. Finch CA, Deubelbeiss K, Cook JD, et al: Ferrokinetics in man. *Medicine (Baltimore)* 49:17, 1970.

173. Chalavelakis G, Clegg JB, Weatherall DJ: Imbalanced globin chain synthesis in heterozygous beta-thalassemic bone marrow. *Proc Natl Acad Sci U S A* 72:3853, 1975.

174. Rund D, Rachmilewitz E: Advances in the pathophysiology and treatment of thalassemia. *Crit Rev Oncol Hematol* 20:237, 1995.

175. Schrier SL: Pathobiology of thalassemic erythrocytes. *Curr Opin Hematol* 4:75, 1997.

176. Fibach E, Rachmilewitz E: The role of oxidative stress in hemolytic anemia. *Curr Mol Med* 8:609, 2008.

177. Yuan J, Angelucci E, Lucarelli G, et al: Accelerated programmed cell death (apoptosis) in erythroid precursors of patients with severe beta-thalassemia (Cooley's anemia). *Blood* 82:374, 1993.

178. Ager JAM, Lehmann H: Observations on some "fast" haemoglobins: K, J, N, and "Bart's." *Br Med J* 1:929, 1958.

179. Rigas DA, Kohler RD, Osgood EE: New hemoglobin possessing a higher electrophoretic mobility than normal adult hemoglobin. *Science* 121:372, 1955.

180. Gabuzda TG, Nathan DG, Gardner FH: The turnover of hemoglobins A, F, and A(2) in the peripheral blood of three patients with thalassemia. *J Clin Invest* 42:1678, 1963.

181. Loukopoulos D, Fessas P: The distribution of hemoglobin types in thalassemic erythrocyte. *J Clin Invest* 44:231, 1965.

182. Nathan DG, Gunn RB: Thalassemia: The consequences of unbalanced hemoglobin synthesis. *Am J Med* 41:815, 1966.

183. Rees DC, Porter JB, Clegg JB, Weatherall DJ: Why are hemoglobin F levels increased in HbE/beta thalassemia? *Blood* 94:3199, 1999.

184. Thein SL, Weatherall DJ: A non-deletion hereditary persistence of fetal hemoglobin (HPFH) determinant not linked to the β-globin gene complex, in *Hemoglobin Switching, Part B: Cellular and Molecular Mechanisms*, edited by Stamatoyannopoulos G, Nienhuis AW, p 97. Alan R. Liss, New York, 1989.

185. O'Donnell A, Premawardhena A, Arambepola M, et al: Age-related changes in adaptation to severe anemia in childhood in developing countries. *Proc Natl Acad Sci U S A* 104:9440, 2007.

186. Multicentre study on prevalence of endocrine complications in thalassemia major. Italian Working Group on Endocrine Complications in Non-endocrine Diseases. *Clin Endocrinol (Oxf)* 42:581, 1995.

187. Wood JC, Enriquez C, Ghugre N, et al: Physiology and pathophysiology of iron cardiomyopathy in thalassemia. *Ann N Y Acad Sci* 1054:386, 2005.

188. Ganz T, Nemeth E: Iron metabolism: Interactions with normal and disordered erythropoiesis. *Cold Spring Harb Perspect Med* 2:a011668, 2012.

189. Olivieri NF, Brittenham GM: Iron-chelating therapy and the treatment of thalassemia. *Blood* 89:739, 1997.

190. Singer ST, Ataga KI: Hypercoagulability in sickle cell disease and beta-thalassemia. *Curr Mol Med* 8:639, 2008.

191. Morris CR, Kuypers FA, Kato GJ, et al: Hemolysis-associated pulmonary hypertension in thalassemia. *Ann N Y Acad Sci* 1054:481, 2005.

192. Weatherall DJ: Phenotype-genotype relationships in monogenic disease: Lessons from the thalassaemias. *Nat Rev Genet* 2:245, 2001.

193. Weatherall DJ, Pressley L, Wood WG, et al: The molecular basis for mild forms of homozygous beta thalassaemia. *Lancet* 1:527, 1981.

194. Wainscoat JS, Old JM, Weatherall DJ, Orkin SH: The molecular basis for the clinical diversity of beta thalassaemia in Cypriots. *Lancet* 1:1235, 1983.

195. Labie D, Pagnier J, Lapoumeroulie C, et al: Common haplotype dependency of high G gamma-globin gene expression and high Hb F levels in beta-thalassemia and sickle cell anemia patients. *Proc Natl Acad Sci U S A* 82:2111, 1985.

196. Thein SL, Sampietro M, Old JM, et al: Association of thalassaemia intermedia with a beta-globin gene haplotype. *Br J Haematol* 65:370, 1987.

197. Thein SL, Hesketh C, Wallace RB, Weatherall DJ: The molecular basis of thalassaemia major and thalassaemia intermedia in Asian Indians: Application to prenatal diagnosis. *Br J Haematol* 70:225, 1988.

198. Ho PJ, Hall GW, Luo LY, et al: Beta thalassaemia intermedia: Is it possible to predict phenotype from genotype? *Br J Haematol* 100:70, 1998.

199. Rund D, Oron-Karni V, Filon D, et al: Genetic analysis of beta-thalassemia intermedia in Israel: Diversity of mechanisms and unpredictability of phenotype. *Am J Hematol* 54:16, 1997.

200. Rund D, Fucharoen S: Genetic modifiers in hemoglobinopathies. *Curr Mol Med* 8:600, 2008.

201. Wonke B, Hoffbrand AV, Bouloux P, et al: New approaches to the management of hepatitis and endocrine disorders in thalassaemia. *Ann N Y Acad Sci* 850:232, 1998.

202. Girot R, Lefrére JJ, Schettini F, et al: HIV infection and AIDS in thalassemia, in *Thalassemia 1990: 5th Annual Meeting of the COOLEY-CARE Group*, edited by Rebulla P, Fessas P, p 69. Centro Trasfusionale Ospedale Maggiore Policlinico Dio Milano, Athens, 1991.

203. Choudhury NV, Dubey ML, Jolly JG, et al: Post-transfusion malaria in thalassaemia patients. *Blut* 61:314, 1990.

204. Chatterjee R, Katz M, Cox TF, Porter JB: Prospective study of the hypothalamic-pituitary axis in thalassaemic patients who developed secondary amenorrhoea. *Clin Endocrinol (Oxf)* 39:287, 1993.

205. Premawardhena A, Arambepola M, Katugaha N, et al: Is the beta thalassaemia trait of clinical importance? *Br J Haematol* 141:407, 2008.

206. Liang ST, Wong VCW, So WWK, et al: Homozygous alpha-thalassaemia: Clinical presentation, diagnosis and management: A review of 46 cases. *Br J Obstet Gynaecol* 92:680, 1985.

207. Beaudry MA, Ferguson DJ, Pearse K, et al: Survival of a hydropic infant with homozygous alpha-thalassaemia-1. *J Pediatr* 108:713, 1986.

208. Bianchi DW, Beyer EC, Stark AR, et al: Normal long-term survival with alpha thalassemia. *J Pediatr* 108:716, 1986.

209. Gouttas A, Fessas P, Tsevrenis H, Xefteri E: Description d'une nouvelle variete d'anemie hemolytique congenitale. *Sang* 26:911, 1955.

210. Rigas DA, Koler RD, Osgood EE: Hemoglobin H: Clinical, laboratory, and genetic studies of a family with a previously undescribed hemoglobin. *J Lab Clin Med* 48:51, 1956.

211. Wasi P: Hemoglobinopathies in southeast Asia, in *Distribution and Evolution of the Hemoglobin and Globin Loci*, edited by Bowman JE, p 179. Elsevier, New York, 1983.

212. Kattamis C, Tzotzos S, Kanavakis E, et al: Correlation of clinical phenotype to genotype in haemoglobin H disease. *Lancet* 1:442, 1988.

213. Galanello R, Pirastu M, Melis MA, et al: Phenotype-genotype correlation in haemoglobin H disease in childhood. *J Med Genet* 20:425, 1983.

214. Fucharoen S, Winichagoon P, Pootrakul P, et al: Differences between two types of Hb H disease, alpha-thalassemia 1/alpha-thalassemia 2 and alpha-thalassemia 1/Hb constant spring. *Birth Defects Orig Artic Ser* 23:309, 1988.

215. Styles L, Foote DH, Kleman KM, et al: Hemoglobin H-Constant Spring disease: An under recognized, severe form of alpha thalassemia. *Int J Pediatr Hematol Oncol* 4:69, 1977.

216. Lie-Injo LE, Ganesan J, Clegg JB, Weatherall DJ: Homozygous state for Hb Constant Spring (slow-moving Hb X components). *Blood* 43:251, 1974.

217. Derry S, Wood WG, Pippard MJ, et al: Hematologic and biosynthetic studies in homozygous hemoglobin Constant Spring. *J Clin Invest* 73:1673, 1984.

218. Higgs DR, Pressley L, Clegg JB, et al: Detection of alpha thalassaemia in Negro infants. *Br J Haematol* 46:39, 1980.

219. Higgs DR, Lamb J, Aldridge BE, et al: Inadequacy of Hb Bart's as an indicator of alpha-thalassaemia. *Br J Haematol* 48:177, 1982.

220. Silvestroni E, Bianco I, Reitano G: Three cases of homozygous delta beta-thalassemia (or microcythemia) with high haemoglobin F in a Sicilian family. *Acta Haematol* 40:220, 1968.

221. Ramot BN, Ben-Bassat I, Gafni D, Zaanoon R: A family with three delta beta-thalassemia homozygotes. *Blood* 35:158, 1970.

222. Tsistrakis GA, Amarantos SP, Konkouris LL: Homozygous beta delta-thalassaemia. *Acta Haematol* 51:185, 1974.

223. Efremov GD: Hemoglobins Lepore and anti-Lepore. *Hemoglobin* 2:197, 1978.

224. Charache S, Clegg JB, Weatherall DJ: The Negro variety of hereditary persistence of fetal haemoglobin is a mild form of thalassaemia. *Br J Haematol* 34:527, 1976.

225. Huisman TH, Miller A, Schroeder WA: A G gamma type of hereditary persistence of fetal hemoglobin with beta chain production in cis. *Am J Hum Genet* 27:765, 1975.

226. Higgs DR, Clegg JB, Wood WG, Weatherall DJ: G gamma beta + type of hereditary persistence of fetal haemoglobin in association with Hb C. *J Med Genet* 16:288, 1979.

227. Fessas P, Stamatoyannopoulos G: Hereditary persistence of fetal hemoglobin in Greece: A study and a comparison. *Blood* 24:223, 1964.

228. Sofroniadou K, Wood WG, Nute PE, Stamatoyannopoulos G: Globin chain synthesis in Greek type (A gamma) of hereditary persistence of fetal haemoglobin. *Br J Haematol* 29:137, 1975.

229. Clegg JB, Metaxatou-Mavromati A, Kattamis C, et al: Occurrence of G gamma Hb F in Greek HPFH: Analysis of heterozygotes and compound heterozygotes with beta thalassaemia. *Br J Haematol* 43:521, 1979.

230. Camaschella C, Oggiano L, Sampietro M, et al: The homozygous state of G to A–117A gamma hereditary persistence of fetal hemoglobin. *Blood* 73:1999, 1989.

231. Weatherall DJ, Cartner R, Clegg JB, et al: A form of hereditary persistence of fetal haemoglobin characterized by uneven cellular distribution of haemoglobin F and the production of haemoglobins A and A2 in homozygotes. *Br J Haematol* 29:205, 1975.

232. Silvestroni E, Bianco I: *La Malattia Microdrepanocitica*. Il Pensiero Scientifico, Rome, 1955.

233. Serjeant GR: *Sickle Cell Disease*, 3rd ed. Oxford University Press, New York, 2001.

234. Fucharoen S, Winichagoon P: Hemoglobinopathies in southeast Asia: Molecular biology and clinical medicine. *Hemoglobin* 21:299, 1997.

235. Agarwal S, Gulati R, Singh K: Hemoglobin E-beta thalassemia in Uttar Pradesh. *Indian Pediatr* 34:287, 1997.

236. Khanh NC, Thu LT, Truc DB, et al: Beta-thalassaemia/haemoglobin E disease in Vietnam. *J Trop Pediatr* 36:43, 1990.

237. De Silva S, Fisher CA; Members of the Sri Lanka Thalassaemia Study, et al: Thalassaemia in Sri Lanka: Implications for the future health burden of Asian populations. *Lancet* 355:786, 2000.

238. Olivieri NF, Muraca GM, O'Donnell A, et al: Studies in haemoglobin E beta-thalassaemia. *Br J Haematol* 141:388, 2008.

239. Premawardhena A, Fisher CA, Olivieri NF, et al: Haemoglobin E beta thalassaemia in Sri Lanka. *Lancet* 366:1467, 2005.

240. Fisher CA, Premawardhena A, De Silva S, et al: The molecular basis for the thalassaemias in Sri Lanka. *Br J Haematol* 121:1, 2003.

241. Sonakul D, Suwanagool P, Sirivaidyapong P, Fucharoen S: Distribution of pulmonary thromboembolic lesions in thalassemic patients, in *Thalassemia: Pathophysiology and Management*, Part A, edited by Fucharoen S, Rowley PT, Paul NW, p 375. Alan R. Liss, New York, 1988.

242. Kattamis C, Metaxotou-Mavromati A, Wood WG, et al: The heterogeneity of normal Hb A2-beta thalassaemia in Greece. *Br J Haematol* 42: 109, 1979.

243. Schwartz E: The silent carrier of beta thalassemia. *N Engl J Med* 281:1327, 1969.

244. Bianco I, Graziani B, Carboni C: Genetic patterns in thalassemia inter-media (constitutional microcytic anemia): Familial, hematologic and biosynthetic studies. *Hum Hered* 27:257, 1977.

245. Pirastu M, Ristaldi MS, Loudianos G, et al: Molecular analysis of atypical beta-thalassemia heterozygotes. *Ann N Y Acad Sci* 612:90, 1990.

246. Olds RJ, Sura T, Jackson B, et al: A novel delta 0 mutation in cis with Hb Knossos: A study of different interactions in three Egyptian families. *Br J Haematol* 78:430, 1991.

248. Schokker RC, Went LN, Bok J: A new genetic variant of beta-thalassaemia. *Nature* 209:44, 1966.

248. Ohta Y, Yamaoka K, Sumida I, et al: Homozygous delta-thalassemia first discovered in Japanese family with hereditary persistence of fetal hemoglobin. *Blood* 37:706, 1971.

249. Vella F, Wells RMC, Ager JAM: A haemoglobinopathy involving haemoglobin H and a new (Q) haemoglobin. *Br Med J* 1:752, 1958.

250. Lie-Injo LE, Pillay RP, Thuraisingham V: Further cases of Hb-Q-H disease (Hb Q-alpha-thalassemia). *Blood* 28:830, 1966.

251. Milner PF, Huisman THJ: Studies on the proportion and synthesis of haemoglobin G Philadelphia in red cells of heterozygotes, a homozygote, and a heterozygote for both haemoglobin G and alpha thalassaemia. *Br J Haematol* 34:207, 1976.

252. Rieder RF, Woodbury DH, Rucknagel DL: The interaction of alpha-thalassaemia and haemoglobin G Philadelphia. *Br J Haematol* 32:159, 1976.

253. Pich P, Saglio G, Camaschella C, et al: Interaction between Hb Hasharon and alpha thalassemia: An approach to the problem of the number of human alpha loci. *Blood* 51:339, 1978.

254. Higgs DR, Aldridge BE, Lamb J, et al: The interaction of alpha-thalassaemia and homozygous sickle cell disease. *N Engl J Med* 306:1441, 1982.

255. Embury SH, Dozy AM, Miller J, et al: Concurrent sickle-cell anemia and alpha-thalassemia. *N Engl J Med* 306:270, 1982.

256. Olivieri N, Weatherall DJ: Clinical aspects of β thalassemia and related disorders, in *Disorders of Hemoglobin*, 2nd ed, edited by Steinberg MH, Forget BG, Higgs DR, Weatherall DJ, p 357. Cambridge University Press, Cambridge, UK, 2009.

257. Cazzola M, Borgna-Pignatti C, Locatelli F, et al: A moderate transfusion regimen may reduce iron loading in beta-thalassemia major without producing excessive expansion of erythropoiesis. *Transfusion* 37:135, 1997.

258. Propper RD, Cooper B, Rufo RR, et al: Continuous subcutaneous administration of deferoxamine in patients with iron overload. *N Engl J Med* 297:418, 1977.

259. Pippard MJ, Callender ST, Letsky EA, Weatherall DJ: Prevention of iron loading in transfusion-dependent thalassaemia. *Lancet* 1:1178, 1978.

260. Pippard MJ, Callender ST, Weatherall DJ: Intensive iron-chelation therapy with desferrioxamine in iron loading patients. *Clin Sci Mol Med* 54:99, 1978.

261. Nienhuis AW: Safety of intensive chelation therapy. *N Engl J Med* 296:114, 1977.

262. Olivieri NF, Bunic JR, Chew E, et al: Visual and auditory neurotoxicity in patients receiving subcutaneous deferoxamine infusions. *N Engl J Med* 314:869, 1986.

263. Porter JB, Jawson MS, Huehns ER, et al: Desferrioxamine ototoxicity: Evaluation of risk factors in thalassaemia patients and guidelines for safe dosage. *Br J Haematol* 73:403, 1989.

264. Olivieri NF, Basran RK, Talbot AL, et al: Abnormal growth in thalassemia major associated with deferoxamine-induced destruction of spinal cartilage and compromise of sitting height. *Blood* 86:482a, 1995.

265. Porter JB: Practical management of iron overload. *Br J Haematol* 115:239, 2001.

266. Nisbet-Brown E, Olivieri NF, Giardina PJ, et al: Effectiveness and safety of ICL670 in iron-loaded patients with thalassaemia: A randomized, double-blind, placebo-controlled dose-escalation trial. *Lancet* 361:1597, 2003.

267. Olivieri NF, Brittenham GM: Management of the thalassemias. *Cold Spring Harb Perspect Med* 3:a011767, 2013.

268. Olivieri NF, Nathan DG, MacMillan JH, et al: Survival in medically treated patients with homozygous beta-thalassemia. *N Engl J Med* 331:574, 1994.

269. Brittenham GM, Griffith PM, Nienhuis AW, et al: Efficacy of deferoxamine in preventing complications of iron overload in patients with thalassemia major. *N Engl J Med* 331:567, 1994.

270. Borgna-Pignatti C, Rugolotto S, De Stefano P, et al: Survival and complications in patients with thalassemia major treated with transfusion and deferoxamine. *Haematologica* 89:1187, 2004.

271. St Pierre TG, Clark PR, Chua-Anusorn W: Measurement and mapping of liver iron concentrations using magnetic resonance imaging. *Ann N Y Acad Sci* 1054:379, 2005.

272. Pennell DJ: T2* magnetic resonance and myocardial iron in thalassemia. *Ann N Y Acad Sci* 1054:373, 2005.

273. Lucarelli G, Giardini C, Baronciani D: Bone marrow transplantation in beta-thalassemia. *Semin Hematol* 32:297, 1995.

274. Lucarelli G, Giardini C, Baronciani D: Bone marrow transplantation in thalassemia. *Semin Hematol* 32:297, Review, 1995.

275. Di Bartolomeo P, Di Girolamo G, Olioso P, et al: The Pescara experience of allogenic bone marrow transplantation in thalassemia. *Bone Marrow Transplant* 19(Suppl 2):48, 1997.

276. Argiolu F, Sanna MA, Addari MC, et al: Bone marrow transplantation in thalassemia: The experience of Cagliari. *Bone Marrow Transplant* 19(Suppl 2):65, 1997.

277. Gaziev D, Polchi P, Galimberti M, et al: Graft-versus-host disease following bone marrow transplantation for thalassemia: An analysis of incidence and risk factors. *Transplantation* 63:854, 1997.

278. Lucarelli G, Isgro A, Sodani P, Gaziev J: Hematopoietic stem cell transplantation in thalassemia and sickle cell anemia. *Cold Spring Harb Perspect Med* 2:a011825, 2012.

279. Olivieri NF, Weatherall DJ: The therapeutic reactivation of fetal haemoglobin. *Hum Mol Genet* 7:1655, 1998.

280. Swank RA, Stamatoyannopoulos G: Fetal gene reactivation. *Curr Opin Genet Dev* 8:366, 1998.

281. Weatherall DJ: Pharmacological treatment of monogenic disease. *Pharmacogenomics J* 3:264, 2003.

282. Quek L, Thein SL: Molecular therapies in beta-thalassaemia. *Br J Haematol* 136:353, 2007.

283. Olivieri NF, Rees DC, Ginder GD, et al: Treatment of thalassemia major with phenylbutyrate and hydroxyurea. *Lancet* 350:491, 1997.

284. Sadelain M: Genetic treatment of the haemoglobinopathies: Recombinations and new combinations. *Br J Haematol* 98:248, 1997.

285. Dominski Z, Kole R: Restoration of correct splicing in thalassemic pre-mRNA by antisense oligonucleotides. *Proc Natl Acad Sci U S A* 90:8673, 1993.

286. Lan N, Howrey RP, Lee S-W, et al: Ribozyme-mediated repair of sickle beta-globin mRNAs in erythrocyte precursors. *Science* 280:1593, 1998.

287. Rivella S, Sadelain M: Therapeutic globin gene delivery using lentiviral vectors. *Curr Opin Mol Ther* 4:505, 2002.

288. Persons DA, Nienhuis AW: Gene therapy for the hemoglobin disorders. *Curr Hematol Rep* 2:348, 2003.

289. Nienhuis AW, Persons DA: Development of gene therapy for thalassemia. *Cold Spring Harb Perspect Med* 2:a011833, 2012.

290. WHO Working Group: Hereditary anemias: Genetic basis, clinical features, diagnosis and treatment. *Bull World Health Organ* 60:543, 1982.

291. Stamatoyannopoulos G: Problems of screening and counseling in the hemoglobinopathies, in *Proceedings of the IV International Conference on Birth Defects*, p 268. Exerpta Medica, Vienna, 1974.

292. Alter BP: Antenatal diagnosis: Summary of results. *Ann N Y Acad Sci* 612:237, 1990.

293. Kazazian HH, Phillips JAI, Boehm CD, et al: Prenatal diagnosis of beta-thalassemia by amniocentesis: Linkage analysis of multiple polymorphic restriction endonuclease sites. *Blood* 56:926, 1980.

294. Old JM, Ward RH, Petrou M, et al: First trimester diagnosis for haemoglobinopathies: Three cases. *Lancet* 2:1413, 1982.

295. Old JM, Fitches A, Heath C, et al: First trimester fetal diagnosis for haemoglobinopathies: Report on 200 cases. *Lancet* 2:763, 1986.

296. Cao A, Galanello R, Rosatelli MC: Prenatal diagnosis and screening of the haemoglobinopathies. *Clin Haematol* 11:215, 1998.

297. Modell B, Petrou M, Layton M, et al: Audit of prenatal diagnosis for haemoglobin disorders in the United Kingdom: The first 20 years. *BMJ* 315:779, 1997.

298. Cheung MC, Goldberg JD, Kan YW: Prenatal diagnosis of sickle cell anemia and thalassemia by analysis of fetal cells in maternal blood. *Nat Genet* 14:264, 1996.

299. Hung EC, Chiu RW, Lo YM: Detection of circulating fetal nucleic acids: A review of methods and applications. *J Clin Pathol* 62:308, 2009.

300. Kuliev A, Rechitsky S, Verlinsky O, et al: Preimplantation diagnosis of thalassemias. *J Assist Reprod Genet* 15:219, 1998.

301. Kuliev A, Rechitsky S, Verlinsky O, et al: Birth of healthy children after preimplantation diagnosis of thalassemia. *J Assist Reprod Genet* 16:201, 1999.

302. Cao A, Kan YW: The prevention of thalassemia. *Cold Spring Harb Perspect Med* 3:a011775, 2013.

303. Weatherall DJ, Akinyanju O, Fucharoen S, et al: Inherited disorders of hemoglobin, in *Disease Control Priorities in Developing Countries*, 2nd ed, edited by Jamison DT, Breman JG, Measham AR, Alleyne G, Claeson M, Evans DB, Jha P, Mills A, Musgrove P, p 663. Oxford University Press and the World Bank, New York, 2006.

304. A database of human hemoglobin variants and thalassemias. http://globin.bx.psu.edu/hbvar/

CHAPTER 49
DISORDERS OF HEMOGLOBIN STRUCTURE: SICKLE CELL ANEMIA AND RELATED ABNORMALITIES

Kavita Natrajan and Abdullah Kutlar

SUMMARY

Hemoglobinopathies are the most common inherited red cell disorders worldwide. Among these disorders, sickle cell syndromes and thalassemias constitute a major public health problem. A glutamic acid to valine substitution at the sixth amino acid of the β-globin chain of human hemoglobin (HbA) results in formation of sickle hemoglobin (HbS). Sickle cell disease results from homozygosity for this mutation, or from a compound heterozygosity for sickle hemoglobin and β-thalassemia or another β-globin variant such as HbC, HbD, HbE, or HbO_{Arab}. The sickle mutation renders the hemoglobin molecule insoluble upon deoxygenation; thus red blood cells containing deoxy HbS polymer are rigid and have impaired rheologic properties. The downstream effects of the sickling process include: membrane changes leading to potassium loss and cellular dehydration, interaction of sickle hemoglobin with microvascular endothelium, neutrophils, and monocytes, hemolysis, nitric oxide depletion, release of inflammatory proteins and activation of coagulation. These processes lead to a hemolytic anemia, an inflammatory state, painful vasoocclusive episodes, and damage to multiple organ systems with a resultant shortened life expectancy.

Acronyms and Abbreviations: ACS, acute chest syndrome; ADMA, asymmetric dimethylarginine; AHSCT, allogeneic hematopoietic stem cell transplantation; BMP, bone morphogenic protein; 2,3-BPG, 2,3-bisphosphoglycerate; CO_2, carbon dioxide; CSSCD, Cooperative Study of Sickle Cell Disease; eNOS, endothelial nitric oxide synthase; Hb, hemoglobin; HbAS, sickle cell trait; HbF, fetal hemoglobin; HbS, sickle hemoglobin; HbSC, sickle cell–HbC disease; HIF, hypoxia-inducible factor; HLA human leukocyte antigen; HPLC, high-performance liquid chromatography; IL, interleukin; iNKT cells, invariant natural killer T cells; K+, potassium; LDH, lactate dehydrogenase; MCHC, mean cell hemoglobin concentration; MCV, mean corpuscular volume; MPs, microparticles; MRI, magnetic resonance imaging; NO, nitric oxide; NT-pro-BNP, N-terminal pro–brain natriuretic peptide; O_2, oxygen; P_{50}, point at which hemoglobin is one-half saturated with oxygen; PCV7, pneumococcal polyvalent conjugate 7; PH, pulmonary hypertension; PIGF, placenta growth factor; P_{O_2}, partial pressure of oxygen; R state, relaxed oxy; SCD, sickle cell disease; SCT, stem cell transplantation; sPLA$_2$, secretory phospholipase A$_2$; STOP, Stroke Prevention Trial in Sickle Cell Disease; T state, tense, deoxy; TCD, transcranial Doppler; TF, tissue factor; TGF-β, transforming growth factor-beta; TNF-α, tumor necrosis factor-alpha; UDP, uridine diphosphate; UGT1A1, UDP glucuronosyltransferase 1 family; VOE, vasoocclusive episode; VTE, venous thromboembolism.

There is considerable heterogeneity in the severity of the disease; the best known modifier of the disease is an elevated level of fetal hemoglobin (HbF), which exerts a potent antisickling effect. Concomitant α-thalassemia is also a modifier, which leads to a decrease in hemolysis. There is an interest in nonglobin genetic modifiers of sickle cell disease. Over the past 3 decades, advances in supportive care and implementation of disease-modifying therapies, such as anti-γ to β-globin switching therapies, which result in increased HbF and less HbS synthesis, and have led to an increase in life expectancy. Hydroxyurea has emerged as an effective disease-modifying agent that has been approved by the FDA for use in adults with sickle cell disease. Although its main mechanism of action is to enhance HbF production, other effects such as a decrease in neutrophils, platelets, and decreased expression of adhesion molecules contribute to its efficacy. Novel antiswitching agents, most notably, DNA methyltransferase 1 inhibitors (5′-azacytidine and decitabine) and histone deacetylase inhibitors (butyrate derivatives and others) are now in clinical trials. Evolving therapies include antiadhesive therapies to prevent interaction of sickle cells with microvascular endothelium, antiinflammatory approaches, and modulation of hemoglobin–oxygen affinity to prevent sickling. To date, the only curative therapy remains allogeneic hematopoietic stem cell transplantation.

Sickle trait, the heterozygous state for sickle hemoglobin, affects approximately 8 percent of Americans of African descent, and with rare exceptions is asymptomatic. HbC is associated with target cells and spherocytes in the blood film and splenomegaly. HbD disease is essentially asymptomatic. HbE is very common in Southeast Asia, and because of large population movements from this area, it has become a prevalent hemoglobinopathy in other regions of the world. HbE is a thalassemic variant and its coinheritance with β^0-thalassemia mutations can result in severe transfusion-dependent thalassemia major. Unstable hemoglobin variants appear as rare, sporadic cases and are characterized by a Heinz body hemolytic anemia. Variants that alter the oxygen affinity of the Hb molecule lead to erythrocytosis (high oxygen affinity variants) or anemia (low oxygen affinity variants) and are rare causes of these syndromes.

● THE STRUCTURE AND FUNCTION OF NORMAL HEMOGLOBIN

The red protein hemoglobin (Hb) serves to transport oxygen from the lungs to the tissues and carbon dioxide (CO_2) from the tissues to the lungs. Hb also binds the physiologically important nitric oxide (NO) molecule. The protein has evolved to perform its gas transport functions in a highly efficient manner. The oxygen affinity of Hb permits nearly complete saturation with oxygen in the lungs, as well as efficient oxygen unloading in the tissues because of its sigmoid oxygen dissociation curve. This curve results from the fact that Hb is a four-subunit, allosteric molecule; its conformation, and hence the oxygen affinity, changes as each successive molecule of oxygen is bound. Hb also plays an important role in acid–base balance: deoxyhemoglobin binds protons and oxyhemoglobin releases protons. Regulation of the oxygen dissociation curve to meet the needs of the body is remarkable. Hypoxic tissues become acidotic acutely, and the protons released produce a shift in the oxygen dissociation curve that enables more oxygen to be delivered to the tissue. However, longer-term acidosis or alkalosis (as occurs at high altitudes) is counteracted by modulation of red cell 2,3-bisphosphoglycerate (2,3-BPG), serving to decrease hemoglobin–oxygen affinity (Chap. 47).

Normal mammalian Hbs contain two pairs of related polypeptide chains: one chain of each pair is α or α-like and the other is non-α (β, γ, or δ). The α-chains of all human Hbs encountered after early embryogenesis are the same. The non-α chains include the β-chain of normal adult Hb ($\alpha_2\beta_2$), the γ-chain of fetal Hb ($\alpha_2\gamma_2$), and the δ-chain of the minor adult Hb (HbA$_2$ [$\alpha_2\delta_2$]), which accounts for 2.5 percent of the Hb of normal adults. Chapter 48 discusses the regulation of production of the globin chains.

Certain residues in the amino acid sequence of each polypeptide chain appear to be critical to stability and function. Such residues are usually the same (invariant) in α or β chains. The NH$_2$-terminal valines of the β chains are important in 2,3-BPG interactions. The C-terminal residues are important in the salt bridges that characterize the unliganded

molecules. Areas of contact between chains and between heme and globin tend to contain invariant residues. The non-α (β, γ, δ, or ε) chains are all 146 amino acids in length. The γ-chain of fetal Hb (HbF) differs from the β-chain by 39 residues. The γ genes are duplicated: one codes for glycine ($^{G}\gamma$) and the other for alanine ($^{A}\gamma$)[7] at residue 136, giving rise to two kinds of γ chains. In addition, a common polymorphism, the substitution of threonine for isoleucine, is frequently found at residue 75 of the $^{A}\gamma$-chain.

Approximately 75 percent of the amino acids in α and β chains are in a helical arrangement. All Hbs studied have a similar helical content (Fig. 49–1A). Eight helical areas, lettered A to H, occur in the β chains.

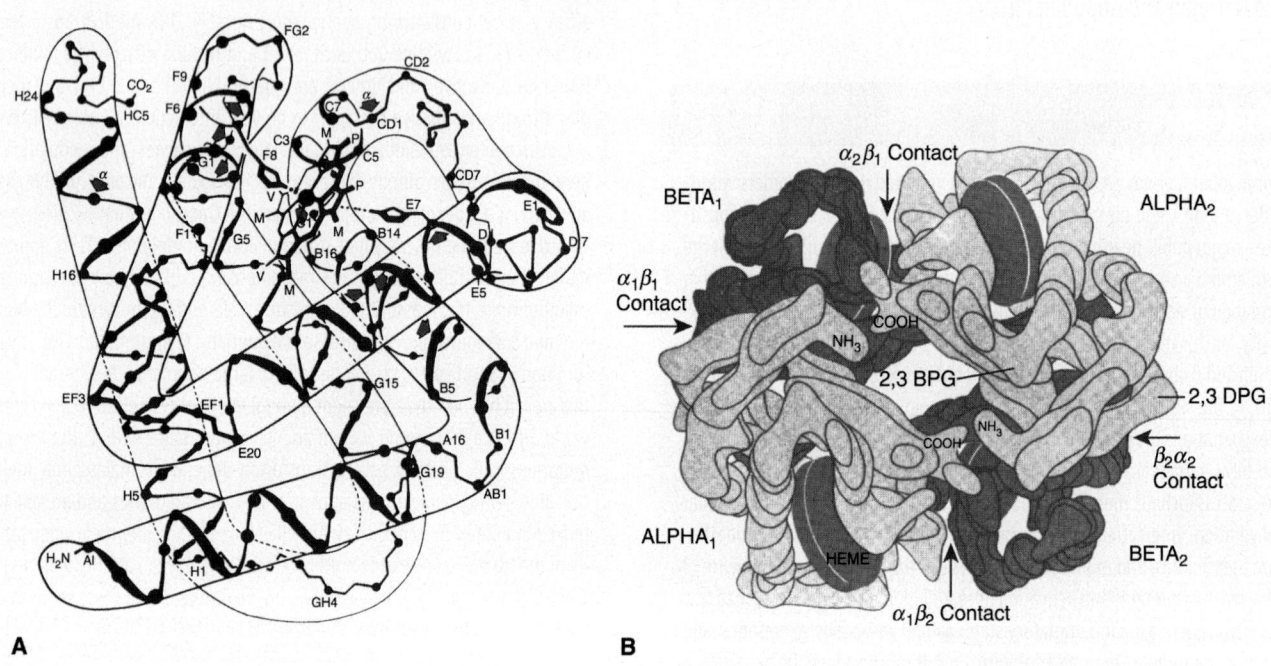

A

B

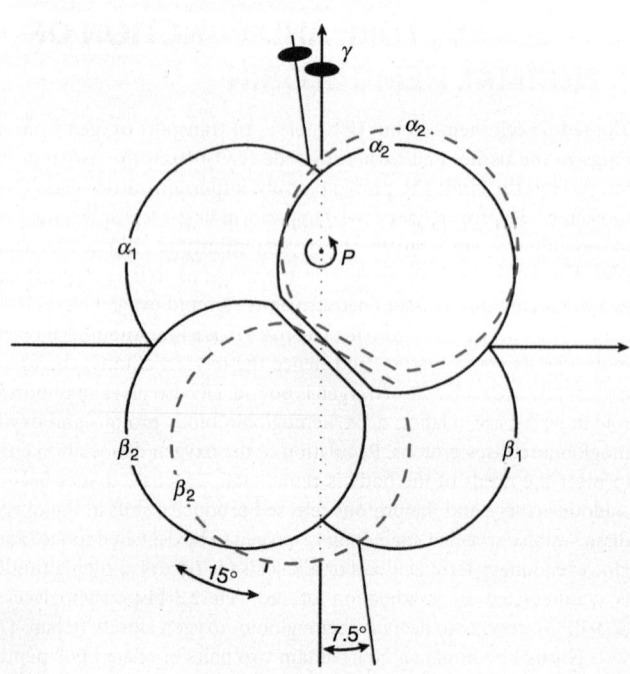

C

Figure 49–1. A. Representation of the structure of β chains. *Arrows* indicate sites of substitutions in a number of unstable hemoglobins. **B.** The hemoglobin molecule, as deduced from x-ray diffraction studies, shown from above. The molecule is composed of four subunits: two identical α chains (*light blocks*) and two identical β chains (*dark blocks*). 2,3-BPG binds to the two β chains in the deoxyhemoglobin molecule. **C.** Schematic of rotation of $\alpha_2\beta_2$ dimer relative to $\alpha_1\beta_1$ in quaternary structure change from deoxyhemoglobin (*solid lines*) to carboxyhemoglobin (*dashed lines*). *(Modified from Baldwin J, Chothia C: Haemoglobin: The structural changes related to ligand binding and its allosteric mechanism. J Mol Biol 129(2):175–220, 1979.)*

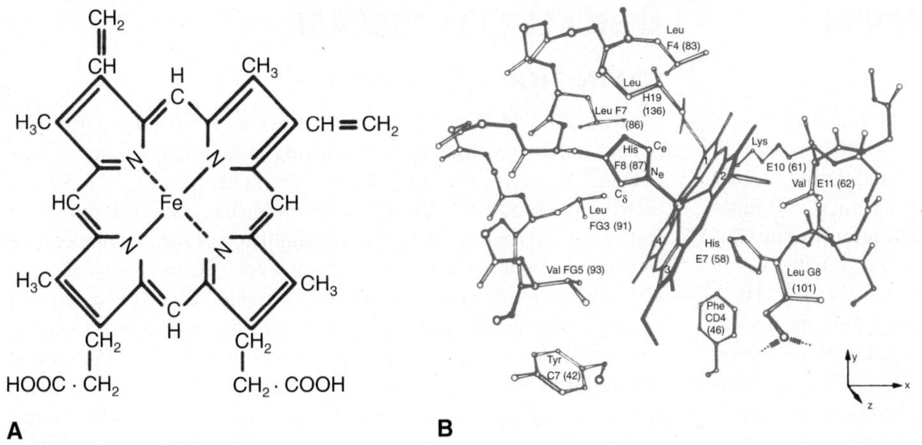

Figure 49–2. A. Structure of heme (ferro-protoporphyrin IX). **B.** Heme group and its environment in the unliganded α-chain. Only selected side chains are shown; the heme 4-propionate is omitted. *(Reproduced from Gelin BR, Lee AW, Karplus M: Hemoglobin tertiary structural change on ligand binding. J Mol Biol 25;171(4):489–559, 1983.)*

Hb nomenclature specifies that amino acids within helices are designated by the amino acid number and the helix letter, whereas amino acids between helices bear the number of the amino acid and the letters of the two helices. Thus, residue EF3 is the third residue of the segment connecting the E and F helices, whereas residue F8 is the eighth residue of the F helix. Alignment according to helical designation makes homology evident: Residue F8 is the proximal heme linked histidine, and the histidine on the distal side of the heme is E7.

Figure 49-1B show the tertiary structure of the α and β chains. The prosthetic group of Hb is heme (ferroprotoporphyrin IX); Fig. 49–2A shows its structure. The heme group is located in a crevice between the E and F helices in each chain (Fig. 49–2B). The highly polar propionate side chains of the heme are on the surface of the molecule and are ionized at physiologic pH. The rest of the heme is inside the molecule, surrounded by nonpolar residues except for two histidines. The iron atom is linked by a coordinate bond to the imidazole nitrogen (N) of histidine F8. The E7 *distal* histidine, on the other side of the heme plane, is not bonded to the iron atom, but is very close to the ligand-binding site.

The sigmoid oxygen dissociation curve is a function of the change of the conformation of the molecule from the liganded to the unliganded state (Table 49–1). In the deoxy state, the Hb tetramer is held together by intersubunit salt bonds (Fig. 49–3) and intersubunit hydrophobic contacts (see Fig. 49–1B), in addition to a certain number of hydrogen bonds. In deoxyhemoglobin, 2,3-BPG is situated in the central cavity between the two β chains (see Fig. 49–1B). The change in conformation of the Hb molecule is brought about by a complex, coordinated series of changes in the structure of the molecule as heme binds oxygen. The oxygen dissociation curve can be linearized by a transformation known as the Hill plot:

$$\log[y/(1-y)] = \log K + n \log P_{O_2}$$

where K is an empiric overall constant without physicochemical basis. The slope n is taken as a convenient measure of cooperativity. Values of n in noninteracting Hbs that exhibit hyperbolic, not sigmoid, oxygen dissociation curves (e.g., myoglobin) are approximately 1. In a normal tetrameric Hb with four oxygen-reactive sites, the maximum value for n is 4.0; however, n values of 2.7 to 3.0 are found in normal Hb.

The point at which the Hb is one-half saturated with oxygen (P_{50}) is the usual measurement of oxygen affinity. It depends upon pH (the Bohr effect), temperature, and 2,3-BPG concentration. In common practice, P_{50} is standardized at 37°C and pH 7.20. P_{50} of freshly drawn blood is approximately 26.7 torr under standard conditions, but the partial pressure of oxygen (P_{O_2}) of Hb from which 2,3-BPG has been removed is only approximately 13 torr. Although fetal and newborn red cells have 2,3-BPG levels similar to those of adults, their oxygen dissociation curve is left shifted (increased oxygen affinity) with a P_{50} of approximately 23 torr because HbF does not react as strongly with 2,3-BPG as does HbA.

TABLE 49–1. Nomenclature of Hemoglobin Quaternary Structures

Liganded (Oxygen Bound)	Unliganded (Reduced)
Oxy	Deoxy
R-state	T-state
Relaxed	Tense
High affinity	Low affinity

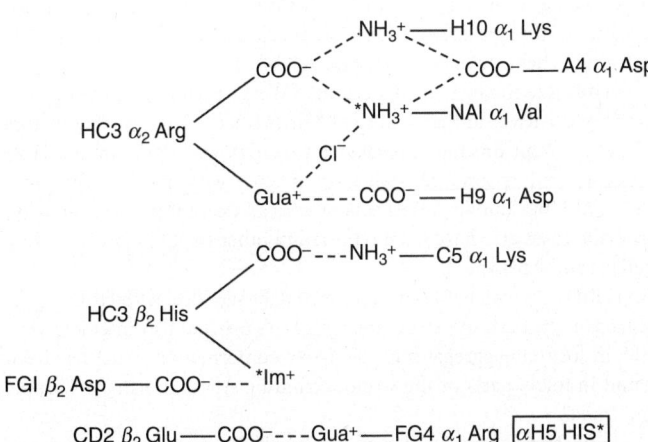

Figure 49–3. Salt bridges in deoxyhemoglobin (* = ionizable group less protonated at pH 9.0 than at pH 7.0). These groups account for 60% of the alkaline Bohr effect. The remainder is due to αH5 His. *(Data from Perutz MF, Wilkinson AJ, Paoli M, et al: The stereochemical mechanism of the cooperative effects in hemoglobin revisited, Annu Rev Biophys Biomol Struct 1998;27:1-34.)*

NOMENCLATURE OF ABNORMAL HEMOGLOBINS

Following the molecular characterization of HbS by Ingram and colleagues in 1956, there has been a rapid and exponential increase in the number of variant or "abnormal" Hbs.[1] This number now exceeds 1000. A detailed description of variant Hbs, their chemical and functional properties, and population distribution can be found on the Globin Gene Server website (http://globin.cse.psu.edu/). Initially, newly described variants were designated by letters of the alphabet (e.g., HbC, HbD, HbE, HbJ). When the letters of the alphabet were exhausted, the practice of naming the variant Hbs after the geographic location where they were first described was adapted (e.g., Hb_{Koln}, Hb_{Zurich}). Variants with electrophoretic or functional properties similar to previously described abnormal Hbs were designated with the letter and the geographic location (e.g., HbD_{Punjab}, $HbE_{Saskatoon}$, $HbM_{Hyde Park}$). Some alphabetic designations were also used to indicate electrophoretic properties of certain variants; for example, there are a number of HbDs (D_{Punjab}, D_{Iran}, D_{Ibadan}). All of these variants share the electrophoretic properties of HbS-like mobility on alkaline (cellulose acetate) electrophoresis, whereas they move with HbA at acidic pH (citrate agar electrophoresis). Similarly, HbEs have HbC-like mobility on alkaline electrophoresis and move with HbA on citrate agar electrophoresis.

The vast majority of Hb variants arise as a result of single nucleotide mutations, leading to an amino acid change in either α-, β-, δ-, or γ-globin subunits of the Hb tetramer resulting in variants of HbA (α or β), HbA2 (δ), or HbF (γ). Other mechanisms include small deletions or insertions, elongated chains, and fusions (for a detailed description of Hb variants and associated clinical syndromes, see "Other Abnormal Hemoglobins" below.

The coinheritance of HbS with some other variant Hbs or β-thalassemia mutations results in a number of sickling syndromes. In the United States, the most common sickling disorder is homozygous HbS (HbSS, sickle cell anemia), which is now commonly referred to as sickle cell disease (SCD). This is followed by sickle cell-HbC disease (HbSC), sickle cell–β^+-thalassemia (HbS–β^+-thalassemia), and sickle cell–β^0-thalassemia (HbS–β^0-thalassemia). Other rarer forms include $HbSD_{Punjab}$, $HbSO_{Arab}$, HbS_{Lepore}, and HbSE diseases. Coinheritance of a large number of β-chain variants with HbS does not result in a symptomatic sickling disorder; rather, they are clinically and hematologically indistinguishable from sickle cell trait (HbAS).

HbC is found in 17 to 28 percent of West Africans, particularly east of the Niger River in the vicinity of North Ghana. The selective factors that account for this high prevalence are unknown at present, but HbC probably confers some resistance to infection with malaria. The prevalence of HbC among Americans of African descent is 2 to 3 percent. Sporadic cases also have been reported in other populations, including Italians and Afrikaners.

HbD_{Punjab}, which is now recognized to be identical with $HbD_{Los Angeles}$ because both have the structure $\alpha_2\beta_2$121 Glu→Gln, also interacts with HbS in forming aggregates in the deoxy conformation. HbD has been found in many parts of the world, including Africa, northern Europe, and India.

HbE is so prevalent that it may be the most common abnormal Hb or second in prevalence only to HbS. HbE is found principally in Burma, Thailand, Laos, Cambodia, Malaysia, and Indonesia. In some areas, HbE is found with a carrier rate of 30 percent. On the other hand, it is not prevalent among Chinese. Studies of restriction length polymorphisms in the β-globin cluster indicate the HbE mutation has arisen several times independently. It, too, probably confers some resistance to infection with malaria.

SICKLE CELL DISEASE

DEFINITION AND HISTORY

The first case of SCD, reported in 1910, was that of a dental student from Grenada, Walter Clement-Noel, studying in Chicago. Dr. James Herrick and his intern, Dr. Ernest Irons, were in charge of Mr. Noel's care between 1904 and 1907, during which time he had several bouts of fever and cough and a history of leg ulcers, jaundice, and exercise intolerance. Herrick and Irons made astute clinical observations and prepared blood films and photomicrographs of nucleated red blood cells and of red cells having a "slender sickle shape" (Fig. 49–4).[2] During the next decade, two more cases of this unusual anemia were reported. In 1915, Cook and Meyer raised the question of a genetic basis for the disorder based on the family history of the third reported case. In 1917, Victor Emmel used *in vitro* culture to show that sickle red cells represented a physical alteration of morphologically normally appearing red cells and were not released from the marrow as sickle cells.[3] He also demonstrated that morphologically normal red cells of the father of a patient became sickle shaped after *in vitro* culture. Vernon Mason, who reported the fourth case in 1922, coined the term *sickle cell anemia* after observing the similarities between all the cases reported up to that time. In 1923, Sydenstricker and Huck noted "latent-sicklers" among relatives of the diagnosed patients, confirming and expanding on Emmel's finding. In 1927, Hahn and Gillespie showed that sickling was related to low oxygen tension and low pH. In 1933, Diggs distinguished the difference of symptomatic cases called sickle cell anemia, from asymptomatic cases that were termed *sickle cell trait*, and he found that approximately 8 percent of Americans of African descent had the sickle cell trait.[4]

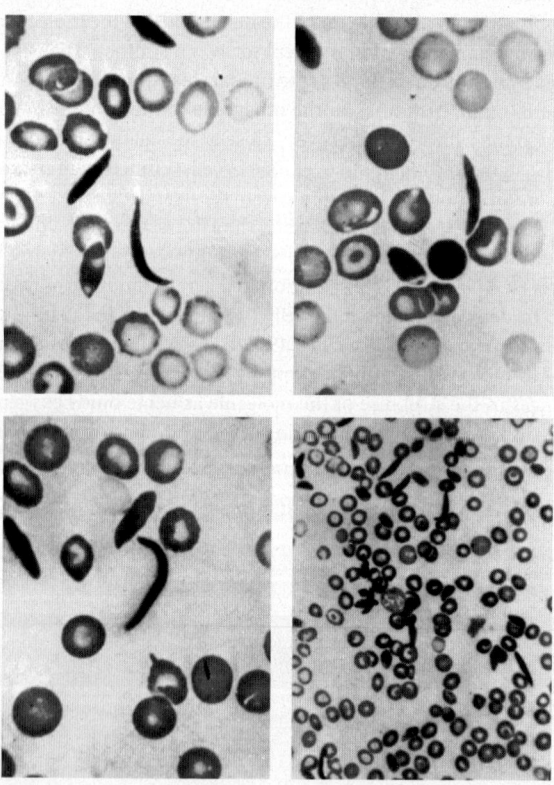

Figure 49–4. Peculiar elongated and sickle-shaped red cells from the first report of sickle cell anemia with depiction of sickle cells. *(Reproduced with permission from Herrick JB: Peculiar elongated and sickle-shaped red corpuscles in a case of severe anemia. Arch Intern Med 6:517, 1910.)*

Irving Sherman, while a medical student at Johns Hopkins, showed that sickled red cells were birefringent under a polarizing microscope and that this finding was reversible with oxygenation of the cells. This observation ultimately led Linus Pauling to study sickle Hb after being advised of this property of sickle cell by William Castle, a noted research hematologist. Indeed, in 1949, Pauling and his colleagues demonstrated electrophoretic differences between Hbs from normal, sickle cell trait, and sickle cell anemia subjects and hypothesized that there must be chemical differences, thus establishing sickle cell anemia as the first molecular disease described. In the late 1950s, Hunt and Ingram sequenced the globin peptide and linked the abnormality to a change in the amino acid composition of the β-globin chain (replacement of glutamic acid by valine at residue 6). In 1977, Marotta and coworkers showed that the corresponding change in codon 6 of the β-globin gene was GAG→GTG. The discovery of a variant fragment in HbS versus HbA during restriction endonuclease mapping of amniotic fluid cells by Y. W. Kan paved the way for antenatal diagnosis of SCD and opened the way for modern genetics using recombinant DNA technology.[5]

The history of sickle cell anemia serves as an inspiring reminder of the power of clinical and laboratory observations, and in an era of mechanistic basic science research, serves to highlight the importance of bedside to bench and bench to bedside research integration.[6–9]

EPIDEMIOLOGY

The observation that sickle cell trait may have a survival advantage against some environmental factors was first suggested by Dr. Alan Raper in East Africa in 1949. Drs. Mackey and Vivarelli suggested that the environmental influence might be malaria. It was subsequently noted that blood from sickle cell trait persons contained less malarial parasites and that the sickle trait conferred some protection against malaria in early childhood. Data suggest that sickle trait is maximally protective against severe malaria as opposed to asymptomatic parasitemia or mild disease.[10] The mechanism of such a protection has been the matter of much debate. Plausible mechanisms include selective sickling of parasitized red blood cells, resulting in more effective removal by the monocyte-macrophage system, and inhibitory effect on parasite growth by increased red cell potassium loss, decreased red cell pH, and increased endothelial adherence of parasitized sickle red cells.

Thus, the prevalence of sickle cell anemia closely mirrors the worldwide distribution of falciparum malaria; however, as a result of migration of peoples to the industrialized Western countries, SCD has become more prevalent in areas where malaria is not endemic.

The World Health Organization estimated in 2006 that 5 percent of the world population carries a gene for a hemoglobinopathy. Sickle cell anemia is highly prevalent in sub-Saharan and equatorial Africa with lesser but significant prevalence in the Middle East, India, and the Mediterranean region. Incidence of SCD in sub-Saharan African countries ranges between 1 and 2 percent, which translates into approximately 500,000 cases per year. In the Jamaican cohort study, newborn screening in 100,000 consecutive vaginal deliveries resulted in the finding of sickle cell trait in 10 percent of newborns.[11]

In the United States, the Centers for Disease Control and Prevention estimates that sickle cell anemia is present in 1 in 500 livebirths among Americans of African descent; 1 in 12 American of African descent have the trait, and approximately 100,000 Americans largely of African descent live with the disease. In Americans of Hispanic descent, the rate of SCD is 1 in 36,000 livebirths. Accurate population statistics of SCD are difficult to obtain in the United States because of a lack of standardized data collection and central reporting.[12]

As of 2002, in the United States, more than one billion dollars are spent per year on hospitalizations for SCD.[13] Data from a single state Medicaid program estimated a lifetime cost of care of $500,000 per patient with SCD. In this patient population, cost increased with increasing age, including cost of non-SCD health issues. The majority of the costs were for inpatient healthcare utilization.[14]

Previously, speculation existed as to whether the sickle mutation arose once and gained worldwide distribution or whether the mutation had arisen independently in different regions of the world. The non-random association of restriction endonuclease polymorphisms in the β-globin cluster define the β-globin haplotype. The β-globin gene cluster yields five distinct haplotypes associated with sickle cell mutations (Chap. 9).[15–17] Four of the five patterns occur in Africa and are designated as the Senegal, Benin, Bantu, and Cameroon haplotypes, whereas the fifth arose on the Indian subcontinent.[18] These findings indicate that the sickle mutation arose independently at five different times.

PATHOPHYSIOLOGY

The *sine qua non* of sickle cell anemia is a Glu→Val substitution in the sixth amino acid of the β-globin gene. However, the pathophysiologic processes that result in the clinical phenotype extend beyond the red cell (Fig. 49–5). There is marked clinical heterogeneity from one patient to another and in the same patient over time. The heterogeneity for the same genotypic abnormality therefore implies that a multitude of other factors must contribute to the pathology of sickle cell anemia. The pathology is now far removed from the simplistic theory of hypoxia-induced microvascular occlusion. Sickle cell anemia is a chronic inflammatory state punctuated by acute increase in inflammation wherein the endothelium, neutrophils and monocytes, platelets, coagulation pathways, several plasma proteins, adhesion molecules, and derangements in NO metabolism interact in concert with the abnormality in Hb polymerization described several decades ago (Fig. 49–6). Abnormal adenosine signaling and activation of invariant natural killer T (iNKT) cells have been implicated in disease pathophysiology. Added to that are the complex differences in tissue-specific vascular beds and differences in various parts of the vasculature in the same organ. Also, variation in several genes other than the β-globin gene that modify the milieu in which organ damage occurs may play a role.

The pathophysiology of sickle cell anemia is described in separate sections; however, because no single, dominant pathway explains the multitude of manifestations, no single therapeutic modality serves to abrogate all of the pathology. Most experiments are in isolation in animal models or relatively simplistic experimental conditions with few *in vivo* studies in humans and thus do not replicate the complexity of this disorder.

Hemoglobin Polymerization

Aggregation of deoxy HbS molecules into polymers occurs when aggregates reach a thermodynamically critical size. This process is termed *homogenous nucleation*, and the smallest aggregate formed that favors polymer growth is called the critical nucleus.[19–24] Addition of subsequent deoxy HbS molecules to already formed polymers is termed *heterogenous nucleation*, which results in polymer branching. Polymer growth is, therefore, an exponential process wherein there is a delay time between presence of deoxy HbS molecules and polymer formation. This delay time is inversely proportional to the concentration of HbS molecules. Polymer formation alters the rheologic properties of the red cell.

The quaternary structure of oxy HbS cannot maintain axial and lateral hydrophobic contacts unlike that in the deoxygenated state, thus explaining the unsickling phenomenon upon reoxygenation.[25–28] The sickling process that is initially reversible with oxygenation of deoxy HbS eventually leads to the formation of sickle-shaped red cells that

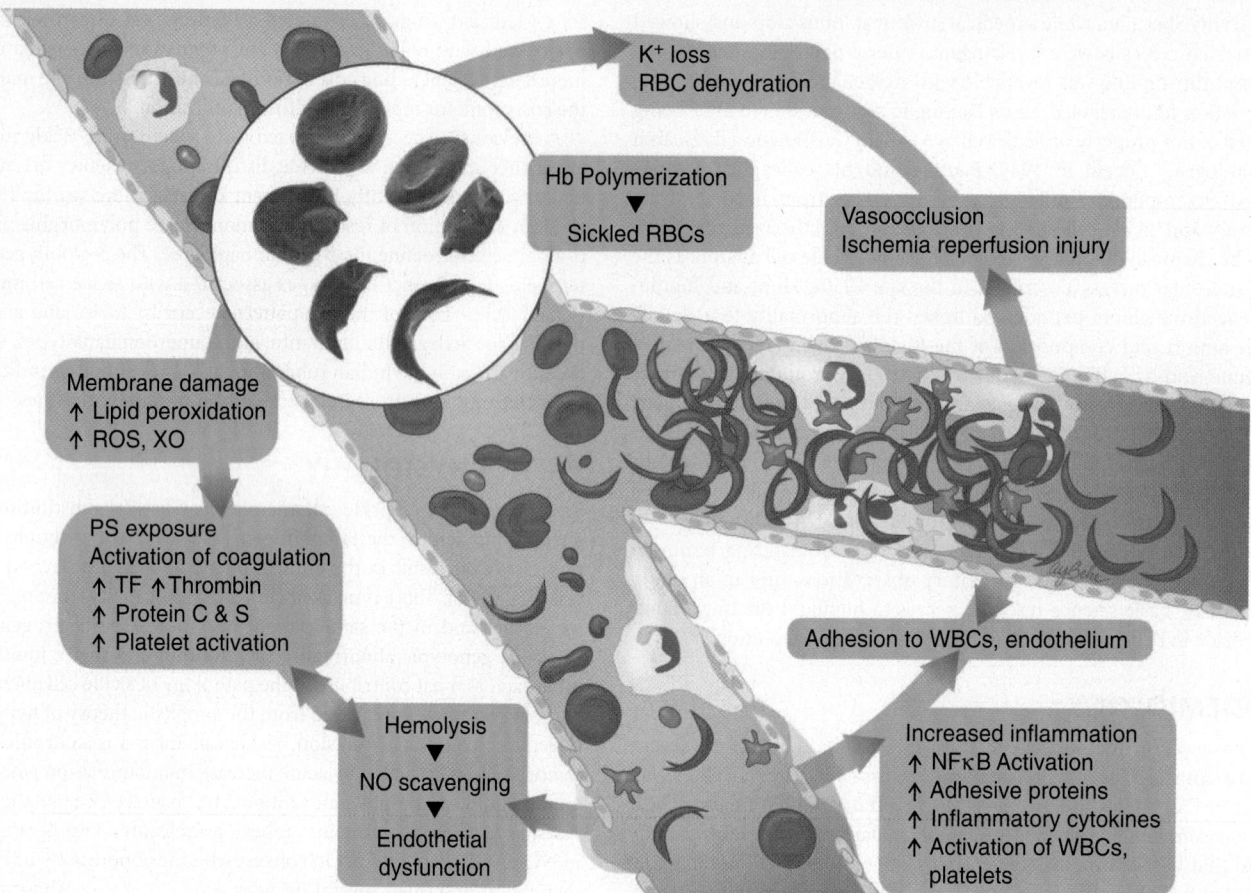

K+ loss
RBC dehydration

Hb Polymerization
▼
Sickled RBCs

Vasoocclusion
Ischemia reperfusion injury

Membrane damage
↑ Lipid peroxidation
↑ ROS, XO

PS exposure
Activation of coagulation
↑ TF ↑Thrombin
↑ Protein C & S
↑ Platelet activation

Adhesion to WBCs, endothelium

Hemolysis
▼
NO scavenging
▼
Endothelial
dysfunction

Increased inflammation
↑ NFκB Activation
↑ Adhesive proteins
↑ Inflammatory cytokines
↑ Activation of WBCs,
   platelets

Figure 49–5. Schema summarizing the pathophysiology of sickle cell anemia. K+, potassium; NO, nitric oxide; PS, phosphatidylserine; RBC, red blood cell; ROS, reactive oxygen species; TF, tissue factor; WBC, white blood cell; XO, xanthine oxidase.

fail to return to their normal discoid shape with oxygenation because of membrane damage imparted by repeated cycles of sickling and unsickling in the circulation. These cells are then termed *irreversibly sickled cells*. The rate and extent of polymerization is dependent on several factors, including intracellular Hb concentration, presence of Hbs other than HbS, blood oxygen saturation, pH, temperature, and 2,3-BPG levels.[29] Microvascular occlusion by sickle red cells containing polymers is favored by prolonged transit times through the microcirculation, rapid deoxygenation and increased numbers of dense sickle red cells that contain polymers even at oxygen saturation levels found in the arterial circulation.[29–32] Arguments against HbS polymerization as the major determinant of sickle cell pathophysiology include lack of clinically significant events despite constant sickling of red cells, the association of neutrophilia with vasoocclusive episodes (VOEs), and clinical features that imply macrovascular rather than microvascular perturbation, for example, large-vessel stroke.[33]

Cellular Dehydration

Membrane injury in HbSS red cells results in impaired cation homeostasis with decreased ability to maintain intracellular potassium concentrations. The calcium-activated potassium (K+) channel (Gardos channel), potassium-chloride cotransport channel, and a sickling-induced nonselective cation leak pathway have been implicated in sickle red cell dehydration. The net result is loss of intracellular potassium and water resulting in cellular dehydration.[34–39] This change effectively increases the red cell Hb concentration, favoring sickling.

Hemolysis and Nitric Oxide Scavenging

NO is a key component of the vascular endothelium that has vasodilatory, antiinflammatory, and antiplatelet properties.[40] NO is a soluble gas synthesized from L-arginine by endothelial nitric oxide synthase (eNOS).[41] Red cell L-arginase released as a consequence of sickle red cell hemolysis converts arginine to ornithine, thereby limiting L-arginine availability for NO synthesis. Decreased NO production because of elevated levels of endogenous nitric oxide synthase (NOS) inhibitors, especially asymmetric dimethylarginine (ADMA) and reduced L-arginine, have been documented in SCD especially during VOE.[42–46] Reduced plasma arginine levels and elevated ADMA levels also result in NOS coupling causing production of reactive oxygen species rather than NO.[47,48] Chronic hemolysis with release of plasma free Hb results in scavenging of NO with consequent endothelial dysfunction, which may favor sickle cell adherence.[49,50]

Abnormal Cell Adhesiveness

Seminal work by several groups showed that sickle red cells adhere to stimulated endothelium unlike their normal counterparts.[51,52] Newly released red cells, called *reticulocytes*, express high levels of adhesion molecules, integrin $\alpha_4\beta_1$, and CD36, and are more adherent than dense sickle red cells.[53,54] Increased endothelial reticulocyte adhesion as compared to dense red cell adhesion is thought to be secondary to deformable red cells adhering to the endothelium behind which the dense red cells are trapped, leading to microvascular occlusion.[29] Other molecules involved in sickle red cell-endothelium interactions include vascular

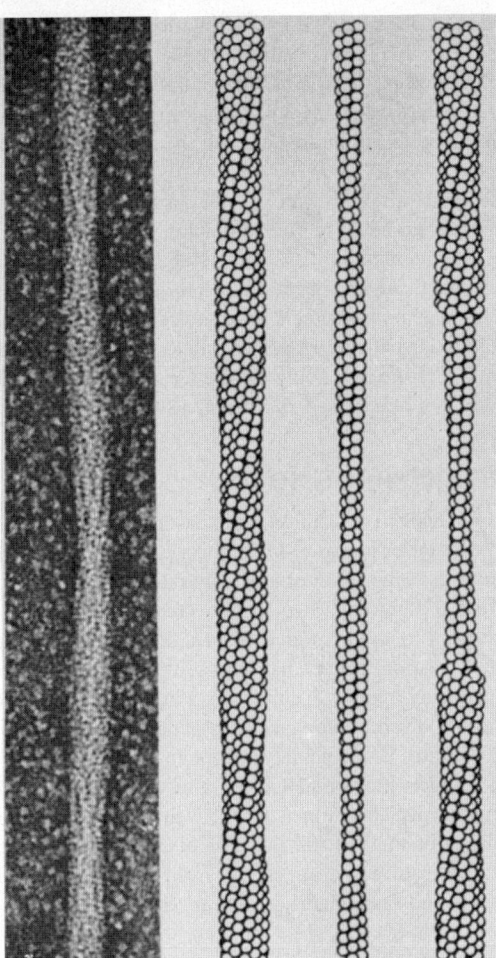

Figure 49–6. Electron micrograph of negatively stained fiber of HgS and the structure deduced by three-dimensional image reconstruction. The reconstructed fiber is presented as ball models, with each ball representing a HgS tetramer. The models are presented as the outer sheath *(left)*, the inner core *(center)*, and a combination of both inner and outer filaments *(right)*. *(Reproduced with permission from the University of Texas Medical Branch.)*

cell adhesion molecule (VCAM)-1, integrin $\alpha_V\beta_3$, P-selectin, P-selectin glycoprotein ligand (PSGL)-1, E-selectin, Lutheran blood group antigen, and thrombospondin.[55–60] The site of adhesion is purported to be the postcapillary venule at which site sickle red cells appear to interact with white cells adherent to the endothelium rather than engaging the endothelium directly.[31]

Neutrophilia is an adverse prognostic factor in sickle cell anemia. Because of their larger size, adherent leukocytes cause a greater decrease in vessel caliber than red cells. Diapedesis occurs in postcapillary venules, a site of vasoocclusion in sickle cell anemia.[31,61–63] Neutrophil integrin $\alpha_M\beta_2$ microdomains capture sickle red cells causing vascular occlusion in sickle cell mouse models. Monocytes are also highly activated in sickle cell anemia, and they promote increased endothelial activation by increased production of tumor necrosis factor (TNF)-α and interleukin (IL)-1β.[60] Expression of leukocyte adhesion molecules, L-selectin, and integrin $\alpha_M\beta_2$, are associated with a severe clinical phenotype.[61,64]

Inflammation and Chronic Vasculopathy

Sickle cell anemia is characterized by chronic leukocytosis, abnormal activation of neutrophils and monocytes, and an increase in several proinflammatory mediators including TNF-α, IL-6, and IL-1β. Several

adhesion molecules are upregulated, including VCAM, selectins, integrins, the acute phase reactants C-reactive protein, secretory phospholipase A$_2$ (sPLA$_2$), and coagulation factors are activated.[64–76] Placenta growth factor (PIGF) released from erythrocytes activates monocytes to produce inflammatory cytokines and upregulates endothelin-1 signaling via the endothelin B receptor. Endothelin-1 is a potent vasoconstrictor and upregulation is associated with adverse outcomes in SCD. Placental growth factor has independently been shown to be correlated with disease severity as well.[77,78] Hemin has been demonstrated to activate PIGF in mice via the erythroid Kruppel-like factor; consequently, PIGF may play an important role in the pathophysiology of iron overload as well.[79] It is an open question whether inflammation is caused by abnormally adhesive red cells to the vascular endothelium or whether inflammation causes abnormal red cell adhesiveness. It is likely both occur, given that red cell adhesiveness incites endothelial activity, and infection-induced inflammation precipitates clinically significant vascular events in patients.

The vascular beds in sickle cell anemia display changes akin to atherosclerotic vascular disease: large vessel intimal hyperplasia and smooth muscle proliferation.[80,81] However, the characteristic lipid laden plaques of atherosclerotic vascular disease are not present.[64]

Ischemia–Reperfusion Injury

Akin to other disease states, such as myocardial infarction, resolution of vasoocclusion results in reperfusion injury characterized by increased oxygen free radical formation via activation of xanthine oxidase, generation of oxidant stress, lipid peroxidation, upregulation of cellular adhesion molecules, and nuclear factor-κB, a key player in the inflammatory process.[64,82,83] iNKT cells propagate the inflammatory cascade in ischemia reperfusion injury and are increased and activated in patients with SCD. Agonists to adenosine 2A receptor (A$_{2A}$R) on iNKT cells downregulate their activation and attenuate inflammation in mouse models of SCD.[84]

Activation of the Coagulation System

The initiator of coagulation, tissue factor (TF), is elevated in patients with sickle cell anemia.[40,74,85–87] Microparticles (MPs) expressing TF derived from monocytes, macrophages, neutrophils and endothelial cells have been described in SCD.[58,68,74,88] Conflicting results exist in the literature on the presence and contribution of TF bearing MPs. There is a lack of correlation between TF bearing MPs and procoagulant activity in SCD. Erythrocyte and platelet MPs are TF-negative and are the major component of MPs in SCD. Activation of the intrinsic pathway of coagulation by TF-negative, red cell, and platelet MPs through a phosphatidylserine-dependent mechanism appears to be the major contributor of MP-dependent coagulation activation in SCD. Perivascular TF interaction with plasma coagulation factors made possible by increased vascular permeability and phosphatidylserine exposure on the surface of red cells secondary to repeated cycles of sickling provide an impetus for the coagulation process.[89] Heightened thrombin generation, platelet activation, and decreased protein C and S levels favor a procoagulant state.[69,90,91] Increased plasma levels of D-dimers, thrombin–antithrombin complexes, prothrombin fragment 1.2, and plasmin–antiplasmin complexes are indicative of increased thrombin-mediated coagulation with subsequent fibrinolysis.[92] Plasma from sickle cell patients contains increased ultralarge von Willebrand factor multimers as a result of increased endothelial cell secretion and impaired cleavage by ADAMTS13 (a disintegrin and metalloprotease with a thrombospondin type 1 motif member 13).[93]

Adenosine Signaling

Cellular stress leads to the degradation of adenine nucleotides, resulting in the generation of adenosine. Adenosine homeostasis is maintained by two enzymes: adenosine kinase, which phosphorylates adenosine to adenosine monophosphate and adenosine deaminase, which converts adenosine to inosine. Adenosine signals through four different receptors that have differing functions. Signaling via the $A_{2A}R$ expressed on most leukocyte and platelets results in an antiinflammatory effect; however, signaling via the $A_{2B}R$ was shown to cause priapism in SCD mice via hypoxia-inducible factor (HIF)-1–mediated decrease of phosphodiesterase 5. Signaling via $A_{2B}R$ also leads to increased 2,3-BPG in red cells causing decreased oxygen binding affinity of Hb, which promotes sickling. Pegylated adenosine deaminase treatment of sickle mice resulted in decreased hemolysis and hypoxia reoxygenation injury.[94,95]

SICKLE CELL TRAIT

Inheritance of only one HbS allele is termed *sickle cell trait* (HbAS). An estimated 300 million people carry the trait worldwide.[96] The percentage of HbA is always higher (~60 percent) than HbS (~40 percent) in sickle cell trait.

HbAS is considered a generally asymptomatic state with HbA in the cell preventing sickling except in the most unusual circumstances. HbAS cells sickle at O_2 tension of approximately 15 torr.[97]

Plasma myeloperoxidase and red cell sickling have been reported to increase during exercise with fluid restriction in HbAS subjects.[98] Plasma levels of VCAM-1 are higher in HbAS subjects and remain elevated following exercise compared to normal controls or HbAS with concomitant α-thalassemia, which is suggestive of subtle microcirculatory dysfunction in this population.[99] Skeletal muscle capillary structures are different in HbAS subjects compared to controls. There is a 30-fold increased risk of sudden death in black army recruits with HbAS.[100] Although controversial, in 2009 the National Collegiate Athletic Association recommended mandatory testing for HbAS for all its student athletes.[101]

Renal abnormalities are among the most common manifestations of HbAS. Anoxia, hyperosmolarity, and low pH of the renal medulla predisposes to sickling. Microscopic or gross hematuria from renal papillary necrosis is usually painless. Renal neoplasm or stones should be excluded in those with persistent gross hematuria. Isosthenuria may be seen in and may contribute to exercise induced rhabdomyolysis and sudden death.[102] Renal medullary carcinoma is a rare but serious complication of HbAS. Risk of urinary tract infection is higher in females with HbAS, especially during pregnancy. End-stage renal disease occurs at an earlier age for HbAS patients with polycystic kidney disease and HbAS may contribute to erythropoietin resistance.[103]

Splenic infarction occurs under extreme environmental conditions in persons with HbAS; most resolve spontaneously.[104,105] Caution and immediate intervention is also warranted in those HbAS individuals who develop traumatic hyphema.[106] The risk of venous thromboembolism is increased twofold in HbAS subjects compared to those without the trait. The risk appears to be greater for pulmonary embolism than for deep vein thrombosis.[101,105] HbAS patients do not have increased perioperative morbidity or mortality. The life span of patients with HbAS is normal.[107]

LABORATORY FEATURES

Sickle cell anemia is characterized by a laboratory profile of evidence of hemolytic anemia with increases in lactate dehydrogenase (LDH), indirect bilirubin, reticulocyte count, and a decrease in serum haptoglobin. Anemia is usually normochromic, normocytic with a steady-state Hb level between 5 and 11 g/dL.[1,108] The red cell density is increased with a normal mean cell Hb concentration (MCHC).[109] Serum erythropoietin level is decreased relative to the degree of anemia.[110] Elevated neutrophil and platelet levels are observed even in asymptomatic patients reflective of persistent low-grade inflammation.[111–113]

Plasma tocopherol and zinc levels are low.[114–116] Serum ferritin is increased, especially in iron overloaded patients. Elevated brain natriuretic peptide is seen in patients with pulmonary hypertension (PH) and congestive heart failure. Morphologically, classic sickle red cells are seen on blood film examination, and the marrow shows erythroid hyperplasia.

Sickle cell anemia can be accurately diagnosed with high-performance liquid chromatography (HPLC) and isoelectric focusing.[117] Rapid methods, such as solubility testing and sickling of red cells using sodium metabisulfite, are less-reliable tests.[118] Polymerase chain reaction is the method of choice for prenatal diagnosis.[119] No HbA is found in patients with HbSS, HbSC, or HbSβ⁰ diseases. Varying amounts of HbA (depending on the severity of the β-thalassemia mutation) are found in HbS–β⁺-thalassemia subjects.

COURSE AND PROGNOSIS

Mortality from SCD in the United States has declined since 1968, coinciding with the introduction of pneumococcal polyvalent conjugate 7 (PVC7) vaccine. Comparison of mortality rates between 1979 to 1998 and 1999 to 2009 showed a 61 percent decrease in infants, 67 percent in children ages 1 to 4 years, and 35 percent decrease in children ages 5 to 19 years. Transition from pediatric to adult medical care showed an increased mortality trend with similar rises in rates during the decades of comparison.[120] Average life expectancy of patients with HbSS disease in the United States is 42 and 48 years for males and females, respectively.[121] In Jamaica, the population has a median survival of 53 years and 58 years for men and women, respectively, with 44 percent of individuals born prior to 1943 still living as of 2009.[122] As the sickle cell population ages, causes of death change from an infectious etiology to those related to end-organ damage, such as renal failure.

CLINICAL FEATURES AND MANAGEMENT

The reader is referred to the National Institutes of Health, National Heart, Lung and Blood Institute's guidelines from 2002 for an extensive review on the topic; revised guidelines were released in the fall of 2014 at http://www.nhlbi.nih.gov/health-pro/guidelines/sickle-cell-disease-guidelines/.[123] General approaches to SCD management and pain management are described separately (Table 49–2).

Sickle Cell Crises

The typical course for a sickle cell patient is that of periods of relatively normal functioning despite chronic anemia and ongoing vasoocclusion, punctuated by periods of increased pain, and serial changes in various laboratory parameters that is termed "a sickle cell crisis." Crises have typically been classified as VOEs, aplastic crises, sequestration crises, and hyperhemolytic crises.

Vasoocclusive Crises   The hallmark of SCD is the VOE. It is the most common clinical manifestation but occurs with varying frequency in different individuals. It results from increasing vasoocclusion causing tissue hypoxia, which manifests as pain. Vasoocclusion may affect any tissue, but patients typically have pain in the chest, lower back, and extremities. Abdominal pain may mimic acute abdomen from other causes. Different patients display different patterns of painful sites during a VOE, but each patient's recurrences usually mimic the same pattern of pain. Fever is often present, even in the absence of infection. Episodes may be precipitated by dehydration, infection, and cold weather although in about most cases no precipitating factor is found.[124]

Figure 49–7 illustrates the phases of VOEs.[125] Crises requiring readmission within 1 week occur in approximately 20 percent of patients after hospital discharge.[125]

TABLE 49–2. Pathophysiologic Mechanisms and Potential Therapeutic Targets in Sickle Cell Disease

Pathophysiology/ Complication	Therapeutic Interventions
Sickle hemoglobin (HbS) polymerization	Fetal hemoglobin (HbF) induction
Cellular dehydration	Gardos channel inhibition
	Potassium-chloride cotransport channel inhibition
Adhesion to endothelium	
Red blood cell	Antiselectin
	Antiintegrin
White blood cell	Antiselectin
	Intravenous immunoglobulin
	Hydroxyurea (HU)
Inflammation	Nuclear factor-κB inhibition
	Immunomodulatory drugs
	HU
	Statins
Nitric oxide (NO) scavenging	NO donor (NO, HU, tetrahydrobiopterin)
	Phosphodiesterase 5 inhibition
	Modulation of hemolysis
Coagulation	Tissue factor inhibition
	Antiplatelet therapy
	Anticoagulation
Hyposplenism/infection	Penicillin prophylaxis
Ischemia–reperfusion	Xanthine oxidase inhibition
	Myeloperoxidase inhibition
Iron overload	Chelation

The characterization of crisis phases has implications for clinical research, especially in pain management, wherein interventions early in the course of a crisis could result in better outcomes for patients.

Aplastic Crises Aplastic crises in sickle cell anemia result when there is a marked reduction in red cell production in the face of ongoing hemolysis, causing an acute, severe drop in Hb level. The characteristic laboratory finding is a reticulocyte count less than 1 percent. The most common causative agent is parvovirus B19, which attaches to the P antigen receptor on erythroid progenitor cells, causing a temporary arrest in red cell production (Chap. 36). Recurrent aplastic crises by parvovirus B19 are rare because of the development of protective antibodies. Other rare complications associated with parvovirus B19 include acute splenic and/or hepatic sequestration, acute chest syndrome, marrow necrosis, and renal dysfunction. Patients usually recover within 2 weeks; however, those with severe symptomatic anemia need red cell transfusion. Siblings of SCD patients with parvovirus infections should be monitored closely for aplastic crisis given high secondary attack rates (>50 percent). Patients need to be isolated from pregnant individuals given increased risk of hydrops fetalis with parvovirus B19 infection.[126]

Sequestration Crises This type of crisis is characterized by sudden, massive pooling of red cells, typically in the spleen and less commonly in the liver.[127] Splenic sequestration is typically seen in children (younger than 5 years of age) prior to autoinfarction of the spleen, but can be seen in adults with HbSC disease or HbS–β-thalassemia with persisting splenomegaly.[128–130] A minor sequestration episode is usually accompanied by a Hb of more than 7 g/dL, and a major episode usually is one in which the Hb is less than 7 g/dL or the Hb has decreased by 3 g/dL from baseline.[131]

Acute splenic and hepatic sequestration crises can present with rapidly enlarging spleen or liver, pain, hypoxemia, and hypovolemic shock. Treatment consists of red cell transfusion. Transfusion carries the risk of hyperviscosity when the sequestration crisis resolves and the sequestered red cells are returned to the general circulation. Splenic sequestration crisis has a high rate of recurrence, especially in children. Splenectomy to prevent recurrence is debated in very young children. Some report chronic red cell exchange transfusion as a means of delaying splenectomy until the child is older while others did not see any benefit to this treatment. Patients younger than 2 years of age can be placed on chronic transfusion until they are older, at which time splenectomy should be considered. Splenectomy is recommended after the first episode of life-threatening splenic sequestration crisis or chronic hypersplenism. Partial splenectomy and emergency splenectomy during a crisis is not recommended. Parental education is important for early recognition of the problem so they can seek medical care promptly.[126]

Hyperhemolytic Crisis The term *hyperhemolytic crisis* is used to describe the occurrence of episodes of accelerated rates of hemolysis characterized by decreased blood Hb, increasing reticulocytes, and other markers of hemolysis (hyperbilirubinemia, increased LDH). Hyperhemolysis can occur during resolution of a VOE, at which time irreversibly sickled and dense red cells are rapidly destroyed, as well as from an acute or delayed hemolytic transfusion reactions.[126,132]

Pain Control

Patients with SCD have acute pain, chronic pain, or both. As a symptom, pain is often underrated in its intensity and undertreated by caregivers, especially inexperienced physicians. Patients are often perceived as drug-seekers or drug addicts, when in fact less than 10 percent of patients are addicted, a number comparable to other disease states. Unsatisfactory relief of pain drives patients to behaviors that appear to healthcare givers as signs of addiction—a state termed *pseudoaddiction*. A study comparing sickle cell anemia patients who use the emergency department frequently or infrequently found significant impairment in quality of life and increased markers of disease severity in those who use the emergency department frequently, dispelling the myth that frequent emergency department use indicates narcotic-addicted individuals when, in fact, they may have more severe disease.[3,133–137] The landmark *Pain in Sickle Cell Epidemiology Study* revealed that adult SCD patients have pain at home approximately 55 percent of the time, which contrasts sharply to pain studies in children, who report at-home pain approximately 9 percent of the time.[138,139]

Acute pain is managed with opioids, nonsteroidal antiinflammatory drugs, acetaminophen, or a combination of these medications. Immediate pain assessment and frequent reassessment with appropriate application of medications until pain relief is obtained is important. For adults and children weighing more than 50 kg, morphine can be started at a dose of 0.1 to 0.15 mg/kg. The hydromorphone dose should be 0.015 to 0.020 mg/kg intravenously. These are recommended doses for opioid-naïve patients and are at the lower end of the dosing range.[123,140,141] The use of meperidine has declined because of neurologic side effects, especially in patients with renal failure, who are at risk for the serotonin syndrome in conjunction with use of other medications.[142–144] However, the use of morphine is not benign and concerns of increased association of acute chest syndrome, dysphoria, and neuroexcitatory

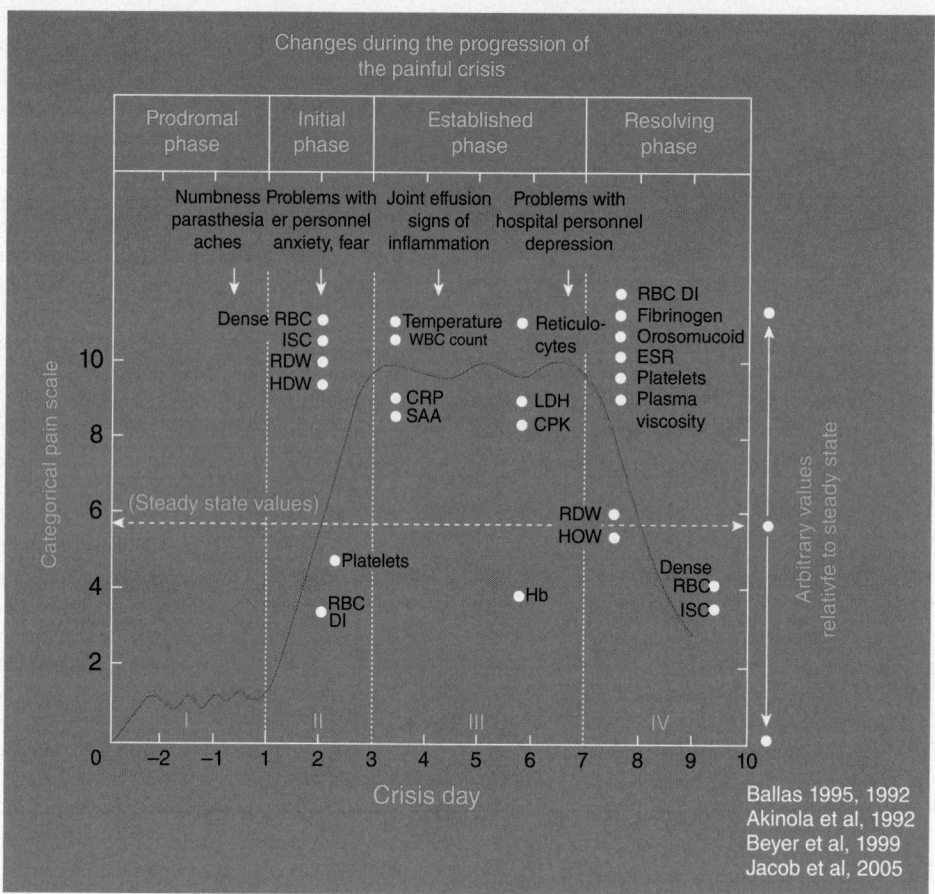

Figure 49–7. A typical profile of the events that develop during the evolution of a severe sickle cell painful crisis in an adult in the absence of overt infection or other complications. Such events are usually treated in the hospital with an average stay of 9 to 11 days. Pain becomes most severe by day 3 of the crisis and starts decreasing by day 6 or 7. The Roman numerals refer to the phase of the crisis: I indicates prodromal phase; II, initial phase; III, established phase; and IV, resolving phase. Dots on the x-axis indicate the time when changes became apparent; and dots on the y-axis, the relative value of change compared with the steady state indicated by the horizontal dashed line. Arrows indicate the time when certain clinical signs and symptoms may become apparent. Values shown are those reported at least twice by different investigators; values that were anecdotal, unconfirmed, or that were not reported to occur on a specific day of the crisis are not shown. CPK, creatinine phosphokinase; CRP, C-reactive protein; ESR, erythrocyte sedimentation rate; HDW, hemoglobin distribution width; ISC, irreversibly sickled cells; LDH, lactate dehydrogenase; RBC DI, red cell deformability index; RDW, red cell distribution width; SAA, serum amyloid A. *(Reproduced with permission from SK Ballas, K Gupta, P Adams-Graves: Sickle cell pain: A critical reappraisal.* Blood *120(18):3647–3656, 2012.)*

side effects have been raised.[125] Prior use of opioid therapy should be taken into consideration when deciding initial opioid doses as patients may be tolerant and require higher doses. Caution should be exercised with nonsteroidal antiinflammatory drugs and acetaminophen if there is renal or hepatic dysfunction. Patients with acute pain are better managed in a setting dedicated to sickle cell patients.[145] A multidisciplinary approach is needed for pain management, especially if chronic pain is present.[146,147] Opioid side effects should be anticipated and managed. Antidepressants, anticonvulsants, and clonidine can be used for neuropathic pain. Occasionally, severe, unrelenting pain may require red cell transfusion to decrease sickle Hb below 30 percent in the blood.[148]

There is a paucity of data regarding optimal management of pain in SCD. A randomized trial of optimizing patient controlled analgesia strategy was closed because of poor accrual.[149] A trial looking at NO inhalation for treatment of VOE did not show improvement in pain.[150]

Pulmonary Manifestations

Acute Chest Syndrome The acute chest syndrome (ACS) is a constellation of signs and symptoms in patients with SCD that includes a new infiltrate on chest radiograph defined by alveolar consolidation

but not atelectasis, chest pain, fever, tachypnea, wheezing, or cough, and hypoxia (Fig. 49–8).[151] However, respiratory findings on clinical examination in the absence of radiographic findings should trigger high suspicion for ACS and warrants close monitoring. ACS is the leading cause of mortality in patients with SCD.[121] Etiology varies depending on age, with viral and bacterial infections dominating in the pediatric age group and fat embolization resulting from marrow necrosis during VOE dominating in adults.[152,153] Important pathogens include *Chlamydia pneumoniae*, *Mycoplasma pneumoniae*, *Streptococcus pneumoniae*, *Staphylococcus aureus*, parvovirus B19, respiratory syncytial virus, and influenza. Regardless of the triggering factor, the pathogenesis of ACS involves increased intrapulmonary sickling, intrapulmonary inflammation with increased microvascular permeability, and alveolar consolidation. ACS can rapidly evolve with bilateral infiltrates and consolidation leading to acute respiratory failure requiring intubation and ventilatory assistance.

Independent risk factors for respiratory failure are age older than 20 years, platelet count less than $20 \times 10^9/L$, multilobar lung involvement, and a history of cardiac disease.[152] Thrombocytopenia is an independent predictor of neurologic complications during hospitalization

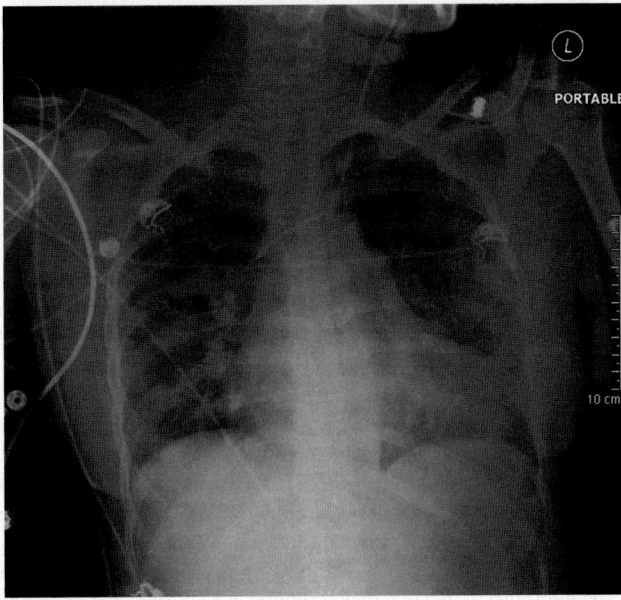

Figure 49–8. Anteroposterior view of chest radiograph depicting bilateral, patchy, lung infiltrates in a 30-year-old female with sickle cell disease and evolving acute chest syndrome.

for ACS, which was seen in 22 percent of adult patients in the National Acute Chest Syndrome study.[154]

The treatment of ACS includes oxygenation, incentive spirometry, adequate pain control to avoid chest splinting, antimicrobial therapy that always covers atypical bacteria and influenza when indicated, avoidance of overhydration, use of bronchodilators, and red cell transfusion to decrease intrapulmonary sickling.[152,155-160] The use of glucocorticoids may attenuate the course of ACS; however, its use is not well established and readmission rates for VOE after ACS resolution are increased.[153] sPLA$_2$ has been recognized as a predictor of ACS; however, a clinical trial investigating early transfusion based on sPLA$_2$ elevation closed because of poor accrual. Hydroxyurea therapy should be offered to all patients with a history of ACS because it reduces the incidence by 50 percent in adults and 73 percent in children.[161]

Pulmonary Hypertension PH, defined by a resting mean pulmonary arterial pressure of 25 torr or higher on right-heart catheterization, is seen in 6 to 11 percent of SCD patients. An elevated tricuspid regurgitant velocity of 2.5 m/s has a positive predictive value of 25 percent for PH in SCD and is seen in one-third of these patients. PH, as defined by right-heart catheterization, elevated tricuspid regurgitant jet velocity of 2.5 m/s or higher, and a serum N-terminal pro–brain natriuretic peptide (NT-pro-BNP) level of 160 pg/mL or higher, confers an increased mortality risk.[162]

Abnormalities in NO metabolism, hemolysis, and inflammation contribute to the pathophysiology of PH.[162] Parenchymal lung disease from repeated episodes of ACS and thromboembolism are other causal factors.

Clinical symptoms of PH include fatigue, dizziness, and dyspnea on exertion, chest pain, and syncope. These may be unrecognized as being related to PH, as PH is often undiagnosed in patients with SCD.

PH should be treated following guidelines set for the treatment of primary PH unrelated to SCD. Two trials looking at bosentan (endothelin receptor antagonist) in SCD patients closed because of sponsor withdrawal. A trial of sildenafil was halted early because of increased incidence of VOE. Patients who have venous thromboembolism in the setting of PH should be considered for indefinite anticoagulation.

Hydroxyurea should be offered to all patients with any of the risk factors for increased mortality described above.[162]

Asthma, Abnormal Pulmonary Function Tests, and Airway Hyperreactivity. Asthma is a common comorbidity with higher-than-average prevalence in patients with SCD and is associated with increased risk of ACS, VOE, stroke, and mortality. Airway hyperreactivity as evidenced by a positive bronchodilator response on pulmonary function testing, irrespective of baseline function, and in response to cold air or methacholine challenge, is seen in approximately two-thirds of SCD patients. Inflammation, hypoxemia, and increased oxidative stress associated with asthma may contribute to the vasculopathy of SCD.[163]

Pulmonary function tests collected as part of the Cooperative Study of Sickle Cell Disease (CSSCD) revealed abnormalities in 90 percent of the 310 patients, with the majority having restrictive lung disease.

Asthma treatment follows general treatment guidelines as in the non-SCD populations.[164,165]

Cardiac Manifestations

Anemia in SCD results in an elevated cardiac output secondary to an increased stroke volume with minimal increase in heart rate.[166,167] Clinical manifestations of a hyperdynamic circulation include a forceful precordial apical impulse, systolic and diastolic flow murmurs, and tachycardia that may increase during periods of increased hemodynamic stress. Diastolic left ventricular dysfunction may begin in early childhood and is an independent risk factor for death, with even greater risk of mortality in those having PH. Left ventricular hypertrophy is common and progressive with age; left ventricular dysfunction is a late event. Myocardial infarction is an underrecognized problem in SCD. Epicardial coronary artery disease is rare; microvascular ischemia is likely causative. Sudden cardiac death has been reported in 40 percent of patients in an autopsy series.[168-170] Previously sudden cardiac death was ascribed to narcotic overdose; currently, it is thought to be secondary to cardiopulmonary causes in the majority of cases. QTc prolongation, atrial and ventricular arrhythmias, nonspecific ST-T wave changes are common in SCD patients. Patients presenting with chest pain should have a thorough evaluation to rule out cardiac disease. Cardiac magnetic resonance may be a good modality to image microvascular flow and quantitate cardiac iron overload.[171,172] Blood pressure in patients with SCD is significantly lower than age-, sex-, and race-matched controls, partly secondary to anemia.[173] Relative hypertension is associated with end-organ damage. Diuretics may be used, keeping in mind that SCD patients have obligate hyposthenuria and are prone to dehydration, which can precipitate a VOE.

Central Nervous System

Originally thought to be a small vessel disease, stroke in SCD is a macrovascular phenomenon with devastating consequences that affects approximately 11 percent of patients younger than 20 years of age.[174,175] Risk is highest in the first decade of life followed by a second smaller peak after age 29 years. Ischemic stroke is most common in children and older adults, whereas hemorrhagic stroke predominates in the third decade of life.[175] Recurrent stroke is most common in the first 2 years following the primary event.[176] Silent infarcts, defined as an increased T2 signal abnormality on magnetic resonance imaging (MRI), begins in infancy and has a cumulative incidence of 37 percent by age 14 years. They occur in watershed areas of the brain, are not predicted by abnormal transcranial Doppler (TCD) velocity, and may progress despite chronic transfusion.[177-180] There is evidence of neurocognitive decline in asymptomatic adults despite having normal brain imaging that is attributed to anemia and hypoxemia.[154]

Cerebral blood flow is significantly increased in SCD because of chronic anemia and hypoxemia, but does not increase further in response to increased hypoxic stress, thereby predisposing to ischemia.[181,182] Stenosis of large vessels, especially of the circle of Willis, without the classic atherosclerotic plaque occurs in conjunction with a multitude of other factors, including chronic hemolysis, deranged NO metabolism and impaired vascular autoregulation, and can lead to stroke.[182] Rare causes of cerebral vascular disease include fat embolization and venous sinus thrombosis. Moyamoya type fragile collaterals have been reported in more than one-fifth of patients with prior stroke, possibly leading to hemorrhagic stroke in later life.[183–188]

Risk factors for ischemic stroke include transient ischemic attack, recent or recurrent ACS, nocturnal hypoxemia, silent infarcts, hypertension, elevated lactic dehydrogenase, and leukocytosis, whereas anemia, neutrophilia, the use of glucocorticoids, and recent transfusion are independent risk factors for hemorrhagic stroke, especially in children.[175,189–195] Sickle cell genotypes other than HbSS carry a lower risk, as do patients with HbS–α-thalassemia.[175,196,197] The best predictor of stroke risk, however, is an increased blood flow velocity in major intracranial arteries on TCD ultrasonography.[197] Blood flow velocities less than 170 cm/s are considered normal. Velocities between 170 and 200 cm/s are termed *conditional*, and velocities of greater than 200 cm/s are considered high and are associated with a 10-fold increase in ischemic stroke in children 2 to 16 years of age.

There is an increased frequency of stroke among siblings of patients with SCD than would be expected by chance alone, raising the possibility of other modifier genes contributing to stroke risk.[183] The TNF (–308) G/A promoter polymorphism is associated with increased large-vessel stroke risk as is the IL-4–receptor gene 503 S/P variant, although it did not reach statistical significance. The clinical features of stroke in SCD encompass the classic findings of stroke in other disorders, including, but not limited to, hemiparesis, seizures, coma, paresthesias, headaches, and cranial nerve palsies. Neurocognitive deficits in IQ, memory, language, and executive function have been demonstrated.[154,198]

Imaging approaches for acute stroke are the same as those for non-SCD patients and includes MRI and magnetic resonance angiography.

Prevention of Primary Stroke Based on the results from the Stroke Prevention in Sickle Cell Disease (STOP) Study, it is recommended that asymptomatic children with HbSS disease older than two years of age should be screened for stroke risk using TCD.[197] Those with high TCD velocities should be offered a chronic red cell transfusion program for primary stroke prevention. Repeat TCD screenings should be done every 3 to 12 months even in patients who have normal or conditional baseline velocities, because they can evolve into a higher-risk category. Despite obstacles to TCD screening, clinical practice changes based on the STOP study translated into declining stroke rates since 1991.[199,200]

Prevention of Secondary Stroke Patients with SCD who present with a stroke and are not on chronic transfusion should be placed on a transfusion program to prevent secondary strokes. Exchange transfusion may be preferable to periodic red cell transfusion, not only to avoid iron overload, but also to further reduce stroke risk. In a retrospective study, children who received periodic transfusion had a five-fold higher relative risk of a recurrent stroke compared to those on an exchange transfusion regimen.[201] Despite chronic transfusions, patients may have a recurrent stroke, especially in patients with HbS greater than 30 percent.[202] Hydroxyurea was shown to decrease high and conditional TCD velocities in more than 90 percent of patients studied.[203] However, a randomized trial comparing transfusions with iron chelation to hydroxyurea with phlebotomy showed a 10 percent stroke rate in the hydroxyurea arm, thus establishing transfusion as the preferred preventive strategy.[204]

Anticoagulation therapy has not been studied in patients with SCD and, therefore, no recommendations can be made. Treatment guidelines

for intracranial hemorrhage are as those for non-SCD–related intracranial hemorrhage; role of transfusion is less clear in SCD especially when cause of intracranial hemorrhage is unclear. Patients with moyamoya disease who have a particularly poor outcome may benefit from revascularization using encephaloduroarteriosyangiosis.[205,206]

Genitourinary Systems

Renal Failure Sickling of HbSS erythrocytes in the hypoxic, acidic, and hypertonic environment of the renal medulla, oxidative stress, increase in prostaglandins and endothelin-1 in the kidney, and abnormalities of the renin angiotensin system contribute to the pathophysiology of renal disease in SCD.[207] The incidence of renal failure varies between 4 and 20 percent.[208–211] Dehydration is the most common cause of acute renal failure in SCD. Isosthenuria is highly prevalent in SCD, may increase the risk of dehydration, and is irreversible.[212] Glomerular hypertrophy, focal and segmental glomerular sclerosis, and hemosiderin deposition in proximal renal tubular epithelium have been described; however, no single lesion is pathognomonic of sickle cell nephropathy. Cystatin C is an accurate marker of glomerular filtration and therefore is preferable to serum creatinine in estimating renal function.[213,214] Glomerular hyperfiltration, microalbuminuria, and macroalbuminuria occur sequentially in SCD patients starting in infancy and increasing in frequency with age.[122,161,215] Incidence of microalbuminuria is greater than 60 percent in those over age 35 years.[213] End-stage renal disease requiring dialysis carries a poor prognosis and is associated with a median survival of 4 years.[216]

Angiotensin-converting enzyme inhibitors decrease proteinuria and hyperfiltration in SCD; however, large-scale studies are needed to characterize the magnitude of the benefit. Treatment of renal disease follows principles used for non-SCD kidney pathology and includes effective blood pressure control, avoidance of nephrotoxic agents, and treatment of urinary tract infection. A relative decrease in serum erythropoietin levels, proportionate to the degree of anemia is observed; however, erythropoietin treatment, with its resultant increase in Hb may cause an increase in VOEs because of an increase in blood viscosity.[213]

Renal tubular acidosis type IV, secondary to decreased potassium and hydrogen ion in the distal tubule can cause disproportionate acidosis and hyperkalemia in patients with declining renal function.[213]

Hematuria is discussed in the section on sickle cell trait.

Priapism Priapism is prevalent in at least 35 percent of male patients with SCD with devastating psychological consequences; true prevalence may be higher as it is often underreported.[217–219] The mean age of episodes is 15 years and two-thirds of patients have "stuttering priapism" a term used for episodes that last less than 3 hours.[220] Derangements in NO metabolism and adenosine signaling are thought to be the major contributors to priapism in SCD.[94] Greater than 95 percent of priapism is the "low-flow" type resulting from ischemia, is painful, and is a medical emergency.[221]

Aspiration of the corpus cavernosa followed by epinephrine injections, exchange transfusion, and α and β agonists have all been used, but data regarding efficacy are sparse. α-Agonists, etilefrine 50 mg, and ephedrine 15 to 30 mg per day, seem to reduce the incidence of stuttering priapism.[222] Hormonal therapies, including antiandrogens and luteinizing hormone-releasing hormone, reduce nocturnal erections but are associated with loss of libido.[221] Transfusion therapy has resulted in neurologic sequelae termed "the ASPEN syndrome" (Association of Sickle Cell Disease, Priapism, Exchange Transfusion) and is thought to be secondary to hyperviscosity; care, therefore, must be taken not to increase the hematocrit beyond 30 percent.[223] In recalcitrant cases, a shunt is performed but results in permanent impotence.[222] A penile prosthesis is used to ameliorate sexual dysfunction.

Nocturnal Enuresis Nocturnal enuresis is prevalent in 25 to 33 percent of the pediatric sickle cell population, which is higher compared to that of age-matched controls.[224-226] It tends to decrease with age but is still prevalent in adults. Social and environmental factors, decreased functional bladder capacity, and decreased arousal during sleep appear to be contributing factors.

Musculoskeletal System

VOE is commonly manifested by marrow infarction causing musculoskeletal pain, swelling at involved sites, fever, and leukocytosis. Marrow hypercellularity is thought to predispose to this phenomenon by causing a decrease in local blood flow and oxygenation.

Dactylitis Dactylitis is a painful swelling of digits of the hands and feet ("hand-foot syndrome"). It occurs early in infancy as hematopoietic marrow is still present in these bones at this age. Most episodes resolve within in 2 weeks.[227-230] Epiphyseal infarction can result in joint pain and swelling mimicking septic arthritis. Use of hydroxyurea in the BABY HUG trial resulted in significant reduction of rate of dactylitis.[161]

Osteomyelitis, Septic Arthritis, and Bone Infarction Impaired cellular and humoral immunity together with infarction of bone contribute to this complication with an estimated prevalence of 12 percent. Atypical serotypes of *Salmonella*, *S. aureus*, and Gram-negative bacilli are the principal infectious offenders. No single lab or imaging test reliably differentiates osteomyelitis from infarction.[227,229,231-235] Culture results may be nondiagnostic as patients usually receive antibiotics on presentation with fever; therefore, the presence of leukocytes in bone and joint aspirates should evoke a high suspicion for osteomyelitis.[126] Septic arthritis tends to occur in joints involved with avascular necrosis, also seen following hip arthroplasty. Multiple joints may be involved. An elevated C-reactive protein should raise suspicion for septic arthritis and prompt intervention with appropriate antibiotics as needed to prevent joint deterioration and collapse.[227] Vertebral body infarctions with subsequent collapse causes the classic "fish mouth" appearance of vertebrae on radiographs of the spine.

Osteopenia and Osteoporosis Osteopenia and osteoporosis are prevalent (30 to 80 percent) in patients with sickle cell anemia, with a predilection for the lumbar spine. Presence of avascular necrosis with local bone remodeling may lead to false-negative results on a bone mineral density test at the femoral neck.[126] Fractures of the long bones are commonly underdiagnosed and self-reported rates of fractures in young adults with SCD are high. Etiology of osteoporosis is multifactorial with hypogonadism, hypothyroidism, nutritional deficiencies, and iron overload interfering with osteoblast function being the major causes.[126,236-238] More than 50 percent of patients are vitamin D deficient with the majority (>80 percent) having less-than-optimal levels. High doses of vitamin D supplementation have resulted in improvement in chronic pain and higher levels of physical activity.[239]

Avascular Necrosis Vasoocclusion resulting in infarction of articular surfaces of long bone occurs most commonly in the femur followed by the humerus. It was previously thought to occur with increased frequency in HbSC disease as opposed to patients with HbSS. However, with increased longevity of HbSS patients, its prevalence is greater in patients with HbSS.[240-242] As per the CSSCD estimates, 50 percent of patients by age 33 years will have avascular necrosis of the femoral head (Fig. 49–9). The presence of concurrent deletional α-thalassemia ($-\alpha^{3.7}$) and a history of frequent VOEs are classic risk factors for avascular necrosis. Other risk factors include male gender, higher Hb concentration, low fetal Hb, and vitamin D deficiency.[126,243,244] Polymorphisms in *BMP6*, *ANNEXIN A2*, and *KLOTHO* genes are associated with avascular necrosis.[245]

Patients present with chronic joint pain with progressive decrease in range of motion of affected joints. Multiple joints are commonly involved.[246] The vast majority of untreated patients will progress to femoral head collapse within 5 years.[247,248]

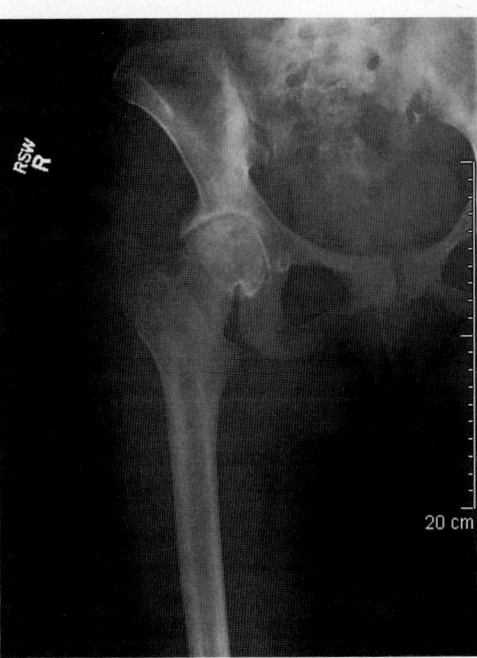

Figure 49–9. Avascular necrosis of the right hip in a 31-year-old female with sickle cell disease depicting a patchy lucency and sclerosis and irregular contour of the femoral head and loss of the joint space.

Avascular necrosis has been treated with a number of modalities including core decompression, osteotomy, bone grafting, surface arthroplasty, and joint replacement. Two randomized trials in avascular necrosis compared core decompression and physical therapy versus physical therapy alone and did not show a difference in outcome between the two arms; however, followup was short, a significant number of stage III hip joints were included in one study, and sample size was limited.[249] In our experience, core decompression is a useful option in early stage avascular necrosis. Several studies associate total hip replacement in SCD with a higher rate of orthopedic and medical complications. However, other studies show a lower rate of orthopedic complications. Structural bone diseases in SCD make joint replacement challenging.[250-252] Hydroxyurea and chronic transfusion therapy have not been shown to reduce the risk of avascular necrosis.[243]

Leg Ulcers

Leg ulcers occur in 2 to 40 percent of cases with SCD and varies geographically with the highest rate being reported in Jamaica.[1,253] In the United States, leg ulcers are seen in 4 to 6 percent of patients with SCD and are most common in patients older than 10 years of age.[254] They occur on the lower extremities, especially on the malleoli, and cause chronic pain and disability. Venous stasis is a predisposing factor while coinheritance of α-thalassemia appears to have a protective effect. The relationship between hydroxyurea use and increased occurrence of leg ulcers is controversial.[255] Polymorphisms in *KLOTHO*, *TEK*, and several other genes in the transforming growth factor (TGF)-β and bone morphogenic protein (BMP) pathways are associated with leg ulcers.[245] Once established, ulcers are recalcitrant and significantly impair quality of life.[256]

Treatment of leg ulcers is largely empiric. Leg elevation, bed rest when practical and feasible, wet-to-dry dressings, gentle debridement, Unna boots, and treatment of infection and topical or systemic antibiotics are commonly used. The peptide encoding integrin-interaction site of many extracellular matrix proteins (RGD peptide) enhanced healing of the ulcers in preliminary studies, but, unfortunately, it never came to clinical practice because of nonmedical reasons.[257] Increases in HbF and transfusions occasionally hasten healing of leg ulcers.[258]

Hepatobiliary Complications

Chronic liver abnormalities in SCD are frequent and of different etiologies that include vasoocclusion, transfusional iron overload, pigmented gallstones with bile duct obstruction, acute or chronic cholecystitis, viral hepatitis, and cholestasis.[259,260] Common clinical manifestations include right upper quadrant pain, fever, hepatomegaly, nausea, and vomiting. Bilirubin levels from chronic hemolysis are usually not above 6 mg/dL, with a majority of it being the indirect fraction.[261] Because some degree of aspartate transaminase elevation is seen with hemolysis, alanine transaminase elevation is a more accurate marker of liver injury.

Vasoocclusion involving the hepatic sinusoids was seen in 39 percent of patients in one study, while previous reports of vasoocclusion involving the liver, termed *acute sickle hepatic crisis*, has been reported in 10 percent of patients. The differing prevalence is the result of varying criteria used to include biochemical and clinical abnormalities.[262] Acute hepatic sequestration crisis characterized by a rapidly enlarging, tender liver and hypovolemia is akin to splenic sequestration but much rarer. It requires prompt treatment with red cell transfusion. Severe intrahepatic cholestasis with serum bilirubin levels as high as 100 mg/dL is a catastrophic situation needing exchange transfusion for resolution; synthetic liver function is lost as characterized by low serum albumin and coagulation protein abnormalities; renal impairment may occur. A more benign form of cholestasis has been described, which resolves with conservative measure.[263–268]

Chronic hemolysis results in an increased burden on the heme catabolic pathway leading to increased unconjugated bilirubin and formation of pigmented gallstones. The incidence of gallstones increases with age, with a reported prevalence of 50 percent at 22 years of age.[269–271] The number of uridine diphosphate (UDP) glucuronosyltransferase 1 family (UGT1A1) promoter (TA) repeats (the polymorphism associated with Gilbert syndrome) is strongly associated with increased incidence of gallstones and bilirubin levels while coinherited α-thalassemia (Chap. 48) decreases bilirubin levels in patients with SCD.[272] Laparoscopic cholecystectomy is recommended in symptomatic patients with cholelithiasis. The treatment of asymptomatic patients with positive findings on abdominal ultrasonography is more controversial. In the Jamaican cohort study, only 7 percent of patients with positive ultrasonograms had symptoms suggestive of biliary tract disease and needed a cholecystectomy. However, patients in the United States appear to be more symptomatic, with the majority of gallbladders removed after only a positive ultrasonogram have pathologic evidence of cholecystitis.[269] Asymptomatic patients with negative screening ultrasonograms should be observed; however, timing and frequency of screening has not been standardized.

Ophthalmic Complications

The microvasculature of the retina with relative hypoxemia facilitates "sickling" akin to several other vascular beds. Microcirculatory obstruction occurs followed by neovascularization and arteriovenous aneurysms. Hemorrhage, scarring, and retinal detachment leading to blindness are the sequelae. Changes occur at the periphery, thereby sparing central vision at earlier stages. The term *sickle cell retinopathy* encompasses nonproliferative and proliferative changes.

Nonproliferative changes include "salmon-patch" hemorrhages, peripheral retinal lesions termed "black sunbursts," and iridescent spots, whereas neovascularization is characteristic of proliferative changes, giving a pattern of vascular lesions resembling a marine invertebrate and is termed as "sea fans."[273]

Increased levels of plasma and intraocular vascular endothelial growth factor have been documented in proliferative sickle cell retinopathy, as have angiopoietin-1 and -2 and von Willebrand factor. Pigment epithelium derived factor, an angiogenesis inhibitor, is increased as well, especially in nonviable "sea fans."[274–276]

Proliferative sickle cell retinopathy may differ from other proliferative retinopathies in that spontaneous regression of neovascularization can occur in up to 60 percent of cases.[277,278] The Jamaican cohort study reported an annual incidence of 0.5 cases per 100 HbSS subjects versus 2.5 cases per 100 HbSC subjects. Prevalence was greater in HbSC subjects as well, with a 43 percent rate in the third decade versus 14 percent for those with HbSS. However, there was a 32 percent incidence of spontaneous regression. Irreversible visual loss occurred only in 2 percent of HbSC subjects up to 26 years of age observed at time of the study.[277]

Central retinal artery occlusion is rare in HbSS disease.[279] Conjunctival vascularity is decreased in SCD patients compared to controls with further decreased vascularity and decreased conjunctival red cell velocities during vasoocclusion.[280–283]

An orbital compression syndrome characterized by fever, headache, orbital swelling, and visual impairment secondary to optic nerve dysfunction can occur in SCD. Orbital marrow infarction is a common cause.[284]

All patients with sickle hemoglobinopathies should have a yearly ophthalmology examination beginning in childhood. The examination should be carried out by an ophthalmologist and should include slit-lamp examination of the anterior chamber and detailed retinal visualization including a fluorescein angiography in addition to visual acuity.

The evaluation and treatment of proliferative sickle retinopathy is complicated by the fact that spontaneous regression may occur. Laser photocoagulation remains the most commonly performed procedure for this finding. Traumatic hyphema needs urgent optical referral because increased sickle red cells can cause obstruction of outflow channels, resulting in acute glaucoma. This vascular obstruction may cause decrease in retinal and optic nerve perfusion causing further visual problems. Unresolved vitreous hemorrhage and retinal detachment may need surgical intervention. Exchange transfusion to keep HbA at more than 50 percent is recommended. Central retinal artery occlusion needs urgent exchange transfusion and an ophthalmology consultation.[277,285–287] Orbital compression syndrome is treated with glucocorticoids with the addition of antibiotics if concomitant infection cannot be ruled out.[126]

Splenic Complications

Functional asplenia defined as impaired mononuclear phagocyte system functions in the spleen occurs in 86 percent of infants with SCD.[288] It is defined by the presence of Howell-Jolly bodies and absence of [99m]Tc (99m-technetium) splenic uptake, even in the presence of a palpable spleen. Slow blood flow in the red pulp of the spleen sets the stage for increased red cell sickling. Repeated splenic infarctions lead to "autosplenectomy." As a consequence, patients are prone to microbial infections, especially with encapsulated microorganisms such as *S. pneumoniae*, *Haemophilus influenzae*, and *Neisseria meningitidis*. Hypertransfusion early in childhood, prior to age 7 years, may lead to reversal of functional asplenia. Marrow transplantation and hydroxyurea have resulted in reversal of functional asplenia in some older subjects. Splenic sequestration occurs in young children.[289–293]

Management during Pregnancy

Differing morbidity and mortality rates have been reported in pregnant women with SCD, some of which is attributed to geographic location and access to healthcare. Although the CSSCD data showed low rates of pregnancy loss and mortality, other studies have shown an increased mortality of 10 to 100 orders of magnitude greater as compared to non-SCD patients.[285–290] Preterm delivery occurs in 30 to 50 percent of SCD patients and two-thirds will have infants with birth weights less than the 50th percentile.[294,295] There is an increased frequency of VOEs reported during pregnancy. In a study looking at pregnancy outcomes in SCD patients compared to non-SCD patients with comorbidities, patients with SCD displayed a significantly increased incidence of venous thromboembolism (VTE), nonhemorrhagic obstetric shock (defined as pulmonary thromboembolism, amniotic fluid embolism, acute uterine inversion, and sepsis), and infection, despite being significantly younger.[296,297] Other studies have shown similar findings, especially the fivefold increased risk of VTE in this population.[295,297,298]

Given increased risk of preeclampsia and eclampsia, patients should have close monitoring of blood pressure and proteinuria after 20 weeks of gestation. Fetal nonstress and umbilical artery Doppler studies should be undertaken after 28 weeks to identify patients who might benefit from early delivery. Studies examining prophylactic red cell transfusions in pregnancy have shown mixed results. Patients should be transfused to a Hb concentration of less than 6 g/dL, because abnormal fetal oxygenation and death have been reported below this Hb level in non-SCD populations. Otherwise, patients should be transfused based on guidelines for the nonpregnant patient with SCD.[294] Based on data from animal models and small reports of spontaneous abortion or fetal death, the use of hydroxyurea is not recommended during pregnancy and breastfeeding.[299,300] Hydroxyurea may decrease spermatogenesis and therefore male patients may need to stop the drug temporarily when their partners are trying to conceive. Narcotics administered for relief of pain have not been shown to cause fetal harm, but babies of mothers exposed to narcotics during pregnancy should be monitored for the neonatal abstinence syndrome.[294]

Despite increased concern for VTE, given insufficient data, contraception advice is similar as for women without SCD.[301]

Management of and Prevention of Infection

Patients with SCD are predisposed to infections for a variety of reasons, including functional asplenia and defective neutrophil responses.[302–306] The magnitude of this problem was highlighted in 1971 in a landmark paper by E. Barrett-Connor.[306] Functional asplenia results in susceptibility to encapsulated microorganisms, particularly to *S. pneumoniae*, especially in children younger than 5 years of age. The CSSCD data reported an eight-per-100-patient-years rate of invasive bacterial infection in children younger than 3 years of age.[307]

Given the high incidence of infection, especially in childhood, infection prevention and rapid diagnosis of established infections is of paramount importance.[308,309] The pneumococcal vaccine (PCV7) can be administered in infancy with effective immunologic response prior to 2 years of age; the American Academy of Pediatrics recommends it be administered at ages 2, 4, 6, 8, and 12 to 15 months. The PCV7 vaccine decreases invasive pneumococcal disease by as much as 80 to 90 percent.[310] The pneumococcal polysaccharide vaccine, PPV23, covers more serotypes but is not immunogenic prior to 24 months and response lasts for 3 years. The first dose is recommended at 24 months with additional doses 3 to 5 years later.[309,311–314] Nonvaccine covered strains of *S. pneumoniae* are emerging as important pathogens; therefore, prompt referral of patients with suspected infection to a healthcare facility is important.[315]

Oral penicillin prophylaxis is recommended at a dose of 125 mg twice a day for children between 0 and 3 years of age and at 250 mg twice a day for children between 3 and 5 years of age.[316] Penicillin prophylaxis beyond 5 years is recommended only for patients with recurrent pneumococcal infections or who have had surgical splenectomy. Patients allergic to penicillin are offered erythromycin.

The meningococcal vaccine covers most invasive isolates of *N. meningitidis* and is recommended by the American Academy of Pediatrics.[317] Standard pediatric immunizations protecting against

H. influenzae and hepatitis B virus should be given. Influenza virus vaccine should be given annually because viral respiratory infection favors invasive bacterial infection.

Parents and caregivers of children should be educated to recognize infections and to seek medical attention early. Diagnosis of established infections varies by site and offending agent. For invasive pneumococcal disease, ceftriaxone remains the drug of choice despite concerns of immune-mediated hemolysis. Infections seen classically in SCD patients include salmonella osteomyelitis and penumonia caused by atypical bacteria like *Chlamydia* and *M. pneumoniae*, which need to be treated with the appropriate antibiotics.

The spectrum of infectious complications in adults may be different. One study reported data on blood infections in adults.[302] Pneumococcal infections were rare. *S. aureus* was the predominant organism. Patients with *S. aureus* had a predilection for bone-joint infection. Those with indwelling venous catheters and a severe disease course appeared to have a high risk for bloodstream infections.

Although the sickle trait confers resistance to malaria, protection is not complete and severe disease and deaths from malaria have been reported in SCD patients. Malaria chemoprophylaxis is recommended for all patients living in or traveling to endemic regions.[318,319]

Management during Anesthesia and Surgery

Patients with SCD should have careful monitoring of Hb concentration, hydration, oxygen, and metabolic studies in the perioperative period. Acute chest syndrome and VOE occur with higher frequency in the perioperative period. Increased age is associated with increased complications.[320–322] Transfusion to keep Hb levels approximately 10 g/dL is recommended. Although a prior randomized trial showed no benefit in decreasing SCD-related complications between patients transfused aggressively to a mean HbS of less than 30 percent versus those transfused to a total Hb of 10 g/dL with mean HbS percent of 59, more recent data show reduction in clinically important events, especially serious complications, in the preoperative transfused group prior to low and moderate risk surgery.[202,323] Care should be taken to avoid transfusion-induced hyperviscosity.

MODIFIERS OF DISEASE SEVERITY

Some patients have a mild course with few problems related to SCD, and survive into the sixth or seventh decade. In contrast, some patients have a difficult course with multiple complications, frequent hospitalizations, severe organ damage, and a significantly shortened life expectancy.[324,325] Inheritance of α-thalassemia trait and a high HbF are two factors that ameliorate many complications of SCD. Genome-wide association studies revealed three major loci associated with HbF levels: The β-globin locus on chromosome 11, an intergenic region between *HBSIL* and *MYB* genes on chromosome 6, and the *BCL11* gene on chromosome 2.[326] Repression of BCL11A results in increased γ-globin gene expression and, consequently, in increased HbF. The exact mechanism of how BCL11A silences γ-globin expression is unclear; its expression seems to be controlled by an erythroid specific transcription factor, KLF1 with decreased expression of BCL11A upon knockdown of *KLF1* gene transcript.[326,327]

Inheritance of α-thalassemia and HbF level do not account for all of the clinical diversity of SCD. The completion of the human genome project has provided the impetus to study polymorphisms in candidate genes as potential modifiers of disease severity. Association of polymorphisms in candidate genes and different features of SCD such as stroke,[328–330] ACS,[331] bilirubin levels and cholelithiasis,[332–335] avascular necrosis,[245] priapism,[336] and leg ulcers,[253] as well as HbF levels,[337–342] and HbF response to hydroxyurea,[343] have been studied in different groups of patients.

Polymorphisms in the TGF-β–BMP pathway, a ubiquitous signaling pathway that is involved in many cellular processes and pathways, have emerged as recurrent findings in many of these studies. Some of the associations have functional consequences; the association of bilirubin levels in polymorphisms in the *UGT1A1* gene promoter is such an example. The 7TA repeat in the promoter leads to a decreased activity of this enzyme and hence a decrease in glucuronidation of bilirubin. Thus, the association of this polymorphism with higher bilirubin levels can be understood. On the other hand, the mechanisms by which polymorphisms in the ubiquitous TGF-β–BMP pathway are associated with various complications of SCD are unknown, and thus a causal relationship cannot yet be established. Functional studies of these variants and genomewide association studies are expected to provide a better insight into genetic modulation of the phenotype of SCD.

GENERAL MANAGEMENT OF SICKLE CELL DISEASE

Pharmacotherapeutics to Increase Fetal Hemoglobin Levels

The observation that HbF results in ameliorating the phenotype of SCD led to research focused on HbF modulation as a therapy for SCD. The γ-chains of HbF are excluded from the deoxy HbS polymer; thus the presence of HbF in sickle red cells exerts a potent antisickling effect. This effect has also been supported by clinical observations; the manifestations of SCD do not become apparent in the first few months of life until the switch from γ-chain production to β-chain production is almost complete in the postnatal period. Additionally, the phenotypes of some compound heterozygous states with HbS and other inherited globin disorders that lead to increased expression of HbF in the adult life ($\delta\beta$-thalassemias, hereditary persistence of HbF) are very mild (Chap. 47). In fact, compound heterozygotes for HbS and deletional hereditary persistence of HbF, in which there is continued high levels of HbF expression (30 to 35 percent) uniformly distributed in all red cells (pancellular), are clinically asymptomatic and hematologically normal. In the late 1970s, further evidence in support of the ameliorating effect of high HbF came from the observation of Saudi Arabian sickle cell anemia patients who had few, if any, symptoms of SCD, had mild anemia, and were not diagnosed until adult age.[344] These individuals had HbF levels in the 20 to 25 percent range as opposed to the African patients or American patients of African descent, the majority of whom had HbF levels of approximately 5 percent. Similar patients were reported from India, and this genetic propensity for high HbF production in SCD patients was linked to a unique β-globin gene cluster haplotype (Saudi Arabian–Indian) that is distinct from those found in Africa. These observations paved the way for intense investigations on the cellular and molecular mechanisms of the fetal to adult (γ to β) switch during the perinatal period and the search for "antiswitching" agents, agents that would facilitate retaining elevated HbF levels. The observation that there is a transient increase in HbF production during recovery from marrow aplasia or suppression provided the rationale for the use of myelosuppressive agents as *antiswitching* therapy (Table 49–3). Antiswitching indicates a mechanism to prevent the switch from γ-globin chains to β-globin chains.

Hydroxyurea Although many myelosuppressive agents have been studied in primates and some have been used in a small number of patients, only one of these, hydroxyurea, has been used, starting in the early 1980s, in large-scale clinical trials. This is largely attributable to its excellent oral bioavailability, relatively short half-life (important from the standpoint of rapid reversibility of toxicity), no evidence that its use leads to an increase in cancer prevalence, and few side effects.

Hydroxyurea is the only FDA-approved agent for the treatment of SCD. It is a ribonucleotide reductase inhibitor and is S-phase specific

TABLE 49–3. Antiswitching Therapies

Drug	Mechanism
Hydroxyurea	Myelosuppression
	Antiinflammatory
	Nitric oxide donor
	Increased cyclic guanosine monophosphate
Decitabine	DNA methyltransferase 1 inhibition, i.e., hypomethylation
5′-Azacitidine	DNA methyltransferase 1 inhibition, i.e., hypomethylation
Butyrate derivatives	Histone deacetylase inhibition
Histone deacetylase inhibitors	Histone deacetylase inhibition
Immunomodulatory drugs	P38 mitogen-activated protein kinase pathway

in the cell cycle. The mechanism by which hydroxyurea increases HbF synthesis is not fully understood; it has been postulated that the myelosuppressive effect leads to the recruitment of early erythroid progenitors that have retained their fetal (γ) globin synthesis capability, giving rise to the production of red cells with a higher HbF content. Some studies show that hydroxyurea acts as a NO donor and increases HbF synthesis via the cyclic guanosine monophosphate (cGMP) pathway.[345] Others suggest it works by reducing the neutrophil count, thereby reducing the contributions of neutrophils to the abnormal vascular adhesion of sickle red cells. It has several other actions that explain its efficacy in SCD other than increasing HbF. These include decrease in platelets and reticulocytes, improvement in red cell hydration, and a decrease in red cell adhesiveness to the vascular endothelium (Fig. 49–10).[346–348]

In the landmark Multicenter Study of Hydroxyurea, hydroxyurea was shown to decrease frequency of painful crises, ACS, hospitalizations, and blood transfusions. Followup showed a 40 percent decrease in mortality in patients randomized to the drug.[160,349] Hydroxyurea is recommended in patients with three or more VOEs or history of ACS. It can be started at a dose of 15 mg/kg given as a single daily dose and escalated by 5 mg/kg per day every 8 weeks until toxicity or a maximum dose of 35 mg/kg is reached. *Maximum tolerated dose* is defined as the dose that targets an absolute neutrophil count of 2 to 4×10^9/L and absolute reticulocyte count 100 to 200×10^9/L.[350,351] Periodic monitoring of blood cell counts and serum chemistries, especially in the first year of treatment is important. Maximal effect on HbF may not be seen until 6 to 12 months of therapy is completed. The dose should be decreased in renal failure. Although not proven to have teratogenic or leukemogenic potential in SCD patients, it is recommended that it not be used in pregnant or breastfeeding patients. Concerns about detrimental effect on spermatogenesis have also been raised based on studies in mice.[352–355]

Patients receiving hydroxyurea who die while on treatment are likely to be older when therapy is initiated, more anemic, likely to have Bantu or Cameron β-globin gene haplotypes, and have impaired renal function.[324]

Several studies have now been published on the use of hydroxyurea in infants and children. Therapy can begin between 6 and 9 months of age, is safe and well tolerated with improved growth rates, preserves organ function, and the additional benefits as seen in adults.[161,351,356,357]

Other Fetal Hemoglobin-Inducing Agents Although significant advances have been made in understanding the basic mechanism(s) of the perinatal switch from γ- to β-globin synthesis, this knowledge is

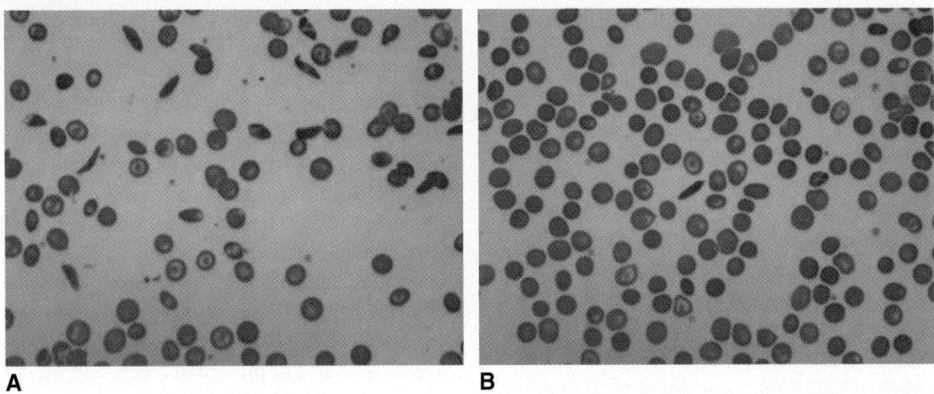

Figure 49–10. Blood film from SCD patients: effect of hydroxyurea therapy. **A.** Blood film before therapy. Note frequent sickled cells. **B.** Marked decrease in sickle cells with therapy. *(Reproduced with permission from Dr. Scott Drury and Dr. Elizabeth Manaloor, Department of Pathology, Medical College of Georgia.)*

far from complete. Certain epigenetic mechanisms (histone deacetylation and DNA methylation) are involved in the silencing of the γ-globin genes postnatally. This has led to the use of agents that target the two common epigenetic silencing mechanisms: histone deacetylase inhibitors and DNA methyltransferase 1 inhibitors.

The histone deacetylase inhibitors that have been most widely used in early phase small clinical trials in SCD and in some patients with β-thalassemia are butyrate derivatives (arginine butyrate, sodium phenyl butyrate, isobutyramide). Arginine butyrate has to be administered by IV infusion; earlier studies suggested that continuous daily infusions of arginine butyrate were not very effective in leading to a sustained increase in HbF.[258] Later, it was shown that daily continuous infusion induced tachyphylaxis and hence the failure to cause a sustained HbF response. An intermittent schedule of administration (4 days, given every 4 weeks) was efficacious in increasing HbF.[358] Although orally administered sodium phenyl butyrate was effective in increasing HbF, the daily doses required for maintaining a HbF response required the administration of a large number of tablets and was impractical.[359] A phase II trial studying the efficacy of oral 2,2-dimethylbutyrate sodium salt (HQK1001) did not show significant increase in HbF and was associated with a trend for increased VOE.[360]

The two DNA methyltransferase inhibitors with antiswitching activity are 5′-azacytidine and decitabine. Both of these agents are myelosuppressive when used in higher doses; however, at low doses, they are potent inhibitors of DNA methyltransferase 1 and have been shown to increase HbF synthesis in baboons and in patients with SCD.[361-368] Unlike 5′-azacytidine, which incorporates into both DNA and RNA, decitabine incorporates only in DNA and is believed to have a better genotoxicity profile. It has been effective in increasing HbF and ameliorating the disease severity in patients with SCD who have been refractory to hydroxyurea.[363]

Immunomodulatory agents (thalidomide and derivatives) increase HbF synthesis in erythroid colonies from SCD patients.[369] Pomalidomide augments HbF in sickle cell mice.[370] Data from use in sickle cell patients is awaited. The finding that the KLF-1–BCL11a axis is the major factor in the switch from β- to γ-globin has made these factors attractive targets for therapy; however, to date, no effective means of targeting these transcription factors has been developed.

Allogeneic Hematopoietic Stem Cell Transplantation
Because SCD is an inherited defect in the hematopoietic stem cell, stem cell transplantation (SCT) is an attractive option to permanently cure the disease rather than managing its sequelae piecemeal. However, the

tremendous phenotypic variability that characterizes the disorder combined with lack of an accurate predictive model to foretell which patients are likely to have a catastrophic disease course, make selecting patients for allogeneic hematopoietic stem cell transplantation (AHSCT) challenging. AHSCT should be done in patients who are likely to have a severe disease course, but should be instituted early, prior to end-organ damage. The risk-to-benefit ratio of the morbidity and mortality associated with AHSCT has to be weighed against the disease severity of a nonmalignant hematologic disorder.

AHSCT is an underused treatment modality in SCD even in eligible patients secondary to lack of donor availability and socioeconomic factors.[371] Human leukocyte antigen (HLA)–matched sibling donor transplant with myeloablative conditioning represents the most common transplant type in SCD. Cerebrovascular disease, recurrent ACS, and frequent VOEs despite adequate hydroxyurea therapy are the most common indications for SCT. Data from approximately 1200 patients worldwide show an overall survival of 95 percent; early or late allograft failure resulting in disease recurrence occurs in 10 to 15 percent of patients.[371,372] The most common myeloablative regimen used is busulfan, cyclophosphamide, and antithymocyte globulin; the addition of antithymocyte globulin resulted in a significant reduction in allograft rejection. Transplant-related mortality ranges between 2 and 8 percent.[372] Acute graft-versus-host disease occurs in approximately 10 to 15 percent of patients, whereas chronic graft-versus-host disease has been reported in 12 to 20 percent of patients. Most series have used cyclosporine alone or in combination with methotrexate for graft-versus-host disease prophylaxis (Chap. 21).

Risk of increased incidence of neurologic complications following transplantation has been ameliorated with the use of prophylactic anticonvulsants, strict control of arterial hypertension, correction of hypomagnesemia, and maintenance of Hb greater than 10 g/dL and platelets greater than 50×10^9/L. Long-term toxicity still remains a concern, especially in relation to growth, reproduction, and secondary malignancies. Followup data on AHSCT in children between 1991 and 2000 show significant gonadal toxicity and infertility, especially in females.[373]

AHSCT in adults is problematic given toxicity of the conditioning regimen. In an attempt to address this issue, reduced-intensity conditioning has been used but has resulted in an increased rate of graft failure. A small cohort of patients who received blood stem cells from HLA-matched siblings and used low-dose total-body radiation plus alemtuzumab as the conditioning regimen followed by sirolimus for graft-versus-host disease prophylaxis had stable engraftment at 30 months of followup.[374]

Cord blood and HLA haploidentical transplantation have been used in a small number of patients with SCD, but graft failure remains a significant issue.[371,375,376]

Transfusion

Red cell transfusions are used frequently in SCD on an acute or chronic basis. The rationale for transfusion in SCD is twofold. Besides increasing Hb concentration, thereby increasing the oxygen-carrying capacity of the blood, transfusion also decreases the percentage of circulating HbS-containing red cells. Hb level alone should not constitute an indication to transfusion as patients adapt to their level, making it important to know the patient's baseline Hb concentration. It is also important to calculate whether the reticulocyte count, a measure of marrow red cell production, is adequate or not.

Indications for red cell transfusion include symptomatic anemia, ACS, stroke, aplastic and sequestration crises, other major organ damage secondary to vasoocclusion, and occurrence of unrelenting priapism. Transfusion is also required prior to major surgery or surgery involving critical organs. The best-established indication for chronic transfusion is stroke and an abnormal TCD velocity. Patients with other chronic or recurrent events are sometimes placed on chronic transfusion as well. Inappropriate indications for transfusion include chronic steady-state anemia, uncomplicated VOE, pregnancy, minor surgeries, infection, and avascular necrosis.[377]

Simple red cell or exchange transfusion can be used.[378] Simple transfusion is easier to perform and is generally associated with fewer complications. Exchange transfusion, however, has the advantage of not raising total Hb, and thereby blood viscosity, while decreasing percentage of circulating sickle cells because sickle cell patients transport less oxygen to their tissues beyond a hematocrit of 30 percent as a result of increased blood viscosity.[379–381] Exchange transfusion has also the advantage of not causing iron overload.

Alloimmunization occurs in 20 to 50 percent of transfused SCD patients.[382–384] In the United States, the majority of blood donors are of European descent, and the majority of SCD patients are of African descent (Chaps. 136 and 138). This results in blood group antigenic disparity, and antibodies to E, C, K, Jkb, S, and Fyb antigens are common. Age at first transfusion, total number of transfusions, transfusion in the context of inflammation, and influence of immunoregulatory genes may affect the rate and extent of alloimmunization.[384] Extended antigen phenotyping (Kell, Duffy, Kidd, Lewis, Lutheran, P, and M&S) in addition to the usual ABO and D antigens (Chaps. 136 and 138) and leukodepletion of blood products are recommended.[378,382,384,385] Delayed hemolytic transfusion reaction complicates 4 to 11 percent[386] of transfusions in SCD and may present as a painful crises. It typically occurs a week after transfusion and is caused by alloantibodies to non-ABO antigens. It can cause the Hb to fall lower than the prior pretransfusion Hb and can be associated with a depressed reticulocyte count and autoantibodies. Alloantibody mediated hemolysis will present as a rapid decrease in the percent of HbA as opposed to HbS. A failure to demonstrate a new alloantibody posttransfusion should not exclude the diagnosis of delayed hemolytic transfusion reaction (Chaps. 136 and 138). Patients should be transfused only if symptomatic under such circumstances as further transfusion can exacerbate the problem.[377,384]

Iron overload and its attendant complications and infection transmission are the other major complications of transfusion.

Iron Overload

Iron overload (Chap. 43) in SCD is similar to other chronically transfused populations.[169,387,388] The multicenter study of the iron overload research group showed that transfused sickle cell patients had increased morbidity and mortality when compared to transfused thalassemic patients and nontransfused SCD patients.[389]

Diagnosing significant iron overload accurately and early can be difficult. Serum ferritin is an easy, widely employed method, but is unreliable in SCD as it is an acute phase reactant. Its measurement can result in over- or underestimation and is poorly correlated to liver iron content.[390] A serum ferritin value of greater than 1000 mg/mL in the steady-state has been used as an indication of iron overload. Liver iron content is the current accepted standard and a value of 7.7 mg/g dry weight is used as indication for treatment.[391] However, noninvasive methods of assessment of iron overload, like superconducting quantum interference device (SQUID) or MRI T2* (Chap. 43), are becoming standard. Transfusion of 120 mL of red blood cells/kg of body weight can also be used as a chelation trigger.[382]

Iron chelation (Chap. 43) was typically carried out with desferrioxamine at a dose of 25 to 40 mg/kg per day given over 8 hours subcutaneously.[392] Desferrioxamine can reverse cardiac iron overload. A once-daily oral iron chelator, deferasirox, is now approved and available for use in the United States. It is a tridentate ligand that binds iron with a high affinity in a 2:1 ratio. It has a half-life of 8 to 16 hours and is metabolized by glucuronidation and excreted in the feces. In an open-label phase II trial of deferasirox versus desferrioxamine in a 2:1 randomization, safety and tolerability were established. Nausea and vomiting, abdominal pain, rash, reversible increase in liver function tests, and stable increases in serum creatinine were reported. Rare cases of anaphylaxis occurring mostly in the first month of starting treatment have also been reported. Postmarketing reports suggest an increased incidence of renal failure, and caution is to be exercised in a patient population where renal insufficiency may not be readily appreciated prior to starting treatment. Postmarketing experience has also reported cases of fatal hepatotoxicity and agranulocytosis. Auditory and ophthalmic side effects occur in less than 1 percent of patients; however, annual eye and auditory examinations are recommended for deferasirox as they are for desferrioxamine. The recommended daily dose is 20 mg/kg body weight; this dose may be adjusted every 3 to 5 months in increments of 5 to 10 mg/kg if the therapeutic goal is not achieved, although the total dose should not exceed 40 mg/kg. Safety in combination with other iron chelators has not been established.[393] Deferiprone is not available in the United States but has been used in other parts of the world. It is orally administered and is considered a better chelator of cardiac iron because of its ability to cross cell membranes.[394] Although iron chelation in SCD follows the general guidelines of iron chelation in other iron overloaded populations, rigorous studies of its effects on morbidity and mortality in SCD are lacking.[394,395]

Evolving Therapies

Given the complex pathophysiology of SCD, numerous therapies targeting different pathways have been tried to ameliorate disease manifestations. Many drugs have failed to show efficacy, especially in phase II/III trials, because of failure to choose appropriate end points or because they were too narrowly focused. Table 49–4 is a comprehensive list of trials and their outcomes. A few of the novel and promising studies are with immunomodulatory agents (thalidomide/pomalidomide), E- and P-selectin inhibitors, iNKT agonists, and Aes-103, and all are in trials as of this writing.

● OTHER ABNORMAL HEMOGLOBINS

The number of Hb variants discovered to the time of writing this chapter totals 1187. The vast majority of these variants are benign, without any significant clinical or hematologic problems, but are of interest to geneticists and biochemists (http://globin.cse.psu.edu). Most of the

TABLE 49–4. Novel Therapies for Sickle Cell Disease

Drug	Mechanism of Action	Pathway Targeted in SCD	Trial Phase/Type	Number Enrolled	Outcomes	Ref.
GMI1070	E-selectin inhibitor	Abnormal cell adhesiveness	I	15	Decrease in coagulation, leukocyte, and endothelial cell activation	412
Aes-103	Allosteric modifier of Hb	RBC sickling, membrane stabilization under shear stress	I/IIa	18	Decrease in pain and markers of RBC sickling	
Regadenoson	iNKT A_2A receptor agonist	Inflammation	I	27	Safety demonstrated; iNKT cells inhibited	413,414
Omega-3 fatty acid	Reduction in oxidative injury	Abnormal cell adhesiveness	RCT	140	Decreased VOE, anemia, and blood transfusion in supplemented group	415
Arginine	Increased NO production	NO signaling	RCT	38	Decreased parenteral opioids use and pain scores	416
Magnesium sulfate	Increased cellular hydration	Cellular dehydration	RCT	106	No difference on LOS, pain scores, or analgesia use	417
Prasugrel	P2Y12 ADP receptor antagonist	Platelet activation	II	62	Pain rate and intensity decreased in intervention; platelet activation biomarkers decreased	418
Eptifibatide	Platelet $\alpha_{IIb}\beta_3$ inhibitor	Platelet activation	RCT	13	Safe but no difference in VOE resolution	419
Senicapoc	Gardos channel inhibitor	Cellular dehydration	III	144	Increased hemoglobin and hematocrit and decreased erythrocytes and reticulocytes	420
Poloxamer 188	Amphipathic copolymer	Tissue oxygenation	III	255	Safe and well tolerated and demonstrated crisis resolution in a percentage of patients (greater in children than adults)	421
TRF-1101	P-selectin inhibitor	Abnormal cell adhesiveness	II	5	Safe and increased microvascular blood flow	422

ADP, adenosine diphosphate; Hb, hemoglobin; iNKT, invariant natural killer T cell; LOS, length of stay; NO, nitric oxide; RBC, red blood cell; RCT, randomized controlled trial; SCD, sickle cell disease; VOE, vasoocclusive episode.

Hb variants are missense mutations in the globin genes (α, β, γ, or δ) resulting from single nucleotide substitutions. Other uncommon mechanisms include deletion or insertion of one or more nucleotides altering the reading frame and fusion of globin genes with deletion of intergenic DNA sequences ($\gamma\beta$ fusion in Hb_{Kenya} and $\delta\beta$ fusion in Hb_{Lepore}), mutations of the termination codon leading to the production of elongated globin chains.

Hb variants that significantly alter the structure, stability, synthesis, or function of the molecule have hematologic and/or clinical consequences. These can be classified in certain categories (Table 49–5). HbS and HbC are two examples of mutations on the surface of the Hb molecule that alter both the charge and the physical/chemical properties of the molecule with polymer formation in the case of deoxyhemoglobin S and crystallization in HbC with profound effects on the function, morphology, rheology, and life span of the red cells. Several mechanisms account for the pathogenesis of unstable Hb variants. The common mechanism involves the precipitation of the unstable Hb molecule within the red cell with attachment to the inner layer of the red cell membrane ("Heinz body" formation); red cells containing

membrane-attached Heinz bodies (see Chap. 31, Fig. 31–11) have impaired deformability and filterability leading to their premature destruction (congenital Heinz body hemolytic anemia). Mutations in certain residues alter the oxygen affinity of the Hb molecule; a stabilization of the R (relaxed, oxy) state will result in high O_2 affinity variants and erythrocytosis. Conversely, a stabilization of the T (tense, deoxy) configuration will result in a variant with low O_2 affinity with enhanced unloading of O_2 to the tissues with resultant cyanosis and anemia in certain cases (because of the suppression of the O_2 sensing pathway) (Chaps. 32 and 50). Mutations of the heme binding site, particularly those affecting the conserved proximal (F8) and distal (E7) histidine residues, lead to the oxidation of the iron atom in heme from ferrous (Fe^{2+}) to ferric (Fe^{3+}) state with resultant methemoglobinemia (M Hbs) and cyanosis (Chap. 50). A group of mutations alter both the structure and the synthetic rate of the globin chain leading to a "thalassemic" phenotype (Chap. 48). These include fusion Hbs (e.g., Hb_{Lepore}, where the 5' δ-globin sequences are fused to 3' β-globin sequences with deletion of the intergenic DNA; this puts the $\delta\beta$-fusion gene under the transcriptional control of the inefficient δ-globin promoter with low expression

TABLE 49–5. Clinically Significant Hemoglobin Variants

I. Altered physical/chemical properties

   A. HbS (deoxyhemoglobin S polymerization): sickle syndromes

   B. HbC (crystallization): hemolytic anemia; microcytosis

II. Unstable hemoglobin variants:

   A. Congenital Heinz body hemolytic anemia (N = 135)

III. Variants with altered oxygen affinity

   A. High-affinity variants: erythrocytosis (N = 92)

   B. Low-affinity variants: anemia, cyanosis

IV. M hemoglobins

   A. Methemoglobinemia, cyanosis (N = 9)

V. Variants causing a thalassemic phenotype (N = 50)

   A. β-Thalassemia

     1. Hb_{Lepore} ($\delta\beta$) fusion (N = 3)

     2. Aberrant RNA processing (HbE, $Hb_{Knossos}$, Hb_{Malay})

     3. Hyperunstable globins (Hb_{Geneva}, $Hb_{Westdale}$, etc.)

   B. α-Thalassemia

     1. Chain termination mutants ($Hb_{Constant\ Spring}$)

     2. Hyperunstable variants ($Hb_{Quong\ Sze}$)

Data from Bunn HF, Forget BG: *Hemoglobin: Molecular, Genetic, and Clinical Aspects.* Philadelphia, PA: WB Saunders; 1986.

of the fusion globin (hence the thalassemic phenotype), mutations that cause both a missense mutation and create an aberrant splice site (such as HbE, $Hb_{Knossos}$, and Hb_{Malay}), and "hyperunstable" globins where the nascent globin chains are highly unstable, undergo rapid proteolytic degradation, and result in a reduction in the affected globin.

Except for the commonly occurring variants (HbS, HbC, HbE, and $HbD_{Los\ Angeles}$), very few abnormal Hbs have been observed in the homozygous state. Variant Hbs are usually found in the heterozygous state. Although γ-chain variants are expressed in fetal life and their level gradually decreases as the γ-globin to β-globin (fetal to adult) switch progresses during the postnatal period, β- and α-chain variants are expressed throughout life. δ-Globin variants are expressed at very low levels and can be detected only after the switch to adult globin synthesis is complete. Because α-globin chains are present in all of the Hbs expressed after the embryonic stage (HbF-$\alpha_2\gamma_2$; HbA-$\alpha_2\beta_2$, and HbA$_2$-$\alpha_2\delta_2$), α-chain variants are associated with the production of variant HbF ($\alpha_2^x\gamma_2$) and HbA$_2$ ($\alpha_2^x\delta_2$) as well. In heterozygous states, β-chain variants constitute 40 to 50 percent of the Hb in red cells; it should, however, be kept in mind that certain factors affect the amount of variant β chains in carriers. These factors include the stability of the variant, the surface charge of the variant β-chain, and the presence of concomitant α- or β-thalassemia (Chap. 48). The more unstable the variant, the lower the quantity. Surface charge of the variant also plays a role in determining the quantity in red cells; this is because the formation of the $\alpha\beta$-dimers ($\alpha_1\beta_1$ and $\alpha_2\beta_2$ contacts) is the critical first step in Hb tetramer formation, and this step is primarily driven by electrostatic interactions between α and β chains. The α-globin chains have a relatively positive surface charge, they interact more readily with relatively negatively charged β-globin variants to form $\alpha\beta$ dimers. This is reflected in the higher percentage of negatively charged β-globin variants such as $HbN_{Baltimore}$ ($\beta95Lys{\rightarrow}Glu$), which is found in approximately 50 percent in heterozygotes compared to β-globin variants with a positive surface charge, HbS ($\beta6Glu{\rightarrow}Val$) or HbC ($\beta6Glu{\rightarrow}Lys$) whose quantity in the

heterozygote is 40 to 45 percent. In the presence of α-thalassemia, negatively charged β-globin variants compete more favorably for the available α-chains; this phenomenon is reflected in even lower percentages of HbS and HbC in heterozygous carriers of these variants in the presence of common deletional forms of α-thalassemia (HbS of 30 to 35 percent in individuals with heterozygous α^+-thalassemia, $-\alpha/\alpha\alpha$; and 25 to 30 percent in homozygous α^+-thalassemia, $-\alpha/-\alpha$).[396,397] Conversely, the amount of a β-globin variant will increase if there is a β-thalassemia allele in *trans*; the percentage of the variant will be inversely proportional to the output of the β-thalassemia allele; thus, the higher the variant the lower the output of the β^+-thalassemia allele. In the case of a β^0-thalassemia allele in *trans*, the variant will amount to greater than 90 percent or more of the Hb in red cells, with HbA$_2$ and HbF constituting the remainder. The quantity of α-globin variants is also variable, depending on the α-globin gene involved, and the presence of concomitant α- or β-thalassemia. Because there are normally four α-globin loci ($\alpha\alpha/\alpha\alpha$) and the upstream 5' α-globin gene (α_2) is expressed at a higher level, some of the variation in the level of α-globin variants depends on which α-globin gene carries the mutation; α_2-globin mutations are usually present at 20 to 25 percent of the total Hb, whereas 3' downstream α_1-globin variants are expressed at a lower level (15 to 20 percent). Concomitant α-thalassemia results in a higher level of expression of α-globin variants. Observations on the different levels of expression of the common α-globin variant, $HbG_{Philadelphia}$ ($\alpha68Asn{\rightarrow}Lys$), is a case in point.[398] Although this variant is found in approximately 25 percent of Northern Italians, its percentages in Americans of African descent can be either 33 or approximately 50 percent. This is clearly related to the different genotypes found in these two distinct populations: In northern Italy and Sardinia, the genotype is $\alpha^G\alpha/\alpha\alpha$, with an expression level of approximately 30 percent, whereas in Americans of African descent, the $HbG_{Philadelphia}$ mutation is commonly found on a hybrid $\alpha_2\alpha_1$ gene associated with the common 3.7 kb α^+-thalassemia deletion ($-\alpha^G/\alpha\alpha$) with approximately 33 percent expression. When there is an α^+-thalassemia deletion in *trans* ($-\alpha^G/-\alpha$ genotype), as expected, the level of $HbG_{Philadelphia}$ will be approximately 50 percent. Coinheritance of α-chain variants with β-thalassemia results in the increase of the α-chain variant.

HEMOGLOBIN C DISEASE

Definition and History

HbC was the second Hb variant described after HbS.[399] Homozygous HbC was described by Spaet and colleagues[400] and Ranney and colleagues.[401] HbC trait is found in 2 percent of Americans of African descent, and approximately one in 6000 have homozygous HbC.[402] Coinheritance of HbC with HbS results in HbSC disease, which is the second most common form of SCD in the United States. There are also rare cases of HbC-β^+-thalassemia and HbC–β^0-thalassemia. HbC is thought to have originated in Central West Africa and in parts of West Africa, where the prevalence of HbC can reach 12.5 percent. The HbC gene was found on three distinct β-globin cluster haplotypes, termed CI, CII, and CIII; the most common is CI, accounting for 70 percent or more of HbC studied.[403]

Etiology and Pathogenesis

HbC is the result of a GAG$\rightarrow$AAG transition in codon 6 of the β-globin gene, which changes the amino acid residue at this position from glutamic acid to lysine (Glu$\rightarrow$Lys). The resultant positively charged Hb variant can easily be distinguished from HbA and HbS by electrophoresis and chromatography, including high-performance liquid chromatography. HbC does not differ from HbA in its solubility; however, purified solutions of HbC form tetragonal crystals in high-molarity phosphate buffer. The Hb in red cells from homozygous HbC individuals also

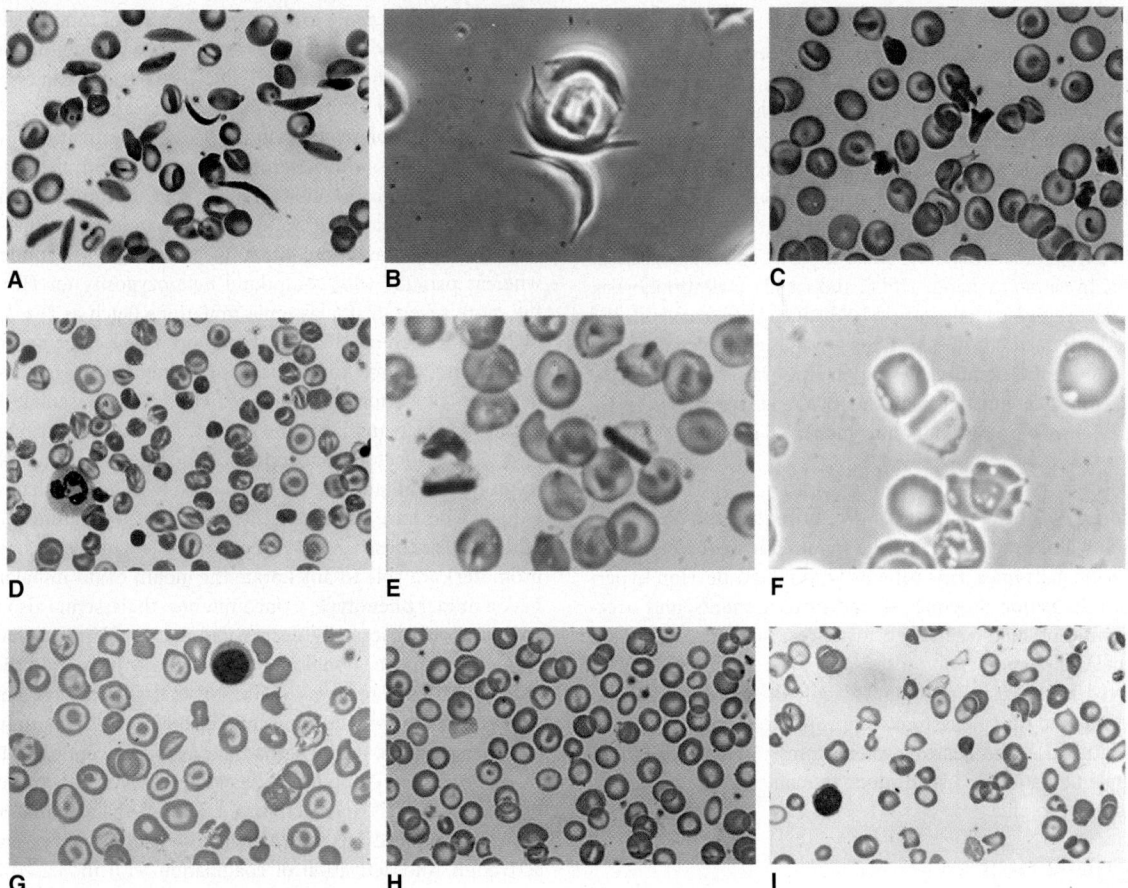

Figure 49–11. Blood cell morphology in patients with structural hemoglobinopathies. **A.** Blood film. Hemoglobin (Hb) SS disease with characteristic sickle-shaped cells and extreme elliptocytes with dense central Hb staining. Both shapes are characteristic of sickled cells. Occasional target cells. **B.** Phase-contrast microscopy of wet preparation. Note the three sickled cells with terminal fine-pointed projections as a result of tactoid formation and occasional target cells. **C.** HbSC disease. Blood film. Note the high frequency of target cells characteristic of HbC and the small dense, irregular, contracted cells reflective of their content of HbS. **D.** HbCC disease. Blood film. Characteristic combination of numerous target cells and a population of dense (hyperchromatic) microspherocytes. Of the nonspherocytic cells, virtually all are target cells. **E.** HbCC disease postsplenectomy. Blood film. Note the rod-like inclusions in two cells as a result of HbC paracrystallization. These cells are virtually all removed in patients with spleens. **F.** HbCC disease postsplenectomy. Phase-contrast microscopy of wet preparation. Note the HbC crystalline rod in a cell. **G.** HbDD disease. Blood film. Note Frequent target cells admixed with population of small spherocytes, poikilocytes, and tiny red cell fragments. **H.** HbEE disease. Blood film. Hypochromia, anisocytosis, and target cells. **I.** HbE thalassemia. Blood film. Marked anisocytosis (primarily microcytes) and poikilocytosis. Hypochromia. *(Reproduced with permission from Lichtman's Atlas of Hematology, www.accessmedicine.com.)*

form crystals when incubated with hypertonic saline; HbC crystals are also observed *in vivo*, particularly in the red cells of splenectomized HbCC patients (Fig. 49–11F). Crystal-containing HbCC red cells have impaired deformability and filterability. HbCC red cells have a propensity for potassium (K⁺) loss, which is followed by water loss; unlike in sickle red cells, this K⁺ leak does not appear to be mediated through either the potassium chloride cotransport or the calcium ion activated K⁺ efflux (Gardos) channel; it is thought to be a volume-stimulated K⁺ efflux.[402] The consequence of this K⁺ loss is dehydrated, often spherocytic, red cells with increased MCHC, and decreased osmotic fragility. These changes result in impaired rheologic properties of HbCC red cells; their life span is reduced to 40 days.

Clinical Features

Mild to moderate splenomegaly is a common feature of homozygous HbC. Like many other chronic hemolytic states, cholelithiasis may be present. HbCC individuals do not suffer from vasoocclusion or episodic pain. Occasionally, abdominal pain may be present and can be a result of splenomegaly and/or cholelithiasis. Pregnancy does not pose an increased risk to women with HbCC. Life expectancy of HbCC individuals is comparable to non-HbC Americans of African descent. In a recent single-institution study, splenomegaly and cholelithiasis occurred in approximately 2.5 percent of patients younger than 8 years of age, but it was far more common (71 percent) in individuals older than 8 years of age.[404]

Laboratory Features

HbCC individuals have a mild to moderate hemolytic anemia. Hb is usually in the 10 to 11 g/dL range. There is associated reticulocytosis usually in the 3 to 4 percent range. There usually is mild microcytosis (mean corpuscular volume [MCV] 70 to 75 fL) and, often, an elevated MCHC. The blood film is characteristic, showing an abundance of target cells, microspherocytes, and HbC red cell crystals, especially in splenectomized patients (see Fig. 49–11F). Indirect bilirubin may be mildly elevated. White cell and platelet counts are normal in the absence of hypersplenism.

Differential Diagnosis

Differential diagnosis is usually achieved by Hb electrophoresis. HbC moves to a cathodic position, comigrating with HbA_2, HbE, and HbO_{Arab} on alkaline pH (cellulose acetate) electrophoresis. The distinction from these Hbs can be made by electrophoresis on citrate agar in acid pH where HbE and HbA_2 comigrate with HbA; HbO_{Arab} has a HbS-like mobility, and HbC has a unique migration pattern. Alternatively, newer diagnostic methods can be used; these include isoelectric focusing, where HbC can readily be distinguished from other Hbs with similar mobility on cellulose acetate electrophoresis. In cation exchange HPLC and capillary electrophoresis, HbC has a distinct elution pattern and can be distinguished from HbE and HbO_{Arab}; these latter methods also have the advantage of separating and quantifying HbA_2 in HbC homozygotes and in HbC trait. This confers the advantage of readily differentiating between HbCC and rare cases of HbC–β^0–thalassemia (where HbA_2 is significantly higher, ~5 percent).

Therapy

The vast majority of HbCC individuals do not require any therapeutic intervention. Cholecystectomy may be required in individuals who have symptomatic gallstones. Few patients with HbCC develop hypersplenism with a reduction in white cell and platelet counts, and occasionally worsening of anemia. In such instances, splenectomy should be considered. Another indication for splenectomy is pain associated with an enlarged spleen. It is important to apply the usual precautions in patients considered for splenectomy (appropriate vaccinations, prophylactic antibiotic use, and delaying splenectomy in young children). Folic acid supplementation, as usually done in many chronic hemolytic states, is of no proven value.

HEMOGLOBIN DISEASE

Definition and History

HbE (β26Glu→Lys) was the fourth abnormal Hb described.[405] It is most commonly found in Southeast Asia; in some areas (in the border between Thailand, Laos, and Cambodia, the so-called HbE triangle) the reported gene frequency may reach as high as 0.50.[406] This high frequency is thought to be from a protective effect against malaria. HbE is also found in other malaria-endemic areas such as Bangladesh, India, and Madagascar. HbE now has a wide distribution as a result of the large population movements from Southeast and South Asia to Western Europe and North America, and may now be the most common Hb variant worldwide.

Etiology and Pathogenesis

The GAG→AAG mutation in codon 26 of the β-globin gene not only leads to a missense mutation (Glu→Lys) at this position, but also activates a cryptic donor splice site at the boundary of exon 1 and intron 1 by increasing the sequence similarity of this site to a consensus splice sequence. The resultant aberrant splicing through this alternate site leads to a decrease in the correctly spliced messenger RNA and hence a β^+-thalassemic phenotype. This is reflected in the fact that heterozygotes for HbE have 25 to 30 percent of the variant; in the presence of concomitant α-thalassemia, this quantity decreases even further. The coinheritance of HbE with a host of other globin mutants (α-thalassemia, β-thalassemia, other Hb variants), which are also common in the populations where HbE is prevalent, results in a wide spectrum of hemoglobinopathies with varying degrees of severity (HbE disorders or HbE syndromes). The most significant of these is HbE–β-thalassemia syndromes. HbE has also been reported in combination with HbS (HbSE disease).

Clinical Features

Individuals with homozygous HbE are asymptomatic. Most patients do not have hepatosplenomegaly or jaundice. They are usually diagnosed during screening programs or family studies of individuals with severe HbE disorders, or on routine evaluation of a blood film with significant microcytosis without anemia. HbE–β-thalassemia is a rather heterogeneous group of disorders varying from a mild thalassemia intermedia like phenotype to severe transfusion dependent thalassemia major (Chap. 48). Part of this heterogeneity results from the type of coinherited β-thalassemia mutation. Patients who are compound heterozygotes for HbE and one of the mild β^+-thalassemia mutations (such as the mild promoter mutation, −28A→G) have a mild to moderate anemia, whereas patients with compound heterozygosity for HbE and one of the more severe β^+-thalassemia mutations (such as IVS I nucleotide 5 or IVS II nucleotide 654 mutations) do have a more severe phenotype with severe anemia and transfusion dependency. There is also a large heterogeneity among patients with HbE–β^0-thalassemia; these patients do not produce any HbA and have only HbE and varying amounts of HbF. Known factors that influence the phenotype include the ability to produce HbF and the presence of concomitant α-thalassemia. Individuals who have the propensity to synthesize significant amounts of HbF (such as those who have the Xmn I C→T mutation in the $^G\gamma$-globin promoter) are able to ameliorate the globin chain imbalance and thus have a milder phenotype. Concomitant α-thalassemia also mitigates the course of the disease by decreasing globin chain imbalance. In some cases, there may be nonglobin modifiers that impact on the phenotype. Patients with severe forms of HbE–β^0-thalassemia have clinical features very similar to β-thalassemia major; they develop complications such as hypersplenism, iron overload, increased susceptibility to infections, thromboembolic complications, and heart failure, and have a shortened life expectancy.[406] Splenectomized HbE–β-thalassemia patients have more pronounced intravascular hemolysis, markers of endothelia cell activation, and activation of coagulation with increased levels of cell free Hb, sE-selectin, sP-selectin, high-sensitivity C-reactive protein, and thrombin–antithrombin complex compared to nonsplenectomized patients.[407]

Laboratory Features

HbE-trait individuals have a borderline microcytosis (MCV in the lower 80s) but are not anemic. Homozygotes for HbE are usually only borderline or mildly anemic (Hb 11 to 13 g/dL), but they are microcytic (MCV ~70 fL). Blood film shows target cells, hypochromia, and microcytosis (see Fig. 49–11H). Osmotic fragility of the red cells is decreased. Hb electrophoresis shows greater than 90 percent HbE and 5 to 10 percent HbF. Certain chromatography techniques that can separate HbE from HbA_2 reveal elevated levels of HbA_2. Patients with mild forms of HbE–β^+-thalassemia (Chap. 48) have Hb levels in the 9.0 to 9.5 g/dL range, whereas those with severe HbE–β^+-thalassemia are more severely anemic (Hb 6.5 to 8.0 g/dL). Individuals with HbE–β^0-thalassemia have varying degrees of anemia, depending on their ability to produce HbF; these patients have HbE in the 40 to 60 percent range, with the remainder being HbF. Patients with higher HbF values are less anemic.

Therapy

HbE homozygotes do not require any therapy. Patients with severe HbE–β^0-thalassemia are similar to thalassemia intermedia or major; most of the latter patients should be on a chronic transfusion regimen aiming at Hb levels of approximately 10 g/dL; iron chelation should be a part of standard therapy. Splenectomy should be considered when hypersplenism develops. Patients with a thalassemia intermedia-like phenotype may require sporadic transfusions. Hydroxyurea can increase HbF levels and decrease ineffective erythropoiesis in HbE–β-thalassemia.[408] AHSCT (including umbilical cord blood–derived stem cells in one patient) has also been used in HbE–β-thalassemia.

Course and Prognosis

The prognosis is dependent upon the clinical phenotype. Patients with milder phenotypes tend to do well. Severe HbE–β-thalassemia patients require chronic red cell transfusion and iron-chelation therapy; this places a great burden on the economies of countries where this disease is prevalent. AHSCT, although potentially curative, will not be available for the vast majority of these patients. Prenatal diagnosis and neonatal screening should be an important part of the strategies to decrease the disease burden and improve care. Long-term use of hydroxyurea and other novel HbF-inducing agents as modifiers of disease (histone deacetylase inhibitors and DNA methyltransferase 1 inhibitors) can be an important addition to therapy.

HEMOGLOBIN D DISEASE

HbD was the third Hb variant identified.[409] The substitution in HbD is a glutamic acid to glutamine at the 121st amino acid of the β-globin chain (β121Glu→Gln). HbD has an S-like mobility on alkaline electrophoresis, but comigrates with HbA on acid pH. Subsequently, a number of other Hb variants with the same electrophoretic properties were discovered and named HbD (HbD$_{Ibadan}$, HbD$_{Gainesville}$, etc.). The most common HbD is HbD$_{Los\ Angeles}$ (β121Glu→Gln), the originally discovered HbD, which is identical to HbD$_{Punjab}$. It is most commonly found in Punjab, India where 2 to 3 percent of the population have the HbD gene. Subsequently, it has also been found in a number of other populations including Europeans of Mediterranean region, and Americans of African descent.[410]

HbD heterozygotes are asymptomatic, are not anemic, and have normal red cell indices. Homozygotes for HbD$_{Los\ Angeles}$ are asymptomatic and are hematologically normal with normal red cell indices. Blood films may show target cells (see Fig. 49–11G). Osmotic fragility may be decreased. Compound heterozygotes for HbD$_{Los\ Angeles}$ and a β^0-thalassemia mutation have mild microcytic anemia and show minimal hemolysis. Coinheritance of HbD$_{Los\ Angeles}$ with HbS results in a severe SCD phenotype not different from homozygous HbS.

HbD$_{Los\ Angeles}$ should be distinguished from HbS. This can be done by a combination of routine alkaline and acid Hb electrophoretic methods. Techniques such as isoelectric focusing, HPLC, and capillary electrophoresis readily provide this distinction. Such methods allow accurate diagnosis of SCD from compound heterozygosity for HbS and HbD$_{Los\ Angeles}$.

UNSTABLE HEMOGLOBINS

Unstable Hbs form an important group of clinically significant Hb variants. Several different mechanisms lead to the generation of unstable variants, which result in a congenital hemolytic anemia with inclusion bodies in red cells (Heinz bodies), hence the term *congenital Heinz body hemolytic anemia*.

Definition and History

Cathie reported a 10-month-old child with hemolytic anemia, jaundice, and splenomegaly in 1952.[411] Splenectomy did not result in improvement. The patient's red cells had large Heinz bodies (Chap. 31). Similar cases were reported from around the world, and the observation that these cases were characterized by the precipitation of their hemolysate upon exposure to heat, suggested a Hb abnormality as the cause. Subsequently, nearly all of similar cases were found to have a variant Hb, and Cathie's case was found to have Hb-Bristol (β67Val→Asp). To date, 146 unstable variants have been reported; the vast majority is sporadic cases reported only once. Few have been observed repeatedly in different populations.

Etiology and Pathogenesis

Several different mechanisms lead to the instability of the globin molecule with precipitation in the red cell leading to hemolysis. These are summarized below.

Substitutions Near the Heme Pocket Heme is inserted into a hydrophobic pocket in each globin molecule where it is in contact with a number of invariant nonpolar amino acid residues (see Fig. 49–2). Substitution of these invariant nonpolar residues will decrease the stability of heme-globin association and ultimately lead to the instability of the globin moiety. Hb$_{Zurich}$ (β63His→Arg), Hb$_{Koln}$ (β98Val→Met), and Hb$_{Hammersmith}$ (β42Phe→Ser) are examples of this group.

Disruption of Secondary Structure (α-Helix) The secondary structure of globin chains is 75 percent in the conformation of an α helix (see Fig. 49–1). Proline residues cannot participate in an α helical conformation. Thus, the substitution of a proline residue for any other amino acid except for the first three residues of an α helix will disrupt the secondary structure and lead to the disruption and precipitation of the mutant globin chain.

Mutations in $\alpha_1\beta_1$ Interface The first step in the assembly of the Hb tetramer is the formation of an $\alpha\beta$ dimer. This structure is stabilized by a secondary structure that exposes the charged amino acids (glutamic acid, aspartic acid, lysine, and arginine) on the surface of the molecule in contact with water and stabilizes the interior of the molecule ($\alpha_1\beta_1$ interface) with hydrophobic interactions. Substitution of a charged (polar) residue for a nonpolar amino acid involved in $\alpha_1\beta_1$ contact will disrupt and destabilize this dimer formation and lead to the precipitation of the Hb molecule.

Amino Acid Deletions Deletion of one or more amino acid residues is expected to disrupt the secondary structure of the globin chains and may lead to instability of the mutant chain. Mutant globins with deletion of one or more residues have been reported. Examples of this type include Hb$_{Leiden}$ (β6 or β7Glu→0), Hb$_{Gun\ Hill}$ (β91-95→0), and Hb$_{Freiburg}$ (β23Val→0).

Elongated Globin Chains Some variants result from either a mutation in the termination codon or a frameshift leading to the synthesis of longer than normal globin chains. These variants tend to be unstable because of the presence of a nonfunctional fragment. Examples include Hb$_{Cranston}$ and Hb$_{Tak}$.

Whatever the underlying mechanism may be, unstable Hb variants precipitate within developing red cell precursors forming hemichromes (intermediate substances in Hb denaturation) and ultimately aggregates that attach to the inner layer of red cell membrane (Heinz bodies). Heinz bodies can be visualized with supravital stains, such as brilliant cresyl blue. Red cells with Heinz bodies have impaired rheologic properties (deformability and filterability) and are trapped in the splenic circulation (Chaps. 6, 34, and 56) with pitting of the membrane attached bodies. Hemolysis ultimately ensues. The degree of hemolysis is proportionate to the quantity and the instability of the variant.

Clinical Features

Patients with unstable Hb variants have varying degrees of hemolytic anemia. This can range from a compensated, asymptomatic hemolytic state to severe, life-threatening hemolysis. Generally, hemolytic anemia is mild to moderate and does not require therapeutic intervention. Typically, hemolysis is exacerbated by increased oxidant stress such as infections and the use of oxidant drugs. Patients may have jaundice and splenomegaly. As is the case with other chronic hemolytic states, gallstones may develop. Hypersplenism can be a problem in some cases. Many unstable Hb variants that are associated with mild, compensated hemolysis are diagnosed fortuitously or during population screening for hemoglobinopathies. Unstable variants are inherited in a mendelian pattern; they usually manifest in the heterozygous state. There are instances of *de novo* mutations without evidence of the variant in parents of an affected individual. Many of the 146 known unstable variants are found in a single individual or in a limited number of instances. However, some unstable variants like Hb$_{Koln}$ (β98Val→Met) and Hb$_{Zurich}$ (β67His→Arg) have been found in many populations around the world.

Laboratory Features

Patients with unstable Hb variants may have varying degrees of anemia. Generally, the anemia is mild and does not require therapeutic intervention. However, exacerbation of anemia during exposure to oxidant stress (such as infections and the use of oxidant drugs) is a common feature. Features of a hemolytic state (reticulocytosis, indirect hyperbilirubinemia, elevated LDH, decreased or undetectable haptoglobin) are present. Red cell morphology shows polychromasia, anisocytosis, poikilocytosis, and occasionally basophilic stippling. A typical feature of this disorder is the presence of Heinz bodies, best visualized with supravital staining with brilliant cresyl blue as membrane attached inclusion bodies in red cells. Hb electrophoresis reveals the presence of an additional abnormal Hb band. The quantity of the variant Hb is variable and inversely proportional to the degree of instability of the abnormal Hb (e.g., the more unstable the variant, the less the quantity). More accurate quantification can be achieved with cation exchange or reversed phase HPLC. The presence of an unstable variant in the hemolysate can be demonstrated by simple tests of stability. The most commonly used tests are heat denaturation and isopropanol precipitation. The heat denaturation test is more cumbersome and time consuming and is seldom used in practice. The isopropanol precipitation test is a simple screening test for unstable variants and involves the incubation of the hemolysate with a 17 percent solution of isopropanol; hemolysates containing unstable Hb variants will form a precipitate, whereas a normal hemolysate will remain clear.

HEMOGLOBINS WITH ALTERED OXYGEN AFFINITY

M Hbs result from mutations around the heme pocket that disrupt the hydrophobic nature of this structure with resultant oxidation of the iron in the heme moiety from ferrous (Fe^{2+}) to ferric (Fe^{3+}) state and cause methemoglobinemia (Chap. 50). Mutations in certain critical areas of the globin molecule alter the affinity of the globin for oxygen. In general, mutations that stabilize the molecule in the T state lead to low O$_2$-affinity variants, which can clinically manifest as cyanosis or mild anemia. Mutations that stabilize the R state or destabilize the T state result in high O$_2$-affinity variants. These variants will cause secondary polycythemia (Chap. 57). The mutations that affect the ligand binding affinity of the Hb molecule are mostly in the $\alpha_1\beta_2$ interface. Rarely, mutations in the $\alpha_1\beta_1$ interface lead to altered O$_2$ affinity. Another mechanism in the generation of high O$_2$ affinity mutants involves mutations that alter the binding of 2,3-BPG.

REFERENCES

1. Beutler E, ed. Disorders of hemoglobin structure: Sickle cell anemai and related abnormalities, in *Williams Hematology*, ed 7, edited by _____, pp ___–___. McGraw-Hill, New York, 2003.
2. Herrick JB: Peculiar elongated and sickle-shaped red corpuscles in a case of severe anemia. *Arch Intern Med* 6:517, 1910.
3. Grahmann PH, Jackson KC 2nd, Lipman AG: Clinician beliefs about opioid use and barriers in chronic nonmalignant pain. *J Pain Palliat Care Pharmacother* 18(2):7–28, 2004.
4. Diggs LW, Ahmann CF, Bibb J: The incidence and significance of the sickle cell trait. *Ann Intern Med* 7:769–778, 1933.
5. Kan YW, Dozy AM: Antenatal diagnosis of sickle-cell anaemia by D.N.A. analysis of amniotic-fluid cells. *Lancet* 2(8096):910–912, 1978.
6. Gormley M: The first "molecular disease": A story of Linus Pauling, the intellectual patron. *Endeavour* 31(2):71–77, 2007.
7. Haller JO, Berdon WE, Franke H: Sickle cell anemia: The legacy of the patient (Walter Clement Noel), the interne (Ernest Irons), and the attending physician (James Herrick) and the facts of its discovery. *Pediatr Radiol* 31(12):889–890, 2001.
8. Serjeant GR: The emerging understanding of sickle cell disease. *Br J Haematol* 112(1):3–18, 2001.
9. Williams VL: Pathways of innovation: A history of the first effective treatment for sickle cell anemia. *Perspect Biol Med* 47(4):552–563, 2004.
10. Goldsmith JC, Bonham VL, Joiner CH, et al: Framing the research agenda for sickle cell trait: Building on the current understanding of clinical events and their potential implications. *Am J Hematol* 87(3):340–346, 2012.
11. Serjeant GR, Serjeant BE, Forbes M, et al: Haemoglobin gene frequencies in the Jamaican population: A study in 100,000 newborns. *Br J Haematol* 64(2):253–262, 1986.
12. Hassell KL: Population estimates of sickle cell disease in the U.S. *Am J Prev Med* 38(4 Suppl):S512–S521, 2010.
13. Okumura MJ, Campbell AD, Nasr SZ, et al: Inpatient health care use among adult survivors of chronic childhood illnesses in the United States. *Arch Pediatr Adolesc Med* 160(10):1054–1060, 2006.
14. Kauf TL, Coates TD, Huazhi L, et al: The cost of health care for children and adults with sickle cell disease. *Am J Hematol* 84(6):323–327, 2009.
15. Kan YW, Dozy AM: Polymorphism of DNA sequence adjacent to human beta-globin structural gene: Relationship to sickle mutation. *Proc Natl Acad Sci U S A* 75(11):5631–5635, 1978.
16. Nagel RL, Fabry ME, Pagnier J, et al: Hematologically and genetically distinct forms of sickle cell anemia in Africa. The Senegal type and the Benin type. *N Engl J Med* 312(14):880–884, 1985.
17. Pagnier J, Mears JG, Dunda-Belkhodja O, et al: Evidence for the multicentric origin of the sickle cell hemoglobin gene in Africa. *Proc Natl Acad Sci U S A* 81(6):1771–1773, 1984.
18. Powars DR: Sickle cell anemia: Beta s-gene-cluster haplotypes as prognostic indicators of vital organ failure. *Semin Hematol* 28(3):202–208, 1991.
19. Dykes GW, Crepeau RH, Edelstein SJ: Three-dimensional reconstruction of the 14-filament fibers of hemoglobin S. *J Mol Biol* 130(4):451–472, 1979.
20. Fronticelli C, Gold R: Conformational relevance of the beta6Glu replaced by Val mutation in the beta subunits and in the beta(1–55) and beta(1–30) peptides of hemoglobin S. *J Biol Chem* 251(16):4968–4972, 1976.
21. Wishner BC, Ward KB, Lattman EE, et al: Crystal structure of sickle-cell deoxyhemoglobin at 5 A resolution. *J Mol Biol* 98(1):179–194, 1975.
22. Ferrone FA, Hofrichter J, Eaton WA: Kinetics of sickle hemoglobin polymerization. I. Studies using temperature-jump and laser photolysis techniques. *J Mol Biol* 183(4):591–610, 1985.
23. Ferrone FA, Hofrichter J, Eaton WA: Kinetics of sickle hemoglobin polymerization. II. A double nucleation mechanism. *J Mol Biol* 183(4):611–631, 1985.
24. Huang Z, Hearne L, Irby CE, et al: Kinetics of increased deformability of deoxygenated sickle cells upon oxygenation. *Biophys J* 85(4):2374–2383, 2003.
25. Carragher B, Bluemke DA, Gabriel B, et al: Structural analysis of polymers of sickle cell hemoglobin. I. Sickle hemoglobin fibers. *J Mol Biol* 199(2):315–331, 1988.
26. Padlan EA, Love WE: Refined crystal structure of deoxyhemoglobin S. II. Molecular interactions in the crystal. *J Biol Chem* 260(14):8280–8291, 1985.
27. Vekilov PG: Sickle-cell haemoglobin polymerization: Is it the primary pathogenic event of sickle-cell anaemia? *Br J Haematol* 139(2):173–184, 2007.
28. Ferrone FA: Polymerization and sickle cell disease: A molecular view. *Microcirculation* 11(2):115–128, 2004.
29. Ballas SK, Mohandas N: Sickle red cell microrheology and sickle blood rheology. *Microcirculation* 11(2):209–225, 2004.
30. Eaton WA, Hofrichter J: Hemoglobin S gelation and sickle cell disease. *Blood* 70(5):1245–1266, 1987.
31. Kaul DK, Fabry ME, Nagel RL: Microvascular sites and characteristics of sickle cell adhesion to vascular endothelium in shear flow conditions: Pathophysiological implications. *Proc Natl Acad Sci U S A* 86(9):3356–3360, 1989.
32. Noguchi CT, Schechter AN: The intracellular polymerization of sickle hemoglobin and its relevance to sickle cell disease. *Blood* 58(6):1057–1068, 1981.
33. Embury SH: The not-so-simple process of sickle cell vasoocclusion. *Microcirculation* 11(2):101–113, 2004.
34. Steinberg MH: Pathophysiologically based drug treatment of sickle cell disease. *Trends Pharmacol Sci* 27(4):204–210, 2006.
35. Stuart MJ, Nagel RL: Sickle-cell disease. *Lancet* 364(9442):1343–1360, 2004.
36. Brugnara C: Sickle cell disease: From membrane pathophysiology to novel therapies for prevention of erythrocyte dehydration. *J Pediatr Hematol Oncol* 25(12):927–933, 2003.
37. Stocker JW, De Franceschi L, McNaughton-Smith GA, et al: ICA-17043, a novel Gardos channel blocker, prevents sickled red blood cell dehydration in vitro and in vivo in SAD mice. *Blood* 101(6):2412–2418, 2003.
38. Bennekou P, Pedersen O, Moller A, et al: Volume control in sickle cells is facilitated by the novel anion conductance inhibitor NS1652. *Blood* 95(5):1842–1848, 2000.
39. Joiner CH, Jiang M, Claussen WJ, et al: Dipyridamole inhibits sickling-induced cation fluxes in sickle red blood cells. *Blood* 97(12):3976–3983, 2001.
40. Aslan M, Freeman BA: Redox-dependent impairment of vascular function in sickle cell disease. *Free Radic Biol Med* 43(11):1469–1483, 2007.

41. Gladwin MT, Schechter AN: Nitric oxide therapy in sickle cell disease. *Semin Hematol* 38(4):333–342, 2001.

42. Enwonwu CO, Xu XX, Turner E: Nitrogen metabolism in sickle cell anemia: Free amino acids in plasma and urine. *Am J Med Sci* 300(6):366–371, 1990.

43. Lopez BL, Barnett J, Ballas SK, et al: Nitric oxide metabolite levels in acute vaso-occlusive sickle-cell crisis. *Acad Emerg Med* 3(12):1098–1103, 1996.

44. Lopez BL, Davis-Moon L, Ballas SK, et al: Sequential nitric oxide measurements during the emergency department treatment of acute vasoocclusive sickle cell crisis. *Am J Hematol* 64(1):15–19, 2000.

45. Morris CR, Kuypers FA, Larkin S, et al: Arginine therapy: A novel strategy to induce nitric oxide production in sickle cell disease. *Br J Haematol* 111(2):498–500, 2000.

46. Morris CR, Kuypers FA, Larkin S, et al: Patterns of arginine and nitric oxide in patients with sickle cell disease with vaso-occlusive crisis and acute chest syndrome. *J Pediatr Hematol Oncol* 22(6):515–520, 2000.

47. Kato GJ, Wang Z, Machado RF, et al: Endogenous nitric oxide synthase inhibitors in sickle cell disease: Abnormal levels and correlations with pulmonary hypertension, desaturation, haemolysis, organ dysfunction and death. *Br J Haematol* 145(4):506–513, 2009.

48. Kato GJ, Taylor JG 6th: Pleiotropic effects of intravascular haemolysis on vascular homeostasis. *Br J Haematol* 148(5):690–701, 2010.

49. Frenette PS, Atweh GF: Sickle cell disease: Old discoveries, new concepts, and future promise. *J Clin Invest* 117(4):850–858, 2007.

50. Reiter CD, Wang X, Tanus-Santos JE, et al: Cell-free hemoglobin limits nitric oxide bioavailability in sickle-cell disease. *Nat Med* 8(12):1383–1389, 2002.

51. Hebbel RP, Yamada O, Moldow CF, et al: Abnormal adherence of sickle erythrocytes to cultured vascular endothelium: Possible mechanism for microvascular occlusion in sickle cell disease. *J Clin Invest* 65(1):154–160, 1980.

52. Hoover R, Rubin R, Wise G, et al: Adhesion of normal and sickle erythrocytes to endothelial monolayer cultures. *Blood* 54(4):872–876, 1979.

53. Barabino GA, McIntire LV, Eskin SG, et al: Rheological studies of erythrocyte-endothelial cell interactions in sickle cell disease. *Prog Clin Biol Res* 240:113–127, 1987.

54. Mohandas N, Evans E: Sickle erythrocyte adherence to vascular endothelium. Morphologic correlates and the requirement for divalent cations and collagen-binding plasma proteins. *J Clin Invest* 76(4):1605–1612, 1985.

55. Kaul DK, Tsai HM, Liu XD, et al: Monoclonal antibodies to alphaVbeta3 (7E3 and LM609) inhibit sickle red blood cell-endothelium interactions induced by platelet-activating factor. *Blood* 95(2):368–374, 2000.

56. Frenette PS: Sickle cell vaso-occlusion: Multistep and multicellular paradigm. *Curr Opin Hematol* 9(2):101–106, 2002.

57. Gee BE, Platt OS: Sickle reticulocytes adhere to VCAM-1. *Blood* 85(1):268–274, 1995.

58. Parsons SF, Lee G, Spring FA, et al: Lutheran blood group glycoprotein and its newly characterized mouse homologue specifically bind alpha5 chain-containing human laminin with high affinity. *Blood* 97(1):312–320, 2001.

59. Swerlick RA, Eckman JR, Kumar A, et al: Alpha 4 beta 1-integrin expression on sickle reticulocytes: Vascular cell adhesion molecule-1-dependent binding to endothelium. *Blood* 82(6):1891–1899, 1993.

60. Udani M, Zen Q, Cottman M, et al: Basal cell adhesion molecule/lutheran protein. The receptor critical for sickle cell adhesion to laminin. *J Clin Invest* 101(11):2550–2558, 1998.

61. Okpala I: The intriguing contribution of white blood cells to sickle cell disease—A red cell disorder. *Blood Rev* 18(1):65–73, 2004.

62. Okpala I: Leukocyte adhesion and the pathophysiology of sickle cell disease. *Curr Opin Hematol* 13(1):40–44, 2006.

63. Tan P, Luscinskas FW, Homer-Vanniasinkam S: Cellular and molecular mechanisms of inflammation and thrombosis. *Eur J Vasc Endovasc Surg* 17(5):373–389, 1999.

64. Hebbel RP, Osarogiagbon R, Kaul D: The endothelial biology of sickle cell disease: Inflammation and a chronic vasculopathy. *Microcirculation* 11(2):129–151, 2004.

65. Steinberg MH, Mohandas N: Laboratory values, in *Sickle Cell Disease: Basic Principles and Clinical Practice*, edited by Embury SH, Hebbel RP,, Mohandas N, , Steinberg MH, pp 469–484. Raven, New York, 1994.

66. Belcher JD, Marker PH, Weber JP, et al: Activated monocytes in sickle cell disease: Potential role in the activation of vascular endothelium and vaso-occlusion. *Blood* 96(7):2451–2459, 2000.

67. Benkerrou M, Delarche C, Brahimi L, et al: Hydroxyurea corrects the dysregulated L-selectin expression and increased H(2)O(2) production of polymorphonuclear neutrophils from patients with sickle cell anemia. *Blood* 99(7):2297–2303, 2002.

68. Fadlon E, Vordermeier S, Pearson TC, et al: Blood polymorphonuclear leukocytes from the majority of sickle cell patients in the crisis phase of the disease show enhanced adhesion to vascular endothelium and increased expression of CD64. *Blood* 91(1):266–274, 1998.

69. Francis R Jr, Hebbel RP: Hemostasis, in *Sickle Cell Disease: Basic Principles and Clinical Practice*, edited by Embury SH, Hebbel RP, Mohandas N, Steinberg MH, pp 299–310. 1994, Raven, New York, 1994..

70. Hofstra TC, Kalra VK, Meiselman HJ, et al: Sickle erythrocytes adhere to polymorphonuclear neutrophils and activate the neutrophil respiratory burst. *Blood* 87(10):4440–4447, 1996.

71. Inwald DP, Kirkham FJ, Peters MJ, et al: Platelet and leucocyte activation in childhood sickle cell disease: Association with nocturnal hypoxaemia. *Br J Haematol* 111(2):474–481, 2000.

72. Lard LR, Mul FP, de Haas M, et al: Neutrophil activation in sickle cell disease. *J Leukoc Biol* 66(3):411–415, 1999.

73. Nath KA, Grande JP, Haggard JJ, et al: Oxidative stress and induction of heme oxygenase-1 in the kidney in sickle cell disease. *Am J Pathol* 158(3):893–903, 2001.

74. Solovey A, Gui L, Key NS, et al: Tissue factor expression by endothelial cells in sickle cell anemia. *J Clin Invest* 101(9):1899–1904, 1998.

75. Solovey A, Lin Y, Browne P, et al: Circulating activated endothelial cells in sickle cell anemia. *N Engl J Med* 337(22):1584–1590, 1997.

76. Wun T, Cordoba M, Rangaswami A, et al: Activated monocytes and platelet-monocyte aggregates in patients with sickle cell disease. *Clin Lab Haematol* 24(2):81–88, 2002.

77. Patel N, Gonsalves CS, Malik P, et al: Placenta growth factor augments endothelin-1 and endothelin-B receptor expression via hypoxia-inducible factor-1 alpha. *Blood* 112(3):856–865, 2008.

78. Perelman N, Selvaraj SK, Batra S, et al: Placenta growth factor activates monocytes and correlates with sickle cell disease severity. *Blood* 102(4):1506–1514, 2003.

79. Wang X, Mendelsohn L, Rogers H, et al: Heme-bound iron activates placenta growth factor in erythroid cells via erythroid Kruppel-like factor. *Blood* 124(6):946–954, 2014.

80. Hillery CA, Panepinto JA: Pathophysiology of stroke in sickle cell disease. *Microcirculation* 11(2):195–208, 2004.

81. Prengler M, Pavlakis SG, Prohovnik I, et al: Sickle cell disease: The neurological complications. *Ann Neurol* 51(5):543–552, 2002.

82. Granger DN, Korthuis RJ: Physiologic mechanisms of postischemic tissue injury. *Annu Rev Physiol* 57:311–332, 1995.

83. Grisham MB, Granger DN, Lefer DJ: Modulation of leukocyte-endothelial interactions by reactive metabolites of oxygen and nitrogen: Relevance to ischemic heart disease. *Free Radic Biol Med* 25(4–5):404–433, 1998.

84. Field JJ, Nathan DG, Linden J: Targeting iNKT cells for the treatment of sickle cell disease. *Clin Immunol* 140(2):177–183, 2011.

85. Eilertsen KE, Osterud B: Tissue factor: (patho)physiology and cellular biology. *Blood Coagul Fibrinolysis* 15(7):521–538, 2004.

86. Key NS, Slungaard A, Dandelet L, et al: Whole blood tissue factor procoagulant activity is elevated in patients with sickle cell disease. *Blood* 91(11):4216–4223, 1998.

87. Krishnaswamy S: The interaction of human factor VIIa with tissue factor. *J Biol Chem* 267(33):23696–23706, 1992.

88. Chantrathammachart P, Pawlinski R: Tissue factor and thrombin in sickle cell anemia. *Thromb Res* 129 Suppl 2:S70–S72, 2012.

89. Setty BN, Kulkarni S, Dampier CD, et al: Fetal hemoglobin in sickle cell anemia: Relationship to erythrocyte adhesion markers and adhesion. *Blood* 97(9):2568–2573, 2001.

90. Kurantsin-Mills J, Ofosu FA, Safa TK, et al: Plasma factor VII and thrombin-antithrombin III levels indicate increased tissue factor activity in sickle cell patients. *Br J Haematol* 81(4):539–544, 1992.

91. Tomer A, Harker LA, Kasey S, et al: Thrombogenesis in sickle cell disease. *J Lab Clin Med* 137(6):398–407, 2001.

92. Sparkenbaugh E, Pawlinski R: Interplay between coagulation and vascular inflammation in sickle cell disease. *Br J Haematol* 162(1):3–14, 2013.

93. Chen J, Hobbs WE, Le J, et al: The rate of hemolysis in sickle cell disease correlates with the quantity of active von Willebrand factor in the plasma. *Blood* 117(13):3680–3683, 2011.

94. Zhang Y, Dai Y, Wen J, et al: Detrimental effects of adenosine signaling in sickle cell disease. *Nat Med* 17(1):79–86, 2011.

95. Zhang Y, Xia Y: Adenosine signaling in normal and sickle erythrocytes and beyond. *Microbes Infect* 14(10):863–873, 2012.

96. Tsaras G, Owusu-Ansah A, Boateng FO, et al: Complications associated with sickle cell trait: A brief narrative review. *Am J Med* 122(6):507–512, 2009.

97. Harris JW, Brewster HH, Ham TH, et al: Studies on the destruction of red blood cells. X. The biophysics and biology of sickle-cell disease. *AMA Arch Intern Med* 97(2):145–168, 1956.

98. Bergeron MF, Cannon JG, Hall EL, et al: Erythrocyte sickling during exercise and thermal stress. *Clin J Sport Med* 14(6):354–356, 2004.

99. Monchanin G, Serpero LD, Connes P, et al: Effects of progressive and maximal exercise on plasma levels of adhesion molecules in athletes with sickle cell trait with or without alpha-thalassemia. *J Appl Physiol* 102(1):169–173, 2007.

100. Weisman IM, Zeballos RJ, Johnson BD: Cardiopulmonary and gas exchange responses to acute strenuous exercise at 1,270 meters in sickle cell trait. *Am J Med* 84(3 Pt 1):377–383, 1988.

101. Key NS, Derebail VK: Sickle-cell trait: Novel clinical significance. *Hematology Am Soc Hematol Educ Program* 2010:418–422, 2010.

102. Gupta AK, Kirchner KA, Nicholson R, et al: Effects of alpha-thalassemia and sickle polymerization tendency on the urine-concentrating defect of individuals with sickle cell trait. *J Clin Invest* 88(6):1963–1968, 1991.

103. Yium J, Gabow P, Johnson A, et al: Autosomal dominant polycystic kidney disease in blacks: Clinical course and effects of sickle-cell hemoglobin. *J Am Soc Nephrol* 4(9):1670–1674, 1994.

104. Kark JA, Ward FT: Exercise and hemoglobin S. *Semin Hematol* 31(3):181–225, 1994.

105. Austin H, Key NS, Benson JM, et al: Sickle cell trait and the risk of venous thromboembolism among blacks. *Blood* 110(3):908–912, 2007.

106. Pastore LM, Savitz DA, Thorp JM Jr: Predictors of urinary tract infection at the first prenatal visit. *Epidemiology* 10(3):282–287, 1999.

107. Heller P, Best WR, Nelson RB, et al: Clinical implications of sickle-cell trait and glucose-6-phosphate dehydrogenase deficiency in hospitalized black male patients. *N Engl J Med* 300(18):1001–1005, 1979.

108. Glader BE, Propper RD, Buchanan GR: Microcytosis associated with sickle cell anemia. *Am J Clin Pathol* 72(1):63–64, 1979.

109. Mohandas N, Johnson A, Wyatt J, et al: Automated quantitation of cell density distribution and hyperdense cell fraction in RBC disorders. *Blood* 74(1):442–447, 1989.
110. Sherwood JB, Goldwasser E, Chilcote R, et al: Sickle cell anemia patients have low erythropoietin levels for their degree of anemia. *Blood* 67(1):46–49, 1986.
111. Boggs DR, Hyde F, Srodes C: An unusual pattern of neutrophil kinetics in sickle cell anemia. *Blood* 41(1):59–65, 1973.
112. Buchanan GR, Glader BE: Leukocyte counts in children with sickle cell disease. Comparative values in the steady state, vaso-occlusive crisis, and bacterial infection. *Am J Dis Child* 132(4):396–398, 1978.
113. Corvelli AI, Binder RA, Kales A: Disseminated intravascular coagulation in sickle cell crisis. *South Med J* 72(4):505–506, 1979.
114. Karayalcin G, Lanzkowsky P, Kazi AB: Zinc deficiency in children with sickle cell disease. *Am J Pediatr Hematol Oncol* 1(3):283–284, 1979.
115. Natta C, Machlin L: Plasma levels of tocopherol in sickle cell anemia subjects. *Am J Clin Nutr* 32(7):1359–1362, 1979.
116. Niell HB, Leach BE, Kraus AP: Zinc metabolism in sickle cell anemia. *JAMA* 242(24):2686–2687, 1979.
117. Mario N, Baudin B, Aussel C, et al: Capillary isoelectric focusing and high-performance cation-exchange chromatography compared for qualitative and quantitative analysis of hemoglobin variants. *Clin Chem* 43(11):2137–2142, 1997.
118. Partington MD, Aronyk KE, Byrd SE: Sickle cell trait and stroke in children. *Pediatr Neurosurg* 20(2):148–151, 1994.
119. Steinberg MH: DNA diagnosis for the detection of sickle hemoglobinopathies. *Am J Hematol* 43(2):110–115, 1993.
120. Hamideh D, Alvarez O: Sickle cell disease related mortality in the United States (1999–2009). *Pediatr Blood Cancer* 60(9):1482–1486, 2013.
121. Platt OS, Brambilla DJ, Rosse WF, et al: Mortality in sickle cell disease. Life expectancy and risk factors for early death. *N Engl J Med* 330(23):1639–1644, 1994.
122. Serjeant GR, Serjeant BE, Mason KP, et al: The changing face of homozygous sickle cell disease: 102 patients over 60 years. *Int J Lab Hematol* 31(6):585–596, 2009.
123. National Heart, Lung, and Blood Institute: *The Management of Sickle Cell Disease*, ed 4, pp 59–74. NIH Publication No. 02-2117. National Institutes of Health, Bethesda, MD, 2002.
124. Yale SH, Nagib N, Guthrie T: Approach to the vaso-occlusive crisis in adults with sickle cell disease. *Am Fam Physician* 61(5):1349–1356, 1363–1364, 2000.
125. Ballas SK, Gupta K, Adams-Graves P: Sickle cell pain: A critical reappraisal. *Blood* 120(18):3647–3656, 2012.
126. Ballas SK, Kesen MR, Goldberg MF, et al: Beyond the definitions of the phenotypic complications of sickle cell disease: An update on management. *ScientificWorldJournal* 2012:949535, 2012.
127. Kinney TR, Ware RE, Schultz WH, et al: Long-term management of splenic sequestration in children with sickle cell disease. *J Pediatr* 117(2 Pt 1):194–199, 1990.
128. Solanki DL, Kletter GG, Castro O: Acute splenic sequestration crises in adults with sickle cell disease. *Am J Med* 80(5):985–990, 1986.
129. Bowcock SJ, Nwabueze ED, Cook AE, et al: Fatal splenic sequestration in adult sickle cell disease. *Clin Lab Haematol* 10(1):95–99, 1988.
130. Koduri PR, Agbemadzo B, Nathan S: Hemoglobin S-C disease revisited: Clinical study of 106 adults. *Am J Hematol* 68(4):298–300, 2001.
131. Vichinsky E, Lubin BH: Suggested guidelines for the treatment of children with sickle cell anemia. *Hematol Oncol Clin North Am* 1(3):483–501, 1987.
132. de Montalembert M, Dumont MD, Heilbronner C, et al: Delayed hemolytic transfusion reaction in children with sickle cell disease. *Haematologica* 96(6):801–807, 2011.
133. Solomon LR: Treatment and prevention of pain due to vaso-occlusive crises in adults with sickle cell disease: An educational void. *Blood* 111(3):997–1003, 2008.
134. Labbe E, Herbert D, Haynes J: Physicians' attitude and practices in sickle cell disease pain management. *J Palliat Care* 21(4):246–251, 2005.
135. Elander J, Lusher J, Bevan D, et al: Understanding the causes of problematic pain management in sickle cell disease: Evidence that pseudoaddiction plays a more important role than genuine analgesic dependence. *J Pain Symptom Manage* 27(2):156–169, 2004.
136. Ballas SK: Ethical issues in the management of sickle cell pain. *Am J Hematol* 68(2):127–132, 2001.
137. Aisiku IP, Smith WR, McClish DK, et al: Comparisons of high versus low emergency department utilizers in sickle cell disease. *Ann Emerg Med* 53(5):587–593, 2009.
138. McClish DK, Smith WR, Dahman BA, et al: Pain site frequency and location in sickle cell disease: The PiSCES project. *Pain* 145(1–2):246–251, 2009.
139. Dampier C, Ely E, Brodecki D, et al: Home management of pain in sickle cell disease: A daily diary study in children and adolescents. *J Pediatr Hematol Oncol* 24(8):643–647, 2002.
140. Rees DC, Olujohungbe AD, Parker NE, et al: Guidelines for the management of the acute painful crisis in sickle cell disease. *Br J Haematol* 120(5):744–752, 2003.
141. Benjamin L, Dampier CD, Jacox, A, et al: *Guideline for Management of Acute Pain in Sickle-Cel Disease.* Glenview, IL, 2001.
142. Ballas SK: Meperidine for acute sickle cell pain in the emergency department: Revisited controversy. *Ann Emerg Med* 51(2):217, 2008.
143. Howland MA, Goldfrank LR: Why meperidine should not make a comeback in treating patients with sickle cell disease. *Ann Emerg Med* 51(2):203–205, 2008.
144. Morgan MT: Use of meperidine as the analgesic of choice in treating pain from acute painful sickle cell crisis. *Ann Emerg Med* 51(2):202–203, 2008.
145. Benjamin LJ, Swinson GI, Nagel RL: Sickle cell anemia day hospital: An approach for the management of uncomplicated painful crises. *Blood* 95(4):1130–1136, 2000.
146. Platt OS, Thorington BD, Brambilla DJ, et al: Pain in sickle cell disease. Rates and risk factors. *N Engl J Med* 325(1):11–16, 1991.
147. Vichinsky EP, Johnson R, Lubin BH: Multidisciplinary approach to pain management in sickle cell disease. *Am J Pediatr Hematol Oncol* 4(3):328–333, 1982.
148. Styles LA, Vichinsky E: Effects of a long-term transfusion regimen on sickle cell-related illnesses. *J Pediatr* 125(6 Pt 1):909–911, 1994.
149. Dampier CD, Smith WR, Wager CG, et al: IMPROVE trial: A randomized controlled trial of patient-controlled analgesia for sickle cell painful episodes: Rationale, design challenges, initial experience, and recommendations for future studies. *Clin Trials* 10(2):319–331, 2013.
150. Gladwin MT, Kato GJ, Weiner D, et al: Nitric oxide for inhalation in the acute treatment of sickle cell pain crisis: A randomized controlled trial. *JAMA* 305(9):893–902, 2011.
151. Gladwin MT, Vichinsky E: Pulmonary complications of sickle cell disease. *N Engl J Med* 359(21):2254–2265, 2008.
152. Vichinsky EP, Neumayr LD, Earles AN, et al: Causes and outcomes of the acute chest syndrome in sickle cell disease. National Acute Chest Syndrome Study Group. *N Engl J Med* 342(25):1855–1865, 2000.
153. Miller ST: How I treat acute chest syndrome in children with sickle cell disease. *Blood* 117(20):5297–5305, 2011.
154. Vichinsky EP, Neumayr LD, Gold JI, et al: Neuropsychological dysfunction and neuroimaging abnormalities in neurologically intact adults with sickle cell anemia. *JAMA* 303(18):1823–1831, 2010.
155. Emre U, Miller ST, Gutierez M, et al: Effect of transfusion in acute chest syndrome of sickle cell disease. *J Pediatr* 127(6):901–904, 1995.
156. Emre U, Miller ST, Rao SP, et al: Alveolar-arterial oxygen gradient in acute chest syndrome of sickle cell disease. *J Pediatr* 123(2):272–275, 1993.
157. Bellet PS, Kalinyak KA, Shukla R, et al: Incentive spirometry to prevent acute pulmonary complications in sickle cell diseases. *N Engl J Med* 333(11):699–703, 1995.
158. Uchida K, Rackoff WR, Ohene-Frempong K, et al: Effect of erythrocytapheresis on arterial oxygen saturation and hemoglobin oxygen affinity in patients with sickle cell disease. *Am J Hematol* 59(1):5–8, 1998.
159. Bernini JC, Rogers ZR, Sandler ES, et al: Beneficial effect of intravenous dexamethasone in children with mild to moderately severe acute chest syndrome complicating sickle cell disease. *Blood* 92(9):3082–3089, 1998.
160. Charache S, Terrin ML, Moore RD, et al: Effect of hydroxyurea on the frequency of painful crises in sickle cell anemia. Investigators of the Multicenter Study of Hydroxyurea in Sickle Cell Anemia. *N Engl J Med* 332(20):1317–1322, 1995.
161. Wang WC, Ware RE, Miller ST, et al: Hydroxycarbamide in very young children with sickle-cell anaemia: A multicentre, randomised, controlled trial (BABY HUG). *Lancet* 377(9778):1663–1672, 2011.
162. Klings ES, Machado RF, Barst RJ, et al: An official American Thoracic Society clinical practice guideline: Diagnosis, risk stratification, and management of pulmonary hypertension of sickle cell disease. *Am J Respir Crit Care Med* 189(6):727–740, 2014.
163. Morris CR: Asthma management: Reinventing the wheel in sickle cell disease. *Am J Hematol* 84(4):234–241, 2009.
164. Klings ES, Wyszynski DF, Nolan VG, et al: Abnormal pulmonary function in adults with sickle cell anemia. *Am J Respir Crit Care Med* 173(11):1264–1269, 2006.
165. Newaskar M, Hardy KA, Morris CR: Asthma in sickle cell disease. *ScientificWorldJournal* 11:1138–1152, 2011.
166. Varat MA, Adolph RJ, Fowler NO: Cardiovascular effects of anemia. *Am Heart J* 83(3):415–426, 1972.
167. Balfour IC, Covitz W, Davis H, et al: Cardiac size and function in children with sickle cell anemia. *Am Heart J* 108(2):345–350, 1984.
168. Fitzhugh CD, Lauder N, Jonassaint JC, et al: Cardiopulmonary complications leading to premature deaths in adult patients with sickle cell disease. *Am J Hematol* 85(1):36–40, 2010.
169. Manci EA, Culberson DE, Yang YM, et al: Causes of death in sickle cell disease: An autopsy study. *Br J Haematol* 123(2):359–365, 2003.
170. Darbari DS, Kple-Faget P, Kwagyan J, et al: Circumstances of death in adult sickle cell disease patients. *Am J Hematol* 81(11):858–863, 2006.
171. Chacko P, Kraut EH, Zweier J, et al: Myocardial infarction in sickle cell disease: Use of translational imaging to diagnose an under-recognized problem. *J Cardiovasc Transl Res* 6(5):752–761, 2013.
172. Voskaridou E, Christoulas D, Terpos E: Sickle-cell disease and the heart: Review of the current literature. *Br J Haematol* 157(6):664–673, 2012.
173. Pegelow CH, Colangelo L, Steinberg M, et al: Natural history of blood pressure in sickle cell disease: Risks for stroke and death associated with relative hypertension in sickle cell anemia. *Am J Med* 102(2):171–177, 1997.
174. Stockman JA, Nigro MA, Mishkin MM, et al: Occlusion of large cerebral vessels in sickle-cell anemia. *N Engl J Med* 287(17):846–849, 1972.
175. Ohene-Frempong K, Weiner SJ, Sleeper LA, et al: Cerebrovascular accidents in sickle cell disease: Rates and risk factors. *Blood* 91(1):288–294, 1998.
176. Steen RG, Xiong X, Langston JW, et al: Brain injury in children with sickle cell disease: Prevalence and etiology. *Ann Neurol* 54(5):564–572, 2003.
177. Webb J, Kwiatkowski J: L. Stroke in patients with sickle cell disease. *Expert Rev Hematol* 6(3):301–315, 2013.
178. Bernaudin F, Verlhac S, Arnaud C, et al: Impact of early transcranial Doppler screening and intensive therapy on cerebral vasculopathy outcome in a newborn sickle cell anemia cohort. *Blood* 117(4):1130–1140; quiz 1436, 2011.

179. DeBaun MR, Sarnaik SA, Rodeghier MJ, et al: Associated risk factors for silent cerebral infarcts in sickle cell anemia: Low baseline hemoglobin, sex, and relative high systolic blood pressure. *Blood* 119(16):3684–3690, 2012.

180. Hulbert ML, McKinstry RC, Lacey JL, et al: Silent cerebral infarcts occur despite regular blood transfusion therapy after first strokes in children with sickle cell disease. *Blood* 117(3):772–779, 2011.

181. Prohovnik I, Pavlakis SG, Piomelli S, et al: Cerebral hyperemia, stroke, and transfusion in sickle cell disease. *Neurology* 39(3):344–348, 1989.

182. Wang WC: The pathophysiology, prevention, and treatment of stroke in sickle cell disease. *Curr Opin Hematol* 14(3):191–197, 2007.

183. Switzer JA, Hess DC, Nichols FT, et al: Pathophysiology and treatment of stroke in sickle-cell disease: Present and future. *Lancet Neurol* 5(6):501–512, 2006.

184. Powars D, Adams RJ, Nichols FT, et al: Delayed intracranial hemorrhage following cerebral infarction in sickle cell anemia. *J Assoc Acad Minor Phys* 1(3):79–82, 1990.

185. Diggs LW, Brookoff D: Multiple cerebral aneurysms in patients with sickle cell disease. *South Med J* 86(4):377–379, 1993.

186. Anson JA, Koshy M, Ferguson L, et al: Subarachnoid hemorrhage in sickle-cell disease. *J Neurosurg* 75(4):552–558, 1991.

187. Oyesiku NM, Barrow DL, Eckman JR, et al: Intracranial aneurysms in sickle-cell anemia: Clinical features and pathogenesis. *J Neurosurg* 75(3):356–363, 1991.

188. Preul MC, Cendes F, Just N, et al: Intracranial aneurysms and sickle cell anemia: Multiplicity and propensity for the vertebrobasilar territory. *Neurosurgery* 42(5):971–977; discussion 977–978, 1998.

189. O'Driscoll S, Height SE, Dick MC, et al: Serum lactate dehydrogenase activity as a biomarker in children with sickle cell disease. *Br J Haematol* 140(2):206–209, 2008.

190. Miller ST, Macklin EA, Pegelow CH, et al: Silent infarction as a risk factor for overt stroke in children with sickle cell anemia: A report from the Cooperative Study of Sickle Cell Disease. *J Pediatr* 139(3):385–390, 2001.

191. Pegelow CH, Macklin EA, Moser FG, et al: Longitudinal changes in brain magnetic resonance imaging findings in children with sickle cell disease. *Blood* 99(8):3014–3018, 2002.

192. Kirkham FJ, Hewes DK, Prengler M, et al: Nocturnal hypoxaemia and central-nervous-system events in sickle-cell disease. *Lancet* 357(9269):1656–1659, 2001.

193. Kinney TR, Sleeper LA, Wang WC, et al: Silent cerebral infarcts in sickle cell anemia: A risk factor analysis. The Cooperative Study of Sickle Cell Disease. *Pediatrics* 103(3):640–645, 1999.

194. Moser FG, Miller ST, Bello JA, et al: The spectrum of brain MR abnormalities in sickle-cell disease: A report from the Cooperative Study of Sickle Cell Disease. *AJNR Am J Neuroradiol* 17(5):965–972, 1996.

195. Strouse JJ, Hulbert ML, DeBaun MR, et al: Primary hemorrhagic stroke in children with sickle cell disease is associated with recent transfusion and use of corticosteroids. *Pediatrics* 118(5):1916–1924, 2006.

196. Adams RJ, Kutlar A, McKie V, et al: Alpha thalassemia and stroke risk in sickle cell anemia. *Am J Hematol* 45(4):279–282, 1994.

197. Adams R, McKie V, Nichols F, et al: The use of transcranial ultrasonography to predict stroke in sickle cell disease. *N Engl J Med* 326(9):605–610, 1992.

198. Berkelhammer LD, Williamson AL, Sanford SD, et al: Neurocognitive sequelae of pediatric sickle cell disease: A review of the literature. *Child Neuropsychol* 13(2):120–131, 2007.

199. Fullerton HJ, Gardner M, Adams RJ, et al: Obstacles to primary stroke prevention in children with sickle cell disease. *Neurology* 67(6):1098–1099, 2006.

200. Fullerton HJ, Adams RJ, Zhao S, et al: Declining stroke rates in Californian children with sickle cell disease. *Blood* 104(2):336–339, 2004.

201. Hulbert ML, Scothorn DJ, Panepinto JA, et al: Exchange blood transfusion compared with simple transfusion for first overt stroke is associated with a lower risk of subsequent stroke: A retrospective cohort study of 137 children with sickle cell anemia. *J Pediatr* 149(5):710–712, 2006.

202. Vichinsky EP, Haberkern CM, Neumayr L, et al: A comparison of conservative and aggressive transfusion regimens in the perioperative management of sickle cell disease. The Preoperative Transfusion in Sickle Cell Disease Study Group. *N Engl J Med* 333(4):206–213, 1995.

203. Zimmerman SA, Schultz WH, Burgett S, et al: Hydroxyurea therapy lowers transcranial Doppler flow velocities in children with sickle cell anemia. *Blood* 110(3):1043–1047, 2007.

204. Ware RE, Helms RW, SWiTCH Investigators: Stroke With Transfusions Changing to Hydroxyurea (SWiTCH). *Blood* 119(17):3925–3932, 2012.

205. Dobson SR, Holden KR, Nietert PJ, et al: Moyamoya syndrome in childhood sickle cell disease: A predictive factor for recurrent cerebrovascular events. *Blood* 99(9):3144–3150, 2002.

206. Hankinson TC, Bohman LE, Heyer G, et al: Surgical treatment of moyamoya syndrome in patients with sickle cell anemia: Outcome following encephaloduroarteriosynangiosis. *J Neurosurg Pediatr* 1(3):211–216, 2008.

207. Nur E, Biemond BJ, Otten HM, et al: Oxidative stress in sickle cell disease; pathophysiology and potential implications for disease management. *Am J Hematol* 86(6):484–489, 2011.

208. Sklar AH, Campbell H, Caruana RJ, et al: A population study of renal function in sickle cell anemia. *Int J Artif Organs* 13(4):231–236, 1990.

209. Falk RJ, Scheinman J, Phillips G, et al: Prevalence and pathologic features of sickle cell nephropathy and response to inhibition of angiotensin-converting enzyme. *N Engl J Med* 326(14):910–915, 1992.

210. Powars DR, Elliott-Mills DD, Chan L, et al: Chronic renal failure in sickle cell disease: Risk factors, clinical course, and mortality. *Ann Intern Med* 115(8):614–620, 1991.

211. Powars DR, Chan LS, Hiti A, et al: Outcome of sickle cell anemia: A 4-decade observational study of 1056 patients. *Medicine (Baltimore)* 84(6):363–376, 2005.

212. Scheinman J: *Sickle Cell Nephropathy*. Williams & Wilkins, Boston, 1994.

213. Sharpe CC, Thein SL: Sickle cell nephropathy—A practical approach. *Br J Haematol* 155(3):287–297, 2011.

214. Huang SH, Sharma AP, Yasin A, et al: Hyperfiltration affects accuracy of creatinine eGFR measurement. *Clin J Am Soc Nephrol* 6(2):274–280, 2011.

215. McKie KT, Hanevold CD, Hernandez C, et al: Prevalence, prevention, and treatment of microalbuminuria and proteinuria in children with sickle cell disease. *J Pediatr Hematol Oncol* 29(3):140–144, 2007.

216. Kanso AA, Hassan NMA, Badr KF: *Microvascular and Macrovascular Diseases of the Kidney*, ed 8. WB Saunders, Philadelphia, 2007.

217. Mantadakis E, Cavender JD, Rogers ZR, et al: Prevalence of priapism in children and adolescents with sickle cell anemia. *J Pediatr Hematol Oncol* 21(6):518–522, 1999.

218. Fowler JE Jr, Koshy M, Strub M, et al: Priapism associated with the sickle cell hemoglobinopathies: Prevalence, natural history and sequelae. *J Urol* 145(1):65–68, 1991.

219. Emond AM, Holman R, Hayes RJ, et al: Priapism and impotence in homozygous sickle cell disease. *Arch Intern Med* 140(11):1434–1437, 1980.

220. Adeyoju AB, Olujohungbe AB, Morris J, et al: Priapism in sickle-cell disease; incidence, risk factors and complications-an international multicentre study. *BJU Int* 90(9):898–902, 2002.

221. Olujohungbe A, Burnett AL: How I manage priapism due to sickle cell disease. *Br J Haematol* 160(6):754–765, 2013.

222. Olujohungbe AB, Adeyoju A, Yardumian A, et al: A prospective diary study of stuttering priapism in adolescents and young men with sickle cell anemia: Report of an international randomized control trial—the priapism in sickle cell study. *J Androl* 32(4):375–382, 2011.

223. Siegel JF, Rich MA, Brock WA: Association of sickle cell disease, priapism, exchange transfusion and neurological events: ASPEN syndrome. *J Urol* 150(5 Pt 1):1480–1482, 1993.

224. Field JJ, Austin PF, An P, et al: Enuresis is a common and persistent problem among children and young adults with sickle cell anemia. *Urology* 72(1):81–84, 2008.

225. Jordan SS, Hilker KA, Stoppelbein L, et al: Nocturnal enuresis and psychosocial problems in pediatric sickle cell disease and sibling controls. *J Dev Behav Pediatr* 26(6):404–411, 2005.

226. Barakat LP, Smith-Whitley K, Schulman S, et al: Nocturnal enuresis in pediatric sickle cell disease. *J Dev Behav Pediatr* 22(5):300–305, 2001.

227. Almeida A, Roberts I: Bone involvement in sickle cell disease. *Br J Haematol* 129(4):482–490, 2005.

228. Kim SK, Miller JH: Natural history and distribution of bone and bone marrow infarction in sickle hemoglobinopathies. *J Nucl Med* 43(7):896–900, 2002.

229. Lonergan G, Cline DB, Abbondanzo SL: Sickle cell anemia. *Radiographics* 21:971–994, 2001.

230. Smith J: Bone disorders in sickle cell disease. *Hematol Oncol Clin North Am* 10:1 345–1356, 1996.

231. Atkins BL, Price EH, Tillyer L, et al: Salmonella osteomyelitis in sickle cell disease children in the east end of London. *J Infect* 34(2):133–138, 1997.

232. Burnett MW, Bass JW, Cook BA: Etiology of osteomyelitis complicating sickle cell disease. *Pediatrics* 101(2):296–297, 1998.

233. William R, Hussein SS, Jeans WD, et al: A prospective study of soft-tissue ultrasonography in sickle cell disease patients with suspected osteomyelitis. *Clin Radiol* 55:307–310, 2000.

234. Umans H, Haramati, N, Flusser G. The diagnostic role of gadolinium enhanced MRI in distinguishing between acute medullary bone infarct and osteomyelitis. *Magn Reson Imaging* 18:255–262, 2000.

235. Neonato M, Guilloud-Bataille M, Beauvais P, et al: Acute clinical events in 299 homozygous sickle cell patients living in France. French study group on sickle cell disease. *Eur J Haematol* 65:155–164, 2000.

236. Guggenbuhl P, Fergelot P, Doyard M, et al: Bone status in a mouse model of genetic hemochromatosis. *Osteoporos Int* 22(8):2313–2319, 2011.

237. Tsay J, Yang Z, Ross FP, et al: Bone loss caused by iron overload in a murine model: Importance of oxidative stress. *Blood* 116(14):2582–2589, 2010.

238. Fung EB, Harmatz PR, Milet M, et al: Fracture prevalence and relationship to endocrinopathy in iron overloaded patients with sickle cell disease and thalassemia. *Bone* 43(1):162–168, 2008.

239. Osunkwo I, Ziegler TR, Alvarez J, et al: High dose vitamin D therapy for chronic pain in children and adolescents with sickle cell disease: Results of a randomized double blind pilot study. *Br J Haematol* 159(2):211–215, 2012.

240. Milner P, Kraus AP, Sebes JJ, et al: Sickle cell disease as a cause of osteonecrosis of the femoral head. *N Engl J Med* 325:1479–1481, 1991.

241. Ware H, Brooks AP, Toye R, Berney SI: Sickle cell disease and silent avascular necrosis of the hip. *J Bone Joint Surg Br* 73:947–949, 1991.

242. Adekile AD, Gupta R, Yacoub F, et al: Avascular necrosis of the hip in children with sickle cell disease and high Hb F: Magnetic resonance imaging findings and influence of alpha-thalassemia trait. *Acta Haematol* 105(1):27–31, 2001.

243. Mahadeo KM, Oyeku S, Taragin B, et al: Increased prevalence of osteonecrosis of the femoral head in children and adolescents with sickle-cell disease. *Am J Hematol* 86(9):806–808, 2011.

244. Akinyoola AL, Adediran IA, Asaleye CM, et al: Risk factors for osteonecrosis of the femoral head in patients with sickle cell disease. *Int Orthop* 33(4):923–926, 2009.

245. Baldwin C, Nolan VG, Wyszynski DF, et al: Association of Klotho, bone morphogenic protein 6, and annexin A2 polymorphisms with sickle cell osteonecrosis. *Blood* 106(1):372–375, 2005.

246. Milner P, Kraus AP, Sebes JJ, et al: Osteonecrosis of the humeral head in sickle cell disease. *Clin Orthop Relat Res* 289:136–143, 1993.

247. Hernigou P, Bachir D, Galacteros F: The natural history of symptomatic osteonecrosis in adults with sickle-cell disease. *J Bone Joint Surg Am* 85-A(3):500–504, 2003.

248. Hernigou P, Habibi A, Bachir D, et al: The natural history of asymptomatic osteonecrosis of the femoral head in adults with sickle cell disease. *J Bone Joint Surg Am* 88(12):2565–2572, 2006.

249. Neumayr LD, Aguilar C, Earles AN, et al: Physical therapy alone compared with core decompression and physical therapy for femoral head osteonecrosis in sickle cell disease. Results of a multicenter study at a mean of three years after treatment. *J Bone Joint Surg Am* 88(12):2573–2582, 2006.

250. Hernigou P, Zilber S, Filippini P, et al: Total THA in adult osteonecrosis related to sickle cell disease. *Clin Orthop Relat Res* 466(2):300–308, 2008.

251. Moran MC, Huo MH, Garvin KL, et al: Total hip arthroplasty in sickle cell hemoglobinopathy. *Clin Orthop Relat Res* (294):140–148, 1993.

252. Acurio MT, Friedman RJ: Hip arthroplasty in patients with sickle-cell haemoglobinopathy. *J Bone Joint Surg Br* 74(3):367–371, 1992.

253. Nolan VG, Adewoye A, Baldwin C, et al: Sickle cell leg ulcers: Associations with haemolysis and SNPs in Klotho, TEK and genes of the TGF-beta/BMP pathway. *Br J Haematol* 133(5):570–578, 2006.

254. Koshy M, Entsuah R, Koranda A, et al: Leg ulcers in patients with sickle cell disease. *Blood* 74(4):1403–1408, 1989.

255. Best PJ, Daoud MS, Pittelkow MR, et al: Hydroxyurea-induced leg ulceration in 14 patients. *Ann Intern Med* 128(1):29–32, 1998.

256. Halabi-Tawil M, Lionnet F, Girot R, et al: Sickle cell leg ulcers: A frequently disabling complication and a marker of severity. *Br J Dermatol* 158(2):339–344, 2008.

257. Wethers DL, Ramirez GM, Koshy M, et al: Accelerated healing of chronic sickle-cell leg ulcers treated with RGD peptide matrix. RGD Study Group. *Blood* 84(6):1775–1779, 1994.

258. Sher GD, Olivieri NF: Rapid healing of chronic leg ulcers during arginine butyrate therapy in patients with sickle cell disease and thalassemia. *Blood* 84(7):2378–2380, 1994.

259. Traina F, Jorge SG, Yamanaka A, et al: Chronic liver abnormalities in sickle cell disease: A clinicopathological study in 70 living patients. *Acta Haematol* 118(3):129–135, 2007.

260. Banerjee S, Owen C, Chopra S: Sickle cell hepatopathy. *Hepatology* 33(5):1021–1028, 2001.

261. West MS, Wethers D, Smith J, et al: Laboratory profile of sickle cell disease: A cross-sectional analysis. The Cooperative Study of Sickle Cell Disease. *J Clin Epidemiol* 45(8):893–909, 1992.

262. Koskinas J, Manesis EK, Zacharakis GH, et al: Liver involvement in acute vaso-occlusive crisis of sickle cell disease: Prevalence and predisposing factors. *Scand J Gastroenterol* 42(4):499–507, 2007.

263. Buchanan GR, Glader BE: Benign course of extreme hyperbilirubinemia in sickle cell anemia: Analysis of six cases. *J Pediatr* 91(1):21–24, 1977.

264. Johnson CS, Omata M, Tong MJ, et al: Liver involvement in sickle cell disease. *Medicine (Baltimore)* 64(5):349–356, 1985.

265. Shao SH, Orringer EP: Sickle cell intrahepatic cholestasis: Approach to a difficult problem. *Am J Gastroenterol* 90(11):2048–2050, 1995.

266. Ahn H, Li CS, Wang W: Sickle cell hepatopathy: Clinical presentation, treatment, and outcome in pediatric and adult patients. *Pediatr Blood Cancer* 45(2):184–190, 2005.

267. Sheehy TW: Sickle cell hepatopathy. *South Med J* 70(5):533–538, 1977.

268. Schubert TT: Hepatobiliary system in sickle cell disease. *Gastroenterology* 90(6):2013–2021, 1986.

269. Suell MN, Horton TM, Dishop MK, et al: Outcomes for children with gallbladder abnormalities and sickle cell disease. *J Pediatr* 145(5):617–621, 2004.

270. Rennels MB, Dunne MG, Grossman NJ, et al: Cholelithiasis in patients with major sickle hemoglobinopathies. *Am J Dis Child* 138(1):66–67, 1984.

271. Bond LR, Hatty SR, Horn ME, et al: Gall stones in sickle cell disease in the United Kingdom. *Br Med J (Clin Res Ed)* 295(6592):234–236, 1987.

272. Vasavda N, Menzel S, Kondaveeti S, et al: The linear effects of alpha-thalassaemia, the UGT1A1 and HMOX1 polymorphisms on cholelithiasis in sickle cell disease. *Br J Haematol* 138(2):263–270, 2007.

273. To KW, Nadel AJ: Ophthalmologic complications in hemoglobinopathies. *Hematol Oncol Clin North Am* 5(3):535–548, 1991.

274. Mohan JS, Lip PL, Blann AD, et al: The angiopoietin/Tie-2 system in proliferative sickle retinopathy: Relation to vascular endothelial growth factor, its soluble receptor Flt-1 and von Willebrand factor, and to the effects of laser treatment. *Br J Ophthalmol* 89(7):815–819, 2005.

275. Aiello LP, Avery RL, Arrigg PG, et al: Vascular endothelial growth factor in ocular fluid of patients with diabetic retinopathy and other retinal disorders. *N Engl J Med* 331(22):1480–1487, 1994.

276. Aiello LP, Northrup JM, Keyt BA, et al: Hypoxic regulation of vascular endothelial growth factor in retinal cells. *Arch Ophthalmol* 113(12):1538–1544, 1995.

277. Downes SM, Hambleton IR, Chuang EL, et al: Incidence and natural history of proliferative sickle cell retinopathy: Observations from a cohort study. *Ophthalmology* 112(11):1869–1875, 2005.

278. Condon PI, Serjeant GR: Behaviour of untreated proliferative sickle retinopathy. *Br J Ophthalmol* 64(6):404–411, 1980.

279. Liem RI, Calamaras DM, Chhabra MS, et al: Sudden-onset blindness in sickle cell disease due to retinal artery occlusion. *Pediatr Blood Cancer* 50(3):624–627, 2008.

280. Paton D: The conjunctival sign of sickle-cell disease. *Arch Ophthalmol* 66:90–94, 1961.

281. Paton D: The conjunctival sign ox sickle-cell disease. Further observations. *Arch Ophthalmol* 68:627–632, 1962.

282. Cheung AT, Chen PC, Larkin EC, et al: Microvascular abnormalities in sickle cell disease: A computer-assisted intravital microscopy study. *Blood* 99(11):3999–4005, 2002.

283. Knisely MH, Bloch EH, Eliot TS, et al: Sludged blood. *Science* 106(2758):431–440, 1947.

284. Curran EL, Fleming JC, Rice K, et al: Orbital compression syndrome in sickle cell disease. *Ophthalmology* 104(10):1610–1615, 1997.

285. Sayag D, Binaghi M, Souied EH, et al: Retinal photocoagulation for proliferative sickle cell retinopathy: A prospective clinical trial with new sea fan classification. *Eur J Ophthalmol* 18(2):248–254, 2008.

286. Fox PD, Minninger K, Forshaw ML, et al: Laser photocoagulation for proliferative retinopathy in sickle haemoglobin C disease. *Eye (Lond)* 7(Pt 5):703–706, 1993.

287. Fox PD, Vessey SJ, Forshaw ML, et al: Influence of genotype on the natural history of untreated proliferative sickle retinopathy—An angiographic study. *Br J Ophthalmol* 75(4):229–231, 1991.

288. Rogers ZR, Wang WC, Luo Z, et al: Biomarkers of splenic function in infants with sickle cell anemia: Baseline data from the BABY HUG Trial. *Blood* 117(9):2614–2617, 2011.

289. Brousse V, Buffet P, Rees D: The spleen and sickle cell disease: The sick(led) spleen. *Br J Haematol* 166(2):165–176, 2014.

290. Pearson HA, Spencer RP, Cornelius EA: Functional asplenia in sickle-cell anemia. *N Engl J Med* 281(17):923–926, 1969.

291. Ferster A, Bujan W, Corazza F, et al: Bone marrow transplantation corrects the splenic reticuloendothelial dysfunction in sickle cell anemia. *Blood* 81(4):1102–1105, 1993.

292. Buchanan GR, McKie V, Jackson EA, et al: Splenic phagocytic function in children with sickle cell anemia receiving long-term hypertransfusion therapy. *J Pediatr* 115(4):568–572, 1989.

293. Claster S, Vichinsky E: First report of reversal of organ dysfunction in sickle cell anemia by the use of hydroxyurea: Splenic regeneration. *Blood* 88(6):1951–1953, 1996.

294. Naik RP, Lanzkron S: Baby on board: What you need to know about pregnancy in the hemoglobinopathies. *Hematology Am Soc Hematol Educ Program* 2012:208–214, 2012.

295. Sun PM, Wilburn W, Raynor BD, et al: Sickle cell disease in pregnancy: Twenty years of experience at Grady Memorial Hospital, Atlanta, Georgia. *Am J Obstet Gynecol* 184(6):1127–1130, 2001.

296. Boulet SL, Okoroh EM, Azonobi I, et al: Sickle cell disease in pregnancy: Maternal complications in a Medicaid-enrolled population. *Matern Child Health J* 17(2):200–207, 2013.

297. Villers MS, Jamison MG, De Castro LM, et al: Morbidity associated with sickle cell disease in pregnancy. *Am J Obstet Gynecol* 199(2):125 e1–e5, 2008.

298. James AH, Jamison MG, Brancazio LR, et al: Venous thromboembolism during pregnancy and the postpartum period: Incidence, risk factors, and mortality. *Am J Obstet Gynecol* 194(5):1311–1315, 2006.

299. Wilson JG, Scott WJ, Ritter EJ, et al: Comparative distribution and embryotoxicity of hydroxyurea in pregnant rats and rhesus monkeys. *Teratology* 11(2):169–178, 1975.

300. Thauvin-Robinet C, Maingueneau C, Robert E, et al: Exposure to hydroxyurea during pregnancy: A case series. *Leukemia* 15(8):1309–1311, 2001.

301. Austin H, Lally C, Benson JM, et al: Hormonal contraception, sickle cell trait, and risk for venous thromboembolism among African American women. *Am J Obstet Gynecol* 200(6):620 e1–3, 2009.

302. Zarrouk V, Habibi A, Zahar JR, et al: Bloodstream infection in adults with sickle cell disease: Association with venous catheters, *Staphylococcus aureus*, and bone-joint infections. *Medicine (Baltimore)* 85(1):43–48, 2006.

303. Mollapour E, Porter JB, Kaczmarski R, et al: Raised neutrophil phospholipase A2 activity and defective priming of NADPH oxidase and phospholipase A2 in sickle cell disease. *Blood* 91(9):3423–3429, 1998.

304. Overturf GD: Infections and immunizations of children with sickle cell disease. *Adv Pediatr Infect Dis* 14:191–218, 1999.

305. Sullivan JL, Ochs HD, Schiffman G, et al: Immune response after splenectomy. *Lancet* 1(8057):178–181, 1978.

306. Barrett-Connor E: Bacterial infection and sickle cell anemia. An analysis of 250 infections in 166 patients and a review of the literature. *Medicine (Baltimore)* 50(2):97–112, 1971.

307. Zarkowsky HS, Gallagher D, Gill FM, et al: Bacteremia in sickle hemoglobinopathies. *J Pediatr* 109(4):579–585, 1986.

308. Leikin SL, Gallagher D, Kinney TR, et al: Mortality in children and adolescents with sickle cell disease. Cooperative Study of Sickle Cell Disease. *Pediatrics* 84(3):500–508, 1989.

309. Adamkiewicz TV, Sarnaik S, Buchanan GR, et al: Invasive pneumococcal infections in children with sickle cell disease in the era of penicillin prophylaxis, antibiotic resistance, and 23-valent pneumococcal polysaccharide vaccination. *J Pediatr* 143(4):438–444, 2003.

310. Gaston MH, Verter JI, Woods G, et al: Prophylaxis with oral penicillin in children with sickle cell anemia. A randomized trial. *N Engl J Med* 314(25):1593–1599, 1986.

311. Halasa NB, Shankar SM, Talbot TR, et al: Incidence of invasive pneumococcal disease among individuals with sickle cell disease before and after the introduction of the pneumococcal conjugate vaccine. *Clin Infect Dis* 44(11):1428–1433, 2007.

312. Kyaw MH, Lynfield R, Schaffner W, et al: Effect of introduction of the pneumococcal conjugate vaccine on drug-resistant *Streptococcus pneumoniae*. *N Engl J Med* 354(14):1455–1463, 2006.

313. Section on Hematology/Oncology Committee on Genetics; American Academy of Pediatrics: Health supervision for children with sickle cell disease. *Pediatrics* 109(3):526–535, 2002.

314. Adamkiewicz TV, Silk BJ, Howgate J, et al: Effectiveness of the 7-valent pneumococcal conjugate vaccine in children with sickle cell disease in the first decade of life. *Pediatrics* 121(3):562–569, 2008.

315. McCavit TL, Quinn CT, Techasaensiri C, et al: Increase in invasive *Streptococcus pneumoniae* infections in children with sickle cell disease since pneumococcal conjugate vaccine licensure. *J Pediatr* 158(3):505–507, 2011.

316. Falletta JM, Woods GM, Verter JI, et al: Discontinuing penicillin prophylaxis in children with sickle cell anemia. Prophylactic Penicillin Study II. *J Pediatr* 127(5):685–690, 1995.

317. Rice TW, Rubinson L, Uyeki TM, et al: Critical illness from 2009 pandemic influenza A virus and bacterial coinfection in the United States. *Crit Care Med* 40(5):1487–1498, 2012.

318. Makani J, Komba AN, Cox SE, et al: Malaria in patients with sickle cell anemia: Burden, risk factors, and outcome at the outpatient clinic and during hospitalization. *Blood* 115(2):215–220, 2010.

319. McAuley CF, Webb C, Makani J, et al: High mortality from *Plasmodium falciparum* malaria in children living with sickle cell anemia on the coast of Kenya. *Blood* 116(10):1663–1668, 2010.

320. Koshy M, Weiner SJ, Miller ST, et al: Surgery and anesthesia in sickle cell disease. Cooperative Study of Sickle Cell Diseases. *Blood* 86(10):3676–3684, 1995.

321. Firth PG, Head CA: Sickle cell disease and anesthesia. *Anesthesiology* 101(3):766–785, 2004.

322. Griffin TC, Buchanan GR: Elective surgery in children with sickle cell disease without preoperative blood transfusion. *J Pediatr Surg* 28(5):681–685, 1993.

323. Howard J, Malfroy M, Llewelyn C, et al: The Transfusion Alternatives Preoperatively in Sickle Cell Disease (TAPS) study: A randomised, controlled, multicentre clinical trial. *Lancet* 381(9870):930–938, 2013.

324. Kutlar A: Sickle cell disease: A multigenic perspective of a single gene disorder. *Hemoglobin* 31(2):209–224, 2007.

325. Steinberg MH: Predicting clinical severity in sickle cell anaemia. *Br J Haematol* 129(4):465–481, 2005.

326. Sankaran VG: Targeted therapeutic strategies for fetal hemoglobin induction. *Hematology Am Soc Hematol Educ Program* 2011:459–465, 2011.

327. Zhou D, Liu K, Sun CW, et al: KLF1 regulates BCL11A expression and gamma- to beta-globin gene switching. *Nat Genet* 42(9):742–744, 2010.

328. Hoppe C, Klitz W, Cheng S, et al: Gene interactions and stroke risk in children with sickle cell anemia. *Blood* 103(6):2391–2396, 2004.

329. Sebastiani P, Ramoni MF, Nolan V, et al: Genetic dissection and prognostic modeling of overt stroke in sickle cell anemia. *Nat Genet* 37(4):435–440, 2005.

330. Taylor JG 6th, Tang DC, Savage SA, et al: Variants in the VCAM1 gene and risk for symptomatic stroke in sickle cell disease. *Blood* 100(13):4303–4309, 2002.

331. Sharan K, Surrey S, Ballas S, et al: Association of T-786C eNOS gene polymorphism with increased susceptibility to acute chest syndrome in females with sickle cell disease. *Br J Haematol* 124(2):240–243, 2004.

332. Adekile A, Kutlar F, McKie K, et al: The influence of uridine diphosphate glucuronosyl transferase 1A promoter polymorphisms, beta-globin gene haplotype, co-inherited alpha-thalassemia trait and Hb F on steady-state serum bilirubin levels in sickle cell anemia. *Eur J Haematol* 75(2):150–155, 2005.

333. Fertrin KY, Melo MB, Assis AM, et al: UDP-glucuronosyltransferase 1 gene promoter polymorphism is associated with increased serum bilirubin levels and cholecystectomy in patients with sickle cell anemia. *Clin Genet* 64(2):160–162, 2003.

334. Haverfield EV, McKenzie CA, Forrester T, et al: UGT1A1 variation and gallstone formation in sickle cell disease. *Blood* 105(3):968–972, 2005.

335. Passon RG, Howard TA, Zimmerman SA, et al: Influence of bilirubin uridine diphosphate-glucuronosyltransferase 1A promoter polymorphisms on serum bilirubin levels and cholelithiasis in children with sickle cell anemia. *J Pediatr Hematol Oncol* 23(7):448–451, 2001.

336. Nolan VG, Baldwin C, Ma Q, et al: Association of single nucleotide polymorphisms in Klotho with priapism in sickle cell anaemia. *Br J Haematol* 128(2):266–272, 2005.

337. Close J, Game L, Clark B, et al: Genome annotation of a 1.5 Mb region of human chromosome 6q23 encompassing a quantitative trait locus for fetal hemoglobin expression in adults. *BMC Genomics* 5(1):33, 2004.

338. Garner CP, Tatu T, Best S, et al: Evidence of genetic interaction between the beta-globin complex and chromosome 8q in the expression of fetal hemoglobin. *Am J Hum Genet* 70(3):793–799, 2002.

339. Lettre G, Sankaran VG, Bezerra MA, et al: DNA polymorphisms at the BCL11A, HBS1L-MYB, and beta-globin loci associate with fetal hemoglobin levels and pain crises in sickle cell disease. *Proc Natl Acad Sci U S A* 105(33):11869–11874, 2008.

340. Thein SL, Menzel S: Discovering the genetics underlying foetal haemoglobin production in adults. *Br J Haematol* 145(4):455–467, 2009.

341. Uda M, Galanello R, Sanna S, et al: Genome-wide association study shows BCL11A associated with persistent fetal hemoglobin and amelioration of the phenotype of beta-thalassemia. *Proc Natl Acad Sci U S A* 105(5):1620–1625, 2008.

342. Wyszynski DF, Baldwin CT, Cleves MA, et al: Polymorphisms near a chromosome 6q QTL area are associated with modulation of fetal hemoglobin levels in sickle cell anemia. *Cell Mol Biol (Noisy-le-grand)* 50(1):23–33, 2004.

343. Wyszynski DF, Baldwin CT, Cleves MA, et al: Genetic polymorphisms associated with fetal hemoglobin response to hydroxyurea in patients with sickle cell anemia. *Blood Coagul Fibrinolysis* 104 (Suppl):34a, 2004.

344. Pembrey ME, Wood WG, Weatherall DJ, et al: Fetal haemoglobin production and the sickle gene in the oases of Eastern Saudi Arabia. *Br J Haematol* 40(3):415–429, 1978.

345. Platt OS: Hydroxyurea for the treatment of sickle cell anemia. *N Engl J Med* 358(13):1362–1369, 2008.

346. Gladwin MT, Shelhamer JH, Ognibene FP, et al: Nitric oxide donor properties of hydroxyurea in patients with sickle cell disease. *Br J Haematol* 116(2):436–444, 2002.

347. Hillery CA, Du MC, Wang WC, et al: Hydroxyurea therapy decreases the *in vitro* adhesion of sickle erythrocytes to thrombospondin and laminin. *Br J Haematol* 109(2):322–327, 2000.

348. Orringer EP, Blythe DS, Johnson AE, et al: Effects of hydroxyurea on hemoglobin F and water content in the red blood cells of dogs and of patients with sickle cell anemia. *Blood* 78(1):212–216, 1991.

349. Steinberg MH, Barton F, Castro O, et al: Effect of hydroxyurea on mortality and morbidity in adult sickle cell anemia: Risks and benefits up to 9 years of treatment. *JAMA* 289(13):1645–1651, 2003.

350. Ware RE: How I use hydroxyurea to treat young patients with sickle cell anemia. *Blood* 115(26):5300–5311, 2010.

351. Ware RE: Hydroxycarbamide: Clinical aspects. *C R Biol* 336(3):177–182, 2013.

352. Brawley OW, Cornelius LJ, Edwards LR, et al: National Institutes of Health Consensus Development Conference statement: Hydroxyurea treatment for sickle cell disease. *Ann Intern Med* 148(12):932–938, 2008.

353. Lanzkron S, Strouse JJ, Wilson R, et al: Systematic review: Hydroxyurea for the treatment of adults with sickle cell disease. *Ann Intern Med* 148(12):939–955, 2008.

354. Shelby MD: National Toxicology Program Center for the Evaluation of Risks to Human Reproduction: Guidelines for CERHR expert panel members. *Birth Defects Res B Dev Reprod Toxicol* 74(1):9–16, 2005.

355. Shelby MD: Center for the Evaluation of Risks to Human Reproduction 2007; Available from: http://cerhr.niehs.nih.gov/chemicals/hydroxyurea/Hydroxyurea_final.pdf.

356. Hankins JS, Ware RE, Rogers ZR, et al: Long-term hydroxyurea therapy for infants with sickle cell anemia: The HUSOFT extension study. *Blood* 106(7):2269–2275, 2005.

357. Kinney TR, Helms RW, O'Branski EE, et al: Safety of hydroxyurea in children with sickle cell anemia: Results of the HUG-KIDS study, a phase I/II trial. Pediatric Hydroxyurea Group. *Blood* 94(5):1550–1554, 1999.

358. Atweh GF, Sutton M, Nassif I, et al: Sustained induction of fetal hemoglobin by pulse butyrate therapy in sickle cell disease. *Blood* 93(6):1790–1797, 1999.

359. Dover GJ, Brusilow S, Charache S: Induction of fetal hemoglobin production in subjects with sickle cell anemia by oral sodium phenylbutyrate. *Blood* 84(1):339–343, 1994.

360. Reid ME, El Beshlawy A, Inati A, et al: A double-blind, placebo-controlled phase II study of the efficacy and safety of 2,2-dimethylbutyrate (HQK-1001), an oral fetal globin inducer, in sickle cell disease. *Am J Hematol* 89(7):709–713, 2014.

361. DeSimone J, Heller P, Schimenti JC, et al: Fetal hemoglobin production in adult baboons by 5-azacytidine or by phenylhydrazine-induced hemolysis is associated with hypomethylation of globin gene DNA. *Prog Clin Biol Res* 134:489–500, 1983.

362. Saunthararajah Y, Hillery CA, Lavelle D, et al: Effects of 5-aza-2'-deoxycytidine on fetal hemoglobin levels, red cell adhesion, and hematopoietic differentiation in patients with sickle cell disease. *Blood* 102(12):3865–3870, 2003.

363. Saunthararajah Y, Molokie R, Saraf S, et al: Clinical effectiveness of decitabine in severe sickle cell disease. *Br J Haematol* 141(1):126–129, 2008.

364. Charache S, Dover G, Smith K, et al: Treatment of sickle cell anemia with 5-azacytidine results in increased fetal hemoglobin production and is associated with nonrandom hypomethylation of DNA around the gamma-delta-beta-globin gene complex. *Proc Natl Acad Sci U S A* 80(15):4842–4846, 1983.

365. DeSimone J, Heller P, Hall L, et al: 5-Azacytidine stimulates fetal hemoglobin synthesis in anemic baboons. *Proc Natl Acad Sci U S A* 79(14):4428–4431, 1982.

366. Ley TJ, DeSimone J, Noguchi CT, et al: 5-Azacytidine increases gamma-globin synthesis and reduces the proportion of dense cells in patients with sickle cell anemia. *Blood* 62(2):370–380, 1983.

367. Lowrey CH, Nienhuis AW: Brief report: Treatment with azacitidine of patients with end-stage beta-thalassemia. *N Engl J Med* 329(12):845–848, 1993.

368. Mavilio F, Giampaolo A, Care A, et al: Molecular mechanisms of human hemoglobin switching: Selective undermethylation and expression of globin genes in embryonic, fetal, and adult erythroblasts. *Proc Natl Acad Sci U S A* 80(22):6907–6911, 1983.

369. Moutouh-de Parseval LA, Verhelle D, Glezer E, et al: Pomalidomide and lenalidomide regulate erythropoiesis and fetal hemoglobin production in human CD34+ cells. *J Clin Invest* 118(1):248–258, 2008.

370. Meiler SE, Wade M, Kutlar F, et al: Pomalidomide augments fetal hemoglobin production without the myelosuppressive effects of hydroxyurea in transgenic sickle cell mice. *Blood* 118(4):1109–1112, 2011.

371. Gluckman E: Allogeneic transplantation strategies including haploidentical transplantation in sickle cell disease. *Hematology Am Soc Hematol Educ Program* 2013:370–376, 2013.

372. Locatelli F, Pagliara D: Allogeneic hematopoietic stem cell transplantation in children with sickle cell disease. *Pediatr Blood Cancer* 59(2):372–376, 2012.

373. Walters MC, Hardy K, Edwards S, et al: Pulmonary, gonadal, and central nervous system status after bone marrow transplantation for sickle cell disease. *Biol Blood Marrow Transplant* 16(2):263–272, 2010.

374. Hsieh MM, Kang EM, Fitzhugh CD, et al: Allogeneic hematopoietic stem-cell transplantation for sickle cell disease. *N Engl J Med* 361(24):2309–2317, 2009.

375. Ruggeri A, Eapen M, Scaravadou A, et al: Umbilical cord blood transplantation for children with thalassemia and sickle cell disease. *Biol Blood Marrow Transplant* 17(9):1375–1382, 2011.

376. Bolanos-Meade J, Fuchs EJ, Luznik L, et al: HLA-haploidentical bone marrow transplantation with posttransplant cyclophosphamide expands the donor pool for patients with sickle cell disease. *Blood* 120(22):4285–4291, 2012.

377. Smith-Whitley K, Thompson AA: Indications and complications of transfusions in sickle cell disease. *Pediatr Blood Cancer* 59(2):358–364, 2012.

378. Telen MJ: Principles and problems of transfusion in sickle cell disease. *Semin Hematol* 38(4):315–323, 2001.

379. Chien S, Usami S, Bertles JF: Abnormal rheology of oxygenated blood in sickle cell anemia. *J Clin Invest* 49(4):623–634, 1970.

380. Morris CL, Gruppo RA, Shukla R, et al: Influence of plasma and red cell factors on the rheologic properties of oxygenated sickle blood during clinical steady state. *J Lab Clin Med* 118(4):332–342, 1991.

381. Schmalzer EA, Lee JO, Brown AK, et al: Viscosity of mixtures of sickle and normal red cells at varying hematocrit levels. Implications for transfusion. *Transfusion* 27(3):228–233, 1987.

382. Vichinsky EP: Current issues with blood transfusions in sickle cell disease. *Semin Hematol* 38(1 Suppl 1):14–22, 2001.

383. Rosse WF, Gallagher D, Kinney TR, et al: Transfusion and alloimmunization in sickle cell disease. The Cooperative Study of Sickle Cell Disease. *Blood* 76(7):1431–1437, 1990.

384. Yazdanbakhsh K, Ware RE and Noizat-Pirenne F: Red blood cell alloimmunization in sickle cell disease: Pathophysiology, risk factors, and transfusion management. *Blood* 120(3):528–537, 2012.

385. Wahl S, Quirolo KC: Current issues in blood transfusion for sickle cell disease. *Curr Opin Pediatr* 21(1):15–21, 2009.

386. Talano JA, Hillery CA, Gottschall JL, et al: Delayed hemolytic transfusion reaction/hyperhemolysis syndrome in children with sickle cell disease. *Pediatrics* 111(6 Pt 1):e661–e665, 2003.

387. Ballas SK: Iron overload is a determinant of morbidity and mortality in adult patients with sickle cell disease. *Semin Hematol* 38(1 Suppl 1):30–36, 2001.

388. Vichinsky E, Butensky E, Fung E, et al: Comparison of organ dysfunction in transfused patients with SCD or beta thalassemia. *Am J Hematol* 80(1):70–74, 2005.

389. Fung EB, Harmatz P, Milet M, et al: Morbidity and mortality in chronically transfused subjects with thalassemia and sickle cell disease: A report from the multi-center study of iron overload. *Am J Hematol* 82(4):255–265, 2007.

390. Brittenham GM, Cohen AR, McLaren CE, et al: Hepatic iron stores and plasma ferritin concentration in patients with sickle cell anemia and thalassemia major. *Am J Hematol* 42(1):81–85, 1993.

391. National Institutes of Health, Division of Blood Diseases and Resources: *The Management of Sickle Cell Disease*, ed 4. NIH Publication No. 02-2117. NIH, Bethesda, MD, 2002. Available at: http://www.nhlbi.nih.gov/health/prof/blood/sickle/sc_mngt.pdf

392. Silliman CC, Peterson VM, Mellman DL, et al: Iron chelation by deferoxamine in sickle cell patients with severe transfusion-induced hemosiderosis: A randomized, double-blind study of the dose-response relationship. *J Lab Clin Med* 122(1):48–54, 1993.

393. Vichinsky E, Onyekwere O, Porter J, et al: A randomised comparison of deferasirox versus deferoxamine for the treatment of transfusional iron overload in sickle cell disease. *Br J Haematol* 136(3):501–508, 2007.

394. Lucania G, Vitrano A, Filosa A, et al: Chelation treatment in sickle-cell-anaemia: Much ado about nothing? *Br J Haematol* 154(5):545–555, 2011.

395. Brittenham GM: Iron-chelating therapy for transfusional iron overload. *N Engl J Med* 364(2):146–156, 2011.

396. Steinberg MH, Adams JG 3rd, Dreiling BJ: Alpha thalassaemia in adults with sickle-cell trait. *Br J Haematol* 30(1):31–37, 1975.

397. Wong SC, Ali MA, Boyadjian SE: Sickle cell traits in Canada. Trimodal distribution of Hb S as a result of interaction with alpha-thalassaemia gene. *Acta Haematol* 65(3):157–163, 1981.

398. Sciarratta GV, Sansone G, Ivaldi G, et al: Alternate organization of alpha G-Philadelphia globin genes among U.S. black and Italian Caucasian heterozygotes. *Hemoglobin* 8(6):537–547, 1984.

399. Itano HA, Neel JV: A new inherited abnormality of human hemoglobin. *Proc Natl Acad Sci U S A* 36(11):613–617, 1950.

400. Spaet TH, Alway RH, Ward G: Homozygous type c hemoglobin. *Pediatrics* 12(5):483–490, 1953.

401. Ranney HM, Larson DL, McCormack GH Jr: Some clinical, biochemical and genetic observations on hemoglobin C. *J Clin Invest* 32(12):1277–1284, 1953.

402. Nagel RL, Steinberg MH: Hb SC disease and Hb C disorders, in *Disorders of Hemoglobin: Genetics, Pathophysiology, and Clinical Management*, edited by Steinberg MH, Forget BG, Higgs DR, Nagel RL, pp 756–785. Cambridge University Press, Cambridge, 2001.

403. Boehm CD, Dowling CE, Antonarakis SE, et al: Evidence supporting a single origin of the beta(C)-globin gene in blacks. *Am J Hum Genet* 37(4):771–777, 1985.

404. Cook CM, Smeltzer MP, Mortier NA, et al: The clinical and laboratory spectrum of Hb C [beta6(A3)Glu—>Lys, GAG>AAG] disease. *Hemoglobin* 37(1):16–25, 2013.

405. Itano HA, Bergren WR, Sturgeon P: Identification of fourth abnormal human hemoglobin. *J Am Chem Soc* 76:2278, 1954.

406. Fucharoen S: Hb E disorders, in *Disorders of Hemoglobin: Genetics, Pathophysiology, and Clinical Management*, edited by Steinberg MH, Forget BG, Higgs DR, Nagel RL, pp 1139–1154. Cambridge University Press, Cambridge, 2001.

407. Atichartakarn V, Chuncharunee S, Archararit N, et al: Intravascular hemolysis, vascular endothelial cell activation and thrombophilia in splenectomized patients with hemoglobin E/beta-thalassemia disease. *Acta Haematol* 132(1):100–107, 2014.

408. Fucharoen S, Siritanaratkul N, Winichagoon P, et al: Hydroxyurea increases hemoglobin F levels and improves the effectiveness of erythropoiesis in beta-thalassemia/hemoglobin E disease. *Blood* 87(3):887–892, 1996.

409. Itano HA: A third abnormal hemoglobin associated with hereditary hemolytic anemia. *Proc Natl Acad Sci U S A* 37(12):775–784, 1951.

410. Huisman THJ, Carver MFH, Efremov GD: *A Syllabus of Human Hemoglobin Variants.* The Sickle Cell Anemia Foundation, Augusta, GA, 1998.

411. Cathie IAB: Apparent idiopathic Heinz body anaemia. *Great Ormond St J* 3:343, 1952.

412. Wun T, Styles L, DeCastro L, et al: Phase 1 study of the E-selectin inhibitor GMI 1070 in patients with sickle cell anemia. *PLoS One* 9(7):e101301, 2014.

413. Nathan DG, Field J, Lin G, et al: Sickle cell disease (SCD), iNKT cells, and regadenoson infusion. *Trans Am Clin Climatol Assoc* 123:312–317; discussion 317–318, 2012.

414. Field JJ, Lin G, Okam MM, et al: Sickle cell vaso-occlusion causes activation of iNKT cells that is decreased by the adenosine A2A receptor agonist regadenoson. *Blood* 121(17):3329–3334, 2013.

415. Daak AA, Ghebremeskel K, Hassan Z, et al: Effect of omega-3 (n-3) fatty acid supplementation in patients with sickle cell anemia: Randomized, double-blind, placebo-controlled trial. *Am J Clin Nutr* 97(1):37–44, 2013.

416. Morris CR, Kuypers FA, Lavrisha L, et al: A randomized, placebo-controlled trial of arginine therapy for the treatment of children with sickle cell disease hospitalized with vaso-occlusive pain episodes. *Haematologica* 98(9):1375–1382, 2013.

417. Goldman RD, Mounstephen W, Kirby-Allen M, et al: Intravenous magnesium sulfate for vaso-occlusive episodes in sickle cell disease. *Pediatrics* 132(6):e1634–e1641, 2013.

418. Wun T, Soulieres D, Frelinger AL, et al: A double-blind, randomized, multicenter phase 2 study of prasugrel versus placebo in adult patients with sickle cell disease. *J Hematol Oncol* 6:17, 2013.

419. Desai PC, Brittain JE, Jones SK, et al: A pilot study of eptifibatide for treatment of acute pain episodes in sickle cell disease. *Thromb Res* 132(3):341–345, 2013.

420. Ataga KI, Reid M, Ballas SK, et al: Improvements in haemolysis and indicators of erythrocyte survival do not correlate with acute vaso-occlusive crises in patients with sickle cell disease: A phase III randomized, placebo-controlled, double-blind study of the Gardos channel blocker senicapoc (ICA-17043). *Br J Haematol* 153(1):92–104, 2011.

421. Orringer EP, Casella JF, Ataga KI, et al: Purified poloxamer 188 for treatment of acute vaso-occlusive crisis of sickle cell disease: A randomized controlled trial. *JAMA* 286(17):2099–2106, 2001.

422. Kutlar A, Ataga KI, McMahon L, et al: A potent oral P-selectin blocking agent improves microcirculatory blood flow and a marker of endothelial cell injury in patients with sickle cell disease. *Am J Hematol* 87(5):536–539, 2012.

CHAPTER 50
METHEMOGLOBINEMIA AND OTHER DYSHEMOGLOBINEMIAS

Archana M. Agarwal and Josef T. Prchal

SUMMARY

Normal hemoglobin can be oxidized to methemoglobin. Methemoglobinemia occurs because of either increased production of oxidized hemoglobin from exposure to environmental agents or diminished reduction of oxidized hemoglobin because of underlying germline mutations. Cyanosis is virtually invariant in patients with methemoglobinemia. Hemoglobin can also bind carbon monoxide and nitric oxide, resulting in the formation of carboxyhemoglobin and nitrosohemoglobin. Sulfhemoglobinemia occurs because of increased production secondary to occupational exposure to sulphur compounds or exposure to oxidant medications. These modified hemoglobins are known as *dyshemoglobins*. Depending upon the severity and individual predisposition, presence of dyshemoglobins can result in varying degree of clinical manifestations. Prompt diagnosis is the key to effective and timely treatment.

● METHEMOGLOBINEMIA

DEFINITION AND HISTORY

A bluish discoloration of the skin and mucous membrane, designated *cyanosis*, has been recognized since antiquity as a manifestation of lung or heart disease; however, in methemoglobinemia and sulfhemoglobinemia, it has a different molecular basis than in hemoglobin oxygen desaturation. Cyanosis resulting from drug administration has also been recognized since before 1890.[1] Toxic methemoglobinemia occurs when various drugs or toxic substances either oxidize hemoglobin (Hb) directly in the circulation or facilitate its oxidation by molecular oxygen.

In 1912, Sloss and Wybauw[2] reported a case of a patient with idiopathic methemoglobinemia. Later Hitzenberger[3] suggested that a hereditary form of methemoglobinemia might exist and, subsequently,

numerous such cases were reported.[4] In 1948, Hörlein and Weber[5] described a family in which eight members over four generations had cyanosis. The absorption spectrum of methemoglobin was abnormal and they demonstrated that the defect must reside in the globin portion of the molecule. Subsequently, Singer[6] proposed that such abnormal hemoglobins be given the designation hemoglobin M. The cause of another form of methemoglobinemia that occurs independently of drug administration and without the existence of any abnormality of the globin portion of hemoglobin was first explained by Gibson,[7] who clearly pointed to the site of the enzyme defect, nicotinamide adenine dinucleotide (reduced form) (NADH) diaphorase, also designated as methemoglobin reductase, and now known as cytochrome b_5 reductase. More than 50 years after Gibson's insightful studies, the genetic disorder that he had predicted was verified at the DNA level.[8]

The existence of abnormal hemoglobins that cause cyanosis through quite another mechanism was first recognized in 1968 with the description of hemoglobin Kansas.[9] Here the cyanosis resulted not from methemoglobin, as occurs in hemoglobin M, but rather from an abnormally low oxygen affinity of the mutant hemoglobin. Thus, at normal oxygen tensions, a large amount of deoxygenated hemoglobin is present in the blood of affected patients.

EPIDEMIOLOGY

Methemoglobinemia occurring as a result of cytochrome b_5 reductase deficiency is more common among Native Americans, both in Alaska and in the continental United States, and among the Evenk people of Yakutia of Russian Siberia than in other ethnic groups.[10–12] Methemoglobinemia resulting from hemoglobin M is inherited and sporadic. The occurrence of methemoglobinemia due to toxic chemicals is acquired, transient, and is also sporadic.

ETIOLOGY AND PATHOGENESIS

Methemoglobinemia decreases the oxygen-carrying capacity of blood because the oxidized iron cannot reversibly bind oxygen. Moreover, when one or more iron atoms have been oxidized, the conformation of hemoglobin is changed so as to increase the oxygen affinity of the remaining ferrous heme groups. In this way methemoglobinemia exerts a dual effect in impairing the supply of oxygen to tissues.[13]

Toxic Methemoglobinemia

Hemoglobin is continuously oxidized *in vivo* from the ferrous to the ferric state. The rate of such oxidation is accelerated by many drugs and toxic chemicals, including sulfonamides, lidocaine and other aniline derivatives, and nitrites. A vast number of chemical substances may cause methemoglobinemia.[14–16] Table 50–1 lists some of the agents that are responsible for clinically significant methemoglobinemia in clinical practice.

The most common offenders include benzocaine and lidocaine.[17–19] In some cases, the patients have been unaware that they have been ingesting one of the drugs known to produce methemoglobinemia; dapsone is apparently used in some "street drugs."[20,21] Nitrates and the nitrites contaminating water supplies or used as preservatives in foods are also common offending agents.[22–30]

Cytochrome b_5 Reductase Deficiency

Cytochrome b_5 reductase, also known as NADH diaphorase, catalyzes a step in the major pathway for methemoglobin reduction. This enzyme reduces cytochrome b_5, using NADH as a hydrogen donor. The reduced cytochrome b_5 reduces, in turn, methemoglobin to hemoglobin. A

TABLE 50–1. Some Drugs That Cause Methemoglobinemia

Phenazopyridine (Pyridium)[163–165]
Sulfamethoxazole[166]
Dapsone[20,167,168]
Aniline[88,89]
Paraquat/monolinuron[169–171]
Nitrate[22–24,81]
Nitroglycerin[163,172]
Amyl nitrite[173]
Isobutyl nitrite[174]
Sodium nitrite[23,82]
Benzocaine[175–177]
Prilocaine[178–180]
Methylene blue[87]
Chloramine[171,181]

steady-state methemoglobin level is achieved when the rate of methemoglobin formation equals the rate of methemoglobin reduction either through the cytochrome b_5 reductase or through a relatively minor auxiliary mechanism such as direct chemical reduction by ascorbate and reduced glutathione. A reduced nicotinamide adenine dinucleotide phosphate (NADPH)-linked enzyme, NADPH diaphorase, does not play a role in methemoglobin reduction except when a linking dye such as methylene blue is supplied (see "Therapy, Course, and Prognosis" below). A marked diminution in the activity of cytochrome $b5$ reductase will result in the accumulation of the brown pigment in circulating erythrocytes.

A balance to methemoglobin formation is antioxidant protein 2 (AOP2), which is present in high concentrations in human and mouse red cells (Chap. 47). This member of the peroxiredoxin protein family binds to hemoglobin and prevents both spontaneous and oxidant-induced methemoglobin formation.[31] Mutations of this gene or its acquired deficiency are theoretical candidates responsible for congenital and acquired methemoglobinemia. Cyanosis resulting from abnormal hemoglobins (both hemoglobin M and low-oxygen affinity hemoglobins) is inherited as an autosomal dominant disorder. In contrast, hereditary methemoglobinemia resulting from cytochrome b_5 reductase deficiency is inherited in an autosomal recessive fashion.

Many mutations of cytochrome b5 reductase that cause methemoglobinemia have been identified at the nucleotide level,[8] and the functional effect of some of these have been deduced from the structure of the enzyme.[32,33] Although most of the mutants have been found in persons of European descent, five unique mutations were found in Chinese,[34] at least three in Thais,[35] two in Americans of African descent,[36] and one in an Asian Indian.[37] In addition, a common polymorphism (allele frequency = 0.023) has been identified in Americans of African descent; it does not appear to impair the activity of the enzyme.[38] Most of the patients with cytochrome b_5 reductase deficiency merely have methemoglobinemia and the enzyme deficiency is limited to the red cells, and these have been classified as having type I disease. In type II cytochrome b_5 reductase deficiency, which represents 10 to 15 percent of cases of enzyme deficient congenital methemoglobinemia, cytochrome $b5$ reductase is decreased in all cells. In addition to cyanosis, severe developmental abnormalities can occur; most affected infants die

in the first year of life.[39,40] Patients with this form of disease are afflicted, in addition to methemoglobinemia, with a progressive encephalopathy and mental retardation. The finding that fatty acid elongation is defective in the platelets and leukocytes of such patients[41] provides a clue to the type of defect that could occur in the central nervous system, where fatty acid elongation plays an important role in myelination. Rare patients with deficiency of cytochrome b5 reductase in nonerythroid cells do not suffer any neurologic disorder, and it has been suggested that they be designated as having type III disease[42]; however, existence of such an entity has been challenged and type III disease likely does not exist.[43]

Heterozygosity for Cytochrome b_5 Reductase Deficiency

Heterozygotes for cytochrome b_5 reductase deficiency are not usually clinically methemoglobinemic or cyanotic. However, under the stress of administration of drugs that normally induce only slight, clinically unimportant, methemoglobinemia, such persons have been reported to become severely cyanotic because of methemoglobinemia.[44] Although in this report the affected patients were Ashkenazi Jews, the prevalence of cytochrome b5 reductase deficiency in 500 unselected Jewish subjects was found to be low.[45] In addition, predisposition to acute toxic methemoglobinemia in heterozygous subjects for cytochrome b5 reductase deficiency seems to be quite uncommon.[43]

Animal models of cytochrome b5 reductase deficiency have been described in dogs, cats, and horses.[46,47]

Infant Susceptibility

A combination of both increased hemoglobin oxidation and decreased methemoglobin reduction also may occur. Because the activity of cytochrome b5 reductase is normally low in newborn infants,[48] they are particularly susceptible to the development of methemoglobinemia. Thus, serious degrees of methemoglobinemia have been observed in infants as a result of toxic materials, such as aniline dyes used on diapers,[49] and the ingestion of nitrate-contaminated water[24,30] and even of beets.[50] Bacterial action in the intestinal tract may reduce nitrates to nitrites, which, in turn, cause methemoglobinemia. In rural areas, fatal methemoglobinuria in infants caused by drinking water from wells contaminated with nitrates still occurs.[51]

Inhaled nitric oxide (NO) is approved for treatment of infants with pulmonary hypertension because of its vasodilatory effect on pulmonary vessels. During the binding and release of NO from hemoglobin, methemoglobin is formed at a higher rate. In one study of 81 premature and 82 term infants, methemoglobin was above 5 percent in preterm infants and between 2.5 and 5 percent in 16 infants.[52]

Methemoglobinemia occurring in acidotic infants with diarrhea is a syndrome that may have a fatal outcome.[53] Such infants have normal red cell cytochrome b5 reductase activity, and the mechanism by which methemoglobinemia occurs is unknown. However, the syndrome seems most common when soy formula is being fed[54] and breastfeeding appears to protect against this.[51]

Cytochrome b5 Deficiency

Rarely, the defect leading to methemoglobinemia may not be in the cytochrome b5 reductase that transfers hydrogen to the cytochrome b5, but rather to a deficiency in the cytochrome b5 itself.[55]

Hemoglobin M

The molecular mechanisms by which hemoglobin binds oxygen and releases it are discussed in Chap. 49. Heme is held in a hydrophobic "heme pocket" between the E and F α-helices of each of the four globin chains. The iron atom in the heme forms four bonds with the pyrrole nitrogen atoms of the porphyrin ring and a fifth covalent bond with the imidazole nitrogen of a histidine residue in the nearby F α-helix (Fig. 50–1).[56]

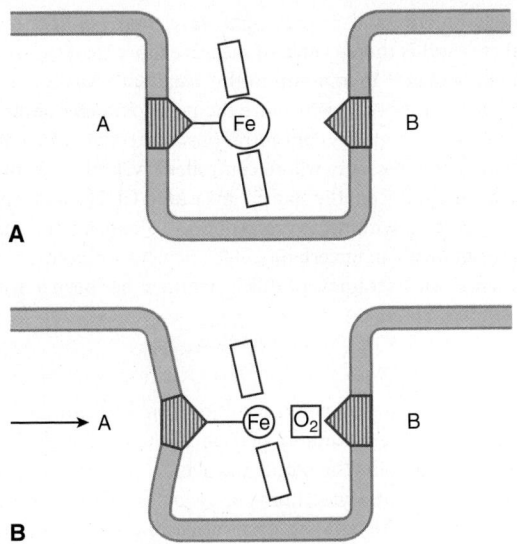

Figure 50–1. Diagrammatic representation of the heme group inserted into the heme pocket. *A,* Proximal histidine; *B,* distal histidine. **A.** In the deoxygenated form the larger ferrous atom lies out of the place of the porphyrin ring. **B.** In the oxygenated form the now smaller "ferric-like" atom can slip into the plane of the porphyrin ring. As a result, the proximal histidine, and helix F into which it is incorporated, are displaced. *(Reproduced with permission from Lehmann H, Huntsman RG: Man's Haemoglobins. Philadelphia PA: Lippincott Williams & Wilkins; 1974.)*

This histidine, residue 87 in the α chain and 92 in the β chain, is designated as the proximal histidine. On the opposite side of the porphyrin ring the iron atom lies adjacent to another histidine residue to which, however, it is not covalently bonded. This distal histidine occupies position 58 in the α chain and position 63 in the β chain. Under normal circumstances oxygen is occasionally discharged from the heme pocket as a superoxide anion, removing an electron from the iron and leaving it in the ferric state. The enzymatic machinery of the red cell efficiently reduces the iron to the divalent form, converting the methemoglobin to hemoglobin (Chap. 47).

In most of the hemoglobins M, tyrosine has been substituted for either the proximal or the distal histidine. Tyrosine can form an iron–phenolate complex that resists reduction to the divalent state by the normal metabolic systems of the erythrocyte. Four hemoglobins M are a consequence of substitution of tyrosine for histidine in the proximal and distal sites of the α and β chains. As Table 50–2 shows, these four hemoglobins M have been designated by the geographic names of their discovery, Boston, Saskatoon, Iwate, and Hyde Park.

Analogous His→Tyr substitutions in the γ chain of fetal hemoglobin have also been documented and have been designated hemoglobin FM$_{Osaka}$[57] and FM$_{Fort Ripley}$.[58]

Another hemoglobin M, HbM$_{Milwaukee}$, is formed by substitution of glutamic acid for valine in the 67th residue of the β chain. The glutamic acid side chain points toward the heme group and its γ-carboxyl group interacts with the iron atom, stabilizing it in the ferric state.

It is rare for methemoglobinemia to occur as a result of hemoglobinopathies other than hemoglobins M, but Hb$_{Chile}$ (β28 Leu→Met) is such a hemoglobin. Producing hemolysis only with drug administration, this unstable hemoglobin is characterized clinically by chronic methemoglobinemia.[59]

TABLE 50–2. Properties of Hemoglobins M				
Hemoglobin	Amino Acid Substitution	Oxygen Dissociation and Other Properties	Clinical Effect	Reference
HbM$_{Boston}$	α58 (E7)His→Tyr	Very low O$_2$ affinity, almost nonexistent heme–heme interaction, no Bohr effect	Cyanosis resulting from formation of methemoglobin	182
HbM$_{Saskatoon}$	β63 (E7)His→Tyr	Increased O$_2$ affinity, reduced heme-heme interaction, normal Bohr effect, slightly unstable	Cyanosis resulting from methemoglobin formation, mild hemolytic anemia exacerbated by ingestion of sulfonamides	182,183
HbM$_{Iwate}$ (HbMKankakee, HbMOldenburg, HbMSendai)	α87 (F8)His→Tyr	Low O$_2$ affinity, negligible heme-heme interaction, no Bohr effect	Cyanosis resulting from formation of methemoglobin	182,184
HbM$_{Hyde Park}$	β92 (F8)His→Tyr	Increased O$_2$ affinity, reduced heme interaction, normal Bohr effect, slightly unstable	Cyanosis resulting from formation of methemoglobin, mild hemolytic anemia	79
Hb M(hyde park)$_{(HbMilwaukee 2)}$				
HbM$_{Akita}$				
HbM$_{Milwaukee}$	β67 (E11)Val →Glu	Low O$_2$ affinity, reduced heme-heme interaction, normal Bohr effect, slightly unstable	Cyanosis resulting from methemoglobin formation	185
HbFM$_{Osaka}$	$^G\gamma$63His→Tyr	Low O$_2$ affinity, increased Bohr effect, methemoglobinemia	Cyanosis at birth	57
HbFM$_{Fort Ripley}$	$^G\gamma$92His→Tyr	Slightly increased O$_2$ affinity	Cyanosis at birth	186

CLINICAL FEATURES

Drug Ingestion

Methemoglobinemia may be chronic or acute and acquired or congenital. Acquired severe acute methemoglobinemia, usually the consequence of drug ingestion or toxic exposure, can produce symptoms of anemia, since methemoglobin lacks the capacity to transport oxygen. Symptoms may include shortness of breath, palpitations, and vascular collapse. Chemicals that induce methemoglobinemia are often also capable of causing hemolysis, and a combination of hemolytic anemia and methemoglobinemia may occur. Chronic methemoglobinemia, whether a result of exposure to drugs or toxins or of hereditary causes, is usually asymptomatic. Cyanosis, even if present, may not be discernable in persons with very dark skin coloration.[60] In instances when the methemoglobin levels are chronically very high (>20 percent of the total pigment), mild erythrocytosis may be noted (Chap. 57).

M Hemoglobins

Patients with hemoglobin M also manifest cyanosis. In the case of α-globin variants, the dusky color of the infants will be noted at birth, but the clinical manifestations of β-globin variants become apparent only after β chains have largely replaced the fetal γ chains at 6 to 9 months of age. In spite of the impaired hemoglobin function, no cardiopulmonary symptoms are observed and there is no clubbing. In the case of $HbM_{Saskatoon}$ and $HbM_{Hyde Park}$, hemolytic anemia with jaundice may be present. The hemolytic state may be exacerbated by administration of sulfonamides.[61]

Cytochrome b5 Reductase Deficiency

Hereditary methemoglobinemia resulting from cytochrome $b5$ reductase deficiency may, as noted above, be associated with mental retardation, failure to thrive and early death. In one case, skeletal anomalies were documented as well.[62]

LABORATORY FEATURES

Toxic Methemoglobinemia

In toxic methemoglobinemia, an elevated level of methemoglobin is found, but the activity of cytochrome $b5$ reductase is normal. Methemoglobin levels are best measured using the change of absorbance of methemoglobin at 630 nm that occurs when cyanide is added, converting the methemoglobin to cyanmethemoglobin, a principle used in the Evelyn–Malloy method.[63,64] Errors in diagnosis are frequently made when automated instruments designed to estimate levels of reduced hemoglobin, oxygenated hemoglobin, methemoglobin, and carboxyhemoglobin (COHb) are used. Most automated instruments do not properly make this distinction.[65,66]

The clinical incidence of methemoglobinemia can be overestimated by cooximeter measurements compared to the more specific Evelyn–Malloy method.[67] Evelyn-Malloy method involves direct spectrophotometric analysis and should be used when methemoglobinemia is suspected. This is achieved by lysing the blood in a slightly acid buffer and measuring the optical density at 630 nm before and after adding a small amount of neutralized cyanide. The absorption of methemoglobin at this wavelength disappears when it is converted to cyanmethemoglobin. Although this method was described in 1938,[63] it remains the most accurate technique for the estimation of methemoglobin in the blood. Details of its performance can be found in an earlier edition of this text[68] and elsewhere.[61]

An eight-wavelength pulse oximeter, Masimo Rad-57 (Rainbow-SET Rad-57 Pulse CO-Oximeter, Masimo Inc, Irvine, CA), has been approved by the FDA for the measurement of both COHb and methemoglobin. The Rad-57 uses eight wavelengths of light instead of the usual two and is thereby able to measure more than two species of human hemoglobin.[69] In addition to the usual SpO_2 value, the Rad-57 displays SpCO and SpMet, which are the pulse oximeter's estimates of COHb and methemoglobin concentrations, respectively. In a study on healthy human volunteers in whom controlled levels of methemoglobin and COHb were induced, the Rad-57 measured COHb with an uncertainty of ±2 percent within the range of 0 to 15 percent and measured methemoglobin with an uncertainty of 0.5 percent within the range of 0 to 12 percent,[69] the usefulness of this instrument has been verified also by other studies.[70,71]

Cytochrome b5 Reductase Deficiency

In hereditary methemoglobinemia resulting from cytochrome $b5$ reductase deficiency, between 8 and 40 percent of the hemoglobin is in the form of methemoglobin. The blood may have a chocolate-brown color and cyanosis is present. Cytochrome $b5$ reductase activity is best measured using ferricyanide as a receptor, measuring the rate of oxidation of NADH.[72,73] The residual level of enzyme activity is usually less than 20 percent of normal in patients with methemoglobinemia resulting from deficiency of this enzyme. An immunoassay has been described,[74] but such an assay would not detect mutants in which enzyme molecules with impaired catalytic activity are present. For unknown reasons, glutathione reductase activity (Chap. 47) is usually also diminished.[75]

Cytochrome b5 Deficiency

Cytochrome $b5$ assays may be useful if cytochrome $b5$ reductase activity is normal, and the presence of hemoglobin M is ruled out.[76]

M Hemoglobins

Optical Spectrum Figure 50-2 illustrates the spectrum of normal methemoglobin A at pH 7.0.[77] Hemoglobins M may be differentiated from methemoglobin formed from hemoglobin A by its absorption spectrum in the range of 450 to 750 nm. Because only some 20 to 35 percent of the total hemoglobin will ordinarily be the hemoglobin M, the mixed spectra of methemoglobin A and the hemoglobin M may be difficult to interpret. Therefore, it is preferable to perform these spectral studies on purified hemoglobin M isolated by electrophoretic or chromatographic means.[56]

Electrophoresis All hemoglobin M samples should be converted to methemoglobin so that any difference found in electrophoresis will be the result of the amino acid substitution and not the different charge of the iron atom. Electrophoresis at pH 7.1 is most useful for separation of hemoglobins M because the imidazole groups of histidine have a net positive charge at this pH, while at higher pH levels the histidines and the substituting tyrosines are both neutral.

Other Biochemical Methods The hemoglobins M differ in their reactivity to cyanide and to azide ions.[78] This property may help to identify the subunit affected, as the iron-phenolate bonds are stronger in the α-chain variants than in the β-chain variants. However, definitive identification of the variant requires peptide or DNA analysis. Hemoglobins that cause cyanosis because of a diminished oxygen affinity may be detected by determining the oxygen dissociation curve of blood, being certain that the 2,3-bisphosphoglycerate (2,3-BPG) level is normal, or by estimating the oxygen dissociation curve of hemoglobin, which has been stripped of 2,3-BPG by extensive dialysis against an appropriate buffer. Many of the hemoglobins with decreased oxygen affinity are unstable (Chap. 49) and will precipitate in the isopropanol stability test.[78] In many laboratories, it may be easier to analyze the coding sequence of the globin chains at the DNA level than to attempt to determine the properties of the hemoglobin.[79]

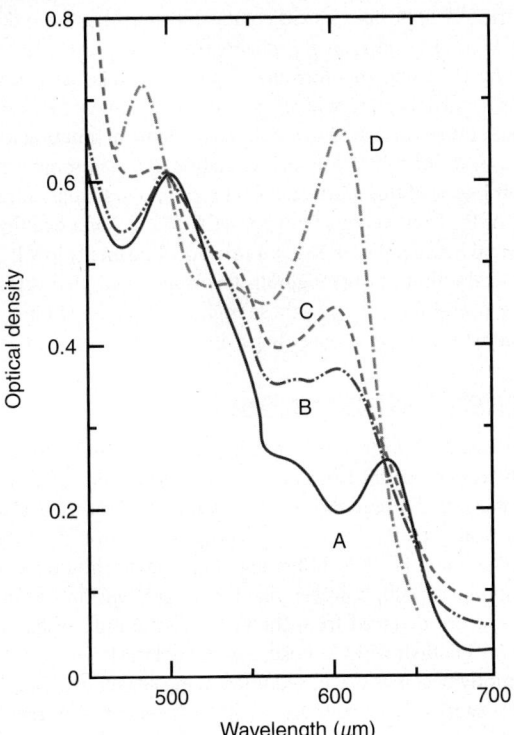

Figure 50–2. Absorption spectra at pH 7.0. *A*, Methemoglobin A; *B*, methemoglobin M$_{Boston}$; *C*, methemoglobin M$_{Saskatoon}$; *D*, methemoglobin A fluoride complex. For purposes of comparison, all the optical densities have been made equal to 0.61 at 500 nm. *(Reproduced with permission from Gerald PS, George P: Second spectroscopically abnormal methemoglobin associated with hereditary cyanosis. Science 1959 Feb 13;129(3346):393-394.)*

TREATMENT AND COURSE

Toxic Methemoglobinemia

Acute toxic methemoglobinemia may represent a serious medical emergency. Because of the loss of oxygen-carrying capacity of the blood and the left shift in the oxygen dissociation curve that occurs when methemoglobin is present in high concentrations,[80] acute methemoglobinemia may be life-threatening when the level of the pigment exceeds one-third of the total circulating hemoglobin. Levels of methemoglobin exceeding 50 percent of the total pigment may be associated with vascular collapse, coma, and death,[81,82] but recovery was documented in one patient with a level as high as 81.5 percent of the total pigment.[83]

Methylene blue[84] is an effective treatment for patients with methemoglobinemia because NADPH formed in the hexose monophosphate pathway can rapidly reduce this dye to leukomethylene blue in a reaction catalyzed by NADPH diaphorase (Chap. 47). Leukomethylene blue, in turn, nonenzymatically reduces methemoglobin to hemoglobin.[85] An exception to the efficacy of this treatment exists in those patients who are glucose-6-phosphate dehydrogenase deficient (Chap. 47). In these subjects, methylene blue would not only fail to give the desired effect on methemoglobin levels, but might compound the patient's difficulty by inducing an acute hemolytic episode[86] or increasing the level of methemoglobin.[87]

In patients with acute toxic methemoglobinemia who are symptomatic or whose methemoglobin level is rising rapidly, the intravenous administration of 1 or 2 mg methylene blue per kilogram body weight over a period of 5 minutes is the preferred treatment because of its very rapid action.[88] Use of excessive amounts of methylene blue should be avoided; the administration of repeated doses of 2 mg methylene blue per kilogram body weight has produced acute hemolysis even in patients with normal glucose-6-phosphate dehydrogenase levels.[89]

The response to treatment is so rapid, with marked lowering or normalization of methemoglobin levels within an hour or two, that no other treatment is usually needed, but the patient should be observed carefully because continued absorption of a toxic substance from the gastrointestinal tract may cause recurrence of the methemoglobinemia. In patients who are in shock, blood transfusion may be helpful. Cimetidine, used as a selective inhibitor of N-hydroxylation, may decrease the methemoglobinemia produced by dapsone in patients with dermatitis herpetiformis.[90]

Hereditary Methemoglobinemia

The course of hereditary methemoglobinemia is generally benign (although not in type II cytochrome *b5* reductase deficiency), but patients with this disorder should be shielded from exposure to aniline derivatives, nitrites, and other agents that may, even in normal persons, induce methemoglobinemia.

Hereditary methemoglobinemia resulting from cytochrome *b5* reductase deficiency is readily treated by the administration of ascorbic acid, 300 to 600 mg orally daily divided into three or four doses. Although intravenously administered methylene blue is very effective in correcting this type of methemoglobinemia, it is not suitable for the long-term therapy that needs to be given if the state is to be treated at all. Riboflavin administration seems to benefit some patients[91] but not others.[92]

The iron phenolate complex that exists in the hemoglobins M prevents the reduction of ferric to ferrous iron. For this reason, the methemoglobinemia does not respond to administration of ascorbic acid or of methylene blue. No effective treatment exists for the cyanosis that is present in patients with abnormal hemoglobins with reduced oxygen affinity.

● SULFHEMOGLOBIN

DEFINITION AND HISTORY

Sulfhemoglobinemia refers to the presence in the blood of hemoglobin derivatives that are defined by their characteristic absorption of light at 620 nm, even in the presence of cyanide. Sulfhemoglobin derives its name from the fact that it can be produced *in vitro* from the action of hydrogen sulfide on hemoglobin[93] and that the feeding of dogs with elemental sulfur has been associated with sulfhemoglobinemia.[94]

ETIOLOGY AND PATHOGENESIS

Sulfhemoglobin may contain one excess sulfur atom. The sulfur atom appears to be bound to a β-pyrrole carbon atom at the periphery of the porphyrin ring.[95-97] Sulfhemoglobinemia has been associated with the ingestion of various drugs, particularly sulfonamides, phenacetin, acetanilid, and phenazopyridine.[65,98] It also occurs independently of drug use, and has been thought to be related to chronic constipation or to purging.[99] Some patients with sulfhemoglobinemia or a past history of this disorder appear to have increased levels of red blood cell reduced glutathione (GSH).[100] The reason for this and its relationship to sulfhemoglobinemia are not clearly understood, but it may be of significance that some of the types of drugs that are associated with sulfhemoglobinemia cause an elevation of red cell GSH levels, probably by activating the enzyme glutathione synthase[101] or by increasing intracellular glutamate levels.[102]

Evidence for the occurrence of hereditary sulfhemoglobinemia is not convincing,[103] and it is likely that the single family reported represents a hemoglobin M hemoglobinopathy.

CLINICAL FEATURES

Sulfhemoglobinemia is characterized by cyanosis. Drugs that cause sulfhemoglobinemia often have the capacity to produce accelerated red cell destruction as well. Thus, mild hemolysis is sometimes observed in patients with sulfhemoglobinemia.

LABORATORY FEATURES

Sulfhemoglobin is detected in the lysate of blood treated with ferricyanide, cyanide, and ammonia by comparing the optical density at 620 nm with that at 540 nm.[63,64]

TREATMENT AND COURSE

Sulfhemoglobinemia is almost always a benign disorder. Unlike methemoglobin, sulfhemoglobin does not produce a left shift in the oxygen dissociation curve; instead, it decreases the affinity of hemoglobin for oxygen.[98] The disorder tends to recur in the same persons after exposure to drugs but does not generally appear to affect their overall health. Unlike methemoglobin, sulfhemoglobin cannot be converted to hemoglobin. Thus, once sulfhemoglobinemia occurs, it will persist until the erythrocytes carrying the abnormal pigment reach the end of their life span.

● LOW-OXYGEN-AFFINITY HEMOGLOBINS: A CAUSE OF CYANOSIS

ETIOLOGY AND PATHOGENESIS

In some hemoglobin variants, the deoxy conformation of the hemoglobin molecule is favored because the angle of the heme is altered from that found normally in deoxyhemoglobin. Such changes occur in $Hb_{Hammersmith}$, $Hb_{Bucuresti}$, Hb_{Torino}, and $Hb_{Peterborough}$. In other instances, the quaternary conformation is changed by mutations involving the $\alpha_1\beta_2$ contact (Hb_{Kansas}, $Hb_{Titusville}$, and $Hb_{Yoshizuka}$). Table 50–3 summarizes the properties of abnormal hemoglobins associated with low oxygen affinity.

CLINICAL FEATURES

In response to the improved tissue oxygen supply brought about by a right-shifted oxygen dissociation curve, the "oxygen sensor" of the body decreases the output of erythropoietin.[104] As a result, the steady-state level of hemoglobin is diminished; mild anemia and cyanosis are characteristics of patients with hemoglobins with a decreased oxygen affinity.

LABORATORY FEATURES

The affinity of hemoglobin with oxygen is expressed as P_{50}, which is the partial pressure of oxygen at which 50 percent of the blood hemoglobin is saturated with oxygen. The venous P_{50} can be measured directly using a cooximeter, which is no longer easily available in either routine or reference laboratories. A mathematical formula has been developed that can be used to calculate P_{50} reliably from a venous blood sample.[105] Calculating P_{50} using this formula requires the following venous gas parameters: partial pressure of oxygen (venous), venous pH, and venous oxygen saturation, and uses an antilog mathematical function that many clinicians find difficult to use for calculation. An electronic version (in Microsoft Excel) of this mathematical formula is available for rapid calculation of P_{50} from venous blood gases.[106] The P_{50} of a healthy person with normal hemoglobin is 26 ± 1.3 torr. An abnormally low P_{50} reflects an increased affinity of hemoglobin for oxygen and vice versa, and is especially useful for detecting those high affinity hemoglobin mutants associated with polycythemia (Chaps. 49 and 57).

DIFFERENTIAL DIAGNOSIS

Cyanosis resulting from methemoglobinemia or sulfhemoglobinemia should be differentiated from cyanosis resulting from cardiac or pulmonary disease, particularly when right-to-left shunting is present. In the latter instances, the arterial oxygen tension will be low, whereas in methemoglobinemia and sulfhemoglobinemia it should be normal. One should be certain, however, that the oxygen tension was measured directly and not deduced from the percent saturation of hemoglobin. Blood from a patient with cyanosis because of arterial oxygen desaturation promptly becomes bright red upon being shaken with air. In addition, these causes of cyanosis are readily differentiated by carrying out quantitative blood methemoglobin and sulfhemoglobin levels. Because of the potential lethal nature of high levels of methemoglobin and because prompt treatment may be life-saving, a high index of suspicion is important. A patient with cyanosis whose arterial blood is brown with an SpO_2 that is found to be normal on blood gas examination is likely to have methemoglobinemia. One should not rely on the readings of a standard pulse oximeter, as false readings may be obtained in the presence of methemoglobin. Rapid examination of a blood sample using an automatic analyzer, such as a cooximeter, is the first step in confirming the diagnosis. Treatment should not be delayed, but, as pointed out in "Laboratory Features" above, direct spectrophotometric analysis should be carried out on the pretreatment sample as soon as possible to distinguish between methemoglobinemia and sulfhemoglobinemia.

A family history, as well as any information as to whether it is acquired or congenital, is helpful in differentiating hereditary methemoglobinemia as a result of cytochrome b5 reductase deficiency from hemoglobin M disease. The former has a recessive mode of inheritance, the latter a dominant mode. Thus, cyanosis in successive generations suggests the presence of hemoglobin M; normal parents but possibly affected siblings implies the presence of cytochrome b5 reductase. Consanguinity is more common in cytochrome b5 reductase deficiency. In cytochrome b5 reductase deficiency, incubation of the blood with small amounts of methylene blue will result in rapid reduction of the methemoglobin; in hemoglobin M disease, such reduction does not take place. The absorption spectra of methemoglobin and its derivatives

TABLE 50–3. Some Abnormal Hemoglobins Associated with Low Oxygen Affinity

Hemoglobin	Amino Acid Substitution	Oxygen Dissociation and Other Properties	Clinical Effect	Reference
$Hb_{Seattle}$	$\beta70$ (E14) Ala→Asp	Decreased O_2 affinity normal heme–heme interaction	Mild chronic anemia associated with reduced urinary erythropoietin; physiologic adaptation to more efficient oxygen release to tissues	104
Hb_{Kansas}	$\beta102$ (G4) Asn→Thr	Very low O_2 affinity, low heme–heme interaction, dissociates into dimers in ligand form	Cyanosis resulting from deoxyhemoglobin, mild anemia	187

are normal in cytochrome *b5* reductase deficiency; they are abnormal in hemoglobin M disease. In the case of toxic methemoglobinemia, cyanosis is generally of relatively recent origin, and a history of exposure to drug or toxin may usually be obtained; in hereditary methemoglobinemia, a history of lifelong cyanosis may usually be elicited.

● OTHER DYSHEMOGLOBINS

CARBON MONOXIDE AND CARBOXYHEMOGLOBIN

Carbon monoxide (CO) is a toxic, odorless, colorless, and tasteless gas. It can be unknowingly inhaled to dangerous levels with serious clinical implications when present in high concentration in the atmosphere.[107]

Epidemiology

Acute CO intoxication is one of the most common causes of morbidity from poisoning in the United States. In the United States, CO poisoning results in approximately 50,000 emergency department visits per year,[108,109] and approximately 500 accidental deaths as a result of CO poisoning occur annually, with the number of intentional CO-related deaths being five to 10 times higher.[110,111] Primary sources of CO are home appliances, and the majority of exposures occur during the fall and winter months and during weather-related disasters.[112,113] During warmer months, boating activities are another source of exposure.[114] The death rate is highest among the elderly and can be attributed to delayed diagnosis because symptoms often resemble those of associated comorbidities.[115,116] The exhaust produced by the typical home-use 5.5-kW generator contains as much CO as that of six idling automobiles.[117]

Chronic CO intoxication is commonly caused by cigarette smoking, which can increase the COHb level up to 15 percent. Houses with defective heating exhaust systems and vehicles that leak CO into the passenger compartment, either because of mechanical failure or driving with the rear hatch-door open, are the second most common cause of chronic CO exposure. Occupations that involve a high risk for CO intoxication include garage work with improper ventilation, toll booth attendants, tunnel workers, fire fighters, and workers exposed to paint remover, aerosol propellant, or organic solvents containing dichloromethane.[118]

Etiology and Pathogenesis

CO binds with high affinity to heme and with lesser affinities to myoglobin and cytochromes at the iron core, a site it shares with O_2.[119]

At equilibrium in physiologic conditions, CO affinity for hemoglobin is approximately 240 times greater than that of O_2. This very high equilibrium constant is the result of reaction kinetics. Contrary to popular belief, CO reacts more slowly than O_2 with the heme of hemoglobin. Once CO is bound to heme, its "off" rate is only 0.015 mol/L per second in contrast to 35 mol/L per second for O_2.[119] This extraordinarily slow-release process produces a very high affinity constant of CO for heme and a life-threatening danger for individuals exposed to high levels of CO. Once two molecules of CO are bound to hemoglobin, the hemoglobin switches to the relaxed (R) state, which increases the affinity of hemoglobin for oxygen. As a consequence of this phenomenon, called the Darling–Roughton effect,[80] the hemoglobin O_2 affinity increases in parallel with increasing CO levels, making tissue delivery of oxygen more difficult.

In the absence of environmental CO, the blood of adults contains approximately 1 to 2 percent COHb. This represents approximately 80 percent of the total body CO, the remainder probably sequestered in myoglobin and other heme binding proteins. This CO is endogenously produced,[120] originating from the degradation of heme by the rate-limiting heme oxygenase–cytochrome P450 complex, which produces CO and biliverdin. Caloric restriction, dehydration, infancy, and the genetic variations reported in Japanese and Native Americans generate higher endogenous levels of CO. Hemolytic anemia (Chap. 33), hematomas, and infection tend to increase CO production up to threefold. Fetuses and newborns have double the normal adult levels of COHb. Drugs such as diphenylhydantoin and phenobarbital, by inducing the cytochrome P450 complex, increase CO production. Normal adult level of COHb is less than 2 percent. Hemolysis can produce COHb levels of more than 2 percent. Levels more than 3 percent must have an exogenous origin, except for rare conditions as occur in carriers of abnormal hemoglobins such as Hb_{Zurich}. The affinity of Hb_{Zurich} for CO is approximately 65 times that of normal hemoglobin.[121]

Pregnant women and fetuses are particularly at risk[122] because they already have higher levels of COHb. CO readily crosses the placenta, and the half-life of CO in the fetus is as much as five times longer than it is in the mother.[123] The O_2 affinity of fetal hemoglobin (HbF) is shifted to the left[124,125] owing to its lack of 2,3-BPG binding, making the Darling–Roughton effect particularly pernicious. This is one of the reasons why cigarette smoking during pregnancy is hazardous to the fetus.

Clinical and Laboratory Features

CO poisoning is a clinical diagnosis that is confirmed by laboratory testing. Signs and symptoms consistent with CO poisoning in certain circumstances should raise the suspicion of CO intoxication. A higher index of suspicion should attend the simultaneous presentation of multiple patients from the same family or housing complex. The eight-wavelength pulse oximeter, Masimo Rad-57 (see paragraphs on "Laboratory features" of methemoglobinemia.) has been reported to be accurate in measuring COHb concentration in normal healthy volunteers,[69] as well as in emergency room patients.[126]

Acute intoxication with CO rapidly affects the central and peripheral nervous systems and cardiopulmonary functions. Cerebral edema is common, as is impairment of the peripheral nervous system. CO induces increased capillary permeability in the lungs, resulting in acute pulmonary edema. Cardiac arrhythmias, generalized hypoxemia, and respiratory failure are the common causes of CO-related death. In survivors, considerable neuropsychological deficits might remain. In a prospective longitudinal study, approximately 45 percent of patients with CO poisoning had cognitive sequelae 6 weeks after poisoning.[127,128] Acute CO intoxication in children[129] sometimes has unique symptomatology resembling gastroenteritis. Surviving children are more likely to have severe sequelae such as leukoencephalopathy and severe myocardial ischemia.[130]

Chronic intoxication in adults might result in irritability, nausea, lethargy, headaches, and sometimes a flu-like condition. Higher COHb levels produce somnolence, palpitations, cardiomegaly, and hypertension, and could contribute to atherosclerosis. Chronic CO poisoning can produce erythrocytosis, the magnitude of which varies with the level of COHb. By increasing red cell production, chronic CO poisoning can mask the mild anemia of acquired or congenital hemolytic disorders.

Therapy, Course, and Prognosis

The most important step in the treatment for CO poisoning is prompt removal of patients from the source of CO, followed by administering 100 percent supplemental O_2 via a tight-fitting mask. The serum elimination half-life of CO is 5 hours when breathing room air and 30 minutes with O_2 therapy (100 percent O_2 at 3 atmospheres).[123]

For mild to moderate cases of CO poisoning, which more often happen with chronic intoxication, removing the patient from the source of environmental CO is usually curative. If the COHb level is high, breathing 100 percent O_2 will increase the rate of CO removal.

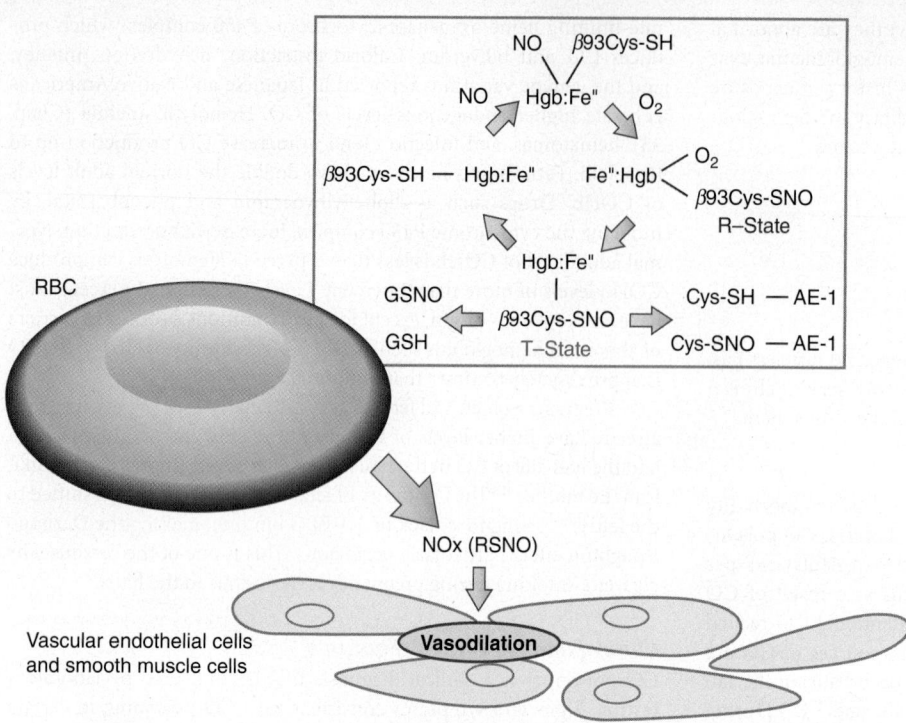

Figure 50–3. *S*-nitrosohemoglobin (SNO-Hb) and hypoxic vasodilation. *(Reproduced with permission from Parker C: SNO-HB a Snow Job? The Hematologist: ASH News and Reports. 6:12;2009.)*

In severe cases of CO poisoning, which more often occur with acute intoxication, after identification and removal of the source of CO, 100 percent O_2 should be administered, with cardiac monitoring. Endotracheal intubation should be done in any patient with impaired mental status, and other interventions should be dictated by the symptomatology.

Because of conflicting evidence, there is no absolute indication for the use of hyperbaric O_2 treatment for patients with CO poisoning. Hyperbaric O_2 might be indicated in patients who have obvious neurologic abnormalities, cardiac dysfunction, persistent symptoms despite normobaric O_2, or metabolic acidosis.[131] Hyperbaric O_2 has complications of its own, such as bronchial irritation and pulmonary edema, and should be reserved for exceptional cases of CO intoxication. Locations of hyperbaric chambers throughout the world and in the United States can be found at the Undersea and Hyperbaric Medical Society website (http://www.uhms.org) under "chamber directory."

Pregnant women exposed to CO are at particularly high risk. CO poisoning is especially dangerous to the fetus because CO readily crosses the placenta and the half-life of CO in the fetus is as much as five times longer than it is in the mother. For these reasons, treatment with hyperbaric O_2 should be carried out during pregnancy when the COHb levels exceed 15 percent. In a limited number of studies done on pregnant patients, hyperbaric O_2 does not seem to adversely affect the fetus.[132,133]

NITRIC OXIDE AND NITRIC OXIDE HEMOGLOBINS

Physiology and Chemistry

NO, a soluble gas, is continuously synthesized in endothelial cells by isoforms of the NO synthase (NOS) enzyme. A functional NOS transfers electrons from NADPH to its heme center, where L-arginine is oxidized to L-citrulline and NO.[134] Vasodilation is caused by diffusion of NO into the smooth muscle cells, wherein NO binds avidly to the heme of soluble guanylyl cyclase, producing cyclic guanosine monophosphate

(cGMP), which activates cGMP-dependent protein kinases and ultimately produces smooth muscle relaxation.[134]

Blood NO levels are set by the balance between the production of NO by NOS and the binding or scavenging of NO by the heme groups of erythrocyte hemoglobin. The half-life of NO in whole blood is extremely short, estimated to be 1.8 milliseconds.[135] The short half-life of NO greatly limits its diffusional distance in blood and only maintains NO as a paracrine vasoregulator.[136,137] This does not explain how hemoglobin is capable of transducing NO bioactivity far from its location of formation.

Interaction of the red blood cells with NO is a complex phenomenon (Fig. 50–3). Two models have been proposed: (1) The first model, an *S*-nitrosohemoglobin (SNO-Hb)–dependent mechanism, proposes that NO binds to heme when the hemoglobin is in the T state (deoxygenated). In the oxygenated state, NO gets transferred from heme to a cysteine residue on the globin portion of hemoglobin, forming SNO-Hb.[138,139] Nitric oxide is transported by red blood cells from the lungs to hypoxic tissues in a protected form as SNO-Hb, and is delivered in the hypoxic microvasculature at the same time as oxygen, coupling hemoglobin deoxygenation to vasodilation. (2) The second model is of deoxyhemoglobin-mediated nitrite reduction to NO.[140] In the blood, deoxygenated hemoglobin functions as the predominant nitrite reductase.[141] Deoxygenated hemoglobin reacts with nitrite to form NO and methemoglobin and causes vasodilation along the physiological oxygen gradient. Although this reaction is experimentally associated with NO generation, kinetic analysis suggests that NO should not be able to escape inactivation in the erythrocyte.[142] This inactivation or scavenging of NO is avoided by the formation of an intermediate species, that is, dinitrogen trioxide (N_2O_3). Products of the nitrite–hemoglobin reaction generate N_2O_3 via a novel reaction of NO and nitrite-bound methemoglobin.[143] N_2O_3 diffuses out of the red cell, later forms NO, and affects vasodilation and/or forms nitrosothiols (Fig. 50–4). According to this paradigm, nitrite, previously thought to be an inert end product of endogenous NO metabolism, is the main stable NO reservoir in blood and tissues.[144,145] Nitrite is formed during normoxic conditions

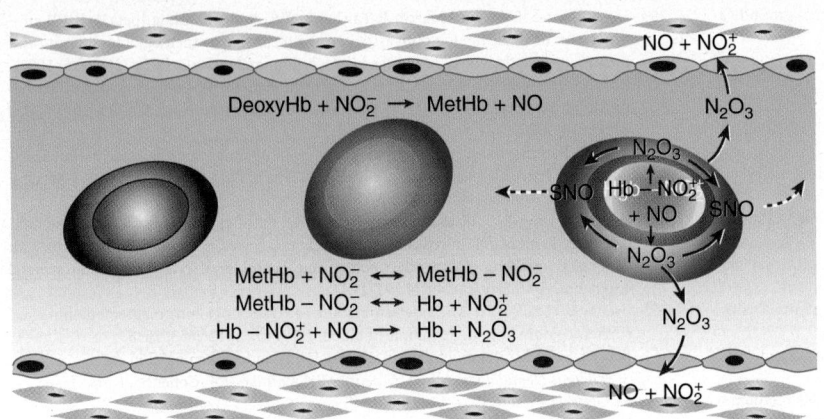

Figure 50–4. Hemoglobin deoxygenation *(purple)* occurs in capillaries. Nitrite reacts with deoxyHb that is oxidized to MetHb and NO. The NO binds to hemes of deoxyHb, and also undergoes dioxygenation to form nitrate and MetHb from oxyHb. MetHb binds nitrite to form an adduct with some Fe(II)-NO$_2$, that is, Hb-NO. This species reacts quickly with NO to form N$_2$O$_3$, which can diffuse out of the red cell forming NO and effecting vasodilation and/or forming nitrosothiols (SNOs). *(Reproduced with permission from Basu S, et al: Catalytic generation of N2O3 by the concerted nitrite reductase and anhydrase activity of hemoglobin, Nature Chemical Biology 2007 Dec;3(12):785-794.)*

and then is reduced to NO and N$_2$O$_3$ along the physiologic oxygen and pH gradient by the heme globins.[143]

Cell free hemoglobin and red cell microparticles formed during hemolytic conditions and long storage of red blood cells (RBCs) lead to NO scavenging 1000 times faster than regular RBCs and to insufficient NO bioavailability.[146] Stored RBCs are also stored in acidic solution that also leads to a decrease in SNO-Hb levels. This has been further substantiated by the fact that renitrosylated RBCs lead to improved oxygen delivery in animal models.[147] This could explain the morbidity and mortality associated with stored RBCs. Moreover, underlying recipient endothelial dysfunction, for example, obesity or hypertension, can also induce increased RBC membrane damage in transfused blood, leading to increased microparticle formation and increased NO scavenging.[148,149]

Pathophysiology and Potential Therapeutic Applications

Nitric oxide was long considered highly toxic. Exogenous administration of NO by inhalation activates cytosolic guanylate cyclase, increasing intracellular levels of cGMP, and resulting in relaxation of the smooth muscles in the pulmonary arteries.

Based on this observation, inhaled NO (iNO) has been used to manage the acute pulmonary hypertension seen in adult respiratory distress syndrome, sickle cell disease, and primary or secondary pulmonary hypertension. Even though NO lowers the pulmonary artery pressure and improves oxygenation in acute respiratory distress syndrome in both adults and children, it has not consistently resulted in an improvement in mortality.

At present, prolonged administration of iNO is not considered as first-line therapy for pulmonary artery hypertension and instead is used only for vasoreactivity testing in these patients.[150] iNO has beneficial effects in animal models, as well as in preliminary human trials of acute vasoocclusive crisis and chest syndrome associated with sickle cell disease.[151-153] Some animal data suggest beneficial effects of iNO therapy in the setting of ischemia–reperfusion injury (lung, heart, and intestine).[154] However, iNO is also associated with multiple side effects, such as methemoglobinemia,[155] left-heart failure,[156] renal insufficiency,[157] and a "rebound" increase in pulmonary artery pressure upon discontinuation of iNO that may result in cardiovascular collapse.[158]

Direct repletion of *S*-nitrosothiol in the lung and blood has the potential to avoid toxicities related to iNO. In a porcine model of acute lung injury, inhaled ethyl nitrite, but not iNO, efficiently repleted lung SNO-Hb, lowered pulmonary vascular resistance, improved oxygenation dose-dependently, and had a protective effect against a decline in cardiac output.[159]

In humans, newborns with persistent pulmonary hypertension showed improved oxygenation and hemodynamics following ethyl

nitrite inhalation.[160] Use of cell free hemoglobin is associated with vasoconstriction and subsequent development of hypertension. Increased vascular resistance and vasoconstriction has been shown to be mediated mainly by the scavenging of NO because of the high affinity of free hemoglobin for NO.[161,162]

REFERENCES

1. Hsieh H, Jaffe ER: The metabolism of methemoglobin in human erythrocytes, in *The Red Blood Cell*, edited by Surgenor DM, p 799. Academic Press, New York. 1975.
2. Sloss A, Wybauw R: Un Cas de methemoglobinemie idiopathique. *Ann Soc R Sci Med Nat Brux* 70:206, 1912.
3. Hitzenberger K: Autotoxic cyanosis due to intraglobular methemoglobinemia. *Wien Arch Med* 23:85, 1932.
4. Jaffe E: Hereditary methemoglobinemias associated with abnormalities in the metabolism of erythrocytes. *Am J Med* 41:786, 1966.
5. Horlein H, Weber G: Über Chronische familiare Methämoglobinamie und eine neue Modification des Methämoglobins. *Dtsch Med Wochenschr* 73:476, 1948.
6. Singer K: Hereditary hemolytic disorders associated with abnormal hemoglobins. *Am J Med* 18(4):633, 1955.
7. Gibson QH: The reduction of methaemoglobin in red blood cells and studies on the cause of idiopathic methaemoglobinaemia. *Biochem J* 42(1):13, 1948.
8. Percy M, Gillespie M, Savage G, et al: Familial idiopathic mutations in NADH-cytochrome b5 reductase. *Blood* 100:3447, 2002.
9. Bonaventura J, Riggs A: Hemoglobin Kansas, a human hemoglobin with a neutral amino acid substitution and an abnormal oxygen equilibrium. *J Biol Chem* 243(5):980, 1968.
10. Scott E, Hoskins D: Hereditary methemoglobinemia in Alaskan Eskimos and Indians. *Blood* 13:795, 1958.
11. Balsamo P, Hardy W, Scott E. Hereditary methemoglobinemia due to diaphorase deficiency in Navajo Indians. *J Pediatr* 65:928, 1964.
12. Burtseva T, Ammosova T, Prchal JT, et al: Type I methemoglobinemia caused by the cytochrome b5 reductase 806C>T mutation is present in the indigenous Evenk people of Yakutia. *ASH Annu Meet* 2009.
13. Sorensen PR: The influence of pH, pCO2 and concentrations of dyshemoglobins on the oxygen dissociation curve (ODC) of human blood determined by non-linear least squares regression analysis. *Scand J Clin Lab Invest Suppl* 203:163, 1990.
14. Bodansky O: Methemoglobinemia and methemoglobin-producing compounds. *Pharmacol Rev* 3(2):144, 1951.
15. Kiese M: The biochemical production of ferrihemoglobin-forming derivatives from aromatic amines and mechanisms of ferrihemoglobin formation. *Pharmacol Rev* 18:1091, 1966.
16. Dean BS, Lopez G, Krenzelok EP: Environmentally-induced methemoglobinemia in an infant. *J Toxicol Clin Toxicol* 30(1):127, 1992.
17. McGuigan MA: Benzocaine-induced methemoglobinemia. *Can Med Assoc J* 125(8):816, 1981.
18. O'Donohue WJ Jr, Moss LM, Angelillo VA: Acute methemoglobinemia induced by topical benzocaine and lidocaine. *Arch Intern Med* 140(11):1508, 1980.
19. Kane GC, Hoehn SM, Behrenbeck TR, et al: Benzocaine-induced methemoglobinemia based on the Mayo Clinic experience from 28,478 transesophageal echocardiograms: Incidence, outcomes, and predisposing factors. *Arch Intern Med* 167(18):1977, 2007.
20. Lee SW, Lee JY, Lee KJ, et al: A case of methemoglobinemia after ingestion of an aphrodisiac, later proven as dapsone. *Yonsei Med J* 40(4):388, 1999.
21. Esbenshade AJ, Ho RH, Shintani A, et al: Dapsone-induced methemoglobinemia: A dose-related occurrence? *Cancer* 117(15):3485, 2011.

22. Johnson CJ, Kross BC: Continuing importance of nitrate contamination of groundwater and wells in rural areas. *Am J Ind Med* 18(4):449, 1990.
23. Chan TY: Food-borne nitrates and nitrites as a cause of methemoglobinemia. *Southeast Asian J Trop Med Public Health* 27(1):189, 1996.
24. Knobeloch L, Proctor M: Eight blue babies. *WMJ* 100(8):43, 2001.
25. Askew GL, Finelli L, Genese CA, et al: Boilerbaisse: An outbreak of methemoglobinemia in New Jersey in 1992. *Pediatrics* 94(3):381, 1994.
26. Bakshi SP, Fahey JL, Pierce LE: Brief recording: Sausage cyanosis—Acquired methemoglobinemic nitrite poisoning. *N Engl J Med* 277(20):1072, 1967.
27. Bradberry SM, Whittington RM, Parry DA, et al: Fatal methemoglobinemia due to inhalation of isobutyl nitrite. *J Toxicol Clin Toxicol* 32(2):179, 1994.
28. Bradberry SM, Gazzard B, Vale JA: Methemoglobinemia caused by the accidental contamination of drinking water with sodium nitrite. *J Toxicol Clin Toxicol* 32(2):173, 1994.
29. Harris JC, Rumack BH, Peterson RG, et al: Methemoglobinemia resulting from absorption of nitrates. *JAMA* 242(26):2869, 1979.
30. Lukens JN: Landmark perspective: The legacy of well-water methemoglobinemia. *JAMA* 257(20):2793, 1987.
31. Stuhlmeier KM, Kao JJ, Wallbrandt P, et al: Antioxidant protein 2 prevents methemoglobin formation in erythrocyte hemolysates. *Eur J Biochem* 270:334, 2003.
32. Bewley M, Marohnic C, Barber M: The structure and biochemistry of NADH-dependent cytochrome b5 reductase are now consistent. *Biochemistry* 40:13574, 2001.
33. Yamada M, Tamada T, Takeda K, et al: Elucidations of the catalytic cycle of NADH-cytochrome b5 reductase by X-ray crystallography: New insights into regulation of efficient electron transfer. *J Mol Biol* 425(22):4295, 2013.
34. Wang Y, Wu Y, Zheng P, et al: A novel mutation in the NADH-cytochrome b5 reductase gene of a Chinese patient with recessive congenital methemoglobinemia. *Blood* 95:3250, 2000.
35. Shotelersuk V, Tosukhowong P, Chotivitayatarakorn P, et al: A Thai boy with hereditary enzymopenic methemoglobinemia type II. *J Med Assoc Thai* 83:1380, 2000.
36. Jenkins MM, Prchal JT: A novel mutation found in the 3′ domain of NADH-cytochrome B5 reductase in an African-American family with type I congenital methemoglobinemia. *Blood* 87(7):2993, 1996.
37. Nussenzveig RH, Lingam HB, Gaikwad A, et al: A novel mutation of the cytochrome-b5 reductase gene in an Indian patient: The molecular basis of type I methemoglobinemia. *Haematologica* 91(11):1542, 2006.
38. Jenkins M, Prchal J: A high frequency polymorphism of NADH-cytochrome b5 reductase in African-Americans. *Hum Genet* 99:248, 1997.
39. Ewenczyk C, Leroux A, Roubergue A, et al: Recessive hereditary methaemoglobinaemia, type II: Delineation of the clinical spectrum. *Brain* 131(Pt 3):760, 2008.
40. Leroux A, Junien C, Kaplan J, et al: Generalised deficiency of cytochrome b5 reductase in congenital methaemoglobinaemia with mental retardation. *Nature* 258(5536):619, 1975.
41. Takeshita M, Tamura M, Kugi M, et al: Decrease of palmitoyl-CoA elongation in platelets and leukocytes in the patient of hereditary methemoglobinemia associated with mental retardation. *Biochem Biophys Res Commun* 148:384, 1987.
42. Tanishima K, Tanimoto K, Tomoda A, et al: Hereditary methemoglobinemia due to cytochrome b5 reductase deficiency in blood cells without associated neurologic and mental disorders. *Blood* 66:1288, 1985.
43. Maran J, Guan Y, Ou CN, et al: Heterogeneity of the molecular biology of methemoglobinemia: A study of eight consecutive patients. *Haematologica* 90(5):687, 2005.
44. Cohen RJ, Sachs JR, Wicker DJ, et al: Methemoglobinemia provoked by malarial chemoprophylaxis in Vietnam. *N Engl J Med* 279(21):1127, 1968.
45. Moore MR, Conrad ME, Bradley EL Jr, et al: Studies of nicotinamide adenine dinucleotide methemoglobin reductase activity in a Jewish population. *Am J Hematol* 12(1):13, 1982.
46. Fine DM, Eyster GE, Anderson LK, et al: Cyanosis and congenital methemoglobinemia in a puppy. *J Am Anim Hosp Assoc* 35(1):33, 1999.
47. Harvey JW, Ling GV, Kaneko JJ: Methemoglobin reductase deficiency in a dog. *J Am Vet Med Assoc* 164(10):1030, 1974.
48. Lo SC, Agar NS: NADH-methemoglobin reductase activity in the erythrocytes of newborn and adult mammals. *Experientia* 42(11–12):1264, 1986.
49. Graubarth J, Bloom CJ, Coleman FC, Solomon, HN. Dye poisoning in the nursery: A review of seventeen cases. *JAMA* 128:1155, 1945.
50. Sanchez-Echaniz J, Benito-Fernandez J, Mintegui-Raso S: Methemoglobinemia and consumption of vegetables in infants. *Pediatrics* 107(5):1024, 2001.
51. Hanukoglu A, Danon PN: Endogenous methemoglobinemia associated with diarrheal disease in infancy. *J Pediatr Gastroenterol Nutr* 23(1):1, 1996.
52. Hamon I, Gauthier-Moulinier H, Grelet-Dessioux E, et al: Methaemoglobinaemia risk factors with inhaled nitric oxide therapy in newborn infants. *Acta Paediatr* 99(10):1467, 2010.
53. Bricker T, Jefferson, LS, Mintz, AA: Methemoglobinemia in infants with enteritis. *J Pediatr* 102(1):161, 1983.
54. Murray KF, Christie DL: Dietary protein intolerance in infants with transient methemoglobinemia and diarrhea. *J Pediatr* 122(1):90, 1993.
55. Hegesh E, Hegesh J, Kaftory A: Congenital methemoglobinemia with a deficiency of cytochrome b5. *N Engl J Med* 314:757, 1986.
56. Lehmann H, Huntsman RG: *Man's Haemoglobins*. Lippincott, Philadelphia, 1974.
57. Hayashi A, Fujita T, Fujimura M, et al: A new abnormal fetal hemoglobin, Hb FM-Osaka (alpha 2 gamma 2 63His replaced by Tyr). *Hemoglobin* 4(3–4):447, 1980.
58. Priest JR, Watterson J, Jones RT, et al: Mutant fetal hemoglobin causing cyanosis in a newborn. *Pediatrics* 83(5):734, 1989.

59. Hojas-Bernal R, McNab-Martin P, Fairbanks VF, et al: Hb Chile [beta28(B10)Leu—>Met]: An unstable hemoglobin associated with chronic methemoglobinemia and sulfonamide or methylene blue-induced hemolytic anemia. *Hemoglobin* 23(2):125, 1999.
60. Prchal JT, Borgese N, Moore MR, et al: Congenital methemoglobinemia due to methemoglobin reductase deficiency in two unrelated American black families. *Am J Med* 89(4):516, 1990.
61. Wild B, Bain BJ: Investigation of abnormal haemoglobins and thalassaemia, in *Dacie and Lewis Practical Haematology*, edited by Lewis S, Bain B, Bates I, p 295. Churchill Livingstone, Philadelphia, 2006.
62. Yawata Y, Ding L, Tanishima K, et al: New variant of cytochrome b5 reductase deficiency (b5RKurashiki) in red cells, platelets, lymphocytes, and cultured fibroblasts with congenital methemoglobinemia, mental and neurological retardation, and skeletal anomalies. *Am J Hematol* 40(4):299, 1992.
63. Evelyn K, Malloy H: Microdetermination of oxyhemoglobin, methemoglobin, and sulfhemoglobin in a single sample of blood. *J Biol Chem* 126:655, 1938.
64. Beutler E: Carboxyhemoglobin, methemoglobin, and sulfhemoglobin determinations, in *Williams Hematology*, edited by Beutler E, Lichtman MA, Coller BS, Kipps TJ, p L50. McGraw-Hill, New York, 1995.
65. Halvorsen SM, Dull WL: Phenazopyridine-induced sulfhemoglobinemia: Inadvertent rechallenge. *Am J Med* 91(3):315, 1991.
66. Watcha MF, Connor MT, Hing AV: Pulse oximetry in methemoglobinemia. *Am J Dis Child* 143(7):845, 1989.
67. Molthrop D, Wheeler R, Hall K, et al: Evaluation of the methemoglobinemia associated with sulofenur. *Invest New Drugs* 12:99, 1994.
68. Beutler E, Gelbart T: Carboxyhemoglobin, methemoglobin, and sulf-hemoglobin determinations, in *Williams Hematology*, 4th ed, edited by Williams WJ, Beutler E, Erslev AJ, Lichtman MA, p 1732. McGraw-Hill, New York, 1990.
69. Barker SJ, Curry J, Redford D, et al: Measurement of carboxyhemoglobin and methemoglobin by pulse oximetry: A human volunteer study. *Anesthesiology* 105:892, 2006.
70. Annabi EH, Barker SJ: Severe methemoglobinemia detected by pulse oximetry. *Anesth Analg* 108(3):898, 2009.
71. Hampson NB: Noninvasive pulse CO-oximetry expedites evaluation and management of patients with carbon monoxide poisoning. *Am J Emerg Med* 30(9):2021, 2012.
72. Beutler E: *Red Cell Metabolism: A Manual of Biochemical Methods*. Grune & Stratton, New York, 1984.
73. Board P: NADH-ferricyanide reductase, a convenient approach to the evaluation of NADH-methaemoglobin reductase in human erythrocytes. *Clin Chim Acta* 109:233, 1981.
74. Lan FH, Tang YC, Huang CH, et al: Antibody-based spot test for NADH-cytochrome b5 reductase activity for the laboratory diagnosis of congenital methemoglobinemia. *Clin Chim Acta* 273(1):13, 1998.
75. Das Gupta A, Vaidya MS, Bapat JP, et al: Associated red cell enzyme deficiencies and their significance in a case of congenital enzymopenic methemoglobinemia. *Acta Haematol* 64(5):285, 1980.
76. Kaftory A, Hegesh E: Improved determination of cytochrome b5 in human erythrocytes. *Clin Chem* 30(8):1344, 1984.
77. Gerald PS, George P: Second spectroscopically abnormal methemoglobin associated with hereditary cyanosis. *Science* 129(3346):393, 1959.
78. Carrell RW, Kay R: A simple method for the detection of unstable haemoglobins. *Br J Haematol* 23(5):615, 1972.
79. Hutt PJ, Pisciotta AV, Fairbanks VF, et al: DNA sequence analysis proves Hb M-Milwaukee-2 is due to beta-globin gene codon 92 (CAC—>TAC), the presumed mutation of Hb M-Hyde Park and Hb M-Akita. *Hemoglobin* 22(1):1, 1998.
80. Darling R, Roughton F: The effect of methemoglobin on the equilibrium between oxygen and hemoglobin. *Am J Physiol* 137:56, 1942.
81. Johnson CJ, Bonrud PA, Dosch TL, et al: Fatal outcome of methemoglobinemia in an infant. *JAMA* 257(20):2796, 1987.
82. Ellis M, Hiss Y, Shenkman L: Fatal methemoglobinemia caused by inadvertent contamination of a laxative solution with sodium nitrite. *Isr J Med Sci* 28(5):289, 1992.
83. Caudill L, Walbridge J, Kuhn G: Methemoglobinemia as a cause of coma. *Ann Emerg Med* 19(6):677, 1990.
84. Clifton J 2nd, Leikin JB: Methylene blue. *Am J Ther* 10(4):289, 2003.
85. Beutler E, Baluda MC: Methemoglobin reduction: Studies of the interaction between cell populations and of the role of methylene blue. *Blood* 22:323, 1963.
86. Rosen PJ, Johnson C, McGehee WG, et al: Failure of methylene blue treatment in toxic methemoglobinemia: Associations with glucose-6-phosphate dehydrogenase deficiency. *Ann Intern Med* 75:83, 1971.
87. Bilgin H, Ozcan B, Bilgin T: Methemoglobinemia induced by methylene blue perturbation during laparoscopy. *Acta Anaesthesiol Scand* 42(5):594, 1998.
88. Kearney TE, Manoguerra AS, Dunford JV Jr: Chemically induced methemoglobinemia from aniline poisoning. *West J Med* 140(2):282, 1984.
89. Harvey J, Keitt A: Studies of the efficacy and potential hazards of methylene blue therapy in aniline-induced methemoglobinemia. *Br J Haematol* 54:29, 1983.
90. Coleman MD, Rhodes LE, Scott AK, et al: The use of cimetidine to reduce dapsone-dependent methaemoglobinaemia in dermatitis herpetiformis patients. *Br J Clin Pharmacol* 34:244, 1992.
91. Kaplan J, Chirouze M: Therapy of recessive congenital methaemoglobinaemia by oral riboflavin. *Lancet* 2:1043, 1978.
92. Beutler E: Important recent advances in the field of red cell metabolism: Practical implications, in *Erythrocytes, Thrombocytes, Leukocytes*, edited by Gerlach E, Moser K, Deutsch E, Wilmanns W, p 123. George Thieme Verlag, Stuttgart, 1973.

93. Lemberg R, Legge, JW: *Hematin Compounds and Bile Pigments*. Inter-science Publishers, New York, 1949.
94. Harrop GJ, Waterfield RL: Sulphemoglobinemia. *JAMA* 95:647, 1930.
95. Nichol A, Hendry I, Movell DB, et al: Mechanism of formation of sulfhemoglobin. *Biochim Biophys Acta* 156:97, 1968.
96. Berzofsky JA, Peisach J, Horecker BL: Sulfheme proteins. IV. The stoichiometry of sulfur incorporation and the isolation of sulfhemin, the prosthetic group of sulfmyoglobin. *J Biol Chem* 247(12):3783, 1972.
97. Berzofsky JA, Peisach J, Blumberg WE: Sulfheme proteins. II. The reversible oxygenation of ferrous sulfmyoglobin. *J Biol Chem* 246: 7366–7372, 1971.
98. Park CM, Nagel RL: Sulfhemoglobinemia. Clinical and molecular aspects. *N Engl J Med* 310(24):1579, 1984.
99. Discombe G: Sulphaemoglobinaemia and glutathione. *Lancet* 2:371, 1960.
100. McCutcheon A: Sulphaemoglobinaemia and glutathione. *Lancet* 2:290, 1960.
101. Paniker NV, Beutler E: The effect of methylene blue and diaminodiphenysulfone on red cell reduced glutathione synthesis. *J Lab Clin Med* 80(4):481, 1972.
102. Smith JE, Mahaffey E, Lee M: Effect of methylene blue on glutamate and reduced glutathione of rabbit erythrocytes. *Biochem J* 168(3):587, 1977.
103. Pandey J, Chellani H, Garg M, et al: Congenital sulfhemoglobin and transient methemoglobinemia secondary to diarrhoea. *Indian J Pathol Microbiol* 39(3):217, 1996.
104. Stamatoyannopoulos G, Parer JT, Finch CA: Physiologic implications of a hemoglobin with decreased oxygen affinity (hemoglobin Seattle). *N Engl J Med* 281(17):916, 1969.
105. Lichtman MA, Murphy MS, Adamson JW: Detection of mutant hemoglobins with altered affinity for oxygen. A simplified technique. *Ann Intern Med* 84(5):517, 1976.
106. Agarwal N, Mojica-Henshaw MP, Simmons ED, et al: Familial polycythemia caused by a novel mutation in the beta globin gene: Essential role of P50 in evaluation of familial polycythemia. *Int J Med Sci* 4(4):232, 2007.
107. Vreman HJ, Mahoney JJ, Stevenson, DK. Carbon monoxide and carboxyhemoglobin. *Adv Pediatr* 42:303–325, 1995.
108. Hampson NB, Weaver LK: Carbon monoxide poisoning: A new incidence for an old disease. *Undersea Hyperb Med* 34(3):163, 2007.
109. Weaver LK: Carbon monoxide poisoning. *Crit Care Clin* 15:297, 1999.
110. Centers for Disease Control and Prevention: Epidemiologic assessment of the impact of four hurricanes—Florida, 2004. *MMWR Morb Mortal Wkly Rep* 54(28):693, 2005.
111. Ernst A, Zibrak JD: Carbon monoxide poisoning. *N Engl J Med* 339:1603, 1998.
112. Chen BC, Shawn LK, Connors NJ, et al: Carbon monoxide exposures in New York City following hurricane Sandy in 2012. *Clin Toxicol (Phila)* 51(9):879, 2013.
113. Centers for Disease Control and Prevention: Carbon monoxide exposures after hurricane Ike—Texas, September 2008. *MMWR Morb Mortal Wkly Rep* 58(31):845, 2009.
114. Centers for Disease Control and Prevention: Unintentional non–fire-related carbon monoxide exposures—United States, 2001–2003. *MMWR Morb Mortal Wkly Rep* 54(2):36, 2005.
115. Mott JA, Wolfe MI, Alverson CJ, et al: National vehicle emissions policies and practices and declining US carbon monoxide-related mortality. *JAMA* 288:988, 2002.
116. Harper A, Croft-Baker J: Carbon monoxide poisoning: Undetected by both patients and their doctors. *Age Ageing* 33(2):105, 2004.
117. U.S. Environmental Protection Agency: *Emission facts: Idling vehicle Emissions*. Publication EPA420-F-98-014. USEPA, Washington, DC, 1998. Available online at: http://www.epa.gov/oms/consumer/f98014.pdf
118. Stewart RD, Fisher TN, Hosko MJ, et al: Carboxyhemoglobin elevation after exposure to dichloromethane. *Science* 176:295, 1972.
119. Antonini E, Brunori M: *Hemoglobin and myoglobin in their reactions with ligands.* Amsterdam: North-Holland, 1971.
120. Sjostrand T: Endogenous formation of carbon monoxide in man. *Nature* 164(4170):580, 1949.
121. Giacometti GM, Brunori M, Antonini E, et al: The reaction of hemoglobin Zurich with oxygen and carbon monoxide. *J Biol Chem* 255(13):6160, 1980.
122. Balster RL, Ekelund LG, Grover RF: Evaluation of subpopulations potentially at risk to carbon monoxide exposure, in *Air Quality Criteria for Carbon Monoxide* edited by the U.S. EPA, p 12-1. EPA No. 600/8-90/045F. U.S. Environmental Protection Agency, Environmental Criteria and Assessment Office, Research Triangle Park, NC, 1991.
123. Hampson NB, Dunford RG, Kramer CC, et al: Selection criteria utilized for hyperbaric oxygen treatment of carbon monoxide poisoning. *J Emerg Med* 13:227, 1995.
124. Benesch RE, Maeda N, Benesch R: 2,3-Diphosphoglycerate and the relative affinity of adult and fetal hemoglobin for oxygen and carbon dioxide. *Biochim Biophys Acta* 257:178, 1972.
125. Engel RR, Rodkey FL, O'Neal JD, et al: Relative affinity of human fetal hemoglobin for CO and O₂. *Blood* 33:37, 1969.
126. Suner S, Partridge R, Sucov A, et al: Non-invasive screening for carbon monoxide toxicity in the emergency department is valuable. *Ann Emerg Med* 49(5):719, 2007.
127. Weaver LK: Clinical practice. Carbon monoxide poisoning. *N Engl J Med* 360(12):1217, 2009.
128. Jasper BW, Hopkins RO, Duker HV, et al: Affective outcome following carbon monoxide poisoning: A prospective longitudinal study. *Cogn Behav Neurol* 18(2):127, 2005.
129. Gemelli F, Cattani R: Carbon monoxide poisoning in childhood. *Br Med J* 291:1197, 1985.
130. Lacey DJ: Neurologic sequelae of acute carbon monoxide intoxication. *Am J Dis Child* 135(2):145, 1981.
131. Buckley NA, Juurlink DN, Isbister G, et al: Hyperbaric oxygen for carbon monoxide poisoning. *Cochrane Database Syst Rev* (4):CD002041, 2011.
132. Elkharrat D, Raphael JC, Korach JM, et al: Acute carbon monoxide intoxication and hyperbaric oxygen in pregnancy. *Intensive Care Med* 17:289, 1991.
133. Koren G, Shara, T, Pastuszak A, et al: A multicenter, prospective study of fetal outcome following accidental carbon monoxide poisoning in pregnancy. *Reprod Toxicol* 5:397, 1991.
134. Ignarro LJ: Nitric oxide. A novel signal transduction mechanism for transcellular communication. *Hypertension* 16(5):477, 1990.
135. Liu X, Miller MJ, Joshi MS, et al: Diffusion-limited reaction of free nitric oxide with erythrocytes. *J. Biol Chem* 273:18709, 1998.
136. Azarov I, Huang KT, Basu S, Gladwin MT, et al: Nitric oxide scavenging by red blood cells as a function of hematocrit and oxygenation. *J Biol Chem* 280:39024, 2005.
137. Kim-Shapiro DB, Schechter AN, Gladwin MT: Unraveling the reactions of nitric oxide, nitrite, and hemoglobin in physiology and therapeutics. *Arterioscler Thromb Vasc Biol* 26:697, 2006.
138. Stamler JS, Jia L, Eu JP, et al: Blood flow regulation by S-nitrosohemoglobin in the physiological oxygen gradient. *Science* 276:2034, 1997.
139. Stamler JS, Singel DJ, Piantadosi CA: SNO-hemoglobin and hypoxic vasodilation. *Nat Med* 14(10):1009, 2008.
140. Vitturi DA, Teng X, Toledo JC, et al: Regulation of nitrite transport in red blood cells by hemoglobin oxygen fractional saturation. *Am J Physiol Heart Circ Physiol* 296(5):H1398, 2009.
141. Gladwin MT, Kim-Shapiro DB. The functional nitrite reductase activity of the hemeglobins. *Blood* 112(7):2636, 2008.
142. Gladwin MT, Schechter AN, Kim-Shapiro DB, et al: The emerging biology of the nitrite anion. *Nat Chem Biol* 1(6):308, 2005.
143. Basu S, Grubina R, Huang J, et al: Catalytic generation of N₂O₃ by the concerted nitrite reductase and anhydrase activity of hemoglobin. *Nat Chem Biol* 3(12):785, 2007.
144. Lauer T, Preik M, Rassaf T, et al: Plasma nitrite rather than nitrate reflects regional endothelial nitric oxide synthase activity but lacks intrinsic vasodilator action. *Proc Natl Acad Sci U S A* 98(22):12814, 2001.
145. Shiva S, Wang X, Ringwood LA, et al: Ceruloplasmin is a NO oxidase and nitrite synthase that determines endocrine NO homeostasis. *Nat Chem Biol* 2(9):486, 2006.
146. Liu C, Zhao W, Christ GJ, et al: Nitric oxide scavenging by red cell microparticles. *Free Radic Biol Med* 65:1164, 2013.
147. Reynolds JD, Bennett KM, Cina AJ, et al: S-nitrosylation therapy to improve oxygen delivery of banked blood. *Proc Natl Acad Sci U S A* 110(28):11529, 2013.
148. Kanias T, Gladwin MT: Nitric oxide, hemolysis, and the red blood cell storage lesion: Interactions between transfusion, donor, and recipient. *Transfusion* 52(7):1388, 2012.
149. Kahn MJ, Maley JH, Lasker GF, et al: Updated role of nitric oxide in disorders of erythrocyte function. *Cardiovasc Hematol Disord Drug Targets* 13(1):83, 2013.
150. Badesch DB, Abman SH, Ahearn GS, et al: Medical therapy for pulmonary arterial hypertension: ACCP evidence-based clinical practice guidelines. *Chest* 126(1 Suppl):35S, 2004.
151. Martinez-Ruiz R, Montero-Huerta P, Hromi J, et al: Inhaled nitric oxide improves survival rates during hypoxia in a sickle cell (SAD) mouse model. *Anesthesiology* 94:1113, 2001.
152. Weiner DL, Hibberd PL, Betit P, et al: Preliminary assessment of inhaled nitric oxide for acute vaso-occlusive crisis in pediatric patients with sickle cell disease. *JAMA* 289:1136, 2003.
153. Sullivan KJ, Goodwin SR, Evangelist J, et al: Nitric oxide successfully used to treat acute chest syndrome of sickle cell disease in a young adolescent. *Crit Care Med* 27:2563, 1999.
154. McMahon TJ, Doctor A: Extrapulmonary effects of inhaled nitric oxide: Role of reversible S-nitrosylation of erythrocytic hemoglobin. *Proc Am Thorac Soc* 3(2):153, 2006.
155. Young JD, Dyar O, Xiong L, et al: Methaemoglobin production in normal adults inhaling low concentrations of nitric oxide. *Intensive Care Med* 20:581, 1994.
156. Loh E, Stamler JS, Hare JM, et al: Cardiovascular effects of inhaled nitric oxide in patients with left ventricular dysfunction. *Circulation* 90:2780, 1994.
157. Lundin S, Mang H, Smithies M, et al: Inhalation of nitric oxide in acute lung injury: Results of a European multicentre study. The European Study Group of Inhaled Nitric Oxide. *Intensive Care Med* 25:911, 1999.
158. Christenson J, Lavoie A, O'Connor M, et al: The incidence and pathogenesis of cardiopulmonary deterioration after abrupt withdrawal of inhaled nitric oxide. *Am J Respir Crit Care Med* 161:1443, 2000.
159. Moya MP, Gow AJ, McMahon TJ, et al: S-nitrosothiol repletion by an inhaled gas regulates pulmonary function. *Proc Natl Acad Sci U S A* 98:5792, 2001.
160. Moya MP, Gow AJ, Califf RM, et al: Inhaled ethyl nitrite gas for persistent pulmonary hypertension of the newborn. *Lancet* 360:141, 2002.
161. Gulati A, Sen AP, Sharma AC, et al: Role of ET and NO in resuscitative effect of diaspirin cross-linked hemoglobin after hemorrhage in rat. *Am J Physiol* 273:H827, 1997.
162. Gibson JB, Maxwell RA, Schweitzer JB, et al: Resuscitation from severe hemorrhagic shock after traumatic brain injury using saline, shed blood, or a blood substitute. *Shock* 17:234, 2002.
163. Paris PM, Kaplan RM, Stewart RD, et al: Methemoglobin levels following sublingual nitroglycerin in human volunteers. *Ann Emerg Med* 15(2):171, 1986.
164. Gavish D, Knobler H, Gottehrer N, et al: Methemoglobinemia, muscle damage and renal failure complicating phenazopyridine overdose. *Isr J Med Sci* 22(1):45, 1986.

165. Christensen CM, Farrar HC, Kearns GL: Protracted methemoglobinemia after phenazopyridine overdose in an infant. *J Clin Pharmacol* 36(2):112, 1996.

166. Damergis JA, Stoker JM, Abadie JL: Methemoglobinemia after sulfametoxazole and trimethoprim. *JAMA* 249(5):590, 1983.

167. Falkenhahn M, Kannan S, O'Kane M: Unexplained acute severe methaemoglobinaemia in a young adult. *Br J Anaesth* 86(2):278, 2001.

168. Wagner A, Marosi C, Binder M, et al: Fatal poisoning due to dapsone in a patient with grossly elevated methaemoglobin levels. *Br J Dermatol* 133(5):816, 1995.

169. Ng LL, Nai KR, Polak A: Paraquat ingestion with methaemoglobinaemia treated with methylene blue. *Br Med J (Clin Res Ed)* 284(6327):1445, 1982.

170. Proudfoot AT: Methaemoglobinaemia due to monolinuron—Not paraquat. *Br Med J (Clin Res Ed)* 285(6344):812, 1982.

171. de Torres JP, Strom JA, Jaber BL, et al: Hemodialysis-associated methemoglobinemia in acute renal failure. *Am J Kidney Dis* 39(6):1307, 2002.

172. Gibson GR, Hunter JB, Raabe DS Jr, et al: Methemoglobinemia produced by high-dose intravenous nitroglycerin. *Ann Intern Med* 96(5):615, 1982.

173. Forsyth RJ, Moulden A: Methaemoglobinaemia after ingestion of amyl nitrite. *Arch Dis Child* 66(1):152, 1991.

174. Guss DA, Normann SA, Manoguerra AS: Clinically significant methemoglobinemia from inhalation of isobutyl nitrite. *Am J Emerg Med* 3(1):46, 1985.

175. Kuschner WG, Chitkara RK, Canfield J Jr, et al: Benzocaine-associated methemoglobinemia following bronchoscopy in a healthy research participant. *Respir Care* 45(8):953, 2000.

176. Abdallah HY, Shah SA: Methemoglobinemia induced by topical benzocaine: A warning for the endoscopist. *Endoscopy* 34(9):730, 2002.

177. Novaro G, Aronow H, Militello M, et al: Benzocaine-induced methemoglobinemia: Experience from a high-volume transesophageal echocardiography laboratory. *J Am Soc Echocardiogr* 16:170, 2003.

178. Nilsson A, Engberg G, Henneberg S, et al: Inverse relationship between age-dependent erythrocyte activity of methaemoglobin reductase and prilocaine-induced methaemoglobinaemia during infancy. *Br J Anaesth* 64(1):72, 1990.

179. Duncan PG, Kobrinsky N: Prilocaine-induced methemoglobinemia in a newborn infant. *Anesthesiology* 59(1):75, 1983.

180. Lloyd CJ: Chemically induced methaemoglobinaemia in a neonate. *Br J Oral Maxillofac Surg* 30(1):63, 1992.

181. Davidovits M, Barak A, Cleper R, et al: Methaemoglobinaemia and haemolysis associated with hydrogen peroxide in a paediatric haemodialysis centre: A warning note. *Nephrol Dial Transplant* 18(11):2354, 2003.

182. Gerald PS, Efron ML: Chemical studies of several varieties of Hb M. *Proc Natl Acad Sci U S A* 47:1758, 1961.

183. Stavem P, Stromme J, Lorkin PA, et al: Haemoglobin M Saskatoon with slight constant haemolysis, markedly increased by sulphonamides. *Scand J Haematol* 9(6):566, 1972.

184. Hayashi N, Motokawa Y, Kikuchi G: Studies on relationships between structure and function of hemoglobin M-Iwate. *J Biol Chem* 241(1):79, 1966.

185. Horst J, Schafer R, Kleihauer E, et al: Analysis of the Hb M Milwaukee mutation at the DNA level. *Br J Haematol* 54(4):643, 1983.

186. Hain RD, Chitayat D, Cooper R, et al: Hb FM-Fort Ripley: Confirmation of autosomal dominant inheritance and diagnosis by PCR and direct nucleotide sequencing. *Hum Mutat* 3(3):239, 1994.

187. Reissmann KR, Ruth WE, Nomura T: A human hemoglobin with lowered oxygen affinity and impaired heme-heme interactions. *J Clin Invest* 40:1826, 1961.

CHAPTER 51
FRAGMENTATION HEMOLYTIC ANEMIA

Kelty R. Baker and Joel Moake

SUMMARY

Erythrocyte fragmentation and hemolysis occur when red cells are forced at high shear stress through partial vascular occlusions or over abnormal vascular surfaces. "Split" red cells, or schistocytes, are prominent on blood films under these conditions, and considerable quantities of lactate dehydrogenase are released into the blood from traumatized red cells. In the high-flow (high-shear) microvascular (arteriolar/capillary) or arterial circulation, partial vascular obstructions are caused by platelet aggregates in the systemic microvasculature during episodes of thrombotic thrombocytopenic purpura by platelet-fibrin thrombi in the renal microvasculature in the hemolytic uremic syndrome; and by malfunction of a cardiac prosthetic valve in valve-related hemolysis. Less-extensive red cell fragmentation, hemolysis, and schistocytosis occur under conditions of more moderate vascular occlusion or endothelial surface abnormalities, sometimes under conditions of lower shear stress. These latter entities include excessive platelet aggregation, fibrin polymer formation, and secondary fibrinolysis in the arterial or venous microcirculation (disseminated intravascular coagulation); in the placental vasculature in preeclampsia/eclampsia and the syndrome of hemolysis, elevated liver enzymes and low platelets (HELLP) in march hemoglobinuria; and in giant cavernous hemangiomas (the Kasabach-Merritt phenomenon).

● PREECLAMPSIA/ECLAMPSIA AND HELLP SYNDROME

DEFINITION AND HISTORY

A life-threatening condition of pregnancy denoted by eclampsia, hemolysis, and thrombocytopenia was first noted in the German literature by Stahnke in 1922.[1] Subsequently, Pritchard and coworkers described three cases in English and suggested that an immunologic process might account for both the preeclampsia or eclampsia and the hematologic abnormalities.[2]

Although initially known as edema-proteinuria-hypertension gestosis type B,[3] a catchier phrase, HELLP syndrome (H for hemolysis, EL for elevated liver function tests, and LP for low platelet counts), was later applied by Louis Weinstein in 1982.[4]

EPIDEMIOLOGY

HELLP syndrome occurs in approximately 0.5 percent of pregnancies overall,[5] in 4 to 12 percent of those complicated by preeclampsia (hypertension + proteinuria), and in 30 to 50 percent of those complicated by eclampsia (hypertension + proteinuria + seizures); however, approximately 15 percent of patients ultimately diagnosed with HELLP syndrome present with neither hypertension nor proteinuria.[6] Two-thirds of HELLP patients are diagnosed antepartum, usually between 27 and 37 weeks. The remaining one-third are diagnosed in the postpartum period, from a few to 48 hours following delivery (occasionally as long as 6 days).[7,8] Risk factors for HELLP syndrome include European ancestry, multiparity, older maternal age (older than age 34 years), and a personal or familial history of the disorder.[5] Although the presence of homozygosity for the 677 (C→T) polymorphism of the methylenetetrahydrofolate reductase gene may be a modest risk factor for the development of preeclampsia, this weak association does not exist for HELLP syndrome.[9] Whether or not the factor V Leiden or prothrombin 20210 gene mutations are risk factors for HELLP syndrome remains controversial.[10–12]

ETIOLOGY AND PATHOGENESIS

A developing embryo must acquire a supply of maternal blood to survive. During a normal pregnancy, the first wave of trophoblastic invasion into the decidua occurs at 10 to 12 days. This is followed by a second wave at 16 to 22 weeks, when these specialized placental epithelial cells replace the endothelium of the uterine spiral arteries and intercalate within the muscular tunica, increasing the vessels' diameters and decreasing their resistance. As a result, the spiral arteries are remodeled into unique hybrid vessels composed of fetal and maternal cells, and the vasculature is converted into a high-flow–low-resistance system resistant to vasoconstrictors circulating in the maternal blood.[13] In a preeclamptic pregnancy, the second wave fails to penetrate adequately the spiral arteries of the uterus, perhaps as a result of reduced placental expression of syncytin and subsequent altered cell fusion processes during placentogenesis.[14] The resultant poorly perfused, hypoxic placenta then releases the extracellular domain (soluble) form of fms-like tyrosine kinase 1 (sFLT-1), also known as soluble vascular endothelial growth factor receptor-1 (sVEGF receptor-1, or sVEGFR-1). sVEGFR-1 functions as an antiangiogenic protein because it binds to vascular endothelial growth factor (VEGF) and placental growth factor (PGF), and prevents their interaction with endothelial cell receptors. The result is glomerular endothelial cell and placental dysfunction.[15–17] Direct and indirect sequelae include increased vascular tone, hypertension, proteinuria, enhanced platelet activation and aggregation, and decreased levels of the vasodilators prostaglandin I$_2$ (PGI$_2$) and nitrous oxide (NO).[5,17] Concurrent activation of the coagulation cascade results in platelet-fibrin deposition in the capillaries, multiorgan microvascular injury, microangiopathic hemolytic anemia, elevated liver enzymes because of hepatic necrosis, and thrombocytopenia because of peripheral consumption of platelets.[5]

Another antiangiogenic molecule, a soluble form of endoglin (sEng), also increases in patient serum during early and severe preeclampsia.[18] Endoglin is part of the transforming growth factor-β (TGF-β) complex, and is expressed on vascular endothelial cells and syncytiotrophoblasts. The shed extracellular domain of endoglin, sEng, is capable of binding to and inactivating the proangiogenic growth factors, TGF-β_1 and TGF-β_3. The presence of elevated serum levels of both sFLT-1 (sVEGFR-1) and sEng may be associated with the progression of preeclampsia to HELLP.[17,18]

CLINICAL FEATURES

Ninety percent of patients with HELLP syndrome present with malaise and right upper quadrant or epigastric pain. Between 45 and 86 percent have nausea or vomiting, 55 to 67 percent have edema, 31 to 50 percent have headache, and a smaller percentage complain of visual changes. Fever is not typically seen. Although hypertension is found in 85 percent of affected patients, 15 percent of those with HELLP syndrome do not develop either hypertension or proteinuria.[6]

LABORATORY FEATURES

There is no consensus regarding the laboratory criteria necessary to diagnose HELLP syndrome, so clinical judgment in conjunction with judicious interpretation of a variety of laboratory tests constitute the diagnostic standard. In 54 to 86 percent of patients, the blood film has schistocytes, helmet cells, and burr cells consistent with microangiopathic hemolytic anemia. Reticulocytosis can be present. Low haptoglobin levels are both sensitive (83 percent) and specific (96 percent) for confirming the presence of hemolysis, and return to normal within 24 to 30 hours postpartum.[6]

Lactate dehydrogenase (LDH) levels are usually above normal. The ratio of LDH-5 (an isoenzyme found specifically in the liver) to total LDH is elevated in proportion to the severity of HELLP. The high LDH seen in HELLP is most likely the result, principally, of liver damage rather than hemolysis. Serum levels of aspartic acid transaminase (AST) and alanine transaminase (ALT) can be more than 100 times normal, whereas alkaline phosphatase values are typically only about twice normal and total bilirubin ranges between 1.2 and 5.0 mg/dL. Liver enzymes usually return to normal within 3 to 5 days postpartum.[6]

The degree of thrombocytopenia has been used in a classification system to predict maternal morbidity and mortality, the rapidity of postpartum recovery, the risk of disease recurrence, and perinatal outcome. This *Mississippi triple-class system* places those patients with platelet counts less than 50×10^9/L in class 1 (approximately 13 percent incidence of bleeding); those with platelet counts between 50 and 100×10^9/L in class 2 (approximately 8 percent incidence of bleeding); and those with a platelet count greater than 100×10^9/L in class 3 (no increased bleeding risk). Patients with class 1 HELLP syndrome suffer the highest incidence of perinatal morbidity and mortality, and have the most protracted recovery periods postpartum.[19] There is a direct correlation between the extent of thrombocytopenia and measurements of liver function,[20] but the same cannot be said for the severity of associated hepatic histopathologic changes.[21] If a marrow aspiration and biopsy are performed, abundant megakaryocytes are found consistent with a consumptive thrombocytopenia causing reduction of the normal platelet life span of approximately 10 days to 3 to 5 days.[19] The platelet count nadir occurs 23 to 29 hours postpartum, with subsequent normalization within 6 to 11 days.[7]

The prothrombin time (PT) and activated partial thromboplastin time (aPTT) are usually within normal limits, although one report cited a prolonged aPTT in 50 percent of patients.[22] Although low fibrinogen levels are inconsistently found, other measures of increased coagulation and secondary fibrinolysis may be present. These include decreased protein C and antithrombin III (AT III) levels, and increased D-dimer and thrombin-AT III values. von Willebrand factor (VWF) antigen levels increase in proportion to the severity of the disease, reflecting the extent

of endothelial damage; however, no unusually large VWF multimers are present in plasma[23] and ADAMTS13 (a disintegrin and metalloproteinase with thrombospondin domains-13) levels are within a broad normal range (ADAMTS13 normally declines moderately during pregnancy).[24,25] This is in contrast to the severe deficiency of ADAMTS13 in familial and autoantibody-mediated types of thrombotic thrombocytopenic purpura (TTP).[26] Unlike TTP, the thrombi found in organs involved in the HELLP syndrome contain increased amounts of fibrin and low levels of VWF.[23]

In patients with severe liver involvement, hepatic ultrasonography shows large, irregular, well-demarcated (or "geographical") areas of increased echogenicity.[27] Liver biopsy shows periportal or focal necrosis, platelet-fibrin deposits in the sinusoids, and vascular microthrombi. As the disease progresses, large areas of necrosis can coalesce and dissect into the liver capsule. This produces a subcapsular hematoma and the risk of hepatic rupture.[5]

DIFFERENTIAL DIAGNOSIS

Other complications of pregnancy that can be confused with HELLP include TTP[28] and the hemolytic uremic syndrome, sepsis, disseminated intravascular coagulation (DIC), connective tissue disease, antiphospholipid antibody syndrome, and acute fatty liver of pregnancy. This latter entity is also seen in the last trimester or postpartum and presents with thrombocytopenia and right upper quadrant pain, but the levels of AST and ALT only rise to 1 to 5 times normal and the PT and partial thromboplastin time (PTT) are both prolonged. Oil-red-O staining of liver biopsies demonstrates fat in the cytoplasm of centrilobular hepatocytes, and routine stains show inflammation and patchy hepatocellular necrosis as a result of the HELLP syndrome. Because it causes right upper quadrant pain and nausea, HELLP has also been misdiagnosed as viral hepatitis, biliary colic, esophageal reflux, cholecystitis, and gastric cancer. Conversely, other conditions misdiagnosed as HELLP syndrome include cardiomyopathy, dissecting aortic aneurysm, acute cocaine intoxication, essential hypertension and renal disease, and alcoholic liver disease.[19]

THERAPY

Supportive care of HELLP includes intravenous administration of magnesium sulfate to control hypertension and prevent eclamptic seizures, management of fluids and electrolytes, judicious transfusion of blood products, stimulation of fetal lung maturation with beclomethasone, and delivery of the fetus as soon as possible.[19] Indications for delivery include a severe disease presentation, maternal DIC, fetal distress, and a gestational age greater than 32 weeks with evidence of lung maturity.[6] Cesarean section under general anesthesia is used in 60 to 97 percent of cases, but vaginal delivery after induction can be attempted if the fetus is older than 32 weeks of age and the mother's cervical anatomy is favorable. Postpartum curettage is helpful in lowering the mean arterial pressure and increasing the urine output and platelet count. Transfusion therapy with packed red cells, platelets, or fresh-frozen plasma is indicated in cases complicated by severe anemia or bleeding because of coagulopathy.

Although previously thought to be beneficial based upon the results of observational studies and small randomized trials, the use of dexamethasone has fallen out of favor after large randomized trials found that it didn't reduce the duration of hospitalization, amount of blood products transfused, maternal complications, or time to normalization of laboratory abnormalities.[29]

Plasma exchange cannot arrest or reverse HELLP syndrome when used antepartum, but may minimize hemorrhage and morbidity when used peripartum. It can also be tried postpartum in the 5 percent of patients who fail to improve within 72 to 96 hours of delivery. These women are more likely to be younger than 20 years of age or nulliparous.[7] Whether or not plasma exchange can effectively lower circulating levels of sVEGF and/or sEng is not known. Liver transplantation may be necessary in occasional patients with HELLP complicated by large hematomas or total hepatic necrosis. It is not yet known if replacement with some (possibly modified) form of VEGF and/or TGF-β may have future therapeutic use in preeclampsia or HELLP. A single case report describes the successful use of eculizumab to prolong by 17 days a pregnancy affected by severe HELLP, without associated maternal or fetal morbidity or mortality.[30]

COURSE AND PROGNOSIS

Most patients stabilize within 24 to 48 hours following delivery; however, maternal death still occurs in 3 to 5 percent even with best supportive care. Mortality rates as high as 25 percent were reported prior to 1980. Events leading to maternal death include cerebral hemorrhage, cardiopulmonary arrest, DIC, adult respiratory distress syndrome, and hypoxic ischemic encephalopathy.[5] Other complications include infection, placenta abruptio, postpartum hemorrhage, intraabdominal bleeding, and subcapsular liver hematomas with resultant rupture (a fatal event in 50 percent of those in whom it occurs).[6] The latter patients complain of right-sided shoulder pain and are found to be in shock with ascites or pleural effusions. The hematoma is usually present in the anterior superior portion of the right lobe of the liver.[5] If the liver remains intact when discovered, abdominal palpation, seizures, and emesis should be avoided or prevented. Emergency surgery is required for hepatic artery embolization or ligation, hepatic lobectomy, or even liver transplantation in patients with total hepatic necrosis.[5,19]

Renal complications of HELLP include acute renal failure, hyponatremia, and nephrogenic diabetes insipidus as a result of impaired hepatic metabolism of vasopressinase and resultant "resistance to vasopressin" (antidiuretic hormone). Pulmonary complications of HELLP include of pleural effusions, pulmonary edema, and adult respiratory distress syndrome. Neurologic sequelae of HELLP not mentioned above include retinal detachment, postictal cortical blindness, and hypoglycemic coma.[31]

Fetal morbidity and mortality are between 9 and 24 percent.[6] Complications arise as a result of prematurity, placental abruption, and intrauterine asphyxia. Intrauterine growth retardation is seen in 39 percent of infants. One-third of all babies born to mothers with HELLP have thrombocytopenia, but intraventricular hemorrhage is seen in only 4 percent of thrombocytopenic infants.[32]

HELLP syndrome complicates 2 to 5 percent of all pregnancies,[5] and can recur in as many as 27 percent of those affected during subsequent pregnancies.[33] Other hypertensive disorders of pregnancy (preeclampsia or pregnancy-induced hypertension) are also relatively common in future pregnancies (27 percent of second and subsequent pregnancies).[34] Women who recover from preeclampsia/HELLP may also be more likely to develop subsequent hypertension and cardiovascular disorders, possibly because of some persistent abnormal balance between proangiogenic and antiangiogenic factors.[17]

● DISSEMINATED MALIGNANCY

DEFINITION AND HISTORY

The association between widespread malignancy and hemolytic anemia associated with pathologic changes in small blood vessels was first noted by Brain and colleagues in 1962.[35]

EPIDEMIOLOGY

Cancer-associated microangiopathic hemolytic anemia (MAHA) has been described in a wide variety of malignancies (Table 51–1). MAHA is more likely to be associated with metastatic malignant disease than with localized cancers or benign tumors.[36] Approximately 80 percent of the tumors are mucinous adenocarcinomas of either the stomach (55 percent), breast (13 percent), or lung (10 percent). The median age at diagnosis is 50 years, with a slight male predominance.[37]

ETIOLOGY AND PATHOGENESIS

MAHA as a result of malignancy can be caused by either of two distinct mechanisms: (1) DIC with intravascular occlusions (often partial) of small vessels by platelet-fibrin thrombi; or (2) intravascular tumor emboli.[35,38] In the first mechanism,[1] intravascular activation of coagulation may occur from excessive exposure of tissue factor on phagocytes, activated endothelial cells, or tumor cells. Alternatively, a protease in the mucin secreted by adenocarcinomas may directly activate factor X.[39] Subsequent activation of coagulation factors, thrombin generation, fibrin polymer deposition, and platelet aggregation result in the formation of intravascular platelet-fibrin thrombi, and the shearing of red cells attempting to maneuver past the partial platelet-fibrin occlusions in the high-flow microvasculature. Also, circulating carcinoma mucins may interact with leukocyte L-selectin and platelet P-selectin, causing the rapid generation of platelet-rich microthrombi.[40] In the second mechanism,[2] intravascular tumor emboli partially occlude small vessels, mechanically or chemically disrupt the endothelium and promote platelet adherence to exposed subendothelium, coagulation activation and fibrin polymer formation, intimal hyperplasia, and vascular hypertrophy.[35,37,38]

TABLE 51–1. Cancers Associated with Microangiopathic Hemolytic Anemia

Gastric (55%)[37,40]

Breast (13%)[129]

Lung (10%)[35]

Other Adenocarcinomas

  Unknown primary[38]

  Prostate[35]

  Colon[38]

  Gallbladder

  Pancreas

  Ovary

Other Malignancies

  Hemangiopericytoma[36]

  Hepatoma

  Melanoma

  Small cell cancer of the lung[130]

  Testicular cancer

  Squamous cell cancer of the oropharynx

  Thymoma

  Erythroleukemia[131]

LABORATORY FEATURES

Patients with cancer-associated DIC/MAHA present with moderate-to-severe anemia. The blood film reveals schistocytes (accounting for approximately 5 to 21 percent of the red cells), burr cells, microspherocytes, reticulocytes/polychromasia, and nucleated red cells.[38] Although the reticulocyte count can be high, it is an unreliable measure of hemolysis because extensive replacement of the marrow by metastatic tumor (Chap. 45) may prevent the reticulocytosis expected with MAHA. Other indicators of hemolysis that could be more reliable include increased levels of serum unconjugated bilirubin and LDH, the presence of plasma hemoglobin, and elevated urine urobilinogen and hemoglobinuria (as $\alpha\beta$ dimers).[37] Absent or low levels of haptoglobin may also be found; however, haptoglobin is an acute-phase reactant that may be increased in malignancy.[38] The direct antiglobulin test is negative.[37,41]

Additional findings in MAHA include thrombocytopenia, with mean platelet counts of approximately 50×10^9/L (range: 3 to 225 × 10^9/L),[37] caused by a shortened platelet life span without demonstrable sequestration of platelets in the liver or spleen. Some patients with malignant tumors, however, may have preexisting thrombocytosis, and so superimposed MAHA may reduce the platelet count only toward "normal" values.[38] A normal-to-high white cell count with immature myeloid precursors may also be seen.[37,38,41] Leukoerythroblastosis caused by marrow invasion (Chap. 45), along with MAHA, is highly suggestive of metastatic malignancy.[38] Marrow aspiration and biopsy will demonstrate erythroid hyperplasia, normal-to-high numbers of megakaryocytes, and (in 55 percent of patients) cancer cells.[41]

Additional laboratory evidence of DIC has been reported in approximately 50 percent of patients with MAHA secondary to malignancy. Findings include reduced levels of fibrinogen (mean: 177 g/dL; range: 8 to 490 mg/dL), increased levels of D-dimers (or fibrin degradation products), and prolonged prothrombin and thrombin times.[37] In the early phase of DIC, aPTTs may be shortened (e.g., to <23 seconds).[42–45] It is not known if shortened aPTT values reflect the presence of activated coagulation factors in the plasma, consumption of coagulation inhibitor proteins faster than their production by hepatic cells (e.g., protein C, protein S, AT, tissue factor pathway inhibitor), or the presence in plasma of a cysteine protease capable of directly activating factor X.[39] Cancer-related DIC has been reported to be associated with a deficiency of the VWF-cleaving protease, ADAMTS13.[46] Although this was disputed by some investigators,[47] ADAMTS13 levels gradually decrease in DIC patients with poor survival rates,[48] perhaps as a result of ADAMTS13 consumption onto the long VWF multimeric strings released from cytokine-stimulated endothelial cells.[49]

DIFFERENTIAL DIAGNOSIS

The most common cause of anemia in malignancy is anemia of chronic disease (Chap. 37). Other diagnostic considerations include blood loss, myelophthisis as a result of disease metastatic to the marrow (Chap. 45), DIC/MAHA (Chap. 129), and autoimmune hemolytic anemia (Chap. 54). The latter is more often found with lymphoproliferative disease (Chap. 95) but is occasionally seen with carcinoma of the stomach, colon, breast, and cervix.[58] The treatment of cancer can also induce anemia by causing myelosuppression, oxidative hemolysis (doxorubicin, pentostatin), autoimmune hemolysis (cisplatin, chlorambucil, cyclophosphamide, melphalan, teniposide, methotrexate), or thrombotic microangiopathic anemia (mitomycin C, cisplatin, gemcitabine, and targeted cancer agents[50]).

THERAPY

Heparin, glucocorticoids, dipyridamole, indomethacin, and ε-aminocaproic acid have all been tried without success for malignancy-associated DIC/MAHA. Plasma infusion and platelet transfusions, sometimes with additional cryoprecipitate containing fibrinogen, may be useful during bleeding episodes associated with prolonged PT and aPTT, low fibrinogen levels, and thrombocytopenia. Control of the underlying metastatic malignancy, if achievable, has been beneficial.[51]

COURSE AND PROGNOSIS

MAHA caused by cancer is usually a preterminal event. Life expectancy following diagnosis is 2 to 150 days, with a mean of 21 days.[37,38]

● HEART VALVE HEMOLYSIS

DEFINITION AND HISTORY

Anemia arising after cardiac valve replacement was first described in 1954,[59] soon after corrective valvular surgery became possible. This anemia was subsequently shown to be caused by erythrocyte shearing and fragmentation as the red cells traversed the turbulent flow through or around the prosthetic valve.[60] Since then, prevention of irreversible red cell injury has been a goal when designing new prostheses; as a result, the incidence of significant valve-associated hemolysis has declined from 5 to 15 percent in the 1960s and 1970s[61,62] to less than 1 percent with newer-generation prostheses.[63] However, compensated hemolysis can occur with any type of valve prosthesis and can be detected in almost every patient when assayed using appropriate methods.[61,64,65] Additionally, intravascular hemolysis can be seen following mitral valve repair[66] and in unoperated patients with native valvular disease[61] and hypertrophic obstructive cardiomyopathy.[67]

EPIDEMIOLOGY

A variety of factors can increase the chance of valvular hemolysis: the presence of central or paravalvular regurgitation,[62,68] placement of small valve prostheses with resultant high transvalvular pressure gradients,[62] and regurgitation because of bioprosthetic valve failure, seen especially once the valve is more than 10 to 15 years old.[68] Patients with ball-and-cage valves,[64] bileaflet valves versus tilting disk valves,[69] mechanical valve prostheses versus xenograft tissue prostheses,[70] and double-valve as compared to single-valve replacement,[69] are more likely to experience clinically significant hemolysis. Some studies have found no difference in the degree of hemolysis when comparing aortic and mitral valve prostheses,[65,69] whereas others have found that the aortic location is associated with slightly greater hemolysis than the mitral location.[71–73]

ETIOLOGY AND PATHOGENESIS

Valve-related hemolysis occurs when red cells are exposed to the shearing stresses created by turbulent blood flow through and around a valve prosthesis, impaction against foreign surfaces or cardiac structures such as the wall of the atrial appendage,[68] or large pressure fluctuations between cardiac chambers. A transvalvular pressure gradient of more than 50 torr can generate shearing forces exceeding 4000 dynes/cm^2, more than the 3000 dynes/cm^2 usually needed to cause red cell fragmentation.[74] In a study looking at malfunctioning mitral valve prostheses, sophisticated computer modeling using transesophageal echocardiography demonstrated a maximal shear value of 6000 dynes/cm^2 when the regurgitant jet was divided by a solid structure such as a loose suture or dehisced annuloplasty ring. A maximal shear rate of 4500 dynes/cm^2 was found when the regurgitant jet was suddenly decelerated by a solid structure like the left atrial appendage, or when the blood was regurgitated through a small orifice (<2 mm in diameter) such as a leaflet perforation or a paravalvular leak.[68] Lack of endothelialization of the prosthetic ring may contribute to the severity of hemolysis following valve repair or replacement, but it is unclear if this is primary or secondary to the high-velocity jet of blood preventing fibrous incorporation of the prosthetic materials.[68,75]

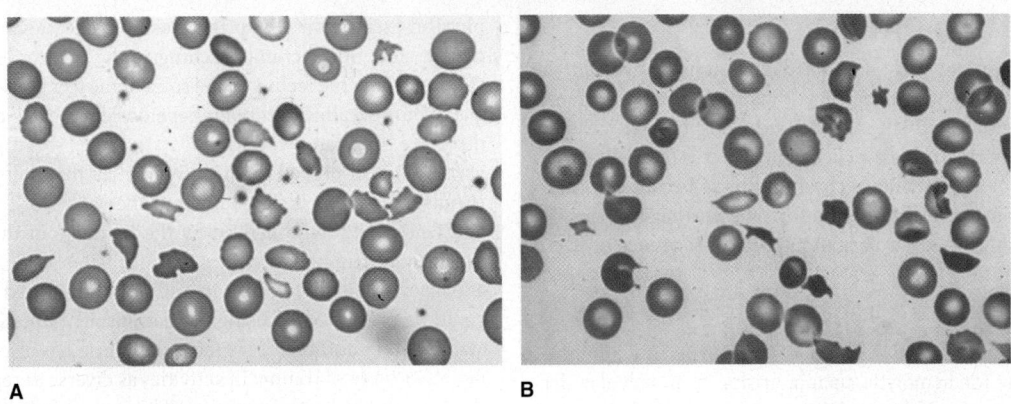

Figure 51–1. Two cases of fragmentation hemolytic anemia as a result of heart valve hemolysis. The red cell shape abnormalities are varied and characteristic of fragmentation hemolysis, although they are not specific for the cause. *(Reproduced with permission from Lichtman's Atlas of Hematology, www.accessmedicine.com.)*

Similarly, lack of endothelialization of the Teflon patch can result in clinically significant hemolysis necessitating reoperation following repair of a ventricular septal defect.[76] These sorts of surface interactions appear to be more important at lower shear-stress values (<1500 dynes/cm²) when the amount of hemolysis depends more directly on the area of the contact surface and the time of exposure.[77] Additionally, excessive wear of the cloth that covers caged-ball prostheses, such as the Starr-Edwards valve, can cause ballooning of the material into the blood jet, with resultant turbulence and hemolysis.[78] A modified Blalock-Taussig shunt also has been reported to cause hemolytic anemia.[79]

CLINICAL FEATURES

Patients with valve-induced hemolysis can present with symptoms caused by anemia or congestive heart failure, pallor, icterus, and dark urine (described variously as red, brown, or black). Urine excreted during periods of physical activity may be darker than that excreted at rest.[80] Similarly, hemolysis can be exacerbated by supraventricular tachycardia or other tachyarrhythmias and regress once normal sinus rhythm is restored.[81] Anecdotally, some patients with severe valve hemolysis complain of chest pain subsequently proven to be caused by esophageal spasm, and one can speculate that the culprit is NO depletion such as that reported in paroxysmal nocturnal hemoglobinuria.[82]

LABORATORY FEATURES

Helpful laboratory studies include review of the blood film, which will reveal moderate poikilocytosis, schistocytosis, and polychromasia

(Fig. 51–1). The red cells are usually normochromic and normocytic but can occasionally be hypochromic and microcytic as a result of long-standing urinary iron loss[61] and increased erythropoiesis caused by ongoing hemolysis.[62] The reticulocyte count, urine hemosiderin, plasma hemoglobin, and serum levels of total and indirect bilirubin, and LDH can be elevated, whereas the serum haptoglobin will be depressed. Both the number of schistocytes in the blood[61,64] and the elevation of LDH[64,65,83,84] correlate with the severity of hemolysis. Hemoglobinuria is usually seen only in those with particularly severe hemolysis and high LDH levels. There is no correlation between the severity of hemolysis and bilirubin levels, however, and whether the reticulocyte count is helpful in assessing the severity of hemolysis is controversial.[64,65] The aforementioned laboratory tests can be used as a means to determine the degree of hemolysis and to help guide management (Table 51–2).[64]

Red cell labeling studies demonstrate that erythrocyte life span is markedly shortened to between 6 and 9 days.[76,80] Measurement of erythrocyte creatine, a relatively simple but not yet widely available assay, can be performed in lieu of red cell labeling studies. Young erythrocytes contain much higher levels of creatine than older cells. Thus, an increase in erythrocyte creatine represents shortened red cell survival and is significantly correlated with total peak flow velocity across the valve and the severity of any associated hemolysis.[85] When performed, marrow aspiration will be remarkable for erythroid hyperplasia.[75,80] As a result of hemosiderin deposition, magnetic resonance imaging of the kidneys will reveal reduced signal intensity of the renal cortex compared with the medulla on T1- and T2-weighted images, both with and without gadolinium enhancement.[86]

TABLE 51–2. Severity of Prosthetic Valve Hemolysis			
	Mild	**Moderate**	**Severe**
Hemosider inuria	Present	Present	Marked
Hemoglobinuria	Absent	Absent	Absent
Schistocytosis	<1%	>1%	>>1%
Reticulocytosis	<5%	>5%	>>5%
Haptoglobin	Decreased	Absent	Absent
LDH	<500 U/L	>500 U/L	>>500 U/L

LDH, lactate dehydrogenase.
Data from Eyster E, Rothchild J, Mychajliw O: Chronic intravascular hemolysis after aortic valve replacement, Circulation 1971 Oct;44(4):657-665.

DIFFERENTIAL DIAGNOSIS

Factors that can promote valve-associated hemolysis or worsen the resultant anemia include iron deficiency (Chap. 43), because anemia increases cardiac output and shear stress and iron-poor red cells are more fragile than normal; folate deficiency (Chap. 41) arising from increased erythropoiesis; anemia of chronic disease because of endocarditis; anticoagulant-induced gastrointestinal hemorrhage (Chaps. 37, 133, and 134); and increased cardiac output as a consequence of strenuous physical exertion.[82]

THERAPY

Appropriate therapy for hemolytic anemia arising from valvular dysfunction consists of iron and folate replacement (if deficient) and surgical repair or replacement of the malfunctioning prosthesis (if indicated).[87] Poor surgical candidates with perivalvular leaks may benefit from percutaneous closure with an Amplatzer occluder device.[88] Adjunctive measures to be tried include β-blockade to slow the velocity of the circulation,[89] erythropoietin therapy to stimulate erythropoiesis further,[90] and pentoxifylline therapy to increase the deformability of red cells.[91]

Although some authors have not found the use of pentoxifylline to be beneficial,[92] several case reports have described amelioration of valve-related hemolysis and resultant decreased need for red cell transfusion in patients receiving pentoxifylline.[93–95] A prospective study of 40 individuals with double (mitral and aortic) valve replacements randomized patients to receive either no treatment or pentoxifylline 400 mg orally three times daily for 120 days. The group who received pentoxifylline had significantly higher hemoglobin and haptoglobin levels, and significantly lower LDH, total and indirect bilirubin, and corrected reticulocyte levels, after 4 months of treatment. Of the nine patients with severe hemolysis (LDH >1500 U/L), six individuals had amelioration or complete resolution of their disease, while three patients' hemolysis persisted unchecked, suggesting that pentoxifylline therapy is beneficial in more than 60 percent of those with valve-related hemolysis.[96]

Between 15 and 30 percent of patients will develop black pigment gallstones following valve surgery, the majority occurring within 6 months of the procedure. Whether this is a result of acute hemolysis associated with use of the heart–lung machine[97] or chronic hemolysis because of the valve replacement itself[98,99] is uncertain; however, therapy with ursodeoxycholic acid 600 mg daily beginning 1 week before surgery significantly decreases the incidence of gallstone formation from approximately 29 percent in those who were left untreated to approximately 8 percent (P <0.01).[100]

COURSE AND PROGNOSIS

Evidence of hemolysis can be seen within days[60] or weeks[64,76,80] following valve surgery. If reoperation is required, reported mortality rates range between 0 and 6 percent,[75,101] and hemolytic anemia can occasionally recur.[60,101]

● OTHER CAUSES OF NONIMMUNE HEMOLYSIS

MARCH HEMOGLOBINURIA

In 1881, Fleischer described a German soldier in whom hemoglobinuria was brought on by marching.[102] Although usually reported in young males, no doubt explained by their more frequent participation in severe and prolonged exertion, it can also be seen in women.[103,104] The presenting complaint is passage of dark urine immediately following physical exertion in the upright position, occasionally accompanied by nausea, abdominal cramps, aching in the back or legs, a "stitch in the side," or a burning feeling in the soles of the feet. Physical examination is usually unrevealing, although hepatosplenomegaly and transient jaundice have been rarely reported.[105]

Davidson proved definitively in 1969 that march hemoglobinuria is caused by red cell trauma within the vessels of the soles of the feet, and its severity is influenced by the hardness of the running surface, the distance run, the heaviness of the running's stride, and the protective adequacy of his footwear.[105] In addition, he showed that the condition could be prevented by using padded insoles, a finding later substantiated by other authors.[106,107] Hemoglobinuria has also been seen following other types of trauma in activities as diverse as repetitive slapping of the forehead,[108] karate exercises,[109] basketball followed by congo drum playing,[110] and kendo (a Japanese martial art where heavily padded combatants strike each other repeatedly with bamboo swords).[103]

Because the estimated quantity of blood hemolyzed in an average paroxysm is only 6 to 40 mL, anemia is uncommon and if present is usually mild[105]; however repeated episodes can cause iron deficiency, which may lead to or accentuate anemia (Chap. 43). Morphologic evidence of red cell damage is not seen, although one patient was found to have poikilocytes and occasional "four-leaf clover" cells after exercise.[111] Renal damage is also not commonly seen, but cases of acute tubular necrosis and resultant acute renal insufficiency have been described.[112–115]

KASABACH-MERRITT PHENOMENON

First described in 1940,[116] the Kasabach-Merritt phenomenon is a syndrome that usually develops in early childhood, and is characterized by thrombocytopenia, MAHA, consumptive coagulopathy, and hypofibrinogenemia caused by an enlarging kaposiform hemangioendothelioma or tufted angioma.[117] Kaposiform hemangioendotheliomas are highly aggressive, vascular tumors that occur equally in males and females, and show little tendency to resolve spontaneously. They can be locally invasive but have never been reported to metastasize.[118] Complications can include hemothorax or pericardial effusion.[118,119] It is postulated that endothelial cell abnormalities and vascular stasis lead to activation of platelets and the coagulation cascade within the tumor's vessels, with subsequent depletion of both platelets and clotting factors. Microangiopathic hemolytic anemia results from mechanical trauma sustained by the erythrocytes traversing the tumor's abnormal, partially thrombosed vascular channels.[120]

Although numerous therapies are used, the mortality rate of Kasabach-Merritt phenomenon can be as high as 30 percent.[121] Even though surgical resection is always followed by normalization of hematologic parameters, many lesions are too large to be resected without severe disfigurement. Other treatments include glucocorticoids, interferon-α, antifibrinolytic agents, and the antiplatelet agents ticlopidine and aspirin, low-molecular-weight heparin, embolization, radiation, laser therapy, and chemotherapy using vincristine, cyclophosphamide, actinomycin D, or methotrexate.[117,118,120,122,123]

MISCELLANEOUS

Microangiopathic hemolytic anemia has also been seen in malignant systemic hypertension, pulmonary hypertension, giant cavernous hemangiomas of the liver,[124] and various vasculitides, including Wegener granulomatosis[125,126] and giant cell arteritis.[127] Osmotically induced hemolysis has occurred when distilled water is used as an irrigant during transurethral resection of the prostate.[128]

REFERENCES

1. Stahnke E: Über das Verhalten der Blutplättchen bei Eklampsie. *Zentralbl Gynakol* 46:391, 1922.

2. Pritchard JA, Weisman R Jr, Ratnoff OD, Vosburgh GJ: Intravascular hemolysis, thrombocytopenia and other hematologic abnormalities associated with severe toxemia of pregnancy. *N Engl J Med* 250:89, 1954.

3. Goodlin RC, Cotton DB, Haesslein HC: Severe edema-proteinuria-hypertension gestosis. *Am J Obstet Gynecol* 132:595, 1978.

4. Weinstein L: Syndrome of hemolysis, elevated liver enzymes, and low platelet count: A severe consequence of hypertension in pregnancy. *Am J Obstet Gynecol* 142:159, 1982.

5. Rahman TM, Wendon J: Severe hepatic dysfunction in pregnancy. *Q J Med* 95:343, 2002.

6. Rath W, Faridi A, Dudenhausen JW: HELLP syndrome. *J Perinat Med* 28:249, 2000.

7. Martin JN Jr, Magann EF, Blake PG, et al: Analysis of 454 pregnancies with severe preeclampsia/eclampsia HELLP syndrome using the 3-class system of classification. *Am J Obstet Gynecol* 68:386, 1993.

8. Sibai BM, Ramadan MK, Usta I, et al: Maternal morbidity and mortality in 442 pregnancies with hemolysis, elevated liver enzymes, and low platelets (HELLP syndrome). *Am J Obstet Gynecol* 169:1000, 1993.

9. Zusterzeel PLM, Visser W, Blom HJ, et al: Methylenetetrahydrofolate reductase polymorphisms in preeclampsia and the HELLP syndrome. *Hypertens Pregnancy* 19:299, 2000.

10. Krauss T, Augustin HG, Osmers R, et al: Activated protein C resistance and factor V Leiden in patients with haemolysis, elevated liver enzymes, low platelets syndrome. *Obstet Gynecol* 92:457, 1998.

11. Bozzo M, Carpani G, Leo L, et al: HELLP syndrome and factor V Leiden. *Eur J Obstet Gynecol Reprod Biol* 95:55, 2001.

12. Benedetto C, Marozio L, Salton L, et al: Factor V Leiden and factor II G20210A in preeclampsia and HELLP syndrome. *Acta Obstet Gynecol Scand* 81:1095, 2002.

13. Zhou Y, McMaster M, Woo K, et al: Vascular endothelial growth factor ligands and receptors that regulate human cytotrophoblast survival are dysregulated in severe preeclampsia and hemolysis, elevated liver enzymes, and low platelets syndrome. *Am J Pathol* 160:1405, 2002.

14. Knerr I, Beinder E, Rascher W: Syncytin, a novel human endogenous retroviral gene in human placenta: Evidence for its dysregulation in preeclampsia and HELLP syndrome. *Am J Obstet Gynecol* 186:210, 2002.

15. Levine RJ, Maynard SE, Qian C, et al: Circulating angiogenic factors and the risk of preeclampsia. *N Engl J Med* 350:672, 2004.

16. Widmer M, Villar J, Beniani A, et al: Mapping the theories of preeclampsia and the role of angiogenic factors: A systematic review. *Obstet Gynecol* 109:168, 2007.

17. Mutter WP, Karumanchi SA: Molecular mechanisms of preeclampsia. *Microvasc Res* 75:1, 2008.

18. Kim YN, Lee DS, Jeong DH, et al: The relationship of the level of circulating antiangiogenic factors to the clinical manifestations of preeclampsia. *Prenat Diagn* 29:464, 2009.

19. Magann EF, Martin JN Jr: Twelve steps to optimal management of HELLP syndrome. *Clin Obstet Gynecol* 42:532, 1999.

20. Thiagarajah S, Bourgeois FJ, Harbert GM, Caudle MR: Thrombocytopenia in preeclampsia: Associated abnormalities and management principles. *Am J Obstet Gynecol* 150:1, 1984.

21. Barton JR, Riely CA, Adamed TA, et al: Hepatic histopathologic condition does not correlate with laboratory abnormalities in HELLP syndrome (hemolysis, elevated liver enzymes, and low platelet count). *Am J Obstet Gynecol* 167:1538, 1992.

22. De Boer K, Büller HR, Ten Cate JW, Treffers PE: Coagulation studies in the syndrome of haemolysis, elevated liver enzymes and low platelets. *Br J Obstet Gynaecol* 98:42, 1991.

23. Thorp JM Jr, Gilbert GC II, Moake JL, Bowes WA Jr: von Willebrand factor multimeric levels and patterns in patients with severe preeclampsia. *Obstet Gynecol* 75:163, 1990.

24. Lattuada A, Rossi E, Calzarossa C, et al: Mild to moderate reduction of a von Willebrand factor cleaving protease (ADAMTS13) in pregnant women with HELLP microangiopathic syndrome. *Haematologica* 88:1029, 2003.

25. Molvarec A, Rigo J, Boze T, et al: Increased plasma von Willebrand factor antigen levels but normal von Willebrand factor cleaving protease (ADAMTS13) activity in preeclampsia. *Thromb Haemost* 101:305, 2009.

26. Moake JL: Thrombotic microangiopathies. *N Engl J Med* 347:589, 2002.

27. Thomas EA, Copplestone JA, Dubbins PA, Friend JR: The radiologist cries "HELLP"! *Br J Radiol* 64:964, 1991.

28. Rehberg JF, Briery CM, Hudson WT, et al: Thrombotic thrombocytopenic purpura masquerading as hemolysis, elevated liver enzymes, low platelets (HELLP) syndrome in late pregnancy. *Obstet Gynecol* 108:817, 2006.

29. Fonseca JE, Mendez F, Catano C. Dexamethasone treatment does not improve the outcome of women with HELLP syndrome: A double-blind, placebo-controlled, randomized clinical trial. *Am J Obstet Gynecol* 193:1591, 2005.

30. Burwick RM, Feinberg BB: Eculizumab for the treatment of preeclampsia/HELLP syndrome. *Placenta* 34:201, 2012.

31. Reubinoff BE, Schenker JG: HELLP syndrome—a syndrome of hemolysis, elevated liver enzymes and low platelet count—complicating preeclampsia-eclampsia. *Int J Gynaecol Obstet* 36:95, 1991.

32. Harms K, Rath W, Herting E, Kuhn W: Maternal hemolysis, elevated liver enzymes, low platelet count, and neonatal outcome. *Am J Perinatol* 12:1, 1995.

33. Sullivan CA, Magann EF, Perry KG Jr, et al: The recurrence risk of the syndrome of hemolysis, elevated liver enzymes, and low platelets: Subsequent pregnancy outcome and long term prognosis. *Am J Obstet Gynecol* 172:125, 1995.

34. van Pampus MG, Wolf H, Mayruhu G, et al: Long-term follow-up in patients with a history of (H)ELLP syndrome. *Hypertens Pregnancy* 20:15, 2001.

35. Brain MC, Dacie JV, Hourihane DO: Microangiopathic haemolytic anemia: The possible role of vascular lesions in pathogenesis. *Br J Haematol* 8:358, 1962.

36. Kupers EC, Friedman NB, Lee S, Wolfstein RS: Metastatic hemangiopericytoma associated with microangiopathic hemolytic anemia: Review and report of a case. *J Am Geriatr Soc* 23:411, 1975.

37. Antman KH, Skarin AT, Mayer RJ, et al: Microangiopathic hemolytic anemia and cancer: A review. *Medicine (Baltimore)* 58:377, 1979.

38. Lohrmann H-P, Adam W, Heymer B, Kubanek B: Microangiopathic hemolytic anemia in metastatic carcinoma. Report of eight cases. *Ann Intern Med* 79:368, 1973.

39. Gordon SG, Cross BA: A factor X-activating cysteine protease from malignant tissue. *J Clin Invest* 67:1665, 1981.

40. Wahrenbrock M, Borsig L, Le D, et al: Selectin-mucin interactions as a probable molecular explanation for the association of Trousseau syndrome with mucinous adenocarcinomas. *J Clin Invest* 112:853, 2003.

41. Lynch EC, Bakken CL, Casey TH, Alfrey CP Jr: Microangiopathic hemolytic anemia in carcinoma of the stomach. *Gastroenterology* 52:88, 1967.

42. Moake JL: Disseminated intravascular coagulation, in *Conn's Current Therapy*, edited by Rakel RE, p 338. WB Saunders, Philadelphia, 1989.

43. Reddy NM, Hall SW, MacKintosh R: Partial thromboplastin time: Prediction of adverse events and poor prognosis by low abnormal values. *Arch Intern Med* 159:2706, 1999.

44. Tripodi A, Chantarangkul V, Martinelli I, et al: A shortened activated partial thromboplastin time is associated with the risk of venous thromboembolism. *Blood* 104:3631, 2004.

45. Lippi G, Favaloro EJ: Activated partial thromboplastin time: New tricks for an old dogma. *Semin Thromb Hemost* 34:604, 2008.

46. Oleksowicz L, Bhagwati N, DeLeon-Fernandez M: Deficient activity of von Willebrand's factor-cleaving protease in patients with disseminated malignancies. *Cancer Res* 59:2244, 1999.

47. Fontana S, Gerritsen HE, Hovinga JK, et al: Microangiopathic haemolytic anaemia in metastasizing malignant tumours is not associated with a severe deficiency of the von Willebrand factor-cleaving protease. *Br J Haematol* 113:100, 2001.

48. Hyun J, Kim HK, Kim JE, et al: Correlation between plasma activity of ADAMTS13 and coagulopathy, and prognosis in disseminated intravascular coagulation. *Thromb Res* 124:75, 2009.

49. Bernardo A, Ball C, Nolasco L, et al: Effects of inflammatory cytokines on the release and cleavage of the endothelial cell-derived ultra-large von Willebrand factor multimers under flow. *Blood* 104:100, 2004.

50. Blake-Haskins JA, Lechleider RJ, Kreitman RJ: Thrombotic microangiopathy with targeted cancer agents. *Clin Cancer Res* 17:5858, 2011.

51. Kayatani H, Matsuo K, Ueda Y, et al: Pulmonary tumor thrombotic microangiopathy diagnosed antemortem and treated with combination chemotherapy. *Intern Med* 51:2767, 2012.

58. Ellis LD, Westerman MP: Autoimmune hemolytic anemia and cancer. *JAMA* 193:962, 1965.

59. Rose JC, Hufnagel CA, Fries ED, et al: The hemodynamic alterations produced by plastic valvular prosthesis for severe aortic insufficiency in man. *J Clin Invest* 33:891, 1954.

60. Rodgers BM, Sabiston DC Jr: Hemolytic anemia following prosthetic valve replacement. *Circulation* 39:155, 1969.

61. Marsh GW, Lewis SM: Cardiac haemolytic anaemia. *Semin Hematol* 6:133, 1969.

62. Kloster FE: Diagnosis and management of complications of prosthetic heart valves. *Am J Cardiol* 35:872, 1975.

63. Iguro Y, Moriyama Y, Yamaoka A, et al: Clinical experience of 473 patients with the Omnicarbon prosthetic heart valve. *J Heart Valve Dis* 8:674, 1999.

64. Eyster E, Rothchild J, Mychajliw O: Chronic intravascular hemolysis after aortic valve replacement. *Circulation* 44:657, 1971.

65. Crexells C, Aerichide N, Bonny Y, et al: Factors influencing hemolysis in valve prosthesis. *Am Heart J* 84:161, 1972.

66. Demirsoy E, Yilmaz O, Sirin G, et al: Hemolysis after mitral valve repair; a report of five cases and literature review. *J Heart Valve Dis* 17:24, 2008.

67. Kubo T, Kitaoka H, Terauchi Y, et al: Hemolytic anemia in a patient with hypertrophic obstructive cardiomyopathy. *J Cardiol* 55:125, 2010.

68. Garcia MJ, Vandervoort P, Stewart WJ, et al: Mechanisms of hemolysis with mitral prosthetic regurgitation. *J Am Coll Cardiol* 27:399, 1996.

69. Skoularigis J, Essop MR, Skudicky D, et al: Frequency and severity of intravascular hemolysis after left-sided cardiac valve replacement with Medtronic Hall and St. Jude Medical prostheses, and influence of prosthetic type, position, size and number. *Am J Cardiol* 71:587, 1993.

70. Chang H, Lin FY, Hung CR, Chu SH: Chronic intravascular hemolysis after valvular surgery. *J Formos Med Assoc* 89:880, 1990.

71. Yacoub MH, Keeling DH: Chronic haemolysis following insertion of ball valve prostheses. *Br Heart J* 30:676, 1968.

72. Falk RH, Mackinnon J, Wainscoat J, et al: Intravascular haemolysis after valve replacement: Comparative study between Starr-Edwards (ball valve) and Bjork-Shiley (disc valve) prosthesis. *Thorax* 34:746, 1979.

73. Febres-Roman PR, Bourg WC, Crone RA, et al: Chronic intravascular hemolysis after aortic valve replacement with Ionescu-Shiley xenograft: Comparative study with Bjork-Shiley prosthesis. *Am J Cardiol* 46:735, 1980.

74. Nevaril CG, Lynch EC, Alfrey CP, et al: Erythrocyte damage and destruction induced by shearing stress. *J Lab Clin Med* 71:784, 1968.

75. Cerfolio RJ, Orszulak TA, Daly RC, Schaff HV: Reoperation for hemolytic anaemia complicating mitral valve repair. *Eur J Cardiothorac Surg* 11:479, 1997.

76. Sayed HM, Dacie JV, Handley DA, et al: Haemolytic anaemia of mechanical origin after open heart surgery. *Thorax* 16:356, 1961.

77. Leverett LB, Hellums JD, Alfrey CP, Lynch EC: Red blood cell damage by shear stress. *Biophys J* 12:257, 1972.

78. Murakami M, Tanaka H, Watanabe M, et al: Severe hemolysis due to cloth wear 23 years after aortic valve replacement on a Starr-Edwards ball valve model 2320. *Cardiovasc Surg* 10:284, 2002.

79. Ryerson LM, Wechsler SB, Ohye RG: Hemolytic anemia secondary to modified Blalock-Taussig shunt. *Pediatr Cardiol* 28:238, 2007.

80. Sears DA, Crosby WH: Intravascular hemolysis due to intracardiac prosthetic devices. *Am J Med* 39:341, 1965.

81. Papadogiannakis A, Xydakis D, Sfakianaki M, et al: An unusual cause of severe hyperkalemia in a dialysis patient. *J Cardiovasc Med (Hagerstown)* 8:541, 2007.

82. Pu JJ, Brodsky RA: Paroxysmal nocturnal hemoglobinuria from bench to bedside. *Clin Transl Sci* 4:219, 2011.

83. Myhre E, Rasmussen K, Andersen A: Serum lactic dehydrogenase activity in patients with prosthetic heart valves: A parameter of intravascular hemolysis. *Am Heart J* 80:463, 1970.

84. Thompson ME, Lewis JH, Prokolab FL, et al: Indexes of intravascular hemolysis quantification of coagulation factors, and platelet survival in patients with porcine heterograft valves. *Am J Cardiol* 51:489, 1983.

85. Okumiya T, Ishikawa-Nishi M, Doi T, et al: Evaluation of intravascular hemolysis with erythrocyte creatine in patients with cardiac valve prostheses. *Chest* 125:2115, 2004.

86. Lee JW, Kim SH, Yoon CJ: Hemosiderin deposition on the renal cortex by mechanical hemolysis due to malfunctioning prosthetic cardiac valve: Report of MR findings in two cases. *J Comput Assist Tomogr* 23:445, 1999.

87. Amidon TM, Chou TM, Rankin JS, Ports TA: Mitral and aortic paravalvular leaks with hemolytic anemia. *Am Heart J* 125:122, 1993.

88. Shapira Y, Hirsch R, Kornowski R, et al: Percutaneous closure of perivalvular leaks with Amplatzer occluders: Feasibility, safety, and short-term results. *J Heart Valve Dis* 16:305, 2007.

89. Okita Y, Miki S, Kusuhara K, et al: Propranolol for intractable hemolysis after open heart operation. *Ann Thorac Surg* 52:1158, 1991.

90. Shapira Y, Bairey O, Vatury M, et al: Erythropoietin can obviate the need for repeated heart valve replacement in high-risk patients with severe mechanical hemolytic anemia: Case reports and literature review. *J Heart Valve Dis* 10:431, 2001.

91. Ward A, Clissold SP: Pentoxifylline: A review of its pharmacodynamic and pharmacokinetic properties, and its therapeutic efficacy. *Drugs* 34:50, 1987.

92. Okita Y, Miki S: Reply to the editor. *Ann Thorac Surg* 54:7, 1992.

93. Jim RT: New therapy for cardiac valve prosthesis caused by microangiopathic hemolytic anemia: A case report. *Hawaii Med J* 47:285, 1988.

94. Golino A, Stassano P, Spampinato N: Hemolysis after open heart operations [letter]. *Ann Thorac Surg* 54:1246, 1992.

95. Geller S, Gelber R: Pentoxifylline treatment for microangiopathic hemolytic anemia caused by mechanical heart valves. *Md Med J* 48:173, 1999.

96. Golbasi I, Turkay C, Timuragaoglu A, et al: The effect of pentoxifylline on haemolysis in patients with double cardiac prosthetic valves. *Acta Cardiol* 58:379, 2003.

97. Azemoto R, Tsuchiya Y, Ai T, et al: Does gallstone formation after open cardiac surgery result only from latent hemolysis by replaced valves? *Am J Gastroenterol* 91:2185, 1996.

98. Merendino KA. Manhas DR: Man-made gallstones: A new entity following cardiac valve replacement. *Ann Surg* 177:694, 1973.

99. Harrison EC, Roschke EJ, Meyers HI, et al: Cholelithiasis: A frequent complication of artificial heart valve replacement. *Am Heart J* 95:483, 1978.

100. Ai T, Azemoto R, Saisho H: Prevention of gallstones by ursodeoxycholic acid after cardiac surgery. *J Gastroenterol* 38:1071, 2003.

101. Lam BK, Cosgrove DM, Bhudia SK, Gillinov AM: Hemolysis after mitral valve repair: Mechanisms and treatment. *Ann Thorac Surg* 77:191, 2004.

102. Fleischer R: Ueber eine neue Form von Haemoglobinurie beim Menschen. *Berl Klin Wschr* 18:691, 1881.

103. Urabe M, Hara Y, Hokama A, et al: A female case of march hemoglobinuria induced by kendo (Japanese fencing) exercise. *Nippon Naika Gakkai Zasshi* 75:1657, 1986.

104. Gilligan A: March hemoglobinuria in a woman. *N Engl J Med* 243:944, 1950.

105. Davidson RJL: March or exertional haemoglobinuria. *Semin Hematol* 6:150, 1969.

106. Buckle RM: Exertional (march) haemoglobinuria: Reduction of haemolytic episodes by use of Sorbo-rubber insoles in shoes. *Lancet* 68:1136, 1965.

107. Sagov SE: March hemoglobinuria treated with rubber insoles: Two case reports. *J Am Coll Health Assoc* 19:146, 1970.

108. Ensor CW, Barrett JOW: Paroxysmal haemoglobinuria of traumatic origin. *Med Chir Trans* 86:165, 1903.

109. Streeton JA: Traumatic haemoglobinuria caused by karate exercises. *Lancet* 2:191, 1967.

110. Schwartz KA, Flessa HC: March hemoglobinuria. Report of a case after basketball and congo drum playing. *Ohio State Med J* 69:448, 1973.

111. Watson EM, Fischer LC: Paroxysmal "march" haemoglobinuria with a report of a case. *Am J Clin Pathol* 5:151, 1935.

112. Pollard TD, Weiss IW: Acute tubular necrosis in a patient with march hemoglobinuria. *N Engl J Med* 283:803, 1970.

113. Susa S, Dumovic B, Pantovic R: March hemoglobinuria associated with acute renal failure. *Vojnosanit Pregl* 29:44, 1972.

114. Ciko Z, Radojicic B, Lazic D: Pathogenesis of acute renal insufficiency in march hemoglobinuria. *Vojnosanit Pregl* 30:198, 1973.

115. Yashpal M, Abdulkader TA, Chatterji JC: Acute tubular necrosis in march haemoglobinuria. *J Assoc Physicians India* 28:145, 1980.

116. Kasabach HH, Merritt KK: Capillary hemangioma with extensive purpura: Report of a case. *Am J Dis Child* 59:1063, 1940.

117. Haisley-Royster C, Enjolras O, Frieden IJ, et al: Kasabach-Merritt phenomenon: A retrospective study of treatment with vincristine. *J Pediatr Hematol Oncol* 24:459, 2002.

118. San Miguel FL, Spurbeck W, Budding C, Horton J: Kaposiform hemangioendothelioma: A rare cause of spontaneous hemothorax in infancy. Review of the literature. *J Pediatr Surg* 43:E37, 2008.

119. Walsh MA, Carcao M, Pope E, Lee K-J: Kaposiform hemangioendothelioma presenting antenatally with a pericardial effusion. *J Pediatr Hematol Oncol* 30:761, 2008.

120. Ortel TL, Onorato JJ, Bedrosian CL, Kaufman RE: Antifibrinolytic therapy in the management of the Kasabach-Merritt syndrome. *Am J Hematol* 29:44, 1988.

121. Esterly NB: Kasabach-Merritt syndrome in infants. *J Am Acad Dermatol* 8:504, 1983.

122. Hall GW: Kasabach-Merritt syndrome: Pathogenesis and management. *Br J Haematol* 112:851, 2001.

123. Hauer J, Graubner U, Konstantopoulos N, et al: Effective treatment of kaposiform hemangioendotheliomas associated with Kasabach-Merritt phenomenon using four-drug regimen. *Pediatr Blood Cancer* 49:852, 2006.

124. Shimizu M, Miura J, Itoh H, Saitoh Y: Hepatic giant cavernous hemangioma with microangiopathic hemolytic anemia and consumption coagulopathy. *Am J Gastroenterol* 85:1411, 1990.

125. Crummy CS, Perlin E, Moquin RB: Microangiopathic hemolytic anemia in Wegener's granulomatosis. *Am J Med* 51:544, 1971.

126. Jordan JM, Manning M, Allen NB: Multiple unusual manifestations of Wegener's granulomatosis: Breast mass, microangiopathic hemolytic anemia, consumptive coagulopathy, and low erythrocyte sedimentation rate. *Arthritis Rheum* 29:1527, 1986.

127. Zauber NP, Echikson AB: Giant cell arteritis and microangiopathic hemolytic anemia. *Am J Med* 73:928, 1982.

128. Chen SS, Lin AT, Chen KK, Chang LS: Hemolysis in transurethral resection of the prostate using distilled water as the irrigant. *J Chin Med Assoc* 69:270, 2006.

129. Stratford EC, Tanaka KR: Microangiopathic hemolytic anemia in metastatic carcinoma. Report of a case and biochemical studies. *Arch Intern Med* 116:346, 1965.

130. Davis S, Rambotti P, Grignani F, Steinhouse K: Microangiopathic hemolytic anemia and pulmonary small-cell carcinoma [letter]. *Ann Intern Med* 103:638, 1985.

131. Atkins JN, Muss HB: Case report: Schistocytes in erythroleukemia. *Am J Med Sci* 289:110, 1985.

CHAPTER 52
ERYTHROCYTE DISORDERS AS A RESULT OF CHEMICAL AND PHYSICAL AGENTS

Paul C. Herrmann

SUMMARY

Erythrocyte disorders from physical or chemical agents occur via such processes as red cell volume expansion within hypotonic solutions, erythrocyte membrane damage from biotoxins, damage to the spectrin skeleton from insults such as heat, and eryptosis associated with oxidizing agents such as oxygen, arsine gas, and chlorates. Erythrocyte damage also can be induced by other agents that lack well defined mechanisms of action (see Table 52–1). These processes include erythrocyte damage caused by lead, copper, and radiation, as well as neocytolysis, a phenomenon once thought unique to microgravity, but subsequently observed in individuals demonstrating altitude induced polycythemia upon transition to normoxic conditions.

● MECHANISTICALLY DESCRIBED ERYTHROCYTE DAMAGE

Chemical and physical agents causing erythrocyte disorders within the context of enzyme deficiency, unstable hemoglobins, cell fragmentation or immune dysfunction are discussed in Chaps. 46 to 51 and 54. The present chapter deals with drugs, toxins, and other physical agents that can cause red cell disorders, which are not discussed elsewhere within this text.

ERYTHROCYTE VOLUME EXPANSION AND HYPOTONIC LYSIS

When large amounts of distilled water gain access to the systemic circulation, either by intravenous injection or when used as an irrigating solution during surgery, hemolysis will occur.[1] Severe hemolysis may also result from water inhalation in near-drowning.[2] Occasionally self-induced hypotonic lysis secondary to water intoxication from polydipsia in the setting of psychiatric illness or hazing rituals occurs.[3] In all cases, hemolysis follows expansion of the erythrocyte volume, transition to a spherical shape and ultimately cell rupture.[4]

DAMAGE TO THE RED BLOOD CELL MEMBRANE

Bee[5,6] and wasp[7–9] stings, as well as contact with caterpillar bristle from *Lonomia obliqua*,[10] are associated with severe hemolysis. In addition,

Abbreviations and Acronyms: AsH₃, arsenic hydride (arsine gas); EDTA, ethylenediaminetetraacetic acid; G6PD, glucose-6-phosphate dehydrogenase; NADPH, reduced nicotinamide adenine dinucleotide phosphate.

spider and scorpion bites occasionally are followed by hemolytic anemia and hemoglobinuria.[11–16] The spiders usually responsible are *Loxosceles laeta* and *Loxosceles recluse*. In such cases, sphingomyelinase D is one of the causative toxins. The venom preferentially hydrolyzes band 3 of the red cell membrane protein.[17] Band 3 has dual functions of ion exchange and anchoring of the cell membrane to the underlying cellular skeleton.[18] It appears disruption of the structural role is responsible for cell lysis.

One of the most intriguing mechanisms of membrane damage is that induced by a class of pore-forming cytotoxins, usually from *Bacillus cereus*.[19] Toxins using similar mechanisms of hemolysis are found in marine organisms including jelly fish (*Chironex fleckeri*),[20] sea cucumbers (*Cucumaria echinata*),[21] and sea anemones (*Stichodactyla helianthus*).[22] X-ray crystallography reveals these toxins to be composed of proteins that associate to span the erythrocyte membrane forming an ion permeable pore.[21] Aged cells appear preferentially damaged.

Additional discussion of hemolysis associated with microorganism-produced toxins, including *Clostridium*-induced spherocytosis and massive hemolysis, is found in Chap. 53.

DAMAGE TO SKELETAL OR STRUCTURAL PROTEINS

Gross hemoglobinemia was observed in 11 of 40 patients with second- and third-degree burns involving 15 to 65 percent of body surface area.[23] Within the first 24 hours following a burn, hemolytic anemia results from the direct effect of heat on circulating erythrocytes. Blood heated to temperatures above 49°C demonstrates morphologically similar damage (Fig. 52–1A), consistent with increased osmotic and mechanical fragility.[24,25]

In addition to acute damage, heat decreases erythrocyte resilience. A normal erythrocyte in liquid behaves physically as a drop of fluid because the flexible membrane allows the surface of the cell to rotate around the intracellular contents.[26] These fluid-like properties couple collisional energy between the erythrocyte membrane and the viscous hemoglobin solution within the cell, allowing dissipation of collisional energy through the entire cell and ultimately protecting the cell membrane. When heated, the spectrin comprising the erythrocyte skeleton melts, and upon cooling becomes rigid. This rigidity prevents collisional energy dissipation, making such cells particularly susceptible to membrane damage.[27] The ensuing damage to the erythrocyte membrane structure results in splenic sequestration and cell removal.[28]

OXIDANT DAMAGE

Although oxygen is a powerful oxidizing agent, quantum mechanical properties of the oxygen molecule prevent spontaneous oxidation of biologic membranes.[29] When bound to hemoglobin, oxygen has significantly different quantum mechanical properties and occasionally, an exceptionally reactive superoxide molecule escapes.[30] It is estimated that 2 to 3 percent of total hemoglobin would be oxidized daily in the absence of enzyme systems to protect against escaped superoxide.[31,32] Although the hemolysis that occurs when these systems are overwhelmed is dealt with in Chap. 47, a few additional examples are briefly described below. Hemolysis following oxidation is thought to occur via eryptosis (Chap. 33). In addition to oxidative stress, osmotic shock and certain toxic ions, including gold and aluminum, may act through eryptosis.[33,34]

Oxygen Gas and Ozone

Hemolytic anemia can occur when ambient oxygen (O_2) concentration is increased markedly.[35] Hyperbaric oxygenation has been associated with acute hemolysis.[36] Ozone (O_3), which has been widely used in

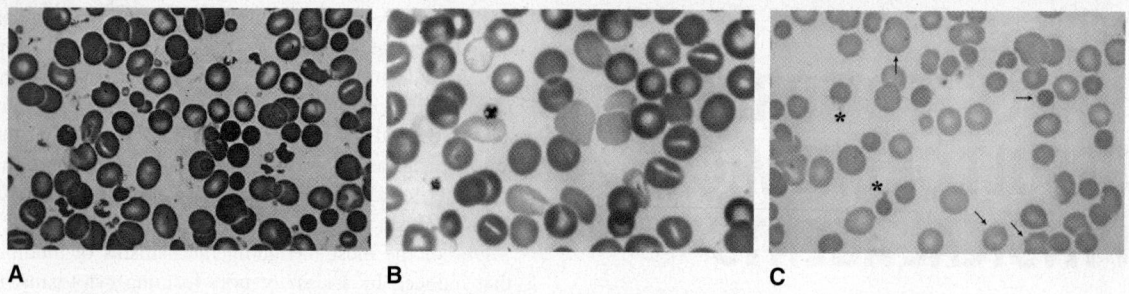

Figure 52–1. A. Blood film prepared at admission from a patient who had suffered severe burn injury involving a large percentage of the body surface. Note the presence of normal erythrocytes (apparently from vessels not exposed to heat damage) along with populations of normocytic and microcytic spherocytes. In addition, there are numerous red cell fragments, some smaller than platelets. **B.** Blood film prepared from a patient exposed to arsenic hydride. Note the very pale red cells resulting from partial hemoglobin loss secondary to membrane damage. An extreme example, represented by the virtual ghost thinly rimmed with scant residual hemoglobin, can be found in the upper left-hand corner. **C.** Wilson disease. In this image from a patient with Wilson disease, there are numerous visible sequelae of oxidative damage caused by excess copper. The striking microspherocytosis indicates damage to the membrane. Damage to hemoglobin is demonstrated by the Heinz bodies projecting from red cells (*asterisks* show two examples). The *horizontal arrow* points to one of several spherocytes. The *vertical arrow* points to a macrocyte (reticulocyte). An occasional cell shows damage to both membrane and hemoglobin. The presence of echinocytes (*oblique arrows* show two examples) suggests that the liver is also affected. *(A & B, reproduced with permission from* Lichtman's Atlas of Hematology, www.accessmedicine.com. *C, used with permission of Barbara J. Bain, Imperial College, London, UK.)*

some countries for a variety of therapeutic purposes, had no apparent effect *in vivo* on red cell enzymes and intermediates at the 30 mcg/mL concentration commonly infused, but did produce some *in vitro* hemolysis at that concentration.[37]

Arsenic Hydride

Arsenic exposure is a major cause of anemia in regions with high environmental concentration. Examples include Bangladesh's tainted water supply, and areas of China where arsenic laden coal is used.[38] Arsine gas (arsenic hydride, AsH_3) is the most erythrotoxic form of arsenic and inhalation of arsine gas is a well-recognized cause of hemolytic anemia (see Fig. 52–1B).[39–41] Arsine is formed during many industrial processes, including the reaction of hydrogen with available arsenic compounds in metallurgic processes. The arsenic is usually a contaminant, so contact with arsenic compounds may not be apparent from the patient's history. The mechanism of erythrocyte damage occurs via oxidation of sulfhydryl groups in the erythrocyte membrane and associated cytoskeleton,[42,43] and decreased levels of reduced glutathione in erythrocytes exposed to AsH_3 are observed.[44]

Chlorates and Chloramines

Sodium and potassium chlorate are oxidative drugs that produce methemoglobinemia, Heinz bodies, and hemolytic anemia.[45] Although it has been presumed that the mechanism of hemolysis is similar to that resulting from other oxidative drugs, enigmatically, no cases have been observed in patients deficient in glucose-6-phosphate dehydrogenase (G6PD). Hemolytic anemia with Heinz body formation has also occurred in patients undergoing dialysis when the water contained a substantial amount of chloramines. Oxidative damage to the red cells of these patients was demonstrated by the presence of Heinz bodies, a positive ascorbate-cyanide test, and methemoglobinemia.[46,47]

Formaldehyde

Leaching of formaldehyde from plastic used in water filters employed for hemodialysis is also a cause of hemolytic anemia. The low level of formaldehyde in the contaminated water does not result in a fixative effect, but instead induces metabolic changes within the red cells.[48]

● CHEMICAL AND PHYSICAL AGENTS NOT DEFINITIVELY DESCRIBED MECHANISTICALLY

A variety of chemical and physical agents cause erythrocyte disorders through unknown or not well-characterized mechanisms. There are isolated reports of hemolytic anemia occurring after the administration of a variety of chemical substances, some of which are listed in Table 52–1. What follows is a collection of miscellaneous erythrocyte damaging agents and processes for which the mechanisms are still largely undefined or disputed.

NEOCYTOLYSIS

Astronauts experience significant anemia after space flight even in the presence of normal or elevated ambient oxygen concentration.[35] The

TABLE 52–1. Drugs and Chemicals That Have Been Reported to Cause Hemolytic Anemia Secondary to Erythrocyte Damage

Chemicals	Drugs
Aniline[86]	Amyl nitrite[94]
Apiol[87]	Mephenesin[95]
Dichlorprop (herbicide)[88]	Methylene blue[96]
Formaldehyde[48]	Omeprazole[97]
Hydroxylamines[89]	Pentachlorophenol[98]
Lysol[90]	Phenazopyridine (Pyridium)[99]
Mineral spirits[91]	Salicylazosulfapyridine (Azulfidine)[100]
Nitrobenzene[92]	Tacrolimus[101]
Resorcin[93]	

mechanism of this anemia remains elusive with intriguing observations of altered erythropoietin levels and radiolabeling studies of astronaut erythrocytes suggesting selective hemolysis of young erythrocytes less than 12 days old.[49] In addition to space flight, neocytolysis has been invoked to explain the anemia resulting when high-altitude dwellers relocate to sea level.[50]

LEAD

Lead poisoning (plumbism) has been recognized since antiquity. The ingestion of beverages containing lead leached from highly soluble lead based glazes or earthenware containers has been blamed for the decline and fall of the Roman aristocracy and is still an occasional cause of lead intoxication.[51] The distillation of alcohol in leaded flasks is another rare cause of plumbism, although the practice was prohibited in 1723 by the Massachusetts Bay Colony after it was noticed that consumption of rum so distilled resulted in abdominal pain known as the "dry gripes."[51] Among the earliest published descriptions of lead poisoning is a letter written in 1786 by Benjamin Franklin.[52]

Lead intoxication in children generally results from ingestion of flaking lead paint or chewing lead-painted articles. Lead poisoning tends to be more severe in iron-deficient children, as a relatively close relationship exists between blood lead levels and hematocrit.[53] In adults, lead poisoning primarily occurs as the result of inhalation of lead compounds from industrial processes such as battery manufacture,[54,55] or ingestion of food having leached lead from pottery or dishes.[56,57] Lead poisoning from restoring tapestries and producing ceramics also has been noted.[58,59]

Generally, the erythrocyte disorder associated with lead intoxication *in vivo* is thought to be a result of interference with normal production of erythrocytes. There is direct evidence that lead inhibits red blood cell (RBC) 5′ nucleotidase and results in basophilic stippling and hemolysis indistinguishable from the morphologic changes observed with inherited deficiency of this enzyme. The other lead-poisoning–associated morphologic changes are observed when chronic lead exposure is associated with sideroblastic anemia, but are not observed in acute lead poisoning.[60,61] In addition, modest shortening of red cell life span is a relatively constant feature of lead intoxication.[62,63] The literature describes a number of tantalizing observations and proposed mechanisms. For instance, *in vitro* treatment of red cells with lead produces membrane damage and inhibition of activity of the hexose monophosphate shunt.[64] Lead interferes with the erythrocyte cation pump,[65,66] possibly by inhibiting membrane adenosine triphosphatase.[67,68] Free radical and Fenton type chemistry around the iron atoms of hemoglobin have also been described.[69]

Microscopic examination of the blood provides the key diagnostic clue to lead poisoning. Complete observations of the acute hematologic changes, including erythrocyte distortion, occurring after the intravenous injection of lead in an attempt to treat malignant disease were first published in 1928.[70] Lead induces normocytic and slightly hypochromic erythrocytes, with the hypochromia possibly resulting from coexisting iron deficiency.[71] Basophilic stippling of the erythrocytes may be fine or coarse, and the number of granules seen in each cell may be quite variable. Blood collected in heparin may most reliably demonstrate basophilic stippling, as storage of red blood cells in ethylenediaminetetraacetic acid (EDTA) is associated with the disappearance of stippling.[72] Young polychromatophilic cells are most likely to be stippled. Electron microscopic studies have demonstrated that the basophilic granules represent abnormally aggregated ribosomes.[73] Ringed sideroblasts are frequently found in the marrow (Chaps. 32 and 59). Iron-laden mitochondria are present, but do not appear to contribute to the basophilic stippling that is observed on light microscopy.[73]

COPPER

Erythrocyte damage has resulted from ingestion of copper sulfate in suicide attempts and from copper accumulation when hemodialysis fluid is contaminated by copper pipes.[74,75] Hemolysis in Wilson disease has been attributed to the elevated plasma copper levels characteristic of that disorder.[76–78] Spherocytic anemia with a hematocrit below 25 percent may be the presenting symptom (see Fig. 52–1C).[79] The pathogenesis may be related to oxidation of intracellular glutathione, hemoglobin, and the reduced nicotinamide adenine dinucleotide phosphate (NADPH), along with inhibition of G6PD by copper.[80] However, the amount of copper required to inhibit G6PD is large. Copper in much lower concentrations inhibits pyruvate kinase, hexokinase, phosphogluconate dehydrogenase, phosphofructokinase, and phosphoglycerate kinase, suggesting a global metabolic insult.[81,82] Plasma exchange successfully prevents hemolytic anemia in Wilson disease.[83]

RADIATION

Although decreased red cell survival is part of the complex series of events occurring after administration of large doses of total body radiation, erythrocytes appear to be very resistant to the direct effects of radiation.[84,85] Shortened red cell survival after radiation is likely related to red cell loss through internal bleeding and various secondary events such as infection.

REFERENCES

1. Landsteiner EK, Finch CA: Hemoglobinemia accompanying transurethral resection of the prostate. *N Engl J Med* 237:310, 1947.
2. Rath CE: Drowning hemoglobinuria. *Blood* 8:1099, 1953.
3. Farrell DJ, Bower L: Fatal water intoxication. *J Clin Pathol* 56:803, 2003.
4. Delano MD: Simple physical constraints in hemolysis. *J Theor Biol* 175:517, 1995.
5. Bresolin NL, Carvalho LC, Goes EC, et al: Acute renal failure following massive attack by Africanized bee stings. *Pediatr Nephrol* 17:625, 2002.
6. Dacie JV: *The Haemolytic Anaemias: Congenital and Acquired*, 2d ed. Grune & Stratton, New York, 1960.
7. Monzon C, Miles J: Hemolytic-anemia following a wasp sting. *J Pediatr* 96:1039, 1980.
8. Schulte KL, Kochen MM: Hemolytic-anemia in an adult after a wasp sting. *Lancet* 2:478, 1981.
9. Vachvanichsanong P, Dissaneewate P, Mitarnun W: Non-fatal acute renal failure due to wasp stings in children. *Pediatr Nephrol* 11:734, 1997.
10. Seibert CS, Santoro ML, Tambourgi DV, et al: *Lonomia obliqua* (Lepidoptera, Saturniidae) caterpillar bristle extract induces direct lysis by cleaving erythrocyte membrane glycoproteins. *Toxicon* 55:1323, 2010.
11. Barretto OC, Cardoso JL, Decillo D: Viscerocutaneous form of loxoscelism and erythrocyte glucose-6-phosphate deficiency. *Rev Inst Med Trop Sao Paulo* 27:264, 1985.
12. Chadha JS, Leviav A: Hemolysis, renal-failure, and local necrosis following scorpion sting. *JAMA* 241:1038, 1979.
13. Madrigal GC, Wenzl JE, Ercolani RL: Toxicity from a bite of brown spider (*Loxosceles reclusus*)—Skin necrosis, hemolytic anemia, and hemoglobinuria in a 9-year-old child. *Clin Pediatr (Phila)* 11:641, 1972.
14. Nance WE: Hemolytic anemia of necrotic arachnidism. *Am J Med* 31:801, 1961.
15. Wasserman GS, Siegel C: Loxoscelism (brown recluse spider bites)—Review of the literature. *Clin Toxicol* 14:353, 1979.
16. Wright SW, Wrenn KD, Murray L, Seger D: Clinical presentation and outcome of brown recluse spider bite. *Ann Emerg Med* 30:28, 1997.
17. Barretto OC, Satake M, Nonoyama K, Cardoso JL: The calcium-dependent protease of *Loxosceles* gaucho venom acts preferentially upon red cell band 3 transmembrane protein. *Braz J Biol Res* 36:309, 2003.
18. Tanner MJ: The structure and function of band 3 (AE1): Recent developments (review). *Mol Membr Biol* 14:155, 1997.
19. Fagerlund A, Lindback T, Storset AK, et al: *Bacillus cereus* Nhe is a pore-forming toxin with structural and functional properties similar to the ClyA (HlyE, SheA) family of haemolysins, able to induce osmotic lysis in epithelia. *Microbiology* 154:693, 2008.
20. Brinkman DL, Konstantakopoulos N, McInerney BV, et al: Chironex fleckeri (box jellyfish) venom proteins: Expansion of a cnidarian toxin family that elicits variable cytolytic and cardiovascular effects. *J Biol Chem* 289:4798, 2014.
21. Uchida T, Yamasaki T, Eto S, et al: Crystal structure of the hemolytic lectin CEL-III isolated from the marine invertebrate *Cucumaria echinata*: Implications of domain structure for its membrane pore-formation mechanism. *J Biol Chem* 279:37133, 2004.

22. Celedon G, Gonzalez G, Barrientos D, et al: Stycholysin II, a cytolysin from the sea anemone *Stichodactyla helianthus* promotes higher hemolysis in aged red blood cells. *Toxicon* 51:1383, 2008.

23. Shen SC, Ham TH, Fleming EM: Studies on the destruction of red blood cells. III. Mechanism and complications of hemoglobinuria in patients with thermal burns: Spherocytosis and increased osmotic fragility of red blood cells. *N Engl J Med* 229:701, 1943.

24. Zarkowsky HS, Mohandas N, Speaker CB, Shohet SB: A congenital haemolytic-anemia with thermal sensitivity of the erythrocyte membrane. *Br J Haematol* 29:537, 1975.

25. Prchal JT, Castleberry RP, Parmley RT, et al: Hereditary pyropoikilocytosis and ellipto-cytosis: Clinical, laboratory, and ultrastructural features in infants and children. *Pediatr Res* 16:484, 1982.

26. Schmid-Schonbein H, Wells R: Fluid drop-like transition of erythrocytes under shear. *Science* 165:288, 1969.

27. Bull BS, Brailsford JD: Red-cell membrane deformability—New data. *Blood* 48:663, 1976.

28. Wagner HN, Gaertner RA, Feagin OT, et al: Removal of erythrocytes from circulation. *Arch Intern Med* 110:90, 1962.

29. Taube H: Mechanisms of oxidation with oxygen. *J Gen Physiol* 49:29, 1965.

30. Collman JP, Hermann PC, Fu L, et al: Aza-crown capped porphyrin models of myoglo-bin: Studies of the steric interactions of gas binding. *J Am Chem Soc* 119:3481, 1997.

31. Harris JW, Kellermeyer RW: *The Red Cell: Production, Metabolism, Destruction: Normal and Abnormal*, rev. ed. Harvard University Press, Cambridge, MA, 1970.

32. Bunn HF, Forget BG: *Hemoglobin—Molecular, Genetic, and Clinical Aspects*. WB Saunders, Philadelphia, 1986.

33. Niemoeller OM, Kiedaisch V, Dreischer P, et al: Stimulation of eryptosis by aluminium ions. *Toxicol Appl Pharmacol* 217:168, 2006.

34. Sopjani M, Foller M, Lang F: Gold stimulates Ca^{2+} entry into and subsequent suicidal death of erythrocytes. *Toxicology* 244:271, 2008.

35. Tavassoli M: Anemia of spaceflight. *Blood* 60:1059, 1982.

36. Mengel CE, Kann HE Jr, Heyman A, Metz E: Effects of *in vivo* hyperoxia on erythro-cytes. II. Hemolysis in a human after exposure to oxygen under high pressure. *Blood* 25:822, 1965.

37. Zimran A, Wasser G, Forman L, et al: Effect of ozone on red blood cell enzymes and intermediates. *Acta Haematol* 102:148, 1999.

38. Biswas D, Banerjee M, Sen G, et al: Mechanism of erythrocyte death in human pop-ulation exposed to arsenic through drinking water. *Toxicol Appl Pharmacol* 230:57, 2008.

39. Mahmud H, Foller M, Lang F: Arsenic-induced suicidal erythrocyte death. *Arch Toxicol* 83:107, 2009.

40. Phoon WH, Chan MO, Goh CH, et al: Five cases of arsine poisoning. *Ann Acad Med Singapore* 13:394, 1984.

41. Romeo L, Apostoli P, Kovacic M, et al; Acute arsine intoxication as a consequence of metal burnishing operations. *Am J Ind Med* 32:211, 1997.

42. Rael LT, Ayala-Fierro F, Carter DE: The effects of sulfur, thiol, and thiol inhibitor com-pounds on arsine-induced toxicity in the human erythrocyte membrane. *Toxicol Sci* 55:468, 2000.

43. Winski SL, Barber DS, Rael LT, Carter DE: Sequence of toxic events in arsine-induced hemolysis in vitro: Implications for the mechanism of toxicity in human erythrocytes. *Fundam Appl Toxicol* 38:123, 1997.

44. Blair PC, Thompson MB, Bechtold M, et al: Evidence for oxidative damage to red blood cells in mice induced by arsine gas. *Toxicology* 63:25, 1990.

45. Eysseric H, Vincent F, Peoc'h M, et al: A fatal case of chlorate poisoning: Confirmation by ion chromatography of body fluids. *J Forensic Sci* 45:474, 2000.

46. Caterson RJ, Savdie E, Raik E, et al: Heinz-body hemolysis in hemodialyzed patients caused by chloramines in Sydney tap water. *Med J Aust* 2:367, 1982.

47. Eaton JW, Kolpin CF, Swofford HS, et al: Chlorinated urban water—Cause of dialysis-induced hemolytic-anemia. *Science* 101:463, 1973.

48. Orringer EP, Mattern WD: Formaldehyde-induced hemolysis during chronic-hemodi-alysis. *N Engl J Med* 294:1416, 1976.

49. Rice L, Alfrey CP: The negative regulation of red cell mass by neocytolysis: Physiologic and pathophysiologic manifestations. *Cell Physiol Biochem* 15:245, 2005.

50. Risso A, Turello M, Biffoni F, Antonutto G: Red blood cell senescence and neocytolysis in humans after high altitude acclimatization. *Blood Cells Mol Dis* 38:83, 2007.

51. Klein M, Namer R, Harpur E, Corbin R: Earthenware containers as a source of fatal lead poisoning—Case study and public-health considerations. *N Engl J Med* 283:669, 1970.

52. Andreasen NJ: Benjamin Franklin: Physicus et medicus. *JAMA* 236:57, 1976.

53. Schwartz J, Landrigan PJ, Baker EL Jr, et al: Lead-induced anemia: Dose-response rela-tionships and evidence for a threshold. *Am J Public Health* 80:165, 1990.

54. Staudinger KC, Roth VS: Occupational lead poisoning. *Am Fam Physician* 57:719, 1998.

55. Froom P, Kristal-Boneh E, Benbassat J, et al: Predictive value of determinations of zinc protoporphyrin for increased blood lead concentrations. *Clin Chem* 44:1283, 1998.

56. Autenrieth T, Schmidt T, Habscheid W: Lead poisoning caused by a Greek ceramic cup. *Dtsch Med Wochenschr* 123:353, 1998.

57. Kakosy T, Hudak A, Naray M: Lead intoxication epidemic caused by ingestion of con-taminated ground paprika. *J Toxicol Clin Toxicol* 34:507, 1996.

58. Fischbein A, Wallace J, Sassa S, et al: Lead poisoning from art restoration and pottery work: Unusual exposure source and household risk. *J Environ Pathol Toxicol Oncol* 11:7, 1992.

59. Vahter M, Counter SA, Laurell G, et al: Extensive lead exposure in children living in an area with production of lead-glazed tiles in the Ecuadorian Andes. *Int Arch Occup Environ Health* 70:282, 1997.

60. Valentine WN, Paglia DE, Fink K, Madokoro G: Lead-poisoning: Association with hemolytic- anemia, basophilic stippling, erythrocyte pyrimidine 5′-nucleotidase deficiency, and intraerythrocytic accumulation of pyrimidines. *J Clin Invest* 58:926, 1976.

61. Paglia DE, Valentine WN, Dahlgren JG: Effects of low-level lead-exposure on pyrim-idine 5′-nucleotidase and other erythrocyte enzymes: Possible role of pyrimidine 5′-nucleotidase in pathogenesis of lead-induced anemia. *J Clin Invest* 56:1164, 1975.

62. Waldron HA: The anaemia of lead poisoning: A review. *Br J Ind Med* 23:83, 1966.

63. Westerman MP, Pfitzer E, Ellis LD, Jensen WN: Concentrations of lead in bone in plumbism. *N Engl J Med* 273:1246, 1965.

64. Lachant NA, Tomoda A, Tanaka KR: Inhibition of the pentose-phosphate shunt by lead—A potential mechanism for hemolysis in lead-poisoning. *Blood* 63:518, 1984.

65. Khalil-Manesh F, Tartaglia-Erler J, Gonick HC: Experimental model of lead nephropa-thy. IV. Correlation between renal functional changes and hematological indices of lead toxicity. *J Trace Elem Electrolytes Health Dis* 8:13, 1994.

66. Vincent PC: The effects of heavy metal ions on the human erythrocyte. I Comparisons of the action of several heavy metals. *Aust J Exp Biol Med Sci* 36:471, 1958.

67. Hasan J, Vihko V, Hernberg S: Deficient red cell membrane/Na$^+$ + K$^+$/-ATPase in lead poisoning. *Arch Environ Health* 14:313, 1967.

68. Hernberg S, Nikkanen J: Enzyme inhibition by lead under normal urban conditions. *Lancet* 1:63, 1970.

69. Casado MF, Cecchini AL, Simao AN, et al: Free radical-mediated pre-hemolytic injury in human red blood cells subjected to lead acetate as evaluated by chemiluminescence. *Food Chem Toxicol* 45:945, 2007.

70. Brookfield RW: Blood changes occurring during the course of treatment of malignant disease by lead, with special reference to punctate basophilia and the platelets. *J Pathol* 31:277, 1928.

71. Clark M, Royal J, Seeler R: Interaction of iron deficiency and lead and the hematologic findings in children with severe lead poisoning. *Pediatrics* 81:247, 1988.

72. White JM, Selhi HS: Lead and the red cell. *Br J Haematol* 30:133, 1975.

73. Jensen WN, Moreno GD, Bessis MC: An electron microscopic description of basophilic stippling in red cells. *Blood* 25:933, 1965.

74. Klein WJ Jr, Metz EN, Price AR: Acute copper intoxication. A hazard of hemodialysis. *Arch Intern Med* 129:578, 1972.

75. Manzler AD, Schreiner AW: Copper-induced acute hemolytic anemia. A new compli-cation of hemodialysis. *Ann Intern Med* 73:409, 1970.

76. Deiss A, Lee GR, Cartwright GE: Hemolytic anemia in Wilson's disease. *Ann Intern Med* 73:413, 1970.

77. Hansen PB: Wilson's disease presenting with severe hemolytic anemia. *Ugeskr Laeger* 150:1229, 1988.

78. McIntyre N, Clink HM, Levi AJ, et al: Hemolytic anemia in Wilson's disease. *N Engl J Med* 276:439, 1967.

79. Grudeva-Popova JG, Spasova MI, Chepileva KG, Zaprianov ZH: Acute hemolytic ane-mia as an initial clinical manifestation of Wilson's disease. *Folia Med (Plovdiv)* 42:42, 2000.

80. Fairbanks VF: Copper sulfate-induced hemolytic anemia. Inhibition of glucose-6-phosphate dehydrogenase and other possible etiologic mechanisms. *Arch Intern Med* 120:428, 1967.

81. Blume KG, Hoffbauer RW, Lohr GW, Rudiger HW: Genetische und biochemische Aspekte der Pyruvatkinase menschlicher Erythrozyten. *Verh Dtsch Ges Inn Med* 75:450, 1969.

82. Boulard M, Beutler E, Blume KG: Effect of copper on red-cell enzyme-activities. *J Clin Invest* 51:459, 1972.

83. Kiss JE, Berman D, Van Thiel D: Effective removal of copper by plasma exchange in fulminant Wilson's disease. *Transfusion* 38:327, 1998.

84. Stohlman F Jr, Brecher G, Schneiderman M, Cronkite EP: The hemolytic effect of ion-izing radiations and its relationship to the hemorrhagic phase of radiation injury. *Blood* 12:1061, 1957.

85. Jin YS, Anderson G, Mintz PD: Effects of gamma irradiation on red cells from donors with sickle cell trait. *Transfusion* 37:804, 1997.

86. Lubash GD, Phillips RE, Bonsnes RW, Shields JD: Acute aniline poisoning treated by hemodialysis—Report of case. *Arch Intern Med* 114:530, 1964.

87. Lowenstein L, Ballew DH: Fatal acute haemolytic anaemia, thrombocytopenic purpura, nephrosis and hepatitis resulting from ingestion of a compound containing apiol. *Can Med Assoc J* 78:195, 1958.

88. Schroder C, Kruger E, Abel J: [Acute poisoning caused by the herbicide dichlorprop (preparation SYS 67 PROP)] [in German]. *Kinderarztl Prax* 59:81, 1991.

89. Martin H, Woerner W, Rittmeister B: Hemolytic anemia by inhalation of hydroxy-lamines, with a contribution to the problem of Heinz body formation. *Klin Wochenschr* 42:725, 1964.

90. Fisher B: The significance of Heinz bodies in anemias of obscure etiology. *Am J Med Sci* 230:143, 1955.

91. Nierenberg DW, Horowitz MB, Harris KM, James DH: Mineral spirits inhalation asso-ciated with hemolysis, pulmonary edema, and ventricular fibrillation. *Arch Intern Med* 151:1437, 1991.

92. Hunter D: Industrial toxicology. *Q J Med* 12:185, 1943.

93. Gasser C: Perakute hämolytische Innenkörperanämie mit Methämoglobinämie nach Behandlung eines Säuglingsekzems mit Resorcin. *Helv Paediatr Acta* 9:285, 1954.

94. Graves TD, Mitchell S: Acute haemolytic anaemia after inhalation of amyl nitrite. *J R Soc Med* 96:594, 2003.

95. Pugh JI, Enderby GEH: Haemoglobinuria after intravenous myanesin. *Lancet* 2:387, 1947.

96. Sills MR, Zinkham WH: Methylene blue-induced Heinz body hemolytic anemia. *Arch Pediatr Adolesc Med* 148:306, 1994.

97. Davidson S, Seldon M, Jones B: Omeprazole and Heinz-body haemolytic anaemia. *Aust N Z J Med* 27:441, 1997.

98. Hassan AB, Seligmann H, Bassan HM: Intravascular haemolysis induced by pentachlorophenol. *Br Med J (Clin Res Ed)* 291:21, 1985.

99. Adams JG, Heller P, Abramson RK, Vaithianathan T: Sulfonamide-induced hemolytic anemia and hemoglobin Hasharon. *Arch Intern Med* 137:1449, 1977.

100. Kaplinsky N, Frankl O: Salicylazosulphapyridine-induced Heinz body anemia. *Acta Haematol* 59:310, 1978.

101. Lin CC, King KL, Chao YW, et al: Tacrolimus-associated hemolytic uremic syndrome: A case analysis. *J Nephrol* 16:580, 2003.

CHAPTER 53
HEMOLYTIC ANEMIA RESULTING FROM INFECTIONS WITH MICROORGANISMS

Marshall A. Lichtman

SUMMARY

Hemolytic anemia is a prominent part of the clinical presentation of patients infected with organisms such as the *Plasmodium* sp., *Babesia*, and *Bartonella*, which directly invade the erythrocyte. Malaria is the most common cause of hemolytic anemia on a worldwide basis, and much has been learned about how the parasite enters the erythrocyte and the mechanism of anemia. Falciparum malaria, in particular, can cause severe and sometimes fatal hemolysis (blackwater fever). Other organisms cause hemolytic anemia by producing a hemolysin (e.g., *Clostridium perfringens*), by stimulating an immune response (e.g., *Mycoplasma pneumoniae*), by enhancing macrophage recognition and hemophagocytosis, or by as yet unknown mechanisms. The many different infections that have been associated with hemolytic anemia are tabulated and references to the original studies provided.

Shortening of erythrocyte life span occurs commonly in the course of inflammatory and infectious diseases. This effect may occur particularly in patients with glucose-6-phosphate dehydrogenase (G6PD) deficiency (Chap. 47), splenomegaly (Chap. 56), and in the microvascular fragmentation syndrome (Chaps. 51 and 132). In some infections, however, rapid destruction of erythrocytes represents a prominent part of the overall clinical picture (Table 53–1).[1–49] This chapter deals only with the latter states.

Several distinct mechanisms may lead to hemolysis during infections.[49] These include direct invasion of or injury to the erythrocytes by the infecting organism, as in malaria, babesiosis, and bartonellosis; elaboration of hemolytic toxins, as by *Clostridium perfringens*; and development of antibodies, either autoantibodies against red cell antigens or deposition of microbial antigens or immune complexes on erythrocytes, which result in hemolytic anemia.[50]

● MALARIA

EPIDEMIOLOGY

Known since antiquity, malaria is the world's most common cause of hemolytic anemia.[36] Human malaria is caused by one of five species of a protozoan, *Plasmodium*. In 2012, an estimated 207 million episodes of malaria occurred worldwide, resulting in approximately 627,000 deaths, mainly children in sub-Saharan Africa.[51] Severe malaria anemia is most commonly seen in young children and pregnant women.[52]

Malaria transmission depends on geography, rainfall patterns, and the breeding sites of the *Anopheles* mosquito, the specific vector. Some regions have conditions that make malaria common throughout the year, so-called endemic areas, whereas in other places there are seasonal peaks, usually the rainy season when mosquito breeding is enhanced. Persons in Africa, Asia, the Middle East, and parts of Europe may be at risk. Travelers to such places are at high risk because of lack of immunity and because when they return home, the diagnosis might not be considered promptly. Malaria may also be transmitted by blood transfusion or organ donation from an infected donor.

LIFE CYCLE

Sporozoites enter the circulation while the female *Anopheles* mosquito takes a blood meal. They invade and multiply in hepatocytes. The latter cells rupture when engorged and release merozoites that invade the red cell. In the red cell, the merozoites also cycle through these stages: trophozoites (ring-forms), which then can convert to schizonts. Mature schizonts burst the red cells and release merozoites that invade other red cells. The bursting and release coincides with the abrupt rises in temperature and related signs and symptoms seen in malaria. A small fraction of merozoites in red cells convert to male and female gametocytes that are ingested when the mosquito bites. In the mosquito, they fuse and form an oocyst that divides asexually into numerous sporozoites. The sporozoites migrate to the mosquito's salivary glands from where they reenter a victim's blood upon the next bite, initiating a malarial infection. *Plasmodium vivax* and *Plasmodium ovale* can persist in the liver in a dormant stage (hypnozoites) and produce relapses months or years later.

ALTERATIONS IN THE INFECTED RED CELL

After the host is bitten by an infected female *Anopheles* mosquito, the sporozoites invade the liver and possibly other internal organs in the asymptomatic tissue stage of malaria. Merozoites, emerging at first from the tissues and later from previously parasitized red cells, use specialized invasion proteins such as the erythrocyte binding-like (EBA) and reticulocyte homology (RH) protein families, which bind to receptors on the erythrocyte surface, including glycophorins A/B/C, CR1 (CD35), and basigin (CD147).[53–55] A complex series of events eventuates in invasion of the interior of the red cell by the parasite.[35,53] Having entered the erythrocyte, the parasite grows intracellularly, nourished by the cell's contents, and modifies the host cell by exporting hundreds of proteins into the cytoplasm, some of which are inserted into the red cell membrane.[56]

Erythrocytes infected with *Plasmodium falciparum* develop surface knobs[57] that contain receptors, especially the *P. falciparum* erythrocyte membrane protein-1 (PfEMP-1), for endothelial proteins. All parasites bind to CD36 antigen (platelet glycoprotein IV) and thrombospondin found on endothelial surfaces, whereas some bind to the intercellular adhesion molecule-1 (ICAM-1), and a few bind to the vascular cell adhesion molecule (VCAM)[58–62] and mediate the

TABLE 53–1. Organisms Causing Hemolytic Anemia

Aspergillus[1]

Bacillus anthracis[2]

Babesia microti and *Babesia divergens*[3]

Bartonella bacilliformis[4,5]

Campylobacter jejuni[6,7]

Clostridium perfringens(Welchii)[8,9]

Coxsackievirus[10]

Cytomegalovirus[11]

Diplococcus pneumoniae[12]

Epstein-Barr virus[13,14]

Escherichia coli[15,16, 123]

Fusobacterium necrophorum[17]

Haemophilus influenzae[12,23]

Hepatitis A[18–20]

Hepatitis B[19,21]

Hepatitis C[22]

Herpes simplex virus[10]

Human immunodeficiency virus[24–26] (Chap. 81)

Influenza A virus[27,28]

Leishmania donovani[30]

Leptospira interrogans serovar *ballum* and/or *Leptospira kirschneri* serovar *butembo*[29]

Mumps virus[31]

Mycobacterium tuberculosis[12,32]

Mycoplasma pneumoniae[33]

Neisseria intracellularis[12]

Parvovirus B19[34]

Plasmodium falciparum[35]

Plasmodium malariae[35]

Plasmodium vivax[36]

Rubella virus[37,38]

Rubeola virus[10]

Salmonella[12,39]

Shigella[40,41,123]

Streptococcus[12,42–45]

Toxoplasma[12]

Trypanosoma brucei[46]

Varicella virus[10,47]

Vibrio cholerae[12]

Yersinia enterocolitica[48]

adherence of parasitized cells to endothelium. Activated endothelium secretes strands of ultralarge von Willebrand factor, which bind platelets, allowing PfEMP-1 to interact with platelet CD36 and this provides an additional means of cytoadherence.[63] Rosetting of parasitized cells with unparasitized cells also occurs through a mechanism mediated by complement receptor-1 (CR1) on uninfected erythrocytes.[64] One of the membrane proteins of *P. falciparum* binds specifically to the spectrin on the inner surface of the red cell membrane.[65] The anemia of falciparum malaria is characteristically normocytic-normochromic anemia with a paucity of reticulocytes (see "Pathogenesis of the Anemia" below). If microcytosis is present, the concomitant presence of α- or β-thalassemia or iron deficiency should be considered.[66] A large number of genetic polymorphisms that interfere with invasion of erythrocytes by parasites and their proliferation have developed in areas where malaria has been a leading cause of death for many generations.[64,67–69] These include G6PD deficiency, Southeast Asian ovalocytosis, CR1 deficiency, the thalassemias, sickle cell anemia (Chaps. 46 to 48), and other hemoglobinopathies.

PLASMODIUM SPECIES AND SEVERITY OF ANEMIA

There are five plasmodial species that cause human malaria: *P. falciparum, P. vivax, Plasmodium malariae, P. ovale* and *Plasmodium knowlesi.* The first two cause the most cases worldwide and are principally associated with hemolytic anemia. *P. vivax* invades only young red cells, whereas *P. falciparum* attacks both young and old cells. Thus, anemia tends to be more severe in the latter form of malaria and is the most deadly type.[35]

PATHOGENESIS OF THE ANEMIA
Hemolytic Mechanisms

Destruction of parasitized red cells appears to occur largely in the spleen, and splenomegaly typically is present in chronic malarial infection. The "pitting" of parasites from infected erythrocytes may also occur in the spleen.[70] The degree of parasitemia, in part, determines the destruction of infected erythrocytes. Low rates of red cell parasitemia may have little effect on the development of anemia, whereas high rates, for example, 10 percent, may have very significant effects.[71] The degree to which anemia develops often seems to be disproportionate to the number of cells infected with the parasite. It is estimated that 10 times the number of uninfected red cells are removed for each infected red cell, dramatically magnifying the hemolytic rate. Osmotic fragility is increased in nonparasitized cells, as well as in cells containing plasmodia.[72] The erythrocyte cation permeability is altered in monkeys with malaria.[73] Hemin accumulation facilitates hemolytic cell loss via a process of programmed cell death, referred to as eryptosis. This suicidal death pathway is mediated by increased cell calcium, increased annexin-V binding, and ceramide formation.[74] Oxidative damage to red cell lipids occurs[75,76] and there is an abnormality in the phosphorylation of membranes of parasitized red cells.[77] *P. falciparum*-infected red cells have a highly irregular surface produced by the intracellular growth of the plasmodium, but nonparasitized cells often have similar surface defects.[78] Activation of hepatosplenic macrophages enhance red cell clearance supported by red cell surface changes in both parasitized and unparasitized cells that foster recognition and erythrophagocytosis by macrophages. Both marked loss of red cell deformability and deposition of immunoglobulin G and complement (C3d), sometimes resulting in a positive direct antiglobulin reaction, may enhance red cell removal by macrophages.[79,80] Parasite products are part of the immune complexes on the red cell surface. The *P. falciparum* ring surface protein 2 (RSP-2) mediates adhesion of infected red cells to endothelial cells and is deposited on uninfected cells, undoubtedly providing a mechanism for removal of these cells by mediating complement-dependent phagocytosis.[66] Splenomegaly further enhances red cell removal from the circulation.

Decrease in Erythropoiesis

P. falciparum also decreases the erythropoietin response, resulting in less erythropoiesis than expected for the degree of anemia, reticulocytopenia, and coincidentally striking dyserythropoiesis with stippling, cytoplasmic vacuolization, nuclear fragmentation and multinuclearity.[66] The inhibition of the erythroid response (anemia of chronic disease) is secondary to release of the cytokines interferon-γ and tumor necrosis factor-α, and the interleukin-10–to–tumor-necrosis-factor ratio, which when low correlates with severe malarial anemia in children (Chap. 37).[66]

BLACKWATER FEVER

The fever associated with malaria, accompanied by rigors, headache, abdominal pain, nausea and vomiting, and extreme fatigue, is characteristically cyclic, varying in frequency according to the malaria type. Although classic periodicity is often absent, febrile paroxysms of *P. vivax* malaria tend to occur every 48 hours; those of *P. malariae* infection occur each 72 hours; and those of *P. falciparum* malaria, daily. In the latter cases, the periodicity is the result the synchronization of schizogony with schizont rupture occurring at regular intervals. It is schizont rupture that accounts for the fever and associated symptoms. Falciparum malaria is occasionally associated with particularly severe

hemolysis, hemoglobinemia, hemoglobinuria, and the passage of dark, almost black, urine. This disorder, also called *blackwater fever*, is no longer common. At one time it was seen frequently among Europeans in Africa and in India, usually after quinine was given to treat malaria. The event seems to be related to the intermittent use of antimalarials.[81]

DIAGNOSTIC METHODS

Diagnosis of malaria depends upon demonstration of the parasites on the blood film, or the presence of antigenic parasite proteins using rapid detection tests (RDTs).[82] Alternative techniques involve polymerase chain reaction (PCR) to demonstrate the appropriate DNA sequences in the blood[83,84] or the use of automated hematology analyzers to identify parasites as part of a routine complete blood count (CBC) investigation.[85] The morphologic differentiation of *P. falciparum* from other forms of malaria, principally *P. vivax*, is clinically important as *P. falciparum* infection may constitute a clinical emergency. If more than 5 percent of the red cells infected contain parasites, the infection is almost certainly with *P. falciparum*. In an infection with this organism, rings are practically the only form of parasite evident on the blood film. The finding of two or more rings within the same red cells is regarded as pathognomonic of *P. falciparum* (Fig. 53–1A and B). In nonimmune

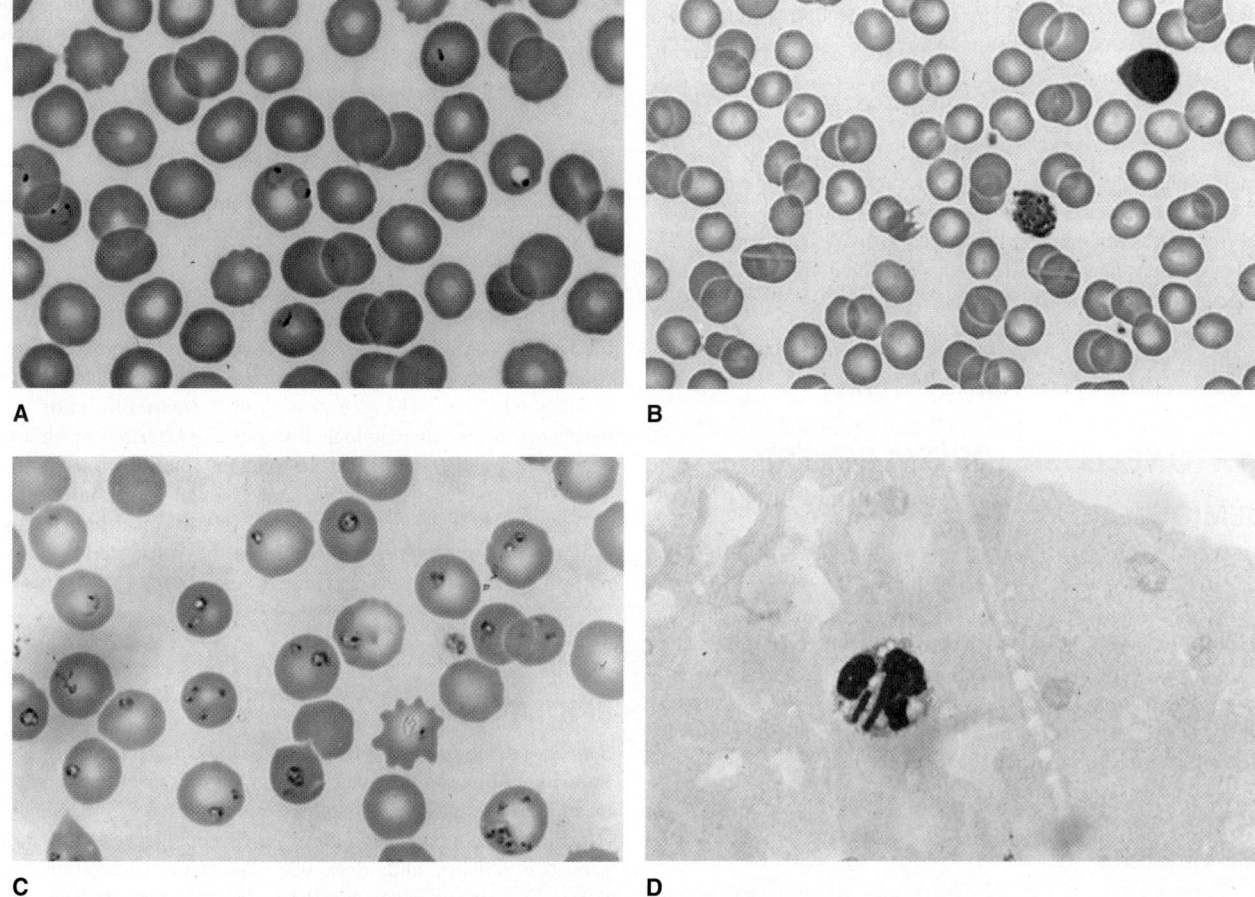

Figure 53–1. A. Blood film from a patient with malaria caused by *Plasmodium falciparum*. Several red cells contain ring forms. Note red cell with double ring form in center of the field, characteristic of *P. falciparum* infection. Note the ring form with double dots at the left edge of figure, suggestive of *P. falciparum* infection. Note also high rate of parasitemia (~10 percent of red cells in this field) characteristic of *P. falciparum* infection. **B.** Blood film from a patient with malaria caused by *Plasmodium vivax*. Note mature schizont. **C.** Blood film from a patient with *Babesia microti* infection. The heavy parasitemia is characteristic of babesiosis (approximately two-thirds of red cells infected). **D.** Blood film from a patient with *Clostridium perfringens* septicemia. Few red cells evident as a result of intense erythrolysis. Neutrophil with two bacilli (*C. perfringens*). (*Reproduced with permission from Lichtman's Atlas of Hematology, www.accessmedicine.com.*)

patients, examination of the blood film for malarial parasites should be made for at least 3 days after onset of symptoms because parasitemia may not reach detectable levels for several days.

TREATMENT

Early treatment is important. The spread of antimalarial therapy has resulted in major problems with drug resistance. Eradication of blood forms can be achieved with individual agents or combinations of antimalarials. Artemisinins are the most effective agents for *P. falciparum*. Numerous studies are in progress to determine the best single agent or combination of agents to be used in the treatment of malaria in different regions.[86] Many such drugs are capable of producing severe hemolysis in patients with G6PD deficiency, which is relevant in areas with endemic malaria (Chap. 47).[87]

PREVENTION

An initial test of a *P. falciparum* sporozoite vaccine, administered intravenously in five doses, has shown efficacy in a small number of experimental subjects. The immunologic responses were closely correlated with vaccine dose. Although a very important step forward, the practical limitations of five intravenous doses will have to be circumvented for extensive application to susceptible populations.[88] Another vaccine, RTS,S, is the first candidate to be tested in phase 3 clinical trials, but the preliminary results have been disappointing. Protection against clinical malaria in infants ranged between 30 and 50 percent and the effect waned after several months.[88a]

COURSE AND PROGNOSIS

When acute, unusually severe hemolysis occurs in the course of falciparum malaria (blackwater fever), the physician should be certain that a hemolytic drug is not being administered to a G6PD-deficient individual. Transfusions may be needed with severe hemolysis, and if renal failure occurs, extracorporeal dialysis may be required. With early institution of therapy the prognosis in malaria is excellent. However, when treatment is delayed or the strain is resistant to the administered agent, *P. falciparum* malaria may follow a rapid, fatal course.

● BARTONELLOSIS (OROYA FEVER)

EPIDEMIOLOGY

In 1885, Daniel A. Carrión, a medical student, inoculated himself with blood obtained from a verrucous node of the skin of a patient with verruca peruviana. He developed a fatal hemolytic anemia with the characteristics of Oroya fever, a disease that had first been observed some years earlier among workers in a railroad construction project near the city of Oroya in the Peruvian Andes. This fatal self-experiment established the identity of the verrucosa form and the hemolytic phase of human bartonellosis, an infection that now bears the name Carrión disease.[5,5a] Human bartonellosis is transmitted by the sandfly.

PATHOGENESIS

After a sandfly bite, the red blood cells become infected with *Bartonella bacilliformis*. It is believed that the organism does not grow within the red cell, but rather adheres to its exterior surface: When infected red cells are washed with citrated plasma, free organisms are found but the red cells are not hemolyzed. In hanging-drop cultures, masses of organisms are clearly seen outside the erythrocytes, while the cells themselves are intact.[89] The osmotic fragility of the red cells is normal.[5] They are rapidly removed from the circulation, apparently both by liver

and spleen. Normal red cells transfused into patients with bartonellosis meet a similar fate.[4] A 130-kDa *Bartonella* protein that causes erythrocytes to acquire trenches, indentations, and invaginations has been purified from culture broths and has been called *deformin*.[90] In addition, two *B. bacilliformis* genes, designated *ialA* and *ialB*, predicted to encode polypeptides of 170 amino acids (20.1 kDa) and of 186 amino acids (19.9 kDa), respectively, greatly enhance the ability of *Escherichia coli* to invade erythrocytes.[91]

CLINICAL FINDINGS

As demonstrated by Carrión's experiment, bartonellosis has two clinical stages. The acute hemolytic anemia, *Oroya fever*, represents the early, invasive stage of a chronic granulomatous disorder, the late stage of which is designated *verruca peruviana*. Most patients manifest no clinical symptoms during the Oroya fever phase, but when anemia does occur, its onset is dramatic. Red counts as low as $750,000/\mu L$ ($0.750 \times 10^{12}/L$) have been documented.[92] In addition to symptoms of anemia, patients manifest thirst, anorexia, sweating, and generalized lymphadenopathy. Spleen and liver enlargement are unusual. Large numbers of nucleated red cells appear in the blood film, and reticulocytosis is often striking. The white cell count is variable. Diagnosis is established by demonstrating the presence of the organism *B. bacilliformis* on the erythrocytes. Giemsa-stained blood films reveal red-violet rods varying in length from 1 to 3 μm and in width from 0.25 to 0.2 μm. Although molecular methods for diagnosis of *Bartonella* species are available,[93] in a person with the clinical picture, the examination of the blood film can be accomplished and therapy initiated, rapidly.

TREATMENT AND COURSE

Oroya fever responds well to treatment with penicillin, streptomycin, chloramphenicol, and the tetracyclines. The mortality rate among untreated patients is very high, but those who do survive undergo a sudden transitional period in which the *Bartonellae* change from an elongated to a coccoid form, the number of parasitized cells decreases, and the red cell count increases. Lymphocytosis and improved neutrophil count are observed with disappearance of the fever and abatement of other symptoms. The second stage of *Bartonella* infection, verruca peruviana, is a nonhematologic disorder characterized by an eruption over the face and extremities developing into bleeding warty tumors.

Other species of *Bartonella* cause human febrile infections such as "cat-scratch fever," or "trench fever," or can infect individuals with acquired immunodeficiency disease, but these disorders are not ordinarily associated with severe hemolytic anemia.[94–96]

● BABESIOSIS

EPIDEMIOLOGY

Babesiae are intraerythrocytic protozoas known as piroplasms. They are transmitted by ticks that may infect many species of wild and domestic animals. Humans occasionally become infected with *Babesia microti* (North America) or *Babesia divergens* (Europe), species that normally parasitize rodents, and, deer, elk, and cattle, respectively.[97] Other *Babesia*-like piroplasms, such as *Babesia WA1*, first isolated from a patient in the state of Washington, and *Babesia MO1*, isolated in Missouri, may also produce human disease.[98] Once thought to be rare, babesiosis is being recognized with increasing frequency.[99,100] The disease is usually tickborne in humans, but has also been transmitted by transfusion.[101–106] Cases of babesiosis, mostly caused by *B. microti* but also by *Babesia WA1* species, have been transmitted by transfusion of blood from asymptomatic infected blood donors. The risk of transfusion-transmitted babesiosis is higher than generally appreciated and represents a threat to the blood supply in endemic areas. Presumably because of the distribution of the vector in the United States, the disease is most common in the northeastern coastal and Great Lakes regions where it became known as "Nantucket fever," but has also been encountered in the Midwest.[107] Infections with *B. divergens* usually occur in splenectomized patients, but this is not the case with *B. microti* infections.[3]

CLINICAL FINDINGS

The symptoms are prompted by reproduction of the organisms in the red cell and subsequent cell lysis. The clinical expression is broad, reflecting the degree of parasitemia. The incubation period ranges from 1 week to 3 months but usually is about 3 weeks. The disease generally has a gradual onset with malaise, anorexia, and fatigue, followed by fever (sometimes as high as 40°C), chills, sweats, and muscle and joint pains. The onset, occasionally, may be fulminant. Hepatic and splenic enlargement may be evident.[108]

A moderate degree of hemolytic anemia is usually present; on occasion it has been sufficiently severe to cause hypotension,[109] and transfusion has occasionally been required.[97] The hemolysis may last a few days, but in asplenic, elderly, or otherwise immunocompromised patients, it can go on for months. Elevation in serum transaminases, lactic dehydrogenase, unconjugated bilirubin, and alkaline phosphatase correlates with the severity of the parasitemia. Thrombocytopenia and leukopenia may occur, which may be the result of inflammatory cytokine release.[108]

DIAGNOSIS

The history may indicate exposure to a tick-infested area, recent blood transfusion, or asplenia. Parasites can be seen in the red cells in Giemsa-stained thin blood films. They appear as darkly stained ring forms with light blue cytoplasm. Merozoites may also be visible. Infrequently, the classical Maltese cross tetrad can be found. This intraerythrocytic structure consists of four daughter cells of *Babesia* connected by cytoplasmic bridges, resembling a Maltese cross. The parasitemia can be very high, affecting more than 75 percent of red cells (see Fig. 53–1C).[108] Immunofluorescent tests for antibodies to *Babesia* are available and PCR-based diagnostic tests are the test of choice for confirmation of an active infection in an individual bearing antibodies to *Babesia* and for following the response to therapy.[108]

The onset of fever and hemolytic anemia after transfusion should lead to the consideration of babesiosis.

TREATMENT AND COURSE

Most mild *B. microti* infections respond without treatment. The infection has responded to drug therapy with clindamycin and quinine,[110] but failure to respond to antibiotics has also been encountered.[102] The two-drug combination can increase rate of clearance of parasites, but they have consequential side effects. A combination of atovaquone and azithromycin has also been proposed as treatment.[98,111] Whole-blood or red cell exchange can result in marked improvement in recalcitrant cases.[108,111]

COINFECTION

In endemic areas two or more parasites may coinfect an individual by a tick bite. *B. microti* and *Borrelia burgdorferi* (Lyme disease) may both enter the human circulation as a result of the *Ixodes* tick bite, as can several other parasites (e.g., human granulocytic ehrlichiosis). Initial signs and symptoms may be similar. Successful early treatment for Lyme disease may leave a residual *B. microti* infection because antibiotic therapy for the former will not eradicate the latter.[108]

● *CLOSTRIDIUM PERFRINGENS* SEPTICEMIA

EPIDEMIOLOGY

C. perfringens (formerly *Clostridium welchii*) sepsis is most likely to occur in patients who have undergone septic abortion. It has also been observed following acute cholecystitis,[112] as a result of an intrahepatic abscess,[9] and, rarely, after amniocentesis (amnionitis).[113]

PATHOGENESIS

C. perfringens are Gram-positive, encapsulated, spore-forming, anaerobic bacilli. The organism causes gas gangrene in soft tissues. The α toxin of *C. perfringens* is a lecithinase C that reacts with lipoprotein complexes at cell surfaces, liberating potent hemolytic substances, lysolecithins. This toxin is the agent that causes intravascular hemolysis and its subsequent effects. It has also been suggested that erythrocyte membrane proteolysis plays an important role in hemolysis.[114]

CLINICAL FEATURES

Severe, often fatal hemolysis occurs in patients with *C. perfringens* septicemia. Striking hemoglobinemia and hemoglobinuria occur. The serum may become a brilliant red, and the urine is a dark-brown mahogany color. The lysis of red cells (decreasing packed red cell volume) and the high plasma hemoglobin can produce a marked dissociation between the blood hemoglobin and hematocrit level. For example, hematocrits approaching zero with blood hemoglobins as high as 8 g/dL can occur. Dehemoglobinized red cells ("ghosts") may be evident on the blood film (see Fig. 53–1D). Microspherocytes are prominent (Chap. 46), and both leukocytosis with a left shift and thrombocytopenia are often present. Acute renal and hepatic failure usually develops, and the prognosis is grave; more than half of the patients die, even with appropriate treatment (Chap. 129).[8,115]

THERAPY AND COURSE

Therapy consists of antibiotic therapy, fluid support, red cell transfusion, and where appropriate surgical debridement.[116] The infection is often of abrupt onset and overwhelming, and the profundity of the hemolysis and secondary organ damage (e.g., renal) results in a high mortality rate.

● OTHER INFECTIONS

A variety of other infections occasionally have been associated with hemolytic anemia. The mechanisms involved vary. Some organisms, among them such common pathogens as *Haemophilus influenzae*, *E. coli*, and *Salmonella* species, can produce red cell agglutination *in vitro*, but it is not known whether this phenomenon is important in initiating *in vivo* hemolysis.[117] Bacteria may also produce destruction of red cells indirectly when bacterial polysaccharides are adsorbed onto erythrocytes. Action of an antibody directed against the antigen-coated cells results in their agglutination[118] or in complement-mediated lysis.[23] The unmasking of T-type antigens by bacteria renders the cell polyagglutinable. This may be a rare cause of hemolysis occurring in the course of bacterial infections.[119,120]

Many different types of microorganisms may play a role in precipitating autoimmune hemolytic disease (Chap. 54). In one study of

234 patients,[10] 55 were found to have an antecedent bacterial infection, 18 of these exhibiting an "unequivocal etiologic relationship" of infection to anemia. However, the principal evidence for such a relationship was a temporal one. A number of viral agents, including measles, cytomegalovirus, varicella, herpes simplex, influenzas A and B, Epstein-Barr, human immunodeficiency virus[24-26] (Chap. 82), and coxsackievirus have also been associated with immune hemolytic disease.[10,121] Various mechanisms have been postulated, including absorption of immune complexes and complement, cross-reacting antigen, and a true autoimmune state with possible loss of tolerance secondary to the infectious organism.[10] Histopathologic and sometimes virologic evidence of infection with cytomegalovirus has been reported in a high percentage of children with lymphadenopathy and hemolytic anemia.[122] A positive antiglobulin reaction was demonstrated in some of these patients, and it has been suggested that some cases of "idiopathic autoimmune hemolytic anemia" are in reality caused by cytomegalovirus infection.[122]

The high cold agglutinin titer that sometimes develops in the course of *Mycoplasma pneumoniae* pneumonia (Chap. 54) may occasionally result in hemolytic anemia[1,33] or compensated hemolysis, although most patients with high cold agglutinin titers do not become anemic. The red cells of a number of patients with kala azar were found to be agglutinated with anticomplement and anti–non-γ-globulin serum.[30] Both splenic and hepatic sequestration of red cells appears to occur in this disease.[13]

Microangiopathic hemolytic anemia is discussed in detail in Chaps. 51 and 129. This disorder may be triggered by a variety of infections, some of which are caused by well-characterized organisms such as Shiga toxin-producing *Escherichia coli*, *Shigella dysenteriae* type 1,[123] *Campylobacter*,[124] and *Aspergillus*.[1]

REFERENCES

1. Robboy SJ, Salisbury K, Ragsdale B, et al: Mechanism of *Aspergillus*-induced microangiopathic hemolytic anemia. *Arch Intern Med* 128:790, 1971.
2. Freedman A, Afonja O, Chang MW, et al: Cutaneous anthrax associated with microangiopathic hemolytic anemia and coagulopathy in a 7-month-old infant. *JAMA* 287:869, 2002.
3. Pruthi RK, Marshall WF, Wiltsie JC, Persing DH: Human babesiosis. *Mayo Clin Proc* 70:853, 1995.
4. Reynafarje C, Ramos J: The hemolytic anemia of human bartonellosis. *Blood* 17:562, 1961.
5. Ricketts WE: *Bartonella bacilliformis* anemia (Oroya fever). A study of thirty cases. *Blood* 3:1025, 1948.
5a. Schultz MG. A history of Bartonellosis (Carrión's disease). *Am J Trop Med Hygiene* 17:503, 1968.
6. Smith MA, Shah NR, Lobel JS, Hamilton W: Methemoglobinemia and hemolytic anemia associated with *Campylobacter jejuni* enteritis. *Am J Pediatr Hematol Oncol* 10:35, 1988.
7. Damani NN, Humphrey CA, Bell B: Haemolytic anaemia in *Campylobacter* enteritis. *J Infect* 26:109, 1993.
8. Rogstad B, Ritland S, Lunde S, Hagen AG: *Clostridium perfringens* septicemia with massive hemolysis. *Infection* 21:54, 1993.
9. Kreidl KO, Green GR, Wren SM: Intravascular hemolysis from a *Clostridium perfringens* liver abscess. *J Am Coll Surg* 194:387, 2002.
10. Pirofsky B: Infectious disease and autoimmune hemolytic anemia, in *Autoimmunization and the Autoimmune Hemolytic Anemias*, p 147. Waverly Press, Baltimore, 1969.
11. van Spronsen DJ, Breed WP: Cytomegalovirus-induced thrombocytopenia and haemolysis in an immunocompetent adult. *Br J Haematol* 92:218, 1996.
12. Dacie JV: Secondary or symptomatic hemolytic anemias, in *The Haemolytic Anaemias, Part III*, edited by JV Dacie, p 908. Grune & Stratton, New York, 1967.
13. Tonkin AM, Mond HG, Alford FP, Hurley TH: Severe acute haemolytic anaemia complicating infectious mononucleosis. *Med J Aust* 2:1048, 1973.
14. Whitelaw F, Brook MG, Kennedy N, Weir WR: Haemolytic anaemia complicating Epstein-Barr virus infection. *Br J Clin Pract* 49:212, 1995.
15. Ludwig K, Ruder H, Bitzan M, et al: Outbreak of *Escherichia coli* O157: H7 infection in a large family. *Eur J Clin Microbiol Infect Dis* 16:238, 1997.
16. Pennings CM, Seitz RC, Karch H, Lenard HG: Haemolytic anaemia in association with *Escherichia coli* O157 infection in two sisters. *Eur J Pediatr* 153:656, 1994.
17. Chand DH, Brady RC, Bissler JJ: Hemolytic uremic syndrome in an adolescent with *Fusobacterium necrophorum* bacteremia. *Am J Kidney Dis* 37:E22, 2001.
18. Gundersen SG, Bjoerneklett A, Bruun JN: Severe erythroblastopenia and hemolytic anemia during a hepatitis A infection. *Scand J Infect Dis* 21:225, 1989.
19. Kanematsu T, Nomura T, Higashi K, Ito M: Hemolytic anemia in association with viral hepatitis. *Nippon Rinsho* 54:2539, 1996.
20. Urganci N, Akyildiz B, Yildirmak Y, Ozbay G: A case of autoimmune hepatitis and autoimmune hemolytic anemia following hepatitis A infection. *Turk J Gastroenterol* 14:204, 2003.
21. Gurgey A, Yuce A, Ozbek N, Kocak N: Acute hemolysis in association with hepatitis B infection in a child with beta-thalassemia trait. *Turk J Pediatr* 36:259, 1994.
22. Etienne A, Gayet S, Vidal F, et al: Severe hemolytic anemia due to cold agglutinin complicating untreated chronic hepatitis C: Efficacy and safety of anti-CD20 (rituximab) treatment. *Am J Hematol* 75:243, 2004.
23. Shurin SB, Anderson P, Zollinger J, Rathbun RK: Pathophysiology of hemolysis in infections with *Haemophilus influenzae* type B. *J Clin Invest* 77:1340, 1986.
24. Rheingold SR, Burnham JM, Rutstein R, Manno CS: HIV infection presenting as severe autoimmune hemolytic anemia with disseminated intravascular coagulation in an infant. *J Pediatr Hematol Oncol* 26:9, 2004.
25. Koduri PR, Singa P, Nikolinakos P: Autoimmune hemolytic anemia in patients infected with human immunodeficiency virus-1. *Am J Hematol* 70:174, 2002.
26. Saif MW: HIV-associated autoimmune hemolytic anemia: An update. *AIDS Patient Care STDS* 15:217, 2001.
27. Watanabe T: Hemolytic uremic syndrome associated with influenza A virus infection. *Nephron* 89:359, 2001.
28. Asaka M, Ishikawa I, Nakazawa T, et al: Hemolytic uremic syndrome associated with influenza A virus infection in an adult renal allograft recipient: Case report and review of the literature. *Nephron* 84:258, 2000.
29. Trowbridge AA, Green JB III, Bonnett JD, et al: Hemolytic anemia associated with leptospirosis. Morphologic and lipid studies. *Am J Clin Pathol* 76:493, 1981.
30. Woodruff AW, Topley E, Knight R, Downie CGB: The anaemia of kala azar. *Br J Haematol* 22:319, 1972.
31. Ozen S, Damarguc I, Besbas N, et al: A case of mumps associated with acute hemolytic crisis resulting in hemoglobinuria and acute renal failure. *J Med* 25:255, 1994.
32. Kuo PH, Yang PC, Kuo SS, Luh KT: Severe immune hemolytic anemia in disseminated tuberculosis with response to antituberculous therapy. *Chest* 119:1961, 2001.
33. Fiala M, Myhre BA, Chinh LT, et al: Pathogenesis of anemia associated with *Mycoplasma pneumoniae*. *Acta Haematol* 51:297, 1974.
34. Chambers LA, Rauck AM: Acute transient hemolytic anemia with a positive Donath-Landsteiner test following parvovirus B19 infection. *J Pediatr Hematol Oncol* 18:178, 1996.
35. Weatherall DJ, Miller LH, Baruch DI, et al: Malaria and the red cell. *Hematology Am Soc Hematol Educ Program* 35, 2002.
36. White NJ: The treatment of malaria. *N Engl J Med* 335:800, 1996.
37. Moriuchi H, Yamasaki S, Mori K, et al: A rubella epidemic in Sasebo, Japan in 1987, with various complications. *Acta Paediatr Jpn* 32:67, 1990.
38. Yoneda S, Yoshikawa H, Yamane Y, et al: A case of rubella complicated by hemolytic anemia. *Kansenshogaku Zasshi* 74:724, 2000.
39. Albaqali A, Ghuloom A, Al Arrayed A, et al: Hemolytic uremic syndrome in association with typhoid fever. *Am J Kidney Dis* 41:709, 2003.
40. Houdouin V, Doit C, Mariani P, et al: A pediatric cluster of Shigella dysenteriae serotype 1 diarrhea with hemolytic uremic syndrome in 2 families from France. *Clin Infect Dis* 38:e96, 2004.
41. Kavaliotis J, Karyda S, Konstantoula T, et al: Shigellosis of childhood in northern Greece: Epidemiological, clinical and laboratory data of hospitalized patients during the period 1971–1996. *Scand J Infect Dis* 32:207, 2000.
42. Shepherd AB, Palmer AL, Bigler SA, Baliga R: Hemolytic uremic syndrome associated with group A beta-hemolytic streptococcus. *Pediatr Nephrol* 18:949, 2003.
43. Apilanez UM, Areses TR, Ruiz Benito MA, et al: Hemolytic uremic syndrome secondary to Streptococcus pneumoniae pulmonary infection. *An Esp Pediatr* 57:378, 2002.
44. Reynolds E, Espinoza M, Monckeberg G, Graf J: Hemolytic-uremic syndrome and Streptococcus pneumoniae. *Rev Med Chil* 130:677, 2002.
45. Brandt J, Wong C, Mihm S, et al: Invasive pneumococcal disease and hemolytic uremic syndrome. *Pediatrics* 110:371, 2002.
46. Wéry M, Mulumba PM, Lambert PH, Kazyumba L: Hematologic manifestations, diagnosis, and immunopathology of African trypanosomiasis. *Semin Hematol* 19:83, 1982.
47. Papalia MA, Schwarer AP: Paroxysmal cold haemoglobinuria in an adult with chicken pox. *Br J Haematol* 109:328, 2000.
48. Von Knorring J, Pettersson T: Haemolytic anaemia complicating *Yersinia enterocolitica* infection. Report of a case. *Scand J Haematol* 9:149, 1972.
49. Berkowitz FE: Hemolysis and infection: Categories and mechanisms of their interrelationship. *Rev Infect Dis* 13:1151, 1991.
50. Seitz RC, Buschermohle G, Dubberke G, et al: The acute infection-associated hemolytic anemia of childhood: Immunofluorescent detection of microbial antigens altering the erythrocyte membrane. *Ann Hematol* 67:191, 1993.
51. World Health Organization: *World Malaria Report 2013*. Available at http://www.who.int/malaria/publications/world_malaria_report_2013/en/ (last accessed 23 January 2015).
52. Greenwood BM: The epidemiology of malaria. *Ann Trop Med Parasitol* 91:763, 1997.
53. Miller LH, Ackerman HC, Su X, Wellems TE: Malaria biology and disease pathogenesis: Insights for new treatments. *Nature* 19:156, 2013.

54. Tham WH, Healer, J Cowman A: Erythrocyte and reticulocyte binding-like proteins of *Plasmodium falciparum. Trends Parasitol* 28:23, 2012.

55. Crosnier C, Bustamante LY, Bartholdson SJ, et al: Basigin is a receptor essential for erythrocyte invasion by Plasmodium falciparum. *Nature* 480:534, 2011.

56. Goldberg D, Cowman A: Moving in and renovating: Exporting proteins from *Plasmodium* into host erythrocytes. *Nat Rev Microbiol* 8:617, 2010.

57. Nakamura K, Hasler T, Morehead K, et al: *Plasmodium falciparum*-infected erythrocyte receptor(s) for CD36 and thrombospondin are restricted to knobs on the erythrocyte surface. *J Histochem Cytochem* 40:1419, 1992.

58. Newbold C, Warn P, Black G, et al: Receptor-specific adhesion and clinical disease in *Plasmodium falciparum. Am J Trop Med Hyg* 57:389, 1997.

59. Baruch DI, Ma XC, Singh HB, et al: Identification of a region of PfEMP1 that mediates adherence of *Plasmodium falciparum* infected erythrocytes to CD36: Conserved function with variant sequence. *Blood* 90:3766, 1997.

60. Sherman IW, Eda S, Winograd E: Cytoadherence and sequestration in *Plasmodium falciparum:* Defining the ties that bind. *Microbes Infect* 5:897, 2003.

61. Udomsangpetch R, Taylor BJ, Looareesuwan S, et al: Receptor specificity of clinical *Plasmodium falciparum* isolates: Nonadherence to cell-bound E-selectin and vascular cell adhesion molecule-1. *Blood* 88:2754, 1996.

62. McCormick CJ, Craig A, Roberts D, et al: Intercellular adhesion molecule-1 and CD36 synergize to mediate adherence of *Plasmodium falciparum*-infected erythrocytes to cultured human microvascular endothelial cells. *J Clin Invest* 100:2521, 1997.

63. Bridges DJ, Bunn J, van Mourik JA, et al: Rapid activation of endothelial cells enables *Plasmodium falciparum* adhesion to platelet-decorated von Willebrand factor strings. *Blood* 115:1472, 2010.

64. Cockburn IA, MacKinnon MJ, O'Donnell A, et al: A human complement receptor 1 polymorphism that reduces *Plasmodium falciparum* rosetting confers protection against severe malaria. *Proc Natl Acad Sci U S A* 101:272, 2004.

65. Herrera S, Rudin W, Herrera M, et al: A conserved region of the MSP-1 surface protein of *Plasmodium falciparum* contains a recognition sequence for erythrocyte spectrin. *EMBO J* 12:1607, 1993.

66. Lamikanra AA, Brown D, Potocnik A, et al: Malarial anemia: Of mice and men. *Blood* 110:18, 2007.

67. Mombo LE, Ntoumi F, Bisseye C, et al: Human genetic polymorphisms and asymptomatic *Plasmodium falciparum* malaria in Gabonese school-children. *Am J Trop Med Hyg* 68:186, 2003.

68. Clegg JB, Weatherall DJ: Thalassemia and malaria: New insights into an old problem. *Proc Assoc Am Physicians* 111:278, 1999.

69. Zimmerman PA, Patel SS, Maier AG, et al: Erythrocyte polymorphisms and malaria parasite invasion in Papua New Guinea. *Trends Parasitol* 19:250, 2003.

70. Angus BJ, Chotivanich K, Udomsangpetch R, White NJ: In vivo removal of malaria parasites from red blood cells without their destruction in acute falciparum malaria. *Blood* 90:2037, 1997.

71. Jakeman GN, Saul A, Hogarth WL, Collins WE: Anaemia of acute malaria infections in non-immune patients primarily results from destruction of uninfected erythrocytes. *Parasitology* 119(Pt 2):127, 1999.

72. George JN, Wicker DJ, Fogel BJ, et al: Erythrocytic abnormalities in experimental malaria. *Proc Soc Exp Biol Med* 124:1086, 1967.

73. Overman RR: Reversible cellular permeability alterations in disease. In vivo studies on sodium, potassium and chloride concentrations in erythrocytes of the malarious monkey. *Am J Physiol* 152:113, 1948.

74. Gatidis S, Föller M, Lang F: Hemin-induced suicidal erythrocyte death. *Ann Hematol* 88:721, 2009.

75. Clark IA, Hunt NH: Evidence for reactive oxygen intermediates causing hemolysis and parasite death in malaria. *Infect Immun* 39:1, 1983.

76. Stocker R, Cowden WB, Tellan RL, et al: Lipids from *Plasmodium vinckei*-infected erythrocytes and their susceptibility to oxidative damage. *Lipids* 22:51, 1987.

77. Yuthavong Y, Limpaiboon T: The relationship of phosphorylation of membrane proteins with the osmotic fragility and filterability of *Plasmodium berghei*-infected mouse erythrocytes. *Biochim Biophys Acta* 929:278, 1987.

78. Balcerzak SP, Arnold JD, Martin DC: Anatomy of red cell damage by *Plasmodium falciparum* in man. *Blood* 40:98, 1972.

79. Jenkins NE, Chakravorty SJ, Urban BC, et al: The effect of *Plasmodium falciparum* infection on expression of monocyte surface molecules. *Trans R Soc Trop Med Hyg* 100:1007, 2006.

80. Helegbe GK, Goka BQ, Kurtzhals JA, et al: Complement activation in Ghanaian children with severe *Plasmodium falciparum* malaria. *Malar J* 6:165, 2007.

81. Price R, van Vugt M, Phaipun L, et al: Adverse effects in patients with acute falciparum malaria treated with artemisinin derivatives. *Am J Trop Med Hyg* 60:547, 1999.

82. Mouatcho JC, Goldring JP. Malaria rapid diagnostic tests: Challenges and prospects. *J Med Microbiol* 62(Pt 10):1491, 2013.

83. Weiss JB: DNA probes and PCR for diagnosis of parasitic infections. *Clin Microbiol Rev* 8:113, 1995.

84. Mangold KA, Manson RU, Koay ES, et al: Real time PCR for detection and identification of *Plasmodium* spp. *J Clin Microbiol* 43: 2435, 2005.

85. Campuzano-Zuluaga G, Hanscheid T, Grobusch MP. Automated haematology analysis to diagnose malaria. *Malar J* 9:346, 2010.

86. Flannery EL, Chatterjee AK, Winzeler EA. Antimalarial drug discovery—Approaches and progress towards new medicines. *Nat Rev Microbiol* 11:849, 2013.

87. Beutler E, Duparc S; G6PD Deficiency Working Group: Glucose-6-phosphate dehydrogenase deficiency and antimalarial drug development. *Am J Trop Med Hyg* 77:779, 2007.

88. Seder RA, Chang LJ, Enama ME, et al: Protection against malaria by intravenous immunization with a nonreplicating sporozoite vaccine. *Science* 341:1359, 2013.

88a. Riley EM, Stewart VA. Immune mechanisms in malaria: New insights in vaccine development. *Nat Med* 19:168, 2013.

89. Aldana L: Bacteriologia de la enfermedad de carrion. *Cron Med* 46:235, 1929.

90. Xu YH, Lu ZY, Ihler GM: Purification of deformin, an extracellular protein synthesized by *Bartonella bacilliformis* which causes deformation of erythrocyte membranes. *Biochim Biophys Acta* 1234:173, 1995.

91. Mitchell SJ, Minnick MF: Characterization of a two-gene locus from *Bartonella bacilliformis* associated with the ability to invade human erythrocytes. *Infect Immun* 63:1552, 1995.

92. Weinman D: Human *Bartonella* infection and African sleeping sickness. *Bull N Y Acad Med* 22:647, 1946.

93. García-Esteban C, Gil H, Rodríguez-Vargas M, et al: Molecular method for *Bartonella* species identification in clinical and environmental samples. *J Clin Microbiol* 46:776, 2008.

94. Dalton MJ, Robinson LE, Cooper J, et al: Use of *Bartonella* antigens for serologic diagnosis of cat-scratch disease at a national referral center. *Arch Intern Med* 155:1670, 1995.

95. Eremeeva ME, Gerns HL, Lydy SL, et al: Bacteremia, fever, and splenomegaly caused by a newly recognized *Bartonella* species. *N Engl J Med* 356:2381, 2007.

96. Koehler JE, Sanchez MA, Tye S, et al: Prevalence of *Bartonella* infection among human immunodeficiency virus-infected patients with fever. *Clin Infect Dis* 37:559, 2003.

97. Reubush TK II, Cassaday PB, Marsh HJ, et al: Human babesiosis on Nantucket Island. *Ann Intern Med* 86:6, 1977.

98. Krause PJ: Babesiosis. *Med Clin North Am* 86:361, 2002.

99. Krause PJ, McKay K, Gadbaw J, et al: Increasing health burden of human babesiosis in endemic sites. *Am J Trop Med Hyg* 68:431, 2003.

100. Herwaldt BL, McGovern PC, Gerwel MP, et al: Endemic babesiosis in another eastern state: New Jersey. *Emerg Infect Dis* 9:184, 2003.

101. Jacoby GA, Hunt JV, Kosinski KS, et al: Treatment of transfusion-transmitted babesiosis by exchange transfusion. *N Engl J Med* 303:1098, 1980.

102. Smith RP, Evans AT, Popovsky M, et al: Transfusion-acquired babesiosis and failure of antibiotic treatment. *JAMA* 256:2726, 1986.

103. Herwaldt BL, Kjemtrup AM, Conrad PA, et al: Transfusion-transmitted babesiosis in Washington State: First reported case caused by a WA1-type parasite. *J Infect Dis* 175:1259, 1997.

104. Nelson R: Blood on demand. *Am Herit Invent Technol* 19:24, 2004.

105. Dobroszycki J, Herwaldt BL, Boctor F, et al: A cluster of transfusion-associated babesiosis cases traced to a single asymptomatic donor. *JAMA* 281:927, 1999.

106. Kjemtrup AM, Lee B, Fritz CL, et al: Investigation of transfusion transmission of a WA1-type babesial parasite to a premature infant in California. *Transfusion* 42:1482, 2002.

107. Steketee RW, Eckman MR, Burgess EC, et al: Babesiosis in Wisconsin. A new focus of disease transmission. *JAMA* 253:2675, 1985.

108. Homer MJ, Aguilar-Delfin I, Telford SR 3rd, et al: Babesiosis. *Clin Microbiol Rev* 13:451, 2000.

109. Cheng D, Yakobi-Shvilli R, Fernandez J: Life-threatening hypotension from babesiosis hemolysis. *Am J Emerg Med* 20:367, 2002.

110. Wittner M, Rowin KS, Tanowitz HB, et al: Successful chemotherapy of transfusion babesiosis. *Ann Intern Med* 96:601, 1982.

111. Weiss LM: Babesiosis in humans: A treatment review. *Expert Opin Pharmacother* 3:1109, 2002.

112. Clancy MT, OBriain S: Fatal *Clostridium welchii* septicaemia following acute cholecystitis. *Br J Surg* 62:518, 1975.

113. Hamoda H, Chamberlain PF: *Clostridium welchii* infection following amniocentesis: A case report and review of the literature. *Prenat Diagn* 22:783, 2002.

114. Simpkins H, Kahlenberg A, Rosenberg A, et al: Structural and compositional changes in the red cell membrane during *Clostridium welchii* infection. *Br J Haematol* 21:173, 1971.

115. Mahn HE, Dantuono LM: Postabortal septicotoxemia due to *Clostridium welchii. Am J Obstet Gynecol* 70:604, 1955.

116. Moustoukas NM, Nichols RL, Voros D: Clostridial sepsis: Unusual clinical presentations. *South Med J* 78:440, 1985.

117. Neter E: Bacterial hemagglutination and hemolysis. *Bacteriol Rev* 20:166, 1956.

118. Ceppellini R, De Gregorio M: Crisi emolitica in animali batterio-immuni transfusi con sangue omologo sensibilizzato in vitro mediante l'antigene batterico specifico. *Boll Ist Sieroter Milan* 32:445, 1953.

119. Dausset J, Moullec J, Bernard J: Acquired hemolytic anemia with polyagglutinability of red blood cells due to a new factor. *Blood* 14:1079, 1959.

120. Klein PJ, Vierbuchen M, Roth B, et al: Hemolytic anemia in infections caused by neuraminidase-producing bacteria. *Verh Dtsch Ges Pathol* 67:415, 1983.

121. McGinniss MH, Macher AM, Rook AH, Alter HJ: Red cell autoantibodies in patients with acquired immune deficiency syndrome. *Transfusion* 26:405, 1986.

122. Zuelzer WW, Stulberg CS, Page RH, et al: The Emily Cooley lecture. Etiology and pathogenesis of acquired hemolytic anemia. *Transfusion* 6:438, 1966.

123. Walker CL, Applegate JA, Black RE. Haemolytic-uraemic syndrome as a sequela of diarrhoeal disease. *J Health Popul Nutr* 30:257, 2012.

124. Dickgiesser A: Campylobacter infection and the hemolytic-uremic syndrome. *Immun Infekt* 11:71, 1983.

CHAPTER 54
HEMOLYTIC ANEMIA RESULTING FROM IMMUNE INJURY

Charles H. Packman

SUMMARY

Autoimmune hemolytic anemia (AHA) is characterized by shortened red blood cell (RBC) survival and the presence of autoantibodies directed against autologous RBCs. Demonstration of antibody and/or complement on RBC membranes, usually by a positive direct antiglobulin test (DAT, also referred to as the Coombs test) is essential for diagnosis. Most patients with AHA (80 percent) exhibit warm-reactive antibodies of the immunoglobulin (Ig) G isotype on their red cells. Most of the remainder of patients exhibit cold-reactive autoantibodies. Two types of cold-reactive autoantibodies to RBCs are recognized: cold agglutinins and cold hemolysins. Cold agglutinins are generally of IgM isotype, whereas cold hemolysins usually are of IgG isotype. The DAT may detect IgG, proteolytic fragments of complement (mainly C3), or both on the RBCs of patients with warm-antibody AHA. In cold-antibody AHA, only complement is detected because the antibody dissociates from the RBCs during washing of the cells. About half of patients with AHA have no underlying associated disease; these cases are termed primary or idiopathic. Secondary cases are associated with underlying autoimmune, malignant, or infectious diseases or with ingestion of certain drugs.

Although most patients do not require transfusion of RBCs, transfusion should not be withheld from those with symptomatic anemia. In warm-antibody AHA, rituximab and glucocorticoids are effective in slowing the rate of hemolysis. Splenectomy is indicated for patients who are refractory to medical therapy or who require an unacceptably high maintenance dose or prolonged administration of glucocorticoids. Intravenous immunoglobulin may provide short-term control of hemolysis. Immunosuppressive drugs and danazol have been used successfully in refractory cases. In cold agglutinin- and cold hemolysin-mediated hemolysis, keeping the patient warm and treating underlying lymphoproliferative disorders usually are effective. Rituximab has been effective in about half of cases of cold AHA. Drug-induced immune hemolytic anemia usually is ameliorated by discontinuation of the offending drug.

Acronyms and Abbreviations: AHA, autoimmune hemolytic anemia; CLL, chronic lymphocytic leukemia; DAF, decay-accelerating factor; DAT, direct antiglobulin test; HLA, human leukocyte antigen; HRF, homologous restriction factor; HS, hereditary spherocytosis; IAT, indirect antiglobulin test; Ig, immunoglobulin; IGHV, immunoglobulin heavy chain variable region; PNH, paroxysmal nocturnal hemoglobinuria; RBC, red blood cell; SLE, systemic lupus erythematosus.

DEFINITION AND HISTORY

The two main features of immune red blood cell (RBC) injury are (1) shortened RBC survival *in vivo* and (2) evidence of host antibodies reactive with autologous RBCs, most frequently demonstrated by a positive direct antiglobulin test (DAT), also known as the Coombs test. Most cases in adults are mediated by warm-reactive autoantibodies. A smaller proportion of patients exhibit cold-reactive autoantibodies or drug-related antibodies.

By the early 20th century, reticulocytes, spherocytes, and osmotic fragility of RBCs had been described. Clinicians could diagnose hemolytic anemia, but the distinction between congenital and acquired forms was imprecise. Some clinicians even doubted the existence of acquired hemolytic anemia.[1] The sera of some patients with hemolytic anemia directly agglutinated saline suspensions of normal or autologous human RBCs. These serum factors, later shown to be specific antibodies (largely of the immunoglobulin [Ig] M class), were termed *direct* or *saline agglutinins*. In a smaller proportion of cases, the patients' sera could mediate lysis of the test RBCs in the presence of fresh serum as a complement source. The heat-stable factors (antibodies) necessary for *in vitro* complement-mediated lysis were called *hemolysins*. However, in the majority of cases of hemolytic anemia, neither direct agglutinins nor hemolysins could be demonstrated. In 1945, Coombs and colleagues[2] reported that RBCs coated with nonagglutinating Rh antibodies (now known to be of the IgG isotype) could be agglutinated by rabbit antiserum to human γ-globulin. That is, the rabbit antiglobulin serum crosslinked IgG antibody-coated RBCs to produce visible agglutination. Addition of rabbit antiglobulin serum to a suspension of washed RBCs isolated from patients with suspected acquired hemolytic anemia produced agglutination in many cases, including those patients lacking saline agglutinins or hemolysins. RBCs from patients with congenital hemolytic anemia did not agglutinate.[3,4] This procedure now is termed the *direct antiglobulin (Coombs) test*. Subsequent studies established that positive direct antiglobulin reactions in autoimmune hemolytic anemia (AHA) are attributable to coating of the RBCs with immunoglobulins (mainly IgG) and/or complement proteins. When the RBCs are coated chiefly with complement proteins, a positive DAT depends upon the presence of anticomplement (principally anti-C3) in the antiglobulin reagent. In warm-antibody AHA, the autoantibodies, chiefly of IgG isotype, bind optimally to RBCs at 37°C. Warm antibodies may or may not activate complement binding to RBCs.

Cryopathic hemolytic syndromes are caused by autoantibodies that bind RBCs optimally at temperatures less than 37°C and usually less than 31°C. Two major types of "cold antibody" may produce AHA. Cold agglutinins, which directly agglutinate RBCs, mediate cold agglutinin disease. The Donath-Landsteiner autoantibody, which is not an agglutinin but a potent hemolysin, mediates paroxysmal cold hemoglobinuria. In both cryopathic syndromes, the complement system plays a major role in RBC injury (Chap. 19); as such, much greater potential exists for direct intravascular hemolysis than in warm-antibody–mediated AHA.

Cold agglutinins were first described by Landsteiner[5] in 1903. However, recognition of the connection among cold agglutinins, hemolytic anemia, and Raynaud-like peripheral vascular phenomena evolved slowly. In 1918, Clough and Richter[6] detected cold agglutinins in a patient with pneumonia. In 1925 and 1926, Iwai and MeiSai[7,8] reported two patients with cold agglutinins and Raynaud phenomenon and showed that flow of blood through capillary tubes *in vitro* or in superficial capillaries *in vivo* was impeded at low temperatures. During the late 1940s and early 1950s, the observations of many investigators gradually established the pathogenic importance of cold agglutinins in RBC injury. Schubothe[9] introduced the term *cold agglutinin disease* in

1953 and clearly distinguished the disorder from other acquired hemolytic syndromes.

In current usage, cold agglutinin disease pertains to patients with chronic AHA in which the autoantibody directly agglutinates human RBCs at temperatures below body temperature, maximally at 0 to 5°C. Fixation of complement to a patient's RBCs by cold agglutinins *in vivo* occurs at higher temperatures but generally less than 37°C. Cold agglutinins typically are IgM, although occasionally they may be immunoglobulins of other isotypes. The cold agglutinins in chronic cold agglutinin disease generally are monoclonal. Most cold agglutinins have specificity for oligosaccharide antigens (I or i) of the RBC (see "Origin of Cold Agglutinins" below).

Donath and Landsteiner first described the cold hemolysin that bears their name in 1904. The Donath-Landsteiner antibody is responsible for complement-mediated hemolysis in paroxysmal cold hemoglobinuria, a rare form of AHA in adults. The disorder is characterized by recurrent episodes of massive hemolysis following cold exposure.[10,11] A related form of hemolytic anemia occurs much more commonly in children (or young adults) as an acute, self-limited hemolytic process following several types of viral syndromes.[10-16] The disease was recognized during the latter half of the 19th century, when the disease was more common because of its association with congenital or tertiary syphilis. With the advent of effective therapy for syphilis, this cause of paroxysmal cold hemoglobinuria has almost disappeared. Now, recurrent paroxysmal cold hemoglobinuria occurs very rarely in a chronic idiopathic form.[10,11] An increasing proportion of Donath-Landsteiner autoantibody-mediated hemolytic anemias occurs as a single postviral episode in children, without recurrent attacks (paroxysms). The prognosis for such cases is excellent. Thus, rather than paroxysmal cold hemoglobinuria, a proposed term for this latter entity is *Donath-Landsteiner hemolytic* anemia.[13,14]

The first example of drug-related immune blood cell destruction was Ackroyd's description of sedormid purpura in 1949.[17] In 1953, Snapper and coworkers[18] described a case of immune hemolysis and pancytopenia in a patient treated with mephenytoin (Mesantoin). Hemolysis ceased upon withdrawal of the drug. In 1956, Harris[19] reported what are now classic studies of a patient who developed immune hemolytic anemia during a second course of stibophen administered for treatment of schistosomiasis. Since then, many drugs have been implicated in the production of positive DATs and accelerated RBC destruction.

CLASSIFICATION

Warm-Reactive versus Cold-Reactive Red Cell Antibody

AHA can be classified in two complementary ways (Table 54–1). The majority of cases (80 to 90 percent in adults) are mediated by warm-reactive autoantibodies[10,11,20] or antibodies displaying optimal reactivity with human RBCs at 37°C. A smaller proportion of cases is attributable to cold-reactive autoantibodies exhibiting greater affinity for RBCs at temperatures less than 37°C. The distinction is important, not only because of differences in the pathophysiology of RBC injury but also in the therapeutic approaches required. An even smaller proportion of patients with AHA exhibit both cold-reactive and warm-reactive autoantibodies,[21,22] which apparently recognize different antigens on the RBC membrane.[23] RBC destruction is generally more severe in mixed cases.

Absence or Presence of an Associated Disease

Classification of AHA based on the presence or absence of underlying diseases also is useful (see Table 54–1). When no recognizable underlying disease is present, the AHA is termed *primary* or *idiopathic*. When AHA appears to be a manifestation or complication of an underlying

TABLE 54–1. Classification of Hemolytic Anemia as a Result of Immune Injury

I. Warm-Autoantibody Type: Autoantibody Maximally Active at Body Temperature (37°C)
   A. Primary or idiopathic warm autoimmune hemolytic anemia (AHA)
   B. Secondary warm AHA
      1. Associated with lymphoproliferative disorders (e.g., Hodgkin lymphoma)
      2. Associated with the rheumatic disorders, particularly systemic lupus erythematosus (SLE)
      3. Associated with certain nonlymphoid neoplasms (e.g., ovarian tumors)
      4. Associated with certain chronic inflammatory diseases (e.g., ulcerative colitis)
      5. Associated with ingestion of certain drugs (e.g., α-methyldopa)

II. Cold-Autoantibody Type: Autoantibody Optimally Active at Temperatures <37°C
   A. Mediated by cold agglutinins
      1. Idiopathic (primary) chronic cold agglutinin disease (usually associated with clonal B-lymphocyte proliferation)
      2. Secondary cold agglutinin hemolytic anemia
         a. Postinfectious (e.g., *Mycoplasma pneumoniae* or infectious mononucleosis)
         b. Associated with malignant B-cell lymphoproliferative disorder
   B. Mediated by cold hemolysins
      1. Idiopathic (primary) paroxysmal cold hemoglobinuria (very rare)
      2. Secondary
         a. Donath-Landsteiner hemolytic anemia, usually associated with an acute viral syndrome in children (relatively common)
         b. Congenital or tertiary syphilis in adults (very rare)

III. Mixed Cold and Warm Autoantibodies
   A. Primary or idiopathic mixed AHA
   B. Secondary mixed AHA
      1. Associated with the rheumatic disorders, particularly SLE

IV. Drug-Immune Hemolytic Anemia
   A. Hapten or drug adsorption mechanism
   B. Ternary (immune) complex mechanism
   C. True autoantibody mechanism

disorder, the term *secondary AHA* is applied. Lymphocytic malignancies, particularly chronic lymphocytic leukemia (CLL) and lymphomas, account for approximately half of all secondary AHA cases and for the majority of AHA cases mediated by cold agglutinins.[24] Systemic lupus erythematosus (SLE) and other autoimmune diseases account for a lesser but considerable proportion of secondary AHA cases. A large proportion of patients with mixed cold and warm autoantibodies have SLE.[21,22] Infectious mononucleosis and *Mycoplasma pneumoniae* occasionally are associated with cryopathic AHA. Despite the frequent occurrence of immune thrombocytopenia and positive DATs in patients infected with HIV, AHA is relatively rare in these patients.[25-27] Table 54–1 lists other associated diseases that are less-commonly reported. The etiologic and pathogenic significance of these associations is poorly understood, but most of the associated diseases involve components of the immune system, either by neoplasia or by aberrant immunopathologic responses.

Drug-Mediated Cases

Certain drugs also mediate immune injury to RBCs, and three general mechanisms are recognized (see Table 54–1 and Fig. 54–1). This classification is based on the effector mechanism of RBC injury, because the induction mechanism for formation of drug-related RBC antibodies is unknown. Two of the mechanisms, hapten-drug adsorption and ternary complex formation, involve drug-dependent antibodies. In the third mechanism, the drugs in question appear to induce formation of true autoantibodies capable of reacting with human RBCs in the absence of the inciting drug. These types of drug-mediated immune injury to RBCs often are referred to collectively as *drug-immune hemolytic anemia* to distinguish them from de novo AHA. Distinguishing among the mechanisms is not always possible, and some cases involve a combination of mechanisms. In addition, drug-related non-immunologic protein adsorption by RBCs may result in a positive DAT without actual RBC injury. This phenomenon should be distinguished from the three forms of drug-immune RBC injury. Table 54–2 lists drugs documented to cause either immune injury or a positive DAT.

● EPIDEMIOLOGY

The annual incidence of warm-antibody AHA is 1 per 75,000 to 80,000 population.[11] Estimates of the frequency of primary (idiopathic) AHA vary from 20 to 80 percent of all types of AHA, depending on the referral patterns of the reporting center.[11,20,118] In general, AHA is considered

secondary (1) when AHA and the underlying disease occur together with greater frequency than can be accounted for by chance alone; (2) when the AHA reverses simultaneously with correction of the associated disease; or (3) when AHA and the associated disease are related by evidence of immunologic aberration.[11] Using these criteria, the frequency of primary warm-antibody AHA probably is closer to 50 percent of all cases. Careful followup of patients with primary AHA is essential, because hemolytic anemia may be the presenting finding in a patient who subsequently develops overt evidence of an underlying disorder. For example, in one series, 18 of 107 patients with AHA developed a malignant lymphoproliferative disorder at a median of 26.5 months after diagnosis of the AHA.[119]

Warm-antibody AHA has been diagnosed in people of all ages, from infants to the elderly. The majority of patients are older than 40 years of age, with peak incidence around the seventh decade. This age distribution probably reflects, in part, the increased frequency of lymphoproliferative malignancies in the elderly, resulting in an age-related increase in the frequency of secondary AHA. Although multiple cases are occasionally observed in families,[120–122] most cases of primary AHA arise sporadically. Development of AHA does not have an apparent association with any particular human leukocyte antigen (HLA) haplotype or other genetic factor.

Cold agglutinin disease is less common than warm-antibody AHA, with a prevalence of approximately 14 per 1 million population,[24] accounting for only 10 to 20 percent of all cases of AHA.[10,11,123] Women are affected more commonly than men.[10,11] No genetic or racial factors are known to contribute to the pathogenesis of this disease.

Secondary cold agglutinin disease is seen most commonly in adolescents or young adults as a self-limited process associated with

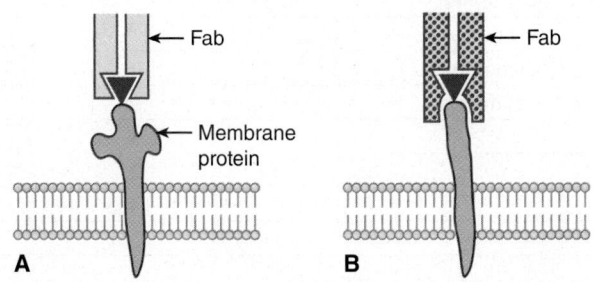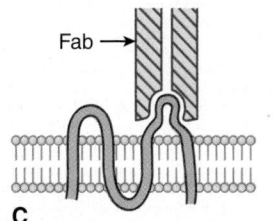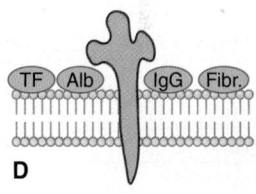

Figure 54–1. Effector mechanisms by which drugs mediate a positive direct antiglobulin test. Relationships of drug, antibody-combining site, and red blood cell membrane protein are shown. Panels **A, B,** and **C** show only a single immunoglobulin Fab region (bearing one combining site). **A.** Drug adsorption/hapten mechanism. The drug (▼) binds avidly to an unknown red blood cell membrane protein *in vivo*. Antidrug antibody (usually immunoglobulin [Ig] G) binds to the protein-bound drug. The membrane protein is not known to be part of the epitope recognized by the antidrug antibody. The direct antiglobulin test (with anti-IgG) detects IgG antidrug antibody on the patient's circulating (drug-coated) red blood cells. The indirect antiglobulin test detects antibody in the patient's serum only when the test red blood cells have been previously coated with the drug by incubation *in vitro*. **B.** Ternary complex mechanism. Drug binds loosely or in undetectable amounts to red blood cell membrane. However, in the presence of appropriate antidrug antibody, a stable trimolecular (ternary) complex is formed by drug, red blood cell membrane protein, and antibody. In general, the antibody-combining site *(Fab)* recognizes both drug and membrane protein components but binds only weakly to either drug or protein unless both are present in the reaction mixture. In this mechanism, the direct antiglobulin test typically detects only red blood cell–bound complement components (e.g., C3 fragments) that are bound covalently and in large number to the patient's red blood cells *in vivo*. The antibody itself escapes detection, possibly because of its low concentration but also because washing of the red cells (in the antiglobulin test procedure) apparently dissociates antibody and drug from the cells, leaving only the covalently bound C3 fragments. The indirect antiglobulin test also detects complement proteins on the test red blood cells when both antibody (patient serum) and a complement source (fresh patient serum or fresh normal serum) are present in the reaction mixture together with the drug. **C.** Autoantibody induction. Some drug-induced antibodies can bind avidly to red blood cell membrane proteins (usually Rh proteins) in the absence of the inducing drug and are indistinguishable from the autoantibodies of patients with autoimmune hemolytic anemia. The direct antiglobulin test detects the IgG antibody on the patient's red blood cells. The indirect antiglobulin test usually detects antibody in the serum of patients with active hemolysis. **D.** Drug-induced nonimmunologic protein adsorption. Certain drugs cause plasma proteins to attach nonspecifically to the red blood cell membrane. The direct antiglobulin test detects nonspecifically bound IgG and complement components. If special antiglobulin reagents are used, other plasma proteins, such as transferrin (TF), albumin (Alb), and fibrinogen (Fibr), also may be detected. In contrast to the other mechanisms of drug-induced red blood cell injury, this mechanism does not shorten red blood cell survival *in vivo*.

TABLE 54–2. Association between Drugs and Positive Direct Antiglobulin Tests

Drug	Reference	Drug	Reference
HAPTEN OR DRUG ADSORPTION MECHANISM			
Penicillins	28–34	Tolbutamide	44, 45
Cephalosporins	35–39	Cianidanol	46
Tetracycline	40, 41	Hydrocortisone	47
6-Mercaptopurine	42	Oxaliplatin	48
Carbromal	43	Cimetidine	49
TERNARY COMPLEX MECHANISM			
Stibophen	19	Cephalosporins	37–39, 64
Quinine	50	Diethylstilbestrol	65
Quinidine	51, 52	Amphotericin B	66
Chlorpropamide	53, 54	Doxepin	67
Metformin	55	Diclofenac	68, 69
Rifampicin	56	Etodolac	70
Antazoline	57	Hydrocortisone	47
Thiopental	58	Oxaliplatin	48
Tolmetin	59	Pemetrexed	71
Probenecid	60	Cimetidine	49
Nomifensine	61–63	Iomeprol	72
AUTOANTIBODY MECHANISM			
Cephalosporins	39	Latamoxef	84
Tolmetin	59	Glafenine	84
Nomifensine	61	Procainamide	85
a-Methyldopa	73–76	Diclofenac	69, 86
L-dopa	78–81	Pentostatin	87
Mefenamic acid	82, 83	Fludarabine	88, 89
Teniposide	84	Cladribine	90
Oxaliplatin	48	Efalizumab	91
Cianidanol	46	Lenalidomide	92
NONIMMUNOLOGIC PROTEIN ADSORPTION			
Cephalosporins	93, 94		
Oxaliplatin	48		
Carboplatin	48		
Cisplatin	48, 95		
UNCERTAIN MECHANISM OF IMMUNE INJURY			
Mesantoin	18	Erythromycin	106
Phenacetin	50	5-fluorouracil	107
Insecticides	96	Nalidixic Acid	108
Chlorpromazine	97	Sulindac	109
Melphalan	98	Omeprazole	110
Isoniazid	99	Temafloxacin	111
p-Aminosalicylic acid	100	Carboplatin	112
Acetaminophen	101	Efavirenz	113
Thiazides	102	Etoricoxib	114
Streptomycin	103	Levofloxacin	115
Ibuprofen	104	Pueraria (Chinese herb)	116
Triamterene	105	Cabergoline	117

The drugs listed above are those which, in the author's opinion, have been documented to cause a positive direct antiglobulin test, with or without immune injury. Other drugs, omitted from this list, have been alleged to cause immune injury but laboratory confirmation is lacking. New drugs will be added to this list in the future. When an association between a drug and hemolysis is suspected, it is important to evaluate for an immune etiology and to document the mechanism, by referral to a reference laboratory if necessary.

M. pneumoniae infections or infectious mononucleosis and, rarely, in children with chickenpox. The term also has been used to describe a chronic disorder occurring in older patients with known malignant lymphoproliferative diseases. On the other hand, idiopathic (primary) chronic cold agglutinin disease has its peak incidence after age 50 years. This disorder, with its characteristic monoclonal IgM cold agglutinins, may be considered a special form of monoclonal gammopathy (Chap. 106). Nearly all of these patients exhibit clonal B lymphocyte proliferation.[24] As with other "essential" or idiopathic monoclonal gammopathies, some patients in this group gradually develop features of a B-cell lymphoproliferative disorder resembling Waldenström macroglobulinemia, CLL, or a B-cell lymphoma. Thus, the distinction between primary and secondary types of chronic cold agglutinin disease is not absolute.

Although the majority of patients with mycoplasma pneumonia have significant cold agglutinin titers, they only infrequently develop clinical hemolytic anemia.[124–126] However, subclinical RBC injury may occur. In *M. pneumoniae* infections, weakly positive direct antiglobulin reactions and/or mild reticulocytosis are often noted in the absence of anemia in a substantial number of cases.[124] Cold agglutinins occur in more than 60 percent of patients with infectious mononucleosis, but again, hemolytic anemia is rare.[127–129]

Medical centers that receive many referrals report that paroxysmal cold hemoglobinuria constitutes 2 to 5 percent of all cases of AHA.[10,11] Among children, however, Donath-Landsteiner hemolytic anemia accounted for 32.4 percent of 68 immune hemolytic syndromes diagnosed over a 4-year period.[15] Commonly, the diagnosis is missed because of lack of physician awareness or failure to perform the proper serologic studies (see "Serologic Features" below).[12,15] Thus, the true incidence may be higher. Although familial occurrence has been reported, no racial or genetic risk factors are known.[10] As noted, most childhood cases follow either specific viral infections or upper respiratory infections of undefined etiology.[10–15]

Older series report that drug-induced immune hemolytic anemia accounts for 12 to 18 percent of immune hemolytic anemias.[11] The disorder is much less common now that α-methyldopa and megaunit doses of penicillin rarely are used. The current incidence of drug-induced immune hemolytic anemia is estimated at 1 per 1 million population, approximately 88 percent of which result from the second- and third-generation cephalosporins, cefotetan, and ceftriaxone.[89,130] Fludarabine has replaced α-methyldopa as the most common cause of drug-induced autoantibodies.[89]

● ETIOLOGY AND PATHOGENESIS

ETIOLOGY

Warm-Antibody Autoimmune Hemolytic Anemia
The etiology of AHA is unknown. In warm-antibody AHA, the autoantibodies that mediate RBC destruction are predominantly (but not exclusively) IgG globulins possessing relatively high binding affinity for human RBCs at 37°C. As a result, the major share of plasma autoantibody is bound to the patient's circulating RBCs. Eluates prepared from the patient's washed, autoantibody-coated RBCs constitute an important source of purified autoantibody for investigation of specificity, immunoglobulin structure, or other properties. In addition, sera from patients with warm AHA often are used in blood banks for crossmatching and for general screening of antibody specificity. The quantity of such autoantibody in serum may be low and in some cases may not reflect the full spectrum of anti-RBC specificity revealed in concurrently prepared RBC eluates.[124]

In patients with primary AHA, erythrocyte autoantibodies are the only recognizable immunologic aberration. Furthermore, the autoantibodies of any one patient often are specific for only a single RBC membrane protein (see "Serologic Features" below). The narrow spectrum of autoreactivity suggests the mechanism underlying AHA development in such patients is not secondary to a generalized defect in immune regulation. Rather, these patients may develop warm-antibody AHA through an aberrant immune response to a self-antigen or to an immunogen that mimics a self-antigen.

In patients with secondary AHA, the disease may be associated with a fundamental disturbance in the immune system, for example, when in the setting of lymphoma, CLL, SLE, primary agammaglobulinemia (common variable immunodeficiency), or hyper-IgM immunodeficiency syndrome. In these settings, warm-antibody AHA most likely arises through an underlying defect in immune regulation, although the contribution of an aberrant immune response to self-antigen cannot be excluded. AHA seems especially frequent in patients with low-grade lymphoma or CLL treated with fludarabine [88,89] or 2-chlorodeoxyadenosine (cladribine).[90] The T-lymphocytopenia induced by these drugs may exacerbate the preexisting tendency of patients to form autoantibodies.

A long-recognized but poorly understood phenomenon, the development of AHA or a positive DAT following RBC transfusion, has received renewed interest lately.[132,133] Although generally transient, the positive DAT may persist for up to 300 days in some transfusion recipients, long after any transfused RBCs have disappeared.[134,135] It is not clear whether this represents true autoimmunity or some other mechanism, for example, microchimerism resulting from temporary engraftment of passenger memory lymphocytes from the RBC donor.[132]

A still unexplained observation is that certain drugs, such as α-methyldopa, can induce warm-reacting IgG anti-RBC autoantibodies in otherwise normal persons. The autoantibodies induced by α-methyldopa have Rh-related serologic and immunochemical[136] specificity similar to that of autoantibodies arising in many patients with "spontaneous" AHA. A critical difference is that the drug-associated autoantibodies subside when the drug is discontinued, suggesting that (1) the latent potential to form this type of anti-RBC autoantibody is present in many immunologically normal individuals, and (2) the steps required to generate such autoantibodies do not necessarily create a sustained autoimmune state. On the other hand, maintenance of chronic idiopathic AHA may be either secondary to a continuing (but unknown) stimulus or induced by a short stimulus to which the patient continues to respond.

Normal subjects sometimes have a positive DAT when they volunteer to donate blood.[137,138] The positive DAT in these normal donors often results from warm-reacting IgG autoantibodies, similar in serologic specificity[131] and in IgG subclass[137] to the autoantibodies occurring in AHA. Although many of these donors remain DAT-positive without developing overt hemolytic anemia, a few have been documented to develop AHA.[137,138] The prevalence of positive DATs in normal blood donors is approximately 1 in 10,000 donors.[137,139] Because blood donation *per se* likely does not contribute to an increased risk of developing autoantibodies, the 1 in 10,000 proportion likely is the approximate frequency of positive DATs in the entire population. A proportion of patients who present with clinically overt primary AHA may come from a subset of asymptomatic individuals who are DAT-positive, but this notion is not established.

Several concepts have been developed to explain immunologic tolerance to self-antigens.[140–143] Relevant to warm-antibody AHA, membrane-bound antigens expressed in a multivalent array at high concentration may induce tolerance by effecting clonal deletion of autoreactive B cells.[144] Both the Rh-related and the non-Rh types of RBC antigens targeted by AHA autoantibodies (see "Serologic Features" below) are expressed normally by human fetal erythrocytes, as early as

10 to 12 weeks of life.[145] However, because new B cells develop daily in the marrow throughout life and because B cells may somatically mutate their Ig receptors, self-tolerance in the B cell compartment is never assured. Analogy to observations in NZB (New Zealand black) mice[146,147] suggests the peritoneal cavity is a privileged compartment that shelters autoreactive B cells from host RBCs, allowing them to escape deletion, later to produce anti-RBC autoantibodies with appropriate T-cell help. The strong predominance of IgG antibodies in AHA suggests B-cell isotype switching, which is consistent with the idea of an antigen-driven process. Moreover, because T-cell help is necessary for inducing B-cell isotype switching, the pathway(s) to autoantibody induction in AHA also may involve an abnormal or unique mode of antigen presentation to T cells.[148]

Origin of Cold Agglutinins

A high proportion of monoclonal IgM cold agglutinins with either anti-I or anti-i specificity have heavy-chain variable regions encoded by IGHV4–34 (immunoglobulin heavy chain variable region), formerly designated IGHV4.21.[143,149–151] IGHV4–34 encodes a distinct idiotype identified by the rat monoclonal antibody 9G4. This idiotype is expressed both by the cold agglutinins themselves and on the surface immunoglobulin of B cells synthesizing cold agglutinins or related immunoglobulins possessing IGHV4–34 sequences.[152] Using the 9G4 monoclonal antibody as a probe, this idiotype was found not only in a very high proportion of circulating B cells and marrow lymphoplasmacytoid cells of patients with lymphoma-associated chronic cold agglutinin disease, but also in a smaller proportion of B cells in the blood and lymphoid tissues of normal adult donors and in the spleens of 15-week human fetuses.[152] These data suggest B cells expressing the IGHV4–34 gene (or a closely related sequence) are present throughout ontogeny. Therefore, chronic cold agglutinin disease may represent a marked, unregulated expansion of a subset (clone) of such B cells.

Light-chain V-region gene use in anti-I cold agglutinins is highly selective. A strong bias toward use of the κ III variable region subgroup (Vκ-III) is observed.[150–153] Light-chain selection among anti-i cold agglutinins, however, is much more variable and includes the λ type.[150–154]

Observations that pathologic cold agglutinins are synthesized with distinct and highly selected V-region sequences must be viewed against the background of two other subsequent observations. First, IGHV4–34 or related IGHV genes also may encode the heavy-chain variable regions of other types of antibodies, such as rheumatoid factor autoantibodies and alloantibodies to a variety of blood group antigens, including polypeptide determinants such as Rh.[155] Second, normal human antibodies to an exogenous carbohydrate antigen, *Haemophilus influenzae* type b capsular polysaccharide, also are encoded by a restricted set of IGHV genes[156] and Ig light-chain V genes.[157] Thus, regulation of Ig gene use for production of anti-I or anti-i cold agglutinins may not differ fundamentally from normal antibody formation to other carbohydrate antigens.

In the setting of B-cell lymphoma or Waldenström macroglobulinemia, cold agglutinins may be produced by the malignant clone itself. Two patients with lymphoma and monoclonal cold agglutinin were identified as having a karyotypically abnormal B-cell clone that produced a cold agglutinin identical to that found in their sera.[158,159] Trisomy 3 has been the most frequently observed karyotypic abnormality in patients with non-Hodgkin lymphoma and cold agglutinins.[158,160]

Normal human sera generally have naturally occurring polyclonal cold agglutinins in low titer (usually 1/64 or less).[10] Otherwise healthy persons may develop elevated titers of cold agglutinins specific for I/i antigens during certain infections (e.g., *M. pneumoniae*, Epstein-Barr virus, cytomegalovirus). In contrast to other forms of cold agglutinin disease, hyperproduction of these postinfectious cold agglutinins is transient. Some evidence indicates postinfectious cold agglutinins may

be less clonally restricted than those occurring in chronic cold agglutinin disease,[161] but this finding is not universal.[162] Whether IGHV4–34 also encodes most heavy-chain variable regions of all naturally occurring or postinfectious cold agglutinins remains to be determined.

The increased production of cold agglutinins in response to infection with *M. pneumoniae* may be secondary to the fact that the oligosaccharide antigens of the I/i type serve as specific *Mycoplasma* receptors.[163] This process may lead to altered antigen presentation involving a complex between a self-antigen (I/i) and a non–self-antigen (*Mycoplasma*). Alternatively, the anti-i cold agglutinins may arise as a consequence of polyclonal B cell activation, as occurs in infectious mononucleosis (Chap. 82).

The mechanism(s) whereby dissimilar infectious agents (e.g., spirochetes and several types of virus) induce the immune system to produce Donath-Landsteiner antibodies with specificity for the human P blood group antigen (see "Serologic Features" below) is not known.

PATHOGENESIS

Pathogenic Effects of Warm Antibodies

Warm autoantibodies to RBCs in AHA are pathogenic. In contrast to autologous RBCs, labeled RBCs lacking the antigen targeted by the autoantibodies may survive normally in patients with warm-antibody AHA.[10,164,165] Furthermore, transplacental passage of IgG anti-RBC autoantibodies from a mother with AHA to the fetus can induce intrauterine or neonatal hemolytic anemia.[166] Finally, despite notable exceptions and differences related to IgG subclass of the autoantibody, in general, an inverse relationship between the quantity of RBC-bound IgG antibody and RBC survival is noted in serial studies performed on animals and patients.[167–172]

In warm-antibody AHA, the patient's RBCs typically are coated with IgG autoantibodies with or without complement proteins. Autoantibody-coated RBCs are trapped by macrophages in the Billroth cords of the spleen and, to a lesser extent, by Kupffer cells in the liver (Chap. 68).[164,167,168,170–174] The process leads to generation of spherocytes and fragmentation and ingestion of antibody-coated RBCs.[175,176] The macrophage has surface receptors for the Fc region of IgG, with preference for the IgG$_1$ and IgG$_3$ subclasses[177,178] and surface receptors for opsonic fragments of C3 (C3b and C3bi) and C4b.[179–181] When present together on the RBC surface, IgG and C3b/C3bi appear to act cooperatively as opsonins to enhance trapping and phagocytosis.[170,171,180–184] Although RBC sequestration in warm-antibody AHA occurs primarily in the spleen,[164,171–173] very large quantities of RBC-bound IgG[167,168,174] or the concurrent presence of C3b on the RBCs[167,170,171] may favor trapping in the liver.

Interaction of a trapped RBC with splenic macrophages may result in phagocytosis of the entire cell. More commonly, a type of partial phagocytosis results in spherocyte formation. As RBCs adhere to macrophages via the Fc receptors, portions of RBC membrane are internalized by the macrophage. Because membrane is lost in excess of contents, the noningested portion of the RBC assumes a spherical shape, the shape with the lowest ratio of surface area to volume.[175,176,185] Spherical RBCs are more rigid and less deformable than normal RBCs. As such, spherical RBCs are fragmented further and eventually destroyed in future passages through the spleen. Spherocytosis is a consistent and diagnostically important hallmark of AHA,[186] and the degree of spherocytosis correlates well with the severity of hemolysis.[10]

Direct complement-mediated hemolysis with hemoglobinuria is unusual in warm-antibody AHA, even though many warm autoantibodies fix complement. The failure of C3b-coated RBCs to be hemolyzed by the terminal complement cascade (C5–C9) has been attributed, at least in part, to the ability of complement regulatory proteins (factors

I and H) in plasma and C3b receptors on the RBC surface to alter the hemolytic function of cell-bound C3b and C4b.[187] Glycosylphosphat-idylinositol-linked erythrocyte membrane proteins, such as decay-accelerating factor (DAF; CD55) and homologous restriction factor (HRF; CD59), may limit the action of autologous complement on auto-antibody-coated RBCs.[188-190] DAF inhibits the formation and function of cell-bound C3-converting enzyme,[188] thus, indirectly limiting forma-tion of C5-converting enzyme. HRF, on the other hand, impedes C9 binding and formation of the C5b–9 membrane attack complex.[189]

Cytotoxic activities of macrophages and lymphocytes also may play a role in the destruction of RBCs in warm-antibody AHA. Monocytes can lyse IgG-coated RBCs *in vitro* independently of phagocytosis.[191,192] Cell-bound complement is neither necessary nor sufficient for such cytotoxicity, but bound C3b/C3d can potentiate the effects of IgG.[192] In one study, cytotoxicity, but not phagocytosis, was inhibited by hydro-cortisone *in vitro*.[191] Lymphocytes also can lyse IgG antibody-coated RBCs *in vitro*.[193-195] The relative contribution of antibody-dependent monocyte- and lymphocyte-mediated cytotoxicity to RBC destruction in patients with warm-antibody AHA is not known.

Pathogenic Effects of Cold Agglutinins and Hemolysins

Most cold agglutinins are unable to agglutinate RBCs at temperatures higher than 30°C. The highest temperature at which these antibodies cause detectable agglutination is termed the *thermal amplitude*. The value varies considerably among patients. Generally, patients with cold agglutinins with higher thermal amplitudes have a greater risk for cold agglutinin disease.[9] For example, active hemolytic anemia has been observed in patients with cold agglutinins of modest titer (e.g., 1:256) and high thermal amplitudes.[196]

The pathogenicity of a cold agglutinin depends upon its ability to bind host RBCs and to activate complement.[10,182,197,198] This process is called *complement fixation*. Although *in vitro* agglutination of the RBCs may be maximal at 0 to 5°C, complement fixation by these antibodies may occur optimally at 20 to 25°C and may be significant at even higher physiologic temperatures.[10,196,197] Agglutination is not required for the process. The great preponderance of cold agglutinin molecules are IgM pentamers, but small numbers of IgM hexamers with cold agglutinin activity are found in patients with cold agglutinin disease. Hexamers fix complement and lyse RBCs more efficiently than do pentamers, sug-gesting that hexameric IgM plays a role in the pathogenesis of hemolysis in these patients.[199]

Cold agglutinins may bind to RBCs in superficial vessels of the extremities, where the temperature generally ranges between 28 and 31°C, depending upon ambient temperature.[200] Cold agglutinins of high thermal amplitude may cause RBCs to aggregate at this temperature, thereby impeding RBC flow and producing acrocyanosis. In addition, the RBC-bound cold agglutinin may activate complement via the classic pathway. Once activated complement proteins are deposited onto the RBC surface, the cold agglutinin need not remain bound to the RBCs for hemolysis to occur. Instead, the cold agglutinin may dissociate from the RBCs at the higher temperatures in the body core and again be capa-ble of binding other RBCs at the lower temperatures in the superficial vessels. As a result, patients with cold agglutinins of high thermal ampli-tude tend toward a sustained hemolytic process and acrocyanosis.[201] In contrast, patients with antibodies of lower thermal amplitude require significant chilling to initiate complement-mediated injury of RBCs. This sequence may result in a burst of hemolysis with hemoglobinuria.[201] Combinations of these clinical patterns also occur. Cold agglutinins of the IgA isotype, an isotype that does not fix complement, may cause acrocyanosis but not hemolysis.[202] Thus, the relative degree of hemolysis or impeded RBC flow is influenced significantly by the properties and quantity of the cold agglutinins in a given patient.

Complement fixation by cold agglutinins may affect RBC injury by two major mechanisms: (1) direct lysis and (2) opsonization for hepatic and splenic macrophages. Both mechanisms probably operate to vary-ing degrees in any patient. Direct lysis requires propagation of the full C1 to C9 sequence on the RBC membrane. If this process occurs to a significant degree, the patient may experience intravascular hemolysis leading to hemoglobinemia and hemoglobinuria. Intravascular hemoly-sis of this severity is relatively rare because phosphatidylinositol-linked RBC membrane proteins (DAF and HRF) protect against injury by autologous complement components. Thus, the complement sequence on many RBCs is completed only through the early steps, leaving opsonic fragments of C3 (C3b/C3bi) and C4 (C4b) on the cell surface. The fragments provide only a weak stimulus for phagocytosis by mono-cytes *in vitro*.[184,203] However, activated macrophages may ingest C3b-coated particles avidly.[204] Accordingly, RBCs heavily coated with C3b (and/or C3bi) may be removed from the circulation by macrophages either in the liver or, to a lesser extent, the spleen.[171,197,205,206] The trapped RBCs may be ingested entirely or released back into the circulation as spherocytes after losing plasma membrane.

In vivo studies of the fate of ^{51}Cr-labeled C3b-coated RBCs[170,197,205,206] indicate many of the erythrocytes trapped in the liver or spleen gradually may reenter the circulation. The released cells generally are coated with the opsonically inactive C3 fragment C3dg. Conversion of cell-bound C3b or C3bi to C3dg results from the action of the naturally occurring complement inhibitor factor I in concert with factor H or CR1 recep-tors.[181] The surviving C3dg-coated RBCs circulate with a near-normal life span[170,197,205,206] and are resistant to further uptake of cold agglutinins or complement.[197,205,207] However, C3dg-coated RBCs also may react *in vitro* with anticomplement (anti-C3) serum in the DAT. In fact, most of the antiglobulin-positive RBCs of patients with cold agglutinin disease are coated with C3dg.

In paroxysmal cold hemoglobinuria, the mechanism of hemolysis probably parallels *in vitro* events (see "Serologic Features" below). Dur-ing severe chilling, blood flowing through skin capillaries is exposed to low temperatures. The Donath-Landsteiner antibody and early acting complement components presumably bind to RBCs at the lowered tem-peratures. Upon return of the cells to 37°C in the central circulation, the cells are lysed by propagation of the terminal complement sequence through C9. The Donath-Landsteiner antibody itself dissociates from the RBCs at 37°C. Erythrocyte membrane proteins that restrict C5b–9 assembly (e.g., HRFs) may be less effective in controlling Donath-Landsteiner antibody-initiated complement activation than that initi-ated by cold agglutinins.

Pathogenesis of Drug-Mediated Immune Injury

Table 54–3 summarizes the three mechanisms of drug-mediated immune injury to RBCs. Drugs also may mediate protein adsorption to RBCs by nonimmune mechanisms, but RBC injury does not occur.

Hapten or Drug Adsorption Mechanism This mechanism applies to drugs that can bind firmly to proteins, including RBC membrane pro-teins. The classic setting is very-high-dose penicillin therapy,[28-34] which is encountered less commonly today than in previous decades.

Most individuals who receive penicillin develop IgM antibodies directed against the benzylpenicilloyl determinant of penicillin, but this antibody plays no role in penicillin-related immune injury to RBCs. The antibody responsible for hemolytic anemia is of the IgG class, occurs less frequently than the IgM antibody, and may be directed against the benzylpenicilloyl,[31] or, more commonly, nonbenzylpenicilloyl determi-nants.[28-30,32] Other manifestations of penicillin sensitivity usually are not present.

All patients receiving high doses of penicillin develop substan-tial coating of RBCs with penicillin. The penicillin coating itself is not

TABLE 54–3. Major Mechanisms of Drug-Related Hemolytic Anemia and Positive Direct Antiglobulin Tests

	Hapten/Drug Adsorption	Ternary Complex Formation	Autoantibody Binding	Nonimmunologic Protein Adsorption
Prototype drug	Penicillin	Quinidine	*a*-Methyldopa	Cephalothin
Role of drug	Binds to red cell membrane	Forms ternary complex with antibody and red cell membrane component	Induces formation of antibody to native red cell antigen	Possibly alters red cell membrane
Drug affinity to cell	Strong	Weak	None demonstrated to intact red cell but binding to membranes reported	Strong
Antibody to drug	Present	Present	Absent	Absent
Antibody class predominating	Immunoglobulin (Ig) G	IgM or IgG	IgG	None
Proteins detected by direct antiglobulin test	IgG, rarely complement	Complement	IgG, rarely complement	Multiple plasma proteins
Dose of drug associated with positive antiglobulin test	High	Low	High	High
Presence of drug required for indirect antiglobulin test	Yes (coating test red cells)	Yes (added to test medium)	No	Yes (added to test medium)
Mechanism of red cell destruction	Splenic sequestration of IgG-coated red cells	Direct lysis by complement plus splenic–hepatic clearance of C3b-coated red cells	Splenic sequestration	None

injurious. If the penicillin dose is very high (10 to 30 × 10⁶ units per day, or less in the setting of renal failure) and promotes cell coating, and if the patient has an IgG antipenicillin antibody, the antibody binds to the RBC-bound penicillin molecules and the DAT with anti-IgG becomes positive (see Fig. 54–1*A*).[29,31,32,51,208] Antibodies eluted from patients' RBCs or present in their sera react in the indirect antiglobulin test (IAT) only against penicillin-coated RBCs. This step is critical in distinguishing these drug-dependent antibodies from true autoantibodies.

Not all patients receiving high-dose penicillin develop a positive DAT reaction or hemolytic anemia because only a small proportion of such individuals produce the requisite antibody. Destruction of RBCs coated with penicillin and IgG antipenicillin antibody occurs mainly through sequestration by splenic macrophages.[30,209] In some patients with penicillin-induced immune hemolytic anemia, blood monocytes and presumably splenic macrophages may lyse the IgG-coated RBCs without phagocytosis.[210] Hemolytic anemia resulting from penicillin typically occurs only after the patient has received the drug for 7 to 10 days and ceases a few days to 2 weeks after the patient discontinues taking the drug.

Low-molecular-weight substances, such as drugs, generally are not immunogenic in their own right. Induction of antidrug antibody is thought to require firm chemical coupling of the drug (as a hapten) to a protein carrier. In the case of penicillin, the carrier protein involved in antibody induction need not be the same as the erythrocyte membrane protein to which penicillin is coupled in the effector phase, that is, when the IgG antipenicillin antibodies bind to penicillin-coated RBCs. In contrast to evidence on the ternary complex mechanism, no evidence indicates the drug-dependent antibodies responsible for RBC injury in this hapten/drug adsorption mechanism also recognize native erythrocyte membrane structures.

Cephalosporins have antigenic cross-reactivity with penicillin[211,213] and bind firmly to RBC membranes, as do semisynthetic penicillins.[33,34] Hemolytic anemia similar to that seen with penicillin has been ascribed to cephalosporins[35–39] and some semisynthetic penicillins.[33,34]

Tetracycline[40,41] and tolbutamide[44,45] also may cause hemolysis by this mechanism. Carbromal causes positive IgG antiglobulin reactions by a similar mechanism,[43] but hemolytic anemia has not been described.

Ternary Complex Mechanism: Drug–Antibody–Target Cell Interaction Many drugs can induce immune injury not only of RBCs but also of platelets or granulocytes by a process that differs in several ways from the mechanism of hapten/drug adsorption (see Table 54–3). First, drugs in this group (see Table 54–2) exhibit only weak direct binding to blood cell membranes. Second, a relatively small dose of drug is capable of triggering destruction of blood cells. Third, cellular injury appears to be mediated chiefly by complement activation at the cell surface. The cytopathic process induced by such drugs previously has been termed the *innocent bystander* or *immune complex mechanism*. The terminology reflected the prevailing notion that, *in vivo*, drug–antibody complexes formed first (immune complexes) and then became secondarily bound to target blood cells as "innocent bystanders," either nonspecifically or possibly via membrane receptors (e.g., Fcγ receptors on platelets or C3b receptors on red cells), with the potential for subsequent activation of complement by bound complexes.

The "immune complex" and "innocent bystander" terminology now seems less appropriate because of models developed from research on analogous drug-dependent platelet injury[214–216] (Chap. 117) and a series of relevant serologic observations on drug-mediated immune hemolytic anemia. These studies suggest blood cell injury is mediated by a cooperative interaction among three reactants to generate a ternary complex (see Fig. 54–1*B*) involving (1) the drug (or drug metabolite in some cases), (2) a drug-binding membrane site on the target cell, and (3) antibody. For example, several patients possessed drug-dependent antibodies that exhibited specificity for RBCs bearing defined alloantigens such as those of the Rh, Kell, or Kidd blood groups. That is, even in the presence of drug, the antibodies were selectively nonreactive with human RBCs lacking the alloantigen in question.[58,84,217–219] In each case, high-affinity drug binding to cell membrane could not be demonstrated. The drug-dependent antibody is thought to bind, through its

Fab domain, to a compound neoantigen consisting of loosely bound drug and a blood group antigen intrinsic to the red cell membrane. Elegant studies on quinidine- or quinine-induced immune thrombocytopenia have demonstrated the IgG antibodies implicated in this disorder bind through their Fab domains, not by their Fc domains to platelet Fcγ receptors.[220,221]

The data elucidate how one patient with quinidine sensitivity may have selective destruction of platelets and another may have selective destruction of RBCs. This process occurs because the pathogenic antibody recognizes the drug only in combination with a particular membrane structure of the RBC (e.g., a known alloantigen) or of the platelet (e.g., α domain of the glycoprotein Ib complex). Therefore, at least in these cases, the target cell does not appear to be purely an innocent bystander. Binding of the drug itself to the target cell membrane is weak until the attachment of the antibody to *both* drug and cell membrane is stabilized. Yet the binding of the antibody is drug dependent. Such a three-reactant interdependent "troika" is unique to this mechanism of immune cytopenia.

The foregoing discussion depicting drugs as creating a "self + non-self" neoantigen on the target cell applies to the effector phase as opposed to the induction phase of the process. However, the same drug-binding membrane protein appears to be involved in forming the immunogen that induces the antibody, as evidenced by drug-dependent antibodies exhibiting selective reactivity with defined red cell alloantigens (carrier specificity).[58,84,217-219] How this process is accomplished in the absence of evidence for strong, covalent binding of the drugs in this group to a host membrane protein remains to be elucidated.

RBC destruction by this mechanism may occur intravascularly after completion of the whole complement sequence, resulting in hemoglobinemia and hemoglobinuria. Some destruction of intact C3b-coated RBCs may be mediated by splenic and liver sequestration via the C3b/C3bi receptors on macrophages. The DAT is positive usually only with anticomplement reagents, but exceptions occur. Sometimes, however, the drug-dependent antibody itself can be detected on the RBCs if the offending drug (or its metabolites) is included in all steps of the antiglobulin test, including washing.[222]

Autoantibody Mechanism A variety of drugs induce the formation of autoantibodies reactive with autologous (or homologous) RBCs in the absence of the instigating drug (see Tables 54–2 and 54–3). The most studied drug in this category has been α-methyldopa, an antihypertensive agent that no longer is commonly used.[73-76] Levodopa and several unrelated drugs also have been implicated.[39,46,59,61,68,77-86] Patients with CLL treated with pentostatin,[87] fludarabine,[88] or cladribine[90] are particularly predisposed to autoimmune hemolysis, which usually is severe and sometimes fatal.

Positive DAT reactions (with anti-IgG reagents) in patients taking α-methyldopa vary in frequency from 8 to 36 percent. Patients taking higher doses of the drug develop positive reactions with greater frequency.[73,75,76] A lag period of 3 to 6 months exists between the start of therapy and development of a positive antiglobulin test. The delay is not shortened when the drug is administered to patients who previously had positive antiglobulin tests while taking α-methyldopa.[75]

In contrast to the frequent observation of positive antiglobulin reactions, less than 1 percent of patients taking α-methyldopa exhibit hemolytic anemia.[74] Development of hemolytic anemia does not depend on drug dose. The hemolysis usually is mild to moderate and occurs chiefly by splenic sequestration of IgG-coated RBCs. α-Methyldopa has been proposed to suppress splenic macrophage function in some patients, and normal survival of antibody-coated RBCs in such patients may be related, in part, to this effect of the drug.[223]

The DAT reaction usually is positive only for IgG.[11] Occasionally, weak anticomplement reactions also are encountered.[11] Patients with

immune hemolytic anemia resulting from α-methyldopa therapy typically exhibit strongly positive DAT reactions and serum antibody, evidenced by the IAT reaction.[11] Antibodies in the serum or eluted from RBC membranes react optimally at 37°C with unaltered autologous or homologous RBCs in the absence of drug (see Fig. 54–1C).[74,76,224] Frequently the autoantibodies are reactive with determinants of the Rh complex,[74,76,224] and at least some appear to target the same 34-kDa Rh-related polypeptide targeted by the autoantibodies in many cases of "spontaneously arising" AHA.[136] Thus, distinguishing these drug-induced antibodies from similar warm-reacting autoantibodies in idiopathic AHA currently is not possible.

The mechanism by which a drug induces formation of an autoantibody is unknown. Radiolabeled α-methyldopa does not react directly with the membranes of intact human RBCs.[76,225] However, both α-methyldopa and levodopa reportedly bind to isolated RBC membranes. Binding of the drug to membranes of intact RBCs is inhibited by RBC superoxide dismutase and probably by hemoglobin.[225,226] Although not formally demonstrated, these drugs probably bind to membrane antigens of cells that are relatively hemoglobin free, for example, cells at the early proerythroblast stage or RBC stroma. In any case, the resulting altered membrane antigens then may induce autoantibodies. The concept that a drug–membrane compound neoantigen could lead to production of an autoantibody is supported by studies of patients receiving drugs unrelated to α-methyldopa. Patients simultaneously developed a drug-dependent antibody and an autoantibody, both of which showed specificity for the same RBC alloantigen.[84] Another hypothesis is that α-methyldopa interacts with human T lymphocytes, resulting in loss of suppressor cell function.[227] Subsequent studies, however, have failed to demonstrate any evidence for such a mechanism.[228]

Patients with CLL treated with the purine analogues fludarabine[88,229,230] or cladribine[90] may develop AHA. Risk factors for hemolysis include previous therapy with a purine analogue, high β_2-microglobulin, a positive DAT prior to therapy, and hypogammaglobulinemia. Purine analogues are potent suppressors of T lymphocytes. These drugs may accelerate the preexisting T-cell immune suppression that normally occurs during progression of CLL, exacerbating the underlying tendency to autoimmunity in CLL. However, the degree of depletion of T-cell subsets is similar in patients who develop hemolysis and in patients who do not.

Nonimmunologic Protein Adsorption Less than 5 percent of patients receiving cephalosporin antibiotics develop positive antiglobulin reactions[11] as a result of nonspecific adsorption of plasma proteins to their RBC membranes.[93,94,231] This process may occur within 1 to 2 days after the drug is instituted. Multiple plasma proteins, including immunoglobulins, complement, albumin, fibrinogen, and others, may be detected on RBC membranes in such cases.[231,232] Hemolytic anemia resulting from this mechanism has not been reported. The clinical importance of this phenomenon is its potential to complicate crossmatch procedures unless the drug history is considered. Cephalosporin antibiotics also may induce RBC injury by the hapten mechanism, by the ternary complex mechanism, and by the autoantibody mechanism. The latter reactions are more serious but apparently occur less frequently than nonimmunologic protein adsorption.

● CLINICAL FEATURES

WARM-ANTIBODY AUTOIMMUNE HEMOLYTIC ANEMIA

Presenting complaints of warm-antibody AHA usually are referable to the anemia itself, although occasionally jaundice is the immediate cause for the patient to seek medical advice. Symptom onset usually is slow and insidious over several months, but occasionally a patient has sudden onset of symptoms of severe anemia and jaundice over a period of a few days. In secondary AHA, the symptoms and signs of the underlying disease may overshadow the hemolytic anemia and associated features.

In idiopathic AHA with only mild anemia, results of physical examination may be normal. Even patients with relatively severe hemolytic anemia may have only modest splenomegaly. However, in very severe cases, particularly those of acute onset, patients may present with fever, pallor, jaundice, hepatosplenomegaly, hyperpnea, tachycardia, angina, or heart failure.

Clinical warm-antibody AHA may be aggravated or first become apparent during pregnancy.[166,233,234] Most cases are mild, however, and the prognosis for the fetus is generally good, provided the mother is treated early.[233]

COLD-ANTIBODY AUTOIMMUNE HEMOLYTIC ANEMIA

Most patients with cold agglutinin hemolytic anemia have chronic hemolytic anemia with or without jaundice. In other patients, the principal feature is episodic, acute hemolysis with hemoglobinuria induced by chilling (see discussion of thermal amplitude in "Pathogenic Effects of Cold Agglutinins and Hemolysins" above). Combinations of these clinical features may occur. Acrocyanosis and other cold-mediated vasoocclusive phenomena affecting the fingers, toes, nose, and ears are associated with sludging of RBCs in the cutaneous microvasculature. Skin ulceration and necrosis are distinctly unusual. Hemolysis occurring in *M. pneumoniae* infections is acute in onset, typically appearing as the patient is recovering from pneumonia and coincident with peak titers of cold agglutinins. The hemolysis is self-limited, lasting 1 to 3 weeks.[11] Hemolytic anemia in infectious mononucleosis develops either at the onset of symptoms or within the first 3 weeks of illness.[128]

Other physical findings are variable, depending upon the presence of an underlying disease. Splenomegaly, a characteristic finding in lymphoproliferative diseases or infectious mononucleosis, may be observed in idiopathic cold agglutinin disease.

In paroxysmal cold hemoglobinuria, constitutional symptoms are prominent during a paroxysm. A few minutes to several hours after cold exposure, the patient develops aching pains in the back or legs, abdominal cramps, and perhaps headaches. Chills and fever usually follow. The first urine passed after onset of symptoms typically contains hemoglobin. The constitutional symptoms and hemoglobinuria generally last a few hours. Raynaud phenomenon and cold urticaria sometimes occur during an attack; jaundice may follow.

DRUG-INDUCED IMMUNE HEMOLYTIC ANEMIA

A careful history of drug exposure should be obtained from all patients with hemolytic anemia and/or a positive DAT. As in idiopathic AHA, the clinical picture in drug-induced immune hemolytic anemia is quite variable. The severity of symptoms largely depends upon the rate of hemolysis. In general, patients with hapten/drug adsorption (e.g., penicillin) and autoimmune (e.g., α-methyldopa) types of drug-induced hemolytic anemia exhibit mild to moderate hemolysis, with insidious onset of symptoms developing over a period of days to weeks. In contrast, the ternary complex mechanism (e.g., cephalosporins or quinidine) often causes sudden, severe hemolysis with hemoglobinuria. In the latter setting, hemolysis can occur after only one dose of the drug in a patient previously exposed to the drug. Acute renal failure may accompany severe hemolysis by the ternary complex mechanism.[39,56,58,62,63,86] Several reports indicate that second- and third-generation cephalosporins may cause severe, even fatal, hemolysis by the ternary complex mechanism.[37–39,64]

● LABORATORY FEATURES

GENERAL FEATURES

By definition, patients with AHA present with anemia, the severity of which ranges from life-threatening to very mild. Patients with warm-antibody AHA may present with hematocrit levels less than 10 percent or may have compensated hemolytic anemia and a near-normal hematocrit. For the latter patients, the predominant laboratory features are an increased reticulocyte count and a positive DAT. Occasionally, the patient has leukopenia and neutropenia.[10,235] Platelet counts typically are normal. Rarely, severe immune thrombocytopenia is associated with warm-antibody AHA. This constellation is termed *Evans syndrome*.[236] In this syndrome, the RBC and platelet antibodies are apparently distinct.[237]

Patients with classic chronic cold agglutinin disease exhibit mild to moderate, fairly stable anemia, with hematocrit levels only occasionally as low as 15 to 20 percent. In contrast, patients with paroxysmal cold hemoglobinuria have hematocrit levels that decrease rapidly during a paroxysm. During a paroxysm, leukopenia is noted early, followed by leukocytosis. Complement titers frequently are depressed because of consumption of complement proteins during hemolysis.

In drug-induced immune hemolytic anemia of the hapten/drug adsorption and true autoantibody types, the hematologic findings are similar to those described for spontaneously occurring warm-antibody AHA. Most patients exhibit anemia and reticulocytosis. Leukopenia and thrombocytopenia may be noted in cases of ternary complex-mediated hemolysis.

Evaluation of the blood film can reveal several features related to all types of AHA (Fig. 54–2). Polychromasia indicates a reticulocytosis, reflecting an increased rate of reticulocyte egress from the marrow. Spherocytes are seen in patients with moderate to severe hemolytic anemia. If hereditary spherocytosis can be excluded, this finding suggests an immune hemolytic process. RBC fragments, nucleated RBCs, and occasionally erythrophagocytosis by monocytes may be seen in severe cases (Fig. 54–2). Most patients have mild leukocytosis and neutrophilia. Additionally, patients with cold-antibody AHA may exhibit RBC autoagglutination in the blood film and in chilled anticoagulated blood (Fig. 54–3).

The reticulocyte count usually is elevated. Nevertheless, early in the course of the disease, more than one-third of all patients may have transient reticulocytopenia despite a normal or hyperplastic erythroid marrow.[238–241] The mechanism is unknown, but autoantibodies reactive against antigens on reticulocytes are speculated to lead to their selective destruction.[239] One unusual patient with warm-antibody AHA, reticulocytopenia, and marrow erythroid aplasia had a serum autoantibody that inhibited erythroid colony formation *in vitro*.[242] The aplastic crisis remitted after the serum IgG level was lowered by immunoadsorption. Reticulocytopenia also may be seen in patients with marrow function compromised by an underlying disease, parvovirus infection, toxic chemicals, or nutritional deficiency. Marrow examination usually reveals erythroid hyperplasia and may provide evidence of an underlying lymphoproliferative disorder.

Hyperbilirubinemia (chiefly unconjugated) is highly suggestive of hemolytic anemia, although its absence does not exclude the diagnosis. Total bilirubin is only modestly increased (up to 5 mg/dL) and, with rare exceptions, the conjugated (direct) fraction constitutes less than 15 percent of the total. Urinary urobilinogen is increased regularly, but bile is not detected in the urine unless serum conjugated bilirubin is increased. Usually, serum haptoglobin levels are low, and lactate dehydrogenase levels are elevated. Hemoglobinuria is encountered in rare patients with warm-antibody AHA and hyperacute hemolysis, more commonly in patients with cold agglutinin disease, and characteristically in patients

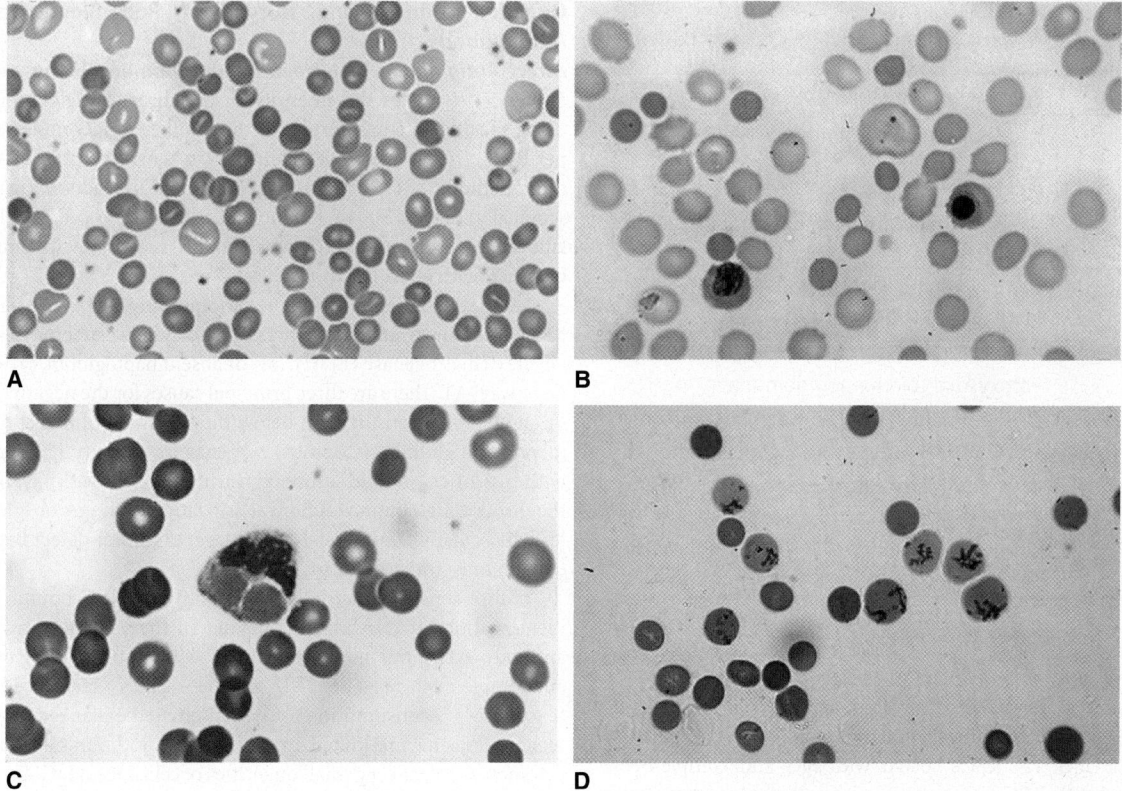

Figure 54–2. A. Blood film. Autoimmune hemolytic anemia. Moderately severe. Note high frequency of microspherocytes (small hyperchromatic RBCs) and the high frequency of macrocytes (putative reticulocytes). **B.** Blood film. Autoimmune hemolytic anemia. Severe. Note the low density of red cells on the film (profound anemia), high frequency of microspherocytes (hyperchromatic), and the large red cells (putative reticulocytes). Note the two nucleated RBCs and the Howell-Jolly body (nuclear remnant) in the macrocyte. Nucleated RBCs and Howell-Jolly bodies may be seen in autoimmune hemolytic anemia with severe hemolysis or after splenectomy. **C.** Blood film. Autoimmune hemolytic anemia. Severe. Monocyte engulfing two red cells (erythrophagocytosis). Note frequent microspherocytes and scant red cell density. **D.** Reticulocyte preparation. Autoimmune hemolytic anemia. Note high frequency of reticulocytes, the large cells with precipitated ribosomes. Remaining cells are microspherocytes. *(Reproduced with permission from Lichtman's Atlas of Hematology, www.accessmedicine.com.)*

with paroxysmal cold hemoglobinuria and with drug-induced immune hemolytic anemia mediated by the ternary complex mechanism.

Direct Antiglobulin Test Pattern

Diagnosis of AHA or drug-induced immune hemolytic anemia requires demonstration of immunoglobulin and/or complement bound to the patient's RBCs. As a screening procedure, use of a "broad-spectrum" antiglobulin (Coombs) reagent—that is, one that contains antibodies directed against human immunoglobulin and complement components (principally C3)—is customary. If agglutination is noted with a broad-spectrum reagent, antisera reacting selectively with IgG (the "gamma" Coombs) or with C3 (the "nongamma" Coombs) are used to define the specific pattern of RBC sensitization. Monospecific antisera to IgM or IgA also have been used in selected cases.

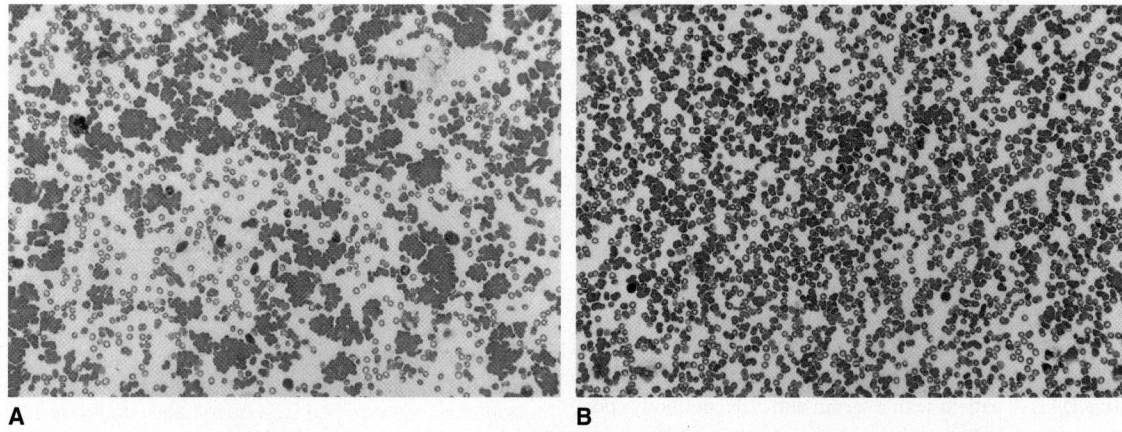

Figure 54–3. Blood films. **A.** Cold-reactive (IgM) antibody. Red cell agglutination at room temperature. **B.** Same blood examined at 37°C. Note marked reduction in agglutination. *(Reproduced with permission from Lichtman's Atlas of Hematology, www.accessmedicine.com.)*

TABLE 54–4. Major Reaction Patterns of the Direct Antiglobulin Test and Associated Types of Immune Injury

Reaction Pattern	Type of Immune Injury
Immunoblobulin (Ig) G alone	Warm-antibody autoimmune hemolytic anemia
	Drug-immune hemolytic anemia: hapten drug adsorption type or autoantibody type
Complement alone	Warm-antibody autoimmune hemolytic anemia with subthreshold IgG deposition
	Cold-agglutinin disease
	Paroxysmal cold hemoglobinuria
	Drug-immune hemolytic anemia: ternary complex type
IgG plus complement	Warm-antibody autoimmune hemolytic anemia
	Drug-immune hemolytic anemia: autoantibody type (rare)

Three possible *major* patterns of direct antiglobulin reaction in AHA and drug-induced immune hemolytic anemia exist: (1) RBCs coated with only IgG, (2) RBCs coated with IgG and complement components, and (3) RBCs coated with complement components without detectable immunoglobulin.[10,123,243,244] In patterns 2 and 3, the complement components most readily detected are C3 fragments (mainly C3dg). Each pattern is associated with accelerated RBC destruction. Positive antiglobulin reactions with anti-IgA or anti-IgM are encountered less commonly, often in association with bound IgG and/or complement.[245-251] Table 54–4 summarizes the diagnostic significance of each of these major patterns (see "Serologic Features" below).

SEROLOGIC FEATURES

Warm-Antibody Autoimmune Hemolytic Anemia

Free versus Bound Autoantibody The autoantibody molecules in patients with warm-antibody AHA exist in a reversible, dynamic equilibrium between RBCs and plasma.[252,253] In addition to the major portion of autoantibody bound to the patient's RBCs (detected by the DAT), "free" autoantibody may be detected in the plasma or serum of these patients by the IAT. In the IAT, the patient's serum or plasma is incubated with normal donor erythrocytes at the appropriate temperature (in this case, 37°C). The cells are washed, suspended in saline solution, and then tested for agglutination by antiglobulin serum. The presence of unbound autoantibody in plasma depends upon the total amount of antibody being produced and the binding affinity of the antibody for RBC antigens. In general, patients whose RBCs are heavily coated with IgG more likely exhibit plasma autoantibody. Protease-modified RBCs are more sensitive than native RBCs in detecting plasma autoantibody, but such data must be interpreted with caution, because alloantibodies, naturally occurring antibodies to cryptic antigens, and other serum components may interact with enzyme-modified RBCs. Patients with a positive IAT as a result of a warm-reactive autoantibody should also have a positive DAT. A patient with a serum anti-RBC antibody (positive IAT) and a negative DAT probably does not have an autoimmune process but rather an alloantibody stimulated by prior transfusion or pregnancy.

Quantity, Affinity, and Isotype of Red Blood Cell–Bound Autoantibody

Direct Antiglobulin Test–Negative Autoimmune Hemolytic Anemia

Figure 54–4 relates the intensity of the direct antiglobulin reaction, using specific anti-IgG serum, to the number of IgG molecules bound per RBC. The latter was determined by a sensitive antibody-consumption method.[254] A trace-positive antiglobulin reaction (read macroscopically) detects 300 to 400 molecules of IgG per cell.[254,255] In another laboratory, a trace-positive antiglobulin reaction with anti-C3 was obtained with 60 to 115 molecules C3 per cell.[182]

Sometimes patients with warm-antibody AHA and many of its hallmarks, for example, anemia, reticulocytosis, spherocytes, elevated lactate dehydrogenase (LDH), low or absent haptoglobin, present with a negative DAT. There are three principal causes for the negative DAT: IgG or complement sensitization below the threshold of detection of commercial antiglobulin (Coombs) reagents; low affinity IgG sensitization with loss of cell-bound antibody during the cell washing steps before the direct antiglobulin reaction; sensitization with IgA or IgM antibodies which many commercial DAT reagents cannot detect because they contain only anti-IgG anti-C3.

More sensitive methods for quantifying RBC-bound IgG allow identification of AHA patients having all the usual features of warm-antibody AHA but a negative DAT with antiimmunoglobulin and anticomplement reagents.[254-256] In these cases, specialized methods (e.g., anti-IgG consumption assays, automated enhanced agglutination techniques, enzyme-linked immunoassays, radioimmunoassays, flow cytometry) detect very small quantities of cell-bound IgG. In such cases, studies with highly concentrated RBC eluates confirm these IgG molecules are warm-reacting anti-RBC autoantibodies.[254] Patients generally have relatively mild hemolysis and often respond favorably to glucocorticoid therapy. By these specialized methods, subthreshold IgG also may be detected in a significant number of patients exhibiting the "complement alone" pattern of direct antiglobulin reaction in the absence of

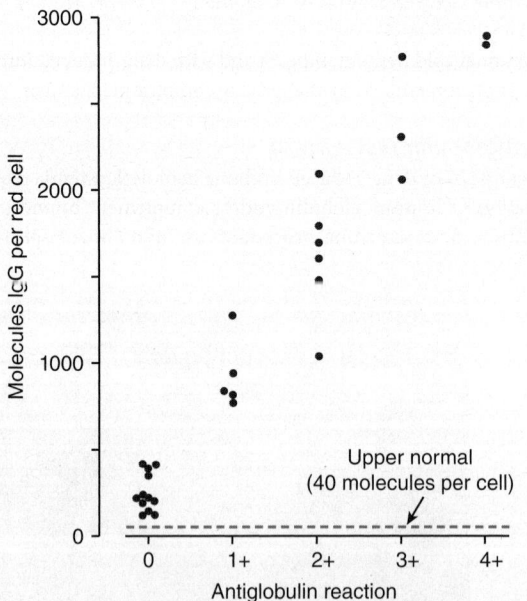

Figure 54–4. Comparison of direct antiglobulin reactions (with anti–immunoglobulin [Ig]G serum) with molecules of red blood cell–bound IgG determined by a quantitative antibody consumption assay (method described by Gilliland and colleagues[247]). The two assays were conducted concurrently on the same blood specimen. The antiglobulin reactions were performed manually and read macroscopically.

drug sensitivity or cold agglutinins. Studies with concentrated RBC eluates suggest subthreshold quantities of bound IgG antibodies are capable of fixing much larger quantities of C3 to the cell membrane.[254] In cases of low-affinity IgG sensitization, detection of IgG bound to RBCs may be accomplished by cold washing (0 to 4°C) or by use of low ionic strength saline in the wash steps prior to the DAT reaction. Cell Bound IgA and IgM may be detected by means of antisera to IgA and IgM. DAT-negative AHA has been reviewed extensively elsewhere.[257–259]

Nature of the Autoantibodies and Red Blood Cell Target Antigens In any series of warm-antibody AHA patients, the correlation between the strength of the antiglobulin reaction (IgG molecules per RBC) and the rate of RBC destruction is variable. The IgG subclass of warm autoantibodies influences the degree to which these antibodies shorten RBC survival. IgG_1 is the most commonly encountered subclass, either alone or in combination with other IgG subclasses.[245,260] IgG_1 and IgG_3 autoantibodies appear to be more effective in decreasing RBC life span than do those of the IgG_2 or IgG_4 subclass.[245,261]

The difference may result from the greater affinity of macrophage Fc receptors for IgG_1 and IgG_3[177,178] and the higher complement-fixing activity of IgG_1 or IgG_3 antibodies relative to the activity of IgG_2 or IgG_4 antibodies.[187]

Autoantibodies eluted from patients' RBCs or present in their plasma typically bind to all the common types of human RBCs represented in test panels used by blood banks and thus might appear to be nonspecific. However, the antibodies of any one patient typically recognize one or more antigenic determinants (epitopes) that are common to almost all human RBCs, that is, "public" antigens. These antibodies have been useful for evaluating RBC membrane structures and for identifying rare RBC phenotypes, namely, RBCs that lack a common blood group antigen(s). Nearly half of all AHA patients have autoantibodies specific for epitopes on Rh proteins.[10,11,131,262,264] The autoantibodies of such patients commonly do not react with human Rh_{null} RBCs, which lack expression of the Rh complex. Occasionally, the anti-Rh autoantibodies have anti-e, anti-E, or anti-c (or, more rarely, anti-D) specificity. Patients who have autoantibodies with selective specificity (e.g., anti-e) nearly always have other autoantibodies reactive with all human RBCs, except Rh_{null}. Autoantibodies with such specificity are designated collectively as Rh related.[136,264]

The remaining patients with warm-antibody AHA have IgG autoantibodies that are fully reactive with Rh_{null} RBCs.[10,11,131,262–264] The exact specificity of the autoantibodies for many of these patients is undefined. However, in other instances, autoantibody specificity for serologically defined blood group antigens outside the Rh system has been identified (using RBCs of appropriate antigen-deficient phenotype) including anti-Wr^b,[131] anti-En^a,[265] anti-LW,[266] anti-U,[267] anti-Ge,[250,268] anti-Sc1,[269] or antibodies to Kell blood group antigens.[270] For ease of reference, the entire group of autoantibodies is designated non-Rh related.[136,264]

Immunochemical studies indicate the autoantibodies from almost any AHA patient react with individual membrane proteins. The major target of Rh-related autoantibodies is a 32- to 34-kDa nonglycosylated polypeptide lacking on Rh_{null} RBCs.[136,271] This polypeptide is similar, if not identical, to the polypeptide expressing the Rh(e) alloantigen. Many α-methyldopa–induced autoantibodies also react with this polypeptide.[136] Autoantibodies with non-Rh serologic specificity react with the band 3 anion transporter[136,272] or with both band 3 and glycophorin A.[136] The latter autoantibodies may react with an epitope formed through the interaction of these two proteins on the RBC membrane.[273] It is interesting to note that anti-RBC autoantibodies in NZB mice exhibit anti–band 3 specificity.[274] Furthermore, naturally occurring anti–band 3 IgG autoantibodies are found in almost all humans.[275,276] These autoantibodies may play a role in the clearance of senescent RBCs by reacting with neoantigens formed on these cells by proteolytic alteration[275] or

aggregation[276] of band 3 proteins. Such neoantigens are not found on younger RBCs. An important but unanswered question concerns the possible relationship between naturally occurring and pathologic anti–band 3 autoantibodies.

Cold-Antibody Hemolytic Anemia

Cold agglutinins are distinguished by their ability to directly agglutinate saline-suspended human RBCs at low temperature, maximally at 0 to 5°C. The reaction is reversible by warming. In chronic cold agglutinin disease, serum titers are commonly 1:1000 or higher and may reach 1:512,000 or more.[11] Cold agglutinins are characteristically IgM. IgA or IgG cold agglutinins have been reported,[11,202,277] sometimes in combination with IgM.[278] In mixed warm- and cold-antibody AHA, warm-reactive IgG autoantibodies are found in association with IgM cold agglutinins.[21]

The DAT result is positive with anticomplement reagents. The antibody itself, however, is not detected by the DAT because the cold agglutinins readily dissociate from the RBCs both *in vivo* and during the washing steps of the standard antiglobulin procedure. In contrast, C4b and C3b are covalently bound to target RBCs via thioester linkages. In one unusual case, a low-titer IgG cold agglutinin could be detected by washing the patient's RBCs in ice-cold saline solution and performing the DAT at 4°C.[277]

The majority of cold agglutinins are reactive with oligosaccharide antigens of the I/i system, which are precursors of the ABH and Lewis blood group substances.[279–281] The I/i determinants are bound to erythrocyte membrane glycoprotein (band 3 anion transporter) or to glycolipids.[280,281] Anti-I and anti-i reportedly bind solubilized RBC glycoproteins at 37°C, suggesting the temperature dependence of cold agglutination of intact RBCs may be a function of temperature-induced conformational effects on the cell surface.[282,283]

I antigens are expressed strongly on adult RBCs but weakly on neonatal (cord) RBCs. The converse is true of i antigens, indicating I/i antigen expression is developmentally regulated.[280] The differences between adult and cord blood RBCs allow evaluation of the serologic specificity of cold agglutinins.[10,11,202] I/i antigens, or structurally related analogues, occur in human saliva, milk, amniotic fluid, and hydatid cyst fluid,[202] and are expressed on human lymphocytes, neutrophils, and monocytes.[284]

Anti-I is the predominant specificity of cold agglutinins in idiopathic cold agglutinin disease, in patients with *M. pneumoniae*, and in some cases of lymphoma. Cold agglutinins with anti-i specificity are found in patients with infectious mononucleosis and in some patients with lymphoma. A small percentage of cold agglutinin-containing sera react equally well with adult and neonatal RBCs. These antibodies recognize antigens outside the I/i system, including Pr antigens, consisting of carbohydrate epitopes of glycophorins that are inactivated by protease treatment[202] and, less commonly, the M or P blood group antigens.[285,286] Most cold agglutinins associated with chickenpox exhibit anti-Pr specificity. A single case with anti-I specificity has been observed.[287] Hemolysis resulting from a cold agglutinin with anti-Pr specificity occurred following an allogeneic marrow transplant.[288]

In hemolytic anemia associated with infectious mononucleosis, the patient's serum may contain IgM anti-i cold agglutinins or cold-reactive nonagglutinating IgG anti-i with IgM cold-reactive anti-IgG antibodies ("rheumatoid factors") that may crosslink the IgG-coated RBCs to produce agglutination.[289]

In paroxysmal cold hemoglobinuria, the direct antiglobulin reaction usually is positive during and briefly following an acute attack because of the coating of surviving RBCs with complement, primarily C3dg fragments. The Donath-Landsteiner antibody is responsible for complement deposition on the cells; it is a nonagglutinating IgG that binds RBCs only in the cold. It readily dissociates from the RBCs at room temperature. In adults subject to recurring episodes in association with cold exposure, the DAT result remains negative between attacks. The antibody is detected by the biphasic Donath-Landsteiner test, in which the patient's fresh serum is incubated with RBCs initially at 4°C and the mixture is then warmed to 37°C.[11] Intense hemolysis occurs. Addition of fresh guinea pig serum or ABO-compatible human serum may be necessary to serve as a source of fresh complement if the patient's serum has been stored or is complement depleted. Antibody titers rarely exceed 1:16. The Donath-Landsteiner antibody typically has specificity for the P blood group antigen, a glycosphingolipid structure.[281] The P antigen also occurs on lymphocytes and skin fibroblasts.[16] The finding of P antigen on skin fibroblasts might be related in some way to the occurrence of cold urticaria in paroxysmal cold hemoglobinuria, a phenomenon that may be transferred passively by serum to normal skin.[10] Antibody specificities for RBC antigens other than the P blood group have been noted.[290]

Drug-Induced Immune Hemolytic Anemia

In the hapten/drug adsorption mechanism of immune injury associated with cephalosporins or penicillin, the patient's drug-coated RBCs bind drug-specific IgG antibody and exhibit positive DAT reactions with anti-IgG. Rarely, both anti-IgG and anti-C3d antisera produce positive DAT reactions. Such cases could have superficial resemblance to warm-antibody AHA. The key serologic difference is that, in this form of drug-induced immune hemolytic anemia, the antibodies in the patient's serum or eluted from the patient's RBCs react *only* with drug-coated RBCs. In contrast, the IgG antibodies in warm-type AHA react with unmodified human RBCs and may show preference for certain known blood groups (e.g., within the Rh complex). Such serologic distinction and the history of exposure to high blood levels of penicillin or a cephalosporin should be instructive.

In hemolysis mediated by the ternary complex mechanism, the DAT is positive with anticomplement serum. Immunoglobulins are only rarely detectable on the patient's RBCs. This pattern is similar to that encountered in AHA mediated by cold agglutinins. Moreover, the brisk type of hemolysis in the ternary complex mechanism also is seen in certain cases of cold-antibody AHA. In the drug-induced cases, however, the cold agglutinin titer and the Donath-Landsteiner test result are normal, and demonstration of serum antibody acting on human RBCs depends upon the presence of the drug in the test system. Thus, the IAT reaction with anticomplement serum may be positive only if the incubation mixture permits interaction of (1) normal RBCs; (2) anti-drug antibody from the patient's serum; (3) the relevant drug, either still in the patient's serum or added *in vitro* in appropriate concentration; and (4) a source of complement, that is, fresh normal serum or the patient's own serum if freshly obtained. A negative result does not necessarily absolve the suspected drug because the critical determinant may be a metabolite of the drug in question. In some cases, use of urine or serum (of the patient or a volunteer taking the drug) as a source of drug metabolite has permitted successful demonstration of a drug-dependent mechanism.[61,218,222,291]

In patients with true autoantibodies as a result of α-methyldopa, the DAT reaction is strongly positive for IgG, but complement only rarely is detected on the patient's RBCs. Autoantibody to RBCs is regularly present in the serum of patients and mediates a positive IAT reaction with unmodified human RBCs, often showing specificity related to the Rh complex. No presently available specific serologic test can separate idiopathic warm-reacting IgG autoantibodies with Rh-related specificities from those induced by α-methyldopa administration. The evidence must be circumstantial, with the helpful knowledge that discontinuation of α-methyldopa, without any form of immunosuppressive therapy,

consistently permits a slow recovery from anemia and a gradual disappearance of anti-RBC antibodies.

Drugs now not known to cause immune RBC injury will be implicated in the future. In any patient with a clinical picture compatible with drug-related immune hemolysis, a reasonable approach is stopping any drug that is suspect while serologic studies are being performed. The patient should be monitored for improvement in hematocrit level, decrease in reticulocytosis, and gradual disappearance of the positive DAT. Repeat challenge with the suspected drug may confirm the diagnosis, but this measure is seldom necessary in patient management and may be unsafe. Therefore, rechallenge to exclude a drug-induced immune hemolytic anemia should be undertaken only for compelling reasons, such as the need to use the specific drug for the patient's illness.

● DIFFERENTIAL DIAGNOSIS

Several nonautoimmune diseases may result in spherocytic anemia, such as hereditary spherocytosis (HS), Zieve syndrome, clostridial sepsis, and the hemolytic anemia preceding Wilson disease. Among the hereditary hemolytic anemias, HS can resemble acquired AHA most closely because the spherocytic anemia associated with HS may be detected first in adulthood (Chap. 46). In addition, splenomegaly may be prominent in both HS and AHA. Family studies of patients with HS, however, usually can identify other affected individuals. Most important, in hereditary hemolytic anemia the DAT is negative.

In hemolytic anemia accompanied by a positive DAT, serologic characterization of the autoantibody may distinguish warm-antibody AHA from cold-reacting autoantibody syndromes. Diagnosis of a drug-induced immune hemolytic anemia depends upon a history of appropriate drug intake supported by compatible serologic findings. In patients who recently received a transfusion, a positive DAT reaction may reflect the binding of a newly formed alloantibody to donor RBCs in the patient's circulation (delayed transfusion reaction; Chap. 138). This finding could lead to a false impression of an autoimmune process.

The venom of the brown recluse spider (*Loxosceles recluse*) may cause severe life-threatening hemolysis.[292,293] The DAT may be positive for IgG and or complement[292,293] and spherocytes and RBC fragments are present on the blood film.[293] The diagnosis should be considered when there is history or evidence by physical examination of a spider bite. The role of IgG and complement in hemolysis is unclear, but the terminal complement inhibitor, eculizumab, inhibits lysis *in vitro*. To date, the clinical use of eculizumab in this population has not been reported.

Recent recipients of allogeneic blood stem cell or solid organ transplantations may develop autoimmune hemolysis.[294] In the former, antibodies are produced by the stem cell graft against RBCs also produced by the stem cell graft; that is, both antibodies and RBCs are of donor origin. In the case of solid-organ transplantations, the recipient's own lymphocytes make antibody against recipient RBCs. In both situations, the autoimmunity is thought to arise from immunosuppressive therapy causing delayed reconstitution or dysfunction of T-cell immunity, leading to development of antibodies autologous to the offended immune system.

Recipients of transplantations may also develop an *allo*immune hemolytic anemia that mimics warm-antibody AHA. The problem is seen in kidney, liver, or hematopoietic stem cell transplantations and usually occurs when an organ from a blood group O donor is transplanted into a blood group A or B recipient. B lymphocytes present in the donated organ or stem cell product form alloantibodies against recipient RBCs.[295–299] Patients of blood group O who receive a stem cell transplant from a donor of blood group A or B may develop a transiently positive DAT and hemolysis of RBCs made by the marrow graft because of temporary persistence of previously synthesized host anti-A or anti-B.[300] Furthermore, some group O stem cell transplantation recipients exhibit mixed hematopoietic chimerism with persistence of host B lymphocytes that can make alloantibodies directed against RBCs made by the stem cell graft.[300] In these settings, the findings of hemolysis and a positive DAT as a result of anti-A and anti-B probably are diagnostic of an alloimmune process, because *auto*antibodies directed against the major blood group antigens A and B are extremely rare.

Other acquired types of hemolytic anemia are less easily confused with either warm- or cold-antibody AHA because spherocytes are not prominent on the blood film and the DAT is negative. Patients with paroxysmal nocturnal hemoglobinuria (PNH) may complain of dark urine (hemoglobinuria). This finding is unusual in patients with warm-antibody AHA but can occur in patients with the cold-antibody syndromes. Decreased levels of CD55 and CD59 on blood cells, detected by flow analysis, are characteristic of PNH but not AHA (Chap. 40). Microangiopathic hemolytic disorders, such as thrombotic thrombocytopenic purpura and hemolytic uremic syndrome, can be distinguished from AHA by examining the blood film. In the microangiopathic hemolytic diseases, the blood film displays marked RBC fragmentation and minimal spherocytosis. In addition, microangiopathic hemolytic anemias more frequently are associated with thrombocytopenia than is either warm- or cold-antibody AHA.

The clinical and laboratory features of chronic cold agglutinin disease are sufficiently distinctive so that the diagnostic possibilities are limited. In general, a high-titer cold agglutinin (>1:512) and a positive DAT with anticomplement serum (but not with anti-IgG) are consistent with cold agglutinin disease. In many instances of drug-induced immune hemolytic anemia, the DAT result also is positive only for complement. The drug history and a low (or absent) cold agglutinin titer, however, help to distinguish drug-induced immune hemolytic anemia from cold agglutinin disease. If the patient has an elevated cold agglutinin level and a positive DAT result with both anti-IgG and anti-C3, then the patient may have a mixed-type AHA. Warm-antibody AHA, hereditary hemolytic disorders, and PNH should be excluded in cases exhibiting primarily a chronic hemolytic anemia. The pattern of antiglobulin reaction, family history, the result of analysis of CD55/CD59 on blood cells provide additional help in difficult cases. When the hemolysis is episodic, paroxysmal cold hemoglobinuria, march hemoglobinuria, and PNH also should be considered. When cold-induced peripheral vasoocclusive symptoms are predominant, the differential diagnosis should include cryoglobulinemia and Raynaud phenomenon, with or without an associated rheumatic disease. Infectious mononucleosis, *M. pneumoniae* infection, and lymphoma can be considered in appropriate clinical settings.

Paroxysmal cold hemoglobinuria must be distinguished from the subset of cases of chronic cold agglutinin disease manifesting episodic hemolysis and hemoglobinuria. This distinction is made primarily in the laboratory. In general, patients with paroxysmal cold hemoglobinuria lack high titers of cold agglutinins. Furthermore, the Donath-Landsteiner antibody is a potent *in vitro* hemolysin, in contrast to most cold agglutinins, which are weak hemolysins. Warm-antibody AHA, march hemoglobinuria, myoglobinuria, and PNH can be distinguished through the history and appropriate laboratory studies.

Immune hemolysis caused by drugs should be distinguished from (1) the warm- or cold-antibody types of idiopathic AHA, (2) congenital hemolytic anemias such as HS, and (3) drug-mediated hemolysis resulting from disorders of red cell metabolism, such as glucose-6-phosphate dehydrogenase deficiency. Patients with drug-induced

immune hemolytic anemia have a positive DAT that distinguishes this group from patients with inherited RBC defects.

● THERAPY

GENERAL

Transfusion

The clinical consequences of AHA or drug-induced immune hemolytic anemia are related to the severity of the anemia and acuity of its onset. Many patients develop anemia over a period sufficient to allow for cardiovascular compensation and hence do not require RBC transfusions. However, RBC transfusions may be necessary and should not be withheld from a patient with an underlying disease complicating the anemia, such as symptomatic coronary artery disease, or a patient who rapidly develops severe anemia with signs and/or symptoms of circulatory failure, as in paroxysmal cold hemoglobinuria or ternary complex drug-induced immune hemolysis.

Transfusion of RBCs in immune hemolytic anemia presents two difficulties: (1) crossmatching and (2) the short half-life of the transfused RBCs (Chap. 138). Finding truly serocompatible donor blood is nearly always impossible except in rare cases when the autoantibody is specific for a defined blood group antigen (see "Serologic Features" above).

It is most important to identify the patient's ABO type so as to avoid a hemolytic transfusion reaction mediated by anti-A or anti-B. This part of the matching process allows for selection of either ABO-identical or -compatible blood for transfusion. With respect to compatibility, the more difficult technical issue relates to the detection of RBC alloantibodies which may be masked by the presence of the autoantibody.

Clinicians often speak of "least incompatible" blood for transfusion, but this term has lately fallen into disrepute because it lacks a precise definition.[301,302] In fact all units will be serologically incompatible but units that are incompatible because of the presence of autoantibody are less dangerous to transfuse than those units that are incompatible because of an alloantibody.

Before transfusing an incompatible unit, the patient's serum must be tested carefully for an alloantibody that could cause a severe hemolytic transfusion reaction against donor RBCs, especially in patients with a history of pregnancy, abortion or prior transfusion.[264,303–305] Patients who have been neither pregnant nor transfused with blood products are unlikely to harbor an alloantibody. Early consultation between the clinician and the blood bank physician is essential. An understanding of the basic aspects of blood compatibility testing, coupled with the knowledge of a patient's pregnancy and transfusion history allow for informed discussion and confident transfusion of mismatched blood if the situation demands.

Once selected, the packed RBCs should be administered slowly and in the case of cold hemolysis syndromes should be brought at least to room temperature. During the transfusion, the patient should be monitored for signs of a hemolytic transfusion reaction (Chap. 138). The transfused cells may be destroyed as fast as or perhaps even faster than the patient's own cells. However, the increased oxygen-carrying capacity provided by the transfused cells may be sufficient to maintain the patient during the acute interval required for other modes of therapy to become effective.

For patients with AHA who require chronic transfusion support, use of prophylactic antigen-matched donor RBCs for transfusion has been proposed as a means of preventing alloimmunization.[306] This process is feasible only in institutions with access to a good selection of phenotyped RBC units and a reference laboratory.[307]

THERAPY OF WARM-ANTIBODY AUTOIMMUNE HEMOLYTIC ANEMIA

Glucocorticoids

Therapy with glucocorticoids has reduced the mortality associated with severe idiopathic warm-antibody AHA. Glucocorticoids were first used for this disorder more than 60 years ago.[308] Glucocorticoids can cause dramatic cessation or marked slowing of hemolysis in about two-thirds of patients.[10,11,123,309,310] Approximately 20 percent of treated patients with warm-antibody AHA achieve complete remission. Approximately 10 percent show minimal or no response to glucocorticoids. The best responses are seen in idiopathic cases or in those related to SLE.

Most patients should be treated with oral prednisone at an initial daily dose of 1 to 1.5 mg/kg (e.g., 50 to 100 mg). Critically ill patients with rapid hemolysis may receive intravenous methylprednisolone 100 to 200 mg in divided doses over the first 24 hours. High doses of prednisone may be required for 10 to 14 days. When the hematocrit stabilizes or begins to increase, the prednisone dose can be decreased in rapid-step dose reductions to approximately 30 mg/day. With continued improvement, the prednisone dose can be further decreased at a rate of 5 mg/day every week, to a dose of 15 to 20 mg/day. These doses should be administered for 2 to 3 months after the acute hemolytic episode has subsided, after which the patient can be weaned from the drug over 1 to 2 months or treatment switched to an alternate-day therapy schedule (e.g., 20 to 40 mg every other day). Alternate-day therapy reduces glucocorticoid side effects but should be attempted only after the patient has achieved stable remission on daily prednisone in the range of 15 to 20 mg/day. Therapy should not be stopped until the DAT becomes negative. Although many patients achieve full remission of their first hemolytic episode, relapses may occur after the glucocorticoids are discontinued. Consequently, patients should be followed for at least several years after treatment. A relapse may require repeat glucocorticoid therapy, splenectomy, or immunosuppression.

Occasionally, patients who present with only a positive DAT, minimal hemolysis, and stable hematocrit require no treatment. However, these patients should be observed for clinical deterioration because the rate of RBC destruction may increase spontaneously.

Glucocorticoids may influence hemolysis in warm-antibody AHA by several mechanisms. Earlier investigators noted that hematologic improvement was often, but not always, accompanied by reduction in the strength of the DAT.[10] The subsequent observation of a decrease in cell-bound and/or free serum autoantibody during stable glucocorticoid-induced remission suggested improved RBC survival following treatment with glucocorticoids resulted from a decrease in synthesis of anti-RBC autoantibodies.[169,252] However, this finding cannot explain why glucocorticoid-treated patients often improve within 24 to 72 hours, a time much shorter than the half-life of anti-RBC autoantibody. Rather, glucocorticoids may suppress RBC sequestration by splenic macrophages.[171,172,183,311] A quantitative decrease in one of the three known classes of Fcγ receptors[170,171] has been observed in the blood monocytes of AHA patients during glucocorticoid therapy.[312]

Splenectomy

Nearly one-third of patients with warm-antibody AHA require prednisone chronically in doses greater than 15 mg/day to maintain an acceptable hemoglobin concentration. These patients are candidates for laparoscopic splenectomy.

Splenectomy removes the primary site of RBC trapping. Investigations in human[169] and animal[171] subjects confirm that maintenance of a given rate of RBC destruction requires 6 to 10 times more RBC-bound IgG in splenectomized subjects than in nonsplenectomized subjects.

Continuation of hemolysis after splenectomy is partly related to persisting high levels of autoantibody, favoring RBC destruction in the liver by hepatic Kupffer cells.[169,171,174]

Several investigators noted the amount of RBC-bound autoantibody decreased in AHA patients following splenectomy.[10,309,313] However, a significant proportion of patients show no change in cell-bound autoantibody following splenectomy. The processes determining the rate of autoantibody production are poorly understood. The beneficial effect of splenectomy may be related to several factors interacting in complex fashion.[314]

A patient's clinical data constitute the best selection criteria for splenectomy. Attempts to select potential responders by ^{51}Cr RBC sequestration studies have been disappointing.[10,309,315] In most cases, a reasonable approach is to continue glucocorticoids for 1 to 2 months while waiting for a maximal response. However, if no response is noted within 3 weeks, the patient's condition deteriorates, or the anemia is very severe, splenectomy should be performed sooner.

Results of splenectomy are variable. Approximately two-thirds of AHA patients have a partial or complete remission following splenectomy.[309,314] However, the relapse rate is disappointingly high. Many patients require further glucocorticoid therapy to maintain acceptable hemoglobin levels, although often at a lower dose than required prior to splenectomy.[10,123,309] Alternate-day therapy is preferable to daily therapy in these cases if adequate control of the anemia can be achieved.

The immediate mortality and morbidity from splenectomy depend upon the presence of underlying disease and the preoperative clinical status but generally are quite low.[316] Following splenectomy, children, more than adults, have an increased risk for developing sepsis as a result of encapsulated organisms.[317] Vaccination against *H. influenzae* type b and pneumococcal and meningococcal organisms is recommended at least 2 weeks prior to surgery (Chap. 56).[318]

Rituximab

Rituximab is a monoclonal antibody directed against the CD20 antigen expressed on B lymphocytes and is used for treatment of B-cell lymphoma. Its use for treatment of AHA is based on the antibody's ability to eliminate B lymphocytes, including, presumably, those making autoantibodies to RBCs. However, the mechanism of action is more complex than that, as the effect of rituximab can occur very early, before the autoantibodies can recede. In fact, sometimes in responding patients, autoantibody levels are not significantly affected.[319,320] Opsonized B lymphocytes may decoy effector monocytes and macrophages from autoantibody complexes and normalize autoreactive T lymphocyte responses.[319]

Rituximab was used initially in refractory AHA either unresponsive to or relapsed after oral glucocorticoid therapy. In a prospective series,[321] 13 of 15 children with warm-antibody AHA responded to rituximab 375 mg/m^2 weekly for 2 to 4 weeks, intravenously. Other case series support the use of similar doses of rituximab in adults, with response rates ranging from 40 to 100 percent.[320,322] Another prospective study in adults exhibited a 100 percent response using rituximab 100 mg/m^2 weekly for 4 weeks along with a short course of oral glucocorticoid as first- or second-line therapy.[323] Sustained responses were observed at 3 years in more than two-thirds of the cases.[324]

A phase 3 randomized controlled trial compared glucocorticoid monotherapy versus glucocorticoid and rituximab 375 mg/m^2 as first-line therapy in patients with warm-antibody AHA.[325] The complete and partial response rates were similar (approximately 50 percent) in the two groups at 3 and 6 months. At 12 and 36 months after randomization the relapse-free survival was superior for the combination of glucocorticoids and rituximab.

Other Immunosuppressive Drugs

Cytotoxic drugs such as cyclophosphamide, 6-mercaptopurine, aza-thioprine, and 6-thioguanine have been given to patients with AHA to suppress synthesis of autoantibody. Direct evidence of such an effect is lacking. Although immunosuppressive therapy is not universally accepted, beneficial responses to immunosuppressive drugs have been observed in some patients who did not respond to glucocorticoids.[11,326] Importantly, the majority of patients with warm-antibody AHA respond to glucocorticoids and/or splenectomy and usually are not candidates for immuno-suppressive therapy. At present, immunosuppressive therapy should be reserved primarily for patients who do not respond to glucocorticoids, rituximab, or splenectomy, or for patients who are poor surgical risks.[326]

The most successful approach used high-dose cyclophosphamide 50 mg/kg ideal body weight per day for 4 consecutive days, intrave-nously, with granulocyte colony-stimulating factor support.[327] Of nine patients, eight of whom had warm autoantibodies, all became trans-fusion independent. All patients had prolonged severe cytopenias and required hospitalization for a median of 21 days. Cyclophosphamide may cause severe hemorrhagic cystitis and sodium 2-mercaptoethane-sulfonate (mesna) 10 mg/kg was given at 3, 6, and 8 hours following each cyclophosphamide dose, to minimize the effect of cyclophos-phamide on the bladder.

For patients who may not tolerate prolonged cytopenias, the drugs of choice are cyclophosphamide 60 mg/m[2] or azathioprine 80 mg/m[2] given daily. If the patient tolerates the drug, continue treatment for up to 6 months while waiting for a response. When response occurs, the patient can be weaned slowly from the drug. If no response is observed, the alternative drug can be tried. Because cyclophosphamide and aza-thioprine suppress hematopoiesis, blood counts, including reticulocyte count, must be monitored with extra care during therapy. Treatment with either agent increases the risk of subsequent neoplasia.

Patients with refractory AHA have been treated effectively with the purine analogue 2-chlorodeoxyadenosine (cladribine)[328] and with mycophenolate mofetil.[329,330] Alemtuzumab was successfully used to treat 5 patients with refractory AHA associated with CLL.[331]

Other Therapies

For patients with chronic compensated hemolysis, treatment with folate at 1 mg/day, orally, is recommended to satisfy the increased demands for the vitamin because of increased red cell production. Plasma exchange or plasmapheresis has been used in patients with warm-antibody AHA. Improvement has been reported in a few cases, but use of the method is controversial.[332,333] A patient with life-threatening warm IgG-mediated AHA refractory to glucocorticoids and splenectomy exhibited rapid clinical improvement following manual whole blood exchange.[334] A patient with severe warm IgM-mediated AHA was successfully treated with C1-esterase inhibitor (C1-inh) resulting in attenuation of comple-ment deposition on RBCs and hemolysis, along with improved recovery of transfused RBCs.[335] Another patient with refractory warm IgM-mediated AHA responded to rituximab and eculizumab.[336] Thymec-tomy has been reported useful in a few children who were refractory to glucocorticoids and splenectomy.[326] Selective injury to splenic macro-phages by administration of vinblastine-loaded, IgG-sensitized platelets reportedly was successful in a few patients.[337] Several anecdotal reports and a case series indicate short-term successful treatment of patients with AHA using high-dose intravenous γ-globulin.[338-341] Uncontrolled studies indicate danazol, a nonvirilizing androgen, may be useful in patients with AHA.[342,343] Danazol may eliminate the need for splenec-tomy when combined with prednisone and may allow for a shorter duration of prednisone therapy.[343] Some patients with ulcerative coli-tis and AHA unresponsive to glucocorticoids and splenectomy may respond to colectomy.[344] In patients with AHA associated with an ovar-ian dermoid cyst, cyst removal produces remission of the hemolysis.[345]

THERAPY OF COLD-ANTIBODY HEMOLYTIC ANEMIA

Keeping the patient warm, particularly the patient's extremities, is moderately effective in providing symptomatic relief. This action may be the only measure required in patients with mild chronic hemoly-sis. In symptomatic patients, rituximab is effective and well tolerated. In two prospective trials, approximately half the patients responded to rituximab 375 mg/m[2] weekly for 4 weeks.[346,347] Patients who relapsed responded to a second course of rituximab at about the same rate. In a prospective trial of rituximab and fludarabine, the response rate was 76 percent, including complete responses in 21 percent with a median response duration of 66 months.[348] In another small study, 60 percent of patients responded to low dose rituximab, 100 mg/m[2], a rate compa-rable to that seen with rituximab 375 mg/m[2].[323] Chlorambucil or cyclo-phosphamide may be helpful for patients with symptomatic chronic cold agglutinin disease.[9-11,349,350] In patients with lymphoma, treatment of the underlying disorder usually results in control of the cold agglu-tinin disease. Single patients with refractory cold agglutinin disease have exhibited responses to eculizumab[351,352] and bortezomib.[353] Results of splenectomy[10,11,354] or use of glucocorticoids[10,11] generally have been disappointing, although exceptions have been reported,[10,196,277,278] par-ticularly in atypical cases. Experimental[171] and clinical[196] bases exist for considering very high doses of glucocorticoids in seriously ill patients. RBC transfusions generally are reserved for patients with severe anemia of rapid onset who are in danger of cardiorespiratory complications. Washed RBCs often are used to avoid replenishing depleted comple-ment components and reactivating the hemolytic process. In critically ill patients, plasma exchange (with replacement by albumin-containing saline solution) may provide transient amelioration of hemolysis.[355-357]

In patients with cold agglutinin disease secondary to infection, spontaneous resolution of the hemolysis is expected in all patients after resolution of the infection. RBC transfusion may be required as a tem-porizing measure and in severe cases, plasma exchange may be bene-ficial. There is little evidence to support the use of glucocorticoids or antiviral therapy.

Most contemporary cases of paroxysmal cold hemoglobinuria are self-limited. Acute attacks in both chronic and transient forms of parox-ysmal cold hemoglobinuria may be prevented by avoiding cold exposure. Glucocorticoid therapy and splenectomy have not been useful. When paroxysmal cold hemoglobinuria is associated with syphilis, effective treatment of the infection may result in complete remission. Antihis-taminic and adrenergic agents may relieve symptoms of cold urticaria.

THERAPY OF DRUG-INDUCED IMMUNE HEMOLYTIC ANEMIA

Discontinuation of the offending drug often is the only treatment needed. This measure is essential and may be lifesaving in patients with severe hemolysis mediated by the ternary complex mechanism.

In the past, high-dose penicillin was not necessarily discontinued because of a positive DAT alone. A change in therapy was considered mainly in the presence of overt hemolytic anemia. For example, lower-ing the penicillin dose and coadministering other antibiotics sometimes allowed continuation of the drug, particularly if hemolysis was not severe. For other drugs causing only mild hemolysis by the hapten-drug adsorption mechanism, in the unlikely event that no alternatives are available, a similar approach may be effective.

In patients taking α-methyldopa in the absence of hemolysis, a positive DAT has not necessarily been an indication for stopping the drug. However, given all the choices available, it is prudent to consider alternative antihypertensive therapy. Because less information on the natural history of autoantibodies induced by drugs other than α-methyldopa is available, discontinuation of the offending drug is advisable unless no suitable alternative exists.

Glucocorticoids are generally unnecessary, and their efficacy is questionable. However, prednisone is effective in patients with CLL and autoimmune hemolysis caused by purine analogues,[88,89] as are cyclosporine, rituximab, and intravenous immunoglobulin.[230] For treatment of CLL, combination of cyclophosphamide with fludarabine, with or without rituximab, seems to reduce the frequency of fludarabine-induced AHA.[229,230] Transfusions should be given in the unusual circumstance of severe, life-threatening anemia. Problems with crossmatching, similar to those encountered in warm-antibody AHA, may occur in patients with a strongly positive IAT, for example, in α-methyldopa–related cases. Patients with hemolytic anemia resulting from the hapten/drug adsorption mechanism should have a compatible crossmatch because the serum antibody reacts only with drug-coated cells. However, if therapy with the offending drug is still in progress, transfused cells may be destroyed at an increased rate as they become coated with drug *in vivo.* Patients with ternary complex–mediated hemolysis will also hemolyze transfused RBCs until the offending drug clears from the plasma.

Several cases of transfusion-associated graft-versus-host disease as a result of purine analogues have been reported in CLL patients transfused for hemolysis.[90,358,359] Such patients, who have an immunodeficiency state secondary to CLL, impairing their ability to eliminate the transfused lymphocytes, should receive irradiated blood products.

● COURSE AND PROGNOSIS

Patients with idiopathic warm-antibody AHA have unpredictable clinical courses characterized by relapses and remissions. No particular feature of the illness has been a consistent predictor of outcome. Despite a rather high initial rate of response to glucocorticoids and splenectomy, the overall mortality rate was significant (up to 46 percent) in several older series, but much lower in more recent studies.[10,11,309,360,361] The actuarial survival at 10 years reportedly is 73 percent.[360]

Pulmonary emboli, infection, and cardiovascular collapse are causes of death. Thromboembolic episodes in the form of deep vein thrombosis or splenic infarcts are relatively common during active phases of the disease.[309,361] In one series, 8 of 30 patients with AHA developed venous thromboembolism; 19 of the patients had antiphospholipid antibodies, including six of the eight patients with thromboembolism.[362] In another retrospective analysis of 36 exacerbations of severe AHA in 28 patients, only six of whom were tested and found negative for antiphospholipid antibodies, venous thromboembolism occurred in 5 of 15 exacerbations without anticoagulation and in 1 of 21 with anticoagulation.[363] The contribution of antiphospholipid antibodies to morbidity and mortality in AHA is not clear from these data. However, it seems prudent to consider prophylactic anticoagulation for patients with AHA and antiphospholipid antibodies or other risk factors for venous thromboembolism.

The prognosis in secondary warm-antibody AHA largely depends upon the course of the underlying disease.

In children, warm-antibody AHA frequently follows an acute infection or immunization.[313,364,365] Most of these patients exhibit a self-limited course and respond rapidly to glucocorticoids. Those who recover from the initial hemolytic episode have a good prognosis and are unlikely to relapse, although exceptions are known. Children with chronic AHA tend to be older.[364,365] The overall mortality rate is lower

than in adults, ranging from 4 to 30 percent,[313,364–369] with higher mortality rates in those with chronic AHA[313,368,369] and associated autoimmune thrombocytopenia (Evans syndrome).[369,370] Evans syndrome was noted in 37 percent of children with AHA in one large study, a much higher frequency than observed in adults.[369]

Patients with idiopathic cold agglutinin disease often have a relatively benign course and survive for many years.[9–11] Occasionally, death results from infection or severe anemia or, not uncommonly, from an underlying lymphoproliferative process.

The postinfectious forms of cold agglutinin disease typically are self-limited. Recovery generally occurs in a few weeks. A few cases with massive hemoglobinuria have been complicated by acute renal failure, requiring temporary hemodialysis.

Postinfectious forms of paroxysmal cold hemoglobinuria terminate spontaneously within a few days to weeks after onset,[12–15] although the Donath-Landsteiner antibody may persist in low titer for several years.[10] Most patients with chronic idiopathic paroxysmal cold hemoglobinuria survive for many years despite occasional paroxysms of hemolysis.

Immune hemolysis in response to drugs usually is mild, and the prognosis is good. Occasional episodes of exceptionally severe hemolysis with renal failure or death have been reported, usually because of drugs operating through the ternary complex mechanism or purine analogues in patients with CLL.[39,56,58,62–65,67,86,108,109] In hemolysis resulting from ternary complex or hapten/drug adsorption mechanisms, the DAT becomes negative shortly after the drug is discontinued, that is, soon after the drug clears from the circulation. In addition, the hemolysis associated with α-methyldopa–induced autoantibodies ceases promptly after drug cessation. However, a positive DAT of gradually diminishing intensity may remain for weeks or months.

REFERENCES

1. Packman C: Historical review: The spherocytic haemolytic anaemias. *Br J Haematol* 112:888, 2001.
2. Coombs RRA, Mourant AE, Race EE: A new test for the detection of weak and incomplete Rh agglutinins. *Br J Exp Pathol* 26:255, 1945.
3. Boorman KE, Dodd BE, Loutit JF: Haemolytic icterus (acholuric jaundice), congenital and acquired. *Lancet* 1:812, 1946.
4. Loutit JF, Mollison PL: Haemolytic icterus (acholuric jaundice), congenital and acquired. *J Pathol Bacteriol* 58:711, 1946.
5. Landsteiner K: Uber Beziehungen zwischen dem Blutserum und den Körperzeller. *Munch Med Wochenschr* 50:1812, 1903.
6. Clough MC, Richter IM: A study of an autoagglutinin occurring in a human serum. *Bull Johns Hopkins Hosp* 29:86, 1918.
7. Iwai S, Mei-Sai N: Etiology of Raynaud's disease: A preliminary report. *Jpn Med World* 5:119, 1925.
8. Iwai S, Mei-Sai N: Etiology of Raynaud's disease. *Jpn Med World* 6:345, 1926.
9. Schubothe H: The cold hemagglutinin disease. *Semin Hematol* 3:27, 1966.
10. Dacie JV: *The Haemolytic Anaemias,* vol 3, *The Autoimmune Haemolytic Anaemias,* 3d ed. Churchill Livingstone, New York, 1992.
11. Petz LD, Garratty G: *Immune Hemolytic Anemias.* Churchill Livingstone, Philadelphia, 2004.
12. Nordhagen R, Stensvold K, Winsnes A, et al: Paroxysmal cold hemoglobinuria. The most frequent autoimmune hemolytic anemia in children? *Acta Paediatr Scand* 73:258, 1984.
13. Wolach B, Heddle N, Barr RD, et al: Transient Donath-Landsteiner hemolytic anemia. *Br J Haematol* 48:425, 1981.
14. Sokol RJ, Hewitt S, Stamps BK: Autoimmune hemolysis associated with Donath-Landsteiner antibodies. *Acta Haematol* 68:268, 1982.
15. Gottsche B, Salama A, Mueller-Eckhardt C: Donath-Landsteiner autoimmune hemolytic anemia in children: A study of 22 cases. *Vox Sang* 58:281, 1990.
16. Fellous M, Gerbal A, Tessier C, et al: Studies on the biosynthetic pathway of human P erythrocyte antigens using somatic cells in culture. *Vox Sang* 26:518, 1974.
17. Ackroyd JF: The pathogenesis of thrombocytopenic purpura due to hypersensitivity to sedormid. *Clin Sci (Lond)* 7:249, 1949.
18. Snapper I, Marks D, Schwartz L, Hollander L: Hemolytic anemia secondary to mesantoin. *Ann Intern Med* 39:619, 1953.
19. Harris JW: Studies on the mechanism of drug-induced hemolytic anemia. *J Lab Clin Med* 47:760, 1956.

20. Sokol RJ, Hewitt S, Stamps BK: Autoimmune haemolysis: An 18-year study of 865 cases referred to a regional transfusion centre. *Br Med J* 282:2023, 1981.

21. Sokol RJ, Hewitt S, Stamps BK: Autoimmune haemolysis: Mixed warm and cold antibody type. *Acta Haematol* 69:266, 1983.

22. Shulman IA, Branch DR, Nelson JM, et al: Autoimmune hemolytic anemias with both cold and warm autoantibodies. *JAMA* 253:1746, 1985.

23. Kajii E, Miura Y, Ikemoto S: Characterization of autoantibodies in mixed-type autoimmune hemolytical anemia. *Vox Sang* 60:45, 1991.

24. Berentsen S, Bo K, Shammas F, et al: Chronic cold agglutinin disease of the "idiopathic" type is a premalignant or low-grade malignant lymphoproliferative disease. *APMIS* 105:354, 1997.

25. Telen MJ, Roberts KB, Bartlett JA: HIV-associated autoimmune hemolytic anemia: Report of a case and review of the literature. *J Acquir Immune Defic Syndr* 3:933, 1990.

26. Rapoport AP, Rowe JM, McMican A: Life-threatening autoimmune hemolytic anemia in patient with acquired immune deficiency syndrome. *Transfusion* 28:190, 1988.

27. Saif M: HIV Associated autoimmune hemolytic anemia: An update. *AIDS Patient Care* 15:217, 2001.

28. VanArsdel PP Jr, Gilliland BC: Anemia secondary to penicillin treatment: Studies on two patients with non-allergic serum hemagglutinins. *J Lab Clin Med* 65:277, 1965.

29. Petz LD, Fudenberg HH: Coombs-positive hemolytic anemia caused by penicillin administration. *N Engl J Med* 274:171, 1966.

30. Swanson MA, Chanmougan D, Schwartz RS: Immuno-hemolytic anemia due to antipenicillin antibodies. *N Engl J Med* 274:178, 1966.

31. Levine B, Redmond A: Immunochemical mechanisms of penicillin-induced Coombs positivity and hemolytic anemia in man. *Int Arch Allergy Appl Immunol* 1:594, 1967.

32. White JM, Brown DL, Hepner GW, Worlledge SM: Penicillin-induced hemolytic anaemia. *Br Med J* 3:26, 1968.

33. Seldon MR, Bain B, Johnson CA, Lennox CS: Ticarcillin-induced immune haemolytic anaemia. *Scand J Haematol* 28:459, 1982.

34. Tuffs L, Manoharan A: Flucloxacillin-induced haemolytic anaemia. *Med J Aust* 144:559, 1986.

35. Gralnick HR, McGinnis MH, Elton W, McCurdy P: Hemolytic anemia associated with cephalothin. *JAMA* 217:1193, 1971.

36. Branch DR, Berkowitz LR, Becker RL, et al: Extravascular hemolysis following the administration of cefamandole. *Am J Hematol* 18:213, 1985.

37. Chambers LA, Donovan BA, Kruskall MS: Ceftazidime-induced hemolysis patient with drug-dependent antibodies reactive by immune complex and drug adsorption mechanisms. *Am J Clin Pathol* 95:393, 1991.

38. Gallagher NI, Schergen AK, Sokol-Anderson ML, et al: Severe immune-mediated hemolytic anemia secondary to treatment with cefotetan. *Transfusion* 32:266, 1992.

39. Garratty G, Nance S, Lloyd M, Domen R: Fatal immune hemolytic anemia due to cefotetan. *Transfusion* 32:269, 1992.

40. Wenz B, Klein RL, Lalezari P: Tetracycline-induced immune hemolytic anemia. *Transfusion* 14:265, 1974.

41. Simpson MB, Pryzbylik J, Innis B, Denham MA: Hemolytic anemia after tetracycline therapy. *N Engl J Med* 312:840, 1985.

42. Pujol M, Fernandez F, Sancho JM, et al: Immune hemolytic anemia induced by 6-mercaptopurine. *Transfusion* 40:75, 2000.

43. Steanini M, Johnson NL: Positive antihuman globulin test in patients receiving carbromal. *Am J Med Sci* 259:49, 1970.

44. Bird GWG, Eccles GH, Litchfield JA, et al: Haemolytic anaemia associated with antibodies to tolbutamide and phenacetin. *Br Med J* 1:728, 1972.

45. Malacarne P, Castaldi G, Bertusi M, Zavagli G: Tolbutamide-induced hemolytic anemia. *Diabetes* 26:156, 1977.

46. Salama A, Mueller-Eckhardt C: Cianidanol and its metabolites bind tightly to red cells and are responsible for the production of auto- and/or drug-dependent antibodies against these cells. *Br J Haematol* 66:263, 1987.

47. Martinengo M, Ardenghi DF, Tripodi G, Reali G: The first case of drug-induced immune hemolytic anemia due to hydrocortisone. *Transfusion* 48:1925, 2008.

48. Arndt P, Garratty G, Isaak E, et al: Positive direct and indirect antiglobulin tests associated with oxaliplatin can be due to drug antibody and or drug-induced nonimmunologic protein adsorption. *Transfusion* 49:711, 2009.

49. Arndt PA, Garratty G, Brasfield FM, et al: Immune hemolytic anemia due to cimetidine: The first example of a cimetidine antibody. *Transfusion* 50:302, 2010.

50. Muirhead EE, Halden ER, Groves M: Drug-dependent Coombs (antiglobulin) test and anemia: Observations on quinine and acetophenetidin (phenacetin). *Arch Intern Med* 101:827, 1958.

51. Croft JD Jr, Swisher SN, Gilliland BC, et al: Coombs test positivity induced by drugs: Mechanisms of immunologic reactions and red cell destruction. *Ann Intern Med* 68:176, 1968.

52. Freedman AL, Barr PS, Brody E: Hemolytic anemia due to quinidine: Observations on its mechanism. *Am J Med* 20:806, 1956.

53. Logue GL, Boyd AE, Rosse WF: Chlorpropamide-induced immune hemolytic anemia. *N Engl J Med* 283:900, 1970.

54. Kopicky JA, Packman CH: The mechanisms of sulfonylurea-induced immune hemolysis. Case report and review of the literature. *Am J Hematol* 23:283, 1986.

55. Kashyap AS, Kashyap S: Hemolytic anemia due to metformin. *Postgrad Med J* 76:125, 2000.

56. Pereira A, Sanz C, Cervantes F, Castillo R: Immune hemolytic anemia and renal failure associated with rifampicin-dependent antibodies with anti-I specificity. *Ann Hematol* 63:56, 1991.

57. Bengtsson U, Staffan A, Aurell M, Kaijser B: Antazoline-induced immune hemolytic anemia, hemoglobinuria and acute renal failure. *Acta Med Scand* 198:223, 1975.

58. Habibi B, Basty R, Chodez S, Prunat A: Thiopental-related immune hemolytic anemia and renal failure. *N Engl J Med* 312:353, 1985.

59. Squires JE, Mintz PD, Clark S: Tolmetin-induced hemolysis. *Transfusion* 25:410, 1985.

60. Sosler SD, Behzad V, Garratty G, et al: Immune hemolytic anemia associated with probenecid. *Am J Clin Pathol* 84:391, 1985.

61. Salama A, Mueller-Eckhardt C: Two types of nomifensine-induced immune haemolytic anaemias: Drug-dependent sensitization and/or auto-immunization. *Br J Haematol* 64:613, 1986.

62. Habibi B, Cartron JP, Bretagne M, et al: Anti-nomifensine antibody causing immune hemolytic anemia and renal failure. *Vox Sang* 40:79, 1981.

63. Fulton JD, Briggs JD, Dominiczak AF, et al: Intravascular haemolysis and acute renal failure induced by nomifensine. *Scott Med J* 31:242, 1986.

64. Garratty G, Postoway N, Schwellenbach J, McMahill PC: A fatal case of ceftriaxone (Rocephin)-induced hemolytic anemia associated with intravascular immune hemolysis. *Transfusion* 31:176, 1991.

65. Rosenfeld CS, Winters SJ, Tedrow HE: Diethylstilbestrol-associated hemolytic anemia with a positive direct antiglobulin test result. *Am J Med* 86:617, 1989.

66. Salama A, Burger M, Mueller-Eckhardt C: Acute immune hemolysis induced by a degradation product of amphotericin B. *Blut* 58:59, 1989.

67. Wolf B, Conradty M, Grohmann R, et al: A case of immune complex hemolytic anemia, thrombocytopenia, and acute renal failure associated with doxepin use. *J Clin Psychiatry* 50:99, 1989.

68. Salama A, Kroll H, Wittmann G, Mueller-Eckhardt C: Diclofenac-induced immune haemolytic anaemia: Simultaneous occurrence of red blood cell autoantibodies and drug-dependent antibodies. *Br J Haematol* 95:640, 1996.

69. Bougie D, Johnson ST, Weitekamp LA, Aster RH: Sensitivity to metabolite of diclofenac as a cause of acute immune hemolytic anemia. *Blood* 90:407, 1997.

70. Cunha PD, Lord RS, Johnson ST, et al: Immune hemolytic anemia caused by sensitivity to a metabolite of etodolac, a nonsteroidal anti-inflammatory drug. *Transfusion* 40:663, 2000.

71. Park GM, Han KS, Chang YH, et al: Immune hemolytic anemia after treatment with pemetrexed for lung cancer. *J Thorac Oncol* 3:196 2008.

72. Mayer B, Leo A, Herziger A, et al: Intravascular hemolysis caused by the contrast medium iomeprol. *Transfusion* 53:2141, 2013.

73. Carstairs KC, Breckenridge A, Dollery CT, Worlledge SM: Incidence of a positive direct Coombs test in patients on alpha-methyldopa. *Lancet* 2:133, 1966.

74. Worlledge SM, Carstairs KC, Dacie JV: Autoimmune haemolytic anaemia associated with α-methyldopa therapy. *Lancet* 2:135, 1966.

75. Breckenridge A, Dollery CT, Worlledge SM, et al: Positive direct Coombs tests and antinuclear factors in patients treated with methyldopa. *Lancet* 2:1265, 1967.

76. Lo Buglio AF, Jandl JH: The nature of alpha-methyldopa red cell antibody. *N Engl J Med* 276:658, 1967.

77. Cotzias GC, Papavasiliou PS: Autoimmunity in patients treated with levodopa. *JAMA* 207:1353, 1969.

78. Henry RE, Goldberg LS, Sturgeon P, Ansel RD: Serologic abnormalities associated with L-dopa therapy. *Vox Sang* 20:306, 1971.

79. Joseph C: Occurrence of positive Coombs test in patients treated with levodopa. *N Engl J Med* 286:1400, 1972.

80. Gabor EP, Goldberg LS: Levodopa-induced Coombs positive haemolytic anaemia. *Scand J Haematol* 11:201, 1973.

81. Territo MC, Peters RW, Tanaka KR: Autoimmune hemolytic anemia due to levodopa therapy. *JAMA* 226:1347, 1973.

82. Scott GL, Myles AB, Bacon PA: Autoimmune haemolytic anaemia and mefenamic acid therapy. *Br Med J* 3:543, 1968.

83. Robertson JH, Kennedy CC, Hill CM: Haemolytic anaemia associated with mefenamic acid. *Ir J Med Sci* 140:226, 1971.

84. Habibi B: Drug-induced red blood cell autoantibodies co-developed with drug-specific antibodies causing a hemolytic anaemia. *Br J Haematol* 61:139, 1985.

85. Kleinman S, Nelson R, Smith L, Goldfinger D: Positive direct antiglobulin tests and immune hemolytic anemia in patients receiving procainamide. *N Engl J Med* 311:809, 1984.

86. Kramer MR, Levene C, Hershko C: Severe reversible autoimmune haemolytic anaemia and thrombocytopenia associated with diclofenac therapy. *Scand J Haematol* 36:118, 1986.

87. Byrd JC, Hertler AA, Weiss RB, et al: Fatal recurrence of autoimmune hemolytic anemia following pentostatin therapy in a patient with a history of fludarabine-associated hemolytic anemia. *Ann Oncol* 6:300, 1995.

88. Weiss R, Freiman J, Kweder S, et al: Hemolytic anemia after fludarabine therapy for chronic lymphocytic leukemia. *J Clin Oncol* 16:1885, 1998.

89. Garratty, G: Immune hemolytic anemia associated with drug therapy. *Blood Rev* 24:143, 2010.

90. Chasty RC, Myint H, Oscier DG, et al: Autoimmune haemolysis in patients with B-CLL treated with chlorodeoxyadenosine (CDA). *Leuk Lymphoma* 29:391, 1998.

91. Kwan JM, Reese AM, Trafeli JP: Delayed autoimmune hemolytic anemia in efalizumab-treated psoriasis. *J Am Acad Dermatol* 58:1053, 2008.

92. Darabi K, Kantamnei S, Weirnik PH: Lenalidomide-induced warm autoimmune hemolytic anemia. *J Clin Oncol* 24:e59, 2006.

93. Gralnick HR, Wright LD, McGinnis MH: Coombs' positive reactions associated with sodium cephalothin therapy. *JAMA* 199:725, 1967.

94. Molthan L, Reidenberg MM, Eichman MF: Positive direct Coombs' tests due to cephalothin. *N Engl J Med* 277:123, 1967.

95. Zeger G, Smith L, McQuiston D, Goldfinger D: Cisplatin-induced nonimmunologic adsorption of immunoglobulin by red cells. *Transfusion* 28:493, 1988.

96. Muirhead EE, Groves M, Guy R, et al: Acquired hemolytic anemia, exposures to insecticides and positive Coombs' test dependent on insecticide preparations. *Vox Sang* 4:277, 1959.

97. Lindberg LG, Norden A: Severe hemolytic reaction to chlorpromazine. *Acta Med Scand* 170:195, 1961.

98. Eyster ME: Melphalan (Alkeran) erythrocyte agglutinin and hemolytic anemia. *Ann Intern Med* 66:573, 1967.

99. Robinson MG, Foadi M: Hemolytic anemia with positive Coombs' test. Association with isoniazid therapy. *JAMA* 208:656, 1969.

100. Mueller-Eckhardt C, Kretschmer V, Coburg KH: Allergic, immunohemolytic anemia due to para-aminosalicylic acid (PAS). Immunohematologic studies of three cases. *Dtsch Med Wochenschr* 97:234, 1972.

101. Manor E, Marmor A, Kaufman S, Leiba H: Massive hemolysis caused by acetaminophen. *JAMA* 236:2777, 1976.

102. Vilal JM, Blum L, Dosik H: Thiazide-induced immune hemolytic anemia. *JAMA* 236:1723, 1976.

103. Letona JM-L, Barbolla L, Frieyro E, et al: Immune haemolytic anaemia and renal failure induced by streptomycin. *Br J Haematol* 35:561, 1977.

104. Korsager S, Sorensen H, Jensen OH, Falk JV: Antiglobulin tests for determination of autoimmunohaemolytic anaemia during long-term treatment with ibuprofen. *Scand J Rheumatol* 10:174, 1981.

105. Takahashi H, Tsukada T: Triamterene-induced immune hemolytic anemia with acute intravascular hemolysis and acute renal failure. *Scand J Haematol* 23:169, 1979.

106. Wong KY, Boose GM, Issitt CH: Erythromycin-induced hemolytic anemia. *J Pediatr* 98:647, 1981.

107. Sandvei P, Nordhagen R, Michaelsen TE, Wolthuis K: Fluorouracil (5-FU) induced acute immune haemolytic anaemia. *Br J Haematol* 65:357, 1987.

108. Tafani O, Mazzoli M, Landini G, Alterini B: Fatal acute immune haemolytic anaemia caused by nalidixic acid. *Br Med J* 285:936, 1982.

109. Angeles ML, Reid ME, Yacob UA, et al: Sulindac-induced immune hemolytic anemia. *Transfusion* 34:255, 1994.

110. Marks DR, Joy JV, Bonheim NA: Hemolytic anemia associated with the use of omeprazole. *Am J Gastroenterol* 86:217, 1991.

111. Blum MD, Graham DJ, McCloskey CA: Temafloxacin syndrome: Review of 95 cases. *Clin Infect Dis* 18:946, 1994.

112. Marani TM, Trich MB, Armstrong KS, et al: Carboplatin-induced immune hemolytic anemia. *Transfusion* 36:1016, 1996.

113. Freercks RJ, Mehta U, Stead DF, Meintjes GA: Haemolytic anaemia associated with efavirenz. *AIDS* 20:1212, 2006.

114. Mayer B, Genth R, Dehner R, Salama A: The first example of a patient with etoricoxib-induced immune hemolytic anemia. *Transfusion* 53:1033, 2013.

115. Sheikh-Taha M, Frenn P: Autoimmune hemolytic anemia induced by levofloxacin. *Case Reports in Infectious Diseases*, 2014. http://dx.doi.org/10.1155/2014/201015

116. Chen F, Liu S, Wu J: Puerarin-induced immune hemolytic anemia. *Int J Hematol* 98:112, 2013

117. Gurbuz F, Yagci-Kupeli B, Kor Y, et al: The first report of cabergoline-induced immune hemolytic anemia in an adolescent with prolactinoma. *J Pediatr Endocrinol Metab* 27:159, 2013.

118. Chaplin H, Avioli LV: Autoimmune hemolytic anemia. *Arch Intern Med* 137:346, 1977.

119. Sallah S, Wan J, Hanrahan L: Future development of lymphoproliferative disorders in patients with autoimmune hemolytic anemia. *Clin Cancer Res* 7:791, 2001.

120. Pirofsky B: Hereditary aspects of autoimmune hemolytic anemia: A retrospective analysis. *Vox Sang* 14:334, 1968.

121. Dobbs CE: Familial auto-immune hemolytic anemia. *Arch Intern Med* 116:273, 1965.

122. Cordova MS, Baez-Villasenor J, Mendez JJ, Campos E: Acquired hemolytic anemia with positive antiglobulin (Coombs' test) in mother and daughter. *Arch Intern Med* 117:692, 1966.

123. Eyster ME, Jenkins DE Jr: Erythrocyte coating substances in patients with positive direct antiglobulin reactions: Correlation of gamma-G globulin and complement coating with underlying diseases, overt hemolysis and response to therapy. *Am J Med* 46:360, 1969.

124. Feizi T: Cold agglutinins, the direct Coombs' test and serum immunoglobulins in *Mycoplasma pneumoniae* infection. *Ann N Y Acad Sci* 143:801, 1967.

125. Jacobson LB, Longstreth GF, Edington TS: Clinical and immunologic features of transient cold agglutinin hemolytic anemia. *Am J Med* 54:514, 1973.

126. Murray HW, Masur H, Senterfit LB, Roberts RB: The protean manifestations of *Mycoplasma pneumoniae* infection in adults. *Am J Med* 58:229, 1975.

127. Rosenfield RE, Schmidt PJ, Calvo RC, McGinniss MH: Anti-i, a frequent cold agglutinin in infectious mononucleosis. *Vox Sang* 10:631, 1965.

128. Worrledge SM, Dacie JV: Haemolytic and other anaemias in infectious mononucleosis, in *Infectious Mononucleosis*, edited by RL Carter, HG Penman, p 82. Blackwell Science, Oxford, 1969.

129. Hossaini AA: Anti-i in infectious mononucleosis. *Am J Clin Pathol* 53:198, 1970.

130. Arndt P, Garratty G: Cross-reactivity of cefotetan and ceftriaxone antibodies, associated with hemolytic anemia, with other cephalosporins and penicillin. *Am J Clin Pathol* 118:256, 2002.

131. Issitt PD, Pavone BG, Goldfinger D, et al: Anti-Wr^b and other autoantibodies responsible for positive direct antiglobulin test in 150 individuals. *Br J Haematol* 34:5, 1976.

132. Garratty G: Autoantibodies induced by blood transfusions. *Transfusion* 44:5, 2004.

133. Young PP, Uzieblo A, Trulock E, et al: Autoantibody formation after alloimmunization: Are blood transfusions a risk factor for autoimmune hemolytic anemia? *Transfusion* 44:67, 2004.

134. Salama A, Mueller-Eckhardt C: Delayed hemolytic transfusion reactions: Evidence for complement activation involving allogeneic and autologous red cells. *Transfusion* 24:188, 1984.

135. Ness PM, Shirey RS, Thoman SK, Buck SA: The differentiation of delayed serologic and delayed hemolytic transfusion reactions: Incidence, long-term serologic findings and clinical significance. *Transfusion* 30:688, 1990.

136. Leddy JP, Falany JL, Kissel GE, et al: Erythrocyte membrane proteins reactive with human (warm-reacting) anti-red cell autoantibodies. *J Clin Invest* 91:1672, 1993.

137. Gorst DW, Rawlinson VI, Merry AH, Stratton F: Positive direct anti-globulin test in normal individuals. *Vox Sang* 38:99, 1980.

138. Bareford D, Langster G, Gilks L, Demick-Torey LA: Follow-up of normal individuals with a positive antiglobulin test. *Scand J Haematol* 35:348, 1985.

139. Worlledge SM: The interpretation of a positive direct antiglobulin test. *Br J Haematol* 39:157, 1978.

140. Nossal GJV: B-cell selection and tolerance. *Curr Opin Immunol* 3:193, 1991.

141. Basten A, Brink R, Peake P, et al: Self-tolerance in the B-cell repertoire. *Immunol Rev* 122:5, 1991.

142. Kroemer G, Martinez-A C: Mechanisms of self-tolerance. *Immunol Today* 13:401, 1992.

143. Leddy JP: Immune hemolytic anemia, in *Clinical Immunology: Principles and Practice*, edited by RR Rich, TA Fleisher, BD Schwartz, WT Shearer, W Strober, p 1273. Mosby, St. Louis, 1996.

144. Hartley SB, Crosbie J, Brink R, et al: Elimination from peripheral lymphoid tissue of self-reactive B lymphocytes recognizing membrane bound antigens. *Nature* 353:765, 1991.

145. Leddy JP: Reactivity of human gamma-G erythrocyte autoantibodies with fetal, autologous and maternal red cells. *Vox Sang* 17:525, 1969.

146. Okamoto M, Murakami M, Shimizu A, et al: A transgenic model of autoimmune hemolytic anemia. *J Exp Med* 175:71, 1992.

147. Murakami M, Tsubata T, Okamoto M, et al: Antigen-induced apoptotic death of Ly-1 B cells responsible for autoimmune disease in transgenic mice. *Nature* 357:77, 1992.

148. Lin RH, Mamula MJ, Hardin JA, Janeway CA: Induction of autoreactive B cells allows priming of autoreactive T cells. *J Exp Med* 173:1433, 1991.

149. Silverman GJ, Carson DA: Structural characterization of human monoclonal cold agglutinins: Evidence for a distinct primary sequence-defined V_H4 idiotype. *Eur J Immunol* 20:351, 1990.

150. Silberstein LE, Jefferies LC, Goldman J, et al: Variable region gene analysis of pathologic human autoantibodies to the related i and I red blood cell antigens. *Blood* 78:2372, 1991.

151. Pascual V, Victor K, Spellerberg M, et al: V_H restriction among human cold agglutinins: The V_H4–21 gene segment is required to encode anti-I and anti-i specificities. *J Immunol* 149:2337, 1992.

152. Stevenson FK, Smith GJ, North J, et al: Identification of normal B-cell counterparts of neoplastic cells which secrete cold agglutinins of anti-I and anti-i specificity. *Br J Haematol* 72:9, 1989.

153. Silverman GJ, Chen PP, Carson DA: Cold agglutinins: Specificity, idiotype and structural analysis, in *Idiotypes in Biology and Medicine: Chemistry and Immunology*, vol 48, edited by DA Carson, PP Chen, TJ Kipps, p 109. Karger, Basel, 1990.

154. Feizi T: Lambda chains in cold agglutinins. *Science* 156:111, 1987.

155. Thompson KM, Sutherland J, Barden G, et al: Human monoclonal antibodies against blood group antigens preferentially express a V_H4–21 variable region gene-associated epitope. *Scand J Immunol* 34:509, 1991.

156. Adderson EE, Shackelford PG, Quinn A, et al: Restricted immunoglobulin VH usage and VDJ combinations in the human response to *Haemophilus influenzae* type b capsular polysaccharide: Nucleotide sequences of monospecific anti-*Haemophilus* antibodies and polyspecific antibodies cross-reacting with self-antigens. *J Clin Invest* 91:2734, 1993.

157. Adderson EE, Shackelford PG, Insel RA, et al: Immunoglobulin light chain variable region gene sequences for human antibodies to *Haemophilus influenzae* type b capsular polysaccharide are dominated by a limited number of V kappa and V lambda segments and VJ combinations. *J Clin Invest* 89:729, 1992.

158. Silberstein LE, Robertson GA, Hannam-Harris AC, et al: Etiologic aspects of cold agglutinin disease: Evidence of cytogenetically defined clones of lymphoid cells and the demonstration that an anti-Pr cold autoantibody is derived from an aberrant B cell clone. *Blood* 67:1705, 1986.

159. Gordon J, Silberstein LE, Moreau L, Nowell PC: Trisomy 3 in cold agglutinin disease. *Cancer Genet Cytogenet* 46:89, 1990.

160. Michaux L, Dierlamm J, Wlodarska I, et al: Trisomy 3q11-q29 is recurrently observed in B-cell non-Hodgkin's lymphomas associated with cold agglutinin syndrome. *Ann Hematol* 76:201, 1998.

161. Harboe M, Lind K: Light chain types of transiently occurring cold haemagglutinins. *Scand J Haematol* 3:269, 1966.

162. Feizi T: Monotypic cold agglutinins in infection by *Mycoplasma pneumoniae*. *Nature* 215:540, 1967.

163. Feizi T, Loveless W: Carbohydrate recognition by *Mycoplasma pneumoniae* and pathologic consequences. *Am J Respir Crit Care Med* 154:S133, 1996.

164. Mollison PL: Measurement of survival and destruction of red cells in haemolytic syndromes. *Br Med Bull* 15:59, 1959.

165. Hollander L: Erythrocyte survival time in a case of acquired haemolytic anaemia. *Vox Sang* 4:164, 1954.

166. Chaplin H, Cohen R, Bloomberg G, et al: Pregnancy and idiopathic autoimmune haemolytic anaemia: A prospective study during 6 months gestation and 3 months "post-partum". *Br J Haematol* 24:219, 1973.

167. Mollison PL, Crome P, Hughes-Jones NC, Rochna E: Rate of removal from the circulation of red cells sensitized with different amounts of antibody. *Br J Haematol* 11:461, 1965.

168. Mollison PL, Hughes-Jones NC: Clearance of Rh-positive red cells by low concentration of Rh antibody. *Immunology* 12:63, 1967.

169. Rosse WF: Quantitative immunology of immune hemolytic anemia: II. The relationship of cell-bound antibody to hemolysis and the effect of treatment. *J Clin Invest* 50:734, 1971.

170. Schreiber AD, Frank MM: Role of antibody and complement in the immune clearance and destruction of erythrocytes: I. *In vivo* effects of IgG and IgM complement-fixing sites. *J Clin Invest* 51:575, 1972.

171. Atkinson JP, Schreiber AD, Frank MM: Effects of corticosteroids and splenectomy on the immune clearance and destruction of erythrocytes. *J Clin Invest* 52:1509, 1973.

172. Atkinson JP, Frank MM: Complement independent clearance of IgG sensitized erythrocytes: Inhibition by cortisone. *Blood* 44:629, 1974.

173. Jandl JH, Richardson-Jones A, Castle WB: The destruction of red cells by antibodies in man: I. Observations on the sequestration and lysis of red cells altered by immune mechanisms. *J Clin Invest* 36:1428, 1957.

174. Jandl JH, Kaplan ME: The destruction of red cells by antibodies in man: III. Quantitative factors influencing the pattern of hemolysis *in vivo*. *J Clin Invest* 39:1145, 1960.

175. Abramson N, LoBuglio AF, Jandl JH, Cotran RS: The interaction between human monocytes and red cells: Binding characteristics. *J Exp Med* 132:1191, 1970.

176. LoBuglio AF, Cotran RS, Jandl JH: Red cells coated with immunoglobulin G: Binding and sphering by mononuclear cells in man. *Science* 158:1582, 1967.

177. Anderson CL, Looney RJ: Human leukocyte IgG Fc receptors. *Immunol Today* 7:264, 1986.

178. Ravetch JV, Kinet J-P: Fc receptors. *Annu Rev Immunol* 9:457, 1991.

179. Gigli I, Nelson RA: Complement-dependent immune phagocytosis: I. Requirements of C1, C4, C2, C3. *Exp Cell Res* 51:45, 1968.

180. Lay WF, Nussenzweig V: Receptors for complement on leukocytes. *J Exp Med* 128:991, 1968.

181. Ross GD: Opsonization and membrane complement receptors, in *Immunobiology of the Complement System*, edited by GD Ross, p 87. Academic Press, Orlando, FL, 1986.

182. Fischer JT, Petz LD, Garratty G, Cooper NR: Correlations between quantitative assay of red cell bound C3, serologic reactions, and hemolytic anemia. *Blood* 44:359, 1974.

183. Schreiber AD, Parsons J, McDermott P, Cooper RA: Effect of corticosteroids on the human monocyte IgG and complement receptors. *J Clin Invest* 56:1189, 1975.

184. Ehlenberger AG, Nussenzweig V: The role of membrane receptors for C3b and C3d in phagocytosis. *J Exp Med* 145:357, 1977.

185. Rosse WF, De Boisfleury A, Bessis M: The interaction of phagocytic cells and red cells modified by immune reactions: Comparison of antibody and complement coated red cells. *Blood Cells* 1:345, 1975.

186. Dameshek W, Schwartz SO: Acute hemolytic anemia (acquired hemolytic icterus, acute type). *Medicine (Baltimore)* 19:231, 1940.

187. Leddy JP, Rosenfeld SI: Role of complement in hemolytic anemia and thrombocytopenia, in *Immunobiology of the Complement System*, edited by GD Ross, p 213. Academic Press, Orlando, FL, 1986.

188. Nicholson-Weller A, Burge J, Fearon DT, et al: Isolation of a human erythrocyte membrane glycoprotein with decay-accelerating activity for C3 convertases of the complement system. *J Immunol* 129:184, 1982.

189. Lachmann PJ: The control of homologous lysis. *Immunol Today* 12:312, 1991.

190. Packman CH: Pathogenesis and management of paroxysmal nocturnal hemoglobinuria. *Blood Rev* 12:1, 1998.

191. Fleer A, Van Schaik ML, von dem Borne AE, Engelfriet CP: Destruction of sensitized erythrocytes by human monocytes *in vitro*: Effects of cytochalasin B, hydrocortisone and colchicine. *Scand J Immunol* 8:515, 1978.

192. Kurlander RJ, Rosse WF, Logue WL: Quantitative influence of antibody and complement coating of red cells on monocyte-mediated cell lysis. *J Clin Invest* 61:1309, 1978.

193. Urbaniak SJ: Lymphoid cell dependent (K-cell) lysis of human erythrocytes sensitized with rhesus alloantibodies. *Br J Haematol* 33:409, 1976.

194. Handwerger BS, Kay NW, Douglas SD: Lymphocyte-mediated antibody-dependent cytolysis: Role in immune hemolysis. *Vox Sang* 34:276, 1978.

195. Milgrom H, Shore SL: Lysis of antibody-coated human red cells by peripheral blood mononuclear cells: Altered effector cell profile after treatment of target cells with enzymes. *Cell Immunol* 39:178, 1978.

196. Schreiber AD, Herskovitz BS, Goldwein M: Low-titer cold-hemagglutinin disease. *N Engl J Med* 296:1490, 1977.

197. Evans RS, Turner E, Bingham M, Woods R: Chronic hemolytic anemia due to cold agglutinins: II. The role of C in red cell destruction. *J Clin Invest* 47:691, 1968.

198. Atkinson JP, Frank MM: Studies on *in vivo* effects of antibody: Interaction of IgM antibody and complement in the immune clearance and destruction of erythrocytes in man. *J Clin Invest* 54:339, 1974.

199. Hughey CT, Brewer JW, Colosia AD, et al: Production of IgM hexamers by normal and autoimmune B cells: Implications for the physiologic role of hexameric IgM. *J Immunol* 161:4091, 1998.

200. Logue GL, Rosse WF, Gockerman JP: Measurement of the third component of complement bound to red blood cells in patients with the cold agglutinin syndrome. *J Clin Invest* 52:493, 1973.

201. Evans RS, Turner E, Bingham M: Studies with radioiodinated cold agglutinins of ten patients. *Am J Med* 38:378, 1965.

202. Roelcke D: Cold agglutination: Antibodies and antigens. *Clin Immunol Immunopathol* 2:266, 1974.

203. Mantovani B, Rabinovitch M, Nussenzweig V: Phagocytosis of immune complexes by macrophages: Different roles of the macrophage receptor sites for complement (C3) and for immunoglobulin (IgG). *J Exp Med* 135:780, 1972.

204. Silverstein SC, Steinman RM, Cohn ZA: Endocytosis. *Annu Rev Biochem* 46:669, 1977.

205. Jaffe CH, Atkinson JP, Frank MM: The role of complement in the clearance of cold agglutinin-sensitized erythrocytes in man. *J Clin Invest* 58:942, 1976.

206. Brown DL, Nelson DA: Surface microfragmentation of red cells as a mechanism for complement-mediated immune spherocytosis. *Br J Haematol* 24:301, 1973.

207. Evans RS, Turner E, Bingham M: Chronic hemolytic anemia due to cold agglutinins: I. The mechanism of resistance of red cells to C hemolysis by cold agglutinins. *J Clin Invest* 46:1461, 1967.

208. Kerr RO, Cardamone J, Dalmasso AP, Kaplan ME: Two mechanisms of erythrocyte destruction in penicillin-induced hemolytic anemia. *N Engl J Med* 287:1322, 1972.

209. Nesmith LW, Davis JW: Hemolytic anemia caused by penicillin. *JAMA* 203:27, 1968.

210. Yust I, Frisch B, Goldsher N: Simultaneous detection of two mechanisms of immune destruction of penicillin-treated human red blood cells. *Am J Hematol* 13:53, 1982.

211. Brandriss MW, Smith JW, Steinman HG: Common antigenic determinants of penicillin G, cephalothin and 6-aminopenicillanic acid in rabbits. *J Immunol* 94:696, 1965.

212. Abraham GN, Petz LD, Fudenberg HH: Immuno-hematological cross-allergenicity between penicillin and cephalothin in humans. *Clin Exp Immunol* 3:343, 1968.

213. Petz LD: Immunologic cross reactivity between penicillins and cephalosporins: A review. *J Infect Dis* 137:S74, 1978.

214. Kunicki TJ, Russell N, Nurten AT, et al: Further studies of the human platelet receptor for quinine- and quinidine-dependent antibodies. *J Immunol* 126:398, 1981.

215. Christie DJ, Aster RH: Drug-antibody-platelet interaction in quinine-and quinidine-induced thrombocytopenia. *J Clin Invest* 70:989, 1982.

216. Berndt MC, Chong BH, Bull HA, et al: Molecular characterization of quinine/quinidine drug-dependent antibody platelet interaction using monoclonal antisera. *Blood* 66:1292, 1985.

217. Sosler SD, Behzad O, Garratty G, et al: Acute hemolytic anemia associated with a chlorpropamide-induced apparent auto-anti-Jk$_a$. *Transfusion* 24:206, 1984.

218. Salama A, Mueller-Eckhardt C: Rh blood group-specific antibodies in immune hemolytic anemia induced by nomifensine. *Blood* 68:1285, 1986.

219. Salama A, Mueller-Eckhardt C: On the mechanisms of sensitization and attachment of antibodies to RBC in drug-induced immune hemolytic anemia. *Blood* 69:1006, 1987.

220. Christie DJ, Mullen PC, Aster RH: Fab-mediated binding of drug-dependent antibodies to platelets in quinidine- and quinine-induced thrombocytopenia. *J Clin Invest* 75:310, 1985.

221. Smith ME, Reid DM, Jones CE, et al: Binding of quinine- and quinidine-dependent drug antibodies to platelets is mediated by the Fab domain of immunoglobulin G and is not Fc dependent. *J Clin Invest* 29:912, 1987.

222. Salama A, Mueller-Eckhardt C: The role of metabolite-specific antibodies in nomifensine-dependent immune hemolytic anemia. *N Engl J Med* 313:469, 1985.

223. Kelton JG: Impaired reticuloendothelial function in patients treated with methyldopa. *N Engl J Med* 313:596, 1985.

224. Bakemeier RF, Leddy JP: Erythrocyte autoantibody associated with alpha-methyldopa: Heterogeneity of structure and specificity. *Blood* 32:1, 1968.

225. Green FA, Jung CY, Rampal A, Lorusso DJ: Alpha-methyldopa and the erythrocyte membrane. *Clin Exp Immunol* 40:554, 1980.

226. Green Fa, Jung CY, Hui H: Modulation of alpha-methyldopa binding to the erythrocyte membrane by superoxide dismutase. *Biochem Biophys Res Commun* 95:1037, 1980.

227. Kirtland HH III, Mohler DN, Horwitz DA: Methyldopa inhibition of suppressor-lymphocyte function. A proposed cause of autoimmune hemolytic anemia. *N Engl J Med* 302:825, 1980.

228. Garratty G, Arndt P, Prince HE, Schulman IA: The effect of methyldopa and procainamide on suppressor cell activity in relation to red cell autoantibody production. *Br J Haematol* 84:310, 1993.

229. Dearden C, Wade R, Else M, et al: The prognostic significance of a positive direct antiglobulin test in chronic lymphocytic leukemia: A beneficial effect of the combination of fludarabine and cyclophosphamide on the incidence of hemolytic anemia. *Blood* 111:1820, 2008.

230. Borthakur G, O'Brien S, Wierda WG, et al: Immune anaemias in patients with chronic lymphocytic leukaemia treated with fludarabine, cyclophosphamide and rituximab-incidence and predictors. *Br J Haematol* 136:800, 2007.

231. Spath P, Garratty G, Petz LD: Studies on the immune response to penicillin and cephalothin in humans: II. Immunohematologic reactions to cephalothin administration. *J Immunol* 107:860, 1971.

232. Garratty G, Petz L: Drug-induced hemolytic anemia. *Am J Med* 58:398, 1975.
233. Sokol RJ, Hewitt S, Stamps BK: Erythrocyte autoantibodies, autoimmune haemolysis and pregnancy. *Vox Sang* 43:169, 1982.
234. Issaragrisil S, Kruatrachue M: An association of pregnancy and auto-immune haemolytic anaemia. *Scand J Haematol* 31:63, 1983.
235. Evans RS, Duane RT: Acquired hemolytic anemia: I. The relation of erythrocyte antibody production to activity of the disease: II. The significance of thrombocytopenia and leukopenia. *Blood* 4:1196, 1949.
236. Evans RS, Takahashi K, Duane RT, et al: Primary thrombocytopenic purpura and acquired hemolytic anemia: Evidence for a common etiology. *Arch Intern Med* 87:48, 1951.
237. Pegels JG, Helmerhorst FM, van Leeuwen EF, et al: The Evans syndrome: Characterization of the responsible autoantibodies. *Br J Haematol* 51:445, 1982.
238. Liesveld JL, Rowe JM, Lichtman MA: Variability of the erythropoietic response in autoimmune hemolytic anemia: Analysis of 109 cases. *Blood* 69:820, 1987.
239. Hegde UM, Gordon-Smith EC, Worlledge SM: Reticulocytopenia and absence of red cell autoantibodies in immune haemolytic anaemia. *Br Med J* 2:1444, 1977.
240. Conley CL, Lippman SM, Ness P: Autoimmune hemolytic anemia with reticulocytopenia: A medical emergency. *JAMA* 244:1688, 1980.
241. Greenberg J, Curtis-Cohen M, Gill FM, Cohen A: Prolonged reticulocytopenia in autoimmune hemolytic anemia of childhood. *J Pediatr* 97:784, 1980.
242. Mangan KF, Besa EC, Shadduck RK, et al: Demonstration of two distinct antibodies in autoimmune hemolytic anemia with reticulocytopenia and red cell aplasia. *Exp Hematol* 12:788, 1984.
243. Leddy JP: Immunological aspects of red cell injury in man. *Semin Hematol* 3:48, 1966.
244. Engelfriet CP, Borne AE vd, Giessen M vd, et al: Autoimmune haemolytic anaemias: I. Serological studies with pure anti-immunoglobulin reagents. *Clin Exp Immunol* 3:605, 1968.
245. Engelfriet CP, Borne AE, Beckers D, van Loghem JJ: Autoimmune haemolytic anaemia: Serological and immunochemical characteristics of the autoantibodies: Mechanisms of cell destruction. *Ser Haematol* 7:328, 1974.
246. Suzuki S, Amano T, Mitsunaga M, et al: Autoimmune hemolytic anemia associated with IgA autoantibody. *Clin Immunol Immunopathol* 21:247, 1981.
247. Wolf CF, Wolf DJ, Peterson P: Autoimmune hemolytic anemia with predominance of IgA autoantibody. *Transfusion* 22:238, 1982.
248. Szymanski IO, Teno R, Rybak ME: Hemolytic anemia due to a mixture of low-titer IgG lambda and IgM agglutinins reacting optimally at 22°C. *Vox Sang* 51:112, 1986.
249. Reusser P, Osterwalder B, Burri H, Speck B: Autoimmune hemolytic anemia associated with IgA: Diagnostic and therapeutic aspects in a case with long-term follow-up. *Acta Haematol* 77:53, 1987.
250. Göttsche B, Salama A, Mueller-Eckhardt C: Autoimmune hemolytic anemia associated with an IgA autoanti-Gerbich. *Vox Sang* 58:211, 1990.
251. Arndt P, Leger RM, Garratty G: Serologic findings in autoimmune hemolytic anemia associated with immunoglobulin M warm autoantibodies. *Transfusion* 49:235, 2009.
252. Evans RS, Bingham M, Boehni P: Autoimmune hemolytic disease: Antibody dissociation and activity. *Arch Intern Med* 108:338, 1961.
253. Evans RS, Bingham M, Turner E: Autoimmune hemolytic disease: Observations of serological reactions and disease activity. *Ann N Y Acad Sci* 124:422, 1965.
254. Gilliland BC, Leddy JP, Vaughan JH: The detection of cell-bound antibody on complement-coated human red cells. *J Clin Invest* 49:898, 1970.
255. Gilliland BC, Baxter E, Evans RS: Red cell antibodies in acquired hemolytic anemia with negative antiglobulin serum tests. *N Engl J Med* 285:252, 1971.
256. Gilliland BC: Coombs-negative immune hemolytic anemia. *Semin Hematol* 13:267, 1976.
257. Segel GB, Lichtman MA: Direct antiglobulin ("Coombs") test-negative autoimmune hemolytic anemia: A review. *Blood Cells Mol Dis* 52:152, 2014.
258. Kamesaki T, Toyotsuji T, Kajii E: Characterization of direct antiglobulin test-negative autoimmune hemolytic anemia: A study of 154 cases. *Am J Hematol* 88:93, 2013.
259. Leger RM, Co P, Hunt G, Garratty G: Attempts to support an immune etiology in 800 patients with direct antiglobulin test-negative hemolytic anemia. *Immunohematol* 26:156, 2010.
260. Sokol RJ, Hewitt S, Booker DJ, Bailey A: Erythrocyte autoantibodies, subclasses of IgG and autoimmune haemolysis. *Autoimmun Rev* 6:99, 1990.
261. von dem Borne AE, Beckers D, van der Meulen FW, Engelfriet CP: IgG₄ autoantibodies against erythrocytes, without increased hemolysis: A case report. *Br J Haematol* 37:137, 1977.
262. Weiner W, Vos GH: Serology of acquired hemolytic anemia. *Blood* 22:606, 1963.
263. Vos GH, Petz L, Funenberg HH: Specificity of acquired haemolytic anaemia autoantibodies and their serological characteristics. *Br J Haematol* 19:57, 1970.
264. Leddy JP, Peterson P, Yeaw MA, Bakemeier RF: Patterns of serologic specificity of human gamma-G erythrocyte autoantibodies. *J Immunol* 105:677, 1970.
265. Bell CA, Zwicker H: Further studies on the relationship of anti-Enᵃ and anti-Wrᵇ in warm autoimmune hemolytic anemia. *Transfusion* 18:572, 1978.
266. Celano MJ, Levine P: Anti-LW specificity in autoimmune acquired hemolytic anemia. *Transfusion* 7:265, 1967.
267. Marsh WL, Reid ME, Scott EP: Autoantibodies of U blood group specificity in autoimmune haemolytic anaemia. *Br J Haematol* 22:625, 1972.
268. Shulman IA, Vengelen-Tyler V, Thompson JC, et al: Autoanti-Ge associated with severe autoimmune hemolytic anemia. *Vox Sang* 59:232, 1990.
269. Owen I, Chowdhury V, Reid ME, et al: Autoimmune hemolytic anemia associated with anti-Sc 1. *Transfusion* 32:173, 1992.
270. Marsh WL, Oyen R, Alicea E, et al: Autoimmune hemolytic anemia and the Kell blood groups. *Am J Hematol* 7:155, 1979.
271. Barker RN, Casswell KM, Reid ME, et al: Identification of autoantigens in autoimmune haemolytic anaemia by a non-radioisotope immunoprecipitation method. *Br J Haematol* 82:126, 1992.
272. Victoria EJ, Pierce SW, Branks MJ, Masouredis SP: IgG red blood cell autoantibodies in autoimmune hemolytic anemia bind to epitopes on red blood cell membrane band 3 glycoprotein. *J Lab Clin Med* 115:74, 1990.
273. Telen MJ, Chasis JA: Relationship of the human erythrocyte Wrᵇ antigen to an interaction between glycophorin A and band 3. *Blood* 76:842, 1990.
274. Barker RN, De la Sa Oliveira GG, Elson CJ, et al: Pathogenic autoantibodies in the NZB mouse are specific for erythrocyte band 3 protein. *Eur J Immunol* 23:1723, 1993.
275. Kay MMB, Marchalonis JJ, Hughes J, et al: Definition of a physiologic aging autoantigen by using synthetic peptides of membrane protein band 3: Localization of the active antigenic sites. *Proc Natl Acad Sci U S A* 87:5734, 1990.
276. Turrini F, Mannu F, Arese P, et al: Characterization of autologous antibodies that opsonize erythrocytes with clustered integral membrane proteins. *Blood* 181:3146, 1993.
277. Curtis BR, Lamon J, Roelcke D, Chaplin H: Life-threatening, antiglobulin test-negative, acute autoimmune hemolytic anemia due to a non-complement-activating IgG1 kappa cold antibody with Prₐ specificity. *Transfusion* 30:838, 1990.
278. Silberstein LE, Berkman EM, Schreiber AD: Cold hemagglutinin disease associated with IgG cold reactive antibody. *Ann Intern Med* 106:238, 1987.
279. Feizi T, Kabat EA, Vicari G, et al: Immunochemical studies on blood groups: XLVII. The I antigen complex precursors in the A, B, H, Leᵃ, and Leᵇ blood group system: Hemagglutination inhibition studies. *J Exp Med* 133:39, 1971.
280. Hakomori S: Blood group ABH and Ii antigens of human erythrocytes: Chemistry, polymorphism, and their developmental change. *Semin Hematol* 18:39, 1981.
281. Marcus DM: A review of the immunogenic and immunomodulatory properties of glycosphingolipids. *Mol Immunol* 21:1083, 1984.
282. Rosse WF, Lauf PK: Reaction of cold agglutinins with I antigen solubilized from human red cells. *Blood* 36:777, 1970.
283. Lauf PK, Rosse WF: The reactivity of red blood cell membrane glycophorin with "cold-reacting" antibodies. *Clin Immunol Immunopathol* 4:1, 1975.
284. Pruzanski W, Shumak KH: Biologic activity of cold-reacting autoantibodies. *N Engl J Med* 297:583, 1977.
285. Chapman J, Murphy MF, Waters AH: Chronic cold hemagglutinin disease due to an anti-M-like autoantibody. *Vox Sang* 42:272, 1982.
286. von dem Borne AEG, Mol JJ, Joustra-Maas N, et al: Autoimmune hemolytic anemia with monoclonal IgM (kappa) anti-P cold autohemolysins. *Br J Haematol* 50:345, 1982.
287. Terada K, Tanaka H, Mori R, et al: Hemolytic anemia associated with cold agglutinin during chickenpox and a review of the literature. *J Pediatr Hematol Oncol* 20:149, 1998.
288. Tamura T, Kanamori H, Yamazaki E, et al: Cold agglutinin disease following allogeneic bone marrow transplantation. *Bone Marrow Transplant* 13:321, 1994.
289. Capra JD, Dowling P, Cook S, Kunkel HG: An incomplete cold-reactive gamma G antibody with i specificity in infectious mononucleosis. *Vox Sang* 16:10, 1969.
290. Shirey RS, Park K, Ness PM, et al: An anti-i biphasic hemolysin in chronic paroxysmal cold hemoglobinuria. *Transfusion* 26:62, 1986.
291. Salama A, Santoso S, Mueller-Eckhardt C: Antigenic determinants responsible for the reactions of drug-dependent antibodies with blood cells. *Br J Haematol* 78:535, 1991.
292. Gehrie EA, Nian H, Young PP: Brown recluse spider bite mediated hemolysis: Clinical features, a possible role for complement inhibitor therapy and reduced RBC surface glycophorin A as a potential biomarker of venom exposure. *PloS One* 8:e76558, 2013.
293. McDade J, Aygun B, Ware RE: Brown recluse spider (*Loxosceles reclusa*) envenomation leading to acute hemolytic anemia in six adolescents. *J Pediatr* 156:155, 2010.
294. Sokol R, Stamps R, Booker D, et al: Posttransplant immune-mediated hemolysis. *Transfusion* 42:198, 2002.
295. Lundgren G, Asaba H, Bergström J, et al: Fulminating anti-A autoimmune hemolysis with anuria in a renal transplant recipient: A therapeutic role of plasma exchange. *Clin Nephrol* 16:211, 1981.
296. Ramsey G, Nusbacher J, Starzl TE, Lindsay GD: Isohemagglutinins of graft origin after ABO-unmatched liver transplantation. *N Engl J Med* 311:1167, 1984.
297. Mangal AK, Growe GH, Sinclair M, et al: Acquired hemolytic anemia due to "auto"-anti-A or "auto"-anti-B induced by group O homograft in renal transplant recipients. *Transfusion* 24:201, 1984.
298. Hazlehurst GR, Brenner MK, Wimperis JZ, et al: Haemolysis after T-cell depleted bone marrow transplantation involving minor ABO incompatibility. *Scand J Haematol* 37:1, 1986.
299. Solheim BG, Albrechtsen D, Egeland T, et al: Auto-antibodies against erythrocytes in transplant patients produced by donor lymphocytes. *Transplant Proc* 6:4520, 1987.
300. Sniecinski IJ, Oien L, Petz LD, Blume KG: Immunohematologic consequences of major ABO-mismatched bone marrow transplantation. *Transplantation* 45:530, 1988.
301. Petz LD: "Least incompatible" units for transfusion in autoimmune hemolytic anemia: Should we eliminate this meaningless term? A commentary for clinicians and transfusion medicine professionals. *Transfusion* 42:1503, 2003.
302. Ness PM: How do I encourage clinicians to transfuse mismatched blood to patients with autoimmune hemolytic anemia in urgent situations? *Transfusion* 46:1859, 2006.

303. Issitt PD: Autoimmune hemolytic anemia and cold hemagglutinin disease: Clinical disease and laboratory findings. *Prog Clin Pathol* 7:137, 1978.

304. Wallhermfechtel MA, Pohl BA, Chaplin H: Alloimmunization in patients with warm autoantibodies: A retrospective study employing three donor alloabsorptions to aid in antibody detection. *Transfusion* 24:482, 1984.

305. Branch DR, Petz LD: Detecting alloantibodies in patients with autoantibodies. *Transfusion* 39:6, 1999.

306. Shirey RS, Boyd JS, Parwani AV, et al: Prophylactic antigen matched donor blood for patients with warm autoantibodies: An algorithm for transfusion management. *Transfusion* 42:1435, 2002.

307. Garratty G, Petz LD: Approaches to selecting blood for transfusion to patients with autoimmune hemolytic anemia. *Transfusion* 42:1390, 2002.

308. Dameshek W, Rosenthal MC, Schwartz SO: The treatment of acquired hemolytic anemia with adrenocorticotrophic hormone (ACTH). *N Engl J Med* 244:117, 1951.

309. Allgood JW, Chaplin H Jr: Idiopathic acquired autoimmune hemolytic anemia: A review of forty-seven cases treated from 1955 to 1965. *Am J Med* 43:254, 1967.

310. Meyer O, Stahl D, Beckhove P, et al: Pulsed high-dose dexamethasone in chronic autoimmune haemolytic anaemia of warm type. *Br J Haematol* 98:860, 1997.

311. Greendyke RM, Bradley EB, Swisher SN: Studies of the effects of administration of ACTH and adrenal corticosteroids on erythrophagocytosis. *J Clin Invest* 44:746, 1965.

312. Fries LF, Brickman CM, Frank MM: Monocyte receptors for the Fc portion of IgG increase in number in autoimmune hemolytic anemia and other hemolytic states and are decreased by glucocorticoid therapy. *J Immunol* 131:1240, 1983.

313. Habibi B, Homberg JC, Schaison G, Salmon C: Autoimmune hemolytic anemia in children: A review of 80 cases. *Am J Med* 56:61, 1974.

314. Christensen BE: The pattern of erythrocyte sequestration in immunohaemolysis: Effects of prednisone treatment and splenectomy. *Scand J Haematol* 10:120, 1973.

315. Parker AC, MacPherson AIS, Richmond J: Value of radiochromium investigation in autoimmune haemolytic anemia. *Br Med J* 1:208, 1977.

316. Schwartz SI, Bernard RP, Adams JT, Bauman AW: Splenectomy for hematologic disorders. *Arch Surg* 101:338, 1970.

317. Eichner ER: Splenic function: Normal, too much and too little. *Am J Med* 66:311, 1979.

318. Centers for Disease Control and Prevention: Recommended adult immunization schedule—United States 2003–2004. *MMWR Morb Mortal Wkly Rep* 52:965, 2003.

319. Taylor RP, Lindorfer MA: Drug insight: The mechanism of action of rituximab in autoimmune disease—The immune complex decoy hypothesis. *Nat Clin Pract Rheumatol* 3:86, 2007.

320. Garvey B: Rituximab in the treatment of autoimmune haematological disorders. *Br J Haematol* 141:149, 2008.

321. Zecca M, Nobili B, Ramenghi U, et al: Rituximab for the treatment of refractory autoimmune hemolytic anemia in children. *Blood* 101:3857, 2003.

322. Bussone G, Ribeiro E, Dechartres A, et al: Efficacy and safety of rituximab in adults' warm antibody autoimmune hemolytic anemia: Retrospective analysis of 27 cases. *Am J Hematol* 84:153, 2009.

323. Barcellini W, Zaja F, Zaninoni A, et al: Low-dose rituximab in adult patients with idiopathic autoimmune hemolytic anemia: Clinical efficacy and biologic studies. *Blood* 119:3691, 2012.

324. Barcellini W, Zaja F, Zaninoni A, et al: Sustained response to low-dose rituximab in idiopathic autoimmune hemolytic anemia. *Eur J Haematol* 91:546, 2013.

325. Birgins H, Frederiksen H, Hasselbalch H, et al: A phase III randomized trial comparing glucocorticoid monotherapy versus glucocorticoid and rituximab in patients with autoimmune hemolytic anaemia. *Br J Haematol* 163:393, 2013.

326. Murphy S, LoBuglio AF: Drug therapy of autoimmune hemolytic anemia. *Semin Hematol* 13:323, 1976.

327. Moyo VM, Smith D, Brodsky I, et al: High-dose cyclophosphamide for refractory autoimmune hemolytic anemia. *Blood* 100:704, 2002.

328. Beutler E: New chemotherapeutic agent: 2-Chlorodeoxyadenosine. *Semin Hematol* 31:40, 1994.

329. Kotb R, Pinganaud C, Trichet C, et al: Efficacy of mycophenolate mofetil in adult refractory auto-immune cytopenias: A single center preliminary study. *Eur J Haematol* 75:60, 2005.

330. Howard J, Hoffbrand AV, Prentice HG, Mehta A: Mycophenolate mofetil for the treatment of refractory auto-immune haemolytic anaemia and auto-immune thrombocytopenic purpura. *Br J Haematol* 117:712, 2002.

331. Karlsson C, Hansson L, Celsing F, Lundin J: Treatment of severe refractory autoimmune hemolytic anemia in B-cell chronic lymphocytic leukemia with alemtuzumab (humanized CD52 monoclonal antibody). *Leukemia* 21:511, 2007.

332. Shumak KH, Rock GA: Therapeutic plasma exchange. *N Engl J Med* 310:762, 1984.

333. Council Report: Current status of therapeutic plasmapheresis and related techniques. *JAMA* 253:819, 1985.

334. Cooling L, Boxer G, Simon R: Life-threatening autoimmune hemolytic anemia treated with manual whole blood exchange with rapid clinical improvement. *J Blood Disord Transfus* 4:163, 2013.

335. Wouters A, Stephan F, Strengers P, et al: C1-esterase inhibitor concentrate rescues erythrocytes from complement-mediated destruction in autoimmune hemolytic anemia. *Blood* 121:1242, 2014.

336. Chao MP, Hong J, Kunder C, et al: Refractory warm IgM-mediated autoimmune hemolytic anemia associated with Churg-Strauss Syndrome responsive to eculizumab and rituximab. *Am J Hematol* 90:78, 2015.

337. Ahn YS, Harrington WJ, Byrnes JJ, et al: Treatment of autoimmune hemolytic anemia with vinca-loaded platelets. *JAMA* 249:2189, 1983.

338. Oda H, Honda A, Sugita K, et al: High-dose intravenous intact IgG infusion in refractory autoimmune hemolytic anemia (Evans syndrome). *J Pediatr* 107:744, 1985.

339. Bussel JB, Cunningham-Rundles C, Abraham C: Intravenous treatment of autoimmune hemolytic anemia with very high dose gammaglobulin. *Vox Sang* 41:264, 1986.

340. Besa EC: Rapid transient reversal of anemia and long-term effects of maintenance intravenous immunoglobulin for autoimmune hemolytic anemia in patients with lymphoproliferative disorders. *Am J Med* 84:691, 1988.

341. Flores G, Cunningham-Rundles C, Newland AC, Bussel JB: Efficacy of intravenous immunoglobulin in the treatment of autoimmune hemolytic anemia: Results in 73 patients. *Am J Hematol* 44:237, 1993.

342. Ahn YS, Harrington WJ, Mylvaganam R, et al: Danazol therapy for autoimmune hemolytic anemia. *Ann Intern Med* 102:298, 1985.

343. Pignon J-M, Poirson E, Rochant H: Danazol in autoimmune haemolytic anaemia. *Br J Haematol* 83:343, 1993.

344. Giannadaki E, Potamianos S, Roussomoustakaki M, et al: Autoimmune hemolytic anemia and positive Coombs' test associated with ulcerative colitis. *Am J Gastroenterol* 92:1872, 1997.

345. Cobo F, Pereira A, Nomdedeu B, et al: Ovarian dermoid cyst-associated autoimmune hemolytic anemia. *Am J Clin Pathol* 105:567, 1996.

346. Berentsen S, Ulvestad E, Gjertsen BT, et al: Rituximab for primary cold agglutinin disease: A prospective study of 37 courses of therapy in 27 patients. *Blood* 103:2925, 2004.

347. Schollkopf, C, Kjeldsen L, Bjerrum OW, et al: Rituximab in chronic cold agglutinin disease: A prospective study of 20 patients. *Leuk Lymphoma* 47:253, 2006.

348. Berentsen S, Randen U, Vagan AM, et al: High response rate and durable remissions following fludarabine and rituximab combination therapy for chronic cold agglutinin disease. *Blood* 116:3180, 2010.

349. Hippe E, Jensen KB, Olesen H, et al: Chlorambucil treatment of patients with cold agglutinin syndrome. *Blood* 35:68, 1970.

350. Evans RS, Baxter E, Gilliland BC: Chronic hemolytic anemia due to cold agglutinins: A 20-year history of benign gammapathy with response to chlorambucil. *Blood* 42:463, 1973.

351. Gupta N, Wang ES: Long-term response of refractory primary cold agglutinin disease to eculizumab therapy. *Ann Hematol* 93:343, 2014.

352. Roth A, Huttmann A, Rother RP, et al: Long-term efficacy of the complement inhibitor eculizumab in cold agglutinin disease. *Blood* 113:3885, 2009.

353. Carson KR, Beckwith LG, Mehta J: Successful treatment of IgM-mediated autoimmune hemolytic anemia with bortezomib. *Blood* 115:915, 2010.

354. Bell CA, Zwicker H, Sacks HJ: Autoimmune hemolytic anemia. *Am J Clin Pathol* 60:903, 1973.

355. Taft EG, Propp RP, Sullivan SA: Plasma exchange for cold agglutinin hemolytic anemia. *Transfusion* 17:173, 1977.

356. Brooks BD, Steane EA, Sheehan RG, Frenkel EP: Therapeutic plasma exchange in the immune hemolytic anemias and immunologic thrombocytopenic purpura. *Prog Clin Biol Res* 106:317, 1982.

357. Silberstein LE, Berkman EM: Plasma exchange in autoimmune hemolytic anemia (AIHA). *J Clin Apher* 1:238, 1983.

358. Zulian GB, Roux E, Tiercy J-M, et al: Transfusion-associated graft-versus-host disease in a patient treated with cladribine (2-chlorodeoxyadenosine): Demonstration of exogenous DNA in various tissue extracts by PCR analysis. *Br J Haematol* 89:83, 1995.

359. Briz M, Cabrera R, Sanjuan I: Diagnosis of transfusion-associated graft-versus-host disease by polymerase chain reaction in fludarabine-treated B-chronic lymphocytic leukaemia. *Br J Haematol* 91:409, 1995.

360. Silverstein MN, Gomes MR, Elveback LR, et al: Idiopathic acquired hemolytic anemia: Survival in 117 cases. *Arch Intern Med* 129:85, 1972.

361. Dausset J, Colombani J: The serology and the prognosis of 128 cases of autoimmune hemolytic anemia. *Blood* 14:1280, 1959.

362. Pullarkat V, Ngo M, Iqbal S, et al: Detection of lupus anticoagulant identifies patients with autoimmune haemolytic anaemia at increased risk of venous thromboembolism. *Br J Haematol* 118:1166, 2002.

363. Hendrick AM: Auto-immune haemolytic anaemia—A high-risk disorder for thromboembolism? *Hematology* 8:53, 2003.

364. Buchanan GR, Boxer LA, Nathan DG: The acute and transient nature of idiopathic immune hemolytic anemia in childhood. *J Pediatr* 88:780, 1976.

365. Zupanska B, Lawkowicz W, Gorska B, et al: Autoimmune haemolytic anemia in children. *Br J Haematol* 34:511, 1976.

366. Heisel MA, Ortega JA: Factors influencing prognosis in childhood autoimmune hemolytic anemia. *Am J Pediatr Hematol Oncol* 5:147, 1983.

367. Carapella de Luca E, Casadei AM, DiPero G, et al: Autoimmune haemolytic anemia in childhood: Follow-up in 29 cases. *Vox Sang* 36:13, 1979.

368. Sokol RJ, Hewitt S, Stamps BK, Hitchen PA: Autoimmune haemolysis in childhood and adolescence. *Acta Haematol* 72:245, 1984.

369. Aladjidi N, Leverger G, Leblanc T, et al: New insights into childhood autoimmune hemolytic anemia: A French national observational study of 265 children. *Haematologica* 96:655, 2011.

370. Wang WC: Evans syndrome in childhood: Pathophysiology, clinical course, and treatment. *Am J Pediatr Hematol Oncol* 10:330, 1988.

CHAPTER 55
ALLOIMMUNE HEMOLYTIC DISEASE OF THE FETUS AND NEWBORN

Ross M. Fasano, Jeanne E. Hendrickson, and Naomi L. C. Luban

SUMMARY

Alloimmune hemolytic disease of the fetus and newborn is caused by the action of transplacentally transmitted maternal immunoglobulin (Ig) G antibodies on paternally inherited antigens present on fetal red cells but absent on the maternal red cells. Maternal IgG antibodies bind to fetal red cells, causing hemolysis or suppression of erythropoiesis. As a consequence, anemia, extramedullary hematopoiesis, and neonatal hyperbilirubinemia may result, with severe cases resulting in fetal loss or neonatal death or disability. Collaboration among maternal–fetal medicine specialists, hematologists, transfusion medicine physicians, radiologists, and neonatologists has substantially reduced perinatal mortality and morbidity resulting from hemolytic disease of the fetus and newborn. Antenatal diagnostic methods identify at risk fetuses, and assess disease severity in affected fetuses. After birth, phototherapy and exchange transfusions prevent serum bilirubin from rising to levels that could produce bilirubin encephalopathy and resultant brain damage (kernicterus), remove maternal antibody, and replace circulating fetal red blood cells with those negative for the implicated antigen(s). RhIg has successfully prevented alloimmune hemolytic disease resulting from rhesus D sensitization in many at risk infants, but no prophylactic therapy exists as of this writing to prevent alloimmune hemolytic disease resulting from other red cell antibodies. Advances in immunohematology and molecular biology may offer new avenues for prevention and treatment in the future.

Alloimmune hemolytic disease of the fetus and newborn (HDFN) is a disorder in which the life span of fetal and/or neonatal red cells is shortened as a result of binding of transplacentally transferred maternal immunoglobulin (Ig) G antibodies on fetal red blood cell (RBC) antigens foreign to the mother, inherited by the fetus from the father.

Acronyms and Abbreviations: AAP, American Academy of Pediatrics; anti-D, antibody against D antigen; ccff-DNA, circulating cell-free fetal DNA; DAT, direct antiglobulin test; ΔOD_{450}, change in optical density at 450 nm; FFP, fresh-frozen plasma; FMH, fetomaternal hemorrhage; HDFN, hemolytic disease of the fetus and newborn; HDN, hemolytic disease of the newborn; IAT, indirect antiglobulin test; Ig, immunoglobulin; IUT, intrauterine transfusion; IVIG, intravenous immunoglobulin G; QT-PCR, quantitative polymerase chain reaction; RBC, red blood cell; Rh, rhesus; rHuEPO, recombinant human erythropoietin; RhIg, Rho(D) immunoglobulin; SGA, small for gestational age; TBV, total blood volume; TSB, total serum bilirubin; WB, whole blood.

The resulting hemolysis or suppression of erythropoiesis may cause fetal and/or neonatal anemia and significant neonatal jaundice. There are three main classes of alloimmune HDFN, based on the antigen(s) involved: Rh (rhesus), minor red cell antigens (i.e., Kell, Duffy, Kidd antigens) and ABO.

Prior to the development of medical interventions in the 1950s, almost half of all newborn infants with Rh HDFN died or were severely handicapped. Although the clinical condition was described in newborn infants as early as the 1600s, it was only in the 1930s and 1940s that the pathophysiology of Rh HDFN was uncovered. In 1932, Diamond and colleagues[1] recognized that the clinical syndromes of stillbirth with unusual erythroblastic activity in the extramedullary sites and blood, fetal hydrops, anemia in the newborn, and "icterus gravis neonatorum" were closely related and likely had the same pathophysiology in the hematopoietic system. In 1938, Ruth Darrow, a pathologist who lost a baby to kernicterus, postulated that hemolysis of fetal RBCs was a result of maternal antibody produced in response to fetal hemoglobin.[2] The discovery of the Rh factor by Landsteiner and Weiner led to elucidation of Rh HDFN by Levine and colleagues who established that erythroblastosis fetalis was caused by immunization of an Rh-negative mother by the red cells from an Rh-positive fetus.[3] Antibodies produced by the sensitized mother crossed the placenta in the next pregnancy and coated the fetal Rh-positive cells, leading to hemolysis, anemia, hydrops, and severe neonatal jaundice.

Neonatal mortality from Rh HDFN decreased considerably with the development of exchange transfusion techniques for correction of severe anemia and hyperbilirubinemia.[4] However, severely affected fetuses continued to die in utero before 34 weeks' gestation. In 1961, Liley demonstrated the prognostic value of amniotic fluid spectrophotometry in identifying fetuses at risk and then showed that intrauterine transfusions (IUTs) could prevent fetal deaths.[5] The most dramatic reduction in the incidence of Rh HDFN was achieved in the 1960s and 1970s with the development of postpartum and antepartum anti-D prophylaxis to prevent maternal Rh sensitization.[6]

Despite these advances, Rh HDFN has not disappeared, and cases of hemolytic disease of the newborn resulting from red cell antibodies directed toward antigens other than the Rh blood group system are being increasingly recognized.[7-11] Furthermore, maternal Rh isoimmunization and Rh hemolytic disease still occur, particularly in developing countries where anti-RhD prophylaxis is not widely available or in infants born outside of medical facilities.[12]

EPIDEMIOLOGY

The epidemiology of HDFN varies in different ethnic and racial groups; the frequency of specific blood group alleles in a given population determines the probability of blood group incompatibility and maternal alloimmunization. Antigen-negative women may have naturally occurring antibodies to certain red cell antigens (anti-A or anti-B) or may develop antibodies as a result of exposure to foreign red cell antigens through blood transfusion or by silent fetomaternal hemorrhage during pregnancy or at delivery. More than 50 different RBC antigens are associated with maternal alloimmunization[7-11,13] and with HDFN of varying severity; however, the vast majority of clinically significant maternal alloantibodies are within the Rh (D, CE), Kell, Duffy, MNS, and Kidd systems (Table 55–1).

Antenatal screening programs detect antibodies to clinically significant Rh or other minor RBC antigens in 0.01 to 0.4 percent of pregnant women,[7-11,13] although these numbers vary by country. Approximately 15 percent of Americans of European descent are RhD-negative, compared to 7 percent of Americans of African descent and Hispanics,

TABLE 55-1. Blood Group Systems Associated with Hemolytic Disease of the Fetus and Newborn

Blood Group System	Antigens
Rhesus	D, C, E, Ce, f, $C_,^w$ $C_,^x$ $E_,^w$ G, Rh29, Rh32 (R^N), Rh42, Go^a, Hr_o, Be^a, Evans, Tar, Sec, JAL, STEM
Kell	K, k, K_o, Kp^a, Kp^b, Js^a, Js^b (and others)
Duffy	Fy^a, Fy^b, Fy3
Kidd	Jk^a, Jk^b, Jk3
MNS	M, N, S, s, U, Mi^a, Mt^a, Vx, Mur, Hil, Hut, En^a, (and others)
Lutheran	Lu^a, Lu^b
Diego	Di^a, Di^b, Wr^a
Others	Co^a, Co^b, Co^3, Ge^3, JFV, Jones, Kg, Lan, Lsa, MAM, PPIPk, Rd (Sc^4), Vel, (and others)

Data from Moise, K.J., Fetal anemia due to non-Rhesus-D red-cell alloimmunization. *Semin Fetal Neonatal Med,* 2008. 13(4): p. 207–14 and Eder, A.F., Update on HDFN: new information on long-standing controversies. *Immunohematology,* 2006. 22(4): p. 188–95.

5 percent of Asian Indians, and 0.3 percent of Chinese people.[14-16] Despite the success of Rh prophylaxis, anti-D antibodies still constitute a large proportion of clinically significant antibodies detected in Europe and the United States. When RhD is excluded, non-D Rh antibodies (c, C, e, E, cc, and Ce) and antibodies belonging to the Kell, Duffy, Kidd, and MNS systems, are most frequently involved[7,13]; Table 55–2 shows representative estimate of antibodies other than anti-D in women referred to a major national Maternal Alloimmunization Program at Wexner Medical Center at the Ohio State University.

TABLE 55-2. Incidence of Maternal Non-D Alloantibodies Associated with Hemolytic Disease of the Fetus and Newborn at a Major U.S. Referral Center*

Alloantibody	1970–1988 N (%)	1989–2006 N (%)
Anti-c	49 (16.6)	89 (10.4)
Anti-C	3 (1.0)	30 (3.5)
Anti-e	8 (2.7)	8 (0.9)
Anti-E	77 (26.1)	198 (23.1)
Anti-Kell†	87 (29.5)	167 (19.5)
Anti-Fy^a	19 (6.4)	61 (7.1)
Anti-Jk^a	1 (0.3)	44 (5.1)
Anti-M	12 (4.1)	197 (23.0)
Anti-S	12 (4.1)	13 (1.5)
Others	27 (9.2)	51 (5.9)
Total:	295	858

*The Ohio State University RBC Alloimmunization Program.

†Incidence of Kell alloimmunization has increased in other reports,[8] which may be explained by geographic variations in gene frequency or transfusion practices.

Used with permission of Richard W. O'Shaughnessy, Alloimmunization Program, Wexner Medical Center at the Ohio State University.

● CLINICAL FEATURES OF HEMOLYTIC DISEASE OF THE FETUS AND NEWBORN

OVERVIEW

Anemia, jaundice, and hepatosplenomegaly are the hallmarks of hemolytic disease of the newborn (HDN). The clinical spectrum of affected infants is highly variable. In Rh HDN, half of the infants have mild disease and do not require intervention. One-fourth of affected infants are born at term with moderate anemia and develop severe jaundice. In the days prior to intrauterine intervention, hydrops developed *in utero* in the remaining one-fourth of infants; half became hydropic prior to 34 weeks' gestation. Hydrops recurs in 90 percent of affected pregnancies, often at an earlier gestation. In Kell HDN, the clinical spectrum of hemolytic disease is less predictable, ranging from mild anemia to frank hydrops; jaundice may be less severe than that seen in Rh HDFN, given the erythroid suppression that anti-Kell alloantibodies may induce. Jaundice is the predominant feature of ABO HDN, but anemia and mild hepatosplenomegaly may also be seen. Severe fetal anemia and hydrops are unusual in ABO hemolytic disease.[17]

HEMOLYTIC ANEMIA

Infants with mild HDN may have cord blood hemoglobin concentrations only slightly lower than the age-related normal range. Hemoglobin values usually continue to fall after birth in all affected infants. Hemolysis continues until all incompatible red cells and/or circulating maternal alloantibody are eliminated from the circulation. Physical examination in infants having moderate to severe anemia reveals pallor, tachypnea, and tachycardia. In cases of severe HDFN, fetal anemia secondary to hemolysis results in compensatory extramedullary hematopoiesis in the liver, spleen, kidneys, and adrenal glands, and an outpouring of immature nucleated RBCs in the fetal circulation due to increased fetal plasma erythropoietin levels.[18] The marked increase in erythropoiesis may be accompanied by down-modulation of platelet and neutrophil production.[19]

After birth, the quantity of maternal antibodies in the neonatal circulation decreases over the next 12 weeks, with a half-life of approximately 25 days. Infants with moderate to severe hemolytic disease may develop significant anemia beyond the immediate neonatal period lasting up to 8 to 12 weeks of life. Delayed anemia is related to continuing hemolysis because of persistence of maternal antibodies and a hyporegenerative component with decreased red cell production from low serum concentrations of erythropoietin.[20-22]

NEONATAL JAUNDICE

Most infants with HDN are not jaundiced at birth because the placenta effectively transports most of the lipid-soluble unconjugated fetal bilirubin. Bilirubin concentrations in amniotic fluid reflect bilirubin concentrations in fetal blood and are influenced by fetal blood and amniotic fluid albumin concentrations.[23] The mechanism of entry of bilirubin into the amniotic fluid compartment has been debated, but of the five possible pathways (excretion through the fetal kidneys, meconium, skin, fetal lung secretions, and transmembranous), transmembranous appears to be most likely.[24]

At birth, the newborn infant's immature liver is incapable of handling the large bilirubin load that results from the ongoing destruction of antibody-coated neonatal red cells, and jaundice usually develops during the first day of life, often in the first few hours of life in severely affected infants. The jaundice progresses in a cephalopedal direction with rising bilirubin levels. In patients with mild disease, the serum indirect bilirubin peaks by the fourth or fifth day and then declines slowly. Premature infants may have higher levels of serum bilirubin for a longer duration because of lower hepatic glucuronyl transferase activity. Conjugated hyperbilirubinemia at birth is sometimes noted in infants who received multiple IUTs. Babies who received IUTs may still have anemia at birth and may still develop significant hyperbilirubinemia in the neonatal period.[25] As discussed later in the section "Postnatal Management", these infants may require intermittent transfusion therapy until 2 to 3 months of age due to persistent anemia.

KERNICTERUS

An important complication of elevated serum levels of indirect bilirubin in the neonate is the development of bilirubin encephalopathy.[26] This disorder, also termed *kernicterus*, is caused by bilirubin pigment deposition in the basal ganglia and brainstem nuclei, leading to neuronal necrosis. Acute bilirubin encephalopathy is initially marked by lethargy, poor feeding, and hypotonia. With increasing severity, the infant develops a high-pitched cry, fever, hypertonia progressing to frank opisthotonos, and irregular respiration. The infants then develop any or all of the classic sequelae of kernicterus: choreoathetoid cerebral palsy, gaze abnormalities, especially in upward gaze, sensorineural hearing loss, and cognitive deficits. The clinical presentation of bilirubin encephalopathy in preterm infants may be less distinctive. Abnormal or absent brainstem auditory evoked potentials and magnetic resonance imaging scans demonstrating the characteristic bilateral lesions of the globus pallidus help confirm the clinical diagnosis of kernicterus.

Infants with HDFN are at higher risk for kernicterus than are other infants with the same bilirubin level from other causes.[27] Heme pigments produced during active hemolysis are hypothesized to inhibit bilirubin–albumin binding. Alternatively, many conditions that potentially compromise the blood–brain barrier, such as prematurity, acidosis, hypoxemia, hypothermia, and hypoglycemia, are present in severely affected infants, making them more vulnerable to bilirubin encephalopathy.

OTHER CLINICAL FEATURES

Extensive extramedullary hemopoiesis in the liver and spleen may cause portal and umbilical venous hypertension, leading to ascites, pleural effusions, and consequent pulmonary hypoplasia.[28] Trophoblastic hypertrophy and placental edema cause impaired placental function. Hypoproteinemia as a result of liver dysfunction leads to generalized edema. "Hydrops fetalis," a state of anasarca, is the end result of a combination of anemia, hypoproteinemia, cardiac failure, elevated venous pressures, increased capillary permeability, and impaired lymphatic clearance. Hepatosplenomegaly is usually present. Cholestatic liver disease, previously believed to be associated with iron overload caused by IUTs, has been shown to occur in 13 percent of neonates with HDFN independent of previous IUT treatment and type of alloimmunization.[29] Hydropic babies may also have respiratory distress as a result of pulmonary hypoplasia, pleural and/or pericardial effusions, or surfactant deficiency.

Although the pathophysiology is not entirely clear, purpura associated with thrombocytopenia is sometimes seen in infants with HDFN. Thrombocytopenia at birth has been occurs in 26 percent of neonates with HDFN, independent of other comorbidities, such as lower gestational age at birth, being small for gestational age (SGA), and previous IUTs.[30] Severe fetal thrombocytopenia (platelet count $<50 \times 10^9$/L) has been reported in 3 percent of all fetal blood samplings and in 23 percent of severely RhD alloimmunized hydropic fetuses in one center when fetal platelet counts were measured prior to IUT.[31] In addition, neutropenia is a common feature of HDN and may be prolonged up to a year

of life, regardless of severity of HDFN, treatment received, or antibody specificity.[32]

OBSTETRIC HISTORY

The course and outcome of prior pregnancies are critically important in the initial evaluation of an alloimmunized pregnancy. A history of early fetal deaths or hydrops is ominous. In Rh alloimmunization, the severity of HDFN typically remains the same or worsens in subsequent affected pregnancies. Hydrops recurs in 90 percent of affected pregnancies, often at an earlier gestation in subsequent pregnancies. Alloimmunized women who report previous neonatal deaths, neonatal exchange transfusions, or IUTs should receive very close fetal surveillance.[33] Jaundice as a result of hemolysis often recurs to the same degree of severity in subsequent affected siblings. The history of prior blood transfusions may be obtained in women sensitized to antigens other than RhD, especially if Kell alloimmunization is detected. Establishment of paternity for each pregnancy is particularly relevant in both Rh and Kell alloimmunization, because the fetus is at risk only if the father is positive for the antigen in question. Unlike Rh and other minor alloantibody HDFN, ABO HDN may affect the first-born ABO-incompatible infant. Although rare, severe ABO HDN may recur in subsequent ABO-incompatible pregnancies.[34]

DIFFERENTIAL DIAGNOSIS

Hydrops fetalis may be secondary to α-thalassemia (Chap. 49) cardiac anomalies or arrhythmias, fetal genetic or metabolic disorders, intrauterine infections such as syphilis or toxoplasmosis, or any of a multitude of causes that lead to severe derangements in fetal homeostasis. These disorders are classified as nonimmune hydrops and are differentiated from the etiologies discussed in this chapter by the absence of any clinically significant red cell alloantibodies in the mother's blood. Parvovirus B19 infection of the mother at any time during gestation can cause nonimmune hydrops, profound fetal anemia, and death.

Neonatal anemia caused by intrinsic red cell defects such as hereditary spherocytosis (Chap. 46), red cell enzyme deficiencies (Chap. 47), and hemoglobinopathies, notably α-thalassemia (Chap. 48) can give a similar clinical picture to HDN. The absence of maternal red cell alloantibodies, a negative direct antiglobulin test (DAT) result, and detection of the specific defect determining the disorder clarify the diagnosis. Disorders of bilirubin metabolism can lead to unconjugated hyperbilirubinemia; however, they are not associated with anemia. Hepatitis or obstructive biliary diseases present with direct hyperbilirubinemia, most often after the first week of life.

● PATHOPHYSIOLOGY

There are three main classes of alloimmune HDFN, based on the antigen(s) involved: (1) Rh, (2) minor red cell antigens (i.e., Kell, Duffy, Kidd antigens), and (3) ABO. Factors affecting the risk to the fetus or neonate not only include the class of antigens involved, but also the titer (i.e., 4 vs. 32) and class/subclass (i.e., IgM vs. IgG_4 vs. IgG_1) of the antibody, the level of antigen expression on fetal RBCs, and the antibody's ability to suppress erythropoiesis (i.e., anti-K).[35,36] Rh HDFN is discussed first because it is archetypal of this condition; however, ABO incompatibility is much more common than Rh HDFN. The distinguishing features of the three classes of HDFN are highlighted below.

RHD HEMOLYTIC DISEASE

The standard nomenclature for designation of one's blood type is ABO and Rh-positive or Rh-negative based on the presence or absence of the

RhD antigen. However, the Rh blood system consists of numerous other antigens, the most common clinically significant include C, c, E, and e, which are encoded on the paired *RHCE* gene. RhD-positive individuals may have one or two copies of *RHD* gene (heterozygous or homozygous RhD-positive, respectively). More than 150 alleles have been defined for *RHD* and more are likely to be revealed as population studies expand.[37] In whites, RhD-negative individuals are homozygous for deletion of the *RHD* gene, which encompasses the whole of *RHD* and part of each of the flanking Rh boxes. The resultant RhD-negative phenotype is characterized by the absence of the whole RhD protein from the red cell membrane; however the *RHCE*-encoded antigens are present. Only 18 percent of RhD-negative Americans of African Descent are homozygous for *RHD* deletion. The majority (66 percent) of RhD-negative Americans of African descent have an inactive *RHD* gene *(RHψ)*, while 15 percent have a hybrid *RHD-CE-D* gene, neither of which produces epitopes of RhD antigen.

A number of *RHD* alleles responsible for RhD protein variants with altered RhD antigen expression have been classified according to their phenotype and molecular variation as partial D, weak D, and DEL. Amino acid substitutions located in extracellular domains result in different forms of partial D phenotype. Women with partial D phenotypes may develop antibodies against D epitopes absent on their cell membranes but present on the fetal RBCs. Amino acid substitutions located in the transmembrane or intracellular segments of the RhD protein result in a weak D phenotype. The expressed RhD antigen is reduced quantitatively but not qualitatively, so carriers are usually not susceptible to anti-D immunization. However, some types of weak D (weak D type 15, weak D type 4.2 or DAR, and weak D type 7) may produce anti-D. DEL is a very weakly expressed D antigen found in 30 percent of RhD-"negative" blood donors in East Asia. Anti-D antibody molecules recognize the epitopes on the external loops of RhD protein (Chap. 136).[37-39]

There currently are no requirements in the United States for blood banks to test for variant RhD on RhD-negative pregnant mothers. However, monoclonal RhD typing sera most commonly used for RhD typing do not detect weak D or partial D phenotypes, which results in reporting patients with variant RhD phenotypes as RhD-negative. Therefore, pregnant women with variant RhD phenotypes are usually treated with anti-D immunoglobulin prophylaxis.

RhD-negative pregnant women who appear to have both anti-D and anti-C, especially if at a similar strengths of reactivity serologically, require special consideration. In this instance, if the pregnant woman is lacking both RhD and RhC antigens, she is also lacking the RhG antigen, a combination antigen in the Rh Blood Group System found on RBCs containing either RhD or RhC antigens. In these situations, the laboratory must determine whether the antibodies are truly anti-D/anti-C rather than an anti-G because a patient who develops anti-C and/or anti-G antibodies but no anti-D should receive anti-D immunoglobulin prophylaxis.[40]

Fetomaternal Hemorrhage and Anti-D Alloimmunization
Asymptomatic transplacental passage of fetal red cells occurs in 75 percent of pregnant women at some time during pregnancy or during labor and delivery.[41] The incidence of fetomaternal transfusion increases with advancing gestation—from 3 percent (first trimester) to 12 percent (second trimester) to 45 percent (third trimester) and to 64 percent at delivery. The average volume of fetal blood in the maternal circulation after delivery is approximately 0.1 mL in most women and less than 1 mL in 96 percent of women.[42] Intrapartum fetomaternal hemorrhage of more than 30 mL may occur in up to 1 percent of deliveries.[43] Massive fetomaternal hemorrhage may present with decreased fetal movement and sinusoidal heart rhythm (undulating wave form alternating with a

flat or smooth baseline fetal heart rate); however, it also may be clinically silent, with no clinical signs differentiating such deliveries from those with minimal fetomaternal hemorrhage.[43,44] Fetomaternal transfusion can also result from obstetric procedures such as chorionic villus sampling, amniocentesis, funipuncture, therapeutic abortion, external cephalic version, cesarean section, and manual removal of the placenta, and from pathologic conditions such as abdominal trauma, spontaneous abortion, or ectopic pregnancy.[42,45-47]

The presence of RhD-positive red cells in an RhD-negative mother initially provokes a weak and slow primary immune response, which develops over 4 weeks and consists of transient elevation of IgM antibodies. Subsequently, approximately 5 to 15 weeks after exposure to the RhD-positive red cells, anti-D IgG antibodies capable of crossing the placenta are produced. The RhD antigen is the most immunogenic of the Rh antigens and, indeed, of all red cell antigens (after ABO).[48] The RhD protein is processed by antigen-processing cells in the spleen and lymphoid tissue of D-negative individuals into multiple short allogeneic linear peptides, which stimulate helper T cells, which then activate B cells to produce IgM and later IgG antibodies. Memory T and B cells that are generated following the initial immune response are long lived, and exposure to the antigen, even years later, results in an accelerated antibody response as a result of rapid proliferation of antigen-specific clones. Repeated exposure to RhD-positive fetal RBCs, as in a second RhD-positive pregnancy in a sensitized RhD-negative woman, produces a brisk secondary immune response marked by rapid production of large amounts of anti-D IgG antibody by maternal memory B lymphocytes.

In the absence of Rho(D) immunoglobulin (RhIg) prophylaxis, sensitization occurs in 7 to 16 percent of RhD-negative women at risk, within 6 months after delivery of the first RhD-positive ABO-compatible fetus. The relatively low rate of 16 percent of primary alloimmunization in Rh-negative women at risk may be a result of the low volume of fetomaternal hemorrhage (FMH) in most women. In fact, as little as 0.03 mL of RhD-positive RBCs has been shown to be sufficient to immunize some RhD-negative individuals.[49]

The potential for immunization of the mother is not only determined by the extent of FMH and the presence of fetomaternal blood group incompatibility, but also by other factors, such as the frequency of fetomaternal transfusion and whether the mother and fetus are ABO compatible. As an example, repetitive exposure to minuscule amounts of RhD-positive red cells in RhD-negative women who abuse intravenous drugs and share needles with RhD-positive partners has been reported to lead to severe Rh sensitization.[50] Fetomaternal ABO incompatibility offers some protection against primary Rh immunization because incompatible fetal red cells are destroyed rapidly by maternal anti-A and anti-B antibodies, reducing maternal exposure to RhD antigenic sites. Primary Rh immunization occurs in 2 to 4 percent of women at risk after delivery of an ABO-incompatible fetus.[51] ABO incompatibility confers no protection against the secondary immune response once sensitization has occurred.[52]

Binding of transplacentally transferred maternal anti-D IgG antibodies to D-antigen sites on the fetal red cell membrane is followed by adherence of the coated red cells to the Fcγ receptors of macrophages with rosette formation, leading to extravascular noncomplement-mediated phagocytosis and lysis, predominantly in the spleen.[51] Although Rh antigens are found on fetal RBCs as early as week 6 of gestation,[39] active transport of IgG across the placenta is slow until 20 to 24 weeks of gestation. The severity of fetal anemia is influenced primarily by the anti-D IgG concentration, but is also by other factors including: the IgG subclass, the rate of transplacental transfer of maternal IgG, the functional maturity of the fetal mononuclear phagocyte system, and the presence of maternal human leukocyte antigen (HLA) antibodies and or maternal–fetal ABO incompatibility.[53] Although IgG anti-D consists mainly of IgG_1 and IgG_3 subclasses, the relative contribution of each of these subclasses to the severity of HDFN remains controversial.[51,54,55]

HEMOLYTIC DISEASE CAUSED BY OTHER RED CELL ANTIBODIES

Although antibodies against RhD tend to be the most clinically significant in terms of fetal outcomes, there are many other RBC antigens capable of inducing alloantibodies after exposure through transfusion or pregnancy. Any alloantibody capable of inducing hemolysis or suppressing erythropoiesis may be clinically significant to developing fetuses. However, the mere presence of antibodies on screening tests may not be clinically significant, because of the unique characteristics of some antibodies. For example, antibodies to Lewis antigens (Le[a], Le[b]) are IgM and do not cross the placenta. Alternatively, Lutheran (Lu[a], Lu[b]) and Chido antigens are poorly expressed on fetal and neonatal red cells and therefore are not susceptible to destruction by maternal antibodies.

Case reports may be biased toward more-severe cases, and there is considerable variability in the clinical spectrum of disease produced by different alloantibodies. With the widespread use of RhIg, anti-Kell has bypassed anti-D as the leading cause of HDFN in some centers.[8] Table 55–1 lists some of the antibodies more commonly associated with HDFN.[13,56] Of note, many cases severe enough to require IUT involve antibodies to RhD, with or without antibodies to other alloantigens being present. Figure 55–1 shows data from 178 pregnancies requiring IUT at Wexner Medical Center, Ohio State University.

Kell

The Kell blood group system consists of at least 28 discrete antigens, of which eight are associated with HDFN. The *KEL* gene is located on chromosome 7q34, and Kell antigens are located on the red cell membrane glycoprotein CD238. Kell is unique in that it spans the RBC membrane once; it has a short N-terminal domain of 47 amino acids in the cytosol and a large C-terminal domain (665 amino acids) outside the membrane. The most common of the K antigens, Kell (also known as KEL1), is expressed by erythroid progenitor cells and mature erythroid cells by 9 percent of people of European ancestry and 1 to 2 percent of people of African ancestry; most KEL1-positive individuals are heterozygous.[57] Alloimmunization to KEL1 can occur through transfusion or through pregnancy.[58,59]

Given the relatively low prevalence of the KEL1 antigen, the likelihood of KEL1 incompatibility between mother and child is less than that of RhD. However, any KEL1-positive fetus being carried by a woman alloimmunized to the KEL1 antigen is at risk of anemia. Between 2.5 and 10 percent of alloimmunized pregnancies result in an affected infant, with fetal hydrops and severe anemia being common presentations of

Kell HDFN.[59-61] In contrast to the hemolysis observed in RhD HDFN, the severe fetal anemia observed because of maternal anti-Kell alloantibodies is largely a result of suppression of erythropoiesis and not to hemolysis. Clinical observations of inappropriately low levels of circulating reticulocytes and normoblasts for the degree of anemia have long been noted in affected fetuses, and suppression of erythropoiesis has been established by *in vitro* studies showing that growth of Kell-positive erythroid progenitor cells is inhibited by monoclonal IgG and IgM anti-Kell antibodies.[62] Furthermore, anti-Kell antibodies are associated with suppression of megakaryocyte and granulocyte colony-forming units with resultant fetal and neonatal thrombocytopenia and pancytopenia.[63,64] As discussed in further detail later in this the section" MATERNAL IMMUNOHEMATOLOGIC TESTING", titers of maternal anti-Kell do not necessarily correlate with the severity of fetal anemia and thus all maternal anti-Kell alloantibodies must be considered to be potentially clinically significant to antigen positive fetuses.

Other Minor Antigens (Non-D, Non-Kell)

Many other minor RBC antigens besides D and Kell are immunogenic in transfusion and pregnancy settings, with some of these alloantibodies having the capacity of being detrimental to developing fetuses. The incidence and prevalence of other minor antigens contributing to HDFN depends in part on the geographical area evaluated, as genetics and local transfusion practices impact alloimmunization. Any IgG that can cross the placenta is, in theory, capable of binding to cognate antigen on fetal RBCs. Antigen copy number, as well as other characteristics of the antigens/antibodies (potentially including IgG subtype), may impact the clinical significance of the alloantibodies.

ABO HEMOLYTIC DISEASE

ABO HDN occurs almost exclusively in infants with blood group A or B who are born to group O mothers, given that group O mothers have naturally occurring antibodies against the A and B antigens that are of the IgG class and are thus capable of crossing the placenta. The fetal reticuloendothelial system may completely remove RBCs bound with IgG, or it may remove portions of the RBCs, resulting in microspherocytes visible on blood film. (Table 55–3 compares ABO and RhD HDN.) Infants with ABO HDN generally have less-severe disease than those with Rh incompatibility. Hydrops fetalis caused by ABO alloimmune HDN is extremely rare. Although infants affected by ABO incompatibility may require phototherapy to treat their jaundice, less than 0.1 percent require exchange transfusion.[17,65] Unlike Rh disease, ABO HDN may affect the firstborn ABO-incompatible infant because anti-A and anti-B IgG antibodies are normally present in group O adults. Antenatal testing of anti-A and anti-B levels in group O mothers has little value in predicting ABO HDN, though the number of fully developed A or B antigens on fetal RBCs may impact disease severity. A recurrence rate of 88 percent has been reported in siblings having the same blood type as the affected index baby, with two-thirds of the affected siblings requiring therapy.[34] A higher incidence and greater severity of jaundice as a result of ABO incompatibility is reported in southeast Asians, Hispanics, Arabs, and South African and Americans of African descent than in whites.[17,66,67] This may be partly a result of the extent of development of A or B antigen sites on fetal RBCs, as well as of the prevalence of Gilbert syndrome in different patient populations.[68]

● ANTENATAL MONITORING

The evaluation and management of HDFN require close collaboration between obstetricians, maternal fetal medicine specialists, radiologists, hematologists, transfusion medicine specialists, and neonatologists.

RBC Alloantibodies in 178 Pregnancies Requiring Intrauterine Transfusions (from the Ohio State Alloimmunization Committee, 1965-2007)

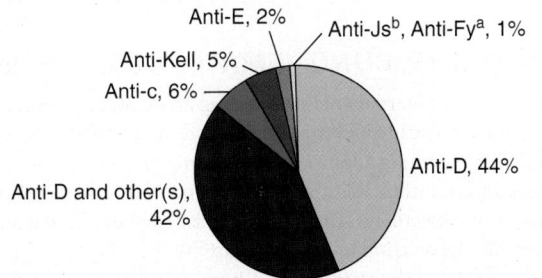

Anti-E, 2%
Anti-Js[b], Anti-Fy[a], 1%
Anti-Kell, 5%
Anti-c, 6%
Anti-D, 44%
Anti-D and other(s), 42%

Figure 55–1. RBC alloantibodies in 178 pregnancies requiring intrauterine transfusions during the period 1965 to 2007. (*Used with permission of Richard W. O'Shaughnessy, Alloimmunization Program, Wexner Medical Center at Ohio State University.*)

TABLE 55–3. Comparison of Rh and ABO Hemolytic Disease of the Newborn

	Rh	ABO
Blood groups		
Mother	Negative	O
Infant	Positive	A or B
Type of antibody	IgG$_1$ and/or IgG$_3$	IgG$_2$
Clinical aspects		
Occurrence in firstborn	5%	40–50%
Predictable severity in subsequent pregnancies	Usually	No
Stillbirth and/or hydrops	Frequent	Rare
Severe anemia	Frequent	Rare
Degree of jaundice	+++	+ to ++
Hepatosplenomegaly	+++	+
Laboratory findings		
Maternal antibodies	Always present	Usually present
Direct antiglobulin test (infant)	+	+ or −
Microspherocytes	−	+
Treatment		
Antenatal measures	Yes	No
Exchange transfusion frequency	Approx. 2/3	Occasional
Donor blood type	Rh-negative, group specific when possible	Group O only
Incidence of late anemia	Common	Rare

Ig, immunoglobulin.

Figure 55–2 is an algorithm for the clinical management of an alloimmunized pregnancy.

DETERMINATION OF PATERNAL ZYGOSITY AND FETAL BLOOD TYPE

When a clinically significant alloantibody is identified, or if there is a history of a previous fetus or neonate affected by HDFN, the next step is to determine if the fetus is at risk because the fetus carries the corresponding antigen. If the father is homozygous for the corresponding antigen, the fetus is at definite risk for HDFN. The child of an antigen-negative mother and a heterozygous antigen-positive father has a 50 percent chance of being antigen-positive and thus being affected by maternal alloimmunization. When the father is heterozygous or paternal zygosity is unknown, determination of fetal blood type early in pregnancy allows early institution of monitoring and therapy in antigen-positive fetuses that are at risk and forestalling invasive and potentially risky procedures in antigen negative fetuses.

Paternal zygosity is determined using serology for all common blood group antigens implicated in HDFN except for D. Alternatively, RBC genotyping can be used when typing for antigen systems where serologic reagents are rare or nonexistent. The probable *RHD* zygosity in RhD-positive persons may be inferred, but not definitively, from serologic phenotyping studies, based on gene frequencies in certain populations and the fact that the C/c and E/e antigens are closely linked to the *RHD* locus.[14,56] Elucidation of the genetic structure of the prevalent *RHD* locus and haplotypes responsible for RhD-negative phenotypes has led to the development of more direct and robust methods of determination of *RHD* zygosity molecularly. *RHD* zygosity testing by quantitative fluorescence polymerase chain reaction (QF-PCR) is commercially available and uses *RHD* (exons 5 and 7) to *RHCE* (exon 7) amplification ratios to determine *RHD* copy number. Although suitable for use in both white and ethnic African individuals, this molecular technique has a false-positive rate of 1 percent as a result of rare *RHD* alleles that are not expressed, and a false-negative rate of 1 percent as a result of rare partial D alleles (i.e., DBT type 1, type 2) which lack *RHD* exons 5 and 7 but still express RhD epitopes.[69,70]

If paternal heterozygosity is suspected or confirmed, determination of fetal blood type is helpful in planning further management. There are several sources of fetal tissue for fetal blood group genotyping. These include blood obtained by cordocentesis, chorionic villus sampling, and cervical tissue obtained by transvaginal lavage; each has risks to the fetus and issues related to quality of sample. Cordocentesis, amniocentesis, and chorionic villus sampling for fetal genetic typing carry a risk of FMH with increased risk of augmenting maternal sensitization and of fetal loss.[45,46] The advent of noninvasive methods of prenatal diagnosis using fetal DNA extracted from maternal plasma as early as the first trimester of pregnancy has obviated those concerns and has dramatically improved the ability to perform molecular testing on fetal tissue.[71]

Circulating cell-free fetal DNA (ccff-DNA) in maternal plasma can be identified as early as 5 weeks of gestation and is derived from apoptotic syncytiotrophoblasts. Fetal DNA used for typing is extracted and then evaluated by real-time quantitative polymerase chain reaction (QT-PCR). Most protocols amplify three exons or more, which include *RHD* exons 4 to 7 and 10, and detect target Psi (ψ) pseudogene sequences in exon 4 to avoid false-positives when the fetus has *RHDψ*.[72,73] Confirmation of detection of nonmaternal markers is required and can be accomplished by testing for the presence of the Y chromosome in male fetuses and/or housekeeping genes such as hemoglobin β-chain, β-actin, albumin, or chemokine receptor 5. A recent meta-analysis reviewed 37 publications describing 44 protocols reporting noninvasive *RHD* genotyping using fetal DNA obtained from more than 3000 maternal blood samples; an accuracy rate of 94.8 percent was reported.[72] Very high accuracy rates (>96 percent) have been reported for noninvasive fetal *RHCE* genotyping from maternal blood as well.[74] *RHD* ccff-DNA testing is commercially available, and is being increasingly used in the United States, United Kingdom, and Europe.[75] Although used more often in non-U.S. countries than in the United States at the present time, ccff-DNA testing may also be used to predict whether infants of alloimmunized women carry the cognate minor RBC antigen and are thus at risk for HDFN.

MATERNAL IMMUNOHEMATOLOGIC TESTING

The dual aims of maternal antenatal testing are to identify women who enter pregnancy already alloimmunized, and to identify those who are at high risk of becoming alloimmunized during pregnancy. The practice guidelines and recommendations for pregnancy-associated immunohematologic and molecular testing were established in the United States by the American Association of Blood Banks.[57]

Every obstetrical patient should have samples obtained between 10 and 16 weeks' gestation and tested for ABO and RhD type; D typing discrepancies must always be investigated and resolved. These maternal samples should also be screened for the presence of red cell alloantibodies. A second sample should be obtained at 28 weeks' gestation to

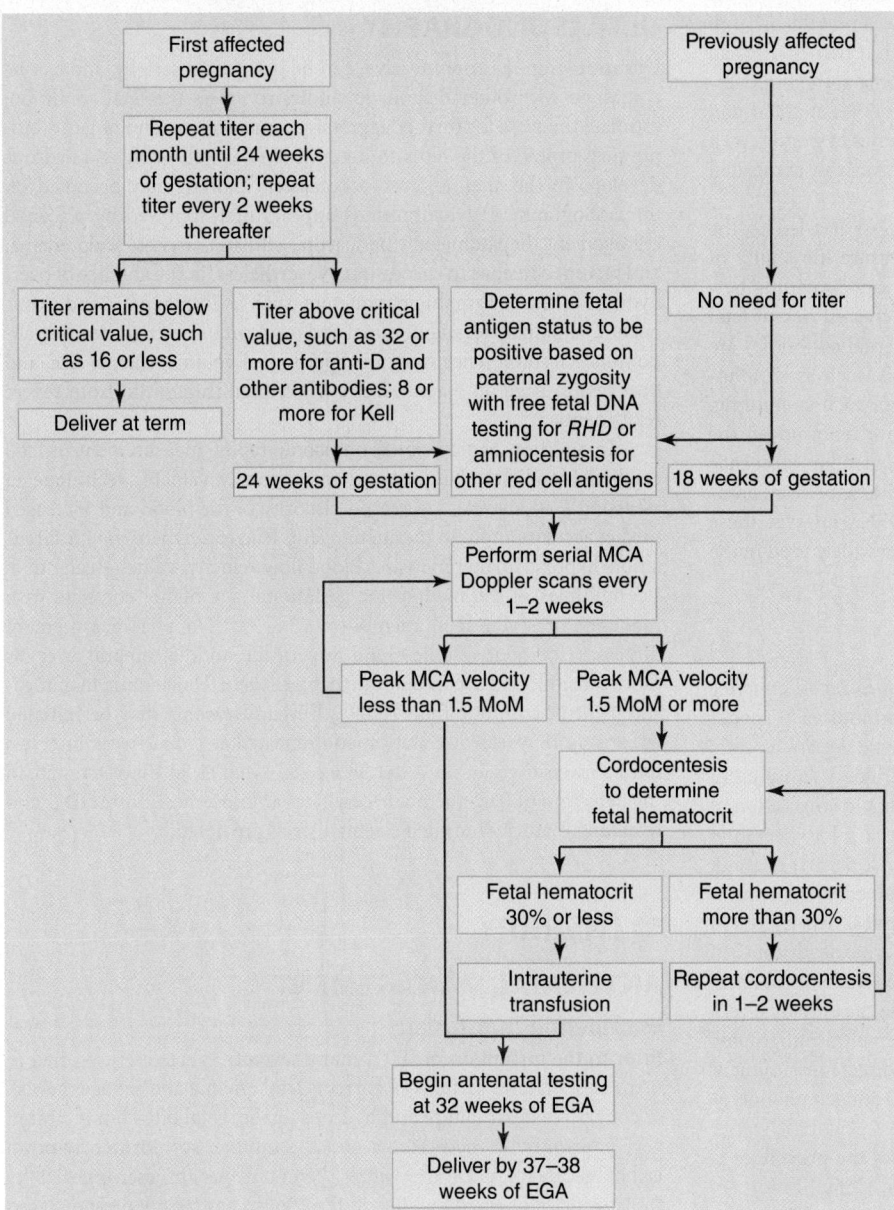

Figure 55–2. Algorithm for the clinical management of an alloimmunized pregnancy. EGA, estimated gestational age; MCA, middle cerebral artery; MoM, multiples of median. *(Modified with permission from Moise KJ Jr: Management of rhesus alloimmunization in pregnancy. Obstet Gynecol 2008 Jul;112(1):164-176.)*

confirm the maternal blood type, and to further evaluate the pregnant mother for other red cell alloantibodies that may have been evanescent or nonexistent earlier in pregnancy. If an unexpected antibody is identified anytime during pregnancy, the specificity, titer, and likelihood of leading to HDFN must be determined. The indirect antiglobulin test (IAT), using reagent red cells expressing C, c, D, E, e, K, k, Fy[a], Fy[b], Jk[a], Jk[b], S, s, M, N, and Le[a], is typically used for maternal antibody screening, Blood samples from women with anti-D alloantibodies should be tested monthly until 28 weeks' gestation and every 2 weeks thereafter.[76] Antibody titers are reported as the reciprocal of the highest dilution step at which agglutination is observed. A difference of two dilutions is considered a significant change. Testing should ideally be performed in parallel with previously frozen samples to minimize the possibility that changes in the titer result from differences in technique or reagent red cell selection.[57] A critical titer is defined as the titer associated with significant risk of fetal anemia or hydrops, and is the threshold at which the fetus will need monitoring. Once the critical titer is reached and a decision is made to monitor the fetus by ultrasonography or amniocentesis,

further antibody titration plays no role in assessment of fetal status. The critical titer varies from 8 to 32 in different laboratories in the United States.[76] In the United Kingdom and Europe, the level of anti-D is compared to an international standard and reported in IU/mL. Anti-D levels of 4 IU/mL or greater prompt referral to a specialist fetomaternal unit for further monitoring; at levels of 4 to 15 IU/mL, there is a potential risk of moderate HDFN; levels greater than 15 IU/mL imply a risk of severe HDN.[77] In the Netherlands, anti-Kell titers as low as 2 prompt referral to a perinatal center,[59] and the critical titer is defined as 16 or greater.[7] When RhIg has been administered during pregnancy, a positive low anti-D antibody titer may be detected (generally 2 to 4). Specific laboratory techniques may be used, if required, to distinguish between passive RhIg and active alloimmunization to D.

The significance of titer levels for antibodies other than D has not been fully defined. Maternal anti-Kell titers, in particular, correlate poorly with fetal outcome.[62] In a review of 156 anti–Kell-positive pregnancies over 37 years, McKenna and colleagues found that all severely affected fetuses had a titer of at least 32.[60] Bowman and colleagues also noted that a titer of 32 or greater was present in 16 of 17 severely affected pregnancies, but 1 patient with a titer of 1:8 had a grossly hydropic fetus at 23 weeks' gestation.[61] Some authors recommend further testing of the fetus if a critical titer of 8 is attained and paternal red cell typing is Kell-positive.[76] In a case series of women with anti-c isoimmunization, a titer of 32 or greater was invariably associated with severe fetal or neonatal disease.[78]

The imperfect predictive value of serologic tests has led to the development of functional cellular assays that measure the ability of maternal antibodies to cause red cell destruction, thus providing better noninvasive differentiation of pregnancies at increased risk of fetal anemia. In these assays, RBCs sensitized with maternal antibodies are incubated with effector cells carrying Fcγ receptors, such as lymphocytes or monocytes, to measure cellular interaction, such as binding, phagocytosis, or cytotoxic lysis.[79] Some authors have reported on the superiority of the monocyte monolayer assay, the chemiluminescence test, and the antibody-dependent cell-mediated cytotoxicity assay, compared to serologic tests, in predicting severity of HDFN. However, these tests are complex, difficult to standardize, and are not widely used in the United States.

FETAL BLOOD SAMPLING

Fetal blood sampling (also called *percutaneous umbilical blood sampling* or *cordocentesis*) allows direct measurement of blood indices to specifically evaluate the degree of severity of fetal hemolytic disease as early as 17 to 18 weeks' gestation.[80] Indications for fetal blood sampling in alloimmunized pregnancies include fetal blood typing, confirmation of severe fetal anemia suspected based on elevated peak middle cerebral artery Doppler velocities, or ultrasonographic evidence of early or frank hydrops Historically, fetal blood samples were obtained when amniocentesis results returned with ΔOD_{450} (change in optical density at 450 nm) measurements in Liley zone 3 or in the "intrauterine death zone" in the Queenan graph.[76,81,82] The procedure is performed under local anesthesia. A 20- to 22-gauge spinal needle is inserted into the umbilical vein at the level of cord insertion into the placenta under ultrasonographic guidance. Specimens of fetal blood are obtained for direct measurement of complete blood count, reticulocyte count, red cell antigen phenotyping, DAT, bilirubin, blood gases, and lactate to assess acid–base status. Blood should be available for immediate IUT when the procedure is being performed for suspected severe fetal anemia. Complications of fetal blood sampling include fetal loss, with procedure-related rates ranging from 0 to 4.9 percent, umbilical cord bleeding, chorioamnionitis, and significant risk of FMH with anamnestic maternal sensitization or the formation of additional alloantibodies.[83,84]

AMNIOTIC FLUID SPECTROPHOTOMETRY

Amniotic fluid spectrophotometry has been used for the last half century using bilirubin as an indicator to measure fetal hemolysis. Although briefly reviewed here for historical perspective, this method has now largely been replaced by noninvasive fetal monitoring techniques.[76,85,86] Elevations of ΔOD_{450} by spectrophotometry reflect the concentration of amniotic fluid bilirubin, which is derived from the fetus.[81] The original Liley chart, from 27 weeks to term, defined three zones: readings in zone 3, the upper zone, indicate severe fetal disease with hydrops or impending fetal death; readings in zone 1, the lowest zone, indicate mild or no hemolytic disease with a 10 percent risk of needing a postnatal exchange transfusion; and readings in zone 2 indicate moderate disease. The Liley chart was later modified by Queenan to include data from 14 to 40 weeks gestation and had 4 zones, with the lowest zone representing unaffected fetuses and the highest zone associated with increased risk of intrauterine death.[81]

ULTRASONOGRAPHY

Ultrasonography is noninvasive, can be performed serially, and can be combined with other diagnostic studies to assess the fetal condition, estimate the need for further aggressive management, and obtain a biophysical profile of the fetus to determine fetal well-being. As hydrops develops in the anemic fetus, a consistent pattern may be noted on ultrasonography. Polyhydramnios appears first, followed by placental enlargement, hepatomegaly, pericardial effusion, ascites, scalp edema, and pleural effusions in succession. Nevertheless, in the absence of overt hydrops, ultrasonographic parameters, such as intrahepatic and extrahepatic vein diameters, abdominal and head circumference, head-to-abdominal-circumference ratio, intraperitoneal volume, splenic size, and liver length have not been reliable in distinguishing mild from severe fetal anemia.[82]

In addition to traditional ultrasonography, measurement of fetal cerebral blood flow has become an extremely valuable technique in assessing fetal anemia. Decreased viscosity of the blood and increased cardiovascular output in the anemic fetus lead to a hyperdynamic circulation; hypoxia further increases blood flow velocity. Values greater than 1.5 multiples of the median for gestational age highly correlate with moderate or severe fetal anemia (Fig. 55–3).[86] Doppler measurement of peak velocity of systolic blood flow in the middle cerebral artery is more sensitive and accurate for detecting severe fetal anemia than measurement of amniotic fluid ΔOD_{450}.[85] Measurements may be initiated as early as 18 weeks of gestation and repeated at 1- to 2-week intervals until 35 weeks' gestation. After 38 weeks, a higher false-positive rate in the detection of fetal anemia necessitates amniocentesis for ΔOD_{450} and fetal lung maturity testing if elevated levels are noted.[76]

●THERAPY

ANTENATAL MANAGEMENT

Intrauterine Transfusion

Prior to the institution of IUTs, many severely affected fetuses died *in utero* or soon after birth. IUT corrects fetal anemia and reduce the risk of congestive heart failure and hydrops fetalis. Fetal bilirubin is cleared very efficiently by the placenta and the mother, so bilirubin removal is not necessary until after birth. Percutaneous intraperitoneal fetal transfusion, pioneered by Liley in the 1960s,[5] has been largely replaced by ultrasound-guided direct intravascular transfusion into the umbilical vein.[80,87] The intravascular technique circumvents the problem of erratic and often poor absorption of RBCs from the peritoneal cavity in such fetuses. However, intraperitoneal transfusions may be necessary when intravascular access is difficult, as in early pregnancy when the umbilical vessels are narrow or later when increased fetal size prevents access to the umbilical cord.[88,89] The first fetal blood sampling with transfusion ideally is performed before hydrops develops. Transfusions are given at fetal hematocrit levels of 25 to 30 percent or less, or if the fetal hemoglobin is 4 to 6 standard deviations below the mean for gestational age. Generally, the hematocrit drops by 1 to 2 percent per day in the transfused hydropic fetus. The fall in hematocrit is rapid in fetuses with severe hemolytic disease, often necessitating a second transfusion within 7 to 14 days. The interval between subsequent transfusions varies, but may be 21 to 28 days. The nonhydropic fetus can tolerate rapid RBC infusions of 5 to 7 mL/min because of the capacitance of the placenta. The hydropic fetus requires slower transfusion rates and can tolerate only smaller, more frequent transfusions. Very low pretransfusion fetal hematocrit levels, rapid large increases in posttransfusion hematocrit level, and increases in umbilical venous pressure during IUTs are associated with fetal death after transfusion.[90,91]

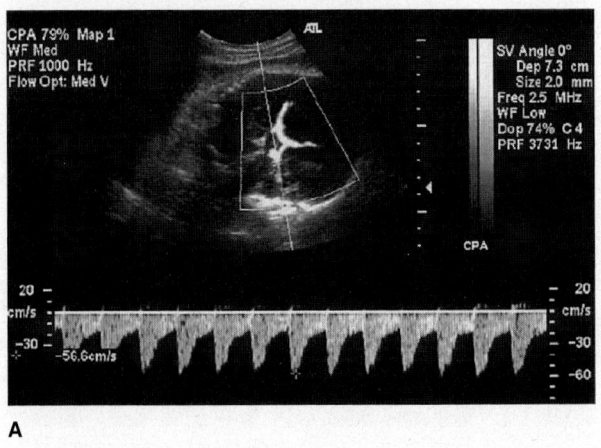

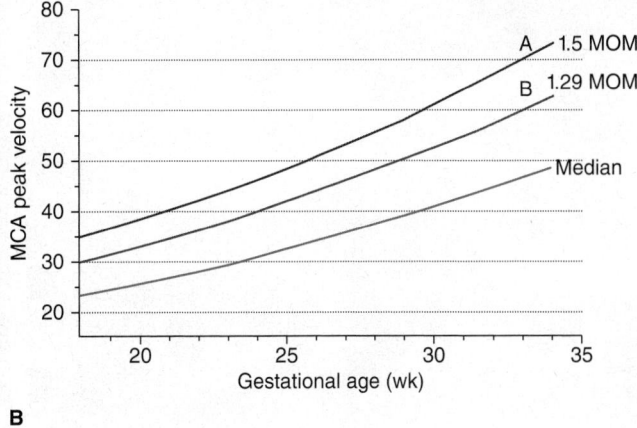

A   **B**

Figure 55–3. Peak velocity of systolic blood flow in the middle cerebral artery can be measured by ultrasound **(A)** and compared to multiples of the median (MoMs) for the prediction of fetal anemia **(B)**. *(A, reproduced with permission from Dukler D, Oepkes D, Seaward G, et al., Noninvasive tests to predict fetal anemia: a study comparing Doppler and ultrasound parameters. Am J Obstet Gynecol 2003 May;188(5):1310–1314. B, reproduced with permission from Moise KJ Jr, Management of rhesus alloimmunization in pregnancy, Obstet Gynecol 2002 Sep;100(3):600–11.)*

RBCs for IUT are typically crossmatch compatible with the mother's plasma and negative for any identified antibody; they should also be irradiated and leukoreduced.[92,93] Many centers do not use RBCs heterozygous for sickle hemoglobin to prevent sickling in the fetus at low oxygen tension although direct evidence of its benefit is lacking, and 5 to 7 days old to maximize circulatory half-life. Obtaining RBCs from a rare donor registry may be required in cases of unusual or combination antibodies. In this circumstance, frozen, deglycerolized RBCs may be the only available product. Some centers use maternal RBCs for IUTs, supporting serial maternal donations with iron and folate therapy.[94] RBC transfusion is calculated to increase the fetal hematocrit to between 40 and 45 percent. The RBCs are often washed free of additive solutions, and packed to a hematocrit of 70 to 85 percent in a volume calculation based on estimated fetal placental blood volume, fetal hematocrit, and hematocrit of donor RBCs. Various normograms and formulas for the calculation of donor blood volume have been published.[95,96] If the hematocrit of the donor unit is approximately 75 percent, multiplying the estimated fetal weight in grams (estimated by ultrasonography) by a factor of 0.02 provides a fairly accurate estimate of the volume of RBCs to be transfused to achieve a fetal hematocrit increment of 10 percent.[97]

Van Kamp and colleagues estimated procedure-related complication rates of 2.9 percent in the absence of hydrops and 3.9 percent in the presence of hydrops in a cohort study of 254 fetuses treated with 740 IUTs in a single center.[98] The most common problem was transient fetal heart rate abnormalities, which occurred in 8 percent of procedures. The procedure-related pregnancy loss rate was calculated to be 1.6 percent per procedure. Fetal distress during or after the procedure may result in emergency cesarean section. Cord accidents such as hemorrhage from the puncture site or rupture of the cord are rare. Additional alloantibodies may develop in already alloimmunized women undergoing IUT; in one study, 25 percent (53 of 212) of "responder" women treated with IUT formed new alloantibodies, 53 percent of which were directed against non-Rh and -K antigens.[99]

Delivery

The decision regarding the appropriate time to deliver the baby is based on gestational age, fetal weight and lung maturity, fetal response to the IUTs, ease of performing the transfusions, and antenatal ultrasonography and Doppler studies for fetal anemia. Transfusions usually are provided up to 35 weeks so as to prolong gestation safely until the risks of preterm birth and its attendant complications are minimized, with delivery once adequate lung maturity has occurred.[76]

Other Therapies

In women with severe alloimmunization and with fetal losses or hydrops very early in pregnancy, a variety of methods have been used to suppress the antibody response and prolong survival of the fetus until IUT becomes technically feasible. Use of intravenous immunoglobulin (IVIG), serial plasmapheresis, or plasmapheresis combined with IVIG have been successful in some cases.[89,100,101] IVIG may cause nonspecific Fc blockade of the fetal reticuloendothelial system.

POSTNATAL MANAGEMENT

Neonatal Monitoring

A sample of cord blood should be collected from all newborns at the time of delivery. However, specific testing of cord blood samples is performed only if the mother is Rh-negative, if the maternal serum contains red cell alloantibodies of potential clinical significance, or if the neonate develops signs of hemolytic disease. Tests should include ABO and Rh typing and a DAT. Many birth hospitals routinely test cord blood for the infant's blood type and DAT if the mother is O Rh-positive in order to predict which infants are at increased risk of hyperbilirubinemia. In severe Rh alloimmunization, high titers of maternal antibody may block Rh-antigenic sites on the neonatal red cells, leading to false-negative Rh typing. Antepartum RhIg given to the mother may cause a weakly positive DAT result in the infant at birth. Contamination of the cord blood sample with Wharton jelly during collection can also result in a false-positive DAT result. Although the DAT usually is positive in all forms of alloimmune HDFN, the test cannot predict reliably the degree of clinical severity.[102,103] This is especially true for cases resulting from ABO sensitization. When fetomaternal ABO incompatibility is present, the presence of maternally derived IgG anti-A or anti-B in the infant's serum may be demonstrated by the IAT to support the diagnosis of ABO hemolytic disease. On the other hand, it is important to bear in mind that hemolysis in ABO-incompatible, DAT-negative infants may result from hematologic causes other than alloimmunization or from red cell membrane defects (Chap. 46).[104] Elution of maternal antibody from the infant's red cells, followed by tests to determine the specificity of the antibody in the eluate, may be useful, particularly when several antibodies are present in the maternal serum or when the maternal antibody screen is negative.[57] Infants who received IUTs may have mild or moderate anemia with little reticulocytosis. Because most of their circulating red cells are transfused antigen-negative cells, the DAT may be negative, but the IAT will be strongly positive.

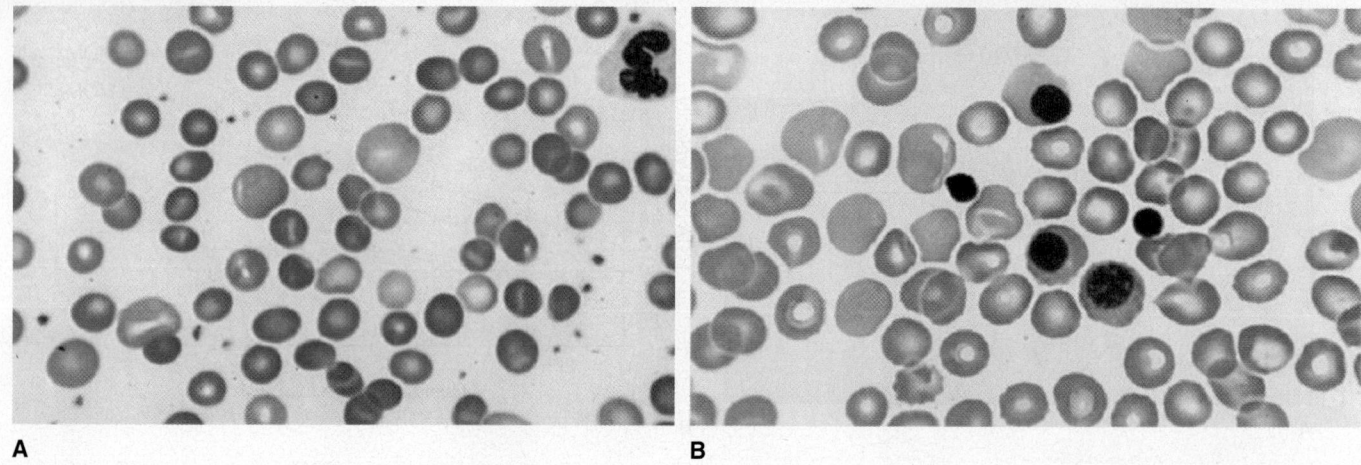

A   **B**

Figure 55–4. Alloimmune hemolytic disease of the newborn. Blood films. **A.** Infant with ABO blood group alloimmune hemolytic anemia. Note the high prevalence of spherocytes and the large polychromatophilic cells, indicative of reticulocytosis. **B.** Infant with Rh blood group alloimmune hemolytic anemia. Note spherocytes, reticulocytes, and the nucleated red cells. The intense erythroblastosis is characteristic of Rh blood group allo-immune hemolytic anemia and is less prominent in ABO blood group alloimmune hemolytic anemia. *(Reproduced with permission from* Lichtman's Atlas of Hematology, *www.accessmedicine.com.)*

Cord blood hemoglobin and indirect bilirubin determinations are useful in determining disease severity. Most infants with cord hemoglobin levels within the age-adjusted normal range do not require exchange transfusion. Usually, a cord hemoglobin level less than 11 g/dL in a term newborn and/or a cord-indirect bilirubin level greater than 4.5 to 5 mg/dL indicate severe hemolysis and often warrant early exchange transfusion. Early exchange transfusion also may be indicated if the rate of rise of bilirubin, measured every 4 to 6 hours, exceeds 0.5 mg/dL per hour. The reticulocyte count usually is greater than 6 percent and may approach 30 to 40 percent in severe Rh disease. The blood film in Rh disease is characterized by increased nucleated RBCs, polychromasia, and anisocytosis. Alternatively, the blood film in ABO HDN is marked by microspherocytes (Fig. 55–4). Severely affected infants may also have thrombocytopenia. Low reticulocyte counts disproportionate to the low hematocrit may be noted in Kell-mediated HDN. Severely affected infants may have hypoglycemia, secondary to hyperinsulinemia. Arterial blood gas analysis may reveal metabolic acidosis and/or respiratory decompensation, and hypoalbuminemia is often present.

Immediate Postnatal Management

Results of antenatal monitoring and obstetric interventions during pregnancy and the history of the outcome of previous pregnancies allow the neonatal team to anticipate the needs of the infant born with hemolytic disease. In infants with severe hemolytic disease without the benefit of IUTs, severe anemia and hydrops are the immediate life-threatening concerns and often are accompanied by perinatal asphyxia, surfactant deficiency, hypoglycemia, acidosis, and thrombocytopenia. Exchange transfusions and phototherapy are the mainstays of treatment.

Resuscitation and stabilization of hydropic infants is challenging. Endotracheal intubation and positive-pressure ventilation with oxygen is usually necessary. Drainage of pleural effusions and ascites may be required to facilitate gas exchange. Metabolic acidosis and hypoglycemia require correction. A partial exchange transfusion may initially be performed using packed red cells to improve hemoglobin levels and oxygenation. A double-volume exchange transfusion is considered only after the initial stabilization.

In a study of 191 infants born alive after IUTs between 1988 and 1999, the hematocrit at birth ranged from 13 to 51 percent.[105] Endotracheal ventilation was required more often in babies who had been

severely hydropic *in utero*, but the requirements for exchange transfusion or simple transfusion did not differ between babies who had been hydropic *in utero* and those without evidence of hydrops. Although some centers report no difference in the frequency of exchange transfusions in babies who have had IUTs compared with babies who have not had IUTs,[105,106] other centers report that infants who received multiple IUTs are usually born closer to term and often require less phototherapy and fewer exchange transfusions in the neonatal period.[25,107] Nonetheless, many infants with severe HDFN require additional RBC transfusions for severe and prolonged hyporegenerative anemia secondary to suppression of fetal erythropoiesis.[21,22,106] Approximately three-quarters of term and near-term infants who had received IUT for Rh HDFN required transfusion within 6 months of age, compared with 26 percent of infants with Rh HDFN who had not received an IUT.[106] Thus, careful monitoring of the baby and the baby's lab values are necessary not only during the initial hospital course but also after hospital discharge.

Exchange Transfusion

Exchange transfusion corrects anemia, removes bilirubin and free maternal antibody in the plasma, and replaces the infant's blood with antigen-negative RBCs that should have normal *in vivo* survival. Neonatal exchange transfusions can be performed by a continuous technique (simultaneous withdrawal and replacement) or discontinuous technique (alternating withdrawal and replacement). Regardless of the technique, the kinetics of exchange are very similar. A double-blood-volume exchange replaces approximately 85 percent of the infant's blood volume with antigen-negative RBCs; however, the amount of bilirubin or maternal alloantibody removed by exchange transfusion is significantly less (25 to 45 percent) reflecting the equilibrating tissue-bound plasma pool. Infusion of albumin prior to the exchange transfusion may help bilirubin binding, thus increasing the amount of bilirubin removed. Equilibration of extravascular and intravascular bilirubin, and continued breakdown of red cells by persisting maternal antibodies, result in a rebound of bilirubin following initial exchange transfusion, sometimes requiring repeated exchange transfusions in severe hemolytic disease.

The ideal volume for an exchange transfusion is twice the infant's blood volume. There is little benefit achieved by exceeding two blood volumes because the efficiency of exchange transfusion declines exponentially as the procedure continues. The volume needed for double-volume exchange depends on the total blood volume (TBV) recognizing differences in term and preterm infants:

- Double-blood-volume exchange volume (term) = 85 mL/kg × 2, or 170 mL/kg
- Double-blood-volume exchange volume (preterm) = 100 mL/kg × 2, or 200 mL/kg

To perform the exchange transfusion, aliquots of the reconstituted whole blood product are administered while equal amounts of the infant's blood are withdrawn. Careful attention not to exceed 2 mL/kg per minute (continuous) or 5 mL/kg at a time over 3 to 10 minutes (discontinuous technique) is required to prevent rapid fluctuations in arterial and intracranial pressure.[108]

The indications for "early" exchange transfusions performed within the first 12 hours of life have remained essentially unchanged over the last 45 years, with minor modifications. Cord hemoglobin levels equal to or less than 11 g/dL, cord bilirubin levels equal to or greater than 5.5 mg/dL, and rapidly rising total serum bilirubin (TSB) equal to or greater than 0.5 mg/dL per hour despite phototherapy are commonly used criteria for early exchange transfusions. Early exchange transfusion has the advantage of replacing sensitized RBCs with normal RBCs, thereby removing not only bilirubin but also the source of future bilirubin. Because bilirubin is distributed in the extracellular fluids, efficiency is enhanced by removing sensitized cells early in the process. Newborns that have been treated with serial IUTs until term often do not require exchange transfusions; however, late anemia is common because of IUT-induced erythropoietic suppression, which may last for many weeks after delivery.[109]

"Late" exchange transfusions are performed when serum bilirubin levels threaten to exceed approximately 20 to 22 mg/dL in term infants. The American Academy of Pediatrics (AAP) Subcommittee on Hyperbilirubinemia provided revised guidelines for exchange transfusion in infants 35 or more weeks' gestation.[110] In view of the fact that bilirubin levels rise steadily from birth and peak at approximately 72 to 96 hours of age, exchange transfusion should be considered if serum bilirubin levels reach 15 mg/dL in an infant of 35 weeks' gestation or 17 mg/dL in an infant of 38 weeks' gestation despite intensive phototherapy. Immediate exchange transfusion is recommended in infants showing signs of acute bilirubin encephalopathy, even if bilirubin levels are falling.[110] Conjugated or direct bilirubin values are not subtracted from total bilirubin levels when considering levels for exchange transfusions. Exchange transfusions are performed at lower bilirubin levels in premature infants, particularly those with hypoxemia, acidosis, and hypothermia, but little data are available to guide intervention in these infants. In infants with birth weights of at least 1500 g, exchange transfusions usually are performed at TSB of 13 to 16 mg/dL but may be considered even at levels as low as 8 to 9 mg/dL in sick babies of 24 weeks' gestation.[111] The bilirubin-to-albumin ratio (mg/dL:g/dL), considered to be a surrogate measure of free bilirubin, may provide additional data in determining the need for exchange transfusion in both term and preterm neonates.[112]

Blood components chosen for the exchange transfusion should be ABO and Rh compatible (Rh-negative in Rh HDN), negative for offending antibody(ies), and crossmatch compatible with maternal serum. In the case of ABO HDN, O RBCs should be chosen for exchange out of concern that the more developed A or B antigens on any transfused adult donor RBCs may more avidly bind maternal anti-A or anti-B and may result in hemolysis. Either reconstituted whole blood (WB) (e.g., RBCs plus fresh-frozen plasma [FFP]) or stored WB if available can be used for neonatal exchange transfusions. The RBCs are reconstituted with AB or compatible plasma to a final hematocrit of 50 to 60 percent. Fresh (<7 days) RBCs should be used. When fresh RBC units are unavailable, some centers wash the RBCs and transfuse as soon as possible after washing to avoid hyperkalemia. Additionally, the RBC units should be leukoreduced, gamma irradiated, and sickle-negative.[113]

Potential complications of exchange transfusion include hypocalcemia, hyperglycemia, hypoglycemia, thrombocytopenia, dilutional coagulopathy, neutropenia, disseminated intravascular coagulation, umbilical venous and/or arterial thrombosis, necrotizing enterocolitis, and infection. Thrombocytopenia and hypocalcemia are reported to be the most common complications (incidence ranging from 29 to 47 percent).[114,115] Thrombocytopenia results from a dilutional effect of replacing platelet rich neonatal WB with platelet-deficient reconstituted WB. Infants who may be thrombocytopenic from severe HDFN or other comorbidities should be monitored closely after an exchange transfusion as they may require platelet transfusion. Hypocalcemia occurs as a result of the citrate load infused, which an immature neonatal liver has difficulties metabolizing. In anticipation of hypocalcemia, ionized calcium levels should be monitored throughout the exchange transfusion procedure, and intravenous calcium replacement may be needed in sick preterm infants. Furthermore, attempts should be made to correct conditions that may potentiate the symptoms of hypocalcemia such as alkalosis, hypothermia, hypomagnesemia, and hyperkalemia.[116]

In a retrospective review of exchange transfusions performed in two neonatal intensive care units between 1981 and 1995, the risk of death or permanent serious sequelae was reported to be as high as 12 percent in sick infants, compared with less than 1 percent in healthy infants. Adverse outcomes were more frequent in exchanges done on preterm infants younger than 32 weeks, infants with other significant comorbidities, and when umbilical catheters were used rather than other means of central venous access.[117] Another center reported no increase in the number of complications and no exchange transfusion–related deaths over a 21-year period, even though there was a decline in the frequency of exchange transfusions performed over the years.[115] Careful clinical judgment is required to balance the potential risk of adverse events from exchange transfusion with the risk of bilirubin encephalopathy in neonates who are premature, sick, or both.

Phototherapy

Phototherapy is the mainstay of treatment for unconjugated hyperbilirubinemia; the objective of treatment is preventing bilirubin neurotoxicity. Exposure of bilirubin to light results in structural and configurational isomerization of bilirubin to less toxic and less lipophilic products that are excreted efficiently without hepatic conjugation. The effectiveness of phototherapy is influenced by the wavelength and irradiance of light, the surface area of exposed skin, and the duration of exposure. Intensive phototherapy involves the use of high levels of irradiance ($\geq 30\ \mu$W/cm^2) in the 430- to 490-nm band, delivered to as much of the infant's surface area as possible. Intensive phototherapy effectively reduces bilirubin levels and decreases the need for exchange transfusions for hyperbilirubinemia in ABO and Rh HDN.[118,119] Early and intensive phototherapy should be initiated in infants with moderate or severe hemolysis or in infants with rapidly rising bilirubin levels (>0.5 mg/dL per hour). In full-term infants (at least 38 weeks' gestation) with HDFN, intensive phototherapy should be initiated if TSB levels are 5 mg/dL or greater at birth, 10 mg/dL at 24 hours after birth, or approximately 13 to 15 mg/dL at 48 to 72 hours after birth.[110] Phototherapy is recommended at lower levels for preterm or sick infants. Therapy often is initiated at TSB less than 5 mg/dL in preterm infants with HDFN so as to avoid potentially risky exchange transfusions.[110,111]

Other Therapies

A number of small studies have reported on the successful administration of high-dose IVIG as an adjuvant treatment to standard therapy for HDN as way to prevent the need for exchange transfusions.[109] The decreased bilirubin levels in infants treated with IVIG is attributed to reduction in hemolysis secondary to blockade of mononuclear phagocyte Fc receptors. A Cochrane meta-analysis of the three largest studies demonstrated that IVIG administration (0.5 to 1.0 g/kg) may prevent exchange transfusion for many term infants with HDN, which contributed to an AAP published recommendation that IVIG be considered in Rh HDN when TSB continues to rise despite aggressive phototherapy or when the TSB is within 2 to 3 mg/dL of the exchange level.[110] However, a prospective randomized control trial showed that prophylactic IVIG (0.75 g/kg) did not decrease the duration of phototherapy, maximum bilirubin levels, need for RBC transfusion or for exchange transfusion in Rh HDN.[120] Although, the majority of the infants included in this study were treated with IUT, IVIG was not effective at reducing the need for exchange transfusion in either the group treated with IUTs or those who were not. Thus, there is no universal approach to the use of IVIG in patients with HDN; it seems justified as a temporizing measure to exchange transfusion in neonates with severe HDN unmodified by IUT or neonates with HDN where a previous sibling had suffered from severe disease requiring exchange transfusion.[109]

Recombinant human erythropoietin (rHuEPO) given subcutaneously at a dose of 200 to 400 U/kg given three times weekly for 2 weeks is sometimes administered to infants in an effort to reduce or prevent transfusion for late-onset anemia from HDN. Some studies show its use to decrease the need for postnatal transfusions in infants with late hyporegenerative anemia of Rh HDN and in neonates with Kell HDN.[21,121,122] In one study of 103 patients with Rh HDN, administration of 200 U/kg of rHuEPO, three times per week for 6 weeks, reduced the number of RBC transfusions to a mean of 1.5, and 55 percent of patients did not require any transfusions.[121] rHuEPO is more effective in decreasing future transfusion needs in neonates that never received IUTs suggesting that IUTs may decrease the neonatal response to rHuEPO.[123] Despite encouraging reports in relatively small numbers of neonates, it remains unclear whether rHuEPO, or the longer-acting analogue darbepoetin, offer a distinct clinical benefit in regard to decreasing donor exposures or improvement of morbidity and/or mortality in this population. rHuEPO has been shown to lessen neurologic sequelae in term infants with hypoxic ischemic encephalopathy, therefore it may have a role as a potential treatment for perinatal brain injury in the future.[124]

● OUTCOME

Perinatal survival rates greater than 90 percent have been achieved with IUT in nonhydropic fetuses with severe HDFN.[98,105] The overall survival rate for hydropic fetuses is lower (78 to 89 percent) despite IUTs.[105,107] An 11-year study (from 1988 to 1999) which examined 80 fetuses with immune-mediated hydrops reported a survival rate for fetuses with mild hydrops of 98 percent, and an intrauterine reversal of hydrops in 88 percent of the fetuses. The outcome in severe fetal hydrops was poor, with reversal of hydrops in 39 percent of cases, and a survival rate of 26 percent for fetuses with persistent hydrops.[105] This study underscores the importance of early diagnosis and treatment of fetal anemia, before hydrops develops. Implementation of a nationwide first trimester screening program for red cell antibodies in the Netherlands in 1998 was associated with increased referrals for suspected fetal anemia, more timely referrals and an increase in perinatal survival in Kell HDFN from 61 to 100 percent.[59]

The neurodevelopmental outcome for infants saved by IUTs has generally been good, with almost 90 percent of survivors being free of disability, even when they have been profoundly anemic *in utero*.[25,107] The LOTUS study evaluated 291 children at a median age of 8.2 years (range: 2 to 17 years) to determine the incidence and risk factors for

neurodevelopmental impairment in children with HDFN treated with IUT. The overall incidence of neurodevelopmental impairment was 4.8 percent with severe developmental delay seen in 3.1 percent of children. Cerebral palsy was detected in 2.1 percent and bilateral deafness in 1 percent of the children. Severe hydrops was identified as a strong predictor for neurodevelopmental impairment.[125]

It is estimated that kernicterus, secondary to bilirubin encephalopathy, is associated with at least 10 percent mortality and 70 percent long-term morbidity.[126] Although the preponderance of kernicterus cases occur in infants with bilirubin levels higher than 20 mg/dL, it has been shown that when treated promptly with phototherapy or exchange transfusion, peak bilirubin levels in the range of 25.0 and 29.9 mg/dL were not associated with adverse neurodevelopmental outcomes in term or near-term infants.[126,127] However, there was an adverse association with IQ among infants with a positive DAT and a TSB level equal to or greater than 25 mg/dL, supporting the AAP recommendations to initiate treatment at lower bilirubin levels for jaundiced infants if they have a positive DAT.[27,110,127]

● PREVENTION

Transfusion of blood phenotypically matched for D and for Kell antigens has been advocated for all premenopausal women to prevent primary RBC alloimmunization.[7,13] RhIg prophylaxis is very effective when administered to women exposed to RhD-positive RBCs either from pregnancy or from transfusion; however, once alloimmunization has occurred, RhIg is not effective for preventing or reducing the severity of HDFN. Unlike RhD, there are no commercially available immune globulin products for prevention of alloimmunization to minor RBC antigens (including non-D Rh antigens). If a nonpregnant woman is found to have a RBC alloantibody, counseling should be provided regarding the potential effects of the antibody on future pregnancies. Interventions which can be applied but are seldom offered to prevent HDFN in high risk maternal-paternal pairs include: artificial insemination with sperm from an antigen-negative donor; pre-implantation genetic diagnosis selecting for antigen-negative embryos; and surrogate pregnancy.[128]

Rh IMMUNOGLOBULIN

Use of RhIg is the standard of care for the prevention of maternal D immunization. Postpartum administration of RhIg to all nonsensitized Rh-negative women who deliver an Rh-positive infant decreases the incidence of Rh isoimmunization from 12 percent to approximately 2 percent. Further reduction in the incidence of Rh-isoimmunization (to 0.1 percent) has been achieved by antepartum RhIg prophylaxis at 28 weeks' gestation. This is the current standard recommendation in the United States.[129] In the United Kingdom, routine antenatal anti-D prophylaxis can be given as two doses of anti-D immunoglobulin of 500 IU (one at 28 weeks' and one at 34 weeks' gestation), as two doses of anti-D immunoglobulin of 1000 to 1650 IU (one at 28 weeks' and one at 34 weeks' gestation), or as a single dose of 1500 IU at 28 weeks' gestation.[130] Although the efficacy of RhIg is clear, its mechanism of action is not. Some of the proposed mechanisms are accelerated clearance and destruction of D-positive red cells from the circulation, antibody-mediated immune suppression, and the production of immunomodulatory cytokines.[51]

RhIg is prepared from plasma pools of screened, sensitized human donors; the plasma is tested using polymerase chain reaction (PCR) and serologic methods for all known transfusion transmitted organisms. Several steps are taken to further inactivate potential infectious organisms, including solvent-detergent treatment, ion exchange chromatography, and nanofiltration. There are at least four formulations of RhIg, including two preparations that may be administered intravenously.[131] A 300 mcg (1500 IU) dose of RhIg affords protection against a fetomaternal transfusion of 15 mL of Rh-positive RBCs or 30 mL of Rh-positive WB. However, FMH in excess of 30 mL may occur in women without predisposing risk factors.[42,43] The blood of all Rh-negative nonimmunized women should be tested for FMH approximately 1 hour after delivery of an Rh-positive baby.[57,129] During the antenatal period, testing is indicated after 20 weeks' gestation if clinical circumstances suggest the possibility of excessive transplacental hemorrhage (e.g., abdominal trauma or abruptio placentae). Screening for FMH can be performed by the rosette test, which detects as little as 2.5 mL of WB. If the rosette test result is positive, the number of fetal red cells in the maternal circulation is quantified more accurately by the Kleihauer-Betke test, which is based on the resistance of fetal hemoglobin to acid elution, unlike adult hemoglobin (Fig. 55–5).[132] False-positive results can be obtained in maternal conditions associated with increased fetal hemoglobin, such as hereditary persistence of fetal hemoglobin, sickle cell disease, or sickle cell trait. Flow cytometric methods are used in some laboratories for both screening and quantification of fetal red cells.

RhIg should be administered as soon as possible, within 72 hours of delivery of an Rh-positive baby. RhIg is thought to be ineffective once alloimmunization to RhD antigen has occurred. RhIg is also indicated following pregnancy termination, miscarriage, amniocentesis, chorionic villus sampling, or other manipulation during pregnancy. A smaller 50-mcg dose is adequate if pregnancy is terminated at less than 12 weeks' gestation.[129] If therapeutic or spontaneous abortion occurs after the first trimester, the standard 300-mcg dose is recommended.[129] If a woman was exposed to more than 30 mL of D-positive blood, the dose of RhIg should be calculated to cover the volume of D-positive cells to prevent immunization (20 mcg of RhIg for 1 mL of D+ RBCs or 2 mL of WB).[57,131,133] Despite the efficacy of RhIg, RhD alloimmunization occurs despite recommended prophylaxis in 0.1 percent of pregnancies, but many cases of preventable Rh alloimmunization continue to occur because of failure to seek medical care or because of failure to implement immunoprophylaxis protocols.

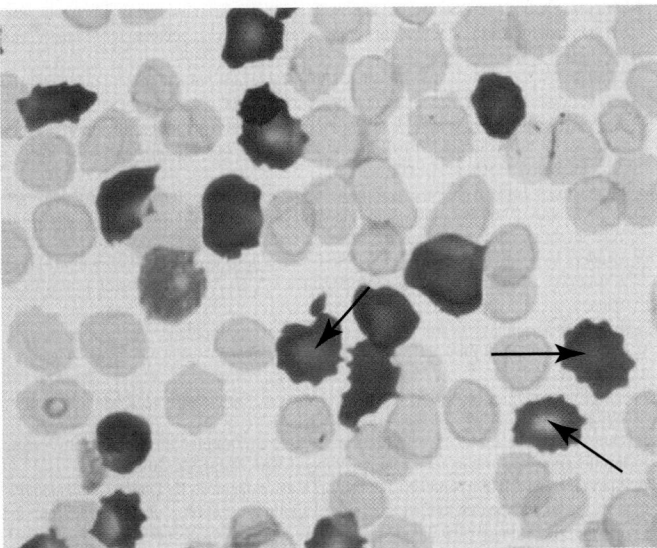

Figure 55–5. Kleihauer-Betke test. Maternal red blood cells appear as pale "ghost cells," whereas fetal red blood cells containing hemoglobin F are resistant to acid denaturation. Crenated red cells *(arrows)* are an artifact of the drying in preparation of the slide. *(Reproduced from Lazarchick J, American Society of Hematology Image bank 2011–2370.)*

● CONCLUSIONS

HDFN is a clinically significant problem that may potentially affect any pregnancy. Although a number of strategies are in place to prevent RhD HDFN, few options exist to prevent the development of non-D HDFN. Researchers continue to investigate strategies to prevent primary maternal RBC alloimmunization to RhD and to non-D antigens, as well as strategies to mitigate the dangers of existing maternal RBC alloantibodies. Over the past decade, the ability to identify pregnancies/ fetuses "at risk" because of maternal RBC alloimmunization has significantly improved. In particular, the use of noninvasive investigations, such as evaluation of fetal RBC antigen zygosity by circulating cell free fetal DNA testing and the evaluation of fetal anemia by middle cerebral artery Doppler ultrasonography, have advanced the care of fetuses at risk for HDFN. Through the continued combined efforts of maternal–fetal medicine specialists, hematologists, transfusion medicine physicians, radiologists, neonatologists, and researchers, in combination with advancements in basic science research involving alloimmunization, the care for infants at risk for HDFN, and their mothers, will likely continue to improve in the years to come.

REFERENCES

1. Diamond L, Blackfan K, Baty J: Erythroblastosis fetalis and its association with universal edema of the fetus, icterus gravis neonatorum and anemia of the newborn. *J Pediatr* 1932(1):269.
2. Darrow R: Icterus gravis (erythroblastosis neonatorum, examination of etiologic considerations). *Arch Pathol* 1938(25):378.
3. Levine P, Katzin E, Burnham L: Isoimmunization in pregnancy: Its possible bearing on the etiology of erythroblastosis fetalis. *JAMA* 116(9):825, 1941.
4. Diamond LK, Allen FH Jr, Thomas WO Jr: Erythroblastosis fetalis. VII. Treatment with exchange transfusion. *N Engl J Med* 244(2):39, 1951.
5. Liley AW: The use of amniocentesis and fetal transfusion in erythroblastosis fetalis. *Pediatrics* 35:836, 1965.
6. Bowman J: Thirty-five years of Rh prophylaxis. *Transfusion* 43(12):1661, 2003.
7. Poole J, Daniels G: Blood group antibodies and their significance in transfusion medicine. *Transfus Med Rev* 21(1):58, 2007.
8. Geifman-Holtzman O, et al: Female alloimmunization with antibodies known to cause hemolytic disease. *Obstet Gynecol* 89(2):272, 1997.
9. Gottvall T, Filbey D: Alloimmunization in pregnancy during the years 1992-2005 in the central west region of Sweden. *Acta Obstet Gynecol Scand* 87(8):843, 2008.
10. Koelewijn JM, Vrijkotte TG, van der Schoot CE, et al: Effect of screening for red cell antibodies, other than anti-D, to detect hemolytic disease of the fetus and newborn: A population study in the Netherlands. *Transfusion* 48(5):941, 2008.
11. Lee CK, Ma ES, Tang M, et al: Prevalence and specificity of clinically significant red cell alloantibodies in Chinese women during pregnancy—A review of cases from 1997 to 2001. *Transfus Med* 13(4):227, 2003.
12. Zipursky A, Paul VK: The global burden of Rh disease. *Arch Dis Child Fetal Neonatal Ed* 96(2):F84, 2011.
13. Moise KJ: Fetal anemia due to non-Rhesus-D red-cell alloimmunization. *Semin Fetal Neonatal Med* 13(4):207, 2008.
14. Garratty G, Glynn SA, McEntire R: ABO and Rh(D) phenotype frequencies of different racial/ethnic groups in the United States. *Transfusion* 44(5):703, 2004.
15. Joseph KS: Controlling Rh haemolytic disease of the newborn in India. *Br J Obstet Gynaecol* 98(4):369, 1991.
16. Mak KH, Yan KF, Cheng SS, Yuen MY: Rh phenotypes of Chinese blood donors in Hong Kong, with special reference to weak D antigens. *Transfusion* 33(4):348, 1993.
17. Ziprin JH, Payne E, Hamidi L, et al: ABO incompatibility due to immunoglobulin G anti-B antibodies presenting with severe fetal anaemia. *Transfus Med* 15(1):57, 2005.
18. Thilaganathan B, Salvesen DR, Abbas A, et al: Fetal plasma erythropoietin concentration in red blood cell-isoimmunized pregnancies. *Am J Obstet Gynecol* 167(5):1292, 1992.
19. Koenig JM, Christensen RD: Neutropenia and thrombocytopenia in infants with Rh hemolytic disease. *J Pediatr* 114(4 Pt 1):625, 1989.
20. Hayde M, Widness JA, Pollak A, et al: Rhesus isoimmunization: increased hemolysis during early infancy. *Pediatr Res* 41(5):716, 1997.
21. al-Alaiyan S, al Omran A: Late hyporegenerative anemia in neonates with rhesus hemolytic disease. *J Perinat Med* 27(2):112, 1999.
22. Pessler F, Hart D: Hyporegenerative anemia associated with Rh hemolytic disease: treatment failure of recombinant erythropoietin. *J Pediatr Hematol Oncol* 24(8):689, 2002.
23. Sikkel E, Pasman SA, Oepkes D, et al: On the origin of amniotic fluid bilirubin. *Placenta* 25(5):463, 2004.

24. Pasman SA, Sikkel E, Le Cessie S, et al: Bilirubin/albumin ratios in fetal blood and in amniotic fluid in rhesus immunization. *Obstet Gynecol* 111(5):1083, 2008.

25. Janssens HM, de Haan MJ, van Kamp IL, et al: Outcome for children treated with fetal intravascular transfusions because of severe blood group antagonism. *J Pediatr* 131(3):373, 1997.

26. Shapiro SM: Definition of the clinical spectrum of kernicterus and bilirubin-induced neurologic dysfunction (BIND). *J Perinatol* 25(1):54, 2005.

27. Kuzniewicz M, Newman TB: Interaction of hemolysis and hyperbilirubinemia on neurodevelopmental outcomes in the collaborative perinatal project. *Pediatrics* 123(3):1045, 2009.

28. Nicolaides KH: Studies on fetal physiology and pathophysiology in rhesus disease. *Semin Perinatol* 13(4):328, 1989.

29. Smits-Wintjens VE, Rath ME, Lindenburg IT, et al: Cholestasis in neonates with red cell alloimmune hemolytic disease: incidence, risk factors and outcome. *Neonatology* 101(4):306, 2012.

30. Rath ME, Smits-Wintjens VE, Oepkes D, et al: Thrombocytopenia at birth in neonates with red cell alloimmune haemolytic disease. *Vox Sang* 102(3):228, 2012.

31. Smits-Wintjens VE, Walther FJ, Lopriore E: Rhesus haemolytic disease of the newborn: Postnatal management, associated morbidity and long-term outcome. *Semin Fetal Neonatal Med* 13(4):265, 2008.

32. Blanco E, Johnston DL: Neutropenia in infants with hemolytic disease of the newborn. *Pediatr Blood Cancer* 58(6):950, 2012.

33. Lobato G, Soncini CS: Relationship between obstetric history and Rh(D) alloimmunization severity. *Arch Gynecol Obstet* 277(3):245, 2008.

34. Katz MA, Kanto WP Jr, Korotkin JH: Recurrence rate of ABO hemolytic disease of the newborn. *Obstet Gynecol* 59(5):611, 1982.

35. Kleinman S: Hemolytic disease of the newborn: RBC alloantibodies in pregnancy and associated serologic issues. UpToDate 2014. http://www.uptodate.com/contents/hemolytic-disease-of-the-newborn-rbc-alloantibodies-in-pregnancy-and-associated-serologic-issues. Last accessed on June 20, 2014.

36. Barss VA, Moise KJ Jr: Significance of minor red blood cell antibodies during pregnancy. UpToDate 2014. http://www.uptodate.com/contents/significance-of-minor-red-blood-cell-antibodies-during-pregnancy. Last accessed on June 20, 2014.

37. Flegel WA: Molecular genetics of RH and its clinical application. *Transfus Clin Biol* 13(1–2):4, 2006.

38. Denomme GA, Wagner FF, Fernandes BJ, et al: Partial D, weak D types, and novel RHD alleles among 33,864 multiethnic patients: implications for anti-D alloimmunization and prevention. *Transfusion* 45(10):1554, 2005.

39. Avent ND, Reid ME: The Rh blood group system: A review. *Blood* 95(2):375, 2000.

40. Shirey RS, Mirabella DC, Lumadue JA, Ness PM: Differentiation of anti-D, -C, and -G: clinical relevance in alloimmunized pregnancies. *Transfusion* 37(5):493, 1997.

41. Bowman JM, Pollock JM, Penston LE: Fetomaternal transplacental hemorrhage during pregnancy and after delivery. *Vox Sang* 51(2):117, 1986.

42. Sebring ES, Polesky HF: Fetomaternal hemorrhage: incidence, risk factors, time of occurrence, and clinical effects. *Transfusion* 30(4):344, 1990.

43. Ness PM, Baldwin ML, Niebyl JR: Clinical high-risk designation does not predict excess fetal-maternal hemorrhage. *Am J Obstet Gynecol* 156(1):154, 1987.

44. Pourbabak S, Rund CR, Crookston KP: Three cases of massive fetomaternal hemorrhage presenting without clinical suspicion. *Arch Pathol Lab Med* 128(4):463, 2004.

45. Jansen MW, Brandenburg H, Wildschut HI, et al: The effect of chorionic villus sampling on the number of fetal cells isolated from maternal blood and on maternal serum alpha-fetoprotein levels. *Prenat Diagn* 17(10):953, 1997.

46. Bowman JM, Pollock JM: Transplacental fetal hemorrhage after amniocentesis. *Obstet Gynecol* 66(6):749, 1985.

47. Bowman JM, Pollock JM, Peterson LE, et al: Fetomaternal hemorrhage following funipuncture: increase in severity of maternal red-cell alloimmunization. *Obstet Gynecol* 84(5):839, 1994.

48. Urbaniak SJ: Alloimmunity to RhD in humans. *Transfus Clin Biol* 13(1–2):19, 2006.

49. Cid J, Lozano M: Risk of Rh(D) alloimmunization after transfusion of platelets from D+ donors to D- recipients. *Transfusion* 45(3):453; author reply 453, 2005.

50. Bowman J, Harman C, Manning F, et al: Intravenous drug abuse causes Rh immunization. *Vox Sang* 61(2):96, 1991.

51. Kumpel BM: On the immunologic basis of Rh immune globulin (anti-D) prophylaxis. *Transfusion* 46(9):1652, 2006.

52. Bowman JM: Fetomaternal ABO incompatibility and erythroblastosis fetalis. *Vox Sang* 50(2):104, 1986.

53. Neppert J, v Witzleben-Schürholz E, Zupanska B, et al: High incidence of maternal HLA A, B and C antibodies associated with a mild course of haemolytic disease of the newborn. Group for the Study of Protective Maternal HLA Antibodies in the Clinical Course of HDN. *Eur J Haematol* 63(2):120, 1999.

54. Palfi M, Hildén JO, Gottvall T, Selbing A: Placental transport of maternal immunoglobulin G in pregnancies at risk of Rh (D) hemolytic disease of the newborn. *Am J Reprod Immunol* 39(5):323, 1998.

55. Lambin P, Debbia M, Puillandre P, Brossard Y: IgG1 and IgG3 anti-D in maternal serum and on the RBCs of infants suffering from HDN: Relationship with the severity of the disease. *Transfusion* 42(12):1537, 2002.

56. Eder AF: Update on HDFN: New information on long-standing controversies. *Immunohematol* 22(4):188, 2006.

57. Kennedy M: Perinatal issues in transfusion practice, in *Technical Manual*, edited by J Roback, M Combs, B Grossman. AABB Press, Bethesda, MD, 2008.

58. Grant SR, Kilby MD, Meer L, et al: The outcome of pregnancy in Kell alloimmunisation. *BJOG* 107(4):481, 2000.

59. Kamphuis MM, Lindenburg I, van Kamp IL, et al: Implementation of routine screening for Kell antibodies: Does it improve perinatal survival? *Transfusion* 48(5):953, 2008.

60. McKenna DS, Nagaraja HN, O'Shaughnessy R: Management of pregnancies complicated by anti-Kell isoimmunization. *Obstet Gynecol* 93(5 Pt 1):667, 1999.

61. Bowman JM, Pollock JM, Manning FA, et al: Maternal Kell blood group alloimmunization. *Obstet Gynecol* 79(2):239, 1992.

62. Vaughan JI, Manning M, Warwick RM, et al: Inhibition of erythroid progenitor cells by anti-Kell antibodies in fetal alloimmune anemia. *N Engl J Med* 338(12):798, 1998.

63. Wagner T, Bernaschek G, Geissler K: Inhibition of megakaryopoiesis by Kell-related antibodies. *N Engl J Med* 343(1):72, 2000.

64. Wagner T, Resch B, Reiterer F, et al: Pancytopenia due to suppressed hematopoiesis in a case of fatal hemolytic disease of the newborn associated with anti-K supported by molecular K1 typing. *J Pediatr Hematol Oncol* 26(1):13, 2004.

65. Sarici SU, Yurdakök M, Serdar MA, et al: An early (sixth-hour) serum bilirubin measurement is useful in predicting the development of significant hyperbilirubinemia and severe ABO hemolytic disease in a selective high-risk population of newborns with ABO incompatibility. *Pediatrics* 109(4):e53, 2002.

66. Lin M, Broadberry RE: ABO hemolytic disease of the newborn is more severe in Taiwan than in white populations. *Vox Sang* 68(2):136, 1995.

67. Miqdad AM, Abdelbasit OB, Shaheed MM, et al: Intravenous immunoglobulin G (IVIG) therapy for significant hyperbilirubinemia in ABO hemolytic disease of the newborn. *J Matern Fetal Neonatal Med* 16(3):163, 2004.

68. Kaplan M, Hammerman C, Renbaum P, et al: Gilbert's syndrome and hyperbilirubinaemia in ABO-incompatible neonates. *Lancet* 356(9230):652, 2000.

69. Pirelli KJ, Pietz BC, Johnson ST, et al: Molecular determination of RHD zygosity: Predicting risk of hemolytic disease of the fetus and newborn related to anti-D. *Prenat Diagn* 30(12-13):1207, 2010.

70. Blood Center of Wisconsin Diagnostics: RhD Zygosity Testing. 2014. Available from: https://www.bcw.edu/cs/groups/public/documents/documents/mdaw/mdaz/~edisp/rhd_zygosity_desc.pdf. Last accessed on May 29, 2015.

71. Lo YM, Bowell PJ, Selinger M, et al: Prenatal determination of fetal RhD status by analysis of peripheral blood of rhesus negative mothers. *Lancet* 341(8853):1147, 1993.

72. Geifman-Holtzman O, Grotegut CA, Gaughan JP: Diagnostic accuracy of noninvasive fetal Rh genotyping from maternal blood—A meta-analysis. *Am J Obstet Gynecol* 195(4):1163, 2006.

73. Daniels G, Finning K, Martin P, Massey E: Noninvasive prenatal diagnosis of fetal blood group phenotypes: Current practice and future prospects. *Prenat Diagn* 29(2):101, 2009.

74. Geifman-Holtzman O, Grotegut CA, Gaughan JP, et al: Noninvasive fetal RhCE genotyping from maternal blood. *BJOG* 116(2):144, 2009.

75. Bombard AT, Akolekar R, Farkas DH, et al: Fetal RHD genotype detection from circulating cell-free fetal DNA in maternal plasma in non-sensitized RhD negative women. *Prenat Diagn* 31(8):802, 2011.

76. Moise KJ Jr: Management of rhesus alloimmunization in pregnancy. *Obstet Gynecol* 112(1):164, 2008.

77. Gooch A, Parker J, Wray J, Qureshi H: Guideline for blood grouping and antibody testing in pregnancy. *Transfus Med* 17(4):252, 2007.

78. Adeniji AA, Fuller I, Dale T, Lindow SW: Should we continue screening rhesus D positive women for the development of atypical antibodies in late pregnancy? *J Matern Fetal Neonatal Med* 20(1):59, 2007.

79. Hadley AG: Laboratory assays for predicting the severity of haemolytic disease of the fetus and newborn. *Transpl Immunol* 10(2–3):191, 2002.

80. Daffos F, Capella-Pavlovsky M, Forestier F: Fetal blood sampling during pregnancy with use of a needle guided by ultrasound: A study of 606 consecutive cases. *Am J Obstet Gynecol* 153(6):655, 1985.

81. Queenan JT, Tomai TP, Ural SH, King JC: Deviation in amniotic fluid optical density at a wavelength of 450 nm in Rh-immunized pregnancies from 14 to 40 weeks' gestation: A proposal for clinical management. *Am J Obstet Gynecol* 168(5):1370, 1993.

82. Dukler D, Oepkes D, Seaward G, et al: Noninvasive tests to predict fetal anemia: a study comparing Doppler and ultrasound parameters. *Am J Obstet Gynecol* 188(5):1310, 2003.

83. Buscaglia M, Ghisoni L, Bellotti M, et al: Percutaneous umbilical blood sampling: indication changes and procedure loss rate in a nine years' experience. *Fetal Diagn Ther* 11(2):106, 1996.

84. Ghidini A, Sepulveda W, Lockwood CJ, Romero R: Complications of fetal blood sampling. *Am J Obstet Gynecol* 168(5):1339, 1993.

85. Oepkes D, Seaward PG, Vandenbussche FP, et al: Doppler ultrasonography versus amniocentesis to predict fetal anemia. *N Engl J Med* 355(2):156, 2006.

86. Mari G, Deter RL, Carpenter RL, et al: Noninvasive diagnosis by Doppler ultrasonography of fetal anemia due to maternal red-cell alloimmunization. Collaborative Group for Doppler Assessment of the Blood Velocity in Anemic Fetuses. *N Engl J Med* 342(1):9, 2000.

87. Oepkes D, Adama van Scheltema P: Intrauterine fetal transfusions in the management of fetal anemia and fetal thrombocytopenia. *Semin Fetal Neonatal Med* 12(6):432, 2007.

88. Howe DT, Michailidis GD: Intraperitoneal transfusion in severe, early-onset Rh isoimmunization. *Obstet Gynecol* 110(4):880, 2007.

89. Fox C, Martin W, Somerset DA, et al: Early intraperitoneal transfusion and adjuvant maternal immunoglobulin therapy in the treatment of severe red cell alloimmunization prior to fetal intravascular transfusion. *Fetal Diagn Ther* 23(2):159, 2008.

90. Radunovic N, Lockwood CJ, Alvarez M, et al: The severely anemic and hydropic isoimmune fetus: Changes in fetal hematocrit associated with intrauterine death. *Obstet Gynecol* 79(3):390, 1992.

91. Hallak M, Moise KJ Jr, Hesketh DE, et al: Intravascular transfusion of fetuses with rhesus incompatibility: Prediction of fetal outcome by changes in umbilical venous pressure. *Obstet Gynecol* 80(2):286, 1992.

92. Wong E, Luban N: Intrauterine, neonatal, and pediatric transfusion, in *Transfusion Therapy: Clinical Principles and Practice*, edited by PD Mintz, p 159. AABB Press, Bethesda, MD, 2005.

93. Gibson BE, Todd A, Roberts I, et al: Transfusion guidelines for neonates and older children. *Br J Haematol* 124(4):433, 2004.

94. Gonsoulin WJ, Moise KJ Jr, Milam JD, et al: Serial maternal blood donations for intrauterine transfusion. *Obstet Gynecol* 75(2):158, 1990.

95. Nicolaides KH, Clewell WH, Rodeck CH: Measurement of human fetoplacental blood volume in erythroblastosis fetalis. *Am J Obstet Gynecol* 157(1):50, 1987.

96. Hoogeveen M, Meerman RH, Pasman S, Egberts J: A new method to determine the feto-placental volume based on dilution of fetal haemoglobin and an estimation of plasma fluid loss after intrauterine intravascular transfusion. *BJOG* 109(10):1132, 2002.

97. Giannina G, Moise KJ Jr, Dorman K: A simple method to estimate volume for fetal intravascular transfusions. *Fetal Diagn Ther* 13(2):94, 1998.

98. Van Kamp IL, Klumper FJ, Oepkes D, et al: Complications of intrauterine intravascular transfusion for fetal anemia due to maternal red-cell alloimmunization. *Am J Obstet Gynecol* 192(1):171, 2005.

99. Schonewille H, Klumper FJ, van de Watering LM, et al: High additional maternal red cell alloimmunization after Rhesus- and K-matched intrauterine intravascular transfusions for hemolytic disease of the fetus. *Am J Obstet Gynecol* 196(2):143.e1, 2007.

100. Ruma MS, Moise KJ Jr, Kim E, et al: Combined plasmapheresis and intravenous immune globulin for the treatment of severe maternal red cell alloimmunization. *Am J Obstet Gynecol* 196(2):138.e1, 2007.

101. Collinet P, Subtil D, Puech F, Vaast P: Successful treatment of extremely severe fetal anemia due to Kell alloimmunization. *Obstet Gynecol* 100(5 Pt 2):1102, 2002.

102. Dinesh D: Review of positive direct antiglobulin tests found on cord blood sampling. *J Paediatr Child Health* 41(9–10):504, 2005.

103. Heddle NM, Wentworth P, Anderson DR, et al: Three examples of Rh haemolytic disease of the newborn with a negative direct antiglobulin test. *Transfus Med* 5(2):113, 1995.

104. Herschel M, Karrison T, Wen M, et al: Isoimmunization is unlikely to be the cause of hemolysis in ABO-incompatible but direct antiglobulin test-negative neonates. *Pediatrics* 110(1 Pt 1):127, 2002.

105. van Kamp IL, Klumper FJ, Bakkum RS, et al: The severity of immune fetal hydrops is predictive of fetal outcome after intrauterine treatment. *Am J Obstet Gynecol* 185(3):668, 2001.

106. De Boer IP, Zeestraten EC, Lopriore E, et al: Pediatric outcome in Rhesus hemolytic disease treated with and without intrauterine transfusion. *Am J Obstet Gynecol* 198(1):54.e1, 2008.

107. Harper DC, Swingle HM, Weiner CP, et al: Long-term neurodevelopmental outcome and brain volume after treatment for hydrops fetalis by in utero intravascular transfusion. *Am J Obstet Gynecol* 195(1):192, 2006.

108. Ramasethu J: Exchange transfusions, in *Atlas of Procedures in Neonatology*, edited by M MacDonald, J Ramasethu, K. Rais-Bahrami, pp 315–323. Lippincott, Williams & Wilkins, Philadelphia, 2013.

109. Murray NA, Roberts IA: Haemolytic disease of the newborn. *Arch Dis Child Fetal Neonatal Ed* 92(2):F83, 2007.

110. American Academy of Pediatrics Subcommittee on Hyperbilirubinemia: Management of hyperbilirubinemia in the newborn infant 35 or more weeks of gestation. *Pediatrics* 114(1):297, 2004.

111. Maisels MJ, Watchko JF: Treatment of jaundice in low birthweight infants. *Arch Dis Child Fetal Neonatal Ed* 88(6):F459, 2003.

112. Hulzebos CV, van Imhoff DE, Bos AF, et al: Usefulness of the bilirubin/albumin ratio for predicting bilirubin-induced neurotoxicity in premature infants. *Arch Dis Child Fetal Neonatal Ed* 93(5):F384, 2008.

113. Fasano R, Luban N: Blood component therapy for the neonate, in *Fanaroff and Martin's Neonatal-Perinatal Medicine: Diseases of the Fetus and Infant*, edited by R Martin, A Fanaroff, M Walsh, pp 1360–1374. Elsevier, St. Louis, MO, 2010.

114. Patra K, et al: Adverse events associated with neonatal exchange transfusion in the 1990s. *J Pediatr* 144(5):626, 2004.

115. Steiner LA, Storfer-Isser A, Siner B, et al: A decline in the frequency of neonatal exchange transfusions and its effect on exchange-related morbidity and mortality. *Pediatrics* 120(1):27, 2007.

116. Fasano RM, Paul WM, Pisciotto PT: Complications of neonatal transfusion, in *Transfusion Reactions*, edited by M Popovsky, pp 471–518. AABB Press, Bethesda, MD, 2012.

117. Jackson JC: Adverse events associated with exchange transfusion in healthy and ill newborns. *Pediatrics* 99(5):E7, 1997.

118. Tan KL, Lim GC, Boey KW: Phototherapy for ABO haemolytic hyperbilirubinaemia. *Biol Neonate* 61(6):358, 1992.

119. Ebbesen F: Evaluation of the indications for early exchange transfusion in rhesus haemolytic disease during phototherapy. *Eur J Pediatr* 133(1):37, 1980.

120. Smits-Wintjens VE, Walther FJ, Rath ME, et al: Intravenous immunoglobulin in neonates with rhesus hemolytic disease: A randomized controlled trial. *Pediatrics* 127(4):680, 2011.

121. Ovaly F: Late anaemia in Rh haemolytic disease. *Arch Dis Child Fetal Neonatal Ed* 88(5):F444; author reply F445, 2003.

122. Dhodapkar KM, Blei F: Treatment of hemolytic disease of the newborn caused by anti-Kell antibody with recombinant erythropoietin. *J Pediatr Hematol Oncol* 23(1):69, 2001.

123. Zuppa AA, Alighieri G, Calabrese V, et al: Recombinant human erythropoietin in the prevention of late anemia in intrauterine transfused neonates with Rh-isoimmunization. *J Pediatr Hematol Oncol* 32(3):e95, 2010.

124. McPherson RJ, Juul SE: Erythropoietin for infants with hypoxic-ischemic encephalopathy. *Curr Opin Pediatr* 22(2):139, 2010.

125. Lindenburg IT, Smits-Wintjens VE, van Klink JM, et al: Long-term neurodevelopmental outcome after intrauterine transfusion for hemolytic disease of the fetus/newborn: the LOTUS study. *Am J Obstet Gynecol* 206(2):141 e1, 2012.

126. Ip S, Chung M, Kulig J, et al: An evidence-based review of important issues concerning neonatal hyperbilirubinemia. *Pediatrics* 114(1):e130, 2004.

127. Newman TB, Liljestrand P, Jeremy RJ, et al: Outcomes among newborns with total serum bilirubin levels of 25 mg per deciliter or more. *N Engl J Med* 354(18):1889, 2006.

128. Moise KJ Jr: Overview of Rhesus (Rh) alloimmunization in pregnancy. UpToDate 2014. http://www.uptodate.com/contents/overview-of-rhesus-rh-alloimmunization-in-pregnancy. Last accessed on June 20, 2014.

129. American College of Obstetrics and Gynecology: ACOG Practice Bulletin, Prevention of Rh(D) Alloimmunization, Number 4, 1999. Clinical Management Guidelines for Obstetricians and Gynecologists. http://www.acog.org/goto/PBListOfTitles.aspx (accessed on 29 May 2015).

130. National Institutes for Health and Clinical Excellence: *Pregnancy (Rhesus Negative Women) Routine Anti-D Review: Final Appraisal Determination*, 2008. Available from: http://www.nice.org.uk/guidance/ta156/documents/pregnancy-rhesus-negative-women-routine-antid-review-final-appraisal-determination2. Last accessed on May 29, 2015.

131. Ayache S, Herman JH: Prevention of D sensitization after mismatched transfusion of blood components: Toward optimal use of RhIG. *Transfusion* 48(9):1990, 2008.

132. Kleihauer E, Braun H, Betke K: [Demonstration of fetal hemoglobin in erythrocytes of a blood smear] [in German]. *Klin Wochenschr* 35(12):637, 1957.

133. Ramsey G: Inaccurate doses of R immune globulin after Rh-incompatible fetomaternal hemorrhage: Survey of laboratory practice. *Arch Pathol Lab Med* 133(3):465, 2009.

134. Moise KJ Jr, Argoti PS: Management and prevention of red cell alloimmunization in pregnancy: A systematic review. *Obstet Gynecol* 120(5):1132, 2012.

135. Moise KJ Jr: Management of rhesus alloimmunization in pregnancy. *Obstet Gynecol* 100(3):600, 2002.

CHAPTER 56
HYPERSPLENISM AND HYPOSPLENISM

Jaime Caro and Srikanth Nagalla

SUMMARY

The spleen culls aged and abnormal cells from the blood; removes intraerythrocytic inclusions through a process called *pitting*; sequesters approximately one-third of the normal intravascular platelet pool; removes bacteria, foreign particles, and tumor cells from the blood; and by virtue of the T and B lymphocytes and macrophages in the white pulp, plays a role in immune surveillance and antibody formation. Splenomegaly can occur as a result of vascular engorgement or cellular infiltration, and it is frequently associated with a combination of neutropenia, thrombocytopenia, and anemia. Hypersplenism is defined as one or more blood cytopenias in the setting of splenomegaly. Hypersplenism can occur with moderate or minimal splenic enlargement as a result of exaggerated removal of physically abnormal (e.g., as in hereditary spherocytosis) or antibody-coated blood cells (e.g., as in autoimmune hemolytic anemia). The presence of splenomegaly in a patient with blood cytopenias is useful to narrow the cause of the cytopenias, although the cause of the blood cytopenias may not be solely or principally as a result of hypersplenism (e.g., as in hairy cell leukemia). Thrombocytopenia in the setting of cirrhosis and splenomegaly is the result of pooling in the enlarged spleen and a relative decrease in thrombopoietin. The role of the spleen in the anemia and neutropenia associated with cirrhosis with splenomegaly is poorly understood, but a relative reduction in erythropoietin levels and decreased marrow myeloid progenitor cells have been proposed. Splenectomy has been used in cases of severe thrombocytopenia requiring chronic platelet transfusions or leading to bleeding. Thrombopoietin receptor agonists are another option in the management of thrombocytopenia, and nonpeptide thrombopoietin receptor agonists have been shown to increase platelet counts in patients with thrombocytopenia associated with hepatitis C virus–related cirrhosis and splenomegaly. Splenectomy may be justified in the case of massive splenomegaly, infarction, or disabling symptoms of pain and compression of neighboring structures. In some circumstances, benefit can be achieved by partial destruction of splenic tissue by embolization using intraarterial infusion of gel microparticles. Hyposplenism can result from agenesis, atrophy, surgical removal of the spleen, or reduction of splenic function by disease. In the latter case, disturbance in splenic circulation disrupts the specific architecture required for the spleen's culling, phagocytic, and pitting functions. Hyposplenism may be suspected by alterations in red cell morphology, such as target cells or acanthocytes; red cell inclusions, specifically Howell-Jolly and Pappenheimer bodies (siderotic granules highlighted with polychrome stains); pitted red cells; or an elevated platelet count. The presence of pitted red cells identified by interference-contrast microscopy is perhaps the most specific blood finding of hyposplenism, followed by Howell-Jolly bodies. The most devastating consequence of hyposplenism is sudden overwhelming sepsis by encapsulated bacteria. Immunizations and prophylactic antibiotics can decrease the risk of sepsis. A high awareness and prompt antibiotic treatment of febrile episodes are warranted.

Acronyms and Abbreviations: G-CSF, granulocyte colony-stimulating factor; Ig, immunoglobulin; TPO-RA, thrombopoietin-receptor agonist.

● HYPERSPLENISM

HISTORY

The spleen has intrigued physicians and philosophers since ancient times[1] and has been assigned mysterious powers, but its association with destruction of blood cells was not elucidated until the turn of the 20th century. The exaggerated and unfounded worry about somatic complaints often reflected by the sense of pain in the spleen (left hypochondrium) led to the term *hypochondriac*. In 1899, Chauffard proposed that increased splenic activity causes hemolysis.[2] This proposal provided the impetus for therapeutic splenectomy, which was performed first in 1910 by Sutherland and Burghard[3] in a patient with splenic anemia (hereditary spherocytosis) and subsequently by Kaznelson[4] in a patient with essential thrombocytopenia (immune thrombocytopenic purpura) in 1916.

DEFINITION

Hypersplenism is defined as blood cytopenias in the setting of splenomegaly. This is usually accompanied by hyperplasia of the affected cell precursors in the marrow. There can be a disproportional decrease in the blood platelets, white cells, and red cells, with thrombocytopenia and leukopenia being disproportionate to the anemia as a result of hypersplenism. Splenomegaly can occur as a result of elevated splenic venous pressures and vascular congestion, histiophagocytic hyperplasia, other cellular infiltration, or because of the inability of physically abnormal red cells, such as sickle cells in infants and children (prior to infarction atrophy), or antibody-coated cells, such as in autoimmune hemolytic anemia, to navigate the circulation or avoid engulfment by the mononuclear phagocyte population of the normal spleen.[5] The blood cytopenias are not generally corrected by relief of portal hypertension.[6,7]

ONTOGENY

The embryonic spleen appears in the first trimester of gestation as a multiply lobulated condensation of highly vascular mesenchymal cell aggregates interposed in the arterial circulation in the dorsal mesogastrium. The full scope of the molecular basis of splenic organogenesis is not known. The *HOX11 and WT1* genes are essential for its formation, and defects in their expression result in hyposplenia or asplenia.[8–10]

The lymphoid compartment, the white pulp, begins its development early in the second trimester of gestation, when mature T cells, principally CD4+ lymphocytes, form a continuous layer along the length of the vessels (periarteriolar sheaths). CD8+ cells reside in splenic cords and a specialized subset of $\gamma\delta$T cells home to the pulp (Chap. 6). Immunoglobulin (Ig) D+ and IgG+ B lymphocytes form localized deposits, the primary lymph follicles. Secondary follicles arise later in life, after exposure to immunologic stimuli, and have a distinctive structure that includes a germinal center, a mantle zone, and a marginal zone containing IgM+ and IgG+ B lymphocytes.[11,12]

STRUCTURE AND FUNCTIONAL ORGANIZATION

The normal adult spleen weighs 135 ± 30 g and has a blood flow that is approximately 5 percent of the cardiac output. In addition to serving as a filter, the spleen plays a role in innate and adaptive immunity and protection against microbes. The spleen is composed of white pulp, a marginal zone, and red pulp. The spleen's principal structure is organized around an arborizing array of arterioles that branch and narrow until they terminate in either (1) the stroma of cords, forming the open circulation, or (2) the sinusoids, forming the closed circulation of the spleen (Chap. 6). The cordal elements include histiocytes, antigen-presenting cells, pericytes, fibroblasts, and other cells necessary to maintain the discontinuous basal lamina that separates cords from sinusoid lumen.[13] Lymphatic tissue is inconspicuous and found in T-cell–rich zones in the periarteriolar lymphoid sheaths.

The arterial vascular tree, which is lined by conventional CD31+ and CD34+ endothelial cells, branches into arterioles that terminate abruptly in caps of cordal macrophages. Blood cells must pass clusters of macrophages to enter the sinusoids.[13] The sinusoids, the origin of the venous circulation, are lined by specialized cells having combined phagocytic and endothelial activities and a distinctive CD31+, CD34–, CD68+, CD8+ phenotype. A principal function of the spleen is to serve as a filter, removing aged or defective red cells and foreign particles by macrophages. This function is facilitated by diverting part of the splenic blood supply into the red pulp, where the blood slowly percolates through the nonendothelialized mesh studded with macrophages. Abnormal or senescent red cells and pathogens undergo phagocytosis by the macrophages. The blood then reenters the circulation through narrow slits, measuring 1 to 3 μm, in the endothelium of the venous sinuses. The bulk of the blood is rapidly channeled through vessels that link the arterioles with the venous sinuses. This blood is not filtered or modified.[14]

Approximately one-third of platelets are normally sequestered in the spleen.[15] In many animals, such as dogs and horses, the red pulp is a reservoir for red cells, and splenic contraction provides the red cell volume with a functionally important boost.[16] In humans, however, the splenic capsule is poorly contractile, and the spleen does not store red cells to any significant degree.[17] Although margination of neutrophils occurs in the spleen, it is unclear to what degree it occurs in that site.[18] Granulocyte colony-stimulating factor (G-CSF) administered to cirrhotic patients caused a rise in the blood neutrophil count; thereafter, indium scans of the spleen were performed, which did not show significant uptake by white cells.[19]

The slow transit of blood through the red pulp permits macrophages to recognize and destroy antibody- or complement-coated red cells and microorganisms, and to ingest poorly deformable red cells or particles retained mechanically by the narrow exit slits in the venous sinuses. The white pulp plays a major role in adaptive immunity. The spleen is involved in the phagocytosis of encapsulated bacteria including *Streptococcus pneumoniae*, *Haemophilus influenzae*, and *Neisseria meningitidis*.

PATHOPHYSIOLOGY

Filtration and elimination of defective cells occur notably in hereditary abnormalities of the red cell membranes, such as spherocytosis, elliptocytosis, or stomatocytosis, or with antibody-coated red cells, neutrophils, or platelets. In these circumstances, cytopenias of varying severity may ensue. The spleen not only removes antibody-coated cells, but also produces antibodies, especially antiplatelet antibodies.[20] Thus, the benefits of splenectomy in immune thrombocytopenic purpura is a result of both the decreased production of antiplatelet antibodies

as well as decreased clearance by macrophages of antibody-coated platelets through the Fc recognition function of its large macrophage population.

Splenomegaly increases the proportion of blood channeled through the red pulp.[13,21] Spleen enlargement may result from expansion of the red pulp compartment with increased blood flow; extramedullary hematopoiesis, notable in primary myelofibrosis; hyperplasia or neoplasia involving the white pulp, such as in infectious mononucleosis or lymphoma; or histiophagocytic hyperplasia.

The increased size of the filtering bed is more pronounced when the splenomegaly is caused by congestion as in portal hypertension than when it is caused by cellular infiltration as in leukemias, extramedullary hematopoiesis, or amyloidosis. Even in space-occupying disorders such as Gaucher disease and primary myelofibrosis, splenomegaly may be associated with hypersplenic sequestration of normal cells.

Splenomegaly increases the vascular surface area and thereby the marginated neutrophil pool.[18,19] Platelets are especially likely to be sequestered in an enlarged spleen. However, sequestered white cells and platelets survive in the spleen and may be available when increased demand requires neutrophils or platelets, although their release may be slow.[22]

Some patients with anemia and splenomegaly have a relative erythropoietin deficiency.[23] In one study of cirrhotic patients, 30 percent had a blunted erythropoietin response to anemia.[24] Dilution of red cells in an expanded plasma volume is another commonly cited cause of a decreased blood hemoglobin concentration,[25] although some studies do not demonstrate hemodilution.[26] Iron deficiency associated with chronic blood loss, folic acid and vitamin B_{12} deficiency, and increased red cell destruction are frequently investigated, although rarely found in patients with liver disease.[27] Red cells are destroyed prematurely in the red pulp in the setting of splenomegaly, but only rarely does this explain the anemia.[28]

Varying amounts of erythrophagocytosis are present, reflecting the normal culling of senescent red cells. Erythrophagocytosis increases as a result of hemolytic anemia and viral infections, and in alloimmunized transfusion recipients. Macrophages within the sinusoids contain red cell fragments. When the process is pronounced, the littoral cells become cuboidal and stand out on the basement membrane ("hobnails"). Sickle cell disease and red cell membrane disorders such as hereditary spherocytosis lead to sequestration of the poorly deformable red cells in the cords but little extrasinusoidal erythrophagocytosis is seen, in contrast to immune hemolytic anemia where macrophage erythrophagocytosis is prominent.[13]

The increased blood flow from an enlarged spleen expands the splenic and portal veins. A significant increase in portal venous pressure may occur when hepatic vessel compliance is decreased, as in cirrhosis or myelofibrosis. This process initiates a vicious cycle in which portal hypertension contributes to splenomegaly, organ enlargement leads to increased arterial blood flow, which, in turn, increases portal pressure.

Table 56–1 lists causes of splenomegaly, and Table 56–2 lists causes of massive splenic enlargement.

CLINICAL FEATURES

Slight to moderate enlargement of the spleen usually does not produce local symptoms. Even massive splenomegaly can be well tolerated if it develops gradually. However, not infrequently, the patient complains of a sagging feeling or other types of abdominal discomfort, early satiety from gastric encroachment, and trouble sleeping on one side. Pleuritic pain in the left upper quadrant or referred to the left shoulder may accompany splenic infarcts, which may be recurrent.

In children with sickle cell anemia or patients with malaria, the spleen may become acutely enlarged and painful as a result of a sudden increase in red cell pooling and sequestration. These sequestration crises are characterized by sudden aggravation of the anemia. Splenic

TABLE 56-1. Classification and Most Common Causes of Splenomegaly

1. Congestive
   a. Right-sided congestive heart failure
   b. Budd-Chiari syndrome (inferior vena cava and hepatic vein thrombosis)
   c. Cirrhosis with portal hypertension
   d. Portal or splenic vein thrombosis
2. Immunologic
   a. Viral infection
      i. Acute HIV infection/chronic Infection
      ii. Acute mononucleosis
      iii. Dengue fever
      iv. Rubella (rare except newborns)
      v. Cytomegalovirus (rare except newborns)
      vi. Herpes simplex (rare except newborns)
   b. Bacterial infection
      i. Subacute bacterial endocarditis
      ii. Brucellosis
      iii. Tularemia
      iv. Melioidosis
      v. Listeriosis
      vi. Plague
      vii. Secondary syphilis
      viii. Relapsing fever
      ix. Psittacosis
      x. Ehrlichiosis
      xi. Rickettsial diseases (scrub typhus, Rocky Mountain spotted fever, Q fever)
      xii. Tuberculosis
      xiii. Splenic abscess (most common organisms are *Enterobacteriaceae*, *Staphylococcus aureus*, *Streptococcus* group D, and anaerobic organisms as part of mixed flora infections)
   c. Fungal infection
      i. Blastomycosis
      ii. Histoplasmosis
      iii. Systemic candidiasis; hepatosplenic candidiasis

   d. Parasitic infection
      i. Malaria
      ii. Kala-Azar
      iii. Leishmaniasis
      iv. Schistosomiasis
      v. Babesiosis
      vi. Coccidioidomycosis
      vii. Paracoccidioidomycosis
      viii. Trypanosomiasis (cruzi, brucei)
      ix. Toxoplasmosis (rare except newborns)
      x. Echinococcosis
      xi. Cysticercosis
      xii. Visceral larva migrans (*Toxocara* infection)
   e. Inflammatory/autoimmune
      i. Systemic lupus erythematosus
      ii. Felty syndrome
      iii. Juvenile rheumatoid arthritis
      iv. Autoimmune lymphoproliferative syndrome (ALP syndrome)
      v. Hemophagocytic syndrome
      vi. Common variable immunodeficiency
      vii. Splenomegaly caused by granulocyte colony-stimulating factor administration
      viii. Anti-D immunoglobulin administration (RhoGAM)
3. Secondary to hemolysis
   a. Thalassemia major
   b. Pyruvate kinase deficiency
   c. Hereditary spherocytosis
   d. Autoimmune hemolytic anemia (uncommon)
   e. Sickle cell disease in early childhood (splenic sequestration)

4. Infiltrative
   a. Nonmalignant
      i. Splenic hematoma (splenic cysts are usually a late complication of a hematoma)
      ii. Littoral cell angioma
      iii. Disorders of sphingolipid metabolism
         1. Gaucher disease
         2. Niemann-Pick disease
      iv. Cystinosis
      v. Amyloidosis (light chain amyloid [AL] and amyloid A protein [AA])
      vi. Multicentric Castleman disease
      vii. Mastocytosis
      viii. Hypereosinophilic syndrome
      ix. Sarcoidosis
   b. Extramedullary hematopoiesis
      i. Primary myelofibrosis
      ii. Osteopetrosis (childhood)
      iii. Thalassemia major
   c. Malignant
      i. Hematologic
         1. Chronic lymphocytic leukemia (especially prolymphocytic variant)
         2. Chronic myeloid leukemia
         3. Polycythemia vera
         4. Hairy cell leukemia
         5. Heavy chain disease
         6. Hepatosplenic lymphoma
         7. Acute leukemia (acute lymphoblastic leukemia/acute myeloid leukemia)
         8. Hodgkin lymphoma
      ii. Nonhematologic
         1. Metastatic carcinoma (rare)
         2. Neuroblastoma
         3. Wilms tumor
         4. Leiomyosarcoma
         5. Fibrosarcoma
         6. Malignant fibrous histiocytoma
         7. Kaposi sarcoma
         8. Hemangiosarcoma
         9. Lymphangiosarcoma
         10. Hemangioendothelial sarcoma

rupture is uncommon but can occur spontaneously with most causes of splenic enlargement or after blunt trauma. Rupture related to the splenic enlargement in infectious mononucleosis is a classic example.

The volume of an enlarged spleen is difficult to assess by palpation and percussion. Children and thin patients with low diaphragms may have a palpable spleen tip without splenomegaly.[29] Generally, a palpable spleen signifies splenomegaly and is measured by the number of centimeters the spleen extends below the left costal margin. Splenic size is most accurately measured with abdominal ultrasound (Fig. 56–1) or

computed tomographic scans (Fig. 56–2). Magnetic resonance imaging is used primarily to identify cysts, abscesses, and infarcts.[30]

SPLENOPTOSIS

A wandering spleen (splenoptosis) is an uncommon phenomenon in which the spleen hangs by a long pedicle of mesentery. The condition may present in three ways: (1) an asymptomatic mass in the pelvis, (2) intermittent abdominal pain with or without gastrointestinal symptoms, or, less often, (3) an acute abdomen resulting from torsion.

TABLE 56–2. Causes of Massive Splenomegaly

1. Myeloproliferative disorders
   a. Primary myelofibrosis
   b. Chronic myeloid leukemia
2. Lymphomas
   a. Hairy cell leukemia
   b. Chronic lymphocytic leukemia (especially prolymphocytic variant)
3. Infectious
   a. Malaria
   b. Leishmaniasis (kala azar)
4. Extramedullary hematopoiesis
   a. Thalassemia major
5. Infiltrative
   a. Gaucher disease

The diagnosis of splenoptosis may be made coincidentally on an imaging study.[31] The condition may be accompanied by signs of hypersplenism, hyposplenism, and often, when developing slowly, is initially mistaken for a pelvic or lower abdominal tumor.

LABORATORY FEATURES

The characteristic features of hypersplenism are splenomegaly, blood cytopenias, and absence of other causes of cytopenias (e.g., anemia caused by bleeding). The blood cell morphology usually is normal, although a few spherocytes may result from metabolic conditioning of red cells during repeated slow transits through the expanded red pulp. Tests, such as epinephrine mobilization, were used in the past to try to distinguish sequestration from ineffective cellular production, but results are difficult to interpret as epinephrine also releases platelets and neutrophils from marginal pools.[32]

Thrombocytopenia is a common finding in patients with hepatic cirrhosis, portal hypertension, and splenomegaly. In a retrospective study, 64 percent of patients with nonalcoholic cirrhosis had thrombocytopenia.[33] Other studies have found that approximately one-third of patients with cirrhosis develop severe thrombocytopenia or neutropenia.[34,35] Decompensated liver disease and history of alcohol consumption are independent risk factors for hypersplenism,[36] but why some patients develop marked blood cytopenias is not clear, although folate deficiency is a factor in some instances. The presence of thrombocytopenia or leukopenia in patients with chronic liver disease is associated with increased mortality.[37]

Ultrasound-guided fine-needle biopsy of the spleen can be useful in circumstances in which the spleen holds the tissue required for diagnosis, such as splenic lymphoma. However, fine-needle aspiration is rarely a definitive diagnostic tool but can indicate monoclonality of splenic lymphocytes, which is helpful and forces further diagnostic evaluation. Aspiration cytology and core biopsy can be obtained with relative safety in experienced hands using image-guided fine needles.[38]

The response to transfusion of blood products, especially platelets, may be significantly impaired in patients with massive splenomegaly.[39]

THERAPY, COURSE, AND PROGNOSIS

Total Splenectomy

Splenectomy is indicated as an emergency procedure after abdominal trauma and partial rupture of the spleen. It also may be indicated when splenic size or infarcts causes sustained left upper abdominal pain or discomfort. Splenectomy has been used for the treatment of functionally significant blood cytopenias.[39] In such circumstances, case reports have described dramatic restoration of blood counts to normal levels within days to weeks after splenectomy; however, the only controlled trial evaluating relief of cytopenias showed no improvement.[6] Orthotopic liver transplant corrects the cytopenias in the majority of patients with cirrhosis.[40]

Hereditary spherocytosis, immune thrombocytopenic purpura, and immune hemolytic anemia are the most common indications for splenectomy. Splenectomy exerts its effect in autoimmune cytopenias by improving cell survival and also by decreasing autoantibody production. In thalassemia major, an improvement in the anemia is well described after splenectomy. In such cases, splenectomy may improve the response to transfusion. Some children with sickle cell anemia may benefit from splenectomy if repeated sequestration crises with abdominal pain occur before autosplenectomy renders the spleen atrophic.[41]

Splenectomy in patients with a massive spleen size (>1500 g), especially in primary myelofibrosis, is accompanied by higher morbidity and mortality than is removal of the spleen for immune blood cytopenia.[42] Possible postoperative complications include extensive adhesions with collateral blood vessels, hepatic or portal vein thrombosis, injury to the tail of the pancreas, operative site infections, and subdiaphragmatic abscesses.

Laparoscopic splenectomy performed by experienced surgeons for suitable hematologic conditions can result in less abdominal trauma

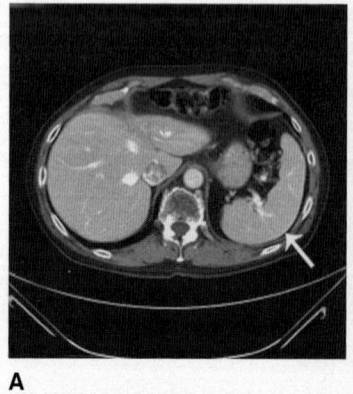 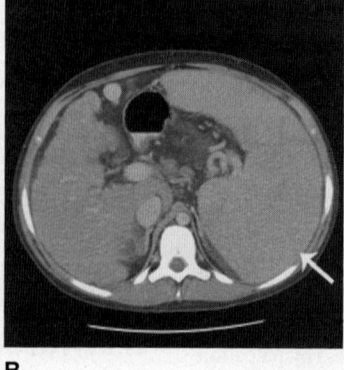 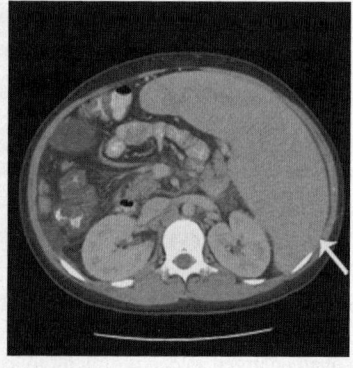

A   B   C

Figure 56–1. A three-way composite of abdominal computerized tomography. **A.** Normal spleen size. **B.** Enlarged spleen. **C.** Massively enlarged spleen at the level of mid-kidney. Normally the spleen would either not be visualized or only a small lower pole would be evident at the level of the mid-kidney. (*White arrow* in each of the three images marks edge of splenic silhouette.) *(Used with permission of Deborah Rubens, MD, The University of Rochester Medical Center.)*

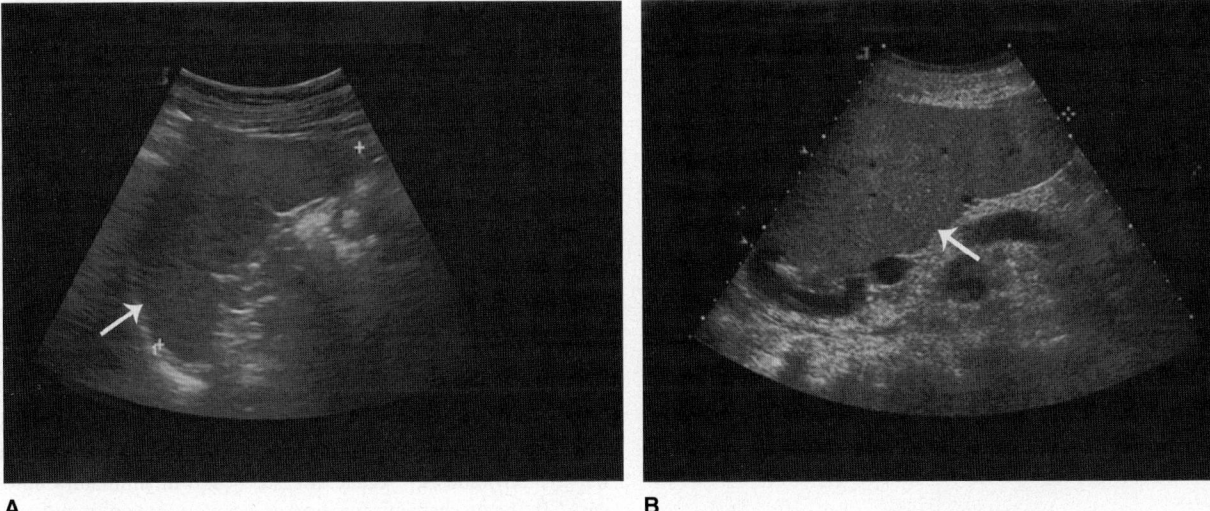

Figure 56–2. A two-way composite of ultrasonography examination for spleen size. **A.** Image of echo indicating normal spleen size with cranial to caudal longitudinal dimension of 10.3 cm. **B.** Image of echo indicating enlarged spleen with cranial to caudal longitudinal dimension of 16.2 cm. (*White arrow* in each image marks edge of splenic silhouette.) The normal spleen is usually less than 13 cm in length but the examiner has to consider other dimensions in assessing spleen size (volume). *(Used with permission of Deborah Rubens, MD, The University of Rochester Medical Center.)*

and pain, shorter hospital stays, and smaller abdominal scars.[43] An advantage of open splenectomy in hematologic conditions such as the treatment of immune thrombocytopenic purpura is the increased ease of searching assiduously for accessory spleens.

Partial Splenectomy

Partial splenectomy has been explored because it may minimize the risks of immediate postsplenectomy thrombocytosis and overwhelming sepsis that may result from a complete absence of splenic function.[44] However, the degree of thrombocytosis after splenectomy wanes to some degree with time postsplenectomy. Reduction of the splenic volume has been performed with ligation of some of the splenic arteries or the intraarterial infusion of Gelfoam particles causing embolization.[45-48] These procedures induce large splenic infarcts and reduce the functional splenic mass. Arterial embolization can be performed percutaneously or intravascularly, but the patients must be observed closely for a number of days to weeks to detect signs of intraabdominal rupture of the splenic infarcts. The long-term results of embolization have been encouraging.[46-48] Treatment with partial arterial embolization for recurrent thrombocytopenia in children temporarily improved the platelet count in approximately 70 percent of patients.[49]

Splenic Radiation

Splenic radiation for treatment of an enlarged spleen is used sparingly. The procedure may be associated with severe cytopenias and especially thrombocytopenia (abscopal effect). It can be used in patients with an absolute contraindication to splenectomy who might benefit symptomatically from reduction of a massively enlarged spleen.[50]

Liver Transplantation

Thrombopoietin synthesis and secretion are impaired in liver failure and this is corrected after liver transplantation.[51,52] However, thrombocytopenia may not be corrected after liver transplant if the splenomegaly persists.

Thrombopoietin Receptor Agonists

After thrombopoietin was cloned[53,54] several thrombopoietin mimetic drugs have been developed and tested. A phase II study reported that

the oral thrombopoietin-receptor agonist (TPO-RA) eltrombopag increases platelet counts in patients with thrombocytopenia as a result of hepatitis C virus–related cirrhosis.[55] A phase III study done in cirrhotic patients who received eltrombopag for 2 weeks prior to elective procedures had to be terminated prematurely because of the increased incidence of portal vein thrombosis in the treatment group compared to the placebo group. Although 72 percent of the eltrombopag patients avoided platelet transfusions compared to 19 percent of the placebo group patients, there was no significant difference in the incidence of major bleeding.[56] A small study using the TPO-RA romiplostim administered subcutaneously in cirrhotic patients demonstrated the usefulness of the drug in reducing platelet transfusions in preparation for an elective surgical procedure.[57]

Erythropoietin and Granulocyte Colony-Stimulating Factor

There are minimal data to support the use of erythropoietic or myeloid growth factors in patients with splenomegaly and blood cytopenias. Patients with cirrhosis who have inappropriately low serum erythropoietin levels may benefit from treatment with exogenous erythropoietin; however, it may increase spleen size. Two reports documented the use of erythropoietin before and after liver transplantation to amplify marrow erythropoiesis in patients who refused blood transfusions for religious reasons.[58,59] These reports demonstrated that liver transplantation in the setting of advanced cirrhosis can be successfully undertaken without the use of blood products.

A rise in the neutrophil count after G-CSF administration was described in patients with cirrhosis and leukopenia. The mean absolute neutrophil count increased from $1300 \pm 200/\mu L$ to $4100 \pm 200/\mu L$ following subcutaneous administration of G-CSF for 7 days.[19] However, the clinical benefit of such treatment is not clear.

● HYPOSPLENISM

DEFINITION

Hyposplenism is the designation for decreased splenic function resulting from diseases that impair function or from the absence of splenic tissue because of agenesis, atrophy (e.g., autoinfarction of sickle cell

TABLE 56–3. Conditions Associated with Hyposplenism

MISCELLANEOUS

Surgical splenectomy

Splenic irradiation

Sickle hemoglobinopathies

Congenital agenesis

Thrombosis of splenic artery or vein

Normal infants

GASTROINTESTINAL AND HEPATIC DISEASES

Celiac disease

Dermatitis herpetiformis

Inflammatory bowel disease

Cirrhosis

AUTOIMMUNE DISORDERS

Systemic lupus erythematosus

Rheumatoid arthritis

Vasculitis

Glomerulonephritis

Hashimoto thyroiditis

Sarcoidosis

HEMATOLOGIC AND NEOPLASTIC DISORDERS

Graft versus host disease

Essential thrombocytosis

Chronic lymphocytic leukemia

Non-Hodgkin lymphoma

Hodgkin lymphoma

Amyloidosis

Advanced breast cancer

Hemangiosarcoma

SEPSIS/INFECTIOUS DISEASES

Malaria

Disseminated meningococcemia

disease), or splenectomy. Splenic hypofunction may be associated with a normal spleen size. In some cases, engorgement of ingested materials impairs the macrophage-dependent functions of the spleen. Impaired filtering function may cause a mild thrombocytosis. Functional or anatomical asplenia, especially after surgical removal in infants and children, increases the risk of an overwhelming bacterial infection. Table 56–3 lists conditions associated with hyposplenism.

CLINICAL FEATURES

The normal neonate and the elderly adult may have findings suggestive of impaired splenic function.[60] These include the presence of Howell-Jolly bodies and erythrocyte pits (see "Laboratory Features" below). However, the clinical significance of functional hyposplenism is uncertain.[61–63]

Sickle cell anemia and surgical splenectomy are the most common causes of hyposplenism. In sickle cell anemia, hyposplenism may

be functional in young children with enlarged spleens and disordered circulation and may be the result of atrophy after repeated infarcts have destroyed splenic tissue in older children and adults. Although the presence of an enlarged spleen usually suggests hypersplenism, spleen size is not a reliable index of splenic function. Complete splenic replacement by cysts, neoplastic tissue, or amyloid is an example of hyposplenic splenomegaly.[64] Acute sequestration crises in children with sickle hemoglobinopathies, and occasionally in patients with malaria, may clog the red cell pulp with cellular debris and lead to hyposplenism.[65,66]

Congenital asplenia may be found in infants with situs inversus and other developmental abnormalities.[38] Autoimmune disorders, such as glomerulonephritis,[67] systemic lupus erythematosus,[68,69] and rheumatoid arthritis,[70] are occasionally associated with laboratory evidence and clinical manifestations (overwhelming sepsis with encapsulated bacteria) of functional hyposplenism. Hyposplenism also occurs in chronic graft-versus-host disease,[71,72] sarcoidosis,[73] alcoholic liver cirrhosis,[74,75] hepatic amyloidosis,[76,77] celiac disease,[78,79] and inflammatory bowel disease.[80,81] The mechanisms for these associations are unknown.

Splenic replacement by neoplastic cells, as in lymphomas and leukemias, usually does not cause hyper- or hyposplenism. Splenic irradiation[82] and vascular obstruction[83] may also lead to functional hyposplenism.

Overwhelming Sepsis

Absence of a functional spleen may lead to life-threatening infections by removal of an efficient filtering bed in which opsonized organisms are engulfed and destroyed by splenic macrophages. The responsible organism is typically an encapsulated bacteria, such as *S. pneumoniae*, *N. meningitidis*, or *H. influenzae*. Unrestrained *in vivo* proliferation of such microorganisms may cause fatal septicemia.[84–86] The risk is greatest among infants whose general immunologic system has not matured enough to counteract bacterial infections, although the risk is present regardless of the patient's age. For this reason, splenectomy in children should be deferred until 5 years of age, if possible. The risk of sepsis varies depending on the reason for the splenectomy. In a child with an underlying immune disorder, such as Wiskott-Aldrich syndrome, the risk is very high. The infectious risk is higher in children with thalassemia than in those with hereditary spherocytosis and lowest in those with splenectomy for splenic trauma. The risk is reduced by the use of pneumococcal and *H. influenzae* vaccines prior to splenectomy and prophylactic penicillin therapy.[87]

Because the spleen is a major component of the mononuclear phagocyte system and has substantial lymphatic tissue in the white pulp, hyposplenism or splenectomy can also reduce antibody synthesis that may be beneficial in the management of autoimmune disorders.

LABORATORY FEATURES

The reduction or absence of normal splenic function is accompanied by a slight to moderate increase in white cell and platelet counts. Howell-Jolly bodies, target cells, Pappenheimer (siderotic) bodies, and occasional acanthocytes often are present in the blood film, but the finding of pitted erythrocytes in wet preparations is the most specific of all the blood findings.[88] Target cells reflecting an increased red cell surface[89] are almost always present in the asplenic state, but only 1 in 100 to 1 in 1000 red cells is affected. A sensitive indication of hyposplenism is the appearance of pits or pocks on the cell surface.[90] These pits consist of submembranous vacuoles and can be seen only in wet preparations of red cells using direct interference-contrast microscopy. Intracellular vesiculation containing hemoglobin is a normal occurrence during aging of the red cell in the circulation. This process is intensified in the last half of the erythrocyte life span and leads to a decreased mean cell

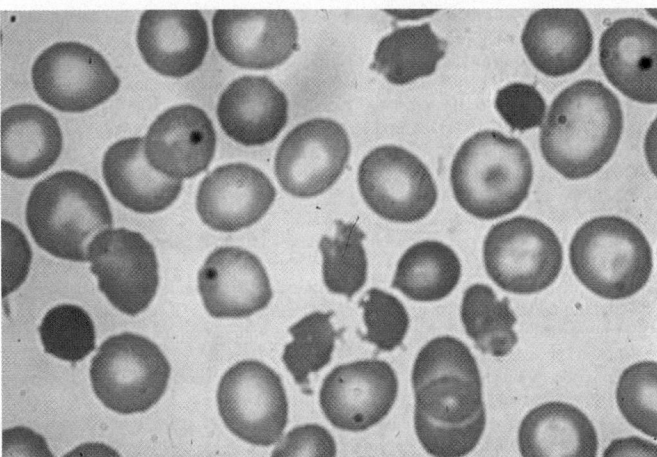

Figure 56–3. Blood film of splenectomized patient showing three red cells with Howell-Jolly bodies (nuclear remnants). Note also the cluster of acanthocytes and scattered spheroacanthocytes and the target cell. These changes are also indicative of postsplenectomy red cell changes. *(Reproduced with permission from* Lichtman's Atlas of Hematology, *www. accessmedicine.com.)*

hemoglobin level as the vesicles are removed (pitted) by the spleen. In asplenic individuals the vesicles are more numerous and enlarge, forming vacuoles that are evident by interference-phase microscopy.[88] This finding is the most specific evidence of hyposplenism, followed by the presence of DNA inclusions in circulating red cells (Howell-Jolly bodies; Fig. 56–3).

Oxidative drugs may produce Heinz bodies even in normal individuals, but the spleen effectively removes these red cell inclusions, as well as Pappenheimer bodies. Heinz bodies may be observed in supravitally stained blood films after splenectomy. Nucleated red cells rarely are seen on blood films after splenectomy, except in patients with hemolytic disorders in whom the number of nucleated red cells may increase dramatically. The reticulocyte count remains within normal values, and the life span of red cells is unchanged as other organs take up the function of removing senescent erythrocytes.

Technetium-99m sulfur-colloid particles are used for spleen scanning, a reliable measure of the capacity of the spleen to clear particulate matter from the bloodstream.[91]

THERAPY, COURSE, AND PROGNOSIS

Vaccination against *H. influenzae*, *N. meningitidis*, and *S. pneumoniae* is recommended in previously unvaccinated individuals prior to splenectomy.[92] Prophylactic immunization has significantly reduced, but not eliminated, the risk of overwhelming infection.[87,93–95] Oral penicillin or a macrolide antibiotic as prophylaxis for asplenic patients is recommended based on publicized guidelines despite problems with compliance and resistance.[96,97] Physicians should advise all asplenic patients that any febrile episode (>38°C) should be considered an emergency requiring immediate medical attention. A febrile asplenic patient must have blood and urine cultures drawn, followed by antibiotic treatment. Patients should be given written information about asplenia and carry a card or medical alert bracelet to alert health professionals of the risk of overwhelming infection.[96,97] Dental work, especially tooth extraction, should be preceded by broad-spectrum antibiotics, such as amoxicillin, if the patient is not taking prophylactic antibiotics. Patients should be educated about risks of travel, including risk of malaria infection or animal bites, which could be deadly unless promptly treated.[96,97]

REFERENCES

1. Crosby WH: The spleen, in *Blood, Pure and Eloquent*, edited by MM Wintrobe, p 96. McGraw-Hill, New York, 1980.
2. Chauffard AME: Des hepatites d'origine splenique. *Semin Med* 19:177, 1899.
3. Sutherland GA, Burghard FF: The treatment of splenic anaemia by splenectomy. *Lancet* 2:1819, 1910.
4. Kaznelson P: Verschwinden der hamorrhagischen Diathesis bei einen falle von "Essentieller Thrombopenia". *Wien Klin Wochenschr* 29:1451, 1916.
5. Crosby WH: Hypersplenism. *Annu Rev Med* 13:127, 1962.
6. Mutchnick MG, Lerner E, Conn HO: Effect of portacaval anastomosis on hypersplenism. *Dig Dis Sci* 25:929, 1980.
7. Jabbour N, Zajko A, Orons P, et al: Does transjugular intrahepatic portosystemic shunt (TIPS) resolve thrombocytopenia associated with cirrhosis? *Dig Dis Sci* 43:2459, 1998.
8. Roberts CW, Shutter JR, Korsmeyer SJ: Hox11 controls the genesis of the spleen. *Nature* 368:747, 1994.
9. Dear TN, Colledge WH, Carlton MB, et al: The Hox11 gene is essential for cell survival during spleen development. *Development* 121:2909, 1995.
10. Roberts CW, Sonder AM, Lumsden A, et al: Developmental expression of HOV11 and specification of splenic cell fate. *Am J Pathol* 146:1089, 1995.
11. Steininger B, Barth P, Herbst B, et al: The species-specific structure of microanatomical compartments in the human spleen. *Immunology* 92:307, 1997.
12. Bourdessoule D, Gaulard P, Mason DY: Preferential localization of human lymphocytes bearing –/– T cell receptors to the red pulp of the spleen. *J Clin Pathol* 43:461, 1990.
13. Kraus MD: Splenic histology and histopathology: An update. *Semin Diagn Pathol* 20:84, 2003.
14. Rosse WF: The spleen as a filter [editorial]. *N Engl J Med* 317:704, 1987.
15. Bowdler AJ: Splenomegaly and hypersplenism. *Clin Haematol* 12:467, 1983.
16. Areas Elenas N, Ewald R, Crosby WH: The reservoir function of the spleen and its relation to postsplenectomy anemia of the dog. *Blood* 24:299, 1964.
17. Wadenvik H, Kutti J: The spleen and pooling of blood cells. *Eur J Haematol* 41:1, 1988.
18. Aster RH: Pooling of platelets in the spleen: Role in the pathogenesis of "hypersplenic thrombocytopenia." *J Clin Invest* 45:645, 1966.
19. Gurakar A, Fagiuoli S, Gavaler JS, et al: The use of granulocyte-macrophage colony-stimulating factor to enhance hematologic parameters of patients with cirrhosis and hypersplenism. *J Hepatol* 21:582, 1994.
20. Karpatkin S: The spleen and thrombocytopenia. *Clin Haematol* 12:591, 1983.
21. Zwiebel WJ, Mountford RA, Halliwell MJ, Wells PN: Splanchnic blood flow in patients with cirrhosis and portal hypertension: Investigation with duplex Doppler US. *Radiology* 194:807, 1995.
22. Brubaker LH, Johnson CA: Correlation of splenomegaly and abnormal neutrophil pooling (margination). *J Lab Clin Med* 92:508, 1978.
23. Siciliano M, Tomasello D, Milani A, et al: Reduced serum levels of immunoreactive erythropoietin in patients with cirrhosis and chronic anemia. *Hepatology* 22:1132, 1995.
24. Vasilopoulos S, Hally R, Caro J, et al: Erythropoietin response to post-liver transplantation anemia. *Liver Transpl* 6:349, 2000.
25. Hess CE, Ayers CR, Sandusky WR, et al: Mechanism of dilutional anemia in massive splenomegaly. *Blood* 47:629, 1976.
26. Zhang B, Lewis SM: Splenic hematocrit and the splenic plasma pool. *Br J Haematol* 66:97, 1987.
27. Jandl JH: The anemia of liver disease: Observations on its mechanism. *J Clin Invest* 34:390, 1955.
28. Christensen BE: Quantitative determination of splenic red cell blood destruction in patients with splenomegaly. *Scand J Haematol* 14:295, 1975.
29. McIntyre OR, Ebaugh FA: Palpable spleens in college freshmen. *Ann Intern Med* 66:301, 1967.
30. Sty JR, Wells RG: Imaging the spleen, in *Disorders of the Spleen: Pathophysiology and Management*, edited by C Pochedly, RH Sills, AD Schwartz, p 355. Marcel Dekker, New York, 1989.
31. Buehner M, Baker MS: The wandering spleen. *Surg Gynecol Obstet* 175:373, 1992.
32. Joyce RA, Boggs DR, Hasiba U, Srodes CH: Marginal neutrophil in the pool size in normal subjects as measured by epinephrine infusion. *J Lab Clin Med* 88:614, 1976.
33. Alvarez OA, Lopera GA, Patel V, et al: Improvement of thrombocytopenia due to hypersplenism after transjugular intrahepatic portosystemic shunt placement in cirrhotic patients. *Am J Gastroenterol* 91:134, 1996.
34. Peck-Radosavljevic M: Hypersplenism. *Eur J Gastroenterol Hepatol* 13:317, 2001.
35. Bashour FN, Teran JC, Mullen KD: Prevalence of peripheral blood cytopenias (hypersplenism) in patients with nonalcoholic chronic liver disease. *Am J Gastroenterol* 95:2936, 2000.
36. Liangpunsakul S, Ulmer BJ, Chalasani N: Predictors and implications of severe hypersplenism in patients with cirrhosis. *Am J Med Sci* 326:111, 2003.
37. Qamar A, Grace N, Groszmann R, et al: Incidence, prevalence and clinical significance of abnormal hematological indices in compensated cirrhosis. *Clin Gastroenterol Hepatol* 7:689, 2009.
38. Civardi G, Vallisa D, Berte R, et al: Ultrasound guided fine needle biopsy of the spleen: High clinical efficacy and low risk in a multicenter Italian study. *Am J Hematol* 67:93, 2001.
39. Pochedly C, Sills RH, Schwartz A: *Disorders of the Spleen: Pathophysiology and Management*. Marcel Dekker, New York, 1989.

40. Yanaga K, Tzakis A, Shimade M, Campbell W, et al: Reversal of hypersplenism following orthotopic liver transplantation. *Ann Surg* 210:180, 1989.

41. Al-Salem AH, Qaisaruddin S, Nasserallah Z, et al: Splenectomy in patients with sickle-cell disease. *Am J Surg* 172:254, 1996.

42. Mohren M, Markman I, Dworschak U, et al: Thromboembolic complications after splenectomy for hematologic diseases. *Am J Hematol* 76:143, 2004.

43. Caprotti R, Porta G, Franciosi C, et al: Laparoscopic splenectomy for hematological disorders. *Int Surg* 83:303, 1998.

44. Bar-Moor JA: Partial splenectomy in Gaucher's disease. *J Pediatr Surg* 28:686, 1993.

45. Banani SA: Partial dearterialization of the spleen in thalassemia major. *J Pediatr Surg* 33:449, 1998.

46. Stanley P, Shen TC: Partial embolization of the spleen in patients with thalassemia. *J Vasc Interv Radiol* 6:137, 1995.

47. Palsson B, Hallen M, Forsberg AM, Alwmark A: Partial splenic embolization: Long-term outcome. *Langenbecks Arch Surg* 387:421, 2003.

48. Petersons A, Volrats O, Bernsteins A: The first experience with nonoperative treatment of hypersplenism in children with portal hypertension. *Eur J Pediatr Surg* 12:299, 2002.

49. Watanabe Y, Todani T, Noda T: Changes in splenic volume after partial splenic embolization in children. *J Pediatr Surg* 31:241, 1996.

50. Paulino AC, Reddy AC: Splenic irradiation in the palliation of patients with lymphoproliferative and myeloproliferative disorders. *Am J Hosp Palliat Care* 13:32, 1996.

51. Peck-Radosavljevic M, Wichlas M, Zacherl J, et al: Thrombopoietin induces rapid resolution of thrombocytopenia after orthotopic liver transplantation through increased platelet production. *Blood* 95:795, 2000.

52. Rios R, Sangro B, Herrero I, et al: The role of thrombopoietin in the thrombocytopenia of patients with liver cirrhosis. *Am J Gastroenterol* 100:1311, 2005.

53. Lok S, Kaushansky K, Holly RD, et al: Cloning and expression of murine thrombopoietin cDNA and stimulation of platelet production *in vivo*. *Nature* 369:565, 1994.

54. de Sauvage FJ, Hass PE, Spencer SD, et al: Stimulation of megakaryocytopoiesis and thrombopoiesis by the c-Mpl ligand. *Nature* 369:533, 1994.

55. McHutchinson JG, Dusheiko G, Shiffman ML, et al: Eltrombopag in patients with cirrhosis associated with hepatitis C. *N Engl J Med* 357:2227, 2007.

56. Afdhal NH, Giannini EG, Tayyab G, et al: Eltrombopag before procedures in patients with cirrhosis and thrombocytopenia. *N Engl J Med* 23;367, 2012.

57. Moussa MM, Mowafy N: Preoperative use of romiplostim in thrombocytopenic patients with chronic hepatitis C and liver cirrhosis. *J Gastroenterol Hepatol* 28(2):335, 2013.

58. Ramos H, Todo S, Kang Y, et al: Liver transplantation without the use of blood products. *Arch Surg* 129:528, 1994.

59. Snook NJ, O'Beirne HA, Enright S, et al: Use of recombinant human erythropoietin to facilitate liver transplantation in a Jehovah's Witness. *Br J Anaesth* 76:740,1996.

60. Freedman RM, Johnston D, Mahoney MJ, et al: Development of splenic reticuloendothelial function in neonates. *J Pediatr* 96:466, 1980.

61. Padmanabhan J, Risemberg HM, Rome RD: Howell-Jolly bodies in the peripheral blood of full-term and premature neonates. *Johns Hopkins Med J* 132:146, 1973.

62. Markus HS, Toghill PJ: Impaired splenic function in elderly people. *Age Ageing* 20:287, 1991.

63. Ravaglia G, Forti P, Biagi F, et al: Splenic function in old age. *Gerontology* 44:91, 1998.

64. Steinberg MH, Gatling RR, Tavassoli M: Evidence of hyposplenism in the presence of splenomegaly. *Scand J Haematol* 31:437, 1983.

65. Looareesuwan S, Ho M, Wallanagoon Y, et al: Dynamic alteration in splenic function during acute falciparum malaria. *N Engl J Med* 317: 675, 1987.

66. Emond AM, Callis R, Darvill D, et al: Acute splenic sequestration in homozygous sickle cell disease: Natural history and management. *J Pediatr* 107:201, 1985.

67. Lawrence SE, Pussell BA, Charlesworth JA: Splenic function in primary glomerulonephritis. *Adv Exp Med Biol* 641:1, 1982.

68. Webster J, Williams BD, Smith AP, et al: Systemic lupus erythematosus presenting as pneumococcal septicemia and septic arthritis. *Ann Rheum Dis* 49:181, 1990.

69. Liote F, Angle J, Gilmore N, Osterland CK: Asplenism and systemic lupus erythematosus. *Clin Rheumatol* 14:220, 1995.

70. Jarolim DR: Asplenia and rheumatoid arthritis [letter]. *Ann Intern Med* 97:61, 1982.

71. Kalhs P, Panzer S, Kletter K, et al: Functional asplenia after bone marrow transplantation. *Ann Intern Med* 109:461, 1988.

72. Cuthbert RJ, Iqbal A, Gates A, et al: Functional hyposplenism following allogeneic bone marrow transplantation. *J Clin Pathol* 48:257, 1995.

73. Stone RW, McDaniel WR, Armstrong EM, et al: Acquired functional asplenia in sarcoidosis. *J Natl Med Assoc* 77:930, 1985.

74. Muller AF, Toghill PJ: Splenic function in alcoholic liver disease. *Gut* 33:1386, 1992.

75. Muller AF, Toghill PJ: Functional hyposplenism in alcoholic liver disease: A toxic effect of alcohol? *Gut* 35:679, 1994.

76. Gertz MA, Kyle RA: Hepatic amyloidosis (primary [AL], immunoglobulin light chain): The natural history in 80 patients. *Am J Med* 85:73, 1988.

77. Powsner RA, Simms RW, Chudnovsky A, et al: Scintigraphic functional hyposplenism in amyloidosis. *J Nucl Med* 39:221, 1998.

78. Robinson PJ, Bullen AW, Hall R, et al: Splenic size and functions in adult coeliac disease. *Br J Radiol* 53:532, 1980.

79. O'Grady JG, Stevens FM, Harding B, et al: Hyposplenism and gluten sensitive enteropathy. *Gastroenterology* 87:1316, 1984.

80. Palmer KR, Sherriff SB, Holdsworth CD, et al: Further experience of hyposplenism in inflammatory bowel disease. *Q J Med* 50:461, 1981.

81. Muller AF, Toghill PJ: Hyposplenism in gastrointestinal disease. *Gut* 36:165, 1995.

82. Dailey MO, Coleman CN, Kaplan HS: Radiation-induced splenic atrophy in patients with Hodgkin disease and non-Hodgkin lymphoma. *N Engl J Med* 302:215, 1990.

83. Spencer RP, Sziklas JJ, Turner JW: Functional obstruction of splenic blood vessel in adults: A radiocolloid study. *Int J Nucl Med Biol* 9:208, 1982.

84. Torres J, Bisno AL: Hyposplenism and pneumococcemia. *Am J Med* 55:851, 1973.

85. Cavenagh JD, Joseph AE, Dilly S, Bevan DH: Splenic sepsis in sickle cell disease. *Br J Haematol* 86:187, 1994.

86. Gopal V, Bisno AL: Fulminant pneumococcal infections in "normal" asplenic hosts. *Arch Intern Med* 137:1526, 1977.

87. Konradsen HB, Henrichsen J: Pneumococcal infections in splenectomized children are preventable. *Acta Paediatr Scand* 80:423, 1991.

88. Corazza GR, Ginaldi L, Zoli G, et al: Howell-Jolly body counting as a measure of splenic function: A reassessment. *Clin Lab Haematol* 12:269, 1990.

89. Holroyde CP, Oski FA, Gardner FH: The "pocked" erythrocytes. *N Engl J Med* 281:516, 1969.

90. Reinhart WH, Chien S: Red cell vacuoles: Their size and distribution under normal conditions and after splenectomy. *Am J Hematol* 27:265, 1988.

91. Rutland MD: Correlation of splenic function with the splenic uptake rate of Tc-colloids. *Nucl Med Commun* 13:843, 1992.

92. Kobel DE, Friedl A, Cerny T, et al: Pneumococcal vaccine in patients with absent or dysfunctional spleen. *Mayo Clin Proc* 75:749, 2000.

93. Ward KM, Celebi JT, Gmyrek R, Grossman ME: Acute infectious purpura fulminans associated with asplenism or hyposplenism. *J Am Acad Dermatol* 47:493, 2002.

94. Sumaraju V, Smith LG, Smith SM: Infectious complications in asplenic hosts. *Infect Dis Clin North Am* 15:551, 2001.

95. Castagnola E, Fioredda F: Prevention of life-threatening infections due to encapsulated bacteria in children with hyposplenia or asplenia: A brief review of current recommendations for practical purposes. *Eur J Haematol* 71:319, 2003.

96. Guidelines for the prevention and treatment of infection in patients with an absent or dysfunctional spleen. *BMJ* 312:430, 1996.

97. Davies JM, Barnes R, Milligan D: Update of guidelines for the prevention and treatment of infection in patients with an absent or dysfunctional spleen. *Clin Med* 2:440, 2002.

CHAPTER 57
PRIMARY AND SECONDARY ERYTHROCYTOSES

Josef T. Prchal

SUMMARY

Increased blood red cell mass can be termed either *polycythemia* or *erythrocytosis;* no clear consensus for either term has been achieved. Primary polycythemias are caused by acquired or inherited mutations causing functional changes within hematopoietic stem cells or erythroid progenitors leading to an accumulation of red cells. The most common primary polycythemia, polycythemia rubra vera, which is a clonal disorder, is discussed in Chap. 84; other primary polycythemias, such as those inherited from mutations in the erythropoietin receptor or congenital disorders of hypoxia sensing, are discussed herein. In contrast, secondary polycythemias are a result of either an appropriate or inappropriate increase in the red cell mass, most often as a result of augmented levels of erythropoietin; these polycythemias can also be either acquired or hereditary. Although the clinical presentations of primary and secondary polycythemias may be similar, distinguishing amongst them is important for accurate diagnoses and proper management.

For example, those secondary polycythemic states that represent an appropriate physiologic compensation to tissue hypoxia, should not be treated by phlebotomies. An occasional patient may experience hyperviscosity symptoms and may benefit from isovolemic reduction of hematocrit. Inappropriate polycythemias are caused by erythropoietin-secreting tumors, self-administration of erythropoiesis-stimulating agents, including androgens, inherited disorders of hypoxia sensing, or, rarely, some endocrine disorders (described in Chap. 38). Correction of hypoxia, discontinuation of erythropoiesis-stimulating agents or resection of erythropoietin-secreting tumors will typically correct the associated polycythemia.

DEFINITION AND HISTORY

The term *polycythemia*, denoting an increased amount of blood cells, has traditionally been applied to those conditions in which the mass of erythrocytes is increased. *Erythrocytosis* is an alternative term that has also been applied to circumstances in which the increased red cell

mass is the singular finding, distinguishing it from polycythemia vera in which, classically, there is an increase in red cells, granulocytes, and platelets. Although this usage has much to recommend it, no consensus about terminology has been reached and the term *polycythemia* is used interchangeably with erythrocytosis by many physicians. In some instances, time-honored terms such as post–renal transplant erythrocytosis or Chuvash polycythemia will be used. A classification of the polycythemias is presented in Chap. 34 in Table 34–2.

PRIMARY POLYCYTHEMIAS

Polycythemia vera (Chap. 84) and *primary familial and congenital polycythemia (PFCP)* are primary polycythemic disorders, which have erythroid progenitors that are hypersensitive to erythropoietin.[1-3] These are caused by somatic (polycythemia vera) or germline (PFCP) mutations wherein erythroid progenitors are intrinsically hyperproliferative by mechanisms other than the presence of increased levels of erythropoietin and have, as shown by *in vitro* assays, an augmented response to erythropoietin. Some congenital polycythemias, as best described in Chuvash polycythemia, have erythroid progenitors that are hypersensitive to erythropoietin, but also may have normal or even increased erythropoietin levels despite the increased red cell volume.[4,5] Thus, some of these rare inherited polycythemias share features of both primary and secondary polycythemias.[6]

SECONDARY POLYCYTHEMIAS/ ERYTHROCYTOSES

The term *secondary polycythemia*, more appropriately *secondary erythrocytosis*, which refers to those conditions in which only erythrocytes are increased in number and volume, describes a group of disorders characterized by an increased red cell mass brought about by enhanced stimulation of red cell production by circulating physiologic mediators, most commonly erythropoietin. Secondary polycythemia may be subdivided into *appropriate polycythemia*, that is, responding normally to tissue hypoxia such as in pulmonary disease, Eisenmenger complex, high-altitude polycythemia and hemoglobins with increased affinity for oxygen (Chaps. 49 and 50), and *inappropriate polycythemia* in which erythropoiesis is being stimulated by the aberrant production of erythropoietin, as in erythropoietin-secreting tumors, by high levels of insulin growth factor 1, by cobalt toxicity, by self-administration of erythropoietin, androgens, or adrenocorticotropic hormone, or by other stimulators of erythropoiesis (as in post–renal transplant erythrocytosis).[7]

In his important monograph on barometric pressure published in 1878, Paul Bert showed that physiologic impairment observed at high altitude was caused by a reduction in the oxygen content of the air.[8] A few years earlier, his friend and mentor, Dennis Jourdanet, had observed an increase in the number of red corpuscles in blood of the highlanders in Mexico,[9] and Bert recognized that such an increase would tend to ameliorate the effect of atmospheric hypoxia. However, neither Bert nor Jourdanet suspected a cause-and-effect relationship. It was not until 1890, when Viault[10] observed a prompt increase in the number of his own red corpuscles after having traveled from Lima, Peru, at sea level, to Morococha, at 4570 m (15,000 ft) above sea level, that altitude erythrocytosis was accepted as a compensatory adaptation to hypoxia.[11] At about the same time, it was observed that many patients with cyanosis were also polycythemic. Both *cardiacos negros*,[12] with severe pulmonary failure and arterial oxygen desaturation, and children with *morbus caeruleus*, or right-to-left shunt through a congenital cardiac malformation, were found to have increased red cell counts.[13] Mechanical or neurogenic hypoventilation as a cause of cyanosis and polycythemia was first popularized in 1956 with the classic description of the pickwickian syndrome by Burwell and colleagues.[14] Polycythemia associated with carboxyhemoglobinemia resulting in hypoxemia as a result of smoking and with tissue hypoxia because of inherited abnormal hemoglobins with high-affinity oxygen binding to hemoglobin was recognized subsequently (Chaps. 49 and 50).[15] Erythrocytosis associated with abnormal hemoglobins with an increased affinity for oxygen also represents an appropriate response to hypoxia first noted by Charache and colleagues[15] in 1966 when they described hemoglobin Chesapeake.

Relative erythrocytosis is the term used to depict enhanced red cell count or blood hemoglobin values resulting from reduced plasma volume, not increased red cell mass. The disorder is, therefore, not a true polycythemia and is designated *apparent, spurious,* or *relative polycythemia.* The cause of the reduced plasma volume and hence relative erythrocytosis is often known, that is, diuretic use, dehydration from excessive sweating, etc. However, there are some patients with mild erythrocytosis in which neither the cause nor the clinical significance is clear. In 1905, Gaisbock reported that a number of hypertensive patients had plethora and an elevated red cell count but no splenomegaly, a condition he termed *polycythemia hypertonica,* sometimes called *Gaisbock syndrome.*[16] In 1952, direct measurement of blood volume in patients with polycythemia led Lawrence and Berlin to identify a subgroup of patients with a normal red cell volume but reduced plasma volume. Although some members of this group were hypertensive, the authors were more impressed by their tense and anxious behavior and coined the term *stress polycythemia.*[17]

● EPIDEMIOLOGY

PRIMARY POLYCYTHEMIAS

Primary Familial and Congenital Polycythemia

This autosomal dominant disorder (designated PFCP) is uncommon but more prevalent than is generally appreciated, as many affected subjects are initially misdiagnosed as having polycythemia vera. Its prevalence is similar to congenital polycythemias because of high oxygen-affinity hemoglobin mutants, and far more common than 2,3-bisphosphoglycerate (2,3-BPG) deficiency.[18]

SECONDARY POLYCYTHEMIAS

Pulmonary Disease with Hypoxia

In one study of 2524 patients with severe chronic obstructive pulmonary disease (COPD), 8.4 percent had a hematocrit higher than 55 percent. In this study, hematocrit was an independent predictor of longer survival, decreased hospital admission rate, and decreased cumulative duration of hospitalization.[19] In another, smaller study of 309 subjects with COPD and chronic respiratory failure, 67 percent had normal hemoglobin levels, 20 percent had anemia, and 18 percent had polycythemia.[20]

Obstructive Sleep Apnea

Although the evidence is largely anecdotal,[21] secondary polycythemia is a widely recognized complication of longstanding obstructive sleep apnea (OSA), being found in 5 to 10 percent of those with nocturnal apnea and hypopnea.[22] The published studies remain controversial; in a study of 263 patients (189 men and 74 women), patients with severe sleep apnea had significantly higher hematocrit values than did patients with mild to moderate sleep apnea or nonapneic controls (p <0.01).[23] In contrast, in other studies, there were no significant differences in hemoglobin levels or hematocrit between subjects with and without

OSA.[24,25] The total number of hours of hypoxia per day may dictate whether the stimulus to erythropoietin production is sufficient to cause erythrocytosis.

Polycythemia Associated with Smoking

Smoking clearly increases hematocrit in COPD compared to controls of comparable pulmonary function. In a study of 2524 patients with severe COPD, 10.2 percent of patients reported as current smokers had significantly higher hematocrit values than did ex-smokers or nonsmokers of comparable pulmonary impairment of both genders, with p <0.02.[20]

Even young male smokers without pulmonary impairment have higher hematocrits. In one study, 1169 subjects (age range: 18.6 to 22.8 years; mean: 19.4 years) were recruited and 25 percent were smokers. Predictably, carboxyhemoglobin was much higher in smokers than in nonsmokers (r = 0.958, p <0.001) and both hemoglobin and hematocrits were also markedly higher in smokers (hemoglobin (p = 0.001), hematocrit (p = 0.004).[26]

High Oxygen Affinity and Hemoglobins

These disorders are reviewed in detail in Chaps. 49 and 50. High oxygen-affinity hemoglobins deliver less oxygen to tissues, which is appropriately compensated by increased erythropoiesis and a higher steady-state hemoglobin concentration. While considered rare, high oxygen affinity has been found, according to one report, in approximately 20 percent of 70 unrelated subjects with otherwise idiopathic polycythemia.[27]

Polycythemia of Eisenmenger Complex

Eisenmenger syndrome, characterized by elevated pulmonary vascular resistance and right-to-left shunting of blood, is usually accompanied by polycythemia.[28] Most patients with the syndrome survive for 20 to 30 years.

Polycythemia of Endocrine Disorders and from Iatrogenic or Self-Administration of Androgens

Erythrocytosis has been reported in Cushing syndrome,[29] primary aldosteronism,[30] and Bartter syndrome (Chap. 38).[31]

In a prospective trial of testosterone use in older men, erythrocytosis (defined as a hematocrit greater than 50 or 52 percent) was three times more likely to occur in the testosterone-treated group compared to placebo.[32] (Refer to Chap. 38 for more details.)

Inappropriate Tissue Elaboration of Erythropoietin

The prevalence of various types of secondary polycythemia is a function of underlying causes, such as geographical location of the patient or presence of a causative neoplasm. Approximately 1 to 3 percent of all patients with pheochromocytoma or paraganglioma have erythrocytosis.[33] Rare patients with congenital erythrocytosis will develop pheochromocytoma or paraganglioma.[34] Uterine leiomyomas in premenopausal women are very common, estimated at 20 to 40 percent, and the occurrence of erythrocytosis ranges from 0.02 to 0.5 percent of cases.[35] Isolated instances of polycythemia have been attributed to myxoma of the atrium,[36] hamartoma of the liver,[37] and focal hyperplasia of the liver.[38] Erythrocytosis and inappropriate secretion of erythropoietin may be found in approximately 15 percent of patients with cerebellar hemangioma.[39,40]

Self-Administration of Erythropoietin

Athletes have attempted for decades to manipulate their blood to gain a competitive advantage either by blood transfusions or erythropoietin. This evolving, but continuous, problem has been the subject of a review.[41]

Polycythemia of High Altitude

Elevation of red cell mass as a response to high altitude hypoxia represents an appropriate adjustment to reduced blood oxygen content and delivery. The exponentially decreasing atmospheric oxygen pressure with altitude stimulates the body to accommodate by an increase in respiratory rate and volume. Such adaptation is possible only in the short-term, because the body may not always be able to adequately enhance respiration. Polycythemia is considered to be a universal, uniform adaptation response to hypoxia that arises in normal individuals, but when it is exaggerated, in some cases it results in chronic mountain sickness with associated symptoms of fatigue, headache, and pulmonary hypertension.[42]

Altitude above sea level should be used as an independent variable for the definition of polycythemia[43] and Centers for Disease Control data lists the appropriate adjustment values.[44]

Post–Renal Transplant Erythrocytosis

This syndrome, defined as a persistent elevation of hematocrit at greater than 51 percent, is a relatively common condition found in approximately 5 to 10 percent of renal allograft recipients.[45,46] Post–renal transplant erythrocytosis usually develops within 8 to 24 months after transplantation, despite persistently good function of the allograft, and resolves spontaneously within 2 years in approximately 25 percent of patients.[47] Factors that increase the likelihood of its development are lack of erythropoietin therapy prior to transplantation, a history of smoking, diabetes mellitus, renal artery stenosis, low serum ferritin levels, and normal or higher pretransplant erythropoietin levels. Post–renal transplant erythrocytosis is also more frequent in patients who are not undergoing graft rejection.

Chuvash Polycythemia

A Russian hematologist, Lydia A. Polyakova, described polycythemia in the Chuvash population (an ethnic isolate in the mid-Volga River region of Russia of Turkish descent) in the early 1960s,[48] and by 1974, 103 cases from 81 families had been described.[48] Since then, more cases have come to light; hundreds of children and adults suffer from this condition, indicating that Chuvash polycythemia is the only known endemic congenital polycythemia in the world.[49] Outside of Chuvashia, Chuvash polycythemia has also been found sporadically in diverse ethnic and racial groups,[50,51] and recently a high prevalence of this disorder has also been reported on the Italian island of Ischia.[52]

● ETIOLOGY AND PATHOGENESIS

PRIMARY POLYCYTHEMIAS

Primary Familial and Congenital Polycythemia

In contrast to polycythemia vera, PFCP is caused by germline rather than acquired somatic mutations. It is congenital and manifests autosomal dominant inheritance[3] and, not infrequently, sporadic occurrence from *de novo* germline mutations. Like polycythemia vera (Chap. 84), it is primary in that the defect changes intrinsic responses of erythroid progenitors, and erythropoietin levels are low.

To date, 12 mutations of the erythropoietin receptor (EPOR) associated with PFCP have been described (Table 57–1). Nine of the 12 result in truncation of the EPOR cytoplasmic carboxyl terminal, and are the only mutations convincingly linked with PFCP. Such truncations lead to a loss in the negative regulatory domain of the EPOR (Chaps. 32 and 34). Three missense *EPOR* mutations have also been described, but these have not been linked to PFCP or any other disease phenotype (Table 57–1).

Erythropoietin-mediated activation of erythropoiesis involves several steps (also see Chap. 32). First, erythropoietin activates its receptor by inducing conformational changes of its dimers (Chap. 17). These changes lead to initiation of an erythroid-specific cascade of events. The first signal is initiated by conformation change-induced activation of Janus-type tyrosine kinase 2 (JAK2) and its phosphorylation and activation of a transcription factor, signal transducer and activator of transcription 5 (STAT5), which regulates erythroid-specific genes. This "on" signal is negated by dephosphorylation of EPOR by hematopoietic cell phosphatase (HCP), also known as SHP1, that is, the "off" signal. EPOR truncations lead to a loss of the negative regulatory domain of the EPOR, a binding site for HCP, explaining the gain-of-function properties of these *EPOR* mutations (Fig. 57–1).

TABLE 57–1. Summary of Erythropoietin Receptor Gene Mutations

Type of Mutation	Mutation	Structural Defect	Association with PFCP	Ref.
Deletion (7bp)	Del5985–5991	Frameshift > ter truncation	Yes	163, 192
Duplication (8 bp)	5968–5975	Frameshift > ter truncation	Yes	222
Nonsense	G6002	Trp439 > ter truncation	Yes	223
Nonsense	5986 *C>T*	Gln435 > ter truncation	Yes	224
Nonsense	5964*C>G*	Tyr426 > ter truncation	Yes	162
Nonsense	5881*C>T*	Glu399 > ter truncation	Yes	225
Nonsense	5959*G>T*	Glu425 > ter truncation	Yes	226
Insertion (G)	5974insG	Frameshift > ter truncation	Yes	227
Insertion (T)	5967insT	Frameshift > ter truncation	Yes	228
Substitution	6148*C>T*	Pro 488 > Ser	No	192, 229
Substitution	6146*A>G*	Asn487 > Ser	No	230
Substitution	2706 *A>T*	Unknown	No	226

Ter, termination codon.

Data from Kralovics R, Indrak K, Stopka T, et al. Two new EPO receptor mutations: truncated EPO receptors are most frequently associated with primary familial and congenital polycythemias. *Blood* 1997 Sep 1;90(5):2057–2061.

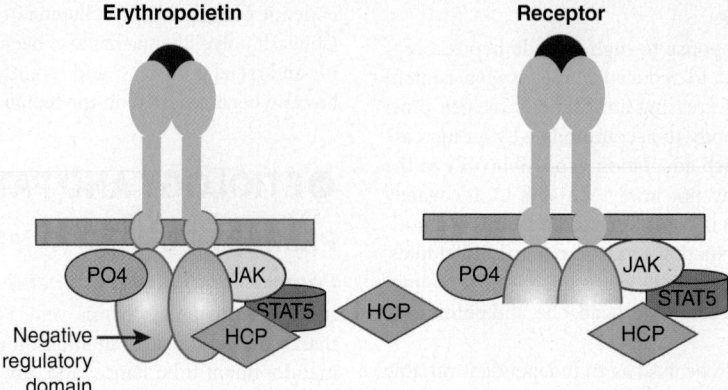

Figure 57–1. *Left panel:* Erythropoietin binding to a normal erythropoietin receptor (EPOR) results in interaction of a protein kinase (JAK) with the receptor. The interaction leads to phosphorylation of the receptor and initiates a cascade of signaling that ultimately results in erythroid progenitor proliferation and differentiation. This process is self-regulatory. Activated signal transduction molecules, hematopoietic cell phosphatase (HCP) binds to the C-terminal of the EPOR, which is a negative regulatory domain. This interaction dephosphorylates the receptor and turns off the signaling resulting in cessation of erythroid progenitor proliferation. *Right panel:* Patients with mutated gain-of-function *EPOR* gene lack the C-terminal portion of the receptor that contains the negative regulatory domain. Erythropoietin binds and the signal transduction pathway is activated by change of configuration of erythropoietin receptor dimer, but because there is there is no structure for HCP to bind on the activated EPOR dimer, the receptor is left in the activated position resulting in unbridled erythroid proliferation and an elevated red cell mass. PO4, phosphate; STAT, signal transducer and activator of transcription.

SECONDARY POLYCYTHEMIAS

The morbidity of primary polycythemias, such as polycythemia vera (Chap. 84), is largely the result of increased activated neutrophils and, perhaps, attendant pathologic platelet–endothelial interactions, whereas in secondary polycythemias it is presumably related to an increase in blood viscosity and, in part, to the resulting increased cardiac work.[53] In most instances, the etiology of morbidity or mortality, such as associated with congenital disorders of hypoxia sensing, is largely unknown.[54] The effect of blood viscosity on oxygen delivery is often oversimplified and the emphasis on the hematocrit alone may lead to ill-advised therapeutic interventions. In the normovolemic state, viscosity increases in a log-linear fashion as hematocrit increases, and the effect is particularly pronounced when the hematocrit rises above 50 percent. The prediction is that oxygen delivery *decreases* as hematocrit rises significantly above 50, as the greatly increased viscosity reduces blood flow, overshadowing the increased oxygen-carrying capacity of blood with a higher concentration of hemoglobin. However, polycythemia is not a normovolemic state, but is accompanied by an increase in blood volume, which, in turn, enlarges the vascular bed and decreases peripheral resistance (Chap. 34). Thus, hypervolemia can increase oxygen transport, and the optimum for oxygen transport occurs at higher hematocrit values than in normovolemic states. Consequently, despite the attendant increase in viscosity, an increase in hematocrit may generally be of benefit in appropriate secondary polycythemias. However, at some point, the high viscosity causes an increase in the work of the heart and a reduction in blood flow to most tissues and may be responsible for cerebral and cardiovascular impairment.

APPROPRIATE POLYCYTHEMIAS

High Altitude Polycythemia

Adaptive adjustments of humans living at high altitude involve a series of steps that reduce the steepness of the oxygen gradient between the atmosphere and mitochondria (Fig. 57–2).[55] The initial oxygen gradient between atmospheric and alveolar air can be reduced by an increase in respiratory rate and volume. Because dead space and water

vapor pressure are constant and acclimatized individuals do not ventilate excessively, the normal sea level gradient of about 60 torr is only reduced to approximately 40 torr at 4540 m (14,900 ft) above sea level.[55] Further reduction can be achieved, and at the top of Mount Everest, extreme hyperventilation reduces the gradient to less than 10 torr. A shift in the oxygen dissociation curve to the right, which represents decreased affinity of hemoglobin for oxygen, may be of benefit for short-term high-altitude acclimatization,[56] but its usefulness for chronic acclimatization has probably been exaggerated.[57] In the unacclimatized subject exposed acutely to high altitude, hyperventilation alkalosis leads initially to a shift of the oxygen dissociation curve to the left, representing an increased affinity of hemoglobin for oxygen, further worsening already present tissue hypoxia. The alkalosis and the hypoxia will, in turn, promote red cell synthesis of 2,3-BPG and cause the oxygen dissociation curve to shift back to a normal or even right-shifted position

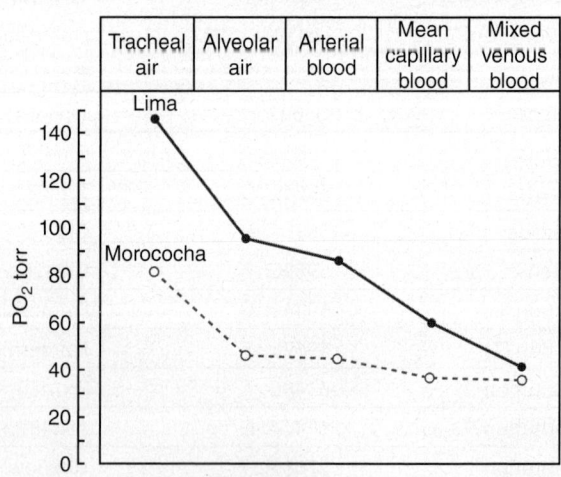

Figure 57–2. The oxygen gradient from atmospheric air to the tissues in individuals living at sea level (Lima, Peru) and in Morococha, Peru, at 4540 m (14,900 ft) above sea level.

(Chap. 49). In chronic acclimatization, blood pH is slightly increased, and when this is taken into account, the dissociation curve is shifted approximately to normal.[58] It is unlikely that a shift to the right would be to the advantage of high-altitude dwellers, except as a partial compensation for respiratory alkalosis.[59] In addition, a right-shifted curve also has a decrease in oxygen loading in the alveolar capillary, minimizing any net gain in off-loading. There is a relationship between higher altitude and hemoglobin concentration response, best studied among Andean highlanders and Europeans in the United States; hemoglobin concentration is almost 10 percent higher in those Andean highlanders living at 5500 m than in those living at 4355 m. Furthermore, native Andean high-altitude dwellers have a gradual increase in their hemoglobin levels with age[60] and body weight.[61] Although it has been postulated that high hemoglobin–oxygen affinity in the setting of extremely low ambient oxygen may be one such adaptive change,[62] increased hemoglobin–oxygen affinity or increased fetal hemoglobin are not adaptive phenotypes of Tibetan or Andean highlanders.[63]

In a subset of Andean high-altitude native dwellers, namely Quechua and Aymara Indians, polycythemia becomes excessive and often results in chronic mountain sickness with its associated constitutional symptoms and pulmonary hypertension.[42,60] This excessive erythrocytosis, called Monge disease or chronic mountain sickness,[42,64] is also described in Han Chinese living in Tibet[65] and occurs in whites living at high altitudes.[66]

The polycythemia encountered in high-altitude dwellers is often considered to be a universal, uniform adaptation process to hypoxia that would arise in all normal individuals. In reality, there is marked variability in erythropoietin level and subsequent polycythemic response to chronic hypoxia,[60,67] suggesting that some of these factors may be genetically determined; the same degree of hypoxia induces substantial differences in erythropoietin production in response to high altitude.[62,68,69] Three distinct adaptations to high altitude appear to have evolved. Andean highlanders have higher oxygen saturation than Tibetans at the same altitudes.[62] Tibetan mean resting ventilation and hypoxic ventilatory response are higher than Andean Aymaras, whereas the mean Tibetan hemoglobin concentration is below the Andean mean. High levels of nitric oxide (NO) in the exhaled breath of Tibetans may represent increased physiologic NO. This effect may improve oxygen delivery by inducing vasodilation and increasing blood flow to tissues, thus making the compensatory increase in red cell volume unnecessary.[70] Another distinct successful pattern of human adaptation in high-altitude dwellers that contrasts with both the Andean "classic" (arterial hypoxemia with polycythemia) and Tibetan (arterial hypoxemia with normal venous hemoglobin concentration) patterns evolved in Ethiopia. While Ethiopian high-altitude dwellers have hemoglobin concentrations that fall in the normal range (15.9 and 15.0 g/dL for males and females, respectively), they have a surprisingly, as-yet-unexplained high (average of 95.3 percent) oxygen saturation of hemoglobin despite their hypoxic environment (reviewed in Ref. 62). Their cerebral circulation is increased but is insensitive to hypoxia, unlike Peruvian high-altitude dwellers.[71] Thus, Ethiopian highlanders maintain venous hemoglobin concentrations and arterial oxygen saturation within the ranges of sea level populations, despite the decrease in ambient oxygen tension at high altitude.[72] Tibetans and Ethiopians have lived as mountain dwellers much longer than the Quechua or Aymara Indians,[73] suggesting that extreme elevation of red cell mass is a maladaptation that Tibetans avoided by evolving a more efficient, or less detrimental, compensatory mechanism than that which causes Monge disease.

With rapid advances in genomics (Chap. 11), progress has been made in identification of the molecular basis of high-altitude adaptation; most of these advances have been in our understanding of Tibetan adaptation. Several studies reported evidence for positive natural selection in genomic regions in Tibetans; not surprisingly, most are haplotypes comprising genes that are components of hypoxia sensing that are mediated by hypoxia-inducible factors (HIFs) (described in Chap. 32). Two of these selected regions include genes that have undergone the strongest genetic selection, and are thus likely the most beneficial for Tibetan adaptation. These two regions encompass the *EPAS1* gene, encoding the α subunit of HIF-2, and the *EGLN1* gene, encoding proline hydroxylase 2 (PHD2). PHD2 is the principal negative regulator of both HIF-1 and HIF-2. Both of these haplotypes were shown to be associated with differences in hemoglobin concentration at high altitude by several independent studies.[74-76] Intriguingly, the *EPAS1* haplotype was previously identified as having the strongest Tibetan positive selection and was found to have an unusual haplotype structure that originated by introgression of DNA from Denisovan or Denisovan-related hominins.[77] Denisovans, a sister group to the Neanderthals, branched off from the human lineage perhaps 600,000 years ago,[78] and available evidence suggests that Denisovan and Neanderthal hominins contributed to the modern *homo sapiens* admixture before their extinction, likely by interbreeding,[79] and that these hominin species provided genetic variations that helped humans adapt to new environments, such as extreme hypoxia associated with high altitude.[77] The first Tibetan adaptation gene mutation identified, which changes the encoded PHD2 protein within the selected haplotype, is a missense variant of the *EGLN1* gene, c.12C>G,[80] that is in near complete linkage disequilibrium with a previously reported missense variant, *EGLN1:c.380G>C*.[80] Both *EGLN1:c.[12C>G; 380G>C]* (PHD2[D4E,C127S]) are in *cis*; that is, the constituting PHD2[D4E,C127S] locus. Analysis of Tibetans and related populations suggests that *12C>G* started on the *380G>C* variant that is not Tibetan specific,[80,81] that PHD2[D4E,C127S] originated from a single individual approximately 8000 years ago,[81] and that now greater than 80 percent of Tibetans carry this PHD2 variant.[81] Functional assessment of homozygous PHD2[D4E,C127S] recombinant proteins showed that the variant protein has increased hydroxylase activity under hypoxic conditions. Furthermore, native homozygous PHD2[D4E,C127S] erythroid progenitors have blunted erythropoietic responses to hypoxia by both erythropoietin-specific and erythropoietin-independent mechanisms.[81] Although this is the first identified variant that contributes to the molecular and cellular basis of Tibetan adaptation to high altitude, there are other evolutionarily selected genomic regions, and elucidation of their functional impact is, at the time of this writing, unknown.

Understanding the etiology of polycythemia of high altitude is made more complex by a study of inhabitants of the Peruvian mining community of Cerro de Pasco (altitude 4280 m) with excessive erythrocytosis (mean hematocrit: 76 percent; range: 66 to 91 percent). About half of those individuals with a hematocrit greater than 75 percent had toxic serum cobalt levels,[82] suggesting that other erythropoiesis promoting factors such as cobalt[83] can augment hypoxia induction of erythropoietin, causing extreme polycythemias (Chap. 32). Most high-altitude dwellers do not have measurable levels or a history of exposure to cobalt or other heavy metals.[84]

Erythrocytosis of Pulmonary Disease

Degrees of arterial hypoxia comparable to those observed in individuals at high altitudes are observed in patients with right-to-left shunting resulting from cardiac or intrapulmonary shunts or to ventilation defects, as in COPD.

Many patients with COPD with severe cyanosis are not polycythemic. This has been attributed to infections and inflammation often present in the lungs, resulting in anemia of chronic inflammation, and to an increase in plasma volume. Why some patients with lung disease and congenital heart disease develop polycythemia, while others do not, is not entirely clear.

Erythrocytosis of Eisenmenger Syndrome

Patients with right-to-left shunting (Eisenmenger syndrome) develop a degree of erythrocytosis comparable to that observed with similar degrees of desaturation at high altitudes.[85] The hematologic changes associated with this syndrome include hyperviscosity caused by erythrocytosis. Erythrocytosis is present in most patients, but excessive phlebotomy may cause microcytosis and some have attributed this effect to the exacerbation of the symptoms of hyperviscosity.[28] In view of recent understanding of physiology of HIF regulation, it may not be the microcytosis, per se, that is detrimental, but the induced iron deficiency that inhibits PHD2 and increases HIF, which then directly causes pulmonary vasoconstriction and enhanced pulmonary vascular pressure (Chaps. 32 and 34).

Obstructive Sleep Apnea-Induced Syndrome

In the colorfully named pickwickian syndrome,[86] polycythemia is characterized by its association with extreme obesity and somnolence. Today, the more widely studied OSA may not always be associated with obesity[87] but can, if severe, cause arterial hypoxemia, hypercapnia, somnolence, and secondary polycythemia.[88]

Smoker's Polycythemia

Heavy smoking will result in the formation of carboxyhemoglobin, which does not transport oxygen (Chap. 50), and causes an increase in oxygen affinity of the remaining normal hemoglobin. Carboxyhemoglobin increases in relationship to the number of cigarettes or cigars smoked each day (Table 57–2). This leads to tissue hypoxia, erythropoietin production, and stimulation of red cell production.[89] Smoking may also cause a reduction in plasma volume.[90] Either augmentation of red cell mass or shrinkage of plasma volume could easily explain the rise in the hematocrit.

Polycythemia Secondary to High-Affinity Hemoglobins

Hemoglobins with certain amino acid substitutions manifest an increased affinity for oxygen, producing tissue hypoxia and compensatory erythrocytosis (Chap. 49). Mutations affecting amino acids of the $\alpha_1\beta_2$-globin chain interface affect normal rotation within molecules and impair the rate of deoxygenation. Changes in the carboxyl terminal and penultimate amino acids also impair intramolecular motion and tend to keep molecules in a high-affinity state. Alterations in the amino acids lining the central cavity of hemoglobin destabilize the binding of 2,3-BPG in this cavity and lead to increased oxygen affinity (Chaps. 47 and 49). Finally, some heme pocket mutations interfere with deoxygenation. Most hemoglobins with a mutation involving amino acids in the heme pocket are unstable and are associated with hemolytic anemia and cyanosis. Inheritance of these disorders is autosomal dominant. High-affinity hemoglobins result from mutations in any of three globin genes; those from α-globin gene mutations are congenital and life-long. β-Globin gene mutations are not apparent at birth but manifest after fetal to adult hemoglobin switching at approximately 6 months of life, while γ-globin gene mutations cause transient increase of hemoglobin concentration at birth lasting only about 6 months.

Polycythemia Secondary to Red Cell Enzyme Deficiencies

Deficiencies of red cell enzymes in early steps of glycolysis sometimes cause a marked decrease in the levels of 2,3-BPG (Chap. 47). Occasionally, mild polycythemia occurs in patients with methemoglobinemia as a result of cytochrome b_5 reductase (methemoglobin reductase) deficiency (Chap. 50).

The same pathophysiology as that seen in high-affinity hemoglobins is also exhibited in mutations of the *2,3-BPG mutase* gene, resulting in low 2,3-BPG. Because these mutations are very rare, with only a single family comprehensively studied,[91] it is not clear if the mode of inheritance is recessive or dominant.

This condition, as well as other high-affinity hemoglobins, can only be conclusively confirmed by direct measurement of a hemoglobin dissociation curve, conveniently expressed as the partial pressure of oxygen required to saturate 50 percent of hemoglobin (p50O$_2$); when equipment for this is not available, p50 can be estimated from pH, pO$_2$ and hemoglobin oxygen saturation of venous blood.[92,93]

Chemically Induced Tissue Hypoxia

A number of chemicals have been suspected of causing histotoxic anoxia and secondary polycythemia, but the only chemical with a predictable capacity to cause erythrocytosis is cobalt.[83] Cobalt administration increases erythropoietin production by increasing HIFs (see Chap. 32).[94]

INAPPROPRIATE POLYCYTHEMIAS

Congenital Disorders of Hypoxia Sensing

Chuvash Polycythemia Chuvash polycythemia is the only known endemic congenital polycythemia. The condition is caused by an abnormality in the oxygen-sensing pathway and causes thrombotic and hemorrhagic vascular complications that lead to early mortality; survival beyond age 65 years is uncommon.[48,95] Inheritance is autosomal recessive, and affected patients tend to have normal blood gases, normal calculated p50, normal to increased erythropoietin levels, absence

TABLE 57–2. Blood Oxygen Capacity in Smokers with Polycythemia

Subject	Hemoglobin (Hgb) (g/dL)	Carboxyhemoglobin (COHb) (g/dL)	Hgb-COHb (g/dL)	Affinity Correction (g/dL)	Adjusted Hgb (g/dL)
Healthy male nonsmokers	16 (14–18)	0.16 (0.08–0.25)	15.8 (14–18)	0	16 (14–18)
Male smokers with increased Hgb concentration	20 (17–23)	2 (1–3)	1816–21	1.5 (0.5–2.0)	16.5 (15–19)

The male smokers include 10 consecutive subjects studied with elevated hematocrit and no evidence for polycythemia vera. The Hgb available for O$_2$ binding in blood is the Hgb-COHb. COHb also influences the residual hemoglobin to bind oxygen more tightly, making it less accessible to tissues. A correction for this effect has been calculated and is labeled *affinity correction*. The adjusted hemoglobin indicates the blood concentrations that would be present in the subjects in the absence of excess carbon monoxide. Thus, the blood hemoglobin in this group of smokers was increased by 3.5 g/dL on the average (from 16.5 [last column] to 20 [first column]) as a result of smoking-induced carboxyhemoglobinemia.

Data from Marshall A. Lichtman, MD.

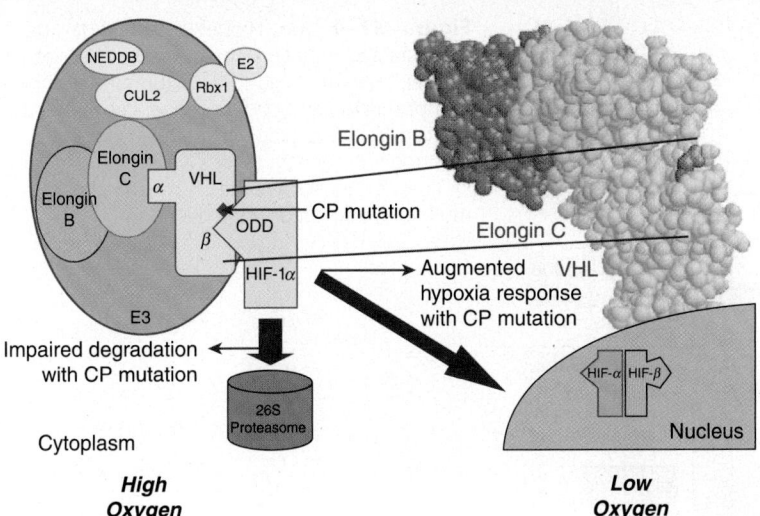

Figure 57–3. Elongins B, C, and proteins Rbx1, Cul2 E2, and NEDD 8 are interacting proteins that facilitate von Hippel-Lindau (VHL) function. Interaction of mutated VHL protein with HIF-1α. The Chuvash VHL mutation leads to the impaired interaction with HIF-1α, which results in impaired degradation in 26S proteasome and augmented hypoxia sensing. CP, Chuvash polycythemia.

of genetic linkage to *erythropoietin* and *EPOR* loci, and no evidence of abnormal hemoglobin.[95] In a study of five multiplex Chuvash families with Chuvash polycythemia, a homozygous mutation of the von Hippel-Lindau (*VHL*) gene (598C>T); that is, *VHL*[R200W], was found in all affected individuals. This mutation impairs the interaction of VHL protein (pVHL) with both HIF-1α and HIF-2α, thus reducing the rate of ubiquitin-mediated destruction of HIF-1α and HIF-2α (Chap. 32). As a result, the level of HIF-1 and HIF-2 heterodimers increases and leads to the increased expression of target genes, including the erythropoietin (*EPO*), vascular endothelial growth factor (*VEGF*), and plasminogen activator inhibitor genes (*PAI-1*), among others.[4,5] Figure 57–3 depicts the effect of this mutation on hypoxic sensing. The role of circulating erythropoietin in the Chuvash polycythemia phenotype is indisputable. However, there must be other factors associated with the Chuvash polycythemia VHL mutation that contribute to the polycythemic phenotype, as the erythroid progenitors of Chuvash polycythemia patients are hypersensitive *in vitro* to extrinsic erythropoietin; the mechanism of this observation is not fully explained.[4,5] Some, but not all, patients with other *VHL* mutations have erythropoietin hypersensitive erythroid colonies[96–98]; in these patients there is also increased expression of the *RUNX1* and *NFE1* genes, which can stimulate erythropoiesis.[6]

Despite increased expression of HIF-1α, HIF-2α, and VEGF in normoxia, Chuvash polycythemia patients do not display a predisposition to tumor formation. Imaging studies of 33 Chuvash polycythemia patients revealed unsuspected cerebral ischemic lesions in 45 percent, but no tumors characteristic of VHL syndrome.[99] There also, is a high prevalence of this disorder on the Italian island of Ischia.[52] The Chuvash *VHL*[R200W] mutation has also been described in whites in the United States and Europe, and in people of Punjabi/Bangladeshi Asian ancestry.[100] Some patients with congenital polycythemia have proved to be compound heterozygotes for the *VHL*[R200W] mutation and other *VHL* mutations. Additionally, two distantly related Croatians with polycythemia are homozygous for *VHL*[H191D], the first example of a homozygous *VHL* germline mutation other than *VHL*[R200W] causing polycythemia.[51,54,101–105]

A small number of cases of congenital polycythemia that appear to have a mutation of only one *VHL* allele confound an obvious pathophysiologic explanation. In a Ukrainian family, two children with polycythemia were heterozygous for *VHL* 376G>T (D126Y), but the father with the same mutation was not polycythemic.[104] An English polycythemic patient was a heterozygote for *VHL* 598C>T[106]; but the inheritance of the deletion of a *VHL* allele, or null *VHL* allele, in a *trans* position was not excluded. Subsequently, two polycythemic *VHL* heterozygous

patients were described in whom a null VHL allele was more rigorously excluded[101,102]; the molecular mechanism of their polycythemic phenotype remains to be elucidated.

To address the question of whether the *VHL* 598C>T substitution occurred in a single founder or resulted from recurrent mutational events, haplotype analysis of eight highly informative single nucleotide polymorphic markers covering 340 kb spanning the *VHL* gene was performed on 101 subjects bearing the *VHL* 598C>T mutation and 447 normal unrelated individuals from Chuvash, Southeast Asian, white, Hispanic, and African American ethnic groups.[49] Polymorphism of the *VHL* locus in normal controls (having a wild *VHL* 598C allele) and subjects bearing Chuvash polycythemia *VHL* 598T were in strong linkage disequilibrium. These studies indicated that, in most individuals, the *VHL* 598C>T mutation arose in a single ancestor between 51,000 and 12,000 years ago. However, this is not the case for a Turkish polycythemic family with a *VHL* 598C>T mutation wherein the *VHL* 598C>T mutation occurred independently.[102]

Chuvash polycythemia homozygotes have decreased survival because of thrombotic and hemorrhagic complications, mostly in the venous circulation,[99] and thus are under negative selection pressure. The high frequency of the mutation in some areas may be the result of random factors ("drift"), but it is also possible that propagation of the *VHL* 598C>T mutation is the result of a survival advantage for heterozygotes. Such an advantage might be related to a subtle improvement of iron metabolism, erythropoiesis, embryonic development, energy metabolism,[106] or some other as yet unknown effect. Indeed, heterozygotes were shown to be less likely to be anemic compared to control subjects.[107] Another potential protective role of a mildly augmented hypoxic response is improved protection against bacterial infections, as the hypoxia-mediated response has been reported to be essential for the bactericidal action of neutrophils.[108]

Classic von Hippel-Lindau Syndrome VHL syndrome is an autosomal dominant genetic abnormality affecting the posttranslational control of HIF-1α.[109–111] The syndrome is characterized by a propensity for developing renal cell carcinomas, retinal hemangioblastomas, cerebellar and spinal hemangioblastomas, pancreatic cysts, and pheochromocytomas. The tumors result from a somatic mutation in addition to the germline mutation, that is, loss-of-heterozygosity. Polycythemia is not part of VHL syndrome but hemangioblastomas of the central nervous system and, less commonly, pheochromocytoma and renal cancer, have been associated with polycythemia mediated by paraneoplastic erythropoietin production.[111] Other patients with VHL syndrome

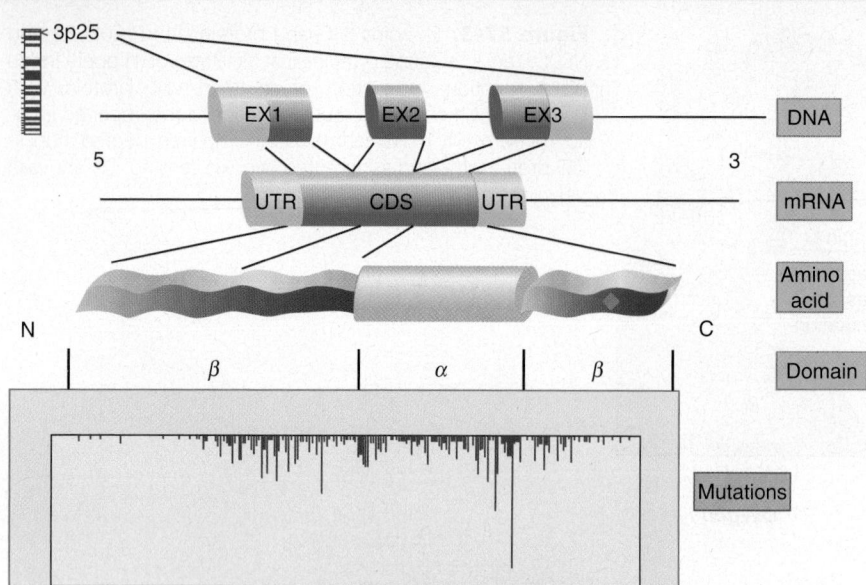

Figure 57–4. von Hippel-Lindau *(VHL)* gene structure and mutation. Three exons of VHL genes are depicted encoding for UTR (untranslated portion of mRNA), and coding sequences (CDs). VHL domains β, α, β are shown. The relative number of reported *VHL* gene mutations are depicted in vertical lines. The location of the Chuvash polycythemia mutation is depicted by the diamond.

also develop acquired polycythemia.[99,111] The *VHL* gene codes for 213 amino acids, and more than 130 germline mutations associated with classic VHL syndrome have been identified, virtually all of them 5′ to the codon 200 position that is mutated in Chuvash polycythemia.[112] Figure 57–4 depicts the schematic effect of the Chuvash polycythemia mutation in the context of other previously found *VHL* mutations.

It is not clear why mutations of a single gene lead to these two diverse phenotypes. It has been suggested that quantitative differences in loss of activity could explain the variable phenotypes among *VHL* mutations,[113] but the *VHL* gene may also have other functions, possibly as a result of interactions with other modifying factors, that can contribute to the onset of disease and that await future clarification. Another plausible explanation of polycythemia versus cancer predisposition syndrome is that almost all polycythemic subjects have germline mutations of both *VHL* alleles, whereas those with VHL cancer predisposition syndrome have only a single germline mutation and then acquire a somatic mutation that is essential for tumor genesis.

***EGLN1* Gene Mutations, Proline Hydroxylase Deficiency** Another principal negative regulator of HIFs is PHD2 (encoded by the *EGLN1* gene), which targets the α subunit of HIF for degradation. The first loss-of-function mutation of PHD2 (PHD2[P317R]) was identified in a family in which heterozygotes had mild or borderline polycythemia.[114] Since then, 25 additional patients with unexplained polycythemia who are heterozygote carriers of different PHD2 mutations have been reported.[115] Almost all patients with PHD2-associated polycythemia have normal erythropoietin levels. Whether the cause of polycythemia in this case is haploinsufficiency or a dominant negative effect remains to be determined.

***EPAS1* (HIF-2α) Gain-of-Function Mutations** Affected patients have heterozygous missense mutations in the coding sequence of the *EPAS1* gene that encodes HIF-2α, and typically have elevated erythropoietin levels.[115,116] There is heterogeneity in these gain-of-function *HIF-2α* mutations, but their existence supports the critical role of HIF-2α in controlling the expression of erythropoietin. Some patients with *EPAS1* mutations, similar to Chuvash polycythemia, have erythropoietin hypersensitive colonies, thus sharing features of both primary and secondary polycythemias.[97]

An explanation for the hypersensitivity of erythroid colonies bearing mutations that augment HIF stabilization remains to be discovered.

It has been proposed that mutated VHL[R200W] protein hinders suppression of cytokine signaling SOCS1-mediated JAK2 degradation, via binding of a negative regulator of erythropoiesis, SOCS1,[117] to the extreme 3′ coding region of the *VHL* gene. Other observations are not consistent with this proposed mechanism: Another closely positioned VHL polycythemia mutation, *VHL*[H191D], is not associated with erythropoietin hypersensitivity,[96] while other, more upstream, mutations such as *VHL*[P138L] are.[80] Furthermore, the hypersensitivity of erythroid colonies is also seen in some *HIF-2α* mutations.[86] Interestingly, in some, but not all, of these families, upregulation of *NFE2*, which enhances erythropoiesis, has been found.[6,118]

Unexplained Congenital Polycythemias with Elevated or Inappropriately Normal Levels of Erythropoietin The majority of patients with congenital polycythemias with inappropriately normal or elevated erythropoietin levels do not have *VHL* mutations, *EGLN1* or *EPAS1* mutations, hemoglobinopathies, or 2,3-BPG deficiency, and the molecular basis of polycythemia in these cases remains to be elucidated. Some such families show dominant inheritance,[119] while in others inheritance is recessive, and in some it is sporadic. Lesions in genes linked to hypoxia independent regulation of HIF, as well as oxygen-dependent gene regulation pathways, are leading candidates for mutation screening in polycythemic patients with normal or elevated erythropoietin without *VHL*, *EGLN1* (proline hydroxylase), or *EPAS1* (HIF-2α) mutations.

Other Inappropriate Secondary Erythrocytoses

Renal Polycythemia and Post–Renal Transplant Erythrocytosis Absolute erythrocytosis has been observed in a considerable number of patients with solitary renal cysts, polycystic renal disease, or hydronephrosis. In most of these cases, erythropoietin assays on cyst fluid, serum, or urine have disclosed the presence of erythropoietin.[120] Patients with polycystic disease have a hematocrit value slightly higher than normal and definitely higher than would have been expected of patients with uremia. In some patients on prolonged dialysis treatment, cystic transformation occurs in the native kidneys. This acquired cystic disease is occasionally associated with marked erythrocytosis.[121] In patients with pheochromocytoma or paraganglioma and erythrocytosis, erythropoietin assays of serum and urine have disclosed higher-than-normal levels, and the erythrocytosis is most likely caused by excessive erythropoietin secretion by the tumor. This assumption has been supported by the presence of erythropoietin mRNA in tumor cells.[122] Wilms tumors[123] and paraganglioma[124] are also occasionally associated with an erythrocytosis. Many of these cases may have a somatic VHL gene mutation that, in combination with a germline mutation of another allele, may constitute an unrecognized VHL syndrome. A patient with congenital erythrocytosis and recurrent paraganglioma with a PHD2 mutation was described. Tumor tissue exhibited a loss of heterozygosity of PHD2 in the tumor, suggesting that PHD2 could be a tumor-suppressor gene.[34]

Partial obstruction of the renal artery would be expected to cause renal tissue hypoxia and a physiologic stimulation of erythropoietin production. Nevertheless, it has proved quite difficult to induce erythrocytosis in laboratory animals by placing a Goldblatt clamp on the renal arteries.[125] Only a few of the many patients who have arteriosclerotic narrowing of the renal arteries have been reported to be polycythemic.[126]

Post–Renal Transplantation Erythrocytosis Although the full molecular basis of post–renal transplant erythrocytosis remains unknown, angiotensin II (Chaps. 32 and 34) plays an important role in its pathogenesis.[127] Increased activity of the angiotensin II–angiotensin receptor 1 pathway makes the erythroid progenitors hypersensitive to angiotensin II.[128,129] Furthermore, angiotensin II can modulate release of erythropoiesis stimulatory factors (Chap. 32) including erythropoietin and insulin-like growth factor (IGF)-1.[130,131] Studies of venous effluents have determined that the native rather than the transplanted kidneys are the source of the inappropriate production of erythropoietin,[132] and in some patients, removal of the native kidneys has led to rapid restoration of normal hematocrit values.[133] The condition is rarely seen in patients with nonrenal solid-organ allografts. The role of angiotensin II in augmenting erythropoiesis was confirmed by anemia in angiotensin-converting enzyme–knockout mice.[134] Prior to the late 1990s when the use of angiotensin-converting enzyme inhibitors increased as a means to reduce proteinuria, the incidence of erythrocytosis in renal transplant patients was approximately 8 to 10 percent within the first 2 years after engraftment.

Polycythemia with Connective Tissue Tumors Occasionally, there is an association of erythrocytosis with large uterine myomas.[35] Usually, the tumor has been huge and extirpation has routinely been followed by a hematologic "cure." The suggestion that the tumor interferes with pulmonary ventilation has not been supported by the normal arterial blood gas findings in the few patients so studied. Another possible mechanism is that the large abdominal mass causes mechanical interference with the blood supply to the kidneys, resulting in renal hypoxia and erythropoietin production. Inappropriate erythropoietin secretion by smooth muscle cells has been demonstrated both in uterine myomas and in one case of cutaneous leiomyoma.[35,135] Rare cases of polycythemia attributed to a myxoma of the atrium,[36] hamartoma of the liver,[37] and focal hyperplasia of the liver[38] have been documented.

Brain Tumors In adequately studied patients with erythrocytosis and cerebellar hemangiomas, arterial blood gas tensions have been normal. That the tumors are directly responsible for the polycythemia can be surmised from the identification of erythropoietin in cyst fluid and stromal cells and from a case in which erythropoietin mRNA was present in the tumor.[136] Although in these cases a mutation of the VHL gene was not sought, it is likely that these tumors were a manifestation of an underlying VHL syndrome as cerebellar hemangiomas are an integral feature of VHL syndrome.

Hepatoma In 1958, McFadzean and coworkers reported that almost 10 percent of patients in Hong Kong with hepatocellular carcinoma developed erythrocytosis.[137] Since then, this association has been recognized as an important clinical clue in the diagnostic consideration of patients with liver disease.[138] The cause of erythrocytosis is probably inappropriate production of erythropoietin by the neoplastic cells.[139]

Normal hepatocytes, and to a lesser degree nonparenchymal liver cells, produce small amounts of erythropoietin, both constitutively and in response to hypoxia.

Congenital Polycythemia and Pheochromocytoma Pheochromocytomas have been described in association with congenital erythrocytosis.[140] In a growing number of reports, several individuals with congenital polycythemia have developed recurrent pheochromocytomas, paragangliomas, and sometimes somatistatinomas.[141–143] The tumors in these patients are heterozygous for gain-of-function mutations of the EPAS1 gene (encoding HIF-2α), and an erythropoietin transcript is present in tumor tissues (Chaps. 32 and 57). Even though these tumors may be recurrent, they bear the same heterozygous mutations of the EPAS1 gene. However, these mutations are generally not found in nontumor tissues, so the etiology of the association of these tumors with polycythemia is not certain; it is also possible that they may be associated with postgonadal genetic mosaicism, wherein the EPAS1 mutation predisposes to tumor development.[141–143] However, in one family the EPAS1 mutation was inherited and also associated with the development of recurrent pheochromocytomas/paragangliomas.[116]

Endocrine Disorders Chapter 38 has additional discussion.

Aldosterone-producing adenomas,[144] Bartter syndrome,[145] and dermoid cyst of the ovary[146] have been described in association with erythrocytosis. Erythropoietin levels were found to be elevated in the serum and returned to normal after extirpation of the tumors. A number of pathogenetic mechanisms have been suggested (Chaps. 32 and 38), including decreased plasma volume; mechanical interference with renal blood supply; hypertensive damage to renal parenchyma; functional interaction between aldosterone, renin, and erythropoietin; and inappropriate secretion of erythropoietin by the tumors. Mild polycythemia may be present in patients with Cushing syndrome, but its pathophysiologic basis is not entirely clear (Chap. 38).

The erythropoietic effect of androgens is of considerable practical importance.[147] For many years, it was assumed that the higher red cell count in males was caused by androgens because the hemoglobin levels of boys and girls were identical up until the time of puberty. It was not until pharmacologic doses of testosterone were administered to women with carcinoma of the breast that the full erythropoietic potency of androgens was appreciated.[148] Since then, various androgen preparations have been used in the treatment of refractory anemia, occasionally causing dramatic erythropoiesis, with hemoglobin values climbing into the polycythemic range (Fig. 57–5).

The mechanism of androgen action on erythropoiesis appears to be complex, related both to their capacity to stimulate erythropoietin production[149] and their capacity to induce differentiation of marrow stem cells directly.[147] These two effects have specific structural requirements. Androgens with the 5α-H configuration stimulate renal and extrarenal erythropoietin production, whereas androgens with the 5β-H configuration enhance the differentiation of stem cells.[149] Testosterone administration is associated with an increase in erythropoietin levels and a decrease in hepcidin levels.[150] Although erythropoietin levels declined with continued testosterone administration, they remained inappropriately high despite improved hemoglobin levels, suggesting a new set point.[150]

Neonatal Polycythemia Polycythemia at birth is a normal physiologic response to intrauterine hypoxia and to the high oxygen affinity of red cells containing very high proportions of hemoglobin F (Chap. 7). It may become excessive and even symptomatic, especially in infants of diabetic mothers, or if the clamping of the cord is delayed, permitting placental blood to boost the blood volume of the infant.[151] Because it is difficult to recognize symptoms of hyperviscosity in the neonate, many pediatricians perform a partial plasma exchange transfusion if the venous hematocrit is above 65 percent at birth.[152]

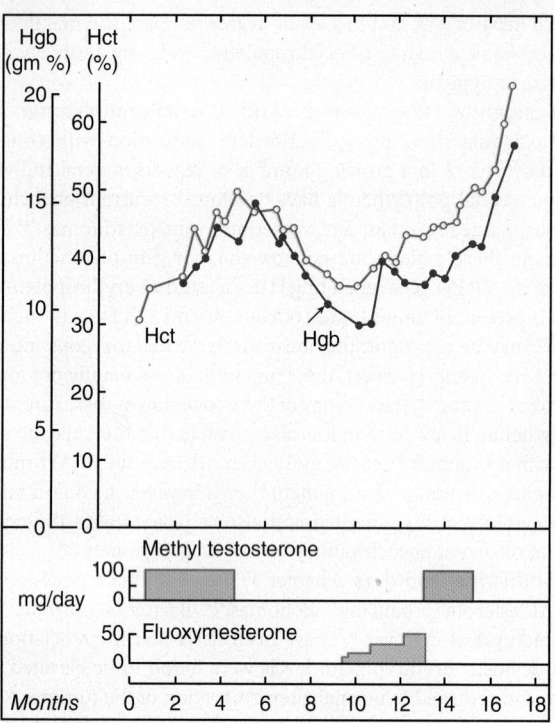

Figure 57–5. Erythropoietic response to testosterone derivatives in a patient with myelofibrosis. Hgb, hemoglobin; Hct, hematocrit.

One study of 25,000 neonates in Utah[153] showed that the average hematocrit at birth would be considered "polycythemic" in adults, while 2 weeks later it has fallen to "anemic" levels. This dramatic decrease of red blood cells in neonates during their first days of life likely contributes to neonatal jaundice (Chap. 33).[154]

APPARENT (RELATIVE) POLYCYTHEMIA

(Refer to section "Secondary Polycythemias/Erythrocytoses" above.)

Some believe that apparent polycythemia is merely a mild absolute polycythemia accentuated by a compensatory reduction in plasma volume. Others suggest that it is caused by a primary reduction in plasma volume and have associated it with hypertension, obesity, and stress. When the red cell mass is documented to be normal, spurious polycythemia is also an appropriate term. Its clinical significance has also been disputed. The high hematocrit with its associated high viscosity is believed by some to be a risk factor heralding cerebral and cardiac complications, while others believe it is merely a well-tolerated anomaly. Because the designation *apparent polycythemia*[155] is noncommittal, it is used here.

The main clinical associations with apparent polycythemia are obesity, hypertension, and smoking. In obese patients, the finding of a normal red cell volume may be spurious because if the volume is expressed in terms of lean body weight, some of these patients would have a significant increase in red cell mass. In hypertensive patients, there is no adequate explanation for the apparent increase in red cell production or decrease in plasma volume. Sleep apnea (common in patients with congestive failure), excessive production of atrial natriuretic factor, increased adrenal activation, decreased aldosterone secretion, and hypoxic vasoconstriction are all factors that have been invoked,[156-158] but with uncertainty. Chronic administration of diuretics to treat hypertension may be a more likely cause.[158]

CLINICAL FEATURES

PRIMARY POLYCYTHEMIA

Primary Familial and Congenital Polycythemia

Although PFCP is uncommon, it is frequently misdiagnosed.[18] Unlike patients with polycythemia vera, patients with PFCP lack splenomegaly, neutrophilia, basophilia, thrombocytosis, and a *JAK2* mutation. Unless exposed to alkylating agents or radioactive phosphorus, as many have been, these patients do not progress to acute leukemia or myelodysplastic syndrome.[159] Generally thought to be benign, this condition predisposes patients to severe cardiovascular problems because of chronic augmented erythropoietin signaling in all tissues bearing *EPOR*.[160] An increased incidence of cardiovascular disease has been observed in affected members of PFCP families.[161] Erythrocytosis may be very severe, with hemoglobin levels that typically exceed 20 g/dL in men and 18 g/dL in women. Headaches are commonly present. Hypertension, coronary artery disease, and strokes have been reported, but do not clearly appear to be related to an elevated hematocrit as they also occur in aggressively phlebotomized patients with normal hematocrits,[162] and are not a constant feature of the disorder.[163]

Chuvash Polycythemia

The recessive polycythemia that is endemic in the Chuvash Autonomous Republic of the Russian Federation is characterized by elevation of the hemoglobin level to a mean of 22.6 with a standard deviation of 1.4 g/L.[95] Some patients are symptomatic, with headache, fatigue, and signs that include clubbing, hemorrhaging, and peptic ulcer. Chuvash polycythemia is also associated with thrombosis, relatively low blood pressure (also seen in heterozygotes), and varicose veins.[4,95,99] As of yet, no significant association of thrombosis with elevated hematocrit and history of phlebotomies has been found.[99] A matched cohort study of 96 patients diagnosed in 1977 (65 spouses and 79 unaffected community members of the same age, sex, and village of birth) found that homozygosity for VHL 598C>T was associated with polycythemia, varicose veins, lower blood pressures, elevated serum VEGF and PAI-1 levels, and premature mortality related to cerebral vascular events and both venous and arterial thromboses.[99]

Because Chuvash polycythemia is characterized by a germline mutation in the *VHL* gene, it was expected that homozygotes for this mutation may develop certain vascular tumors similar to those associated with classic VHL syndrome. However, tumors typical of classic VHL syndrome, such as spinocerebellar hemangioblastomas, renal carcinomas and pheochromocytomas/paragangliomas, were not found, indicating that increased expression of HIF-1α and VEGF is not sufficient for tumorigenesis. Benign vertebral body hemangiomas (a distinct entity from hemangioblastoma) were found in significantly more patients with Chuvash polycythemia compared to controls (55 percent vs. 21 percent). Imaging studies of 33 Chuvash polycythemia patients revealed unsuspected cerebral ischemic lesions in 45 percent of patients.[99] Affected patients have elevated systolic pulmonary artery pressures as estimated by echocardiography compared to controls, and iron deficiency associated with phlebotomy therapy may exacerbate this finding.[164-167]

Other Congenital Disorders of Hypoxia Sensing

Because of their only recent discovery and apparent rarity, reliable clinical information is lacking. However, these disorders, in view of their global deregulation of hypoxia sensing, are expected to also have extra-erythroid manifestation(s). This author is aware of a yet unpublished large family with a gain-of-function *EPAS1* gene mutation wherein affected members appear to have early onset of strokes and cardiovascular disease, which are not prevented by control of their erythrocytosis by phlebotomies.

SECONDARY ACQUIRED POLYCYTHEMIA

High-Altitude Erythrocytosis

Tolerance to high altitudes varies greatly, but most normal individuals have no discomfort at altitudes of up to 2130 m (7000 ft). Above this level, and especially if the ascent is rapid, some manifestations of cerebral hypoxia are common. Headaches, sleeplessness, and palpitations are frequently encountered, and weakness, nausea, vomiting, and mental dullness may be present. More-severe manifestations include pulmonary and cerebral edema that may lead to death. Cheyne-Stokes respiration commonly occurs, especially during sleep. These symptoms constitute the syndrome of *acute mountain sickness*.[168]

Ruddy cyanosis and physiologic emphysema are the two characteristic features of some humans living at high altitudes. Venous and capillary engorgement can be observed readily in the conjunctiva, mucous membranes, and skin, and may contribute to the remarkable capacity of Tibetan Sherpas to walk barefoot and sleep on ice and snow.[169] Asymptomatic retinal hemorrhages are seen frequently at high altitudes, but rarely at altitudes of 3000 m (9000 ft) or less.[170] Splenomegaly and jaundice are unusual, although the sustained erythrocytosis is associated with an increased fractional rate of red cell destruction and bilirubin generation. It has been stated that Monge disease includes low fertility,[42,66] but this may not be universally so. It has been suggested that high-altitude native-resident Tibetans exhibit two distinct genotypes for increased oxygen affinity of hemoglobin, and that women with genotypes for high oxygen saturation have more surviving children[171] suggesting natural selection on the locus for oxygen saturation of hemoglobin.[72,171] However, these conclusions have been based not on measurement of the hemoglobin-oxygen dissociation curve, but on assumptions based on arterial oxygen saturation. In point of fact, when properly measured, Tibetans have normal oxygen affinity of hemoglobin when the hemoglobin-oxygen dissociation curve is rigorously determined.[63]

Erythrocytosis Associated with Pulmonary Disease

The erythrocytosis associated with smoking is generally asymptomatic. There may be an increase in thrombotic events, but this may be from smoking rather than erythrocytosis.

When erythrocytosis is present in patients with COPD, with or without smoking, elevated hematocrit is associated with higher survival rates than anemic and normocythemic subjects.[19,20,175] Furthermore, moderate erythrocytosis has no adverse effect on vascular function in COPD[176] and is not associated with venous thromboembolism.[177]

Large studies of patients with Eisenmenger syndrome[28] and other patients with cyanotic heart disease[178] caution against routine phlebotomy for asymptomatic elevation of the hematocrit; in fact, thrombotic complications were not observed in these studies. Transgenic mice with extreme polycythemia (hematocrit 85 percent) from constitutive overexpression of erythropoietin did not develop the expected thrombotic complications.[179] Adults with cyanotic congenital heart disease are at risk of having cerebrovascular events. This risk is increased in the presence of hypertension, atrial fibrillation, history of phlebotomy, and microcytosis, the latter condition having the strongest significance (p <0.005). The authors of these findings endorsed a more conservative approach toward phlebotomy and more aggressive approach toward treating microcytosis with iron preparations in adults with cyanotic congenital heart disease.[180]

In a prospective cohort of U.S. Veterans Health Administration outpatients with stable COPD (n = 683), polycythemia prevalence was low and, unlike anemia, had no association with worsened outcomes.[175]

Renal Polycythemia and Post–Renal Transplant Erythrocytosis

Although most patients with kidney failure are anemic, a fraction (often with polycystic kidney disease) display erythrocytosis, which, like the post–renal transplant state, can be very severe. Erythrocyte counts may be as high as 8×10^{12} cells/L and associated with hypertension and congestive failure.[181] At higher hematocrit levels (usually >60 percent), thrombotic events may complicate the clinical course.[46,47,182] Comorbidities that are associated with or causative of renal failure are frequently also factors predisposing to thrombosis, and the risk of erythrocytosis-associated thrombosis has not been submitted to rigorous multivariate rigorous statistical analyses. Thus, reports of increased thrombotic risks must be viewed with great caution.

Tumors

The erythrocytosis that occurs with erythropoietin-secreting tumors is generally mild,[136] and the predominating clinical manifestations are those of the tumor itself. Even moderate elevations to a hematocrit of 64 percent have been encountered without symptoms referable to the polycythemia.[38] Resection of the erythropoietin-secreting tumor cures the associated polycythemia.[105]

In the syndrome of congenital polycythemia and pheochromocytoma or paraganglioma (see description in "Etiology" earlier) tumor resection does not lead to normalization of elevated hematocrit.

Neonatal Polycythemia

Of 55 infants with neonatal polycythemia, 47 (85 percent) had signs and symptoms attributed to this disorder. These included "feeding problems" (21.8 percent), plethora (20 percent), lethargy (14.5 percent), cyanosis (14.5 percent), respiratory distress (9.1 percent), jitteriness (7.3 percent), and hypotonia (7.3 percent). Other findings included hypoglycemia (40 percent) and hyperbilirubinemia (21.8 percent). In a larger group of nearly 1000 infants, six had intracranial hemorrhage.[151]

● LABORATORY FEATURES

PRIMARY POLYCYTHEMIA

Primary Familial and Congenital Polycythemia

Characteristic laboratory findings of PFCP are: (1) increased red blood cell mass without increased leukocyte or platelet counts; (2) normal hemoglobin–oxygen dissociation curve; (3) invariably low serum erythropoietin levels; and (4) *in vitro* hypersensitivity of erythroid progenitors to erythropoietin.[5] PFCP is often misdiagnosed as polycythemia vera, although with the advent of a reliable polymerase chain reaction-based test for the *JAK2*[V617F] mutation, this should no longer ever happen. Whereas leukocytes are typically normal, platelet counts are often mildly decreased, presumably by dilution of the normal platelet mass by an often-dramatic increase of red cell and whole-blood volumes. Some patients come to attention because of concurrent medical problems that may cause leukocytosis and secondary thrombocytosis, falsely suggesting the phenotype of polycythemia vera.

Chuvash Polycythemia

Blood profiling in patients with Chuvash polycythemia indicates increased hemoglobin and hematocrit and lower white blood cell and platelet counts than in controls. Erythropoietin ranges from normal (but never close to the lower limits of normal) to elevated, at times exceeding 10 times the mean normal value. In larger studies, hemoglobin-adjusted serum erythropoietin concentrations were approximately 10-fold higher in *VHL* 598C>T homozygotes than in controls.[4,5,99]

Affected subjects have lower CD4 counts, elevated levels of both proinflammatory and antiinflammatory cytokines, and altered plasma thiol levels, with elevated homocysteine and glutathione and low cysteine concentrations.[164,183,184] Their serum PAI-1 and VEGF levels are also increased.[4,95,99] Circulating transferrin receptor levels are higher in Chuvash polycythemia homozygotes as compared to their unaffected relatives and spouses.[4,5,99] Ferritin-adjusted transferrin receptor concentrations were approximately threefold higher in *VHL*

598C>T homozygotes than in unaffected participants (p <0.0005), which is consistent with upregulation by HIF-1.

Chuvash polycythemia is a relatively recently described disorder; thus, additional laboratory findings as a result of augmentation of hypoxia sensing are expected to be described.

Other Congenital Polycythemias from Augmented Hypoxia Sensing

At present, a paucity of data precludes any reliable description of other congenital polycythemias from augmented hypoxia sensing. Some affected subjects have unexpectedly low-normal erythropoietin levels.

SECONDARY ERYTHROCYTOSIS

Characteristically, only the number of erythrocytes in the blood is increased in secondary erythrocytosis. An increase in the leukocyte count and/or splenomegaly may be present as features of the underlying disease, for example, pulmonary infection in COPD with *cor pulmonale*, or as seen in Monge disease among Andean high-altitude dwellers or patients inheriting a high-affinity hemoglobin that is also unstable (Chaps. 34 and 49).

In patients with appropriate erythrocytosis, the underlying defect is usually demonstrable. Arterial hypoxia can be demonstrated in most cases. Some obese patients who, like Mr. Wardle's proverbial boy, Joe, in *The Pickwick Papers* by Charles Dickens, are always half asleep, will be very much awake when exposed to arterial puncture and ventilatory testing, and their apprehensive hyperventilation will result in the disappearance of all abnormalities in arterial oxygen tension. As soon as they return to bed, however, they will go to sleep again and display the characteristic somnolent cyanosis.

In inappropriate erythrocytosis, the laboratory findings will be those of the underlying defect.

● DIFFERENTIAL DIAGNOSIS

Also refer to Chaps. 34 and 59, Table 57–3, and Fig. 57–6.

Distinguishing between polycythemia vera and other polycythemic disorders used to be challenging, but discovery of the *JAK2*[V617F] and *JAK2* exon 12 mutations has made it, in most instances, straightforward. Some of the clinical and laboratory features that can be helpful for differential diagnosis are summarized in Chap. 34, Table 34–2, and in Fig. 57–6.

RED CELL MASS DETERMINATION

Determination of red cell mass is invaluable for differentiation of apparent (spurious) polycythemia from true polycythemic states. Unfortunately, determination of the red cell mass is expensive and, when performed by the inexperienced, often inaccurate.[185] It is not useful in distinguishing polycythemia vera from secondary erythrocytoses, the differentiation that is usually needed, because it is increased in both disorders. Ideally, the red cell mass and plasma volume should be measured separately. Unfortunately, the ^{131}I-labeled albumin necessary to measure the plasma volume is often unavailable. Fortunately, in most cases, the diagnosis of polycythemia vera and other true polycythemic states can be established with confidence without measuring the red cell mass.

ERYTHROID COLONY CULTURES

In vitro assays of erythroid progenitor cells permit the study of their responsiveness to erythropoietin. This can be applied to polycythemia

TABLE 57–3. VHL Mutations Associated with Congenital Polycythemia

VHL Genotype	Ethnicities	References	Clinical Features
235 C>T/586 C>G	White	101	
598 C>T/598 C>T	Chuvash, Danish, U.S. (white), Bangladeshi,, Pakistani, Russian, Turkish	101, 102, 104, 105, 231	Frequent thrombotic complications
598 C>T/574 C>T	U.S. (white)	104	
598 C>T/562 C>G	U.S. (white)	104	
598 C>T/388 G>C	U.S. (white)	105	
571 C>G/571 C>G	Croatian	104	Failure to thrive
311 G>T/wild-type	German (?)	102	
376 G>T/wild-type	Ukrainian	105	?VHL syndrome
598 C>T/wild-type	English, German	102	
523 A>G/wild-type	Portuguese	101	A-T patient
370 A>G/562 C>G	Native American	PMID: 23772956	
376 G>A/376 G>A	Bangladeshi	PMID: 24729484	Fatal pulmonary hypertension
413 C>T/413 C>T	Punjabi	PMID: 23538339	

A-T, ataxia-telangiectasia; VHL, von Hippel-Lindau.

vera and erythroid progenitor burst-forming unit–erythroid (BFU-E) growth without added erythropoietin,[186] referred to as "endogenous erythroid colonies." Detection of endogenous erythroid colonies in cultures of marrow or blood used to be the most specific test for polycythemia vera.[50,187,188] In one study, all patients with polycythemia vera, but none with secondary or other causes of polycythemia, had endogenous erythroid colonies.[189] Rare endogenous erythroid colonies may at times be observed in PFCP, Chuvash polycythemia, and in a single studied subject with the HIF-2α mutation,[190] but unlike the endogenous erythroid colonies of polycythemia vera, these are abrogated by pretreatment with erythropoietin and EPOR-blocking antibodies.[191,192]

In experienced hands, endogenous erythroid colonies is a specific and sensitive means for detecting polycythemia vera and may be useful in diagnosing patients with unusual presentations of polycythemia vera, such as Budd-Chiari syndrome[193–196] or isolated thrombocytosis.[197] However, this test has not been standardized, is expensive and laborious, and technical variations make interlaboratory results difficult to compare.

ERYTHROPOIETIN LEVELS

All patients with PFCP encountered[54] have erythropoietin below normal levels or below levels of detection. Thus, a low erythropoietin level is not pathognomonic of polycythemia vera, as patients with PFCP have as low or even lower erythropoietin levels.[18]

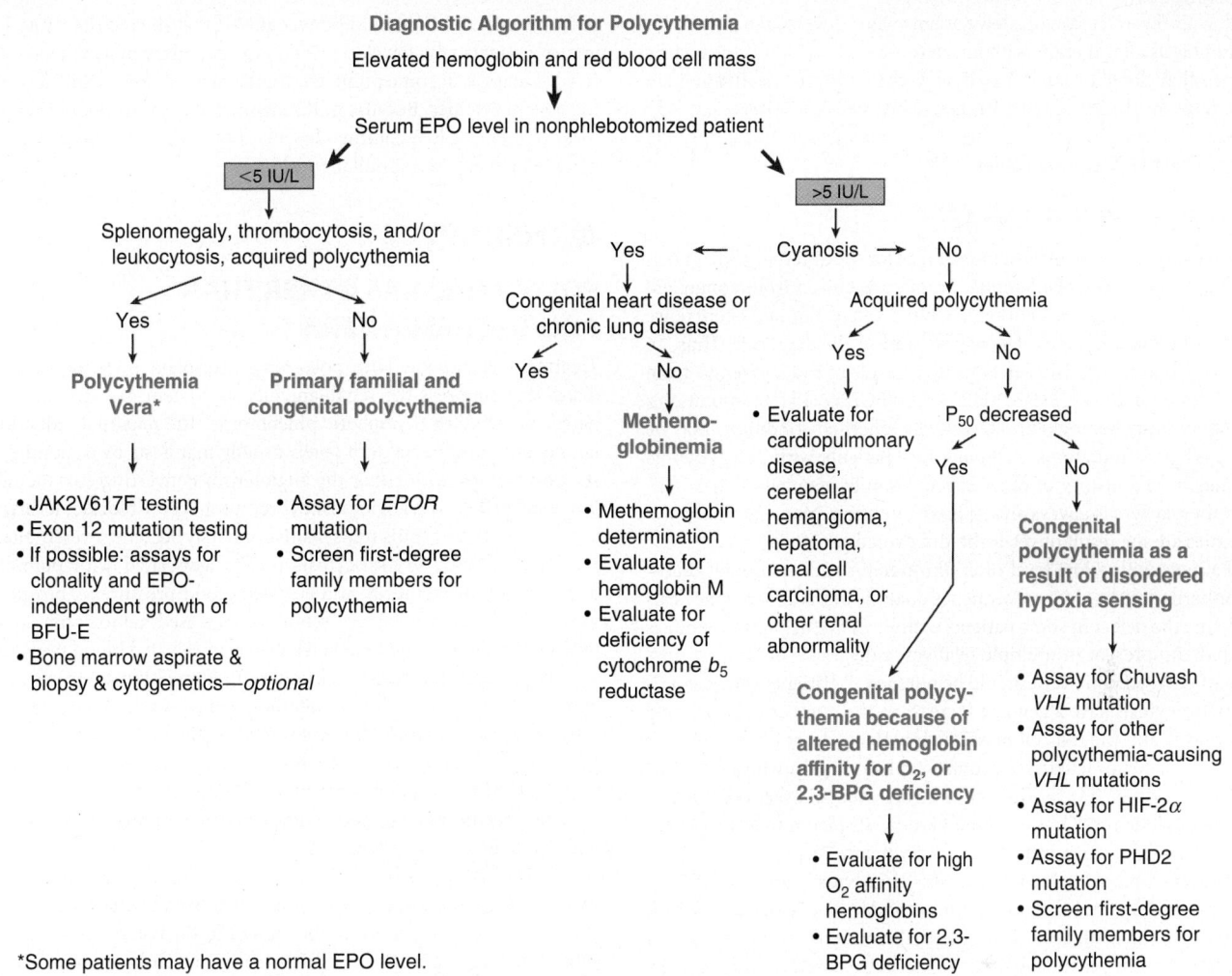

Figure 57–6. Diagnostic algorithm for polycythemia based on erythropoietin (EPO) level. 2,3-BPG, 2,3-bisphosphoglycerate; BFU-E, burst-forming unit–erythroid; *EPOR*, erythropoietin receptor gene; HIF, hypoxia-inducible factor; PHD2, proline hydroxylase 2; *VHL*, von Hippel-Landau gene.

Because polycythemia vera is distinguished by the fact that erythroid cells proliferate even in the absence of substantial levels of erythropoietin, one would expect that at high hematocrit levels the production of erythropoietin would be inhibited and serum levels consequently reduced. Older erythropoietin assays were too insensitive to detect subnormal levels of erythropoietin, but using improved technology, several studies have documented serum erythropoietin levels below the normal reference range in patients with polycythemia vera.[198–200] Erythropoietin levels remain low even after phlebotomy,[198] which increases erythropoietin levels in normal individuals. Erythropoietin levels in Budd-Chiari syndrome may be normal or even increased.[201]

Patients with secondary erythrocytosis usually have normal to elevated erythropoietin levels, although considerable overlap exists in the range of erythropoietin levels between some patients with polycythemia vera and those with secondary erythrocytosis.[199,202]

CLONALITY IN FEMALE SUBJECTS USING ASSAYS EMPLOYING X-CHROMOSOME–BASED POLYMORPHISM ASSAYS

The principal role of the clonality assay is to differentiate polycythemia vera with an incomplete phenotype or atypical presentation from idiopathic, or as-yet undiagnosed erythrocytosis. Polycythemia vera results from an acquired mutation in a pluripotential hematopoietic stem/progenitor cell. Clonality studies based on the phenomenon of X-chromosome inactivation[203] show that red cells, granulocytes, platelets, monocytes, and B lymphocytes are all part of the clone.[204,205] The majority of T lymphocytes and natural killer (NK) cells are polyclonal, but a small proportion of these cells are also derived from the polycythemia vera clone[206]; this is presumed to be a result of the presence of long-lived normal T cells that preceded the development of the clone. Unfortunately, interpretation of publications on the applicability of X-chromosome inactivation for differential diagnosis of polycythemia vera is hampered by the many methodologic and conceptual differences that have drawn conflicting conclusions.[207] Some discrepancies are caused by the fact that two different approaches, which are not comparable, are used to distinguish the active from the inactive X-chromosome; one approach uses X-chromosome differential methylation,[208] typically using the polymorphic CAG repeat in the human androgen-receptor gene *(HUMARA)*,[209] while the other approach uses more biologically sound but more technically demanding transcriptional analysis of the active X-chromosome.[208,210] Furthermore, the wide range of skewing of the X-chromosome allelic usage that is normally present[211] is often misinterpreted as clonality, and the potentially clonal myeloid cells are not compared to the polyclonal control cells of the same origin.[50] In our study of 56 PV female polycythemia vera patients, reticulocytes, platelets, and granulocytes were always clonal, with the exception of a few patients who converted to polyclonal hematopoiesis after therapy with interferon-α.[50] While it was previously reported that clonality assays based on X-chromosome inactivation are not suitable for studies of older women using the HUMARA assay,[212–214] that was not confirmed by studies using quantitative transcriptional analysis of active X-chromosomes.[215,216]

OTHER POLYCYTHEMIAS

Clinical history is of the utmost importance for the differential diagnosis of polycythemic states. Differentiation of an acquired from congenital disorder, and distinction between sporadic versus familial occurrence of polycythemia, when possible, will streamline the diagnosis. Thus, an autosomal dominant disorder is likely a result of polycythemia from gain-of-function EPOR, EPAS1 (HIF-2α) or EGLN1 (PHD2) mutations, or a high-affinity hemoglobin. Recessively inherited conditions may be from VHL gene mutations. Although rare patients with polycythemia vera may have a history of other affected family members (Chap. 84), polycythemia vera is always an acquired condition. Many familial polycythemias are the result of yet-to-be-discovered genetic events.

Patients with a low level of erythropoietin and autosomal dominant inheritance should have sequence analysis of the EPOR gene. This will define the defect in some patients with PFCP; if the polycythemia is acquired and present in multiple relatives, a diagnosis of familial clustering of polycythemia vera should be pursued.[217] Patients with secondary erythrocytosis have a genuine increase in the number of circulating erythrocytes and the red cell mass. Such patients do not typically have increased platelet or leukocyte counts or splenomegaly, which are often seen in polycythemia vera. The lack of involvement of other cell lineages in hematopoietic proliferation should arouse suspicion that the patient may have erythrocytosis other than polycythemia vera.

However, reactive thrombocytosis, leukocytosis, and splenomegaly may occasionally also be present in secondary erythrocytosis, which then renders the distinction from polycythemia vera more difficult. In patients in whom secondary erythrocytosis is caused by lung or cardiac disease, clubbing is often present. In some cases, determining the arterial oxygen saturation will clarify the diagnosis, but modest arterial oxygen desaturation may also be present in polycythemia vera.[85,218] Imaging of the kidneys may reveal a neoplasm or cyst in some patients. Determining the hemoglobin oxygen dissociation curve (Chaps. 32, 34, 50), or estimation of p50 from venous blood[92] will detect abnormalities related to increased oxygen affinity either because of inheritance of a high-affinity hemoglobin (Chap. 49), or because of very rare 2,3-BPG depletion, as in phosphoglyceromutase deficiency (Chap. 47). The mild erythrocytosis associated with hereditary methemoglobinemia (Chap. 50) is readily diagnosed because of coexistent cyanosis.

In patients with elevated erythropoietin, or with erythropoietin levels inappropriately normal for the degree of hemoglobin elevation, analysis of VHL, EGLN1, and EPAS1 genes may be in order; some of these patients may have a history of autosomal recessive inheritance and have a typical history of congenital polycythemia. It may also be useful to determine the carboxyhemoglobin level of the blood if smoker's polycythemia is suspected.

SPURIOUS POLYCYTHEMIA

The erythrocytosis observed in patients with spurious polycythemia (apparent polycythemia, stress polycythemia) is the consequence of a decrease in plasma volume.[155] The observed erythrocytosis does not represent a true increase in the red cell mass. Usually, the increase in hematocrit is very modest. Such patients do not have an increased white blood count, thrombocytosis, splenomegaly, or JAK2 mutation. The arterial oxygen saturation is normal. Estimation of the red cell mass and plasma volume is required to establishing a diagnosis of spurious polycythemia, but it should be recognized that during the natural history of patients who develop primary or secondary polycythemia, their red cell mass is, at some point, within the normal range while it is rising to abnormal values. Because of the significant error rate of red cell mass measurement, it is recommended that both red cell mass and plasma volume be measured simultaneously.

● THERAPY

POLYCYTHEMIAS OTHER THAN POLYCYTHEMIA VERA

Treatment of patients with post–renal transplant erythrocytosis with drugs that suppress the renal–angiotensin system has virtually eliminated the need for therapeutic phlebotomy. The maximal reduction of hemoglobin and hematocrit levels usually manifests by 6 months after starting therapy with either the angiotensin-converting enzyme inhibitor, enalapril, or the angiotensin II receptor type 1 blocker, losartan.[127] Some patients are exquisitely sensitive and may become severely anemic.

High-altitude erythrocytosis is also associated with pulmonary hypertension, proteinuria, and elevated blood pressure. A prospective randomized trial of enalapril reported decreased hemoglobin concentration, proteinuria and beneficial effects on elevated blood pressure.[219]

When erythrocytosis is secondary to a renal tumor or cyst, pheochromocytoma, myoma, or brain tumor, removal of the neoplasm usually results in disappearance of the erythrocytosis, but in the syndrome of congenital polycythemia with pheochromocytoma caused by EPAS1 mutations (see above paragraphs) erythrocytosis persist after tumor resection.

No specific therapy is currently available for polycythemic subjects with VHL, EGLN1, or EPAS1 mutations.

Lowering the hematocrit to a normal or near-normal level by phlebotomy is the usual, but empiric, treatment of secondary erythrocytosis,[220,221] but should always be viewed in the context of a particular subject.[28,178] The appropriate level is that at which the patient becomes asymptomatic. Although cytotoxic agents are sometimes used for this purpose, phlebotomy is preferred, if indeed needed, because of the leukemogenic risk of the agents that are used in polycythemia vera. This author favors, in most instances, benign neglect, unless specific therapy, such as that seen in erythropoietin-secreting tumors or post–renal transplant erythrocytosis, is available. One should phlebotomize only those patients who are symptomatic from the elevated red cell mass and continue to do so cautiously only if symptoms respond promptly to phlebotomy.

● COURSE AND PROGNOSIS

CHUVASH POLYCYTHEMIA

A study compared 96 patients with Chuvash polycythemia diagnosed before 1977 to 65 spouses, and 79 unrelated community members with normal hemoglobin concentration, same age, sex, and village of birth; the estimated survival to 65 years was 31 percent or less for Chuvash polycythemia patients versus 67 percent or greater for spouses and community members (p ≤0.002).[99]

OTHER POLYCYTHEMIAS

The clinical course of secondary erythrocytosis is largely a function of the underlying disorder. In patients with PFCP secondary to mutations of the EPOR gene, coronary artery disease and strokes have been reported,[162] although not in all series.[163] The rarity of patients having mutations of the EPOR, VHL, EGLN1, and EPAS1 genes and polycythemias from globin mutations and or red cell enzyme deficiencies precludes any meaningful prognostic evaluation.

REFERENCES

1. Juvonen E, Ikkala E, Fyhrquist F, et al: Autosomal dominant erythrocytosis caused by increased sensitivity to erythropoietin. *Blood* 78(11):3066, 1991.

2. Perrine GM, Prchal JT, Prchal JF: Study of a polycythemic family. *Blood* 50:134, 1977.

3. Prchal JT, Crist WM, Goldwasser E, et al: Autosomal dominant polycythemia. *Blood* 66(5):1208, 1985.

4. Ang SO, Chen H, Gordeuk VR, et al: Endemic polycythemia in Russia: Mutation in the VHL gene. *Blood Cells Mol Dis* 28(1):57, 2002.

5. Ang SO, Chen H, Hirota K, et al: Disruption of oxygen homeostasis underlies congenital Chuvash polycythemia. *Nat Genet* 32(4):614, 2002.

6. Kapralova K, Lanikova L, Lorenzo F, et al: RUNX1 and NF-E2 upregulation is not specific for MPNs, but is seen in polycythemic disorders with augmented HIF signaling. *Blood* 123(3):391, 2014.

7. Prchal JT, Gregg XT: Erythropoiesis—Genetic abnormalities, in *Erythropoietins and Erythropoiesis*, edited by Graham M, Foote MA, Elliott SG, p 61. Birkhäuser-Verlag AG, Basel, 2009.

8. Bert P: *La Pression Barometrique.* Bailliere, Paris, 1878.

9. Jourdanet D: *De l'anemie des altitudes et de l'anemie en general dans ses rapports avec la pression l'atmorphere.* Bailliere, Paris, 1863.

10. Viault F: Sur l'augmentation considerable du nombre des globules rouges dans le sang chez les habitants des hauts plateaux de l'Amerique du Sud. *CR Acad Sci* 111:917, 1890.

11. Erslev AJ: Blood and mountains, in *Blood, Pure and Eloquent*, edited by MM Wintrobe. McGraw-Hill, New York, 1980.

12. Leopold SS: The etiology of pulmonary arteriosclerosis (Ayerza's syndrome). *Am J Med* 219:152, 1950.

13. Abbott ME: *Atlas of Congenital Heart Disease.* American Heart Association, New York, 1936.

14. Burwell CS, Robin ED, Whaley RD, Bickelman AG: Extreme obesity associated with alveolar hypoventilation: A Pickwickian syndrome. *Am J Med* 21:811, 1956.

15. Charache S, Weatherall DJ, Clegg JB: Polycythemia associated with a hemoglobinopathy. *J Clin Invest* 45(6):813, 1966.

16. Fairbanks VF, Klee GG, Wiseman GA, et al: Measurement of blood volume and red cell mass: Re-examination of ^{51}Cr and ^{125}I methods. *Blood Cells Mol Dis* 22(2):169; discussion 186a, 1996.

17. Lawrence JH, Berlin NI: Relative polycythemia—The polycythemia of stress. *Yale J Biol Med* 24:498, 1952.

18. Prchal JT: Classification and molecular biology of polycythemias (erythrocytoses) and thrombocytosis. *Hematol Oncol Clin North Am* 17(5):1151, vi, 2003.

19. Chambellan A, Chailleux E, Similowski T, et al: Prognostic value of the hematocrit in patients with severe COPD receiving long-term oxygen therapy. *Chest* 128(3):1201, 2005.

20. Kollert F, Tippelt A, Muller C, et al: Hemoglobin levels above anemia thresholds are maximally predictive for long-term survival in COPD with chronic respiratory failure. *Respir Care* 58(7):1204, 2013.

21. Hoffstein V, Mateika S: Differences in abdominal and neck circumferences in patients with and without obstructive sleep apnoea. *Eur Respir J* 5(4):377, 1992.

22. Carlson JT, Hedner J, Fagerberg B, et al: Secondary polycythaemia associated with nocturnal apnoea—A relationship not mediated by erythropoietin? *J Intern Med* 231(4):381, 1992.

23. Choi JB, Loredo JS, Norman D, et al: Does obstructive sleep apnea increase hematocrit? *Sleep Breath* 10(3):155, 2006.

24. Solmaz S, Duksal F, Ganidagli S: Is obstructive sleep apnoea syndrome really one of the causes of secondary polycythaemia? *Hematology* 2014. [Epub ahead of print]

25. King AJ, Eyre T, Littlewood T: Obstructive sleep apnoea does not lead to clinically significant erythrocytosis. *BMJ* 347:f7340, 2013.

26. Kung CM, Wang HL, Tseng ZL: Cigarette smoking exacerbates health problems in young men. *Clin Invest Med* 31(3):E138, 2008.

27. Bento C, Almeida H, Maia TM, et al: Molecular study of congenital erythrocytosis in 70 unrelated patients revealed a potential causal mutation in less than half of the cases (Where is/are the missing gene(s)?). *Eur J Haematol* 91(4):361, 2013.

28. Vongpatanasin W, Brickner ME, Hillis LD, et al: The Eisenmenger syndrome in adults. *Ann Intern Med* 128(9):745, 1998.

29. Plotz CM, Knowlton AI, Ragan C: The natural history of Cushing's syndrome. *Am J Med* 13(5):597, 1952.

30. Mann DL, Gallagher NI, Donati RM: Erythrocytosis and primary aldosteronism. *Ann Intern Med* 66(2):335, 1967.

31. Erkelens DW, Statius van Eps LW: Bartter's syndrome and erythrocytosis. *Am J Med* 55(5):711, 1973.

32. Fernandez-Balsells MM, Murad MH, Lane M, et al: Clinical review 1: Adverse effects of testosterone therapy in adult men: A systematic review and meta-analysis. *J Clin Endocrinol Metab* 95(6):2560, 2010.

33. Thorling EB: Paraneoplastic erythrocytosis and inappropriate erythropoietin production. A review. *Scand J Haematol Suppl* 17:1, 1972.

34. Ladroue C, Carcenac R, Leporrier M, et al: PHD2 mutation and congenital erythrocytosis with paraganglioma. *N Engl J Med* 359(25):2685, 2008.

35. LevGur M, Levie MD: The myomatous erythrocytosis syndrome: A review. *Obstet Gynecol* 86(6):1026, 1995.

36. Levinson JP, Kincaid OW: Myxoma of the right atrium associated with polycythemia. Report of successful excision. *N Engl J Med* 264:1187, 1961.

37. Josephs BN, Robbins G, Levine A: Polycythemia secondary to hamartoma of the liver. *JAMA* 179:867, 1961.

38. Sandler A, Rivlin L, Filler R, et al: Polycythemia secondary to focal nodular hyperplasia. *J Pediatr Surg* 32(9):1386, 1997.

39. Constans JP, Meder F, Maiuri F, et al: Posterior fossa hemangioblastomas. *Surg Neurol* 25(3):269, 1986.

40. Sharma RR, Cast IP, O'Brien C: Supratentorial haemangioblastoma not associated with von Hippel Lindau complex or polycythaemia: Case report and literature review. *Br J Neurosurg* 9(1):81, 1995.

41. Morkeberg J: Blood manipulation: Current challenges from an anti-doping perspective. *Hematology Am Soc Hematol Educ Program* 2013:627, 2013.

42. Monge CC: Life in the Andes and chronic mountain sickness. *Science* 95:79, 1942.

43. Beutler E, Waalen J: The definition of anemia: What is the lower limit of normal of the blood hemoglobin concentration? *Blood* 107(5):1747, 2006.

44. Centers for Disease Control: CDC criteria for anemia in children and childbearing-aged women. *MMWR Morb Mortal Wkly Rep* 38(22):400, 1989.

45. Dagher FJ, Ramos E, Erslev AJ, et al: Are the native kidneys responsible for erythrocytosis in renal allorecipients? *Transplantation* 28(6):496, 1979.

46. Kessler M, Hestin D, Mayeux D, et al: Factors predisposing to post-renal transplant erythrocytosis. A prospective matched-pair control study. *Clin Nephrol* 45(2):83, 1996.

47. Gaston RS, Julian BA, Curtis JJ: Posttransplant erythrocytosis: An enigma revisited. *Am J Kidney Dis* 24(1):1, 1994.

48. Polyakova LA: Familial erythrocytosis among inhabitants of the Chuvash ASSR. *Probl Gematol Pereliv Krovi* 10:30, 1974.

49. Liu E, Percy MJ, Amos CI, et al: The worldwide distribution of the VHL 598C>T mutation indicates a single founding event. *Blood* 103(5):1937, 2004.

50. Liu E, Jelinek J, Pastore YD, et al: Discrimination of polycythemias and thrombocytoses by novel, simple, accurate clonality assays and comparison with PRV-1 expression and BFU-E response to erythropoietin. *Blood* 101(8):3294, 2003.

51. Percy MJ, Beard ME, Carter C, et al: Erythrocytosis and the Chuvash von Hippel-Lindau mutation. *Br J Haematol* 123(2):371, 2003.

52. Perrotta S, Nobili B, Ferraro M, et al: Von Hippel-Lindau-dependent polycythemia is endemic on the island of Ischia: Identification of a novel cluster. *Blood* 107(2):514, 2006.

53. Chetty KG, Light RW, Stansbury DW, et al: Exercise performance of polycythemic chronic obstructive pulmonary disease patients. Effect of phlebotomies. *Chest* 98(5):1073, 1990.

54. Gordeuk VR, Stockton DW, Prchal JT: Congenital polycythemias/erythrocytoses. *Haematologica* 90(1):109, 2005.

55. Hurtado A: Acclimatization of high altitudes, in *Physiological Effects of High Altitude*, edited by Weihe WH. Macmillan, New York, 1964.

56. Moore LG, Brewer GJ: Beneficial effect of rightward hemoglobin-oxygen dissociation curve shift for short-term high-altitude adaptation. *J Lab Clin Med* 98(1):145, 1981.

57. Finch CA, Lenfant C: Oxygen transport in man. *N Engl J Med* 286(8):407, 1972.

58. Winslow RM, Monge CC, Statham NJ, et al: Variability of oxygen affinity of blood: Human subjects native to high altitude. *J Appl Physiol* 51(6):1411, 1981.

59. Eaton JW, Skelton TD, Berger E: Survival at extreme altitude: Protective effect of increased hemoglobin-oxygen affinity. *Science* 183(126):743, 1974.

60. Leon-Velarde F, Gamboa A, Chuquiza JA, et al: Hematological parameters in high altitude residents living at 4,355, 4,660, and 5,500 meters above sea level. *High Alt Med Biol* 1(2):97, 2000.

61. Mejia OM, Prchal JT, Leon-Velarde F, et al: Genetic association analysis of chronic mountain sickness in an Andean high-altitude population. *Haematologica* 90(1):13, 2005.

62. Beall CM: Two routes to functional adaptation: Tibetan and Andean high-altitude natives. *Proc Natl Acad Sci U S A* 104 Suppl 1:8655, 2007.

63. Tashi T, Feng T, Koul P, et al: High altitude genetic adaptation in Tibetans: No role of increased hemoglobin-oxygen affinity. *Blood Cells Mol Dis* 53(1–2):27, 2014.

64. Maignan M, Rivera-Ch M, Privat C, et al: Pulmonary pressure and cardiac function in chronic mountain sickness patients. *Chest* 135(2):499, 2009.

65. Wu TY, Ding SQ, Liu JL, et al: Who should not go high: Chronic disease and work at altitude during construction of the Qinghai-Tibet railroad. *High Alt Med Biol* 8(2):88, 2007.

66. Winslow RM, Monge CC: *Hypoxia, Polycythemia and Chronic Mountain Sickness.* Johns Hopkins University Press, Baltimore, 1987.

67. Chapman RF, Stray-Gundersen J and Levine BD: Epo production at altitude in elite endurance athletes is not associated with the sea level hypoxic ventilatory response. *J Sci Med Sport* 13(6):624, 2010.

68. Winslow RM, Chapman KW, Gibson CC, et al: Different hematologic responses to hypoxia in Sherpas and Quechua Indians. *J Appl Physiol* 66(4):1561, 1989.

69. Zhou ZN, Zhuang JG, Wu XF, et al: Tibetans retained innate ability resistance to acute hypoxia after long period of residing at sea level. *J Physiol Sci* 58(3):167, 2008.

70. Beall CM, Laskowski D, Erzurum SC: Nitric oxide in adaptation to altitude. *Free Radic Biol Med* 52(7):1123, 2012.

71. Claydon VE, Gulli G, Slessarev M, et al: Cerebrovascular responses to hypoxia and hypocapnia in Ethiopian high altitude dwellers. *Stroke* 39(2):336, 2008.

72. Beall CM: High-altitude adaptations. *Lancet* 362 Suppl:s14, 2003.

73. Zhou D, Udpa N, Ronen R, et al: Whole-genome sequencing uncovers the genetic basis of chronic mountain sickness in Andean highlanders. *Am J Hum Genet* 93(3):452, 2013.

74. Simonson TS, Yang Y, Huff CD, et al: Genetic evidence for high-altitude adaptation in Tibet. *Science* 329(5987):72, 2010.
75. Yi X, Liang Y, Huerta-Sanchez E, et al: Sequencing of 50 human exomes reveals adaptation to high altitude. *Science* 329(5987):75, 2010.
76. Beall CM, Cavalleri GL, Deng L, et al: Natural selection on EPAS1 (HIF2alpha) associated with low hemoglobin concentration in Tibetan highlanders. *Proc Natl Acad Sci U S A* 107(25):11459, 2010.
77. Huerta-Sanchez E, Jin X, Asan, et al: Altitude adaptation in Tibetans caused by introgression of Denisovan-like DNA: *Nature* 512(7513):194, 2014.
78. Krause J, Fu Q, Good JM, et al: The complete mitochondrial DNA genome of an unknown hominin from southern Siberia. *Nature* 464(7290):894, 2010.
79. Abi-Rached L, Jobin MJ, Kulkarni S, et al: The shaping of modern human immune systems by multiregional admixture with archaic humans. *Science* 334(6052):89, 2011.
80. Lorenzo FR, Rili G, Simonson T, et al: A novel PHD2 mutation associated with Tibetan genetic adaptation to high altitude hypoxia. ASH 52nd Annual Meeting, Orlando, FL, 2010.
81. Lorenzo FR, Huff C, Myllymaki M, et al: A genetic mechanism for Tibetan high-altitude adaptation. *Nat Genet* 46(9):951, 2014.
82. Jefferson JA, Escudero E, Hurtado ME, et al: Excessive erythrocytosis, chronic mountain sickness, and serum cobalt levels. *Lancet* 359(9304):407, 2002.
83. Goldwasser E, Jacobson LO, Fried W, et al: Mechanism of the erythropoietic effect of cobalt. *Science* 125(3257):1085, 1957.
84. Bernardi L, Roach RC, Keyl C, et al: Ventilation, autonomic function, sleep and erythropoietin. Chronic mountain sickness of Andean natives. *Adv Exp Med Biol* 543:161, 2003.
85. Murray JF: Classification of polycythemic disorders. With comments on the diagnostic value of arterial blood oxygen analysis. *Ann Intern Med* 64:892, 1966.
86. Kuhl W: History of clinical research on the sleep apnea syndrome. The early days of polysomnography. *Respiration* 64 Suppl 1:5, 1997.
87. Block AJ, Boysen PG, Wynne JW, et al: Sleep apnea, hypopnea and oxygen desaturation in normal subjects. A strong male predominance. *N Engl J Med* 300(10):513, 1979.
88. Moore-Gillon JC, Treacher DF, Gaminara EJ, et al: Intermittent hypoxia in patients with unexplained polycythaemia. *Br Med J (Clin Res Ed)* 293(6547):588, 1986.
89. Smith JR, Landaw SA: Smokers' polycythemia. *N Engl J Med* 298(1):6, 1978.
90. Stonesifer LD: How carbon monoxide reduces plasma volume. *N Engl J Med* 299(6):311, 1978.
91. Cartier P, Labie D, Leroux JP, et al: [Familial diphosphoglycerate mutase deficiency: Hematological and biochemical study] [in French]. *Nouv Rev Fr Hematol* 12(3):269, 1972.
92. Lichtman MA, Murphy MS and Adamson JW: Detection of mutant hemoglobins with altered affinity for oxygen. A simplified technique. *Ann Intern Med* 84(5):517, 1976.
93. Agarwal N, Mojica-Henshaw MP, Simmons ED, et al: Familial polycythemia caused by a novel mutation in the beta globin gene: Essential role of P50 in evaluation of familial polycythemia. *Int J Med Sci* 4(4):232, 2007.
94. Xia M, Huang T, Sun Y, et al: Identification of chemical compounds that induce HIF-1 alpha activity. *Toxicol Sci* 112(1):153, 2009.
95. Sergeyeva A, Gordeuk VR, Tokarev YN, et al: Congenital polycythemia in Chuvashia. *Blood* 89(6):2148, 1997.
96. Tomasic NL, Piterkova L, Huff C, et al: The phenotype of polycythemia due to Croatian homozygous VHL (571C>G:H191D) mutation is different from that of Chuvash polycythemia (VHL 598C>T:R200W). *Haematologica* 98(4):560, 2013.
97. Lanikova L, Lorenzo F, Yang C, et al: Novel homozygous VHL mutation in exon 2 is associated with congenital polycythemia but not with cancer. *Blood* 121(19):3918, 2013.
98. Lorenzo FR, Yang C, Lanikova L, et al: Novel compound VHL heterozygosity (VHL T124A/L188V) associated with congenital polycythaemia. *Br J Haematol* 162(6):851, 2013.
99. Gordeuk VR, Sergueeva AI, Miasnikova GY, et al: Congenital disorder of oxygen sensing: Association of the homozygous Chuvash polycythemia VHL mutation with thrombosis and vascular abnormalities but not tumors. *Blood* 103:3924, 2004.
100. Percy MJ, McMullin MF, Jowitt SN, et al: Chuvash-type congenital polycythemia in 4 families of Asian and Western European ancestry. *Blood* 102(3):1097, 2003.
101. Bento MC, Chang KT, Guan Y, et al: Congenital polycythemia with homozygous and heterozygous mutations of von Hippel-Lindau gene: Five new Caucasian patients. *Haematologica* 90(1):128, 2005.
102. Cario H, Schwarz K, Jorch N, et al: Mutations in the von Hippel-Lindau (VHL) tumor suppressor gene and VHL-haplotype analysis in patients with presumable congenital erythrocytosis. *Haematologica* 90(1):19, 2005.
103. Collins TS, Arcasoy MO: Iron overload due to X-linked sideroblastic anemia in an African American man. *Am J Med* 116(7):501, 2004.
104. Pastore Y, Jedlickova K, Guan Y, et al: Mutations of von Hippel-Lindau tumor-suppressor gene and congenital polycythemia. *Am J Hum Genet* 73(2):412, 2003.
105. Pastore YD, Jelinek J, Ang S, et al: Mutations in the VHL gene in sporadic apparently congenital polycythemia. *Blood* 101(4):1591, 2003.
106. Semenza GL: HIF-1 and mechanisms of hypoxia sensing. *Curr Opin Cell Biol* 13(2):167, 2001.
107. Miasnikova GY, Sergueeva AI, Nouraie M, et al: The heterozygote advantage of the Chuvash polycythemia VHLR200W mutation may be protection against anemia. *Haematologica* 96(9):1371, 2011.
108. Cramer T, Yamanishi Y, Clausen BE, et al: HIF-1alpha is essential for myeloid cell-mediated inflammation. *Cell* 112(5):645, 2003.
109. Friedrich CA: Von Hippel-Lindau syndrome. A pleomorphic condition. *Cancer* 86(11 Suppl):2478, 1999.
110. Haase VH, Glickman JN, Socolovsky M, et al: Vascular tumors in livers with targeted inactivation of the von Hippel-Lindau tumor suppressor. *Proc Natl Acad Sci U S A* 98(4):1583, 2001.
111. Krieg M, Marti HH, Plate KH: Coexpression of erythropoietin and vascular endothelial growth factor in nervous system tumors associated with von Hippel-Lindau tumor suppressor gene loss of function. *Blood* 92(9):3388, 1998.
112. Richards FM: Molecular pathology of von Hippel Lindau disease and the VHL tumour suppressor gene. *Expert Rev Mol Med* 2001:1, 2001.
113. Couvé S, Ladroue C, Laine C, et al: Genetic evidence of a precisely tuned dysregulation in the hypoxia signaling pathway during oncogenesis. *Cancer Res* 74(22):6554, 2014.
114. Percy MJ, Zhao Q, Flores A, et al: A family with erythrocytosis establishes a role for prolyl hydroxylase domain protein 2 in oxygen homeostasis. *Proc Natl Acad Sci U S A* 103(3):654, 2006.
115. Bento C, Percy MJ, Gardie B, et al: Genetic basis of congenital erythrocytosis: Mutation update and online databases. *Hum Mutat* 35(1):15, 2014.
116. Lorenzo FR, Yang C, Ng Tang Fui M, et al: A novel EPAS1/HIF2A germline mutation in a congenital polycythemia with paraganglioma. *J Mol Med (Berl)* 91(4):507, 2013.
117. Russell RC, Sufan RI, Zhou B, et al: Loss of JAK2 regulation via a heterodimeric VHL-SOCS1 E3 ubiquitin ligase underlies Chuvash polycythemia. *Nat Med* 17(7):845, 2011.
118. Kaufmann KB, Grunder A, Hadlich T, et al: A novel murine model of myeloproliferative disorders generated by overexpression of the transcription factor NF-E2. *J Exp Med* 209(1):35, 2012.
119. Maran J, Jedlickova K, Stockton D, Prchal JT: Finding the novel molecular defect in a family with high erythropoietin autosomal dominant polycythemia. *Blood* 102:162b, 2003.
120. Hammond D, Winnick S: Paraneoplastic erythrocytosis and ectopic erythropoietins. *Ann N Y Acad Sci* 230:219, 1974.
121. Navarro J, Aguilera A, Liano F, et al: Phlebotomy for polycythemia associated with acquired cystic renal disease in a patient on hemodialysis. *Nephron* 62(1):110, 1992.
122. Da Silva JL, Lacombe C, Bruneval P, et al: Tumor cells are the site of erythropoietin synthesis in human renal cancers associated with polycythemia. *Blood* 75(3):577, 1990.
123. Lal A, Rice A, al Mahr M, et al: Wilms tumor associated with polycythemia: Case report and review of the literature. *J Pediatr Hematol Oncol* 19(3):263, 1997.
124. Grignon DJ, Eble JN: Papillary and metanephric adenomas of the kidney. *Semin Diagn Pathol* 15(1):41, 1998.
125. Fisher JW, Samuels AI: Relationship between renal blood flow and erythropoietin production in dogs. *Proc Soc Exp Biol Med* 125(2):482, 1967.
126. Beebe HG, Chesebro K, Merchant F, et al: Results of renal artery balloon angioplasty limit its indications. *J Vasc Surg* 8(3):300, 1988.
127. Mrug M, Julian BA, Prchal JT: Angiotensin II receptor type 1 expression in erythroid progenitors: Implications for the pathogenesis of postrenal transplant erythrocytosis. *Semin Nephrol* 24(2):120, 2004.
128. Danovitch GM, Jamgotchian NJ, Eggena PH, et al: Angiotensin-converting enzyme inhibition in the treatment of renal transplant erythrocytosis. Clinical experience and observation of mechanism. *Transplantation* 60(2):132, 1995.
129. Mrug M, Stopka T, Julian BA, et al: Angiotensin II stimulates proliferation of normal early erythroid progenitors. *J Clin Invest* 100(9):2310, 1997.
130. Glicklich D, Burris L, Urban A, et al: Angiotensin-converting enzyme inhibition induces apoptosis in erythroid precursors and affects insulin-like growth factor-1 in posttransplantation erythrocytosis. *J Am Soc Nephrol* 12(9):1958, 2001.
131. Gossmann J, Burkhardt R, Harder S, et al: Angiotensin II infusion increases plasma erythropoietin levels via an angiotensin II type 1 receptor-dependent pathway. *Kidney Int* 60(1):83, 2001.
132. Thevenod F, Radtke HW, Grutzmacher P, et al: Deficient feedback regulation of erythropoiesis in kidney transplant patients with polycythemia. *Kidney Int* 24(2):227, 1983.
133. Friman S, Nyberg G, Blohme I: Erythrocytosis after renal transplantation; treatment by removal of the native kidneys. *Nephrol Dial Transplant* 5(11):969, 1990.
134. Cole J, Ertoy D, Lin H, et al: Lack of angiotensin II-facilitated erythropoiesis causes anemia in angiotensin-converting enzyme-deficient mice. *J Clin Invest* 106(11):1391, 2000.
135. Venencie PY, Puissant A, Boffa GA, et al: Multiple cutaneous leiomyomata and erythrocytosis with demonstration of erythropoietic activity in the cutaneous leiomyomata. *Br J Dermatol* 107(4):483, 1982.
136. Trimble M, Caro J, Talalla A, et al: Secondary erythrocytosis due to a cerebellar hemangioblastoma: Demonstration of erythropoietin mRNA in the tumor. *Blood* 78(3):599, 1991.
137. McFadzean AJS, Todd D, Tsang, KC: Polycythemia in primary carcinoma of the liver. *Blood* 13:427, 1958.
138. Davidson CS: Hepatocellular carcinoma and erythrocytosis. *Semin Hematol* 13(2):115, 1976.
139. Muta H, Funakoshi A, Baba T, et al: Gene expression of erythropoietin in hepatocellular carcinoma. *Intern Med* 33(7):427, 1994.
140. Shulkin BL, Shapiro B, Sisson JC: Pheochromocytoma, polycythemia, and venous thrombosis. *Am J Med* 83(4):773, 1987.
141. Zhuang Z, Yang C, Lorenzo F, et al: Somatic HIF2A gain-of-function mutations in paraganglioma with polycythemia. *N Engl J Med* 367(10):922, 2012.

142. Pacak K, Jochmanova I, Prodanov T, et al: New syndrome of paraganglioma and somatostatinoma associated with polycythemia. *J Clin Oncol* 31(13):1690, 2013.

143. Yang C, Sun MG, Matro J, et al: Novel HIF2A mutations disrupt oxygen sensing, leading to polycythemia, paragangliomas, and somatostatinomas. *Blood* 121(13):2563, 2013.

144. Mann DL, Gallagher NI, Donati RM: Erythrocytosis and primary aldosteronism. *Ann Intern Med* 66(2):335, 1967.

145. Erkelens DW, Statius van Eps LW: Bartter's syndrome and erythrocytosis. *Am J Med* 55(5):711, 1973.

146. Ghio R, Haupt E, Ratti M, et al: Erythrocytosis associated with a dermoid cyst of the ovary and erythropoietic activity of the tumour fluid. *Scand J Haematol* 27(2):70, 1981.

147. Shahani S, Braga-Basaria M, Maggio M, et al: Androgens and erythropoiesis: A review. *J Endocrinol Invest* 32(8):704, 2009.

148. Gardner FH, Nathan DG, Piomelli S, et al: The erythrocythaemic effects of androgen. *Br J Haematol* 14(6):611, 1968.

149. Besa EC: Hematologic effects of androgens revisited: An alternative therapy in various hematologic conditions. *Semin Hematol* 31(2):134, 1994.

150. Bachman E, Travison TG, Basaria S, et al: Testosterone induces erythrocytosis via increased erythropoietin and suppressed hepcidin: Evidence for a new erythropoietin/hemoglobin set point. *J Gerontol A Biol Sci Med Sci* 69(6):725, 2014.

151. Wiswell TE, Cornish JD, Northam RS: Neonatal polycythemia: Frequency of clinical manifestations and other associated findings. *Pediatrics* 78(1):26, 1986.

152. Black VD, Lubchenco LO, Koops BL, et al: Neonatal hyperviscosity: Randomized study of effect of partial plasma exchange transfusion on long-term outcome. *Pediatrics* 75(6):1048, 1985.

153. Jopling J, Henry E, Wiedmeier SE, et al: Reference ranges for hematocrit and blood hemoglobin concentration during the neonatal period: Data from a multihospital health care system. *Pediatrics* 123(2):e333, 2009.

154. Christensen RD, Lambert DK, Henry E, et al: Unexplained extreme hyperbilirubinemia among neonates in a multihospital healthcare system. *Blood Cells Mol Dis* 50(2):105, 2013.

155. Pearson TC: Apparent polycythaemia. *Blood Rev* 5(4):205, 1991.

156. Chrysant SG, Frohlich ED, Adamopoulos PN, et al: Pathophysiologic significance of "stress" or relative polycythemia in essential hypertension. *Am J Cardiol* 37(7):1069, 1976.

157. Isbister JP: The contracted plasma volume syndromes (relative polycythaemias) and their haemorheological significance. *Baillieres Clin Haematol* 1(3):665, 1987.

158. Leth A: Changes in plasma and extracellular fluid volumes in patients with essential hypertension during long-term treatment with hydrochlorothiazide. *Circulation* 42(3):479, 1970.

159. Prchal JT: *Personal communication and direct experience with about 100 affected subjects.* 2009.

160. Queisser W, Heim ME, Schmitz JM, et al: [Idiopathic familial erythrocytosis. Report on a family with autosomal dominant inheritance] [in German]. *Dtsch Med Wochenschr* 113(21):851, 1988.

161. Prchal JT, Semenza GL, Prchal J, et al: Familial polycythemia. *Science* 268(5219):1831, 1995.

162. Kralovics R, Sokol L, Prchal JT: Absence of polycythemia in a child with a unique erythropoietin receptor mutation in a family with autosomal dominant primary polycythemia. *J Clin Invest* 102(1):124, 1998.

163. Arcasoy MO, Degar BA, Harris KW, et al: Familial erythrocytosis associated with a short deletion in the erythropoietin receptor gene. *Blood* 89(12):4628, 1997.

164. Bushuev VI, Miasnikova GY, Sergueeva AI, et al: Endothelin-1, vascular endothelial growth factor and systolic pulmonary artery pressure in patients with Chuvash polycythemia. *Haematologica* 91(6):744, 2006.

165. Gladwin MT: Polycythemia, HIF-1alpha and pulmonary hypertension in Chuvash. *Haematologica* 91(6):722, 2006.

166. Smith TG, Brooks JT, Balanos GM, et al: Mutation of von Hippel-Lindau tumour suppressor and human cardiopulmonary physiology. *PLoS Med* 3(7):e290, 2006.

167. Sable CA, Aliyu ZY, Dham N, et al: Pulmonary artery pressure and iron deficiency in patients with upregulation of hypoxia sensing due to homozygous VHL(R200W) mutation (Chuvash polycythemia). *Haematologica* 97(2):193, 2012.

168. Zafren K and Honigman B: High-altitude medicine. *Emerg Med Clin North Am* 15(1):191, 1997.

169. Bishop BC: Wintering in the high Himalayas. *Natl Geogr Mag* 122:503, 1962.

170. Botella de Maglia J, Martinez-Costa R: [High altitude retinal hemorrhages in the expeditions to 8,000 meter peaks. A study of 10 cases] [in Spanish]. *Med Clin (Barc)* 110(12):457, 1998.

171. Beall CM, Song K, Elston RC, et al: Higher offspring survival among Tibetan women with high oxygen saturation genotypes residing at 4,000 m. *Proc Natl Acad Sci U S A* 101(39):14300, 2004.

172. Beall CM: Oxygen saturation increases during childhood and decreases during adulthood among high altitude native Tibetans residing at 3,800-4,200 m. *High Alt Med Biol* 1(1):25, 2000.

173. Beall CM: Tibetan and Andean contrasts in adaptation to high-altitude hypoxia. *Adv Exp Med Biol* 475:63, 2000.

174. Beall CM, Decker MJ, Brittenham GM, et al: An Ethiopian pattern of human adaptation to high-altitude hypoxia. *Proc Natl Acad Sci U S A* 99(26):17215, 2002.

175. Cote C, Zilberberg MD, Mody SH, et al: Haemoglobin level and its clinical impact in a cohort of patients with COPD. *Eur Respir J* 29(5):923, 2007.

176. Boyer L, Chaar V, Pelle G, et al: Effects of polycythemia on systemic endothelial function in chronic hypoxic lung disease. *J Appl Physiol (1985)* 110(5):1196, 2011.

177. Nadeem O, Gui J, Ornstein DL: Prevalence of venous thromboembolism in patients with secondary polycythemia. *Clin Appl Thromb Hemost* 19(4):363, 2013.

178. Thorne SA: Management of polycythaemia in adults with cyanotic congenital heart disease. *Heart* 79(4):315, 1998.

179. Shibata J, Hasegawa J, Siemens HJ, et al: Hemostasis and coagulation at a hematocrit level of 0.85: Functional consequences of erythrocytosis. *Blood* 101(11):4416, 2003.

180. Ammash N, Warnes CA: Cerebrovascular events in adult patients with cyanotic congenital heart disease. *J Am Coll Cardiol* 28(3):768, 1996.

181. Stefenelli T, Silberbauer K, Ulrich W, et al: Cardial decompensation caused by hypertension and polyglobulia associated with multiple renal oncocytomas. *Clin Nephrol* 23(6):307, 1985.

182. Lezaic V, Biljanovic-Paunovic L, Pavlovic-Kentera V, et al: Erythropoiesis after kidney transplantation: The role of erythropoietin, burst promoting activity and early erythroid progenitor cells. *Eur J Med Res* 6(1):27, 2001.

183. Niu X, Miasnikova GY, Sergueeva AI, et al: Altered cytokine profiles in patients with Chuvash polycythemia. *Am J Hematol* 84(2):74, 2009.

184. Sergueeva AI, Miasnikova GY, Okhotin DJ, et al: Elevated homocysteine, glutathione and cysteinylglycine concentrations in patients homozygous for the Chuvash polycythemia VHL mutation. *Haematologica* 93(2):279, 2008.

185. Beutler E: Polycythemia. *Med Grand Rounds* 3:142, 1984.

186. Prchal JF, Axelrad AA: Letter: Bone-marrow responses in polycythemia vera. *N Engl J Med* 290(24):1382, 1974.

187. Kralovics R, Buser AS, Teo SS, et al: Comparison of molecular markers in a cohort of patients with chronic myeloproliferative disorders. *Blood* 102(5):1869, 2003.

188. Weinberg RS: In vitro erythropoiesis in polycythemia vera and other myeloproliferative disorders. *Semin Hematol* 34(1):64, 1997.

189. Shih LY, Lee CT, See LC, et al: In vitro culture growth of erythroid progenitors and serum erythropoietin assay in the differential diagnosis of polycythaemia. *Eur J Clin Invest* 28(7):569, 1998.

190. Prchal JT: *Personal communication.* 2009.

191. Fisher MJ, Prchal JF, Prchal JT, et al: Anti-erythropoietin (EPO) receptor monoclonal antibodies distinguish EPO-dependent and EPO-independent erythroid progenitors in polycythemia vera. *Blood* 84(6):1982, 1994.

192. Kralovics R, Indrak K, Stopka T, et al: Two new EPO receptor mutations: Truncated EPO receptors are most frequently associated with primary familial and congenital polycythemias. *Blood* 90(5):2057, 1997.

193. Acharya J, Westwood NB, Sawyer BM, et al: Identification of latent myeloproliferative disease in patients with Budd-Chiari syndrome using X-chromosome inactivation patterns and in vitro erythroid colony formation. *Eur J Haematol* 55(5):315, 1995.

194. De Stefano V, Teofili L, Leone G, et al: Spontaneous erythroid colony formation as the clue to an underlying myeloproliferative disorder in patients with Budd-Chiari syndrome or portal vein thrombosis. *Semin Thromb Hemost* 23(5):411, 1997.

195. Pagliuca A, Mufti GJ, Janossa-Tahernia M, et al: In vitro colony culture and chromosomal studies in hepatic and portal vein thrombosis—Possible evidence of an occult myeloproliferative state. *Q J Med* 76(281):981, 1990.

196. Valla D, Casadevall N, Lacombe C, et al: Primary myeloproliferative disorder and hepatic vein thrombosis. A prospective study of erythroid colony formation in vitro in 20 patients with Budd-Chiari syndrome. *Ann Intern Med* 103(3):329, 1985.

197. Shih LY, Lee CT: Identification of masked polycythemia vera from patients with idiopathic marked thrombocytosis by endogenous erythroid colony assay. *Blood* 83(3):744, 1994.

198. Birgegard G, Wide L: Serum erythropoietin in the diagnosis of polycythaemia and after phlebotomy treatment. *Br J Haematol* 81(4):603, 1992.

199. Messinezy M, Westwood NB, El-Hemaidi I, et al: Serum erythropoietin values in erythrocytoses and in primary thrombocythaemia. *Br J Haematol* 117(1):47, 2002.

200. Mossuz P, Girodon F, Donnard M, et al: Diagnostic value of serum erythropoietin level in patients with absolute erythrocytosis. *Haematologica* 89(10):1194, 2004.

201. Thurmes PJ, Steensma DP: Elevated serum erythropoietin levels in patients with Budd-Chiari syndrome secondary to polycythemia vera: Clinical implications for the role of JAK2 mutation analysis. *Eur J Haematol* 77(1):57, 2006.

202. Remacha AF, Montserrat I, Santamaria A, et al: Serum erythropoietin in the diagnosis of polycythemia vera. A follow-up study. *Haematologica* 82(4):406, 1997.

203. Beutler E, Yeh M, Fairbanks VF: The normal human female as a mosaic of X-chromosome activity: Studies using the gene for C-6-PD-deficiency as a marker. *Proc Natl Acad Sci U S A* 48:9, 1962.

204. Adamson JW, Fialkow PJ, Murphy S, et al: Polycythemia vera: Stem-cell and probable clonal origin of the disease. *N Engl J Med* 295(17):913, 1976.

205. Prchal JT: Pathogenetic mechanisms of polycythemia vera and congenital polycythemic disorders. *Semin Hematol* 38(1 Suppl 2):10, 2001.

206. Kralovics R, Guan Y, Prchal JT: Acquired uniparental disomy of chromosome 9p is a frequent stem cell defect in polycythemia vera. *Exp Hematol* 30(3):229, 2002.

207. Chen GL, Prchal JT: X-linked clonality testing: Interpretation and limitations. *Blood* 110(5):1411, 2007.

208. Curnutte JT, Hopkins PJ, Kuhl W, et al: Studying X inactivation. *Lancet* 339(8795):749, 1992.

209. Allen RC, Zoghbi HY, Moseley AB, et al: Methylation of HpaII and HhaI sites near the polymorphic CAG repeat in the human androgen-receptor gene correlates with X chromosome inactivation. *Am J Hum Genet* 51(6):1229, 1992.

210. Prchal JT, Guan YL, Prchal JF, et al: Transcriptional analysis of the active X-chromosome in normal and clonal hematopoiesis. *Blood* 81(1):269, 1993.

211. Prchal JT, Prchal JF, Belickova M, et al: Clonal stability of blood cell lineages indicated by X-chromosomal transcriptional polymorphism. *J Exp Med* 183(2):561, 1996.

212. Busque L, Mio R, Mattioli J, et al: Nonrandom X-inactivation patterns in normal females: Lyonization ratios vary with age. *Blood* 88(1):59, 1996.

213. Champion KM, Gilbert JG, Asimakopoulos FA, et al: Clonal haemopoiesis in normal elderly women: Implications for the myeloproliferative disorders and myelodysplastic syndromes. *Br J Haematol* 97(4):920, 1997.

214. Gale RE, Fielding AK, Harrison CN, et al: Acquired skewing of X-chromosome inactivation patterns in myeloid cells of the elderly suggests stochastic clonal loss with age. *Br J Haematol* 98(3):512, 1997.

215. Swierczek SI, Agarwal N, Nussenzveig RH, et al: Hematopoiesis is not clonal in healthy elderly women. *Blood* 112(8):3186, 2008.

216. Swierczek SI, Piterkova L, Jelinek J, et al: Methylation of AR locus does not always reflect X chromosome inactivation state. *Blood* 119(13):e100, 2012.

217. Kralovics R, Stockton DW, Prchal JT: Clonal hematopoiesis in familial polycythemia vera suggests the involvement of multiple mutational events in the early pathogenesis of the disease. *Blood* 102(10):3793, 2003.

218. Lertzman M, Frome BM, Israels LG, et al: Hypoxia in polycythemia vera. *Ann Intern Med* 60:409, 1964.

219. Plata R, Cornejo A, Arratia C, et al: Angiotensin-converting-enzyme inhibition therapy in altitude polycythaemia: A prospective randomised trial. *Lancet* 359(9307):663, 2002.

220. Manglani MV, DeGroff CG, Dukes PP, et al: Congenital erythrocytosis with elevated erythropoietin level: An incorrectly set "erythrostat"? *J Pediatr Hematol Oncol* 20(6):560, 1998.

221. Piccirillo G, Fimognari FL, Valdivia JL, et al: Effects of phlebotomy on a patient with secondary polycythemia and angina pectoris. *Int J Cardiol* 44(2):175, 1994.

222. Watowich SS, Xie X, Klingmuller U, et al: Erythropoietin receptor mutations associated with familial erythrocytosis cause hypersensitivity to erythropoietin in the heterozygous state. *Blood* 94(7):2530, 1999.

223. de la Chapelle A, Traskelin AL and Juvonen E: Truncated erythropoietin receptor causes dominantly inherited benign human erythrocytosis. *Proc Natl Acad Sci U S A* 90(10):4495, 1993.

224. Furukawa T, Narita M, Sakaue M, et al: Primary familial polycythaemia associated with a novel point mutation in the erythropoietin receptor. *Br J Haematol* 99(1):222, 1997.

225. Arcasoy MO, Harris KW, Forget BG: A human erythropoietin receptor gene mutant causing familial erythrocytosis is associated with deregulation of the rates of Jak2 and Stat5 inactivation. *Exp Hematol* 27(1):63, 1999.

226. Kralovics R, Prchal JT: Genetic heterogeneity of primary familial and congenital polycythemia. *Am J Hematol* 68(2):115, 2001.

227. Sokol L, Luhovy M, Guan Y, et al: Primary familial polycythemia: A frameshift mutation in the erythropoietin receptor gene and increased sensitivity of erythroid progenitors to erythropoietin. *Blood* 86(1):15, 1995.

228. Kralovics R, Sokol L, Broxson EH Jr, et al: The erythropoietin receptor gene is not linked with the polycythemia phenotype in a family with autosomal dominant primary polycythemia. *Proc Assoc Am Physicians* 109(6):580, 1997.

229. Sokol L, Prchal JF, D'Andrea A, et al: Mutation in the negative regulatory element of the erythropoietin receptor gene in a case of sporadic primary polycythemia. *Exp Hematol* 22(5):447, 1994.

230. Le Couedic JP, Mitjavila MT, Villeval JL, et al: Missense mutation of the erythropoietin receptor is a rare event in human erythroid malignancies. *Blood* 87(4):1502, 1996.

231. Hultberg B, Sjoblad S and Ockerman PA: Properties of five acid hydrolases in human skin fibroblast cultures. Possible use in the diagnosis of inborn lysosomal diseases. *Acta Paediatr Scand* 62(5):474, 1973.

CHAPTER 58
THE PORPHYRIAS

John D. Phillips and Karl E. Anderson

SUMMARY

Porphyrias are diseases that result from derangements of specific enzymes in the heme biosynthetic pathway that lead to overproduction and accumulation of pathway intermediates and cause neurologic symptoms, photocutaneous symptoms or both. Multiple inherited mutations have been identified in all the porphyrias. However, porphyria cutanea tarda (PCT), which is caused primarily by an acquired deficiency of the fifth enzyme in the heme biosynthetic pathway, specifically in the liver, is usually not associated with a mutation of this enzyme.

Porphyrias can be classified as either hepatic or erythropoietic, depending on the principal site of initial accumulation of excess pathway intermediates. Erythropoietic porphyrias are characterized by childhood onset and a generally stable clinical course. Hepatic porphyrias almost always develop during adult life, and are more variable because of multiple influences of drugs, hormones, and nutritional factors on the heme biosynthetic pathway in the liver.

Porphyrias are also classified as acute or cutaneous. The four acute porphyrias are associated with neurologic manifestations that usually occur as acute attacks. δ-Aminolevulinate dehydratase porphyria (ADP) is an autosomal recessive disorder caused by a deficiency of the second enzyme in the pathway and is the rarest type of porphyria. ADP has been classified as hepatic, but also has erythropoietic features. The three other acute porphyrias, namely acute intermittent porphyria (AIP), hereditary coproporphyria (HCP), and variegate porphyria (VP), are autosomal dominant hepatic porphyrias, and result from deficiencies of the third, sixth, and seventh enzymes in the pathway, respectively. HCP and VP are also classified as cutaneous, because photocutaneous lesions may develop, especially in VP. AIP is the most common acute porphyria and the second most common porphyria. Disease expression is highly variable

in acute porphyrias, and the great majority of individuals who inherit deficiencies of these enzymes remain latent through all or most of their lives. Attacks are produced by factors that increase hepatic heme synthesis, including certain drugs, sex steroid hormones and their metabolites and restriction of dietary calories and carbohydrate. Treatment of acute porphyrias includes glucose loading and hemin infusions, which repress δ-aminolevulinic acid synthase-1, the rate-limiting enzyme of the heme biosynthetic pathway in the liver.

Cutaneous porphyrias are associated with either blistering skin lesions or, in erythropoietic protoporphyria (EPP), with acute nonblistering photosensitivity. Blistering skin manifestations are identical in PCT, HCP, and VP. Similar lesions in congenital erythropoietic porphyria (CEP) are much more severe and often associated with loss of digits and facial mutilation. CEP results from a severe deficiency of the fourth enzyme in the pathway and is inherited in an autosomal recessive fashion. Hemolytic anemia is common, and severe cases may be transfusion dependent, and may even present *in utero* with fetal hydrops. Hematopoietic stem cell transplantation in early childhood is the most effective treatment.

EPP is the third most common porphyria and the most common in children. It is usually caused by a deficiency of the final enzyme in the pathway. In most families, inheritance of EPP is best described as autosomal recessive, with a severe ferrochelatase mutation inherited from one parent and a low-expression variant allele from the other. X-linked protoporphyria (XLP) has the same phenotype as EPP, but is caused by gain-of-function mutations of δ-aminolevulinic acid synthase-2, which is expressed only in erythroblasts and reticulocytes. Protoporphyrin-containing gallstones may develop in EPP and XLP. An uncommon but potentially life-threatening complication is protoporphyric hepatopathy, which is a result of the cholestatic effects of protoporphyrin, and may require liver transplantation. Sequential marrow transplantation can prevent recurrent hepatopathy in the transplanted liver.

PCT is an iron-related hepatic porphyria that usually begins in middle or late adult life. Activity of hepatic uroporphyrinogen decarboxylase (UROD) is reduced in the presence of iron to approximately 20 percent of normal in PCT by a uroporphomethene inhibitor probably derived from uroporphyrinogen. Multiple susceptibility factors, including use of alcohol, smoking, estrogens, hepatitis C and HIV contribute. *HFE* (hemochromatosis gene) mutations that cause excess iron absorption are common in PCT. A minority of patients are heterozygous for UROD mutations and are said to have familial PCT. Polyhalogenated aromatic hydrocarbons cause PCT in laboratory animals and occasionally in humans. PCT responds well to treatment by repeated phlebotomy, which reduces hepatic iron, or low-dose hydroxychloroquine or chloroquine, which mobilizes accumulated hepatic porphyrins. Hepatoerythropoietic porphyria is the homozygous form of familial PCT, and is usually a severe disorder that starts in childhood and resembles CEP clinically.

Acronyms and Abbreviations: ADP, δ-aminolevulinate dehydratase deficiency porphyria; AIP, acute intermittent porphyria; ALA, δ-aminolevulinic acid; ALAD, δ-aminolevulinic acid dehydratase; ALAS, δ-aminolevulinic acid synthase; ALAS1, δ-aminolevulinic acid synthase, housekeeping form; ALAS2, δ-aminolevulinic acid synthase, erythroid-specific form; cDNA, complementary DNA to mRNA template; CEP, congenital erythropoietic porphyria; CPO, coproporphyrinogen oxidase; CPRE, coproporphyrinogen oxidase gene promoter regulatory element; CRIM, cross-reactive immunologic material; CYP, cytochrome P450; EC, enzyme commission; EPP, erythropoietic protoporphyria; FECH, ferrochelatase; HCP, hereditary coproporphyria; HEP, hepatoerythropoietic porphyria; *HFE*, hemochromatosis gene; HMB, hydroxymethylbilane; IRE, iron-responsive element; IRPs, iron-responsive element binding proteins; NRF-1, nuclear regulatory factor 1; PBG, porphobilinogen; PBGD, porphobilinogen deaminase; PCT, porphyria cutanea tarda; PGC-1a, peroxisomal proliferator-activated cofactor 1a; PPO, protoporphyrinogen oxidase; PXR, pregnane X receptor; SCS-βA, β subunit of ATP-specific succinyl coenzyme A synthetase; UROD, uroporphyrinogen decarboxylase; UROS, uroporphyrinogen synthase; VP, variegate porphyria; XLP, X-linked protoporphyria.

DEFINITION AND HISTORY

The porphyrias are a group of metabolic diseases resulting from derangements, usually of a genetic nature, in the activity of specific enzymes in the heme biosynthetic pathway, leading to overproduction and accumulation of pathway intermediates. Symptoms of these diseases can be neurologic, photocutaneous, or both. The intermediates that accumulate include porphyrins and the porphyrin precursors δ-aminolevulinic acid (ALA) and porphobilinogen (PBG) and their derivatives. Patterns of these substances in plasma, erythrocytes, urine, and feces are characteristic for each porphyria, and are the basis for screening tests and more comprehensive biochemical characterization.

Porphyrias are classified as either *erythropoietic* or *hepatic*, depending on the principal site of accumulation of pathway intermediates. The erythropoietic porphyrias are congenital erythropoietic porphyria (CEP), which is very rare, erythropoietic protoporphyria (EPP), the third most common porphyria and the most common in children, and X-linked protoporphyria (XLP), which has the same phenotype as EPP but is less common. Hepatic porphyrias include the acute porphyrias, which cause neurologic symptoms usually in the form of acute attacks, and porphyria cutanea tarda (PCT), which is the most common of the porphyrias, and causes chronic blistering lesions on sun-exposed areas of the skin. The acute porphyrias include ALA dehydratase deficiency porphyria (ADP), acute intermittent porphyria (AIP), hereditary coproporphyria (HCP), and variegate porphyria (VP). VP, and less commonly HCP, can also cause skin manifestations identical to those in PCT.

A type of porphyria is associated with loss-of-function mutations of seven of the eight enzymes in the heme biosynthetic pathway (Table 58–1 and Fig. 58–1) PCT is primarily caused by an acquired deficiency of the fifth pathway enzyme, with heterozygous mutations of that enzyme contributing in some cases. Gain-of-function mutations of ALAS2, the erythroid form of the first pathway enzyme, cause XLP, whereas loss-of-function mutations of this enzyme cause X-linked sideroblastic anemia (Chap. 59). Table 58–2 summarizes the major clinical and laboratory features of the porphyrias.

A case of CEP reported by Schultz in 1874 was the first description of porphyria in the literature. This case was a 33-year-old man with photosensitivity since age 3 months, anemia, splenomegaly, red-wine-colored urine as a result of a pigment resembling hematoporphyrin, and brown-colored bones at autopsy.[1,2] In 1898, T. McCall Anderson described two brothers (ages 23 and 26 years) who most likely had CEP,[3] and suffered from *hydroa aestivale*, with red urine, pruritus and blistering of sun-exposed skin, especially in summer, leading to extensive scarring and mutilation of the ears and nose (see Chap. 58, Fig. 58–5). Using available methods, their urine was also demonstrated to contain a substance related to hematoporphyrin.[4] In 1889, Stokvis first described a case of acute porphyria in an elderly woman who developed dark-red urine and later died after taking sulphonal, a drug related to the barbiturates.[5]

Hans Günther[6] published a monograph on porphyrins in 1911 and classified porphyrias into four groups: (1) those that have an acute onset without association with drug ingestion, (2) those that are caused by sulphonal or trional, (3) hematoporphyria congenita, and (4) chronic hematoporphyria. The first two groups correspond to the acute porphyrias, which may present with attacks sometimes related to ingestion of certain drugs, the second group to CEP and hepatoerythropoietic porphyria (HEP), and the fourth to PCT. In 1923, Archibald Garrod proposed the term *inborn errors of metabolism* for a number of inherited metabolic disorders, including the porphyrias.[7]

Sachs noted an Ehrlich-positive chromogen that was not urobilinogen in urine of patients with acute porphyria in 1931. In the late1930s, Waldenström noted that excretion of this chromogen was an autosomal dominant trait in AIP families, which he identified as PBG in 1939.[8] The classification of porphyrias as erythropoietic and hepatic was proposed in 1954 by Schmid, Schwartz, and Watson.[9] An epidemic of hexachlorobenzene-induced PCT in eastern Turkey in 1957[10,11] provided

TABLE 58–1. Human Porphyrias: Specific Enzymes Affected by Mutations, Modes of Inheritance, Classification, and Major Types of Clinical Features of Each of the Human Porphyrias

Porphyria*	Affected Enzyme	Known Mutations	Inheritance	Classification	Principal Clinical Features
X-linked protoporphyria	δ-Aminolevulinic acid (ALA) synthase–erythroid-specific form (ALAS2)	4 (gain of function)	X-linked recessive	Erythropoietic	Nonblistering photosensitivity
δ-Aminolevulinic acid dehydratase porphyria (ADP)	ALA dehydratase (ALAD)	10	Autosomal recessive	Hepatic†	Neurovisceral
Acute intermittent porphyria (AIP)	PBG deaminase (PBGD)	273	Autosomal dominant	Hepatic	Neurovisceral
Congenital erythropoietic porphyria (CEP)	Uroporphyrinogen III synthase (UROS)	36	Autosomal recessive	Erythropoietic	Neurovisceral
Porphyria cutanea tarda (PCT)	Uroporphyrinogen decarboxylase (UROD)	70 (includes HEP)	Autosomal dominant‡	Hepatic	Blistering photosensitivity
Hepatoerythropoietic porphyria (HEP)	UROD	–	Autosomal recessive	Hepatic†	Blistering photosensitivity
Hereditary coproporphyria (HCP)	Coproporphyrinogen oxidase (CPO)	42	Autosomal dominant	Hepatic	Neurovisceral; blistering photosensitivity (uncommon)
Variegate porphyria (VP)	Protoporphyrinogen oxidase (PPO)	130	Autosomal dominant	Hepatic	Neurovisceral; blistering photosensitivity (common)
Erythropoietic protoporphyria (EPP)	Ferrochelatase (FECH)	90	Autosomal recessive	Erythropoietic	Nonblistering photosensitivity

*Porphyrias are listed in the order of the affected enzyme in the heme biosynthetic pathway.

†These porphyrias also have erythropoietic features, including increases in erythrocyte zinc protoporphyrin.

‡UROD inhibition in PCT is mostly acquired, but an inherited deficiency of the enzyme predisposes in familial (type 2) disease.

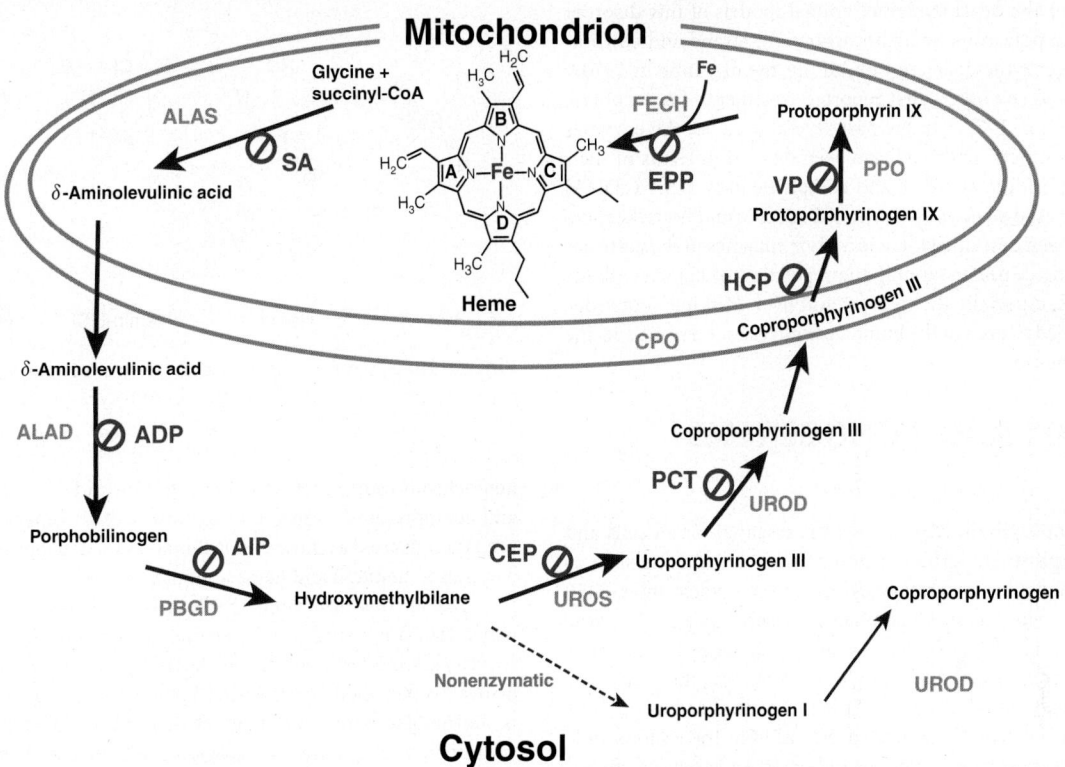

Figure 58–1. Enzymes and intermediates in the heme biosynthetic pathway and the type of porphyria associated with a deficiency of each enzyme (indicated by Ø). Gain-of-function mutation of the erythroid form of ALA synthase is not shown. ADP, ALA dehydratase porphyria; AIP, acute intermittent porphyria; ALA, δ-aminolevulinic acid; ALAD, δ-aminolevulinic acid dehydratase; ALAS, δ-aminolevulinic acid synthase; CEP, congenital erythropoietic porphyria; CoA, coenzyme A; CPO, coproporphyrinogen oxidase; EPP, erythropoietic protoporphyria; FECH, ferrochelatase; HCP, hereditary coproporphyria; PBG, porphobilinogen; PBGD, porphobilinogen deaminase; PCT, porphyria cutanea tarda; PPO, protoporphyrinogen oxidase; SA, sideroblastic anemia; UROD, uroporphyrinogen decarboxylase; UROS, uroporphyrinogen III synthase; VP, variegate porphyria.

TABLE 58–2. Biochemical Findings Including Major Increases in Porphyrins and Porphyrin Precursors in the Human Porphyrias

Porphyria	Erythrocytes	Plasma	Urine	Stool
XLP	Metal-free and zinc protoporphyrin§	Protoporphyrin (~634 nm)‡	¶	Protoporphyrin*
ADP	Zinc protoporphyrin	ALA*	ALA, coproporphyrin III	*
AIP	Decreased PBGD activity (most cases)*	ALA, PBG* (~620 nm, some cases)†	ALA, PBG, uroporphyrin	*
CEP	Uroporphyrin I; coproporphyrin I	Uroporphyrin I, coproporphyrin I (~620 nm)†	Uroporphyrin I; coproporphyrin I	Coproporphyrin I
PCT and HEP	Zinc protoporphyrin (in HEP)	Uroporphyrin, heptacarboxyl porphyrin (~620 nm)†	Uroporphyrin, heptacarboxyl porphyrin	Heptacarboxyl porphyrin, isocoproporphyrins
HCP	*	‡(~620 nm, some cases)†	ALA, PBG, coproporphyrin III	Coproporphyrin III
VP	*	Protoporphyrin (~628 nm)†	ALA, PBG, coproporphyrin III	Coproporphyrin III, protoporphyrin
EPP	Metal-free protoporphyrin§	Protoporphyrin (~634 nm)†	¶	Protoporphyrin*

ADP, δ-aminolevulinate dehydratase deficiency porphyria; AIP, acute intermittent porphyria; ALA, δ-aminolevulinic acid; CEP, congenital erythropoietic porphyria; EPP, erythropoietic protoporphyria; HCP, hereditary coproporphyria; HEP, hepatoerythropoietic porphyria; PBG, porphobilinogen; PCT, porphyria cutanea tarda; VP, variegate porphyria; XLP, X-linked protoporphyria.

*Porphyrin levels normal or slightly increased.

†Fluorescence emission peak of diluted plasma at neutral pH.

‡Plasma porphyrins usually normal, but increased when blistering skin lesions develop.

§Zinc protoporphyrin ≤15 percent of total in EPP, but 15 to 50 percent in XLP.

¶Increase in urine porphyrins (especially coproporphyrin) only with hepatopathy.

the foundation for the development of animal models of this disorder using halogenated polyaromatic hydrocarbons.[12,13] Strand and coworkers described the enzyme deficiency in AIP for the first time in 1970,[14] and Bonkovsky and coworkers first reported treatment of a porphyria patient with hemin in 1971.[15] In the past several decades, the enzymes of the heme biosynthetic pathway have been defined in terms of their amino acid composition, genomic and complementary DNA (cDNA) sequences, and crystal structures. Erythroid-specific and housekeeping transcripts have been described for at least four enzymes in the pathway, and progress made in understanding the regulation of heme synthesis in specific tissues, especially the marrow and liver. Multiple mutations have been described in each of the human porphyrias, and some specific treatments introduced.

● ETIOLOGY AND PATHOGENESIS

HEME

Heme (iron protoporphyrin IX; Fig. 58–2) is essential for all cells and functions as the prosthetic group of numerous hemoproteins such as hemoglobin, myoglobin, respiratory cytochromes, cytochromes P450 (CYPs), catalase, peroxidase, tryptophan pyrrolase, and nitric oxide synthase. Approximately 85 percent of heme is synthesized in the marrow to meet the requirement for hemoglobin formation; the remainder is synthesized largely in the liver.[16] Most heme synthesized in the liver is required for CYPs, which are located primarily in the endoplasmic reticulum where they turn over rapidly and oxidize a variety of chemicals, including drugs, environmental carcinogens, endogenous steroids, vitamins, fatty acids, and prostaglandins.[17]

The term *heme* may refer more specifically to ferrous protoporphyrin IX, and is readily oxidized *in vitro* to hemin, that is, ferric protoporphyrin IX. Hemin has one residual positive charge and is usually isolated as a halide, most commonly as the chloride. In alkaline solution the halide is replaced by a hydroxyl ion to form hematin (Fig. 58–3). Heme can form further hexacoordinated complexes with nitrogenous bases to form a *hemochrome* or *hemochromogen;* for example, pyridine

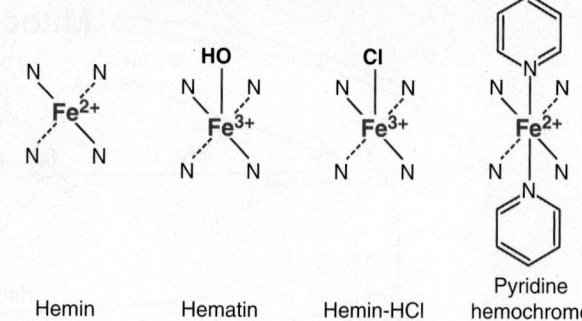

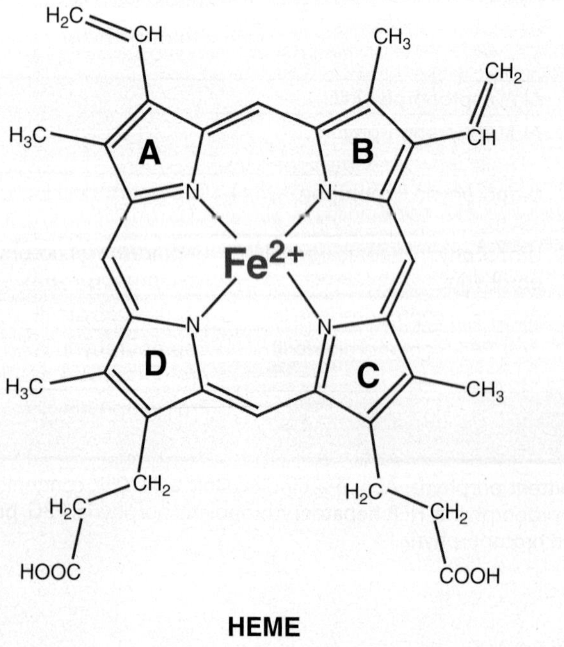

Figure 58–3. Forms of iron protoporphyrin IX. The porphyrin macrocycle is represented only by its pyrrole nitrogen atoms.

hemochromogen is useful for identification and quantification of heme and hemoproteins. In medicine, hemin is also a generic term for heme preparations used as intravenous therapies for acute porphyrias, such as lyophilized hematin and heme arginate.

The ferrous iron atom (Fe^{2+}) in heme has six electron pairs, of which four are bound to the pyrrolic nitrogens of the porphyrin macrocycle, leaving two unoccupied electron pairs, one above and the other below the plane of the porphyrin ring. In hemoglobin, one of these pairs is coordinated with a histidine residue of the globin chain. The other coordination site in deoxyhemoglobin is protected from oxidation by the nonpolar environment of surrounding amino acid residues, and is available to bind molecular oxygen for transport from the lung to other tissues. To reversibly bind oxygen, the iron in hemoglobin must be in the ferrous state. Methemoglobin (oxidized hemoglobin) that is generated in erythrocytes is continuously reduced to ferrous hemoglobin by the reduced form of nicotinamide adenine dinucleotide–cytochrome b_5 reductase–cytochrome b_5 system (Chap. 50).

Heme Biosynthesis

Figure 58–4 shows the enzymatic steps involved in heme biosynthesis in eukaryotic cells. The first and last three enzymes are mitochondrial and the intermediate four are cytosolic. Erythroid heme synthesis occurs in marrow erythroblasts and reticulocytes, which contain mitochondria. Circulating erythrocytes lack mitochondria and no longer synthesize heme. They contain residual cytosolic enzymes of the heme biosynthetic pathway, zinc protoporphyrin and a small amount of metal-free protoporphyrin. These enzyme activities and protoporphyrin decline during the life span of erythrocytes in the circulation.

δ-Aminolevulinate Synthase (Succinyl Coenzyme A: Glycine C-Succinyl Transferase; Enzyme Commission (EC) 2.3.1.37) The first enzyme in the heme biosynthetic pathway catalyzes the condensation of glycine and succinyl coenzyme A (CoA) to form ALA (see Fig. 58–4, *step 1*), and requires pyridoxal 5′-phosphate as a cofactor. δ-Aminolevulinic acid synthase (ALAS) in mammalian cells is localized to the mitochondrial matrix.[18] The enzyme is synthesized as a precursor protein in the cytosol and transported into mitochondria. Two separate ALAS genes encode housekeeping (tissue nonspecific) and erythroid-specific forms of the enzyme (ALAS1 and ALAS2, respectively).[19] The gene locus for human ALAS1 is at 3p.21, and for ALAS2 it is at Xp11.2.[19] The human ALAS2 gene encodes a precursor of 587 amino acids, with an Mr of 64,600 Da. Nucleotide sequences for the ALAS2 and the ALAS1 isoforms are approximately 60 percent similar. No homology is observed between the aminoterminal regions, whereas high homology (approximately 73 percent) is seen after residue 197 of the housekeeping form.[21] The two human ALAS genes appear to have evolved by duplication of a common ancestral gene that encoded a primitive catalytic

HEME

Figure 58–2. Structure of heme. The pyrrole rings are labeled A through D, according to the nomenclature of Hans Fischer.

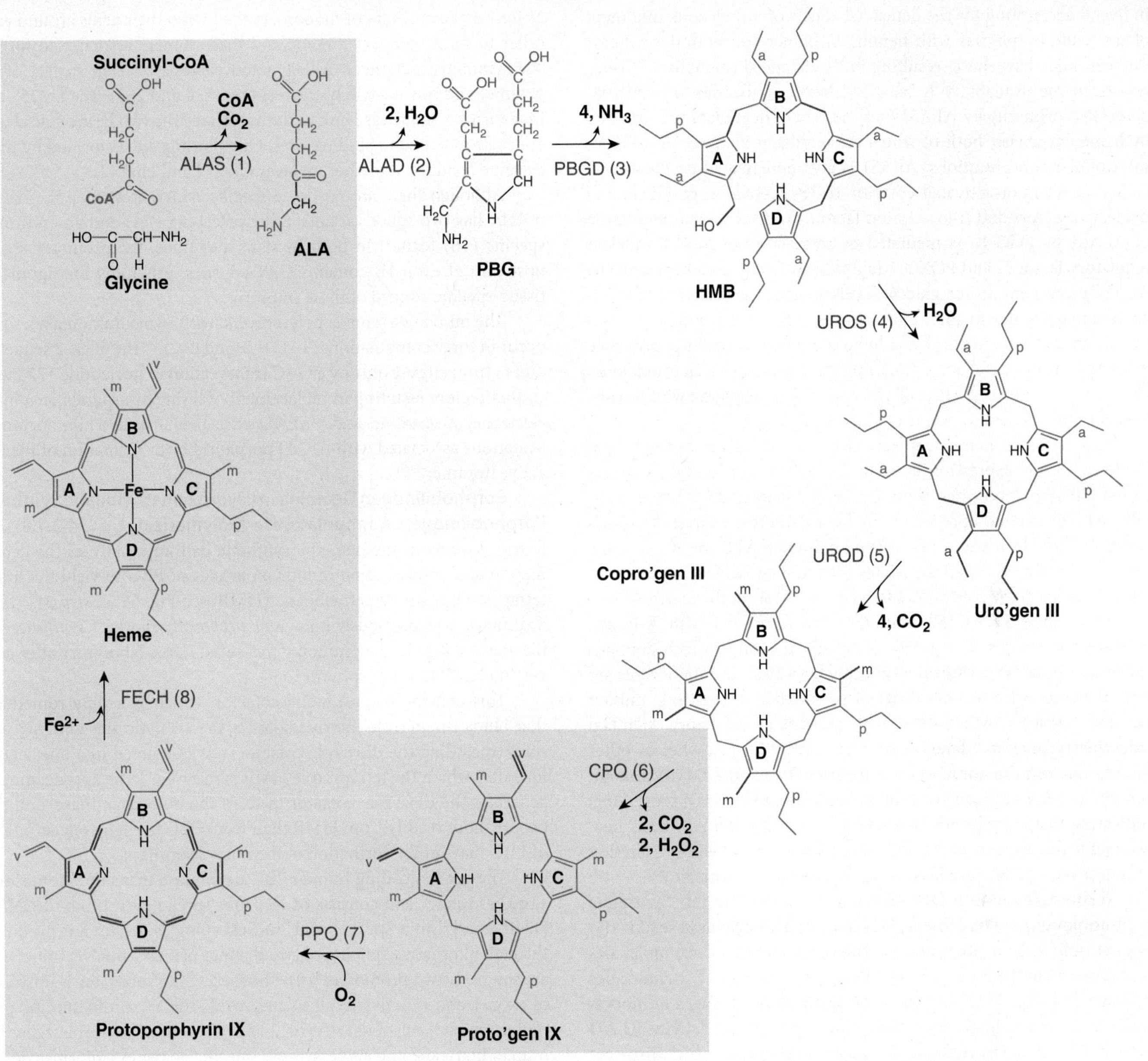

Figure 58–4. The heme biosynthetic pathway. The subcellular distribution of the eight enzymes and their substrates and intermediates are shown; enzymes within the light blue shading are located in the mitochondrion, and the others in the cytosol. The substrate positions that are changed are shown in blue, bold lines. ALA, δ-aminolevulinic acid; Copro'gen, coproporphyrinogen; HMB, hydroxymethylbilane; PBG, porphobilinogen; Proto'gen, protoporphyrinogen; Uro'gen, uroporphyrinogen. a, $-CH_2COOH$; p, $-CH_2-CH_2-COOH$; m, $-CH_3$; v, $-CH=CH_2$; carbon groups shown in red, carbon atom derived from the α-carbon of glycine; *, location of the α-carbon atom from glycine in the pyrrole ring that undergoes reversion. *Step 1*, ALA synthase (ALAS); *step 2*, ALA dehydratase (ALAD); *step 3*, PBG deaminase (PBGD); *step 4*, uro'gen III cosynthase (UROS); *step 5*, uro'gen decarboxylase (UROD); *step 6*, copro'gen oxidase (CPO); *step 7*, proto'gen oxidase (PPO); *step 8*, ferrochelatase (FECH).

site. Subsequently the DNA sequences were modified to encode gene-specific regulatory regions, functioning mostly at the amino termini.[22]

The promoter in the human ALAS2 gene contains several putative erythroid-specific *cis*-acting elements including both a GATA-1 and an NF-E2 binding site.[22,23] Both GATA-1 and NF-E2 are erythroid transcription factors that also bind other DNA sites, such as the promoters of the human β-globin, porphobilinogen deaminase (PBGD), and uroporphyrinogen synthase (UROS) genes.[24] Thus, expression of ALAS2 is under the regulatory influence of erythroid transcription factors such as GATA-1 and is coordinated with expression of other genes involved in hemoglobin synthesis. Additionally, ALAS2 mRNA

contains an iron-responsive element in its 5′-untranslated region,[23] similar to mRNAs encoding ferritin and the transferrin receptor (Chap. 42).[25] Gel retardation analysis shows that the iron-responsive element in ALAS2 mRNA is functional and suggests that translation of the erythroid-specific mRNA is directly linked to the availability of iron, or heme, in erythroid cells.[26]

In the liver, synthesis of ALAS1 is induced by a variety of chemicals, including drugs and steroids that increase the demand for hepatic CYPs. Upstream enhancer elements in the ALAS1 gene and certain hepatic CYP genes respond to inducing chemicals and interact with the pregnane X receptor (PXR).[27] Hemin represses synthesis of ALAS1 in liver,[28] accounting for the beneficial effects of intravenous treatment of the acute porphyrias with hemin. At higher concentrations, heme induces heme oxygenase, resulting in its enhanced catabolism.[29] Thus, hepatic heme availability is balanced between the rate of synthesis controlled primarily by ALAS1 and the rate of degradation controlled by heme oxygenase, both of which are regulated by heme at different intracellular concentrations. ALAS1 is also upregulated by the peroxisomal proliferator-activated cofactor 1α (PGC-1α),[30] a coactivator of nuclear receptors and transcription factors. Transcriptional regulation of ALAS1 by PGC-1α is mediated by interaction of NRF-1 (nuclear regulatory factor 1) and FOXO-1 (a forkhead family member) with the ALAS1 promoter.[31] When glucose levels are low, transcription of PGC-1α is upregulated,[32] in turn increasing ALAS1, which might precipitate an attack of acute porphyria in an individual with the appropriate inherited enzyme deficiency. Thus, upregulation of PGC-1α provides an explanation for the induction of acute attacks of porphyria with fasting, as well as the therapeutic value of glucose loading.

Regulation of heme synthesis in erythroid cells is distinct from the liver. ALAS2 expression in erythroid cells is increased during erythroid differentiation when heme synthesis is increased.[33,34] Experimentally, ALAS2 is often upregulated by heme, whereas in liver ALAS1 is downregulated by heme. The β subunit of human ATP-specific succinyl CoA synthetase (SCS-βA) associates with human ALAS2 but not with ALAS1, and thereby contributes to heme synthesis in the marrow.[35]

More than 20 ALAS2 mutations are associated with X-linked sideroblastic anemia (Chap. 59); many are in exon 9, which contains the binding site for pyridoxal 5′-phosphate (K391), and these cases are typically responsive to high doses of pyridoxine. At least one mutant enzyme (D190V) in a patient with pyridoxine-refractory X-linked sideroblastic anemia,[36] failed to associate with SCS-βA, whereas other ALAS2 mutants did not have this property. The mature D190V mutant protein, but not its precursor protein, underwent abnormal processing; indicating that appropriate association of SCS-βA and ALAS2 is necessary for functioning of ALAS2 in mitochondria.[36] Gain-of-function mutations of ALAS2 have been identified in patients with XLP.[37]

δ-Aminolevulinate Dehydratase (Porphobilinogen Synthase; δ-Aminolevulinate Hydrolase; EC 4.2.1.24) ALA dehydratase (ALAD) is a cytosolic enzyme that catalyzes the condensation of two molecules of ALA to form the monopyrrole PBG, with removal of two molecules of water (see Fig. 58–4, *step 2*). The enzyme functions as a homooctamer, and requires intact sulfhydryl groups and zinc for activity. ALAD activity is inhibited by sulfhydryl reagents[38] and by lead, which displaces zinc.[39] In lead poisoning (Chap. 52), erythrocyte ALAD activity is markedly inhibited, urinary ALA and coproporphyrin excretion increased, erythrocyte zinc protoporphyrin elevated, and neurologic symptoms resemble those seen in acute porphyrias.[40] 4,6-Dioxoheptanoic acid (succinylacetone) is a substrate analogue and potent inhibitor of ALAD,[41,42] and is a byproduct of the enzyme deficiency in hereditary tyrosinemia type I. This substance is found in urine and blood of patients with this disease, who may also have increased ALA and symptoms resembling acute porphyrias.[43]

Human ALAD mRNA has an open-reading frame of 990 bp, encoding a protein with an Mr of 36,274.[44] Sequences known to be essential for enzymatic activity, are those for the active site lysine residues and for the cysteine- and histidine-rich zinc binding sites. The gene for human ALAD is localized to chromosome 9p34.[45]

Studies using [^{14}C]-ALA have shown that of the two ALA molecules used as substrate, the ALA molecule contributing the propionic acid side is initially bound to the enzyme.[38] The tertiary structure of the yeast ALAD has been solved to 2.3-Å resolution, revealing that each subunit adopts a triosephosphate isomerase barrel fold with a 39-residue

N-terminal arm. Pairs of monomers then wrap their arms around each other to form compact dimers, and these dimers associate to form a 422 symmetric octamer.[46] All eight active sites are on the surface of the octamer and possess two lysine residues (210 and 263). The Lys263 residue forms a Schiff base link to the substrate. The two lysine side chains are close to two zinc binding sites. One binding site is formed by three cysteine residues; the other involves Cys234 and His142.

Although there are no tissue-specific ALAD isozymes, the ALAD mRNA has two splice variants, a housekeeping (1A) and an erythroid-specific (1B) form.[45] In both humans and mice, the promoter region upstream of exon 1B contains GATA-1 sites, providing for significant tissue-specific control of these transcripts.[47]

The human enzyme is polymorphic with two common alleles that occur in three combinations (1–1, 1–2, and 2–2).[44] The allele 2 sequence differs from allele 1 only by a G→C transversion of nucleotide 177 in the coding region, resulting in replacement of lysine by asparagine, a more electronegative amino acid.[48] ALAD exists primarily as a homooctamer. Mutations associated with ALAD porphyria favor formation of the less active hexamer.[49,50]

Porphobilinogen Deaminase (Hydroxymethylbilane Synthase; Porphobilinogen Ammonia-Lyase [Polymerizing], EC 4.3.1.8) The fourth enzyme in the heme biosynthetic pathway catalyzes the deamination and condensation of four molecules of PBG to yield the linear tetrapyrrole hydroxymethylbilane (HMB; see Fig. 58–4, *step 3*).[51] PBG deaminase was previously known as *uroporphyrinogen I synthase*, and the enzyme activity is commonly measured in the laboratory after converting HMB to uroporphyrin I.

This enzyme has a unique cofactor, which is a dipyrromethane that binds the pyrrole intermediates at the catalytic site until six pyrroles (including the dipyrrole cofactor) are assembled in a linear fashion, after which the tetrapyrrole HMB is released.[52] The apo-deaminase generates the dipyrrole cofactor to form the holo-deaminase, and this occurs more readily from HMB than from PBG.[53] High concentrations of PBG may inhibit formation of the holo-deaminase.

The gene encoding human PBG deaminase maps to chromosome 11q23→11qter,[54] and consists of 15 exons spread over 10 kb of DNA.[55] Distinct erythroid-specific and housekeeping isoforms are produced through alternative splicing of two distinct primary mRNA transcripts arising from two promoters.[56] The housekeeping promoter is upstream of exon 1 and is active in all tissues, while the erythroid-specific promoter, which is upstream of exon 2, is active only in erythroid cells. The human housekeeping and erythroid-specific enzymes isoforms contain 361 and 344 amino acid residues, respectively.[57] Of the additional 17 residues at the N-terminal end of the housekeeping form, 11 are encoded by exon 1, and 6 by a short segment of exon 3 that immediately precedes a methionine codon that initiates translation of the erythroid isoform. Erythroid-specific *trans*-acting factors, such as GATA-1 and NF-E2, recognize sequences in the erythroid promoter.[58] A 1320-bp stretch of perfect identity is present between the erythroid and the nonerythroid PBG deaminase, but with a mismatch in the first exon at their 5′ extremities. An additional inframe AUG codon present 51 bp upstream from the initiating codon of the erythroid cDNA accounts for the additional 17 amino acid residues at the N-terminus of the housekeeping isoform. Accordingly, a splice site mutation at the last position of exon 1, or a base transition in intron 1, in certain patients with AIP results in decreased PBG deaminase expression in nonerythroid tissues including the liver, but not in erythroid cells, because transcription of the gene in erythroid cells starts downstream of the site of the genetic lesion.[59]

Uroporphyrinogen III Synthase (Uroporphyrinogen III Cosynthase; EC 4.2.1.75) UROS, a cytosolic enzyme, catalyzes the formation of uroporphyrinogen III from HMB. The process involves an intramolecular rearrangement that affects only ring D of the porphyrin macrocycle (see Fig. 58–4, *step 4*).[51] In the absence of this enzyme, HMB spontaneously forms the ring structure uroporphyrinogen I, which, like the III isomer, is a substrate for uroporphyrinogen decarboxylase (UROD). However, because coproporphyrinogen I is not a substrate for coproporphyrinogen oxidase (CPO) the type I porphyrinogen isomers are not further metabolized, and only the type III isomers are precursors of heme.

The UROS cDNA has an open-reading frame of 798 bp, and the predicted protein product consists of 263 amino acid residues, with an Mr of 28,607 Da.[20] The amino acid compositions of the hepatic and the purified erythrocyte enzyme are essentially identical, and no tissue-specific isoforms have been described.

The interspecies homology for the UROS proteins is below 10 percent, depending on the number and divergence of the species being compared. However, the crystal structures of uroporphyrinogen III synthase from human and *Thermus thermophilus* have been solved and are very similar.[60,61] The structure supports a mechanism that includes the formation of a spirolactam intermediate by positioning the A and D rings such that the noncatalytic closure, to form uroporphyrinogen I, is not possible.[61]

Uroporphyrinogen Decarboxylase (EC 4.1.1.37) UROD is a cytosolic enzyme that catalyzes the sequential removal of the four carboxylic groups of the carboxymethyl side chains in uroporphyrinogen to yield coproporphyrinogen (see Fig. 58–4, *step 5*). The four successive decarboxylation reactions yield 7-, 6-, 5-, and 4-carboxylated porphyrinogens. Increased amounts of these intermediates can be identified as the corresponding oxidized porphyrins in liver, plasma, urine and stool in human PCT and in laboratory animal models in which hepatic UROD is inhibited. An inhibitor of UROD activity, a partially oxidized substrate molecule,[62] is produced in liver of experimental animals in response to halogenated polycyclic aromatic hydrocarbons such as hexachlorobenzene, dioxin, and polychlorinated biphenyls, as well as other compounds able to activate the Ah receptor.[63] This porphomethene compound is believed to explain UROD inhibition in human PCT.[62] Human UROD is a 42-kDa polypeptide encoded by a single gene containing 10 exons spread over 3 kb and functions as a homodimer.[64] The gene has been mapped to chromosome 1p34.[65]

Although the UROD gene contains two initiation sites, both sites are used with the same frequencies in all tissues, and the gene is transcribed into a single mRNA.[66] Recombinant human UROD purified to homogeneity has been crystallized, and its crystal structure was determined at 1.60-Å resolution.[67] The purified protein is a dimer with a dissociation constant of 0.1 μM.[67] The 40.8-kDa polypeptide forms a single domain with a distorted $(\beta/\alpha)_8$-barrel fold, and a distinctive deep cleft for the enzyme's active site is formed by loops at the C-terminal ends of the barrel strands. The protein forms a homodimer with one active-site cleft per monomer located adjacent to its neighbor in the dimer. The structure creates a single extended cleft that is large enough to accommodate two substrate molecules in close proximity. Although both uroporphyrinogen I and III are metabolized by UROD, only the coproporphyrinogen III isomer is further metabolized to heme.[68]

Coproporphyrinogen Oxidase (EC 4.1.1.37) CPO is located on the outer surface of the inner mitochondrial membrane in mammalian cells.[69] The enzyme catalyzes the removal of the carboxyl group and two hydrogens from the propionic groups of pyrrole rings A and B, forming vinyl groups at these positions (see Fig. 58–4, *step 6*). The enzyme is isomer specific for coproporphyrinogen III, yielding protoporphyrinogen IX (see Fig. 58–4, *step 6*). The gene for human CPO has been assigned to chromosome 3q12, spans approximately 14 kb, and consists of seven exons and six introns.[70] cDNA cloning for this enzyme was first reported in mouse erythroleukemia cells.[71] The predicted mouse protein comprises

354 amino acid residues (Mr = 40,647 Da), with a putative leader sequence of 31 amino acid residues. The result is a mature protein consisting of 323 amino acid residues (Mr = 37,225 Da).[71] Potential regulatory elements exist in the GC-rich promoter region of the gene, such as six Sp1, four GATA-1, one CACCC site, and the *CPO* gene promoter regulatory element (CPRE).[72] CPRE binds specifically to a CPRE-binding protein, which has a leucine-zipper-like structure and serves as a DNA sequence-specific transcription factor that regulates gene expression.[72] Tissue-specific expression of CPO is significant. For example, binding proteins to the Spl-like element, CPRE and GATA-1, cooperatively function in *CPO* gene expression in erythroid cells. The CPRE-binding protein by itself plays a principal role in basal expression of CPO in nonerythroid cells.[73] *CPO* mRNA increases during erythroid cell differentiation.[74]

Newly synthesized human CPO contains a 110-amino-acid N-terminal signal peptide,[74] which is removed during transport into the intermembrane space of mitochondria, yielding a mature protein of 354 amino acid residues (Mr = 36,842 Da). A five-base insertional mutation in the middle of this presequence has been described in one patient with HCP.[75]

Protoporphyrinogen Oxidase (EC 1.3.3.4) The penultimate step in heme biosynthesis is the oxidation of protoporphyrinogen IX to protoporphyrin IX, with removal of six hydrogen atoms. This reaction is mediated by the mitochondrial enzyme protoporphyrinogen oxidase (PPO; see Fig. 58–4, *step 7*). Human PPO cDNA has been cloned.[76] The gene is present as a single copy per haploid genome, at chromosome 1q22.[77] PPO consists of 477 amino acids with an Mr of 50,800 Da. The deduced protein exhibits a high degree of homology over its entire length to the amino acid sequence of PPO encoded by the *HEMY* gene of *Bacillus subtilis*. PPO has been crystallized and the structure shows that the enzyme is a homodimer.[78] Sequences required for import into the mitochondria have been identified.[79] Expression of PPO is upregulated, approximately fourfold, in the developing erythron from two GATA-1 binding sites located in exon 1.[80]

Ferrochelatase (Protoheme-Ferrolyase; EC 4.99.1.1) The final step of heme biosynthesis is the insertion of iron into protoporphyrin IX. This reaction is catalyzed by the mitochondrial enzyme ferrochelatase (FECH; see Fig. 58–4, *step 8*). The enzyme uses protoporphyrin IX, rather than its reduced form, as substrate, but requires the reduced ferrous form of iron.[81] The gene encoding human FECH has been assigned to chromosome 18q.[82] Two FECH mRNA species, approximately 2.5 kb and approximately 1.6 kb in size, are derived from the utilization of two alternative polyadenylation sites in the mRNA. The human FECH gene contains a total of 11 exons and has a minimum size of approximately 45 kb. A major site of transcription initiation is at an adenine, 89 bp upstream from the translation-initiating ATG. The promoter region contains a potential binding site for several transcription factors, Sp1, NF-E2, and GATA-1, but not a typical TATA or CAAT sequence. The transcripts are identical in all tissues examined.

The crystal structure of *B. subtilis* FECH has been determined at 1.9-Å resolution.[83] Subsequently the structure of human FECH was solved and the location of the substrate binding site determined. The enzyme functions as a homodimer and associates with the inside of the inner mitochondrial membrane.[83] The mechanism of catalysis has not been identified nor has a function been assigned to the ^2Fe-^2S cluster that is present in human FECH. Lead inhibits FECH, and a structure of the protein-lead complex has been solved indicating a critical role for the pi helix in catalysis.[84] FECH seems to have a structurally conserved core region that is common to the enzyme from bacteria, plants, and mammals.

Control of Heme Synthesis in the Liver and Erythroid Cells

Tissue-specific aspects of heme synthesis have been studied mostly in erythroid cells and hepatocytes, as the marrow and liver have the greatest requirements for heme. The rate of heme synthesis in the liver is largely regulated by ALAS1 activity. The synthesis of ALAS1, in turn, is under feedback control by heme, which regulates ALAS1 at the levels of transcription, translation, and transfer into mitochondria. Many chemicals, hormones, and drugs increase the synthesis of hepatic CYPs, which increases the demand for heme and lead to induction of ALAS1. In addition, the ALAS1 gene contains upstream enhancer elements that are responsive to inducing chemicals and interact with the PXR. Therefore, ALAS1 and CYPs are subject to direct induction by xenobiotics and certain steroids.[27] Chemical exposures that induce hepatic heme oxygenase and accelerate the destruction of hepatic heme, or inhibit heme formation, can also induce hepatic ALAS1.

ALAS2 is not inducible in erythroid cells by drugs that induce ALAS1 in hepatocytes.[85] The synthesis of ALAS2 is uninfluenced, or often upregulated, by hemin, at both the transcriptional and the translational levels. Hemin treatment of marrow cultures increases erythroid colony-forming units,[86] whereas hemin treatment of hepatocytes inhibits synthesis of ALAS1 and CYPs. An additional distinct difference in these ALAS isoforms is that SCS-βA associates with ALAS2 but not with ALAS1, suggesting a tissue-specific difference in mitochondrial transport of these isoforms.

● ERYTHROPOIETIC PORPHYRIAS

There are two major erythropoietic porphyrias in humans. CEP is caused by mutations of the *UROS* gene. It is one of the least-common porphyrias, but is well known as a result of its long history and the severe photomutilation of exposed areas such as the face and fingers that is a dramatic feature in many cases (Fig. 58–5). EPP, which is caused by *FECH* mutations, is the third most common porphyria, and the most common in children, but was not well described until 1965. XLP is much less common, has the same phenotype as EPP, but normal FECH activity. In 2008, the discovery of gain-of-function mutations in the last exon of ALAS2 provided an explanation for the increased level of erythrocyte protoporphyrin seen in this type of protoporphyria.[37] Characteristics in most patients with erythropoietic porphyrias that are distinct from the hepatic porphyrias include childhood onset, stable symptoms and levels of porphyrins over time, and severity largely determined by genotype rather than factors that affect the heme pathway, primarily in the liver. Substantial increases in erythrocyte zinc protoporphyrin in ADP and homozygous forms of other hepatic porphyrias, such as HEP (the homozygous form of familial PCT), AIP, HCP, and VP, suggest that an erythropoietic component may be important in these conditions.[87]

CONGENITAL ERYTHROPOIETIC PORPHYRIA

Definition and History

CEP is caused by a deficiency of UROS (see Fig. 58–4, *step 4*), is an autosomal recessive condition, and is also known as Günther disease. It results in accumulation and excretion of isomer I porphyrins, especially uroporphyrin I and coproporphyrin I (see Table 58–1 and Fig. 58–1). Characteristic manifestations of CEP include chronic, severe photosensitivity and hemolytic anemia evident in early childhood. Atypical presentations include milder disease that resembles PCT, and onset during adult life often in association with a myeloproliferative disorder.[88] Early case descriptions of CEP appeared in 1874 and 1898,[3] and approximately 130 cases were reported up to 1997.[89] However, some of these patients may have had HEP, which has very similar clinical features. Perhaps the most well-known patient was Mathias Petry, who survived until age 34, and beginning in 1915, worked with the porphyrin chemist Hans Fisher, providing samples for early studies of porphyrin chemistry.[90]

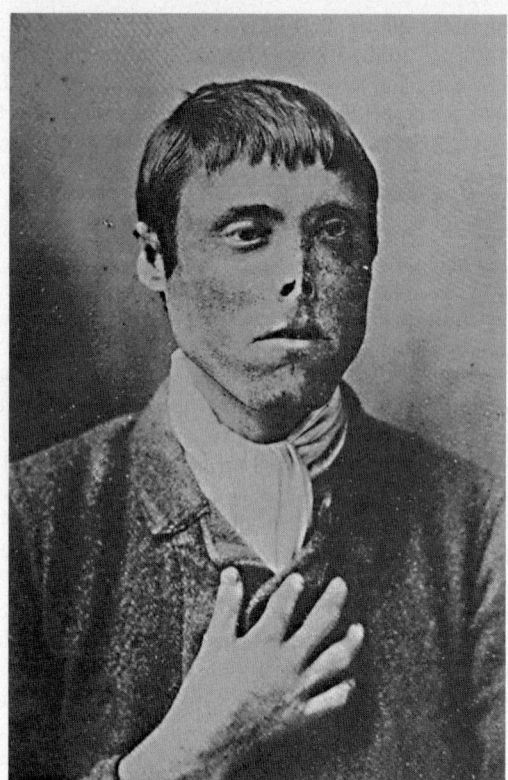

Figure 58–5. A 23-year-old Scottish fisherman with congenital erythropoietic porphyria and scarring and mutilation of the face, ears, and digits as a consequence of repeated sun exposure. He was described in 1898 as having red urine containing excess porphyrins and "hydroa aestivale," because the symptoms, which began at age 3 years, worsened in early summer. A 26-year-old brother was similarly affected. *(Reproduced with permission from Anderson TM: Hydroa aestivale in two brothers, complicated with the presence of haematoporphyrin in the urine.* Br J Dermatol *10:1, 1898.)*

Pathophysiology

The uroporphyrinogen III synthase defects in CEP are remarkably heterogeneous at the molecular level, with at least 46 different mutations of the *UROS* gene, and one *GATA-1* mutation reported as of this writing.[87] The UROS mutations include deletions, insertions, rearrangements, splicing abnormalities, and both missense and nonsense mutations.

The missense mutations are well distributed throughout the gene. Of the 12 single-base substitutions, four (T228M, G225S, A66V, A104V) were hotspot mutations, occurring at CpG dinucleotides.[91] The identification of a mutation that altered the penultimate nucleotide in exon 4, resulting in an E81D mutation, also produced exon skipping on approximately 85 percent of the transcripts from that allele. With the exception of V82F, all CEP missense mutations occurred in amino acid residues that are conserved in both the mouse and the human enzyme.

Genotype–phenotype correlation in CEP was studied by prokaryotic expression of mutant *UROS* cDNAs. Mean activities of the mutant enzymes expressed in *Escherichia coli* ranged from 0 to 36 percent of the activity expressed by the normal cDNA. The majority of the mutant cDNAs expressed polypeptides with no enzymatic activity. However, V82F, E81D, A66V, A104V, and V99A showed 36, 30, 15, 8, and 6 percent enzyme activity, respectively, compared with the normal control. A66V and V82F were thermodynamically unstable mutants.[91] Homoallelism for C73R, the most common mutation, found in five patients, was associated clinically with the most severe phenotypes, such as hydrops fetalis and transfusion dependency from birth.

Pathogenesis of the Clinical Findings

Porphyrins in their oxidized state are reddish, fluorescent, and photo-sensitizing, whereas porphyrin precursors and the reduced porphyrinogens are colorless and nonfluorescent. Most marrow normoblasts in CEP display marked fluorescence as a result of porphyrin accumulation (located principally in the nuclei, probably because of fixation artifact).[92] Anemia and the excess production and excretion of porphyrins is largely accounted for by ineffective erythropoiesis in the marrow. Porphyrin concentrations are also increased in circulating erythrocytes, and intravascular hemolysis may result from exposure to light in the dermal capillaries, causing erythrocyte damage and lysis or uptake by the spleen. Splenomegaly is very common in CEP and is presumed to be secondary to the hemolytic process. The excess porphyrins that are produced by the marrow or released by hemolysis are transported in plasma to the skin, leading to photosensitivity.

Clinical Features

Severe cutaneous photosensitivity is noted soon after birth in most cases. The disease may be recognized even earlier as a cause of hydrops fetalis. Phototherapy for hyperbilirubinemia may cause severe cutaneous burns and scarring in newborns with unrecognized CEP. Brown staining of the teeth by porphyrins (erythrodontia) is evident when the teeth erupt. Blistering and scarring resemble those found in PCT, but are usually much more severe, reflecting the much higher plasma porphyrin levels observed in CEP. Some cases are relatively mild, and can closely mimic PCT. Late-onset cases are often associated with myeloproliferative disorders, with expansion of a clone of erythroid cells bearing a somatic mutation and displaying UROS deficiency.[88]

Subepidermal bullous lesions are characteristic, and progress to crusted erosions that heal with scarring and areas of hyper- and hypopigmentation. Also common is hypertrichosis, which is sometimes severe, and alopecia. Loss of facial features and digits are common and result from recurrent blisters, infection, and scarring. Fingers may be shortened and tapered as a consequence of scarring and contraction of the skin during childhood growth. Erythrodontia, with brown staining and red fluorescence of the teeth under long-wave ultraviolet light is characteristic, and results from deposition of porphyrins in the developing deciduous and permanent teeth *in utero*. Porphyrins are also deposited in bone. The skeleton is also affected by expansion of the marrow, leading to pathologic fractures, vertebral compression, short stature, and osteolytic and sclerotic lesions. Vitamin D deficiency resulting from avoiding sunlight might also contribute.

Anemia may be severe and lead to transfusion dependence in the more severe cases. Uncorrected anemia can increase erythropoiesis, which, in turn, is a stimulus to porphyrin production by the abnormal erythropoietic cells in the marrow. Erythrocytes exhibit polychromasia, poikilocytosis, anisocytosis, and basophilic stippling, and reticulocytes and nucleated red blood cells are increased.[93]

Diagnosis

CEP may be suspected even before birth if a sibling is known to have CEP. However, the family history is often negative. CEP should be suspected as a cause of hydrops fetalis, as the disease can be diagnosed and treated *in utero*. Aspirated amniotic fluid is dark brown in color and contains large amounts of porphyrins. The diagnosis of CEP is often made after birth when pink to dark-brown staining of the diapers, with red fluorescence under long-wave ultraviolet light, is noted. Cutaneous vesicles and bullae on sun-exposed areas may be severe, with scarring.

Urinary porphyrin excretion is markedly increased, and often in the range of 50 to 100 mg/day (normal: up to ~0.3 mg/day). Uroporphyrin I and coproporphyrin I account for most of the increase, although the III isomers and hepta-, hexa-, pentacarboxylate porphyrins are also increased. Fecal porphyrins are increased, and are predominantly coproporphyrin I. Plasma total porphyrins are markedly increased as well, with a pattern of individual porphyrins similar to that in urine. Markedly increased erythrocyte porphyrins are predominantly uroporphyrin I and coproporphyrin I, although protoporphyrin IX may predominate especially in milder cases.

CEP must be distinguished by biochemical testing from other causes of blistering skin lesions. HEP can present with photosensitivity in early childhood. Mild cases of CEP may be misdiagnosed as PCT.

The diagnosis should be confirmed in all cases by DNA studies, which can identify causative mutations in almost all cases. This is especially important for genetic counseling and for prenatal diagnosis in subsequent pregnancies. Demonstration of a GATA-1 mutation in one case, illustrates that on occasion a genetic defect outside the heme biosynthetic pathway can cause CEP.[93]

Therapy

Patients should be advised that to avoid severe scarring and loss of facial features and digits it is essential to avoid sunlight, trauma to the skin, and infections. Topical sunscreens that block long-wave ultraviolet light (ultraviolet A light) and oral treatment with β-carotene are somewhat helpful,[94] but are marginally beneficial in most cases. Erythrocyte transfusions are essential in patients with severe anemia.[95] Transfusions to maintain the hematocrit above 35 percent, with an iron chelator to avoid iron overload, has been beneficial in some cases.[96] Hydroxyurea to reduce erythropoiesis and porphyrin production may also be considered.[97] Splenectomy has provided short-term benefit. Oral charcoal reportedly was quite effective in one patient,[98] and ascorbic acid and α-tocopherol improved anemia in another.[89] Unaffected infants born to mothers with CEP may have erythrodontia as a result of exposure to maternal porphyrins before birth.[99]

Hematopoietic stem cell transplantation is the treatment of choice when a suitable donor is available, especially for young patients.[100] When transplantation is successful, there is marked clinical improvement and reduction in porphyrin levels, even if these are not completely normalized. Gene therapy is being explored using retroviral and lentiviral vectors and hematopoietic stem cells from patients with CEP.[101,102]

ERYTHROPOIETIC PROTOPORPHYRIA

Definition and History

EPP is caused by a partial deficiency of FECH (see Fig. 58–4, *step 8*) activity, which results in the accumulation of the substrate protoporphyrin in the marrow. XLP has the same phenotype but is much less common, and is a result of ALAS2 gain-of-function mutations (ALAS; see Fig. 58–1).[37] EPP and XLP are characterized by onset of nonblistering cutaneous photosensitivity in early childhood. EPP is the most common porphyria in children and the third most common in adults. Reported prevalence varies between 5 and 15 cases per 1 million individuals.[103–105] Protoporphyric hepatopathy is a potentially fatal complication estimated to occur in less than 5 percent of patients.

Pathophysiology

In most families, EPP is best described as an autosomal recessive disease, in which a severe *FECH* mutation is inherited from one parent and a low-expression (hypomorphic) *FECH* allele from the other. More than 75 different severe mutations, including nonsense, missense, and splice-site mutations, and deletions, insertions, and rearrangements have been described. Splicing mutations are most common. Recombinant human FECH, when engineered to have individual exon skipping for exons 3 through 11, lacks significant enzyme activity when expressed in *E. coli* and almost all such variants lacked the [²Fe-²S] cluster.[106]

EPP was usually described in the past as an autosomal dominant disorder, with variable penetrance. However, it was noted that EPP patients have only 30 percent or less of normal FECH activity, rather than 50 percent, which would be expected in an autosomal dominant condition. It was then shown that, in addition to a severe *FECH* mutation, a low-expression (hypomorphic) intronic polymorphism (a −23C→T transition) is found in the other *FECH* allele of patients with EPP, which is inherited from the other parent.[107-109] This transition favors the use of a cryptic acceptor splice site 63 bases upstream of the normal splice site. The aberrantly spliced mRNA contains a premature stop codon and is degraded by a nonsense-mediated decay mechanism.[109] The result is a lower steady-state level of wild-type *FECH* mRNA. Coinheritance of the hypomorphic allele in *trans* to a loss-of-function mutant allele was found in 98 percent of French cases with EPP,[110] and with a similar frequency in South African patients.[105] The frequency of the IVS3–48C hypomorphic allele is common in the white population, and by itself has no phenotype. Its frequency varies widely in different populations and relates to the observed differences in the prevalence of EPP.[103-105]

Other underlying genetic mechanisms must be considered in newly identified EPP families. In a few families, a severe *FECH* mutation, at least one of which must produce some FECH enzyme, is inherited from each parent and the hypomorphic allele is not present. Interestingly, EPP in such families is sometimes associated with seasonal palmar keratoderma, unusual neurologic symptoms, less-than-expected increases in erythrocyte protoporphyrin and absence of liver dysfunction.[111]

XLP was first perceived as a variant form of EPP in which *FECH* mutations were absent. After family studies suggested sex-linked inheritance, gain-of-function mutations of *ALAS2* (the only heme pathway enzyme found on the X chromosome) were discovered.[37] This is the only porphyria caused by mutations of ALAS, the first enzyme in the pathway.

EPP can develop late in life in patients with clonal hematologic disorders and expansion of a clone of hematopoietic cells with mutations of a *FECH* allele.[112,113] For example, a patient with a myeloproliferative disorder later developed severe EPP because of clonal expansion of a cell of erythropoietic lineage with a *FECH* deletion and the IVS3–48C/T polymorphism, and died of EPP-induced liver disease.[114]

Pathogenesis of the Clinical Findings

Marrow reticulocytes are thought to be the primary source of the excess protoporphyrin in EPP.[115,116] Most of the excess erythrocyte protoporphyrin in circulating erythrocytes is found in younger cells as metal-free protoporphyrin (i.e., not complexed with zinc), in contrast to other conditions associated with increased erythrocyte protoporphyrin content. Metal-free protoporphyrin declines much more rapidly with red cell age than it does zinc protoporphyrin.[115,116] Metal-free protoporphyrin, but not zinc protoporphyrin, is released from erythrocytes following solar irradiation, which may explain why lead intoxication and iron deficiency, which are associated with elevated erythrocyte zinc protoporphyrin levels, are not associated with photosensitivity.[117] Excess metal-free protoporphyrin enters plasma from reticulocytes, as well as from circulating erythrocytes, and is taken up by hepatocytes, excreted in bile and feces, and may undergo enterohepatic recirculation. Hepatocytes may also provide a limited additional source of excess protoporphyrin in this disease.

Light-excited protoporphyrin in EPP generates free radicals and singlet oxygen,[118] which in EPP can lead to peroxidation of lipids[119] and crosslinking of membrane proteins. Skin irradiation in EPP patients leads to complement activation and polymorphonuclear chemotaxis, which contributes to the development of skin pathology.[120] Skin histopathology is not specific but may include thickened capillary walls in the papillary dermis surrounded by amorphous hyaline-like deposits,

immunoglobulin, complement, and periodic acid-Schiff–positive mucopolysaccharides.[121] Basement membrane abnormalities are less marked than in other forms of porphyria.[122]

Protoporphyric hepatopathy is a feared complication that develops in less than 5 percent of patients, and is attributed to the cholestatic effects of excess protoporphyrin presented to the liver. This complication may begin with chronic abnormalities in liver function tests and then progress rapidly as a vicious cycle of increasing protoporphyrin levels in plasma and erythrocytes and worsening liver function and photosensitivity. Hepatopathy is sometimes precipitated by another cause of liver dysfunction such as viral or alcoholic hepatitis. Protoporphyrin is cholestatic, and can form crystalline structures in hepatocytes and impair mitochondrial function, leading to decreased hepatic bile formation and flow.[123,124] Accumulated protoporphyrin may appear as brown pigment in hepatocytes, Kupffer cells, and biliary canaliculi, and these deposits are doubly refractive with a Maltese cross appearance under polarizing microscopy.[125] DNA microarray studies in explanted livers of patients with hepatopathy revealed significant changes in expression of several genes involved in wound-healing, organic anion transport, and oxidative stress.[126]

Clinical Features

Photosensitivity is present from early childhood in almost all cases. Parents may observe that an affected infant cries and develops skin swelling and erythema when exposed to sunlight. Although EPP is the most common porphyria in children, there is often considerable delay in diagnosis.

Cutaneous photosensitivity in EPP is acute and nonblistering, which is distinctly different from the more chronic, blistering skin manifestations of the other cutaneous porphyrias. Table 58–3 tabulates symptoms in a series of 32 patients with EPP. Skin symptoms are usually worse during spring and summer and affect light-exposed areas, especially of the face and hands. Characteristically, stinging or burning pain develops within 1 hour of sunlight exposure, and if exposure continues is followed by erythema and edema—described as solar urticaria, sometimes with petechiae, and less commonly purpura. Blistering and crusted lesions are uncommon. Artificial lights may contribute to photosensitivity.[127] Patients typically avoid sunlight and may display no objective cutaneous signs. Repeated light exposure can lead to chronic changes including leathery hyperkeratotic skin especially on the dorsa of the hands and finger joints, mild scarring, and separation of the nail plate (onycholysis).

TABLE 58–3. Common Clinical Features of Erythropoietic Protoporphyria from a Series of 32 Cases

Symptoms and Signs	Incidence (% of Total)
Burning	97
Edema	94
Itching	88
Erythema	69
Scarring	19
Vesicles	3
Anemia	27
Cholelithiasis	12
Abnormal liver function results	4

Data from Bloomer J, Wang Y, Singhal A, et al: Molecular studies of liver disease in erythropoietic protoporphyria, *J Clin Gastroenterol* 2005 Apr;39(4 Suppl 2):S167–S175.

Mild anemia with microcytosis, hypochromia, reduced iron stores, but usually normal serum iron, and serum transferrin receptor-1, is a common feature of EPP,[115,128,129,130,131] but there is little evidence for impaired erythropoiesis or abnormal iron metabolism,[129,130] and hemolysis is absent or very mild.[131,153] Iron accumulation in erythroblasts and ring sideroblasts have been noted in marrow in some patients.[132] Findings in XLP are similar. Also, iron is proposed to have a role in splicing of FECH mRNA, where decreased iron leads to an increase in incorrect splicing of the mRNA.[133] Binding of iron-responsive elements binding proteins (IRPs) to the 5′-iron-responsive element (IRE) in *ALAS2* mRNA, in low iron conditions, prevents translation of *ALAS2* mRNA. When iron is supplemented, the IRPs no longer have high affinity for the ALAS2 5′-IRE, leading to increased translation, import into the mitochondria, and enhanced production of ALA.[134]

Precipitating factors that are important in the hepatic porphyrias do not appear to play an important role in EPP. Although more long-term followup studies are needed, porphyrin levels and symptoms typically do not change over time, unless liver dysfunction develops. Concurrent iron deficiency or other marrow problems might also lead to further increases in porphyrin levels and photosensitivity. Pregnancy is reported to lower erythrocyte protoporphyrin levels somewhat and increase tolerance to sunlight.[135]

Neurovisceral manifestations are absent in uncomplicated EPP. Patients with severe protoporphyric hepatopathy may develop a severe motor neuropathy similar to that seen in the acute porphyrias.[136] Autosomal recessive EPP associated with palmar keratoderma has also been associated with unexplained neurologic symptoms.[111]

Gallstones containing large amounts of protoporphyrin are common, and may require cholecystectomy at an unusually early age.[137] Liver function and liver protoporphyrin content are usually normal in EPP. Protoporphyric hepatopathy, which is the most life-threatening complication of EPP, results from the cholestatic effects of protoporphyrin presented in excess amounts to the liver. It can be the major presenting feature of EPP,[138] and may be chronic or progress rapidly to death from liver failure. Unnecessary surgery for suspected biliary obstruction can be detrimental and should be avoided.[124] Operating room lights during liver transplantation or other surgery, especially in patients with hepatopathy, can cause marked photosensitivity with extensive burns of the skin and peritoneum and photodamage of circulating erythrocytes.[139]

Diagnosis

Painful, nonblistering photosensitivity suggests the diagnosis. A substantial elevation of erythrocyte protoporphyrin is expected, but is not specific, as erythrocyte zinc protoporphyrin is predominantly increased in conditions such as homozygous porphyrias (other than most cases of CEP), iron deficiency, lead poisoning, anemia of chronic disease,[140] hemolytic conditions,[141] and many other erythrocyte disorders. A unique finding in EPP is increased erythrocyte protoporphyrin with a predominance of metal-free rather than zinc protoporphyrin. This occurs because FECH, which can utilize metals in addition to iron, catalyzes the formation of zinc protoporphyrin, and this activity is deficient in EPP. Because FECH is not deficient in XLP, erythrocytes contain increased amounts of both zinc and metal-free protoporphyrin, although the latter still predominates in most cases.

Consequently, the diagnosis of EPP requires demonstration of an increase in metal-free protoporphyrin in red cells. Amounts of metal-free and zinc protoporphyrin in erythrocytes can be measured by ethanol or acetone extraction or high-performance liquid chromatography. There is confusion about terminology used by different laboratories. For example, the term "free erythrocyte protoporphyrin," refers to protoporphyrin results measured with a hematofluorometer as an indicator of lead exposure, but actually refers to zinc protoporphyrin rather than

metal-free or total protoporphyrin. At this writing, we are aware of only two laboratories in the United States (Mayo Clinic Laboratories and the Porphyria Laboratory at the University of Texas Medical Branch), that reliably report the amounts of total, metal-free, and zinc protoporphyrin, as is needed for confirmation of a diagnosis of EPP. The proportions of metal-free and zinc protoporphyrin can also usually distinguish XLP (50 to approximately 85 percent metal-free protoporphyrin) from EPP (>85 percent metal-free protoporphyrin).

The plasma porphyrin concentration is almost always at least mildly increased in EPP, but often less than in other cutaneous porphyrias, and may be normal in mild cases. Plasma porphyrins in EPP are particularly subject to photodegradation during sample processing unless great care is taken to shield the sample from natural or fluorescent light.[142] For these reasons, measurement of erythrocyte rather than plasma porphyrin should be relied upon for diagnosis of EPP and XLP.

Fecal porphyrins are normal or somewhat increased, and consist mostly of protoporphyrin. Urine porphyrins are normal, except after hepatopathy develops, which causes increases in urinary coproporphyrin as is typical for other forms of liver diseases.

Therapy

Avoidance of the sunlight exposure is important, and often requires changes in lifestyle and the working environment. Topical sunscreens that absorb ultraviolet A and sunblocks containing zinc oxide or titanium dioxide may be helpful. Orally administered β-carotene, which probably quenches activated oxygen radicals,[143,144] may afford some protection after 1 to 3 months of therapy, but results are variable. A daily dose of 120 to 180 mg or higher is recommended to achieve a serum β-carotene level of 600 to 800 mcg/dL.[127] Oral cysteine may also quench excited oxygen species and increase tolerance to sunlight in EPP.[145] Other treatments that aim to either increase skin pigmentation or scavenge activated oxygen species have been reviewed[144] and include dihydroxyacetone/Lawsone, vitamin C and narrow-wave ultraviolet B phototherapy to increase melanin.[146] Afamelanotide, an α-melanocyte–stimulating hormone analogue that increases skin melanin, has shown benefit in clinical trials.[147]

It is advisable to monitor liver function tests at least yearly, and avoid severe caloric restriction and drugs or hormone preparations that impair hepatic excretory function.[148,149] Because iron deficiency might be detrimental by further limiting heme synthesis and increasing protoporphyrin accumulation, ferritin levels should be followed in EPP and XLP patients, keeping in mind that ferritin in the lower part of the normal range (especially for women) may indicate depleted iron stores. Iron supplementation has been reported to worsen photosensitivity in some cases (although increases in protoporphyrin levels were not documented) and to correct microcytosis without increasing porphyrin levels in others. Therefore, at present iron supplementation in EPP and XLP is controversial, and systematic studies are needed. Because patients avoid sunlight exposure, vitamin D supplementation is recommended.

Management of protoporphyric liver disease is difficult. The condition may resolve spontaneously especially if another reversible cause of liver dysfunction, such as viral hepatitis or alcohol, is contributing.[122,150] Cholestyramine,[124,151,152] ursodeoxycholic acid,[153] vitamin E, red blood cell transfusions,[154] plasma exchange, and intravenous hemin may be given in combination to bridge patients until liver transplantation or there is spontaneous improvement.[155] Success of liver transplantation is comparable to that in other liver diseases, even though protoporphyric hepatopathy may recur in the new liver, a result of the continued erythrocyte protoporphyrin release by the marrow.[156] Acute motor neuropathy has developed in some patients with protoporphyric liver disease after transfusion[157] or liver transplantation,[158,159] and is sometimes reversible.[158]

Marrow transplantation can achieve remission in human EPP,[160] as well in murine models of protoporphyria.[161] Sequential liver and marrow transplantation can correct the overproduction of protoporphyrin by the marrow and prevent recurrence of liver disease.[162] Promising studies in murine models suggest a future role for gene therapy in human EPP.[163,165]

ACUTE PORPHYRIAS

The acute porphyrias are comprised of four disorders caused by different enzyme deficiencies, and are distinctive for neurologic symptoms that usually occur as acute exacerbations during adult life. Similar symptoms occur in lead poisoning, hereditary tyrosinemia type I, and in some reported cases of porphyria with dual enzyme deficiencies.

δ-AMINOLEVULINIC ACID DEHYDRATASE PORPHYRIA

Definition and History

ADP is an autosomal recessive disorder resulting from severe deficiency of ALAD activity (see Table 58–1 and Fig. 58–1). This is the rarest of the porphyrias, with only six cases documented at the molecular level.[50,168]

Pathophysiology

All reported cases were males.[164,166–169] Compound heterozygosity for two distinct ALAD mutations was documented in five cases (see Fig. 58–4, *step 2*).[167,168] Four (three in Germany and one in the United States) experienced onset of symptoms in their teens, whereas one Swedish case developed severe symptoms in infancy.[166] The sixth patient was a Belgian male who developed ADP at age 63 years and was found to have two inherited base transitions in one allele, and was therefore heterozygous for ALAD deficiency.[164,169] He also developed polycythemia vera and his erythrocyte ALAD activity was less than 1 percent of normal, while lymphocyte ALAD activity was greater than 20 percent of normal. Heterozygous ALAD deficiency was apparently clinically silent in this patient until there was expansion of a clone of erythroid cells that carried the mutant ALAD allele.[169]

Thus ADP is highly heterogeneous at the molecular level, with a total of 11 mutant alleles identified in these 6 patients.[168] An additional mutation was found in a healthy Swedish girl with markedly decreased ALAD activity (12% of normal), which was detected by ALAD measurement during neonatal screening for hereditary tyrosinemia.[170] The same mutation was found in a U.S. male patient with acute porphyria who also had a *CPO* mutation and an unusual pattern of porphyrin precursors and porphyrins reflecting dual enzyme deficiencies.[171] Thus, heterozygous ALAD deficiency may rarely be combined with another enzyme deficiency, or may itself cause porphyria if a marrow disorder leads to clonal expansion of the mutant *ALAD* allele.

Human ALAD consists of eight identical oligomers, each with two zinc-binding sites. Lead can bind at least one of these sites and impair enzyme activity. Some mutations found in ADP may affect zinc binding, or favor assembly of a hexameric enzyme with decreased activity. Thus ADP has been described as a conformational disease.[50]

ADP is classified as one of the hepatic porphyrias because it closely resembles the other acute porphyrias. However, the site of overproduction of ALA is not established, and the Swedish infant with severe, early onset disease did not benefit from liver transplantation.[172] Substantial increase in erythrocyte zinc protoporphyrin also suggests an erythroid component. The excess urinary coproporphyrin III in ADP may originate from metabolism of ALA to porphyrinogens in a tissue other than the site of ALA overproduction. Indeed, ALA loading in normal

subjects was shown to cause substantial coproporphyrinuria.[173] The pathogenesis of the neurologic symptoms is poorly understood, as in other acute porphyrias.

Clinical Features

The four adolescent males had intermittent symptoms resembling other acute porphyrias, including abdominal pain, vomiting, extremity pain, and motor neuropathy, although exacerbating factors were less evident.[168,174] Two German cases had initial acute attacks and then remained well during 20 years of followup.[175] The third German case[176] and the U.S. case[168] had further attacks and were maintained on prophylactic hemin infusions. The Swedish infant had more severe neurologic disease, including failure to thrive, and died after liver transplantation.[177] The 63-year-old man in Belgium, developed an acute motor polyneuropathy concurrently with a myeloproliferative disorder.[88,164,178]

Diagnosis

A biochemical diagnosis of ADP includes demonstration of markedly deficient erythrocyte ALAD activity, marked elevation in urinary ALA and coproporphyrin III and erythrocyte zinc protoporphyrin, with little or no increase in urinary PBG. Erythrocyte ALAD activity is approximately half-normal in both parents. Lead poisoning is differentiated by increased blood lead and restoration of ALAD activity *in vitro* by reduced glutathione or dithiothreitol.[167,179] Although biochemical measurements can strongly suggest ADP, the diagnosis must be confirmed by DNA studies.

Patients with hereditary tyrosinemia type I may also have ALAD inhibition and increased excretion of ALA.[43] Dioxoheptanoic acid (succinylacetone), a structural analogue of ALA and a potent ALAD inhibitor, accumulates as a result of an inherited deficiency of fumarylacetoacetate hydrolase in these patients. The presence of this inhibitor can be demonstrated in urine by measuring ALAD activity in normal blood after addition of a patient's urine. ALAD protein is not reduced in this disease.[180]

Therapy

Because few cases have been documented, treatment recommendations are based on limited experience. Hemin was beneficial in the four male patients, but there was little or no response to glucose. A long-term preventive hemin regimen was effective in two of these patients. The Swedish infant did not respond to glucose or hemin, and did not improve greatly after liver transplantation.[172] Whether transplantation would benefit less severe cases is unknown. Hemin produced a biochemical response but no clinical improvement in the late-onset case in Belgium, who had a peripheral neuropathy but no acute attacks.[178]

ACUTE INTERMITTENT PORPHYRIA

Definition and History

AIP is an autosomal dominant disorder caused by a partial deficiency of PBG deaminase (see Table 58–1 and Fig. 58–1). Symptoms usually occur as acute attacks and are neurologic in origin. In most countries this is the most common acute porphyria and the second most common porphyria. Most individuals who inherit the enzyme deficiency (probably more than 90 percent) never develop symptoms, but are at some risk to develop symptoms after puberty. The first case of acute porphyria was described in 1889 by Stokvis[5] who noted a relationship of the symptoms to the drug sulfonal, which is related to the barbiturates.

Prevalence of AIP was estimated to be 1 to 2 per 100,000 population in Europe,[181] and 2.4 per 100,000 population in Finland.[182] Up to 300 *PBGD* mutations have been described in AIP, with many found in only one or a few families.[183,184] The disease occurs in all races, but clusters as a result of founder effects occur in some countries. A founder mutation in northern Sweden is associated with a disease prevalence of 1 per 1500 population.[185] The prevalence of low PBG deaminase activity, which includes latent gene carriers of AIP, is as high as 1 per 500 in the general population of Finland.[186] Based on DNA studies, the minimal prevalence of the AIP-associated genes in France has been calculated to be 1 per 1675 population.[187]

Pathophysiology

PBG deaminase is also known as HMB synthase, and formerly as uroporphyrinogen I synthase. *PBGD* mutations have been classified based in part on the presence or absence of cross-reactive immunologic material (CRIM), which indicates the presence of inactive enzyme protein. *Type I* mutations are CRIM-negative, with reduction of both enzyme activity and protein to approximately 50 percent of normal in heterozygotes. *Type II* mutations are associated with reduced PBGD activity only in nonerythroid tissue. These patients with "variant AIP" comprise less than 5 percent of AIP patients, and have normal erythrocyte PBGD activity and decreased hepatic activity because, as explained earlier in the section on hydroxymethylbilane synthase, transcription of the gene to form the erythroid-specific enzyme starts downstream of the site of the mutation. *Type III* are CRIM-positive mutations that result in decreased activity with structurally abnormal enzyme protein.[188]

Pathogenesis of the Clinical Findings

A partial deficiency of PBGD rarely causes clinical expression of AIP, and most individuals who inherit this enzyme deficiency remain healthy with normal porphyrin precursor excretion throughout life. Certain drugs and hormones that exacerbate AIP can directly induce ALAS[27] and also increase the demand for heme by inducing CYP enzymes, which turn over rapidly and use most of the heme synthesized in the liver.[189]

When heme synthesis is stimulated, the partial enzyme deficiency in AIP apparently impairs heme synthesis sufficiently to compromise negative feedback by the regulatory heme pool, which controls synthesis of the rate-limiting enzyme ALAS1. This leads to marked induction of ALAS1 and overproduction of ALA, PBG and porphyrins in the liver.

It is generally accepted, although not proven, that hepatic PBGD remains constant at approximately 50 percent of normal activity during exacerbations and remissions of AIP, as in erythrocytes. An early report suggested that the enzyme activity is considerably less than half-normal in liver during an acute attack,[14] but additional data is lacking. It has been suggested that once the disease becomes activated, excess PBG may interfere with assembly of the dipyrromethane cofactor for this enzyme.

Clinical improvement and normalization of porphyrin precursor excretion after liver transplantation in patients with severe AIP is a clear indication that the liver plays an essential role in neuropathic processes in the acute porphyrias.[190] Proposed explanations for neurologic dysfunction in the acute porphyrias include the following. (1) Heme pathway intermediates or products derived from them may be neurotoxic. This hypothesis is most favored, although the evidence is not conclusive. (2) PBG deaminase deficiency in the nervous system tissues may limit heme synthesis and formation of important hemoproteins. For example, decreased activity of the hemoprotein nitric oxide synthase might decrease production of nitric oxide and cause vasospasm, which might account for some cerebral manifestations of AIP,[191,192] and possibly compromise intestinal blood flow.[193] However, regulation of heme and hemoprotein synthesis in nervous tissue and blood vessels is difficult to study, and convincing evidence is lacking. (3) Impaired hepatic heme synthesis during an attack may lead to decreased activity of hepatic tryptophan pyrrolase, which might increase levels of

tryptophan in plasma and brain, leading to increased synthesis of the neurotransmitter 5-hydroxytryptamine.

ALA is increased in a number of disorders with similar neurologic manifestations, including all four of the acute porphyrias, lead poisoning, and hereditary tyrosinemia type I, which favors a neuropathic role for this porphyrin precursor or perhaps a derivative. ALA can enter cells readily and be converted to porphyrins, which, in turn, may have toxic potential.[194] ALA is also structurally similar to γ-aminobutyric acid and can interact with γ-aminobutyric acid receptors.[195,196] However, studies of ALA loading have not shown adverse effects.

Impaired motor function with ataxia develops in mice with PBGD deficiency resulting from compound heterozygous or homozygous mutations induced by gene targeting.[197] Induction of hepatic CYPs is impaired in these animals and corrected by heme.[198] But motor neuropathy can develop even with normal or only slightly increased ALA in plasma and urine, suggesting a primary role for heme deficiency in porphyric neuropathy in this murine model.[199]

Precipitating Factors Acute attacks are precipitated in some heterozygotes by various endogenous or exogenous factors that are additive. Additional unknown genetic factors are also likely to contribute. Some individuals remain susceptible to repeated attacks even after avoidance of known precipitants. Many precipitating factors cause *induction of hepatic ALAS1*, which is closely associated with induction of CYPs and leads to overproduction of ALA and other pathway intermediates.

Drugs and Other Exogenous Chemicals Most drugs that are harmful in acute porphyrias are known inducers of hepatic CYPs. These drugs increase *de novo* heme synthesis, thereby derepressing hepatic ALAS1, and also directly induce this rate-limiting enzyme.[27] Table 58–4 identifies some drugs that are known to be harmful or safe. Information regarding safety of many drugs in clinical practice is uncertain or lacking. More extensive drug safety databases are available at the websites of the American Porphyria Foundation (www.porphyriafoundation.com) and the European Porphyria Initiative (www.porphyria-europe.com). These drug classifications are often based on limited evidence and may be controversial. Ethanol and other alcohols are inducers of hepatic ALAS1 and some CYPs.[200] Smoking is known to increase CYPs in humans, probably from effects of polycyclic aromatic hydrocarbons, and has been associated with more frequent symptoms of acute porphyria.[201]

Endocrine Factors Rarity of symptoms before puberty and more common clinical expression in women point to hormonal factors as important contributors in AIP. Although estrogens are considered harmful, it is likely that progesterone is mostly responsible for cyclic premenstrual attacks that occur in some women. Progesterone, certain metabolites of testosterone, and synthetic progestins are potent inducers of ALAS1. Thus administration of progestational agents should be avoided. Diabetes mellitus is not known to precipitate attacks of porphyria, and has been observed to decrease the frequency of attacks and lower porphyrin precursor levels, possibly in relation to high circulating glucose levels.[202]

Pregnancy Pregnancy is usually well tolerated.[203] Attacks during pregnancy are sometimes a result of harmful drugs or reduced caloric intake. Metoclopramide, considered at least by some a contraindicated drug, is associated with exacerbation of the disease when used to treat hyperemesis gravidarum.[204,205] But for reasons that are not clear, some women experience attacks during pregnancy even when harmful factors are avoided.

Nutrition Reduced intake of calories and carbohydrate can exacerbate acute porphyrias. This may occur from efforts to lose weight, bariatric surgery or from metabolic stress from an illness or surgery. Under these conditions, upregulation of PGC-1α can lead to induction of ALAS1, increases in ALA and PBG, and symptoms of

TABLE 58–4. A Partial List of Drugs Known to Be Unsafe or Safe in the Acute Porphyrias

Unsafe		Safe
Alcohol	Meprobamate* (also mebutamate*, tybamate*)	Acetaminophen
Barbiturates*		Aspirin
Carbamazepine*	Methyprylon	Atropine
Carisoprodol*	Metoclopramide*	Bromides
Clonazepam (high doses)	Phenytoin*	Cimetidine
Danazol*	Primidone*	Erythropoietin*,†
Diclofenac* and possibly other NSAIDs	Progesterone and synthetic progestins*	Gabapentin
Ergots		Glucocorticoids
Estrogens*,‡	Pyrazinamide*	Insulin
Ethchlorvynol*	Pyrazolones (aminopyrine, antipyrine)	Narcotic analgesics
Glutethimide*	Rifampin*	Penicillin and derivatives
Griseofulvin*	Succinimides (ethosuximide, methsuximide)	Phenothiazines
Mephenytoin		Ranitidine*,†
	Sulfonamide antibiotics*	Streptomycin
	Valproic acid*	Vigabatrin

NSAIDs, nonsteroidal antiinflammatory drugs.

*Porphyria is listed as a contraindication, warning, precaution, or adverse effect in U.S. labeling for these drugs.

†Although porphyria is listed as a precaution in U.S. labeling, these drugs are regarded as safe by other sources.

‡Estrogens are unsafe for porphyria cutanea tarda, but can be can be used with caution in the acute porphyrias.

NOTE: More complete sources, such as the websites of the American Porphyria Foundation (www.porphyriafoundation.com) and the European Porphyria Initiative (www.porphyria-europe.com) should be consulted before using drugs not listed here, keeping in mind that classifications may not be supported by high-quality evidence.

acute porphyria, and these effects are reversed by administration of carbohydrate.[30,206] Starvation, may also induce hepatic heme oxygenase,[207] which may deplete hepatic heme and contribute to ALAS1 induction.

Stress Various forms of physical or psychological stress may exacerbate acute porphyrias, although the mechanisms are not well defined. Medical illnesses, fever, infections, alcoholic excess, and surgery may decrease food intake and contribute to induction of hepatic ALAS1 and heme oxygenase. Psychological stress may also lead to decreased food intake and have other metabolic effects.

Clinical Features

Symptoms are almost never seen before puberty, and most commonly develop in women in the third or fourth decade of life. Acute attacks are life-threatening but rarely fatal if promptly recognized and treated. Frequently recurring attacks and chronic symptoms can develop and be disabling. Although the most prominent symptoms are a result of effects on the nervous system, liver and kidney damage may be important in the long-term. In very rare homozygous cases, severe neurologic manifestations are seen early in childhood, and acute attacks are not prominent.[207a,209]

Symptoms and signs are nonspecific and highly variable. Abdominal pain is the most common symptom, occurring in 85 to 95 percent of cases.[210] It is usually severe, steady, and poorly localized, but may be cramping, and is often accompanied by nausea, vomiting, constipation, and abdominal distention because of ileus. Pain in the chest and extremities are also common. Tachycardia is the most common physical sign, occurring in up to 80 percent of acute attacks,[211] and often accompanied by hypertension, sweating, tremors, and other effects of sympathetic overactivity and excess catecholamine production. There is little or no abdominal tenderness, fever, or leukocytosis because inflammation is not prominent. Bowel sounds are usually decreased, but are sometimes increased with diarrhea. The urine is often dark (because of porphobilin, a degradation product of PBG) or reddish (because of porphyrins, including uroporphyrin formed nonenzymatically from PBG). Urinary hesitancy and dysuria may occur as a consequence of bladder dysfunction. Acute mental symptoms may include insomnia, anxiety, restlessness, disorientation, paranoia, and hallucinations.

Paresis because of peripheral motor neuropathy usually occurs with prolonged, severe attacks, but is sometimes an early or even initial manifestation.[212,213] Porphyric neuropathy is primarily motor and results from axonal degeneration, which may be followed by demyelinization.[214] Muscle weakness may not be detected until it is quite advanced because it usually begins in the proximal muscles of the upper extremities. Paresis is usually symmetrical, but may be asymmetrical or focal. Course tremors, clonus and increased reflexes are sometimes prominent. Magnetic resonance imaging may demonstrate cortical densities resembling the posterior reversible encephalopathy syndrome.[192] Sensory loss may develop, especially in the distal extremities. Cranial nerve involvement and cortical blindness have been described.

Motor neuropathy may progress to respiratory and bulbar paralysis and death especially if diagnosis and treatment are delayed and harmful drugs continued. Death may also result from respiratory arrest or cardiac arrhythmia.[214,215] Most attacks treated promptly resolve within days or even hours. Advanced neuropathy from a severe attack is potentially completely reversible, with improvement continuing for up to 1 to 2 years.[216]

Hyponatremia is common during severe attacks and is sometimes a result of hypothalamic involvement and the syndrome of inappropriate antidiuretic hormone secretion. However, hyponatremia may be accompanied by reductions in blood volume,[217] indicating that increased antidiuretic hormone secretion in this setting is an appropriate physiologic response.[215] Hyponatremia may sometimes result from gastrointestinal loss, poor intake, and excess renal sodium loss.[215,218] A possible nephrotoxic effect of ALA may explain renal tubular sodium loss and impaired renal function in some patients.[218] Other electrolyte abnormalities may include hypomagnesemia and hypercalcemia.[219] Seizures may result from hyponatremia or represent a neurologic effect of acute porphyria.

Chronic mental symptoms, such as depression, are difficult to attribute to AIP. But chronic pain accompanied by depression develops in some patients after frequent exacerbations, and risk for suicide is increased. The disease also predisposes to chronic arterial hypertension and impaired renal function.[203,220,221] The latter may progress and require renal transplantation.[222,223]

Mild abnormalities in serum transaminases are common in AIP.[224] More advanced liver disease may develop and the risk of hepatocellular carcinoma is greatly increased (60- to 70-fold) in AIP, and is not related to specific *PBGD* mutations. Serum α-fetoprotein was not increased and the uninvolved liver was not cirrhotic in most acute porphyria cases with liver cancer reported as of this writing. Increased serum thyroxin levels because of increased thyroxin-binding globulin occurs in some patients with AIP, and occasionally hyperthyroidism and porphyria occur together.[225] Elevated low-density lipoprotein cholesterol is apparently less commonly observed in this disorder than in the past.[226]

Diagnosis

A high index of suspicion and knowing when to suspect these diseases contributes to making an *initial diagnosis* of acute porphyria. Because the disease so often remains latent, there is often no family history of porphyria. Acute porphyria should be considered in patients with unexplained abdominal pain or other characteristic symptoms when initial evaluation does not suggest another more common explanation, and ruled in or out by rapid assessment of urinary PBG, which is both sensitive and specific. A substantial increase in PBG, which can be determined rapidly by a commercial kit,[227] establishes that a patient has either AIP, HCP, or VP. Consensus recommendations are that all major medical centers should retain the capacity for rapid urinary PBG testing on single-void urine specimens, as collection of 24 hour urines and reliance on outside laboratories for screening can greatly delay diagnosis and treatment. The urine specimen should be saved for later quantitative measurement of PBG, ALA, and total porphyrin levels. If PBG is substantially increased, samples of plasma, erythrocytes and feces should also be obtained prior to treatment with hemin. This approach provides for rapid initial diagnosis of AIP, HCP, and VP, subsequent biochemical differentiation of these conditions and diagnosis of ADP. In patients with renal failure, PBG can be measured in serum by a specialized laboratory. Figure 58–6 presents a diagnostic flow chart for use when acute porphyria is suspected.

PBG excretion is generally 50 to 200 mg/day (normal range: 0 to ~4 mg/day) during acute attacks of AIP. Excretion of ALA is usually about half that of PBG (expressed as mg/day). Increases in ALA and PBG can persist for prolonged periods between attacks, especially in AIP. Increases in ALA and PBG are less striking during acute attacks of HCP and VP and often decrease more rapidly.

The diagnosis of an acute attack is largely clinical, and is not based on a specific level of ALA or PBG. Levels of ALA and PBG during an acute attack may be increased compared to baseline levels, which fluctuate considerably and can be difficult to establish between attacks. Intravenous hemin causes dramatic, rapid but often transient decreases in these levels.

Urinary porphyrins are increased in AIP, are predominantly uroporphyrin and account for reddish urine (ALA and PBG are colorless). Uroporphyrin can form nonenzymatically from PBG in urine even prior to excretion. However, there is evidence that porphyrins in this condition are predominantly type III, which may be formed enzymatically,[228] perhaps from ALA transported to tissues other than the liver.[194] Total fecal porphyrins and plasma porphyrins are normal or slightly increased in AIP, and erythrocyte zinc protoporphyrin concentrations may be nonspecifically increased.

Erythrocyte PBGD activity is approximately half-normal in most (70 to 80 percent) patients with AIP. However, this measurement is not definitive for confirming or excluding the diagnosis. As described earlier, some PBGD mutations cause the enzyme to be deficient only in nonerythroid tissues. Moreover, the ranges of activity for normals and AIP are wide and overlapping, and the erythrocyte enzyme is highly age-dependent, such that an increase in the proportion of younger cells in the circulation can raise the activity into the normal range in AIP patients with a concurrent condition such as hemolytic anemia or hepatic disease.[229,230] A decrease in this enzyme also does not distinguish between latent and active disease. For these reasons, and because it does not detect other acute porphyrias, erythrocyte PBGD measurement in not useful for initial diagnosis of ill patients.

Once the diagnosis of AIP is established by biochemical methods, the underlying *PBGD* mutation should be identified. This confirms the diagnosis and, most importantly, enables reliable and definitive identification of other gene carriers by DNA testing. Erythrocyte PBGD

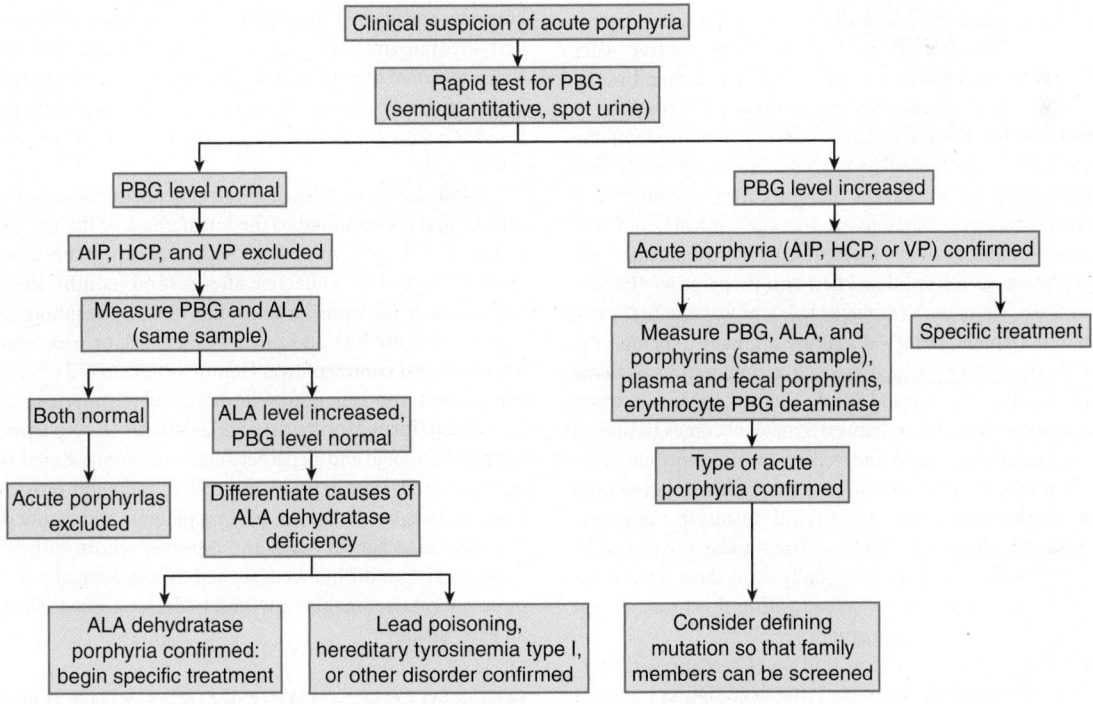

Figure 58–6. Recommended laboratory evaluation of patients with concurrent symptoms suggesting an acute porphyria, indicating how the diagnosis is established or excluded by biochemical testing and when specific therapy should be initiated. This schema is not applicable to patients who were recently treated with hemin or who have recovered from past symptoms suggestive of porphyria. Levels of δ-aminolevulinic acid (ALA) and porphobilinogen (PBG) may be less increased in hereditary coproporphyria (HCP) and variegate porphyria (VP) and decrease more quickly with recovery than in acute intermittent porphyria (AIP). Mutation detection provides confirmation and greatly facilitates detection of relatives with latent porphyria.

measurement is useful for screening of asymptomatic family members if a known case in the family has low erythrocyte enzyme activity, but is less dependable than DNA testing. PBGD deficiency can be documented in the fetus by measuring the enzyme activity or by identifying the maternal or paternal mutation in amniotic fluid cells. However, prenatal diagnosis is usually not indicated because the great majority of heterozygous carriers of PBGD mutations have a good prognosis.

Therapy

Hospitalization is usually required for treatment of attacks, although well-characterized patients with frequently recurring attacks that respond rapidly to treatment are sometimes managed as outpatients. Hospitalization facilitates treatment of severe symptoms, intravenous therapies and monitoring of respiration, electrolytes and nutritional status. Admission to intensive care is warranted if the vital capacity is impaired. Harmful drugs should be discontinued whenever possible. Pain, nausea, and vomiting are generally severe and require narcotic analgesics, chlorpromazine or another phenothiazine, or ondansetron. Low doses of short-acting benzodiazepines are probably safe for anxiety and insomnia. β-Adrenergic blocking agents may be useful to control tachycardia and hypertension, but may be hazardous in patients with hypovolemia or incipient cardiac failure.[231] Seizures are treated by correcting hyponatremia, if present. Almost all anticonvulsant drugs have at least some potential for exacerbating acute porphyrias. Clonazepam may be less harmful than phenytoin, barbiturates, or valproic acid.[232,233] Bromides, gabapentin, and vigabatrin are safe.

Carbohydrate Loading Glucose and other carbohydrates repress hepatic ALAS1 and reduce porphyrin precursor excretion, but the effects are weak compared to those of hemin. Attacks with mild pain and without severe manifestations such as paresis and hyponatremia may be treated with carbohydrate loading. Oral glucose polymer solutions may be given if tolerated. Intravenous treatment with 300 to 500 g of intravenous glucose, usually administered as a 10 percent solution, is recommended. However, the dilutional effects of a large volume of free water may increase risk of hyponatremia. A more complete parenteral nutrition regimen may be needed if oral or enteral feeding is not possible.

Intravenous Hemin Hemin is much more potent in reducing levels of ALA and PBG compared to glucose. Although controlled clinical trials are lacking for all current therapies for acute attacks of porphyria, consensus recommendations are that the clinical benefits of hemin are superior to other available therapies.[234,235,243a] Hemin is available in the United States as a lyophilized hematin preparation (Panhematin, Recordati Rare Diseases, Northfield, IL), and was the first drug approved under the Orphan Drug Act. Heme arginate (Normosang, Orphan Europe, Paris, France), which is a stable preparation of heme and arginine, is available in Europe and South Africa.[235,236] Hemin, when infused intravenously as hematin or heme arginate, becomes bound to circulating hemopexin and albumin and is then taken up primarily by hepatocytes. It then enters and reconstitutes the regulatory heme pool and represses the synthesis of hepatic ALAS1. This results in a dramatic reduction in porphyrin precursor excretion. The standard regimen for treatment of acute attacks is 3 to 4 mg/kg daily for 4 days. Treatment may be extended if a response is not observed within this time. Hemin has been administered safely during pregnancy.[235,236,243a]

Product labeling recommends reconstitution of hematin with sterile water. But it was subsequently discovered that degradation products of hematin begin to form immediately upon reconstitution with water, and these are responsible for phlebitis at the site of infusion, which occurs frequently and can lead to loss of venous access with repeated dosing, and a transient anticoagulant effect.[236a] Stabilization of hematin with 25 percent human albumin can prevent these adverse effects,[238] and is currently recommended.[239] Uncommon side effects include fever,

aching, malaise, hemolysis, anaphylaxis, and circulatory collapse.[240,241] Excessive dosing caused reversible acute renal tubular damage in one case.[242]

Controlled trials comparing initial treatment with either glucose or hemin are lacking, except for one randomized, double-blind, placebo-controlled trial of heme arginate for acute attacks of porphyria, which was underpowered (only 12 patients). Although treatment with hemin was delayed for 2 days, striking decreases in urinary PBG and trends in clinical benefit were noted.[243] In contrast, a larger uncontrolled study enrolled 22 patients who had 51 acute attacks, and heme arginate was initiated within 24 hours of admission in 37 attacks (73 percent); all patients responded and hospitalization was less than 7 days in 90 percent of cases.[235] Therefore, based on this and numerous other uncontrolled clinical studies, it is now recommended that most acute attacks of porphyria be treated promptly with intravenous hemin, without an initial trial of intravenous glucose.[235,243a] Response to hemin may be delayed or incomplete when there is advanced neurologic damage. Subacute or chronic symptoms are unlikely to respond.

Liver Transplantation Liver transplantation has been highly effective in several patients who were disabled by recurrent attacks of AIP.[190] This may be an option for severely affected patients.

Other Therapies Cimetidine has been recommended for human acute porphyrias based on uncontrolled observations in small numbers of patients.[244,245] This drug inhibits hepatic CYPs, and can prevent experimental forms of porphyria induced by agents such as allylisopropylacetamide that undergo activation by these enzymes.[246] However, these mechanisms are not immediately relevant to inherited porphyrias in humans. Therefore, cimetidine cannot be recommended as an alternative to hemin.

Prevention of Acute Attacks Multiple inciting factors must be avoided especially in patients who continue to have repeated attacks. Consultation with a dietitian may be useful to identify dietary indiscretions, and to help maintain a well-balanced diet somewhat high in carbohydrate (60 to 70 percent of total calories). There is little evidence that additional dietary carbohydrate helps further in preventing attacks. Iron deficiency, if present, should be corrected. Patients who wish to lose excess weight should do so gradually and when they are clinically stable.

Gonadotropin-releasing hormone analogues can prevent repeated attacks that are confined to the luteal phase of the menstrual cycle,[247,248] but are less effective in patients with attacks partially associated with the cycle. If treatment is effective after several months, low-dose estradiol, preferably by the transdermal route, or a bisphosphonate may be added to prevent bone loss and other side effects, or treatment changed to a low-dose oral contraceptive. Hemin administered once or twice weekly can prevent frequent, noncyclic attacks of porphyria in some patients.[249]

Long-Term Monitoring Patients with acute porphyrias are at risk for renal damage and hepatocellular carcinoma. Renal function should be monitored, hypertension controlled, and nephrotoxic drugs avoided. Current recommendations are that patients with acute porphyrias who are older than age 50 years, and especially those with continued elevations of ALA and PBG, be screened at least annually by ultrasonogram or an alternative imaging method to detect hepatocellular carcinoma at an early stage.[243a]

HEREDITARY COPROPORPHYRIA AND VARIEGATE PORPHYRIA

Definition

These closely related hepatic porphyrias are caused by deficiencies of CPO and PPO, the sixth and seventh enzymes of the heme biosynthetic pathway. They present with neurovisceral symptoms, as in AIP, or with blistering skin lesions identical to those seen in PCT. Cutaneous manifestations are much more common in VP than in HCP. The enzyme deficiency in each is inherited as an autosomal dominant trait with variable penetrance (see Table 58–1 and Fig. 58–1). As in AIP, most individuals who inherit the trait remain asymptomatic. Both disorders are less common and generally less severe than AIP in most countries. The incidence of HCP was estimated to be 2 per 1,000,000 population in Denmark,[250] and the incidence of VP in Finland reported at 1.3 per 100,000 population.[251]

Because of a founder effect, VP is especially common among whites of Dutch descent in South Africa, where almost all cases share the same *PPO* mutation (R59W). The incidence of VP in that country was estimated at 3 per 1000 population.[252] Very rare cases of homozygous HCP and VP are manifested by severe neurologic impairment early in life, but not acute attacks, and severe photosensitivity.[253]

Pathophysiology

Like other porphyrias, HCP and VP are heterogeneous at the molecular level. At least 43 *CPO* mutations, mostly missense mutations, have been identified in HCP,[254] and 130 *PPO* mutations in VP (see Table 58–1). Clinical expression is variable and onset of neurologic manifestations is influenced by the same factors that are important in AIP.

CPO catalyzes the two-step decarboxylation of coproporphyrinogen III to yield protoporphyrinogen IX, with intermediate formation of harderoporphyrinogen, a tricarboxyl porphyrinogen. A single active site carries out both decarboxylations, and most of the harderoporphyrinogen formed is not released before being further decarboxylated to protoporphyrinogen IX. However, a variant form of HCP, termed *harderoporphyria*, is a result of *CPO* mutations that favor premature release of harderoporphyrinogen from the enzyme.[255]

Clinical Features

Neurovisceral manifestations are identical to those in other acute porphyrias. Although both HCP and VP are generally less severe than AIP, attacks may be life-threatening. Blistering skin lesions may be seen, and are much more common in VP than in HCP. Factors that contribute to attacks, including drugs, hormones, and dietary factors, are also the same as in AIP. Oral contraceptives may precipitate cutaneous manifestations of VP. Risk of chronic hypertension, renal disease, and hepatocellular carcinoma are increased, as in AIP.

Diagnosis

Urinary PBG is elevated during acute attacks, and usually is the basis for diagnosis of these acute porphyrias. However, increases in PBG may be less than in AIP, and more transient. Levels of coproporphyrin III are markedly increased in urine and feces, whereas in AIP fecal porphyrins are normal or only slightly increased. Fecal porphyrins in HCP are almost entirely coproporphyrin III, whereas in VP both coproporphyrin III and protoporphyrin are approximately equally increased. The fecal coproporphyrin III:I ratio is sensitive for diagnosis of HCP, even in asymptomatic stages of the disease.[256] Plasma porphyrin concentration is commonly increased in VP, seldom increased in HCP unless there are cutaneous manifestations, and are normal or only slightly increased in AIP. A characteristic plasma porphyrin fluorescence maximum observed at neutral pH is a very specific marker for VP, and is believed to represent protoporphyrin bound covalently to plasma proteins.[257] The fluorescence maximum as at approximately 626 nm in VP, approximately 634 in EPP, and approximately 620 in other porphyrias. This fluorometric method is more effective than examination of fecal porphyrins for detecting asymptomatic VP,[257] and is useful for rapidly differentiating VP and PCT. Erythrocyte PBG deaminase activity is normal in HCP and VP, and usually deficient in AIP. Assays for CPO and

PPO are not widely available. DNA studies are most reliable for identifying asymptomatic carriers, once the mutation affecting the family is identified.

Harderoporphyria is a variant form of HCP that results from a homozygous defect of a structurally altered CPO, such that harderoporphyrinogen is released prematurely from the enzyme. This variant is identified by finding a predominance of harderoporphyrin in urine and feces. Neonatal hemolytic anemia is a distinctive feature of this condition.[258] Increases in porphyrin precursors and porphyrins may be more severe in homozygous HCP and VP, with substantial increases in erythrocyte zinc protoporphyrin.

Therapy

The identification and avoidance of precipitating factors is essential. Treatment of acute attacks is the same as in AIP. Treatment of the phototoxic manifestations is not satisfactory. Although the lesions are identical to the blistering skin lesions seen in PCT, there is no response in HCP and VP to phlebotomies or low-dose chloroquine or hydroxychloroquine. Therefore, avoidance of sunlight and use of protective clothing is most important. Yearly screening for hepatocellular carcinoma by imaging is recommended after age 50 years, especially in individuals with persistent increases in porphyrin precursors or porphyrins.

PORPHYRIA CUTANEA TARDA AND HEPATOERYTHROPOIETIC PORPHYRIA

Definition

PCT is caused by a deficiency of hepatic UROD activity and is manifested by the development of chronic, blistering skin lesions on the dorsal aspects of the hands and other sun-exposed areas of skin in middle or late life. This iron-related disorder is the most common and readily treated form of porphyria (see Table 58–1 and Fig. 58–1). The enzyme deficiency develops specifically in the liver as a result of generation of a UROD inhibitor in the presence of multiple susceptibility factors. The disease has been classified as types 1 to 3, based on the presence or absence of heterozygous *UROD* mutations and other unknown inherited factors. Patients with familial (type 2) PCT are heterozygous for *UROD* mutations, which are inherited as an autosomal dominant trait with low penetrance. HEP is the homozygous (or compound heterozygous) form of familial (type 2) PCT, which usually presents in childhood and resembles CEP clinically. Rarely, hepatocellular carcinomas may secrete porphyrins and simulate PCT; however the enzyme defect was not established in such cases.[259]

PCT must be differentiated from other porphyrias that cause identical blistering skin lesions and from pseudoporphyria (also known as pseudo-PCT). The latter is a poorly understood condition that presents with lesions that closely resemble PCT, but with plasma porphyrins that are not significantly increased. Potentially photosensitizing drugs, such as nonsteroidal antiinflammatory agents, are sometimes implicated.

Pathophysiology

UROD sequentially decarboxylates uroporphyrinogen (which has eight carboxyl side chains) to yield coproporphyrinogen (with four carboxyl groups). When hepatic UROD is profoundly inhibited, the substrate and the intermediate and final products of the reaction accumulate as the oxidized porphyrins in the liver (mostly uroporphyrin and heptacarboxylporphyrin), and then appear in plasma and urine. Photosensitivity results from activation of porphyrins in the skin by long-wave ultraviolet light and generation of reactive oxygen species.

Hepatic UROD activity is inhibited to less than approximately 20 percent of normal in all patients with PCT. Types 1, 2, and 3 are not fundamentally different or clinically distinguished from each other. Patients with type 1 or "sporadic" PCT have no *UROD* mutations and no family history of PCT. Approximately 80 percent of patients fall into this category. Type 2 or "familial" PCT comprises approximately 20 percent of cases who are heterozygous for *UROD* mutations; but because the penetrance of this trait is low there are usually no other documented cases in the family. In families with type 3, which is rare, more than one member has PCT, but there is no *UROD* mutation; these familial cases presumably share other inherited or environmental susceptibility factors.

Although hepatic UROD activity must be reduced to approximately 20 percent of normal for PCT to be manifest, the amount of enzyme protein, when measured immunochemically in liver, remains at its genetically determined level, which in type 2 cases is approximately 50 percent of normal.[260] Mice heterozygous for mutant *UROD* alleles are much more sensitive to porphyrinogenic stimuli than wild-type animals.[261] In heterozygous mice that display porphyric phenotypes, hepatic UROD protein is half normal, but the catalytic activity of the enzyme is reduced to approximately 20 percent, suggesting the existence of an inhibitor of hepatic UROD.[261]

Although iron does not directly inhibit UROD, there is considerable evidence that PCT is an iron-related disease, with hepatic siderosis seen in many cases. This explains why *HFE* (hemochromatosis gene) mutations that lead to increased intestinal iron absorption predispose to development of PCT (Chap. 42). Individuals who inherit a *UROD* mutation have approximately 50 percent of normal enzyme activity from birth, such that a UROD inhibitor can more readily reduce enzyme activity to less than approximately 20 percent of normal. How iron and other known or suspected susceptibility factors such as alcohol, smoking, estrogens, hepatitis C, HIV, hepatic steatosis, and other suspected factors contribute to the development of PCT is less-well understood, but these may act in part by increasing oxidative stress in hepatocytes. A deficiency of ascorbic acid,[261a] and perhaps other antioxidants,[263] may play a role in some patients. Smoking may also act by inducing hepatic CYPs, including CYP1A2, which is essential for causing uroporphyria in rodent models,[264,265] and may produce a UROD inhibitor, which has been characterized as a uroporphomethene. This substance is a product of partial oxidation of uroporphyrinogen, and is found in the liver of mice that are heterozygous for a *UROD* mutation, homozygous for an *HFE* mutation (C282Y), and develop uroporphyria spontaneously.[62] Other potential mechanisms for lowering of hepatic UROD activity in PCT, such as oxidative damage to UROD active site residues, are less favored but have not been excluded.[266]

At least 70 different *UROD* mutations have been identified in type 2 PCT and HEP (see Table 58–1). These reduce UROD activity and immunoreactivity to approximately 50 percent of normal in all tissues from birth. Most are missense mutations, with each occurring in one or a few families. Homozygosity for a null *UROD* mutation is lethal in early neonatal life. Therefore, in HEP at least one of the mutant *UROD* alleles must preserve at least some catalytic activity. Knowledge of the crystal structure of UROD allows mapping of specific mutations and prediction of their impact on enzyme structure and function. Expression studies in eukaryotic cells suggest that some mutations may destabilize the enzyme protein in a tissue-specific manner.[267]

Pathogenesis of the Clinical Findings

A distinctive feature of PCT is massive accumulation of porphyrins in the liver. As a result, fresh hepatic tissue shows strong red fluorescence on exposure to long-wave ultraviolet light. Microscopic, birefringent, needle-like inclusions are found in lysosomes, and paracrystalline inclusions in mitochondria. Increased stainable iron is very common. Other nonspecific hepatic findings are probably partly a result of the disease itself, although the effects of associated factors such as alcohol and hepatitis C are difficult to differentiate. Liver histopathology includes

hepatocyte necrosis, inflammation, increased iron, and increased fat. Mild abnormalities in liver function tests, especially serum transaminases and γ-glutamyltranspeptidase, are present in almost all cases, but cirrhosis is unusual. The risk of hepatocellular carcinoma is increased, especially in those with more prolonged disease, cirrhosis, or other risk factors such as hepatitis C or alcoholic liver disease.[268–270]

Excess porphyrins are transported in plasma from the liver. Skin histopathology includes subepidermal blistering and deposition of periodic acid-Schiff–positive material around blood vessels and fine fibrillar material in the upper dermis and at the dermoepithelial junction. Immunoglobulin G, other immunoglobulins, and complement are deposited around dermal blood vessels and at the dermoepithelial junction. Splits in the lamina lucida of the basement membrane lead to formation of fluid-containing bullae.[271] These histologic changes are found in other cutaneous porphyrias, as well as pseudoporphyria, and are not diagnostic for PCT. Activation of the complement system after irradiation has been demonstrated in PCT patients both *in vivo* and *in vitro* in sera,[272] and is thought to result from generation of reactive oxygen species.

Susceptibility Factors PCT is a highly heterogeneous disease, with multiple susceptibility factors expected in the individual patient.[273] Multiple factors are important in familial as well as sporadic PCT, because heterozygosity for a *UROD* mutation is a susceptibility factor that does not of itself reduce hepatic enzyme activity sufficiently to cause the disease. The environmental, infectious, and inherited factors discussed below, none of which is invariably present, are known or suspected to play an important role. Their prevalence may show considerable geographic variation in PCT patients as well as healthy subjects.

Alcohol PCT has long been associated with excess alcohol use. Alcohol and its metabolites may induce ALAS1 and CYP2E1, generate active oxygen species that contribute to oxidative damage, cause mitochondrial injury, deplete reduced glutathione and other antioxidant defenses, increase production of endotoxin, activate Kupffer cells, decrease the iron regulatory hormone hepcidin[274] and increase iron absorption.

Smoking and Cytochrome P450 Enzymes Smoking is less extensively studied as a risk factor but is commonly associated with alcohol use in PCT.[273] Smoking may increase oxidative stress in hepatocytes, and induces CYP1A2, which is essential to the development of uroporphyria in rodent models. CYP levels have been found to be increased in liver in human PCT, but it is not clear which CYP might be important in pathogenesis of the human disease. A study of caffeine metabolism did not find evidence for increased CYP1A2 activity *in vivo* in PCT, even when smokers and nonsmokers were analyzed separately.[275] However, a more inducible polymorphism of CYP1A2 has been found to be more common in PCT than in normal subjects.[276]

Estrogens Estrogen use is very common in women with PCT.[273,277,278] In the past, some men developed the disease after treatment of prostate cancer with estrogens.[277] Female rats or males treated with estrogens are more susceptible to development of chemically induced uroporphyria than untreated males.[279] The mechanism is not established, although estrogens can generate reactive oxygen species in some experimental systems.[266]

Hepatitis C Reported prevalence of hepatitis C in PCT has ranged from 21 to 92 percent in various countries, and greatly exceeds the prevalence of this viral infection in healthy subjects, which shows considerable geographic variation. Hepatitis C is associated with excess fat, some iron accumulation, mitochondrial dysfunction, and oxidative stress in hepatocytes, which may contribute to the development of PCT. Dysregulation of hepcidin may contribute to iron accumulation in hepatitis C.[280]

Human Immunodeficiency Virus PCT is less commonly associated with HIV infection than with hepatitis C.[281] Occasionally PCT is the initial manifestation of this infection. The mechanism is unknown.

Iron and *HFE* Mutations Mild to moderate iron overload is found in most patients with PCT, and iron deficiency is protective. The importance of iron has been confirmed in animal models, such as rodents treated with hexachlorobenzene and other halogenated polyaromatic hydrocarbons.[266] Mice with disruption of one *UROD* allele (*UROD[+/−]*) and two disrupted *HFE* alleles (*HFE[−/−]*) develop uroporphyria without administration of exogenous chemicals.[261] Prevalence of the *C282Y* mutation of the *HFE* gene, which is the major cause of hemochromatosis in whites, is increased in both sporadic and familial PCT, and 10 to 20 percent of patients may be *C282Y* homozygotes (Chap. 43).[282] In southern Europe, where the *C282Y* is less prevalent, the *H63D* mutation is more commonly associated with PCT.[283] Excess iron may contribute to UROD inhibition by providing an oxidative environment that is apparently needed for generation of a UROD inhibitor. Hepatic hepcidin expression is reduced in hemochromatosis, and is also reduced in PCT patients without hemochromatosis genotypes when compared to patients without PCT and comparable iron overload, suggesting that reduced expression of this peptide is important in causing hepatic siderosis in PCT.[274]

Antioxidants Substantial reductions in plasma levels of ascorbate and carotenoids have been noted in some patients with PCT.[263] Ascorbate deficiency in rodents enhances susceptibility to development or uroporphyria, and ascorbate decreases uroporphyrin accumulation except in animals treated with large amounts of iron.[262]

A large outbreak of PCT occurred during a period of food shortage in a population in eastern Turkey in the 1950s from consumption of seed wheat treated with the fungicide hexachlorobenzene.[11] Smaller outbreaks and individual cases have occurred after exposures to other chemicals such as 2,3,7,8-tetrachlorodibenzo-*p*-dioxin (TCDD, dioxin).[284] These chemicals were subsequently shown to cause hepatic UROD deficiency and biochemical features resembling PCT in laboratory animals, and many studies that followed have greatly increased our understanding of this acquired enzyme deficiency.[266,285] But such exposures are rarely identified in PCT patients in current clinical practice.

Clinical Features

Disease onset is usually in the fourth or fifth decade of life, and is more common in men. Onset may occur earlier in familial (type 2) disease or

in cases with the C282Y/C282Y *HFE* genotype.[286] Fluid-filled vesicles develop most commonly on the backs of the hands (Fig. 58–7A). Skin friability is increased and blisters often follow minor trauma. These also occur on the forearms, face, ears, neck, legs, and feet. The blisters often rupture, crust over, and are prone to infection before healing slowly. Milia may precede or follow vesicle formation. Facial hypertrichosis and hyperpigmentation are particularly noticed by female patients (Fig. 58–7B). Severe thickening of affected areas of skin is termed *pseudoscleroderma* and resembles systemic scleroderma.

Blistering skin lesions in VP and HCP are identical to those in PCT. Those in CEP and HEP resemble PCT but are usually much more severe and mutilating. Mild or moderate erythrocytosis is common in PCT, and is not well explained. Chronic lung disease from smoking may contribute.

Drugs that exacerbate the acute porphyrias are only occasionally reported to play a role in PCT.[287] PCT may occur with other conditions predisposing to iron overload such as myelofibrosis[288,289] and end-stage renal disease,[290] and with diabetes mellitus[270] and cutaneous and systemic lupus erythematosus. PCT associated with end-stage renal disease is usually more severe, sometimes with severe mutilation. Lack of urinary porphyrin excretion in these patients leads to much higher concentrations of porphyrins in plasma, and the excess porphyrins are poorly dialyzable.[290] The disease occasionally develops during pregnancy, perhaps related to effects of estrogen.

The clinical manifestations of HEP usually resemble CEP, with onset of blistering skin lesions, hypertrichosis, scarring, and red urine in infancy or childhood. Sclerodermoid skin changes are sometimes prominent. Excess porphyrins originate mostly from the liver in this condition. Unusually mild cases have been described.[291]

Diagnosis

A diagnosis of PCT is established by finding a substantial elevation of porphyrins in urine or plasma, with a predominance of highly carboxylated porphyrins (uroporphyrin and hepta-, hexa-, and pentacarboxylporphyrins); coproporphyrins are also increased. Levels of PBG are normal, and urinary ALA is normal or slightly increased. The pattern of porphyrins in feces is complex, and includes heptacarboxylporphyrins and isocoproporphyrins. The latter are overproduced in the presence of UROD deficiency because pentacarboxylporphyrinogen is a substrate

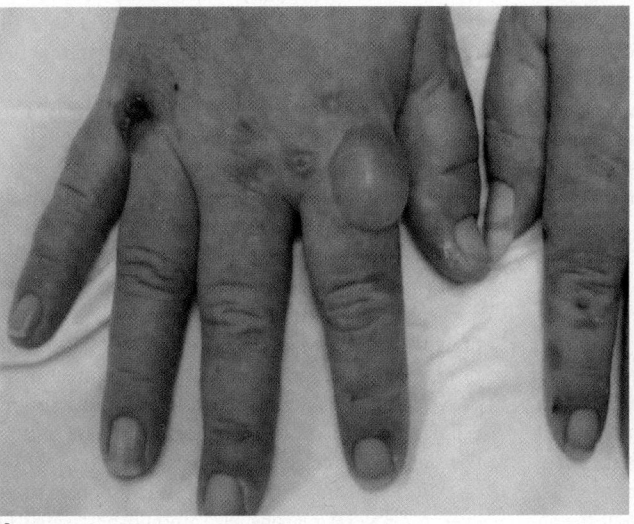 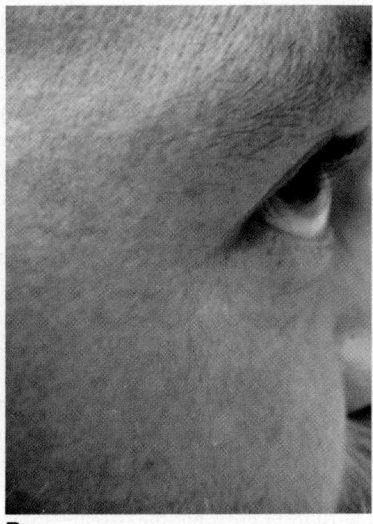

Figure 58–7. Cutaneous findings in porphyria cutanea tarda include **(A)** bullous lesions most commonly on the dorsal aspects of the hands and fingers, which rupture and crust over, and **(B)** facial hirsutism most noticeable on the upper cheeks.

for CPO, leading to formation of dehydroisocoproporphyrinogen, which is excreted in bile and undergoes oxidation by intestinal bacteria to isocoproporphyrins.[292]

Measurement of plasma porphyrins and determination of the fluorescence emission peak at neutral pH is especially useful for screening patients with blistering skin lesions. A substantial increase with a peak at approximately 620 nm is most commonly caused by PCT, and excludes VP and pseudoporphyria, which are the most common conditions that mimic PCT clinically.[292a] Plasma porphyrin measurements are essential for diagnosis of PCT in patients with advanced renal disease; the reference range is higher in patients with renal failure than in normals.[293]

Erythrocyte porphyrins are substantially increased in CEP and HEP, but are normal or only modestly increased in PCT. Rare cases of HCP with blistering lesions are identified by a predominance of coproporphyrin III in urine and especially feces. Familial (type 2) cases are identified by half-normal erythrocyte UROD activity or preferably by DNA studies to identify a *UROD* mutation. Erythrocyte UROD activity is 5 to 30 percent of normal in HEP, and DNA studies reveal that a *UROD* mutation is inherited from each parent.

Biochemical findings in HEP resemble PCT, with predominant accumulation and excretion of highly carboxylated porphyrins and isocoproporphyrins. However, in contrast to PCT, erythrocyte zinc protoporphyrin is substantially increased. At least one genotype may be associated with predominant excretion of pentacarboxylporphyrin.[291]

Therapy

Treatment is highly effective but specific in both sporadic and familial PCT, and therefore should be initiated only after the diagnosis is well established. It is sometimes reasonable to start treatment after PCT is validated with a plasma porphyrin screen and excludes VP and pseudoporphyria (see "Diagnosis" above). Patients should be questioned and tested for all known susceptibility factors, including use of alcohol, tobacco, and estrogens, hepatitis C, HIV, *HFE* mutations, and inherited UROD deficiency (erythrocyte UROD activity or, preferably, *UROD* mutations), because their presence influences management. Serum ferritin should be measured before starting treatment. Patients are advised to stop drinking and smoking and to discontinue estrogens. A nutritionally adequate intake of ascorbic acid and other nutrients should be assured, but this vitamin should not be administered as primary therapy.

Improvement may occur after removing one or more susceptibility factor, but without phlebotomy or low-dose hydroxychloroquine recovery is unpredictable or slow.[294] Repeated phlebotomy is the preferred treatment at most centers. The original rationale proposed by Ippen in 1961 was to decrease the commonly associated mild or moderately increased hemoglobin, stimulate erythropoiesis, and perhaps channel excess heme pathway intermediates to hemoglobin synthesis.[295] However, the oxidized porphyrins that accumulate in PCT cannot reenter the heme biosynthetic pathway and be converted to heme, and it is now understood that phlebotomy is effective by reducing body iron stores and liver iron content. Treatment with an iron chelator such as desferrioxamine is less efficient than phlebotomies in reducing iron, but may be tried when the latter are contraindicated.[296]

Approximately 450 mL of blood is removed, usually at 2-week intervals. In one series an average of 5.4 phlebotomies was required for remission, but many more are needed in some patients with coexisting hemochromatosis and marked increases in serum ferritin levels. Hemoglobin or hematocrit levels are followed as safety (not therapeutic) targets, to prevent symptomatic anemia. Usually, the hemoglobin should not fall below 10 to 11 g/dL, but the baseline value and the age and clinical condition of the patient are also considered. The therapeutic target is a serum ferritin near 15 ng/mL, which is close to the lower limit of normal and associated with tissue iron depletion but usually not

anemia. Additional iron depletion is not beneficial, and causes anemia. Treatment is also guided by plasma (or serum) porphyrin levels, which are more convenient to measure repeatedly than urine porphyrins, and fall more slowly than the serum ferritin. Plasma porphyrins usually decline from initial levels of 10 to 25 mcg/dL during treatment, to below the upper limit of normal (~1 mcg/dL) within weeks after phlebotomies are completed.[297] New skin lesions are generally decreased at the end of treatment, but some may occur for a few weeks after plasma porphyrin levels become normal. Severe sclerodermatous changes and liver function abnormalities can also improve.

After a remission, continued phlebotomies are generally not needed. However, relapses may occur, especially in patients who resume use of alcohol, and are treated by another course of phlebotomies. For patients with the *C282Y/C282Y* or *C282Y/H63D HFE* genotypes, management guidelines for hemochromatosis should be followed. Continued phlebotomies as needed to maintain a serum ferritin below approximately 50 ng/mL may also be beneficial in patients who have experienced recurrences of PCT, although published experience is limited. It is also advisable to follow porphyrin levels and reinstitute phlebotomies promptly if porphyrin levels begin to rise. Liver imaging and a serum α-fetoprotein determination should be repeated as screening for hepatocellular carcinoma. After remission, transdermal estrogen can be resumed in women, if needed, with little risk for recurrence of PCT.[275]

A low-dose regimen of hydroxychloroquine or chloroquine is also effective,[266,298–303] and most appropriate when phlebotomy is contraindicated or poorly tolerated, if iron overload is not severe. However, this treatment is preferred at some centers because it is more convenient and much less expensive. These 4-aminoquinoline antimalarials do not appear to deplete hepatic iron, and the mechanism for their effect in PCT is not fully understood. Full therapeutic doses of these drugs exacerbate photosensitivity in PCT, induce fever, malaise, and nausea, markedly increase urinary and plasma porphyrins, and increase serum transaminases, other liver function tests, and ferritin. This reaction can even unmask previously unrecognized PCT.[304] Although these adverse effects, which are unique to PCT, are followed by complete remission,[305] they should be avoided by a low-dose treatment regimen (hydroxychloroquine 100 mg or chloroquine 125 mg—one-half of a standard tablet—twice weekly) at least until plasma or urine porphyrins are normalized.[298,301,302] However, some patients may respond poorly and require later treatment with larger doses, or phlebotomy.[305] There is a small risk of retinopathy,[306] which may be lower with hydroxychloroquine. A recent prospective study found that time to biochemical remission with low-dose hydroxychloroquine was comparable to that with phlebotomy.[307] In a retrospective study, low-dose chloroquine was ineffective in patients homozygous for the *C282Y* mutation of the *HFE* gene,[308] which suggests that the degree of excess hepatic iron may influence response to this treatment.

These 4-aminoquinolines are not effective in other porphyrias, and do not mobilize all types of porphyrins from liver and other tissues.[309] Chloroquine may form complexes with a variety of porphyrins, which might promote their mobilization from liver,[310,311] but this does not appear to explain the effects in PCT. It was suggested that mobilization of hepatic iron may be important,[302,312,313] but serum ferritin concentrations do not change significantly during treatment. Most likely, these drugs colocalize with excess porphyrins in lysosomes and other intracellular organelles and promote their release by a process that involves transient cell damage.

PCT may improve after treatment of coexisting hepatitis C. However, for several reasons PCT should be treated first and hepatitis C later in most cases. First, PCT is usually more symptomatic and can be treated more quickly and effectively. Second, there is some evidence that treatment of hepatitis C may be more effective after iron reduction.

Third, interferon and ribavirin commonly cause anemia, which usually precludes phlebotomy for PCT. Hydroxychloroquine may be an option during treatment with interferon and ribavirin, but initial worsening of liver function tests, even with a low-dose regimen, may cause concern. It is reasonable to consider continuing low-dose hydroxychloroquine after PCT is in remission to avoid a reoccurrence of PCT during treatment of hepatitis C, but there is little experience with this approach. Reports that PCT patients are often resistant to treatment of hepatitis C,[314,315] contrast with reports of successful treatment, and prospective studies are needed. Studies are needed with newer and more effective agents for hepatitis C as these become available.

Treatment of PCT associated with end-stage renal disease is more difficult, as phlebotomy is often contraindicated by anemia. Erythropoietin administration can correct anemia, mobilize iron, and support phlebotomy in many cases.[290,316,317] High-flux hemodialysis may remove porphyrins from plasma and provide some benefit.[318] PCT is not a contraindication to renal transplantation, which is likely to lead to remission[319] partly because of resumption of endogenous erythropoietin production. The level of plasma porphyrins are often especially high in these patients, and should be assessed prior to surgery, because there may be some risk of skin and peritoneal burns from exposure to operating room lights.

Management of HEP emphasizes avoiding sunlight, as in CEP. Oral charcoal was helpful in a severe case associated with dyserythropoiesis.[98] Phlebotomy has shown little or no benefit. Retrovirus-mediated gene transfer can correct porphyria in cell lines from patients with this disease, which suggests that gene therapy may be applicable in the future.[320]

REFERENCES

1. Moore MR, McColl KE: *Disorders of Porphyrin Metabolism.* Plenum, New York, 1987.
2. Schultz J: *Ein fall von pemphigus, kompliziert durch lepra visceralis,* in *Medicine.* Greifswald University, Greifswald, Germany, 1874.
3. Anderson TM: Hydroa aestivale in two brothers, complicated with the presence of haematoporphyrin in the urine. *Br J Dermatol* 10:1, 1898.
4. Harris DF: Haematoporphyrinuria and its relations to the source of urobilin. *J Anat Physiol* 31:383, 1897.
5. Stokvis BJ: Over Twee Zeldsame Kleuerstoffen in Urine van Zicken. *Ned Tijdschr Geneeskd* 13:409, 1889.
6. Günther H: Die haematoporphyrie. *Deutsche Archiv für Klinische Medizin* 105:89, 1911.
7. Garrod AE: *Inborn Errors of Metabolism.* Hodder & Stoughton, London, 1923.
8. Waldenström J, Vahlquist BC: Studien uber die entstehung der roten harnpigmente (uroporphyrin und porphobilin) bein der akuten porphyrie aus iher farblosen vorstufe (porphobilinogen). *Hoppe Seylers Z Physiol Chem* 260:189, 1939.
9. Schmid R, Schwartz S, Watson CJ: Porphyrin content of bone marrow and liver in the various forms of porphyria. *Arch Intern Med* 93:167, 1954.
10. Cam C, Nigogosyan G: Acquired toxic porphyria cutanea tarda due to hexachlorobenzene. *JAMA* 183(2):90, 1963.
11. Schmid R: Cutaneous porphyria in Turkey. *N Engl J Med* 263:397, 1960.
12. Ockner RK, Schmid R: Acquired porphyria in man and rat due to hexachlorobenzene intoxication. *Nature* 189:499, 1961.
13. Schmid R: Acquired porphyria. *JAMA* 183:133, 1963.
14. Strand LJ, Felsher BF, Redeker AG, et al: Heme biosynthesis in intermittent acute porphyria: Decreased hepatic conversion of porphobilinogen to porphyrins and increased delta-aminolevulinic acid synthetase activity. *Proc Natl Acad Sci U S A* 67:1315, 1970.
15. Bonkowsky HL, Tschudy DP, Collins A, et al: Repression of the overproduction of porphyrin precursors in acute intermittent porphyria by intravenous infusions of hematin. *Proc Natl Acad Sci U S A* 68(11):2725, 1971.
16. Granick S, Sassa S: δ-Aminolevulinic acid synthase and the control of heme and chlorophyll synthesis, in *Metabolic Regulation,* edited by Vogel HJ, p 77. Academic Press, New York, 1971.
17. Sassa S, Kappas A: Genetic, metabolic and biochemical aspects of the porphyrias, in *Advances in Human Genetics,* edited by Harris H, Hirschhorn K, p 121. Plenum Publications, New York, 1981.
18. McKay R, Druyan R, Getz GS, et al: Intramitochondrial localization of delta-aminolaevulate synthetase and ferrochelatase in rat liver. *Biochem J* 114(3):455, 1969.
19. Riddle RD, Yamamoto M, Engel JD: Expression of delta-aminolevulinate synthase in avian cells: Separate genes encode erythroid-specific and nonspecific isozymes. *Proc Natl Acad Sci U S A* 86(3):792, 1989.
20. Tsai SF, Bishop DF, Desnick RJ: Human uroporphyrinogen III synthase: Molecular cloning, nucleotide sequence, and expression of a full-length cDNA. *Proc Natl Acad Sci U S A* 85(19):7049, 1988.
21. Bishop DF: Two different genes encode delta-aminolevulinate synthase in humans: Nucleotide sequences of cDNAs for the housekeeping and erythroid genes. *Nucleic Acids Res* 18(23):7187, 1990.
22. Cox TC, Bawden MJ, Martin A, et al: Human erythroid 5-aminolevulinate synthase: Promoter analysis and identification of an iron-responsive element in the mRNA. *EMBO J* 10(7):1891, 1991.
23. Aziz N, Munro HN: Iron regulates ferritin mRNA translation through a segment of its 5′ untranslated region. *Proc Natl Acad Sci U S A* 84(23):8478, 1987.
24. Lowry JA, Mackay JP: GATA-1: One protein, many partners. *Int J Biochem Cell Biol* 38(1):6, 2006.
25. Casey JL, Di Jeso B, Rao K, et al: The promoter region of the human transferrin receptor gene. *Ann N Y Acad Sci* 526:54, 1988.
26. Melefors O, Goossen B, Johansson HE, et al: Translational control of 5-aminolevulinate synthase mRNA by iron-responsive elements in erythroid cells. *J Biol Chem* 268(8):5974, 1993.
27. Podvinec M, Handschin C, Looser R, et al: Identification of the xenosensors regulating human 5-aminolevulinate synthase. *Proc Natl Acad Sci U S A* 101(24):9127, 2004.
28. Elferink CJ, Srivastava G, Maguire DJ, et al: A unique gene for 5-aminolevulinate synthase in chickens. Evidence for expression of an identical messenger RNA in hepatic and erythroid tissues. *J Biol Chem* 262(9):3988, 1987.
29. Kitchin KT: Regulation of rat hepatic delta-aminolevulinic acid synthetase and heme oxygenase activities: Evidence for control by heme and against mediation by prosthetic iron. *Int J Biochem* 15(4):479, 1983.
30. Handschin C, Lin J, Rhee J, et al: Nutritional regulation of hepatic heme biosynthesis and porphyria through PGC-1alpha. *Cell* 122(4):505, 2005.
31. Virbasius JV, Scarpulla RC: Activation of the human mitochondrial transcription factor A gene by nuclear respiratory factors: A potential regulatory link between nuclear and mitochondrial gene expression in organelle biogenesis. *Proc Natl Acad Sci U S A* 91(4):1309, 1994.
32. Scassa ME, Guberman AS, Ceruti JM, et al: Hepatic nuclear factor 3 and nuclear factor 1 regulate 5-aminolevulinate synthase gene expression and are involved in insulin repression. *J Biol Chem* 279(27):28082, 2004.
33. Dandekar T, Stripecke R, Gray NK, et al: Identification of a novel iron-responsive element in murine and human erythroid delta-aminolevulinic acid synthase mRNA. *EMBO J* 10(7):1903, 1991.
34. Fujita H, Yamamoto M, Yamagami T, et al: Erythroleukemia differentiation. Distinctive responses of the erythroid-specific and the nonspecific delta-aminolevulinate synthase mRNA. *J Biol Chem* 266(26):17494, 1991.
35. Furuyama K, Sassa S: Interaction between succinyl CoA synthetase and the heme-biosynthetic enzyme ALAS-E is disrupted in sideroblastic anemia. *J Clin Invest* 105(6):757, 2000.
36. Furuyama K, Fujita H, Nagai T, et al: Pyridoxine refractory X-linked sideroblastic anemia caused by a point mutation in the erythroid 5-aminolevulinate synthase gene. *Blood* 90(2):822, 1997.
37. Whatley SD, Ducamp S, Gouya L, et al: C-terminal deletions in the ALAS2 gene lead to gain of function and cause X-linked dominant protoporphyria without anemia or iron overload. *Am J Hum Genet* 83(3):408, 2008.
38. Sassa S: Delta-aminolevulinic acid dehydratase assay. *Enzyme* 28(2–3):133, 1982.
39. Tsukamoto I, Yoshinaga T, Sano S: The role of zinc with special reference to the essential thiol groups in delta-aminolevulinic acid dehydratase of bovine liver. *Biochim Biophys Acta* 570(1):167, 1979.
40. Granick JL, Sassa S, Kappas A: Some biochemical and clinical aspects of lead intoxication, in *Advances in Clinical Chemistry,* edited by Bodansky O, Latner AL, p 287. Academic Press, New York, 1978.
41. Sassa S, Kappas A: Hereditary tyrosinemia and the heme biosynthetic pathway. Profound inhibition of delta-aminolevulinic acid dehydratase activity by succinylacetone. *J Clin Invest* 71(3):625, 1983.
42. Tschudy DP, Hess RA, Frykholm BC: Inhibition of delta-aminolevulinic acid dehydrase by 4,6-dioxoheptanoic acid. *J Biol Chem* 256(19):9915, 1981.
43. Lindblad B, Lindstedt S, Steen G: On the enzymic defects in hereditary tyrosinemia. *Proc Natl Acad Sci U S A* 74(10):4641, 1977.
44. Wetmur JG, Bishop DF, Cantelmo C, et al: Human delta-aminolevulinate dehydratase: Nucleotide sequence of a full-length cDNA clone. *Proc Natl Acad Sci U S A* 83(20):7703, 1986.
45. Potluri VR, Astrin KH, Wetmur JG, et al: Human delta-aminolevulinate dehydratase: Chromosomal localization to 9q34 by in situ hybridization. *Hum Genet* 76(3):236, 1987.
46. Erskine PT, Senior N, Awan S, et al: X-ray structure of 5-aminolaevulinate dehydratase, a hybrid aldolase. *Nat Struct Biol* 4(12):1025, 1997.
47. Bishop TR, Miller MW, Beall J, et al: Genetic regulation of delta-aminolevulinate dehydratase during erythropoiesis. *Nucleic Acids Res* 24(13):2511, 1996.
48. Wetmur JG, Kaya AH, Plewinska M, et al: Molecular characterization of the human delta-aminolevulinate dehydratase 2 (ALAD2) allele: Implications for molecular screening of individuals for genetic susceptibility to lead poisoning. *Am J Hum Genet* 49(4):757, 1991.
49. Inoue R, Akagi R: Co-synthesis of human delta-aminolevulinate dehydratase (ALAD) mutants with the wild-type enzyme in cell-free system-critical importance of conformation on enzyme activity. *J Clin Biochem Nutr* 43(3):143, 2008.

50. Jaffe EK, Stith L: ALAD porphyria is a conformational disease. *Am J Hum Genet* 80(2):329, 2007.

51. Battersby AR, Fookes CJ, Matcham GW, et al: Biosynthesis of the pigments of life: Formation of the macrocycle. *Nature* 285(5759):17, 1980.

52. Jordan PM: The biosynthesis of 5-aminolevulinic acid and its transformation into coproporphyrinogen in animals and bacteria, in *Biosynthesis of Heme and Chlorophylls*, edited by Dailey HA, p 55. McGraw-Hill, New York, 1990.

53. Awan SJ, Siligardi G, Shoolingin-Jordan PM, et al: Reconstitution of the holoenzyme form of *Escherichia coli* porphobilinogen deaminase from apoenzyme with porphobilinogen and preuroporphyrinogen: A study using circular dichroism spectroscopy. *Biochemistry* 36(30):9273, 1997.

54. Wang AL, Arredondo-Vega FX, Giampietro PF, et al: Regional gene assignment of human porphobilinogen deaminase and esterase A4 to chromosome 11q23 leads to 11qter. *Proc Natl Acad Sci U S A* 78(9):5734, 1981.

55. Chretien S, Dubart A, Beaupain D, et al: Alternative transcription and splicing of the human porphobilinogen deaminase gene result either in tissue-specific or in housekeeping expression. *Proc Natl Acad Sci U S A* 85(1):6, 1988.

56. Grandchamp B, De Verneuil H, Beaumont C, et al: Tissue specific expression of porphobilinogen deaminase. Two isoenzymes from a single gene. *Eur J Biochem* 162:105, 1987.

57. Raich N, Romeo PH, Dubart A, et al: Molecular cloning and complete primary sequence of human erythrocyte porphobilinogen deaminase. *Nucleic Acids Res* 14(15):5955, 1986.

58. Mignotte V, Eleouet JF, Raich N, et al: Cis- and trans-acting elements involved in the regulation of the erythroid promoter of the human porphobilinogen deaminase gene. *Proc Natl Acad Sci U S A* 86(17):6548, 1989.

59. Grandchamp B, Picat C, De Rooij FWM, et al: Molecular analysis of acute intermittent porphyria in a Finnish family with normal erythrocyte porphobilinogen deaminase. *Eur J Clin Invest* 19:415, 1989.

60. Mathews MA, Schubert HL, Whitby FG, et al: Crystal structure of human uroporphyrinogen III synthase. *EMBO J* 20(21):5832, 2001.

61. Schubert HL, Phillips JD, Heroux A, et al: Structure and mechanistic implications of a uroporphyrinogen III synthase-product complex. *Biochemistry* 47(33):8648, 2008.

62. Phillips JD, Bergonia HA, Reilly CA, et al: A porphomethene inhibitor of uroporphyrinogen decarboxylase causes porphyria cutanea tarda. *Proc Natl Acad Sci U S A* 104(12):5079, 2007.

63. Smith AG, Clothier B, Robinson S, et al: Interaction between iron metabolism and 2,3,7,8-tetrachlorodibenzo-p-dioxin in mice with variants of the Ahr gene: A hepatic oxidative mechanism. *Mol Pharmacol* 53(1):52, 1998.

64. Romana M, Dubart A, Beaupain D, et al: Structure of the gene for human uroporphyrinogen decarboxylase. *Nucleic Acids Res* 15(18):7343, 1987.

65. de Verneuil H, Grandchamp B, Foubert C, et al: Assignment of the gene for uroporphyrinogen decarboxylase to human chromosome 1 by somatic cell hybridization and specific enzyme immunoassay. *Hum Genet* 66(2–3):202, 1984.

66. Romeo PH, Raich N, Dubart A, et al: Molecular cloning and nucleotide sequence of a complete human uroporphyrinogen decarboxylase cDNA. *J Biol Chem* 261(21):9825, 1986.

67. Whitby FG, Phillips JD, Kushner JP, et al: Crystal structure of human uroporphyrinogen decarboxylase. *EMBO J* 17(9):2463, 1998.

68. Phillips JD, Whitby FG, Kushner JP: Structural basis for tetrapyrrole coordination by uroporphyrinogen decarboxylase. *EMBO J* 22(23):6225, 2003.

69. Rhee HW, Zou P, Udeshi ND, et al: Proteomic mapping of mitochondria in living cells via spatially restricted enzymatic tagging. *Science* 339(6125):1328, 2013.

70. Cacheux V, Martasek P, Fougerousse F, et al: Localization of the human coproporphyrinogen oxidase gene to chromosome band 3q12. *Hum Genet* 94(5):557, 1994.

71. Kohno H, Furukawa T, Yoshinaga T, et al: Coproporphyrinogen oxidase. Purification, molecular cloning, and induction of mRNA during erythroid differentiation. *J Biol Chem* 268(28):21359, 1993.

72. Takahashi S, Furuyama K, Kobayashi A, et al: Cloning of a coproporphyrinogen oxidase promoter regulatory element binding protein. *Biochem Biophys Res Commun* 273(2):596, 2000.

73. Takahashi S, Taketani S, Akasaka JE, et al: Differential regulation of coproporphyrinogen oxidase gene between erythroid and nonerythroid cells. *Blood* 92(9):3436, 1998.

74. Conder LH, Woodard SI, Dailey HA: Multiple mechanisms for the regulation of haem synthesis during erythroid cell differentiation. Possible role for coproporphyrinogen oxidase. *Biochem J* 275(Pt 2):321, 1991.

75. Lamoril J, Deybach JC, Puy H, et al: Three novel mutations in the coproporphyrinogen oxidase gene. *Hum Mutat* 9(1):78, 1997.

76. Nishimura K, Taketani S, Inokuchi H: Cloning of a human cDNA for protoporphyrinogen oxidase by complementation in vivo of a hemG mutant of *Escherichia coli*. *J Biol Chem* 270(14):8076, 1995.

77. Taketani S, Inazawa J, Abe T, et al: The human protoporphyrinogen oxidase gene (PPOX): Organization and location to chromosome 1. *Genomics* 29(3):698, 1995.

78. Koch M, Breithaupt C, Kiefersauer R, et al: Crystal structure of protoporphyrinogen IX oxidase: A key enzyme in haem and chlorophyll biosynthesis. *EMBO J* 23(8):1720, 2004.

79. Morgan RR, Errington R, Elder GH: Identification of sequences required for the import of human protoporphyrinogen oxidase to mitochondria. *Biochem J* 377(Pt 2):281, 2004.

80. de Vooght KM, van Wijk R, van Solinge WW: GATA-1 binding sites in exon 1 direct erythroid-specific transcription of PPOX. *Gene* 409(1–2):83, 2008.

81. Porra RJ, Jones OT: Studies on ferrochelatase. 1. Assay and properties of ferrochelatase from a pig-liver mitochondrial extract. *Biochem J* 87:181, 1963.

82. Whitcombe DM, Carter NP, Albertson DG, et al: Assignment of the human ferrochelatase gene (FECH) and a locus for protoporphyria to chromosome 18q22. *Genomics* 11(4):1152, 1991.

83. Medlock A, Swartz L, Dailey TA, et al: Substrate interactions with human ferrochelatase. *Proc Natl Acad Sci U S A* 104(6):1789, 2007.

84. Medlock AE, Dailey TA, Ross TA, et al: A pi-helix switch selective for porphyrin deprotonation and product release in human ferrochelatase. *J Mol Biol* 373(4):1006, 2007.

85. Wada O, Sassa S, Takaku F, et al: Different responses of the hepatic and erythropoietic delta-aminolevulinic acid synthetase of mice. *Biochim Biophys Acta* 148(2):585, 1967.

86. Sassa S, Nagai T: The role of heme in gene expression. *Int J Hematol* 63(3):167, 1996.

87. Erwin A, Balwani M, Desnick RJ: *Congenital Erythropoietic Porphyria*. University of Washington, Seattle, 2013.

88. Sassa S, Akagi R, Nishitani C, et al: Late-onset porphyrias: What are they? *Cell Mol Biol (Noisy-le-grand)* 48(1):97, 2002.

89. Fritsch C, Bolsen K, Ruzicka T, et al: Congenital erythropoietic porphyria. *J Am Acad Dermatol* 36(4):594, 1997.

90. Günther H: in *Handbuch der Krankheiten des Blutes und der Blutbildenden Organe*, vol 2, edited by Schittenhelm A. Springer-Verlag, Berlin, 1925.

91. Desnick RJ, Glass IA, Xu W, et al: Molecular genetics of congenital erythropoietic porphyria. *Semin Liver Dis* 18(1):77, 1998.

92. Watson CJ, Perman V, Spurrell FA, et al: Some studies of the comparative biology of human and bovine porphyria erythropoietica. *Trans Assoc Am Physicians* 71:196, 1958.

93. Phillips JD, Steensma DP, Pulsipher MA, et al: Congenital erythropoietic porphyria due to a mutation in GATA1: The first trans-acting mutation causative for a human porphyria. *Blood* 109(6):2618, 2007.

94. Seip M, Thune PO, Eriksen L: Treatment of photosensitivity in congenital erythropoietic porphyria (CEP) with beta-carotene. *Acta Derm Venereol* 54(3):239, 1974.

95. Haining RG, Cowger ML, Labbe RF, et al: Congenital erythropoietic porphyria. II. The effects of induced polycythemia. *Blood* 36(3):297, 1970.

96. Piomelli S, Poh-Fitzpatrick MB, Seaman C, et al: Complete suppression of the symptoms of congenital erythropoietic porphyria by long-term treatment with high-level transfusions. *N Engl J Med* 314(16):1029, 1986.

97. Guarini L, Piomelli S, Poh-Fitzpatrick MB: Hydroxyurea in congenital erythropoietic porphyria [letter]. *N Engl J Med* 330:1091, 1994.

98. Pimstone NR, Gandhi SN, Mukerji SK: Therapeutic efficacy of oral charcoal in congenital erythropoietic porphyria. *N Engl J Med* 316(7):390, 1987.

99. Hallai N, Anstey A, Mendelsohn S, et al: Pregnancy in a patient with congenital erythropoietic porphyria. *N Engl J Med* 357(6):622, 2007.

100. Dupuis-Girod S, Akkari V, Ged C, et al: Successful match-unrelated donor bone marrow transplantation for congenital erythropoietic porphyria (Gunther disease). *Eur J Pediatr* 164(2):104, 2005.

101. Geronimi F, Richard E, Lamrissi-Garcia I, et al: Lentivirus-mediated gene transfer of uroporphyrinogen III synthase fully corrects the porphyric phenotype in human cells. *J Mol Med (Berl)* 81(5):310, 2003.

102. Kauppinen R, Glass IA, Aizencang G, et al: Congenital erythropoietic porphyria: Prolonged high-level expression and correction of the heme biosynthetic defect by retroviral-mediated gene transfer into porphyric and erythroid cells. *Mol Genet Metab* 65(1):10, 1998.

103. Holme SA, Anstey AV, Finlay AY, et al: Erythropoietic protoporphyria in the U.K.: Clinical features and effect on quality of life. *Br J Dermatol* 155(3):574, 2006.

104. Marko PB, Miljkovic J, Gorenjak M, et al: Erythropoietic protoporphyria patients in Slovenia. *Acta Dermatovenerol Alp Pannonica Adriat* 16(3):99, 104, 2007.

105. Parker M, Corrigall AV, Hift RJ, et al: Molecular characterization of erythropoietic protoporphyria in South Africa. *Br J Dermatol* 159(1):182, 2008.

106. Nakahashi Y, Fujita H, Taketani S, et al: The molecular defect of ferrochelatase in a patient with erythropoietic protoporphyria. *Proc Natl Acad Sci USA.* 89(1):281-285, 192.

107. Gouya L, Deybach JC, Lamoril J, et al: Modulation of the phenotype in dominant erythropoietic protoporphyria by a low expression of the normal ferrochelatase allele. *Am J Hum Genet* 58(2):292, 1996.

108. Gouya L, Puy H, Lamoril J, et al: Inheritance in erythropoietic protoporphyria: A common wild-type ferrochelatase allelic variant with low expression accounts for clinical manifestation. *Blood* 93(6):2105, 1999.

109. Gouya L, Puy H, Robreau AM, et al: The penetrance of dominant erythropoietic protoporphyria is modulated by expression of wildtype FECH. *Nat Genet* 30(1):27, 2002.

110. Gouya L, Martin-Schmitt C, Robreau AM, et al: Contribution of a common single-nucleotide polymorphism to the genetic predisposition for erythropoietic protoporphyria. *Am J Hum Genet* 78(1):2, 2006.

111. Holme SA, Whatley SD, Roberts AG, et al: Seasonal palmar keratoderma in erythropoietic protoporphyria indicates autosomal recessive inheritance. *J Invest Dermatol* 129(3):599, 2009.

112. Aplin C, Whatley SD, Thompson P, et al: Late-onset erythropoietic porphyria caused by a chromosome 18q deletion in erythroid cells. *J Invest Dermatol* 117(6):1647, 2001.

113. Shirota T, Yamamoto H, Hayashi S, et al: Myelodysplastic syndrome terminating in erythropoietic protoporphyria after 15 years of aplastic anemia. *Int J Hematol* 72(1):44, 2000.

114. Goodwin RG, Kell WJ, Laidler P, et al: Photosensitivity and acute liver injury in myeloproliferative disorder secondary to late-onset protoporphyria caused by deletion of a ferrochelatase gene in hematopoietic cells. *Blood* 107(1):60, 2006.

115. Bottomley SS, Tanaka M, Everett MA: Diminished erythroid ferrochelatase activity in protoporphyria. *J Lab Clin Med* 86(1):126, 1975.

116. Piomelli S, Lamola AA, Poh-Fitzpatrick MF, et al: Erythropoietic protoporphyria and lead intoxication: The molecular basis for difference in cutaneous photosensitivity. I. Different rates of disappearance of protoporphyrin from the erythrocytes, both in vivo and in vitro. *J Clin Invest* 56(6):1519, 1975.

117. Sandberg S, Brun A, Hovding G, et al: Effect of zinc on protoporphyrin induced photohaemolysis. *Scand J Clin Lab Invest* 40(2):185, 1980.

118. Spikes JD: Porphyrins and related compounds as photodynamic sensitizers. *Ann N Y Acad Sci* 244:496, 1975.

119. Goldstein BD, Harber LC: Erythropoietic protoporphyria: Lipid peroxidation and red cell membrane damage associated with photohemolysis. *J Clin Invest* 51(4):892, 1972.

120. Lim HW, Poh-Fitzpatrick MB, Gigli I: Activation of the complement system in patients with porphyrias after irradiation in vivo. *J Clin Invest* 74(6):1961, 1984.

121. Ryan EA: Histochemistry of the skin in erythropoietic protoporphyria. *Br J Dermatol* 78(10):501, 1966.

122. Poh-Fitzpatrick MB. The erythropoietic porphyrias. *Dermatol Clin* 4(2):291, 1986.

123. Berenson MM, Kimura R, Samowitz W, et al: Protoporphyrin overload in unrestrained rats: Biochemical and histopathologic characterization of a new model of protoporphyric hepatopathy. *Int J Exp Pathol* 73(5):665, 1992.

124. Bloomer JR: The liver in protoporphyria. *Hepatology* 8(2):402, 1988.

125. Bloomer JR, Enriquez R: Evidence that hepatic crystalline deposits in a patient with protoporphyria are composed of protoporphyrin. *Gastroenterology* 82(3):569, 1982.

126. Bloomer J, Wang Y, Singhal A, et al: Molecular studies of liver disease in erythropoietic protoporphyria. *J Clin Gastroenterol* 39(4 Suppl 2):S167, 2005.

127. Mathews-Roth MM: Systemic photoprotection. *Dermatol Clin* 4(2):335, 1986.

128. De Leo VA, Poh-Fitzpatrick M, Mathews-Roth M, et al: Erythropoietic protoporphyria. 10 years experience. *Am J Med* 60:8, 1976.

129. Delaby C, Lyoumi S, Ducamp S, et al: Excessive erythrocyte ppix influences the hematologic status and iron metabolism in patients with dominant erythropoietic protoporphyria. *Cell Mol Biol (Noisy-le-grand)* 55(1):45, 2009.

130. Turnbull A, Baker H, Vernon-Roberts B, et al: Iron metabolism in porphyria cutanea tarda and in erythropoietic protoporphyria. *Q J Med* 42:341, 1973.

131. Holme SA, Worwood M, Anstey AV, et al: Erythropoiesis and iron metabolism in dominant erythropoietic protoporphyria. *Blood* 110(12):4108, 2007.

132. Rademakers LH, Koningsberger JC, Sorber CW, et al: Accumulation of iron in erythroblasts of patients with erythropoietic protoporphyria. *Eur J Clin Invest* 23(2):130, 1993.

133. Barman-Aksözen J, Beguin C, Dogar AM, et al: Iron availability modulates aberrant splicing of ferrochelatase through the iron- and 2-oxoglutarate dependent dioxygenase Jmjd6 and U2AF(65). *Blood Cells Mol Dis* 51(3):151, 2013.

134. Barman-Aksözen J, Minder EI, Schubiger C, et al: In ferrochelatase-deficient protoporphyria patients, ALAS2 expression is enhanced and erythrocytic protoporphyrin concentration correlates with iron availability. *Blood Cells Mol Dis* 2014.

135. Poh-Fitzpatrick MB: Human protoporphyria: Reduced cutaneous photosensitivity and lower erythrocyte porphyrin levels during pregnancy. *J Am Acad Dermatol* 36(1):40, 1997.

136. Rank JM, Carithers R, Bloomer J: Evidence for neurological dysfunction in end-stage protoporphyric liver disease. *Hepatology* 18(6):1404, 1993.

137. Doss MO, Frank M: Hepatobiliary implications and complications in protoporphyria, a 20-year study. *Clin Biochem* 22:223, 1989.

138. Singer JA, Plaut AG, Kaplan MM: Hepatic failure and death from erythropoietic protoporphyria. *Gastroenterology* 74(3):588, 1978.

139. Key NS, Rank JM, Freese D, et al: Hemolytic anemia in protoporphyria: Possible precipitating role of liver failure and photic stress. *Am J Hematol* 39:202, 1992.

140. Hastka J, Lasserre JJ, Schwarzbeck A, et al: Zinc protoporphyrin in anemia of chronic disorders. *Blood* 81:1200, 1993.

141. Anderson KE, Sassa S, Peterson CM, et al: Increased erythrocyte uroporphyrinogen-I-synthetase, d-aminolevulinic acid dehydratase and protoporphyrin in hemolytic anemias. *Am J Med* 63:359, 1977.

142. Poh-Fitzpatrick MB, DeLeo VA: Rates of plasma porphyrin disappearance in fluorescent vs. red incandescent light exposure. *J Invest Dermatol* 69(6):510, 1977.

143. Mathews-Roth MM, Pathak MA, Fitzpatrick TB, et al: Beta carotene therapy for erythropoietic protoporphyria and other photosensitivity diseases. *Arch Dermatol* 113(9):1229, 1977.

144. Minder EI, Schneider-Yin X, Steurer J, et al: A systematic review of treatment options for dermal photosensitivity in erythropoietic protoporphyria. *Cell Mol Biol (Noisy-le-grand)* 55(1):84, 2009.

145. Mathews-Roth MM, Rosner B: Long-term treatment of erythropoietic protoporphyria with cysteine. *Photodermatol Photoimmunol Photomed* 18(6):307, 2002.

146. Warren LJ, George S: Erythropoietic protoporphyria treated with narrow-band (TL-01) UVB phototherapy. *Australas J Dermatol* 39(3):179, 1998.

147. Harms J, Lautenschlager S, Minder CE, et al: An alpha-melanocyte-stimulating hormone analogue in erythropoietic protoporphyria. *N Engl J Med* 360(3):306, 2009.

148. Gordeuk VR, Brittenham GM, Hawkins CW, et al: Iron therapy for hepatic dysfunction in erythropoietic protoporphyria. *Ann Intern Med* 105:27, 1986.

149. Mercurio MG, Prince G, Weber FL, et al: Terminal hepatic failure in erythropoietic protoporphyria. *J Am Acad Dermatol* 29:829, 1993.

150. Bonkovsky HL, Schned AR: Fatal liver failure in protoporphyria. Synergism between ethanol excess and the genetic defect. *Gastroenterology* 90(1):191, 1986.

151. Bloomer JR: Pathogenesis and therapy of liver disease in protoporphyria. *Yale J Biol Med* 52(1):39, 1979.

152. Kniffen JC: Protoporphyrin removal in intrahepatic porphyrastasis. *Gastroenterology* 58:1027, 1970.

153. Gross U, Frank M, Doss MO: Hepatic complications of erythropoietic protoporphyria. *Photodermatol Photoimmunol Photomed* 14(2):52, 1998.

154. Bechtel MA, Bertolone SJ, Hodge SJ: Transfusion therapy in a patient with erythropoietic protoporphyria. *Arch Dermatol* 117(2):99, 1981.

155. Van Wijk HJ, Van Hattum J, Delafaille HB, et al: Blood exchange and transfusion therapy for acute cholestasis in protoporphyria. *Dig Dis Sci* 33:1621, 1988.

156. McGuire BM, Bonkovsky HL, Carithers RL Jr, et al: Liver transplantation for erythropoietic protoporphyria liver disease. *Liver Transpl* 11(12):1590, 2005.

157. Todd DJ, Callender ME, Mayne EE, et al: Erythropoietic protoporphyria, transfusion therapy and liver disease. *Br J Dermatol* 127:534, 1992.

158. Muley SA, Midani HA, Rank JM, et al: Neuropathy in erythropoietic protoporphyrias. *Neurology* 51(1):262, 1998.

159. Nordmann Y: Erythropoietic protoporphyria and hepatic complications. *J Hepatol* 16(1-2):4, 1992.

160. Poh-Fitzpatrick MB, Wang X, Anderson KE, et al: Erythropoietic protoporphyria: Altered phenotype after bone marrow transplantation for myelogenous leukemia in a patient heteroallelic for ferrochelatase gene mutations. *J Am Acad Dermatol* 46:861, 2002.

161. Fontanellas A, Mazurier F, Landry M, et al: Reversion of hepatobiliary alterations by bone marrow transplantation in a murine model of erythropoietic protoporphyria. *Hepatology* 32(1):73, 2000.

162. Rand EB, Bunin N, Cochran W, et al: Sequential liver and bone marrow transplantation for treatment of erythropoietic protoporphyria. *Pediatrics* 118(6):e1896, 2006.

163. Richard E, Robert E, Cario-Andre M, et al: Hematopoietic stem cell gene therapy of murine protoporphyria by methylguanine-DNA-methyltransferase-mediated in vivo drug selection. *Gene Ther* 11(22):1638, 2004.

164. Hassoun A, Verstraeten L, Mercelis R, et al: Biochemical diagnosis of an hereditary aminolaevulinate dehydratase deficiency in a 63-year-old man. *J Clin Chem Clin Biochem* 27(10):781, 1989.

165. Pawliuk R, Tighe R, Wise RJ, et al: Prevention of murine erythropoietic protoporphyria-associated skin photosensitivity and liver disease by dermal and hepatic ferrochelatase. *J Invest Dermatol* 124(1):256, 2005.

166. Plewinska M, Thunell S, Holmberg L, et al: Delta-aminolevulinate dehydratase deficient porphyria: Identification of the molecular lesions in a severely affected homozygote. *Am J Hum Genet* 49(1):167, 1991.

167. Sassa S: ALAD porphyria. *Semin Liver Dis* 18(1):95, 1998.

168. Akagi R, Kato N, Inoue R, et al: delta-Aminolevulinate dehydratase (ALAD) porphyria: The first case in North America with two novel ALAD mutations. *Mol Genet Metab* 87:329, 2006.

169. Akagi R, Nishitani C, Harigae H, et al: Molecular analysis of delta-aminolevulinate dehydratase deficiency in a patient with an unusual late-onset porphyria. *Blood* 96(10):3618, 2000.

170. Akagi R, Yasui Y, Harper P, et al: A novel mutation of delta-aminolaevulinate dehydratase in a healthy child with 12% erythrocyte enzyme activity. *Br J Haematol* 106(4):931, 1999.

171. Akagi R, Inoue R, Muranaka S, et al: Dual gene defects involving delta-aminolaevulinate dehydratase and coproporphyrinogen oxidase in a porphyria patient. *Br J Haematol* 132:237, 2006 [erratum in: *Br J Haematol* 132(5):662, 2006].

172. Thunell S, Henrichson A, Floderus Y, et al: Liver transplantation in a boy with acute porphyria due to aminolaevulinate dehydratase deficiency. *Eur J Clin Chem Clin Biochem* 30(10):599, 1992.

173. Shimizu Y, Ida S, Naruto H, et al: Excretion of porphyrins in urine and bile after the administration of delta-aminolevulinic acid. *J Lab Clin Med* 92:795, 1978.

174. Doss M, von Tiepermann R, Schneider J, et al: New type of hepatic porphyria with porphobilinogen synthase defect and intermittent acute clinical manifestation. *Klin Wochenschr* 57(20):1123, 1979.

175. Gross U, Sassa S, Jacob K, et al: 5-Aminolevulinic acid dehydratase deficiency porphyria: A twenty-year clinical and biochemical follow-up. *Clin Chem* 44(9):1892, 1998.

176. Doss MO, Stauch T, Gross U, et al: The third case of Doss porphyria (delta-amino-levulinic acid dehydratase deficiency) in Germany. *J Inherit Metab Dis* 27(4):529, 2004.

177. Thunell S, Holmberg L, Lundgren J: Aminolaevulinate dehydratase porphyria in infancy. A clinical and biochemical study. *J Clin Chem Clin Biochem* 25(1):5, 1987.

178. Mercelis R, Hassoun A, Verstraeten L, et al: Porphyric neuropathy and hereditary delta-aminolevulinic acid dehydratase deficiency in an adult. *J Neurol Sci* 95:39, 1990.

179. Fujita H, Sato K, Sano S: Increase in the amount of erythrocyte delta-aminolevulinic acid dehydratase in workers with moderate lead exposure. *Int Arch Occup Environ Health* 50(3):287, 1982.

180. Sassa S, Fujita H, Kappas A: Succinylacetone and delta-aminolevulinic acid dehydratase in hereditary tyrosinemia: Immunochemical study of the enzyme. *Pediatrics* 86(1):84, 1990.

181. Goldberg A, Moore MR, McColl KEL, et al: Porphyrin metabolism and the porphyrias, in *Oxford Textbook of Medicine*, edited by Ledingham DA, Warrell DA, Wetherall DJ, p 9136. Oxford University Press, Oxford, 1987.

182. Mustajoki P, Koskelo P: Hereditary hepatic porphyrias in Finland. *Acta Med Scand* 200(3):171, 1976.

183. Grandchamp B: Acute intermittent porphyria. *Semin Liver Dis* 18(1):17, 1998.

184. Kauppinen R, von und zu Fraunberg M: Molecular and biochemical studies of acute intermittent porphyria in 196 patients and their families. *Clin Chem* 48(11):1891, 2002.

185. Wetterberg L: *A Neuropsychiatric and Genetical Investigation of Acute Intermittent Porphyria.* Scandinavian University Books, Stockholm, 1967.

186. Mustajoki P, Kauppinen R, Lannfelt L, et al: Frequency of low erythrocyte porphobilinogen deaminase activity in Finland. *J Intern Med* 231(4):389, 1992.

187. Nordmann Y, Puy H, Da Silva V, et al: Acute intermittent porphyria: Prevalence of mutations in the porphobilinogen deaminase gene in blood donors in France. *J Intern Med* 242(3):213, 1997.

188. Grandchamp B, Picat C, de Rooij F, et al: A point mutation G—A in exon 12 of the porphobilinogen deaminase gene results in exon skipping and is responsible for acute intermittent porphyria. *Nucleic Acids Res* 17(16):6637, 1989.

189. Anderson KE, Freddara U, Kappas A: Induction of hepatic cytochrome P-450 by natural steroids: Relationships to the induction of delta-aminolevulinate synthase and porphyrin accumulation in the avian embryo. *Arch Biochem Biophys* 217:597, 1982.

190. Soonawalla ZF, Orug T, Badminton MN, et al: Liver transplantation as a cure for acute intermittent porphyria. *Lancet* 363(9410):705, 2004.

191. Kauppinen R, Mustajoki P: Prognosis of acute porphyria: Occurrence of acute attacks, precipitating factors, and associated diseases. *Medicine (Baltimore)* 71(1):1, 1992.

192. Kuo HC, Huang CC, Chu CC, et al: Neurological complications of acute intermittent porphyria. *Eur Neurol* 66(5):247, 2011.

193. Lithner F: Could attacks of abdominal pain in cases of acute intermittent porphyria be due to intestinal angina? *J Intern Med* 247(3):407, 2000.

194. Anderson KE, Drummond GS, Freddara U, et al: Porphyrogenic effects and induction of heme oxygenase in vivo by delta-aminolevulinic acid. *Biochim Biophys Acta* 676:289, 1981.

195. Brennan MJW, Cantrill RC: Delta-aminolaevulinic acid is a potent agonist for GABA autoreceptors. *Nature* 280:514, 1979.

196. Müller WE, Snyder SH: Delta-aminolevulinic acid: Influences on synaptic GABA receptor binding may explain CNS symptoms of porphyria. *Ann Neurol* 2:340, 1977.

197. Meyer UA, Schuurmans MM, Lindberg RLP: Acute porphyrias: Pathogenesis of neurological manifestations. *Semin Liver Dis* 18(1):43, 1998.

198. Jover R, Hoffmann F, Scheffler-Koch V, et al: Limited heme synthesis in porphobilinogen deaminase-deficient mice impairs transcriptional activation of specific cytochrome P450 genes by phenobarbital. *Eur J Biochem* 267(24):7128, 2000.

199. Lindberg RL, Martini R, Baumgartner M, et al: Motor neuropathy in porphobilinogen deaminase-deficient mice imitates the peripheral neuropathy of human acute porphyria. *J Clin Invest* 103(8):1127, 1999.

200. Louis CA, Sinclair JF, Wood SG, et al: Synergistic induction of cytochrome-P450 by ethanol and isopentanol in cultures of chick embryo and rat hepatocytes. *Toxicol Appl Pharmacol* 118:169, 1993.

201. Lip GY, McColl KE, Goldberg A, Moore MR: Smoking and recurrent attacks of acute intermittent porphyria. *Br Med J* 302:507, 1991.

202. Andersson C, Bylesjo I, Lithner F: Effects of diabetes mellitus on patients with acute intermittent porphyria. *J Intern Med* 245(2):193, 1999.

203. Kauppinen R: *Prognosis of Acute Porphyrias and Molecular Genetics of Acute Intermittent Porphyria in Finland* [thesis]. University of Helskinki, Helsinki, 1992.

204. Milo R, Neuman M, Klein C, et al: Acute intermittent porphyria in pregnancy. *Obstet Gynecol* 73(3 Pt 2):450, 1989.

205. Shenhav S, Gemer O, Sassoon E, et al: Acute intermittent porphyria precipitated by hyperemesis and metoclopramide treatment in pregnancy. *Acta Obstet Gynecol Scand* 76(5):484, 1997.

206. Welland FH, Hellman ES, Gaddis EM, et al: Factors affecting the excretion of porphyrin precursors by patients with acute intermittent porphyria. I. The effect of diet. *Metabolism* 13:232, 1964.

207. Thaler MM, Dawber NH: Stimulation of bilirubin formation in liver of newborn rats by fasting and glucagon. *Gastroenterology* 72(2):312, 1977.

207a. Anderson KE, Bloomer JR, Bonkovsky HL, et al: Recommendations for the diagnosis and treatment of the acute porphyrias. *Ann Intern Med* 142:439, 2005

208. Bernstein HD, Rapport TA, Walter P: Cytosolic protein translocation factors. Is SRP Still unique? *Cell* 58:1017, 1989.

209. Picat C, Delfau MH, De Rooij FWM, et al: Identification of the mutations in the parents of a patient with a putative compound heterozygosity for acute intermittent porphyria. *J Inherit Metab Dis* 13:684, 1990.

210. Bonkovsky HL, Maddukuri VC, Yazici C, et al: Acute porphyrias in the USA: Features of 108 subjects from Porphyrias Consortium. *Am J Med* 127(12):1233, 2014.

211. Stein JA, Tschudy DP: Acute intermittent porphyria. A clinical and biochemical study of 46 patients. *Medicine (Baltimore)* 49(1):1, 1970.

212. Barohn RJ, Sanchez JE, Anderson KE: Acute peripheral neuropathy due to hereditary coproporphyria. *Muscle Nerve* 17:793, 1994.

213. Greenspan GH, Block AJ: Respiratory insufficiency associated with acute intermittent porphyria. *South Med J* 74(8):954, 959, 1981.

214. Ridley A: Porphyric neuropathy, in *Peripheral neuropathy*, edited by Dyck PJ, Thomas PK, Lambert EH, Bunge R, p 1704. WB Saunders, Philadelphia, 1984.

215. Stein JA, Curl FD, Valsamis M, et al: Abnormal iron and water metabolism in acute intermittent porphyria with new morphologic findings. *Am J Med* 53:784, 1972.

216. Goldberg A: Acute intermittent porphyria. A study of 50 cases. *Q J Med* 28:183, 1959.

217. Bloomer JR, Berk PD, Bonkowsky HL, et al: Blood volume and bilirubin production in acute intermittent porphyria. *N Engl J Med* 284:17, 1971.

218. Eales L, Dowdle EB, Sweeney GD: The acute porphyric attack. I. The electrolyte disorder of the acute porphyric attack and the possible role of delta-aminolevulinic acid. *S Afr Med J* Sep 25:89, 1971.

219. Tschudy DP, Valsamis M, Magnussen CR: Acute intermittent porphyria: Clinical and selected research aspects. *Ann Intern Med* 83(6):851, 1975.

220. Andersson C, Wikberg A, Stegmayr B, et al: Renal symptomatology in patients with acute intermittent porphyria. A population-based study. *J Intern Med* 248(4):319, 2000.

221. Church SE, McColl KE, Moore MR, et al: Hypertension and renal impairment as complications of acute porphyria. *Nephrol Dial Transplant* 7(10):986, 1992.

222. Barone GW, Gurley BJ, Anderson KE, et al: The tolerability of newer immunosuppressive medications in a patient with acute intermittent porphyria. *J Clin Pharmacol* 41(1):113, 2001.

223. Nunez DJ, Williams PF, Herrick AL, et al: Renal transplantation for chronic renal failure in acute porphyria. *Nephrol Dial Transplant* 2:271, 1987.

224. Ostrowski J, Kostrzewska E, Michalak T, et al: Abnormalities in liver function and morphology and impaired aminopyrine metabolism in hereditary hepatic porphyrias. *Gastroenterology* 85:1131, 1983.

225. Hollander CS, Scott RL, Tschudy DP, et al: Increased protein bound iodine and thyroxine binding globulin in acute intermittent porphyria. *N Engl J Med* 277:995, 1967.

226. Mustajoki P, Nikkila EA: Serum lipoproteins in asymptomatic acute porphyria: No evidence for hyperbetalipoproteinemia. *Metabolism* 33:266, 1984.

227. Deacon AC, Peters TJ: Identification of acute porphyria: Evaluation of a commercial screening test for urinary porphobilinogen. *Ann Clin Biochem* 35(Pt 6):726, 1998.

228. Minder EI: Coproporphyrin isomers in acute-Intermittent porphyria. *Scand J Clin Lab Invest* 53:87, 1993.

229. Blum M, Koehl C, Abecassis J: Variations in erythrocyte uroporphyrinogen I synthetase activity in non porphyrias. *Clin Chim Acta* 87:119, 1978.

230. Kostrzewska E, Gregor A: Increased activity of porphobilinogen deaminase in erythrocytes during attacks of acute intermittent porphyria. *Ann Clin Res* 18:195, 1986.

231. Bonkowsky HL, Tschudy DP: Hazard of propranolol in treatment of acute porphyria [letter]. *Br Med J* 4:47, 1974.

232. Bonkowsky HL, Sinclair PR, Emery S, et al: Seizure management in acute hepatic porphyria: Risks of valproate and clonazepam. *Neurology* 30(6):588, 1980.

233. Larson AW, Wasserstrom WR, Felsher BF, et al: Posttraumatic epilepsy and acute intermittent porphyria: Effects of phenytoin, carbamazepine, and clonazepam. *Neurology* 28:824, 1978.

234. Harper P, Wahlin S: Treatment options in acute porphyria, porphyria cutanea tarda, and erythropoietic protoporphyria. *Curr Treat Options Gastroenterol* 10(6):444, 2007.

235. Mustajoki P, Nordmann Y: Early administration of heme arginate for acute porphyric attacks. *Arch Intern Med* 153(17):2004, 1993.

236. Tenhunen R, Mustajoki P: Acute porphyria: Treatment with heme. *Semin Liver Dis* 18(1):53, 1998.

237. Jones RL: Hematin-derived anticoagulant. Generation in vitro and in vivo. *J Exp Med* 163:724, 1986.

238. Bonkovsky HL, Healey JF, Lourie AN, et al: Intravenous heme-albumin in acute intermittent porphyria: Evidence for repletion of hepatic hemoproteins and regulatory heme pools. *Am J Gastroenterol* 86(8):1050, 1991.

239. Anderson KE, Bonkovsky HL, Bloomer JR, et al: Reconstitution of hematin for intravenous infusion. *Ann Intern Med* 144(7):537, 2006.

240. Daimon M, Susa S, Igarashi M, et al: Administration of heme arginate, but not hematin, caused anaphylactic shock. *Am J Med* 110(3):240., 2001.

241. Khanderia U: Circulatory collapse associated with hemin therapy for acute intermittent porphyria. *Clin Pharm* 5(8):690, 1986.

242. Jeelani Dhar G, Bossenmaier I, Cardinal R, et al: Transitory renal failure following rapid administration of a relatively large amount of hematin in a patient with acute intermittent porphyria in clinical remission. *Acta Med Scand* 203:437, 1978.

243. Herrick AL, McColl KE, Moore MR, et al: Controlled trial of haem arginate in acute hepatic porphyria. *Lancet* 1(8650):1295, 1989.

243a. Anderson KE, Bloomer JR, Bonkovsky HL, et al: Recommendations for the diagnosis and treatment of the acute porphyrias. *Ann Intern Med* 142:439, 2005.

244. Cherem JH, Malagon J, Nellen H: Cimetidine and acute intermittent porphyria. *Ann Intern Med* 143(9):694, 2005.

245. Horie Y, Tanaka K, Okano J, et al: Cimetidine in the treatment of porphyria cutanea tarda. *Intern Med* 35(9):717, 1996.

246. Marcus DL, Nadel H, Lew G, et al: Cimetidine suppresses chemically induced experimental hepatic porphyria. *Am J Med Sci* 300:214, 1990.

247. Anderson KE, Spitz IM, Bardin CW, et al: A GnRH analogue prevents cyclical attacks of porphyria. *Arch Intern Med* 150:1469, 1990.

248. Yamamori I, Asai M, Tanaka F, et al: Prevention of premenstrual exacerbation of hereditary coproporphyria by gonadotropin-releasing hormone analogue. *Intern Med* 38(4):365, 1999.

249. Anderson KE, Egger NG, Goeger DE: Heme arginate for prevention of acute porphyric attacks [abstract]. *Acta Haematol* 98(Suppl 1):120, 1997.

250. With TK: Hereditary coproporphyria and variegate porphyria in Denmark. *Dan Med Bull* 30(2):106, 1983.

251. Mustajoki P: Variegate porphyria. Twelve years' experience in Finland. *Q J Med* 49(194):191, 1980.

252. Eales L, Day RS, Blekkenhorst GH: The clinical and biochemical features of variegate porphyria: An analysis of 300 cases studied at Groote Schuur Hospital, Cape Town. *Int J Biochem* 12(5–6):837, 1980.

253. Grandchamp B, Phung N, Nordmann Y: Homozygous case of hereditary coproporphyria. *Lancet* 2(8052–8053):1348, 1977.

254. To-Figueras J, Badenas C, Enriquez MT, et al: Biochemical and genetic characterization of four cases of hereditary coproporphyria in Spain. *Mol Genet Metab* 85(2):160, 2005.

255. Nordmann Y, Grandchamp B, de Verneuil H, et al: Harderoporphyria: A variant hereditary coproporphyria. *J Clin Invest* 72(3):1139, 1983.

256. Blake D, McManus J, Cronin V, et al: Fecal coproporphyrin isomers in hereditary coproporphyria. *Clin Chem* 38:96, 1992.

257. Hift RJ, Davidson BP, van der Hooft C, et al: Plasma fluorescence scanning and fecal porphyrin analysis for the diagnosis of variegate porphyria: Precise determination of sensitivity and specificity with detection of protoporphyrinogen oxidase mutations as a reference standard. *Clin Chem* 50(5):915, 2004.

258. Lamoril J, Puy H, Gouya L, et al: Neonatal hemolytic anemia due to inherited harderoporphyria: Clinical characteristics and molecular basis. *Blood* 91(4):1453, 1998.

259. Tio TH, Leijnse B, Jarrett A, et al: Acquired porphyria from a liver tumor. *Clin Sci Mol Med* 16:517, 1959.

260. Elder GH, Urquhart AJ, de Salamanca RE, et al: Immunoreactive uroporphyrinogen decarboxylase in the liver in porphyria cutanea tarda. *Lancet* 2:229, 1985.

261. Phillips JD, Jackson LK, Bunting M, et al: A mouse model of familial porphyria cutanea tarda. *Proc Natl Acad Sci U S A* 98(1):259, 2001.

261a. Sinclair PR, Gorman N, Shedlofsky SI, et al: Ascorbic acid deficiency in porphyria cutanea tarda. *J Lab Clin Med* 130:197–201, 1997.

262. Gorman N, Zaharia A, Trask HS, et al: Effect of iron and ascorbate on uroporphyria in ascorbate-requiring mice as a model for porphyria cutanea tarda. *Hepatology* 45(1):187, 2007.

263. Rocchi E, Casalgrandi G, Masini A, et al: Circulating pro- and antioxidant factors in iron and porphyrin metabolism disorders. *Ital J Gastroenterol Hepatol* 31(9):861, 1999.

264. Sinclair PR, Gorman N, Walton HS, et al: CYP1A2 is essential in murine uroporphyria caused by hexachlorobenzene and iron. *Toxicol Appl Pharmacol* 162(1):60, 2000.

265. Smith AG, Francis JE, Walters DG, et al: Protection against iron-induced uroporphyria in C57BL/10ScSn mice by the peroxisome proliferator nafenopin. *Biochem Pharmacol* 40(11):2564, 1990.

266. Elder GH: Porphyria cutanea tarda and related disorders, in *Porphyrin Handbook, Part II*, edited by Kadish KM, Smith K, Guilard R, p 67. Academic Press, San Diego, 2003.

267. Phillips JD, Parker TL, Schubert HL, et al: Functional consequences of naturally occurring mutations in human uroporphyrinogen decarboxylase. *Blood* 98(12):3179, 2001.

268. Cassiman D, Vannoote J, Roelandts R, et al: Porphyria cutanea tarda and liver disease. A retrospective analysis of 17 cases from a single centre and review of the literature. *Acta Gastroenterol Belg* 71(2):237, 2008.

269. Gisbert JP, Garcia-Buey L, Alonso A, et al: Hepatocellular carcinoma risk in patients with porphyria cutanea tarda. *Eur J Gastroenterol Hepatol* 16(7):689, 2004.

270. Rossmann-Ringdahl I, Olsson R: Porphyria cutanea tarda in a Swedish population: Risk factors and complications. *Acta Derm Venereol* 85(4):337, 2005.

271. Dabski C, Beutner EH: Studies of laminin and type IV collagen in blisters of porphyria cutanea tarda and drug-induced pseudoporphyria. *J Am Acad Dermatol* 25(1 Pt 1):28, 1991.

272. Pigatto PD, Polenghi MM, Altomare GF, et al: Complement cleavage products in the phototoxic reaction of porphyria cutanea tarda. *Br J Dermatol* 114(5):567, 1986.

273. Jalil S, Grady JJ, Lee C, Anderson KE: Associations among behavior-related susceptibility factors in porphyria cutanea tarda. *Clin Gastro Hepatol* 8:297–302, 2010.

274. Ajioka RS, Phillips JD, Weiss RB, et al: Down-regulation of hepcidin in porphyria cutanea tarda. *Blood* 112(12):4723, 2008.

275. Bulaj ZJ, Franklin MR, Phillips JD, et al: Transdermal estrogen replacement therapy in postmenopausal women previously treated for porphyria cutanea tarda. *J Lab Clin Med* 136(6):482, 2000.

276. Wickliffe JK, Abdel-Rahman SZ, Lee C, et al: CYP1A2*1F and GSTM1 alleles are associated with susceptibility to porphyria cutanea tarda. *Molec Med* 17:241-247, 2011.

277. Grossman ME, Bickers DR, Poh-Fitzpatrick MB, et al: Porphyria cutanea tarda. Clinical features and laboratory findings in 40 patients. *Am J Med* 67(2):277, 1979.

278. Sixel-Dietrich F, Doss M: Hereditary uroporphyrinogen-decarboxylase deficiency predisposing porphyria cutanea tarda (chronic hepatic porphyria) in females after oral contraceptive medication. *Arch Dermatol Res* 278(1):13, 1985.

279. Legault N, Sabik H, Cooper SF, et al: Effect of estradiol on the induction of porphyria by hexachlorobenzene in the rat. *Biochem Pharmacol* 54(1):19, 1997.

280. Fujita N, Sugimoto R, Motonishi S, et al: Patients with chronic hepatitis C achieving a sustained virological response to peginterferon and ribavirin therapy recover from impaired hepcidin secretion. *J Hepatol* 49(5):702, 2008.

281. Wissel PS, Sordillo P, Anderson KE, et al: Porphyria cutanea tarda associated with the acquired immune deficiency syndrome. *Am J Hematol* 25(1):107, 1987.

282. Roberts AG, Whatley SD, Nicklin S, et al: The frequency of hemochromatosis-associated alleles is increased in British patients with sporadic porphyria cutanea tarda. *Hepatology* 25(1):159, 1997.

283. Dereure O, Aguilar-Martinez P, Bessis D, et al: HFE mutations and transferrin receptor polymorphism analysis in porphyria cutanea tarda: A prospective study of 36 cases from southern France. *Br J Dermatol* 144(3):533, 2001.

284. Calvert GM, Sweeney MH, Fingerhut MA, et al: Evaluation of porphyria cutanea tarda in U.S. workers exposed to 2,3,7,8-tetrachlorodibenzo-p-dioxin. *Am J Ind Med* 25(4):559, 1994.

285. Smith A: Porphyria caused by chlorinated AH receptor ligands and associated mechanisms of liver injury and cancer, in *Porphyrin Handbook, Part II*, edited by Kadish KM, Smith K, Guilard RR, p 169. Academic Press, San Diego, 2003.

286. Brady JJ, Jackson HA, Roberts AG, et al: Co-inheritance of mutations in the uroporphyrinogen decarboxylase and hemochromatosis genes accelerates the onset of porphyria cutanea tarda. *J Invest Dermatol* 115(5):868, 2000.

287. Barzilay D, Orion E, Brenner S: Porphyria cutanea tarda triggered by a combination of three predisposing factors. *Dermatology* 203(2):195, 2001.

288. Au WY, Tam SC, Ho KM, et al: Hypertrichosis due to porphyria cutanea tarda associated with blastic transformation of myelofibrosis. *Br J Dermatol* 141(5):932, 1999.

289. Lee SC, Yun SJ, Lee JB, et al: A case of porphyria cutanea tarda in association with idiopathic myelofibrosis and CREST syndrome. *Br J Dermatol* 144(1):182-5, 2001.

290. Anderson KE, Goeger DE, Carson RW, et al: Erythropoietin for the treatment of porphyria cutanea tarda in a patient on long-term hemodialysis. *N Engl J Med* 322:315, 1990.

291. Armstrong DK, Sharpe PC, Chambers CR, et al: Hepatoerythropoietic porphyria: A missense mutation in the UROD gene is associated with mild disease and an unusual porphyrin excretion pattern. *Br J Dermatol* 151(4):920, 2004.

292. Elder GH: The metabolism of porphyrins of the isocoproporphyrin series. *Enzyme* 17(1):61, 1974.

292a. Poh-Fitzpatrick MB, Lamola AA: Direct spectrophotometry of diluted erythrocytes and plasma: A rapid diagnostic method in primary and secondary porphyrinemias. *J Lab Clin Med* 87:362, 1976.

293. Poh-Fitzpatrick MB, Sosin AE, Bemis J: Porphyrin levels in plasma and erythrocytes of chronic hemodialysis patients. *J Am Acad Dermatol* 7:100, 1982.

294. Topi GC, Amantea A, Griso D: Recovery from porphyria cutanea tarda with no specific therapy other than avoidance of hepatic toxins. *Br J Dermatol* 111(1):75, 1984.

295. Ippen H: Treatment of porphyria cutanea tarda by phlebotomy. *Semin Hematol* 14:253, 1977.

296. Rocchi E, Cassanelli M, Ventura E; High weekly intravenous doses of desferrioxamine in porphyria cutanea tarda. *Br J Dermatol* 117:393, 1987.

297. Ratnaike S, Blake D, Campbell D, et al: Plasma ferritin levels as a guide to the treatment of porphyria cutanea tarda by venesection. *Australas J Dermatol* 29:3, 1988.

298. Ashton RE, Hawk JLM, Magnus IA: Low-dose oral chloroquine in the treatment of porphyria cutanea tarda. *Br J Dermatol* 3:609, 1984.

299. Bruce AJ, Ahmed I: Childhood-onset porphyria cutanea tarda: Successful therapy with low-dose hydroxychloroquine (Plaquenil). *J Am Acad Dermatol* 38(5 Pt 2):810, 1998.

300. Freesemann A, Frank M, Sieg I, et al: Treatment of porphyria cutanea tarda by the effect of chloroquine on the liver. *Skin Pharmacol* 8(3):156, 1995.

301. Kordac V, Semradova M: Treatment of porphyria cutanea tarda with chloroquine. *Br J Dermatol* 90(1):95, 1974.

302. Taljaard JJF, Shanley BC, Stewart-Wynne EG, et al: Studies on low dose chloroquine therapy and the action of chloroquine in symptomatic porphyria. *Br J Dermatol* 87:261, 1972.

303. Timonen K, Niemi KM, Mustajoki P: Skin morphology in porphyria cutanea tarda does not improve despite clinical remission. *Clin Exp Dermatol* 16(5):355, 1991.

304. Thornsvard CT, Guider BA, Kimball DB: An unusual reaction to chloroquine-primaquine. *JAMA* 235:1719, 1976.

305. Sweeney GD, Jones KG: Porphyria cutanea tarda: Clinical and laboratory features. *Can Med Assoc J* 120:803, 1979.

306. Malkinson FD, Levitt L: Hydroxychloroquine treatment of porphyria cutanea tarda. *Arch Dermatol* 116(10):1147, 1980.

307. Singal AK, Kormos-Hallberg C, Lee C, et al: Low-dose hydroxychloroquine is as effective as phlebotomy in treatment of patients with porphyria cutanea tarda. *Clin Gastroenterol Hepatol* 10(12):1402, 2012.

308. Stolzel U, Kostler E, Schuppan D, et al: Hemochromatosis (HFE) gene mutations and response to chloroquine in porphyria cutanea tarda. *Arch Dermatol* 139(3):309, 2003.

309. Egger NG, Goeger DE, Anderson KE: Effects of chloroquine in hematoporphyrin-treated animals. *Chem Biol Interact* 102:69, 1996.

310. Cohen SN, Phifer KO, Yielding KL: Complex formation between chloroquine and ferrihaemic acid *in vitro*, and its effect on the antimalarial action of chloroquine. *Nature* 202:805, 1964.

311. Scholnick PL, Epstein J, Marver HS: The molecular basis of the action of chloroquine in porphyria cutanea tarda. *J Invest Dermatol* 61(4):226, 1973.

311a. Solis C, Martinez-Bermejo A, Naidich TP, et al: Acute intermittent porphyria: Studies of the severe homozygous dominant disease provides insights into the neurologic attacks in acute porphyrias. *Arch Neurol* 61:1764, 2004.

312. Chlumska A, Chlumsky J, Malina L: Liver changes in porphyria cutanea tarda patients treated with chloroquine. *Br J Dermatol* 102:261, 1980.

313. Vizethum W, Dahlmann D, Bolsen K, et al: Influence of chloroquine (Resochin) on hexachlorobenzene (HCB) induced porphyria of the rat. *Arch Dermatol Res* 264:125, 1979.

314. Fernandez I, Castellano G, de Salamanca RE, et al: Porphyria cutanea tarda as a predictor of poor response to interferon alfa therapy in chronic hepatitis C. *Scand J Gastroenterol* 38(3):314, 2003.

315. Rossini A, Contessi GB, Leali C, et al: Efficacy of iron depletion and antiviral therapy in patients with porphyria cutanea tarda (PCT) and hepatitis C virus (HCV) chronic infection [abstract]. *Hepatology* 40(Suppl 1):320A, 2004.

316. Shieh S, Cohen JL, Lim HW: Management of porphyria cutanea tarda in the setting of chronic renal failure: A case report and review. *J Am Acad Dermatol* 42(4):645, 2000.

317. Yaqoob M, Smyth J, Ahmad R, et al: Haemodialysis-related porphyria cutanea tarda and treatment by recombinant human erythropoietin. *Nephron* 60:428, 1992.

318. Carson RW, Dunnigan EJ, DuBose TDJ, et al: Removal of plasma porphyrins with high-flux hemodialysis in porphyria cutanea tarda associated with end-stage renal disease. *J Am Soc Nephrol* 2:1445, 1992.

319. Stevens BR, Fleischer AB, Piering F, et al: Porphyria cutanea tarda in the setting of renal failure: Response to renal transplantation. *Arch Dermatol* 129:337, 1993.

320. Fontanellas A, Mazurier F, Moreau-Gaudry F, et al: Correction of uroporphyrinogen decarboxylase deficiency (hepatoerythropoietic porphyria) in Epstein-Barr virus-transformed B-cell lines by retrovirus-mediated gene transfer: Fluorescence-based selection of transduced cells. *Blood* 94(2):465, 1999.

CHAPTER 59
POLYCLONAL AND HEREDITARY SIDEROBLASTIC ANEMIAS

Prem Ponka and Josef T. Prchal

SUMMARY

Sideroblastic anemias are characterized by the presence of ring sideroblasts in the marrow. These cells are erythroid precursors that have accumulated abnormal amounts of mitochondrial iron. A variety of abnormalities of porphyrin metabolism in affected erythroid cells have been documented. Hereditary sideroblastic anemias are usually X linked, as the result of mutations in the erythroid form of 5-aminolevulinic acid synthase. Inherited autosomal and mitochondrial forms are seen, occasionally. Acquired sideroblastic anemias can occur as a result of the ingestion of drugs, alcohol, or toxins such as lead or zinc, or copper deficiency. Patients with acquired sideroblastic macrocytic anemia and variable degrees of thrombocytopenia and leukopenia from copper deficiency have been recognized more frequently; the hematologic abnormalities typically resolve after copper replacement. Ring sideroblasts are also a feature of myelodysplastic neoplasms, and are discussed in Chap. 87. Some patients with sideroblastic anemia may respond to pharmacologic doses of pyridoxine. Iron loading is common in the sideroblastic anemias and can be treated by phlebotomy when the anemia is mild or with iron chelators (Chap. 43) when it is more severe.

● DEFINITION AND HISTORY

Sideroblastic anemias are a heterogeneous group of disorders that have as a common feature the presence of: (1) large numbers of pathologic sideroblasts in the marrow, which characteristically display abnormal mitochondrial iron accumulation is in a circumnuclear position in erythroblasts; these are referred to as ringed sideroblasts; (2) ineffective erythropoiesis; (3) increased levels of tissue iron; and (4) varying proportions of hypochromic erythrocytes in the blood. They may be acquired or hereditary (Table 59–1).[1,2]

Acquired monoclonal sideroblastic anemia is a neoplastic disease; that is, a clonal cytopenia or oligoblastic myelogenous leukemia that can progress to acute leukemia. This subject is considered in Chap. 87,

Myeloid Neoplasms, in which ringed sideroblasts are a common phenotypic feature. Acquired polyclonal sideroblastic anemia may also develop as a result of the administration of certain drugs, exposure to toxins, or coincident to neoplastic or inflammatory disease. Hereditary sideroblastic anemias include X-linked, autosomal, and mitochondrial entities. Occasionally, a patient with familial disease develops a myelodysplastic syndrome later,[1,2] but with these rare exceptions, the disorders are distinct and do not coexist or evolve one from the other.

Although the perinuclear distribution of siderotic granules in the erythroblasts of patients with various types of anemia was described in 1947,[3,4] the concept of sideroblastic anemia as a generic designation was not generally accepted until the publications of Björkman,[5] Dacie,[6] Heilmeyer,[7,8] Bernard,[9] and Mollin.[10] After these descriptions of the acquired, "*primary adult form of refractory sideroblastic anemia*,"[5,6] similarity to the morphologic and erythrokinetic changes in hereditary (sex-linked) hypochromic anemia was recognized. Cooley[11] described a patient with an anemia with ovalocytosis who was shortly thereafter shown to have inherited a hereditary sex-linked disorder[12] that we now know resulted from the mutation of erythroid-specific aminolevulinic acid (ALA) synthase, ALAS2.[13] Autosomally inherited cases were also described,[14] and prominent sideroblastic changes of the marrow were found in Pearson marrow-pancreas syndrome (Chap. 36), a disorder that is caused by mutations of mitochondrial DNA.[15-19] Sideroblastic anemia can also be associated with a wide variety of diseases,[20] therapy with antituberculosis drugs,[21,22] and lead intoxication.[23-26] In some patients, the anemia responded to large doses of pyridoxine and was designated "pyridoxine-responsive anemia."[10,27-29] These "secondary" acquired disorders were then incorporated into the classification.

● EPIDEMIOLOGY

All of the hereditary forms are rare, and no particular ethnic predilection is known. Drug-induced forms occur sporadically among subjects taking the drugs listed in Table 59–1.

● ETIOLOGY AND PATHOGENESIS

MORPHOLOGIC ASPECTS: THE SIDEROBLASTS

Sideroblasts are erythroblasts containing aggregates of non–heme iron that appear as one or more Prussian blue–positive granules on light microscopy.[30] The morphology of these cells in normal and abnormal states is discussed in detail in Chap. 31. In normal marrow, virtually every erythroblast has siderosomes, iron-containing organelles that are demonstrable by transmission electron microscopy. Light microscopy of Prussian blue–stained marrow aspirates or biopsy sections is a relatively insensitive method to identify these structures. One can usually identify approximately 25 to 35 percent of erythroblasts with one to three very fine Prussian blue–stained granules in the cytoplasm of a well-prepared marrow sample. Pathologic sideroblasts may be of two types: erythroblasts with a marked increase in the number and size of siderotic granules in the cytoplasm, compared to normal erythroblasts, or ringed sideroblasts. Ringed sideroblasts are the hallmark of the sideroblastic anemias. In contrast to the normal cytoplasmic location of siderotic granules, the pathologic sideroblasts in the sideroblastic anemias have large amounts of iron deposited as dust- or plaque-like ferruginous micelles between the cristae of mitochondria (Fig. 59–1).[31] The iron-loaded mitochondria are distorted and swollen, their cristae are indistinct, and identification of mitochondria may itself be difficult. In humans, the mitochondria of the erythroblast are distributed perinuclearly,[23] which accounts for the distinctive "ringed" sideroblast identified by Prussian blue staining

TABLE 59–1. Classification of Sideroblastic Anemias

I. Acquired
  A. Primary sideroblastic anemia (myelodysplastic syndromes) (Chap. 88)
    1. Subunit 1 of the mitochondrial cytochrome oxidase[54,55]
  B. Sideroblastic anemia secondary to:
    1. Isoniazid[21,22]
    2. Pyrazinamide[21,22]
    3. Cycloserine[149]
    4. Chloramphenicol[149]
    5. Ethanol[118]
    6. Lead[24]
    7. Chronic neoplastic disease (Chap. 8)
    8. Zinc-induced copper deficiency[124,125]
II. Hereditary
  A. X chromosome linked
  B. Autosomal
    1. Defects in the erythroid specific mitochondrial carrier family protein SLC25A38[47]
    2. Mitochondrial myopathy and sideroblastic anemia (*PSU1* mutations)[57,108,109]
  C. Mitochondrial
    1. Pearson marrow-pancreas syndrome[15–19]

when mitochondrial iron overload is present (Fig. 59–1). The morphologic features that characterize pathologic sideroblasts in various disorders have been summarized.[32]

PATHOGENESIS

The pathogenesis of most of the sideroblastic anemias is not well understood.[33,34] It is not clear whether the basic mechanism by which abnormal accumulations of intramitochondrial iron occurs is the same in inherited and acquired forms of the disease. However, it seems appropriate, given the present state of knowledge, to discuss both forms together. The pathogenesis of the disorder may be viewed from two standpoints: the underlying biochemical lesions and the mechanism(s) of the anemia itself.

Biochemical Lesions and Genetics
In the search for the biochemical lesions responsible for the development of sideroblastic anemia, attention has been focused upon an intramitochondrial defect in heme synthesis and on possible disturbances in pyridoxine metabolism.

Defects in Heme Synthesis
The role of defects in heme biosynthesis have occupied central stage since the early studies of Garby and colleagues,[35] who postulated that such a defect might exist; they demonstrated that the level of free erythrocyte protoporphyrin was decreased. Subsequently, a variety of abnormalities of the levels of precursors and of their rate of incorporation into heme was documented (Chap. 58).[36–41] However, the findings have not all been consistent, as levels of free erythrocyte protoporphyrin have often been increased,[42,43] not diminished. The role of mitochondria in the etiology of sideroblastic anemia gained further credence when mutations of the mitochondrial genome were found in patients with Pearson syndrome.[15–19]

Hereditary Sideroblastic Anemias
Shortly after the identification of erythroid-specific ALA synthase (ALAS2, the first enzyme in heme synthesis; Fig. 59–2), it became apparent that most patients with hereditary X-linked sideroblastic anemias (XLSAs) had mutations in the *ALAS2* gene.[44–46] However, a proportion of patients with congenital sideroblastic anemia had autosomal recessive inheritance. At least some such patients have a defect in the gene encoding the erythroid-specific mitochondrial carrier protein, SLC25A38.[47] This transporter is important for the biosynthesis of heme in eukaryotes and it was proposed that this protein may be translocating glycine into mitochondria (Fig. 59–2).[47] Hence, SLC25A38 defects would be expected to generate a phenotype identical to that seen in patients with defects in ALAS2. One can speculate that, in erythroid cells, a common control mechanism exists that regulates acquisition of the two substrates for heme synthesis (iron and glycine).

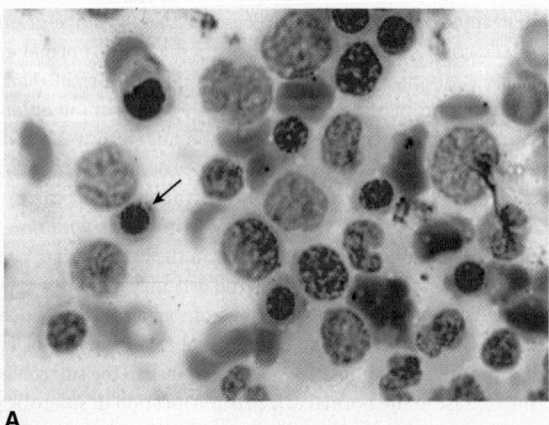
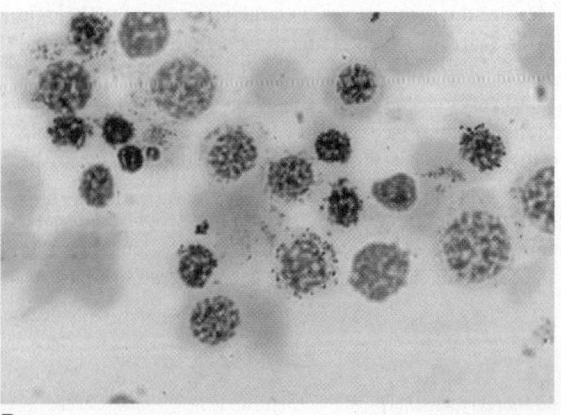

A   B

Figure 59–1. Marrow films. **A.** Normal marrow stained with Prussian blue. Note several erythroblasts without apparent siderotic (blue-stained) granules. The *arrow* indicates erythroblast with several very small cytoplasmic blue-stained granules. It is very difficult to see siderosomes in most erythroblasts in normal marrow because they are often below the resolution of the light microscope. **B.** Sideroblastic anemia. Note the florid increase in Prussian blue–staining granules in the erythroblasts, most with circumnuclear locations. These are classic examples of ringed sideroblast, which are by definition pathologic changes in the red cell precursors. In some cases, cytoplasmic iron granules are also increased in size and number, also a pathologic change. *(Reproduced with permission from Lichtman's Atlas of Hematology, www.accessmedicine.com.)*

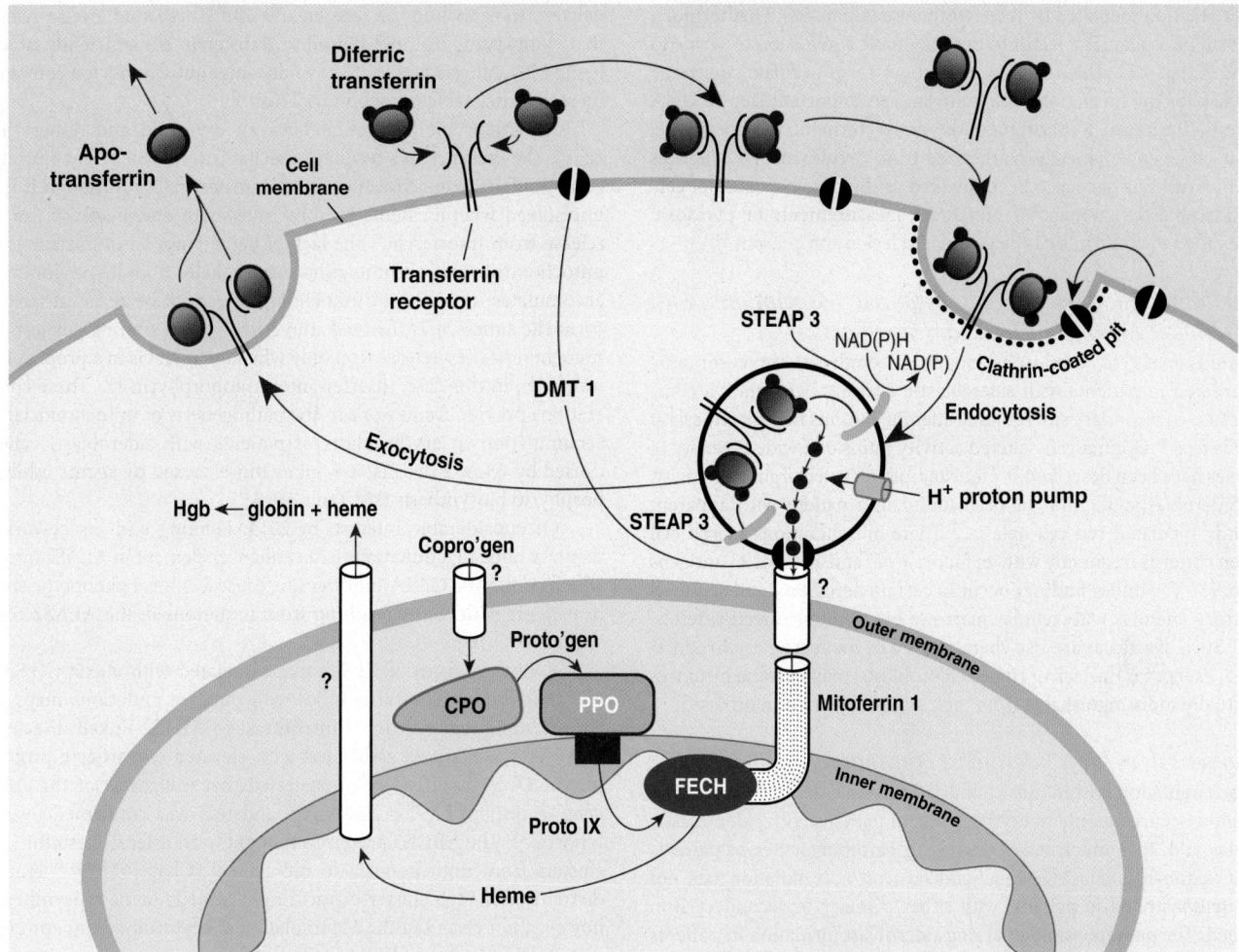

Figure 59–2. Schematic of iron uptake from transferrin and its delivery to the hemoglobin (Hgb) molecule. Extracellular differic transferrin is bound by the membrane-bound transferrin receptor (TfR) and internalized via receptor-mediated endocytosis into an endosome. Iron is released from transferrin by a decrease in pH (~pH 5.5), reduced by STEAP 3 (six-transmembrane epithelial antigen of prostate 3-ferric reductase), following which the metal is transported through the endosomal membrane by DMT 1. In erythroid cells, more than 90 percent of iron must enter mitochondria wherein ferrochelatase (FECH), the enzyme that inserts Fe^{2+} into protoporphyrin IX (Proto IX), resides on the inner leaflet of the inner mitochondrial membrane. The transport of coproporphyrinogen (Copro'gen) into mitochondria is not fully understood. Neither mechanisms nor the regulation of the transport of heme from mitochondria to globin polypeptides are known; however, it has been proposed that a carrier protein, heme binding protein 1 (gene: *HEBP1*), is involved in this process. CPO, coproporphyrinogen oxidase; NAD(P), nicotinamide adenine dinucleotide phosphate; NAD(P)H reduced form of nicotinamide adenine dinucleotide phosphate; PPO, protoporphyrinogen oxidase. *(Reproduced with permission from Anderson GJ, McLaren G: Iron Physiology and Pathophysiology in Humans. New York, NY: Humana Press; 2012.)*

Hereditary sideroblastic anemia with spinocerebellar degeneration with ataxia is a rare X-linked syndrome that appears to be distinct from the other forms of sideroblastic anemia.[48–51] It is caused by mutation of ATP-binding cassette (ABCB7).[48,52,53]

Heteroplasmic point mutations in subunit 1 of the mitochondrial cytochrome oxidase have been documented in some patients with sideroblastic anemia.[54–56]

Rare autosomal forms of inherited sideroblastic anemia have also been reported,[57,58] including those with a deficiency of uroporphyrinogen decarboxylase[59,60] and ferrochelatase (FECH)[36,41,61–63] enzymes, both necessary for the synthesis of heme (Chap. 58). The other reported defects of ferrochelatase could result from the inhibitory effect of mitochondrial iron overload on enzyme activity.[41] A defect in coproporphyrinogen oxidase (CPO) could not be confirmed by direct measurement.[64]

An unusual phenotype with of inherited sideroblastic anemia, developmental delay with variable neurologic defects and B-cell lymphopenia with hypogammaglobulinemia was reported of yet unknown etiology.[65]

Pyridoxine Metabolism

A role for pyridoxine has been supported by the demonstration that pyridoxine deficiency in animals is a prototype of sideroblastic anemia.[31] Sideroblastic anemia can be induced by drugs that reduce the level of pyridoxal phosphate in blood, which decreases the ALAS2 activity in normoblasts.[22,36,40] Moreover, certain sideroblastic disorders, although not a result of pyridoxine deficiency, are nonetheless responsive to pharmacologic doses of pyridoxine.[44,66–68] Pyridoxal phosphate is a necessary coenzyme for the initial reaction of protoporphyrin synthesis, the condensation of glycine and succinyl coenzyme A to form

ALA, a reaction mediated by ALA synthetase (Chap. 58). Furthermore, pyridoxal phosphate is a factor in the enzymatic conversion of serine to glycine (Chap. 41). This reaction generates a form of folate coenzyme necessary for the formation of thymidylate, an important step in DNA synthesis. Pyridoxal 5′-phosphate, the active form of the coenzyme, must itself be enzymatically synthesized from pyridoxine. Deficiencies in its biosynthesis have also been invoked as the possible cause of certain sideroblastic anemias,[27,69] but direct measurements of pyridoxal kinase failed to confirm that the postulated lesion was present.[70]

Other Metabolic Defects and Acquired Associations with Sideroblastic Anemia of Uncertain Significance

Increased levels of uroporphyrinogen 1 synthase are commonly encountered in patients with sideroblastic anemias.[39] Alcohol, a common cause of secondary sideroblastic anemia, inhibits heme synthesis at several steps.[38] Dramatically altered activity ratios of a wide diversity of enzymes have been described,[71,72] for example, elevated arginase activity.

Sideroblastic anemia has been found in a patient with apparent antibody-mediated red cell aplasia.[73] There are alterations in red cell antigen patterns frequently with an increase of i and a loss of A_1 antigens (Chap. 136).[74] Similar findings occur in certain hereditary and acquired refractory anemias with cellular marrows but without ringed sideroblasts.[72] Such dyscrasias are also characterized by ineffective erythropoiesis and, except for the lack of ringed sideroblasts, may in some instances be virtually indistinguishable from their sideroblastic counterparts.[75]

Pathogenesis of Ring Sideroblast Formation

Iron accumulation within mitochondria is an unusual pathologic phenomenon occurring only in erythroblasts of patients with sideroblastic anemias and, to a much lesser degree, in cardiomyocytes of patients with Friedreich ataxia.[76,77] Mitochondrial iron accumulation has not been demonstrated in patients with either primary or secondary iron overload. The pathophysiology of ring sideroblast formation in patients with ALAS2 defects and those resulting from inhibitors of porphyrin biosynthesis (see Table 59–1) is likely because of the unique aspects of the regulation of iron metabolism and heme synthesis in erythroid cells (Chap. 58).[78] These differences can account for the accumulation of non–heme iron in erythroid mitochondria of sideroblastic anemia patients. In hemoglobin-synthesizing cells, iron is specifically targeted toward mitochondria that avidly take up iron even when the synthesis of protoporphyrin IX is suppressed (Chap. 58).[79–82] In contrast, non-erythroid cells store iron in excess of metabolic needs within ferritin.[83] Hence, erythroid-specific mechanisms and controls are involved in the transport of iron into mitochondria in erythroid cells, but the nature of these processes, including the role of mitoferrin 1 (Chap. 42); an inner mitochondrial membrane protein, which presumably provides Fe^{2+} to FECH,[84] is poorly understood. The transferrin-bound iron is used for hemoglobin synthesis[78,82] with a high degree of efficiency and is targeted into erythroid mitochondria (Chap. 52), and because no intermediate for cytoplasmic iron transport has ever been identified in erythroid cells, the following hypothesis of intracellular iron trafficking in developing red cells has been proposed (see Fig. 59-2 from Chap. 52). This model postulates that iron released from transferrin in the endosome is passed directly from protein to protein until it reaches FECH, which incorporates Fe^{2+} into protoporphyrin IX[85] in the mitochondrion. Such a transfer bypasses the cytosol, as the movement of iron between proteins could be mediated by a direct interaction of the endosome with the mitochondrion.[78,86] The results of supporting experiments revealed that (1) iron, delivered to mitochondria via the transferrin–transferrin receptor (TfR) pathway, is unavailable to cytoplasmic chelators[87,88]; (2) transferrin-containing endosomes move to and contact mitochondria in erythroid cells; and (3) endosomal movement is required for iron

delivery to mitochondria (see Fig. 59–2).[87] These studies also revealed that cytoplasmic iron not bound to transferrin is inefficiently used for heme biosynthesis and that the endosome–mitochondrion interaction increases chelatable mitochondrial iron.[87]

An important distinction between erythroid and nonerythroid cells is the presence of a feedback mechanism in which "uncommitted" heme inhibits iron acquisition from transferrin.[89–92] Although it is still unresolved whether heme inhibits transferrin endocytosis[89,90] or iron release from transferrin,[92] the lack of heme plays an important role in mitochondrial iron accumulation. Additionally, non–heme iron, which accumulates in erythroid mitochondria, cannot be released from the organelle unless it is inserted into heme.[82] This finding suggests that mitochondria can release iron only when the metal is in a proper chemical form, in this case, inserted into protoporphyrin IX. These considerations provide framework to the pathogenesis of mitochondrial iron accumulation in erythroblasts of patients with sideroblastic anemia caused by ALAS2 defects, as well as those caused by agents inhibiting porphyrin biosynthesis (see Table 59–1).

Of considerable interest, in 2014, Fleming and his coworkers[93] demonstrated that mutations in an enhancer element in ALAS2 intron 1, which contains a GATA-binding site, cause a clinical phenotype similar to patients with XLSA resulting from mutations in the ALAS2 coding sequence itself.

A distinct form of XLSA, that associated with ataxia (XLSA/A), was described in several families with putative mutations mapped to chromosome region Xq13.[50] In contrast to ALAS2-linked disease, the XLSA/A syndrome is associated with elevated erythrocyte protoporphyrin IX levels. It was demonstrated that mutations of the *ABCB7* gene is responsible for XLSA/A,[48] and this was confirmed by other reports.[52,94] The ABCB7 protein is thought to transfer iron-sulfur (Fe-S) clusters from mitochondria to the cytosol (Chap. 42).[76,95,96] How the disruption of Fe-S cluster export might impede heme biosynthesis is, however, not clear, but the accumulation of erythrocyte zinc–protoporphyrin IX is found in XLSA/A.[48,50,52] Additionally, mouse erythrocytes with mutated (E433K) ABCB7 have an increase in zinc–protoporphyrin IX-to-heme ratios.[97] Because the formation of zinc–protoporphyrin IX requires FECH, ABCB7 mutations cannot interfere with the activity of this enzyme. Instead, the loss of function of ABCB7 may, by a yet-to-be-defined mechanism, diminish the availability of reduced iron (the only substrate of iron for FECH) required for the assembly of heme from protoporphyrin IX. In XLSA, as in ALAS2-associated sideroblastic anemia, decreased levels of heme likely contribute to the pathogenesis of ring sideroblast formation.

Another type of hereditary hypochromic anemia was described in *shiraz* (*sir*) zebra fish mutants.[98] These mutants have a deficiency of glutaredoxin 5 (GLRX5) encoded by a gene (*GLRX5*) whose product is required for Fe-S cluster assembly. This study demonstrated that the loss of the Fe-S cluster in the iron-regulatory protein 1 (IRP1) blocked ALAS2 translation by binding to the iron-responsive element (IRE) located in the 5′-untranslated region of ALAS2 mRNA. Subsequently, a case of GLRX5 deficiency in an anemic male with iron overload and a low number of ringed sideroblasts was reported.[99] As in zebra fish with *shiraz* mutants, ferritin levels were low and TfR levels were high in the patient's cells; this can be explained by increased IRP1 binding to IREs in mRNAs of these two proteins. However, erythroblasts from zebra fish *shiraz* mutants were not found to contain iron-loaded mitochondria.

Primary Acquired Sideroblastic Anemia (Refractory Anemia with Ring Sideroblasts—Myelodysplastic Syndrome)

The pathophysiology of acquired idiopathic sideroblastic anemias associated with myelodysplastic syndrome is distinct from the above discussed XLSAs. In these patients there is no evidence for a decrease in the formation protoporphyrin IX levels; instead, the amount of protoporphyrin IX is moderately increased.[43] Impaired iron reduction could cause intramitochondrial iron accumulation in patients with myelodysplastic syndromes. The ferric reductase, STEAP 3 (six-transmembrane epithelial antigen of prostate 3-ferric reductase), is involved in the reduction of Fe^{3+} to Fe^{2+} in endosomes.[100] Based on the model of the direct interorganellar transfer of iron (see Fig. 59–2), it can be assumed that there is only one reduction step during the path of iron from endosomes to FECH. However, the efficient insertion of ferrous ions into protoporphyrin IX may still require a reducing environment in mitochondria that would be provided by an uninterrupted respiratory chain. This proposal is compatible with the fact that sideroblastic anemia accompanying Pearson marrow-pancreas syndrome[101] is caused by deletions of mitochondrial DNA genes, products of these are involved in electron transport.[102] Indeed, there are at least some myelodysplasia-associated sideroblastic anemia patients described caused by acquired mutations in cytochrome oxidase, encoded by mitochondrial DNA.[54,55,103–105] However, a rigorous study failed to find cytochrome oxidase mutations in 10 patients with myelodysplasia-associated sideroblastic anemia.[106] Alternatively, these is some evidence that *ABCB7* (see the above discussion on XLSA/A) could be a possible candidate gene for the formation of ringed sideroblasts in refractory anemia with ring sideroblasts.[107]

Mitochondrial Myopathy and Sideroblastic Anemia

There are some similarities and some dissimilarities between Pearson marrow-pancreas syndrome and patients with mitochondrial myopathy and sideroblastic anemia (MLASA).[57,108,109] In both cases, there are defects in the mitochondrial electron transport chain, likely creating an environment that retards iron access to FECH in the reduced form. Both disorders are hereditary, but Pearson syndrome is caused by large deletions of mitochondrial DNA, whereas MLASA results from a homozygous missense mutation in the genomic DNA of pseudouridine synthase 1, encoded by *PUS1* gene.[108] It has been proposed that deficient pseudouridylation of mitochondrial transfer RNAs (tRNAs) explains the pathogenesis of MLASA type of sideroblastic anemia.[108]

Mitochondrial Ferritin Mitochondrial ferritin is a ferritin isoform with ferroxidase activity that is expressed only in mitochondria (Chap. 42). This protein is encoded by an intronless nuclear gene and can store iron within a shell of homopolymers.[110–112] Although the function and regulation of expression of this protein is not fully understood, the induction of mitochondrial ferritin causes the transfer of iron from cytosolic ferritin to mitochondrial ferritin.[113] The mitochondrial ferritin has a very low expression in all tissues except testis.[110,112] Although mitochondrial ferritin is not expressed in normal erythroblasts, it is expressed in ring sideroblasts of patients with sideroblastic anemias,[114] caused by ALAS2 defects, as well as those associated with myelodysplastic syndromes. In both, iron is sequestered within mitochondrial ferritin.[114] Because mitochondrial ferritin has ferroxidase activity, it likely protects mitochondria by converting the toxic ferrous iron to ferric iron that is stored. Further research is needed to explain the mechanism of mitochondrial ferritin induction in erythroblasts of patients with sideroblastic anemias, both hereditary and acquired. Whether the mitochondrial ferritin also accumulates iron in ring sideroblasts of patients with XLSA/A has not yet been studied.

Mechanism of Anemia

The dominant factor that determines anemia is ineffective erythropoiesis (intramedullary apoptosis); the rate of red cell destruction is usually near-normal or only moderately accelerated to levels for which a normally functioning marrow can compensate.[115] The half-time of disappearance of intravenously injected tracer doses of radioactive iron is usually is rapid (25 to 50 minutes; normal mean: 90 to 100 minutes) but in some patients may be normal. The plasma iron turnover tends to be increased (1.5 to 5.9 mg/dL of blood per day; normal: approximately 0.30 to 0.70 mg/dL per day), but incorporation of radioactive iron into heme and its delivery to the blood as newly synthesized hemoglobin are depressed (15 to 30 percent of tracer dose; normal: 70 to 90 percent). Red cell survival ranges between 40 and 120 days, indicating some cases have moderate or only very slightly shortened red cell life-span, whereas in other cases red cell survival is normal. As in other kinds of anemia characterized by ineffective erythropoiesis, the fecal stercobilin excreted per day may be greater than can be accounted for by the daily catabolism of circulating hemoglobin.

● CLINICAL AND LABORATORY FEATURES

PRIMARY ACQUIRED (CLONAL) SIDEROBLASTIC ANEMIA

The primary acquired sideroblastic anemia is described in Chap. 87. Anemia is present in more than 90 percent of patients. Patients may be asymptomatic or, if anemia is more severe, have the nonspecific symptoms of anemia including pallor, weakness, loss of a sense of well-being, and exertional dyspnea. A small proportion of patients have infections related to severe granulocytopenia or hemorrhage related to severe thrombocytopenia at the time of diagnosis; however, this variant of myelodysplastic syndrome has the lowest probability of symptomatic neutropenia, thrombocytopenia, and acute leukemic transformation among all myelodysplastic syndromes (Chap. 87). Hepatomegaly or splenomegaly occurs also rarely in this type of myelodysplastic syndrome. Iron overloading regularly accompanies this disorder, usually in those who have a large requirement for transfusion, and may be the cause of death (Chap. 87).

SECONDARY ACQUIRED SIDEROBLASTIC ANEMIA

Drugs and Alcohol

The administration of certain drugs and the ingestion of alcohol may cause sideroblastic anemia (see Table 59–1). The drugs that are most commonly associated with this type of anemia are isonicotinic acid hydrazide,[116] pyrazinamide,[21,22,117] and cycloserine,[21,22,117] all pyridoxine antagonists. Although plasma pyridoxal phosphate levels are often low in alcoholic patients, there is no correlation between these levels and the appearance of ringed sideroblasts in the marrow.[118]

Anemia secondary to drugs may be quite severe, even necessitating transfusion,[22] but characteristically the anemia improves rapidly when the patient is given pyridoxine and/or when administration of the offending drug is discontinued. The red cells are hypochromic, and a dimorphic appearance of the erythrocytes in the blood film may be notable, that is, two populations of red cells can be distinguished; hypochromic and anisocytic, along with normochromic and normocytic. The reticulocyte count is low or normal.[119] In rare instances, a sideroblastic anemia first observed during the course of drug administration has progressed in the face of discontinuing the putative offending drug. In such cases, the patient presumably was suffering from an unmasked underlying myelodysplastic neoplasm.

Copper Deficiency

In 1974, two patients with sideroblastic anemia, one also with neutropenia, following extensive bowel surgery and long-term parenteral nutrition were described.[120] In 2002, another patient was described who developed progressive macrocytic anemia, thrombocytopenia, and leukopenia with ringed sideroblasts after gastroduodenal bypass (Billroth II procedure). This patient also had optic neuritis and other neurologic abnormalities.[121] The hematologic abnormalities, but not neurologic defects, resolved fully with copper therapy. Since that time numerous similar cases, with and without neurologic abnormalities, have been reported.[122,123] A similar hematologic picture can be seen with zinc-induced copper deficiency.[124,125]

HEREDITARY SIDEROBLASTIC ANEMIA

Hereditary sideroblastic anemia is very uncommon. More instances of the X-chromosome linked varieties than of apparently autosomally inherited cases have been documented.[126] The disorder is heterogeneous. The variant with ataxia is characterized by neurologic impairment and typically mild anemia in males. The neurologic symptoms include ataxia, dysmetria, dysdiadochokinesis, dysarthria, and intention tremor that are referred to as spinocerebellar syndrome. A mild intellectual impairment may be also seen.

In some of the cases of hereditary iron-loading anemia that are cited below, the presence of the sideroblasts in the marrow or the hereditary nature of the disorder is documented, whereas in others it is presumed but not clearly documented.

Anemia is usually apparent during the first few months[127] or years[35,37] of life; it may even occur prenatally.[103] However, there are patients in whom microcytic anemia first became evident in the eighth and ninth decade of life and were found to have a microcytic, pyridoxine response anemia apparently related to inherited mutations of the *ALAS2* gene.[128,129]

Pallor is the most prominent physical finding; splenomegaly may be present,[130] but not universally so.[35,127] The anemia is characteristically microcytic and hypochromic, and prominent dimorphism of the red cell population has been noted in carrier females of the sex-linked form of the anemia.[12,127,131] This has been regarded as evidence of X-inactivation affecting the locus responsible for this disorder,[37,127,131,132] but it is notable that marked dimorphism sometimes is seen in the red cells of affected males as well,[12,35] and in autosomal forms of the disease.[133] The degree of anisocytosis and poikilocytosis is usually striking. Sometimes the anemia can be macrocytic,[2,134] especially in mitochondrial forms of the disease. The red cells show marked heterogeneity with respect to resistance to osmotic lysis: a flattened curve indicates that cells with both increased and decreased resistance to lysis are present.[35,135] The white cell count is usually normal or slightly decreased, unless splenectomy has been performed. Then it may be greatly elevated.[136] Splenomegaly is present in most cases.[136] In one family, a platelet function abnormality resembling a storage pool defect was noted,[137] but this could have been an independently inherited disorder.

Pearson marrow-pancreas syndrome is a refractory sideroblastic anemia with vacuolization of marrow precursors and exocrine pancreatic dysfunction (Chap. 36).[56,138] It is often fatal in infancy or early childhood, is characterized by marrow failure with macrocytic sideroblastic anemia, which is typically transfusion dependent. Neutropenia and thrombocytopenia may also be present. However, the invariable dysfunction of the exocrine pancreas from fibrosis and acinar atrophy resulting in chronic malabsorption and diarrhea may, in some affected patients, be dominant features of morbidity and mortality of Pearson syndrome. Lactic acidosis, caused by a defect in oxidative phosphorylation and other organ dysfunction, including liver impairment, is also common. The usual causes of death are bacterial sepsis from neutropenia, metabolic crisis, and hepatic failure. Most patients die in infancy, although there is considerable phenotypic variation, presumably depending upon the number of mitochondria affected and their tissue distribution.

● TREATMENT

Many patients with hereditary sideroblastic anemia have some response to treatment with pyridoxine in doses of 50 to 200 mg/day,[12,127,131,136,139–141] but failures have also been observed.[8,35,42] Some patients have responded to doses as low as 2.5 mg/day.[136] An additional effect may be achieved by the administration of folic acid.[127] Very rarely, patients have been reported to respond to a crude liver extract, and tryptophan may be an active principle, enhancing the effect of pyridoxine.[142,143] Responses to pyridoxine may result in an increase in the steady-state hemoglobin level of the blood or a decrease in the transfusion requirement, but normalization of the hemoglobin level does not usually occur and the anemia relapses when pyridoxine administration is discontinued.

Iron overloading regularly accompanies this disorder and may be the cause of death (Chap. 43).[41] Iron storage may be enhanced when any of the mutations of hereditary hemochromatosis are coinherited.[144] If the anemia is not too severe or if it can be partially corrected by the administration of pyridoxine, phlebotomy may be used to diminish the iron burden.[145,146] Otherwise, it may be advisable to attempt to decrease the amount of body iron by iron chelation (Chap. 43).

Marrow transplantation, both ablative[147] and nonmyeloblative,[148] has been used on rare occasions to treat patients with severe hereditary sideroblastic anemia.

REFERENCES

1. Kardos G, Veerman AJ, de Waal FC, et al: Familial sideroblastic anemia with emergence of monosomy 5 and myelodysplastic syndrome. *Med Pediatr Oncol* 26(1):54–56, 1996.
2. Tuckfield A, Ratnaike S, Hussein S, et al: A novel form of hereditary sideroblastic anaemia with macrocytosis. *Br J Haematol* 97(2):279–285, 1997.
3. Dacie JV, Doniach I: The basophilic property of the iron-containing granules in siderocytes. *J Pathol Bacteriol* 59(4):684–686, 1947.
4. McFadzean AJ, Davis LJ: Iron-staining erythrocyte inclusions with special reference to acquired haemolytic anaemia. *Glasgow Med J* 28(9):237, 1947.
5. Bjorkman SE: Chronic refractory anemia with sideroblastic bone marrow; a study of four cases. *Blood* 11(3):250–259, 1956.
6. Dacie JV, Smith MD, White JC, et al: Refractory normoblastic anaemia: A clinical and haematological study of seven cases. *Br J Haematol* 5(1):56–82, 1959.
7. Heilmeyer L, Emmrich J, Hennemann HH, et al: [Chronic hypochromic anemia in two siblings based on iron metabolism disorders (anemia hypochromica sideroachrestica hereditaria)] [in German]. *Folia Haematol (Frankf)* 2(1):61–75, 1958.
8. Heilmeyer L, Keiderling W, Bilger R, et al: [Chronic refractory anemia with sideroblastic bone marrow (Anemia refractoria sideroblastica)] [in German]. *Folia Haematol (Frankf)* 2(1):49–60, 1958.
9. Bernard J, Lortholary P, Levy JP, et al: [Primary sideroblastic normochromic anemia] [in French]. *Nouv Rev Fr Hematol* 71:723–748, 1963.
10. Mollin DL: Sideroblasts and sideroblastic anaemia. *Br J Haematol* 11:41–48, 1965.
11. Cooley TB: A severe type of hereditary anemia with elliptocytosis. Interesting sequence of splenectomy. *Am J Med Sci* 209, 1945.
12. Rundles R: Hereditary (sex-linked) anemia. *Am J Med Sci* 211(Jun):641–658, 1946.
13. Cotter PD, Rucknagel DL, Bishop DF: X-linked sideroblastic anemia: Identification of the mutation in the erythroid-specific delta-aminolevulinate synthase gene (ALAS2) in the original family described by Cooley. *Blood* 84(11):3915–3924, 1994.
14. Kasturi J, Basha HM, Smeda SH, et al: Hereditary sideroblastic anaemia in 4 siblings of a Libyan family—autosomal inheritance. *Acta Haematol* 68(4):321–324, 1982.
15. Cormier V, Rotig A, Quartino AR, et al: Widespread multi-tissue deletions of the mitochondrial genome in the Pearson marrow-pancreas syndrome. *J Pediatr* 117(4):599–602, 1990.
16. Danse PW, Jakobs C, Rotig A, et al: [Pearson's syndrome: A multi-system disorder based on a mt-DNA deletion] [in Dutch]. *Tijdschr Kindergeneeskd* 59(6):196–202, 1991.
17. Gurgey A, Rotig A, Gumruk F, et al: Pearson's marrow-pancreas syndrome in 2 Turkish children. *Acta Haematol* 87(4):206–209, 1992.
18. McShane MA, Hammans SR, Sweeney M, et al: Pearson syndrome and mitochondrial encephalomyopathy in a patient with a deletion of mtDNA. *Am J Hum Genet* 48(1):39–42, 1991.
19. Rotig A, Cormier V, Blanche S, et al: Pearson's marrow-pancreas syndrome. A multisystem mitochondrial disorder in infancy. *J Clin Invest* 86(5):1601–1608, 1990.
20. Macgibbon BH, Mollin DL: Sideroblastic anaemia in man: Observations on seventy cases. *Br J Haematol* 11:59–69, 1965.
21. Hines JD, Grasso JA: The sideroblastic anemias. *Semin Hematol* 7(1):86–106, 1970.
22. Verwilghen R, Reybrouck G, Callens L, et al: Antituberculous drugs and sideroblastic anaemia. *Br J Haematol* 11:92–98, 1965.

23. Bessis MC, Jensen WN: Sideroblastic anaemia, mitochondria and erythroblastic iron. *Br J Haematol* 11:49–51, 1965.
24. Griggs RC: Lead poisoning: Hematologic aspects. *Prog Hematol* 4:117–137, 1964.
25. Jensen WN, Moreno G: [The ribosomes and basophilic granulations of erythrocytes in lead poisoning] [in French]. *C R Hebd Seances Acad Sci* 258:3596–3597, 1964.
26. Jensen WN, Moreno GD, Bessis MC: An electron microscopic description of basophilic stippling in red cells. *Blood* 25:933–943, 1965.
27. Gehrmann G: Pyridoxine-responsive anaemias. *Br J Haematol* 11:86–91, 1965.
28. Harris JW, Whittington RM, Weisman R Jr, et al: Pyridoxine responsive anemia in the human adult. *Proc Soc Exp Biol Med* 91(3):427–432, 1956.
29. Horrigan DL, Harris JW: Pyridoxine-responsive anemias in man. *Vitam Horm* 26:549–571, 1968.
30. Cartwright GE, Deiss A: Sideroblasts, siderocytes, and sideroblastic anemia. *N Engl J Med* 292(4):185–193, 1975.
31. Hammond E, Deiss A, Carnes WH, et al: Ultrastructural characteristics of siderocytes in swine. *Lab Invest* 21(4):292–297, 1969.
32. Koc S, Harris JW: Sideroblastic anemias: Variations on imprecision in diagnostic criteria, proposal for an extended classification of sideroblastic anemias. *Am J Hematol* 57(1):1–6, 1998.
33. Fleming MD: The genetics of inherited sideroblastic anemias. *Semin Hematol* 39(4):270–281, 2002.
34. Furuyama K, Sassa S: Multiple mechanisms for hereditary sideroblastic anemia. *Cell Mol Biol (Noisy-le-grand)* 48(1):5–10, 2002.
35. Garby L, Sjolin S, Vahlquist B: Chronic refractory hypochromic anaemia with disturbed haem-metabolism. *Br J Haematol* 3(1):55–67, 1957.
36. Konopka L, Hoffbrand AV: Haem synthesis in sideroblastic anaemia. *Br J Haematol* 42(1):73–83, 1979.
37. Lee GR, MacDiarmid WD, Cartwright GE, et al: Hereditary, X-linked, sideroachrestic anemia. The isolation of two erythrocyte populations differing in Xga blood type and porphyrin content. *Blood* 32(1):59–70, 1968.
38. McColl KE, Thompson GG, Moore MR, et al: Acute ethanol ingestion and haem biosynthesis in healthy subjects. *Eur J Clin Invest* 10(2 Pt 1):107–112, 1980.
39. Pasanen AV, Vuopio P, Borgstrom GH, et al: Haem biosynthesis in refractory sideroblastic anaemia associated with the preleukaemic syndrome. *Scand J Haematol* 27(1):35–44, 1981.
40. Tanaka M, Bottomley SS: Bone marrow delta-aminolevulinic acid synthetase activity in experimental sideroblastic anemia. *J Lab Clin Med* 84(1):92–98, 1974.
41. Vogler WR, Mingioli ES: Porphyrin synthesis and heme synthetase activity in pyridoxine-responsive anemia. *Blood* 32(6):979–988, 1968.
42. Heilmeyer L: *Disturbances in Heme Synthesis.* Charles C. Thomas, Springfield, IL, 1966.
43. Kushner JP, Lee GR, Wintrobe MM, et al: Idiopathic refractory sideroblastic anemia: Clinical and laboratory investigation of 17 patients and review of the literature. *Medicine (Baltimore)* 50(3):139–159, 1971.
44. Cotter PD, Baumann M, Bishop DF: Enzymatic defect in "X-linked" sideroblastic anemia: Molecular evidence for erythroid delta-aminolevulinate synthase deficiency. *Proc Natl Acad Sci U S A* 89(9):4028–4032, 1992.
45. Bottomley SS: Congenital sideroblastic anemias. *Curr Hematol Rep* 5(1):41–49, 2006.
46. Fleming MD: Congenital sideroblastic anemias: Iron and heme lost in mitochondrial translation. *Hematology Am Soc Hematol Educ Program* 2011:525–531, 2011.
47. Guernsey DL, Jiang H, Campagna DR, et al: Mutations in mitochondrial carrier family gene SLC25A38 cause nonsyndromic autosomal recessive congenital sideroblastic anemia. *Nat Genet* 41(6):651–653, 2009.
48. Allikmets R, Raskind WH, Hutchinson A, et al: Mutation of a putative mitochondrial iron transporter gene (ABC7) in X-linked sideroblastic anemia and ataxia (XLSA/A). *Hum Mol Genet* 8(5):743–749, 1999.
49. Hellier KD, Hatchwell E, Duncombe AS, et al: X-linked sideroblastic anaemia with ataxia: Another mitochondrial disease? *J Neurol Neurosurg Psychiatry* 70(1):65–69, 2001.
50. Pagon RA, Bird TD, Detter JC, et al: Hereditary sideroblastic anaemia and ataxia: An X-linked recessive disorder. *J Med Genet* 22(4):267–273, 1985.
51. Raskind WH, Wijsman E, Pagon RA, et al: X-linked sideroblastic anemia and ataxia: Linkage to phosphoglycerate kinase at Xq13. *Am J Hum Genet* 48(2):335–341, 1991.
52. Maguire A, Hellier K, Hammans S, et al: X-linked cerebellar ataxia and sideroblastic anaemia associated with a missense mutation in the ABC7 gene predicting V411L. *Br J Haematol* 115(4):910–917, 2001.
53. Shimada Y, Okuno S, Kawai A, et al: Cloning and chromosomal mapping of a novel ABC transporter gene (hABC7), a candidate for X-linked sideroblastic anemia with spinocerebellar ataxia. *J Hum Genet* 43(2):115–122, 1998.
54. Broker S, Meunier B, Rich P, et al: MtDNA mutations associated with sideroblastic anaemia cause a defect of mitochondrial cytochrome c oxidase. *Eur J Biochem* 258(1):132–138, 1998.
55. Gattermann N, Retzlaff S, Wang YL, et al: Heteroplasmic point mutations of mitochondrial DNA affecting subunit I of cytochrome c oxidase in two patients with acquired idiopathic sideroblastic anemia. *Blood* 90(12):4961–4972, 1997.
56. Seneca S, De Meirleir L, De Schepper J, et al: Pearson marrow pancreas syndrome: A molecular study and clinical management. *Clin Genet* 51(5):338–342, 1997.
57. Casas K, Bykhovskaya Y, Mengesha E, et al: Gene responsible for mitochondrial myopathy and sideroblastic anemia (MSA) maps to chromosome 12q24.33. *Am J Med Genet A* 127A(1):44–49, 2004.
58. Jardine PE, Cotter PD, Johnson SA, et al: Pyridoxine-refractory congenital sideroblastic anaemia with evidence for autosomal inheritance: Exclusion of linkage to ALAS2 at Xp11.21 by polymorphism analysis. *J Med Genet* 31(3):213–218, 1994.
59. Goodman JR, Hall SG: Accumulation of iron in mitochondria of erythroblasts. *Br J Haematol* 13(3):335–340, 1967.
60. Kushner JP, Barbuto AJ, Lee GR: An inherited enzymatic defect in porphyria cutanea tarda: Decreased uroporphyrinogen decarboxylase activity. *J Clin Invest* 58(5):1089–1097, 1976.
61. Chauhan MS, Dakshinamurti K: Fluorometric assay of B6 vitamers in biological material. *Clin Chim Acta* 109(2):159–167, 1981.
62. Lee GR, Cartwright GE, Wintrobe MM: The response of free erythrocyte protoporphyrin to pyridoxine therapy in a patient with sideroachrestic (sideroblastic) anemia. *Blood* 27(4):557–567, 1966.
63. Pasanen AV, Salmi M, Vuopio P, et al: Heme biosynthesis in sideroblastic anemia. *Int J Biochem* 12(5–6):969–974, 1980.
64. Pasanen AV, Eklof M, Tenhunen R: Coproporphyrinogen oxidase activity and porphyrin concentrations in peripheral red blood cells in hereditary sideroblastic anaemia. *Scand J Haematol* 34(3):235–237, 1985.
65. Wiseman DH, May A, Jolles S, et al: A novel syndrome of congenital sideroblastic anemia, B-cell immunodeficiency, periodic fevers, and developmental delay (SIFD). *Blood* 122(1):112–123, 2013.
66. Barton JR, Shaver DC, Sibai BM: Successive pregnancies complicated by idiopathic sideroblastic anemia. *Am J Obstet Gynecol* 166(2):576–577, 1992.
67. Pignon JM, Breton-Gorius J, Bachir D, Rochant H: Congenital sideroblastic anemia without clinical iron overload. A case report. *Nouv Rev Fr Hematol* 32(4):281–284, 1990.
68. Murakami R, Takumi T, Gouji J, et al: Sideroblastic anemia showing unique response to pyridoxine. *Am J Pediatr Hematol Oncol* 13(3):345–350, 1991.
69. Mason DY, Emerson PM: Primary acquired sideroblastic anaemia: Response to treatment with pyridoxal-5-phosphate. *Br Med J* 1(5850):389–390, 1973.
70. Chillar RK, Johnson CS, Beutler E: Erythrocyte pyridoxine kinase levels in patients with sideroblastic anemia. *N Engl J Med* 295(16):881–883, 1976.
71. Nishibe H, Yamagata K, Goto H: A case of sideroblastic anaemia associated with marked elevation of erythrocytic arginase activity. *Scand J Haematol* 15(1):17–21, 1975.
72. Valentine WN, Konrad PN, Paglia DE: Dyserythropoiesis, refractory anemia, and "preleukemia:" metabolic features of the erythrocytes. *Br J Haematol* 24(6):857–875, 1973.
73. Ritchey AK, Hoffman R, Dainiak N, et al: Antibody-mediated acquired sideroblastic anemia: Response to cytotoxic therapy. *Blood* 54(3):734–741, 1979.
74. Rochant H, Dreyfus B, Bouguerra M, Tont-Hat H: Hypothesis: Refractory anemias, preleukemic conditions, and fetal erythropoiesis. *Blood* 39(5):721–726, 1972.
75. Geschke W, Beutler E: Refractory sideroblastic and nonsideroblastic anemia: A review of 27 cases. *West J Med* 127(2):85–92, 1977.
76. Napier I, Ponka P, Richardson DR: Iron trafficking in the mitochondrion: Novel pathways revealed by disease. *Blood* 105(5):1867–1874, 2005.
77. Pandolfo M: Frataxin deficiency and mitochondrial dysfunction. *Mitochondrion* 2(1–2):87–93, 2002.
78. Ponka P: Tissue-specific regulation of iron metabolism and heme synthesis: Distinct control mechanisms in erythroid cells. *Blood* 89(1):1–25, 1997.
79. Adams ML, Ostapiuk I, Grasso JA: The effects of inhibition of heme synthesis on the intracellular localization of iron in rat reticulocytes. *Biochim Biophys Acta* 1012(3):243–253, 1989.
80. Borova J, Ponka P, Neuwirt J: Study of intracellular iron distribution in rabbit reticulocytes with normal and inhibited heme synthesis. *Biochim Biophys Acta* 320(1):143–156, 1973.
81. Ponka P, Wilczynska A, Schulman HM: Iron utilization in rabbit reticulocytes. A study using succinylacetone as an inhibitor or heme synthesis. *Biochim Biophys Acta* 720(1):96–105, 1982.
82. Richardson DR, Ponka P, Vyoral D: Distribution of iron in reticulocytes after inhibition of heme synthesis with succinylacetone: Examination of the intermediates involved in iron metabolism. *Blood* 87(8):3477–3488, 1996.
83. Harrison PM, Arosio P: The ferritins: Molecular properties, iron storage function and cellular regulation. *Biochim Biophys Acta* 1275(3):161–203, 1996.
84. Shaw GC, Cope JJ, Li L, et al: Mitoferrin is essential for erythroid iron assimilation. *Nature* 440(7080):96–100, 2006.
85. Ajioka RS, Phillips JD, Kushner JP: Biosynthesis of heme in mammals. *Biochim Biophys Acta* 1763(7):723–736, 2006.
86. Ponka P, Sheftel AD, Zhang AS: Iron targeting to mitochondria in erythroid cells. *Biochem Soc Trans* 30(4):735–738, 2002.
87. Sheftel AD, Zhang AS, Brown C, et al: Direct interorganellar transfer of iron from endosome to mitochondrion. *Blood* 110(1):125–132, 2007.
88. Zhang AS, Sheftel AD, Ponka P: Intracellular kinetics of iron in reticulocytes: Evidence for endosome involvement in iron targeting to mitochondria. *Blood* 105(1):368–375, 2005.
89. Cox TM, O'Donnell MW, Aisen P, et al: Hemin inhibits internalization of transferrin by reticulocytes and promotes phosphorylation of the membrane transferrin receptor. *Proc Natl Acad Sci U S A* 82(15):5170–5174, 1985.
90. Iacopetta B, Morgan E: Heme inhibits transferrin endocytosis in immature erythroid cells. *Biochim Biophys Acta* 805(2):211–216, 1984.
91. Ponka P, Neuwirt J: Regulation of iron entry into reticulocytes. I. Feedback inhibitory effect of heme on iron entry into reticulocytes and on heme synthesis. *Blood* 33(5):690–707, 1969.

92. Ponka P, Schulman HM, Martinez-Medellin J: Haem inhibits iron uptake subsequent to endocytosis of transferrin in reticulocytes. *Biochem J* 251(1):105–109, 1988.

93. Campagna DR, de Bie CI, Schmitz-Abe K, et al: X-linked sideroblastic anemia due to ALAS2 intron 1 enhancer element GATA-binding site mutations. *Am J Hematol* 89(3):315–319, 2014.

94. Bekri S, Kispal G, Lange H, et al: Human ABC7 transporter: Gene structure and mutation causing X-linked sideroblastic anemia with ataxia with disruption of cytosolic iron-sulfur protein maturation. *Blood* 96(9):3256–3264, 2000.

95. Csere P, Lill R, Kispal G: Identification of a human mitochondrial ABC transporter, the functional orthologue of yeast Atm1p. *FEBS Lett* 441(2):266–270, 1998.

96. Lill R, Muhlenhoff U: Iron-sulfur protein biogenesis in eukaryotes: Components and mechanisms. *Annu Rev Cell Dev Biol* 22:457–486, 2006.

97. Pondarre C, Campagna DR, Antiochos B, et al: Abcb7, the gene responsible for X-linked sideroblastic anemia with ataxia, is essential for hematopoiesis. *Blood* 109(8):3567–3569, 2007.

98. Wingert RA, Galloway JL, Barut B, et al: Deficiency of glutaredoxin 5 reveals Fe-S clusters are required for vertebrate haem synthesis. *Nature* 436(7053):1035–1039, 2005.

99. Camaschella C, Campanella A, De Falco L, et al: The human counterpart of zebrafish shiraz shows sideroblastic-like microcytic anemia and iron overload. *Blood* 110(4):1353–1358, 2007.

100. Ohgami RS, Campagna DR, Greer EL, et al: Identification of a ferrireductase required for efficient transferrin-dependent iron uptake in erythroid cells. *Nat Genet* 37(11):1264–1269, 2005.

101. Pearson HA, Lobel JS, Kocoshis SA, et al: A new syndrome of refractory sideroblastic anemia with vacuolization of marrow precursors and exocrine pancreatic dysfunction. *J Pediatr* 95(6):976–984, 1979.

102. Fontenay M, Cathelin S, Amiot M, et al: Mitochondria in hematopoiesis and hematological diseases. *Oncogene* 25(34):4757–4767, 2006.

103. Andersen K, Kaad PH: Congenital sideroblastic anaemia with intrauterine symptoms and early lethal outcome. *Acta Paediatr* 81(8):652–653, 1992.

104. Gattermann N: From sideroblastic anemia to the role of mitochondrial DNA mutations in myelodysplastic syndromes. *Leuk Res* 24(2):141–151, 2000.

105. Inoue S, Yokota M, Nakada K, et al: Pathogenic mitochondrial DNA-induced respiration defects in hematopoietic cells result in anemia by suppressing erythroid differentiation. *FEBS Lett* 581(9):1910–1916, 2007.

106. Shin MG, Kajigaya S, Levin BC, et al: Mitochondrial DNA mutations in patients with myelodysplastic syndromes. *Blood* 101(8):3118–3125, 2003.

107. Boultwood J, Pellagatti A, Nikpour M, et al: The role of the iron transporter ABCB7 in refractory anemia with ring sideroblasts. *PLoS One* 3(4):e1970, 2008.

108. Bykhovskaya Y, Casas K, Mengesha E, et al: Missense mutation in pseudouridine synthase 1 (PUS1) causes mitochondrial myopathy and sideroblastic anemia (MLASA). *Am J Hum Genet* 74(6):1303–1308, 2004.

109. Casas KA, Fischel-Ghodsian N: Mitochondrial myopathy and sideroblastic anemia. *Am J Med Genet A* 125A(2):201–204, 2004.

110. Drysdale J, Arosio P, Invernizzi R, et al: Mitochondrial ferritin: A new player in iron metabolism. *Blood Cells Mol Dis* 29(3):376–383, 2002.

111. Levi S, Arosio P: Mitochondrial ferritin. *Int J Biochem Cell Biol* 36(10):1887–1889, 2004.

112. Levi S, Corsi B, Bosisio M, et al: A human mitochondrial ferritin encoded by an intronless gene. *J Biol Chem* 276(27):24437–24440, 2001.

113. Nie G, Sheftel AD, Kim SF, et al: Overexpression of mitochondrial ferritin causes cytosolic iron depletion and changes cellular iron homeostasis. *Blood* 105(5):2161–2167, 2005.

114. Cazzola M, Invernizzi R, Bergamaschi G, et al: Mitochondrial ferritin expression in erythroid cells from patients with sideroblastic anemia. *Blood* 101(5):1996–2000, 2003.

115. Singh AK, Shinton NK, Williams JD: Ferrokinetic abnormalities and their significance in patients with sideroblastic anaemia. *Br J Haematol* 18(1):67–77, 1970.

116. Sharp RA, Lowe JG, Johnston RN: Anti-tuberculous drugs and sideroblastic anaemia. *Br J Clin Pract* 44(12):706–707, 1990.

117. Harriss EB, Macgibbon BH, Mollin DL: Experimental sideroblastic anaemia. *Br J Haematol* 11:99–106, 1965.

118. Pierce HI, McGuffin RG, Hillman RS: Clinical studies in alcoholic sideroblastosis. *Arch Intern Med* 136(3):283–289, 1976.

119. McCurdy PR, Donohoe RF: Pyridoxine-responsive anemia conditioned by isonicotinic acid hydrazide. *Blood* 27(3):352–362, 1966.

120. Dunlap WM, James GW 3rd, Hume DM: Anemia and neutropenia caused by copper deficiency. *Ann Intern Med* 80(4):470–476, 1974.

121. Gregg XT, Reddy V, Prchal JT: Copper deficiency masquerading as myelodysplastic syndrome. *Blood* 100(4):1493–1495, 2002.

122. Fong T, Vij R, Vijayan A, et al: Copper deficiency: An important consideration in the differential diagnosis of myelodysplastic syndrome. *Haematologica* 92(10):1429–1430, 2007.

123. Kumar N, Elliott MA, Hoyer JD, et al: "Myelodysplasia," myeloneuropathy, and copper deficiency. *Mayo Clin Proc* 80(7):943–946, 2005.

124. Broun ER, Greist A, Tricot G, et al: Excessive zinc ingestion. A reversible cause of sideroblastic anemia and bone marrow depression. *JAMA* 264(11):1441–1443, 1990.

125. Patterson WP, Winkelmann M, Perry MC: Zinc-induced copper deficiency: Megamineral sideroblastic anemia. *Ann Intern Med* 103(3):385–386, 1985.

126. Nusbaum NJ: Concise review: Genetic bases for sideroblastic anemia. *Am J Hematol* 37(1):41–44, 1991.

127. Weatherall DJ, Pembrey ME, Hall EG, et al: Familial sideroblastic anaemia: Problem of Xg and X chromosome inactivation. *Lancet* 2(7676):744–748, 1970.

128. Cotter PD, May A, Fitzsimons EJ, et al: Late-onset X-linked sideroblastic anemia. Missense mutations in the erythroid delta-aminolevulinate synthase (ALAS2) gene in two pyridoxine-responsive patients initially diagnosed with acquired refractory anemia and ringed sideroblasts. *J Clin Invest* 96(4):2090–2096, 1995.

129. Furuyama K, Harigae H, Kinoshita C, et al: Late-onset X-linked sideroblastic anemia following hemodialysis. *Blood* 101(11):4623–4624, 2003.

130. Buchanan GR, Bottomley SS, Nitschke R: Bone marrow delta-aminolaevulinate synthase deficiency in a female with congenital sideroblastic anemia. *Blood* 55(1):109–115, 1980.

131. Prasad AS, Tranchida L, Konno ET, et al: Hereditary sideroblastic anemia and glucose-6-phosphate dehydrogenase deficiency in a Negro family. *J Clin Invest* 47(6):1415–1424, 1968.

132. Beutler E: The distribution of gene products among populations of cells in heterozygous humans. *Cold Spring Harb Symp Quant Biol* 29:261–271, 1964.

133. van Waveren Hogervorst GD, van Roermund HP, Snijders PJ: Hereditary sideroblastic anaemia and autosomal inheritance of erythrocyte dimorphism in a Dutch family. *Eur J Haematol* 38(5):405–409, 1987.

134. Fitzsimons EJ, May A: The molecular basis of the sideroblastic anemias. *Curr Opin Hematol* 3(2):167–172, 1996.

135. Seip M, Gjessing LR, Lie SO: Congenital sideroblastic anaemia in a girl. *Scand J Haematol* 8(6):505–512, 1971.

136. Horrigan DL, Harris JW: Pyridoxine-responsive anemia: Analysis of 62 cases. *Adv Intern Med* 12:103–174, 1964.

137. Soslau G, Brodsky I: Hereditary sideroblastic anemia with associated platelet abnormalities. *Am J Hematol* 32(4):298–304, 1989.

138. Smith OP, Hann IM, Woodward CE, et al: Pearson's marrow/pancreas syndrome: Haematological features associated with deletion and duplication of mitochondrial DNA. *Br J Haematol* 90(2):469–472, 1995.

139. Bishop RC, Bethell FH: Hereditary hypochromic anemia with transfusion hemosiderosis treated with pyridoxine: Report of a case. *N Engl J Med* 261:486–489, 1959.

140. Harris JW, Horrigan DL: Pyridoxine-responsive anemia—Prototype and variations on the theme. *Vitam Horm* 22:721–753, 1964.

141. Vogler WR Mingioli ES. Heme synthesis in pyridoxine responsive anemia. *N Engl J Med* 273, 1965.

142. Albahary C, Boiron M: [Primary refractory anemia with medullary and hepatic hypersiderosis of blood in a woman] [in French]. *Acta Med Scand* 163(5):429–438, 1959.

143. Horrigan DL: Pyridoxine-responsive anemia: Influence of tryptophan on pyridoxine responsiveness. *Blood* 42(2):187–193, 1973.

144. Yaouanq J, Grosbois B, Jouanolle AM, et al: Haemochromatosis Cys282Tyr mutation in pyridoxine-responsive sideroblastic anaemia. *Lancet* 349(9063):1475–1476, 1997.

145. French TJ, Jacobs P: Sideroblastic anaemia associated with iron overload treated by repeated phlebotomy. *S Afr Med J* 50(15):594–596, 1976.

146. Weintraub LR, Conrad ME, Crosby WH: Iron-loading anemia. Treatment with repeated phlebotomies and pyridoxine. *N Engl J Med* 275(4):169–176, 1966.

147. Urban C, Binder B, Hauer C, et al: Congenital sideroblastic anemia successfully treated by allogeneic bone marrow transplantation. *Bone Marrow Transplant* 10(4):373–375, 1992.

148. Medeiros BC, Kolhouse JF, Cagnoni PJ, et al: Nonmyeloablative allogeneic hematopoietic stem cell transplantation for congenital sideroblastic anemia. *Bone Marrow Transplant* 31(11):1053–1055, 2003.

149. Yunis AA, Salem Z: Drug-induced mitochondrial damage and sideroblastic change. *Clin Haematol* 9(3):607–619, 1980.

Part VII Neutrophils, Eosinophils, Basophils, and Mast Cells

60. Structure and Composition of Neutrophils, Eosinophils, and Basophils 925

61. Production, Distribution, and Fate of Neutrophils 939

62. Eosinophils and Related Disorders . . . 947

63. Basophils, Mast Cells, and Related Disorders 965

64. Classification and Clinical Manifestations of Neutrophil Disorders 983

65. Neutropenia and Neutrophilia 991

66. Disorders of Neutrophil Function 1005

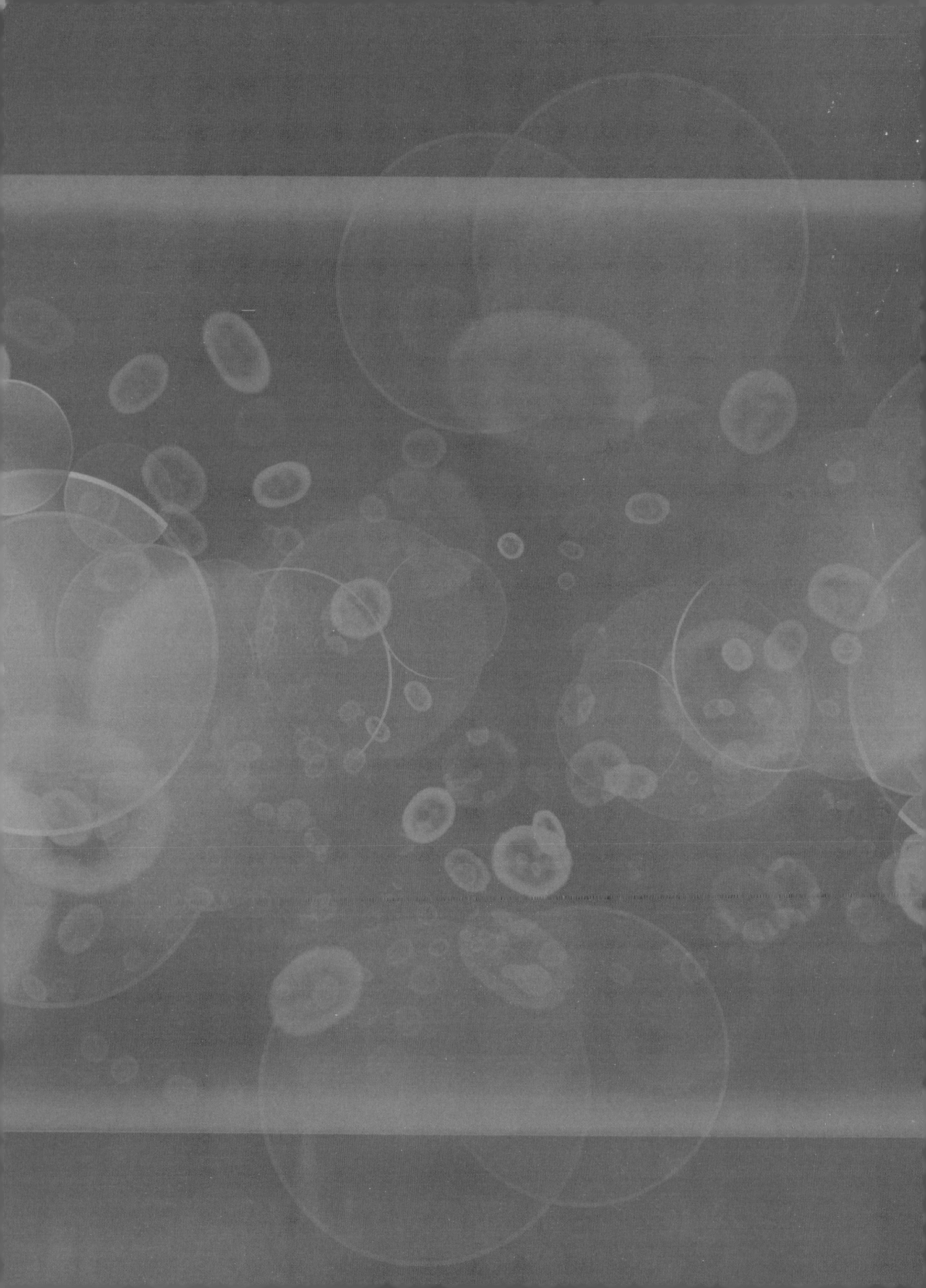

CHAPTER 60
STRUCTURE AND COMPOSITION OF NEUTROPHILS, EOSINOPHILS, AND BASOPHILS

C. Wayne Smith

SUMMARY

Early in precursor development in the marrow, cells destined to be leukocytes of the granulocytic series—neutrophils, eosinophils, and basophils—synthesize proteins and store them as cytoplasmic granules. The synthesis of primary or azurophilic granules defines the conversion of the myeloblast, a virtually agranular, primitive cell that is the earliest granulocyte precursor identifiable by light microscopy, into the promyelocyte, which is rich in azurophilic granules. Synthesis and accumulation of secondary or specific granules follows. The appearance of specific granules marks the progression of the promyelocyte to neutrophilic, eosinophilic, or basophilic myelocytes. Thereafter, the cell continues maturation into an amitotic cell with a segmented nucleus, capable of chemotaxis, phagocytosis and microbial killing. The mature granulocytes also develop cytoplasmic and surface structures that permit them to attach to and penetrate the wall of venules. The mature granulocytes enter the blood from the marrow, circulate briefly, and move to the tissues to carry out their major function of host defense. Blood neutrophils exhibit the capacity for changes in phenotypic characteristics and life span depending on the stimulating milieu of cytokines and chemokines. Gene expression profiling studies indicate the neutrophil is a transcriptionally active cell, responsive to environmental stimuli, and capable of a complex series of early and late changes in gene expression.

Acronyms and Abbreviations: AML1, AML2, AML3, transcription factor for various hematologic lineages; C3a, serum complement fragment 3a; C5a, serum complement fragment 5a; CBFA1, CBFA2, core-binding factor subunit α-1 or -2; CCR, C-C chemokine receptor; C/EBPε, regulating factor of gene expression; CD11b/CD18, Mac-1 or integrin $\alpha_m\beta_2$; ECP, eosinophil cationic protein; EDN, eosinophil-derived neurotoxin; FcγRIIIB, receptor IIIB for the Fc region of IgG; GATA-1, lineage-specific transcription factor; G-CSF, granulocyte colony-stimulating factor; GM-CSF, granulocyte-macrophage colony-stimulating factor; GRO, growth-regulated protein; IFN, interferon; Ig, immunoglobulin; IL, interleukin; IP-10, interferon-γ–induced protein 10; JAK2, Janus-associated kinase 2; LPS, lipopolysaccharide; MBP, major basic protein; MMP-8, metalloproteinase-8, also called collagenase; MMP-9, metalloproteinase-9, also called gelatinase B; NADPH, reduced form of nicotinamide adenine dinucleotide phosphate; PAF, platelet-activating factor; PMN, polymorphonuclear neutrophil; RUNX1, RUNX2, RUNX3, runt-related transcription factor 1, 2, or 3; SNAP, soluble NSF (N-ethylmaleimide-sensitive factor) attachment protein; TGF, transforming growth factor; TNF, tumor necrosis factor; VAMP, vesicle-associated membrane protein.

In the normal adult human, the life of granulocytes is spent in three environments: marrow, blood, and tissues. Marrow is the site of differentiation of hematopoietic stem cells into granulocyte progenitors and of proliferation and terminal maturation (Fig. 60–1). Precursor cell proliferation, which consists of approximately five divisions, occurs only during the first three stages of maturation (blast, promyelocyte, and myelocyte). After the myelocyte stage, the cells are no longer capable of mitosis and enter a large marrow storage pool from which they are released into the blood where they circulate for a few hours before entering tissues.

● NEUTROPHILS

LIGHT MICROSCOPY AND ELECTRON MICROSCOPY

The Myeloblast

The myeloblast is an immature cell with a large, oval nucleus, sizable nucleoli, and few or no granules. As the earliest precursor in the evolution of the neutrophil from the colony forming unit, it is an immature cell with a large nucleus and multiple nucleoli (Fig. 60–2). The nucleolus is the site of assembly of ribosomal proteins and ribosomal RNA, and is a prominent feature of early maturing cells. The scant cytoplasm contains reaction product for peroxidase within the rough-surfaced endoplasmic reticulum and Golgi cisternae and, sometimes, in early developing azurophilic granules. The dense product of the peroxidase reaction serves as a marker of azurophilic granules in human marrow and blood cells for electron and for light microscopy.[1-4]

The Promyelocyte

In the promyelocyte stage, the azurophilic or primary granules, large peroxidase-positive granules that stain metachromatically (reddish-purple) with a polychromatic stain such as Wright stain, are formed. Figure 60–3 shows that the promyelocyte produces and accumulates a large population of peroxidase-positive granules. Most of the granules are spherical and have a diameter of 500 nm, but ellipsoid, crystalline forms and small granules connected by filaments also are present.[5] As with other secretory cells, peroxidase is present throughout the secretory apparatus of the promyelocyte, including cisternae of the rough endoplasmic reticulum, all Golgi cisternae, some vesicles, and all developing granules.[2]

The Neutrophilic Myelocyte

During the myelocyte stage of maturation, the specific or secondary granules, which are peroxidase negative, are formed (see Fig. 60–2). At the end of the promyelocyte stage, peroxidase abruptly disappears from rough endoplasmic reticulum and Golgi cisternae, and the production of azurophilic granules ceases. The myelocyte stage begins with production of peroxidase-negative specific granules.[2]

The only peroxidase-positive elements at this stage are the azurophilic granules. The specific granules are formed by the Golgi complex. The granules vary in size and shape but typically are spherical (approximately 200 nm) or rod shaped (130 × 1000 nm). Figure 60–4 shows the cell also labeled with immunogold particles to illustrate the presence of lactoferrin, a specific granule marker. Approximately three cell divisions occur at this stage of maturation. Mitoses can be observed (Fig. 60–5), and the two types of granules appear to be distributed to the daughter cells in fairly equal numbers.

Metamyelocyte, Band, and Mature Neutrophil

The metamyelocyte and band neutrophils are nonproliferating cells that precede the development of the mature neutrophil (see Fig. 60–2).

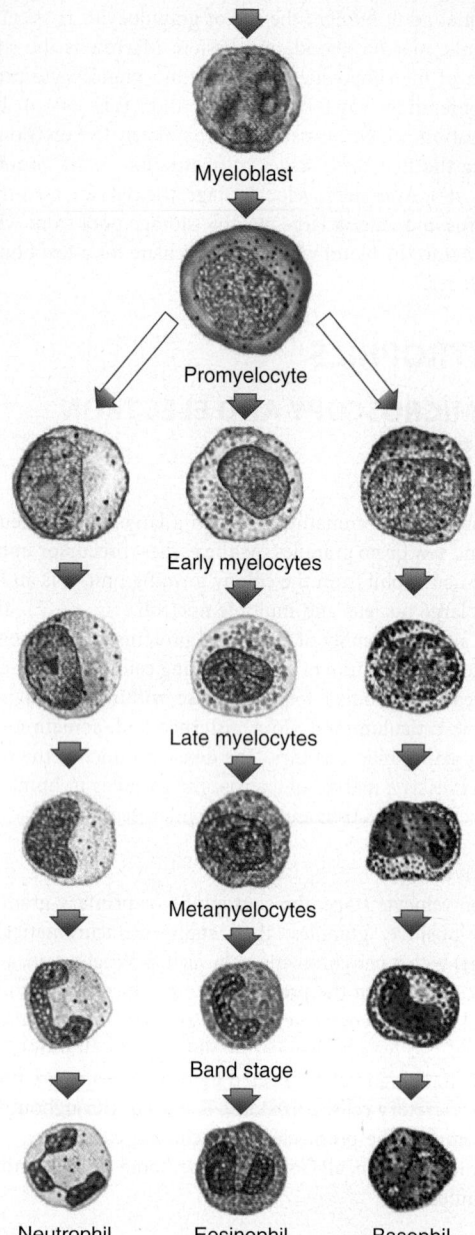

Figure 60–1. Diagrammatic representation of neutrophil (polymorphonuclear neutrophil [PMN]) and stages of maturation (see text for discussion). Of every 100 nucleated cells in marrow, 0.5 percent are myeloblasts, 5 percent are promyelocytes, 12 percent are myelocytes, 22 percent are metamyelocytes and bands, and 20 percent are maturing and mature neutrophilic cells, yielding a total of approximately 60 percent of cells representing developing neutrophils in normal human marrow. *(Reproduced with permission from* Lichtman's Atlas of Hematology. *www.accessmedicine.com.)*

The mature, segmented neutrophilic cells contain primary, peroxidase-positive granules and specific peroxidase-negative granules in a 1:2 ratio. The nucleus of the circulating neutrophil is segmented, usually into two to four interconnected lobes. The late stages of maturation consist of nondividing cells that can be distinguished by their nuclear morphology, mixed granule populations, small Golgi regions, and accumulations of glycogen particles. On average, an electron micrograph of a neutrophil displays 200 to 300 granules, and approximately one-third are peroxidase-positive (Fig. 60–6).

The violet-colored granules seen with light microscopy in mature neutrophils on Wright-stained blood films are azurophilic granules whose staining characteristics altered during maturation (Fig. 60–7). Therefore, with light microscopy, the most reliable method for identifying azurophilic granules on blood films is staining the cells for peroxidase. The size of most of the peroxidase-negative granules (approximately 200 nm) is at the limit of resolution of the light microscope. The granules cannot be distinguished individually but are responsible for the pink background color of neutrophil cytoplasm during and after the myelocyte stage.

Peroxidase-negative granules are more numerous than peroxidase-positive granules during the myelocyte stage because peroxidase granule formation ceases after the promyelocyte stage, the number of oxidase-positive granules per cell is reduced by mitoses, and peroxidase-negative granules continue to be produced by each myelocyte generation.[1]

The purpose of nuclear segmentation is not known. Fluorescence *in situ* hybridization with chromosome-specific probes has shown that chromosomes are randomly distributed among the nuclear lobes.[6] Some mature neutrophils in women have drumstick- or club-shaped nuclear appendages. These appendages contain the inactivated X chromosome. An X-chromosome–specific nucleic acid probe has confirmed the position of the X chromosomes in the drumstick structure of leukocyte nuclei by *in situ* hybridization.[7]

● NEUTROPHIL GRANULES

The diversity of neutrophil granules appears to be linked to the timing of biosynthesis during myelopoiesis. The hypothesis is that the different subsets of granules are the result of differences in the biosynthetic windows of the various granule proteins during maturation[7] and not the result of specific sorting between individual granule subsets (Chap. 66). The control of biosynthesis is exerted by transcription factors that control the expression of the genes for the various granule proteins. Several transcription factors identified as important in the timing of granule protein synthesis, including the lineage-specific transcription factor GATA-1, the lineage-specific transcription factor PU.1, transcription factor for various hematologic lineages, AML1 (also known as runt-related transcription factor 1 [RUNX1] or core-binding factor subunit alpha-2 [CBFA2]), AML2 (also known as RUNX3), and AML3 (also known as RUNX2 or CBFA1), and regulating factor of gene expression C/EBPε.[7-9] The importance of C/EBPε has been emphasized by the recognition of mutations in this protein in patients with the rare syndrome called "specific granule deficiency,"[10-12] a condition that leads to increased susceptibility to bacterial infections. In neutrophils from these patients, total cellular content and release of the secondary and tertiary granule markers (e.g., lactoferrin, B_{12} binding protein, and lysozyme) are diminished, although levels of primary granule constituents (e.g., myeloperoxidase, β-glucuronidase) generally are normal.

The granular constituents are released from the membrane-enclosed granules into phagosomes or transported to the cell surface by a process of exocytosis following stimulation of the neutrophil.[13] The signal cascade following stimulation of specific receptors on the cytoplasmic membrane results in elevated intracellular Ca^{2+}, lipid remodeling, and protein kinase activation, which culminate in fusion of granules with phagosomes or the cell surface membrane. The process is rapid, highly efficient, and involves families of docking proteins related to those found in neurons (e.g., vesicle-associated membrane protein [VAMP]-2, syntaxin-4, soluble NSF (N-ethylmaleimide-sensitive factor)-attachment protein [SNAP]-23).[14]

The granule subsets appear to have a significant differential sensitivity to undergo exocytosis, ranging from secretory vesicles to tertiary,

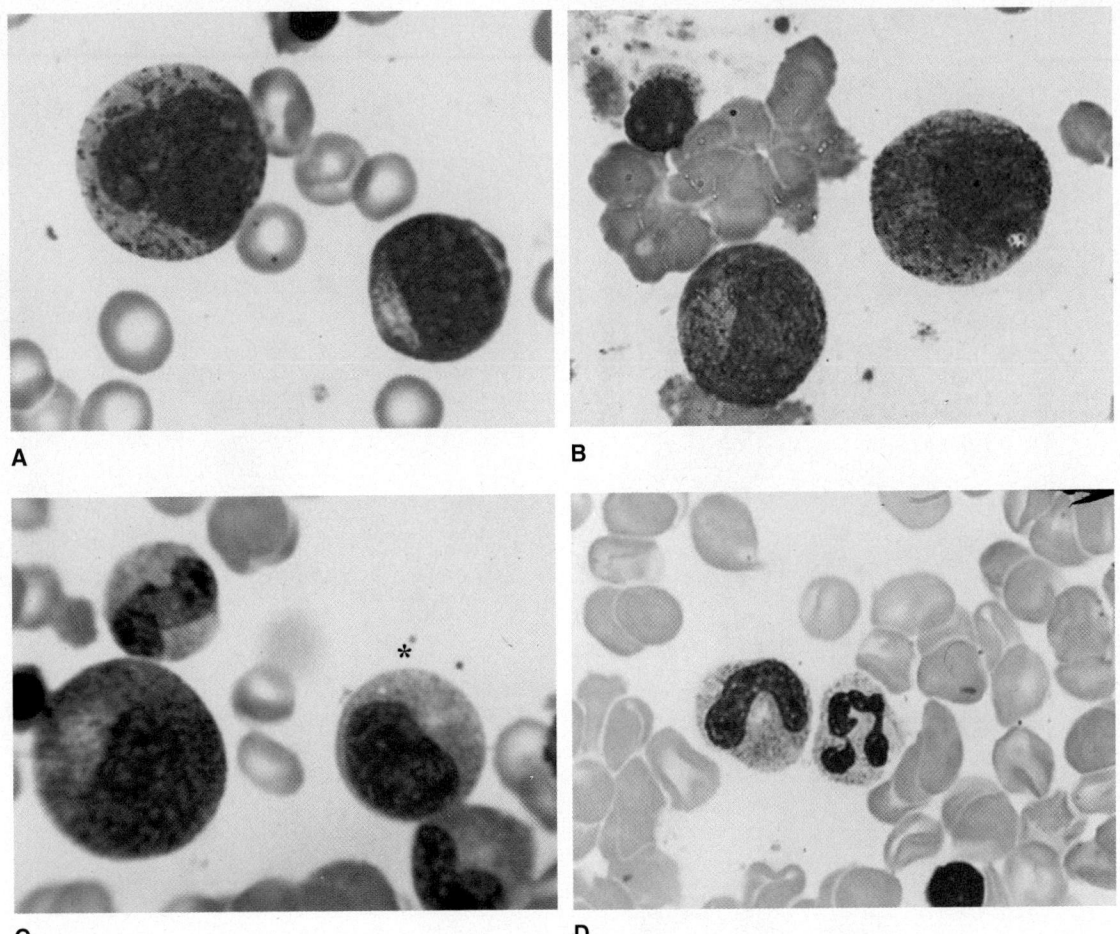

Figure 60–2. Marrow films. **A.** Myeloblast is the smaller cell to the lower right. It is the first recognizable precursor in the granulocytic series. Relatively high nuclear-to-cytoplasmic ratio. Note nucleoli and agranular cytoplasm. Promyelocyte in upper left. This cell is the largest granulocyte precursor in the marrow. It often has overt nucleoli, usually more cytoplasm, and azurophilic (primary) granules scattered throughout the cytoplasm and overlying the nucleus. **B.** Two very early neutrophilic myelocytes. They are very similar to the promyelocyte in appearance with nucleoli and scattered azurophilic granules throughout the cytoplasm. The distinguishing feature is the burst of tan coloring at the site of the Golgi zone, indicating the initial synthesis of neutrophilic granules. **C.** Large cell to the left is an early neutrophilic myelocyte with more neutrophilic granules evident spreading from the Golgi zone at the hilus of the nucleus. It still has some features of the promyelocyte. The cell beneath the asterisk is a late neutrophilic myelocyte. The cell has decreased in size, the nuclear chromatin has condensed. Nucleoli are not evident and the cytoplasm is nearly filled with neutrophilic granules. Below the neutrophilic myelocyte is a neutrophilic metamyelocyte, characterized by its reniform nucleus and cytoplasm filled with neutrophilic granules. The cell above the large early myelocyte on the left is a band neutrophil. The nucleus has reached the shape of a sausage and is about equal in diameter through its length. **D.** A band neutrophil *(left)* and a segmented neutrophil *(right)*. Neutrophilic granules, because of their small size, are not resolvable by the light microscope and are inferred by the characteristic tan staining quality of the cytoplasm. *(Reproduced with permission from* Lichtman's Atlas of Hematology. *www.accessmedicine.com.)*

secondary, and primary granules, with primary granules being most resistant. The significance of this differential release is incompletely understood, but some aspects are apparent in the functions of the constituents within the granules and granular membranes. For example, secretory vesicles and tertiary granules contain receptors, such as CD11b/CD18 (adhesion molecule, Mac-1), formyl peptide receptor (chemotactic receptor), FcγRIIIB (Fc receptor), and gelatinase (metalloproteinase [MMP]-9), which potentially enhance extracellular interactions of the neutrophil. Primary granules contain microbicidal proteins and acid hydrolases, and the acidic environment of the phagolysosome creates an optimal pH for these enzymes.

BIOACTIVE FACTORS IN GRANULES

Neutrophil granules are particularly rich in factors with antimicrobial activity. Some (e.g., myeloperoxidase) function in conjunction with

the reduced form of nicotinamide adenine dinucleotide phosphate (NADPH) oxidase, whereas others (e.g., defensins) exhibit activity independent of the oxidative burst. Table 60–1 lists the principal contents of the four granule types in neutrophils: primary (azurophilic), secondary (specific), tertiary, and secretory vesicles.[15-56]

● EOSINOPHILS

LIGHT MICROSCOPY OF EOSINOPHILS IN MARROW AND BLOOD FILMS

The earliest morphologically identifiable form of an eosinophilic leukocyte is as a late myeloblast or early promyelocyte (see Fig. 60–1). This cell is approximately 15 μm in diameter and has a large nucleus with nucleoli and a few blue or azurophilic granules in intensely basophilic

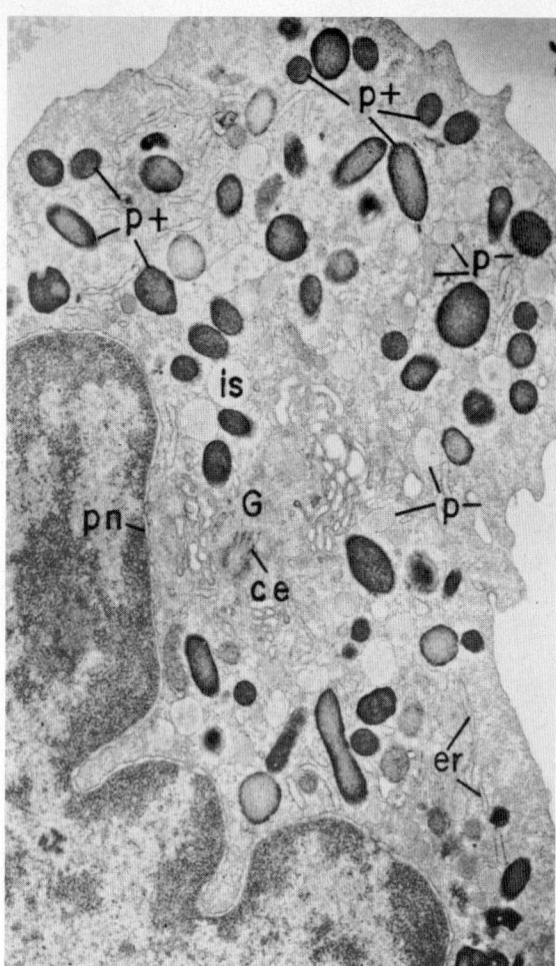

Figure 60–3. Electron micrograph of a neutrophilic promyelocyte from normal human marrow reacted for peroxidase. This cell is the largest of the neutrophilic series. It has a sizable, slightly indented nucleus with a nucleolus, a prominent Golgi region (G), centriole (ce), and cytoplasm packed with dense peroxidase-positive (p+) azurophilic granules of varying shapes and sizes. Peroxidase reaction product is visible in less concentrated form within all compartments of the secretory apparatus—endoplasmic reticulum (er), perinuclear cisterna (pn), and Golgi cisternae (G), and there are peroxidase negative granules (p–). No reaction product is apparent in the cytoplasmic matrix or mitochondria. (×8000).

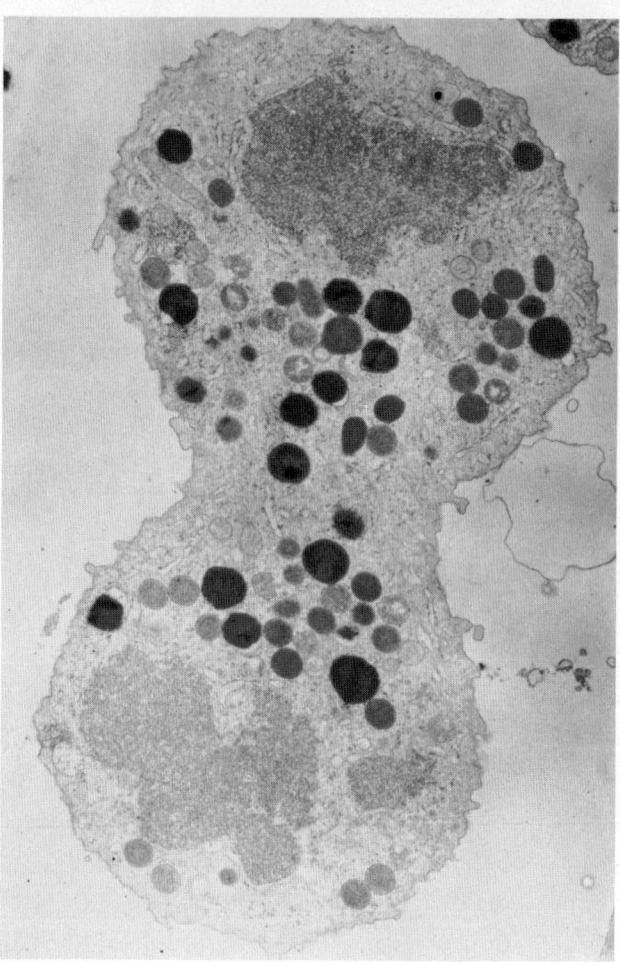

Figure 60–4. Portion of cytoplasm stained for peroxidase to mark the azurophil granules and then immunolabeled with gold particles to detect lactoferrin. The peroxidase-positive (p+) azurophil granules contain dense reaction product, whereas the lighter specific granules are peroxidase negative. Many of the peroxidase-negative granules (arrows) have gold label within their matrix (×70,000).

cytoplasm. The later eosinophilic promyelocyte and myelocyte contain mostly acidophilic granules. A lineage-committed eosinophil progenitor has recently been identified that expresses high levels of interleukin (IL)-5 receptor α and is negative for myeloperoxidase.[57] The fully mature eosinophilic leukocyte has a bilobed nucleus (see Fig. 60–7), and its cytoplasm is filled with large eosinophilic granules whose rims stain for peroxidase and Sudan black. Multilobed nuclei, comparable to those of neutrophils, are rare. Eosinophils are susceptible to mechanical damage during preparation of blood films.

ELECTRON MICROSCOPY AND CYTOCHEMISTRY

Eosinophils of the promyelocyte and myelocyte stages stain positively for peroxidase in all cisternae of the rough-surfaced endoplasmic reticulum, including transitional elements and the perinuclear cisterna;

clusters of smooth vesicles at the periphery of the Golgi complex; all cisternae of the Golgi complex; and all immature- and mature-specific granules.[4,58] Mature granules are completely filled with peroxidase except in areas occupied by centrally located crystals.

In the later stages of development, after granule formation has ceased, the eosinophils contain few of the organelles associated with the synthesis and packaging of secretory proteins. The endoplasmic reticulum is sparse or virtually nonexistent. The Golgi complex is small and inconspicuous. The cytoplasm of the mature eosinophil (Fig. 60–8) primarily contains granules and glycogen. Most of the granules are specific granules with crystals, which usually are centrally located. After the myelocyte stage, peroxidase can no longer be detected in the endoplasmic reticulum or Golgi elements of the eosinophil by any of the enzyme procedures; however, peroxidase can be found in the matrix of granules.[1,58]

GRANULES

Contents

As with neutrophils, eosinophils contain distinct granular organelles: primary granules, crystalloid granules, small granules and secretory vesicles.[59] The crystalloid granules (see Fig. 60–8)

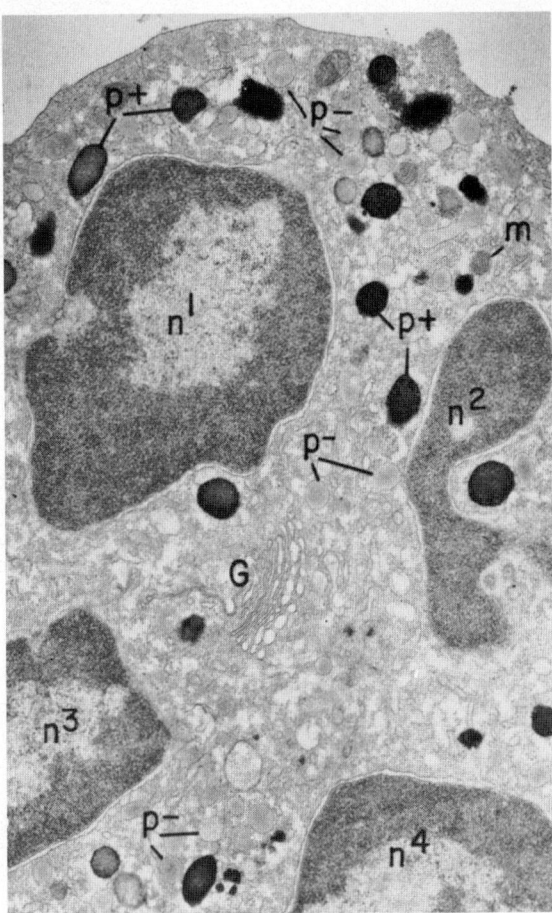

Figure 60–5. Myelocyte from rabbit marrow in the late stage of mitosis. This myelocyte is in telophase. Note that the granules are relatively equally distributed to the daughter cells (×15,000).

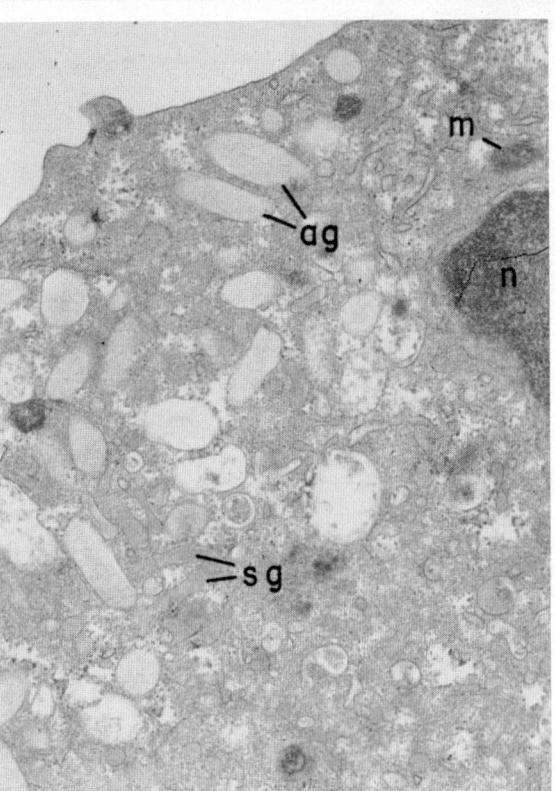

Figure 60–6. Mature neutrophil from normal human marrow reacted for peroxidase. The cytoplasm is filled with granules of the two basic types: (1) the smaller, pale, peroxidase-negative granules (p–) and (2) the large, dense, peroxidase-positive granules (p+). The nucleus is condensed and lobulated (n¹–n⁴), the Golgi region (G) is small and without any forming granules, the endoplasmic reticulum is scant, and mitochondria (m) are few (×21,000).

are the largest, 0.5 to 0.8 μm in diameter, and contain much of the granular protein. The proteins packaged in these granules are highly basic proteins, with the crystalline core being mostly major basic protein (MBP).[60,61] The granule matrix contains eosinophil peroxidase, eosinophil cationic protein (ECP), and eosinophil-derived neurotoxin (EDN). The primary granules contain Charcot-Leyden crystals. Charcot-Leyden crystals are bipyramidal crystals observed in fluids in association with eosinophilic inflammatory reactions. They possess lysophospholipase activity and compose

7 to 10 percent of total eosinophil protein.[62,63] The ultrastructural localization of this protein is in a large, crystal-free granule and supports the presence of a distinct primary granule population in mature eosinophils.[4,63,64] MBP consists of two homologues and is an abundant granular protein, 5 to 10 pg per cell. Mature eosinophils can no longer express this protein so all MBP is stored during development.[65] Eosinophil peroxidase is an abundant heme-containing protein (approximately 15 pg per cell) that catalyzes the peroxidation of halides together with hydrogen peroxide forming

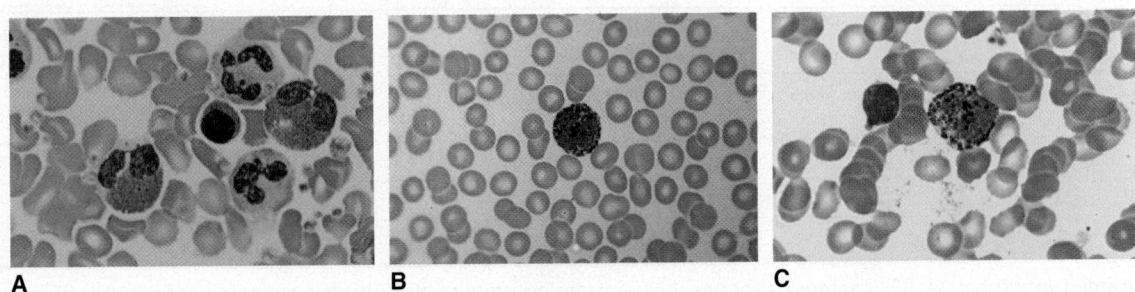

Figure 60–7. Images of granulocytes in blood films. **A.** Image shows two neutrophils, two eosinophils with bilobed nuclei, and a single neutrophil. **B** and **C.** The images are of basophils showing densely stained metachromatic cytoplasmic granules. *(Reproduced with permission from Lichtman's Atlas of Hematology. www.accessmedicine.com.)*

TABLE 60–1. Neutrophil Granules

Granules	Membrane Markers	NADPH Oxidase	Receptors	Antimicrobial	Enzymes	Other Factors
Primary (azurophilic)	CD63			BPI-protein	Elastase	Acid mucopoly-saccharide
	CD68			Defensins (HNP 1–4)	Cathepsin G	α_1-Antitrypsin
	V-type H$^+$-ATPase			CAP37	Proteinase 3	
				Myeloperoxidase	α-Mannosidase	
				Lysozyme	β-Glucuronidase	
					β-Glycerophos-phatase	
					Sialidase	
					N-Acetyl-β-glucosaminidase	
Secondary (specific)	CD15	gp91phox	Formyl peptide R	Lactoferrin	Gelatinase B (MMP-9)	β_2-Microglobulin
	CD66	p22phox	CR3 (CD11b/CD18)	Lysozyme	Histaminase	Vitamin B$_{12}$-binding protein
	CD67	Rap1A	Fibronectin R	hCAP-18	Sialidase	Plasminogen activator
	CD11b/CD18	Rap2	G-protein α-subunit		Collagenase (MMP-8)	
			Laminin R		Heparinase	NGAL (lipocalin)
			Thrombospon-din R			
			TNF R			
			uPAR			
			VAMP-2			
			Vitronectin R			
Tertiary	CD11b/CD18	gp91phox	Formyl peptide R	Lysozyme	Gelatinase B (MMP-9)	β_2-Microglobulin
	V-type H$^+$-ATPase	p22phox	CR3 (CD11b/CD18)		Acetyltransferase	Oncostatin M
		Rap1A	uPAR		Diacylglycerol-deacylating enzyme	
			VAMP-2			
Secretory vesicles	CD11b/CD18	gp91phox	Formyl peptide R	CAP37	Proteinase 3	Plasma proteins (e.g., albumin)
	CD10	p22phox	CR1 (CD35)			
	CD13	Rap1A	CR3 (CD11b/CD18)			Decay accelerat-ing factor
	CD45		CR4 (CD11c/CD18)			
	CD35		C1qR			
	CD14		FcγRIIIB (CD16)			
			uPAR			

ATPase, adenosine triphosphatase; BPI, bactericidal/permeability-increasing protein; hCAP, human cationic peptide; HNP, human neutrophil peptide; MMP-9, metalloproteinase-9; NGAL, neutrophil gelatinase-associated lipocalin; TNF, tumor necrosis factor; uPAR, urokinase plasmino-gen activator receptor, VAMP, vesicle-associated membrane protein.

Data regarding antimicrobial factors from Refs. 15 to 41. Data regarding enzymes from Refs. 42 to 56.

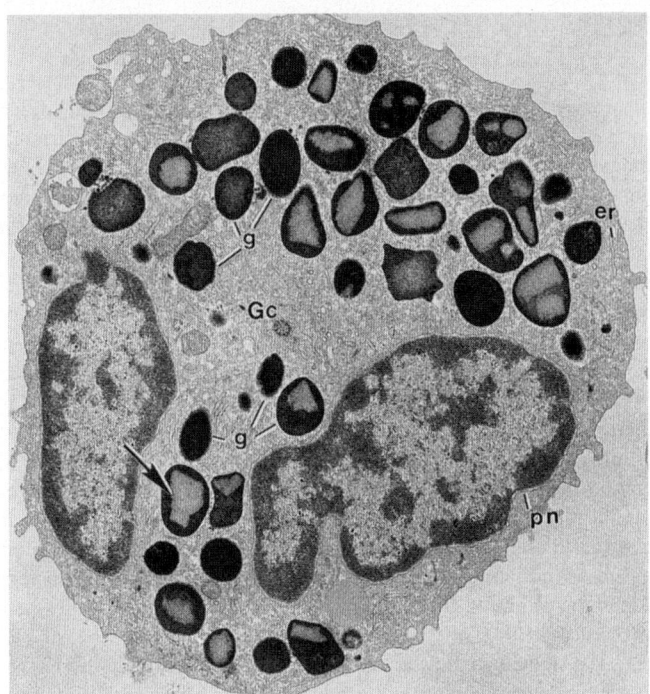

Figure 60–8. Human mature eosinophil incubated for peroxidase. Reaction product is present only in granules (g). The rough endoplasmic reticulum (er), including the perinuclear cisterna (pn) and the Golgi cisternae (Gc), does not contain reaction product. Most of the granules *(arrow)* contain the distinctive crystalline bar (×8000).

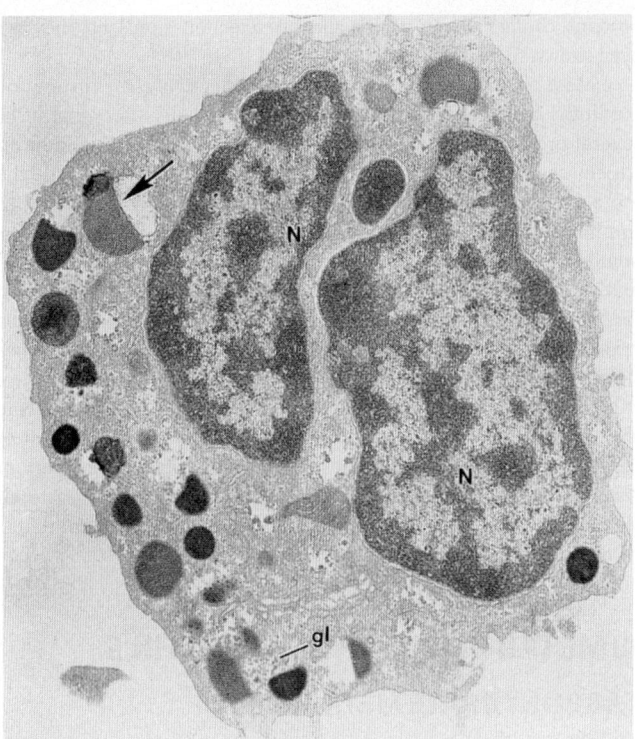

Figure 60–9. Mature basophil from human blood reacted for peroxidase. Note the unusually large nucleus (N) and scattered glycogen particles (gl). Human basophil granules contain peroxidase, as illustrated by their density (as a result of the presence of reaction product) in this type of preparation. They usually are spherical, difficult to fix, and may be speckled in appearance *(arrow)* (×17,000).

bactericidal hypohalous acids.[66,67] ECP is a bactericidal protein exists in two isoforms (ECP-1 and ECP-2) with activity toward helminthic parasites. EDN shares high sequence homology with ECP and is abundant, approximately 10 pg per cell. Other granule-stored proteins include several enzymes of potential importance in inflammation, including acid phosphatase, collagenase (MMP-8), matrix metalloproteases, histaminase, catalase, and phospholipase D.[68-70] Chapter 62 discusses the functional aspects of these granular proteins. In addition, mature eosinophils retain the ability to synthesize a diverse array of proteins including cytokines and chemokines,[71,72] adhesion molecules,[73-76] receptors for cytokines, complement components, lipid mediators, and immunoglobulins.[77-82]

BASOPHILS AND MAST CELLS

Basophils (see Fig. 60–7) and mast cells were considered to be derived from distinct lineages, but recent data indicates a common basophil-mast cell progenitor exists from which mast cells exit the marrow as immature precursors and terminally differentiate in tissues; basophils mature in the marrow before entering the circulation.[83-86] This common progenitor is derived from the granulocyte–monocyte progenitor. The granules of the two cell types stain metachromatically but are distinct when examined by electron microscopy (Figs. 60–9 and 60–10). Identification of basophils in tissue at the light microscopic level is difficult without the use of cell specific antibodies.[87] Basophils and mast cells express the FcεR1 receptor. The cells can phagocytose sensitized red cells but are less active phagocytes than the other granulocytes. They lack significant amounts of antibacterial or lysosomal enzymes. Basophils are found in small numbers in blood (0.5 percent) and can be seen in tissues in which inflammation resulting from hypersensitivity to

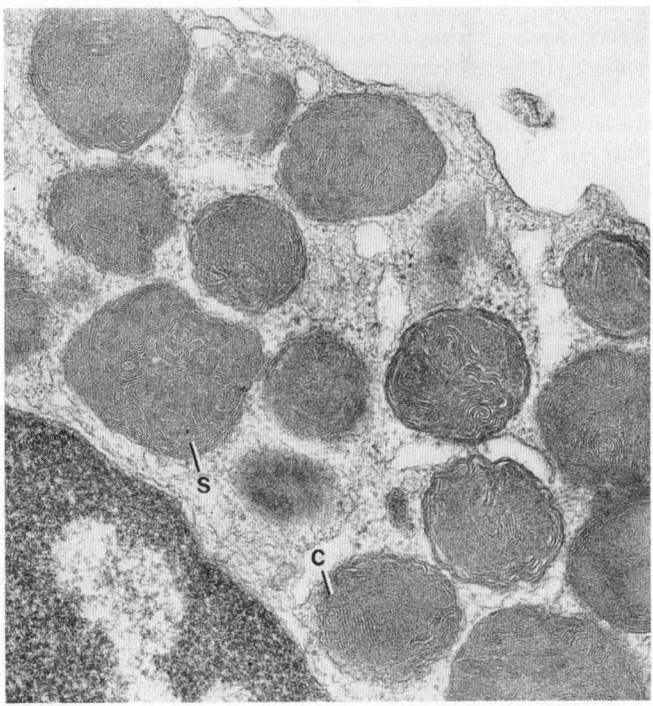

Figure 60–10. Portion of a mast cell from human marrow. Note the granules are filled with scroll-like (s) and crystal (c) images and are distinct from human basophil granules (see Fig. 60–9) in fine structural morphology (×50,000).

proteins, contact allergy, or skin allograft rejection is present. They have been shown to be rich sources of IL-4 and IL-13.[83,84,88]

Mast cells are normal residents of connective tissue throughout the body. Mast cell granules contain various substances, including several preformed biologically active substances such as histamine, which causes increased vascular permeability; eosinophil chemotactic factor of anaphylaxis; and heparin, which has antithrombin activity.[89-92] This accounts for the metachromatic staining quality of the granules. The generation of anaphylatoxin (C3a, C5a) or the interaction of allergen with immunoglobulin (Ig) E receptors of plasma membrane can stimulate extracellular release of these granule contents and of several newly formed substances, such as slow-reacting substance of anaphylaxis, a leukotriene that causes contraction of human bronchioles and increased vascular permeability, and platelet-activating factor (PAF), which causes platelet aggregation and the subsequent release of serotonin. This phenomenon is called IgE-mediated mast cell degranulation.[90] Mast cells also have been implicated in various diseases that are accompanied by neovascularization (Chap. 63).

● METABOLISM OF NEUTROPHILS

CARBOHYDRATE METABOLISM

Glycolysis

Glycolytic (Embden-Meyerhof) Pathway The main energy-producing pathway in the neutrophil is glycolysis, resulting in the conversion of glucose to lactate.[93-95] When intact or homogenized leukocytes are incubated with glucose uniformly labeled with ^{14}C, approximately 80 percent of the radioactivity is recovered in lactic acid. Glycolysis is inhibited by cortisol.[96,97] In some cases, the conditions under which the neutrophils are disrupted have a significant effect on the activities measured.[98] Hexokinase is the rate-limiting enzyme of glycolysis in normal neutrophils.[94] The rate of glycolysis is not altered during phagocytosis,[95] but ATP levels, normally 1.9 nmol/10^6 cells, fall to 0.8 nmol/10^6 cells. Both the glycogen stores of neutrophils and the glucose of the plasma can serve as the source of glucose. Galactose, mannose, and fructose can also be metabolized by leukocytes.[99] Table 60–2 shows the glycolytic and other principal enzymes of the neutrophil.

Hexose Monophosphate Shunt Pathway

Neutrophils also metabolize glucose by way of the hexose monophosphate shunt,[100-102] thus accounting for some of the oxygen consumption of the cells. In resting cells, the amount of glucose metabolized via this route amounts to only 2 to 3 percent of the total glucose consumed by the cell.[101-103] The operation of the hexose monophosphate shunt, however, is of special importance to the neutrophil, because this pathway provides the NADPH needed for generation of microbicidal oxidants.

Glycogen Metabolism

Neutrophils contain a large quantity of glycogen arising mostly from glucose. Little net synthesis from substrates occurs at the triose phosphate level. Glycogen turnover increases when these cells are deprived of glucose, especially if they are engaged in phagocytosis, but resynthesis occurs when adequate glucose is added.[95,104,105] During phagocytosis by glucose-starved cells, glycogen phosphorylase activity rises, but phosphorylase kinase and glycogen synthase levels remain unchanged.[105] Glycogen first appears in myelocytes and increases with cell maturation.[106]

PROTEIN SYNTHESIS BY MATURE NEUTROPHILS

Mature neutrophils have been classically viewed as terminally differentiated cells without the ability to synthesize proteins. This view has changed as a result of numerous investigations *in vitro* and *in vivo* showing that neutrophils can synthesize numerous proteins (e.g., cytokines, chemokines, growth factors, interferons) potentially important to the inflammatory process and the regulation of immune reactions. Table 60–3 lists some of the proteins expressed by mature neutrophils. The database for these observations has been extensively reviewed,[107,108] and some potentially important concepts are discussed here. As is evident from this list, the diversity is impressive, but the extent of production of each protein by individual neutrophils is limited when compared to mononuclear cells. However, because neutrophils make up the majority of infiltrating cells early in an acute inflammatory process, often emigrating in massive numbers, their aggregate synthetic ability may be significant to the course of the inflammatory or healing response. *In vitro*, an array of stimuli have been used to induce protein expression, including lipopolysaccharide (LPS), cytokines, chemotactic factors, adhesive ligands, opsonized particles, and modulatory cytokines such as IL-10 and IL-4.

The signaling pathways leading to new protein synthesis are subjects of extensive studies and are briefly described here. Granulocyte colony-stimulating factor (G-CSF), granulocyte-macrophage colony-stimulating factor (GM-CSF), and IL-10 have the ability to activate signal transducer and activator of transcription (STAT) proteins in neutrophils. Both STAT-1 and STAT-3 and the upstream kinase Janus-associated kinase 2 (JAK2) are rapidly tyrosine phosphorylated.[109,110] Neutrophils express nuclear factor κB-1 (NFκB1)/p50, p65/RelA, and c-Rel. Tumor necrosis factor-α (TNF-α), IL-1β, and IL-15 lead to the rapid loss of IκBα and the concomitant nuclear accumulation of NFκB/Rel proteins. This pathway is not activated by G-CSF, GM-CSF, IL-8, or IL-10. PU.1 is expressed in mature neutrophils and constitutively binds DNA, and the AP-1 transcription factor is evident. Several of the inflammatory mediators produced by mature neutrophils are AP-1 driven (e.g., TNF, IL-1, IL-8, intercellular adhesion molecule [ICAM]).[68] Production of the CXC chemokine IL-8 by neutrophils has been extensively studied, and a wide range of stimuli can induce its expression.[111] Cytokines such as TNF-α, IL-15, IL-1β, and GM-CSF; chemotactic factors such as C5a, PAF, and leukotriene B$_4$ (LTB$_4$); particles such as monosodium urate crystals; microbial products such as LPS and zymosan; interaction with antibody and complement opsonized bacteria and yeasts; and interactions with extracellular matrix molecules such as laminin and fibronectin, all have been shown to induce synthesis of IL-8 by neutrophils. In most studies, release of significant amounts of protein from the neutrophils and synthesis of mRNA have been demonstrated. Immunocytochemistry and *in situ* hybridization studies have provided evidence of IL-8 production in neutrophils infiltrating inflammatory sites.

Some of the stimuli that induce expression of IL-8 also stimulate production by mature neutrophils of other proinflammatory agents, such as growth-regulated protein (GRO)-α, TNF-α, IL-1β, oncostatin M, and C-C chemokines. In addition, neutrophils may produce antiinflammatory agents such as IL-1RA and transforming growth factor (TGF)-β, and of interest is the observation that cytokines such as IL-10 may have some selectivity with regard to induction of antiinflammatory factors in neutrophils. Thus, considerable evidence exists for protein synthesis capability in neutrophils, but because this field of study is relatively new, much work remains to define the importance of the various proteins to inflammation, immune reactions and healing, the selectivity of the conditions, and disease states linked to the synthetic activities of neutrophils. In keeping with its critical role in the inflammatory

TABLE 60-2. Glycolytic and Related Enzyme Activities in Neutrophils

Enzyme	Activity at 37°C in Neutrophils*	Activity at 30°C in Neutrophils†	Activity at 25°C in Mixed Leukocytes‡
Hexokinase	78 ± 14	39.6 ± 27.3	—
Phosphofructokinase	36 ±2	—	—
Aldolase	76 ± 7	118.7 ± 27.4	123
Glucosephosphate isomerase	4930 ± 716	—	—
Triosephosphate isomerase	7853 ± 323	—	2189
Glyceraldehyde dehydrogenase	3683 ± 124	—	242
Monophosphoglycerate mutase	508 ± 35	—	—
Phosphoglycerate kinase	3744 ± 197	—	890
Enolase	136 ± 17	—	734
Pyruvate kinase	173 ± 11	4125 ± 549	976
Lactate dehydrogenase	1128 ± 51	2981 ± 893	1165
Glucose-6-phosphate dehydrogenase	517 ± 11	596 ± 116.6	176
6-Phosphogluconate dehydrogenase	287 ± 5	—	—
Glutathione reductase	63 ± 7	—	—
Glutathione peroxidase	17 ± 3	—	—
Glutamic oxaloacetic transaminase	25 ± 2	—	43
Adenylate kinase	32 ± 2	163 ± 9.9	149
α-Glycerophosphate dehydrogenase	—	—	23
Isocitric dehydrogenase	—	—	47
Fructose 1,6-diphosphatase	—	0.76 ± 0.18	—
Isocitrate dehydrogenase	—	44.1 ± 6.4	—
Citrate synthase	—	32.0 ± 5.4	—
Malate dehydrogenase	—	482 ± 62.6	—
Transketolase	—	0.99 ± 0.27	—
Phosphorylase A	—	9.60 ± 2.66	—
Lipoamide dehydrogenase	—	29.7 ± 13.8	—
Ca^{2+} ATPase	—	—	28
Mg^{2+} ATPase	—	—	30

ATPase, adenosine triphosphatase.

*IU/mg protein. †IU/L. ‡Calculated as units/10^{11} leukocytes, assuming a protein content of 7.4 mg/10^{11} leukocytes.

TABLE 60-3. Proteins Synthesized by Neutrophils

Cytokines	Receptors	Chemokines	Growth Factors	Miscellaneous
TNF-α	IL-1 receptor antagonist (IL-1RA)	IL-8	G-CSF	Fas ligand
IL-1β		GRO-α	M-CSF	CD40
IL-12	TGF-β	GRO-β	GM-CSF	CD83
IFN-α		IP-10	IL-3	CCR6
IL-6		MIP-1α	VEGF	CCR2
Oncostatin M		MIP-1β	TGF-β	HLA-DR
		MCP-1		

CCR, C-C chemokine receptor; CD, cluster of differentiation; G-CSF, granulocyte colony-stimulating factor; GM-CSF, granulocyte-monocyte colony-stimulating factor; GRO, growth-related oncogene; HLA-DR, human leukocyte antigen-D–related; IFN, interferon; IL, interleukin; IP, interferon-inducible protein; MCP, membrane cofactor protein; M-CSF, monocyte colony-stimulating factor; MIP, macrophage inflammatory protein; TGF, transforming growth factor; TNF, tumor necrosis factor; VEGF, vascular endothelial growth factor.

TABLE 60–4. Neutrophil Adhesion Molecules

Neutrophil Receptor	Classification	Ligands
L-selectin (CD62L)	Selectin family	PSGL-1, E-selectin
PSGL-1 (CD162)	Mucin family	E-selectin, P-selectin
sLe^x glycoproteins	Various glycoproteins	E-selectin
LFA-1 (CD11a/CD18)	$\alpha_L\beta_2$-Integrin	ICAM-1, ICAM-3
Mac-1 (CD11b/CD18)	$\alpha_M\beta_2$-Integrin	ICAM-1, GPIbα, factor X, fibrinogen, iC3b
CR4 (CD11c/CD18)	$\alpha_X\beta_2$-Integrin	Fibrinogen, iC3b
VLA-2 (CD49b/CD29)	$\alpha_2\beta_1$-Integrin	Collagen, laminin
VLA-3 (CD49c/CD29)	$\alpha_3\beta_1$-Integrin	Collagen, laminin, fibronectin, tenascin
VLA-4 (CD49d/CD29)	$\alpha_4\beta_1$-Integrin	VCAM-1, fibronectin
VLA-5 (CD49e/CD29)	$\alpha_5\beta_1$-Integrin	Fibronectin
VLA-6 (CD49f/CD29)	$\alpha_6\beta_1$-Integrin	Laminin
VLA-9	$\alpha_9\beta_1$-Integrin	VCAM-1, tenascin
$\alpha_v\beta_3$ (CD51/CD61)	β_3-Integrin	Vitronectin

GPIbα, glycoprotein Ibα; ICAM, intercellular adhesion molecule; LFA, leukocyte function-associated antigen; PSGL, P-selectin glycoprotein ligand; sLe^x, sialyl Lewis X; VCAM-1, vascular cell adhesion molecule-1; VLA, very-late antigen.

TABLE 60–5. Chemotactic Receptors on Human Neutrophils

Receptor	Ligands
Formyl peptide receptor (FPR) (high affinity)	f-met-leu-phe (fMLP), other f-met peptides of bacterial origin
Formyl peptide receptor-like 1 (FPRL-1) (low affinity)	f-met peptides, LXA$_4$, SAA, HIV envelope domains
C5aR (high affinity)	C5a complement fragment
CXCR1 (high affinity)	IL-8 (CXCL8)
CXCR2 (high affinity)	GRO-α (CXCL1), GRO-β (CXCL2), ENA-78 (CXCL5)
CXCR4 in marrow (high affinity)	SDF-1α (CXCL12)
CCR2 (induced; high affinity)	MCP-1 (CCL2)
CCR6 (induced; high affinity)	LARC (CCL20), β-defensin
Platelet-activating factor R (low and high affinity)	Platelet-activating factor
BLT1 (high affinity)	LTB$_4$
BLT2 (low affinity)	LTB$_4$, other eicosanoids

CCR, C-C chemokine receptor; CXCR, chemokine-related receptor; GRO, growth-regulated protein; IL, interleukin; LTB$_4$, leukotriene B$_4$; MCP, monocyte chemoattractant protein; SDF, stromal cell-derived factor.

process, the neutrophil's movement from blood to tissues requires surface adhesion molecules (Table 60–4), chemotactic receptors (Table 60–5), and the requirement to phagocytize microorganisms through opsonin receptors (Table 60–6).

PHENOTYPIC CHANGES

Phenotypic changes occur in neutrophils under specific conditions.[112,113] Degranulation results in marked changes in surface expression of an array of proteins arriving at the surface from the storage pools of granules (e.g., CD11b/CD18, CD66, some β_1-integrins). These phenomena can be seen in degrees in circulating neutrophils. Exposure of neutrophils to activating factors results in surface and functional changes as a result of new synthesis (e.g., Fc region of IgG [FcγR]I following elevations in interferon [IFN]-γ) or shedding (e.g., loss of L-selectin), also seen in circulating neutrophils. Cytokines (e.g., IL-15, IL-1, TNF) induce *de novo* synthesis of proteins (as noted in Table 60–1) to various degrees in blood neutrophils. Substantial changes occur once the neutrophil leaves the vasculature, increasing its expression of β_1-integrins, C-C chemokine receptors (CCRs), and protein synthesis.

Evidence indicates that in response to specific combinations of cytokines (e.g., GM-CSF, TNF-α, IFN-γ), neutrophils can acquire phenotypic and functional characteristics of immature dendritic antigen-presenting cells.[112] Thus, any consideration of the "composition" of neutrophils requires a detailed understanding of the stage of development and the environment to which the neutrophil is exposed *in vivo*. The neutrophil is a remarkably versatile cell.

TABLE 60–6. Opsonic Receptors on Neutrophils

Receptor	Characteristics	Ligand
FcγRI (CD64)	72 kDa, transmembrane, induced by IFN-γ	IgG$_1$, high affinity
FcγRIIA (CD32)	40 kDa, transmembrane, constitutive, A isoform associates with CR3	IgG$_3$ > IgG$_1$, low affinity, binds polymeric IgG
FcγRIIIB (CD16)	50 kDa, GPI-linked, constitutive, associates with CR3	IgG$_1$, low affinity, binds polymeric IgG
FcαR (CD89)	60 kDa, transmembrane, constitutive	IgA, polymeric (e.g., sIgA)
CR1 (CD35)	160–250 kDa, transmembrane, constitutive	C3b, C4b
CR3 (CD11b/CD18)	165/90 kDa, transmembrane, heterodimer, storage pool in granules	iC3b
CR4 (CD11c/CD18)	145/90 kDa transmembrane, heterodimer	iC3b

CR, complement receptor; FcγR, Fc region of IgG; GPI, glycosyl phosphatidylinositol; IFN, interferon; Ig, immunoglobulin; sIgA, secretory immunoglobulin A.

Gene expression profiling has provided rich insights into the capacity of the mature neutrophil to change in response to environmental stimuli. Following exposure to 10 ng/mL *Escherichia coli* LPS, 307 genes are activated or repressed.[114] These changes include transcription factors, cytokines, chemokines, interleukins, surface antigens, toll-like receptors, and members of immune mediator gene families. Major changes in gene expression occur following LPS,[115] migration in wounds,[116] activation by phagocytosis,[117] or during the processes of apoptosis.[118] These findings indicate that the neutrophil is a transcriptionally active cell responsive to environmental stimuli and capable of a complex series of both early and late changes in gene expression.

● OTHER BIOCHEMICAL FEATURES OF NEUTROPHILS.

The neutrophil is particularly rich in glycogen. The concentration of this complex polysaccharide has been reported to average 7.36 mg/10^9 cells.[119-121] The rate of glucose metabolism by neutrophils is affected by insulin in diabetics but not in normal subjects.[122,123] Inflammatory activation of normal neutrophils stimulates glucose uptake. The plasma membrane and the membranes of the intracellular organelles are rich in lipids. Five percent of the wet weight of neutrophils is lipid, which is distributed among various classes, as shown in Table 60–7.[124,125] The rare polyphosphoinositides are of special interest as sources of inositol 1,4,5-trisphosphate (a calcium-releasing mediator) and diacylglycerol (which activates protein kinase C).[126,127] The main glycolipid of neutrophils is lactosylceramide.[128]

The reduced glutathione content of neutrophils is 9.8 nmol/10^7 cells.[129] The protein content of the neutrophil is 74.2 ± 3.1 (mean ± 1 SE [standard error]) mg/10^9 cells. These proteins include those of the structural matrix of the neutrophil; proteins required for its locomotion, chemotactic properties, and adhesiveness; and the many granule proteins with bactericidal, hydrolytic, and inflammatory functions. Table 60–8 summarizes the unbound amino acid concentration in neutrophils.

Table 60–9 summarizes the levels of nucleotides in the neutrophils.[130,131] Neutrophils contain all the forms of RNA needed for protein synthesis.[132,133] The DNA content of neutrophils is identical to that of all other haploid cells, at 0.7 pg DNA phosphorus per cell.[134]

TABLE 60–8. Unbound Amino Acid Concentrations in Leukocytes (Lymphocytes Included)

Amino Acid	μmol/kg Water*
Alanine	2881 ± 256
Arginine	<290
Ergothioneine	<300
Ethanolamine	<250
Glutamic acid	2745 ± 251
Glutamine	2650 ± 251
Histidine	762 ± 70
Leucine plus isoleucine	1999 ± 195
Lysine	2111 ± 216
Methionine	391 ± 54
O-phosphoethanolamine	2651 ± 389
Ornithine	1767 ± 113
Phenylalanine	647 ± 105
Proline	862 ± 79
Serine plus glycine	13,021 ± 1480
Taurine	28,683 ± 2726
Threonine	2345 ± 174
Tryptophan	222 ± 31
Tyrosine	480 ± 97
Valine	1335 ± 132

*Mean ± 1 SD.

The average folic acid content of the leukocytes of normal subjects is 0.1 mcg/mL of packed leukocytes. Approximately 20 percent of the folic acid is free and the remainder conjugated. The cocarboxylate content of neutrophils is 340 mcg/10^{11} cells,[135] pyridoxal phosphate 0.24 to 0.38 ng/10^6 cells,[136] thiamine 67.5 ± 4.1 mcg/100 mL,[137] ascorbic acid 16.5 ± 5.1 mg/100 mL,[137] and folate 92 ng/mL.[138]

TABLE 60–7. Lipid Composition of Neutrophils

Lipid	Content (%)
Phospholipid	35
Phosphatidylcholine	12
Phosphatidylethanolamine	12
Sphingomyelin	6.5
Phosphatidylserine	1.5
Phosphatidylinositol	1.5
Phosphatidic acid	1.5
Triglyceride	20
Glycolipid	16
Cholesterol	10

Data from DiScipio RG, Schraufstatter I U: The role of the complement anaphylatoxins in the recruitment of eosinophils. *Int Immunopharmacol* 7:1909, 2007 and Sullivan BM, Locksley RM: Basophils: a nonredundant contributor to host immunity. *Immunity* 30:12, 2009.

TABLE 60–9. Nucleotides in Leukocytes (Lymphocytes Included)

Nucleotide	nmol/10^9 Cells (Mean ± SE)
NAD (nicotinamide adenine dinucleotide)	32 ± 2.0
NADH (reduced form of nicotinamide adenine dinucleotide)	25 ± 2.3
NADP (nicotinamide adenine dinucleotide phosphate)	8 ± 1.5
NADPH (reduced form of nicotinamide adenine dinucleotide phosphate)	24 ± 39
ATP	8800
ADP (adenosine diphosphate)	1600
AMP (adenosine monophosphate)	6100

REFERENCES

1. Bainton DF, Farquhar MG: Origin of granules in polymorphonuclear leukocytes. Two types derived from opposite faces of the Golgi complex in developing granulocytes. *J Cell Biol* 28:277, 1966.
2. Bainton DF, Ullyot JL, Farquhar MG: The development of neutrophilic polymorphonuclear leukocytes in human bone marrow. *J Exp Med* 134:907, 1971.
3. Bainton DF: Distinct granule populations in human neutrophils and lysosomal organelles identified by immuno-electron microscopy. *J Immunol Methods* 232:153, 1999.
4. Bainton DF, Farquhar MG: Segregation and packaging of granule enzymes in eosinophilic leukocytes. *J Cell Biol* 45:54, 1970.
5. Pryzwansky KB, Breton-Gorius J: Identification of a subpopulation of primary granules in human neutrophils based upon maturation and distribution. Study by transmission electron microscopy cytochemistry and high voltage electron microscopy of whole cell preparations. *Lab Invest* 53:664, 1985.
6. Aquiles SJ, Karni RJ, Wangh LJ: Fluorescent in situ hybridization (FISH) analysis of the relationship between chromosome location and nuclear morphology in human neutrophils. *Chromosoma* 106:168, 1997.
7. Borregaard N, Sorensen OE, Theilgaard-Monch K: Neutrophil granules: A library of innate immunity proteins. *Trends Immunol* 28:340, 2007.
8. Gombart AF, Kwok SH, Anderson KL, et al: Regulation of neutrophil and eosinophil secondary granule gene expression by transcription factors C/EBP epsilon and PU.1. *Blood* 101:3265, 2003.
9. Lekstrom-Himes JA: The role of C/EBP(epsilon) in the terminal stages of granulocyte differentiation. *Stem Cells*, 19:125, 2001.
10. Shiohara M, Gombart AF, Sekiguchi Y, et al: Phenotypic and functional alterations of peripheral blood monocytes in neutrophil-specific granule deficiency. *J Leukoc Biol* 75:190, 2004.
11. Lekstrom-Himes JA, Dorman SE, Kopar P, et al: Neutrophil-specific granule deficiency results from a novel mutation with loss of function of the transcription factor CCAAT/enhancer binding protein epsilon. *J Exp Med* 189:1847, 1999.
12. Gallin JI: Neutrophil specific granule deficiency. *Annu Rev Med* 36:263, 1985.
13. Brumell JH, Volchuk A, Sengelov H, et al: Subcellular distribution of docking/fusion proteins in neutrophils, secretory cells with multiple exocytic compartments. *J Immunol* 155:5750, 1995.
14. Mollinedo F, Calafat J, Janssen H, et al: Combinatorial SNARE complexes modulate the secretion of cytoplasmic granules in human neutrophils. *J Immunol* 177:2831, 2006.
15. Soehnlein O, Lindbom L: Neutrophil-derived azurocidin alarms the immune system. *J Leukoc Biol* 85:344, 2009.
16. Dalli J, Norling LV, Renshaw D, et al: Annexin 1 mediates the rapid anti-inflammatory effects of neutrophil-derived microparticles. *Blood* 112:2512, 2008.
17. Cocucci E, Racchetti G, Meldolesi J: Shedding microvesicles: Artefacts no more. *Trends Cell Biol* 19:43, 2009.
18. Rocha-Pereira P, Santos-Silva A, Rebelo I, et al: The inflammatory response in mild and in severe psoriasis. *Br J Dermatol* 150:917, 2004.
19. Levy O: Impaired innate immunity at birth: Deficiency of bactericidal/permeability-increasing protein (BPI) in the neutrophils of newborns. *Pediatr Res* 51:667, 2002.
20. Nupponen I, Turunen R, Nevalainen T, et al: Extracellular release of bactericidal/permeability-increasing protein in newborn infants. *Pediatr Res* 51:670, 2002.
21. Schultz H, Weiss J, Carroll SF, et al: The endotoxin-binding bactericidal/permeability-increasing protein (BPI): A target antigen of autoantibodies. *J Leukoc Biol* 69:505, 2001.
22. Watorek W: Azurocidin—Inactive serine proteinase homolog acting as a multifunctional inflammatory mediator. *Acta Biochim Pol* 50:743, 2003.
23. Gonzalez ML, Ruan X, Kumar P, et al: Functional modulation of smooth muscle cells by the inflammatory mediator CAP37. *Microvasc Res* 67:168, 2004.
24. Lee TD, Gonzalez ML, Kumar P, et al: CAP37, a neutrophil-derived inflammatory mediator, augments leukocyte adhesion to endothelial monolayers. *Microvasc Res* 66:38, 2003.
25. Tapper H, Karlsson A, Morgelin M, et al: Secretion of heparin-binding protein from human neutrophils is determined by its localization in azurophilic granules and secretory vesicles. *Blood* 99:1785, 2002.
26. Gray PW, Flaggs G, Leong SR, et al: Cloning of the cDNA of a human neutrophil bactericidal protein. Structural and functional correlations. *J Biol Chem* 264:9505, 1989.
27. Boman HG: Antibacterial peptides: Basic facts and emerging concepts. *J Intern Med* 254:197, 2003.
28. Niyonsaba F, Ogawa H, Nagaoka I: Human beta-defensin-2 functions as a chemotactic agent for tumour necrosis factor-alpha-treated human neutrophils. *Immunology* 111:273, 2004.
29. Oppenheim JJ, Biragyn A, Kwak LW, et al: Roles of antimicrobial peptides such as defensins in innate and adaptive immunity. *Ann Rheum Dis* 62 Suppl 2:ii17, 2003.
30. Nizet V, Gallo RL: Cathelicidins and innate defense against invasive bacterial infection. *Scand J Infect Dis* 35:670, 2003.
31. Zanetti M: Cathelicidins, multifunctional peptides of the innate immunity. *J Leukoc Biol* 75:39, 2004.
32. Murakami M, Lopez-Garcia B, Braff M, et al: Postsecretory processing generates multiple cathelicidins for enhanced topical antimicrobial defense. *J Immunol* 172:3070, 2004.
33. Elssner A, Duncan M, Gavrilin M, et al: A novel P2X7 receptor activator, the human cathelicidin-derived peptide LL37, induces IL-1 beta processing and release. *J Immunol* 172:4987, 2004.
34. Davidson DJ, Currie AJ, Reid GS, et al: The cationic antimicrobial peptide LL-37 modulates dendritic cell differentiation and dendritic cell-induced T cell polarization. *J Immunol* 172:1146, 2004.
35. Ibrahim HR, Aoki T, Pellegrini A: Strategies for new antimicrobial proteins and peptides: Lysozyme and aprotinin as model molecules. *Curr Pharm Des* 8:671, 2002.
36. Ganz T, Gabayan V, Liao HI, et al: Increased inflammation in lysozyme M-deficient mice in response to *Micrococcus luteus* and its peptidoglycan. *Blood* 101:2388, 2003.
37. Ganz T: Antimicrobial polypeptides. *J Leukoc Biol* 75:34, 2004.
38. Quinn MT, Gauss KA: Structure and regulation of the neutrophil respiratory burst oxidase: Comparison with nonphagocyte oxidases. *J Leukoc Biol* 76:760, 2004.
39. Klebanoff SJ: Myeloperoxidase. *Proc Assoc Am Physicians* 111:383, 1999.
40. Hampton MB, Kettle AJ, Winterbourn CC: Inside the neutrophil phagosome: Oxidants, myeloperoxidase, and bacterial killing. *Blood* 92:3007, 1998.
41. Wheeler MA, Smith SD, Garcia-Cardena G, et al: Bacterial infection induces nitric oxide synthase in human neutrophils. *J Clin Invest* 99:110, 1997.
42. Pham CT: Neutrophil serine proteases fine-tune the inflammatory response. *Int J Biochem Cell Biol* 40:1317, 2008.
43. Kawabata K, Hagio T, Matsuoka S: The role of neutrophil elastase in acute lung injury. *Eur J Pharmacol* 451:1, 2002.
44. Aprikyan AA, Liles WC, Boxer LA, et al: Mutant elastase in pathogenesis of cyclic and severe congenital neutropenia. *J Pediatr Hematol Oncol* 24:784, 2002.
45. Horwitz M, Benson KF, Duan Z, et al: Role of neutrophil elastase in bone marrow failure syndromes: Molecular genetic revival of the chalone hypothesis. *Curr Opin Hematol* 10:49, 2003.
46. Belaaouaj A: Neutrophil elastase-mediated killing of bacteria: Lessons from targeted mutagenesis. *Microbes Infect* 4:1259, 2002.
47. Hirche TO, Atkinson JJ, Bahr S, et al: Deficiency in neutrophil elastase does not impair neutrophil recruitment to inflamed sites. *Am J Respir Cell Mol Biol* 30:576, 2004.
48. Sennstrom MB, Brauner A, Bystrom B, et al: Matrix metalloproteinase-8 correlates with the cervical ripening process in humans. *Acta Obstet Gynecol Scand* 82:904, 2003.
49. Balbin M, Fueyo A, Tester AM, et al: Loss of collagenase-2 confers increased skin tumor susceptibility to male mice. *Nat Genet* 35:252, 2003.
50. Opdenakker G, Van den Steen PE, Dubois B, et al: Gelatinase B functions as regulator and effector in leukocyte biology. *J Leukoc Biol* 69:851, 2001.
51. Schonbeck U, Mach F, Libby P: Generation of biologically active IL-1 beta by matrix metalloproteinases: A novel caspase-1-independent pathway of IL-1 beta processing. *J Immunol* 161:3340, 1998.
52. Peppin GJ, Weiss SJ: Activation of the endogenous metalloproteinase, gelatinase, by triggered human neutrophils. *Proc Natl Acad Sci U S A* 83:4322, 1986.
53. Ogata Y, Enghild JJ, Nagase H: Matrix metalloproteinase 3 (stromelysin) activates the precursor for the human matrix metalloproteinase 9. *J Biol Chem* 267:3581, 1992.
54. Van den Steen PE, Husson SJ, Proost P, et al: Carboxyterminal cleavage of the chemokines MIG and IP-10 by gelatinase B, neutrophil collagenase. *Biochem Biophys Res Commun* 310:889, 2003.
55. Van den Steen PE, Wuyts A, Husson SJ, et al: Gelatinase B/MMP-9 and neutrophil collagenase/MMP-8 process the chemokines human GCP-2/CXCL6, ENA-78/CXCL5 and mouse GCP-2/LIX and modulate their physiological activities. *Eur J Biochem* 270:3739, 2003.
56. Pelus LM, Bian H, King AG, et al: Neutrophil-derived MMP-9 mediates synergistic mobilization of hematopoietic stem and progenitor cells by the combination of G-CSF and the chemokines GRObeta/CXCL2 and GRObetaT/CXCL2delta4. *Blood* 103:110, 2004.
57. Mori Y, Iwasaki H, Kohno K, et al: Identification of the human eosinophil lineage-committed progenitor: revision of phenotypic definition of the human common myeloid progenitor. *J Exp Med* 206:183, 2009.
58. Bainton DF: Developmental biology of neutrophils and eosinophils, in *Inflammation: Basic Principles and Clinical Correlates*, 2nd ed, edited by Gallin JI, Goldstein R, Snyderman R, p13. Raven Press, New York, 1992.
59. Hogan SP, Rosenberg HF, Moqbel R, et al: Eosinophils: Biological properties and role in health and disease. *Clin Exp Allergy* 38:709, 2008.
60. Gleich GJ, Loegering DA, Maldonado JE: Identification of a major basic protein in guinea pig eosinophil granules. *J Exp Med* 137:1459, 1973.
61. Melo RC, Spencer LA, Perez SA, et al: Vesicle-mediated secretion of human eosinophil granule-derived major basic protein. *Lab Invest* 2009.
62. Calafat J, Janssen H, Knol EF, et al: Ultrastructural localization of Charcot-Leyden crystal protein in human eosinophils and basophils. *Eur J Haematol* 58:56, 1997.
63. Dvorak AM, Ackerman SJ, Weller PF: Subcellular morphological and biochemistry of eosinophils, in *Blood Cell Biochemistry, Megakaryocytes, Platelets, Macrophages, and Eosinophils*, vol 2, edited by Harris JR. Plenum Press, New York, 1990.
64. Dvorak AM, Letourneau L, Login GR, et al: Ultrastructural localization of the Charcot-Leyden crystal protein (lysophospholipase) to a distinct crystalloid-free granule population in mature human eosinophils. *Blood* 72:150, 1988.
65. Popken-Harris P, Checkel J, Loegering D, et al: Regulation and processing of a precursor form of eosinophil granule major basic protein (ProMBP) in differentiating eosinophils. *Blood* 92:623, 1998.
66. Ten RM, Pease LR, McKean DJ, et al: Molecular cloning of the human eosinophil peroxidase. Evidence for the existence of a peroxidase multigene family. *J Exp Med* 169:1757, 1989.
67. Weiss SJ, Test ST, Eckmann CM, et al: Brominating oxidants generated by human eosinophils. *Science* 234:200, 1986.

68. Ohno I, Ohtani H, Nitta Y, et al: Eosinophils as a source of matrix metalloproteinase-9 in asthmatic airway inflammation. *Am J Respir Cell Mol Biol* 16:212, 1997.

69. Gauthier MC, Racine C, Ferland C, et al: Expression of membrane type-4 matrix metalloproteinase (metalloproteinase-17) by human eosinophils. *Int J Biochem Cell Biol* 35:1667, 2003.

70. Wiehler S, Cuvelier SL, Chakrabarti S, Patel KD: p38 MAP kinase regulates rapid matrix metalloproteinase-9 release from eosinophils. *Biochem Biophys Res Commun* 315:463, 2004.

71. Lacy P, Moqbel R: Eosinophil cytokines. *Chem Immunol* 76:134, 2000.

72. Moqbel R, Lacy P: Eosinophil cytokines, in *Inflammatory Mechanisms in Asthma*, edited by Busse WW, Holgate ST, pp 227–246. Marcel Dekker, New York, 1998.

73. Georas SN, McIntyre BW, Ebisawa M, et al: Expression of a functional laminin receptor (alpha 6 beta 1, very late activation antigen-6) on human eosinophils. *Blood* 82:2872, 1993.

74. Grayson MH, Van der Vieren M, Sterbinsky SA, et al: alphadbeta2 integrin is expressed on human eosinophils and functions as an alternative ligand for vascular cell adhesion molecule 1 (VCAM-1). *J Exp Med* 188:2187, 1998.

75. Tachimoto H, Bochner BS: The surface phenotype of human eosinophils. *Chem Immunol* 76:45, 2000.

76. Bochner BS, Busse WW: Allergy and asthma. *J Allergy Clin Immunol* 115:953, 2005.

77. Phillips RM, Stubbs VE, Henson MR, et al: Variations in eosinophil chemokine responses: An investigation of CCR1 and CCR3 function, expression in atopy, and identification of a functional CCR1 promoter. *J Immunol* 170:6190, 2003.

78. Elsner J, Dulkys Y, Gupta S, et al: Differential pattern of CCR1 internalization in human eosinophils: Prolonged internalization by CCL5 in contrast to CCL3. *Allergy* 60:1386, 2005.

79. Ponath PD, Qin S, Post TW, et al: Molecular cloning and characterization of a human eotaxin receptor expressed selectively on eosinophils. *J Exp Med* 183:2437, 1996.

80. Lee JH, Chang HS, Kim JH, et al: Genetic effect of CCR3 and IL5RA gene polymorphisms on eosinophilia in asthmatic patients. *J Allergy Clin Immunol* 120:1110, 2007.

81. Takatsu K, Kouro T, Nagai Y: Interleukin 5 in the link between the innate and acquired immune response. *Adv Immunol* 101:191, 2009.

82. DiScipio RG, Schraufstatter IU: The role of the complement anaphylatoxins in the recruitment of eosinophils. *Int Immunopharmacol* 7:1909, 2007.

83. Sullivan BM, Locksley RM: Basophils: A nonredundant contributor to host immunity. *Immunity* 30:12, 2009.

84. Gurish MF, Boyce JA: Mast cells: Ontogeny, homing, and recruitment of a unique innate effector cell. *J Allergy Clin Immunol* 117:1285, 2006.

85. Arinobu Y, Iwasaki H, Gurish MF, et al: Developmental checkpoints of the basophil/mast cell lineages in adult murine hematopoiesis. *Proc Natl Acad Sci U S A* 102:18105, 2005.

86. Arinobu Y, Iwasaki H, Akashi K: Origin of basophils and mast cells. *Allergol Int* 58:21, 2009.

87. Falcone FH, Haas H, Gibbs BF: The human basophil: A new appreciation of its role in immune responses. *Blood* 96:4028, 2000.

88. Gessner A, Mohrs K, Mohrs M: Mast cells, basophils, and eosinophils acquire constitutive IL-4 and IL-13 transcripts during lineage differentiation that are sufficient for rapid cytokine production. *J Immunol* 174:1063, 2005.

89. Siracusa MC, Wojno ED, Artis D: Functional heterogeneity in the basophil cell lineage 1. *Adv Immunol* 115:141, 2012.

90. Wedemeyer J, Tsai M, Galli SJ: Roles of mast cells and basophils in innate and acquired immunity. *Curr Opin Immunol* 12:624, 2000.

91. Marone G, Galli SJ, Kitamura Y: Probing the roles of mast cells and basophils in natural and acquired immunity, physiology and disease. *Trends Immunol* 23:425, 2002.

92. Dvorak AM: Histamine content and secretion in basophils and mast cells. *Prog Histochem Cytochem* 33:III, 1998.

93. Beck WS, Valentine WN: The aerobic carbohydrate metabolism of leukocytes in health and leukemia. I. Glycolysis and respiration. *Cancer Res* 12:818, 1952.

94. Beck WS: A kinetic analysis of the glycolytic rate and certain glycolytic enzymes in normal and leucemic leucocytes. *J Biol Chem* 216:333, 1955.

95. Borregaard N, Herlin T: Energy metabolism of human neutrophils during phagocytosis. *J Clin Invest* 70:550, 1982.

96. Lane TA, Beutler E, West C, Lamkin G: Glycolytic enzymes of stored granulocytes. *Transfusion* 24:153, 1984.

97. Fauth U, Schlechtriemen T, Heinrichs W, et al: The measurement of enzyme activities in the resting human polymorphonuclear leukocyte—Critical estimate of a method. *Eur J Clin Chem Clin Biochem* 31:5, 1993.

98. McKinney GR, Martin SP, Rundles RW, Green R: Respiratory and glycolytic activities of human leukocytes in vitro. *J Appl Physiol* 5:335, 1953.

99. Stjernholm RL, Burns CP, Hohnadel JH: Carbohydrate metabolism by leukocytes. *Enzyme* 13:7, 1972.

100. Sbarra AJ, Karnovsky ML: The biochemical basis of phagocytosis. I. Metabolic changes during the ingestion of particles by polymorphonuclear leukocytes. *J Biol Chem* 234:1355, 1959.

101. Beck WS: Occurrence and control of the phosphogluconate oxidation pathway in normal and leukemic leukocytes. *J Biol Chem* 232:271, 1958.

102. Stjernholm RL, Manak RC: Carbohydrate metabolism in leukocytes. XIV. Regulation of pentose cycle activity and glycogen metabolism during phagocytosis. *J Reticuloendothel Soc* 8:550, 1970.

103. Wood HG, Katz J, Landau BR: Estimation of pathways of carbohydrate metabolism. *Biochem Z* 338:809, 1963.

104. Scott RB: Glycogen in human peripheral blood leukocytes. I. Characteristics of the synthesis and turnover of glycogen in vitro. *J Clin Invest* 47:344, 1968.

105. Borregaard N, Juhl H: Activation of the glycogenolytic cascade in human polymorphonuclear leucocytes by different phagocytic stimuli. *Eur J Clin Invest* 11:257, 1981.

106. Wachstein M: The distribution of histochemically demonstrable glycogen in human blood and bone marrow cells. *Blood* 4:54, 1949.

107. Cassatella MA: Neutrophil-derived proteins: Selling cytokines by the pound. *Adv Immunol* 73:369, 1999.

108. Scapini P, Lapinet-Vera JA, Gasperini S, et al: The neutrophil as a cellular source of chemokines. *Immunol Rev* 177:195, 2000.

109. Boneberg EM, Hartung T: Molecular aspects of anti-inflammatory action of G-CSF. *Inflamm Res* 51:119, 2002.

110. Cloutier A, McDonald PP: Transcription factor activation in human neutrophils. *Chem Immunol Allergy* 83:1, 2003.

111. Cheng SS, Kunkel SL: The evolving role of the neutrophil in chemokine networks. *Chem Immunol Allergy* 83:81, 2003.

112. Gonzalez AL, El Bjeirami W, West JL, et al: Transendothelial migration enhances integrin-dependent human neutrophil chemokinesis. *J Leukoc Biol* 81(3):686–95, 2007.

113. Girard D: Phenotypic and functional change of neutrophils activated by cytokines utilizing the common cytokine receptor gamma chain. *Chem Immunol Allergy* 83:64, 2003.

114. Tsukahara Y, Lian Z, Zhang X, et al: Gene expression in human neutrophils during activation and priming by bacterial lipopolysaccharide. *J Cell Biochem* 89:848, 2003.

115. Malcolm KC, Arndt PG, Manos EJ, et al: Microarray analysis of lipopolysaccharide-treated human neutrophils. *Am J Physiol Lung Cell Mol Physiol* 284:L663, 2003.

116. Theilgaard-Monch K, Knudsen S, Follin P, Borregaard N: The transcriptional activation program of human neutrophils in skin lesions supports their important role in wound healing. *J Immunol* 172:7684, 2004.

117. Kobayashi SD, Voyich JM, Braughton KR, et al: Gene expression profiling provides insight into the pathophysiology of chronic granulomatous disease. *J Immunol* 172:636, 2004.

118. Kobayashi SD, Voyich JM, Braughton KR, DeLeo FR: Down-regulation of proinflammatory capacity during apoptosis in human polymorphonuclear leukocytes. *J Immunol* 170:3357, 2003.

119. Scott RB: Glycogen in human peripheral blood leukocytes. I. Characteristics of the synthesis and turnover of glycogen *in vitro*. *J Clin Invest* 47:344, 1968.

120. Scott RB, Still WJ: Glycogen in human peripheral blood leukocytes. II. The macromolecular state of leukocyte glycogen. *J Clin Invest* 47:353, 1968.

121. Esman V: The glycogen content of WBC from diabetic and nondiabetic subjects. *Scand J Clin Lab Invest* 13:134, 1961.

122. Rauch HC, Loomis ME, Johnson ME, et al: *In vitro* suppression of polymorphonuclear leukocyte and lymphocyte glycolysis by cortisol. *Endocrinology* 68:375, 1961.

123. Martin SP, McKinney GR, Green R, et al: The influence of glucose, fructose, and insulin on the metabolism of leukocytes of healthy and diabetic subjects. *J Clin Invest* 32:1171, 1953.

124. Gottfried EL: Lipids of human leukocytes: Relation to cell type. *J Lipid Res* 8:321, 1967.

125. Gottfried EL: Lipid patterns of leukocytes in health and disease. *Semin Hematol* 9:241, 1972.

126. Nishizuka Y: Studies and perspectives of protein kinase C. *Science* 233:305, 1986.

127. Berridge MJ, Irvine RF: Inositol trisphosphate, a novel second messenger in cellular signal transduction. *Nature* 312:315, 1984.

128. Symington FW, Murray WA, Bearman SI, et al: Intracellular localization of lactosylceramide, the major human neutrophil glycosphingolipid. *J Biol Chem* 262:11356, 1987.

129. Thornalley PJ, Bellavite P: Modification of the glyoxalase system during the functional activation of human neutrophils. *Biochim Biophys Acta* 931:120, 1987.

130. Silber R, Gabrio BW, Huennekens FM: Studies on normal and leukemic leukocytes. III. Pyridine nucleotides. *J Clin Invest* 41:230, 1962.

131. Willoughby HW, Waisman HA: Nucleic acid precursors and nucleotides in normal and leukemic blood. I. Comparison of formic acid chromatograms. *Cancer Res* 17:942, 1957.

132. Silber R, Unger KW, Ellman L: RNA metabolism in normal and leukaemic leucocytes: Further studies on RNA synthesis. *Br J Haematol* 14:261, 1968.

133. Tryfiates GP, Laszlo J: Human leukemic polyribosomes. *Proc Soc Exp Biol Med* 124:1125, 1967.

134. Garcia AM, Iorio R: Studies on DNA in leukocytes and related cells of mammals. V. The fast green-histone and the Feulgen-DNA content of rat leukocytes. *Acta Cytol* 12:46, 1968.

135. Smits G, Florijn E: The aneurinpyrophosphate content of red and white blood corpuscles in the rat and in man, in various states of aneurin provision and in disease. *Biochim Biophys Acta* 3:44, 1949.

136. Boxer GE, Pruss MP, Goodhart RS: Pyridoxal-5-phosphoric acid in whole blood and isolated leukocytes of man and animals. *J Nutr* 63:623, 1957.

137. Barkhan P, Howard AN: Distribution of ascorbic acid in normal and leukaemic human blood. *Biochem J* 70:163, 1958.

138. Hoffbrand AV, Newcombe BF: Leucocyte folate in vitamin B12 and folate deficiency and in leukaemia. *Br J Haematol* 13:954, 1967.

CHAPTER 61
PRODUCTION, DISTRIBUTION, AND FATE OF NEUTROPHILS

C. Wayne Smith

SUMMARY

Blood neutrophil levels are maintained in a normal steady state by hematopoiesis in the marrow, the distribution of neutrophils between the marginated pool in the microvasculature and the freely circulating pool in the blood, and the rate of egress from blood to tissues. Marrow production of neutrophils is regulated by three principal glycoprotein hormones, or cytokines: interleukin-3, granulocyte-monocyte colony-stimulating factor, and granulocyte colony-stimulating factor (G-CSF), but only the genetic elimination of G-CSF has a measurable effect on blood neutrophil levels. The latter two cytokines are available as recombinant pharmaceutical products that can be administered therapeutically to ameliorate certain causes of neutropenia. Neutrophil interaction with endothelium is mediated by selectins, glycoproteins with sugar-binding sites that support shear-dependent rolling on endothelium, and by integrins on the neutrophil binding to ligands on the endothelial cells, permitting firm attachment to endothelium and emigration into tissues. Neutrophils have a short life span in blood, with a disappearance half-time of approximately 7 hours. The process can be accelerated when inflammation is present and highlights the need for a sustained rate of production to maintain a normal blood neutrophil count. The pathogenesis of neutropenia is more complex to analyze kinetically than anemia or thrombocytopenia because at least four compartments are involved: marrow storage pool, circulating pool, marginated pool, and tissue pool. The latter is particularly difficult to assay. Measurements can be further complicated in the nonsteady state, when dramatic increases in turnover rates and distribution among the four principal pools are in disequilibrium, as occurs during acute inflammatory states.

Acronyms and Abbreviations: β_2-Integrin, a member of family of receptors that mediate attachment between a cell and the tissues surrounding it; C5a, chemotactic fragment of complement component C5; CD, one of the cluster of differentiation antigens; CSF, colony-stimulating factor; DF^{32}P, diisopropyl fluorophosphate; G-CSF, granulocyte colony-stimulating factor; GM-CSF, granulocyte-monocyte colony-stimulating factor; IL, interleukin; L-selectin (and other selectins), a member of selectin family of proteins, which are leukocyte cell-adhesion molecules; Mr, relative molecular mass; NTR, neutrophil turnover rate; T$_{1/2}$, half-time; TBNP, total blood neutrophil pool; TNF-a, tumor necrosis factor-a.

DEFINITION AND HISTORY

Neutrophils are produced in the marrow, where they arise from progenitor and precursor cells by a process of cellular proliferation and maturation. They differentiate from the pluripotential stem cell[1,2] through a series of progressively more committed progenitor or colony-forming units, including the granulocyte-monocyte colony-forming unit and the granulocyte colony-forming unit, which give rise to neutrophils.[3,4] The early progenitor cells cannot be recognized under the microscope but can be identified retrospectively by the type of colony formed in culture of marrow cells (Chap. 18). The earliest morphologically recognizable neutrophil precursor is the myeloblast. From there, the formal sequence of precursor development is myeloblast → promyelocyte → myelocyte → metamyelocyte → band neutrophil → segmented neutrophil (Chap. 60). The term *granulocyte* often is loosely used to refer to neutrophils but strictly speaking includes eosinophils and basophils. Eosinophilic (Chap. 62) and basophilic granulocytes (Chap. 63) develop from progenitors in a manner analogous to the neutrophils, although commitment to neutrophilic, eosinophilic, or basophilic development probably is established at an early progenitor stage, and are dependent on the cytokines interleukin (IL)-5 and stem cell factor, respectively.

The normal human neutrophil production rate is 0.85 to 1.6×10^9 cells/kg per day. Mature neutrophils are stored in the marrow before they are released into the blood. In the absence of an inflammatory focus, they leave the circulation randomly, with a half-disappearance time of approximately 7 hours. The cells then enter the tissues and probably function for 1 or 2 days before their death or loss into the gastrointestinal tract through mucosal surfaces.

The marrow has an impressive capacity to produce neutrophils, yet it is carefully regulated both at steady state and in times of heightened demand. This chapter outlines current concepts of neutrophil production, distribution, and survival. For detailed data and methods, the reader is referred to original articles and reviews on neutropoiesis and neutrophil kinetics.[5–17]

REGULATION OF NEUTROPHILIC GRANULOPOIESIS

Although the primary cellular manifestation of commitment is the expression of receptors for lineage-specific hematopoietic growth factors, the "decision" for a stem cell to self-renew is, at least partially, a stochastic event.[1,18] On the other hand, stromal elements, collectively referred to as the *hematopoietic microenvironment*, release short-range signals that regulate the process of commitment from multipotential stem cell pools. Although many details of hematopoietic stem cell regulation (Chap. 18) remain to be elucidated, much is known regarding the interaction of hematopoietic cytokines with their receptors and actions on the committed granulocyte progenitor cells and their mature progeny.[19–24]

HUMORAL REGULATORS

The humoral regulators involved in granulopoiesis have been defined by *in vitro* culture systems.[20,21] Originally identified by their ability to stimulate colony formation from marrow progenitor cells, the hemopoietic cytokines were initially termed *colony-stimulating factors* (CSFs) based on this assay system.[25] With regard to neutrophil production, at least four human CSFs have been defined. Granulocyte-monocyte colony-stimulating factor (GM-CSF) is a

22,000 relative molecular mass (Mr) glycoprotein that stimulates the production of neutrophils, monocytes, and eosinophils. Granulocyte colony-stimulating factor (G-CSF) has a Mr of 20,000 and stimulates exclusively the production of neutrophils. IL-3, or multi-CSF, also has a Mr of 20,000 and acts relatively early in hematopoiesis, affecting pluripotential stem cells. Finally, stem cell factor (also known as c-*kit* ligand or steel factor), with a Mr of 28,000, acts in combination with IL-3 and/or GM-CSF to stimulate the proliferation of the early hematopoietic progenitor cells, basophils and mast cells.

In addition to their effects on neutrophil precursors, G-CSF and GM-CSF act directly on the neutrophil, enhancing its function. These cytokines regulate the production, survival, and functional activity of neutrophils.[21,22,26,27] In a murine model of severe bacterial infection, endothelial cells translate pathogen signals into G-CSF–driven marrow neutrophil production.[28] The mature neutrophil lacks IL-3 receptors and thus is not affected by IL-3. In fact, the genetic elimination of IL-3 obliterates delayed type hypersensitivity. However, IL-3 receptors are present on mature eosinophils and monocytes. IL-3 is produced by activated T lymphocytes and thus is expected to have a physiologic role in circumstances of cell-mediated immunity. GM-CSF also is produced by activated lymphocytes. However, like G-CSF, it also is elaborated by mononuclear phagocytes and endothelial and mesenchymal cells when these cell types are stimulated by certain cytokines, including IL-1 and tumor necrosis factor, or bacterial products, such as endotoxin.[29–31] Stem cell factor is secreted by a variety of cells, including marrow stromal cells,[32,33] and affects the development of several kinds of tissues.[32,34]

The activities of exogenously administered biosynthetic (recombinant) human G-CSF and GM-CSF in humans are well documented.[22,27,35–37] G-CSF administration rapidly induces neutrophilia, whereas GM-CSF causes an increase in neutrophils, eosinophils, and monocytes. GM-CSF cannot be detected easily in normal plasma; thus, its role as a day-to-day, long-range modulator of neutrophil production is uncertain. Mice in which the GM-CSF gene is "knocked out" have generally normal hematopoiesis, but show macrophage abnormalities, pulmonary alveolar proteinosis, and decreased resistance to microbial challenge.[38–41] However, G-CSF appears to be a critical regulator of neutrophil development, as giving an animal an antibody to G-CSF leads to profound neutropenia.[42] The G-CSF knockout mouse shows severe neutropenia.[43] Neutropenia that results from a production disturbance, such as exposure to cytotoxic drugs, is associated with high circulating serum concentrations of G-CSF.[44]

NEUTROPHIL KINETICS

Methods used to study granulocyte kinetics can be categorized as follows: (1) neutrophil depletion or destruction to determine the size and rate of mobilization of reserves and the level of compensatory neutrophil production; (2) use of radioactive tracers to study neutrophil distribution, production rates, and survival times; (3) mitotic indices of marrow granulocytic cells to assess proliferative activity and cell cycle times; and (4) induced inflammatory lesions to study cell movement into the tissues. Of these categories, the most popular has been the use of radioactive tracers.

Neutrophil production and neutrophil kinetics usually are analyzed by describing neutrophil movement through a number of interconnected compartments. These compartments can be arranged into three major groups: the marrow, the blood, and the tissue (Fig. 61–1). The complexities of analyzing these compartments are covered in several recent reviews.[45–48]

The Marrow

Marrow neutrophils can be divided into the mitotic, or proliferative, compartment and the maturation storage compartment. Myeloblasts, promyelocytes, and myelocytes are capable of replication and constitute the mitotic compartment. Earlier progenitor cells are few in number, not morphologically identifiable, and usually neglected in kinetic studies. Metamyelocytes, bands, and mature neutrophils, none of which replicate, constitute the maturation storage compartment.

The average number of cell divisions from the myeloblast to the myelocyte stage in the proliferative compartment has been estimated between four and five.[49] Data obtained using radioactive diisopropyl fluorophosphate (DF^{32}P) suggest the existence of three divisions at the myelocyte stage, but the number of cell divisions at each step may not be constant. The major increase in neutrophil number probably occurs at the myelocyte level, because the myelocyte pool is at least four times the size of the promyelocyte pool. Because of the difficulties in measuring human intramarrow neutrophil kinetics, a precise model of the dynamics of the mitotic compartment is not available.

Table 61–1 lists the estimated sizes of the marrow neutrophil compartments and the transit times and cell-cycle stages of the cells in the various compartments. Precise studies have measured a postmitotic pool of $(5.59 \pm 0.9) \times 10^9$ cells/kg and a mitotic pool (promyelocytes and myelocytes) of $(2.11 \pm 0.36) \times 10^9$ cells/kg. These studies led to a

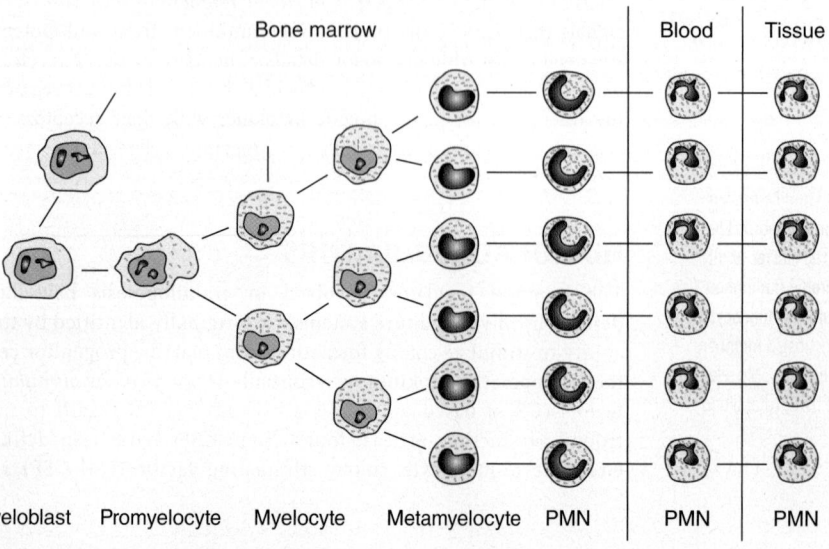

	Bone marrow				Blood	Tissue
Myeloblast	Promyelocyte	Myelocyte	Metamyelocyte	PMN	PMN	PMN

Figure 61–1. Scheme of maturation of neutrophil precursor cells. The myeloblast is the first recognizable precursor of neutrophils. Myeloblasts undergo division and maturation into promyelocytes and thereafter into neutrophilic myelocytes after which stage mitotic capability is lost. The major compartments of precursor proliferation and distribution are indicated across the top of the figure: marrow, blood, and tissues. The marrow precursor compartment is made up of the proliferating compartment (myeloblasts through myelocytes) and the maturation and storage compartment (metamyelocytes to mature polymorphonuclear neutrophils [PMN]). Under normal conditions, cells do not return from the tissue compartment to the blood or marrow.

TABLE 61–1. Marrow Neutrophil Kinetics

	Fraction in Mitosis (Mitotic Index)	Fraction in DNA Synthesis (S Phase)	Transit Time Range (h)	Total Cells (× 0⁹/kg)
Mitotic compartment				
Myeloblast	0.025	0.85	23	0.14
Promyelocyte	0.015	0.65	26–78	0.51
Myelocyte	0.011	0.33	17–126	1.95
Maturation storage compartment				
Metamyelocyte			8–108	2.7
Band			12–96	3.6
Polymorphonuclear neutrophil			0–120	2.5

calculated normal marrow neutrophil production of 0.85×10^9 cells/kg per day. Radioautographic studies with [³H]thymidine support the concept of an orderly progression from metamyelocytes to mature neutrophils within the maturation storage compartment. These studies also suggest a "first in, first out" pattern for cells leaving this compartment and entering the blood. Several labeling techniques indicate the myelocyte-to-blood transit time is 5 to 7 days.[12,50] Previous studies with DF³²P reported a range from 8 to 14 days.[9,49] During infections, however, the myelocyte-to-blood transit time may be as short as 48 hours.[51]

Whether the production of neutrophils in the mitotic compartment exactly equals the neutrophil turnover rate (NTR) is not known with certainty. Studies in dogs suggest some immature neutrophils die in the marrow ("ineffective granulopoiesis").[52] Ineffective granulopoiesis has not been shown in normal humans,[14,53] although ineffective granulopoiesis occurs in some pathologic states, including the myelodysplastic syndromes,[54] myelofibrosis, and some of the idiopathic neutropenic disorders. At present, however, no convenient means of quantitating ineffective granulopoiesis is available.

On completion of maturation, the neutrophils are stored in the marrow and are referred to as the *mature neutrophil reserve*. The reserve contains many more cells than are normally circulating in the blood. Table 61–2 lists comparative data on the characteristics of the maturation storage compartment. Under stress, maturation time may be shortened, divisions may be skipped, and release into the blood may occur prematurely.

The Blood

Neutrophils leave the marrow storage compartment and enter the blood without significant reentry into the marrow. The total blood neutrophil pool (TBNP) consists of all the neutrophils in the vascular spaces. Some of these neutrophils are free in the circulation (the circulating pool), while others roll along the endothelium of small vessels or

are temporarily sequestered in the alveolar capillaries of the lung (the marginated pool).[55,56] Cells in the two pools are freely exchangeable. When neutrophils labeled with DF³²P are injected into normal subjects, approximately half can be accounted for in the circulating pool; the remainder enters the marginated pool.[5–7] Neutrophils shift from the marginated to the circulating pool with exercise, epinephrine injection, or stress, but eventually the neutrophils leave the blood and enter the tissues. Once the neutrophils enter the tissues, they do not normally return to the blood. The flow of cells is unidirectional.

DF³²P-labeled neutrophils disappear from the circulation with a half-time ($T_{1/2}$) of 6.7 hours.[7,57,58] These data are supported by the finding that more than half of Pelger-Huët cells infused into a normal individual disappeared after 6 to 8 hours.[59] Data obtained with ⁵¹Cr-labeled neutrophils give substantially longer half-times.[60] The exponential disappearance of cells from the blood suggests the cells leave in a random manner. Thus, neutrophils newly released from the marrow are as likely to leave the blood as are neutrophils that have been circulating for several hours. Neutrophils also are eliminated by programmed cell death and disposed of by the macrophage system.[51,61–64]

Direct observations of blood vessels have revealed some degree of leukocyte rolling along the endothelium (first observed many years ago by Atherton and Born[60]). Although the observation has been clearly confirmed by numerous laboratories in different species of animals, the extent to which this phenomenon contributes to the marginated pool of neutrophils is uncertain.

A more compelling concept of the marginated pool is derived from investigations of the vascular bed of the lung. A distinctive characteristic of this tissue is the complex interconnecting network of short capillary segments where the path from arteriole to venule crosses several alveolar walls (often more than eight) and often contains more than 50 capillary segments.[65–69] Compared to blood in the large vessels of most vascular beds, the blood in this complex network

TABLE 61–2. Comparative Data on Marrow Maturation Storage Compartment

Size (Cells × 10⁹ kg)	Transit Time (Days)	Measurement Technique	Reference
6.5–13	4–8	[³H]thymidine, *in vitro* DF³²P	5
3–23	8–14	*In vivo* and *in vitro* DF³²P	45
5.6	6.6	⁵⁹Fe and neutrophil/erythroid ratio	14

DF³²P, diisopropyl fluorophosphate.

contains approximately 50-fold more neutrophils and even more lymphocytes and monocytes.[70] Videomicroscopic study of these vessels in animal models has revealed the transit of neutrophils through this network required a median time of 26 seconds and mean time of 6.1 seconds.[71,72] In contrast, the transit times of red blood cells ranges from 1.4 to 4.2 seconds. The increased transit time results primarily from the time neutrophils are stopped within this vascular network. The longer time required for the neutrophils to pass through this bed apparently accounts for their increased concentration.

Recruitment of neutrophils into the lungs through the alveolar capillary network contrasts with the recruitment of neutrophils through postcapillary venules at sites of inflammation in a number of important ways. The tethering mechanisms required to capture neutrophils from flowing blood in larger vessels apparently are not necessary in the alveolar capillary bed. The diameters of spherical neutrophils (6 to 8 μm) are larger than the diameters of many capillary segments (2 to 15 μm). Approximately 50 percent of the capillary segments would require neutrophils to change their shape in order to pass through.[72–75] Given the large number of capillary segments through which a neutrophil must pass (often more than 50), most neutrophils must change shape during transit from arteriole to venule. Morphometric analysis of neutrophils in the alveolar capillary beds has revealed significant deviation from spherical shape.[72,73] Computational models of the capillary bed describing flow, hematocrit, pressure gradients, and the effects of deformation on the capillary transit times of neutrophils support the concept that the structure of the capillary bed and the deformation of neutrophils are critical under normal conditions. Thus, the enormous lung vascular bed contains a substantial number of neutrophils that can be mobilized into the systemic circulation with stimuli such as epinephrine or exercise.

During inflammation, much of the sequestration and infiltration occur through vessels so narrow that physical tapping is sufficient to stop the flowing neutrophil.[68,72,76,77] Binding of mediators such as chemotactic factors (e.g., C5a, the chemotactic fragment of complement component C5) to neutrophil receptors induces a transient resistance of the cells to deformation.[78–83] Because neutrophils must deform to pass through the capillary bed, leukocyte activation by inflammatory mediators could affect further concentration of neutrophils at the alveolar walls.[65,76] The role of mechanical factors in the initial sequestration of neutrophils in the alveolar capillaries is supported by evidence that neither L-selectin nor β_2-integrins are required.[76,84,85] In contrast, both selectins and β_2-integrins are required for localization of neutrophils in postcapillary venules at sites of inflammation.

The events following the initial sequestration of neutrophils within alveolar capillary beds are influenced by adhesion molecules. For example, simple systemic activation of neutrophils by intravenous injection of chemotactic factors (e.g., IL-8 or C5a) results in rapid (<1 minute) neutropenia with massive sequestration of neutrophils within alveolar capillaries. This event is not dependent on L-selectin or β_2-integrins, but the retention times within this capillary bed are influenced by these adhesion molecules.[76,85] Adhesion likely is an interaction of leukocyte adhesion molecules and endothelial adhesion molecules. Blockade of the adhesive mechanism (e.g., using blocking monoclonal antibodies) results in release of neutrophils from the lungs.[76,84,86–88] Mediator-induced decreases in deformability are temporally correlated with upregulation of β_2-integrins (e.g., both occurring within approximately 1 minute of exposure to IL-8). This allows both physical trapping and sticking to the vascular wall within the alveolar capillary bed. A similar phenomenon occurs in the liver where sequestration is the result of physical trapping and liver injury is heavily dependent on adhesion of leukocytes through the β_2-integrins.[89]

Assuming a random loss of neutrophils from the blood, NTR can be calculated from $T_{1/2}$ and TBNP: NTR = $0.693 \times$ TBNP/$T_{1/2}$. In the

steady state, NTR measures the rate of effective neutrophil production. Table 61–3 lists the definitions and calculations related to blood neutrophil kinetics. Table 61–4 lists data for normal human blood neutrophil kinetics. The high production rate of neutrophils under normal conditions is remarkable, especially given that the rate may increase several fold in response to inflammatory stimuli.

Glucocorticoids increase TBNP by increasing influx from the marrow and decreasing efflux from the circulation. Five hours after a pharmacologic dose of glucocorticoid, the neutrophil count increases by approximately 4000/μL because of release from the marrow, demargination, and prolongation of $T_{1/2}$ to approximately 10 hours.[90–92] Consistent with the increase in $T_{1/2}$, prednisone reduces the accumulation of neutrophils at induced sites of skin inflammation.[75] With alternate-day, single-dose prednisone, neutrophil counts and kinetics are normal 24 hours after administration and during the day off.[93] Endotoxin causes a prompt neutropenia as a result of cell margination and sequestration, followed in 2 to 4 hours by a rebound neutrophilia as a result of cell release from the marrow. The size of the neutrophilic response correlates with the functional marrow reserves.[94–97] After epinephrine administration, a peak leukocytosis occurs in 5 to 10 minutes and rarely lasts more than 20 minutes. This finding reflects a shift of cells from the marginated to the circulating pool.

MIGRATION OF NEUTROPHILS INTO TISSUES

The migration of neutrophils from blood into tissue at sites of inflammation involves a series of sequential adhesive steps proceeding from tethering (rolling adhesion) on endothelium under shear conditions in

TABLE 61–3. Definitions and Calculations Relating to Blood Neutrophil Kinetics

Circulating neutrophil pool (CNP) = Blood neutrophil concentration × blood volume
Total blood neutrophil pool (TBNP) = All neutrophils in the circulation
Marginal neutrophil pool (MNP) = TBNP − CNP
Blood clearance half-time ($T_{1/2}$) = Disappearance time of half the labeled neutrophils from circulation
Neutrophil turnover rate (NTR) = $\dfrac{0.693 \times \text{TBNP}}{T_{1/2}}$

TABLE 61–4. Data for Human Blood Neutrophil Kinetics

Pool	Mean Pool Size × 10^7 kg	95% Limits
TBNP	70	14–160
CNP	31	11–46
MNP	39	0–85
	Mean Value	**95% Limits**
Blood clearance $T_{1/2}$	6.7 h	4–10 h
NTR	63×10^7 kg/day	$50–340 \times 10^7$ kg/day

CNP, circulating neutrophil pool; MNP, marginal neutrophil pool; NTR, neutrophil turnover rate; $T_{1/2}$, half-time; TBNP, total blood neutrophil pool.

postcapillary venules.[98] This model has been investigated in a variety of vascular beds[99] and *in vitro* with monolayers of endothelial cells in parallel plate flow chambers.[98] The tethering event in this model depends on adhesion molecules in the selectin family, E-selectin and P-selectin on the endothelium, L-selectin on the neutrophil, and ligands for the selectins expressed on both cell types. These adhesion molecules are necessary to efficiently initiate the cascade of adhesive steps ultimately leading to firm attachment of the neutrophils to endothelium. The cascade appears to be necessary for neutrophils to move from blood to tissues because the unstimulated neutrophil is not adhesive to endothelium.[98,100] The integrins necessary for firm adhesion and cell locomotion require stimulation to promote sufficient increases in avidity or affinity to support these functions (Chap. 19).

LIFE SPAN OF NEUTROPHILS

After emigrating into tissue, the life span of neutrophils can be significantly prolonged (24 to 48 hours).[101] Programmed cell death (apoptosis) accounts for significant removal of tissue neutrophils through phagocytosis by macrophages. The constitutive rate of apoptosis of neutrophils is altered by inflammatory cytokines and chemokines. For example, tumor necrosis factor-α (TNF-α) accelerates the rate, but endotoxin, G-CSF, GM-CSF, IL-15, and IL-3 inhibit the rate of apoptosis. The balance of these effects at specific inflammatory sites is poorly understood, but the functional life of neutrophils in tissue appears to be controlled by the rate of apoptosis. Apoptotic neutrophils lose the ability to release granular enzymes in response to external stimuli (see below), and marked changes in cell surface proteins occur (e.g., CD16, CD43, CD62L are greatly reduced). Although the loss of responsiveness may contribute to resolution of the inflammatory process, evidence indicates macrophages also are altered by the phagocytosis of apoptotic neutrophils. In contrast to the macrophage response to phagocytosis of microbes, where secretion of proinflammatory cytokines (e.g., IL-1β) and chemokines (e.g., IL-8) is stimulated, phagocytosis of apoptotic neutrophils fails to provoke secretion of proinflammatory factors; instead, phagocytosis stimulates release of factors that may suppress inflammatory responses (e.g., transforming growth factor-β and prostaglandin E$_2$). Macrophage recognition of apoptotic neutrophils is partially understood to involve the vitronectin receptor $\alpha_v\beta_3$ and the thrombospondin receptor CD36 on the macrophage surface. In addition, phosphatidylserine residues on the neutrophil are involved.[98]

Neutrophils are capable of phenotypic changes depending on the tissue and cytokine/chemokine milieu at the time of their migration into tissue (Chap. 60). Because our understanding of neutrophil physiology is relatively new, knowing the extent of this phenomenon on neutrophil life span in tissues is not possible at present.

● EVALUATION OF ADEQUACY OF NEUTROPHIL RESERVES

WHITE CELL COUNT AND MARROW CELLULARITY

White cell and absolute neutrophil counts are the most widely used guides to the status of neutrophil production. They are useful in evaluating the effects of cytotoxic chemotherapy, although they do not provide quantitative information on the rate of neutrophil production or destruction, the status of marrow reserves, or the presence of abnormalities in cell distribution.

Gauging neutrophil production by the appearance of marrow films, clot sections, or biopsies suffers from the limitations of sampling

error and relatively poor correlation with kinetics, as measured by other techniques.[68] For example, the morphologic findings in the marrow of a "maturation arrest," with little neutrophil development beyond the promyelocyte or myelocyte stage, does not distinguish between a defect in precursor cell maturation and rapid mobilization of postmitotic cells from the marrow. Similarly, distinguishing by purely morphologic means neutropenic conditions resulting from ineffective neutrophil production from conditions caused by peripheral destruction of neutrophils often is difficult. However, despite these limitations, when the absolute neutrophil count and marrow cellularity are used together, they provide a useful guide in most clinical settings. If the absolute neutrophil count is less than 1.0×10^9/L and multiple marrow aspirations and/or biopsies are hypocellular, the patient almost invariably has impaired production of marrow neutrophils. Very low neutrophil counts predispose to infections by bacteria and certain fungi (e.g., *Candida* and *Aspergillus*). Such infections become especially troublesome as the neutrophil count falls below 0.5×10^9/L (Chap. 65). Unfortunately, the converse is not true. The finding of cellular marrow and neutrophil count >1.0×10^9/L does not mean production is normal. Nevertheless, when marrow cellularity and absolute neutrophil count are considered together, they provide the most clinically useful assessment of neutrophil production.

FUNCTIONAL EVALUATION

Several agents that increase neutrophil numbers in circulation, including glucocorticoids, endotoxin, and etiocholanolone, have been used to evaluate neutrophil reserves in a clinical setting. These agents have been supplanted by recombinant human G-CSF, a remarkably nontoxic cytokine that, when given in therapeutic doses (5 to 8 mcg/kg), increases the blood neutrophil count by stimulating neutrophil production and accelerating neutrophil release from the marrow storage compartment (Chap. 65). The increase in neutrophil production results from a threefold increase in the number of cell divisions in the mitotic compartment and shortening of the maturation time from myelocyte to neutrophil from 4 to 5 days to less than 1 day.[102,103] Thus, as a byproduct of its therapeutic action, G-CSF administration directly tests an individual's capacity to produce neutrophils. This effect of G-CSF makes obsolete most of the older methods for evaluating neutrophil compartments.

G-CSF does not test the distribution of neutrophils between the marginated and circulating pools. On the rare occasions when such information is desirable, epinephrine stimulation can be used to assess the distribution. For this purpose, epinephrine 0.1 mg infused intravenously over 5 minutes has been used, and blood for white counts is obtained before and 1, 3, and 5 minutes after completion of the epinephrine infusion. Normally the neutrophils increase by approximately 50 percent after epinephrine infusion.[104]

REFERENCES

1. Kondo M, Wagers AJ, Manz MG, et al: Biology of hematopoietic stem cells and progenitors: Implications for clinical application. *Annu Rev Immunol* 21:759, 2003.
2. Spangrude GJ: When is a stem cell really a stem cell? *Bone Marrow Transplant* 32 Suppl 1:S7, 2003.
3. Smaaland R, Sothern RB, Laerum OD, Abrahamsen JF: Rhythms in human bone marrow and blood cells. *Chronobiol Int* 19:101, 2002.
4. Metcalf D: Hematopoietic stem cells: Old and new. *Biomed Pharmacother* 55:75, 2001.
5. Athens JW: Neutrophilic granulocyte kinetics and granulopoiesis, in *Regulation of Hematopoiesis*, edited by Gordon AS, p 1143. Appleton-Century-Crofts, New York, 1961.
6. Athens JW, Raab SO, Haab OP, et al: Leukokinetic studies. III. The distribution of granulocytes in the blood of normal subjects. *J Clin Invest* 40:159, 1961.
7. Athens JW, Haab OP, Raab SO, et al: Leukokinetic studies. IV. The total blood, circulating and marginal granulocyte pools and the granulocyte turnover rate in normal subjects. *J Clin Invest* 40:989, 1961.

8. Boggs DR: The kinetics of neutrophilic leukocytes in health and in disease. *Semin Hematol* 4:359, 1967.

9. Cartwright GE, Athens JW, Boggs DR, Wintrobe MM: The kinetics of granulopoiesis in normal man. *Ser Haematol* 1:1, 1965.

10. Cronkite EP: Kinetics of granulocytopoiesis. *Clin Haematol* 8:351, 1979.

11. Cronkite EP, Fliedner TM: Granulocytopoiesis. *N Engl J Med* 270:1347, 1964.

12. Vincent PC: The measurement of granulocyte kinetics. *Br J Haematol* 36:1, 1977.

13. Donohue DM, Gabrio BW, Finch CA: Quantitative measurement of hematopoietic cells of the marrow. *J Clin Invest* 37:1564, 1958.

14. Dancey JT, Deubelbeiss KA, Harker LA, Finch CA: Neutrophil kinetics in man. *J Clin Invest* 58:705, 1976.

15. Dresch C, Faille A, Rain JD, Najean Y: [Granulopoiesis: Comparison of several methods for studying production and bone marrow cellularity (author's transl)]. *Nouv Rev Fr Hematol* 15:31, 1975.

16. Simon HU: Neutrophil apoptosis pathways and their modifications in inflammation. *Immunol Rev* 193:101, 2003.

17. Kuijpers TW: Clinical symptoms and neutropenia: The balance of neutrophil development, functional activity, and cell death. *Eur J Pediatr* 161 Suppl 1:S75, 2002.

18. Ogawa M: Changing phenotypes of hematopoietic stem cells. *Exp Hematol* 30:3, 2002.

19. Friedman AD: Transcriptional regulation of myelopoiesis. *Int J Hematol* 75:466, 2002.

20. Metcalf D: Hematopoietic regulators: Redundancy or subtlety? *Blood* 82:3515, 1993.

21. Metcalf D: Neutrophilic granulocytes and macrophages: Molecular, cellular, and clinical aspects, in *Regulation of Hematopoiesis*, edited by Gordon AS, p 1143. Appleton-Century-Crofts, New York, 1970.

22. Lieschke GJ, Burgess AW: Granulocyte colony-stimulating factor and granulocyte-macrophage colony-stimulating factor (1). *N Engl J Med* 327:28, 1992.

23. Kaushansky K, Karplus PA: Hematopoietic growth factors: Understanding functional diversity in structural terms. *Blood* 82:3229, 1993.

24. Groopman JE, Molina JM, Scadden DT: Hematopoietic growth factors. Biology and clinical applications. *N Engl J Med* 321:1449, 1989.

25. Barreda DR, Hanington PC, Belosevic M: Regulation of myeloid development and function by colony stimulating factors. *Dev Comp Immunol* 28:509, 2004.

26. Welte K, Gabrilove J, Bronchud MH, et al: Filgrastim (r-metHuG-CSF): The first 10 years. *Blood* 88:1907, 1996.

27. Anderlini P, Przepiorka D, Champlin R, Korbling M: Biologic and clinical effects of granulocyte colony-stimulating factor in normal individuals. *Blood* 88:2819, 1996.

28. Boettcher S, Gerosa R, Radpour R, et al. Endothelial cells translate pathogen signals into G-CSF-driven emergency granulopoiesis. *Blood* 124:1393, 2014.

29. Munker R, Gasson J, Ogawa M, Koeffler HP: Recombinant human TNF induces production of granulocyte-monocyte colony-stimulating factor. *Nature* 323:79, 1986.

30. Zucali JR, Dinarello CA, Oblon DJ, et al: Interleukin 1 stimulates fibroblasts to produce granulocyte-macrophage colony-stimulating activity and prostaglandin E2. *J Clin Invest* 77:1857, 1986.

31. Metcalf D, Nicola NA, Mifsud S, Di Rago L: Receptor clearance obscures the magnitude of granulocyte-macrophage colony-stimulating factor responses in mice to endotoxin or local infections. *Blood* 93:1579, 1999.

32. Akin C, Metcalfe DD: The biology of Kit in disease and the application of pharmacogenetics. *J Allergy Clin Immunol* 114:13, 2004.

33. Heissig B, Werb Z, Rafii S, Hattori K: Role of c-kit/Kit ligand signaling in regulating vasculogenesis. *Thromb Haemost* 90:570, 2003.

34. Wehrle-Haller B: The role of Kit-ligand in melanocyte development and epidermal homeostasis. *Pigment Cell Res* 16:287, 2003.

35. Lalami Y, Paesmans M, Aoun M, et al: A prospective randomised evaluation of G-CSF or G-CSF plus oral antibiotics in chemotherapy-treated patients at high risk of developing febrile neutropenia. *Support Care Cancer* 12:725, 2004.

36. De Waele M, Renmans W, Asosingh K, et al: Growth factor receptor profile of CD34 cells in normal bone marrow, cord blood and mobilized peripheral blood. *Eur J Haematol* 72:193, 2004.

37. Crawford J: Neutrophil growth factors. *Curr Hematol Rep* 1:95, 2002.

38. LeVine AM, Reed JA, Kurak KE, et al: GM-CSF-deficient mice are susceptible to pulmonary group B streptococcal infection. *J Clin Invest* 103:563, 1999.

39. Dranoff G, Crawford AD, Sadelain M, et al: Involvement of granulocyte-macrophage colony-stimulating factor in pulmonary homeostasis. *Science* 264:713, 1994.

40. Stanley E, Lieschke GJ, Grail D, et al: Granulocyte/macrophage colony-stimulating factor-deficient mice show no major perturbation of hematopoiesis but develop a characteristic pulmonary pathology. *Proc Natl Acad Sci U S A* 91:5592, 1994.

41. Huffman JA, Hull WM, Dranoff G, Mulligan RC, Whitsett JA: Pulmonary epithelial cell expression of GM-CSF corrects the alveolar proteinosis in GM-CSF-deficient mice. *J Clin Invest* 97:649, 1996.

42. Hammond WP, Csiba E, Canin A, et al: Chronic neutropenia. A new canine model induced by human granulocyte colony-stimulating factor. *J Clin Invest* 87:704, 1991.

43. Lieschke GJ, Grail D, Hodgson G, et al: Mice lacking granulocyte colony-stimulating factor have chronic neutropenia, granulocyte and macrophage progenitor cell deficiency, and impaired neutrophil mobilization. *Blood* 84:1737, 1994.

44. Mempel K, Pietsch T, Menzel T, et al: Increased serum levels of granulocyte colony-stimulating factor in patients with severe congenital neutropenia. *Blood* 77:1919, 1991.

45. Tak T, Tesselaar K, Pillay J, et al: What's your age again? Determination of human neutrophil half-lives revisited. *J Leukoc Biol* 94:595, 2013.

46. Tofts PS, Chevassut T, Cutajar M, et al: Doubts concerning the recently reported human neutrophil lifespan of 5.4 days. *Blood* 117:6050, 2011.

47. Geering B, Stoeckle C, Conus S, Simon HU: Living and dying for inflammation: Neutrophils, eosinophils, basophils. *Trends Immunol* 34:398, 2013.

48. Timar CI, Lorincz AM, Ligeti E: Changing world of neutrophils. *Pflugers Arch* 465:1521, 2013.

49. Warner HR, Athens JW: An analysis of granulocyte kinetics in blood and bone marrow. *Ann N Y Acad Sci* 113:523, 1964.

50. Dresch C, Faille A, Bauchet J, Najean Y: Granulopoiesis: Comparison of different methods for studying maturation time and bone marrow storage. *Nouv Rev Fr Hematol* 13:5, 1973.

51. Fliedner TM, Cronkite EP, Robertson JS: Granulocytopoiesis. I. Senescence and random loss of neutrophilic granulocytes in human beings. *Blood* 24:402, 1964.

52. Patt HM, Maloney MA: Kinetics of neutrophil balance, in *The Kinetics of Cellular Proliferation*, edited by Stohlman F, p 201. Grune and Stratton, New York, 1959.

53. Cronkite EP: Enigmas underlying the study of hemopoietic cell proliferation. *Fed Proc* 23:649, 1964.

54. Raza A, Cruz R, Latif T, et al: The biology of myelodysplastic syndromes: Unity despite heterogeneity. *Hematol Rep* 2:e4, 2010.

55. Doerschuk CM: Mechanisms of leukocyte sequestration in inflamed lungs. *Microcirculation* 8:71, 2001.

56. Schwab AJ, Salamand A, Merhi Y, et al: Kinetic analysis of pulmonary neutrophil retention in vivo using the multiple-indicator-dilution technique. *J Appl Physiol* 95:279, 2003.

57. Mauer AM, Athens JW, Ashenbrucker H, et al: Leukokinetic studies: II. A method for labeling granulocytes in vitro with radioactive diisopropylfluorophosphate (DFP32). *J Clin Invest* 39:1481, 1960.

58. Bishop CR, Rothstein G, Ashenbrucker HE, Athens JW: Leukokinetic studies. XIV. Blood neutrophil kinetics in chronic, steady-state neutropenia. *J Clin Invest* 50:1678, 1971.

59. Rosse WF, Gurney CW: The Pelger-Huet anomaly in three families and its use in determining the disappearance of transfused neutrophils from the peripheral blood. *Blood* 14:170, 1959.

60. Dresch C, Najean Y, Bauchet J: Kinetic studies of 51Cr and DF32P labelled granulocytes. *Br J Haematol* 29:67, 1975.

61. Maianski NA, Maianski AN, Kuijpers TW, Roos D: Apoptosis of neutrophils. *Acta Haematol* 111:56, 2004.

62. Edwards SW, Moulding DA, Derouet M, Moots RJ: Regulation of neutrophil apoptosis. *Chem Immunol Allergy* 83:204, 2003.

63. Cassatella MA: *The Neutrophil. An Emerging Regulator of Inflammatory and Immune Response.* Karger, Verona, 2003.

64. Fadeel B, Kagan VE: Apoptosis and macrophage clearance of neutrophils: Regulation by reactive oxygen species. *Redox Rep* 8:143, 2003.

65. Hogg JC: Neutrophil kinetics and lung injury. *Physiol Rev* 67:1249, 1987.

66. Staub NC, Schultz EL: Pulmonary capillary length in dogs, cat and rabbit. *Respir Physiol* 5:371, 1968.

67. Ambrus CM, Ambrus JL, Johnson GC, et al: Role of the lungs in regulation of the white blood cell level. *Am J Physiol* 178:33, 1954.

68. Doerschuk CM, Allard MF, Martin BA, et al: Marginated pool of neutrophils in rabbit lungs. *J Appl Physiol* 63:1806, 1987.

69. Lien DC, Wagner WW Jr, Capen RL, et al: Physiological neutrophil sequestration in the lung: Visual evidence for localization in capillaries. *J Appl Physiol* 62:1236, 1987.

70. Doerschuk CM, Downey GP, Doherty DE, et al: Leukocyte and platelet margination within microvasculature of rabbit lungs. *J Appl Physiol* 68:1956, 1990.

71. Presson RG Jr, Graham JA, Hanger CC, et al: Distribution of pulmonary capillary red blood cell transit times. *J Appl Physiol* 79:382, 1995.

72. Gebb SA, Graham JA, Hanger CC, et al: Sites of leukocyte sequestration in the pulmonary microcirculation. *J Appl Physiol* 79:493, 1995.

73. Doerschuk CM, Beyers N, Coxson HO, et al: Comparison of neutrophil and capillary diameters and their relation to neutrophil sequestration in the lung. *J Appl Physiol* 74:3040, 1993.

74. Martin BA, Wright JL, Thommasen H, Hogg JC: Effect of pulmonary blood flow on the exchange between the circulating and marginating pool of polymorphonuclear leukocytes in dog lungs. *J Clin Invest* 69:1277, 1982.

75. Hogg JC, McLean T, Martin BA, Wiggs B: Erythrocyte transit and neutrophil concentration in the dog lung. *J Appl Physiol* 65:1217, 1988.

76. Doerschuk CM: The role of CD18-mediated adhesion in neutrophil sequestration induced by infusion of activated plasma in rabbits. *Am J Respir Cell Mol Biol* 7:140, 1992.

77. Downey GP, Worthen GS, Henson PM, Hyde DM: Neutrophil sequestration and migration in localized pulmonary inflammation. Capillary localization and migration across the interalveolar septum. *Am Rev Respir Dis* 147:168, 1993.

78. Brown GM, Brown DM, Donaldson K, Drost E, MacNee W: Neutrophil sequestration in rat lungs. *Thorax* 50:661, 1995.

79. Buttrum SM, Drost EM, MacNee W, et al: Rheological response of neutrophils to different types of stimulation. *J Appl Physiol* 77:1801, 1994.

80. Downey GP, Doherty DE, Schwab B III, et al: Retention of leukocytes in capillaries: Role of cell size and deformability. *J Appl Physiol* 69:1767, 1990.

81. Downey GP, Worthen GS: Neutrophil retention in model capillaries: Deformability, geometry, and hydrodynamic forces. *J Appl Physiol* 65:1861, 1988.

82. Erzurum SC, Downey GP, Doherty DE, et al: Mechanisms of lipopolysaccharide-induced neutrophil retention. Relative contributions of adhesive and cellular mechanical properties. *J Immunol* 149:154, 1992.

83. Worthen GS, Schwab B III, Elson EL, Downey GP: Mechanics of stimulated neutrophils: Cell stiffening induces retention of capillaries. *Science* 245:183, 1989.
84. Doyle NA, Bhagwan SD, Meek BB, et al: Neutrophil margination, sequestration, and emigration in the lungs of L-selectin-deficient mice. *J Clin Invest* 99:526, 1997.
85. Kubo H, Doyle NA, Graham L, et al: L- and P-selectin and CD11/CD18 in intracapillary neutrophil sequestration in rabbit lungs. *Am J Respir Crit Care Med* 159:267, 1999.
86. Doerschuk CM, Mizgerd JP, Kubo H, et al: Adhesion molecules and cellular biomechanical changes in acute lung injury: Giles F. Filley Lecture. *Chest* 116:37S, 1999.
87. Doerschuk CM, Quinlan WM, Doyle NA, et al: The role of P-selectin and ICAM-1 in acute lung injury as determined using blocking antibodies and mutant mice. *J Immunol* 157:4609, 1996.
88. Gamble JR, Skinner MP, Berndt MC, Vadas MA: Prevention of activated neutrophil adhesion to endothelium by soluble adhesion protein GMP140. *Science* 249:414, 1990.
89. Jaeschke H, Farhood A, Fisher MA, Smith CW: Sequestration of neutrophils in the hepatic vasculature during endotoxemia is independent of β2 integrins and intercellular adhesion molecule-1. *Shock* 6:351, 1996.
90. Bishop CR, Athens JW, Boggs DR, et al: Leukokinetic studies. 13. A non-steady-state kinetic evaluation of the mechanism of cortisone-induced granulocytosis. *J Clin Invest* 47:249, 1968.
91. Dale DC, Fauci AS, Guerry D IV, Wolff SM: Comparison of agents producing a neutrophilic leukocytosis in man. Hydrocortisone, prednisone, endotoxin, and etiocholanolone. *J Clin Invest* 56:808, 1975.
92. Stausz I, Barcsak J, Kekes E, Szebeni A: Prednisone-induced acute changes in circulating neutrophil granulocytes: I. In cases of normal granulocyte reserves. *Haematologia (Budap)* 1:319, 1993.
93. Dale DC, Fauci AS, Wolff SM: Alternate-day prednisone. Leukocyte kinetics and susceptibility to infections. *N Engl J Med* 291:1154, 1974.
94. Craddock CG Jr, Perry S, Ventzke LE, Lawrence JS: Evaluation of marrow granulocytic reserves in normal and disease states. *Blood* 15:840, 1960.
95. Marsh JC, Perry S: The granulocyte response to endotoxin in patients with hematologic disorders. *Blood* 23:581, 1964.
96. DeConti RC, Kaplan SR, Calabresi P: Endotoxin stimulation in patients with lymphoma: Correlation with the myelosuppressive effects of alkylating agents. *Blood* 39:602, 1972.
97. Korbitz BC, Toren FA, Davis HL Jr, et al: The Piromen test: A useful assay of bone marrow granulocyte reserves. *Curr Ther Res Clin Exp* 11:491, 1969.
98. Smith CW: Possible steps involved in the transition to stationary adhesion of rolling neutrophils: A brief review. *Microcirculation* 7:385, 2000.
99. Kubes P, Kerfoot SM: Leukocyte recruitment in the microcirculation: The rolling paradigm revisited. *News Physiol Sci* 16:76, 2001.
100. Ley K: Pathways and bottlenecks in the web of inflammatory adhesion molecules and chemoattractants. *Immunol Res* 24:87, 2001.
101. Haslett C: Granulocyte apoptosis and its role in the resolution and control of lung inflammation. *Am J Respir Crit Care Med* 160:S5, 1999.
102. Buescher ES, Gallin JI: Leukocyte transfusions in chronic granulomatous disease: Persistence of transfused leukocytes in sputum. *N Engl J Med* 307:800, 1982.
103. Lord BI, Gurney H, Chang J, Thatcher N, et al: Haemopoietic cell kinetics in humans treated with rGM-CSF. *Int J Cancer* 50:26, 1992.
104. Buchanan MR, Crowley CA, Rosin RE, et al: Studies on the interaction between GP-180 deficient neutrophils and vascular endothelium. *Blood* 60:160, 1982.

CHAPTER 62
EOSINOPHILS AND RELATED DISORDERS

Andrew J. Wardlaw

SUMMARY

Eosinophils continue to be studied intensively, in large part, as a result of their potential role in the pathogenesis of asthma. The concept of the eosinophil as a cell that has protective effects against helminthic parasite infection, but can cause tissue damage when inappropriately activated, remains intact, although the evidence for both these roles is circumstantial. Eosinophil production and function are profoundly influenced by interleukin (IL)-5; and, thus, eosinophilia is associated with diseases characterized by T-helper (Th)2-mediated immune responses, including infections by helminthic parasites and extrinsic asthma. However, eosinophilia also occurs in diseases not obviously associated with Th2 dominance, such as intrinsic asthma, hypereosinophilic syndromes (HESs), and inflammatory bowel disease. Thus, IL-5 and other eosinophil mediators can be generated in various types of inflammatory response.

The eosinophil, like other leukocytes, can generate proinflammatory mediators. Eosinophil-specific granule proteins are toxic for a range of mammalian cells and parasitic larvae. Eosinophils, like mast cells, produce sulfidopeptide leukotrienes, as well as other lipid mediators, such as platelet-activating factor (PAF). Cytokine production by eosinophils broadens their potential functions, for example in wound healing through their generation of transforming growth factor (TGF)-α. Synthesis of TGF-β may explain the propensity of eosinophils to be associated with fibrotic reactions such as endomyocardial fibrosis, characteristic of HES, and fibrosing alveolitis.

Considerable effort has gone into trying to unravel the molecular basis of eosinophil tissue recruitment. The selective accumulation of eosinophils is the result of a concerted and integrated series of events involving their production in the marrow and egress therefrom, adhesion to endothelium, selective chemotaxis, and prolonged survival in tissues. These events are controlled, either directly or indirectly, by production of IL-4, IL-5, and IL-13.

The discovery that a proportion of patients with HES have either a clonal myeloid neoplasm resulting from an acquired mutation that generates a constitutively active, novel tyrosine kinase (FIP1L1-PDGFRα [F/P]) or a T-cell lymphoproliferative disease causing a reactive eosinophilia has offered the prospect of new and more effective treatments for these conditions, as well as giving new insights into the control of eosinophil production. There has long been a debate about the extent to which eosinophils cause tissue damage, are innocent bystanders, or even help to ameliorate the condition. This is now being resolved with data showing that specific reduction in eosinophils using anti–IL-5 monoclonal antibody is beneficial in eosinophilic airway disease and HES.

Acronyms and Abbreviations: AAV, ANCA-associated vasculitides; AHR, airway hyperresponsiveness; ANCA, antineutrophil cytoplasmic antibodies; BAL, bronchoalveolar lavage; BSA, bovine serum albumin; CCL, chemokine (C-C motif) ligand; CCR, chemokine receptor; CEL, chronic eosinophilic leukemia; CLC, Charcot-Leyden crystal; CLM-1, CMRF35-like molecule-1; CMPD, chronic myeloproliferative disease; ECP, eosinophil cationic protein; EDN, eosinophil-derived neurotoxin; EGPA, eosinophilic granulomatosis with polyangiitis; EM, electron microscopic; EMR, mucin-like hormone receptor; FEV_1, forced expiratory volume in 1 second; FISH, fluorescence *in situ* hybridization; GM-CSF, granulocyte-monocyte colony-stimulating growth factor; GPA, granulomatosis with polyangiitis; HES, hypereosinophilic syndrome; HLA, human leukocyte antigen; ICAM, intercellular adhesion molecule; iHES, idiopathic hypereosinophilic syndrome; IL, interleukin; ILC, innate lymphoid cell; LAMP, lysosome-associated membrane protein; LIMP, lysosome integral membrane protein; LT, leukotriene; mAb, monoclonal antibody; MBP, major basic protein; MPA, microscopic polyangiitis; NADPH, nicotinamide adenine dinucleotide phosphate oxidase; NO, nitric oxide; ORMDL3, orosomucoid-like 3; PAF, platelet-activating factor; PIN1, peptidylprolyl isomerase; PSGL, P-selectin glycoprotein ligand; Siglec, sialic acid-recognizing animal lectin; SNARE, soluble *N*-ethylmaleimide–sensitive factor attachment protein receptor complex; TGF, transforming growth factor; Th, T-helper; TRAIL, tumor necrosis factor-related apoptosis-inducing ligand; T_{REG}, T-regulatory cell; TSLP, thymic stromal lymphopoietin; TXB_2, thromboxane B_2; VCAM, vascular cell adhesion molecule; VIP, vasoactive intestinal peptide; VLA, very-late antigen; WHO, World Health Organization.

● BIOLOGY OF EOSINOPHILS

EOSINOPHIL MORPHOLOGY AND RECEPTOR PHENOTYPE

Eosinophils are spherical, end-stage, nondividing leukocytes, approximately 8 μm in diameter derived from the marrow.[1] *In vitro* granulocyte-monocyte colony-stimulating factor (GM-CSF), interleukin (IL)-3 and IL-5 stimulate colony growth; additionally, IL-5 is a critical eosinopoietic factor *in vivo* involved in late differentiation.[2] The electron microscopic (EM) morphology of the mature eosinophil has been well described (Fig. 62–1).[3,4] The relatively specific features which distinguish the eosinophil from other leukocytes are the bilobed nucleus, the specific granules with an electron dense core, the paucity of mitochondria (approximately 20 per cell) and endoplasmic reticulum, and the dense network of cytoplasmic tubulovesicular structures or secretory vesicles that contain albumin and cytochrome b_{558} and are therefore thought to be involved in superoxide production. Eosinophils also contain lipid bodies, which are the major site of eicosanoid synthesis, primary granules, and small granules.[5] Small granules are particularly prominent in tissue eosinophils and contain arylsulphatase B, acid phosphatase, and catalase. They may be derived from specific granules and act as a lysosomal compartment since specific granules express lysosome-associated membrane proteins (LAMP) 1 and 2, as well as lysosome integral membrane protein (LIMP, CD63) 1.[6] Eosinophils also contain multilaminar bodies that contain transforming growth factor (TGF)–α. Eosinophil precursors derived from cord blood can be first identified morphologically when specific core containing granules appear, although expression of Charcot Leyden crystal (CLC) protein and the basic granules proteins can be detected by immunohistochemistry or mRNA expression at the promyelocyte stage where they are found in the endoplasmic reticulum, Golgi apparatus and large round coreless granules, most of which develop

Lipid Mediators
LTC$_4$/D$_4$
PAF
15 HETE
TBX-B2
PGE 1&2

Eosinophil Basic Proteins
MBP:EDN:EPO:ECP

Superoxide

CLC protein

Cytokines
IL-1–6, 9–12, 13, 17
TGF α/β
GM-CSF

Chemokines
CXCL8
CCL3
CCL5
CXCL10

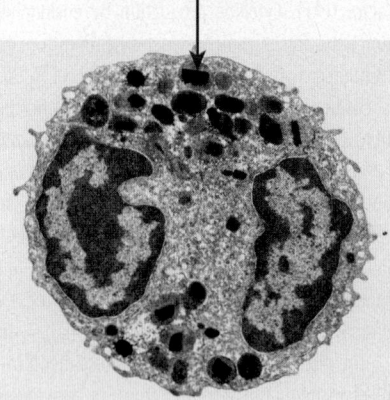

Growth Factors
Nerve GF:PDGF:VEGF:stem cell factor
Heparin-binding epidermal GF-like
binding protein

Enzymes
Phospholipase D
Arylsulfatase
Histaminase
Catalase
Acid phosphatase
Nonspecific esterases
Glycosaminoglycans
hexosaminidase

Figure 62–1. Transmission electron micrograph (×10,000) of an eosinophil showing the characteristic specific granules with their electron dense core and various mediators, receptors and granule proteins produced by eosinophils. CLC, Charcot-Leyden crystal; ECP, eosinophil cationic protein; EDN, eosinophil-derived neurotoxin; EPO, eosinophil peroxidase; GF, growth factor; GM-CSF, granulocyte-monocyte colony-stimulating growth factor; HETE, hydroxyeicosatetraenoic acid; LT, leukotriene; MBP, major basic protein; PAF, platelet-activating factor; PDGF, platelet-derived growth factor; PG, prostaglandin; PSGL, P-selectin glycoprotein ligand; TBX, thromboxane; TGF-β, transforming growth factor-β; VEGF, vascular endothelial growth factor. *(Used with permission of Dr. A. Dewar, National Heart and Lung Institute.)*

into specific granules. Electron microscopy can distinguish activated from resting blood eosinophils by the increased number of lipid bodies, primary and small granules, secretory vesicles, and endoplasmic reticulum. Cytoplasmic crystals of CLC protein may also be present. Eosinophils are relatively inefficient phagocytes, although they can ingest opsonized zymosan, which gets taken up into phagolysosomes formed in part by fusion with specific granules. The eosinophil also degranulates onto large opsonized surfaces such as a Sephadex bead or parasitic larvae in a process called *frustrated phagocytosis.*

The ultrastructure of *in vitro* activated and tissue-infiltrating eosinophils has suggested three potential mechanisms of degranulation: necrosis or cytolytic degranulation, exocytosis or "classical degranulation," and piecemeal degranulation.[7] Cytolytic degranulation is associated with loss of eosinophil plasma membrane integrity and results in the release of clusters of free membrane-bound granules (termed *Cfegs*). This is commonly observed in eosinophilic inflammation and is particularly marked in severe disease, such as fatal attacks of asthma in which large quantities of basic proteins can be detected in the tissue by immunohistochemistry often with relatively few intact eosinophils.[8] Exocytosis or classical degranulation occurs in mast cells and basophils after crosslinking of immunoglobulin (Ig) E receptors. It describes a process by which granules migrate to the plasma membrane and fuse with it leading to the extrusion of membrane free granule contents. This phenomenon has been described for eosinophils in the gut, but not the airway mucosa. Piecemeal degranulation has been described in cord blood derived eosinophils[9] and refers to the appearance of empty or partially empty granules together with small vesicles in the cytoplasm which transport the granule proteins to the cell surface where they are released.[10] These appearances are common in tissue eosinophils in asthma and other allergic diseases.

Many studies have used a mouse model involving ovalbumin challenge to generate a lung eosinophilia and increased airway hyperresponsiveness (AHR). A striking feature of this model is that lung eosinophils do not have the appearance of having undergone degranulation by either cytolysis or piecemeal degranulation.[11] Immunostaining of the mouse lung in this model locates all the basic proteins within intact eosinophils and bronchoalveolar lavage (BAL) contains no free major basic protein (MBP).[12] This is quite unlike human disease in which the

cell free basic proteins can be readily detected in both tissue and BAL. Consistent with this observation, mice in which the gene for eosinophil peroxidase or MBP has been deleted had the same phenotype as wild-type mice.[13] However some degranulation may be seen in the airway lumen.[14] Mice were genetically modified using two approaches to completely delete eosinophils, one by inserting an eosinophil toxic gene into the lineage (PHIL) and one by deleting a high-affinity binding site in the GATA-1 promoter.[15,16] The GATA mice still developed AHR and mucus secretion but not airway remodeling, which is consistent with evidence for their role in asthma. In contrast, the PHIL mouse did not develop AHR and mucus hypersecretion after airway challenge. Two other strains of mice, iPHIL and eoCRE, have been developed. iPHIL can induce eosinophil cell death at any point in the life of the mouse using diphtheria toxin and eoCRE can be used to selectively induce gene expression in eosinophils. These flexible "knock-in" strains of mice have revealed unexpected complexity in the role of the eosinophil in the allergic immune response.[17] Apoptotic eosinophils are small cells with a shrunken nucleus and condensed chromatin but an intact plasma membrane. They are readily identifiable in aged cell populations *in vitro* and in cells from the airway lumen such as sputum, but are more difficult to identify in tissue. This has led some investigators to argue that the majority of airway eosinophils, at least in asthma and rhinitis, are removed through luminal entry rather than by undergoing apoptosis in tissue.[7]

Like all leukocytes, eosinophils express a large number of membrane receptors which allow them to interact with the extracellular environment (Tables 62–1 and 62–2). These include receptors required for locomotion, activation, growth and mediator release. Most of the receptors are shared to some extent with other leukocytes but some have a degree of specificity in terms of level of expression and function. An important feature of tissue eosinophils is that they express a different pattern of receptors, compared to blood eosinophils, consistent with a more activated phenotype. This includes induction of expression of CD69, intercellular adhesion molecule (ICAM)-1 and FcγR1 and increased expression of human leukocyte antigen (HLA)-DR and Mac-1. Changes in expression can be induced *in vitro* by culture with cytokines such as IL-5, but also occur to some extent as the result of transmigration through endothelium.[18] A major difference between eosinophils and neutrophils that has been exploited to purify eosinophils

TABLE 62–1. Eosinophil Adhesion Receptors

Receptor	Ligand	
	Endothelial	Matrix Protein
INTEGRINS		
$\alpha_4\beta_1$ (VLA-4)	VCAM-1	Fibronectin
$\alpha_4\beta_6$		Laminin
$\alpha_4\beta_7$	MAdCAM-1	Fibronectin
LFA-1 ($\alpha_N\beta_2$)	ICAM-1-3	
Mac-1 ($\alpha_M\beta_2$)	ICAM-1	
P150,95 ($\alpha_x\beta_2$)		
$\alpha_d\beta_2$	VCAM-1 (ICAM-3?)	
SELECTINS AND LIGANDS		
PSGL-1	P-selectin(E-selectin)	
L-Selectin	Gly-CAM-1, CD34, Podocalyxin	
OTHER		
CD44		Hyaluronate
ICAM-3		
PECAM	PECAM	

ICAM, intercellular cell adhesion molecule; MAdCAM-1, mucosal addressin cell adhesion molecule; PECAM: platelet endothelial cell adhesion molecule; PSGL-1, P-selectin glycoprotein 1; VCAM-1, vascular cell adhesion molecule.

by immunomagnetic selectin is the expression of CD16 by neutrophils but not eosinophils. Another important difference is the expression of VLA-4 by eosinophils, but not to any great extent in neutrophils. Sialic acid-recognizing animal lectin (Siglec) 8 has been identified as a receptor expressed only by eosinophils, mast cells, and basophils.[19–21] Siglecs are of the immunoglobulin superfamily. Eosinophils, as well as monocytes and a subset of dendritic cells, also express Siglec 10.[22] In contrast, neutrophils express Siglec 9.[23] Siglec 8 is important in triggering eosinophil apoptosis.[24,25] Epidermal growth factor-like module containing mucin-like hormone receptor 1 (EMR1) is expressed exclusively on eosinophils and has the potential to be a therapeutic target for eosinophilic disorders.[26] Eosinophils express both CD48 and its ligand CD244 (2B4), both members of the IgG superfamily. Crosslinking of CD48 causes eosinophil degranulation.[27] Eosinophils also express a number of inhibitory receptors including CMRF35-like molecule-1 (CLM-1) that negatively regulate eotaxin-induced eosinophil responses.[28]

TABLE 62–2. Eosinophil Adhesion Receptors

Immunoglobulin receptors: Fcγ R11 (CD32); Fcα R;

Receptors for mediators: CCR3*; CCR1; PAF-R; LTC4/D4/E4-R; LTB4-R; C5aR; C3aR; IL-5R*; IL-3R; IL-4R; IL-13R; CRTh2

Receptors induced by cytokine stimulation: Fcγ RIII (CD16); Fcγ R1 (CD69); HLA-DR; ICAM-1; CD25; CD4

Well-expressed miscellaneous receptors: CD9; CD45; CR1; CD154 (CD40 ligand); CD95 (Fas); Siglec 8*; ERM1*; CLM-1

*Relatively selectively expressed by eosinophils.

EOSINOPHIL PRODUCTION

Eosinophils are nondividing, end-stage cells that, like other leukocytes, differentiate from the hematopoietic stem cell in the marrow. They share a progenitor with basophils before further differentiation separates the lineages. GATA-1 is a particularly important transcription factor for eosinophil development with deletion of the high-affinity binding site in GATA-1 resulting in specific loss of the eosinophil lineage.[29] The F/P receptor mutation which is responsible for a myeloproliferative form of hypereosinophilic syndrome (HES)/chronic eosinophilic leukemia (CEL) works through cEBPα and GATA-2, as well as GATA-1, showing that these transcription factors are also important in eosinophil development.[30] Eosinophilopoiesis requires the combined expression of MBP and eosinophil peroxidase.[31]

Eosinophils migrate into the blood, where they circulate with a half-life of about 18 hours before entering the tissues. Eosinophils are primarily tissue-dwelling cells, and it has been estimated that there are approximately 100 tissue eosinophils for each eosinophil in the blood, although relatively few studies have been performed on eosinophil kinetics and even fewer have compared eosinophil turnover in health and disease. However, studies demonstrate that eosinophils can be tracked *in vivo* using radiolabeling and that the kinetics of migration through the lung, spleen, and marrow are distinct from that of neutrophils.[32,33] Normal human adult marrow contains approximately 3 percent eosinophils of which one-third are mature and two-thirds are precursors.

Eosinophilia is often T-cell dependent. Characterization of T-cell–derived supernatants led to the characterization of IL-5 and awareness of the pivotal role that this cytokine plays in eosinophil development.[34] IL-3 and GM-CSF are also important in eosinophil development. The three cytokines bind to receptors that share a common β chain but have distinct α chains. IL-5 seems to be a rate-limiting step for eosinophil production in that administration of IL-5 either exogenously or through transgenic manipulation in mice results in a marked eosinophilia[35] and anti–IL-5 in humans dramatically diminishes the blood eosinophil count in asthma.[36] Increased eosinophilopoiesis as a result of increased IL-5 synthesis appears to be a feature of a number of diseases, including parasitic and allergic diseases. For example, pulmonary eosinophilia caused by *Necator americanus* infection in mice is IL-5–dependent[37] and both the eosinophilia and host defense to filariasis and *Trichinella spiralis* is markedly impaired in IL-5–deficient mice.[38] In asthma, IL-5 mRNA can be detected in increased amounts in the airways in asthma.[39] However, IL-5 gene-deleted mice have a baseline eosinophilia and can develop pulmonary eosinophilia after infection with paramyxovirus, demonstrating that other late differentiation factors such as chemokine (C-C motif) ligand (CCL)-3 may be involved.[40,41] It is therefore an accepted paradigm that a blood and tissue eosinophilia in IgE-mediated diseases, such as atopic asthma and helminthic parasite infections, are a result of antigen-dependent activation of T-helper (Th)-2 cells leading to IL-5 production and increased eosinophilopoiesis and tissue recruitment of eosinophils. The control of development of Th2 and Th1 cells is beyond the scope of this chapter, but may relate to the cytokine milieu at the time of sensitization, genetically regulated transcriptional control of IL-4, or the route of sensitization and the way in which the antigen is presented (Chap. 76).[42,43] The HLA haplotype of individuals responsive to certain allergens has also been investigated. A degree of restriction has been observed, particularly to simple allergens, with, for example, the phenotype DR2.2 being overrepresented in individuals atopic to the ragweed allergen Amb a V. However, with the majority of allergens, no clear pattern has emerged. Although HLA haplotypes may influence responses to individual allergens, it is unlikely to provide a universal explanation for Th2-type responsiveness.

Many eosinophilic diseases, including many cases of pulmonary eosinophilia, are not associated with atopy and IgE production and therefore do not entirely fit with the Th2-driven eosinophilic paradigm. Intrinsic asthma is generally assumed to be associated with IL-5-producing T cells; however, the evidence for this is limited. One model for non–IgE-associated eosinophilic disease is those cases of eosinophilic esophagitis caused by a defined food allergen in which there is no specific IgE.[44] In some of these cases, the patients are patch-test–positive to the food allergen concerned, which raises the possibility of a Th2 type of type IV cell-mediated immunity, but this is still unexplored.

There is increasing interest in the role of T regulatory cells (T_{REG}) in controlling inappropriate immune responses including those associated with Th2 cell activation.[45] T_{REG} were first identified as mediating some aspects of immune tolerance and were then found to play an important role in suppressing immune-mediated inflammatory bowel disease in mice. Three types of T_{REG} cells have been identified: CD4+/CD25+ cells which require direct contact to mediate their immunosuppressive effects, T_{REG} cells producing TGF-β and T_{REG} cells producing IL-10.[46–48] A current idea is that the increase in allergic disease that is also paralleled by an increase in autoimmune disease is not caused by a Th1 to Th2 switch, but by a failure to develop T_{REG} responses, which leads to enhancement of both Th1 and Th2 immunity.[49–51] IL-10 producing T_{REG} is of particular interest in the context of pulmonary eosinophilia because of evidence that immunotherapy works by inducing expansion of an antigen specific IL-10 producing T_{REG} cells.[52] In addition, regulatory T cells were able to suppress ovalbumin-induced pulmonary eosinophilia in mice.[53]

EOSINOPHIL HETEROGENEITY

Blood eosinophils from normal individuals are relatively dense cells that can be separated from other leukocytes by density-gradient centrifuge. For many years these differences were the basis for the standard method of purifying eosinophils. This method has now been largely superseded by negative immunomagnetic selection based on the expression of the low affinity (Fcγ RIII, CD16) IgG receptor by neutrophils but not eosinophils. This latter technique has the advantage of improved purity and cell yields as well as enabling purification of eosinophils from individuals with low eosinophil counts, A proportion of eosinophils from individuals with elevated eosinophil counts are less dense than eosinophils from normal subjects. So-called hypodense eosinophils appear to be vacuolated and contain smaller granules, although in equal numbers to normal-density eosinophils. The mechanism for this heterogeneity is unclear; although a correlation with eosinophil activation has been a favored hypothesis, the evidence to support this hypothesis is contradictory.[54]

EOSINOPHIL TRAFFICKING AND TISSUE ACCUMULATION

Eosinophils are not normally found in tissues other than the gut and the appearance of increased numbers of these cells can be a notable feature of the pathology of a number of diseases. The normal pattern of gut homing of eosinophils is likely to be mediated by CCL-11 (eotaxin 1), which is constitutively expressed in the gut, and the integrin $\alpha_4\beta_7$ binding to mucosal addressin cell adhesion molecule (MAdCAM)-1, which is selectively expressed in the intestine.[55] Type 2 innate lymphoid cells are central to this process, constitutively producing IL-5, which generates an eosinophilia, and IL-13, which stimulates production of eotaxin. Activation of innate lymphoid cell (ILC)-2 was modulated by nutrient intake and circadian rhythms, which may explain the circadian cycling of blood eosinophils.[56] Although an eosinophilia can accompany a

general inflammatory response, as for example in idiopathic pulmonary fibrosis where increased numbers of eosinophils and neutrophils can be seen in the BAL fluid, it often occurs without a marked increase in other leukocytes raising the question of the mechanism behind the specific tissue accumulation of these picturesque leukocytes. Selective eosinophil accumulation occurs as a result of the coordinated effect of a number of adhesion, chemotactic and growth/survival orientated signals at each stage in the life cycle of the cell. Generally speaking, these events are controlled by mediators associated with Th2 cells, in particular the cytokines IL-4, IL-5, IL-13, and possibly IL-9.[57,58] Another group of epithelial derived cytokines—IL-25, IL-33, and thymic stromal lymphopoietin (TSLP)—play a key role in the development of eosinophilic inflammation through the activation of a newly described class of innate immune cells called ILC2.[59]

As well as being crucial for differentiation, IL-5 is also important in promoting emigration from the marrow. In particular, it acts as a priming factor for specific chemoattractants such as eotaxin.[60] The observation that eotaxin decreased adhesion to vascular cell adhesion molecule (VCAM)-1 while increasing adhesion to the CD18 ligand bovine serum albumin (BSA) may be a mechanism for promoting egress from the marrow.[61] Localized inflammatory responses can cause systemic effects after allergen challenge in mice in which IL-5–producing cells (both T cells and non–T cells), increase in the marrow.[62]

Accumulation of leukocytes in tissue is a highly regulated process with the aim of being able to respond effectively to noxious insults without causing an inappropriate inflammatory response. An obligate step in the migration of all leukocytes from the systemic circulation into tissue is their capture by endothelium as they flow at high shear rates through the postcapillary endothelium. A key receptor mediating eosinophil capture is P-selectin, whose low-level surface expression is selectively induced on endothelium by IL-4 and IL-13. Eosinophils express higher levels of P-selectin glycoprotein ligand (PSGL)-1 (the primary receptor for P-selectin) than other leukocytes and this results in increased avidity for P-selectin compared to neutrophils, especially at the low levels of expression induced by Th2 cytokines.[63] Increased expression of PSGL-1 leading to enhanced recruitment has also been reported in allergic disease.[64] IL-4 and IL-13 can also induce low levels of VCAM-1 expression which can bind eosinophils through very-late antigen (VLA)-4 and also capture flowing cells albeit at lower shear stresses. VLA-4/VCAM-1 and PSGL-1/P-selectin cooperate as a major endothelial control point for selective eosinophil migration.[65] Once captured, eosinophils roll along the surface of the blood vessel until they are activated, which allows the CD18 integrins binding to ICAM-1 and ICAM-2 to nonselectively promote transmigration. VLA-4/VCAM-1 can also exert selective pressure at this stage.[66] In mice, this process is dependent on the intracellular RAC-binding protein SWAP-70.[67] The activation step mediated by chemoattractants expressed on the endothelial surface is another potential point of eosinophil selection, as shown by the effect of exogenously added chemoattractants such as eotaxin, but the identity of the endogenous chemoattractant involved and the extent to which it is selectively expressed in eosinophilic inflammation remains to be conclusively resolved. Orosomucoid-like 3 (ORMDL3), a molecule that has been identified by genetic epidemiology to be associated with asthma, is expressed by eosinophils and gene deletion in a mouse model resulted in reduced adhesion and recruitment into the lung.[68]

Once the eosinophil has transmigrated through the endothelium it has to migrate through the basement membrane and into the tissue. Chemokines as well as other eosinophil chemoattractants are likely to be central to this process (Table 62–3). Many eosinophil-active chemokines bind to the chemokine receptor (CCR)-3 and deletion of this gene severely impairs eosinophil migration into the lung in the mouse asthma model. The three specific eosinophil chemokines, eotaxins 1 to 3, appear

TABLE 62–3. Eosinophil Chemokine Receptors and Their Ligands

Receptor	Chemokine
CCR1*	CCL3 (Mip-1a); CCL5 (RANTES)
CCR3	CCL11 (eotaxin 1); CCL24 (eotaxin 2); CCL26 (eotaxin 3); CCL7, -8, -13 (MCP2–4); CCL5
CXCR1, -2	CXCL8 (IL-8†)

*Only expressed on eosinophils from some donors.

†Only active on *in vivo*–activated or cytokine-primed eosinophils (may be indirect effect via neutrophils).

to play overlapping roles in eosinophil migration into the lung in mice.[69] However, a potent CCR3 antagonist had no effect on eosinophil migration into the airways in human asthma, questioning the physiologic relevance of the mouse data in human disease.[70]

Apoptosis is the universal mechanism by which cells undergo cell senescence in a manner that allows them to be efficiently removed by macrophages without inducing an inflammatory response. Morphologic observations have indicated that eosinophil apoptosis is an unusual event in tissue and that most eosinophils either die by cytolysis or migrate into the lumen where they do become apoptotic.[7] A slow rate of apoptosis in tissues is consistent with the survival signals delivered to eosinophils by the extracellular matrix as part of normal homeostasis as well as increased production of eosinophil growth factors during Th2-mediated inflammation.[71,72] The importance of prolonged survival of eosinophils in tissue as a mechanism for selective accumulation has been emphasized by studies using anti–IL-5, which effectively inhibits blood and sputum eosinophil numbers but has a much-less-marked effect on tissue eosinophils.[73] Unlike neutrophils, where they prolong survival, glucocorticoids directly enhance the rate of eosinophil apoptosis, an effect inhibited by IL-5.[74] Tumor necrosis factor-related apoptosis-inducing ligand (TRAIL), another family of survival modulating mediators related to tumor necrosis factor (TNF)-α, prolongs eosinophil survival, both *in vitro* and *ex vivo*, after allergen challenge.[75]

The biochemical mechanism by which growth factors mediate eosinophil survival is dependent on both new protein synthesis and phosphorylation events. The survival effects of IL-5 are dependent on activation of the Ras-Raf-MEC pathway and the Jak-2 Stat 1 and Stat 5 pathways, and involve LYN kinase, which binds to the IL-5Rα chain.[76] The roles of p38 and phosphatidylinositide (PI) 3 kinase are less clear, and wortmannin, which blocks PI3 kinase, had no effect on eosinophil apoptosis, although it did inhibit IL-5 enhancement of adhesion to fibrinogen. Eosinophils express significant amounts of the proapoptotic BAX and the antiapoptotic BCL-xl, but very little Bad or BCL-2. As in other cell types, both spontaneous and FAS-induced eosinophil apoptosis is associated with the migration of BAX into the mitochondria. This event led to loss of mitochondrial membrane potential, cytochrome c release, and activation of downstream caspases. These events are all inhibited by IL-5, demonstrating that IL-5 works by blocking BAX translocation.[77,78] Inhibition of BAX activation prevents eosinophil apoptosis even in the absence of cytokine. Treatment of eosinophils with dexamethasone also leads to loss of mitochondrial permeability.[79] GM-CSF–activated ERK1/2, which phosphorylates BAX at Thr167, facilitates interaction with peptidylprolyl isomerase (PIN1). If interaction with PIN1 is prevented, BAX is activated and translocated to the mitochondria, resulting in apoptosis. It appears, therefore, that the eosinophil growth factors exert their antiapoptotic effects through fostering the PIN1–BAX interaction.[80] IL-5–mediated eosinophil survival is

also regulated by the balance between the signaling through two paired immunoglobulin-like receptors, PIR-A and PIR-B, with PIR-B counteracting the proapoptotic effect of PIR-A.[81]

Another potential mechanism involved in eosinophil tissue accumulation is *in situ* differentiation from eosinophil precursors. Eosinophil precursors can be identified in an IL-5Rα⁺CD34⁺ population in blood, increased after allergen challenge and in atopic disease. These cells have also been found in asthmatic airways.[82]

Of equal importance as endothelial interactions to the kinetics of eosinophil migration are the factors controlling the fate of the eosinophil once it enters the tissue. There are three possible outcomes. The eosinophil can remain in the tissue interacting with matrix proteins, other leukocytes, or structural cells such as, in the bronchial mucosa, the epithelium, airway smooth muscle, mucus glands, and nerves; alternatively, the cell can migrate into the lumen of the gut or airway where it is likely to undergo apoptosis and be removed; or it can return to the circulation via the lymphatics. The length of time that eosinophils remain in tissue before migrating into the lumen is unclear as there are virtually no studies of the kinetics of eosinophil migration *in vivo* in humans. An anti–IL-5 completely inhibited migration into the lumen, which suggests that transepithelial migration is IL-5–dependent. However, it only inhibited tissue numbers by at best 50 percent, emphasizing that different compartments are controlled by different mechanisms.[73] In the mouse model of asthma, eosinophil migration into the lumen does not occur in the MMP-2 gene-deleted mouse, and the lack of migration causes the mouse to asphyxiate.[83] As with senescent neutrophils, when tissue eosinophils become senescent they start to alter their receptor phenotype in a way that inhibits tissue retention and promotes migration into the lumen.[84] The factors controlling the retention and survival of eosinophils in tissue are likely to involve the integration of chemoattractant, adhesive, and survival signals delivered by interactions with matrix proteins and structural cells. Studies modeling eosinophil migration in a tissue context using collagen gels have shown a different pattern to standard Boyden chamber assays with a much greater, albeit random, migratory response to growth factors than to chemoattractants.[85] This observation suggests that migration into the lumen requires both a growth factor and a chemotactic stimulus.

ANIMAL MODELS OF EOSINOPHILIC DISEASE

Animal models, particularly the mouse model of ovalbumin challenge, which results in a selective and marked pulmonary eosinophilia, have been used extensively to analyze the molecular basis of eosinophil trafficking and the pathologic consequences of this movement.[86] The majority of studies have focused on the role of eosinophilic inflammation in asthma.[87] The combination of transgenic, gene-deletion, and antibody-based manipulations in the mouse make this a powerful tool for analyzing the biology of eosinophil migration, although the relevance of the findings to human disease should be treated with caution. Generally speaking, these studies support the concept of eosinophil migration as being caused by a series of interlinked and obligate steps with IL-5 necessary for providing a pool of circulating eosinophils, priming eosinophils for chemotactic responsiveness, and prolonging eosinophil survival. IL-4 and IL-13 control adhesion-related events in the endothelium and enhance the release of eosinophil chemoattractants, particularly CCR3-binding chemokines from mesenchymal cells within the airway.[58] However, there are a number of other studies that look at other aspects of the immune response and as a result challenge this neat concept, in particular showing potential roles for innate immunity as well as other inflammatory mediators.[88-90] Our understanding of the role of eosinophils in health and disease, using mouse models of disease, has been summarized.[17]

EOSINOPHIL FUNCTIONS

The eosinophil exerts its effects largely through its mediators (see Fig. 62–1). These chemicals are either newly generated, as is the case with leukotrienes and other lipid mediators, or stored preformed in various compartments within the cytoplasm and released when the eosinophil receives a degranulating stimulus. The eosinophil is relatively biosynthetically inactive and, although new protein synthesis does occur, the majority of its protein mediators are stored. Although the eosinophil can phagocytose particles its interactions with larval forms of helminthic parasites have formed the model by which eosinophil function has been described. In this situation, the eosinophil adheres tightly to the organism and releases its granule contents in local, high concentrations onto the surface in a process described as frustrated phagocytosis. The paradigm of eosinophil effector function in host defense was developed from the observation that the basic granule proteins, in particular, were highly toxic for larval parasites. This observation was extended to include a proinflammatory role in which they were also shown to be toxic for bronchial epithelium and, therefore, associated with the epithelial desquamation which is a well-established feature of severe asthma. Eosinophils are not thought to play a major role in bacterial host defense and, indeed, bacterial sepsis causes an eosinopenia; however, eosinophils can release mitochondrial DNA which has antibacterial properties.[91] Eosinophils can also release a plethora of cytokines and chemokines although many of these are generated in low amounts compared to other cells and the extent to which they are important in eosinophil function is not clear.[92]

Role in Immunoregulation

Most research into the role of eosinophils has focused on host defense against helminthic parasites and as effector cells in asthma. However, since 2010 there has been groundbreaking research emphasizing a potential homeostatic role for eosinophils in a number of areas, including antigen presentation, tissue repair, adipogenesis and glucose homeostasis, and B-cell development.[93] There has been evidence for many years that eosinophils can present antigen to T cells, although the physiologic relevance of this function in the context of an intact dendritic cell antigen-presenting capacity remains uncertain.[94] Type 2 immunity is necessary for the regeneration of skeletal muscle after injury. Muscle damage resulted in the rapid recruitment of eosinophils, which secretes IL-4 and activates muscle resident stem cells.[95] Similarly, eosinophil-derived IL-4 was necessary for liver regeneration.[96] A role in adipose tissue and glucose homeostasis was first suggested in 2011 when it was demonstrated that eosinophils, through the production of IL-4, were necessary for the maintenance of adipose tissue associated alternatively activated macrophages, which, in turn, were necessary to control glucose metabolism and body fat.[97] This same pathway in concert with ILC2 cells is involved in the development of cold-induced, beige fat, which provides a defense against cold and obesity.[98,99] Long-lived plasma cells, which survive in specialized niches in the marrow, do so as a result of growth factors (APRIL and IL-6) supplied by colocalized eosinophils.[100] Eosinophils are also important in gut immune homeostasis, with eosinophil deficiency resulting in a reduction in IgA+ plasma cells and secreted IgA, as well as defects in the intestinal mucous shield, alteration in the gut microbiota, and the formation of CD103+ Tr and dendritic cells.[101] B-cell development was also shown to be regulated by eosinophils in mice and humans.[102] These studies were almost exclusively undertaken in mice, but they are potentially clinically relevant as a number of biologic therapies targeted at the Th2 pathway, including specific antieosinophil therapies, are in the late stages of clinical development for asthma and other eosinophilic diseases. So far, these drugs appear relatively free of serious adverse effects, so it is possible that the relatively modest effects of these drugs on the tissue eosinophilia means that the homeostatic role of eosinophils will not be perturbed.

Mediator Release

Eosinophils can release a number of lipid mediators and are one of the relatively few sources of suliphidopeptide leukotrienes, although per cell they release approximately 10-fold less than mast cells and basophils.[103] This is in contrast to neutrophils that produce large amounts of leukotriene (LT)B$_4$, but little, if any, LTC$_4$. LTC$_4$ generation by human eosinophils also occurs after stimulation with opsonized zymosan and beads coated with IgG. Eosinophils can also generate substantial quantities of 15-HETE (hydroxyeicosatetraenoic acid) via 15-lipoxygenase. Eosinophils also generate platelet-activating factor (PAF) after stimulation with either calcium ionophore or IgG-coated beads. Eosinophils can also generate mediators of the cyclooxygenase pathway, including prostaglandins E$_1$ and E$_2$, thromboxane B$_2$ (TXB$_2$), and prostaglandin D$_2$.[104] The principal sites of eicosanoid formation in eosinophils are the lipid bodies, which contain large amounts of arachidonic acid and enzymes required for eicosanoid synthesis, including 5-lipoxygenase, LTC$_4$ synthase, and cyclooxygenase.[105] Eosinophils release significant amounts of TGF–β and TGF–α and this has stimulated interest in a potential role in causing airway remodeling. There is evidence that TGF–β released by eosinophils can promote the generation of fibromyocytes and anti–IL-5 reduced the amount of tenascin in the reticular subepithelial membrane.[106,107] Thickening of this membrane is closely associated with eosinophilic airway inflammation, although not with AHR or airflow obstruction.[108] Vasoactive intestinal peptide (VIP) has been detected in eosinophils in granulomas from mice infected with schistosomes and the eosinophil contains a number of granule-stored enzymes, whose roles in eosinophil function are not clear. These enzymes include acid phosphatase, collagenase, arylsulfatase B, histaminase, phospholipase D, catalase, nonspecific esterases, vitamin B$_{12}$–binding proteins, and glycosaminoglycans. Eosinophils can undergo a respiratory burst with release of superoxide ion and H$_2$O$_2$ in response to stimulation, with both particulate stimuli, such as opsonized zymosan, and soluble mediators, such as leukotriene and phorbolmyristate acetate. Eosinophils are twice as chemoluminescent as neutrophils.

Eosinophil Granule Proteins

A specific and important feature of eosinophils is the large amounts of basic proteins they contain within their specific granules. These are MBP, eosinophil cationic protein (ECP), eosinophil peroxidase, and eosinophil derived neurotoxin (EDN).[109] MBP has a molecular mass of 13.8 kDa and an isoelectric point (pI) of 10.9. Its 17 arginine residues account for its alkalinity. It is initially synthesized as an acidic proprotein that is stored in the eosinophil granule. MBP becomes toxic only after it is released and processed into its final form. Purified MBP is cytotoxic for the schistosomula of *Schistosoma mansoni*, and adherence of eosinophils to IgG-coated schistosomula results in the secretion of MBP onto the tegument of the larvae, resulting in loss of viability.[110] MBP at concentrations as low as 10 mg/mL is toxic for both guinea pig and human respiratory epithelial cells, as well as for rat and human pneumocytes. The mechanism of action of MBP on epithelial cells is mediated through inhibition of adenosine triphosphatase (ATPase) activity. MBP and eosinophil peroxidase are strong agonists for platelet activation as well as activation of mast cells, basophils, and neutrophils.[111] The mechanisms of action of MBP is likely to be related to its hydrophobicity and strong negative charge. Basophils also contain MBP but only approximately 2 percent that of eosinophils.

Eosinophil peroxidase is a heme-containing protein that is synthesized as a single protein and then cleaved into 14- and 58-kDa subunits. The molecule shares a 68 percent identity in amino acid sequence with human neutrophil myeloperoxidase as well as other peroxidase enzymes. The protein is toxic for parasites, respiratory epithelium, and pneumocytes, either alone, or (more potently) when combined with H$_2$O$_2$ and halide, the preferred ion *in vivo* being bromide.

ECP is an arginine-rich protein. The complementary DNA (cDNA) encodes for a 27-amino-acid leader sequence and a 133-amino-acid mature polypeptide with a molecular mass of 15.6 kDa. ECP has 66 percent amino-acid-sequence homology with EDN and 31 percent homology with human pancreatic ribonuclease, but it has low ribonuclease activity compared to EDN. ECP is toxic for helminthic parasites, isolated myocardial cells, and guinea pig tracheal epithelium. ECP also inhibits lymphocyte proliferation *in vitro*. Both ECP and EDN produce neurotoxicity (the Gordon phenomenon) when injected into the cerebrospinal fluid of experimental animals. ECP may damage cells by a colloid osmotic process, as it can induce non–ion-selective pores in both cellular and synthetic membranes.

EDN, also called *EPX*, is a 16-kDa, glycosylated protein possessing marked ribonuclease activity. The cDNA predicts a 134-amino-acid, mature polypeptide that is identical to human urinary ribonuclease. Like ECP, it is a member of a ribonuclease multigene family. EDN expression is not restricted to eosinophils, as it is found in mononuclear cells and possibly neutrophils. It is also probably secreted by the liver. It does not appear to be toxic to parasites or mammalian cells, and its only known effect, other than its ribonuclease activity, is neurotoxicity.

A major constituent of eosinophil is CLC protein, which is a lysophospholipase. It constitutes up to 10 percent of eosinophil protein and is also found in large quantities in basophils. It was thought to possess lysophospholipase activity, but this is not the case. It is a member of the galactin family (galectin 10).[112] Its function is unknown.

EOSINOPHIL SECRETION AND ACTIVATION

A striking feature of eosinophil-rich inflammatory reactions is the high concentration of granule proteins, often in the presence of relatively small numbers of intact eosinophils. Sometimes free granules can be seen independent of eosinophils.[113] This may occur as part of a cytolytic nonapoptotic process involving nicotinamide adenine dinucleotide phosphate oxidase (NADPH) and the formation of extracellular DNA traps.[114,115] Mediator secretion can be triggered physiologically by engagement of immunoglobulin Fc receptors, especially after eosinophil activation has been primed with soluble mediators such as PAF, IL-5, and GM-CSF. Priming by GM-CSF involves phosphorylation of L-plastin and PKCβII.[116] The eosinophil expresses receptors for IgG, IgA, and IgD. The eosinophil also binds IgE, and eosinophils can undertake a number of IgE-dependent functions, including killing of schistosomes opsonized with specific IgE. The receptor involved is unclear as the accumulated evidence now suggests that eosinophils do not express either the low-affinity (FcϵRII) or high-affinity (FcϵRI) IgE receptor to any degree although they do express high intracellular levels of the α chain of FcϵRI.[117]

Three receptors for IgG have been described: the high-affinity receptor FcγR1 (CD64), and two low-affinity receptors FcγRII (CDw32) and FcγRIII (CD16). CD16 is expressed both as a transmembrane form and a form with a phosphatidylinositol anchor, transcribed from two distinct genes. Only FcγRII is constitutively expressed by eosinophils to any significant degree. A number of eosinophil functions are mediated via this receptor, including schistosomula killing, phagocytosis, secretion of granule proteins, and generation of newly formed, membrane-derived lipid mediators such as PAF and LTC$_4$. After stimulation for 2 days *in vitro* with interferon (IFN)-γ, eosinophils express CD16 and CD64 as well as CD32. Perhaps the most potent stimulus for eosinophil degranulation is crosslinking of IgA receptors, especially when the cells have been primed with growth factors. Consistent with the preference of eosinophils to secrete their mediators onto a large surface, Fc-mediated degranulation is enhanced if the eosinophils are adherent to a protein-coated surface via integrin $\alpha_M\beta_2$.[118] Eosinophils are particularly

effective in generating reactive oxygen species with about 1.7-fold greater generation than neutrophils after stimulation with PMA (phorbol myristate acetate), possibly as a result of a 10-fold greater expression of the voltage-gated channel Hv1.[119]

The killing of schistosomula opsonized with nonimmune serum is presumed to be mediated via the complement receptors, CR1 and CR3. Incubation of eosinophils with serum-coated beads results in the release of 15 percent of ECP. Similarly, opsonized zymosan interacts with eosinophils, causing generation of hydrogen peroxide and the phagocytosis of the zymosan. Soluble mediators, such as PAF, LTB$_4$, and 5-oxoeicosatetraenoate, can elicit the direct secretion of both granule proteins and lipid mediators, although only with highly activated eosinophils or when used in conjunction with cytochalasin B, which inhibits microtubule assembly. Eosinophils release their granule components by exocytosis, with individual granules fusing with the plasma membrane. This process involves a guanosine triphosphate (GTP)-binding protein and is modulated by the intracellular calcium concentration. In common with other secretory cells degranulation is controlled by soluble *N*-ethylmaleimide–sensitive factor attachment protein (SNAP) receptor complex (SNARE) proteins that guide the granules to the cell surface. Vesicular SNAREs expressed on granules bind to target SNAREs expressed on the plasma membrane. The SNARE proteins VAMP 2 and VAMP 7 are important in eosinophil secretion from granules and their function in eosinophils is regulated by cyclin-dependent kinase 5.[120]

● EOSINOPHILS IN DISEASE

MEASUREMENT OF EOSINOPHILS IN THE BLOOD

Eosinophils can be enumerated in the blood either by "wet counts" in modified Neubauer chambers, differential counts on dried films, or by automated cell counting by flow cytometry. Automated counting that uses detection of eosinophil peroxidase is the most accurate method, followed by counting in a cell chamber. Counting on films is least accurate because of the tendency for eosinophils to congregate at the margins of the slide. Common wet stains for eosinophils include eosin in acetone, phloxine, and Kimura stain, which was originally developed to stain basophils.[121] Many stains, including May-Grunewald-Giemsa, Romanowsky, chromotrope 2R, and Biebrich scarlet, will identify eosinophils in blood films, cytospin preparations, or tissues.

The eosinophil count should preferentially be evaluated in absolute numbers rather than as a percentage of white cells, as the latter will depend on the total white cell count. The normal eosinophil count is generally taken as less than 0.4×10^9/L, although healthy medical students in the United States had a range of 0.015 to 0.65×10^9/L.[122] Eosinophil counts are higher in neonates (Chap. 7). Clinical trials of anti-Th2 therapies are using a lower cut off in the region of 0.3×10^9/L to identify patients with eosinophilic asthma suggesting that the "normal" eosinophil count in people without allergic disease is below this level. The eosinophil count varies with age, time of day, exercise status, and environmental stimuli, particularly allergen exposure. Blood eosinophil counts undergo diurnal variation, being lowest in the morning and highest at night. This effect results in a greater than 40 percent variation and may be related to the reciprocal diurnal variation in cortisol levels, which are highest in the morning. The factors that control blood eosinophil counts in health are imperfectly understood. Concentrations of eosinophil growth factors are likely to be important, but other factors may be involved, including an element of genetic control.[123] Normal counts vary by up to 40-fold, and, in populations where eosinophilia is common, such as endemically parasitized areas, there are marked variations in the blood eosinophil level, independent of the degree of infection. This variation is comparable to variations in IgE levels. There are no differences between ethnic groups in eosinophil counts.

The eosinophil count in hospitalized patients is less than 0.01×10^9/L in only 0.1 percent of patients, and in virtually all patients the eosinopenia can be ascribed to glucocorticoids or to disease activity. Acute infection, or treatment with glucocorticoids or adrenaline, decreases eosinophil counts. In contrast, β-blockers inhibit adrenaline-induced eosinopenia and can cause a rise in the eosinophil count.

There have been several isolated case reports of patients with absent eosinophils in the blood and marrow.[124] A rare disorder, eosinophil peroxidase deficiency, may be brought to light by automatic counting that uses detection of eosinophil peroxidase to count eosinophils. Eosinophil peroxidase deficiency does not have any adverse clinical consequences.

CAUSES OF AN EOSINOPHILIA

An eosinophilia accompanies a discrete number of diseases and a high eosinophil count is always a clinically notable observation that requires explanation, although this is not always forthcoming.[125] The causes of eosinophilia can be classified according to the degree and frequency of occurrence (Table 62–4). Division of eosinophil counts is arbitrary, but a mild eosinophilia could be regarded as less than 1.0×10^9/L, a moderate elevation as 1.0 to 5.0×10^9/L, and a high count as greater than 5.0×10^9/L. The most common cause of an eosinophilia worldwide is infection with helminthic parasites, which can often result in a very high eosinophil count. The most common cause of an eosinophilia in industrialized countries is the atopic allergic diseases, seasonal and perennial rhinitis, atopic dermatitis, and asthma. Allergic disease generally results in only a mild increase in eosinophil counts. A moderate or high eosinophil count in asthma, especially outside a severe exacerbation, raises the possibility of a complication such as eosinophilic granulomatosis with polyangiitis (EGPA, formerly Churg-Strauss syndrome), allergic fungal airway disease, or eosinophilic pneumonia.[126] Drug allergy is not always straightforward to diagnose as a cause of an eosinophilia and less-common causes include Addison disease (although the eosinophilia is not usually marked).

THE ROLE OF EOSINOPHILS

For years eosinophils were thought to ameliorate inflammatory responses, a view that is possibly coming back into vogue as noted above (see "Role in Immunoregulation" above); then through the 1980s and 1990s they were believed to cause tissue damage in some situations. The subsequent use of anti–IL-5 and tyrosine kinase inhibitors to inhibit eosinophil production has suggested a complex interaction between eosinophilic inflammation and target organ damage.[127] Eosinophils, in part through release of cytokines such as TGF-α, may also have a homeostatic role in certain circumstances, such as wound healing and mammary gland development.[128,129] Eosinophils can certainly cause severe tissue damage under certain circumstances. Chronically high eosinophil counts from many causes, including drug reactions, parasitic infections, eosinophilic leukemia, and HES, are associated with endomyocardial fibrosis. The observation in the mid-1970s that eosinophils could kill parasite targets led to the hypothesis that the principal role of eosinophils was to counter parasitic infection, although this remains a controversial area.[130] Eosinophils in a mouse model had a protective effects against fungal growth in the lungs and eosinophils have also been demonstrated in mice to protect against lethal respiratory virus infection.[131,132] Eosinophils are therefore associated with a number of different types of pathologic and reparative processes ranging from the permanent tissue damage seen in HES, the partly reversible tissue damage seen in asthma and pulmonary eosinophilia, and tissue repair characteristic of wound healing. The factors that determine which role the eosinophil adopts are unclear.

EOSINOPHILS AND ASTHMA

The relationship between airway inflammation and asthma is complex. In particular, there is no close relationship between the severity of eosinophilic airway inflammation and either the severity of symptoms, AHR, or abnormalities in forced expiratory volume in 1 second (FEV$_1$).[133] The potential dissociation between an airway smooth muscle dysfunctional phenotype, which leads to many of the symptoms and physiologic abnormalities in asthma, and an eosinophilic inflammation-predominant phenotype more closely associated with severe exacerbations was demonstrated in an examination of asthma heterogeneity using cluster analysis techniques.[134] This dissociation was further illustrated by clinical trials of mepolizumab, an anti–IL-5 monoclonal antibody (mAb), which markedly reduced eosinophils in the blood and sputum but had no effect, either on AHR or lung function in patients with mild asthma, or on the late response to allergen challenge.[36] The interpretation of this study and others using the anti–IL-5 antibody was complicated by the observation that anti–IL-5 only partially decreases the tissue eosinophilia.[73] A dissociation between AHR and eosinophilia has also been seen in animal models of allergen challenge. For example, anti–VLA-4 mAb was able to block ovalbumin-induced AHR, but not airway eosinophilia when given by aerosol to mice.[135] Strikingly, in a condition called *eosinophilic bronchitis* in which patients have an eosinophilic airway inflammation but no evidence of asthma (no AHR or variable airflow obstruction), the asthma phenotype correlated with the number of mast cells in the airway smooth muscle and the tissue eosinophilia did not differ between the asthmatic and eosinophilic bronchitis groups.[108] Large numbers of eosinophils and mononuclear cells are found in and around the bronchi of patients who have died of asthma, and their bronchial tissue contains large amounts of MBP.[8] The pathology of asthma deaths is at the extreme end of the pathology of asthma exacerbations. There is increasing evidence that an airway eosinophilia is closely associated with the risk of having severe exacerbations. There is now definitive evidence from two studies using mepolizumab that eosinophils are directly causal in the pathogenesis of severe exacerbations of asthma. Asthmatics with documented eosinophil airway inflammation were treated for up to a year with the drug with the primary outcome of a reduction in severe exacerbations in one study and dose of corticosteroids in another. Both demonstrated that mepolizumab was an effective form of treatment with response correlating with the effect on reducing eosinophils.[136,137] These observations were confirmed in phase II and III clinical trials and mepolizumab is now going through the licensing procedure for the treatment of asthma.[138,139] Of note, a dose of mepolizumab that was suboptimal for suppressing the airway eosinophilia was as effective in preventing exacerbations as a higher dose that did suppress sputum eosinophils. Both doses effectively suppressed the blood eosinophilia, suggesting this is a better biomarker of response. The exact mechanism by which mepolizumab prevents exacerbations of asthma is therefore not entirely clear, especially as it does not obviously suppress eosinophil activation in the airway lumen.[140]

EOSINOPHILS AND THE SKIN

A large number of skin conditions are associated with infiltration of the skin by eosinophils.[141] The normal skin contains few eosinophils, so their presence is usually associated with pathology. The commonest causes of eosinophilic infiltration of the skin is atopic dermatitis where, as with asthma, the relationship to pathogenesis remains contentious.[142]

TABLE 62-4. Causes of an Eosinophilia

Disease	Frequency of Cause of Eosinophilia	Usual Degree of Eosinophilia	Comment
INFECTIONS			
Parasitic disease	Common worldwide	Moderate to high	
Bacterial	Rare		Almost invariably causes an eosinopenia
Mycobacterial	Rare		Secondary to drug therapy
Invasive fungal	Unusual		Apart from allergic responses which are common and coccidiomycosis, in which as many as 88% of patients have an eosinophilia
Rickettsial infections	Rare		
Yeast	Rare		Cryptococcus reported as causing cerebrospinal fluid eosinophilia
Viral infections	Rare		Occasional case reports of an eosinophilia in a variety of viral infections, including herpes and HIV infection
ALLERGIC DISEASES			
Allergic rhinitis	Common	Mild	
Atopic dermatitis	Common especially children	Mild to moderate	
Urticaria/angioedema	Common	Mild	Eosinophils seen in skin even with normal count
Fungal allergy	Common	Mild to high	Immunoglobulin (Ig) E sensitization to thermotolerant colonizing yeast (e.g., *Candida albicans*) and molds, e.g., *Aspergillus fumigatus* is a common cause of an eosinophilia
Asthma	Common	Mild	Syndrome of intrinsic asthma, nasal polyps, and aspirin intolerance associated with higher-than-usual eosinophil counts
DRUG REACTIONS			
Many drugs	Uncommon	Mild to high	Antibiotics, nonsteroidal antiinflammatory drug, and antipsychotics commonest groups; count should return to normal on stopping drug
NEOPLASMS			
Acute eosinophil leukemia	Rare	High	
Chronic eosinophilic leukemia	Rare	high	See text on hypereosinophilic syndrome
Myeloid leukemia	Uncommon	Moderate to high	Raised eosinophil counts can be seen in chronic myeloid leukemia
Lymphomas	Uncommon	Moderate	Often intense tissue eosinophilia with moderate blood eosinophil count; Hodgkin disease commonest type
Histiocytosis X	Rare	Mild	Intense tissue eosinophilia in eosinophilic granuloma but blood eosinophilia unusual
Solid tumors	Uncommon	Mild to high	Many different tumors reported
MUSCULOSKELETAL			
Rheumatoid arthritis	Rare	Mild to high	Occasional case reports. More usually secondary to therapy
Eosinophilic fasciitis	Rare	Moderate	
GASTROINTESTINAL			
Eosinophilic gastroenteritis	Rare	Mild to moderate	Characterized by irritable bowel syndrome–like symptoms; mucosal biopsies often normal
Eosinophilic esophagitis	Increasingly recognized	mild	Marked tissue eosinophilia with mild or absent blood eosinophilia
Celiac disease	Uncommon	Normal	Tissue eosinophilia
Inflammatory bowel disease			Eosinophils seen in biopsies in both Crohn and ulcerative colitis, but blood eosinophilia unusual
Allergic gastroenteritis	Rare	Mild to high	Young children

(continued)

TABLE 62–4. Causes of an Eosinophilia (Continued)

Disease	Frequency of Cause of Eosinophilia	Usual Degree of Eosinophilia	Comment
RESPIRATORY TRACT (FOR *ASTHMA* SEE *ALLERGIC DISEASES*)			
Eosinophilic granulomatosis with polyangiitis	Rare	Moderate to high	Syndrome of eosinophilic vasculitis and asthma
Chronic eosinophilic pneumonia	Uncommon	Mild to high	Syndrome of eosinophilia and chest x-ray shadowing
Bronchiectasis/cardiac failure	Common	Mild	Often associated with asthma or allergic fungal airway disease
SKIN DISEASES (FOR *ATOPIC DERMATITIS* SEE *ALLERGIC DISEASES*)			
Bullous pemphigoid	Uncommon	Moderate	
Eosinophilic cellulitis	Uncommon	Moderate to high	High eosinophil count distinguishes from bacterial cause
Skin lymphoma (Sézary syndrome: mycosis fungoides)	Uncommon	Moderate	
MISCELLANEOUS CAUSES			
Interleukin (IL)-2 therapy	Rare	Moderate to high	For renal cell carcinoma.
Hypereosinophilic syndrome	Rare	Moderate to high	
Endomyocardial fibrosis	Rare	High	Secondary to any cause of a high eosinophil count
Hyper-IgE syndrome	Rare	Moderate to high	Possibly caused by fungal allergy
Eosinophilia/myalgia and toxic oil syndrome	Rare	High	Two related conditions, one caused by poisoning with contaminated cooking oil in Spain and the other by a batch of tryptophan
Graft-vs.-host disease	Uncommon	Mild to moderate	
DOCK8 (dedicator of cytokinesis 8) deficiency	Rare	Mild	May be caused by fungal allergy
Olmsted syndrome	Rare		
Kimura disease	Rare		
Angiolymphoid hyperplasia	Rare		
Addison disease	Uncommon		

The skin is one of the most commonly effected organs in HES with pruritus being the commonest symptom, although ulceration also occurs.[143]

EOSINOPHILS AND THE GASTROINTESTINAL TRACT

Eosinophils are present in the normal gastrointestinal tract as a result of constitutive expression of eotaxin and MAdCAM1 (mucosal addressin cell adhesion molecule-1) the receptor for $\alpha_4\beta_7$ which is expressed by eosinophils.[55] A number of diseases are associated with a gastrointestinal eosinophilia, including eosinophilic esophagitis, eosinophilic gastroenteritis, and inflammatory bowel disease, although this latter condition does not result in a blood eosinophilia.[144] Eosinophilic esophagitis is an increasingly recognized condition in both children and adults. It is associated with food allergy often in the absence of specific IgE. It is another condition characterized by a marked tissue eosinophilia without a marked blood eosinophil count.[145]

EOSINOPHILS AND PARASITIC DISEASE

The role of eosinophils in parasitic disease is complex and still incompletely understood.[130] Table 62–5 and reference 146 summarize the most common helminthic causes of an eosinophilia. Eosinophils have

been shown *in vitro* to be able to kill a number of opsonized parasites, including newborn larvae of *Trichinella spiralis*, larvae of *Nippostrongylus brasiliensis*, a gut parasite in the rat, and larvae of *Fasciola hepatica*, as well as shistosomulae of *Schistosoma mansoni*. *In vivo*, parasite larvae become opsonized with both specific IgG and IgE antibodies and components of the complement cascade such as C3bi, which can promote adhesion and activation of eosinophils. Dead larvae of *Schistosoma haematobium* and other parasites have been detected in the skin surrounded by eosinophils and eosinophil granule products. Adult worms, both *in vitro* and *in vivo*, appear resistant to eosinophil-mediated damage. Despite the circumstantial evidence of eosinophils being involved in host defense against parasites, there remains doubt about their role. A number of experiments have been carried out in animal models of helminthic infection using IL-5 gene deletion, IL-5 transgenics, and anti–IL-5 antibodies to ablate the tissue eosinophilia. These studies have suggested that eosinophils may have a protective role in *Strongyloides* and *Filariasis* but not in *Schistosoma*, *Nippostrongylus*, and *Trichuris* infections. For example, treatment of mice infected with *N. brasiliensis* or *S. mansoni* with neutralizing anti–IL-5 mAbs abolished the eosinophilia without modulating the disease process.[146] In contrast, using diffusion chambers eosinophils were conclusively shown to be involved in killing the larvae of *Strongyloides stercoralis*.[147] In *Trichinella spiralis* infections, eosinophils prolonged larval survival during the primary

TABLE 62–5. Helminthic Causes of an Eosinophilia

Parasite	Comment
NEMATODES	
Ascariasis	Higher eosinophil counts in children. Larvae migrate from intestine to lungs where they cause Loeffler syndrome, a form of pulmonary eosinophilia.
Toxocara canis	Infective eggs are present in feces of puppies and pregnant bitches. Larvae in hosts such as chicken. Eosinophilia seen mainly in children younger than 9 years of age. Can migrate to eye and cause blindness. Serologic evidence suggests infection not uncommon in industrialized countries.
Filariasis	Common. Invariably result in marked eosinophilia, especially Loa Loa infection. Filariasis causes tropical pulmonary eosinophilia as a result of migration of adult worms to the lung, elephantiasis because of the involvement of lymphatics (*Wuchereria bancrofti* and *Brugia malayi*), and river blindness (*Onchocerca volvulus*). Treatment can result in systemic reaction called *Mazzotti reaction*, possibly a result of massive eosinophil degranulation.
Ancylostomiasis	Hookworm infection. *Ancylostoma duodenale* and *Necator americanus*. One of the main causes of eosinophilia in patients returning from tropical countries. Counts in region of 2.0×10^9/L.
Strongyloidiasis	Subclinical infection can persist for longer than 20 years. Stool examinations often negative. Cause of eosinophilia in ex-servicemen who spent time in tropics. If strongyloides infection is not considered and these patients are given steroids for suspected hypereosinophilic syndrome or as trial of therapy, they can develop disseminated disease.
Trichinosis	Caused by ingestion of encysted muscle larvae of *Trichinella spiralis*. Most prominent eosinophilia seen during early stages of infection when larvae migrating into striated muscle via the blood. Fatal cases reported of which only 20% were noted to have an eosinophilia.
Others	Other nematodes that can cause eosinophilia include *Trichuris trichiura*, *Capillaria*, and *Gnathostomiasis*. The thread worm *Enterobius vermicularis* occasionally causes an eosinophilia when they invade tissues.
TREMATODES	
Schistosomiasis (Bilharzia)	Infection with one of the *Schistosoma* (blood flukes)— *Schistosoma mansoni*, *Schistosoma haematobium*, and *Schistosoma japonicum*—is perhaps the commonest cause of a moderate to high eosinophilia worldwide, with 200 million people being infected. Infection is nearly always associated with an eosinophilia.
Fascioliasis	Adult worms of *Fasciola hepatica* reside in the bile ducts, where they are associated with abnormal liver function tests and an eosinophilia.
CESTODES	
Echinococcus	Eosinophilia occurs in 25–50% of patients with hydatid disease.

infection by producing IL-10 which led to a reduction in nitric oxide (NO) synthase expression and protected the intracellular larvae from NO-mediated killing.[148] In contrast, eosinophils were protective for host with a secondary infection.[149] The mechanism of eosinophilia in parasitic disease is thought to be similar to allergic disease, with a Th2-type response mediated by both adaptive Th2 cells and innate lymphoid type 2 cells to helminthic antigens resulting in increased production of eosinophil growth factors, in particular IL-5.[150] Recruitment of eosinophils to the site of parasite infection may involve nematode induced production of LTB_4 by eosinophils.[151]

HYPEREOSINOPHILIC SYNDROMES

Idiopathic Hypereosinophilic Syndrome

Definition and History Idiopathic hypereosinophilic syndrome (iHES) is a rare and potentially fatal disorder first described as a distinct entity by Hardy and Anderson in 1968.[152] It is defined as a persistent eosinophilia of greater than 1.5×10^9 cells/L for more than 6 months with no other explanation after comprehensive investigation and evidence of end-organ damage.[153] Patient series have consistently shown that the major target organs for tissue damage are the skin, heart, and nervous system.[154] The definition and classification of HES is unsatisfactory as conditions such as EGPA, eosinophilic pneumonia, eosinophilic gastroenteritis, and other more organ-specific conditions are arbitrarily excluded. Attempts have been made to create a more comprehensive and less arbitrary system although this requires more data on specific etiologies.[155,156] The World Health Organization (WHO) takes the view that all myeloproliferative variants of HES are malignant conditions. It previously classified them under chronic myeloproliferative diseases (CMPDs) with CEL/HES as a subcategory. In WHO's 2008 revision they have called CMPD myeloproliferative neoplasms. Where there is no defined genotypic abnormality the condition has been termed CEL-NOS (not otherwise specified), and where there is a defined mutation such as F/P they fall into a new category of their own.[157]

Epidemiology HES is a rare disorder with an estimated prevalence (although there are limited data on this), in the region of one in 50,000. It occurs sporadically and there appears to be no geographic or environmental influences. For unknown reasons the myeloproliferative form has a strong male bias.

Differential Diagnosis The commonest causes are allergic disease and in particular allergy to thermotolerant colonizing fungi such as *Aspergillus fumigatus* and *Candida albicans*, chronic infection with helmintic parasites (see Table 62–5), severe asthma, chronic eosinophilic pneumonia, drug allergy, malignancy, EGPA, and eosinophilic gastroenteritis (which could be regarded as part of the HES spectrum).

Etiology and Pathogenesis New insights into both the pathophysiology and management of HES have been offered by the use of anti–IL-5 and the tyrosine kinase inhibitor imatinib mesylate to treat the disease. HES appears to be a heterogenous condition with some patients having evidence of abnormal T-cell clones, some of which overproduce IL-5 and some cases being because of somatic mutations leading to constitutively active tyrosine kinases. This finding has led to the proposal that there are two broad variants of HES: myeloid and lymphoid.[158] The myeloid variant has features in common with myeloproliferative neoplasms, including raised serum vitamin B_{12} and serum tryptase, elevated neutrophil alkaline phosphatase score, clonal chromosomal abnormalities, anemia and thrombocytopenia, splenomegaly, and circulating blast cells. The cardiac and neurologic involvement that is a poor prognostic factor in HES is found mainly, but far from exclusively, in this group. A small proportion of these patients go on to develop acute eosinophilic or myeloid leukemia (see Chaps. 88 and 89). Demonstration of eosinophil clonality has been difficult but there is compelling evidence that these patients have chromosomal abnormalities leading to constitutive activation of growth factor associated tyrosine kinases. In particular, an interstitial deletion on 4q12 resulting in the encoding of a fusion protein consisting of the products of the F/P oncogene, which has constitutive tyrosine kinase activity, was found in eight of 15 patients with iHES, all of whom responded to treatment with the tyrosine kinase inhibitor imatinib.[159] This mutation caused the Ba/F3 cell line to become IL-3–independent and was found in the EOL-1 cell line derived from a patient with eosinophilic leukemia.[160] The presence of this mutation and the response to treatment with imatinib has been confirmed by other groups and is now recognized as the most common clonal abnormality in CEL/myeloid HES.[161] Imatinib has also been effective in other patients with iHES without this particular mutation.[159,162] A number of other rare mutated tyrosine kinases also cause the condition, including the JAK2 V617F point mutation usually associated with polycythemia vera,[163] other partners for *PDGFRα*, the *PDGFRβ* gene, and rearrangements in the *FGFR1* gene at 8p11 in which most patients progress to an aggressive leukemia or lymphoma.[164,165] Karyotyping can identify these mutations, except the F/P mutation. The F/P mutation can be identified by fluorescence *in situ* hybridization (FISH) studies (Chap. 89). A number of other tyrosine kinase inhibitors with activity against CEL are in clinical development.[166] Serum tryptase appears to be a good, though not perfect, marker of this variant of iHES, suggesting that mast cells are also affected by the mutation.[167] It is, however, clinically distinct from systemic mastocytosis.[167] The lymphoid variant of HES clinically generally follows a more benign course than m-HES (myeloproliferative HES) and there is less sex bias.[168] Patients tend to respond well to glucocorticoids and do not develop the cardiac fibrosis and other severe complications of the disease. The lymphoid variant of HES variant is presumed to be a result of the overproduction of eosinophil-related growth factors by aberrant T cells. The eosinophils are, therefore, normal, unlike the m-HES variant. A number of different patterns of T cell abnormality have been found in association with HES the most common being a CD3– CD4+ CD5 subset of T cells[169–172] (reviewed in Ref. 173). In many cases, these clones secrete increased amounts of eosinophil-related cytokines such as IL-5, IL-4, and IL-13. Clonality of the phenotypically aberrant T cells has been demonstrated in many cases and some progress to frank malignancy.

Clinical Features HES has a heterogeneous presentation with the marked and persistent blood eosinophilia being the obvious hallmark.[158,173,174] It is a chronic disease that usually presents in the third or fourth decade but can present at any age, including (rarely) in childhood.

It varies from being relatively asymptomatic to an aggressive disease leading to death within a few years if left untreated. The more severe complications are generally found in the myeloproliferative variant of the disease. HES can present with nonspecific symptoms such as general malaise, weight loss, aches and pains, and sweating attacks, or with one of the organ-specific features. Cardiac complications are common in the myeloproliferative variant of the disease, in particular endomyocardial fibrosis, which leads to a restrictive cardiomyopathy and left ventricular failure. Mitral incompetence can occur. Thromboembolic complications of large and small vessels are common in more severe disease some of which originate from endomyocardial clot. Many of the central neurologic features are embolic in origin. Respiratory symptoms, including cough that is (usually) productive of only small amounts of sputum and breathlessness, are common. Although airflow obstruction occurs there is a limited response to bronchodilators and AHR is often absent. Wheezing is not a prominent symptom. Pulmonary shadowing including alveolar infiltration and nodules may be present. Skin symptoms are common, particularly pruritus. which is sometimes associated with erythematous papules and urticaria. A variant of HES is Gleich syndrome in which patients have recurring episodes of angioedema. Eosinophilic cellulitis may also be a feature.[175] As well as embolic events, HES can be associated with confusion, loss of memory, and ataxia. Peripheral nervous system symptoms can include mononeuritis multiplex, sensorimotor neuropathy, multifocal neuropathy, and radiculopathy. The differential diagnosis with EGPA can be difficult and may be semantic.[176] Patients can develop mucosal ulcerations but as with the renal system, severe complications are not usually prominent.

Laboratory Features Investigations to exclude a reactive cause for the eosinophilia need to be undertaken (see "Differential Diagnosis" below), if the neoplastic nature of the eosinophilia is not evident. Examination of stools for parasites in patients with chronic eosinophilia is an insensitive investigation and serology is only available for common helminths such as *Strongyloides*, schistosomiasis, and filariasis. Empirical treatment with broad-spectrum antihelminths can sometimes be justified if there is high clinical suspicion with exposure and a high total IgE. Occult fungal allergy is another common cause of hypereosinophilia and specific IgE for thermotolerant fungi which can colonize the host, such as *A. fumigatus, C. albicans, Penicillium chrysogenum,* and *Malassezia* species, should be routinely undertaken. A scheme for stepwise investigation of patients with iHES has been suggested.[173] These are mainly aimed at determining if there is evidence of clonality, or an abnormal T-cell clone. They include a complete blood count with examination of a blood film. Serum immunoglobulins, serum vitamin B_{12} and tryptase, examination of a marrow aspirate and biopsy, lymphocyte phenotyping and, if available, analysis of cytokine production, T-cell receptor gene rearrangement, karyotyping and analysis of the presence of the F/P fusion protein by reverse transcription polymerase chain reaction or FISH analysis. A chest radiograph, spirometry, biochemical profile, troponin, cortisol, echocardiogram and abdominal ultrasound should also be considered as well as neurologic investigations such as electromyography studies, if prior studies have not uncovered the explanation for the HES. Depending on the major site of organ damage, more detailed organ-specific investigations, such as cardiac magnetic resonance imaging, chest computerized tomography, full lung function tests, and gastrointestinal endoscopy, may be required.

Differential Diagnosis Table 62–4 lists the reactive causes of a marked eosinophilia, which causes should be excluded with appropriate investigations. Once these causes have been excluded the differential diagnosis includes familial eosinophilia, which is a rare condition that has been mapped to a region of chromosome 5q31-q33,[177] CEL, eosinophilia secondary to malignancy, EGPA, and chronic eosinophilic pneumonia. Some patients also appear to have a raised eosinophil count without any evidence of organ damage, a so-called benign eosinophilia.

Treatment The rarity of HES means that there are few clinical trials and most agents are used on the basis of anecdotal experience, the opinion of the HES community or experience with related diseases.[154] However, the use of imatinib mesylate for some patients with the myeloproliferative variant and the potential use of anti–IL-5 for T cell-driven disease offers new promise to patients with HES.[178] The mainstay of treatment has been glucocorticoids, which in many cases, particularly those caused by something other than myeloproliferative disease, are effective at controlling both the eosinophil count and the target organ damage, albeit at the risk of long-term side effects. In patients with a myeloproliferative neoplasm, the eosinophil count is not completely controlled with glucocorticoids, although these drugs can still limit organ damage. In patients where glucocorticoids are not sufficiently effective, hydroxyurea is a useful second-line agent. Other cytotoxic drugs, such as vincristine and cyclophosphamide, are less commonly used than in the past. Interferon-α has also been used with some success. As discussed above, imatinib mesylate has resulted in remission in patients with the F/P mutation, usually at doses well below those used in chronic myeloid leukemia and some patients remain in remission when the treatment is stopped.[179] In the absence of the F/P mutation in patients with myeloproliferative features, a trial of imatinib is indicated as occasionally F/P-negative patients have responded[180,181] and this form of CEL carries a poor prognosis.[182] Response to imatinib at a dose of 400 mg a day should be rapid (within several weeks) and result in a return of the eosinophil count to within the normal range if the cause of the eosinophilia is an imatinib-responsive tyrosine kinase mutation. Resistance to imatinib treatment has emerged in some cases as it does when used for chronic myeloid leukemia.[183] In one patient who developed resistance an alternative PDGFRα inhibitor was effective.[184] Treatment with imatinib has caused acute left ventricular failure in some cases and cardiac troponin has been suggested to be useful in monitoring response.[185] Another novel approach to treatment has been the use of anti–IL-5 mAb. This approach has resulted in a dramatic response in some patients, even in the absence of raised serum IL-5 concentrations.[186,187] In a double-blind, placebo-controlled trial of F/P-negative HES, patients requiring 20 mg or more of prednisolone, mepolizumab, a humanized mAb that binds IL-5, allowed a reduction below 10 mg of oral prednisone in 84 percent of patients, compared to 43 percent given a placebo, without any increase in the activity of the HES.

Course and Prognosis The outlook for patients with HES was poor with a series in 1973 reporting a 3-year survival of only 12 percent with cardiac failure accounting for much of the morbidity.[153] In a later report, the outlook had improved with a survival of 80 percent at 5 years.[188]

Toxic Oil Syndrome

In 1981, more than 20,000 cases of a syndrome manifested by fever, cough, dyspnea, leukocytosis, neutrophilia, and an eosinophil count greater than 0.75×10^9/L were reported in Spain.[189] Occasionally, the eosinophil count rose above normal only after the onset of the pulmonary symptoms. Eosinophil degranulation was seen in the effected tissues. Pulmonary infiltrates were evident on x-rays of the chest. Pleural effusion was common, and hypoxemia was frequent. There were 1500 deaths in the cohort. Approximately half of the patients went on to a chronic course that mimicked the eosinophilia-myalgia syndrome, with myalgias, eosinophilia, peripheral neuritis, scleroderma-like skin lesions, hair loss, and a sicca syndrome. Most patients improved from the acute or chronic symptoms and signs, but some residual nerve, muscle, or skin damage persisted. Endothelial

cell proliferation, mononuclear cell infiltrates around blood vessels (vasculitis), and perineural inflammatory infiltrates were identified histopathologically. Glucocorticoid therapy may have decreased the pulmonary symptomatology. The disease was thought to be a response to an unlabeled food oil, aniline-denatured rapeseed oil, marketed as pure olive oil.

Reactive Hypereosinophilia and Neoplasms

Eosinophilia is associated with a 2.4-fold increase of developing a hematologic malignancy over 4 years of observation compared with subjects with a normal eosinophil count.[190] Exaggerated tissue and blood eosinophilia has been reported in association with a variety of lymphoid and solid tumors particularly lymphoma of various types including Hodgkin and non-Hodgkin lymphoma, cutaneous T-cell lymphoma, and marginal zone lymphoma.[191] In these cases, the eosinophilia is thought to be the result of an increase in IL-5 and other cytokines or chemokines elaborated by the tumor cells. Unlike other types of reactive eosinophilia, the blood eosinophil count may not be suppressed by glucocorticoids. The eosinophilia may precede the clinical diagnosis of the tumor but usually occurs concomitantly. There is evidence that eosinophils slow the rate of progression of solid tumors, presumably by being cytotoxic to tumor cells with the extent peritumoral eosinophils predicting recurrence of colon cancer although other studies have raised the possibility of a tumor promoting role.[192,193]

Eosinophilic Granulomatosis with Polyangiitis

Clinical Features EGPA, formerly Churg-Strauss syndrome, is a rare disorder of unknown etiology characterized by eosinophilic asthma, chronic rhinosinusitis, and small vessel vasculitis. It is one of the three antineutrophil cytoplasmic antibodies (ANCA)-associated vasculitides (AAV), alongside microscopic polyangiitis (MPA) and granulomatosis with polyangiitis (GPA, formerly Wegener disease). Patients with EGPA are ANCA positive in approximately 40 percent of cases and generally this is of the perinuclear-ANCA antimyeloperoxidase type compared to GPA which is generally proteinase-3 positive.[194] ANCA titers do not appear to correlate well with disease activity. Patients who are ANCA-positive have a different profile of disease compared to those who are ANCA-negative in that vasculitic features are more prominent and renal disease more common, but there is less cardiac disease, although there is considerable overlap.[195,196] The vasculitic process leads to a multisystem presentation commonly affecting the respiratory system, heart, skin, and peripheral nerves, although it can cause damage to any organ.[197] A marked blood eosinophilia is a prominent feature as are lethargy, general malaise, and weight loss. Mononeuritis multiplex is a particularly characteristic feature that sometimes leads to rapid onset of a peripheral neuropathy, which can be permanent, causing considerable morbidity. Cardiac disease with valvular damage or endomyocarditis is one of the most serious complications. The epidemiology of EGPA is not precise, but the point prevalence of new cases is approximately 1:1,000,000 with an accumulated prevalence of approximately 1:50,000, with precise numbers depending on the diagnostic criteria used. The condition generally presents in middle age and is very rare in children. The adult onset in people with preexisting asthma has led to speculation that EGPA is the result of an inflammatory stimulus on the background of a respiratory eosinophilia leading to systemic eosinophilic activation.[176] Consistent with this, case-control studies suggest a link with various environmental exposures, including farming, silica, and solvents, but no single trigger has been identified.[198] There is no obvious gender, geographic, ethnic or socio-economic predilection. There are case reports of family clusters, but in most cases there is no evidence of an inherited cause. The syndrome is heterogeneous in its presentation depending on the main organ affected and the description of the disease in case series is influenced by the medical discipline of the reporting team. In the past, EGPA carried a poor prognosis with a 10 percent 1-year survival, but currently 5-year survival is greater than 90 percent. In most cases, patients go into remission with high-dose oral glucocorticoids, although guidelines recommend the use of other immunosuppressants, such as cyclophosphamide or azathioprine, to induce remission where there is evidence of life-threatening organ involvement.[199,200] Once remission is achieved the patient often requires lifelong oral glucocorticoids to maintain remission. Relapse is not uncommon and this, together with the adverse effects of medication, result in significant morbidity.

There are no universally accepted criteria for the diagnosis of EGPA. The widely used American College of Rheumatology criteria were for classification purposes rather than to aid diagnosis. They were based on comparing 20 patients with EGPA against 787 control patients with other forms of vasculitis.[201] Six criteria were specified (1) asthma (2) eosinophilia of greater than 10% (3) mononeuropathy (4) fleeting pulmonary shadows (5) paranasal sinus abnormality (6) a biopsy containing a blood vessel with extravascular eosinophils. Because there was no comparison with asthma or other eosinophilic disorders, the criteria lack specificity. The differential diagnosis of EGPA includes, on the one hand, other vasculitic conditions, and on the other hand, severe adult-onset eosinophilic asthma and HES. The diagnostic hallmark is evidence of an eosinophilic vasculitis with granuloma on biopsy, but in many cases it is not possible to obtain tissue and the diagnosis is based on clinical assessment.

Putative Biomarkers Other than the blood eosinophil count and ANCA, which is used as a subgrouping biomarker for disease with more vasculitic features, there are no biomarkers that are helpful in the diagnosis or management of this condition. All patients with suspected EGPA should undergo detailed investigations to exclude other causes of a hypereosinophilia (>1.5×10^9/L), to determine the type of vasculitis present, and to assess the extent of organ damage.[125] A subset of patients with aggressive hypereosinophilic disease have either mastocytosis in which there is a genetic defect in the KIT mast cell growth factor receptor or CEL. Both these possibilities need to be excluded with genetic testing. To identify novel biomarkers, a retrospective audit of patients who had been investigated at a tertiary center for an unexplained eosinophilia were studied. Twenty-nine patients with EGPA, 20 patients with HES and asthma, 16 patients with HES without asthma, and eight normal subjects were compared. An extensive range of cytokine and chemokine biomarkers were assayed. CCL-17 and soluble IL-2 receptor were raised but tracked with eosinophilia (demonstrating the importance of the eosinophilia control groups), but not with disease category.[202] However, these patients were all ANCA-negative and findings in ANCA-positive EGPA may differ.

Eosinophilic Fasciitis

This rare syndrome may occur at any age in either sex and is characterized by stiffness, pain, and swelling of the arms, forearms, thighs, legs, hands, and feet in descending order of frequency. Malaise, fever, weakness, and weight loss also occur.[203] Eosinophilia greater than 1×10^9/L is present in most patients, but may be intermittent. A biopsy, usually required for the diagnosis, shows inflammation, edema, thickening, and fibrosis of the involved fascia. Synovial tissue may show similar changes. Aplastic anemia, isolated cytopenias, pernicious anemia, and acute myelogenous leukemia have been associated with eosinophilic fasciitis and in the late 1980s a series of cases was described in association with ingestion of a particular batch of L-tryptophan.[204] Glucocorticoids are the first-line of treatment but other immunosuppressant therapy, such as methotrexate, may be required.[205]

Eosinophiluria and Eosinophilorrachia

The urinary excretion of eosinophils is seen in several inflammatory disorders of the kidney but most often in urinary tract infection or acute interstitial nephritis.[206] Hansel stain is superior to Wright stain in identifying eosinophils in a stained urinary sediment. Cerebrospinal fluid eosinophilia may occur with infection, shunts, and allergic reactions involving the meninges.[207]

REFERENCES

1. Lee JJ, Rosenberg HF: *Eosinophils in Health and Disease.* Elsevier, Philadelphia, 2012.
2. Gauvreau GM, Ellis AK, Denburg JA: Haemopoietic processes in allergic disease: Eosinophil/basophil development. *Clin Exp Allergy* 39:1297–1306, 2009.
3. Egesten A, Calafat J, Janssen H, et al: Granules of human eosinophilic leukocytes and their mobilization. *Clin Exp Allergy* 31:1173–1188, 2001.
4. Dvorak AM, Weller PF: Ultrastructural analysis of human eosinophils. *Chem Immunol* 76:1–28, 2000.
5. Melo RC, Weller PF: Unraveling the complexity of lipid body organelles in human eosinophils. *J Leukoc Biol* 96:703–712, 2014.
6. Persson T, Calafat J, Janssen H, et al: Specific granules of human eosinophils have lysosomal characteristics: Presence of lysosome-associated membrane proteins and acidification upon cellular activation. *Biochem Biophys Res Commun* 291:844–854, 2002.
7. Erjefalt JS, Persson CG: New aspects of degranulation and fates of airway mucosal eosinophils. *Am J Respir Crit Care Med* 161:2074–2085, 2000.
8. Filley WV, Holley KE, Kephart GM, et al: Identification by immunofluorescence of eosinophil granule major basic protein in lung tissues of patients with bronchial asthma. *Lancet* 2:11–16, 1982.
9. Dvorak AM, Furitsu T, Letourneau L, et al: Mature eosinophils stimulated to develop in human cord blood mononuclear cell cultures supplemented with recombinant human interleukin-5. Part I. Piecemeal degranulation of specific granules and distribution of Charcot-Leyden crystal protein. *Am J Pathol* 138:69–82, 1991.
10. Duffy SM, Lawley WJ, Kaur D, et al: Inhibition of human mast cell proliferation and survival by tamoxifen in association with ion channel modulation. *J Allergy Clin Immunol* 112:965–972, 2003.
11. Malm-Erjefalt M, Persson CG, Erjefalt JS: Degranulation status of airway tissue eosinophils in mouse models of allergic airway inflammation. *Am J Respir Cell Mol Biol* 24:352–359, 2001.
12. Denzler KL, Borchers MT, Crosby JR, et al: Extensive eosinophil degranulation and peroxidase-mediated oxidation of airway proteins do not occur in a mouse ovalbumin-challenge model of pulmonary inflammation. *J Immunol* 167:1672–1682, 2001.
13. Denzler KL, Farmer SC, Crosby JR, et al: Eosinophil major basic protein-1 does not contribute to allergen- induced airway pathologies in mouse models of asthma. *J Immunol* 165:5509–5517, 2000.
14. Clark K, Simson L, Newcombe N, et al: Eosinophil degranulation in the allergic lung of mice primarily occurs in the airway lumen. *J Leukoc Biol* 75:1001–1009, 2004.
15. Humbles AA, Lloyd CM, McMillan SJ, et al: A critical role for eosinophils in allergic airways remodeling. *Science* 305:1776–1779, 2004.
16. Lee JJ, Dimina D, Macias MP, et al: Defining a link with asthma in mice congenitally deficient in eosinophils. *Science* 305:1773–1776, 2004.
17. Jacobsen EA, Lee NA, Lee JJ: Re-defining the unique roles for eosinophils in allergic respiratory inflammation. *Clin Exp Allergy* 44:1119–1136, 2014.
18. Yamamoto H, Sedgwick JB, Vrtis RF, et al: The effect of transendothelial migration on eosinophil function. *Am J Respir Cell Mol Biol* 23:379–388, 2000.
19. Floyd H, Ni J, Cornish AL, et al: Siglec-8. A novel eosinophil-specific member of the immunoglobulin superfamily. *J Biol Chem* 275:861–866, 2000.
20. Kikly KK, Bochner BS, Freeman SD, et al: Identification of SAF-2, a novel siglec expressed on eosinophils, mast cells, and basophils. *J Allergy Clin Immunol* 105:1093–1100, 2000.
21. Aizawa H, Plitt J, Bochner BS: Human eosinophils express two Siglec-8 splice variants. *J Allergy Clin Immunol* 109:176, 2002.
22. Munday J, Kerr S, Ni J, et al: Identification, characterization and leucocyte expression of Siglec-10, a novel human sialic acid-binding receptor. *Biochem J* 355:489–497, 2001.
23. Swystun VA, Gordon JR, Davis EB, et al: Mast cell tryptase release and asthmatic responses to allergen increase with regular use of salbutamol. *J Allergy Clin Immunol* 106:57–64, 2000.
24. Kiwamoto T, Brummet ME, Wu F, et al: Mice deficient in the St3gal3 gene product alpha2,3 sialyltransferase (ST3Gal-III) exhibit enhanced allergic eosinophilic airway inflammation. *J Allergy Clin Immunol* 133:240–247.e1–e3, 2014.
25. Kano G, Almanan M, Bochner BS, et al: Mechanism of Siglec-8-mediated cell death in IL-5-activated eosinophils: Role for reactive oxygen species-enhanced MEK/ERK activation. *J Allergy Clin Immunol* 132:437–445, 2013.
26. Legrand F, Tomasevic N, Simakova O, et al: The eosinophil surface receptor epidermal growth factor-like module containing mucin-like hormone receptor 1 (EMR1): A novel therapeutic target for eosinophilic disorders. *J Allergy Clin Immunol* 133:1439–1447.e1–e8, 2014.
27. Munitz A, Bachelet I, Finkelman FD, et al: CD48 is critically involved in allergic eosinophilic airway inflammation. *Am J Respir Crit Care Med* 175:911–918, 2007.

28. Moshkovits I, Shik D, Itan M, et al: CMRF35-like molecule 1 (CLM-1) regulates eosinophil homeostasis by suppressing cellular chemotaxis. *Mucosal Immunol* 7:292–303, 2014.
29. Yu C, Cantor AB, Yang H, et al: Targeted deletion of a high-affinity GATA-binding site in the GATA-1 promoter leads to selective loss of the eosinophil lineage *in vivo. J Exp Med* 195:1387–1395, 2002.
30. Fukushima K, Matsumura I, Ezoe S, et al: FIP1L1-PDGFRalpha imposes eosinophil lineage commitment on hematopoietic stem/progenitor cells. *J Biol Chem* 284:7719–7732, 2009.
31. Doyle AD, Jacobsen EA, Ochkur SI, et al: Expression of the secondary granule proteins major basic protein 1 (MBP-1) and eosinophil peroxidase (EPX) is required for eosinophilopoiesis in mice. *Blood* 122:781–790, 2013.
32. Farahi N, Singh NR, Heard S, et al: Use of 111-Indium-labeled autologous eosinophils to establish the in vivo kinetics of human eosinophils in healthy subjects. *Blood* 120:4068–4071, 2012.
33. Lukawska JJ, Livieratos L, Sawyer BM, et al: Real-time differential tracking of human neutrophil and eosinophil migration *in vivo. J Allergy Clin Immunol* 133:233–239.e1, 2014.
34. Takatsu K, Kouro T, Nagai Y: Interleukin 5 in the link between the innate and acquired immune response. *Adv Immunol* 101:191–236, 2009.
35. van Rensen EL, Stirling RG, Scheerens J, et al: Evidence for systemic rather than pulmonary effects of interleukin-5 administration in asthma. *Thorax* 56:935–940, 2001.
36. Leckie MJ, ten Brinke A, Khan J, et al: Effects of an interleukin-5 blocking monoclonal antibody on eosinophils, airway hyper-responsiveness, and the late asthmatic response. *Lancet* 356:2144–2148, 2000.
37. Culley FJ, Brown A, Girod N, et al: Innate and cognate mechanisms of pulmonary eosinophilia in helminth infection. *Eur J Immunol* 32:1376–1385, 2002.
38. Martin C, Al-Qaoud KM, Ungeheuer MN, et al: IL-5 is essential for vaccine-induced protection and for resolution of primary infection in murine filariasis. *Med Microbiol Immunol* 189:67–74, 2000.
39. Humbert M, Corrigan CJ, Kimmitt P, et al: Relationship between IL-4 and IL-5 mRNA expression and disease severity in atopic asthma. *Am J Respir Crit Care Med* 156:704–708, 1997.
40. Domachowske JB, Bonville CA, Easton AJ, et al: Pulmonary eosinophilia in mice devoid of interleukin-5. *J Leukoc Biol* 71:966–972, 2002.
41. Fulkerson PC, Schollaert KL, Bouffi C, et al: IL-5 triggers a cooperative cytokine network that promotes eosinophil precursor maturation. *J Immunol* 193:4043–4052, 2014.
42. Finotto S, Neurath MF, Glickman JN, et al: Development of spontaneous airway changes consistent with human asthma in mice lacking T-bet. *Science* 295:336–338, 2002.
43. Neurath MF, Finotto S, Glimcher LH: The role of Th1/Th2 polarization in mucosal immunity. *Nat Med* 8:567–573, 2002.
44. Rothenberg ME, Mishra A, Collins MH, et al: Pathogenesis and clinical features of eosinophilic esophagitis. *J Allergy Clin Immunol* 108:891–894, 2001.
45. Ozdemir C, Akdis M, Akdis CA: T regulatory cells and their counterparts: Masters of immune regulation. *Clin Exp Allergy* 39:626–639, 2009.
46. McHugh RS, Shevach EM: The role of suppressor T cells in regulation of immune responses. *J Allergy Clin Immunol* 110:693–702, 2002.
47. Levings MK, Sangregorio R, Sartirana C, et al: Human CD25(+)CD4(+) T suppressor cell clones produce transforming growth factor beta, but not interleukin 10, and are distinct from type 1 T regulatory cells. *J Exp Med* 196:1335–1346, 2002.
48. Curotto de Lafaille MA, Lafaille JJ: CD4(+) regulatory T cells in autoimmunity and allergy. *Curr Opin Immunol* 14:771–778, 2002.
49. Yazdanbakhsh M, Kremsner PG, van Ree R: Allergy, parasites, and the hygiene hypothesis. *Science* 296:490–494, 2002.
50. Wills-Karp M, Santeliz J, Karp CL: The germless theory of allergic disease: Revisiting the hygiene hypothesis. *Nat Rev Immunol* 1:69–75, 2001.
51. Umetsu DT, Akbari O, Dekruyff RH: Regulatory T cells control the development of allergic disease and asthma. *J Allergy Clin Immunol* 112:480–487; quiz 488, 2003.
52. Akdis CA, Blaser K: Mechanisms of interleukin-10-mediated immune suppression. *Immunology* 103:131–136, 2001.
53. Finlay CM, Walsh KP, Mills KH: Induction of regulatory cells by helminth parasites: Exploitation for the treatment of inflammatory diseases. *Immunol Rev* 259:206–230, 2014.
54. Wardlaw A: Eosinophil density: What does it mean? *Clin Exp Allergy* 25:1145–1149, 1995.
55. Mishra A, Hogan SP, Brandt EB, et al: Enterocyte expression of the eotaxin and interleukin-5 transgenes induces compartmentalized dysregulation of eosinophil trafficking. *J Biol Chem* 277:4406–4412, 2002.
56. Nussbaum JC, Van Dyken SJ, von Moltke J, et al: Type 2 innate lymphoid cells control eosinophil homeostasis. *Nature* 502:245–248, 2013.
57. Bochner BS: Road signs guiding leukocytes along the inflammation superhighway. *J Allergy Clin Immunol* 106:817–828, 2000.
58. Rosenberg HF, Phipps S, Foster PS: Eosinophil trafficking in allergy and asthma. *J Allergy Clin Immunol* 119:1303–1310; quiz 1311–1312, 2007.
59. Mjosberg J, Eidsmo L: Update on innate lymphoid cells in atopic and non-atopic inflammation in the airways and skin. *Clin Exp Allergy* 44:1033–1043, 2014.
60. Palframan RT, Collins PD, Williams TJ, et al: Eotaxin induces a rapid release of eosinophils and their progenitors from the bone marrow. *Blood* 91:2240–2248, 1998.
61. Tachimoto H, Burdick MM, Hudson SA, et al: CCR3-active chemokines promote rapid detachment of eosinophils from VCAM-1 in vitro. *J Immunol* 165:2748–2754, 2000.
62. Tomaki M, Zhao LL, Lundahl J, et al: Eosinophilopoiesis in a murine model of allergic airway eosinophilia: Involvement of bone marrow IL-5 and IL-5 receptor alpha. *J Immunol* 165:4040–4050, 2000.
63. Edwards BS, Curry MS, Tsuji H, et al: Expression of P-selectin at low site density promotes selective attachment of eosinophils over neutrophils. *J Immunol* 165:404–410, 2000.
64. Dang B, Wiehler S, Patel KD: Increased PSGL-1 expression on granulocytes from allergic-asthmatic subjects results in enhanced leukocyte recruitment under flow conditions. *J Leukoc Biol* 72:702–710, 2002.
65. Woltmann G, McNulty CA, Dewson G, et al: Interleukin-13 induces PSGL-1/P-selectin-dependent adhesion of eosinophils, but not neutrophils, to human umbilical vein endothelial cells under flow. *Blood* 95:3146–3152, 2000.
66. Johansson MW: Activation states of blood eosinophils in asthma. *Clin Exp Allergy* 44:482–498, 2014.
67. Bahaie NS, Hosseinkhani MR, Ge XN, et al: Regulation of eosinophil trafficking by SWAP-70 and its role in allergic airway inflammation. *J Immunol* 188:1479–1490, 2012.
68. Ha SG, Ge XN, Bahaie NS, et al: ORMDL3 promotes eosinophil trafficking and activation via regulation of integrins and CD48. *Nat Commun* 4:2479, 2013.
69. Pope SM, Zimmermann N, Stringer KF, et al: The eotaxin chemokines and CCR3 are fundamental regulators of allergen-induced pulmonary eosinophilia. *J Immunol* 175:5341–5350, 2005.
70. Neighbour H, Boulet LP, Lemiere C, et al: Safety and efficacy of an oral CCR3 antagonist in patients with asthma and eosinophilic bronchitis: A randomized, placebo-controlled clinical trial. *Clin Exp Allergy* 44:508–516, 2014.
71. Simon HU, Yousefi S, Schranz C, et al: Direct demonstration of delayed eosinophil apoptosis as a mechanism causing tissue eosinophilia. *J Immunol* 158:3902–3908, 1997.
72. Anwar AR, Moqbel R, Walsh GM, et al: Adhesion to fibronectin prolongs eosinophil survival. *J Exp Med* 177:839–843, 1993.
73. Flood-Page PT, Menzies-Gow AN, Kay AB, et al: Eosinophil's role remains uncertain as anti-interleukin-5 only partially depletes numbers in asthmatic airway. *Am J Respir Crit Care Med* 167:199–204, 2003.
74. Brode S, Farahi N, Cowburn AS, et al: Interleukin-5 inhibits glucocorticoid-mediated apoptosis in human eosinophils. *Thorax* 65:1116–1117, 2010.
75. Robertson NM, Zangrilli JG, Steplewski A, et al: Differential expression of TRAIL and TRAIL receptors in allergic asthmatics following segmental antigen challenge: Evidence for a role of TRAIL in eosinophil survival. *J Immunol* 169:5986–5996, 2002.
76. Adachi T, Alam R: The mechanism of IL-5 signal transduction. *Am J Physiol* 275:C623–C633, 1998.
77. Dewson G, Cohen GM, Wardlaw AJ: Interleukin-5 inhibits translocation of Bax to the mitochondria, cytochrome c release, and activation of caspases in human eosinophils. *Blood* 98:2239–2247, 2001.
78. Letuve S, Druilhe A, Grandsaigne M, et al: Involvement of caspases and of mitochondria in Fas ligation-induced eosinophil apoptosis: Modulation by interleukin-5 and interferon-gamma. *J Leukoc Biol* 70:767–775, 2001.
79. Letuve S, Druilhe A, Grandsaigne M, et al: Critical role of mitochondria, but not caspases, during glucocorticosteroid-induced human eosinophil apoptosis. *Am J Respir Cell Mol Biol* 26:565–571, 2002.
80. Oh J, Malter JS: Pin1-FADD interactions regulate Fas-mediated apoptosis in activated eosinophils. *J Immunol* 190:4937–4945, 2013.
81. Ben Baruch-Morgenstern N, Shik D, Moshkovits I, et al: Paired immunoglobulin-like receptor A is an intrinsic, self-limiting suppressor of IL-5-induced eosinophil development. *Nat Immunol* 15:36–44, 2014.
82. Robinson DS, Damia R, Zeibecoglou K, et al: CD34(+)/interleukin-5Ralpha messenger RNA+ cells in the bronchial mucosa in asthma: Potential airway eosinophil progenitors. *Am J Respir Cell Mol Biol* 20:9–13, 1999.
83. Corry DB, Rishi K, Kanellis J, et al: Decreased allergic lung inflammatory cell egression and increased susceptibility to asphyxiation in MMP2-deficiency. *Nat Immunol* 3:347–353, 2002.
84. Martin C, Burdon PC, Bridger G, et al: Chemokines acting via CXCR2 and CXCR4 control the release of neutrophils from the bone marrow and their return following senescence. *Immunity* 19:583–593, 2003.
85. Muessel MJ, Scott KS, Friedl P, et al: CCL11 and GM-CSF differentially use the Rho GTPase pathway to regulate motility of human eosinophils in a three-dimensional microenvironment. *J Immunol* 180:8354–8360, 2008.
86. Daubeuf F, Frossard N: Eosinophils and the ovalbumin mouse model of asthma. *Methods Mol Biol* 1178:283–293, 2014.
87. Lambrecht BN, Hammad H: The immunology of asthma. *Nat Immunol* 16:45–56, 2014.
88. Gwinn WM, Damsker JM, Falahati R, et al: Novel approach to inhibit asthma-mediated lung inflammation using anti-CD147 intervention. *J Immunol* 177:4870–4879, 2006.
89. Uller L, Mathiesen JM, Alenmyr L, et al: Antagonism of the prostaglandin D2 receptor CRTH2 attenuates asthma pathology in mouse eosinophilic airway inflammation. *Respir Res* 8:16, 2007.
90. Sturm EM, Schratl P, Schuligoi R, et al: Prostaglandin E2 inhibits eosinophil trafficking through E-prostanoid 2 receptors. *J Immunol* 181:7273–7283, 2008.
91. Yousefi S, Gold JA, Andina N, et al: Catapult-like release of mitochondrial DNA by eosinophils contributes to antibacterial defense. *Nat Med* 14:949–953, 2008.
92. Lacy P, Moqbel R: Eosinophil cytokines. *Chem Immunol* 76:134–155, 2000.

93. Lee JJ, Jacobsen EA, McGarry MP, et al: Eosinophils in health and disease: The LIAR hypothesis. *Clin Exp Allergy* 40:563–575, 2010.

94. Akuthota P, Wang HB, Spencer LA, et al: Immunoregulatory roles of eosinophils: A new look at a familiar cell. *Clin Exp Allergy* 38:1254–1263, 2008.

95. Heredia JE, Mukundan L, Chen FM, et al: Type 2 innate signals stimulate fibro/adipogenic progenitors to facilitate muscle regeneration. *Cell* 153:376–388, 2013.

96. Goh YP, Henderson NC, Heredia JE, et al: Eosinophils secrete IL-4 to facilitate liver regeneration. *Proc Natl Acad Sci U S A* 110:9914–9919, 2013.

97. Wu D, Molofsky AB, Liang HE, et al: Eosinophils sustain adipose alternatively activated macrophages associated with glucose homeostasis. *Science* 332:243–247, 2011.

98. Lee M, Odegaard JI, Mukundan L, et al: Activated type 2 innate lymphoid cells regulate beige fat biogenesis. *Cell* 160:74–87, 2015.

99. Qiu Y, Nguyen KD, Odegaard JI, et al: Eosinophils and type 2 cytokine signaling in macrophages orchestrate development of functional beige fat. *Cell* 157:1292–1308, 2014.

100. Chu VT, Frohlich A, Steinhauser G, et al: Eosinophils are required for the maintenance of plasma cells in the bone marrow. *Nat Immunol* 12:151–159, 2011.

101. Chu VT, Beller A, Rausch S, et al: Eosinophils promote generation and maintenance of immunoglobulin-A-expressing plasma cells and contribute to gut immune homeostasis. *Immunity* 40:582–593, 2014.

102. Wong TW, Doyle AD, Lee JJ, et al: Eosinophils regulate peripheral B cell numbers in both mice and humans. *J Immunol* 192:3548–3558, 2014.

103. Bandeira-Melo C, Weller PF: Eosinophils and cysteinyl leukotrienes. *Prostaglandins Leukot Essent Fatty Acids* 69:135–143, 2003.

104. Luna-Gomes T, Magalhaes KG, Mesquita-Santos FP, et al: Eosinophils as a novel cell source of prostaglandin D2: Autocrine role in allergic inflammation. *J Immunol* 187:6518–6526, 2011.

105. Bozza PT, Yu W, Penrose JF, et al: Eosinophil lipid bodies: Specific, inducible intracellular sites for enhanced eicosanoid formation. *J Exp Med* 186:909–920, 1997.

106. Flood-Page P, Menzies-Gow A, Phipps S, et al: Anti-IL-5 treatment reduces deposition of ECM proteins in the bronchial subepithelial basement membrane of mild atopic asthmatics. *J Clin Invest* 112:1029–1036, 2003.

107. Phipps S, Ying S, Wangoo A, et al: The relationship between allergen-induced tissue eosinophilia and markers of repair and remodeling in human atopic skin. *J Immunol* 169:4604–4612, 2002.

108. Brightling CE, Bradding P, Symon FA, et al: Mast-cell infiltration of airway smooth muscle in asthma. *N Engl J Med* 346:1699–1705, 2002.

109. Acharya KR, Ackerman SJ: Eosinophil granule proteins: Form and function. *J Biol Chem* 289:17406–17415, 2014.

110. Butterworth AE, Sturrock RF, Houba V, et al: Eosinophils as mediators of antibody-dependent damage to schistosomula. *Nature* 256:727–729, 1975.

111. Gleich GJ: Mechanisms of eosinophil-associated inflammation. *J Allergy Clin Immunol* 105:651–663, 2000.

112. Ackerman SJ, Liu L, Kwatia MA, et al: Charcot-Leyden crystal protein (galectin-10) is not a dual function galectin with lysophospholipase activity but binds a lysophospholipase inhibitor in a novel structural fashion. *J Biol Chem* 277:14859–14868, 2002.

113. Persson C, Uller L: Theirs but to die and do: Primary lysis of eosinophils and free eosinophil granules in asthma. *Am J Respir Crit Care Med* 189:628–633, 2014.

114. Ueki S, Melo RC, Ghiran I, et al: Eosinophil extracellular DNA trap cell death mediates lytic release of free secretion-competent eosinophil granules in humans. *Blood* 121:2074–2083, 2013.

115. Simon D, Hoesli S, Roth N, et al: Eosinophil extracellular DNA traps in skin diseases. *J Allergy Clin Immunol* 127:194–199, 2011.

116. Pazdrak K, Young TW, Straub C, et al: Priming of eosinophils by GM-CSF is mediated by protein kinase CbetaII-phosphorylated L-plastin. *J Immunol* 186:6485–6496, 2011.

117. Seminario MC, Saini SS, MacGlashan DW Jr, et al: Intracellular expression and release of Fc epsilon RI alpha by human eosinophils. *J Immunol* 162:6893–6900, 1999.

118. Kaneko M, Horie S, Kato M, et al: A crucial role for beta 2 integrin in the activation of eosinophils stimulated by IgG. *J Immunol* 155:2631–2641, 1995.

119. Kovacs I, Horvath M, Kovacs T, et al: Comparison of proton channel, phagocyte oxidase, and respiratory burst levels between human eosinophil and neutrophil granulocytes. *Free Radic Res* 48:1190–1199, 2014.

120. Odemuyiwa SO, Ilarraza R, Davoine F, et al: Cyclin-dependent kinase 5 regulates degranulation in human eosinophils. *Immunology*. 144(4):641–648, 2015.

121. Kimura I, Moritani Y, Tanizaki Y: Basophils in bronchial asthma with reference to reagin-type allergy. *Clin Allergy* 3:195–202, 1973.

122. Krause JR, Boggs DR: Search for eosinopenia in hospitalized patients with normal blood leukocyte concentration. *Am J Hematol* 24:55–63, 1987.

123. Gudbjartsson DF, Bjornsdottir US, Halapi E, et al: Sequence variants affecting eosinophil numbers associate with asthma and myocardial infarction. *Nat Genet* 41:342–347, 2009.

124. Juhlin L, Michaelsson G: A new syndrome characterised by absence of eosinophils and basophils. *Lancet* 1:1233–1235, 1977.

125. Roufosse F, Weller PF: Practical approach to the patient with hypereosinophilia. *J Allergy Clin Immunol* 126:39–44, 2010.

126. Wechsler ME: Pulmonary eosinophilic syndromes. *Immunol Allergy Clin North Am* 27:477–492, 2007.

127. Bochner BS: Verdict in the case of therapies versus eosinophils: The jury is still out. *J Allergy Clin Immunol* 113:3–9; quiz 10, 2004.

128. Todd R, Donoff BR, Chiang T, et al: The eosinophil as a cellular source of transforming growth factor alpha in healing cutaneous wounds. *Am J Pathol* 138:1307–1313, 1991.

129. Gouon-Evans V, Rothenberg ME, Pollard JW: Postnatal mammary gland development requires macrophages and eosinophils. *Development* 127:2269–2282, 2000.

130. Klion AD, Nutman TB: The role of eosinophils in host defense against helminth parasites. *J Allergy Clin Immunol* 113:30–37, 2004.

131. Percopo CM, Dyer KD, Ochkur SI, et al: Activated mouse eosinophils protect against lethal respiratory virus infection. *Blood* 123:743–752, 2014.

132. Lilly LM, Scopel M, Nelson MP, et al: Eosinophil deficiency compromises lung defense against *Aspergillus fumigatus. Infect Immun* 82:1315–1325, 2014.

133. Gonem S, Raj V, Wardlaw AJ, et al: Phenotyping airways disease: An A to E approach. *Clin Exp Allergy* 42:1664–1683, 2012.

134. Haldar P, Pavord ID, Shaw DE, et al: Cluster analysis and clinical asthma phenotypes. *Am J Respir Crit Care Med* 178:218–224, 2008.

135. Henderson WR Jr, Chi EY, Albert RK, et al: Blockade of CD49d (alpha4 integrin) on intrapulmonary but not circulating leukocytes inhibits airway inflammation and hyperresponsiveness in a mouse model of asthma. *J Clin Invest* 100:3083–3092, 1997.

136. Nair P, Pizzichini MM, Kjarsgaard M, et al: Mepolizumab for prednisone-dependent asthma with sputum eosinophilia. *N Engl J Med* 360:985–993, 2009.

137. Haldar P, Brightling CE, Hargadon B, et al: Mepolizumab and exacerbations of refractory eosinophilic asthma. *N Engl J Med* 360:973–984, 2009.

138. Pavord ID, Korn S, Howarth P, et al: Mepolizumab for severe eosinophilic asthma (DREAM): A multicentre, double-blind, placebo-controlled trial. *Lancet* 380:651–659, 2012.

139. Ortega HG, Liu MC, Pavord ID, et al: Mepolizumab treatment in patients with severe eosinophilic asthma. *N Engl J Med* 371:1198–1207, 2014.

140. Johansson MW, Gunderson KA, Kelly EA, et al: Anti-IL-5 attenuates activation and surface density of beta(2)-integrins on circulating eosinophils after segmental antigen challenge. *Clin Exp Allergy* 43:292–303, 2013.

141. Leiferman KM, Gleich GJ: Hypereosinophilic syndrome: Case presentation and update. *J Allergy Clin Immunol* 113:50–58, 2004.

142. Simon D, Braathen LR, Simon HU: Eosinophils and atopic dermatitis. *Allergy* 59:561–570, 2004.

143. Leiferman KM, Gleich GJ, Peters MS: Dermatologic manifestations of the hypereosinophilic syndromes. *Immunol Allergy Clin North Am* 27:415–441, 2007.

144. Rothenberg ME: Eosinophilic gastrointestinal disorders (EGID). *J Allergy Clin Immunol* 113:11–28; quiz 29, 2004.

145. Abonia JP, Rothenberg ME: Eosinophilic esophagitis: Rapidly advancing insights. *Annu Rev Med* 63:421–434, 2012.

146. Sher A, Coffman RL, Hieny S, et al: Ablation of eosinophil and IgE responses with anti-IL-5 or anti-IL-4 antibodies fails to affect immunity against Schistosoma mansoni in the mouse. *J Immunol* 145:3911–3916, 1990.

147. Herbert DR, Lee JJ, Lee NA, et al: Role of IL-5 in innate and adaptive immunity to larval Strongyloides stercoralis in mice. *J Immunol* 165:4544–4551, 2000.

148. Huang L, Gebreselassie NG, Gagliardo LF, et al: Eosinophil-derived IL-10 supports chronic nematode infection. *J Immunol* 193:4178–4187, 2014.

149. Huang L, Gebreselassie NG, Gagliardo LF, et al: Eosinophils mediate protective immunity against secondary nematode infection. *J Immunol* 194:283–290, 2015.

150. Neill DR, Wong SH, Bellosi A, et al: Nuocytes represent a new innate effector leukocyte that mediates type-2 immunity. *Nature* 464:1367–1370, 2010.

151. Patnode ML, Bando JK, Krummel MF, et al: Leukotriene B4 amplifies eosinophil accumulation in response to nematodes. *J Exp Med* 211:1281–1288, 2014.

152. Hardy WR, Anderson RE: The hypereosinophilic syndromes. *Ann Intern Med* 68:1220–1229, 1968.

153. Chusid MJ, Dale DC, West BC, et al: The hypereosinophilic syndrome: Analysis of fourteen cases with review of the literature. *Medicine (Baltimore)* 54:1–27, 1975.

154. Ogbogu PU, Bochner BS, Butterfield JH, et al: Hypereosinophilic syndrome: A multicenter, retrospective analysis of clinical characteristics and response to therapy. *J Allergy Clin Immunol* 124:1319–1325.e3, 2009.

155. Valent P, Klion AD, Horny HP, et al: Contemporary consensus proposal on criteria and classification of eosinophilic disorders and related syndromes. *J Allergy Clin Immunol* 130:607–612.e9, 2012.

156. Simon HU, Rothenberg ME, Bochner BS, et al: Refining the definition of hypereosinophilic syndrome. *J Allergy Clin Immunol* 126:45–49, 2010.

157. Gotlib J: World Health Organization-defined eosinophilic disorders: 2014 update on diagnosis, risk stratification, and management. *Am J Hematol* 89:325–337, 2014.

158. Sheikh J, Weller PF: Advances in diagnosis and treatment of eosinophilia. *Curr Opin Hematol* 16:3–8, 2009.

159. Cools J, DeAngelo DJ, Gotlib J, et al: A tyrosine kinase created by fusion of the PDGFRA and FIP1L1 genes as a therapeutic target of imatinib in idiopathic hypereosinophilic syndrome. *N Engl J Med* 348:1201–1214, 2003.

160. Griffin JH, Leung J, Bruner RJ, et al: Discovery of a fusion kinase in EOL-1 cells and idiopathic hypereosinophilic syndrome. *Proc Natl Acad Sci U S A* 100:7830–7835, 2003.

161. Fletcher S, Bain B: Diagnosis and treatment of hypereosinophilic syndromes. *Curr Opin Hematol* 14:37–42, 2007.

162. Musto P, Perla G, Minervini MM, et al: Imatinib-mesylate for all patients with hypereosinophilic syndrome? *Leuk Res* 28:773–774, 2004.

163. Helbig G, Stella-Holowiecka B, Majewski M, et al: Interferon alpha induces a good molecular response in a patient with chronic eosinophilic leukemia (CEL) carrying the JAK2V617F point mutation. *Haematologica* 92:e118–e119, 2007.

164. Noel P: Eosinophilic myeloid disorders. *Semin Hematol* 49:120–127, 2012.

Chapter 62: Eosinophils and Related Disorders 963

165. Arefi M, Robledo C, Penarrubia MJ, et al: Genomic analysis of clonal eosinophils by CGH arrays reveals new genetic regions involved in chronic eosinophilia. *Eur J Haematol* 93:422–428, 2014.

166. Sadovnik I, Lierman E, Peter B, et al: Identification of Ponatinib as a potent inhibitor of growth, migration, and activation of neoplastic eosinophils carrying FIP1L1-PDGFRA. *Exp Hematol* 42:282–293.e4, 2014.

167. Klion AD, Noel P, Akin C, et al: Elevated serum tryptase levels identify a subset of patients with a myeloproliferative variant of idiopathic hypereosinophilic syndrome associated with tissue fibrosis, poor prognosis, and imatinib responsiveness. *Blood* 101:4660–4666, 2003.

168. Lefevre G, Copin MC, Staumont-Salle D, et al: The lymphoid variant of hypereosinophilic syndrome: Study of 21 patients with CD3-CD4+ aberrant T-cell phenotype. *Medicine (Baltimore)* 93:255–266, 2014.

169. Roufosse F, Cogan E, Goldman M: Lymphocytic variant hypereosinophilic syndromes. *Immunol Allergy Clin North Am* 27:389–413, 2007.

170. Cogan E, Schandene L, Crusiaux A, et al: Brief report: Clonal proliferation of type 2 helper T cells in a man with the hypereosinophilic syndrome. *N Engl J Med* 330:535–538, 1994.

171. Simon HU, Plotz SG, Dummer R, et al: Abnormal clones of T cells producing interleukin-5 in idiopathic eosinophilia. *N Engl J Med* 341:1112–1120, 1999.

172. Roufosse F, Schandene L, Sibille C, et al: Clonal Th2 lymphocytes in patients with the idiopathic hypereosinophilic syndrome. *Br J Haematol* 109:540–548, 2000.

173. Roufosse F, Cogan E, Goldman M: Recent advances in pathogenesis and management of hypereosinophilic syndromes. *Allergy* 59:673–689, 2004.

174. Spry CJF: The idiopathic hypereosinophilic syndrome, in *Eosinophils, Biological and Clinical Aspects*, edited by Makino S, Fukuda T. CRC Press, Boca Raton, FL, 1991.

175. Davis RF, Dusanjh P, Majid A, et al: Eosinophilic cellulitis as a presenting feature of chronic eosinophilic leukaemia, secondary to a deletion on chromosome 4q12 creating the FIP1L1-PDGFRA fusion gene. *Br J Dermatol* 155:1087–1089, 2006.

176. Khoury P, Grayson PC, Klion AD: Eosinophils in vasculitis: Characteristics and roles in pathogenesis. *Nat Rev Rheumatol* 10:474–483, 2014.

177. Klion AD, Law MA, Riemenschneider W, et al: Familial eosinophilia: A benign disorder? *Blood* 103:4050–4055, 2004.

178. Gleich GJ, Leiferman KM: The hypereosinophilic syndromes: Current concepts and treatments. *Br J Haematol* 145:271–285, 2009.

179. Legrand F, Renneville A, Macintyre E, et al: The spectrum of FIP1L1-PDGFRA-associated chronic eosinophilic leukemia: New insights based on a survey of 44 cases. *Medicine (Baltimore)*. 92(5):E1–E9, 2013.

180. Metzgeroth G, Walz C, Erben P, et al: Safety and efficacy of imatinib in chronic eosinophilic leukaemia and hypereosinophilic syndrome: A phase-II study. *Br J Haematol* 143:707–715, 2008.

181. Jain N, Cortes J, Quintas-Cardama A, et al: Imatinib has limited therapeutic activity for hypereosinophilic syndrome patients with unknown or negative PDGFRalpha mutation status. *Leuk Res* 33:837–839, 2009.

182. Helbig G, Soja A, Bartkowska-Chrobok A, et al: Chronic eosinophilic leukemia-not otherwise specified has a poor prognosis with unresponsiveness to conventional treatment and high risk of acute transformation. *Am J Hematol* 87:643–645, 2012.

183. Salemi S, Yousefi S, Simon D, et al: A novel FIP1L1-PDGFRA mutant destabilizing the inactive conformation of the kinase domain in chronic eosinophilic leukemia/hypereosinophilic syndrome. *Allergy* 64:913–918, 2009.

184. Cools J, Stover EH, Boulton CL, et al: PKC412 overcomes resistance to imatinib in a murine model of FIP1L1-PDGFRalpha-induced myeloproliferative disease. *Cancer Cell* 3:459–469, 2003.

185. Pitini V, Arrigo C, Azzarello D, et al: Serum concentration of cardiac Troponin T in patients with hypereosinophilic syndrome treated with imatinib is predictive of adverse outcomes. *Blood* 102:3456–3457; author reply 3457, 2003.

186. Garrett JK, Jameson SC, Thomson B, et al: Anti-interleukin-5 (mepolizumab) therapy for hypereosinophilic syndromes. *J Allergy Clin Immunol* 113:115–119, 2004.

187. Klion AD, Law MA, Noel P, et al: Safety and efficacy of the monoclonal anti-interleukin-5 antibody SCH55700 in the treatment of patients with hypereosinophilic syndrome. *Blood* 103:2939–2941, 2004.

188. Gotlib J, Cools J, Malone JM 3rd, et al: The FIP1L1-PDGFRalpha fusion tyrosine kinase in hypereosinophilic syndrome and chronic eosinophilic leukemia: Implications for diagnosis, classification, and management. *Blood* 103:2879–2891, 2004.

189. Posada de la Paz M, Philen RM, Borda AI: Toxic oil syndrome: The perspective after 20 years. *Epidemiol Rev* 23:231–247, 2001.

190. Andersen CL, Siersma VD, Hasselbalch HC, et al: Association of the blood eosinophil count with hematological malignancies and mortality. *Am J Hematol* 90:225–229, 2015.

191. Davis BP, Rothenberg ME: Eosinophils and cancer. *Cancer Immunol Res* 2:1–8, 2014.

192. Harbaum L, Pollheimer MJ, Kornprat P, et al: Peritumoral eosinophils predict recurrence in colorectal cancer. *Mod Pathol* 28:403–413, 2015.

193. Wong DT, Bowen SM, Elovic A, et al: Eosinophil ablation and tumor development. *Oral Oncol* 35:496–501, 1999.

194. Sable-Fourtassou R, Cohen P, Mahr A, et al: Antineutrophil cytoplasmic antibodies and the Churg-Strauss syndrome. *Ann Intern Med* 143:632–638, 2005.

195. Kallenberg CG: Churg-Strauss syndrome: Just one disease entity? *Arthritis Rheum* 52:2589–2593, 2005.

196. Comarmond C, Pagnoux C, Khellaf M, et al: Eosinophilic granulomatosis with polyangiitis (Churg-Strauss): Clinical characteristics and long-term followup of the 383 patients enrolled in the French Vasculitis Study Group cohort. *Arthritis Rheum* 65:270–281, 2013.

197. Mouthon L, Dunogue B, Guillevin L: Diagnosis and classification of eosinophilic granulomatosis with polyangiitis (formerly named Churg-Strauss syndrome). *J Autoimmun* 48–49:99–103, 2014.

198. Lane SE, Watts RA, Bentham G, et al: Are environmental factors important in primary systemic vasculitis? A case-control study. *Arthritis Rheum* 48:814–823, 2003.

199. Guillevin L, Pagnoux C, Seror R, et al: The five-factor score revisited: Assessment of prognoses of systemic necrotizing vasculitides based on the French Vasculitis Study Group (FVSG) cohort. *Medicine (Baltimore)* 90:19–27, 2011.

200. Kallenberg CG: Key advances in the clinical approach to ANCA-associated vasculitis. *Nat Rev Rheumatol* 10:484–493, 2014.

201. Masi AT, Hunder GG, Lie JT, et al: The American College of Rheumatology 1990 criteria for the classification of Churg-Strauss syndrome (allergic granulomatosis and angiitis). *Arthritis Rheum* 33:1094–1100, 1990.

202. Khoury P, Zagallo P, Talar-Williams C, et al: Serum biomarkers are similar in Churg-Strauss syndrome and hypereosinophilic syndrome. *Allergy* 67:1149–1156, 2012.

203. Pinal-Fernandez I, Selva-O'Callaghan A, Grau JM: Diagnosis and classification of eosinophilic fasciitis. *Autoimmun Rev* 13:379–382, 2014.

204. Martin RW, Duffy J, Lie JT: Eosinophilic fasciitis associated with use of L-tryptophan: A case-control study and comparison of clinical and histopathologic features. *Mayo Clin Proc* 66:892–898, 1991.

205. Berianu F, Cohen MD, Abril A, et al: Eosinophilic fasciitis: Clinical characteristics and response to methotrexate. *Int J Rheum Dis.* 18(1):91–98, 2015.

206. Corwin HL, Bray RA, Haber MH: The detection and interpretation of urinary eosinophils. *Arch Pathol Lab Med* 113:1256–1258, 1989.

207. Hughes PA, Magnet AD, Fishbain JT: Eosinophilic meningitis: A case series report and review of the literature. *Mil Med* 168:817–821, 2003.

CHAPTER 63
BASOPHILS, MAST CELLS, AND RELATED DISORDERS

Stephen J. Galli, Dean D. Metcalfe,

Daniel A. Arber, and Ann M. Dvorak*

SUMMARY

Basophils and mast cells share biochemical and functional characteristics, but they are not identical. In humans, basophils are the least frequent of the three granulocytes, typically accounting for less than 0.5 percent of blood leukocytes. Basophils circulate as mature cells and can be recruited into tissues, particularly at sites of immunologic or inflammatory responses, but they ordinarily do not reside in tissues. By contrast, mast cells typically are derived from blood precursors that lack many of the characteristic features of the mature cells and complete their maturation in the tissues. The mature mast cells can reside in tissues for long periods of time. Mast cells are particularly abundant near blood vessels and nerves and in connective tissues beneath surfaces that are exposed to the external environment, such as the skin, gastrointestinal and urogenital tracts, and respiratory system. Tissue mast cell numbers can increase at sites of parasite infection or in association with certain chronic allergic diseases or other forms of pathology, by recruitment and local maturation of blood precursors and by proliferation of resident mast cells.

Mast cells and basophils express the high-affinity receptor for immunoglobulin (Ig) E (FcεRI) on their surface. Both cell types can be triggered to release potent mediators in response to activation via FcεRI, for example, when their cell-bound IgE recognizes bivalent or multivalent allergens. Accordingly, mast cells and basophils have long been regarded as important effector cells in asthma, hay fever, and other allergic disorders. The cells' cytoplasmic granule-associated preformed mediators, including histamine and certain proteases, their lipid mediators (such as prostaglandin D_2 and leukotriene C_4), which are generated upon activation of the cells, and their cytokines, growth factors, and chemokines contribute to many of the characteristic signs and symptoms of these diseases. However, several lines of evidence indicate mast cells and basophils also contribute to protective host responses associated with IgE production, especially those directed against parasites. In mice, mast cells can enhance innate and acquired (IgE-dependent) defense against animal venoms and also can contribute to host defense in innate immune responses to certain bacterial infections. Mast cells and basophils also may express positive and negative immunoregulatory functions through cytokine production and other mechanisms.

Although a variety of systemic disorders are associated with changes in the numbers of blood basophils and many pathologic processes can be associated with changes in the numbers of tissue mast cells, patients with primary deficiencies in basophils appear to be exceedingly rare (if they exist at all). Patients with a primary deficiency of tissue mast cells have not been reported. By contrast, neoplastic processes can affect both of the lineages. Increased numbers of basophils may be present in association with myeloproliferative neoplasms and several forms of myeloid leukemia. Increased numbers of basophils, sometimes to levels of 20 to 90 percent of blood leukocytes, occur in virtually all patients with chronic myelogenous leukemia. The basophils associated with both chronic myelogenous and acute myeloid leukemias are themselves part of the neoplastic clone. The management of patients with "basophilic leukemia" can be complicated by shock as a result of massive release of histamine and other mediators in association with acute cytolysis.

Disorders of mast cell hyperplasia/neoplasia include solitary mastocytomas, the pathogenesis of which is uncertain, the spectrum of disorders encompassed in the term *mastocytosis*, in which significantly increased numbers of mast cells occur in the skin and/or other organs, and mast cell leukemia. The most common form of mastocytosis, indolent systemic mastocytosis, typically presents with urticaria pigmentosa involving the skin, although other organs may be involved. Patients with indolent systemic mastocytosis have the best prognosis and can expect a normal life span. The prognosis of systemic mastocytosis with associated clonal, hematologic non–mast-cell-lineage disease depends on the course of the associated disease. Patients with aggressive systemic mastocytosis have a guarded prognosis because of complications arising from rapid increases in tissue mast cell numbers. Patients with mast cell leukemia, who often present with large numbers of immature mast cells in the blood at the time of diagnosis, have a fulminant and rapidly fatal course. Most adult patients with mastocytosis have gain-of-function mutations affecting *KIT*, which encodes the receptor for the major mast cell growth factor stem cell factor (also known as *kit ligand* and *mast cell growth factor*). Some pediatric patients with mastocytosis reportedly have the same Asp816Val gain-of-function *KIT* mutation observed in most adult patients. Some pediatric patients have a dominant inactivating *KIT* mutation, whereas others lack *KIT* mutations entirely.

Acronyms and Abbreviations: AML, acute myeloid leukemia; ASM, aggressive systemic mastocytosis; CML, chronic myelogenous leukemia; CPA3, carboxypeptidase A3; DEXA, dual-energy x-ray absorptiometry; ET-1, endothelin-1; FcεRI, high-affinity receptor for IgE; gp120, glycoprotein 120; H&E, hematoxylin and eosin; HLA, human leukocyte antigen; IFN-*a*, interferon *a*; Ig, immunoglobulin; IL, interleukin; ISM, indolent systemic mastocytosis; MCAS, mast cell activation syndrome; MCL, mast cell leukemia; MCP, mast cell–committed progenitor; MCS, mast cell sarcoma; MMAS, monoclonal mast cell activation syndrome; mMCP, mouse mast cell protease; PUVA, psoralen ultraviolet A; qPCR, quantitative polymerase chain reaction; SCF, stem cell factor; SCT, stem cell transplantation; SM-AHNMD, systemic mastocytosis with associated clonal hematologic non–mast-cell-lineage disease; Th, T-helper; TLR, toll-like receptor; TNF-*a*, tumor necrosis factor *a*; UP, urticaria pigmentosa; VEGF, vascular endothelial growth factor; VIP, vasoactive intestinal polypeptide.

*Acknowledgment: This work was in part supported by the Division of Intramural Research, NIAID.

● DISTINGUISHING FEATURES OF BASOPHILS AND MAST CELLS

BASOPHILS

Despite certain similarities in biochemistry and function, mammalian basophils and mast cells are not identical (Fig. 63–1).[1–5] The distinction was appreciated by Paul Ehrlich, who described the histochemical staining characteristics of these cells in the late 19th century. Much evidence indicates that basophils share a common precursor with other granulocytes and monocytes.[1–5] Basophils have a short life span[5,6] and retain granulocytic features even after emigrating into tissues (Fig. 63–1C).[7]

The basophil is the least-common granulocyte in human blood, with a prevalence of approximately 0.5 to 0.6 percent of total leukocytes and approximately 0.3 percent of nucleated marrow cells.[8,9] The basophil's prominent metachromatic cytoplasmic granules allow unmistakable identification in Wright-Giemsa–stained films of blood (see Fig. 63–1B) or marrow, but accurate enumeration requires absolute counting methods.[9,10] Differential counts of blood films yield valid results only if the percentage of basophils is substantially elevated or many thousands of leukocytes are counted.

Interleukin (IL)-3 promotes the production and survival of human basophils *in vitro*[3,11] and induces basophilia *in vivo*.[12] Findings in IL-3 –/– mice indicate IL-3 is not necessary for the development of normal numbers of marrow or blood basophils, but is important for the marrow and blood basophilia associated with certain T-helper (Th) 2 cell-associated immunologic responses.[13,14] Basophils also express receptors for several other cytokines (Table 63–1).[5,15] IL-3 and many of these other cytokines, including IL-33, can modulate basophil function, for example, by inducing mediator release directly and/or by augmenting the cells' ability to release mediators in response to immunoglobulin (Ig) E-dependent challenge.[3,5,12]

MAST CELLS

Mast cells normally reside in the connective tissue, particularly beneath epithelial surfaces and around blood vessels, and, in some species, in serous cavities.[1,4,16,17] Mast cells are derived from hematopoietic

precursors.[16–21] Except for a numerically minor population of mast cells residing in the marrow (see Fig. 63–1A),[8] this lineage completes its program of maturation in other tissues.[16–21] Unlike basophils, mast cells can be long-lived. At least some mast cells can proliferate in the tissues during a variety of inflammatory or reparative processes.[1,16,17] Studies in mice, rats, nonhuman primates, and humans indicate many aspects of mast cell development are critically regulated by stem cell factor (SCF), the ligand for the KIT receptor tyrosine kinase.[17,22–24] SCF is produced in membrane-associated and soluble forms, both of which are biologically active (Chap. 18).[17,24] Beside promoting the migration, survival, proliferation, and maturation of cells in the mast cell lineage, SCF can directly promote mast cell mediator release[23,25–27] and, at even lower concentrations, can augment mast cell mediator release in response to stimulation by IgE and antigen.[25,26] Abnormalities affecting *KIT* are involved in the pathogenesis of certain types of mastocytosis (see "Disorders Affecting Mast Cells" below). Alterations in the production of SCF by fibroblasts and other cells may contribute to the changes in mast cell numbers that occur during many chronic inflammatory conditions and other pathologic responses.[17,22,28]

MAST CELL AND BASOPHIL HETEROGENEITY

Variation in the morphologic, biochemical, and/or functional characteristics of mast cells from different anatomic locations or from the same organ or site has been reported in several mammalian species, including humans.[16,17,21,29,30] This phenomenon, often referred to as *mast cell heterogeneity*, raises the possibility that mast cells of different phenotype express different functions in health or disease and may exhibit different sensitivities to pharmacologic manipulation. At least four mechanisms may account for phenotypic variation in mast cell populations: (1) factors promoting branching within the mast cell lineage; (2) factors influencing differentiation and maturation (within a single pathway or, if they occur, within multiple pathways); (3) factors modulating mast cell function; and (4) factors influencing local concentrations of exogenous substances not derived from mast cells but taken up and stored in mast cell granules. Of these four mechanisms, experimental evidence has been obtained for all but the first.[21,30] Basophils can exhibit

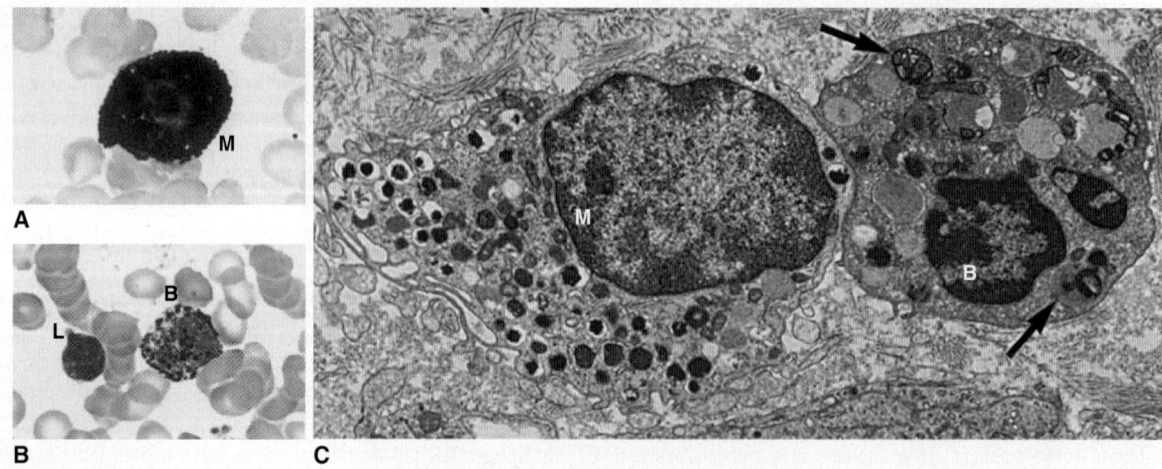

Figure 63–1. A. Mast cell *(M)* in a Wright-Giemsa–stained marrow aspirate. **B.** A basophil *(B)* and lymphocyte *(L)* in a Wright-Giemsa-stained film prepared from the buffy coat of blood from a normal donor. **C.** Transmission electron micrograph illustrating a mast cell *(M)* and basophil *(B)* in the ileal submucosa of a patient with Crohn disease. The mast cell is a larger, mononuclear cell with a more complex plasma membrane surface and cytoplasmic granules that are smaller and more numerous than those of the basophil. In this section plane, the basophil exhibits two nuclear lobes. Several basophil cytoplasmic granules contain whorls of membranes *(arrows)*. Osmium collidine uranyl *en bloc* processing. *(C, reproduced with permission from Dvorak AM, Monahan RA, Osage JE, et al: Crohn's disease: Transmission electron microscopic studies. II. Immunologic inflammatory response. Alterations of mast cells, basophils, eosinophils, and the microvasculature. Hum Pathol 11(6):606–619, 1980.)*

TABLE 63–1. Natural History, Major Mediators, and Surface Membrane Structures of Human Mast Cells and Basophils

Characteristics	Basophils	Mast Cells
NATURAL HISTORY		
Origin of precursor cells	Marrow	Marrow
Site of maturation	Marrow	Connective tissue (a few in marrow)
Mature cells in circulation	Yes (usually <1% of blood leukocytes)	No
Mature cells recruited into tissues from circulation	Yes (during immunologic, inflammatory responses)	No
Mature cells normally residing in connective tissues	No (not detectable by microscopy)	Yes
Proliferative ability of morphologically mature cells	None reported	Yes (limited; under certain circumstances)
Life span	Days (like other granulocytes)	Weeks to months (according to studies in rodents)
Major growth factor	IL-3	SCF
MEDIATORS		
Major mediators stored preformed in cytoplasmic granules	Histamine, chondroitin sulfates, tryptase,* chymase,* carboxypeptidase A,* neutral protease with bradykinin-generating activity, β-glucuronidase, elastase, cathepsin G-like enzyme, major basic protein, Charcot-Leyden crystal protein	Histamine, heparin,* chondroitin sulfates,* chymase,* tryptase,* cathepsin G,* carboxypeptidases, major basic protein, acid hydrolases, peroxidase, phospholipases
Major lipid mediators produced on appropriate activation	Leukotriene C_4	Leukotriene B_4, prostaglandin D_2, leukotriene C_4, platelet-activating factor
Cytokines released on appropriate activation	IL-4, IL-6, IL-13, GM-CSF, VEGF-A, leptin	TNF, TGF-β, IFN-α, VEGF-A–D, IL-6, IL-11, IL-13, IL-16, IL-18, GM-CSF, NGF, PDGF (mouse and human mast cells can secrete many more; see text)
Chemokines	IL-8 (CXCL-8), MIP-1α (CCL3), Eotaxin (CCL-11), MIP-5 (CCL15)	IL-8 (CXCL-8), I-309 (CCL-1), MCP-1 (CCL2), MIP-1α (CCL3), MIP-1β (CCL-4), MCP-3 (CCL-7), RANTES (CCL-5), Eotaxin (CCL-11)
SURFACE STRUCTURES		
Ig receptors	FcεRI, FcγRIIA, FcγRIIB	FcεRI, FcγRI (after IFNγ exposure), FcγRIIA
Cytokine or growth factor receptors for:	IL-1, IL-2 (CD25), IL-3, IL-4, IL-5, IL-6, IL-8, and IL-33; chemokines (CCR1, -2, -3, -5; CXCR1, -2, -4); and interferons; SCF (basophils express variable numbers of the SCF receptor, Kit)	SCF (ligand for Kit), IFN-γ, IL-4, IL-5, IL-6, IL-9, and IL-33; chemokines (CCR1, -3, -4, -5, -7; CXCR1, -2, -3, -4, -6); thrombopoietin receptor (CD110), GM-CSF, NGF
TLRs	TLR-2, -4 (but lack CD14)	TLR-1, -2, -3, -4, -5, -6, -7, -9

IFN, interferon; Ig, immunoglobulin; IL, interleukin; GM-CSF, granulocyte-macrophage colony-stimulating factor; MCP, monocyte chemotactic protein; MIP, macrophage inflammatory protein; NGF, nerve growth factor; PDGF, platelet-derived growth factor; RANTES, regulated on activation, normal T-cell expressed, presumed secreted; SCF, stem cell factor; TNF, tumor necrosis factor; TGF, transforming growth factor; TLR, toll-like receptor; VEGF, vascular endothelial growth factor.

*Basophil and mast cell content of these (and perhaps other) mediators vary, for example, in different subjects and tissues; and/or in association with certain inflammatory diseases.[15]

NOTE: Expression of these and other surface structures, including chemokine receptors, and production of individual cytokines and chemokines, can vary in different *in vitro* or *in vivo* derived basophil or mast cell populations.

Data Modified from Galli SJ, Dvorak AM, Dvorak HF: Basophils and mast cells: morphologic insights into their biology, secretory patterns, and function. *Prog Allergy* 34:1–141, 1984 and Valent P: Immunophenotypic characterization of human basophils and mast cells. *Chem Immunol* 61:34–48, 1995.

some variation in phenotypic characteristics also, such as immunoreactivity for tryptase, chymase, and carboxypeptidase A,[15] or levels of expression of surface structures, including human leukocyte antigen (HLA)-DR, CD32 (FcγRII), and receptors for cytokines.[5,31] Such variation in basophil mediator content and/or cell surface phenotype may reflect individual differences among different subjects and/or the effects of disease processes[15] or the consequences of immunotherapy.[31]

RELATIONSHIP BETWEEN BASOPHILS AND MAST CELLS

Mature basophils and mast cells differ in morphology, natural history, tissue distribution, mediator production, cell-surface phenotype, growth factor requirements, and responses to drugs (see Fig. 63–1 and Table 63–1).[1-5] Nevertheless, certain similarities of the two cells, taken together with evidence indicating that tissue mast cells are derived from circulating marrow-derived precursors,[16,18] had suggested to some investigators that basophils might be circulating precursors of mast cells. However, the following evidence strongly favors the view that mature basophils represent terminally differentiated granulocytes and not circulating mast cell precursors: (1) no evidence has been presented, in any species, indicating that mature circulating basophils are capable of either mitosis or differentiation into mast cells; (2) rare reports of patients with hereditary or acquired abnormalities affecting basophil numbers or morphology indicate that eosinophils also may be affected in these disorders but not mast cells[32–34]; (3) morphologically identifiable human tissue mast cells can exhibit mitotic activity,[35] indicating that mast cells can replicate independently of a stage resembling that of basophils, and (4) in mice, evidence indicates that a mast cell–committed progenitor (MCP) present in the marrow is developmentally distinct during hematopoiesis from a Sca-1[lo] granulocyte-macrophage progenitor.[19,20] Evidence for a committed bipotential precursor of mast cells and basophils during hematopoiesis in the mouse has been reported by some studies[36,37] but not others.[19,20,38]

MORPHOLOGY OF BASOPHILS AND MAST CELLS

Routine histologic methods are poorly suited for demonstrating basophils and mast cells. Optimal visualization is achieved in appropriately prepared 1 μm sections or by electron microscopy.[1,2] By ultrastructure, human basophils are 5 to 7 μm in spherical diameter, exhibit a segmented or unsegmented nucleus with marked condensation of nuclear chromatin, and contain round or oval cytoplasmic granules surrounded by a membrane and containing a substructure of dense particles, less-dense matrix, and, in some granules, membrane whorls and Charcot-Leyden crystals (see Fig. 63–1C).[1,2] A minor population of small, uniform granules is characteristically located near the nucleus.[39] The cytoplasm of mature human basophils also contains glycogen particles, mitochondria, free ribosomes, and small membrane-bound vesicles. Lipid bodies are rarely present. Other organelles are inconspicuous.

In tissue sections, mast cells typically appear as either round or elongated cells, usually with a nonsegmented nucleus with moderate condensation of nuclear chromatin, and contain prominent cytoplasmic granules. Mast cell granules are smaller, more numerous, and generally more variable in appearance than in basophils and contain scroll-like structures, particles, and crystals, alone or in combination (see Fig. 63–1C).[1,2] In contrast to the irregularly spaced blunt surface projections of basophils, mast cells are covered by uniformly distributed thin surface processes. Mast cells also differ from basophils in having many more cytoplasmic filaments and lacking cytoplasmic glycogen deposits. Human mast cells can contain numerous cytoplasmic lipid bodies.

BIOCHEMISTRY AND ROLE IN IMMUNOGLOBULIN E-ASSOCIATED IMMUNE RESPONSES

Mediators

The cytoplasmic granules of basophils and mast cells contain proteoglycans, consisting of sulfated glycosaminoglycans covalently linked to a protein core.[40] These substances can be stained metachromatically with basic dyes (see Fig. 63–1A and B). In humans and murine species, individual mast cell populations can contain variable mixtures of heparin and chondroitin sulfate proteoglycans.[29,40] Although the sulfated glycosaminoglycans of normal human blood basophils have not yet been characterized, two studies of the proteoglycans synthesized by blood leukocytes (containing 10 to 75 percent basophils) of five patients with myeloid leukemia indicate that such cells may produce solely

chondroitin sulfates[41] or a mixture of chondroitin sulfates (50 to 84 percent) and heparin (8 to 43 percent).[42] Although the biologic functions of basophil and mast cell proteoglycans are not fully understood, in mice, heparin is required for normal packaging of certain neutral proteases in mast cell cytoplasmic granules.[40,43] Both human mast cells and basophils synthesize and store histamine.[1,4] Basophils represent the source of most (if not all) of the histamine present in normal human blood.[44] Although macrophages,[45] neutrophils,[46] and platelets,[47] as well as basophils,[44] can produce histamine, mast cells represent the source of virtually all the histamine stored in normal tissues in mice, with the notable exceptions of the glandular stomach and parts of the central nervous system.[48]

In addition to proteoglycans and histamine, basophils and mast cells generate many other products that can influence the course of inflammatory processes (see Table 63–1).[1,3–5,49–51] These substances are either preformed and granule associated (e.g., histamine, neutral proteases, proteoglycans) or produced during activation of the cell (e.g., prostaglandin D_2, leukotrienes and other metabolites of arachidonic acid, and platelet-activating factor). Appropriately stimulated mouse or human mast cells can release the cytokine tumor necrosis factor α (TNF-α),[52,53] and many other cytokines, chemokines, and growth factors with effects on inflammation, immunity, hematopoiesis, tissue remodeling, and many other biologic processes.[1,3–5,49–51] By contrast, the spectrum of basophil-derived cytokines appears to be more limited but includes IL-4 and IL-13, vascular endothelial growth factor (VEGF)-A,[54] certain chemokines, and, at least in mice, IL-6, TNF-α, and thymic stromal lymphopoietin (TSLP).[4,5,55–57]

ROLE IN ACUTE REACTIONS

Basophils and mast cells have specific, high-affinity plasma membrane receptors for the Fc region of IgE (FcϵRI).[58,59] When IgE antibodies bound to FcϵRI on the basophil or mast cell surface are bridged by specific divalent or multivalent antigens, anaphylactic degranulation is triggered.[57,58] The critical signal in this event is the aggregation of FcϵRI on the plasma membrane.[57,58] Anaphylactic degranulation involves the fusion of plasma membranes with the membranes delimiting individual cytoplasmic granules or with groups of granules whose membranes have undergone fusion, leading to rapid noncytolytic release of granule contents, such as histamine and other preformed mediators.[1,2] The complex sequence of biochemical events associated with anaphylactic degranulation, the signaling mechanisms that positively and negatively regulate this response, and the rationale for the pharmacologic manipulation of these processes have been reviewed.[57,58]

The sudden, massive release of mediators from basophils and mast cells provokes many of the clinical manifestations of acute immediate hypersensitivity reactions in disorders such as certain forms of bronchial asthma (including fatal asthma, in which basophils can be prominent[60]); urticaria; allergic rhinitis; and anaphylaxis to foods, drugs, insect stings, and other antigens.[1,5,49,50,55–57] Both mast cells and basophils can bind IgG antibodies (as well as IgE), and the binding of IgG or IgG immune complexes can contribute to the activation of these cells (in certain mouse models of anaphylaxis) or, in other circumstances, to the downregulation of their activation (e.g., via Fcγ RIIB).[5,55–57,61–64] Other diverse stimuli, including certain complement fragments (anaphylatoxins), neutrophil lysosomal proteins, a variety of basic peptides and peptide hormones, components of insect or reptile venoms, radiocontrast solutions, cold, calcium ionophores, and certain drugs such as narcotics and muscle relaxants, also may initiate rapid release of mediators from basophils and/or mast cells, independently of IgE.[1,4,5,48,49,54–56] The clinical reactions provoked by these agents can closely mimic those of immediate hypersensitivity. Basophils activated via FcϵRI or other mechanisms can exhibit increased surface levels of

CD63, CD69, and CD203c, and the clinical value of using such findings to monitor basophil activation *in vivo* (e.g., in the setting of allergic disorders or antigen-specific immunotherapy) is under investigation.[65]

ROLE IN LATE-PHASE REACTIONS

Mast cells and basophils also can contribute to late-phase reactions. Late-phase reactions occur when antigen challenge is followed, hours after initial IgE-dependent mast cell activation, by recurrence of signs (e.g., cutaneous edema) and symptoms (e.g., bronchoconstriction).[49,50] Much of the morbidity associated with chronic allergic conditions, including allergic asthma, is widely believed to reflect the actions of leukocytes that are recruited to sites of late-phase reactions.[49,50] Studies in mast cell–deficient and mast cell knockin mice (genetically mast cell–deficient mice that have been selectively repaired of their mast cell deficiency) indicate mast cells are responsible for virtually all of the vascular permeability changes and leukocyte infiltration associated with IgE-dependent cutaneous late-phase reactions[66,67] and that TNF-α can, importantly, contribute to these responses.[66] The extent to which mast cells (or TNF-α) contribute to late-phase reactions in humans, in which such reactions may have components that are either IgE or T-cell dependent (and in which it has been suggested that certain IgE-dependent mechanisms may not involve mast cells[63]), is not yet clear.[68,69] However, the lymphocytes, basophils, eosinophils, and other leukocytes that are recruited to these reactions likely produce cytokines and other mediators that regulate further development and, ultimately, resolution of these reactions.[4,5,49,50]

ROLE IN CHRONIC CHANGES ASSOCIATED WITH ALLERGIC DISORDERS

Studies in mice (see "Genetic Approaches for Analyzing Basophil and Mast Cell Function" below) indicate that mast cells can contribute importantly to many of the features of asthma, as observed in certain mouse models of chronic allergic inflammation involving the lungs. The features include the development of airway hyperreactivity to immunologically nonspecific agonists of bronchoconstriction such as methacholine; infiltration of the airways and lung interstitium with inflammatory cells, including eosinophils, neutrophils, and T cells; increased deposition of collagen in the lungs and hyperplasia and/or hypertrophy of airway smooth muscle; and induction of increased numbers of mucus-producing goblet cells in the large airways.[50,70,71] Thus, such mouse models indicate mast cells and their products can promote the development of much of the pathology and pathophysiologic changes observed in longstanding asthma in humans.[50,70,71] Studies in mice indicate that basophils also can enhance the development of IgE-dependent chronic inflammation of the skin, even in the absence of mast cells or T cells.[56,67]

IMMUNOGLOBULIN E-DEPENDENT UPREGULATION OF FcεRI EXPRESSION AND FcεRI-DEPENDENT FUNCTION

As plasma levels of IgE increase (as often occurs in subjects with allergic diseases or parasite infections), levels of FcεRI expression on the surface of basophils and mast cells also increase.[72,73] Compared with cells with low "baseline" levels of FcεRI expression, such cells can bind more IgE, release mediators in response to lower concentrations of allergens, and produce significantly larger amounts of preformed and lipid mediators and cytokines.[74] Thus, basophils and mast cells in subjects with high levels of IgE may have significantly

enhanced ability to express IgE-dependent and/or immunoregulatory functions.[49,74] Exposure of mouse mast cells to certain monoclonal IgE antibodies, in the absence of exposure to the antigen for which the IgE is known to have specificity, can enhance the survival of the cells and, in some cases, induce the cells to release all three classes of mediators (preformed, lipid, cytokines).[74] Exposure to IgE in the absence of known antigen also can induce enhanced survival and cytokine and chemokine release in *in vitro* derived human mast cells.[75] Although the mechanisms responsible for these intriguing findings are not fully understood, some types of IgE antibodies appear to induce aggregation of FcεRI in the absence of known antigen.[74,76] The clinical implications of these findings, if any, remain to be defined.

ROLES IN T-CELL–DEPENDENT RESPONSES NOT INVOLVING IMMUNOGLOBULIN E

Mast cell activation and/or infiltration of affected tissues with circulating basophils can occur during a variety of T-cell–dependent immunologic responses in both humans and experimental animals.[1,5,49,55–57,63,64,77–79] However, despite years of study, the importance of the contributions of mast cells or basophils in such settings is not fully understood. In part this may reflect differences in the types of mast cell–deficient mice used to investigate such responses and/or the strain background of such mice, and in part this may reflect differences in the details of the experimental models used to probe the roles of mast cells and basophils in these settings (see "Genetic Approaches for Analyzing Basophil and Mast Cell Function" below). In some of the models of T-cell–dependent responses tested, authors have concluded that mast cell can either enhance or suppress features of the responses, and in some settings evidence has been reported that mast cells can enhance the features of relatively weak responses and suppress features of strong responses.[63,64] It also has been proposed that mast cells and basophils might have immunomodulatory effects on the development or magnitude of certain acquired immune responses (e.g., positive effects via mast cell–dependent enhancement of dendritic cell migration or activation or negative effects *via* the production of IL-10 by mast cells).[5,55–57,63,64,78–80] However, some of the findings in this area are considered controversial.[5,63,64,79]

BIOLOGIC FUNCTIONS OF BASOPHILS AND MAST CELLS

Roles in Host Defense

Parasites Basophils and mast cells may have critical roles in the expression of host resistance to certain parasites. Whether basophils, mast cells, or both represent major effector cell types in these responses appears to vary according to factors such as species of parasite, species of host, and site of infection. Thus, in the guinea pig, basophils appear to be required for expression of immune resistance to infestation of the skin by larval ixodid *Amblyomma americanum* ticks,[77,81] whereas expression of IgE-dependent immune resistance to the cutaneous infestation of larval *Haemaphysalis longicornis* ticks in mice is dependent on mast cells and basophils, and IgE.[57,82] Such findings support the notion that basophils and mast cells express similar or complementary functions as effector cells in host defense against parasites and other agents.

Bacterial Infections Studies in mast cell–deficient and "mast cell knockin mice" (see "Genetic Approaches for Analyzing Basophil and Mast Cell Function" below) or in mice that lack TNF-α or certain mast cell–associated proteases indicate that mast cells can contribute to "innate" host defense against some experimental bacterial infections.[63,64,83] Depending on the model system tested, the beneficial role of the mast cell in such models of "innate immunity" in mice may partly reflect complement-dependent, toll-like receptor (TLR) 4-dependent, endothelin-1–dependent, or neurotensin-dependent activation of mast cells, inducing the release of mast cell–derived mediators, which, in turn, can contribute to enhanced local recruitment or activation of neutrophils and enhanced clearance of bacteria, or which may reduce harmful levels of TNF-α.[63,64,83] Studies in mice indicate mast cells can phagocytose bacteria,[83] and mouse and human mast cells can produce antimicrobial peptides (cathelicidin LL-37 in humans).[84] However, mast cells also may contribute to survival during bacterial infection in mice by additional mechanisms, such as protease-dependent degradation of endothelin-1,[85,86] neurotensin,[87] and perhaps other endogenous peptides that are produced during infections and which contribute to the pathology associated with the disorders.[63] On the other hand, some mast cell functions that may be expressed during bacterial infections in mice, such as the ability of mast cells to degrade IL-6 via dipeptidyl peptidase 1[88] or to produce IL-10 that suppresses host acquired immunity,[89] may have detrimental consequences. Thus, mast cells may have complex roles in innate immune responses, with some actions promoting host defense and survival and others enhancing the pathology associated with the response.

Viral Infections

Mast cell progenitors[90–92] and basophils[93] can become infected with "M tropic" strains of HIV. Although mature mast cells appear to be resistant to such infection, mast cells that matured from infected progenitors while harboring latent infection exhibited enhanced viral replication upon stimulation with ligands for TLR2, TLR4, or TLR9,[91,92] or via an IgE-dependent mechanism.[92] At least one HIV-derived protein, glycoprotein 120 (gp120), can induce mast cell or basophil mediator release (histamine and, in basophils, IL-4 and IL-13) by binding to and crosslinking cell-surface-bound IgE.[93] Many patients infected with HIV develop high levels of IgE and can exhibit exacerbation of the symptoms and signs of their allergic disorders.[93] However, the clinical significance of such findings in HIV-infected patients remains to be determined. Many potential secreted products of mast cells or basophils may have effects that enhance (or suppress) host responses to a variety of viruses or contribute to the pathology associated with the infections.[94] However, the extent to which mast cells contribute to host defense or pathology during viral infections is not clear.

Venoms The venoms of many animals contain substances that can activate mast cells via innate mechanisms and/or can induce specific IgE responses to venom components.[95,96] Many humans have IgE antibodies against components of honeybee or wasp venom, but only a small fraction of such "venom-sensitized" individuals have a history of anaphylaxis or other serious clinical response to such venoms.[97] Work in mast cell–deficient, mast cell knockin, and mast cell protease-deficient mice indicates that mast cells can enhance the resistance of mice to diverse animal venoms and/or their toxic components, including the venoms of three poisonous snakes,[96] the honey bee,[96,98] the Gila monster,[99] and two species of scorpions,[99] as well as to sarafotoxin 6b, a major toxin in Israeli mole viper snake venom[86] and helodermin, a toxin in Gila monster venom.[99]

Notably, carboxypeptidase A3 (CPA3) or mouse mast cell protease (mMCP-4, the functional counterpart in the mouse to human chymase) appeared to account for much or all of the protective effects against various venoms that were attributable to mast cells.[86,96,98,99] CPA3 and mMCP-4 can degrade both endogenous biologically active peptides (endothelin-1 [ET-1][86,96] and vasoactive intestinal polypeptide [VIP],[99] respectively) and similar peptides present in animal venoms (sarafotoxin 6b and helodermin, respectively), which are thought to act in mammals via the same receptors that bind the similar endogenous

peptides. Work in mice deficient in mast cells, IgE, or components of the FcεRI suggests that mast cells also can contribute to the IgE antibody- and FcεRI-dependent enhanced resistance to challenge with potentially lethal amounts of honeybee venom that is observed in animals after an initial exposure to a sublethal amount of that venom.[98] Indeed, it has been hypothesized that the ability to participate in innate and acquired immune defenses against components of venoms and other toxins are important functions of mast cells and, in the case of acquired immunity, of IgE antibodies.[95,96,100]

GENETIC APPROACHES FOR ANALYZING BASOPHIL AND MAST CELL FUNCTION

Factors capable of inducing basophil infiltration, mast cell proliferation, and/or basophil or mast cell activation are generated during a wide variety of immunologic or pathologic processes, including immune responses to parasites.[1,5,30,49–51,55–57,77] As a result, speculation is considerable that basophils and mast cells express critical roles in diverse biologic responses. On the other hand, the precise functions of basophils and mast cells in most of the biologic responses in which the cells have been implicated are obscure. Studies of basophil function in guinea pigs[81] and mice[55–57] have employed antibodies to deplete basophils, and such approaches also have been used to deplete mast cells in mice[101]; however, the antibodies used may also influence other cell types.[5,55–57,63,64,79] Various mutant or transgenic mice that exhibit constitutive or inducible depletion of some or all mast cell populations, as well as mast cell–deficient mice that have been selectively engrafted with wild-type or genetically altered mast cells (so-called mast cell knockin mice), have been used in efforts to define and quantify the contributions of mast cells to many different biologic responses.[63,64,79] Transgenic mice also are now available that exhibit constitutive or inducible depletion of basophils, or that lack certain mast cell–associated products either globally or in selected cell populations.[5,55–57,63,64,79] As has been extensively reviewed,[5,54–56,74–76] the availability of such models has the potential to advance substantially our understanding of the roles of mast cells and basophils in health and disease in mice, including ascertaining the importance of strain background on some of the findings. In evaluating the results of such studies, one should keep in mind that such genetic models can have various advantages and disadvantages, and that even very strong evidence that mast cells or basophils have particular roles in mice does not prove that the cells have identical functions in humans.

No humans devoid of mast cells have been reported. In addition, the clinical findings in the rare patients who express a deficiency of basophils are not easy to interpret. One patient with a profound basopenia experienced persistent and severe infestation with scabies,[32] a finding that might be viewed as consistent with the role of basophils in resisting ectoparasites in humans. However, that patient also had eosinopenia, IgA deficiency, and multiple other clinical problems.[32] A second basophil-deficient patient had a history of recurrent bacterial and viral infections.[34] However, this patient also had a deficiency of eosinophils, hypogammaglobulinemia, abnormal suppressor T-cell function *in vitro*, and a thymoma.[34]

● BLOOD BASOPHIL COUNT

The normal blood basophil count is difficult to define precisely, but several studies place the normal range between approximately 14 to 20 and 80 to 90/μL (approximately 0.014 to 0.020 and 0.080 to 0.090 × 10^9/L).[8–10,102] The blood basophil count reportedly varies by age,[103] gender (in one study[103] but not in another[9]), and season.[104]

BASOPHILOPENIA

Because numbers of blood basophils can be very low even in apparently normal individuals,[8–10,102] determining whether examples of *basophilopenia* reflect pathologic processes as opposed to normal variation can be difficult. Nevertheless, reduced numbers of circulating basophils have been reported in several disorders (Table 63–2). Basophilopenia has been recorded in association with urticaria and anaphylaxis,[105,106] but the extent to which the latter finding represents a loss of metachromatic staining of circulating degranulated cells rather than a true decrease in the number of cells is undetermined. Basophilopenia occurs in conditions that also are associated with eosinophilopenia. These conditions often are associated with increased secretion of adrenal glucocorticoids.[102,107,108] Basophil counts may diminish, sometimes markedly, during leukocytosis accompanying infection, inflammatory states, immunologic reactions, neoplasia, or hemorrhage.[107] Basophil counts also are diminished in thyrotoxicosis or after pharmacologic administration of thyroid hormones. Conversely, basophil counts may be increased in myxedema or after ablation of thyroid function.[107] A rapid

TABLE 63–2. Conditions Associated with Alterations in Numbers of Blood Basophils

I. Decreased Numbers (Basopenia)
  A. Hereditary absence of basophils (very rare)
  B. Elevated levels of glucocorticoids
  C. Hyperthyroidism or treatment with thyroid hormones
  D. Ovulation
  E. Hypersensitivity reactions
    1. Urticaria
    2. Anaphylaxis
    3. Drug-induced reactions
  F. Leukocytosis (in association with diverse disorders)
II. Increased Numbers (Basophilia)
  A. Allergy or inflammation
    1. Ulcerative colitis
    2. Drug, food, inhalant hypersensitivity
    3. Erythroderma, urticaria
    4. Juvenile rheumatoid arthritis
  B. Endocrinopathy
    1. Diabetes mellitus
    2. Estrogen administration
    3. Hypothyroidism (myxedema)
  C. Infection
    1. Chicken pox
    2. Influenza
    3. Smallpox
    4. Tuberculosis
  D. Iron deficiency
  E. Exposure to ionizing radiation
  F. Neoplasia
    1. "Basophilic leukemia" (see text)
  G. Myeloproliferative neoplasms (especially chronic myelogenous leukemia; also polycythemia vera, primary myelofibrosis, essential thrombocythemia)
  H. Carcinoma

and significant drop in blood basophil levels of up to 50 percent has been documented at ovulation.[108] A few patients with an apparent total lack of basophils have been reported.[32,34]

A morphologic abnormality expressed in the majority of eosinophils and basophils but not in other leukocytes or mast cells has been described as an autosomal dominant condition affecting four members of a family.[33] Cytoplasmic inclusions and crystals in basophils resembling the May-Hegglin anomaly have occurred in healthy individuals.

BASOPHILIA

Table 63–2 lists conditions associated with increased numbers of blood basophils (*basophilia*).

Inflammatory and Immunologic Responses

An increased number of basophils is commonly associated with chronic, IgE-associated hypersensitivity disorders. These disorders often are accompanied by increased levels of IgE. Although serum IgE levels and basophil numbers are not directly related,[109] increased IgE levels are associated with increased expression of FcεRI on the surfaces of both basophils and mast cells.[72,73,110] Moreover, basophils can be recruited into tissues at sites of IgE-associated and other immunologic responses.[1,4,5,55–57,77] Basophil levels may be elevated in ulcerative colitis[111] and juvenile rheumatoid arthritis,[112] whereas many inflammatory conditions that cause a leukocytosis are associated with basophilopenia. Basophilia can occur in subjects exposed to ionizing radiation.[113]

Clonal Myeloid Diseases

Myeloproliferative Neoplasms The concentration of blood basophils is slightly increased in many patients with polycythemia vera (Chap. 84), primary myelofibrosis (Chap. 86), and essential thrombocythemia (Chap. 85). A slight increase in the absolute basophil count may be a useful early sign of a myeloproliferative neoplasm. An increased absolute basophil count occurs in virtually all patients with chronic myelogenous leukemia (CML).[114–116] In some patients, basophils can represent 20 to 90 percent of blood leukocytes (Chap. 89). Exaggerated basophilia of this type is a poor prognostic sign and may herald transformation to the accelerated phase of CML.[117] The basophil in myeloproliferative neoplasms is derived from the malignant clone and in CML can contain the Philadelphia (Ph) chromosome.[118] The basophils in CML exhibit a variety of ultrastructural and biochemical abnormalities.[119,120] In some cases, the abnormalities obscure the typical distinctions between basophils and mast cells.[121–124] Release of basophil-associated histamine can lead to episodes of flushing, pruritus, and hypotension in occasional patients with basophilic CML.[125,126] Severe peptic ulcer of the stomach and duodenum can occur in association with hypersecretion of gastric acid and pepsin.[127,128] Ph chromosome–positive acute basophilic leukemia may be a presenting manifestation of CML.[129]

Basophilic Leukemias The basis for designating some cases as basophilic leukemias as opposed to examples of other more typical myelogenous leukemias with an associated pronounced basophilia is not always clear. Accordingly, we refer to these conditions herein as *leukemias associated with basophilia.* Table 63–3 lists the leukemias associated with basophilia. In addition to extreme basophilia in the chronic phase CML or as a manifestation of the accelerated phase of CML, acute basophilic leukemia can rarely occur *de novo.*[130–136] Thus, acute basophilic leukemia is included in the World Health Organization classification of acute myeloid leukemias (AMLs),[137] but the entity is poorly defined.[135,136,138] Some cases are recognized only by electron microscopy, a procedure not used routinely in the diagnosis or classification of leukemias. One report suggests that the detection

TABLE 63–3. Leukemias Associated with Basophilia

Chronic myelogenous leukemia with exaggerated basophilia

Blast transformation, including acute basophilic transformation, of chronic myelogenous leukemia

Acute myelogenous leukemia with t(9;22), t(6;9), t(3;6) or 12p abnormalities and marrow basophilia

Acute basophilic leukemia with t(X;6)(p11.2;q23.3); *MYB-GATA1*

"Acute basophilic leukemia"

of a CD123-positive, CD203c-positive, and CD117-negative blast cell immunophenotype may be useful in making a diagnosis of acute basophilic leukemia.[139] The best defined entity of acute basophilic leukemia appears to occur in male infants and is associated with t(X;6) (p11.2;q23.3), resulting in the fusion of *MYB* and *GATA1*.[140,141]

Other types of AML that have an associated increase in basophils are more prevalent than acute basophilic leukemia. Such acute leukemias most commonly have t(9;22), t(6;9), t(3;6), or 12p abnormalities.[142–145] The t(9;22) AMLs have features similar to blast crisis of CML, but studies show that *de novo* cases are associated with deletion of antigen receptor genes.[146] The t(6;9) AML often is associated with erythroid hyperplasia and dysplasia, a high frequency of *FLT3* mutations, and poor prognosis.[147–149]

AML with inv(16) or t(16;16) are characteristically associated with cells having large basophilic granules, but the cells containing these granules are generally thought to represent abnormal eosinophils rather than basophils.[150]

Although the clinical and pathologic features of acute basophilic leukemia are largely similar to those of AML, affected patients occasionally exhibit symptoms that result from release of mediators (especially histamine) from degranulating or dying basophils.[125,126,132,151] Remission induction therapy is similar to the therapy used for other types of AML, but management can be complicated by shock resulting from massive release of histamine and other mediators associated with acute cytolysis.

Chapter 88 provides further details on the acute leukemias associated with basophilia.

● DISORDERS AFFECTING MAST CELLS

NORMAL MAST CELL LEVELS

Mast cells cannot be identified in the blood of healthy individuals using standard techniques. However, mast cells can be observed in the blood of monkeys that have been treated chronically with large amounts of the *KIT* ligand SCF[22] and in the blood of some patients with systemic mastocytosis.[152] Increases in tissue mast cells can occur by a combination of enhanced progenitor influx and proliferation of resident mast cells in tissues.[16,153] Human mast cells have been classified according to their content of neutral proteases as MC_T, because the granules contain tryptase but not detectable chymase, and MC_{TC}, whose secretory granules contain both enzymes.[29] The former mast cell type ordinarily predominates in lung and gastrointestinal mucosal tissues, and the latter type in dermis and submucosal tissues.[154–156] Mast cells that express chymase but little or no tryptase (MC_C) also have been described.[157]

SECONDARY CHANGES IN MAST CELL NUMBERS

Although long-term treatment with glucocorticoids (particularly topical treatment of the skin) can result in diminished mast cell numbers,[158] no clinical disorder whose primary feature is a reduction in levels of

tissue mast cells has been reported. Studies of small numbers of patients indicate that certain mast cell populations, namely, the MC_T mast cells in the gastrointestinal mucosa, can be strikingly reduced in numbers in subjects with genetically determined or acquired (HIV-induced) immunodeficiency.[159] Human mast cell precursors can be infected *in vitro* with so-called M tropic strains of HIV[90,91,93]; and *in vivo* may comprise a long-lived inducible reservoir of persistent HIV.[92] Whether mast cell infection with HIV contributes to the reduction in gastrointestinal mast cells observed in some subjects with HIV infection remains to be determined.

A number of disorders are associated with small to up to several fold increases in mast cell numbers in or near the tissues affected by the disorder (Table 63–4). Tissues at sites of recurrent allergic reactions often exhibit increases in mast cell numbers, to levels as high as approximately fourfold normal.[154,160] Small increases in mast cell numbers have been observed at sites of pathology in rheumatoid arthritis, psoriatic arthritis, scleroderma, and systemic lupus erythematosus.[154,160–162] Mast cells are reported to be increased in osteoporosis,[163] but the extent to which this increase reflects decreases in other cell types and/or a decrease in bone matrix is unclear. Numbers of marrow mast cells can be increased in patients with chronic liver or renal diseases.[164] Increases in mast cells also have been documented in infectious diseases, particularly at sites

TABLE 63–4. Conditions Associated with Secondary Changes in Mast Cell Numbers

I. Decreased Numbers

  A. Long-term treatment with glucocorticoids

  B. Primary or acquired immunodeficiency disorders (certain mast cell populations; see text and reference 159)

II. Increased Numbers

  A. Immunoglobulin E–associated disorders

    1. Allergic rhinitis

    2. Asthma

    3. Urticaria

  B. Connective tissue disorders

    1. Rheumatoid arthritis

    2. Psoriatic arthritis

    3. Scleroderma

    4. Systemic lupus erythematosus

  C. Infectious diseases

    1. Tuberculosis

    2. Syphilis

    3. Parasitic diseases

  D. Neoplastic disorders

    1. Lymphoproliferative diseases* (lymphoplasmacytic lymphoma/Waldenström macroglobulinemia, lymphoma, chronic lymphocytic leukemia)

    2. Hematopoietic stem cell diseases* (acute or chronic myelogenous leukemias, myelodysplastic syndromes, idiopathic refractory sideroblastic anemia)

  E. Lymph nodes draining areas of tumor growth

  F. Osteoporosis*

  G. Chronic liver disease*

  H. Chronic renal disease*

*Can include increases in numbers of mast cells in the marrow.

of infection with parasites such as *Strongyloides*, in which a greater than fourfold increase in mast cell numbers can occur.[165] In such settings, mast cell numbers return toward normal upon resolution of the infection. Finally, mast cell numbers can be increased several-fold in lymph nodes draining areas of tumor growth[164,166] and in subjects with stem cell diseases and lymphoproliferative diseases, including lymphoma in the marrow and in association with CML.[164,167–169]

DISORDERS OF MAST CELLS: HYPERPLASIA AND NEOPLASIA

DEFINITION AND HISTORY

A group of systemic disorders associated with significant increases in mast cell numbers in the skin and internal organs have been brought together under the term *mastocytosis*. The first report of a primary mast cell disorder is attributed to Unna[170] who, in 1887, reported that the skin lesions of urticaria pigmentosa (UP)[171,172] contained numerous mast cells. Ellis[173] recognized the systemic nature of the disorder in 1949. In addition to the systemic disorders classified as mastocytosis, localized cutaneous aggregates of mast cells, ranging from *mast cell nevi* and *mastocytomas* in infants and children to multiple nodules in older children, may occur.[174,175]

The clinical pattern of disease in mastocytosis and its prognosis can vary substantially among patients (see "Course and Prognosis" below). A consensus classification for mastocytosis has been developed to address the issue and to provide guidelines regarding prognosis and treatment (Table 63–5).[176] Patients with indolent disease, who compose the great majority of subjects with mastocytosis, can expect a normal life span. Patients with systemic mastocytosis with associated clonal, hematologic non–mast-cell-lineage disease (SM-AHNMD) have a prognosis determined by the associated hematologic disorder. Patients with aggressive systemic mastocytosis (ASM) generally have a 3- to 5-year survival. Mast cell leukemia (MCL) is often rapidly fatal.

ETIOLOGY AND PATHOGENESIS

Activating mutations in *KIT*, which encodes the SCF receptor, a member of the type III receptor tyrosine kinase family, have been documented in patients with mastocytosis. Several lines of evidence indicate such mutations can be involved in the pathogenesis of the disease. The most common of these mutations (Asp816Val), which results in

TABLE 63–5. World Health Organization Classification of Systemic Mastocytosis
Cutaneous mastocytosis (CM)
Urticaria pigmentosa (UP)/maculopapular cutaneous mastocytosis (MPCM)
Diffuse cutaneous mastocytosis
Solitary mastocytoma of skin
Indolent systemic mastocytosis (ISM)
Systemic mastocytosis with associated clonal, hematologic non–mast-cell-lineage disease (SM-AHNMD)
Aggressive systemic mastocytosis (ASM)
Mast cell leukemia (MCL)
Mast cell sarcoma (MCS)
Extracutaneous mastocytoma

Modified with permission from Horny HP, Metcalfe DD, Bennett JM, et al: Mastocytosis, in *WHO Classification of Tumours of Haematopoietic and Lymphoid Tissues* edited by Swerdlow SH, Campo E, Harris NL, Jaffe ES, Pileri SA, Stein H, Thiele J, Vardiman JW. p 54. IARC Press, Lyon, 2008.

ligand-independent activation of the *KIT* receptor, was first identified in a long-term cell line derived from a patient with MCL.[177] It then was detected in mononuclear cells in the blood of patients with mastocytosis who had an associated hematologic disorder,[178] as a somatic mutation in lesional tissue obtained from one patient with an aggressive form of mastocytosis and from a second patient with an indolent form of UP,[179] and in the skin, but not the marrow and blood, of an 11-month-old child with mastocytosis.[180]

Together these findings suggest the mutation occurs initially in a mast cell progenitor and that, as the clone expands, it becomes detectable in the marrow, blood, and skin lesions. The Asp816Val mutation, or similar 816 activating mutations that result in the substitution of phenylalanine or tyrosine for aspartate, now are believed to occur in more than 90 percent of adult patients with mastocytosis.[181] Mutations at codon 816 have been identified in a subset of pediatric patients, whereas other pediatric patients exhibit *KIT* mutations elsewhere, including within the extracellular domain. These other mutations also cause constitutive activation in *KIT* to a varying degree.[181]

The extent to which the presence of various *KIT* mutations, and the anatomical distribution of the affected cells, can be used to predict prognosis or disease severity in patients with mastocytosis remains under investigation. Moreover, additional "gain-of-function" mutations of *KIT* in human subjects with mastocytosis have been reported. For example, a novel form of mastocytosis with a *KIT* mutation in the transmembrane domain (Phe522Cys) has been described.[182] In a second example, a *PRKG2-PDGFRB* fusion was identified in a patient presenting with increased numbers of mast cells and peripheral basophilia.[183] The latter case falls within the World Health Organization category of myeloid neoplasms with *PDGFRB* rearrangements, rather than being categorized as a subvariant of mastocytosis. Gain-of-function mutations of *KIT* also have been reported in gastrointestinal stromal tumors.[184] Additional genetic lesions have been reported in aggressive mastocytosis and in patients with SM-AHNMD, including mutations in *JAK2*, *TET2*, *NRAS*, and *KRAS*.[185]

CLINICAL FEATURES

The organs most frequently involved in systemic mastocytosis are the skin, lymph nodes, liver, spleen, marrow, and gastrointestinal tract.

The Skin

The usual presenting lesion of mastocytosis in the skin is UP/maculopapular cutaneous mastocytosis. UP lesions appear as small yellowish-tan to reddish-brown macules or slightly raised papules (Fig. 63–2), which can exhibit the Darier sign, that is, urticaria after mild friction of the skin.[174] The palms, soles, face, and scalp generally remain free of lesions. In many cases, UP develops before age 2 years and subsides by puberty. Adults with UP usually have extracutaneous involvement by mastocytosis. However, some patients, particularly those with SM-AHNMD, ASM, or MCL, lack cutaneous lesions. In such cases, other organs must be biopsied to make the diagnosis. Diffuse cutaneous mastocytosis is an unusual manifestation of mastocytosis.[175,186] The skin appears yellowish-brown and is thickened. Young children with cutaneous disease may have bullous eruptions with hemorrhage.[175] Some adults develop prominent vascularity in association with the skin lesions, a condition that has been termed *telangiectasia macularis eruptiva perstans*.[175]

Lymph Nodes

In one series, peripheral lymphadenopathy occurred in 26 percent and central lymphadenopathy in 19 percent of patients at diagnosis.[187] Lymphadenopathy is most prominent in patients with SM-AHNMD or ASM. Mast cell infiltrates are observed in the node's

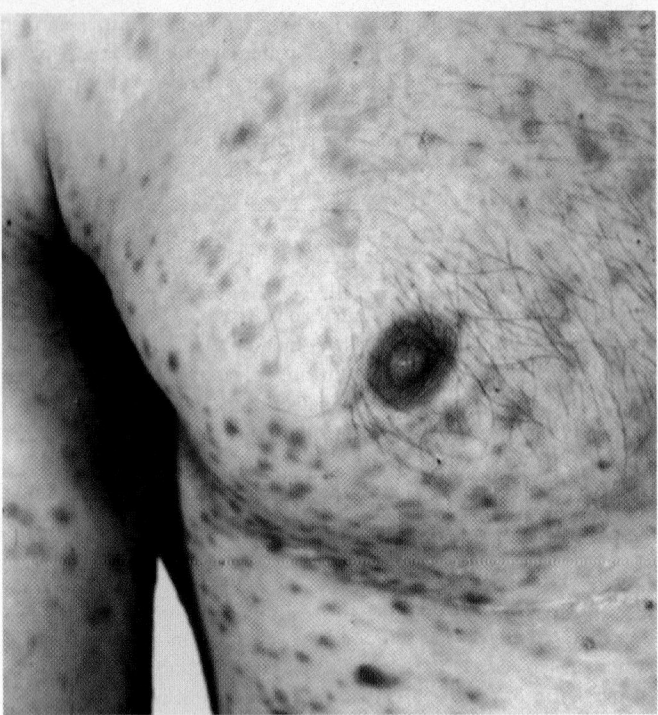

Figure 63–2. Urticaria pigmentosa in an adult man with indolent systemic mastocytosis. Multiple pigmented macules are present. If local pressure is applied to the skin, individual lesions show urtication and become raised, pruritic, and erythematous.

paracortex, follicles, medullary cords, and sinuses. Additional findings include infiltrates of eosinophils, blood vessel proliferation in association with mast cells in the paracortical areas, and extramedullary hematopoiesis. In hematoxylin-and-eosin (H&E)–stained sections, mast cell infiltrates in the lymph nodes may resemble T-cell lymphomas in their pericortical distribution, the clear cytoplasm that is sometimes exhibited by the mast cells, and the associated vascular proliferation and eosinophilia.[187] Alternatively, when mast cells replace lymphoid follicles, the pattern may resemble follicular hyperplasia or follicular lymphoma.[187] Fibrosis may be observed in lymph nodes involved by mast cell infiltrates.

Liver

Patients frequently exhibit infiltration of the liver with mast cells. Many of these individuals have some associated liver pathology, but severe liver disease is uncommon. When severe liver disease does occur, it typically affects patients with SM-AHNMD or ASM. In one series of 41 patients, 61 percent had some liver disease.[188] Elevated serum levels of alkaline phosphatase, aminotransaminases, 5′-nucleotidase, or γ-glutamyl transpeptidase was detected in approximately half of the patients. Hepatomegaly, prominent infiltration of the liver with mast cells, and hepatic fibrosis are positively correlated with elevated levels of alkaline phosphatase and were observed more frequently in patients with aggressive disease; some of these patients also had ascites or portal hypertension. Portal fibrosis was observed in 68 percent and was positively correlated with hepatic inflammation and mast cell infiltrates. Venopathy and associated venoocclusive disease was observed in four patients, all of whom had an associated hematologic disorder.

Spleen

Splenic involvement at diagnosis has been reported in approximately half of patients with systemic disease.[187,189] Mast cells most commonly occurred in a paratrabecular distribution, followed by perifollicular, follicular, and diffuse infiltrates. Trabecular and capsular fibrosis and eosinophilic infiltration also were observed, and extramedullary hematopoiesis was present in most cases. On H&E stained sections, the infiltrates of mast cells produced lesions that may resemble those of T-cell lymphoma, follicular hyperplasia, follicular lymphoma, myeloproliferative neoplasms, hairy cell leukemia, or a granulomatous process. Splenomegaly has also been reported in the absence of infiltration of the spleen by mast cells.[190] Increased splenic weights greater than 700 g generally occurred in patients within unfavorable categories of mastocytosis.

Marrow

The majority of adults with systemic mast cell disease have focal mast cell lesions in the marrow,[189,191–194] typically appearing as foci of spindle-shaped mast cells in a fibrotic background (Fig. 63–3), sometimes with associated eosinophils and T and B lymphocytes. These focal mast cell lesions are the major criterion in the diagnosis of systemic mastocytosis (Table 63–6).[176] Reticulin staining may be increased, and Masson trichome staining may reveal collagen deposition. In specimens extensively involved by mast cell lesions, the bony trabeculae may be moderately to markedly thickened. Aggressive variants of mastocytosis, such as MCL, should be considered if the percentage of mast cells in the marrow aspirate film exceeds 20 percent of all nucleated cells. In the typical leukemic variant of MCL, mast cells account for 10 percent or more of blood leukocytes.[176] This type of MCL should be distinguished from an aleukemic variant of MCL where circulating mast cells account for less than 10 percent of white blood cells.[195]

In H&E–stained sections, the mast cells typically exhibit a spindle-shaped or oval nucleus (see Fig. 63–3A and B), and fine eosinophilic granules are apparent in the cytoplasm at high-power magnification (see Fig. 63–3B). Mast cells with bilobed nuclei may be seen in these lesions and is a finding associated with a poor prognosis.[189] Mast cells stain positively for chloroacetate esterase and aminocaproate esterase, and for mast cell tryptase by immunohistochemistry (see Fig. 63–3D). The latter is the procedure of choice for visualizing mast cells. Mast cells exhibit immunoreactivity for a variety of paraffin section markers.[196] The more specific mast cell markers in paraffin sections are CD117 (KIT) (see Fig. 63–3C) and mast cell tryptase (see Fig. 63–3D). Strong CD117 membrane staining is equally sensitive for mast cells as tryptase but is less specific.

Films of marrow aspirates or clot sections alone cannot be used to diagnose mast cell disease in the marrow. Although increased numbers of mast cells may be present in marrow aspirate films of patients with systemic mast cell diseases, similar findings have been reported in patients without mast cell disorders or in patients with a reactive increase in marrow mast cells. However, mast cells in reactive lesions usually are not spindle shaped, nor do they typically exhibit evidence of degranulation. On marrow films, a normal mast cell has a round or oval shape, a round and centrally located, nonlobated nucleus, and a fully granulated cytoplasm. Mast cells from patients with mastocytosis may exhibit phenotypic aberrations, such as a spindle shape, cytoplasmic projections, and hypogranulation. A multilobular and/or eccentrically located nucleus may be observed.[176] If at least 25 percent of all mast cells on aspirate smears have aberrant morphology, the findings are considered to support the diagnosis of systemic mastocytosis (minor criterion).[176] An aberrant mast cell phenotype also may be detected on flow cytometric analysis of the marrow aspirate. In patients with mastocytosis, mast cells may express CD2, CD25 (minor criterion), and CD33.[197]

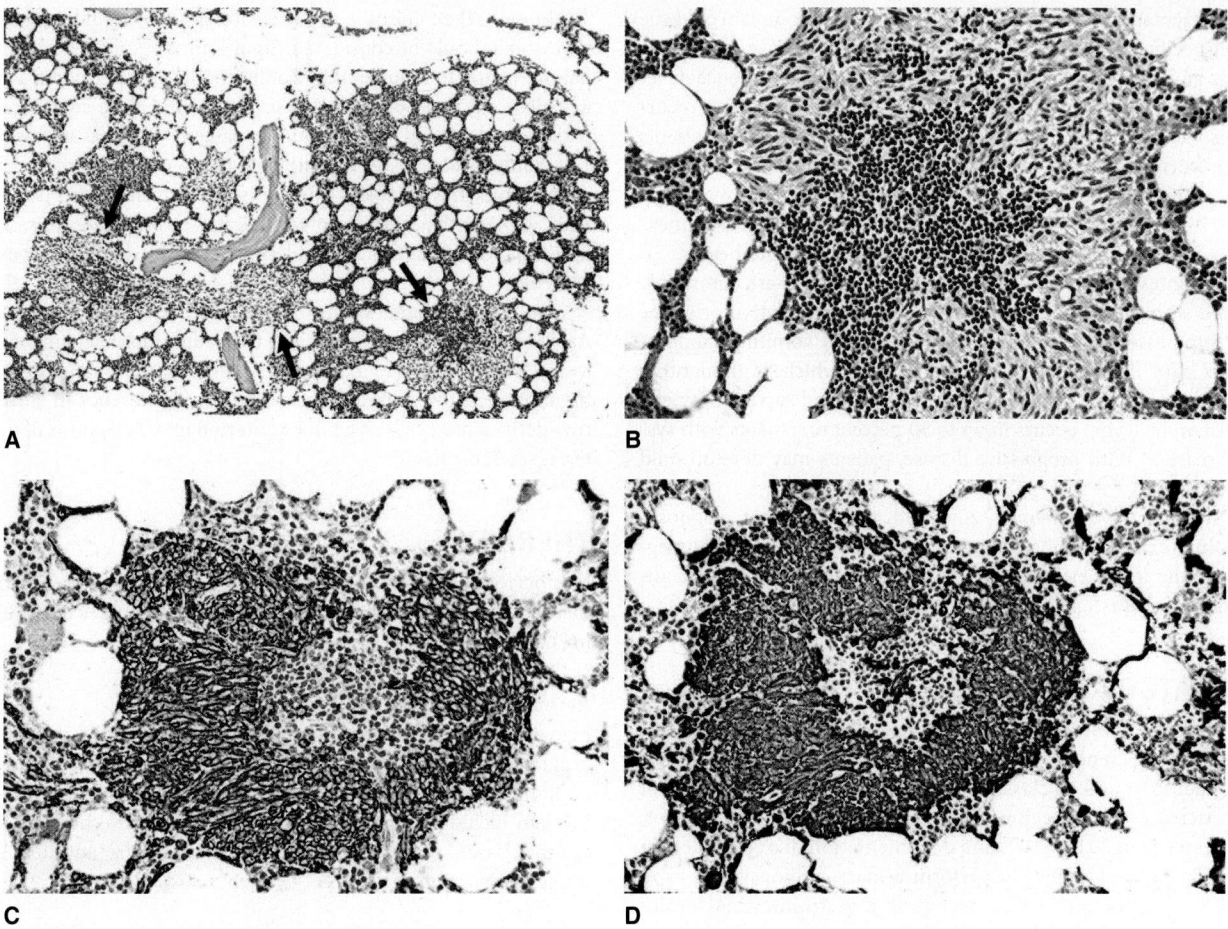

Figure 63–3. Marrow sections. Marrow biopsy from an adult with indolent systemic mastocytosis showing characteristic focal aggregates of mast cells, some of which are spindle-shaped, with admixed eosinophils and numerous small lymphocytes; different areas of the specimen were stained by hematoxylin and eosin (H&E) (**A**, **B**; ×40 and ×200, respectively) or with an antibody to human CD117 (**C**; ×200) or tryptase (**D**; ×200). Areas that contain many mast cells are depicted with *arrows* in **A**.

TABLE 63–6. Diagnostic Criteria for Systemic Mastocytosis

Major Criterion

Multifocal, dense infiltrates of mast cells (≥15 mast cells in an aggregate) detected in sections of marrow and/or other extracutaneous organ(s)

Minor Criteria

a. In biopsy sections of marrow or other extracutaneous organs, >25% of the mast cells in the infiltrate are spindle shaped or have atypical morphology, or, of all mast cells in marrow aspirate smears, >25% are immature or atypical mast cells

b. Detection of a point mutation in *KIT* at codon 816 in marrow, blood, or other extracutaneous organ

c. Mast cells in marrow, blood, or other extracutaneous organs that coexpress CD117 with CD2 and/or CD25

d. Serum total tryptase persistently >20 ng/mL (if there is an associated myeloid disorder, this criterion is not valid)

The diagnosis of systemic mastocytosis can be made if one major and one minor criterion are present or if three minor criteria are met.

Marrow involvement is much less common in children. In a study of 17 children with cutaneous or disseminated mast cell disease, small focal mast cell lesions were observed in marrow biopsies in 10 individuals, and increased mast cells in marrow aspirate films were noted in 5.[193] The focal lesions found in children usually are small and perivascular.

Progression of marrow involvement in systemic mast cell disease is variable. Some adults with indolent disease appear to have stable, or even decreasing, marrow involvement over time.[189] In contrast, a progressive increase in focal mast cell lesions is more commonly observed in patients with more aggressive patterns of disease.

CLINICAL PRESENTATION

Even though individuals may differ in the specific pathogenesis of their disease, all patients within a given category of mastocytosis (see Table 63–5) tend to exhibit similar clinical features. Manifestations of the disease largely reflect the local and systemic consequences of mediator release from tissue mast cells. Effects caused by disruption of normal structures by local collections of mast cells also may be seen.

At presentation, patients with mastocytosis may complain of vague and nonspecific constitutional symptoms, such as fatigue, weakness, flushing, and musculoskeletal pain. Some patients experience fever and/or weight loss.[152,186] A subset of patients may present with recurrent episodes of unexplained anaphylaxis.[198] However, most patients with mastocytosis and a hematologic disorder are diagnosed based on marrow biopsy findings, during the investigation of their hematologic disease.[187,189] Patients with aggressive disease often present with unexplained lymphadenopathy and splenomegaly and/or hepatomegaly.

Gastrointestinal disease and associated symptoms are commonly associated with systemic mastocytosis, either at presentation or as the disease progresses.[174,199] Findings include nausea, vomiting, abdominal pain, and diarrhea. Peptic ulcer disease, which is thought to reflect, at least in part, the promotion of gastric acid secretion by elevated histamine levels, occurs in up to 50 percent of patients with systemic disease.[199] With progressive disease, patients may develop mild malabsorption.[199]

If systemic involvement is advanced at the time of diagnosis, patients may exhibit lymphadenopathy, hepatomegaly, and splenomegaly during the initial evaluation.[152] Because osteoporosis may accompany systemic disease, pathologic fractures may occur.

LABORATORY FEATURES

When systemic mastocytosis is suspected in patients based on a combination of: reports of symptoms consistent with mediator release, identification of classical skin lesions showing a 10-fold or greater increase in mast cell numbers, an elevation in serum tryptase of greater than 20 ng/mL[200] and documentation of organomegaly, an appropriate next step is to perform a marrow biopsy and aspirate.[152,176,201] Additional studies, including a gastrointestinal evaluation involving radiographic studies of the upper gastrointestinal tract and small intestines, computed tomographic scan of the abdomen, and endoscopy, also may be justified.

Plasma and/or urinary histamine levels may be increased in systemic mastocytosis.[186] However, the isolated findings of increased levels of histamine or histamine metabolites may reflect a number of other situations, including anaphylaxis. Furthermore, the accuracy of laboratory measurement of histamine depends on the assay used. Urine histamine levels may be falsely elevated as a result of bacterial contamination, pharmacologic agents and their metabolites excreted in the urine, or diets rich in histamine or histamine precursors. Similarly, serum tryptase may be elevated after anaphylaxis. Thus, no single laboratory test showing an elevation in a mast cell mediator is diagnostic of mastocytosis. Rather, the demonstration of such mediators in blood or urine should prompt the clinician to investigate further for the presence of mastocytosis.

There are patients who have symptoms of mediator release but no mastocytosis in the skin or organomegaly. Some of these patients may have experienced venom-induced anaphylaxis. These patients may also exhibit elevations in tryptase but below the 20 ng/mL which is used as a minor diagnostic criterion. In such situations, reports have suggested the detection of the D816V mutation in blood using a highly sensitive allele-specific quantitative polymerase chain reaction (qPCR) may be useful as a diagnostic parameter.[201] At the time of writing of this chapter, this test is not widely available and it is being used largely in referral centers.

DIFFERENTIAL DIAGNOSIS

The differential diagnosis of systemic mastocytosis includes allergic diseases; hereditary or acquired angioneurotic edema; idiopathic flushing, urticaria, and anaphylaxis; carcinoid tumor; and idiopathic capillary leak

syndrome. When episodic hypertension is a major finding, pheochromocytoma should be considered. Significant unexplained gastroduodenal ulcer disease requires that Zollinger-Ellison gastrinoma syndrome be ruled out. *Helicobacter pylori* infection should be considered in all patients with ulcer disease, including patients with mastocytosis.

Some diseases have hematologic findings that overlap with those of systemic mastocytosis. These disorders include tryptase-positive AML, CML with accumulation of tryptase-positive cells, primary myelofibrosis with mast cell accumulation, and acute or chronic basophilic leukemia.

A somatic mutation in *KIT* at codon 816 (most commonly Asp816Val) is associated especially with adult-onset systemic mastocytosis. Demonstration of a codon 816 gain-of-function mutation, where the most sensitive approach is to look for its presence in sorted marrow-derived mast cells, is a minor criterion in the diagnosis of mastocytosis (see Table 63–6).

THERAPY

Mastocytosis currently has no cure.[202] In addition, no evidence indicates that symptomatic therapy significantly alters the course of the underlying disease.

Avoiding Triggers

Management of mastocytosis includes instructing the patient on the avoidance of factors that may trigger symptoms (presumably by direct or indirect activation of mast cell mediator production). Such factors can include temperature extremes, physical exertion, or, in some unusual cases, ingestion of ethanol, nonsteroidal antiinflammatory drugs, or opiate analgesics.[174]

Epinephrine and H_1 or H_2 Antihistamines

Anaphylaxis may follow insect stings, even in the absence of evidence of allergic sensitivity.[198] Epinephrine-filled syringes and instructions on their use can be given to patients considered at risk for such a reaction. Patients with mast cell disease and a history of anaphylaxis should be advised to carry epinephrine-filled syringes, instructed on their use, and taught to self-medicate, if necessary. These patients also may benefit from the concurrent use of H_1 and H_2 antihistamines prophylactically. Patients may experience severe reactions to iodinated contrast materials. Thus, consideration should be given to premedicating mastocytosis patients with H_1 and H_2 antihistamines and prednisone. Nonsedative H_1 antihistamines decrease skin irritability and pruritus.[186,202] Pruritus may be relieved by approaches that maintain skin hydration. H_2 antihistamines, including ranitidine and famotidine, are used to treat the gastritis and peptic ulcer disease associated with mastocytosis.[186,202–204] H_2 antihistamines may be titrated based on symptom control or to a particular level of gastric secretion. Proton pump inhibitors are useful for management of gastric hypersecretion.[199,204]

OTHER DRUG THERAPY

Disodium Cromoglycate; Ketotifen

Oral administration of disodium cromoglycate may be useful for treatment of gastrointestinal cramping and diarrhea.[186,202,205] The agent has been beneficial in cutaneous mast cell disease in children and infants.[186] Other symptoms, including headache, have improved with administration of cromolyn sodium. Ketotifen reportedly has been effective in relieving pruritus and wheal formation in cutaneous mastocytosis.[206] By contrast, one pediatric study found ketotifen was no more effective than hydroxyzine.[207]

Bisphosphonates

Osteoporosis in patients with mastocytosis may be unrecognized and thus undertreated, especially in patients with milder forms of disease. It is thus important to utilize dual-energy x-ray absorptiometry (DEXA) scanning in the evaluation of those with mastocytosis. Recommended approaches for the treatment of osteoporosis include calcium supplementation, consideration of estrogen replacement in postmenopausal women, and use of bisphosphonates.[204]

Nonsteroidal Antiinflammatory Agents

Nonsteroidal antiinflammatory agents have been useful in some patients whose primary manifestations are recurrent episodes of flushing, syncope, or both.[202,204] It should be noted that these agents may exacerbate ulcer disease. Patients with a history of aspirin sensitivity should not be placed on this therapy unless they first undergo desensitization.

Glucocorticoids; Methoxypsoralen

Cutaneous lesions have been treated with either glucocorticoids[208] or 8-methoxypsoralen plus ultraviolet A (PUVA),[209] largely to reduce pruritus or for cosmetic improvement. No evidence indicates such approaches alter the progression of systemic disease. Relapses 3 to 6 months after cessation of PUVA therapy are common. Patients may experience a decrease in the intensity of lesions after exposure to natural sunlight. Repeated or extensive application of glucocorticoids may result in cutaneous atrophy or adrenocortical suppression.[208]

Systemic glucocorticoids are used to decrease significant malabsorption and ascites[210] in patients with advanced disease. In adults, oral prednisone (40 to 60 mg/day) usually results in decreased symptoms over a 2- to 3-week period. After initial improvement, steroids usually can be tapered to an alternate-day regimen. However, with time, the ascites frequently recurs. Such patients reportedly can benefit from a portacaval shunt.

Interferon-α Cladribine

Patients with more advanced categories of systemic mastocytosis may be candidates for approaches directed at reducing the mast cell burden. None of these approaches has resulted in cure of the disease. For severe disease, some limited success has been reported for interferon α (IFN-α) and it is often considered to be a first-line drug of choice along with cladribine.[204,211,212] It is presumed to act by restricting the proliferation of hematopoietic progenitor cells. Studies with IFN-α, often in combination with glucocorticoids, have reported variable success, with unchanged or modest reductions in marrow infiltration with mast cells, and in tryptase levels. Many patients do report symptomatic benefits. Resolutions of ascites and increased bone remineralization also have been reported. Use of IFN-α is often limited by side effects such as fever, fatigue, and cytopenias. Its use is not routinely recommended for patients with indolent systemic disease, unless there is concomitant severe osteoporosis.

Cladribine (2-chlorodeoxyadenosine), a nucleoside analogue, does not require cells in active cell cycle to exert its cytotoxic activity and may be beneficial in slowly progressing neoplastic processes. The drug has myelosuppressive and immunosuppressive properties and thus cannot be recommended for patients with indolent disease.[204]

Hematopoietic Stem Cell Transplantation

Allogeneic stem cell transplantation (SCT) has been employed as a treatment option for patients with advanced categories of mastocytosis associated with poor survival. SCT has been used to treat a hematologic disorder associated with mastocytosis in relatively few cases.[213–216] Although these studies reported favorable responses of the associated hematologic disorders, complete remission of the mast cell disease was reported in only one study, which used non–T-cell-depleted blood SCT in a patient with an associated myeloproliferative neoplasm.[215] The value of allogeneic SCT in mastocytosis may result from the immunotherapeutic effects of the donor marrow rather than the myeloablative conditioning regimen.[213] One study using nonmyeloablative blood SCT for treatment of advanced systemic mastocytosis in three patients with advanced mastocytosis reported no effect on mastocytosis progression despite the induction of a graft-versus-mast-cell response.[216] Perhaps performing targeted therapy directed at the mast cell compartment before transplantation would improve outcome.

Tyrosine Kinase Inhibitors

The availability of low-molecular-weight inhibitors of tyrosine kinases suggested the mutated KIT tyrosine kinases in mastocytosis as a therapeutic target. Imatinib mesylate (Gleevec; Novartis, Basel, Switzerland) currently is the only such drug available. It has a specific inhibition profile that includes ABL1, KIT, and PDGFR (platelet-derived growth factor receptor) tyrosine kinases.[217,218] Although the drug inhibits wild-type KIT and KIT bearing juxtamembrane-activating mutations similar to those found in gastrointestinal stromal tumors, it does not inhibit KIT bearing the codon 816 mutations associated with most common forms of systemic mastocytosis.[219,220] This finding is attributed to a conformational change in KIT bearing the codon 816 mutation, which interferes with the association of the drug with the ATP-binding domains of the receptor. Consistent with these observations, imatinib mesylate showed a strong *in vitro* cytotoxic effect on mast cells bearing wild-type KIT. Mast cells bearing a codon 816 mutation isolated from marrow of patients with mastocytosis were fairly resistant to the drug.[221] These studies suggest imatinib mesylate is unlikely to be an effective therapy for patients who carry codon 816 mutations. However, the drug appears to be of value when there is an imatinib-sensitive mutation or in KIT816-unmutated patients. For example, a patient with an unusual form of systemic mastocytosis associated with a KIT mutation (Phe-522Cys) affecting the transmembrane region of the receptor responded to treatment with imatinib.[182] Accordingly, a careful mutational analysis of a sample enriched for lesional mast cells appears to be essential in patients with mastocytosis before contemplating imatinib therapy. Other tyrosine kinase inhibitors that decrease the activity of KIT with codon 816 mutations including midostaurin (PKC412) and dasatinib are in clinical trials.[222,223] Studies to date suggest that midostaurin may produce significant decreases in mast cell burden in some patients.[222]

Some patients with a variant of chronic eosinophilic leukemia (clonal hypereosinophilic syndrome) and FIPIL1-PDGFRA fusions exhibit elevated serum tryptase levels, increased numbers of mast cells in the marrow, some of which can appear atypical and spindle shaped, tissue fibrosis, and, like other patients who have the FIPIL1-PDGFRA fusion gene, are responsive to imatinib mesylate.[224,225] Such cases are classified within the World Health Organization category of myeloid and lymphoid neoplasms with eosinophilia and abnormalities of PDGFRA, PDGFRB, or FGFR1.

Monoclonal Mast Cell Activation Syndrome

Monoclonal mast cell activation syndrome (MMAS) is a term adopted by a consensus conference to be applied to patients who are found to have one or two minor diagnostic criteria for mastocytosis but lack the full diagnostic criteria for systemic disease.[226] Patients with such findings have been identified within groups of patients diagnosed with idiopathic anaphylaxis and patients with anaphylaxis to stinging insects. It is possible that these studies are identifying patients with a progressive clonal mast cell disorder that may one day meet the diagnostic criteria for systemic mastocytosis. For now, such patients are treated symptomatically and for anaphylaxis. Followup at yearly intervals is recommended to determine if there is evidence of an expanding mast cell compartment.

Mast Cell Activation Syndrome

The term *mast cell activation syndrome* (MCAS) is sometimes applied as a diagnosis for patients with episodic allergic-like signs and symptoms, including flushing, urticaria, diarrhea, and wheezing, involving two or more organ systems; and where an extensive medical evaluation has failed to identify an etiology.[227,228] The assumption is that individuals to whom this diagnosis is applied are having episodes caused by release of mediators associated with hyperreactivity of mast cells that then activate spontaneously.

Diagnostic criteria have been proposed to separate this proposed entity from other causes of such clinical findings. These criteria include response to antimediator therapy and an elevation in a marker of mast cell activation, such as serum tryptase, with an episode.[227] Primary (clonal) and other clinical disorders associated with mast cell activation, as well as other conditions associated with vasoactive mediator release, must be eliminated as possible causes of the clinical findings, including allergic diseases, mast cell activation associated with chronic inflammatory or neoplastic disorders and chronic autoimmune urticaria. Once the diagnostic criteria are met, therapy is symptomatic. Patients must be followed regularly in the event that one of the diagnoses eliminated during the initial evaluation reaches the level of diagnosis.

Splenectomy

Splenectomy has been performed on patients with severe aggressive mastocytosis in an attempt to improve their limiting cytopenias.[229] Based on comparisons to historical controls, splenectomy increased survival by an average of 12 months. Patients who had undergone splenectomy appeared to be better able to tolerate chemotherapy. Splenectomy is of no value in the management of indolent mast cell disease.

COURSE AND PROGNOSIS

The prognosis of adult patients with mast cell disorders is related to the disease category. The vast majority of patients who present with UP and indolent systemic mastocytosis (ISM) have a chronic protracted course that responds to symptomatic medical management. A normal life span is expected. Few of these patients progress to more severe forms of the disease; some patients may even experience a diminution in the severity of skin lesions in later years, while their marrow findings remain unchanged.[230] However, elevated serum lactate dehydrogenase levels, a late age of onset, and, in patients with SM-AHNMD, presence of a significant hematologic abnormality (such as a myeloproliferative or myelodysplastic disorder or, more rarely, overt leukemia) are indicators of a poor prognosis and shortened survival.[189] The prognosis for patients with SM-AHNMD depends on the course of the associated hematologic disorder.

Mast Cell Leukemia

MCL is relatively rare and prognosis is poor.[195,222] A major differential diagnosis to MCL is myelomastocytic leukemia (MML).[231] Patients with MCL may have fever, anorexia, weight loss, fatigue, severe abdominal cramping, nausea, vomiting, diarrhea, flushing, hypotension, pruritus, or bone pain. Peptic ulcer and gastrointestinal bleeding, hepatomegaly, splenomegaly, and lymph node enlargement are frequent findings. Anemia is a constant feature, and thrombocytopenia is nearly always present. The total leukocyte count varies from 10,000 to 150,000/μL (10 to 150 × 10^9/L), and mast cells compose 10 to 90 percent of leukocytes. Marrow biopsy shows a striking increase in mast cells, sometimes up to 90 percent of marrow cells, although the leukemic mast cells often are hypogranular or agranular.[195,231]

Mast Cell Sarcoma

This is an exceedingly rare tumor, characterized by nodules at various cutaneous and mucosal sites.[164,176]

REFERENCES

1. Galli SJ, Dvorak AM, Dvorak HF: Basophils and mast cells: Morphologic insights into their biology, secretory patterns, and function. *Prog Allergy* 34:1–141, 1984.
2. Dvorak AM. *Basophil and Mast Cell Degranulation and Recovery*, vol. 4. Springer, New York, 1991.
3. Valent P: Immunophenotypic characterization of human basophils and mast cells. *Chem Immunol* 61:34–48, 1995.
4. Metz M, Brockow K, Metcalfe D, et al: Mast cells, basophils and mastocytosis, in *Clinical Immunology: Principles and Practice* edited by Rich RR, Fleisher TA, Shearer WT, Schroeder HW Jr, Frew AJ, Weyand CM, p 285. Elsevier Saunders, Philadelphia, 2013.
5. Voehringer D: Protective and pathological roles of mast cells and basophils. *Nat Rev Immunol* 13:362–375, 2013.
6. Murakami M, Izumi H, Morimoto S, et al: Thalassemia intermedia complicated by hemochromatosis: Clinical and autopsy report of a case. *Nihon Ketsueki Gakkai Zasshi* 32:336–352, 1969.
7. Dvorak AM, Monahan RA, Osage JE, et al: Crohn's disease: Transmission electron microscopic studies. II. Immunologic inflammatory response. Alterations of mast cells, basophils, eosinophils, and the microvasculature. *Hum Pathol* 11:606–619, 1980.
8. Juhlin L: Basophil leukocyte differential in blood and bone marrow. *Acta Haematol* 29:89–95, 1963.
9. Ducrest S, Meier F, Tschopp C, et al: Flow cytometric analysis of basophil counts in human blood and inaccuracy of hematology analyzers. *Allergy* 60:1446–1450, 2005.
10. Gilbert HS, Ornstein L: Basophil counting with a new staining method using Alcian blue. *Blood* 46:279–286, 1975.
11. Ishizaka T, Iwata M, Ishizaka K: Release of histamine and arachidonate from mouse mast cells induced by glycosylation-enhancing factor and bradykinin. *J Immunol* 134:1880–1887, 1985.
12. Ganser A, Lindemann A, Seipelt G, et al: Effects of recombinant human interleukin-3 in aplastic anemia. *Blood* 76:1287–1292, 1990.
13. Lantz CS, Boesiger J, Song CH, et al: Role for interleukin-3 in mast-cell and basophil development and in immunity to parasites. *Nature* 392:90–93, 1998.
14. Lantz CS, Min B, Tsai M, et al: IL-3 is required for increases in blood basophils in nematode infection in mice and can enhance IgE-dependent IL-4 production by basophils in vitro. *Lab Invest* 88:1134–1142, 2008.
15. Li L, Li Y, Reddel SW, et al: Identification of basophilic cells that express mast cell granule proteases in the peripheral blood of asthma, allergy, and drug-reactive patients. *J Immunol* 161:5079–5086, 1998.
16. Kitamura Y: Heterogeneity of mast cells and phenotypic change between subpopulations. *Annu Rev Immunol* 7:59–76, 1989.
17. Galli SJ, Zsebo KM, Geissler EN: The kit ligand, stem cell factor. *Adv Immunol* 55:1–96, 1994.
18. Rodewald HR, Dessing M, Dvorak AM, et al: Identification of a committed precursor for the mast cell lineage. *Science* 271:818–822, 1996.
19. Chen CC, Grimbaldeston MA, Tsai M, et al: Identification of mast cell progenitors in adult mice. *Proc Natl Acad Sci U S A* 102:11408–11413, 2005.
20. Franco CB, Chen CC, Drukker M, et al: Distinguishing mast cell and granulocyte differentiation at the single-cell level. *Cell Stem Cell* 6:361–368, 2010.
21. Galli SJ, Borregaard N, Wynn TA: Phenotypic and functional plasticity of cells of innate immunity: Macrophages, mast cells and neutrophils. *Nat Immunol* 12:1035–1044, 2011.
22. Galli SJ, Iemura A, Garlick DS, et al: Reversible expansion of primate mast cell populations in vivo by stem cell factor. *J Clin Invest* 91.148–152, 1993.
23. Costa JJ, Demetri GD, Harrist TJ, et al: Recombinant human stem cell factor (kit ligand) promotes human mast cell and melanocyte hyperplasia and functional activation in vivo. *J Exp Med* 183:2681–2686, 1996.
24. Smith MA, Court EL, Smith JG: Stem cell factor: Laboratory and clinical aspects. *Blood Rev* 15:191–197, 2001.
25. Bischoff SC, Dahinden CA: C-kit ligand: A unique potentiator of mediator release by human lung mast cells. *J Exp Med* 175:237–244, 1992.
26. Columbo M, Horowitz EM, Botana LM, et al: The human recombinant c-kit receptor ligand, rhSCF, induces mediator release from human cutaneous mast cells and enhances IgE-dependent mediator release from both skin mast cells and peripheral blood basophils. *J Immunol* 149:599–608, 1992.
27. Wershil BK, Tsai M, Geissler EN, et al: The rat c-*kit* ligand, stem cell factor, induces c-*kit* receptor-dependent mouse mast cell activation in vivo. Evidence that signaling through the c-*kit* receptor can induce expression of cellular function. *J Exp Med* 175:245–255, 1992.
28. Finotto S, Mekori YA, Metcalfe DD: Glucocorticoids decrease tissue mast cell number by reducing the production of the c-kit ligand, stem cell factor, by resident cells: In vitro and in vivo evidence in murine systems. *J Clin Invest* 99:1721–1728, 1997.
29. Irani AA, Schechter NM, Craig SS, et al: Two types of human mast cells that have distinct neutral protease compositions. *Proc Natl Acad Sci U S A* 83:4464–4468, 1986.
30. Galli SJ: New insights into "the riddle of the mast cells": Microenvironmental regulation of mast cell development and phenotypic heterogeneity. *Lab Invest* 62:5–33, 1990.

31. Siegmund R, Vogelsang H, Machnik A, et al: Surface membrane antigen alteration on blood basophils in patients with Hymenoptera venom allergy under immunotherapy. *J Allergy Clin Immunol* 106:1190–1195, 2000.

32. Juhlin L, Michaelsson G: A new syndrome characterised by absence of eosinophils and basophils. *Lancet* 1:1233–1235, 1977.

33. Tracey R, Smith H: An inherited anomaly of human eosinophils and basophils. *Blood Cells* 4:291–300, 1978.

34. Mitchell EB, Platts-Mills TA, Pereira RS, et al: Basophil and eosinophil deficiency in a patient with hypogammaglobulinemia associated with thymoma. *Birth Defects Orig Artic Ser* 19:331, 1983.

35. Dvorak AM, Mihm MC Jr, Dvorak HF: Morphology of delayed-type hypersensitivity reactions in man. II. Ultrastructural alterations affecting the microvasculature and the tissue mast cells. *Lab Invest* 34:179–191, 1976.

36. Arinobu Y, Iwasaki H, Gurish MF, et al: Developmental checkpoints of the basophil/mast cell lineages in adult murine hematopoiesis. *Proc Natl Acad Sci U S A* 102:18105–18110, 2005.

37. Qi X, Hong J, Chaves L, et al: Antagonistic regulation by the transcription factors C/EBPα and MITF specifies basophil and mast cell fates. *Immunity* 39:97–110, 2013.

38. Mukai K, BenBarak MJ, Tachibana M, et al: Critical role of P1-Runx1 in mouse basophil development. *Blood* 120:76–85, 2012.

39. Hastie R: A study of the ultrastructure of human basophil leukocytes. *Lab Invest* 31:223–231, 1974.

40. Ronnberg E, Melo FR, Pejler G: Mast cell proteoglycans. *J Histochem Cytochem* 60:950–962, 2012.

41. Rothenberg ME, Caulfield JP, Austen KF, et al: Biochemical and morphological characterization of basophilic leukocytes from two patients with myelogenous leukemia. *J Immunol* 138:2616–2625, 1987.

42. Metcalfe DD, Bland CE, Wasserman SI: Biochemical and functional characterization of proteoglycans isolated from basophils of patients with chronic myelogenous leukemia. *J Immunol* 132:1943–1950, 1984.

43. Porter JF, Mitchell RG: Distribution of histamine in human blood. *Physiol Rev* 52:361–381, 1972.

44. Wernersson S, Pejler G: Mast cell secretory granules: Armed for battle. *Nat Rev Immunol* 14:478–494, 2014.

45. Oh C, Suzuki S, Nakashima I, et al: Histamine synthesis by non-mast cells through mitogen-dependent induction of histidine decarboxylase. *Immunology* 65:143–148, 1988.

46. Xu X, Zhang D, Zhang H, et al: Neutrophil histamine contributes to inflammation in mycoplasma pneumonia. *J Exp Med* 203:2907–2917, 2006.

47. Saxena SP, Brandes LJ, Becker AB, et al: Histamine is an intracellular messenger mediating platelet aggregation. *Science* 243:1596–1599, 1989.

48. Galli SJ, Kitamura Y: Genetically mast-cell-deficient W/W^v and Sl/Sl^d mice. Their value for the analysis of the roles of mast cells in biologic responses *in vivo*. *Am J Pathol* 127:191–198, 1987.

49. Galli SJ, Kalesnikoff J, Grimbaldeston MA, et al: Mast cells as "tunable" effector and immunoregulatory cells: Recent advances. *Annu Rev Immunol* 23:749–786, 2005.

50. Galli SJ, Tsai M, Piliponsky AM: The development of allergic inflammation. *Nature* 454:445–454, 2008.

51. Galli SJ, Grimbaldeston M, Tsai M: Immunomodulatory mast cells: Negative, as well as positive, regulators of immunity. *Nat Rev Immunol* 8:478–486, 2008.

52. Gordon JR, Galli SJ: Mast-cells as a source of both preformed and immunologically inducible TNF-α cachectin. *Nature* 346:274–276, 1990.

53. Walsh LJ, Trinchieri G, Waldorf HA, et al: Human dermal mast cells contain and release tumor necrosis factor α, which induces endothelial leukocyte adhesion molecule 1. *Proc Natl Acad Sci U S A* 88:4220–4224, 1991.

54. de Paulis A, Prevete N, Fiorentino I, et al: Expression and functions of the vascular endothelial growth factors and their receptors in human basophils. *J Immunol* 177:7322–7331, 2006.

55. Min B: Basophils: What they "can do" versus what they "actually do". *Nat Immunol* 9:1333–1339, 2008.

56. Sullivan BM, Liang HE, Bando JK, et al: Genetic analysis of basophil function *in vivo*. *Nat Immunol* 12:527–535, 2011.

57. Karasuyama H, Mukai K, Obata K, et al: Nonredundant roles of basophils in immunity. *Annu Rev Immunol* 29:45–69, 2011.

58. Rivera J, Gilfillan AM: Molecular regulation of mast cell activation. *J Allergy Clin Immunol* 117:1214–1225; quiz 1226, 2006.

59. Kraft S, Kinet JP: New developments in FcεRI regulation, function and inhibition. *Nat Rev Immunol* 7:365–378, 2007.

60. Koshino T, Teshima S, Fukushima N, et al: Identification of basophils by immunohistochemistry in the airways of post-mortem cases of fatal asthma. *Clin Exp Allergy* 23:919–925, 1993.

61. Finkelman FD: Anaphylaxis: Lessons from mouse models. *J Allergy Clin Immunol* 120:506–515; quiz 516–517, 2007.

62. Jonsson F, Daeron M: Mast cells and company. *Front Immunol* 3:16, 2012.

63. Galli SJ, Tsai M, Marichal T, et al: Approaches for analyzing the roles of mast cells and their proteases *in vivo*. *Adv Immunol* 125:45–127, 2015.

64. Reber LL, Marichal T, Galli SJ: New models for analyzing mast cell functions *in vivo*. *Trends Immunol* 33:613–625, 2012.

65. Ebo DG, Bridts CH, Hagendorens MM, et al: Basophil activation test by flow cytometry: Present and future applications in allergology. *Cytometry B Clin Cytom* 74:201–210, 2008.

66. Wershil BK, Wang ZS, Gordon JR, et al: Recruitment of neutrophils during IgE-dependent cutaneous late phase reactions in the mouse is mast cell-dependent. Partial inhibition of the reaction with antiserum against tumor necrosis factor-alpha. *J Clin Invest* 87:446–453, 1991.

67. Mukai K, Matsuoka K, Taya C, et al: Basophils play a critical role in the development of IgE-mediated chronic allergic inflammation independently of T cells and mast cells. *Immunity* 23:191–202, 2005.

68. Ong YE, Menzies-Gow A, Barkans J, et al: Anti-IgE (omalizumab) inhibits late-phase reactions and inflammatory cells after repeat skin allergen challenge. *J Allergy Clin Immunol* 116:558–564, 2005.

69. Conner E, Bochner BS, Brummet M, et al: The effect of etanercept on the human cutaneous allergic response. *J Allergy Clin Immunol* 121:258–260, 2008.

70. Yu M, Tsai M, Tam SY, et al: Mast cells can promote the development of multiple features of chronic asthma in mice. *J Clin Invest* 116:1633–1641, 2006.

71. Yu M, Eckart MR, Morgan AA, et al: Identification of an IFN-γ/mast cell axis in a mouse model of chronic asthma. *J Clin Invest* 121:3133–3143, 2011.

72. MacGlashan DW Jr, Bochner BS, Adelman DC, et al: Down-regulation of FcεRI expression on human basophils during in vivo treatment of atopic patients with anti-IgE antibody. *J Immunol* 158:1438–1445, 1997.

73. Yamaguchi M, Lantz CS, Oettgen HC, et al: IgE enhances mouse mast cell FcεRI expression in vitro and in vivo: Evidence for a novel amplification mechanism in IgE-dependent reactions. *J Exp Med* 185:663–672, 1997.

74. Kawakami T, Galli SJ: Regulation of mast-cell and basophil function and survival by IgE. *Nat Rev Immunol* 2:773–786, 2002.

75. Matsuda K, Piliponsky AM, Iikura M, et al: Monomeric IgE enhances human mast cell chemokine production: IL-4 augments and dexamethasone suppresses the response. *J Allergy Clin Immunol* 116:1357–1363, 2005.

76. James LC, Roversi P, Tawfik DS: Antibody multispecificity mediated by conformational diversity. *Science* 299:1362–1367, 2003.

77. Galli SJ, Askenase PW. Cutaneous basophil hypersensitivity, in *The Reticuloendothelial System: A Comprehensive Treatise*, edited by Abramoff P, Phililps S, Escobar N, p 321. Plenum, New York, 1986.

78. Galli SJ, Nakae S, Tsai M: Mast cells in the development of adaptive immune responses. *Nat Immunol* 6:135–142, 2005.

79. Rodewald HR, Feyerabend TB: Widespread immunological functions of mast cells: Fact or fiction? *Immunity* 37:13–24, 2012.

80. McLachlan JB, Shelburne CP, Hart JP, et al: Mast cell activators: A new class of highly effective vaccine adjuvants. *Nat Med* 14:536–541, 2008.

81. Brown SJ, Galli SJ, Gleich GJ, et al: Ablation of immunity to Amblyomma americanum by anti-basophil serum: Cooperation between basophils and eosinophils in expression of immunity to ectoparasites (ticks) in guinea pigs. *J Immunol* 129:790–796, 1982.

82. Matsuda H, Watanabe N, Kiso Y, et al: Necessity of IgE antibodies and mast cells for manifestation of resistance against larval *Haemaphysalis longicornis* ticks in mice. *J Immunol* 144:259–262, 1990.

83. Abraham SN, St John AL: Mast cell-orchestrated immunity to pathogens. *Nat Rev Immunol* 10:440–452, 2010.

84. Di Nardo A, Vitiello A, Gallo RL: Cutting edge: Mast cell antimicrobial activity is mediated by expression of cathelicidin antimicrobial peptide. *J Immunol* 170:2274–2278, 2003.

85. Maurer M, Wedemeyer J, Metz M, et al: Mast cells promote homeostasis by limiting endothelin-1-induced toxicity. *Nature* 432:512–516, 2004.

86. Schneider LA, Schlenner SM, Feyerabend TB, et al: Molecular mechanism of mast cell mediated innate defense against endothelin and snake venom sarafotoxin. *J Exp Med* 204:2629–2639, 2007.

87. Piliponsky AM, Chen CC, Nishimura T, et al: Neurotensin increases mortality and mast cells reduce neurotensin levels in a mouse model of sepsis. *Nat Med* 14:392–398, 2008.

88. Mallen-St Clair J, Pham CT, Villalta SA, et al: Mast cell dipeptidyl peptidase I mediates survival from sepsis. *J Clin Invest* 113:628–634, 2004.

89. Chan CY, St John AL, Abraham SN: Mast cell interleukin-10 drives localized tolerance in chronic bladder infection. *Immunity* 38:349–359, 2013.

90. Bannert N, Farzan M, Friend DS, et al: Human mast cell progenitors can be infected by macrophagetropic human immunodeficiency virus type 1 and retain virus with maturation in vitro. *J Virol* 75:10808–10814, 2001.

91. Sundstrom JB, Little DM, Villinger F, et al: Signaling through Toll-like receptors triggers HIV-1 replication in latently infected mast cells. *J Immunol* 172:4391–4401, 2004.

92. Sundstrom JB, Ellis JE, Hair GA, et al: Human tissue mast cells are an inducible reservoir of persistent HIV infection. *Blood* 109:5293–5300, 2007.

93. Li Y, Li LX, Wadley R, et al: Mast cells/basophils in the peripheral blood of allergic individuals who are HIV-1 susceptible due to their surface expression of CD4 and the chemokine receptors CCR3, CCR5, and CXCR4. *Blood* 97:3484–3490, 2001.

94. St John AL, Rathore AP, Yap H, et al: Immune surveillance by mast cells during dengue infection promotes natural killer (NK) and NKT-cell recruitment and viral clearance. *Proc Natl Acad Sci U S A* 108:9190–9195, 2011.

95. Profet M: The function of allergy: Immunological defense against toxins. *Q Rev Biol* 66:23–62, 1991.

96. Metz M, Piliponsky AM, Chen CC, et al: Mast cells can enhance resistance to snake and honeybee venoms. *Science* 313:526–530, 2006.

97. Haftenberger M, Laussmann D, Ellert U, et al: [Prevalence of sensitisation to aeroallergens and food allergens: Results of the German Health Interview and Examination Survey for Adults (DEGS1)] [in German]. *Bundesgesundheitsblatt Gesundheitsforschung Gesundheitsschutz* 56:687–697, 2013.

98. Marichal T, Starkl P, Reber LL, et al: A beneficial role for immunoglobulin E in host defense against honeybee venom. *Immunity* 39:963–975, 2013.

99. Akahoshi M, Song CH, Piliponsky AM, et al: Mast cell chymase reduces the toxicity of Gila monster venom, scorpion venom, and vasoactive intestinal polypeptide in mice. *J Clin Invest* 121:4180–4191, 2011.

100. Palm NW, Rosenstein RK, Medzhitov R: Allergic host defences. *Nature* 484:465–472, 2012.

101. Brandt EB, Strait RT, Hershko D, et al: Mast cells are required for experimental oral allergen-induced diarrhea. *J Clin Invest* 112:1666–1677, 2003.

102. Shelley WB, Parnes HM: The absolute basophil count. *JAMA* 192:368–370, 1965.

103. Thonnard-Neumann E: Studies of basophils, variations with age and sex. *Acta Haematol* 30:221–228, 1963.

104. Chavance M, Herbeth B, Kauffmann F: Seasonal patterns of circulating basophils. *Int Arch Allergy Appl Immunol* 86:462–464, 1988.

105. Shelley WB, Juhlin L: A new test for detecting anaphylactic sensitivity: The basophil reaction. *Nature* 191:1056–1058, 1961.

106. Grattan CE, Dawn G, Gibbs S, et al: Blood basophil numbers in chronic ordinary urticaria and healthy controls: Diurnal variation, influence of loratadine and prednisolone and relationship to disease activity. *Clin Exp Allergy* 33:337–341, 2003.

107. Juhlin L: Basophil and eosinophil leukocyted in various internal disorders. *Acta Med Scand* 174:249–254, 1963.

108. Juhlin L: The effect of corticotrophin and corticosteroids on the basophil and eosinophil granulocytes. *Acta Haematol* 29:157–165, 1963.

109. Malveaux FJ, Conroy MC, Adkinson NF Jr, et al: IgE receptors on human basophils. Relationship to serum IgE concentration. *J Clin Invest* 62:176–181, 1978.

110. Lantz CS, Yamaguchi M, Oettgen HC, et al: IgE regulates mouse basophil FcεRI expression in vivo. *J Immunol* 158:2517–2521, 1997.

111. Juhlin L: Basophil leukocytes in ulcerative colitis. *Acta Med Scand* 173:351–359, 1963.

112. Athreya BH, Moser G, Raghavan TE: Increased circulating basophils in juvenile rheumatoid arthritis. A preliminary report. *Am J Dis Child* 129:935–937, 1975.

113. Fredericks RE, Moloney WC: The basophilic granulocyte. *Blood* 14, 1959.

114. Spiers AS, Bain BJ, Turner JE: The peripheral blood in chronic granulocytic leukaemia. Study of 50 untreated Philadelphia-positive cases. *Scand J Haematol* 18:25–38, 1977.

115. Kamada N, Uchino H: Chronologic sequence in appearance of clinical and laboratory findings characteristic of chronic myelocytic leukemia. *Blood* 51:843–850, 1978.

116. Drewinko B, Bollinger P, Brailas C, et al: Flow cytochemical patterns of white blood cells in human haematopoietic malignancies. II. Chronic leukaemias. *Br J Haematol* 67:157–165, 1987.

117. Denburg JA, Browman G: Prognostic implications of basophil differentiation in chronic myeloid leukemia. *Am J Hematol* 27:110–114, 1988.

118. Goh KO, Anderson FW: Cytogenetic studies in basophilic chronic myelogenous leukemia. *Arch Pathol Lab Med* 103:288–290, 1979.

119. Denburg JA, Wilson WE, Goodacre R, et al: Chronic myeloid leukaemia: Evidence for basophil differentiation and histamine synthesis from cultured peripheral blood cells. *Br J Haematol* 45:13–21, 1980.

120. Parkin JL, McKenna RW, Brunning RD: Philadelphia chromosome-positive blastic leukaemia: Ultrastructural and ultracytochemical evidence of basophil and mast cell differentiation. *Br J Haematol* 52:663–677, 1982.

121. Zucker-Franklin D: Ultrastructural evidence for the common origin of human mast cells and basophils. *Blood* 56:534–540, 1980.

122. Soler J, O'Brien M, de Castro JT, et al: Blast crisis of chronic granulocytic leukemia with mast cell and basophilic precursors. *Am J Clin Pathol* 83:254–259, 1985.

123. Weil SC, Hrisinko MA: A hybrid eosinophilic-basophilic granulocyte in chronic granulocytic leukemia. *Am J Clin Pathol* 87:66–70, 1987.

124. Gabriel LC, Escribano LM, Marie JP, et al: Peroxidase activity in circulating mast cells in blast crisis of chronic granulocytic leukemia. Comparative studies with basophils and cutaneous mast cells. *Am J Clin Pathol* 86:212–219, 1986.

125. Youman JD, Taddeini L, Cooper T: Histamine excess symptoms in basophilic chronic granulocytic leukemia. *Arch Intern Med* 131:560–562, 1973.

126. Rosenthal S, Schwartz JH, Canellos GP: Basophilic chronic granulocytic leukaemia with hyperhistaminaemia. *Br J Haematol* 36:367–372, 1977.

127. Valimaki M, Vuopio P, Salaspuro M: Plasma histamine and serum pepsinogen I concentrations in chronic myelogenous leukaemia. *Acta Med Scand* 217:89–93, 1985.

128. Anderson W, Helman CA, Hirschowitz BI: Basophilic leukemia and the hypersecretion of gastric acid and pepsin. *Gastroenterology* 95:195–198, 1988.

129. Xue YQ, Guo Y, Lu DR, et al: A case of basophilic leukemia bearing simultaneous translocations t(8;21) and t(9;22). *Cancer Genet Cytogenet* 51:215–221, 1991.

130. Cecio A, Dini E, Quattrin N: Initial electron microscopy studies in 2 cases of acute basophilic leukaemia. *Boll Soc Ital Biol Sper* 46:459–462, 1970.

131. Dvorak AM, Dickersin GR, Connell A, et al: Degranulation mechanisms in human leukemic basophils. *Clin Immunol Immunopathol* 5:235–246, 1976.

132. Quattrin N: Follow-up of sixty two cases of acute basophilic leukemia. *Biomedicine* 28:72–79, 1978.

133. Wick MR, Li CY, Pierre RV: Acute nonlymphocytic leukemia with basophilic differentiation. *Blood* 60:38–45, 1982.

134. Lertprasertsuke N, Tsutsumi Y: An unusual form of chronic myeloproliferative disorder. Aleukemic basophilic leukemia. *Acta Pathol Jpn* 41:73–81, 1991.

135. Peterson LC, Parkin JL, Arthur DC, et al: Acute basophilic leukemia. A clinical, morphologic, and cytogenetic study of eight cases. *Am J Clin Pathol* 96:160–170, 1991.

136. Shvidel L, Shaft D, Stark B, et al: Acute basophilic leukaemia: Eight unsuspected new cases diagnosed by electron microscopy. *Br J Haematol* 120:774–781, 2003.

137. Arber DA, Brunning RD, Orazi A, et al: Acute myeloid leukaemia, not otherwise specified, in *WHO Classification of Tumours of Haematopoietic and Lymphoid Tissues*, edited by Swerdlow SH, Campo E, Harris NL, Jaffe ES, Pileri SA, Stein H, Thiele J, Vardiman JW. p 130. IARC Press, Lyon, 2008.

138. Staal-Viliare A, Latger-Cannard V, Rault JP, et al: A case of de novo acute basophilic leukaemia: Diagnostic criteria and review of the literature. *Ann Biol Clin (Paris)* 64:361–365, 2006.

139. Staal-Viliare A, Latger-Cannard V, Didion J, et al: CD203c+/CD117–, an useful phenotype profile for acute basophilic leukaemia diagnosis in cases of undifferentiated blasts. *Leuk Lymphoma* 48:439–441, 2007.

140. Dastugue N, Duchayne E, Kuhlein E, et al: Acute basophilic leukaemia and translocation t(X;6)(p11;q23). *Br J Haematol* 98:170–176, 1997.

141. Quelen C, Lippert E, Struski S, et al: Identification of a transforming MYB-GATA1 fusion gene in acute basophilic leukemia: A new entity in male infants. *Blood* 117:5719–5722, 2011.

142. Pearson MG, Vardiman JW, Le Beau MM, et al: Increased numbers of marrow basophils may be associated with a t(6;9) in ANLL. *Am J Hematol* 18:393–403, 1985.

143. Horsman DE, Kalousek DK: Acute myelomonocytic leukemia (AML-M4) and translocation t(6;9)(p23;q34): Two additional patients with prominent myelodysplasia. *Am J Hematol* 26:77–82, 1987.

144. Matsuura Y, Sato N, Kimura F, et al: An increase in basophils in a case of acute myelomonocytic leukaemia associated with marrow eosinophilia and inversion of chromosome 16. *Eur J Haematol* 39:457–461, 1987.

145. Hoyle CF, Sherrington P, Hayhoe FG: Translocation (3;6)(q21;p21) in acute myeloid leukemia with abnormal thrombopoiesis and basophilia. *Cancer Genet Cytogenet* 30:261–267, 1988.

146. Nacheva EP, Grace CD, Brazma D, et al: Does BCR/ABL1 positive acute myeloid leukaemia exist? *Br J Haematol* 161:541–550, 2013.

147. Alsabeh R, Brynes RK, Slovak ML, et al: Acute myeloid leukemia with t(6;9) (p23;q34): Association with myelodysplasia, basophilia, and initial CD34 negative immunophenotype. *Am J Clin Pathol* 107:430–437, 1997.

148. Slovak ML, Gundacker H, Bloomfield CD, et al: A retrospective study of 69 patients with t(6;9)(p23;q34) AML emphasizes the need for a prospective, multicenter initiative for rare "poor prognosis" myeloid malignancies. *Leukemia* 20:1295–1297, 2006.

149. Oyarzo MP, Lin P, Glassman A, et al: Acute myeloid leukemia with t(6;9)(p23;q34) is associated with dysplasia and a high frequency of flt3 gene mutations. *Am J Clin Pathol* 122:348–358, 2004.

150. Le Beau MM, Larson RA, Bitter MA, et al: Association of an inversion of chromosome 16 with abnormal marrow eosinophils in acute myelomonocytic leukemia. A unique cytogenetic-clinicopathological association. *N Engl J Med* 309:630–636, 1983.

151. Lewis RA, Goetzl EJ, Wasserman SI, et al: The release of four mediators of immediate hypersensitivity from human leukemic basophils. *J Immunol* 114:87–92, 1975.

152. Travis WD, Li CY, Bergstralh EJ, et al: Systemic mast cell disease. Analysis of 58 cases and literature review. *Medicine (Baltimore)* 67:345–368, 1988.

153. Tsai M, Shih LS, Newlands GF, et al: The rat c-kit ligand, stem cell factor, induces the development of connective tissue-type and mucosal mast cells in vivo. Analysis by anatomical distribution, histochemistry, and protease phenotype. *J Exp Med* 174:125–131, 1991.

154. Irani AA, Garriga MM, Metcalfe DD, et al: Mast cells in cutaneous mastocytosis: Accumulation of the MCTC type. *Clin Exp Allergy* 20:53–58, 1990.

155. Schwartz LB, Metcalfe DD, Miller JS, et al: Tryptase levels as an indicator of mast-cell activation in systemic anaphylaxis and mastocytosis. *N Engl J Med* 316:1622–1626, 1987.

156. Weidner N, Horan RF, Austen KF: Mast-cell phenotype in indolent forms of mastocytosis. Ultrastructural features, fluorescence detection of avidin binding, and immunofluorescent determination of chymase, tryptase, and carboxypeptidase. *Am J Pathol* 140:847–857, 1992.

157. Weidner N, Austen KF: Heterogeneity of mast-cells at multiple body sites-fluorescent determination of avidin binding and immunofluorescent determination of chymase, tryptase, and carboxypeptidase content. *Pathol Res Pract* 189:156–162, 1993.

158. Lavker RM, Schechter NM: Cutaneous mast cell depletion results from topical corticosteroid usage. *J Immunol* 135:2368–2373, 1985.

159. Irani AM, Craig SS, DeBlois G, et al: Deficiency of the tryptase-positive, chymase-negative mast cell type in gastrointestinal mucosa of patients with defective T lymphocyte function. *J Immunol* 138:4381–4386, 1987.

160. Garriga MM, Friedman MM, Metcalfe DD: A survey of the number and distribution of mast cells in the skin of patients with mast cell disorders. *J Allergy Clin Immunol* 82:425–432, 1988.

161. Malone DG, Irani AM, Schwartz LB, et al: Mast cell numbers and histamine levels in synovial fluids from patients with diverse arthritides. *Arthritis Rheum* 29:956–963, 1986.

162. Malone DG, Wilder RL, Saavedra-Delgado AM, et al: Mast cell numbers in rheumatoid synovial tissues. Correlations with quantitative measures of lymphocytic infiltration and modulation by antiinflammatory therapy. *Arthritis Rheum* 30:130–137, 1987.

163. Frame B, Nixon RK: Bone-marrow mast cells in osteoporosis of aging. *N Engl J Med* 279:626–630, 1968.

164. Lennert K, Parwaresch MR: Mast cells and mast cell neoplasia: A review. *Histopathology* 3:349–365, 1979.

165. Barrett KE, Neva FA, Gam AA, et al: The immune response to nematode parasites: Modulation of mast cell numbers and function during *Strongyloides stercoralis* infections in nonhuman primates. *Am J Trop Med Hyg* 38:574–581, 1988.

166. Bowers HM Jr, Mahapatro RC, Kennedy JW: Numbers of mast cells in the axillary lymph nodes of breast cancer patients. *Cancer* 43:568–573, 1979.

167. Yoo D, Lessin LS, Jensen WN: Bone-marrow mast cells in lymphoproliferative disorders. *Ann Intern Med* 88:753–757, 1978.

168. Yoo D, Lessin LS: Bone marrow mast cell content in preleukemic syndrome. *Am J Med* 73:539–542, 1982.

169. Fohlmeister I, Reber T, Fischer R: Bone marrow mast cell reaction in preleukaemic myelodysplasia and in aplastic anaemia. *Virchows Arch A Pathol Anat Histopathol* 405:503–509, 1985.

170. Unna PG: Beitrage zur anatomic und pathogenese der urticaria simplex und pigmentosa. *Mscch Prakt Dermatol* 6:EH1, 1887.

171. Nettleship E, Tay W, Med J: Rare forms of urticaria. *Br Med J* 2:323–330, 1869.

172. Sangster A: An anomalous mottled rash, accompanied by pruritus, factious urticaria and pigmentation, "urticaria pigmentosa (?)." *Trans Clin Soc Lond* 11:161, 1878.

173. Ellis JM: Urticaria pigmentosa; a report of a case with autopsy. *Arch Pathol* 48:426–435, 1949.

174. Carter MC, Metcalfe DD, Komarow HD: Mastocytosis. *Immunol Allergy Clin North Am* 34:181–196, 2014.

175. Soter NA: Mastocytosis and the skin. *Hematol Oncol Clin North Am* 14:537–555, vi, 2000.

176. Horny HP, Metcalfe DD, Bennett JM, et al: Mastocytosis, in *WHO Classification of Tumours of Haematopoietic and Lymphoid Tissues* edited by Swerdlow SH, Campo E, Harris NL, Jaffe ES, Pileri SA, Stein H, Thiele J, Vardiman JW. p 54. IARC Press, Lyon, 2008.

177. Furitsu T, Tsujimura T, Tono T, et al: Identification of mutations in the coding sequence of the proto-oncogene c-*kit* in a human mast cell leukemia cell line causing ligand-independent activation of c-*kit* product. *J Clin Invest* 92:1736–1744, 1993.

178. Nagata H, Worobec AS, Oh CK, et al: Identification of a point mutation in the catalytic domain of the protooncogene c-*kit* in peripheral blood mononuclear cells of patients who have mastocytosis with an associated hematologic disorder. *Proc Natl Acad Sci U S A* 92:10560–10564, 1995.

179. Longley BJ, Tyrrell L, Lu SZ, et al: Somatic c-*KIT* activating mutation in urticaria pigmentosa and aggressive mastocytosis: Establishment of clonality in a human mast cell neoplasm. *Nat Genet* 12:312–314, 1996.

180. Nagata H, Okada T, Worobec AS, et al: C-*kit* mutation in a population of patients with mastocytosis. *Int Arch Allergy Immunol* 113:184–186, 1997.

181. Valent P: Mastocytosis: A paradigmatic example of a rare disease with complex biology and pathology. *Am J Cancer Res* 3:159–172, 2013.

182. Akin C, Fumo G, Yavuz AS, et al: A novel form of mastocytosis associated with a transmembrane c-kit mutation and response to imatinib. *Blood* 103:3222–3225, 2004.

183. Lahortiga I, Akin C, Cools J, et al: Activity of imatinib in systemic mastocytosis with chronic basophilic leukemia and a PRKG2-PDGFRB fusion. *Haematologica* 93:49–56, 2008.

184. Hirota S, Isozaki K, Moriyama Y, et al: Gain-of-function mutations of c-kit in human gastrointestinal stromal tumors. *Science* 279:577–580, 1998.

185. Schwaab J, Schnittger S, Sotlar K, et al: Comprehensive mutational profiling in advanced systemic mastocytosis. *Blood* 122:2460–2466, 2013.

186. Castells M, Metcalfe DD, Escribano L: Diagnosis and treatment of cutaneous mastocytosis in children: Practical recommendations. *Am J Clin Dermatol* 12:259–270, 2011.

187. Travis WD, Li CY: Pathology of the lymph node and spleen in systemic mast cell disease. *Mod Pathol* 1:4–14, 1988.

188. Mican JM, Di Bisceglie AM, Fong TL, et al: Hepatic involvement in mastocytosis: Clinicopathologic correlations in 41 cases. *Hepatology* 22:1163–1170, 1995.

189. Lawrence JB, Friedman BS, Travis WD, et al: Hematologic manifestations of systemic mast cell disease: A prospective study of laboratory and morphologic features and their relation to prognosis. *Am J Med* 91:612–624, 1991.

190. Horny HP, Ruck MT, Kaiserling E: Spleen findings in generalized mastocytosis. A clinicopathologic study. *Cancer* 70:459–468, 1992.

191. Horny HP, Parwaresch MR, Lennert K: Bone marrow findings in systemic mastocytosis. *Hum Pathol* 16:808–814, 1985.

192. Ridell B, Olafsson JH, Roupe G, et al: The bone marrow in urticaria pigmentosa and systemic mastocytosis. Cell composition and mast cell density in relation to urinary excretion of tele-methylimidazoleacetic acid. *Arch Dermatol* 122:422–427, 1986.

193. Kettelhut BV, Parker RI, Travis WD, et al: Hematopathology of the bone marrow in pediatric cutaneous mastocytosis. A study of 17 patients. *Am J Clin Pathol* 91:558–562, 1989.

194. Parker RI: Hematologic aspects of systemic mastocytosis. *Hematol Oncol Clin North Am* 14:557–568, 2000.

195. Valent P, Sotlar K, Sperr WR, et al: Refined diagnostic criteria and classification of mast cell leukemia (MCL) and myelomastocytic leukemia (MML): A consensus proposal. *Ann Oncol* 25:1691–1700, 2014.

196. Yang F, Tran TA, Carlson JA, et al: Paraffin section immunophenotype of cutaneous and extracutaneous mast cell disease: Comparison to other hematopoietic neoplasms. *Am J Surg Pathol* 24:703–709, 2000.

197. Escribano L, Diaz-Agustin B, Lopez A, et al: Immunophenotypic analysis of mast cells in mastocytosis: When and how to do it. Proposals of the Spanish Network on Mastocytosis (REMA). *Cytometry B Clin Cytom* 58:1–8, 2004.

198. Brockow K, Jofer C, Behrendt H, et al: Anaphylaxis in patients with mastocytosis: A study on history, clinical features and risk factors in 120 patients. *Allergy* 63:226–232, 2008.

199. Cherner JA, Jensen RT, Dubois A, et al: Gastrointestinal dysfunction in systemic mastocytosis. A prospective study. *Gastroenterology* 95:657–667, 1988.

200. Akin C, Soto D, Brittain E, et al: Tryptase haplotype in mastocytosis: Relationship to disease variant and diagnostic utility of total tryptase levels. *Clin Immunol* 123:268–271, 2007.

201. Kristensen T, Vestergaard H, Bindslev-Jensen C, et al: Sensitive KIT D816V mutation analysis of blood as a diagnostic test in mastocytosis. *Am J Hematol* 89:493–498, 2014.

202. Siebenhaar F, Akin C, Bindslev-Jensen C, et al: Treatment strategies in mastocytosis. *Immunol Allergy Clin North Am* 34:433–447, 2014.

203. Frieri M, Alling DW, Metcalfe DD: Comparison of the therapeutic efficacy of cromolyn sodium with that of combined chlorpheniramine and cimetidine in systemic mastocytosis. Results of a double-blind clinical trial. *Am J Med* 78:9–14, 1985.

204. Robyn J, Metcalfe DD: Systemic mastocytosis. *Adv Immunol* 89:169–243, 2006.

205. Soter NA, Austen KF, Wasserman SI: Oral disodium cromoglycate in the treatment of systemic mastocytosis. *N Engl J Med* 301:465–469, 1979.

206. Czarnetzki BM: A double-blind cross-over study of the effect of ketotifen in urticaria pigmentosa. *Dermatologica* 166:44–47, 1983.

207. Kettelhut BV, Berkebile C, Bradley D, et al: A double-blind, placebo-controlled, crossover trial of ketotifen versus hydroxyzine in the treatment of pediatric mastocytosis. *J Allergy Clin Immunol* 83:866–870, 1989.

208. Barton J, Lavker RM, Schechter NM, et al: Treatment of urticaria pigmentosa with corticosteroids. *Arch Dermatol* 121:1516–1523, 1985.

209. Kolde G, Frosch PJ, Czarnetzki BM: Response of cutaneous mast cells to PUVA in patients with urticaria pigmentosa: Histomorphometric, ultrastructural, and biochemical investigations. *J Invest Dermatol* 83:175–178, 1984.

210. Reisberg IR, Oyakawa S: Mastocytosis with malabsorption, myelofibrosis, and massive ascites. *Am J Gastroenterol* 82:54–60, 1987.

211. Kluin-Nelemans HC, Jansen JH, Breukelman H, et al: Response to interferon alfa-2b in a patient with systemic mastocytosis. *N Engl J Med* 326:619–623, 1992.

212. Lim KH, Pardanani A, Tefferi A: KIT and mastocytosis. *Acta Haematol* 119:194–198, 2008.

213. Gromke T, Elmaagacli AH, Ditschkowski M, et al: Delayed graft-versus-mast-cell effect on systemic mastocytosis with associated clonal haematological non-mast cell lineage disease after allogeneic transplantation. *Bone Marrow Transplant* 48:732–733, 2013.

214. Fodinger M, Fritsch G, Winkler K, et al: Origin of human mast cells: Development from transplanted hematopoietic stem cells after allogeneic bone marrow transplantation. *Blood* 84:2954–2959, 1994.

215. Przepiorka D, Giralt S, Khouri I, et al: Allogeneic marrow transplantation for myeloproliferative disorders other than chronic myelogenous leukemia: Review of forty cases. *Am J Hematol* 57:24–28, 1998.

216. Nakamura R, Chakrabarti S, Akin C, et al: A pilot study of nonmyeloablative allogeneic hematopoietic stem cell transplant for advanced systemic mastocytosis. *Bone Marrow Transplant* 37:353–358, 2006.

217. Buchdunger E, Cioffi CL, Law N, et al: Abl protein-tyrosine kinase inhibitor STI571 inhibits in vitro signal transduction mediated by c-kit and platelet-derived growth factor receptors. *J Pharmacol Exp Ther* 295:139–145, 2000.

218. Druker BJ, Tamura S, Buchdunger E, et al: Effects of a selective inhibitor of the Abl tyrosine kinase on the growth of Bcr-Abl positive cells. *Nat Med* 2:561–566, 1996.

219. Ma Y, Zeng S, Metcalfe DD, et al: The c-*KIT* mutation causing human mastocytosis is resistant to STI571 and other KIT kinase inhibitors; kinases with enzymatic site mutations show different inhibitor sensitivity profiles than wild-type kinases and those with regulatory-type mutations. *Blood* 99:1741–1744, 2002.

220. Zermati Y, De Sepulveda P, Feger F, et al: Effect of tyrosine kinase inhibitor STI571 on the kinase activity of wild-type and various mutated c-kit receptors found in mast cell neoplasms. *Oncogene* 22:660–664, 2003.

221. Akin C, Brockow K, D'Ambrosio C, et al: Effects of tyrosine kinase inhibitor STI571 on human mast cells bearing wild-type or mutated c-kit. *Exp Hematol* 31:686–692, 2003.

222. Pardanani A: Systemic mastocytosis in adults: 2013 update on diagnosis, risk stratification, and management. *Am J Hematol* 88:612–624, 2013.

223. Ustun C, DeRemer DL, Akin C: Tyrosine kinase inhibitors in the treatment of systemic mastocytosis. *Leuk Res* 35:1143–1152, 2011.

224. Klion AD, Noel P, Akin C, et al: Elevated serum tryptase levels identify a subset of patients with a myeloproliferative variant of idiopathic hypereosinophilic syndrome associated with tissue fibrosis, poor prognosis, and imatinib responsiveness. *Blood* 101:4660–4666, 2003.

225. Maric I, Robyn J, Metcalfe DD, et al: KIT D816V-associated systemic mastocytosis with eosinophilia and FIP1L1/PDGFRA-associated chronic eosinophilic leukemia are distinct entities. *J Allergy Clin Immunol* 120:680–687, 2007.

226. Valent P, Akin C, Escribano L, et al: Standards and standardization in mastocytosis: Consensus statements on diagnostics, treatment recommendations and response criteria. *Eur J Clin Invest* 37:435–453, 2007.

227. Akin C, Valent P, Metcalfe DD: Mast cell activation syndrome: Proposed diagnostic criteria. *J Allergy Clin Immunol* 126:1099–104 e4, 2010.

228. Valent P, Akin C, Arock M, et al: Definitions, criteria and global classification of mast cell disorders with special reference to mast cell activation syndromes: A consensus proposal. *Int Arch Allergy Immunol* 157:215–225, 2012.

229. Friedman B, Darling G, Norton J, et al: Splenectomy in the management of systemic mast cell disease. *Surgery* 107:94–100, 1990.

230. Brockow K, Scott LM, Worobec AS, et al: Regression of urticaria pigmentosa in adult patients with systemic mastocytosis: Correlation with clinical patterns of disease. *Arch Dermatol* 138:785–790, 2002.

231. Valentini CG, Rondoni M, Pogliani EM, et al: Mast cell leukemia: A report of ten cases. *Ann Hematol* 87:505–508, 2008.

CHAPTER 64
CLASSIFICATION AND CLINICAL MANIFESTATIONS OF NEUTROPHIL DISORDERS

Marshall A. Lichtman

SUMMARY

Neutrophil disorders can be grouped into deficiencies, or neutropenia, excesses, or neutrophilia, and qualitative abnormalities. Neutropenia can have the severe consequence of predisposing to infection, whereas neutrophilia usually is a manifestation of an underlying inflammatory or neoplastic disease: the neutrophilia, per se, having no specific consequences. Qualitative disorders of neutrophils may lead to infection as a result of defective cell translocation to an inflammatory site or defective microbial killing. Neutropenia may reflect an inherited disease that is evident in childhood (such as congenital [hereditary] severe neutropenia), but more often it is acquired. A common cause of neutropenia is the adverse effect of a drug. Some cases of neutropenia have no evident cause. The health consequence of neutropenia is a function of the mechanism of the neutropenia, the abruptness and severity of the decrease in the blood neutrophil count, and the duration of the decrease. Neutrophils have also been identified as mediators of vascular or tissue injury. Table 64–1 provides a comprehensive categorization of quantitative and qualitative neutrophil disorders.

CLASSIFICATION

Table 64–1 lists disorders that result from a primary deficiency in neutrophil numbers or function. Neutropenia or neutrophilia also occurs as part of a disorder that affects multiple blood cell lineages, as in infiltrative diseases of the marrow, or intrinsic disorders of multipotential marrow hematopoietic cells, or removal of several blood cell types in the circulation. These diseases are not included in this classification and are discussed in other chapters of this text. This classification and chapter considers disorders in which the neutrophil either is the only cell type affected or the dominant cell type affected.

A pathophysiologic classification of neutrophil disorders has proved elusive. Techniques for measuring mechanisms of (1) impaired production resulting from hypoplasia or exaggerated apoptosis of marrow precursors (ineffective neutropoiesis) or (2) accelerated destruction of neutrophils are more difficult and complex than the techniques used to measure decreases in red cells or platelet concentrations. The low concentration of blood neutrophils, accentuated in neutropenic states, makes radioactive-labeling techniques for studying the kinetics of autologous cells in neutropenic subjects difficult, if not impossible.

Acronyms and Abbreviations: CD, cluster of differentiation; G-CSF, granulocyte colony-stimulating factor; HLA-DR, human leukocyte antigen-D related.

The two compartments of neutrophils in the blood (cells marginated along vascular beds as distinct from cells circulating and counted in the blood neutrophil count [Chap. 65]), the random disappearance of neutrophils from the circulation, the short circulation time of neutrophils, the absence of practical techniques for measuring the size of the tissue neutrophil compartment, and the disappearance of neutrophils by apoptosis or excretion from the tissue compartment also make multicompartmental kinetic analysis difficult. Also, neutropenic disorders are uncommon, and few laboratories are able, or prepared, to undertake the studies necessary to define the mechanisms of their development in sporadic cases. Therefore, efforts to understand the pathophysiology and kinetics of neutropenia have been of more limited success than that of red cells or platelets. Hence, the classification of neutrophil disorders is partly pathophysiologic and partly descriptive (see Table 64–1). Classification, although imperfect, does provide a language for communication and a basis for rectification as knowledge of the cause and mechanism of each entity advances.

The classification is self-explanatory except in two areas. First, certain childhood (congenital or hereditary) syndromes listed under decreased neutrophilic granulopoiesis could have been listed under chronic hypoplastic neutropenia or chronic idiopathic neutropenia; however, they seem to hold a special interest. Their unique status and their pathogenesis have become further clarified as the mutations linked to each are identified. Three childhood syndromes that are associated with neutropenia are omitted because the neutropenia is part of a more global suppression of hematopoiesis: Pearson syndrome,[1,2] Fanconi anemia,[3,4] and dyskeratosis congenita (Chap. 35).[5,6]

A second area requiring explanation is the chronic idiopathic neutropenias. This group includes (1) cases with normocellular marrows but an inadequate compensatory increase in granulopoiesis for the degree of neutropenia and (2) cases with hyperplastic granulopoiesis that apparently is ineffective as a result of apoptosis of marrow neutrophils and late precursors. Unlike hypoplastic neutropenia in which the granulocyte precursors are markedly reduced or absent, precursors are present in the marrow in the idiopathic neutropenias, but the extent of effective granulopoiesis probably is low. A variety of mutations have been discovered that are causal for inherited or sporadic neutropenia syndromes. For example, mutation of the serine protease neutrophil elastase 2 gene (ELANE) is found in 70 percent of cases of the autosomal dominant form of severe congenital neutropenia and in most cases of cyclic neutropenia.[7] Kostmann syndrome is the autosomal recessive form of severe congenital neutropenia and is caused by mutations in the HAX1 gene.[8] Some cases of severe congenital neutropenia have been related to mutations in GPI1, G6PC3, and others.[9–11] There is evidence that these mutations result in apoptotic loss of marrow neutrophil precursors as a result of downregulation of the BCL-2 family of antiapoptotic proteins, the upregulation of the proapoptotic FAS receptor, or other apoptosis-enhancing pathways, described more fully in Chap. 65. A comprehensive listing of the genetic mutations found in monogenic congenital neutropenia and the extra hematopoietic manifestations of those disorders can be found in a publication of the Service d'Hémato Oncologie Pédiatrique Registre des neutropénies.[12]

Qualitative disorders of neutrophils affect their ability to enter the circulation, to leave the circulation, enter inflammatory exudates, or to ingest or kill microorganisms. Chapter 66 describes these abnormalities in more detail.

CLINICAL MANIFESTATIONS

The clinical manifestations of decreased concentrations or abnormal function of neutrophils principally result from infection. The combined deficit of neutrophils and monocytes characteristic of aplastic anemia,

TABLE 64–1. Classification of Neutrophil Disorders

I. Quantitative Disorders of Neutrophils
  A. Neutropenia[12,13]
    1. Decreased neutrophilic granulopoiesis
      a. Congenital severe neutropenias (Kostmann syndrome and related disorders)[14,15,]
      b. Reticular dysgenesis (congenital aleukocytosis)[16,17]
      c. Neutropenia and exocrine pancreas dysfunction (Shwachman-Diamond syndrome)[13,18]
      d. Neutropenia and immunoglobulin abnormality (e.g., hyperimmunoglobulin M syndrome)[19–21]
      e. Neutropenia and disordered cellular immunity (cartilage hair hypoplasia)[22,23]
      f. Mental retardation, anomalies, and neutropenia (Cohen syndrome)[24,25]
      g. X-linked cardioskeletal myopathy and neutropenia (Barth syndrome)[26,27]
      h. Myelokathexis[28,29]
      i. Warts, hypogammaglobulinemia, infection, myelokathexis (WHIM) syndrome[30,31]
      j. Neonatal neutropenia and maternal hypertension[32,33]
      k. Griscelli syndrome[34]
      l. Glycogen storage disease 1b[35]
      m. Hermansky-Pudlak syndrome 2[36,37]
      n. Wiskott-Aldrich syndrome[38]
      o. Chronic hypoplastic neutropenia
        (1) Drug-induced[39–42]
        (2) Cyclic[43,44]
        (3) Branched-chain aminoacidemia[45]
      p. Acute hypoplastic neutropenia
        (1) Drug-induced[39,46,47]
        (2) Infectious[48]
      q. Chronic idiopathic neutropenia
        (1) Benign
          (a) Familial[49]
          (b) Sporadic[50]
        (2) Symptomatic[51–53]

    2. Accelerated neutrophil destruction
      a. Alloimmune neonatal neutropenia[54–56]
      b. Autoimmune neutropenia[57–59]
        (1) Idiopathic[59]
        (2) Drug-induced[59,60]
        (3) Felty syndrome[61–63]
        (4) Systemic lupus erythematosus[64,65]
        (5) Other autoimmune diseases[66–71]
        (6) Complement activation-induced neutropenia[72]
        (7) Pure white cell aplasia[71,73–75]
    3. Maldistribution of neutrophils
      a. Pseudoneutropenia[76–78]
  B. Neutrophilia
    1. Increased neutrophilic granulopoiesis
      a. Hereditary neutrophilia[79]
      b. Trisomy 13 or 18[80]
      c. Chronic idiopathic neutrophilia[81]
        (1) Asplenia[82]
      d. Neutrophilia or neutrophilic leukemoid reactions
        (1) Inflammation[83,84]
        (2) Infection[83–85]
        (3) Acute hemolysis or acute hemorrhage[83]
        (4) Cancer, including granulocyte colony-stimulating factor (G-CSF)-secreting tumors[86–89]
        (5) Drugs (e.g., glucocorticoids, lithium, granulocyte- or granulocyte-monocyte colony-stimulating factor, tumor necrosis factor-α)[83,90–94]
        (6) Ethylene glycol exposure[83]
        (7) Exercise[95,96]
      e. Sweet syndrome[97,98]
      f. Cigarette smoking[99,100]
      g. Cardiopulmonary bypass[101]
    2. Decreased neutrophil circulatory egress
      a. Drugs (e.g., glucocorticoids)[102]
    3. Maldistribution of neutrophils
      a. Pseudoneutrophilia[103]

II. Qualitative Disorders of Neutrophils
  A. Defective adhesion of neutrophils
    1. Leukocyte adhesion deficiency[104,105]
    2. Drug-induced[106]
  B. Defective locomotion and chemotaxis
    1. Actin polymerization abnormalities[107–110]
    2. Neonatal neutrophils[111]
    3. Interleukin-2 administration[112]
    4. Cardiopulmonary bypass[101]
  C. Defective microbial killing
    1. Chronic granulomatous disease[113,114]
    2. RAC-2 deficiency[115,116]
    3. Myeloperoxidase deficiency[117,118]
    4. Hyperimmunoglobulin E (Job) syndrome[119,120]
    5. Glucose-6-phosphate dehydrogenase deficiency[121,122]
    6. Extensive burns[123,124]
    7. Glycogen storage disease Ib[125,126]
    8. Ethanol toxicity[127,128]
    9. End-stage renal disease[129]
    10. Diabetes mellitus[130]
  D. Abnormal structure of the nucleus or of an organelle
    1. Hereditary macropolycytes[131]
    2. Hereditary hypersegmentation[135]
    3. Specific granule deficiency[136–138]
    4. Pelger-Huët anomaly[139,140]
    5. Alder-Reilly anomaly[141]
    6. May-Hegglin anomaly[142–144]
    7. Chédiak-Higashi disease[145,146]
III. Neutrophil-Induced Vascular or Tissue Damage[147–149]
  A. Pulmonary disease[150–155]
  B. Transfusion-related lung injury[156,157]
  C. Renal disease[158,159]
  D. Arterial occlusion[160,161]
  E. Venous occlusion[162]
  F. Myocardial infarction[157–163,167]
  G. Ventricular function[164–168]
  H. Stroke[157,169]
  I. Neoplasia[170–172]
  J. Sickle cell vasoocclusive crisis[157,173]

RAC-2, RAS-Related C3 botulinum toxin substrate 2.

hairy cell leukemia, and cytotoxic therapy leads to susceptibility to a broader spectrum of infectious agents. Increased concentrations of normal neutrophils per se are usually not associated with clinical manifestations; although, increased concentrations of leukemic neutrophil precursors can produce clinical manifestations of microcirculatory leukostasis (Chap. 83). Neutrophils also play a role in deleterious vascular or tissue effects, as noted in the last entries in Table 64–1 (see "Neutrophilia" below).

NEUTROPENIA

The lower limit of the normal neutrophil count is approximately 1800/μL (1.8 × 10⁹/L) in subjects of European descent and 1400/μL (1.4 × 10⁹/L) in subjects of African descent.[174–177] An additional small proportion (~5 percent) of persons of African descent have neutrophil counts between 1000/μL (1.0 × 10⁹/L) and 1400 (1.4 × 10⁹/L) without evidence of associated abnormalities and this finding also may represent "ethnic neutropenia." These findings have not been explained by exaggerated margination of neutrophils.[176] Neutropenia is especially striking in Yemenite Jews, another ethnic group with very low "normal" neutrophil counts,[178] and has been reported in West Africans, Caribbean inhabitants of African descent, Ethiopians, and some Arab groups.[176,177] Persons of African descent do not have the increase of neutrophil count seen in Europeans who smoke or are administered glucocorticoids; however, they have an appropriate increase of neutrophils in response to infection. Americans of Mexican descent have a slightly elevated neutrophil count.[176] A decrement in neutrophil concentration to 1000/μL (1.0 × 10⁹/L) usually poses little threat in the individual with an intact immune system. If the neutrophil count drops farther, the risk of infection may increase, if the decrease reflects a decrease in flux rate into the tissues. Subjects who are chronically neutropenic, as a result of severe marrow cell production abnormalities, with counts less than 500 neutrophils/μL (0.5 × 10⁹/L) may be at heightened risk for developing recurrent infections.[179]

The relationship of frequency or type of infection to neutrophil concentration is imperfect. The cause of the neutropenia, the coincidence of monocytopenia or lymphopenia, concurrent use of alcohol or glucocorticoids, exposure to nosocomial infections, and other factors influence the likelihood of infection. A breakdown in the barrier function of the skin or circumstances such as indwelling catheters, also, increase the risk of infection in severely neutropenic subjects. Lower neutrophil counts in African (Malawian) mothers infected with HIV were associated with an increased risk of HIV in their newborns.[180]

Infections in neutropenic subjects who are not otherwise compromised usually result from Gram-positive cocci and usually are superficial, involving skin, oropharynx, bronchi, anal canal, or vagina. However, any site can become infected and Gram-negative organisms, viruses, or opportunistic organisms can be involved.

A decrease in neutrophil count can occur abruptly or gradually (Chap. 65). One type of drug-induced neutropenia is distinguished by the rapidity of onset. Abrupt-onset neutropenia more likely is severe and leads to symptoms. If the neutrophil count approaches zero (agranulocytosis), high fever; chills; necrotizing, painful oral ulcers (agranulocytic angina), and prostration may occur, presumably as a result of sepsis.[181] As the disease progresses, headache, stupor, and rash may develop. In the preantibiotic era, persistent agranulocytosis had a fatality rate approaching 100 percent. Even with bactericidal, broad-spectrum antibiotics, severe, sustained neutropenia or agranulocytosis is a serious illness with a high fatality rate.

Pus formation decreases in patients with severe neutropenia.[182] The failure to suppurate can mislead the clinician and delay identification of the infection site because minimal physical or radiographic findings

develop. For example, lack of pneumonic consolidation is characteristic of pneumonia in granulocytopenic subjects. An exudate, swelling, heat, and regional adenopathy are much less prevalent in granulocytopenic patients. Fever is common, and local pain, tenderness, and erythema nearly always are present despite a marked reduction in neutrophils.[181]

The mechanism of neutropenia and the severity of the deficiency of cells play roles in clinical manifestations. Chronic idiopathic (benign) neutropenia is associated with apparent normal granulopoiesis in the marrow and is asymptomatic even when the neutropenia has been present for prolonged periods, sometimes in the face of neutrophil counts approaching zero for prolonged periods.[50] Presumably the delivery of neutrophils from marrow to tissues is sufficient to prevent infection despite the low blood pool size. Monocyte counts are normal, which may aid in host defenses because monocytes are effective phagocytes.

Chronic idiopathic (symptomatic) neutropenia often is associated with pyoderma and otitis media in children. The former usually is caused by *Staphylococcus aureus, Escherichia coli*, and *Pseudomonas* species, and the latter usually results from infection by pneumococci or *Pseudomonas aeruginosa*. Unexplained chronic gingivitis may be a manifestation of chronic neutropenia. Pneumonia, lung abscesses, stomatitis, hepatic abscesses, or infections in other sites can occur.

Chronic cyclic neutropenia is characterized by periodic oscillations in the number of neutrophils, with the nadir occurring at approximately 3-week intervals.[43] During a period of neutropenia, patients develop malaise; fever; buccal, labial, or lingual ulcers; and cervical adenopathy. Furuncles, carbuncles, cellulitis, infected cuts with lymphangitis, chronic gingivitis, and abscesses of the axilla or groin may occur. Although severe infections may be fatal, life-threatening complications are uncommon. The cycling involves other hematopoietic cells as well, but the neutropenia is the most consequential functionally (Chap. 65).

Some individuals have neutropenia because a larger fraction of their blood neutrophils is in the marginal rather than the circulating pool. The total blood neutrophil pool is normal, and infections do not result from this atypical distribution of neutrophils. This alteration has been called *pseudoneutropenia*.[76–78]

NEUTROPHILIA

An increased neutrophil count can accompany virtually any cause of inflammation, especially inflammation caused by bacterial or fungal organisms, and a variety of cancers, especially if metastatic. Certain drugs, such as glucocorticoids or hematopoietic growth factors and minocycline, can induce neutrophilia, as can ethylene glycol intoxication (see Table 64–1). Acute hemolysis or acute hemorrhage may also result in neutrophilia. A notable cause of neutrophilia is cancers that elaborate granulocyte-colony stimulating factor (G-CSF). Numerous cancers are associated with neutrophilia and, in many cases, elaboration of very high concentrations of G-CSF has been documented. In these cases, neutrophil counts exceeding 100,000 μL (100 × 10⁹/L) are common. Neutrophilia exceeding 50,000 neutrophils/μL (50 × 10⁹/L) has been designated a "leukemoid reaction" and reflects an underlying inflammatory (e.g., pancreatitis), infectious (e.g., pneumococcal pneumonia), or neoplastic (e.g., carcinoma of the lung) cause. A leukemoid reaction can mimic rare types of chronic myelogenous or chronic neutrophilic leukemia. The leukemoid reaction classically (1) is composed largely of mature neutrophils with a low proportion of bands and myelocytes, (2) has increased leukocyte alkaline phosphatase reaction in neutrophils, (3) has increased granulopoiesis with normal maturation and morphology of cells in the marrow, (4) has normal cytogenetics of marrow cells, (5) has polyclonal-derived cells in women in whom such studies can be conducted (using the human androgen receptor gene assay), and (6) has cytometric analysis of neutrophils indicating a cluster of differentiation (CD) 13 and CD15 phenotype with absent expression of human leukocyte antigen-D related (HLA-DR) and CD34.

QUALITATIVE NEUTROPHIL ABNORMALITIES

Neutrophil function depends on the ability of neutrophils to exit the marrow, adhere to vascular endothelium, move, respond to chemotactic gradients, ingest microorganisms, and kill ingested pathogens. Loss of any of these functions can predispose to infection (Chap. 66). Defects in each step of the neutrophil's participation in the inflammatory response have been identified. Defects in adhesion molecules, cytoplasmic contractile proteins, granule synthesis or contents, or intracellular enzymes may underlie a movement, ingestion, or killing defect. These defects may be inherited or acquired. Chronic granulomatous disease[113,114] and Chédiak-Higashi disease[145,146] are two examples of inherited defects. Among the acquired disorders are those extrinsic to the cell, as in the movement, chemotactic, or phagocytic defects of diabetes mellitus, the effects of alcohol abuse, or glucocorticoid excess. Acquired intrinsic disorders usually are manifestations of clonal hematopoietic (myeloid) disorders such as acute myelogenous leukemia (Chap. 85).

Severe defects in bacterial killing, as occur in chronic granulomatous disease, result in *S. aureus, Klebsiella-Aerobacter, E. coli*, and other catalase-positive bacterial infections. Suppurative lymphadenitis, pneumonia, dermatitis, hepatic abscesses, osteomyelitis, and stomatitis occur, and chronic granulomatous reactions in these sites give the disease its name. Fatality rates have been high. Functional disorders may be severe, as in chronic granulomatous disease. Mild functional disorders predispose to infections that occur infrequently and respond readily to antibiotics. Severe functional disorders result in suppurative lesions because neutrophil influx into inflammatory foci is not impaired, whereas agranulocytosis is associated with nonsuppurative lesions.

NEUTROPHIL-INDUCED VASCULAR OR TISSUE DAMAGE

An overabundance of neutrophils does not result in specific clinical manifestations. Neutrophils, however, can transiently occlude capillaries, as determined by supravital microscopy, and such occlusions may reduce local blood flow transiently and contribute to the development of ischemia. Impairment of reperfusion of the coronary microcirculation has been thought to be dependent, in part, on neutrophil plugging of myocardial capillaries, but these effects can occur at normal neutrophil concentrations. An elevated neutrophil count is a feature of sickle cell disease and is a prognostic variable, increasing the likelihood of vasoocclusive events. Neutrophil adhesion to the vascular wall is an intrinsic part of the vasoocclusive events and the salutary effect of hydroxyurea is related to the decrease in neutrophil concentration that accompanies its use.[157,173] In patients with ischemic vascular disease, an increased neutrophil count is associated with an increased probability of acute thrombotic episodes and the severity of chronic atherosclerosis.[183]

Neutrophil products may contribute to the pathogenesis of inflammatory skin, bowel, synovial, glomerular, and bronchial and interstitial pulmonary diseases (see Table 64–1). Diabetic retinopathy has been ascribed in part to the effects of hyperadhesive neutrophils on retinal capillaries.[157] Neutrophils may act as mediators of tissue injury in stroke and myocardial infarction.[157] Highly reactive oxygen products of neutrophils may be mutagens that increase the risk of neoplasia. This action may explain, for example, the development of carcinoma of the bowel in patients with chronic ulcerative colitis and the relationship between elevated leukocyte count and the occurrence of lung cancer, independent

of the effect of cigarette usage. The oxidants, especially hypochlorous acid and chloramines, released by the neutrophil are extremely short lived and may play a role in tissue injury by inactivating several protease inhibitors in tissue fluids, permitting proteases, especially elastase, collagenase, and gelatinase, to cause tissue injury. Thrombogenesis also has been ascribed to leukocyte products.

REFERENCES

1. Pearson HA, Lobel JS, Kocoshis SA, et al: A new syndrome of refractory sideroblastic anemia with vacuolization of marrow precursors and exocrine pancreatic dysfunction. *J Pediatr* 95:976, 1979.
2. Jacobs LJ, Jongbloed RJ, Wijburg FA, et al: Pearson syndrome and the role of deletion dimers and duplications in the mtDNA. *J Inherit Metab Dis* 27:47, 2004.
3. Bagby GC Jr: Genetic basis of Fanconi anemia. *Curr Opin Hematol* 10:68, 2003.
4. Taniguchi T, D'Andrea AD: Molecular pathogenesis of Fanconi anemia: Recent progress. *Blood* 107:4223, 2006.
5. Srinavin C, Trowbridge A: Dyskeratosis congenita: Clinical features and genetic aspects. *J Med Genet* 12:339, 1975.
6. Walne AJ, Dokal I: Dyskeratosis congenita: A historical perspective. *Mech Ageing Dev* 129:48, 2008.
7. Tidwell T, Wechsler J, Nayak RC, et al. Neutropenia-associated *ELANE* mutations disrupting translation initiation produce novel neutrophil elastase isoforms. *Blood* 123:562, 2014.
8. Klein C, Grudzien M, Appaswamy G, et al. *HAX1* deficiency causes autosomal recessive severe congenital neutropenia (Kostmann disease). *Nat Genet* 39:86, 2007.
9. Person RE, Li FQ, Duan Z, et al. Mutations in proto-oncogene *GFI1* cause human neutropenia and target *ELA2*. *Nat Genet* 34:308, 2003.
10. Boztug K, Appaswamy G, Ashikov A, et al. A syndrome with congenital neutropenia and mutations in G6PC3. *N Engl J Med* 360:32, 2009.
11. Boztug K, Klein C: Genetics and pathophysiology of severe congenital neutropenia syndromes unrelated to neutrophil elastase. *Hematol Oncol Clin North Am* 27:43, 2013.
12. Donadieu J, Fenneteau O, Beaupain B, et al. Congenital neutropenia: Diagnosis, molecular bases and patient management. *Orphanet J Rare Dis* 6:26, 2011
13. Bouma G, Ancliff PJ, Thrasher AJ, Burns SO. Recent advances in the understanding of genetic defects of neutrophil number and function. *Br J Haematol* 151:312, 2010.
14. Ward AC, Dale DC: Genetic and molecular diagnosis of severe congenital neutropenia. *Curr Opin Hematol* 16:9, 2009.
15. Ishikawa N, Okada S, Miki M, et al: Neurodevelopmental abnormalities associated with severe congenital neutropenia due to the R86X mutation in the HAX1 gene. *J Med Genet* 45:802, 2008.
16. Levinsky RJ, Tiedman K: Successful bone-marrow transplantation for reticular dysgenesis. *Lancet* 1:671, 1983.
17. Calhoun DA, Christensen RD: Recent advances in the pathogenesis and treatment of nonimmune neutropenias in the neonate. *Curr Opin Hematol* 5:37, 1998.
18. Shimamura A: Shwachman-Diamond syndrome. *Semin Hematol* 43:178, 2006.
19. Lonsdale D, Doedhar SD, Mercer RD: Familial granulocytopenia associated with immunoglobulin abnormality. *J Pediatr* 71:760, 1967.
20. Kozlowski C, Evans DIK: Neutropenia associated with X-linked agammaglobulinemia. *J Clin Pathol* 44:388, 1991.
21. Lougaris V, Badolato R, Ferrari S, Plebani A: Hyper immunoglobulin M syndrome due to CD40 deficiency: Clinical, molecular, and immunological features. *Immunol Rev* 203:48, 2005.
22. Lux SE, Johnston RB Jr, August CS, et al: Chronic neutropenia and abnormal cellular immunity in cartilage-hair hypoplasia. *N Engl J Med* 282:231, 1970.
23. Trojak JE, Polmar SH, Winkelstein JA: Immunologic studies of cartilage-hair hypoplasia in the Amish. *Johns Hopkins Med J* 148:157, 1981.
24. Olivieri O, Lombardi S, Russo C, Corrocher R: Increased neutrophil adhesive capability in Cohen syndrome, an autosomal recessive disorder associated with granulocytopenia. *Haematologica* 83:778, 1998.
25. Kolehmainen J, Black GC, Saarinen A, et al: Cohen syndrome is caused by mutations in a novel gene, COH1, encoding a transmembrane protein with a presumed role in vesicle-mediated sorting and intracellular protein transport. *Am J Hum Genet* 72:1359, 2003.
26. Barth PG, Scholte HR, Berden JA, et al: An X-linked mitochondrial disease affecting cardiac muscle, skeletal muscle and neutrophil leukocytes. *J Neurol Sci* 62:327, 1983.
27. Yen TY, Hwu WL, Chien YH, et al: Acute metabolic decompensation and sudden death in Barth syndrome: Report of a family and a literature review. *Eur J Pediatr* 167:941, 2008.
28. Bassan R, Viero P, Minetti B, et al: Myelokathexis: A rare form of chronic benign neutropenia. *Br J Haematol* 58:115, 1984.
29. Wetzler M, Talpaz M, Kellagher MJ, et al: Myelokathexis. *JAMA* 267:2179, 1992.
30. Beaussant Cohen S, Fenneteau O, Plouvier E, et al: Description and outcome of a cohort of 8 patients with WHIM syndrome from the French Severe Chronic Neutropenia Registry. *Orphanet J Rare Dis* 7:71, 2012.
31. Balabanian K, Levoye A, Klemm L, et al: Leukocyte analysis from WHIM syndrome patients reveals a pivotal role for GRK3 in CXCR4 signaling. *J Clin Invest* 118:1074, 2008.

32. Koenig JM, Christensen RD: Incidence, neutrophil kinetics and natural history of neonatal neutropenia associated with maternal hypertension. *N Engl J Med* 321:557, 1989.

33. Tsao PN, Teng RJ, Tang JR, Yau KI: Granulocyte colony-stimulating factor in the cord blood of premature neonates born to mothers with pregnancy-induced hypertension. *J Pediatr* 135:56, 1999.

34. Menasche G, Fischer A, de Saint Basile G: Griscelli syndrome types 1 and 2. *Am J Hum Genet* 71:1237, 2002.

35. Kuijpers TW, Maianski NA, Tool AT, et al: Apoptotic neutrophils in the circulation of patients with glycogen storage disease type 1b (GSD1b). *Blood* 101:5021, 2003.

36. Shotelersuk V, Dell'Angelica EC, Hartnell L, et al: A new variant of Hermansky-Pudlak syndrome due to mutations in a gene responsible for vesicle formation. *Am J Med* 108:423, 2000.

37. Huizing M, Scher CD, Strovel E, et al: Nonsense mutations in ADTB3A cause complete deficiency of the beta3A subunit of adaptor complex-3 and severe Hermansky-Pudlak syndrome type 2. *Pediatr Res* 51:150, 2002.

38. Devriendt K, Kim AS, Mathijs G, et al: Constitutively activating mutation in WASP causes X-linked severe congenital neutropenia. *Nat Genet* 27:313, 2001.

39. Vial T, Gallant C, Choqu-Kastylevsky G, Descotes J: Treatment of drug-induced agranulocytosis with haematopoietic growth factors: A review of the clinical experience. *BioDrugs* 11:185, 1999.

40. Andersohn F, Konzen C, Garbe E: Systematic review: Agranulocytosis induced by nonchemotherapy drugs. *Ann Intern Med* 146:657, 2007.

41. Crawford J, Dale DC, Kuderer NM, et al: Risk and timing of neutropenic events in adult cancer patients receiving chemotherapy: The results of a prospective nationwide study of oncology practice. *J Natl Compr Canc Netw* 6:109, 2008.

42. Flanagan RJ, Dunk L: Haematological toxicity of drugs used in psychiatry. *Hum Psychopharmacol* 23(Suppl 1):27, 2008.

43. Dale DC, Hammond WP: Cyclic neutropenia: A clinical review. *Blood Rev* 2:178, 1988.

44. Horwitz MS, Duan Z, Korkmaz B, et al: Neutrophil elastase in cyclic and severe congenital neutropenia. *Blood* 109:1817, 2007.

45. Hutchinson R, Bunnell K, Thorne J: Suppression of granulopoietic progenitor cell proliferation by metabolites of the branched-chain amino acids. *J Pediatr* 106:62, 1985.

46. Andrès E, Maloisel F: Idiosyncratic drug-induced agranulocytosis or acute neutropenia. *Curr Opin Hematol* 15:15, 2008.

47. Andrès E, Federici L, Weitten T, et al: Recognition and management of drug-induced blood cytopenias: The example of drug-induced acute neutropenia and agranulocytosis. *Expert Opin Drug Saf* 7:481, 2008.

48. Chuang VW, Wong TY, Leung YH, et al: Review of dengue fever cases in Hong Kong during 1998 to 2005. *Hong Kong Med J* 14:170, 2008.

49. Cutting HO, Lange JE: Familial-benign chronic neutropenia. *Ann Intern Med* 61:876, 1964.

50. Kyle RA: Natural history of chronic idiopathic neutropenia. *N Engl J Med* 302:908, 1970.

51. Yilmaz D, Ritchey AK: Severe neutropenia in children: A single institutional experience. *J Pediatr Hematol Oncol* 29:513, 2007.

52. Vlacha V, Feketea G: The clinical significance of non-malignant neutropenia in hospitalized children. *Ann Hematol* 86:865, 2007.

53. Wlodarski MW, Nearman Z, Jiang Y, et al: Clonal predominance of CD8(+) T cells in patients with unexplained neutropenia. *Exp Hematol* 36:293, 2008.

54. Maheshwari A, Christensen RD, Calhoun DA: Immune neutropenia in the neonate. *Adv Pediatr* 49:317, 2002.

55. Williams BA, Fung YL: Alloimmune neonatal neutropenia: Can we afford the consequences of a missed diagnosis? *J Paediatr Child Health* 42:59, 2006.

56. Bux J: Human neutrophil alloantigens. *Vox Sang* 94:277, 2008.

57. Marmont AM: The autoimmune myelopathies. *Semin Hematol* 28:269, 1991.

58. Bux J, Behrens G, Jaeger G, Welte K: Diagnosis and clinical course of autoimmune neutropenia in infancy: Analysis of 240 cases. *Blood* 91:181, 1998.

59. Capsoni F, Sarzi-Puttini P, Zanella A: Primary and secondary autoimmune neutropenia. *Arthritis Res Ther* 7:208, 2005.

60. Winkelstein A, Kiss JE: Immunohematologic disorders. *JAMA* 278:1982, 1997.

61. Bowman SJ: Hematological manifestations of rheumatoid arthritis. *Scand J Rheumatol* 31:251, 2002.

62. Burks EJ, Loughran TP Jr: Pathogenesis of neutropenia in large granular lymphocyte leukemia and Felty syndrome. *Blood Rev* 20:245, 2006.

63. Prochorec-Sobieszek M, Rymkiewicz G, Makuch-asica H, et al: Characteristics of T-cell large granular lymphocyte proliferations associated with neutropenia and inflammatory arthropathy. *Arthritis Res Ther* 10:R55, 2008.

64. Beyan E, Beyan C, Turan M: Hematological presentation in systemic lupus erythematosus and its relationship with disease activity. *Hematology* 12:257, 2007.

65. Chen M, Zhao MH, Zhang Y, Wang H: Antineutrophil autoantibodies and their target antigens in systemic lupus erythematosus. *Lupus* 13:584, 2004.

66. Mathieson PW, O'Neill JH, Durrant STS, et al: Antibody-mediated pure neutrophil aplasia, recurrent myasthenia gravis and previous thymoma. *Q J Med* 74:57, 1990.

67. Brito-Zerón P, Soria N, Muñoz in S, et al: Prevalence and clinical relevance of autoimmune neutropenia in patients with primary Sjögren's syndrome. *Semin Arthritis Rheum* 38:389, 2009.

68. Cuadrado A, Aresti S, Cortés MA, et al: Autoimmune hepatitis and agranulocytosis. *Dig Liver Dis* 41:e14, 2009.

69. Stevens C, Peppercorn MA, Grand RJ: Crohn's disease associated with autoimmune neutropenia. *J Clin Gastroenterol* 13:328, 1991.

70. Ogershok PR, Hogan MB, Welch JE, et al: Spectrum of illness in pediatric common variable immunodeficiency. *Ann Allergy Asthma Immunol* 97:653, 2006.

71. Tamura H, Okamoto M, Yamashita T, et al: Pure white cell aplasia: Report of the first case associated with primary biliary cirrhosis. *Int J Hematol* 85:97, 2007.

72. Zachee P, Daeleans R, Pollaris P, et al: Neutrophil adhesion molecules in chronic hemodialysis patients. *Nephron* 68:192, 1994.

73. Levitt LJ, Ries CA, Greenberg PL: Pure white-cell aplasia. Antibody-mediated autoimmune inhibition of granulopoiesis. *N Engl J Med* 308:1141, 1983.

74. Chakupurakal G, Murrin RJ, Neilson JR: Prolonged remission of pure white cell aplasia (PWCA), in a patient with CLL, induced by rituximab and maintained by continuous oral cyclosporin. *Eur J Haematol* 79:271, 2007.

75. Marmont AM, Dominietto A, Gualandi F, et al: Pure white cell aplasia (PWCA) relapsing after allogeneic BMT and successfully treated with nine DLIs. *Biol Blood Marrow Transplant* 12:987, 2006.

76. Joyce RA, Boggs DR, Hasiba U, Srodes CH: Marginal neutrophil pool size in normal subjects and neutropenic patients as measured by epinephrine infusion. *J Lab Clin Med* 88:614, 1976.

77. Carr ME, Whitehead J, Carlson P, et al: Case report: Immunoglobulin M-mediated, temperature-dependent neutrophil agglutination as a cause of pseudoneutropenia. *Am J Med Sci* 311:92, 1996.

78. Esposito D, Chouinard G, Hardy P, Corruble E: Successful initiation of clozapine treatment despite morning pseudoneutropenia. *Int J Neuropsychopharmacol* 9:489, 2006.

79. Herring WB, Smith LG, Walker RI, Herion JC: Hereditary neutrophilia. *Am J Med* 56:729, 1974.

80. Wiedmeier SE, Henry E, Christensen RD: Hematological abnormalities during the first week of life among neonates with trisomy 18 and trisomy 13: Data from a multi-hospital healthcare system. *Am J Med Genet A* 146:312, 2008.

81. Ward HN, Reinhard EH: Chronic idiopathic leukocytosis. *Ann Intern Med* 75:193, 1971.

82. Joyce RA, O'Donnell J, Sanghvi J, Westerman MP: Asplenia and abnormal neutrophil kinetics in chronic idiopathic neutrophilia. *Am J Med* 69:633, 1980.

83. Sakka V, Tsiodras S, Giamarellos-Bourboulis EJ, Giamarellou H: An update on the etiology and diagnostic evaluation of a leukemoid reaction. *Eur J Intern Med* 17:394, 2006.

84. Reding MT, Hibbs JR, Morrison VA, et al: Diagnosis and outcome of 100 consecutive patients with extreme granulocytic leukocytosis. *Am J Med* 104:12, 1998.

85. Marsh JC, Boggs DR, Cartwright GE, Wintrobe MM: Neutrophil kinetics in acute infection. *J Clin Invest* 46:1943, 1967.

86. Jardin F, Vasse M, Debled M, et al: Intense paraneoplastic neutrophilic leukemoid reaction related to a G-CSF-secreting lung sarcoma. *Am J Hematol* 80:243, 2005.

87. Nara T, Hayakawa A, Ikeuchi A, et al: Granulocyte colony-stimulating factor-producing cutaneous angiosarcoma with leukaemoid reaction arising on a burn scar. *Br J Dermatol* 149:1273, 2003.

88. Sato T, Omura M, Saito J, et al: Neutrophilia associated with anaplastic carcinoma of the thyroid. *Thyroid* 10:1113, 2000.

89. Sevastos N, Theodossiades G, Malaktari S, Archimandritis AJ: Persistent neutrophilia as a preceding symptom of pheochromocytoma. *J Clin Endocrinol Metab* 90:2472, 2005.

90. Bishop CR: Leukokinetic studies: XIII. A non-steady state kinetic evaluation of the mechanism of cortisone-induced granulocytosis. *J Clin Invest* 47:249, 1968.

91. Crockard AD, Boylan MT, Droogan AG, et al: Methylprednisolone-induced neutrophil leukocytosis-down-modulation of neutrophil L-selectin and Mac-1 expression and induction of colony-stimulating factor. *Int J Clin Lab Res* 28:110, 1998.

92. Murphy DL, Goodwin FK, Bunney WE: Leukocytosis during lithium treatment. *Am J Psychiatry* 127:135, 1971.

93. Salloum E, Stoessel KM, Cooper DL: Hyperleukocytosis and retinal hemorrhages after chemotherapy and filgrastim administration for peripheral blood progenitor cell mobilization. *Bone Marrow Transplant* 21:835, 1998.

94. de Oliveira JP, Levy A, Morel P, Guibal F: Severe neutrophilia induced by infliximab for psoriasis. *Br J Dermatol* 158:200, 2008.

95. Kratz A, Lewandrowski KB, Siegel AJ: Effect of marathon running on hematologic and biochemical laboratory parameters, including cardiac markers. *Am J Clin Pathol* 118:856, 2002.

96. Laing SJ, Jackson AR, Walters R, et al: Human blood neutrophil responses to prolonged exercise with and without a thermal clamp. *J Appl Physiol* 104:20, 2008.

97. Cohen PR: Sweet's syndrome—A comprehensive review of an acute febrile neutrophilic dermatosis. *Orphanet J Rare Dis* 2:34, 2007.

98. Ratzinger G, Burgdorf W, Zelger BG, Zelger B: Acute febrile neutrophilic dermatosis: A histopathologic study of 31 cases with review of literature. *Am J Dermatopathol* 29:125, 2007.

99. Petitti DB, Kipp H: The leukocyte count: Association with intensity of smoking and persistence of effect after quitting. *Am J Epidemiol* 123:89, 1986.

100. Iho S, Tanaka Y, Takauji R, et al: Nicotine induces human neutrophils to produce IL-8 through the generation of peroxynitrate and subsequent activation of NF-kappaB. *J Leukoc Biol* 74:942, 2003.

101. Fung YL, Silliman CC, Minchinton RM, et al: Cardiopulmonary bypass induces enduring alterations to host neutrophil physiology: A single-centre longitudinal observational study. *Shock* 30:642, 2008.

102. Bishop CR, Athens JW, Boggs DR, et al: Leukokinetic studies XIII. A non-steady-state kinetic evaluation of the mechanism of cortisone-induced granulocytosis. *J Clin Invest* 47:249, 1968.

103. Athens JW, Haab OP, Raab SO, et al: Leukokinetic studies: IV. The total blood, circulating and marginal granulocyte pools and the granulocyte turnover rate in normal subjects. *J Clin Invest* 40:989, 1961.

104. Kuijpers TW, Van Lier RA, Hamann D, et al: Leukocyte adhesion deficiency type 1 (LAD-1)/variant. A novel immunodeficiency syndrome characterized by dysfunctional beta2 integrins. *J Clin Invest* 100:1725, 1997.

105. Etzioni A, Tonetti M: Leukocyte adhesion deficiency II—From A to almost Z. *Immunol Rev* 178:138, 2000.

106. MacGregor RR, Spagnulo PJ, Lentnek AL: Inhibition of granulocyte adherence by ethanol, prednisone, and aspirin, measured with an assay system. *N Engl J Med* 291:642, 1974.

107. Boxer LA, Hedley-White ET, Stossel TP: Neutrophil actin dysfunction and abnormal neutrophil behavior. *N Engl J Med* 291:1043, 1974.

108. Coates TD, Torkildson JC, Torres M, et al: An inherited defect of neutrophil motility and microfilamentous cytoskeleton associated with abnormalities in 47-Kd and 89-Kd proteins. *Blood* 78:1338, 1991.

109. Nunoi H, Yamazaki T, Kanegasaki S: Neutrophil cytoskeletal disease. *Int J Hematol* 74:119, 2001.

110. Hill HR, Augustine NH, Jaffe HS: Human recombinant interferon gamma enhances neonatal PMN activation and movement increases free intracellular calcium. *J Exp Med* 173:767, 1991.

111. Al-Hertani W, Yan SR, Byers DM, Bortolussi R: Human newborn polymorphonuclear neutrophils exhibit decreased levels of MyD88 and attenuated p38 phosphorylation in response to lipopolysaccharide. *Clin Invest Med* 30:E44, 2007.

112. Klempner MS, Noring R, Meir JW, Atkins MB: An acquired chemo-tactic defect in neutrophils from patients receiving interleukin-2 immunotherapy. *N Engl J Med* 322:959, 1990.

113. Kannengiesser C, Gérard B, El Benna J, et al: Molecular epidemiology of chronic granulomatous disease in a series of 80 kindreds: Identification of 31 novel mutations. *Hum Mutat* 29:E132, 2008.

114. Stasia MJ, Li XJ: Genetics and immunopathology of chronic granulomatous disease. *Semin Immunopathol* 30:209, 2008.

115. Gu Y, Williams DA: RAC2 GTPase deficiency and myeloid cell dysfunction in human and mouse. *J Pediatr Hematol Oncol* 24:791, 2002.

116. Williams DA, Tao W, Yang Y, et al: Dominant negative mutation of the hematopoietic-specific Rho GTPase, Rac2, is associated with a human phagocyte immunodeficiency. *Blood* 96:1646, 2000.

117. Nauseef WM. Diagnostic assays for myeloperoxidase deficiency. *Methods Mol Biol* 412:525, 2007.

118. Goedken M, McCormick S, Leidal KG, et al: Impact of two novel mutations on the structure and function of human myeloperoxidase. *J Biol Chem* 282:27994, 2007.

119. Minegishi Y, Karasuyama H: Hyperimmunoglobulin E syndrome and tyrosine kinase 2 deficiency. *Curr Opin Allergy Clin Immunol* 7:506, 2007.

120. Holland SM, DeLeo FR, Elloumi HZ, et al: STAT3 mutations in the hyper-IgE syndrome. *N Engl J Med* 357:1608, 2007.

121. Cooper MR, DeChatelet LR, McCall CE: Complete deficiency of leukocyte glucose-6-phosphate dehydrogenase with defective bactericidal activity. *J Clin Invest* 51:769, 1972.

122. Vives Corrons JL, Feliu E, Pujades MA, et al: Severe-glucose-6-phosphate dehydrogenase (G6PD) deficiency associated with chronic hemolytic anemia, granulocyte dysfunction, and increased susceptibility to infections: Description of a new molecular variant (G6PD Barcelona). *Blood* 59:428, 1982.

123. Arturson G: Neutrophil granulocyte functions in severely burned patients. *Burns Incl Therm Inj* 11:309, 1985.

124. Ahmed S el-D, el-Shahat AS, Saad SO: Assessment of certain neutrophil receptors, opsonophagocytosis and soluble intercellular adhesion molecule-1 (ICAM-1) following thermal injury. *Burns* 25:395, 1999.

125. Lesma E, Riva E, Giovannini M, et al: Amelioration of neutrophil membrane function underlies granulocyte-colony stimulating factor action in glycogen storage disease 1b. *Int J Immunopathol Pharmacol* 18:297, 2005.

126. Kim SY, Jun HS, Mead PA, et al: Neutrophil stress and apoptosis underlie myeloid dysfunction in glycogen storage disease type Ib. *Blood* 111:5704, 2008.

127. Tamura DY, Moore EE, Patrick DA, et al: Clinically relevant concentrations of ethanol attenuate primed neutrophil bactericidal activity. *J Trauma* 44:320, 1998.

128. Breitmeier D, Becker N, Weilbach C, et al: Ethanol-induced malfunction of neutrophils respiratory burst on patients suffering from alcohol dependence. *Alcohol Clin Exp Res* 32:1708, 2008.

129. Porter CJ, Burden RP, Morgan AG, et al: Impaired bacterial killing and hydrogen peroxide production by polymorphonuclear neutrophils in end-stage renal failure. *Nephron* 77:479, 1997.

130. Hopps E, Camera A, Caimi G: [Polimorphonuclear leukocytes and diabetes mellitus] [in Italian]. *Minerva Med* 99:197, 2008.

131. Davidson WM, Milner RDG, Lawlor SD: Giant neutrophil leukocytes: An inherited anomaly. *Br J Haematol* 6:339, 1960.

135. Undritz VE: Eine neue Sippe mit Erblich—Konstitutioneller Hochsegmentierung der Neutrophilenkerne. *Schweiz Med Wochenschr* 94:1365, 1964.

136. Uzel G, Holland SM: White blood cell defects: Molecular discoveries and clinical management. *Curr Allergy Asthma Rep* 2:385, 2002.

137. Lekstrom-Himes JA, Dorman SE, Kopar P, et al: Neutrophil-specific granule deficiency results from a novel mutation with loss of function of the transcription factor CCAAT/enhancer binding protein. *J Exp Med* 189:1847, 1999.

138. Gombart AF, Koeffler HP: Neutrophil specific granule deficiency and mutations in the gene encoding transcription factor C/EBP (epsilon). *Curr Opin Hematol* 9:36, 2002.

139. Hoffmann K, Dreger CK, Olins AL, et al: Mutations in the gene encoding the laminin B receptor produce an altered nuclear morphology in granulocytes (Pelger-Hüet anomaly). *Nat Genet* 31:410, 2002.

140. Worman HJ, Bonne G: "Laminopathies": A wide spectrum of human diseases. *Exp Cell Res* 313:2121, 2007.

141. Brunning RD: Morphologic alterations in nucleated blood and marrow cells in genetic disorders. *Hum Pathol* 1:99, 1970.

142. Oski FA, Naiman JL, Allen DM, Diamond LK: Leukocytic inclusions—Döhle bodies-associated with platelet abnormality (the May-Hegglin anomaly): Report of a family and review of the literature. *Blood* 20:657, 1962.

143. Pecci A, Panza E, Pujol-Moix N, et al: Position of nonmuscle myosin heavy chain IIA (NMMHC-IIA) mutations predicts the natural history of MYH9-related disease. *Hum Mutat* 29:409, 2008.

144. Seri M, Pecci A, Di Bari F, et al: MYH9-related disease: May-Hegglin anomaly, Sebastian syndrome, Fechtner syndrome, and Epstein syndrome are not distinct entities but represent a variable expression of a single illness. *Medicine (Baltimore)* 82:203, 2003.

145. Westbroek W, Adams D, Huizing M, et al: Cellular defects in Chediak-Higashi syndrome correlate with the molecular genotype and clinical phenotype. *J Invest Dermatol* 127:2674, 2007.

146. Lazarchick J, McRae B: Chediak-Higashi syndrome. *Blood* 105:4162, 2005.

147. Schmid-Schönbein GN: Leukocyte kinetics in the microcirculation. *Biorheology* 24:139, 1987.

148. Smedly LA, Tonnesen MG, Sandhaus RA, et al: Neutrophil-mediated injury to endothelial cells: Enhancement by endotoxin and essential role of neutrophil elastase. *J Clin Invest* 77:1233, 1986.

149. Weiss SJ: Tissue destruction by neutrophils. *N Engl J Med* 320:365, 1989.

150. Swank DW, Moore SB: Roles of the neutrophil and other mediators in adult respiratory distress syndrome. *Mayo Clin Proc* 64:1118, 1989.

151. MacNee W, Wiggs B, Balzberg AS, Hogg JC: The effect of cigarette smoking on neutrophil kinetics in human lungs. *N Engl J Med* 321:924, 1989.

152. Martin TR, Pistorese BP, Hudson LD, Maunder RJ: The function of lung and blood neutrophils in patients with the adult respiratory distress syndrome. Implication for the pathogenesis of lung infections. *Am Rev Respir Dis* 144:254, 1991.

153. Godek JE: Adverse effects of neutrophils on the lung. *Am J Med* 92(Suppl 6A):27S, 1992.

154. Palmgren MS, deShazo RO, Cater RM, et al: Mechanisms of neutrophil damage to human alveolar extracellular matrix: The role of serine and metalloproteases. *J Allergy Clin Immunol* 89:905, 1992.

155. Weiss ST, Segal MR, Sparrow D, Wager C: Relation of FEV1 and peripheral blood leukocyte count to total mortality. *Am J Epidemiol* 142:493, 1995.

156. Fung YL, Goodison KA, Wong JK, Minchinton RM: Investigating transfusion-related acute lung injury (TRALI). *Intern Med J* 33:286, 2003.

157. Segel GB, Halterman MW, Lichtman MA. The paradox of the neutrophil's role in tissue injury. *J Leukoc Biol* 89:359, 2011.

158. Boventre JV, Colvin RB: Adhesion molecules in renal disease. *Curr Opin Nephrol Hypertens* 5:254, 1996.

159. Kitching AR, Holdsworth SR, Hickey MJ: Targeting leukocytes in immune glomerular diseases. *Curr Med Chem* 15:448, 2008.

160. Chibber R, Ben-Mahmud BM, Chibber S, Kohner EM: Leukocytes in diabetic retinopathy. *Curr Diabetes Rev* 3:3, 2007.

161. Fadlon E, Vordermeier S, Pearson TC, et al: Blood polymorphonuclear leukocytes from the majority of sickle cell patients in the crisis phase of the disease show adhesion to vascular endothelium and increased expression of CD64. *Blood* 91:266, 1998.

162. Schaub RG, Yamashita A, Simmons CA, et al: Leukocyte-mediated large vein injury and thrombosis: Pharmacologic intervention with lipoxygenase inhibitors, in *Leukocyte Emigration and Its Sequelae*, edited by Morat HZ, p 62. Karger, Basel, 1987.

163. Ranjadayalan K, Umachandran V, Daviews SW, et al: Thrombolytic treatment in acute myocardial infarction: Neutrophil activation, peripheral leucocyte responses, and myocardial injury. *Br Heart J* 66:10, 1991.

164. Welbourn CRB, Goldman G, Paterson IS, et al: Pathophysiology of ischaemia reperfusion injury: Central role of the neutrophil. *Br J Surg* 78:651, 1991.

165. Kassirer M, Zeltser D, Gluzman B, et al: The appearance of L-selectin (low) polymorphonuclear leukocytes in the circulating pool of peripheral blood during myocardial infarction correlates with neutrophilia and the size of the infarct. *Clin Cardiol* 22:721, 1999.

166. Takahashi T, Hiasa Y, Ohara Y, et al: Relationship of admission neutrophil count to microvascular injury, left ventricular dilation, and long-term outcome in patients treated with primary angioplasty for acute myocardial infarction. *Circ J* 72:867, 2008.

167. Takahashi T, Hiasa Y, Ohara Y, et al: Relation between neutrophil counts on admission, microvascular injury, and left ventricular functional recovery in patients with an anterior wall first acute myocardial infarction treated with primary coronary angioplasty. *Am J Cardiol* 100:35, 2007.

168. Kyne L, Hausdorff JM, Knight E, et al: Neutrophilia and congestive heart failure after acute myocardial infarction. *Am Heart J* 139:32, 2000.

169. Buck BH, Liebeskind DS, Saver JL, et al: Early neutrophilia is associated with volume of ischemic tissue in acute stroke. *Stroke* 39:355, 2008.

170. Trush MA, Seed JL, Kensler TW: Oxidant-dependent metabolic activation of polycyclic aromatic hydrocarbons by phorbol ester-stimulated human polymorphonuclear leukocytes: Possible link between inflammation and cancer. *Proc Natl Acad Sci U S A* 82:5194, 1985.

171. Weitzman SA, Weitburg AB, Clark EP, Stossel TP: Phagocytes as carcinogens: Malignant transformation produced by human neutrophil. *Science* 227:1231, 1985.

172. Phillips AN, Neaton JD, Cook DG, et al: The leukocyte count and risk of lung cancer. *Cancer* 69:680, 1992.

173. Segel GB, Simon W, Lichtman MA. Should we still be focused on red cell hemoglobin F as the principal explanation for the salutary effect of hydroxyurea in sickle cell disease? *Pediatr Blood Cancer* 57:8, 2011.

174. Reed WW, Diehl LF: Leukopenia, neutropenia, and reduced hemoglobin levels in healthy American Blacks. *Arch Intern Med* 151:501, 1991.

175. Beutler E, West C: Hematologic differences between African-Americans and whites: The roles of iron deficiency and alpha-thalassemia on hemoglobin levels and mean corpuscular volume. *Blood* 106:740, 2005.

176. Hsieh MM, Everhart JE, Byrd-Holt DD, et al: Prevalence of neutropenia in the U.S. population: Age, sex, smoking status, and ethnic differences. *Ann Intern Med* 146:486, 2007.

177. Grann VR, Bowman N, Joseph C, et al: Neutropenia in six ethnic groups from the Caribbean and the U.S. *Cancer* 113:854, 2008.

178. Berliner S, Shapira I, Toker S, et al: Benign hereditary leukopenia-neutropenia does not result from lack of low grade inflammation. A new look in the era of microinflammation. *Blood Cells Mol Dis* 34:135, 2005.

179. Bodey GP, Buckley M, Sathe YS: Quantitative relationships between circulating leukocytes and infection in patients with acute leukemia. *Ann Intern Med* 64:328, 1966.

180. Kourtis AP, Hudgens, MG, Kayira D, for the BAN study team. Neutrophil count in African mothers and newborns and HIV transmission. *N Engl J Med* 367:23, 2012.

181. Sickles EA, Green WH, Wiernick PH: Clinical presentation of infection in granulocytopenic patients. *Arch Intern Med* 135:715, 1975.

182. Dale DC, Wolff SM: Skin window studies of the acute inflammatory responses of neutropenic patients. *Blood* 38:138, 1971.

183. Coller B: Leukocytosis and ischemic vascular disease morbidity and mortality. Is it time to intervene? *Arterioscler Thromb Vasc Biol* 25:658, 2005.

CHAPTER 65
NEUTROPENIA AND NEUTROPHILIA

David C. Dale and Karl Welte

SUMMARY

Neutropenia designates a blood absolute neutrophil count that is less than 2 SD below the mean of a normal population. Neutropenia can be inherited or acquired. It usually results from decreased production of neutrophil precursor cells in the marrow. Neutropenia also can result from a shift of neutrophils from the circulating into the marginated cell pools in the circulation. Less commonly, neutropenia results from accelerated destruction of neutrophils or increased egress of neutrophil from the circulation into the tissues. When neutropenia is the sole or dominant abnormality, the condition is called "selective" or isolated" neutropenia, such as severe congenital neutropenia, chronic idiopathic neutropenia, or drug-induced neutropenia. Neutropenia can occur in other inherited or acquired marrow failure syndromes, such as severe aplastic anemia or Fanconi anemia, in which the condition is a bicytopenia or pancytopenia. In some diseases, several cell lineages are mildly affected but the reduction in neutrophil is the most severe, such as Felty syndrome. Neutropenia may be an indicator of an underlying systemic disease, such as early vitamin B$_{12}$ or transcobalamin deficiency. Neutropenia, particularly severe neutropenia (neutrophil counts <0.5 × 10⁹/L [500/μL]), increases susceptibility to bacterial or fungal infections and impairs the resolution of these infections. Therapy with the hormone primarily responsible for neutrophil production, granulocyte colony-stimulating factor, can increase blood neutrophil counts for most types of neutropenia, although whether its administration makes a clinically useful impact is dependent on the origin, duration and severity of the neutropenia. Clinical guidelines have been published on the rational use of the drug.

Neutrophilia is an increase in the absolute neutrophil count to a concentration greater than 2 SD above the normal population mean value. Neutrophilia contributes to the inflammatory response and to resolution of infections. Inflammatory and infectious diseases are the most frequent causes of neutrophilia. Bacterial infections usually produce neutrophilia, whereas viral infections may not produce neutrophilia or may raise the neutrophil count only slightly. Solid tumors occasionally engender striking neutrophilia. Hereditary neutrophilia can be caused by activating mutations within the CSF3R gene. When the neutrophil count is very high, it may be referred to as a leukemoid reaction. The rare neutrophilic variants of chronic myeloid leukemia and chronic neutrophilic leukemia may result in striking neutrophilia. Demargination of neutrophils or rapid release of neutrophils from a large marrow pool may transiently increase the blood neutrophil count. Sustained increased require increased production of these cells.

Acronyms and Abbreviations: ANA, antinuclear antibody; BTH, Bruton tyrosine kinase; G-CSF, granulocyte colony-stimulating factor; GM-CSF, granulocyte-macrophage colony-stimulating factor; Ig, immunoglobulin; IL, interleukin; TRAIL, tumor necrosis factor-related apoptosis-inducing ligand.

● NEUTROPENIA

Neutropenia refers to an absolute blood neutrophil count (total leukocyte count per microliter × percent of neutrophils) that is less than 2 SD below the normal mean of the population. The terms *leukopenia*, a reduced total white blood cell count, and *granulocytopenia*, reduced numbers of blood granulocytes (neutrophils, eosinophils, and basophils), sometimes are imprecisely used as synonyms for neutropenia. *Agranulocytosis* literally means a complete absence of blood granulocytes, but this term often is used to indicate severe neutropenia, that is, counts less than 0.5×10^9/L (0.5×10^3/μL).

The concentration of neutrophils in blood is influenced by age, activity, and genetic and environmental factors (Chap. 2). For children from 1 month to 10 years old, neutropenia is defined as a blood neutrophil count less than 1.5×10^9/L. For individuals older than age 10 years, neutropenia is defined as a count less than approximately 1.8×10^9/L (see Chap. 7 regarding levels in newborns). Healthy older persons have the same blood neutrophil counts as younger individuals (Chap. 9). Some racial and ethnic groups, such as Africans, African Americans, and Yemenite Jews, have lower mean neutrophil counts than persons of Asian or European ancestry (see Chap. 2, Table 2–2). The mean differences in neutrophils are modest and have no recognized health consequences.[1,2]

Severe neutropenia is a predisposing factor for infections. The organisms normally are found on the skin, in the nasopharynx, and as part of the intestinal flora. The risk of infections is inversely related to the severity of the neutropenia (Chap. 24). Individuals with neutrophil counts of 1.0 to 1.8×10^9/L are at little risk of infection. In general, neutrophil counts between 0.5 and 1.0×10^9/L are associated with only slight risk of infection unless other contributing factors are present. Individuals with neutrophil counts less than 0.5×10^9/L are at substantially greater risk, but the frequency of infections varies considerably, depending on the cause and duration of neutropenia. Severe acute neutropenia (i.e., developing over a few hours or days) usually is associated with greater risk of infection than severe chronic neutropenia (usually present for months or years). Neutropenia resulting from disorders of production that affect early hematopoietic precursor cells (e.g., aplastic anemia, severe congenital neutropenia) leads to greater susceptibility to infections than do conditions with adequate neutrophil precursors in the marrow and neutropenia attributed to accelerated turnover in the blood (e.g., rheumatoid arthritis, Felty syndrome, autoimmune neutropenia). For patients made severely neutropenic by cancer chemotherapy, the risk is greater when the neutrophils are decreasing than with similar counts when neutrophils are increasing. Neutropenia accompanied by monocytopenia, lymphocytopenia, or hypogammaglobulinemia is more serious than isolated neutropenia. Other factors, such as the integrity of the skin and mucous membranes, the vascular supply to tissues, and the nutritional status of the patient, also influence the risk of infections.

PATHOPHYSIOLOGIC MECHANISMS
General Mechanisms

Neutropenia occurs because of (1) hypoplastic neutropoiesis, (2) ineffective neutropoiesis (resulting from exaggerated apoptosis of late precursors), (3) accelerated removal or utilization of circulating neutrophils, (4) shifts of cells from the circulating to the marginal blood pools, or (5) a combination of these mechanisms (Fig. 65–1). Some production disorders are caused by intrinsic abnormalities of hematopoietic progenitor cells (Chap. 83). Other disorders in cell production are caused by extrinsic factors, including changes in the marrow environment, such as tumor infiltration, fibrosis, or irradiation (Chap. 45).

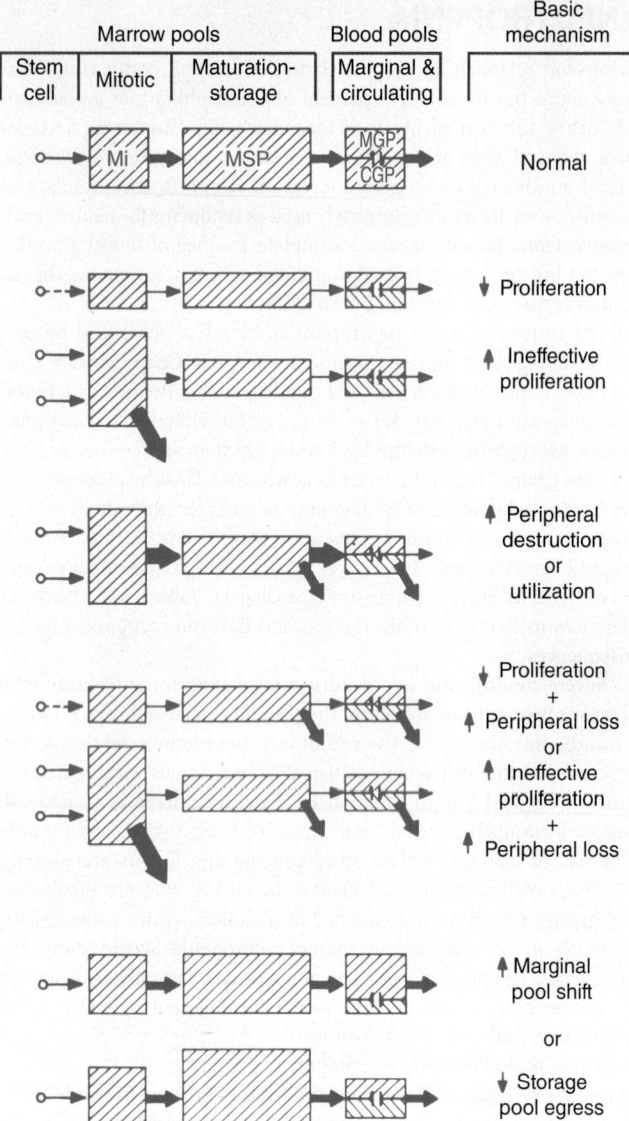

Figure 65–1. Mechanisms of neutropenia are shown schematically. The size of each pool is represented by the size of the *cross-hatched areas*. The rate of flow of cells through each compartment is represented by the size of the *arrows*. CGP, circulating granulocyte (neutrophil) pool; MGP, marginated granulocyte (neutrophil) pool; Mi, mitotic; MSP, maturation (marrow storage) pool

Myelotoxic chemotherapeutic drugs commonly cause neutropenia because of the high proliferative activity of neutrophil precursors in the marrow and short half-life (4 to 8 hours) of neutrophils in the blood. Production of neutrophils is defined as ineffective when, under a steady state of hematopoiesis, a relative abundance of early neutrophil precursors, a paucity of late-maturing cells, and neutropenia occur. This condition has often been referred to as "maturation arrest," but it is almost always explained by either the apoptotic loss of late precursors in the marrow as an intrinsic defect in cell maturation or rapid release of segmented neutrophils because of exaggerated tissue demands.

Accelerated neutrophil utilization occurs with autoimmune neutropenia and acute bacterial infections. When rapid neutrophil utilization and impaired production occur, acute severe neutropenia often develops. The condition is illustrated by the abrupt and sustained fall

in neutrophils when an alcoholic patient develops pneumococcal pneumonia. Alcohol suppresses the marrow, and the infection consumes the available neutrophil supply. After myelotoxic cancer chemotherapy, the abrupt fall in blood neutrophils at the onset of infections reflects a similar mechanism: high demand and limited supply. With idiosyncratic drug-induced neutropenia, the counts may fall abruptly because both blood and marrow cells are simultaneously damaged. Acute neutropenia that develops because of a shift of blood neutrophils from the circulating to the marginal blood pools, that is, increased margination (e.g., after injection of endotoxin, with exposure of blood to dialysis membranes, or after intravenous granulocyte colony-stimulating factor [G-CSF] or granulocyte-macrophage colony-stimulating factor [GM-CSF]) usually is a transient event. The marginated cells reenter the circulating pool, and the blood supply of neutrophils is rapidly restored from the large reserves of marrow neutrophils entering the blood.

Cellular and Molecular Mechanisms of Neutropenia

Our understanding of the mechanisms of neutropenia at the cellular and molecular levels is increasing rapidly because of advances in molecular genetics and cell biology. For many inherited forms of neutropenia, the genetic mutations causing these diseases are now known, and the mutant protein products have been identified. Some mutations and acquired defects shorten the survival of the precursor cells, that is, they accelerate apoptosis. This form of cell loss now is thought to be the mechanism for "maturation arrest" in several diseases. Examples of increased apoptosis causing neutropenia include vitamin B_{12} or transcobalamin deficiency,[3] clonal cytopenias (myelodysplasia),[4] myelokathexis,[5] congenital and cyclic neutropenia,[6,7] and the Shwachman-Diamond syndrome.[8] Neutrophils also can be depleted from the blood and the marrow as a result of extrinsic factors such as antineutrophil antibodies and toxic cytokines generated by other cells.[9,10] Some disorders that cause neutropenia also perturb neutrophil function, such as glycogen storage disease type 1b,[11] Chédiak-Higashi syndrome,[12] and HIV infection.[13] Susceptibility to infection in these conditions relates to the combination of defects.

CAUSES OF NEUTROPENIA

Causes of neutropenia are classified physiologically as disorders of production, distribution, or turnover. Not every condition fits neatly into this scheme, but it provides a framework for understanding these diverse disorders.

Disorders of Production

Cytotoxic drugs given for cancer chemotherapy and as immunosuppressive agents regularly cause neutropenia by decreasing cell production (Chap. 22). These drugs now are probably the most frequent cause of neutropenia in the United States. Neutropenia as a result of impaired production is a common feature of several diseases affecting hematopoietic stem cells, such as acute leukemia (Chaps. 88 and 91), the myelodysplastic syndromes (Chap. 87), and aplastic anemia (Chap. 35). The selective causes of impaired production, progressing from disorders of early precursors to disorders presumed to involve defective maturation (ineffective production), are described briefly as follows.

Congenital Neutropenias (Kostmann Syndrome and Related Disorders In 1956, Kostmann described congenital neutropenia (agranulocytosis) as an autosomal recessive disease occurring in an extended family in northern Sweden.[14] Phenotypically similar sporadic cases and families with autosomal dominant congenital neutropenia have been reported.[15,16] In severe congenital neutropenia, symptoms and signs of otitis, gingivitis, pneumonia, enteritis, peritonitis, and bacteremia usually begin in the first months of life. At diagnosis,

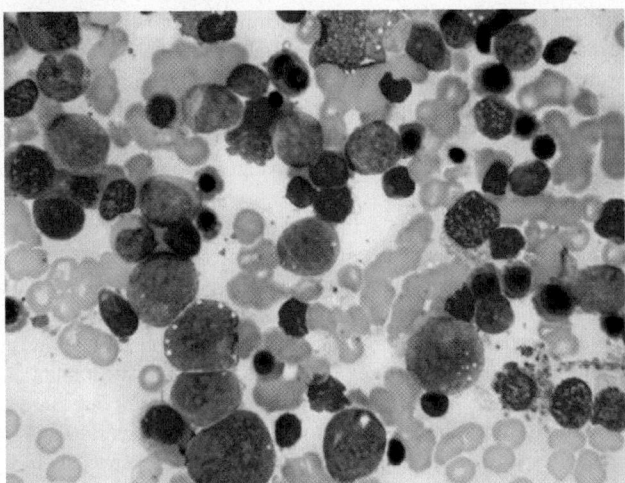

Figure 65–2. Morphology of a marrow sample from a patient with congenital neutropenia showing the maturation arrest at the level of promyelocytes.

the neutrophil count usually is less than 0.2×10^9/L.[17] Monocytosis, mild anemia, thrombocytosis, and splenomegaly frequently are present. Characteristically, the marrow shows early neutrophil precursors (myeloblasts, promyelocytes) but few or no myelocytes or mature neutrophils (Fig. 65–2). Marrow eosinophilia is common. *In vitro* marrow culture studies show poor growth in response to various growth factors and with reduced numbers of marrow neutrophil and monocyte progenitor cell colonies.[18] Usually blood lymphocyte numbers are normal, immunoglobulin levels are normal or increased, and lymphocyte functions are intact.

The majority of patients with sporadic or autosomal dominant severe congenital neutropenia have heterozygous mutations of the gene for neutrophil elastase (also called *ELANE*). Its product is a protease found normally in the neutrophil's primary granules and lead to the induction of the unfolded protein response in the endoplasmatic reticulum.[15,19,20] A variety of mutations in exons 2 through 5 as well as in introns III and IV are the cause of this disease.[20–23] In the original Kostmann family, and some other families with autosomal recessive disease, neutropenia is caused by mutations in the *HAX-1* gene.[24] HAX-1 is a mitochondrial protein, and the mutations lead to accelerated apoptosis of myeloid cells, as well as neurologic abnormalities. In addition, mutations in HAX-1 lead to defective G-CSF receptor signaling via HCLS1 and LEF-1.[25] Mutations in the gene for glucose-6-phosphatase catalytic subunit 3 *(G6PC3)* also cause severe neutropenia as a result of apoptosis of neutrophil precursors, as well as congenital cardiac and urogenital abnormalities.[26] Additional autosomal-dominant, autosomal-recessive, X-linked, and sporadic forms have been described, with mutations in other genes, including *GFI1*,[27] *WAS*,[28] *p14*,[29] *TAZ*,[30] *JAGN1*,[31] *TCIRG1*,[32] and many others, although the genetic causes in many patients with severe congenital neutropenia remain unidentified.

Mutations in the gene for the receptor for G-CSF also occur in patients with severe congenital neutropenia[33,34]; however, most of these receptor mutations have caused truncations of the distal portion of the cytoplasmic domain of the receptor, an abnormality associated with altered sensitivity to G-CSF. G-CSF receptor mutations are part of the evolution to myelodysplasia or acute myelogenous leukemia and are not the primary cause of this neutropenia. An exception may be a patient identified with a mutation in the external domain of the G-CSF receptor who responded to treatment with G-CSF and glucocorticoids and has not developed leukemia over several years of observation.[35] There are

rare cases of biallelic mutations within the extracellular domain of the G-CSF receptor which lead to nonresponse to treatment with G-CSF.[36]

G-CSF is a very effective therapy for all of the recognized subtypes of severe congenital neutropenia, increasing the neutrophil counts and reducing recurrent fevers and infections.[37] G-CSF acts to increase the neutrophil counts by enhancing expression of a critical transcription factor for granulopoiesis, C/EBPβ (CCAAT/enhancer binding protein β), and the "emergency" pathway of myelopoiesis (as during steady state C/EBPα is not functional).[38] Approximately 5 percent of patients do not respond to G-CSF. Hematopoietic transplantation is the only other therapy known to improve the clinical course for these patients.[39,40] Untreated patients and patients treated with G-CSF are at risk for developing acute myelogenous leukemia. The risk increases with time on treatment with G-CSF, particularly in poorly responsive patients.[41] A novel molecular pathway of leukemogenesis was recently identified: mutations in the hematopoietic cytokine receptor (G-CSFR) in combination with the second mutations in the downstream hematopoietic transcription factor (RUNX1), which could be used as a marker for identifying severe congenital neutropenia patients with a high risk of progressing to leukemia or myelodysplastic syndrome.[42]

Congenital Immunodeficiency Diseases Neutropenia is a feature of the congenital immunodeficiency diseases and a contributing factor to their susceptibility to infections (Chap. 80). In most of these conditions, neutropenia is attributed to a production disorder based largely on histologic examination of the marrow. In X-linked agammaglobulinemia, which is attributed to defective B-cell development and a mutation in a cytoplasmic (Bruton) tyrosine kinase *(BTK)*, severe neutropenia is present in approximately 25 percent of patients.[43] Children with common variable immunodeficiency often have neutropenia associated with thrombocytopenia and hemolytic anemia.[43] Neutropenia occurs in almost half of patients with the X-linked hyperimmunoglobulin-M syndrome, a disorder caused by a mutation in the gene encoding the CD40 ligand.[44] In severe combined immunodeficiency, neutropenia is not always present. The neutropenia varies over time in individual patients. Neutropenia is particularly prominent in the rare immunodeficiency state, reticular dysgenesis.[43] Neutropenia is a less-common feature of adenosine deaminase deficiency, the T−B+, T−B−, Wiskott-Aldrich, and Omenn syndromes.[43,45,46] Neutropenia also occurs on an autoimmune basis in some cases of the Wiskott-Aldrich syndrome.[34,46] Mutations in the genes for growth factor independent protein-1 *(GFI 1)* can also cause neutropenia.[47]

G-CSF therapy is effective in most patients with neutropenia associated with these immunodeficiency syndromes.

Cartilage Hair Hypoplasia Syndrome This rare autosomal recessive disorder is characterized by short-limbed dwarfism, hyperextensible digits, very fine hair, neutropenia, lymphopenia, and recurrent infections.[43] The genetic locus is at 9p13 and affects a gene coding for an endoribonuclease. The degree of neutropenia is variable, with blood counts ranging from 0.1 to 2.0×10^9/L. An accompanying defect in T-cell proliferation results from an abnormality in the transition from the G_0 to the G_1 phase of the mitotic cycle. Patients have frequent bacterial and viral respiratory infections. Hematopoietic stem cell transplantation can correct the neutropenia and immune deficiency.[48,49]

Shwachman-Diamond Syndrome This autosomal recessive disorder combines short stature, pancreatic exocrine deficiency, and marrow failure with neutropenia beginning early in the neonatal period.[50–53] Thrombocytopenia and anemia may be severe (Chap. 35). The chromosomal locus of the mutation is at 7qll, and the mutation affects the *SBDS* gene.[50] The mutation causes a proliferative defect and increased apoptosis of early myeloid progenitor cells.[51] A chemotactic defect also occurs in mature neutrophils.[52] The patients are malnourished, but the neutropenia is not corrected by improving the patients' nutritional status.

Treatment with G-CSF raises blood neutrophil levels, and hematopoietic stem cell transplantation corrects the hematologic abnormalities.[53] Without transplantation, the risk of evolution to myelodysplastic syndrome and acute myelogenous leukemia is 20 percent or greater.[53]

Diamond-Blackfan Syndrome Neutropenia is a rare complication of hereditary hypoplastic anemia.[54] Other features include congenital anomalies of the head and upper limbs. Two genetic loci have been identified: 19q13.2 and 8p23.[55,56] The varying severity of neutropenia may reflect genetic heterogeneity among patients with this diagnosis (Chap. 36).

Griscelli Syndrome This rare autosomal recessive disorder is characterized by pigmentary dilution and variable degrees of cellular immunodeficiency. The syndrome consists of three types. Neutropenia is a feature of type 2 but not types 1 or 3. In type 2, the neutropenia is relatively mild and associated with pancytopenia. These hematologic abnormalities are attributable to a mutation located at 15q21 affecting the *RAB27a* gene.[57] The gene product is a guanosine triphosphatase (GTPase). The mutation also causes abnormal release of granule proteins and hematophagocytosis.[58] As in the Chédiak-Higashi syndrome (Chap. 66), type 2 patients may develop an acute phase of uncontrolled lymphocyte and macrophage activation leading rapidly to death.[59] Hematopoietic stem cell transplantation can correct the hematologic features. Evolution to myelodysplasia has been reported.[60]

Chédiak-Higashi Syndrome This rare autosomal recessive disorder is characterized by partial oculocutaneous albinism, giant granules in many cells (including granulocytes, monocytes, and lymphocytes), neutropenia, and recurrent infections (Chap. 66). This syndrome now is attributable to a chromosomal mutation at 1q43 affecting the *LYST* gene.[61] The product of this gene regulates lysosomal trafficking. In Chédiak-Higashi syndrome, the neutropenia usually is mild, and susceptibility to infection is attributed to neutropenia and defective microbicidal activity of the phagocytes.[62]

Myelokathexis, WHIM, and Related Syndromes Myelokathexis is a rare autosomal dominant or sporadically occurring disorder in which patients have severe neutropenia and lymphocytopenia, with total white cell counts often less than $1.0 \times 10^9/L$.[63] WHIM syndrome, characterized by *w*arts, *h*ypogammaglobulinemia, *i*nfections, and *m*yelokathexis, now is attributable to a mutation in the gene encoding the receptor for the CXC chemokine CXCL12 (previously termed stromal cell-derived factor-1), termed CXCR-4.[64,65] The ligand–receptor pair CXCL-12/CXCR-4 is important for regulating the trafficking of all type of blood and marrow cells, including hematopoietic stem cells, from the marrow to the blood and tissues. In these syndromes, the marrow usually shows abundant precursors and developing neutrophils. Neutrophils in the marrow and the blood show hypersegmentation with pyknotic nuclei and cytoplasmic vacuoles. These morphologic changes and some molecular studies suggest cell loss in the marrow and blood caused by accelerated apoptosis. Favorable responses to G-CSF and GM-CSF occur, as does evolution to the myelodysplastic syndrome. A myelokathexis-like variant of myelodysplastic syndrome has been reported.[66]

Cohen Syndrome Cohen syndrome is another rare cause of neutropenia. Mental retardation, postnatal microcephaly, facial dysmorphism, pigmentary retinopathy, myopia, and intermittent neutropenia are characteristic features. Patients with Cohen syndrome of diverse origins have mutations in the *COH1* gene.[67] Current studies suggest that *COH1* plays a role in vesicle-mediated sorting and transport of proteins within many types of cells.

Glycogen Storage Diseases These autosomal recessive disorders are characterized by hypoglycemia, hepatosplenomegaly, seizures, and failure to thrive in infants. Only type 1b is associated with neutropenia.[68] The genetic defect in type 1b maps to chromosome 11q23 and is attributed to a defect in an intracellular transport protein for glucose.[69] The marrow appears normal despite severely reduced blood neutrophils. The neutrophils have a reduced oxidative burst when stimulated and defective chemotaxis.[70,71] Treatment with G-CSF is effective for correcting the neutropenia and improving the associated inflammatory bowel disease, but has been associated with evolution to acute myelogenous leukemia.[72]

Cyclic Neutropenia Cyclic neutropenia is an autosomal dominant or sporadically occurring disease characterized by regularly recurring episodes of severe neutropenia, usually every 21 days.[73] Regular oscillations of other white cells, reticulocytes, and platelets are sometimes observed. Cyclic neutropenia now is attributable to mutations in the gene for neutrophil elastase *(ELANE)* at locus 19q3. Most mutations in the *ELANE* gene are in the regions of exons 4 and 5, but there are also mutations in exons 2 and 3, as well as in the introns II and IV.[74,23] The diagnosis usually is made in the first year of life, especially in the presence of a family history of the condition.[75] The neutropenic periods last for 3 to 6 days and often are accompanied by fever, malaise, anorexia, mouth ulcers, and cervical lymphadenopathy. A few cases of acquired cyclic neutropenia in adults, some of whom have an associated clonal proliferation of large granular lymphocytes (Chap. 94), have been reported.[76]

The diagnosis of cyclic neutropenia can be made only by serial differential white cell counts, at least two or three times per week for a minimum of 6 weeks. Sequencing of the gene may be helpful in confirming the diagnosis.[77] Most affected children survive to adulthood, with symptoms often milder after puberty. Fatal clostridial bacteremia has been reported in several cases, and careful observation is warranted with each neutropenic period in untreated patients. Treatment with G-CSF is very effective.[78] G-CSF does not abolish cycling, but it shortens the neutropenic periods sufficiently to prevent symptoms and infections. In contrast to severe congenital neutropenias, cyclic neutropenia patients have no risk to develop leukemias.

Other Inherited Neutropenia Neutropenia caused by genetic defects of folate, cobalamin, and transcobalamin IIA varieties of congenital disorders lead to disturbed function of methylmalonyl coenzyme A mutase and methionine synthetase, the two cobalamin-requiring enzymes. Each of these disorders causes neutropenia, anemia, and thrombocytopenia as a result of ineffective hematopoiesis (Chap. 41).[79–81]

Several disorders, currently with only descriptive names, may be genetically determined forms of neutropenia. These cases often are called familial (benign) neutropenia and probably are autosomal dominant disorders.[82–84] Some cases of chronic benign neutropenia of childhood (usually a negative family history) may represent new mutations, and patients with chronic idiopathic neutropenia of adulthood may be childhood cases escaping early detection. Until better information is available, these conditions probably are best referred to as "idiopathic neutropenias."

Acquired Disorders Neutropenia in Neonates of Hypertensive Mothers Hypertensive women often have low-birth-weight infants with low neutrophil counts, attributed to decreased production.[84] The neutropenia often is severe with a high risk of infection, particularly during the first few weeks of life. The neutropenia usually resolves within a few weeks. G-CSF elevates the neutrophil count in this form of neonatal neutropenia, but the clinical benefit of treatment remains to be determined.[85]

Neutropenia Resulting from Nutritional Deficiencies Neutropenia is an early and consistent feature of megaloblastic anemias resulting from vitamin B_{12} or folate deficiency. When present it usually is accompanied by macrocytic anemia and mild thrombocytopenia (Chap. 41). Copper deficiency can cause neutropenia in patients on total parenteral nutrition, with a history of gastrectomy, and in malnourished children[86-88] and the bicytopenia or tricytopenias with a marrow showing dysplastic precursors can masquerade as myelodysplastic syndrome.

Neutropenia Resulting from Immune Suppression of Production Pure white cell aplasia is a rare acquired disorder causing severe selective neutropenia. The marrow is devoid or nearly devoid of neutrophils and their precursors.[89] Ibuprofen, chlorpropamide, excessive zinc, and various infectious and inflammatory diseases are considered possible causes of this syndrome. Differential diagnosis includes aplastic anemia, myelodysplasia, hairy cell leukemia, and neutropenia associated with the large granular lymphocyte syndrome. Immunosuppressive therapy with antithymocyte globulin, glucocorticoids, and cyclosporine has been used in individual cases.

Chronic Idiopathic Neutropenia in Adults This is a distinct syndrome predominantly affecting young adult women ages 18 to 35 years; the female-to-male ratio is approximately 8:1.[90] The medical history (lack of episodes of fever, gingivitis, mouth sores, or other infections) and previous blood counts suggest the condition is acquired in most cases. Erythrocyte, reticulocyte, and platelet counts usually are normal. Mild leukopenia and lymphocytopenia may be present, and the spleen is normal or only minimally enlarged. The patients have no chromosomal abnormalities or other evidence of myelodysplasia.[91,92] Marrow examinations show a spectrum of abnormalities, ranging from normal cellularity to selective hypoplasia of the neutrophilic series. In most cases, quantitative marrow studies show the ratio of immature to mature cells is increased, suggesting loss of cells during the maturation process, that is, ineffective granulocytopoiesis.[93] Antineutrophil antibodies, autoantibodies, including antinuclear or antimitochondrial antibodies, are absent.[94] Chronic idiopathic neutropenia in adults is the result of accelerated apoptosis of neutrophils and their precursors mediated via the Fas ligand or interferon-γ.[95] The disease mechanism, that is, activation of the extracellular apoptotic pathway, is similar to the mechanism described for patients with systemic lupus erythematosus.[96]

For most patients, the clinical course can be predicted from the level of blood neutrophils, marrow examination, and prior history of fevers and infections. In general, patients with the lowest levels of blood and marrow neutrophils have the most frequent problems. Long-term observations show, however, that some patients have very low blood neutrophil levels for long periods with few or no infections. Evolution to acute leukemia or aplastic anemia generally does not occur. G-CSF increases neutrophils in most patients and is a useful therapy for patients with recurrent fever and infections.[37,97]

DISORDERS AFFECTING NEUTROPHIL UTILIZATION AND TURNOVER

Mechanisms of Immune Neutropenia

Immune disorders primarily alter the distribution of neutrophils in the blood and accelerate neutrophil turnover. Antineutrophil antibodies cause transfusion reactions, alloimmune neonatal neutropenia, and autoimmune neutropenia. Antigen–antibody complexes, autoantibodies, and cytokine-mediated cellular injury are possible contributors to neutropenia of systemic lupus erythematosus and Felty syndrome. The association of neutropenia with increased numbers of circulating large granular lymphocytes demonstrates that cellular and humoral immune mechanisms can cause neutropenia (Chap. 94).

Neutrophils share surface antigens with other tissues including the i-I antigens and human leukocyte antigens (HLAs). They also have some specific antigens, including NA-1, NA-2 (now recognized as isotypes of FcγRIII or CD16), NB-1, NC-1, and NC-9a.[98-100] A number of other

antigens can be identified on neutrophils and neutrophil precursors with monoclonal antibodies. The clearest associations of autoantibodies and neutropenia are with NA-1 and NA-2.[101]

Several tests are available for detecting antineutrophil antibodies, including agglutination and microagglutination, cytotoxicity, direct and indirect immunofluorescence, direct and indirect antiglobulin assays, and tests involving the binding of staphylococcal protein A to immunoglobulins on the surface of cells.[101] The agglutination tests are the oldest methods and depend on the propensity of immunoglobulin-coated cells to aggregate. Immunofluorescence tests utilize antihuman γ-globulin tagged with a fluorescein label. These tests can be adapted for quantitative studies with fluorescence-activated cell sorting. Immunofluorescence and staphylococcal protein A–binding tests also can be adapted for examining immunoglobulins bound to single cells, including marrow cells. Direct methods are used to detect the antibodies on the patient's neutrophils. Indirect methods are used to test the patient's plasma or serum against panels of normal cells. Use of paraformaldehyde to expose antigens and to preserve the neutrophils for multiple tests has been especially helpful. Appropriate controls are essential for proper interpretation of these studies. Measurements of apoptosis and cytokine-mediated cellular injury are done through research laboratories.

Causes of Immune-Mediated Neutropenia

Alloimmune Neonatal Neutropenia Newborn infants may have neutropenia for a variety of reasons.[102] In some cases, the disorder results from transplacental passage of maternal immunoglobulin (Ig) G antibodies that bind to the infant's neutrophil-specific antigens, usually the FcγRIIIb (HNA1 or CD16b) isotype inherited from the infant's father.[103,104] Other antigens, such as NB1 glycoprotein (NB1 or CD177), HNA-3a(5b), HLA, and unknown antigens, also may be involved.[101] Overall, this disorder occurs in approximately 1 in 2000 neonates. The disorder usually lasts 2 to 4 months until the passively acquired antibody is lost.

Immune neonatal neutropenia may be severe or relatively mild. It often is not recognized until bacterial infections occur in an otherwise healthy infant. The hematologic picture usually consists of severe neutropenia with normal to increased lymphocytes and normal monocytes, erythrocytes, and platelets. Marrow cellularity is normal or increased, with reduced numbers of mature neutrophils. Alloimmune neonatal neutropenia may be confused with neonatal sepsis because the latter condition also causes severe neutropenia. The diagnosis of alloimmune neutropenia usually is made using neutrophil agglutination or immunofluorescence tests. Treatment should be conservative; antibiotics are used only when necessary. Exchange transfusions to decrease antibody titers or neutrophil transfusions from the patient's mother are rarely needed.

Autoimmune Neutropenia Neutrophil autoantibodies can decrease neutrophil survival and impair neutrophil production. From a clinical perspective, however, distinguishing autoimmune neutropenia from chronic idiopathic neutropenia often is difficult.[105] Patients diagnosed with autoimmune neutropenia have one or more positive tests for antineutrophil antibodies. Their cytopenia is selective; other blood cell counts are normal or near normal. Marrow morphology (Fig. 65–3), colony forming cells, and other tests, including antinuclear antibody tests, are normal. In general, therapy should be conservative and expectant. Intravenous γ-globulin may transiently increase neutrophils, but the therapy is expensive and relatively ineffective. The response to glucocorticoid therapy is unpredictable. Daily or alternate-day G-CSF is effective but should be reserved for patients with recurrent infections. Spontaneous remissions appear to occur much more commonly in children than adults.[106,107]

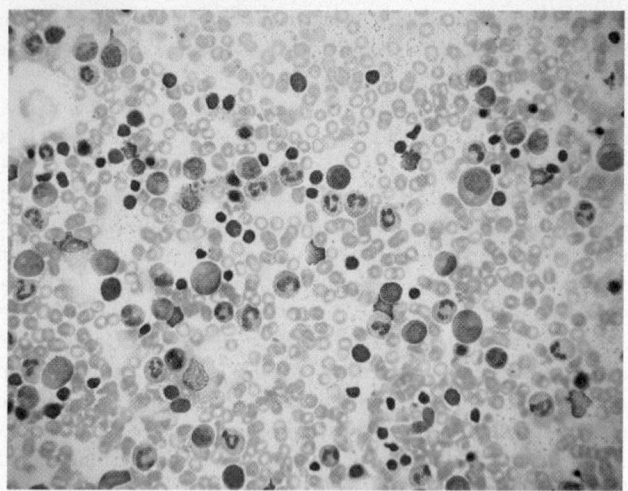

Figure 65–3. Morphology of a marrow sample from a patient with autoimmune neutropenia, demonstrating a normal maturation of neutrophil precursors.

Systemic Lupus Erythematosus Total leukocyte counts usually are between 2 and 5×10^9/L and neutrophils are less than 1.8×10^9/L in approximately 50 percent of patients with systemic lupus erythematosus.[108–110,123] Mild neutropenia often is accompanied by monocytopenia and lymphocytopenia, anemia, thrombocytopenia, and mild degrees of splenomegaly. Marrow cellularity and maturation of cells usually are normal. An increased amount of IgG is present on the surface of neutrophils, and immune complexes are increased within the neutrophils.[110] Fas and tumor necrosis factor–related apoptosis-inducing ligand (TRAIL) mediate many of the clinical features of autoimmune diseases, including apoptosis of neutrophils in systemic lupus erythematosus. Glucocorticoids, G-CSF, and GM-CSF elevate neutrophils in most patients with lupus, including patients on immunosuppressive therapies, but the mild neutropenia of these patients usually does not require treatment.[110]

Rheumatoid Arthritis, Sjögren Syndrome, and Felty Syndrome Leukopenia in association with rheumatoid arthritis is unusual, occurring in less than 3 percent of large series of patients.[124] Approximately 1 percent of patients with rheumatoid arthritis develop additional features of Felty syndrome (splenomegaly, deforming rheumatoid arthritis, and leukopenia). Usually, these patients have had active, deforming arthritis and very high rheumatoid factor titers. The neutropenia may be moderate to severe; occasionally patients are seen with no circulating neutrophils. The marrow usually is normal or hypercellular but occasionally is hypocellular. Granulopoiesis usually is marked by sufficient precursors but few band or segmented neutrophils. No clear relationship between spleen size and the neutrophil count is evident.

The incidence of bacterial infections in patients with Felty syndrome is low until the neutrophil count is less than 0.2×10^9/L, which has long suggested that neutrophils are made but that their blood kinetics are altered. The altered kinetics may result from high levels of circulating and intracellular immune complexes and IgG on the surface of neutrophils. Cellular injury via Fas-mediated apoptosis is an additional mechanism for cell loss from the marrow and blood.[125]

In Sjögren syndrome, approximately 30 percent of patients have moderate leukopenia. The total leukocyte count usually is 2 to 5×10^9/L with a normal differential count.[115,126] Rarely, severe neutropenia occurs in association with recurrent bacterial infections.

Therapeutic options for management of neutropenia in these autoimmune disorders include methotrexate, glucocorticoids, G-CSF, GM-CSF, splenectomy, and biologic agents such as rituximab and tocilizumab.[116,117] Results with these therapies are unpredictable.[122,127] Many specialists prefer weekly methotrexate because of its ease of administration, efficacy, and low toxicity.[118] G-CSF or GM-CSF can increase neutrophils but may exacerbate arthralgias.[119] Combinations of these agents is another good alternative. Splenectomy is followed by a rapid increase in counts in approximately two-thirds of cases, but approximately two-thirds of patients who respond to splenectomy have recurrence of neutropenia.[120] A subset of patients with Felty syndrome have a high blood concentration of large granular lymphocytes with a phenotype characteristic of immature natural killer cells.[121] These patients tend to respond poorly to therapies directed toward increasing neutrophil levels but may respond to combinations of methotrexate and G-CSF. Several factors in addition to neutropenia predispose these patients to infections, including monocytopenia, hypocomplementemia, circulating immune complexes, and treatment with glucocorticoids or cytotoxic drugs. In general, treatments to correct neutropenia should be reserved for patients with documented infections.

Other Causes of Neutropenia Associated with Splenomegaly In 1942, Wiseman and Doan[122] described a disorder they called primary splenic neutropenia. Since then, a variety of diseases have been recognized as also possibly causing this type of neutropenia, or pseudoneutropenia. Diseases associated with splenomegaly and neutropenia include sarcoidosis, lymphoma, tuberculosis, malaria, kala azar, and Gaucher disease. Usually thrombocytopenia and anemia are present as well. Immune mechanisms in patients with inflammatory diseases are similar to the mechanisms observed in patients with systemic lupus erythematosus and Felty syndrome may be operative. In other patients, sluggish blood flow through the spleen with passive trapping of neutrophils in the congested red pulp probably is the primary cause. For the most part, the neutropenia in these patients is not sufficiently severe to be of clinical consequence. Removal of the spleen to raise the neutrophil count is rarely indicated.

DRUG-INDUCED NEUTROPENIA

Idiosyncratic drug reactions cause neutropenia with an estimated annual frequency of three to 12 cases per 1 million population.[123–125] In 1922, Schultz[128] reported six cases of severe sore throat and prostration with absent blood neutrophils, which led rapidly to sepsis and death. A few years later, this syndrome was associated with the coal tar–derived drug aminopyrine.[127] Over the past 50 years, scores of other drugs have been recognized to cause this syndrome.

Two main types of idiosyncratic drug-induced neutropenia are recognized.[128,129] One type is a dose-related toxicity resulting from interference of the drug with protein synthesis or cell replication. This effect often is nonselective. It can involve the hematopoietic stem cell and highly proliferative cells in other organs, such as the epithelial cells of the gastrointestinal tract. Prototype drugs for this type of reaction include phenothiazines, antithyroid drugs, chloramphenicol, and clozapine.[130,131] Similar effects on marrow cells may be mediated through free radicals and drug metabolites. Patients receiving multiple drugs and patients having high plasma concentration of drugs as a result of the dose administered, slow metabolism, or renal excretory impairment are more prone to these reactions.[130]

A second type of drug-induced neutropenia may not be dose related. The neutropenia is thought to be allergic or immunologic in origin, similar to drug-induced skin reactions and drug-initiated, antibody-mediated erythrocyte destruction. Many drugs can trigger this form of neutropenia.[132] Women are affected more often than men. Older patients are affected more frequently than younger patients. Patients with a history of allergies, including allergies to other drugs, are affected more often than individuals without allergies. Neutropenia may occur at any time, but tends to occur relatively early in the course of treatment with drugs to which the patient has been previously exposed.

Our basic understanding of drug-induced neutropenia is limited, partly because of the unpredictable occurrence of cases, the myriad agents involved, and the lack of good animal models for research. Clinical studies suggest the rate of recovery can be roughly predicted from the degree of marrow hypoplasia present when neutropenia is discovered. In patients with sparse marrow neutrophils but normal-appearing precursor cells (promyelocytes and myelocytes), neutrophils reappear in the blood approximately 4 to 7 days after the offending drug is stopped. Often an increase in the blood monocyte count heralds marrow recovery, and an "overshoot" with marked neutrophilia follows. When early precursor cells are severely depleted, recovery may require considerably more time.

Symptomatic patients with drug-induced neutropenia usually present with fever, myalgia, and sore throat, but usually no rash or evidence of allergy elsewhere.[127] Blood examination shows few or absent neutrophils. Mild lymphopenia may be observed, but other cell counts usually are normal. A high level of suspicion and careful clinical history are critical to identifying the offending drug. Differential diagnosis includes acute viral infections, particularly infectious mononucleosis and infectious hepatitis, and acute bacterial sepsis. If other hematologic abnormalities also are present, acute leukemia and aplastic anemia should be considered. Treatment usually consists of supportive care, including broad-spectrum antibiotics for febrile patients. Hematopoietic growth factors such as G-CSF or GM-CSF may be beneficial, but their use in this setting has not been established in randomized trials.[130] An alternative to discontinuing drugs such as clozapine is the addition of G-CSF treatment,[127-129] although it is usually preferable to discontinue the suspected offending agent.

Table 65–1 lists some of the drugs frequently implicated in neutropenia. Given the rapidity of introduction of new agents, consult the manufacturer, a drug information center, or a poison control center when questions arise to learn if a drug can cause neutropenia.

NEUTROPENIA WITH INFECTIOUS DISEASES

Neutropenia can result from acute or chronic bacterial, viral, parasitic, or rickettsial diseases. Several mechanisms are involved. Certain viral infections, such as infectious mononucleosis, infectious hepatitis, Kawasaki disease, and HIV infection, may cause severe or protracted neutropenia and pancytopenia resulting from infection of hematopoietic precursor cells. Other agents, such as *Rickettsia* and *Bartonella*, can infect endothelial cells. These agents may cause leukopenia, neutropenia, thrombocytopenia, and anemia as part of a generalized vasculitic process. Increased neutrophil adherence to altered endothelial cells may occur in dengue, measles, and other viral infections. With severe Gram-negative bacterial infections, neutropenia probably results from increased adherence to the endothelium and increased utilization at the site of infection. Some chronic infections causing splenomegaly, such as tuberculosis, brucellosis, typhoid fever, malaria, and kala azar, probably cause neutropenia because of splenic sequestration and marrow invasion and suppression.

CLINICAL APPROACH TO THE PATIENT PRESENTING WITH NEUTROPENIA

Ordinarily, patients with acute onset of severe neutropenia present with fever, sore throat, and evidence of inflammation beneath the skin or mucous membranes. New respiratory or abdominal symptoms should heighten concern of an urgent clinical situation. Immediate investigation should include a careful history with particular attention to drugs. The physical examination should give careful attention to the oropharynx, sinuses, chest, abdomen, bones for evidence of tenderness, and size of the lymph nodes and spleen. Prompt blood counts and microbial cultures, institution of intravenous fluids, antibiotics, and other supportive measures may be lifesaving. In this situation, fever and infections usually result from surface bacteria sensitive to numerous broad-spectrum agents, unless the patient has been treated recently with antibiotics. A complete blood count should be obtained and a marrow examination considered, particularly if the cause of acute neutropenia is not known. The marrow may reveal fibrosis, selective or nonselective hypoplasia of marrow precursors, excessive blasts, or atypical cells. With this information in hand and supportive care started, further diagnostic tests can be considered.

Chronic neutropenia often is discovered as a chance finding at a routine examination or during the course of investigation of a patient with recurrent fevers and infections. Determining if the neutropenia is chronic or cyclic and the mean level of blood cell counts when the patient is afebrile and relatively well is useful. Other important hematologic and immunologic data include the absolute monocyte, lymphocyte, eosinophil, and platelet counts; hematocrit or hemoglobin determination; and immunoglobulin levels. Patients with hypergammaglobulinemia usually have chronic and recurrent inflammation; patients with hypogammaglobulinemia and neutropenia usually are very susceptible to recurrent infections. Morphologic examination of the blood and marrow can identify some causes of benign neutropenia in children, the Chédiak-Higashi syndrome, and myelokathexis. The marrow examination is most useful for ruling out leukemia and myelodysplastic disorders and assessing the severity of the marrow defect.

In patients with chronic neutropenia, measurement of antinuclear antibodies (ANA) and rheumatoid factor titers and other serologic tests for autoimmune diseases may be useful. Usually, neutropenia associated with these disorders occurs in patients with obvious and severe disease, but occasionally patients are seen with occult splenomegaly, high ANA and rheumatoid factor titers, and a few other symptoms. Examination of the blood and marrow for large granular lymphocytes may be helpful. Infectious and nutritional causes of chronic neutropenia are rare and usually are evident at the time of patient evaluation. In adults, differentiation between chronic idiopathic neutropenia and the myelodysplastic syndromes may be the most difficult. Abnormalities in other cell lines (e.g., anemia with poikilocytosis, anisocytosis, basophilic stippling, and thrombocytopenia, pseudo–Pelger-Huët cells), low proportions of blast cells in the marrow, dysmorphic granulocyte and erythroid precursors, and clonal chromosomal abnormalities indicate myelodysplasia, particularly in older patients. Investigations of the mechanism of neutropenia with marrow and blood kinetic studies, *in vitro* marrow cultures, measurements of marrow granulocyte reserves, and indirect measurements of marrow proliferative activity may be useful in defining mechanisms of neutropenia, but are not widely available.

● NEUTROPHILIA

Neutrophilia is defined as an increase in the absolute blood neutrophil count to a level greater than 2 SD above the mean value for normal individuals. For children age 1 month or older and adults of all ages, this level is approximately 7.5×10^9/L, combining bands and mature neutrophils (Chap. 2). At birth the mean neutrophil count is 12×10^9/L, and counts as high as 26×10^9/L are regarded as normal (Chap. 7).

Several terms are used almost synonymously with neutrophilia, including *neutrophilic leukocytosis, polymorphonuclear leukocytosis,* and *granulocytosis. Leukocytosis* is used because an elevated number of

TABLE 65-1. Classification of Widely Used Drugs Associated with Idiosyncratic Neutropenia

ANALGESICS AND ANTIINFLAMMATORY AGENTS	ANTIMALARIALS
Indomethacin*	Amodiaquine
Gold salts	Chloroquine
Pentazocine	Dapsone
Para-aminophenol derivatives*	Pyrimethamine
Acetaminophen	Quinine
Phenacetin	ANTITHYROID DRUGS*
Pyrazolone derivatives*	Carbimazole
Aminopyrine	Methimazole
Dipyrone	Propylthiouracil
Oxyphenbutazone	CARDIOVASCULAR DRUGS
Phenylbutazone	Captopril
ANTIBIOTICS	Disopyramide
Cephalosporins	Hydralazine
Chloramphenicol*	Methyldopa
Clindamycin	Procainamide
Gentamicin	Propranolol
Isoniazid	Quinidine
Para-aminosalicylic acid	Tocainide
Penicillins and semisynthetic penicillins*	DIURETICS
Rifampin	Acetazolamide
Streptomycin	Chlorthalidone
Sulfonamides*	Chlorothiazide
Tetracyclines	Ethacrynic acid
Trimethoprim-sulfamethoxazole	Hydrochlorothiazide
Vancomycin	HYPOGLYCEMIC AGENTS
ANTICONVULSANTS	Chlorpropamide
Carbamazepine	Tolbutamide
Mephenytoin	HYPNOTICS AND SEDATIVES
Phenytoin	Chlordiazepoxide and other benzodiazepines
ANTIDEPRESSANTS	
Amitriptyline	Meprobamate
Amoxapine	PHENOTHIAZINES*
Desipramine	Chlorpromazine
Doxepin	Phenothiazines
Imipramine	OTHER DRUGS
ANTIHISTAMINES—H$_2$ BLOCKERS	Allopurinol
Cimetidine	Clozapine
Ranitidine	Levamisole
	Penicillamine
	Ticlopidine

*More frequently reported to cause neutropenia in epidemiologic studies.

NOTE: Documentation of the role of specific drugs in the causation of neutropenia is dependent on either (1) the frequency of the occurrence among patients, (2) the timing of the event in relationship to drug use, (3) the absence of alternative explanations, or (4) the inadvertent or intentional reuse of the drug (rechallenges) with a similar response. Readers who require supplementary lists of putative drugs involved in the development of neutropenia or wish to read original references for these interactions are referred to Refs. 123 and 124

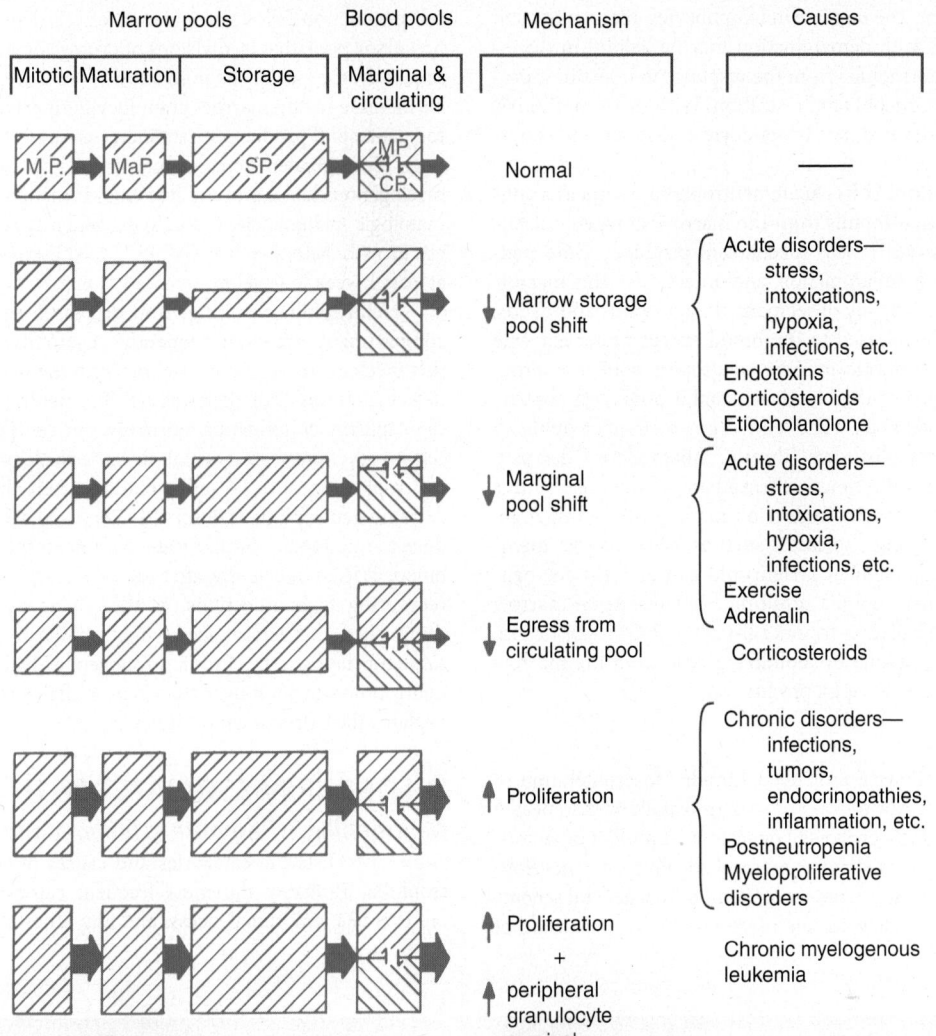

Figure 65–4. Mechanisms of neutrophilia are shown schematically. The rate of flow of cells through each compartment is represented by the size of the *arrows*. CP, circulating neutrophil pool; MaP, maturation (postmitotic) pool; M.P., mitotic pool; MP, marginated neutrophil pool; SP, storage pool (marrow reserves).

neutrophils is the most frequent cause of an increased total white cell count. *Granulocytosis* is less specific than neutrophilia, because granulocytes include eosinophils and basophils as well as neutrophils. Extreme neutrophilia often is referred to as a *leukemoid reaction* because the height of the white cell count may suggest leukemia. This exaggerated reaction may be the result of segmented neutrophils or may be associated with band neutrophils, metamyelocytes, and myelocytes in smaller proportions.

In normal individuals, the neutrophil count follows a diurnal pattern of variation, with peak counts in the late afternoon. Neutrophil counts also rise slightly after meals, with erect posture, and with emotional stimuli. Ordinarily these changes are not sufficient to cause neutrophilia.[134]

MECHANISMS OF NEUTROPHILIA

Under normal circumstances, neutrophils follow an orderly progression from the marrow through the blood to tissue sites of utilization.[135] Mild neutrophilia may occur by several mechanisms: increased cell production, accelerated release of cells from the marrow into the blood, shift within the circulation from the marginal to the circulating pool,

reduced egress of neutrophils from the blood to tissues, or a combination of these mechanisms. The time required for these events varies substantially. Shifts between the marginal and circulating pools take only a few minutes. Shifts of neutrophils from the marrow to the blood occur within a few hours. Increases in the production of neutrophils, even with intense stimulation, may take at least a few days (Fig. 65–4). With sustained moderate to marked neutrophilia the cause is virtually always increased production of neutrophils.

Acute Neutrophilia

Pseudoneutrophilia (Demargination) Vigorous exercise and acute physical and emotional stress can increase the number of blood neutrophils within a few minutes.[136] The response is mimicked by infusion of epinephrine and other catecholamines that increase heart rate and cardiac output.[137] The response is caused by a shift of cells from the marginal to the circulating pool; hence, it frequently is referred to as *demargination*. This response in humans is dependent partially on release of neutrophils from the spleen,[138] but redistribution from other vascular beds, particularly the pulmonary capillaries, is quantitatively more important. This mechanism can account for about a doubling in neutrophil count. Greater elevations in neutrophils cannot be ascribed solely to this mechanism. The increase in lymphocytes, monocytes, and neutrophils that occurs with demargination may be helpful in distinguishing this type of neutrophilia from the response to infections, protracted stress, or glucocorticoid administration. With these conditions, neutrophil counts are elevated, but lymphocyte and monocyte counts generally are depressed.

Marrow Storage Pool Shift Acute neutrophilia occurs as a consequence of release of neutrophils from the marrow storage pool, the *marrow neutrophil reserves.*[139] This mechanism produces acute neutrophilia in response to inflammation and infections. The marrow reserve pool consists principally of segmented neutrophils and bands. Metamyelocytes are not released to the blood except under extreme circumstances. The postmitotic marrow neutrophil pool is approximately 10 times the size of the blood neutrophil pool, and approximately half of these cells are band and segmented neutrophils.[135] In neutrophil production disorders, chronic inflammatory diseases, and malignancies, and with cancer chemotherapy, the size of this pool is reduced and the capacity to develop neutrophilia is impaired. Exposure of blood to foreign surfaces, such as hemodialysis membranes, activates the complement system and causes transient neutropenia, followed by neutrophilia resulting from release of marrow neutrophils. Colony-stimulating factors (G-CSF and GM-CSF) cause acute and chronic neutrophilia by mobilizing cells from the marrow reserves and stimulating neutrophil production.[140,141]

Chronic Neutrophilia

Chronic neutrophilia follows a prolonged stimulus to proliferation of neutrophil precursors. It can be studied experimentally with repeated doses of endotoxin, glucocorticoids, or colony-stimulating factors. Although the details of the mediators and mechanisms for the development of chronic neutrophilia are not understood fully, a general scheme for this response is now widely accepted (see Fig. 65–4). Expansion of

cell production follows stimulation of cell divisions within the mitotic precursor pool, that is, divisions of promyelocytes and myelocytes. Subsequently, the size of the postmitotic pool increases. The changes cause an increase in the marrow granulocytic to erythroid ratio. In humans, the neutrophil production rate increases severalfold with chronic infections. Even greater increases may occur in polycythemia vera, chronic myelogenous leukemia, and leukemoid reactions in response to nonhematologic malignancies[142] and to exogenously administered hematopoietic growth factors such as G-CSF,[140,141] with a maximum response taking at least 1 week to develop.

Neutrophilia resulting from decreased egress from the vascular compartment occurs infrequently. A prototype disorder illustrating this mechanism occurs in patients with the neutrophil cell membrane defect CD11a/CD18 deficiency.[143] The neutrophils do not adhere to the capillary endothelium normally, but cell production and marrow release apparently are normal. Because these patients cannot mobilize neutrophils to sites of inflammation when they develop infections, extreme neutrophilia is observed (Chap. 66). Glucocorticoids may produce a functionally similar state, with neutrophils accumulating in the blood, at least transiently, after each dose is administered.[144] In patients recovering from infections, as the "tissue demand" for neutrophils diminishes, the persistence of neutrophilia may be attributed to this same mechanism. In chronic myelogenous leukemia, accumulation of neutrophils with a longer than normal half-life in the blood partially explains the extreme neutrophilia.[145]

DISORDERS ASSOCIATED WITH NEUTROPHILIA
Neutrophilia in Response to Inflammation and Stress
Table 65–2 lists the categories and causes of acute and chronic neutrophilia. Probably the most frequent causes of acute neutrophilia are exercise, emotional stress, and any other circumstance that raises

TABLE 65–2. Major Causes of Neutrophilia

Acute Neutrophilia	Chronic Neutrophilia
Physical stimuli	Infections
Cold, heat, exercise, convulsions, pain, labor, anesthesia, surgery	Persistence of infections that cause acute neutrophilia
Emotional stimuli	Inflammation
Panic, rage, severe stress, depression	Most acute inflammatory reactions, such as colitis, dermatitis, drug-sensitivity reactions, gout, hepatitis, myositis, nephritis, pancreatitis, periodontitis, rheumatic fever, rheumatoid arthritis, vasculitis, thyroiditis, Sweet syndrome
Infections	
Many localized and systemic acute bacterial, mycotic, rickettsial, spirochetal, and certain viral infections	Tumors
Inflammation or tissue necrosis	Gastric, bronchogenic, breast, renal, hepatic, pancreatic, uterine, and squamous cell cancers; rarely Hodgkin lymphoma, lymphoma, brain tumors, melanoma, and multiple myeloma
Burns, electric shock, trauma, infarction, gout, vasculitis, antigen-antibody complexes, complement activation	Drugs, hormones, and toxins
Drugs, hormones, and toxins	Continued exposure to many substances that produce acute neutrophilia, lithium; rarely as a reaction to other drugs
Colony-stimulating factors, epinephrine, etiocholanolone, endotoxin, glucocorticoids, smoking tobacco, vaccines, venoms	Metabolic and endocrinologic disorders
	Eclampsia, thyroid storm, overproduction of adrenocorticotropic hormone
	Hematologic disorders
	Rebound from agranulocytosis or therapy of megaloblastic anemia, chronic hemolysis or hemorrhage, asplenia, myeloproliferative disorders, chronic idiopathic leukocytosis
	Hereditary and congenital disorders
	Down syndrome, congenital

endogenous epinephrine, norepinephrine, or cortisol levels. Acute neutrophilia occurs in pregnant patients and may be especially notable at the time of entering labor. Acute neutrophilia occurs with induction of general or epidural anesthesia, with all types of surgery, and with other acute events such as seizures, gastrointestinal hemorrhage, subarachnoid hemorrhage, or other internal bleeding.

Neutrophilia occurs with many acute bacterial infections. It occurs less predictably with infections caused by viruses, fungi, and parasites. Many aspects of the complex interactions of microbes with the infected host are not fully understood. Most patients with Gram-positive infections, such as pneumococcal pneumonia, staphylococcal abscesses, and streptococcal pharyngitis, have neutrophilia. Infections caused by Gram-negative bacteria, particularly those resulting in bacteremia or septic shock, may cause neutropenia or extreme neutrophilia.[146] Increased circulating levels of activated complement components, G-CSF, tumor necrosis factor, and interleukin (IL)-1, IL-6, and IL-8 may cause this response. Bacterial infections that have an insidious onset and cause splenomegaly, such as typhoid fever and brucellosis, characteristically do not show neutrophilia except in the initial or disseminated phase. Miliary tuberculosis is an important cause of leukemoid reactions. Neutrophilia is far less common with viral infections. In general, neutrophilia is seen in infections producing substantial tissue injury, evoked by toxins produced by the infecting organisms. Damage to host tissues also is the presumed mechanism of neutrophilia in thermal burns, electric shock, myocardial infarction, pulmonary embolism, sickle cell crisis, and systemic vasculitis.

Many chronic noninfectious conditions cause neutrophilia. Probably the most frequent cause is cigarette smoking.[147,148] Neutrophil counts of smokers are increased in proportion to the amount of exposure. Neutrophil counts of smokers inhaling two packs of cigarettes per day average twice the normal levels. Chronic inflammatory diseases, including dermatitis, bronchitis, rheumatoid arthritis, osteomyelitis, ulcerative colitis, and gout, may cause a persistent neutrophilia. Sweet syndrome is an unusual dermatologic condition manifested as intense neutrophil accumulation in the skin and persistent neutrophilia.[149]

Neutrophilia in Association with Cancer or Heart Disease

Neutrophilia is associated with many nonhematologic malignancies, such as lung and gastrointestinal malignancies, particularly when they metastasize to the liver and lung.[150] In some cases, tumor cells produce colony-stimulating factors that presumably cause the neutrophilia by direct marrow stimulation. Tumor necrosis and superinfections are other possible mechanisms. Neutrophilia is unusual in brain tumors, melanoma, prostate cancer, and lymphocytic malignancies.

Neutrophilia is a marker for the occurrence and severity of a variety of illnesses. Neutrophilia is associated with an increased incidence and severity of coronary heart disease, independent of smoking status.[151,152] Similarly, elevated white cell counts have been associated with increased cancer mortality, independent of smoking history. In patients with cancer, subarachnoid hemorrhage, and other serious inflammatory conditions, neutrophilia portends a less favorable prognosis.

Hereditary Neutrophilia and Neutrophilia as a Manifestation of a Hematologic Disorder

In addition to the myeloproliferative neoplasms, including chronic neutrophilic leukemia and neutrophilic chronic myelogenous leukemia (Chap. 89), several unusual hematologic conditions may be associated with neutrophilia. The mechanisms for most of these disorders remain obscure. In Down syndrome, transient neonatal leukemoid reactions resembling chronic myelogenous leukemia may occur.[153] This type of neutrophilia may be related to a defect in regulation of neutrophil

production caused by chromosome 21 trisomy, but the precise mechanism is unknown. Idiopathic neutrophilic leukocytosis with a negative family history and a similar condition of hereditary neutrophilia with an autosomal dominant pattern of inheritance have been reported[154,155] but are very rare. An inherited activating mutation in the G-CSF receptor (CSF3R) gene induces chronic hereditary neutrophilia.[156] Careful clinical examination and followup almost always reveal the cause of the neutrophilia.

Neutrophilia Associated with Drugs

Many drugs cause neutropenia, but neutrophilia in response to drugs is uncommon except for the well-known effects of epinephrine, other catecholamines, and glucocorticoids. Lithium salts cause sustained neutrophilia.[157] The counts return to normal when the drug is discontinued. The drug increases levels of colony-stimulating factor. Cases of neutrophilia have been reported with ranitidine and quinidine therapy, but such reactions are very uncommon.

CLINICAL APPROACH TO PATIENTS WITH NEUTROPHILIA

In most instances, the finding of neutrophilia, band neutrophils, and toxic granules in the mature cells can be related to an obvious ongoing inflammatory condition. Often the finding of neutrophilia helps confirm the diagnosis of appendicitis, cholecystitis, or bacterial pharyngitis. When the cause of neutrophilia is not readily apparent, especially if the neutrophilia is associated with fever or other signs of inflammation, more subtle infections such as tuberculosis or osteomyelitis should be considered. In addition, a history of smoking and evidence for a chronic anxiety state or an occult malignancy should be sought. If neutrophilia is accompanied by myelocytes and promyelocytes, increased basophils, and unexplained splenomegaly, the diagnosis of a myeloproliferative disease (e.g., chronic myelogenous leukemia, idiopathic myelofibrosis, or polycythemia vera) should be considered. Measurement of leukocyte alkaline phosphatase activity can be a useful screening test in cases of moderate neutrophilia (15 to 25×10^9/L). Ordinarily the values are elevated with inflammation of any cause and in subjects receiving glucocorticoid therapy. The values are low in chronic myelogenous leukemia and variable with other myeloproliferative neoplasms. Serum vitamin B_{12} levels and B_{12}-binding proteins are elevated in both benign neutrophilia and chronic myelogenous leukemia. In unexplained neutrophilia, testing for the cytogenetic alterations and the BCR gene rearrangement (Chap. 89) and JAK2 gene mutations (Chap. 84) are important in the diagnostic evaluation. Chapter 89 discusses the diagnosis of chronic myelogenous leukemia and other chronic myelogenous leukemia disorders with prominent neutrophilia.

Epidemiologic studies show an association of neutrophilia with adverse effects of smoking, obesity, coronary artery disease, cerebral vascular disease and malignancies.[158–162] In myeloproliferative neoplasms, neutrophilia is a predictor of thrombotic events.[163–165] In patients with sickle cell disease, neutrophilia correlates with increased complications and severity of the disease.[166,167] In these patients, treatment with hydroxyurea lowers the blood neutrophil counts, and has been shown in randomized trials to reduce some of the complications of the disease. In some inflammatory diseases, glucocorticoids, which raise blood neutrophils, and immunosuppressive therapies, which lower blood neutrophils, are used to reduce inflammation; this is because both of these classes of drugs reduce the deployment of neutrophils and other leukocytes to tissue sites of inflammation. For instance, glucocorticoids usually suppress the inflammation of the skin in Sweet syndrome. In most clinical settings, therapies to reduce the neutrophil count are generally not indicated.

REFERENCES

1. Haddy TB, Rana SR, Castro O: Benign ethnic neutropenia: What is a normal absolute neutrophil count? *J Lab Clin Med* 133:15, 1999.
2. Denic S, Showqi S, Klein C, et al: Prevalence, phenotype and inheritance of benign neutropenia in Arabs. *BMC Blood Disord* 9:3, 2009.
3. Koury MJ, Price JO, Hicks GG: Apoptosis in megaloblastic anemia occurs during DNA synthesis by a p53-independent, nucleoside-reversible mechanism. *Blood* 96:3249, 2000.
4. Kerbauy DB, Deeg HJ: Apoptosis and antiapoptotic mechanisms in the progression of myelodysplastic syndrome. *Exp Hematol* 35:1739, 2007.
5. Kawai T, Malech HL: WHIM syndrome: Congenital immune deficiency disease. *Curr Opin Hematol* 16:20, 2009.
6. Aprikyan AA, Liles WC, Rodger E, et al: Impaired survival of bone marrow hematopoietic progenitor cells in cyclic neutropenia. *Blood* 97:147, 2001.
7. Ward AC, Dale DC: Genetic and molecular diagnosis of severe congenital neutropenia. *Curr Opin Hematol* 16:9, 2009.
8. Watanabe K, Ambekar C, Wang H, et al: SBDS-deficiency results in specific hypersensitivity to Fas stimulation and accumulation of Fas at the plasma membrane. *Apoptosis* 14:77, 2009.
9. Bux J: Molecular nature of antigens implicated in immune neutropenias. *Int J Hematol* 76:399, 2002.
10. Palmblad J, Papadaki HA: Chronic idiopathic neutropenias and severe congenital neutropenia. *Curr Opin Hematol* 15:8, 2008.
11. Melis D, Fulceri R, Parenti G, et al: Genotype/phenotype correlation in glycogen storage disease type 1b: A multicentre study and review of the literature. *Eur J Pediatr* 164:501, 2005.
12. Kaplan J, De Domenico I, Ward DM: Chediak-Higashi syndrome. *Curr Opin Hematol* 15:22, 2008.
13. Kaul D, Coffey MJ, Phare SM, Kazanjian PH: Capacity of neutrophils and monocytes from human immunodeficiency virus-infected patients and healthy controls to inhibit growth of *Mycobacterium bovis*. *J Lab Clin Med* 141:330, 2003.
14. Kostmann R: Infantile genetic agranulocytosis; agranulocytosis infantilis hereditaria. *Acta Paediatr* 45:1, 1956.
15. Dale DC, Link DC: The many causes of severe congenital neutropenia. *N Engl J Med* 360:3, 2009.
16. Zeidler C, Germeshausen M, Klein C: Clinical implications of ELA2-, HAX1- and G-CSF-receptor (CSF3R) mutations in severe congenital neutropenia. *Br J Haematol* 144:459, 2009.
17. Welte K, Zeidler C, Dale DC: Severe congenital neutropenia. *Semin Hematol* 43:189, 2006.
18. Konishi N, Kobayashi M, Miyagawa S: Defective proliferation of primitive myeloid progenitor cells in patients with severe congenital neutropenia. *Blood* 94:4077, 1999.
19. Dale DC, Person RE, Bolyard AA, et al: Mutations in the gene encoding neutrophil elastase in congenital and cyclic neutropenia. *Blood* 96:2317, 2000.
20. Köllner I, Sodeik B, Schreek S, et al: Mutations in neutrophil elastase causing congenital neutropenia lead to cytoplasmic protein accumulation and induction of the unfolded protein response. *Blood* 108:493, 2006.
21. Bellanne-Chantelot C, Clauin S, Leblanc T, et al: Mutations in the ELA2 gene correlate with more severe expression of neutropenia: A study of 81 patients from the French Neutropenia Register. *Blood* 103:4119, 2004.
22. Ancliff PJ, Gale RE, Linch DC: Neutrophil elastase mutations in congenital neutropenia. *Hematology* 8:165, 2003.
23. Makaryan V, Zeidler C, Bolyard AA, et al: The diversity of mutations and clinical outcomes for ELANE-associated neutropenia. *Curr Opin Hematol* 22:3, 2015.
24. Klein C, Grudzien M, Appaswamy G, et al: HAX1 deficiency causes autosomal recessive severe congenital neutropenia (Kostmann disease). *Nat Genet* 39:86, 2007.
25. Skokowa J, Klimiankou M, Klimenkova O, et al: Interactions among HCLS1, HAX1 and LEF-1 proteins are essential for G-CSF-triggered granulopoiesis. *Nat Med* 18:1550, 2012.
26. Boztug K, Appaswamy G, Ashikov A, et al: A syndrome with congenital neutropenia and mutations in G6PC3. *N Engl J Med* 360:32, 2009.
27. Person RE, Li FQ, Duan Z, Benson KF: Mutations in proto-oncogene GFI1 cause human neutropenia and target ELA2. *Nat Genet* 34:308, 2003.
28. Devriendt K, Kim AS, Mathijs G, et al: Constitutively activating mutation in WASP causes X-linked severe congenital neutropenia. *Nat Genet* 27:313, 2001.
29. Bohn G, Allroth A, Brandes G, et al: A novel human primary immunodeficiency syndrome caused by deficiency of the endosomal adaptor protein p14. *Nat Med* 13:38, 2007.
30. Barth PG, Valianpour F, Bowen VM, et al: X-linked cardioskeletal myopathy and neutropenia (Barth syndrome): An update. *Am J Med Genet A* 126:349, 2004.
31. Boztug K, Järvinen PM, Salzer E, et al: JAGN1 deficiency causes aberrant myeloid cell homeostasis and congenital neutropenia. *Nat Genet* 46:1021, 2014.
32. Makaryan V, Rosenthal EA, Bolyard AA, et al: TCIRG1-associated congenital neutropenia. *Hum Mutat* 35:824, 2014.
33. Dong F, Brynes RK, Tidow N, et al: Mutations in the gene for the granulocyte colony-stimulating-factor receptor in patients with acute myeloid leukemia preceded by severe congenital neutropenia. *N Engl J Med* 333:487, 1995.
34. Germeshausen M, Ballmaier M, Welte K. Incidence of CSF3R mutations in severe congenital neutropenia and relevance for leukemogenesis: Results of a long-term survey. *Blood* 109:93, 2007.

35. Dror Y, Ward AC, Touw IP, Freedman MH: Combined corticosteroid/granulocyte colony-stimulating factor (G-CSF) therapy in the treatment of severe congenital neutropenia unresponsive to G-CSF: Activated glucocorticoid receptors synergize with G-CSF signals. *Exp Hematol* 28:1381, 2000.
36. Triot A, Järvinen PM, Arostegui JI, et al: Inherited biallelic CSF3R mutations in severe congenital neutropenia. *Blood* 123:3811, 2014.
37. Skokowa J, Lan D, Thakur BK, et al: NAMPT is essential for the G-CSF-induced myeloid differentiation via a NAD(+)-sirtuin-1-dependent pathway. *Nat Med* 15:151, 2009.
38. Dale DC, Bolyard AA, Schwinzer BG, et al: The Severe Chronic Neutropenia International Registry: 10-Year follow-up report. *Support Cancer Ther* 3:220, 2006.
39. Zeidler C, Welte K, Barak Y, et al: Stem cell transplantation in patients with severe congenital neutropenia without evidence of leukemic transformation. *Blood* 95:1195, 2000.
40. Choi SW, Boxer LA, Pulsipher MA, et al: Stem cell transplantation in patients with severe congenital neutropenia with evidence of leukemic transformation. *Bone Marrow Transplant* 35:473, 2005.
41. Rosenberg PS, Alter BP, Bolyard AA, et al: The incidence of leukemia and mortality from sepsis in patients with severe congenital neutropenia receiving long-term G-CSF therapy. *Blood* 107:4628, 2006.
42. Skokowa J, Steinemann D, Katsman-Kuipers JE, et al: Cooperativity of RUNX1 and CSF3R mutations in severe congenital neutropenia: A unique pathway in myeloid leukemogenesis. *Blood* 123:2229, 2014.
43. Cham B, Bonilla MA, Winkelstein J: Neutropenia associated with primary immunodeficiency syndromes. *Semin Hematol* 39:107, 2002.
44. Rezaei N, Aghamohammadi A, Ramyar A, et al: Severe congenital neutropenia or hyper-IgM syndrome? A novel mutation of CD40 ligand in a patient with severe neutropenia. *Int Arch Allergy Immunol* 147:255, 2008.
45. Albert MH, Notarangelo LD, Ochs HD. Clinical spectrum, pathophysiology and treatment of the Wiskott-Aldrich syndrome. *Curr Opin Hematol* 18:42, 2011.
46. Dupuis-Girod S, Medioni J, Haddad E, et al: Autoimmunity in Wiskott-Aldrich syndrome: Risk factors, clinical features, and outcome in a single-center cohort of 55 patients. *Pediatrics* 111:e622, 2003.
47. Horman SR, Velu CS, Chaubey A, et al: Gfi1 integrates progenitor versus granulocytic transcriptional programming. *Blood* 113:5466, 2009.
48. Berthet F, Siegrist CA, Ozsahin H, et al: Bone marrow transplantation in cartilage-hair hypoplasia: Correction of the immunodeficiency but not of the chondrodysplasia. *Eur J Pediatr* 155:286, 1996.
49. Ammann RA, Duppenthaler A, Bux J, et al: Granulocyte colony-stimulating factor-responsive chronic neutropenia in cartilage-hair hypoplasia. *J Pediatr Hematol Oncol* 26:379, 2004.
50. Boocock GR, Morrison JA, Popovic M, et al: Mutations in SBDS are associated with Shwachman-Diamond syndrome. *Nat Genet* 33:97, 2003.
51. Dror Y, Freedman MH: Shwachman-Diamond syndrome marrow cells show abnormally increased apoptosis mediated through the Fas pathway. *Blood* 97:3011, 2001.
52. Orelio C, Kuijpers TW: Shwachman-Diamond syndrome neutrophils have altered chemoattractant-induced F-actin polymerization and polarization characteristics. *Haematologica* 94:409, 2009.
53. Shimamura A: Shwachman-Diamond syndrome. *Semin Hematol* 43:178, 2006.
54. Willig TN, Gazda H, Sieff CA: Diamond-Blackfan anemia. *Curr Opin Hematol* 7:85, 2000.
55. Orfali KA, Ohene-Abuakwa Y, Ball SE: Diamond Blackfan anaemia in the UK: Clinical and genetic heterogeneity. *Br J Haematol* 125:243, 2004.
56. Campagnoli MF, Garelli E, Quarello P, et al: Molecular basis of Diamond-Blackfan anemia: New findings from the Italian registry and a review of the literature. *Haematologica* 89:480, 2004.
57. Griscelli C, Durandy A, Guy-Grand D, et al: A syndrome associating partial albinism and immunodeficiency. *Am J Med* 65:691, 1978.
58. Menasche G, Pastural E, Feldmann J, et al: Mutations in RAB27A cause Griscelli syndrome associated with haemophagocytic syndrome. *Nat Genet* 25:173, 2000.
59. Sanal O, Ersoy F, Tezcan I, et al: Griscelli disease: Genotype-phenotype correlation in an array of clinical heterogeneity. *J Clin Immunol* 22:237, 2002.
60. Baumeister FA, Stachel D, Schuster F, et al: Accelerated phase in partial albinism with immunodeficiency (Griscelli syndrome): Genetics and stem cell transplantation in a 2-month-old girl. *Eur J Pediatr* 159:74, 2000.
61. Barbosa MD, Nguyen QA, Tchernev VT, et al: Identification of the homologous beige and Chediak-Higashi syndrome genes. *Nature* 382:262, 1996.
62. Introne W, Boissy RE, Gahl WA: Clinical, molecular, and cell biological aspects of Chediak-Higashi syndrome. *Mol Genet Metab* 68:283, 1999.
63. Kawai T, Malech HL: WHIM syndrome: Congenital immune deficiency disease. *Curr Opin Hematol* 16:20, 2009.
64. Gorlin RJ, Gelb B, Diaz GA, et al: WHIM syndrome, an autosomal dominant disorder: Clinical, hematological, and molecular studies. *Am J Med Genet* 91:368, 2000.
65. Hernandez PA, Gorlin RJ, Lukens JN, et al: Mutations in the chemokine receptor gene CXCR4 are associated with WHIM syndrome, a combined immunodeficiency disease. *Nat Genet* 34:70, 2003.
66. Rassam SM, Roderick P, al-Hakim I, Hoffrand AV: A myelokathexis-like variant of myelodysplasia. *Eur J Haematol* 42:99, 1989.
67. Seifert W, Holder-Espinasse M, Kühnisch J, et al: Expanded mutational spectrum in Cohen syndrome, tissue expression, and transcript variants of COH1. *Hum Mutat* 30:E404, 2009.
68. Kannourakis G: Glycogen storage disease. *Semin Hematol* 39:103, 2002.

69. Annabi B, Hiraiwa H, Mansfield BC, et al: The gene for glycogen-storage disease type 1b maps to chromosome 11q23. *Am J Hum Genet* 62:400, 1998.

70. Visser G, Rake JP, Fernandes J, et al: Neutropenia, neutrophil dysfunction, and inflammatory bowel disease in glycogen storage disease type Ib: Results of the European Study on Glycogen Storage Disease type I. *J Pediatr* 13:187, 2000.

71. Schroten H, Wendel U, Burdach S, et al: Colony-stimulating factors for neutropenia in glycogen storage disease Ib. *Lancet* 337:736, 1991.

72. Schroeder T, Hildebrandt B, Mayatepek E, et al: A patient with glycogen storage disease type Ib presenting with acute myeloid leukemia (AML) bearing monosomy 7 and translocation t(3;8)(q26;q24) after 14 years of treatment with granulocyte colony-stimulating factor (G-CSF): A case report. *J Med Case Reports* 2:319, 2008.

73. Dale DC, Bolyard AA, Aprikyan A: Cyclic neutropenia. *Semin Hematol* 39:89, 2002.

74. Horwitz M, Benson KF, Person RE, et al: Mutations in ELA2, encoding neutrophil elastase, define a 21-day biological clock in cyclic haematopoiesis. *Nat Genet* 23:433, 1999.

75. Palmer SE, Stephens K, Dale DC: Genetics, phenotype, and natural history of autosomal dominant cyclic hematopoiesis. *Am J Med Genet* 66:413, 1996.

76. Dale DC, Hammond WP IV: Cyclic neutropenia: A clinical review. *Blood Rev* 2:178, 1998.

77. Makaryan V, Zeidler C, Bolyard AA, et al: The diversity of mutations and clinical outcomes for ELANE-associated neutropenia. *Curr Opin Hematol* 22:3-11,2015.

78. Hammond WP IV, Price TH, Souza LM, Dale DC: Treatment of cyclic neutropenia with granulocyte colony-stimulating factor. *N Engl J Med* 320:1306, 1989.

79. Fowler B: Genetic defects of folate and cobalamin metabolism. *Eur J Pediatr* 157:S60, 1998.

80. Monagle PT, Tauro GP: Long-term follow up of patients with transcobalamin II deficiency. *Arch Dis Child* 72:237, 1995.

81. Quadros, EV. Advances in the understanding of cobalamin assimilation and metabolism. *Br J Haematol* 148:195, 2010.

82. Dale DC, Guerry D 4th, Wewerka JR, et al: Chronic neutropenia. *Medicine (Baltimore)* 58:128, 1979.

83. Juul SE, Haynes JW, McPherson RJ: Evaluation of neutropenia and neutrophilia in hospitalized preterm infants. *J Perinatol* 24:150, 2004.

84. James RM, Kinsey SE: The investigation and management of chronic neutropenia in children. *Arch Dis Child* 91:852, 2006.

85. Juul SE, Christensen RD: Effect of recombinant granulocyte colony-stimulating factor on blood neutrophil concentrations among patients with "idiopathic neonatal neutropenia": A randomized, placebo-controlled trial. *J Perinatol* 23:493, 2003.

86. Percival SS: Neutropenia caused by copper deficiency: Possible mechanisms of action. *Nutr Rev* 53:59, 1999.

87. Olivares M, Uauy R: Copper as an essential nutrient. *Am J Clin Nutr* 63:791S, 1996.

88. Gregg XT, Reddy V, Prchal JT: Copper deficiency masquerading as myelodysplastic syndrome. *Blood* 100:1493, 2002.

89. Levitt LJ: Chlorpropamide-induced pure white cell aplasia. *Blood* 69:394, 1987.

90. Kyle RA: Natural history of chronic idiopathic neutropenia. *N Engl J Med* 302:908, 1980.

91. Palmblad JE, von dem Borne AE: Idiopathic, immune, infectious, and idiosyncratic neutropenias. *Semin Hematol* 39:113, 2002.

92. Papadaki HA, Palmblad J, Eliopoulos GD: Non-immune chronic idiopathic neutropenia of adult: An overview. *Eur J Haematol* 67:35, 2001.

93. Price TH, Lee MY, Dale DC, Finch CA: Neutrophil kinetics in chronic neutropenia. *Blood* 54:581, 1979.

94. Logue GL, Shastri KA, Laughlin M, et al: Idiopathic neutropenia: Antineutrophil antibodies and clinical correlations. *Am J Med* 90:211, 1991.

95. Palmblad J, Papadaki HA: Chronic idiopathic neutropenias and severe congenital neutropenia. *Curr Opin Hematol* 15:8, 2008.

96. Matsuyama W, Yamamoto M, Higashimoto I, et al: TNF-related apoptosis-inducing ligand is involved in neutropenia of systemic lupus erythematosus. *Blood* 104:184, 2004.

97. Dale DC, Bonilla MA, Davis MW, et al: A randomized controlled phase III trial of recombinant human granulocyte colony-stimulating factor (filgrastim) for treatment of severe chronic neutropenia. *Blood* 81:2496, 1993.

98. Lalezari P, Radel E: Neutrophil-specific antigens: Immunology and clinical significance. *Semin Hematol* 11:281, 1974.

99. Bux J: Molecular nature of antigens implicated in immune neutropenias. *Int J Hematol* 76(Suppl 1):399, 2002.

100. Stroncek D: Neutrophil alloantigens. *Transfus Med Rev* 16:67, 2002.

101. Bux J: Human neutrophil alloantigens. *Vox Sang* 94:277, 2008.

102. Maheshwari A, Christensen RD, Calhoun DA: Immune neutropenia in the neonate. *Adv Pediatr* 49:317, 2002.

103. Puig N, de Haas M, Kleijer M, et al: Isoimmune neonatal neutropenia caused by Fc gamma RIIIb antibodies in a Spanish child. *Transfusion* 35:683, 1995.

104. Maslanka K, Guz K, Uhrynowska M, Zupanska B: Isoimmune neonatal neutropenia due to anti-Fc(gamma) RIIIb antibody in a mother with an Fc(gamma) RIIIb deficiency. *Transfus Med* 11:111, 2001.

105. Maheshwari A, Christensen RD, Calhoun DA: Immune-mediated neutropenia in the neonate. *Acta Paediatr Suppl* 91:98, 2002.

106. Taniuchi S, Masuda M, Hasui M, et al: Differential diagnosis and clinical course of autoimmune neutropenia in infancy: Comparison with congenital neutropenia. *Acta Paediatr* 91:1179, 2002.

107. Bux J, Behrens G, Jaeger G, Welte K. Diagnosis and clinical course of autoimmune neutropenia in infancy: Analysis of 240 cases. *Blood* 91:181, 1998.

108. Nossent JC, Swaak AJ: Prevalence and significance of haematological abnormalities in patients with systemic lupus erythematosus. *Q J Med* 80:605, 1991.

109. Bowman SJ: Hematological manifestations of rheumatoid arthritis. *Scand J Rheumatol* 31:251, 2002.

110. Starkebaum G: Chronic neutropenia associated with autoimmune disease. *Semin Hematol* 39:121, 2002.

111. Martinez-Baños D, Crispin JC, Lazo-Langner A, Sánchez-Guerror J: Moderate and severe neutropenia in patients with systemic lupus erythematosus. *Rheumatology* 45:994, 2006.

112. Campion G, Maddison PJ, Goulding N, et al: The Felty syndrome: A case-matched study of clinical manifestations and outcome, serologic features, and immunogenetic associations. *Medicine (Baltimore)* 69:69, 1990.

113. Liu JH, Wei S, Lamy T, Epling-Burnette PK, et al: Chronic neutropenia mediated by Fas ligand. *Blood* 95:3219, 2000.

114. Starkebaum G, Dancey JT, Arend WP: Chronic neutropenia: Possible association with Sjögren's syndrome. *J Rheumatol* 8:679, 1981.

115. Coppo P, Sibilia J, Maloisel F, et al: Primary Sjögren's syndrome associated agranulocytosis: A benign disorder? *Ann Rheum Dis* 62:476, 2003.

116. Chandra PA, Margulis Y, Schiff C: Rituximab is useful in the treatment of Felty's syndrome. *Am J Ther* 15:321, 2008.

117. Patel AM, Moreland LW: Tocilizumab versus methotrexate in moderate to severe rheumatoid arthritis. *Curr Rheumatol Rep* 11:313, 2009.

118. Wiseman BK, Doan CA: A newly recognized granulopenic syndrome caused by excessive splenic leukolysis and successfully treated by splenectomy. *Ann Intern Med* 16:1097, 1942.

119. Kracke RR: Relation of drug therapy to neutropenic states. *JAMA* 111:1255, 1938.

120. Wassenberg S, Herborn G, Rau R: Methotrexate treatment in Felty's syndrome. *Br J Rheumatol* 37:908, 1998.

121. Hellmich B, Schnabel A, Gross WL: Treatment of severe neutropenia due to Felty's syndrome or systemic lupus erythematosus with granulocyte colony-stimulating factor. *Semin Arthritis Rheum* 29:82, 1999.

122. Rashba EJ, Rowe JM, Packman CH: Treatment of the neutropenia of Felty syndrome. *Blood Rev* 10:177, 1996.

123. Bowman SJ, Geddes GC, Corrigall V, et al: Large granular lymphocyte expansions in Felty's syndrome have an unusual phenotype of activated CD45RA+ cells. *Br J Rheumatol* 35:1252, 1996.

124. van Staa TP, Boulton F, Cooper C, et al: Neutropenia and agranulocytosis in England and Wales: Incidence and risk factors. *Am J Hematol* 72:248, 2003.

125. Andres E, Noel E, Kurtz JE, et al: Life-threatening idiosyncratic drug-induced agranulocytosis in elderly patients. *Drugs Aging* 21:427, 2004.

126. Andrès E, Maloisel F: Idiosyncratic drug-induced agranulocytosis or acute neutropenia. *Curr Opin Hematol* 15:15, 2008.

127. Curtis BR: Drug-induced immune neutropenia/agranulocytosis. *Immunohematology* 30:95, 2014.

128. Khan AA, Harvey J, Sengupta S. Continuing clozapine with granulocyte colony-stimulating factor in patients with neutropenia. *Ther Adv Psychopharmacol* 3:266, 2013.

129. Schulz W: Ueber digenartige Halserkrankungen. *Dtsch Med Wochenschr* 48:1495, 1922.

130. Uetreicht JP: Reactive metabolites and agranulocytosis. *Eur J Haematol Suppl* 60:33, 1996.

131. Claas FH: Immune mechanisms leading to drug-induced blood dyscrasias. *Eur J Haematol Suppl* 60:64, 1996.

132. Carey PJ: Drug-induced myelosuppression: Diagnosis and management. *Drug Saf* 26:691, 2003.

133. Mauri MC, Rudelli R, Bravin S, et al: Clozapine metabolism rate as a possible index of drug induced granulocytopenia. *Psychopharmacology (Berl)* 35:459, 1998.

134. Garrey WE, Bryan WR: Variations in white blood cell counts. *Physiol Rev* 15:597, 1935.

135. Dancey JT, Deubelbeiss KA, Harker LA, Finch CA: Neutrophil kinetics in man. *J Clin Invest* 58:705, 1976.

136. Quindry JC, Stone WL, King J, Broeder CE: The effects of acute exercise on neutrophils and plasma oxidative stress. *Med Sci Sports Exerc* 35:1139, 2003.

137. Benschop RJ, Rodriquez-Feuerhahn M, Schedlowski M: Catecholamine-induced leukocytosis: Early observations, current research, and future directions. *Brain Behav Immun* 10:77, 1996.

138. Toft P, Helbo-Hansen HS, Tonnesen E, et al: Redistribution of granulocytes during adrenaline infusion and following administration of cortisol in healthy volunteers. *Acta Anaesthesiol Scand* 38:254, 1994.

139. Dale DC, Fauci, AS, Gerry D IV, Wolff SM: Comparison of agents producing neutrophilic leukocytosis in man. *J Clin Invest* 56:808, 1975.

140. Price TH, Chatta GS, Dale DC: The effect of recombinant granulocyte-colony stimulating factor on neutrophil kinetics in normal young and elderly humans. *Blood* 88:335, 1996.

141. Dale DC, Liles WC, Llewellyn C, Price TH: The effects of granulocyte macrophage colony stimulating factor (GM-CSF) on neutrophil kinetics and function in normal human volunteers. *Am J Hematol* 57:7, 1998.

142. Reding MT, Hibbs JR, Morrison VA, et al: Diagnosis and outcome of 100 consecutive patients with extreme granulocytic leukocytosis. *Am J Med* 104:12, 1998.

143. Etzioni A, Tonetti M: Leukocyte adhesion deficiency II—From A to almost Z. *Immunol Rev* 178:138, 2000.

144. Bishop CR, Athens JW, Boggs DR, et al: Leukokinetic studies: XIII. A non-steady state kinetic evaluation of the mechanism of cortisone-induced granulocytosis. *J Clin Invest* 47:249, 1968.

145. Cartwright GE, Athens JW, Haab OP, et al: Blood granulocyte kinetics in conditions associated with granulocytosis. *Ann N Y Acad Sci* 11:963, 1964.

146. Alves-Filho JC, de Freitas A, Spiller F, et al: The role of neutrophils in severe sepsis. *Shock* 30 (Suppl 1):3, 2008.

147. Parry H, Cohen S, Schlarb JE, et al: Smoking, alcohol consumption, and leukocyte counts. *Am J Clin Pathol* 107:64, 1997.

148. Miki K, Miki M, Nakamura Y, et al: Early-phase neutrophilia in cigarette smoke-induced acute eosinophilic pneumonia. *Intern Med* 42:839, 2003.

149. Weenig RH, Bruce AJ, McEvoy MT, et al: Neutrophilic dermatosis of the hands: Four new cases and review of the literature. *Int J Dermatol* 43:95, 2004.

150. Shoenfeld Y, Tal A, Berliner S, Pinkhas J: Leukocytosis in nonhematological malignancies—A possible tumor-associated marker. *J Cancer Res Clin Oncol* 111:54, 1986.

151. Zalokar JB, Richard JL, Claude JR: Leukocyte count, smoking, and myocardial infarction. *N Engl J Med* 304:465, 1981.

152. Kirtane AJ, Bui A, Murphy SA, et al: Association of peripheral neutrophilia with adverse angiographic outcomes in ST-elevation myocardial infarction. *Am J Cardiol* 93:532, 2004.

153. Al-Kasim F, Doyle JJ, Massey GV, et al: Incidence and treatment of potentially lethal diseases in transient leukemia of Down syndrome: Pediatric Oncology Group Study. *J Pediatr Hematol Oncol* 24:9, 2002.

154. Ward HN, Reinhard EH: Chronic idiopathic leukocytosis. *Ann Intern Med* 75:193, 1971.

155. Herring WB, Smith LB, Walker R, Herion JC: Hereditary neutrophilia. *Am J Med* 56:729, 1974.

156. Plo I, Zhang Y, Le Couédic JP, et al: An activating mutation in the CSF3R gene induces a hereditary chronic neutrophilia. *J Exp Med* 206:1701, 2009.

157. Focosi D, Azzarà A, Kast RE, et al: Lithium and hematology: Established and proposed uses. *J Leukoc Biol* 85:20, 2009.

158. Herishanu Y, Rogowski O, Polliack A, Marilus R: Leukocytosis in obese individuals: Possible link in patients with unexplained persistent neutrophilia. *Eur J Haematol* 76:516, 2006.

159. Loimaala A, Rontu R, Vuori I, et al: Blood leukocyte count is a risk factor for intima-media thickening and subclinical carotid atherosclerosis in middle-aged men. *Atherosclerosis* 188:363, 2006.

160. Prasad A, Stone GW, Stuckey TD, et al: Relation between leucocyte count, myonecrosis, myocardial perfusion, and outcomes following primary angioplasty. *Am J Cardiol* 99:1067, 2007.

161. Kruk M, Przyuski J, Kaliczuk L, et al: Hemoglobin, leukocytosis and clinical outcomes of ST-elevation myocardial infarction treated with primary angioplasty: ANIN Myocardial Infarction Registry. *Circ J* 73:323, 2009.

162. Brown DW, Ford ES, Giles WH, et al: Associations between white blood cell count and risk for cerebrovascular disease mortality: NHANES II Mortality Study, 1976–1992. *Ann Epidemiol* 14:425, 2004.

163. Landolfi R, Di Gennaro L, Barbui T, et al: European Collaboration on Low-Dose Aspirin in Polycythemia Vera (ECLAP). Leukocytosis as a major thrombotic risk factor in patients with polycythemia vera. *Blood* 109:2446, 2007.

164. Caramazza D, Caracciolo C, Barone R, et al: Correlation between leukocytosis and thrombosis in Philadelphia-negative chronic myeloproliferative neoplasms. *Ann Hematol* 2009.

165. Marchetti M, Falanga A: Leukocytosis, JAK2V617F mutation, and hemostasis in myeloproliferative disorders. *Pathophysiol Haemost Thromb* 36:148, 2009.

166. Quinn CT, Lee NJ, Shull EP, et al: Prediction of adverse outcomes in children with sickle cell anemia: A study of the Dallas Newborn Cohort. *Blood* 111:544, 2008.

167. Litos M, Sarris I, Bewley S, et al: White blood cell count as a predictor of the severity of sickle cell disease during pregnancy. *Eur J Obstet Gynecol Reprod Biol* 133:169, 2007.

CHAPTER 66
DISORDERS OF NEUTROPHIL FUNCTION

Niels Borregaard

SUMMARY

The neutrophil circulates in blood as a quiescent cell. Its main function as a phagocytic and bactericidal cell is performed outside the circulation in tissues where microbial invasion takes place. Neutrophil function is traditionally viewed as chemotaxis, phagocytosis, and bacterial killing. Although these conceptually represent distinct entities, they are functionally related, and rely to a large extent on the same intracellular signal transduction mechanisms that result in localized rises in intracellular Ca^{2+}, changes in organization of the cytoskeleton, assembly of the nicotinamide adenine dinucleotide phosphate (NADPH) oxidase from its cytosolic and membrane integrated subunits, and fusion of granules with the phagosome or neutrophil plasma membrane. Clinical disorders of the neutrophil may arise from impairment of these normal functions. The clinical presentation of a patient who has a qualitative neutrophil abnormality may be similar to that of one who has an antibody, complement, or toll-like receptor disorder. In general, evaluation for phagocyte cell disorders should be initiated among those patients who have at least one of the following clinical features: (1) two or more systemic bacterial infections in a relatively short time period; (2) frequent, serious respiratory infections, such as pneumonia or sinusitis, or otitis media, or lymphadenitis; (3) infections present at unusual sites (liver or brain abscess); and (4) infections associated with unusual pathogens (e.g., *Aspergillus* pneumonia, disseminated candidiasis, or infections with *Serratia marcescens*, *Nocardia* species, or *Burkholderia cepacia*).

NEUTROPHIL STRUCTURE AND FUNCTION

CHEMOTAXIS AND MOTILITY

The similarity between neutrophil locomotion and that of amebas was noted long ago.[1] Neutrophils respond to spatial gradients of chemotaxins with differences in concentration of chemotaxin of as little as 1 percent across the cell,[2] although there has been contention as to whether chemotaxis also requires temporal, as well as spatial, sensing.[3] Even with populations of cells as "homogenous" as neutrophils, a broad range of responsiveness is found.[4] During locomotion toward a chemotactic source, neutrophils acquire a characteristic asymmetric shape (Fig. 66–1). In the front of the cell is a pseudopodium, referred to as the *lamellipodium*, that advances before the body of the cell containing the nucleus and the cytoplasmic granules. At the rear of the moving cell is a knob-like tail, the uropod. The lamellipodium undulates or "ruffles" as the neutrophil moves, at a rate of up to 50 $\mu m/min$. The membrane lipids also flow during locomotion,[5] and enhanced cytosolic Ca^{2+} is observed along the membrane margin.[6] The lamellipodium, which is very thin, forms immediately when the cell encounters a gradient of chemotactic factor. As the cell moves, the cytoplasm behind the lamellipodium streams forward, almost obliterating it. At this point, some granules appear to contact the cell periphery and release granule contents in response to chemotactic agents. The lamellipodium extends again and the process repeats itself. A flow of cortical materials, composed particularly of actin filaments, has been proposed to account for chemotaxis as well as other cellular movements.[7] This may also account for changes in cell viscosity. Polarity and movement is orchestrated by the cytoskeleton through signals generated from receptor associated G-proteins in an intricate network that regulates both direction and intensity of movement.[8–11]

INGESTION

When a neutrophil comes in contact with a particle, the pseudopodium flows around the particle, its extensions fuse, and it thereby encompasses the particle within the phagosome.[1] The ingestion phase can be

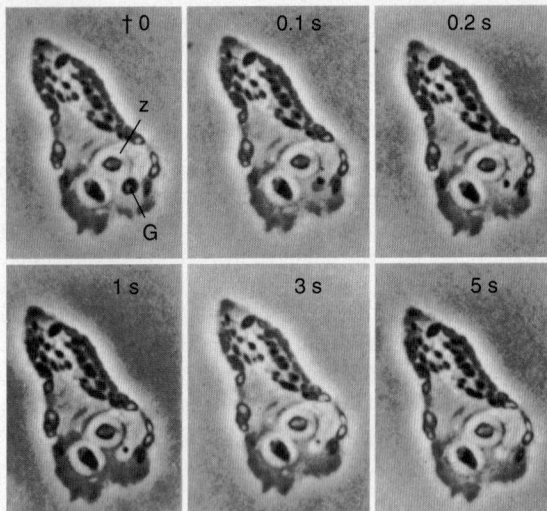

Figure 66–1. Cinemicrophotographic observation of granule lysis of a chicken neutrophil following phagocytosis of zymosan particles. Note the lysis of the cytoplasmic granule (G) against one of two ingested zymosan particles (Z). The dense body of the granule disappears from view in the interval of 5 s (original magnification ×1200). *(Reproduced with permission from Hirsch JG: Cinemicrophotographic observations on granule lysis in polymorphonuclear leucocytes during phagocytosis.* J Exp Med 116:827–834,1962.)

said to extend from recognition to the end of pseudopodium fusion. The particle thus becomes enclosed within a phagosome into which granules are rapidly discharged, as illustrated in Fig. 66–1. As with locomotion, phagocytosis results in Ca^{2+} being released in the vicinity of the active membranes.[6] The number of ingested particles may be eventually limited by the availability of plasma membrane.[7] Locomotion is not a prerequisite for ingestion: If neutrophils collide with a particle not secreting a chemotactic substance, pseudopodia form abruptly at the contact point and envelop the particle.[12]

The formation of a lamellipodium is essential for neutrophil locomotion and is also required for ingestion. When dissolution of the lamellipodium occurs, the interior contents of the cell are allowed to contact the cell membrane. Granule discharge may occur. Fusion of membranes is a common feature of (1) ingestion, where pseudopodia fuse; (2) degranulation, where granules fuse with the phagosome; and possibly (3) locomotion, where some granules may fuse with the plasma membrane. Pseudopodia form whether neutrophils are suspended in liquid medium or are attached to a surface, but the cell can only move translationally when fixed to a surface; thus it crawls but does not swim. Such "stickiness" is also a phase of ingestion.[7] The neutrophil membrane adheres firmly to particles they ingest, presumably to provide the frictional force needed to move pseudopodia around the particles. Thus, the formation of pseudopodia, membrane fusion, and membrane adhesiveness are all characteristics associated with the functional responses of neutrophils.

ADHESION

The dual neutrophil functions of immune surveillance and *in situ* elimination of microorganisms or cellular debris require rapid transition between a circulating nonadherent state to an adherent state, allowing the cells to migrate into tissues when necessary. Initially neutrophils appear at sites on the endothelium adjacent to the site of inflammation. Adhesion molecules on endothelium are induced by the inflammatory mediators tumor necrosis factor (TNF)-α and interleukin (IL)-1.

Lipopolysaccharide (LPS), released by local activated macrophages and microorganisms, results in local extravasation of the neutrophil. In postcapillary venules or in pulmonary capillaries the slow rate of blood flow, further reduced by vessel dilatation at sites of inflammation, permits a loose and somewhat transient adhesion referred to as "tethering," and results in the rolling of the neutrophil along the endothelium.[13] Extensions from the rear of the neutrophil wraps around the rolling neutrophils as so called slings and provide "crawler tracks" at their front that assists in adhesion to the endothelium.[14] During this tethering step, neutrophils respond to ligands, primarily chemokines dispatched on the endothelial surface by a signaling event that acts to reorganize the neutrophil surface membrane, thereby exposing adhesion molecules, which, in turn, lead to sustained adhesion and spreading (Chap. 19).

NEUTROPHIL MICROVILLI AND THEIR DYNAMICS

Circulating neutrophils contain surface microvilli of a diameter of 0.3 μm.[15] Moesin, ezrin, and p205 radixin are actin-binding proteins associated with neutrophil plasma membranes and are important for organization of microvilli on the surface of the cell.[16,17] These actin binding proteins tether the primary adhesion proteins exposed on the microvilli, L-selectin and P-selectin glycoprotein ligand 1 (PSGL-1).[18] L-selectin and PSGL-1 are filamentous glycosylated proteins protruding from the tips of the microvilli. E-selectin ligand 1 (ESL-1) located in the side of microvilli,[19] and CD44, located on the cell body, both serve a ligands for E-selectin.[20] L-selection, like the other selectins, including P-selectin, which is expressed on platelets and endothelial Weibel-Palade bodies, and E-selectin, which is expressed in endothelial cells, bind with a variable affinity to sialyl fucosylated oligosaccharides including sialyl Lewis X (sLe^x), which is present on multiple specific glycolipids and glycoproteins on leukocytes and inflamed endothelial cells.[21] When binding to their ligands, L-selectin, PSGL-1, ESL-1, and CD44 recruit Syk (spleen tyrosine kinase), a tyrosine kinase, which binds to the immunoreceptor tyrosine-based activation motif (ITAM). ITAMs are present in the cytoplasmic domains of surface membrane proteins, and Syk then orchestrates the further signaling to initiate cell activation.[22–25]

ROLLING AND TETHERING

P-selectin is mobilized rapidly to the endothelial cell surface following stimulation by thrombin, histamine, or oxygen radicals and interacts with neutrophil PSGL-1 to initiate neutrophil rolling.[21] Rolling subsequently involves newly expressed E-selectin, which appears on endothelial cells 1 to 2 hours after cell stimulation by IL-1, TNF-α, or LPS. E-selectin counterreceptors include PSGL-1, ESL-1, and CD44.[19,24] Both P- and L-selectin contribute sequentially to leukocyte rolling, but L-selectin is involved in the prolonged neutrophil sequestration on inflamed microvasculature. L-selectin is constitutively present on neutrophils and its binding capacity is rapid and transiently increased after neutrophil activation, possibly via receptor oligomerization. Activation of ADAM17, a matrix metalloproteinase expressed at the neutrophil surface, severs L-selectin from the surface of neutrophils and impairs their recruitment to endothelium.[26,27] Thus far, only one inducible L-selectin counterreceptor has been identified on inflamed endothelium.[28] In addition to its binding to endothelial ligands, neutrophil PSGL-1 is a counterreceptor for L-selectin, which permits previously adherent neutrophils to recruit other neutrophils to inflamed endothelium (Chap. 19).[13,21]

NEUTROPHIL ADHESION AND SPREADING

Figure 66–2 shows a sequence of molecular and biophysical events leading to neutrophil activation and increased adherence during acute

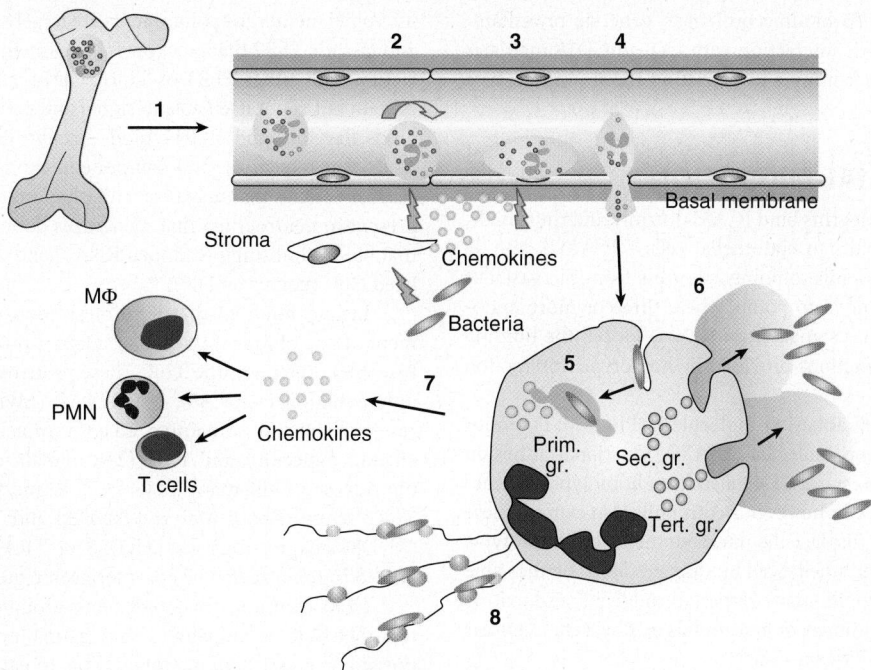

Figure 66–2. Neutrophil-mediated inflammatory response. (1) Egress of mature neutrophils from marrow to circulation. (2) Initial tethering and rolling are dominantly mediated by selectins present both on neutrophils and endothelial cells and their ligands. Invasion by bacteria stimulates tissues macrophages to secrete inflammatory cytokines, interleukin (IL)-1 and tumor necrosis factor, which, in turn, activate endothelial cells to express E- and P-selectin and IL-8. E- and P-selectin serve as counterreceptors for the neutrophil P-selectin glycoprotein ligand-1. (3) Activated endothelial cells express intercellular adhesion molecule (ICAM)-1 and ICAM-2, which serve as ligands for the neutrophil β_2 integrins. The β_2 integrins mediate tight adhesion and arrest of the leukocytes in cooperation with the selectins. Localized activation of neutrophils by juxtacrine signaling molecules or chemoattractants that bind to surface receptors is critical for inside-out signaling of β_2 integrins, making them adhesive for the ICAM ligands on the endothelium. (4) Neutrophil invasion through the vascular basement membrane with release of proteases and reactive oxidative intermediates that cause local destruction of the extracellular matrix which allows for migration of the neutrophils into tissues. (5, 6) Uptake of microorganisms into the phagocytic vacuole with concomitant degranulation both into the phagocytic vacuole (azurophil granules and specific granules) and to the exterior (specific granules and gelatinase granules). (7) A burst of transcriptional activity is initiated during diapedesis of neutrophils and during phagocytosis, which results in generation of chemokines such as IL-8, monocyte chemoattractant protein-1, macrophage inflammatory protein-1α, and IL-1β that may recruit additional cells of the immune system.[58] (8) Formation of neutrophil extracellular traps by extrusion of chromatin and cationic bactericidal granule proteins.[262] MΦ, macrophages; PMN, polymorphonuclear neutrophil.

inflammatory response *in vivo*. The inflamed endothelium produces chemoattractants such as platelet-activating factor (PAF), leukotriene B_4 (LTB$_4$), and various chemokines, immobilized by proteoglycans on the luminal surface of endothelial cells.[29] Among these chemokines, IL-8 specifically attracts neutrophils. IL-8 is synthesized by endothelial cells in response to IL-1, TNF-α, or LPS, and is stored in Weibel-Palade bodies; IL-8 can be released by histamine or thrombin.[30] Additionally, IL-8 can be internalized by endothelial cells and transcytosed from the abluminal surface via vesicular caveolae, and presented to the tips of microvilli of the endothelial cell luminal surface.[31] The binding of signaling molecules such as PAF and IL-8 to surface receptors on the leukocytes activates them in a juxtacrine fashion and triggers changes in affinity or avidity of β_2 integrins, leukocyte function-associated antigen (LFA)-1 (CD11a/CD18), which is constitutively expressed on neutrophil plasma membranes, and Mac-1 (CD11b/CD18), which becomes incorporated in the neutrophil plasma membrane from secretory vesicles.[13,21,32] β_2 Integrins are recognized by counterligands on endothelial cells, including members of the intercellular adhesion molecule (ICAM) family such as ICAM-1 and ICAM-2. The ICAM glycoproteins are induced by cytokines that include TNF and IL-1. The relative affinity of the β_2 integrins for ICAM is increased by exposure of neutrophils to numerous stimuli, including C5a, N-formylated bacterial peptides, IL-8, and LTB$_4$. The extracellular domains of unactivated integrins are

in a bent position and not able to bind ligands. Intracellular signals, such as those generated via Syk as discussed above, can transform the integrins into an extended but not fully open conformation, capable of ligand binding with weak affinity permitting the integrin (LFA-1) to participate in rolling[33] and an extended and fully open form capable of ligand binding with strong affinity, mediating firm adhesion. The molecular mechanisms have been worked out in great detail. In essence, tailins and kindlins are recruited and bound to membrane near phosphotyrosine (NPxY and NxxY) motifs present on the integrin β chains and twist the cytoplasmic domains of the α and β chains. This changes the conformation of the extracellular domains from the bent to the open state, thereby permitting binding to ligands, and in so doing transmit signals from outside to inside.[21,34–36] Neutrophils integrate the signals of integrin engagement and those delivered simultaneously by inflammatory cytokines or chemoattractants to activate a cascade of intracellular events resulting in cell spreading (Fig. 66–2). The CD11b/CD18 integrin (MAC-1) is known to interact in *cis* fashion with glycosylphosphatidylinositol (GPI)-anchored membrane proteins such as FcγRIIIB (CD16), the LPS receptor CD14, and the urokinase plasminogen activator receptor (uPAR; CD87). Integrins behave as transducers mediating signals transferred by these GPI-linked receptors.[37] For instance, FcγRIIIB interaction with CD11b/CD18 promotes antibody-dependent phagocytosis, whereas CD14 interaction with CD11b/CD18 occurs in the presence of LPS and LPS-binding protein to generate proinflammatory mediators, and uPAR interaction with CD11b/CD18 mediates neutrophil migration by recruiting and activating the urokinase-type plasminogen activator.[29]

TRANSENDOTHELIAL MIGRATION

Fully extended and open integrins bind ICAM-1 firmly and thus mediate attachment of neutrophils to endothelial cells.[38] ICAM-1 and -2 direct the motion of neutrophils to points of egress from the vascular lining. The majority are guided to points where three or more endothelial cells join. Intracellular signals from ICAMs loosen the binding between endothelial cell junctions provided by homotypic interaction of VE-cadherins.[39]

Platelet endothelial cell adhesion molecule 1 (PECAM-1), endothelial cell-selective adhesion molecule (ESAM), junctional adhesion molecule A, B, and C (JAMs), and CD99 also form homotypic interactions between endothelial cells; however, neutrophils also express these adhesion proteins and may displace the interendothelial cell homotypic binding with neutrophil–endothelial cell binding mediated by the same proteins. In this way neutrophils can "zipper" through[40–42] and exit by this paracellular route. A minority of neutrophils exit by a transcellular route through so-called endothelial cups.[42]

Pericytes are perivascular contractile cells that interact with endothelial cells and regulate vascular permeability. Neutrophils exit the vascular wall through gaps between pericytes.[43] Pericytes adopt different morphologies and distributions in different tissues. Such may explain differences in neutrophil recruitment to viscera.[44]

Once out in tissues the forefront neutrophils generate IL-8 and LTB$_4$ in order to recruit an additional swarm of neutrophils to the area and recruit later incoming monocytes and macrophages.[45]

NEUTROPHIL SURFACE PROTEINS

Several proteins associated with the surface of the neutrophil function in the normal housekeeping activities such as Na$^+$/K$^+$ adenosine triphosphatase (ATPase), but others serve specific functions such as L-selectin, PSGL-1, and integrins. The surface of neutrophils is highly dynamic as a result of the incorporation of membrane from intracellular vesicles and granules, a process that is known to add significantly to the total cell surface measured by an increase in electric capacitance.[46] A number of membrane-bound receptors are localized to secretory vesicles and incorporated into the surface membrane when secretory vesicles fuse with the plasma membrane, as occurs during diapedesis. This enhances the ability of neutrophils to respond to the signals presented by endothelial cells or present in the extravascular tissue.

Receptors for Recognition of Microbes

Neutrophils and other cells of the innate immune system recognize microbes through germline-encoded receptors, which recognize molecular patterns that are relative unique to pathogens and shared among groups of pathogens, so-called pathogen-associated molecular patterns (PAMPs). These pattern-recognition receptors (PRRs) include the membrane-bound toll-like receptors (TLRs) and C-type lectin receptors (CLRs), and the cytosolic nucleotide-binding oligomerization domain (NOD)-like receptors (NLRs) and RIG-like receptors (RLRs).[47–50] Although PRRs are highly expressed in myeloid cells, they are also widely expressed in cells that are regularly exposed to microorganisms, particularly in epithelial cells.

TLRs are type 1 transmembrane signaling receptors that are activated by dimerization induced by ligand binding.[51] The TLRs may dimerize both as homodimers and heterodimers. TLRs that recognize microbial membrane components are largely present on the cell surface, and include TLR2 that recognizes lipoproteins and lipopeptides in association with either TLR1 or TLR6. CD14 is known as an LPS-binding protein but is not itself able to signal and presents LPS to TLR4.[51] TLR5 binds flagellin, and TLR11 binds profilin-like proteins of protozoa.[52] TLRs that recognize viral components are largely expressed on intracellular vesicles that may fuse with phagosomes and include TLR3 (not present in neutrophils) that recognizes double-stranded RNA, TLR7/8 that binds viral single-stranded RNA,[53] and TLR9 that binds unmethylated GpC regions on DNA.[54]

Ligand binding, that is, dimerization of TLRs leads to recruitment of one of four intracellular adaptor proteins to the TIR (toll/IL-1 receptor) domain of the TLR. These proteins include MyD88 (myeloid differentiation factor 88), Mal/TIRAP (MyD88-adaptor-like/toll-IL 1 receptor domain containing adaptor protein), TRAM (TRIF-related adaptor molecule), and TRIF (TIR domain-containing adaptor inducing IFN-β). While many TLRs (5, 7, 8, and 9) exclusively use MyD88, TLR2 requires both Mal and MyD88 and TLR4 can use either Mal (MyD88-adaptor-like) and MyD88 or TRAM and TRIF to signal to NF-κB (nuclear factor-κB) or interferon regulatory factor (IRF)-3.[55,56,47]

CLRs comprise a heterogeneous group of *trans*-membrane receptors that bind carbohydrates such as mannose, fucose, and β-glucans present on a variety of microbes, fungi in particular. They signal largely via their cytosolic ITAMs and Syk to activate NF-κB, nuclear factor of activated T cell (NFAT), and microtubule-associated protein kinases (MAPKs) resulting in production of proinflammatory cytokines.[48]

NLR proteins are cytosolic proteins that are divided into five subfamilies, NLRA, NLRB, NLRC, NLRP, and NLRX.[50] Their N terminus contains either a caspase activation and recruitment domain (CARD) or a pyrin domain (PYD). The NLRC members NOD1 and NOD2 recognize peptidoglycans of both Gram-positive and Gram-negative bacteria and signal to activate the NF-κB pathway. Other members of the NLRC and NLRP subfamily are essential in organizing the inflammasome. The NLRs multimerize through their CARDs into inflammasomes,[50] cytoplasmic structures that activate caspase-1, which, in turn, convert pro–IL-1 and pro–IL-18 to the mature proinflammatory cytokines that are secreted.[57]

A variety of chemokine receptors are found on the surface of the neutrophil. These are in general G-protein–coupled receptors. Other G-protein–coupled receptors on neutrophils are the purine receptors for adenosine diphosphate (ADP) and ATP, the PAF receptor C5a, and formyl-methionyl-leucyl-phenylalanine (fMLP) receptors. Receptors not belonging to the G-protein–coupled receptor family include receptors for IL-1, IL-10, and TNF-α, and the growth factors receptors for granulocyte colony-stimulating factor (G-CSF) and granulocyte-macrophage colony-stimulating factor (GM-CSF). Both growth factor receptors are important for myeloid development, and play an important role in enhancing neutrophil function and gene transcription in mature neutrophils. A burst of transcriptional activity is associated with the diapedesis of neutrophils into tissues, which results in downregulation of proapoptotic genes and upregulation of genes coding for antiapoptotic proteins, upregulation of genes encoding chemokines and cytokines that may recruit macrophages, T cells and additional neutrophils, and downregulation of genes encoding chemokine receptors (see Fig. 66–2).[58]

Surface Components for Phagocytosis

Neutrophils express the Fc α receptor (CD89) for immunoglobulin (Ig) A and IgG receptors, FcγRIIA (CD32), and FcγRIII (CD16). Neutrophils also express receptors for the complement components, including CD1qR, CR1 (CD35), CR3 (CD11/CD18), and CR4. CR1 binds CD3b, C4b, and C3bi with decreasing affinity. CR3 recognizes

C3bi (a proteolytic fragment of C3b). Of particular importance is that both Fcγ receptors and GPI-coupled receptors appear to be localized to lipid rafts. Lipid rafts are important, but elusive structures that facilitate signal transduction leading to phagocytosis by promoting several membrane protein interactions. Initially the rafts were conceptionally associated with caveolae, which are structures identified on endothelial cells and thought to be important for transendothelial cell traffic. The caveolae were identified by their high content of cholesterol lipids and the presence of the structural protein, caveolin. Rafts were subsequently identified on neutrophils, but these cells are devoid of caveolin.[59] Rafts are perhaps best viewed as patches of surface membrane that attract many hydrophobic proteins including signaling molecules such as tyrosine kinases and phosphatases. Other membrane protein receptors that are not normally associated with rafts may change their conformation and subsequently associate with rafts upon binding their ligands. This is particularly true for the Fcγ and GPI-coupled receptors.

SECRETORY VESICLES

Secretory vesicles are small intracellular vesicles that were discovered during the search for the structural basis for upregulation of a variety of surface molecules on neutrophils in response to nanomolar concentrations of fMLP and other chemotactic stimuli. They were initially identified by "latent" alkaline phosphatase.[60] Secretory vesicles of neutrophils should not be confused with the vesicles that carry cargo from endoplasmic reticulum and Golgi in the constitutive secretory pathway of other cells and that are sometimes also named secretory vesicles. Secretory vesicles of neutrophils are specialized endocytosis vesicles that are formed in the final stages of neutrophil maturation in the marrow. They contain plasma proteins, seemingly without any selectivity. Albumin thus serves as a marker for secretory vesicles and has allowed the identification of these as small intracellular vesicles that are scattered throughout the cytoplasm of neutrophils as is true for neutrophil granules. The plasma proteins inside secretory vesicles show no sign of degradation, thus no fusion takes place with lysosomal structures.[61] Secretory vesicles behave like the traditional neutrophil granules. They require a specific signal for mobilization.[62] Secretory vesicles are not important for their cargo (plasma proteins), but for their membrane which becomes fully incorporated into the plasma membrane of the neutrophil upon stimulation.[61,63–66] Secretory vesicles host most of the neutrophil chemotactic and GPI-coupled receptors, TLRs, and one of the early acting downstream effectors, phospholipase D.[67] They enrich the plasma membrane with receptors for adhesion and signaling, and can be seen as the structural basis for transition of neutrophils from circulating quiescent cells that do not respond well to stimuli such as chemoattractants and objects to be phagocytosed, to highly responsive cells capable of establishing firm contact with endothelium. The signals generated by tethering of selectins or PSGL-1 to the endothelium are sufficient to mobilize secretory vesicles. Secretory vesicles are completely mobilized *in vivo* during neutrophil diapedesis.[21,66]

The first identified marker of secretory vesicles, latent alkaline phosphatase, is known to be elevated in chronic myeloproliferative disorders except for chronic myelogenous leukemia (CML), but the content of secretory vesicles in neutrophils from patients with chronic myeloproliferative disorders is not different from normal neutrophils.[68–70] The best marker for secretory vesicles is CD35, a transmembrane protein of 160 to 250 kDa that binds complement components C3b and C4b, because CD35, in contrast to alkaline phosphatase, is absent from the plasma membrane of unstimulated neutrophils, and because it is absent from granules (in contrast to $\alpha_M\beta_2$).[32,65,71] It is not known whether secretory vesicles contain lipid rafts, but most GPI-linked proteins are raft-associated[72] and are localized to secretory vesicles in neutrophils.

GRANULES

Nomenclature of Neutrophil Granules

The neutrophil is known for its granules. When Paul Ehrlich introduced aniline dyes in histochemistry and discovered the different subsets of leukocytes, the neutrophil granules were divided into those that took up the azure dye, the azurophilic granules, and the others, the specific granules.[73,74] When the peroxidase reaction was introduced, the azurophil granules were found to be peroxidase-positive as a result of the presence of the major myeloid cell protein, myeloperoxidase (MPO), and the specific granules were thus named peroxidase-negative granules.[75,76] Because the azurophil granules are formed first, in the promyelocyte, and the specific granules later, in the myelocyte, these are also termed primary and secondary granules, respectively. A tertiary granule subset was identified in human neutrophils and shown to contain gelatinase,[77] but the ultrastructure was not determined until the issue of the neutrophil gelatinase (matrix metalloproteinase [MMP]-9) as a possible complex with neutrophil gelatinase-associated lipocalin (NGAL) was identified.[78,79]

Granules were initially viewed of as small bags that emptied their content of bactericidal substances onto the ingested microorganisms when granules fuse with the phagocytic vacuole during phagocytosis, but it later became clear that granules are not only important for their cargo, but also for their membranes, as they contain proteins that become incorporated into the membrane of the phagocytic vacuole and into the surface membrane when the granules are mobilized.[80,81] If granules were classified by their content, both of matrix proteins and membrane proteins, the number of different granule subsets that exists in neutrophils would be meaninglessly high. Yet nature has provided a beautiful setting that allows the neutrophil to fine tune its response to a specific task. *A priori*, there would be two reasons for having different subsets of granules: One would be to ensure that proteins, which cannot coexist, are segregated; that is, protease-sensitive proteins are separated from proteases. The other reason would be to have proteins whose service is needed at one time separated from proteins whose service is needed at a different time.

Heterogeneity of Neutrophil Granules

Among the peroxidase-positive granules, subsets can be identified that are rich in defensins as well as some that are not.[82,83] Functionally, no difference has been identified in terms of the regulation of exocytosis of these peroxidase-positive granule subsets.[84] Other constituents include the serine proteases elastase, cathepsin G, proteinase 3, and neutrophil serine protease 4 (NSP4), and the inactive serine protease azurocidin (aka CAP 37), the antimicrobial proteins BPI (bacterial permeability-increasing protein), lysozyme, and the α defensins, which are the dominating species.[80] Defensins are also named HNPs (human neutrophil peptides). The membrane of the azurophil granules contains CD63 (granulophysin) and CD68, but their role in neutrophil function remains unclear.[85,86] Many of the proteins present in peroxidase granules are proteolytically processed both at the N-terminus and the C-terminus to the active mature forms, which are stored in the granule matrix.

Peroxidase-negative granules can be divided into three subsets based on the distribution of the two marker proteins lactoferrin and gelatinase: granules that contain lactoferrin, but no gelatinase (15 percent of peroxidase-negative granules), granules that contain both proteins (60 percent), and granules that are rich in gelatinase, but low (or absent) in lactoferrin (25 percent).[87] The latter are named gelatinase granules or tertiary granules, whereas those that contain lactoferrin are called specific or secondary granules. It is a characteristic of peroxidase-negative granules that the proteins present in their matrix are not proteolytically processed. The MMPs of peroxidase-negative granules are stored as a proform,[88] as is the major bactericidal protein hCAP-18.[89,90] No major differences have been identified in the content of membrane proteins of the peroxidase-negative granule subsets. All contain the flavocytochrome $p22^{phox}/gp91^{phox}$ complex that is part of the nicotinamide adenine dinucleotide phosphate (NADPH) oxidase, and all contain the major β_2-integrin $\alpha_M\beta_2$—and these are even shared with the membrane of secretory vesicles.[32,91,92] The divalent cation transporter Nramp1 is localized only to gelatinase granules,[93] and the membrane MMP leukolysin (MMP-25)[94] is shared between gelatinase granules and secretory vesicles. However, the subsets differ markedly in their propensity for exocytosis. Following neutrophil stimulation, gelatinase granules are exocytosed to a larger extent than granules containing both lactoferrin and gelatinase, and these are more readily mobilized than granules containing lactoferrin but lacking gelatinase. These, in turn, are mobilized more readily than peroxidase-positive granules.[62,66,79,87,95] This organization of granule subsets with different content and different set points to trigger exocytosis allows the neutrophil to mobilize MMPs and integrins necessary for movement through the basal membrane and tissue before the bactericidal peptides and serine protease are called to play, but it puts an enormous task on the organization of the biosynthetic apparatus to secure that the right granule proteins are targeted to the granules with a given trigger for exocytosis.

The content of isolated granules has been mapped by proteome analysis.[96] High-resolution mass spectrometry has identified 1300 proteins associated with neutrophil granules, plasma membranes and secretory vesicles and confirmed that localization is largely determined by time of biosynthesis.[97]

Targeting by Biosynthetic Timing

The extreme heterogeneity of neutrophil granules and their individual control of exocytosis can be explained simply by timing of their biosynthesis (Fig. 66–3). Granule proteins are synthesized during myelopoiesis from myeloblasts to band cells and segmented neutrophils in the marrow.[75,76,98] The window of biosynthesis of each granule protein is highly controlled by combinations of transcription factors that change as the cells differentiate and mature.[99,100] If all granule proteins are targeted to granules during synthesis, the content of newly formed granules would change as the cell matures because the profile of biosynthesis changes. A global view of the change in transcriptional activity of neutrophil precursors during maturation in the marrow confirmed the association between granule localization and transcriptional activity.[101] This simple mechanism largely explains the heterogeneity of granules[102] and their contents, but it does not account for the differences in exocytotic rates among individualized subsets. By timing the biosynthesis of the proteins essential for fusion[103,104] to granule membranes during maturation, it is possible to regulate the rates of exocytosis. Indeed, the v-SNARE (SNAP receptor), vesicle-associated membrane protein (VAMP)-2 is present in a higher density on gelatinase granules than on specific granules and is most highly expressed on secretory vesicles,[105,106] which correlates with the ease of releasing granule subsets from the neutrophil following activation.

Sorting between the Constitutive and Regulated Exocytotic Pathway

Although the sorting by timing can explain the granule heterogeneity of neutrophil granules, it does not provide any clues to the mechanisms

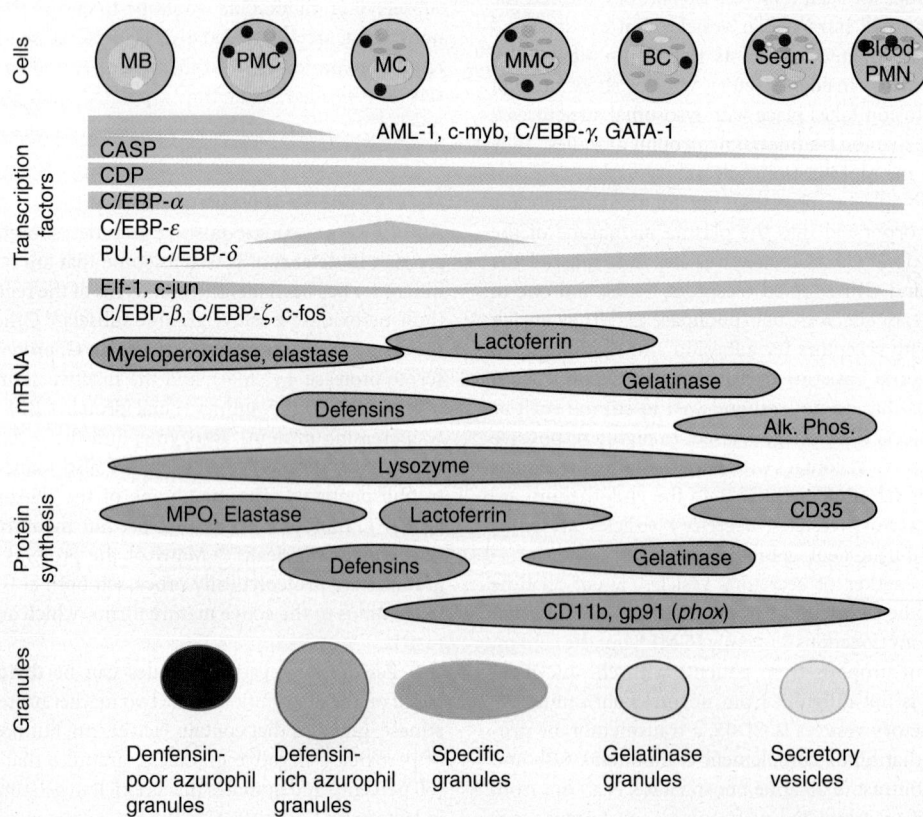

Figure 66–3. Formation of granule subsets during myelopoiesis and regulation of granule protein transcription. Difference in the appearance and disappearance of transcription factors regulate the individual window of granule protein gene transcription and translation into protein that is targeted to forming granules, explaining the heterogeneity of neutrophil granules.

responsible for diverting newly synthesized proteins to granules as opposed to immediate (constitutive) secretion. Not all granule proteins are equally efficiently directed to granules. Lysozyme is poorly retained during biosynthesis.[107] This explains the high concentration of lysozyme in plasma.[108] MPO is efficiently retained and the plasma level of MPO is consequently very low. A particularly interesting observation pertains to α defensins. These are localized exclusively to azurophil granules, but their window of biosynthesis is very similar to that of lactoferrin,[107,100] and defensins and lactoferrin are both controlled by the transcription factor C/EBPε (CCAAT/enhancer binding protein ε), which is absolutely required for biosynthesis of specific granule proteins.[109,110] The absence of defensins from specific granules, despite an active biosynthesis when other specific granule proteins are formed, is explained by a complete lack of sorting of defensins to granules in myelocytes.[99,100,107] Only defensins synthesized at the late promyelocytic stage are routed to granules, whereas defensins synthesized at the myelocyte stage are secreted from cells after biosynthesis[107] and is present in relatively high concentrations in plasma.[111] The defensins that are targeted to granules are processed to mature defensins, whereas the defensins that are secreted remain unprocessed. Processing of defensins removes a charge neutralizing propiece, sorting of defensins and other granule proteins to granules may depend on their ability to interact with negatively charged proteoglycans that are present in the matrix of granules.[112–114] Serglycin, an intracellular proteoglycan is present in Golgi and immature granules of promyelocytes and disappears as the cells mature.[115] Serglycin is absolutely critical for confining a variety of mast cell proteins to the mast cell granules.[116] Granulocytes from mice with a targeted disruption of the serglycin gene are morphologically normal and contain normal levels of granule proteins except elastase.[117] CD63 was demonstrated to be involved in sorting of elastase to azurophil granules,[118] but this may be indirectly via serglycin. An N-terminal sorting domain has been identified in serglycin and was shown to be essential for routing of serglycin to mast cell granules.[119] No common denominator has been identified that can fully explain why neutrophil proteins are sorted to granules. Perhaps the lack of efficient sorting to granules may not solely be taken as inefficiency, but may be a way to secure a desirable level of antibiotic protein such as lysozyme[108] and hCAP-18[120] in plasma which renders the myeloid cells of the marrow a major secretory organ.

Control of Neutrophil Granule Protein Expression

The biosynthesis of neutrophil granule proteins is controlled at the transcriptional and not the translational level (see Fig. 66–3).[98–100] Not all transcription factors that are responsible for biosynthesis of granule protein have been identified, and the role of an individual transcription factor may be difficult to identify from gene knockout studies as transcription factors may work at multiple stages during myelopoiesis. The transcription factor PU.1 is essential for myelopoiesis because knockout mice do not form myeloid progenitors beyond myeloblasts[121,122]; but this does not preclude PU.1 from regulating transcription of individual granule proteins at a later stage of development.[123–126] Figure 66–3 shows the profile of important myeloid transcription factors during maturation of normal myeloid cells in the marrow *in vivo*. *RUNX1* (AML-1), *c-MYB*, *CASP*, *C/EBPα*, *C/EBPγ*, *GATA-1*, and *ELF-1* gene products are all strongly expressed in the myeloblast and promyelocyte, and some of these are required for azurophil granule protein expression. Then *c-MYB*, *AML-1*, *GATA-1*, and *ELF-1* gene products are downregulated as the cells enter the myelocyte stage, heralded by a brisk and transient upregulation of C/EBPε to initiate expression of peroxidase-negative granule proteins[99] in agreement with the lack of specific granules in C/EBPε –/– mice and with the observation of a *C/EBPε* mutation in patients with a rare specific granule deficiency.[109,110,127,128] PU.1, C/EBPβ, and C/EBPδ also appear at the promyelocyte myelocyte

transition, but in contrast to C/EBPε, continue to increase as the cells mature to neutrophils. ELF-1 reappears at the metamyelocyte stage followed by C/EBPξ, c-Jun, and c-fos that are expressed at the band cell stage and increase in content as the cells mature.[99]

MicroRNA

MicroRNAs (miRNAs) are important regulators of protein synthesis. In general, they bind to the 3′-end of mRNA and inhibit translation. Just like genes for granule proteins, mRNAs are expressed during maturation of neutrophils in the marrow depending on the stage of neutrophil maturation and can be classified into six groups, each with its characteristic expression profile.[129] So far, miRNAs have been shown to regulate proteins of importance for proliferation but not (yet) expression of individual granule proteins. Expression of the myeloid-specific miRNA-223 increases during maturation of neutrophils in the marrow, and after their release into the circulating. One of the targets of miRNA-223 is the Mef2c transcription factor. Mice that lack miRNA-223 expand granulopoiesis and the mature neutrophils mount an enhanced respiratory burst in response to phorbol myristate acetate (PMA), indicating that miRNA-223 acts as a negative regulator of granulopoiesis and neutrophil activation.[130] miRNA-130a is highly expressed in myeloblasts and promyelocytes and targets SMAD4, which, despite a high level of mRNA in promyelocytes, is not expressed at the protein level, and the cells are consequently insensitive to growth inhibition by transforming growth factor β (TGF-β)–induced growth inhibition. miRNA-130a also inhibits C/EBPε which induces exit from cell cycle and growth arrest at the myelocyte stage. Hence, miRNA-130a seems important for the expansion of myeloblasts, promyelocytes and early myelocytes.[131,132]

FUNCTION OF INDIVIDUAL GRANULE PROTEINS AND THEIR ROLE IN OXIDATIVE AND NONOXIDATIVE MICROBIAL KILLING

Proteins of Azurophil Granules

Table 66–1 lists the physical-chemical and functional properties of neutrophil granules.

The protein MPO is a marker of azurophil granules. It is formed as a 90-kDa precursor with an internal disulphide bridge that forms a link between the 57- and 13.5-kDa subunits that are generated by the proteolytic processing that takes place during routing to granules. The heme group, which is necessary for the reduction-oxidation (redox) functions of MPO, associates with the 90-kDa subunit.[133] This seems to be a necessary prerequisite for subsequent processing.[134] MPO reacts with H_2O_2, formed by the NADPH oxidase, and increases the toxic potential of this oxidant. Through oxidation of chloride, tyrosine, and nitrite, the hydrogen peroxide (H_2O_2)-MPO system induces formation of hypochlorous acid (HOCl), other chlorination products, tyrosine radicals, and reactive nitrogen intermediates, each of which can attack the surface membrane of microorganisms.[135,136] MPO may be found on endothelial cells during inflammation and can inactivate nitric oxide (NO).[137] In addition to the activities of MPO itself, MPO is known for the anti-MPO autoantibodies that are characteristic of the pANCAs (perinuclear antineutrophil cytoplasmic antibodies) that are found in vasculitides, in particular those that primarily affect kidneys.[138,139]

BPI is a 55-kDa protein with high homology to the LPS-binding protein of plasma. It is organized into two largely symmetrical subdomains, one of which is responsible for the binding of LPS and for the antimicrobial activity against Gram-negative microorganisms. In contrast to LPS-binding protein, which presents endotoxin to CD14 and elicits a proinflammatory response, BPI binds LPS independent of CD14 and neutralizes the effects of LPS.[140] A transgene expressing

TABLE 66–1. Physical-Chemical and Functional Properties of Neutrophil Granules

Granule Protein	Localization	Physicochemical Properties	Function
Myeloperoxidase	Azurophil granule (AG)	Heme protein, 90-kDa proform with an internal disulphide bond between the 57- and the 13.5-kDa subunits, generated by proteolytic processing that takes place during routing to granules	The MPO–halide–H_2O_2 system generates hypochlorous acid (HÓCl), other chlorination products, tyrosine radicals, and reactive nitrogen intermediates, each of which can attack the surface membrane of microorganisms
Bacterial permeability-increasing (BPI) protein	AG	55-kDa protein with high homology to the LPS-binding protein of plasma	BPI is organized into two largely symmetrical subdomains one of which is responsible for the binding of lipopolysaccharide (LPS) and for the antimicrobial activity against Gram-negative microorganisms
Defensins: three a-defensins; human neutrophil peptides (HNPs) 1–3	AG	7-kDa proforms processed by proteolytic cleavage to mature 3-kDa defensins that share a characteristic three disulfide bond motif: 1–6, 2–4, 3–5	Defensins are small, amphipathic, pore-forming, antibacterial cationic peptides with a broad spectrum of antibacterial activity
Serine proteases of azurophil granules: elastase, cathepsin G, proteinase 3, and neutrophil serine protease 4 (NSP4); azurocidin (CAP37 or heparin-binding protein [HBP]) is enzymatically inactive	AG	28-kDa proforms, processed to active proteases en route to azurophil granules	Serine proteases, but both elastase and cathepsin G have direct antibacterial activities that are not dependent on their enzymatic activity; proteinase 3 liberates the antibacterial peptide LL37 from hCAP-18; HBP is chemotactic for monocytes; HBP may open endothelial cell tight junctions
Lysozyme	AG ~30%; specific granules (SG) ~50%; gelatinase granules (GG) ~20%	Cationic antimicrobial peptide of 14 kDa; in contrast to many neutrophil granule proteins, lysozyme is inefficiently targeted to granules and circulates free in plasma in a substantial quantity that reflects the normal myelopoietic activity	Lysozyme cleaves peptidoglycan-polymers of bacterial cell walls and displays bactericidal activity toward the nonpathogenic Gram-positive bacteria *Bacillus subtilis*; a particular high serum level is characteristic for the myelomonocytic leukemias
Lactoferrin	SG	78-kDa iron chelator; member of the transferrin protein family with a high affinity for iron and similar iron-binding characteristics as ferritin	The antibacterial activity of lactoferrin does not depend exclusively on its ability to sequester iron. Proteolytic fragments, some of which are known as lactoferricin, are directly bactericidal
Neutrophil gelatinase-associated lipocalin (NGAL) or siderochelin	SG	25-kDa N-glycosylated member of the lipocalin protein family	NGAL is the first known siderophore-binding eukaryotic protein; NGAL binds enterochelin/enterobactin with high affinity, and blocks growth of *Escherichia coli* by sequestering siderophore–iron complexes
hCAP-18	SG	18 kDa; only human member of the cathelicidin protein family	Stored and released intact; binds endotoxin; C-terminal antibactericidal peptide, LL-37 released by proteinase 3; active mainly against Gram-positive bacteria, is chemotactic for T cells, monocytes, and neutrophils, and has angiogenetic properties
Neutrophil collagenase	SG	75-kDa matrix metalloproteinase 8 (MMP-8); like other MMPs, MMP-8 is stored inactive and must be N-terminally trimmed to remove the inhibitory peptide	Active against types I, II, and III collagen
Olfactomedin 4 (OLFM4)	SG	65-kDa protein that forms multimers by disulfide bonding	Function is unknown, but OLFM4 is present only in a subset (25%) of neutrophils
Gelatinase	GG	92-kDa MMP-9; stored inactive	Active against type IV collagen
Leukolysin, which is distributed among of resting neutrophils	SG ~10%; GG ~40%; secretory vesicles (SV) ~30%; plasma membranes (PM) ~20%	Leukolysin is a 56-kDa glycosyl-phosphatidylinositol (GPI)-anchored membrane-bound MMP (MT6-MMP/MMP-25)	Active against fibronectin, chondroitin sulfate proteoglycan, dermatan sulfate proteoglycan

(continued)

TABLE 66–1. Physical-Chemical and Functional Properties of Neutrophil Granules (Continued)

Granule Protein	Localization	Physicochemical Properties	Function
Cytochrome b$_{558}$, (gp91^{phox}, p22^{phox})	SG ~60%; GG ~25%; SV ~15%	Heterodimeric flavoheme protein; 91-kDa glycoprotein subunit (heme-flavin binding); 22-kDa protein subunit, possibly heme binding	Together with p47^{phox}, p67^{phox}, and p40^{phox}, cytochrome b$_{558}$ constitutes the superoxide generating nicotinamide adenine dinucleotide phosphate (NADPH) oxidase of phagocytes
CD11b/CD18 (Mac-1, Mo1, CR3, $a_M\beta_2$)	SG ~60%; GG ~25%; SV ~15%	Most prominent β_2-integrin in neutrophils; CD11B = a_M and is a glycoprotein of 170 kDa; CD18 = β_2 and is a glycoprotein of 95 kDa	Multifunctional integrin that functions as an adhesion receptor binding to members of the immunoglobulin family intercellular adhesion molecule (ICAM)-1, to fibronectin, collagen; is important in mediating firm adhesion to vascular endothelial cells; functions as a phagocytosis receptor for C3bi-coated particles
Pentraxin-3	SG	Pentamer of 47-kDa subunits	Binds complement C1q, selected microorganisms
Ficolin-1	GG	Multimer of 32-kDa subunits	Binds acetylated carbohydrates on microorganisms; may activate mannose-binding lectin-associated serine proteases
Arginase 1	GG	37-kDa glycoprotein	Degrades arginine, the substrate for nitric oxide (NO) synthase

high levels of BPI has enhanced resistance against endotoxin.[141] Important effects not related to LPS have been described, such as chemotaxis, opsonization, and dendritic cell function, as reviewed in Ref. 142.

Defensins are small antibacterial cationic peptides with a broad spectrum of antibacterial activity.[143] They share a characteristic three-disulfide-bond motif.[82,144,145] Based on this, mammalian defensins are divided into α defensins, β defensins, and the cyclical θ defensins.[146] Only α defensins are found in human neutrophils, and reside exclusively in azurophil granules. They are by far the dominating proteins of azurophil granules, yet are only expressed in a subset of granules that are formed late in the promyelocyte stage.[83,100,107] Three defensins have been isolated from azurophil granules, HNP-1 to HNP-3.[82] Large amounts of unprocessed defensing, that is, prodefensin, are secreted from late promyelocytes and myelocytes in the marrow and may serve as a marker of normal myelopoietic activity.[111] In contrast to lysozyme and MPO, prodefensins are not expressed by acute leukemia cells. A rise of prodefensin in plasma precedes detectable neutrophils by 6 days and is a measure of normal granulopoiesis which may be of clinical use in the setting of myeloablative treatment for acute leukemia.[111]

The serine proteases of azurophil granules include elastase, cathepsin G, proteinase-3, and NSP4.[147,148] Azurocidin, which is also named CAP37 or heparin-binding protein (HBP), is an enzymatically inactive serine protease.[149-153] Both elastase and cathepsin G have direct antibacterial activities that are not dependent on their enzymatic activity. Proteinase 3 expression leads to autoantibodies against itself in Wegener granulomatosis, which is known as cANCA (cytoplasmic antineutrophil cytoplasmic antibody).[154] Proteinase 3 is also bound to the surface of circulating neutrophils at levels that vary considerably amongst individuals but are highly constant throughout life in a given individual. The binding is mediated by the NB1 antigen (CD177).[155,156] A secreted precursor of proteinase 3 has been suggested to inhibit normal myelopoiesis[157] and to play a role in regulation of myelopoiesis. So far, the only specific substrate of proteinase 3 identified is the cathelicidin of specific granules hCAP-18. Proteinase 3 activates hCAP-18 by removing the cathelicidin part, and unleashing the antibacterial activity of the C-terminal LL-37 peptide.[90] Cathepsin C, also known as dipeptidyl

peptidase 1, removes two inhibitory N-terminal amino acids from the serine proteases prior to their storage in granules.[158] Patients with the Papillon-Lefèvre syndrome lack cathepsin C activity and are not able to store serine proteases in their neutrophils.[159] The condition is characterized by severe juvenile periodontitis and keratosis in hands and feet, but not by major systemic infections,[160] arguing against the notion the serine proteases are important for immune defense.[161]

The membrane of azurophil granules contains CD63 (granulophysin), which is implicated in transmembrane signaling with the β_2 integrins in the activated neutrophil.[85,86,162] Also, the CD68 antigen[100,163] and presenilin appear localized exclusively to the membrane of azurophil granules,[164] whereas stromatin is found in the membrane of all granules[165] and the vacuolar-type H$^+$-ATPase is shared between azurophil, gelatinase granules and secretory vesicles.[166] These membrane proteins will translocate to the phagocytic vacuole or to the plasma membrane when neutrophils are activated and engaged in phagocytosis.

Proteins of Peroxidase-Negative Granules

For an overview, see Table 66–1.

Lactoferrin is the dominating protein of specific granules.[167] It is a 78-kDa iron-chelator, member of the transferrin protein family with a high affinity for iron and similar binding characteristics as ferritin.[168,169] The antibacterial activity of lactoferrin does not depend exclusively on its ability to sequester iron because proteolytic fragments of lactoferrin, some of which are known as lactoferricin, are directly bactericidal.[170,171]

NGAL, or lipocalin 2, is a 25-kDa N-glycosylated member of the lipocalin protein family.[79] Lipocalins are transport proteins that bind small and often lipophilic substances in their canonical lipocalin pocket.[172] Some NGAL is associated with gelatinase (MMP-9) in a subset of specific granules,[173] but the majority is present either as a monomer or as a homodimer in specific granules. NGAL interferes with the activation and stability of MMPs,[174] but the major function of NGAL is to bind and sequester siderophores. NGAL binds enterochelin/enterobactin with high affinity, and blocks growth of *Escherichia coli* by sequestering siderophore-iron complexes,[175] which might not be only a neutrophil-specific antibacterial defense because NGAL can be induced in a variety of epithelial cells during inflammation by IL-1.[176] NGAL has been demonstrated to play a protective role in infections against *E. coli*,[177] *Klebsiella pneumoniae*,[178] *Salmonella typhimurium*,[179] and *Mycobacterium tuberculosis*.[180] NGAL has effects not explained by sequestering bacterial siderophores and was shown to worsen the outcome of pneumococcal pneumonia by deactivating macrophages.[181] It is possible that the ability of NGAL to bind endogenous siderophore-like structures and transport iron may explain some of these effects.[182] Nramp1, the cation transporter, was initially identified first in macrophages as an essential resistance factor against mycobacterial infection. It is present in membranes of both specific and gelatinase-containing neutrophil granules.[93,183]

Lysozyme is a cationic antimicrobial peptide of 14 kDa.[184] In agreement with its biosynthetic profile, lysozyme is present in all granule subsets, with peak concentrations in specific granules.[100,108] Lysozyme cleaves peptidoglycan polymers of bacterial cell walls and displays bactericidal activity toward the nonpathogenic Gram-positive bacteria *Bacillus subtilis*.[185] Lysozyme also binds LPS[186] and reduces cytokine production and mortality caused by LPS in a murine model system of septic shock.[187] In contrast to many neutrophil granule proteins, lysozyme is inefficiently targeted to granules and circulates free in plasma in a substantial quantity that reflects the granulopoietic activity.[107,108] Lysozyme is also secreted from activated macrophages,[188] and a particular elevated serum level is characteristic of the leukemias with a large proportion of monocytes.[189]

hCAP-18,[89] also known as LL-37[190] or CAMP, is the only human member of a family of antimicrobial peptides known as cathelicidins. Cathelicidins are typically found in peroxidase-negative granules of mammalian neutrophils.[191] hCAP-18 is a prominent protein of neutrophil specific granules present in equimolar concentrations with lactoferrin.[192] It is also present in plasma at a substantial concentration bound to lipoproteins.[120] In general, cathelicidins are proantibiotic peptides that share a common and highly conserved 14-kDa N-terminal region known as the cathelin region, whereas the C-terminal regions vary extensively among the different cathelicidins. The C-terminal peptides must be liberated from the cathelin domain by proteolysis to become antibacterial. In most species this is carried out by elastase, but in human neutrophils this is done by proteinase 3 from azurophil granules. The liberated C-terminal peptide is known as LL-37.[90,190] Like several other neutrophil proteins, hCAP-18 is formed by cells in other tissues, particularly epithelial cells.[90,193–195] It is constitutively expressed in the testis and present in semen. Here, the activating protease is gastricin, a prostate protease that is active at low pH. This cleaves hCAP-18 to ALL-38, which has the same antibacterial spectrum as LL-37.[196] The cathelin part, which is released has some protease inhibitory activity by itself.[197] The LL-37 stimulates neutrophil, monocyte, and T-cell chemotaxis via the formyl peptide receptor-like-1.[198] In addition, hCAP-18/LL-37 has angiogenic[199] and endotoxin-neutralizing properties.[200]

Three MMPs have been identified in neutrophils: neutrophil collagenase (MMP-8, 75 kDa), which is localized to specific granules,[201] gelatinase (MMP-9, 92 kDa), which resides predominantly in gelatinase granules,[78,202] and leukolysin (MT6-MMP/MMP-25, 56 kDa), which is distributed among specific granules (approximately 10 percent), gelatinase granules (approximately 40 percent), secretory vesicles (approximately 30 percent), and the plasma membrane (approximately 20 percent) of resting neutrophils.[94,203] The MMPs are stored as inactive proforms that are proteolytically activated following exocytosis. Together, the MMPs are capable of degrading major structural components of the extracellular matrix, including collagens, fibronectin, proteoglycans, and laminin, and they are believed to be of central importance for the degradation of vascular basal membranes and interstitial structures during neutrophil extravasation and migration.

Two pattern-recognition molecules, pentraxin 3 and ficolin1, are found in specific granules and gelatinase granules, respectively. Pentraxin 3, a member of the long pentraxins family, is synthesized in myelocytes and metamyelocytes and stored in specific granules of neutrophils. Pentraxin-3 binds the complement component C1q and mediates activation of the classical complement cascade. In addition, pentraxin-3 binds *K. pneumoniae* outer membrane protein A (KpOmpA) from Gram-negative bacteria, especially the *Enterobacteriaceae* species, and binds *Aspergillus fumigatus* conidia. Pentraxin-3 was shown to play a major role in uptake and killing of *A. fumigatus* conidia by neutrophils in a mouse model.[204,205]

Ficolin-1 is present in gelatinase granules. Ficolin-1 binds acetylated carbohydrate structures on Gram-positive bacteria and can recruit mannose-binding lectin-associated serine proteases (MASPs) and activate the lectin complement cascade.[206]

Arginase-1 is a constituent of gelatinase granules[207] and may participate in regulation of T-cell activities by removing arginine, the essential substrate for inducible nitrous oxide synthase. The product, proline, is essential for collagen synthesis and arginase-1 from neutrophils may thus support wound healing.

Olfactomedin 4, a 65-kDa specific granule protein, forms huge multimers, but only in approximately 25 percent of neutrophils, ranging from 5 to 40 percent between individuals and constant in each individual. The functional consequence is unknown.[208,209]

Membrane proteins of peroxidase-negative granules are shared among the subsets of peroxidase-negative granules that can be distinguished based on their matrix proteins; that is, specific and azurophil granules. Two exceptions are Nramp1 and MMP-25, which are both present, predominantly in the membrane of gelatinase granules and secretory vesicles.[93,94] Cytochrome b_{558}, which is comprised of gp91^{phox} and p22^{phox}, forms the membrane component of the NADPH oxidase and is a prominent membrane protein of peroxidase-negative granules.[81,210] It codistributes with the major β_2-integrin of neutrophils CD11b/CD18, with the major segment in specific granules, some in gelatinase granules, and some in secretory vesicles. Secretory vesicles are rapidly mobilized, and even though only 15 percent of the total cytochrome b_{588} and CD11b localizes to secretory vesicles, this is the fraction that is primarily translocated to the plasma membrane during neutrophil diapesis.[66,32] Hv1is a voltage-gated proton channel situated in the plasma membrane and membranes of peroxidase-negative granules.[211] Hv1 associates with nascent phagosomes, and neutralizes the negative charge induced by transport of electrons by the NADPH oxidase.[212,213] The CD66 antigens found in the membrane of specific granules may play a role as bacterial receptors (galectin receptors) and generate signals to activate the NADPH oxidase.[214,215]

STIMULUS-RESPONSE COUPLING BY NEUTROPHILS

Stimulus-response coupling by neutrophils has been the subject of intense research for many years. This work has been fruitful in illuminating some of the underlying causes of defects in cell activation. Studies of neutrophil degranulation and oxidative metabolism have also revealed transduction mechanisms common to a wide variety of other important secretory cell types, thereby greatly expanding the relevance of this work. This chapter considers next our current understanding of the activation process, which is shown schematically in Fig. 66–4.

RECEPTOR–LIGAND INTERACTIONS
Formyl Peptide Receptor
Neutrophil responses can be evoked by a variety of particulate and soluble stimuli. Opsonized particles, immune complexes, and

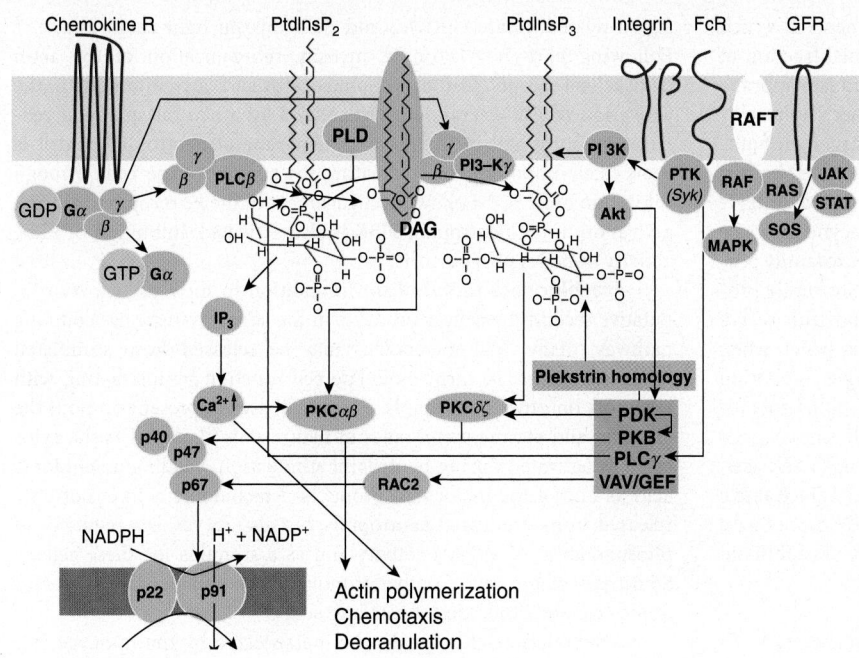

Figure 66–4. Signal transduction in neutrophils. G-protein–coupled receptors are seven transmembrane receptors that couple to heterotrimeric guanosine triphosphate (GTP)-binding (G) proteins. Agonist binding to the receptor triggers exchange of guanine diphosphate (GDP) for guanine triphosphate (GTP) on the Gα subunit of the G-protein, and consequently, the disassociation of the α subunit for the βg-dimer. Both subunits can regulate the activity of multiple effectors such as phospholipase Cβ (PLCβ). PLCβ cleaves an endogenous lipid, namely phosphatidylinositol bisphosphate (PtdInsP$_2$), yielding diacylglycerol (DAG) and inositol trisphosphate (IP$_3$). IP$_3$ is known to liberate calcium from bound intracellular stores leading to a rise in intracellular-free calcium (Ca^{2+})i. The increase in intracellular Ca^{2+} is augmented by an influx of Ca^{2+} from the extracellular space. Increased DAG, in concert with elevated Ca^{2+} can activate protein kinase isozymes α and β (PKC$\alpha\beta$) leading to their translocation to membranous sites. Phospholipase D (PLD) can be activated by PKC converting phosphatidylcholine to phosphatidic (PA) acid. Elevations in PA can mobilize the cytosolic proteins, p47, p67^{phox}, and p40^{phox} to bind to the membrane-bound proteins gp91^{phox} and p22^{phox}, which then reduces O$_2$ to O$_{2-}$ in the presence of NADPH.

chemokine and chemotactic factors produced during the inflammatory process activate neutrophils by binding to specific cell-surface receptors. Of the neutrophil chemotactic receptors, the *N*-formyl peptide receptor is the best characterized. *N*-formyl peptide, the synthetic analogues of bacterial *N*-formyl peptide products, induces a variety of neutrophil responses and has been extensively employed as activating stimuli. Specific receptors for the chemotactic peptide, fMLP, have been identified on the neutrophil surface,[216] and binding of the formyl peptide to its receptor correlates with its ability to induce chemotaxis and degranulation.[217] The formyl peptide receptor,[218] like the receptors for C5a, IL-8, LTB$_4$, and PAF, belongs to a family of seven *trans*-membrane–spanning domain proteins (7TMRs) that are coupled to heterotrimeric G-proteins (containing G α and β,γ subunits).[219,213] Upon ligand binding, guanine diphosphate (GDP) bound to the Gα subunit is exchanged with guanine triphosphate (GTP) and the β,γ subunits dissociate from the receptor and mediate downstream signaling. Phosphorylation of the receptors then augments their affinity for β arrestins. The association with β arrestins block association with β,γ subunits and mediate internalization of the receptors, but may also induce additional signals via β arrestins.[220,221] The formyl peptide receptor has been studied in most detail in neutrophils. The receptor is highly glycosylated and has a relative molecular mass (Mr) of 50 to 70 kDa. It has been identified on the membranes of gelatinase granules and secretory vesicles, and shown to be mobilized to the cell surface following stimulation.[222]

C5a Receptor

Activation of the complement system generates C5a, a derivative of C5 and the most potent of the chemotactic proteins. C5a induces neutrophil chemotaxis, degranulation, and superoxide generation.[222,223] Responses to C5a result from interactions with specific receptors on the cell surface.[222,224] The receptor was identified as a single polypeptide in the plasma membrane with an apparent mass of 40 to 48 kDa.[222,225] Binding studies show that there are 50,000 to 113,000 receptor sites per cell with a dissociation constant (Kd) of 2×10^{-9} M. The C5a receptor has been isolated and cloned, and is a member of the seven transmembrane-spanning class of G-protein–coupled receptors.[226]

Three other important G-protein–coupled receptors are for PAF, IL-8, and LTB$_4$. PAF and IL-8 receptors have been cloned.[227,228] Their intracellular stores and signal transduction mechanisms are largely similar to those used by other G-protein–coupled receptors (e.g., fMLP).[227] IL-8 has two related receptors, for which slightly different signal transduction pathways have been detected.[229]

C3 Receptors

Neutrophils also express receptors for the complement-derived chemotactic factors C3b and C3bi. Receptors for C3b and C3bi (also known as CR1 and CR3, respectively) are sparse on resting neutrophils, but increase significantly in numbers following activation with several stimuli because of incorporation from secretory vesicles (CR1 and CR3) and gelatinase and specific granules (CR3, which is the integrin Mac-1).[32,71] The C3b receptor (CR1) is a glycoprotein with a molecular weight of 205 kDa and is located in secretory vesicles.[65,71]

Integrins

CD11/CD18 integrins also play an important role in cell signaling. The adhesion of cells to surfaces or to other cells can either activate neutrophils directly or "prime" them for an enhanced response to other stimuli. For example, the oxidative burst of neutrophils is very different in cells that are suspended versus those that are adherent to surfaces.[230] H$_2$O$_2$ production in response to chemotaxins is influenced by monoclonal antibodies to CD11b, but not CD11a.[231]

Fc Receptors

Neutrophils possess three different receptors for immunoglobulins. Unstimulated cells express FcγRIIA and FcγRIII, also known as CD32 and CD16, respectively. Functionally, the most important of the two is the FcγRIII for clearing immune complexes,[232] and it is attached to the membrane by a GPI linkage.[232] The linkage is relatively labile, so the amount of FcγRIII on the membrane reflects a balance between shedding and mobilization from intracellular stores. FcγRIIA is a protein that spans the plasma membrane.[233] The signal transduction pathways initiated by FcγRIII can crosstalk with the formyl peptide receptor, with CR3, and even with each other. A direct physical linkage between

CD11b and FcγRIIIB has been demonstrated by experiments in which capping of one receptor results in co-capping a substantial fraction of the other receptor. CD11b can also interact with the transmembrane FcγRII, and both of these molecules can modify each other's signals.[234]

The tyrosine kinase Syk, plays a critical role in the phagocytic pathway mediated by FcγRIIA.[235] A cytoplasmic amino acid motif, known as ITAM, is present on FcγRIIA and FcγRI/γ (a receptor found on IFN-γ–stimulated myeloid cells) and is essential for the phagocytic response during crosslinking of these two Fc receptors. Binding of Src family protein tyrosine kinases to the ITAM leads to activation of Src family protein tyrosine kinases and ITAM tyrosine phosphorylation. This serves to recruit phosphatidylinositol 3′-kinase (PI3K) and Syk, which when activated phosphorylates multiple substrates, including neighboring ITAMs. Syk is recruited from the cytosolic pool. The essential role for Syk-affecting signal transduction is reflected by ITAM-dependent activation of actin assembly. Other tyrosine kinases, including Src kinases, especially Lyn, facilitate the formation of the phagosome.[236] Once active microfilaments are formed, they enhance the activity of phospholipase D (PLD) to generate phosphatidic acid (PA), a necessary phospholipid for phagocytosis to ensue.[237,238]

Phospholipid Metabolism and Tyrosine Kinase Activation

The next step in signal transduction can be attributed to interactions of receptor-activated G proteins or through FcγRIIA and tyrosine kinases with phospholipases.[239,240] For instance, a membrane-associated phosphoinositide-specific phospholipase is activated upon stimulation with chemotactic stimuli. In particular, phospholipase C (PLC) hydrolyzes phosphatidylinositol-4,5-bisphosphate (PIP_2) and phosphatidyl inositol-4-monophosphate (PIP_1) to the putative second-messenger products inositol 1,4,5-trisphosphate (IP_3) and 1,2-diacylglycerol (DAG) (see Fig. 66–4).[241] In neutrophils, IP_3 interacts with a specific intracellular receptor and stimulates the release of Ca^{2+}, as well as opens Ca^{2+} channels on the plasma membrane, resulting in rises in intracellular Ca^{2+}.[242] Activation of the small GTP-binding proteins of the Rac, Rho, and Cdc42 families regulates actin-dependent processes such as membrane ruffling, formation of pseudopodia, and stress fibers leading to cell adhesion and motility, and appears critical in neutrophil function,[243,244] while working in concert with the phospholipases.

Even in the absence of PLC metabolism, there is a significant increase in DAG and Ca^{2+} intracellularly that accompanies phagocytosis.[245] Ca^{2+} is necessary for granule phagosome fusion and DAG has been linked to both particle ingestion and degranulation.[246] Both can be formed by the activation of PLD, which hydrolyzes phosphatidylcholine to produce PA and choline. Activation of PLD is mediated by Rho and/or ADP-ribosylation factor (ARF).[247] Diacylglycerol is then generated by PA phosphohydrolase, which catalyzes the dephosphorylation of PA. The hallmark of the phosphatidylcholine-derived DAG is the presence of 1-O-alkyl linkages. During PA formation by the action of PLD on phosphatidylcholine, PA can act as a Ca^{2+} ionophore, thereby initiating fusogenic activity.[248] Thus, the phosphatidylcholine acid generated during phagocytosis may promote fusion of neutrophil granules with newly formed phagosomes.

Another downstream target of DAG in phagocytosis is the activation of protein kinase C (PKC), particularly PKCδ, a Ca^{2+}-independent isozyme of PKC found in neutrophils.[237] PKCδ is one of four PKC isozymes that translocate to the plasma membrane during phagocytosis. During phagocytosis, PKCδ is translocated from the cytosol to the plasma membrane. Accompanying the translocation of PKCδ to the membrane, RAF-1 translocation is promoted. Following translocation of these two key components, mitogen-activated extracellular signal-regulated kinase (MEK) activation occurs, which is followed by activation of mitogen-activated protein (MAP) kinase/extracellular

signal-related kinase (ERK)-2 and then myosin light-chain kinase.[240] Following phosphorylation of myosin, reorganization of the actin cytoskeletal occurs leading to phagocytosis. Concomitant with the activation of PLD, ceramide is generated by a neutral sphingomyelinase activity found in the plasma membrane of neutrophils and it is most likely important in attenuating the activity of the cells through inhibition of PLD.[240] Following engagement of the Fc receptors and Syk activation in the neutrophil, PI3K is also activated. Inhibition of PI3K activity impedes phagocytosis.[237]

Arachidonate Metabolism In addition to their participation as putative second-messenger products in the stimulus–response coupling pathway, many lipid metabolites may be released from stimulated neutrophils, and, in turn, modulate cell function by interacting with receptors on other neutrophils. Phospholipase A_2, present on both the granules and plasma membranes of neutrophils,[249] as well as the cytosol,[250] is activated during neutrophil stimulation, yielding arachidonic acid as one of the major end products. Arachidonic acid is not only released from stimulated neutrophils, but also serves as a regulator of phospholipase A_2 (PLA_2) activity and as a stimulus for these cells.[251] Sensitivity of the cells to other stimuli can be enhanced with arachidonic acid and other long-chain fatty acids.[252]

Arachidonic acid can also be metabolized by the lipoxygenase pathway to produce hydroxyeicosatetraenoic acids (HETEs), including 5-HETE, 12-HETE, and 5,12-diHETE.[253] These compounds have also been shown to induce several neutrophil responses.[254] Stimulated neutrophils also produce the diHETE LTB_4 through the lipoxygenase pathway. LTB_4 and other leukotrienes can be released in response to a variety of stimuli.[255] Receptors for LTB_4 have been partially purified, and their activation serves as a potent stimulus for chemotaxis and adherence.[256]

Another potent mediator of inflammation produced by stimulated neutrophils is 1-O-alkyl-2-acetyl-sn-glyceryl-3-phosphoryl choline, also known as PAF.[21] Not only is PAF synthesized by neutrophils and activated endothelial cells, but it induces degranulation, aggregation, and superoxide generation.[29] Inflamed endothelium generates PAF, which serves to immobilize neutrophils on the luminal surface of the endothelial cells, thereby facilitating the interaction of the neutrophil integrin receptors with the ICAM ligands on the endothelial cells.

Degranulation and Membrane Fusion

In stimulated cells the signal transduction cascade activates G proteins, followed by enhanced intracellular Ca^{2+}, lipid remodeling, and protein kinase activation. These events culminate in secretion. This ultimate event—the fusion of granule membranes with phagosomes or the plasma membrane—occurs rapidly and is highly efficient.

Fusion Proteins Over the past 20 years the SNARE (soluble *N*-ethylmaleimide-sensitive factor attachment protein receptor) hypothesis has become the reigning paradigm for fusion of biomembranes.[104] The hypothesis is centered around the protein that is sensitive to *N*-ethylmaleimide (designated *NEM-sensitive fusion protein* or *NSF*) and several SNAREs on the participating membranes. The SNAREs are divided into the v-SNAREs, being found on vesicles or granules, and t-SNAREs, being found on the target plasma membranes. The SNARE hypothesis has proven to have great predictive value as the constellation of fusion proteins and their interactions appears in almost all species and tissues. Initial docking of granules with the membrane to which they fuse is likely mediated by Rab-GTPases. Once docking is obtained, SNAREs are recruited to both membranes and interact and mediate actual fusion assisted by SNARE-interacting proteins such as sSec1/Munc18 proteins and a local rise in Ca^{2+}. Disassembly of the fusion complex is mediated by NSF in an ATP-dependent process.[257] The t-SNARE

VAMP-2 is localized to the membranes of specific and gelatinase granule and secretory vesicles in resting human neutrophils,[105,106] and the t-SNARE syntaxin 4 is associated with the plasma membrane as shown by immunoelectron microscopy. Munc18–3 may interact with syntaxin 4 and regulate fusion of secondary and gelatinase granules. VAMP-7 is associated with azurophil granule fusion and Munc18–2 may interact with syntaxin 3 and regulate azurophil granule fusion.[258,259]

Neutrophil Extracellular Traps

What previously was considered pus was identified as a highly bactericidal structure composed of strands of chromatin and bactericidal neutrophil granule proteins attached.[260,261] These NETs (see Fig. 66–2) are extruded from neutrophils in a process called *netosis* and represent one of three death programs of neutrophils: apoptosis, necrosis, and netosis. Neutrophils only undergo netosis if they have mounted a respiratory burst.[262] Elastase and MPO are also required for netosis.[263] The NADPH oxidase activity of stimulated neutrophils thus serves two purposes, namely to generate reactive oxygen species for microbial killing and to induce formation of the bactericidal NETs after the intact neutrophil has ceased to function. This, in turn, means that patients with defective NADPH oxidase assembly (patients with chronic granulomatous disease [CGD]) lack both the ability to generate microbicidal oxygen species and the ability to form the NETs. Patients with the Papillon-Lefèvre syndrome (PLS) lack elastase and are incapable of generating NETs. PLS patients do not have a major immune defect and their symptoms are largely related to periodontal infections, in contrast to CGD patients. Negative effects of NETs have been noted as NETs may induce thrombosis.[264] Neutrophils are able to generate NETs and maintain their structural integrity as an anucleate cell still capable of migration and phagocytosis.[265]

● CLINICAL DISORDERS OF NEUTROPHIL FUNCTION

CLASSIFICATION

Neutrophil dysfunction may arise from (1) the absence of antibodies or complement components required to opsonize microorganisms, an interaction that provides a chemotactic signal; (2) the abnormalities of cytoplasmic and granule movement that alter the chemotactic response or that result in abnormalities of the plasma membrane affecting the cells in terms of capability to modulate movement; and (3) defective microbicidal capability. Comprehensive reviews of these syndromes are available to the interested reader.[266–268]

ABNORMALITIES OF THE SIGNAL MECHANISM AS A RESULT OF ANTIBODY AND COMPLEMENT DEFECTS OR IMPAIRMENT OF PATTERN RECEPTOR RECOGNITION

Because the synergistic action of immunoglobulins and complement proteins creates the opsonins that coat microorganisms and stimulate the development of chemotactic factors, a deficiency of either one may result in impaired neutrophil function. The most profound disturbances arise from abnormalities in C3, because this protein is the focal point for generation of opsonins and chemotactic factors (Chap. 19).[269–271] Opsonins such as C3b, generated from cleavage of C3, serve to coat bacteria. Opsonization in general refers to the coating of pathogens by serum proteins such that they are more likely to be ingested. Activation of C3 can occur in the absence of an antibody or the classical complement components C1, C2, and C4; thus, disorders of these latter molecules result in less-severe clinical conditions. C3 deficiency is inherited as an autosomal recessive disorder. Homozygotes have undetectable serum levels of C3 and suffer from recurrent severe pyrogenic infections, whereas asymptomatic heterozygotes have half the normal values.

A functional deficiency of C3 protease resulting in severe pyrogenic infections also is seen in patients with a deficiency in C3b inactivator, a protein inhibitor of the alternative complement pathway. Unchecked activation of this pathway leads to hypercatabolism of C3 and factor B.[272] Properidin deficiency also results in a functional deficiency in C3.[273] Properidin is a serum protein that belongs to the alternative complement pathway; it is involved in the stabilization of the enzyme complex C3bBb. The protein is a multimeric glycoprotein with a subunit Mr of 56,000, the gene of which has been cloned.[274] Absence of properidin is associated with severe, often fatal, pyrogenic infections, often with meningococci.

Approximately 5 percent of the population have low serum levels of mannose-binding lectin (MBL),[275] a serum lectin secreted by the liver that binds mannose sugars present and on the surface of bacteria, fungi, and some viruses. MBL is one of the soluble collectin effector proteins that contribute to the basic armamentarium of innate immunity. MBL can function as an opsonin when bound to the surfaces by activating the complement cascade. A deficiency of MBL has been reported in infants with frequent unexplained infection, chronic diarrhea, and otitis media.[275] Other studies have identified an increased susceptibility to infection by specific pathogens in MBL-deficient individuals, including human immunodeficiency virus, *Plasmodium falciparum*, *Cryptosporidium parvum*, and *Neisseria meningitidis*.[276] The deficiency in MBL largely results from three relatively common single-point mutations in exon 1 of the gene, which leads to the failure of MBL to activate complement.[277] In addition, the protein also modulates disease severity, at least in part through complex, dose-dependent influences on cytokine production.

Phagocytes, including neutrophils, express a large number of cell surface proteins that play crucial functional roles in their biology. Microbial PRRs are an essential component of innate immunity, in which they recognize and detect PAMPs, resulting in activation of neutrophils and other phagocytes. The mammalian TLR family comprises an important class of PRRs, which recognize a wide range of microbial pathogens and pathogen-related products. At least 12 different TLRs that can be found on mononuclear phagocytes have been described.[278] TLRs signal via MyD88, an adapter protein. MyD88 deficiency in humans can lead to recurrent infections with both Gram-positive and Gram-negative infections, thereby indicating a role for both mononuclear cells and neutrophils in host defense in the MyD88-deficient state.[279]

Because a large number of chemoattractants are generated during inflammation, it is difficult to establish the relative significance of a given individual component. Furthermore, chemotactic factors and opsonins are involved in the activity of both neutrophils and mononuclear phagocytes. Therefore, it is not clear whether the clinical consequences of disorders involving these substances are unique to one or the other of these phagocytic cells. Patients with antibody- or complement-deficient syndromes suffer mainly from infections with encapsulated pathogens such as *Haemophilus influenzae*, pneumococci, streptococci, and meningococci.[280] Furthermore, splenectomized individuals deprived of an organ rich in mononuclear phagocytes have a small, but finite risk of sepsis because of the same microorganisms. Encapsulated pathogens characteristically are not associated with neutropenic states. Antibody coating of encapsulated organisms facilitates their ingestion by mononuclear phagocytes, but may be less important for their ingestion by neutrophils.

ABNORMALITIES OF THE CELLULAR RESPONSES AS THE RESULTS OF DEFECTS IN CYTOPLASMIC MOVEMENT

Degranulation Abnormalities

Chédiak-Higashi Syndrome

Definition and History This rare autosomal recessive disease was initially recognized as one in which neutrophils, monocytes, and lymphocytes contained giant cytoplasmic granules.[281] Chédiak-Higashi syndrome (CHS) is now recognized as a disorder of generalized cellular dysfunction characterized by increased fusion of cytoplasmic granules.[282] Pigmentary dilution affecting the hair, skin, and ocular fundi results from pathologic aggregation of melanosomes and is associated with failure of decussation of the optic and auditory nerves (Table 66–2).[283] Patients with this syndrome exhibit an increased susceptibility to infection, which begins in infancy. Infections most commonly involve the skin and respiratory systems. The susceptibility to infection can be explained in part through defects in neutrophil chemotaxis, degranulation, and bactericidal activity.[281] The presence of giant granules in the neutrophil interferes with their ability to traverse narrow passages between endothelial cells. Other features of the disease include neutropenia, thrombocytopathy,[284] natural killer cell abnormalities,[281,285] and peripheral neuropathies.[286] Similar genetic syndromes have been described in mice, mink, cats, rats, cattle, and killer whales.[286]

Although CHS carries the names of Moises Chédiak and Ototaka Higashi, the disorder was first described by Béguez César, a Cuban pediatrician in 1943. Initially characterized by neutropenia and abnormal granules in leukocytes, the syndrome was further delineated in 1948 by Steinbrinck's description of a second case.[287] In 1952, Chédiak reported the hematologic characteristics of the disorder,[288] and in 1953 Higashi emphasized the giant peroxidase-containing granules within patients' neutrophils.[289] Besides the susceptibility to infections, patients often suffer a fatal lymphohistiocytic infiltration known as the accelerated phase occurring months from birth to several years later.[290]

Epidemiology By 2008, 300 cases worldwide had been described, with concentrations in the United States, Japan, northern Europe, and Latin America.[286] Patients of African descent have also been described.

Etiology and Pathogenesis CHS is caused by a fundamental defect in granule morphogenesis that results in abnormally large granules in multiple tissues.[282,291] Giant granules are seen in Schwann cells, leukocytes, and macrophages of the liver and spleen, and certain cells of the pancreas, gastric mucosa, kidney, adrenal gland, and pituitary gland.[286] Giant melanosomes form and prevent the even distribution of melanin, which results in pigmentary dilution of the hair, skin, iris, and optic fundus. Although the giant lysosomes are the primary morphologic feature of the disorder, only cells relying on the secretion by these lysosomes manifest pathologic defects. In the early stages of myelopoiesis some of the normal-size azurophil granules coalesce to form giant granules that result in large secondary lysosomes that contain reduced content of hydrolytic enzymes, including proteinases, elastase, and cathepsin G.[281] Many of the myeloid precursors die in the marrow, resulting in a moderate neutropenia, with white cell counts of about 2.5×10^9/L and absolute neutrophil counts ranging from 0.5 to 2.0×10^9/L.[290] The marrow itself appears normal to hypercellular. In spite of the normal ingestion of particles and active oxygen metabolism, these neutrophils kill microorganisms relatively slowly. This delay reflects a slow and inconsistent delivery of diluted amounts of hydrolytic enzymes from the giant granules into the phagosomes, which may predispose the host to bacterial infection.[291,292] In this syndrome, monocytes have the same functional derangements as neutrophils,[281] and in an analogous fashion perforin-deficient natural killer (NK) cells show profoundly impaired cytotoxic activity and are unable to kill many targets.[293]

The CHS blood cell membranes are more fluid than cells of normal individuals,[281,294] and the altered membrane structure could lead to defective regulation of membrane activation, as well as promoting fusion of neutrophil azurophilic granules with each other. Conceivably, changes in membrane fluidity may affect cell function by reducing expression of Mac-1 (CD11b/CD18). The altered membrane fluidity could result in elevated levels of intracellular cyclic adenosine monophosphate, which appears in this disorder and is reflected in the reduced chemotactic responses.[281]

The gene that is mutated in CHS is *CHS1* (syn. *LYST*) found on chromosome 1q. Its size indicates a protein of more than 400 kDa is encoded.[295] During early development, granule biogenesis is normal; with perforin in NK cells and granule enzymes in myeloid cells synthesized and routed correctly to the granules. However, once formed the granules fuse to form giant organelles.[296] Several studies led to the suggestion that the enlarged lysosomes found in CHS cells are the results of abnormalities in membrane fusion, which could occur during the biogenesis of the lysosomes. It has been hypothesized that this CHS1 protein interacts with attachment proteins on lysosomes (v-SNAREs) and that this mutated protein leads to indiscriminate interactions with v-SNARE to yield uncontrolled fusion of lysosomes with each other.[297]

Clinical Features Characteristically patients with CHS have light skin and silvery hair. They frequently complain of solar sensitivity and photophobia. Other eye findings can include horizontal or rotatory nystagmus. Infections are common and involve the mucous membranes, skin, and respiratory tract. They are susceptible to both Gram-positive and Gram-negative bacteria, as well as fungi, with *Staphylococcus aureus* being the most common infecting organism.[266] Attenuated NK function probably contributes to the increased susceptibility to infection as well. Neurologic signs and symptoms are variable in CHS and may include a peripheral and cranial neuropathy, autonomic dysfunction, weakness, and sensory deficit; and ataxia may also be a prominent feature.

Patients with CHS have prolonged bleeding times with normal platelet counts, resulting from impaired platelet aggregation associated with a deficiency of the storage pools of ADP and serotonin.[284] Electron micrographs reveal normal numbers of α granules in platelets, but decreased numbers of platelet dense bodies.[286]

The accelerated phase of CHS is characterized by lymphocytic proliferation in the liver, spleen, marrow, and central nervous system. The accelerated phase may occur at any age and is now recognized as a genetic form of hemophagocytic lymphohistiocytosis (HLH).[298] Typically, the patient develops hepatosplenomegaly and high fever in the absence of bacterial sepsis. The pancytopenia becomes worse at this stage, producing hemorrhage and an increased susceptibility to infection. The onset of the accelerated phase may be related to the inability of these patients to contain and control the Epstein-Barr virus (EBV) leading to HLH (Chap. 70). The lymphocyte expansion into the tissue is associated with excessive cytokine production and massive tissue necrosis and organ failure leading to the propensity to recurrent bacterial and viral infections, fever, and prostration usually resulting in death.[298] At autopsy, the lymphohistiocytic infiltrates in the liver, spleen, and lymph nodes are extensive, but not neoplastic by histopathologic criteria.[298]

Laboratory Features The laboratory test diagnostic for CHS is examination of granular cell morphology. The pathognomonic feature is giant peroxidase-positive granules that can be seen in neutrophils.[289] A microscopic examination of hair shafts reveal large, speckled pigment clumps as opposed to the normal pattern of finally divided pigment of melanin spread along the length of the shaft.[286] Similar giant granules can occasionally be present in CML and acute myelocytic leukemia.[286] Molecular diagnosis of CHS remains difficult and is not commercially available. Heterozygotes for CHS are considered completely normal and cannot be detected clinically or biochemically.

TABLE 66–2. Clinical Disorders of Neutrophil Function

Disorder	Etiology	Impaired Function	Clinical Consequence
DEGRANULATION ABNORMALITIES			
Chédiak-Higashi syndrome	Autosomal recessive; disordered coalescence of lysosomal granules; responsible gene is *CHSI/LYST* which encodes a protein hypothesized to regulate granule fusion	Decreased neutrophil chemotaxis; degranulation and bactericidal activity; platelet storage pool defect; impaired NK function, failure to disperse melanosomes	Neutropenia; recurrent pyogenic infections, propensity to develop marked hepatosplenomegaly as a manifestation of the hemophagocytic syndrome
Specific granule deficiency	Autosomal recessive; functional loss of myeloid transcription factor arising from a mutation or arising from reduced expression of Gfi-1 or C/EBPε, which regulates specific granule formation	Impaired chemotaxis and bactericidal activity; bilobed nuclei in neutrophils; defensins, gelatinase, collagenase, vitamin B_{12}-binding protein, and lactoferrin	Recurrent deep-seated abscesses
ADHESION ABNORMALITIES			
Leukocyte adhesion deficiency I	Autosomal recessive; absence of CD11/CD18 surface adhesive glycoproteins (β_2 integrins) on leukocyte membranes most commonly arising from failure to express CD18 mRNA	Decreased binding of C3bi to neutrophils and impaired adhesion to ICAM-1 and ICAM-2	Neutrophilia; recurrent bacterial infection associated with a lack of pus formation
Leukocyte adhesion deficiency II	Autosomal recessive; loss of fucosylation of ligands for selectins and other glycol conjugates arising from mutations of the GDP-fucose transporter	Decreased adhesion to activated endothelium expressing ELAM	Neutrophilia; recurrent bacterial infection without pus
Leukocyte adhesion deficiency III (LAD-1 variant syndrome)	Autosomal recessive; impaired integrin function arising from mutations of *FERMT3* which encodes kindlin-3 in hematopoietic cells; kindlin-3 binds to β-integrin and thereby transmits integrin activation	Impaired neutrophil adhesion and platelet activation	Recurrent infections, neutropenia, bleeding tendency
DISORDERS OF CELL MOTILITY			
Enhanced motile responses; FMF	Autosomal recessive gene responsible for FMF on chromosome 16, which encodes for a protein called "pyrin"; pyrin regulates caspase-1 and thereby IL-1β secretion; mutated pyrin may lead to heightened sensitivity to endotoxin, excessive IL-1β production, and impaired monocyte apoptosis	Excessive accumulation of neutrophils at inflamed sites which may be the result of excessive IL-1β production	Recurrent fever, peritonitis, pleuritis, arthritis, and amyloidosis
DEPRESSED MOTILE RESPONSES			
Defects in the generation of chemotactic signals	IgG deficiencies; C3 and properdin deficiency can arise from genetic or acquired abnormalities; mannose-binding protein deficiency predominantly in neonates	Deficiency of serum chemotaxis and opsonic activities	Recurrent pyogenic infections
Intrinsic defects of the neutrophil, e.g., leukocyte adhesion deficiency, Chédiak-Higashi syndrome, specific granule deficiency, neutrophil actin dysfunction, neonatal neutrophils; direct inhibition of neutrophil mobility, e.g., drugs	In the neonatal neutrophil there is diminished ability to express β_2 integrins and there is a qualitative impairment in β_2-integrin function; ethanol, glucocorticoids, cyclic AMP	Diminished chemotaxis; impaired locomotion and ingestion; impaired adherence	Propensity to develop pyogenic infections; possible cause for frequent infections; neutrophilia seen with epinephrine arises from cyclic AMP release from endothelium
Immune complexes	Bind to Fc receptors on neutrophils in patients with rheumatoid arthritis, systemic lupus erythematosus, and other inflammatory states	Impaired chemotaxis	Recurrent pyogenic infections

(continued)

TABLE 66–2. Clinical Disorders of Neutrophil Function (Continued)

Disorder	Etiology	Impaired Function	Clinical Consequence
Hyperimmunoglobulin-E syndrome	Autosomal dominant; responsible gene is *STAT3*	Impaired chemotaxis at times; impaired regulation of cytokine production	Recurrent skin and sinopulmonary infections, eczema, mucocutaneous candidiasis, eosinophilia, retained primary teeth, minimal trauma fractures, scoliosis, and characteristic facies
Hyperimmunoglobulin-E syndrome	Autosomal recessive; more than one gene likely contributes to its etiology	High IgE levels, impaired lymphocyte activation to staphylococcal antigens	Recurrent pneumonia without pneumatoceles sepsis, enzyme, boils, mucocutaneous candidiasis, neurologic symptoms, eosinophilia
MICROBICIDAL ACTIVITY			
Chronic granulomatous disease	X-linked and autosomal recessive; failure to express functional gp91^{phox} in the phagocyte membrane in p22^{phox} (autosomal recessive); other autosomal recessive forms of CGD arise from failure to express protein p47^{phox} or p67^{phox}	Failure to activate neutrophil respiratory burst leading to failure to kill catalase-positive microbes	Recurrent pyogenic infections with catalase-positive microorganisms
G6PD deficiency	Less than 5% of normal activity of G6PD	Failure to activate NADPH-dependent oxidase, and hemolytic anemia	Infections with catalase-positive microorganisms
Myeloperoxidase deficiency	Autosomal recessive; failure to process modified precursor protein arising from missense mutation	H_2O_2-dependent antimicrobial activity not potentiated by myeloperoxidase	None
Rac-2 deficiency	Autosomal dominant; dominant negative inhibition by mutant protein of Rac-2–mediated functions	Failure of membrane receptor–mediated O_2 generation and chemotaxis	Neutrophilia, recurrent bacterial infections
Deficiencies of glutathione reductase and glutathione synthetase	Autosomal recessive; failure to detoxify H_2O_2	Excessive formation of H_2O_2	Minimal problems with recurrent pyogenic infections

AMP, adenosine monophosphate; C, complement; CD, cluster designation; CGD, chronic granulomatous disease; ELAM, endothelial-leukocyte adhesion molecule; FMF, familial Mediterranean fever; G6PD, glucose-6-phosphate dehydrogenase; GDP, glucose diphosphate; ICAM, intracellular adhesion molecule; Ig, immunoglobulin; IL, interleukin; LAD, leukocyte adhesion deficiency; NADPH, nicotinamide adenine dinucleotide phosphate; NK, natural killer.

Data from Remington JS Swartz MN: *Current Clinical Topics in Infectious Disease,* 6th ed. New York, NY: McGraw-Hill; 1985.

Differential Diagnosis The diagnosis of CHS should be considered in individuals with partial albinism, exaggerated bleeding, and recurrent infections. Patients with CHS must be distinguished from those patients with Griscelli syndrome (GS) and Hermansky-Pudlak syndrome (HPS).

GS is a rare disorder, arising from mutations in the *RAB27A* gene, and is defined by partial ocular and cutaneous albinism, variable cellular and humeral immunodeficiency, variable neurologic involvement, and the development of the accelerated phase. Individuals with GS lack giant granules in neutrophils and have large pigment clumps in hair shafts.[286] HPS is a disorder of ocular and cutaneous albinism, bleeding diathesis arising from platelet dysfunction, and deposition of ceroid lipofuscin in various organs (Chap. 120). In contrast to CHS, HPS cells lack giant granules and the patients are not predisposed to recurrent infections.[286]

Therapy High-dose ascorbic acid (200 mg/day for infants, 2 g/day for adults) improves the clinical status of some patients with CHS in the stable phase.[281] Although there is controversy regarding the efficacy

of ascorbic acid, given the safety of the vitamin,[286] it is reasonable to administer it to all patients. CHS presents a therapeutic dilemma, particularly when the accelerated phase begins. Prophylactic antibiotics do not prevent infections. The only potential for curative therapy for preventing the accelerated phase is marrow transplantation.[299] Marrow transplantation reconstitutes normal hematopoietic and immunologic function and corrects the NK deficiency in patients before entering the accelerated phase.[299] On the other hand, if the patient is actively in the accelerated phase, stem cell transplantation from a matched unrelated donor is associated with a poor prognosis.[299] Ocular and cutaneous albinism are not corrected after transplantation, nor does transplantation prevent progressive neuropathies from occurring.[300]

Specific Granule Deficiency Specific granule deficiency (SGD) has been described in patients of both sexes and is inherited as an autosomal recessive disorder (see Table 66–2).[281] Besides the absence of specific granules, the nuclei of the neutrophils are bilobed. Patients are afflicted with recurrent infections primarily involving the skin and lungs. *S. aureus* and *Pseudomonas aeruginosa* have been the most commonly observed pathogens, although *Candida albicans* also has been isolated. Specific granule-deficient neutrophils lack gelatinolytic activity in the tertiary granules; vitamin B_{12}-binding protein, lactoferrin, hCAP-18, and collagenase in the specific granules; and defensins in the primary granules.[301-303] This disorder also extends to eosinophils that lack the characteristic eosinophil granule proteins: major basic protein, eosinophilic cationic protein, and eosinophil-derived neurotoxin (Chap. 62).[304] Thus, the disorder is a global defect in phagocytic granules rather than limited to specific granules, as suggested by its name. Neutrophils from these patients are defective in chemotaxis, possibly related to the absence of the intracellular pool of leukocyte adhesion molecules that normally reside in the tertiary and specific granules, and exhibit a mild defect in bactericidal activity, possibly related to the deficiency of the granule constituents, lactoferrin and defensins.[301,305] The impairment in granule protein synthesis affecting the granulocytic cells appears secondary to the functional loss of the myeloid transcription factor, C/EBPε, which was identified in two patients.[109,306] In another case of SGD, the expression of the transcription factor growth factor independence-1 (Gfi-1) was markedly reduced along with a heterozygous mutation of C/EBPε gene.[307] It was suggested that the combined abnormalities blocked specific granule expression leading to the expression of the SGD phenotype. The defect is restricted to blood cells, as normal lactoferrin secretion has been demonstrated in the nasal secretions of an SGD patient despite the abnormality demonstrated in his neutrophils.[302] The diagnosis of SGD is suggested by the presence of neutrophils devoid of specific granules but containing azurophilic granules on the blood film.[281] The diagnosis can be confirmed by demonstrating a severe deficiency in either lactoferrin or hCAP-18. An acquired form of SGD can be observed in thermally injured patients or in individuals with myelodysplasia.[281,308] Treatment of SGD is symptomatic, with the administration of parenteral antibiotics for acute infections and surgical drainage of refractory infections. With aggressive medical management, patients may survive into their adult years.

Adhesion Abnormalities

Leukocyte Adhesion Deficiency

Definition and History Leukocyte adhesion deficiency type I (LAD-1) is a rare autosomal recessive disorder of leukocyte function (see Table 66–2). More than 100 cases have been reported worldwide. The disease is characterized clinically by recurrent soft-tissue infections, delayed wound healing, and severely impaired pus formation despite striking blood neutrophilia.[309] Individuals with this disorder have decreased or absent expression of a family of structurally and functionally related leukocyte surface glycoproteins designated CD11/CD18 complex (also referred to as the β_2-integrin family of leukocyte adhesive proteins; Table 66–3). These proteins include LFA-1 (CD11a/CD18), Mo-1 or Mac-1 (CD11b/CD18), p150,95 (CD11c/CD18), and p160,95 (CD11d/CD18).[309] The CD11 subunits are integral membrane glycoproteins, each spanning the plasma membrane only once. They are approximately 40 percent homologous, suggesting that they arise from a common primordial gene.[309] The three distinct genes encoding the α subunits occur in a cluster on chromosome 16, whereas the gene for the β subunit is located on chromosome 21.[310]

The initial clinical description in 1979 described six children and two families with findings of delayed separation of the umbilical cord and delayed healing at the site of detachment of the cord, recurrent infections despite neutrophilia, neutrophilia persisting during

---

TABLE 66–3. Biologic and Clinical Features of Leukocyte Adherence Deficiencies 1 and 2

	Genetic Defect	Leukocyte Functional Abnormalities	Clinical Features	Diagnosis
LAD-1	Molecular mutations affecting expression of the β_2-integrin CD18	Neutrophils; adherence spreading, homotypic aggregation, chemotaxis receptor CR3 activities: C3bi binding affecting phagocytosis, respiratory burst, and degranulation in response to C3bi-coated particles*	Autosomal recessive; delayed umbilical cord separation; neutrophilia; defective neutrophil migration into tissue; recurrent bacterial infections; impaired wound healing	Flow cytometry for expression of CD11b/CD18 (Mac-1)
		Monocytes; adherence, CR3 activities		
		Lymphocytes; cytotoxic		
		T-lymphocyte activities; NK cytotoxic activities; blastogenesis		
LAD-2 (CDG-IIc)	Mutations affecting function of GDP-fucose transporter 1 resulting in defective glycosylation expression at the $\alpha_{1,3}$-position of selectin ligands including sLe^x and other fucosylated proteins requiring fucosylation	Neutrophils; rolling mediated by sLe^x to endothelium; neutrophilia[†]	Autosomal recessive; recurrent bacterial infections; periodontitis; growth retardation; developmental retardation; Bombay red cell phenotype	Flow cytometry for leukocyte sLe^x (CD15)

CDG-11c, congenital disorder of glycosylation type IIc; GDP, glucose diphosphate; NK, natural killer; sLe^x, sialyl Lewis X.

*These functional abnormalities and clinical features are a consequence of lack of the CD11b/CD18, which includes CD11a, CD11b, CD11c, and CD11d markers of four different α chains and the common β_2-chain CD18 of Mr 95 kDa.

[†]These functional abnormalities and clinical features are a consequence of lack of sLe^x expression on leukocytes.

infection-free periods, and impaired neutrophil chemotaxis.[311] The molecular basis for LAD-1 was first suggested when neutrophils from a patient with the disorder was found to lack a high-molecular-weight membrane glycoprotein.[312] This finding suggested that the lack of the membrane protein impaired the neutrophil's functional responses. In 1982, another patient was evaluated and it was confirmed that the membrane glycoprotein with a Mr of 150 kDa was missing.[313] The normal parents and siblings of the proband exhibited intermediate quantities of the glycoprotein, which suggested the existence of a heterozygous carrier state. The disorder then became known as LAD. Subsequently, in 1984, a glycoprotein 150 was identified as one subunit of a glycoprotein that had two subunits that served as a receptor for a plasma complement component.[314] This was followed by other investigations that found that two other related leukocyte membrane glycoproteins also were deficient. Each of the three glycoproteins was then determined to be heterodimers with one common subunit and one subunit unique to each glycoprotein.[315] Synthesis of a defective subunit common to the three glycoproteins of CD11/CD18 complex resulted in loss of expression of all heterodimers.[316] This observation provided the molecular explanation for the cellular defect. In 1985, the extent of clinical severity and magnitude of the cellular abnormalities were correlated with the degree of CD11/CD18 deficiency, thereby laying the groundwork for the direct relationship between the glycoprotein deficiency and the clinical presentation.[315]

Etiology and Pathogenesis Each of these molecules contains an α and a β subunit noncovalently associated in an $\alpha\beta$ structure. They all have the same β subunit and are distinguished by their α subunits, which have different isoelectric points, molecular weights, and cell distribution (see Table 66–3).[315] The structure of CD11/CD18 has been deduced from molecular cloning of the various subunits.[315] The x-ray crystal structure and nuclear magnetic resonance analysis also reveal that activation signals lead to the separation of the α and β subunit cytoplasmic tails, thereby converting the bent conformation of each integrin with its headpiece near the plasma membrane into fully extended high-affinity structures in a switchblade-like movement.[317] These studies establish that the CD11/CD18 heterodimers are members of a large gene family involved in cell–cell and cell–matrix adhesion (integrins). Several subfamilies of integrins are described and classified according to the type of their highly homologous β subunits. The α subunits are also homologous to each other, but to a lesser degree than are the associated β subunits. Within each subfamily, a single β subunit usually is shared by several α subunits. Certain α subunits often share more than one β subunit, which alters their specificity for various ligands.[315] The molecular defect involves all four members of the CD11 integrin subfamily. In patients with LAD-1 who have been evaluated at the molecular level, absent, diminished, or structurally abnormal β subunits (CD18) were identified.[315] A heterogeneous group of mutations that are confined to the gene on chromosome 21q22.3 also was identified.[315] Many patients have point mutations that result in single amino acid substitutions in CD18, which predominantly reside between amino acids 111 and 361.[315] This peptide domain is highly conserved among all β subunits and appears to be important for interaction with the α subunit. Several affected individuals are compound heterozygotes for two different mutant alleles, whereas others are homozygotes for a single mutant allele. Messenger RNA splicing abnormalities that have been described in two kindreds can result in either deletion or insertion of amino acids in the conserved extracellular domain of CD18. Small deletions within the coding sequences of the CD18 gene disrupting the reading frame or a nucleotide substitution resulting in a premature termination signal has been described. Mutations in CD18 disrupt the association in the $\alpha\beta$ subunits so that maturation, intracellular transport, and all cell surface assembly of functionally active $\alpha\beta$ molecules fail to occur.[315]

Approximately half of patients exhibit a low level of CD11/CD18 cell surface molecules and moderate disease, with the remainder having totally absent surface expression of these proteins, which accounts for a profound impairment of neutrophil and monocyte adherence and adhesion-dependent functions *in vitro*, including cell migration, phagocytosis, and complement- or antibody-dependent cytotoxicity.[315,316]

The bulk of the neutrophil Mac-1 glycoprotein is stored inside the cell in the membrane of neutrophil specific and gelatinase granules and in secretory vesicles.[32,318] Exposure of neutrophils to degranulating stimuli results in a 5- to 10-fold increase in the number of Mac-1 molecules on the cell surface, which parallels the fusion of granules to the plasma membrane.[318] Neutrophils from these patients fail to augment their surface adhesive glycoproteins, as the defect in β-subunit synthesis affects both membrane and granule pools of Mac-1.[319] In contrast to Mac-1 and p150,95, LFA-1 is predominantly confined to the neutrophil plasma membrane. Consequently, the cell surface levels of LFA-1 are not enhanced by neutrophil degranulation.

Lymphocytes deficient in CD11/CD18 are able to adhere to endothelial surfaces via the expression on lymphocytes of very-late antigen-4 (VLA-4) integrin (synonym: integrin $\alpha_4\beta_1$) receptors, which bind to the vascular cell adhesion molecule 1 (VCAM-1), found on the endothelial cells.[320] This residual adhesion may account for the paucity of clinical symptoms related to lymphocyte function. The patients are not unusually susceptible to viral infection, although three patients had one or more episodes of aseptic meningitis.[315]

The failure of the LAD-1 neutrophils to migrate to the sites of inflammation outside of the lung and peritoneum arises from their inability to adhere firmly to surfaces and undergo transendothelial migration from venules.[321-323] Failure of Mac-1–deficient neutrophils to undergo transendothelial migration occurs because β_2 integrins bind to ICAM-1 (CD54) and ICAM-2 expressed on inflamed endothelial cells.[309,324] LAD-1 neutrophils are able to accumulate in the lung, perhaps through a process of movement mediated by "chimneying," which does not require functional integrins.[325] Chemotaxis that occurs despite blockade of CD11/CD18 under special *in vitro* conditions has been dubbed "chimneying." The neutrophils that do arrive at inflammatory sites in the inflamed lung by CD11/CD18-independent processes fail to recognize microorganisms coated with the opsonic complement fragment C3bi (an important stable opsonin formed by the cleavage of C3b by C3b inactivator).[313,326] Other neutrophil functions, such as degranulation and oxidative metabolism, normally triggered by C3bi binding are also diminished and markedly compromised in neutrophils from LAD-1.[309] Similarly, the urokinase-plasminogen activator-receptor and the FcγRIII receptors, both phosphatidylinositol-linked proteins, are defective in their functions because these receptors transduce their signals through CD11/CD18.[234,327] Monocyte function is also impaired. Monocytes of affected individuals have poor fibrinogen-binding function, an activity promoted by the CD11/CD18 complex[309,328]; consequently, such cells are not able to participate effectively in wound healing. Thus, impairment in neutrophil function underlies the propensity to recurrent infections, which is the clinical expression of this disease. Similar genetic syndromes have been discovered in Irish Setter dogs and Holstein cattle.[315] A CD11/CD18-deficient mouse with 2 to 6 percent of normal β_2-integrin expression has been produced by gene targeting.[321,329]

Clinical Features Activated leukocytes of patients with the most-severe clinical form express less than 0.3 percent of the normal amount of the β_2 integrins, whereas those of patients with the moderate phenotype may express 2 to 7 percent of normal numbers of β_2-integrin molecules.[309] The severely affected patients suffer from recurrent and chronic or even gangrenous soft-tissue infections (subcutaneous tissues or mucous membranes), generally by bacterial or fungal microorganisms such as *S. aureus*, *Pseudomonas* spp. and other Gram-negative enteric rods, or *Candida* spp. Patients with the moderate phenotype have fewer and less-severe infections. Infectious susceptibility and impaired wound healing are related to diminished or delayed infiltration of neutrophils and monocytes into extravascular inflammatory sites. In all patients surviving infancy, severe progressive generalized periodontitis is present. Individuals who are clinically well, but who are heterozygous carriers of LAD have been identified. Their stimulated neutrophils express approximately 50 percent of the normal amount of the Mac-1 α subunit and the common β subunit.[309] The diagnosis of LAD-1 should be considered in infants with a paucity of neutrophils at sites of infection despite blood neutrophilia and have a history of delayed separation of the umbilical cord.

Laboratory Features The diagnosis is made most readily by flow cytometric measurement of surface CD11b in stimulated and unstimulated neutrophils using monoclonal antibodies directed against CD11b (Fig. 66–5). Assessment of neutrophil and monocyte adherence, aggregation, chemotaxis, C3bi-mediated phagocytosis, and cytotoxicity generally demonstrates striking abnormalities that are directly related to the molecular deficiency. Delayed-type hypersensitivity reactions are normal, and most individuals have normal specific antibody synthesis. The ability of lymphocytes to generate specific antibodies explains the self-limited course of varicella or viral respiratory infections. However, some patients have impaired T-lymphocyte–dependent antibody responses, for example, to repeat vaccination with tetanus toxoid, diphtheria toxoid, and polio virus.

Patients with LAD-1 usually have blood neutrophil counts of 15 to 60×10^9/L. However, during infectious episodes, they commonly have neutrophil counts in excess of 100×10^9/L and sometimes as high as 160×10^9/L. Granulocytic hyperplasia is a feature of the marrow examination which may relate to excessive production of IL-17 and G-CSF as a result of decreased uptake of apoptotic neutrophils by tissue macrophages.[319,330] Despite elevated blood counts, there is a paucity of neutrophils in inflammatory skin windows and biopsies of infected tissues.

Differential Diagnosis Eight patients (four Arab, two Turkish, one Pakistani, one Brazilian) who had neutrophilia, recurrent bacterial infections, and an inability to form pus have been described.[13,331,332] The patients also had the Bombay blood phenotype (deficiency in H blood group integrins), severe mental retardation, unusual facial appearance, microcephaly, cortical atrophy, seizures, hypotonia, and short stature (see Table 66–2). Functionally, the neutrophils were unable to adhere to E-selectin or cytokine-activated endothelial cells and exhibited impaired chemotaxis and an inability to roll on postcapillary venules *in vivo*. The patients are now classified as having LAD-2 or congenital disorder of glycosylation type IIc (CDG-IIc).[333] In contrast to LAD-1, the patients' NK cell activity is normal. The LAD-2 neutrophils express normal levels of CD18 integrins, but are deficient in the carbohydrate structure sLe^x, which renders the cells unable to roll on activated endothelial

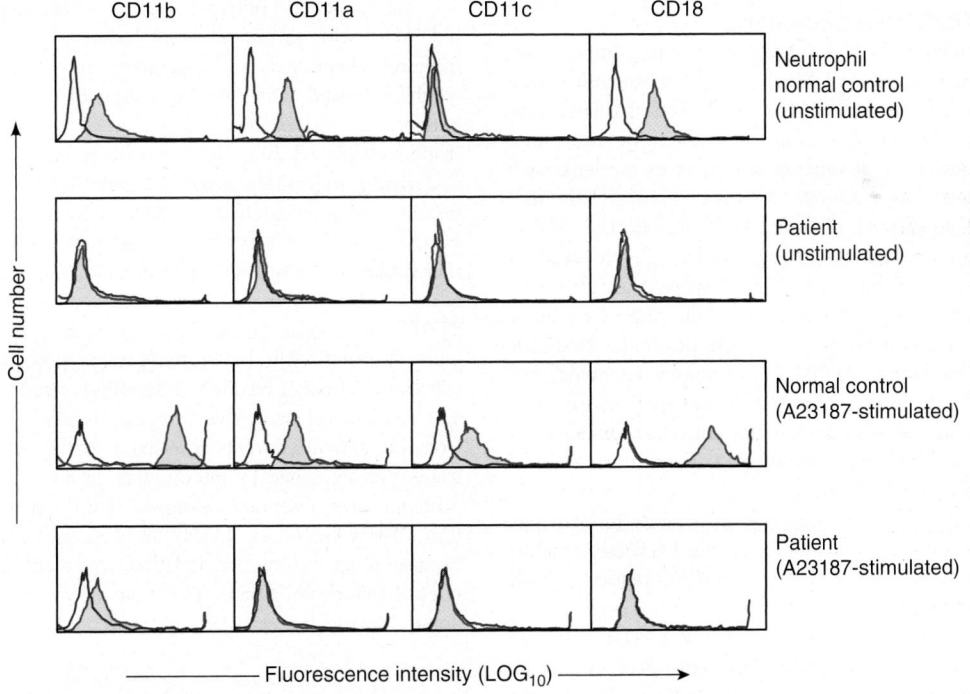

Figure 66–5. Specific diagnosis of CD11/CD18 glycoprotein deficiency by indirect immunofluorescence flow cytometric analysis. Blood neutrophils of a pediatric patient suspected of having CD11/CD18 glycoprotein deficiency and those of an abnormal individual were subjected to immunofluorescence staining for the expression of the CD11b, CD11a, CD11c, and CD18 epitope (crosshatched histograms) as compared with the background immunofluorescence staining by isotype-identical negative-control antibodies (open histograms). Neutrophils were either stained immediately after purification by Ficoll-Hypaque density centrifugation (unstimulated) or after exposure to calcium ionophore A23187 (1 mM) for 15 minutes at 37°C (A23187-stimulated). A23187 stimulation causes significant increase in CD11b and CD18 epitope staining (surface MO1 expression) by normal neutrophils as compared with unstimulated normal cells. A23187 stimulation also causes a small increase in the CD11b-epitope expression of patient cells (the CD11b crosshatched histogram becomes distinguishable from background staining after A23187 stimulation), suggesting that this patient has a "moderate" form of the disorder (capable of expressing small but detectable quantities of CD11/CD18 glycoproteins). Flow cytometric analysis was performed on a Coulter Electronics EPICS F C Flow Cytometer with a logarithmic amplifier. *(Reproduced with permission from Todd R, Freyer DR: The CD11/CD18 leukocyte glycoprotein deficiency,* Hematol Oncol Clin North Am *1988 Mar;2(1):13-31.)*

cells expressing E-selectin (see Table 66–3). Thus, the neutrophils from the patients categorized as having a LAD-2 phenotype are unable to tether to inflamed venules, which is necessary for subsequent activation (Chap. 19). The LAD-2 can be explained by a congenital disorder of fucosylation of ligands for selectins and other glycoconjugates. Each of the three selectins binds with variable affinity to sialylated and fucosylated oligosaccharides, including sLe^x, which is present on multiple specific glycolipids and glycoproteins on leukocytes and activated endothelial cells.[13] Neutrophils from LAD-2 subjects lack sLe^x, which leads to impaired neutrophil rolling on endothelial cells. Other fucosylated determinants, including the H, Lewis, and secretor blood group antigens, are lacking as well, suggesting a global defect in fucosylation. The diminished fucosylation arises from impaired transport of GDP-fucose from the cytoplasm to the Golgi lumen.[331] A human GDP-fucose transporter (GFTP) that localizes to the Golgi apparatus has been demonstrated to be defective secondary to distinct mutations in the *SLC35C1* gene encoding the transporter.[13] When fibroblasts and lymphoblastoid cells derived from a LAD-2 patient were grown in the presence millimolar concentrations of fucose, cell-surface fucosylation could be restored. Following this observation oral administration of L-fucose to two Turkish patients led to normalization of neutrophil counts and functional E- and P-selectin ligands on myeloid cells accompanied by abatement of fevers and infections.[13] Two Arab patients, in contrast to the Turkish patients who have different mutations of the gene encoding the putative GFTP, did not respond to oral fucose.[332] A Brazilian LAD-2 patient, like the Turkish patients, initially benefited from oral fucose; but, following expression of sLe^x on the myeloid cells, the patient developed autoimmune neutropenia.[334] The diagnosis of LAD-2 can be made by flow cytometry analysis of CD15s (sLe^x) expression.

LAD-3, also known as LAD-1 variant syndrome, compromises two major hallmarks: a moderate LAD-1–like syndrome and severe Glanzmann-like bleeding diathesis (Chap. 120). Four patients have been described in whom the inheritance appears to be autosomal recessive and is associated with functional defects of the leukocyte and platelet integrins arising from intracellular signaling.[335] The disease initially presents in early childhood and consists of the inability to form pus at sites of microbial infections, as well as a severe bleeding tendency. The neutrophils from the patients display defective adhesion and chemotaxis and are unable to undergo the respiratory burst when triggered by unopsonized zymosan. The molecular basis for LAD-3 arises from mutations in *FERMT3*, which encodes kindlin-3 in hematopoietic cells. Kindlin-3 binds to regions of the β-integrin tails and constitutes an essential element for transition of integrins from the bent and inactive to the extended an active conformation.[336] Marrow transplantation can be curative.

Another rare cause of neutrophilia and an inability to form pus was observed in a patient with a mutation in the Rac2 GTPase, which is discussed below. The neutrophils from the patient had defects in both adhesion and chemotaxis (see Table 66–2).

Therapy, Course, and Prognosis Treatment of LAD-1 is largely supportive.[309,315] Patients with a history of recurrent infections can be maintained on prophylactic trimethoprim-sulfamethoxazole. Marrow transplantation with human leukocyte antigen (HLA)-compatible siblings or parental donors has resulted in engraftment and restoration of neutrophil function and remains the treatment of choice for patients with a severe phenotype.[337]

The restoration of CD11/CD18 expression in CD34 peripheral stem cells from LAD-1 following transduction with a retrovirus bearing CD18 and induced to differentiate into neutrophils with growth factors indicates that LAD-1 is caused by a defective CD18 gene and provides a basis for somatic gene therapy, which was accomplished

in a dog model.[338,339] Not only did the neutrophils express the integrins, but the cells demonstrated improvement in their functional responses, such as adhesion and the respiratory burst when challenged with ligands for CD11/CD18. These results indicate that *ex vivo* of the transfer gene for CD18 into LAD-1 CD34+ cells followed by reinfusion of the transfused cells may represent a therapeutic approach for LAD.

The severity of infectious complications correlates with the degree of β_2 deficiency. Patients with severe deficiency may die in infancy, and those surviving infancy have a susceptibility to severe, life-threatening, systemic infections. In patients with moderate deficiency, life-threatening infections are infrequent and survival relatively long.[319] LAD-1 can be diagnosed by prenatal screening.

Neutrophil Actin Dysfunction

These patients, like patients with LAD, have recurrent pyogenic infections from birth as a result of defective chemotactic and phagocytic response (see Table 66–2). In one patient, actin isolated from blood and neutrophils could not polymerize under conditions that fully polymerized the actin of neutrophils from normal individuals.[340] Subsequent studies on the index patient's family confirmed that partial actin dysfunction was present in the parents and one sister.[341] One of the parents was found to be a heterozygote for LAD, and the other was not, but further studies established that LAD was not generally associated with defective actin filament assembly.[342,343] The basis of the defective polymerization of actin in the index patient remains unknown, but this disorder of phagocytes is distinct from LAD.

Defective actin polymerization has been described in a 2-month-old infant with severe recurrent bacterial infections associated with impaired chemotaxis and phagocytic response.[344] The patient's neutrophils showed increased expression of CD11b, distinguishing the patient's clinical problem from LAD-1. Morphologically, the neutrophils displayed thin, filamentous projections of membrane with an underlying abnormal cytoskeletal structure. Subsequently, a 47-kDa protein was purified that inhibited actin polymerization *in vitro*.[345] Further biochemical studies revealed a markedly defective actin polymerization in the patient's neutrophils along with a severe deficiency of an 89-kDa protein and an elevated level of the 47-kDa protein. The 47-kDa protein was identified as LSP-1 (lymphocyte-specific protein-1), which is an actin-binding protein present in normal neutrophils. Overexpression of LSP-1 resulted in bundling of actin in cells, leading to an abnormal cytoskeletal structure and motility defects.[346] Neutrophils from the patient's parents revealed a partial defect in actin polymerization accompanied by intermediate levels of LSP-1 and the 89-kDa protein. These observations suggest that the neutrophil actin dysfunction (NAD) known as NAD47/89 is an autosomal recessive disorder. Because actin dysfunction is lethal, treatment requires restoration of normal neutrophil function by marrow replacement from a normal donor. Marrow transplantation was successful.[347,344]

DISORDERS OF NEUTROPHIL MOTILITY

Familial Mediterranean Fever

Definition and History Familial Mediterranean fever (FMF) is an autosomal recessive disease that primarily affects populations surrounding the Mediterranean basin. The disease is characterized by acute limited attacks of fever often accompanied by pleuritis, peritonitis, arthritis, pericarditis, inflammation of the tunica vaginalis of the testes, and erysipelas-like skin disease (see Table 66–2). The initial description occurred in 1908, identifying a Jewish girl who had episodic abdominal pain and fever.[348] Subsequently additional cases were identified,[349] but it took nearly a half century to establish this disorder as familial Mediterranean fever.[350]

Epidemiology More than 10,000 patients worldwide are affected with FMF. It occurs predominantly in Sephardic Jews, Arabs, Turks, Italians, and Armenians.[348] The disorder can occur in other populations, but it is unusual. The frequency of the susceptibility gene varies widely; it is very high among Armenians (ratio of persons with the gene to those without it is 1:7) and Sephardic Jews (1:5 to 1:16), but is lower in Ashkenazi Jews (1:135).

Etiology and Pathogenesis The pathologic findings in FMF are those of nonspecific acute inflammation affecting serosal tissues such as the pleura, peritoneum, and synovium. Neutrophilic infiltration predominates in the affected tissues. Physical and emotional stress, menstruation, and a high-fat diet may trigger the attacks.[351]

The gene responsible for FMF has been identified to be located on chromosome 16. It encodes for a 781-amino-acid protein called *pyrin* or *marenostrin*.[352] The gene *(MEFV)* is predominantly expressed in neutrophils, eosinophils, monocytes, dendritic cells, and synovial and peritoneal fibroblasts, and its expression is upregulated by IFN-γ and TNF, and by the process of myeloid differentiation itself.[353] Nearly all the 50 mutations in the *MEFV* gene are missense changes, most of which are clustered in on exon 2 and 10.[354] Founder effects in FMF have been established, and the two most common mutations, V726A and M694V, originated in common ancestors who lived about 2500 years ago in the Middle East.[352]

Pyrin plays a role in controlling the activity of inflammasomes (see "Neutrophil Surface Receptors"). PYRIN, one of the four domains of pyrin, bears homology to a number of proteins involved in apoptosis and in inflammation, and is similar to a member of the six-helix-bundle death-domain superfamily that includes death domains and death effector domains known as CARDs.[355] The PYD appears to allow for the interaction of macromolecular complexes by PYRIN–PYRIN interactions. This interaction has led to the identification of pyrin's ability to interact specifically with another PYRIN-domain protein termed *apoptosis-associated speck-like protein with a CARD* (ASC).[356] Besides the aminoterminal PYD, ASC has a C-terminal CARD domain that allows binding to the CARD of procaspase-1 (IL-1β–converting enzyme), which results in procaspase-1 autoactivation.[355] Activated caspase-1 then converts proininterleukin-1β to IL-1β, which is, in turn, secreted and interacts with the IL-1 receptor to mediate inflammation. It has been suggested that pyrin may act as an antiinflammatory molecule by inhibiting ASC-induced IL-1 processing, which, in turn, could be defective in FMF. This hypothesis is supported by observing increased IL-1 processing and heightened sensitivity to LPS and impaired apoptosis in peritoneal macrophages from pyrin knockout mice. The puzzle, however, remains as to why serosal tissues are the main targets of inflammation in FMF.

Clinical Features Febrile episodes in FMF may begin in infancy, but by age 20 years, 90 percent of patients have had their first attack. The duration and frequency of attacks may vary considerably, even in the same patient.[351] Acute attacks frequently last 24 to 48 hours and recur once or twice a month. In some patients, attacks may recur as frequently as several times a week, or as infrequently as once a year, and symptoms may persist as long as a week during individual episodes. Some patients experience spontaneous remission that persists for years, followed by recurrence of frequent attacks. Peritonitis caused by FMF may resemble an acute abdomen, thereby leading to potential uncertainties about the clinical management of the acute abdominal episode. Attacks of pleuritic pain occur in approximately 25 to 80 percent of patients. Symptoms of pleuritis may sometimes precede abdominal pain, and some patients experience pleuritic attacks

without abdominal symptoms. Recurrent pericarditis is rare. The course of peritonitis in FMF is similar to attacks at other serosal sites; however, it tends to appear at a late stage of the disease. Mild arthralgia is a common feature of febrile attacks, and monoarticular or oligoarticular arthritis may occur. Arthritis usually affects large joints, the knees in particular, and effusions are common. As many as one-third of the patients experience transient erysipelas-like skin lesions that appear typically on the lower leg, ankle, or dorsum of the foot. These lesions are circumscribed, painful, erythematous areas of swelling, which usually subsides within 24 to 48 hours.

In approximately 25 percent of affected patients, a form of renal amyloidosis develops in which the amyloid derives from a normal serum protein called serum amyloid A (amyloidosis of the AA type; Chap. 108). The amyloidosis progresses over a period of years to renal failure in almost all cases, and the cause of death in patients with FMF is usually attributed to this complication. It appears that polymorphisms in the gene for serum amyloid A increase the susceptibility to renal amyloidosis and that polymorphisms in a gene for the major histocompatibility complex class 1 α-chain influence the severity of the disease.[350]

Laboratory Features Laboratory findings in FMF are nonspecific. Nonspecific findings include increases in inflammatory mediators such as amyloid A, fibrinogen, and C-reactive protein during febrile attacks.[350] Proteinuria greater than 0.5 g of protein per 24 hours in patients with FMF may suggest amyloidosis.

The cloning of the FMF gene now allows a reliable diagnostic test. Five founder mutations account for 74 percent of FMF carrier chromosomes from typical populations known to harbor the disease.[357] Carrier rates for FMF mutations may be as high as 1:3 in some populations, suggesting that the disease is often underdiagnosed. Some amino acids that cause human disease are often present in wild-type in primates.[358]

Differential Diagnosis The TNF receptor–associated periodic syndrome (TRAPS) was first described in 1982 in a large Irish family.[359] The affected family members had recurrent fever with localized myalgia and painful erythema. Differentiating this disorder from FMF was its response to corticosteroids and the autosomal dominant inheritance of the disorder. Affected patients can have attacks that last for at least 1 or 2 days, but prolonged attacks lasting longer than a week are common. Localized pain and tightness in one muscle group and a migratory pattern of the symptoms are prominent features. The disorder may be associated with colicky abdominal pain, diarrhea or constipation, nausea, and or vomiting. Painful conjunctivitis, periorbital edema, or both are common as well as chest pain secondary to sterile pleuritis.[350] During febrile attacks, painless skin lesions may develop on the trunk or extremities and may migrate distally. Missense mutations in the gene for the type-1 TNF 55-kDa cell membrane receptor, which is required for diagnosis, have been identified. Patients with TRAPS respond dramatically to high doses of oral prednisone (>20 mg). In time, however, the responses wane, requiring higher doses of corticosteroids. Standard doses of a p75:Fc fusion protein, etanercept, administrated subcutaneously twice weekly decreases the frequency, duration, and severity of attacks; thus, etanercept may provide a safer, more effective alternative then corticosteroids in controlling the disease.

Therapy Colchicine treatment is effective in FMF and may prevent the development of amyloidosis.[351] Prophylactic colchicine, 0.6 mg orally, two to three times a day, prevents or substantially reduces the acute attacks of FMF in most patients. Some patients can abort attack with intermittent doses of colchicine beginning at the onset of attacks (0.6 mg orally every hour for 4 hours, then every 2 hours for four doses, and then every 12 hours for 2 days). In general, patients who benefit from intermittent colchicine therapy are those who experience a recognizable prodrome before developing fever and clear-cut acute symptoms.

Course and Prognosis The prognosis for normal longevity for patients has been excellent since the recognition that colchicine is an effective treatment of this disease. Most patients can be maintained almost entirely symptom-free. However, if amyloidosis develops, it may be followed by the nephrotic syndrome or uremia. Unless the patient receives a renal transplant, the likelihood of eventual death from renal failure is high.

Other Disorders of Neutrophil Motility

The directed migration of neutrophils from the circulation to an inflammatory site is a consequence of chemotaxis and leads to the accumulation of an exudate. For normal chemotaxis to occur, a complex series of events must be coordinated. Chemotactic factors must be generated in sufficient quantities to establish a chemotactic gradient. The neutrophils must have receptors for the chemotactic agents and mechanisms for discerning the direction of the chemotactic gradient. Depressed neutrophil chemotaxis has been observed in a wide variety of clinical conditions (see Table 66–2).[360] These can be stratified as follows: (1) defects in the generation of chemotactic signals; (2) intrinsic defects of the neutrophil; and (3) direct inhibitors of neutrophil motility in response to chemotactic factors.

Older patients with chemotactic disorders may be infected by a variety of microorganisms, including fungi and Gram-positive or Gram-negative bacteria. *S. aureus* is the most frequent bacterial offender. Typically, the skin, gingival mucosa, and regional lymph nodes are involved. Respiratory tract infections are frequent, but sepsis is rare. Delayed or inappropriate signs and symptoms of inflammation are common. Although the cells move slowly in Boyden chambers or other chemotactic assays, they do accumulate in sufficient numbers in inflammatory sites to produce pus. However, detection of patients with neutrophils that have profound defects in chemotaxis usually is accomplished through other phagocytic assays.

Patients with the hereditary deficiency of complement factors C3, C5, or properidin exhibit an increased incidence of bacterial infections because they are unable to form the chemotactic peptide C5a.[361] The degree to which defective chemotaxis plays a role in C3 deficiency is unclear because opsonization and ingestion rates also are abnormal in these disorders. Frequently, chemotactic disorders are associated with other impaired neutrophil functions. For instance, both glycogen storage disease type 1b[362] and Shwachman-Diamond syndrome[363] are chemotactic disorders frequently associated with an absolute neutrophil count below 0.5×10^9/L. Following restoration of a normal neutrophil count with G-CSF, the patients no longer are predisposed to recurrent bacterial infections in spite of a persistent chemotactic defect. Thus, a chemotactic defect observed *in vitro* does not correlate invariably with decreased resistance to bacterial infections *in vivo*.

Among the impaired defense mechanisms of the neonate is neutrophil adherence and chemotaxis, as demonstrated by the *in vitro* response of neonatal neutrophils to a variety of chemotactic factors.[322] The impaired motility of the neonatal neutrophils in part arises from the diminished ability to mobilize neutrophil β_2 integrins following neutrophil activation.[364] Additionally, the neonatal neutrophil may have a qualitative defect in β_2-integrin function, resulting in impaired neutrophil transendothelial migration for up to 1 month after birth.

At the other end of the spectrum, neutrophils from elderly loose focus during chemotaxis while their motility is unimpaired. This is caused by increased activity of PI3-K and results in less efficient bacterial killing and enhanced release of tissue destructive proteases. Inhibition of PI3K activity reverts this condition *in vitro*.[365]

Drugs and Extrinsic Agents That Impair Neutrophil Motility

Although many pharmacologic agents can influence neutrophil function, few drugs used in clinical medicine affect neutrophil behavior *in vivo*. Ethanol, an inhibitor of PLD, in concentrations that occur in human blood can inhibit neutrophil locomotion and ingestion.[366] Glucocorticoids, especially at high and sustained doses, inhibit neutrophil locomotion, ingestion, and degranulation.[367] Administration of glucocorticoids on alternate days does not interfere with neutrophil movement.[368] Epinephrine does not have a direct effect on neutrophil adhesion but cyclic adenosine monophosphate (cAMP), which is released from endothelial cells following exposure to epinephrine, can depress neutrophil adherence.[369] Similarly, elevated cAMP levels following epinephrine administration may impair neutrophil adherence, leading to diminished neutrophil margination and apparent neutrophilia. Immune complexes, as seen in patients with rheumatoid arthritis or other autoimmune diseases, also can inhibit neutrophil movement by binding to neutrophil Fc receptors.

Hyperimmunoglobulin E Syndrome

Definition and History Autosomal dominant hyperimmunoglobulin E syndrome (HIES) is a disorder characterized by markedly elevated serum IgE levels, chronic dermatitis, and serious recurrent bacterial infections.[370] The skin infections in these patients are remarkable for their absence of surrounding erythema, leading to the formation of "cold abscesses." The neutrophils and monocytes from patients with this syndrome exhibit a variable, but at times profound, chemotactic defect that appears extrinsic to the neutrophil (see Table 66–2).[371]

The syndrome was originally described in 1966 in two red-headed, fair-skinned females who had "cold abscesses" and hyperextensible joints, which led to the appellation "Job's syndrome."[370] Subsequently Buckley and coworkers documented the association of levels of immunoglobulin E with undue susceptibility to infection.[372]

Epidemiology Reports of more than 200 cases have been documented.[372,373] HIES occurs in persons from diverse ethnic backgrounds and does not seem to be more common in any specific population.

Etiology and Pathogenesis Both males and females have been affected, as well as members of succeeding generations, indicating that the disorder is autosomal dominant with an incomplete penetrance form of inheritance.[370] STAT3 mutations cause most, if not all cases of autosomal dominant HIES. All mutations have been missense mutations or in-frame deletions, leading to the formation of full-length mutant STAT3 protein, which exerts a dominant negative effect. STAT3 is a major transduction protein affecting pathways involving wound healing angiogenesis, immunity, and cancer. The more rare autosomal recessive form is caused by mutations in dedicator of cytokinesis 8 (DOCK8), a guanine nucleotide exchange factor.[374]

The mechanism of the immune deficiencies in HIES remains clouded. Several reports with limited numbers of patients have conflicted results as to whether a chemotactic defect exists and whether there is a T-helper 1/T-helper 2 cytokine imbalance.

Clinical Features HIES may begin as early as day 1 after birth.[372] The syndrome is characterized by chronic eczematoid rashes, which are typically papular and pruritic. The rash generally involves the face and extensor surfaces of arms and legs; skin lesions are frequently sharply demarcated and usually lack surrounding erythema. By 5 years of age all patients have had a history of recurrent skin abscess formation with recurrent pneumonias, along with chronic otitis media and sinusitis. Patients may also develop septic arthritis, cellulitis, or osteomyelitis. The major offending pathogen is generally *S. aureus*. Other pathogens commonly infecting patients are *C. albicans*, *H. influenzae*, and pneumococci. Other associated features include coarse facial features, including a prominent forehead, deep set eyes, a broad nasal bridge, a wide fleshly nasal tip, mild prognathism facial asymmetry, and hemihypertrophy.[370] There is a high incidence of scoliosis, hyperextensible joints, and delayed shedding of the primary teeth.[370] Occasionally, unexplained osteopenia presents, which is often complicated by recurrent bone fractures. Additionally, there is an increased risk of both Hodgkin and non-Hodgkin lymphoma.

Laboratory Features Blood and sputum eosinophilia have been a consistent finding in all patients.[370] Patient serum IgE levels range from three to 80 times the upper limit of normal. The serum IgE usually rises above 2000 IU/mL and often is elevated at birth. Upon reaching adulthood the IgE may decline over years, despite the clinical abnormalities of STAT3 deficiency. Usually patients have normal concentrations of IgG, IgA, and IgM, and may have elevated levels of IgD. Patients often have abnormally low anamnestic antibody response and poor antibody and cell-mediated responses to neoantigens. At times the neutrophils and monocytes of patients have a profound chemotactic defect.

Differential Diagnosis Autosomal recessive-HIES (AR-HIES) is a distinct clinical entity manifested by elevated IgE ligands, and recurrent skin and cutaneous viral infections and mutations in *DOCK8*.[370,375]

Fatal sepsis occurs in AR-HIES from both Gram-positive and Gram-negative bacteria. Patients with AR-HIES have more symptomatic neurologic disease than STAT3 deficiency. Autoimmune hemolytic anemia may occur, but neutrophil chemotaxis is normal. The genetic mutation underlying AR-HIES remain unclear. Therapy remains supportive.

Therapy No known therapy is curative, and management decisions are based on the clinical findings. Prophylactic trimethoprim-sulfamethoxazole is effective in reducing infections with *S. aureus*.[370] Type and route of antibiotic therapy are dictated by the results of the Gram stain and culture in patients with acute bacterial infections. Incision and drainage are essential for the management of abscesses, including superinfected pneumatoceles. Eczematoid dermatitis can be controlled with topical glucocorticoids to reduce inflammation and antihistamines to control pruritus. Intravenous immunoglobulin may decrease the number of infections for some patients. Attention needs to be paid to the scoliosis, fractures and degenerative joints by orthopedists. Retention of primary teeth requires dental expertise.

Course and Prognosis If the hyperimmunoglobulin E is recognized early in life and the patient is maintained on chronic anti-*Staphylococcal* antibiotic therapy, the prognosis remains good. Many such patients have reached maturity, indicating that the syndrome is compatible with prolonged survival. Conversely, if the diagnosis is delayed and the patient develops infected giant pneumatoceles, secondary fungal infections may occur, leading to a morbid state.

DEFECTS IN MICROBICIDAL ACTIVITY

Chronic Granulomatous Disease

Definition and History CGD is a genetic disorder affecting the function of neutrophils and monocytes. These phagocytic cells are able to ingest, but not kill, catalase-positive microorganisms because of an inability to generate antimicrobial oxygen metabolites (see Table 66–2). It is caused by mutations involving one of several genes encoding a component of the NADPH oxidase.[376]

In 1957, two pediatric groups caring for six male infants reported a clinical disorder of chronic suppurative lymphadenitis and recurrent fevers leading to premature deaths in the children.[377,378] In the same time period, three observations assisted in providing the framework to understand the defect in the phagocytes of patients with CGD. Scientists described first that a striking increase in oxygen consumption

was found upon particle ingestion by phagocytes, which was not related to mitochondrial oxygen metabolism.[379] Next, it was found that the process of phagocytosis was accompanied by the formation of large quantities of H_2O_2 in the cell.[380] Subsequently, it was reported that homogenates of phagocytes consume oxygen when incubated with pyridine nucleotides.[381] These observations indicated that an oxidase enzyme or enzymes in the phagocytes were activated during phagocytosis to convert molecular oxygen into H_2O_2. It was then established that phagocytes from patients with CGD could ingest, but could not kill, the catalase-positive organisms.[381] Building on previous studies that a neutrophil oxidase mediates the increase in oxygen consumption, a pyridine-dependent oxidase was found to be deficient in neutrophils of patients with CGD, which led to their inability to reduce the dye nitroblue tetrazolium (NBT) during phagocytosis of particles.[382] Collectively, these studies laid the groundwork for subsequent studies to unravel the biochemical and genetic defects in CGD.

Epidemiology The incidence of CGD in the United States is 1 per 200,000 livebirths, based on data from the National Institutes of Allergy and Infectious Disease Registry.[383] Data from the Registry indicates that 86 percent of patients are male and 14 percent female; 80 percent are classified as white, 11 percent as black patients, and 3 percent Asians or mixed-race patients. Of the 340 patients in the Registry with adequate information for determination genetic transmission, 70 percent had the X-linked recessive form of the disease.

Etiology and Pathogenesis Several laboratory tests are used to classify forms of CGD and aid in understanding its pathogenesis (Table 66–4). The diagnosis of CGD is based on a compatible clinical history and demonstration of a defective respiratory burst. Several methods detect the production of reactive oxidants. The NBT method relies on the intracellular reduction of NBT by superoxide anion to a blue formazan precipitate that can be seen microscopically.[376] More sensitive methods rely on the reaction of oxidants with specific chemiluminescent and fluorescent probes. The patients with CGD may have heterogeneous array of regular symptoms and severity, depending on which subunit is defective and on the nature of the genetic mutation.

Nicotinamide Adenine Dinucleotide Phosphate-Oxidase Function Engulfment of microbes by phagocytic cells is associated with a burst of oxygen consumption that is important for microbicidal killing and digestion. The respiratory burst is accompanied, not by mitochondrial respiration, but by a unique electron transport chain called the NADPH oxidase. Prior to stimulation, the components of the oxidase are physically separated into two major subcellular locations (Fig. 66–6). The membrane-bound portion of the NADPH oxidase contains a heterodimeric cytochrome b$_{558}$ composed of a large, heavily glycosylated subunit with a Mr of 91 kDa, known as a gp91^{phox} (91-kDa glycoprotein of the phagocyte oxidase), and a 22-kDa protein known as p22^{phox}.[376,384] Eighty to 90 percent of the cytochrome b$_{558}$ is found in specific and gelatinase granules and secretory vesicles of the neutrophil and following neutrophil activation translocates to the plasma membrane.[66,318] The heavy chain of cytochrome b contains sites for heme binding, flavin adenine dinucleotide (FAD) groups, and NADPH binding.[385-388] The three-dimensional structure of cytochrome b$_{558}$ indicates that the carboxyl-terminal half of the peptide contains sequences for flavin and NADPH binding.[389] The amino half of the molecule is hydrophobic and contains the histidines that coordinate heme binding.[390] The p22^{phox} also contains a site for heme binding.[385] The synthesis of the p22^{phox} peptide is absolutely required for stability of gp91^{phox} and for oxidase activity in the membrane.[376] The p22^{phox} also contains proline-rich regions that display consensus protein–protein interactions that provide a binding site for p47^{phox}.[391] Three other proteins vital to the function

TABLE 66–4. Diagnostic Classification of Chronic Granulomatous Disease

Affected Component	Inheritance	Subtype	Membrane-Bound Cytochrome b$_{558}$*	Cytosol p47^{phox}*	Cytosol p67^{phox}*
gp91^{phox}	X	X91^0	Not detectable	Normal	Normal
		X91$^+$	Normal quantity, but nonfunctional	Normal	Normal
		X91$^-$	Defective gp91^{phox}, which is poorly functional or expressed in a small fraction of phagocytes	Normal	Normal
p22^{phox}	A	A22^0	Not detectable	Normal	Normal
		A22$^+$	Normal quantity, but nonfunctional	Normal	Normal
p47^{phox}	A	A47^0	Normal quantity	Not detectable	Normal
p67^{phox}	A	A67^0	Normal	Normal	Not detectable

*Detected by spectral analysis or immunoblotting. In this nomenclature, the first letter represents the mode of inheritance (-linked [X] or autosomal recessive [A]). The number indicates the phox component, which is genetically affected. The superscript symbols indicate whether the level of protein of the affected component is undetectable (0), diminished (−), or normal (+) as measured by immunoblot or spectral analysis.

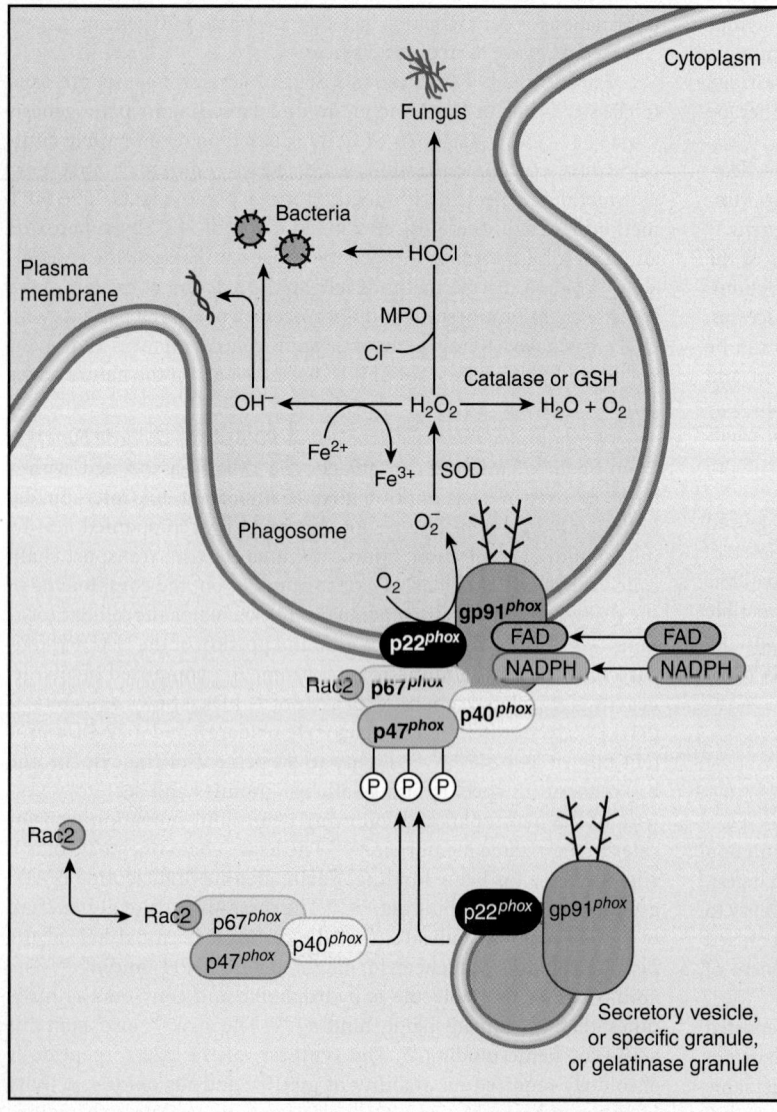

Figure 66–6. Possible mechanisms for the production of superoxide anion in neutrophils. Oxygen is reduced to superoxide (O_2^-) by an nicotinamide adenine dinucleotide phosphate (NADPH) oxidase. The oxidase is a composite of (1) a 47-kDa cytosolic protein (p47); (2) a 67-kDa cytosolic protein (p67); (3) a 40-kDa cytosolic protein (p40); (4) a low-molecular-weight cytosolic G-protein, Rac2; and (5) a membrane-bound cytochrome b$_{558}$. Cytochrome b consists of a 22-kDa protein subunit (p22) and a 91-kDa glycoprotein subunit (gp91), both of which contain heme. The gp91 subunit is a flavin adenine dinucleotide (FAD)-dependent flavoprotein that contains the NADPH binding site and ultimately shuttles electrons to molecular oxygen, forming O_2^-, and (6) the cytosol components translocate to the membrane and may serve to alter the tertiary structure of cytochrome b, to permit the flow of electrons from NADPH to O_2. The p47 subunit (p47) is phosphorylated upon activation of the neutrophil. The p40^{phox} component stabilizes the preactivation complex of p67^{phox}. The unstable superoxide anion (O_2^-) is converted to hydrogen peroxide (H_2O_2), either spontaneously or by the enzyme superoxide dismutase (SOD). H_2O_2 in the presence of myeloperoxidase (MPO) converts H_2O_2 to hypochlorous acid (HOCl). Both H_2O_2 and O_2^- can be transformed into hydroxyl radical (OH$^-$). H_2O_2 can be reduced to H_2O and O_2 by the enzyme catalase or by glutathione (GSH), a product of the hexose-monophosphate shunt. These reactive oxygen species are responsible for microbial killing. Normal oxidative function of the NADPH complex requires fully functional individual components.

of this oxidase system reside in the cytosol of the resting phagocyte. Upon stimulation, translocation of p47^{phox} takes place. Phosphorylated p47^{phox} together with two other cytoplasmic components of the oxidase, p67^{phox}, and a low-molecular-weight guanosine triphosphate Rac-2, translocate to the membrane, where they interact with cytoplasmic domains of the transmembrane cytochrome b$_{558}$ to form the active oxidase.[391,392] Both p47^{phox} and p67^{phox} contain SH3 (Src homology 3) domains that may participate in intramolecular and intermolecular binding with consensus proline-rich regions in p47^{phox}.[392] Phosphorylation, which occurs on serines in the cationic C-terminal region of p47^{phox}, serves to disrupt this intermolecular interaction, making the SH3 regions available for binding to p22^{phox}. Another cytoplasmic component with homology to p47^{phox} has been identified as p40^{phox}. p40^{phox}, like p47^{phox}, contains a PX domain, a motif that supports the binding to phosphoinositides on the cytosolic side of membranes.[393] The p40^{phox} component stabilizes the cytoplasmic complexes of p67^{phox} and p47^{phox} on phagosomes. Its binding of phosphatidylinositol 3 phosphate also potentiates superoxide production upon neutrophil activation.[394] Cytochrome b$_{558}$ spans the membrane, permitting NADPH to be oxidized at the cytoplasmic surface and oxygen to be reduced to form O$_2^-$ on the outer surface of the plasma membrane or on the inner surface of the phagosomal membrane.[395]

Genetic Alterations Affecting Cytochrome b The most frequent form of CGD occurs in 70 percent of patients and is caused by mutations in the gp91^{phox} gene, termed *CYBB*, which is located on chromosome Xp21.1.[376,396] These mutations lead to the X-linked form of the disease. Large interstitial deletions causing other X-linked disorders such as retinitis pigmentosa, Duchenne muscular dystrophy, McLeod hemolytic anemia, and ornithine transcarbamylase deficiency, have been reported in a few patients with X-linked CGD.[383,397–399] Mutation analysis of the gene encoding gp91 and a large group of X-linked CGD kindreds has documented many distinct defects, including point mutations, inversions, deletions, or insertions that disrupt the reading frame and nonsense mutations that create a premature stop codon.[396] Some splice-site defects have also been identified. In this situation, short deletions in gp91^{phox} mRNA are caused by point mutations that produce partial or complete exon skipping during mRNA splicing.[400] This abnormality is a common cause of X-linked CGD. In the remaining patients, point mutations have been identified that generate either premature stop codons or amino acid substitutions that apparently disrupt protein stability or function and lead to a complete lack of detectable cytochrome b$_{558}$ protein in phagocytic cells in most patients with X-linked CGD. In some situations, low levels of functional cytochrome b are present, whereas in others, normal levels of dysfunctional cytochrome b$_{558}$ occur.[401] In the latter situation there is some clustering of defects in regions of known function, such as the NADPH- or flavin-binding consensus regions.[402] Approximately 10 to 15 percent of X-linked CGD arises from new germline mutations.[403]

A similar array of mutations has been identified in the 5 percent of CGD patients who have abnormalities in the p22^{phox} gene, termed *CYBA*, which is located on chromosome 16q24.[376,402,404] In this autosomal disorder, mutations in the p22^{phox} gene result in deletions, frameshifts, and/or missense mutations. Patients with a defective p22^{phox} gene do not express the other cytoplasmic unit polypeptide. In one patient, p22^{phox} peptide was associated with normal amounts of cytochrome b with normal heme spectrum, but p47^{phox} translocation membrane did not occur and there was no oxidase activation because the mutation affected a proline-rich region thought to mediate binding to one of the SH3 domains of p47^{phox}. In gp91^{phox}-deficient patients, p22^{phox} mRNA is present, but it is not translated, which is consistent with the notion that either cytochrome subunit polypeptide is dependent upon the stable expression of the other subunit.[376]

Genetic Alterations Affecting Cytosolic Proteins Two other proteins have been identified as being vital to the function of the NADPH-oxidase system. Their absence results in the syndrome of CGD.[405] These proteins have molecular masses of 47 kDa and 67 kDa, respectively, and are located in the cytosol of resting cells. Defects in the genes for p47^{phox}, termed *NCF1*, which is found on chromosome 7q11, are responsible for the majority of all cases of autosomal recessive CGD, whereas inherited defects for the gene for neutrophil p67^{phox}, termed *NCF2*, account for a small subgroup of autosomal recessive CGD.[376] The function of p47^{phox} and p67^{phox} in regulating the respiratory burst oxidase is thought to involve activation of the electron transport function of cytochrome b$_{558}$. The mutation analysis in patients with p47^{phox}-deficient forms of CGD reveals an unusual pattern, in that more than 90 percent of mutant alleles have guanine-thymine dinucleotide deletion at the start of exon 2, resulting in frameshift and premature stop.[402,406] The truncated protein is unstable in that it cannot be detected immunologically. The majority of patients appear to be homozygous for this mutation without any history of consanguinity. The p47^{phox} gene occurs in an area of chromosome 7 that has a high degree of evolutionary duplication in normal individuals because a pseudogene highly homologous to the normal p47^{phox} gene exists in the normal genome in this region of duplication. The pseudogene contains the same GT deletion associated with most cases of p47^{phox} CGD. This implies that recombination of the normal gene and pseudogene with conversion of the normal gene to partial pseudotype sequence in that region may be responsible for the high relative rate of this specific mutation in diverse racial groups, which proved to be the case.[407]

A second rare form of CGD is caused by mutations in the gene for the p67^{phox} cytosolic component.[401] The p67^{phox} gene, which has been mapped to the long arm of chromosome 1, spans 37 kb and contains 16 exons. The mutations identified in p67^{phox}-deficiency CGD have included missense mutations and spliced junction mutations affecting mRNA processing, which led to nondetectable p67^{phox} protein by immunologic means.[402]

Mutation of *NCF4*, the gene encoding p40^{phox}, was reported in a child with granulomatous colitis. One allele had a frameshift mutation with a premature stop codon. The other had a missense mutation predicting an R105Q substitution in the PX domain which is responsible for binding to phosphatidylinositol 3 phosphate. The functional defect was inability to assemble the NADPH oxidase in the membrane of phagosomes but not on the plasma mambrane.[408]

Predisposition to Infection Mutations in the gene for cytochrome b$_{558}$ or the cytosolic factors involved in activating the cytochrome are associated with the CGD phenotype. Figure 66–7 shows schematically the manner in which the metabolic deficiency of the CGD neutrophil predisposes the host to infection. Normal neutrophils accumulate H$_2$O$_2$ and other oxygen metabolites in the phagosomes containing ingested microorganisms. MPO is delivered to the phagosome by degranulation and in this setting H$_2$O$_2$ acts as a substrate for MPO to oxidize halide to HOCl and chloramines, which kill the microbes. The quantity of H$_2$O$_2$ produced by the normal neutrophils is sufficient to exceed the capacity of catalase, a H$_2$O$_2$-catabolizing enzyme produced by many aerobic microorganisms, including *S. aureus*, most Gram-negative enteric bacteria, *C. albicans*, and *Aspergillus* spp. In contrast, H$_2$O$_2$ is not produced by CGD neutrophils, and any generated by the microbes themselves may be destroyed by their own catalase. Thus, catalase-positive microbes can multiply inside CGD neutrophils, where they are protected from most circulating antibiotics, and can be transported to

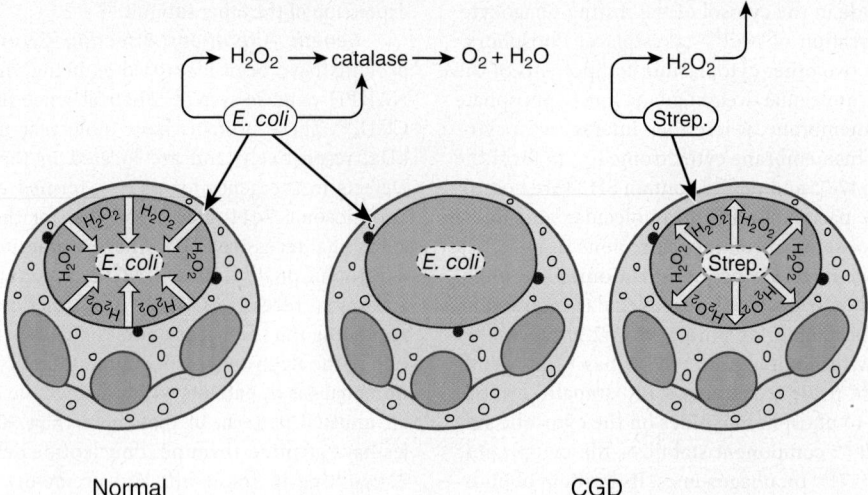

Figure 66–7. The pathogenesis of chronic granulomatous disease (CGD). The manner in which the metabolic deficiency of the CGD neutrophil predisposes the host to infection is shown schematically. Normal neutrophils accumulate hydrogen peroxide (H_2O_2) in the phagosome containing ingested *Escherichia coli*. Myeloperoxidase is delivered to the phagosome by degranulation, as indicated by the closed circles, and in this setting, H_2O_2 acts as a substrate for myeloperoxidase to oxidize halide to hypochlorous acid and chloramines, which kill the microbes. The quantity of H_2O_2 produced by the normal neutrophils is sufficient to exceed the capacity of catalase, a H_2O_2-catabolizing enzyme of many aerobic microorganisms, including most Gram-negative enteric bacteria, *Staphylococcus aureus*, *Candida albicans*, and *Aspergillus* spp. When organisms such as *E. coli* gain entry into the CGD neutrophils, they are not exposed to H_2O_2 because the neutrophils do not produce it, and the H_2O_2 generated by microbes themselves is destroyed by their own catalase. When CGD neutrophils ingest streptococci (Strep.) or pneumococci, these organisms generate enough H_2O_2 to result in a microbicidal effect. On the other hand, as indicated in the middle figure, catalase-positive microbes, such as *E. coli*, can survive within the phagosome of the CGD neutrophil.

distant sites and released to establish new foci of infection.[405] Activation of the oxidase also has a pronounced effect on the pH within the phagocytic vacuole. It is controversial whether activation of the respiratory burst is associated with an alkaline phase, but the pH of the phagocytic vacuole becomes more acidic in CGD patients than in normal patients.[161,409] The alkaline phase may be important for the antimicrobial and digestive functions of the neutral hydrolases released from the cytoplasmic granules into the vacuole upon phagocytosis. In CGD, the phagocytic vacuoles remain acidic and the bacteria are not digested properly.[410] The impairment in the respiratory burst by CGD neutrophils leads to delayed neutrophil apoptosis and subsequent impaired clearance of degenerating neutrophils by CGD macrophages, which, in turn, predisposes the host to enhanced inflammation.[411] CGD neutrophils are incapable of generating NETs and cannot trap microorganisms by this mechanism.[412] The CGD macrophage is unable to clear CGD neutrophils because of a deficiency of intrinsic IL-4 production, which occurs because of defective phosphatidylserine exposure on CGD neutrophils, that is a necessary requirement to engage CGD macrophage phosphatidylserine membrane receptors and subsequent macrophage activation.[411] In hematoxylin-and-eosin-stained sections from patients, macrophages eventually may contain a golden pigment, which reflects the abnormal accumulation of ingested material and also contributes to the diffuse granulomata that give CGD its descriptive name.[413] On the other hand, when CGD neutrophils ingest pneumococci or streptococci, these organisms generate enough H_2O_2 to result in a microbicidal effect.

Clinical Features Although the clinical presentation is variable, several clinical features suggest the diagnosis of CGD.[376] Any patient with recurrent lymphadenitis should be considered to have CGD. Additionally, patients with bacterial hepatic abscesses, osteomyelitis at multiple sites or in the small bones of the hands and feet, a family history of recurrent infections, or unusual catalase-positive microbial infections all require clinical evaluation for this disorder. Table 66–5 lists the most

common clinical infections that afflict CGD patients and Table 66–6 cites their prevalence.

Among the various infections, only perirectal abscess, suppurative adenitis, and bacteremia/fungemia differ significantly in prevalence in the X-linked recessive and autosomal recessive CGD patients.[383] Each of these conditions was twice as common in the X-linked form.

The onset of clinical signs and symptoms may occur from early infancy to young adulthood. Although the majority of patients with CGD (76 percent) are diagnosed before the age of 5 years, approximately 10 percent are not diagnosed until the second decade of life, and on rare occasions, not until the third decade or later.[383] The organisms infecting CGD patients have changed considerably from those initially reported between 1957 and 1976. *Staphylococcus* caused most of the infections in the initial cases; *Klebsiella* and *E. coli* were then the next most common pathogens. Now *Aspergillus* is the prominent organism causing pneumonia and is the leading cause of death in patients.[376] Invasive aspergillosis can occur in the first few months of life in healthy infants as well as in those with CGD. Although aspergillosis is the most common infecting fungus in CGD, *Candida* and several other fungal strains have been invasive in this disorder. *Burkholderia cepacia* is another leading cause of death in patients with CGD. *Serratia marcescens* is the third leading organism that commonly infects patients with CGD. Infections are characterized by microabscesses and granuloma formation. The presence of pigmented histiocytes is helpful in establishing the diagnosis. Patients may suffer from the consequences of chronic infections including the anemia of chronic disease, lymphadenopathy, hepatosplenomegaly, chronic purulent dermatitis, restrictive lung disease, gingivitis, hydronephrosis, and gastroenteric narrowing.[383] Patients with CGD are also at risk for developing colitis and chorioretinitis, and discoid lupus erythematosus.[383]

Several mothers of patients in whom X-linked inheritance was established had an illness resembling systemic lupus erythematosus.[383] Both X-linked and autosomal recessive patients with CGD also have a

TABLE 66–5. Common Infecting Organisms Isolated from Chronic Granulomatous Disease Patients

Infection Type	Organism	X-Linked Recessive (%)	Autosomal Recessive (%)
Pneumonia	Aspergillus spp.	41	29
	Staphylococcus spp.	11	13
	Burkholderia cepacia	7	11
	Nocardia spp.	6	13
	Serratia spp.	4	5
Abscess			
Subcutaneous	Staphylococcus spp.	28	21
	Serratia spp.	19	9
	Aspergillus spp.	7	0
Liver	Staphylococcus spp.	52	52
	Serratia spp.	6	4
	Candida spp.	12	0
Lung	Aspergillus spp.	27	18
Perirectal	Staphylococcus spp.	9	15
Brain	Aspergillus spp.	75	25
Suppurative adenitis	Staphylococcus spp.	29	12
	Serratia spp.	9	15
	Candida spp.	7	4
Osteomyelitis	Serratia spp.	32	12
	Aspergillus spp.	25	18
Bacteremia/fungemia	Salmonella spp.	20	13
	Burkholderia cepacia	13	0
	Candida spp.	9	25
	Staphylococcus spp.	11	0

Data from Segal BH, Leto TL, Gallin JI, et al: Genetic, biochemical, and clinical features of chronic granulomatous disease, *Medicine* (Baltimore) 2000 May;79(3):170–200.

TABLE 66–6. Prevalence of Infectious Complication of Chronic Granulomatous Disease Patients

Infection Type	X-Linked Recessive (%)	Autosomal Recessive (%)
Pneumonia	80	77
Abscess (all)	68	70
Subcutaneous	43	42
Liver	26	33
Lung	16	14
Brain	3	5
Perirectal	17	7
Suppurative adenitis	59	32
Osteomyelitis	27	21
Bacteremia/fungemia	21	10
Cellulitis	7	5

Data from Segal BH, Leto TL, Gallin JI, et al: Genetic, biochemical, and clinical features of chronic granulomatous disease, *Medicine* (Baltimore) 2000 May;79(3):170–200.

similar disorder.[414] It may be that these mothers' and patients' cells are unable to clear immune complexes sufficiently, which is a characteristic feature of CGD cells *in vitro*.[415] Variant alleles of MBL and FcγRIIA especially in combination are associated with rheumatologic disorders in patients with CGD.[416]

Laboratory Findings The defect in the respiratory burst is best determined by measuring superoxide or H_2O_2 production in response to both soluble and particulate stimuli.[417] A test that is being employed is the use of flow cytometry using dihydrorhodamine-123 fluorescence.[418] Dihydrorhodamine-123 fluorescence detects oxidant production because it increases fluorescence upon oxidation.[418] In most cases there is no detectable superoxide or H_2O_2 generation with either type of stimulus. In the variant form of CGD, however, superoxide may be produced at rates between 0.5 and 10 percent of control.[419]

An alternative method for measuring respiratory burst activity is the NBT test. This assay is performed by microscopically assessing the ability of individual cells to reduce NBT to purple formazan crystals following stimulation. Commonly there is no NBT reduction with most forms of CGD. In some of the variant forms, however, a high percentage of cells may contain some formazan, a finding indicative of a greatly diminished respiratory burst in most of the neutrophils. This test also permits detection of the carrier state in X-linked CGD when as few as 5 to 10 percent of the cells are NBT-negative.[420]

Most sophisticated procedures can identify the molecular defect. Cytochrome b content can be measured in extracts of detergent-disrupted neutrophils by a spectrophotometric assay.[420] Once the diagnosis of CGD is made, the genotype can be determined. A mosaic population of oxidation that has positive and negative neutrophils in a male patient's mother and sister strongly suggests X-linked CGD. Lack of a mosaic pattern among female relatives does not rule out the X-linked mode of inheritance because the defect can arise spontaneously. Prenatal diagnosis of CGD is established by analysis of DNA from amniocytes or chorionic villus samples.

Differential Diagnosis Leukocytes from patients with CGD have normal glucose-6-phosphate dehydrogenase (G6PD) activity. However, a few individuals with apparent CGD have been described who have neutrophils that lack or are almost lacking in G6PD activity.[421,422] The erythrocytes of these patients also lack the enzyme, and the patients have chronic hemolysis. In the cases of severe neutrophil G6PD deficiency, an attenuated respiratory burst progressively decreases as a result of the depletion of intracellular NADPH, the primary substrate for the respiratory burst oxidase. CGD and G6PD deficiency can be distinguished from each other by the hemolytic anemia seen in the latter disorder and by the fact that erythrocyte G6PD activity is normal in CGD and markedly reduced in G6PD deficiency.[401] A variety of studies indicate that the small GTPase Rac-2 plays an essential role in activity of the NADPH and the actin cytoskeleton in human neutrophils.[383] A toddler has been described as presenting with a perirectal abscess at 5 weeks of age. This patient subsequently had necrosis of the periumbilical skin and fascia, and his surgical wounds did not heal properly. Functionally his neutrophils had multiple defective components; for example, adhesion to ligands for sLe^x, chemotaxis, release of primary azurophil granules upon stimulation with chemotactic peptide, and failure to undergo the respiratory burst using the same stimulus.[423,424] Molecular analysis identified the asparagine for aspartic acid mutation at amino acid 57 of one allele of the Rac-2 gene.[423,424] Mutant Rac-2 did not bind GTP and it inhibited and behaved as a dominant negative to impair Rac-2–mediated activation of the respiratory burst.[424] Fortunately, the youngster was successfully transplanted with marrow from a HLA-identical older brother.[424]

Therapy, Course, and Prognosis Allogeneic hematopoietic stem cell transplantation is the only recognized curative treatment for CGD. Reduced intensity conditioning stem cell transplantation from HLA-matched donors performed in 56 patients with intractable infections and severe inflammation carried a 2-year overall survival of 96 percent.[425] However, vigorous supportive care along with the use of recombinant IFN continues to be the foundation of treatment.[376] Cultures must be obtained as soon as infection is suspected, as unusual organisms are commonly the source of infection and may grow promptly *in vitro*. Most abscesses require surgical drainage for therapeutic and diagnostic purposes, and prolonged use of antibiotics is often required. If fever occurs, it is advisable to obtain certain studies that aid in the management of septic episodes. These include roentgenograms of the chest and skeleton and a computed tomography (CT) scan of the liver because of the frequency of pneumonia, osteomyelitis, and liver abscesses.[383] Arrangements should be made for prompt medical attention at the first signs of infection. With early intervention, many lesions can be managed by conservative medical means. For example, enlarging lymph nodes often regress when treated with local heat and orally administered antistaphylococcal antibiotics. It is particularly important to obtain a microbiologic diagnosis, and fine-needle aspiration may be helpful in this regard. In general, antibiotic therapy for the offending organisms is indicated and purulent masses should be drained. The cause of fever and prostration cannot always be established, and empiric

treatment with broad-spectrum parenteral antibiotics is required. Often it is necessary to treat with antibiotics for a prolonged time until the initially elevated sedimentation rate approaches normal values. *Aspergillus* spp. infection requires treatment with amphotericin B or, in refractory cases, with granulocyte transfusions.[376] Glucocorticoids also may be useful in the treatment of patients with antral and urethral obstruction. The risk of *Aspergillus* infection can be reduced by avoiding marijuana smoke and decaying plant material, such as mulch and hay, both of which contain numerous fungal spores.[426] Long-term oral prophylaxis with trimethoprim-sulfamethoxazole (5 mg/kg per day of trimethoprim) is an accepted practice in the management of patients with CGD.[376] Patients have prolonged infection-free periods, which result from the prevention of infections caused by *S. aureus*, without increasing the incidence of fungal infections. The use of itraconazole prophylactically has reduced the development of fungal infections.[427,428]

IFN-γ (50 mcg/m^2, three times per week, subcutaneously) can reduce the number of serious bacterial and fungal infections.[427,429] IFN-γ–enhanced neutrophil function *in vitro* has not been correlated with improvement in the activity of the neutrophil respiratory burst in patients totally lacking the ability to generate superoxide. On the other hand, its use increases the neutrophil expression of the high-affinity Fcγ receptor 1, as well as monocyte expression of FcγRI, FcγRII, FcγRIII, CD11/CD18, and HLA-DR.[430] The IFN-γ protective effect in patients with CGD may involve improved microbial clearance, as suggested by the enhanced phagocytic activity by neutrophils of opsonized *S. aureus*. In rare, X-linked CGD patients able to generate some superoxide, IFN-γ programs granulocyte cells to increase their expression of cytochrome b, which results in normal superoxide generation.[431] With the use of current prophylactic treatments, the mortality in CGD has been reduced to two patient deaths per year per 100 patients followed.[376]

CGD patients with mutations that result in 5 to 10 percent of normal-functioning amounts of NADPH have a mild phenotype and better clinical prognosis than do patients with complete absence of any NADPH-oxidase activity.[432] Similarly, female carriers of X-linked CGD who have only 3 to 5 percent oxidase-normal neutrophils rarely get serious infections suggestive of the CGD clinical phenotype.[433] Thus, even low levels or partial correction by gene therapy of CGD is likely to provide clinical benefits. In support of that hypothesis, mouse models of X-linked and p47^{phox}-deficient CGD have been developed by gene targeting.[434,435] Studies in the gp91^{phox}- and the p47^{phox}-deficient mouse models of CGD show that retrovirus-mediated gene-therapy-targeting of marrow progenitor cells *ex vivo* can result in the correction of defects in oxidant production *in vivo* in blood neutrophils after radiation conditioning and transplantation of marrow stem cells.[436,437] Protection from infection challenge occurred even when the oxidase-corrected cells comprised less than 10 percent of circulating neutrophils. These promising results suggest that somatic gene therapy can be employed to correct defective phagocyte oxidase function in selected patients with CGD. In a phase I clinical trial, gene therapy for p47^{phox}-deficiency CGD, five adult patients received intravenous infusions of autologous blood stem cells that were *ex vivo* transduced using a retrovirus encoding normal p47^{phox}.[438] Although conditioning therapy was not given prior to the stem cell infusion, functionally corrected neutrophils were detectable in blood for several months.[339] In another study, long-term high-level clinical beneficial correction in *ex vivo* gene therapy of X-linked CGD occurred in two adult patients.[439] Nonablative busulfan conditioning was used to augment gene therapy correction. There needs to be caution regarding the long-term stability and safety of gene therapy. For instance, there are concerns about gene insertion rendering patients vulnerable to developing an hematological malignancy.

Myeloperoxidase Deficiency

The functional and immunochemical absence of the enzyme MPO from granules of neutrophils and monocytes, but not eosinophils, is inherited as an autosomal recessive trait, with a prevalence of 1:2000.[440] MPO, an enzyme that catalyzes the production of HOCl in the phagosome. In MPO deficiency, the microbicidal activity of the neutrophils is reduced early after ingestion of microorganisms (see Table 66–2). However, normal microbicidal activity is observed in approximately 1 hour after a variety of organisms are ingested.[440] Thus, the MPO-deficient neutrophil uses an MPO-independent system for killing bacteria that is slower than the MPO–H_2O_2–halide system, but that is eventually effective in eliminating bacteria. MPO-deficient neutrophils accumulate more H_2O_2 than do normal neutrophils; the higher peroxide concentration improves the bactericidal activity of the affected neutrophils. In contrast to the retardation of bactericidal activity, candidacidal activity in MPO-deficient neutrophils is absent.[440] The most significant clinical manifestation in a few patients with diabetes mellitus and MPO deficiency has been severe infection with *C. albicans*. Because this is such a common disorder of phagocytes, it is important to note that the vast majority of patients with this genetic disorder have not been unusually susceptible to pyogenic infections and do not require therapy.

The complementary DNA encoding human MPO has been cloned and the gene structure, including promoter and regulatory elements, delineated.[440] The gene consists of 12 exons and 11 introns and is located on the long arm of chromosome 17, and its expression is finely coordinated with expression of genes encoding other lysosomal proteins. Expression of genes for human neutrophil elastase and MPO is very similar; it is low in myeloblasts, peaks during the promyelocyte stage, and eventually drops to low levels in myelocytes. MPO is a symmetric molecule composed of four peptides, where each half consists of a heavy- and a light-chain heterodimer.[440] Each heavy- and light-chain heterodimer starts as a single peptide that is cleaved during the posttranslational process to yield the heavy and light chains that form half of the mature molecules. The two halves of the molecule are associated by a disulfide linkage between heavy-subunit residues at their residue C319.

The primary translation product of the gene is a single-chain peptide of 80 kDa that undergoes cotranslational glycosylation at several asparagine residues, followed by a series of modifications of these oligosaccharides. The apopromyeloperoxidase exists for a prolonged time in the endoplasmic reticulum, where it associates reversibly with several endoplasmic reticulum–resident proteins known as molecular chaperones.[440] Subsequent to heme insertion, the enzymatically active promyeloperoxidase undergoes proteolytic cleavage of the pro region. Then, in a prelysosomal compartment, the single peptide is cleaved into the heavy and light subunits, which remain linked. During final sorting within the azurophil lysosome compartment, there is dimerization of half-molecules to form the mature MPO.

Most patients with MPO deficiency have a missense mutation in the gene that results in replacement of arginine 569 with tryptophan.[440] The mutation results in a precursor that associates with molecular chaperones, but does not incorporate heme, resulting in a maturational arrest during processing at the stage of an inactive enzymatic apopromyeloperoxidase. Other patients are heterozygotes with one allele bearing the common mutation and the other being normal, resulting in a partial deficiency.[441] To date, four genotypes have been reported to cause inherited MPO deficiency, each of which results in missense mutations. In the genotype Y173C, a missense mutation results in replacement of a tyrosine at codon 173 with a cysteine residue resulting in the mutant precursor being retained in the endoplasmic reticulum by virtue of its prolonged interaction with the chaperone calnexin, and eventually undergoing degradation in a proteasome.[440] In this way, the quality control system operating in the endoplasmic reticulum retrieves misfolded MPO precursors from the biosynthetic pathway and creates the biochemical phenotype of MPO deficiency. In another patient, a missense mutation resulted in an intact MPO molecule that acquired heme but failed to undergo proteolytic processing to a mature molecule.

Acquired disorders are associated with MPO deficiency. Reported states include lead intoxication, ceroid lipofuscinosis, myelodysplastic syndromes, and acute myelogenous leukemia.[442] One-half of untreated patients with acute myelogenous leukemia and 20 percent of patients with CML may have MPO deficiency.[442]

Deficiencies of Glutathione Reductase and Glutathione Synthetase

Neutrophils contain enzymes capable of inactivating potentially damaging reduced oxygen byproducts. Disposal of superoxide anion is accomplished through superoxide dismutase, a soluble enzyme that converts superoxide to a H_2O_2. H_2O_2 is detoxified by catalase and by the glutathione peroxidase–glutathione reductase system, which converts H_2O_2 to water and oxygen.[443] In addition to the soluble enzymes, cellular vitamin E serves as an antioxidant to prevent damage to the surface of activated neutrophils when releasing H_2O_2.[443] Single cases of profound deficiencies in glutathione reductase[444] and glutathione synthetase[443] have been associated with impaired neutrophil bactericidal activity (see Table 66–2). Both deficiencies are associated with hemolysis under conditions of oxidative stress (Chap. 48). Glutathione synthetase deficiency also has been associated with intermittent neutropenia during times of mild infection. Vitamin E has been employed to ameliorate the hemolysis and improve neutrophil function in a patient with glutathione synthetase deficiency.[445] Like patients with MPO-deficient neutrophils, the patients with glutathione reductase deficiency and glutathione synthetase deficiency are not unusually susceptible to bacterial infections.

● DIAGNOSTIC APPROACH TO THE PATIENT WITH SUSPECTED NEUTROPHIL DYSFUNCTION

An increased susceptibility to pyogenic infections must be viewed in light of a number of factors: (1) adequacy of host defense; (2) the microbes to which the host is exposed; and (3) the conditions of the exposure. It is not always easy to establish a diagnosis of a specific neutrophil dysfunction on clinical grounds alone. Patients with recurrent pyogenic infections often yield no clues as to why they are afflicted, and patients with established deficiency of a defense mechanism may have an unimpressive clinical history. On the other hand, patients may be suspected of having a neutrophil dysfunction if they have a history of frequent bacterial or severe infections. Recurrent pulmonary infections, hepatic abscesses, and perirectal abscesses also should alert the clinician to consider further diagnostic evaluation of neutrophil function. For example, the identification of unusual catalase-positive bacteria and fungi, such as *B. cepacia*, *S. marcescens*, *Nocardia*, and *Aspergillus*, could be indicative of CGD.

Because many of the tests of neutrophil function are bioassays with great variability, the results of the tests must be interpreted in light of the patient's clinical condition. For instance, isolated chemotactic defects usually do not explain the propensity for a patient to have recurrent severe infections. Furthermore, variation in bioassays is often intensified by inflammation or infection. Figure 66–8 is an algorithm for evaluation of the patient with recurrent infection.

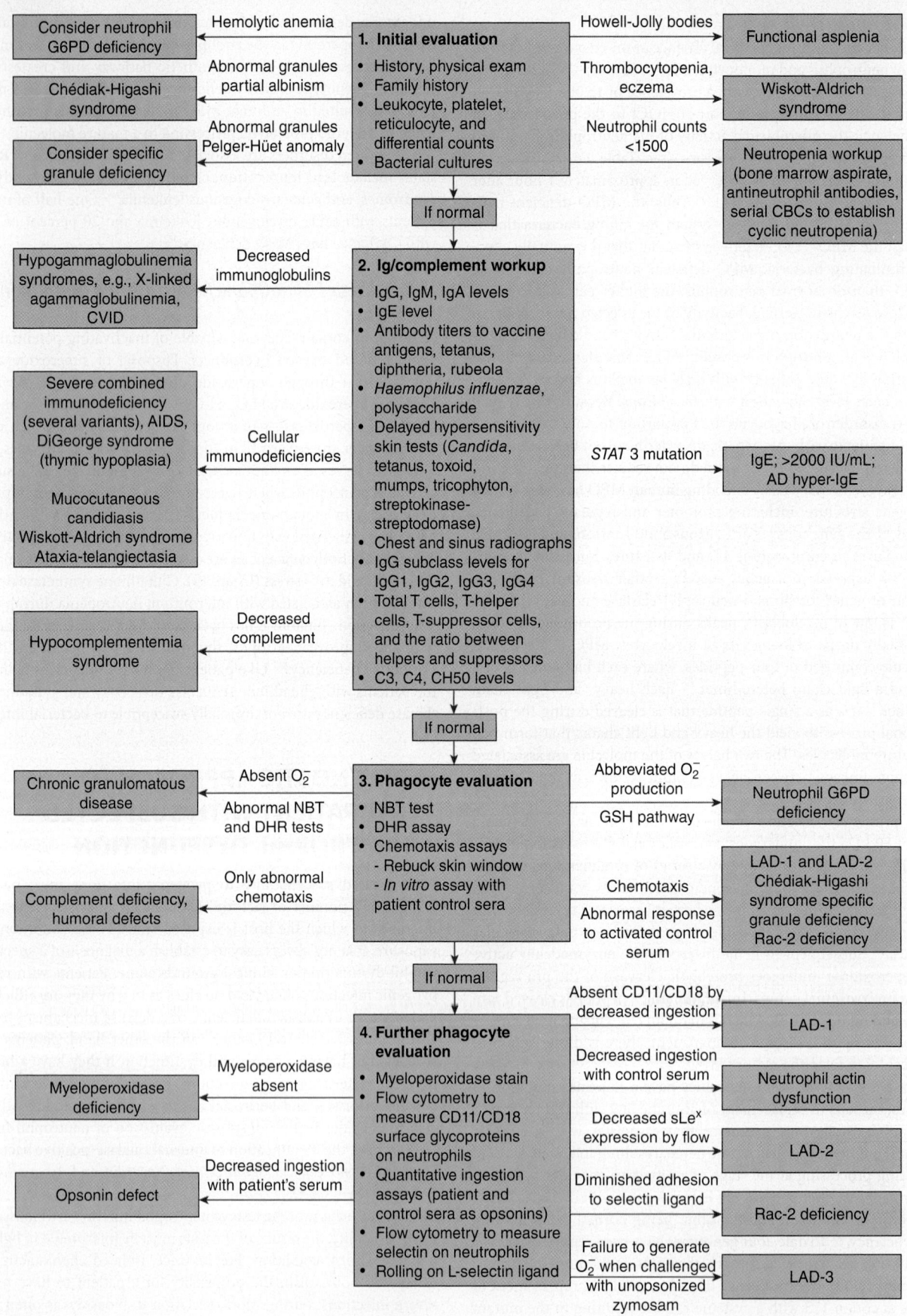

Figure 66–8. Algorithm for the workup of patients with recurrent infections. AD, autosomal dominant; CBC, complete blood count; CVID, common variable immunodeficiency; DHR, delayed hypersensitivity reaction; G6PD, glucose-6-phosphate dehydrogenase; GSH, glutathione; Ig, immunoglobulin; LAD, leukocyte adhesion deficiency; NBT, nitroblue tetrazolium; sLe^x, sialyl Lewis X.

REFERENCES

1. Mudd S, McCutcheon S, Lucké B: Phagocytosis. *Physiol Rev* 14:210, 1934.
2. Zigmond SH: Ability of polymorphonuclear leukocytes to orient in gradients of chemotactic factors. *J Cell Biol* 75:606, 1977.
3. Foxman EF, Campbell JJ, Butcher EC: Multistep navigation and the combinatorial control of leukocyte chemotaxis. *J Cell Biol* 139:1349, 1997.
4. Quitt M, Torres M, McGuire W, et al: Neutrophil chemotactic heterogeneity to N-formyl-methionyl-leucyl-phenylalanine detected by the under-agarose assay. *J Lab Clin Med* 115:159, 1990.
5. Lee J, Gustafsson M, Magnusson KE, et al: The direction of membrane lipid flow in locomoting polymorphonuclear leukocytes. *Science* 247:1229, 1990.
6. Marks PW, Maxfield FR: Local and global changes in cytosolic free calcium in neutrophils during chemotaxis and phagocytosis. *Cell Calcium* 11:181, 1990.
7. Stossel TP, Hartwig JH, Janmey PA, et al: Cell crawling two decades after Abercrombie. *Biochem Soc Symp* 65:267, 1999.
8. Sasawatari S, Yoshizaki M, Taya C, et al: The Ly49Q receptor plays a crucial role in neutrophil polarization and migration by regulating raft trafficking. *Immunity* 32:200, 2010.
9. Kamakura S, Nomura M, Hayase J, et al: The cell polarity protein mInsc regulates neutrophil chemotaxis via a noncanonical G protein signaling pathway. *Dev Cell* 26:292, 2013.
10. Damoulakis G, Gambardella L, Rossman KL, et al: P-Rex1 directly activates RhoG to regulate GPCR-driven Rac signalling and actin polarity in neutrophils. *J Cell Sci* 127:2589, 2014.
11. Ku CJ, Wang Y, Weiner OD, et al: Network crosstalk dynamically changes during neutrophil polarization. *Cell* 149:1073, 2012.
12. Berlin RD, Fera JP, Pfeiffer JR: Reversible phagocytosis in rabbit polymorphonuclear leukocytes. *J Clin Invest* 63:1137, 1979.
13. Bunting M, Harris ES, McIntyre TM, et al: Leukocyte adhesion deficiency syndromes: Adhesion and tethering defects involving beta 2 integrins and selectin ligands. *Curr Opin Hematol* 9:30, 2002.
14. Sundd P, Gutierrez E, Koltsova EK, et al: "Slings" enable neutrophil rolling at high shear. *Nature* 488:399, 2012.
15. Shao JY, Ting-Beall HP, Hochmuth RM: Static and dynamic lengths of neutrophil microvilli. *Proc Natl Acad Sci U S A* 95:6797, 1998.
16. Yonemura S, Tsukita S, Tsukita S: Direct involvement of ezrin/radixin/moesin (ERM)-binding membrane proteins in the organization of microvilli in collaboration with activated ERM proteins. *J Cell Biol* 145:1497, 1999.
17. Pestonjamasp K, Amieva MR, Strassel CP, et al: Moesin, ezrin, and p205 are actin-binding proteins associated with neutrophil plasma membranes. *Mol Biol Cell* 6:247, 1995.
18. Bruehl RE, Moore KL, Lorant DE, et al: Leukocyte activation induces surface redistribution of P-selectin glycoprotein ligand-1. *J Leukoc Biol* 61:489, 1997.
19. Steegmaier M, Borges E, Berger J, et al: The E-selectin-ligand ESL-1 is located in the Golgi as well as on microvilli on the cell surface. *J Cell Sci* 110:687, 1997.
20. Buscher K, Riese SB, Shakibaei M, et al: The transmembrane domains of L-selectin and CD44 regulate receptor cell surface positioning and leukocyte adhesion under flow. *J Biol Chem* 285:13490, 2010.
21. McIntyre TM, Prescott SM, Weyrich AS, et al: Cell-cell interactions: Leukocyte-endothelial interactions. *Curr Opin Hematol* 10:150, 2003.
22. Urzainqui A, Serrador JM, Viedma F, et al: ITAM-based interaction of ERM proteins with Syk mediates signaling by the leukocyte adhesion receptor PSGL-1. *Immunity* 17:401, 2002.
23. Green CE, Pearson DN, Christensen NB, et al: Topographic requirements and dynamics of signaling via L-selectin on neutrophils. *Am J Physiol Cell Physiol* 284:C705, 2003.
24. Yago T, Shao B, Miner JJ, et al: E-selectin engages PSGL-1 and CD44 through a common signaling pathway to induce integrin $\alpha_L\beta_2$-mediated slow leukocyte rolling. *Blood* 116:485, 2010.
25. Mocsai A, Ruland J, Tybulewicz VL: The SYK tyrosine kinase: A crucial player in diverse biological functions. *Nat Rev Immunol* 10:387, 2010.
26. Li Y, Brazzell J, Herrera A, et al: ADAM17 deficiency by mature neutrophils has differential effects on L-selectin shedding. *Blood* 108:2275, 2006.
27. Long C, Hosseinkhani MR, Wang Y, et al: ADAM17 activation in circulating neutrophils following bacterial challenge impairs their recruitment. *J Leukoc Biol* 92:667, 2012.
28. Shigeta A, Matsumoto M, Tedder TF, et al: An L-selectin ligand distinct from P-selectin glycoprotein ligand-1 is expressed on endothelial cells and promotes neutrophil rolling in inflammation. *Blood* 112:4915, 2008.
29. Witko-Sarsat V, Rieu P, Descamps-Latscha B, et al: Neutrophils: Molecules, functions and pathophysiological aspects. *Lab Invest* 80:617, 2000.
30. Wolff B, Burns AR, Middleton J, et al: Endothelial cell "memory" of inflammatory stimulation: Human venular endothelial cells store interleukin 8 in Weibel-Palade bodies. *J Exp Med* 188:1757, 1998.
31. Middleton J, Neil S, Wintle J, et al: Transcytosis and surface presentation of IL-8 by venular endothelial cells. *Cell* 91:385, 1997.
32. Sengelov H, Kjeldsen L, Diamond MS, et al: Subcellular localization and dynamics of Mac-1 $\alpha_M\beta_2$ in human neutrophils. *J Clin Invest* 92:1467, 1993.
33. Kuwano Y, Spelten O, Zhang H, et al: Rolling on E- or P-selectin induces the extended but not high-affinity conformation of LFA-1 in neutrophils. *Blood* 116:617, 2010.
34. Abram CL, Lowell CA: The ins and outs of leukocyte integrin signaling. *Annu Rev Immunol* 27:339, 2009.
35. Evans R, Patzak I, Svensson L, et al: Integrins in immunity. *J Cell Sci* 122:215, 2009.
36. Svensson L, Howarth K, Mcdowall A, et al: Leukocyte adhesion deficiency-III is caused by mutations in KINDLIN3 affecting integrin activation. *Nat Med* 15:306, 2009.
37. Petty HR, Kindzelskii AL, Adachi Y, et al: Ectodomain interactions of leukocyte integrins and pro-inflammatory GPI-linked membrane proteins. *J Pharm Biomed Anal* 15:1405, 1997.
38. Woodfin A, Voisin MB, Nourshargh S: Recent developments and complexities in neutrophil transmigration. *Curr Opin Hematol* 17:9, 2010.
39. Broermann A, Winderlich M, Block H, et al: Dissociation of VE-PTP from VE-cadherin is required for leukocyte extravasation and for VEGF-induced vascular permeability in vivo. *J Exp Med* 208:2393, 2011.
40. Borregaard N: Neutrophils, from marrow to microbes. *Immunity* 33:657, 2010.
41. Woodfin A, Voisin MB, Beyrau M, et al: The junctional adhesion molecule JAM-C regulates polarized transendothelial migration of neutrophils in vivo. *Nat Immunol* 12:761, 2011.
42. Kolaczkowska E, Kubes P: Neutrophil recruitment and function in health and inflammation. *Nat Rev Immunol* 13:159, 2013.
43. Stark K, Eckart A, Haidari S, et al: Capillary and arteriolar pericytes attract innate leukocytes exiting through venules and "instruct" them with pattern-recognition and motility programs. *Nat Immunol* 14:41, 2013.
44. Rossaint J, Zarbock A: Tissue-specific neutrophil recruitment into the lung, liver, and kidney. *J Innate Immun* 5:348, 2013.
45. Lammermann T, Afonso PV, Angermann BR, et al: Neutrophil swarms require LTB4 and integrins at sites of cell death in vivo. *Nature* 498:371, 2013.
46. Booth JW, Trimble WS, Grinstein S: Membrane dynamics in phagocytosis. *Semin Immunol* 13:357, 2001.
47. Kawai T, Akira S: Toll-like receptors and their crosstalk with other innate receptors in infection and immunity. *Immunity* 34:637, 2011.
48. Osorio F, Reis e Sousa C: Myeloid C-type lectin receptors in pathogen recognition and host defense. *Immunity* 34:651, 2011.
49. Loo YM, Gale M Jr: Immune signaling by RIG-I-like receptors. *Immunity* 34:680, 2011.
50. Elinav E, Strowig T, Henao-Mejia J, et al: Regulation of the antimicrobial response by NLR proteins. *Immunity* 34:665, 2011.
51. Jin MS, Lee JO: Structures of the toll-like receptor family and its ligand complexes. *Immunity* 29:182, 2008.
52. West AP, Koblansky AA, Ghosh S: Recognition and signaling by toll-like receptors. *Annu Rev Cell Dev Biol* 22:409, 2006.
53. Diebold SS: Recognition of viral single-stranded RNA by Toll-like receptors. *Adv Drug Deliv Rev* 60:813, 2008.
54. Kindrachuk J, Potter J, Wilson HL, et al: Activation and regulation of toll-like receptor 9: CpGs and beyond. *Mini Rev Med Chem* 8:590, 2008.
55. Akira S, Sato S: Toll-like receptors and their signaling mechanisms. *Scand J Infect Dis* 35:555, 2003.
56. Gay NJ, Gangloff M: Structure and function of Toll receptors and their ligands. *Annu Rev Biochem* 76:141, 2007.
57. Bakele M, Joos M, Burdi S, et al: Localization and functionality of the inflammasome in neutrophils. *J Biol Chem* 289:5320, 2014.
58. Theilgaard-Monch K, Knudsen S, Follin P, et al: The transcriptional activation program of human neutrophils in skin lesions supports their important role in wound healing. *J Immunol* 172:7684, 2004.
59. Sengelov H, Voldstedlund M, Vinten J, et al: Human neutrophils are devoid of the integral membrane protein caveolin. *J Leukoc Biol* 63:563, 1998.
60. Borregaard N, Miller LJ, Springer TA: Chemoattractant-regulated mobilization of a novel intracellular compartment in human neutrophils. *Science* 237:1204, 1987.
61. Borregaard N, Kjeldsen L, Rygaard K, et al: Stimulus-dependent secretion of plasma proteins from human neutrophils. *J Clin Invest* 90:86, 1992.
62. Sengelov H, Kjeldsen L, Borregaard N: Control of exocytosis in early neutrophil activation. *J Immunol* 150:1535, 1993.
63. Chaudhuri S, Kumar A, Berger M: Association of ARF and Rabs with complement receptor type-1 storage vesicles in human neutrophils. *J Leukoc Biol* 70:669, 2001.
64. Dahlgren C, Karlsson A, Sendo F: Neutrophil secretory vesicles are the intracellular reservoir for GPI-80, a protein with adhesion-regulating potential. *J Leukoc Biol* 69:57, 2001.
65. Kumar A, Wetzler E, Berger M: Isolation and characterization of complement receptor type 1 (CR1) storage vesicles from human neutrophils using antibodies to the cytoplasmic tail of CR1. *Blood* 89:4555, 1997.
66. Sengelov H, Follin P, Kjeldsen L, et al: Mobilization of granules and secretory vesicles during in vivo exudation of human neutrophils. *J Immunol* 154:4157, 1995.
67. Morgan CP, Sengelov H, Whatmore J, et al: ADP-ribosylation-factor-regulated phospholipase D activity localizes to secretory vesicles and mobilizes to the plasma membrane following N-formylmethionyl-leucyl-phenylalanine stimulation of human neutrophils. *Biochem J* 325:581, 1997.
68. Borregaard N, Kjeldsen L, Sengelov H: Mobilization of granules in neutrophils from patients with myeloproliferative disorders. *Eur J Haematol* 50:189, 1993.
69. Dotti G, Garattini E, Borleri G, et al: Leucocyte alkaline phosphatase identifies terminally differentiated normal neutrophils and its lack in chronic myelogenous leukaemia is not dependent on p210 tyrosine kinase activity. *Br J Haematol* 105:163, 1999.

70. Rambaldi A, Masuhara K, Borleri GM, et al: Flow cytometry of leucocyte alkaline phosphatase in normal and pathologic leucocytes. *Br J Haematol* 96:815, 1997.

71. Sengelov H, Kjeldsen L, Kroeze W, et al: Secretory vesicles are the intracellular reservoir of complement receptor 1 in human neutrophils. *J Immunol* 153:804, 1994.

72. Muniz M, Riezman H: Intracellular transport of GPI-anchored proteins. *EMBO J* 19:10, 2000.

73. Ehrlich P: Beiträge zur kenntniss der anilinfärbunden und ihrer verwendung in der mikroskopizchen technik. *Arch Mikrosk Anat* 13:263, 1878.

74. Ehrlich P: Über die specifischen granulationen des blutes. *Arch Anat Physiol* 571 Supplementum, 1879.

75. Bainton DF, Farquhar MG: Origin of granules in polymorphonuclear leukocytes. Two types derived from opposite faces of the Golgi complex in developing granulocytes. *J Cell Biol* 28:277, 1966.

76. Bainton DF, Ullyot JL, Farquhar MG: The development of neutrophilic polymorphonuclear leukocytes in human bone marrow. *J Exp Med* 134:907, 1971.

77. Dewald B, Bretz U, Baggiolini M: Release of gelatinase from a novel secretory compartment of human neutrophils. *J Clin Invest* 70:518, 1982.

78. Kjeldsen L, Sengelov H, Lollike K, et al: Isolation and characterization of gelatinase granules from human neutrophils. *Blood* 83:1640, 1994.

79. Kjeldsen L, Johnsen AH, Sengelov H, et al: Isolation and primary structure of NGAL, a novel protein associated with human neutrophil gelatinase. *J Biol Chem* 268:10425, 1993.

80. Borregaard N, Cowland JB: Granules of the human neutrophilic polymorphonuclear leukocyte. *Blood* 89:3503, 1997.

81. Borregaard N, Heiple JM, Simons ER, et al: Subcellular localization of the b-cytochrome component of the human neutrophil microbicidal oxidase: Translocation during activation. *J Cell Biol* 97:52, 1983.

82. Ganz T, Selsted ME, Szklarek D, et al: Defensins. Natural peptide antibiotics of human neutrophils. *J Clin Invest* 76:1427, 1985.

83. Rice WG, Ganz T, Kinkade JM Jr, et al: Defensin-rich dense granules of human neutrophils. *Blood* 70:757, 1987.

84. Faurschou M, Sorensen OE, Johnsen AH, et al: Defensin-rich granules of human neutrophils: Characterization of secretory properties. *Biochim Biophys Acta* 1591:29, 2002.

85. Cham BP, Gerrard JM, Bainton DF: Granulophysin is located in the membrane of azurophilic granules in human neutrophils and mobilizes to the plasma membrane following cell stimulation. *Am J Pathol* 144:1369, 1994.

86. Skubitz KM, Campbell KD, Iida J, et al: CD63 associates with tyrosine kinase activity and CD11/CD18, and transmits an activation signal in neutrophils. *J Immunol* 157:3617, 1996.

87. Kjeldsen L, Bainton DF, Sengelov H, et al: Structural and functional heterogeneity among peroxidase-negative granules in human neutrophils: Identification of a distinct gelatinase-containing granule subset by combined immunocytochemistry and subcellular fractionation. *Blood* 82:3183, 1993.

88. Kjeldsen L, Bjerrum OW, Hovgaard D, et al: Human neutrophil gelatinase: A marker for circulating blood neutrophils. Purification and quantitation by enzyme linked immunosorbent assay. *Eur J Haematol* 49:180, 1992.

89. Cowland JB, Johnsen AH, Borregaard N: hCAP-18, a cathelin/pro-bactenecin-like protein of human neutrophil specific granules. *FEBS Lett* 368:173, 1995.

90. Sorensen OE, Follin P, Johnsen AH, et al: Human cathelicidin, hCAP-18, is processed to the antimicrobial peptide LL-37 by extracellular cleavage with proteinase 3. *Blood* 97:3951, 2001.

91. Borregaard N, Kjeldsen L, Sengelov H, et al: Changes in subcellular localization and surface expression of L-selectin, alkaline phosphatase, and Mac-1 in human neutrophils during stimulation with inflammatory mediators. *J Leukoc Biol* 56:80, 1994.

92. Borregaard N, Lollike K, Kjeldsen L, et al: Human neutrophil granules and secretory vesicles. *Eur J Haematol* 51:187, 1993.

93. Canonne-Hergaux F, Calafat J, Richer E, et al: Expression and subcellular localization of NRAMP1 in human neutrophil granules. *Blood* 100:268, 2002.

94. Kang T, Yi J, Guo A, et al: Subcellular distribution and cytokine- and chemokine-regulated secretion of leukolysin/MT6-MMP/MMP-25 in neutrophils. *J Biol Chem* 276:21960, 2001.

95. Kjeldsen L, Bjerrum OW, Askaa J, et al: Subcellular localization and release of human neutrophil gelatinase, confirming the existence of separate gelatinase-containing granules. *Biochem J* 287(Pt 2):603, 1992.

96. Lominadze G, Powell DW, Luerman GC, et al: Proteomic analysis of human neutrophil granules. *Mol Cell Proteomics* 4:1503, 2005.

97. Rorvig S, Ostergaard O, Heegaard NH, et al: Proteome profiling of human neutrophil granule subsets, secretory vesicles, and cell membrane: Correlation with transcriptome profiling of neutrophil precursors. *J Leukoc Biol* 94:711, 2013.

98. Borregaard N, Sehested M, Nielsen BS, et al: Biosynthesis of granule proteins in normal human bone marrow cells. Gelatinase is a marker of terminal neutrophil differentiation. *Blood* 85:812, 1995.

99. Bjerregaard MD, Jurlander J, Klausen P, et al: The in vivo profile of transcription factors during neutrophil differentiation in human bone marrow. *Blood* 101:4322, 2003.

100. Cowland JB, Borregaard N: The individual regulation of granule protein mRNA levels during neutrophil maturation explains the heterogeneity of neutrophil granules. *J Leukoc Biol* 66:989, 1999.

101. Theilgaard-Monch K, Jacobsen LC, Borup R, et al: The transcriptional program of terminal granulocytic differentiation. *Blood* 105:1785, 2005.

102. Le Cabec V, Cowland JB, Calafat J, Borregaard N: Targeting of proteins to granule subsets is determined by timing and not by sorting: The specific granule protein NGAL is localized to azurophil granules when expressed in HL-60 cells. *Proc Natl Acad Sci U S A* 93:6454, 1996.

103. Goda Y: SNAREs and regulated vesicle exocytosis. *Proc Natl Acad Sci U S A* 94:769, 1997.

104. Rothman JE: Mechanisms of intracellular protein transport. *Nature* 372:55, 1994.

105. Brumell JH, Volchuk A, Sengelov H, et al: Subcellular distribution of docking/fusion proteins in neutrophils, secretory cells with multiple exocytic compartments. *J Immunol* 155:5750, 1995.

106. Mollinedo F, Martin-Martin B, Calafat J, et al: Role of vesicle-associated membrane protein-2, through Q-soluble N-ethylmaleimide-sensitive factor attachment protein receptor/R-soluble N-ethylmaleimide-sensitive factor attachment protein receptor interaction, in the exocytosis of specific and tertiary granules of human neutrophils. *J Immunol* 170:1034, 2003.

107. Arnljots K, Sorensen O, Lollike K, et al: Timing, targeting and sorting of azurophil granule proteins in human myeloid cells. *Leukemia* 12:1789, 1998.

108. Lollike K, Kjeldsen L, Sengelov H, et al: Lysozyme in human neutrophils and plasma. A parameter of myelopoietic activity. *Leukemia* 9:159, 1995.

109. Gombart AF, Shiohara M, Kwok SH, et al: Neutrophil-specific granule deficiency: Homozygous recessive inheritance of a frameshift mutation in the gene encoding transcription factor CCAAT/enhancer binding protein—epsilon. *Blood* 97:2561, 2001.

110. Verbeek W, Wachter M, Lekstrom-Himes J, et al: C/EBPepsilon −/− mice: Increased rate of myeloid proliferation and apoptosis. *Leukemia* 15:103, 2001.

111. Emmertsen F, Glenthoj A, Sonderskov J, et al: ProHNPs are specific markers of normal myelopoiesis. *Blood Cancer J* 4:e193, 2014.

112. Liu L, Ganz T: The pro region of human neutrophil defensin contains a motif that is essential for normal subcellular sorting. *Blood* 85:1095, 1995.

113. Lemansky P, Gerecitano-Schmidek M, Das RC, et al: Targeting myeloperoxidase to azurophilic granules in HL-60 cells. *J Leukoc Biol* 74:542, 2003.

114. Glenthoj A, Cowland JB, Heegaard NH, et al: Serglycin participates in retention of alpha-defensin in granules during myelopoiesis. *Blood* 118:4440, 2011.

115. Niemann CU, Cowland JB, Klausen P, et al: Localization of serglycin in human neutrophil granulocytes and their precursors. *J Leukoc Biol* 76:406, 2004.

116. Abrink M, Grujic M, Pejler G: Serglycin is essential for maturation of mast cell secretory granule. *J Biol Chem* 279:40897, 2004.

117. Niemann CU, Abrink M, Pejler G, et al: Neutrophil elastase depends on serglycin proteoglycan for localization in granules. *Blood* 109:4478, 2007.

118. Kallquist L, Hansson M, Persson AM, et al: The tetraspanin CD63 is involved in granule targeting of neutrophil elastase. *Blood* 112:3444, 2008.

119. Braga T, Ringvall M, Tveit H, et al: Reduction with dithiothreitol causes serglycin-specific defects in secretory granule integrity of bone marrow derived mast cells. *Mol Immunol* 46:422, 2009.

120. Sorensen O, Bratt T, Johnsen AH, et al: The human antibacterial cathelicidin, hCAP-18, is bound to lipoproteins in plasma. *J Biol Chem* 274:22445, 1999.

121. Anderson KL, Smith KA, Conners K, et al: Myeloid development is selectively disrupted in PU.1 null mice. *Blood* 91:3702, 1998.

122. Fisher RC, Lovelock JD, Scott EW: A critical role for PU.1 in homing and long-term engraftment by hematopoietic stem cells in the bone marrow. *Blood* 94:1283, 1999.

123. Eklund EA, Jalava A, Kakar R: PU.1, interferon regulatory factor 1, and interferon consensus sequence-binding protein cooperate to increase gp91(phox) expression. *J Biol Chem* 273:13957, 1998.

124. Gombart AF, Kwok SH, Anderson KL, et al: Regulation of neutrophil and eosinophil secondary granule gene expression by transcription factors C/EBP epsilon and PU.1. *Blood* 101:3265, 2003.

125. Oelgeschlager M, Nuchprayoon I, Luscher B, et al: C/EBP, c-Myb, and PU.1 cooperate to regulate the neutrophil elastase promoter. *Mol Cell Biol* 16:4717, 1996.

126. Simon MC, Olson M, Scott E, et al: Terminal myeloid gene expression and differentiation requires the transcription factor PU.1. *Curr Top Microbiol Immunol* 211:113, 1996.

127. Yamanaka R, Barlow C, Lekstrom-Himes J, et al: Impaired granulopoiesis, myelodysplasia, and early lethality in CCAAT/enhancer binding protein epsilon-deficient mice. *Proc Natl Acad Sci U S A* 94:13187, 1997.

128. Morosetti R, Park DJ, Chumakov AM, et al: A novel, myeloid transcription factor, C/EBP epsilon, is upregulated during granulocytic, but not monocytic, differentiation. *Blood* 90:2591, 1997.

129. Larsen MT, Hother C, Hager M, et al: MicroRNA profiling in human neutrophils during bone marrow granulopoiesis and in vivo exudation. *PLoS One* 8:e58454, 2013.

130. Johnnidis JB, Harris MH, Wheeler RT, et al: Regulation of progenitor cell proliferation and granulocyte function by microRNA-223. *Nature* 451:1125, 2008.

131. Hager M, Pedersen CC, Larsen MT, et al: MicroRNA-130a-mediated down-regulation of Smad4 contributes to reduced sensitivity to TGF-beta1 stimulation in granulocytic precursors. *Blood* 118:6649, 2011.

132. Larsen MT, Hager M, Glenthoj A, et al: MiRNA-130a regulates C/EBP-epsilon expression during granulopoiesis. *Blood* 123:1079, 2014.

133. Arnljots K, Olsson I: Myeloperoxidase precursors incorporate heme. *J Biol Chem* 262:10430, 1987.

134. Nauseef WM, McCormick S, Yi H: Roles of heme insertion and the mannose-6-phosphate receptor in processing of the human myeloid lysosomal enzyme, myeloperoxidase. *Blood* 80:2622, 1992.

135. Klebanoff SJ: Myeloperoxidase. *Proc Assoc Am Physicians* 111:383, 1999.

136. Klebanoff SJ, Nathan CF: Nitrite production by stimulated human polymorphonuclear leukocytes supplemented with azide and catalase. *Biochem Biophys Res Commun* 197:192, 1993.

137. Eiserich JP, Baldus S, Brennan ML, et al: Myeloperoxidase, a leukocyte-derived vascular NO oxidase. *Science* 296:2391, 2002.

138. Savige J, Davies D, Falk RJ, et al: Antineutrophil cytoplasmic antibodies and associated diseases: A review of the clinical and laboratory features. *Kidney Int* 57:846, 2000.

139. Tervaert JW, Goldschmeding R, Elema JD, et al: Association of autoantibodies to myeloperoxidase with different forms of vasculitis. *Arthritis Rheum* 33:1264, 1990.

140. Levy O, Elsbach P: Bactericidal/permeability-increasing protein in host defense and its efficacy in the treatment of bacterial sepsis. *Curr Infect Dis Rep* 3:407, 2007.

141. Alexander S, Bramson J, Foley R, et al: Protection from endotoxemia by adenoviral-mediated gene transfer of human bactericidal/permeability-increasing protein. *Blood* 103:93, 2004.

142. Balakrishnan A, Marathe SA, Joglekar M, et al: Bactericidal/permeability increasing protein: A multifaceted protein with functions beyond LPS neutralization. *Innate Immun* 19:339, 2013.

143. Ganz T: Defensins: Antimicrobial peptides of innate immunity. *Nat Rev Immunol* 3:710, 2003.

144. Selsted ME, Harwig SS, Ganz T, et al: Primary structures of three human neutrophil defensins. *J Clin Invest* 76:1436, 1985.

145. Selsted ME, Tang YQ, Morris WL, et al: Purification, primary structures, and antibacterial activities of beta-defensins, a new family of antimicrobial peptides from bovine neutrophils. *J Biol Chem* 268:6641, 1993.

146. Tang YQ, Yuan J, Osapay G, et al: A cyclic antimicrobial peptide produced in primate leukocytes by the ligation of two truncated alpha-defensins. *Science* 286:498, 1999.

147. Perera NC, Wiesmuller KH, Larsen MT, et al: NSP4 is stored in azurophil granules and released by activated neutrophils as active endoprotease with restricted specificity. *J Immunol* 191:2700, 2013.

148. Perera NC, Schilling O, Kittel H, et al: NSP4, an elastase-related protease in human neutrophils with arginine specificity. *Proc Natl Acad Sci U S A* 109:6229, 2012.

149. Almeida RP, Vanet A, Witko-Sarsat V, et al: Azurocidin, a natural antibiotic from human neutrophils: Expression, antimicrobial activity, and secretion. *Protein Expr Purif* 7:355, 1996.

150. Campanelli D, Detmers PA, Nathan CF, et al: Azurocidin and a homologous serine protease from neutrophils. Differential antimicrobial and proteolytic properties. *J Clin Invest* 85:904, 1990.

151. Flodgaard H, Ostergaard E, Bayne S, et al: Covalent structure of two novel neutrophile leucocyte-derived proteins of porcine and human origin. Neutrophile elastase homologues with strong monocyte and fibroblast chemotactic activities. *Eur J Biochem* 197:535, 1991.

152. Gautam N, Olofsson AM, Herwald H, et al: Heparin-binding protein (HBP/CAP37): A missing link in neutrophil-evoked alteration of vascular permeability. *Nat Med* 7:1123, 2001.

153. Tapper H, Karlsson A, Morgelin M, et al: Secretion of heparin-binding protein from human neutrophils is determined by its localization in azurophilic granules and secretory vesicles. *Blood* 99:1785, 2002.

154. Goldschmeding R, Tervaert JW, Dolman KM, et al: ANCA: A class of vasculitis-associated autoantibodies against myeloid granule proteins: Clinical and laboratory aspects and possible pathogenetic implications. *Adv Exp Med Biol* 297:129, 1991.

155. von Vietinghoff S, Tunnemann G, Eulenberg C, et al: NB1 mediates surface expression of the ANCA antigen proteinase 3 on human neutrophils. *Blood* 109:4487, 2007.

156. von Vietinghoff S, Eulenberg C, Wellner M, et al: Neutrophil surface presentation of the anti-neutrophil cytoplasmic antibody-antigen proteinase 3 depends on N-terminal processing. *Clin Exp Immunol* 152:508, 2008.

157. Skold S, Rosberg B, Gullberg U, et al: A secreted proform of neutrophil proteinase 3 regulates the proliferation of granulopoietic progenitor cells. *Blood* 93:849, 1999.

158. Salvesen G, Enghild JJ: An unusual specificity in the activation of neutrophil serin proteinase zymogens. *Biochemistry* 29:5304, 1990.

159. Pham CT, Ivanovich JL, Raptis SZ, et al: Papillon-Lefevre syndrome: Correlating the molecular, cellular, and clinical consequences of cathepsin C/dipeptidyl peptidase I deficiency in humans. *J Immunol* 173:7277, 2004.

160. Dalgic B, Bukulmez A, Sari S: Eponym: Papillon-Lefevre syndrome. *Eur J Pediatr* 170:689, 2011.

161. Segal AW: How neutrophils kill microbes. *Annu Rev Immunol* 23:197, 2005.

162. Skubitz KM, Campbell KD, Skubitz AP: CD63 associates with CD11/CD18 in large detergent-resistant complexes after translocation to the cell surface in human neutrophils. *FEBS Lett* 469:52, 2000.

163. Saito N, Pulford KA, Breton-Gorius J, et al: Ultrastructural localization of the CD68 macrophage-associated antigen in human blood neutrophils and monocytes. *Am J Pathol* 139:1053, 1991.

164. Mirinics ZK, Calafat J, Udby L, et al: Identification of the presenilins in hematopoietic cells with localization of presenilin 1 to neutrophil and platelet granules. *Blood Cells Mol Dis* 28:28, 2002.

165. Feuk-Lagerstedt E, Samuelsson M, Mosgoeller W, et al: The presence of stomatin in detergent-insoluble domains of neutrophil granule membranes. *J Leukoc Biol* 72:970, 2002.

166. Nanda A, Brumell JH, Nordstrom T, et al: Activation of proton pumping in human neutrophils occurs by exocytosis of vesicles bearing vacuolar-type H+-ATPases. *J Biol Chem* 271:15963, 1996.

167. Masson PL, Heremans JF, Schonne E: Lactoferrin, an iron-binding protein in neutrophilic leukocytes. *J Exp Med* 130:643, 1969.

168. Baveye S, Elass E, Mazurier J, et al: Lactoferrin: A multifunctional glycoprotein involved in the modulation of the inflammatory process. *Clin Chem Lab Med* 37:281, 1999.

169. Farnaud S, Evans RW: Lactoferrin—A multifunctional protein with antimicrobial properties. *Mol Immunol* 40:395, 2003.

170. Aguilera O, Ostolaza H, Quiros LM, et al: Permeabilizing action of an antimicrobial lactoferricin-derived peptide on bacterial and artificial membranes. *FEBS Lett* 462:273, 1999.

171. Nibbering PH, Ravensbergen E, Welling MM, et al: Human lactoferrin and peptides derived from its N terminus are highly effective against infections with antibiotic-resistant bacteria. *Infect Immun* 69:1469, 2001.

172. Flower DR: The lipocalin protein family: Structure and function. *Biochem J* 318:1, 1996.

173. Kjeldsen L, Bainton DF, Sengelov H, et al: Identification of neutrophil gelatinase-associated lipocalin as a novel matrix protein of specific granules in human neutrophils. *Blood* 83:799, 1994.

174. Yan L, Borregaard N, Kjeldsen L, et al: The high molecular weight urinary matrix metalloproteinase (MMP) activity is a complex of gelatinase B/MMP-9 and neutrophil gelatinase-associated lipocalin (NGAL). Modulation of MMP-9 activity by NGAL. *J Biol Chem* 276:37258, 2001.

175. Goetz DH, Holmes MA, Borregaard N, et al: The neutrophil lipocalin NGAL is a bacteriostatic agent that interferes with siderophore-mediated iron acquisition. *Mol Cell* 10:1033, 2002.

176. Cowland JB, Muta T, Borregaard N: IL-1beta-specific up-regulation of neutrophil gelatinase-associated lipocalin is controlled by IkappaB-zeta. *J Immunol* 176:5559, 2006.

177. Flo TH, Smith KD, Sato S, et al: Lipocalin 2 mediates an innate immune response to bacterial infection by sequestrating iron. *Nature* 432:917, 2004.

178. Chan YR, Liu JS, Pociask DA, et al: Lipocalin 2 is required for pulmonary host defense against Klebsiella infection. *J Immunol* 182:4947, 2009.

179. Nairz M, Theurl I, Schroll A, et al: Absence of functional Hfe protects mice from invasive Salmonella enterica serovar Typhimurium infection via induction of lipocalin-2. *Blood* 114:3642, 2009.

180. Saiga H, Nishimura J, Kuwata H, et al: Lipocalin 2-dependent inhibition of mycobacterial growth in alveolar epithelium. *J Immunol* 181:8521, 2008.

181. Warszawska JM, Gawish R, Sharif O, et al: Lipocalin 2 deactivates macrophages and worsens pneumococcal pneumonia outcomes. *J Clin Invest* 123:3363, 2013.

182. Bao G, Clifton M, Hoette TM, et al: Iron traffics in circulation bound to a siderocalin (Ngal)-catechol complex. *Nat Chem Biol* 6:602, 2010.

183. Cellier M, Govoni G, Vidal S, et al: Human natural resistance-associated macrophage protein: CDNA cloning, chromosomal mapping, genomic organization, and tissue-specific expression. *J Exp Med* 180:1741, 1994.

184. Fleming A: On a remarkable bacteriolytic element found in tissues and excretions. *Proc R Soc Lond B Biol Sci* 93:306, 1922.

185. Selsted ME, Martinez RJ: Lysozyme: Primary bactericidin in human plasma serum active against Bacillus subtilis. *Infect Immun* 20:782, 1978.

186. Tanida N, Onho N, Adachi Y, et al: Binding of lysozyme to synthetic monosaccharide lipid A analogue, GLA60. *Biol Pharm Bull* 16:288, 1993.

187. Takada K, Ohno N, Yadomae T: Binding of lysozyme to lipopolysaccharide suppresses tumor necrosis factor production in vivo. *Infect Immun* 62:1171, 1994.

188. Keshav S, Chung P, Milon G, et al: Lysozyme is an inducible marker of macrophage activation in murine tissues as demonstrated by in situ hybridization. *J Exp Med* 174:1049, 1991.

189. Sexton C, Buss D, Powell B, et al: Usefulness and limitations of serum and urine lysozyme levels in the classification of acute myeloid leukemia: An analysis of 208 cases. *Leuk Res* 20:467, 1996.

190. Gudmundsson GH, Agerberth B, Odeberg J, et al: The human gene FALL39 and processing of the cathelin precursor to the antibacterial peptide LL-37 in granulocytes. *Eur J Biochem* 238:325, 1996.

191. Zanetti M: Cathelicidins, multifunctional peptides of the innate immunity. *J Leukoc Biol* 75:39, 2004.

192. Sorensen O, Arnljots K, Cowland JB, et al: The human antibacterial cathelicidin, hCAP-18, is synthesized in myelocytes and metamyelocytes and localized to specific granules in neutrophils. *Blood* 90:2796, 1997.

193. Frohm NM, Sandstedt B, Sorensen O, et al: The human cationic antimicrobial protein (hCAP18), a peptide antibiotic, is widely expressed in human squamous epithelia and colocalizes with interleukin-6. *Infect Immun* 67:2561, 1999.

194. Heilborn JD, Nilsson MF, Kratz G, et al: The cathelicidin anti-microbial peptide LL-37 is involved in re-epithelialization of human skin wounds and is lacking in chronic ulcer epithelium. *J Invest Dermatol* 120:379, 2003.

195. Sorensen OE, Cowland JB, Theilgaard-Monch K, et al: Wound healing and expression of antimicrobial peptides/polypeptides in human keratinocytes, a consequence of common growth factors. *J Immunol* 170:5583, 2003.

196. Sorensen OE, Gram L, Johnsen AH, et al: Processing of seminal plasma hCAP-18 to ALL-38 by gastricsin: A novel mechanism of generating antimicrobial peptides in vagina. *J Biol Chem* 278:28540, 2003.

197. Zaiou M, Nizet V, Gallo RL: Antimicrobial and protease inhibitory functions of the human cathelicidin (hCAP18/LL-37) prosequence. *J Invest Dermatol* 120:810, 2003.

198. De Y, Chen Q, Schmidt AP, et al: LL-37, the neutrophil granule- and epithelial cell-derived cathelicidin, utilizes formyl peptide receptor-like 1 (FPRL1) as a receptor to chemoattract human peripheral blood neutrophils, monocytes, and T cells. *J Exp Med* 192:1069, 2000.

199. Koczulla R, von DG, Kupatt C, et al: An angiogenic role for the human peptide antibiotic LL-37/hCAP-18. *J Clin Invest* 111:1665, 2003.

200. Scott MG, Davidson DJ, Gold MR, et al: The human antimicrobial peptide LL-37 is a multifunctional modulator of innate immune responses. *J Immunol* 169:3883, 2002.

201. Murphy G, Reynolds JJ, Bretz U, et al: Collagenase is a component of the specific granules of human neutrophil leucocytes. *Biochem J* 162:195, 1977.

202. Murphy G, Bretz U, Baggiolini M, et al: The latent collagenase and gelatinase of human polymorphonuclear neutrophil leucocytes. *Biochem J* 192:517, 1980.

203. Pei D: Leukolysin/MMP25/MT6-MMP: A novel matrix metalloproteinase specifically expressed in the leukocyte lineage. *Cell Res* 9:291, 1999.

204. Jaillon S, Peri G, Delneste Y, et al: The humoral pattern recognition receptor PTX3 is stored in neutrophil granules and localizes in extracellular traps. *J Exp Med* 204:793, 2007.

205. Mantovani A, Garlanda C, Doni A, et al: Pentraxins in innate immunity: From C-reactive protein to the long pentraxin PTX3. *J Clin Immunol* 28:1, 2008.

206. Aoyagi Y, Adderson EE, Rubens CE, et al: L-Ficolin/mannose-binding lectin-associated serine protease complexes bind to group B streptococci primarily through N-acetylneuraminic acid of capsular polysaccharide and activate the complement pathway. *Infect Immun* 76:179, 2008.

207. Jacobsen LC, Theilgaard-Monch K, Christensen EI, et al: Arginase 1 is expressed in myelocytes/metamyelocytes and localized in gelatinase granules of human neutrophils. *Blood* 109:3084, 2007.

208. Clemmensen SN, Bohr CT, Rorvig S, et al: Olfactomedin 4 defines a subset of human neutrophils. *J Leukoc Biol* 91:495, 2012.

209. Welin A, Amirbeagi F, Christenson K, et al: The human neutrophil subsets defined by the presence or absence of OLFM4 both transmigrate into tissue in vivo and give rise to distinct NETs in vitro. *PLoS One* 8:e69575, 2013.

210. Ginsel LA, Onderwater JJ, Fransen JA, et al: Localization of the low-Mr subunit of cytochrome b558 in human blood phagocytes by immunoelectron microscopy. *Blood* 76:2105, 1990.

211. Petheo GL, Orient A, Barath M, et al: Molecular and functional characterization of Hv1 proton channel in human granulocytes. *PLoS One* 5:e14081, 2010.

212. El CA, Okochi Y, Sasaki M, et al: VSOP/Hv1 proton channels sustain calcium entry, neutrophil migration, and superoxide production by limiting cell depolarization and acidification. *J Exp Med* 207:129, 2010.

213. Ramsey IS, Ruchti E, Kaczmarek JS, et al: Hv1 proton channels are required for high-level NADPH oxidase-dependent superoxide production during the phagocyte respiratory burst. *Proc Natl Acad Sci U S A* 106:7642, 2009.

214. Feuk-Lagerstedt E, Jordan ET, Leffler H, et al: Identification of CD66a and CD66b as the major galectin-3 receptor candidates in human neutrophils. *J Immunol* 163:5592, 1999.

215. Karlsson A, Follin P, Leffler H, et al: Galectin-3 activates the NADPH-oxidase in exudated but not peripheral blood neutrophils. *Blood* 91:3430, 1998.

216. Williams LT, Snyderman R, Pike MC, et al: Specific receptor sites for chemotactic peptides on human polymorphonuclear leukocytes. *Proc Natl Acad Sci U S A* 74:1204, 1977.

217. Schiffmann E, Aswanikumar S, Venkatasubramanian K, et al: Some characteristics of the neutrophil receptor for chemotactic peptides. *FEBS Lett* 117:1, 1980.

218. Boulay F, Tardif M, Brouchon L, et al: The human N-formylpeptide receptor. Characterization of two cDNA isolates and evidence for a new subfamily of G-protein-coupled receptors. *Biochemistry* 29:11123, 1990.

219. Polakis PG, Uhing RJ, Snyderman R: The formylpeptide chemoattractant receptor copurifies with a GTP-binding protein containing a distinct 40-kDa Pertussis toxin substrate. *J Biol Chem* 263:4969, 1988.

220. Min J, Defea K: Beta-arrestin-dependent actin reorganization: Bringing the right players together at the leading edge. *Mol Pharmacol* 80:760, 2011.

221. Shukla AK, Xiao K, Lefkowitz RJ: Emerging paradigms of beta-arrestin-dependent seven transmembrane receptor signaling. *Trends Biochem Sci* 36:457, 2011.

222. Sengelov H, Boulay F, Kjeldsen L, et al: Subcellular localization and translocation of the receptor for N-formylmethionyl-leucyl-phenylalanine in human neutrophils. *Biochem J* 299:473, 1994.

223. Hugli TE: Structure and function of the anaphylatoxins. *Springer Semin Immunopathol* 7:193, 1984.

224. Chenoweth DE, Hugli TE: Demonstration of specific C5a receptor on intact human polymorphonuclear leukocytes. *Proc Natl Acad Sci U S A* 75:3943, 1978.

225. Rollins TE, Springer MS: Identification of the polymorphonuclear leukocyte C5a receptor. *J Biol Chem* 260:7157, 1985.

226. Boulay F, Mery L, Tardif M, et al: Expression cloning of a receptor for C5a anaphylatoxin on differentiated HL-60 cells. *Biochemistry* 30:2993, 1991.

227. Didsbury JR, Uhing RJ, Tomhave E, et al: Receptor class desensitization of leukocyte chemoattractant receptors. *Proc Natl Acad Sci U S A* 88:11564, 1991.

228. Nakamura M, Honda Z, Izumi T, et al: Molecular cloning and expression of platelet-activating factor receptor from human leukocytes. *J Biol Chem* 266:20400, 1991.

229. Jones SA, Wolf M, Qin S, et al: Different functions for the interleukin 8 receptors (IL-8R) of human neutrophil leukocytes: NADPH oxidase and phospholipase D are activated through IL-8R1 but not IL-8R2. *Proc Natl Acad Sci U S A* 93:6682, 1996.

230. Nathan CF: Neutrophil activation on biological surfaces. Massive secretion of hydrogen peroxide in response to products of macrophages and lymphocytes. *J Clin Invest* 80:1550, 1987.

231. Shappell SB, Toman C, Anderson DC, et al: Mac-1 (CD11b/CD18) mediates adherence-dependent hydrogen peroxide production by human and canine neutrophils. *J Immunol* 144:2702, 1990.

232. Kew RR, Grimaldi CM, Furie MB, et al: Human neutrophil Fc gamma RIIIB and formyl peptide receptors are functionally linked during formyl-methionyl-leucyl-phenylalanine-induced chemotaxis. *J Immunol* 149:989, 1992.

233. Leeuwenberg JF, Van de Winkel JG, Jeunhomme TM, et al: Functional polymorphism of IgG FcRII (CD32) on human neutrophils. *Immunology* 71:301, 1990.

234. Sehgal G, Zhang K, Todd RF, III, et al: Lectin-like inhibition of immune complex receptor-mediated stimulation of neutrophils. Effects on cytosolic calcium release and superoxide production. *J Immunol* 150:4571, 1993.

235. Indik ZK, Park JG, Hunter S, et al: The molecular dissection of Fc gamma receptor mediated phagocytosis. *Blood* 86:4389, 1995.

236. Strzelecka-Kiliszek A, Kwiatkowska K, Sobota A: Lyn and Syk kinases are sequentially engaged in phagocytosis mediated by Fc gamma R. *J Immunol* 169:6787, 2002.

237. Raeder EM, Mansfield PJ, Hinkovska-Galcheva V, et al: Syk activation initiates downstream signaling events during human polymorphonuclear leukocyte phagocytosis. *J Immunol* 163:6785, 1999.

238. Kusner DJ, Barton JA, Wen KK, et al: Regulation of phospholipase D activity by actin. Actin exerts bidirectional modulation of mammalian phospholipase D activity in a polymerization-dependent, isoform-specific manner. *J Biol Chem* 277:50683, 2002.

239. Dusi S, Donini M, Della BV, et al: Tyrosine phosphorylation of phospholipase C-gamma 2 is involved in the activation of phosphoinositide hydrolysis by Fc receptors in human neutrophils. *Biochem Biophys Res Commun* 201:1100, 1994.

240. Mansfield PJ, Shayman JA, Boxer LA: Regulation of polymorphonuclear leukocyte phagocytosis by myosin light chain kinase after activation of mitogen-activated protein kinase. *Blood* 95:2407, 2000.

241. Cockcroft S, Baldwin JM, Allan D: The Ca2+-activated polyphosphoinositide phosphodiesterase of human and rabbit neutrophil membranes. *Biochem J* 221:477, 1984.

242. Favre CJ, Lew DP, Krause KH: Rapid heparin-sensitive Ca2+ release following Ca(2+)-ATPase inhibition in intact HL-60 granulocytes. Evidence for Ins(1,4,5)P3-dependent Ca2+ cycling across the membrane of Ca2+ stores. *Biochem J* 302:155, 1994.

243. Cox D, Chang P, Zhang Q, et al: Requirements for both Rac1 and Cdc42 in membrane ruffling and phagocytosis in leukocytes. *J Exp Med* 186:1487, 1997.

244. Roberts AW, Kim C, Zhen L, et al: Deficiency of the hematopoietic cell-specific Rho family GTPase Rac2 is characterized by abnormalities in neutrophil function and host defense. *Immunity* 10:183, 1999.

245. Mansfield PJ, Hinkovska-Galcheva V, Carey SS, et al: Regulation of polymorphonuclear leukocyte degranulation and oxidant production by ceramide through inhibition of phospholipase D. *Blood* 99:1434, 2002.

246. Blackwood RA, Smolen JE, Transue A, et al: Phospholipase D activity facilitates Ca2+-induced aggregation and fusion of complex liposomes. *Am J Physiol* 272:C1279, 1997.

247. Mansfield PJ, Carey SS, Hinkovska-Galcheva V, et al: Ceramide inhibition of phospholipase D and its relationship to RhoA and ARF1 translocation in GTP gamma S-stimulated polymorphonuclear leukocytes. *Blood* 103:2363, 2004.

248. English D, Cui Y, Siddiqui RA: Messenger functions of phosphatidic acid. *Chem Phys Lipids* 80:117, 1996.

249. Diez E, Balsinde J, Mollinedo F: Subcellular distribution of fatty acids, phospholipids and phospholipase A2 in human neutrophils. *Biochim Biophys Acta* 1047:83, 1990.

250. Pessach I, Leto TL, Malech HL, et al: Essential requirement of cytosolic phospholipase A(2) for stimulation of NADPH oxidase-associated diaphorase activity in granulocyte-like cells. *J Biol Chem* 276:33495, 2001.

251. Naccache PH, Showell HJ, Becker EL, et al: Arachidonic acid induced degranulation of rabbit peritoneal neutrophils. *Biochem Biophys Res Commun* 87:292, 1979.

252. Hardy SJ, Robinson BS, Ferrante A, et al: Polyenoic very-long-chain fatty acids mobilize intracellular calcium from a thapsigargin-insensitive pool in human neutrophils. The relationship between Ca2+ mobilization and superoxide production induced by long- and very-long-chain fatty acids. *Biochem J* 311:689, 1995.

253. Borgeat P, Hamberg M, Samuelsson B: Transformation of arachidonic acid and homo-gamma-linolenic acid by rabbit polymorphonuclear leukocytes. Monohydroxy acids from novel lipoxygenases. *J Biol Chem* 251:7816, 1976.

254. Naccache PH, Sha'afi RI, Borgeat P, et al: Mono- and dihydroxyeicosatetraenoic acids alter calcium homeostasis in rabbit neutrophils. *J Clin Invest* 67:1584, 1981.

255. Palmer RM, Salmon JA: Release of leukotriene B4 from human neutrophils and its relationship to degranulation induced by N-formyl-methionyl-leucyl-phenylalanine, serum-treated zymosan and the ionophore A23187. *Immunology* 50:65, 1983.

256. Palmblad J, Malmsten CL, Uden AM, et al: Leukotriene B4 is a potent and stereospecific stimulator of neutrophil chemotaxis and adherence. *Blood* 58:658, 1981.

257. Wickner W, Schekman R: Membrane fusion. *Nat Struct Mol Biol* 15:658, 2008.

258. Brochetta C, Vita F, Tiwari N, et al: Involvement of Munc18 isoforms in the regulation of granule exocytosis in neutrophils. *Biochim Biophys Acta* 1783:1781, 2008.

259. Logan MR, Lacy P, Odemuyiwa SO, et al: A critical role for vesicle-associated membrane protein-7 in exocytosis from human eosinophils and neutrophils. *Allergy* 61:777, 2006.

260. Brinkmann V, Reichard U, Goosmann C, et al: Neutrophil extracellular traps kill bacteria. *Science* 303:1532, 2004.

261. Brinkmann V, Zychlinsky A: Beneficial suicide: Why neutrophils die to make NETs. *Nat Rev Microbiol* 5:577, 2007.

262. Fuchs TA, Abed U, Goosmann C, et al: Novel cell death program leads to neutrophil extracellular traps. *J Cell Biol* 176:231, 2007.

263. Papayannopoulos V, Metzler KD, Hakkim A, et al: Neutrophil elastase and myeloperoxidase regulate the formation of neutrophil extracellular traps. *J Cell Biol* 191:677, 2010.

264. Fuchs TA, Brill A, Duerschmied D, et al: Extracellular DNA traps promote thrombosis. *Proc Natl Acad Sci U S A* 107:15880, 2010.

265. Yipp BG, Petri B, Salina D, et al: Infection-induced NETosis is a dynamic process involving neutrophil multitasking in vivo. *Nat Med* 18:1386, 2012.

266. Lekstrom-Himes JA, Gallin JI: Immunodeficiency diseases caused by defects in phago-cytes. *N Engl J Med* 343:1703, 2000.

267. Dinauer MC: Disorders of neutrophil function: An overview. *Methods Mol Biol* 1124:501, 2014.

268. Dale DC, Boxer L, Liles WC: The phagocytes: Neutrophils and monocytes. *Blood* 112:935, 2008.

269. Mollnes TE, Jokiranta TS, Truedsson L, et al: Complement analysis in the 21st century. *Mol Immunol* 44:3838, 2007.

270. Botto M, Fong KY, So AK, et al: Molecular basis of hereditary C3 deficiency. *J Clin Invest* 86:1158, 1990.

271. Frank MM: Complement deficiencies. *Pediatr Clin North Am* 47:1339, 2000.

272. Alper CA, Abramson N, Johnston RB Jr, et al: Studies in vivo and in vitro on an abnor-mality in the metabolism of C3 in a patient with increased susceptibility to infection. *J Clin Invest* 49:1975, 1970.

273. Densen P, Weiler JM, Griffiss JM, et al: Familial properdin deficiency and fatal menin-gococcemia. Correction of the bactericidal defect by vaccination. *N Engl J Med* 316:922, 1987.

274. Nolan KF, Schwaeble W, Kaluz S, et al: Molecular cloning of the cDNA coding for properdin, a positive regulator of the alternative pathway of human complement. *Eur J Immunol* 21:771, 1991.

275. Super M, Thiel S, Lu J, et al: Association of low levels of mannan-binding protein with a common defect of opsonisation. *Lancet* 2:1236, 1989.

276. Jack DL, Klein NJ, Turner MW: Mannose-binding lectin: Targeting the microbial world for complement attack and opsonophagocytosis. *Immunol Rev* 180:86, 2001.

277. Turner MW: The role of mannose-binding lectin in health and disease. *Mol Immunol* 40:423, 2003.

278. Trinchieri G, Sher A: Cooperation of Toll-like receptor signals in innate immune defence. *Nat Rev Immunol* 7:179, 2007.

279. von Bernuth H, Picard C, Jin Z, et al: Pyogenic bacterial infections in humans with MyD88 deficiency. *Science* 321:691, 2008.

280. Buckley RH: Immunodeficiency diseases. *JAMA* 258:2841, 1987.

281. Boxer LA, Smolen JE: Neutrophil granule constituents and their release in health and disease. *Hematol Oncol Clin North Am* 2:101, 1988.

282. Ward DM, Shiflett SL, Kaplan J: Chediak-Higashi syndrome: A clinical and molecular view of a rare lysosomal storage disorder. *Curr Mol Med* 2:469, 2002.

283. Creel D, Boxer LA, Fauci AS: Visual and auditory anomalies in Chediak-Higashi syn-drome. *Electroencephalogr Clin Neurophysiol* 55:252, 1983.

284. Boxer GJ, Holmsen H, Robkin L, et al: Abnormal platelet function in Chediak-Higashi syndrome. *Br J Haematol* 35:521, 1977.

285. Abo T, Roder JC, Abo W, et al: Natural killer (HNK-1+) cells in Chediak-Higashi patients are present in normal numbers but are abnormal in function and morphology. *J Clin Invest* 70:193, 1982.

286. Introne W, Boissy RE, Gahl WA: Clinical, molecular, and cell biological aspects of Che-diak-Higashi syndrome. *Mol Genet Metab* 68:283, 1999.

287. Steinbrinck W: Über ene neue granulations anomalie der leukocyten. *Dtsch Arch Klin Med* 193:577, 1948.

288. Chediak MM: New leukocyte anomaly of constitutional and familial character. *Rev Hematol* 7:362, 1952.

289. Higashi O: Congenital gigantism of peroxidase granules; the first case ever reported of qualitative abnormality of peroxidase. *Tohoku J Exp Med* 59:315, 1954.

290. Blume RS, Bennett JM, Yankee RA, et al: Defective granulocyte regulation in the Che-diak-Higashi syndrome. *N Engl J Med* 279:1009, 1968.

291. White JG, Clawson CC: The Chediak-Higashi syndrome; the nature of the giant neu-trophil granules and their interactions with cytoplasm and foreign particulates. I. Progressive enlargement of the massive inclusions in mature neutrophils. II. Manifesta-tions of cytoplasmic injury and sequestration. III. Interactions between giant organelles and foreign particulates. *Am J Pathol* 98:151, 1980.

292. Andrews T, Sullivan KE: Infections in patients with inherited defects in phagocytic function. *Clin Microbiol Rev* 16:597, 2003.

293. Trambas CM, Griffiths GM: Delivering the kiss of death. *Nat Immunol* 4:399, 2003.

294. Ingraham LM, Burns CP, Boxer LA, et al: Fluidity properties and liquid composition of erythrocyte membranes in Chediak-Higashi syndrome. *J Cell Biol* 89:510, 1981.

295. Barbosa MD, Barrat FJ, Tchernev VT, et al: Identification of mutations in two major mRNA isoforms of the Chediak-Higashi syndrome gene in human and mouse. *Hum Mol Genet* 6:1091, 1997.

296. Stinchcombe JC, Page LJ, Griffiths GM: Secretory lysosome biogenesis in cytotoxic T lymphocytes from normal and Chediak Higashi syndrome patients. *Traffic* 1:435, 2000.

297. Tchernev VT, Mansfield TA, Giot L, et al: The Chediak-Higashi protein interacts with SNARE complex and signal transduction proteins. *Mol Med* 8:56, 2002.

298. Filipovich AH: Hemophagocytic lymphohistiocytosis and related disorders. *Curr Opin Allergy Clin Immunol* 6:410, 2006.

299. Eapen M, DeLaat CA, Baker KS, et al: Hematopoietic cell transplantation for Chedi-ak-Higashi syndrome. *Bone Marrow Transplant* 39:411, 2007.

300. Tardieu M, Lacroix C, Neven B, et al: Progressive neurologic dysfunctions 20 years after allogeneic bone marrow transplantation for Chediak-Higashi syndrome. *Blood* 106:40, 2005.

301. Ganz T, Metcalf JA, Gallin JI, et al: Microbicidal/cytotoxic proteins of neutrophils are deficient in two disorders: Chediak-Higashi syndrome and "specific" granule defi-ciency. *J Clin Invest* 82:552, 1988.

302. Lomax KJ, Gallin JI, Rotrosen D, et al: Selective defect in myeloid cell lactoferrin gene expression in neutrophil specific granule deficiency. *J Clin Invest* 83:514, 1989.

303. Johnston JJ, Boxer LA, Berliner N: Correlation of messenger RNA levels with protein defects in specific granule deficiency. *Blood* 80:2088, 1992.

304. Rosenberg HF, Gallin JI: Neutrophil-specific granule deficiency includes eosinophils. *Blood* 82:268, 1993.

305. Gallin JI, Fletcher MP, Seligmann BE, et al: Human neutrophil-specific granule defi-ciency: A model to assess the role of neutrophil-specific granules in the evolution of the inflammatory response. *Blood* 59:1317, 1982.

306. Lekstrom-Himes JA, Dorman SE, Kopar P, et al: Neutrophil-specific granule deficiency results from a novel mutation with loss of function of the transcription factor CCAAT/ enhancer binding protein epsilon. *J Exp Med* 189:1847, 1999.

307. Khanna-Gupta A, Sun H, Zibello T, et al: Growth factor independence-1 (Gfi-1) plays a role in mediating specific granule deficiency (SGD) in a patient lacking a gene-inacti-vating mutation in the C/EBPepsilon gene. *Blood* 109:4181, 2007.

308. Kuriyama K, Tomonaga M, Matsuo T, et al: Diagnostic significance of detecting pseu-do-Pelger-Huet anomalies and micro-megakaryocytes in myelodysplastic syndrome. *Br J Haematol* 63:665, 1986.

309. Arnaout MA: Leukocyte adhesion molecules deficiency: Its structural basis, patho-physiology and implications for modulating the inflammatory response. *Immunol Rev* 114:145, 1990.

310. Corbi AL, Larson RS, Kishimoto TK, et al: Chromosomal location of the genes encod-ing the leukocyte adhesion receptors LFA-1, Mac-1 and p150,95. Identification of a gene cluster involved in cell adhesion. *J Exp Med* 167:1597, 1988.

311. Hayward AR, Harvey BA, Leonard J, et al: Delayed separation of the umbilical cord, widespread infections, and defective neutrophil mobility. *Lancet* 1:1099, 1979.

312. Crowley CA, Curnutte JT, Rosin RE, et al: An inherited abnormality of neutrophil adhesion. Its genetic transmission and its association with a missing protein. *N Engl J Med* 302:1163, 1980.

313. Arnaout MA, Pitt J, Cohen HJ, et al: Deficiency of a granulocyte-membrane glycopro-tein (gp150) in a boy with recurrent bacterial infections. *N Engl J Med* 306:693, 1982.

314. Dana N, Todd RF, III, Pitt J, et al: Deficiency of a surface membrane glycoprotein (Mo1) in man. *J Clin Invest* 73:153, 1984.

315. Anderson DC, Smith CW: Leukocyte adhesion deficiencies, in *The Metabolic and Molecular Basis of Inherited Disease*, 8th ed, edited by Scriver C, Beaudet A, Sly W, Valle D, Childs B, Kinzler K, Vogelstein B, p 4829. McGraw-Hill, New York, 2001.

316. Springer TA, Thompson WS, Miller LJ, et al: Inherited deficiency of the Mac-1, LFA-1, p150,95 glycoprotein family and its molecular basis. *J Exp Med* 160:1901, 1984.

317. Wagner DD, Frenette PS: The vessel wall and its interactions. *Blood* 111:5271, 2008.

318. Petrequin PR, Todd RF, III, Devall LJ, et al: Association between gelatinase release and increased plasma membrane expression of the Mo1 glycoprotein. *Blood* 69:605, 1987.

319. Anderson DC, Springer TA: Leukocyte adhesion deficiency: An inherited defect in the Mac-1, LFA-1, and p150,95 glycoproteins. *Annu Rev Med* 38:175, 1987.

320. Schwartz BR, Wayner EA, Carlos TM, et al: Identification of surface proteins mediating adherence of CD11/CD18-deficient lymphoblastoid cells to cultured human endothe-lium. *J Clin Invest* 85:2019, 1990.

321. Mizgerd JP, Kubo H, Kutkoski GJ, et al: Neutrophil emigration in the skin, lungs, and peritoneum: Different requirements for CD11/CD18 revealed by CD18-deficient mice. *J Exp Med* 186:1357, 1997.

322. Anderson DC, Rothlein R, Marlin SD, et al: Impaired transendothelial migration by neonatal neutrophils: Abnormalities of Mac-1 (CD11b/CD18)-dependent adherence reactions. *Blood* 76:2613, 1990.

323. Mulligan MS, Varani J, Dame MK, et al: Role of endothelial-leukocyte adhesion molecule 1 (ELAM-1) in neutrophil-mediated lung injury in rats. *J Clin Invest* 88:1396, 1991.

324. Wertheimer SJ, Myers CL, Wallace RW, et al: Intercellular adhesion molecule-1 gene expression in human endothelial cells. Differential regulation by tumor necrosis fac-tor-alpha and phorbol myristate acetate. *J Biol Chem* 267:12030, 1992.

325. Malawista SE, de Boisfleury CA, Boxer LA: Random locomotion and chemotaxis of human blood polymorphonuclear leukocytes from a patient with leukocyte adhe-sion deficiency-1: Normal displacement in close quarters via chimneying. *Cell Motil Cytoskeleton* 46:183, 2000.

326. Arnaout MA: Structure and function of the leukocyte adhesion molecules CD11/ CD18. *Blood* 75:1037, 1990.

327. Cao D, Mizukami IF, Garni-Wagner BA, et al: Human urokinase-type plasminogen activator primes neutrophils for superoxide anion release. Possible roles of complement receptor type 3 and calcium. *J Immunol* 154:1817, 1995.

328. Altieri DC, Bader R, Mannucci PM, et al: Oligospecificity of the cellular adhesion receptor Mac-1 encompasses an inducible recognition specificity for fibrinogen. *J Cell Biol* 107:1893, 1988.

329. Wilson RW, Ballantyne CM, Smith CW, et al: Gene targeting yields a CD18-mutant mouse for study of inflammation. *J Immunol* 151:1571, 1993.

330. Stark MA, Huo Y, Burcin TL, et al: Phagocytosis of apoptotic neutrophils regulates granulopoiesis via IL-23 and IL-17. *Immunity* 22:285, 2005.

331. Yakubenia S, Wild MK: Leukocyte adhesion deficiency II. Advances and open ques-tions. *FEBS J* 273:4390, 2006.

332. Helmus Y, Denecke J, Yakubenia S, et al: Leukocyte adhesion deficiency II patients with a dual defect of the GDP-fucose transporter. *Blood* 107:3959, 2006.

333. Aebi M, Helenius A, Schenk B, et al: Carbohydrate-deficient glycoprotein syndromes become congenital disorders of glycosylation: An updated nomenclature for CDG. First International Workshop on CDGS. *Glycoconj J* 16:669, 1999.

334. Hidalgo A, Ma S, Peired AJ, et al: Insights into leukocyte adhesion deficiency type 2 from a novel mutation in the GDP-fucose transporter gene. *Blood* 101:1705, 2003.

335. Kuijpers TW, van BR, Kamerbeek N, et al: Natural history and early diagnosis of LAD-1/variant syndrome. *Blood* 109:3529, 2007.

336. Kuijpers TW, van de V, Weterman MA, et al: LAD-1/variant syndrome is caused by mutations in FERMT3. *Blood* 113:4740, 2009.

337. Fischer A, Lisowska-Grospierre B, Anderson DC, et al: Leukocyte adhesion deficiency: Molecular basis and functional consequences. *Immunodefic Rev* 1:39, 1988.

338. Bauer TR Jr, Hickstein DD: Gene therapy for leukocyte adhesion deficiency. *Curr Opin Mol Ther* 2:383, 2000.

339. Malech HL, Hickstein DD: Genetics, biology and clinical management of myeloid cell primary immune deficiencies: Chronic granulomatous disease and leukocyte adhesion deficiency. *Curr Opin Hematol* 14:29, 2007.

340. Boxer LA, Hedley-Whyte ET, Stossel TP: Neutrophil action dysfunction and abnormal neutrophil behavior. *N Engl J Med* 291:1093, 1974.

341. Southwick FS, Dabiri GA, Stosse TP: Neutrophil actin dysfunction is a genetic disorder associated with partial impairment of neutrophil actin assembly in three family members. *J Clin Invest* 82:1525, 1988.

342. Malech HL, Gallin JI: Current concepts: Immunology neutrophils in human diseases. *N Engl J Med* 317:687, 1987.

343. Southwick FS, Howard TH, Holbrook T, et al: The relationship between CR3 deficiency and neutrophil actin assembly. *Blood* 73:1973, 1989.

344. Coates TD, Torkildson JC, Torres M, et al: An inherited defect of neutrophil motility and microfilamentous cytoskeleton associated with abnormalities in 47-kD and 89-kD proteins. *Blood* 78:1338, 1991.

345. Howard T, Li Y, Torres M, et al: The 47-kD protein increased in neutrophil actin dysfunction with 47-and 89-kD protein abnormalities is lymphocyte-specific protein. *Blood* 83:231, 1994.

346. Howard TH, Hartwig J, Cunningham C: Lymphocyte-specific protein 1 expression in eukaryotic cells reproduces the morphologic and motile abnormality of NAD 47/89 neutrophils. *Blood* 91:4786, 1998.

347. Camitta BM, Quesenberry PJ, Parkman R, et al: Bone marrow transplantation for an infant with neutrophil dysfunction. *Exp Hematol* 5:109, 1977.

348. Samuels J, Aksentijevich I, Torosyan Y, et al: Familial Mediterranean fever at the millennium. Clinical spectrum, ancient mutations, and a survey of 100 American referrals to the National Institutes of Health. *Medicine (Baltimore)* 77:268, 1998.

349. Siegal S: Benign paroxysmal peritonitis. *Gastroenterology* 12:234, 1949.

350. Drenth JP, van der Meer JW: Hereditary periodic fever. *N Engl J Med* 345:1748, 2001.

351. Ben-Chetrit E, Levy M: Familial Mediterranean fever. *Lancet* 351:659, 1998.

352. Ancient missense mutations in a new member of the RoRet gene family are likely to cause familial Mediterranean fever. The International FMF Consortium. *Cell* 90:797, 1997.

353. Centola M, Wood G, Frucht DM, et al: The gene for familial Mediterranean fever, MEFV, is expressed in early leukocyte development and is regulated in response to inflammatory mediators. *Blood* 95:3223, 2000.

354. Ryan JG, Kastner DL: Fevers, genes, and innate immunity. *Curr Top Microbiol Immunol* 321:169, 2008.

355. Hull KM, Shoham N, Chae JJ, et al: The expanding spectrum of systemic autoinflammatory disorders and their rheumatic manifestations. *Curr Opin Rheumatol* 15:61, 2003.

356. Richards N, Schaner P, Diaz A, et al: Interaction between pyrin and the apoptotic speck protein (ASC) modulates ASC-induced apoptosis. *J Biol Chem* 276:39320, 2001.

357. Touitou I: The spectrum of Familial Mediterranean Fever (FMF) mutations. *Eur J Hum Genet* 9:473, 2001.

358. Schaner P, Richards N, Wadhwa A, et al: Episodic evolution of pyrin in primates: Human mutations recapitulate ancestral amino acid states. *Nat Genet* 27:318, 2001.

359. Williamson LM, Hull D, Mehta R, et al: Familial Hibernian fever. *Q J Med* 51:469, 1982.

360. Lakshman R, Finn A: Neutrophil disorders and their management. *J Clin Pathol* 54.7, 2001.

361. Perlmutter DH, Colten HR: Molecular basis of complement deficiencies. *Immunodefic Rev* 1:105, 1989.

362. Kannourakis G: Glycogen storage disease. *Semin Hematol* 39:103, 2002.

363. Smith OP: Shwachman-Diamond syndrome. *Semin Hematol* 39:95, 2002.

364. Jones DH, Schmalstieg FC, Dempsey K, et al: Subcellular distribution and mobilization of MAC-1 (CD11b/CD18) in neonatal neutrophils. *Blood* 75:488, 1990.

365. Sapey E, Greenwood H, Walton G, et al: Phosphoinositide 3-kinase inhibition restores neutrophil accuracy in the elderly: Toward targeted treatments for immunosenescence. *Blood* 123:239, 2014.

366. Brayton RG, Stokes PE, Schwartz MS, et al: Effect of alcohol and various diseases on leukocyte mobilization, phagocytosis and intracellular bacterial killing. *N Engl J Med* 282:123, 1970.

367. Oseas RS, Allen J, Yang HH, et al: Mechanism of dexamethasone inhibition of chemotactic factor induced granulocyte aggregation. *Blood* 59:265, 1982.

368. Dale DC, Fauci AS, Wolff SM: Alternate-day prednisone. Leukocyte kinetics and susceptibility to infections. *N Engl J Med* 291:1154, 1974.

369. Boxer LA, Allen JM, Baehner RL: Diminished polymorphonuclear leukocyte adherence. Function dependent on release of cyclic AMP by endothelial cells after stimulation of beta-receptors by epinephrine. *J Clin Invest* 66:268, 1980.

370. Freeman AF, Holland SM: The hyper-IgE syndromes. *Immunol Allergy Clin North Am* 28:277, 2008.

371. Engelich G, Wright DG, Hartshorn KL: Acquired disorders of phagocyte function complicating medical and surgical illnesses. *Clin Infect Dis* 33:2040, 2001.

372. Buckley RH: The hyper-IgE syndrome. *Clin Rev Allergy Immunol* 20:139, 2001.

373. Grimbacher B, Holland SM, Gallin JI, et al: Hyper-IgE syndrome with recurrent infections—An autosomal dominant multisystem disorder. *N Engl J Med* 340:692, 1999.

374. Zhang Q, Davis JC, Lamborn IT, et al: Combined immunodeficiency associated with DOCK8 mutations. *N Engl J Med* 361:2046, 2009.

375. Yong PF, Freeman AF, Engelhardt KR, et al: An update on the hyper-IgE syndromes. *Arthritis Res Ther* 14:228, 2012.

376. Segal BH, Leto TL, Gallin JI, et al: Genetic, biochemical, and clinical features of chronic granulomatous disease. *Medicine (Baltimore)* 79:170, 2000.

377. Berendes H, Bridges RA, Good RA: A fatal granulomatosus of childhood: The clinical study of a new syndrome. *Minn Med* 40:309, 1957.

378. Landing BH, Shirkey HS: A syndrome of recurrent infection and infiltration of viscera by pigmented lipid histiocytes. *Pediatrics* 20:431, 1957.

379. Sbarra AJ, Karnovsky ML: The biochemical basis of phagocytosis. I. Metabolic changes during the ingestion of particles by polymorphonuclear leukocytes. *J Biol Chem* 234:1355, 1959.

380. Iyer GYN, Islam MF, Quastel JH: Biochemical aspects of phagocytosis. *Nature* 192:535, 1961.

381. Iyer GY, Quastel JH: NADPH and NADH oxidation by guinea pig polymorphonuclear leucocytes. *Can J Biochem Physiol* 41:427, 1963.

382. Baehner RL, Nathan DG: Quantitative nitroblue tetrazolium test in chronic granulomatous disease. *N Engl J Med* 278:971, 1968.

383. Winkelstein JA, Marino MC, Johnston RB Jr, et al: Chronic granulomatous disease. Report on a national registry of 368 patients. *Medicine (Baltimore)* 79:155, 2000.

384. Parkos CA, Allen RA, Cochrane CG, et al: Purified cytochrome b from human granulocyte plasma membrane is comprised of two polypeptides with relative molecular weights of 91,000 and 22,000. *J Clin Invest* 80:732, 1987.

385. Quinn MT, Mullen ML, Jesaitis AJ: Human neutrophil cytochrome b contains multiple hemes. Evidence for heme associated with both subunits. *J Biol Chem* 267:7303, 1992.

386. Rotrosen D, Yeung CL, Leto TL, et al: Cytochrome b558: The flavin-binding component of the phagocyte NADPH oxidase. *Science* 256:1459, 1992.

387. Segal AW, West I, Wientjes F, et al: Cytochrome b-245 is a flavocytochrome containing FAD and the NADPH-binding site of the microbicidal oxidase of phagocytes. *Biochem J* 284:781, 1992.

388. Sumimoto H, Sakamoto N, Nozaki M, et al: Cytochrome b558, a component of the phagocyte NADPH oxidase, is a flavoprotein. *Biochem Biophys Res Commun* 186:1368, 1992.

389. Zhen L, Yu L, Dinauer MC: Probing the role of the carboxyl terminus of the gp91phox subunit of neutrophil flavocytochrome b558 using site-directed mutagenesis. *J Biol Chem* 273:6575, 1998.

390. Shatwell KP, Dancis A, Cross AR, et al: The FRE1 ferric reductase of Saccharomyces cerevisiae is a cytochrome b similar to that of NADPH oxidase. *J Biol Chem* 271:14240, 1996.

391. Deleo FR, Quinn MT: Assembly of the phagocyte NADPH oxidase: Molecular interaction of oxidase proteins. *J Leukoc Biol* 60:677, 1996.

392. Segal AW: The NADPH oxidase and chronic granulomatous disease. *Mol Med Today* 2:129, 1996.

393. Kanai F, Liu H, Field SJ, et al: The PX domains of p47phox and p40phox bind to lipid products of PI(3)K. *Nat Cell Biol* 3:675, 2001.

394. Chen J, He R, Minshall RD, et al: Characterization of a mutation in the Phox homology domain of the NADPH oxidase component p40phox identifies a mechanism for negative regulation of superoxide production. *J Biol Chem* 282:30273, 2007.

395. Cross AR, Jones OT: Enzymic mechanisms of superoxide production. *Biochim Biophys Acta* 1057:281, 1991.

396. Heyworth PG, Curnutte JT, Rae J, et al: Hematologically important mutations: X linked chronic granulomatous disease (second update). *Blood Cells Mol Dis* 27:16, 2001.

397. Francke U, Ochs HD, de MB, et al: Minor Xp21 chromosome deletion in a male associated with expression of Duchenne muscular dystrophy, chronic granulomatous disease, retinitis pigmentosa, and McLeod syndrome. *Am J Hum Genet* 37:250, 1985.

398. Royer-Pokora B, Kunkel LM, Monaco AP, et al: Cloning the gene for an inherited human disorder—chronic granulomatous disease—on the basis of its chromosomal location. *Nature* 322:32, 1986.

399. Frey D, Machler M, Seger R, et al: Gene deletion in a patient with chronic granulomatous disease and McLeod syndrome: Fine mapping of the Xk gene locus. *Blood* 71:252, 1988.

400. de Boer M., Bolscher BG, Dinauer MC, et al: Splice site mutations are a common cause of X-linked chronic granulomatous disease. *Blood* 80:1553, 1992.

401. Curnutte JT, Orkin S, Dinauer MC: Genetic disorders of phagocyte function, in *The Molecular Basis of Blood Diseases*, 2nd ed, edited by Stammatoyannopoulos G, p 493. WB Saunders, Philadelphia, 1994.

402. Roos D, de BM, Kuribayashi F, et al: Mutations in the X-linked and autosomal recessive forms of chronic granulomatous disease. *Blood* 87:1663, 1996.

403. Rae J, Newburger PE, Dinauer MC, et al: X-Linked chronic granulomatous disease: Mutations in the CYBB gene encoding the gp91-phox component of respiratory-burst oxidase. *Am J Hum Genet* 62:1320, 1998.

404. Dinauer MC, Pierce EA, Bruns GA, et al: Human neutrophil cytochrome b light chain (p22-phox). Gene structure, chromosomal location, and mutations in cytochrome-negative autosomal recessive chronic granulomatous disease. *J Clin Invest* 86:1729, 1990.

405. Segal AW: Biochemistry and molecular biology of chronic granulomatous disease. *J Inherit Metab Dis* 15:683, 1992.

406. Casimir CM, Bu-Ghanim HN, Rodaway AR, et al: Autosomal recessive chronic granulomatous disease caused by deletion at a dinucleotide repeat. *Proc Natl Acad Sci U S A* 88:2753, 1991.

407. Roos D: X-CGDbase: A database of X-CGD-causing mutations. *Immunol Today* 17:517, 1996.

408. Matute JD, Arias AA, Wright NA, et al: A new genetic subgroup of chronic granulomatous disease with autosomal recessive mutations in p40 phox and selective defects in neutrophil NADPH oxidase activity. *Blood* 114:3309, 2009.

409. Jankowski A, Scott CC, Grinstein S: Determinants of the phagosomal pH in neutrophils. *J Biol Chem* 277:6059, 2002.

410. Reeves EP, Lu H, Jacobs HL, et al: Killing activity of neutrophils is mediated through activation of proteases by K+ flux. *Nature* 416:291, 2002.

411. Fernandez-Boyanapalli RF, Frasch SC, McPhillips K, et al: Impaired apoptotic cell clearance in CGD due to altered macrophage programming is reversed by phosphatidylserine-dependent production of IL-4. *Blood* 113:2047, 2009.

412. Bianchi M, Hakkim A, Brinkmann V, et al: Restoration of NET formation by gene therapy in CGD controls aspergillosis. *Blood* 114:2619, 2009.

413. Johnston RB Jr, Baehner RL: Chronic granulomatous disease: Correlation between pathogenesis and clinical findings. *Pediatrics* 48:730, 1971.

414. Johnston RB Jr: Clinical aspects of chronic granulomatous disease. *Curr Opin Hematol* 8:17, 2001.

415. Petty HR, Francis JW, Boxer LA: Deficiency in immune complex uptake by chronic granulomatous disease neutrophils. *J Cell Sci* 90:425, 1988.

416. Foster CB, Lehrnbecher T, Mol F, et al: Host defense molecule polymorphisms influence the risk for immune-mediated complications in chronic granulomatous disease. *J Clin Invest* 102:2146, 1998.

417. Wolach B, Scharf Y, Gavrieli R, et al: Unusual late presentation of X-linked chronic granulomatous disease in an adult female with a somatic mosaic for a novel mutation in CYBB. *Blood* 105:61, 2005.

418. Crockard AD, Thompson JM, Boyd NA, et al: Diagnosis and carrier detection of chronic granulomatous disease in five families by flow cytometry. *Int Arch Allergy Immunol* 114:144, 1997.

419. Newburger PE, Luscinskas FW, Ryan T, et al: Variant chronic granulomatous disease: Modulation of the neutrophil defect by severe infection. *Blood* 68:914, 1986.

420. Curnutte JT: Chronic granulomatous disease: The solving of a clinical riddle at the molecular level. *Clin Immunol Immunopathol* 67:S2, 1993.

421. Cooper MR, DeChatelet LR, McCall CE, et al: Complete deficiency of leukocyte glucose-6-phosphate dehydrogenase with defective bactericidal activity. *J Clin Invest* 51:769, 1972.

422. Vives Corrons JL, Feliu E, Pujades MA, et al: Severe-glucose-6-phosphate dehydrogenase (G6PD) deficiency associated with chronic hemolytic anemia, granulocyte dysfunction, and increased susceptibility to infections: Description of a new molecular variant (G6PD Barcelona). *Blood* 59:428, 1982.

423. Ambruso DR, Knall C, Abell AN, et al: Human neutrophil immunodeficiency syndrome is associated with an inhibitory Rac2 mutation. *Proc Natl Acad Sci U S A* 97:4654, 2000.

424. Williams DA, Tao W, Yang F, et al: Dominant negative mutation of the hematopoietic-specific Rho GTPase, Rac2, is associated with a human phagocyte immunodeficiency. *Blood* 96:1646, 2000.

425. Gungor T, Teira P, Slatter M, et al: Reduced-intensity conditioning and HLA-matched haemopoietic stem-cell transplantation in patients with chronic granulomatous disease: A prospective multicentre study. *Lancet* 383:436, 2014.

426. Chusid MJ, Gelfand JA, Nutter C, et al: Letter: Pulmonary aspergillosis, inhalation of contaminated marijuana smoke, chronic granulomatous disease. *Ann Intern Med* 82:682, 1975.

427. Seger RA: Modern management of chronic granulomatous disease. *Br J Haematol* 140:255, 2008.

428. Gallin JI, Alling DW, Malech HL, et al: Itraconazole to prevent fungal infections in chronic granulomatous disease. *N Engl J Med* 348:2416, 2003.

429. A controlled trial of interferon gamma to prevent infection in chronic granulomatous disease. The International Chronic Granulomatous Disease Cooperative Study Group. *N Engl J Med* 324:509, 1991.

430. Schiff DE, Rae J, Martin TR, et al: Increased phagocyte Fc gammaRI expression and improved Fc gamma-receptor-mediated phagocytosis after in vivo recombinant human interferon-gamma treatment of normal human subjects. *Blood* 90:3187, 1997.

431. Woodman RC, Erickson RW, Rae J, et al: Prolonged recombinant interferon-gamma therapy in chronic granulomatous disease: Evidence against enhanced neutrophil oxidase activity. *Blood* 79:1558, 1992.

432. Kuhns DB, Alvord WG, Heller T, et al: Residual NADPH oxidase and survival in chronic granulomatous disease. *N Engl J Med* 363:2600, 2010.

433. Malech HL, Bauer TR Jr, Hickstein DD: Prospects for gene therapy of neutrophil defects. *Semin Hematol* 34:355, 1997.

434. Pollock JD, Williams DA, Gifford MA, et al: Mouse model of X-linked chronic granulomatous disease, an inherited defect in phagocyte superoxide production. *Nat Genet* 9:202, 1995.

435. Jackson SH, Gallin JI, Holland SM: The p47phox mouse knock-out model of chronic granulomatous disease. *J Exp Med* 182:751, 1995.

436. Mardiney M, III, Jackson SH, Spratt SK, et al: Enhanced host defense after gene transfer in the murine p47phox-deficient model of chronic granulomatous disease. *Blood* 89:2268, 1997.

437. Bjorgvinsdottir H, Ding C, Pech N, et al: Retroviral-mediated gene transfer of gp91phox into bone marrow cells rescues defect in host defense against Aspergillus fumigatus in murine X-linked chronic granulomatous disease. *Blood* 89:41, 1997.

438. Malech HL, Maples PB, Whiting-Theobald N, et al: Prolonged production of NADPH oxidase-corrected granulocytes after gene therapy of chronic granulomatous disease. *Proc Natl Acad Sci U S A* 94:12133, 1997.

439. Ott MG, Schmidt M, Schwarzwaelder K, et al: Correction of X-linked chronic granulomatous disease by gene therapy, augmented by insertional activation of MDS1-EVI1, PRDM16 or SETBP1. *Nat Med* 12:401, 2006.

440. Hansson M, Olsson I, Nauseef WM: Biosynthesis, processing, and sorting of human myeloperoxidase. *Arch Biochem Biophys* 445:214, 2006.

441. Nauseef WM: Insights into myeloperoxidase biosynthesis from its inherited deficiency. *J Mol Med (Berl)* 76:661, 1998.

442. Nauseef WM: Myeloperoxidase deficiency. *Hematol Pathol* 4:165, 1990.

443. Boxer LA: The role of antioxidants in modulating neutrophil functional responses. *Adv Exp Med Biol* 262:19, 1990.

444. Roos D, Weening RS, Voetman AA, et al: Protection of phagocytic leukocytes by endogenous glutathione: Studies in a family with glutathione reductase deficiency. *Blood* 53:851, 1979.

445. Boxer LA, Oliver JM, Spielberg SP, et al: Protection of granulocytes by vitamin E in glutathione synthetase deficiency. *N Engl J Med* 301:901, 1979.

Part VIII Monocytes and Macrophages

67. Structure, Receptors, and Functions of Monocytes and Macrophages 1045

68. Production, Distribution, and Activation of Monocytes and Macrophages. 1075

69. Classification and Clinical Manifestations of Disorders of Monocytes and Macrophages 1089

70. Monocytosis and Monocytopenia 1095

71. Inflammatory and Malignant Histiocytosis 1101

72. Gaucher Disease and Related Lysosomal Storage Diseases 1121

CHAPTER 67
STRUCTURE, RECEPTORS, AND FUNCTIONS OF MONOCYTES AND MACROPHAGES

Steven D. Douglas and Anne G. Douglas

SUMMARY

The monocyte is a spherical cell with prominent surface ruffles and blebs when examined by scanning electron microscopy. As the monocyte enters the tissue and differentiates into a macrophage, the cell volume and number of cytoplasmic granules increase. Cell shape varies, depending on the tissue in which the macrophage resides (e.g., lung, liver, spleen, brain). A characteristic feature of macrophages is their prominent electron-dense membrane-bound lysosomes, which can be seen fusing with phagosomes to form secondary lysosomes. The latter contain ingested cellular and noncellular material in different stages of degradation. A broad range of surface receptors for many ligands, including the Fc portion of immunoglobulin, complement proteins, cytokines, chemokines, lipoproteins, and others, are on the cell surface. Macrophages differ in appearance, biochemistry, and function based on the environment in which they mature from monocytes. These differences are exemplified by the diversity among dendritic cells of lymph nodes, histiocytes of connective tissue, osteoclasts of bone, Kupffer cells of liver, microglia of the central nervous system, and macrophages of the serosal surfaces, each fashioned to meet the local needs of the mononuclear phagocyte system, which plays a role in inflammation and host defense against microbes. Modern cell biologic methods refined our knowledge of surface receptors, endocytosis, and lysosomal

Acronyms and Abbreviations: APC, antigen-presenting cell; CD, cluster of differentiation; CR, complement receptor; CSF, colony-stimulating factor; DC, dendritic cell; EGF, epidermal growth factor; EGF-TM7, epidermal growth factor–seven transmembrane; EMR2, epidermal growth factor–like module containing mucin-like hormone receptor–like 2; FcR, Fc receptor; GM-CSF, granulocyte-monocyte colony-stimulating factor; GPCR, G-protein–coupled receptor; HLA, human leukocyte antigen; IBD, inflammatory bowel disease; IFN, interferon; Ig, immunoglobulin; IL, interleukin; IMP, intramembrane particle; IRAK, interleukin receptor-associated kinase; LFA, lymphocyte function–associated antigen; LPS, lipopolysaccharide; m-ϕ, macrophage; MARCO, macrophage receptor with collagenous structure; M-CSF, macrophage colony-stimulating factor; MHC, major histocompatibility complex; MPO, myeloperoxidase; NF, nuclear factor; NLR, NOD-like receptor; NOD, nucleotide-binding oligomerization domain; PI3K, phosphatidylinositol 3-kinase; PS, phosphatidylserine; SR, scavenger receptor; TGF, transforming growth factor; TLR, toll-like receptor.

degradation, with emphasis on membrane flow and secretion. These pioneering studies culminated in the discovery of dendritic cells as potent, specialized antigen-presenting cells. Subsequent development of monoclonal antibodies and molecular cloning of surface proteins and cytokines, followed by microarray analysis and genomics, provided the sensitive and specific tools to analyze macrophage functions *in vitro* and *in vivo*. These studies have brought insights into macrophage cytotoxic and antimicrobial activities and, to a lesser extent, their trophic, homeostatic functions in the body. Macrophages play a major role in innate as well as adaptive immunity.

MONONUCLEAR PHAGOCYTE SYSTEM OVERVIEW

Modern study of mammalian phagocytes began with Metchnikoff in the 19th century. An understanding of the ontogeny, kinetics, and function of phagocytic cells in animals led to the concept of the mononuclear phagocyte system.[1,2] Kinetic studies indicate that marrow monoblasts and monocytes develop from the common myeloid progenitor, a derivative of the hematopoietic stem cell, and that tissue macrophages develop from monocytes that have migrated from the blood pool in response to chemotactic stimuli (Table 67-1 and Chap. 18). Tissue macrophages share many functional characteristics, such as phagocytic and microbial killing capabilities and adherence to glass or plastic surfaces *in vitro*. Vascular endothelium, reticular cells, and dendritic cells of lymphoid germinal centers usually are not included in the mononuclear phagocyte system, although the now obsolete term *reticuloendothelial system*[3] denoted those cells as playing some complementary part with mononuclear phagocytes. In addition to developing the multitude of types of tissue macrophages, monocytes can differentiate into myeloid-derived dendritic cells.[4,5]

STRUCTURE

The blood monocyte is a medium to large motile cell that can marginate along vessel walls and has a propensity for adherence to surfaces. Monocytes respond to inflammation and chemotactic stimuli by active diapedesis across vessel walls into inflammatory foci, where they can mature into macrophages, with greater phagocytic capacity and increased content of hydrolytic enzymes. Free macrophages also are present in mammary glands, alveolar spaces, pleura, peritoneum, and synovia. The somewhat less-motile fixed-tissue macrophages are found in different tissues and serous cavities. The functions of mononuclear phagocytes include phagocytosis, killing, and digestion of microorganisms, particulate material, or tissue debris; secretion of chemical mediators and regulators of the inflammatory response; interaction (as dendritic cells) with antigen and lymphocytes in the generation of the immune response; cytotoxicity, such as killing of some tumor cells; and other functions specific for macrophages of particular tissues.

The development of techniques to isolate monocytes from blood of adult human subjects led to the discovery that monocytes are heterogeneous with regard to cell volumes. Isolation of purified monocytes by adherence to glass substrates or to gelatin-coated flasks or by centrifugal elutriation reveals distinct populations of monocytes.[1,2] In addition to the usual 12- to 15-μm diameter (when measured on a dried blood film) monocyte, so-called regular monocytes, a somewhat smaller cell that is less active than its larger, more mature counterpart has been identified. This cell is referred to as a small immature monocyte, but its functional significance is not clear.

TABLE 67–1. Distribution of Mononuclear Phagocytes

Marrow	Tissues
Monoblasts	Liver (Kupffer cells)
Promonocytes	Lung (alveolar macrophages)
Monocytes	Connective tissue (histiocytes)
Macrophages	Spleen (red pulp macrophages)
Blood	Lymph nodes
Monocytes	Thymus
Body cavities	Bone (osteoclasts)
Pleural macrophages	Synovium (type A cells)
Peritoneal macrophages	Mucosa-associated lymphoid tissue
Inflammatory tissues	Gastrointestinal tract
Epithelioid cells	Genitourinary tract
Exudate macrophages	Endocrine organs
Multinucleate giant cells	Central nervous system (microglia)
	Skin (histiocyte/dendritic cells)

Data from Lewis, C, McGee, JD: *The Macrophage*, 2nd ed., Oxford University Press, New York, NY, 1992; Gordon S, Fraser I, Nath D. et al: Macrophages in tissues and in vitro. *Curr Opin Immunol* 4:25-32, 1992; Lasser A: The mononuclear phagocytic system: A review. *Hum Pathol* 14:108-26, 1983.

Monocytes continuously emigrate from the blood into tissue, with a half-life in the blood of approximately 1 day in mice.[6] Nondividing monocytes can be induced to differentiate into dendritic like cells in vitro. However, this process requires culture of the cells for 7 to 10 days with exogenous cytokines, typically interleukin (IL)-4 and granulocyte-monocyte colony-stimulating factor (GM-CSF).[7] The major lineage regulator of nearly all macrophages is monocyte/macrophage colony-stimulating factor (M-CSF; also termed CSF-1) and its receptor (M-CSF R). The M-CSF R is a class III transmembrane tyrosine kinase receptor, which is expressed on most mononuclear phagocytes.[8] In the presence of endothelial cells grown on an extracellular matrix, monocytes differentiate along two distinct pathways: toward dendritic cells or macrophages. Monocytes that migrate across endothelium in an abluminal to luminal direction differentiate into dendritic cells. In contrast, monocytes that remain in the subendothelial matrix differentiate into macrophages.

MORPHOLOGY OF MONOCYTE PRECURSORS

Monoblasts and promonocytes are the precursors of monocytes, bearing finely dispersed nuclear chromatin and nucleoli when observed in the stained film of the marrow. The monoblast is a very-low-prevalence marrow cell, indistinguishable by light microscopy from the myeloblast. Promonocytes are 12 to 18 μm in diameter (as measured on dried blood films) and have characteristic deeply indented, irregularly shaped nuclei with condensed chromatin, and numerous cytoplasmic microfilaments.

In animal studies, a small percentage of marrow cells are phagocytic, synthesize DNA, adhere to glass surfaces, and contain nonspecific esterases.[9] These cells have been referred to as *promonocytes* and are considered as intermediate between monoblasts and the monocytes of the blood.[9] Cytochemical studies identify the promonocyte in normal human marrow. Promonocytes have deeply indented and irregularly shaped nuclei and bundled and scattered single filaments in the cytoplasm. These morphologic features distinguish the promonocyte

from the progranulocyte.[10,11] Peroxidase is present throughout the cell secretory apparatus in all cisternae of the rough-surfaced endoplasmic reticulum, the Golgi complex, associated vesicles, and all immature and mature granules. Cytochemical reaction products for acid phosphatase and arylsulfatase also are deposited throughout the secretory apparatus of the promonocyte.

MORPHOLOGY OF MONOCYTES

Light Microscopy

The morphology of monocytes has been investigated by light and phase-contrast optics,[12] scanning and transmission electron microscopy, and freeze-fracture and freeze-etch procedures.[13]

On the stained blood film the monocyte has a diameter of 12 to 15 μm (Fig. 67–1). The monocyte nucleus occupies approximately half the area of the cell and usually is eccentrically placed. The nucleus most often is reniform, but may be round or irregular. It contains a characteristic chromatin net with fine strands bridging small chromatin clumps. Chromatin aggregates are arranged along the internal side of the nuclear membrane. The cytoplasm is spread out, stains grayish-blue with Wright stain, and contains a variable number of fine, pink-purple granules, which at times are sufficiently numerous to give the entire cytoplasm a pink hue. Clear cytoplasmic vacuoles and a variable number of larger azurophilic granulations often are encountered in these cells.

Phase Microscopy

The monocyte nucleus has a distinct chromatin pattern on a cloudy background when examined by phase-contrast microscopy. The cytoplasm is clear gray. Mitochondria are extremely fine and occasionally form a small, juxtanuclear rosette surrounding the centrosome. The phase-dense cytoplasmic granules, varying in number, are generally at the limit of resolution of light microscopy and appear as fine intracytoplasmic dust. Monocytes contain several types of cytoplasmic vacuoles. The reniform nucleus with a juxtanuclear depression filled by a centrosome and its active undulating movement similar to that of other leukocytes are characteristic of the monocyte. The locomotion of the monocyte has the same pattern of undulating cytoplasmic veils seen in macrophages. The monocyte generally assumes a triangular shape as it moves, with one point trailing behind and the other two points advancing before the cell. Blood monocytes undergo adherence and cytoplasmic spreading following attachment to glass surfaces.[14] The extent of spreading increases in the presence of antigen–antibody complexes, certain divalent metals, and proteolytic enzymes.[14,15] The spread form of the monocyte reveals that the nucleus and granules are located centrally and the abundant hyaloplasm is in the periphery of the cell, terminating in a fringed border that displays undulating movement. The small monocyte may be difficult to distinguish from the large lymphocyte when examined by phase-contrast microscopy.

A striking feature on phase-contrast microscopy is the ruffled plasma membrane that forms prominent phase-dense folds at the cell surface and edges. Some cells have a dense thickening at the edge of the cytoplasm, with microextensions on the thickened edge.

Scanning Electron Microscopy

The monocyte surface has very prominent ruffles and small surface blebs.[16,17] Extensive ruffling on the monocyte plasma membrane is of functional significance. The monocyte is both motile and phagocytic, and these functions require physical contact with particles or cell surfaces. Reduction in the radius of curvature of the cell surface

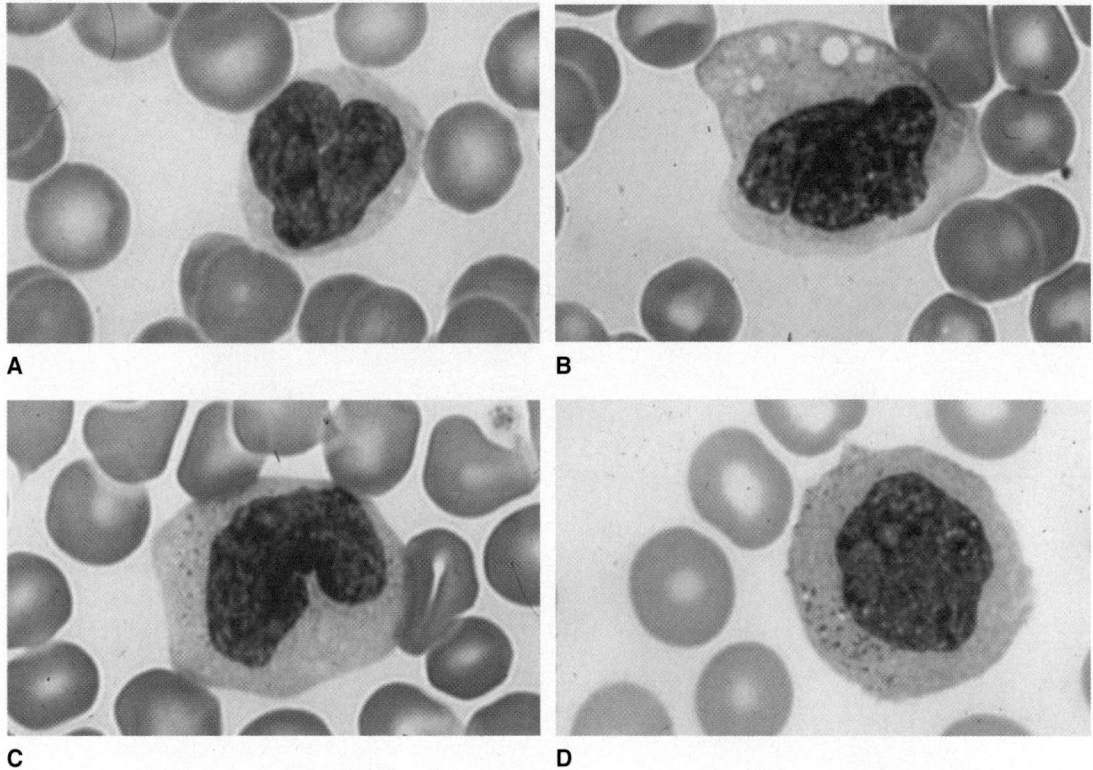

Figure 67–1. Blood films. This composite shows four examples of normal monocytes with different nuclear configurations. **A.** In this case, the nucleus is contorted on itself and the nuclear-to-cytoplasmic ratio is a bit higher than the average case. **B.** Another contorted nucleus with a lower nuclear-to-cytoplasmic ratio. Scattered vacuoles are common in monocytes collected in ethylenediaminetetraacetic acid (EDTA)-anticoagulated blood before film preparation. **C.** Characteristic reniform nuclear shape. **D.** Circular nuclear shape. Azurophilic granules are evident in the cytoplasm of monocytes. *(Reproduced with permission from* Lichtman's Atlas of Hematology, *www.accessmedicine.com.)*

by formation of ruffles or microvilli may reduce repulsive forces when surface negative-charge groups on the cell approach and contact a negatively charged substratum or cell. In addition, redundancy of the cell membrane may provide reserve membrane required for locomotion and phagocytosis.

Transmission Electron Microscopy

The nucleus of the monocyte contains one or two small nucleoli surrounded by nucleolar-associated chromatin (Fig. 67–2).[18] The cytoplasm contains a relatively small quantity of endoplasmic reticulum and a variable quantity of ribosomes and polysomes. The mitochondria are numerous, small, and elongated. The Golgi complex is well developed and is situated about the centrosome within the nuclear indentation. Centrioles and filamentous centriolar satellites are often visualized in this region. Microtubules are numerous, and microfibrils are found in bundles surrounding the nucleus. In cultured macrophages, collections of microfilaments are present underneath the plasma membrane near sites of cell attachment either to a substratum or to phagocytosable particles.[19] The cell surface is characterized by numerous microvilli and vesicles of micropinocytosis. The cytoplasmic granules resemble the small granules found in the granulocytic series, measuring approximately 0.05 to 0.2 μm in diameter. They are dense and homogeneous and are surrounded by a limiting membrane. These granules, as with the lysosomal granules of other leukocytes, are packaged by the Golgi apparatus after their enzymatic content has been produced by the ribosomal complex of the cell.[10,11] These cytoplasmic granules contain acid phosphatase and arylsulfatase and, therefore, are primary lysosomes. After endocytosis, lysosomes fuse with the phagosome, forming secondary lysosomes.

Some monocyte granules stain positive for peroxidase, whereas others are peroxidase negative.[10,11]

Freeze-Fracture Microscopy

In this technique, a cell suspension is frozen, placed in a high-vacuum chamber, and struck with a blunt edge, thus producing a fracture that propagates through the frozen specimen. The utility of the procedure comes from the remarkable finding that when the fracture encounters a cell, the fracture tends to propagate along the interior of the plasma membrane and thus split the lipid bilayer into its two constituent layers. After fracture, the specimen is coated with platinum, which is electron dense when viewed with transmission electron microscopy. All cell types examined thus far by the freeze-fracture technique reveal intramembrane particles (IMPs) as the predominant topographic feature of the interior of the bilayer. Studies of the erythrocyte show that at least some particles contain intercalated membrane proteins, and this is assumed to be the case for nucleated cells as well. The distribution of IMPs is dramatically altered in a number of cell systems by physiologic stimuli, for example, hormonal stimulation.

Profound changes in the distribution of IMPs on mononuclear phagocytes occur following binding of antibody-coated erythrocytes.[13] Because redistribution of IMPs also occurs in some nonphagocyte Fc receptor (FcR)–bearing cells[13] and after exposure to aggregated immunoglobulin (Ig) G, this alteration in IMPs presumably reflects interaction with FcR. Freeze-etch electron micrographs of the monocyte show nuclear pores traversing both lamellae of the nuclear membrane and contours of cytoplasmic lysosomes and mitochondria (Fig. 67–3).

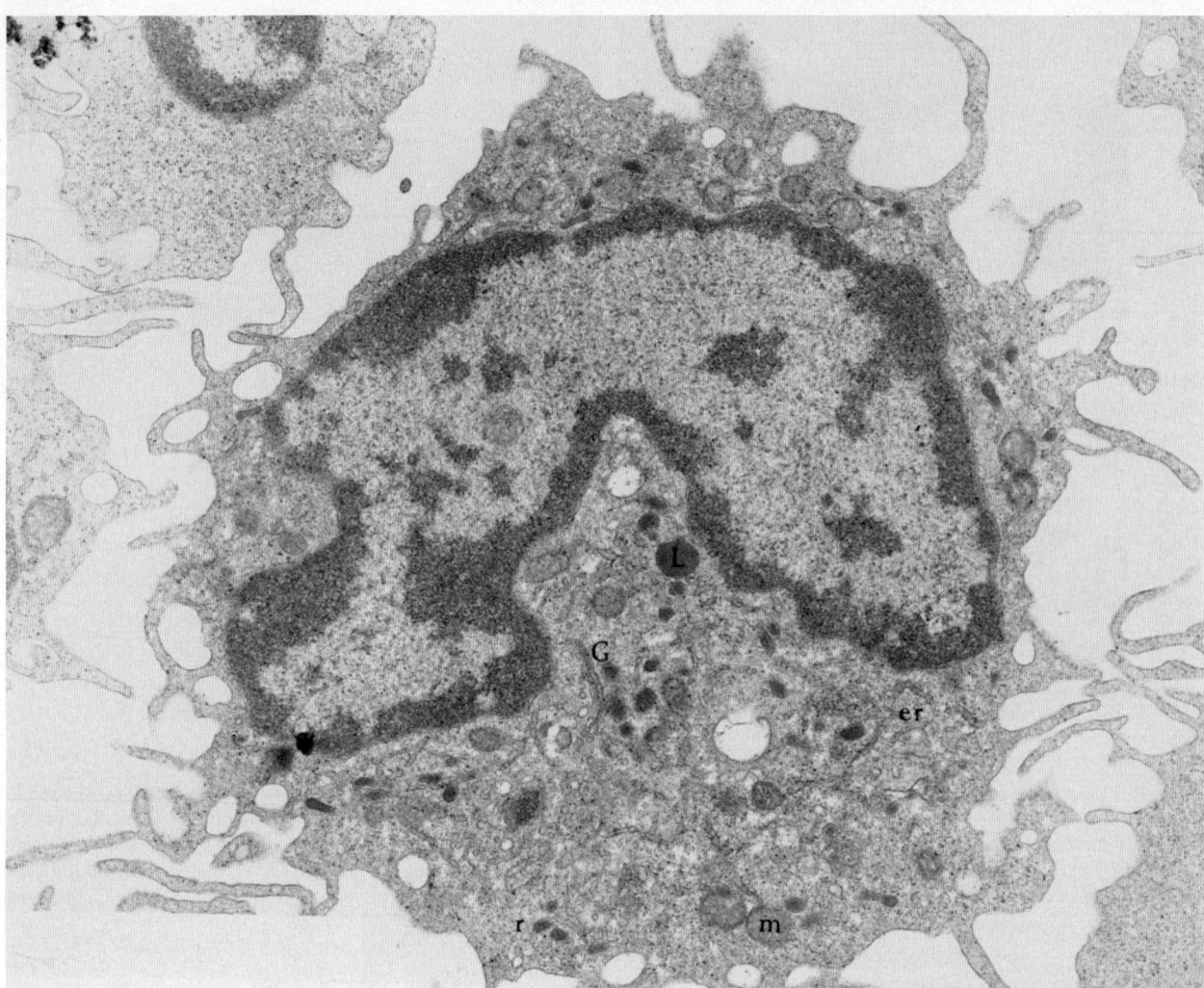

Figure 67–2. Transmission electron micrograph of a monocyte. The eccentric reniform nucleus has a thinly dispersed chromatin pattern. The Golgi complex (G) is in a juxtanuclear position. Small electron-dense granules can be seen evolving in the Golgi complex. Small amounts of rough endoplasmic reticulum (er) and polyribosomes (r) are present, particularly about the cell periphery. Mitochondria (m) are concentrated in the region of the Golgi apparatus; they also are scattered in the cell periphery. Lysosomes (L) are small, electron-dense granules surrounded by a limiting membrane. The irregular ruffled cell margin is apparent with numerous microprojections (×24,000).

HISTOCHEMISTRY OF MONOCYTES

Table 67–2 compares the hydrolytic enzyme contents of monocytes, neutrophils, and lymphocytes. Monocytes also give a weak but positive periodic acid–Schiff reaction (for polysaccharides) and Sudan black B reaction (for lipids). Nonspecific esterase[20–22] is frequently used as a marker for monocytes. Monocyte esterases are inhibited by sodium fluoride, whereas the esterases of the granulocytic series are not. The nonspecific esterase reaction is positive in promyelocytes and myelocytes; therefore, analysis of fluoride inhibition is necessary to distinguish marrow monocytes from early myelocytes. Monocyte granules, although heterogeneous in size (0.3 to 0.6 μm), are not separable into populations by routine electron microscopic criteria. Identification of monocyte granule populations has depended on subcellular localization of monocyte enzymes by electron microscopic cytochemistry.[10] Human marrow promonocytes and blood monocytes contain granules that comprise two functionally distinct populations.[10,11] One population contains the enzymes acid phosphatase, arylsulfatase, and peroxidase. These granules are modified primary lysosomes and are analogous to the azurophil granules of the neutrophil. The monocyte azurophil granule population is heterogeneous in cytochemical reactivity for peroxidase, acid phosphatase, and arylsulfatase.[23,24] Moreover, primary granules that are morphologically identical with other vesicles can be identified as lysosomes cytochemically. The other population of monocyte granules lacks alkaline phosphatase[23] and is not strictly analogous to the specific granules of neutrophils.

MORPHOLOGY OF MACROPHAGES

Macrophage characteristics are heralded by a significant increase in cell size, increase in the number of cytoplasmic granules, increase in the heterogeneity of cell size and shape, and increase in the number of cytoplasmic clear vacuoles in comparison to monocytes.

Light and Phase-Contrast Microscopy

In vitro culture of monocytes purified from adult human blood has provided an opportunity to observe the maturation of these cells into mature macrophages. The macrophages of the pulmonary alveoli,

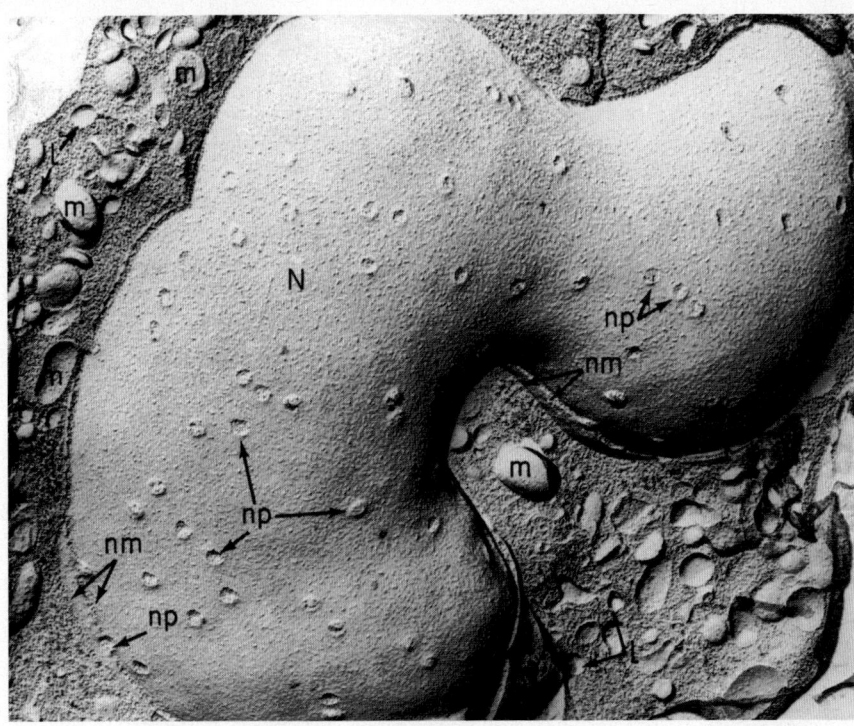

Figure 67–3. Freeze-etch electron micrograph of a monocyte. Fracture plane displays the large nucleus (N), with multiple nuclear pores (np) and the two lamellae of the fractured nuclear membrane (nm) evident in some regions. Membrane and cleaved surfaces of mitochondria (m) and lysosomal granules (L) can be identified in the cytoplasm.

peritoneal and pleural cavities, and inflammatory exudates are hypermature cells that have undergone *in vivo* stimulation and maturation. This process results in enhanced bactericidal activity[1,2] because of augmentation of lysosome number and acid hydrolase content. Macrophages display attributes of morphologic specialization specific to their location and function. The fixed macrophages of the spleen (littoral cells) are involved in the sequestration and destruction of effete or abnormal red cells and exhibit stages of erythrophagocytosis and intracytoplasmic aggregates of ferritin (Chap. 6). The macrophages of the marrow, the "nurse cells" of the erythroblastic island, play a similar role in erythrophagocytosis and iron storage and transfer (Chaps. 5 and 31). Hepatic macrophages (Kupffer cells), found in liver sinusoids, also phagocytize red cells and other cellular elements and are important sites of iron storage. Macrophages of the pulmonary alveoli, the lamina propria of the gastrointestinal tract, and the peritoneal and pleural fluids reflect in their morphology a specific function of phagocytosis of microorganisms, cells, and cellular and noncellular debris, characteristic of the specific organ location.

Most macrophages are 25 to 50 μm in diameter on Wright or hematoxylin-and-eosin–stained films (Fig. 67–4). They have an eccentrically placed reniform or fusiform nucleus with one or two distinct nucleoli and finely dispersed, loosely stranded nuclear chromatin that tend to clump in the nuclear interior and along the internal aspect of the nuclear membrane (Fig. 67–5A). A juxtanuclear clear zone (Golgi complex) is well defined when the Wright stain is used. The cytoplasm shows fine granules and multiple pink-purple, large azurophil granules. The cytoplasmic borders are irregularly serrated. Cytoplasmic vacuoles are present near the cell periphery, reflecting the active pinocytosis in these cells.

The surface antigen CD68, also known as *macrosialin*, is commonly used as a macrophage marker. Figure 67–5B shows an immunohistochemistry micrograph of a macrophage in a lymph node. The cytoplasm of the macrophage is intensely positive for CD68, while the surrounding lymphocytes are negative.

On phase-contrast microscopy, living macrophages are large cells with a propensity to adhere to and spread on glass surfaces. Thus, the cell organelles are concentrated within the central portion of the cell and clear veils of hyaloplasm spread about the cell, with intense ruffling of the membrane borders. Vesicles and contractile vacuoles are seen about the cell periphery and in the cell interior. The juxtanuclear clear zone bearing the centrosome and the Golgi complex is particularly dynamic and displays an undulating motion.

TABLE 67–2. Cytochemical Reactions of Leukocyte Enzymes

Chemical	Monocytes	Neutrophils	Lymphocytes
Acid phosphatase	+ +	+	+
β-Glucuronidase	+ +	+	0 to +
Sulfatase	+	+	0
N-Acetylglucosaminidase	+ +	+ +	0
Lysozyme*	++	+ +	0
Naphthylamidase	+ +	+	0 to +
α-Naphthylbutyrate esterase†	+ +	0 to +	0
Naphthol AS-D chloro-acetate esterase	0 to +	+ +	0
Peroxidase	+	+ +	0
Alkaline phosphatase	0	0 to +	0

*Most lysozyme produced by mononuclear phagocytes is secreted rather than stored intracellularly.

†α-Naphthylacetate and α-naphthylbutyrate esterase activities may appear in human T lymphocytes under certain conditions.

Data from Braunsteiner H, Schmalzl F: Cytochemistry of monocytes and macrophages. In *Mononuclear Phagocytes*, edited by R van Furth, p 62. Blackwell, Oxford, England, 1970; Li CY, Lam KW, Yam LT: Esterases in human leukocytes. *J Histochem Cytochem* 21:1-12, 1973.

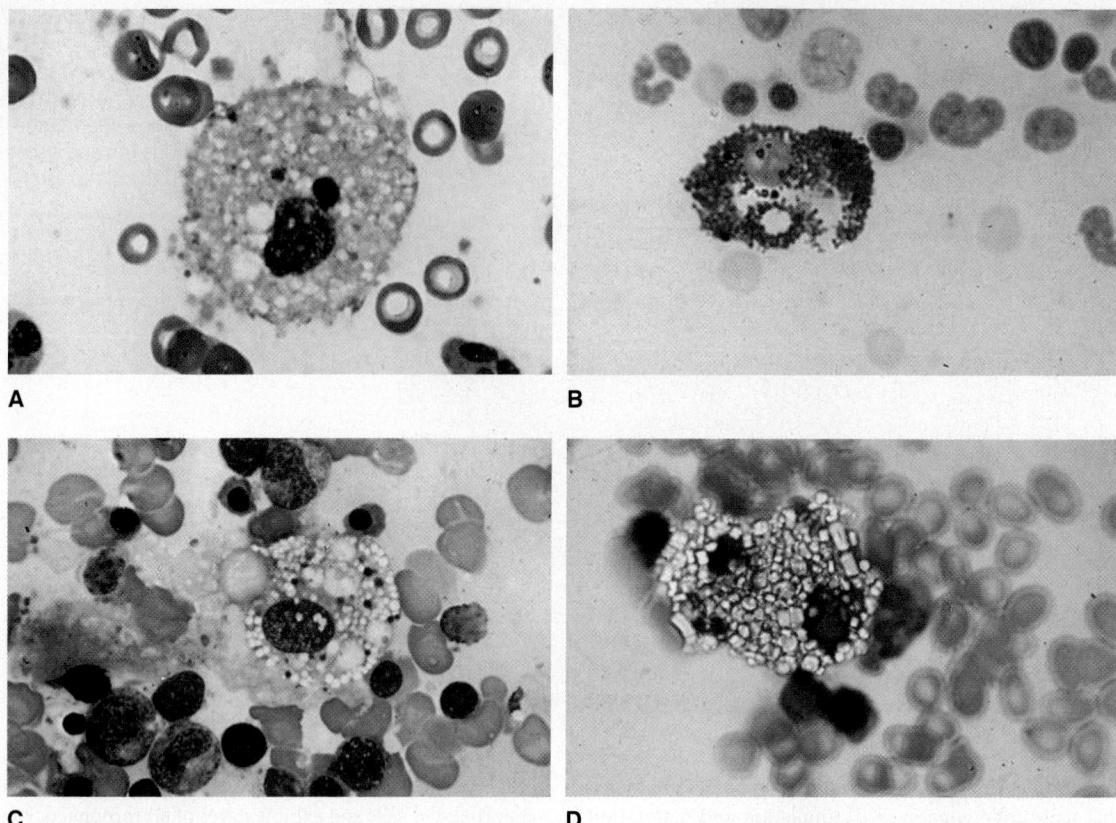

A

B

C

D

Figure 67–4. Marrow films. Macrophages. These cells characteristically have a circular, sometimes centrally placed and sometimes eccentrically placed nucleus dwarfed by a very large expanse of cytoplasm. **A**. Activated macrophage, full of cytoplasmic vacuoles and some residual ingested cellular debris. **B**. Macrophage stained with Prussian blue showing cytoplasmic iron granules. **C**. Macrophage with erythrophagocytosis. Note pale red cells (partially dehemoglobinized) undergoing hemolysis and destruction. The highly vacuolated cytoplasm is presumably the site of red cell degradation. **D**. Macrophage in a patient with cystinosis engorged with cystine crystals. *(Reproduced with permission from Lichtman's Atlas of Hematology, www.accessmedicine.com.)*

Electron Microscopy

Scanning electron micrographs of macrophages adherent to glass surface show membrane ruffling and pseudopodia (Fig. 67–6). Transmission electron microscopy of monocyte-derived macrophages show a variable degree of differentiation, nuclear "maturity," ribosomes, mitochondria, and lysosome content, and the nucleus varies in shape from horseshoe to fusiform (Fig. 67–7). Clear spaces between membrane-fixed chromatin aggregates mark the sites of nuclear pores that are relatively abundant on freeze-etch electron micrographs of macrophages and monocytes (see Fig. 67–3). Polyribosomes and scant smooth

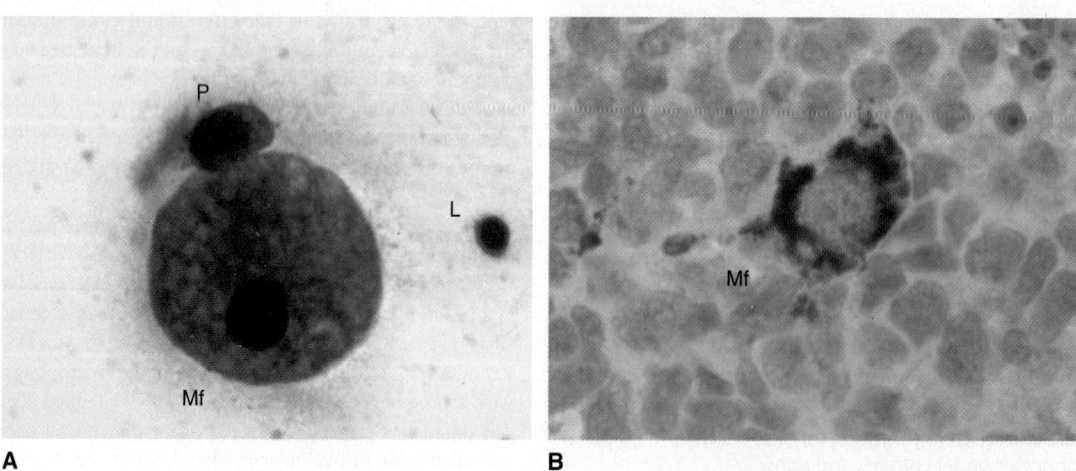

A

B

Figure 67–5. Micrographs of macrophages (Mf). **A.** Hematoxylin-and-eosin stain of cytology smear (×400) showing a macrophage, a plasma cell (P), and a lymphocyte (L). **B.** Immunohistochemistry stain for the macrophage marker CD68 of a lymph node (×400). Numerous lymphocytes with blue nuclei surround a macrophage with brown-red cytoplasm. *(Used with permission of Dr. Madalina Tuluc, Thomas Jefferson University Hospital, Philadelphia, PA.)*

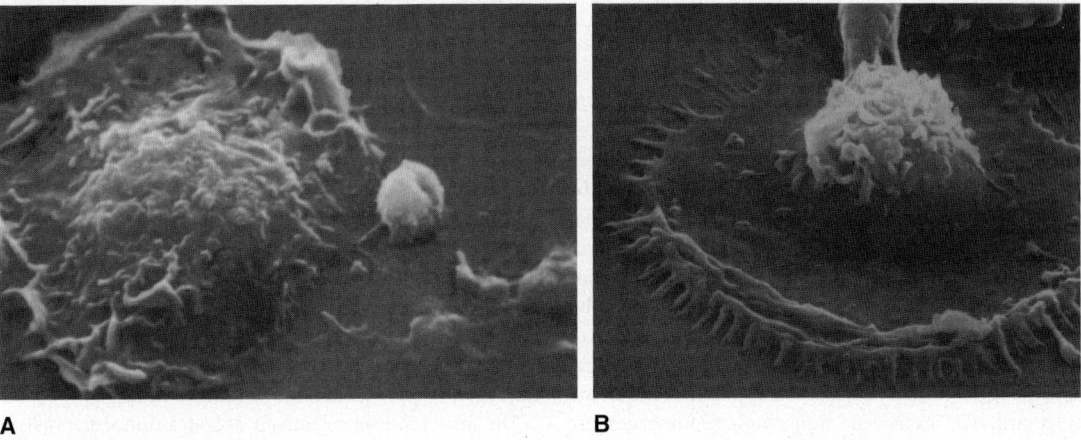

A   **B**

Figure 67–6. Scanning electron micrograph of cultured macrophages on coverglasses coated with (**A**) bovine serum albumin (BSA) or (**B**) with immune complexes (BSA–anti-BSA). The macrophage develops prominent peripheral membrane ruffling and numerous microadhesion points to the surface coated with immune complexes.

and rough endoplasmic reticulum are seen about the cell periphery. A well-developed Golgi complex is in a juxtanuclear location. It often is multicentric and contains a concentration of vesicles, some with dense inclusions that mark them as early lysosomes. A relatively constant feature of cells engaged in endocytosis is the large number of microvilli at the cell surface. The degree of development of this surface adaptation is related to the phagocytic activity of the cell and its rate of pinocytosis. The number and size of mitochondria vary with the phagocytic and hence metabolic activity of the cell. Mitochondria tend to be grouped about the region of the Golgi complex, although several usually are seen dispersed about the cell periphery, presumably supplying energy for the active endocytic processes occurring there.

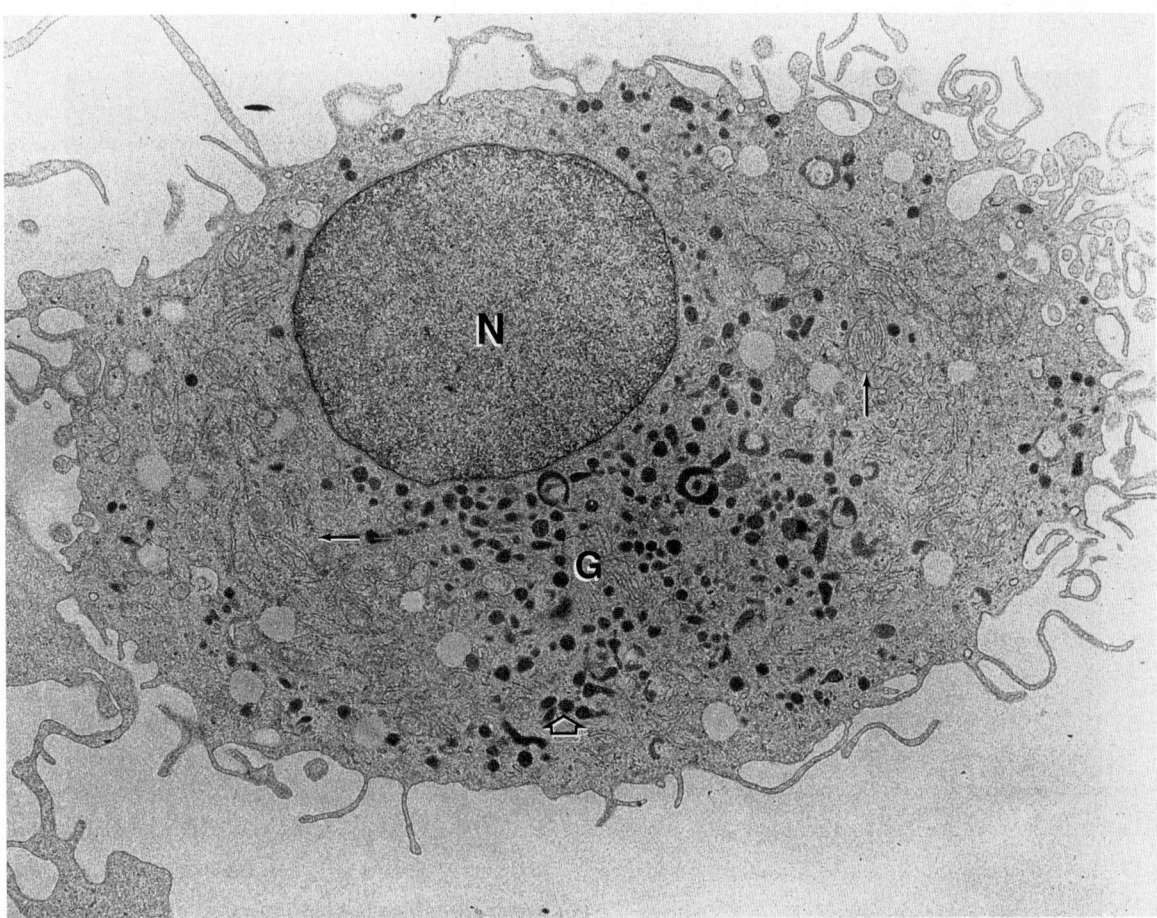

Figure 67–7. Electron micrograph of monocyte-derived macrophage cultured *in vitro* for 9 days. G, Golgi zone; N, nucleus. *Arrow on right* indicates endoplasmic reticulum; *arrow on left* indicates mitochondria; *open arrow* indicates lysosomes (×7600).

The most constant and characteristic ultrastructural features of macrophages are the electron-dense membrane-bound lysosomes that often can be seen fusing with phagosomes to form secondary lysosomes. Within the secondary lysosomes, ingested cellular, bacterial, and non-cellular material can be seen in various stages of degradation, often recognizable as degenerating mitochondria or nuclear material. These secondary lysosomes also contain partially degraded material from the late stages of the endocytic process, often appearing as multilamellar lipid bodies. Microtubules and microfilaments are prominent in macrophages. Actin- and myosin-like proteins have been isolated from monocytes and partially characterized. Resting macrophages have irregular cell borders and pseudopodia pushed out in all directions. Their cytoplasm has rough endoplasmic reticulum and Golgi complex in the perinuclear area. Lipid globules, primary lysosomes, and mitochondria are characteristically prominent. Activated monocytes/macrophages are motile cells that extend a leading pseudopod as they move forward.[25]

● RECEPTORS

MEMBRANE RECEPTORS AND OTHER SURFACE PROTEINS OF MONOCYTES AND MACROPHAGES

Monocyte/macrophage cells have surface receptors that have been characterized by their binding to specific monoclonal antibodies. These receptors (Fig. 67–8) are markers for origin, growth, differentiation,[26] activation, recognition, migration, and function of the monocyte/macrophage. Monocytes have been classified into distinct subtypes based on surface expression of CD14 and CD16, molecules that form part of the lipopolysaccharide (LPS) toll-like receptor (TLR) and one of the immunoglobulin FcRs, respectively. These include CD14+-bright/CD16– monocytes, CD14+-dim/CD16+ monocytes, and CD14-dim/CD16+ monocytes. Monocyte heterogeneity was initially divided into the CD14+-bright/CD16-negative cells, which comprise 90 to 95 percent of total circulating monocytes (classical monocyte)[27]—CD14-bright or dim refer to the fluorescence magnitude of staining using a specific CD14 monoclonal antibody. The minor subset is CD14-dim, CD16-positive, and less phagocytic than the classical monocyte. The classical monocyte produces reactive oxygen species (ROS) and cytokines in response to TLR engagement. The minor subset selectively secretes tumor necrosis factor (TNF)-α, IL-13, and CCL2 in response to viruses and immune complexes containing nucleic acids via TLR-7, TLR-8, MyD88-MEK (myeloid differentiation factor 88–MAPK kinase), and AHD.[28] This minor subset, CD14-dim,[29] is competent in (SR [scavenger receptor]) function of vascular, intraluminal debris and uptake of immune complexes.[30] In addition, their phenotype is related to the ability to produce and secrete select cytokines.[31]

Macrophages are proficient at endocytosis (both fluid phase and receptor-mediated) and are highly professional phagocytes of particulates of all origin, organic (cellular, microbial) as well as inorganic foreign materials.[32] In contrast, when dendritic cells (DCs) mature into antigen-presenting cells (APCs), they have reduced uptake capacity

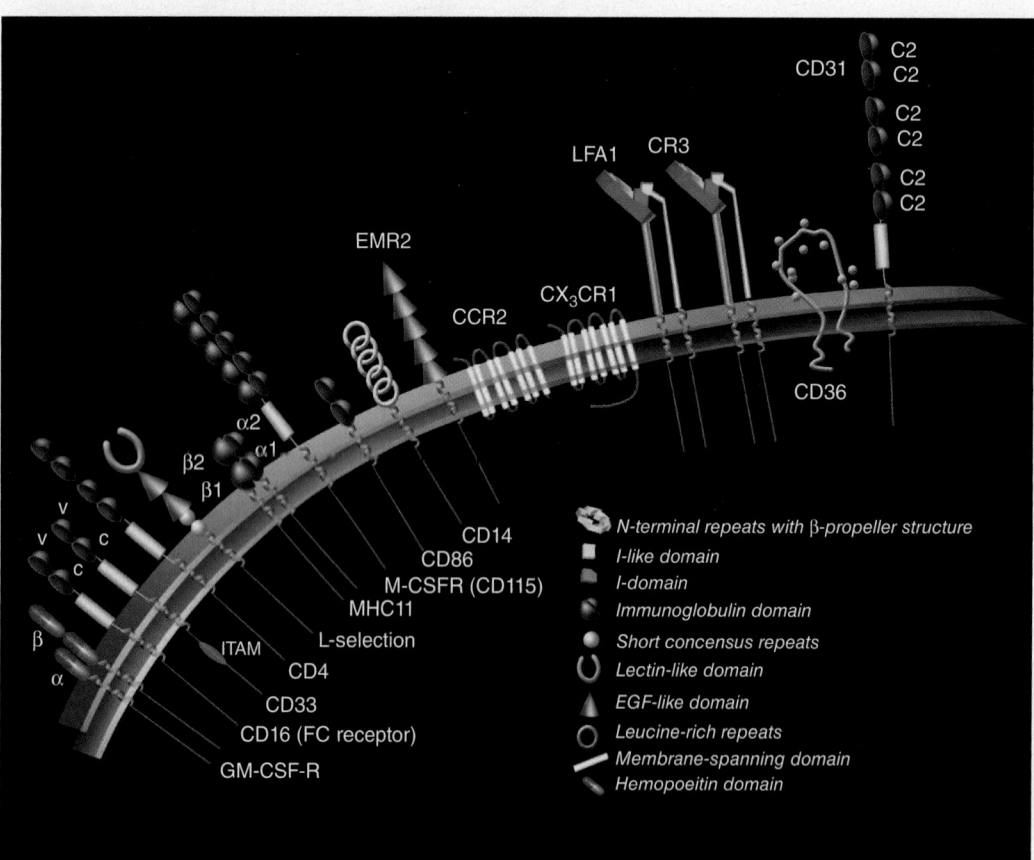

Figure 67–8. Schematic of selected molecules of varied structure and functions of monocyte receptors and surface antigens. *(Used with permission of S. Seif, GraphisMedica, 2014.)*

and induce an adaptive immune response or tolerance. Immature DCs display active macropinocytosis and capture exogenous materials for cross-presentation.[33] It is convenient to classify plasma membrane uptake receptors as opsonic and nonopsonic TLRs and non–TLR-dependent. The latter category includes a range of SRs[34,35] and a family of lectin-like, carbohydrate recognition molecules.[36,37] Given the complex ligands presented on the surface of microorganisms and damaged host cells, or generated within the vacuolar system after uptake, these receptors frequently cooperate with one another.

Fc Receptors

FcRs for IgG are expressed on the surface of mononuclear cells, macrophages, granulocytes, and platelets.[38,39] FcRs are divided into three distinct classes: FcRI, FcRII, and FcRIII (Fig. 67–9). These receptors have broad ranges of expression on different cells. The first IgG receptor, FcRI (CD64), is a receptor found on monocytes, macrophages, and activated neutrophils. This receptor binds monomeric IgG through the Fc portion of the molecule. This Ig receptor has increased

expression on activated monocytes and macrophages. CD64 allows for receptor-mediated endocytosis of IgG–antigen complexes for presentation to T cells, can trigger the release of cytokines and ROS, and can play a role in granulocyte-mediated antibody-dependent cytotoxicity. The second IgG receptor, FcRII (CD32), is a widely distributed receptor present on many cell types, including monocytes, platelets, neutrophils, B cells, some T cells, and some capillary endothelium. This receptor can bind complexed IgG rather than monomeric IgG. This FcR regulates B-cell function when coengaged with the B-cell receptor for antigen, namely, surface Ig. It also can induce mediator release from myeloid cells and phagocytosis of Ig-coated particles *in vitro*. Finally, this FcR also can target antigen into presenting pathways. The third IgG receptor, FcRIII (CD16), is expressed by neutrophils, natural killer cells, and tissue macrophages.[40] This receptor can bind Ig in immune complexes and Ig bound to cell-surface membranes. It is the main FcR responsible for antibody-dependent cellular cytotoxicity. All three FcRs specifically bind the human IgG subclasses IgG_1 and IgG_3 (Chap. 75). The interaction of FcR on

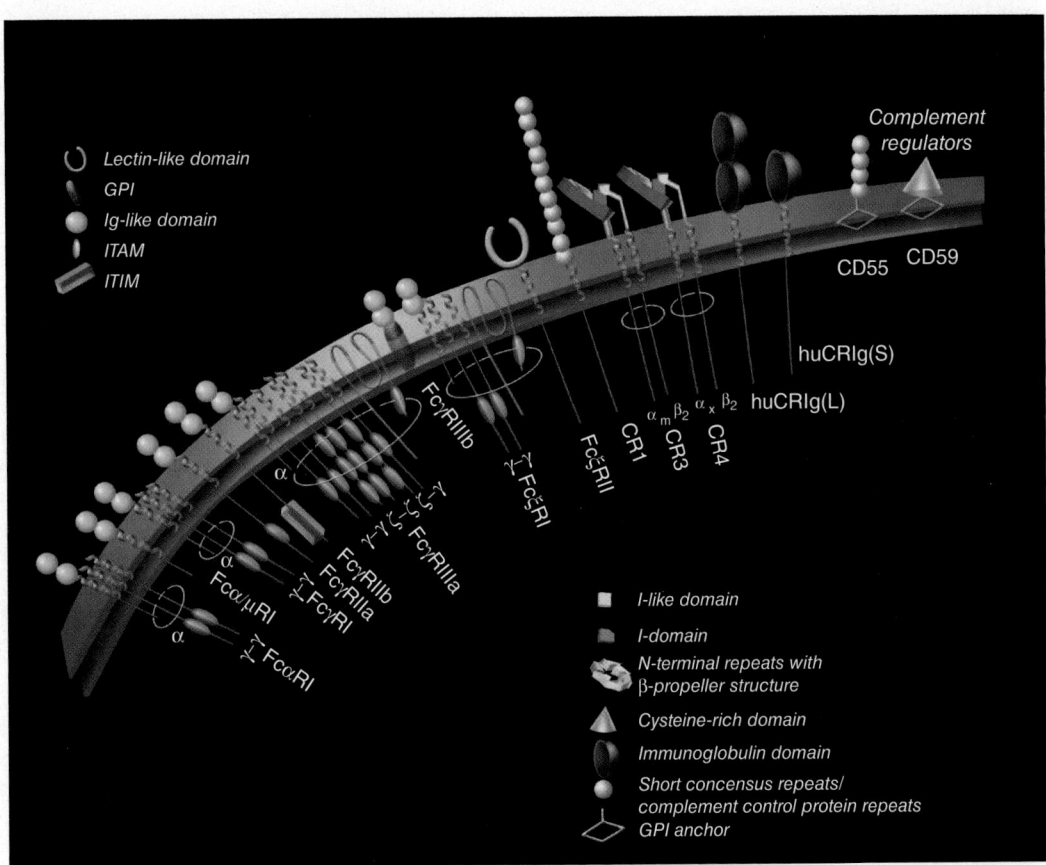

Figure 67–9. Human Fc receptors and complement. Myeloid cells express a range of classical Fc receptors that initiate a variety of cellular responses, including phagocytosis, antibody-dependent cell-mediated toxicity, antigen presentation, respiratory burst, and release of inflammatory mediators. Immunoglobulin (Ig) subclasses are bound by extracellular domains; signaling via cytoplasmic immunoreceptor tyrosine-based activation motif (ITAM) or immunoreceptor tyrosine-based inhibition motif (ITIM) is mediated by associated membrane-spanning polypeptides. Activation and inhibitory receptors are usually coexpressed on the cell surface and function in concert, determining the magnitude of effector cell responses. Complement receptors (CRs) and membrane regulators are expressed by m-φ-CR. CR1 is broadly expressed by nucleated cells, acting as a "sink" for activated complement. CR3 (CD11b/CD18), a phagocytic receptor for C3bi-coated particles, and CR4 (CD11c/CD18) are β_2 integrins, which, together with lymphocyte function-associated antigen (LFA)-1 (CD11a/CD18), mediate adhesion of myeloid cells to endothelium and extracellular matrix and migration. Human CR immunoglobin (huCRIg) are long (L) and short (S) forms of the complement-binding receptor on Kupffer cells that mediate uptake of opsonized bacteria. CD55 and CD59 are glycosylphosphatidylinositol (GPI)-anchored regulators of complement activation. (*Used with permission of S. Seif, GraphisMedica, 2014.*)

macrophages with immune complexes results in cell "activation," with an increase in phagocytosis, superoxide production, and prostaglandin and leukotriene release.

Complement Receptors

Activation of the complement system results in liberation of numerous ligands that bind to specific receptors on mononuclear phagocytes. Four receptors that bind fragments of the complement component C3 have been identified (see Fig. 67–9).[41] Complement receptor (CR) 1 (or CD35) binds dimeric C3bi and is found on both monocytes and macrophages. CR3 (or CD11b) binds the complement fragment C3b. CR3 is a heterodimeric glycoprotein that is composed of two noncovalently linked polypeptides. The α chain of the polypeptide has an Mr of 185,000, and the β subunit has an Mr of 95,000. This receptor and the leukocyte antigens lymphocyte function–associated antigen (CD11a) and alpha-X integrin chain (CD11c) compose a family of heterodimers that share a common β subunit (CD18).[42] This family is designated the *leukocyte integrin (β_2)* subfamily.[43] These heterodimers are involved in cell–cell interactions, including leukocyte trafficking into the tissues, binding of opsonized particles and plasma proteins, and attachment to various substrates. They also may modulate intercellular adhesion. Elimination of the integrin β_2 subunit causes leukocyte adhesion deficiency.[44]

The classical opsonins, which promote the uptake of particles, are antibody, IgG complexed with antigens, and complement, activated by the classical pathway (antibody-dependent IgM or IgG) or recognized directly via the lectin-carbohydrate–stimulated alternative pathway. Fc and CRs are heterogeneous in structure, expression, and function, activating or inhibiting macrophage responses,[45,46] as illustrated in Fig. 67–9. Other opsonins include fibronectin and milk-fat globulin.[47] Through their expression of various opsonic receptors, monocytes, macrophages, and DCs perform versatile roles in innate and adaptive immunity,[48] in antigen clearance and destruction, in autoimmunity, and in pathogenesis of a range of inflammatory and infectious disorders. Genetic polymorphisms influence the expression and functions of FcRs in homeostasis and disease. Although prominent in host protection, invading microorganisms may be able to exploit, even subvert these receptors to facilitate their entry and survival.[49] Opsonic receptors play an important role in clearance of hematopoietic cells, for example, antibody-coated platelets, giving rise to thrombocytopenia, and in therapeutic antibody treatment, for example, to facilitate engraftment. Antibody engineering has provided novel therapeutic agents to minimize undesirable consequences, such as cell activation. The initiation or avoidance of complement activation in particular controls an important effector pathway in tissue injury and repair.

Toll-Like Receptors

The family of TLRs, identified on macrophages in mammals, is a pattern-recognition receptor that bind structurally conserved molecules derived from microorganisms, including endotoxins (LPS) and viral nucleic acids. TLRs are now considered key molecules responsible for alerting the immune system to the presence of microbial infections. For example, TLR4 is part of a recognition couple for LPS. Pathogen recognition by TLRs activates the innate immune system through the signaling pathway and provokes inflammatory responses, such as cytokine production.[50] These are shown schematically in Fig. 67–10 to illustrate their diverse structures and signaling pathways.

The discovery of TLR has transformed the study of innate immunity, inflammation, and adjuvant actions on APC.[51–53] Receptor structures, heterogeneity of expression, microbial and endogenous ligands, and signaling have been defined, and knowledge of their regulation

has begun to offer agents to manipulate TLR signaling in humans. The discovery of inborn errors, such as the interleukin receptor–associated kinase (IRAK)-4 deficiency,[54] and the role of toll-interleukin receptor adaptor protein (TIRAP) function in *Plasmodium falciparum* infection,[55] for example, have illustrated their role in human disease. Several concepts have emerged. From the original studies on LPS recognition and signaling by the multiprotein complex formed by CD14, LPS binding protein, and MD2, and the clarification of the distinct adaptor pathways (MyD88 [myeloid differentiation factor 88], TIRAP/MAL [MyD88 adaptor-like], TRIF [TIR domain-containing adaptor inducing interferon (IFN)-β], and TRAM [TRIF-related adaptor molecule]), the recognition and sensing of TLR ligands have become clear. The tertiary structure of TLR4 has been reported.[56] TLRs are expressed either on the plasma membrane of myeloid and other cells, or within the vacuole, especially in the case of TLRs 3, 7, and 9, which are implicated in viral nucleic acid recognition. Crosstalk among nuclear factor (NF) κB, IFN, and mitogen-activated protein kinase (MAPK) kinase pathways has also become apparent.[57] TLRs collaborate with other recognition receptors,[58] such as dectin-1. Furthermore, a role has been proposed for TLR signaling in nontranscriptional activities, such as the kinetics of phagosome maturation in macrophages.[59]

Non–Toll-Like, Nonopsonic Receptors

The study of lectins and SRs has lagged behind that of the above receptors, but is gaining ground, documenting receptor expression and ligands, mainly in mouse models of inflammation and infection.[35,60,61] These receptors are present on macrophages and DCs, and variably on monocytes and neutrophils. They are implicated in the recognition and uptake of microbial and host ligands, and vary in their ability to activate host defense functions. Figure 67–11 and Table 67–3 illustrate the functional attributes of these receptor systems. The mannose receptor is mainly involved in endocytosis, with a predominant intracellular localization.[62,63] The multilectin mannose receptor displays dual functions, contributing to the clearance of mannose-terminal lysosomal hydrolases and of neutrophil granule glycoproteins such as MPO, as well as of hormones (e.g., thyroglobulin) and exocrine secretion products (e.g., amylase). It plays a role in the capture and transport of mannose-terminal glycoproteins to targets in spleen (marginal metallophilic macrophages) and in lymph nodes (subcapsular sinus macrophages) that express sulfated receptors for its cysteine-rich domain. The outcome of such targeting is either silent disposal or, if combined with TLR stimulation, induction of an immune response.[64] In common with several other nonopsonic receptors, it can play dual, even opposing actions in host protection or in pathogenesis, as shown by ongoing studies in mice.

Dectin 1 is a lectin-like receptor that is widely expressed on myeloid cells, with a single immunoreceptor tyrosine-based activation motif (ITAM)–like motif in its cytoplasmic tail.[65] It recognizes β glucans, abundant in fungal walls, including bioactive zymosan particles, and has been implicated in innate resistance to fungal infection. Dectin-1 activates syk and caspase activation and recruitment domain (CARD)-9, regulating various effector pathways such as TNF-α, leukotriene production, and T-helper (Th) 17 cell activation, with heterogeneity in responses by macrophages and DCs. Dectin-1 collaborates with TLR 2/6 in the response to zymosan. Other lectins expressed by macrophages include sialic acid recognition molecules, Siglec-1 (sialoadhesin),[66] an extended Ig superfamily plasma membrane protein implicated in cell–cell interactions (Chap. 68 discusses a possible role in the hematopoietic system).

SRs are a diverse family of structurally unrelated, promiscuous receptors, with a predilection for polyanionic ligands, expressed by

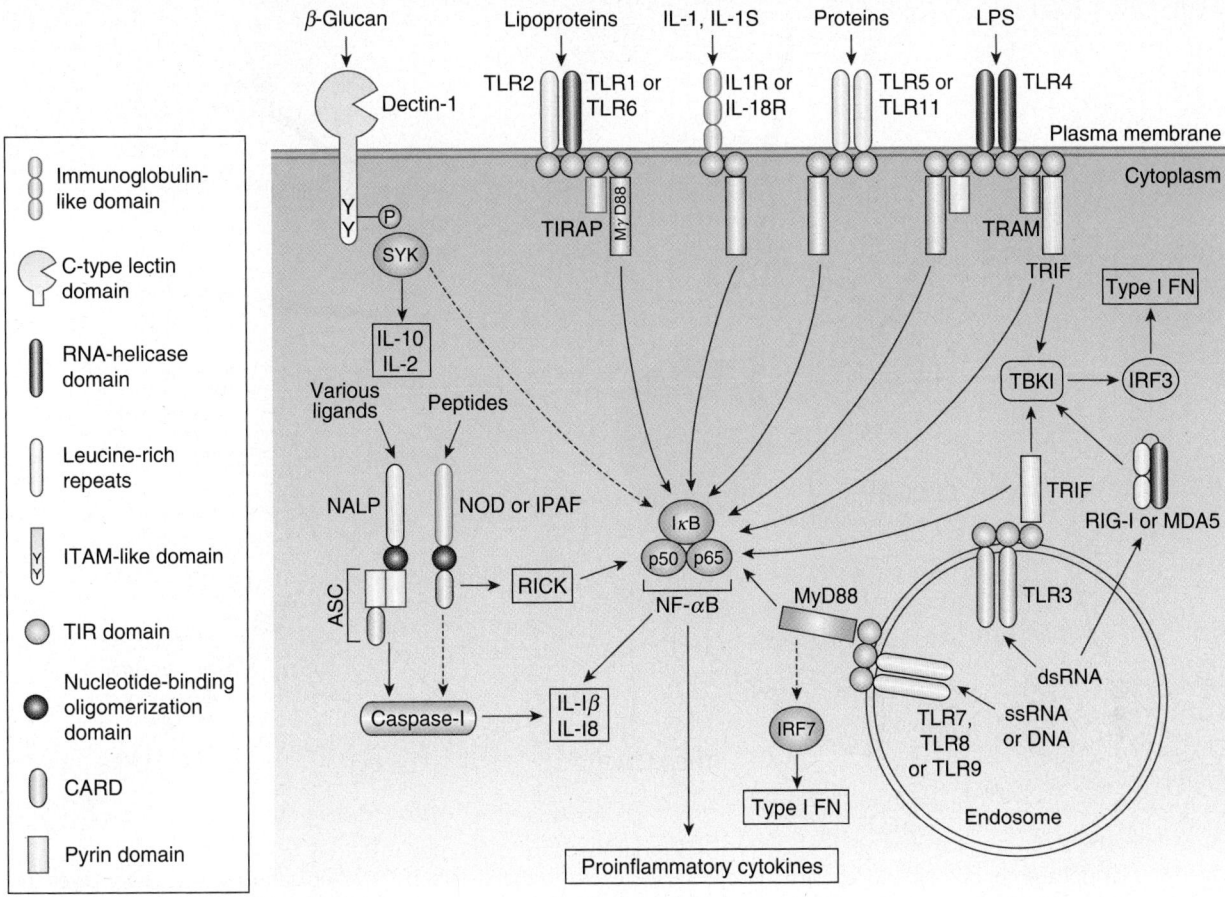

Figure 67–10. The main toll-like receptor (TLR) signaling pathways and adaptor molecules. The pathways that are activated by the different receptors are multiple and complex. For example, TLR signaling involves not only nuclear factor-κB (NF-κB) activation, but also mitogen-activated protein kinases, phosphatidylinositol 3-kinase, and several other pathways that markedly affect the overall biologic response to the activation of TLRs. Dectin-1 (a β-glucan receptor) is shown as an example of various signaling-competent cell-surface pattern-recognition receptors. ASC, apoptosis-associated speck-like protein containing a caspase activation and recruitment domain; CARD, caspase activation and recruitment domain; ds, double-stranded; type I IFN, type I interferon; IFN, interferon; IκB, inhibitor of NF-κB; IL, interleukin; IPAF, interleukin-1β–converting enzyme-protease activating factor; IRF, IFN-regulatory factor; LPS, lipopolysaccharide; MDA5, melanoma differentiation-associated gene 5; MyD88, myeloid differentiation primary response gene 88; NACHT, domain present in NAIP, CIITA, HET-E, and TP-1; NALP, NACHT leucine-rich repeat and pyrin-domain-containing protein; NOD, nucleotide-binding oligomerization domain; RICK, receptor-interacting serine/threonine kinase; RIG-I, retinoic acid-inducible gene I; ss, single-stranded; TBK1, TANK-binding kinase 1; TIRAP, toll/IL-1R (TIR) domain-containing adaptor protein; TRAM, TRIF-related adaptor molecule; TRIF, TIR domain-containing adaptor protein inducing IFN-β; SYK, spleen tyrosine kinase. See text for further details. *(Reproduced with permission from Trinchieri G, Sher A: Cooperation of Toll-like receptor signals in innate immune defence. Nat Rev Immunol 2007 Mar;7(3):179-190.)*

diverse microorganisms, apoptotic cells, and modified host lipoproteins.[34] SR-A I/II and MARCO (macrophage receptor with collagenous structure) (class A SR) are collagenous transmembrane receptors that mediate endocytosis, phagocytosis, and cell adhesion. SR-A I/II is upregulated by M-CSF and MARCO by TLR and MyD88-dependent microbial ligands, triggers of innate immune activation.[67] A number of naturally occurring ligands for SR-A have been identified, including apolipoprotein A₁ and *Neisserial* outer-surface proteins,[68] as well as previously described lipid A, lipoteichoic acid, and modified (acetylated) low-density lipoproteins, among others. After initial interest primarily in its role in atherogenesis (Chap. 134), attention has also focused on innate immune functions in bacterial infection.

Class B SRs, such as CD36 and SR-BI, have distinct structures and have been implicated in mycobacterial recognition as well as in the uptake and exchange of lipids.[69,70] CD36, together with thrombospondin,

plays a role in apoptotic cell uptake[47] and has been implicated in macrophage fusion. Other SRs, expressed on a variety of cells as well as macrophages, have similar roles in clearance.

Human Leukocyte Antigen Class II Receptors

Monocytes and macrophages serve an important function as APCs. They bear the class II glycoproteins of the major histocompatibility gene complex, human leukocyte antigen (HLA)-DR, HLA-DP, and HLA-DQ. Expression of major histocompatibility complex (MHC) class II antigens on macrophages from different tissues varies widely. Splenic macrophages contain a high percentage of HLA-DR–positive cells (50 percent), whereas peritoneal macrophages have relatively few (10 to 20 percent).[71] The proportion of Ia-positive alveolar macrophages is only approximately 5 percent.[72] Lymphokines, primarily IFN-γ, can induce macrophages to express higher levels of MHC class II antigens,

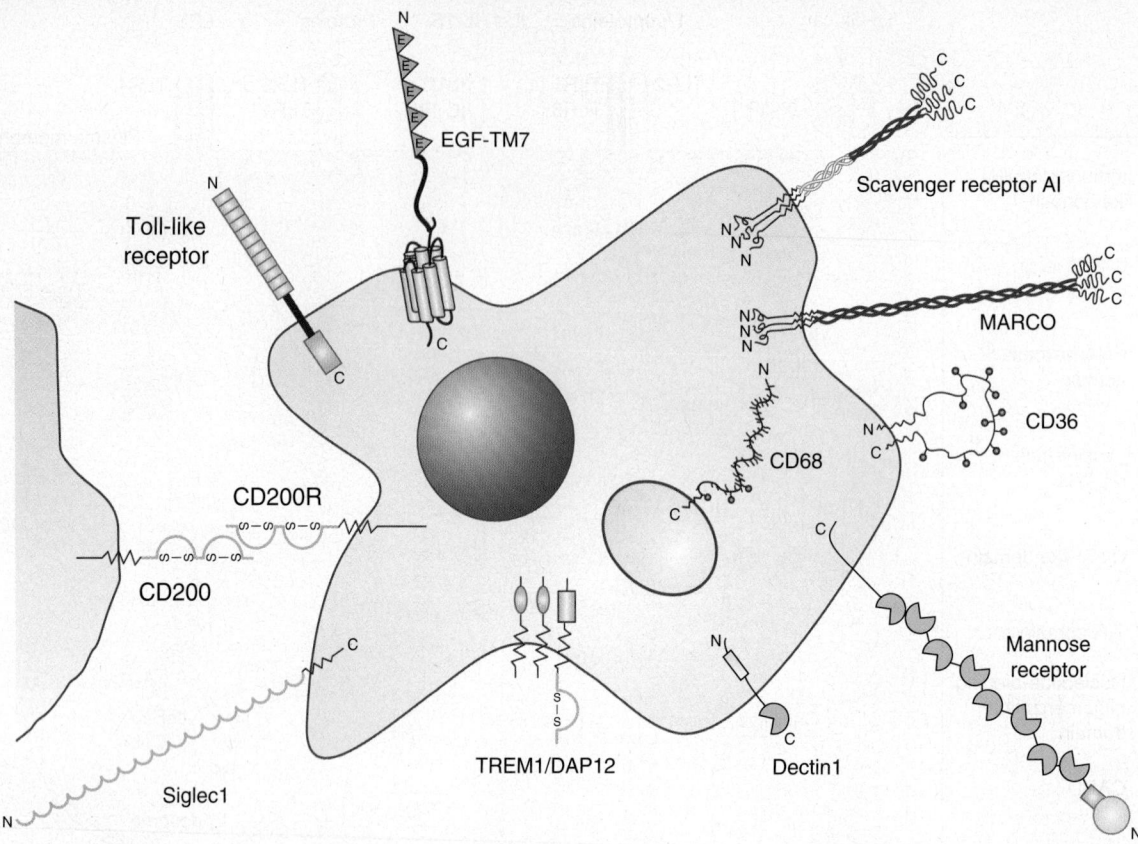

Figure 67–11. Macrophage nonopsonic and regulatory receptors. See text for further details. EGF-TM7, epidermal growth factor-seven transmembrane; MARCO, macrophage receptor with collagenous structure; Siglec, sialic acid-binding immunoglobulin-like lectin.

whereas prostaglandin E, α-fetoprotein, and glucocorticoids downregulate HLA-DR antigen expression on macrophages.

CD11

CD11 defines a family of three accessory adhesion surface glycoproteins: CD11a, CD11b, and CD11c. These proteins are distinct α subunits for three heterodimeric surface glycoproteins, each sharing a common β subunit, designated CD18. The α subunits have different isoelectric points, molecular weights, and cell distribution (Chap. 15).[73] Whereas CD11a is expressed on all leukocytes, CD11b and CD11c are expressed predominantly on monocytes and macrophages, a minor subset of B lymphocytes, and most polymorphonuclear leukocytes. CD11b is expressed on more than 95 percent of fresh human monocytes and macrophages but declines rapidly on cells maintained *in vitro*. Antibodies specific for CD11b, such as OKM1 or Mo1, may block this CR's ability to bind to CD3bi.[74] Accordingly, these antibodies strongly inhibit CR-mediated rosetting of erythrocyte–IgM antibody–complement complexes.

CD14 and CD16

The CD14 molecule is one of the most characteristic surface antigens of the monocyte lineage. It is a polypeptide of 356 amino acids that is anchored to the plasma membrane by a phosphoinositol linkage.[75] It is expressed strongly on the surface of monocytes and weakly on the surface of granulocytes and most tissue macrophages. It can be detected on some nonmyeloid cells (e.g., hepatocytes and some epithelial cells). CD14 functions as a receptor for endotoxin (LPS). LPS binds to a serum protein, LPS-binding protein, which facilitates the binding of LPS to CD14. The coreceptor MD2 and TLR4 also are vital in this process. When LPS binds to CD14/MD-2/TLR4 expressed by monocytes or neutrophils, the cells become activated and release cytokines such as TNF and upregulate cell surface molecules, including adhesion molecules. *In vitro*, soluble CD14 binds to LPS, and the complex stimulates cells that do not express CD14 to secrete cytokines and coregulate adhesion molecules.[76]

A subset of human blood monocytes that express low levels of CD14 molecules and high levels of the Fcγ receptor III (FcγRIII) CD16 has been identified.[77,78] These CD14+CD16+ monocytes resemble alveolar but not peripheral macrophages. CD14+CD16+ monocytes represent 5 to 10 percent of blood monocytes in normal individuals and can be dramatically expanded in pathologic conditions, such as sepsis, HIV infection, and cancer. CD16+ monocytes produce high levels of proinflammatory cytokines.

CD4

T lymphocytes express several surface receptors. The surface antigen CD4 is expressed primarily in T-helper lymphocytes (Chap. 76). CD4 and its corresponding messenger RNA have been demonstrated on monocytes, macrophages, and the monocyte-like cell line U-937.[79,80] Although CD4 is present at low concentrations in blood monocytes, the proportion of cells that display this plasma membrane determinant ranges from less than 5 percent to 90 percent. The CD4 molecule is involved in induction of T-lymphocyte helper functions (T_4) and T proliferative responses to antigen stimulation; however, its role

TABLE 67–3. Ligands for Selected Nonopsonic, Non–Toll-Like Receptors

Class	Receptor	Microbial Ligands	Endogenous Ligands	Function
Scavenger receptors	SR-A I/II	Gram+/− bacteria	Apoptotic cells	Phagocytosis
		Lipoteichoic acid	Modified low- and high-density lipoproteins (LDL, HDL, apolipoprotein A₁, apolipoprotein E)	Endocytosis
		Lipid A	AGE-modified proteins	Foam cell formation
		Neisserial surface proteins	β-Amyloid	Adhesion
	MARCO	Gram+/− bacteria	Marginal zone B lymphocytes	Adhesion
		Trehalose dimycolate	Uteroglobin-related protein	Phagocytosis
		Neisserial surface proteins		Innate activation
	CD36	Diacylated lipopeptide from Gram+ bacteria	Apoptotic cells (with thrombospondin and vitronectin receptor)	Uptake, exchange of lipids, adhesion
		Plasmodium falciparum-parasitized erythrocytes	HDL	
			Outer rod segments	
Lectins	Dectin-1	β-Glucan	T lymphocytes (noncarbohydrate)	Fungal uptake and immunomodulation
	DC-SIGN	Mannosyl/fucosyl glyco-conjugates viruses (e.g., HIV-1, Dengue)	ICAM 2/3	Adhesion
			T lymphocytes	Endocytosis
	Mannose receptor	Mannosyl/fucosyl	Lysosomal hydrolases	Endocytosis
	C-type lectin domains	Glycoconjugates on bacteria, viruses, fungi, parasites	Thyroglobulin	Adhesion
	Cysteine-rich domain		Ribonuclease B	Antigen targeting
	Fibronectin type II domain		Amylase	Adhesion
			Sulfated carbohydrates in marginal zone (spleen) and subcapsular sinus (lymph node)	
			Collagens	

AGE, advanced glycation end product; DC-SIGN, dendritic cell–specific intercellular adhesion molecule-3–grabbing nonintegrin; ICAM, intercellular adhesion molecule; MARCO, macrophage receptor with collagenous structure; SR, scavenger receptor.

Data from Fogelman AM, Van Lenten BJ, Warden C, et al: Macrophage lipoprotein receptors. *J Cell Sci* (Suppl 9):135-49, 1988; Adams DO, Hamilton TA: Phagocytic cells: Cytotoxic activities of macrophages. In *Inflammation: Basic Principles and Clinical Correlates* 2 edition, edited by J.I. Gallin & R. Snyderman, p. 471. Raven Press, New York, NY, 1992; Werb, Z. & Goldstein, I.: Phagocytic cells: Chemotactic and effector functions of macrophages and granulocytes, 7th ed., in Basic and Clinical Immunology, edited by D. Stites & A. Terr, p. 96. Appleton and Lange, Norwalk, CT, 1991; Papadimitriou, J.M. & Ashman, R.B.: Macrophages: current views on their differentiation, structure, and function. *Ultrastruct Pathol* 13:343-72, 1989; Gordon, S., Perry, V.H., Rabinowitz, S., Chung, L.P. & Rosen, H.: Plasma membrane receptors of the mononuclear phagocyte system. J Cell Sci Suppl 9:1-26, 1988; Law, S.K.: C3 receptors on macrophages. *J Cell Sci* Suppl 9:67-97, 1988; Hume, D.A. et al.: The mononuclear phagocyte system revisited. *J Leukoc Biol* 72:621–7, 2002.

in the function of monocyte/macrophages has not been determined. An important aspect of the monocyte/macrophage phenotype is the presence of CD4 molecules on the surface of monocytes that can act as receptors for HIV type 1 (HIV-1). HIV-1 uses the CD4 receptors as an entry pathway for infection of monocyte/macrophages.[79,80]

Chemokine Receptors

Chemokines mediate their activities by binding to target cell surface chemokine receptors that belong to a large family of G-protein–coupled, seven transmembrane domain receptors. Human monocytes/macrophages express several chemokine receptors (Table 67–4). The chemokine receptor CCR5 has been implicated in HIV-1 infection of monocytes/macrophages.[81–85] CCR5 is a major coreceptor on monocytes/macrophages for M-tropic HIV-1 infection. At least one copy of a 32-nucleotide deletion within the *CCR5* gene (CCR5Δ32) has been found in approximately 4 to 16 percent of individuals, depending on their background; when in the homozygous state, individuals are highly protected against acquisition of HIV.[86,87]

TABLE 67–4. Surface Receptors of Monocytes and Macrophages

Fc Receptors	Transferrin and Lactoferrin Receptors
IgG$_{2a}$, IgG$_{2b}$/IgG$_1$, IgG$_3$, IgA, IgE	Lipoprotein lipid receptors
Complement receptors	Anionic low-density lipoproteins
C3b, C3bi, C5a, C1q	PGE$_2$, LTB$_4$, LTC$_4$, PAG
LPS receptors	Apolipoproteins B and E (chylomicron remnants, VLDL)
CD14	
Cytokine receptors	Receptors for coagulants and anticoagulants
MIF, MAF, LIF, CF, MFF, TNF-α, IL-1, IL-2, IL-3, IL-4, IL-10, IL-18, INF-α, INF-β, INF-γ, GM-CSF, M-CSF/CSF-1	Fibrinogen/fibrin
	Coagulation factor VII
Chemokine receptors	α_1-Antithrombin
CCR1, CCR2A, CCR2B, CCR3, CXCR4, CCR5	Heparin
Macrophage growth factor receptors	Integrins (CD11b, CD18)
M-CSF, GM-CSF	Fibronectin receptors
Receptors for peptides and small molecules	Laminin receptors
Neurokinin-1	Mannosyl, fucosyl, galactosyl residue
H$_1$, H$_2$, 5-HT	α_2-Macroglobulin-proteinase complex receptors
1,2,5-Dihydroxy vitamin D$_3$	Toll-like receptors
N-formylated peptides	TLR2, TLR4, TLR5, TLR9
Enkephalins/endorphins	Others
Substance P	Cholinergic agonists
Hemokinin-1	α_1-Adrenergic agonists
Arg-vasopressin	β_2-Adrenergic agonists
Hormone receptors	
Insulin	
Glucocorticoids	
Angiotensin	

C, complement; GM, granulocyte macrophage; H$_1$, histamine; 5-HT, 5-hydroxytryptamine; Ig, immunoglobulin; IL, interleukin; INF, interferon; LIF, leukocyte migration inhibition factor; LT, leukotriene; MAF, macrophage-activating factor; MFF, macrophage fusion factor; MIF, macrophage inhibitory factor; PAG, platelet-activating factor; PG, prostaglandin; TNF, tumor necrosis factor; VLDL, very-low-density lipoprotein.

Data from Lewis C, McGee JD: *The Macrophage*, 2nd ed. Oxford University Press, New York, 1992; Fogelman AM, Van Lenten BJ, Warden C, et al: Macrophage lipoprotein receptors. *J Cell Sci* Suppl 9:135–149, 1988; Adams DO, Hamilton TA: Phagocytic cells: *Cytotoxic activities of macrophages, in Inflammation: Basic Principles and Clinical Correlates*, 2nd ed., edited by Gallin JI, Snyderman R, p 471. Raven Press, New York, 1992; Werb Z, Goldstein I: *Phagocytic cells: Chemotactic and effector functions of macrophages and granulocytes, in Basic and Clinical Immunology*, 7th ed., edited by Stites D, Terr A, p 96. Appleton and Lange, Norwalk, CT, 1991; Papadimitriou JM, Ashman RB: Macrophages: Current views on their differentiation, structure, and function. *Ultrastruct Pathol* 13:343–372, 1989; Gordon S, Perry VH, Rabinowitz S, et al: Plasma membrane receptors of the mononuclear phagocyte system. *J Cell Sci Suppl* 9:1–26, 1988; Law SK: C3 receptors on macrophages. *J Cell Sci* Suppl 9:67–97, 1988. Hume DA, Ross IL, Himes SR, et al: The mononuclear phagocyte system revisited. *J Leukoc Biol* 72:621–627, 2002.

To illustrate the dynamic interaction of macrophages and virus, a video showing an HIV-1 infected human macrophage sensing its environment was captured from a spinning disk confocal microscope using a 100× objective by Raphael Gaudin (see http://www.cellimagelibrary.org/images/41568#.VAR6eNcDfRo.email).

FUNCTION

Monocytes respond to activating signals, for example, chemokines, through chemokine receptors, setting in motion a series of adhesion and migration events associated with diapedesis.[88] They play a direct role in sepsis and in more poorly defined changes associated with intravascular coagulation and platelet activation. Their phagocytic potential is mainly expressed after adherence to the vascular endothelium. Monocytes are relatively resistant to virus infection, compared with more differentiated macrophages. These cells selectively adhere to lipid- and platelet-activated endothelium, a precursor to atherogenesis.[89] Although metabolic, microbial, or environmental stimuli are normally required to induce monocyte activation, once activated monocytes express a greater potential for cytotoxicity and antimicrobial functions than resident tissue macrophages.

Figure 67–11 schematically shows select surface receptors related to monocyte function. These include chemokine recognition, adhesion, and immunoregulatory molecules. Receptors involved in microbial recognition and innate immunity (e.g., cluster of differentiation [CD]14),[90] phagocytosis (e.g., FcR, CR), secretory, and killing mechanisms are described, as are cytokine production and responses. Intracellular granule contents of monocytes include myeloperoxidase (MPO) and lysozyme, although these are less studied than in neutrophils.

MOTILITY OF MONOCYTES AND MACROPHAGES

An effective monocyte response to infection is predicated upon the ability to migrate and accumulate at sites of inflammation and infection. Monocytes are capable of both random and directed movement. Random migration is nondirected movement that occurs in the absence of attracting substances. Directed movement, as a result of chemotaxis, refers to monocyte migration that occurs in response to soluble factors or stimuli and that is mediated by different types of receptors on phagocyte cell surfaces. A number of different methods have been used to study macrophage movement both *in vivo*[91] and *in vitro*.[92]

Monocytes and macrophages are unusual among hematopoietic cells in that they are motile (ameboid type), migratory, yet capable of sessile, "fixed" life in tissues as resident and more newly recruited cells. Although not as motile as neutrophils, and more difficult to study in physiologically relevant assays *in vitro*, they display lineage-specific, as well as shared, yet distinct properties with DCs, which can be considered as more motile, less-adherent cells specialized for antigen capture and delivery to naïve and primed lymphocytes.[93] They also share receptors and cytoskeletal properties with fibroblasts. Apart from diapedesis in response to endothelial and extravascular signals, monocytes and their progeny display polarization and specialized adhesion structures, most evident in the tight seal of osteoclasts to bone surfaces, so as to localize secretion of powerful catabolic products.

Adhesion is a defining event in the differentiation of monocytes, profoundly influencing the organization of the cell, its plasma membrane, cytoplasm, and nuclear transcription machinery, as well as regulating posttranslational modification of the proteome. Monocytes express diverse integrins, implicated in outside-in as well as inside-out signaling.[94] Particularly important are the β_2-integrin heterodimers, restricted to myeloid cells, as opposed to β_1 and β_3 integrins shared with mesenchymal and other cells. The β_2 integrins, lymphocyte function–associated antigen (LFA)-1 (CD11a/CD18), CR3 (CD11b/CD18), and CD11c/CD18, have been of great value in studies of monocyte/macrophage adhesion. Inhibitory and stimulatory monoclonal antibodies have been generated, and rare inborn errors of metabolism, such as the leukocyte adhesion deficiency syndrome, caused by a genetic deficiency of the common β_2 chain, result in defective myeloid cell recruitment to inflammatory stimuli.

The well-known sequence paradigm of rolling (mediated by L-selectin), more stable adhesion (mediated by β_2 integrins), and diapedesis has been extensively studied in neutrophils (Chap. 19), and is thought to be similar for monocyte recruitment in response to chemokines, as described in Chap. 68. Monocyte-specific and constitutive migration through different tissue compartments (marrow, blood, tissues) are still poorly understood. An unresolved question is whether circulating monocytes are already "bar coded" for entry to special tissues, such as the CNS, or whether cells enter tissues stochastically from blood.

The control of monocyte motility in relation to chemotaxis continues to be studied.[95] In particular, the energetics and role of mitochondria in aerobic and hypoxic conditions deserve further study. Mitochondria are prominent in DCs and play a wider role than anticipated in innate

resistance to viral infection and in cytosolic stress. Several well-known G-protein–coupled receptors (GPCRs), including the array of selective, shared, even redundant chemokine receptors, β-adrenergic receptors, and others contribute to the regulation of directed migration and other cellular functions (Table 67–5).[96,97] In addition, a newly defined family of GPCR with large extracellular domains, includes myeloid-restricted members of the epidermal growth factor–seven transmembrane (EGF-TM7) subfamily with multiple EGF (epidermal growth factor) repeats. EMR2 (epidermal growth factor–like module containing mucin-like hormone receptor–like 2) and CD97, structurally related to the F4/80 antigen marker discussed in Chap. 68, likely support additional important monocyte functions.[97] Their ligands include complement regulatory molecules (CD55, associated with paroxysmal nocturnal hemoglobinuria; Chap. 40) and chondroitin sulphate B, a matrix component. EMR2 expression on myeloid cells is upregulated by septic shock, its ligation on neutrophils potentiates a range of cellular responses.

The roles of phosphoinositide metabolism, diacylglycerol generation, calcium fluxes, and phosphorylation/dephosphorylation in regulating actin assembly have been studied in human and mouse cells, using mainly neutrophils as a prototype.[95] Genetic models of value for macrophage studies include src kinase knockout animals and the Wiskott-Aldrich syndrome. Small guanosine triphosphatases (GTPases; rac, rho, cdc42) have been implicated in diverse myeloid functions, including cell spreading and membrane ruffling. Specialized adhesion structures that deserve further study in macrophages include focal adhesion, podocyte formation (particularly prominent in osteoclasts) and possible participation in tight junctions; hemiconnexons have been reported in macrophages in marrow stroma. CR3 contributes to divalent cation-dependent adhesion of monocytes and macrophages to artificial, serum-coated substrates, such as bacteriologic plastic and the class A SR and MARCO (see "Non–Toll-Like, Nonopsonic Receptors" above), which mediate divalent cation-independent adhesion to serum-coated tissue culture plastic *in vitro*. However, the basis of the remarkable, even unique, protease-resistant adhesion of macrophages to foreign materials remains mysterious. Improved imaging studies, combined with genetic manipulations, will bring further insights into the regulation of monocyte/macrophage adhesion and migration *in vivo*.

INTERACTION WITH COAGULATION CASCADE

Monocytes and resident macrophages line the sinusoids of liver (Kupffer cells) and spleen and readily recognize activated platelets, binding them for clearance and destruction. In addition, monocytes produce potent procoagulants, such as tissue factor, initiating a clotting cascade which, if dysregulated, can lead to diffuse intravascular coagulation during septic shock. Following injury and inflammation, monocytes/macrophages produce urokinase, to generate plasmin, in concert with endothelial cell-derived tissue plasminogen activator.[98] Macrophage production of urokinase is regulated by phagocytic and other stimuli, and the active enzyme can bind to receptors (urokinase plasminogen activator receptor) on the cell surface in a complex interaction with protease–antiprotease complexes, thus localizing fibrinolysis, which is important in wound repair.

The nature and source of the lipid tissue factor produced by monocytes is not well characterized. The cells also produce a complex mix of lipid metabolites, consisting of labile prostaglandins, leukotrienes, and thromboxanes, by utilization of arachidonate-derived precursors and substrates for phospholipase and cyclooxygenase-processing enzymes, among others.

TABLE 67–5. Selected G-Protein–Coupled Receptors Implicated in Functions of Monocytes and Macrophages

Chemotaxis	Adhesion/Cell–Cell Contact	Activation and Resolution of Inflammation	Alternative Activation	Survival
Chemokine receptors	EGF-TM7 receptors	BAI-1	Purinergic receptors GPR86, GPR105, P2Y8, P2Y11, and P2Y12	Sphingosine-1-phosphate receptors
C5a receptor	Sphingosine-1-phosphate receptors			
Leukotriene B_4 receptor		Formyl peptide receptors	Chemokine receptors	
Formyl peptide receptors	CX_3CR1	Chemokine receptors		
Platelet-activating factor receptor		C5a receptor		
		EMR2		
EMR2		Protease-activated receptors		
Neuropeptide Y receptor		Platelet-activating factor receptor		
		Leukotriene B_4 receptor		
		Neurokinin receptors		
		Neuropeptide Y receptor		
		Vasoactive intestine peptide receptor		
		Prostaglandin receptors		
		Resolvin		

BAI-1, brain-specific angiogenesis inhibitor 1; EGF-TM7, epidermal growth factor–seven transmembrane; EMR2, epidermal growth factor–like module containing mucin-like hormone receptor–like 2.

Data from Lattin, J.E. et al.: Expression analysis of G Protein-Coupled Receptors in mouse macrophages. *Immunome Res* 4:5, 2008; Yona, S., Lin, H.H., Siu, W.O., Gordon, S. & Stacey, M.: Adhesion-GPCRs: emerging roles for novel receptors. *Trends Biochem Sci* 33:491-500, 2008; Lattin, J. et al.: G-protein-coupled receptor expression, function, and signaling in macrophages. *J Leukoc Biol* 82:16–32, 2007.

RECOGNITION AND CLEARANCE OVERVIEW

Resident macrophages of the liver and marrow, as well as in lung and other nonhematopoietic tissues, play a major role in the recognition, phagocytosis, and endocytosis of foreign particles and macromolecules, as well as of modified host components. Clearance can be silent, even suppressing inflammation, mediated by transforming growth factor (TGF)-β generation, as observed after the uptake of apoptotic cells by macrophages.[99] Production of hematopoietic cells is balanced by their programmed senescence and increased destruction, which can be enhanced in response to microbial and other toxic substances. Macrophages initiate and perpetuate inflammation, both acute and chronic, as a result of their biosynthetic and secretory responses to injurious particles. Uptake and vacuole formation sequester the membrane-enclosed contents for digestion and possible antigen processing and presentation, a specialized property of DCs after their further differentiation from active endocytic to APCs.[33] Specialized studies show that blood-derived monocytes have unique functions. For example, in the human disorder multiple sclerosis and the model experimental autoimmune encephalitis, monocyte-derived macrophages initiate demyelination at nodes of Ranvier; whereas, microglia derived from yolk-sac progenitors during embryogenesis are relatively inert at disease onset.[31] To illustrate the role of macrophages in the recognition and clearance of foreign substances, images of macrophage spreading and engulfment of erythrocytes can be visualized by scanning electron microscopy, and the sequence of engulfment by phase-contrast optics (see video talk on macrophage phagocytosis at http://hstalks.com/?t=BL1473311).

In addition, interest has grown explosively in cytosolic recognition systems, designed to protect the cell from various infectious and lytic agents.[100-102] The process of autophagy shares aspects with both membrane-bound and cytoplasmic organelle injury, and has become of great current interest because of its contribution to pathogenesis of infectious, malignant, and inflammatory syndromes.[103]

APOPTOSIS

Macrophages take up large numbers of naturally dying cells, hematopoietic and others, through a complex mechanism involving multiple, often redundant nonopsonic receptors.[47,99] A possible role for complement has also been proposed. Figure 67–12 illustrates receptors and ligands that have been implicated. Apart from the SRs already discussed, they include receptors for opsonins and for milk-fat globulin, as well as for the vitronectin receptor. Phosphatidylserine (PS) expressed on the outer leaflet of apoptotic cells, contributes to apoptotic cell recognition, but its role is probably more complex as apparently healthy cells can express patches of PS on their surface and PS recognition plays a role in CD36-dependent macrophage–macrophage fusion.[104] The recognition

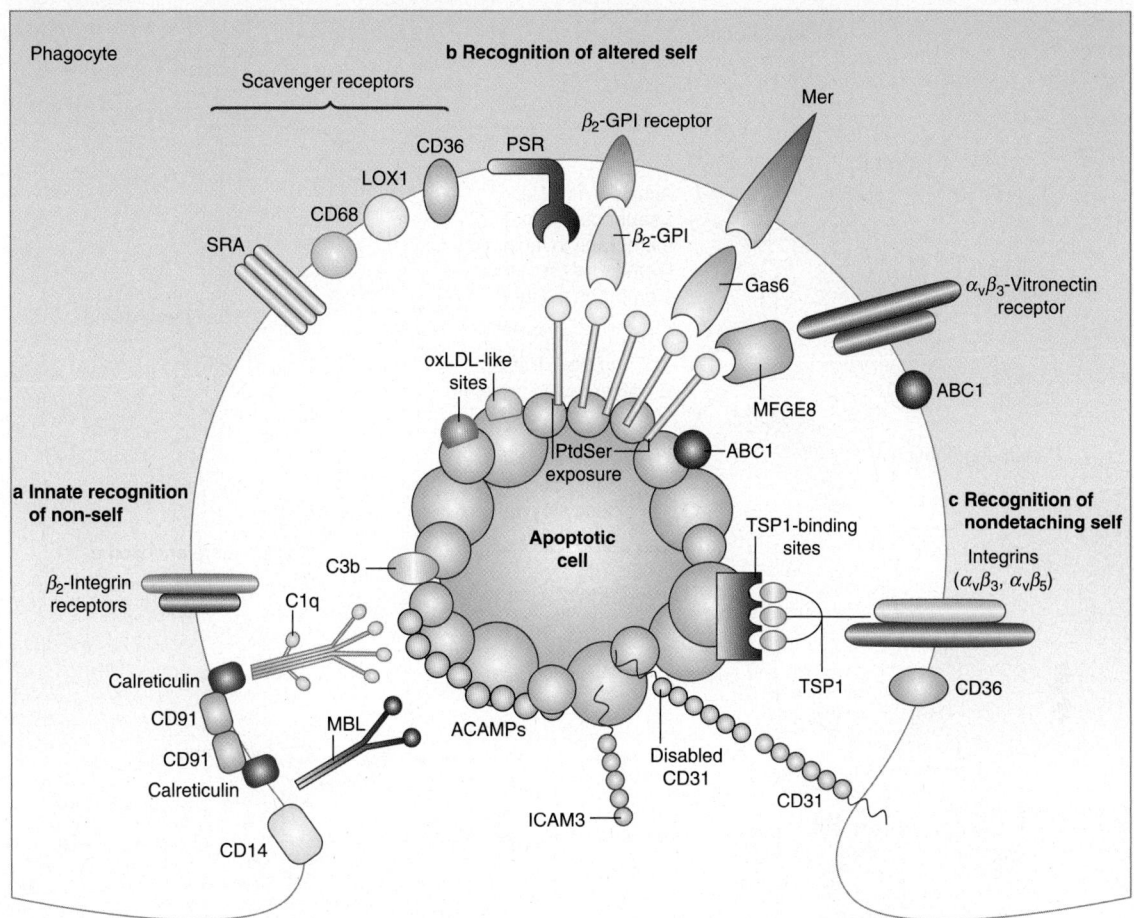

Figure 67–12. Phagocytic receptors for apoptotic cell phagocytosis. Macrophages and immature myeloid dendritic cells (DCs) are the main immune cells involved in the clearance of apoptotic cells. They express broadly similar multiple receptors that can bind directly or via opsonic-soluble proteins, for example, mannose-binding lectins (MBLs) to ligands. Phosphatidylserine (PS) becomes exposed on the outer surface of the apoptotic cell and a receptor for this ligand has been long sought. A new receptor (TIM4, and related TIM1) was discovered on resident mϕ, with specificity for PS. Other mϕ populations utilize MFGE8 (a milk-fat globulin protein secreted by mϕ) as an opsonin. Discrimination of non-self and altered self may involve combinations of different phagocyte receptors. Apoptotic cell uptake results in an antiinflammatory response by mϕ (e.g., release of transforming growth factor [TGF]-β and prostaglandin E$_2$), but has also been implicated in cross-presentation by DCs. For further details see Ref. 47. (*Reproduced with permission of Savill J, Dransfield I, Gregory C, et al: A blast from the past: clearance of apoptotic cells regulates immune responses. Nat Rev Immunol 2002 Dec;2(12):965-975.*)

mechanisms for uptake of necrotic cells and enucleated erythroblast nuclei by macrophages are not clear (Chap. 15).

ENDOCYTOSIS, PHAGOCYTOSIS, AND KILLING

Apart from the above ligands, macrophages express receptors for endocytosis of growth factors, cytokines, peptides, and lipids. Macrophages express a functional folate receptor that is induced during activation and can be used to target drugs or tracers to macrophages *in situ*.[105] Hemoglobin–haptoglobin complexes are internalized by CD163, a glucocorticoid-regulated receptor with a remarkable SR-cysteine extracellular domain structure.[106] CD163 is also upregulated by substance P.[107]

The cell biology of endocytosis and of phagocytosis is illustrated in Figs. 67–13 and 67–14. Apart from size and resultant involvement of the cytoskeleton, they have much in common; vesicle/phagosome formation, falling pH and initial digestion, fusion with secretory vesicles derived from the Golgi, and maturation to form secondary lysosomes/

phagolysosomes with a more acidic pH, and further digestion.[108,109] Apart from selective fusion with intracellular vesicles, there is extensive membrane flow, recycling, and fusion. Small GTPases play an important role in the control of membrane traffic.[110] Early estimates revealed that a substantial fraction of surface membrane is internalized constitutively by endocytosis.

Studies that used opsonic receptors to examine the uptake mechanism of antibody-coated erythrocytes via opsonic receptors gave rise to the zipper hypothesis: local segmental engagement of FcR, and circumferential flow of macrophage pseudopodia around the particle, followed by fusion at the tip, closure, and ingestion. Subsequent studies by several groups documented the role of phosphatidylinositol 3-kinase (PI3K) and phosphoinositides in the initial fusion and subsequent associations between the actin cytoskeleton and cellular membranes.[111] Latex has provided a useful test particle to isolate latex-containing phagolysosomes by flotation. Proteomic analyses[112] demonstrated the protein composition of phagosomes and drew attention to functional constituents in the phagolysosomal membrane.

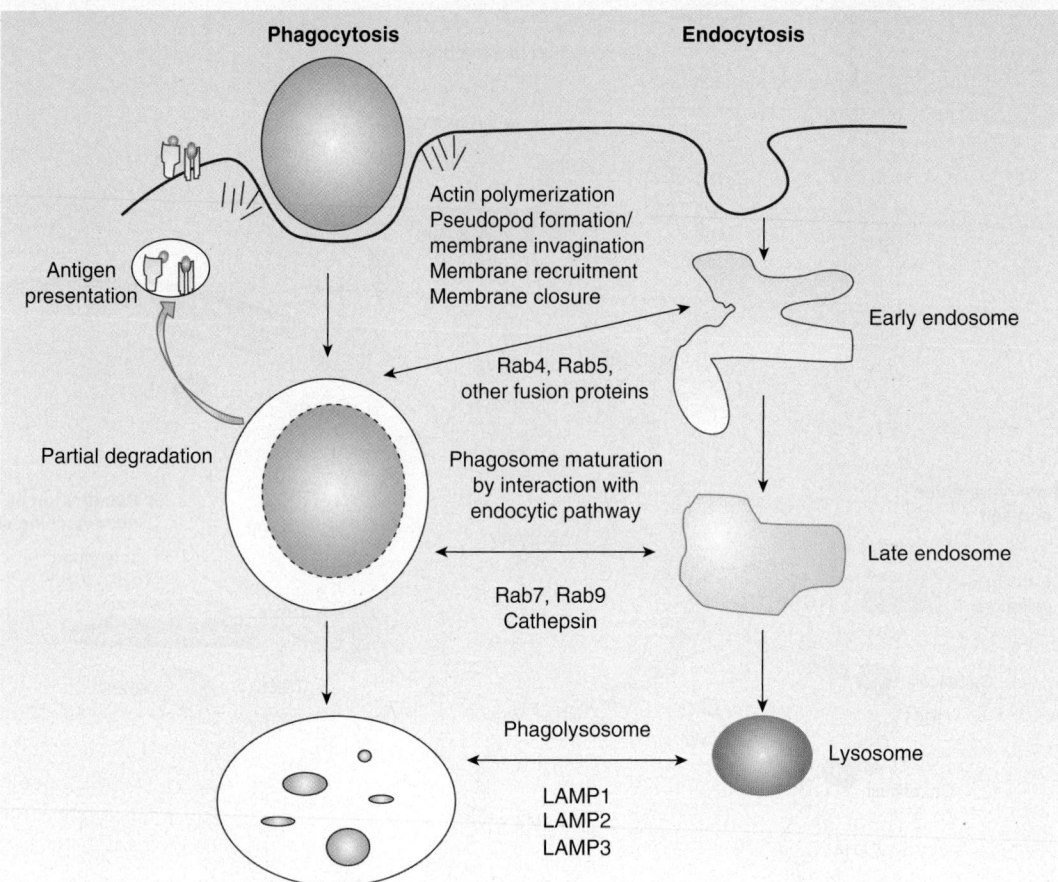

Figure 67–13. Phagocytosis and endocytosis pathways. Particulates are taken up by actin-dependent sequential maturation processes, involving membrane fusion and fission, which intersect with the endocytic pathway at several stages. Cytosolic small guanosine triphosphatases (rabs) determine organelle-specific interactions. Membrane is recycled to the plasma membrane, with processed antigen. Progressive acidification and delivery of lysosomal hydrolases result in terminal degradation. Compartment membranes express marker proteins such as lysosomal-associated membrane protein (LAMP)-1; the pan-macrophage CD68 antigen is associated with late endosomes and lysosomes.

These observations have provided the basis for numerous investigations regarding the interactions of diverse microorganisms with the vacuolar system, which are often necessary for pathogen survival and establishment of intracellular infection (Fig. 67–15). Organisms can inhibit acidification and fusion (*Mycobacterium*),[101,113] multiply within secondary lysosomes (*Leishmania*),[114] escape free into the cytosol (*Listeria*),[115] or translocate their genomes into the cytoplasm by fusion (enveloped viruses); other organisms induce variations on this theme; for example, *Brucella* seeks out the endoplasmic reticulum after entry and *Legionella* can enter macrophages by inducing a phagosome membrane of unusual composition.[116] Nonpathogenic organisms or pathogens taken up via opsonic receptors or after IFN-γ activation undergo a different fate, with killing and destruction.

The zipper mechanism, with tight apposition of membrane to the particle's surface ligands, does not apply to all forms of ingestion. For example, complement opsonized particles seem to sink into the cytoplasm, and other phagosomes can be spacious. A number of key methods of visualization[109] illustrate the dynamic nature of phagocytosis. Figure 67–14 illustrates some of the signaling pathways that control the cytoskeleton.

Macrophages are rich in lysosomal digestive enzymes,[33] activated by a falling pH of approximately 6.5 within the mature vacuole. Unless captured as peptides by MHC molecules, a feature of antigen processing by DCs, macromolecular substrates can be degraded to their constituent amino acids, sugars, or nucleic acid bases. Early studies[117] probed the permeability of the lysosomal vacuolar membrane. If the

content cannot be fully degraded because of its nature (e.g., sucrose), overload (e.g., lipid), or owing to a genetic deficiency in a catabolic enzyme (lysosomal storage diseases), it accumulates within residual lysosomes, altering macrophage gene expression and secretory output, thus mediating chronic inflammation or metabolic forms of modified inflammation, such as atherosclerosis, foam cell formation and Gaucher disease. Figure 67–16A illustrates the uptake of senescent erythrocytes, the breakdown of heme and storage of Fe^{2+}.[118] Figure 67–16B shows how phagocytosis by DCs can bring about processing and cross-presentation of exogenous antigens.[119] By comparison (Fig. 67–16C), autophagy is the envelopment of damaged intracellular organelles and cytoplasm by cytoplasmic membrane, and sequestration within a digestive vacuole, resembling heterophagy (Chap. 15).[116] Its biochemical and cellular basis has become of interest because of its apparent relevance to cancer, infections such as tuberculosis and Legionnaire disease, and inflammatory syndromes such as inflammatory bowel disease (IBD).

Although the phagocytic mechanism has been investigated in depth, we do not understand fully how the process of internalization is controlled. For example, ingestion can be thwarted by attempts to ingest too large a particle or foreign surface, or by close apposition of plasma membrane to noninternalizable immune complexes. This results in redirecting secretory vesicles to the surface, reminiscent of osteoclast adhesion. In other circumstances, as in response to foreign bodies, and especially mycobacteria, and in the presence of

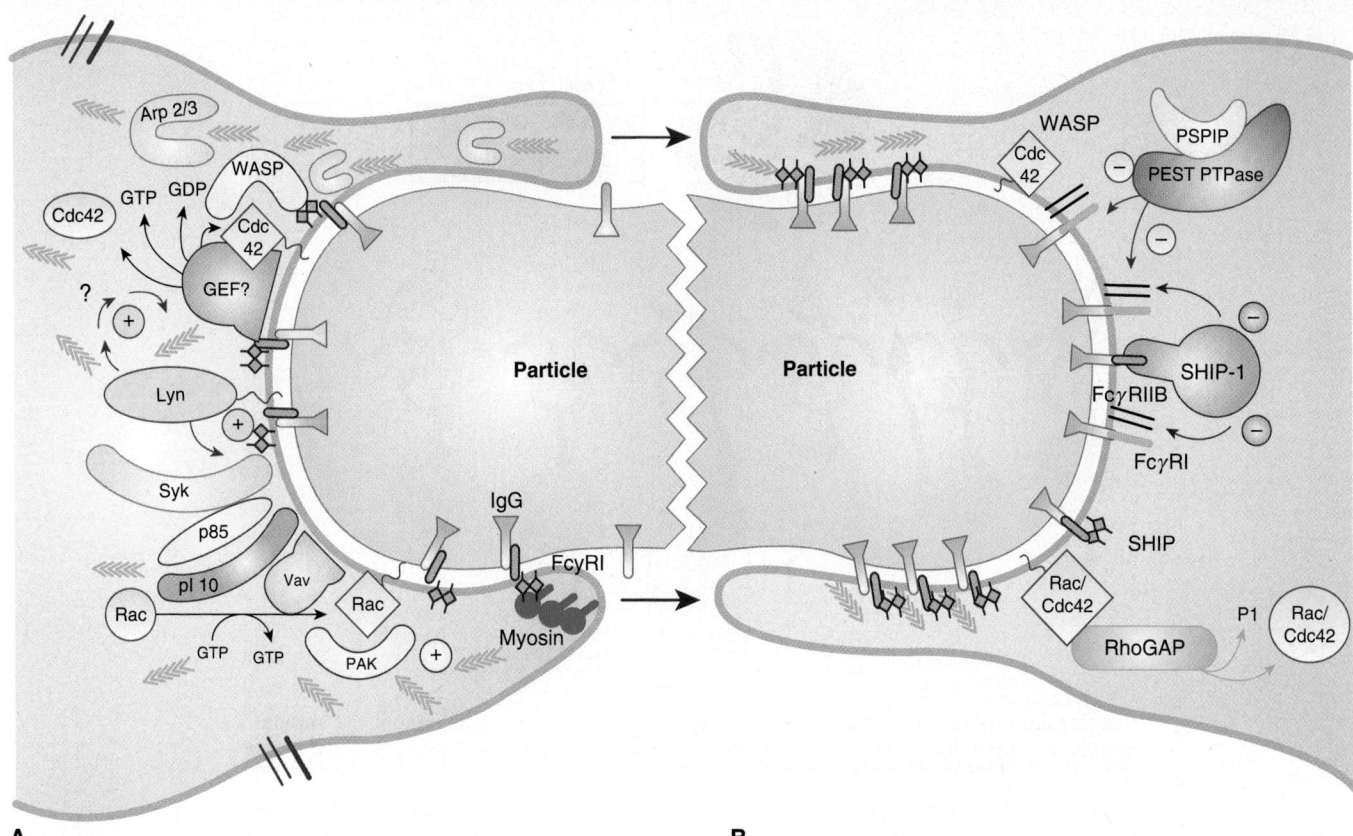

Figure 67-14. A model for FcγR-mediated phagocytosis. **A.** Signaling upstream and downstream of Rho guanosine triphosphatases during FcγR-mediated phagocytosis. Immunoglobulin (Ig) G bound to antigen on the particle binds to FcγRI receptors at the surface of the mφ and induces their aggregation (shown in *red*). This activates a Src family tyrosine kinase (probably Lyn). Lyn phosphorylates the receptor γ chain (phosphotyrosine residues in the γ chains are depicted as *red diamonds*) and Syk. Syk is activated and recruited to the phosphotyrosine residues of the γ chain through its two SH2 (Src homology 2) domains. Cdc42 activation by an unknown guanine–nucleotide exchange factor (GEF) allows the recruitment of WASP (Wiskott-Aldrich syndrome protein). In turn, WASP activates the Arp2/3 complex that triggers actin polymerization to generate the protrusive force for pseudopod extension *(red arrowheads)*. Activation of a Rac1 GEF, possibly Vav, by tyrosine phosphorylation in conjunction with PI3 kinase products (PIP$_3$) promotes GDP/GTP (guanosine diphosphate/guanosine triphosphate) exchange on Rac1. GTP-bound Rac1 interacts with and activates the serine/threonine kinase Pak1, which may induce the actinomyosin contractility involved in phagosome closure. **B.** In the next step, FcγRI is rapidly down-modulated and returned to an inactive state (shown in *blue*), resulting in actin filament disassembly. According to this model, actin assembly proceeds as a wave at the distal rim of the pseudopodia, while actin depolymerization occurs rearward. Polyphosphoinositide phosphatases such as the SH2 domain-containing SHIP, which selectively hydrolyze PIP$_3$, may contribute to down-modulation. Modulation of FcγRI activation may also involve tyrosine phosphatases such as SHP-1, which associates with FcγRIIb, a member of the FcγR family that may be coligated with FcγRI. In addition, PEST family phosphotyrosine phosphatases (PTPases) may contribute to dephosphorylation by interacting with PSPIP, a cytoskeletal protein that interacts with WASP. GAPs may also contribute to down-modulation by returning Cdc42/Rac1 to the inactive, GDP-bound state. Eventually, cytoskeletal proteins are shed from the ingestion site to leave the phagosome free in the cytosol (not shown here). *(Reproduced with permission from Chimini G, Chavrier P: Function of Rho family proteins in actin dynamics during phagocytosis and engulfment. Nat Cell Biol 2000 Oct;2(10):E191-E196.)*

the Th2 cytokines IL-4 and/or IL-13, individual macrophages can fuse to form giant cells, with a common cytoplasm and multinucleation. Several fusogenic surface molecules have been identified and DNAX-activating protein (DAP) 12 expression and signaling is important in generating a fusogenic differentiation phenotype in macrophages.[120]

INFLAMMASOME

The recognition of the multiprotein inflammasome complex[101] has stimulated intense interest in the recognition by cytosolic proteins of foreign nucleic acid, uric acid-induced injury, and breakdown products of microbial walls, for example, muramyl dipeptide. More complex peptidoglycan structures can also be recognized

by surface receptors in *Drosophila*. Several reviews chart the rapid growth in our knowledge of inflammasome function in health and disease.[100,102,121,122] Figure 67-17 illustrates selected nucleotide-binding oligomerization domain (NOD)-like and related receptors (NLRs) with nucleotide oligomerization and other characteristic domains. Mutations in NLR have been implicated in IBD, in periodic familial Mediterranean fever, and in a range of autohyperinflammatory syndromes.[123] More specifically, NOD-2 has been implicated in Crohn disease.[124,125] Excessive caspase activation and IL-1β release can be countered therapeutically with IL-1 receptor antagonists. Figure 67-18 illustrates the role of inflammasome activation in intracellular infection. Antiviral production of IFN-α and -β involves retinoid-inducible gene (RIG)-I–like helicases, indicating a role for mitochondria in cytosolic sensing.

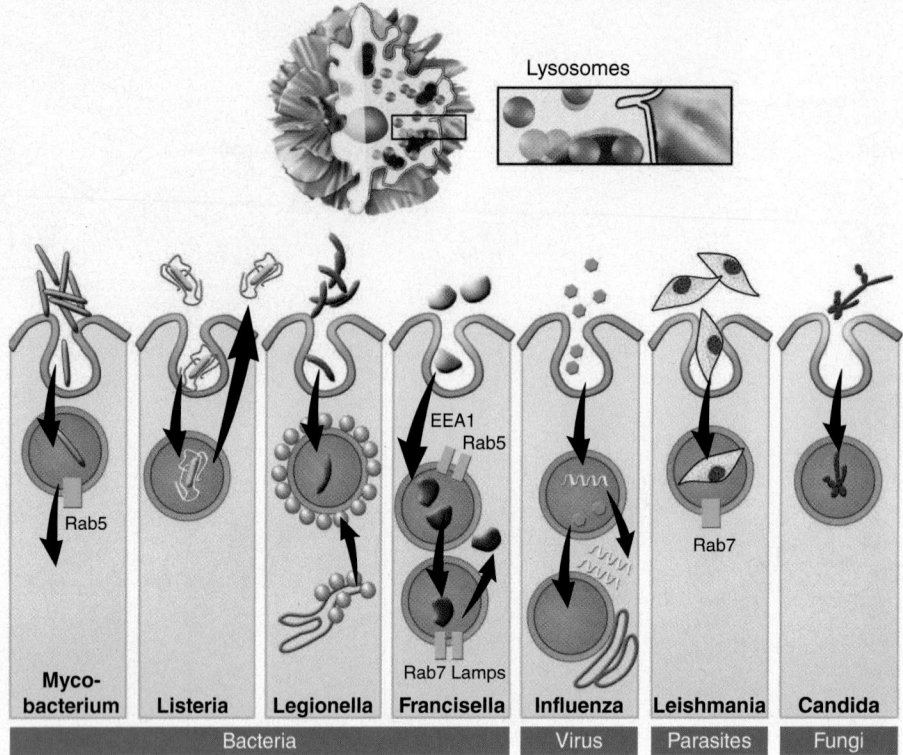

Figure 67–15. Selected pathogens evade distinct phagocytic mechanisms. Pathogens have developed several mechanisms to enter and survive inside macrophages. *Legionella pneumophila* resides and multiplies in a vacuole studded with ribosomes as a result of interaction with the rough endoplasmic reticulum. The organism secretes effector molecules via its type IV secretion system into the cell, which inhibit phagosome/lysosome fusion. The *Francisella tularensis* phagosome acquires the early endosome markers EEA1 and Rab5 and then matures into a late endosome defined by the presence of the markers Lamp1, Lamp2, and Rab7. The late endosome does not acidify and the phagosomal membrane is disrupted, releasing the bacteria into the cytosol. The *Mycobacterium tuberculosis* phagosome acquires the early endosome marker Rab5 but excludes the late endosomal Lamps and Rab7. This organism also produces molecules that block fusion with the lysosome and resides and replicates in this early endosome. Acidification of the *Listeria monocytogenes* phagosome is essential for the perforation of the phagosomal membrane and escape of the bacteria into the cytosol. Here they mobilize the actin polymerization machinery to move within the cell and then from cell to cell. *Candida albicans* undergoes a conversion from a unicellular form to a multicellular hyphal form, which allows this fungus to escape the macrophage. The *Leishmania mexicana* phagosome develops into an acidic phagolysosome containing Rab7 where the parasite is able to survive and replicate. Viruses such as the influenza virus are able to inhibit the activation of antiviral mechanisms, such as the activation of IFN regulatory function proteins that induce IFN production upon viral infection, and enter the nucleus. Cytomegalovirus (not shown) incapacitates a range of major histocompatibility complex-antigen presenting pathways. *(Used with permission of S. Seif, GraphisMedica, 2014.)*

GENE EXPRESSION, SYNTHESIS, AND SECRETION

The development of microarray technology has had a dramatic impact on the analysis of macrophage gene expression in response to a wide range of stimuli, including microbial ligands, cytokines, and immunomodulators. Macrophages are able to express a large number of genes and are extremely versatile in their responses to environmental cues. It has been possible to discern signatures of particular agonists, for example, IFN-α and -β and IL-4, but many caveats remain in the interpretation of such data. Heterogeneity of cellular origin, differentiation stage, and populations from diverse origins, as well as substantial species differences, make it difficult to compare results within and among experiments. Validation of more quantitative messenger RNA analysis of protein synthesis and modification is difficult, although proteomic analysis is gaining ground. The study of macrophage chromatin organization in relation to gene expression is in its infancy.

There is extensive crosstalk between the secretory and endocytic pathways.[126] Table 67–6 is a selected list of secretory products. This includes lysozyme, a major myelomonocytic product that is

constitutively expressed *in vitro*, but upregulated in granulomata *in vivo*. The secretion pathway of lysozyme in monocytes and macrophages has not been defined. The well-known pro- and antiinflammatory cytokines are better characterized, both in terms of regulation and the secretion pathway.[109] The response to IL-6 and TNF-α secretion in model systems shows a more complex pathway than previously recognized.[127,128] In addition to these and other important growth and differentiation factors that regulate angiogenesis, for example, macrophages are able to produce and secrete enzymes and proenzymes for a range of activities, as well as their inhibitors, for example, proteinases and antiproteinases. Although the amounts of complement proteins produced, for example, are relatively small, they can be significantly concentrated in a local microenvironment. In addition, macrophages can produce a range of antimicrobial peptides and lytic agents, but their most important killing mechanisms depend on oxygen[129] and nitrogen metabolites,[109,114] which are illustrated in Figs. 67–19 and 67–20. Regulation of the nicotinamide adenine dinucleotide phosphate oxidase and of inducible nitric oxide synthase has been studied extensively in mice and humans through biochemical and genetic approaches. Apart from their antimicrobial activity, nitrogen metabolites contribute to signaling pathways.[130] IFN-α and -β play

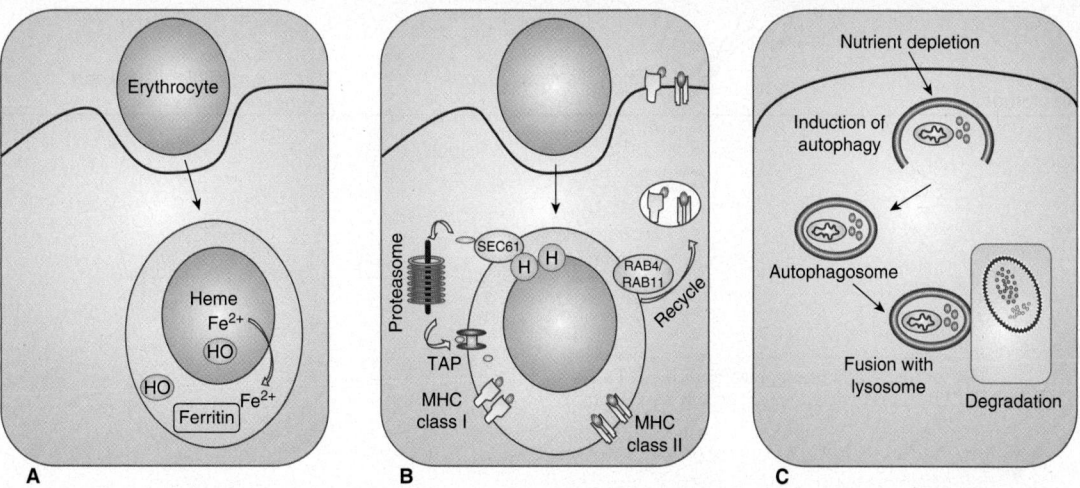

Figure 67–16. A. Macrophages have an important role in iron metabolism by processing effete erythrocytes, internalized by phagocytosis, and returning iron to the blood (through ferritin) for reuse. Dissociation of iron linked to heme on erythrocytes requires the action of heme oxygenase (HO), an enzyme present in the endoplasmic reticulum (ER). The process allowing the transfer of heme oxygenase from the ER to the phagosome lumen is so far unknown. **B.** Presentation of antigens from intracellular pathogens is mainly carried out by major histocompatibility complex (MHC) class II molecules loaded in phagosomes. Presentation of some pathogen antigens could also involve MHC class I molecules. Current models indicate that antigens generated by hydrolases in the phagosome lumen could use SEC61 for translocation to the cytoplasm. After processing by the proteasome, antigens could be translocated to the phagosome lumen through the transporter for antigen processing (TAP) complex where loading onto MHC class I or MHC class II molecules would occur. Transport to the cell surface from the phagosome lumen could take place by using the existing membrane recycling machinery, involving the small guanosine triphosphatases Rab4 and Rab11. **C.** Autophagy is a conserved membrane traffic pathway that equips eukaryotic cells to capture cytoplasmic components within a double-membrane vacuole, or autophagosome, for delivery to lysosomes. Although best known as a mechanism to survive starvation, autophagy is now recognized as a mechanism to combat infection by a variety of intracellular microbes.

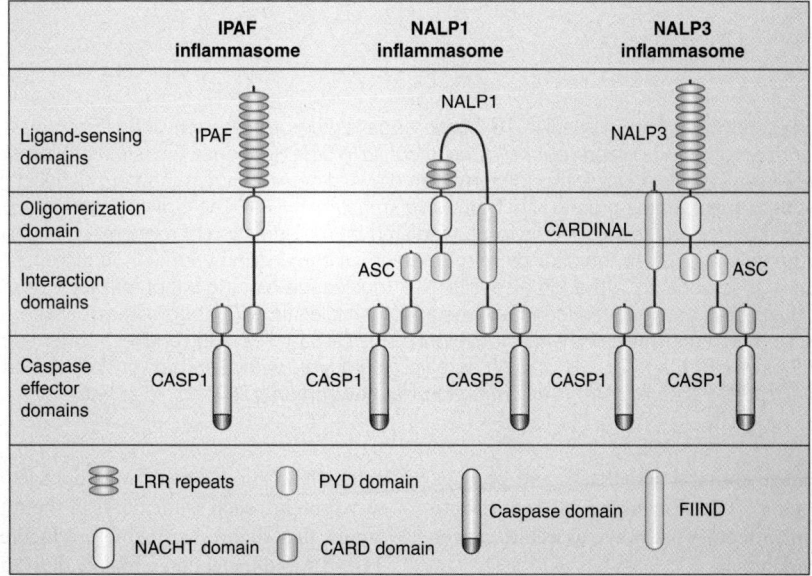

Figure 67–17. Nucleotide-binding and oligomerization domain (NOD)–leucine-rich repeat (LRR) and inflammasome structures. NOD-like receptors (NLRs) have three structural domains: The LRR domain at the C-terminus, the NACHT (domain present in NAIP, CIITA, AHD, HET-E, TP-1) domain, and the N-terminal domain that can be a pyrin domain (PYD), a caspase activation and recruitment domain (CARD), or a baculovirus inhibitor-of-apoptosis protein repeat domain (BIR). The LRR domain is considered as the ligand-sensing motif, thus involved in the interaction with pathogen-associated molecular patterns (PAMPs), in analogy to toll-like receptors (TLRs). The NACHT domain is responsible for the oligomerization and activation of NLRs. The PYD or CARD domain of NLR is the link to downstream adaptors (such as apoptosis-associated speck-like protein containing a CARD [ASC]) or effectors (such as caspase-1). The BIR domain is proposed to act as caspase inhibitor. During NACHT LRR protein (NALP) and NALP1 inflammasome activation, NALP3 or NALP1 interact through PYD–PYD homotypic interactions with ASC, resulting in its activation. Subsequently, the CARD domain of ASC interacts with the CARD domain of caspase-1 and mediates its activation. NALP1 may also activate directly the caspase-5 through its C-terminal CARD domain. In contrast, NALP3 does not simultaneously activate caspase-5, but NALP3 can recruit a second capsase-1 through the CARD domain of CARD inhibitor of nuclear factor-κB–activating ligand (CARDINAL), a component of the NALP3 inflammasome. Interleukin-1β–converting enzyme (ICE)-protease activating factor (IPAF), that can on its own sense PAMPs, possesses a CARD domain at the N-terminal and thus may directly activate caspase-1 without ASC recruitment ("IPAF inflammasome"). *(Reproduced with permission of Sidiropoulos PI, Goulielmos G, Voloudakis GK, et al: Inflammasomes and rheumatic diseases: evolving concepts. Ann Rheum Dis 2008 Oct;67(10):1382-1389.)*

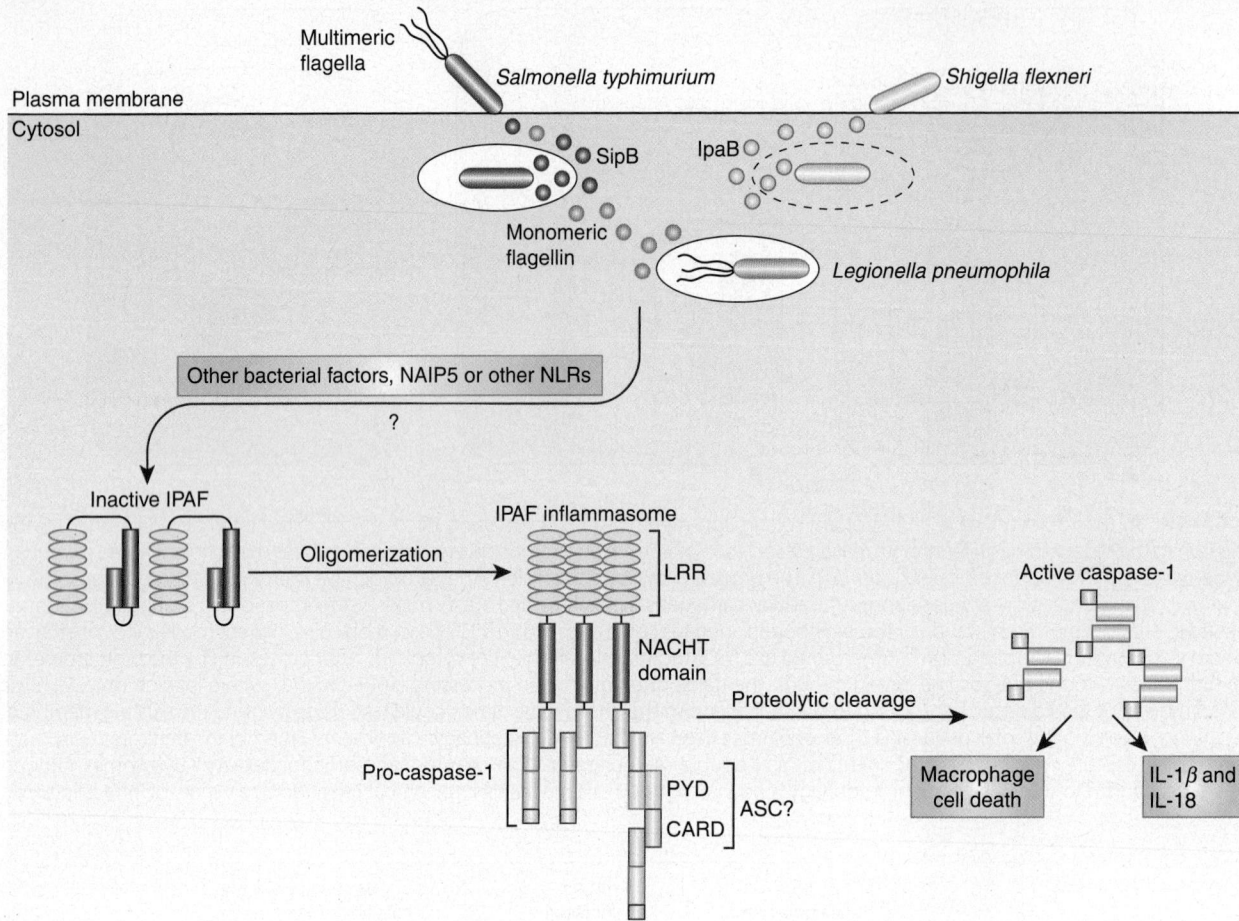

Figure 67–18. Knockout studies show that IPAF (interleukin-1β–converting enzyme-protease activating factor) is essential for the activation of caspase-1 by *Salmonella typhimurium*, *Shigella flexneri*, and *Legionella pneumophila* in order to induce the release of interleukin (IL)-1β, IL-18, and macrophage cell death. Sensing intracellular *S. typhimurium* seems to be mediated by the detection of monomeric flagellin that is secreted by the bacterial type III secretion system (and is dependent on the protein SipB from *S. typhimurium*) by IPAF. The type III secretion system protein IpaB is involved in sensing *S. flexneri*. Sensing intracellular *L. pneumophila* seems to be mediated by the detection of monomeric flagellin that is secreted by the type IV secretion system by NAIP5 (neuronal apoptosis inhibitor protein 5), which, in conjunction with IPAF, induces caspase-1 activation and restricts the growth of these pathogens in macrophages. Although a specific NLR (nucleotide-binding oligomerization domain-like receptor) protein that detects cytosolic *Francisella tularensis* has not yet been identified, the adaptor molecule ASC (apoptosis-associated speck-like protein containing a CARD) seems to be essential for counteracting infections with *F. tularensis*. CARD, caspase activation and recruitment domain; LRR, leucine-rich repeat; NACHT, domain present in NAIP, CIITA, HET-E, and TP-1; PYD, pyrin domain. *(Reproduced with permission of Mariathasan S, Monack DM: Inflammasome adaptors and sensors: intracellular regulators of infection and inflammation.* Nat Rev Immunol 2007 Jan;7(1):31-40.)

an important role in macrophage antiviral activities[131] and perhaps in the cellular response to bacteria.[132] These cytokines also contribute significantly to immune and inflammatory pathways, as well as cancer immunoediting[133] and autoimmunity.[134]

Macrophages may be able to produce IFN-γ, for example, under particular circumstances, but *in vivo* most of the cytokine derives from other sources. IFN-γ has a major impact on macrophage function (the initial name of IFN-γ was macrophage activating factor), including priming of biosynthetic and functional responses associated with cytotoxicity and inflammation in cell-mediated immunity (Fig. 67–21).[135] Table 67–7 summarizes the markers and functions associated with various forms of macrophage activation and deactivation, as described in Chap. 68.[136] Intracellular GTPases have been implicated in cell activation by IFN-γ, for example, and in relation to IBD.[121,124,125] Similarly, the Th2 cytokines IL-4 and IL-13 induce characteristic changes in macrophage phenotype, which are associated with an alternative activation pathway. The cellular biology of alternatively activated macrophages is modified

extensively (Fig. 67–22).[137] Macrophages also express a range of inhibitory proteins, such as members of the suppressor of cytokine signaling family, that suppress cytokine production, in addition to IL-10[138] and TGF-β. Lipid metabolites, mainly derived from arachidonate and other lipid precursors, provide another potent source of inflammatory and immunomodulatory products.[139] The suppressive functions of monocytes and macrophages in chronic infections and experimental tumors require further study, including the development of new phenotypic markers in mice and humans.

CELLULAR INTERACTIONS

In addition to cytokine and other soluble afferent and efferent responses, macrophages are able to directly interact among themselves, with all other cell types in the body, both viable and injured, as well as with all kinds of microorganisms. Their interactions are reciprocal and regulated, contributing to homeostasis and to pathogenesis, both

TABLE 67–6. Selected Secretion Products of Macrophages

Proteins	Product	Comment
Enzymes	Lysozyme	Bulk product
	Urokinase-type plasminogen activator	Regulated by inflammation
	Collagenase	Regulated by inflammation
	Elastase	Regulated by inflammation
	Metalloproteinases	Also inhibitors
	Complement	All components and regulators
	Arginase	Alternative activation
	Angiotensin-converting enzyme	Induced glucocorticoids, granulomas
	Chitotriosidase	Gaucher disease, lysosomal storage
Inhibitors	Acid hydrolases	All classes (mainly intracellular)
	TIMP	
Chemokines	Many C-C, C-X-C, CX_3C; e.g., MCP, RANTES, IL-8	Initiates acute and chronic recruitment of myeloid and lymphoid cells
Cytokines	IL-1β, TNF-α	Pro- and antiinflammatory
	IL-6, IL-10, IL-12, IL-17, IL-18, IL-23	Also antagonists, e.g., IL-1Ra
	Type I IFN	Autocrine and paracrine amplification
Apolipoproteins	Apolipoprotein E	Local source, marrow origin after adoptive transfer
Growth/differentiation factors	TGF-β	Also other family members (activins), myeloid growth and differentiation
	M-CSF	
	GM-CSF	
	FGF	Fibrosis
	PDGF	Repair
	VEGF	Angiogenesis
Opsonins	Fibronectin, pentraxin (PTX3)	Also uncharacterized receptor on Mϕ
Soluble receptors	Mannose receptor	Soluble mannose receptor
Cationic peptides	Defensins	Subpopulations and species variation
Lipids	Procoagulant	Initiation clotting
	Arachidonate metabolites:	Pro- and antiinflammatory mediators
	Prostaglandins	
	Leukotrienes	
	Thromboxanes	
	Resolvins	
Metabolites	Reactive oxygen intermediates	
	Reactive nitrogen intermediates	
	Haem breakdown (bile pigments)	
	Iron, B_{12}-binding protein	
	Vitamin D metabolites	

FGF, fibroblast growth factor; GM-CSF, granulocyte-macrophage colony-stimulating factor; IFN, interferon; IL, interleukin; MCP, monocyte chemotactic protein; M-CSF, macrophage colony-stimulating factor; PDGF, platelet-derived growth factor; RANTES, regulated on activation, normal T-cell expressed, presumed secreted; TGF, transforming growth factor; TIMP, tissue inhibitor of metalloproteinase; TNF, tumor necrosis factor; VEGF, vascular endothelial growth factor.

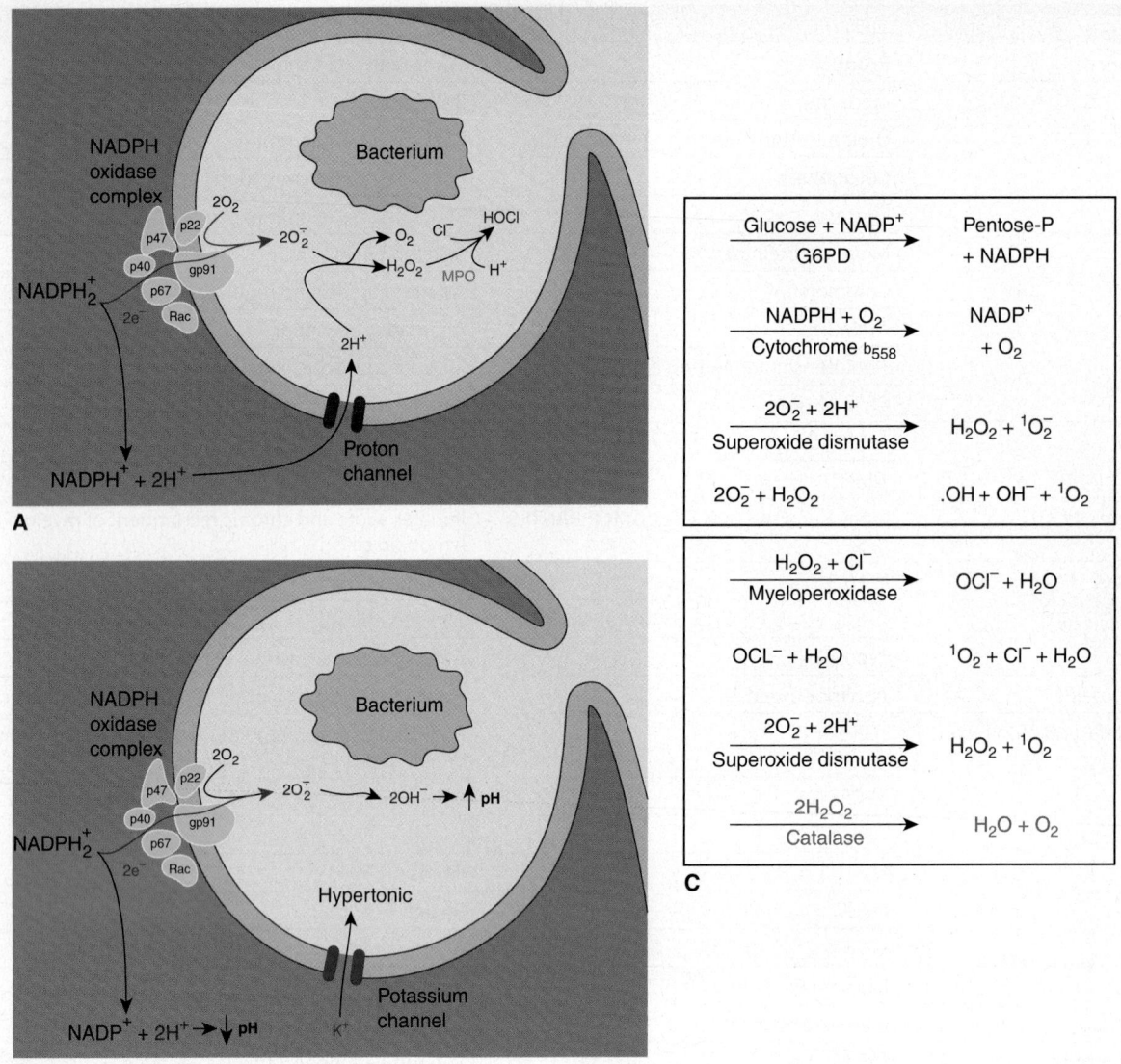

The reactions shown in the figure include:

$$\frac{\text{Glucose} + \text{NADP}^+}{\text{G6PD}} \longrightarrow \text{Pentose-P} + \text{NADPH}$$

$$\frac{\text{NADPH} + \text{O}_2}{\text{Cytochrome } b_{558}} \longrightarrow \text{NADP}^+ + \text{O}_2$$

$$\frac{2\text{O}_2^- + 2\text{H}^+}{\text{Superoxide dismutase}} \longrightarrow \text{H}_2\text{O}_2 + {}^1\text{O}_2^-$$

$$2\text{O}_2^- + \text{H}_2\text{O}_2 \quad .\text{OH} + \text{OH}^- + {}^1\text{O}_2$$

$$\frac{\text{H}_2\text{O}_2 + \text{Cl}^-}{\text{Myeloperoxidase}} \longrightarrow \text{OCl}^- + \text{H}_2\text{O}$$

$$\text{OCL}^- + \text{H}_2\text{O} \quad {}^1\text{O}_2 + \text{Cl}^- + \text{H}_2\text{O}$$

$$\frac{2\text{O}_2^- + 2\text{H}^+}{\text{Superoxide dismutase}} \longrightarrow \text{H}_2\text{O}_2 + {}^1\text{O}_2$$

$$\frac{2\text{H}_2\text{O}_2}{\text{Catalase}} \longrightarrow \text{H}_2\text{O} + \text{O}_2$$

Figure 67–19. The respiratory burst in a phagocyte is triggered when a bacterium is phagocytosed. During the phagocytosis of bacteria by macrophages and neutrophils, the phagosome membrane pinches off and the microbe is endocytosed along with a small volume of extracellular fluid. The mechanisms discussed here are based on studies in neutrophils and are still controversial.[112] Electrons are removed from nicotinamide adenine dinucleotide phosphate (NADPH) in the cytoplasm and transferred through the gp91*phox* component (which includes flavin adenine dinucleotide and two hemes) across the membrane, where they reduce extracellular (or intraphagosomal) O_2 to O_2^-. Protons left behind in the cell are extruded through voltage-gated proton channels *(red)*. Some of the reactive oxygen species (ROS) derived from O_2^- are indicated. Spontaneous or superoxide dismutase–catalyzed disproportionation of O_2^- produces hydrogen peroxide (H_2O_2), which may be converted to HOCl (hypochlorous acid, or household bleach) by myeloperoxidase (MPO). **A.** Traditional view of the respiratory burst with charge compensation by proton channels. A perfect match of one proton per electron results in no change in membrane potential, intracellular pH (pHi), or external pH (pHo) and little change in ionic strength. Because proton channels are separate molecules and for the most part operate independently of NADPH oxidase, perfect 1:1 stoichiometry is not obligatory. The large depolarization that occurs during the respiratory burst in intact neutrophils and eosinophils is likely the most important factor that causes proton channels to open, although both pHi and pHo tend to change in a direction that causes proton channels to open. That depolarization occurs demonstrates unequivocally that proton efflux initially lags behind electron efflux. **B.** If any fraction of the total charge compensation were mediated by K+ efflux, pHi would fall, pHo (or phagosomal pH) would increase, and the osmolality of the phagosomal contents would increase. In this model, the elevated pH and osmolality of the phagosomal contents are crucial to activating proteolytic enzymes that actually kill bacteria, as opposed to ROS, which are said to be inert. **C.** Respiratory burst reactions. During phagocytosis glucose is metabolized via the pentose monophosphate shunt and NADPH is formed. Cytochrome b_{588}, which was part of the specific granule, combines with the plasma membrane NADPH oxidase and activates it. The activated NADPH oxidase uses oxygen to oxidize the NADPH. The result is the production of superoxide anion. Some of the superoxide anion is converted to H_2O_2 and singlet oxygen by superoxide dismutase. In addition, superoxide anion can react with H_2O_2 resulting in the formation of hydroxyl radical and more singlet oxygen. The result of all of these reactions is the production of the toxic oxygen compounds superoxide anion (O_2^-), H_2O_2, singlet oxygen (${}^1\text{O}_2$) and hydroxyl radical (OH•). As the azurophilic granules fuse with the phagosome, myeloperoxidase is released into the phagolysosome. Myeloperoxidase uses H_2O_2 and halide ions (usually Cl–) to produce hypochlorite, a highly toxic substance. Some of the hypochlorite can spontaneously break down to yield singlet oxygen. The result of these reactions is the production of toxic hypochlorite (Ocl–) and singlet oxygen (${}^1\text{O}_2$). *(A and B, modified with permission from Decoursey TE: Voltage-gated proton channels and other proton transfer pathways,* Physiol Rev *2003 Apr;83(2):475-579.)*

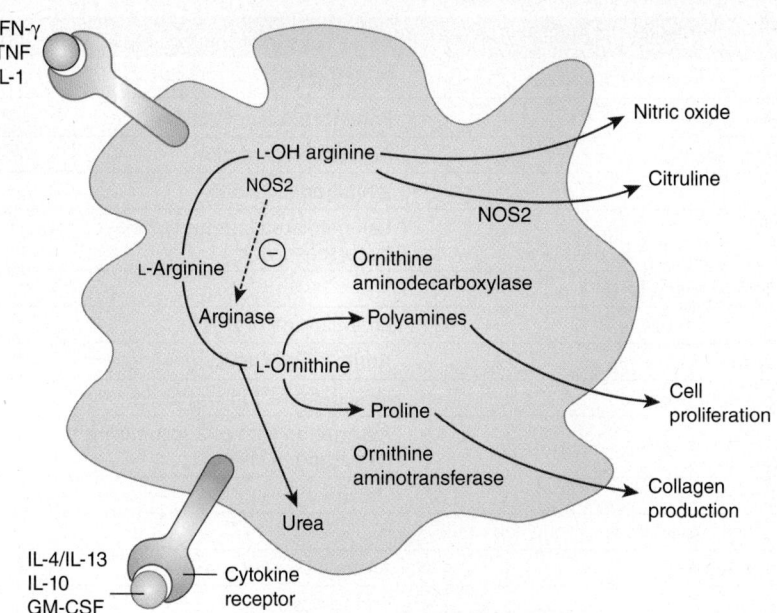

Figure 67–20. The role of nitrogen metabolism in mφ function. Interferon-γ (IFN-γ) enhances the activity of nitric oxide synthase 2 (NOS2) to generate nitric oxide, and inhibits arginase. Interleukin (IL)-4 and IL-13 promote arginase-dependent formation of L-ornithine and, ultimately, fibroblast proliferation and collagen production. GM-CSF, granulocyte-macrophage colony-stimulating factor; TNF, tumor necrosis factor. *(Adapted with permission from Hesse M1, Modolell M, La Flamme AC, et al: Differential regulation of nitric oxide synthase-2 and arginase-1 by type 1/type 2 cytokines in vivo: granulomatous pathology is shaped by the pattern of L-arginine metabolism. J Immunol 2001 Dec 1;167(11):6533-6544.)*

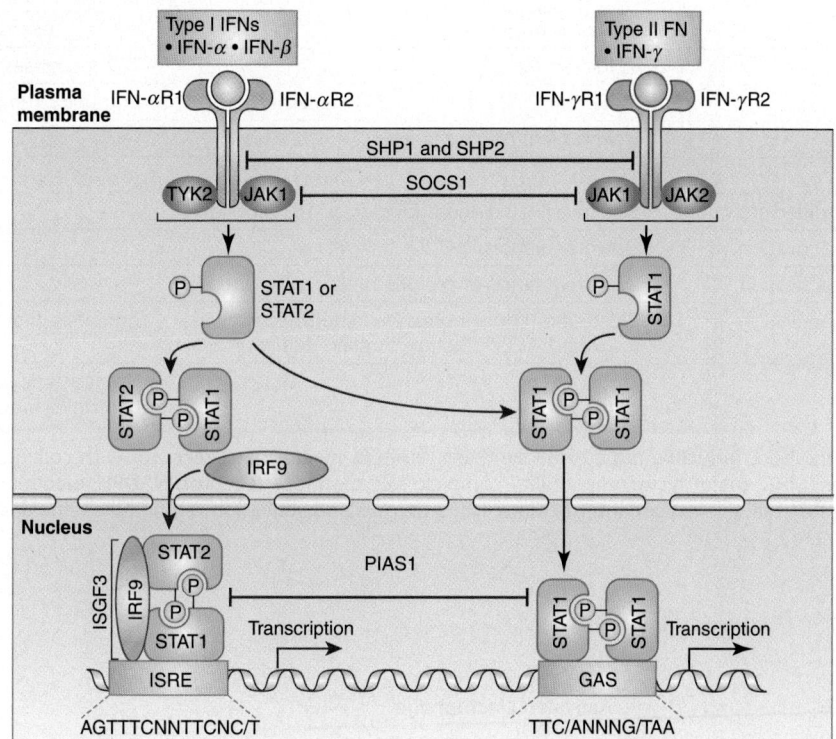

Figure 67–21. Signaling pathways induced by type I and type II interferon (IFN). The type I IFNs (IFN-α and IFN-β) bind a receptor that consists of the subunits IFN-α receptor (IFN-αR)-1 and IFN-αR2, which are constitutively associated with tyrosine kinase 2 (TYK2) and Janus kinase (JAK) 1, respectively. Type I IFN-induced JAK-STAT (signal transducer and activator of transcription) signaling is propagated similarly to IFN-γ–induced JAK-STAT signaling (below). Activated TYK2 and JAK1 phosphorylate STAT1 or STAT2. Type I IFN-induced signaling then induces homodimerization of STAT1 and heterodimerization of STAT1 and STAT2. STAT1 and STAT2 associate with the cytosolic transcription factor IFN-regulatory factor 9 (IRF9), forming a trimeric complex known as IFN-stimulated gene factor 3 (ISGF3). On entering the nucleus, ISGF3 binds IFN-stimulated response elements (ISREs). Studies of gene-targeted mice have shown that JAK1, STAT1, STAT2, and IRF9 are required for signaling through the type I IFN receptor. TYK2 is required for optimal type I IFN-induced signaling. IFN-γ signaling: IFN-γ induces reorganization of the IFN-γR subunits, IFN-γR1 and IFN-γR2, activating the Janus kinases JAK1 and JAK2, which are constitutively associated with each subunit, respectively. The JAKs phosphorylate a crucial tyrosine residue of IFN-γR1, forming a STAT1-binding site; they then tyrosine phosphorylate receptor-bound STAT1, which homodimerizes through Src homology 2 (SH2) domain–phosphotyrosine interactions and is fully activated by serine phosphorylation. STAT1 homodimers enter the nucleus and bind promoters at IFN-γ–activated sites (GASs) and induce gene transcription in conjunction with coactivators, such as CBP (cyclic adenosine monophosphate-responsive–element-binding protein [CREB]), p300, and minichromosome maintenance-deficient 5 (MCM5). IFN-γ–mediated signaling is controlled by several mechanisms: by dephosphorylation of IFN-γR1, JAK1, and STAT1 (mediated by SH2 domain-containing protein tyrosine phosphatase 2 [SHP2]); by inhibition of the JAKs (mediated by suppressor of cytokine signaling 1 [SOCS1]); by proteasomal degradation of the JAKs; and by inhibition of STAT1 (mediated by protein inhibitor of activated STAT1 [PIAS1]). *(Reproduced with permission from Platanias LC: Mechanisms of type-I- and type-II-interferon-mediated signalling. Nat Rev Immunol 2005 May;5(5):375-386.)*

TABLE 67–7. Immunomodulation of Macrophage Phenotype

Stimulus	Category	Markers	Function
Microbial (bacterial)	Innate activation	Induction of MARCO	Enhanced phagocytosis
		Costimulatory molecules	Antigen presentation
		CD200	Inhibition (CD200R)
IFN-γ	Classical activation	Induction MHC II	Cell-mediated immunity/delayed-type hypersensitivity
		Potentiation innate markers	
		- TNF-α	Proinflammatory
		- iNOS induction	Antimicrobial (NO) signaling
		- NADPH, respiratory burst	Host defense, inflammation
		LGP47 induction	Association with phagosome/intracellular pathogen killing
		Downregulation of MR	Unknown
		Modulation of FcR expression	
		Proteasomal composition	Antigen presentation
IL-4/IL-13	Alternative activation	Enhanced MR	Endocytosis
		Induction arginase	Humoral immunity
		Induction YM1, FIZZ1 (mouse)	Th2-responses, allergy, antiparasitic
		Induction CCL17 (MDC) and CCL22 (TARC)	Immunity, repair/fibrosis
		Fusion, giant cell formation	
	Upregulation	CD23 (FcRε)	
Immune complexes	Modified activation	Selective IL-12 downregulation, IL-10 induction	
IL-10	Deactivation	Downregulation MHC II	
TGF-β	Deactivation	Downregulation of proinflammatory NO and ROI	
Glucocorticoids	Deactivation	CD163 induction, monocyte recruitment downregulated, ACE induction, Stabilin induction	Antiinflammatory
			Homeostatic clearance of hemoglobin/haptoglobin complexes

IFN, interferon; IL, interleukin; iNOS, inducible nitric oxide synthase; MARCO, macrophage receptor with collagenous structure; MDC, macrophage-derived chemokine; MHC, major histocompatibility complex; MR, mannose receptor; NADPH, nicotinamide adenine dinucleotide phosphate; NO, nitric oxide; ROI, reactive oxygen intermediate; TARC, thymus and activation-regulated chemokine; TGF, transforming growth factor; TNF, tumor necrosis factor.

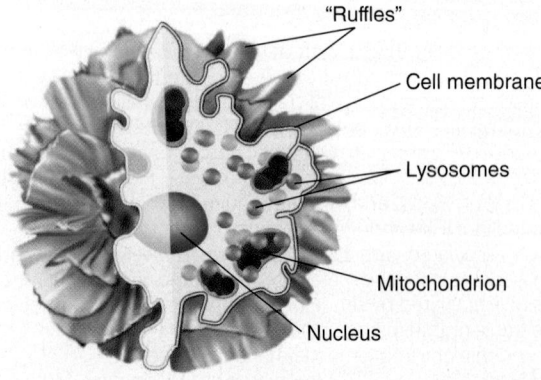

Figure 67–22. Schematic cross-section of "activated" macrophage, showing ruffling of cell membrane and cellular organelles (also see Fig. 67–15). *(Used with permission of S. Seif, GraphisMedica, 2014.)*

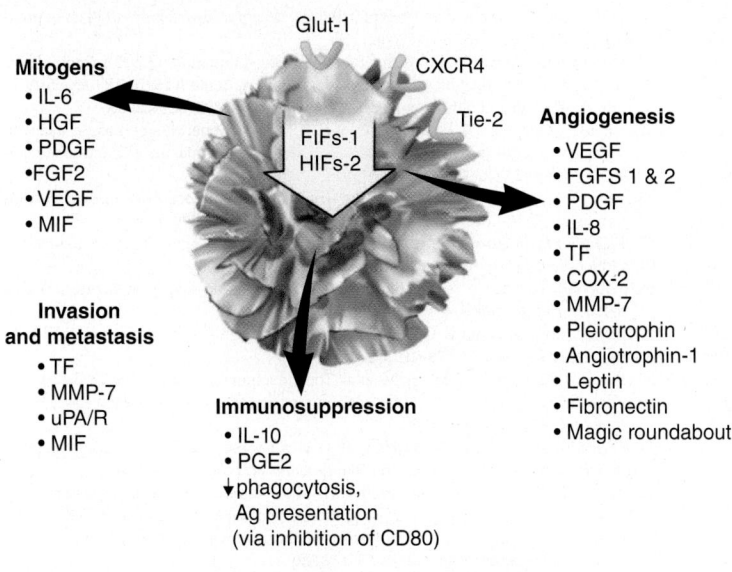

Glut-1

CXCR4

Mitogens
• IL-6
• HGF
• PDGF
• FGF2
• VEGF
• MIF

FIFs-1
HIFs-2

Tie-2

Angiogenesis
• VEGF
• FGFS 1 & 2
• PDGF
• IL-8
• TF
• COX-2
• MMP-7
• Pleiotrophin
• Angiotrophin-1
• Leptin
• Fibronectin
• Magic roundabout

**Invasion
and metastasis**
• TF
• MMP-7
• uPA/R
• MIF

Immunosuppression
• IL-10
• PGE2
↓phagocytosis,
 Ag presentation
 (via inhibition of CD80)

Figure 67–23. Hypoxia induces marked changes in the phenotype of macrophages. Macrophages upregulate hypoxia-inducible transcription factor (HIF)-1 and HIF-2 in hypoxia, which translocate to the nucleus to induce the expression of a wide array of target genes. Several important cell-surface receptors are upregulated in hypoxia, including the glucose receptor GLUT-1 (for increased glucose uptake as the cell switches to anaerobic glycolysis to make ATP in the absence of oxygen), the chemokine stromal cell-derived factor-1 (SDF-1) receptor CXCR4, and the angiopoietin receptor Tie-2. Hypoxia also stimulates the expression of a wide array of other protumor cytokines, enzymes, and receptors, grouped here according to their known function in tumors. Downregulation of a factor or tumor-associated macrophage function is indicated by an *arrow*. Ag, antigen; COX, cyclooxygenase; FGF, fibroblast growth factor; HGF, hepatocyte growth factor; MIF, macrophage migration inhibitory factor; MMP, matrix metalloproteinase; PDGF, platelet-derived growth factor; PGE_2, prostaglandin E_2; TF, tissue factor; uPA/R, urokinase-type plasminogen activator receptor; VEGF, vascular endothelial growth factor. (*Modified with permission from Lewis CE, Hughes R: Inflammation and breast cancer. Microenvironmental factors regulating macrophage function in breast tumours: hypoxia and angiopoietin-2. Breast Cancer Res 2007;9(3):209.)*

acutely and following persistent injury, to chronic inflammation. Storage of poorly degraded materials in lysosomes, for example, results in sustained production of degradation products, whereas massive, acute responses have a profound impact on the systemic circulation, endocrine and nervous systems, and on metabolic pathways. Short-range interactions include giant cell formation during granulomatous inflammation, and also contact-dependent immunoregulation by surface molecules such as CD200/CD200R and SIRPα/CD47.[140] Matrix and other surface interactions regulate the induction or suppression of adaptive immune responses, as well of other functions. The availability of oxygen plays an important role in macrophage interactions with a range of other cells, both normally and in a range of pathologies inducing inflammation, repair, and malignancy (Fig. 67–23).

RELEVANCE TO HEMATOPOIETIC FUNCTIONS AND DISORDERS

In addition to their essential role in host defense (innate and acquired immunity), inflammation, and repair, macrophages contribute to hematopoiesis, as well as to the turnover of hematopoietic cells and their products. Macrophages can be induced to take up folate, sense and respond to oxygen levels, and promote vascular growth, regulating the integrity of the hematopoietic microenvironment. However, they also play a central effector role in pathogenesis. Their surface expression and secretion of TNF-α, other proinflammatory cytokines, enzymes, and metabolites contribute to vascular injury and increased permeability of the microvasculature, as well as to local and systemic catabolic effects associated with chronic inflammation. In this regard, anti–TNF-α therapy is of considerable value in selected inflammatory conditions and has been extended to the treatment of cancer and rheumatologic conditions.[141–144] Stromal and other resident macrophage populations provide a niche for acute and persistent infections in marrow and elsewhere, and these macrophages also contribute to trophic support of hematopoietic malignancies, such as multiple myeloma. The macrophage, therefore, provides an important target cell for selective therapeutic intervention, without undue enhancement of vulnerability to infection. Additional molecular targets are needed, based on more detailed

analysis of macrophage functions within their native hematopoietic tissue environment. A deeper understanding of macrophage physiologic functions and of their role in a broad range of diseases should lead to the development of fresh insights into the pathogenesis and management of hematologic disorders.

REFERENCES

1. van Furth R: *Mononuclear Phagocytes: Characteristics, Physiology, Function.* M. Nijhoff, The Hague, 1985.
2. Lewis C, McGee JD: *The Macrophage,* 2nd ed. Oxford University Press, New York, 1992.
3. Aschoff L: Das reticulo-endotheliale system. *Ergeb Inn Med Kinderheilkd* 26, 1924.
4. Randolph GJ, Beaulieu S, Lebecque S, et al: Differentiation of monocytes into dendritic cells in a model of transendothelial trafficking. *Science* 282:480–483, 1998.
5. Steinman RM: The dendritic cell system and its role in immunogenicity. *Annu Rev Immunol* 9:271–296, 1991.
6. van Furth R, Cohn ZA: The origin and kinetics of mononuclear phagocytes. *J Exp Med* 128:415–435, 1968.
7. Sallusto F, Lanzavecchia A: Efficient presentation of soluble antigen by cultured human dendritic cells is maintained by granulocyte/macrophage colony-stimulating factor plus interleukin 4 and downregulated by tumor necrosis factor alpha. *J Exp Med* 179:1109–1118, 1994.
8. Wynn TA, Chawla A, Pollard JW: Macrophage biology in development, homeostasis and disease. *Nature* 496:445–455, 2013.
9. van Furth R: Phagocytic cells: Development and distribution of mono-nuclear phagocytes in normal steady state and inflammation, 2nd ed., in *Inflammation: Basic Principles and Clinical Correlates,* edited by Gallin JI, Snyderman R, p 325–329. Raven Press, New York, 1992.
10. Nichols BA, Bainton DF, Farquhar MG: Differentiation of monocytes. Origin, nature, and fate of their azurophil granules. *J Cell Biol* 50:498–515, 1971.
11. Nichols BA, Bainton DF: Differentiation of human monocytes in bone marrow and blood. Sequential formation of two granule populations. *Lab Invest* 29:27–40, 1973.
12. Ploem J: Reflection contrast microscopy as a tool in investigations of the attachment of living cells to a glass surface, in *Mononuclear Phagocytes in Immunity, Infection, and Pathology,* edited by Furth R van, p 405. Blackwell, Oxford, England, 1975.
13. Douglas SD: Alterations in intramembrane particle distribution during interaction of erythrocyte-bound ligands with immunoprotein receptors. *J Immunol* 120:151–157, 1978.
14. Rabinovitch M, DeStefano MJ: Macrophage spreading in vitro. I. Inducers of spreading. *Exp Cell Res* 77:323–334, 1973.
15. Douglas SD: Human monocyte spreading in vitro—Inducers and effects on Fc and C3 receptors. *Cell Immunol* 21:344–349, 1976.
16. Ackerman SK, Douglas SD: Purification of human monocytes on microexudate-coated surfaces. *J Immunol* 120:1372–1374, 1978.
17. Zuckerman SH, Ackerman SK, Douglas SD: Long-term human peripheral blood monocyte cultures: Establishment, metabolism and morphology of primary human monocyte-macrophage cell cultures. *Immunology* 38:401–411, 1979.

18. Sutton JS, Weiss L: Transformation of monocytes in tissue culture into macrophages, epithelioid cells, and multinucleated giant cells. An electron microscope study. *J Cell Biol* 28:303–332, 1966.

19. Reaven EP, Axline SG: Subplasmalemmal microfilaments and microtubules in resting and phagocytizing cultivated macrophages. *J Cell Biol* 59:12–27, 1973.

20. Wachstein M, Wolf G: The histochemical demonstration of esterase activity in human blood and bone marrow smears. *J Histochem Cytochem* 6:457, 1958.

21. Braunsteiner H, Schmalzl F: Cytochemistry of monocytes and macrophages, in *Mononuclear Phagocytes*, edited by Furth R van, p 62. Blackwell, Oxford, England, 1970.

22. Li CY, Lam KW, Yam LT: Esterases in human leukocytes. *J Histochem Cytochem* 21:1–12, 1973.

23. Bodel PT, Nichols BA, Bainton DF: Appearance of peroxidase reactivity within the rough endoplasmic reticulum of blood monocytes after surface adherence. *J Exp Med* 145:264–274, 1977.

24. Nichols BA, Bainton DF: Ultrastructure and cytochemistry of mono-nuclear phagocytes, in *Mononuclear Phagocytes in Immunity, Infection, and Pathology*, edited by Furth R van, p 17. Blackwell, Oxford, England, 1975.

25. Fawcett DW: *Bloom & Fawcett Textbook of Histology*. Chapman and Hall, New York, New York, 1994.

26. Russell SW, Gordon S: *Macrophage Biology and Activation*, Springer-Verlag, Berlin, 1992.

27. Passlick B, Flieger D, Ziegler-Heitbrock HW: Identification and characterization of a novel monocyte subpopulation in human peripheral blood. *Blood* 74:2527–2534, 1989.

28. Cros J, Cagnard N, Woollard K, et al: Human CD14dim monocytes patrol and sense nucleic acids and viruses via TLR7 and TLR8 receptors. *Immunity* 33:375–386, 2010.

29. Collison J, Carlin L, Geissmann F, Peakman M: Migratory behavior of human CD14 dim CD16+ monocytes on human macro- and micro-vascular endothelia: An in vitro approach (P5144). *J Immunol* 190 (Meeting Abstract Supplement):26, 2013.

30. Gomez Perdiguero E, Geissmann F: Myb-independent macrophages: A family of cells that develops with their tissue of residence and is involved in its homeostasis. *Cold Spring Harb Symp Quant Biol* 78:91–100, 2013.

31. Yamasaki R, Lu H, Butovsky O, et al: Differential roles of microglia and monocytes in the inflamed central nervous system. *J Exp Med* 211:1533–1549, 2014.

32. Rabinovitch M: Professional and non-professional phagocytes: An introduction. *Trends Cell Biol* 5:85–87, 1995.

33. Delamarre L, Pack M, Chang H, et al: Differential lysosomal proteolysis in antigen-presenting cells determines antigen fate. *Science* 307:1630–1634, 2005.

34. Pluddemann A, Mukhopadhyay S, Gordon S: The interaction of macrophage receptors with bacterial ligands. *Expert Rev Mol Med* 8:1–25, 2006.

35. Pluddemann A, Hoe JC, Makepeace K, et al: The macrophage scavenger receptor A is host-protective in experimental meningococcal septicaemia. *PLoS Pathog* 5:e1000297, 2009.

36. Taylor PR, Martinez-Pomares L, Stacey M, et al: Macrophage receptors and immune recognition. *Annu Rev Immunol* 23:901–944, 2005.

37. van Kooyk Y, Rabinovich GA: Protein-glycan interactions in the control of innate and adaptive immune responses. *Nat Immunol* 9:593–601, 2008.

38. Metzger H: *Fc Receptors and the Action of Antibodies*. American Society for Microbiology, Washington, DC, 1990.

39. Anderson CL, Guyre PM, Whitin JC, et al: Monoclonal antibodies to Fc receptors for IgG on human mononuclear phagocytes. Antibody characterization and induction of superoxide production in a monocyte cell line. *J Biol Chem* 261:12856–12864, 1986.

40. Looney RJ, Abraham GN, Anderson CL: Human monocytes and U937 cells bear two distinct Fc receptors for IgG. *J Immunol* 136:1641–1647, 1986.

41. Wright SD, Griffin FM Jr: Activation of phagocytic cells' C3 receptors for phagocytosis. *J Leukoc Biol* 38:327–339, 1985.

42. Kishimoto TK, Hollander N, Roberts TM, et al: Heterogeneous mutations in the beta subunit common to the LFA-1, Mac-1, and p150,95 glycoproteins cause leukocyte adhesion deficiency. *Cell* 50:193–202, 1987.

43. Hynes RO: Integrins: A family of cell surface receptors. *Cell* 48:549–554, 1987.

44. Etzioni A, Doerschuk CM, Harlan JM: Of man and mouse: Leukocyte and endothelial adhesion molecule deficiencies. *Blood* 94:3281–3288, 1999.

45. Carroll MC: The complement system in regulation of adaptive immunity. *Nat Immunol* 5:981–986, 2004.

46. Nimmerjahn F, Ravetch JV: Fcgamma receptors as regulators of immune responses. *Nat Rev Immunol* 8:34–47, 2008.

47. Savill J, Dransfield I, Gregory C, Haslett C: A blast from the past: Clearance of apoptotic cells regulates immune responses. *Nat Rev Immunol* 2:965–975, 2002.

48. Medzhitov R: Origin and physiological roles of inflammation. *Nature* 454:428–435, 2008.

49. Areschoug T, Gordon S: Pattern recognition receptors and their role in innate immunity: Focus on microbial protein ligands. *Contrib Microbiol* 15:45–60, 2008.

50. Athman R, Philpott D: Innate immunity via Toll-like receptors and Nod proteins. *Curr Opin Microbiol* 7:25–32, 2004.

51. Gazzinelli R, Fitzgerald K, Golenbock D: Toll-like receptors, in *Phagocyte–Pathogen Interactions: Macrophages and the Host Response to Infection*, edited by Russell DG, Gordon S, p 107. ASM Press, Washington, DC, 2009.

52. McCoy CE, O'Neill LA: The role of toll-like receptors in macrophages. *Front Biosci* 13:62–70, 2008.

53. O'Neill LA: The interleukin-1 receptor/toll-like receptor superfamily: 10 years of progress. *Immunol Rev* 226:10–18, 2008.

54. Davidson DJ, Currie AJ, Bowdish DM, et al: IRAK-4 mutation (Q293X): Rapid detection and characterization of defective post-transcriptional TLR/IL-1R responses in human myeloid and non-myeloid cells. *J Immunol* 177:8202–8211, 2006.

55. Khor CC, Chapman SJ, Vannberg FO, et al: A Mal functional variant is associated with protection against invasive pneumococcal disease, bacteremia, malaria and tuberculosis. *Nat Genet* 39:523–528, 2007.

56. Park BS, Song DH, Kim HM, et al: The structural basis of lipopolysaccharide recognition by the TLR4-MD-2 complex. *Nature* 458:1191–1195, 2009.

57. Kagan JC, Su T, Horng T, et al: TRAM couples endocytosis of toll-like receptor 4 to the induction of interferon-beta. *Nat Immunol* 9:361–368, 2008.

58. Trinchieri G, Sher A: Cooperation of toll-like receptor signals in innate immune defence. *Nat Rev Immunol* 7:179–190, 2007.

59. Blander JM, Medzhitov R: On regulation of phagosome maturation and antigen presentation. *Nat Immunol* 7:1029–1035, 2006.

60. Rosas M, Liddiard K, Kimberg M, et al: The induction of inflammation by dectin-1 in vivo is dependent on myeloid cell programming and the progression of phagocytosis. *J Immunol* 181:3549–3557, 2008.

61. Taylor PR, Tsoni SV, Willment JA, et al: Dectin-1 is required for beta-glucan recognition and control of fungal infection. *Nat Immunol* 8:31–38, 2007.

62. Taylor PR, Gordon S, Martinez-Pomares L: The mannose receptor: Linking homeostasis and immunity through sugar recognition. *Trends Immunol* 26:104–110, 2005.

63. Gazi U, Martinez-Pomares L: Influence of the mannose receptor in host immune responses. *Immunobiology* 214:554–561, 2009.

64. McKenzie EJ, Taylor PR, Stillion RJ, et al: Mannose receptor expression and function define a new population of murine dendritic cells. *J Immunol* 178:4975–4983, 2007.

65. Brown GD: Dectin-1: A signalling non-TLR pattern-recognition receptor. *Nat Rev Immunol* 6:33–43, 2006.

66. Crocker PR, Paulson JC, Varki A: Siglecs and their roles in the immune system. *Nat Rev Immunol* 7:255–266, 2007.

67. Mukhopadhyay S, Gordon S: The role of scavenger receptors in pathogen recognition and innate immunity. *Immunobiology* 209:39–49, 2004.

68. Peiser L, Makepeace K, Plüddemann A, et al: Identification of Neisseria meningitidis nonlipopolysaccharide ligands for class A macrophage scavenger receptor by using a novel assay. *Infect Immun* 74:5191–5199, 2006.

69. Hoebe K, Georgel P, Rutschmann S, et al: CD36 is a sensor of diacylglycerides. *Nature* 433:523–527, 2005.

70. Means TK, Mylonakis E, Tampakakis E, et al: Evolutionarily conserved recognition and innate immunity to fungal pathogens by the scavenger receptors SCARF1 and CD36. *J Exp Med* 206:637–653, 2009.

71. Cowing C, Schwartz BD, Dickler HB: Macrophage Ia antigens. I. macrophage populations differ in their expression of Ia antigens. *J Immunol* 120:378–384, 1978.

72. Unanue ER, Allen PM: The basis for the immunoregulatory role of macrophages and other accessory cells. *Science* 236:551–557, 1987.

73. Sanchez-Madrid F, Nagy JA, Robbins E, et al: A human leukocyte differentiation antigen family with distinct alpha-subunits and a common beta-subunit: The lymphocyte function-associated antigen (LFA-1), the C3bi complement receptor (OKM1/Mac-1), and the p150,95 molecule. *J Exp Med* 158:1785–1803, 1983.

74. Beller DI, Springer TA, Schreiber RD: Anti-Mac-1 selectively inhibits the mouse and human type three complement receptor. *J Exp Med* 156:1000–1009, 1982.

75. Haziot A, Chen S, Ferrero E, et al: The monocyte differentiation antigen, CD14, is anchored to the cell membrane by a phosphatidylinositol linkage. *J Immunol* 141:547–552, 1988.

76. Yu B, Hailman E, Wright SD: Lipopolysaccharide binding protein and soluble CD14 catalyze exchange of phospholipids. *J Clin Invest* 99:315–324, 1997.

77. Ziegler-Heitbrock HW, Fingerle G, Ströbel M, et al: The novel subset of CD14+/CD16+ blood monocytes exhibits features of tissue macrophages. *Eur J Immunol* 23:2053–2058, 1993.

78. Ziegler-Heitbrock HW: Heterogeneity of human blood monocytes: The CD14+ CD16+ subpopulation. *Immunol Today* 17:424–428, 1996.

79. Kazazi F, Mathijs JM, Foley P, Cunningham AL: Variations in CD4 expression by human monocytes and macrophages and their relationships to infection with the human immunodeficiency virus. *J Gen Virol* 70(Pt 10):2661–2672, 1989.

80. Collman R, Godfrey B, Cutilli J, et al: Macrophage-tropic strains of human immunodeficiency virus type 1 utilize the CD4 receptor. *J Virol* 64:4468–4476, 1990.

81. Alkhatib G, Combadiere C, Broder CC, et al: CC CKR5: A RANTES, MIP-1alpha, MIP-1beta receptor as a fusion cofactor for macrophage-tropic HIV-1. *Science* 272:1955–1958, 1996.

82. Hill CM, Littman DR: Natural resistance to HIV? *Nature* 382:668–669, 1996.

83. Deng H, Liu R, Ellmeier W, et al: Identification of a major co-receptor for primary isolates of HIV-1. *Nature* 381:661–666, 1996.

84. Huang Y, Paxton WA, Wolinsky SM, et al: The role of a mutant CCR5 allele in HIV-1 transmission and disease progression. *Nat Med* 2:1240–1243, 1996.

85. Dragic T, Litwin V, Allaway GP, et al: HIV-1 entry into CD4+ cells is mediated by the chemokine receptor CC-CKR-5. *Nature* 381:667–673, 1996.

86. Samson M, Libert F, Doranz BJ, et al: Resistance to HIV-1 infection in caucasian individuals bearing mutant alleles of the CCR-5 chemokine receptor gene. *Nature* 382:722–725, 1996.

87. Liu R, Paxton WA, Choe S, et al: Homozygous defect in HIV-1 coreceptor accounts for resistance of some multiply-exposed individuals to HIV-1 infection. *Cell* 86:367–377, 1996.

88. Williams T, Rankin S: Chemokines and phagocyte trafficking, in *Phagocyte–Pathogen Interactions: Macrophages and the Host Response to Infection*, edited by Russell DG, Gordon S, p 93. ASM Press, Washington, DC, 2009.

89. Ross R: Atherosclerosis—An inflammatory disease. *N Engl J Med* 340:115–126, 1999.

90. Janeway CA Jr, Medzhitov R: Innate immune recognition. *Annu Rev Immunol* 20:197–216, 2002.

91. Rebuck JW, Crowley JH: A method of studying leukocytic functions in vivo. *Ann N Y Acad Sci* 59:757–805, 1955.

92. Boyden S: The chemotactic effect of mixtures of antibody and antigen on polymorphonuclear leucocytes. *J Exp Med* 115:453–466, 1962.

93. Jiang A, Bloom O, Ono S, et al: Disruption of E-cadherin-mediated adhesion induces a functionally distinct pathway of dendritic cell maturation. *Immunity* 27:610–624, 2007.

94. Hazenbos W, Brown E: Integrins on phagocytes, in *Phagocyte–Pathogen Interactions: Macrophages and the Host Response to Infection*, edited by Russell DG, Gordon S, p 137. ASM Press, Washington, DC, 2009.

95. Wheeler A, Ridley A: Leukocyte chemotaxis, in *Phagocyte–Pathogen Interactions: Macrophages and the Host Response to Infection*, edited by Russell DG, Gordon S, p 183. ASM Press, Washington, DC, 2009.

96. Lattin JE, Schroder K, Su AI, et al: Expression analysis of G Protein-Coupled Receptors in mouse macrophages. *Immunome Res* 4:5, 2008.

97. Yona S, Lin HH, Siu WO, et al: Adhesion-GPCRs: Emerging roles for novel receptors. *Trends Biochem Sci* 33:491–500, 2008.

98. Gordon S, Unkeless JC, Cohn ZA: Induction of macrophage plasminogen activator by endotoxin stimulation and phagocytosis: Evidence for a two-stage process. *J Exp Med* 140:995–1010, 1974.

99. Henson P, Bratton D: Recognition and removal of apoptotic cells, in *Phagocyte–Pathogen Interactions: Macrophages and the Host Response to Infection*, edited by Russell DG, Gordon S, p 341. ASM Press, Washington, DC, 2009.

100. Mariathasan S, Monack DM: Inflammasome adaptors and sensors: Intracellular regulators of infection and inflammation. *Nat Rev Immunol* 7:31–40, 2007.

101. Martinon F, Burns K, Tschopp J: The inflammasome: A molecular platform triggering activation of inflammatory caspases and processing of proIL-beta. *Mol Cell* 10:417–426, 2002.

102. Martinon F, Mayor A, Tschopp J: The inflammasomes: Guardians of the body. *Annu Rev Immunol* 27:229–265, 2009.

103. Deretic V: Autophagy: A fundamental cytoplasmic sanitation process operational in all cell types including macrophages, in *Phagocyte–Pathogen Interactions: Macrophages and the Host Response to Infection*, edited by Russell DG, Gordon S, p 419. ASM Press, Washington, DC, 2009.

104. Helming L, Winter J, Gordon S: The scavenger receptor CD36 plays a role in cytokine-induced macrophage fusion. *J Cell Sci* 122:453–459, 2009.

105. Xia W, Hilgenbrink AR, Matteson EL, et al: A functional folate receptor is induced during macrophage activation and can be used to target drugs to activated macrophages. *Blood* 113:438–446, 2009.

106. Kristiansen M, Graversen JH, Jacobsen C, et al: Identification of the haemoglobin scavenger receptor. *Nature* 409:198–201, 2001.

107. Tuluc F, Meshki J, Spitsin S, Douglas SD: HIV infection of macrophages is enhanced in the presence of increased expression of CD163 induced by substance P. *J Leukoc Biol* 96:143–150, 2014.

108. Chimini G, Chavrier P: Function of Rho family proteins in actin dynamics during phagocytosis and engulfment. *Nat Cell Biol* 2:E191–E196, 2000.

109. Russell DG, Gordon S: *Phagocyte–Pathogen Interactions: Macrophages and the Host Response to Infection*. ASM Press, Washington, DC, 2009.

110. Ridley AJ, Hall A: Snails, Swiss, and serum: The solution for Rac 'n' Rho. *Cell* 116:S23–S25, 2 p following S25, 2004.

111. Swanson JA: Shaping cups into phagosomes and macropinosomes. *Nat Rev Mol Cell Biol* 9:639–649, 2008.

112. Jutras I, Desjardins M: Phagocytosis: At the crossroads of innate and adaptive immunity. *Annu Rev Cell Dev Biol* 21:511–527, 2005.

113. Rohde K, Yates RM, Purdy GE, Russell DG: Mycobacterium tuberculosis and the environment within the phagosome. *Immunol Rev* 219:37–54, 2007.

114. Bogdan C: Mechanisms and consequences of persistence of intracellular pathogens: Leishmaniasis as an example. *Cell Microbiol* 10:1221–1234, 2008.

115. Portnoy DA, Auerbuch V, Glomski IJ: The cell biology of Listeria monocytogenes infection: The intersection of bacterial pathogenesis and cell-mediated immunity. *J Cell Biol* 158:409–414, 2002.

116. Swanson MS: Autophagy: Eating for good health. *J Immunol* 177:4945–4951, 2006.

117. Steinman RM, Moberg CL: Zanvil Alexander Cohn 1926–1993. *J Exp Med* 179:1–30, 1994.

118. Ganz T: Iron in innate immunity: Starve the invaders. *Curr Opin Immunol* 21:63–67, 2009.

119. Giodini A, Rahner C, Cresswell P: Receptor-mediated phagocytosis elicits cross-presentation in nonprofessional antigen-presenting cells. *Proc Natl Acad Sci U S A* 106:3324–3329, 2009.

120. Helming L, Tomasello E, Kyriakides TR, et al: Essential role of DAP12 signaling in macrophage programming into a fusion-competent state. *Sci Signal* 1:ra11, 2008.

121. Sidiropoulos PI, Goulielmos G, Voloudakis GK, et al: Inflammasomes and rheumatic diseases: Evolving concepts. *Ann Rheum Dis* 67:1382–1389, 2008.

122. Ye Z, Ting JP: NLR, the nucleotide-binding domain leucine-rich repeat containing gene family. *Curr Opin Immunol* 20:3–9, 2008.

123. Ryan JG, Kastner DL: Fevers, genes, and innate immunity. *Curr Top Microbiol Immunol* 321:169–184, 2008.

124. Ogura Y, Inohara N, Benito A, et al: Nod2, a Nod1/Apaf-1 family member that is restricted to monocytes and activates NF-kappaB. *J Biol Chem* 276:4812–4818, 2001.

125. Inohara N, Ogura Y, Fontalba A, et al: Host recognition of bacterial muramyl dipeptide mediated through NOD2. Implications for Crohn's disease. *J Biol Chem* 278:5509–5512, 2003.

126. Kzhyshkowska J, Krusell L: Cross-talk between endocytic clearance and secretion in macrophages. *Immunobiology* 214:576–593, 2009.

127. Lieu ZZ, Lock JG, Hammond LA, et al: A trans-Golgi network golgin is required for the regulated secretion of TNF in activated macrophages in vivo. *Proc Natl Acad Sci U S A* 105:3351–3356, 2008.

128. Stow JL, Low PC, Offenhauser C, Sangermani D: Cytokine secretion in macrophages and other cells: Pathways and mediators. *Immunobiology* 214:601–612, 2009.

129. McPhail LC: SH3-dependent assembly of the phagocyte NADPH oxidase. *J Exp Med* 180:2011–2015, 1994.

130. O'Shea JJ, Murray PJ: Cytokine signaling modules in inflammatory responses. *Immunity* 28:477–487, 2008.

131. Garcia-Sastre A, Biron CA: Type 1 interferons and the virus-host relationship: A lesson in detente. *Science* 312:879–882, 2006.

132. Bogdan C, Mattner J, Schleicher U: The role of type I interferons in non-viral infections. *Immunol Rev* 202:33–48, 2004.

133. Dunn GP, Koebel CM, Schreiber RD: Interferons, immunity and cancer immunoediting. *Nat Rev Immunol* 6:836–848, 2006.

134. Sharif MN, Tassiulas I, Hu Y, et al: IFN-alpha priming results in a gain of proinflammatory function by IL-10: Implications for systemic lupus erythematosus pathogenesis. *J Immunol* 172:6476–6481, 2004.

135. Herrero C, Hu X, Li WP, et al: Reprogramming of IL-10 activity and signaling by IFN-gamma. *J Immunol* 171:5034–5041, 2003.

136. Martinez FO, Helming L, Gordon S: Alternative activation of macrophages: An immunologic functional perspective. *Annu Rev Immunol* 27:451–483, 2009.

137. Varin A, Gordon S: Alternative activation of macrophages: Immune function and cellular biology. *Immunobiology* 214:630–641, 2009.

138. Kaiser F, O'Garra A: Cytokines and macrophages and dendritic cells: Key modulators of immune response, in *Phagocyte–Pathogen Interactions: Macrophages and the Host Response to Infection*, edited by Russell DG, Gordon S, p281–299. ASM Press, Washington, DC, 2009.

139. Lin DA, Boyce JA: Lysophospholipids as mediators of immunity. *Adv Immunol* 89:141–167, 2006.

140. Barclay AN, Wright GJ, Brooke G, Brown MH: CD200 and membrane protein interactions in the control of myeloid cells. *Trends Immunol* 23:285–290, 2002.

141. Feldmann M: Development of anti-TNF therapy for rheumatoid arthritis. *Nat Rev Immunol* 2:364–371, 2002.

142. Palladino MJ, Bower JE, Kreber R, Ganetzky B: Neural dysfunction and neurodegeneration in Drosophila Na+/K+ ATPase alpha subunit mutants. *J Neurosci* 23:1276–1286, 2003.

143. Balkwill F: Tumour necrosis factor and cancer. *Nat Rev Cancer* 9:361–371, 2009.

144. Bongartz T, Sutton AJ, Sweeting MJ, et al: Anti-TNF antibody therapy in rheumatoid arthritis and the risk of serious infections and malignancies: Systematic review and meta-analysis of rare harmful effects in randomized controlled trials. *JAMA* 295:2275–2285, 2006.

145. Gordon S, Fraser I, Nath D, et al: Macrophages in tissues and in vitro. *Curr Opin Immunol* 4:25–32, 1992.

146. Lasser A: The mononuclear phagocytic system: A review. *Hum Pathol* 14:108–126, 1983.

147. Fogelman AM, Van Lenten BJ, Warden C, et al: Macrophage lipoprotein receptors. *J Cell Sci Suppl* 9:135–149, 1988.

148. Adams DO, Hamilton TA: Phagocytic cells: Cytotoxic activities of macrophages, in *Inflammation: Basic Principles and Clinical Correlates*, 2nd ed., edited by Gallin JI, Snyderman R, p 471. Raven Press, New York, 1992.

149. Werb Z, Goldstein I: Phagocytic cells: Chemotactic and effector functions of macrophages and granulocytes, in *Basic and Clinical Immunology*, 7th ed., edited by Stites D, Terr A, p 96. Appleton and Lange, Norwalk, CT, 1991.

150. Papadimitriou JM, Ashman RB: Macrophages: Current views on their differentiation, structure, and function. *Ultrastruct Pathol* 13:343–372, 1989.

151. Gordon S, Perry VH, Rabinowitz S, et al: Plasma membrane receptors of the mononuclear phagocyte system. *J Cell Sci Suppl* 9:1–26, 1988.

152. Law SK: C3 receptors on macrophages. *J Cell Sci Suppl* 9:67–97, 1988.

153. Hume DA, Ross IL, Himes SR, et al: The mononuclear phagocyte system revisited. *J Leukoc Biol* 72:621–627, 2002.

154. Gordon S: Mononuclear phagocytes in rheumatic diseases, in *Kelley's Textbook of Rheumatology*, edited by Firestein G, Budd RC, Harris ED Jr, McInnes IB, Ruddy S, Sergent JS, pp 135–154. WB Saunders, Philadelphia, 2008.

CHAPTER 68

PRODUCTION, DISTRIBUTION, AND ACTIVATION OF MONOCYTES AND MACROPHAGES

Steven D. Douglas and Anne G. Douglas

SUMMARY

Monocytes and macrophages play an important role in human biology, both as a component of the hematopoietic system and within the stroma and tissue microenvironment where they contribute trophic and clearance functions. They constitute a widely dispersed cellular system throughout the body, interacting with host cells and foreign invaders through their versatile biosynthetic and secretory responses, to maintain physiologic homeostasis. They are specialized migratory or sessile phagocytes, present within the circulation and extravascular tissue compartment, contributing to diverse pathologic processes directly and through their production of bioactive products. Because of their extensive heterogeneity and plasticity, the centrality of monocytes and their progeny has not always been recognized by hematologists. The origin, life span, and functions of the monocyte are the focus of this chapter, including their relevance to health and disease in humans, based on current understanding of their properties. The relationship of monocytes and macrophages to dendritic cells, and monocyte-derived cells with a specialized immunologic role in T-lymphocyte activation, are described. Together, macrophages and dendritic cells are major antigen-presenting cells, contributing to host defense, innate and acquired immunity, and inflammation, as well as noninfectious disease processes, both within and outside the lymphohematopoietic organs.

METHODS OF MONOCYTE AND MACROPHAGE STUDY

There has been a resurgence of interest in the *in situ* analysis of macrophages.[1] Genetic/ribonucleic acid interference manipulation, more recently with macrophage-specific/restricted promoters, has been

Acronyms and Abbreviations: CR, complement receptor; DC, dendritic cell; DC-SIGN, dendritic cell–specific intercellular adhesion molecule-3–grabbing nonintegrin; EMR, epidermal growth factor module-containing mucin-like hormone receptor; FACS, fluorescence-activated cell sorting; FcR, Fc receptor; GM-CSF, granulocyte-macrophage colony-stimulating factor; IFN-γ, interferon-γ; IL, interleukin; LPS, lipopolysaccharide; M-CSF, macrophage colony-stimulating factor; MARCO, macrophage receptor with a collagenous structure; MR, mannose receptor; PRR, pattern recognition receptor; Sn, sialoadhesin; SR-A, scavenger receptor A; TGF, transforming growth factor; TLR, toll-like receptor; TNF-a, tumor necrosis factor-a.

used to knock down macrophage genes or messenger RNA, and to mark cells with fluorescent labels such as green fluorescent protein. Of particular value in tracing their origins and distribution has been the use of fractalkine receptor-transgenics,[2] and myeloid-specific lysozyme-Cre for targeted ablation.[3] Random chemical mutagenesis has been spectacularly successful in validating known, and discovering novel, gene targets that affect macrophage functions.[4,5] A wider range of experimental models (*Drosophila*, zebra fish) have facilitated interspecies comparisons of macrophage migration and phagocytosis *in vivo*.[6,7] The analysis of microRNA expression[8] and functions is still in its infancy and is likely to generate important insights into monocyte/macrophage gene expression in health and disease. Combined with improved imaging methods (fluorescent, nuclear magnetic resonance imaging-based, 2-photon microscopy), new insights have been obtained regarding the dynamic behavior of macrophages and dendritic cells (DCs) *in vivo*.[9] There has been progress in provoking embryonic and induced pluripotent stem cell differentiation into macrophages and DCs *in vitro*, opening the possibility of introducing mutations into human genes, to complement the naturally occurring material derived from human inborn errors and resultant genetic diseases.[10]

Although individual-labeled cells can be followed in accessible tissues or *ex vivo*, the resolution, isolation, and characterization of important embedded macrophage populations are limiting. Methods of isolation from solid organs, for example, brain and even liver and gut, are prone to artifact, and macrophages are profoundly affected by removal from their natural tissue environment. Many of the genetic manipulations introduced by transgenesis are leaky and not uniform, not surprising in the light of macrophage heterogeneity. Although the fate of recently recruited cells from blood into tissues can be tracked more easily, the slowly turning over resident populations are less easily accessed, resulting in bias. Finally, there are intrinsic difficulties with human experimentation *in vivo*. Induced skin blisters, for example, make it possible to collect fluid and cells from sites of inflammation.[11] However, the low frequency of monocytes compared with neutrophils limits the use of *ex vivo* indium-labeled cells for transfer studies *in vivo*.

PRODUCTION

DEVELOPMENT OF MONOCYTES AND MACROPHAGES

Macrophages and related amoeboid phagocytic cells, ancient in the evolution of multicellular organisms, are the main leukocytes responsible for innate immunity and tissue remodeling, as documented by Metchnikoff in his pioneering studies on invertebrates,[12] and confirmed by contemporary studies on *Drosophila melanogaster*.[7] In mammals, much of our knowledge of macrophage ontogeny derives from studies in the mouse. After origins from an aortic mesonephric site, the best understood phases of macrophage development occur during midfetal development, in the yolk sac, followed by fetal liver, spleen, and marrow, before and after birth.[13] The association of macrophages with definitive erythropoiesis is a striking feature of fetal liver hematopoiesis from approximately day 12 of mouse development; macrophages then, for the first time, become intimately associated with nucleated erythroblasts, reaching a peak of hematopoietic cluster formation at day 14. The role of stromal macrophages in hematopoiesis within the adult is illustrated and discussed further in this chapter.

The association of macrophages with erythroblasts is mediated by surface adhesion molecules,[14] including a poorly characterized divalent cation-dependent receptor and the sialic acid-binding molecule sialoadhesin (Siglec1).[15] The potential trophic functions of stromal macrophages in marrow erythropoietic islands is poorly understood, as is the considerable role of macrophages in iron and heme metabolism. Macrophages interact with cells in numerous ways; however, during erythropoiesis a special phagocytic process allows for the removal of pyknotic erythroid nuclei during the final stages of erythropoiesis. The mechanism of recognition of membrane-bound erythroid nuclei is not clear, nor its relationship to the uptake of apoptotic cells elsewhere during development. The production of granulocytes from progenitors also involves macrophage–myeloblast clusters and similar adhesion receptors. Once fetal liver hematopoiesis declines before and after birth, the macrophages in the liver adopt the features of resident Kupffer cells. The stromal macrophages associate with developing blood cells within islands of clustered cells, a feature of hematopoiesis throughout life.[16] During fetal life, monocytes and macrophages are distributed through the developing vasculature, providing amoeboid, phagocytic cells implicated in tissue remodeling, for example, sculpting of digits,[17] and growth of the central nervous system.[18] Blood monocytes seed resident tissue macrophage populations throughout the organism, and these cells proliferate more readily in the fetus than in later life; the adhesion molecules, chemotactic signals, and receptors involved during this constitutive phase of distribution are poorly defined, but it is independent of the β_2-integrin CD11b/CD18, which plays a role in myelomonocytic cell recruitment induced by inflammation in the adult.[19] The appearance of macrophages during development has been correlated with fibrous scar formation after injury.[17] In sum, macrophages play a major role during development, both in hematopoiesis and in extravascular tissues, and much remains to be learned regarding their properties in the fetus.

Growth, Differentiation, and Turnover

Figure 68–1 gives an overview of differentiation of monocytic cells in the adult.[20] The origins of monocytes from multipotential (progenitors colony-forming units, spleen [CFU-S]) and committed hematopoietic precursors (colony-forming units, culture [CFU-C]) and the role of lineage-restricted growth factors such as monocyte/macrophage colony-stimulating factor (M-CSF; also termed CSF-1) and granulocyte-macrophage (GM)-CSF have been studied extensively, but new details are still emerging. Both transcription factor c-Myb and receptor FLT3, M-CSF–dependent myeloid lineages (monocyte and dendritic) occur. These cell types may have different responses to tissue damage and infection.[20] Monocytes share precursors with other hematopoietic cells and are closely related to granulocytes. Monocytic precursors are the source of adult tissue macrophages, as well as of myeloid DCs and osteoclasts. Their relationship to B lymphocytes and to plasmacytoid DCs is still unclear, as plasmacytoid DCs express a range of myeloid as well as lymphoid markers. There is a considerable body of knowledge about the specific growth factors and their receptors, and growing knowledge of the nature and role of transcription factors involved in monocyte/macrophage differentiation.[21] Genetic and cellular abnormalities in growth and differentiation pathways underlie myeloid leukemogenesis, though rarely giving rise to monocytic leukemia.

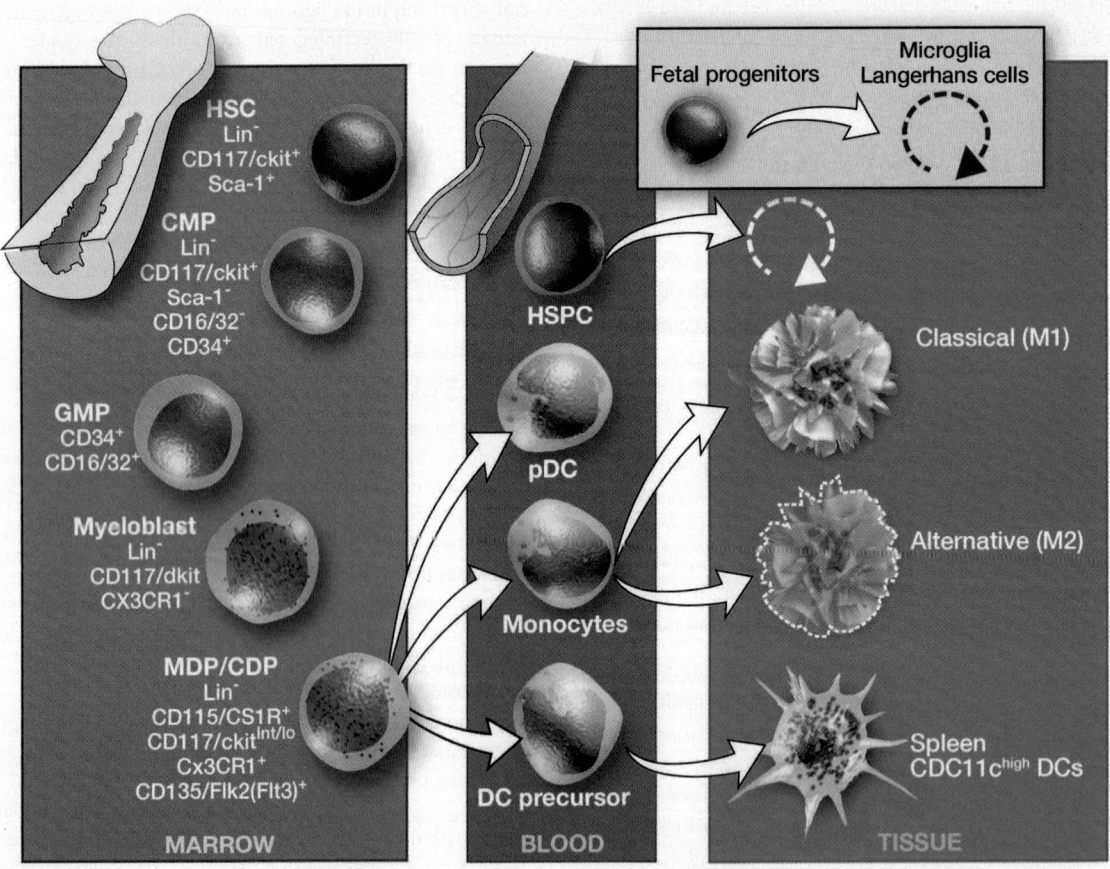

Figure 68–1. Differentiation of the macrophage/dendritic cell (DC) progenitor and origin of macrophage and DC subsets. CDP, common dendritic cell precursor; CMP, common myeloid progenitor; GMP, granulocyte/macrophage progenitor; HSC, hematopoietic stem cell; HSPCs, hematopoietic stem and progenitor cells; MDP, macrophage/DC progenitor; pDC, plasmacytoid dendritic cell. For further details see Ref. 20. *(Used with permission of S. Seif, GraphisMedica, 2014.)*

MATURATION AND DIFFERENTIATION OF MONOCYTES AND MACROPHAGES

The classic studies of Lewis and Lewis[22] in 1926, Maximow[23] in 1932, and Ebert and Florey[24] in 1939, showed that monocytes transform into macrophages and multinucleated giant cells *in vitro*. Macrophages can be produced from monocytes or hematopoietic progenitor cells culture in cytokines, such as GM-CSF or M-CSF.

The alterations of ultrastructure during transformation into macrophages, epithelioid cells, and giant cells have been described using purified populations of monocytes and *in vitro* culture techniques.[25] As the monocyte matures into the macrophage, the cell enlarges in size, and the lysosomal content and the amount of hydrolytic enzymes within the lysosomes (e.g., phosphatases, esterases, β-glucuronidase, lysozyme, arylsulfatase) increase. At the time, the size and number of mitochondria increase, their energy metabolism increases concomitantly. Production of lactate also increases. The Golgi complex, which packages lysosomes, increases in size and vesicle complexity (Chap. 67). Several stimuli induce formation of multinucleated giant cells from monocytes.[26]

Growth Factors

M-CSF and GM-CSF are the major growth factors implicated in monocyte and macrophage differentiation. Other cytokines, such as interleukin (IL)-3 and IL-4, result in minimal monocyte proliferative expansion, and their genetic elimination has no effect on the lineage. M-CSF promotes survival as well as growth and differentiation of macrophages, exclusively, acting through a specific receptor (CSF-1R), encoded by the protooncogene *c-FMS*, which has been extensively used as a lineage marker for fluorescence-activated cell sorting (FACS) analysis (CD115) and transgenesis.[27,28] The role of M-CSF has been reviewed[29] and its role in macrophage and osteoclast development is illustrated in Fig. 68–2. The naturally occurring mouse mutant, *op/op*, gives rise to M-CSF deficiency and osteopetrosis, with marked or partial deficiency in monocyte and selected tissue macrophage populations; DC numbers are unaffected.[30] Unlike PU.1 deficiency, the op/op mouse is viable, though its reproductive ability is impaired, because M-CSF also plays an important role in the reproductive system. Uterine epithelium is a rich source of M-CSF, inducing monocyte-macrophage recruitment, growth and differentiation, and upregulating scavenger receptor (SR) expression, cell adhesion, and endocytosis of modified low-density lipoproteins and other polyanionic ligands. M-CSF is produced in a soluble and membrane-bound forms, is present in plasma, and has been implicated in atherosclerosis and tumor-dependent recruitment of monocytes and macrophages. The size of the growth burst induced by M-CSF depends on the stage of differentiation of the target cell, decreasing markedly as the precursors mature into monocytes and macrophages. Adhesion and inflammatory stimuli enhance the response to growth factors and can result in macrophage proliferation at peripheral sites, for example, in granulomata.

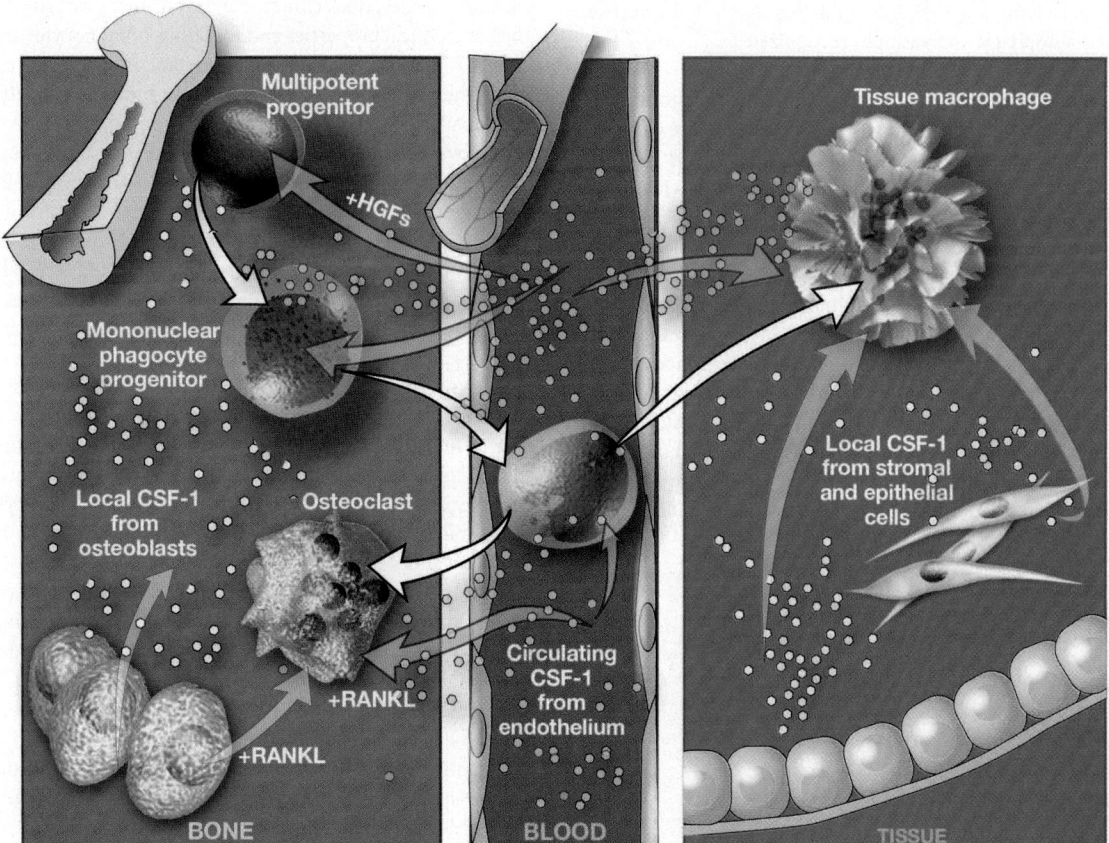

Figure 68–2. Regulation of macrophage and osteoclast development by macrophage colony-stimulating factor (M-CSF). Circulating M-CSF, produced by endothelial cells in blood vessels, together with locally produced M-CSF regulates the survival, proliferation, and differentiation of mononuclear phagocytes and osteoclasts. The cytokine synergizes with other hematopoietic growth factors (HGFs) to generate mononuclear progenitor cells from multipotent progenitors, and with receptor activator of nuclear factor-κB ligand (RANKL) to generate osteoclasts from mononuclear phagocytes. *Brown arrows* indicate cell differentiation steps; *blue arrows* indicate cytokine regulation. *(Used with permission of S. Seif, GraphisMedica, 2014.)*

GM-CSF has a broader myeloid target profile. It is produced by many cells, including macrophages themselves, especially after inflammatory stimuli such as lipopolysaccharide (LPS), and it enhances production of monocytes and macrophages with a different morphology to that induced by M-CSF. GM-CSF is required for myeloid DC differentiation *in vitro* and has been widely used, alone and in combination with cytokines such as IL-4 or transforming growth factor (TGF)-β, to produce DC from mouse marrow or from human monocytes in cell culture.[31,32] Its targeted deletion in mice or genetic loss of function mutants of its specific receptor chain in humans results in pulmonary alveolar proteinosis, associated with defective alveolar macrophage metabolism of pulmonary surfactant.[33]

Survival, Differentiation, and Turnover Overview

Once the cells have acquired the characteristics of mature monocytes/macrophages, they display considerable heterogeneity in morphology and phenotypic plasticity. In general, their proliferative potential is limited, and their life span can vary from less than 1 day to many months, depending on their microenvironment, infections, and other stimuli. Although terminally differentiated, macrophages remain extremely active in messenger RNA and protein synthesis, with complex, often characteristic profiles of gene expression, depending on innate and acquired immune stimuli and cellular interactions. Tissue macrophages are relatively resistant to apoptosis, compared with neutrophils, but this feature changes during infection. Their active membrane turnover and endocytosis make them susceptible to toxic agents, making them targets for clearance by surviving macrophages. Sublethal injury and infection can also induce autophagy, increasingly recognized as an important component of inflammatory and infectious diseases.

The remarkable ability of macrophages to undergo homotypic cell–cell fusion results in giant cell formation. This is a feature of osteoclast differentiation, depending on M-CSF and the tumor necrosis factor (TNF) family member receptor activator of nuclear factor-κB ligand (RANKL), which act on monocytic precursors to yield catabolic cells able to excavate and remodel living bone. Local adhesion and ruffling of their plasma membrane are associated with focal, polarized release of H+ and hydrolytic enzymes by monocyte-derived osteoclasts. The attempted uptake of non- or poorly degradable foreign materials induces "foreign-body giant cells," with distinct properties; macrophage-derived giant cells are also characteristic of granulomatous diseases such as tuberculosis (Langerhans giant cells; Fig. 68–3) and parasitic infections (e.g., schistosomiasis). Mycobacterial and ill-defined host lipids are able to induce giant cell formation *in vitro*. The mechanism of fusion involves cellular differentiation to induce a fusogenic phenotype and

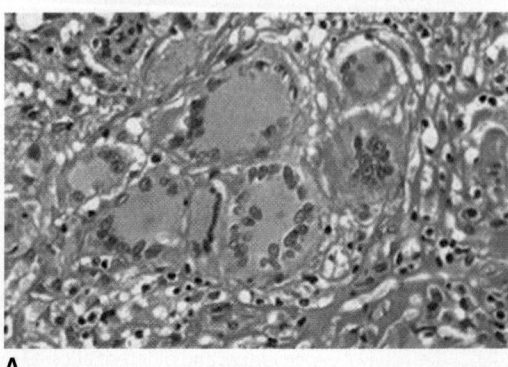

A

Figure 68–3. Microscopic image of Langhans giant cells, tuberculosis induced. (*Reproduced with permission from Y Rosen,* Atlas of Granulomatous Diseases, *at http://granuloma.homestead.com.*)

surface glycoprotein interactions with a selected substratum; T-helper type 2 (Th2) cytokines, such as IL-4 and IL-13, act through a common receptor chain and signaling pathway to enhance macrophage fusion.[34] DNA synthesis, a feature of high-turnover granulomata associated with infection, can result in abortive cell division and cell death. These macrophage-derived giant cells are distinct from syncytia induced by fusogenic virus infection, especially paramyxoviruses and retroviruses such as the human immunodeficiency virus.

HETEROGENEITY

Monocytes are defined as the population of differentiated cells present in the circulation, with classical morphologic features (Chap. 67), and include the less-well defined precursors able to give rise to myeloid DCs and osteoclasts. Because of their ready availability from human blood and the sensitive methods now available to analyze their phenotype *ex vivo* (FACS, microarray, immunochemistry, and cytochemistry), human monocytes have been more amenable to study, whereas in the mouse, analysis of precursor–product relationship and tissue distribution have provided new insights into the fate and heterogeneity of the circulating population. The number of monocytes in the circulation depends on constitutive, steady-state production and delivery from marrow, possibly from marginated pools in spleen, as well as adhesion and diapedesis in response to unknown stimuli and enhanced recruitment in response to peripheral stimuli such as infection and inflammation. M-CSF and glucocorticoids affect their level and phenotype, as do metabolic stimuli; Chap. 70 describes clinical conditions that give rise to monocytosis. The biochemical properties and functions of monocytes are described in Chap. 67. They are relatively radioresistant once entering the circulation, where they persist for 12 to 48 hours as motile cells, with an ability to engulf particles and to adhere transiently or more stably to arterial as well as microvascular endothelium, thus modulating their phagocytic ability. Depending on interactions with the vessel wall and local differentiation, monocytes are able to crawl along and patrol the intravascular surface utilizing CD11a, a β2-integrin–dependent property.[20] Mature macrophages lining the endothelium can also detach and recirculate, for example, filled with lipid stores as foam cells in atherosclerosis, and circulate heavily laden with erythroid breakdown products in malaria.

The presence of significant numbers of immune cells and molecules in adipose tissue suggest vibrant interactions between the immune and metabolic systems. In obesity, the inflammatory infiltrate and activation state of macrophages in adipose tissue may contribute to insulin resistance. The cellular localization and inflammatory potentials of macrophages,[35] as well as the ratio of macrophages to adipocytes,[36] differ in obese and lean mice. In lean mice, macrophages in the adipose tissue have the alternate or M2 phenotype (ARG1+CD206+CD301+), are uniformly distributed, and serve a protective function as they are less inflammatory and promote insulin sensitivity by producing IL-10; however, in obese mice, macrophages distribute around necrotic adipocytes, and induce inflammation and insulin resistance.[35,37] CC-chemokine receptor 2 (CCR2) and its ligand (CCL2) are critical for macrophage recruitment to adipose tissue.[38] Metabolic disease can be viewed as maladaptive consequence of inflammation-induced insulin resistance, which may beneficially conserve energy resources for the immune system combatting infection for brief periods.[39–43]

The precursors of myeloid DC and osteoclasts may represent a subpopulation of monocytes, whose further differentiation depends on cytokines and local factors in the vessel wall, marrow, and other tissues. *Ex vivo* substantial numbers of monocytes give rise to myeloid DC after treatment with GM-CSF and IL-4.[32] Monocytes that differentiate into macrophages do not recirculate for the most part, but persist for varying times as "resident" tissue cells that turn over locally, especially in lymph

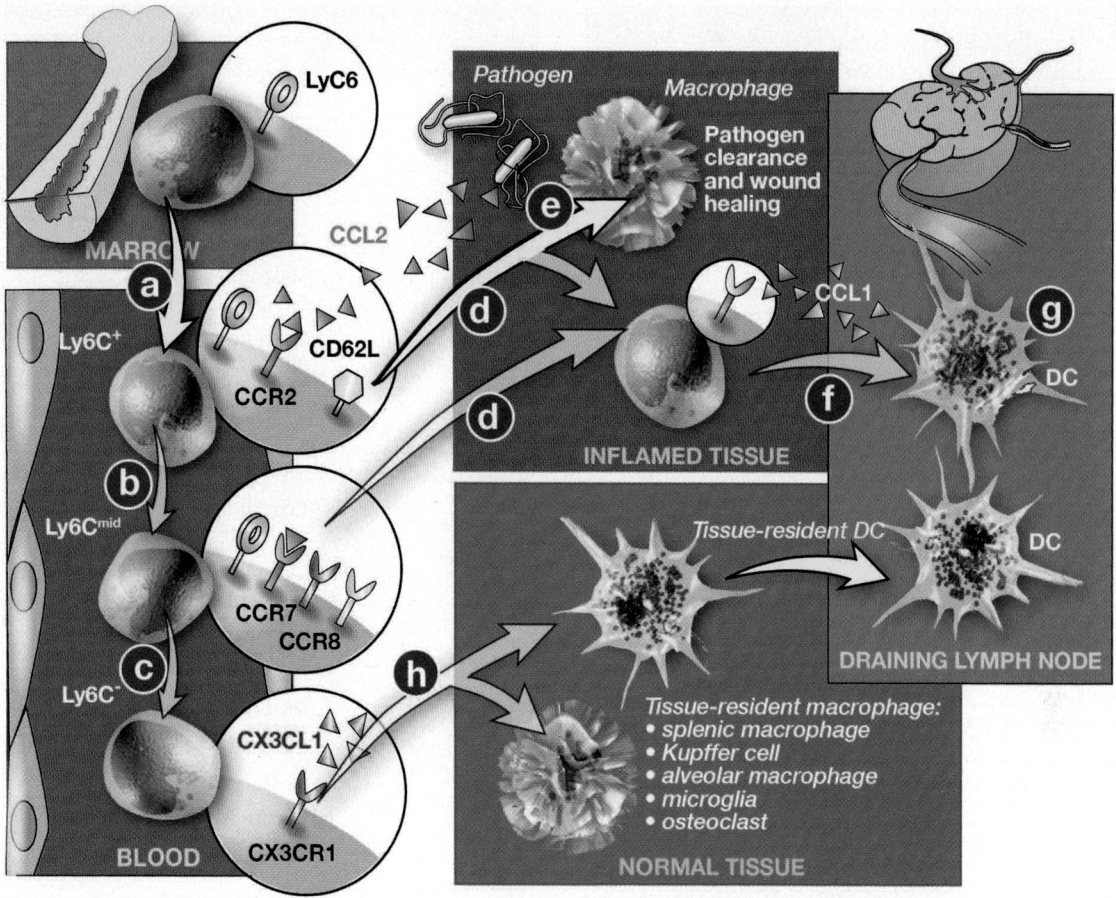

Figure 68–4. Heterogeneity of monocytes in blood and the contribution of different subsets to resident and inflammatory macrophages DCs in tissues. For further details see Ref. 34. *(Used with permission of S. Seif, GraphisMedica, 2014.)*

nodes. It is not known if the constitutive exit from blood is a stochastic process or specific to particular tissues.

Phenotypic heterogeneity of monocyte populations has become a topic of intense interest, thanks to the availability of surface antigens/receptors such as CD14, CD16 (human), and Ly6C (mouse), and analysis of chemokine/receptor expression, especially fractalkine receptor (CX$_3$CR) and CCR2.[34] Figure 68–4 illustrates the subsets and tissue progeny established by the use of genetically manipulated mice and Table 68–1 compares expression of markers to characterize monocyte subsets in mouse and human blood. The relationship of monocyte precursor subsets that give rise to inflammatory tissue macrophages and DCs is better defined than is that of those that give rise to resident cells, which turn over more slowly. Current studies aim to elucidate the subset origin of other recruited populations, for example, in atherosclerosis, normal CNS, and tumors, and in response to metabolic, traumatic, or degenerative injury. Conceptually, it is still not clear how stable these apparently distinct subsets are or whether they represent part of a continuous phenotypic spectrum, arising by modulation of subpopulations rather than irreversible, true differentiation. Separation and microarray analysis of freshly isolated monocytes will yield further information regarding this question, providing novel markers and diagnostic signatures. Removal from an *in vivo* environment, as well as *in vitro* artifacts, can profoundly alter the phenotype and function of monocytes in such studies. Imaging and *in situ* analysis may enable single-cell direct studies of their fate.

Monocyte/macrophages have a major role in the development and progression of cardiovascular disease.[44,45] In acute myocardial infarction

macrophages with an M1 proinflammatory profile migrate to the cardiac tissue and are involved in cardiac remodeling (Chap. 134).[46]

In atherogenesis, there is recruitment of monocytes into the vascular wall at sites of turbulent flow. Once within the subendothelial tissue, the monocytes differentiate into macrophages and engulf oxidized low-density lipoprotein accumulated in arteries, leading to foam cell formation, atheroma development, and the secretion of profibrotic agents by adjacent vascular smooth muscle cells, resulting in a fibrous cap formation. Thus, vascular wall macrophages are key factors in initiating the atherosclerotic lesion. Moreover, macrophages activate the coagulation cascade (Chap. 67) inducing thrombus formation and vascular occlusion.

Resident Macrophage Populations in Adult Tissues Overview

It is important to describe first the nature of those macrophages present throughout the body as resident populations, in the absence of overt inflammation, before considering the altered monocyte-derived macrophages recruited to local sites by infectious or sterile inflammatory (e.g., metabolic) stimuli. The properties of such elicited macrophages are well established and are described in Chap. 67. However the functions of resident macrophages, especially in different organs, are still mysterious and are considered in outline here, with further details in Chap. 67.

The use of differentiation antigens such as F4/80 and cd68 (mouse) and CD68 (human) has made it possible to define resident macrophage populations in mouse tissues,[47] and to compare their anatomic relationships in the two species (Table 68–2). F4/80 (EMR1), a member of a family of epidermal growth factor-7 transmembrane (EGF-TM7)

TABLE 68–1. Selected Markers of Different Monocyte Subsets in Mouse and Human Blood

Antigen	Human CD14hi CD16–	Human CD14+ CD16+	Mouse CCR2+ CX₃CR1low	Mouse CCR2– CX₃CR1hi
CHEMOKINE RECEPTORS				
CCR1	+	–	ND	ND
CCR2	+	–	+	–
CCR4	+	–	ND	ND
CCR5	–	+	ND	ND
CCR7	+	–	ND	ND
CXCR1	+	–	ND	ND
CXCR2	+	–	ND	ND
CXCR4	+	++	ND	ND
CX₃CR1	+	++	+	++
OTHER RECEPTORS				
CD4	+	+	ND	ND
CD11a	ND	ND	+	++
CD11b	++	++	++	++
CD11c	++	+++	–	+
CD14	+++	+	ND	ND
CD31	+++	+++	++	+
CD32	+++	+	ND	ND
CD33	+++	+	ND	ND
CD43	ND	ND	–	+
CD49b	ND	ND	+	–
CD62L	++	–	+	–
CD86	+	++	ND	ND
CD115	++	++	++	++
CD116	++	++	++	++
F4/80	ND	ND	+	+
Ly6C	ND	ND	+	–
7/4	ND	ND	+	–
MHC class II	+	++	–	–

MHC, major histocompatibility complex.

Adapted with permssion from Gordon S. & Taylor PR: Monocyte and macrophage heterogeneity. *Nat Rev Immunol* 5(12):953–964, 2005.

TABLE 68–2. Selected Markers of Mononuclear Phagocytes and Related Cells

Cell Type	Antigen Markers	Other Properties
Monocytes/ macrophages	F4/80 (mouse) EMR2 (human) CD68 CR3 (CD11b) Sialoadhesin (Siglec-1) Scavenger receptors (SR-A, MARCO) Mannose receptor M-CSF receptor	Opsonic phagocytosis; lysozyme secretion; abundant acid hydrolases
Myeloid dendritic cells	MHC II Costimulatory molecules CD11c CD8a+/– DEC205 DC-SIGN DC-LAMP	Activation of naïve CD4 T lymphocytes
Plasmacytoid dendritic cells	CD123 B220 Lectin-like receptors (Siglec-H)	Type I interferon production; *in vitro* growth by flt-3 ligand
Osteoclasts	CD68 TRAP Calcitonin receptor α_vβ_3	Vacuolar H⁺ ATPase; proteinase K; resorption of living bone

ATPase, adenosine triphosphatase; DC, dendritic cell; DC-LAMP, dendritic cell lysosomal-associated membrane protein; DC-SIGN, dendritic cell–specific intercellular adhesion molecule-3–grabbing nonintegrin; EMR, epidermal growth factor module-containing mucin-like hormone receptor; M-CSF, macrophage colony-stimulating factor; MARCO, macrophage receptor with collagenous structure; MHC, major histocompatibility complex; TRAP, tartrate-resistant acid phosphatase.

NOTE: Marker expression is variable, depending on cell localization, maturation, and activation. Some markers are also present on other myeloid cells, e.g., polymorphonuclear cells, and selected endothelial cells.

plasma membrane molecules, is broadly present and almost exclusive to macrophages (Fig. 68–5A to C).[48,49] It is related to G-protein–coupled chemokine receptors in structure, but has a large epidermal growth factor (EGF) domain extracellular extension, thought to be involved in adhesion to extracellular matrix. The human members of this family are more broadly present on myeloid cells; EGF module-containing mucin-like hormone receptor 2 (EMR2) is a useful tissue marker for human macrophages, although it is also present in neutrophils and immature DCs (Fig. 68–5A). Additional macrophage antigen markers useful for immunocytochemical and FACS analysis include Siglec1 (Fig. 68–5D), a sialic acid-binding lectin, the β₂ integrins

CD11b/CD18 (Mac1, CR3), and CD11c, present on DCs and selected, especially alveolar, macrophages.[50] Receptor antigen markers include SR-A,[51] a broadly expressed macrophage receptor additionally found on sinusoidal endothelium, whereas MARCO (macrophage receptor with collagenous structure), a related collagenous SR, is more restricted in expression.[52] Additional markers include lectins such as the macrophage mannose/fucose receptor (MR; Fig. 68–5E).[53] CD163, a receptor for hemoglobin–haptoglobin complexes, is induced by glucocorticoids,[54] IL-10,[54] and substance P.[55] Complement receptors (CRs) and Fc receptors (FcRs) are described in Chap. 67.

The resident macrophages in tissues constitute a major dispersed organ system, responsive to endogenous and exogenous stimuli; they are highly active in uptake of particles and soluble ligands, providing not only sentinels for defense at portals of entry, but also mediating the

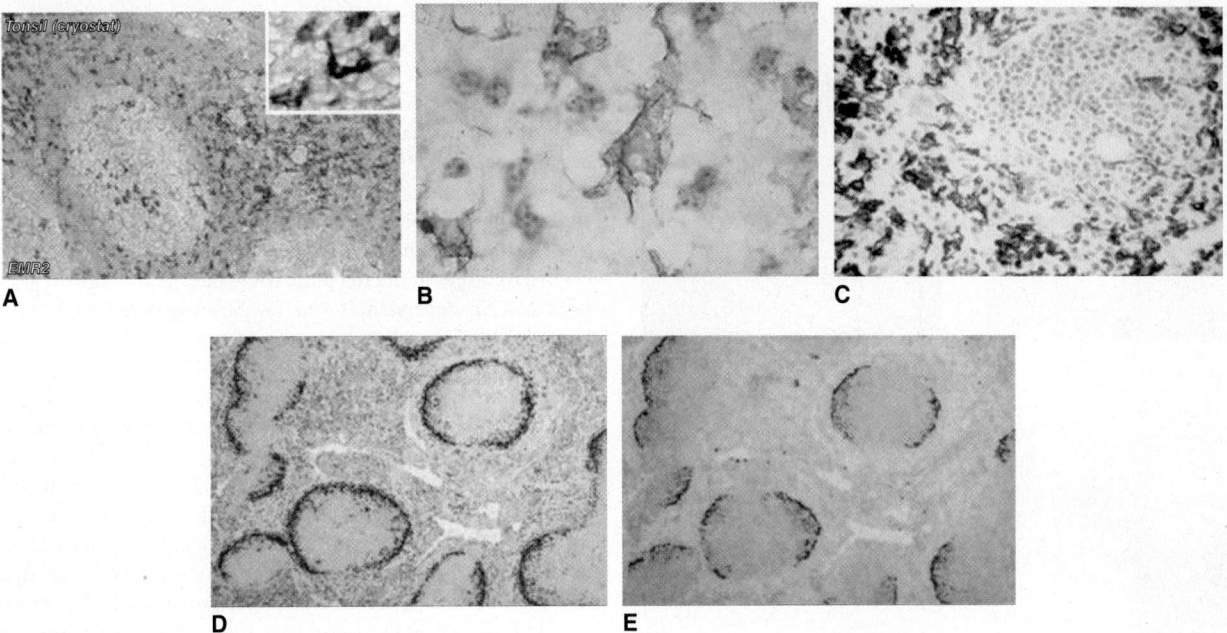

Figure 68–5. Immunocytochemical detection of macrophages in human (**A**) and mouse (**B** to **E**) lymphohematopoietic tissues. **A.** Tonsil. EMR2-positive macrophages are scattered throughout follicles and interfollicular areas. **B.** Liver. Kupffer cells are F4/80+, unlike sinusoidal endothelium and hepatocytes. **C** to **E.** Spleen. **C.** Red pulp macrophages express F4/80, unlike marginal zone cells. Macrophages in T-cell area are F4/80–, except for periarteriolar processes. **D.** Marginal metallophilic macrophages express sialoadhesin (Siglec1) strongly; red pulp macrophages are weakly positive. **E.** A subset of marginal metallophils binds a chimeric protein probe of the cysteine-rich domain of the MR-human Fc. For details see Ref. 91. *(A, used with permission from of T. Marafioti. B to E, reproduced with permission from Taylor PR, Zamze S, Stillion RJ, et al: Development of a specific system for targeting protein to metallophilic macrophages. Proc Natl Acad Sci USA 101(7):1963–1968, 2004.)*

clearance of damaged or dying cells and modulating the properties of viable neighboring cells. In sum, these cells provide a homeostatic, trophic function that is often overlooked in considering their role in cytotoxicity and antimicrobial host defense. The properties of macrophages in hematolymphoid organs and other tissues, with special relevance to hematologic aspects, are discussed in detail.

● DISTRIBUTION

HEMATOPOIETIC ORGANS

Marrow

It is often overlooked that mature macrophages are important constituents of the hematopoietic stroma,[56] along with fibroblastic mesenchymal cells, osteoblasts, and endothelial cells, contributing to hematopoiesis beyond their own differentiation (Figs. 68–6A to E and 68–7). Stromal macrophages in hematopoietic island clusters associate with developing erythroid and other granulocytic cells through nonphagocytic, cell–cell adhesion receptors, such as sialoadhesin and a divalent cation-dependent receptor, as described for fetal liver. The potential trophic functions provided by stromal macrophages are ill-defined but include surface-expressed and secreted growth factors and cytokines. Stromal macrophages are actively endocytic and clear erythroid nuclei and apoptotic hematopoietic cells as required, rapidly degrading them for possible reutilization of iron and other nutrients. Stromal macrophages also interact with less-differentiated hematopoietic precursors through release of potent secretory products, such as IL-1, and with lymphocytic populations, including plasma cells, through IL-6. They are targets for infectious agents, for example, mycobacteria, lentiviruses, and retroviruses, and serve as reservoirs in many chronic infections, while

expressing a reduced killing capacity, as demonstrated for other resident macrophage populations.

Several monocyte and macrophage populations coexist in the marrow compartment; a network of stromal macrophages, clustered in hematopoietic islands, the developing monocytes, as well as osteoclasts and isolated macrophages in apposition to bone surfaces. Mature macrophages in human marrow contain prominent inclusions in storage disorders, such as Gaucher disease and hemosiderosis. Hemophagocytosis, a consequence of perforin deficiency in some patients, and seen in genetic syndromes and postviral infection, is a striking manifestation of excessive macrophage cytopathic activity in the marrow.[57,58] Uptake of opsonized platelets by macrophage FcR and CRs in stromal and other resident tissue macrophages are important features of thrombocytopenic syndromes.

The hematopoietic stem cell lineage which gives rise to monocyte-macrophages and myeloid DCs also leads to production of the osteoclast lineage.[59,60] Following interaction via Stat4 and RANKL (regulator of activation of nuclear factor-κB), a member of the superfamily of TNF, cells undergo differentiation, fusion, attachment to bone as osteoclasts and then function in bone remodeling.[61]

A common marrow progenitor cell that gives rise to both monocytes and DCs has been defined,[20] including both classical DCs and the plasmacytoid DCs.[62,63] This common marrow progenitor cell circulates in the blood and seeds lymphatic tissues.[62,63] These short-lived, migratory cells modify T-cell responses and, unlike Langerhans cells, are replaced by bloodborne precursors.[41,42] The central activity of immature classical DCs is phagocytosis, while that of mature classical DCs is cytokine production.[62,63]

Dendritic cells that occur in lymphoid and nonlymphoid organs have a major role in processing and presenting antigens, leading to

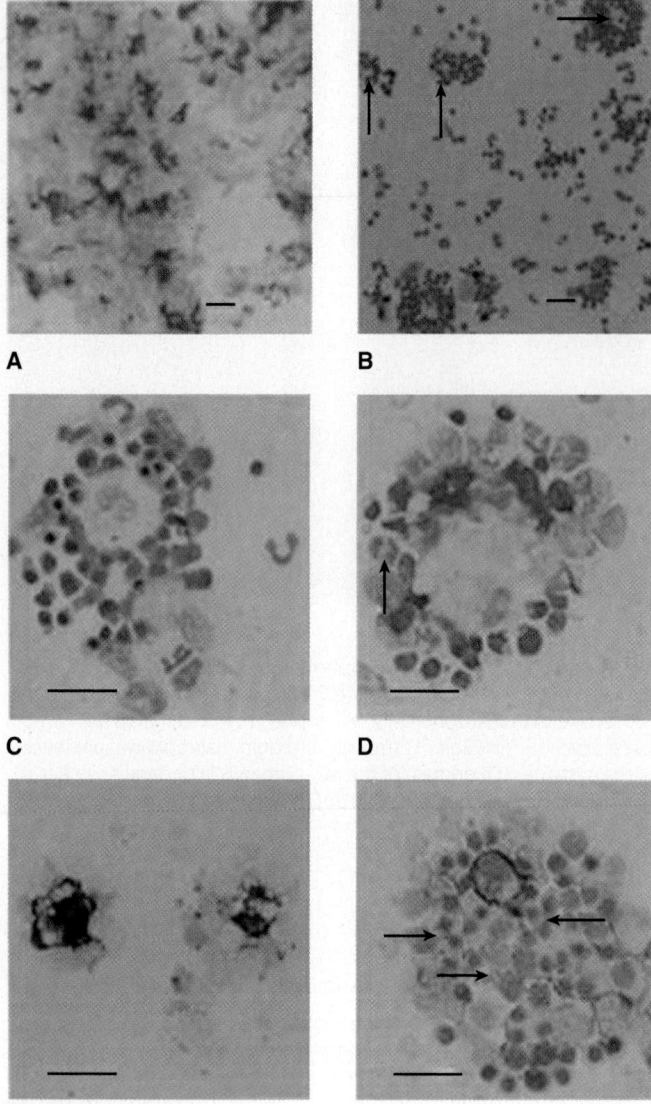

Figure 68–6. Stromal macrophages in human marrow associate with developing hematopoietic cells in islands/clusters. Immunocytochemical staining with antimacrophage monoclonal antibody Y1/82A of marrow section reveals a network of arborizing stromal macrophages uniformly distributed throughout the marrow interstitium (alkaline phosphatase–antialkaline phosphatase [APAAP] stain; hematoxylin counterstain). **B.** Marrow cells depleted of red cells and other single cells are enriched for cell clusters, most of which are erythroid clusters with a central stromal macrophage (*arrows*; Giemsa). **C.** Isolated erythroid cluster with intermediate and late normoblasts surrounding a central stromal macrophage (Giemsa). **D.** Isolated mixed cluster with both myeloid and erythroid cells attached to a central stromal macrophage. A dividing cell (*arrow*) is seen (Giemsa). **E.** Isolated erythroid clusters from a pathologic marrow sample show intense staining for hemosiderin of stromal macrophages with cellular processes extending between attached erythroblasts (Perl acid ferrocyanide reaction; counterstain neutral red). **F.** Immunocytochemical stain with antibody Y1/82A of isolated erythroid cluster. Both the stromal macrophage cell body and processes (*arrows*) between attached erythroblasts are visible (APAAP stain; hematoxylin counterstain). Bar = 50 μm. (*Reproduced with permission from Lee, S.H. et al.: Isolation and immunocytochemical characterization of human bone marrow stromal macrophages in hemopoietic clusters. J Exp Med 168(3):1193–1198, 1988.*)

unique T cell function. The "classical" DC develops from a precursor which is dependent on the growth factor receptor.[62–64]

Spleen

From the macrophage point of view, the spleen is the most complex organ in the body.[65,66] Our knowledge is based mainly on the mouse and we know there is considerable species variation,[67] as well as constitutive hematopoiesis in mouse spleen. Subpopulations observed in the mouse by marker and genetic knockout experiments include (1) macrophages in the red pulp, white pulp, and in the marginal zone, itself M-CSF dependent,[30] and (2) heterogeneous, more phagocytic "metallophilic" macrophages in the outer marginal zone. Characteristic phenotypic markers are available to identify macrophages in mouse spleen (see Fig. 68–5C to E). The F4/80 antigen and the mannose receptor (MR) are restricted to mature macrophages in the red pulp, whereas CD68 is a marker for all macrophages, as well as DCs, although the mainly intracellular expression of CD68 is less prominent in DCs. There are several well-characterized markers for mouse metallophilic macrophages, including sialoadhesin (Sn), a poorly characterized protein recognized by the MOMA-1 monoclonal antibody, and ligands for MR cysteine-rich domain-Fc chimeric proteins (see Fig. 68–5E). The splenic marginal zone macrophage population develops postnatally,[68] in parallel with antipolysaccharide responses to encapsulated bacteria. Functions of splenic marginal zone macrophages include clearance of senescent erythrocytes and neutrophils (red pulp), targeting of circulating antigens and pathogens (marginal zone), interferon (IFN) production, induction of secondary adaptive immune responses, regulation of hematopoiesis, and iron storage. Markers for the outer marginal zone macrophages include MARCO and SIGNR1, a mouse homologue of dendritic cell–specific intercellular adhesion molecule-3–grabbing nonintegrin (DC-SIGN). The spleen is also a site for storage and rapid deployment of monocytes, which participate in wound healing and play a role regulation of inflammation.[69]

Lymph Nodes

Lymph node macrophages are also heterogeneous, with distinctive Sn subcapsular cells, corresponding to marginal metallophils in their marker expression, and F4/80+ macrophages in germinal follicles and in the hilus. Macrophages in T-lymphocyte–rich areas are F4/80– or dim, as in T-cell areas in spleen, but express CD68. It is thought that antigen enters lymph nodes via afferent lymphatics and two photon experiments have defined the possible transfer of viral and other antigens and immune complexes to B lymphocytes after capture by the subcapsular sinus macrophages.[70] Their contributions to the initiation of adaptive immune responses, compared with DCs, are unclear. Tingible body macrophages arise from the clearance of apoptotic B cells in germinal centers, as in the spleen.

Nonlymphohematopoietic Organs

In bulk, the gastrointestinal tract represents the largest accumulation of F4/80+ macrophages in the body, extending throughout the upper and lower gut. The small intestine is essentially sterile, and the abundant F4/80+ resident macrophages in the lamina propria express a distinct phenotype, ascribed to TGF-β production by adjacent cells.[56,71–73] The liver contains an abundant population of sinusoidal F4/80+ Kupffer cells, which share some properties (FcR, MR, SR-A) with sinusoidal endothelium, which lacks F4/80. The skin has F4/80+ epidermal Langerhans cells and F4/80+ dermal macrophages, which can migrate to draining lymph nodes and differentiate into antigen-presenting DCs.[74,75] The lung has a distinctive F4/80– or dim alveolar macrophage population, as well as interstitial F4/80+ macrophages. Alveolar macrophages are CD11c+ and express a range of nonopsonic phagocytic

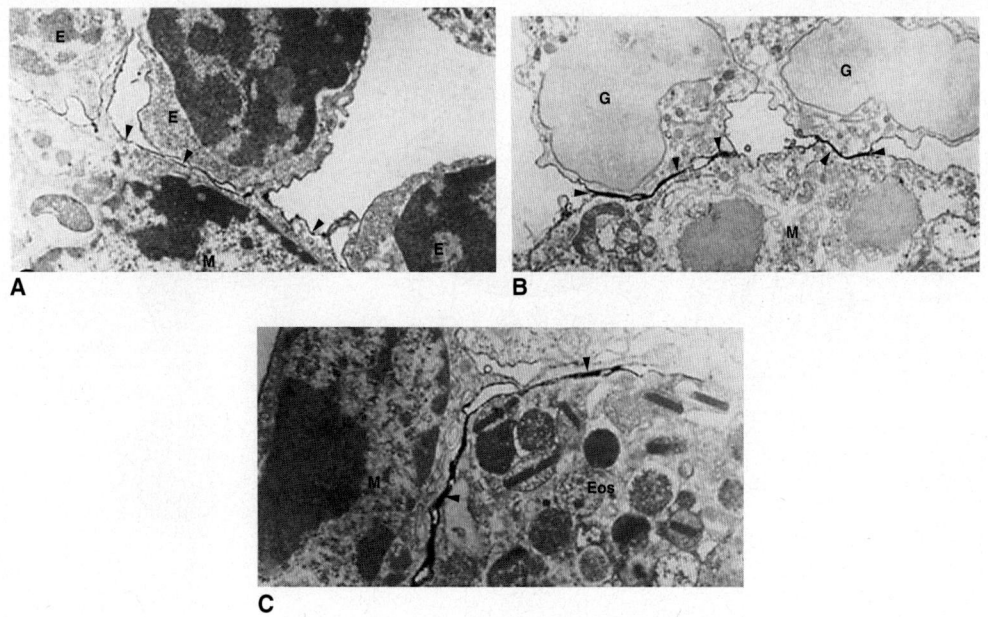

Figure 68–7. Sialoadhesin (Siglec1) *(arrowheads)* is clustered at sites of stromal macrophage adhesion to developing cells (**B**, granulocytes; **C**, eosinophils) but diffusely present in association with erythroblasts **(A)**. For details see Ref. 93. *(Reproduced with permission from Crocker PR, Werb Z, Gordon S, et al: Ultrastructural localization of a macrophage-restricted sialic acid binding hemagglutinin, SER, in macrophage-hematopoietic cell clusters. Blood 76(6):1131–1138, 1990.)*

receptors (MR, SR-A), as well as FcR, but lack CR3. These cells also contain particle debris, cigarette smoke residue, and abundant lysozyme, because of exposure to irritants and uptake of carbon and dust particles, as well as of mucosal secretions in the airway.

The central nervous system contains an extensive network of F4/80+ CR3+ microglia, derived from monocytes during development, when they remove apoptotic neurons.[18] They differentiate into characteristic membrane-rich arborized forms within the neuropil and persist throughout adult life. Their function is obscure but may involve homeostasis and catabolism of neurotransmitters. In addition, there are perivascular F4/80+ macrophages (also MR+ SR-A+) and other F4/80+ populations in the meningeal space and choroid plexus. The endocrine, exocrine, reproductive, and urinary tracts all contain macrophage populations at sites of phagocytosis (ovary, testes) and hormonal metabolism (adrenal, thyroid, for example).[71] Precise characterization of these cell types using monoclonal antibodies with specificity for human cell types in tissue requires further analysis.

● ACTIVATION STATE

RECRUITMENT OF MONOCYTES IN RESPONSE TO INFLAMMATION AND TUMORS

The stimuli that give rise to induced recruitment of monocytes, with or without accompanying myeloid and/or lymphoid cells, and the mechanisms involved are better understood than those of constitutive tissue localization. Bacterial infections induce enhanced myelomonocytic cell recruitment and follow the stages established for neutrophils, transient arrest, and rolling on the microvascular endothelium, mediated by L-selectin, and initiated by chemotactic stimuli acting via G-protein-coupled chemokine receptors (Fig. 68–8). The β_2 integrins CD11a/CD18 and CD11b/CD18 mediate more stable adhesion. This is followed by diapedesis and interactions with CD31. Receptors implicated in subsequent extravascular migration are less defined but may include the fractalkine receptor, and intravascularly, β_1- and β_2-integrin, CD44, and

EMR2. The evidence for an important role of L-selectin and β_2 integrins in human phagocyte recruitment to inflammatory stimuli comes from human inborn error syndromes, mouse genetic experiments, and antibody inhibition. The role of the common β_2-integrin chain (CD18) and definition of leukocyte adhesion deficiency syndrome provided a powerful paradigm for further experimental study of CD11/CD18.[76,77] Cellular signaling gives rise to dynamic changes in migration/adhesion and cytoskeletal reorganization outlined further in Chap. 67. Studies of tumor-associated macrophages (TAMs) in mouse model systems, particularly mammary cancer, have identified a population of unique macrophages. The TAMs develop from marrow-derived macrophages that are inflammatory phenotypes and are recruited to the tumor.[78,79]

Mononuclear cell recruitment without that of other myeloid cells is a feature of viral infection and modified forms of inflammation observed in metabolic diseases, atherosclerosis, storage disorders, autoimmunity, and tumors. Different chemokine receptors and cell adhesion molecules account, in part, for more selective monocytic recruitment, although some are shared. The phenotypic heterogeneity in monocyte subsets is characterized by quantitative differences in expression of plasma membrane molecules resulting in differential recruitment of subsets in response to different stimuli. Once in the tissues, their subsequent fate also varies markedly, depending on the local environment, where newly recruited monocytes respond to tissue-specific factors. A striking example is that observed in the neutrophil, where monocytes can differentiate over a few days into highly arborized, activated microglia, resembling locally reactivated resident microglia.[18] Thus, it becomes progressively more difficult to distinguish newly recruited from initially resident cells through marker analysis. Direct observation by fluorescent imaging *in vivo* may define precursor–product relationships more clearly. Similar issues arise in other organs, for example, lung, liver, gut, and even in skin, where static observations can be misleading. There are also common features of recruited cells irrespective of the local tissue environment, including the expression of CD11b/CD18 and monocytic adhesion molecules, and metabolic markers, such as the ability to undergo a respiratory burst and an increased proliferative potential and

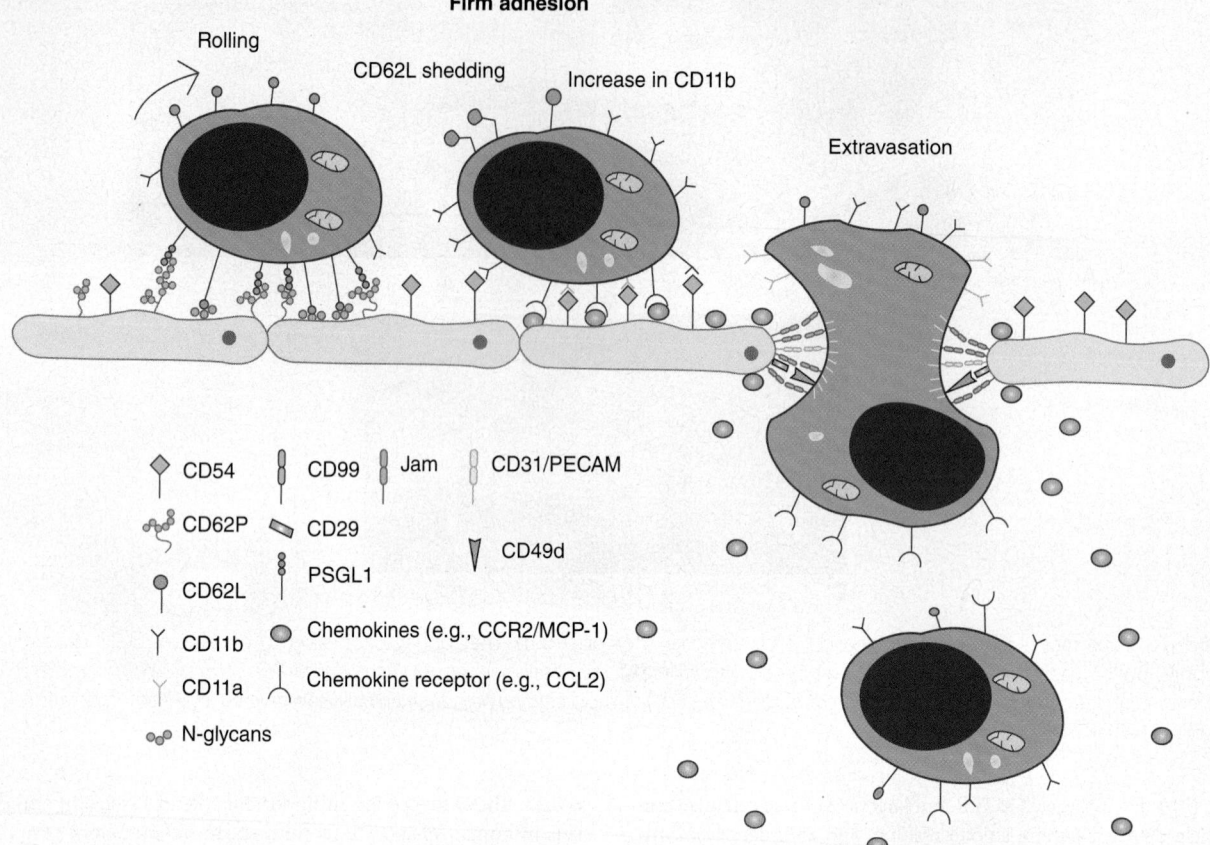

Figure 68–8. Recruitment. Stages of monocyte adherence to endothelium and diapedesis, induced by inflammatory stimuli. The model is mainly based on the recruitment of neutrophils, with which it shares many features, although monocyte-specific chemokines, receptors, and adhesion ligands exist, especially in constitutive and noninfectious, metabolic forms of inflammation. PECAM, platelet endothelial cell adhesion molecule.

high cell turnover rate. These monocytic markers tend to decline upon further macrophage differentiation, and in the case of myeloperoxidase may not be renewed after degranulation.

HETEROGENEITY OF MACROPHAGES IN TISSUES: IMMUNOMODULATION

Characterization of the macrophages found in tissues has yielded insights into their versatility in response to microbial constituents and cytokines produced by lymphoid, other immune and nonimmune cells. Adhesion to extracellular matrix, metabolites, vascular, and hormonal changes all influence the macrophage phenotype. This variety of stimuli can selectively activate or deactivate macrophage gene and protein expression, regulating their function. Figure 68–9 illustrates some of the stereotypic signature phenotypes, and Chap. 67 further describes the innate recognition mechanisms and functional responses.

Broadly considered, it is convenient to distinguish several clusters of activation properties; innate, classical, and alternative activation, and deactivation. The definition of activation has a long and confusing history, has mainly been based on limited models of analysis, typically peritoneal macrophages *in vivo* and *in vitro*, and on studies with macrophage-like cell lines. The advent of microarrays and of proteomics and systems biology has generated increasingly detailed information. It makes sense to schematize the interactions of monocytes and macrophages with microorganisms, microbial products, and Th1/Th2 lymphocytes, although this is subject to revision as CD4 T-lymphocyte

heterogeneity continues to grow in complexity, with the description of Th17, FoxP3+, and other regulatory T cells. Further details are given in Chap. 67.

INNATE ACTIVATION

For this discussion, innate activation is defined as direct microbial stimulation by intact bacteria or their constituents, such as LPS acting via toll-like receptor (TLR) sensors, in the absence of the major Th1/2 cytokines. For example, ethanol-killed *Neisseria meningitidis*, a potent immunomodulator with adjuvant-like properties, stimulates the expression of two useful markers on macrophages: MARCO and CD200. Expression of MARCO, a class A SR, is remarkably specific for macrophages (and DCs) and is regulated developmentally on the outer marginal zone macrophages, but it is inducible on most macrophage populations by TLR and myeloid differentiation factor 88 (MyD88)-dependent bacterial stimuli. It is a phagocytic and adhesion receptor providing an adaptive, enhanced ability to take up *Neisseria* and other bacteria, after innate activation. CD200, an immunoglobulin (Ig) superfamily member, is widely expressed on many cells, but not on resident macrophages, and part of an immunoregulatory receptor pair with CD200 R, is also induced on macrophages by innate stimuli.

Lectins, such as Dectin-1, control innate activation of macrophages by β glucans in fungal walls,[80] in collaboration with TLR pathways, as discussed in Chap. 67. TLR-independent innate activation by viruses, parasites, and other pathogen-associated stimuli requires further study.

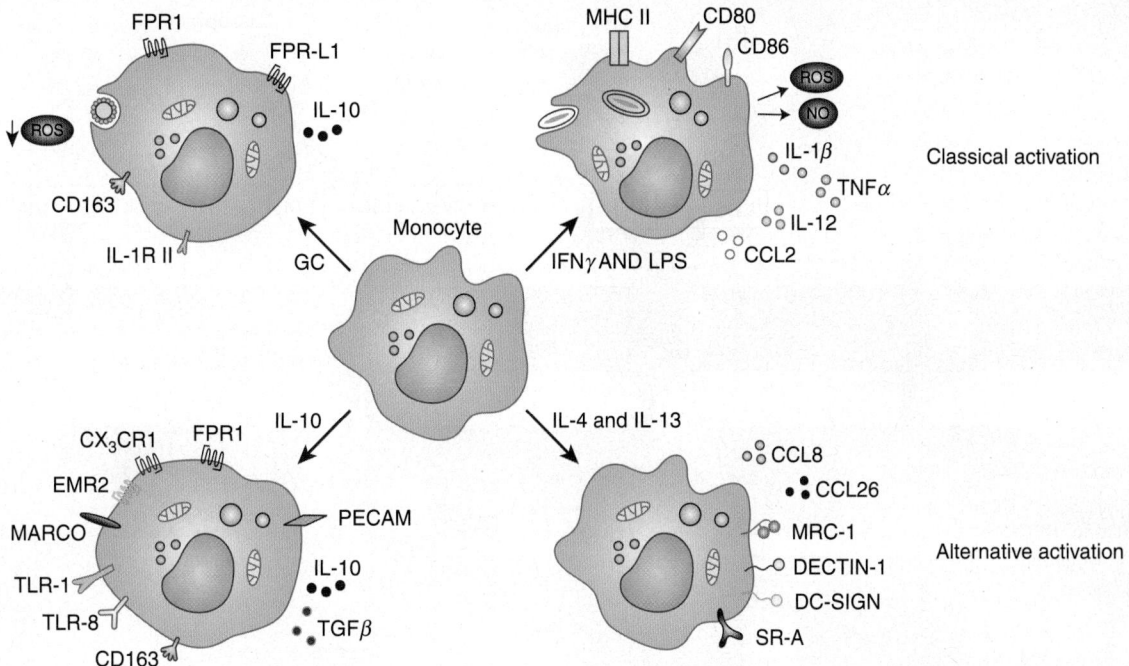

Figure 68–9. Immunomodulation of macrophage phenotype by cytokines, microbial constituents, and glucocorticosteroids. CCL, chemokines; CR, complement receptor; DC-SIGN, dendritic cell–specific intercellular adhesion molecule-3–grabbing nonintegrin; EMR, epidermal growth factor module-containing mucin-like hormone receptor; FPR1, formyl-peptide receptor 1; FPRL-1, formyl-peptide receptor-like 1; GC, glucocorticoids; IL, interleukin; INFγ, interferon-γ; LPS, lipopolysaccharide; MARCO, macrophage receptor with a collagenous structure; MRC-1, mannose receptor C-type 1; NO, nitric oxide; PECAM, platelet endothelial cell adhesion molecule-1; ROS, reactive oxygen species; SR-A, scavenger receptor A; TLR, toll-like receptor; TNF-α, tumor necrosis factor-α. Further details on innate modulation of phenotype by microbial products are given in Chap. 67. (*Adapted with permission from Yona, S. & Gordon, S.: Inflammation: Glucocorticoids turn the monocyte switch.* Immunol Cell Biol 85(2):81–82, 2007.)

CYTOKINE-INDUCED PRIMING AND ACTIVATION: CLASSICAL AND ALTERNATIVE ACTIVATION

Investigations in normal humans, pathologic states, and animal models have led to the characterization of different states of macrophage polarization (Fig. 68–10).[81] The terms macrophage "activation and "polarization" require well-defined nomenclature and experimental guidelines. It has been recommended that the term "activation" be used to refer to perturbation of macrophages with exogenous agents the same way that many authors use "polarization."[82] Studies of *in vitro*, *ex vivo*, and *in vivo* cells from animals and humans have led to descriptions of complex cellular structural, biochemical, and functional activation states of macrophages. Consequently, it is essential to describe the properties of the macrophage its activation/polarization state. There are various nomenclatures and Fig. 68–10 indicates the major features of the M1–M2 dichotomy. This dichotomy, however, is more of a continuum and there are transitional states. The most useful approach is to describe the spectrum of activation states by cell isolation technique, membrane receptors, cytokines, chemokines, and metabolic markers, and when possible, genetic modifications producing shifts in activation phenotype. This approach is essential for deciphering the role of monocyte–macrophages in disease pathogenesis.

Macrophage polarization usually is driven by unique pattern recognition receptors (PRRs). Classical activation of macrophages or M1 in general[83] have a proinflammatory profile. This pathway is triggered by IFN-γ followed by a microbial stimulus, LPS. The M1 macrophage is characterized by high antigen presentation and production of IL-12, IL-23, nitric oxide, and proinflammatory cytokines, including IL-1, TNF-α, IL-6, and CXCL-1, -2, -3, -5, -8, -9, and -10. The pathway to the

alternative M2 macrophage is mediated by IL-4, IL-10, and IL-13. These cells demonstrate enhanced expression of Dectin-1, MR C1 (CD206), CD163, CCR2, CXCR1, CXCR2, and DC-SIGN.[84] M2 produce high levels of IL-10 and low-levels of IL-12.[85] IFN-γ, produced mainly by natural killer cells and activated Th1 CD4+ and CD8+ cytotoxic lymphocytes, induces a set of macrophage biosynthetic and effector responses, known as classical activation, because of its well-established role in enhanced macrophage functions in cell-mediated immunity, inflammation, and host defense, particularly against intracellular pathogens. Full activation of effector functions, such as the respiratory burst and generation of oxidative nitrogen metabolites, depends on a two-stage mechanism of priming by the cytokine, via specific IFN-γ receptors, followed by a local stimulus, LPS, or other TLR ligands. Although essential for host defense, including against opportunistic pathogens such as found in patients with the acquired immunodeficiency syndrome, classical activation is responsible for tissue injury and its consequences in inflammatory bowel disease, tuberculosis, and rheumatoid arthritis, although additional immunopathogenic agents, such as immune complexes, also contribute. Biochemical and cellular aspects of classical activation are described in Chap. 67.

The Th2 cytokines IL-4 and IL-13, acting via a common receptor chain as well as distinct receptors, induce a characteristic signature of altered gene expression in macrophages known as alternative activation.[86,87] Such primed macrophages can be induced to respond further to local, TLR-dependent phagocytic stimuli to secrete enhanced levels of proinflammatory cytokines, analogous to classically activated macrophages. Alternative activation is associated with allergy and parasitic infection, and has been implicated in humoral immunity, control of Th1-dependent inflammation, and host defense to extracellular pathogens, such as helminths. It can promote repair or, if excessive, fibrosis.

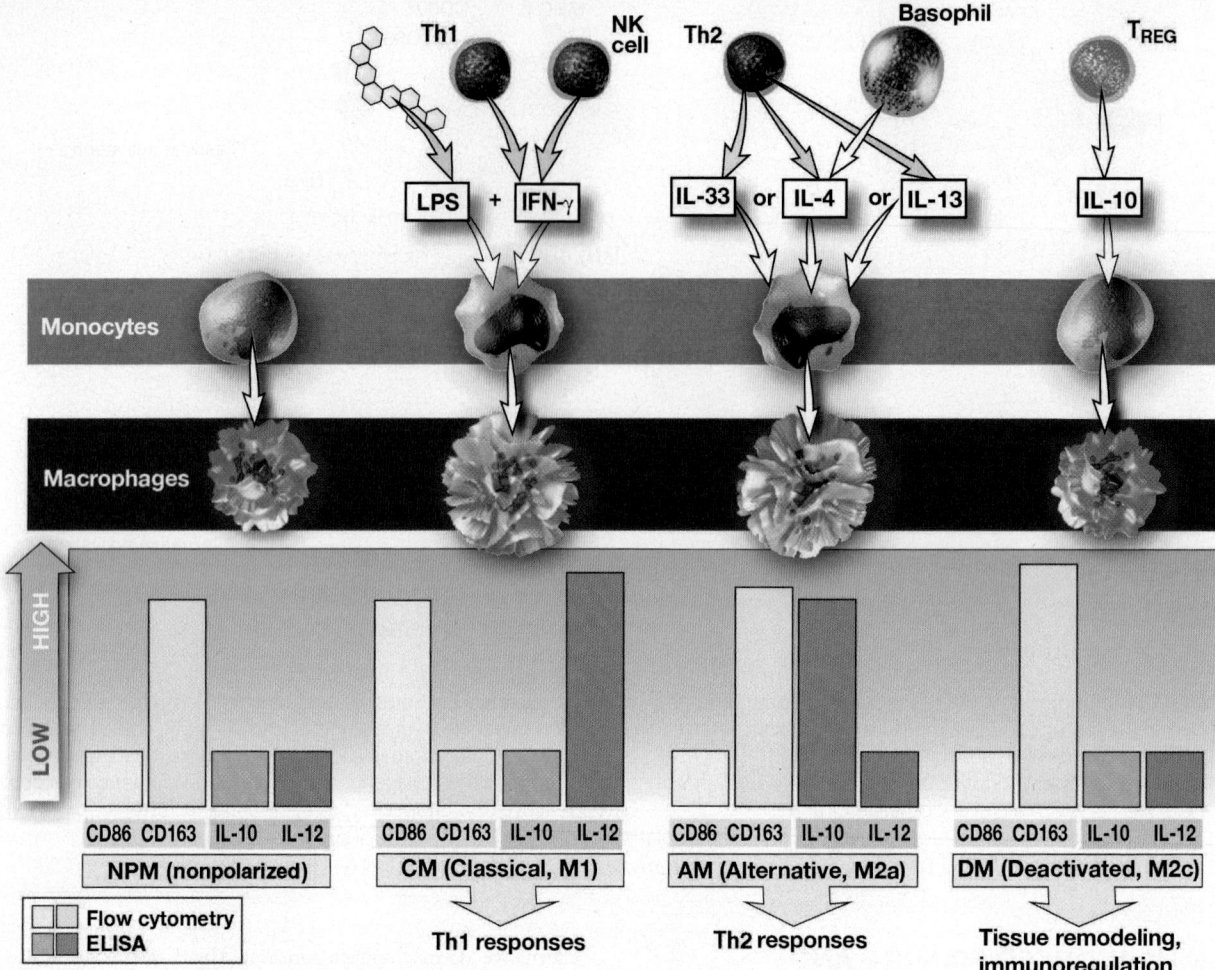

Figure 68-10. Schema of states of monocyte-macrophage activation. AM, alternative M2A; CM, classical (M) activation; DM, M2C deactivated; NPM, nonpolarized. Membrane markers expression in yellow. Flow cytometry and cytokines enzyme-linked immunosorbent assay (ELISA) in blue. IFN-γ, interferon-γ; IL, interleukin; LPS, lipopolysaccharide; NK, natural killer; Th1/Th2, T-helper type 1/2; T_{REG}, T regulatory cell. *(Used with permission of S. Seif, GraphisMedica, 2014.)*

Other forms of alternative activation have been described after stimulation of macrophages by immune complexes, acting via FcR. A major G-protein–coupled receptor that is important in macrophage activation is the Neurokinin-1 receptor.[88] This receptor, which has a full-length form and a truncated splice variant, is important in macrophage signaling and calcium fluxes.[89,90] An important caveat is that there are substantial species differences in the marker changes depending on the differentiation and prior activation state of the macrophages.

IL-10 is a major deactivating cytokine for macrophages, produced by the macrophages themselves, as well as by Th2 lymphocytes and other sources. Acting through its own receptor, it counteracts IFN-γ, and can potentiate IL-4–induced actions. Other antiinflammatory regulators of macrophages activation include glucocorticoids and prostaglandin E_2. Although less-well defined, the overall gene and protein expression profiles of macrophages are also markedly influenced by the extracellular matrix, hormones, and other immunomodulators, so that modified forms of inflammation are associated with macrophages present in lipid-rich environments, tumors, and metabolic diseases. Finally, cell–cell interactions, as well as intracellular regulatory networks, profoundly influence the functions of macrophages, and are described in Chap. 67.

REFERENCES

1. Gordon S: The macrophage: Past, present and future. *Eur J Immunol* 37 (Suppl 1):S9–S17, 2007.
2. Jung S, Aliberti J, Graemmel P, et al: Analysis of fractalkine receptor CX(3)CR1 function by targeted deletion and green fluorescent protein reporter gene insertion. *Mol Cell Biol* 20:4106–4114, 2000.
3. Herbert DR, Hölscher C, Mohrs M, et al: Alternative macrophage activation is essential for survival during schistosomiasis and downmodulates T helper 1 responses and immunopathology. *Immunity* 20:623–635, 2004.
4. Beutler B, Casanova JL: New frontiers in immunology. Workshop on the road ahead: Future directions in fundamental and clinical immunology. *EMBO Rep* 6:620–623, 2005.
5. Georgel P, Du X, Hoebe K, Beutler B: ENU mutagenesis in mice. *Methods Mol Biol* 415:1–16, 2008.
6. Herbomel P, Levraud JP: Imaging early macrophage differentiation, migration, and behaviors in live zebrafish embryos. *Methods Mol Med* 105:199–214, 2005.
7. Lemaitre B, Hoffmann J: The host defense of *Drosophila melanogaster*. *Annu Rev Immunol* 25:697–743, 2007.
8. Frankel LB, Christoffersen NR, Jacobsen A, et al: Programmed cell death 4 (PDCD4) is an important functional target of the microRNA miR-21 in breast cancer cells. *J Biol Chem* 283:1026–1033, 2008.
9. Egen JG, Rothfuchs AG, Feng CG, et al: Macrophage and T cell dynamics during the development and disintegration of mycobacterial granulomas. *Immunity* 28:271–284, 2008.
10. Karlsson KR, Cowley S, Martinez FO, et al: Homogeneous monocytes and macrophages from human embryonic stem cells following coculture-free differentiation in M-CSF and IL-3. *Exp Hematol* 36:1167–1175, 2008.

11. Day RM, Harbord M, Forbes A, Segal AW: Cantharidin blisters: A technique for investigating leukocyte trafficking and cytokine production at sites of inflammation in humans. *J Immunol Methods* 257:213–220, 2001.

12. Gordon S: Elie Metchnikoff: Father of natural immunity. *Eur J Immunol* 38:3257–3264, 2008.

13. Crocker PR, Morris L, Gordon S: Novel cell surface adhesion receptors involved in interactions between stromal macrophages and haematopoietic cells. *J Cell Sci Suppl* 9:185–206, 1988.

14. Fabriek BO, Polfliet MM, Vloet RP, et al: The macrophage CD163 surface glycoprotein is an erythroblast adhesion receptor. *Blood* 109:5223–5229, 2007.

15. Crocker PR, Gordon S: Mouse macrophage hemagglutinin (sheep erythrocyte receptor) with specificity for sialylated glycoconjugates characterized by a monoclonal antibody. *J Exp Med* 169:1333–1346, 1989.

16. Bessis M, Mize C, Prenant M: Erythropoiesis: Comparison of *in vivo* and *in vitro* amplification. *Blood Cells* 4:155–174, 1978.

17. Redd MJ, Cooper L, Wood W, et al: Wound healing and inflammation: Embryos reveal the way to perfect repair. *Philos Trans R Soc Lond B Biol Sci* 359:777–784, 2004.

18. Perry VH, Andersson PB, Gordon S: Macrophages and inflammation in the central nervous system. *Trends Neurosci* 16:268–273, 1993.

19. Hughes DA, Gordon S: Expression and function of the type 3 complement receptor in tissues of the developing mouse. *J Immunol* 160:4543–4552, 1998.

20. Auffray C, Sieweke MH, Geissmann F: Blood monocytes: Development, heterogeneity, and relationship with dendritic cells. *Annu Rev Immunol* 27:669–692, 2009.

21. Glass CK, Ogawa S: Combinatorial roles of nuclear receptors in inflammation and immunity. *Nat Rev Immunol* 6:44–55, 2006.

22. Lewis M, Lewis W: Transformation of mononuclear blood-cells into macrophages, epithelioid cells, and giant cells in hanging-drop blood-cultures from lower vertebrates. *Contrib Embryol* 18:95, 1926.

23. Maximow A: The macrophages or histiocytes, in *Special Cytology: The Form and Functions of the Cell in Health and Disease,* edited by Cowdry E, p 711. Hoeber-Harper, New York, 1932.

24. Ebert RF, Florey HW: The extravascular development of the monocyte observed *in vitro. Br J Exp Pathol* 20:341, 1939.

25. Sutton JS, Weiss L: Transformation of monocytes in tissue culture into macrophages, epithelioid cells, and multinucleated giant cells. An electron microscope study. *J Cell Biol* 28:303–332, 1966.

26. Hassan NF, Kamani N, Meszaros MM, Douglas SD: Induction of multinucleated giant cell formation from human blood-derived monocytes by phorbol myristate acetate in in vitro culture. *J Immunol* 143:2179–2184, 1989.

27. Hume DA: Macrophages as APC and the dendritic cell myth. *J Immunol* 181:5829–5835, 2008.

28. Yu W, Chen J, Xiong Y, et al: CSF-1 receptor structure/function in MacCsf1r-/- macrophages: Regulation of proliferation, differentiation, and morphology. *J Leukoc Biol* 84:852–863, 2008.

29. Pixley FJ, Stanley ER: CSF-1 regulation of the wandering macrophage: Complexity in action. *Trends Cell Biol* 14:628–638, 2004.

30. Witmer-Pack MD, Hughes DA, Schuler G, et al: Identification of macrophages and dendritic cells in the osteopetrotic (op/op) mouse. *J Cell Sci* 104:1021–1029, 1993.

31. Inaba K, Swiggard WJ, Steinman RM, Romani N, Schuler G: Isolation of dendritic cells. *Curr Protoc Immunol* Chapter 3:Unit 3.7, 2001.

32. Sallusto F, Lanzavecchia A: Efficient presentation of soluble antigen by cultured human dendritic cells is maintained by granulocyte/macrophage colony-stimulating factor plus interleukin 4 and downregulated by tumor necrosis factor alpha. *J Exp Med* 179:1109–1118, 1994.

33. Dranoff G, Mulligan RC: Activities of granulocyte-macrophage colony-stimulating factor revealed by gene transfer and gene knockout studies. *Stem Cells* 12 (Suppl 1):173–182; discussion 182–184, 1994.

34. Gordon S, Taylor PR: Monocyte and macrophage heterogeneity. *Nat Rev Immunol* 5:953–964, 2005.

35. Lumeng CN, DelProposto JB, Westcott DJ, Saltiel AR: Phenotypic switching of adipose tissue macrophages with obesity is generated by spatiotemporal differences in macrophage subtypes. *Diabetes* 57:3239–3246, 2008.

36. Weisberg SP, McCann D, Desai M, et al: Obesity is associated with macrophage accumulation in adipose tissue. *J Clin Invest* 112:1796–1808, 2003.

37. Lumeng CN, Bodzin JL, Saltiel AR: Obesity induces a phenotypic switch in adipose tissue macrophage polarization. *J Clin Invest* 117:175–184, 2007.

38. Weisberg SP, Hunter D, Huber R, et al: CCR2 modulates inflammatory and metabolic effects of high-fat feeding. *J Clin Invest* 116:115–124, 2006.

39. Hotamisligil GS: Inflammation and metabolic disorders. *Nature* 444:860–867, 2006.

40. Olefsky JM, Glass CK: Macrophages, inflammation, and insulin resistance. *Annu Rev Physiol* 72:219–246, 2010.

41. Shoelson SE, Lee J, Goldfine AB: Inflammation and insulin resistance. *J Clin Invest* 116:1793–1801, 2006.

42. Odegaard JI, Chawla A: Mechanisms of macrophage activation in obesity-induced insulin resistance. *Nat Clin Pract Endocrinol Metab* 4:619–626, 2008.

43. Ferrante AW Jr: Obesity-induced inflammation: A metabolic dialogue in the language of inflammation. *J Intern Med* 262:408–414, 2007.

44. Fernandez-Velasco M, Gonzalez-Ramos S, Bosca L: Involvement of monocytes/macrophages as key factors in the development and progression of cardiovascular diseases. *Biochem J* 458:187–193, 2014.

45. Epelman S, Lavine KJ, Randolph GJ: Origin and functions of tissue macrophages. *Immunity* 41:21–35, 2014.

46. Anzai A, Anzai T, Nagai S, et al: Regulatory role of dendritic cells in postinfarction healing and left ventricular remodeling. *Circulation* 125:1234–1245, 2012.

47. Taylor PR, Martinez-Pomares L, Stacey M, et al: Macrophage receptors and immune recognition. *Annu Rev Immunol* 23:901–944, 2005.

48. Yona S, Gordon S: Inflammation: Glucocorticoids turn the monocyte switch. *Immunol Cell Biol* 85:81–82, 2007.

49. Yona S, Lin HH, Siu WO, et al: Adhesion-GPCRs: Emerging roles for novel receptors. *Trends Biochem Sci* 33:491–500, 2008.

50. Holt PG, Oliver J, Bilyk N, et al: Downregulation of the antigen presenting cell function(s) of pulmonary dendritic cells *in vivo* by resident alveolar macrophages. *J Exp Med* 177:397–407, 1993.

51. Fraser I, Hughes D, Gordon S: Divalent cation-independent macrophage adhesion inhibited by monoclonal antibody to murine scavenger receptor. *Nature* 364:343–346, 1993.

52. van der Laan LJ, Kangas M, Döpp EA, et al: Macrophage scavenger receptor MARCO: *In vitro* and *in vivo* regulation and involvement in the anti-bacterial host defense. *Immunol Lett* 57:203–208, 1997.

53. Taylor PR, Gordon S, Martinez-Pomares L: The mannose receptor: Linking homeostasis and immunity through sugar recognition. *Trends Immunol* 26:104–110, 2005.

54. Kristiansen M, Graversen JH, Jacobsen C, et al: Identification of the haemoglobin scavenger receptor. *Nature* 409:198–201, 2001.

55. Tuluc F, Meshki J, Spitsin S, Douglas SD: HIV infection of macrophages is enhanced in the presence of increased expression of CD163 induced by substance P. *J Leukoc Biol* 96:143–150, 2014.

56. Hume DA, Robinson AP, MacPherson GG, Gordon S: The mononuclear phagocyte system of the mouse defined by immunohistochemical localization of antigen F4/80. Relationship between macrophages, Langerhans cells, reticular cells, and dendritic cells in lymphoid and hematopoietic organs. *J Exp Med* 158:1522–1536, 1983.

57. Chu T, Jaffe R: The normal Langerhans cell and the LCH cell. *Br J Cancer Suppl* 23:S4–S10, 1994.

58. Favara BE, Jaffe R, Egeler RM: Macrophage activation and hemophagocytic syndrome in Langerhans cell histiocytosis: Report of 30 cases. *Pediatr Dev Pathol* 5:130–140, 2002.

59. Moreno JL, Kaczmarek M, Keegan AD, Tondravi M: IL-4 suppresses osteoclast development and mature osteoclast function by a STAT6-dependent mechanism: Irreversible inhibition of the differentiation program activated by RANKL. *Blood* 102:1078–1086, 2003.

60. Edwards JR, Mundy GR: Advances in osteoclast biology: Old findings and new insights from mouse models. *Nat Rev Rheumatol* 7:235–243, 2011.

61. Mori G, D'Amelio P, Faccio R, Brunetti G: The interplay between the bone and the immune system. *Clin Dev Immunol* 2013:720504, 2013.

62. Liu K, Victora GD, Schwickert TA, et al: *In vivo* analysis of dendritic cell development and homeostasis. *Science* 324:392–397, 2009.

63. Geissmann F, Manz MG, Jung S, et al: Development of monocytes, macrophages, and dendritic cells. *Science* 327:656–661, 2010.

64. Steinman RM: Decisions about dendritic cells: Past, present, and future. *Annu Rev Immunol* 30:1–22, 2012.

65. Martinez-Pomares L, Kosco-Vilbois M, Darley E, et al: Fc chimeric protein containing the cysteine-rich domain of the murine mannose receptor binds to macrophages from splenic marginal zone and lymph node subcapsular sinus and to germinal centers. *J Exp Med* 184:1927–1937, 1996.

66. Mebius RE, Kraal G: Structure and function of the spleen. *Nat Rev Immunol* 5:606–616, 2005.

67. Martinez-Pomares L, Hanitsch LG, Stillion R, et al: Expression of mannose receptor and ligands for its cysteine-rich domain in venous sinuses of human spleen. *Lab Invest* 85:1238–1249, 2005.

68. Morris L, Crocker PR, Hill M, Gordon S: Developmental regulation of sialoadhesin (sheep erythrocyte receptor), a macrophage-cell interaction molecule expressed in lymphohemopoietic tissues. *Dev Immunol* 2:7–17, 1992.

69. Swirski FK, Nahrendorf M, Etzrodt M, et al: Identification of splenic reservoir monocytes and their deployment to inflammatory sites. *Science* 325:612–616, 2009.

70. Martinez-Pomares L, Gordon S: Antigen presentation the macrophage way. *Cell* 131:641–643, 2007.

71. Hume DA, Halpin D, Charlton H, Gordon S: The mononuclear phagocyte system of the mouse defined by immunohistochemical localization of antigen F4/80: Macrophages of endocrine organs. *Proc Natl Acad Sci U S A* 81:4174–4177, 1984.

72. Smythies LE, Maheshwari A, Clements R, et al: Mucosal IL-8 and TGF-beta recruit blood monocytes: Evidence for cross-talk between the lamina propria stroma and myeloid cells. *J Leukoc Biol* 80:492–499, 2006.

73. Smythies LE, Sellers M, Clements RH, et al: Human intestinal macrophages display profound inflammatory anergy despite avid phagocytic and bacteriocidal activity. *J Clin Invest* 115:66–75, 2005.

74. Haniffa M, Ginhoux F, Wang XN, et al: Differential rates of replacement of human dermal dendritic cells and macrophages during hematopoietic stem cell transplantation. *J Exp Med* 206:371–385, 2009.

75. McKenzie EJ, Taylor PR, Stillion RJ, et al: Mannose receptor expression and function define a new population of murine dendritic cells. *J Immunol* 178:4975–4983, 2007.

76. Arnaout MA: Leukocyte adhesion molecules deficiency: Its structural basis, pathophysiology and implications for modulating the inflammatory response. *Immunol Rev* 114:145–180, 1990.

77. Luo BH, Carman CV, Springer TA: Structural basis of integrin regulation and signaling. *Annu Rev Immunol* 25:619–647, 2007.

78. Franklin RA, Liao W, Sarkar A, et al: The cellular and molecular origin of tumor-associated macrophages. *Science* 344:921–925, 2014.

79. Gomez Perdiguero E, Geissmann F: Cancer immunology. Identifying the infiltrators. *Science* 344:801–802, 2014.

80. Brown GD: Dectin-1: A signalling non-TLR pattern-recognition receptor. *Nat Rev Immunol* 6:33–43, 2006.

81. Wynn TA, Chawla A, Pollard JW: Macrophage biology in development, homeostasis and disease. *Nature* 496:445–455, 2013.

82. Murray PJ, Allen JE, Biswas SK, et al: Macrophage activation and polarization: Nomenclature and experimental guidelines. *Immunity* 41:14–20, 2014.

83. Herbein G, Varin A: The macrophage in HIV-1 infection: From activation to deactivation? *Retrovirology* 7:33, 2010.

84. Labonte AC, Tosello-Trampont AC, Hahn YS: The role of macrophage polarization in infectious and inflammatory diseases. *Mol Cells* 37:275–285, 2014.

85. Cassetta L, Cassol E, Poli G: Macrophage polarization in health and disease. *ScientificWorldJournal* 11:2391–2402, 2011.

86. Gordon S: Alternative activation of macrophages. *Nat Rev Immunol* 3:23–35, 2003.

87. Martinez FO, Helming L, Gordon S: Alternative activation of macrophages: An immunologic functional perspective. *Annu Rev Immunol* 27:451–483, 2009.

88. Douglas SD, Leeman SE: Neurokinin-1 receptor: Functional significance in the immune system in reference to selected infections and inflammation. *Ann N Y Acad Sci* 1217:83–95, 2011.

89. Lai JP, Ho WZ, Kilpatrick LE, et al: Full-length and truncated neurokinin-1 receptor expression and function during monocyte/macrophage differentiation. *Proc Natl Acad Sci U S A* 103:7771–7776, 2006.

90. Lai JP, Lai S, Tuluc F, et al: Differences in the length of the carboxyl terminus mediate functional properties of neurokinin-1 receptor. *Proc Natl Acad Sci U S A* 105: 12605–12610, 2008.

91. Taylor PR, Zamze S, Stillion RJ, et al: Development of a specific system for targeting protein to metallophilic macrophages. *Proc Natl Acad Sci U S A* 101:1963–1968, 2004.

92. Lee SH, Crocker PR, Westaby S, et al: Isolation and immunocytochemical characterization of human bone marrow stromal macrophages in hemopoietic clusters. *J Exp Med* 168:1193–1198, 1988.

93. Crocker PR, Werb Z, Gordon S, Bainton DF: Ultrastructural localization of a macrophage-restricted sialic acid binding hemagglutinin, SER, in macrophage-hematopoietic cell clusters. *Blood* 76:1131–1138, 1990.

CHAPTER 69

CLASSIFICATION AND CLINICAL MANIFESTATIONS OF DISORDERS OF MONOCYTES AND MACROPHAGES

Marshall A. Lichtman

SUMMARY

Disorders that exclusively result in abnormalities of monocytes, macrophages, or dendritic cells are uncommon and usually are referred to, pathologically, as histiocytosis. These disorders can be inherited, such as familial hemophagocytic lymphohistiocytosis; inflammatory, such as infectious hemophagocytic lymphohistiocytic syndrome; or clonal (neoplastic), such as Langerhans cell histiocytosis. They can result from an inherited enzyme insufficiency in macrophages that lead to exaggerated storage of macromolecules, such as in Gaucher disease. Monocytes are critical sources for proinflammatory and inflammatory cytokines and, when inappropriately activated, can result in the lymphohistiocytic hemophagocytic syndrome with fever, intravascular coagulation, and organ pathology. A variety of hematopoietic neoplasms may have a phenotype characterized by a large proportion of monocytes. Idiopathic (clonal) monocytosis is a rare manifestation of a myelodysplastic syndrome. Some cases of myelogenous leukemia have progenitor cells that mature preferentially into leukemic monocytes, including acute monoblastic or monocytic leukemia, chronic myelomonocytic leukemia, and juvenile myelomonocytic leukemia. Two acquired diseases, hairy cell leukemia and aplastic anemia, result in a severe depression of blood monocytes (along with other blood cell types). Mutations in GATA2 are associated with severe monocytopenia and mycobacterial infections (the MonoMAC syndrome). Inherited disorders affecting white cells, such as chronic granulomatous disease and Chédiak-Higashi syndrome, result in impaired monocyte function. Monocyte dysfunction may accompany a variety of severe illnesses, such as sepsis, trauma, and cancer. Monocytes also contribute to a variety of diseases, such as Crohn disease and rheumatoid arthritis, by virtue of their being a principal source of tumor necrosis factor. Monocytes play a pathogenetic role in other complex, acquired disorders, such as thrombosis and atherogenesis. Table 69–1 catalogues the qualitative and quantitative abnormalities of monocytes, macrophages, and dendritic cells.

Acronyms and Abbreviations: CD, cluster of differentiation; GM-CSF, granulocyte-macrophage colony-stimulating factor; HLA-DR, human leukocyte antigen-D related; IL, interleukin; MonoMAC, monocytopenia and mycobacterial infections syndrome; TNF, tumor necrosis factor.

● CLASSIFICATION

Classification of monocytic disorders is difficult because few abnormalities result solely in a disturbance of monocytes or macrophages. However, the presence of monocytopenia, monocytosis, histiocytosis, or qualitative disorders of monocytes may be an important diagnostic feature or contribute to the functional abnormality in the patient.

The terms *histiocyte* and *macrophage* are synonymous. The latter term is customary when discussing the biology of the cells of the *mononuclear phagocyte system*, which is the total pool of marrow, blood, and tissue monocytes and macrophages, formerly referred to as the *reticuloendothelial system*. In disease nosology, the terms *histiocyte* and *histiocytosis* continue to be used for diseases that principally involve cells derived from blood monocytes, that is, macrophages and monocyte-derived dendritic cells.

The physician should consider the absolute monocyte count and not the percent of cells that are monocytes when evaluating the differential blood cell count before concluding that there is an inappropriate content of blood monocytes (Chap. 70).

Table 69–1 lists a classification of monocyte and macrophage disorders of relevance to hematologists.

MONOCYTOPENIA

Table 69–1 contains several important causes of monocytopenia. Two notable examples of disorders accompanied by severe monocytopenia are aplastic anemia and hairy cell leukemia. Pancytopenia is usual in both conditions, but the predisposition to serious infection is heightened by the deficiency in monocyte production. In hairy cell leukemia, the severe monocytopenia represents an important diagnostic clue because of its constancy. A syndrome of profound monocytopenia, often amonocytosis, associated with susceptibility to mycobacterial avian complex, fungal, and disseminated papilloma virus infections, and subsequent development of myelodysplasia or acute myelogenous leukemia in some cases, was first described in 2010 (see Table 69–1). It is accompanied by blood B-cell lymphopenia and decreased circulating and tissue dendritic cells, but not by hypogammaglobulinemia or a deficiency of tissue macrophages or skin Langerhans (dendritic) cells. It is the result of mutations of *GATA2* that impair transcription of its mRNA and is usually inherited as an autosomal recessive or can occur sporadically. The mutations of *GATA2* were found in germline and hematopoietic tissues, adding it to the familial leukemia genes, as well as to a slow onset (sometimes decades), complex immunodeficiency state.

MONOCYTOSIS AND HISTIOCYTOSIS

Table 69–1 contains a comprehensive list of causes of monocytosis. Monocytosis is often the manifestation of an inflammatory or a neoplastic disease. Certain hematopoietic tumors, especially acute monocytic and chronic myelomonocytic leukemia, have as their principal manifestation a predominance of monocytic cells in marrow and blood. Occasionally, chronic monocytosis can precede the onset of acute myelogenous leukemia, representing an uncommon manifestation of the myelodysplastic syndromes. Dendritic cell variants of acute myelogenous leukemia have also been discovered since the advent of immunophenotyping and genotyping of acute leukemias. The precise derivation of these myeloid dendritic cells is uncertain (i.e., granulocytic or monocytic). In some cases of monocytic leukemia, the malignant clone does not appear to include progenitors of red cells and platelets. Such cases are not likely to be the result of a mutation of a multipotential hematopoietic cell. This type of progenitor cell monocytic leukemia and other histiocytic or dendritic cell tumors support the concept that primitive

TABLE 69–1. Disorders of Monocytes and Macrophages

I. Monocytopenia
  A. Aplastic anemia[1]
  B. Hairy cell leukemia[2]
  C. MonoMAC syndrome[3-7]
  D. Glucocorticoid therapy[8,9]
II. Monocytosis
  A. Benign
    (1) Reactive monocytosis[10]
    (2) Exercise-induced[11]
  B. Clonal monocytosis
      Indolent
    (1) Chronic idiopathic monocytosis[12]
    (2) Oligoblastic myelogenous leukemia (myelodysplasia)[13]
      Progressive
    (1) Acute monocytic leukemia[14-16]
    (2) Dendritic cell leukemia[17-19]
    (3) Progenitor cell monocytic leukemia[20]
    (4) Chronic myelomonocytic leukemia[21,22]
    (5) Juvenile myelomonocytic leukemia[23]
III. Macrophage Deficiency
  A. Osteopetrosis (isolated osteoclast deficiency)[24,25]
IV. Inflammatory Histiocytosis (Chap. 71)
  A. Primary hemophagocytic lymphohistiocytosis[26-28]
    (1) Familial
    (2) Sporadic
  B. Other inherited syndromes with hemophagocytosis lymphohistiocytosis: Chédiak-Higashi, X-linked lymphoproliferative, Gracelli[29]
  C. Infectious hemophagocytic histiocytosis[30,31]
  D. Tumor-associated hemophagocytic histiocytosis[31,32]
  E. Drug-associated hemophagocytic histiocytosis[33]
  F. Disease-associated hemophagocytic histiocytosis[29-32]
  G. Juvenile rheumatoid arthritis (macrophage activation syndrome)[33,34]
  H. Sinus histiocytosis with massive lymphadenopathy[35,36]
V. Storage Histiocytosis (Chap. 72)
  A. Gaucher disease[37]
  B. Niemann-Pick disease[38]
  C. Gangliosidosis[39]
  D. Sea-blue histiocytosis syndrome[40]

VI. Clonal (Neoplastic) Histiocytosis (Chap. 71)
  A. Langerhans cell histiocytosis[41,42]
    (1) Localized
    (2) Systemic
  B. Tumors or sarcomas of histiocytes and dendritic cells[43]
    (1) Histiocytic sarcoma
    (2) Langerhans cell sarcoma
    (3) Interdigitating dendritic cell sarcoma
    (4) Follicular dendritic cell sarcoma
VII. Monocyte and Macrophage Dysfunction[44-46]
  A. α_1-Proteinase inhibitor deficiency[47,48]
  B. Chédiak-Higashi syndrome[49]
  C. Chronic granulomatous disease[50,51]
  D. Chronic lymphocytic leukemia[52,53]
  E. Disseminated mucocutaneous candidiasis[54,55]
  F. Glucocorticoid therapy[56,57]
  G. Kawasaki disease[58,59]
  H. Malakoplakia[60]
  I. Mycobacteriosis syndrome[61-63]
  J. Leprosy[64]
  K. Posttraumatic[65,66]
  L. Septic shock-induced[67-69]
  M. Critically ill subjects[70]
  N. Solid tumors[71,72]
  O. Tobacco smoking[73,74]
  P. Marijuana smoking or cocaine inhalation[75,76]
  Q. Whipple disease[77,78]
  R. Human interleukin (IL)-10 effects; Epstein-Barr virus IL-10–like gene product (vIL-10)[79,80]
VIII. Atherogenesis[81-85]
IX. Thrombogenesis[85-88]
X. Obesity[89]
XI. Aging[90-92]

cells, committed to the monocyte-macrophage lineage, can undergo malignant transformation (Chaps. 83 and 88).

Several uncommon types of histiocytosis are serious systemic diseases that may masquerade as malignant disease. However, in such cases the cytopathologic changes in monocytes or macrophages do not constitute a malignant transformation and are not monoclonal. Familial and sporadic hemophagocytic lymphohistiocytosis, infection-induced hemophagocytic syndromes, and sinus histiocytosis with massive lymphadenopathy are among such disorders (Chap. 71). Infectious hemophagocytic histiocytosis caused by Epstein-Barr virus may be a

hybrid disease because of the association with an underlying monoclonal or oligoclonal proliferation of virus-infected lymphocytes. The striking activation of macrophages and the resulting cytokine elaboration and organ pathology seen in some patients with juvenile rheumatoid arthritis, referred to as the "macrophage-activation syndrome," is closely related to other types of hemophagocytic syndromes (Chap. 71). Pediatric rheumatologists refer to the hemophagocytic syndrome in patients with juvenile rheumatoid arthritis as the "macrophage activation syndrome," but the clinical expression is closely analogous to other acquired hemophagocytic lymphohistiocytic syndromes. In these hemophagocytic syndromes, it is currently thought that the inherited or acquired inability of natural killer cells and cytotoxic T lymphocytes to modulate and, eventually, abrogate the immune response is responsible for the pathologic events of cytokine storm, fever, intravascular coagulation, organ dysfunction, and intense hemophagocytosis. Tumors of histiocytes (or dendritic cells) are rare, but can be classified into several groups with a combination of morphologic and immunophenotypic markers (Chap. 71).

QUALITATIVE DISORDERS OF MONOCYTES

Inherited abnormalities can result in dysfunctional macrophages (see Table 69–1). In these situations the abnormality is usually shared by other leukocytes, as in chronic granulomatous disease, which results from a defect in oxygen-dependent microbial killing. In Chédiak-Higashi disease, defective macrophages result from an abnormality in their cell and granule membranes (Chap. 66). An indomethacin-sensitive monocyte-killing defect in children is associated with a predisposition to atypical mycobacterial disease. Also, inherited or enzyme deficiencies in macrophages can result in accumulation of undegraded macromolecules, leading to various types of storage diseases. A classic example is Gaucher disease, a disorder that results from an inherited deficiency of the enzyme glucocerebrosidase, in which tissue damage results from the engorgement of macrophages with the enzyme substrate. Recombinant glucocerebrosidase, which enters macrophage lysosomes by endocytosis, can ameliorate this macrophagic disease (Chap. 72).

Acquired functional abnormalities of monocytes occur in a variety of diseases and circumstances (see "VII. Monocyte and Macrophage Dysfunction" in Table 69–1). Monocyte dysfunction occurs after severe trauma, sepsis, in other critically ill patients, and in patients with metastatic cancer. Monocyte production of interleukin (IL)-12 or maturation to dendritic cells also can be impaired in cases of severe trauma, critical illness, or metastatic cancer.

Some factors, such as IL-10, impair monocyte functions. A viral IL-10–like molecule encoded by the Epstein-Barr virus *BCRF1* gene also might play a role in the pathogenesis of that virus infection, and may act, in part, by inhibiting monocyte function. Tobacco smoking and marijuana smoking can result in impairment of alveolar macrophage function. In several diseases, including chronic lymphocytic leukemia, Kawasaki disease, Whipple disease, and malakoplakia, specific abnormalities of monocyte function play a significant role in the immune impairment in each disorder.

CLINICAL MANIFESTATIONS OF MONOCYTE DISORDERS

MONOCYTOPENIA OR MONOCYTE DYSFUNCTION

Isolated monocytopenia in the absence of any other blood cell deficiency or immune deficiency has not been reported. The manifestations of such a clinical state (pure amonocytosis) must be inferred. Neutrophils, endothelial cells, and other cell types can substitute, in part, for some monocyte functions. Monocytes have antibacterial, antiviral, antifungal, and antiparasitic capabilities. They are effective phagocytes that are involved in the ingestion and inactivation of microbes, such as mycobacteria, *Listeria*, *Brucella*, trypanosomes, and other granuloma-producing organisms. Thus, their deficiency

or functional abnormality predisposes to such infections. In association with the amonocytosis of the MonoMAC (monocytopenia and mycobacterial infections) syndrome, opportunistic infections with mycobacteria, fungi, and viral organisms are characteristic. Macrophages can serve as a reservoir for the human immunodeficiency virus and are the principal locus for the virus in the brain and in neural tissue.

Deficiency in a specific subset of macrophages, the osteoclasts, results in *osteopetrosis*, an imbalance in bone metabolism that favors accretion. Osteoclasts normally play a key role in the closely regulated process of bone resorption and accretion, mediating the former process. Monocyte derivatives are, thereby, involved in the development of osteoporosis and other metabolic bone diseases in which the balance tips toward resorption. Bisphosphonates can inhibit osteoclast action by interfering with its function of bone resorption and by inhibiting the mevalonate pathway to geranylgeranyl diphosphate, which prevents the transformation of monocytes to osteoclasts. Thus, the deleterious clinical manifestations of macrophages are being subdued by making the monocyte a target of therapy, in this case the prevention and amelioration of postmenopausal osteoporosis, tumor-induced bone lysis, and Paget disease, as well as of others.

Macrophages and their derivatives, monocyte-derived dendritic cells, process and present antigens and play a role in immune regulation. In complex systems, such as that of antibody production, abnormal macrophages might lead to defects in humoral immunity. Activated monocytes secrete more than 50 chemical mediators or monokines, which, among other things, play a vital role in cellular immunity and inflammation. In effect, they are a critical endocrine (hormone-elaborating) apparatus. The absence of monocytes from the inflammatory response and the failure to elaborate, or the inappropriate elaboration, of monokines such as IL-1, α_1-proteinase inhibitor, prostaglandins, leukotrienes, plasminogen activator, elastase, tumor necrosis factor (TNF), IL-6, IL-12, and other cytokines, may cause or contribute to disease manifestations. A deficiency or impairment of monocytes has the potential of influencing several functions and systems, because monocytes are such important sources of inflammatory cytokines (Chap. 67). In contrast, the unregulated activation of monocytes can lead to deleterious cytokine elaboration. Central to this process is TNF. The monocyte is a major source of TNF, which is a principal proinflammatory cytokine, triggering the elaboration of IL-1, IL-6, and others. Monocyte-derived TNF is also the primary chemical inducer of granuloma formation. The appreciation of its latter roles resulted in therapy to sequester TNF by antibody neutralization or receptor blockade and has resulted in substantial therapeutic effects in adult and juvenile rheumatoid arthritis, psoriasis, psoriatic arthritis, and Crohn disease. The side effects of such therapy confirm the key role of TNF in suppression of intracellular pathogens, such as *Mycobacterium tuberculosis* (potentiation of microbial diseases by TNF sequestrants), and in the role of the monocyte in modulating demyelinization (exacerbation of multiple sclerosis in patients treated with anti-TNF). The therapeutic administration of granulocyte-monocyte colony-stimulating factor (GM-CSF) also activates monocytes to elaborate cytokines, and this effect is being used to augment cancer vaccine therapy.

Monocytopenia and decreased monocyte entry into inflammatory sites occur after glucocorticoid administration. This may explain why patients treated with glucocorticoids are predisposed to infections in which monocytes play a protective role, such as those resulting from fungal, mycobacterial, and other opportunistic organisms. Dysfunctional monocytes, incapable of killing ingested microorganisms, are present in chronic granulomatous disease (Chap. 66), as well as in hematopoietic stem cell diseases, such as monocytic variants of acute myelogenous leukemia.

TISSUE EFFECTS OF MONOCYTOSIS

Benign monocytosis is not associated with specific clinical manifestations. All forms of myelogenous leukemia with a predominance of monocytes are associated with a predisposition to troublesome tissue infiltrates, especially in the skin, gingiva, lymph nodes, meninges, and anal canal. The higher the monocyte count and the higher the proportion of leukemic monocytes, the more prevalent is tissue infiltration. In some cases, the tissue infiltration of leukemic monocytes can produce symptoms: lung dysfunction, laryngeal obstruction, and intracranial vessel rupture, as well as others. Release of procoagulants leading to intravascular coagulation also occurs in myelogenous leukemia with a high proportion of monocytes. The hyperleukocytic syndrome can occur in acute monocytic leukemia with markedly elevated white cell counts (Chaps. 83 and 88).

EFFECTS OF HISTIOCYTOSIS

Hemophagocytic lymphohistiocytosis usually refers to the accumulation of activated macrophages (histiocytes) in tissue sites. The cells become intensely cytophagocytic; ingestion of red cells and occasionally of leukocytes, platelets, erythroblasts in marrow, or cells in other tissue sites is an important feature of these inflammatory histiocytoses (Chap. 71). Because morphology has been misleading, the diagnosis of histiocytosis requires identification of specific cell markers. A histiocytosis may be inflammatory (polyclonal) or neoplastic (clonal). Because tissue macrophages can take on highly specialized phenotypes and localize in different tissues, histiocytosis is further defined by whether they carry markers of these cell types (e.g., Langerhans cells, interdigitating dendritic cells; Chap. 71).

THROMBOATHEROGENESIS

The complex interrelationships among monocytes, atherogenesis, and coagulation are discussed in several other chapters in the text (Chaps. 115 and 134). Monocytes may play a central role in the pathologic aspects of both processes, as a repository for tissue factor, inflammatory cytokines, and a key element in the inflammatory precursor lesions of atheroma formation (Table 69–1, sections VIII and IX).

BLOOD DENDRITIC CELLS

Dendritic cells and macrophages belong to a family of antigen-presenting cells and in the laboratory can be generated from a common precursor. So-called monocyte-derived dendritic cells are easily produced in the culture vessel by the appropriate cytokines. Indeed, the use of GM-CSF as an adjuvant in cancer vaccines may relate in part to the cytokine's ability to activate monocytes and foster conversion to dendritic (antigen-presenting) cells *in vivo* (Chaps. 26 and 27). Dendritic cells can be defined by phenotype into two principal types—myeloid and lymphoid (plasmacytoid) dendritic cells—of which there are likely subtypes. Monocyte-derived dendritic cells are a subset of the myeloid type (Chap. 20).

Flow cytometry using cluster of differentiation (CD) markers and antidendritic cell surface antibodies have permitted the enumeration of myeloid (human leukocyte antigen-D related [HLA-DR]+, CD11c+, CD123–) and lymphocytic-plasmacytoid (HLA-DR+, CD11c–, CD123+, CD303+) dendritic cells in human blood in normal subjects and subjects with disease. Their centrality in the immune response as premier antigen-presenting cells may result in nonspecific alterations in their blood concentration or function in many generalized or localized inflammatory, infectious, and neoplastic diseases. Plasmacytoid dendritic cells may be decreased in numbers with aging, further impairing the immune response of older individuals (Chap. 9). Dendritic cells are also profoundly decreased in patients with hairy cell leukemia and are dysfunctional in patients with chronic lymphocytic leukemia.

REFERENCES

1. Twomey JJ, Douglas CC, Sharkey O Jr: The monocytopenia of aplastic anemia. *Blood* 41:187, 1973.
2. Bourguin-Plonquet A, Rouard H, Roudot-Thoraval F: Severe decrease in peripheral blood dendritic cells in hairy cell leukaemia. *Br J Haematol* 116:595, 2002.
3. Hsu AP, Sampaio EP, Khan J, et al: Mutations in GATA2 are associated with the autosomal dominant and sporadic monocytopenia and mycobacterial infection (MonoMAC) syndrome. *Blood* 118:2653, 2011.
4. Camargo JF, Lobo SA, Hsu AP, et al: MonoMAC syndrome in a patient with a GATA2 mutation: Case report and review of the literature. *Clin Infect Dis* 57:697, 2013.
5. Spinner MA, Sanchez LA, Hsu AP, et al: GATA2 deficiency: A protean disorder of hematopoiesis, lymphatics and immunity. *Blood* 123:809, 2014.
6. Cuellar-Rodriguez J, Gea-Banacloche J, Freeman AF, et al: Successful allogeneic hematopoietic stem cell transplantation for GATA2 deficiency. *Blood* 118:3715, 2011.
7. Dickinson RE, Milne P, Jardine L, et al: The evolution of cellular deficiency in GATA2 mutation. *Blood* 123:863, 2014.
8. Fauci AS, Dale DC: The effect of in vivo hydrocortisone on subpopulations of human lymphocytes. *J Clin Invest* 53:240, 1974.
9. Viegas LR, Hoijman E, Beato M, Pecci A: Mechanisms involved in tissue-specific apoptosis regulated by glucocorticoids. *J Steroid Biochem Mol Biol* 109:273, 2008.
10. Maldonado GE, Hanlon DG: Monocytosis. *Mayo Clin Proc* 40:248, 1965.
11. Lippi G, Banfi G, Montagnana M, et al: Acute variation of leucocytes counts following a half-marathon run. *Int J Lab Hematol* 32:117, 2010.
12. Jaworkowsky LI, Solovey DY, Rhausova LY, Udris OY: Monocytosis as a sign of subsequent leukemia in patients with cytopenias (preleukemia). *Folia Haematol Int Mag Klin Morphol Blutforsch* 110:395, 1983.
13. Rigolin GM, Cuneo A, Roberti MG, et al: Myelodysplastic syndrome with monocytic component: Hematologic and cytologic characterization. *Haematologica* 82:25, 1997.
14. Haferlach T, Schoch C, Schnittger S, et al: Distinct genetic patterns can be identified in acute monoblastic leukaemia (FAB AML M5a and M5b): A study of 124 patients. *Br J Haematol* 118:426, 2002.
15. Villeneuve P, Kim DT, Xu W, et al: The morphological subcategories of acute monocytic leukemia (M5a and M5b) share similar immunophenotypic and cytogenetic features and clinical outcomes. *Leuk Res* 32:269, 2008.
16. de Fonseca LM, Brunetti IL, Campa A, et al: Assessment of monocytic component in acute myelomonocytic and monocytic/monoblastic leukemias by a chemoluminescence assay. *Hematol J* 4:26, 2003.
17. Ferran M, Gallardo F, Ferrer AM, et al: Acute myeloid dendritic cell leukaemia with specific cutaneous involvement: A diagnostic challenge. *Br J Dermatol* 158:1129, 2008.
18. Santiago-Schwartz F, Coppock DL, Hindenberg AA, Kern J: Identification of a malignant counterpart of the monocytic-dendritic cell progenitor in an acute myeloid leukemia. *Blood* 84:3054, 1994.
19. Srivastava HI, Srivistava A, Srivastava MD: Phenotype, genotype and cytokine production in acute leukemia involving progenitors of dendritic Langerhans' cell. *Leuk Res* 18:499, 1994.
20. Ferraris AM, Broccia G, Meloni T, et al: Clonal origin of cells restricted to monocytic differentiation in acute nonlymphocytic leukemia. *Blood* 64:817, 1984.
21. Beran M: Chronic myelomonocytic leukemia. *Cancer Treat Res* 142:107, 2008.
22. Onida F, Kantarjian HM, Smith TL, et al: Prognostic scoring factors and scoring systems in chronic myelomonocytic leukemia: A retrospective analysis of 213 patients. *Blood* 99:840, 2002.
23. Kratz CP, Niemeyer CM: Juvenile myelomonocytic leukemia. *Hematology* 1.100, 2005.
24. Del Fattore A, Capparriello A, Teti A: Genetics, pathogenesis and complications of osteopetrosis. *Bone* 42:19, 2008.
25. Helfrich MH: Osteoclast diseases. *Microsc Res Tech* 61:514, 2003.
26. Aricò M, Janka G, Fischer A, et al, for the FHL Study Group of the Histiocyte Society: Hemophagocytic lymphohistiocytosis. Report of 122 children from the international registry. *Leukemia* 10:197, 1996.
27. Janka GE: Familial and acquired hemophagocytic lymphohistiocytosis. *Eur J Pediatr* 166:95, 2007.
28. Filipovich AH: Hemophagocytic lymphohistiocytosis and related disorders. *Curr Opin Allergy Clin Immunol* 6:410, 2006.
29. Rosado FG, Kim AS: Hemophagocytic lymphohistiocytosis: An update on diagnosis and pathogenesis. *Am J Clin Pathol* 139:713, 2013.
30. Rouphael NG, Talati NJ, Vaughan C, et al: Infections associated with haemophagocytic syndrome. *Lancet Infect Dis* 7:814, 2007.
31. Mehta RS, Smith RE: Hemophagocytic lymphohistiocytosis (HLH): A review of literature. *Med Oncol* 30:740, 2013.
32. Janka GE: Hemophagocytic syndromes. *Blood Rev* 21:245, 2007.
33. Imashuku S: Clinical features and treatment strategies of Epstein-Barr virus-associated hemophagocytic lymphohistiocytosis. *Crit Rev Oncol Hematol* 44:259, 2002.
34. Grom AA: Macrophage activation syndrome and reactive hemophagocytic lymphohistiocytosis: The same entities? *Curr Opin Rheumatol* 15:587, 2003.

35. Foucar E, Rosai J, Dorfman RF: Sinus histiocytosis with massive lymphadenopathy. *Cancer* 54:1834, 1984.

36. Pauli M, Bergamashi G, Tonon L, et al: Evidence of a polyclonal nature of the cell infiltrate in sinus histiocytosis with massive lymphadenopathy (Rosai-Dorfman disease). *Br J Haematol* 91:415, 1995.

37. Beutler E: Gaucher disease: Multiple lessons from a single gene disorder. *Acta Paediatr Suppl* 95:103, 2006.

38. Schuchman EH: The pathogenesis and treatment of acid sphingomyelinase-deficient Niemann-Pick disease. *J Inherit Metab Dis* 30:654, 2007.

39. Brunetti-Pierri N, Scaglia F: GM(1) gangliosidosis: Review of clinical, molecular, and therapeutic aspects. *Mol Genet Metab* 94:391, 2008.

40. Hirayama Y, Kohada K, Andoh M, et al: Syndrome of the sea-blue histiocyte. *Intern Med* 35:419, 1996.

41. Chang KL, Snyder DS: Langerhans cell histiocytosis. *Cancer Treat Res* 142:383, 2008.

42. Bechan GI, Egeler RM, Arceci RJ: Biology of Langerhans cells and Langerhans cell histiocytosis. *Int Rev Cytol* 254:1, 2006.

43. Jaffe ES, Harris NL, Stein H, Vardiman JW: Tumors of haematopoietic and lymphoid tissues. Histiocytic and dendritic cell neoplasms, in *World Health Organization Classification of Tumors*, pp 273–289. IARC Press, Lyon, 2001.

44. Lopez-Berestein G, Klostergaard J, editors: *Mononuclear Phagocytes in Cell Biology*. CRC Press, Boca Raton, FL, 1993.

45. Cline MJ: Histiocytes and histiocytosis. *Blood* 84:2840, 1994.

46. Asherson GL, Zembala M: Monocyte abnormalities in disease, in *Human Monocytes*, edited by Zembala M, Asherson GL, pp 395–415. Academic Press, London, 1989.

47. Abboud RT, Vimalanathan S: Pathogenesis of COPD. Part I. The role of protease-antiprotease imbalance in emphysema. *Int J Tuberc Lung Dis* 12:361, 2008.

48. Aldonyte R, Jansson L, Piitulainen E, Janciauskiene S: Circulating monocytes from healthy individuals and COPD patients. *Respir Res* 4:11, 2003.

49. Kaplan J, De Domenico I, Ward DM: Chediak-Higashi syndrome. *Curr Opin Hematol* 15:22, 2008.

50. Davis WC, Huber H, Douglas SD, Fudenberg HH: A defect in circulating mononuclear phagocytes in chronic granulomatous disease of childhood. *J Immunol* 101:1093, 1968.

51. Stasia MJ, Li XJ: Genetics and immunopathology of chronic granulomatous disease. *Semin Hematol* 30:209, 2008.

52. Orsini E, Guarini A, Chiaretti S, et al: The circulating dendritic cell compartment in patients with chronic lymphocytic leukemia is severely defective and unable to stimulate an effective T cell response. *Cancer Res* 63:4497, 2003.

53. Mami NB, Mohty M, Aurran-Schleinitz T, et al: Blood dendritic cells in patients with chronic lymphocytic leukaemia. *Immunobiology* 213:493, 2008.

54. Snyderman R, Altman LC, Frankel A, Blaese RM: Defective mononuclear leukocyte chemotaxis. *Ann Intern Med* 78:509, 1973.

55. Komiyama A, Ichikawa M, Kanda H, et al: Defective interleukin 1 production in a familial monocyte disorder with a combined abnormality of mobility and phagocytosis-killing. *Clin Exp Immunol* 73:500, 1988.

56. Bhavsar PK, Sukkar MB, Khorasani N, et al: Glucocorticoid suppression of CX3CL1 (fractalkine) by reduced gene promoter recruitment of NF-kappaB. *FASEB J* 22:1807, 2008.

57. Ehrchen J, Steinmüller L, Barczyk K, et al: Glucocorticoids induce differentiation of a specifically activated, anti-inflammatory subtype of human monocytes. *Blood* 109:1265, 2007.

58. Nomura I, Abe J, Noma S, et al: Adrenomedullin is highly expressed in blood monocytes associated with acute Kawasaki disease: A microarray gene expression study. *Pediatr Res* 57:49, 2005.

59. Matsubara T, Ichiyama T, Furukawa S: Immunological profile of peripheral blood lymphocytes and monocytes/macrophages in Kawasaki disease. *Clin Exp Immunol* 141:381, 2005.

60. Van Crevel R, Curfs J, van der Ven AJ et al: Functional and morphological monocyte abnormalities in a patient with malakoplakia. *Am J Med* 105:74, 1998.

61. Ridgeway D, Wolff LJ, Wall M, Bouzy MS, et al: Indomethacin-sensitive monocyte killing defect in a child with disseminated atypical mycobacterial disease. *J Clin Immunol* 11:357, 1991.

62. Onwubalili JK: Defective monocyte chemotactic responsiveness in patients with active tuberculosis. *Immunol Lett* 16:39, 1987.

63. Welin A, Winberg ME, Abdalla H, et al: Incorporation of *Mycobacterium tuberculosis* lipoarabinomannan into macrophage membrane rafts is a prerequisite for the phagosomal maturation block. *Infect Immun* 76:2882, 2008.

64. Murray RA, Siddiqui MR, Mendillo M, et al: *Mycobacterium leprae* inhibits dendritic cell activation and maturation. *J Immunol* 178:338, 2007.

65. Spolarics Z, Siddiqi M, Siegel JH, et al: Depressed interleukin-12-producing activity by monocytes correlates with adverse clinical course and a shift toward Th2-type

66. De AK, Laudanski K, Miller-Graziano CL: Failure of monocytes of trauma patients to convert to immature dendritic cells is related to preferential macrophage-colony-stimulating factor-driven macrophage differentiation. *J Immunol* 170:6355, 2003.

67. Venet F, Tissot S, Debard AL, et al: Decreased monocyte human leukocyte antigen-DR expression after severe burn injury: Correlation with severity and secondary septic shock. *Crit Care Med* 35:1910, 2007.

68. Pachot A, Cazalis MA, Venet F, et al: Decreased expression of the fractalkine receptor CX3CR1 on circulating monocytes as new feature of sepsis-induced immunosuppression. *J Immunol* 180:6421, 2008.

69. Tsujimoto H, Ono S, Efron PA, et al: Role of Toll-like receptors in the development of sepsis. *Shock* 29:315, 2008.

70. Albaiceta GM, Pedreira PR, García-Prieto E, Taboada F: Therapeutic implications of immunoparalysis in critically ill patients. *Inflamm Allergy Drug Targets* 6:191, 2007.

71. Sica A, Schioppa T, Mantovani A, Allavena P: Tumour-associated macrophages are a distinct M2 polarised population promoting tumour progression: Potential targets of anti-cancer therapy. *Eur J Cancer* 42:717, 2006.

72. Allavena P, Sica A, Solinas G, et al: The inflammatory micro-environment in tumor progression: The role of tumor-associated macrophages. *Crit Rev Oncol Hematol* 66:1, 2008.

73. Ryder MI, Saghizadeh M, Ding Y, et al: Effects of tobacco smoke on secretion of interleukin 1-beta, tumor necrosis factor-alpha, and transforming growth-beta from peripheral blood mononuclear cells. *Oral Microbiol Immunol* 17:331, 2002.

74. Chen H, Cowan MJ, Hasday JD, et al: Tobacco smoking inhibits expression of proinflammatory cytokines and activation of IL-1R-associated kinase, p38, and NF-kappaB in alveolar macrophages stimulated with TLR2 and TLR4 agonists. *J Immunol* 179:6097, 2007.

75. Shay AH, Choi R, Whittaker K, et al: Impairment of antimicrobial activity and nitric acid production by alveolar macrophages from smokers of marijuana and cocaine. *J Infect Dis* 187:700, 2003.

76. Klein TW, Cabral GA: Cannabinoid-induced immune suppression and modulation of antigen-presenting cells. *J Neuroimmune Pharmacol* 1:50, 2006.

77. Marth T, Neurath M, Cuccherini BA, Strober W: Defects of monocyte interleukin 12 production an humoral immunity in Whipple's disease. *Gastroenterology* 113:442, 1997.

78. Desnues B, Ihrig M, Raoult D, Mege JL: Whipple's disease: A macrophage disease. *Clin Vaccine Immunol* 13:170, 2006.

79. Moore KW, de Waal Maleyt R, Coffman RL, O'Garra A: Interleukin-10 and the interleukin 10 receptor. *Annu Rev Immunol* 19:683, 2001.

80. Dobrovolskaia MA, Vogel SN: Toll receptors, CD14, and macrophage activation and deactivation by LPS. *Microbes Infect* 4:903, 2002.

81. Tousoulis D, Davies G, Stefanadis C, et al: Inflammatory and thrombotic mechanisms in coronary atherosclerosis. *Heart* 89:993, 2003.

82. Oliveira RT, Mamoni RL, Souza JR, et al: Differential expression of cytokines, chemokines and chemokine receptors in patients with coronary artery disease. *Int J Cardiol* 24:17, 2009.

83. Murphy AJ, Woollard KJ, Hoang A, et al: High-density lipoprotein reduces the human monocyte inflammatory response. *Arterioscler Thromb Vasc Biol* 28:2071, 2008.

84. Jawie J: New insights into immunological aspects of atherosclerosis. *Pol Arch Med Wewn* 118:127, 2008.

85. Brambilla M, Camera M, Colnago D, et al: Tissue factor in patients with acute coronary syndromes: Expression in platelets, leukocytes, and platelet-leukocyte aggregates. *Arterioscler Thromb Vasc Biol* 28:947, 2008.

86. Martin J, Collot-Teixeira S, McGregor L, McGregor JL: The dialogue between endothelial cells and monocytes/macrophages in vascular syndromes. *Curr Pharm Des* 13:1751, 2007.

87. Napoleone E, di Santo A, Peri G, et al: The long pentraxin PTX3 up-regulates tissue factor in activated monocytes: Another link between inflammation and clotting activation. *J Leukoc Biol* 76:203, 2004.

88. Key NS: Platelet tissue factor: How did it get there and is it important? *Semin Hematol* 45(Suppl 1):S16, 2008.

89. Weisberg SP, McCann D, Desai M, et al: Obesity is associated with macrophage accumulation in adipose tissue. *J Clin Invest* 112:1796, 2003.

90. Giannelli S, Taddeo A, Presicce P, et al: A six-color flow cytometric assay for the analysis of peripheral blood dendritic cells. *Cytometry B Clin Cytom* 74:349, 2008.

91. Koga Y, Matsuzaki A, Suminoe A, et al: Expression of cytokine-associated genes in dendritic cells (DCs): Comparison between adult peripheral blood- and umbilical cord blood-derived DCs by cDNA microarray. *Immunol Lett* 116:55, 2008.

92. Pérez-Cabezas B, Naranjo-Gómez M, Fernández MA, et al: Reduced numbers of plasmacytoid dendritic cells in aged blood donors. *Exp Gerontol* 42:1033, 2007.

lymphocyte pattern in severely injured male trauma patients. *Crit Care Med* 31:1722, 2003.

CHAPTER 70
MONOCYTOSIS AND MONOCYTOPENIA

Marshall A. Lichtman

SUMMARY

The blood monocyte is in transit between the marrow and tissues where it transforms (matures) into a macrophage. In tissues, the monocyte develops a phenotype characteristic of the specific tissue of residence (e.g., Kupffer cells of liver, microglia of brain, osteoclasts of bone). Because the monocyte participates in virtually all inflammatory and immune reactions, its concentration in the blood may be increased in many such conditions, including autoimmune diseases, gastrointestinal disorders, sarcoidosis, and several viral and bacterial infections. Monocytosis, an increase in the blood absolute monocyte count to more than 800/μL (0.8 × 10⁹/L), may occur in some patients with cancer and several unrelated conditions, such as postsplenectomy states, inflammatory bowel disease, and some chronic infections (e.g., bacterial endocarditis, tuberculosis, and brucellosis). The inconsistency and unpredictability in the blood monocyte concentration among patients with the same disease is a function of its relatively small blood pool size, the damping effect of a large tissue pool, its relatively long life span, the number and complexity of effectors in the relevant cytokine network that can influence the response, and the ability to expand macrophage numbers by local mitosis in tissues. The most striking increase in blood monocyte concentration occurs with hematopoietic malignancies, especially clonal monocytosis, and monocytic or myelomonocytic leukemia. Depression, myocardial infarction, parturition, thermal injuries, and marathon competition are closely associated with monocytosis. Table 70–1 is a comprehensive list of causes of monocytosis. Monocytopenia is notable in patients with aplastic anemia or hairy cell leukemia as a feature of pancytopenia. Although other cytopenias accompany the monocytopenia, the latter contributes significantly to the predisposition to infection and in hairy cell leukemia is an aid to diagnosis because of its constancy. The MonoMAC syndrome, the result of *GATA2* mutations, is associated with extreme monocytopenia and amonocytosis.

The blood monocyte is a cell in transit from marrow to tissues.[1] There are two major populations of blood monocytes based on physical properties: a smaller population thought to represent a less-mature stage, has a higher buoyant density, a smaller cell volume, lacks Fc receptors,

and has greater tumoricidal activity; the larger population represents a more-mature stage, has a lower buoyant density, has a larger cell volume, displays Fc receptors, expresses more peroxidase activity, secretes larger amounts of interleukin (IL)-1, presents antigen, and mediates antibody-dependent cell-mediated cytotoxicity more efficiently. The larger population, classical monocytes that are highly phagocytic and proinflammatory, composes approximately 90 percent of blood monocytes, and strongly expresses CD14 (lipopolysaccharide receptor) but does not express CD16 (FcγRIII), designated the CD14⁺⁺CD16⁻ subset. These monocytes carry chemokine receptors CCR2^hiCX3CR1^lo. Of the remaining monocyte population, approximately 5 percent exhibit strong expression of CD14 and modest expression of CD16, the CD14⁺⁺CD16⁺ "intermediate" subset, which expresses the chemokine receptors CCR2^midCX3CR1^hiCCR5^mid, are proinflammatory and less phagocytic, and the "nonclassical" subset, which exhibits strong expression of CD16, the CD14⁺CD16⁺⁺ subset, which expresses the chemokines CCR^loCX3CR1^hi, the so-called patrolling subset.[2] The latter subset contains dendritic cell precursors.[3] The major subsets can each be further stratified based on the expression of CD64 (FcγRI) (Chaps. 67 and 68).[4]

In tissues the monocyte is capable of transformation, under the influence of local environmental factors, into a macrophage. The monocyte plays an important role in acute and chronic inflammatory reactions, including granulomatous inflammation; immunologic reactions, including those involved in delayed hypersensitivity; tissue repair and reorganization; atheroma and thrombus formation; and the reaction to neoplasia and allografts. Because of the key role of monocytes in a variety of pathophysiologic reactions, a modest elevation in blood monocyte count can occur in many disparate conditions. In addition, in circumstances in which large increases in the number of macrophages are required in tissue sites, the demand may be met by local proliferation of macrophages and not be reflected either in an increased transit of monocytes through the blood compartment from marrow to tissue or in an increased concentration of blood monocytes.[5] Occasionally, T-cell clones release only macrophage/monocyte colony-stimulating factor (M-CSF), which can stimulate the growth of macrophage colonies, providing a model for local control of macrophage proliferation.[6]

NORMAL BLOOD MONOCYTE CONCENTRATION

In the first 2 weeks of life, the average absolute blood monocyte count is approximately 1000/μL (1 × 10⁹/L; Chap. 7). There is a gradual decline in the normal monocyte count to a mean of 400/μL (0.4 × 10⁹/L) in adulthood, at which time monocytes constitute 1 to 9 percent (mean: 4 percent) of blood leukocytes (Chap. 2). Monocytosis is present when the absolute count exceeds 800/μL (0.8 × 10⁹/L) in adults. Men tend to have slightly higher monocyte counts than women.[7] Increments in the number of blood monocytes correlate directly with increases in the total blood monocyte pool and the monocyte turnover rate.[8] The blood monocyte count cycles with a periodicity of 5 days.[9] Older persons have a decrease in the proportion of CD14⁺⁺CD16⁻ to CD14⁺CD16⁺ monocytes as compared to younger persons, although the functional significance of this difference has not been established.[10]

DISORDERS ASSOCIATED WITH MONOCYTOSIS

Table 70–1 outlines the diseases reported to be associated with monocytosis. In one review, hematologic disorders represented more than 50 percent, collagen vascular diseases approximately 10 percent, and malignant disease approximately 8 percent of cases of monocytosis.[11]

TABLE 70-1. Disorders Associated with Monocytosis

I. Hematologic Disorders
  A. Myeloid neoplasms
    1. Myelodysplastic syndromes[12–16]
    2. Primary myelofibrosis[17]
    3. Acute monocytic leukemia[18,19]
    4. Acute myelomonocytic leukemia[20]
    5. Acute monocytic leukemia with histiocytic features[21]
    6. Acute myeloid dendritic cell leukemia[22–24]
    7. Chronic myelomonocytic leukemia[25–27]
    8. Juvenile myelomonocytic leukemia[28]
    9. Chronic myelogenous leukemia (m-*BCR*–positive type)[29,30]
    10. Polycythemia vera[11]
    11. Primary myelofibrosis[17]
  B. Chronic neutropenias[31–36]
  C. Drug-induced neutropenia[37–39]
  D. Postagranulocytic recovery[40,41]
  E. Lymphocytic neoplasms
    1. Lymphoma[43]
    2. Hodgkin lymphoma[44,45]
    3. Myeloma[46,47]
    4. Macroglobulinemia[48]
    5. T-cell lymphoma[49,50]
    6. Chronic lymphocytic leukemia[51]
  F. Drug-induced pseudolymphoma[52]
  G. Immune hemolytic anemia[11]
  H. Idiopathic thrombocytopenic purpura[11]
  I. Postsplenectomy state[53,54]
II. Inflammatory and Immune Disorders
  A. Connective tissue diseases
    1. Rheumatoid arthritis[55]
    2. Systemic lupus erythematosus[56]
    3. Temporal arteritis[11]
    4. Myositis[11]
    5. Polyarteritis nodosa[11]
    6. Sarcoidosis[57,58]
  B. Infections
    1. Mycobacterial infections[59–62]
    2. Subacute bacterial endocarditis[63–65]
    3. Brucellosis[66]
    4. Dengue hemorrhagic fever[67]
    5. Resolution phase of acute bacterial infections[68]
    6. Syphilis[69,70]
    7. Cytomegalovirus infection[71]
    8. Varicella-zoster virus[72]
    9. Influenza[73]
III. Gastrointestinal Disorders
  A. Alcoholic liver disease[74]
  B. Inflammatory bowel disease[75]
  C. Sprue[11]
IV. Nonhematopoietic Malignancies[76–79]
V. Exogenous Cytokine Administration[80–86]
VI. Myocardial Infarction[87–90]
VII. Cardiac Bypass Surgery[91]
VIII. Miscellaneous Conditions
  A. Tetrachloroethane poisoning[92]
  B. Parturition[93,94]
  C. Glucocorticoid administration[95–98]
  D. Depression[99–101]
  E. Thermal injury[102,103]
  F. Marathon running[104,105]
  G. Holoprosencephaly[106]
  H. Kawasaki disease[107]
  I. Wiskott-Aldrich syndrome[108]
  J. Hemodialysis[109]

HEMATOLOGIC DISORDERS

Approximately 25 percent of patients with a myelodysplastic syndrome have an increase in the absolute monocyte count.[12–16] Occasional patients with a myelodysplastic syndrome may develop an absolute monocyte count as high as 30,000/μL (30 × 10^9/L). Chronic monocytosis may be the principal feature of a clonal myeloid disease and precede by years the development of acute myelogenous leukemia. Patients with myelodysplasia and monocytosis have a high propensity to evolve into acute or chronic myelomonocytic leukemia. Monocytosis, as a feature of primary myelofibrosis, may be a harbinger of rapid progression.[17] The number of promonocytes and monocytes in blood and marrow may be increased in patients with acute myelogenous leukemia of the monocytic[18,19] or myelomonocytic type.[20] Acute myelogenous leukemic cells with a histiocytic (macrophagic)[21] or dendritic cell phenotype have been described.[22–24] Patients with chronic myelomonocytic leukemia

have, by definition, an increased absolute number of monocytes in the blood (≥1.0 × 10^9/L). The monocytosis may be more striking in some cases.[25–27] Juvenile myelomonocytic leukemia, also, is defined in part by the increased number of monocytes in the blood and marrow.[28] In some cases of acute monocytic leukemia, the monocytes are immature and have features of monoblasts or promonocytes, but in some cases they are indistinguishable by light microscopy from normal blood monocytes. Some automated instruments are dependent on the α-naphthol acetate esterase reaction to detect the proportion of monocytes in white cell differential counts. These instruments may underestimate leukemic monocytes counts, especially in cases of chronic myelomonocytic leukemia, because the leukemic monocytes have a decreased activity of the enzyme.[25] An uncommon variant of Ph-positive chronic myelogenous leukemia (CML), expressing a p190 BCR-ABL transcript, is associated with a striking monocytosis in approximately 50 percent of cases.[29,30]

Monocytosis occurs in a number of neutropenic states: cyclic neutropenia,[31] chronic granulocytopenia of childhood,[32] familial benign chronic neutropenia,[33] infantile genetic agranulocytosis[34,35] and chronic hypoplastic neutropenia.[36] In human cyclic neutropenia, monocyte oscillation is reciprocal to the neutrophil cycle; the peak monocytosis, which often exceeds 2000/μL (2.0 × 10^9/L), occurs at the end of the neutropenic period. Monocytes often stay above 500/μL (0.5 × 10^9/L) throughout the cycle. In the variety of other neutropenias mentioned, monocytopoiesis often is preserved in the face of neutropenia. Transient elevations of the monocyte count have been reported in the acute phases of drug-induced agranulocytosis.[37-39] Monocytosis characteristically appears later in the recovery phase of agranulocytosis and may be a harbinger of recovery.[37,40,41] Some observers dispute the validity of the latter observation.[42]

Monocytosis can occur with lymphomas and can increase with exacerbation of disease activity.[43] Monocytosis has been noted in approximately 25 percent of cases of Hodgkin lymphoma, although it does not correlate with prognosis.[43,44] In contrast, one treatise on the disease reports the hematologic values of patients with Hodgkin lymphoma at the time of diagnosis; only 4 of 100 have nominal increases in absolute blood monocyte counts.[45] A statistically significant increase in blood monocyte concentration has been reported in myeloma and has been correlated with the presence of λ light-chain-containing monoclonal immunoglobulin.[46,47] Rare cases of M-CSF secreting lymphoid tumors have been associated with monocytosis.[48,49] Monocytosis at diagnosis has been correlated with decreased survival in several lymphoma types and chronic lymphocytic leukemia.[50,51] Pseudolymphoma syndrome, induced by drugs such as carbamazepine, phenytoin, phenobarbital, and valproic acid, is associated with monocytosis.[52]

SPLENECTOMY

Monocytosis is a common feature in individuals who have had splenectomy.[53,54]

INFLAMMATORY AND IMMUNE DISORDERS

Connective tissue diseases, including rheumatoid arthritis,[55] systemic lupus erythematosus, temporal arteritis, myositis, and periarteritis nodosa, may be associated with monocytosis, although monocytosis is not common in these diseases.[11] The usual alterations of the white cell count in systemic lupus erythematosus, for example, are neutropenia and lymphopenia, but 10 percent of patients have a mild monocytosis.[56] An elevation of the blood monocyte count occurs in sarcoidosis[57] and is inversely related to a reduction in circulating T lymphocytes.[58]

Infectious diseases are an uncommon cause of monocytosis. Only a few instances of infection were noted in a comprehensive review of causes of monocytosis, including tonsillitis, dental infection, recurrent liver abscesses, candidiasis, and one instance of tuberculous peritonitis.[11] Tuberculosis was once a leading cause of monocytosis, because of the role of monocytes in granuloma (tubercle) formation. Neither the monocyte count nor the ratio of monocytes to lymphocytes correlates with the stage or activity of tuberculosis.[59-61] *Mycobacterium fortuitum* infection, usually in the setting of AIDS, also is associated with monocytosis.[62]

Monocytosis is found in 15 to 20 percent of patients with subacute bacterial endocarditis,[63,64] but is not correlated with the presence of blood macrophages, which may be present in this disease.[65]

A number of infections formerly thought to be associated with monocytosis are not, when examined systematically. These include rickettsial diseases, leishmaniasis, typhoid fever, malaria, and disseminated candidiasis, brucellosis,[66] and dengue hemorrhagic fever.[67]

A monocytosis in the resolution phase of acute infections has been noted,[68] and monocytosis occurs in cases of neonatal, primary, and secondary syphilis.[69,70] Certain viruses, especially cytomegalovirus varicella-zoster virus, and influenza virus induce an increase in blood monocytes.[71-73]

GASTROINTESTINAL DISEASES

Sprue, ulcerative colitis, regional enteritis, and alcoholic liver disease are associated with monocytosis.[11,74,75]

NONHEMATOPOIETIC MALIGNANCIES

Sixty percent of patients with nonhematologic malignancy exhibit a monocytosis that is independent of the presence or absence of metastatic disease.[76] An inverse relationship of monocyte count (elevated) and T-lymphocyte concentration (decreased) has also been noted in patients with malignant disease.[77] Reports of hematologic values in metastatic colon cancer and soft-tissue sarcoma have emphasized the frequency of monocytosis in patients with cancer.[78,79] Consequently, if *unexplained* monocytosis persists, malignancy should be considered.

EXOGENOUS CYTOKINE ADMINISTRATION

The administration of granulocyte-macrophage colony-stimulating factor (GM-CSF),[80] IL-10,[81] or granulocyte colony-stimulating factor (G-CSF)[82,83] may result in mild increases in blood monocyte counts. Administration of M-CSF[84,85] results in an invariable increase in blood monocytes. Doses of 40 to 120 mcg/kg per day result in the peak increase, which may reach three- to fourfold baseline, in approximately 8 days. Administration of human macrophage inflammatory protein-1α to patients or normal volunteers is associated with a brief monocytopenia followed by a monocytosis that is proportional to the dose administered.[86]

MYOCARDIAL INFARCTION

Monocytosis occurs after myocardial infarction, reaching a peak on day 3. A correlation exists between serum creatine kinase activity and monocyte count, suggesting a relationship between extent of infarction and monocytosis.[87] After myocardial infarction, persistent monocytosis is correlated with pump failure.[88-90] Monocytosis is a frequent finding after cardiopulmonary bypass surgery.[91] In the latter circumstance, CD14 (lipopolysaccharide [LPS] receptor) is markedly decreased on the monocyte surface and plasma-soluble CD14 is increased, changes compatible with monocyte activation.

MISCELLANEOUS CONDITIONS

Other disorders associated with monocytosis include tetrachloroethane poisoning.[92] Monocytosis is a frequent finding at the time of parturition.[93,94] An increase in blood monocytes occurs in healthy volunteers[95,96] and in patients with myelodysplastic syndrome (MDS)[97,98] who are given moderately high, therapeutic-level doses of glucocorticoids. Psychiatric depression is associated with a conjoint increase in neutrophils and monocytes.[99-101] The monocytosis in depressive and anxiety disorders is associated with high plasma levels of β endorphins and dysfunctional (hypophagocytic) monocytes.[101] Thermal injury is accompanied by monocytosis.[102,103] Competitive marathon runners have a monocytosis associated with elevated plasma levels of several cytokines, including M-CSF.[104,105] An increase in blood monocytes accompanies several rare syndromes: holoprosencephaly,[106] Kawasaki disease,[107] and Wiskott-Aldrich.[108]

BLOOD MONOCYTE SUBSET COUNTS IN DISEASE

Differential monocyte subset responses (CD14++CD16− vs. CD14+CD16+) without deviation of total monocyte counts outside the normal range have been observed in older subjects and those with sepsis, AIDS, allergic disorders, dermatitides, hemodialysis, and atherosclerosis.[4,10,91,109] These monocytic subset variations usually are not measured in clinical laboratories and, as yet, have little diagnostic or prognostic importance.

DISORDERS ASSOCIATED WITH MONOCYTOPENIA

Table 70–2 lists the disorders associated with monocytopenia. Although monocytopenia may occur in any hematopoietic multipotential cell disease associated with pancytopenia (e.g., acute myelogenous leukemia), a decrease in monocytes is notable and constant in aplastic anemia[110] and hairy cell leukemia,[111] in which monocytopenia can be a helpful diagnostic clue and also a contributor to the predisposition to infection, which is an important, morbid feature of the disease. Monocytopenia occurs in a small proportion of patients with chronic lymphocytic leukemia and these patients may have a higher frequency of infections, especially by viruses.[112] Severe thermal injuries also can result in monocytopenia.[113] Cyclic neutropenia is also notable for intermittent periods of monocytopenia.[114] Rare cases of conjoint severe neutropenia and monocytopenia occur.[115] Transient monocytopenia is a feature of hemodialysis, but monocyte counts return to normal within hours after the procedure ends.[109]

In contrast, to reports of monocytosis noted above in "Inflammatory and Immune Disorders," automated blood cell counts in large numbers of subjects find that a decreased absolute monocyte count is frequent in patients with rheumatoid arthritis[116] or systemic lupus erythematosus,[117] and in those with human immunodeficiency virus infection.[118] One has to presume that these contrasting results relate to stage or activity of disease at the time of measurement.

In 2010, a disease was described in which extreme monocytopenia, and sometimes amonocytosis, was the most striking abnormality in the blood counts.[119] It has been named the *MonoMAC syndrome* because of the monocytopenia (mono) and the frequency of *Mycobacterium avium* complex (MAC) opportunistic infections, although persistent fungal and viral infections (especially papillomavirus), also occur. Marked decreases in blood B-cell, natural killer (NK)-cell, and dendritic cell counts are characteristic.[120,121] The disease is the result of mutations in the *GATA2* gene that decrease transcription of the gene message.[122] It may present as an atypical type of MDS with a hypocellular marrow, but with striking dysmorphic megakaryocytes and micromegakaryocytes,

or with acute myelogenous leukemia.[123] Because of the *GATA2* gene product's role in the development of the vascular and lymphatic systems, some cases may have the triad of lymphedema, monosomy 7, and myelodysplasia or acute myelogenous leukemia, designated the Emberger syndrome.[124-127] Hematopoietic stem cell transplantation has been successful in restoring normal immunohematopoiesis in some of the patients so treated.[128]

Glucocorticoid hormones produce a monocytopenia, transiently, approximately 6 hours after administration to human volunteers[129,130] or to patients.[95] Administration of interferon-α and tumor necrosis factor-α may also cause monocytopenia.[131] Monocytopenia may follow radiotherapy.[132]

BLOOD DENDRITIC CELL COUNTS

Blood dendritic cells are composed of two phenotypic subtypes: myeloid-derived (HLA-DR+CD11c+CD123+) and lymphoid-plasmacytoid-derived (HLA-DR+CD11c−CD123+). The total blood dendritic cell count can be measured by flow cytometry.[133-135] Dendritic cells make up approximately 0.6 percent of blood cells (range: 0.15 to 1.30 percent) and represent 14×10^6 cells/L (range: 3 to 30×10^6 cells/L). Approximately one-third of these cells are a lymphoid-plasmacytoid–derived type and two-thirds are a myeloid-derived type.[135-137] Fluctuations in blood dendritic cells are often independent of changes in total blood monocyte count. Blood dendritic cell counts decrease with aging[138] and increase with surgical stress[137] (and presumably other stressful reactions) in relation to plasma cortisol levels.

REFERENCES

1. Turpin JA, Lopez-Bernstein G: Differentiation, maturation, and activation of monocytes and macrophages: Functional activity is controlled by a continuum of activation, in *Mononuclear Phagocytes in Cell Biology*, edited by Lopez-Berestein G, Klostergaard J, p 71. CRC Press, Boca Raton, FL, 1993.
2. Zeigler-Heitbrock HW: Heterogeneity of human blood monocytes: The CD14+ CD16+ subpopulation. *Immunol Today* 17:424, 1996.
3. Yang J, Zhang L, Yu C, et al: Monocyte and macrophage differentiation: Circulating inflammatory monocyte as biomarker for inflammatory diseases. *Biomark Res* 2:1, 2014.
4. Grage-Griebenow E, Flad H-D, Ernst M: Heterogeneity of peripheral blood monocyte subsets. *J Leukoc Biol* 69:11, 2001.
5. Hume DA, Ross IL, Himes SR, et al: The mononuclear phagocyte system revisited. *J Leukoc Biol* 72:621, 2001.
6. Griffin JD, Meuer SC, Schlossman SF, Reinherz EL: T-cell regulation of myelopoiesis: Analysis at a clonal level. *J Immunol* 133:1863, 1984.
7. Munan L, Kelly A: Age-dependent changes in blood monocyte populations in man. *Clin Exp Immunol* 35:161, 1979.
8. Meuret G, Hoffman G: Monocyte kinetic studies in normal and disease states. *Br J Haematol* 24:275, 1973.
9. Meuret G, Bremer C, Bammert J, Ewen J: Oscillation of blood monocyte counts in healthy individuals. *Cell Tissue Kinet* 7:223, 1974.
10. Sadeghi HM, Schnelle JF, Thoma JK, et al: Phenotypic and functional characteristics of circulating monocytes of elderly persons. *Exp Gerontol* 34:959, 1999.
11. Maldonado JE, Hanlon DG: Monocytosis: A current appraisal. *Mayo Clin Proc* 40:248, 1965.
12. Rigolin GM, Cuneo A, Roberti MG, et al: Myelodysplastic syndromes with monocytic component: Hematologic and cytogenetic characterization. *Haematologia (Budap)* 82:25, 1997.
13. Cunningham I, MacCallum SJ, Nicholls MD, et al: The myelodysplastic syndromes: An analysis of prognostic factors in 226 cases from a single institution. *Br J Haematol* 90:602, 1995.
14. Castaldi G, Rigolin GM: The monocytic component in myelodysplastic syndromes. *Cancer Treat Res* 108:81, 2001.
15. Jaworkowsky LI, Solovey DY, Rhausova LY, Udris OY: Monocytosis as a sign of subsequent leukemia in patients with cytopenias (preleukemia). *Folia Haematol Int Mag Klin Morphol Blutforsch* 110:395, 1983.
16. Ruggiero GM, Sica M, Luciano L, et al: A case of myelodysplastic syndrome associated with CD14(+)CD56(+) monocytosis, expansion of NK lymphocytes and defect of HLA-E expression. *Leuk Res* 33:181, 2009.
17. Boiocchi L, Espinal-Witter R, Geyer JT, et al: Development of monocytosis in patients with primary myelofibrosis indicates an accelerated phase of the disease. *Mod Pathol* 26:204, 2013.

TABLE 70–2. Disorders Associated with Monocytopenia

I. Any cause of severe leukopenia

  A. Aplastic anemia[110]

  B. Hairy cell leukemia[111]

  C. Other myeloid or lymphoid malignancies resulting in suppression of monocytopoiesis

II. MonoMAC syndrome[120-123] and Emberger syndrome[124,125] (*GATA2* gene mutations)

III. Miscellaneous conditions (see section "Disorders Associated with Monocytopenia")

18. Haferlach T, Schoch C, Schnittger S, et al: Distinct genetic patterns can be identified in acute monoblastic leukaemia (FAB AML M5a and M5b): A study of 124 patients. *Br J Haematol* 118:426, 2002.

19. Villeneuve P, Kim DT, Xu W, et al: The morphological subcategories of acute monocytic leukemia (M5a and M5b) share similar immunophenotypic and cytogenetic features and clinical outcomes. *Leuk Res* 32:269, 2008.

20. Sun X, Zhang W, Ramdas L, et al: Comparative analysis of genes regulated in acute myelomonocytic leukemia with and without inv(16)(p13q22) using microarray techniques, real-time PCR, immunohistochemistry, and flow cytometry immunophenotyping. *Mod Pathol* 20:811, 2007.

21. Laurencet FM, Chapius B, Roux-Lombard P, et al: Malignant histiocytosis in the leukaemic stage: A new entity (M5c-AML) in the FAB classification? *Leukemia* 8:502, 1994.

22. Ferran M, Gallardo F, Ferrer AM, et al: Acute myeloid dendritic cell leukaemia with specific cutaneous involvement: A diagnostic challenge. *Br J Dermatol* 158:1129, 2008.

23. Santiago-Schwartz F, Coppock DL, Hindenberg AA, Kern J: Identification of a malignant counterpart of the monocytic-dendritic cell progenitor in an acute myeloid leukemia. *Blood* 84:3054, 1994.

24. Lichtman MA, Segel GB: Uncommon phenotypes of acute myelogenous leukemia: Basophilic, mast cell, eosinophilic, and myeloid dendritic cell subtypes: A review. *Blood Cells Mol Dis* 35:370, 2005.

25. Frew ME, Donaldson K: Monocyte analysis in chronic myelomonocytic leukaemia. *Br J Biomed Sci* 54:244, 1997.

26. Onida F, Kantarjian HM, Smith TL, et al: Prognostic scoring factors and scoring systems in chronic myelomonocytic leukemia: A retrospective analysis of 213 patients. *Blood* 99:840, 2002.

27. Xu Y, McKenna RW, Karandikar NJ, et al: Flow cytometric analysis of monocytes as a tool for distinguishing chronic myelomonocytic leukemia from reactive monocytosis. *Am J Clin Pathol* 124:799, 2005.

28. Kratz CP, Niemeyer CM: Juvenile myelomonocytic leukemia. *Hematology* 1:100, 2005.

29. Ohsaka A, Shiina S, Kobayashi M, et al: Philadelphia chromosome-positive chronic myeloid leukemia expressing p190(BCR-ABL). *Intern Med* 41:1092, 2002.

30. Hur M, Song HM, Kang SH, et al: Lymphoid predominance and the absence of basophilia and splenomegaly are frequent in m-bcr-positive chronic myelogenous leukemia. *Ann Hematol* 81:219, 2002.

31. Wright D, Dale DC, Fauci AS, Wolff SM: Human cyclic neutropenia: Clinical review and long-term follow-up of patients. *Medicine (Baltimore)* 60:1, 1981.

32. Zuelzer WW, Bajoghli M: Chronic granulocytopenia in childhood. *Blood* 23:359, 1964.

33. Cutting HO, Lang JE: Familial benign chronic neutropenia. *Ann Intern Med* 61:876, 1964.

34. Krill CE, Mauer AM: Congenital agranulocytosis. *J Pediatr* 68:361, 1966.

35. Lang JE, Cutting HO: Infantile genetic agranulocytosis. *Pediatrics* 35:596, 1965.

36. Spaet TH, Dameshek W: Chronic hypoplastic neutropenia. *Am J Med* 13:35, 1952.

37. Robinson RL, Burk MS, Raman S: Fever, delirium, autonomic instability, and monocytosis associated with olanzapine. *J Postgrad Med* 49:96, 2003.

38. Graf M, Tarlov A: Agranulocytosis with monohistiocytosis associated with ampicillin therapy. *Ann Intern Med* 69:91, 1968.

39. Thöne J, Kessler E: Monocytosis subsequent to ziprasidone treatment: A possible side effect. *Prim Care Companion J Clin Psychiatry* 9:465, 2007.

40. Reznikoff P: The etiologic importance of fatigue and the prognostic significance of monocytosis in neutropenia (agranulocytosis). *Am J Clin Pathol* 6:205, 1936.

41. Rosenthal N, Abel HA: The significance of the monocytes in agranulocytosis (leukopenic infectious agranulocytosis). *Am J Clin Pathol* 6:205, 1936.

42. Pretty HM, Gosselin G, Colprian G, Long LA: Agranulocytosis: A report of 30 cases. *Can Med Assoc J* 93:1058, 1965.

43. Rosenberg SA, Diamond HD, Jaslowitz B, Craver LF: Lymphosarcoma: A review of 1269 cases. *Medicine (Baltimore)* 40:31, 1961.

44. Ultmann JE: Clinical features and diagnosis of Hodgkin's disease. *Cancer* 9:297, 1966.

45. Kaplan HS: *Hodgkin's Disease*, 2nd ed, Table 4.1, pp 127–128. Harvard University Press, Cambridge, MA, 1980.

46. Sewell RL: Lymphocyte abnormalities in myeloma. *Br J Haematol* 36:545, 1977.

47. Blom J, Nielsen H, Larsen SO, et al: A study of certain functional parameters of monocytes from patients with multiple myeloma: Comparison with monocytes from healthy individuals. *Scand J Haematol* 33:425, 1984.

48. Nakajima H, Mori S, Takeuchi T, et al: Monocytosis and high serum macrophage colony-stimulating factor in Waldenström's macroglobulinemia. *Blood* 86:2863, 1995.

49. Tokioka T, Shimamoto Y, Motoyoshi K, Yamaguchi M: Clinical significance of monocytosis and human monocytic colony stimulating factor in patients with adult T-Cell leukaemia/lymphoma. *Haematologia (Budap)* 26:1, 1994.

50. Bari A, Tadmor T, Sacchi S, et al: Monocytosis has adverse prognostic significance and impacts survival in patients with T-cell lymphomas. *Leuk Res* 37:619, 2013.

51. Mazumdar R, Evans P, Culpin R, et al: The automated monocyte count is independently predictive of overall survival from diagnosis in chronic lymphocytic leukaemia and of survival following first-line chemotherapy. *Leuk Res* 37:614, 2013.

52. Choi TS, Doh KS, Kim SH, et al: Clinicopathological and genotypic aspects of anticonvulsant-induced pseudolymphoma syndrome. *Br J Dermatol* 148:730, 2003.

53. Durig M, Landmann RMA, Harder F: Lymphocyte subsets in human peripheral blood after splenectomy and autotransplantation of splenic tissue. *J Lab Clin Med* 104:110, 1984.

54. Lanng Nielson J, Romer FK, Ellegaard J: Serum angiotensin-converting enzyme and blood monocytes in splenectomized individuals. *Acta Haematol* 67:132, 1982.

55. Buchan GS, Palmer DG, Gibbins BL: The response of human peripheral blood mononuclear phagocytes to rheumatoid arthritis. *J Leukoc Biol* 37:221, 1985.

56. Budman DR, Steinberg AD: Hematologic aspects of systemic lupus erythematosus. Current concepts. *Ann Intern Med* 86:220, 1977.

57. Goodwin JS, DeHaratius R, Israel H, et al: Suppressor cell function in sarcoidosis. *Ann Intern Med* 90:169, 1979.

58. Daniele RP, Dauber JH, Rossman MD: Immunologic abnormalities in sarcoidosis. *Ann Intern Med* 92:406, 1980.

59. Stobie W, England NJ, McMenemy WH: The interpretation of haemograms in pulmonary tuberculosis. *Am Rev Tuberc* 46:1, 1942.

60. Flinn JW: A study of the differential blood count in 1000 cases of active pulmonary tuberculosis. *Ann Intern Med* 2:622, 1929.

61. Singh KJ, Ahluwalia G, Sharma SK, et al: Significance of haematological reactions in patients with tuberculosis. *J Assoc Physicians India* 49:788, 2001.

62. Smith MB, Schnadig VJ, Boyars MC, Woods GL: Clinical and pathological features of Mycobacterium fortuitum infections: An emerging pathogen in patients with AIDS. *Am J Clin Pathol* 116:225, 2001.

63. Daland GA, Gottlieb L, Wallerstein RO, et al: Hematologic observations in bacterial endocarditis. *J Lab Clin Med* 48:827, 1956.

64. Myhre EB, Braconier JH, Sjögren U: Automated cytochemical differential leukocyte count in patients hospitalized with acute bacterial infections. *Scand J Infect Dis* 17:201, 1985.

65. Hill RW, Bayrd ED: Phagocytic reticuloendothelial cells in subacute bacterial endocarditis with negative cultures. *Ann Intern Med* 52:310, 1960.

66. Tsolia M, Drakonaki S, Messaritaki A, et al: Clinical features, complications and treatment outcome of childhood brucellosis in central Greece. *J Infect* 44:257, 2002.

67. Khan E, Siddiqi J, Shakoor S, et al: Dengue outbreak in Karachi, Pakistan, 2006: Experience at a tertiary care center. *Trans R Soc Trop Med Hyg* 101:1114, 2007.

68. Hickling RA: The monocytes in pneumonia: A clinical and hematologic study. *Arch Intern Med* 40:594, 1927.

69. Rosahn PD, Pearce L: The blood cytology in untreated and treated syphilis. *Am J Med Sci* 187:88, 1934.

70. Karyalcin G, Khanijou A, Kim KY, et al: Monocytosis in congenital syphilis. *Am J Dis Child* 131:782, 1977.

71. Klemola E: Cytomegalovirus infection in previously healthy adults. *Ann Intern Med* 79:267, 1973.

72. Tsukahara T, Yogushi A, Horiuchi Y: Significance of monocytosis in varicella herpes zoster. *J Dermatol* 19:94, 1992.

73. McClain MT, Park LP, Nicholson B, et al: Longitudinal analysis of leukocyte differentials in peripheral blood of patients with acute respiratory viral infections. *J Clin Virol* 58:689, 2013.

74. McKeever UM, O'Mahoney C, Lawlor E, et al: Monocytosis: A feature of alcoholic liver disease. *Lancet* 2:1492, 1983.

75. Mees AS, Berney J, Jewell DP: Monocytes in inflammatory bowel disease: Absolute monocyte counts. *J Clin Pathol* 33:917, 1980.

76. Barrett O Jr: Monocytosis in malignant disease. *Ann Intern Med* 73:991, 1970.

77. Wood GW, Neff JE, Stephens R: Relationship between monocytosis and T-lymphocyte function in human cancer. *J Natl Cancer Inst* 63:587, 1979.

78. Melichar B, Touskova M, Vesely P: Effect of irinotecan on the phenotype of peripheral blood leukocyte populations in patients with metastatic colorectal cancer. *Hepatogastroenterology* 49:967, 2002.

79. Ruka W, Rutkowski p, Kaminska J, et al: Alterations of routine blood tests in adult patients with soft tissue sarcomas: Relationships to cytokine serum levels and prognostic significance. *Ann Oncol* 12:1423, 2001.

80. Schmitz LL, McClure JS, Litz CE, et al: Morphologic and quantitative changes in blood and marrow cells following growth factor therapy. *Am J Clin Pathol* 101:67, 1994.

81. Chernoff AE, Granowitz EV, Shapiro L, et al: A randomized controlled trial of IL-10 in humans. *J Immunol* 154:5492, 1995.

82. Ranaghan L, Drake M, Humphreys MW, Morris TC: Leukaemoid monocytosis in M4 AML following chemotherapy: G-CSF. *Clin Lab Haematol* 20:49, 1998.

83. Liu CZ, Persad R, Inghirami G, et al: Transient atypical monocytosis mimic acute myelomonocytic leukemia in post-chemotherapy patients receiving G-CSF: Report of two cases. *Clin Lab Haematol* 26:359, 2004.

84. Weiner LM, Li W, Holmes M, et al: Phase I trial of recombinant macrophage colony-stimulating factor and recombinant gamma-interferon: Toxicity, monocytosis, and clinical effects. *Cancer Res* 54:4084, 1994.

85. Minasian LM, Yao TJ, Steffens TA, et al: A phase I study of anti-GD3 ganglioside monoclonal antibody R24 and recombinant human macrophage-colony stimulating factor in patients with metastatic melanoma. *Cancer* 75:2251, 1995.

86. Marshall E, Howell AH, Powles R, et al: Clinical effects of human macrophage inflammatory protein-1 alpha MIP-1 alpha (LD78) administration in humans. *Eur J Cancer* 34:1023, 1998.

87. Meisel SR, Panzner H, Schecter M, et al: Peripheral monocytosis following myocardial infarction. *Cardiology* 90:52, 1998.

88. Maekawa Y, Anzai T, Yoshikawa T, et al: Prognostic significance of peripheral monocytosis after reperfusion acute myocardial infarction: Possible role for left ventricular remodeling. *J Am Coll Cardiol* 16:241, 2002.

89. Gibson WJ, Gibson CM: The association of impaired myocardial perfusion and monocytosis with late recovery of left ventricular function following primary percutaneous coronary intervention. *Eur Heart J* 27:2487, 2006.

90. Hong YJ, Jeong MH, Ahn Y, et al: Relationship between peripheral monocytosis and nonrecovery of left ventricular function in patients with left ventricular dysfunction complicated with acute myocardial infarction. *Circ J* 71:1219, 2007.

91. Fingerle-Rowson G, Auers J, Kreuzer E, et al: Down-regulation of surface monocyte lipopolysaccharide-receptor CD14 in patients on cardiopulmonary bypass undergoing aorta-coronary bypass operation. *J Thorac Cardiovasc Surg* 115:1172, 1998.

92. Minot GR, Smith LW: The blood in tetrachloroethane poisoning. *Arch Intern Med* 28:687, 1921.

93. Siegal I, Gleichner N: Peripheral white blood cells alterations in early labor. *Diagn Gynecol Obstet* 3:123, 1981.

94. Buchan GS, Gibbins BL, Griffin JFT: The influence of parturition on peripheral blood mononuclear phagocyte subpopulation in pregnant women. *J Leukoc Biol* 37:231, 1985.

95. Rinehard JJ, Sagone AL, Balcerzak SP, et al: Effects of corticosteroid therapy on human monocyte function. *N Engl J Med* 292:236, 1975.

96. Shoenfeld Y, Gurewich Y, Gallant LA, et al: Prednisone-induced leukocytosis. *Am J Med* 71:773, 1981.

97. Morales M, Wilkes J, Lowder JN: Monocytic leukemoid reaction, glucocorticoid therapy, and myelodysplastic syndrome. *Cleve Clin J Med* 6:571, 1990.

98. Barker S, Scott M, Chan GT. Corticosteroids and monocytosis. *N Z Med J* 125:76, 2012.

99. Maes M, VanDerPlanken M, Stevens WJ, et al: Leukocytosis, monocytosis and neutrophilia: Hallmarks of severe depression. *J Psychiatr Res* 26:125, 1992.

100. Maes M, Lambrechts J, Suy E, et al: Absolute number and percentage of circulating natural killer, non-MHC-restricted T cytotoxic, and phagocytic cells in unipolar depression. *Neuropsychobiology* 29:157, 1994.

101. Castilla-Cortazar I, Castilla A, Gurpegui M: Opioid peptides and immunodysfunction in a patient with major depression and anxiety disorders. *J Physiol Biochem* 54:203, 1998.

102. Santangelo S, Gamelli RL, Shankar R: Myeloid commitment shifts toward monocytopoiesis after thermal injury and sepsis. *Ann Surg* 233:97, 2001.

103. Lovell R, Madden L, McNaughton LR, Carroll S: Effects of active and passive hyperthermia on heat shock protein 70 (HSP70). *Amino Acids* 34:203, 2008.

104. Kratz A, Lewandrowski KB, Siegel AJ, et al: Effect of marathon running on hematologic and biochemical laboratory parameters, including cardiac markers. *Am J Clin Pathol* 118:856, 2002.

105. Suzuki K, Nakaji S, Yamadi M, et al: Impact of a competitive marathon race on systemic cytokine and neutrophil responses. *Med Sci Sports Exerc* 35:348, 2003.

106. Jubinsky PT, Shanske AL, Pixley FJ, et al: A syndrome of holoprosencephaly, recurrent infections, and monocytosis. *Am J Med Genet A* 140:2742, 2006.

107. Kuo HC, Wang CL, Liang CD, et al: Persistent monocytosis after intravenous immunoglobulin therapy correlated with the development of coronary artery lesions in patients with Kawasaki disease. *J Microbiol Immunol Infect* 40:395, 2007.

108. Watanabe N, Yoshimi A, Kamachi Y, et al: Wiskott-Aldrich syndrome is an important differential diagnosis in male infants with juvenile myelomonocytic leukemia like features. *J Pediatr Hematol Oncol* 29:836, 2007.

109. Nockher WA, Wiemer J, Scherberich JE: Hemodialysis monocytopenia: Differential sequestration kinetics of CD14+CD16+ and CD14++ blood monocyte subsets. *Clin Exp Immunol* 123:49, 2001.

110. Twormey JJ, Douglas CC, Sharkey O Jr: The monocytopenia of aplastic anemia. *Blood* 41:187, 1973.

111. den Ottolander GJ, van der Burgh FJ, Lopes Cardozo P, et al: The Hemalog D automated differential counter in the diagnosis of hairy cell leukemia. *Leuk Res* 7:309, 1983.

112. DeRossi G, Mauro FR, Ialongo P, et al: Monocytopenia and infections in chronic lymphocytic leukemia (CLL). *Eur J Haematol* 46:119, 1991.

113. Peterson V, Hensbrough J, Buerk C, et al: Regulation of granulopoiesis following severe thermal injury. *J Trauma* 23:19, 1983.

114. Adams WH, Liu YK: Periodic neutropenia and monocytopenia. *Am J Hematol* 13:73, 1982.

115. Marinone G, Roncoli B, Marinone MG Jr: Pure white cell aplasia. *Semin Hematol* 28:298, 1991.

116. Isenberg DA, Martin P, Hajirousou V, et al: Haematological reassessment of rheumatoid arthritis using an automated method. *Br J Rheumatol* 25:152, 1986.

117. Isenberg DA, Patterson KG, Todd-Pokropek A, et al: Haematological aspects of systemic lupus erythematosus: A reappraisal using automated methods. *Acta Haematol* 67:242, 1982.

118. Treacy M, Lai L, Costello C, et al: Peripheral blood and bone marrow abnormalities in patients with HIV related disease. *Br J Haematol* 65:289, 1987.

119. Vinh DC, Patel SY, Uzel G, et al: Autosomal dominant and sporadic monocytopenia with susceptibility to mycobacteria, fungi, papillomaviruses, and myelodysplasia. *Blood* 115:1519, 2010.

120. Camargo JF, Lobo SA, Hsu AP, et al: MonoMAC syndrome in a patient with a GATA2 mutation: Case report and review of the literature. *Clin Infect Dis* 57:697, 2013.

121. Hsu AP, Sampaio EP, Khan J, Calvo KR, et al: Mutations in GATA2 are associated with the autosomal dominant and sporadic monocytopenia and mycobacterial infection (MonoMAC) syndrome. *Blood* 118:2653, 2011.

122. Hsu AP, Johnson KD, Falcone EL, et al: GATA2 haploinsufficiency caused by mutations in a conserved intronic element leads to MonoMAC syndrome. *Blood* 121:3830, 2013.

123. Calvo KR, Vinh DC, Maric I, et al: Myelodysplasia in autosomal dominant and sporadic monocytopenia immunodeficiency syndrome: Diagnostic features and clinical implications. *Haematologica* 96:1221, 2011.

124. Ostergaard P, Simpson MA, Connell FC et al: Mutations in GATA2 cause primary lymphedema associated with a predisposition to acute myeloid leukemia (Emberger syndrome). *Nat Genet* 43:929, 2011.

125. Kazenwadel J, Secker GA, Liu YJ, et al: Loss-of-function germline GATA2 mutations in patients with MDS/AML or MonoMAC syndrome and primary lymphedema reveal a key role for GATA2 in the lymphatic vasculature. *Blood* 119:1283, 2012.

126. Spinner MA, Sanchez LA, Hsu AP, et al: GATA2 deficiency: A protean disorder of hematopoiesis, lymphatics, and immunity. *Blood* 123:809, 2014.

127. Dickinson RE, Milne P, Jardine L, et al: The evolution of cellular deficiency in GATA2 mutation. *Blood* 123:863, 2014.

128. Cuellar-Rodriguez J, Gea-Banacloche J, Freeman AF, et al: Successful allogeneic hematopoietic stem cell transplantation for GATA2 deficiency. *Blood* 118:3715, 2011.

129. Steer JH, Vuong Q, Joyce DA: Suppression of human monocyte tumor necrosis factor-alpha release by glucocorticoid therapy: Relationship to systemic monocytopenia and cortisol suppression. *Br J Clin Pharmacol* 43:383, 1997.

130. Fauci AS, Dale DC: Monocytopenia after prednisone. *N Engl J Med* 292:928, 1975.

131. Aulitzky WE, Tilg H, Vogel W, et al: Acute hematologic effects of interferon alpha, interferon gamma, tumor necrosis factor alpha and interleukin 2. *Ann Hematol* 62:25, 1991.

132. Rotman M, Ansley H, Rogow L, et al: Monocytosis: A new observation during radiotherapy. *Int J Radiat Oncol Biol Phys* 2:117, 1977.

133. Fearnley DB, Whyte LF, Carnoutosis SA, et al: The monitoring of human blood dendritic cell numbers. *Blood* 93:728, 1999.

134. Szabolcs P, Park K-D, Reese M, et al: Absolute values of dendritic cell subsets in bone marrow, cord blood, and peripheral blood enumerated by a novel method. *Stem Cells* 21:269, 2003.

135. Giannelli S, Taddeo A, Presicce P, et al: A six-color flow cytometric assay for the analysis of peripheral blood dendritic cells. *Cytometry B Clin Cytom* 74:349, 2008.

136. Koga Y, Matsuzaki A, Suminoe A, et al: Expression of cytokine-associated genes in dendritic cells (DCs): Comparison between adult peripheral blood- and umbilical cord blood-derived DCs by cDNA microarray. *Immunol Lett* 116:55, 2008.

137. Ho CSK, López JA, Vuckovic S, et al: Surgical and physical stress increases circulatory blood dendritic cell counts independently of monocyte counts. *Blood* 98:140, 2001.

138. Pérez-Cabezas B, Naranjo-Gómez M, Fernández MA, et al: Reduced numbers of plasmacytoid dendritic cells in aged blood donors. *Exp Gerontol* 42:1033, 2007.

CHAPTER 71
INFLAMMATORY AND MALIGNANT HISTIOCYTOSIS

Kenneth L. McClain and Carl E. Allen

SUMMARY

Diseases of the histiocyte (i.e., macrophage or dendritic cell) lineage can be divided into four groups based upon the final maturation steps from their myeloid progenitor cells: (1) Langerhans cell histiocytosis (LCH), (2) malignant histiocytoses or dendritic cell sarcomas, (3) juvenile xanthogranuloma/Erdheim-Chester disease, Rosai-Dorfman disease, and (4) hemophagocytic lymphohistiocytosis syndromes. Storage diseases of macrophages are discussed in Chap. 72. The distinction among these diseases is based upon clinical characteristics and histopathologic staining for unique surface markers. LCH may present at birth or in adulthood with skin rash, bone pain, draining ears, oral ulcers, gingivitis, pulmonary dysfunction, chronic diarrhea, diabetes insipidus, and marrow or liver failure. Therapy for LCH in children has been studied in clinical trials by the Histiocyte Society. Treatment for adults is based primarily on case series. Although relapses are not typically rapidly fatal, they are associated with a higher risk of endocrine and central nervous system complications. The diagnostic criteria for the malignant histiocytosis have been clarified by cell-surface marker studies. Treatment options and prognosis vary widely. Erdheim-Chester disease and juvenile xanthogranuloma are phenotypically similar, but are treated differently. Erdheim-Chester disease is found almost exclusively in adults and juvenile xanthogranuloma occurs primarily in children. Rosai-Dorfman disease presents with massive cervical lymphadenopathy in most patients, but may also involve other parts of the body. There are several treatment options for Rosai-Dorfman disease, Erdheim-Chester disease, and juvenile xanthogranuloma, but no clinical trials of specific drugs have been published. Hemophagocytic lymphohistiocytosis (HLH) is characterized by pathologic inflammation and may present with infections, hepatitis, meningitis, or autoimmune diseases. Without therapy, HLH is almost universally fatal. Most patients who receive prompt diagnosis and treatment with immune suppression therapy survive.

Acronyms and Abbreviations: AHSCT, allogeneic hematopoietic stem cell transplantation; ALL, acute lymphoblastic leukemia; ATG, antithymocyte globulin; CD, cluster designation; CT, computed tomography; DC, dendritic cell; DI, diabetes insipidus; DLCO, diffusing capacity in lung for carbon dioxide; ECD, Erdheim-Chester disease; FEV$_1$, forced expiratory volume in 1 second; HLA-DR, human leukocyte antigen-D related; HLH, hemophagocytic lymphohistiocytosis; IFN, interferon; IL, interleukin; JXG, juvenile xanthogranuloma; LC, Langerhans cell; LCH, Langerhans cell histiocytosis; M-CSF, macrophage colony-stimulating factor; MRI, magnetic resonance imaging; NK, natural killer; PET, positron emission tomography; RDD, Rosai-Dorfman disease.

CLASSIFICATION OF THE HISTIOCYTOSES

The general description of cells in the monocyte-macrophage system (mononuclear phagocyte system) has been largely clarified (Chaps. 67 to 69), although some ambiguity remains. Nomenclature committees remain loyal to the term "histiocyte," a designation assigned in the 19th century to tissue macrophages, although the "histiocytosis" umbrella includes functional and neoplastic disorders of a broad range of cells in the monocyte, macrophage, and dendritic cell (DC) lineages. The distinctions among diseases in this category are determined by (1) clinical findings, (2) histopathology, (3) immunocytology to define the antigens on the surface of the pathologic cells, and (4) cytogenetic or genetic features (Table 71–1).

The histiocytic disorders have been classified based upon whether they are (1) DC related, (2) monocyte-macrophage related, or (3) malignancies of macrophages or DCs (Table 71–2).[1,2] Evolving understanding of myelomonocytic differentiation, as well as cellular origins of histiocytic disorders, will likely necessitate revision of these classifications in the near future.

The pathologic cells in Langerhans cell histiocytosis (LCH) lesions have phenotypic similarity to epidermal Langerhans cells (LCs), which has led to the hypothesis that LCH is derived from aberrant activation and/or neoplastic transformation of the epidermal LCs.[3] LCH originates from aberrant proliferation and differentiation of myelomonocytic precursors.[4,5] Regardless of ontogeny, LCH lesions are characterized by pathologic DCs with phenotypic similarity to epidermal LCs, including positive staining with anti-CD207 (antilangerin) and the presence of Birbeck granules identified by electron microscopy.[6,7] Birbeck granules are racket-shaped inclusions that are thought to be involved in antigen processing. Cells staining with anti-CD207 and/or anti-CD1a are required for the diagnosis of LCH. Other antigens, such as S100 or HLA-DR (human leukocyte antigen-D related) are not specific for LCH. The histiocytes in Erdheim-Chester disease (ECD) and juvenile xanthogranuloma (JXG) have phenotypic similarity to the dermal–interstitial dendrocyte that stains with antibodies to CD68, fascin, and factor XIIIa. However, the DCs in these disorders also express surface CD163 that is characteristic of macrophages.

Malignant histiocytosis (or "histiocytic sarcoma") has evolved as a diagnosis of exclusion involving malignant histiocytes that lack markers for anaplastic large cell lymphoma or other hematologic malignancies. Malignant histiocytosis represents a spectrum of malignancies that presumably derive from DCs of different lineages at different stages of differentiation. Human DCs are defined as hematopoietic cells expressing high levels of major histocompatibility complex II (MCHII) and CD11c while lacking other specific lineage markers. Under normal conditions, these cells reside in tissue or circulate in the blood. Once stimulated by antigen, they migrate to lymphoid tissue and interact with effector or suppressor T cells. Malignant histiocytoses are variable and share surface markers with DC subsets: follicular DC "sarcoma" (CD21+, CD35+), interdigitating DC "sarcoma" (CD14+), and Langerhans cell "sarcoma" (CD1a+).

The monocyte-macrophage disorders include Rosai-Dorfman disease (RDD) and hemophagocytic lymphohistiocytosis (HLH). RDD, also known as sinus histiocytosis with massive lymphadenopathy, has the telltale histopathologic finding of intact lymphocytes in the cytoplasm of macrophages (emperipolesis), a feature that must be present to diagnose this disorder. HLH is distinct among the diseases discussed in this chapter in that the macrophages are nonneoplastic, otherwise normal histiocytes, characterized by a pathologic reaction to aberrant stimuli.

TABLE 71-1. Differentiating Characteristics of Histiocytes*

Histologic Features	LCH	Malignant Histiocytosis	ECD/JXG	HLH	RDD
HLH-DR	++	+	−	+	+
CD1a	++	+/−	−	−	−
CD14	−	+/−	++	++	++
CD68	+/−	+/−	++	++	++
CD163	−	−	+	++	++
CD207 (Langerin)	+++	+/−	−	−	−
Factor XIIIa	−	−	++	−	−
Fascin	−	+/−	++	+/−	+
Birbeck granules	+	+/−	−	−	−
Hemophagocytosis	+/−	−	−	+/−	−
Emperipolesis	−	−	−	−	+

CD, cluster of differentiation; ECD, Erdheim-Chester disease; HLH, hemophagocytic lymphohistiocytosis; JXG, Juvenile Xanthogranuloma; LCH, Langerhans cell histiocytosis; RDD, Rosai-Dorfman disease.

Data from Jaffe R: The diagnostic histopathology of Langerhans cell histiocytosis, in *Histiocytic Disorders of Children and Adults. Basic Science Clinical Features, and Therapy,* edited by Weitzman S, Egeler RM, pp 14–39. Cambridge University Press, Cambridge, UK, 2005; Chikwava K, Jaffe R: Langerin (CD207) staining in normal pediatric tissues, reactive lymph nodes, and childhood histiocytic disorders. *Pediatr Dev Pathol* 7:607–614, 2004; and Lau SK, Chu PG, Weiss LM: Immunohistochemical expression of Langerin in Langerhans cell histiocytosis and non-Langerhans cell histiocytic disorders. *Am J Surg Pathol* 32:615–619, 2008.

TABLE 71-2. Classification of Histiocytic Disorders

1. Disorders of varying biologic behavior, lacking cytologic atypia
   a. Dendritic-cell-related
      Langerhans cell histiocytosis
      Juvenile xanthogranuloma
      Erdheim-Chester disease
   b. Monocyte-macrophage related
      Hemophagocytic lymphohistiocytosis
         Familial and/or with identified dysfunctional gene mutation
      Secondary hemophagocytic syndromes
         Infection-associated
         Malignancy-associated
         Autoimmune-associated
         Other
      Sinus histiocytosis with massive lymphadenopathy (Rosai-Dorfman disease)
      Solitary histiocytoma of macrophage phenotype
2. Malignant disorders
   Dendritic cell related
   Histiocytic sarcoma
   Monocyte-macrophage related
   Leukemias: monocytic M5A and M5B, myelomonocytic M4, chronic myelomonocytic leukemia

Data from Jaffe R: The diagnostic histopathology of Langerhans cell histiocytosis, in *Histiocytic Disorders of Children and Adults. Basic Science Clinical Features, and Therapy,* edited by Weitzman S, Egeler RM, pp 14–39. Cambridge University Press, Cambridge, UK, 2005 and Favara BE, Feller AC, Pauli M et al: Contemporary classification of histiocytic disorders. The WHO Committee On Histiocytic/Reticulum Cell Proliferations. Reclassification Working Group of the Histiocyte Society. Med Pediatr Oncol 29:157–166, 1997.

● LANGERHANS CELL HISTIOCYTOSIS

HISTORY

LCH has a complicated history that underlies the current clinicopathologic approach to the disease. What has come to be identified as LCH was first described in case reports and series in the early 1900s.[8] By the 1950s, patterns of clinical presentations had been categorized as Hand-Schüller-Christian (multifocal eosinophilic granulomas) and Letterer-Siwe (disseminated disease including marrow, spleen and liver). However, these apparently disparate entities were found to share the same histopathology: histiocytes with abundant cytoplasm and reniform nuclei among an inflammatory infiltrate that could include lymphocytes, eosinophils and macrophages. Lichtenstein hypothesized that these clinical disorders must be linked by a common etiology, and proposed the designation "Histiocytosis X," with "X" indicating incomplete knowledge of pathogenesis and cell of origin. Two decades later, Birbeck granules, which had previously been identified only in epidermal LCs, were identified in DCs of LCH lesions by electron microscopy. Nezelof and colleagues therefore extended Lichtenstein's hypothesis that this spectrum of disorders arises from the epidermal Langerhans cell.[3] Histiocytosis X has since been regarded as "Langerhans cell histiocytosis."

EPIDEMIOLOGY AND INHERITANCE

The incidence of LCH is 2 to 10 cases per 1 million children younger than age 15 years.[9–11] A survey of LCH patients in France revealed an incidence of 4 to 6 per 1 million in children younger than age 15 years. The male-to-female ratio is close to 1 and the median age of presentation is 30 months, although patients may present with the disease from birth through the ninth decade. Identical and fraternal twins with early onset of LCH have been described. There are occasional reports of affected nontwin siblings and multiple cases in one family, although it is not clear if this is significantly greater than one would expect by chance.[12]

The relatively high rate of high-risk multisystem LCH in identical twins compared to presumed fraternal twins may be explained by shared precursor cells as well as the possibility of shared genes. An increased frequency of family members with thyroid disease,[13] family members with other cancers,[14] *in vitro* fertilization,[15] and parental exposure to metal[16] have also been reported as potential associations. Although inheritance of penetrant mendelian "LCH genes" in the majority of cases seems unlikely, it remains possible that there are inherited genes associated with increased risk of developing LCH.

Molecular Pathology

The focus of studies and reviews on LCH over the past decades has been on either an immune or a neoplastic disorder. The competing models have been (1) an inappropriate activation of an otherwise normal epidermal LC or (2) a neoplastic transformation of the epidermal LC. Twenty years ago, CD1a+ cells from LCH lesions were described as clonal, based on non–random X inactivation.[17,18] Subsequently, somatic activating mutations in the *BRAF* oncogene were reported in 57 percent of LCH histopathologic specimens,[19] with subsequent studies validating the recurrent *BRAF*[V600E] mutation at high frequency.[5,20–22] BRAF is the central kinase of the RAS/RAF/MEK/ERK pathway, which is essential to numerous cell functions and is frequently mutated in cancer cells.[23] Significance of *BRAF*[V600E] as a driver mutation in LCH is supported by early reports of clinical responses to BRAF inhibition in adults with combined LCH and ECD.[24] Other recurrent somatic mutations in LCH may be uncovered.

Cell of Origin

The cell of origin of LCH has been assumed to be the epidermal LC based on phenotypic similarities discussed above. However, the transcriptome of CD207+ cells from LCH lesions is more consistent with an immature myeloid DC phenotype than with the transcriptome of epidermal LCs.[4] Furthermore, DC maturation may be heterogeneous within lesions, with variable CD1a+/CD207– populations.[25,26] Immunohistochemical staining antibodies specific for BRAF[V600E] revealed that the mutations are not limited to CD207+ cells within LCH lesions, but also are found in CD207-negative subpopulations.[21] Using the BRAF[V600E] mutation as a "bar code," cells that carry the mutation were identified in circulating myelomonocytic precursors in blood and in hematopoietic stem cells in marrow aspirates of patients with clinical high-risk LCH, but not in patients with single-lesion low-risk LCH. The functional significance of this observation was supported by the ability of forced expression of BRAF[V600E] in myelomonocytic precursors (CD11c+ cells) to induce a disseminated LCH-like phenotype in mice.[5] We therefore hypothesize that the state of differentiation of the cell in which LCH arises determines the clinical manifestations of the disease; pathologic ERK (extracellular signal-regulated kinase) activation in stem cell or early myelomonocytic precursor resulted in disseminated high-risk disease whereas ERK activation in tissue-restricted precursor resulted in localized disease. These observations define LCH as a myeloid neoplasm.

Inflammation and Langerhans Cell Histiocytosis

Although ERK hyperactivation may drive differentiation and proliferation of myelomonocytic precursors in LCH, the mechanisms that drive inflammation in the LCH lesions are not currently understood. The LCH DCs make up a median of 8 percent of the cells within lesions.[5] Like physiologically activated DCs, they express high levels of T-cell costimulatory molecules and proinflammatory cytokines.[4,27,28] The LCH lesion's inflammatory infiltrate includes lymphocytes, macrophages, and eosinophils in variable proportions, with enrichment of regulatory CD4+CD25+ T cells (T regs).[29] Dozens of cytokines, chemokines,

and cytokine and chemokine receptors have been hypothesized to play roles in LCH pathogenesis, creating a local "cytokine storm" as well as increased circulating proinflammatory cytokines, including tumor necrosis factor α, soluble interleukin (IL)-2 receptor α, RANKL (receptor activator of nuclear factor-κB ligand), osteoprotegerin, and osteopontin.[4,30,31] Although MAPK (mitogen-activated protein kinase) pathway activation in maturing DCs may drive differentiation of LCH DCs, inflammation likely plays a role in the clinical manifestations and possibly also in tumor maintenance: A unique phenomenon in LCH is that disruption of solitary LCH lesions often results in spontaneous resolution, even without clean margins.

CLINICAL FEATURES

LCH usually presents with a skin rash or painful bone lesion. Systemic symptoms of fever, weight loss, diarrhea, edema, dyspnea, polydipsia, and polyuria may also occur.

In LCH, involvement of specific organs at the time of diagnosis determines the designation "high-risk" or "low-risk." Organs that indicate high-risk of progression include liver, spleen, and marrow. Organs that indicate low-risk of progression include skin, bone, lung, lymph nodes, and pituitary gland. Patients may present with disease in one site or organ (single site or single system) or in multiple sites or organs (multisystem). Treatment decisions for patients are based on whether or not organs that indicate high-risk or low-risk of progression are involved, and if LCH presents as a single site or as a multisystem disease. Patients can have LCH of the skin, bone, lymph nodes, and pituitary in any combination and still be considered to have a low-risk of progression.

Single-Site Disease Presentation

In this situation the disease presents with involvement of one site, which can be skin, oral mucosa, bone, lymph nodes, pituitary, or thymus.

Skin Lesions simulating seborrheic dermatitis of the scalp may be mistaken for prolonged "cradle cap" in infants. The lesions may be localized to intertriginous areas or may be diffuse (Fig. 71–1). The most common skin flexures affected are the groin, the perianal area, back of the ears, the neck, the armpits, and, in women, the crease below the breasts. Infants may also present with brown to purplish papules over any part of their body. This latter manifestation may be self-limited as

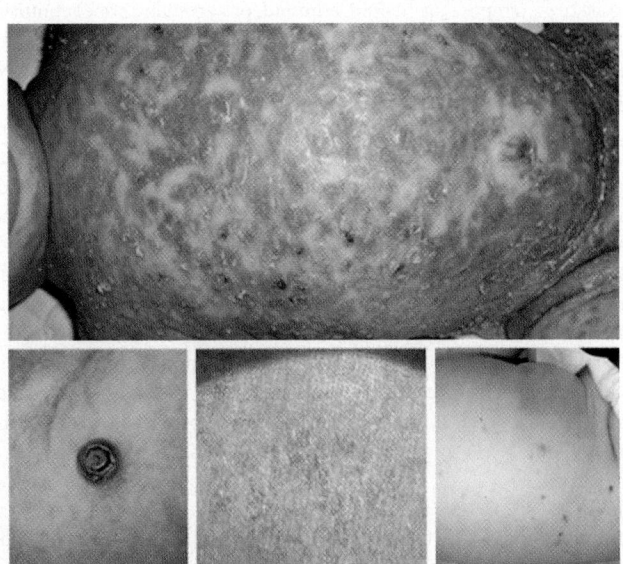

Figure 71–1. Photographs demonstrate variability in clinical presentations of Langerhans cell histiocytosis skin lesions.

the lesions often disappear during the first year of life with no therapy. However, these patients should be evaluated for other sites of disease which may coexist with skin lesions as multisystem LCH. Some reports describe multisystem LCH arising after presenting with lesions limited to the skin,[32,33] although infants with skin lesions were not observed to develop disseminated disease in a relatively large institutional series.[34] In a report of 61 neonatal LCH cases, nearly 60 percent had multisystem disease and 72 percent had high-risk organ involvement.[35] The overall survival was poorer in neonates with high-risk organ involvement compared to infants and children with the same extent of disease. Response to therapy at 12 weeks was more important than patient age in determining outcome. A review of 71 children with skin involvement revealed that those without other organ systems involved had nearly a 90 percent progression-free survival after initial therapy or observation. Often dermatologists or general practitioners who see a patient with skin LCH do not perform a complete evaluation searching for LCH in other sites. Thus, we found that 40% of patients referred for apparent "skin only" LCH did have other sites of disease when a complete evaluation was done.[34]

Isolated skin involvement is rarely observed in children older than 18 months of age.[34] Children and adults may develop red papular lesions in the scalp, skin of the groin, abdomen, back, or chest that resemble the diffuse rash of *Candida* infection. Seborrhea-like involvement of the scalp may be mistaken for a severe case of dandruff in older individuals. Ulcerative lesions behind the ears, involving the scalp, skin of the genitalia, or perianal region are often misdiagnosed as bacterial or fungal infections.

Oral Mucosa Presenting symptoms include gingival hypertrophy, ulcers of the soft or hard palate, buccal mucosa, or on the tongue and lips. Lesions of the oral mucosa may precede evidence of LCH elsewhere.[36]

Bone The most frequent site of LCH in children is a lytic lesion of the skull which may be asymptomatic or painful.[37] LCH can occur in any bone. The most frequently involved sites are skull, femur, ribs, vertebrae, and humerus. Spine lesions are most often located in the cervical vertebrae and are frequently associated with other bone lesions. Proptosis from a LCH mass in the orbit mimics rhabdomyosarcoma, neuroblastoma, and benign fatty tumors of the eye. Some skull lesions are not only lytic but may have an accompanying mass that impinges on the dura. Whether or not this affects risk of progression or not is unknown. Lesions of the facial bones (orbit, mastoid), or anterior or middle cranial fossae (e.g., temporal, sphenoid, ethmoid, or zygomatic bone) comprise the "CNS-risk" sites. These patients have a threefold increased risk for developing diabetes insipidus (DI) and an increased risk of other CNS disease (see "Central Nervous System and Endocrine System" below).

Lymph Nodes and Thymus Cervical nodes are the ones most frequently involved and may be soft or hard-matted masses with accompanying lymphedema. An enlarged thymus or mediastinal node involvement can mimic lymphoma or an infectious process and may cause asthma-like symptoms. Biopsy of the node or mass with histologic examination and microbial cultures is helpful even in patients with known LCH as lymphadenopathy may represent LCH, coexisting neoplastic disease, or infection.[38]

Pituitary Gland The posterior pituitary gland can be affected in LCH patients causing central DI (see "Endocrine System" below). Anterior pituitary involvement may result in impaired growth and sexual maturation.

Multisystem Disease

In multisystem LCH, the disease presents in multiple organs or body systems, including liver and spleen, marrow (high-risk sites) or bones, lungs, skin, lymph nodes endocrine system, gastrointestinal system (low-risk sites), and CNS (intermediate-risk site depending on extent).

Liver and Spleen Patients with liver and spleen involvement have a significantly increased risk of death from LCH. Hence, these are considered "high-risk organs."[39] Hepatic infiltration by LCH lesions can be accompanied by dysfunction, leading to hypoalbuminemia with ascites, hyperbilirubinemia, and clotting factor deficiencies. Sonographic imaging, computed tomography (CT), or magnetic resonance imaging (MRI) of the liver may show hypoechoic or low-signal intensity along the portal veins or biliary tracts when the liver is involved.[40] One of the most serious complications of hepatic LCH is cholestasis and progressive sclerosing cholangitis.[41] The median age of children with hepatic LCH is 23 months. Patients generally present with hepatomegaly with or without splenomegaly, elevated alkaline phosphatase, liver transaminases, and γ-glutamyl transpeptidase. Biopsies may or may not show CD207+ DCs.[42] A classic histologic feature is the collection of lymphocytes around bile ducts. Seventy-five percent of children with sclerosing cholangitis do not respond to chemotherapy and ultimately require liver transplantation.[41]

Massive splenomegaly may lead to consumptive cytopenias and respiratory compromise. Splenectomy may ameliorate severe thrombocytopenia, but the effect is generally not sustained with progressive hepatomegaly and inflammation in the setting of uncontrolled disseminated LCH.

Lung The lungs were once considered a high-risk organ; however, review of a large series of patients shows that the treatment outcome for patients with lung and bone involvement is not statistically different from those with only bone LCH.[43] The lungs are less frequently involved in children (13 percent) than in adults (60 percent), in whom smoking is a key etiologic factor.[44] In young children with diffuse disease, therapy can halt tissue destruction and normal repair mechanisms may restore some lung parenchyma and function. "Spontaneous" pneumothorax can be the first sign of LCH in the lung. Patients also present with cough, tachypnea, or dyspnea. Ultimately, widespread fibrosis and destruction of lung tissue leads to severe pulmonary insufficiency. Declining diffusion capacity may also herald the onset of pulmonary hypertension.[45] Chest radiographs may show a nonspecific interstitial infiltrate. A high-resolution CT image of the chest is needed to visualize the cystic and nodular pattern of LCH that leads to the destruction of lung tissue.

Marrow Involvement of the marrow is considered an indicator of high risk. Most patients with marrow involvement are young children who also have diffuse disease in the liver, spleen, lymph nodes, and skin with significant thrombocytopenia or neutropenia, though some may also have scattered marrow involvement with more mild cytopenias.[46,47] An institutional study found patients with high-risk LCH with the *BRAF*[V600E] mutation to have 0.2 to 2.1 percent of cells from the marrow aspirate carry the mutation, with only four of seven cases being reported as having abnormal histology.[5] LCH patients sometimes present with hemophagocytosis in the marrow.[48] The presence of CD1a+/CD207+ in the marrow or at other sites identifies hemophagocytic syndrome as secondary to LCH rather than from primary HLH (discussed in the section "Hemophagocytic Lymphohistiocytosis" below).

Endocrine System DI is the most frequent endocrine manifestation of LCH. Patients may present with an apparent "idiopathic" DI and sometimes with an enlarged pituitary gland or stalk before other LCH lesions are identified. Approximately half of these patients will have other lesions diagnostic of LCH within a year of identifying the DI.[49] A review of patients with DI and enlarged pituitary glands found the three most likely diagnoses were germinoma, LCH, and lymphoma.[50] DI followed the initial LCH diagnosis at other sites by a mean of 1 year and growth hormone deficiency occurred on the average 5 years later. Historically, the 10-year risk of pituitary involvement has been reported as 24 percent.[51] In one series, this incidence of DI did not decrease in chemotherapy-treated patients (see "Central Nervous System and Diabetes Insipidus" below). In another study the incidence of DI decreased from 40 to 20 percent after 6 months of treatment with vinblastine and prednisone for patients at risk for CNS involvement.[52] However, after a year of this treatment, the incidence of DI was decreased to 12 percent.[39]

Craniofacial Lesions Patients with multisystem disease and craniofacial involvement at the time of diagnosis, particularly of the ear, eye, and oral region, carried a significantly increased risk of developing DI (relative risk: 4.6).[53] This risk increased when the disease remained active for a longer period of time or reactivated. The risk for development of DI in this population was 20 percent at 15 years after diagnosis. Up to 56 percent of DI patients will develop anterior pituitary hormone deficiencies (growth, thyroid, or gonad-stimulating hormones) within 10 years of the onset of DI.[54]

Gastrointestinal System A few patients with diarrhea, hematochezia, perianal fistulas, or malabsorption have been reported.[55,56] Diagnosing gastrointestinal lesions in LCH is difficult because of the patchy involvement. Endoscopic evaluation may reveal CD1a+/CD207+ cells in the intestinal mucosa, though LCH involvement may be patchy and require multiple biopsies to detect.

Central Nervous System and Diabetes Insipidus DI (considered both an endocrine and a CNS manifestation of LCH) can present as an early or late condition. DI caused by damage to the posterior pituitary is the most frequent initial sign (and early manifestation) of LCH in the CNS. Pituitary biopsies are rarely done and only if the stalk is larger than 6.5 mm or there is a hypothalamic mass. The pituitary enlargement may spontaneously decrease or respond to chemotherapy.[57] However, a review of 22 patients with pituitary enlargement of 6.5 mm or greater revealed that despite regression of the mass with therapy, all had anterior pituitary deficiencies as well as MRI evidence of the CNS neurodegenerative syndrome (see "Other Chronic Central Nervous System Disease Manifestations" below) and 17 (77 percent) developed clinical signs of neurodegeneration.[58] Most often the diagnosis of LCH is established by biopsy of skin, bone, or lymph node of a patient who also has the pituitary abnormalities.

Other Chronic Central Nervous System Disease Manifestations LCH patients may develop mass lesions of the choroid plexus, or gray or white matter.[59] These lesions may contain CD1a+ DCs as well as CD8+ lymphocytes.[60] A chronic CNS problem that develops in 1 to 4 percent of LCH patients is the "LCH CNS neurodegenerative syndrome" manifested by dysarthria, ataxia, dysmetria, and, sometimes, behavior changes.[61,62] The brain MRI in these patients shows hyperintensity of the dentate nucleus and white matter of the cerebellum on fluid-attenuated inversion recovery (FLAIR) and T2-weighted images or hyperintense lesions of the basal ganglia on T1-weighted images (Fig. 71–2). Atrophy of the cerebellum also may be seen.[59] The radiologic findings may precede the onset of symptoms by many years or can be found coincidently. Among 83 LCH patients who had at least two MRI studies of the brain for evaluation of craniofacial lesions, DI, other endocrine deficiencies, or neuropsychological symptoms, 57 percent had radiologic neurodegenerative changes at a median time of 34 months after diagnosis. Of these patients, one-quarter had clinical neurologic deficits develop 3 to 15 years after LCH diagnosis.[62]

LABORATORY FEATURES

LCH is defined by characteristic inflammatory lesions including histiocytes expressing CD1a and CD207 (Fig. 71–3).[1] Patients with high-risk disease may present with anemia and thrombocytopenia caused by marrow involvement and/or inflammation.[46,47] An elevated sedimentation rate and thrombocytosis has been reported to correlate with active

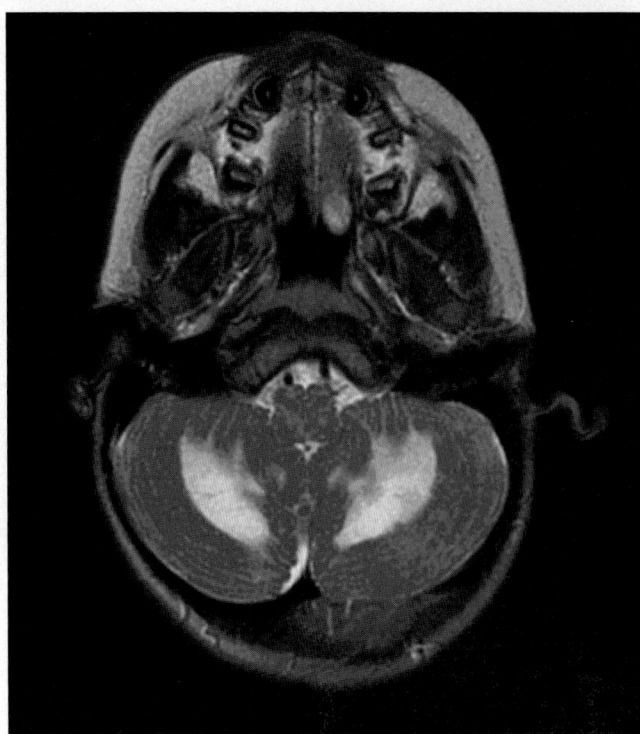

Figure 71–2. Radiologic evidence of Langerhans cells histiocytosis and CNS neurodegenerative syndrome. T2-weighted magnetic resonance image of the brain of a patient with Langerhans cells histiocytosis showing hyperintense changes of the cerebellar white matter.

LCH, but these associations are variable.[63] When the liver is involved hypoalbuminemia, elevated liver enzymes, and elevated bilirubin may be observed. Intestinal involvement may also cause hypoalbuminemia. Lytic lesions of the bone are identified by plain films, CT imaging, MRI, bone scan, or positron emission tomography (PET) scan. PET scans are useful for detecting lesions not found by bone scan or plain films and comparison PET scans are particularly good for providing evidence of healing after 6 to 12 weeks of therapy.[64] An institutional series found the presence of the somatic mutation in LCH lesions to correlate with

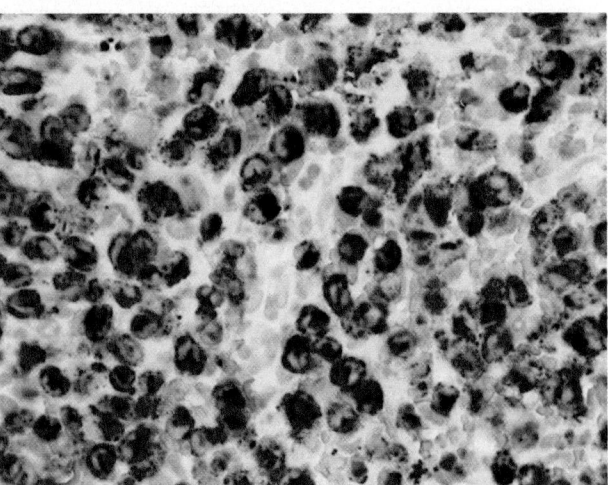

Figure 71–3. Biopsy of a bone lesion in a patient with Langerhans cell histiocytosis. Langerhans cells cytoplasm and membrane stain positively for CD207 (immunoperoxidase stain with hematoxylin and eosin [H&E] counterstain).

higher risk of initial treatment failure, and circulating cells with the *BRAF*[V600E] mutation to correlate with active disease, though these observations remain to be validated in prospective trials.[5]

DIFFERENTIAL DIAGNOSIS

It is not unusual for infants with LCH skin lesions to have symptoms for longer than 1 year prior to having a diagnostic biopsy.[34] The varied cutaneous presentations of LCH may mimic a fungal diaper rash, seborrheic scalp rash or cradle cap, congenital viral infections, neuroblastoma, contact dermatitis, or psoriasis (see Fig. 71–1). Women or men with genital lesions may be thought to have a sexually transmitted disease or other infection. Oral lesions mimic other ulcerative conditions, gingival infections, or dental caries. Copious white or green discharge from the ears resembles otitis externa. Lytic bone lesions are often thought to be evidence of a malignancy such as neuroblastoma, rhabdomyosarcoma, or Ewing sarcoma. Collapsed vertebrae from LCH may mimic tuberculosis bone disease, trauma, or osteomyelitis. The interstitial infiltrates found in LCH patients with pulmonary involvement may resemble a viral pneumonia. An enlarged thymus or mediastinal lymph nodes can cause respiratory distress and wheezing similar to asthma. Enlarged lymph nodes from LCH mimic any infiltrative condition such as lymphomas, other histiocytic diseases, infections, or immune-related conditions. Likewise, hepatosplenomegaly of LCH patients can result from the same conditions. Chronic diarrhea in LCH patients may initially be considered to be an infectious or inflammatory bowel disease. Isolated DI with enlargement of the pituitary may suggest a germinoma, lymphoma, or hypophysitis. LCH should be strongly considered when symptoms of other more common conditions do not respond to therapy.

Occasionally infiltrates of LC are found in various malignancies and as such represent an attempt of the immune system to respond to that disease.[65–67] Similarly LCH may be found in the thymus of patients with myasthenia gravis.[68]

TREATMENT

Pediatric Patients

The current optimal treatment of childhood and adults LCH patients, as with other rare conditions, is on clinical trials. The U.S. National Cancer Institute website (http://www.cancer.gov/cancertopics/pdq/treatment/lchistio/HealthProfessional) and the Histiocytosis Association (http://www.histio.org; 1–856–589–6606) also may be useful resources.

Patients with only skin LCH, some single-bone lesions (non–CNS-risk), and isolated DI have not been studied in Histiocyte Society clinical trials, but are discussed in this section.

Skin-Limited Lesions Skin-limited lesions may require therapy if they are symptomatic. One approach is topical glucocorticoids,[33] although rarely effective. Other approaches with reported efficacy include oral methotrexate (20 mg/m² weekly)[69] or oral thalidomide (50 to 200 mg daily).[70] Topical application of nitrogen mustard may be effective for cutaneous LCH that is resistant to oral therapies, but is contraindicated for large areas of skin.[71] Psoralen plus long-wave ultraviolet A radiation (PUVA) has been used as well.[72] The approach is limited by the severity and distribution of the skin involvement.

Single Skull Lesions of the Frontal, Parietal, or Occipital Regions, or Single Lesions of Any Other Bone Curettage or curettage plus injection of methylprednisolone may be used.[73]

Vertebral or Femoral Bone Lesions at Risk for Collapse Isolated radiation therapy is indicated for patients with single bone lesions of a vertebrae or the femoral neck, which are at risk of collapse.[74,75] When instability of the cervical vertebrae and neurologic symptoms are present, bracing or spinal fusion may be needed.[76] Certain skull lesions, not in the CNS-risk region, could also be considered for radiation therapy.

Skull Lesions in the Mastoid, Temporal, Orbital or Base of Skull Bones (CNS-Risk Lesions) The purpose of treating these patients with systemic therapy is to decrease the risk of developing DI. In a large series of patients with CNS-risk lesions who received little or no chemotherapy there was a 20 to 50 percent incidence of DI compared to incidence rates of 10 percent in patients treated with systemic chemotherapy.[52] The current standard of care, based on the LCH-III study, is to treat patients with single or multifocal lesions in CNS risk sites for 12 months with intravenous vinblastine and oral prednisone: weekly intravenous vinblastine (6 mg/m²) for 7 weeks, with daily oral prednisone (40 mg/m²) for 4 weeks followed by a 2-week taper. If there is a good response by 6 weeks, then vinblastine frequency is decreased to every 3 weeks. After the first 6 weeks, oral prednisone is given for 5 days at 40 mg/m² every 3 weeks with the vinblastine intravenous. Patients with suboptimal responses by 6 weeks are given an additional 6 weeks of weekly intravenous vinblastine.[39]

Multiple Bone Lesions or Combinations of Skin, Lymph Node, or Pituitary Gland Involvement with or Without Bone Lesions Patients should be treated for 12 months with intravenous vinblastine and oral prednisone as outlined for the CNS-risk lesions. Both shorter (<6 months) treatment strategies and treatment with only a single agent (e.g., prednisone) are associated with inferior outcomes. A 37 percent reactivation rate with a two-drug regimen has been reported, versus 50 to 80 percent with only surgery or single-drug treatments.[39,53,77]

Spleen, Liver, or Marrow (May or May Not Include Skin, Bone, Lymph Node, or Pituitary Gland Involvement) The standard therapy used for LCH in high-risk organs (spleen, liver, and/or marrow) is based upon the LCH-III results in which oral mercaptopurine was added to intravenous vinblastine/oral prednisone regimen, outlined for the low-risk patients above.[39] The addition of oral or intravenous methotrexate did not improve the overall survival or risk of reactivation. Another more intensive regimen (JLSG-96) has been reported that includes intravenous cytarabine, intravenous vincristine, oral prednisolone, and methotrexate for good responders or a salvage therapy with intravenous daunorubicin, intravenous cyclophosphamide, intravenous vincristine, and oral prednisolone for poor responders.[78] Both treatments lasted 7.5 months. Table 71–3 compares the results of the LCH-III and JLSG-96 trials.

Central Nervous System Treatment of mass lesions, including enlargement of the hypothalamic–pituitary axis, parenchymal mass lesions, and leptomeningeal involvement, with cladribine has been effective. Doses of cladribine ranged from 5 to 13 mg/m² given intravenously at varying frequencies.[79]

TABLE 71–3. Comparison of Treatment Outcomes in High-Risk Langerhans Cell Histiocytosis Patients

	LCH-III*	JLSG-96
Number of patients	235	59
Median age at diagnosis	1.1	0.9
Therapy duration (mo)	12	7.5
Initial response	70–72*	76
Reactivations	25–29	45
Survival	88	97

LCH-III, Histiocyte Society Langerhans cell histiocytosis treatment protocol III; JLSG-96, Japan Langerhans Cell Histiocytosis Study Group protocol 96.

*Arm A (velban/prednisone) vs. Arm B (velban/prednisone/methotrexate).

Reports for treatment of the CNS neurodegenerative syndrome have been limited to case series and pilot studies. Strategies include oral dexamethasone, intravenous cladribine, oral all-*trans* retinoic acid, intravenous immunoglobulin, and intravenous cytarabine.[80–82] All-*trans* retinoic acid was given at a dose of 45 mg/m^2 daily, orally, for 6 weeks, then 2 weeks a month for 1 year. Intravenous immunoglobulin, 400 mg/m^2 monthly. Some investigators have given chemotherapy along with the IVIG. The chemotherapy plan was prednisolone 2 mg/kg 5 days a month with or without oral or IV methotrexate 20 mg/m^2 one day every 2 weeks, daily oral 6-mercaptopurine 1.5 mg/kg/day, or monthly vinblastine 6 mg/m^2/dose once monthly for a year. MRI findings were stable, but clinical efficacy was difficult to judge as patients were reported to have no progression in their neurologic symptoms. Intravenous cytarabine with or without intravenous vincristine was effective in decreasing neurologic symptoms and improving the MRI images in five of eight patients who were stable for longer than 8 years.

Recurrent, Refractory, or Progressive Childhood Langerhans Cell Histiocytosis

Recurrent "Low-Risk" Organ Involvement The optimal therapy for patients with relapsed or recurrent disease has not been determined. Patients with recurrent bone disease who reoccur more than 6 months after stopping vinblastine and prednisone can benefit from treatment with a "reinduction" of intravenous vinblastine, weekly, and daily oral prednisone for 6 weeks. If there is no active disease, or at least very little evidence of active disease, then treatment can be changed to every 3 weeks with the addition of oral methotrexate weekly and oral 6-mercaptopurine nightly. Three approaches (1) intravenous cladribine, (2) intravenous vincristine and intravenous cytarabine, and (3) intravenous clofarabine are effective regimens for patients with recurrent bone disease.[83–85]

A phase II trial of oral thalidomide for LCH patients (10 low-risk patients; 6 high-risk patients) who failed primary and at least one secondary regimen showed a complete response in 4 of 10 and partial responses in 3 of 10 low-risk patients. However, dose-limiting toxicities and extraordinary cost limit the overall usefulness of thalidomide.[70]

Recurrent High-Risk Organ Involvement A new treatment plan is indicated when a patient with multisystem involvement progresses after 6 weeks of standard treatment, or has not had a partial response by 12 weeks. Data from the LCH-III study showed only 57 percent survival for this group. A prospective trial with cladribine (5 mg/m^2 per day, intravenously, for 5 days monthly for 6 months) had high rates of response in patients with recurrent and refractory low-risk, but not high-risk, LCH.[85] Another regimen for patients with refractory high-risk LCH is treatment with a highly intensive strategy based on acute myelogenous leukemia protocols. Treatment with high-dose cladribine (9 mg/m^2 per day) coupled with cytarabine (1 g/m^2 per day) for 5 days for at least 2 months resulted in increased overall survival and cure in previously refractory patients. However, there was also a relatively high treatment-related mortality.[86] Institutional case series with intravenous clofarabine (25 mg/m^2/day for 5 days/month) have promising results in patients who have failed multiple previous strategies with manageable toxicities.[87–89] There is considerable interest in use of the BRAF inhibitors for treatment of refractory and recurrent LCH in patients with the *BRAF*^{V600E} mutation. There are pediatric and phase I studies for several anti-*BRAF* compounds. Concern for more widespread use in the setting of pediatric LCH is tempered by of the toxicity profile that includes high incidence of squamous cell carcinoma in melanoma patients.[90] There is only one published report on use of oral vemurafenib for two adult patients who had LCH and ECD with positive responses.[91]

Allogeneic hematopoietic stem cell transplantation (AHSCT) has been used for patients with multisystem high-risk organ involvement that is refractory to chemotherapy. Reduced-intensity conditioning regimens are curative and associated with less toxicity and improved survival.[92]

Options No Longer Considered Effective Treatments for LCH in any location that have been used in the past but are no longer recommended include cyclosporine and interferon (IFN)-α. Extensive surgery is also not indicated. It is critical that LCH bone lesions (especially skull and mandible) not be treated by excision with wide margins. Even large defects may remodel to near normal architecture following resolution of LCH follow chemotherapy and/or curettage. Similarly, surgical resection or radiotherapy of groin or genital lesions is contraindicated as chemotherapy can heal skin lesions.

COURSE AND PROGNOSIS

LCH patients with low-risk disease treated with vinblastine and prednisone have a 99 percent chance of survival, but more than 50 percent fail to be cured with initial therapy. Nearly 100 percent of these patients are ultimately cured of LCH, though many require multiple courses of salvage therapy. Patients with high-risk disease who do not respond adequately by 12 weeks of treatment now have an 87 percent chance of long-term survival, but also often require salvage therapy as described earlier.

PERMANENT CONSEQUENCES AND LATE EFFECTS OF TREATMENT

Disease-associated sequelae remain a major challenge for patients with LCH, with risk of complications increasing with multisystem, high-risk, and prolonged duration of active disease. Children with low-risk organ involvement (skin, bones, lymph nodes, or pituitary gland) treated for 6 months have a 24 percent chance of developing long-term sequelae.[93] Those with DI are at risk for panhypopituitarism and should be monitored carefully for adequacy of growth and development. In a retrospective review of 141 patients with LCH and DI, 43 percent developed growth hormone deficiency.[54] The 5- and 10-year risks of growth hormone deficiency among children with LCH and DI were 35 percent and 54 percent, respectively. There was no increased reactivation of LCH in patients who received replacement growth hormone compared to those who did not.

Patients treated before 2000 with multisystem involvement had a 71 percent incidence of long-term problems.[93,94] Hearing loss has been found in 13 percent of children treated for LCH. Neurologic symptoms secondary to vertebral compression of cervical lesions have been reported in LCH patients with spinal lesions. Cognitive defects and MRI abnormalities may develop in some long-term survivors with CNS-risk skull lesions.[95] Some patients have markedly abnormal cerebellar function and behavior abnormalities, while others have subtle deficits in brain stem–evoked potentials and short-term memory.[96]

Orthopedic problems from lesions of the spine, femur, tibia, or humerus may be seen in 20 percent of patients. These problems include vertebral collapse or instability of the spine that may lead to scoliosis, and facial or limb asymmetry.

Diffuse pulmonary disease may result in poor lung function with higher risk for infections and decreased exercise tolerance. These patients should be followed with pulmonary function testing including the diffusing capacity of carbon monoxide and ratio of residual volume to total lung capacity.[45]

Liver disease may lead to sclerosing cholangitis which responds to chemotherapy in only 25 percent of cases and liver transplantation usually is indicated.[41]

Dental problems characterized by loss of teeth have been significant for some patients, usually related to overly aggressive dental surgery.[93]

Marrow failure secondary to LCH or from therapy is rare but is associated with a higher risk of malignancy. Patients with LCH may have a higher than normal risk of developing secondary cancers.[97] Leukemia (usually acute myelogenous) occurs after treatment as does lymphoblastic lymphoma. Concurrent LCH and a malignancy have been reported in a few patients, and some patients have had their malignancy initially followed by development of LCH. Three patients with T-cell acute lymphoblastic leukemia (T-ALL) and aggressive LCH, for which the two disorders had shared clonal markers have been reported.[98,99] Two cases had clonality of the same T-cell receptor genotype. The authors considered the plasticity of lymphocytes permitting development into LCs. The other patient with LCH after T-ALL had the same T-cell receptor gene rearrangements and activating mutations of the NOTCH1 gene in the patient's DCs and acute lymphoblastic leukemia (ALL) blasts. A series of four patients with acute leukemia of ambiguous or myeloid lineage with intermingling LCH cells have been reported.[100] The authors speculated the two diseases shared a common hematopoietic stem cell as had been suggested earlier during investigation of the BRAF[V600E] mutation in the marrow of LCH patients.[6]

ADULT LANGERHANS CELL HISTIOCYTOSIS

Incidence

It is estimated that one to two adult cases of LCH occur per 1 million population.[101] The true incidence of this disease is difficult to assess because large published studies usually are from referral centers and the disorder often is underdiagnosed. A survey from Germany reported that 66 percent of the adult LCH patients were women with an average age of 43.5 years.[102]

Pathogenesis

There are no studies to compare the biology of LCH in adults and children. The association of adult pulmonary LCH with smoking and evidence that the incidence of BRAF[V600E] mutations in adult LCH tissue is not the same as in the pediatric population indicates some differences. The LCs in adult lung lesions are mature DCs expressing high levels of the accessory molecules CD80 and CD86, unlike LCs found in other lung disorders.[103] Molecular studies have shown pulmonary LCH in adults is primarily a reactive process, rather than a clonal proliferation as seen in childhood LCH.[104] Subsequent investigations by this group with the Ion AmpliSeq technology showed two of five adult pulmonary LCH patients had the BRAF[V600E] mutation.[105] An analysis of BRAF[V600E] expression by immunohistochemistry (IHC) and molecular techniques (allele-specific polymerase chain reaction [PCR] and Sanger sequencing) has also been reported for a series of adults with isolated pulmonary LCH and others with nonpulmonary lesions.[106] Of the pulmonary LCH cases 7 of 25 (28 percent) were positive for BRAF[V600E] expression by IHC. The cumulative pack-years of smoking was significantly higher in the BRAF-positive adult pulmonary LCH patients than in the wild-type BRAF cases. Only 19 of 54 (35.2 percent) of the nonpulmonary cases had the BRAF mutation. The frequency of BRAF[V600E] mutation in North American pediatric series ranged from 57 to 65 percent based on deep sequencing and quantitative PCR.[5,19] It is possible that technical differences in sensitivity underlie the relatively decreased reported frequency of BRAF[V600E] in adult cases of LCH. Further studies in adult patients will be needed to determine if age or ethnicity influence the role of BRAF mutations in LCH pathogenesis.

Clinical Findings

Adult LCH patients may have symptoms and signs for many months before a definitive diagnosis is made and treatment instituted. LCH in adults is often similar to that in children, except that isolated adult pulmonary LCH is closely associated with smoking. Presenting symptoms are (in order of decreasing frequency) dyspnea or tachypnea, polydipsia and polyuria, bone pain, lymphadenopathy, weight loss, fever, gingival hypertrophy, ataxia, and memory problems. Among the signs of LCH are skin rash, scalp nodules, soft-tissue swelling near bone lesions, lymphadenopathy, gingival hypertrophy, hepatosplenomegaly. Patients who present with isolated DI should be carefully observed for onset of other symptoms or signs characteristic of LCH. At least 80 percent of patients with DI had involvement of other organ systems: bone (68 percent), skin (57 percent), lung (39 percent), and lymph nodes (18 percent).[107]

Many patients have a papular rash with brown, red, or crusted areas ranging in size from a pinhead to a dime. In the scalp the rash is similar to seborrhea. Skin in the inguinal region, genitalia, or around the anus may have open ulcers that do not heal after antibacterial or antifungal therapy. In the mouth, swollen gums or ulcers along the cheeks, roof of the mouth, or tongue occur. In a series of 18 patients with skin LCH collected from 5 centers in the Netherlands followup revealed 5 developed malignancies which included 2 with myelomocytic leukemia, 1 with histiocytic sarcoma, and 2 with lymphomas. A literature review produced 6 additional cases of adults who had skin LCH and subsequently developed hematologic malignancies.[108]

The sites of bone involvement in adults differ from that of children. Lesions in the mandible occur in 30 percent of adults versus in 7 percent of children, and skull lesions in occur 21 percent of adults versus in 40 percent of children.[102,109] The frequency of LCH lesions in the vertebrae (13 percent), pelvis (13 percent), extremities (17 percent), and ribs (6 percent) of adults is similar to that found in children.

Pulmonary LCH is slightly more prevalent in smokers than in nonsmokers and the male-to-female ratio may be near unity depending on the incidence of smoking in the population studied.[44,102,110] Patients with pulmonary LCH usually present with cough, dyspnea, or chest pain, although nearly 20 percent of adults with lung involvement have no symptoms.[111] The sudden onset of chest pain may indicate a spontaneous pneumothorax. The most frequent pulmonary function abnormality finding (80 percent of patients) with pulmonary LCH is a reduced carbon monoxide diffusing capacity.[112,113] A long-term retrospective study of 49 pulmonary LCH patients showed that lung function deteriorated within 2 years in 60 percent of patients and the forced expiratory volume in 1 second (FEV_1) and diffusing capacity in lung for carbon dioxide (DLCO) were the parameters that most often declined.[114] Airway obstruction was the most important functional pattern observed, which correlated with the percent predicted FEV_1. In this series, the investigators found pulmonary function tests much better than serial CTs for following the disease course and response to therapy. A high-resolution CT scan can uncover cysts and nodules, usually in the upper lobes characteristic of LCH. Despite the typical CT findings, a lung biopsy is needed to confirm the diagnosis.[115] The presence of cystic abnormalities on high-resolution CT scans does not predict which patients will have progressive disease.[116] Adults with pulmonary LCH can have multisystem disease, including bone (18 percent) or skin (13 percent) lesions and DI (5 percent).

Therapy

Although adult patients have been treated with vinblastine and prednisone, vinblastine often causes significant neuropathy in adults when given weekly for 6 weeks, and glucocorticoids are not tolerated as well by adults as children. Alternative approaches in adults for initial therapy include either intravenous cytarabine or intravenous cladribine. The latter is effective for adults with skin, bone, lymph node, and probably pulmonary and mass lesions in the CNS.[79,117,118] A review of 58 adults with bone lesions compared the efficacy and toxicity of intravenous vinblastine plus oral prednisone to intravenous cladribine or cytarabine.[119] In this retrospective review, cytarabine had the best outcomes, with 21 percent of treated patients unresponsive and 20 percent with grades 3 to 4 hematologic toxicity as opposed to intravenous vinblastine plus oral prednisone after which there was an 84 percent of patients without a satisfactory response and 75 percent grades 3 to 4 neurotoxicity. Patients receiving cladribine had an inadequate response 59 percent of the time and had a 37 percent incidence of hematologic toxicity. The relatively promising efficacy and safety of cytarabine in adults with LCH should be confirmed in a prospective study.

As in pediatric cases, extensive or mutilating surgery to remove skin lesions, teeth or jaw bones is not indicated. Systemic chemotherapy will cause bone lesions to regress and the involved teeth and jaw bones can reform. Oral thalidomide and oral methotrexate have also been effective in adults with skin disease.[69,70] Anecdotal reports have described the successful use of the intravenous bisphosphonate pamidronate in controlling severe bone pain in patients with multiple osteolytic lesions.[120,121]

A consensus document authored by experts treating adults with LCH with guidelines for evaluation and management has been published.[122] A clinical trial for adults with LCH was conducted for an agent that inhibited AKT signaling activity, with responses in some patients.[123] There are no current clinical trials for adult LCH patients, although some studies enrolling patients for treatment with MAPK pathway inhibitors may include LCH among the diagnoses being studied.

Adult Langerhans Cell Histiocytosis Patients with Lung Disease and Who Smoke Cigarettes Most adult patients with LCH have gradual disease progression with continued smoking. The disease may regress or progress with the cessation of smoking.[124] Lung transplantation may be necessary for adults with extensive pulmonary destruction from LCH.[125] A multicenter study documented a 54 percent survival at 10 years after lung transplantation, with 20 percent of patients having recurrent LCH, which did not impact on survival, but longer followup of these patients is needed.

● MALIGNANT HISTIOCYTIC DISEASES

DEFINITION AND HISTORY

The original description of this group of malignant histiocytosis is attributed to Scott and Robb-Smith who, in 1939, reported cases of a rapidly fatal disease with jaundice, lymphadenopathy, anemia, leucopenia, and hepatosplenomegaly that they called *histiocytic medullary reticulosis*.[126] They believed the malignant cell was a histiocyte based upon the accepted morphologic criteria of that time. Advanced immunohistochemical techniques resulted in identifying cells as either lymphocytes or histiocytes. The disease was labeled *giant cell reticulosis* and the cells *reticulum cells* based upon their large size, but revealed little as to the place of these cells in the immune system. Later, Rappaport introduced the term *malignant histiocytosis*,[127] as he believed the morphologic characteristics identified the histiocyte as the malignant cell. There has been considerable debate about the identity of malignancies of LC histiocytes as the majority of patients with "histiocytic lymphoma or malignant histiocytosis" reported in the literature had one of the variants of large cell lymphoma.[128,129] By excluding patients with anaplastic large cell lymphomas and other T- or B-lineage large cell lymphomas, the resulting number with malignancies of histiocytes becomes very small. Favara and colleagues suggested that such diseases should be considered sarcomas of histiocytic or macrophage-related lineage. An updated review of the histologic features of these neoplasms based upon the 2008 World Health Organization (WHO) Classification has been published.[130] One of the major changes is that the 2001 WHO definition of histiocytic sarcoma (HS) stated that the neoplasms could not have

clonal B/T-cell receptor gene rearrangements. Now because more cases of "transdifferentiation" between lymphoid malignancies and HS are being recognized, these gene rearrangements are being included among HS. Among the prior or subsequent malignancies associated with HS are B- or T-lymphoblastic lymphoma/leukemia, mature B-cell lymphomas, follicular lymphoma,[100,131] chronic lymphocytic leukemia with *BRAF*^V600E mutation in both malignancies,[100,132] mantle cell lymphoma, extranodal marginal zone lymphoma of mucosa-associated lymphoid tissue, splenic marginal zone lymphoma, and diffuse large B-cell lymphoma. A series of four cases of HS with acute leukemia of ambiguous or myeloid lineage have also been reported.[100]

Acute myelogenous leukemias with a dominant monocytic phenotype represent the other group of malignant disorders involving monocytic cells. Descriptions of the clinical presentation, biology, and treatment of the monocytic leukemias and large cell lymphomas are presented elsewhere in this book (Chaps. 88 and 98, respectively).

Histologically, the tumors consist of large, overtly malignant-appearing cells in a diffuse, noncohesive array often in the lymph node sinuses or paracortical areas. They are round to oval and sometimes spindle shaped. Hemophagocytosis may be seen. The nuclei may be oval, indented, convoluted, or irregular, and may display mild to severe atypia.[130]

The markers most specific for histiocytic cells include monocyte/macrophage colony-stimulating factor (M-CSF) receptor, lysozyme, Ki-M8, S100+, Ki-M4, cathepsins D and E, CD21−, and CD35−. If a dendritic-histiocytic cell proliferation meets a combination of criteria as "malignant," such as having a clonal cytogenetic abnormality, aneuploid DNA profile, malignant histocytomorphology, other evidence of monoclonality, and an aggressive clinical course, it is classified as a HS.

An international panel of experts carefully reviewed 61 cases of tumors of histiocytes and accessory DCs.[133] Seventeen cases (27 percent) were classified as HS and were CD68+, lysozyme+, CD1a−, S100−/+, CD21−, and CD35−. LC tumors (24 cases, 38 percent) were CD68+, lysozyme−/+, CD1a+, S100+, and CD21/35−. Interdigitating DC sarcomas (four cases, 7 percent) were CD68+/−, lysozyme−, CD1a−, S100−/+, and CD21/35−. Follicular DC tumors (13 cases, 21 percent) were CD68+/−, lysozyme−, CD1a−, S100−/+, and CD21/35+. Four cases were unclassifiable. The 2008 WHO classification added immunostaining with anti-CD163, a hemoglobin scavenger receptor, as a criterion, which identifies monocytes and histiocytes and is more specific than anti-CD68. HS found with or subsequent to B-cell lymphomas may have that tumor's immunophenotype and particular features such as BCL6 nuclear staining and BCL2 protein expression. *BRAF*^V600E mutations were reported in five of eight patients with HS and 5 of 27 with follicular DC sarcoma by Sanger sequencing and quantitative PCR.[100,134]

EPIDEMIOLOGY

Although malignant dendritic/histiocytic cell tumors affect all age groups, the median age is 33 years.[133] Males are affected more often than females and most patients had HSs and LC tumors. One review of more than 2000 lymphoma cases found eight patients (0.4 percent) with HSs.[135] Another review found 1 percent of all hematolymphoid neoplasms to be HS with a median age at diagnosis of 46 years.[130]

CLINICAL FEATURES

Systemic symptoms of fever, headache, malaise, weight loss, dyspnea, and sweating occur in patients with diffuse disease.[133,135,136] Lymphadenopathy is the most common presenting feature, but involvement of the spleen, gastrointestinal tract, skin, and soft tissue are common. Marrow involvement occurs in approximately 25 percent of the patients.

Dendritic or Langerhans Cell Sarcomas

Histologic differentiation of dendritic-LC sarcomas from HS include long DC processes, convoluted nuclei, more intense S100 staining and weaker CD68 staining. These patients may have fever or weight loss. They usually present with erythematous nodules or a skin rash, and may also have involvement of bone, lymph nodes, lung, liver, or brain.[137,138] A series of histiocytic-DC sarcomas in patients with follicular lymphomas showed a clonal evolution from the B-cell lymphoma to myeloid-derived sarcomas.

Extranodal Histiocytic Sarcomas

These tumors occur equally in males and females and present at a median age of 55 years.[139] Tumors are found in the soft tissue of extremities, the gastrointestinal tract, the nasal cavity, and the lung, sometimes with involvement of regional lymph nodes. Gastrointestinal masses were usually painful. Extremity tumors often present as painless masses. Patients had symptoms or signs for 1 month to 2 years before diagnosis. Most tumors are localized at the time of diagnosis.

Interdigitating Dendritic Cell Sarcomas

Interdigitating DC sarcomas may occur as extranodal tumors in children and primarily affect lymph nodes in adults.[140] A report of four pediatric cases had involvement of the chest wall, vertebrae, lymph nodes, marrow, and pelvic space. Of the other seven pediatric and 26 adult cases, 17 had extranodal presentations. Many of the 17 cases had intestinal or mediastinal tumors. These tumors were very aggressive in a third of cases.[141,142]

Follicular Dendritic Cell Tumors

The malignant cells in these patients are spindle to ovoid forming fascicles, storiform patterns and whorls which stain with CD21, CD23, and CD35. These malignancies affect males and females equally and present at a median age of 47 years (range: 14 to 77 years).[141] Nodal and extranodal sites can be affected. Most frequent nodal presentations are cervical, axillary, and supraclavicular; mediastinal and mesenteric nodes can also be affected. These tumors are usually slow growing and painless. Although local invasion is common, metastasis to sites other than the lungs is uncommon.

LABORATORY FINDINGS

Patients with diffuse disease may have pancytopenia, although leukocytosis occurs in some as a secondary response. Hemophagocytosis is occasionally seen in the marrow. An elevated lactate dehydrogenase and erythrocyte sedimentation rate may be found.

DIFFERENTIAL DIAGNOSIS

A diagnostic biopsy with a full immunophenotype panel should be done for these rare tumors, which have been mistaken for Hodgkin lymphoma, anaplastic large cell lymphoma, or large cell lymphomas of T- or B-cell subtypes. The DC neoplasms do not express T- or B-lymphocyte markers and do not have rearrangements of immunoglobulin or T-cell receptor genes.[133,142,143] Malignant fibrous histiocytoma, fibrosarcoma, leiomyosarcoma, rhabdomyosarcoma, or melanoma may simulate interdigitating DC sarcoma, as well as inflammatory pseudotumor. Although follicular DC sarcoma and histiocytic lymphoma may have a similar presentation, the specific immunophenotype of the tumors helps differentiate them from interdigitating DC sarcoma. Thymomas, meningiomas, and malignant fibrous histiocytomas can mimic follicular DC sarcoma, but they lack CD21 and CD35.

TREATMENT, COURSE, AND PROGNOSIS

Therapy for dendritic and LC sarcomas has usually been unsuccessful.[144] However, case reports of long-term remissions with oral thalidomide,[145,146] intravenous alemtuzumab,[147] or intravenous MAID (mesna, doxorubicin [Adriamycin], ifosfamide, and dacarbazine)[148] have been published. In some instances, surgical resection of a localized mass with radiotherapy has been successful.

Interdigitating DC sarcomas, also, have been treated successfully with surgery alone or a combination of surgery and radiotherapy, when the tumor is localized.[140] Patients with stage III/IV tumors generally do not respond to multidrug chemotherapy, such as intravenous cyclophosphamide, doxorubicin, and vincristine and oral prednisone with or without the addition of intravenous actinomycin D.

● MALIGNANT FIBROUS HISTIOCYTOMA AND GIANT CELL TUMOR OF THE BONE

Gene-profiling experiments have shown that these tumors are not derived from histiocytes, but are poorly differentiated fibrosarcomas, myosarcomas, fibromyxosarcomas, or liposarcomas.[149–151] They are treated with a similar approach as are osteosarcomas.[152–154]

● ERDHEIM-CHESTER DISEASE

DEFINITION AND HISTORY

In 1930, two cases of "lipid granulomatosis" were described by William Chester and Jakob Erdheim and later designated as *Erdheim-Chester disease.*[155] The histopathologic characteristics of ECD overlap xanthogranuloma and distinctions between the two are made on the basis of clinical and radiologic findings. Lipid-laden histiocytes with foamy or eosinophilic cytoplasm infiltrate bones and various organs and generate a fibroblastic response that leads to critical organ failure. The histiocytes are CD68+, CD163+, factor XIIIa+, CD1a−, and S100−, and do not contain Birbeck granules. Touton-like giant cells are commonly found.

EPIDEMIOLOGY/ETIOLOGY

This disease primarily affects adults (mean age: 53 years; range: 7 to 84 years) with a predominance of males (73 percent).[156] There is no known etiology. Cells from ECD biopsies have been found to be clonal in three of five cases tested and polyclonal in two.[157–159] Elevated levels of osteopontin in ECD tissue have been found at diagnosis, which then declined after treatment with prednisolone.[160] It is difficult to judge the exact role of osteopontin in ECD as it has many functions as a noncollagenous, extracellular matrix protein that may affect cell adhesion, migration, and other functions. Immunohistochemical staining of ECD tissue shows expression of CCL2 (monocyte chemotactic protein 1), CCL4 (macrophage inflammatory protein-1β [MIP-1β]), CCL5 (RANTES [regulated upon activation, normal T-cell expressed and secreted]), CCL20 (MIP-3α), and CCL19 (MIP-3β), along with their receptors CCR1, CCR2, CCR3, CCR5, CCR6, and CCR7.[161] Elevated expression of an IFN-γ–inducible protein, IL-6, and RANKL has been described. The latter two factors are important for bone remodeling. Biopsies of 32 of 37 patients with ECD had prominent staining for the platelet-derived growth factor receptor-β. The inflammatory nature of ECD is indicated by an elevation of cytokines in a cohort of 37 patients. A T-helper type 1 (Th1)-associated signature in ECD patients was associated with elevation of IFN-α, IL-12, monocyte chemotactic protein-1 (MCP-1), IL-4, and IL-7, but there was little difference in the levels of these before and after treatment with IFN-α.

Discovery of $BRAF^{V600E}$ mutations in LCH and ECD has opened important research initiatives as well as the possibility of targeted therapy. Thirteen of 24 (54 percent) ECD patients and 38 percent of LCH patients had this mutation.[162] An *NRAS* mutation has also been found in ECD, further documenting the importance of the MAPK pathway.[163] The frequent occurrence of lesions classified as LCH and ECD in the same patient, along with common finding of $BRAF^{V600E}$ mutation, suggests a common cell of origin in some patients.[164]

CLINICAL FEATURES

A consensus paper on the evaluation and treatment of ECD has been published with helpful summaries of clinical, laboratory, and radiologic findings.[165] Many patients have fever, weakness, and weight loss. The clinical findings include CNS symptoms (50 percent), bone pain (40 percent), xanthelasma (27 percent), exophthalmos (27 percent), and DI (22 percent).[166] Some patients have cerebellar signs and focal neurologic deficits.[167] Fifty percent of patients have extraskeletal disease. It is unusual for lymph nodes, liver, spleen, or axial skeleton to be affected, whereas these areas are frequently affected in LCH and RDD. Retroperitoneal and renal involvement occurs in one-third of ECD patients and causes abdominal pain, dysuria, and hydronephrosis. Pulmonary involvement may present in 20 percent of patients and results in dyspnea. Skin manifestations of ECD include xanthomatous lesions that may begin as reddish-brown papules similar to xanthoma disseminatum. Cardiac dysfunction occurs because of circumferential sheathing of the aorta, and aortic branches, including coronary arteries, but often is not symptomatic. There may also be endocardial, myocardial, or pericardial involvement, leading to pericardial effusions with the risk of tamponade.[168,169]

CNS involvement may occur in up to 50 percent of ECD patients. Cerebellar and pyramidal symptoms are the most frequent, but headaches, neuropsychiatric or cognitive difficulties, and cranial nerve palsies are reported.[170] Parenchymal CNS lesions causing disability are a poor prognostic indicator.[171] ECD may infiltrate any CNS location within or outside the neuraxis, including the pachymeninges, and are similar to meningiomas, sarcoidosis, Wegener granulomatosis, RDD, or LCH. Orbital involvement causes proptosis and pituitary infiltration leads to DI in nearly 25 percent of patients.

LABORATORY FEATURES

There are no specific laboratory findings, but elevated sedimentation rate and alkaline phosphatase have been reported in approximately one-fifth of cases. The consensus publication on ECD provides a list of baseline radiologic tests which include PET/CT, MRI brain with contrast and attention to the pituitary, cardiac MRI, and when indicated clinically, MRI of the orbits with contrast, renal artery ultrasound, high-resolution CT of the chest, pulmonary function tests, testicular ultrasound, and electromyography. Radiographs show bilateral patchy osteosclerosis of the metaphysis and diaphysis of the femur, proximal tibia, and fibula in nearly 100 percent of patients. Lytic lesions are found in approximately one-third of patients. Chest CT imaging findings include diffuse interstitial infiltrates, and pleural and interlobular septal thickening.[169] Perirenal infiltration, extending through the fat of the anterior or posterior pararenal spaces, leading to the classic "hairy kidney" appearance (>60 percent of patients) and circumferential sheathing of the aorta (>60 percent of patients), as well as retroperitoneal

fibrosis-like infiltrates (20 percent), can be seen on an abdominal CT scan and MRI of the heart.

DIFFERENTIAL DIAGNOSIS

Although histologically distinct, the clinical features may suggest LCH, RDD, JXG, or xanthoma disseminatum. Some clinical features overlap with sarcoidosis, amyloidosis, Paget disease, Ormond disease (idiopathic retroperitoneal fibrosis), and Whipple disease (intestinal lipodystrophy). The histologic features can be confused with Gaucher disease, Niemann-Pick disease, mucopolysaccharidosis, or malakoplakia.[172]

THERAPY

Subcutaneous IFN-α and pegylated IFN-α are considered the first-line treatments for ECD.[173] Survival has been improved using doses of 3 million units, 3 times a week.[174-178] When the standard dose is ineffective, increasing the IFN-α dose to greater than 18 million units per week or use of pegylated IFN-α to a dose greater than 180 mcg/wk is recommended. Treatments have been extended for as long as 3 years. Patients treated with the high-dose regimens had a stabilization of CNS disease in 64 percent and of cardiac involvement in 79 percent.

Earlier published treatment results include a review of 37 patients treated with glucocorticoids, usually 1 mg/kg per day, orally, resulting in decreased exophthalmos or general symptoms in 20 patients.[156] Among these patients, glucocorticoids were effective in six patients, transiently effective in four, and ineffective in eight. Of eight patients treated with a variety of chemotherapy agents and glucocorticoids, four had improvement. Radiation was ineffective for orbital masses, but transiently relieved bone pain. A series of six patients treated with oral imatinib mesylate reported two had stable disease and one an initial response before worsening.[179] Some patients have been treated effectively with intravenous cladribine.[180] Anticytokine treatments with anakinra, infliximab, and tocilizumab have had varying degrees of success in a limited number of patients. Anakinra is given at 1 to 2 mg/kg per day, intravenously, and may work best for patients with bone pain and other systemic symptoms.[181-183] However, it seems to be less effective than IFN-α. The same can be said for the anti–tumor necrosis factor α drugs, intravenous infliximab and intravenous etanercept.

Clinical trials currently open to open to ECD patients include:

- NCTT01524978 Vemurafenib: anti-$BRAF^{V600E}$
- NCT01727206 Tocilizumab: anti–IL-6 (phase II clinical trial)
- ACTRN12613001321730: Sirolimus and prednisone (prospective trial)

COURSE AND PROGNOSIS

Nearly 60 percent of ECD patients die of their disease; 36 percent die within 6 months. The mean survival duration is less than 3 years. Cardiac, pulmonary, and renal failure are the primary causes of death.

● JUVENILE XANTHOGRANULOMA

DEFINITION AND HISTORY

JXG is a histiocytic disorder that affects the skin with multiple nodules in the head, neck, and trunk primarily in children, although adults can also be affected.[184] The lesional cells are derived from dermal dendrocytes. Systemic involvement occurs in a few cases. Rudolf Virchow may have been the first to describe a child with what he called "cutaneous xanthomas" in 1871.

EPIDEMIOLOGY

Children with solitary lesions have a median age of onset of 2 years with a male-to-female ratio of 1.5:1. Children with multiple lesions have a median age of onset of 5 months and have a male-to-female ratio of 12:1. No population study of JXG has been reported, so the precise incidence is unknown. However, a review of JXG from the Kiel Pediatric Tumor Registry recorded 129 (0.52 percent) cases of JXG and 800 (3.3 percent) cases of LCH among 24,600 children over a 36-year period.

ETIOLOGY AND PATHOGENESIS

There is no known cause of JXG. Patients with JXG and neurofibromatosis types 1 and 2, as well as the triad of the aforementioned diseases with juvenile chronic myelogenous leukemia, have been reported.[185–187] These and other cases have suggested an increased risk of leukemia in neurofibromatosis patients with JXG, but there is no rigorous proof for this association.[188,189]

CLINICAL FEATURES

The majority of patients are children younger than 2 years of age who have solitary skin nodules on their head, neck, or trunk.[184,190] The lesion is most often the same color as surrounding skin, but may be erythematous or yellowish. Rarely, nodules may be in the subcutaneous fat, deep soft tissue, or skeletal muscle. Organ involvement is rare, but has been reported in the soft tissue, CNS, bone, lung, liver, spleen, pancreas, adrenal, intestines, kidneys, lymph nodes, marrow, and heart.[184,190,191] Systemic symptoms and signs occur only if these organ systems are involved.

LABORATORY FEATURES

Immunohistochemical staining of biopsies is necessary to differentiate JXG from other histiocytic lesions. JXG classically stains with a macrophage marker such as antibodies to CD68 or Ki-M1P, factor XIIIa, fascin, vimentin, and often CD4. They are negative for S100 and anti-CD1a. There are three characteristic histologic patterns: early JXG, classic JXG, and transitional JXG.[190] Early JXG is characterized by small- to intermediate-size mononuclear histiocytes in sheet-like infiltrates. The cells in this category have only small quantities of lipid in the cytoplasm and Touton-type giant cells are absent. This type has relatively more mitoses than the others, but there is no cytologic atypia. Classic JXG exhibits abundant vacuolated, foamy histiocytes with Touton giant cells (lipid-laden histiocytes with multiple nuclei and a small amount of centrally oriented cytoplasm). Transitional JXG has a predominance of spindle-shaped cells resembling benign fibrous histiocytoma with foamy histiocytes and occasional giant cells.[190] Biopsies also contain lymphocytes, eosinophils, and occasionally Charcot-Leyden crystals. If the marrow is involved, patients may have cytopenias. Liver infiltration may cause elevation of liver enzymes, hypoalbuminemia, and an elevated erythrocyte sedimentation rate. Pituitary involvement may lead to DI. Hypercalcemia has been reported. CNS lesions can lead to hydrocephalus, seizures, and developmental delay.

DIFFERENTIAL DIAGNOSIS

LCH is the disease most often confused with JXG. Other disorders to be considered include fibrohistiocytic lesion not otherwise specified, reticulohistiocytoma, hemangioendothelioma, Spitz nevus, malignant fibrous histiocytoma, and rhabdomyosarcoma or other malignancies.

THERAPY

Patients with a single or only a few lesions need no therapy. An excisional biopsy can be used, if desired for cosmetic reasons. For the rare patients who have systemic disease and require treatment a wide variety of chemotherapy and radiotherapy regimens have been reported.[191–193] Inclusion of a vinca alkaloid and a glucocorticoid is associated with better overall response rates than single agents. A child with CNS JXG who failed to respond to vinblastine was successfully treated with cladribine.[194] A series of four children with systemic and CNS JXG were successfully treated with clofarabine.[84]

COURSE AND PROGNOSIS

Patients with only skin or soft-tissue involvement all survive and in a majority of cases, the lesions spontaneously disappear over time. Infants with large retroperitoneal masses, liver, marrow, or CNS involvement usually survive with chemotherapy treatment. Two of 17 patients with multisystem JXG reported in the literature died despite multiagent chemotherapy.[192]

● SINUS HISTIOCYTOSIS WITH MASSIVE LYMPHADENOPATHY (ROSAI-DORFMAN DISEASE)

DEFINITION AND HISTORY

Rosai and Dorfman recognized this nonmalignant proliferation of histiocytes as a unique histopathologic entity, which is part of the differential diagnosis of massive lymphadenopathy.[195] Although this disease is self-limited in some patients, others with airway obstruction, multiple bone lesions, orbital or brain tumors require therapy.[84,196]

EPIDEMIOLOGY

RDD is found throughout the world as a disease of children and young adults (mean age: 20.6 years). Most of our knowledge about it is the result of analysis of the 423 cases in the registry developed by Rosai and Dorfman in which there was no gender, ethnic, or socioeconomic predilection. Persons of African and European descent are equally represented; people of Asian descent less so. In cases of digestive system disease, males and persons of African descent were more commonly affected.[197] Intracranial disease is found in patients with a mean age of 37.5 years. There is an apparent increase in rheumatologic disorders and hemolytic anemia among these patients.[198,199] Germline mutations in the nucleoside transporter SLC29A3 have been described in patients with rare familial syndromes that include lymphadenopathy characteristic of RDD.[200]

ETIOLOGY AND PATHOGENESIS

Although associations with various herpes virus infections have been reported, these most likely represent detection of lymphocytes or macrophages harboring these viruses with no relation to etiology. A model for the key histopathologic finding, emperipolesis of lymphocytes by macrophages, has been proposed.[201] These authors hypothesized that macrophage-activating cytokines could stimulate the macrophages to ingest lymphocytes. The cells in the lesions of this disorder are polyclonal.[202]

CLINICAL FEATURES

Massive, painless bilateral cervical adenopathy is the presenting finding in 87 percent of patients. Some have fever, night sweats, malaise, and weight loss. A few patients have polyarthralgia, rheumatoid arthritis, glomerulonephritis, asthma, and diabetes mellitus. Painless maculopapular eruptions, sometimes reddish or bluish, or yellow xanthomatous rashes occur in 16 percent of patients. Subcutaneous nodules can be found anywhere in the body. Another 16 percent of patients have nasal cavity and paranasal sinus involvement with obstruction of the airways, epistaxis, septal displacement, and mass lesions infiltrating the sinuses. Ten percent have eyelid or orbital masses with proptosis. Unlike patients with LCH, patients with RDD uncommonly (10 percent) have osteolytic bone lesions. These have irregular borders, but may have sclerotic margins. Bilateral parotid or submandibular gland swelling may also be present. Less than 10 percent of patients have CNS, intracranial, epidural, or dural masses, as solitary or multiple lesions leading to headaches, nerve palsies, or syncope. Other organ system involvement in 1 to 3 percent of cases includes the kidney, genitourinary tract, lungs, larynx, liver, tonsil, breast, gastrointestinal tract, and heart. Up to 43 percent of patients have lymphadenopathy coupled with extranodal involvement of the skin, soft tissue, upper respiratory tract, bone, eye, or retroorbital tissue.[203]

LABORATORY FEATURES

Patients may have a hemolytic anemia or anemia of chronic disease, elevated erythrocyte sedimentation rate, and polyclonal hyperimmunoglobulinemia. Elevation of liver enzymes and other laboratory abnormalities depend on the organs involved.[204] Hepatic features include capsular and pericapsular fibrosis. The lymph node sinuses are enlarged by a proliferation of histiocytes with large round or oval vesicular nuclei and a prominent nucleolus. Mitoses are rare. The cytoplasm is pale and eosinophilic, although some may have a foamy cytoplasm. The key diagnostic finding is intact lymphocytes in macrophages (active ingestion, or emperipolesis, the penetration of a smaller cell into larger one). Because the lymphocytes are inside vacuoles, they are not degraded. Accompanying the histiocytes are numerous plasma cells. The pathologic macrophages in this disease infiltrate the sinuses of lymph nodes and are phagocytosing lymphocytes and plasma cells as well as erythrocytes. Although the histiocytes are S100-positive, they are CD1a-negative, unlike the LCs, which are positive for both markers. The macrophages express CD68, CD14, CD15, lysozyme, transferrin receptor, IL-2 receptor, and CD163.[196]

DIFFERENTIAL DIAGNOSIS

Any other cause of lymphadenopathy, such as infections, lymphomas, leukemias, Gaucher disease, melanoma, and other malignancies, should be ruled out by a biopsy. The massive cervical lymph nodes are strikingly similar to those of patients with the autoimmune lymphoproliferative syndrome.[205] Inflammatory pseudotumor and RDD have been found in the same patient suggesting a histologic continuum.[206]

Clinicians should be aware that the sinuses of many reactive lymph nodes contain macrophages (histiocytes) and pathologists will report that presence as "sinus histiocytes or sinus histiocytosis." This is not evidence for RDD because in those cases the sinus histiocytes do not have lymphocytes within their cytoplasm.

THERAPY

Many cases are self-limited and do not require therapy. Surgery may be useful for symptomatic treatment of local large lymph nodes. Multiorgan involvement or dysfunction, and association with immune dysfunction are poor prognostic indicators and indicate the necessity of treatment.[207] Several therapies have been used, including glucocorticoids and chemotherapy, with success in some cases. Several case reports have described improvement or cure of patients with the disease

with oral dexamethasone, oral methotrexate, oral 6-mercaptopurine, intravenous cladribine, or intravenous vinorelbine plus methotrexate.[208–211] Intravenous clofarabine may be the best therapy for patients with bone and CNS involvement.[84]

COURSE AND PROGNOSIS

Most patients will have a slow but steady decrease in the size of their lymph nodes over months to years. For those patients requiring treatment because of impingement on vital organs responses are variable. Because no clinical trials have been done, treatment has been based on anecdotal reports.

● HEMOPHAGOCYTIC LYMPHOHISTIOCYTOSIS

DEFINITION AND HISTORY

Farquhar and Claireux first described this disease in siblings in 1952.[212] Although many case reports using several eponyms ensued, Henter and Elinder provided a logical organization of the diverse clinical presentations.[213] HLH is an aggressive and potentially fatal syndrome that results from inappropriate prolonged activation of lymphocytes and macrophages. The name describes the characteristic (but not diagnostic) pathologic finding of macrophages engulfing all types of blood cells in marrow, lymph nodes, spleen, or liver biopsies (see Fig. 71–3). HLH is also known as autosomal recessive familial HLH, familial erythrophagocytic lymphohistiocytosis, viral-associated hemophagocytic syndrome, and infection-associated hemophagocytosis. "Primary" or "familial" HLH has been used to describe young children with HLH with known gene mutations or a family history of HLH. Older children with HLH, or children without identifiable mutations, are sometimes described as having "secondary" or "acquired" HLH with the assumption that the condition is caused by infection or other stimulus and not a result of genetic predisposition. The same mutations may be present in both situations, and there is no rapid and definitive gene-testing strategy to distinguish the two groups. In general, presentation and outcome are the same for primary and acquired HLH.[214] Hypomorphic mutations in HLH-associated genes and compound heterozygous mutations have been described in patients who develop HLH at an older age or in the context of autoimmune disease.[215,216] Thus, this distinction is not clinically useful in the acute setting as they both must be diagnosed promptly and treated aggressively.

EPIDEMIOLOGY

The incidence of HLH in Sweden was estimated at 1.2 children per 1 million children per year, or 1 in 50,000 livebirths with equal sex distribution.[213] At the Texas Children's Hospital, HLH was diagnosed in 1 of 3000 inpatient admissions in a 2-year study.[217] The incidence in adults is unknown and the outcomes may be worse than for children.[218] Many adult patients with HLH also have lymphoma.[219]

ETIOLOGY AND PATHOGENESIS

Defects in the function of natural killer (NK) cells and cytotoxic T cells have been found in HLH patients. This results in the inappropriate activation of T cells and macrophages, which produce proinflammatory cytokines, including IFN-γ, tumor necrosis factor-α, IL-6, IL-10, IL-12, and soluble IL-2 receptor-α (sCD25).[220,221] In an animal model, perforin deficiency leads to inability to "prune" antigen-presenting DCs, resulting in increased activation of cytotoxic CD8+ T cells.[222] The hypercytokinemia and pathologic activation of T cells and macrophages result in multiorgan dysfunction that can rapidly lead to death.

Perforin Expression

Perforin was identified as a candidate HLH gene by gene mapping and was confirmed by poor expression of perforin in NK cells and cytotoxic T lymphocytes of HLH patients.[223,224] Some HLH characteristics were reproducible in *PRF1* knockout mice.[225] Perforin is secreted from NK cells and cytotoxic T cells upon activation by target cells and introduces pores in the target cell membrane, allowing granzyme to enter and trigger apoptosis.[226]

Other Defects Causing Hemophagocytic Lymphohistiocytosis

Mutations in other genes encoding proteins involved in NK and cytotoxic T-cell–mediated killing of target cells also have been discovered in patients with HLH, including *UNC13D* (encodes MUNC13-4), *STX11* (encodes syntaxin 11), and *UNC18B* (encodes STXBP2).[227] Mutations in the gene that encodes RAB27a (protein that controls secretion of lytic granules) have also been identified in patients with Griscelli syndrome.[228]

Immune Deficiencies Associated with Hemophagocytic Lymphohistiocytosis

Patients with other immune deficiencies associated with lysosomal trafficking defects (e.g., Chédiak-Higashi syndrome, Hermansky-Pudlak syndrome type II) also have a high frequency of HLH.[229] HLH, often associated with infection by the Epstein-Barr virus, is the most common fatal complication of X-linked lymphoproliferative disease (XLP1/*SH2D1A* and XLP2/*XIAP*).[230]

CLINICAL FEATURES

Initial signs and symptoms of HLH mimic more common problems (e.g., fever of unknown origin or sepsis).[231] Confounding diagnoses such as infection, autoimmune disease, hepatitis, multisystem organ failure, encephalitis, and malignancy do not exclude a diagnosis of HLH. Important clues include an acutely ill patient with unexplained fever, rash, or neurologic symptoms. A medical history of immune deficiency should bring HLH to mind. Family history of consanguinity, recurrent spontaneous abortions, or HLH in siblings (or symptoms suggesting undiagnosed HLH) may be suggestive of a risk for HLH.

Prominent early clinical signs in one study included fever (91 percent), hepatomegaly (90 percent), splenomegaly (84 percent), neurologic signs (47 percent), rash (43 percent), and lymphadenopathy (42 percent).[232] Another study found 75 percent of patients with HLH to have CNS symptoms that may mimic encephalitis.[233] Patients with HLH develop liver failure with markedly elevated conjugated bilirubin, pancytopenia, coagulopathy, renal failure heralded by hyponatremia, and pulmonary failure similar to acute respiratory distress syndrome with interstitial infiltrates on chest radiography.[231]

Diagnostic Criteria

The cumulative experiences from the first prospective international treatment protocol sponsored by the Histiocyte Society, HLH-94, as well as other observations and studies, have led to the Histiocyte Society treatment protocol HLH-2004, which includes diagnostic guidelines (Table 71–4).[234] The HLH criteria are derived from retrospective analysis of patients treated on HLH-94 and describe patients with extreme pathologic inflammation and associated defects in cytotoxic immune function.

Biallelic mutations in HLH-associated (or monoallelic in case of X-linked genes) are diagnostic for HLH, but generally not helpful for acute management although genetic results are becoming available more quickly. More rapid flow cytometry studies can identify absence of protein expression of PRF1, SAP (XLP1), or XIAP (XLP2).[235] Flow

---

TABLE 71–4. Clinical Criteria for Diagnosis of Hemophagocytic Lymphohistiocytosis

Hemophagocytic lymphohistiocytosis (HLH) diagnosis is established with at least five of the following:

- Fever
- Splenomegaly
- Cytopenias in at least two cell lines:
  Hemoglobin <90 g/L
  Platelets <100 × 10^9/L
  Neutrophils <1 × 10^9/L
- Hypertriglyceridemia and/or hypofibrinogenemia:
  Fasting triglycerides >3 mmol/L (>265 mg/dL)
  Fibrinogen <1.5 g/L
- Hemophagocytosis in marrow or spleen or lymph nodes
- Low or absent activity of natural killer cells (specialized laboratory test)
- Ferritin >500 mcg/L (>2000 mcg/L may be more specific)
- Soluble cD25 (soluble interleukin-2 receptor) >2400 U/mL

or

- HLH-associated gene mutations

---

cytometry degranulation assays that measure membrane CD107a are also effective for identifying patients with lymphocytes with impaired cytotoxic function.[236]

Hemophagocytosis is sometimes misunderstood as pathognomonic and necessary for the diagnosis of HLH, but biopsies fail to demonstrate hemophagocytosis in approximately one-third of patients (Fig. 71-4).[237] HLH changes over time such that the cytokine stimulation resulting in hemophagocytosis may be modest early in the disease, or the marrow may progress to become aplastic with few macrophages available to engage in hemophagocytosis. Repeat marrow aspirates and biopsies, as well as lymph node or liver biopsies, may be helpful. Finding hemophagocytosis is highly suggestive of HLH, but is neither necessary nor sufficient to make the diagnosis. Cerebrospinal fluid should be tested in patients with signs of CNS abnormalities; pleocytosis, hyperproteinemia and hemophagocytosis support HLH with CNS involvement.

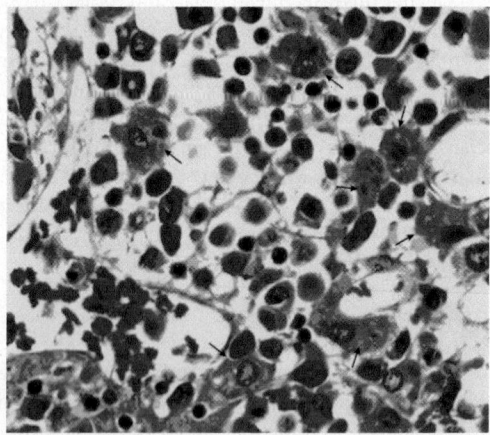

Figure 71–4. Hemophagocytosis by macrophages. Marrow aspirate treated with Wright-Giemsa stain illustrating prominent hemophagocytosis of multiple cell types by macrophages *(arrows)* in the marrow of a patient with hemophagocytic lymphohistiocytosis.

LABORATORY FEATURES

Ferritin

Although no one diagnostic criterion is sufficient to make the diagnosis of HLH, a highly elevated serum ferritin along with four other criteria is strongly indicative. A ferritin concentration of greater than 500 mcg/L was included in the HLH-2004 diagnostic criteria because a survey found that most children with infectious diseases had levels less than that level and those with rheumatologic diagnoses only rarely had higher levels. Ferritin concentrations greater than 500 mcg/L were 100 percent sensitive for HLH in a retrospective review over a 2-year period.[217] However, at this level there is considerable overlap with other disorders. Ferritin concentrations more than 10,000 mcg/L were 90 percent sensitive and 96 percent specific for HLH with very minimal overlap with sepsis, infections, and liver failure. Analysis of ferritin values in an extended cohort suggests that 2000 mcg/L may be a more appropriate measure for diagnosis of HLH than 500 mcg/L.[238]

The following tests should be done on a previously healthy patient who presents with persistent fevers, hepatosplenomegaly, and cytopenia of at least two cell lines: serum ferritin, aspartate aminotransferase/alanine aminotransferase, lactate dehydrogenase, bilirubin, coagulation studies, fibrinogen, triglycerides. A marrow biopsy and aspirate is needed, as well as a lumbar puncture for spinal fluid examination. NK cell function, perforin expression of T cells and NK cells, and sCD25 concentrations should be evaluated, usually requiring access to specialty laboratories, if there is clinical suspicion for HLH. Following daily serum ferritin levels is useful because rapidly rising ferritin is a strong indicator of HLH, and inferior outcomes are associated with slow normalization.[239] It may be necessary to repeat the marrow biopsy or biopsy an enlarged liver or lymph nodes, if the first marrow biopsy fails to show hemophagocytosis and clinical suspicion of HLH is high.

DIFFERENTIAL DIAGNOSIS

Patients with fever of unknown origin, moderate infections, sepsis, multiorgan dysfunction, hepatitis, anemia and thrombocytopenia, and autoimmune phenomena such as Kawasaki disease, lupus erythematosus, or rheumatoid arthritis may present with features that overlap the diagnostic criteria for HLH. These may represent alternative or concurrent diagnoses. One must consider HLH if no clear diagnosis is established of the above mentioned entities is evident and the patient is deteriorating. Identification of an underlying immune deficiency such as X-linked lymphoproliferative disease (Chap. 80), Griscelli syndrome (Chap. 80), or Chédiak-Higashi syndrome (Chap. 80) should increase the suspicion of HLH. Epstein-Barr virus, cytomegalovirus, and other herpes virus infections are the most frequent viral infections associated with HLH. A wide variety of bacterial fungal and protozoal infections may also lead to HLH.

THERAPY

Before treatment with immune-modulating therapy fewer than 10 percent of patients with HLH survived.[240] After case reports and case series described patients successfully treated with strategies that included aggressive immune suppression, podophyllotoxin derivatives, or a combination of immune suppression with etoposide, a prospective treatment protocol was developed that included induction therapy with oral or intravenous dexamethasone and intravenous etoposide, followed by continuous treatment with oral cyclosporine and pulses of dexamethasone and intravenous etoposide.[241-243] Patients with CNS symptoms or cerebrospinal fluid lymphocytosis or pleocytosis also received intrathecal methotrexate. Patients with resistant disease, recurrent disease, or familial HLH underwent AHSCT. The overall estimated 3-year survival

on the HLH-94 protocol was 55 percent.[243] In a study of patients with Epstein-Barr virus–associated HLH, early administration of intravenous etoposide was associated with improved outcomes.[244] Etoposide was recently demonstrated to have specific cytotoxicity to activated T cells, which may explain why it is effective in HLH.[245]

A second protocol, HLH-2004, containing minor modifications from the first included starting oral cyclosporine at the onset of induction therapy, adding glucocorticoids to intrathecal therapy in patients with CNS disease, adding etoposide to conditioning in patients who undergo AHSCT, and considering depletion of T cells in patients who receive stem cells from unrelated donors.[243] At this time, we consider HLH-94 the standard of care. Data are not yet available to evaluate the benefits of early cyclosporine, and it has known risks including increasing susceptibility to posterior reversible encephalopathy syndrome (PRES).[246]

Intravenous antithymocyte globulin (ATG) has been used as a primary treatment of 38 cases of familial HLH.[247] It was intended that all of these patients undergo AHSCT, which ultimately cured 16 of 19 cases. ATG was ineffective for patients who had been previously treated with etoposide, dexamethasone, and cyclosporine and who had relapsed while on therapy.

A study that is open as of this writing, hybrid immunotherapy for HLH (HIT-HLH; clinicaltrials.gov: NCT01104025) combines strategies of early immune suppression with ATG and prolonged immune suppression with etoposide.

A significant number of patients with HLH will fail to respond to initial therapy or will develop recurrent episodes of inflammation while awaiting AHSCT. Treatment failures and recurrences are associated with very high rates of mortality. Escalation of dexamethasone and etoposide is a typical first step for patients with recurrence. Additional salvage strategies that have been reported include infliximab, dalizumab, anakinra, and other agents.[231] A retrospective multiinstitutional study reported that 77 percent of patients who received alemtuzumab therapy for refractory or recurrent HLH survived to AHSCT.[248] A clinical trial is currently open to test the efficacy and safety of inhibition of IFN-γ in patients with HLH with recurrent inflammation (clinicaltrial.gov: NCT01818492).

AHSCT may be indicated for patients with familial HLH or with gene defects, CNS disease, or who relapse either on or off HLH therapy. Long-term survival was 50 to 65 percent with myeloablative conditioning, but patients experience significant treatment-related morbidity and mortality.[214,249] Institutional series have demonstrated improved survival and decreased treatment-associated complications with reduced intensity conditioning (RIC) strategies that include alemtuzumab. RIC strategies are associated with improved survival.[248,250] A multicenter clinical trial (Reduced Intensity Conditioning for Children and Adults with Hemophagocytic Syndromes or Selected Primary Immune Deficiencies [RICHI]) is currently testing the safety and efficacy of RIC with "intermediate" timed alemtuzumab.[251] (clinicaltrials.gov:NCT01998633)

Patients with HLH are generally acutely ill, and therapies for HLH may exacerbate cytopenias and susceptibility to opportunistic infections. Patients may require multiple transfusions of red cells, platelets, and fresh frozen plasma. Prophylaxis against *Pneumocystis carinii* infection with sulfamethoxazole and against fungi with fluconazole is necessary. Newly diagnosed HLH patients should have human leukocyte antigen typing done and a donor search initiated in case AHSCT is required for therapy.

Macrophage Activation Syndrome

This nomenclature describes patients with symptoms and signs of HLH in the setting of juvenile rheumatoid arthritis or systemic lupus erythematosus.[252] Similar to classic HLH, macrophage activation is characterized by proliferation of macrophages and T cells. Patients present with continuous fever, purpura, hepatosplenomegaly, mental status changes, cytopenias, coagulopathy, and hypofibrinogenemia. Laboratory findings may include defective NK cell function and low perforin expression, as seen in HLH. In the setting of pathologic inflammation driven by autoimmune disease, patients may be successfully treated with therapy targeted against the underlying autoimmune disease.[253] Treatment with dexamethasone and etoposide therapy is recommended if patients fail to improve after a brief trial of therapy appropriate for rheumatologic disease.

COURSE AND PROGNOSIS

Patients with HLH are often critically ill, functionally immunosuppressed, and receive toxic chemotherapy. They should be treated at institutions familiar with the complications of chemotherapy and immune suppression. Splenectomy is recommended only in the case of life-threatening respiratory compromise. Some patients have an initial good response to therapy with etoposide and dexamethasone, but then have progressive disease as evidenced by elevation of the serum ferritin, worsening coagulopathy, or need for increased respiratory, blood pressure, or renal support. Although it may seem counterintuitive to treat critically ill patients with immune suppression, patients with HLH require this approach to have a chance to survive to clear the inflammatory trigger or overcome inherited immune defects with AHSCT.

REFERENCES

1. Jaffe R: The diagnostic histopathology of Langerhans cell histiocytosis, in *Histiocytic Disorders of Children and Adults. Basic Science Clinical Features, and Therapy*, edited by Weitzman S, Egeler RM, pp 14–39. Cambridge University Press, Cambridge, UK, 2005.
2. Favara BE, Feller AC, Pauli M, et al: Contemporary classification of histiocytic disorders. The WHO Committee On Histiocytic/Reticulum Cell Proliferations. Reclassification Working Group of the Histiocyte Society. *Med Pediatr Oncol* 29:157–166, 1997.
3. Nezelof C, Basset F, Rousseau MF: Histiocytosis X histogenetic arguments for a Langerhans cell origin. *Biomedicine (Taipei)* 18:365–371, 1973.
4. Allen CE, Li L, Peters TL, et al: Cell-specific gene expression in Langerhans cell histiocytosis lesions reveals a distinct profile compared with epidermal Langerhans cells. *J Immunol* 184:4557–4567, 2010.
5. Berres ML, Lim KP, Peters T, et al: BRAF-V600E expression in precursor versus differentiated dendritic cells defines clinically distinct LCH risk groups. *J Exp Med* 211:669–683, 2014.
6. Chikwava K, Jaffe R: Langerin (CD207) staining in normal pediatric tissues, reactive lymph nodes, and childhood histiocytic disorders. *Pediatr Dev Pathol* 7:607–614, 2004.
7. Lau SK, Chu PG, Weiss LM: Immunohistochemical expression of Langerin in Langerhans cell histiocytosis and non-Langerhans cell histiocytic disorders. *Am J Surg Pathol* 32:615–619, 2008.
8. Arceci RJ: The histiocytoses: The fall of the Tower of Babel. *Eur J Cancer* 35:747–767, 1999.
9. Guyot-Goubin A, Donadieu J, Barkaoui M, et al: Descriptive epidemiology of childhood Langerhans cell histiocytosis in France, 2000–2004. *Pediatr Blood Cancer* 51:71–75, 2008.
10. Salotti JA, Nanduri V, Pearce MS, et al: Incidence and clinical features of Langerhans cell histiocytosis in the UK and Ireland. *Arch Dis Child* 94:376–380, 2009.
11. Stalemark H, Laurencikas E, Karis J, et al: Incidence of Langerhans cell histiocytosis in children: A population-based study. *Pediatr Blood Cancer* 51:76–81, 2008.
12. Arico M, Nichols K, Whitlock JA, et al: Familial clustering of Langerhans cell histiocytosis. *Br J Haematol* 107:883–888, 1999.
13. Bhatia S, Nesbit ME Jr, Egeler RM, et al: Epidemiologic study of Langerhans cell histiocytosis in children. *J Pediatr* 130:774–784, 1997.
14. Egeler RM, Neglia JP, Arico M, et al: The relation of Langerhans cell histiocytosis to acute leukemia, lymphomas, and other solid tumors. The LCH-Malignancy Study Group of the Histiocyte Society. *Hematol Oncol Clin North Am* 12:369–378, 1998.
15. Akefeldt SO, Finnstrom O, Gavhed D, Henter JI: Langerhans cell histiocytosis in children born 1982–2005 after in vitro fertilization. *Acta Paediatr* 101:1151–1155, 2012.
16. Venkatramani R, Rosenberg S, Indramohan G, Jeng M, Jubran R: An exploratory epidemiological study of Langerhans cell histiocytosis. *Pediatr Blood Cancer* 59:1324–1326, 2012.
17. Willman CL, Busque L, Griffith BB, et al: Langerhans'-cell histiocytosis (histiocytosis X)—a clonal proliferative disease. *N Engl J Med* 331:154–160, 1994.
18. Yu RC, Chu C, Buluwela L, Chu AC: Clonal proliferation of Langerhans cells in Langerhans cell histiocytosis. *Lancet* 343:767–768, 1994.
19. Badalian-Very G, Vergilio JA, Degar BA, et al: Recurrent BRAF mutations in Langerhans cell histiocytosis. *Blood* 116:1919–1923, 2010.
20. Haroche J, Charlotte F, Arnaud L, et al: High prevalence of BRAF V600E mutations in Erdheim-Chester disease but not in other non-Langerhans cell histiocytoses. *Blood* 120:2700–2703, 2012.
21. Sahm F, Capper D, Preusser M, et al: BRAFV600E mutant protein is expressed in cells of variable maturation in Langerhans cell histiocytosis. *Blood* 120:e28–e34, 2012.
22. Satoh T, Smith A, Sarde A, et al: B-RAF mutant alleles associated with Langerhans cell histiocytosis, a granulomatous pediatric disease. *PLoS One* 7:e33891, 2012.
23. Davies H, Bignell GR, Cox C, et al: Mutations of the BRAF gene in human cancer. *Nature* 417:949–954, 2002.
24. Haroche J, Cohen-Aubart F, Emile JF, et al: Dramatic efficacy of vemurafenib in both multisystemic and refractory Erdheim-Chester disease and Langerhans cell histiocytosis harboring the BRAF V600E mutation. *Blood* 121:1495–1500, 2013.
25. Coury F, Annels N, Rivollier A, et al: Langerhans cell histiocytosis reveals a new IL-17A-dependent pathway of dendritic cell fusion. *Nat Med* 14:81–87, 2008.
26. Peters TL, McClain KL, Allen CE: Neither IL-17A mRNA nor IL-17A protein are detectable in Langerhans cell histiocytosis lesions. *Mol Ther* 19:1433–1439, 2011.
27. Geissmann F, Lepelletier Y, Fraitag S, et al: Differentiation of Langerhans cells in Langerhans cell histiocytosis. *Blood* 97:1241–1248, 2001.
28. Laman JD, Leenen PJ, Annels NE, Hogendoorn PC, Egeler RM: Langerhans-cell histiocytosis 'insight into DC biology'. *Trends Immunol* 24:190–196, 2003.
29. Senechal B, Elain G, Jeziorski E, et al: Expansion of regulatory T cells in patients with Langerhans cell histiocytosis. *PLoS Med* 4:e253, 2007.
30. Rosso DA, Roy A, Zelazko M, Braier JL: Prognostic value of soluble interleukin 2 receptor levels in Langerhans cell histiocytosis. *Br J Haematol* 117:54–58, 2002.
31. Rosso DA, Ripoli MF, Roy A, et al: Serum levels of interleukin-1 receptor antagonist and tumor necrosis factor-alpha are elevated in children with Langerhans cell histiocytosis. *J Pediatr Hematol Oncol* 25:480–483, 2003.
32. Stein SL, Paller AS, Haut PR, Mancini AJ: Langerhans cell histiocytosis presenting in the neonatal period: A retrospective case series. *Arch Pediatr Adolesc Medicine (Baltimore)* 155:778–783, 2001.
33. Lau L, Krafchik B, Trebo MM, Weitzman S: Cutaneous Langerhans cell histiocytosis in children under one year. *Pediatr Blood Cancer* 46:66–71, 2006.
34. Simko SJ, Garmezy B, Abhyankar H, et al: Differentiating skin-limited and multisystem Langerhans cell histiocytosis. *J Pediatr* 2014; in press.
35. Minkov M, Prosch H, Steiner M, et al: Langerhans cell histiocytosis in neonates. *Pediatr Blood Cancer* 45:802–807, 2005.
36. Hicks J, Flaitz CM: Langerhans cell histiocytosis: Current insights in a molecular age with emphasis on clinical oral and maxillofacial pathology practice. *Oral Surg Oral Med Oral Pathol Oral Radiol Endod* 2005;100:S42–S66.
37. Jubran RF, Marachelian A, Dorey F, Malogolowkin M: Predictors of outcome in children with Langerhans cell histiocytosis. *Pediatr Blood Cancer* 45:37–42, 2005.
38. Ducassou S, Seyrig F, Thomas C, et al: Thymus and mediastinal node involvement in childhood Langerhans cell histiocytosis: Long-term follow-up from the French national cohort. *Pediatr Blood Cancer* 60:1759–1765, 2013.
39. Gadner H, Minkov M, Grois N, et al: Therapy prolongation improves outcome in multisystem Langerhans cell histiocytosis. *Blood* 121:5006–5014, 2013.
40. Wong A, Ortiz-Neira CL, Reslan WA, et al: Liver involvement in Langerhans cell histiocytosis. *Pediatr Radiol* 36:1105–1107, 2006.
41. Braier J, Ciocca M, Latella A, et al: Cholestasis, sclerosing cholangitis, and liver transplantation in Langerhans cell Histiocytosis. *Med Pediatr Oncol* 38:178–182, 2002.
42. Jaffe R: Liver involvement in the histiocytic disorders of childhood. *Pediatr Dev Pathol* 7:214–225, 2004.
43. Ronceray L, Potschger U, Janka G, Gadner H, Minkov M: Pulmonary involvement in pediatric-onset multisystem Langerhans cell histiocytosis: Effect on course and outcome. *J Pediatrics* 161:129–133, 2012.
44. Vassallo R, Ryu JH, Colby TV, Hartman T, Limper AH: Pulmonary Langerhans'-cell histiocytosis. *N Engl J Med* 342:1969–1978, 2000.
45. Bernstrand C, Cederlund K, Henter JI: Pulmonary function testing and pulmonary Langerhans cell histiocytosis. *Pediatr Blood Cancer* 49:323–328, 2007.
46. McClain K, Ramsay NK, Robison L, Sundberg RD, Nesbit M Jr: Bone marrow involvement in histiocytosis X. *Med Pediatr Oncol* 11:167–171, 1983.
47. Minkov M, Potschger U, Grois N, Gadner H, Dworzak MN: Bone marrow assessment in Langerhans cell histiocytosis. *Pediatr Blood Cancer* 49:694–698, 2007.
48. Favara BE, Jaffe R, Egeler RM: Macrophage activation and hemophagocytic syndrome in langerhans cell histiocytosis: Report of 30 cases. *Pediatr Dev Pathol* 5:130–140, 2002.
49. Prosch H, Grois N, Prayer D, et al: Central diabetes insipidus as presenting symptom of Langerhans cell histiocytosis. *Pediatr Blood Cancer* 43:594–599, 2004.
50. Robison NJ, Prabhu SP, Sun P, et al: Predictors of neoplastic disease in children with isolated pituitary stalk thickening. *Pediatr Blood Cancer* 60:1630–1635, 2013.
51. Donadieu J, Rolon MA, Thomas C, et al: Endocrine involvement in pediatric-onset Langerhans' cell histiocytosis: A population-based study. *J Pediatr* 144:344–350, 2004.
52. Grois N, Potschger U, Prosch H, et al: Risk factors for diabetes insipidus in langerhans cell histiocytosis. *Pediatr Blood Cancer* 46:228–233, 2006.
53. Titgemeyer C, Grois N, Minkov M, et al: Pattern and course of single-system disease in Langerhans cell histiocytosis data from the DAL-HX 83- and 90-study. *Med Pediatr Oncol* 37:108–114, 2001.

54. Donadieu J, Rolon MA, Pion I, et al: Incidence of growth hormone deficiency in pediatric-onset Langerhans cell histiocytosis: Efficacy and safety of growth hormone treatment. *J Clin Endocrinol Metab* 89:604–609, 2004.

55. Geissmann F, Thomas C, Emile JF, et al: Digestive tract involvement in Langerhans cell histiocytosis. The French Langerhans Cell Histiocytosis Study Group. *J Pediatr* 129:836–845, 1996.

56. Hait E, Liang M, Degar B, Glickman J, Fox VL: Gastrointestinal tract involvement in Langerhans cell histiocytosis: Case report and literature review. *Pediatrics* 2006;118:e1593–e1599.

57. Grois N, Prayer D, Prosch H, et al: Course and clinical impact of magnetic resonance imaging findings in diabetes insipidus associated with Langerhans cell histiocytosis. *Pediatr Blood Cancer* 43:59–65, 2004.

58. Fahrner B, Prosch H, Minkov M, et al: Long-term outcome of hypothalamic pituitary tumors in Langerhans cell histiocytosis. *Pediatr Blood Cancer* 58:606–610, 2012.

59. Prayer D, Grois N, Prosch H, Gadner H, Barkovich AJ: MR imaging presentation of intracranial disease associated with Langerhans cell histiocytosis. *AJNR Am J Neuroradiol* 25:880–891, 2004.

60. Grois N, Prayer D, Prosch H, Lassmann H: Neuropathology of CNS disease in Langerhans cell histiocytosis. *Brain* 128:829–838, 2005.

61. Grois N, Fahrner B, Arceci RJ, et al: Central nervous system disease in Langerhans cell histiocytosis. *J Pediatrics* 2010;156:873–81, 881.

62. Wnorowski M, Prosch H, Prayer D, et al: Pattern and course of neurodegeneration in Langerhans cell histiocytosis. *J Pediatrics* 153:127–132, 2008.

63. Calming U, Henter JI: Elevated erythrocyte sedimentation rate and thrombocytosis as possible indicators of active disease in Langerhans' cell histiocytosis. *Acta Paediatr* 87:1085–1087, 1998.

64. Phillips M, Allen C, Gerson P, McClain K: Comparison of FDG-PET scans to conventional radiography and bone scans in management of Langerhans cell histiocytosis. *Pediatr Blood Cancer* 52:97–101, 2009.

65. Almanaseer IY, Kosova L, Pellettiere EV: Composite lymphoma with immunoblastic features and Langerhans' cell granulomatosis (histiocytosis X). *Am J Clin J Pathol* 85:111–114, 1986.

66. Burns BF, Colby TV, Dorfman RF: Langerhans' cell granulomatosis (histiocytosis X) associated with malignant lymphomas. *Am J Surg. J Pathol* 7:529–533, 1983.

67. Egeler RM, Neglia JP, Arico M, et al: The relation of Langerhans cell histiocytosis to acute leukemia, lymphomas, and other solid tumors. The LCH-Malignancy Study Group of the Histiocyte Society. *Hematol Oncol Clin North Am* 12:369–378, 1998.

68. Bramwell NH, Burns BF: Histiocytosis X of the thymus in association with myasthenia gravis. *Am J Clin J Pathol* 86:224–227, 1986.

69. Steen AE, Steen KH, Bauer R, Bieber T: Successful treatment of cutaneous Langerhans cell histiocytosis with low-dose methotrexate. *Br J Dermatol* 145:137–140, 2001.

70. McClain KL, Kozinetz C: A phase II trial using thalidomide for Langerhans cell histiocytosis. *Pediatr Blood Cancer* 48(1):44–49, 2007.

71. Hoeger PH, Nanduri VR, Harper JI, Atherton DA, Pritchard J: Long term follow up of topical mustine treatment for cutaneous langerhans cell histiocytosis. *Arch Dis Child* 82:483–487, 2000.

72. Kwon OS, Cho KH, Song KY: Primary cutaneous Langerhans cell histiocytosis treated with photochemotherapy. *J Dermatology* 24:54–56, 1997.

73. Nauert C, Zornoza J, Ayala A, Harle TS: Eosinophilic granuloma of bone: Diagnosis and management. *Skeletal Radiol* 10:227–235, 1983.

74. Nesbit ME, Kieffer S, D'Angio GJ: Reconstitution of vertebral height in histiocytosis X: A long-term follow-up. *J Bone Joint Surg Am* 51:1360–1368, 1969.

75. Womer RB, Raney RB Jr, D'Angio GJ: Healing rates of treated and untreated bone lesions in histiocytosis X. *Pediatrics* 76:286–288, 1985.

76. Mammano S, Candiotto S, Balsano M: Cast and brace treatment of eosinophilic granuloma of the spine: Long-term follow-up. *J Pediatr Orthop* 17:821–827, 1997.

77. Raney RB Jr, D'Angio GJ: Langerhans' cell histiocytosis (histiocytosis X): Experience at the Children's Hospital of Philadelphia, 1970–1984. *Med Pediatr Oncol* 17:20–28, 1989.

78. Morimoto A, Ikushima S, Kinugawa N, et al: Improved outcome in the treatment of pediatric multifocal Langerhans cell histiocytosis: Results from the Japan Langerhans Cell Histiocytosis Study Group-96 protocol study. *Cancer* 107:613–619, 2006.

79. Dhall G, Finlay JL, Dunkel IJ, et al: Analysis of outcome for patients with mass lesions of the central nervous system due to Langerhans cell histiocytosis treated with 2-chlorodeoxyadenosine. *Pediatr Blood Cancer* 50:72–79, 2008

80. Idbaih A, Donadieu J, Barthez MA, et al: Retinoic acid therapy in "degenerative-like" neuro-langerhans cell histiocytosis: A prospective pilot study. *Pediatr Blood Cancer* 43:55–58, 2004.

81. Imashuku S, Okazaki N, Nakayama M, et al: Treatment of neurodegenerative CNS disease in Langerhans cell histiocytosis with a combination of intravenous immunoglobulin and chemotherapy. *Pediatr Blood Cancer* 50:308–311, 2008.

82. Allen CE, Flores R, Rauch K, et al: Neurodegenerative central nervous system Langerhans cell histiocytosis and coincident hydrocephalus treated with vincristine/cytosine arabinoside. *Pediatr Blood Cancer* 54:416–423, 2010.

83. Egeler RM, de KJ, Voute PA: Cytosine-arabinoside, vincristine, and prednisolone in the treatment of children with disseminated Langerhans cell histiocytosis with organ dysfunction: Experience at a single institution. *Med Pediatr Oncol* 21:265–270, 1993.

84. Simko SJ, Tran HD, Jones J, et al: Clofarabine salvage therapy in refractory multifocal histiocytic disorders, including Langerhans cell histiocytosis, juvenile xanthogranuloma and Rosai-Dorfman disease. *Pediatr Blood Cancer* 61:479–487, 2014.

85. Weitzman S, Braier J, Donadieu J, et al: 2'-Chlorodeoxyadenosine (2-CdA) as salvage therapy for Langerhans cell histiocytosis (LCH). Results of the LCH-S-98 protocol of the Histiocyte Society. *Pediatr Blood Cancer* 53:1271–1276, 2009.

86. Bernard F, Thomas C, Bertrand Y, et al: Multi-centre pilot study of 2-chlorodeoxyadenosine and cytosine arabinoside combined chemotherapy in refractory Langerhans cell histiocytosis with haematological dysfunction. *Eur J Cancer* 41:2682–2689, 2005.

87. Simko SJ, Tran HD, Jones J, et al: Clofarabine salvage therapy in refractory multifocal histiocytic disorders, including Langerhans cell histiocytosis, juvenile xanthogranuloma and Rosai-Dorfman disease. *Pediatr Blood Cancer* 61:479–487, 2014.

88. Abraham A, Alsultan A, Jeng M, Rodriguez-Galindo C, Campbell PK: Clofarabine salvage therapy for refractory high-risk langerhans cell histiocytosis. *Pediatr Blood Cancer* 2013;60:E19–E22.

89. Rodriguez-Galindo C, Jeng M, Khuu P, McCarville MB, Jeha S: Clofarabine in refractory Langerhans cell histiocytosis. *Pediatr Blood Cancer* 51:703–706, 2008.

90. Pratilas CA, Xing F, Solit DB: Targeting oncogenic BRAF in human cancer. *Curr Top Microbiol Immunol* 355:83–98, 2012.

91. Haroche J, Cohen-Aubart F, Emile JF, et al: Dramatic efficacy of vemurafenib in both multisystemic and refractory Erdheim-Chester disease and Langerhans cell histiocytosis harboring the BRAF V600E mutation. *Blood* 121:1495–1500, 2013.

92. Cooper N, Rao K, Goulden N, et al: The use of reduced-intensity stem cell transplantation in haemophagocytic lymphohistiocytosis and Langerhans cell histiocytosis. *Bone Marrow Transplant* 2008;42 Suppl 2:S47–S50.

93. Haupt R, Nanduri V, Calevo MG, et al: Permanent consequences in Langerhans cell histiocytosis patients: A pilot study from the Histiocyte Society-Late Effects Study Group. *Pediatr Blood Cancer* 42:438–444, 2004.

94. Willis B, Ablin A, Weinberg V, et al: Disease course and late sequelae of Langerhans' cell histiocytosis: 25-year experience at the University of California, San Francisco. *J Clin Oncol* 14:2073–2082, 1996.

95. Nanduri VR, Lillywhite L, Chapman C, et al: Cognitive outcome of long-term survivors of multisystem langerhans cell histiocytosis: A single-institution, cross-sectional study. *J Clin Oncol* 21:2961–2967, 2003.

96. Mittheisz E, Seidl R, Prayer D, et al: Central nervous system-related permanent consequences in patients with Langerhans cell histiocytosis. *Pediatr Blood Cancer* 48:50–56, 2007.

97. Egeler RM, Neglia JP, Puccetti DM, Brennan CA, Nesbit ME: Association of Langerhans cell histiocytosis with malignant neoplasms. *Cancer* 71:865–873, 1993.

98. Feldman AL, Berthold F, Arceci RJ, et al: Clonal relationship between precursor T-lymphoblastic leukaemia/lymphoma and Langerhans-cell histiocytosis. *Lancet Oncol* 6:435–437, 2005.

99. Rodig SJ, Payne EG, Degar BA, et al: Aggressive Langerhans cell histiocytosis following T-ALL: Clonally related neoplasms with persistent expression of constitutively active NOTCH1. *Am J Hematol* 83:116–121, 2008.

100. Yohe SL, Chenault CB, Torlakovic EE, Asplund SL, McKenna RW: Langerhans cell histiocytosis in acute leukemias of ambiguous or myeloid lineage in adult patients: Support for a possible clonal relationship. *Mod Pathol* 27:651–656, 2014.

101. Baumgartner I, von HA, Baumert B, Luetolf U, Follath F: Langerhans'-cell histiocytosis in adults. *Med Pediatr Oncol* 28:9–14, 1997.

102. Gotz G, Fichter J: Langerhans'-cell histiocytosis in 58 adults. *Eur J Med Res* 9:510–514, 2004.

103. Tazi A, Moreau J, Bergeron A, et al: Evidence that Langerhans cells in adult pulmonary Langerhans cell histiocytosis are mature dendritic cells: Importance of the cytokine microenvironment. *J Immunol* 163:3511–3515, 1999.

104. Yousem SA, Colby TV, Chen YY, Chen WG, Weiss LM: Pulmonary Langerhans' cell histiocytosis: Molecular analysis of clonality. *Am J Surg Pathol* 25:630–636, 2001.

105. Yousem SA, Dacic S, Nikiforov YE, Nikiforova M: Pulmonary Langerhans cell histiocytosis: Profiling of multifocal tumors using next-generation sequencing identifies concordant occurrence of BRAF V600E mutations. *Chest* 143:1679–1684, 2013.

106. Roden AC, Hu X, Kip S, et al: BRAF V600E expression in Langerhans cell histiocytosis: Clinical and immunohistochemical study on 25 pulmonary and 54 extrapulmonary cases. *Am J Surg Pathol* 38:548–551, 2014.

107. Kaltsas GA, Powles TB, Evanson J, et al: Hypothalamo-pituitary abnormalities in adult patients with Langerhans cell histiocytosis: Clinical, endocrinological, and radiological features and response to treatment. *J Clin Endocrinol Metab* 85:1370–1376, 2000.

108. Edelbroek JR, Vermeer MH, Jansen PM, et al: Langerhans cell histiocytosis first presenting in the skin in adults: Frequent association with a second haematological malignancy. *Br J Dermatol Dermatology* 167:1287–1294, 2012.

109. Slater JM, Swarm OJ: Eosinophilic granuloma of bone. *Med Pediatr Oncol* 8:151–164, 1980.

110. Schonfeld N, Frank W, Wenig S, et al: Clinical and radiologic features, lung function and therapeutic results in pulmonary histiocytosis X. *Respiration* 60:38–44, 1993.

111. Travis WD, Borok Z, Roum JH, et al: Pulmonary Langerhans cell granulomatosis (histiocytosis X). A clinicopathologic study of 48 cases. *Am J Surg Pathol* 17:971–986, 1993.

112. Crausman RS, Jennings CA, Tuder RM, et al: Pulmonary histiocytosis X: Pulmonary function and exercise pathophysiology. *Am J Respir Crit Care Med* 153:426–435, 1996.

113. Delobbe A, Durieu J, Duhamel A, Wallaert B: Determinants of survival in pulmonary Langerhans' cell granulomatosis (histiocytosis X). Groupe d'Etude en Pathologie Interstitielle de la Societe de Pathologie Thoracique du Nord. *Eur Respir J* 9:2002–2006, 1996.

114. Tazi A, Marc K, Dominique S, et al: Serial computed tomography and lung function testing in pulmonary Langerhans' cell histiocytosis. *Eur Respir J* 40:905–912, 2012.

115. Diette GB, Scatarige JC, Haponik EF, et al: Do high-resolution CT findings of usual interstitial pneumonitis obviate lung biopsy? Views of pulmonologists. *Respiration* 72:134–141, 2005.

116. Soler P, Bergeron A, Kambouchner M, et al: Is high-resolution computed tomography a reliable tool to predict the histopathological activity of pulmonary Langerhans cell histiocytosis? *Am J Respir Crit Care Med* 162:264–270, 2000.

117. Pardanani A, Phyliky RL, Li CY, Tefferi A: 2-Chlorodeoxyadenosine therapy for disseminated Langerhans cell histiocytosis. *Mayo Clin Proc* 78:301–306, 2003.

118. Saven A, Foon KA, Piro LD: 2-Chlorodeoxyadenosine-induced complete remissions in Langerhans-cell histiocytosis. *Ann Intern Med* 121:430–432, 1994.

119. Cantu MA, Lupo PJ, Bilgi M, et al: Optimal therapy for adults with Langerhans cell histiocytosis bone lesions. *PLoS One* 7:e43257, 2012.

120. Brown RE: Bisphosphonates as antialveolar macrophage therapy in pulmonary Langerhans cell histiocytosis? *Med Pediatr Oncol* 36:641–643, 2001.

121. Farran RP, Zaretski E, Egeler RM: Treatment of Langerhans cell histiocytosis with pamidronate. *J Pediatr Hematol Oncol* 23:54–56, 2001.

122. Girschikofsky M, Arico M, Castillo D, et al: Management of adult patients with Langerhans cell histiocytosis: Recommendations from an expert panel on behalf of Euro-Histio-Net. *Orphanet J Rare Dis* 8:72, 2013.

123. Arceci RJ, Allen CE, Dunkel I, et al: Evaluation of afuresertib, an oral pan-AKT inhibitor, in patients with Langerhans cell histiocytosis. 55th *Blood* 122(21):2907, 2013.

124. Mogulkoc N, Veral A, Bishop PW, et al: Pulmonary Langerhans' cell histiocytosis: Radiologic resolution following smoking cessation. *Chest* 115:1452–1455, 1999.

125. Shah RJ, Kotloff RM: Lung transplantation for obstructive lung diseases. *Semin Respir Crit Care Med* 34:288–296, 2013.

126. Robb-Smith AHT. Before our time: Half a century of histiocytic medullary reticulosis: A T-cell teaser? *Histopathology* 1990279.

127. Rappaport H: *Tumors of the hematopoietic system.* Atlas of Tumor Pathology, Section III, Fascicle 8, 49–63. Washington DC: Armed Forces Institute of Pathology. 1966.

128. Fonseca R, Tefferi A, Strickler JG: Follicular dendritic cell sarcoma mimicking diffuse large cell lymphoma: A case report. *Am J Hematol* 55:148–155, 1997.

129. Wilson MS, Weiss LM, Gatter KC, et al: Malignant histiocytosis. A reassessment of cases previously reported in 1975 based on paraffin section immunophenotyping studies. *Cancer* 66:530–536, 1990.

130. Takahashi K, Nakamura S: Histiocytic sarcoma: An updated literature review based on the 2008 WHO classification. *J Clin Exp Hematop* 53:1–8, 2013.

131. West DS, Dogan A, Quint PS, et al: Clonally related follicular lymphomas and Langerhans cell neoplasms: Expanding the spectrum of transdifferentiation. *Am J Surg Pathol* 37:978–986, 2013.

132. Chen W, Jaffe R, Zhang L, et al: Langerhans cell sarcoma arising from chronic lymphocytic lymphoma/small lymphocytic leukemia: Lineage analysis and BRAF V600E mutation study. *N Am J Med Sci* 5:386–391, 2013.

133. Pileri SA, Grogan TM, Harris NL, et al: Tumours of histiocytes and accessory dendritic cells: An immunohistochemical approach to classification from the International Lymphoma Study Group based on 61 cases. *Histopathology* 41:1–29, 2002.

134. Go H, Jeon YK, Huh J, et al: Frequent detection of BRAF mutations in histiocytic and dendritic cell neoplasms. *Histopathology* 65:261–272, 2014.

135. Lauritzen AF, Delsol G, Hansen NE, et al: Histiocytic sarcomas and monoblastic leukemias. A clinical, histologic, and immunophenotypical study. *Am J Clin Pathol* 102:45–54, 1994.

136. Kamel OW, Gocke CD, Kell DL, et al: True histiocytic lymphoma: A study of 12 cases based on current definition. *Leuk Lymphoma* 18:81–86, 1995.

137. Julg BD, Weidner S, Mayr D: Pulmonary manifestation of a Langerhans cell sarcoma: Case report and review of the literature. *Virchows Arch* 448:369–374, 2006.

138. Newman B, Hu W, Nigro K, Gilliam AC: Aggressive histiocytic disorders that can involve the skin. *J Am Acad Dermatol* 56:302–316, 2007.

139. Hornick JL, Jaffe ES, Fletcher CD: Extranodal histiocytic sarcoma: Clinicopathologic analysis of 14 cases of a rare epithelioid malignancy. *Am J Surg Pathol* 28:1133–1144, 2004.

140. Pillay K, Solomon R, Daubenton JD, Sinclair-Smith CC. Interdigitating dendritic cell sarcoma: A report of four paediatric cases and review of the literature. *Histopathology* 44:283–291, 2004.

141. Kairouz S, Hashash J, Kabbara W, et al: Dendritic cell neoplasms: An overview. *Am J Hematol* 82:924–928, 2007.

142. Porter DW, Gupte GL, Brown RM, et al: Histiocytic sarcoma with interdigitating dendritic cell differentiation. *J Pediatr Hematol Oncol* 26:827–830, 2004.

143. Soriano AO, Thompson MA, Admirand JH, et al: Follicular dendritic cell sarcoma: A report of 14 cases and a review of the literature. *Am J Hematol* 82:725–728, 2007.

144. Feldman AL, Arber DA, Pittaluga S, et al: Clonally related follicular lymphomas and histiocytic/dendritic cell sarcomas: Evidence for transdifferentiation of the follicular lymphoma clone. *Blood* 111:5433–5439, 2008.

145. Abidi MH, Tove I, Ibrahim RB, Maria D, Peres E: Thalidomide for the treatment of histiocytic sarcoma after hematopoietic stem cell transplant. *Am J Hematol* 82:932–933, 2007.

146. Bailey KM, Castle VP, Hummel JM, et al: Thalidomide therapy for aggressive histiocytic lesions in the pediatric population. *J Pediatr Hematol Oncol* 34:480–483, 2012.

147. Shukla N, Kobos R, Renaud T, et al: Successful treatment of refractory metastatic histiocytic sarcoma with alemtuzumab. *Cancer* 118:3719–3724, 2012.

148. Uchida K, Kobayashi S, Inukai T, et al: Langerhans cell sarcoma emanating from the upper arm skin: Successful treatment by MAID regimen. *J Orthop Sci* 13:89–93, 2008.

149. Gazziola C, Cordani N, Wasserman B, et al: Malignant fibrous histiocytoma: A proposed cellular origin and identification of its characterizing gene transcripts. *Int J Oncol* 23:343–351, 2003.

150. Lee Y, John M, Edwards S: Molecular classification of synovial sarcomas, leiomyosarcomas and malignant fibrous histiocytomas by gene expression profiling. *Br J Cancer* 88:510–515, 2003.

151. Nakayama R, Nemoto T, Takahashi H, et al: Gene expression analysis of soft tissue sarcomas: Characterization and reclassification of malignant fibrous histiocytoma. *Mod Pathol* 20:749–759, 2007.

152. Bramwell VH, Steward WP, Nooij M, et al: Neoadjuvant chemotherapy with doxorubicin and cisplatin in malignant fibrous histiocytoma of bone: A European Osteosarcoma Intergroup study. *J Clin Oncol* 17:3260–3269, 1999.

153. Daw NC, Billups CA, Pappo AS, et al: Malignant fibrous histiocytoma and other fibrohistiocytic tumors in pediatric patients: The St. Jude Children's Research Hospital experience. *Cancer* 97:2839–2847, 2003.

154. Picci P, Bacci G, Ferrari S, Mercuri M: Neoadjuvant chemotherapy in malignant fibrous histiocytoma of bone and in osteosarcoma located in the extremities: Analogies and differences between the two tumors. *Ann Oncol* 8:1107–1115, 1997.

155. Jaffe HS: *Metabolic, Degenerative, and Inflammatory Diseases of Bones and Joints.* Lea and Febiger, Philadelphia, 1972.

156. Veyssier-Belot C, Cacoub P, Caparros-Lefebvre D, et al: Erdheim-Chester disease. Clinical and radiologic characteristics of 59 cases. *Medicine (Baltimore)* 75:157–169, 1996.

157. Al-Quran S, Reith J, Bradley J, Rimsza L: Erdheim-Chester disease: Case report, PCR-based analysis of clonality, and review of literature. *Mod Pathol* 15:666–672, 2002.

158. Chetritt J, Paradis V, Dargere D, et al: Chester-Erdheim disease: A neoplastic disorder. *Hum Pathol* 30:1093–1096, 1999.

159. Loddenkemper K, Hoyer B, Loddenkemper C, et al: A case of Erdheim-Chester disease initially mistaken for Ormond's disease. *Nat Clin Pract Rheumatol* 4:50–55, 2008.

160. Taguchi T, Iwasaki Y, Asaba K, et al: Erdheim-Chester disease: Report of a case with PCR-based analysis of the expression of osteopontin and survivin in Xanthogranulomas following glucocorticoid treatment. *Endocr J* 55:217–223, 2008.

161. Stoppacciaro A, Ferrarini M, Salmaggi C, et al: Immunohistochemical evidence of a cytokine and chemokine network in three patients with Erdheim-Chester disease: Implications for pathogenesis. *Arthritis Rheum* 54:4018–4022, 2006.

162. Haroche J, Charlotte F, Arnaud L, et al: High prevalence of BRAF V600E mutations in Erdheim-Chester disease but not in other non-Langerhans cell histiocytoses. *Blood* 120:2700–2703, 2012.

163. Diamond EL, Abdel-Wahab O, Pentsova E, et al: Detection of an NRAS mutation in Erdheim-Chester disease. *Blood* 122:1089–1091, 2013.

164. Hervier B, Haroche J, Arnaud L, et al: Association of both Langerhans cell histiocytosis and Erdheim-Chester disease linked to the BRAFV600E mutation: A multicenter study of 23 cases. *Blood* 124:1119–1126, 2014.

165. Diamond EL, Dagna L, Hyman DM, et al: Consensus guidelines for the diagnosis and clinical management of Erdheim-Chester disease. *Blood* 124:483–492, 2014.

166. Arnaud L, Hervier B, Neel A, et al: CNS involvement and treatment with interferon-alpha are independent prognostic factors in Erdheim-Chester disease: A multicenter survival analysis of 53 patients. *Blood* 117:2778–2782, 2011.

167. Caparros-Lefebvre D, Pruvo JP, Remy M, et al: Neuroradiologic aspects of Chester-Erdheim disease. *AJNR Am J Neuroradiol* 16:735–740, 1995.

168. Dion E, Graef C, Haroche J, et al: Imaging of thoracoabdominal involvement in Erdheim-Chester disease. *AJR Am J Roentgenol* 183:1253–1260, 2004.

169. Gupta A, Kelly B, McGuigan JE: Erdheim-Chester disease with prominent pericardial involvement: Clinical, radiologic, and histologic findings. *Am J Med Sci* 324:96–100, 2002.

170. Lachenal F, Cotton F, smurs-Clavel H, et al: Neurological manifestations and neuroradiological presentation of Erdheim-Chester disease: Report of 6 cases and systematic review of the literature. *J Neurol* 253:1267–1277, 2006.

171. Drier A, Haroche J, Savatovsky J, et al: Cerebral, facial, and orbital involvement in Erdheim-Chester disease: CT and MR imaging findings. *Radiology* 255:586–594, 2010.

172. Caputo R, Marzano AV, Passoni E, Berti E: Unusual variants of non-Langerhans cell histiocytoses. *J Am Acad Dermatol* 57:1031–1045, 2007.

173. Diamond EL, Dagna L, Hyman DM, et al: Consensus guidelines for the diagnosis and clinical management of Erdheim-Chester disease. *Blood* 124:483–492, 2014.

174. Braiteh F, Boxrud C, Esmaeli B, Kurzrock R: Successful treatment of Erdheim-Chester disease, a non-Langerhans-cell histiocytosis, with interferon-alpha. *Blood* 106:2992–2994, 2005.

175. Esmaeli B, Ahmadi A, Tang R, Schiffman J, Kurzrock R: Interferon therapy for orbital infiltration secondary to Erdheim-Chester disease. *Am J Ophthalmol* 132:945–947, 2001.

176. Haroche J, Amoura Z, Trad SG, et al: Variability in the efficacy of interferon-alpha in Erdheim-Chester disease by patient and site of involvement: Results in eight patients. *Arthritis Rheum* 54:3330–3336, 2006.

177. Hervier B, Arnaud L, Charlotte F, et al: Treatment of Erdheim-Chester disease with long-term high-dose interferon-alpha. *Semin Arthritis Rheum* 41:907–913, 2012.

178. Suzuki HI, Hosoya N, Miyagawa K, et al: Erdheim-Chester disease: Multisystem involvement and management with interferon-alpha. *Leuk Res* 34:e21–e24, 2010.

179. Haroche J, Amoura Z, Charlotte F, et al: Imatinib mesylate for platelet-derived growth factor receptor-beta-positive Erdheim-Chester histiocytosis. *Blood* 111:5413–5415, 2008.

180. Myra C, Sloper L, Tighe PJ, et al: Treatment of Erdheim-Chester disease with cladribine: A rational approach. *Br J Ophthalmol* 88:844–847, 2004.

181. Aouba A, Georgin-Lavialle S, Pagnoux C, et al: Rationale and efficacy of interleukin-1 targeting in Erdheim-Chester disease. *Blood* 116:4070–4076, 2010.

182. Aubert O, Aouba A, Deshayes S, et al: Favorable radiological outcome of skeletal Erdheim-Chester disease involvement with anakinra. *Joint Bone Spine* 80:206–207, 2013.

183. Tran TA, Pariente D, Lecron JC, et al: Treatment of pediatric Erdheim-Chester disease with interleukin-1-targeting drugs. *Arthritis Rheum* 63:4031–4032, 2011.

184. Dehner LP: Juvenile xanthogranulomas in the first two decades of life: A clinicopathologic study of 174 cases with cutaneous and extracutaneous manifestations. *Am J Surg Pathol* 27:579–593, 2003.

185. Iyengar V, Golumb CA, Schachner L: Neurilemmomatosis, NF2, and juvenile xanthogranuloma. *J Am Acad Dermatol* 5 pt 2:831–834, 1998.

186. Tan HH, Tay YK: Juvenile xanthogranuloma and neurofibromatosis 1. *Dermatology* 197:43–44, 1998.

187. van Leeuwen RL, Berretty PJ, Knots E, Tan-Go I. Triad of juvenile xanthogranuloma, von Recklinghausen's neurofibromatosis and trisomy 21 in a young girl. *Clin Exp Dermatol* 21:248–249, 1996.

188. Gutmann DH, Gurney JG, Shannon KM: Juvenile xanthogranuloma, neurofibromatosis 1, and juvenile chronic myeloid leukemia. *Arch Dermatol* 132:1390–1391, 1996.

189. Zvulunov A, Barak Y, Metzker A: Juvenile xanthogranuloma, neurofibromatosis, and juvenile chronic myelogenous leukemia. World statistical analysis. *Arch Dermatol* 131:904–908, 1995.

190. Janssen D, Harms D: Juvenile xanthogranuloma in childhood and adolescence: A clinicopathologic study of 129 patients from the kiel pediatric tumor registry. *Am J Surg Pathol* 29:21–28, 2005.

191. Freyer DR, Kennedy R, Bostrom BC, et al: Juvenile xanthogranuloma: Forms of systemic disease and their clinical implications. *J Pediatr* 129:227–237, 1996.

192. Stover DG, Alapati S, Regueira O, et al: Treatment of juvenile xanthogranuloma. *Pediatr Blood Cancer* 51:130–133, 2008.

193. Vijapura CA, Fulbright JM: Use of radiation in treatment of central nervous system juvenile xanthogranulomatosis. *Pediatr Hematol Oncol* 29:440–445, 2012.

194. Rajendra B, Duncan A, Parslew R, Pizer BL: Successful treatment of central nervous system juvenile xanthogranulomatosis with cladribine. *Pediatr Blood Cancer* 52:413–415, 2009.

195. Rosai J, Dorfman RF: Sinus histiocytosis with massive lymphadenopathy. A newly recognized benign clinicopathological entity. *Arch Pathol* 87:63–70, 1969.

196. McClain KL, Natkunam Y, Swerdlow SH: Atypical cellular disorders. *Hematology Am Soc Hematol Educ Program* 283–296, 2004.

197. Lauwers GY, Perez-Atayde A, Dorfman RF, Rosai J: The digestive system manifestations of Rosai-Dorfman disease (sinus histiocytosis with massive lymphadenopathy): Review of 11 cases. *Hum Pathol* 31:380–385, 2000.

198. Deodhare SS, Ang LC, Bilbao JM: Isolated intracranial involvement in Rosai-Dorfman disease: A report of two cases and review of the literature. *Arch Pathol Lab Med* 122:161–165, 1998.

199. Grabczynska SA, Toh CT, Francis N, et al: Rosai-Dorfman disease complicated by autoimmune haemolytic anaemia: Case report and review of a multisystem disease with cutaneous infiltrates. *Br J Dermatol* 145:323–326, 2001.

200. Morgan NV, Morris MR, Cangul H, et al: Mutations in SLC29A3, encoding an equilibrative nucleoside transporter ENT3, cause a familial histiocytosis syndrome (Faisalabad histiocytosis) and familial Rosai-Dorfman disease. *PLoS Genet* 6:e1000833, 2010.

201. Jadus MR, Sekhon S, Barton BE, Wepsic HT: Macrophage colony stimulating factor-activated bone marrow macrophages suppress lymphocytic responses through phagocytosis: A tentative in vitro model of Rosai-Dorfman disease. *J Leukoc Biol* 57:936–942, 1995.

202. Paulli M, Bergamaschi G, Tonon L, et al: Evidence for a polyclonal nature of the cell infiltrate in sinus histiocytosis with massive lymphadenopathy (Rosai-Dorfman disease). *Br J Haematol* 91:415–418, 1995.

203. Foucar E, Rosai J, Dorfman R: Sinus histiocytosis with massive lymphadenopathy (Rosai-Dorfman disease): Review of the entity. *Semin Diagn Pathol* 7:19–73, 1990.

204. Chow CP, Ho HK, Chan GC, et al: Congenital Rosai-Dorfman disease presenting with anemia, thrombocytopenia, and hepatomegaly. *Pediatr Blood Cancer* 52:415–417, 2009.

205. Price S, Shaw PA, Seitz A, et al: Natural history of autoimmune lymphoproliferative syndrome associated with FAS gene mutations. *Blood* 123:1989–1999, 2014.

206. Govender D, Chetty R: Inflammatory pseudotumour and Rosai-Dorfman disease of soft tissue: A histological continuum? *J Clin Pathol* 50:79–81, 1997.

207. Pulsoni A, Anghel G, Falcucci P, et al: Treatment of sinus histiocytosis with massive lymphadenopathy (Rosai-Dorfman disease): Report of a case and literature review. *Am J Hematol* 69:67–71, 2002.

208. Horneff G, Jurgens H, Hort W, et al: Sinus histiocytosis with massive lymphadenopathy (Rosai-Dorfman disease): Response to methotrexate and mercaptopurine. *Med Pediatr Oncol* 27:187–192, 1996.

209. Perry R, Penk J, Kapoor N, Shah A: Vinorelbine and methotrexate for the treatment of Rosai-Dorfman Disease in children. *Pediatr Blood Cancer* 200584–85.

210. Rodriguez-Galindo C, Helton KJ, Sanchez ND, et al: Extranodal Rosai-Dorfman disease in children. *J Pediatr Hematol Oncol* 26:19–24, 2004.

211. Stine KC, Westfall C: Sinus histiocytosis with massive lymphadenopathy (SHML) prednisone resistant but dexamethasone sensitive. *Pediatr Blood Cancer* 44:92–94, 2005.

212. Farquhar JW, MacGregor AR, Richmond J: Familial haemophagocytic reticulosis. *Br Med J* 2:1561–1564, 1958.

213. Henter JI, Elinder G, Soder O, Ost A: Incidence in Sweden and clinical features of familial hemophagocytic lymphohistiocytosis. *Acta Paediatr Scand* 80:428–435, 1991.

214. Henter JI, Samuelsson-Horne A, Arico M, et al: Treatment of hemophagocytic lymphohistiocytosis with HLH-94 immunochemotherapy and bone marrow transplantation. *Blood* 100:2367–2373, 2002.

215. Zhang K, Biroschak J, Glass DN, et al: Macrophage activation syndrome in patients with systemic juvenile idiopathic arthritis is associated with MUNC13-4 polymorphisms. *Arthritis Rheum* 58:2892–2896, 2008.

216. Zhang K, Chandrakasan S, Chapman H, et al: Synergistic defects of different molecules in the cytotoxic pathway lead to clinical familial hemophagocytic lymphohistiocytosis. *Blood* 124:1331–1334, 2014.

217. Allen CE, Yu X, Kozinetz CA, McClain KL: Highly elevated ferritin levels and the diagnosis of hemophagocytic lymphohistiocytosis. *Pediatr Blood Cancer* 50:1227–1235, 2008.

218. Parikh SA, Kapoor P, Letendre L, et al: Prognostic factors and outcomes of adults with hemophagocytic lymphohistiocytosis. *Mayo Clin Proc* 89:484–492, 2014.

219. Li F, Li P, Zhang R, et al: Identification of clinical features of lymphoma-associated hemophagocytic syndrome (LAHS): An analysis of 69 patients with hemophagocytic syndrome from a single-center in central region of China. *Med Oncol* 31:902, 2014.

220. Henter JI, Elinder G, Soder O, et al: Hypercytokinemia in familial hemophagocytic lymphohistiocytosis. *Blood* 78:2918–2922, 1991.

221. Imashuku S, Hibi S, Sako M, et al: Heterogeneity of immune markers in hemophagocytic lymphohistiocytosis: Comparative study of 9 familial and 14 familial inheritance-unproved cases. *J Pediatr Hematol Oncol* 20:207–214, 1998.

222. Terrell CE, Jordan MB: Perforin deficiency impairs a critical immunoregulatory loop involving murine CD8(+) T cells and dendritic cells. *Blood* 121:5184–5191, 2013.

223. Feldmann J, Le DF, Ouachee-Chardin M, et al: Functional consequences of perforin gene mutations in 22 patients with familial haemophagocytic lymphohistiocytosis. *Br J Haematol* 117:965–972, 2002.

224. Kogawa K, Lee SM, Villanueva J, et al: Perforin expression in cytotoxic lymphocytes from patients with hemophagocytic lymphohistiocytosis and their family members. *Blood* 99:61–66, 2002.

225. Jordan MB, Hildeman D, Kappler J, Marrack P: An animal model of hemophagocytic lymphohistiocytosis (HLH): CD8+ T cells and interferon gamma are essential for the disorder. *Blood* 104:735–743, 2004.

226. de Saint BG, Menasche G, Fischer A: Molecular mechanisms of biogenesis and exocytosis of cytotoxic granules. *Nat Rev Immunol* 10:568–579, 2010.

227. zu Stadt U, Rohr J, Seifert W, et al: Familial hemophagocytic lymphohistiocytosis type 5 (FHL-5) is caused by mutations in Munc18-2 and impaired binding to syntaxin 11. *Am J Human Genetics* 85:482–492, 2009.

228. zur Stadt U, Beutel K, Kolberg S, et al: Mutation spectrum in children with primary hemophagocytic lymphohistiocytosis: Molecular and functional analyses of PRF1, UNC13D, STX11, and RAB27A. *Hum Mutat* 27:62–68, 2006.

229. Chandrakasan S, Filipovich AH: Hemophagocytic lymphohistiocytosis: Advances in pathophysiology, diagnosis, and treatment. *J Pediatr* 163:1253–1259, 2013.

230. Marsh RA, Bleesing JJ, Filipovich AH: Using flow cytometry to screen patients for X-linked lymphoproliferative disease due to SAP deficiency and XIAP deficiency. *J Immunol Methods* 362:1–9, 2010.

231. Jordan MB, Allen CE, Weitzman S, et al: How I treat hemophagocytic lymphohistiocytosis. *Blood* 118:4041–4052, 2011.

232. Janka GE, Belohradsky BH, Daumling S, et al: Familial lymphohistiocytosis. *Haematol Blood Transfus* 27:245–253, 1981.

233. Horne A, Trottestam H, Arico M, et al: Frequency and spectrum of central nervous system involvement in 193 children with haemophagocytic lymphohistiocytosis. *Br J Haematol* 140:327–335, 2008.

234. Henter JI, Horne A, Arico M, et al: HLH-2004: Diagnostic and therapeutic guidelines for hemophagocytic lymphohistiocytosis. *Pediatr Blood Cancer* 48:124–131, 2007.

235. Marsh RA, Bleesing JJ, Filipovich AH: Using flow cytometry to screen patients for X-linked lymphoproliferative disease due to SAP deficiency and XIAP deficiency. *J Immunol Methods* 362:1–9, 2010.

236. Bryceson YT, Pende D, Maul-Pavicic A, et al: A prospective evaluation of degranulation assays in the rapid diagnosis of familial hemophagocytic syndromes. *Blood* 119:2754–2763, 2012.

237. Gupta A, Weitzman S, Abdelhaleem M: The role of hemophagocytosis in bone marrow aspirates in the diagnosis of hemophagocytic lymphohistiocytosis. *Pediatr Blood Cancer* 50:192–194, 2008.

238. Lehmberg K, McClain KL, Janka GE, Allen CE: Determination of an appropriate cutoff value for ferritin in the diagnosis of hemophagocytic lymphohistiocytosis. *Pediatr Blood Cancer* 61:2101–2103, 2014.

239. Lin TF, Ferlic-Stark LL, Allen CE, et al: Rate of decline of ferritin in patients with hemophagocytic lymphohistiocytosis as a prognostic variable for mortality. *Pediatr Blood Cancer* 56:154–155, 2011.

240. Janka GE, Lehmberg K: Hemophagocytic lymphohistiocytosis: Pathogenesis and treatment. *Hematology Am Soc Hematol Educ Program* 2013:605–611, 2013.

241. Ambruso DR, Hays T, Zwartjes WJ, et al: Successful treatment of lymphohistiocytic reticulosis with phagocytosis with epipodophyllotoxin VP 16–213. *Cancer* 45:2516–2520, 1980.

242. Fischer A, Virelizier JL, Arenzana-Seisdedos F, et al: Treatment of four patients with erythrophagocytic lymphohistiocytosis by a combination of epipodophyllotoxin, steroids, intrathecal methotrexate, and cranial irradiation. *Pediatrics* 76:263–268, 1985.

243. Henter JI, Samuelsson-Horne A, Arico M, et al: Treatment of hemophagocytic lympho-histiocytosis with HLH-94 immunochemotherapy and bone marrow transplantation. *Blood* 100:2367–2373, 2002.

244. Imashuku S: Treatment of Epstein-Barr virus-related hemophagocytic lymphohistiocy-tosis (EBV-HLH); update 2010. *J Pediatr Hematol Oncol* 33:35–39, 2011.

245. Johnson TS, Terrell CE, Millen SH, et al: Etoposide selectively ablates activated T cells to control the immunoregulatory disorder hemophagocytic lymphohistiocytosis. *J Immunol* 192:84–91, 2014.

246. Thompson PA, Allen CE, Horton T, et al: Severe neurologic side effects in patients being treated for hemophagocytic lymphohistiocytosis. *Pediatr Blood Cancer* 52:621–625, 2009.

247. Mahlaoui N, Ouachee-Chardin M, de Saint BG, et al: Immunotherapy of familial hemophagocytic lymphohistiocytosis with antithymocyte globulins: A single-center retrospective report of 38 patients. *Pediatrics* 120:e622–e628, 2007.

248. Marsh RA, Allen CE, McClain KL, et al: Salvage therapy of refractory hemophagocytic lymphohistiocytosis with alemtuzumab. *Pediatr Blood Cancer* 60:101–109, 2013.

249. Horne A, Janka G, Maarten ER, et al: Haematopoietic stem cell transplantation in hae-mophagocytic lymphohistiocytosis. *Br J Haematol* 129:622–630, 2005.

250. Cooper N, Rao K, Goulden N, et al: The use of reduced-intensity stem cell transplanta-tion in haemophagocytic lymphohistiocytosis and Langerhans cell histiocytosis. *Bone Marrow Transplant* 42 Suppl 2:S47–S50, 2008.

251. Marsh RA, Kim MO, Liu C, et al: An intermediate alemtuzumab schedule reduces the incidence of mixed chimerism following reduced-intensity conditioning hematopoi-etic cell transplantation for hemophagocytic lymphohistiocytosis. *Biol Blood Marrow Transplant* 19:1625–1631, 2013.

252. Grom AA, Mellins ED: Macrophage activation syndrome: Advances towards under-standing pathogenesis. *Curr Opin Rheumatol* 22:561–566, 2010.

253. Schulert GS, Grom AA: Macrophage activation syndrome and cytokine-directed ther-apies. *Best Pract Res Clin Rheumatol* 28:277–292, 2014.

254. Lau SK, Chu PG, Weiss LM: Immunohistochemical expression of Langerin in Langer-hans cell histiocytosis and non-Langerhans cell histiocytic disorders. *Am J Surg Pathol* 32:615–619, 2008.

CHAPTER 72
GAUCHER DISEASE AND RELATED LYSOSOMAL STORAGE DISEASES

Ari Zimran and Deborah Elstein

SUMMARY

Gaucher disease and Niemann-Pick disease are the two lipid storage disorders that are most likely to be encountered by the hematologist because both may cause hepatosplenomegaly and cytopenias.

Gaucher disease is a common autosomal recessive lipid storage disorder, with an increased prevalence among Ashkenazi Jews, in whom the estimated birth occurrence is 1 in 850. Deficiency of the enzyme β-glucocerebrosidase results in accumulation of the sphingolipid glucocerebroside in the cells of the macrophage-monocyte system. Patients with the most prevalent form, type 1, have no primary neuronopathic symptoms, whereas there is involvement of the central nervous system in type 2 and type 3. Diagnosis of Gaucher disease depends on demonstration of decreased enzymatic activity of β-glucocerebrosidase combined with identification of mutations in the β-glucocerebrosidase gene at the DNA level, usually with elevation of biomarkers, such as chitotriosidase as ancillary confirmation and means of followup. Disease manifestations include hepatosplenomegaly, thrombocytopenia, anemia, osteopenia/osteoporosis with pathologic fractures and osteonecrosis, and, less commonly, pulmonary infiltration. Many patients, especially those homozygous for the common N370S mutation, are putatively protected against neurologic involvement, albeit there is evidence of a genetic risk factor for Parkinson disease. Generally, many patients with type 1 may be asymptomatic or so mildly affected that they may not present until their fifth or sixth decade and do not require disease-specific therapy, whereas for those with more severe signs and symptoms, enzyme replacement therapy (currently three infusible enzymes) is available. Substrate reduction therapy is an oral modality but is associated with a more problematic safety profile. Pharmacological chaperones and oral enzyme are being tested.

Niemann-Pick disease is a heterogeneous group of autosomal recessive disorders. Type A and type B result from deficiency of the enzyme sphingomyelinase, whereas type C results from mutations in the NPC1 or NPC2 gene, which appears to be involved in cholesterol trafficking and resulting in accumulation of cholesterol as well as sphingomyelin. Type A is a lethal infantile form with marked progressive neurologic involvement. Type B is a later-onset form with no neurologic involvement but hepatosplenomegaly in many patients. Patients with type C disease manifest progressive neurologic involvement and hepatosplenomegaly, but may survive into adulthood. The marrow of these

Acronyms and Abbreviations: cDNA, complementary DNA; ERT, enzyme replacement therapy; MRI, magnetic resonance imaging; PC, pharmacologic chaperone; SRT, substrate reduction therapy.

patients contains typical foam cells with small droplets in the cytoplasm and sea-blue histiocytes. Substrate reduction therapy was approved for patients with type C disease in 2008 in Europe; pharmacologic chaperone therapy is being attempted.

Fabry disease, Wolman/cholesteryl ester storage disease (CESD), and GM$_1$-gangliosidoses are other lipid storage diseases characterized by hepatosplenomegaly; GM$_2$-gangliosidosis by hepatomegaly only. CESD patients may result in anemia and have sea-blue histiocytes. They are usually not cared for by hematologists and will not be discussed in this chapter.

● DEFINITION OF GLYCOLIPID STORAGE DISEASES

The glycolipid storage diseases are hereditary disorders in which one or more tissues become engorged with specific lipids, because of deficiencies of the lysosomal enzymes required for hydrolysis of one of the glycosidic bonds. Figure 72–1 shows the catabolic pathway of glycosphingolipids and lists the diseases that are involved in impaired degradation because of specific enzyme deficiencies. The type of lipid and its tissue distribution have a characteristic pattern in each disorder. This chapter deals mainly with Gaucher disease, in which glucocerebroside is stored. It is a common lysosomal storage disorder and also the one with the most hematologic features. The second storage disorder with some hematologic features is Niemann-Pick disease, in which the accumulated material is sphingomyelin and/or cholesterol. The remaining lysosomal diseases (Fabry disease, Wolman/cholesteryl ester storage disease, and GM$_1$- and GM$_2$-gangliosidoses), in which there is hepatosplenomegaly but few hematologic abnormalities, are not reviewed in this chapter.

● GAUCHER DISEASE

HISTORY AND DEFINITION

Gaucher disease was first described by P.C.E. Gaucher in 1882, who thought that the large splenic cells of a young woman seen postmortem were evidence of a primary neoplasm.[1] The term *Gaucher disease* appeared first in 1905, when the autosomal recessive genetic nature of the disorder was elucidated.[2] In 1934, it was shown that glucocerebroside is the storage material in Gaucher disease,[3] and in 1965, the primary defect was recognized as a deficiency of glucocerebrosidase resulting in an impairment of degradation of glucocerebroside.[4,5] Enzymatic purification ultimately led to the cloning of the gene in 1985,[6,7] unraveling of its structure, and identification of many glucocerebrosidase mutations.[8] Disease-specific enzyme replacement therapy (ERT) was first introduced in 1991.[9]

EPIDEMIOLOGY

Gaucher disease is inherited as an autosomal recessive disorder. Although panethnic, type 1 is most common among the Ashkenazi Jews, with a carriership prevalence of 1 in 17 and an expected frequency of the disease in 1 in 850 livebirths.[10] Two distinct forms of Gaucher disease, type 3b and type 3c, are also relatively common in Norrbottnia in northern Sweden,[11] and near the Palestinian town of Jenin, respectively.[12] In the general population, the estimated frequency (based on large-scale neonatal screening projects in three countries is in the range of 1 in 50,000 to 1 in 100,000 persons.[13]

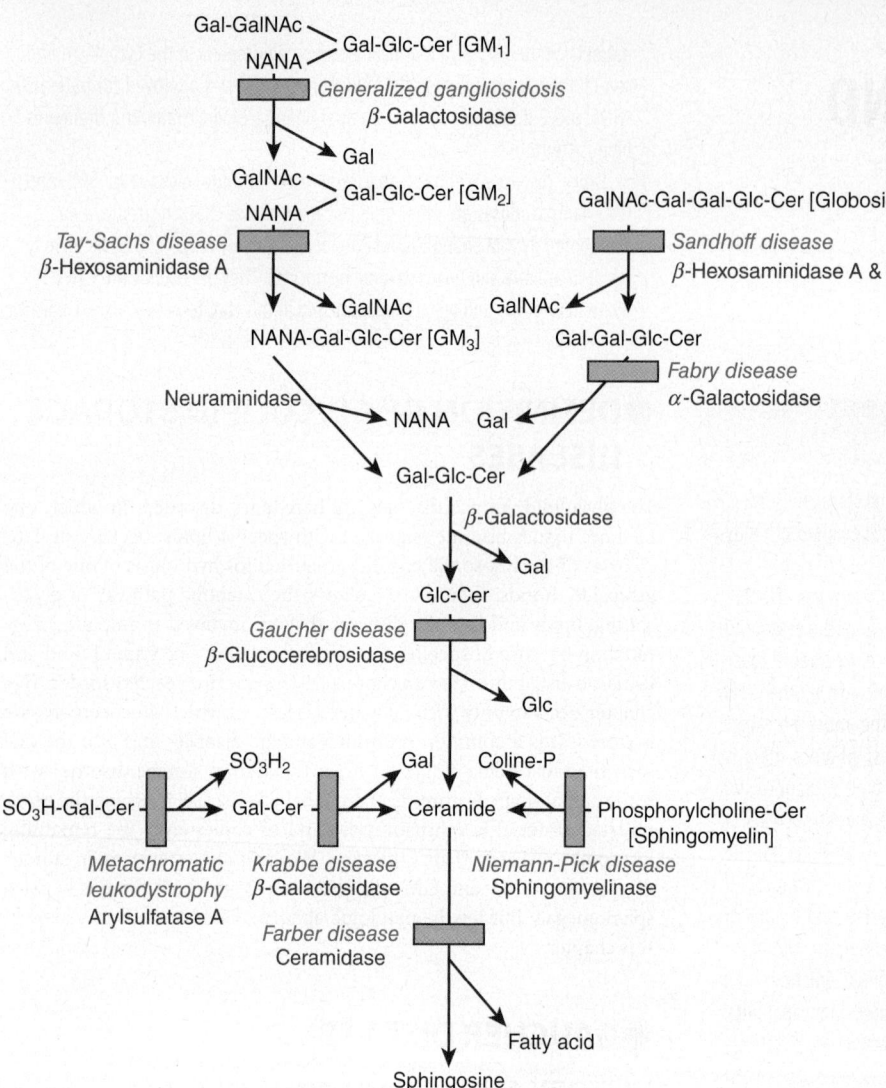

Figure 72–1. The catabolic pathways of selected glycosphingolipids involved in some of the glycolipid storage diseases. *Solid squares* depict the blocked pathways caused by specific inherited deficiencies of enzymes, which give rise to the accumulation of the respective substrates. The names of the various diseases are shown above the names of the deficient enzymes. *(Reproduced with permission from* Lichtman's Atlas of Hematology, www.accessmedicine.com.)

The high prevalence of at least two Gaucher mutation, N370S and 84GG (and possibly R496H[14] and others), among Ashkenazi Jews, and the existence of other lysosomal diseases within this ethnic group, may reflect, in addition to a founder effect, a selective advantage. However, a selective advantage because of greater resistance to tuberculosis[15] or superior intelligence[16] has not been proven. Animal studies suggest that the selective advantage may be the higher circulating serum levels of glucocerebroside that have antiinflammatory and beneficial immunomodulary effects.[17]

ETIOLOGY AND PATHOGENESIS

Enzymatic Basis

During normal growth, development, and senescence, parts of or whole cells are continually replaced. Breakdown of complex constituents of cells requires sequential enzymatic degradation. Such degradation occurs largely in secondary lysosomes, organelles formed by the fusion of primary lysosomes with phagocytic vacuoles containing ingested material.

Gaucher disease is the result of a hereditary deficiency in the activity of a lysosomal enzyme, glucocerebrosidase, required for glycolipid degradation. The reduced activity of glucocerebrosidase results in accumulation of glucocerebroside in macrophages engorgement with

glucocerebroside induces increased cell size and cytoplasmic striations, leading to the formation of "Gaucher cells" (see Fig. 72–1). Inherent in subsequent lysosomal dysfunction is a dysregulation of metabolites and the consequent lack of coordination of cellular metabolism. These changes may explain the elaboration of various cytokines and other biomarkers because of engorgement of macrophages.

Accumulating evidence indicates that in addition to the glucocerebrosidase enzyme (GBA1), a second, nonlysosomal glucocerebrosidase, GBA2, a cytosolic protein that tightly associates with cellular membranes, may be integral to the pathogenesis of Gaucher disease, affecting its phenotype by potentially interacting with GBA1.[18–20]

In rare instances, severe forms of Gaucher disease are associated with deficiency of saposin C, a heat-stable glucocerebrosidase co-factor.[21,22]

GENETIC BASIS OF GAUCHER DISEASE

The glucocerebrosidase gene is located on chromosome 1q21. A pseudogene, with 96 percent sequence homology, has been identified approximately 16 kb downstream from the functional gene. Nearly 300 point mutations causing Gaucher disease have been described[8,23]; most are point mutations, missense, nonsense, frameshift, and splice-site mutations, but there are also insertions, deletions, and recombinant alleles.

Some mutations result from recombinant events between the functional gene and its pseudogene.[8] Since 2000, approximately 20 of these mutated enzymes have undergone crystallography showing the divergence of ligands in the active site and with various degrees of glycosylation.[23]

Among Ashkenazi Jews, the predominant mutation is N370S which accounts for approximately 75 percent of mutant alleles among Jewish patients and approximately 30 percent of the alleles among non-Jewish patients. Homozygosity for N370S is characterized by relatively milder phenotypes (although the phenotype is very heterogenous and severe cases are seen[24]). N370S has heretofore been considered "protective" against the development of neuronopathic features. The second common mutation found almost exclusively among Ashkenazi Jews is one that usually causes a severe phenotype. Five or six common mutations account for approximately 97 percent of alleles among Jews, but account for less than 75 percent of alleles among non-Jews.[8,25-27] Although controversial, premarital/prenatal screening for common mutations has become frequent among Ashkenazi Jews.[28,29,]

The second most common mutation is L444P, which when homozygous accounts for most patients with the neuronopathic type 3 disease, and is the most prevalent mutation in Asians, Arabs, and Norrbottnians. Patients with the unique variant of progressive calcifications of cardiac valves, type 3c, are uniformly homozygous for a point mutation D409H.[12]

Despite some relationship between specific mutations and the clinical course, genotype–phenotype correlation is imperfect. Elucidation of the three-dimensional structure of the glucocerebrosidase by crystallography has also not improved prediction of disease severity based on the location of mutations in the native protein.[30]

The majority of the mutations cause glucocerebrosidase misfolding, which may lead to early degradation of the enzyme in the endoplasmic reticulum.[31,32] The investigation of the proteotoxic effect of the misfolded mutant enzyme in the endoplasmic reticulum has led to the development of the new therapeutic modality of pharmacologic chaperones (PCs). PCs are targeted to stabilize the mutated glucocerebrosidase and allow its appropriate trafficking from endoplasmic reticulum to Golgi and, finally, to the lysosome.

CLINICAL FEATURES

Three major types of Gaucher disease are differentiated clinically based on absence (type 1) or presence of neurologic features (types 2 and 3).[33] Table 72–1 summarizes key clinical, genetic, and demographic features. Although it has been suggested that there is a phenotypic continuum,[34,35] it is still useful to think of Gaucher disease as three distinct forms to facilitate genetic counseling and management decisions.

There is variability in disease severity of all types of Gaucher disease. Type 1 disease may be asymptomatic and be discovered in the course of population surveys of Ashkenazi Jews,[28] or incidentally during evaluation of an unrelated hematologic disorder.

Fatigue

Fatigue is a common complaint, usually not invariably related to anemia, but also quite common in nonanemic patients and may be a result of elevated inflammatory cytokines.[36]

Organomegaly

In symptomatic patients, the spleen is typically enlarged,[37] whether barely palpable or massively enlarged causing positional symptoms, such as early satiety or abdominal discomfort. Splenic infarction and subcapsular hematoma are uncommon. Hepatomegaly is usually asymptomatic, but it may cause abdominal discomfort and in splenectomized

TABLE 72–1. Characteristics of the Three Types of Gaucher Disease

	TYPE 1		TYPE 2		TYPE 3		
Subtype	Asymptomatic	Symptomatic	Neonatal	Infantile	3a	3b	3c
Common genotype	N370S/N370S or 2 mild mutations	N370S/other or 2 mild mutations	Two null or recombinant mutations	One null and one severe mutations	None	L444P/L444P	D409H/D409H
Ethnic predilection	Ashkenazi Jews	Ashkenazi Jews	None	None	None	Norrbottnians, Asians, Arabs	Palestinian Arabs, Japanese
Common presenting features	None	Hepatosplenomegaly, hypersplenism, bleeding, bone pains	Hydrops fetalis; congenital ichthyosis	SNGP, strabismus, opisthotonus, trismus	SNGP; myoclonic seizures	SNGP; hepatosplenomegaly growth retardation	SNGP; cardiac valves' calcifications
CNS involvement	None	None	Lethal	Severe	SNGP; slowly progressive neurologic deterioration	SNGP; gradual cognitive deterioration	SNGP; brachycephalus
Bone involvement	None	Mild to severe (variable)	None	None	Mild	Moderate to severe; kyphosis (gibbus)	Minimal
Lung involvement	None	None to (rarely) severe	Severe	Severe	Mild to moderate	Moderate to severe	Minimal
Life Expectancy	Normal	Normal/near-normal	Neonatal death	Death before age 3 years	Death during childhood	Death in mid-adulthood	Death in early adulthood

SNGP, supranuclear gaze palsy.

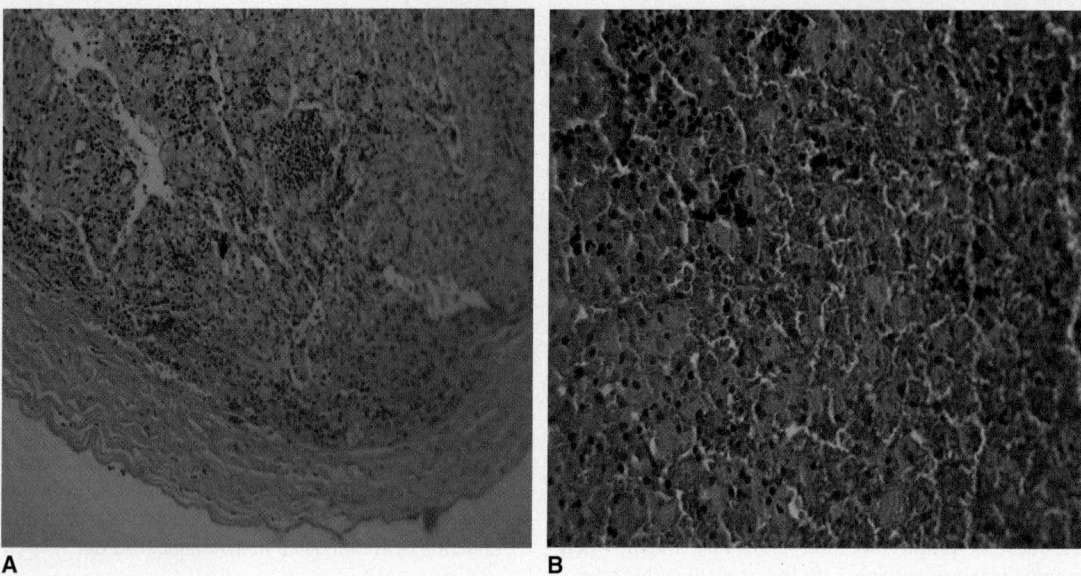

Figure 72–2. A. Histologic section of "Gaucheroma" showing hemorrhagic mass with nucleated red blood cells covered by a fibrous capsule. **B.** Histologic section at a higher magnification showing nucleated red blood cells admixed with numerous Gaucher cells. *(Used with permission of Prof. Eliezer Rosenmann, Shaare Zedek Medical Center, Jerusalem, Israel.)*

patients or others with very severe disease, liver fibrosis and later cirrhosis,[38] with or without portal hypertension, may occur; hepatocellular carcinoma may evolve.[39] An increased incidence of nonalcoholic fatty liver disease has been observed.[40]

Lymphadenopathy

Lymphadenopathy has been described,[41] including a severe protein-losing form,[42] which is a clinical management problem.

Hemorrhagic Events

Epistaxis, easy bruising, and hemorrhage after surgical or dental procedures and bleeding during labor are common presenting symptoms. These manifestations usually are related to thrombocytopenia as the result of hypersplenism or marrow replacement by Gaucher cells, but platelet dysfunction and decreased levels of coagulation factors have also been described and hence should be assessed prior to surgical procedure or before delivery.[43–45] Coagulation factor deficiencies may result from liver disease or consumption coagulopathy.

Anemia

Reduced hemoglobin levels are also primarily a result of hypersplenism and marrow replacement by Gaucher cells, but additional causes include iron deficiency, vitamin B_{12} deficiency, and autoimmune hemolysis.[46,47]

Gaucheromas

"Gaucheromas" (Fig. 72–2), which are possibly extraosseous in origin[48] and/or may mimic a malignant process,[49,50] appear idiosyncratically, but possibly after some invasive procedure such as hip surgery; these have been described to be at increased risk of hemorrhaging when manipulated.

Pulmonary Disease

Severe pulmonary disease with cyanosis and clubbing occurs in some patients with advanced liver involvement, and is usually a consequence of hepatopulmonary syndrome with or without infiltration of the lungs by Gaucher cells.[51,52] Mild pulmonary hypertension may be detected by echocardiography,[53] but may (rarely) be severe especially among

splenectomized patients[54]; it has not been reported in children.[55] Pulmonary function tests may reveal abnormalities, such as reduced diffusion capacity in approximately two-thirds of patients.[56]

Bone Disease

Bone involvement is usually the main cause of morbidity in symptomatic patients and can occur in any long bone.[57] Patchy areas of bone demineralization and infarction are seen (Fig. 72–3A), and asymptomatic widening of the distal femur known as *Erlenmeyer flask* deformity is very common (Fig. 72–3B). Bone metabolism markers indicate that bone resorption predominates,[58] but the overall mechanisms underlying development of bone lesions are poorly understood. Children may have delayed bone age and delayed eruption of the teeth.[59] Bone pain is probably the most troublesome symptom of Gaucher disease. Bone pain may be related to the pathologic processes evident by radiography, magnetic resonance imaging (MRI), and computerized tomography, or have the character of a "crisis," which is a self-limiting, albeit exquisitely painful event, associated with signs of acute local and/or systemic inflammation (Fig. 72–3D). Aseptic necrosis of large joints, mainly the femoral heads but also the shoulders and knees (and rarely even in smaller joints) and vertebral collapse are particularly common typically among untreated patients with genotypes resulting in more severe phenotypes (Fig. 72–3C and E).

Gynecologic Manifestations and Fertility

Gynecologic and obstetric problems are common and are mainly related to bleeding tendency,[60] which may explain why females are more likely to be diagnosed. Delayed menarche and menorrhagia are common, and increased risk of recurrent abortions has been reported.[61] Fertility is unaffected in males and females.

Ophthalmologic Disorders

Organs other than the spleen, liver, bones, and lungs may be affected. Many patients have pinguecula and a few a pterygium at the corneoscleral limbus.[62] Additional findings include uveitis and preretinal white spots in rare cases.[63]

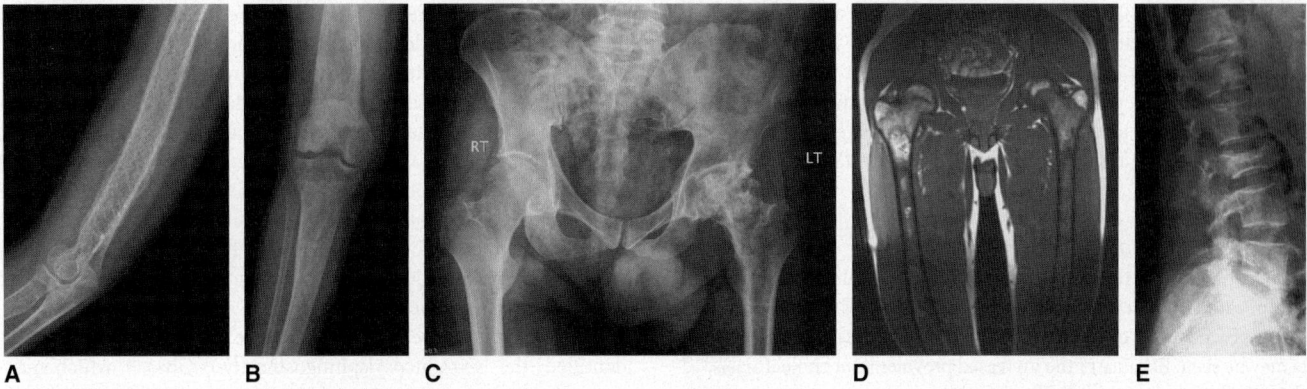

Figure 72–3. Gaucher-related skeletal involvement including **(A)** humerus with chevron or herring-bone pattern; **(B)** Erlenmeyer flask deformity of the proximal femur; **(C)** plain radiograph of osteonecrosis of the left hip; **(D)** magnetic resonance image of pelvis and thighs that was performed 2 weeks after bone crisis of the right thigh. Bone edema is seen in the upper part of the femur at the level of lesser trochanter. Chronic marrow signal changes are seen in both femurs; **(E)** vertebral collapse. *(Used with permission of Dr. Ehud Lebel, Shaare Zedek Medical Center, Jerusalem, Israel.)*

Kidney Disease

Renal manifestations are rare and limited to case reports of nephrotic syndrome and renal cell carcinoma.[64] Nonetheless, many patients seem to have benign urinary hyperfiltration.[65]

Neurologic Findings

Neurologic symptoms constitute the hallmark of types 2 and 3 diseases.[66] Particularly notable and pathognomonic are oculomotor abnormalities, especially supranuclear gaze palsy (SNGP), which is typically noted horizontally,[67] but might occur in the vertical plane as well. Patients with type 2 disease develop hypertonia of the neck muscles with extreme arching of the neck (opisthotonus), bulbar signs, limb rigidity, seizures, and sometimes choreoathetoid movements. In these patients, the SNGP becomes a fixed convergent squint, often facilitating differentiating between type 2 patients, who are terminal by 2 to 3 years of age, and the severe type 3a patients, who may survive longer. Patients with type 3a disease exhibit progressive neurologic abnormalities such as myoclonus and dementia.[68] Patients with type 3b disease display aggressive visceral and skeletal involvement but neurologic manifestations are largely limited to horizontal SNGP.[68] Patients with type 3c disease exhibit SNGP, mild visceral involvement, and fatally progressive calcifications of mitral and tricuspid valves and of the large arteries.[12,68–70]

Several neurologic abnormalities have been observed in patients with type 1 disease, including peripheral neuropathy[71,72] and an increased prevalence of Parkinson disease (the latter also among carriers of a single mutation).[73–77] Carriers of severe mutations (e.g., null alleles) were reported to have a 13.6-fold increased risk of Parkinson disease compared to controls, whereas carriers of the more benign mutations have a 2.2-fold increased risk.[78] A meta-analysis of patients with Parkinson disease has confirmed this strong association between mutations in the glucocerebrosidase gene and Parkinson disease, which is marked by an earlier age of onset and higher prevalence of cognitive changes.[78,79]

Predisposition to Infections

An increased tendency to infections is sometimes seen, occurring among splenectomized patients or severely affected patients, some of whom may have defective neutrophil chemotaxis.[80,81] Bacterial osteomyelitis is most often iatrogenic following surgical intervention at the site of a bone crisis. In children, linear growth retardation is common regardless of disease severity,[82] but a compensatory "catch-up" growth may occur by early adulthood.[83]

Predisposition to Neoplasia

There is a higher prevalence of neoplastic disorders in patients with Gaucher disease.[84,85] Myeloma has been established to be more prevalent.[84,85] Other hematologic malignancies,[86] hepatocellular carcinoma, and renal cell carcinoma, may also have increased prevalence.[87] Although elevated levels of interleukin-6 in patients with Gaucher disease may link Gaucher disease and myeloma,[88] there is no explanation at present for increased incidence of other types of cancer. Some malignancies may be less common.[87] The impact of ERT on either an increased or decreased development of malignancies has not been determined.

LABORATORY FEATURES

Blood Counts

The complete blood count in patients with Gaucher disease may be normal or may reflect the effects of hypersplenism. A normocytic, normochromic anemia is frequently present, but hemoglobin levels only rarely fall below 8 g/dL. A modest reticulocytosis is often present in anemic patients. The white cell count may be decreased to as low as 1.0×10^9/L, but milder degrees of leukopenia are more common. The differential count is normal, but splenectomized patients tend to show a lymphocytosis. A defect of leukocyte chemotaxis which may be corrected by ERT,[89] and in some patients is associated with a tendency to bacterial infections[80]; monocyte dysfunction has also been reported.[81] Thrombocytopenia is typically more prominent than anemia.[46] In an anemic patient with an intact spleen and normal range platelet counts, there is probably an alternative reason for the low hemoglobin level, unrelated to Gaucher disease. Thrombocytopenia may be quite severe, even in an otherwise mildly affected patient. In splenectomized patients, anemia is more likely in the absence of thrombocytopenia; white cell count and platelet counts are usually higher than normal. Severe anisocytosis and poikilocytosis also occur in splenectomized patients, with many target cells, some nucleated red cells and Howell-Jolly bodies. During bone crises, leukocytosis, thrombocytosis, and elevated erythrocyte sedimentation are seen. Other markers of inflammation have been noted regardless of disease severity: elevated fibrinogen levels, elevated high-sensitivity C-reactive protein, and increased adhesion and aggregation of red blood cells.[90,91]

Other Hematologic Findings

Clotting factor abnormalities may be induced by activated macrophages[41,42] or may be found when there is liver involvement. Factor IX deficiency may be a laboratory artifact related to the effect of accumulated lipid on platelet membranes.[92] Factor XI deficiency is common among Ashkenazi Jewish patients because of its high coincidental prevalence in this ethnic group.[93]

Bleeding tendency may also result from defective aggregation or adhesion of platelets[33] and therefore platelet function and/or thromboelastography should be tested before surgical and dental procedures and labor.[44,94]

Biochemical and Immunologic Findings

In most patients, liver function tests are within normal limits but in conjunction with more severe disease, splenectomy, and/or comorbidities (hepatitic B and/or C, or autoimmune diseases) abnormal liver function tests may be seen. Because of the increased prevalence of cholelithiasis,[95,96] cholestatic findings may occur. Renal function tests are usually normal.[64]

Many patients present with polyclonal gammopathies. Monoclonal gammopathies are found in 1 to 20 percent of patients, particularly older patients.[79–82] Increased levels of autoantibodies have been reported,[97] and may indicate coincide with autoimmune diseases such as Hashimoto thyroiditis, rheumatoid arthritis, or immune hemolytic anemia.

Biochemical abnormalities have been used as surrogate markers in Gaucher disease. In the past, increased activities of serum acid phosphatase, angiotensin-converting enzyme, serum ferritin, and other hydrolases, such as β-hexosaminidase or β-glucuronidase, were used.

Other biomarkers correlate better with the extent of glucocerebroside storage. The most widely used biomarker is chitotriosidase,[98] which is undetectable in healthy subjects (its physiologic role is unknown), but is elevated, often several thousand-fold, in patients with Gaucher disease. Chitotriosidase measurement is useful for monitoring both untreated patients, to assess stability *versus* deterioration, and treated patients, to assess response to therapy. A change in chitotriosidase levels rather than absolute values is used for monitoring. In approximately 6 percent of people, it is undetectable, and for those patients, measurements of chemokine CCL18/PARC which is predominantly produced by Gaucher cells, can be used.[99]

A potentially more sensitive and more specific biomarker has been identified: the lyso-glucosylsphingosine (lyso-Gb1),[100] which may be preferred as a more reproducible biomarker, using a more operator-friendly assay.

Serum iron levels may be low in patients because of iron deficiency related to bleeding or chronic inflammation. Deficiencies of vitamin B$_{12}$[101] and vitamin D[102] have been described, albeit these are also very common in the general population. Serum ferritin levels are usually elevated.

Gaucher Cells

Gaucher cells, found mainly in the marrow, spleen, and liver (Fig. 72–4), have small, usually eccentrically placed nuclei and cytoplasm with

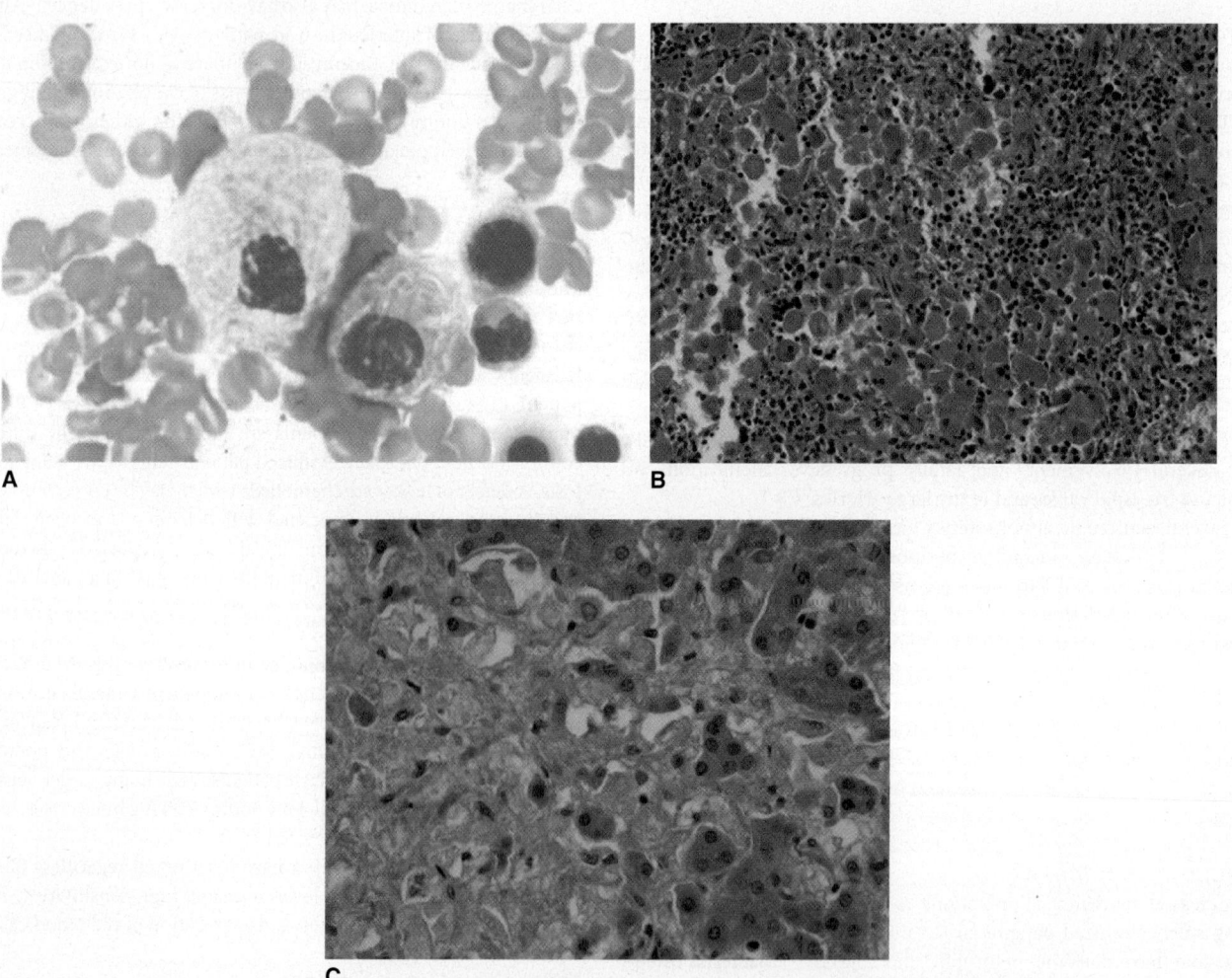

Figure 72–4. A. "Gaucher cell" from the marrow of a patient with Gaucher disease. **B.** Histomicrograph of a Gaucher spleen with marked infiltration of the red pulp by Gaucher cells. **C.** Liver infiltrated by Gaucher cells (the pale pink cells). *(Marrow image used with permission of Prof. Chaim Hershko, Shaare Zedek Medical Center, Jerusalem, Israel; spleen and liver images used with permission of Prof. Gail Amir, Hadassah Medical Center, Jerusalem, Israel.)*

characteristic crinkles or striations. The cytoplasm is stained by the periodic acid-Schiff technique. Electron microscopy demonstrates cytoplasmic spindle- or rod-shaped, membrane-bound inclusion bodies 0.6 to 4 μm in diameter, consisting of numerous small tubules, 130 to 750 Å in diameter, that are composed of twisted multilayers in negatively stained preparations.[103]

DIFFERENTIAL DIAGNOSIS

Diagnosis

The diagnosis of Gaucher disease should be considered in (1) any patient who presents with unexplained splenomegaly, thrombocytopenia, frequent nosebleeds, anemia, acute or chronic bone pain; (2) children with short stature for their age; and (3) nontraumatic avascular necrosis of a large joint at any age, especially if is associated with any of the above features.

A definitive diagnosis requires a reduced enzymatic activity of β-glucocerebrosidase in leukocytes,[104,105] cultured fibroblasts, or amniocytes obtained during prenatal diagnosis. Measurement of glucocerebrosidase levels is supplemented by mutational analysis. This is important for prognosis, particularly in children, and for detection of carriers among affected families. While rapid polymerase chain reaction-based tests are often performed for five or seven common mutations, especially among Ashkenazi Jews as a "first-pass," it is highly recommended to perform whole-genome sequencing[106] to rigorously establish the molecular diagnosis.

Marrow aspiration as a means of diagnosis is only indicated when other hematologic diseases must be considered.[94,105] Gaucher cells are often sparse and thorough examination under low-power may be required to find them. Cells indistinguishable by light microscopy from typical Gaucher cells may also be seen in patients with other disorders such as chronic myelogenous leukemia, Hodgkin lymphoma, myeloma, and acquired immunodeficiency syndrome. The latter patients do not lack the ability to catabolize glucocerebroside, but the great inflow of globoside into phagocytic cells exceeds their capacity to hydrolyze glucocerebroside, forming "pseudo-Gaucher cells."

Prenatal diagnosis can be established by examining cultured amniocytes obtained by amniocentesis for measurement of glucocerebrosidase activity[104] or by examining amniocytes or chorionic villi DNA for known mutations.

Heterozygote Detection

Heterozygotes for Gaucher disease have neither Gaucher cells in their marrow nor stigmata of Gaucher disease (other than the increased risk of Parkinson disease). Existence of a carrier state can be demonstrated by reduced glucocerebrosidase activity to approximately 50 percent of normal values. However, regardless of methodology, enzyme activity among heterozygotes overlaps the normal range and hence definitive diagnosis of heterozygous status only can be made by mutational analysis. Currently various methodologies are being developed to allow noninvasive prenatal diagnosis of monogenic diseases like Gaucher disease; the most promising of these is molecular analysis of cell-free fetal DNA.[107]

THERAPY

Symptomatic Treatment

Symptoms and signs related to massive enlargement of the spleen (e.g., pancytopenia, early satiety, abdominal discomfort, and growth retardation in children) can be resolved by splenectomy. However, because of the efficacy of ERT, splenectomy should only be a last resort as it often induces progressive liver and bony complications, and increases

the risk of infection with encapsulated organisms. Partial splenectomy has not proved useful, with both regrowth of the remnant and risk of osteonecrosis.

When bone lesions result in fractures or osteonecrosis (see Fig. 72–3D), orthopedic procedures may be required. Joint replacement is generally uneventful, with good functional outcome and quality of life. The success of arthroplasties is enhanced by adherence to preoperative protocols including assessment of bleeding tendency, prophylactic use of antibiotic therapy, particularly in splenectomized patients, and early post-operative ambulation.[108]

Deficiencies of iron, vitamin B_{12}, or vitamin D should be corrected and calcium supplementation is recommended in patients with osteoporosis receiving bisphosphonates.[109] Use of erythropoietin may be required for management of anemia because of marrow failure.[110]

Enzyme Replacement Therapy

The use of alglucerase,[9] the first mannose-terminated, placental-derived enzyme, was approved in 1991, and the recombinant form, imiglucerase, albeit with one amino acid R495H that differs from the wild-type protein owing to a cloning artifact in the original complementary DNA (cDNA), was introduced in 1994.[111] Two intravenous preparations, one with the perfect native-enzyme sequence developed in a human cell line, velaglucerase alfa,[112] and the other, a carrot root cell-derived with the imiglucerase core sequence, taliglucerase alfa,[113] have completed phase 3 clinical trials and are available. Phase 2 clinical trials with taliglucerase alfa are currently underway in which the same carrot cells, expressing taliglucerase alfa, are used as vehicle for oral delivery of the enzyme.

The response to ERTs is most gratifying.[9,111–116] Decreased spleen and liver volumes and increased hemoglobin levels and platelet counts usually occur within 6 months of therapy with biweekly doses between 15 and 60 U/kg. Platelet counts in patients with massively enlarged spleens may require longer periods to respond, but improvement continues within the first 2 years of therapy. Thereafter, patients treated with imiglucerase stabilize even while on the same dose.[116]

The bone response is slower and less predictable. Osteonecrosis and lytic lesions do not respond to ERT. Quantitative chemical shift imaging, a sensitive modality to show changes in the marrow, including response to ERT (Fig. 72–5),[117] is a resource available in only one site worldwide and, hence, various other imaging modalities, especially MRI-based modalities, but also bone densitometry and plain radiographs, are used as needed to document skeletal status.

ERT may or may not improve pathologic pulmonary findings. Because the enzyme is a large molecule, it does not cross the blood–brain barrier, and hence, does not impact neuronopathic features.[118,119]

All ERTs are safe, having few side effects that are usually transient.[112,113,120] Hypersensitivity reactions have been reported with each type of ERT, but only rare cases of anaphylaxis. Most patients with such reactions may continue ERT with or without premedication; it is advisable to avoid the administration of glucocorticoids for this purpose because of an increased risk of osteonecrosis. For each ERT there is a different percent of patients who may develop antibodies either shortly after initiation of treatment or over time.

Another side effect is weight gain with some concerns about changes in insulin resistance and the development of metabolic syndrome,[121] including steatohepatitis. Because of the excellent safety profile, many patients receive therapy at home[122] and many female patients are comfortable continuing with ERT during pregnancy and lactation.[123,124] The effects of treatment are unaffected by switching from imiglucerase to velaglucerase alfa[125] or taliglucerase alfa.[126]

The two major disadvantages of ERTs are the apparent lifetime dependency on intravenous infusions and the extremely high cost.

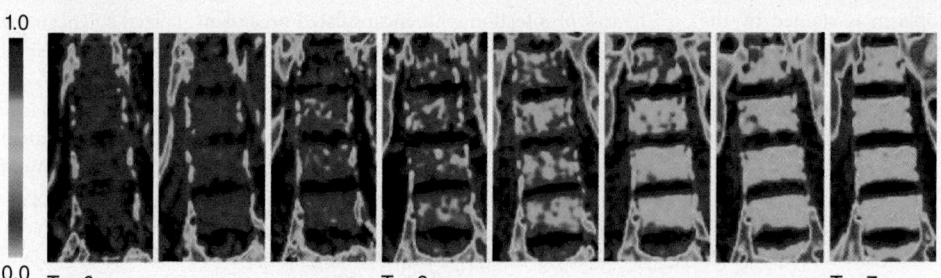

Figure 72–5. Color-coded fat fraction measurements using quantitative chemical shift imaging in an adult patient with type 1 Gaucher disease. Annual measurements show increase in fat fraction with specific therapy (mean value in 1994 = 0.11; mean value in 2001 = 0.45). (*Used with permission of Dr. Mario Maas, Academic Medical Center, Amsterdam, The Netherlands.*)

Guidelines and/or expert opinions usually recommend the use of relatively high doses.[127,128] Yet, it is evident that for most symptomatic patients, there is no justification for doses higher than 30 to 60 U/kg per month, and for patients with asymptomatic type 1 disease, ERT should not be encouraged.[129]

Substrate Reduction Therapy

The possibility that decreasing the formation of glucocerebroside from ceramide and glucose, referred to as *substrate reduction therapy* (SRT),[130] might favorably impact disease parameters was proposed in the 1970s.[131] Oral miglustat (*N*-butyldeoxynojirimycin),[130] a glucose analogue that inhibits glucocerebroside synthase, has been licensed for treatment of patients for whom ERT is not suitable or not a therapeutic option according to the two preeminent regulatory authorities' definitions. This circumscribed approval stems from inferior efficacy of miglustat relative to ERT and a problematic safety profile including peripheral neuropathies, tremor, and memory impairment. Miglustat is effective in reducing hepatosplenomegaly in Gaucher disease when given as 100 mg, three times daily.[132] Response to miglustat is dose-dependent; lower doses yield suboptimal improvement without reducing frequency of side effects.[133] Miglustat has also been studied as maintenance therapy in patients previously treated with imiglucerase.[133] A practical advantage was that it could be considered in type 3 patients because as a small molecule it crosses the blood–brain barrier and impacts neurologic signs. Unfortunately, a clinical trial failed to achieve the end points and, hence, there is no indication for this drug in neuronopathic Gaucher disease.

Another SRT, a ceramide analogue, eliglustat tartrate,[134] has been granted FDA approval. However, it has a more problematic safety profile compared to ERT (including cardiac events), the efficacy parameters.[135] The robust database derived from long-term followup from phase 2 and from three different phase 3 clinical trials[136] indicates it can be useful. However, unlike miglustat, it cannot cross the blood–brain barrier and should be targeted to type 1 patients only.

Pharmacologic Chaperones

A new approach to lysosomal storage diseases is "chaperone therapy." PC therapy is based on *in vitro* experiments showing that some misfolded mutants of glucocerebrosidase are destroyed prior to their export from the endoplasmic reticulum to the lysosome.[137,138] Under these circumstances, a reversible inhibitor stabilizes the mutant enzyme, enabling its passage to the lysosome without losing activity. Clinical trials with the first PC for Gaucher disease, isofagomine tartrate which had been shown to increase mutant enzyme activity in cells, tissues,[139] and healthy volunteers during the phase 1 trial, failed in the phase 2 clinical trial when only 1 of 18 patients with type 1 showed a beneficial effect.[140]

Another PC, ambroxol, an expectorant that is available without prescription in many countries and has decades-long safety experience,

was administered in a pilot study to adult type 1 patients[141]; clinical trials in type 3 patients are planned.

Organ Transplantation

Because the macrophage is a derived from hematopoietic stem cells, allogeneic hematopoietic stem cell transplantation should cure Gaucher disease. Although some enthusiasm was expressed for this approach, the short-term risks of transplantation markedly limit the number of suitable candidates. Effective ERT further limits the appropriateness of transplantation. Liver transplantation has been performed in a few patients with severe hepatic failure.[142]

COURSE AND PROGNOSIS

Age of onset, severity of clinical manifestations, and degree of progression are partially related to genotype. Patients homozygous for the N370S mutation tend to present with symptoms and signs at an older age with relatively milder manifestations, and usually have a relatively stable disease. By contrast, compound heterozygotes for N370S and a "severe" mutation (such as N370S/84GG or N370S/L444P) usually present with the disease during childhood, and if untreated, progress continuously with both visceral and skeletal complications.[108,143,144] Patients homozygous for the L444P mutation will develop neuronopathic disease with deteriorating neurologic signs and symptoms and their life span is reduced.[65]

Although the genotype of the patient provides a benchmark for prognosis, there is much variability in patients with the same genotype, including between siblings with the same genotype. The availability of ERT has changed the natural course of the disease allowing normal growth and development in most patients, even in those with "severe" genotypes. Nevertheless, some patients still develop skeletal complications despite ERT and there is concern regarding development of associated diseases, such as myeloma, other malignancies, or Parkinson disease.[120]

Prior to the availability of ERT, patients with severe type 1 or type 3, died at an early age because of liver disease, bleeding, or sepsis. With the advent of ERT, typical causes of death are malignancy, cardiovascular disease, and cerebrovascular disease.[145] In type 2 disease, death usually results from neurologic complications within the first 4 years of life[65]; there is also a lethal neonatal variant. Total absence of glucocerebrosidase may not be compatible with life.

● NIEMANN-PICK DISEASE

HISTORY AND CLASSIFICATION

In 1914, Niemann, a Berlin pediatrician, reported the case of an infant who died at age 18 months with a disorder that seemed atypical for Gaucher disease because of its early onset and rapid course.[146] In 1927, Pick identified this as a unique disorder of rapid, progressive neurodegeneration in infants.[147] The first adult patients identified had massive hepatosplenomegaly but no neurologic involvement. The predominant phospholipid accumulating in this disorder is sphingomyelin. In 1966, a deficiency of sphingomyelinase activity was demonstrated in a patient with Niemann-Pick disease.[148] Niemann-Pick is not a single entity; it comprises a group of disorders in which sphingomyelin storage occurs. Type A and type B disease, the classic forms of the disorder, represent an infantile neuronopathic and a later-onset nonneuronopathic form, respectively.[149] Type C, the most common form of Niemann-Pick disease, is a neuronopathic disorder, usually with an onset in early childhood, that results from an abnormality in cholesterol transport.[150] The sphingomyelinase gene is normal in type C disease, but mutations occur in one of two genes which have been designated *NPC1* and *NPC2;* the proteins they code may function in closely related steps of cholesterol transport. The designation type D disease was once applied to a population isolate in Nova Scotia[151] but because these individuals also have an *NPC1* mutation, this term is no longer used.

EPIDEMIOLOGY

Niemann-Pick type A and type B diseases, also referred to as acid-sphingomyelinase deficiency, are panethnic disorders. There is a relatively high prevalence of type A disease among Ashkenazi Jews with a carrier rate of approximately 1 in 90.[152] Three mutations account for 90 percent of Ashkenazi Jewish patients. Type B is common among individuals from the Maghreb region and the Arabian peninsula,[153] with three and two mutations accounting for 75 percent and 85 percent of Turkish and Arabic patients, respectively. Type C disease is relatively common in a Nova Scotia isolate,[151] in a Hispanic population from the Upper Rio Grande Valley in the United States,[154] and in Western Europe.[155] The prevalence of Niemann-Pick type C disease in European populations is estimated to be 1 in 120,000 to 1 in 150,000 Europeans.[156]

ETIOLOGY AND PATHOGENESIS

Type A and type B are autosomal recessive diseases caused by loss of function mutations in the gene for sphingomyelinase,[157] which is required for cleaving the bond between ceramide and phosphorylcholine (see Fig. 72–1). Nonsense mutations seem to cause the more severe type A disease, while missense mutations are found in the milder type B disorder.[157] Although sphingomyelinase is believed to be a part of an apoptosis-signaling pathway by generating ceramide from sphingomyelin,[158] no relationship between disease severity and this pathway has been established.

Type C disease also is an autosomal recessive disorder and is caused by mutations in either the *NPC1*[159,160] or *NPC2*[160] gene. The function of the proteins encoded by these genes is unknown, but was suggested to be related to intracellular cholesterol transport.[160,161] The *NPC1* gene encodes for a multi-pass transmembrane protein that localizes to the late endosome. The *NPC2* protein is soluble. The *NPC1* mutations account for more than 95 percent of cases.[161] There are only a few cases of *NPC2* mutations manifested in neonates by severe liver and lung involvement, and progressive neurologic involvement leading to death by 4 years of age; there is a juvenile form in which there seems to be good genotype–phenotype correlation.[162] *NPC1* deficiency is associated with induction of autophagy by the class III-P13K (phosphatidylinositide 3′-kinase)/beclin-1 complex.[163] A naturally occurring murine model of the disease exists.[164]

PATHOLOGY AND CLINICAL MANIFESTATIONS

The most characteristic histopathologic feature of the various forms of Niemann-Pick disease is the presence of foam histiocytes (Fig. 72–6), mainly in lymphoid tissues, but these may be present throughout the body. The foam cells contain largely sphingomyelin and cholesterol, the storage of cholesterol being more prominent in type C disease.

Type A disease presents in infancy. During the first months of life, affected infants gain weight at a diminished rate, the abdomen enlarges, and development is delayed. The patients usually cannot sit and lose physical capabilities already achieved and become blind and deaf. Some infants have a protracted course of jaundice of unknown cause. During the second year of life, the child lies still with nearly flaccid hyporeflexic extremities; there is massive hepatosplenomegaly, mild lymphadenopathy, and often a fine xanthomatous rash. Bone lesions may occur.

Type B disease usually presents in the first decade of life with hepatosplenomegaly, but may not be noted until adulthood. Neurologic manifestations are usually absent. Pulmonary infiltrates are common. The absence of a cherry-red spot in the macula and longer life expectancy differentiate type B from type A. Sea-blue histiocytes are sometimes found in the marrow, and a number of patients had been diagnosed as having sea-blue histiocytosis before a deficiency in sphingomyelinase was demonstrated.[165]

Patients with type C disease often have neonatal jaundice, normal early childhood, and then develop hypotonia, dementia, ataxia, dysarthria, dystonia, seizures, gelastic cataplexy, and cognitive decline.[165] Hepatosplenomegaly is common.[149] Presentation may be at any age, even in the seventh decade,[165] but the "classic" description is of

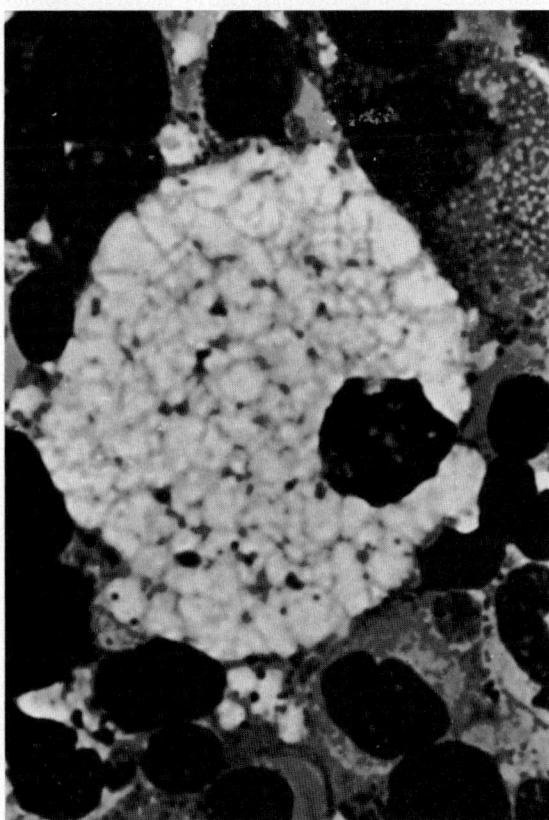

Figure 72–6. Typical foam cell from the marrow of a patient with Niemann-Pick disease.

juvenile dystonic lipidosis with neonatal icterus and hepatosplenomegaly. In infants and toddlers, hepatosplenomegaly may be the only sign. In patients with a later-onset, there are variable presentations, but psychiatric signs and symptoms (disinhibition and deteriorating executive function) predominate.[165]

LABORATORY FEATURES AND DIFFERENTIAL DIAGNOSIS

Hemoglobin values may be normal, or mild anemia may be present. Approximately 75 percent of lymphocytes contain one to nine vacuoles with a diameter of 2 μm. Electron microscopy reveals that these vacuoles are lipid-filled lysosomes.[166] The marrow contains typical foam cells whose diameter ranges between 20 and 100 μm. Small droplets are scattered throughout the cytoplasm (see Fig. 72–6). The cytoplasm of these cells stains only very faintly with the periodic acid-Schiff reagent. Phase microscopy of unstained preparations clearly reveals droplets in the cytoplasm of Niemann-Pick foam cells that distinguish them from Gaucher cells. Sea-blue histiocytes may be present in the spleen and marrow.[158,164]

Type A and type B disease can be distinguished from other disorders by identification of the lipid as sphingomyelin and by demonstration of sphingomyelinase deficiency in leukocytes or cultured fibroblasts.[166,167] Patients with type A disease have acid sphingomyelinase activity levels less than 5 percent of normal in *in vitro* cultures of lymphoblasts or fibroblasts. In type B disease, acid sphingomyelinase activity levels range between 2 and 10 percent of normal levels. Monospecific antibodies against sphingomyelinase are used to differentiate between type A and type B disease.[168] Heterozygotes may be detected by measurement of sphingomyelinase activity of cultured fibroblasts.[169] For patients with type C disease, the presence of foam cells is the only indication of the disease.

Prenatal diagnosis of the three types of the disease is possible, but is difficult in type C.[170]

TREATMENT

There is no effective treatment for types A and B disease, but there has been an announcement of a successful phase 1b trial with ERT for type B disease and plans for continuation into a phase 2 trial.[171]

Splenectomy is only rarely required, because death usually occurs from other manifestations of the disease before hypersplenism becomes clinically important. Liver transplantation in type A disease corrects hepatic pathology but has little long-term benefit[172]; similarly, allogeneic hematopoietic stem cell transplantation does not ameliorate the neurologic deterioration in type B disease,[173] nor does it affect the course of type C disease.[174] Somatic cell gene therapy has been attempted in knockout type B mice[175] and was effective in ameliorating visceral signs but had no effect on neurologic signs.

SRT was attempted in a patient with type C disease.[176] Depletion of glycosphingolipids by miglustat[130] despite having no direct effect on cholesterol metabolism, corrected abnormal lipid trafficking[177] and indicated that glycosphingolipid accumulation is a primary pathogenetic event in type C disease.

A clinical trial using miglustat at a dose of 200 mg three times daily in an open-label 12-month trial with extension to 66 months in juvenile and adult patients with type C disease and in some children, resulted in improvement or stabilization.[177] Subsequent long-term exposure in adults, and some children[179] led to its commercial approval and use clinically in many countries. Miglustat improved neurologic manifestations such as ambulation, manipulation, speech, and swallowing; there are some gastrointestinal side effects.[177–179]

COURSE AND PROGNOSIS

The prognosis in type A Niemann-Pick disease is dire; death nearly always occurs before the third year of life. Patients with type B disease may survive into childhood or longer and there is now hope for a disease-specific ERT. Patients with type C disease usually die in the second decade of life, but some patients with mild disease have a normal life span. New hope for patients with type C emanates from the potential for identification of disease-specific oxysterols as both biomarkers[180] of the disease and as harbingers of PC therapy for misfolded variants.[181]

REFERENCES

1. Gaucher PCE: *De l'epithelioma Primitif de la Rate, Hypertrophie Idiopathique del la Rate San Leucemie*. University of Paris, Paris, 1882.
2. Brill N, Mandelbaum F, Libman E: Primary splenomegaly-Gaucher type. Report on one of four cases occurring in a single generation in a family. *Am J Med Sci* 129:491, 1905.
3. Aghion H: *La maladie de Gaucher dans l'enfance* [PhD thesis]. Paris, 1934.
4. Brady RO, Kanfer JN, Shapiro D: Metabolism of glucocerebrosides: II. Evidence of an enzymatic deficiency in Gaucher's disease. *Biochem Biophys Res Commun* 18:221, 1965.
5. Patrick AD: Short communications: A deficiency of glucocerebrosidase in Gaucher's disease. *Biochem J* 97:17C, 1965.
6. Sorge J, West C, Westwood B, Beutler ED: Molecular cloning and nucleotide sequence of human glucocerebrosidase cDNA. *Proc Natl Acad Sci U S A* 82:7289, 1985.
7. Horowitz M, Wilder S, Horowitz Z, et al: The human glucocerebrosidase gene and pseudogene: Structure and evolution. *Genomics* 4:87, 1989.
8. Hruska KS, LaMarca ME, Scott CR, Sidransky E: Gaucher disease: Mutations and polymorphism spectrum in the glucocerebrosidase gene (GBA). *Hum Mutat* 29:567, 2008.
9. Barton NW, Brady RO, Dambrosia JM, et al: Replacement therapy for inherited enzyme deficiency—Macrophage-targeted glucocerebrosidase for Gaucher's disease. *N Engl J Med* 324:1464, 1991.
10. Beutler E, Nguyen NJ, Henneberger MW, et al: Gaucher disease: Gene frequencies in the Ashkenazi Jewish population. *Am J Hum Genet* 52:85, 1993.
11. Svennerholm L, Erikson A, Groth CG, et al: Norrbottnian type of Gaucher disease—Clinical, biochemical and molecular biology aspects: Successful treatment with bone marrow transplantation. *Dev Neurosci* 13:345, 1991.
12. Abrahamov A, Elstein D, Gross-Tsur V, et al: Gaucher's disease variant characterized by progressive calcification of heart valves and unique genotype. *Lancet* 346:1000, 1995.
13. Meikle PJ, Fuller M, Hopwood JJ: Gaucher Disease: Epidemiology and screening policy, in *Gaucher Disease*, edited by AH Futerman, A Zimran, p 321. CRC Press, Boca Raton, FL, 2007.
14. Bronstein S, Karpati M, Peleg L: An update of Gaucher mutations distribution among Ashkenazi Jewish population: Prevalence and country of origin of the mutation R496H. *Isr Med Assoc J* 16:683, 2014.
15. Kannai R, Elstein D, Weiler-Razell D, Zimran A: The selective advantage of Gaucher's disease: TB or not TB? *Isr Med Assoc J* 30:911, 1994.
16. Cochran G, Hardy J, Harpending H: Natural history of Ashkenazi intelligence. *J Biosoc Sci* 38:659, 2006.
17. Ilan Y, Elstein D, Zimran A: Glucocerebroside-an evolutionary advantage for patients with Gaucher disease: A new immunomodulatory agent. *Immunol Cell Biol* 3:407, 2009.
18. Boot RG, Verhoek M, Donker-Koopman W, et al: Identification of the non-lysosomal glucosylceramidase as beta-glucosidase 2. *J Biol Chem* 282:1305, 2007.
19. Yildiz Y, Hoffmann P, Vom Dahl S, et al: Functional and genetic characterization of the non-lysosomal glucosylceramidase 2 as a modifier for Gaucher disease. *Orphanet J Rare Dis* 8:151, 2013.
20. Mistry PK, Liu J, Sun L, et al: Glucocerebrosidase 2 gene deletion rescues type 1 Gaucher disease. *Proc Natl Acad Sci U S A* 111:4934, 2014.
21. Schnabel D, Schröder M, Sandhoff K: Mutation in the sphingolipid activator protein 2 in a patient with a variant of Gaucher disease. *FEBS Lett* 284:57, 1991.
22. Tylki-Szymaska A, Czartoryska B, Vanier MT, et al: Non-neuronopathic Gaucher disease due to saposin C deficiency. *Clin Genet* 72:538, 2007.
23. Lieberman RL: A guided tour of the structural biology of Gaucher disease: Acid-β-glucosidase and saposin C. *Enzyme Res* 2011:973231, 2011.
24. Fairley C, Zimran A, Phillips M, et al: Phenotypic heterogeneity of N370S homozygotes with type I Gaucher disease: An analysis of 798 patients from the ICGG Gaucher Registry. *J Inherit Metab Dis* 31:738, 2008.
25. Beutler E, Gelbart T, Kuhl W, et al: Mutations in Jewish patients with Gaucher disease. *Blood* 79:1662, 1992.
26. Beutler E, Gelbart T: Gaucher disease mutations in non-Jewish patients. *Br J Haematol* 85:401, 1993.
27. Horowitz M, Pasmanik-Chor M, Borochowitz Z, et al: Prevalence of glucocerebrosidase mutations in the Israeli Ashkenazi Jewish population. *Hum Mutat* 12:240, 1998.
28. Zuckerman S, Lahad A, Shmueli A, et al: Carrier screening for Gaucher disease: Lessons for low-penetrance, treatable diseases. *JAMA* 298:1281, 2007.
29. Falcone D, Wood EM, Mennuti M, et al: Prenatal healthcare providers' Gaucher disease carrier screening practices. *Genet Med* 14:844, 2012.

30. Brumshtein B, Salinas P, Peterson B, et al: Characterization of gene-activated human acid-beta-glucosidase: Crystal structure, glycan composition, and internalization into macrophages. *Glycobiology* 20:24, 2010.

31. Sawkar AR, Adamski-Werner SL, Cheng WC, et al: Gaucher disease-associated glucocerebrosidases show mutation-dependent chemical chaperoning profiles. *Chem Biol* 12:1235, 2005.

32. Ron I, Horowitz M: ER retention and degradation as the molecular basis underlying Gaucher disease heterogeneity. *Hum Mol Genet* 15:2387, 2005.

33. Zimran A, Elstein D: Lipid storage diseases, in: *Williams Hematology*, 8th ed, edited by MA Lichtman, T Kipps, U Seligsohn, K Kaushansky, JT Prchal JT, p 1065. McGraw-Hill, New York, 2010.

34. Sidransky E: Gaucher disease: Complexity in a "simple" disorder. *Mol Genet Metab* 83:6, 2004.

35. Chérin P, Sedel F, Mignot C, et al: Neurological manifestations of type 1 Gaucher's disease: Is a revision of disease classification needed? *Rev Neurol* (Paris) 162:1076, 2006.

36. Pandey MK, Rani R, Zhang W, et al: Immunological cell type characterization and Th1-Th17 cytokine production in a mouse model of Gaucher disease. *Mol Genet Metab* 106:310, 2012.

37. Elstein D, Abrahamov A, Hadas-Halpern I, Zimran A: Gaucher's disease. *Lancet* 358:324, 2001.

38. Bohte AE, van Dussen L, Akkerman EM, et al: Liver fibrosis in type I Gaucher disease: Magnetic resonance imaging, transient elastography and parameters of iron storage. *PLoS One* 8:e57507, 2013.

39. Xu R, Mistry P, McKenna G, Emre S, et al: Hepatocellular carcinoma in type 1 Gaucher disease: A case report with review of the literature. *Semin Liver Dis* 25:226, 2005.

40. Grabowski GA: Gaucher disease and other storage disorders. *Hematology Am Soc Hematol Educ Program* 2012:13, 2012.

41. Burrow TA, Cohen MB, Bokulic R, et al: Gaucher disease: Progressive mesenteric and mediastinal lymphadenopathy despite enzyme therapy. *J Pediatr* 150:202, 2007.

42. Lee BH, Kim DY, Kim GH, et al: Progressive mesenteric lymphadenopathy with protein-losing enteropathy; a devastating complication in Gaucher disease. *Mol Genet Metab* 105:522, 2012.

43. Gillis S, Hyam E, Abrahamov A, et al: Platelet function abnormalities in Gaucher disease patients. *Am J Hematol* 61:103, 1999.

44. Hollak CE, Levi M, Berends F, et al: Coagulation abnormalities in type 1 Gaucher disease are due to low-grade activation and can be partly restored by enzyme supplementation therapy. *Br J Haematol* 96:470, 1997.

45. Zimran A, Altarescu G, Rudensky B, et al: Survey of hematological aspects of Gaucher disease. *Hematology* 10:151, 2005.

46. Zimran A, Altarescu G, Rudensky B, et al: Survey of hematological aspects of Gaucher disease. *Hematology* 10:151, 2005.

47. Hughes D, Cappellini MD, Berger M, et al: Recommendations for the management of the haematological and onco-haematological aspects of Gaucher disease. *Br J Haematol* 138:676, 2007.

48. Poll, LW: Type I Gaucher disease: Extraosseous extension of skeletal disease. *Skeletal Radiol* 29: 15, 2000.

49. Hermann G, Shapiro R, Abdelwahab IF, et al: Extraosseous extension of Gaucher cell deposits mimicking malignancy. *Skeletal Radiol* 23:253, 1994.

50. Kaloterakis A, Cholongitas E, Pantelis E, et al: Type I Gaucher disease with severe skeletal destruction, extraosseous extension and monoclonal gammopathy. *Am J Hematol* 77:377, 2004.

51. Lee RE: The pathology of Gaucher disease, in *Gaucher Disease: A Century of Delineation and Research*, edited by Desnick RJ, Gatt S, Grabowski GA, p 177. Alan R. Liss, New York, 1982.

52. Amir G, Ron N: Pulmonary pathology in Gaucher's disease. *Hum Pathol* 30:666, 1999.

53. Elstein D, Klutstein MW, Lahad A, et al: Echocardiographic assessment of pulmonary hypertension in Gaucher's disease. *Lancet* 351:1544, 1998.

54. Mistry PK, Sirrs S, Chan A, et al: Pulmonary hypertension in type I Gaucher's disease: Genetic and epigenetic determinants of phenotype and response to therapy. *Mol Genet Metab* 77:91, 2002.

55. Rosengarten D, Abrahamov A, Nir A, et al: Outcome of ten years' echocardiographic follow-up in children with Gaucher disease. *Eur J Pediatr* 166:549, 2007.

56. Kerem E, Elstein D, Abrahamov A, et al: Pulmonary function abnormalities in type I Gaucher disease. *Eur Respir J* 9:340, 1996.

57. Itzchaki M, Lebel E, Dweck A, et al: Orthopedic considerations in Gaucher disease since the advent of enzyme replacement therapy. *Acta Orthop Scand* 75:641, 2004.

58. Ciana G, Martini C, Leopaldi A, et al: Bone marker alterations in patients with type 1 Gaucher disease. *Calcif Tissue Int* 72:185, 2003.

59. Carter LC, Fischman SL, Mann J, et al: The nature and extent of jaw involvement in Gaucher disease: Observations in a series of 28 patients. *Oral Surg Oral Med Oral Pathol Oral Radiol Endod* 85:233, 1999.

60. Simchen MJ, Oz R, Shenkman B, et al: Impaired platelet function and peripartum bleeding in women with Gaucher disease. *Thromb Haemost* 105:509, 2011.

61. Granovsky-Grisaru S, Belmatoug N, vom Dahl S, et al: The management of pregnancy in Gaucher disease. *Eur J Obstet Gynecol Reprod Biol* 156:3, 2011.

62. Petrohelos M, Tricoulis D, Kotsiras I, et al: Ocular manifestations of Gaucher's disease. *Am J Ophthalmol* 80:1006, 1975.

63. Wollstein G, Elstein D, Zimran A: Ocular findings in adult patients with type I Gaucher disease. *Haema, J Hellen Soc Hematol* 6:217, 2003.

64. Arends M, van Dussen L, Biegstraaten M, Hollak CE: Malignancies and monoclonal gammopathy in Gaucher disease; a systematic review of the literature. *Br J Haematol* 161:832, 2013.

65. Becker-Cohen R, Elstein D, Abrahamov A, et al: A comprehensive assessment of renal function in patients with Gaucher disease. *Am J Kidney Dis* 46:837, 2005.

66. Brady RO, Barton NW, Grabowski GA: The role of neurogenetics in Gaucher disease. *Arch Neurol* 50:1212, 1993.

67. Harris CM, Taylor DS, Vellodi A: Ocular motor abnormalities in Gaucher disease. *Neuropediatrics* 30:289, 1999.

68. Uyama E, Takahashi K, Owada M, et al: Hydrocephalus, corneal opacities, deafness, valvular heart disease, deformed toes and leptomeningeal fibrous thickening in adult siblings: A new syndrome associated with beta-glucocerebrosidase deficiency and a mosaic population of storage cells. *Acta Neurol Scand* 86:407, 1992.

69. Chabas A, Cormand B, Grinberg D, et al: Unusual expression of Gaucher's disease: Cardiovascular calcifications in three sibs homozygous for the D409H mutation. *J Med Genet* 32:740, 1995.

70. Mistry PK: Genotype/phenotype correlations in Gaucher's disease. *Lancet* 346:982, 1995.

71. Pastores GM, Barnett NL, Bathan P, et al: A neurological symptom survey of patients with type I Gaucher disease. *J Inherit Metab Dis* 26:641, 2003.

72. Biegstraaten M, van Schaik IN, Aerts JM, Hollak CE: "Non-neuronopathic" Gaucher disease reconsidered. Prevalence of neurological manifestations in a Dutch cohort of type I Gaucher disease patients and a systematic review of the literature. *J Inherit Metab Dis* 31:337, 2008.

73. Neudorfer O, Giladi N, Elstein D, et al: Occurrence of Parkinson's syndrome in type I Gaucher disease. *Q J Med* 89:691, 1996.

74. Tayebi N, Callahan M, Madike V, et al: Gaucher disease and parkinsonism: A phenotypic and genotypic characterization. *Mol Genet Metab* 73:313, 2001.

75. Aharon-Peretz J, Rosenbaum H, Gershoni-Baruch R: Mutations in the glucocerebrosidase gene and Parkinson's disease in Ashkenazi Jews. *N Engl J Med* 351:1972, 2004.

76. Sidransky E, Nalls MA, Aasly JO, et al: Multicenter analysis of glucocerebrosidase mutations in Parkinson's disease. *N Engl J Med* 361:1651, 2009.

77. Gan-Or Z, Giladi N, Rozovski U, et al: Genotype-phenotype correlations between GBA mutations and Parkinson disease risk and onset. *Neurology* 70:2277, 2008.

78. Chetrit EB, Alcalay RN, Steiner-Birmanns B, et al: Phenotype in patients with Gaucher disease and Parkinson disease. *Blood Cells Mol Dis* 50:218, 2013.

79. Alcalay RN, Dinur T, Quinn T, et al: Comparison of Parkinson risk in Ashkenazi Jewish patients with Gaucher Disease and GBA heterozygotes. *JAMA Neurol* 71:752, 2014.

80. Aker M, Zimran A, Abrahamov A, et al: Abnormal neutrophil chemotaxis in Gaucher disease. *Br J Haematol* 83:187, 1993.

81. Liel Y, Rudich A, Nagauker-Shriker O, et al: Monocyte dysfunction in patients with Gaucher disease: Evidence for interference of glucocerebroside with superoxide generation. *Blood* 83:2646-53, 1994.

82. Zevin S, Abrahamov A, Hadas-Halpern I, et al: Adult-type Gaucher disease in children: Genetics, clinical features and enzyme replacement therapy. *Q J Med* 86:565, 1993.

83. Kauli R, Zaizov R, Lazar L, et al: Delayed growth and puberty in patients with Gaucher disease type 1: Natural history and effect of splenectomy and/or enzyme replacement therapy. *Isr Med Assoc J* 2:158, 2000.

84. Zimran A, Liphshitz I, Barchana M, et al: Incidence of malignancies among patients with type I Gaucher disease from a single referral clinic. *Blood Cells Mol Dis* 34:197, 2005.

85. Rosenbloom BE, Weinreb NJ, Zimran A, et al: Gaucher disease and cancer incidence: A study from the Gaucher registry. *Blood* 105:4569, 2005.

86. Lo SM, Choi M, Liu J, et al: Phenotype diversity in type 1 Gaucher disease: Discovering the genetic basis of Gaucher disease/hematologic malignancy phenotype by individual genome analysis. *Blood* 119:4731, 2012.

87. Weinreb NJ, Lee RE: Causes of death due to hematological and non-hematological cancers in 57 US patients with type 1 Gaucher Disease who were never treated with enzyme replacement therapy. *Crit Rev Oncog* 18(3):177, 2013.

88. Allen MJ, Myer BJ, Khokher AM, et al: Pro-inflammatory cytokines and the pathogenesis of Gaucher's disease: Increased release of interleukin-6 and interleukin-10. *Q J Med* 90:19, 1997.

89. Zimran A, Abrahamov A, Aker M, et al: Correction of neutrophil chemotaxis defect in patients with Gaucher disease by low-dose enzyme replacement therapy. *Am J Hematol* 43:69, 1993.

90. Zimran A, Bashkin A, Elstein D, et al: Rheological determinants in patients with Gaucher disease and internal inflammation. *Am J Hematol* 75:190, 2004.

91. Rogowski O, Shapira I, Zimran A, et al: Automated system to detect low-grade underlying inflammatory profile: Gaucher disease as a model. *Blood Cells Mol Dis* 34:26, 2005.

92. Boklan BF, Sawitsky A: Factor IX deficiency in Gaucher disease. An in vitro phenomenon. *Arch Intern Med* 136:489, 1976.

93. Berrebi A, Malnick SDH, Vorst EJ, et al: High incidence of factor XI deficiency in Gaucher's disease. *Am J Hematol* 40:153, 1992.

94. Hughes D, Cappellini MD, Berger M, et al: Recommendations for the management of the haematological and onco-haematological aspects of Gaucher disease. *Br J Haematol* 138:676, 2007.

95. Rosenbaum H, Sidransky E: Cholelithiasis in patients with Gaucher disease. *Blood Cells Mol Dis* 28:21, 2002.

96. Ben Harosh-Katz M, Patlas M, Hadas-Halpern I, et al: Increased prevalence of cholelithiasis in Gaucher disease: Association with splenectomy but not with gilbert syndrome. *J Clin Gastroenterol* 38:586, 2004.

97. Shoenfeld Y, Beresovski A, Zharhary D, et al: Natural autoantibodies in sera of patients with Gaucher's disease. *J Clin Immunol* 15:363, 1995.

98. Hollak CE, van Weely S, van Oers MH, Aerts JM: Marked elevation of plasma chitotriosidase activity. A novel hallmark of Gaucher disease. *J Clin Invest* 93:1288, 1994.

99. Boot RG, Verhoek M, de Fost M: Marked elevation of the chemokine CCL18/PARC in Gaucher disease: A novel surrogate marker for assessing therapeutic intervention. *Blood* 103:33, 2004.

100. Rolfs A, Giese AK, Grittner U, et al: Glucosylsphingosine is a highly sensitive and specific biomarker for primary diagnostic and follow-up monitoring in Gaucher disease in a non-Jewish, Caucasian cohort of Gaucher disease patients. *PLoS One* 8:e79732, 2013.

101. Gielchinsky Y, Elstein D, Green R: High prevalence of low serum vitamin B12 in a multi-ethnic Israeli population. *Br J Haematol* 115:707, 2001.

102. Mikosch P, Reed M, Stettner H, et al: Patients with Gaucher disease living in England show a high prevalence of vitamin D insufficiency with correlation to osteodensitometry. *Mol Genet Metab* 96:113, 2009.

103. Beutler E, Kuhl W: The diagnosis of the adult type of Gaucher's disease and its carrier state by demonstration of deficiency of beta-glucosidase activity in peripheral blood leukocytes. *J Lab Clin Med* 76:747, 1970.

104. Rudensky B, Paz E, Altarescu G, Raveh D et al: Fluorescent flow cytometric assay: A new diagnostic tool for measuring beta-glucocerebrosidase activity in Gaucher disease. *Blood Cells Mol Dis* 30:97, 2003.

105. Beutler E, Saven A: Misuse of marrow examination in the diagnosis of Gaucher disease. *Blood* 76:646, 1990.

106. Zhang CK, Stein PB, Liu J, et al: Genome-wide association study of N370S homozygous Gaucher disease reveals the candidacy of CLN8 gene as a genetic modifier contributing to extreme phenotypic variation. *Am J Hematol* 87:377, 2012.

107. Lun FM, Tsui NB, Chan KC, et al: Noninvasive prenatal diagnosis of monogenic diseases by digital size selection and relative mutation dosage on DNA in maternal plasma. *Proc Natl Acad Sci U S A* 105:19920-5, 2008.

108. Itzchaki M, Lebel E, Dweck A, et al: Orthopedic considerations in Gaucher disease since the advent of enzyme replacement therapy. *Acta Orthop Scand* 75:641, 2004.

109. Wenstrup RJ, Bailey L, Grabowski GA, et al: Gaucher disease: Alendronate disodium improves bone mineral density in adults receiving enzyme therapy. *Blood* 104:1253, 2004.

110. Rodgers GP, Lessin LS: Recombinant erythropoietin improves the anemia associated with Gaucher's disease. *Blood* 73:2228, 1989.

111. Grabowski GA, Barton NW, Pastores G, et al: Enzyme therapy in type 1 Gaucher disease: Comparative efficacy of mannose-terminated glucocerebrosidase from natural and recombinant sources. *Ann Intern Med* 122:33, 1995.

112. Zimran A, Altarescu G, Phillips M, et al: Phase I/II and extension study of velaglucerase alfa (Gene-Activated™ Human Glucocerebrosidase) replacement therapy in adults with type 1 Gaucher disease: 48 Month experience. *Blood* 115:4651, 2010.

113. Zimran A, Brill-Almon E, Chertkoff R, et al: Pivotal trial with plant-cell-expressed recombinant glucocerebrosidase, taliglucerase alfa, a novel enzyme replacement therapy for Gaucher disease. *Blood* 118:5767, 2011.

114. Weinreb NJ, Charrow J, Andersson HC, et al: Effectiveness of enzyme replacement therapy in 1028 patients with type 1 Gaucher disease after 2 to 5 years of treatment: A report from the Gaucher Registry. *Am J Med* 113:112, 2002.

115. Zimran A, Bembi B, Pastores G: Enzyme replacement therapy for type I Gaucher disease, in *Gaucher Disease*, edited by Futerman AH, Zimran A, p 341. CRC Press, Boca Raton, FL, 2007.

116. Grabowski GA, Kacena K, Cole JA, et al: Dose-response relationships for enzyme replacement therapy with imiglucerase/alglucerase in patients with Gaucher disease type 1. *Genet Med* 11:92, 2009.

117. Maas M, Hollak CE, Akkerman EM, et al: Quantification of skeletal involvement in adults with type I Gaucher's disease: Fat fraction measured by Dixon quantitative chemical shift imaging as a valid parameter. *AJR Am J Roentgenol* 179:961, 2002.

118. Altarescu G, Hill S, Wiggs E, et al: The efficacy of enzyme replacement therapy in patients with chronic neuronopathic Gaucher's disease. *J Pediatr* 138:539, 2001.

119. Zimran A, Elstein D: No justification for very high-dose enzyme therapy for patients with type III Gaucher disease. *J Inherit Metab Dis* 30:843, 2007.

120. Starzyk K, Richards S, Yee J, et al: The long-term international safety experience of imiglucerase therapy for Gaucher disease. *Mol Genet Metab* 90:157, 2007.

121. Langeveld M, de Fost M, Aerts JM, et al: Overweight, insulin resistance and type II diabetes in type I Gaucher disease patients in relation to enzyme replacement therapy. *Blood Cells Mol Dis* 40:428, 2008.

122. Zimran A, Hollak CEM, Abrahamov A, et al: Home treatment with intravenous enzyme replacement therapy for Gaucher disease: An international collaborative study of 33 patients. *Blood* 82:1107, 1993.

123. Granovsky-Grisaru S, Belmatoug N, vom Dahl S, et al: The management of pregnancy in Gaucher disease. *Eur J Obstet Gynecol Reprod Biol* 156:3, 2011.

124. Elstein D, Hughes D, Goker-Alpan O, et al: Outcome of pregnancies in women receiving velaglucerase alfa for Gaucher disease. *J Obstet Gynaecol Res* 40:968, 2014.

125. Zimran A, Pastores GM, Tylki-Szymanska A, et al: Safety and efficacy of velaglucerase alfa in Gaucher disease type 1 patients previously treated with imiglucerase. *Am J Hematol* 88:172, 2013.

126. Pastores GM, Petakov M, Giraldo P, et al: A Phase 3, multicenter, open-label, switchover trial to assess the safety and efficacy of taliglucerase alfa, a plant cell-expressed recombinant human glucocerebrosidase, in adult and pediatric patients with Gaucher disease previously treated with imiglucerase. *Blood Cells Mol Dis* 2014 Jun 17 [Epub ahead of print]

127. Weinreb NJ, Aggio MC, Andersson HC, et al; International Collaborative Gaucher Group (ICGG): Gaucher disease type 1: Revised recommendations on evaluations and monitoring for adult patients. *Semin Hematol* 41:15, 2004.

128. Sidransky E, Pastores GM, Mori M: Dosing enzyme replacement therapy for Gaucher disease: Older, but are we wiser? *Genet Med* 11:90, 2009.

129. Zimran A, Ilan Y, Elstein D: Enzyme replacement therapy for mild patients with Gaucher disease. *Am J Hematol* 84:202, 2009.

130. Cox T, Lachmann R, Hollak C, et al: Novel oral treatment of Gaucher's disease with N-butyldeoxynojirimycin (OGT 918) to decrease substrate biosynthesis. *Lancet* 355:1481, 2000.

131. Radin NS: Chemical models and chemotherapy in the sphingolipidoses, in *Current Trends in Sphingolipidoses and Allied Disorders*, edited by Volk BW, Schneck L, p 453. Plenum Press, New York, 1976.

132. Heitner R, Elstein D, Aerts J, et al: Low-dose N-butyldeoxynojirimycin (OGT 918) for type I Gaucher disease. *Blood Cells Mol Dis* 28:127, 2003.

133. Elstein D, Dweck A, Attias D, et al: Oral maintenance clinical trial with miglustat for type I Gaucher disease: Switch from or combination with intravenous enzyme replacement. *Blood* 110:2296, 2007.

134. Lukina E, Watman N, Arreguin EA, et al: A phase 2 study of eliglustat tartrate (Genz-112638), an oral substrate reduction therapy for Gaucher disease type 1. *Blood* 116:893, 2010.

135. Lukina E, Watman N, Arreguin EA, et al: Improvement in hematological, visceral, and skeletal manifestations of Gaucher disease type 1 with oral eliglustat tartrate (Genz-112638) treatment: 2-year results of a phase 2 study. *Blood* 116:4095, 2010.

136. Lukina E, Watman N, Dragosky M, et al: Eliglustat, an investigational oral therapy for Gaucher disease type 1: Phase 2 trial results after 4 years of treatment. *Blood Cells Mol Dis* 53:274, 2014.

137. Fan JQ: A contradictory treatment for lysosomal storage disorders: Inhibitors enhance mutant enzyme activity. *Trends Pharmacol Sci* 24:355, 2003.

138. Ron I, Horowitz M: ER retention and degradation as the molecular basis underlying Gaucher disease heterogeneity. *Mol Genet Metab* 93:426, 2008.

139. Sun Y, Liou B, Xu YH, et al: Ex vivo and in vivo effects of isofagomine on acid β-glucosidase variants and substrate levels in Gaucher disease. *J Biol Chem* 287:4275, 2012.

140. Goker-Alpan O: Commentary on "Pilot study using ambroxol as a pharmacological chaperone in type 1 Gaucher disease" by Zimran et al. *Blood Cells Mol Dis* 50:138, 2013.

141. Zimran A, Altarescu G, Elstein D: Pilot study using ambroxol as a pharmacological chaperone in type 1 Gaucher disease. *Blood Cells Mol Dis* 50:134, 2013.

142. Ayto RM, Hughes DA, Jeevaratnam P, et al: Long-term outcomes of liver transplantation in type 1 Gaucher disease. *Am J Transplant* 10:1934, 2010.

143. Mistry P, Zimran A: Type I Gaucher disease—Clinical features, in *Gaucher Disease*, edited by Futerman AH, Zimran A, p 155. CRC Press, Boca Raton, FL, 2007.

144. Taddei TH, Kacena KA, Yang M, et al: The underrecognized progressive nature of N370S Gaucher disease and assessment of cancer risk in 403 patients. *Am J Hematol* 84:208, 2009.

145. Weinreb NJ, Deegan P, Kacena KA, et al: Life expectancy in Gaucher disease type 1. *Am J Hematol* 83:896, 2008.

146. Niemann A: Ein unbekanntes Krankheitsbild. *Jahrbuch Kinderheilkunde* 79:1, 1914.

147. Pick L: Uber die lipoidzellige Splenhepatomegalie Typus Niemann-Pick als Stoffwechselerkrankung. *Med Klin* 23:1483, 1927.

148. Brady RO, Kanfer JN, Mock MB, et al: The metabolism of sphingomyelin II. Evidence of an enzymatic deficiency in Niemann-Pick disease. *Proc Natl Acad Sci U S A* 55:366, 1966.

149. Schuchman EH, Desnick RJ: Niemann-Pick disease types A and B: Acid sphingomyelinase deficiencies, in *The Metabolic and Molecular Bases of Inherited Disease*, 7th ed, edited by Scriver CR, Beaudet AL, Sly WS, Valle D, p 2601. McGraw-Hill, New York, 1995.

150. Pentchev PG, Vanier MT, Suzuki K, et al: Niemann-Pick disease type C: A cellular cholesterol lipidosis, in *The Metabolic and Molecular Bases of Inherited Disease*, 7th ed, edited by Scriver CR, Beaudet AL, Sly WS, Valle D, p 2625. McGraw-Hill, New York, 1995.

151. Greer WL, Riddell DC, Murty S, et al: Linkage disequilibrium mapping of the Nova Scotia variant of Niemann-Pick disease. *Clin Genet* 55:248, 1999.

152. Schuchman EH, Miranda SR: Niemann-Pick disease: Mutation update, genotype/phenotype correlations, and prospects for genetic testing. *Genet Test* 1:13, 1997.

153. Simonaro CM, Desnick RJ, McGovern MM, et al: The demographics and distribution of type B Niemann-Pick disease: Novel mutations lead to new genotype/phenotype correlations. *Am J Hum Genet* 71:1413, 2002.

154. Wenger DA, Barth G, Githens JH: Nine cases of sphingomyelin lipidosis, a new variant in Spanish-American children. Juvenile variant of Niemann-Pick Disease with foamy and sea-blue histiocytes. *Am J Dis Child* 131:955, 1977.

155. Millat G, Marçais C, Rafi MA, et al: Niemann-Pick C1 disease: The I1061T substitution is a frequent mutant allele in patients of Western European descent and correlates with a classic juvenile phenotype. *Am J Hum Genet* 65:1321, 1999.

156. Patterson MC, Vanier MT, Suzuki K, et al: Niemann-Pick disease type C: A lipid trafficking disorder, in *The Metabolic and Molecular Bases of Inherited Disease*, 8th ed, edited by Scriver CR, Beaudet AL, Sly WS, Valle D, Childs B, Kinzler KW, Vogelstein B, p 3611. McGraw-Hill, New York, 2001.

157. Takahashi T, Suchi M, Desnick RJ, et al: Identification and expression of five mutations in the human acid sphingomyelinase gene causing types A and B Niemann-Pick disease. Molecular evidence for genetic heterogeneity in the neuronopathic and non-neuronopathic forms. *J Biol Chem* 267:12552, 1992.

158. De Maria R, Rippo MR, Schuchman EH, et al: Acidic sphingomyelinase (ASM) is necessary for fas-induced GD3 ganglioside accumulation and efficient apoptosis of lymphoid cells. *J Exp Med* 187:897, 1998.

159. Carstea ED, Morris JA, Coleman KG, et al: Niemann-Pick C1 disease gene: Homology to mediators of cholesterol homeostasis. *Science* 277:228, 1997.

160. Park WD, O'Brien JF, Lundquist PA, et al: Identification of 58 novel mutations in Niemann-Pick disease type C: Correlation with biochemical phenotype and importance of PTC1-like domains in NPC1. *Hum Mutat* 22:313, 2003.

161. Millat G, Chikh K, Naureckiene S, et al: Niemann-Pick disease type C: Spectrum of HE1 mutations and genotype/phenotype correlations in the NPC2 group. *Am J Hum Genet* 69:1013, 2001.

162. Verot L, Chikh K, Freydière E, et al: Niemann-Pick C disease: Functional characterization of three NPC2 mutations and clinical and molecular update on patients with NPC2. *Clin Genet* 71:320, 2007.

163. Pacheco CD, Kunkel R, Lieberman AP: Autophagy in Niemann-Pick C disease is dependent upon Beclin-1 and responsive to lipid trafficking defects. *Hum Mol Genet* 16:1495, 2007.

164. Loftus SK, Morris JA, Carstea ED, et al: Murine model of Niemann-Pick C disease: Mutation in a cholesterol homeostasis gene. *Science* 277:232, 1997.

165. Golde DW, Schneider EL, Bainton EL, et al: Pathogenesis of one variant of sea-blue histiocytosis. *Lab Invest* 33:371, 1975.

166. Patterson MC: A riddle wrapped in a mystery: Understanding Niemann-Pick disease, type C. *Neurologist* 9:301, 2003.

167. Lazarus SS, Vethamany VG, Schneck L, et al: Fine structure and histochemistry of peripheral blood cells in Niemann-Pick disease. *Lab Invest* 17:155, 1967.

168. Brady RO: Sphingomyelin lipidoses: Niemann-Pick disease, in *The Metabolic Basis of Inherited Disease*, edited by JB Stanbury, JB Wyngaarden, DS Fredrickson, JL Goldstein, MS Brown, p 831. McGraw-Hill, New York, 1983.

169. Gal AE, Brady RO, Hibberg SR, et al: A practical chromogenic procedure for the detection of homozygotes and heterozygous carriers of Niemann-Pick disease. *N Engl J Med* 293:632, 1975.

170. Vanier MT. Prenatal diagnosis of Niemann-Pick diseases types A, B and C. *Prenat Diagn* 22:630, 2002.

171. Mount Sinai International Center for Types A and B Niemann-Pick Disease: http://www.mssm.edu/niemann-pick

172. Daloze P, Delvin EE, Glorieux FH, et al: Replacement therapy for inherited enzyme deficiency: Liver orthotopic transplantation in Niemann-Pick disease type A. *Am J Med Genet* 1:229, 1977.

173. Victor S, Coulter JB, Besley GT, et al: Niemann-Pick disease: Sixteen-year follow-up of allogeneic bone marrow transplantation in a type B variant. *J Inherit Metab Dis* 26:775, 2003.

174. Hsu YS, Hwu WL, Huang SF, et al: Niemann-Pick disease type C (a cellular cholesterol lipidosis) treated by bone marrow transplantation. *Bone Marrow Transplant* 24:103, 1999.

175. Miranda SR, Erlich S, Friedrich VL Jr, et al: Hematopoietic stem cell gene therapy leads to marked visceral organ improvements and a delayed onset of neurological abnormalities in the acid sphingomyelinase deficient mouse model of Niemann-Pick disease. *Gene Ther* 7:1768, 2000.

176. Lachmann RH, te Vruchte D, Lloyd-Evans E, et al: Treatment with miglustat reverses the lipid-trafficking defect in Niemann-Pick disease type C. *Neurobiol Dis* 16:654, 2004.

177. Patterson MC, Vecchio D, Prady H, et al: Miglustat for treatment of Niemann-Pick C disease: A randomised controlled study. *Lancet Neurol* 6:765, 2007.

178. Wraith JE, Vecchio D, Jacklin E, et al: Miglustat in adult and juvenile patients with Niemann-Pick disease type C: Long-term data from a clinical trial. *Mol Genet Metab* 99:351, 2010.

179. Patterson MC, Vecchio D, Jacklin E, et al: Long-term miglustat therapy in children with Niemann-Pick disease type C. *J Child Neurol* 25:300, 2010.

180. Jiang X, Sidhu R, Porter FD, et al: A sensitive and specific LC-MS/MS method for rapid diagnosis of Niemann-Pick C1 disease from human plasma. *J Lipid Res* 52:1435, 2011.

181. Ohgane K, Karaki F, Dodo K, Hashimoto Y: Discovery of oxysterol-derived pharmacological chaperones for NPC1: Implication for the existence of second sterol-binding site. *Chem Biol* 20:391, 2013.

Part IX Lymphocytes and Plasma Cells

73. The Structure of Lymphocytes and
    Plasma Cells 1137

74. Lymphopoiesis 1149

75. Functions of B Lymphocytes and
    Plasma Cells in Immunoglobin
    Production 1159

76. Functions of T Lymphocytes: T-Cell
    Receptors for Antigen............. 1175

77. Functions of Natural Killer Cells.... 1189

78. Classification and Clinical
    Manifestations of Lymphocyte and
    Plasma Cell Disorders 1195

79. Lymphocytosis and
    Lymphocytopenia 1199

80. Immunodeficiency Diseases....... 1211

81. Hematologic Manifestations of
    Acquired Immunodeficiency
    Syndrome 1239

82. Mononucleosis Syndromes........ 1261

CHAPTER 73
THE STRUCTURE OF LYMPHOCYTES AND PLASMA CELLS

Natarajan Muthusamy and Michael A. Caligiuri*

SUMMARY

Lymphocytes are a heterogeneous population of blood cells that can be distinguished from other leukocytes by their characteristic morphology and structural features. Mature lymphocytes can be divided into several functional types and subtypes based on their organs of development and function. The major classes of lymphocytes include T cells, B cells, and natural killer (NK) cells. T lymphocytes develop in the thymus (Chaps. 6, 74, and 76) and are exported to the blood and lymphoid organs. They are responsible for cell-mediated cytotoxic reactions and for delayed hypersensitivity responses (Chap. 76). T lymphocytes also produce the cytokines that regulate immune responses and provide helper activity for B cells. B lymphocytes can capture, internalize, and present antigens to T cells and are the precursors of immunoglobulin-secreting plasma cells (Chap. 75). NK cells account for innate immunity against infectious agents and transformed cells that have altered expression of transplantation antigens (Chap. 77). Blood T and B lymphocytes are indistinguishable by light and electron microscopy. NK cells tend to be larger cells with relatively large granules scattered in their cytoplasm. B cells can mature into plasma cells upon activation by engagement with antigen or with certain B cell mitogens. Although the different lymphocyte subpopulations appear similar by morphology they have distinct surface and intracellular protein expression patterns. These subpopulations, as defined by antigen expression, reflect different functional subsets, maturation stages, and activation stages. This chapter describes the light and transmission electron microscopic structures of lymphocytes and plasma cells and the major structural features reflected by surface antigens that are characteristic of each lymphocyte type. The chapter also provides information on biophysical and biochemical features of human lymphocytes.

Acronyms and Abbreviations: ADAM, a disintegrin and a metalloprotease; BTK, Bruton tyrosine kinase; CD, cluster of differentiation; Ig, immunoglobulin; lck, leukocyte tyrosine kinase; LGL, large granular lymphocyte; MHC, major histocompatibility complex; NK, natural killer; TCR, T-cell receptor; TdT, terminal deoxynucleotidyl transferase; T_{FH}, follicular helper T cells; Th, T helper cells; T_{REG}, T-regulatory cell; ZAP-70, zeta-associated protein of 70 kDa.

*This chapter was written by H. Elizabeth Broome in the 8th edition and some of the text and images have been retained.

DEFINITION AND HISTORY

Lymphocytes and plasma cells first were described in 1774 and 1875, respectively.[1] Studies during the subsequent 75 years with improved histologic techniques and light microscope optics furthered understanding of the lymphoid organs and the distribution of lymphocytes.[2-6] By the mid-20th century, awareness that the immune system had at least two components—one governing humoral immunity and one governing cellular immunity—led to early concepts of different lymphocyte subsets. Also, at the same time came the discovery that the thymus and bursa of Fabricius in birds were the source of what came to be known as T (thymic-derived) and B (bursa-derived) lymphocytes, respectively, and that the marrow was the bursa equivalent in humans (human B cells therefore could represent marrow-derived cells). This discovery coupled with descriptions of inherited absence of the thymus leading to loss of cellular immunity but retention of humoral immunity and cases of retention of cellular immunity in children who were deficient in antibody production, eventually led to our current understanding of the division of labor among what originally appeared to be a common lymphocyte pool, morphologically. The later advent of monoclonal antibodies against numerous surface antigens coupled with flow cytometry, in vitro functional assays, molecular techniques to distinguish between B cells and T cells, and experiments using inbred strains of mice brought us to our current state of knowledge of the immune response and its abnormalities.

Flow cytometry identifies a multitude of lymphocyte subsets based on antigen expression patterns. These immunophenotypic subsets correlate closely with function as determined by in vitro and in vivo testing. T lymphocytes, B lymphocytes, and natural killer (NK) cells represent three major blood lymphocyte functional subsets. The marrow and thymus contain precursor cells that resemble lymphocytes but lack function without differentiation and maturation into various lymphocyte subsets. Plasma cells are terminally differentiated B lymphocytes that produce immunoglobulin and mostly reside in marrow, lymph nodes, and other lymphoid tissues. (Chap. 6).

MICROSCOPY AND HISTOCHEMISTRY OF NORMAL BLOOD LYMPHOCYTES

LIGHT MICROSCOPY

Classic studies of blood and tissues defined lymphocytes as spherical and/or ovoid cells that have diameters from 6 to 15 μm when flattened on glass slides.[4] Some of these studies described two separate broad types of lymphocytes based on size: small lymphocytes with diameters of 6 to 9 μm and large lymphocytes with diameters of 9 to 15 μm. Patients with acute viral illnesses have increased numbers of circulating large, "reactive," lymphocytes. Other illnesses, such as infection with Bordetella pertussis and autoimmune disorders, can cause blood to have increased small lymphocytes or lymphocytes with plasma cell-like morphology (Chap. 78). The mean absolute number of circulating small lymphocytes in normal adults is 2.5×10^9/L (Chap. 2).[7] Children have higher lymphocyte counts that trend downward until they reach adult levels at approximately 8 to 10 years of age (Chap. 7).[8]

Most lymphocytes in normal blood are small with an ovoid or kidney-shaped nucleus that stains purple, has densely packed nuclear chromatin, and occupies approximately 90 percent of the cell area (Fig. 73–1A and B) by Romanowsky polychromatic stains (e.g., Giemsa or Wright) of air-dried films. A small rim of cytoplasm stains light blue. Nucleoli rarely are observed in Wright-stained films, but nucleoli in these cells may become visible in certain preparations, such as cytospin slides, or after prolonged storage in anti-coagulated blood collection tubes.

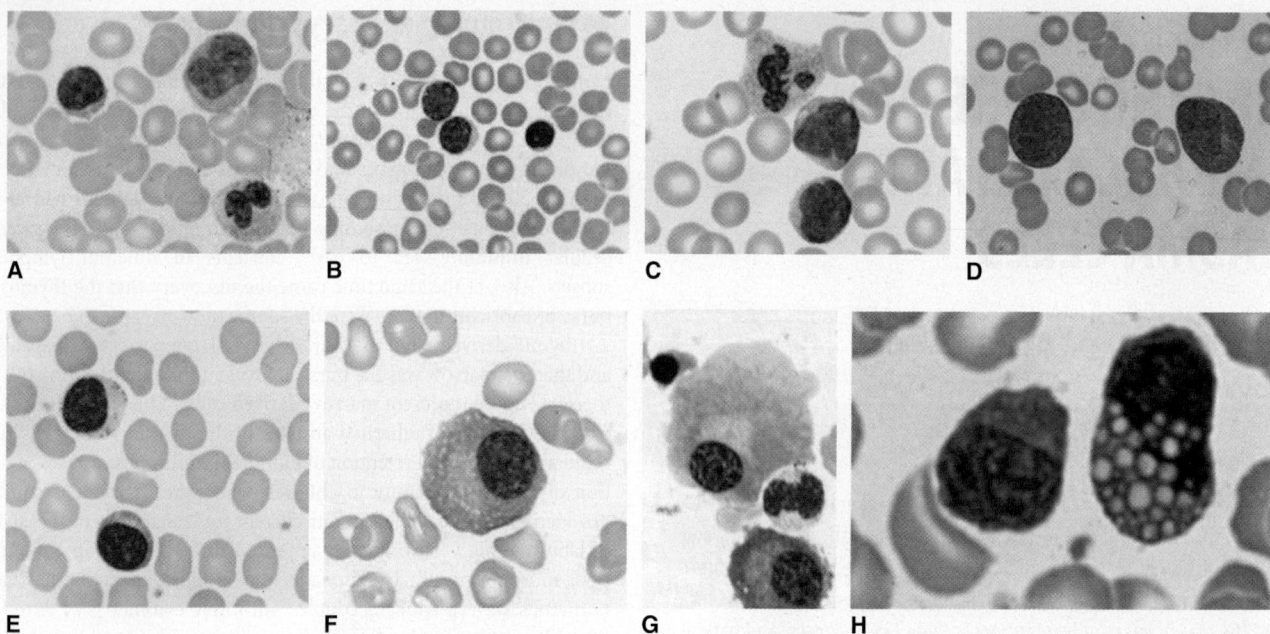

Figure 73–1. Wright-Giemsa stained blood films showing **(A)** a normal, small lymphocyte, monocyte, and segmented neutrophil; **(B)** normal small lymphocyte and two medium-sized lymphocytes; **(C)** neutrophil and two lymphocytes with morphologic features characteristic of *Bordetella pertussis* infection (small size, cleaved nuclei, and scant cytoplasm); **(D)** reactive lymphocytes; and **(E)** large granular lymphocyte and small lymphocyte. Wright-Giemsa stained marrow films showing **(F)** normal plasma cell; **(G)** two normal plasma cells, one nucleated red cell, and one neutrophil; and **(H)** two plasma cells with one containing many Russell bodies.

A minority of lymphocytes in normal blood have morphology that defines them as large granular lymphocytes (LGLs).[9] These LGLs are slightly larger than most lymphocytes, having an increased area of light blue or clear cytoplasm. LGL cytoplasm contains a number of coarse pink granules, usually 5 to 15 per cell, and occasional clear vacuoles. In a normal adult, approximately 5 percent but up to 10 to 15 percent of blood lymphocytes are LGLs (see Fig. 73–1E).[9] The LGLs in blood are composed of NK cells and a subset of cluster of differentiation (CD) 8+ T lymphocytes, indistinguishable by their morphology.

PHASE-CONTRAST MICROSCOPY

Active movement of lymphocytes is studied by phase-contrast, or interference-contrast, microscopy. Lymphocytes move slowly with a "hand mirror" appearance. Cytoplasmic spreading does not occur. However, during cell movement, a thickening occurs in the cytoplasmic rim, which houses most of the cell's organelles, including the Golgi apparatus.

TRANSMISSION ELECTRON MICROSCOPY AND CYTOCHEMISTRY

The blood lymphocyte measures approximately 5 μm in spherical diameter as visualized by transmission electron microscopy.[10] The nucleus has an abundance of electron-dense, condensed heterochromatin, a feature characteristic of nonproliferating cells. The nucleoli are round in section, approximately 0.5 to 1.4 μm in diameter. They are composed of three distinct and concentrically arranged structural units: the central region or agranular zone; the middle, fibrillar region; and the granular zone, which contains intranucleolar chromatin. The lymphocyte's nuclear membrane contains nuclear pores and a perinuclear space.

The cytoplasmic organelles of the lymphocytes are characteristic of eukaryotic cells. Some organelles, such as the Golgi zone, are poorly developed. The cytoplasm contains free ribosomes, occasional

ribosome clusters, and strands of rough-surfaced endoplasmic reticulum (Fig. 73–2). Centrioles, mitochondria, microtubules (diameter approximately 0.25 μm), and microfilaments (diameter approximately 0.07 μm) are present in the cytoplasm adjacent to the cell membrane. The cytoplasm also contains lysosomes, which are approximately 0.4 μm in diameter, are electron opaque, and contain classic lysosomal enzymes (e.g., acid phosphatase, β-glucuronidase, and acid ribonuclease).[11] The lymphocyte plasma membrane stains with colloidal iron, a marker for membrane sialic acid. Lymphocyte cell membranes and cell coat glycoproteins are shown with other electron-dense markers, including phosphotungstic acid, lanthanum colloid, and ruthenium red.

Most T lymphocytes have a localized "dot" pattern when stained for acid phosphatase, acid and neutral nonspecific esterases, β-glucuronidase, and N-acetyl-β-glucosaminidase.[12] LGLs stain for acid hydrolases with a dispersed, granular reaction pattern.[13] B lymphocytes either lack esterase and acid phosphatase or show minimal scattered granular staining.

SCANNING ELECTRON MICROSCOPY

Scanning electron microscopy provides three-dimensional information.[14] However, the resolution achieved with scanning electron microscopy, approximately 0.1 μm, is considerably less than that possible with transmission electron microscopy, generally 0.002 to 0.0039 μm. Normal blood lymphocytes, washed and collected on silver membranes and fixed in glutaraldehyde, have a spherical topography with varying numbers of stubby or finger-like microvilli (Fig. 73–3).[15] In contrast, monocytes are much larger, have few microvilli, and display ruffled membranes and ridge-like profiles (Chap. 67).

Lymphocyte microvilli contain parallel bundles of actin filaments that undergo continuous assembly and disassembly.[16] The function of lymphocyte microvilli probably includes segregating surface receptors involved in extravasation. Two receptors involved in the initial rolling phase of extravasation, L-selectin and $\alpha_4\beta_7$ integrin,[17] localize to microvillar tips. In contrast, the β_2 integrins that mediate stable adhesion

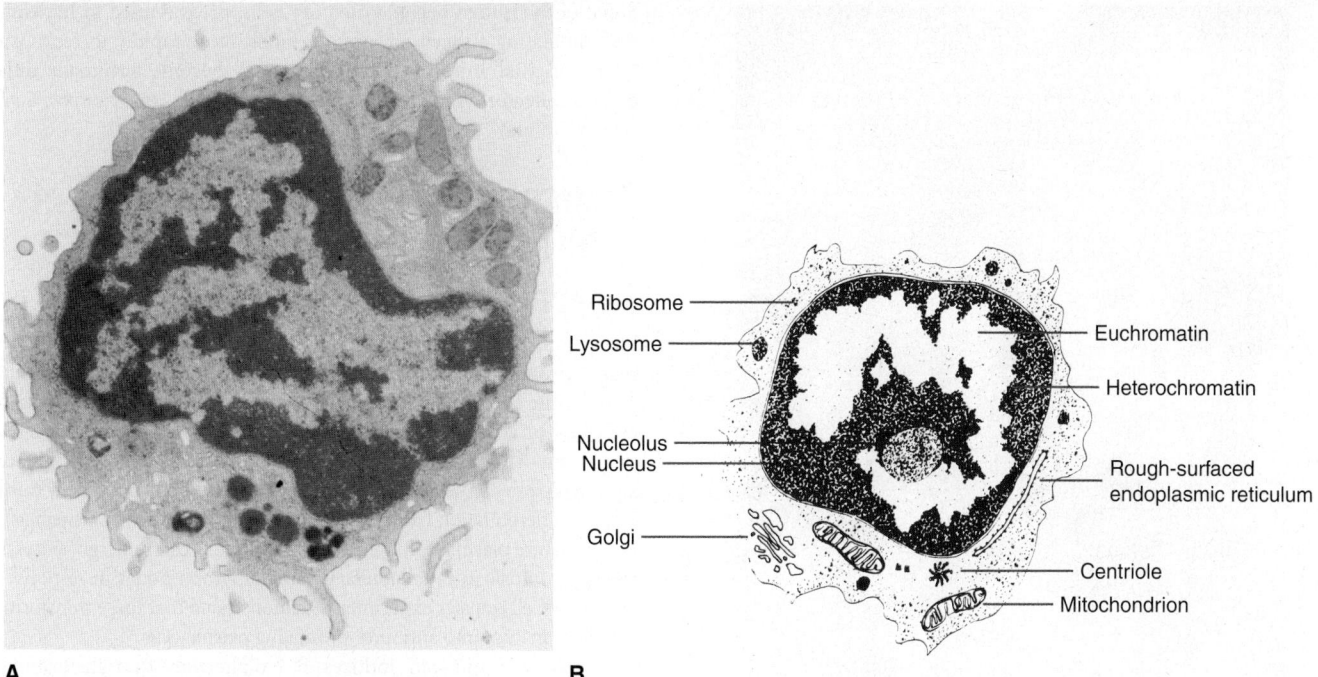

Figure 73–2. A. Transmission electron micrograph of normal human blood lymphocyte (×12,000). **B.** Diagrammatic representation of normal blood lymphocyte, with organelles labeled.

and diapedesis localize to nonprotrusive regions of the cell surface. This spatial separation of surface receptors might enable a temporal segregation of adhesive function during extravasation. Lymphocytes expressing chimeric L-selectin constructs that no longer localize to microvilli do not roll on L-selectin ligands, supporting this hypothesis.[18]

MORPHOLOGIC CHANGES ASSOCIATED WITH ACTIVATION

Lymphocyte stimulation is associated with a complex sequence of morphologic and biochemical events. Activation of B and T lymphocytes results in the transformation of the small, resting lymphocyte into proliferating large cells with abundant highly basophilic cytoplasm, irregularly condensed or smudgy chromatin, and round to slightly irregular

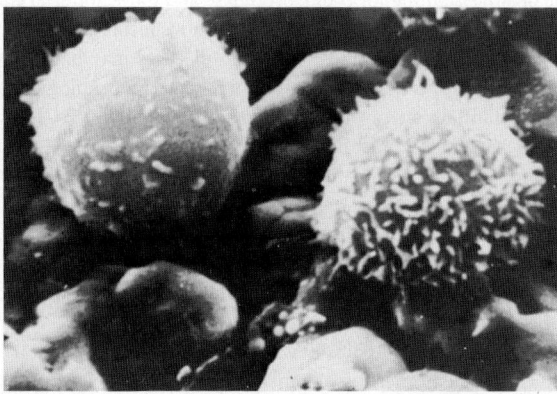

Figure 73–3. Scanning electron micrograph of normal blood lymphocytes separated by the Ficoll-Hypaque method. Cells show varying numbers of microvilli (×5000). *(Used with permission of Dr. Aaron Polliack of the Department of Hematology, Hebrew University Hadassah Medical School, Jerusalem, Israel.)*

nuclear outlines (see Fig. 73–1D). Nucleoli may be evident by light microscopy in these cells, but they usually are not prominent. Infection with B. pertussis causes an increase in blood lymphocytes with a particular activated morphology characterized by small size, scant cytoplasm, and cleaved nuclei with mature chromatin (see Fig. 73–1C).

Activated lymphocytes proliferate and mature into effector lymphocytes and memory cells. Effector cells include helper T cells, cytolytic T cells, and plasma cells (see Figs. 73–1F and G, 73–4, and 73–5). In vitro, plant lectins, bacterial products, polymeric substances, and enzymes activate lymphocytes and cause mitosis. Such agents are called mitogens. Some mitogens are specific for either B or T lymphocytes, whereas other mitogens stimulate both.[19]

Approximately 4 hours after mitogen stimulation, lymphocytes show increased nucleolar size and an increase in the number and concentration of granules in the granular zone. These changes are followed by an increase in fibrillar zones and increased intranucleolar chromatin. Nucleolar chromatin becomes more electron lucent or dispersed. From 48 to 72 hours following the addition of phytohemagglutinin, the volume of the cytoplasm increases. In addition, the cytoplasm contains an increased number of ribosomal clusters and more rough-surfaced endoplasmic reticulum. The activated cell has increased numbers of lysosomes and a larger Golgi complex with more components.[20] Under some circumstances (e.g., cultures of human lymphocytes stimulated for 7 to 10 days with pokeweed mitogen), some B cells form well-developed Golgi and plasmacytoid features.[21] Similar plasmacytoid cells are observed in antigen-stimulated lymph nodes, during graft rejection in vivo, and in some in vitro systems, including the mixed lymphocyte culture. In lymph nodes, the stimulated lymphoid cells may be referred to by various pathologists as lymphoblasts, immunoblasts, centroblasts, or large lymphoid cells. Morphologic criteria for these cells overlap.

Following stimulation with antigen or mitogens, the lymphocyte enters the cell cycle. The fate and function of lymphocytes that traverse the cell cycle can be divided into two pathways. Some lymphocytes undergo several mitotic cycles and then return to the G_0 phase, indistinguishable in morphology from the original nonactivated cells.

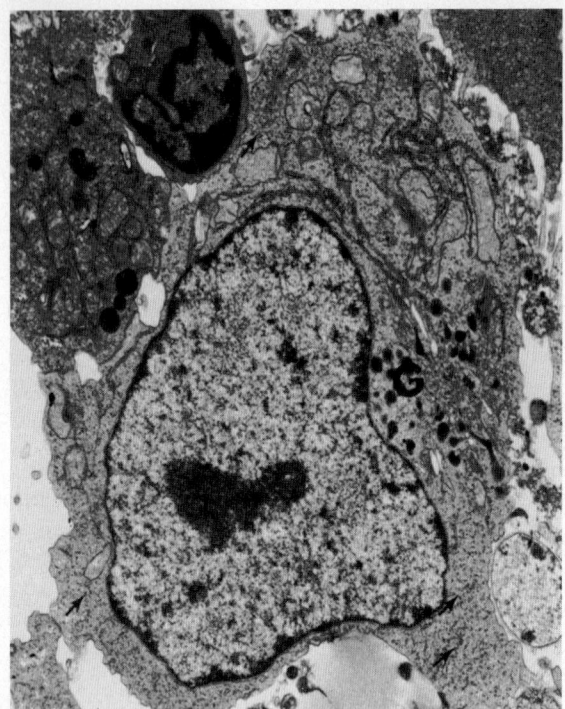

Figure 73–4. Transmission electron micrograph of lymphocyte from normal individual incubated with phytohemagglutinin[20] for 3 days. The transformed cell has a large Golgi zone *(G)* and many ribosomal aggregates *(arrows)*. The nucleus is euchromatic (×7500).

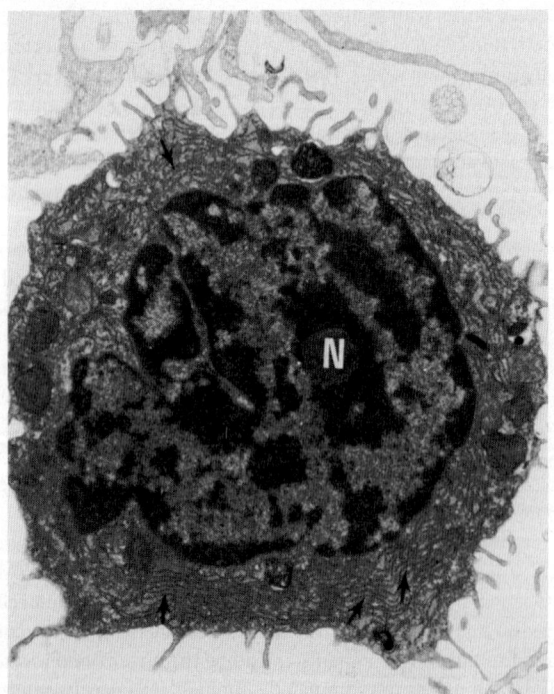

Figure 73–5. Transmission electron micrograph of plasmacytoid cell present in culture of lymphocytes from a patient with chronic lymphocytic leukemia incubated with pokeweed mitogen for 7 days. The nucleolus *(N)* and rough-surfaced endoplasmic reticulum *(arrows)* are evident (×9000). *(Reproduced with permission from Cohnen G, Douglas SD, Konig E, Brittinger G: Pokeweed mitogen response of lymphocytes in chronic lymphocytic leukemia: A fine structural study, Blood 1973 Oct;42(4):591-600)*

Some of them then become memory cells, programmed to remember the stimulating antigen and thus respond more rapidly to reexposure to the original antigen. Alternatively, they become terminally differentiated effector lymphocytes, such as plasma cells or cytotoxic T cells (Chaps. 75 and 76).

● MICROSCOPY AND HISTOCHEMISTRY OF PLASMA CELLS

MORPHOLOGIC STUDIES

Plasma cells derive from small B lymphocytes after activation in the correct environment. The characteristic feature of plasma cells is abundant cytoplasmic and secretory immunoglobulin (Ig). A fully mature plasma cell lacks surface Ig expression. Each plasma cell has the same clonal rearrangement of its V(D)J (variable diversity joining) Ig genes as its predecessor B lymphocyte (Chap. 75). Several mitotic divisions may occur during cellular differentiation from the resting lymphocyte to the plasmablast to the immature plasma cell. Immature plasma cells can undergo successive waves of mitosis in the medullary cords of lymph nodes in response to antigen.[22] Cell transfer experiments demonstrated that these transformed cells later mature into antibody-producing plasma cells.[23]

Pokeweed mitogen induces B lymphocytes to transform into plasma cells after 7 to 10 days of culture.[24] These plasma cells infrequently contain large electron-dense inclusions (Russell bodies), which may measure 2 to 3 μm in diameter (see Fig. 73–1*H*).[25] Russell bodies, cytoplasmic Ig in the endoplasmic reticulum, sometimes are dissolved during the staining procedure. They usually occur in pathologic states but may be found in plasma cells from normal lymph nodes or marrow.

LIGHT MICROSCOPY, HISTOCHEMISTRY, AND ELECTRON MICROSCOPY

The mature plasma cell has a characteristic basophilic cytoplasm and an eccentric nucleus when treated with a polychrome stain. The nuclear polarity is attributable to a large paranuclear zone, which corresponds to the Golgi apparatus. The typical mature plasma cell spread on a slide usually is round or oval and has a diameter of 9 to 20 μm, with a mean cell diameter of 14 μm and a mean nuclear diameter of 8.5 μm (see Fig. 73–1*F* and *G*).[26] The nuclear heterochromatin is coarse and distributed in a pattern that sometimes resembles the spokes of a wheel (cartwheel nucleus) on paraffin sections. Normal plasma cells may occasionally have two or more nuclei. Cytochemical features of plasma cells include positive staining for β-glucuronidase and mitochondrial enzyme markers. They do not stain for peroxidase or nonspecific esterase.[27]

Plasma cells in patients with certain diseases may have different histochemical properties. Plasma cell size and morphology may be altered substantially in myeloma and macroglobulinemia (Chaps. 107 and 109, respectively). Plasma cells with two or three nuclei are more frequent in marrows from patients with plasma cell dyscrasias. Periodic acid-Schiff stains may reveal cytoplasmic or nuclear inclusions in clonal plasma cells.[28] Under some circumstances, amyloid inclusions in plasma cells have been detected by electron microscopy.[29] In hemochromatosis and hemosiderosis, plasma cells may contain hemosiderin when examined by electron microscopy.[30]

The plasma cell is packed with a rough-surfaced endoplasmic reticulum having numerous attached ribosomes as seen by electron microscopy. A large, circumscribed Golgi zone forms a paranuclear halo when observed by light microscopy. The nucleus has dense areas of heterochromatin. The Golgi zone contains lamellae, vesicles, vacuoles, and a number of granules. Mitochondria are located between the strands of endoplasmic reticulum.[31]

ANTIGENS OF HUMAN LYMPHOCYTES

B LYMPHOCYTE ANTIGENS

Figure 73–6 summarizes the expression of antigens on cells of the B-lymphocyte lineage, including committed progenitor B cells and pre-B cells. Chapter 74 discusses these cells and the maturation stages they represent. Figure 73–6 also lists antigens that are expressed or increased upon B-cell activation. Of the B-cell–associated antigens that are commonly used, only a few are restricted to cells of the B lineage. Of these antigens, only CD20, CD22, and Pax 5 are not found on other cell types. Pax 5, a transcription factor, is a "master regulator" of B-cell development[32,33] that is expressed from the precursor stage through all B-cell maturation until it is lost at the plasma cell stage. Demonstration of monoclonal surface Ig allows diagnosis of clonal, neoplastic B cells. CD20 is the target of rituximab, a monoclonal antibody commonly used for treatment of B-cell neoplasms. CD19 is restricted mostly to B cells, but may be expressed weakly by follicular dendritic cells. CD19 is expressed by B cells at all stages of maturation, including the committed B-cell progenitor and most normal plasma cells. As such, it is the best-defined pan–B-cell surface antigen.

In addition to the CD antigens and Igs, B cells express the three major histocompatibility complex (MHC) class II antigens: DR, DP, DQ. These antigens are heterodimers of heavy chains and light chains that are encoded by genes within the D complex of the human leukocyte antigen (HLA) complex (Chap. 137). MHC class I antigens are expressed on all nucleated cells.

B-1 B Cells and CD5+ B Cells

B-1 B cells have distinctive activation requirements and high levels of CD44 and interleukin (IL)-5 receptor α (IL-5Rα). They proliferate more rapidly than other B cells to stimuli such as IgM crosslinking, possibly because of having constitutively activated nuclear signal transducer and activator of transcription 3 (STAT3).[34] Many, but not all, B-1 cells express CD5, a 67-kDa transmembrane glycoprotein that is more brightly expressed by T cells. These cells are designated CD5 B cells.[35] B-1 B cells do not express other T-cell markers but do express all other pan–B-cell surface antigens. Various agents modulate B-cell expression of CD5.[36] B-1 B cells are found in umbilical cord blood,[37] adult blood, the pleura and peritoneum, and all major secondary lymphoid organs; they are rare in the marrow.[38] These cells apparently are enriched for cells that spontaneously produce polyreactive autoantibodies.[39-41]

Plasma Cells

Many B cell differentiation antigens are not expressed by the mature plasma cell, including CD20, Pax-5, surface Ig, and HLA class II antigens (see Fig. 73–6). Of the cells of the B lineage, plasma cells are distinctive in that they express CD138 and bright CD38.[42] Clonal plasma cell neoplasms usually have antigen expression distinct from normal plasma cells including aberrant expression of CD20, CD28, CD56, and CD117. Clonal plasma cells usually aberrantly lack expression of CD19 and CD27.[43]

T-LYMPHOCYTE AND NATURAL KILLER CELL ANTIGENS

Figure 73–7 and Table 73–1 summarize the expression of antigens on cells of the T-lymphocyte and NK lineages. All lymphocyte progenitors originate in the marrow, but T lymphocytes have their own special organ for maturation—the thymus—whereas NK cells appear to differentiate in secondary lymphoid tissue (Chap. 6).

Thymocyte

The thymus promotes the development of antigen-specific T lymphocytes and eliminates self-reactive T lymphocytes. There are three general stages of thymocyte maturation based on the surface CD4 and CD8 expression: double negative, double positive, and single positive. These stages have corresponding anatomic localization within the thymus with the least-mature double-negative cells located in the subcapsular area and the most-mature single-positive cells located in the medulla (Chap. 6). The most immature T lymphocytes in the thymus populate the subcapsular areas and express CD2, CD5, and CD7, antigens present on T lymphocytes of all stages. Capsular, "double-negative" thymocytes also express CD1a, cytoplasmic CD3, and terminal deoxynucleotidyl transferase (TdT). The majority of thymocytes are at the "double-positive" stage within the cortical area. These are the cells undergoing positive selection. Once the thymocytes achieve their "education" without dying, they mature to the single-positive stage in the medulla. These varying stages of immature T-cell maturation in the thymus have corresponding cell phenotypes in T-lymphoblastic leukemia/lymphoma.

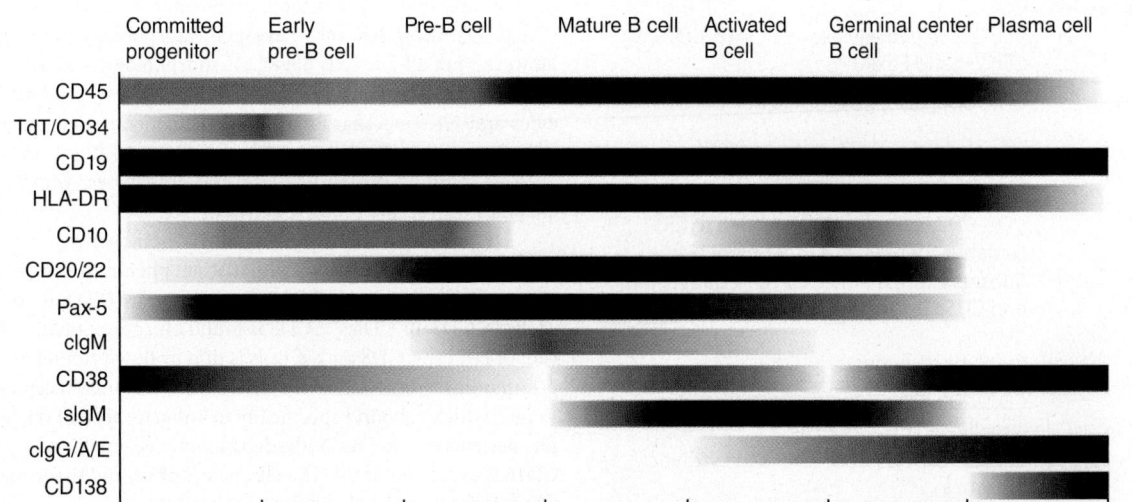

Figure 73–6. Clinically useful antigens expressed during B-lymphocyte maturation. The intensity of the antigen expression at each stage of B-lymphocyte maturation is depicted by gradient density of bars on the graph. c, cytoplasmic; s, surface.

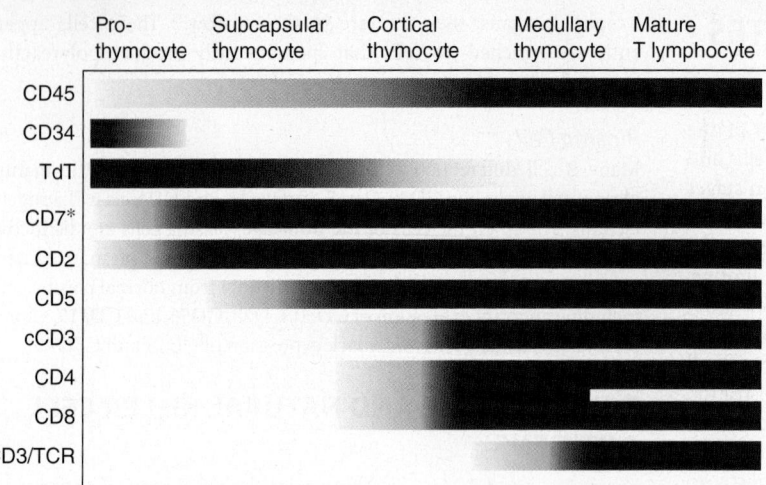

Figure 73–7. Clinically useful antigens expressed during T-lymphocyte maturation. The intensity of the antigen expression at each stage of T-lymphocyte maturation is depicted by gradient density of bars on the graph.

*CD7 is expressed on most, but not all, mature T lymphocytes.

Mature T Lymphocytes

Small, mature T lymphocytes are the most common lymphocytes in blood. T lymphocytes recognize antigen in the context of the MHC through binding with the T-cell receptor (TCR). Signaling from the TCR involves many membrane proteins, including CD3, a three-subunit complex expressed by early thymocytes and mature T cells.[44] It is tightly linked to the T-cell antigen receptor (Chap. 76). Most T lymphocytes have the α/β TCR on their surface, but a few percent of blood lymphocytes have the γ/δ TCR.

CD4 and CD8 Lymphocyte Subsets

Mature T cells express either CD4 or CD8, but not both. CD4, a member of the Ig supergene family, is a single-chain transmembrane glycoprotein.[45] CD8 is a 34-kDa dimeric transmembrane glycoprotein.[46] Most T cells express the α and β subunits of CD8. CD4 and CD8 act as coreceptors during T-cell activation by antigen. CD4 recognizes MHC II and CD8 recognizes MHC class I (Chap. 76). CD4 also is a coreceptor for the

human immunodeficiency virus[47] (Chap. 81), as are CCR5 (chemokine receptor 5) and CXCR4 (chemokine-related receptor). The majority of CD8 cells are cytolytic when appropriately activated.

Subsets of CD4+ T cells have helper function for activation and maturation of cytolytic cells or B cells. Other CD4 subsets have regulatory activity including the T-regulatory (T_{REG}) cells that induce immune tolerance, and follicular T-helper (T_{FH}) cells that promote B cell maturation and differentiation in germinal centers. T_{REG} and T_{FH} cells have unique phenotypes. T_{REG} cells express the low affinity receptor for IL-2 (CD25); and the transcription factor forkhead box P3 (FoxP3).[48] Follicular helper T-T_{FH} cells express CD10 and CD57. Malignant counterparts to both subsets occur. Adult T-cell leukemia/ lymphoma expresses both CD25 and FoxP3 and is associated with marked immunosuppression.[49] Angioimmunoblastic T-cell lymphoma has characteristic clonal T cells that express CD10 and CD57 just like T_{FH} cells, and this lymphoma is associated with polyclonal hypergammaglobulinemia and the expansion and proliferation of both B cells and CD21+ follicular dendritic cells.[50] T-helper-17 (Th17) cells that secrete IL-17 exhibit critical roles in mucosal defense and in autoimmune disease pathogenesis.[51]

Natural Killer Cells

The NK cell is defined as an effector cell that is not MHC restricted and has the capacity for spontaneous cytotoxicity toward various target cells (Chap. 77). Most NK cells have LGL morphology (see Fig. 73–1E).[52] However, not all NK cells have LGL morphology, and not all LGL cells are NK cells. Many are cytolytic T lymphocytes. Cytolytic T lymphocytes and NK cells share many granule contents that can be detected by immunohistochemistry or flow cytometry. These include TIA-1, an RNA binding protein, and several granzymes, which are granule enzymes with serine protease activity.

Despite their relative morphologic homogeneity, NK cells comprise several subpopulations with distinct phenotypes. Human NK cells characteristically express CD16 (FcγRIII) and CD56 but not TCRα/β or TCRγ/δ, CD3, or CD4.[53,54] CD8 is found on approximately 30 to 50 percent of NK cells. CD8 on NK cells is dim by flow cytometry and is of the β-homodimer form. CD16 (FcγRIII) is a low-affinity receptor that binds to IgG, which is bound specifically to antigens present on cells targeted for destruction in antibody-dependent cell-mediated cytotoxicity.[55] CD16 is expressed on all NK cells, neutrophils, and tissue macrophages. CD56 is the neural cell adhesion molecule and is seen on most NK cells in either low ("dim") or high ("bright") density.[53,56] This 200-kDa protein is expressed at higher levels following activation.

TABLE 73–1. Mature Natural Killer and T-Lymphocyte Subsets

NK or T-Cell Subset	Antigens
CD4+ helper T cells	CD2, CD3, CD4, CD5, CD7, and TCR α/β Subsets selectively express CD10, CD25,[49] CD57,[99] and FoxP3[100]
CD8+ cytolytic T cells	CD2, CD3, CD5, CD7, CD8, and TCR α/β Subsets selectively express CD16,[55] CD56, CD57, cytolytic enzymes[101]
NK cells	CD2, CD7, KIRs (multiple), NKp46 (NCR1) Negative for CD3, TCR (α/β or γ/δ) Subsets express either CD16-negative, dim and CD56 bright, or CD16 bright and CD56 dim[54] Cytolytic enzymes
γ/δ T cells	CD2, CD3, CD7, TCR γ/δ Usually negative for CD4 Subsets express CD5, CD8, and cytolytic enzymes

CD, cluster of differentiation; KIR, killer cell immunoglobulin-like receptor; NK, natural killer; TCR, T cell receptor.

LYMPHOCYTE SURFACE ANTIGENS

Lymphocyte subsets generally cannot be distinguished from one another by morphology. Most resting lymphocytes appear as small round cells with a dense nucleus and little cytoplasm. However, this homogeneous appearance is deceptive, as these cells comprise many functionally distinct subpopulations.

These subsets can be distinguished through the differential expression of cell-surface proteins, each of which can be recognized by a specific monoclonal antibody. Coupled with the biochemical analyses of the surface molecules that are recognized by each of these antibodies, many lymphocyte surface antigens have been defined.

Typically, it is necessary to monitor for coexpression of two or more cell-surface proteins to define a functional subset of lymphocytes. The same cell-surface protein is often expressed by more than one cell subset. For example, both helper and cytotoxic T cells express CD3, the proteins associated with the TCR for antigen (Chap. 76). Expression of both CD3 and CD4 helps to distinguish mature Th cells from cytotoxic T cells that express CD3 and CD8, and from other cells, such as dendritic cells, that express CD4 but lack expression of CD3 (Chap. 76). As noted above (see "CD4 and CD8 Lymphocyte Subsets"), T_{REG} cells are defined by the coexpression of CD3, CD4, CD25, and cytoplasmic FoxP3.[48] For these and other types of lymphocytes, it is the expression of a characteristic constellation of surface and cytoplasmic molecules, rather than the expression of any one particular marker, that generally helps to distinguish one subset of lymphocytes from another.

Fluorescent probes also can be used to identify antigen-specific lymphocytes.[57] Each clone of B lymphocytes expresses Ig capable of binding a particular antigen (Chap. 75). The frequencies of B cells specific for one antigen are estimated to range from 1 in 100,000 to 1 in 1,000,000 cells or less. Populations of lymphocytes enriched for B cells binding to a specific antigen can be stained using antigen coupled to probes, allowing for the detection and isolation of antigen-specific B cells using flow cytometry.[58] Alternatively, flow-based techniques can be used to monitor for antigen-specific B cells that are activated by contact with antigen.[59] T lymphocytes, however, generally recognize antigen in the form of peptides nestled into molecules of the MHC (Chap. 76). Thus identification and isolation of antigen-specific T cells require more complex probes using multimeric complexes comprised of specific peptide antigen complexed with the relevant MHC molecule.[57]

● COMPOSITION OF LYMPHOCYTES

Unfortunately, few studies of the composition and biochemistry of lymphocytes have used purified lymphocyte subpopulations. Because mature helper T cells are the predominant blood lymphocyte of normal adults, many reported biochemical parameters are most relevant to this subpopulation.

ION AND WATER CONTENT

The resting blood lymphocyte has a mean cell volume of 200 μm^3 and contains 71 ± 1.2 percent by weight of water.[60] The total lymphocyte cation content is 35 femtomoles (fmol) per cell, of which 22 to 28 fmol per cell is potassium, and 7.9 ± 3.2 fmol per cell is sodium.[60] Lymphocyte membranes have both voltage-gated and calcium-activated potassium channels that regulate cell volume. Pharmacologic inhibition of these channels blocks T-cell activation. The calcium content of resting lymphocytes has been estimated at 580 to 800 $pmol/10^6$ cells.[61] Cytosolic free calcium concentrations are relatively low in resting lymphocytes (approximately 0.1 μM) but increase severalfold after activation.[62]

LYMPHOCYTE MEMBRANE

The lymphocyte plasma membrane is composed of equal parts of weight of protein and glycosphingolipids and 6 percent by weight of carbohydrate.[63] The molar ratio of cholesterol to phospholipid is approximately 0.5.[64,65] Phosphatidylcholine is the predominant phospholipid in the lymphocyte plasma membrane, but phosphatidylethanolamine, phosphatidylinositol, phosphatidylserine, and sphingomyelin are also present. Approximately half the membrane fatty acids are saturated. The membrane proteins are usually glycosylated.

The glycosphingolipids and protein receptors of lymphocytes often are organized in glycolipoprotein microdomains termed *lipid rafts*.[66,67] Such lipid rafts sequester various protein receptors, coreceptors, and accessory molecules that together are involved in lymphocyte cell signaling, cytoskeletal reorganization, and/or membrane trafficking.[68] As such, the surface molecules on lymphocytes are not randomly distributed.

Extracellular Membrane-Associated Enzymes (Ectoenzymes)

Exposed on the exterior surface of lymphocytes are several enzymes called *ectoenzymes* (Table 73–2). Generally, the number of surface enzyme molecules is low compared with that of other surface molecules, such as those involved in lymphocyte adhesion. This probably reflects the fact that these molecules are catalytic and have a higher functional specific activity than do molecules involved in adhesion events, where multiple interactions over large surface areas are required. As such, it is possible that many more enzymes are present than the ones currently recognized because they are expressed at levels that are not detectable by conventional methods using monoclonal antibodies and flow cytometry.

Some of the surface enzymes are involved in nucleotide metabolism (see Table 73–2). For example, CD73 is an ecto-5′-nucleotidase that catalyzes the 5′ dephosphorylation of purine and pyrimidine ribo- and deoxyribonucleoside monophosphates to nucleosides that can be taken up by transport systems.[69] This ecto-5′-nucleotidase is attached to the plasma membrane by a glycerol phosphatidylinositol anchor. In addition, lymphocytes express CD26,[70] which is a membrane protein that can associate with adenosine deaminase, the levels of which are increased after activation.[71] The shedding of adenosine deaminase by stimulated cells may explain why plasma levels of this enzyme are increased in early HIV infection and in other diseases associated with immune activation.[72]

The ectoenzymes of nucleotide metabolism may regulate lymphocyte and granulocyte function at sites of inflammation. Activated T lymphocytes can release ATP, which, in turn, can bind to specific plasma membrane ATP receptors.[73] In addition, CD38 can catalyze the transient formation of cyclic adenosine 5′-diphosphate-ribose, a new second-messenger molecule directly involved in the control of calcium homeostasis by means of receptor-mediated release of calcium from ryanodine-sensitive intracellular stores.[74] The consequent increase in calcium mobilization and phospholipid breakdown can provoke activation or death, depending on the target cell. Subsequently, the dephosphorylation of ATP generates adenosine, which can interact with A2 receptors on the plasma membranes of neutrophils, monocytes, and lymphocytes.[75] The engagement of A2 receptors elevates adenosine 3′,5′-cyclic phosphate levels, counteracting the effects of ATP on cell activation. The deamination of adenosine permits the cycle to begin anew.

The ectodomains of several other surface antigens can possess proteolytic activity. For example, CD10 (or CALLA) also has neutral endopeptidase activity,[76] and CD26 has dipeptidyl peptidase IV activity.[77] These enzymes may play a role in modulating the binding of lymphocytes to other cells and to the extracellular matrix. In addition, inhibition of the

TABLE 73–2. Ectoenzymes Expressed by Lymphocytes

Surface Molecule	Enzymatic Activity	Function	Reference
CD10	Neutral endopeptidase, EC 3.4.24.11	Metalloproteinase that may also play a role in the metabolic stability of glucagon-like peptide-1	76
CD13	Aminopeptidase N, EC 3.4.11.2	Aminopeptidase involved in trimming peptides bound to major histocompatibility complex class II molecules and cleaving macrophage inflammatory protein (MIP)-1 chemokine to alter target cell specificity. Also served as Rc for coronavirus	102
CD26	Dipeptidylpeptidase IV, EC 3.4.14.5	Serine peptidase that may be involved in T-cell signaling and T-cell activation	77
CD38	ADP ribosyl cyclase, EC 3.4.14.5	Ectoenzyme with NAD glycohydrolase, ADP ribosyl cyclase, and cyclic ADP ribose hydrolase activities	74
CD39	Ecto (Ca^{2+}, Mg^{2+})-apyrase (ecto-ATPase)	Ectoenzyme with ADPase and ATPase activities that plays a role in regulating platelet aggregation	103
CD73	Ecto-5′-nucleotidase	Ecto-5′-nucleotidase that may play a role in T-cell signaling	69
CD143	Peptidyl-dipeptide hydrolase (angiotensin-converting enzyme)	Peptidyl-dipeptide hydrolase that is involved in the metabolism of vasoactive peptides angiotensin II and bradykinin	104
CD156a	ADAM8 metalloprotease	Matrix metalloprotease that may play a role in leukocyte extravasation	78
CD156b	ADAM17 metalloprotease	Metalloprotease that cleaves membrane-bound tumor necrosis factor and transforming growth factor-a to release the soluble cytokine	79
CD157	ADP ribosyl cyclase and cyclic ADP ribose hydrolase	ADP ribosyl cyclase and cyclic ADP ribose hydrolase that may play a role in lymphocyte development. Like CD38, this enzyme also is involved in the metabolism of NAD	105
CD224	γ-Glutamyltranspeptidase, EC2.3.2.2	γ-Glutamyltranspeptidase role in γ-glutamyl cycle involving the degradation and neosynthesis of glutathione	106

ADAM, a disintegrin and a metalloprotease; ADP, adenosine 5′-diphosphate; ADPase, adenosine 5′-diphosphatase; ATPase, adenosine 5′-triphosphate; CD, cluster of differentiation; NAD, nicotinamide adenine dinucleotide.

catalytic activity of CD26 can provoke many cellular effects, including induction of tyrosine phosphorylation and p38 mitogen-activated protein kinase activation, as well as suppression of DNA synthesis and reduced production of various cytokines. As such, these ectoenzymes could play an important role in lymphocyte activation.

Some membrane-bound proteases have a disintegrin and a metalloprotease domain, termed ADAM (a disintegrin and a metalloprotease).[78] One such member of this family of proteins is the tumor necrosis factor-α converting enzyme, otherwise known as ADAM17 (CD156b).[79] These enzymes cleave other surface molecules, such as tumor necrosis factor, thereby releasing the soluble active cytokine. In addition, they may play an important role in modifying the activity of cytokines or other cell-surface molecules that are present in the vicinity of the plasma membrane.

Intracellular Membrane-Associated Enzymes

Transmembrane proteins that have cytoplasmic regions with kinase or phosphatase activities are common in biology although relatively few of these are restricted to lymphocytes. Nevertheless, many cytoplasmic domains of transmembrane proteins interact directly with enzymes that are restricted or preferentially expressed by lymphocytes or lymphocyte subsets (Chaps. 75 and 76). B lymphocytes, for example, selectively express Bruton tyrosine kinase (BTK), a tyrosine kinase that plays a critical role in signal transduction via surface Ig receptors.[80] Moreover, mutations that disrupt the function of such kinases can impair B-cell development, leading to dysregulated B-cell function or immune deficiency.[81] On the other hand, T-cell development and function rely heavily on cytoplasmic receptor-associated tyrosine kinases, such as the

zeta-associated protein of 70 kDa (ZAP-70), leukocyte tyrosine kinase (lck), or fyn. ZAP-70 interacts with the ζ-chain (CD247) of the TCR for antigen,[82] whereas the latter enzymes, lck and fyn, are Src family tyrosine kinases that interact with cytoplasmic domains of various accessory molecules, including CD2, CD4, CD8, CD44, CD50, and/or CD137.[83] Through such interactions, these receptor protein tyrosine kinases play important roles in signal transduction following immune recognition and/or cognate intercellular immune interactions.

In addition, lymphocytes possess an important class of intracellular molecules, known collectively as adapter proteins, that have no intrinsic enzymatic activity.[84] These adaptor proteins can serve as a scaffolding for the assembly of kinases and other signaling molecules following antigen-receptor ligation. One important adaptor protein expressed in B lymphocytes is B-cell linker protein (BLNK; Chap. 75).[85] On the other hand, T cells use a distinct adaptor protein called linker for activation of T cells (LAT).[86] These molecules couple proximal biochemical events initiated by surface-receptor ligation with more distal signaling pathways by recruiting other cytosolic proteins (Chaps. 75 and 76).

●CYTOPLASMIC STRUCTURES

CYTOMATRIX

Beneath the lymphocyte's plasma membrane is a fully developed cytomatrix with several different structural and mechanical proteins, including tubulin, actin, myosin, tropomyosin, α-actinin, filamin, and a spectrin-like molecule, which are important in the formation of the immunologic synapse that forms during cognate intercellular interactions.[87] These are arranged into typical microfilaments, microtubules, and intermediate filaments. Lymphocyte activation by antigens or mitogens can lead to changes in the interaction of membrane components with the cytoskeleton, allowing for antigen processing, Ig secretion, or cell-mediated cytotoxic reactions.[88]

ORGANELLES

In large part the composition and metabolism of long-lived blood T lymphocytes reflect their resting state. The T cells have a high nuclear-to-cytoplasmic ratio, few ribosomes or mitochondria, and scant endoplasmic reticulum. Glycogen stores are meager. The DNA content of the resting small lymphocyte, 8 pg per cell, is the same amount in other diploid cells. In contrast, the RNA content averages 2.5 pg per cell, yielding an RNA-to-DNA ratio of approximately 0.32.[89] This value is less than in most other human cells, as a result of the small amount of ribosomal RNA in most lymphocytes.

In contrast to most lymphocytes, however, plasma cells have a high RNA-to-DNA ratio. These cells are the end products of B-cell differentiation and are committed to the synthesis, assembly, and secretion of Ig. Accordingly, these cells have a well-developed rough endoplasmic reticulum and Golgi apparatus, but lack many of the surface receptors found on most lymphocytes. Mature plasma cells are probably terminally differentiated and have a low rate of DNA synthesis and abundant RNA, reflecting the plasma cell's high-level synthesis of Ig.

Lysosomes

The few lysosomes in blood lymphocytes contain several different acid hydrolases, including acid phosphatase, β-glucuronidase, β-galactosidase, β-hexosaminidase, α-arabinosidase, α-galactosidase, α-mannosidase, α-glucosidase, and β-glucosidase.[90-92] Acid hydrolase activities are generally higher in T cells than in non-T lymphocytes. Lysosomal acid esterase, assayed histochemically with α-naphthyl acetate as substrate, has a characteristic punctate appearance in mature T lymphocytes.[93] Secretory lysosomes are specialized organelles that combine catabolic functions of conventional lysosomes with the capacity to be secreted upon induction.[94] An example of such secretory lysosomes are the specialized cytoplasmic granules of T cells and NK cells that are responsible for the cytotoxic effector function of these cells.

Cytoplasmic Granules

In contrast to other lymphocytes, cytotoxic T lymphocytes and NK cells possess abundant cytoplasmic granules. These contain a pore-forming proteolytic enzyme, termed *perforin*, and a series of serine proteinases with specific proapoptotic activity, called *granzymes*.[95] To protect against possible autolysis by granule contents, cytotoxic lymphocytes possess serine-proteinase inhibitors, termed *serpins*.[96] As an additional safeguard, the granzymes of resting lymphocytes are stored as inactive proenzymes.

Cytotoxic lymphocytes rely primarily on the perforin/granzyme system to kill their targets.[97] Upon contact with its target cell, the cytotoxic lymphocyte converts the granzymes into active forms by a lysosomal cysteine protease called dipeptidyl peptidase I.[98] Then perforin introduces a pore in the membrane, allowing the activated granzymes and other granule contents to pass into the cytoplasm and then the nucleus of the cell targeted for destruction.[95] *In vitro* studies indicate that granzyme nuclear import is independent of ATP, cannot be inhibited by nonhydrolyzable guanosine triphosphate analogues, and involves binding within the nucleus, unlike conventional signal-dependent nuclear protein import. The perforin-dependent nuclear entry of granzymes precedes the nuclear events of apoptosis, such as DNA fragmentation and breakdown of the nuclear envelope (Chap. 15).

ACKNOWLEDGMENTS

This chapter was adapted from "Morphology of Lymphocytes and Plasma Cells" by H. Elizabeth Broome and "Composition and Biochemistry of Lymphocytes and Plasma Cells" by Thomas J. Kipps in the earlier edition.

REFERENCES

1. Hewson WJ: No.72, Pauls Church Yard London, 1774, in *Lymphatics, Lymph, and Lymphomyeloid Complex*, edited by Yoffey JF, Courtice FC, p 3. Harvard University Press, Cambridge, MA, 1970.
2. Ackerman GA: Structural studies of the lymphocyte and lymphocyte development, in *Regulation of Hematopoiesis*, edited by Gordon AS, p 1297. Appleton Century Crofts, New York, 1970.
3. Everett NB, Caffrey RW, Rieke WO: Recirculation of lymphocytes. *Ann N Y Acad Sci* 113:887–897, 1964.
4. Ford WI, Gowans JL: The traffic of lymphocytes. *Semin Hematol* 6:67, 1969.
5. Miller RG: *Physical Separation of Lymphocytes and Lymphocyte Structure and Function*. Marcel Dekker, New York, 1977.
6. Nossal GJ, Makela O: Elaboration of antibodies by single cells. *Annu Rev Microbiol* 16:53–74, 1962.
7. Bain BJ: *Blood Cells, A Practical Guide*. Blackwell Science, London, 1995.
8. Cranendonk E, van Gennip AH, Abeling NG, Behrendt H: Numerical changes in the various peripheral white blood cells in children as a result of antineoplastic therapy. *Acta Haematol* 72:315–325, 1984.
9. Timonen T, Ortaldo JR, Herberman RB: Characteristics of human large granular lymphocytes and relationship to natural killer and K cells. *J Exp Med* 153:569–582, 1981.
10. Tanaka T, Goodman JR: *Electron Microscopy of Human Blood Cells*. Harper and Row, New York, 1972.
11. Brittinger G, Hirschhorn R, Douglas SD, Weissmann G: Studies on lysosomes. XI. Characterization of a hydrolase-rich fraction from human lymphocytes. *J Cell Biol* 37:394–411, 1968.
12. Basso G, Cocito MG, Semenzato G, et al: Cytochemical study of thymocytes and T lymphocytes. *Br J Haematol* 44:577–582, 1980.
13. Landay A, Clement LT, Grossi CE: Phenotypically and functionally distinct subpopulations of human lymphocytes with T cell markers also exhibit different cytochemical patterns of staining for lysosomal enzymes. *Blood* 63:1067–1071, 1984.
14. Hayes TL: Scanning electron microscope techniques in biology, in *Advanced Techniques in Biological Electron Microscopy*, edited by Koehler JK, p 153. Springer, New York, 1973.
15. Polliack A, Lampen N, Clarkson BD, et al: Identification of human B and T lymphocytes by scanning electron microscopy. *J Exp Med* 138:607–624, 1973.
16. Majstoravich S, Zhang J, Nicholson-Dykstra S, et al: Lymphocyte microvilli are dynamic, actin-dependent structures that do not require Wiskott-Aldrich syndrome protein (WASp) for their morphology. *Blood* 104:1396–1403, 2004.
17. Berlin C, Bargatze RF, Campbell JJ, et al: Alpha 4 integrins mediate lymphocyte attachment and rolling under physiologic flow. *Cell* 80:413–422, 1995.
18. von Andrian UH, Hasslen SR, Nelson RD, et al: A central role for microvillous receptor presentation in leukocyte adhesion under flow. *Cell* 82:989–999, 1995.
19. Handwerger BS, Douglas SD: The cell biology of blastogenesis, in *Handbook of Inflammation*, edited by Weissman G, p 609. Elsevier, North Holland, 1980.
20. Douglas SD, Cohnen G, Konig E, Brittinger G: Ultrastructural features of phytohemagglutinin and concanavalin A-responsive lymphocytes in chronic lymphocytic leukemia. *Acta Haematol* 50:129–142, 1973.
21. Douglas SD, Fudenberg HH: *In vitro* development of plasma cells from lymphocytes following pokeweed mitogen stimulation: a fine structural study. *Exp Cell Res* 54:277–279, 1969.
22. Sainte-Marie G: Study on plasmocytopoiesis. I. Description of plasmocytes and of their mitoses in the mediastinal lymph nodes of ten-week-old rats. *Am J Anat* 114:207–233, 1964.
23. Sainte-Marie G, Coons AH: Studies on antibody production X. Mode of formation of plasmocytes in cell transfer experiments. *J Exp Med* 119:743–760, 1964.
24. Parkhouse RM, Janossy G, Greaves MF: Selective stimulation of IgM synthesis in mouse B lymphocytes by pokeweed mitogen. *Nat New Biol* 235:21–23, 1972.
25. Welsh RA: Electron microscopic localization of Russell bodies in the human plasma cell. *Blood* 16:1307–1312, 1960.
26. Sacchetti C: [Plasma cells of the bone marrow in normal and pathological states; quantitative, cytometric and auxological research] [article in undetermined language]. *Haematologica* 35:13–53, 1951.
27. Suzuki A, Shibata A, Onodera S: Histochemical study on plasma cells. *Tohoku J Exp Med* 97:1, 1969.
28. Quaglino D, Torelli U, Sauli S, Mauri C: Cytochemical and autoradiographic investigations on normal and myelomatous plasma cells. *Acta Haematol* 38:79–94, 1967.
29. Franklin EC, Zucker-Franklin D: Current concepts of amyloid. *Adv Immunol* 15:249–304, 1972.
30. Lerner RG, Parker JW: Dysglobulinemia and iron in plasma cells. Ferrokinetics and electron microscopy. *Arch Intern Med* 121:284–287, 1968.

31. Bessis MC: Ultrastructure of lymphoid and plasma cells in relation to globulin and antibody formation. *Lab Invest* 10:1040–1067, 1961.
32. Adams B, Dörfler P, Aguzzi A, et al: Pax-5 encodes the transcription factor BSAP and is expressed in B lymphocytes, the developing CNS, and adult testis. *Genes Dev* 6: 1589–1607, 1992.
33. Urbanek P, Wang ZQ, Fetka I, et al: Complete block of early B cell differentiation and altered patterning of the posterior midbrain in mice lacking Pax5/BSAP. *Cell* 79: 901–912, 1994.
34. Karras JG, Wang Z, Huo L, et al: Signal transducer and activator of transcription-3 (STAT3) is constitutively activated in normal, self-renewing B-1 cells but only inducibly expressed in conventional B lymphocytes. *J Exp Med* 185:1035–1042, 1997.
35. Kipps TJ: The CD5 B cell. *Adv Immunol* 47:117–185, 1989.
36. Defrance T, Vanbervliet B, Durand I, et al: Proliferation and differentiation of human CD5+ and CD5− B cell subsets activated through their antigen receptors or CD40 antigens. *Eur J Immunol* 22:2831–2839, 1992.
37. Durandy A, Thuillier L, Forveille M, Fischer A: Phenotypic and functional characteristics of human newborns' B lymphocytes. *J Immunol* 144:60–65, 1990.
38. Caligaris-Cappio F, Gobbi M, Bofill M, Janossy G: Infrequent normal B lymphocytes express features of B-chronic lymphocytic leukemia. *J Exp Med* 155:623–628, 1982.
39. Casali P, Prabhakar BS, Notkins AL: Characterization of multireactive autoantibodies and identification of Leu-1+ B lymphocytes as cells making antibodies binding multiple self and exogenous molecules. *Int Rev Immunol* 3:17–45, 1988.
40. Hayakawa K, Hardy RR, Honda M, et al: Ly-1 B cells: Functionally distinct lymphocytes that secrete IgM autoantibodies. *Proc Natl Acad Sci U S A* 81:2494–2498, 1984.
41. Sthoeger ZM, Wakai M, Tse DB, et al: Production of autoantibodies by CD5-expressing B lymphocytes from patients with chronic lymphocytic leukemia. *J Exp Med* 169: 255–268, 1989.
42. Anderson KC, Park EK, Bates MP, et al: Antigens on human plasma cells identified by monoclonal antibodies. *J Immunol* 130:1132–1138, 1983.
43. Rawstron AC: Immunophenotyping of plasma cells. *Curr Protoc Cytom* Chapter 6: Unit6.23, 2006.
44. Keegan AD, Paul WE: Multichain immune recognition receptors: Similarities in structure and signaling pathways. *Immunol Today* 13:63–68, 1992.
45. Maddon PJ, Littman DR, Godfrey M, et al: The isolation and nucleotide sequence of a cDNA encoding the T cell surface protein T4: A new member of the immunoglobulin gene family. *Cell* 42:93–104, 1985.
46. Snow PM, Terhorst C: The T8 antigen is a multimeric complex of two distinct subunits on human thymocytes but consists of homomultimeric forms on peripheral blood T lymphocytes. *J Biol Chem* 258:14675–14681, 1983.
47. Dalgleish AG, Beverley PC, Clapham PR, et al: The CD4 (T4) antigen is an essential component of the receptor for the AIDS retrovirus. *Nature* 312:763–767, 1984.
48. Sakaguchi S, Yamaguchi T, Nomura T, Ono M: Regulatory T cells and immune tolerance. *Cell* 133:775–787, 2008.
49. Roncador G, Brown PJ, Maestre L, et al: Analysis of FOXP3 protein expression in human CD4+CD25+ regulatory T cells at the single-cell level. *Eur J Immunol* 35:1681–1691, 2005.
50. Grogg KL, Attygalle AD, Macon WR, et al: Expression of CXCL13, a chemokine highly upregulated in germinal center T-helper cells, distinguishes angioimmunoblastic T-cell lymphoma from peripheral T-cell lymphoma, unspecified. *Mod Pathol* 19:1101–1107, 2006.
51. Yang Y, Torchinsky MB, Gobert M, et al: Focused specificity of intestinal TH17 cells towards commensal bacterial antigens. *Nature* 510:152–156, 2014.
52. Timonen T, Saksela E: Isolation of human NK cells by density gradient centrifugation. *J Immunol Methods* 36:285–291, 1980.
53. Hercend T, Griffin JD, Bensussan A, et al: Generation of monoclonal antibodies to a human natural killer clone. Characterization of two natural killer-associated antigens, NKH1A and NKH2, expressed on subsets of large granular lymphocytes. *J Clin Invest* 75:932–943, 1985.
54. Cooper MA, Fehniger TA, Caligiuri MA: The biology of human natural killer-cell subsets. *Trends Immunol* 22:633–640, 2001.
55. Björkström NK, Gonzalez VD, Malmberg KJ, et al: Elevated numbers of Fc gamma RIIIA+ (CD16+) effector CD8 T cells with NK cell-like function in chronic hepatitis C virus infection. *J Immunol* 181:4219–4228, 2008.
56. Lanier LL, Le AM, Phillips JH, et al: Subpopulations of human natural killer cells defined by expression of the Leu-7 (HNK-1) and Leu-11 (NK-15) antigens. *J Immunol* 131:1789–1796, 1983.
57. Thiel A, Scheffold A, Radbruch A: Antigen-specific cytometry—New tools arrived! *Clin Immunol* 111:155–161, 2004.
58. Kodituwakku AP, Jessup C, Zola H, Roberton DM: Isolation of antigen-specific B cells. *Immunol Cell Biol* 81:163–170, 2003.
59. Kinoshita K, Ozawa T, Tajiri K, et al: Identification of antigen-specific B cells by concurrent monitoring of intracellular Ca2+ mobilization and antigen binding with microwell array chip system equipped with a CCD imager. *Cytometry A* 75:682–687, 2009.
60. Segel GB, Cokelet GR, Lichtman MA: The measurement of lymphocyte volume: importance of reference particle deformability and counting solution tonicity. *Blood* 57: 894–899, 1981.
61. Lichtman AH, Segel GB, Lichtman MA: An ultrasensitive method for the measurement of human leukocyte calcium: Lymphocytes. *Clin Chim Acta* 97:107–121, 1979.
62. Komada H, Nakabayashi H, Nakano H, et al: Measurement of the cytosolic free calcium ion concentration of individual lymphocytes by microfluorometry using quin 2 or fura-2. *Cell Struct Funct* 14:141–150, 1989.
63. Crumpton MJ, Snary D: Preparation and properties of lymphocyte plasma membrane. *Contemp Top Mol Immunol* 3:27–56, 1974.
64. Goppelt M, Eichhorn R, Krebs G, Resch K: Lipid composition of functional domains of the lymphocyte plasma membrane. *Biochim Biophys Acta* 854:184–190, 1986.
65. Johnson SM, Robinson R: The composition and fluidity of normal and leukaemic or lymphomatous lymphocyte plasma membranes in mouse and man. *Biochim Biophys Acta* 558:282–295, 1979.
66. Jury EC, Flores-Borja F, Kabouridis PS: Lipid rafts in T cell signalling and disease. *Semin Cell Dev Biol* 18:608–615, 2007.
67. Gupta N, DeFranco AL: Lipid rafts and B cell signaling. *Semin Cell Dev Biol* 18: 616–626, 2007.
68. Landry A, Xavier R: Isolation and analysis of lipid rafts in cell-cell interactions. *Methods Mol Biol* 341:251–282, 2006.
69. Colgan SP, Eltzschig HK, Eckle T, Thompson LF: Physiological roles for ecto-5′-nucleotidase (CD73). *Purinergic Signal* 2:351–360, 2006.
70. Havre PA, Abe M, Urasaki Y, et al: The role of CD26/dipeptidyl peptidase IV in cancer. *Front Biosci* 13:1634–1645, 2008.
71. Kameoka J, Tanaka T, Nojima Y, et al: Direct association of adenosine deaminase with a T cell activation antigen, CD26. *Science* 261:466–469, 1993.
72. Ohtsuki T, Tsuda H, Morimoto C: Good or evil: CD26 and HIV infection. *J Dermatol Sci* 22:152–160, 2000.
73. Swennen EL, Coolen EJ, Arts IC, et al: Time-dependent effects of ATP and its degradation products on inflammatory markers in human blood *ex vivo*. *Immunobiology* 213:389–397, 2008.
74. Partida-Sanchez S, Rivero-Nava L, Shi G, Lund FE: CD38: An ecto-enzyme at the crossroads of innate and adaptive immune responses. *Adv Exp Med Biol* 590:171–183, 2007.
75. Kumar V, Sharma A: Adenosine: An endogenous modulator of innate immune system with therapeutic potential. *Eur J Pharmacol* 616:7–15, 2009.
76. Plamboeck A, Holst JJ, Carr RD, Deacon CF: Neutral endopeptidase 24.11 and dipeptidyl peptidase IV are both involved in regulating the metabolic stability of glucagon-like peptide-1 *in vivo*. *Adv Exp Med Biol* 524:303–312, 2003.
77. Ohnuma K, Takahashi N, Yamochi T, et al: Role of CD26/dipeptidyl peptidase IV in human T cell activation and function. *Front Biosci* 13:2299–2310, 2008.
78. Yamamoto S, Higuchi Y, Yoshiyama K, et al: ADAM family proteins in the immune system. *Immunol Today* 20:278–284, 1999.
79. Black RA: Tumor necrosis factor-alpha converting enzyme. *Int J Biochem Cell Biol* 34:1–5, 2002.
80. Lindvall JM, Blomberg KE, Väliaho J, et al: Bruton's tyrosine kinase: Cell biology, sequence conservation, mutation spectrum, siRNA modifications, and expression profiling. *Immunol Rev* 203:200–215, 2005.
81. Kurosaki T, Hikida M: Tyrosine kinases and their substrates in B lymphocytes. *Immunol Rev* 228:132–148, 2009.
82. Au-Yeung BB, Deindl S, Hsu LY, et al: The structure, regulation, function of ZAP-70. *Immunol Rev* 228:41–57, 2009.
83. Salmond RJ, Filby A, Qureshi I, et al: T-cell receptor proximal signaling via the Src-family kinases, Lck and Fyn, influences T-cell activation, differentiation, and tolerance. *Immunol Rev* 228:9–22, 2009.
84. Leo A, Schraven B: Adapters in lymphocyte signalling. *Curr Opin Immunol* 13:307–316, 2001.
85. Tsukada S, Baba Y, Watanabe D: Btk and BLNK in B cell development. *Adv Immunol* 77:123–162, 2001.
86. Aguado E, Martinez-Florensa M, Aparicio P: Activation of T lymphocytes and the role of the adapter LAT. *Transpl Immunol* 17:23–26, 2006.
87. Rey M, Sanchez-Madrid F, Valenzuela-Fernandez A: The role of actomyosin and the microtubular network in both the immunological synapse and T cell activation. *Front Biosci* 12:437–447, 2007.
88. Miletic AV, Swat M, Fujikawa K, Swat W: Cytoskeletal remodeling in lymphocyte activation. *Curr Opin Immunol* 15:261–268, 2003.
89. Glen AC: Measurement of DNA and RNA in human peripheral blood lymphocytes. *Clin Chem* 13:299–313, 1967.
90. Beaumelle BD, Gibson A, Hopkins CR: Isolation and preliminary characterization of the major membrane boundaries of the endocytic pathway in lymphocytes. *J Cell Biol* 111:1811–1823, 1990.
91. Casey TM, Meade JL, Hewitt EW: Organelle proteomics: Identification of the exocytic machinery associated with the natural killer cell secretory lysosome. *Mol Cell Proteomics* 6:767–780, 2007.
92. Qu P, Du H, Wilkes DS, Yan C: Critical roles of lysosomal acid lipase in T cell development and function. *Am J Pathol* 174:944–956, 2009.
93. Kulenkampff J, Janossy G, Greaves MF: Acid esterase in human lymphoid cells and leukaemic blasts: A marker for T lymphocytes. *Br J Haematol* 36:231–240, 1977.
94. Lettau M, Schmidt H, Kabelitz D, Janssen O: Secretory lysosomes and their cargo in T and NK cells. *Immunol Lett* 108:10–19, 2007.
95. Chavez-Galan L, Arenas-Del Angel MC, Zenteno E, et al: Cell death mechanisms induced by cytotoxic lymphocytes. *Cell Mol Immunol* 6:15–25, 2009.
96. Bots M, Medema JP: Serpins in T cell immunity. *J Leukoc Biol* 84:1238–1247, 2008.
97. Trapani JA, Smyth MJ: Functional significance of the perforin/granzyme cell death pathway. *Nat Rev Immunol* 2:735–747, 2002.
98. Pham CT, Ley TJ: Dipeptidyl peptidase I is required for the processing and activation of granzymes A and B *in vivo*. *Proc Natl Acad Sci U S A* 96:8627–8632, 1999.

99. Maeda T, Yamada H, Nagamine R, et al: Involvement of CD4+, CD57+ T cells in the disease activity of rheumatoid arthritis. *Arthritis Rheum* 46:379–384, 2002.

100. Fontenot JD, Gavin MA, Rudensky AY: Foxp3 programs the development and function of CD4+CD25+ regulatory T cells. *Nat Immunol* 4:330–336, 2003.

101. Chattopadhyay PK, Betts MR, Price DA, et al: The cytolytic enzymes granzyme A, granzyme B, and perforin: Expression patterns, cell distribution, and their relationship to cell maturity and bright CD57 expression. *J Leukoc Biol* 85:88–97, 2009.

102. Tani K, Ogushi F, Huang L, et al: CD13/aminopeptidase N, a novel chemoattractant for T lymphocytes in pulmonary sarcoidosis. *Am J Respir Crit Care Med* 161:1636–1642, 2000.

103. Schulte am Esch J 2nd, Sévigny J, Kaczmarek E, et al: Structural elements and limited proteolysis of CD39 influence ATP diphosphohydrolase activity. *Biochemistry* 38:2248–2258, 1999.

104. Bauvois B: Transmembrane proteases in cell growth and invasion: New contributors to angiogenesis? *Oncogene* 23:317–329, 2004.

105. Ortolan E, Vacca P, Capobianco A, et al: CD157, the Janus of CD38 but with a unique personality. *Cell Biochem Funct* 20:309–322, 2002.

106. Stark AA, Porat N, Volohonsky G, et al: The role of gamma-glutamyl transpeptidase in the biosynthesis of glutathione. *Biofactors* 17:139–149, 2003.

CHAPTER 74
LYMPHOPOIESIS

Christopher S. Seet and Gay M. Crooks

SUMMARY

Lymphopoiesis refers to the process by which the cellular components of the immune system (i.e., T cells, B cells, and natural killer cells, and certain dendritic cells) are produced during hematopoietic differentiation. This process begins with the hematopoietic stem cell and continues through progenitor stages down a series of mostly diverging lineage pathways, ultimately resulting in the remarkable diversity and flexibility of the immune system. Although the more terminal events in lymphocyte differentiation and function have been defined in detail (Chaps. 75 to 77), the earliest events during which hematopoietic stem cells undergo lymphoid lineage commitment are less-well understood and still controversial. Although the conceptual framework for the questions of lymphoid commitment has been established largely on studies in the mouse, experimental systems now exist to better understand how such events are controlled in humans. This chapter summarizes what is known about the ontogeny of lymphoid development and the control of lymphoid differentiation, and discusses some of the persisting controversies in the field.

● LYMPHOPOIESIS DURING PRENATAL DEVELOPMENT

Blood is formed from a succession of sites during embryonic and fetal development, beginning outside the embryo in the yolk sac. Soon afterward, hematopoiesis begins in the embryo proper, initially in the para-aortic splanchnopleura (PAS) and aorto-gonad-mesonephros (AGM) regions, then the fetal liver, spleen, and finally the fetal marrow (Chap. 7). With each change of anatomical site, the range of hematopoiesis becomes progressively more complex and similar to that of the adult (Fig. 74–1).

When assigning hematopoietic function to each developmental stage, it is important to distinguish the lineage "potential" of stem and progenitor cells that arise from certain areas (i.e., the ability to generate specific lineages *in vitro* from immature cells removed from a region) from the spontaneous physiologic production of lineages in each region. With this distinction in mind, the onset of lymphopoiesis

Acronyms and Abbreviations: AGM, aorto-gonad-mesonephros; BM, bone marrow; BCR, B-cell receptor; CLP, common lymphoid progenitor; CT, computed tomography; DC, dendritic cell; DN, double negative; E, days of gestation; EBF, early B-cell factor; FACS, fluorescence-activated cell sorting; FLT3, Fms-like tyrosine kinase 3; HSC, hematopoietic stem cell; Ig, immunoglobulin; IL, interleukin; JAK3, Janus kinase 3; LMPP, lymphoid-primed multipotent progenitor; LSK, lin^neg^sca-1+c-kit+; NK, natural killer; PAS, para-aortic splanchnopleura; SCID, severe combined immunodeficiency.

during embryogenesis lags behind development of the myeloid and erythroid lineages. Although myeloid, erythroid, and natural killer (NK) cells can be produced from all extraembryonic and embryonic sites, B and T lymphocytes are predominantly generated from so-called definitive hematopoietic stem cells (HSCs) in the embryo proper.[1]

MURINE HEMATOPOIETIC DEVELOPMENT

Most of the studies exploring embryonic and fetal hematopoiesis have been performed using mouse models. Although the timing of each developmental stage has been carefully mapped, it has long been a source of controversy as to whether hematopoiesis in the embryo is initiated from colonizing precursors from the extraembryonic yolk sac, or whether the embryonic sites of hematopoiesis arise independently from the yolk sac.[2-6] This debate has implications for understanding the lineages generated at different sites of hematopoiesis and thus for tracing the ancestry of the lymphoid cells that are produced in the mammalian embryo. One reason for the difficulty in assigning the exact organ in which lineages are generated, is that each site of hematopoiesis is active during overlapping periods (see Fig. 74–1). In addition, once circulation has been established, it is difficult to rule out the possibility that stem cells and progenitors found in one location did not migrate from another. However studies using *Ncx1*^-/-^ mice, which lack both heartbeat and circulation,[7,8] are beginning to dissect the autonomous lineage potentials of these distinct embryonic hematopoietic tissues.

The first wave of hematopoiesis in the mouse begins in the extraembryonic tissue of the yolk sac by 7.5 days of gestation (E7.5), before circulation is established.[9,10] This initial stage of so-called primitive hematopoiesis produces mostly erythrocytes and macrophages. Although lymphocytes are not detectable at this time,[10] the contribution of first-wave progenitors to downstream fetal lymphopoiesis has been suggested by the identification of a lymphomyeloid progenitor in the E9.5 yolk sac, which expresses Rag-1, one of the earliest lymphoid-specific events,[11] as well as of a distinct progenitor with B-1/marginal zone B cell potential.[12] Further studies have identified both thymic-repopulating and multipotent potential in the yolk sac,[13,14] indicating emerging changes to our understanding of primitive hematopoiesis. The murine placenta has also been identified as an autonomous source of multipotent hematopoietic cells as early as E8.5[8]; however, the direct contribution of either yolk sac or placental progenitors to definitive lymphoid development remains to be determined. Definitive HSCs that are capable of generating all lymphohematopoietic lineages first appear in the PAS/AGM region at E8.5 to E9.[3,10] High-level, multilineage reconstituting activity typical of definitive HSC can be found in the murine AGM region by E10.5. However, although AGM cells can produce all lineages, including T and B lymphocytes *in vitro*, lymphocytes do not spontaneously develop in the fetus until hematopoiesis has begun in the fetal liver. Rag-1 expression, one of the earliest lymphoid-specific events, can be found in the E11 murine fetal liver.[10] T-cell potential has been identified in the yolk sac and PAS as early as E8.25 to E9.5 of murine gestation[13]; however, T-cell differentiation *in vivo* begins with the colonization of the thymus around E11 by stem or progenitor cells that migrate to the thymus from the AGM, fetal liver, and, later still, the fetal marrow.[15,16]

HUMAN HEMATOPOIETIC DEVELOPMENT

Hematopoietic cells have been identified in the human yolk sac as early as day 18 of embryonic life, at which time, like the mouse, they are almost exclusively comprised of erythrocytes and, to a lesser extent, monocytes and macrophages (see Fig. 74–1).[17] Although no lymphocytes are seen in the yolk sac, yolk sac progenitors do have NK cell potential under certain *in vitro* conditions.[17,18] The same yolk sac progenitors, however,

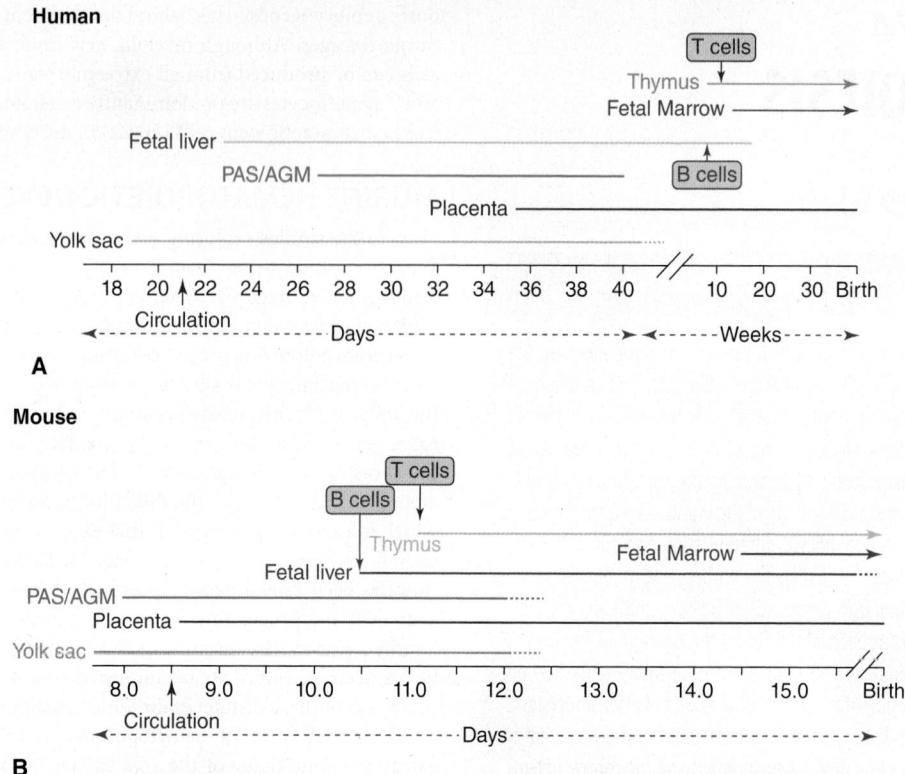

Figure 74–1. Timing of lymphohematopoiesis during prenatal development. Shown is the timeline for activity in each site of hematopoiesis in the embryo and fetus of **(A)** human and **(B)** mouse. B and T cells are first detected *in vivo* in fetal liver and thymus, respectively, at times shown. AGM, aorto-gonad-mesonephros; PAS, para-aortic splanchnopleura.

do not possess the capacity for B- or T-cell development, even when placed in culture conditions that permit lymphoid differentiation.[18]

As in the mouse, definitive hematopoiesis develops first in the AGM region derived from the splanchnopleura, as evidenced by the finding that the AGM is the site where CD34+ cells with the capacity for full lymphoid and myeloid differentiation are first found in the human embryo.[18,19] The AGM develops at day 27 of gestation in the human, when human HSCs are generated as clusters of two or three cells arising from the endothelium specifically on the ventral surface of the preumbilical region of the aorta. These cells are clonogenic and highly proliferative, rapidly increasing to several thousand in number and spreading further along the aorta. However, hematopoiesis exists only transiently in the AGM, disappearing entirely by day 40.[17] Although lymphoid cells can be produced in culture from cells extracted from the AGM,[17,18] the HSC of the AGM do not produce mature cells *in situ*; instead their role is to migrate and colonize the fetal liver, producing the next wave of hematopoiesis. As in the mouse, recent studies have also detected multipotent progenitors with lymphoid potential in the human placenta. These reports suggest that hematopoietic stem/progenitor cells may also be generated *de novo* from the large vessels of the chorionic plate as early as week 5 of gestation, with multipotent HSC detectable at 15 weeks.[20,21] However, the contribution of placental HSC to fetal liver or marrow colonization remains unclear.

Although blood cells are first detectable in the human fetal liver as early as day 23, they exist at this time only as erythroid and myeloid cells associated with hepatic sinusoids. These erythroid cells consist of megaloblasts expressing embryonic hemoglobins (globin chains ζ and ε), and no CD34+ cells are seen in the fetal liver during this early phase. It is likely that this first stage of fetal liver hematopoiesis is secondary to colonization of more mature cells from the yolk sac. By day 30, AGM-derived

CD34+ cells appear in the fetal liver,[22] and by day 32, these cells are able to maintain long-term hematopoiesis *in vitro*.[22] Erythroid cells in the fetal liver at this later stage of definitive hematopoiesis consist of enucleated macrocytes producing fetal hemoglobin (globin chains α and γ). In normal development, as with the yolk sac and AGM, hematopoiesis in the fetal liver is transient, disappearing by 20 weeks of gestation.[1]

The final wave of hematopoietic development takes place in the fetal marrow, starting around 11 weeks of gestation. The initial cells seen in the marrow are CD15+ myeloid cells and glycophorin A+ erythroid cells, and hematopoiesis is again associated with the endothelium, taking place in the medullary sinusoids before osteoblast formation.[23] Eventually, CD34+ cells are found in the fetal marrow and behave functionally as true HSC, generating B, T, NK, and myeloid and erythroid lineages.[1] HSC have found their final niche, and lifelong, self-renewing lymphohematopoiesis resides permanently in the marrow thereafter.

THYMIC DEVELOPMENT

The human thymic microenvironment begins to develop at approximately 4 weeks' gestation and then undergoes three developmental phases.[24] The first phase occurs between 4 and 8 weeks' gestation, with the appearance of thymic epithelium arising as a product of the third and fourth pharyngeal pouches[25] and the expansion of thymic epithelial cells. The second phase occurs between 9 and 15 weeks' gestation and is characterized by the development of subcapsular, cortical, and medullary regions.[24] Thymic colonization by fetal liver-derived progenitors and lymphocyte production begins at approximately week 9.[25] The ability of thymocytes to respond to the mitogen phytohemagglutinin is detectable as early as 10 weeks' gestation,[26] and alloreactive, phenotypically mature T cells can be found by 13 to 16 weeks' gestation.[27]

The third phase occurs from 16 weeks' gestation until age 1 to 2 years and is characterized by robust intrathymic T-cell maturation (Chaps. 6 and 76).

An exhaustive study of 136 human postnatal thymuses ranging from neonatal life to more than 90 years old, found that essentially all postnatal thymic growth (based on weight and volume) occurs during the first postnatal year, mostly in the first few months of life.[28] From the age of 12 months, the human thymus undergoes steady involution, with a reduction of thymocytes and thymic epithelium, particularly the medulla, and a corresponding increase in fatty infiltration of the perivascular space.[28]

Whereas mice lose approximately 90 percent of the wet weight of the thymus during life, the increasing fatty infiltration in the perivascular space in the aging human thymus maintains the total size of the thymus in healthy people into late life.[28] Radiologic studies using computed tomography (CT) scans have confirmed that total thymic size remains stable in humans throughout life although parenchymal tissue atrophies dramatically (~95 percent; Chaps. 6 and 9).[29]

B-CELL DEVELOPMENT

The hallmark characteristic of a mature B cell circulating in blood or residing in secondary lymphoid tissue is the expression of cell-surface immunoglobulin (Ig). The cell-surface Ig consists of μ, δ, γ, α, or ε heavy chains disulfide-linked to κ or λ light chains (Chap. 75). The cell-surface Ig and the associated signaling molecules Igα (CD79a) and Igβ (CD79b) are referred to as the *B-cell receptor* (BCR). Progenitor (pro-) B cells are defined by the absence of both cytoplasmic μ heavy chains and cell-surface BCR. Precursor (pre-) B cells are defined by the presence of cytoplasmic μ heavy chains in the absence of cell-surface BCR. This minimal definition of pro-B, pre-B, and B cells forms the basis of the current detailed model of human B-cell development.[30] B-cell development can be divided into two stages: an antigen-independent stage that occurs primarily in fetal liver and fetal and adult marrow, and an antigen-dependent stage that occurs primarily in secondary lymphoid tissue, such as spleen and lymph node.

The first B cells detectable in the human fetus are found in the fetal liver[25] at approximately 8 weeks' gestation, with the appearance of cytoplasmic IgM+ pre-B cells; by 10 to 12 weeks, surface IgM+ B cells are seen in the fetal liver[31] and fetal omentum.[32] B-cell and IgM production move to the fetal marrow and spleen by 17 weeks of gestation (Chaps. 6, 7, and 75).[33,34] From the end of the second trimester throughout adult life, marrow is the exclusive origin of B-cell development.[35] The frequency of early B-lineage cells as a percentage of the total nucleated lymphohematopoietic cell pool is higher in fetal than in adult marrow. However, the ratio between pro-B, pre-B, and immature B cells and the mitotic activity within these fractions is relatively constant.[36]

In murine B-cell development, two functionally and immunophenotypically distinct types of B cells, B-1 and B-2, have been described.[31] Most B cells in adult mice are B-2 cells, which form part of the adaptive immune system by their ability to interact with T cells and undergo immunoglobulin heavy chain class switching. The B-1 cells make up approximately 5 percent of adult murine lymphocytes, but demonstrate a far less diverse immunoglobulin repertoire than the B-2 cells, responding to carbohydrate antigens and other T-cell–independent immunogens and forming part of the innate immune system. Murine B-1 cells are marked by their expression of CD11b, and are found in multiple sites, including the spleen, intestine, and the pleural and peritoneal cavities.[37,38] The B-1 cells can be further divided into B-1a cells (which secrete immunoglobulins spontaneously) and B-1b cells (in which immunoglobulin production is induced) based on the expression of the marker CD5. The demonstration of a B-1a/marginal zone B-cell–restricted progenitor in the E9 extraembryonic yolk sac suggests the B-1

lineage may emerge prior to the development of the adaptive immune system.[12] At present, there is no clear evidence that humans have similar subpopulations of B-1 and B-2 cells during development.[31]

NATURAL KILLER CELL DEVELOPMENT

Functional NK cells can be detected in the human fetal liver as early as 9 to 10 weeks of gestation,[26] but NK cell differentiation can be induced *in vitro* from progenitors derived at all stages of hematopoietic development, even those from the yolk sac.[1,17,18] Thus, the onset of NK potential is not equivalent to the full lymphoid potential of definitive hematopoiesis, as NK potential can be assigned to a range of progenitor types that exist at different stages, including primitive hematopoiesis. NK cell production can be considered as providing an essential defense mechanism for the developing mammalian embryo prior to development of more complex pathways of adaptive immunity.

DENDRITIC CELL DEVELOPMENT

Dendritic-like cells which express class II major histocompatibility (MHC) antigens are produced at all stages of embryonic and fetal hematopoiesis, being first detected in the human yolk sac and mesenchyme as early as 4 to 8 weeks, before development of the fetal marrow or thymus.[31] Dendritic cells (DCs) are detectable at each site of hematopoiesis as soon as they become active, in the human fetal thymus at 11 to 14 weeks, marrow at 14 to 17 weeks, spleen at 16 weeks, and tonsils at 23 weeks.[39,40] DC and macrophages are closely related and phenotypically similar (Chap. 67), both expressing MHC class II. Thus, clear discrimination of these two cell types can be difficult, particularly as many studies that provided information on human DC development were conducted before all the molecular and antibody tools for analysis of DC were available.

● DIFFERENTIATION PATHWAYS FOR LYMPHOCYTE PRODUCTION

The conceptual framework for how the lymphocyte lineages are generated from HSC was developed largely from studies using genetically engineered mice and murine transplant models. Although necessary and useful as a starting point, caution should be exercised in translating the results of the murine studies to human lymphopoiesis, or in assuming for any species that only one pathway to lymphopoiesis exists at all stages of ontogeny.[41,42] Additionally, the conclusions about lineage relationships of isolated populations are influenced by limitations inherent in any of the *in vitro* or *in vivo* assays employed to examine differentiation potential.[43]

For several decades, our understanding of hematopoiesis has been built on a hierarchical schema in which all the pathways of differentiation lead away from a multipotent HSC, and progress through discrete progenitor stages that mark each branch-point of lineage commitment (Chap. 18). In the classical paradigm, the earliest differentiation "decision" made by an HSC is to enter one of two pathways, marked by either a common lymphoid progenitor (CLP) or a common myeloid progenitor (CMP), which has full myeloid and erythromegakaryocytic differentiation potential (Fig. 74–2).[44] With each successive stage of differentiation, lineage-specific cell-surface markers and transcription factors are upregulated, and alternative lineage potentials are lost. Consequently, the CLP is defined as a single cell that can give rise to all lymphoid lineages (B, T, and NK), but cannot generate myeloid, erythroid, or megakaryocytic lineages. The concept of progenitor populations marking two mutually exclusive differentiation pathways, one limited to myeloid and erythromegakaryocytic potential and the second defining

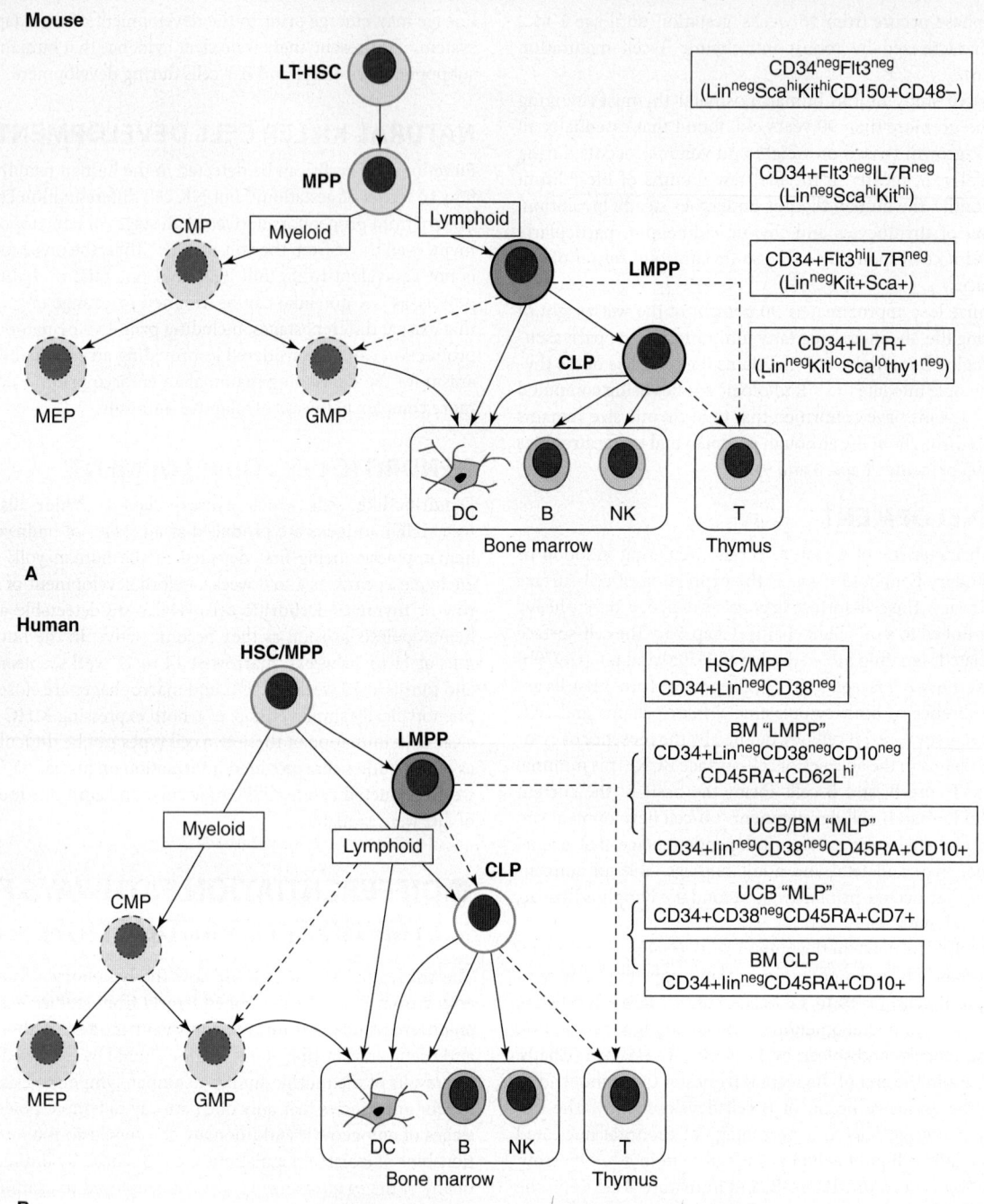

Figure 74–2. Postnatal pathways of lymphopoiesis in mice and humans. The key immunophenotype used to isolate each population is shown in boxes on the right. In parentheses under the main immunophenotypes are other markers also associated with each population. The exact relationship between lymphoid-primed multipotential progenitors (LMPPs) and common lymphoid progenitors (CLPs), and between LMPPs and myeloid progenitors remains controversial, as does the main cell type that initiates thymopoiesis (all shown as dashed lines). In both mice and humans, dendritic cells (DCs) can be produced *in vitro* from all prospectively identified lymphoid progenitors as well as myeloid progenitors. **A.** Murine lymphoid progenitor pathways. Populations with multilineage potential include long-term hematopoietic stem cells (LT-HSCs) and multipotential progenitors (MPPs). FLT3+ LMPPs, have full lymphoid (T-, B-, and natural killer [NK] cell developmental potential) and limited myeloid (nonclonogenic, mostly monocyte) potential. In the CLP, all myeloid potential is lost and full lymphoid potential remains. **B.** Human lymphoid progenitor pathways. Populations with multilineage potential include HSC and LMPP (aka multilymphoid progenitor [MLP]), which have full lymphoid (T-, B-, and NK cell developmental potential) and limited myeloid (mostly monocyte) potential. The CD10+ CLP has predominantly B, and some NK and T potential and is almost devoid of myeloid potential. Alternative phenotypic markers reported for each progenitor type with similar lineage potential are shown. BM, marrow; GMP, granulocyte-macrophage progenitor; MEP, megakaryocyte-erythroid progenitor.

lymphoid commitment, was held long before cells that satisfied the criteria of CLP were identified.[45–47] In contrast, the existence of single clonogenic cells with myeloid, erythroid, and megakaryocyte lineages was shown more than three decades ago through the use of *in vitro* clonal assays to demonstrate so-called colony-forming unit-granulocyte erythromyeloid megakaryocyte,[48] and later confirmed using markers to prospectively isolate such cells in mice[49] and humans.[50] The lymphocyte lineages were assumed to be closely related because of a number of associations, for example, common anatomical sites of T and B lymphopoiesis (spleen, lymph nodes; Chap. 6), similar molecular mechanisms that regulate T-cell receptor and B-cell immunoglobulin rearrangements (Chaps. 75 and 76), and severe B- and T-lymphoid defects that result from single genetic mutations in mice (Chap. 80).[51]

Development of flow cytometry (synonym: fluorescence-activated cell sorting [FACS]) made possible the isolation of rare hematopoietic cell populations and the subsequent interrogation of lineage potential using *in vitro* cultures and *in vivo* reconstitution studies (Chap. 18). Primitive multilymphoid progenitors with little or no clonogenic myeloid or erythroid potential have now been isolated from human tissue using flow cytometry with combinations of various cell-surface markers.[52–54] However, it seems likely that lineage relationships are less-strictly organized than once believed. Studies in mice show that the erythroid and megakaryocytic lineages can branch off at an earlier point in hematopoiesis, and that lymphoid (i.e., T, B, and NK) and myeloid (or at least monocytic) lineages can arise from the same pathway through a so-called lymphoid-primed multipotent progenitor (LMPP).[55] It remains unclear which of these lineage differentiation pathways are most physiologically significant during steady-state hematopoiesis, but it is likely that more than one pathway can exist simultaneously and alternative pathways may predominate during different stages of ontogeny and from different sites of hematopoiesis.

MURINE LYMPHOID PROGENITORS

In 1997, investigators working with murine marrow cells, isolated progenitors that possessed no myeloid or erythromegakaryocytic potential, but when transplanted into irradiated recipients could rapidly restore T-, B-, and NK cell lineages.[56] Clonal *in vitro* and *in vivo* studies showed that all lymphoid lineages were derived from a single common progenitor, thus proving the existence of the long-assumed CLP and supporting the classical model of lymphopoiesis. This study isolated cells based in part on expression of interleukin-7 receptor alpha (IL-7Rα).[56] The IL-7Rα+ CLP do not express hematopoietic markers associated with fully differentiated lineages (they are called "lineage negative" or "lin^neg" cells). As an indication that they are more differentiated than multilineage HSCs, expression of certain HSC-related cell-surface markers (Sca-1, Thy-1, c-kit) is downregulated.[56] Thus the full immunophenotype assigned to the murine CLP is Lin^neg IL-7Rα+ Thy-1^neg Sca-1^lo c-kit^lo. This contrasts the murine CLP immunophenotype with that of the murine HSC, which is found within the Lin^neg IL-7Rα^neg Thy-1^lo Sca-1^hi c-kit^hi population.[56]

Work with murine marrow has prompted a reexamination of when the lymphoid lineage pathways diverge from those of the myeloid and erythroid lineages (see Fig. 74–2). A population from murine marrow cells, defined largely by expression of the receptor FLT3 (Fms-like tyrosine kinase 3), has been shown to possess full lymphoid and some myeloid potential, but not erythroid or megakaryocytic potential.[55,57] These lin^negsca-1+c-kit+CD34+FLT3^hi (synonym: LSK CD34+FLT3^hi) cells are primed for lymphoid commitment in that they have downregulated genes involved in erythromegakaryocytic differentiation and upregulated lymphoid-associated genes.[58] They have thus been termed LMPPs.[55,58] Although they are able to generate monocytes and granulocytes *in vitro*, their differentiation potential is nonetheless skewed

heavily to lymphoid cells; after transplantation into irradiated recipients, LSK CD34+FLT3^hi cells rapidly reconstitute B and T lymphopoiesis. However, unlike the multipotent LSK CD34+FLT3^neg cells, reconstitution of myeloid lineages *in vivo* from LSK CD34+FLT3^hi is very limited, and importantly lacks granulocytic potential.[55] Indeed, subsequent *in vivo* fate-mapping studies have questioned the physiologic importance of a lymphomyeloid differentiation pathway to steady-state myeloid development, both in the marrow and thymus.[59,60]

One confusing factor in defining lineage potential is the ability of both myeloid and lymphoid progenitor populations to differentiate into DCs, at least *in vitro* (Chap. 21).[61–63] As *in vitro*-derived DC express many cell-surface markers common to myeloid antigen-presenting cells, irrespective of the lineage of origin, the extent to which identification of *in vitro* myeloid potential is confounded by a DC program is unclear.

HUMAN LYMPHOID PROGENITORS

The CD34 cell-surface marker is expressed on human HSCs and on a variety of different types of hematopoietic progenitors, including those restricted to lymphoid development (Chap. 18).[64,65] CD34 has been combined with additional cell-surface markers to identify human multilymphoid progenitors, for example, CD10,[52,66] CD7,[53,54,67,68] and CD45RA.[52,67] Similar to the mouse CLP, in addition to the upregulation of expression of the aforementioned markers, lymphoid commitment is accompanied by downregulation of certain HSC cell-surface markers, such as c-kit and Thy-1.[41]

As in murine studies, no one marker used in isolation is able to define a human lymphoid progenitor.[65] For example, although the expression of CD7 can be used to define a subset of CD34+lin^negCD38^neg cells in cord blood that are multilymphoid progenitors without myeloid or erythroid potential,[53,54] CD34+lin^negCD38+CD7+ cells from cord blood have full lineage (lymphoid, myeloid, and erythroid) potential. Furthermore, when comparing the progenitor populations identified in human studies with those described from murine experiments it is important to recognize that species differences exist between cell-surface markers.[41] For example, IL-7Rα expression is used to define murine CLP,[56] but CD34+lin^negCD38^negCD7+ multilymphoid progenitors in human cord blood do not express IL-7Rα,[53] and CD34+lin^negCD38+IL-7Rα+ cells in human cord blood have both myeloid, lymphoid and even some erythroid potential. A different ontogeny and source of hematopoietic cells will also introduce unexpected variations of progenitor immunophenotype and function.[41] Whereas most murine studies have been conducted with adult murine marrow, most human studies have been performed with umbilical cord blood, a more logistically available source containing progenitors that are significantly more proliferative than marrow.[69] Again using the example of the CD34+lin^negCD38^negCD7+ multilymphoid progenitor, although this immunophenotype can be used to identify multilymphoid progenitors in cord blood,[53] the same markers cannot be used in human marrow because CD34+lin^negCD38^neg marrow cells do not express CD7. Two candidates for the human equivalent of the murine LMPP have been described, both of which coexpress FLT3: one in the marrow identified as CD34+lin^negCD38+CD45RA+ and high expression of CD62L (L-selectin)[70]; and another in the marrow and cord blood characterized as a CD34+lin^negCD38^negThy-1^lo/negCD45RA+ multilymphoid progenitor (MLP).[71] The hierarchical relationship of these two populations to each other, or to the marrow CD34+lin^negCD38+CD45RA+CD10+ CLP is unclear; and as in the murine system, the physiologic contributions of a lymphomyeloid developmental pathway to steady-state hematopoiesis has yet to be determined. Adding to the concept of possible independence of dendritic cell development, DC potential has been found in all the primitive human lymphoid progenitors reported.[52,53,67,70–72]

THYMIC PROGENITORS

It was long assumed that lymphoid commitment in the marrow precedes thymic seeding and T-cell development. However, despite the clear existence of lymphoid-committed progenitors within the marrow, the dominant cell type that migrates from the marrow and seeds the thymus to initiate thymopoiesis is still a matter of controversy. As described above, a variety of marrow-derived lymphoid-restricted progenitors and LMPPs are each able to generate T cells *in vitro* and *in vivo*. However, careful examination of the thymus has revealed primitive progenitors that have not only lymphoid, but also myeloid and erythroid potential. Such rare cells have been identified in murine thymus, where they are referred to as early thymic progenitors (ETP),[73] and also in human thymus, where they have the phenotype CD34+lin^neg^CD1a^neg^ CD7^neg^.[74,75] The lineage potential of such cells as well as the sharing of many cell-surface markers and similar gene expression profile to HSCs, suggest strongly that HSCs or at least multipotent progenitors are able to seed the thymus directly without a preceding stage of lymphoid commitment in the marrow. Which of these alternative progenitor types are dominant in terms of their contribution to steady-state thymopoiesis is yet to be determined[76]; however, it is likely that early thymic progenitor lineage potential is itself dynamic, based on colonization of the murine thymus with temporally distinct waves of both lymphoid-restricted and multipotent thymic-seeding progenitors during embryonic development.[77]

CHALLENGES IN FUNCTIONAL CHARACTERIZATION OF LYMPHOID PROGENITORS

The accurate assignment of lineage potential to immunophenotypically defined progenitors requires clonal analysis. Although clonal assays for myelo-erythromegakaryocytic progenitors have existed for more than 30 years,[48] the ability to differentiate HSCs along lymphoid pathways has been relatively recent, particularly for human studies.[43] *In vitro* assays for human lymphoid potential became available when it was observed that selected murine stromal cell lines were capable of supporting B-cell, NK cell, and DC differentiation from primitive human HSCs.[78–80] T-cell differentiation systems are more complex, requiring an *in vitro* model that recapitulates the unique environment of the thymus. Originally this was only possible using the fetal thymic organ culture method, a system in which large numbers of murine or human progenitors are seeded into whole thymic lobes in so-called hanging drop cultures.[81] A more efficient *in vitro* system for studying murine and human T-cell differentiation has been developed using a murine stromal monolayer that expresses the Notch ligand Delta-like 1 ("OP9-DL1 stroma").[82] However, none of the *in vitro* T-cell culture systems simultaneously support B-cell development, making proof of full T- and B-lymphoid potential at a clonal level technically problematic. *In vivo* transplantation of a single murine HSC can prove multilineage potential at a clonal level, but this also is technically difficult, especially when studying progenitor populations that are not self-renewing. *In vivo* studies with human cells are particularly challenging as they rely on xenogeneic transplant models with low engraftment efficiency.[41,43]

● REGULATION OF LYMPHOPOIESIS

CYTOKINES IN LYMPHOPOIESIS

The many cytokine pathways that regulate lymphoid development, differentiation, and function are too numerous and complex for a full description here. However, the cytokine receptors of the common gamma (γ_c) chain family should be mentioned particularly because

of their biologic importance in lymphopoiesis and their clinical relevance in primary immune deficiency disease. The γ_c subunit is a signaling component of six different cytokine receptors, interleukin (IL)-2,[83] IL-4,[84,85] IL-7,[86,87] IL-9,[88] IL-15,[89] and IL-21,[90] all of which act on different stages and pathways involved in lymphopoiesis.[51,91,92] All six γ_c-dependent receptors are unique in their activation of the Janus kinase 3 (JAK3) tyrosine kinase, a molecule that directly interacts with γ_c to mediate signaling.[93] In addition to the γ_c subunit, each of these receptors are comprised of an α subunit through which specific ligands bind; IL-2R and IL-15R also share a common β subunit.[51]

Null mutations of γ_c result in severe combined immunodeficiency (SCID) syndromes in mice and humans. However differences in the specific lineages affected reveal important species differences in cytokine dependency.[51] The most important of these differences is in the requirement for IL-7 signaling in human and murine B-cell development. Adult murine B-cell development has an absolute requirement for IL-7 to IL-7R interaction and subsequent downstream signaling involving the γ_c subunit of the IL-7R and JAK3.[94] In contrast, IL-7 is not essential for human B-cell development. X-linked SCID patients with mutations in the γ_c cytokine-receptor subunit exhibit profound thymic hypoplasia and an absence of NK cells but normal or elevated numbers of B cells.[51] SCID patients with mutations in JAK3[95,96] or the IL-7R[97] also have normal numbers of blood B cells. Although B-cell numbers are normal, B-cell function in patients with γ_c-deficient SCID is not normal and patients are hypogammaglobulinemic, presumably partly as a result of the role of IL-4 in B-cell function and the absence of T-cell interactions in antibody production. These collective results indicate IL-7 is not essential for at least the numerically normal development of human B cells.

NK cells are absent in patients with γ_c-deficient and JAK3-deficient SCID, but are normal in IL-7Rα deficiency.[65,97,98] NK cells are also absent in mice deficient in IL-15,[99] IL-15Rα,[100] or IL-2Rβ (a subunit shared by IL-2R and IL-15R),[101] demonstrating the essential role of IL-15, but not IL-7, in NK cell development. Although no null mutations for IL-15 or its receptor have been described in humans, a familial NK cell deficiency has been described in humans in which the response to IL-15 and IL-2 appears to be subnormal.[102]

The production of both B and NK cells in patients with IL-7Rα deficiency, shows that in humans IL-7 is not required for the earliest stages of lymphoid commitment or growth of CLPs. This point is further supported with the finding that multilymphoid CD34+CD38^neg^CD7+ progenitors in human cord blood do not express IL-7Rα,[53] and that early lymphoid progenitor subsets are preserved in the marrow of γ_c and JAK3-deficient patients.[103] In contrast to B cells and NK cells, however, T-cell development is absolutely dependent on IL-7 in both mice and humans.[91] In both species, mutations of any portion of the IL-7 signaling pathway, that is, γ_c, IL-7Rα, or JAK3, completely prevents T-cell development.[51] IL-2, in contrast, although an important cytokine in proliferation and function of mature T cells, is not essential for thymopoiesis; mutations in IL-2,[104] IL-2Rα, or IL2Rβ[105] result in functional T-cell defects, but T cells are not absent.

TRANSCRIPTIONAL REGULATION IN LYMPHOPOIESIS

The hierarchical differentiation pathways that lead irreversibly to the diverse array of functionally specialized mature lymphocytes are regulated by groups of genes expressed and repressed in a complex, precisely orchestrated sequence. As with cytokine regulation, our understanding of which transcriptional factors control each stage of differentiation has been developed using a combination of gene expression analyses in isolated progenitors and precursors, and an examination of the functional consequences of genetic mutations in mice and humans. The review in this chapter focuses on genes that regulate the earliest commitment decisions in the production of lymphoid progenitors; regulation of later differentiation stages in each lineage is discussed in Chaps. 75 to 77, respectively.

The complex interplay between groups of genes involved in hematopoietic differentiation has been likened to a multidimensional network whose "regulatory space" is formed by a dynamic balance between certain transcriptional regulators.[106] Expression analysis of multiple genes in defined progenitor populations demonstrates levels of promiscuity at early stages of hematopoiesis, that preclude assignment of any unique gene expression pattern to each stage.[106–108] As differentiation proceeds, a more specific "genetic fingerprint" for each lineage develops.

Regulation of Early Lymphoid Commitment

Ikaros Although no single gene has been identified as a lymphoid-specific master regulator, several transcription factors have been shown to be essential for the early stages of lymphopoiesis. The gene *Ikaros*, which encodes a family of DNA-binding zinc finger proteins, was identified in murine knockout studies as essential for all fetal lymphopoiesis.[109,110] However, in the postnatal setting, the role of Ikaros is more complex and less specific. Adult Ikaros[null] mice completely lack B cells, and although T cells are produced, their differentiation is abnormal.[111] A murine study has suggested that Ikaros is not required for the initial lymphomyeloid versus myeloerythroid commitment decision, and that not only lymphoid differentiation, but also certain fate choices in the myeloerythroid pathway are affected by Ikaros.[112] As the expression of two key lymphoid cytokine receptors, FLT3 and IL-7Rα, is dependent on Ikaros, and as these markers are used to isolate murine LMPP and CLP, respectively, it is still not completely clear at which exact lymphoid progenitor stage Ikaros exerts its effects.[112] In addition to lymphoid progenitors, Ikaros isoforms are also expressed in HSCs, and myeloid lineages in mice[112–116] and humans.[116,117] Although Ikaros may act as a typical transcription factor in some settings, Ikaros also affects gene expression through its role in chromatin formation.[118]

Pu.1 The transcription factor PU.1 is essential for normal B- and T-lymphocyte development, but its effects are highly dose dependent. At high levels of PU.1, key myeloid regulatory genes are upregulated and macrophage differentiation is induced preferentially over lymphoid differentiation.[119] Low-level expression of PU.1, however, is essential for lymphopoiesis.[120,121] Mice in which PU.1 is completely absent lack B cells and have abnormal fetal thymopoiesis. However, studies with mice in which PU.1 is deleted specifically in B-lineage cells show that PU.1 is not essential for B-cell differentiation beyond the pre-B stage.[122] It is likely that the critical role for PU.1 in murine lymphopoiesis lies in its upregulation of expression of the receptor for IL-7, which as mentioned above, is a key cytokine in both B and T lymphopoiesis in mice.[120]

E2A E2A (encoded by *TCF3*) generates two basic helix-loop-helix proteins, E12 and E47, through differential splicing.[123] Murine studies suggest that E2A is necessary for lymphoid priming of multipotent progenitors and that the E2A proteins prime expression of a number of lymphoid-associated genes.[124] There is a dose-dependent requirement for E2A expression in the development of LMPP and CLP.[124] Both B- and T-lineage commitment are severely reduced in the absence of E2A, but Ikaros and PU.1 expression are normal.[124–126] E2A affects B lymphopoiesis in part through upregulation of early B-cell factor (EBF)[127] and T lymphopoiesis through upregulation of expression and function of the key T-cell specification factor Notch 1.[128]

Regulation of B-Cell Commitment

The transcription factors Ikaros, PU.1, E2A, EBF, and Pax5 are essential for normal B-cell differentiation. Mice that have functional deletions in any one of these genes have severely abnormal B-cell development; however, of these genes, only EBF and Pax5 are B-cell specific within the hematopoietic system.

Pax5 Pax5 is expressed specifically in B-lineage–committed progenitors and is required for normal expression of the B-lineage genes CD19 and CD79a.[121] Pax5-/- mice are blocked at the pro-B cell stage, but express most early B-cell–related genes.[129] Although Pax5 can activate a small subset of B-lineage genes, its main function in B-cell differentiation appears to be the suppression of T-cell and myeloid transcriptional programs at the murine pro-B-cell stage, thus enforcing commitment to the B lineage.[121,129,130] Consistent with this role, PU.1, E2A, and EBF function earlier than Pax5 in B lymphopoiesis, and forced expression of Pax5 does not rescue the B-cell defect seen in EBF-/- mice or PU.1-/- mice.[121]

Ebf EBF (encoded by *EBF1*) is a helix-loop-helix zinc finger protein that activates a B-lineage transcriptional program, and induces B lymphoid in preference to myeloid development, in part by antagonizing the expression of genes encoding alternative lineages such as C/EBPα (CCAAT/enhancer binding protein), Id2, and PU.1,[131] and, in part, by inducing Pax5 expression.[121] *Ebf1*-/- lymphoid progenitor populations from mice lack the ability to generate B cells but retain the ability to generate T, NK, and myeloid cells.[131] Overexpression of EBF in multipotent progenitors promotes B-cell production at the expense of myeloid differentiation.[131] EBF and E2A function cooperatively in early B lymphopoiesis[124]; however, overexpression of EBF can rescue B-cell differentiation in E2A-deficient mice, including activation of Pax5.[132] Pax5 overexpression however cannot rescue the B-cell defect in EBF-/- mice,[121] demonstrating a critical, Pax5-independent role of EBF in early B-cell fate decisions.

Regulation of T-Cell Commitment

Notch Upon arrival into the thymus, multipotent progenitors from the marrow become rapidly committed to the T- and NK-cell pathways. The most important environmental cue for T-cell commitment is delivered by the thymic epithelium in the form of the Notch ligands, Delta-like 1 (*DLL1*) and Delta-like 4 (*DLL4*).[133] Binding of one of these ligands to the Notch 1 receptor expressed on the surface of thymocyte precursors causes activation of intracellular Notch and a series of transcriptional programs turn on to switch lineage fate toward the T lineage at the expense of B-cell development.[133] In mice, Notch is absolutely required for T-cell differentiation and proliferation, including β selection.[134] Analogous to control of early B cell differentiation by E2A, Notch signaling activates a transcriptional network which includes factors critical for lineage specification (GATA-3, TCF-1), and commitment (BCL11b).[135] However, although Notch signaling is necessary for murine thymopoiesis it is not sufficient for activation of the full complement of T-cell genes.[136] The ability of hematopoietic progenitors to respond to Notch signaling and commit to T-lineage fate depends on a balance between positive and negative regulators. Combinations of at least four other transcription factors are required to initiate T-cell development: PU.1, Ikaros, Runx family factors, and E2A.[124,133] In addition, leukemia-lymphoma–related factor (LRF/Pokemon, encoded by *Zbtb7a*) must be downregulated to allow Notch signaling to induce T-cell fate decisions.[137] Notch signaling also plays important roles at later stages of thymocyte differentiation.[133]

The effects of Notch signaling have been extensively studied in mice, but the exact stages and processes regulated by Notch appear to differ between mice and humans. For example, using *in vitro* studies of human T-cell development, it appears that while Notch is essential for early thymocyte proliferation, it is not required for β selection or T-cell receptor αβ differentiation.[138,139] As with so much of the information described in this chapter, the most important challenge that lies ahead is to translate the detailed mechanistic framework developed from murine studies into careful investigations of human lymphopoiesis.

GATA-3   GATA-3 is a key transcriptional factor for T-cell development, and is essential at various stages of differentiation. However, in addition to T cells, GATA-3 is also expressed in uncommitted HSCs, CLPs, and even in nonhematopoietic cells, and its effects are complex and highly dose-dependent.[33,135,140]

Tcf-1   TCF-1 (encoded by the *TCF7* gene) is a transcription factor essential for T-cell development, and is directly activated by Notch signaling.[141,142] In ETPs, TCF-1 promotes cell survival as well as activation of T-lineage specific genes, including *Gata3* and *Bcl11b*.[141,142] Induction of a T-cell specific transcriptional program by TCF-1 can occur even in the absence of Notch signaling; however, it cannot activate the essential T-lineage gene *Ptcra*,[142] indicating that, as in B-cell development, T-cell specification occurs through both hierarchical and combinatorial transcription factor interactions.

Bcl11b   BCL11B was identified as a transcription factor required for the normal generation of $\alpha\beta$ T cells during β selection; however, upregulation of Bcl11b first occurs at the earlier CD4^{neg}CD8^{neg} (double negative)-2 (DN2) stage, likely through transcriptional activation by TCF-1.[135] In DN2 cells, Bcl11b appears to contribute minimally to the T-lineage specification program governed by Notch/E2A/GATA-3/TCF-1 activity, but rather is required for the suppression of stem/multipotent progenitor-associated genes, which marks the loss of myeloid potential and final commitment to the T-cell lineage.[143]

REFERENCES

1. Tavian M, Peault B: Embryonic development of the human hematopoietic system. *Int J Dev Biol* 49:243, 2005.
2. Ueno H, Weissman IL: Stem cells: Blood lines from embryo to adult. *Nature* 446:996, 2007.
3. Medvinsky A, Dzierzak E: Definitive hematopoiesis is autonomously initiated by the AGM region. *Cell* 86:897, 1996.
4. Yoder MC, Hiatt K, Mukherjee P: *In vivo* repopulating hematopoietic stem cells are present in the murine yolk sac at day 9.0 postcoitus. *Proc Natl Acad Sci U S A* 94:6776, 1997.
5. Yoder MC, Hiatt K, Dutt P, et al: Characterization of definitive lymphohematopoietic stem cells in the day 9 murine yolk sac. *Immunity* 7:335, 1997.
6. Yoder MC, Hiatt K: Engraftment of embryonic hematopoietic cells in conditioned newborn recipients. *Blood* 89:2176, 1997.
7. Koushik SV1, Wang J, Rogers R, et al: Targeted inactivation of the sodium-calcium exchanger (Ncx1) results in the lack of a heartbeat and abnormal myofibrillar organization. *FASEB J* 15:1209, 2001.
8. Rhodes KE, Gekas C, Wang Y, et al: The emergence of hematopoietic stem cells is initiated in the placental vasculature in the absence of circulation. *Cell Stem Cell* 2:252, 2008.
9. Palis J, Yoder MC: Yolk-sac hematopoiesis: The first blood cells of mouse and man. *Exp Hematol* 29:927, 2001.
10. Yokota T: Tracing the first waves of lymphopoiesis in mice. *Development* 133:2041, 2006.
11. Böiers C, Carrelha J, Lutteropp M, et al: Lymphomyeloid contribution of an immune-restricted progenitor emerging prior to definitive hematopoietic stem cells. *Cell Stem Cell* 13:535, 2013.
12. Yoshimoto M, Montecino-Rodriguez E, Ferkowicz MJ, et al: Embryonic day 9 yolk sac and intra-embryonic hemogenic endothelium independently generate a B-1 and marginal zone progenitor lacking B-2 potential. *Proc Natl Acad Sci U S A* 108:1468, 2011.
13. Yoshimoto M, Porayette P, Glosson NL, et al: Autonomous murine T-cell progenitor production in the extra-embryonic yolk sac before HSC emergence. *Blood* 119:5706, 2012.
14. Inlay MA, Serwold T, Mosley A, et al: Identification of multipotent progenitors that emerge prior to hematopoietic stem cells in embryonic development. *Stem Cell Reports* 2:457, 2014.
15. Auerbach R: Experimental analysis of the origin of cell types in the development of the mouse thymus. *Dev Biol* 3:336, 1961.
16. Owen JJ, Ritter MA: Tissue interaction in the development of thymus lymphocytes. *J Exp Med* 129:431, 1969.
17. Oberlin E, Tavian M, Blazsek I, Péault B: Blood-forming potential of vascular endothelium in the human embryo. *Development* 129:4147, 2002.
18. Tavian M, Robin C, Coulombel L, Péault B: The human embryo, but not its yolk sac, generates lympho-myeloid stem cells: Mapping multipotent hematopoietic cell fate in intraembryonic mesoderm. *Immunity* 15:487, 2001.
19. Tavian M, Coulombel L, Luton D, et al: Aorta-associated CD34+ hematopoietic cells in the early human embryo. *Blood* 87:67, 1996.
20. Robin C, Bollerot K, Mendes S, et al: Human placenta is a potent hematopoietic niche containing hematopoietic stem and progenitor cells throughout development. *Cell Stem Cell* 5:385, 2009.
21. Lee LK, Ueno M, Van Handel B, Mikkola HK: Placenta as a newly identified source of hematopoietic stem cells. *Curr Opin Hematol* 17:313, 2010.
22. Tavian M, Hallais MF, Peault B: Emergence of intraembryonic hematopoietic precursors in the pre-liver human embryo. *Development* 126:793, 1999.
23. Charbord P, Tavian M, Humeau L, Péault B: Early ontogeny of the human marrow from long bones: An immunohistochemical study of hematopoiesis and its microenvironment. *Blood* 87:4109, 1996.
24. Haynes BF: The human thymic microenvironment. *Adv Immunol* 36:87, 1984.
25. Hayward AR: Development of lymphocyte responses and interactions in the human fetus and newborn. *Immunol Rev* 57:39, 1981.
26. Toivanen P, Uksila J, Leino A: Development of mitogen responding T cells and natural killer cells in the human fetus. *Immunol Rev* 57:89, 1981.
27. Renda MC, Fecarotta E, Dieli F, et al: Evidence of alloreactive T lymphocytes in fetal liver: Implications for fetal hematopoietic stem cell transplantation. *Bone Marrow Transplant* 25:135, 2000.
28. Steinmann GG: Changes in the human thymus during aging. *Curr Top Pathol* 75:43, 1986.
29. Moore AV, Korobkin M, Olanow W, et al: Age-related changes in the thymus gland: CT-pathologic correlation. *AJR Am J Roentgenol* 141:241, 1983.
30. LeBien TW: Fates of human B-cell precursors. *Blood* 96:9, 2000.
31. Dorshkind K, Montecino-Rodriguez E: Fetal B-cell lymphopoiesis and the emergence of B-1-cell potential. *Nat Rev Immunol* 7:213, 2007.
32. Solvason N, Kearney JF: The human fetal omentum: A site of B cell generation. *J Exp Med* 175:397, 1992.
33. Hofman FM, Danilovs J, Husmann L, Taylor CR: Ontogeny of B cell markers in the human fetal liver. *J Immunol* 133:1197, 1984.
34. Gathings WE, Lawton AR, Cooper MD: Immunofluorescent studies of the development of pre-B cells, B lymphocytes and immunoglobulin isotype diversity in humans. *Eur J Immunol* 7:804, 1977.
35. Nunez C, Nishimoto N, Gartland GL, et al: B cells are generated throughout life in humans. *J Immunol* 156:866, 1996.
36. Rossi MI, Yokota T, Medina KL, et al: B lymphopoiesis is active throughout human life, but there are developmental age-related changes. *Blood* 101:576, 2003.
37. Kroese FG, Ammerlaan WA, Deenen GJ: Location and function of B-cell lineages. *Ann N Y Acad Sci* 651:44, 1992.
38. Kantor AB, Herzenberg LA: Origin of murine B cell lineages. *Annu Rev Immunol* 11:501, 1993.
39. Janossy G, Bofill M, Poulter LW, et al: Separate ontogeny of two macrophage-like accessory cell populations in the human fetus. *J Immunol* 136:4354, 1986.
40. Hofman FM, Danilovs JA, Taylor CR: HLA-DR (Ia)-positive dendritic-like cells in human fetal nonlymphoid tissues. *Transplantation* 37:590, 1984.
41. Payne KJ, Crooks GM: Immune-cell lineage commitment: Translation from mice to humans. *Immunity* 26:674, 2007.
42. Kincade PW, Owen JJ, Igarashi H, et al: Nature or nurture? Steady-state lymphocyte formation in adults does not recapitulate ontogeny. *Immunol Rev* 187:116, 2002.
43. Payne KJ, Crooks GM: Human hematopoietic lineage commitment. *Immunol Rev* 187:48, 2002.
44. Reya T, Morrison SJ, Clarke MF, Weissman IL: Stem cells, cancer, and cancer stem cells. *Nature* 414:105, 2001.
45. Hakoda M, Hirai Y, Shimba H, et al: Cloning of phenotypically different human lymphocytes originating from a single stem cell. *J Exp Med* 169:1265, 1989.
46. Gore SD, Kastan MB, Civin CI: Normal human bone marrow precursors that express terminal deoxynucleotidyl transferase include T-cell precursors and possible lymphoid stem cells. *Blood* 77:1681, 1991.
47. Terstappen LW, Huang S, Picker LJ: Flow cytometric assessment of human T-cell differentiation in thymus and bone marrow. *Blood* 79:666, 1992.
48. Johnson GR, Metcalf D: Pure and mixed erythroid colony formation in vitro stimulated by spleen conditioned medium with no detectable erythropoietin. *Proc Natl Acad Sci U S A* 74:3879, 1977.
49. Akashi K, Traver D, Miyamoto T, Weissman IL: A clonogenic common myeloid progenitor that gives rise to all myeloid lineages. *Nature* 404:193, 2000.
50. Manz MG, Miyamoto T, Akashi K, Weissman IL: Prospective isolation of human clonogenic common myeloid progenitors. *Proc Natl Acad Sci U S A* 99:11872, 2002.
51. Leonard WJ: Cytokines and immunodeficiency diseases. *Nat Rev Immunol* 1:200, 2001.
52. Galy A, Travis M, Cen D, Chen B: Human T, B, natural killer, and dendritic cells arise from a common bone marrow progenitor cell subset. *Immunity* 3:459, 1995.
53. Hao QL, Zhu J, Price MA, et al: Identification of a novel, human multilymphoid progenitor in cord blood. *Blood* 97:3683, 2001.
54. Hoebeke I, De Smedt M, Stolz F, et al: T-, B- and NK-lymphoid, but not myeloid cells arise from human CD34(+)CD38(–)CD7(+) common lymphoid progenitors expressing lymphoid-specific genes. *Leukemia* 21:311, 2007.
55. Adolfsson J, Månsson R, Buza-Vidas N, et al: Identification of Flt3+ lympho-myeloid stem cells lacking erythro-megakaryocytic potential a revised road map for adult blood lineage commitment. *Cell* 121:295, 2005.
56. Kondo M, Weissman IL, Akashi K: Identification of clonogenic common lymphoid progenitors in mouse bone marrow. *Cell* 91:661, 1997.

57. Yang L, Bryder D, Adolfsson J, et al: Identification of Lin(−)Sca1(+)kit(+)CD34(+) Flt3-short-term hematopoietic stem cells capable of rapidly reconstituting and rescuing myeloablated transplant recipients. *Blood* 105:2717, 2005.

58. Luc S, Buza-Vidas N, Jacobsen SE: Biological and molecular evidence for existence of lymphoid-primed multipotent progenitors. *Ann N Y Acad Sci* 1106:89, 2007.

59. Boyer SW, Schroeder AV, Smith-Berdan S, Forsberg EC: All hematopoietic cells develop from hematopoietic stem cells through Flk2/Flt3-positive progenitor cells. *Cell Stem Cell* 9:64, 2011.

60. Schlenner SM, Madan V, Busch K, et al: Fate mapping reveals separate origins of T cells and myeloid lineages in the thymus. *Immunity* 32:426, 2010.

61. Wu L, Liu YJ: Development of dendritic-cell lineages. *Immunity* 26:741, 2007.

62. Wu L, Vandenabeele S, Georgopoulos K: Derivation of dendritic cells from myeloid and lymphoid precursors. *Int Rev Immunol* 20:117, 2001.

63. Manz MG, Traver D, Miyamoto T, et al: Dendritic cell potentials of early lymphoid and myeloid progenitors. *Blood* 97:3333, 2001.

64. Civin CI, Gore SD: Antigenic analysis of hematopoiesis: A review. *J Hematother* 2:137, 1993.

65. Blom B, Spits H: Development of human lymphoid cells. *Annu Rev Immunol* 24:287, 2006.

66. Six EM, Bonhomme D, Monteiro M, et al: A human postnatal lymphoid progenitor capable of circulating and seeding the thymus. *J Exp Med* 204:3085, 2007.

67. Canque B, Camus S, Dalloul A, et al: Characterization of dendritic cell differentiation pathways from cord blood CD34(+)CD7(+)CD45RA(+) hematopoietic progenitor cells. *Blood* 96:3748, 2000.

68. Storms RW, Goodell MA, Fisher A, et al: Hoechst dye efflux reveals a novel CD7 (+) CD34(−) lymphoid progenitor in human umbilical cord blood. *Blood* 96:2125, 2000.

69. Hao QL, Shah AJ, Thiemann FT, et al: A functional comparison of CD34+ CD38− cells in cord blood and bone marrow. *Blood* 86:3745, 1995.

70. Kohn LA, Hao QL, Sasidharan R, et al: Lymphoid priming in human bone marrow begins before expression of CD10 with upregulation of L-selectin. *Nat Immunol* 13:963, 2012.

71. Doulatov S, Notta F, Eppert K, et al: Revised map of the human progenitor hierarchy shows the origin of macrophages and dendritic cells in early lymphoid development. *Nat Immunol* 11:585, 2010.

72. Bjorck P, Kincade PW: CD19+ pro-B cells can give rise to dendritic cells in vitro. *J Immunol* 161:5795, 1998.

73. Allman D, Sambandam A, Kim S, et al: Thymopoiesis independent of common lymphoid progenitors. *Nat Immunol* 4:168, 2003.

74. Hao QL, George AA, Zhu J, et al: Human intrathymic lineage commitment is marked by differential CD7 expression: Identification of CD7− lympho-myeloid thymic progenitors. *Blood* 111:1318, 2008.

75. Weerkamp F, Baert MR, Brugman MH, et al: Human thymus contains multipotent progenitors with T/B lymphoid, myeloid, and erythroid lineage potential. *Blood* 107: 3131, 2006.

76. Bhandoola A, Sambandam A, Allman D, et al: Early T lineage progenitors: New insights, but old questions remain. *J Immunol* 171:5653, 2003.

77. Ramond C, Berthault C, Burlen-Defranoux O, et al: Two waves of distinct hematopoietic progenitor cells colonize the fetal thymus. *Nat Immunol* 15:27, 2014.

78. Rawlings DJ, Quan S, Hao QL, et al: Differentiation of human CD34+CD38− cord blood stem cells into B cell progenitors in vitro. *Exp Hematol* 25:66, 1997.

79. Berardi AC, Meffre E, Pflumio F, et al: Individual CD34+CD38lowCD19−CD10− progenitor cells from human cord blood generate B lymphocytes and granulocytes. *Blood* 89:3554, 1997.

80. Miller JS, McCullar V, Punzel M, et al: Single adult human CD34(+)/Lin−/CD38(−) progenitors give rise to natural killer cells, B-lineage cells, dendritic cells, and myeloid cells. *Blood* 93:96, 1999.

81. Plum J, De Smedt M, Verhasselt B, et al: Human T lymphopoiesis. *In vitro* and *in vivo* study models. *Ann N Y Acad Sci* 917:724, 2000.

82. Awong G, Herer E, Surh CD, et al: Characterization *in vitro* and engraftment potential *in vivo* of human progenitor T cells generated from hematopoietic stem cells. *Blood* 114:972, 2009.

83. Noguchi M, Yi H, Rosenblatt HM, et al: Interleukin-2 receptor gamma chain mutation results in X-linked severe combined immunodeficiency in humans. *Cell* 73:147, 1993.

84. Kondo M, Takeshita T, Ishii N, et al: Sharing of the interleukin-2 (IL-2) receptor gamma chain between receptors for IL-2 and IL-4. *Science* 262:1874, 1993.

85. Russell SM, Keegan AD, Harada N, et al: Interleukin-2 receptor gamma chain: A functional component of the interleukin-4 receptor. *Science* 262:1880, 1993.

86. Noguchi M, Nakamura Y, Russell SM, et al: Interleukin-2 receptor gamma chain: A functional component of the interleukin-7 receptor. *Science* 262:1877, 1993.

87. Kondo M, Takeshita T, Higuchi M, et al: Functional participation of the IL-2 receptor gamma chain in IL-7 receptor complexes. *Science* 263:1453, 1994.

88. Kimura Y, Takeshita T, Kondo M, et al: Sharing of the IL-2 receptor gamma chain with the functional IL-9 receptor complex. *Int Immunol* 7:115, 1995.

89. Giri JG, Ahdieh M, Eisenman J, et al: Utilization of the beta and gamma chains of the IL-2 receptor by the novel cytokine IL-15. *EMBO J* 13:2822, 1994.

90. Asao H, Okuyama C, Kumaki S, et al: Cutting edge: The common gamma-chain is an indispensable subunit of the IL-21 receptor complex. *J Immunol* 167:1, 2001.

91. Kang J, Der SD: Cytokine functions in the formative stages of a lymphocyte's life. *Curr Opin Immunol* 16:180, 2004.

92. Di Santo JP, Kuhn R, Muller W: Common cytokine receptor gamma chain (gamma c)-dependent cytokines: Understanding in vivo functions by gene targeting. *Immunol Rev* 148:19, 1995.

93. Russell SM, Johnston JA, Noguchi M, et al: Interaction of IL-2R beta and gamma c chains with Jak1 and Jak3: Implications for XSCID and XCID. *Science* 266:1042, 1994.

94. Candeias S, Muegge K, Durum SK: IL-7 receptor and VDJ recombination: Trophic versus mechanistic actions. *Immunity* 6:501, 1997.

95. Macchi P, Villa A, Giliani S, et al: Mutations of Jak-3 gene in patients with autosomal severe combined immune deficiency (SCID). *Nature* 377:65, 1995.

96. Russell SM, Tayebi N, Nakajima H, et al: Mutation of Jak3 in a patient with SCID: Essential role of Jak3 in lymphoid development. *Science* 270:797, 1995.

97. Puel A, Ziegler SF, Buckley RH, Leonard WJ: Defective IL7R expression in T(−) B(+) NK(+) severe combined immunodeficiency. *Nat Genet* 20:394, 1998.

98. Giliani S, Mori L, de Saint Basile G, et al: Interleukin-7 receptor alpha (IL-7Ralpha) deficiency: Cellular and molecular bases. Analysis of clinical, immunological, and molecular features in 16 novel patients. *Immunol Rev* 203:110, 2005.

99. Kennedy MK, Glaccum M, Brown SN, et al: Reversible defects in natural killer and memory CD8 T cell lineages in interleukin 15-deficient mice. *J Exp Med* 191:771, 2000.

100. Lodolce JP, Boone DL, Chai S, et al: IL-15 receptor maintains lymphoid homeostasis by supporting lymphocyte homing and proliferation. *Immunity* 9:669, 1998.

101. Suzuki H, Kündig TM, Furlonger C, et al: Deregulated T cell activation and autoimmunity in mice lacking interleukin-2 receptor beta. *Science* 268:1472, 1995.

102. Eidenschenk C, Jouanguy E, Alcaïs A, et al: Familial NK cell deficiency associated with impaired IL-2– and IL-15–dependent survival of lymphocytes. *J Immunol* 177:8835, 2006.

103. Kohn LA, Seet CS, Scholes J, et al: Human lymphoid development in the absence of common γ-chain receptor signaling. *J Immunol* 192:5050, 2014.

104. Weinberg K, Parkman R: Severe combined immunodeficiency due to a specific defect in the production of interleukin-2. *N Engl J Med* 322:1718, 1990.

105. Gilmour KC, Fujii H, Cranston T, et al: Defective expression of the interleukin-2/interleukin-15 receptor beta subunit leads to a natural killer cell-deficient form of severe combined immunodeficiency. *Blood* 98:877, 2001.

106. Warren LA, Rothenberg EV: Regulatory coding of lymphoid lineage choice by hematopoietic transcription factors. *Curr Opin Immunol* 15:166, 2003.

107. Akashi K, He X, Chen J, et al: Transcriptional accessibility for genes of multiple tissues and hematopoietic lineages is hierarchically controlled during early hematopoiesis. *Blood* 101:383, 2003.

108. Miyamoto T, Iwasaki H, Reizis B, et al: Myeloid or lymphoid promiscuity as a critical step in hematopoietic lineage commitment. *Dev Cell* 3:137, 2002.

109. Georgopoulos K, Bigby M, Wang JH, et al: The Ikaros gene is required for the development of all lymphoid lineages. *Cell* 79:143, 1994.

110. Wang JH, Nichogiannopoulou A, Wu L, et al: Selective defects in the development of the fetal and adult lymphoid system in mice with an Ikaros null mutation. *Immunity* 5:537, 1996.

111. Georgopoulos K, Winandy S, Avitahl N: The role of the Ikaros gene in lymphocyte development and homeostasis. *Annu Rev Immunol* 15:155, 1997.

112. Yoshida T, Ng SY, Zuniga-Pflucker JC, Georgopoulos K: Early hematopoietic lineage restrictions directed by Ikaros. *Nat Immunol* 7:382, 2006.

113. Nichogiannopoulou A, Trevisan M, Neben S, et al: Defects in hemopoietic stem cell activity in Ikaros mutant mice. *J Exp Med* 190:1201, 1999.

114. Wu L, Nichogiannopoulou A, Shortman K, Georgopoulos K: Cell-autonomous defects in dendritic cell populations of Ikaros mutant mice point to a developmental relationship with the lymphoid lineage. *Immunity* 7:483, 1997.

115. Klug CA, Morrison SJ, Masek M, et al: Hematopoietic stem cells and lymphoid progenitors express different Ikaros isoforms, and Ikaros is localized to heterochromatin in immature lymphocytes. *Proc Natl Acad Sci U S A* 95:657, 1998.

116. Payne KJ, Huang G, Sahakian E, et al: Ikaros isoform x is selectively expressed in myeloid differentiation. *J Immunol* 170:3091, 2003.

117. Payne KJ, Nicolas JH, Zhu JY, et al: Cutting edge: Predominant expression of a novel Ikaros isoform in normal human hemopoiesis. *J Immunol* 167:1867, 2001.

118. Cobb BS, Smale ST: Ikaros-family proteins: In search of molecular functions during lymphocyte development. *Curr Top Microbiol Immunol* 290:29, 2005.

119. DeKoter RP, Walsh JC, Singh H: PU.1 regulates both cytokine-dependent proliferation and differentiation of granulocyte/macrophage progenitors. *EMBO J* 17:4456, 1998.

120. DeKoter RP, Lee HJ, Singh H: PU.1 regulates expression of the interleukin-7 receptor in lymphoid progenitors. *Immunity* 16:297, 2002.

121. Medina KL, Ponqubala JM, Reddy KL, et al: Assembling a gene regulatory network for specification of the B cell fate. *Dev Cell* 7:607, 2004.

122. Polli M, Dakic A, Light A, et al: The development of functional B lymphocytes in conditional PU.1 knock-out mice. *Blood* 106:2083, 2005.

123. Murre C: Helix-loop-helix proteins and lymphocyte development. *Nat Immunol* 6:1079, 2005.

124. Dias S, Månsson R, Gurbuxani S, et al: E2A proteins promote development of lymphoid-primed multipotent progenitors. *Immunity* 29:217, 2008.

125. Bain G, Engel I, Robanus Maandag EC, et al: E2A deficiency leads to abnormalities in alphabeta T-cell development and to rapid development of T-cell lymphomas. *Mol Cell Biol* 17: 4782, 1997.

126. Bain G, Robanus Maandag EC, te Riele HP, et al: Both E12 and E47 allow commitment to the B cell lineage. *Immunity* 6:145, 1997.

127. Kee BL, Murre C: Induction of early B cell factor (EBF) and multiple B lineage genes by the basic helix-loop-helix transcription factor E12. *J Exp Med* 188:699, 1998.

128. Ikawa T, Kawamoto H, Goldrath AW, Murre C: E proteins and Notch signaling cooperate to promote T cell lineage specification and commitment. *J Exp Med* 203:1329, 2006.

129. Nutt SL, Heavey B, Rolink AG, Busslinger M: Commitment to the B-lymphoid lineage depends on the transcription factor Pax5. *Nature* 401:556, 1999.

130. Cobaleda C, Schebesta A, Delogu A, Busslinger M: Pax5: The guardian of B cell identity and function. *Nat Immunol* 8:463, 2007.

131. Pongubala JM, Northrup DL, Lancki DW, et al: Transcription factor EBF restricts alternative lineage options and promotes B cell fate commitment independently of Pax5. *Nat Immunol* 9:203, 2008.

132. Seet CS, Brumbaugh RL, Kee BL: Early B cell factor promotes B lymphopoiesis with reduced interleukin 7 responsiveness in the absence of E2A. *J Exp Med* 199:1689, 2004.

133. Rothenberg EV, Moore JE, Yui MA: Launching the T-cell-lineage developmental programme. *Nat Rev Immunol* 8:9, 2008.

134. Maillard I, Tu L, Sambandam A, et al: The requirement for Notch signaling at the beta-selection checkpoint *in vivo* is absolute and independent of the pre-T cell receptor. *J Exp Med* 203:2239, 2006.

135. Rothenberg EV: Transcriptional drivers of the T-cell lineage program. *Curr Opin Immunol* 24:132, 2012.

136. Taghon TN, David ES, Zúñiga-Pflücker JC, Rothenberg EV: Delayed, asynchronous, and reversible T-lineage specification induced by Notch/Delta signaling. *Genes Dev* 19:965, 2005.

137. Maeda T, Merghoub T, Hobbs RM, et al: Regulation of B versus T lymphoid lineage fate decision by the proto-oncogene LRF. *Science* 316:860, 2007.

138. Taghon T, Van de Walle I, De Smet G, et al: Notch signaling is required for proliferation but not for differentiation at a well-defined beta-selection checkpoint during human T-cell development. *Blood* 113:3254, 2009.

139. Van de Walle I, De Smet G, De Smedt M, et al: An early decrease in Notch activation is required for human TCR-alphabeta lineage differentiation at the expense of TCR-gammadelta T cells. *Blood* 113:2988, 2009.

140. Taghon T, Yui MA, Rothenberg EV: Mast cell lineage diversion of T lineage precursors by the essential T cell transcription factor GATA-3. *Nat Immunol* 8:845, 2007.

141. Germar K, Dose M, Konstantinou T, et al: T-cell factor 1 is a gatekeeper for T-cell specification in response to Notch signaling. *Proc Natl Acad Sci U S A* 108:20060, 2011.

142. Weber BN, Chi AW, Chavez A, et al: A critical role for TCF-1 in T-lineage specification and differentiation. *Nature* 476:63, 2011.

143. Li L, Leid M, Rothenberg EV: An early T cell lineage commitment checkpoint dependent on the transcription factor Bcl11b. *Science* 329:89, 2010.

CHAPTER 75
FUNCTIONS OF B LYMPHOCYTES AND PLASMA CELLS IN IMMUNOGLOBULIN PRODUCTION

Thomas J. Kipps

SUMMARY

Much of our immune defense against invading organisms is predicated upon the tremendous diversity of immunoglobulin molecules. Immunoglobulins are glycoproteins produced by B lymphocytes and plasma cells. These molecules can be considered receptors because the primary function of the immunoglobulin molecule is to bind antigen. A single person can synthesize 10 to 100 million different immunoglobulin molecules, each having a distinct antigen-binding specificity. The great diversity in this so-called humoral immune system allows us to generate antibodies specific for a variety of substances, including synthetic molecules not naturally present in our environment. Despite the diversity in the specificities of antibody

Acronyms and Abbreviations: ADCC, antibody-dependent cellular cytotoxicity; AID, activation-induced deaminase; BACH2, basic leucine zipper transcription factor 2; BCL-6, B-cell chronic lymphocytic leukemia/lymphoma 6; BiP, immunoglobulin-binding protein; Blimp-1, B-lymphocyte-induced maturation protein-1; BLNK, B-cell linker protein; BTK, Bruton tyrosine kinase; C, constant; CDR, complementarity determining region; CRI, cross-reactive idiotype; CSR, class switch recombination; D, diversity; DLBCL, diffuse large B-cell lymphoma; DNA-PK, DNA protein kinase; E2F1, E2F transcription factor 1; EBF1, early B-cell factor 1; ERGIC, ER-Golgi-intermediate compartment; FR, framework region; H, heavy; HMG, high-mobility group protein; Ig, immunoglobulin; IL, interleukin; IRF4, interferon regulatory factor 4; ITAM, immunoreceptor tyrosine-based activation motif; κ, immunoglobulin kappa light chain; Kde, kappa-deleting element; λ, immunoglobulin lambda light chain; L, light; MITF, microphthalmia-associated transcription factor; MYBL1 and 2, v-myb myeloblastosis viral oncogene homologues 1 and 2; NHEJ, nonhomologous DNA end-joining; PAX5, paired box gene 5; PDI, protein disulphide isomerase; PLC, phospholipase C; POU2AF1, Pou domain, class 2, associating factor 1; POU2F2, Pou domain, class 2, factor 2; PRDM1, positive regulatory domain 1-binding factor-1; *RAG*, recombination-activating gene; RSS, recombination signal sequence; SCID, severe combined immunodeficiency; SHP-1, Src homology 2 domain-containing protein tyrosine phosphatase-1; SHIP-1, phosphatidylinositol-3,4,5-trisphosphate 5-phosphatase 1; TCFE2A, transcription factor E2a; UNG, uracil-DNA glycosylase; V, variable-region gene; V(D)J, exon created by a rearranged immunoglobulin heavy-chain variable-region gene, diversity gene segment, and joining gene segment; XBP1, X-box binding protein-1.

molecules, the binding of antibody to antigen initiates a limited series of biologically important effector functions, such as complement activation and/or adherence of the immune complex to receptors on leukocytes. The eventual outcome is the clearance and degradation of the foreign substance. This chapter describes the structure of immunoglobulins and outlines the mechanisms by which B cells produce molecules of such tremendous diversity with defined effector functions.

● IMMUNOGLOBULIN STRUCTURE AND FUNCTION

BASIC STRUCTURE

All naturally occurring immunoglobulin molecules are composed of one or several basic units consisting of two identical heavy (H) chains and two identical light (L) chains (Fig. 75–1).[1] The four polypeptides are held in a symmetrical, Y-shaped structure by disulfide bonds and noncovalent interactions.[2–4] The internal disulfide bonds of the heavy and light chains cause the polypeptides to fold into compact globe-shaped regions called domains, each containing approximately 110 to 120 amino acid residues. Each domain is composed of β-pleated sheets that are stabilized by a conserved disulfide bond (Fig. 75–1). The light chains have two domains; the heavy chains have four or five domains. The aminoterminal domains of the heavy and light chains are designated the variable (V) regions because their primary structure varies markedly among different immunoglobulin molecules. The carboxyterminal domains are referred to as constant (C) regions because their primary structure is the same among immunoglobulins of the same class or subclass. The amino acids in the light- and heavy-chain variable regions interact to form an antigen-binding site. Each four-chain immunoglobulin basic unit has two identical binding sites. The constant-region domains of the heavy and light chains provide stability for the immunoglobulin molecule. The heavy-chain constant regions also mediate the specific effector functions of the different immunoglobulin classes (Table 75–1).

LIGHT CHAINS

Immunoglobulin light chains have an approximate Mr of 23,000. They are divided into two types, κ and λ, based upon multiple amino acid sequence differences in the single constant-region domain.[5] The λ chains are divided further into subclasses. The proportion of κ-to-λ chains in adult human plasma is approximately 2:1. The immunoglobulin light-chain constant region has no known effector function. Its main purpose may be to allow for proper assembly and release of an intact immunoglobulin molecule. Soon after synthesis, the antibody light-chain constant region associates with the nascent immunoglobulin heavy chain (see Fig. 75–1), releasing the latter from the immunoglobulin-binding protein (BiP). BiP is a heat shock protein that, in the absence of antibody light chain, binds the first constant-region domain of the newly synthesized heavy chain, thereby retaining the heavy-chain polypeptide in the cell's endoplasmic reticulum.[6]

HEAVY CHAINS

Immunoglobulin heavy chains have an Mr of 50,000 to 70,000, depending upon the number and length of the constant-region domains. The five major isotypes of heavy chains—γ, α, μ, δ, and ε—determine the five corresponding classes of immunoglobulin (Ig): IgG, IgA, IgM, IgD, and IgE. The individual immunoglobulin molecules of each isotype may contain either κ or λ light chains, but not both. Tables 75–1 and 75–2

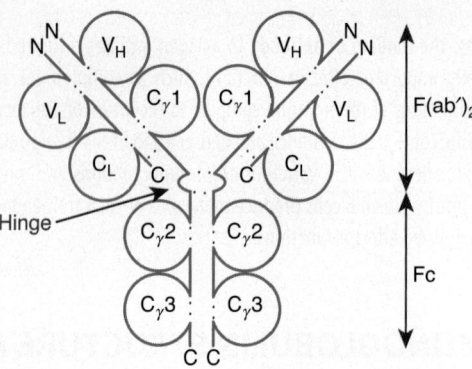

Figure 75–1. Model of an immunoglobulin (Ig) G molecule. The light-chain domains V_L and C_L and the heavy-chain domains V_H, Cγ1 (or C_H1), Cγ2 (or C_H2), and Cγ3 (or C_H3) are labeled inside the respective immunoglobulin domain. Dotted red colored lines indicate intrachain and interchain disulfide bonds. The aminoterminus (N) and carboxyl-terminus (C) of each polypeptide are indicated. The hinge region also is indicated. Digestion by pepsin cleaves the molecule at the carboxyl side of the hinge region, which generates Fc and F(ab')₂ fragments, as indicated on the *right*. The F(ab')₂ fragment is bivalent, as it is held together by the disulfide bridges in the hinge region. On the other hand, digestion of the molecule by papain degrades the Fc portion and generates monovalent Fab fragments, as the cleavage site for papain is on the aminoterminal side of the disulfide bridges of the hinge region.

summarize the distinct physical and functional properties of the human immunoglobulin classes.

IgG

Approximately 80 percent of the immunoglobulins in adult plasma are IgG. The IgG molecule is composed of the basic 150-kDa immunoglobulin four-chain structure plus approximately 3 percent carbohydrate. Near the junction of the two arms of the Y-shaped immunoglobulin molecule, the two heavy chains interact to form a flexible "hinge" region (see Fig. 75–1). Exposed between constant-region globular domains, the hinge region is attacked readily by the proteolytic enzyme papain or pepsin. Figure 75–1 shows the cleavage sites. Digestion of IgG with papain yields three fragments. The single Fc piece contains the carboxy-terminal region of both heavy chains. The two identical F(ab) pieces contain the entire light chain and the aminoterminal portion

of the heavy chain. The Fc-regions also contain a binding epitope for the neonatal Fc receptor (FcRn), responsible for the extended half-life, placental transport, and bidirectional transport of IgG to mucosal surfaces.[7] As such, IgG molecules effectively penetrate extravascular spaces and readily cross the placental barrier to provide passive immunity to the newborn.

IgG is the predominant antibody produced during the secondary immune response to antigen. The average half-life of circulating IgG molecules is approximately 21 days, although the exact value varies among the IgG subclasses (Table 75–3). Within the IgG class are four major subclasses, designated IgG_1, IgG_2, IgG_3, and IgG_4.[7] The most abundant subclass is IgG_1, which constitutes 60 percent of the total IgG in plasma. All IgG subclasses have a similar molecular mass except for IgG_3, which has a much longer hinge region than any other IgG subclass. The IgG_3 hinge region is approximately four times as long as the IgG_1 hinge, containing up to 62 amino acids (including 21 prolines and 11 cysteines), forming a polyproline helix with limited flexibility. Because of this, IgG_3 myeloma protein may aggregate spontaneously to produce a hyperviscosity syndrome.

Each subclass has a distinct heavy-chain constant region and mediates different effector functions (see Table 75–3). Whereas IgG_1 and IgG_3 proteins activate complement via the classic pathway, IgG_2 molecules fix complement poorly and IgG_4 proteins not at all.

Antibody responses to soluble protein antigens and membrane proteins primarily induce IgG_1, but also lower levels of the other subclasses, mostly IgG_3 and IgG_4. On the other hand, IgG antibody responses to bacterial capsular polysaccharide antigens typically are restricted to IgG_2; IgG_2 deficiency can result in the virtual absence of IgG anticarbohydrate antibodies. Viral infections generally induce IgG antibodies of the IgG_1 and IgG_3 subclasses, with IgG_3 antibodies appearing first in the course of the infection. The IgG_4 subclass typically is produced in response to allergens. Because IgG4 has relatively low affinity to activating FcγRIII, but relatively high affinity to the inhibiting FcγRII, it may serve to prevent excessive immune responses against sterile antigens, such as bee venom, which do not pose infectious threats. As such, IgG_4 has been called a "blocking antibody" in the context of allergy, where it may compete with IgE for allergen binding.

For antigens found on pathogens, the bound IgG can: (1) tag the pathogen for ingestion and destruction by phagocytes, a process called *opsonization*; (2) activate complement; and/or (3) direct antibody-dependent cell-mediated cytotoxicity (ADCC). Either aggregated IgG

TABLE 75–1. Physical Properties of Human Immunoglobulins					
	IgG	IgA	IgM	IgD	IgE
Heavy-chain class	γ	α	μ	δ	ε
Heavy chain subclass	$γ_1, γ_2, γ_3, γ_4$	$α_1, α_2$	—	—	—
No. of heavy-chain domains	4	4	5	4	5
Secretory form	Monomer	Monomer, dimer	Pentamer	Monomer	Monomer
Molecular mass (Da)	150,000	160,000 (monomer) 400,000 (secretory)	900,000	184,000	188,000
Antigen-binding valency	2	2 (monomer) 4 (secretory)	10	2	2
Serum concentration (mg/mL)	8–16	1.4–4.0	0.5–2.0	0–0.4	17–450 ng/mL
Percent of total immunoglobulin	80	13	6	1	0.002
Electrophoretic mobility	γ	Fast γ to β	Slow γ	Fast γ	Fast γ
Percent carbohydrate	3	8	12	13	12

TABLE 75–2. Biologic Properties of Human Immunoglobulins

	IgG	IgA	IgM	IgD	IgE
Percent of body pool in intravascular space	45	42	76	75	51
Percent of intravascular pool catabolized per day	6.7	25	18	37	89
Normal synthetic rate (mg/kg per day)	33	24	6.7	0.4	0.02
Serum half-life (days)	21	5.8	10	2.8	2.3
Placental transfer	Yes	No	No	No	No
Cytophilic for mast cells and basophils	No	No	No	No	Yes
Binding to macrophages and other phagocytes	Yes	No	No	No	Yes
Reactivity with staphylococcal protein A	Yes	No	No	No	No
Antibody-dependent cell-mediated cytotoxicity	Yes	No	No	No	No
Complement fixation					
Classic pathway	Yes	No	Yes	No	No
Alternative pathway	No	Yes	No	No	No

TABLE 75–3. Characteristics of Major IgG Subclasses

	IgG$_1$	IgG$_2$	IgG$_3$	IgG$_4$
Heavy chain subclass	γ_1	γ_2	γ_3	γ_4
Molecular mass (kDa)	146	146	170	146
Serum concentration (mg/mL)	7	4	0.5	0.6
Relative abundance (%)	60	32	4	4
Serum half-life (days)	21	21	7-21[a]	21
Placental Transfer	++++	++	++/++++ *	+++
Complement fixation (C1q binding)	++	+	+++	–
FcR Binding				
FcγRI (CD64)	+++	–	++++	++
FcγRIIa$_{H131}$ (CD32)[†]	+++	++	++++	++
FcγRIIa$_{R131}$ (CD32)[†]	+++	+	++++	++
FcγRIIb/c (CD32)	+	–	++	+
FcγRIIIa$_{F158}$ (CD16)[‡]	++	–	++++	–
FcγRIIIa$_{V158}$ (CD16)[‡]	+++	+	++++	–
FcγRIIIb (CD16)	+++	–	++++	++
FcγRn (at pH <6.5)	+++	–	++++	–
Antibody-dependent cell-mediated cytotoxicity	+	–	+	–
Heterologous skin sensitization	+	–	+	+

*Depending on the IgG$_3$ allotype.

[†]Two allotypic variants of FcγRIIa exist: H131 and R131.

[‡]Two allotypic variants of FcγRIIIa exist: F158 and V158.

or antigen–antibody complexes may bind to specific receptors for the Fc fragment, designated FcγRI (CD64), FcγRII (CD32), and FcγRIII (CD16). Of the IgG subclasses, IgG$_1$ binds best to FcγRI (CD64) and FcγRII (CD32), with affinities (dissociation constant [Kd]) of 10 nM and 50 μM, respectively (see Table 75–3). IgG$_1$ and IgG$_3$ bind equally well to FcγRIII (CD16), with a Kd of 2 μM (see Table 75–3). This is the Fc receptor expressed by natural killer (NK) cells (or K cells), which mediate ADCC. Proteins of the IgG$_4$ or IgG$_2$ subclass bind poorly to FcγRI (CD64) and bind not at all to FcγRIII (CD16) (see Table 75–3). IgG$_1$ is the most proficient subclass at directing ADCC. For this reason, most of the therapeutic monoclonal antibodies are of the IgG$_1$ subclass, which can be modified further to enhance their capacity to direct ADCC.[8]

IgA

IgA composes only approximately 13 percent of plasma immunoglobulin (see Table 75–1), even though the production of IgA exceeds that of any other immunoglobulin isotype, accounting for 60 to 70 percent of antibodies produced each day.[9] The relatively low amount in plasma is a result of the high amount of IgA secreted into the gastrointestinal tract. It is estimated that a normal 70-kg adult secretes approximately 2 g of IgA per day.[9] IgA also circulates in the plasma as a monomer, dimer, or higher polymer containing approximately 8 percent carbohydrate. Within the IgA class are two major subclasses, designated IgA$_1$ and IgA$_2$. The most abundant subclass is IgA$_1$, which constitutes approximately 85 percent of the total IgA in plasma. The half-life of circulating IgA of either subclass is approximately 6 days.

The primary role for IgA is in mucosal immunity.[10] Plasma cells in the lamina propria secrete IgA as a dimer that is held together by a J (joining) chain. The secreted IgA can bind to a *poly-Ig receptor*, which is an integral membrane glycoprotein expressed on the basal membrane of mucosal cells. Following the binding of IgA, the mucosal epithelial cells mediate endocytosis and transport of the IgA–poly-Ig receptor complex

in vesicles that are exported to the epithelial luminal surface. Here the poly-Ig receptor is proteolytically cleaved, releasing the extracellular domain, which remains complexed with the secreted IgA as a 70-kDa *secretory protein* that can protect the secreted IgA molecule from proteolytic digestion by enzymes in the intestinal lumen. This modified form of IgA, comprised of an IgA dimer bound to the J chain and secretory protein, is the principal antibody in saliva, tears, colostrum, and the fluids of the gastrointestinal, respiratory, and urinary tracts.

IgA can direct various effector functions by cells that bear specific Fc receptors for IgA (FcαR). FcαRI is the principal myeloid IgA receptor and is responsible for directing various IgA-mediated effector responses, such as respiratory burst, degranulation, and phagocytosis by granulocytes, monocytes, or macrophages. Another IgA receptor specific for the secretory protein can elicit powerful effector responses from eosinophils.[11] On the other hand, IgA antibodies do not cross the placenta, fix complement via the classic pathway, or bind efficiently to cell surfaces. Their main function may be to prevent foreign substances from adhering to mucosal surfaces and entering the blood.

Defective glycosylation of IgA$_1$ can lead to the most common form glomerulonephritis, namely *Berger disease* or *IgA nephropathy*. This is an autoimmune disorder in which neoepitopes caused by defective galactosylation of O-linked glycans in the hinge region of human IgA$_1$ are recognized by antiglycan IgG or IgA$_1$ antibodies.[12] Some of the resultant immune complexes in the circulation escape normal clearance mechanisms, deposit in the renal mesangium, and induce glomerular injury.[13]

Another nephritis associated with glomerular IgA deposits is *Henoch-Schönlein purpura*, a condition that most commonly presents with a characteristic pruritic skin rash, arthritis, and abdominal pain in children or young adults (Chap. 122).

IgM

In a normal adult, approximately 6 percent of the total plasma immunoglobulins belong to the IgM class (see Tables 75–1 and 75–2). IgM molecules classically are termed macroglobulins because of their large molecular weight. Circulating IgM molecules contain 12 percent carbohydrate and are formed through the linkage of five identical immunoglobulin units by disulfide bonds and by a J chain (Fig. 75–2).[14] IgM represents the predominant immunoglobulin class formed during a primary immune response. IgM macroglobulins do not penetrate easily into extravascular spaces or readily cross the placenta. Compared to monomeric IgG antibodies, pentavalent IgM antibodies fix complement more efficiently. A single IgM molecule on the surface of a red blood cell can initiate complement-mediated hemolysis. IgM is catabolized rapidly, with a plasma half-life of only 6 days. The monomeric form of IgM, with only two heavy and two light chains, is the major immunoglobulin expressed on the B-cell surface (Fig. 75–3). The IgM monomer represents the ligand-binding part of the receptor. The component that is responsible for signal transduction consists of two glycoproteins, CD79a and CD79b. The cytoplasmic domains of CD79a (Ig-α) and CD79b (Ig-β) contain tyrosine motifs responsible for transduction of signal from the receptor.[15]

IgD

IgD is a trace serum protein that composes less than 1 percent of plasma immunoglobulins. IgD is expressed on most peripheral B cells, as is IgM, where it may function as a B-cell membrane receptor for antigen that facilitates recruitment of B cells into specific antigen-driven responses. The molecule has the basic four-chain constant region and contains 11 percent carbohydrate (see Tables 75–1 and 75–2). IgD antibodies are sensitive to proteolytic degradation. They do not penetrate extravascular spaces efficiently, cross the placental barrier, or fix complement via the classic pathway. However, circulating IgD may bind to

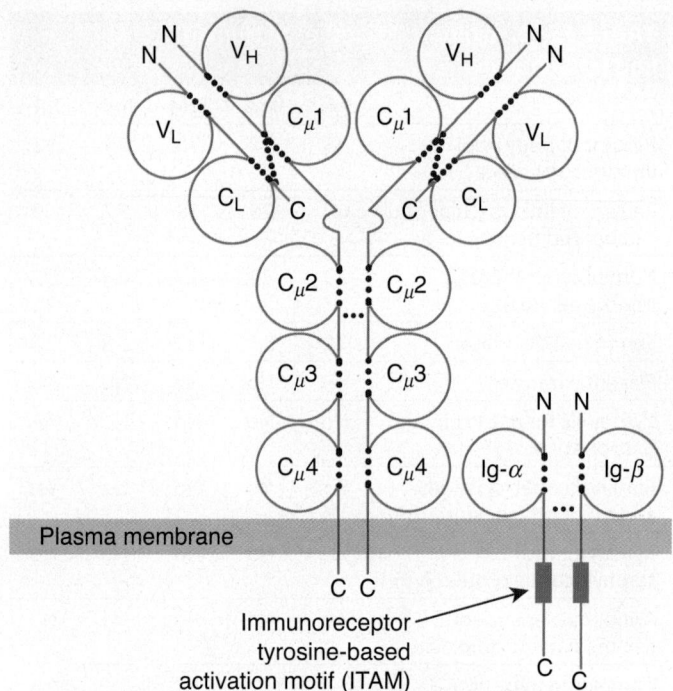

Figure 75–3. Schematic of membrane IgM and its associated accessory proteins Ig-α (CD79a) and Ig-β (CD79b). The light-chain domains V_L and C_L and the heavy-chain domains V_H, Cμ1 (or C_H1), Cμ2 (or C_H2), Cμ3 (or C_H3), and Cμ4 (or C_H4) are labeled inside the respective immunoglobulin domain. Each of the cytoplasmic domains of Ig-α (CD79a) and Ig-β (CD79b) has an immunoreceptor tyrosine-based activation motif (ITAM) depicted by a green rectangle. These ITAMs play a critical role in the signaling events that are initiated by ligation of surface immunoglobulin by antigen. Dotted red colored lines indicate intrachain and interchain disulfide bonds.

basophils through a calcium-mobilizing receptor, which, upon crosslinking, can trigger antimicrobial, proinflammatory responses.[16] Moreover, crosslinking of basophil-bound IgD also could induce basophils to produce interleukin (IL)-4, IL-13, B-cell activating factor (BAFF, CD272), and a proliferation inducing-ligand (APRIL, CD276), factors that, in turn, could enhance B-cell activation and isotype switching. This might explain why mice made deficient in IgD have fewer B cells, delayed affinity maturation, and weaker production of immunoglobulin isotypes, such as IgE, which are highly dependent on such cytokines.[17]

IgE

Although four human IgE isoforms can be produced by alternative splicing of the epsilon primary transcript,[18] each isoform appears to have similar function. IgE has been called reaginic antibody to denote its association with immediate hypersensitivity. It normally constitutes only 0.004 percent of total plasma immunoglobulin (see Tables 75–1 and 75–2). In patients with parasitic infestation and in some children with atopic diseases, plasma IgE levels may rise to 5 to 20 times normal. The IgE molecule consists of a four-chain basic unit plus 12 percent carbohydrate. Monomeric IgE binds via the Fc region to high-affinity receptors on the surface membranes of basophils and mast cells. When bound to tissue mast cells, IgE has a much longer half-life than in plasma, in which its half-life is only approximately 2 days (see Table 75–2). Crosslinking of cell-bound IgE antibody by antigen induces the release of vasoactive amines, lipid-derived inflammatory mediators, proteases, proteoglycans, and cytokines, such as tumor necrosis factor-α (cachectin), interferon-γ, granulocyte-macrophage

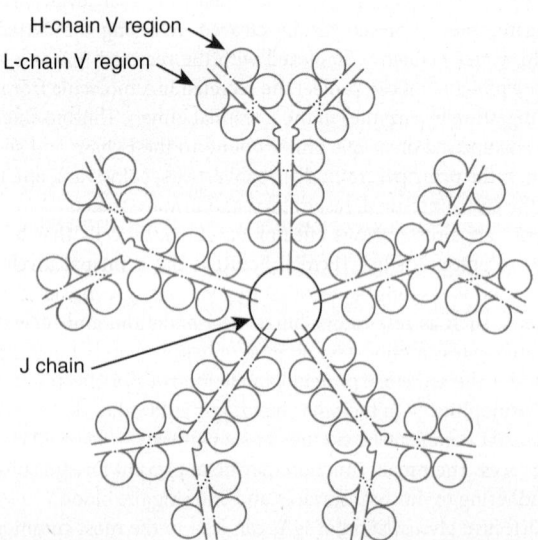

Figure 75–2. Schematic of an IgM pentamer. IgM has 10 binding sites for antigen, each composed of a heavy-chain variable region (H-chain V region) and a light-chain variable region (L-chain V region). Five bivalent IgM molecules are held together by the single joining (J) chain. Broken red colored lines indicate intrachain and interchain disulfide bonds.

colony-stimulating factor, and IL-1, IL-3, IL-4, IL-5, and IL-6. These substances act on adjacent cells and may regulate the metabolism of the connective tissue extracellular matrix. These lipid mediators and biogenic amines may produce the rapid components of immediate hypersensitivity, such as vascular leakage, vasodilation, and bronchoconstriction. The released cytokines, on the other hand, are responsible for the late phase of the immediate hypersensitivity response. The physiologic function of this response is not clear. Instead, the immediate hypersensitivity response may represent a pathologic systemic exaggeration of a local physiologic process that ordinarily contributes to the inflammatory response to invading organisms.

SURFACE IMMUNOGLOBULIN

Any one of the immunoglobulin isotypes may serve as a B-cell membrane receptor for antigen.[15] However, most B cells express surface IgM with or without IgD. Each immunoglobulin is expressed on the surface membrane as a monomer complexed noncovalently with disulfide-linked heterodimeric glycoproteins that, together with surface immunoglobulin, form the B-cell antigen–receptor complex (see Fig. 75–3). For surface IgM, each heterodimer is composed of CD79a, an IgM α-chain of 33 kDa, complexed with CD79b, an Ig β-chain of 37 kDa. CD79a interacts with the transmembrane domain and C_H4 domain of the immunoglobulin molecule, which mediates B-cell receptor clustering and signaling in response to antigen (see Fig. 75–3).[19] The CD79a chain is a product of the human mb-1 gene (designated *CD79a*) located at 19q13.2, whereas CD79b is the product of *CD79b* located on a different chromosome at 17q23. B cells that lack expression of CD79a or CD79b cannot express surface immunoglobulin. CD79a/CD79b are necessary, not only for transport of the assembled immunoglobulin to the cell surface but also for signal transduction following surface immunoglobulin-receptor crosslinking by antigen. Patients with inherited defects in CD79a have an immune deficiency that is indistinguishable from that of classic X-linked agammaglobulinemia (Chap. 80).[20] The cytoplasmic tails of CD79a and CD79b each contain immunoreceptor tyrosine-based activation motifs (ITAMs). Such motifs are found in the cytoplasmic domains of several immune system signaling molecules, including those of the T-cell receptor complex (Chap. 76).

B cells can become activated following ligation of their surface immunoglobulin receptors by antigen, which typically is presented on the surface of dendritic cells or macrophages.[21–24] This can cause microclustering of the immunoglobulin receptor complex into the *immunologic synapse*, which accumulates src family tyrosine kinases (e.g., Lyn, Blk, and Fyn), which can phosphorylate tyrosine residues in the ITAMs of CD79a and CD79b. In turn, the phosphorylated ITAM binds cytoplasmic signaling molecules, the most important of which is p72^{syk}, a 72-kDa tyrosine kinase. Following its recruitment to the activated immunoglobulin receptor complex, p72^{syk} itself becomes activated through phosphorylation, allowing it to phosphorylate the cytosolic adapter protein BLNK (B-cell linker protein, also known as SLP-65, BASH, or BCA).[25] BLNK serves as a docking site for a number of important signaling molecules, including Bruton tyrosine kinase (BTK), Vav-1, Vav-2, and phospholipase C gamma (PLCγ).[26] Dual phosphorylation and activation of PLCγ by BTK and p72^{syk} allows PLCγ to effect hydrolysis of the polyphosphoinositides into inositol-1,4,5-trisphosphate and diacylglycerol, which, in turn, increase intracellular Ca^{2+} and activate protein kinase C and Ras, respectively. The importance of these activation events in B-cell signaling and development is underscored by patients with inherited defects in BTK, who lack B-cell development and have X-linked agammaglobulinemia (Chap. 80). Furthermore, inhibitors of BTK demonstrate

clinical activity in the treatment of patients with various B-cell malignancies, which appear dependent upon constitutive signaling via the immunoglobulin receptor.[27]

To mitigate the problem of accidental initiation of signal transduction, the signaling cascade is subject to negative controls. The quantity and quality of immunoglobulin receptor signaling are modulated by several transmembrane proteins that are associated with the immunoglobulin–CD79a/CD79b receptor complex.[28] These associated proteins can be either costimulatory (e.g., CD19) or inhibitory (e.g., CD22, CD32 [FcγRII], CD72). In contrast to CD79a and CD79b, CD22 and CD72 have cytoplasmic domains with immunoreceptor tyrosine-based inhibitory motifs. When immunoreceptor tyrosine-based inhibitory motifs are phosphorylated by activated Lyn kinase, the domains recruit Src homology 2 (SH2) domain-containing protein tyrosine phosphatase 1 (SHP-1), otherwise known as protein tyrosine phosphatase 1c,[29,30] or phosphatidylinositol-3,4,5-triphosphate 5-phosphatase (SHIP-1).[31] Bound SHP-1 or SHIP-1 can remove the phosphate group from the phosphorylated (and thereby activated) tyrosine kinases, returning these kinases to their inactive state so that they no longer trigger B-cell activation. The importance of SHP-1 in limiting B cell activation is demonstrated by mutant mice that lack this phosphatase.[32] The B lymphocytes of such animals are stimulated by much lower concentrations of antigen than the B lymphocytes of normal mice, causing excessive B-cell proliferation, autoimmune disease, and early mortality.

● GENETICS OF IMMUNOGLOBULINS

IMMUNOGLOBULIN GENE COMPLEXES

Immunoglobulin genes are inherited in three unlinked gene complexes: one for the heavy-chain classes, one for κ light chains, and one for λ light chains. The immunoglobulin heavy-chain gene complex is located at band q32 of the long arm of chromosome 14. This complex is composed of 39 functional heavy-chain variable-region (V_H) genes, more than 120 nonfunctional V_H pseudogenes, 25 functional diversity (D) segments, six functional J_H minigenes, and exons encoding the constant regions for each of the immunoglobulin heavy-chain isotypes (Fig. 75–4).[33] The κ light-chain gene complex is contained within band p12 on the short arm of chromosome 2. This gene complex consists of approximately 40 functional κ light-chain variable-region genes (Vκ genes), more than 30 nonfunctional Vκ pseudogenes, five Jκ segments, one constant-region exon, and one kappa-deleting element (Kde) (Fig. 75–5). Many of the Vκ genes in the so-called p region most proximal to the Jκ segments are in the opposite orientation of the Jκ segments, thus requiring that the Vκ exons in the proximal region to undergo inversion during immunoglobulin gene rearrangement (Fig. 75–5). The λ light-chain gene complex is located at band q11.2 on the long arm of chromosome 22, 6 Mb from the centromere.[34] This gene complex consists of approximately 41 functional λ light-chain variable-region genes (Vλ genes), more than 30 Vλ pseudogenes, four functional λ constant-region genes (Cλ1, Cλ2, Cλ3, Cλ7), and three λ constant-region pseudogenes (Cλ4, Cλ5, Cλ6), each associated with one Jλ segment (Fig. 75–5). The constant-region elements of the heavy-chain gene complex are proximal to variable-region segments on chromosome 14, whereas the constant-region segments of the two light chains are in the opposite orientation, telomeric to the variable-region genes.

Each germline V gene, D element, and J segment is flanked by recognition sequences that are necessary to direct site-specific recombination (Fig. 75–6). Such sequences consist of a highly conserved palindromic heptamer (5′-CACAGTG-3′) a nonconserved spacer of 12 or 23 bp, and a conserved nonamer (5′ACAAAAACC-3′).[35]

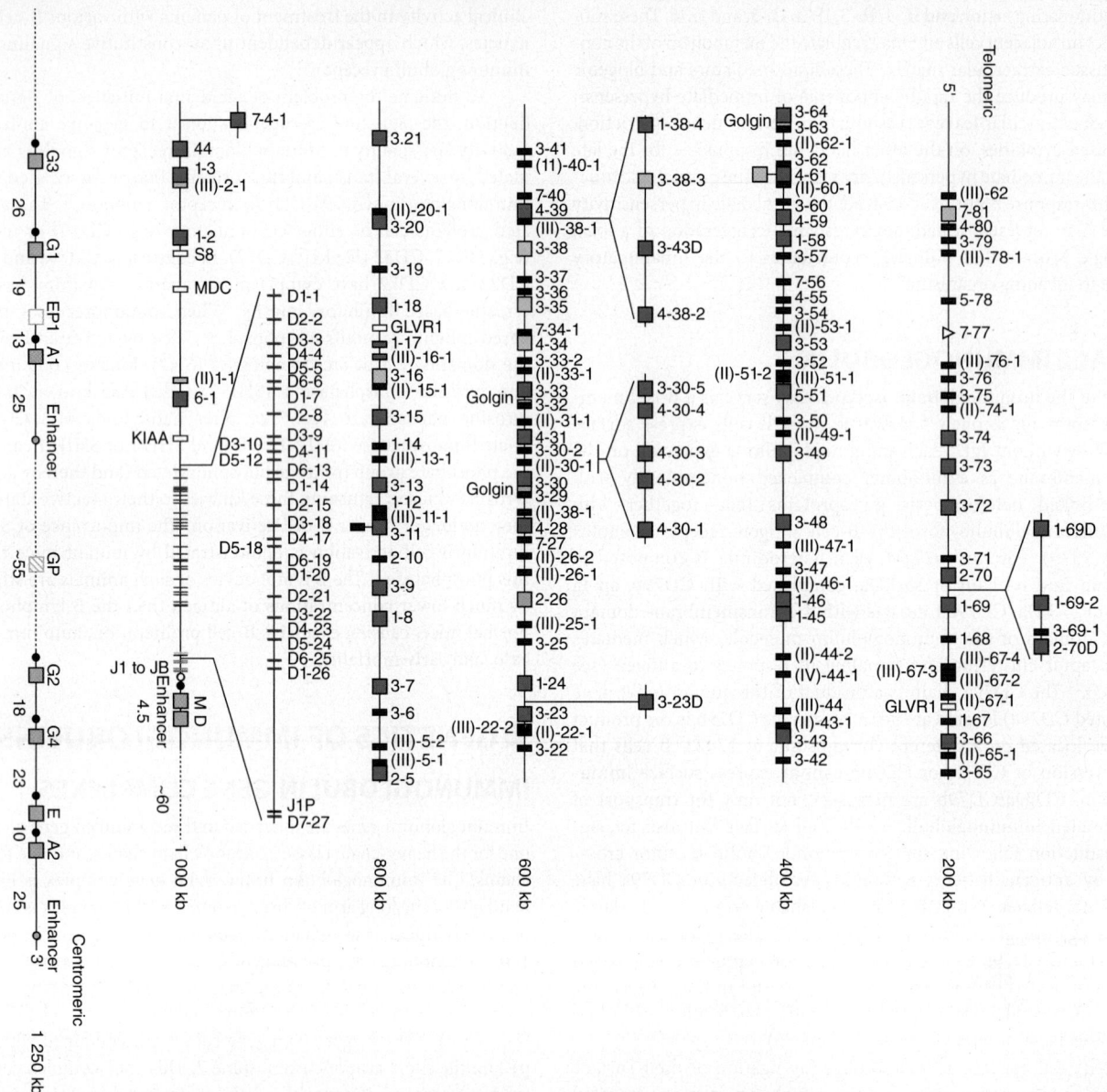

Figure 75–4. Immunoglobulin heavy-chain (IGHC) gene complex. The heavy-chain genes encoding the constant regions are represented by *blue boxes*. Switch regions are represented by a *filled circle* upstream of the IGHC genes. Enhancers are represented by *light blue circles*. Each *IGHV, IGHD* and *IGJH* gene is labeled on the right of each symbol. Functional *IGHV, IGHD*, and *IGHJ* genes are represented by *green boxes* or *blue* and yellow lines, respectively. IGHV, IGJH, and IGHC pseudogenes are represented by red, orange boxes, or blue open boxes, respectively. IGHV and IGHC open-reading frames are represented by *yellow* and *blue dashed boxes*, respectively. Unrelated pseudogenes are represented by *purple open boxes*. Colors are according to IMGT color menu for genes. *(Used with permission of Marie-Paule Lefranc. IMGT®, the international ImMunoGeneTics information system® http://www.imgt.org.)*

Joining usually occurs only between segments flanked by recognition sequences with unequal spacers.[36] Each recognition sequence consists of a dyad symmetric heptamer, an A/T-rich nonamer, and a spacer region of conserved length, either 12 bp or 23 bp ± 1 bp. This sequence is referred to as the 12/23 joining rule.[37] The consensus sequences for the heptamer (CACAGTG) and nonamers (ACAAAAACC) are optimal for rearrangement, but considerable deviation from the consensus sequence is observed and tolerated. Each spacer varies in sequence, but its length is conserved and corresponds to one or two turns of the DNA double helix. Each spacer brings the heptamer and nonamer sequences to one side of the DNA helix, where they are bound by the

Rag-1/Rag-2 protein complex that catalyzes recombination (Fig. 75–6). Similar recognition sequences flank the elements that rearrange to form the T-cell antigen receptor (Chap. 76). Because all segments of a particular type (e.g., Vκ gene segments) are flanked by one type of signal sequence and all the segments to which they should be joined (e.g., Jκ segments) are flanked by the opposite type of signal sequence, the 12/23 rule ensures that the joining is restricted to events that could be biologically productive. Such heptamer-spacer-nonamer sequences, often called recombination signal sequences (RSSs), are targets of lymphocyte-specific enzymes encoded by recombination activating genes *RAG1* and *RAG2*.[36]

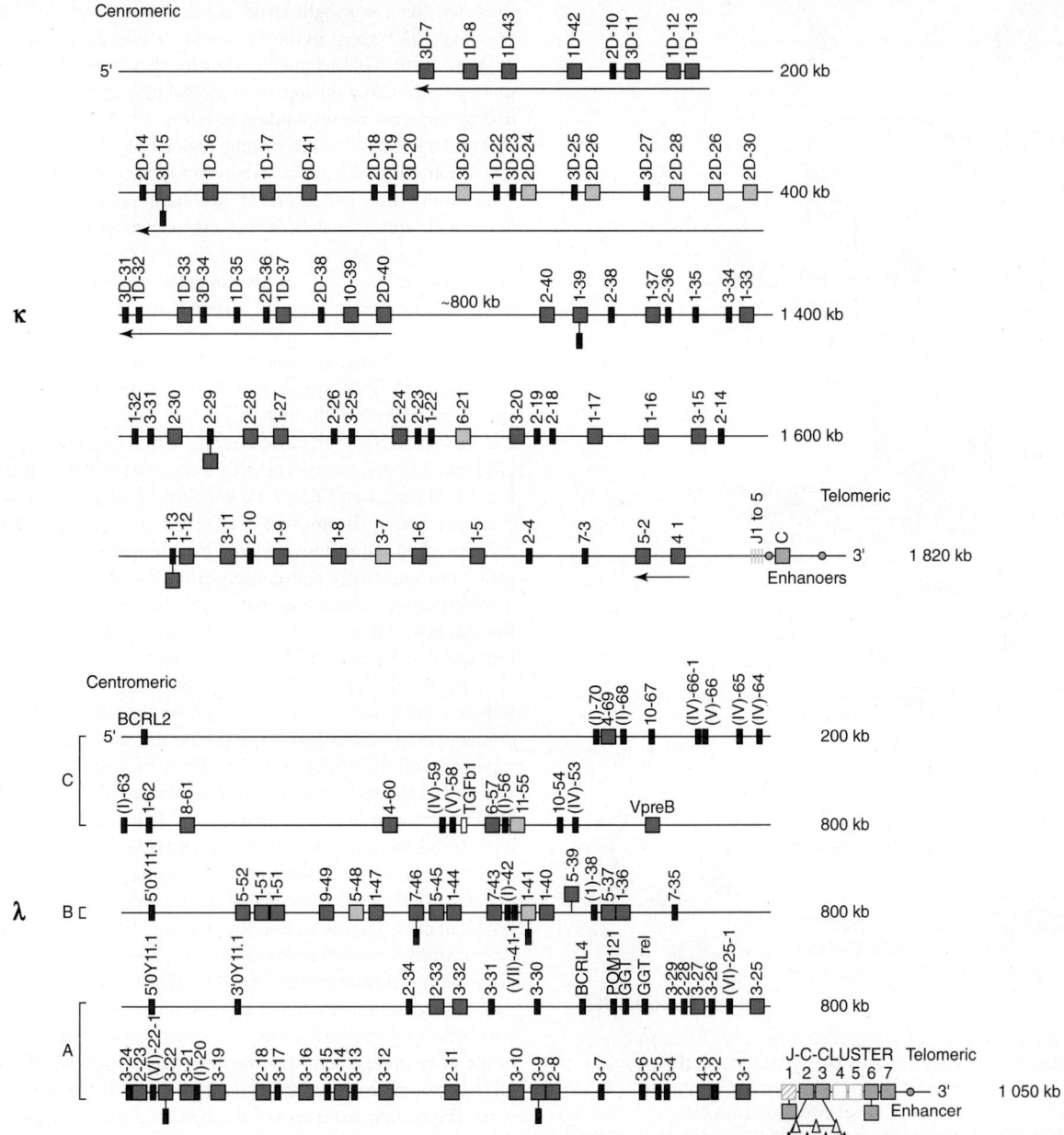

Figure 75–5. Immunoglobulin light-chain gene complexes. The *top panel* depicts the κ light-chain gene complex on chromosome 2p11-12. The *blue box* represents functional *IGLC* gene. The IGKJ gene segments are indicated by *yellow lines* labeled "J1 to 5." The κ light-chain enhancers are represented by *light blue circles*. IGKV functional genes, pseudogenes, and open-reading frames are indicated by *green, red,* and *yellow boxes*, respectively. The *IGKV* genes of the *p region* are designated by a number for the subgroup, followed by a hyphen and a number for the localization from 3' to 5' in the locus. The *IGKV* genes of the *d region* are designated by the same numbers as the corresponding genes in the *p region*, with the letter D added. *Arrows* show the *IGKV* genes whose orientation is opposite to that of the IGKJ gene segments. The *bottom panel* depicts the λ light-chain gene complex on chromosome 22q11.2. The *blue boxes* represent functional IGLJ and IGLC gene segments, whereas the *blue open boxes* represent IGLJ and IGLC pseudogenes. *IGLV* functional genes, pseudogenes, and open-reading frames are indicated by *green, red,* and *yellow boxes*, respectively. IGLV pseudogenes that could not be assigned to subgroups with functional genes are represented by *red boxes* and designated by a roman number between parentheses, corresponding to the clans, followed by a dash and a number for the localization from 3' to 5' in the locus. The *IGLV* genes are organized into three clusters, designated A, B, and C, which are indicated to the *left* of each cluster. Unrelated pseudogenes are represented by *purple open boxes*. The λ light-chain enhancer is represented by a *light blue circle*. Colors are according to IMGT color menu for genes. *(Used with permission of Marie-Paule Lefranc. IMGT®, the international ImMunoGeneTics information system® http://www.imgt.org.)*

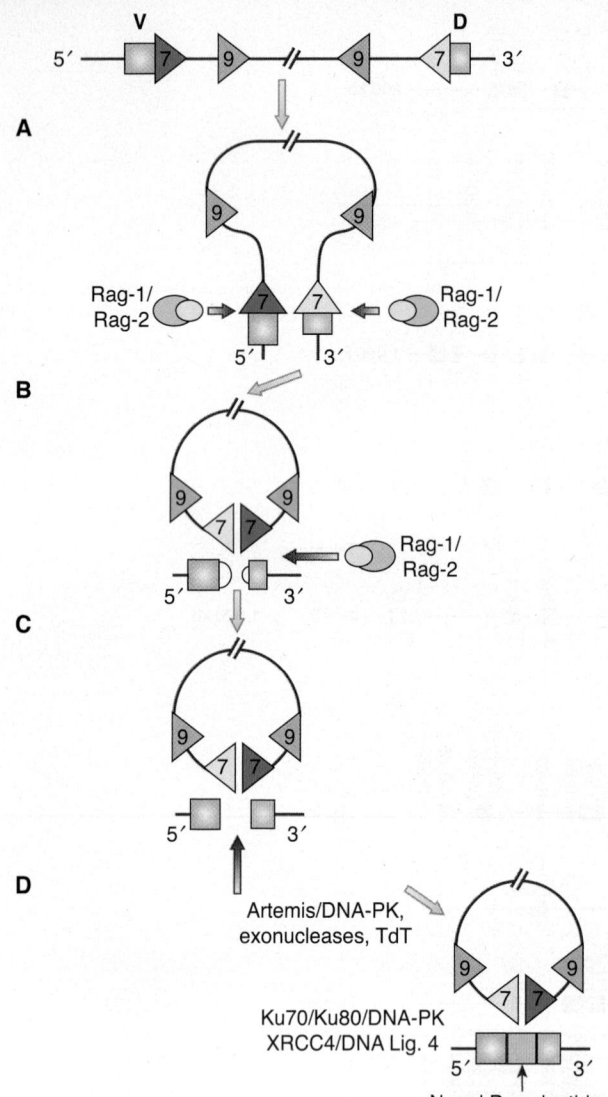

A

B

Rag-1/
Rag-2   Rag-1/
Rag-2

C

Rag-1/
Rag-2

D

Artemis/DNA-PK,
exonucleases, TdT

Ku70/Ku80/DNA-PK
XRCC4/DNA Lig. 4

N and P nucleotides

Figure 75–6. Schematic depicting the process of V(D)J recombination. The Rag-1/Rag-2 complex mediates **(A)** synapsis and **(B)** cleavage of the DNA at the boundaries of the heptamer/coding segments. **C.** The Artemis/DNA-PK (DNA protein kinase) endonuclease opens the hairpin and **(D)** the broken ends are then repaired by the proteins that mediate nonhomologous end-joining, namely the complex of Ku70, Ku80, DNA-PK, XRCC4, and Lig4.

IMMUNOGLOBULIN GENE REARRANGEMENT AND EXPRESSION DURING B-CELL DEVELOPMENT

IMMUNOGLOBULIN GENE REARRANGEMENT

During B-cell ontogeny, the first immunoglobulin gene rearrangements generally occur within the heavy-chain gene complex (Fig. 75–7A). One or more D segments may rearrange and become juxtaposed with a single J_H element, generating a DJ_H complex that then may rearrange with one of the 39 functional V_H genes. Subsequently, gene rearrangements occur in the light-chain loci (Fig. 75–7B). One of the 40 functional Vκ genes can rearrange with any one of five Jκ segments. Should these gene rearrangements fail to generate a functional Vκ Jκ exon, the Kde may rearrange to a site in or immediately downstream of the Vκ Jκ exon,

thus deleting the κ light-chain constant-region exon.[38] Many of the proximal *IGKV* genes in the so-named *p region* are in the opposite orientation of the IGKJ segments, requiring that the V exons in this region undergo inversion during immunoglobulin gene rearrangement. A 650-bp sequence corresponding to DNase I hypersensitive sites HS1–2 within the IGKV-IGKJ intervening region binds a CCCTC-binding factor, which directs locus contraction and long-range *IGKV* gene usage; its deletion results in a sevenfold increase in proximal *IGKV* gene usage along with approximately 50 percent reduction in overall locus contraction.[39] Subsequent to κ light-chain gene rearrangement, one of the 41 functional Vλ exons can rearrange with any one of the four functional JλCλ exons to generate a gene that can encode a λ light chain (Fig. 75–7C).

Somatic V-region gene recombination involves introduction of double-strand DNA breaks at RSS, juxtaposition of the broken ends, and then religation through a process called *nonhomologous DNA end-joining* (NHEJ). The first cleavage step requires a specialized heterodimeric endonuclease complex comprised of Rag-1 and Rag-2 (see Fig. 75–6). Rag-1 and Rag-2 are encoded by adjacent genes located on the short arm of chromosome 11 (11p13–p12). Mice with either *RAG* gene knocked out cannot undergo immunoglobulin or T-cell receptor gene rearrangements and consequently fail to produce mature B or T lymphocytes.[40] Mutations that impair, but do not completely abolish, the function of Rag-1 or Rag-2 in humans result in a form of combined immune deficiency termed *Omenn syndrome*.[41]

The process of somatic DNA recombination is initiated when the Rag (recombination activating gene) endonuclease introduces DNA double-strand breaks (DSBs) at the border of two recombining gene segments and their flanking RSSs.[42] DNA cleavage by Rag leads to four broken DNA ends that are repaired and joined through a process called NHEJ to form coding and signal joints.[43,44] Occasionally these DSBs can be repaired aberrantly, leading to the formation of chromosomal lesions such as translocations, deletions, or inversions,[45,46] often found in B-cell neoplasms. If the breakpoints of these chromosomal lesions lie near potential oncogenes or tumor-suppressor genes, they can lead to cellular transformation and lymphoid tumors. The mechanism of DNA rearrangement is similar for the heavy- and light-chain loci. However, only one joining event is needed to generate a light-chain gene, whereas two are needed to generate a complete heavy-chain gene. The most common mode of rearrangement involves the looping out and deletion of the DNA between two gene segments on the same chromosome; this occurs when the coding sequences of the two gene segments are in the same orientation in the DNA.[47] The 12- and 23-mer-spaced RSSs are brought together by interactions between proteins that specifically recognize the length of the spacer between the heptamer and nonamer signals, thus accounting for the 12/23 joining rule.[36,48] The two DNA molecules then are broken and rejoined in a different configuration. By joining precisely in a head-to-head configuration, the ends of the heptamer sequences form a signal joint in a circular piece of extrachromosomal DNA that then is lost from the genome when the cell divides. However, the DNA that lies between the two gene segments is retained in an inverted orientation when a second mode of recombination occurs between two gene segments with opposite transcriptional orientations. Although this mode of recombination is less common, such rearrangements account for about half of all IGKV-to-IGKJ joins, as the transcriptional orientation of half of the human IGKV gene segments is opposite to that of the IGKJ gene segments.

The Rag-1/Rag-2 endonuclease complex recognizes either the 12-mer–spaced or 23-mer–spaced RSS and then introduces double-stranded DNA breaks (see Fig. 75–6). After introducing these breaks, the Rag-1/Rag-2 complex remains bound to the DNA.[49] Mutations that affect the ability of the Rag proteins to bind and maintain the broken

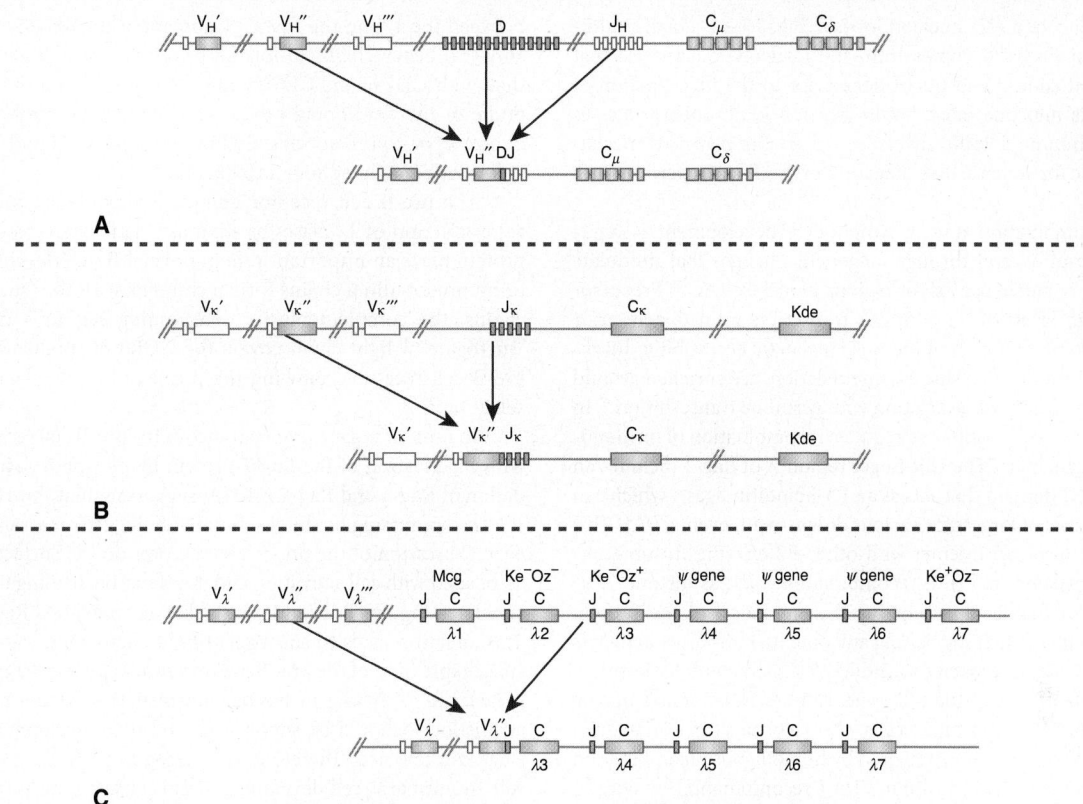

Figure 75–7. Immunoglobulin gene complexes and rearrangement. *Diagonal gold double lines* indicate a large DNA distance between the flanking genes depicted as *rectangular boxes* (not drawn to scale). The upper diagrams in **(A)**, **(B)**, and **(C)** show the germline DNA configuration of the immunoglobulin heavy-chain genes, κ light-chain genes, and λ light-chain genes, respectively. Exemplary immunoglobulin heavy-chain variable-region genes (V_H', V_H'', V_H'''), immunoglobulin κ light-chain genes (Vκ′, Vκ″, Vκ‴), and immunoglobulin λ light-chain variable-region genes (Vλ′, Vλ″, Vλ‴) are depicted on the left side of each immunoglobulin gene complex. D denotes the diversity gene segments of the antibody heavy-chain locus. J_H, Jκ, and Jλ indicate the joining gene segments of the antibody heavy chain, κ light chain, and λ light chain, respectively. $C\mu$ and $C\delta$ denote the constant-region exons of the μ and δ heavy chains, respectively. Below each is a possible immunoglobulin gene rearrangement composed of a V(D)J for the antibody heavy chain or a Vκ Jκ or VλJλ for the κ or λ light-chain gene, respectively. Below the representative λ constant-region loci in **(C)** are listed the names of the λ nonallelic genetic markers Mcg, Ke−Oz−, Ke−Oz+, and Ke+Oz− on Cλ1, Cλ2, Cλ3, and Cλ7, respectively. As indicated, Cλ4, Cλ5, and Cλ6 are pseudogenes (ψ gene) that do not encode protein.

ends in a stable postcleavage complex can lead to misrepair of the DSBs, thereby enhancing the risk for oncogenic chromosomal aberrations.[50]

Several proteins are involved in the processing and juxtaposition of the DSBs, including high-mobility group protein-1 (HMG1) and high-mobility group protein 2 (HMG2). HMG1 and HMG2 are widely expressed, abundant nuclear proteins that bind and bend DNA without sequence specificity, thereby playing an important role in the assembly of nucleoprotein complexes involved in DNA repair and transcription. HMG1 facilitates the bending of the DNA to allow the components of one DSB–Rag complex to bind and cleave the DNA at a different RSS,[51] thus bringing together two disparate RSSs in accordance with the 12/23 joining rule.[52]

The DSB–Rag complex also binds several other proteins, including Artemis, DNA-dependent protein kinase (DNA-PK), Ku70, Ku80, the human protein *X-ray repair complementing defective repair in Chinese hamster cells 4* (XRCC4), and DNA ligase IV (Lig4) (see Fig. 75–6).[43] DNA protein kinase (DNA-PK) is a serine-threonine protein kinase that is activated by DNA DSBs and is essential for the normal repair of DNA breaks induced by ionizing radiation, chemical agents, and during V(D)J (exon created by a rearranged immunoglobulin heavy-chain variable-region gene, diversity gene segment, and joining gene segment) recombination.[53] Mice deficient in DNA-PK can make only trivial amounts of immunoglobulin or T-cell receptors and are called severe combined immunodeficiency

(SCID) mice.[54] Mice deficient in Artemis have a "leaky" SCID phenotype and develop some T and B cells in later life.[55] Ku-deficient mice also are deficient in T and B cells but have a small stature and other nonimmunologic defects, suggesting that these proteins also play important roles in normal development.[56] Defects resulting from mutation in Ku, XRCC4, Lig4, Artemis, or DNA-PK predispose to lymphomagenesis in mice.[57] The initial recognition and recruitment of these repair proteins to DSBs is heavily dependent on phosphorylation events (e.g., kinase activity and autophosphorylation of DNA-PK), but the downstream repair events appear more dependent on E3-ubiquitin ligases.[58]

The process of recombination allows for generation of "junctional diversity" in the sequence of the rearranged gene segments. DNA ends generated by the Rag-1/Rag-2 endonuclease cleavage reaction each is fused by the NHEJ pathway involving the proteins mentioned in the preceding paragraph. The hairpinned termini of gene segments that give rise to the coding joint each is subsequently cleaved at random sites by an exonuclease. Cleavage of a hairpin away from its apex generates an overhanging flap that, if incorporated into the joint, results in addition of palindromic (P) nucleotides that contribute to junctional diversity (see Fig. 75–6). The opened hairpin ends can be modified further by nucleases that can remove a self-complementary overhang or cut further into the original coding sequence. In addition, a lymphocyte-specific enzyme, terminal deoxynucleotidyl transferase, can add non–template-encoded (N) nucleotides (see Fig. 75–6). Finally, additional junctional diversity comes from the nucleolytic activities that remove potential coding end nucleotides prior to the final ligation of the DNA breaks into one intact recombination joint. Such processes contribute to immunoglobulin diversity and are the principal mechanism responsible for somatic diversification of the T-cell repertoire (see Chap. 76).

V(D)J recombination during lymphocyte development is regulated via transcription and through epigenetic changes that modulate the accessibility of particular loci or regions of loci to RAG.[59] Precursor B cells have high-levels of V_H germline transcripts immediately prior to V-to-DJ_H recombination.[60] Numerous epigenetic accessibility markers, such as the histone H3 lysine 4 trimethylation, are enriched around IGHJ in early pro-B cells in association with germline transcription.[61] In addition, ubiquitination events can regulate recombination of immunoglobulin gene segments.[62] The zinc finger region A of Rag-1 includes an N-terminal RING domain that acts as an E3-ubiquitin ligase, which can ubiquitinate a panel of targets for various downstream events.[37,63–66] This region of Rag-1 also can interact with other E2 enzymes to ubiquinate substrates involved in V(D)J recombination, such as histone 3.[63,64] Ubiquitination of Rag-2 allows for rapid degradation of the protein upon entering S phase, thereby halting any potential off-target activities of Rag and limiting its capacity to induce V(D)J recombination during inappropriate phases of the cell cycle. Indeed, DNA breaks during S-phase are potentially harmful for cells, as such breaks can lead to deleterious translocations when misrepaired by homologous recombination (HR). It is therefore crucial to limit V(D)J recombination activity to cells within G_1 phase; this restriction appears to be controlled by Rag-2 degradation.[67]

Under normal conditions, a B-lymphocyte or plasma cell synthesizes only one species of light chain and heavy chain, even though the cell has two different sets of immunoglobulin gene complexes that initially undergo seemingly independent immunoglobulin gene rearrangements. The specificity of the humoral immune response depends upon antigenic selection of unique clones of B cells, each clone expressing a homogeneous set of immunoglobulin receptors. Such restriction is achieved by limiting a given B cell to functional rearrangement and expression of only a single heavy-chain allele and a single light-chain allele. This phenomenon is called *allelic exclusion*. Although occasional neoplastic B-cell populations lack allelic exclusion and express both immunoglobulin alleles, allelic exclusion generally is observed with most B-cell tumors.[68]

SURROGATE λ LIGHT CHAINS

Precursor B cells that only have rearranged D and J_H elements are referred to as progenitor B cells or "pro-B cells." The term *pre-B cells* is reserved for precursor B cells that have completed immunoglobulin heavy-chain gene rearrangement and have a functional V(D)J complex. Both pro-B cells and pre-B cells have immunoglobulin light-chain loci in germline configuration.

Pre-B cells express some immunoglobulin μ chains in association with "surrogate" λ light chains. One of these proteins, called $λ_5$, has similarity with known Cλ light-chain domains. Another protein is called *VpreB* because it resembles a V domain but bears an extra N-terminal protein sequence. Both proteins are encoded by genes located on chromosome 22. The $λ_5$ gene is situated within a λ-like locus that is telomeric to the true λ light-chain locus. The gene encoding VpreB (VPREB1) is located within the cluster of immunoglobulin Vλ genes (see Fig. 75–5), defined by breakpoints of chromosomal translocations found in a few leukemias and lymphomas. Together, VpreB and $λ_5$ pair with the μ heavy chains. Subsequent covalent linkages via an S-S bond

between the $λ_5$ and the first C_H1 domain of the μH chain allow VpreB and $λ_5$ μ heavy chains to form a primitive immunoglobulin receptor that, with CD79a and CD79b, may be expressed on the surface membrane of the developing pre-B cell. Monoclonal antibodies that recognize $λ_5$ or VpreB specifically bind to pre-B cells and can react with B-lineage acute lymphocytic leukemia.[69]

The pre-B cell receptor complex is expressed only transiently, as production of $λ_5$ ceases as soon as it is formed. Nevertheless, this protein plays an important role in normal B-cell development. When immunoglobulin μ chains form a complex with the "surrogate" λ light chains, the complementarity determining region 3 (CDR3) of the "surrogate" λ light chain covers the CDR3 of the heavy chain in the pre-B-cell receptor, allowing the pre-B cell to avoid antigen-specific selection.[70]

In normal mice, the appearance of the pre-B cell receptor coincides with inactivation of the Rag-2 protein by phosphorylation and degradation of Rag-1 and Rag-2 mRNA, suggesting that this receptor plays a role in suppressing further immunoglobulin gene rearrangement. However, expression of the pre–B-cell receptor on the surface membrane is associated with cell activation and proliferation, leading to generation of small, resting pre-B daughter cells that again express Rag-1 and Rag-2. This situation leads to subsequent light-chain gene rearrangement. As such, expression of the pre–B-cell receptor appears to signal that a complete μ heavy-chain gene has been formed, that further rearrangements at this locus should be suppressed, and that development to the next stage can proceed. Therefore, the surrogate light chains play a critical role in normal B-cell development. This observation is underscored by studies on transgenic mice that lack functional $λ_5$ genes. In these mice, B-cell development in the marrow is blocked at the pre–B-cell stage, thereby markedly reducing the numbers of functional mature B lymphocytes in the blood and lymphoid tissues.[71] Similarly, humans who have inactivating mutations in the $λ_5$ genes on both alleles of chromosome 22 have agammaglobulinemia and markedly reduced numbers of B cells.[72]

HEAVY-CHAIN CLASS SWITCHING

During differentiation, a single B lymphocyte can synthesize heavy chains with different constant regions coupled to the same variable region through process called *class switch recombination*, which shares features of V(D)J recombination.[73] As pre-B cells develop into mature B cells, intact IgM monomers are inserted into the plasma membrane, followed by IgD molecules with the same antigen-binding specificity. The IgM and IgD constant-region genes are closely linked in embryonic DNA (see Fig. 75–4) and may be transcribed together. The differential splicing of the transcript allows simultaneous synthesis of the two immunoglobulin heavy chains from a single species of mRNA. As such, the expression of IgD that occurs during B cell maturation only rarely involves deletion of Cμ.

The switch from IgM to IgG, IgA, or IgE requires active transcription of the downstream constant-region exons encoding the future immunoglobulin isotype. This process requires prior interaction of B lymphocytes with antigen or mitogen and ligation of CD40 via the ligand for CD40 (CD154) expressed by activated T cells. Patients with inherited defects in CD40 or CD154 have an immune deficiency (hyper-IgM syndrome type I) characterized by normal to high serum levels of IgM with extremely low serum levels of other immunoglobulin isotypes (Chap. 80).[74] Interleukins provided by antigen-reactive T lymphocytes strongly influence (1) which B cells differentiate into IgM-secreting plasma cells and (2) which B cells switch to synthesizing the heavy chain of another immunoglobulin isotype, such as IgG and IgA. Isotype switching to IgA occurs most efficiently in mucosal lymphoid tissue, particularly in Peyer patches and mesenteric lymph nodes (Chap. 6).[75] Also, class-switched IgA plasmablasts have a propensity to migrate to the lamina propria of the intestine and to other mucosal sites.[76]

Immunoglobulin class switch recombination (CSR) occurs in or near the switch region located in the intron between the rearranged V(D)J$_H$ sequence and the μ gene and any one of similar regions located upstream of the C genes encoding each of the other heavy-chain isotypes, with the exception of the δ gene (see Fig. 77–4). The μ switch region, designated Sμ, consists of approximately 150 repeats of the sequence (GAGCT)$_n$ (GGGGGT), where n is generally 3 but can be as many as 7. The sequences of the other switch regions (Sλ, Sδ, Sϵ) are similar in that they also contain repeats of the GAGCT and GGGGGT sequences. The switch in heavy-chain classes results from DNA recombination between Sμ, and Sλ, Sδ, or Sϵ, accompanied by the deletion of intervening DNA segments and the apposition of the previously rearranged variable-region gene next to the new constant-region gene.

In contrast to V(D)J recombination, which mostly occurs in the G$_0$ and/or G$_1$ stage of the cell cycle, CSR seems to require DNA replication.[77] Also, unlike V(D)J recombination, CSR requires expression of activation-induced deaminase (AID), an enzyme expressed in activated B cells that also is required for somatic hypermutation.[78] Patients with inherited defects in AID have an immune deficiency (hyper-IgM syndrome type II) characterized by relatively high serum levels of IgM and negligible serum levels of other immunoglobulin isotypes.[79] Specific inactivation of the C-terminal AID domain, encoded by exon 5 (E5), allows very efficient deamination of the AID target regions, but greatly impacts the efficiency and quality of subsequent DNA repair. Specifically eliminating E5 not only precludes CSR, but also causes an atypical, enzymatic activity-dependent, dominant-negative effect on CSR. This explains the autosomal dominant inheritance of AID variants with truncated E5 in patients with hyper-IgM syndrome type II and establishes that AID, through the E5 domain, provides a link between DNA damage and repair during CSR.[80]

AID is expressed in germinal centers of peripheral lymphoid organs, the site where CSR occurs in B cells activated in response to antigen. AID most likely deaminates the closely positioned cytosines (dC) in the S-region DNA, converting the dC to uracils (dU), which, in turn, are removed by uracil-DNA glycosylase (UNG). The importance of UNG is underscored by patients who have inherited defects in this enzyme, resulting in an autosomal recessive form of the hyper-IgM immunodeficiency syndrome similar to that of patients with inherited defects in AID (see Chap. 80).[81] The abasic sites generated by UNG are cleaved by AP endonuclease, resulting in closely positioned staggered nicks in the DNA that may result in double-stranded DNA breaks. The end processing, repair, and joining mechanisms for these DNA breaks apparently involve mechanisms and proteins similar to those involved in NHEJ used for V(D)J recombination. Because the CSR occurs in the intron between the variable-region exon and the exon encoding the first constant-region domain, this process does not generate mutations in the regions encoding the variable or constant regions of the newly generated immunoglobulin heavy chain.

MECHANISMS FOR GENERATING ANTIBODY DIVERSITY

Several mechanisms contribute to the generation of diversity among immunoglobulin polypeptide variable regions. The mechanisms are (1) the presence in the germline DNA of multiple different V, J, and D gene segments; (2) the random joining of these DNA segments to produce a complete variable-region exon; (3) junctional diversity; (4) the coming together of the heavy- and light-chain polypeptides to produce a complete immunoglobulin monomer capable of binding antigen; and (5) somatic mutations within the rearranged DNA segments themselves. Somatic mutations occurs through a process called somatic hypermutation.

Somatic hypermutation is not active in all B cells and cannot be triggered merely by mitogen-induced B-cell activation. However, during discrete stages of B-cell differentiation, expressed immunoglobulin V genes may incur new mutations at rates as high as 10^{-3} base substitutions per base pair per generation over several cell divisions, particularly during the secondary humoral immune response to antigen.[82] Hypermutations begin on the 5' end of rearranged V genes downstream of the transcription initiation site and continue through the V gene and into the 3' flanking region before tapering off. As such, the mutations are clustered in the region spanning from 300 bp 5' of the rearranged variable-region exon to approximately 1 kb 3' of the rearranged mini-gene J segment. A high frequency of mutations are clustered around "hotspots" defined by the primary DNA sequence. The sequence RGYW (R = purine, A or G; Y = pyrimidine, C or T; W = A/T) and its complement, for example, is a hotspot for mutation that is conserved among species.[83]

The process of somatic hypermutation requires the activity of AID through a process that has some similarly with CSR.[84,85] In addition to having the hyper-IgM immunodeficiency syndrome type II, patients who have inherited defects in AID have B cells that lack the capacity to undergo somatic hypermutation (Chap. 80).[79,86] As with CSR, somatic hypermutation requires active transcription of the genes undergoing mutation. AID most likely deaminates the cytosines in the region encompassing the rearranged variable-region gene, converting the dC to dU, which are converted to T after DNA replication, giving rise to C/G to T/A transitions. Alternatively, the dU are removed by UNG, resulting in abasic sites that subsequently are cleaved by AP endonuclease. This process generates staggered nick cleavage of the DNA. Repair of these staggered nicks may involve low-fidelity DNA synthesis, giving rise to frequent mutations. DNA cleaving enzymes and DNA repair enzymes (e.g., mismatch repair enzymes, base-excision repair enzymes, proteins involved in NHEJ) form a complex called the *mutasome*, which also apparently binds the target DNA to reduce its tendency to incur complete double-stranded DNA breaks.

Immunoglobulin enhancers may account in part for the preferential somatic hypermutation of immunoglobulin genes. Combinations of immunoglobulin enhancers target somatic mutation to immunoglobulin genes by recruiting AID and/or by making the immunoglobulin genes better substrates for mutation.[87] In addition, posttranslation AID ubiquitination has an important regulatory role during CSR and somatic hypermutation.[88,89] Unlike Rag-2, AID protein stability is not associated with phases of the cell cycle, but rather with subcellular localization. In mouse B cells nuclear AID is subjected to rapid turnover upon polyubiquitination.[88]

As a consequence somatic hypermutation, mostly transitional mutations are introduced at high frequency in the expressed immunoglobulin V genes and in other transcriptionally active genes with "hotspots," which can serve as a substrate for AID, UNG, and the mutasome.[90] Subsequent selection of the B cell and its daughter cells that express mutated V genes encoding an immunoglobulin variable region with improved fitness for binding antigen allows for "affinity maturation" of the antibodies expressed during the immune response to antigen, which typically is retained on follicular dendritic cells.[91] Such selection enhances the frequency of nonconservative base substitutions in the DNA sequences encoding the CDR that serves as the contact site for antigen binding.[84]

IMMUNOGLOBULIN VARIABLE-REGION STRUCTURE

IMMUNOGLOBULIN VARIABLE-REGION SUBGROUPS

Despite the large number of different immunoglobulin variable regions that can be generated through the mechanisms just described, each antibody polypeptide can be assigned to one of a relatively small number of variable-region subgroups.[5] Comparisons of the amino acid sequences of a large number of different monoclonal immunoglobulin proteins reveal four segments of limited amino acid sequence diversity between different antibody heavy- or light-chain variable regions. Each of these segments is designated as an immunoglobulin variable-region framework region (FR), see Fig. 75-7. Each immunoglobulin polypeptide can be assigned to one of a relatively small number of variable-region subgroups based upon the primary structure of its first three FRs. Moreover, each subgroup has characteristic FRs that distinguish it from other variable-region subgroups.

Satisfying expectations that immunoglobulin subgroups defined families of highly related antibody V genes, variable-region amino acid subgroup homologies extend to the nucleic acid sequence level.[92-94] Cloned immunoglobulin V genes whose deduced amino acid sequences belong to a given subgroup generally share greater than 80 percent nucleic acid sequence homology. The human heavy-chain variable regions can be grouped into seven subgroups, whereas κ or λ light chains can be divided into six and 11 subgroups, respectively.

Crystallographic data of immunoglobulin variable regions indicate that amino acids within the first and third FRs of either the light or heavy chain form β bonds on the external surface of the molecule. These regions form relatively compact structures on the external solvent-accessible face of the antibody molecule that are not adjacent to the classic antibody-combining site for antigen. Accordingly, amino acid differences noted between the different variable-region subgroups are amenable to recognition by antisubgroup antibodies.

IMMUNOGLOBULIN IDIOTYPES

Antisubgroup antibodies must be distinguished from antiidiotypic antibodies. Positioned between the FRs are three segments of extreme hypervariability in both light- and heavy-chain sequences.[2] The third hypervariable region is generated through the recombinatorial process that joins the antibody light-chain V gene with the J segment of the light chain or the V_H gene with the somatically generated DJ_H segment of the antibody heavy chain. The diversity in first and second hypervariable regions in part reflects germline DNA-encoded differences between disparate antibody V genes, a diversity often noted even between V genes of the same subgroup.[5,33] During an immune response, somatic hypermutation subsequent to V gene rearrangement also may play an important role in increasing the amino acid sequence diversity noted within these regions. These hypervariable regions on both chains fold together to form the antigen-combining site.[3,4] Hence, each of these regions of hypervariability is designated a CDR (see Fig. 75–7).

During secondary immune responses, extensive amino acid substitutions may occur in the CDRs. In contrast, amino acid replacement mutations occur much less frequently in the FRs than would be anticipated if the nucleic acid substitutions were occurring randomly. As a consequence, the subgroup determinants that characterize an entire variable-region subgroup may be relatively resilient to somatic hypermutation. On the other hand, the CDRs may form determinants of unique specificity that contribute to the epitopes recognized by antiidiotypic antibodies.

Despite the tremendous potential for diversity in Ig V gene expression and genetic polymorphism, antibodies produced by B-cell malignancies or normal B cells of unrelated persons may share common idiotypic determinants.[95] These common idiotypes, designated crossreactive idiotypes (CRIs), were defined initially on IgM autoantibodies, such as rheumatoid factors. However, CRIs may be found on antibodies that do not have anti–self-reactivity. Molecular studies demonstrate that several of these CRIs represent serologic markers for expression of conserved immunoglobulin variable-region genes with little or no somatic mutation.

IMMUNOGLOBULIN ALLOTYPES

HEAVY-CHAIN ALLOTYPES

Human immunoglobulins have inherited differences in structure, termed allotypes. These genetic markers usually are detected with agglutinating sera from individuals naturally immunized through transfusion or pregnancy. These antibodies recognize minor amino acid sequence variations in the constant regions of γ, α, and κ chains.[96] No definite allotypic differences have been detected on μ, δ, or λ chains. On ε chains, a monoclonal antibody to IgE defined an allotype that was common to persons of all races except for a few individuals of Asian or Melanesian background.

The α-chain allotypes, designated Am allotypes, are on the heavy chains of the IgA$_2$ subclass. The γ-chain allotypes are on the heavy chains of the IgG$_1$, IgG$_2$, and IgG$_3$ subclasses and are designated G$_1$m, G$_2$m, and G$_3$m, respectively. More than 24 Gm allotypic markers have been identified serologically. All the heavy-chain constant-region genes reside on chromosome 14. Therefore, different combinations of heavy-chain allotype markers are inherited as haplotypic units, in an autosomal codominant manner. The frequency of the various allelic markers differs among ethnic groups.[4,96,97]

Particular immunoglobulin allotypes have been associated with susceptibility or resistance to infectious diseases or the relative immune response to particular vaccines.[98,99] This could reflect linkage disequilibrium between particular polymorphic immunoglobulin variable region genes and constant region genes encoding particular immunoglobulin allotypes. Also, most humanized IgG$_1$ monoclonal antibodies licensed for therapy have κ light chains of the Km(3) allotype and γ_1 heavy chains of the G$_1$m$_{17}$ or G$_1$m$_3$ allotype.[96] As such, patients lacking such allotypes, who are treated with such monoclonal antibodies, may develop antiallotypic antibodies against G$_1$m or Km(3) determinants, respectively found on the heavy or light chain of the therapeutic antibody.[100]

LIGHT-CHAIN ALLOTYPES

The κ light-chain allotypes are designated Km allotypes (formerly called inv). At least three major Km allotypes exist, designated Km(1), 1 Km(1,2), and Km(3), which may be recognized serologically or via molecular techniques.[98] Patients with B-cell malignancies who are treated with allogeneic hematopoietic stem cell transplantation have been noted to have better survival outcomes when there is disparity in the κ light-chain allotypes between donor and recipient, presumably because of an enhanced capacity to mount a graft-versus-leukemia effect.[101]

Seven Jλ-Cλ gene segments are telomeric to the upstream Vλ genes, but only four such segments are functional, namely Jλ1-Cλ1, Jλ2-Cλ2, Jλ3-Cλ3, and Jλ7-Cλ7 (see Fig. 75–5). These segments respectively encode the four identified isotypes of λ light chains, termed Mcg$^+$Ke$^+$Oz$^-$, Mcg$^-$Ke$^-$Oz$^-$, Mcg$^-$Ke$^-$Oz$^+$, and Mcp$^+$Ke$^+$Oz$^-$, which were defined based on their reactivity with the Oz, Kern, Mcg, and Mcp antisera raised against λ Bence Jones proteins and that reflect minor non-allelic amino acid differences in the λ light-chain constant regions.[102] A fifth type of λ light-chain, termed Mcg⁻Ke⁺Oz⁻ is highly homologous to Mcg⁻Ke⁻Oz⁻ and actually results from a polymorphic gene amplification in a functional polymorphic Cλ2 segment.[102]

IMMUNOGLOBULIN SYNTHESIS AND SECRETION

IMMUNOGLOBULIN SYNTHESIS

The total IgG content of the adult human body is approximately 75 g, of which 2.2 g is synthesized each day. Most immunoglobulin is produced by mature plasma cells, which have abundant rough endoplasmic reticulum, a well-developed Golgi apparatus, and high-level transcription of the immunoglobulin genes. The final mRNAs for immunoglobulin light and heavy chains are derived by the processing of large nuclear RNA transcripts. In plasma cells, the rearranged and spliced mRNA molecules for the heavy-chain and light-chain polypeptides are translated on separate ribosomal complexes.

The folding and assembly of intact immunoglobulin molecules occur in the endoplasmic reticulum (ER), which contains a large set of redox catalysts and chaperones that guide the folding of nascent proteins.[103] First, an aminoterminal leader peptide approximately 18 to 30 residues long is cleaved prior to the release of the completed light and heavy chains in the cisternae of the ER. The ER harbors a single prominent and highly conserved HSP70 family member, BiP, along with over 20 protein-disulphide-isomerase (PDI) oxidoreductases with CXXC active site motifs.[104,105] The heavy-chain immunoglobulin polypeptides interact via their C_H1 domains with BiP that allows for proper folding of the heavy-chain polypeptide and prevents its transport into the Golgi. The nascent immunoglobulin polypeptides also bind the various ER or ER-Golgi-intermediate compartment (ERGIC) proteins transiently, some shorter and some for longer periods, either simultaneously or in sequence, to allow for the proper folding and assembly of the IgM chains. For example, early in the process, GRP94 binds the nascent heavy chain after BiP to promote folding of H chains and assembly with L chains to HL "hemimers," whereas much later, ERGIC53 acts after ERp44, when they assist assembly of H_2L_2 monomers into multimers.[106] The nascent immunoglobulin light chains can displace BiP and then spontaneously combine with the heavy chain to form immunoglobulin half molecules that are stabilized by disulfide bonds.[107] The process also requires the reduction-oxidation (redox) conditions generated by redox catalysts within ER, a requirement that has handicapped efforts to produce immunoglobulin in prokaryotic cell-free expression systems.[108] The joining of two identical half molecules by disulfide bonds yields a basic four-chain immunoglobulin unit, which then is allowed to transport to the Golgi for glycosylation.

Glycosyltransferase enzymes add a defined sequence of sugars to the assembled immunoglobulin unit to form branched-chain oligosaccharides composed of N-acetyl-glucosamine, mannose, galactose, fructose, and sialic acid. The oligosaccharides are attached covalently to the immunoglobulin heavy chain at several sites. The carbohydrate facilitates the transport of the antibody molecule across the plasma membrane and into the extracellular space and increases the solubility of the secreted protein.[109] Specific types of glycosylation also may improve the clinical activity of therapeutic monoclonal antibodies.[7,110]

Five monomeric units of IgM combine to form a pentameric macroglobulin linked by disulfide bonds and a single J-chain polypeptide. Usually polymerization immediately precedes or occurs simultaneously with IgM secretion. Similarly, IgA molecules form dimers and polymers linked by the J chain just prior to secretion from the plasma cell.

REGULATION OF IMMUNOGLOBULIN SYNTHESIS

GENERATION OF PLASMA CELLS

A normal adult has some preexisting B lymphocytes that can produce immunoglobulin that can bind almost any foreign antigen. Such B cells can be recruited to the immune response against the antigen. In the presence of accessory T-follicular helper cells (T_{FH}; Chap. 76), an antigen-binding clone of B lymphocytes may transform into antibody-secreting plasma cells.[111]

Transcription factors regulate this differentiation of B cells into antibody-secreting plasma cells. An important factor in plasma cell differentiation is the *B-lymphocyte-induced maturation protein-1* (Blimp-1),[112] which also is called the *positive regulatory domain 1-binding factor-1* (PRDM1) because it initially was identified by its ability to bind to the positive regulatory domain I of the human interferon-β promoter.[113] Blimp-1 is a zinc finger-containing transcription factor encoded by *PRDM1* on human chromosome 6q21 that represses expression of genes encoding transcription factors that inhibit plasma-cell differentiation (e.g., *MYC*, B-cell chronic lymphocytic leukemia/lymphoma 6 [*BCL-6*], paired box gene 5 [*PAX5*], microphthalmia-associated transcription factor [*MITF*], and basic leucine zipper transcription factor 2 [*BACH2*]).[112] On the other hand, Blimp-1 directly or indirectly induces expression of other transcription factors that control genes encoding other transcription factors or proteins responsible for plasma-cell differentiation and/or immunoglobulin secretion (e.g., X-box binding protein-1 [*XBP1*], E2F transcription factor 1 [*E2F1*], v-myb myeloblastosis viral oncogene homologues 1 and 2 [*MYBL1/MYBL2*], early B-cell factor 1 [*EBF1*], Pou domain, class 2, factor 2, or associating factor 1 [*POU2F2/POU2AF1*], and transcription factor E2a [*TCFE2A*]). This capacity of Blimp-1 to repress and to activate expression of a variety of different transcription factors accounts for its capacity to orchestrate the dramatic changes in B-cell morphology and function associated with plasma-cell differentiation and high-level secretion of immunoglobulin protein. Mice with a conditional deletion of *PRDM1* encoding Blimp-1 in the B lineage demonstrate the critical requirement of Blimp-1 in plasma cell development.[114] Although such mice have normal numbers of B cells and develop germinal centers in response to T-dependent antigens, they fail to generate plasma cells or to secrete normal levels of immunoglobulin in response to either T-independent or T-dependent antigens. Furthermore, other studies found that expression of Blimp-1 is required for the maintenance of long-lived plasma cells in the marrow and the long-term expression of antigen-specific immunoglobulin in the plasma.[115]

Some diffuse large B-cell lymphomas (DLBCLs) have deletions or inactivating mutations in *PRDM1*, suggesting that this gene also might act as a tumor suppressor.[116] However, *PRDM1* mutations are not found in other lymphoid or myeloid leukemias, and myeloma cells and some DLBCLs express abundant levels of Blimp-1, making it appear unlikely that Blimp-1 suppresses tumor development *per se*.[117] Moreover, the DLBCL cases that expressed Blimp-1 lacked detectable plasmacytic features and actually displayed more aggressive behavior.[118] As such, B-cell expression of Blimp-1 appears necessary but not sufficient for plasma-cell differentiation.

The expression of Blimp-1 in B cells is regulated primarily at the level of *PRDM1* transcription, which requires activation by the transcription factor *interferon regulatory factor 4* (IRF4).[112] Transgenic mice that have B cells with a conditional deletion of *IRF4* fail to generate immunoglobulin-secreting plasma cells.[119] Substances that activate toll-like receptor 4 (TLR4) or toll-like receptor 9 (TLR9), such as lipopolysaccharide or CpG oligonucleotides, respectively, also can activate expression of Blimp-1.[112,120] Mice lacking such toll-like receptors cannot mount effective antibody responses,[121] except under certain conditions.[122] Several cytokines, including IL-2, IL-5, IL-6, IL-10, and IL-21, also can induce expression of Blimp-1 when applied in the proper context. Indeed, such cytokines can have positive or negative effects on B-cell differentiation and/or survival depending upon the presence or absence of other signals. IL-21, for example, can induce expression of Blimp-1 and plasma cell differentiation primarily in memory B cells or B cells that previously had been activated via ligation of its B-cell receptor, namely surface immunoglobulin, when in the context of receiving T-cell helper signals, such as that caused by ligation of CD40.[123,124] On the other hand, IL-21 can induce apoptosis of B cells that are activated via ligation of its surface immunoglobulin receptor in the absence of such T-cell helper signals.[124]

MEMORY B CELLS

Following a T-cell dependent immune response to antigen, B cells that express high-affinity immunoglobulin for antigen also can differentiate into memory B cells.[125] Memory B cells differ from plasma cells in morphology and function. In contrast to plasma cells, memory B cells do not secrete immunoglobulin, but rather express surface immunoglobulin that can bind antigen and can be induced to differentiate rapidly into immunoglobulin secreting plasma cells after secondary challenge with antigen. Also, memory B cells may reengage the germinal center to undergo additional rounds of somatic hypermutation to enhance further the Ig repertoire.[126]

Human memory B cells can be distinguished by their expression of CD27 and CD148.[127] Memory B cells also have increased expression of immune costimulatory molecules CD80 and CD86,[128] particularly following immune activation, which enhances their capacity to induce immune coactivation of T-helper cells (Chap. 76). In addition, memory B cells have high-level expression of antiapoptotic genes *BCL2* and *BCL-XL*,[129] which help enhance their long-term survival. Finally, memory B cells lack expression of *BCL-6*, which actually can repress memory B-cell development.[130] Because *BCL-6* also can repress expression of *PRDM1*, the lack of *BCL-6* expression makes memory B cells particularly amenable to stimulation by factors that induce expression of Blimp-1,[119] thereby enhancing the capacity of memory B cells that express antigen-binding immunoglobulin to undergo rapid differentiation into plasma cells during the secondary immune response to antigen.[131]

REFERENCES

1. Edelman GM: Antibody structure and molecular immunology. *Scand J Immunol* 34:1, 1991.
2. Schroeder HW Jr, Cavacini L: Structure and function of immunoglobulins. *J Allergy Clin Immunol* 125:S41, 2010.
3. Alamyar E, Giudicelli V, Duroux P, Lefranc MP: Antibody V and C domain sequence, structure, and interaction analysis with special reference to IMGT(R). *Methods Mol Biol* 1131:337, 2014.
4. Lefranc MP: Immunoglobulin and T cell receptor genes: IMGT((R)) and the birth and rise of immunoinformatics. *Front Immunol* 5:22, 2014.
5. Kabat E, Wu TT, Perry HM, et al: *Sequences of proteins of immunological interest.* U.S. Department of Health and Human Services, Bethesda, MD, 1991.
6. Lee YK, Brewer JW, Hellman R, Hendershot LM: BiP and immunoglobulin light chain cooperate to control the folding of heavy chain and ensure the fidelity of plasmoglobulin assembly. *Mol Biol Cell* 10:2209, 1999.
7. Vidarsson G, Dekkers G, Rispens T: IgG subclasses and allotypes: From structure to effector functions. *Front Immunol* 5:520, 2014.
8. Niwa R, Natsume A, Uehara A, et al: IgG subclass-independent improvement of antibody-dependent cellular cytotoxicity by fucose removal from Asn297-linked oligosaccharides. *J Immunol Methods* 306:151, 2005.
9. Macpherson AJ, McCoy KD, Johansen FE, Brandtzaeg P: The immune geography of IgA induction and function. *Mucosal Immunol* 1:11, 2008.
10. Horton RE, Vidarsson G: Antibodies and their receptors: Different potential roles in mucosal defense. *Front Immunol* 4:200, 2013.
11. Wines BD, Hogarth PM: IgA receptors in health and disease. *Tissue Antigens* 68:103, 2006.
12. Novak J, Julian BA, Tomana M, Mestecky J: IgA glycosylation and IgA immune complexes in the pathogenesis of IgA nephropathy. *Semin Nephrol* 28:78, 2008.
13. Sanders JT, Wyatt RJ: IgA nephropathy and Henoch-Schönlein purpura nephritis. *Curr Opin Pediatr* 20:163, 2008.
14. Yoo EM, Coloma MJ, Trinh KR, et al: Structural requirements for polymeric immunoglobulin assembly and association with J chain. *J Biol Chem* 274:33771, 1999.
15. Brezski RJ, Monroe JG: B-cell receptor. *Adv Exp Med Biol* 640:12, 2008.
16. Chen K, Xu W, Wilson M, et al: Immunoglobulin D enhances immune surveillance by activating antimicrobial, proinflammatory and B cell-stimulating programs in basophils. *Nat Immunol* 10:889, 2009.
17. Roes J, Rajewsky K: Immunoglobulin D (IgD)-deficient mice reveal an auxiliary receptor function for IgD in antigen-mediated recruitment of B cells. *J Exp Med* 177:45, 1993.
18. Lyczak JB, Zhang K, Saxon A, Morrison SL: Expression of novel secreted isoforms of human immunoglobulin E proteins. *J Biol Chem* 271:3428, 1996.
19. Tolar P, Hanna J, Krueger PD, Pierce SK: The constant region of the membrane immunoglobulin mediates B cell-receptor clustering and signaling in response to membrane antigens. *Immunity* 30:44, 2009.
20. Wang Y, Kanegane H, Sanal O, et al: Novel Igalpha (CD79a) gene mutation in a Turkish patient with B cell-deficient agammaglobulinemia. *Am J Med Genet* 108:333, 2002.
21. Carrasco YR, Batista FD: B cell recognition of membrane-bound antigen: An exquisite way of sensing ligands. *Curr Opin Immunol* 18:286, 2006.
22. Qi H, Egen JG, Huang AY, Germain RN: Extrafollicular activation of lymph node B cells by antigen-bearing dendritic cells. *Science* 312:1672, 2006.
23. Phan TG, Grigorova I, Okada T, Cyster JG: Subcapsular encounter and complement-dependent transport of immune complexes by lymph node B cells. *Nat Immunol* 8:992, 2007.
24. Junt T, Moseman EA, Iannacone M, et al: Subcapsular sinus macrophages in lymph nodes clear lymph-borne viruses and present them to antiviral B cells. *Nature* 450:110, 2007.
25. Wu JN, Koretzky GA: The SLP-76 family of adapter proteins. *Semin Immunol* 16:379, 2004.
26. Weber M, Treanor B, Depoil D, et al: Phospholipase C-gamma2 and Vav cooperate within signaling microclusters to propagate B cell spreading in response to membrane-bound antigen. *J Exp Med* 205:853, 2008.
27. Ysebaert L, Michallet AS: Bruton's tyrosine kinase inhibitors: Lessons learned from bench-to-bedside (first) studies. *Curr Opin Oncol* 26:463, 2014.
28. Depoil D, Weber M, Treanor B, et al: Early events of B cell activation by antigen. *Sci Signal* 2:pt 1, 2009.
29. Baba T, Fusaki N, Aoyama A, et al: Dual regulation of BCR-mediated growth inhibition signaling by CD72. *Eur J Immunol* 35:1634, 2005.
30. Zhu C, Sato M, Yanagisawa T, et al: Novel binding site for Src homology 2-containing protein-tyrosine phosphatase-1 in CD22 activated by B lymphocyte stimulation with antigen. *J Biol Chem* 283:1653, 2008.
31. Fournier EM, Siberil S, Costes A, et al: Activation of human peripheral IgM+ B cells is transiently inhibited by BCR-independent aggregation of Fc gammaRIIB. *J Immunol* 181:5350, 2008.
32. Shultz LD, Rajan TV, Greiner DL: Severe defects in immunity and hematopoiesis caused by SHP-1 protein-tyrosine-phosphatase deficiency. *Trends Biotechnol* 15:302, 1997.
33. Matsuda F, Ishii K, Bourvagnet P, et al: The complete nucleotide sequence of the human immunoglobulin heavy chain variable region locus. *J Exp Med* 188:2151, 1998.
34. Dunham I, Shimizu N, Roe BA, et al: The DNA sequence of human chromosome 22. *Nature* 402:489, 1999.
35. Bassing CH, Alt FW, Hughes MM, et al: Recombination signal sequences restrict chromosomal V(D)J recombination beyond the 12/23 rule. *Nature* 405:583, 2000.
36. Gellert M: Recent advances in understanding V(D)J recombination. *Adv Immunol* 64:39, 1997.
37. Schatz DG, Swanson PC: V(D)J recombination: Mechanisms of initiation. *Annu Rev Genet* 45:167, 2011.
38. Das S, Nikolaidis N, Nei M: Genomic organization and evolution of immunoglobulin kappa gene enhancers and kappa deleting element in mammals. *Mol Immunol* 46:3171, 2009.
39. Xiang Y, Park SK, Garrard WT: Vkappa gene repertoire and locus contraction are specified by critical DNase I hypersensitive sites within the Vkappa-Jkappa intervening region. *J Immunol* 190:1819, 2013.
40. Shinkai Y, Rathbun G, Lam KP, et al: RAG-2-deficient mice lack mature lymphocytes owing to inability to initiate V(D)J rearrangement. *Cell* 68:855, 1992.
41. Villa A, Notarangelo LD, Roifman CM: Omenn syndrome: Inflammation in leaky severe combined immunodeficiency. *J Allergy Clin Immunol* 122:1082, 2008.
42. Gellert M: V(D)J recombination: RAG proteins, repair factors, and regulation. *Annu Rev Biochem* 71:101, 2002.

43. Lieber MR: The mechanism of double-strand DNA break repair by the nonhomologous DNA end-joining pathway. *Annu Rev Biochem* 79:181, 2010.

44. Rooney S, Chaudhuri J, Alt FW: The role of the non-homologous end-joining pathway in lymphocyte development. *Immunol Rev* 200:115, 2004.

45. Gostissa M, Alt FW, Chiarle R: Mechanisms that promote and suppress chromosomal translocations in lymphocytes. *Annu Rev Immunol* 29:319, 2011.

46. Nussenzweig A, Nussenzweig MC: Origin of chromosomal translocations in lymphoid cancer. *Cell* 141:27, 2010.

47. Helmink BA, Sleckman BP: The response to and repair of RAG-mediated DNA double-strand breaks. *Annu Rev Immunol* 30:175, 2012.

48. Steen SB, Gomelsky L, Speidel SL, Roth DB: Initiation of V(D)J recombination in vivo: Role of recombination signal sequences in formation of single and paired double-strand breaks. *EMBO J* 16:2656, 1997.

49. Jones JM, Simkus C: The roles of the RAG1 and RAG2 "non-core" regions in V(D)J recombination and lymphocyte development. *Arch Immunol Ther Exp (Warsz)* 57:105, 2009.

50. Tsai CL, Drejer AH, Schatz DG: Evidence of a critical architectural function for the RAG proteins in end processing, protection, and joining in V(D)J recombination. *Genes Dev* 16:1934, 2002.

51. Ciubotaru M, Trexler AJ, Spiridon LN, et al: RAG and HMGB1 create a large bend in the 23RSS in the V(D)J recombination synaptic complexes. *Nucleic Acids Res* 41:2437, 2013.

52. Schatz DG, Spanopoulou E: Biochemistry of V(D)J recombination. *Curr Top Microbiol Immunol* 290:49, 2005.

53. Goodarzi AA, Jeggo PA: The repair and signaling responses to DNA double-strand breaks. *Adv Genet* 82:1, 2013.

54. Khanna KK, Jackson SP: DNA double-strand breaks: Signaling, repair and the cancer connection. *Nat Genet* 27:247, 2001.

55. Le Deist F, Poinsignon C, Moshous D, et al: Artemis sheds new light on V(D)J recombination. *Immunol Rev* 200:142, 2004.

56. Gu Y, Sekiguchi J, Gao Y, et al: Defective embryonic neurogenesis in Ku-deficient but not DNA-dependent protein kinase catalytic subunit-deficient mice. *Proc Natl Acad Sci U S A* 97:2668, 2000.

57. Surucu B, Bozulic L, Hynx D, et al: In vivo analysis of protein kinase B (PKB)/Akt regulation in DNA-PKcs-null mice reveals a role for PKB/Akt in DNA damage response and tumorigenesis. *J Biol Chem* 283:30025, 2008.

58. Al-Hakim A, Escribano-Diaz C, Landry MC, et al: The ubiquitous role of ubiquitin in the DNA damage response. *DNA Repair (Amst)* 9:1229, 2010.

59. Johnson K, Chaumeil J, Skok JA: Epigenetic regulation of V(D)J recombination. *Essays Biochem* 48:221, 2010.

60. Sleckman BP, Oltz EM: Preparing targets for V(D)J recombinase: Transcription paves the way. *J Immunol* 188:7, 2012.

61. Subrahmanyam R, Sen R: Epigenetic features that regulate IgH locus recombination and expression. *Curr Top Microbiol Immunol* 356:39, 2012.

62. Chao J, Rothschild G, Basu U: Ubiquitination events that regulate recombination of immunoglobulin Loci gene segments. *Front Immunol* 5:100, 2014.

63. Grazini U, Zanardi F, Citterio E, et al: The RING domain of RAG1 ubiquitylates histone H3: A novel activity in chromatin-mediated regulation of V(D)J joining. *Mol Cell* 37:282, 2010.

64. Jones JM, Bhattacharyya A, Simkus C, et al: The RAG1 V(D)J recombinase/ubiquitin ligase promotes ubiquitylation of acetylated, phosphorylated histone 3.3. *Immunol Lett* 136:156, 2011.

65. Kassmeier MD, Mondal K, Palmer VL, et al: VprBP binds full-length RAG1 and is required for B-cell development and V(D)J recombination fidelity. *EMBO J* 31:945, 2012.

66. Simkus C, Bhattacharyya A, Zhou M, et al: Correlation between recombinase activating gene 1 ubiquitin ligase activity and V(D)J recombination. *Immunology* 128:206, 2009.

67. Jiang H, Chang FC, Ross AE, et al: Ubiquitylation of RAG-2 by Skp2-SCF links destruction of the V(D)J recombinase to the cell cycle. *Mol Cell* 18:699, 2005.

68. Rassenti LZ, Kipps TJ: Lack of allelic exclusion in B cell chronic lymphocytic leukemia. *J Exp Med* 185:1435, 1997.

69. Tsuganezawa K, Kiyokawa N, Matsuo Y, et al: Flow cytometric diagnosis of the cell lineage and developmental stage of acute lymphoblastic leukemia by novel monoclonal antibodies specific to human pre-B-cell receptor. *Blood* 92:4317, 1998.

70. Bankovich AJ, Raunser S, Juo ZS, et al: Structural insight into pre-B cell receptor function. *Science* 316:291, 2007.

71. Corcos D, Dunda O, Butor C, et al: Pre-B-cell development in the absence of lambda 5 in transgenic mice expressing a heavy-chain disease protein. *Curr Biol* 5:1140, 1995.

72. Minegishi Y, Coustan-Smith E, Wang YH, et al: Mutations in the human lambda5/14.1 gene result in B cell deficiency and agammaglobulinemia. *J Exp Med* 187:71, 1998.

73. Stavnezer J, Guikema JE, Schrader CE: Mechanism and regulation of class switch recombination. *Annu Rev Immunol* 26:261, 2008.

74. Ferrari SPlebani A: Cross-talk between CD40 and CD40L: Lessons from primary immune deficiencies. *Curr Opin Allergy Clin Immunol* 2:489, 2002.

75. Cerutti A: The regulation of IgA class switching. *Nat Rev Immunol* 8:421, 2008.

76. Mora JR, von Andrian UH: Differentiation and homing of IgA-secreting cells. *Mucosal Immunol* 1:96, 2008.

77. Yamane A, Robbiani DF, Resch W, et al: RPA accumulation during class switch recombination represents 5′-3′ DNA-end resection during the S-G2/M phase of the cell cycle. *Cell Rep* 3:138, 2013.

78. Dudley DD, Chaudhuri J, Bassing CH, Alt FW: Mechanism and control of V(D)J recombination versus class switch recombination: Similarities and differences. *Adv Immunol* 86:43, 2005.

79. Revy P, Muto T, Levy Y, et al: Activation-induced cytidine deaminase (AID) deficiency causes the autosomal recessive form of the hyper-IgM syndrome (HIGM2). *Cell* 102:565, 2000.

80. Zahn A, Eranki AK, Patenaude AM, et al: Activation induced deaminase C-terminal domain links DNA breaks to end protection and repair during class switch recombination. *Proc Natl Acad Sci U S A* 111:E988, 2014.

81. Imai K, Slupphaug G, Lee WI, et al: Human uracil-DNA glycosylase deficiency associated with profoundly impaired immunoglobulin class-switch recombination. *Nat Immunol* 4:1023, 2003.

82. Kaji T, Furukawa K, Ishige A, et al: Both mutated and unmutated memory B cells accumulate mutations in the course of the secondary response and develop a new antibody repertoire optimally adapted to the secondary stimulus. *Int Immunol* 25:683, 2013.

83. Michael N, Martin TE, Nicolae D, et al: Effects of sequence and structure on the hypermutability of immunoglobulin genes. *Immunity* 16:123, 2002.

84. Di Noia JM, Neuberger MS: Molecular mechanisms of antibody somatic hypermutation. *Annu Rev Biochem* 76:1, 2007.

85. Peled JU, Kuang FL, Iglesias-Ussel MD, et al: The biochemistry of somatic hypermutation. *Annu Rev Immunol* 26:481, 2008.

86. Muramatsu M, Kinoshita K, Fagarasan S, et al: Class switch recombination and hypermutation require activation-induced cytidine deaminase (AID), a potential RNA editing enzyme. *Cell* 102:553, 2000.

87. Buerstedde JM, Alinikula J, Arakawa H, et al: Targeting of somatic hypermutation by immunoglobulin enhancer and enhancer-like sequences. *PLoS Biol* 12:e1001831, 2014.

88. Aoufouchi S, Faili A, Zober C, et al: Proteasomal degradation restricts the nuclear lifespan of AID. *J Exp Med* 205:1357, 2008.

89. Delker RK, Zhou Y, Strikoudis A, et al: Solubility-based genetic screen identifies RING finger protein 126 as an E3 ligase for activation-induced cytidine deaminase. *Proc Natl Acad Sci U S A* 110:1029, 2013.

90. Storb U, Shen HM, Michael N, Kim N: Somatic hypermutation of immunoglobulin and non-immunoglobulin genes. *Philos Trans R Soc Lond B Biol Sci* 356:13, 2001.

91. Allen CD, Cyster JG: Follicular dendritic cell networks of primary follicles and germinal centers: Phenotype and function. *Semin Immunol* 20:14, 2008.

92. Cook GP, Tomlinson IM: The human immunoglobulin VH repertoire. *Immunol Today* 16:237, 1995.

93. Kipps TJ: Human B cell biology. *Int Rev Immunol* 15:243, 1997.

94. Frippiat JP, Williams SC, Tomlinson IM, et al: Organization of the human immunoglobulin lambda light-chain locus on chromosome 22q11.2. *Hum Mol Genet* 4:983, 1995.

95. Kipps TJ, Carson DA: Autoantibodies in chronic lymphocytic leukemia and related systemic autoimmune diseases. *Blood* 81:2475, 1993.

96. Jefferis R, Lefranc MP: Human immunoglobulin allotypes: Possible implications for immunogenicity. *MAbs* 1:332, 2009.

97. Schanfield MS, Ferrell RE, Hossaini AA, et al: Immunoglobulin allotypes in Southwest Asia: Populations at the crossroads. *Am J Hum Biol* 20:671, 2008.

98. Pandey JP: Immunoglobulin GM and KM allotypes and vaccine immunity. *Vaccine* 19:613, 2000.

99. Muratori P, Sutherland SE, Muratori L, et al: Immunoglobulin GM and KM allotypes and prevalence of anti-LKM1 autoantibodies in patients with hepatitis C virus infection. *J Virol* 80:5097, 2006.

100. Magdelaine-Beuzelin C, Vermeire S, Goodall M, et al: IgG1 heavy chain-coding gene polymorphism (G1m allotypes) and development of antibodies-to-infliximab. *Pharmacogenet Genomics* 19:383, 2009.

101. Etto TL, Stewart LA, Muirhead J, et al: Kappa immunoglobulin light chain polymorphisms and survival after allogeneic transplantation for B-cell malignancies: A potential graft-vs-leukaemia target. *Tissue Antigens* 69:56, 2007.

102. van der Burg M, Barendregt BH, van Gastel-Mol EJ, et al: Unraveling of the polymorphic C lambda 2-C lambda 3 amplification and the Ke+Oz– polymorphism in the human Ig lambda locus. *J Immunol* 169:271, 2002.

103. Shimizu Y, Hendershot LM: Organization of the functions and components of the endoplasmic reticulum. *Adv Exp Med Biol* 594:37, 2007.

104. Appenzeller-Herzog C, Ellgaard L: The human PDI family: Versatility packed into a single fold. *Biochim Biophys Acta* 1783:535, 2008.

105. van Anken E, Pena F, Hafkemeijer N, et al: Efficient IgM assembly and secretion require the plasma cell induced endoplasmic reticulum protein pERp1. *Proc Natl Acad Sci U S A* 106:17019, 2009.

106. Anelli T, Ceppi S, Bergamelli L, et al: Sequential steps and checkpoints in the early exocytic compartment during secretory IgM biogenesis. *EMBO J* 26:4177, 2007.

107. Reddy PS, Corley RB: The contribution of ER quality control to the biologic functions of secretory IgM. *Immunol Today* 20:582, 1999.

108. Frey S, Haslbeck M, Hainzl O, Buchner J: Synthesis and characterization of a functional intact IgG in a prokaryotic cell-free expression system. *Biol Chem* 389:37, 2008.

109. Rudd PM, Elliott T, Cresswell P, et al: Glycosylation and the immune system. *Science* 291:2370, 2001.

110. Jefferis R: Glycosylation as a strategy to improve antibody-based therapeutics. *Nat Rev Drug Discov* 8:226, 2009.

111. Johnston RJ, Poholek AC, DiToro D, et al: Bcl6 and Blimp-1 are reciprocal and antagonistic regulators of T follicular helper cell differentiation. *Science* 325:1006, 2009.

112. Martins G, Calame K: Regulation and functions of Blimp-1 in T and B lymphocytes. *Annu Rev Immunol* 26:133, 2008.

113. Keller AD, Maniatis T: Identification and characterization of a novel repressor of beta-interferon gene expression. *Genes Dev* 5:868, 1991.

114. Shapiro-Shelef M, Lin KI, McHeyzer-Williams LJ, et al: Blimp-1 is required for the formation of immunoglobulin secreting plasma cells and pre-plasma memory B cells. *Immunity* 19:607, 2003.

115. Shapiro-Shelef M, Lin KI, Savitsky D, et al: Blimp-1 is required for maintenance of long-lived plasma cells in the bone marrow. *J Exp Med* 202:1471, 2005.

116. Tam W, Gomez M, Chadburn A, et al: Mutational analysis of PRDM1 indicates a tumor-suppressor role in diffuse large B-cell lymphomas. *Blood* 107:4090, 2006.

117. Garcia JF, Roncador G, Sanz AI, et al: PRDM1/BLIMP-1 expression in multiple B and T-cell lymphoma. *Haematologica* 91:467, 2006.

118. Pasqualucci L, Compagno M, Houldsworth J, et al: Inactivation of the PRDM1/BLIMP1 gene in diffuse large B cell lymphoma. *J Exp Med* 203:311, 2006.

119. Klein U, Casola S, Cattoretti G, et al: Transcription factor IRF4 controls plasma cell differentiation and class-switch recombination. *Nat Immunol* 7:773, 2006.

120. Lin KI, Kao YY, Kuo HK, et al: Reishi polysaccharides induce immunoglobulin production through the TLR4/TLR2-mediated induction of transcription factor Blimp-1. *J Biol Chem* 281:24111, 2006.

121. Pasare C, Medzhitov R: Control of B-cell responses by Toll-like receptors. *Nature* 438:364, 2005.

122. Nemazee D, Gavin A, Hoebe K, Beutler B: Immunology: Toll-like receptors and antibody responses. *Nature* 441:E4; discussion E4, 2006.

123. Ettinger R, Sims GP, Fairhurst AM, et al: IL-21 induces differentiation of human naive and memory B cells into antibody-secreting plasma cells. *J Immunol* 175:7867, 2005.

124. Konforte D, Simard N, Paige CJ: IL-21: An executor of B cell fate. *J Immunol* 182:1781, 2009.

125. Tarlinton D: B-cell memory: Are subsets necessary? *Nat Rev Immunol* 6:785, 2006.

126. Bende RJ, van Maldegem F, Triesscheijn M, et al: Germinal centers in human lymph nodes contain reactivated memory B cells. *J Exp Med* 204:2655, 2007.

127. Tangye SG, Liu YJ, Aversa G, et al: Identification of functional human splenic memory B cells by expression of CD148 and CD27. *J Exp Med* 188:1691, 1998.

128. Liu YJ, Barthelemy C, de Bouteiller O, et al: Memory B cells from human tonsils colonize mucosal epithelium and directly present antigen to T cells by rapid up-regulation of B7-1 and B7-2. *Immunity* 2:239, 1995.

129. Klein U, Tu Y, Stolovitzky GA, et al: Transcriptional analysis of the B cell germinal center reaction. *Proc Natl Acad Sci U S A* 100:2639, 2003.

130. Kuo TC, Shaffer AL, Haddad J Jr, et al: Repression of BCL-6 is required for the formation of human memory B cells *in vitro*. *J Exp Med* 204:819, 2007.

131. Good KL, Avery DT, Tangye SG: Resting human memory B cells are intrinsically programmed for enhanced survival and responsiveness to diverse stimuli compared to naive B cells. *J Immunol* 182:890, 2009.

CHAPTER 76
FUNCTIONS OF T LYMPHOCYTES: T-CELL RECEPTORS FOR ANTIGEN

Fabienne McClanahan and John Gribben*

SUMMARY

All T cells express a receptor for antigen that is formed by two polymorphic polypeptides that invariably are associated with a collection of invariant proteins, namely CD3γ, CD3δ, CD3ε, and CD247. These invariant proteins are necessary for surface expression and signaling by the T-cell receptor. The two polypeptides that form the T-cell receptor on most T cells are termed α and β. A small subset of T cells has receptors formed by different polypeptides termed γ and δ. The polypeptides of the T-cell receptor have a diversity that is comparable to that estimated for immunoglobulin molecules. However, unlike immunoglobulins, the T-cell receptors recognize small fragments of antigen only if they are presented to them by defined major histocompatibility complex molecules on the plasma membrane of another cell, the antigen-presenting cell. The response of the T cell to antigen depends on the intensity of the signal generated by ligation of the T-cell receptor, and is modified by the simultaneous ligation of other accessory molecules. Interactions at the contact sites between T-cells and antigen-presenting cells are organized in the immunologic synapse. The outcome of T-cell antigen recognition can range from immune activation and T-cell proliferation to specific T-cell tolerance and/or programmed cell death.

Acronyms and Abbreviations: AP-1, activation protein-1; APC, antigen-presenting cell; CTLA-4, cytotoxic T-lymphocyte antigen 4; ERK, extracellular receptor-activated kinase; FOXP3, forkhead box P3; ICAM, intercellular adhesion molecule; IFN-γ, interferon-gamma; IL, interleukin; IPEX syndrome, immune dysregulation, polyendocrinopathy, enteropathy, X-linked syndrome; ITAM, immunoreceptor tyrosine-based activation motif; ITIM, immunoreceptor tyrosine-based inhibitory motif; iT_{REG}, induced regulatory T cell; JNK, c-Jun N-terminal kinase; LAT, linker of activation of T cells; LFA, lymphocyte function associated; MAP, mitogen-activated protein; MHC, major histocompatibility complex; NFAT, nuclear factor of activated T cell; PKC, protein kinase C; PLC-$γ_1$, phospholipase C-1 gamma; RORγt, retinoic acid-related orphan receptor γ thymus isoform; SAPK, stress-activated protein kinase; SH2 domain, Src homology 2 domain; SH3 domain, Src homology 3 domain; STAT, signal transducer and activator of transcription; T_{FH} cell, follicular helper T cell; TGF-β, transforming growth factor beta; Th17, CD4+ T-cell subset that produces cytokines of the interleukin-17 family; T_{REG}, CD4+CD25+ regulatory T cells; V-like, variable-region-like; VLA, very-late activation; ZAP-70, zeta-associated protein of 70 kDa.

*This chapter was written by Thomas J. Kipps, M.D., Ph.D. in the 8th edition and portions of that chapter have been retained.

T-LYMPHOCYTE ANTIGEN RECEPTORS

T-CELL RECEPTOR HETERODIMERS

The structural basis of T-cell recognition of antigen has been known since the 1990s, when a plethora of studies demonstrated that the proteins of the T-cell antigen receptor are structurally related to immunoglobulin molecules.[1] The T-cell receptor is formed by a heterodimer, that is, two disulfide-bond-linked polypeptides that are expressed on the cell surface and are associated with a collection of coreceptor accessory and invariant CD3 proteins. In contrast to immunoglobulins, the T-cell receptor is not secreted and also remains membrane bound throughout the activation process. In the majority of T cells, the T-cell receptor heterodimer consists of an α and a β chain, but a small subset of T cells expresses a γδ heterodimer. Following the rule of allelic exclusion, each individual T cell expresses a single α and a single β chain (or a single γ or δ chain, respectively), and can either be αβ or γδ. Each chain is composed of a *variable region,* consisting of a hydrophobic leader sequence of 18 to 29 amino acids and an aminoterminal domain of 102 to 119 amino acids, and a *constant region* with a carboxyl-terminal region segment of 87 to 113 amino acids. The variable region is responsible for the variation in the primary structure among different T-cell receptor polypeptides and represents the antigen-binding site, while the constant region is invariant among chains of the same class. Similar to other surface-membrane receptors, each chain is followed by a small connecting peptide, a transmembrane region of 20 to 24 amino acids, and a small cytoplasmic region of 5 to 12 residues at the carboxyl terminus anchoring the polypeptide in the cell membrane. The T-cell receptor chains fold into tertiary structures that are very similar to that of the light and heavy chains of the immunoglobulin molecule. Overall, the structural similarities between the T-cell receptor and immunoglobulins place the genes encoding these receptor proteins in the so-called immunoglobulin supergene family.

αβ Heterodimers

More than 90 percent of mature T cells express an αβ heterodimer, making this the major class of T-cell receptor. Without glycan side chains, each α or β polypeptide has a respective size of only 27 kDa or 32 kDa. However, within minutes after being translated into protein, both chains are glycosylated and assembled into a heterodimer composed of a single acidic α glycoprotein of 39 to 46 kDa linked to a more basic 40- to 44-kDa β-glycoprotein via a disulfide bond between the constant regions of the two chains (Fig. 76–1).

γδ Heterodimers

Less than 10 percent of blood T cells and thymocytes exclusively express a γδ heterodimer. Within the γδ T-cell population, specific γδ T-cell subsets can be defined by their T-cell receptor gene element usage, and their functionally distinct responses to infections with certain organisms such as *Listeria monocytogenes*.[2] Alternatively, γδ T cells can be grouped according to their tissue location. In secondary lymphoid tissues, only 1 to 5 percent of the CD3-positive T cells express γδ receptors. Murine studies demonstrate that many epithelial tissues, such as the epidermis, the intestine, the lung, and the uterus, are enriched for γδ-expressing T cells, indicating that γδ T cells are involved in the surveillance of body barriers.[3]

The amino acid sequence of the γ chain resembles the T-cell receptor β chain, whereas the amino acid sequence of the δ chain resembles the α chain. Like the homologous αβ heterodimer, the γδ heterodimer is also associated with the CD3 complex and is capable of initiating T-cell activation upon binding of specific ligands. Despite the similarities in chain structure and size, however, the tertiary structure of variable

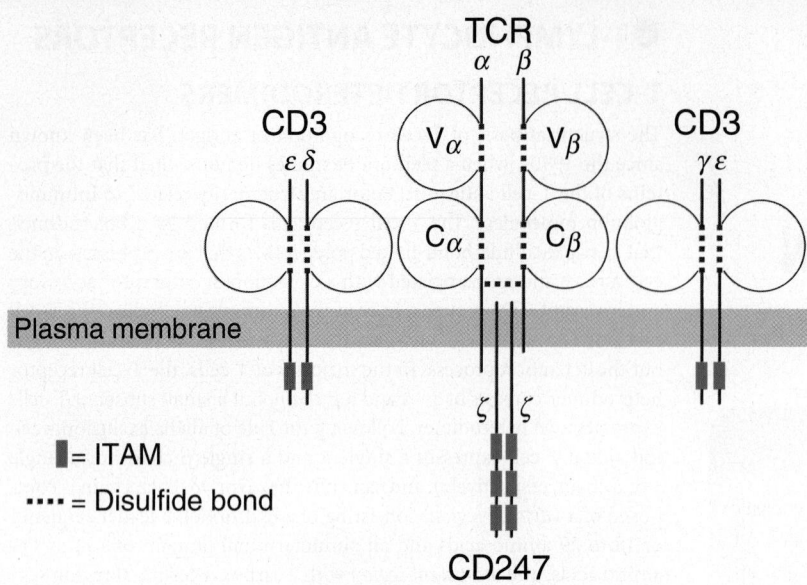

Figure 76–1. Schematic of the T-cell receptor (TCR) complex. The TCR is composed of the $\alpha\beta$ heterodimer, assembled by an α and a β chain, each of which consists of a variable (V) and a constant (C) domain. Both chains form loops and structurally resemble immunoglobulins. The TCR is accompanied by the invariant CD3 molecule, consisting of CD3ε, CD3δ, CD3γ, and CD3. For clarity, CD3ε/CD3δ and CD3γ/CD3ε are depicted separately. An additional component of the CD3 molecule is the ζ chain (CD247) homodimer, which associates with the α and β chain upon stimulation. The *dotted lines* represent intrachain or interchain disulfide bridges, as indicated in the legend in the *lower left-hand* corner. The plasma membrane spanned by each of these chains is indicated. The boxes indicate the immunoreceptor tyrosine-based activation motifs (ITAMs) in the cytoplasmic domains of the CD3 polypeptides and the ζ chain.

regions of $\gamma\delta$ T-cell receptors has a closer resemblance to immunoglobulin variable regions than to the variable regions of $\alpha\beta$ T-cell receptors.

T-CELL RECEPTOR HETERODIMER GENE REARRANGEMENT

Similar to immunoglobulin genes, each chain of the T-cell receptors is encoded by distinct genetic elements that rearrange during development generating a diverse T-cell repertoire (Fig. 76–2).[4] Located at band q35 on the long arm of chromosome 7, the β-chain complex has two closely linked genes, each capable of encoding the β-chain constant region. Each constant region gene is associated with a cluster of functional Jβ-gene segments and a single Dβ segment. The functional gene encoding the variable region of the β chain is constructed from the rearrangement of any of approximately 50 variable region gene segments to either one of the two Dβ regions and one of 13 Jβ regions.

The α-chain complex is located at band q11.2 on the long arm of chromosome 14 and thus is linked to the immunoglobulin heavy-chain complex. The α-chain gene complex consists of one constant region gene and at least 50 different variable region gene segments. The functional gene encoding the α-chain variable region is derived from the juxtaposition of any one of the variable region gene segments with one of the many Jα segments through rearrangement that generally involves the deletion of the intervening DNA.

The organization of the γ and δ genes is similar to that of the α and β genes, but some significant differences exist. First, the gene complex encoding the δ genes is located entirely within the α-chain gene complex between the Vα and Jα gene segments. Consequently, any rearrangement of the α-chain genes inactivates the genes encoding the δ chain. Second, there are fewer V gene segments in the γ and δ gene complexes than at either the T-cell receptor α or β gene loci. The γ-gene complex on band p15 on the short arm of chromosome 7, for example, has only approximately 12 Vγ gene segments, two virtually identical Jγ segments, and two constant region gene segments. Moreover, there are only approximately four Vδ gene segments, three Dδ gene segments, three Jδ gene segments, and a single constant region gene in the δ gene complex. Consequently, most of the variability in the γ and δ chains is found in the junctional region formed during the process of $\gamma\delta$ T-cell receptor gene rearrangement. The amino acids encoded by this region form the center of the T-cell receptor-binding site.

The identification of TCR gene rearrangements is also widely used for diagnostic and therapeutic purposes: In suspected lymphoproliferative disorders, PCR-based clonality testing has been standardized and guidelines and consensus reporting systems have been established.[5] Moreover, the molecular analysis for clonal T-cell receptor gene rearrangements can be used to detect minimal residual disease in patients treated for clonal T-cell disorders, such as T-cell acute lymphoblastic

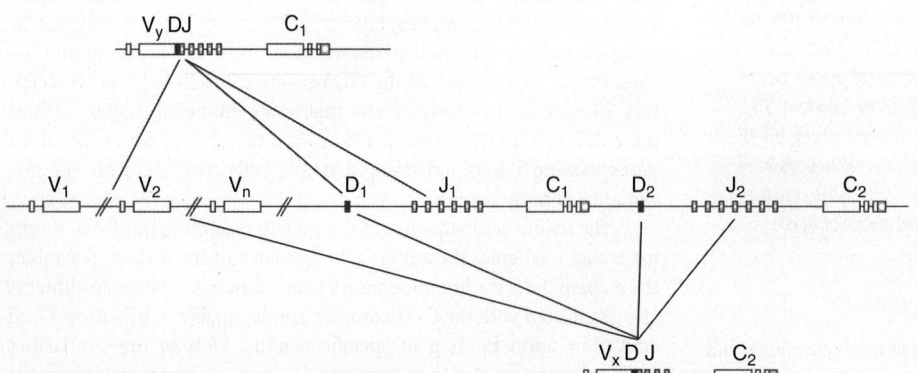

Figure 76–2. Schematic of possible rearrangements of the T-cell receptor (TCR)-β–chain genes. The TCR-β–chain genes in the germline DNA configuration are depicted in the *middle*. Possible recombination of either the first constant region (C$_1$, *above*) or the second constant region (C$_2$, *below*) with the variable region (V), diversity (D), or joining (J) segments are indicated by the *lines*.

leukemia (T-ALL), and guide clinical decision making and provide prognostic information.[6,7]

ANTIGEN PRESENTATION TO T-CELL RECEPTOR HETERODIMERS

Despite their similarities in structure, there are important differences in the way that T-cell receptors and immunoglobulins recognize antigen: immunoglobulins can bind antigens directly, while T-cell receptors generally require that peptide antigens are bound to a molecule of the major histocompatibility complex (MHC) on the surface of another cell.[8,9] MHC molecules, also known as histocompatibility antigens, are highly polymorphic glycoproteins, and have immunoglobulin-like structures themselves. There are two basic classes of MHC molecules: Class I MHC molecules generally bind and present *intracellular* proteins, that is, peptides that are derived from proteins synthesized and degraded in the cytoplasm of the cell. Class II MHC molecules generally bind peptides that are derived from *exogenous* proteins and degraded in intracellular vesicles. The human histocompatibility antigens HLA-A, HLA-B, and HLA-C are class I molecules, whereas HLA-D antigens DP, DQ, and DR are examples of class II molecules.

MHC class I molecules bind peptides that are usually 8 to 10 amino acids long. Their binding is stabilized by contacts in the free amino and carboxyl termini of the peptide and the peptide-binding groove of all MHC class I molecules. In addition, the peptide-binding groove is closed at both ends. The corresponding binding groove on class II molecules is open at either end, and peptides that bind to MHC class II molecules are generally at least 13 amino acids long. For both class I and class II molecules, the peptide binding groove is located in the central cleft between the two α helices of the MHC molecule. Steric factors, hydrogen bonding, and hydrophobic interactions between the peptide and the MHC molecule stabilize the peptide within this cleft and generate a tertiary structure that is further modified by amino acid residues of both the MHC and the peptide antigen.

MHC molecules are encoded by a family of MHC genes, which are located on chromosome 6 in humans (Chap. 137). MHC genes can be divided into three subgroups, with antigen presentation being encoded by class I (i.e., HLA-A, -B, -C) and class II (i.e., HLA-DP, DQ, DR) genes. Each of these gene loci exists in different alleles, and both maternal and paternal alleles are expressed concomitantly. The particular combination of class I and class II MHC alleles found on an individual chromosome is known as the MHC haplotype. Therefore, the number of different MHC molecules is greatly increased not only by MHC gene polymorphism, but also by codominant expression of MHC gene products. The resulting differences within MHC molecules are primarily found in the amino acids lining the clefts that hold the peptide antigen, allowing the MHC molecules encoded by each allele to bind a distinctive array of different peptides.

Structural studies show that the T-cell receptor can recognize both the MHC-bound peptide and the polymorphic amino acid residues themselves that surround the peptide-binding pocket.[10] The specificity of a T-cell receptor (TCR) is defined both by the peptide it recognizes and by the MHC molecule binding it, and TCRs are therefore likely to engage a composite peptide/MHC receptor.[11,12] Additional TCR–MHC binding parameters, such as ligands per cell or dissociation time defined by the affinity of antigen, also have an effect on subsequent T-cell activation, but their exact relationship remains largely controversial.[13]

Some T cells, however, do not recognize MHC-bound peptides. Instead they recognize antigens that are presented by MHC class I-like molecules encoded by genes that map outside the MHC region. One such family of molecules is called CD1. Despite structural similarities

with MHC class I molecules, CD1 molecules present larger extracellular peptides in a MHC class II-like fashion, and are also able to present glycolipids to T cells. Glycolipids are components of mycobacterial membranes; in cells infected with mycobacteria, the CD1 molecules are therefore able to bind and present membrane components such as lipoarabinomannan or mycolic acid. T cells that recognize these complexes play an important role in the immune response to *Mycobacterium tuberculosis*.[14,15]

As discussed above, structural studies show that $\gamma\delta$ TCRs assume a different tertiary structure than $\alpha\beta$ TCRs. As a consequence, $\gamma\delta$ TCRs are able to recognize a wider variety of ligands, such as bacterial phosphoantigens, nonclassical MHC-I molecules and unprocessed proteins, which distinguishes them from the great majority of $\alpha\beta$ T cells.[16] Other $\gamma\delta$ receptors can recognize determinants presented by CD1 molecules.[17] A number of studies have described increased numbers of $\gamma\delta$ T cells in a variety of infectious and autoimmune diseases. Therefore, it is speculated that $\gamma\delta$ T cells link innate and adaptive immune responses under infectious and inflammatory conditions. In addition, it is hypothesized that $\gamma\delta$ T cells might play a role in novel T-cell-based immunotherapy strategies.[18,19]

GENERATION OF T-CELL RECEPTOR DIVERSITY

TCR diversity is achieved by several mechanisms, some of which are the same as those that generate diversity among immunoglobulin molecules (Chap. 75). The joining of different V (variable), D (diversity), and J (joining) elements to produce a complete V gene, the presence of uncorrected errors made during the recombination of these genetic elements, and the combinatorial diversity afforded by the random pairing of two chains encoded by separated gene complexes all function to enhance the diversity of the T-cell antigen receptor repertoire. An important difference between T cells and B cells, however, is that B cells are capable of undergoing somatic hypermutation (Chap. 75). This process requires expression of activation-induced deaminase (AID) along with other enzymes expressed primarily by B cells within the germinal center of secondary lymphoid tissue during the immune response to antigen (Chaps. 6 and 75).

TCRs do not undergo somatic mutation, probably because of the central role they play in directing host immune defenses: During differentiation, immature $\alpha\beta$ T-cell precursors pass through the thymus, where they are educated to distinguish self from non-self by cell-surface proteins of the MHC (Chaps. 6 and 74). Because the ligand for the $\alpha\beta$ TCR is processed antigen presented by MHC molecules, close interaction with the MHC might be lost if the variable region of the TCR were allowed to diverge significantly from the inherited germline repertoire. Furthermore, somatic mutation of expressed TCR variable region genes may lead to constitutive T-cell activation to processed self-antigen presented by self-MHC molecules, which could lead to a breakdown in tolerance to self-antigens and autoimmunity.

● THE INVARIANT CHAINS OF THE T-CELL RECEPTOR COMPLEX

COMPOSITION OF THE T-CELL RECEPTOR COMPLEX

The CD3 complex of polypeptides and CD247, also known as the zeta chain (ζ chain) of the TCR, are closely associated with and required for the surface expression of the polypeptide heterodimer.[20] Unlike the TCR heterodimers, these polypeptides are invariant and are found on all T cells that express $\alpha\beta$ or $\gamma\delta$ heterodimers. The CD3 polypeptides are designated CD3γ, CD3δ, and CD3ε. The CD3ε chain couples with either the CD3γ or the CD3δ chain to generate heterodimers that each form a tight association with the $\alpha\beta$ (or $\gamma\delta$) receptor heterodimer on the T-cell surface (see Fig. 76–1). Each CD3 polypeptide has a negatively charged amino acid in the central portion of the hydrophobic transmembrane region that stabilizes the CD3 complex with the two chains of the TCR. The ζ chain (CD247), on the other hand, forms a disulfide-like homodimer that primarily associates with the two TCR chains and only weakly associates with the CD3 complex. As such, it cannot be coimmunoprecipitated easily with antibodies to the CD3 polypeptides. In addition, the ζ chain lacks a significant extracellular domain (see Fig. 76–1).

MOLECULAR FEATURES OF THE T-CELL RECEPTOR COMPLEX

The genes encoding CD3γ, CD3δ, or CD3ε chains are clustered on the long arm of chromosome 11 in band q23. CD3γ has a 16-kDa polypeptide backbone that is heavily glycosylated to assume a final molecular mass of 25 to 28 kDa. CD3δ and CD3ε are each 20 kDa in molecular mass. The CD3δ is a glycoprotein consisting of 30 percent carbohydrate. In contrast, CD3ε is not glycosylated. CD3δ and CD3γ are highly homologous at both the protein and nucleic acid sequence level. The nucleic acid sequence of each predicts CD3δ and CD3γ to have typical signal peptides, respective hydrophilic extracellular domains of 79 to 89 amino acids, hydrophobic transmembrane regions of 27 amino acids, and hydrophilic intracellular domains of 44 to 55 amino acids. CD3ε is similar, with a 22-residue signal peptide, an extracellular domain of 104 amino acids, a transmembrane domain, and a comparatively long intracellular domain of 81 amino acids. Each CD3 polypeptide has one immunoglobulin-like domain in its extracellular domain that is defined by an intrachain disulfide bond (see Fig. 76–1), indicating that these polypeptides are members of the immunoglobulin superfamily. However, unlike the $\alpha\beta$ or $\gamma\delta$ chains of the TCR, there is no variability in the extracellular domains of the CD3 proteins, indicating that these molecules do not contribute to the specificity of antigen recognition.

The ζ chain has no sequence or structural homology to the other three CD3 chains. It is a nonglycosylated protein of 16-kDa molecular mass that is encoded by a gene found on chromosome 1. The ζ chain has only a very short extracellular domain of 6 to 9 amino acids, a transmembrane domain of 21 amino acids, and a long intracellular domain of 113 amino acids.

The cytoplasmic domains of all the CD3 polypeptides and the ζ chain each contain sequences termed immunoreceptor tyrosine-based activation motifs (ITAMs). Each ITAM contains two copies of the sequence tyrosine-X-X-leucine separated by six to eight amino acid residues, in which X represents an unspecified amino acid. The cytoplasmic domains of each CD3 polypeptide contain one ITAM, whereas each ζ chain contains three ITAMs (see Fig. 76–1). These sequences allow the CD3 proteins to associate with cytosolic protein tyrosine kinases following TCR ligation, thus transducing a signal to the interior of the T cell. The cytoplasmic domains of CD3ε and CD3ζ are particularly important in this regard.

SIGNAL TRANSDUCTION VIA THE T-CELL RECEPTOR COMPLEX

Although the major components of the TCR signaling machinery have been identified and mapped, key components continue to be discovered, adding to the complex network of TCR signal transduction. Signal transduction from the TCR heterodimer to intracellular proteins is mediated by the CD3 polypeptides and the ζ chain. Their spatial

organization and the mechanisms by which this is regulated are, however, still poorly understood.[21] Upon binding to a specific ligand, the TCR $\alpha\beta$ (or $\gamma\delta$) heterodimer undergoes steric changes that result in the phosphorylation of the ITAMs of the ζ chain and each of the CD3 polypeptides (see Fig. 76–1). When tyrosine residues in the ITAMs become phosphorylated, they can act as docking sites for adapter proteins or tyrosine kinases, such as the zeta-associated protein of 70 kDa (ZAP-70), which possesses a Src homology 2 (SH2) domain and a Src homology 3 (SH3) domain. Following ligation of the TCR, Src family protein tyrosine kinases (e.g., Lck) are recruited and become activated. This differentially phosphorylates the ITAMs of the accessory molecules in the TCR complex.[22] ZAP-70 is recruited to the phosphorylated ITAMs of the ζ chain via its SH2 and SH3 domains, and subsequently becomes activated. Activated ZAP-70 phosphorylates tyrosine residues in the intracytoplasmic segments of surface CD6 and membrane-anchored adapter protein called linker of activation of T cells (LAT), both of which constitute a device for the amplification and diversification of signals that are responsible for most of the responses that result from engagement of the TCR.[23]

The network of proteins that interact with the LAT signalosome includes SLP-76, phospholipase Cγ_1 (PLC-γ_1) and GRAP2. Activated PLC-γ_1 mediates hydrolysis of phosphatidylinositol-(4,5)-bisphosphate at the cell membrane, which generates the second messengers inositol-(1,4,5)-trisphosphate and polyunsaturated diacyglycerols, leading to a rapid increase in cytosolic free calcium and activation of the θ isoform of protein kinase C (PKC). Cytosolic free calcium binds to calmodulin, an ubiquitous calcium-dependent regulatory protein. The calcium-calmodulin complex activates the cytoplasmic phosphatase calcineurin, which, in turn, catalyzes the removal of an inhibitory phosphate group on the nuclear factor of activated T cells (NFATs) that retains NFAT proteins in the cytoplasm. Removal of the phosphates from NFAT1 and NFAT2 by activated calcineurin allows these transcription factors to translocate into the nucleus, where they enhance transcription of several activation-induced genes, including those encoding interleukin (IL)-2, IL-4, and tumor necrosis factor.[24] The importance of this pathway in T-cell activation is underscored by the strong immunosuppressive activity of calcineurin inhibitors such as cyclosporine and FK506, which are commonly administered in the clinic to treat autoimmune diseases and to prevent graft rejection.

In parallel, diacylglycerol in the plasma membrane recruits RasGRP1, a guanine nucleotide-exchange factor (GEF), which acts on Ras to activate extracellular receptor-activated kinase 1 and 2 (ERK1/2). Activated ERK phosphorylates Elk, which, in turn, stimulates transcription of Fos, a component of the activation protein-1 (AP-1) factor that is a necessary component of the transcription-factor complex required for expression of IL-2 and other critical T-cell proteins. LAT-bound SLP-76 also interacts with Nck and with Vav1 to promote reorganization of the actin cytoskeleton, and with FYB to increase the binding of the integrin CD58 (LFA-1) to its ligand intercellular adhesion molecule (ICAM)-1. DYN2, a member of the dynamin superfamily of large guanosine triphosphatases (GTPases), is also recruited by phosphorylated LAT molecules and participates in the generation of filamentous actin. Dedicator of cytokinesis 2 (DOCK2), another GEF, also activates GTPases of the Rac family, which, in turn, activate another mitogen-activated protein (MAP) kinase called p38, and initiate a parallel enzymatic cascade resulting in the activation of yet another MAP kinase called c-Jun N-terminal kinase (JNK), otherwise known as stress-activated protein kinase (SAPK). Activated JNK phosphorylates c-Jun, the second component of the AP-1 transcription factor required for IL-2 transcription. The guanosine triphosphate (GTP)-bound form of Rac also induces cytoskeletal reorganization, thereby facilitating the clustering of the TCR complex, accessory molecules, and other accessory proteins at the site of contact between the T cell and the antigen-presenting cell (APC).

CD4 AND CD8

STRUCTURE OF CD4 AND CD8

CD4 and CD8 are glycoproteins that share structural features of other immunoglobulin superfamily receptor molecules. CD8 has two isoforms with different expression patterns and presumably different functions, and is expressed as a CD8α/CD8β heterodimer or as a CD8α/CD8α homodimer.[25] These chains are encoded by genes that are linked closely to the immunoglobulin κ light-chain locus at band p12 on the short arm of chromosome 2. The protein sequence of the aminoterminal domains of each CD8 chain shares greater than 28 percent homology with κ light-chain variable regions. Therefore, these domains are called the variable-region-like (V-like) domains. Following this V-like domain, the CD8 molecule has a short region rich in prolines, threonines, and serines that resembles the immunoglobulin hinge region. This region also contains sites for O-linked glycosylation. A hydrophobic transmembrane region anchors the hinge-like region. The CD8 molecule has a 25-amino-acid cytoplasmic tail consisting of highly basic residues. Two cysteines within the V-like domain form a disulfide bridge that stabilizes the immunoglobulin-like fold. An additional cysteine residue is located each within the V-like domain, the hinge region, the transmembrane segment, and the cytoplasmic domain. These cysteines form intermolecular disulfide bridges between two CD8 molecules, thereby stabilizing the CD8α/CD8β heterodimers or CD8α/CD8α homodimers on the T-cell surface. The cell surface CD8 heterodimer shares structural geometry with the heterodimers formed by the pairing of immunoglobulin light and heavy chains.

CD4, on the other hand, is expressed as a monomer on the surface of a subset of peripheral T cells, mononuclear phagocytes and some blood-derived dendritic cells. It is a 55-kDa monomeric glycoprotein that is encoded by a gene that maps to the short arm of chromosome 12. It consists of 5 external domains, a stretch of hydrophobic transmembrane residues, and a highly basic cytoplasmic tail of 38 residues. Similar to CD8, the aminoterminal domain of CD4 also has extensive homology to immunoglobulin light-chain variable regions. However, following this immunoglobulin-like domain is a domain of 270 amino acids that bears little resemblance to other proteins of the immunoglobulin superfamily.

The cytoplasmic regions of CD4 and CD8 are conserved among vertebrates, suggesting that they are essential for the function of these molecules. The cytoplasmic region of CD4 contains five serines and threonines, one or more of which is phosphorylated by PKC upon activation of T cells by phorbol esters or exposure to antigen. Subsequent to phosphorylation, the CD4 glycoprotein is internalized concomitant with T-cell activation. Similarly, the CD8 protein also possesses a highly charged and conserved cytoplasmic domain that may be involved in transmembrane signal transduction.

FUNCTION OF CD4 AND CD8

In addition to MHC antigen presentation, TCRs generally require activation via CD4 and CD8 as coreceptors. Imaging studies and affinity measurements have demonstrated that CD4 and CD8 molecules associate on the plasma membrane with components of the TCR and contribute to antigen recognition and stabilization of TCR–MHC interactions.[26] The adhesion between the CD3/TCR complex and the MHC glycoproteins expressed by an APC or target cell is more than 100-fold enhanced by CD8 or CD4, probably by focusing MHC molecules of the APC or target cell onto the T-cell surface, allowing for

specific recognition of "processed" antigen that is cradled within the MHC glycoproteins. However, CD4 and CD8 differ in their expression patterns (see section "Helper and Cytotoxic T Cells and CD4+ T Cell Subsets" below) and MHC-binding specificities: CD8 binds to the nonpolymorphic $α_3$ domain of the HLA class I molecule (HLA-A, -B, or -C), whereas CD4 binds to the nonpolymorphic $β_2$ domain of HLA class II molecules (HLA-DP, -DQ, and -DR).[27] Therefore, T cells expressing CD4 or CD8 generally recognize antigens presented by class II or class I MHC glycoproteins, respectively. This selectivity is underscored by studies on knockout mice that lack expression of either of these accessory molecules. Mice lacking CD4 or CD8 fail to develop class II-restricted or class I-restricted T cells, respectively, indicating that these coreceptors play essential roles in the maturation of T cells in the thymus. A similar defect is observed in patients with the bare lymphocyte syndrome who have a congenital immune deficiency caused by genetic defects in their capacity to make MHC class II molecules.[28] Although patients have normal numbers of B cells and T cells, they have markedly reduced numbers of CD4+ T cells, thus accounting in part for their profound immune deficiency.

In addition to serving as coreceptors, CD4 or CD8 molecules enhance antigen responsiveness by transducing a signal either directly or in concert with the CD3/TCR complex. This is mediated through their interaction with the SRC family tyrosine kinase Lck.[29] Lck is noncovalently associated with the cytoplasmic tails of CD4 and/or CD8. When a T cell recognizes a peptide presented by an appropriate MHC antigen, the interaction of CD4 or CD8 with the MHC molecule brings Lck close to the TCR complex. Lck then phosphorylates the tyrosine residues in the ITAMs of CD3 polypeptides and the ζ chain, thereby initiating the receptor signaling required for T-cell activation.

Finally, CD4 also is a cellular coreceptor for HIV.[30] Binding of CD4 along with chemokine receptors such as CCR5 or CXCR4 facilitates entry of the virus into host T cells and stimulates them in an antigen-driven immune response.[31] Targeting HIV entry/fusion by specific monoclonal antibodies and/or inhibitors is, therefore, an important therapeutic approach in HIV.[32] Additionally, CD4 is also of prognostic relevance, as disease progression correlates with depletion of blood T cells that express CD4 (Chap. 81).

T-CELL SUBSETS

PRECURSOR THYMOCYTES

T lymphocytes develop in the marrow from a common lymphoid progenitor that also gives rise to B lymphocytes. While B-lymphocyte precursors remain in the marrow, T-cell precursors migrate to the thymus, where they undergo distinct maturation steps and immunologic education. This is accompanied by characteristic TCR gene and surface expression changes of the CD3 complex, CD4, and CD8. At the early stage, thymocytes are double-negative and express neither CD4 nor CD8. This is a highly heterogeneous population, which includes γδ T cells, αβ T cells that also express the NK1.1 receptor commonly found on natural killer (NK) cells, and immature thymocytes that do not yet express a complete TCR molecule, but are thought to be precursors to the αβ lineage. The latter start to express CD8 and CD4 and enter the double-positive stage, where they undergo positive/negative selection events and CD4/CD8 cell fate choice. This results in the generation of mature thymocytes and peripheral T cells that express either CD4 or CD8, but not both (Chap. 74).[33]

HELPER AND CYTOTOXIC T CELLS

The mutually exclusive expression of CD4 or CD8 on mature T cells defines two major blood T-cell subsets: blood T cells that express CD8 normally constitute 25 to 35 percent of the peripheral T-cell population. They recognize antigens presented by MHC class I molecules and differentiate into cytotoxic CD8 T cells. Their main function is lysis of the target cell bearing the surface antigens for which a cytotoxic T cell is specific. Within this subset, there are a range of phenotypes defined both by function and expression of markers with an immunoregulatory function. Blood T cells that solely express the CD4 surface antigen are designated helper T cells. They normally comprise approximately 65 percent of blood T cells. Generally, their function is the production of lymphokines upon activation by foreign antigens presented by MHC class II molecules, regulating and/or assisting in the active immune response. Helper T cells can differentiate into several subtypes, each secreting different cytokines to facilitate a different type of immune response.

CD4+ T-CELL SUBSETS

Th1 and Th2 Cells

Based on distinct cytokine patterns upon activation, mature CD4+ T cells may be divided into subsets–the first of which identified were named *T-helper type 1 (Th1)* and *T-helper type 2 (Th2)*.[34] In general, Th1 cells are a major source of interferon-γ (IFN-γ), and also the major T-cell population involved in activating macrophages and clearing intracellular pathogens. Th2 cells are a major source of IL-4 and are important for the generation of immunoglobulin (Ig) E, the production of eosinophils, and the immune defense against infections by parasites. Both subsets are produced from a noncommitted population of precursor T cells. The process by which commitment develops is called *polarization.*

In addition to IFN-γ, Th1 cells produce lymphotoxin β, IL-2, and IL-12, whereas Th2 cells also produce IL-5, IL-13, and IL-25. Human Th1 and Th2 cells can also differ in the array of surface antigens or cytokine receptors they express. Th1 cells preferentially express CD26, membrane IFN-γ, the chemokine receptors CCR1 (CD191), CCR2 (CD192), CCR5 (CD195), CXCR3 (CD183), and CXCR6 (CD186), and the receptor for IL-12 (IL-12R or CD212). Higher levels of the lymphocyte activation gene 3 (LAG-3 or CD223), a ligand for MHC class II antigens that is structurally related to CD4, have also been described. Th2 cells preferentially express CD62L, the α chain of the IL-4 receptor (IL-4Rα), the α chain of the IL-33 receptor (IL-33Rα), CD30, and the chemokine receptors CCR3 (CD193), CCR4 (CD194), CCR8 (CDw198), and, to some extent, CXCR4 (CD184).[35–37] Distinctive expression levels of these cytokine and chemokine receptors, along with distinctive binding activities for various endothelial selectins, most likely account for the differences in the response to cytokines and tissue-specific migration of these helper T-cell subsets.

The cytokines produced by each subset also stimulate polarization of additional T cells to the same subset, while inhibiting the polarization of the other subset. In naïve CD4+ T cells, the Th1 cytokine IFN-γ induces or activates the signal transducer and activator of transcription (STAT) 1, STAT4, and the T-box transcription factor T-BET, while simultaneously modulating IL-2 and Th2 cytokines, resulting in an attenuation of Th2 cell development (Fig. 76–3).[38] Several other studies demonstrate that T-BET also physically interacts with other transcription factors important for alternative T helper cell developmental decisions to functionally repress the opposing subtype specific gene expression programs and promote Th1 development.[39] Similarly, IL-4 activates or enhances the expression STAT5, STAT6, and GATA3, transcription factors that play important roles in Th2 cell development (Fig. 76–3).[40] Another Th2 cytokine, IL-10, inhibits Th1 cell activation, thereby limiting the production of Th1-type cytokines. Because of these self-amplifying and mutually excluding feedback loops, an immune response becomes increasingly polarized once it develops along a Th1 or Th2 pathway, particularly upon protracted stimulation by chronic infection or prolonged exposure to environmental antigens. Other factors that drive polarization are chemokines (explaining the differential expression of chemokine receptors on Th1/Th2 cells), eicosanoids, oxygen free radicals, various inflammatory mediators, and direct cell-to-cell interaction with APCs.

Functionally, Th1 cells predominantly drive cellular immunity to fight viruses and other intracellular pathogens, eliminate cancerous cells, and stimulate delayed-type hypersensitivity (DTH) skin reactions. This is mostly achieved by stimulating macrophage Fc receptor expression, phagocytosis, and antigen presentation, enhancing the capacity of macrophages to kill intracellular pathogens. Th2 cells drive humoral immunity and upregulate antibody production to fight extracellular organisms. They initiate the antibody response to antigen by activating naïve antigen-specific B cells to produce IgM antibodies, subsequently stimulate the production of switched immunoglobulin isotypes, including IgA, IgE, and neutralize and/or weakly opsonize subtypes of IgG (Chap. 75), probably via IL-4 as a B-cell stimulatory/growth factor. In addition to stimulating the production of IgE antibodies, the cytokines made by Th2 cells induce differentiation of mast cells and eosinophils.[34]

Several studies have indicated that Th2 polarization and accumulation at inflammatory sites is likely to trigger the hypersensitivity reaction in allergic diseases.[41] On the other hand, these responses are protective against metazoan parasite infections such as helminths: Th2 responses are host protective while extracellular parasites migrate through the body, and reduce the number of parasites either through direct killing in the tissues or expulsion from the intestines.[42] Other studies demonstrate that eosinophilia and elevated IgE that accompany infection with *Schistosoma mansoni* are caused by the induction of Th2-type cells in the immune response to parasite ova.[43] The Th2 polarization in these diseases/conditions is most likely a result of minimal IL-4 secretion during initial activation. If an antigen is present at high concentrations but does not trigger acute inflammation and attendant production of IL-12, the local concentration of IL-4 increases over time and induces a Th2 polarization of cells. On the other hand, pathogens that induce acute inflammation and/or engage toll-like receptors on accessory cells and macrophages can promote production of IFN-γ and IL-12, thereby stimulating development of the immune response along the Th1 pathway.[38] Immune responses restricted to Th1 cells, for example, are observed in patients with leprosy who have developed cellular immunity to *Mycobacterium leprae*[44] or *M. tuberculosis*,[45] in patients with *Yersinia enterocolitica*[46] or arthritis triggered by infection with *Borrelia burgdorferi*.[47]

However, it is probably overly simplistic to view the Th1 pathway as being the more aggressive of the two, generating acute organ-specific autoimmune diseases and inflammations, while the Th2 pathway predisposes to atopic diseases and systemic autoimmune disease. For example, *Helicobacter pylori*-associated peptic ulcer can be regarded as a Th1-driven immunopathologic response to some *H. pylori* antigens, while deregulated and exhaustive *H. pylori*-induced T-cell–dependent B-cell activation can support the onset of low-grade B-cell lymphoma.[48] In addition, many chronic inflammatory and autoimmune conditions such as rheumatoid arthritis (RA), type 1 diabetes, and multiple sclerosis (MS) are mixed Th1/Th2 conditions, and a clear Th1/Th2 bias has also not been identified yet for many types of cancer.[34]

CD4+CD25+ Regulatory T Cells

Another type of CD4 cells that suppresses rather than provides helper activity are regulatory T (T_{REG}) cells. T_{REG}s possess potent suppressive capacity and can exert diverse suppressive mechanisms allowing them

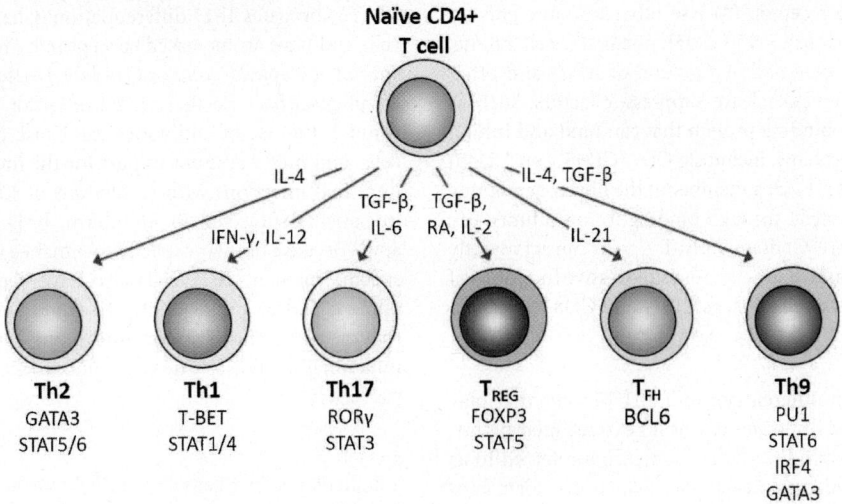

Figure 76–3. Differentiation of CD4+ T-cell subsets. During the course of the immune response, a naïve CD4+ T cell (*top of figure*) can differentiate into any one of several distinctive CD4+ T cells, as indicated beneath each differentiated cell type. Beneath the name of each T-cell subset is listed the transcription factor (if known) that is critical for the differentiation and maintenance of the subset. Interleukin (IL)-4 is critical for development of T-helper (Th)-2 cells (*green*), which triggers activation and/or induction of signal transducer and activator of transcription (STAT)5, STAT6, and GATA3, transcription factors that are important in Th2 differentiation. On the other hand, interferon-γ (IFN-γ) and IL-12 pattern the development of Th1 cells (*light red*) through the activation and/or induction of transcription factors STAT1, STAT4, and T-BET. IL-6 along with transforming growth factor beta (TGF-β) can induce blood CD4+ T cells to express the transcription factors STAT3 and RORγt (retinoic acid-related orphan receptor γ thymus isoform), which programs differentiation into Th17 cells, whereas TGF-β, retinoic acid (RA), and IL-2 induces these cells to express the transcription factors fork-head box P3 (FOXP3) and STAT5, which are required for differentiation into CD4+CD25+ regulatory T cells (T$_{REG}$) cells (*red*). IL-21 favors differentiation of naïve CD4 T cells into follicular helper T cells (T$_{FH}$ [*gold*]). Th9 cells (*dark blue*) are induced by IL-4 and TGF-β, express a combination of transcription factors and secrete IL-9. There is some plasticity in these differentiated T-cell subsets. IL-6 in combination may induce T$_{REG}$ cells to differentiate into Th17 cells, whereas B cells stimulated via CD40-CD40-ligand (CD40L or CD154) may induce their differentiation into T$_{FH}$ cells, as indicated by the *dashed horizontal arrows.*

to influence a very broad range of cell populations in a variety of anatomical locations and disease scenarios, both by direct cell–cell contact and the secretion of cytokines.[49] The cardinal phenotypic features of CD4+ T$_{REG}$ cells include their constitutive expression of the transcription factor forkhead box P3 (FOXP3), their cell surface expression of CD25 (the low-affinity receptor for IL-2 and their cell surface and cytoplasmic expression of the coinhibitory receptor cytotoxic T-lymphocyte antigen 4 (CTLA-4 or CD152).[50]

FOXP3 is an essential transcription factor required to manifest the T$_{REG}$ cell phenotype,[51] but it does not function alone and requires the expression of additional transcription factors to define the T$_{REG}$ cell phenotype and to establish its characteristic transcriptional programme.[52] Patients with the *immune dysregulation, polyendocrinopathy, enteropathy, X-linked syndrome* (IPEX syndrome) are found to have germline mutations in the gene encoding FOXP3, which maps to the long arm of the X chromosome at Xp11.23 (Chap. 80).[53] T$_{REG}$ developmental deficiency or dysfunction is a hallmark of IPEX, leading to severe, multiorgan, autoimmune phenomena. Patients typically have autoimmune skin conditions, such as bullous pemphigoid or alopecia universalis, and autoimmune endocrinopathies similar to those seen in patients with the *autoimmune polyendocrine candidiasis ectodermal dystrophy syndrome* (APECED syndrome), which is associated with genetic defects in the autoimmune regulator *(AIRE)* gene responsible for the generation of T-cell tolerance in the thymus (Chaps. 6 and 80).[54,55] The IPEX syndrome demonstrates the importance of T$_{REG}$ cells in maintaining tolerance to self-antigens and in preventing runaway immune responses to environmental antigens that might evolve into cross-reactive autoimmunity.

Additional key factors and signals required for T$_{REG}$ cell development and survival include IL-2, transforming growth factor-β (TGFβ) and co-stimulatory molecules.[56] It is also becoming clear that unique epigenetic changes that are partly induced by TCR signalling are typical of the T$_{REG}$ cell lineage, and that they can be used to differentiate T$_{REG}$ subpopulations such as thymus-derived T$_{REG}$ (tT$_{REG}$) cells and peripherally derived T$_{REG}$ (pT$_{REG}$) cells.[57,58] These terms have replaced "natural FOXP3+ T$_{REG}$ cells" and "induced or adaptive T$_{REG}$ cells" to more accurately describe the anatomical location of their differentiation. tT$_{REG}$ cells differentiate from CD4+CD8– T cells that have undergone positive and negative selection to self-antigens presented in the thymus (Chap. 6) and are thought to play a role in maintaining tolerance to self-antigens. pT$_{REG}$ cells, on the other hand, differentiate upon antigen encounter under certain conditions and during normal homeostasis of the gut.[59] As such, pT$_{REGs}$ are thought to play an important role in the development and maintenance of mucosal immune tolerance and in the control of severe chronic allergic inflammation and "altered" self-antigens of inflamed tissues or neoplastic cells. They are also required to minimize tissue damage in inflammatory settings such as viral infection[60] or mediate tolerance to allografts.[61] tT$_{REG}$ and pT$_{REG}$ cells have subtle differences in the methylation status of conserved noncoding sequence 2 (CNS2; also known as the T$_{REG}$ cell-specific demethylated region [TSDR]) in the *FOXP3* locus, potentially influencing the stability of the cells under inflammatory or pathogenic conditions.[62]

T$_{REG}$ cells can specifically suppress immune responses via contact-dependent and cytokine-mediated mechanisms.[63] Upon activation through their TCR, T$_{REGs}$ can (1) produce antiinflammatory cytokines (e.g., IL-10, TGF-β, or IL-35), (2) reduce the availability of IL-2 via absorption by the CD25 receptor, (3) lyse other immune effector cells via granzyme secretion or CD95-CD95L–mediated cell killing, (4) modulate the activation state and/or function of APCs and other immune effector cells, and/or (5) release suppressor factors, such as galectin-1[64] (a β-galactoside–binding protein that can bind and inhibit the function of many glycoproteins, including CD7, CD43, and CD45) and fibrinogen-like protein 2 (FGL2; a member of the fibrinogen family that mediates it suppressive effect through binding to low affinity Fcγ receptors expressed on APCs).[65] Consequently, T_{REG} cells can act directly against specific target antigens, while activating suppressive functions of other types of immune effector cells such as CD4+ and CD8+ cells.

Th17 T Cells

Naïve CD4+ T cells also can differentiate into Th17 T cells that play an important role in immune responses to certain extracellular pathogens and fungi.[66] These cells produce IL-17 (sometimes referred to as IL-17A) and a closely related cytokine, IL-17F, which can form biologically active homodimers or heterodimers and induce substantial tissue reactions because of the broad distribution of the IL-17 and IL-22 receptors. Principal cytokines involved in the differentiation of naïve blood CD4+ T cells into Th17 cells are IL-23 and IL-1β (see Fig. 76–3), but a combination of TCR stimulation and the cytokines TGF-β and IL-6 are also required.[67] Prostaglandins, most notably prostaglandin E_2, can synergize with IL-23 and IL-1β to drive differentiation of CD4+ T cells into Th17 cells.[68] These cytokines and factors can induce activation and/or expression of transcription factors that are distinct from those used by Th1 or Th2 cells, including the retinoic acid-related orphan receptor γ (RORγt) and STAT3 (see Fig. 76–3),[69,70] which, in turn, can induce expression of IL-17 and IL-17F.[71,72] However, for full commitment of precursors to the Th17 lineage, RORγt and STAT3 must act in cooperation with other transcription factors, including RORα, interferon regulatory factor 4 (IRF4), and runt-related transcription factor 1 (RUNX1). Th17 cells also express high levels of the IL-23R, CCR4, CCR6, CXCR4, CD161, and multiple CD49 integrins, but not CCR2, CCR5, or CCR7.[37,73,74] In contrast to Th1 or Th2 cells, Th17 cells do not elaborate IFN-γ or IL-4, both of which can inhibit expression of IL-17.[75]

Th17 cells play a central role in inflammation and defense against intestinal bacteria, extracellular pathogens, and fungal infections, mostly via activation of neutrophils. Common pathogens that induce mainly Th17 responses include Gram-positive *Propionibacterium acnes*, gram-negative *Citrobacter, Klebsiella pneumoniae, bacteroides* and *Borrelia* species, and fungi such as *Candida albicans*.[76] Th17 cells are abundantly found in the intestinal lamina propria, where they are induced and stimulated by commensal bacteria, maintain epithelial integrity, and clear extracellular pathogens.[77]

Th17 cells are the principal producers of IL-17 in response to specific immune stimulation, but NK and natural killer T (NKT) cells are also able to produce IL-17. IL-17 is a proinflammatory cytokine that has pleiotropic effects on multiple target cells, resulting in enhanced antigen presentation, antibody production, macrophage activation, cellular extravasation, and neutrophil migration.[78] In addition to IL-17 and IL-17F, Th17 cells elaborate other proinflammatory factors, including chemokines (e.g., CXCL8 [IL-8] and CCL20), cytokines (e.g., IL-6, tumor necrosis factor-α, IL-21, and IL-22), growth factors (e.g., granulocyte colony-stimulating factor and granulocyte-macrophage colony-stimulating factor), acute phase proteins (e.g., C-reactive protein), and antimicrobial peptides and mucins.[76]

The importance of Th17 cells in the defense against certain microorganisms is reflected in the rare primary immunodeficiency disorder called *autosomal dominant hyper-IgE syndrome*, in which a mutation in STAT3 abrogates Th17 differentiation (Chap. 80).[79,80] Patients lack Th17 cells and have an increased susceptibility to infection with the various species of *Staphylococcus* or *Candida*. Furthermore, the loss of intestinal commensal bacteria that are essential for the induction of Th17 cells through the use of antibiotics can cause depletion in intestinal Th17 cells, and might account in part for the increased incidence of gastrointestinal infections with *C. albicans* or *Clostridium difficile* observed in patients subjected to long-term, broad-spectrum antibiotic therapy.[81] Because of their capacity to enhance inflammation in an antigen-specific manner, Th17 cells also have been implicated in the development and/or propagation of several autoimmune disease, such as rheumatoid arthritis,[82] systemic lupus erythematosus (SLE),[83] MS,[84] inflammatory bowel disease,[85] glucocorticoid-resistant asthma,[86] and psoriasis.[87]

T_{FH} Cells

T follicular helper cells (T_{FH} cells) constitute another subset of CD4+ T cells that regulates the development of antigen-specific B-cell immunity in the germinal center of secondary lymphoid follicles. T_{FH} cells express the CXCR5 chemokine receptor, allowing them to home to the CXCL13-rich B-cell zones of lymphoid follicles where they engage antigen-specific B cells in cognate intercellular interactions, and cell-surface proteins such as programmed cell death-1 (PD-1), inducible T-cell costimulator (iCOS), B- and T-lymphocyte attenuator (BTLA), and CD40L, which allow them to form stable contacts with antigen-primed B cells.[88] Such interactions play a critical role in B-cell differentiation into plasma cells or memory B cells in response to antigenic stimulation. In addition, T_{FH} cells secrete cytokines such as IL-4, IFN-γ, IL-10, and/or IL-21, which partly overlap with cytokines characteristic of other T-effector cells, helping to modify the differentiation fate of B lymphocytes (Chap. 75).

T_{FH} cells also express the cytoplasmic adaptor protein signal lymphocyte activation molecule (SLAM)-associated protein (SAP), required for lymphocyte interactions, and the transcription factor B-cell lymphoma 6 (BCL-6), required for T_{FH} cell differentiation. Several lines of evidence suggest that T_{FH} differentiation is a multistage process, but that dendritic cells (DCs) are crucial for CD4+ T cell priming and initial acquisition of T_{FH} cell characteristics, including the induction of BCL-6 expression.[89] The flexibility and plasticity of T_{FH} cells, which is mostly mediated by chromatin modifications, is underlined by the expression of a constellation of transcription factors, including BCL-6, BATF, STAT3, IRF4, c-Maf, and GATA-3, many of which are expressed by other Th effector subsets (see Fig. 76–3).

Th9 Cells

Another helper T-cell subset that has recently emerged are Th9 cells. In contrast to Th17 cells and T_{REGs}, they are induced by the combination of TGF-β and IL-4 and regulated by the transcription factors PU.1, STAT6, IRF4, and GATA-3.[90] They primarily produce IL-9, IL-10, and IL-21.[91] Functionally, Th9 cells appear to be effector rather than regulatory, and they have been implicated in the development of allergic reactions, particularly in the lungs.[92] Recent data indicates that Th9 cells *in vivo* might be implicated in tumor immunity in melanoma.[93,94]

MEMORY T CELLS

Following a successful immune response to antigen including the exposure to and recognition of antigen, expansion of T-cell subsets and exertion of effector function, both naïve CD4+ and CD8+ T-cells can develop into long-lived memory T cells that provide enhanced protection from re-exposure to the same or a related pathogen.[95,96] Memory

T-cell populations maintain the ability to both survive independently of cognate antigen[97] and self-renew in response to external homeostatic signals such as IL-15 and IL-7, hence maintaining themselves at stable levels for many years.[98] In addition, they have less-stringent requirements for activation and an enhanced capacity for lymphokine production upon rechallenge with the same antigen, and require a lower level of costimulatory factors.

Memory CD4+ or CD8+ T lymphocytes can also be distinguished from naïve cells based on their surface phenotypes of CD45 isoforms, rate of cycling, and migration. CD45, also known as leukocyte common antigen or T200, consists of a family of membrane glycoproteins, ranging from 180 to 220 kDa, that are expressed on all leukocytes.[99] Each member is the product of a single complex gene on chromosome 1 that contains 34 exons. Exons 3 through 7 may be spliced differently at the RNA transcript level to generate several distinct messenger RNA and protein products. The deduced amino acid sequences of these protein products have extracellular domains ranging from 391 to 552 amino acids, a transmembrane region, and a highly conserved cytoplasmic domain of 705 amino acids. This large cytoplasmic domain contains an intrinsic tyrosine phosphatase activity that is important in the regulation of various activation pathways involving tyrosine kinase activity, such as those involved in signal transduction via the TCR for antigen.[100] Different isoforms of CD45, designated as CD45R, have distinct expression patterns during lymphocyte ontogeny and activation. Therefore, cell subsets can be readily characterized by flow cytometry approaches using specific monoclonal antibodies. Naïve CD4+ T cells express CD45RA, whereas memory CD4+ T cells and CD8+ T cells express CD45RO. CD45RB can also be useful for distinguishing memory T cells. Within the CD4+ memory T-cell population, for example, there is an increase of helper activity associated with the shift from a CD45RB^{bright} to a CD45RB^{dim} phenotype.[101]

In addition, the distinct expression of chemokine receptors (CCRs) or homing molecules can be used to characterize T-cell subsets: relative to naïve T cells, memory T cells express lower levels of L-selectin (CD62L) and higher levels of CD29 and CD44.[102] More recent studies demonstrate that memory cells can be further subdivided into CD44+CD62L+CCR7+ central memory T cells (T$_{CM}$ cells) and CD44+CD62L−CCR7− effector memory T cells (T$_{EM}$ cells).[103] Because of their constitutive expression of CCR7 and CD62L, T$_{CM}$ cells home to secondary lymphoid organs, where they have little or no immediate effector function, but show greater sensitivity to antigenic stimulation in comparison to naïve T cells, are less dependent on costimulation, and upregulate CD40L to a greater extent. However, upon recognition of their cognate antigen, they have a high proliferative potential and can rapidly differentiate into large numbers of effector cells. T$_{EM}$ cells, in contrast, have higher migratory potential and display immediate effector function. Therefore, T$_{CM}$ cells are predominantly found in the CD4 lineage and are enriched in lymph nodes and tonsils, whereas T$_{EM}$ cells are more frequent in the CD8 compartment in lung, liver, and intestines. Accordingly, CD8+ T$_{EM}$ cells carry large amounts of perforin, and both CD4+ and CD8+ T$_{EM}$ cells can produce IFN-γ, IL-4, and IL-5 within hours after following antigenic stimulation.

It has long been controversial whether memory T cells arise during the contraction phase and develop directly from effector cells, or whether they diverge early during an immune response, and arise in parallel with short-lived effector cells. Recent studies, however, have provided evidence for an early delineation of the effector versus memory T-cell fates regulated through specific transcription factors and cytokines, such as IL-7 receptor α-chain (IL-7R) expression, IL-2, IL-12, and T-BET, EOMES, and BLIMP-1.[104,105]

●T-CELL ACCESSORY MOLECULES

IMMUNE MODULATORY MOLECULES

CD28

CD28 is a 44-kDa disulfide-linked homodimer that is expressed on most resting T cells and plasma cells. Mature thymocytes have higher levels of CD28 than immature cells. Among human peripheral T cells, more than 90 percent of CD4+ cells and approximately 50 percent of CD8 T cells express CD28. In general, activation of T cells induces enhanced expression of CD28, but ligation of CD28 leads to its transient downregulation.[106] CD28 is another member of the immunoglobulin superfamily and binds to both CD80 and CD86 using a highly conserved motif (MYPPPY) in a loop that resembles the third complementarity-determining region of immunoglobulin molecules. CD28 binds to CD80 with relatively low affinity (dissociation constant [Kd] = 4 μM) and dissociates very rapidly (K$_{off}$ = 1.6 s^{-1}),[107] and its binding to CD86 may be even weaker.[108]

CD28 functions as a major costimulatory molecules that is essential for T-cell activation, probably in the context of TCR/CD28 microcluster formation.[109] Ligation of CD28 by CD80 or CD86 or by anti-CD28 antibodies activates distinct signaling pathways that function together with the signals induced by ligation of the TCR to allow for T-cell activation and proliferation.[110] Following coligation of CD28, the Src kinases Lck and Fyn may phosphorylate a tyrosine within an ITAM found in the cytoplasmic domain of CD28, allowing the latter to bind and to activate phosphatidylinositide 3-kinase via its SH2 domains. CD28 signaling also facilitates GTP/guanosine diphosphate (GDP) exchange on Ras, resulting in activation of the MAP kinase pathway, activation of Akt kinase, and activation of the adapter protein Vav and the associated Rac pathway. These signals enhance the transcription of IL-2 and the stability of IL-2 transcripts, thereby stimulating T-cell proliferation.[111] Although mice lacking CD28 can mount effective T-cell responses, they are defective in T-cell–dependent antibody responses, suggesting that CD28 is necessary for T-cell–B-cell interactions and the proficient generation of antibody responses to antigen.[112]

The requirement for the same cell to present both the specific antigen and the costimulatory signal is crucial to prevent destructive autoimmune responses to self-tissues. This restricts the initiation of T-cell responses to APCs that express both the peptide antigen in the context of self-MHC molecules and the ligands for CD28, namely, CD80 and CD86. This is particularly important as not all self-reactive T cells undergo deletion in the thymus because not all self-peptides are presented in the thymus (Chap. 6). This is especially true for specialized tissues that express proteins that are never expressed in the thymus. If simultaneous ligation of the TCR and CD28 was not required, then T cells that recognize the self-peptide expressed by the MHC of such specialized tissues could become activated, leading to autoimmune rejection of the specialized tissue. Instead, ligation of the TCR in the absence of CD28 ligation leads to a state of hyporesponsiveness or anergy, in which the T cell expressing that receptor becomes refractory to activation.[113] Anergized T-cell clones produce only negligible amounts of IL-2, which is crucial for clonal expansion following T-cell activation. Interestingly, clonal T-cell anergy was found not to be a terminal fate, as the addition of exogenous IL-2 during restimulation could reverse the phenotype.[114] These characteristics are not limited to T cells, as anergic B cells also demonstrate some of the hallmark features, such as reduced proliferation and effector function. Anergy is an important basis for development of peripheral tolerance for self-antigens that are not expressed in the thymus (Chaps. 6 and 74).

CTLA-4 (CD152)

CTLA-4 (CD152) is another receptor for CD80 and CD86. It is a 50-kDa disulfide-linked homodimer that shares 31 percent identity with CD28. The gene encoding this receptor is closely linked with that encoding CD28 on the long arm of chromosome 2 at 2q33–q34. However, in contrast to the constitutive expression of CD28, T cells—with the exception of T_{REGs}—express CD152 only upon activation. Expression of CD152 peaks at approximately 24 hours after activation and then subsides by 72 hours but is always approximately 30- to 50-fold lower than that of CD28. CD28 ligation is particularly effective in inducing CD152.

CD152 binds to both CD80 and CD86 using the same highly conserved motif (MYPPPY) used by CD28, which, like CD28, is also in a loop that resembles the third complementarity-determining region of immunoglobulin molecules. However, despite its lower expression levels, CD152 binds to CD80 and CD86 approximately 20 times more avidly than CD28, with a Kd of 0.4 and 2.2 μM, respectively.[107,108] In contrast to CD28, ligation of CD152 transmits a negative signal to T-cell activation.[110] Instead of an ITAM, CD152 possesses an immunoreceptor tyrosine inhibitory motif (ITIM) in its cytoplasmic domain. Ligation of CD152 induces tyrosine phosphorylation of the ITIM, which, in turn, recruits the tyrosine phosphatase SHP-2 that can deactivate the phosphorylated ITAMs of the ζ chains of the TCR complex. Mice made genetically deficient in CD152 develop a fatal lymphoproliferative disorder that is characterized by massive cell activation and infiltration into tissues, indicating that CD152 serves as an important brake on unregulated T-cell activation.[115] Mice that are genetically modified to express only the extracellular domain of CD152 allowing the binding of CD80 or CD86, however, are protected from organ infiltration by T cells, suggesting that modulation of CD28 signals by competitive sequestration of its ligands can regulate tissue infiltration by autoreactive T cells.[116]

Moreover, anti-CD152 monoclonal antibodies that block the interaction of CD152 with CD80 and CD86 can enhance T-cell responses *in vitro* and *in vivo*. This has prompted their evaluation as immune-enhancing agents in models of autoimmune disease and in transplantation models,[117] and more recently in clinical vaccine studies and trials in combination with the blockade of other immunomodulatory molecules.[118,119]

Other Members of the CD28 Receptor Family

Homology-based cloning strategies have identified other proteins that are structurally related to CD28/CTLA-4 or its ligands CD80/CD86. These proteins are categorized as members of the CD28 or CD80 (B7) families, respectively, which belong to the immunoglobulin superfamily, a structurally and functionally highly heterogeneous family of T-cell cosignaling molecules.[120]

Two other important members of the CD28 family are iCOS (CD278) and PDCD1 (CD279, PD-1). Whereas CD278 is found primarily on activated T cells, CD279 can be found on activated T cells, B cells, some myeloid cells, and NK cells. CD278 and CD279, respectively, bind to the iCOS-ligand (iCOS-L or CD275) and the PD-ligands PD-L1 (CD274) or PD-L2 (CD273).[121] CD273, CD274, and CD275 belong to the CD80 (B7) family of surface molecules and are found or can be induced on B cells, APCs, and other nonhematopoietic tissues. CD278 primarily functions as a costimulatory molecule for cells bearing CD275.[122] CD279 plays a negative regulatory role on activated T cells and modifies T cell/APC contact durations by inhibiting TCR stop signals.[121] Like CD152, CD279 possesses an ITIM motif in its cytoplasmic tail that, upon phosphorylation, can recruit the tyrosine phosphatase SHP-2.[123] In this regard, CD279 may play a role similar to that of CD152, helping to brake cellular activation when bound to its ligands CD273 or CD274.

In general, the molecular mechanisms of T-cell costimulation and coinhibition are viewed as an evolving concept, as receptors and ligands exhibit great diversity in their expression, structure and function, and this is likely to be dependent on the context of anatomical location and the existence of underlying healthy and pathological immune responses.[120]

T-CELL ADHESION MOLECULES

In addition to CD3/TCR molecules and CD4 or CD8, several other surface proteins are required for efficient T-cell antigen recognition.[124] Some of these surface proteins are termed adhesion molecules, as they facilitate the adhesion of the T cell to its appropriate APC or target cell (Fig. 76–4). Their main function is to permit the T-cell antigen receptor complex to interact better with the MHC glycoproteins of the other cell, allowing for efficient T-cell antigen recognition and activation. Each member of this group of accessory molecules has distinctive affinities for the surface molecules expressed by the APC or target cell, which is reflected by differential expression patterns on specific T-cell subsets. Adhesion and antigen response are largely considered the final step of the multi-stage T-cell trafficking process that involves migration, adhesion, and signaling.

Lymphocyte Function-Associated Glycoproteins

The lymphocyte function-associated (LFA) molecules are an important family of glycoproteins that facilitate efficient cell–cell adhesion.[124] The family consists of the three major surface molecules LFA-1, LFA-2 (CD2), and LFA-3 (CD58). LFA-1 belongs to a family of three related glycoproteins LFA-1, MAC-1 (CD11b/CD18), and gp150,95 (CD11c/CD18). These proteins also are called "integrins" because they are hypothesized to coordinate the binding of cells to other cell types and to extracellular proteins. Each protein consists of a distinct α subunit noncovalently associated with the β_2 subunit glycoprotein of 95 kDa, designated as CD18. Because they share a common β_2 subunit, these molecules also are referred to as the β_2 integrins. The α subunit of LFA-1, designated CD11a, is a 180-kDa glycoprotein. Coupled together with the common β_2 subunit, this 180-kDa molecule is expressed on more than one-third of all marrow cells, all T cells, all B cells, and all NK cells. The α subunit of MAC-1 is a glycoprotein of 170 kDa, designated CD11b. MAC-1 is expressed on NK cells, monocytes, macrophages, granulocytes, and small subpopulations of T and B cells. The α subunit of p150,95, designated CD11c, is a 150-kDa glycoprotein that is not expressed by T lymphocytes.

The shared β_2 subunit (CD18) has extensive sequence homology to the β_3 subunit (CD61) of the platelet adhesion receptor glycoprotein IIb/IIIa (CD41/CD61) and the β_1 subunit (CD29) of a family of related adhesion proteins, termed very-late-activation (VLA) antigens. Many of these receptors function in cell–cell interactions and recognize their ligands at sites that contain the amino acid sequence Arg-Gly-Asp. In addition, the α subunit provides some selectivity. LFA-1, because of its α subunit, binds best to cell-surface ligands called ICAMs, namely, ICAM-1 (CD54), ICAM-2 (CD102), and ICAM-3 (CD50). CD54 and CD102 are expressed on endothelial cells as well as APCs. The binding of LFA-1 on lymphocytes to these molecules allows lymphocytes to migrate through blood vessel walls. CD50 is expressed only on leukocytes, including T cells, and is thought to play an important role in the adhesion of T cells with LFA-1 expressed on APCs (see Fig. 76–4). The LFA glycoproteins are essential for proper T-cell function and host immunity, and integrin gene defects leading to leukocyte adhesion deficiencies result in severe immune deficiencies. In humans, three LADs (LAD I to III) have been described.[125]

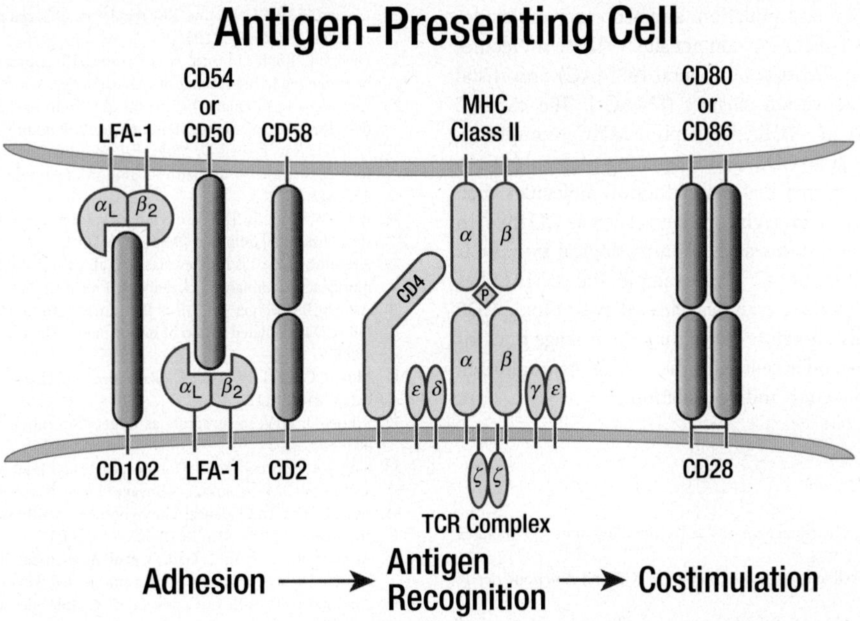

Antigen-Presenting Cell

Figure 76–4. Schematic of a T-cell interactions with an antigen-presenting cell. The *thick green lines* depict the plasma membranes of the interacting cells. The molecules of the antigen-presenting cell, namely, lymphocyte function-associated antigen (LFA)-1, intercellular adhesion molecule (ICAM)-1 or ICAM-3, LFA-3, major histocompatibility complex (MHC) class II, and CD80 or CD86, are displayed on *top*, while the T-cell antigens, ICAM-2, LFA-1, CD2, CD4, the T-cell receptor (TCR) complex, and CD28, are shown on the *bottom* of the diagram. *Thin lines* connecting the stick figures indicate disulfide bridges. The TCR complex consists of the $\alpha\beta$ heterodimer that is noncovalently coupled with the δ, ε, γ, and ζ chains of CD3, as indicated. This complex can recognize peptide antigen (designated by the *diamond labeled P*) that is cradled by the α and β chains of the MHC class II molecule of the antigen-presenting cell. The avidity of this interaction is enhanced by CD4 on the T-cell surface that interacts with nonpolymorphic determinants on the MHC class II molecule. The interaction steps between the T cell and the antigen-presenting cell are listed at the *bottom* of the figure. T-cell molecules ICAM-2 (CD102), LFA-1 (CD11a/CD18), and CD2 bind to LFA-1, ICAM-1 (CD54) or ICAM-3 (CD50), and LFA-3 (CD58), respectively, that are present on the surface of the antigen-presenting cell. These molecules provide for better adhesion between the T cell and the antigen-presenting cell (adhesion), allowing for time for the TCR complex to find the MHC molecule bearing a specific peptide antigen (antigen recognition). Should the antigen-presenting cell express CD80 or CD86, then simultaneous ligation of CD28 will occur (costimulation), leading to activation of the reactive T cell.

Although clinically distinct, they exhibit several common features including recurrent bacterial infections and leukocytosis.

LFA-1, CD2, and CD50 binding partners are CD54, CD102, LFA-1, and CD58 on the APC (see Fig. 76–4). Binding prolongs the time the T cell is exposed to antigen, and allows to sample large numbers of MHC molecules on the plasma membrane of the APC for the presence of specific peptide antigen. When a naïve T cell recognizes its specific peptide in the context of the MHC, signaling through the TCR induces a conformational change in LFA-1 that greatly increases its affinity for CD54 and CD102. This stabilizes the association between the antigen-specific T cell and the APC. This association can last for several days during which time the naïve T cell proliferates, forming daughter cells that also adhere to the APC and that differentiate into armed effector T cells.

Very-Late-Activation Antigens

VLAs received this terminology because the first identified VLA molecules, namely VLA-1 and VLA-2, initially were found on T cells only weeks after repetitive stimulation *in vitro*.[126] VLA molecules are β_1 integrins and share a common β_1 unit (CD29) that is paired with any one of six different α chains (α_1 to α_6), designated CD49a to CD49f. CD49a, CD49b, CD49c, CD49d, CD49e, and CD49f form molecules called VLA-1, VLA-2, VLA-3, VLA-4, VLA-5, and VLA-6, respectively, when paired with CD29. Despite their nomenclature, some of these VLA molecules, most notably VLA-4, are also expressed constitutively by some T cells and are rapidly induced on others. VLA-4 plays an important role in facilitating the attachment of cells that bear this molecule to the endothelium through its binding to vascular cell adhesion molecule-1

(VCAM-1), designated CD106. CD106 can be upregulated by various proinflammatory cytokines, allowing VLA-4 to play an important role in facilitating the homing of T cells to endothelium at sites of inflammation.

CD2

CD2 is a glycoprotein of approximately 50 kDa found on all T lymphocytes, large granular lymphocytes, and thymocytes.[127] CD2 facilitates cell–cell adhesion by binding to CD58, a 55- to 70-kDa surface glycoprotein that is expressed on erythrocytes and leukocytes as well as on endothelial, epithelial, and connective tissue cells (see Fig. 76–4). Monoclonal antibodies that bind CD2 may inhibit a variety of T-lymphocyte functions, including antigen-specific T-lymphocyte proliferative responses to lectins, alloantigens, and soluble antigens. Anti-CD2 inhibits cytotoxic T-lymphocyte–mediated cell killing by binding to the T cell rather than to the target, which generally does not express CD2. On the other hand, antibodies directed against CD58 inhibit cytotoxic T-lymphocyte–mediated cell killing by binding to CD58 on the target cell, thus blocking interaction of CD2 with CD58.

●THE IMMUNOLOGICAL SYNAPSE

T-cell antigen recognition following the principles described above takes place within a contact zone termed the immunological synapse, which organizes the involved membrane proteins at the interface between the T cell and the APC. Immune synapse formation involves polymerization of F-actin and polarization of the cytoskeleton, resulting in the redistribution of TCRs, costimulation, and accessory molecules into the region beneath the T-cell:APC contact site.[128] These molecules are segregated into central (cSMAC), peripheral (pSMAC) and distal (dSMAC) supramolecular activation clusters (SMACs). The cSMAC contains a concentration of TCR:CD3:peptide:MHC complexes, costimulatory molecules such as CD28, and signaling molecules such as PKCθ, while the pSMAC is enriched with adhesion molecules such as LFA-1. The dSMAC contains large glycoproteins such as CD45.[129] In addition to priming of T-cell responses, the immunological synapse is also important for effector functions.[130] For example, the pSMAC has been suggested to polarize cytotoxic granules released by cytotoxic CD8 T cells toward the target cells, therefore preventing the leakage of cyto-lytic granule contents to bystander cells, and the cSMAC is implicated as a site for receptor internalization and degradation.

REFERENCES

1. Garcia KC, Teyton L, Wilson IA: Structural basis of T cell recognition. *Annu Rev Immunol* 17:369–397, 1999.
2. O'Brien RL, Born WK: γδ T cell subsets: A link between TCR and function? *Semin Immunol* 22:193–198, 2010.
3. Chodaczek G, Papanna V, Zal MA, Zal T: Body-barrier surveillance by epidermal γδ TCRs. *Nat Immunol* 13:272–282, 2012.
4. Krangel MS: Mechanics of T cell receptor gene rearrangement. *Curr Opin Immunol* 21:133–139, 2009.
5. Langerak AW, Groenen PJTA, Bruggemann M, et al: EuroClonality/BIOMED-2 guide-lines for interpretation and reporting of Ig/TCR clonality testing in suspected lymph-oproliferations. *Leukemia* 26:2159–2171, 2012.
6. van der Velden VHJ, Cazzaniga G, Schrauder A, et al: Analysis of minimal residual disease by Ig//TCR gene rearrangements: Guidelines for interpretation of real-time quantitative PCR data. *Leukemia* 21:604–611, 2007.
7. Schrappe M, Valsecchi MG, Bartram CR, et al: Late MRD response determines relapse risk overall and in subsets of childhood T-cell ALL: Results of the AIEOP-BFM-ALL 2000 study. *Blood* 118:2077–2084, 2011.
8. Zinkernagel RM, Doherty PC: Immunological surveillance against altered self com-ponents by sensitised T lymphocytes in lymphocytic choriomeningitis. *Nature* 251:547–548, 1974.
9. Zinkernagel RM, Doherty PC: Restriction of *in vitro* T cell-mediated cytotoxicity in lymphocytic choriomeningitis within a syngeneic or semiallogeneic system. *Nature* 248:701–702, 1974.
10. Garcia KC, Degano M, Stanfield RL, et al: An alphabeta T cell receptor structure at 2.5 A and its orientation in the TCR-MHC complex. *Science* 274:209–219, 1996.
11. Baker BM, Scott DR, Blevins SJ, Hawse WF: Structural and dynamic control of T-cell receptor specificity, cross-reactivity, and binding mechanism. *Immunol Rev* 250:10–31, 2012.
12. Wang J-H, Reinherz EL: The structural basis of αβ T-lineage immune recognition: TCR docking topologies, mechanotransduction, and co-receptor function. *Immunol Rev* 250:102–119, 2012.
13. Lever M, Maini PK, van der Merwe PA, Dushek O: Phenotypic models of T cell activa-tion. *Nat Rev Immunol* 14:619–629, 2014.
14. Barral DC, Brenner MB: CD1 antigen presentation: How it works. *Nat Rev Immunol* 7:929–941, 2007.
15. Cohen NR, Garg S, Brenner MB: Antigen presentation by CD1: Lipids, T Cells, and NKT cells in microbial immunity, in *Advances in Immunology*, edited by Frederick WA, pp 1–94.: Academic Press, 102:1–94, 2009.
16. Ferreira LM: Gammadelta T cells: Innately adaptive immune cells? *Int Rev Immunol* 32:223–248, 2013.
17. Godfrey DI, Rossjohn J, McCluskey J: The fidelity, occasional promiscuity, and versatil-ity of T cell receptor recognition. *Immunity* 28:304–314, 2008.
18. Norell H, Moretta A, Silva-Santos B, Moretta L: At the bench: Preclinical rationale for exploiting NK cells and γδ T lymphocytes for the treatment of high-risk leukemias. *J Leukoc Biol* 94:1123–1139, 2013.
19. Bonneville M, O'Brien RL, Born WK: γδ T cell effector functions: A blend of innate programming and acquired plasticity. *Nat Rev Immunol* 10:467–478, 2010.
20. Wucherpfennig KW, Gagnon E, Call MJ, et al: Structural biology of the T-cell receptor: Insights into receptor assembly, ligand recognition, and initiation of signaling. *Cold Spring Harb Perspect Biol* 2:a005140, 2010.
21. Chakraborty AK, Weiss A: Insights into the initiation of TCR signaling. *Nat Immunol* 15:798–807, 2014.
22. Guirado M, de Aós I, Orta T, et al: Phosphorylation of the N-terminal and C-terminal CD3-ε-ITAM tyrosines is differentially lygulated in T cells. *Biochem Biophys Res Commun* 291:574–581, 2002.
23. Malissen B, Gregoire C, Malissen M, Roncagalli R: Integrative biology of T cell activa-tion. *Nat Immunol* 15:790–797, 2014.
24. Macian F: NFAT proteins: Key regulators of T-cell development and function. *Nat Rev Immunol* 5:472–484, 2005.
25. Devine L, Kieffer LJ, Aitken V, Kavathas PB: Human CD8β, but not mouse CD8β, can be expressed in the absence of CD8α as a ββ homodimer. *J Immunol* 164:833–838, 2000.
26. Zhu C, Jiang N, Huang J, et al: Insights from in situ analysis of TCR-pMHC recogni-tion: Response of an interaction network. *Immunol Rev* 251:49–64, 2013.
27. Gao GF, Rao Z, Bell JI: Molecular coordination of αβ T-cell receptors and corecep-tors CD8 and CD4 in their recognition of peptide-MHC ligands. *Trends Immunol* 23:408–413, 2002.
28. Reith W, Mach B: The bare lymphocyte syndrome and the regulation of MHC expres-sion. *Annu Rev Immunol* 19:331–373, 2001.
29. Artyomov MN, Lis M, Devadas S, et al: CD4 and CD8 binding to MHC molecules pri-marily acts to enhance Lck delivery. *Proc Natl Acad Sci U S A* 107:16916–16921, 2010.
30. Ashorn PA, Berger EA, Moss B: Human immunodeficiency virus envelope glycopro-tein/CD4-mediated fusion of nonprimate cells with human cells. *J Virol* 64:2149–2156, 1990.
31. Moir S, Chun T-W, Fauci AS: Pathogenic mechanisms of HIV disease. *Annu Rev Pathol* 6:223–248, 2011.
32. Schols D: HIV co-receptors as targets for antiviral therapy. *Curr Top Med Chem* 4:883–893, 2004.
33. Singer A, Adoro S, Park J-H: Lineage fate and intense debate: Myths, models and mech-anisms of CD4- versus CD8-lineage choice. *Nat Rev Immunol* 8:788–801, 2008.
34. Kidd P: Th1/Th2 balance: The hypothesis, its limitations, and implications for health and disease. *Altern Med Rev* 8:223–246, 2003.
35. Annunziato F, Cosmi L, Galli G, et al: Assessment of chemokine receptor expression by human Th1 and Th2 cells *in vitro* and *in vivo. J Leukoc Biol* 65:691–699, 1999.
36. Annunziato F, Galli G, Cosmi L, et al: Molecules associated with human Th1 or Th2 cells. *Eur Cytokine Netw* 9:12–16, 1998.
37. Bachelerie F, Ben-Baruch A, Burkhardt AM, et al: International Union of Pharmacol-ogy. LXXXIX. Update on the extended family of chemokine receptors and introducing a new nomenclature for atypical chemokine receptors. *Pharmacol Rev* 66:1–79, 2014.
38. Zhu J, Paul WE: Peripheral CD4+ T-cell differentiation regulated by networks of cytok-ines and transcription factors. *Immunol Rev* 238:247–262, 2010.
39. Oestreich KJ, Weinmann AS: Transcriptional mechanisms that regulate T helper 1 cell differentiation. *Curr Opin Immunol* 24:191–195, 2012.
40. Yagi R, Zhu J, Paul WE: An updated view on transcription factor GATA3-mediated regulation of Th1 and Th2 cell differentiation. *Int Immunol* 23:415–420, 2011.
41. Maggi E: The TH1/TH2 paradigm in allergy. *Immunotechnology* 3:233–244, 1998.
42. Allen JE, Sutherland TE: Host protective roles of type 2 immunity: Parasite killing and tissue repair, flip sides of the same coin. *Semin Immunol* 26:329–340, 2014.
43. Schramm G, Haas H: Th2 immune response against *Schistosoma mansoni* infection. *Microbes Infect* 12:881–888, 2010.
44. Singh RP: Immunoregulation of cytokines in infectious diseases (leprosy), future strat-egies. *Nihon Hansenbyo Gakkai Zasshi* 67:263–268, 1998.
45. Lienhardt C, Azzurri A, Amedei A, et al: Active tuberculosis in Africa is associated with reduced Th1 and increased Th2 activity *in vivo. Eur J Immunol* 32:1605–1613, 2002.
46. Galindo CL, Rosenzweig JA, Kirtley ML, Chopra AK: Pathogenesis of *Y. enterocolitica* and *Y. pseudotuberculosis* in human yersiniosis. *J Pathog* 2011:16, 2011.
47. Steere AC, Drouin EE, Glickstein LJ: Relationship between Immunity to *Borrelia burg-dorferi* outer-surface protein A (OspA) and Lyme arthritis. *Clin Infect Dis* 52:s259–s265, 2011.
48. D'Elios MM, Amedei A, Benagiano M, et al: *Helicobacter pylori*, T cells and cytokines: The "dangerous liaisons." *FEMS Immunol Med Microbiol* 44:113–119, 2005.
49. Vignali DA, Collison LW, Workman CJ: How regulatory T cells work. *Nat Rev Immunol* 8:523–532, 2008.
50. Sakaguchi S, Yamaguchi T, Nomura T, Ono M: Regulatory T cells and immune toler-ance. *Cell* 133:775–787, 2008.
51. Rudensky AY: Regulatory T cells and Foxp3. *Immunol Rev* 241:260–268, 2011.
52. Fu W, Ergun A, Lu T, et al: A multiply redundant genetic switch "locks in" the transcrip-tional signature of regulatory T cells. *Nat Immunol* 13:972–980, 2012.
53. d'Hennezel E, Bin Dhuban K, Torgerson T, Piccirillo C: The immunogenetics of immune dysregulation, polyendocrinopathy, enteropathy, X linked (IPEX) syndrome. *J Med Genet* 49:291–302, 2012.
54. Aaltonen J, Bjorses P, Perheentupa J, et al: An autoimmune disease, APECED, caused by mutations in a novel gene featuring two PHD-type zinc-finger domains. *Nat Genet* 17:399–403, 1997.
55. Capalbo D, Giardino G, Martino LD, et al: Genetic basis of altered central tolerance and autoimmune diseases: A lesson from AIRE mutations. *Int Rev Immunol* 31:344–362, 2012.
56. Fontenot JD, Rasmussen JP, Gavin MA, Rudensky AY: A function for interleukin 2 in Foxp3-expressing regulatory T cells. *Nat Immunol* 6:1142–1151, 2005.
57. Ohkura N, Hamaguchi M, Morikawa H, et al: T cell receptor stimulation-induced epigenetic changes and Foxp3 expression are independent and complementary events required for Treg cell development. *Immunity* 37:785–799, 2012.
58. Abbas AK, Benoist C, Bluestone JA, et al: Regulatory T cells: Recommendations to sim-plify the nomenclature. *Nat Immunol* 14:307–308, 2013.
59. Curotto de Lafaille MA, Lafaille JJ: Natural and adaptive Foxp3+ regulatory T cells: More of the same or a division of labor? *Immunity* 30:626–635, 2009.
60. Veiga-Parga T, Sehrawat S, Rouse BT: Role of regulatory T cells during virus infection. *Immunol Rev* 255:182–196, 2013.

61. Waldmann H, Hilbrands R, Howie D, Cobbold S: Harnessing FOXP3+ regulatory T cells for transplantation tolerance. *J Clin Invest* 124:1439–1445, 2014.
62. Rubtsov YP, Niec RE, Josefowicz S, et al: Stability of the regulatory T cell lineage *in vivo*. *Science* 329:1667–1671, 2010.
63. Sakaguchi S, Miyara M, Costantino CM, Hafler DA: FOXP3+ regulatory T cells in the human immune system. *Nat Rev Immunol* 10:490–500, 2010.
64. Garín MI, Chu C-C, Golshayan D, et al: Galectin-1: A key effector of regulation mediated by CD4+CD25+ T cells. *Blood* 109:2058–2065, 2007.
65. Liu H, Yang PS, Zhu T, et al: Characterization of fibrinogen-like protein 2 (FGL2): Monomeric FGL2 has enhanced immunosuppressive activity in comparison to oligomeric FGL2. *Int J Biochem Cell Biol* 45:408–418, 2013.
66. Korn T, Bettelli E, Oukka M, Kuchroo VK: IL-17 and Th17 Cells. *Annu Rev Immunol* 27:485–517, 2009.
67. McGeachy MJ, Chen Y, Tato CM, et al: The interleukin 23 receptor is essential for the terminal differentiation of interleukin 17-producing effector T helper cells *in vivo*. *Nat Immunol* 10:314–324, 2009.
68. Boniface K, Bak-Jensen KS, Li Y, et al: Prostaglandin E2 regulates Th17 cell differentiation and function through cyclic AMP and EP2/EP4 receptor signaling. *J Exp Med* 206:535–548, 2009.
69. Ivanov II, McKenzie BS, Zhou L, et al: The orphan nuclear receptor RORγt directs the differentiation program of proinflammatory IL-17+ T helper cells. *Cell* 126:1121–1133, 2006.
70. Yang XO, Panopoulos AD, Nurieva R, et al: STAT3 regulates cytokine-mediated generation of inflammatory helper T cells. *J Biol Chem* 282:9358–9363, 2007.
71. Bettelli E, Carrier Y, Gao W, et al: Reciprocal developmental pathways for the generation of pathogenic effector TH17 and regulatory T cells. *Nature* 441:235–238, 2006.
72. Mangan PR, Harrington LE, O'Quinn DB, et al: Transforming growth factor-beta induces development of the T(H)17 lineage. *Nature* 441:231–234, 2006.
73. Annunziato F, Cosmi L, Santarlasci V, et al: Phenotypic and functional features of human Th17 cells. *J Exp Med* 204:1849–1861, 2007.
74. Kryczek I, Banerjee M, Cheng P, et al: Phenotype, distribution, generation, and functional and clinical relevance of Th17 cells in the human tumor environments. *Blood* 114:1141–1149, 2009.
75. Harrington LE, Hatton RD, Mangan PR, et al: Interleukin 17-producing CD4+ effector T cells develop via a lineage distinct from the T helper type 1 and 2 lineages. *Nat Immunol* 6:1123–1132, 2005.
76. Miossec P, Korn T, Kuchroo VK: Interleukin-17 and type 17 helper T cells. *N Engl J Med* 361:888–898, 2009.
77. Ouyang W, Kolls JK, Zheng Y: The biological functions of T helper 17 cell effector cytokines in inflammation. *Immunity* 28:454–467, 2008.
78. Iwakura Y, Nakae S, Saijo S, Ishigame H: The roles of IL-17A in inflammatory immune responses and host defense against pathogens. *Immunol Rev* 226:57–79, 2008.
79. Milner JD, Brenchley JM, Laurence A, et al: Impaired TH17 cell differentiation in subjects with autosomal dominant hyper-IgE syndrome. *Nature* 452:773–776, 2008.
80. Ma CS, Chew GY, Simpson N, et al: Deficiency of Th17 cells in hyper IgE syndrome due to mutations in STAT3. *J Exp Med* 205:1551–1557, 2008.
81. Abou Chakra CN, Sirard S, Valiquette L: Risk factors for recurrence, complications and mortality in Clostridium difficile infection: A systematic review. *PLoS One* 9:e98400, 2014.
82. Furst DE, Emery P: Rheumatoid arthritis pathophysiology: Update on emerging cytokine and cytokine-associated cell targets. *Rheumatology* 53:1560–1569, 2014.
83. Martin JC, Baeten DL, Josien R: Emerging role of IL-17 and Th17 cells in systemic lupus erythematosus. *Clin Immunol* 154:1–12, 2014.
84. Sie C, Korn T, Mitsdoerffer M: Th17 cells in central nervous system autoimmunity. *Exp Neurol* 262 Pt A:18–27, 2014.
85. Troncone E, Marafini I, Pallone F, Monteleone G: Th17 cytokines in inflammatory bowel diseases: Discerning the good from the bad. *Int Rev Immunol* 32:526–533, 2013.
86. Newcomb DC, Peebles RS Jr: Th17-mediated inflammation in asthma. *Curr Opin Immunol* 25:755–760, 2013.
87. Elloso MM, Gomez-Angelats M, Fourie AM: Targeting the Th17 pathway in psoriasis. *J Leukoc Biol* 92:1187–1197, 2012.
88. Crotty S: Follicular helper CD4 T cells (TFH). *Annu Rev Immunol* 29:621–663, 2011.
89. Liu X, Yan X, Zhong B, et al: Bcl6 expression specifies the T follicular helper cell program in vivo. *J Exp Med* 209:1841–1852, 2012.
90. Kaplan MH: Th9 cells: Differentiation and disease. *Immunol Rev* 252:104–115, 2013.
91. Jager A, Kuchroo VK: Effector and regulatory T-cell subsets in autoimmunity and tissue inflammation. *Scand J Immunol* 72:173–184, 2010.
92. Jones CP, Gregory LG, Causton B, et al: Activin A and TGF-β promote T(H)9 cell-mediated pulmonary allergic pathology. *J Allergy Clin Immunol* 129:1000–1010.e3, 2012.
93. Purwar R, Schlapbach C, Xiao S, et al: Robust tumor immunity to melanoma mediated by interleukin-9-producing T cells. *Nat Med* 18:1248–1253, 2012.
94. Lu Y, Hong S, Li H, et al: Th9 cells promote antitumor immune responses in vivo. *J Clin Invest* 122:4160–4171, 2012.
95. Williams MA, Bevan MJ: Effector and memory CTL differentiation. *Annu Rev Immunol* 25:171–192, 2007.
96. Lees JR, Farber DL: Generation, persistence and plasticity of CD4 T-cell memories. *Immunology* 130:463–470, 2010.
97. Murali-Krishna K, Lau LL, Sambhara S, et al: Persistence of memory CD8 T cells in MHC class I-deficient mice. *Science* 286:1377–1381, 1999.
98. van Leeuwen EMM, Sprent J, Surh CD: Generation and maintenance of memory CD4+ T Cells. *Curr Opin Immunol* 21:167–172, 2009.
99. Plebanski M, Saunders M, Burtles SS, et al: Primary and secondary human in vitro T-cell responses to soluble antigens are mediated by subsets bearing different CD45 isoforms. *Immunology* 75:86–91, 1992.
100. Alexander DR: The CD45 tyrosine phosphatase: A positive and negative regulator of immune cell function. *Semin Immunol* 12:349–359, 2000.
101. Tortorella C, Schulze-Koops H, Thomas R, et al: Expression of CD45RB and CD27 identifies subsets of CD4+ memory T cells with different capacities to induce B cell differentiation. *J Immunol* 155:149–162, 1995.
102. Clement LT: Functional and phenotypic properties of "naive" and "memory" CD4+ T cells in the human. *Immunol Res* 10:189–195, 1991.
103. Sallusto F, Lenig D, Forster R, et al: Two subsets of memory T lymphocytes with distinct homing potentials and effector functions. *Nature* 401:708–712, 1999.
104. Huster KM, Busch V, Schiemann M, et al: Selective expression of IL-7 receptor on memory T cells identifies early CD40L-dependent generation of distinct CD8+ memory T cell subsets. *Proc Natl Acad Sci U S A* 13:5610–5615, 2004.
105. Kallies A: Distinct regulation of effector and memory T-cell differentiation. *Immunol Cell Biol* 86:325–332, 2008.
106. Lenschow DJ, Walunas TL, Bluestone JA: CD28/B7 system of T cell costimulation. *Annu Rev Immunol* 14:233–258, 1996.
107. van der Merwe PA, Bodian DL, Daenke S, et al: CD80 (B7-1) binds both CD28 and CTLA-4 with a low affinity and very fast kinetics. *J Exp Med* 185:393–404, 1997.
108. Greene JL, Leytze GM, Emswiler J, et al: Covalent dimerization of CD28/CTLA-4 and oligomerization of CD80/CD86 regulate T cell costimulatory interactions. *J Biol Chem* 271:26762–26771, 1996.
109. Yokosuka T, Saito T: The immunological synapse, TCR microclusters, and T cell activation, in *Immunological Synapse*, edited by Saito T, Batista FD, pp 81–107. Springer, Berlin, 2010.
110. Rudd CE, Taylor A, Schneider H: CD28 and CTLA-4 coreceptor expression and signal transduction. *Immunol Rev* 229:12–26, 2009.
111. Powell JD, Ragheb JA, Kitagawa-Sakakida S, Schwartz RH: Molecular regulation of interleukin-2 expression by CD28 co-stimulation and anergy. *Immunol Rev* 165:287–300, 1998.
112. Lumsden JM, Williams JA, Hodes RJ: Differential requirements for expression of CD80/86 and CD40 on B cells for T-dependent antibody responses in vivo. *J Immunol* 170:781–787, 2003.
113. Fathman CG, Lineberry NB: Molecular mechanisms of CD4+ T-cell anergy. *Nat Rev Immunol* 7:599–609, 2007.
114. Beverly B, Kang S-M, Lenardo MJ, Schwartz RH: Reversal of in vitro T cell clonal anergy by IL-2 stimulation. *Int Immunol* 4:661–671, 1992.
115. Ise W, Kohyama M, Nutsch KM, et al: CTLA-4 suppresses the pathogenicity of self antigen-specific T cells by cell-intrinsic and cell-extrinsic mechanisms. *Nat Immunol* 11:129–135, 2010.
116. Masteller EL, Chuang E, Mullen AC, et al: structural analysis of CTLA-4 function in vivo. *J Immunol* 164:5319–5327, 2000.
117. Maltzman JS, Turka LA: T-cell costimulatory blockade in organ transplantation. *Cold Spring Harb Perspect Med* 3:a015537, 2013.
118. Duraiswamy J, Kaluza KM, Freeman GJ, Coukos G: Dual blockade of PD-1 and CTLA-4 combined with tumor vaccine effectively restores T-cell rejection function in tumors. *Cancer Res* 73:3591–3603, 2013.
119. Wolchok JD, Kluger H, Callahan MK, et al: Nivolumab plus ipilimumab in advanced melanoma. *N Engl J Med* 369:122–133, 2013.
120. Chen L, Flies DB: Molecular mechanisms of T cell co-stimulation and co-inhibition. *Nat Rev Immunol* 13:227–242, 2013.
121. Pardoll DM: The blockade of immune checkpoints in cancer immunotherapy. *Nat Rev Cancer* 12:252–264, 2012.
122. Wang S, Zhu G, Chapoval AI, et al: Costimulation of T cells by B7-H2, a B7-like molecule that binds ICOS. *Blood* 96:2808–2813, 2000.
123. Nishimura H, Nose M, Hiai H, et al: Development of lupus-like autoimmune diseases by disruption of the PD-1 gene encoding an ITIM motif-carrying immunoreceptor. *Immunity* 11:141–151, 1999.
124. Chen W, Zhu C: Mechanical regulation of T-cell functions. *Immunol Rev* 256:160–176, 2013.
125. Schmidt S, Moser M, Sperandio M: The molecular basis of leukocyte recruitment and its deficiencies. *Mol Immunol* 55:49–58, 2013.
126. Shimizu Y, van Seventer GA, Horgan KJ, Shaw S: Roles of adhesion molecules in T-cell recognition: Fundamental similarities between four integrins on resting human T cells (LFA-1, VLA-4, VLA-5, VLA-6) in expression, binding, and costimulation. *Immunol Rev* 114:109–143, 1990.
127. Davis SJ, Ikemizu S, Wild MK, Van der Merwe PA: CD2 and the nature of protein interactions mediating cell–cell recognition. *Immunol Rev* 163:217–236, 1998.
128. Huppa JB, Davis MM: T-cell-antigen recognition and the immunological synapse. *Nat Rev Immunol* 3:973–983, 2003.
129. Grakoui A, Bromley SK, Sumen C, et al: The immunological synapse: A molecular machine controlling T cell activation. *Science* 285:221–227, 1999.
130. Dustin ML, Depoil D: New insights into the T cell synapse from single molecule techniques. *Nat Rev Immunol* 11:672–684, 2011.

CHAPTER 77
FUNCTIONS OF NATURAL KILLER CELLS

Giorgio Trinchieri, Richard W. Childs, and Lewis L. Lanier

SUMMARY

Natural killer (NK) cells, with a predominant morphology of large granular lymphocytes, represent a lineage of lymphoid cells with constitutive ability to mediate cytotoxicity toward pathologic target cells and secrete cytokines. NK cells participate in the innate resistance to microbial pathogens and malignancies; opposing effects of activating and inhibitory receptors regulate NK cell activity. Malignant expansions of NK cells, either acute or chronic, are rare, but represent well-identified clinical entities.

● IDENTIFICATION AND DEFINITION OF NATURAL KILLER CELLS

DEFINITION

Natural killer (NK) cells were identified in the blood and lymphoid organs of humans and experimental animals as cells capable of killing tumors, virus-infected cells, and, in some instances, normal cells, in the absence of previous deliberate or known sensitization.[1,2] NK cells are now considered to belong to the cellular subgroup that is characterized by the production of interferon (IFN)-γ within the family of innate lymphoid cells (ILCs), a family of developmentally related cells involved in innate immunity and tissue development.[3] NK cells are defined as cytotoxic cells with the predominant morphology of large granular lymphocytes (LGLs) that: (1) neither productively rearrange any of the genes encoding the T-cell receptor (TCR) chains nor express on their surface the CD3-TCR complex; (2) express the CD56 (N-CAM), CD335 (NKp46), and CD16 (FcγRIIIA), antigens in humans, the NK1.1 (NKR-P1C), NKp46, and DX5 (VLA-2/CD49d) antigens in mice, and the NKR-P1 antigen in rats; and (3) can kill cells not expressing major

Acronyms and Abbreviations: ADCC, antibody-dependent cell-mediated cytotoxicity; AML, acute myelogenous leukemia; CAR, chimeric antigen receptor; CTL, cytotoxic T lymphocyte; GM-CSF, granulocyte-macrophage colony-stimulating factor; HLA, human leukocyte antigen; IFN, interferon; Ig, immunoglobulin; IL, interleukin; ILC, innate lymphoid cell; iNKT, invariant natural killer T cell; ITIM, immunoreceptor tyrosine-based inhibitory motif; KIR, killer cell Ig-like receptor; LCMV, lymphocytic choriomeningitis virus; LGL, large granular lymphocyte; MCMV, mouse cytomegalovirus; MHC, major histocompatibility complex; NK, natural killer; TCR, T-cell antigen receptor; TNF, tumor necrosis factor; TRAIL, TNF-related apoptosis-inducing ligand.

histocompatibility complex (MHC) class I or class II antigens. Thus, target-cell recognition by NK cells is distinct from cytotoxic T lymphocytes (CTLs), which recognize specific antigenic peptides bound to MHC class I molecules. Nonetheless, the presence of MHC class I on target cells affects NK cell recognition, in some cases inhibiting a NK cell response.

Certain T lymphocytes that express either $\alpha\beta$ or a $\gamma\delta$ TCR may exhibit, particularly upon activation, TCR-independent cytolytic activity that resembles that of NK cells and often express many of the same surface receptors as NK cells. Among the T lymphocytes in humans and mice that coexpress many of the NK cell antigens, invariant natural killer T (iNKT) cells express an invariant TCR that recognizes glycolipids presented by CD1d, a nonclassical MHC molecule, and upon stimulation rapidly produce large amounts of IFN-γ, granulocyte-macrophage colony-stimulating factor (GM-CSF), interleukin (IL)-4, and IL-13.[4]

MORPHOLOGY

Human LGLs are medium- to large-size lymphocytes with round or indented nuclei, condensed chromatin, and usually prominent nucleoli. The cytoplasm is abundant and contains a variety of organelles and granules (primary lysosomes) that, in addition to lysosomal enzymes, contain proteins important for cytotoxic function, such as serine esterases (granzymes) and pore-forming proteins (perforin).[5] Although many NK cells have the morphology typical of LGL, a significant proportion of NK cells are agranular and indistinguishable from other lymphocytes.[6]

ORIGIN AND TISSUE DISTRIBUTION

NK cells originate in the marrow from the common lymphoid progenitor cell.[7] Most have a life span ranging from a few days to a few weeks,[8] but some may persist for months after exposure to viral challenge.[9] In mice, the cytokine IL-15 plays a particularly important role in the differentiation and expansion of NK cells.[10] NK cell differentiation does not require the thymus, although NK cell progenitors can differentiate in the thymus from precursors expressing IL-7Rα CD127.[11] Secondary lymphoid tissues may also be a site of NK cell development in humans.[12] The increased number of NK cells and altered anatomical distribution in response to infection or other stimuli are the result of increased NK cell production in the marrow and proliferation of peripheral NK cells.

NK cells represent approximately 5 to 20 percent of blood lymphocytes.[13] Immature NK cells express high amounts of CD56, lack CD16, and have low cytolytic capacity, whereas mature NK cells in blood express low amounts of CD56, high levels of CD16, and mediate potent lytic activity.[14] NK cells are present in the red pulp of the spleen and are found at a low frequency in other lymphoid organs and marrow.[2] NK cells with a phenotype resembling the CD56^high peripheral subset have been detected in lymph nodes.[15] Small numbers of NK cells can be identified in the liver (pit cells), lung, and intestinal mucosa.[16,17] In response to type I IFN or viral or bacterial infections, NK cells accumulate in organs in which they normally are rare, particularly the liver, marrow, and lymph nodes where they may produce large amounts of cytokines.[18] CD56^bright CD16^- NK cells are the predominant cell type present in the human early pregnancy decidua.[19] Decidual NK cells produce cytokines that have tissue remodeling capacity, facilitate embryonic implantation, monitor mucosal integrity throughout the menstrual cycle, control trophoblast invasion during pregnancy, and modulate the maternal immune response against embryo antigens.[19]

● MECHANISMS OF NATURAL KILLER CELL FUNCTIONS

CELL-MEDIATED CYTOTOXICITY

Cytotoxicity mediated by NK cells depends on binding to the target cells, followed by activation of the lytic mechanism, which usually involves release of perforin and granzymes from the granules.[5] Cytotoxicity can also be mediated through the interaction of surface molecules, for example, the interaction of Fas ligand, membrane tumor necrosis factor (TNF), or TNF-related apoptosis-inducing ligand (TRAIL) on NK cells with their death-inducing receptors on target cells. Lysis of the target cells results from alteration of membrane permeability and induction of apoptosis.[5]

Several surface molecules on NK cells have been identified that activate the cytotoxic mechanism and induce cytokine secretion (Fig. 77–1).[20] One of these molecules is the low-affinity receptor for the Fc fragment of immunoglobulin (Ig) G (FcγRIIIA or CD16), which is expressed on most human circulating NK cells in association with the signal-transducing CD3ξ or FcεRIγ chains. When CD16 is cross-linked by IgG antibodies bound to a target cell surface, it triggers antibody-dependent cell-mediated cytotoxicity (ADCC). Natural killing can also be activated by several other receptors that recognize relevant ligands on the potential target cell. NKG2D, a receptor expressed on all NK cells, has been implicated in NK cell recognition of transformed and virus-infected cells.[21] This receptor recognizes a family of MHC class I-related glycoproteins (including MICA, MICB, ULBP1–ULBP6), which are absent or expressed at only low levels on healthy cells but are induced or upregulated upon cell transformation or viral infection.[21] Viruses, such as cytomegalovirus, have devised strategies to prevent the expression of NKG2D ligands in the infected cells,[22] presumably to escape NK cell-mediated immunity. NK cells express many other activating receptors that have been implicated in their recognition of tumors, including DNAM-1 (CD226) and the "natural cytotoxicity" receptors NKp30, NKp44, and NKp46.[20]

NK cells preferentially kill certain tumor cells lacking expression of MHC class I molecules.[23] NK cells are regulated by positive signals initiated by activating receptors and negative signals transmitted by interactions between inhibitory receptors for MHC class I on the NK cells and autologous MHC class I molecules on potential target cells. NK cells may mediate immune surveillance against cells that lose expression of MHC class I. Numerous viruses inhibit the synthesis or transport of MHC class I proteins, presumably to avoid detection by CTL.[24] In addition, frequent loss of MHC class I expression on tumor cells has been documented.[25] However, NK cells are capable of killing cells expressing MHC class I if they receive sufficiently strong activation signals.

Two families of NK cell receptors for MHC class I have been identified in humans. The Killer cell Ig-like receptors (KIRs) are encoded by approximately 15 genes present on human chromosome 19q13.4.[26] *KIR* genes are highly polymorphic and evolve rapidly, diversifying by gene duplication and conversion events. Certain KIRs bind human leukocyte antigen (HLA)-C ligands, whereas other KIRs recognize certain alleles of HLA-B or HLA-A. Another class of NK cell receptors for MHC class I are heterodimeric glycoproteins composed of a CD94 subunit that is disulfide bonded to an NKG2A molecule.[20] The genes encoding CD94 (*KLRD1*) and NKG2A (*KLRC1*) are on human chromosome 12p12-p13 and are members of the C-type lectin superfamily. The CD94-NKG2A receptors bind to HLA-E, a unique MHC class I protein that displays peptides derived from leader segments from HLA-A, HLA-B, HLA-C, or HLA-G proteins.[27] When synthesis of HLA-A, HLA-B, HLA-C, or HLA-G is disrupted, possibly by viral infection or transformation of the host cell, HLA-E cannot be transported to the cell surface for presentation to the CD94-NKG2A receptor. The various KIR and CD94-NKG2A receptors are expressed on overlapping subsets within the NK cell population and on certain memory T cells, usually CD8+ T cells, although a minor subset of CD4+ T cells also express KIR. The inhibitory KIR and CD94-NKG2A receptors have an immunoreceptor tyrosine-based inhibitory motif (ITIM) sequence in their cytoplasmic domains, which binds to the cytoplasmic tyrosine phosphatase SHP-1, resulting in suppression of cytotoxicity and cytokine secretion.[20] Therefore, the functional behavior of NK and T cells expressing KIR or CD94-NKG2A is regulated by the balance of positive signals transmitted by a variety of activating receptors and negative signals provided by the inhibitory MHC class I receptors. Although the expression of NK cell inhibitory receptors is variegated and polymorphic, most NK cells express at least one inhibitory receptor recognizing self MHC and thus are not self-reactive. This is accomplished at least in part by the requirement of interaction of an inhibitory receptor with its ligands during NK cell development for full functional maturation and possibly expansion (NK cell "licensing").[28]

Certain receptors of the KIR and CD94-NKG2 families do not possess ITIM sequences and activate, rather than suppress, NK- and T-cell responses.[20] These receptors noncovalently associate with the homodimeric adapter protein DAP12.[29] Like the CD3ξ and the FcεRIγ subunits, DAP12 contains an immunoreceptor tyrosine-based activation motif (ITAM) in the cytoplasmic domain. Upon receptor ligation, DAP12 becomes tyrosine phosphorylated, recruits the ZAP70 and Syk cytoplasmic tyrosine kinases, and induces cellular activation.[29] The physiologic role of activating NK cell receptors for MHC class I has not been determined, but these receptors may have consequences in allogeneic marrow transplantation. In mice, an activating receptor in the Ly49 family (the functional counterpart of KIRs in humans) has been shown to recognize a viral glycoprotein encoded by cytomegalovirus and protects the mice from this pathogen.[30,31] This finding suggests that certain activating KIRs in humans may also recognize pathogens.

Although resting blood NK cells are cytotoxic, their activity can be greatly enhanced both *in vivo* and *in vitro* by exposure to cytokines such

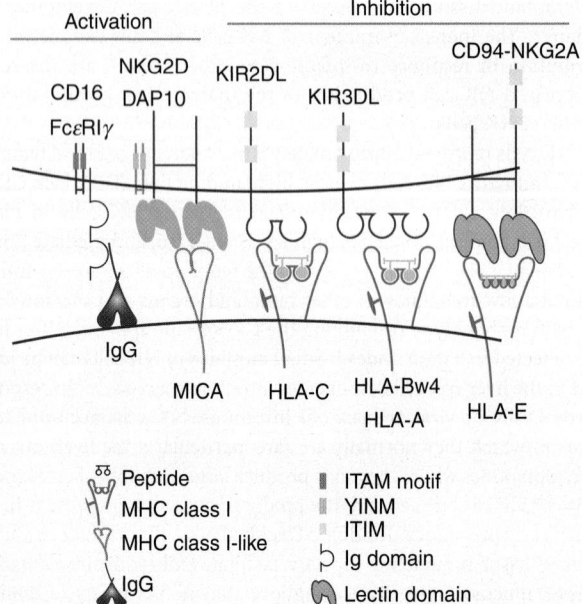

Figure 77–1. Schematic of selected inhibitory and activating natural killer (NK) cell receptors regulating NK cell responses.

as IFN-α/β, IL-2, IL-12, IL-15, and IL-18.[32-34] Resting NK cells constitutively express intermediate-affinity IL-2 receptors, and IL-2 induces the progression of most NK cells into the cell cycle.[35]

PRODUCTION OF CYTOKINES

Many of the physiologic functions of NK cells are mediated at least partly by their ability to secrete cytokines. NK cells are powerful producers of IFN-γ and GM-CSF, and other cytokines and chemokines. Stimulation by cytokines, such as IL-2, IL-12, IL-18, TNF-α, and IL-1,[2,33,36,37] and triggering by activating receptors, such as CD16 interacting with immune complexes, are among the stimuli that, acting individually or often in synergistic combination, induce NK cells to produce cytokines.[2,38,39]

⬤ PHYSIOLOGIC ROLES OF NATURAL KILLER CELLS

INNATE RESISTANCE

Together with myeloid cells, NK cells are effectors of the innate or natural resistance, which represents the first line of defense against infection (Fig. 77–2). The ability of NK cells to participate in the resistance against infection by certain viruses is well documented in experimental animals and is strongly suggested by the recurrent viral infections in the rare patients with a selective deficiency of NK cells.[40] NK cells selectively kill virus-infected cells by a mechanism that is at least partly dependent on the production of IFN-α, a potent stimulator of NK cell activity.[41,42] In vivo viral infection and type I IFN production usually are accompanied by rapid activation of, and increase in the number of, NK cells.[18] The NK cell response to virus infection is followed by an antigen-specific T helper and CTL response, which peaks 7 to 9 days after infection.[18] The early NK cell response induces a significant reduction in the titer of certain viruses, including mouse cytomegalovirus (MCMV).[43] NK cell

activation induced by viral infection may have beneficial or pathogenic effects.[44] After expansion in response to MCMV infection, NK cells expressing the activating Ly49H receptor persist for several months and respond rapidly to rechallenge with MCMV, thus possessing immunologic memory.[9] Similarly, a subset of liver-resident NK cells can mediate antigen-specific contact hypersensitivity responses and immunologic memory.[45,46]

NK cells enhance the response of phagocytic cells to microorganisms, especially intracellular bacteria and parasites, by producing high levels of the phagocyte-activating cytokines IFN-γ and GM-CSF in response to the microorganisms themselves or to factors, such as IL-12 and TNF-α, produced by infected phagocytic cells.[47,48]

REGULATION OF ADAPTIVE IMMUNITY

NK cells, by interacting with infectious agents and antigens early during the immune response, have either stimulatory or inhibitory effects on the function of B and T cells and antigen-presenting cells.[2] Evidence for an enhancing effect of NK cells on B-cell responses has been shown both in vitro and in vivo by studies demonstrating that NK cells in the absence of T cells support antigen-specific B-cell responses, partly by producing IFN-γ.[49,50] In certain infections, NK cells may be necessary for optimal induction of both a CD4+ and CD8+ T-cell response.[51,52] NK cells stimulated by microorganisms or by cytokines, such as IL-12 and IL-18, produce large amounts of IFN-γ and other cytokines that facilitate T-helper cell type 1 development.[53,54] The reciprocal activating interaction between NK cells and the antigen-presenting dendritic cells is important for the regulation of both innate resistance and the downstream adaptive response to pathogens.[55,56]

MODULATION OF HEMATOPOIESIS

Experimental and clinical studies have demonstrated that NK cells are involved in the regulation of hematopoiesis.[57] The effect of NK cells

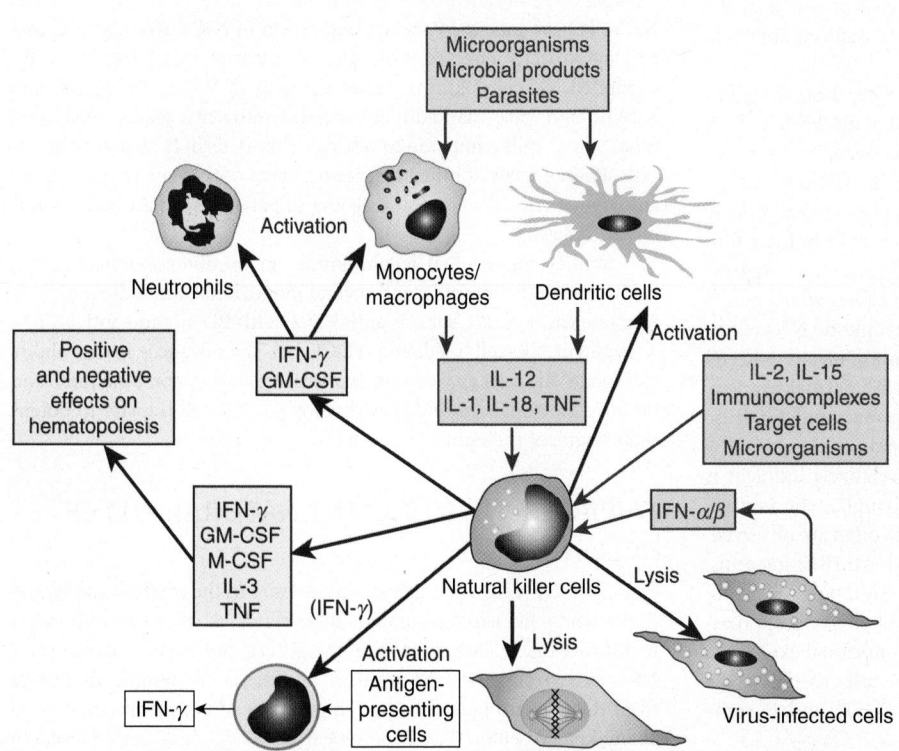

Figure 77–2. Schematic of some of the functions and regulatory pathways of natural killer (NK) cells as effector cells of natural resistance. In addition to mediating cytotoxicity, NK cells exert their physiologic roles by releasing several cytokines that affect the functions of other cell types, including hematopoietic progenitor cells. NK cell activity also is regulated by cytokines. Cytokines interferon (IFN)-α/β, interleukin (IL)-2, IL-15, and IL-12 enhance NK-cell–mediated cytotoxicity. IL-2, IL-12, IL-15, IL-18, tumor necrosis factor (TNF), and IL-1 induce NK cell lymphokine production. IL-2 and IL-12 induce NK cell proliferation. Blue arrows indicate conditions that activate NK cells whereas the red arrows indicate innate, proinflammatory, and immunoregulatory functions of NK cells. GM-CSF, granulocyte-macrophage colony-stimulating factor; M-CSF, macrophage colony-stimulating factor.

is mostly mediated by secretion of soluble factors. NK cells, constitutively or upon activation, produce several lymphokines, some with mostly inhibitory effects on hematopoiesis, such as TNF and IFN-γ, and some with mostly stimulatory effects, such as GM-CSF.[36,58] The effector role of NK cells in rejection of parental marrow graft in irradiated F1 mice[59] and in suppressing erythropoiesis and phagocytopoiesis in mice infected with lymphocytic choriomeningitis virus (LCMV)[60] demonstrate that *in vivo* activated NK cells can affect both allogeneic and syngeneic hematopoietic progenitor cells. Because of the ability of NK cells to kill transformed hematopoietic cells, NK cells have been postulated to play an important role in the graft-versus-leukemia reaction in allogeneic marrow transplantation but only a modest, if any, role in graft-versus-host disease.[61] In haploidentical or mismatched hematopoietic transplantation, the presence on donor NK cells of the KIR not recognizing inhibiting ligands on host hematopoietic and malignant cells results in protection from leukemia relapse.[62] A reduced incidence of graft-versus-host disease has also been observed and thought to result from the elimination of recipient antigen-presenting cells by donor NK cells.[62]

PATHOLOGIC ALTERATIONS IN NATURAL KILLER CELL NUMBER AND FUNCTIONS

NK cell function and NK cell numbers are often decreased in pathologic conditions, including cancer and AIDS.[63,64] The reduced activity or number of NK cells may contribute to disease pathology by decreasing the innate resistance against tumor growth and metastasis in cancer patients or against opportunistic infections in AIDS patients. NK cell (and cytotoxic T-cell) hyporesponsiveness is observed in patients with Chédiak-Higashi syndrome,[65] a rare autosomal recessive disease associated with cellular dysfunction, including fusion of cytoplasmic granules and defective degranulation of neutrophil lysosomes. NK cell numbers are normal in these patients, but the NK cells present a single, large granule in the cytoplasm and have a severely reduced ability to mediate cytotoxicity.[65]

Malignant acute expansion of NK cells is rare, more frequent in Asians than in whites, and often associated with Epstein-Barr virus infection.[66] Extranodal NK cell lymphomas occur in both the nasopharyngeal region and in nonnasal areas as an NK cell (CD2+, CD3-, CD56+, CD16-, CD57-) leukemia or lymphoma that mostly affects extranodal tissues.[67] It affects predominantly men in their fifth decade and usually has an extremely aggressive clinical course. Aggressive NK cell leukemia is a catastrophic disease that affects young adults and is characterized by the systemic presence of neoplastic NK cells in blood and marrow.[67] An entity previously known as "blastic NK cell lymphoma," characterized by CD4+, CD56+ cells with dermal tropism, is now recognized to represent an expansion of plasmacytoid dendritic cells rather than NK cells.[67] A chronic monoclonal proliferative disorder of LGL with a clinical course that is often relatively indolent is more commonly observed.[68] Most patients have lymphocytic infiltration of the marrow. Severe neutropenia and anemia often are observed. Associated diseases, most commonly rheumatoid arthritis, hepatitis, or cancer, are present in up to half of patients.[68] Although cells from all these patients are characterized by a LGL morphology, in approximately two-thirds of the cases they represent a monoclonal expansion of CD8+ T cells, and in only less than one-third of cases they have the typical phenotype and genotype of CD3-, CD56+, CD57+, and, in some patients, CD16+ NK cells.[68]

NATURAL KILLER CELL THERAPY TO TREAT CANCER

TARGETING NK CELL RECEPTORS

Data showing recipients of KIR-incompatible donors have reduced relapse of acute myelogenous leukemia (AML) following mismatched allogeneic stem cell transplantation remain the most compelling evidence to support the antitumor activity of NK cells.[61] Further, studies in mice showing Ly49-incompatible NK cells mediate graft-versus-tumor effects have led to clinical trials exploring adoptively infused allogeneic NK cells in patients with cancer. In humans, pilot studies have shown that adoptive transfer of IL-2-activated MHC-mismatched allogeneic NK cells can proliferate in vivo and can induce tumor regression in patients with AML and solid tumors.[69]

A strategy to disrupt inhibitory KIRs to enhance NK tumor killing involves blocking KIRs with monoclonal antibodies or genetically silencing their expression. IPH2101 is a fully human IgG$_4$ antibody that binds to KIR2D, thus blocking its ability to suppress NK cell function. Studies in a mouse model showing that IPH2101 enhances NK-cell killing of KIR ligand-matched tumor cells has led to phase I studies evaluating the efficacy of IPH2101-mediated KIR2D blockade in patients with AML and other hematologic disorders.[70] Genetic disruption of the inhibitory receptor NKG2A has been shown to enhance NK cell killing of HLA-E–expressing tumors *ex vivo* and *in vivo* following their infusion into tumor-bearing mice.[71]

ADOPTIVE NATURAL KILLER CELL TRANSFER

Recently, methods have been developed to expand large numbers of human NK cells *ex vivo*, which provides the opportunity to study the efficacy of adoptive NK-cell immunotherapy in patients with cancer.[72] Most expansion cultures utilize irradiated feeder cells such as Epstein-Barr virus–transformed lymphoblastoid cell lines or the human erythromyeloblastoid leukemia cell line K562 cells genetically modified to express membrane bound 4–1BB ligand, IL-15, or IL-21. Expanded NK cells have increased surface expression of NK activating receptors and cytotoxicity effector molecules. Compared to resting NK cells, expanded NK cells express higher amounts of IFN-γ, Fas ligand, and TRAIL, and have markedly enhanced cytotoxicity against K562 and other tumor cells compared to resting or short-term IL-2–activated NK cells. Phase I trials of infusing large numbers of these *ex vivo* expanded autologous NK cells are now ongoing in patients with a variety of different cancers.[73]

Studies suggest that lenalidomide, an immunomodulatory drug derived from thalidomide, and several monoclonal antibodies blocking immune checkpoints, such as anti–PD-1, anti–PD-L1, and anti–CTLA-4, augment NK-cell–mediated ADCC.[74,75] The advances in our ability to expand NK cells *ex vivo* now makes it feasible to combine these and other monoclonal antibodies with adoptive NK cell transfer to potentially augment their antitumor effects.

OVERCOMING DEFICIENT NATURAL KILLER CELL HOMING

Expanded NK cells are inefficient at homing to the marrow and lymph nodes where hematologic malignancies reside. A variety of techniques to improve NK cell homing to these target organs have been described.[72] NK cell trogocytosis (the transfer of plasma membrane fragments from the presenting cell to the lymphocyte) of the membrane-bound chemokine receptor CCR7 expressed on K562 cells can be used to increase NK cell CCR7 surface expression, improving their homing into the lymph nodes of athymic mice.[76] Nicotinamide, a specific inhibitor of nicotinamide adenine dinucleotide–dependent enzymes, substantially increases surface expression of CD62L on NK cells when added to cell cultures, improving their homing into the spleens and marrow of immunodeficient mice.

Recruitment of leukocytes to marrow is largely dependent on E-selectin binding.[77] *Ex vivo* expanded NK cells primarily express nonglycosylated ligands for E-selectin, potentially limiting their homing ability to the marrow. *Ex vivo* forced fucosylation of NK cells with fucosyltransferase VI enhances their E-selectin binding capacity *in vitro* and in mice improves their homing to the marrow.[72] Forced fucosylation of NK cells is currently being studied as a novel approach to improve NK homing to the marrow to enhance NK cell killing of hematologic malignancies.

AUGMENTING NATURAL KILLER CELL TUMOR KILLING

Exposing tumors to drugs that enhance caspase activity or upregulate death receptors for the apoptosis-inducing ligands TRAIL or Fas-L is an alternative strategy to bolster the antitumor effects of NK cells.[78] The proteasome inhibitor bortezomib upregulates surface expression of the TRAIL receptor DR5, enhancing tumor susceptibility to NK-cell TRAIL-mediated apoptosis *in vitro* and *in vivo*.[79] In mice, eradicating regulatory T cells prior to adoptive NK cell infusions further potentiates this antitumor effect. Clinical trials evaluating the antitumor activity of *ex vivo* expanded adoptively infused NK cells following bortezomib treatment are ongoing.

Methods to transfect chimeric antigen receptors (CARs) into NK cells have been optimized to induce tumor-specific NK cell killing in clinical applications. CARs specific for antigens expressed on tumors such as CD19 on B-cell malignancies, HER2/ErbB2 on breast carcinomas, and GD2 on neuroblastoma tumors when transduced into NK cells enhance tumor killing by autologous NK cells.[72,80] These findings, as well as studies showing the efficacy of T-cell based CAR therapy targeting CD19 in B-cell malignancies, suggest CAR-modified NK cells are worthy of exploration in the clinic (Chap. 26).

REFERENCES

1. Takasugi M, Mickey MR, Terasaki PI: Reactivity of lymphocytes from normal persons on cultured tumor cells. *Cancer Res* 33:2898–2902, 1973.
2. Trinchieri G: Biology of natural killer cells. *Adv Immunol* 47:187–376, 1989.
3. Spits H, Artis D, Colonna M, et al: Innate lymphoid cells—A proposal for uniform nomenclature. *Nat Rev Immunol* 13:145–149, 2013.
4. Tupin E, Kinjo Y, Kronenberg M: The unique role of natural killer T cells in the response to microorganisms. *Nat Rev Microbiol* 5:405–417, 2007.
5. Chowdhury D, Lieberman J: Death by a thousand cuts: Granzyme pathways of programmed cell death. *Annu Rev Immunol* 26:389–420, 2008.
6. Ortaldo JR, Winkler-Pickett R, Kopp W, et al: Relationship of large and small CD3– CD56+ lymphocytes mediating NK-associated activities. *J Leukoc Biol* 52:287–295, 1992.
7. Vosshenrich CA, Di Santo JP: Developmental programming of natural killer and innate lymphoid cells. *Curr Opin Immunol* 25:130–138, 2013.
8. Jamieson AM, Isnard P, Dorfman JR, et al: Turnover and proliferation of NK cells in steady state and lymphopenic conditions. *J Immunol* 172:864–870, 2004.
9. Sun JC, Beilke JN, Lanier LL: Adaptive immune features of natural killer cells. *Nature* 457:557–561, 2009.
10. Kennedy MK, Glaccum M, Brown SN, et al: Reversible defects in natural killer and memory CD8 T cell lineages in interleukin 15-deficient mice. *J Exp Med* 191:771–780, 2000.
11. Di Santo JP, Vosshenrich CA: Bone marrow versus thymic pathways of natural killer cell development. *Immunol Rev* 214:35–46, 2006.
12. Freud AG, Caligiuri MA: Human natural killer cell development. *Immunol Rev* 214:56–72, 2006.
13. Perussia B, Acuto O, Terhorst C, et al: Human natural killer cells analyzed by B73.1, a monoclonal antibody blocking Fc receptor functions. II. Studies of B73.1 antibody-antigen interaction on the lymphocyte membrane. *J Immunol* 130:2142–2148, 1983.
14. Caligiuri MA: Human natural killer cells. *Blood* 112:461–469, 2008.
15. Fehniger TA, Cooper MA, Nuovo GJ, et al: CD56bright natural killer cells are present in human lymph nodes and are activated by T cell-derived IL-2: A potential new link between adaptive and innate immunity. *Blood* 101:3052–3057, 2003.
16. Bouwens L, Wisse E: Pit cells in the liver. *Liver* 12:3–9, 1992.
17. Weissler JC, Nicod LP, Lipscomb MF, et al: Natural killer cell function in human lung is compartmentalized. *Am Rev Respir Dis* 135:941–949, 1987.
18. Biron CA, Nguyen KB, Pien GC, et al: Natural killer cells in antiviral defense: Function and regulation by innate cytokines. *Annu Rev Immunol* 17:189–220, 1999.
19. Kitaya K: Accumulation of uterine CD16(–) natural killer (NK) cells: Friends, foes, or Jekyll-and-Hyde relationship for the conceptus? *Immunol Invest* 37:467–481, 2008.
20. Vivier E, Raulet DH, Moretta A, et al: Innate or adaptive immunity? The example of natural killer cells. *Science* 331:44–49, 2011.
21. Raulet DH, Gasser S, Gowen BG, et al: Regulation of ligands for the NKG2D activating receptor. *Annu Rev Immunol* 31:413–441, 2013.
22. Champsaur M, Lanier LL: Effect of NKG2D ligand expression on host immune responses. *Immunol Rev* 235:267–285, 2010.
23. Karre K, Ljunggren HG, Piontek G, et al: Selective rejection of H-2-deficient lymphoma variants suggests alternative immune defence strategy. *Nature* 319:675–678, 1986.
24. Hansen TH, Bouvier M: MHC class I antigen presentation: Learning from viral evasion strategies. *Nat Rev Immunol* 9:503–513, 2009.
25. Garcia-Lora A, Algarra I, Garrido F: MHC class I antigens, immune surveillance, and tumor immune escape. *J Cell Physiol* 195:346–355, 2003.
26. Parham P, Moffett A: Variable NK cell receptors and their MHC class I ligands in immunity, reproduction and human evolution. *Nat Rev Immunol* 13:133–144, 2013. .
27. Braud VM, Allan DS, O'Callaghan CA, et al: HLA-E binds to natural killer cell receptors CD94/NKG2A, B and C. *Nature* 391:795–799, 1998.
28. Jonsson AH, Yokoyama WM: Natural killer cell tolerance licensing and other mechanisms. *Adv Immunol* 101:27–79, 2009.
29. Lanier LL, Corliss BC, Wu J, et al: Immunoreceptor DAP12 bearing a tyrosine-based activation motif is involved in activating NK cells. *Nature* 391:703–707, 1998.
30. Brown MG, Dokun AO, Heusel JW, et al: Vital involvement of a natural killer cell activation receptor in resistance to viral infection. *Science* 292:934–937, 2001.
31. Arase H, Mocarski ES, Campbell AE, et al: Direct recognition of cytomegalovirus by activating and inhibitory NK cell receptors. *Science* 296:1323–1326, 2002.
32. Trinchieri G, Santoli D: Anti-viral activity induced by culturing lymphocytes with tumor-derived or virus-transformed cells. Enhancement of human natural killer cell activity by interferon and antagonistic inhibition of susceptibility of target cells to lysis. *J Exp Med* 147:1314–1333, 1978.
33. Trinchieri G, Matsumoto-Kobayashi M, Clark SC, et al: Response of resting human peripheral blood natural killer cells to interleukin 2. *J Exp Med* 160:1147–1169, 1984.
34. Kobayashi M, Fitz L, Ryan M, et al: Identification and purification of Natural Killer cell stimulatory factor (NKSF), a cytokine with multiple biologic effects on human lymphocytes. *J Exp Med* 170:827–846, 1989.
35. London L, Perussia B, Trinchieri G: Induction of proliferation in vitro of resting human natural killer cells: IL 2 induces into cell cycle most peripheral blood NK cells, but only a minor subset of low density T cells. *J Immunol* 137:3845–3854, 1986.
36. Cuturi MC, Anegon I, Sherman F, et al: Production of hematopoietic colony-stimulating factors by human natural killer cells. *J Exp Med* 169:569–583, 1989.
37. Peritt D, Robertson S, Gri G, et al: Differentiation of human NK cells into NK1 and NK2 subsets. *J Immunol* 161:5821–5824, 1998.
38. Anegon I, Cuturi MC, Trinchieri G, et al: Interaction of Fc receptor (CD16) ligands induces transcription of interleukin 2 receptor (CD25) and lymphokine genes and expression of their products in human natural killer cells. *J Exp Med* 167:452–472, 1988.
39. Chan SH, Perussia B, Gupta JW, et al: Induction of interferon gamma production by natural killer cell stimulatory factor: Characterization of the responder cells and synergy with other inducers. *J Exp Med* 173:869–879, 1991.
40. Orange JS: Human natural killer cell deficiencies. *Curr Opin Allergy Clin Immunol* 6:399–409, 2006.
41. Santoli D, Trinchieri G, Koprowski H: Cell-mediated cytotoxicity in humans against virus-infected target cells. II. Interferon induction and activation of natural killer cells. *J Immunol* 121:532–538, 1978.
42. Bandyopadhyay S, Perussia B, Trinchieri G, et al: Requirement for HLA-DR positive accessory cells in natural killing of cytomegalovirus-infected fibroblasts. *J Exp Med* 164:180–195, 1986.
43. Bukowski JF, Woda BA, Habu S, et al: Natural killer cell depletion enhances virus synthesis and virus-induced hepatitis in vivo. *J Immunol* 131:1531–1538, 1983.
44. Waggoner SN, Cornberg M, Selin LK, et al: Natural killer cells act as rheostats modulating antiviral T cells. *Nature* 481:394–398, 2011.
45. O'Leary JG, Goodarzi M, Drayton DL, von Andrian UH: T cell- and B cell-independent adaptive immunity mediated by natural killer cells. *Nat Immunol* 7:507–516, 2006.
46. Paust S, Gill HS, Wang BZ, et al: Critical role for the chemokine receptor CXCR6 in NK cell-mediated antigen-specific memory of haptens and viruses. *Nat Immunol* 11:1127–1135, 2010.
47. Bancroft GJ, Schreiber RD, Bosma GC, et al: A T-cell-independent mechanism of macrophage activation by interferon-gamma. *J Immunol* 139:1104–1107, 1987.

48. Gazzinelli RT, Hieny S, Wynn TA, et al: Interleukin 12 is required for the T-lymphocyte-independent induction of interferon gamma by an intracellular parasite and induces resistance in T-cell-deficient hosts [see comments]. *Proc Natl Acad Sci U S A* 90:6115–6119, 1993.

49. Mond JJ, Brunswick M: A role for IFN-gamma and NK cells in immune response to T cell-regulated antigens types 1 and 2. *Immunol Rev* 99:105–118, 1987.

50. Yuan D, Wilder J, Dang T, et al: Activation of B lymphocytes by NK cells. *Int Immunol* 4:1373–1380, 1992.

51. Goldszmid RS, Bafica A, Jankovic D, et al: TAP-1 indirectly regulates CD4+ T cell priming in Toxoplasma gondii infection by controlling NK cell IFN-gamma production. *J Exp Med* 204:2591–2602, 2007.

52. Scharton TM, Scott P: Natural killer cells are a source of interferon gamma that drives differentiation of CD4+ T cell subsets and induces early resistance to Leishmania major of mice. *J Exp Med* 178:567–577, 1993.

53. Trinchieri G: Interleukin-12 and the regulation of innate resistance and adaptive immunity. *Nat Rev Immunol* 3:133–146, 2003.

54. Goldszmid Romina S, Caspar P, Rivollier A, et al: NK cell-derived interferon-γ orchestrates cellular dynamics and the differentiation of monocytes into dendritic cells at the site of infection. *Immunity* 36:1047–1059, 2012.

55. Gerosa F, Gobbi A, Zorzi P, et al: The reciprocal interaction of NK cells with plasmacytoid or myeloid dendritic cells profoundly affects innate resistance functions. *J Immunol* 174:727–734, 2005.

56. Moretta A: Natural killer cells and dendritic cells: Rendezvous in abused tissues. *Nat Rev Immunol* 2:957–964, 2002.

57. Trinchieri G: Natural killer cells in hematopoiesis, in *The Natural Immune System: Natural Killer Cells* edited by Lewis CE and James O'D. IRL Press at Oxford University Press, Oxford, New York, pp 41–65. 1992.

58. Murphy WJ, Keller JR, Harrison CL, et al: Interleukin-2-activated natural killer cells can support hematopoiesis in vitro and promote marrow engraftment *in vivo. Blood* 80:670–677, 1992.

59. Cudkowicz G, Hochman PS: Do natural killer cells engage in regulated reaction against self to ensure homeostasis? *Immunol Rev* 44:13–41, 1979.

60. Randrup-Thomsen A, Pisa P, Bro-Jorgensen K, et al: Mechanisms of lymphocytic choriomeningitis virus-induced hemopoietic dysfunction. *J Virol* 59:428–433, 1986.

61. Velardi A: Natural killer cell alloreactivity 10 years later. *Curr Opin Hematol* 19:421–426, 2012.

62. Velardi A, Ruggeri L, Alessandro, et al: NK cells: A lesson from mismatched hematopoietic transplantation. *Trends Immunol* 23:438–444, 2002.

63. Vesely MD, Kershaw MH, Schreiber RD, et al: Natural innate and adaptive immunity to cancer. *Annu Rev Immunol* 29:235–271, 2011.

64. Jost S, Altfeld M: Control of human viral infections by natural killer cells. *Annu Rev Immunol* 31:163–194, 2013.

65. Haliotis T, Roder J, Klein M, et al: Chediak-Higashi gene in humans. I. Impairment of natural-killer function. *J Exp Med* 151:1039–1048, 1980.

66. Kanavaros P, Lescs MC, Briere J, et al: Nasal T-cell lymphoma: A clinicopathologic entity associated with peculiar phenotype and with Epstein-Barr virus. *Blood* 81:2688–2695, 1993.

67. Liang X, Graham DK: Natural killer cell neoplasms. *Cancer* 112:1425–1436, 2008.

68. Reynolds CW, Foon KA: Tgamma-lymphoproliferative disorders in man and experimental animals: A review of the clinical, cellular and functional characteristics. *Blood* 64:1146–1158, 1984.

69. Bachanova V, Cooley S, Defor TE, et al: Clearance of acute myeloid leukemia by haploidentical natural killer cells is improved using IL-2 diphtheria toxin fusion protein. *Blood* 123:3855–3863, 2014.

70. Korde N, Carlsten M, Lee MJ, et al: A phase II trial of pan-KIR2D blockade with IPH2101 in smoldering multiple myeloma. *Haematologica* 99:e81–e83, 2014.

71. Furutani E, Smith A, Uchida N, et al: SiRNA inactivation of the inhibitory receptor NKG2A augments the anti-tumor effects of adoptively transferred NK cells in tumor-bearing hosts. *ASH Annu Meet Abstr* 1015, 2010.

72. Childs RW, Berg M: Bringing natural killer cells to the clinic: *Ex vivo* manipulation. *Hematology Am Soc Hematol Educ Program* 2013:234–246, 2013.

73. Berg M, Lundqvist A, McCoy P Jr, et al: Clinical-grade *ex vivo*-expanded human natural killer cells up-regulate activating receptors and death receptor ligands and have enhanced cytolytic activity against tumor cells. *Cytotherapy* 11:341–355, 2009.

74. Zhu D, Corral LG, Fleming YW, et al: Immunomodulatory drugs Revlimid (R) (lenalidomide) and CC-4047 induce apoptosis of both hematological and solid tumor cells through NK cell activation. *Cancer Immunol Immunother* 57:1849–1859, 2008.

75. Benson DM Jr, Bakan CE, Mishra A, et al: The PD-1/PD-L1 axis modulates the natural killer cell versus multiple myeloma effect: A therapeutic target for CT-011, a novel monoclonal anti-PD-1 antibody. *Blood* 116:2286–2294, 2010.

76. Somanchi SS, Somanchi A, Cooper LJ, et al: Engineering lymph node homing of ex vivo-expanded human natural killer cells via trogocytosis of the chemokine receptor CCR7. *Blood* 119:5164–5172, 2012.

77. Sackstein R: The lymphocyte homing receptors: Gatekeepers of the multistep paradigm. *Curr Opin Hematol* 12:444–450, 2005.

78. Srivastava S, Lundqvist A, Childs RW: Natural killer cell immunotherapy for cancer: A new hope. *Cytotherapy* 10:775–783, 2008.

79. Lundqvist A, Yokoyama H, Smith A, et al: Bortezomib treatment and regulatory T-cell depletion enhance the antitumor effects of adoptively infused NK cells. *Blood* 113:6120–6127, 2009.

80. Boissel L, Betancur M, Lu W, et al: Comparison of mRNA and lentiviral based transfection of natural killer cells with chimeric antigen receptors recognizing lymphoid antigens. *Leuk Lymphoma* 53:958–965, 2012.

CHAPTER 78
CLASSIFICATION AND CLINICAL MANIFESTATIONS OF LYMPHOCYTE AND PLASMA CELL DISORDERS

Yvonne A. Efebera and Michael A. Caligiuri*

SUMMARY

This chapter outlines the major categories of lymphocyte and plasma cell disorders. The disorders are classified into three main groups. The first is composed of diseases caused by defects intrinsic to lymphoid cells. The second is caused by disorders that result from factors extrinsic to lymphoid cells. The third is composed of disorders caused by neoplastic or preneoplastic lymphoid cells and are outlined in Chap. 90 using the World Health Organization classification of tumors of lymphoid tissues. The clinical manifestations of diseases in any one of the three groups may be difficult to distinguish, but this grouping can provide a framework with which to proceed in evaluating patients with known or suspected lymphocyte and plasma cell disorders. This chapter introduces the framework and presents a roadmap to other chapters in this book that discuss each of the disorders in greater detail.

CLASSIFICATION

Lymphocyte and plasma cell disorders can be classified into three major groups (Table 78–1). The first group, listed under "primary disorders," is composed of lymphocyte disorders caused by intrinsic defects in lymphoid cells that result in functional abnormalities of marrow-derived (B) lymphocytes, thymic-derived (T) lymphocytes, combined T and B (impaired humoral and cellular immunity), or natural killer (NK) cells. These disorders primarily result from inborn errors in lymphocyte metabolism (Chaps. 73 to 77 and 80) and/or receptor–ligand expression (Chaps. 17 and 80). The second group, listed under "acquired disorders," consists of disorders caused by factors extrinsic to lymphocytes resulting in immune dysfunction. These conditions most commonly result from infection with viruses, or other cellular pathogens (Chaps. 79, 81, and 82), but they also may be caused by bacteria, drugs or systemic disease of nonlymphoid cells. The third group of diseases is composed of preneoplastic and neoplastic lymphocyte disorders and is discussed in detail in Chap. 90.

Acronyms and Abbreviations: GVHD, graft-versus-host disease; Ig, immunoglobulin; NK, natural killer; SCID, severe combined immune deficiency; Th, T helper; T_{REG}, CD4+ regulatory T cell.

---

*This chapter was prepared by Thomas J. Kipps in the 8th edition and much of the text has been retained.

Some categories of lymphocyte and plasma cell disorders may be difficult to distinguish clinically because lymphocyte disorders can have many clinical manifestations that are not restricted to cells of the immune system and disparate disorders can have similar clinical manifestations, with any one disorder associated with a diverse array of clinical pathologies.

In some cases, the classification of lymphocyte disorders is influenced by the manifestations of the disease. For example, autoimmune hemolytic disease (Chap. 54) and autoimmune thrombocytopenia (Chap. 117) are caused by inappropriate secretion of autoantibodies by B lymphocytes. The blood cell that is coated with autoantibody presumably is normal, yet we classify the disease that can result from hemolytic autoantibodies as an acquired hemolytic anemia because that aspect of the disease is more visible and better understood than is the inappropriate synthesis of antierythrocyte antibody by the disturbed lymphocyte population(s). These disorders are not considered here.

Many diseases, especially infection (e.g., tuberculous adenitis), inflammatory states (e.g., rheumatoid arthritis), autoimmune disease (e.g., systemic lupus erythematosus), and metastatic carcinoma can involve lymph nodes or the spleen as a secondary alteration. These disorders also may be associated with abnormal production of antibodies, such as those resulting in the lupus anticoagulant (Chap. 131). These disorders also are not considered here because the primary disease is not generally considered a lymphocyte disorder.

CLINICAL MANIFESTATIONS

B LYMPHOCYTE DISORDERS

Immunoglobulin Deficiency

The clinical manifestations of B-lymphocyte disorders include the consequences of B-lymphocyte deficiency, dysfunction, or malignant transformation. The manifestations may consist of a specific deficiency of one of the immunoglobulin (Ig) isotypes or of several or all Ig molecules (panhypogammaglobulinemia; see Chap. 75). Inability to synthesize or secrete antibodies impairs the clearance of pathogens because of the inability to opsonize microorganisms for phagocytosis, resulting in immune dysregulation and dysfunction (Chap. 80).

Abnormal Immunoglobulin Production

Primary defect in the B-cell clone or expansion of a clone in response to chronic antigen stimulation can result in excess production of Ig that in turn produces a monoclonal gammopathy (Chap. 106). Monoclonal gammopathy can result in B-cell neoplastic disease, such as plasma cell myeloma (Chap. 107), Waldenström macroglobulinemia (Chap. 109) or chronic lymphocytic leukemia (Chap. 92). Production of abnormal Ig molecules or Ig fragments can also be seen in association with chronic infection, leading to development of Ig heavy-chain disease (Chap. 110). Deposition of Ig or Ig fragments can contribute to primary amyloid formation (Chap. 108). Reactivity of the Ig with self-antigen(s), such as those found on the red cell membrane (Chap. 54), can result in systemic autoimmune disease.

T LYMPHOCYTE DISORDERS

Impaired Immunoregulation

The clinical manifestations of deficiencies or excesses of T-lymphocytes depend on the subset of T-lymphocytes involved. Delayed hypersensitivity normally is mediated by CD4+ helper T cells (Th cells) and, more specifically, Th1-type cells (Chap. 76). A deficit or functional disturbance in these T-cells can impair the cellular immune response to mycobacteria, *Listeria*, *Brucella*, fungi, or other intracellular

TABLE 78–1. Classification of Disorders of Lymphocytes and Plasma Cells

I. Primary disorders

A. B-lymphocyte deficiency or dysfunction (Chap. 80)[1,2]

1. Agammaglobulinemia

a. Acquired agammaglobulinemia[3]

b. Associated with plasma cell myeloma, heavy chain disease, light chain amyloid, Waldenström macroglobulinemia, or chronic lymphocytic leukemia (Chaps. 92 and 107–110)[4,5]

c. Associated with celiac disease[6]

d. X-linked agammaglobulinemia[7,8]

e. Autosomal recessive agammaglobilinemia[9]

f. Common variable immunodeficiency[10]

g. Transient hypogammaglobulinemia of infancy[11]

h. Bloom syndrome[12]

i. Comel-Netherton syndrome[13]

2. Selective agammaglobulinemia (Chap. 80)

a. Immunoglobulin (Ig) M deficiency

1. Selective IgM deficiency[14]

2. Wiskott-Aldrich syndrome[15]

b. Selective IgG deficiency (Chap. 80)

c. Selective IgA deficiency[16,17]

d. IgA and IgM deficiency[18]

e. IgA and IgG deficiency[19,20]

1. CD40/CD40L deficiency

2. Activation-induced cytidine deaminase (AID) (uracil-DNA glycosylate [UNG], hyper-IgM$_4$) deficiency

3. *PMS2* deficiency

3. Hyper-IgA[21,22]

4. Hyper-IgD[23–26]

5. Hyper-IgE syndrome (HIES; Chap. 80)[27]

6. Hyper-IgE associated with HIV infection[28]

7. Hyper-IgM immunodeficiency (Chap. 80)[19,20,29]

8. X-linked lymphoproliferative disease[30–32]

B. T-lymphocyte deficiency or dysfunction (Chap. 80)[33,34]

1. Cartilage-hair hypoplasia (Chap. 80)[35,36]

2. Lymphocyte function antigen-1 deficiency[37]

3. Thymic aplasia (DiGeorge syndrome)[38,39]

4. Thymic dysplasia (Nezelof syndrome)[40]

5. Thymic hypoplasia[41,42]

6. CD8 deficiency[43]

7. CD3γ deficiency[44]

8. Winged helix deficiency (Nude)[45]

9. Interleukin-2 receptor α chain (CD25) deficiency[46]

10. Signal transducer and activator of transcription 5b (STAT 5b) deficiency[47]

11. Schimke syndrome[48]

12. Janus kinase 3(JAK3) deficiency[49]

13. γc Deficiency

14. Wiskott-Aldrich syndrome (Chaps. 80 and 120)[15,50]

15. Zeta-associated protein of 70 kDa (ZAP-70) deficiency (Chap. 80)[51,52]

16. Purine nucleoside phosphorylase deficiency (Chap. 80)

17. Interleukin-7 receptor deficiency (Chap. 80)

18. Major histocompatibility complex class I or II deficiency (Chap. 80)

19. Coronin-1A deficiency (Chap. 80)

20. IPEX (immune dysregulation, polyendocrinopathy, enteropathy, X-linked) syndrome caused by mutations in FoxP3 that cause a deficiency of CD4+ regulatory T cells (T$_{REGs}$) (Chaps. 76 and 80)

21. APECED (autoimmune polyglandular, candidiasis, and ectodermal dystrophy) syndrome caused by mutations in the autoimmune regulator gene (AIRE) gene (Chaps. 6, 76, and 80)

22. Autoimmune lymphoproliferative syndrome (Chap. 80)

C. Combined T- and B-cell deficiency or dysfunction (Chap. 80)

1. Ataxia-telangiectasia[53]

2. Combined immunodeficiency syndrome (Chap. 80)[54]

a. Adenosine deaminase deficiency[55,56]

b. Thymic alymphoplasia[57]

c. CD45 deficiency[58]

d. X-linked severe combined immunodeficiency syndrome[59]

3. Major histocompatibility complex class II deficiency— bare lymphocyte syndrome (Chap. 80)[60]

4. IgG and IgA deficiencies and impaired cellular immunity (type I dysgammaglobulinemia)[61]

5. Thymoma-associated immunodeficiency[62]

6. Pyridoxine deficiency[63]

7. Reticular agenesis (congenital aleukocytosis)[64]

8. Omenn syndrome (Chap. 80)[65]

9. Warts, hypogammaglobulinemia, infections, myelokathexis (WHIM) syndrome resulting from mutation in the *CXCR4* gene (Chap. 80)

D. Natural killer cells (Chaps. 77 and 94)

1. Chronic natural killer cell lymphocytosis[72–74]

II. Acquired disorders

A. AIDS (Chap. 81)

B. Reactive lymphocytosis or plasmacytosis (Chap. 79)

1. *Bordetella pertussis* lymphocytosis (Chap. 79)

2. Cytomegalovirus mononucleosis (Chap. 82)

3. Drug-induced lymphocytosis[75]

4. Stress-induced lymphocytosis[76]

5. Persistent polyclonal B-cell lymphocytosis[77]

6. Postsplenectomy lymphocytosis[78]

7. Epstein-Barr virus mononucleosis (Chap. 82)

8. Inflammatory (secondary) plasmacytosis of marrow

9. Large granular lymphocytosis (Chap. 94)

10. Other viral mononucleosis (Chap. 82)

11. Polyclonal lymphocytosis (Chap. 79)

(Continued)

TABLE 78–1. Classification of Disorders of Lymphocytes and Plasma Cells (*Continued*)

12. Serum sickness[79]	C. T-lymphocyte dysfunction or depletion associated with systemic disease
13. T-cell lymphocytosis associated with thymoma (Chap. 79)	1. B-cell chronic lymphocytic leukemia (Chap. 92)
14. *Toxoplasma gondii* mononucleosis (Chap. 82)	2. Hodgkin lymphoma (Chap. 97)
15. Trypanosoma cruzi[80]	3. Leprosy[82]
16. Viral infectious lymphocytosis (Chap. 79)	4. Lupus erythematosus[83]
17. Cat-scratch and other chronic bacterial infection[81]	5. Sjögren syndrome[84]
	6. Sarcoidosis[85]

organisms associated with formation of immune granulomas. Th2-type CD4+ Th cells, on the other hand, appear better suited to induce B-cell responses to antigen and direct the immune response against parasitic infestations (Chap. 76). Deficiency or defects in CD4+ regulator T cells (T_{REGs}) can result in autoimmune disease, whereas depletion or deficiency of Th17 cells can result in impaired resistance to opportunistic infection (Chap. 76). Depletion of CD4+ T cells in patients infected with human immunodeficiency virus accounts in large part for the acquired immune deficiency that develops in patients infected with the virus (Chap. 81).

T lymphocytes within a marrow allograft are responsible for initiation of the graft-versus-host disease (GVHD) (Chap. 23). Acute GVHD can lead to severe dermatitis, gastroenteritis, and hepatitis. Chronic GVHD can encompass a collage of connective tissue diseases, such as scleroderma, xerophthalmia, xerostomia, and pulmonary insufficiency, specifically bronchiolitis obliterans. Eosinophilia, hypergammaglobulinemia, development of autoantibodies, and plasmacytosis can occur. Infection with classic or opportunistic pathogens is a common complication of both acute and chronic GVHD. A similar qualitative reaction, albeit more limited, is seen in mononucleosis resulting from Epstein-Barr virus infection (Chap. 82).

COMBINED T- AND B-CELL DISORDERS

Combined T- and B-cell deficiency and dysfunction can result in heterogeneous group of disorders that affect both cellular and humoral immunity. The disorder can be severe (severe combined immune deficiency [SCID]) or mild depending on whether the defect is partial (hypomorphic defects) or complete (null or amorphic defects). Complete defects can result in early death, typically during the first year of life, from uncontrolled infection. An extreme form of SCID is the T-cell–negative, B-cell–negative, NK-cell–positive phenotype with children presenting early in life with severe infections, failure to thrive, and low-to-absent T-and B-cell numbers and function. Advances in gene therapy and allogeneic stem cell transplantation offer hope in some cases (Chap. 80).

NATURAL KILLER CELL DISORDERS

Chronic NK cell lymphocytosis is a rare proliferative disorder that can be distinguished from NK cell leukemia and lymphoma by its indolent nature (Chap. 77). Patients typically have neutropenia, anemia, vasculitic syndromes, fever of unknown origin, constitutional symptoms, cutaneous lesions and autoimmune disorders, including rheumatoid arthritis, Sjögren syndrome, and/or polymyalgia rheumatica. Studies seeking to define this condition as a clonal disorder using X-linked gene analysis have not yielded consistent findings (Chap. 77).

REFERENCES

1. International Union of Immunological Societies Expert Committee on Primary I; Notarangelo LD, Fischer A, et al: Primary immunodeficiencies: 2009 update. *J Allergy Clin Immunol* 124:1161–1178, 2009.
2. Conley ME, Dobbs AK, Farmer DM, et al: Primary B cell immunodeficiencies: Comparisons and contrasts. *Annu Rev Immunol* 27:199–227, 2009.
3. Ballow M: Primary immunodeficiency disorders: Antibody deficiency. *J Allergy Clin Immunol* 109:581–591, 2002.
4. Kyrtsonis MC, Mouzaki A, Maniatis A: Mechanisms of polyclonal hypogammaglobulinaemia in multiple myeloma (MM). *Med Oncol* 16:73–77, 1999.
5. Pritsch O, Maloum K, Dighiero G: Basic biology of autoimmune phenomena in chronic lymphocytic leukemia. *Semin Oncol* 25:34–41, 1998.
6. Halfdanarson TR, Litzow MR, Murray JA: Hematologic manifestations of celiac disease. *Blood* 109:412–421, 2007.
7. Conley ME, Rohrer J, Minegishi Y: X-linked agammaglobulinemia. *Clin Rev Allergy Immunol* 19:183–204, 2000.
8. Schiff C, Lemmers B, Deville A, et al: Autosomal primary immunodeficiencies affecting human bone marrow B-cell differentiation. *Immunol Rev* 178:91–98, 2000.
9. Conley ME, Dobbs AK, Quintana AM, et al: Agammaglobulinemia and absent B lineage cells in a patient lacking the p85alpha subunit of PI3K. *J Exp Med* 209:463–470, 2012.
10. Sneller MC, Strober W, Eisenstein E, et al: NIH conference. New insights into common variable immunodeficiency. *Ann Intern Med* 118:720–730, 1993.
11. Dalal I, Reid B, Nisbet-Brown E, Roifman CM: The outcome of patients with hypogammaglobulinemia in infancy and early childhood. *J Pediatr* 133:144–146, 1998.
12. Payne M, Hickson ID: Genomic instability and cancer: Lessons from analysis of Bloom's syndrome. *Biochem Soc Trans* 37:553–559, 2009.
13. Di WL, Mellerio JE, Bernadis C, et al: Phase I study protocol for *ex vivo* lentiviral gene therapy for the inherited skin disease, Netherton syndrome. *Hum Gene Ther Clin Dev* 24:182–190, 2013.
14. Louis AG, Gupta S: Primary selective IgM deficiency: An ignored immunodeficiency. *Clin Rev Allergy Immunol* 46:104–111, 2014.
15. Buchbinder D, Nugent DJ, Fillipovich AH: Wiskott-Aldrich syndrome: Diagnosis, current management, and emerging treatments. *Appl Clin Genet* 7:55–66, 2014.
16. Yel L: Selective IgA deficiency. *J Clin Immunol* 30:10–16, 2010.
17. Latiff AH, Kerr MA: The clinical significance of immunoglobulin A deficiency. *Ann Clin Biochem* 44:131–139, 2007.
18. Schroeder HW Jr, Schroeder HW 3rd, Sheikh SM: The complex genetics of common variable immunodeficiency. *J Investig Med* 52:90–103, 2004.
19. Davies EG, Thrasher AJ: Update on the hyper immunoglobulin M syndromes. *Br J Haematol* 149:167–180, 2010.
20. Lanzi G, Ferrari S, Vihinen M, et al: Different molecular behavior of CD40 mutants causing hyper-IgM syndrome. *Blood* 116:5867–5874, 2010.
21. Klasen IS, Goertz JH, van de Wiel GA, et al: Hyper-immunoglobulin A in the hyperimmunoglobulinemia D syndrome. *Clin Diagn Lab Immunol* 8:58–61, 2001.
22. Bermejo JF, Carbone J, Rodriguez JJ, et al: Macroamylasaemia, IgA hypergammaglobulinaemia and autoimmunity in a patient with Down syndrome and coeliac disease. *Scand J Gastroenterol* 38:445–447, 2003.
23. Drenth JP, Haagsma CJ, van der Meer JW: Hyperimmunoglobulinemia D and periodic fever syndrome. The clinical spectrum in a series of 50 patients. International Hyper-IgD Study Group. *Medicine (Baltimore)* 73:133–144, 1994.
24. Stoffels M, Simon A: Hyper-IgD syndrome or mevalonate kinase deficiency. *Curr Opin Rheumatol* 23:419–423, 2011.
25. Korppi M, Van Gijn ME, Antila K: Hyperimmunoglobulinemia D and periodic fever syndrome in children. Review on therapy with biological drugs and case report. *Acta Paediatr* 100:21–25, 2011.
26. Yoshimura K, Wakiguchi H: Hyperimmunoglobulinemia D syndrome successfully treated with a corticosteroid. *Pediatr Int* 44:326–327, 2002.
27. Yong PF, Freeman AF, Engelhardt KR, et al: An update on the hyper-IgE syndromes. *Arthritis Res Ther* 14:228, 2012.
28. Burastero SE, Paolucci C, Breda D, et al: Immunological basis for IgE hyper-production in enfuvirtide-treated HIV-positive patients. *J Clin Immunol* 26:168–176, 2006.

29. Cabral-Marques O, Klaver S, Schimke LF, et al: First report of the Hyper-IgM syndrome Registry of the Latin American Society for Immunodeficiencies: Novel mutations, unique infections, and outcomes. *J Clin Immunol* 34:146–156, 2014.

30. Engel P, Eck MJ, Terhorst C: The SAP and SLAM families in immune responses and X-linked lymphoproliferative disease. *Nat Rev Immunol* 3:813–821, 2003.

31. Gilmour KC, Gaspar HB: Pathogenesis and diagnosis of X-linked lymphoproliferative disease. *Expert Rev Mol Diagn* 3:549–561, 2003.

32. Marsh RA, Bleesing JJ, Chandrakasan S, et al: Reduced-intensity conditioning hematopoietic cell transplantation is an effective treatment for patients with SLAM-associated protein deficiency/X-linked lymphoproliferative disease type 1. *Biol Blood Marrow Transplant* 20:1641–1645, 2014.

33. Elder ME: T-cell immunodeficiencies. *Pediatr Clin North Am* 47:1253–1274, 2000.

34. Edgar JD: T cell immunodeficiency. *J Clin Pathol* 61:988–993, 2008.

35. Notarangelo LD, Roifman CM, Giliani S: Cartilage-hair hypoplasia: Molecular basis and heterogeneity of the immunological phenotype. *Curr Opin Allergy Clin Immunol* 8:534–539, 2008.

36. Maida Y, Yasukawa M, Furuuchi M, et al: An RNA-dependent RNA polymerase formed by TERT and the RMRP RNA. *Nature* 461:230–235, 2009.

37. Smith A, Stanley P, Jones K, et al: The role of the integrin LFA-1 in T-lymphocyte migration. *Immunol Rev* 218:135–146, 2007.

38. Saitta SC, Harris SE, Gaeth AP, et al: Aberrant interchromosomal exchanges are the predominant cause of the 22q11.2 deletion. *Hum Mol Genet* 13:417–428, 2004.

39. McLean-Tooke A, Spickett GP, Gennery AR: Immunodeficiency and autoimmunity in 22q11.2 deletion syndrome. *Scand J Immunol* 66:1–7, 2007.

40. Nezelof C: Thymic pathology in primary and secondary immunodeficiencies. *Histopathology* 21:499–511, 1992.

41. Lima K, Abrahamsen TG, Foelling I, et al: Low thymic output in the 22q11.2 deletion syndrome measured by CCR9+CD45RA+ T cell counts and T cell receptor rearrangement excision circles. *Clin Exp Immunol* 161:98–107, 2010.

42. Sullivan KE, McDonald-McGinn D, Zackai EH: CD4(+) CD25(+) T-cell production in healthy humans and in patients with thymic hypoplasia. *Clin Diagn Lab Immunol* 9:1129–1131, 2002.

43. de la Calle-Martin O, Hernandez M, Ordi J, et al: Familial CD8 deficiency due to a mutation in the CD8 alpha gene. *J Clin Invest* 108:117–123, 2001.

44. Recio MJ, Moreno-Pelayo MA, Kilic SS, et al: Differential biological role of CD3 chains revealed by human immunodeficiencies. *J Immunol* 178:2556–2564, 2007.

45. Frank J, Pignata C, Panteleyev AA, et al: Exposing the human nude phenotype. *Nature* 398:473–474, 1999.

46. Roifman CM: Human IL-2 receptor alpha chain deficiency. *Pediatr Res* 48:6–11, 2000.

47. Kofoed EM, Hwa V, Little B, et al: Growth hormone insensitivity associated with a STAT5b mutation. *N Engl J Med* 349:1139–1147, 2003.

48. Hunter KB, Lucke T, Spranger J, et al: Schimke immunoosseous dysplasia: Defining skeletal features. *Eur J Pediatr* 169:801–811, 2010.

49. Roberts JL, Lengi A, Brown SM, et al: Janus kinase 3 (JAK3) deficiency: Clinical, immunologic, and molecular analyses of 10 patients and outcomes of stem cell transplantation. *Blood* 103:2009–2018, 2004.

50. Bosticardo M, Marangoni F, Aiuti A, et al: Recent advances in understanding the pathophysiology of Wiskott-Aldrich syndrome. *Blood* 113:6288–6295, 2009.

51. Kim VH, Murguia L, Schechter T, et al: Emergency treatment for zeta chain-associated protein of 70 kDa (ZAP70) deficiency. *J Allergy Clin Immunol* 131:1233–1235, 2013.

52. Picard C, Dogniaux S, Chemin K, et al: Hypomorphic mutation of ZAP70 in human results in a late onset immunodeficiency and no autoimmunity. *Eur J Immunol* 39:1966–1976, 2009.

53. Jayadev S, Bird TD: Hereditary ataxias: Overview. *Genet Med* 15:673–683, 2013.

54. Pai SY, Logan BR, Griffith LM, et al: Transplantation outcomes for severe combined immunodeficiency, 2000–2009. *N Engl J Med* 371:434–446, 2014.

55. Cassani B, Mirolo M, Cattaneo F, et al: Altered intracellular and extracellular signaling leads to impaired T cell functions in ADA SCID patients. *Blood* 111:4209–4219, 2008.

56. Candotti F: Gene transfer into hematopoietic stem cells as treatment for primary immunodeficiency diseases. *Int J Hematol* 99:383–392, 2014.

57. Buckley RH: Immunodeficiency diseases. *JAMA* 268:2797–2806, 1992.

58. Tchilian EZ, Wallace DL, Wells RS, et al: A deletion in the gene encoding the CD45 antigen in a patient with SCID. *J Immunol* 166:1308–1313, 2001.

59. Buckley RH: Molecular defects in human severe combined immunodeficiency and approaches to immune reconstitution. *Annu Rev Immunol* 22:625–655, 2004.

60. Reith W, Mach B: The bare lymphocyte syndrome and the regulation of MHC expression. *Annu Rev Immunol* 19:331–373, 2001.

61. Sutor G, Fabel H: Sarcoidosis and common variable immunodeficiency. A case of a malignant course of sarcoidosis in conjunction with severe impairment of the cellular and humoral immune system. *Respiration* 67:204–208, 2000.

62. Vitiello L, Masci AM, Montella L, et al: Thymoma-associated immunodeficiency: A syndrome characterized by severe alterations in NK, T and B-cells and progressive increase in naive CD8+ T Cells. *Int J Immunopathol Pharmacol* 23:307–316, 2010.

63. Trakatellis A, Dimitriadou A, Trakatelli M: Pyridoxine deficiency: New approaches in immunosuppression and chemotherapy. *Postgrad Med J* 73:617–622, 1997.

64. Small TN, Wall DA, Kurtzberg J, et al: Association of reticular dysgenesis (thymic alymphoplasia and congenital aleukocytosis) with bilateral sensorineural deafness. *J Pediatr* 135:387–389, 1999.

65. Poliani PL, Facchetti F, Ravanini M, et al: Early defects in human T-cell development severely affect distribution and maturation of thymic stromal cells: Possible implications for the pathophysiology of Omenn syndrome. *Blood* 114:105–108, 2009.

66. Zhang Q, Davis JC, Lamborn IT, et al: Combined immunodeficiency associated with DOCK8 mutations. *N Engl J Med* 361:2046–2055, 2009.

67. Moshous D, Callebaut I, de Chasseval R, et al: Artemis, a novel DNA double-strand break repair/V(D)J recombination protein, is mutated in human severe combined immune deficiency. *Cell* 105:177–186, 2001.

68. Enders A, Fisch P, Schwarz K, et al: A severe form of human combined immunodeficiency due to mutations in DNA ligase IV. *J Immunol* 176:5060–5068, 2006.

69. Villa A, Sobacchi C, Notarangelo LD, et al: V(D)J recombination defects in lymphocytes due to RAG mutations: Severe immunodeficiency with a spectrum of clinical presentations. *Blood* 97:81–88, 2001.

70. Noordzij JG, Verkaik NS, van der Burg M, et al: Radiosensitive SCID patients with Artemis gene mutations show a complete B-cell differentiation arrest at the pre–B-cell receptor checkpoint in bone marrow. *Blood* 101:1446–1452, 2003.

71. Buck D, Malivert L, de Chasseval R, et al: Cernunnos, a novel nonhomologous end-joining factor, is mutated in human immunodeficiency with microcephaly. *Cell* 124:287–299, 2006.

72. Morice WG, Leibson PJ, Tefferi A: Natural killer cells and the syndrome of chronic natural killer cell lymphocytosis. *Leuk Lymphoma* 41:277–284, 2001.

73. Chee CE, Warrington KJ, Tefferi A: Chronic natural killer-cell lymphocytosis successfully treated with alemtuzumab. *Blood* 114:3500–3502, 2009.

74. Rabbani GR, Phyliky RL, Tefferi A: A long-term study of patients with chronic natural killer cell lymphocytosis. *Br J Haematol* 106:960–966, 1999.

75. Kano Y, Shiohara T: The variable clinical picture of drug-induced hypersensitivity syndrome/drug rash with eosinophilia and systemic symptoms in relation to the eliciting drug. *Immunol Allergy Clin North Am* 29:481–501, 2009.

76. Teggatz JR, Parkin J, Peterson L: Transient atypical lymphocytosis in patients with emergency medical conditions. *Arch Pathol Lab Med* 111:712–714, 1987.

77. Troussard X, Mossafa H, Valensi F, et al: [Polyclonal lymphocytosis with binucleated lymphocytes. Morphological, immunological, cytogenetic and molecular analysis in 15 cases] [in French]. *Presse Med* 26:895–899, 1997.

78. Juneja S, Januszewicz E, Wolf M, Cooper I: Post-splenectomy lymphocytosis. *Clin Lab Haematol* 17:335–337, 1995.

79. Virella G: Immune complex diseases. *Immunol Ser* 50:395–414, 1990.

80. Gao W, Pereira MA: Trypanosoma cruzi trans-sialidase potentiates T cell activation through antigen-presenting cells: Role of IL-6 and Bruton's tyrosine kinase. *Eur J Immunol* 31:1503–1512, 2001.

81. Spach DH, Koehler JE: Bartonella-associated infections. *Infect Dis Clin North Am* 12:137–155, 1998.

82. Im JS, Kang TJ, Lee SB, et al: Alteration of the relative levels of iNKT cell subsets is associated with chronic mycobacterial infections. *Clin Immunol* 127:214–224, 2008.

83. Wenzel J, Gerdsen R, Uerlich M, et al: Lymphocytopenia in lupus erythematosus: Close in vivo association to autoantibodies targeting nuclear antigens. *Br J Dermatol* 150:994–998, 2004.

84. Mandl T, Bredberg A, Jacobsson LT, et al: CD4+ T-lymphocytopenia—A frequent finding in anti-SSA antibody seropositive patients with primary Sjögren's syndrome. *J Rheumatol* 31:726–728, 2004.

85. Gentil B, Cottin V, Girard P, Cordier JF: Ambivalence of CD4 lymphocytopenia in sarcoidosis. *Sarcoidosis Vasc Diffuse Lung Dis* 20:74–75, 2003.

CHAPTER 79
LYMPHOCYTOSIS AND LYMPHOCYTOPENIA

Sumithira Vasu and Michael A. Caligiuri

SUMMARY

Lymphocytosis is defined as an absolute lymphocyte count exceeding 4×10^9/L, whereas *lymphocytopenia* is defined as a total lymphocyte count less than 1.0×10^9/L. Lymphocytosis can be categorized as either polyclonal or monoclonal. *Monoclonal lymphocytosis* reflects an underlying clonal lymphoid disease in which the numbers of lymphocytes are increased because of the acquisition of somatic mutations resulting in clonal expansion of a lymphocyte progenitor. This expansion can be stable, such as monoclonal B-cell lymphocytosis or a progressive malignancy such as acute lymphocytic leukemia, whereas *polyclonal lymphocytosis* is most commonly the result of stimulation or a reaction to factors extrinsic to lymphocytes, generally infections and/or inflammation. Lymphocytopenia, on the other hand, typically reflects depletion of T cells, the most abundant lymphocyte subtype in the blood. The most common cause of such T-cell depletion is a viral infection, such as infection with the human immunodeficiency virus, although other causes exist. This chapter outlines the conditions associated with abnormalities in the numbers of circulating lymphocytes in the blood. It also serves as a useful road map to other chapters in the book that describe in detail those conditions that commonly are associated with abnormalities in the absolute numbers of circulating lymphocytes.

⬤ LYMPHOCYTOSIS

DEFINITION

Lymphocytosis is defined as an absolute lymphocyte count exceeding 4×10^9/L, although somewhat higher threshold values (e.g., >5.0×10^9/L) are sometimes used. The normal absolute lymphocyte count is significantly higher in childhood. Chapter 2 describes the methods for determining the absolute lymphocyte count and the normal range for such counts in older children and adults (see Chap. 2, Tables 2–1 and 2–2). Tables 7–3 and 7–4 in Chapter 7, provide the lymphocyte counts and lymphocyte subset counts in newborns and infants.

The blood film of patients with lymphocytosis should be evaluated for a predominance of reactive lymphocytes associated with infectious

mononucleosis (Chap. 82), large granular lymphocytes associated with large granular lymphocytic leukemia (Chap. 94), smudge cells associated with chronic lymphocytic leukemia (CLL; Chap. 92), or blasts of acute lymphocytic leukemia (Chap. 91). Chapter 73 provides a description of normal lymphocyte morphology.

Characterization of cell-surface markers is valuable in distinguishing primary lymphocytosis (leukemic) from secondary lymphocytosis (reactive). Improvements in flow cytometric techniques and reagents have allowed clinical laboratories to perform flow cytometric immunophenotyping to distinguish benign from neoplastic lymphoproliferative disease.[1] Analysis for immunoglobulin or T-cell receptor gene rearrangement also may provide evidence for monoclonal B-cell or T-cell proliferation, respectively.[1,2]

PRIMARY LYMPHOCYTOSIS

Primary lymphocytosis defines conditions associated with an increase in the absolute number of lymphocytes secondary to an intrinsic defect in the expanded lymphocyte population (Table 79–1). These conditions also are referred to as *lymphoproliferative disorders* and most commonly are secondary to the neoplastic accumulation of monoclonal B cells, T cells, natural killer (NK) cells, or less fully differentiated cells of the lymphoid lineage. Table 79–1 lists the chapters describing each of these conditions.

Although patients with lymphocytosis secondary to lymphoproliferative disease generally maintain abnormal lymphocyte counts that rise over time, this finding is not invariable. Patients with large granular lymphocytic leukemia (Chap. 94) may have only transient lymphocytosis that is induced by stress or exercise.

Monoclonal B-Cell Lymphocytosis

The advent of multiparameter flow cytometric and molecular diagnostic techniques has identified a syndrome in patients who have expanded populations of monoclonal B cells without other associated clinical signs or symptoms.[3] This condition, monoclonal B-cell lymphocytosis (MBL) has generated a series of clinical and biologic studies investigating the prognosis and implications of this condition. An absolute B-cell count of less than 5.0×10^9/L rather than the absolute lymphocyte count is used to distinguish MBL from CLL (Chap. 92).[4] This threshold is essentially arbitrary and is not based on objective clinical outcome data. MBL could be diagnosed in two situations: in subjects with a normal lymphocyte count via a screening assay (screening MBL) or during a clinical evaluation of lymphocytosis (clinical MBL).[5–8] Screening MBL, also commonly referred to as low-count MBL (<500 monoclonal B cells per μL) is diagnosed when high-sensitivity flow cytometric techniques are used in unaffected sibling families with a genetic predisposition to CLL.[9] Prevalence of screening MBL increases with age from 2.1 percent in individuals between 40 and 60 years of age up to 5 percent in individuals older than age 60 years.[10] Single-cell analysis in familial CLL kindreds showed oligoclonality, suggesting a model of stepwise progression to CLL.[11] MBL also has been detected in blood donors, with a prevalence of 6.0 to 8.3 percent in donors age 45 years or older.[12] This study detected presence of a MBL clone in 149 of 2098 donors, showing that MBL prevalence is much higher in blood donors than previously reported.[13] This finding has generated interest given a meta-analysis showing higher risk of non-Hodgkin lymphoma and CLL in patients who received blood transfusions.[14] Individuals with known clinical MBL should not be considered suitable for blood donation. Whether this applies to screening MBL is a matter of investigation. The 10 percent prevalence of screening MBL among relatives of patients with CLL has led to questions concerning their suitability as stem cell donors for patients with CLL requiring allogeneic stem cell transplantation.[15]

TABLE 79–1.   Causes of Lymphocytosis

I. Primary lymphocytosis
  A. Lymphocytic malignancies
    1. Acute lymphocytic leukemia (Chap. 91)
    2. Chronic lymphocytic leukemia and related disorders (Chap. 92)
    3. Prolymphocytic leukemia (Chap. 92)
    4. Hairy cell leukemia (Chap. 93)
    5. Adult T-cell leukemia (Chaps. 92 and 104)
    6. Leukemic phase of B-cell lymphomas (Chap. 95)
    7. Large granular lymphocytic leukemia (Chap. 94)
      a. Natural killer (NK) cell leukemia (Chap. 104)
      b. CD8+ T-cell large granular lymphocytic leukemia
      c. CD4+ T-cell large granular lymphocytic leukemia
      d. γ/δ T-cell large granular lymphocytic leukemia
  B. Monoclonal B-cell lymphocytosis[17] (Chap. 92)
  C. Persistent polyclonal B cell lymphocytosis[26,29]
II. Reactive lymphocytosis
  A. Mononucleosis syndromes (Chap. 82)
    1. Epstein-Barr virus[55]
    2. Cytomegalovirus[58]
    3. HIV[164] (Chap. 81)
    4. Herpes simplex virus type II
    5. Rubella virus[165]
    6. *Toxoplasma gondii*[117]
    7. Adenovirus
    8. Infectious hepatitis virus[166]
    9. Dengue fever virus[167,168]
    10. Human herpes virus type 6 (HHV-6)[169]
    11. Human herpes virus type 8 (HHV-8)[170]
    12. Varicella zoster virus[165]
  B. *Bordetella pertussis*[62]
  C. NK cell lymphocytosis[72]
  D. Stress lymphocytosis (acute)[91]
    1. Cardiovascular collapse[171]
      a. Acute cardiac failure
      b. Myocardial infarction
    2. Staphylococcal toxic shock syndrome[172]
    3. Drug-induced[89]
    4. Major surgery
    5. Sickle cell crisis[173]
    6. Status epilepticus
    7. Trauma
  E. Hypersensitivity reactions
    1. Insect bite[101]
    2. Drugs[102–104]
  F. Persistent lymphocytosis (subacute or chronic)
    1. Cancer[112]
    2. Cigarette smoking[51]
    3. Hyposplenism[116]
    4. Chronic infection
      a. Leishmaniasis[174]
      b. Leprosy
      c. Strongyloidiasis[75]
    5. Thymoma[109,111]

Clinical MBL is more commonly encountered in clinical practice when patients are evaluated for lymphocytosis. A prospective study evaluated classic and new prognostic markers (*IGHV* mutational status and chromosomal abnormalities) in patients with clinical MBL and Rai stage 0 CLL.[16] No significant differences were found either in *IGHV/IGHD/IGHJ* usage between the two patient groups. Similar gene and microRNA (miRNA) signatures were seen in both groups suggesting that the two conditions have an indistinguishable biologic profile but differ only in the initial size of the monoclonal population.[17] This condition is biologically indistinguishable from CLL. Given the seriousness of a diagnosis of CLL, investigators have sought to evaluate how the B-cell clone relates to the clinical outcome of development into CLL.[16,18] The consensus is that the risk of progression requiring CLL-specific treatment among individuals with clinical MBL is 1 to 2 percent per year compared to 5 to 7 percent per year for individuals with Rai stage 0 CLL.[6,10,19–22] In contrast to this quantifiable progression for clinical MBL, progression to CLL is extremely rare among individuals with screening MBL.[23] In addition, a cohort study showed that clinical MBL was an independent risk factor for hospitalization for infection after controlling for age and gender compared to a control cohort.[24] Thus, individuals with clinical MBL should be followed with a physical examination and complete blood counts by a hematologist every 6 to 12 months, while longer followup intervals of 12 to 18 months are recommended in screening MBL. Clinical MBL should also be counseled about screening for second primary malignancies. Table 79–2 lists the features of screening MBL and clinical MBL.

Persistent Polyclonal Lymphocytosis of B Lymphocytes

Persistent polyclonal B-cell lymphocytosis (PPBL) is defined as a chronic, moderate increase in absolute lymphocyte counts (>4 × 10⁹/L) without evidence for infection or other conditions that can increase the lymphocyte count.[25] This type of lymphocytosis is a rare disorder that mostly affects middle-age women and is associated with smoking. It is characterized by the persistent expansion of CD27+immunoglobulin (Ig) M+IgD+ B cells, the presence of circulating binucleated lymphocytes and increased IgM serum levels.[26,27] Such patients have an accumulation of polyclonal B cells that have an unusual binucleated appearance on the blood film.[28] Specific morphologic features predictive of the diagnosis include basophilic vacuolated cytoplasm and monocytoid changes.[28,29] These lymphocytes typically have low-to-negligible expression of CD5 or CD23 found in patients with CLL and are polyclonal with respect to light-chain expression and immunoglobulin heavy-chain gene rearrangements (Fig. 79–1).[30,31]

The B cells commonly express relatively high levels of IgD and CD27, a phenotype shared with that of memory B cells (Chap. 75).[32] Consistent with this phenotype, the immunoglobulin variable-region

TABLE 79–2. Characteristics of Clinical and Screening Monoclonal B-Cell Lymphocytosis

	Clinical MBL	Screening MBL
Risk of transformation to CLL-requiring therapy	1–2% per year	Extremely rare
Hematologic followup interval	6–12 months	12–18 months
Risk of infections	Yes	No
Eligible for blood donation	No	Yes
Eligible for stem-cell donation	No	No

CLL, chronic lymphocytic leukemia; MBL, monoclonal B-cell lymphocytosis.

Adapted with permission from Molica S, Mauro FR, Molica M, et al: Monoclonal B-cell lymphocytosis: a reappraisal of its clinical implications. *Leuk Lymphoma* 53(9):1660–1665, 2012.

genes used by the B cells most commonly have evidence of somatic mutations, implying that the expanded B cells have undergone germinal center maturation in an immune response(s) to antigen(s).[33,34] Analyses of the immunoglobulin variable-region genes expressed by memory-type B cells of patients failed to reveal evidence of positive antigenic selection, suggesting that inappropriate clearance of B cells expressing low-affinity immunoglobulin receptors plays a role in this disorder.[35]

The cause(s) of this type of lymphocytosis is unknown. Gender and genotype may be important in the pathogenesis, as the patients most commonly are young to middle-age women who often are human

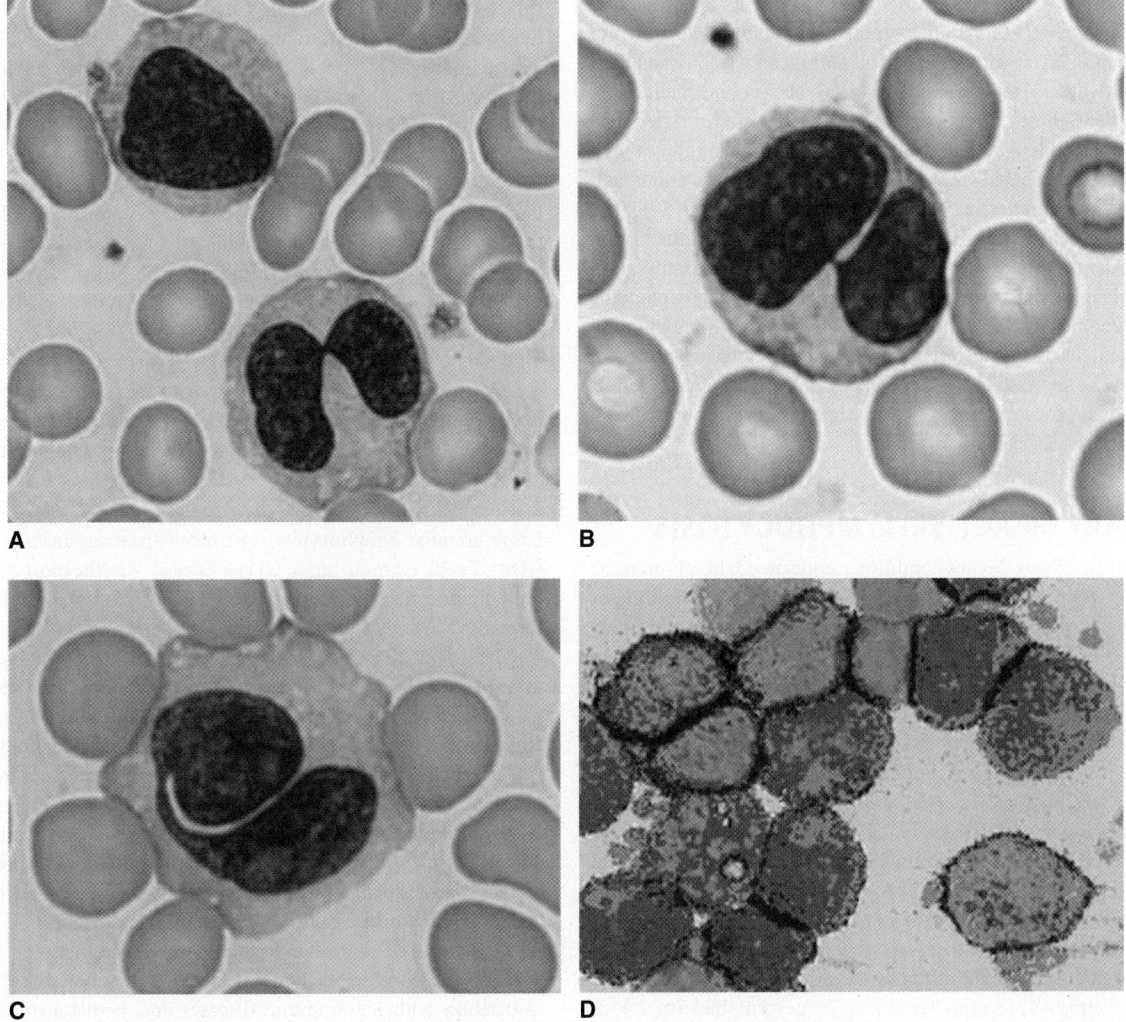

Figure 79–1. Persistent polyclonal lymphocytosis of B lymphocytes. Blood film. **A** to **C.** Examples of the nuclear abnormality of lymphocytes in this disorder. The lymphocyte nucleus may be bilobed or segmented although not fully bilobed. Some are monolobed. **D.** Light chain analysis. Immunoenzymatic method. Cytocentrifuge cell preparation. Antikappa immunoglobulin light chain tagged with peroxidase and antilambda light chain tagged with alkaline phosphatase. Note polyclonal reactivity of lymphocytes; some cells with surface κ light chains *(brownish)* and some with surface λ light chains *(reddish)*. Molecular studies did not show immunoglobulin gene rearrangement. *(Reproduced with permission from Lichtman's Atlas of Hematology, www.accessmedicine.com.)*

leukocyte antigen (HLA)-DR7 positive.[36] In addition, there are shared cases among identical twins and in families.[37,38] Moreover, evaluation of first-degree relatives of individuals with this type of lymphocytosis may identify new patients who have all the criteria for its diagnosis or have slight increases in serum IgM, suggesting a possible hereditary or genetic contribution to the pathogenesis.[39]

Patients can have features resembling those of patients with various monoclonal B-cell malignancies. Patients may have mild splenomegaly.[40] Histologic examination of marrow and secondary lymphoid tissues from patients with progressive splenomegaly can reveal features resembling marginal zone B-cell lymphoma (Chap. 101).[41] In possibly another manifestation of this syndrome, first identified in Japan as hairy B-cell lymphoproliferative disorder, the patients can present with anemia, thrombocytopenia, and splenomegaly and have an excess of polyclonal B lymphocytes that appear similar in morphology and immune phenotype to the neoplastic B cells in hairy cell leukemia (Chap. 93).[42,43]

Although the lymphocytosis generally is not progressive, most patients have small numbers of blood B cells with chromosomal abnormalities. These abnormalities can include an additional isochromosome +i(3q) and premature chromosome condensation, and/or the t(14;18) translocation involving the *BCL-2* and immunoglobulin heavy-chain loci that typically is found in the neoplastic B cells of patients with follicular lymphoma (Chap. 99).[44–47] In another study of 43 patients, two-thirds of patients had lymphocytes with independent chromosomal abnormalities, such as del(6q), +der, +8, or other polyploidy karyotypic abnormalities.[48,49] In any one patient, these chromosomal abnormalities are restricted to B lymphocytes independent of their expression of immunoglobulin or light chains.[50] For cases associated with smoking, these cytogenetic abnormalities apparently persist after the discontinuation of tobacco use.[36,51] The finding of such chromosome abnormalities is consistent with the notion that this disorder represents a preneoplastic state. Extensive proliferation of CD27+ IgM+IgD+ cells have been noted as well, which may explain the finding of splenomegaly.[26] Occasional reports of clonal immunoglobulin gene rearrangements in this disorder suggest that polyclonal expansion in some cases may be followed by the emergence of one predominant clone.[40] Moreover, a small proportion of patients ultimately develop monoclonal B-cell lymphoma or B-cell leukemia.[40,52,53]

SECONDARY (REACTIVE) LYMPHOCYTOSIS

Secondary lymphocytosis defines conditions associated with an increase in the absolute number of lymphocytes secondary to a physiologic or pathophysiologic response to infection, toxins, cytokines, or unknown factors.

Infectious Mononucleosis

The most common reactive lymphocytosis is infectious mononucleosis (see Table 79–1). In cases of mononucleosis secondary to infection with Epstein-Barr virus (EBV), the atypical lymphocytes commonly consist of polyclonal populations of CD8+ T cells, γ/δ T cells, and CD16+CD56+ NK cells that are stimulated in response to EBV-infected B cells (see Chap. 82, Fig. 82–1).[54] A study prospectively evaluated university students to determine the incidence, risk factors, and virologic and immune correlates of disease severity.[55] During a median of 3 years of observation of EBV antibody-negative students, 66 subjects experienced primary infection. Of these, 77 percent had infectious mononucleosis, 12 percent had atypical symptoms, and 11 percent were asymptomatic. Although viremia was transient, median oral shedding was 175 days. Increases were observed in numbers of NK cells and CD8+ T cells but not in numbers of CD4+ T cells during acute infection. Severity of illness correlated with both blood EBV load (P = 0.015) and CD8+ lymphocytosis (P = 0.0003).

Acute Infection Lymphocytosis

Acute infection lymphocytosis is a disorder that occurs in children usually between the ages of 2 and 10 years. It is characterized by an increase in blood lymphocytes, often to 20 to 30×10^9/L[56] and occasionally as high as 100×10^9/L, which might be mistaken for acute leukemia.[57] The lymphocytes may vary in size but are otherwise similar to normal blood lymphocytes (Fig. 79–2). Patients usually are asymptomatic but may have fever, abdominal pain, or diarrhea. Lymph node enlargement and splenomegaly do not occur, and the patient's serum usually is negative for heterophile antibodies found in patients with infectious mononucleosis caused by EBV. In this regard, the disease resembles infectious mononucleosis caused by viruses other than EBV, such as cytomegalovirus (CMV; Chap. 82).[58–60] Clinical symptoms last for a few days, but the lymphocytosis may persist for several weeks. Eosinophilia may be present. Examination of marrow from a few patients has shown minimal increases in lymphocytes, but marked infiltration with lymphocytes also has been observed. In some cases, the lymphocytosis has been found in association with acute infection by coxsackievirus B2.[61]

Bordetella pertussis

A marked increase in the number of lymphocytes occurs in patients infected with the Gram-negative bacterium *Bordetella pertussis*.[62] Absolute lymphocyte counts range from 8 to 70×10^9/L, with a mean of approximately 30×10^9/L, involving all lymphocyte subsets.[63] A notable proportion of lymphocytes have cleaved nuclei, characteristic of the cells in cases of pertussis (see Chap. 73, Fig. 73–1C).

Lymphocytosis primarily results from failure of lymphocytes to leave the blood because of *pertussis toxin*, which is released by the bacteria.[64] Pertussis toxin is an adenosine diphosphate ribosylase that modifies G proteins in mammalian lymphocytes. This inhibits the capacity of lymphocytes to traffic from blood into lymphoid tissues, primarily through inhibition of chemokine receptors. Pertussis toxin also may stimulate egress of maturing T cells from the thymus and may bind to neuraminic acid residues of T-cell surface glycoproteins to induce T-cell activation.[65,66] Despite high levels of vaccination, recent epidemics have been noted primarily as a result of waning immunity in adults who subsequently serve as a source of infection to household infants.[67]

Large Granular Lymphocytosis

Large granular lymphocytosis can result from expansions of NK cells, CD8+ T cells, or, more rarely, CD4+ T cells.[68,69] In the most common form, the lymphocytosis is secondary to CD3–CD16+CD56+ NK cells and is termed *NK lymphocytosis*, in which NK cell counts typically approximate 4×10^9/L, but can sometimes exceed 15×10^9/L.[70] The blood lymphocytes of patients with T-cell large granular lymphocytosis should be evaluated for clonal rearrangements in the T-cell receptor genes (Chap. 76),[51] which would be indicative of T-cell large granular lymphocytic leukemia (LGLL); LGLL is a heterogeneous disorder characterized by an increase in the number of blood large granular lymphocytes between 2 and 20×10^9/L for more than 6 months without a clearly identified cause (see Chap. 94, Fig. 94–1).[71] Currently NK cell lymphoproliferative disorder is considered as a provisional entity, distinct from T-LGLL and NK-LGLL in the 2008 WHO (World Health Organization) classification. A retrospective review compared clinical and pathologic features between patients with T-LGLL and chronic NK lymphocytosis.[72] They noted that median age, association with autoimmune diseases and hematologic malignancies were similar between the two groups. However, neutropenia and association with rheumatoid arthritis was less prevalent in NK cell lymphoproliferative disorder than in T-LGLL.

Large granular lymphocytosis has been observed in 20 percent of allogeneic stem cell transplant recipients for a variety of malignancies with a median onset of 312 days from transplant.[73] CMV-seropositive

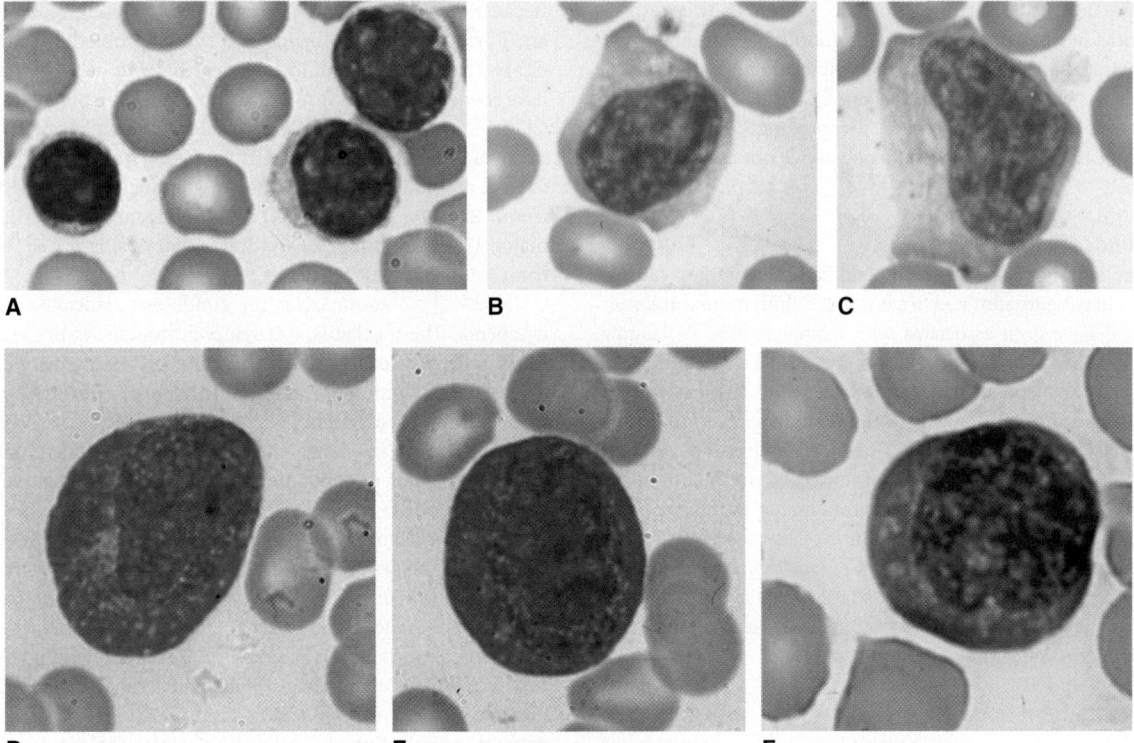

Figure 79–2. Blood films. **A.** Acute infectious lymphocytosis. The lymphocytosis in this disorder of childhood is composed of normal-appearing lymphocytes, which may vary somewhat in size as shown in the blood of this case. Note typical small lymphocyte with dense chromatin pattern and scant rim of cytoplasm and somewhat two larger lymphocytes with less-dense chromatin pattern. **B, C.** Reactive lymphocytes. Large lymphocytes with an increased proportion of cytoplasm with basophilic cytoplasmic edges, often engaging neighboring red cells. Nucleoli may occasionally be evident. This variation in lymphocyte appearance can occur in a variety of disorders that provoke an immunologic response, including viral illnesses. They are indistinguishable in appearance by light microscopy from the reactive lymphocytes seen in infectious mononucleosis, viral hepatitis, or other conditions such as Dengue fever. **D** to **F.** Plasmacytoid lymphocytes. In this type of reactive lymphocytosis, the lymphocytes are large and have deep blue-colored cytoplasm, approaching the coloration of plasma cell cytoplasm, but they retain the nuclear appearance, cell shape, and cell size of a medium-size lymphocyte, and they do not develop a prominent paranuclear clear zone or markedly eccentric nuclear position as do most plasma cells. They may be seen in a variety of situations including infections, drug hypersensitivity, and serum-sickness-type reactions. *(Reproduced with permission from* Lichtman's Atlas of Hematology, *www.accessmedicine.com.)*

recipients and patients who developed CMV reactivation and chronic graft-versus-host disease (GVHD) were more likely to develop large granular lymphocytosis. GVHD is a condition occurring after allogeneic hematopoietic stem cell transplantation when alloreactive T lymphocytes from the graft attack host organs, resulting in protean manifestations in multiple organs, and can cause severe debilitation. Surprisingly, presence of large granular lymphocytosis was associated with an overall survival advantage (86.2 percent vs. 53.8 percent, p<0.0001), lower nonrelapse mortality (3.2 percent vs. 27.3 percent, p<0.0001) and lower relapse incidence (9.6 percent vs. 29.4 percent, p<0.0001).

Expansion of NK cells or T cells may represent an exaggerated response to systemic infection and/or immune deregulation. T-cell large granular lymphocytosis may be secondary to an exaggerated cellular immune response to infection with human CMV.[74] Also, there is an association between NK lymphocytosis and strongyloidiasis.[75]

Patients with NK lymphocytosis frequently have recurrent cutaneous lesions, such as livedoid vasculopathy, urticarial vasculitis, or complex recurrent aphthous stomatitis.[76,77] Other reports noted an association between NK lymphocytosis and various cytopenias, including severe aplastic anemia.[70,78] Large granular lymphocytosis also may be associated with rheumatoid arthritis. Occurring in less than 0.6 percent of patients with rheumatoid arthritis, large granular lymphocytic lymphocytosis almost invariably is associated with neutropenia in the absence of splenomegaly and thus may represent a subset of

Felty syndrome.[79,80] Patients with autoimmune pure red cell aplasia or immune thrombocytopenia also may have large granular lymphocytosis secondary to expanded numbers of polyclonal T cells or NK cells.[81,82]

Drug-Induced Lymphocytosis

Dasatinib and ibrutinib are associated with lymphocytosis when used for chronic myelogenous leukemia (CML) and CLL, respectively. In patients receiving dasatinib, expansion of highly differentiated CD8+ T lymphocytes or NK cells have been noted.[83–85] Some studies associate oligoclonal expansions of these cells to clinical effects such as CMV reactivation and pleural effusion.[86] Clonal lymphocytosis usually has LGLL morphology and also show late differentiated (CD27–CD57+) phenotypes that seem predisposed to apoptosis and reduced NK-cell cytotoxicity. In addition to lymphocytosis, plasma levels of interleukin (IL)-6, monokines induced by interferon-γ (IFN-γ) and IL-2R were significantly increased in LGLL patients. IFN-γ is a soluble cytokine critical for innate and adaptive immunity against viral, bacterial and protozoal infections. IL-2 is also a cytokine that has effects on T lymphocytes and has key functions in tolerance and immunity. Some studies suggest that lymphocytosis after dasatinib is associated with a favorable response in CML.[87]

Ibrutinib targets B-cell receptor signaling and has been approved for use in CLL.[88] After just one dose of ibrutinib, increases in the absolute lymphocyte count of up to 66 percent can occur, representing egress of lymphocytes from nodal compartments.[89] Although this resolves within 8 months in most patients, a small minority has sustained lymphocytosis lasting more than a year. Biologic characterization of the lymphocytosis has shown that the persistent CLL cells do not proliferate and do not represent clonal evolution. The prolonged lymphocytosis likely represents a persistent quiescent clone and is not associated with a risk of relapse.[90]

Stress Lymphocytosis

Transient stress lymphocytosis has been identified as a common cause of lymphocytosis in patients admitted to a hospital.[91] Both trauma and nontraumatic stress have been associated with lymphocytosis.[92,93] Trauma, surgery, acute cardiac failure, septic shock, myocardial infarction, sickle cell crisis, or status epilepticus may be associated with an elevated lymphocyte count, often greater than 5×10^9/L, which may revert to normal or below-normal levels within hours.[94,95] The increased lymphocyte count appears promptly after the event and appears secondary to lymphocyte redistribution affecting all major lymphocyte subsets.[92] A transient lymphocytosis can be induced by the redistribution of leukocyte subsets after both physical and psychological stress.[96,97] Characteristically, two phases are recognized after catecholamine administration: a quick (<30 minutes) mobilization of lymphocytes, followed by an increase in granulocyte numbers with decreasing lymphocyte numbers.[98,99]

Hypersensitivity Reactions

Delayed hypersensitivity reactions to insect bites, especially mosquitos, may be associated with a large granular lymphocytic lymphocytosis and adenopathy.[100] These delayed hypersensitivity reactions can be associated with EBV-NK lymphocytosis.[101] Idiosyncratic drug reactions also may be associated with subacute lymphocytosis, typically developing 2 to 8 weeks after initiating administration of the responsible drug.[102–107] An infectious mononucleosis-like syndrome can be induced in some patients by salazosulfapyridine or sulfasalazine (see Fig. 79–2).[108]

Persistent Lymphocytosis

Patients may have subacute or chronic lymphocytosis, termed *persistent lymphocytosis*, in association with a variety of clinical conditions (see Table 79–1).

Patients with lymphocytosis may have underlying neoplastic disease. Most notably, patients with malignant thymoma may have a polyclonal T-cell lymphocytosis thought to be secondary to the aberrant release of thymic hormones by the neoplastic thymic epithelium.[109–111] A reactive lymphocytosis or plasmacytosis may be detected in patients with acute myeloid leukemia or systemic mastocytosis.[112–114] Patients with solid tumors also may develop lymphocytosis following cancer chemotherapy.

Patients may develop polyclonal lymphocytosis following splenectomy.[76,115,116] An absolute lymphocyte count ranging from 4.0 to 8.7×10^9/L often is noted 4 to 242 (median: 70) months after splenectomy and can persist for prolonged periods (e.g., longer than 50 months).

Chronic Infections A reactive lymphocytosis commonly is associated with many viral and certain bacterial infections, which, if protracted, can result in subacute or chronic lymphocytosis (see Table 79–1).[117]

●LYMPHOCYTOPENIA

DEFINITION

Chapter 2 presents the methods for determining the absolute lymphocyte count and the normal range for such counts. *Lymphocytopenia* is defined as a total lymphocyte count less than 1.0×10^9/L, but some consider the lower limit of normal to be 1.5×10^9/L (1500/μL).

Because approximately 80 percent of normal adult blood lymphocytes are T lymphocytes and nearly two-thirds of blood T lymphocytes are CD4+ (helper) T lymphocytes, most patients with lymphocytopenia have reductions in the absolute numbers of T lymphocytes, particularly CD4+ T lymphocytes. The average absolute number of T lymphocytes in normal adult blood is 1.9×10^9/L, ranging from 1.0 to 2.3×10^9/L. The average absolute number of CD4+ T lymphocytes is 1.1×10^9/L, ranging from 7.2 to 14×10^8/L. The average absolute number of cells of the other major T-cell subgroup, CD8+ T lymphocytes, is 6.5×10^8/L, ranging from 3.8 to 9.7×10^8/L.

Table 79–3 summarizes the conditions associated with lymphocytopenia. The mechanism of lymphocytopenia is not established for many of these disorders, and several possible mechanisms exist. Further discussion of lymphocytes and of the diseases associated with lymphocytopenia are presented in the cited reports (see Table 79–3).

The relative incidence of each of these conditions varies, depending upon the patient population. In one New Zealand survey of patients who had significant lymphocytopenia (<0.6×10^9/L), the patients fell into several categories with some overlap.[118] In order of decreasing frequency, the factors associated with lymphocytopenia were bacterial or fungal sepsis (250 patients), major surgery (228 patients), definite (153 patients) or suspected (53 patients) glucocorticoid therapy, malignancy (180 patients), cytotoxic therapy and/or radiotherapy (90 patients), recent trauma or hemorrhage (86 patients), renal allograft (38 patients), marrow allograft (35 patients), "viral infections" other than HIV (26 patients), or infection with HIV (13 patients). Only one patient was suspected of having idiopathic CD4+ T lymphocytopenia.

INHERITED CAUSES

Patients with inherited immunodeficiency diseases may have associated lymphocytopenia (see Table 79–3 and see Chap. 80, Table 80–2). Inherited immunodeficiency disorders may have a quantitative or qualitative stem cell abnormality, resulting in ineffective lymphopoiesis (see references cited in Table 79–3). Moreover, mutations in the genes that are critical for T-cell development can result in severe combined immunodeficiency and lymphocytopenia as a consequence of the inability to generate mature T cells (Chap. 76).[119] Other immune deficiencies, such as the Wiskott-Aldrich syndrome, have associated lymphopenia because of premature destruction of T cells secondary to a defect in the lymphocyte cytoskeleton.[120] Studies have reported that certain ethnic groups have lower CD4+ T-cell counts in the absence of other identified factors, for example, Ethiopians and Chukotka natives.[121,122]

ACQUIRED LYMPHOCYTOPENIA

Acquired lymphocytopenia defines syndromes associated with depletion of blood lymphocytes that are not secondary to inherited disease.

Infectious Diseases

The most common infectious disease associated with lymphopenia is AIDS caused by HIV (Chap. 81). The lymphocytopenia results in part from destruction and/or clearance of CD4+ T cells infected with HIV-1 or HIV-2.[123,124]

Other viral and bacterial diseases may be associated with lymphocytopenia (see Table 79–3). Patients presenting with active tuberculosis often have lymphocytopenia, even if they are HIV negative and this usually resolves 2 weeks after initiating appropriate antimicrobial therapy.[125–127] Patients with severe acute respiratory syndrome resulting from infection with coronavirus typically have lymphocytopenia that resolves following recovery.[128,129] Several other common viral diseases, such as measles, typically are associated with transient lymphocytopenia during the acute phases of infection, which in turn is thought to contribute to

TABLE 79–3. Causes of Lymphocytopenia

I. Inherited causes
  A. Congenital immunodeficiency diseases (Chap. 80)
    1. Severe combined immunodeficiency disease[175]
      a. Aplasia of lymphopoietic stem cells
      b. Adenosine deaminase deficiency[176]
      c. Absence of histocompatibility antigens
      d. Absence of CD4+ helper cells
      e. Thymic alymphoplasia with aleukocytosis (reticular dysgenesis)[177]
      f. Mutations in genes required for T-cell development
    2. Common variable immune deficiency[154]
    3. Ataxia-telangiectasia[178]
    4. Wiskott-Aldrich syndrome
    5. Immunodeficiency with short-limbed dwarfism (cartilage-hair hypoplasia)[179]
    6. Immunodeficiency with thymoma[180]
    7. Purine nucleoside phosphorylase deficiency[181]
    8. Immunodeficiency with venoocclusive disease of the liver[182]
  B. Lymphopenia resulting from genetic polymorphism[121]
II. Acquired causes
  A. Aplastic anemia[183] (Chap. 35)
  B. Infectious diseases
    1. Viral diseases
      a. Acquired immunodeficiency syndrome[184] (Chap. 81)
      b. Severe acute respiratory syndrome[128]
      c. West Nile encephalitis[158,185]
      d. Hepatitis[186]
      e. Influenza[187]
      f. Herpes simplex virus[188]
      g. Herpes virus type 6 (HHV-6)[189]
      h. Herpes virus type 8 (HHV-8)[190]
      i. Measles virus[191]
      j. Other[192]
    2. Bacterial diseases
      a. Tuberculosis[193]
      b. Typhoid fever[194]
      c. Pneumonia[195]
      d. Rickettsiosis[196]
      e. Ehrlichiosis[197]
      f. Sepsis[131]
    3. Parasitic diseases
      a. Acute phase of malaria infection

  C. Iatrogenic
    1. Immunosuppressive agents
      a. Antilymphocyte globulin therapy[198]
      b. Alemtuzumab (Campath 1-H)[199]
      c. Glucocorticoids[198]
    2. High-dose psoralen plus ultraviolet A treatment[200]
    3. Stevens-Johnson syndrome[201]
    4. Chemotherapy
    5. Renal transplant[202]
    6. Radiation[203]
    7. Major surgery[116]
    8. Extracorporeal bypass circulation[204]
    9. Hematopoietic stem cell transplant[205]
    10. Thoracic duct drainage[139]
    11. Hemodialysis[206]
    12. Pheresis for donor lymphocyte infusion[140]
  D. Systemic disease associated
    1. Autoimmune diseases
      a. Systemic lupus erythematosus[207]
      b. Sjögren syndrome[142]
      c. Myasthenia gravis[208]
      d. Systemic vasculitis[209]
      e. Behçet-like syndrome[210]
      f. Dermatomyositis[211]
      g. Wegener granulomatosis[212]
    2. Hodgkin lymphoma[213] (Chap. 99)
    3. Carcinoma[214]
    4. Idiopathic myelofibrosis[215]
    5. Protein-losing enteropathy[216,217]
    6. Heart failure[145]
    7. Sarcoidosis[218]
    8. Thermal injury[144]
    9. Severe acute pancreatitis[219]
    10. Strenuous exercise[220]
    11. Silicosis[221]
    12. Celiac disease[222]
  E. Nutritional and dietary
    1. Ethanol abuse[149]
    2. Zinc deficiency[148]
III. Idiopathic
  A. Idiopathic CD4+ T lymphocytopenia[153]

a disease course-related immunodeficiency that can predispose patients to infection with opportunistic infectious agents (see Table 79–3).[130] The prognostic value of lymphocytopenia as a consequence of sepsis has been evaluated.[131] In a single-center retrospective study, persistent lymphopenia on the fourth day after the diagnosis of sepsis predicted both 28-day and 1-year survival. Lymphopenia is considered a surrogate marker for sepsis-induced immunosuppression. In patients hospitalized with decompensated heart failure, relative lymphocytopenia

(decrease in percent of lymphocytes, not absolute lymphocyte count) was frequently noted.[132]

Iatrogenic

Radiotherapy, cytotoxic chemotherapy, glucocorticoids, or administration of antilymphocyte globulin or alemtuzumab (Campath-1H) each can lead to lymphocytopenia by destroying circulating lymphocytes (see Table 79–3). Long-term treatment of psoriasis with psoralen and ultraviolet A irradiation may result in T-lymphocyte lymphopenia, possibly through destruction of cells circulating through the cutaneous vasculature.[133] The mechanism by which glucocorticoids cause lymphocytopenia is not clear, but may be secondary to a glucocorticoid-induced redistribution of lymphocytes in addition to induced cell destruction.[134-136] Redistribution also may be responsible for the lymphocytopenia occurring after surgery.[137,138] In thoracic duct drainage, the lymphocytes are lost from the body.[139] Platelet or stem cell apheresis similarly lowers the lymphocyte count because of inadvertent removal of lymphocytes with the platelets.[140]

Systemic Disease Associated with Lymphocytopenia

Patients with systemic autoimmune disease can have lymphocytopenia, secondary to either the underlying disease or therapy. Patients who present with systemic lupus erythematosus may have autoantibody-mediated lymphocytopenia prior to therapy and the presence of antilymphocyte antibodies was independently associated with disease activity and lupus nephritis.[141] Similarly, patients with primary Sjögren syndrome sometimes have lymphocytopenia even prior to therapy and an association between lymphocytopenia and risk of developing lymphoma has been observed.[142,143] In conditions such as protein-losing enteropathy, lymphocytes may be lost from the body. Severe thermal injury may result in profound T-cell lymphopenia secondary to redistribution of blood T cells to the tissues.[144] Lymphopenia has also been noted to be an independent predictor of poor outcomes in heart failure patients requiring hospitalization. Patients with low lymphocyte counts tend to be older with higher rates of comorbid diseases such as diabetes, renal disease, atrial fibrillation and have high levels of brain natriuretic peptides (BNPs) and wide QRS intervals on electrocardiography. After adjusting for multiple known clinical risk factors, lymphocytopenia remains a strong predictor of all-cause or cardiovascular mortality.[145]

Nutritional or Dietary

Zinc is essential for normal T-cell development and function.[146,147] Low zinc levels have been observed in critically ill children within 72 hours of admission to an intensive care unit.[148] Zinc therapy corrects the lymphocytopenia of zinc deficiency, and lymphocytic function is restored. Excessive intake of ethanol and/or chronic ethanol use may result in impaired lymphocyte proliferative responses and lymphopenia, which may resolve with abstinence from alcohol.[149] Concerns over whether the soy isoflavones found in soy protein can factor in the development of lymphocytopenia appear unjustified.[150]

● IDIOPATHIC CD4+ T LYMPHOCYTOPENIA

The advent of immunophenotyping and HIV serologic testing has identified a syndrome of isolated CD4+ T-cell depletion in the absence of evidence for retroviral infection.[151] The syndrome, termed *idiopathic CD4+ T lymphocytopenia* by the Centers for Disease Control and Prevention in 1993, is defined by the WHO as a CD4+ T-lymphocyte count less than 0.3×10^9/L on two separate occasions in patients without serologic or virologic evidence of HIV-1 or HIV-2 infection.[152] Unlike HIV infection, the decrease in the CD4 cell counts of patients with idiopathic CD4+ T lymphocytopenia is generally slow.[153] It is important to exclude congenital immunodeficiency diseases, such as common variable immunodeficiency, which may lead to altered CD4+ T-cell counts that are recognized in later life (Chap. 80).[123,154]

Although some patients with idiopathic CD4+ T lymphocytopenia do not have any clinical manifestations, more than half of all reported cases had prior opportunistic infections indicative of a cellular immunodeficiency (e.g., recurrent herpes zoster, pulmonary *Mycobacterium avium*, *Mycobacterium tuberculosis*, *Pneumocystis carinii* pneumonia,

toxoplasmosis, neuroinvasive West Nile disease, progressive multifocal leukoencephalopathy, or cryptococcal infections).[155-159] The WHO classifies such patients as having idiopathic CD4+ T lymphocytopenia and severe unexplained HIV-seronegative immune suppression.[123]

Several observations have helped understand the pathogenesis of idiopathic lymphocytopenia. Lymphocyte-specific kinases (LCKs) play a key role in initiation of signaling from the T-cell receptor (TCR). TCR activates LCK through the adaptor protein, uncoordinated 119 (UNC119).[160] Consequently a mutation of human UNC119 impairs LCK activation resulting in diminished T-cell responses to TCR stimulation and clinically manifests as lymphopenia and opportunistic infections. A heterozygous mutation of UNC119 has been noted in patients with Idiopathic CD4+ T-lymphocytopenia.[161] IL-7 and IL-2 signaling have been shown to be impaired in this condition, which may explain for the loss of CD4+ T-lymphocyte homeostasis.[162] The exact proportion of patients with this disorder is unknown because patients who are not affected clinically by the isolated CD4+ T-cell depletion may not come to medical attention. In conclusion, idiopathic CD4+ T lymphocytopenia is a heterogeneous condition diagnosed typically in middle age and is associated with multiple opportunistic infections and autoimmune diseases. Experimental cytokine therapies with IL-2 have been evaluated in these patients.[163]

REFERENCES

1. Johansson U, Bloxham D, Couzens S, et al: Guidelines on the use of multicolour flow cytometry in the diagnosis of haematological neoplasms. British Committee for Standards in Haematology. *Br J Haematol* 165(4):455–488, 2014.
2. Rockman SP: Determination of clonality in patients who present with diagnostic dilemmas: A laboratory experience and review of the literature. *Leukemia* 11(6): 852–862, 1997.
3. Ghia P, Caligaris-Cappio F: Monoclonal B-cell lymphocytosis: Right track or red herring? *Blood* 119(19):4358–4362, 2012.
4. Hallek M, Cheson BD, Catovsky D, et al: Guidelines for the diagnosis and treatment of chronic lymphocytic leukemia: A report from the International Workshop on Chronic Lymphocytic Leukemia updating the National Cancer Institute-Working Group 1996 guidelines. *Blood* 111(12):5446–5456, 2008.
5. Nieto WG, Almeida J, Romero A, et al: Increased frequency (12%) of circulating chronic lymphocytic leukemia-like B-cell clones in healthy subjects using a highly sensitive multicolor flow cytometry approach. *Blood* 114(1):33–37, 2009.
6. Rawstron AC, Bennett FL, O'Connor SJ, et al: Monoclonal B-cell lymphocytosis and chronic lymphocytic leukemia. *N Engl J Med* 359(6):575–583, 2008.
7. Marti GE, Faguet G, Bertin P, et al: CD20 and CD5 expression in B-chronic lymphocytic leukemia. *Ann N Y Acad Sci* 651:480–483, 1992.
8. Marti GE, Faguet GB, Stewart C, et al: Evolution of leukemic heterogeneity of human B-CLL lymphocytes between and within patients. *Curr Top Microbiol Immunol* 182: 303–311, 1992.
9. Crowther-Swanepoel D, Corre T, Lloyd A, et al: Inherited genetic susceptibility to monoclonal B-cell lymphocytosis. *Blood* 116(26):5957–5960, 2010.
10. Shanafelt T, Hanson CA: Monoclonal B-cell lymphocytosis: Definitions and natural history. *Leuk Lymphoma* 50(3):493–497, 2009.
11. Lanasa MC, Allgood SD, Volkheimer AD, et al: Single-cell analysis reveals oligoclonality among "low-count" monoclonal B-cell lymphocytosis. *Leukemia* 24(1):133–140, 2010.
12. Shim YK, Rachel JM, Ghia P, et al: Monoclonal B-cell lymphocytosis in healthy blood donors: An unexpectedly common finding. *Blood* 123(9):1319–1326, 2014.
13. Rachel JM, Zucker ML, Fox CM, et al: Monoclonal B-cell lymphocytosis in blood donors. *Br J Haematol* 139(5):832–836, 2007.
14. Castillo JJ, Dalia S, Pascual SK: Association between red blood cell transfusions and development of non-Hodgkin lymphoma: A meta-analysis of observational studies. *Blood* 116(16):2897–2907, 2010.
15. Del Giudice I, Mauro FR, De Propris MS, et al: Identification of monoclonal B-cell lymphocytosis among sibling transplant donors for chronic lymphocytic leukemia patients. *Blood* 114(13):2848–2849, 2009.
16. Morabito F, Mosca L, Cutrona G, et al: Clinical monoclonal B lymphocytosis versus Rai 0 chronic lymphocytic leukemia: A comparison of cellular, cytogenetic, molecular, and clinical features. *Clin Cancer Res* 19(21):5890–5900, 2013.
17. Molica S, Mauro FR, Molica M, et al: Monoclonal B-cell lymphocytosis: A reappraisal of its clinical implications. *Leuk Lymphoma* 53(9):1660–1665, 2012.
18. Henriques A, Rodriguez-Caballero A, Nieto WG, et al: Combined patterns of IGHV repertoire and cytogenetic/molecular alterations in monoclonal B lymphocytosis versus chronic lymphocytic leukemia. *PLoS One* 8(7):e67751, 2013.

19. Molica S, Mauro FR, Giannarelli D, et al: Differentiating chronic lymphocytic leukemia from monoclonal B-lymphocytosis according to clinical outcome: On behalf of the GIMEMA chronic lymphoproliferative diseases working group. *Haematologica* 96(2):277–283, 2011.

20. Shanafelt TD, Kay NE, Jenkins G, et al: B-cell count and survival: Differentiating chronic lymphocytic leukemia from monoclonal B-cell lymphocytosis based on clinical outcome. *Blood* 113(18):4188–4196, 2009.

21. Shanafelt TD, Kay NE, Rabe KG, et al: Brief report: Natural history of individuals with clinically recognized monoclonal B-cell lymphocytosis compared with patients with Rai 0 chronic lymphocytic leukemia. *J Clin Oncol* 27(24):3959–3963, 2009.

22. Rossi D, Sozzi E, Puma A, et al: The prognosis of clinical monoclonal B cell lymphocytosis differs from prognosis of Rai 0 chronic lymphocytic leukaemia and is recapitulated by biological risk factors. *Br J Haematol* 146(1):64–75, 2009.

23. Fazi C, Scarfo L, Pecciarini L, et al: General population low-count CLL-like MBL persists over time without clinical progression, although carrying the same cytogenetic abnormalities of CLL. *Blood* 118(25):6618–6625, 2011.

24. Moreira J, Rabe KG, Cerhan JR, et al: Infectious complications among individuals with clinical monoclonal B-cell lymphocytosis (MBL): A cohort study of newly diagnosed cases compared to controls. *Leukemia* 27(1):136–141, 2013.

25. Deplano S, Nadal-Melsio E, Bain BJ: Persistent polyclonal B lymphocytosis. *Am J Hematol* 89(2):224, 2014.

26. Berkowska MA, Grosserichter-Wagener C, Adriaansen HJ, et al: Persistent polyclonal B-cell lymphocytosis: Extensively proliferated CD27+IgM+IgD+ memory B cells with a distinctive immunophenotype. *Leukemia* 28(7):1560–1564, 2014.

27. Chevalier C, Husson B, Detry G: Polyclonal B lymphocytosis with binucleated lymphocytes in a man. *Am J Hematol* 88(1):86, 2013.

28. Lesesve JF, Troussard X: Persistent polyclonal B-cell lymphocytosis. *Blood* 118(25):6485, 2011.

29. Lesesve JF, Gressot AL, Troussard X, et al: Morphologic features of binucleated lymphocytes to assess the diagnosis of persistent B-cell polyclonal lymphocytosis or other mature B-cell neoplasms. *Leuk Lymphoma* 55(7):1551–1556, 2014.

30. Delage R, Roy J, Jacques L, et al: Multiple bcl-2/Ig gene rearrangements in persistent polyclonal B-cell lymphocytosis. *Br J Haematol* 97(3):589–595, 1997.

31. Schmidt-Hieber M, Burmeister T, Weimann A, et al: Combined automated cell and flow cytometric analysis enables recognition of persistent polyclonal B-cell lymphocytosis (PPBL), a study of 25 patients. *Ann Hematol* 87(10):829–836, 2008.

32. Himmelmann A, Gautschi O, Nawrath M, et al: Persistent polyclonal B-cell lymphocytosis is an expansion of functional IgD(+)CD27(+) memory B cells. *Br J Haematol* 114(2):400–405, 2001.

33. Loembe MM, Neron S, Delage R, Darveau A: Analysis of expressed V(H) genes in persistent polyclonal B cell lymphocytosis reveals absence of selection in CD27+IgM+ IgD+ memory B cells. *Eur J Immunol* 32(12):3678–3688, 2002.

34. Salcedo I, Campos-Caro A, Sampalo A, et al: Persistent polyclonal B lymphocytosis: An expansion of cells showing IgVH gene mutations and phenotypic features of normal lymphocytes from the CD27+ marginal zone B-cell compartment. *Br J Haematol* 116(3):662–666, 2002.

35. Roussel M, Roue G, Sola B, et al: Dysfunction of the Fas apoptotic signaling pathway in persistent polyclonal B-cell lymphocytosis. *Haematologica* 88(2):239–240, 2003.

36. Troussard X, Mossafa H, Salaun V: Persistent polyclonal lymphocytosis (PPLB). *Leukemia* 13(3):497–498, 1999.

37. Carr R, Fishlock K, Matutes E: Persistent polyclonal B-cell lymphocytosis in identical twins. *Br J Haematol* 96(2):272–274, 1997.

38. Delage R, Jacques L, Massinga-Loembe M, et al: Persistent polyclonal B-cell lymphocytosis: Further evidence for a genetic disorder associated with B-cell abnormalities. *Br J Haematol* 114(3):666–670, 2001.

39. Wolowiec D, Nowak J, Majewski M, et al: High incidence of ancestral HLA haplotype 8.1 and monoclonal incomplete DH-JH immunoglobulin heavy chain gene rearrangement in persistent polyclonal B-cell lymphocytosis. *Ann Hematol* 87(7):597–598, 2008.

40. Feugier P, De March AK, Lesesve JF, et al: Intravascular bone marrow accumulation in persistent polyclonal lymphocytosis: A misleading feature for B-cell neoplasm. *Mod Pathol* 17(9):1087–1096, 2004.

41. Del Giudice I, Pileri SA, Rossi M, et al: Histopathological and molecular features of persistent polyclonal B-cell lymphocytosis (PPBL) with progressive splenomegaly. *Br J Haematol* 144(5):726–731, 2009.

42. Okamoto A, Inaba T, Fujita N: The role of interleukin-6 in a patient with polyclonal hairy B-cell lymphoproliferative disorder: A case report. *Lab Hematol* 13(4):124–127, 2007.

43. Machii T, Yamaguchi M, Inoue R, et al: Polyclonal B-cell lymphocytosis with features resembling hairy cell leukemia-Japanese variant. *Blood* 89(6):2008–2014, 1997.

44. Mossafa H, Malaure H, Maynadie M, et al: Persistent polyclonal B lymphocytosis with binucleated lymphocytes: A study of 25 cases. Groupe Francais d'Hematologie Cellulaire. *Br J Haematol* 104(3):486–493, 1999.

45. Callet-Bauchu E, Renard N, Gazzo S, et al: Distribution of the cytogenetic abnormality +i(3)(q10) in persistent polyclonal B-cell lymphocytosis: A FICTION study in three cases. *Br J Haematol* 99(3):531–536, 1997.

46. Espinet B, Florensa L, Sole F, et al: Isochromosome +i(3)(q10) in a new case of persistent polyclonal B-cell lymphocytosis (PPBL). *Eur J Haematol* 64(5):344–346, 2000.

47. Samson T, Mossafa H, Lusina D, et al: Dicentric chromosome 3 associated with binucleated lymphocytes in atypical B-cell chronic lymphoproliferative disorder. *Leuk Lymphoma* 43(9):1749–1754, 2002.

48. Granados E, Llamas P, Pinilla I, et al: Persistent polyclonal B lymphocytosis with multiple bcl-2/IgH rearrangements: A benign disorder. *Haematologica* 83(4):369–375, 1998.

49. Mossafa H, Tapia S, Flandrin G, Troussard X: Chromosomal instability and ATR amplification gene in patients with persistent and polyclonal B-cell lymphocytosis (PPBL). *Leuk Lymphoma* 45(7):1401–1406, 2004.

50. Lancry L, Roulland S, Roue G, et al: No BCL-2 protein over expression but BCL-2/IgH rearrangements in B cells of patients with persistent polyclonal B-cell lymphocytosis. *Hematol J* 2(4):228–233, 2001.

51. Dasanu CA, Codreanu I: Persistent polyclonal B-cell lymphocytosis in chronic smokers: More than meets the eye. *Conn Med* 76(2):69–72, 2012.

52. Bassan R, Spinelli O, Rambaldi A, Barbui T: The course of monoclonal "villous" lymphocytosis over 15 years of follow-up: Progression to SLVL or spontaneous clinical but not molecular remission. *Leukemia* 17(11):2243–2244, 2003.

53. Cornet E, Lesesve JF, Mossafa H, et al: Long-term follow-up of 111 patients with persistent polyclonal B-cell lymphocytosis with binucleated lymphocytes. *Leukemia* 23(2):419–422, 2009.

54. Hudnall SD, Patel J, Schwab H, Martinez J: Comparative immunophenotypic features of EBV-positive and EBV-negative atypical lymphocytosis. *Cytometry B Clin Cytom* 55(1):22–28, 2003.

55. Balfour HH Jr, Odumade OA, Schmeling DO, et al: Behavioral, virologic, and immunologic factors associated with acquisition and severity of primary Epstein-Barr virus infection in university students. *J Infect Dis* 207(1):80–88, 2013.

56. Horwitz MS, Moore GT: Acute infectious lymphocytosis. An etiologic and epidemiologic study of an outbreak. *N Engl J Med* 279(8):399–404, 1968.

57. Yetgin S, Kuskonmaz B, Aytac S, Tavil B: An unusual case of reactive lymphocytosis mimicking acute leukemia. *Pediatr Hematol Oncol* 24(2):129–135, 2007.

58. Kunno A, Abe M, Yamada M, Murakami K: Clinical and histological features of cytomegalovirus hepatitis in previously healthy adults. *Liver* 17(3):129–132, 1997.

59. Labalette M, Salez F, Pruvot FR, et al: CD8 lymphocytosis in primary cytomegalovirus (CMV) infection of allograft recipients: Expansion of an uncommon CD8+ CD57– subset and its progressive replacement by CD8+ CD57+ T cells. *Clin Exp Immunol* 95(3):465–471, 1994.

60. Labalette M, Salez F, Pruvot FR, et al: Successive emergence of two CD8 subsets in primary CMV infection of allograft recipients. *Transpl Int* 7 (Suppl 1):S611–S617, 1994.

61. Arnez M, Cizman M, Jazbec J, Kotnik A: Acute infectious lymphocytosis caused by coxsackievirus B2. *Pediatr Infect Dis J* 15(12):1127–1128, 1996.

62. Ferronato AE, Gilio AE, Vieira SE: Respiratory viral infections in infants with clinically suspected pertussis. *J Pediatr (Rio J)* 89(6):549–553, 2013.

63. Hodge G, Hodge S, Markus C, Lawrence A, Han P: A marked decrease in L-selectin expression by leucocytes in infants with Bordetella pertussis infection: Leucocytosis explained? *Respirology* 8(2):157–162, 2003.

64. Verschueren H, Dewit J, Van der Wegen A, et al: The lymphocytosis promoting action of pertussis toxin can be mimicked in vitro. Holotoxin but not the B subunit inhibits invasion of human T lymphoma cells through fibroblast monolayers. *J Immunol Methods* 144(2):231–240, 1991.

65. Suzuki G, Sawa H, Kobayashi Y, et al: Pertussis toxin-sensitive signal controls the trafficking of thymocytes across the corticomedullary junction in the thymus. *J Immunol* 162(10):5981–5985, 1999.

66. Witvliet MH, Vogel ML, Wiertz EJ, Poolman JT: Interaction of pertussis toxin with human T lymphocytes. *Infect Immun* 60(12):5085–5090, 1992.

67. Kwon HJ, Yum SK, Choi UY, et al: Infant pertussis and household transmission in Korea. *J Korean Med Sci* 27(12):1547–1551, 2012.

68. Lima M, Almeida J, Dos Anjos Teixeira M, et al: TCRalphabeta+/CD4+ large granular lymphocytosis: A new clonal T-cell lymphoproliferative disorder. *Am J Pathol* 163(2):763–771, 2003.

69. Moura J, Rodrigues J, Santos AH, et al: Chemokine receptor repertoire reflects mature T-cell lymphoproliferative disorder clinical presentation. *Blood Cells Mol Dis* 42(1):57–63, 2009.

70. Rabbani GR, Phyliky RL, Tefferi A: A long-term study of patients with chronic natural killer cell lymphocytosis. *Br J Haematol* 106(4):960–966, 1999.

71. O'Malley DP: T-cell large granular leukemia and related proliferations. *Am J Clin Pathol* 127(6):850–859, 2007.

72. Poullot E, Zambello R, Leblanc F, et al: Chronic natural killer lymphoproliferative disorders: Characteristics of an international cohort of 70 patients. *Ann Oncol* 25(10):2030–2035, 2014.

73. Kim D, Al-Dawsari G, Chang H, et al: Large granular lymphocytosis and its impact on long-term clinical outcomes following allo-SCT. *Bone Marrow Transplant* 48(8):1104–1111, 2013.

74. Rossi D, Franceschetti S, Capello D, et al: Transient monoclonal expansion of CD8+/CD57+ T-cell large granular lymphocytes after primary cytomegalovirus infection. *Am J Hematol* 82(12):1103–1105, 2007.

75. Myers R, Speight EL, Huissoon AP, Davies JM: Natural killer-cell lymphocytosis and strongyloides infection. *Clin Lab Haematol* 22(4):237–238, 2000.

76. Granjo E, Lima M, Fraga M, et al: Abnormal NK cell lymphocytosis detected after splenectomy: Association with repeated infections, relapsing neutropenia, and persistent polyclonal B-cell proliferation. *Int J Hematol* 75(5):484–488, 2002.

77. Vanness ER, Davis MD, Tefferi A: Cutaneous findings associated with chronic natural killer cell lymphocytosis. *Int J Dermatol* 41(12):852–857, 2002.

78. Kaito K, Otsubo H, Ogasawara Y, et al: Severe aplastic anemia associated with chronic natural killer cell lymphocytosis. *Int J Hematol* 72(4):463–465, 2000.

79. Agarwal V, Sachdev A, Lehl S, Basu S: Unusual haematological alterations in rheumatoid arthritis. *J Postgrad Med* 50(1):60–61, 2004.

80. Prochorec-Sobieszek M, Chelstowska M, Rymkiewicz G, et al: Biclonal T-cell receptor gammadelta+ large granular lymphocyte leukemia associated with rheumatoid arthritis. *Leuk Lymphoma* 49(4):828–831, 2008.

81. Grossi A, Nozzoli C, Gheri R, et al: Pure red cell aplasia in autoimmune polyglandular syndrome with T lymphocytosis. *Haematologica* 83(11):1043–1045, 1998.

82. Garcia-Suarez J, Prieto A, Reyes E, et al: Persistent lymphocytosis of natural killer cells in autoimmune thrombocytopenic purpura (ATP) patients after splenectomy. *Br J Haematol* 89(3):653–655, 1995.

83. Kreutzman A, Juvonen V, Kairisto V, et al: Mono/oligoclonal T and NK cells are common in chronic myeloid leukemia patients at diagnosis and expand during dasatinib therapy. *Blood* 116(5):772–782, 2010.

84. Kreutzman A, Ladell K, Koechel C, et al: Expansion of highly differentiated CD8+ T-cells or NK-cells in patients treated with dasatinib is associated with cytomegalovirus reactivation. *Leukemia* 25(10):1587–1597, 2011.

85. Tanaka H, Nakashima S, Usuda M: Rapid and sustained increase of large granular lymphocytes and rare cytomegalovirus reactivation during dasatinib treatment in chronic myelogenous leukemia patients. *Int J Hematol* 96(3):308–319, 2012.

86. Nagata Y, Ohashi K, Fukuda S, et al: Clinical features of dasatinib-induced large granular lymphocytosis and pleural effusion. *Int J Hematol* 91(5):799–807, 2010.

87. Awan FT, Johnson AJ, Lapalombella R, et al: Thalidomide and lenalidomide as new therapeutics for the treatment of chronic lymphocytic leukemia. *Leuk Lymphoma* 51(1):27–38, 2010.

88. Byrd JC, O'Brien S, James DF: Ibrutinib in relapsed chronic lymphocytic leukemia. *N Engl J Med* 369(13):1278–1279, 2013.

89. Herman SE, Niemann CU, Farooqui M, et al: Ibrutinib-induced lymphocytosis in patients with chronic lymphocytic leukemia: Correlative analyses from a phase II study. *Leukemia* 2014.

90. Woyach JA, Smucker K, Smith LL, et al: Prolonged lymphocytosis during ibrutinib therapy is associated with distinct molecular characteristics and does not indicate a suboptimal response to therapy. *Blood* 123(12):1810–1817, 2014.

91. Karandikar NJ, Hotchkiss EC, McKenna RW, Kroft SH: Transient stress lymphocytosis: An immunophenotypic characterization of the most common cause of newly identified adult lymphocytosis in a tertiary hospital. *Am J Clin Pathol* 117(5):819–825, 2002.

92. Thommasen HV, Boyko WJ, Montaner JS, et al: Absolute lymphocytosis associated with nonsurgical trauma. *Am J Clin Pathol* 86(4):480–483, 1986.

93. Pinkerton PH, McLellan BA, Quantz MC, Robinson JB: Acute lymphocytosis after trauma—Early recognition of the high-risk patient? *J Trauma* 29(6):749–751, 1989.

94. Bosch JA, Berntson GG, Cacioppo JT, et al: Acute stress evokes selective mobilization of T cells that differ in chemokine receptor expression: A potential pathway linking immunologic reactivity to cardiovascular disease. *Brain Behav Immun* 17(4):251–259, 2003.

95. Benschop RJ, Jacobs R, Sommer B, et al: Modulation of the immunologic response to acute stress in humans by beta-blockade or benzodiazepines. *FASEB J* 10(4):517–524, 1996.

96. Mignini F, Traini E, Tomassoni D, et al: Leucocyte subset redistribution in a human model of physical stress. *Clin Exp Hypertens* 30(8):720–731, 2008.

97. Anane LH, Edwards KM, Burns VE, et al: Mobilization of gammadelta T lymphocytes in response to psychological stress, exercise, and beta-agonist infusion. *Brain Behav Immun* 23(6):823–829, 2009.

98. Toft P, Tonnesen E, Svendsen P, et al: The redistribution of lymphocytes during adrenaline infusion. An in vivo study with radiolabelled cells. *APMIS* 100(7):593–597, 1992.

99. Tonnesen E, Hohndorf K, Lerbjerg G, et al: Immunological and hormonal responses to lung surgery during one-lung ventilation. *Eur J Anaesthesiol* 10(3):189–195, 1993.

100. Roh EJ, Chung EH, Chang YP, et al: A case of hypersensitivity to mosquito bite associated with Epstein-Barr viral infection and natural killer cell lymphocytosis. *J Korean Med Sci* 25(2):321–323, 2010.

101. Satwani P, Bhatia M, Garvin JH Jr, et al: A Phase I study of gemtuzumab ozogamicin (GO) in combination with busulfan and cyclophosphamide (Bu/Cy) and allogeneic stem cell transplantation in children with poor-risk CD33+ AML: A new targeted immunochemotherapy myeloablative conditioning (MAC) regimen. *Biol Blood Marrow Transplant* 18(2):324–329, 2012.

102. Geyer MB, Jacobson JS, Freedman J, et al: A comparison of immune reconstitution and graft-versus-host disease following myeloablative conditioning versus reduced toxicity conditioning and umbilical cord blood transplantation in paediatric recipients. *Br J Haematol* 155(2):218–234, 2011.

103. Neier M, Jin Z, Kleinman C, et al: Pericardial effusion post-SCT in pediatric recipients with signs and/or symptoms of cardiac disease. *Bone Marrow Transplant* 46(4):529–538, 2011.

104. Shah N, Martin-Antonio B, Yang H, et al: Antigen presenting cell-mediated expansion of human umbilical cord blood yields log-scale expansion of natural killer cells with anti-myeloma activity. *PLoS One* 8(10):e76781, 2013.

105. Hillmen P, Young NS, Schubert J, et al: The complement inhibitor eculizumab in paroxysmal nocturnal hemoglobinuria. *N Engl J Med* 355(12):1233–1243, 2006.

106. Krishnan SK, Hill A, Hillmen P, et al: Improving cytopenia with splenic artery embolization in a patient with paroxysmal nocturnal hemoglobinuria on eculizumab. *Int J Hematol* 98(6):716–718, 2013.

107. Hillmen P, Muus P, Roth A, et al: Long-term safety and efficacy of sustained eculizumab treatment in patients with paroxysmal nocturnal haemoglobinuria. *Br J Haematol* 162(1):62–73, 2013.

108. Satwani P, van de Ven C, Ayello J, et al: Interleukin (IL)-15 in combination with IL-2, fms-like tyrosine kinase-3 ligand and anti-CD3 significantly enhances umbilical cord blood natural killer (NK) cell and NK-cell subset expansion and NK function. *Cytotherapy* 13(6):730–738, 2011.

109. Kato T, Yoshida H, Sadfar K, et al: Steroid-free induction and preemptive antiviral therapy for liver transplant recipients with hepatitis C: A preliminary report from a prospective randomized study. *Transplant Proc* 37(2):1217–1219, 2005.

110. Ortega M, Rovira M, Almela M, et al: Bacterial and fungal bloodstream isolates from 796 hematopoietic stem cell transplant recipients between 1991 and 2000. *Ann Hematol* 84(1):40–46, 2005.

111. Choi CM, Schmaier AH, Snell MR, Lazarus HM: Thrombotic microangiopathy in haematopoietic stem cell transplantation: Diagnosis and treatment. *Drugs* 69(2):183–198, 2009.

112. Lapalombella R, Andritsos L, Liu Q, et al: Lenalidomide treatment promotes CD154 expression on CLL cells and enhances production of antibodies by normal B cells through a PI3-kinase-dependent pathway. *Blood* 115(13):2619–2629, 2010.

113. Janik-Moszant A, Barc-Czarnecka M, van der Burg M, et al: Concomitant EBV-related B-cell proliferation and juvenile myelomonocytic leukemia in a 2-year-old child. *Leuk Res* 32(1):181–184, 2008.

114. Horny HP, Lange K, Sotlar K, Valent P: Increase of bone marrow lymphocytes in systemic mastocytosis: Reactive lymphocytosis or malignant lymphoma? Immunohistochemical and molecular findings on routinely processed bone marrow biopsy specimens. *J Clin Pathol* 56(8):575–578, 2003.

115. Juneja S, Januszewicz E, Wolf M, Cooper I: Post-splenectomy lymphocytosis. *Clin Lab Haematol* 17(4):335–337, 1995.

116. Domingo P, Fuster M, Muniz-Diaz E, et al: Spurious post-splenectomy CD4 and CD8 lymphocytosis in HIV-infected patients. *AIDS* 10(1):106–107, 1996.

117. Vidal MA, Sebastianes C, Eizaga R, et al: [Activated recombinant factor VII for bleeding after a kidney transplant] [in Spanish]. *Rev Esp Anestesiol Reanim* 52(10):638–639, 2005.

118. Castelino DJ, McNair P, Kay TW: Lymphocytopenia in a hospital population—What does it signify? *Aust N Z J Med* 27(2):170–174, 1997.

119. Kalman L, Lindegren ML, Kobrynski L, et al: Mutations in genes required for T-cell development: IL7R, CD45, IL2RG, JAK3, RAG1, RAG2, ARTEMIS, and ADA and severe combined immunodeficiency: HuGE review. *Genet Med* 6(1):16–26, 2004.

120. Molina IJ, Kenney DM, Rosen FS, Remold-O'Donnell E: T cell lines characterize events in the pathogenesis of the Wiskott-Aldrich syndrome. *J Exp Med* 176(3):867–874, 1992.

121. Wolday D, Tsegaye A, Messele T: Low absolute CD4 counts in Ethiopians. *Ethiop Med J* 40 (Suppl 1):11–16, 2002.

122. Gyrgolkay LA, Nikitin YP: Leukogram and white blood cells count in native people of Chukotka. *Int J Circumpolar Health* 60(4):534–539, 2001.

123. Laurence J: T-cell subsets in health, infectious disease, and idiopathic CD4+ T lymphocytopenia. *Ann Intern Med* 119(1):55–62, 1993.

124. Portman MD: Routinely test for HIV in everyone presenting with unexplained lymphopenia. *BMJ* 348:g2433, 2014.

125. Skogmar S, Schon T, Balcha TT, et al: CD4 cell levels during treatment for tuberculosis (TB) in Ethiopian adults and clinical markers associated with CD4 lymphocytopenia. *PLoS One* 8(12):e83270, 2013.

126. Mhmoud NA, Fahal AH, van de Sande WW: CD4+ T-lymphocytopenia in HIV-negative tuberculosis patients in Sudan. *J Infect* 65(4):370–372, 2012.

127. Al-Aska A, Al-Anazi AR, Al-Subaei SS, et al: CD4+ T-lymphopenia in HIV negative tuberculous patients at King Khalid University Hospital in Riyadh, Saudi Arabia. *Eur J Med Res* 16(6):285–288, 2011.

128. Panesar NS: What caused lymphopenia in SARS and how reliable is the lymphokine status in glucocorticoid-treated patients? *Med Hypotheses* 71(2):298–301, 2008.

129. Assiri A, Al-Tawfiq JA, Al-Rabeeah AA, et al: Epidemiological, demographic, and clinical characteristics of 47 cases of Middle East respiratory syndrome coronavirus disease from Saudi Arabia: A descriptive study. *Lancet Infect Dis* 13(9):752–761, 2013.

130. Okada H, Kobune F, Sato TA, et al: Extensive lymphopenia due to apoptosis of uninfected lymphocytes in acute measles patients. *Arch Virol* 145(5):905–920, 2000.

131. Drewry AM, Samra N, Skrupky LP, et al: Persistent lymphopenia after diagnosis of sepsis predicts mortality. *Shock* 42(5):383–391, 2014.

132. Ali S, Shahbaz AU, Nelson MD, et al: Reduced relative lymphocyte count in African-Americans with decompensated heart failure. *Am J Med Sci* 337(3):156–160, 2009.

133. Borroni G, Zaccone C, Vignati G, et al: Lymphopenia and decrease in the total number of circulating CD3+ and CD4+ T cells during "long-term" PUVA treatment for psoriasis. *Dermatologica* 183(1):10–14, 1991.

134. Braat MC, Oosterhuis B, Koopmans RP, et al: Kinetic-dynamic modeling of lymphocytopenia induced by the combined action of dexamethasone and hydrocortisone in humans, after inhalation and intravenous administration of dexamethasone. *J Pharmacol Exp Ther* 262(2):509–515, 1992.

135. Buysmann S, van Diepen FN, Yong SL, et al: Mechanism of lymphocytopenia following administration of corticosteroids. *Transplant Proc* 27(1):871–872, 1995.

136. Bloemena E, Weinreich S, Schellekens PT: The influence of prednisolone on the recirculation of peripheral blood lymphocytes in vivo. *Clin Exp Immunol* 80(3):460–466, 1990.

137. Hauser GJ, Chan MM, Casey WF, et al: Immune dysfunction in children after corrective surgery for congenital heart disease. *Crit Care Med* 19(7):874–881, 1991.

138. Menges P, Kessler W, Kloecker C, et al: Surgical trauma and postoperative immune dysfunction. *Eur Surg Res* 48(4):180–186, 2012.

139. Ueo T, Tanaka S, Tominaga Y, et al: The effect of thoracic duct drainage on lymphocyte dynamics and clinical symptoms in patients with rheumatoid arthritis. *Arthritis Rheum* 22(12):1405–1412, 1979.

140. Strauss RG: Risks of clinically significant thrombocytopenia and/or lymphocytopenia in donors after multiple plateletpheresis collections. *Transfusion* 48(7):1274–1278, 2008.

141. Li C, Mu R, Lu XY, et al: Antilymphocyte antibodies in systemic lupus erythematosus: Association with disease activity and lymphopenia. *J Immunol Res* 2014:672126.

142. Mandl T, Bredberg A, Jacobsson LT, et al: CD4+ T-lymphocytopenia—a frequent finding in anti-SSA antibody seropositive patients with primary Sjogren's syndrome. *J Rheumatol* 2004;31(4):726–728, 2014.

143. Ismail F, Mahmoud A, Abdelhaleem H, et al: Primary Sjögren's syndrome and B-non-Hodgkin lymphoma: Role of CD4+ T lymphocytopenia. *Rheumatol Int* 33(4):1021–1025, 2013.

144. Maldonado MD, Venturoli A, Franco A, Nunez-Roldan A: Specific changes in peripheral blood lymphocyte phenotype from burn patients. Probable origin of the thermal injury-related lymphocytopenia. *Burns* 17(3):188–192, 1991.

145. Vaduganathan M, Ambrosy AP, Greene SJ, et al: Predictive value of low relative lymphocyte count in patients hospitalized for heart failure with reduced ejection fraction: Insights from the EVEREST trial. *Circ Heart Fail* 5(6):750–758, 2012.

146. John E, Laskow TC, Buchser WJ, et al: Zinc in innate and adaptive tumor immunity. *J Transl Med* 8:118.

147. Taylor CG, Giesbrecht JA: Dietary zinc deficiency and expression of T lymphocyte signal transduction proteins. *Can J Physiol Pharmacol* 2000;78(10):823–828, 2010.

148. Heidemann SM, Holubkov R, Meert KL, et al: Baseline serum concentrations of zinc, selenium, and prolactin in critically ill children. *Pediatr Crit Care Med* 14(4):e202–e206, 2013.

149. Kapasi AA, Patel G, Goenka A, et al: Ethanol promotes T cell apoptosis through the mitochondrial pathway. *Immunology* 108(3):313–320, 2003.

150. Soung DY, Devareddy L, Khalil DA, et al: Soy affects trabecular microarchitecture and favorably alters select bone-specific gene expressions in a male rat model of osteoporosis. *Calcif Tissue Int* 78(6):385–391, 2006.

151. Ho DD, Cao Y, Zhu T, et al: Idiopathic CD4+ T-lymphocytopenia—immunodeficiency without evidence of HIV infection. *N Engl J Med* 328(6):380–385, 1993.

152. Smith DK, Neal JJ, Holmberg SD: Unexplained opportunistic infections and CD4+ T-lymphocytopenia without HIV infection. An investigation of cases in the United States. The Centers for Disease Control Idiopathic CD4+ T-lymphocytopenia Task Force. *N Engl J Med* 328(6):373–379, 1993.

153. Zonios DI, Falloon J, Bennett JE, et al: Idiopathic CD4+ lymphocytopenia: Natural history and prognostic factors. *Blood* 112(2):287–294, 2008.

154. al-Attas RA, Rahi AH, Ahmed el FE: Common variable immunodeficiency with CD4+ T lymphocytopenia and overproduction of soluble IL-2 receptor associated with Turner's syndrome and dorsal kyphoscoliosis. *J Clin Pathol* 50(10):876–879, 1997.

155. Regent A, Autran B, Carcelain G, et al: Idiopathic CD4 lymphocytopenia: Clinical and immunologic characteristics and follow-up of 40 patients. *Medicine (Baltimore)* 93(2):61–72, 2014.

156. Said J, Alkhateeb H, Cooper CJ, et al: Idiopathic CD4+ lymphocytopenia in Hispanic male: Case report and literature review. *Int Med Case Rep J* 7:117–120, 2014.

157. Pavic I, Cekinovic D, Begovac J, et al: Cryptococcus neoformans meningoencephalitis in a patient with idiopathic CD4+ T lymphocytopenia. *Coll Antropol* 37(2):619–623, 2013.

158. McBath A, Stafford R, Antony SJ: Idiopathic CD4 lymphopenia associated with neuroinvasive West Nile disease: Case report and review of the literature. *J Infect Public Health* 7(2):170–173, 2014.

159. Delgado-Alvarado M, Sedano MJ, Gonzalez-Quintanilla V, et al: Progressive multifocal leukoencephalopathy and idiopathic CD4 lymphocytopenia. *J Neurol Sci* 327(1–2):75–79, 2013.

160. Gorska MM, Alam R: Consequences of a mutation in the UNC119 gene for T cell function in idiopathic CD4 lymphopenia. *Curr Allergy Asthma Rep* 12(5):396–401, 2012.

161. Gorska MM, Alam R: A mutation in the human Uncoordinated 119 gene impairs TCR signaling and is associated with CD4 lymphopenia. *Blood* 119(6):1399–1406, 2012.

162. Bugault F, Benati D, Mouthon L, et al: Altered responses to homeostatic cytokines in patients with idiopathic CD4 lymphocytopenia. *PLoS One* 8(1):e55570, 2013.

163. Kovacs JA, Lempicki RA, Sidorov IA, Adelsberger JW, Sereti I, Sachau W, et al: Induction of prolonged survival of CD4+ T lymphocytes by intermittent IL-2 therapy in HIV-infected patients. *J Clin Invest* 115(8):2139–2148, 2005.

164. Yoo J, Baumstein D, Kuppachi S, et al: Diffuse infiltrative lymphocytosis syndrome presenting as reversible acute kidney injury associated with Gram-negative bacterial infection in patients with newly diagnosed HIV infection. *Am J Kidney Dis* 57(5):752–755, 2011.

165. Buyukcavci M, Tan H, Keskin Z: Profound lymphocytosis preceding chickenpox. *Pediatr Infect Dis J* 23(7):693.

166. Carmack S, Taddei T, Robert ME, et al: Increased T-cell sinusoidal lymphocytosis in liver biopsies in patients with chronic hepatitis C and mixed cryoglobulinemia. *Am J Gastroenterol* 2008;103(3):705–711, 2004.

167. Jameel T, Mehmood K, Mujtaba G, et al: Changing haematological parameters in dengue viral infections. *J Ayub Med Coll Abbottabad* 24(1):3–6, 2012.

168. Ewalt MD, Abeynayake J, Waggoner JJ, et al: Profound plasmacytosis in a patient with dengue. *Int J Hematol* 98(5):518–519, 2013.

169. Tsaparas YF, Brigden ML, Mathias R, et al: Proportion positive for Epstein-Barr virus, cytomegalovirus, human herpesvirus 6, Toxoplasma, and human immunodeficiency virus types 1 and 2 in heterophile-negative patients with an absolute lymphocytosis or an instrument-generated atypical lymphocyte flag. *Arch Pathol Lab Med* 124(9):1324–1330, 2000.

170. Bernit E, Veit V, Zandotti C, et al: Chronic lymphadenopathies and human herpes virus type 8. *Scand J Infect Dis* 34(8):625–626, 2002.

171. Teggatz JR, Parkin J, Peterson L: Transient atypical lymphocytosis in patients with emergency medical conditions. *Arch Pathol Lab Med* 111(8):712–714, 1987.

172. Carulli G, Lagomarsini G, Azzara A, et al: Expansion of TcRalphabeta+CD3+CD4–CD8– (CD4/CD8 double-negative) T lymphocytes in a case of staphylococcal toxic shock syndrome. *Acta Haematol* 111(3):163–167, 2004.

173. Groom DA, Kunkel LA, Brynes RK, et al: Transient stress lymphocytosis during crisis of sickle cell anemia and emergency trauma and medical conditions. An immunophenotyping study. *Arch Pathol Lab Med* 114(6):570–576, 1990.

174. Rai ME, Muhammad Z, Sarwar J, Qureshi AM: Haematological findings in relation to clinical findings of visceral Leishmaniasis in Hazara Division. *J Ayub Med Coll Abbottabad* 20(3):40–43, 2008.

175. Stray-Pedersen A, Jouanguy E, Crequer A, et al: Compound heterozygous CORO1A mutations in siblings with a mucocutaneous-immunodeficiency syndrome of epidermodysplasia verruciformis-HPV, molluscum contagiosum and granulomatous tuberculoid leprosy. *J Clin Immunol* 34(7):871–890, 2014.

176. Nakaoka H, Kanegane H, Taneichi H, et al: Delayed onset adenosine deaminase deficiency associated with acute disseminated encephalomyelitis. *Int J Hematol* 95(6):692–696, 2012.

177. Poliani PL, Facchetti F, Ravanini M, et al: Early defects in human T-cell development severely affect distribution and maturation of thymic stromal cells: Possible implications for the pathophysiology of Omenn syndrome. *Blood* 114(1):105–108, 2009.

178. Carney EF, Srinivasan V, Moss PA, Taylor AM: Classical ataxia telangiectasia patients have a congenitally aged immune system with high expression of CD95. *J Immunol* 189(1):261–268, 2012.

179. Kainulainen L, Lassila O, Ruuskanen O: Cartilage-hair hypoplasia: Follow-up of immunodeficiency in two patients. *J Clin Immunol* 34(2):256–259, 2014.

180. Akinosoglou K, Melachrinou M, Siagris D, et al: Good's syndrome and pure white cell aplasia complicated by cryptococcus infection: A case report and review of the literature. *J Clin Immunol* 34(3):283–288, 2014.

181. Myers LA, Hershfield MS, Neale WT, Escolar M, Kurtzberg J: Purine nucleoside phosphorylase deficiency (PNP-def) presenting with lymphopenia and developmental delay: Successful correction with umbilical cord blood transplantation. *J Pediatr* 145(5):710–712, 2004.

182. Etzioni A, Benderly A, Rosenthal E, et al: Defective humoral and cellular immune functions associated with veno-occlusive disease of the liver. *J Pediatr* 110(4):549–554, 1987.

183. Solomou EE, Rezvani K, Mielke S, et al: Deficient CD4+ CD25+ FOXP3+ T regulatory cells in acquired aplastic anemia. *Blood* 110(5):1603–1606, 2007.

184. Lederman MM, Funderburg NT, Sekaly RP, et al: Residual immune dysregulation syndrome in treated HIV infection. *Adv Immunol* 119:51–83, 2013.

185. Cunha BA, McDermott BP, Mohan SS: Prognostic importance of lymphopenia in West Nile encephalitis. *Am J Med* 117(9):710–711, 2004.

186. Nagai S, Yoshida A, Kohno K, et al: Peritransplant absolute lymphocyte count as a predictive factor for advanced recurrence of hepatitis C after liver transplantation. *Hepatology* 59(1):35–45, 2014.

187. Boonnak K, Vogel L, Feldmann F, et al: Lymphopenia associated with highly virulent H5N1 virus infection due to plasmacytoid dendritic cell-mediated apoptosis of T cells. *J Immunol* 192(12):5906–5912, 2014.

188. Wollenberg A, Zoch C, Wetzel S, et al: Predisposing factors and clinical features of eczema herpeticum: A retrospective analysis of 100 cases. *J Am Acad Dermatol* 49(2):198–205, 2003.

189. Yoshikawa T, Ihira M, Asano Y, et al: Fatal adult case of severe lymphocytopenia associated with reactivation of human herpesvirus 6. *J Med Virol* 66(1):82–85, 2002.

190. Niino D, Tsukasaki K, Torii K, et al: Human herpes virus 8-negative primary effusion lymphoma with BCL6 rearrangement in a patient with idiopathic CD4 positive T-lymphocytopenia. *Haematologica* 93(1):e21–e23, 2008.

191. Avota E, Gassert E, Schneider-Schaulies S: Measles virus-induced immunosuppression: From effectors to mechanisms. *Med Microbiol Immunol* 199(3):227–237, 2010.

192. Kim SK, Welsh RM: Comprehensive early and lasting loss of memory CD8 T cells and functional memory during acute and persistent viral infections. *J Immunol* 172(5):3139–3150, 2004.

193. Okamura K, Nagata N, Wakamatsu K, et al: Hypoalbuminemia and lymphocytopenia are predictive risk factors for in-hospital mortality in patients with tuberculosis. *Intern Med* 52(4):439–444, 2013.

194. Abdool Gaffar MS, Seedat YK, Coovadia YM, Khan Q: The white cell count in typhoid fever. *Trop Geogr Med* 44(1–2):23–27, 1992.

195. Kemp K, Bruunsgaard H, Skinhoj P, Klarlund Pedersen B: Pneumococcal infections in humans are associated with increased apoptosis and trafficking of type 1 cytokine-producing T cells. *Infect Immun* 70(9):5019–5025, 2002.

196. Jensenius M, Fournier PE, Hellum KB, et al: Sequential changes in hematologic and biochemical parameters in African tick bite fever. *Clin Microbiol Infect* 9(7):678–683, 2003.

197. Ismail N, Walker DH, Ghose P, Tang YW: Immune mediators of protective and pathogenic immune responses in patients with mild and fatal human monocytotropic ehrlichiosis. *BMC Immunol* 13:26, 2012.

198. Schatz DA, Riley WJ, Silverstein JH, Barrett DJ: Long-term immunoregulatory effects of therapy with corticosteroids and anti-thymocyte globulin. *Immunopharmacol Immunotoxicol* 11(2–3):269–287, 1989.

199. Zhang X, Tao Y, Chopra M, et al: Differential reconstitution of T cell subsets following immunodepleting treatment with alemtuzumab (anti-CD52 monoclonal antibody) in patients with relapsing-remitting multiple sclerosis. *J Immunol* 191(12):5867–5874, 2013.

200. Moroff G, Wagner S, Benade L, Dodd RY: Factors influencing virus inactivation and retention of platelet properties following treatment with aminomethyltrimethylpsoralen and ultraviolet A light. *Blood Cells* 18(1):43–54; discussion 54-56, 1992.

201. Wang L, Hong KC, Lin FC, Yang KD: Mycoplasma pneumoniae-associated Stevens-Johnson syndrome exhibits lymphopenia and redistribution of CD4+ T cells. *J Formos Med Assoc* 102(1):55–58, 2003.

202. Hutchinson P, Chadban SJ, Atkins RC, Holdsworth SR: Laboratory assessment of immune function in renal transplant patients. *Nephrol Dial Transplant* 18(5):983–989, 2003.

203. Spary LK, Al-Taei S, Salimu J, et al: Enhancement of T cell responses as a result of synergy between lower doses of radiation and T cell stimulation. *J Immunol* 192(7):3101–3110, 2014.

204. Tayama E, Hayashida N, Oda T, et al: Recovery from lymphocytopenia following extracorporeal circulation: Simple indicator to assess surgical stress. *Artif Organs* 23(8):736–740, 1999.

205. Puissant-Lubrano B, Huynh A, Attal M, Blancher A: Evolution of peripheral blood T lymphocyte subsets after allogenic or autologous hematopoietic stem cell transplantation. *Immunobiology* 219(8):611–618, 2014.

206. Chen P, Sun Q, Huang Y, et al: Blood dendritic cell levels associated with impaired IL-12 production and T-cell deficiency in patients with kidney disease: Implications for post-transplant viral infections. *Transpl Int* 27(10):1069–1076, 2014.

207. Newman K, Owlia MB, El-Hemaidi I, Akhtari M: Management of immune cytopenias in patients with systemic lupus erythematosus-Old and new. *Autoimmun Rev* 12(7):784–791, 2013.

208. Gerli R, Paganelli R, Cossarizza A, et al: Long-term immunologic effects of thymectomy in patients with myasthenia gravis. *J Allergy Clin Immunol* 103(5 Pt 1):865–872, 1999.

209. Goupil R, Brachemi S, Nadeau-Fredette AC, et al: Lymphopenia and treatment-related infectious complications in ANCA-associated vasculitis. *Clin J Am Soc Nephrol* 8(3):416–423, 2013.

210. Venzor J, Hua Q, Bressler RB, et al: Behcet's-like syndrome associated with idiopathic CD4+ T-lymphocytopenia, opportunistic infections, and a large population of TCR alpha beta+ CD4– CD8– T cells. *Am J Med Sci* 313(4):236–238, 1997.

211. Marie I, Menard JF, Hachulla E, et al: Infectious complications in polymyositis and dermatomyositis: A series of 279 patients. *Semin Arthritis Rheum* 41(1):48–60, 2011.

212. Morton M, Edmonds S, Doherty AM, et al: Factors associated with major infections in patients with granulomatosis with polyangiitis and systemic lupus erythematosus treated for deep organ involvement. *Rheumatol Int* 32(11):3373–3382, 2012.

213. Porrata LF, Ristow K, Colgan JP, et al: Peripheral blood lymphocyte/monocyte ratio at diagnosis and survival in classical Hodgkin's lymphoma. *Haematologica* 97(2):262–269, 2012.

214. Mehrazin R, Uzzo RG, Kutikov A, et al: Lymphopenia is an independent predictor of inferior outcome in papillary renal cell carcinoma. *Urol Oncol* 189(2):454–461, 2014. [Epub ahead of print]

215. Cervantes F, Hernandez-Boluda JC, Villamor N, et al: Assessment of peripheral blood lymphocyte subsets in idiopathic myelofibrosis. *Eur J Haematol* 65(2):104–108, 2000.

216. Law ST, Ma KM, Li KK: Clinical characteristics of concurrent and sequentially presented lupus-related protein-losing enteropathy: What are their differences? *Rheumatol Int* 33(1):85–92, 2013.

217. Law ST, Ma KM, Li KK: Protein-losing enteropathy associated with or without systemic autoimmune disease: What are the differences? *Eur J Gastroenterol Hepatol* 24(3):294–302, 2012.

218. Crouser ED, Lozanski G, Fox CC, et al: The CD4+ lymphopenic sarcoidosis phenotype is highly responsive to anti-tumor necrosis factor-α therapy. *Chest* 137(6):1432–1435, 2010.

219. Takeyama Y, Takas K, Ueda T, et al: Peripheral lymphocyte reduction in severe acute pancreatitis is caused by apoptotic cell death. *J Gastrointest Surg* 4(4):379–387, 2000.

220. Kruger K, Mooren FC: Exercise-induced leukocyte apoptosis. *Exerc Immunol Rev* 20:117–134, 2014.

221. Subra JF, Renier G, Reboul P, et al: Lymphopenia in occupational pulmonary silicosis with or without autoimmune disease. *Clin Exp Immunol* 126(3):540–544, 2001.

222. Di Sabatino A, D'Alo S, Millimaggi D, et al: Apoptosis and peripheral blood lymphocyte depletion in coeliac disease. *Immunology* 103(4):435–440, 2001.

CHAPTER 80
IMMUNODEFICIENCY DISEASES

Hans D. Ochs and Luigi D. Notarangelo

SUMMARY

Primary immune deficiency diseases (PIDDs) are characterized by increased susceptibility to infections, often associated with autoimmunity and inflammation and an increased risk of malignancies because of impaired immune homeostasis and surveillance. Depending on the nature of the immune defect, the clinical presentation of PIDD may vary and may include recurrence of upper and lower respiratory tract infections, invasive bacterial infections, purulent lymphadenitis, skin or deep abscesses, infections sustained by poorly virulent or opportunistic pathogens (*Pneumocystis jirovecii*, cytomegalovirus, environmental mycobacteria, *Cryptosporidium*, *Giardia lamblia*), persistent or recurrent candidiasis, narrow susceptibility to a selective type of pathogens, autoimmunity, increased susceptibility to malignancies, and may be associated with typical signs of specific immunodeficiency syndromes.

With the exception of immunoglobulin (Ig) A deficiency and DiGeorge syndrome, PIDDs are generally rare, with a prevalence of approximately 1 in 10,000 to 1 in 50,000 of the general population. However, prompt recognition of PIDD is of importance, because diagnostic delay is associated with increased risk of death and of irreversible complications. Most forms of PIDD follow mendelian inheritance; however, some, like common variable immunodeficiency (CVID), have a multifactorial origin. In most cases, PIDDs present in childhood, but late presentations may occur or even predominate in some forms, such as CVID.

The diagnostic approach to PIDD is based on a detailed family and clinical history, physical examination and appropriate laboratory tests. Lymphopenia is characteristic of severe combined immune deficiency. Abnormalities affecting neutrophils can be observed in patients with disorders of neutrophil production (e.g., congenital neutropenia, leukocyte adhesion deficiency; Chap. 65) or function (e.g., chronic granulomatous disease; Chap. 66), respectively. Evaluation of serum immunoglobulin levels and of antibody responses to immunization antigens is of value for patients with a history of recurrent infections.

Acronyms and Abbreviations: AD, autosomal dominant; ADA, adenosine deaminase; AD-HIES, autosomal dominant hyperimmunoglobulin E syndrome; aHSCs, autologous hematopoietic stem cells; AID, activation-induced cytosine deaminase; AIRE, autoimmune regulator; ALPS, autoimmune lymphoproliferative syndrome; APECED, autoimmune polyendocrinopathy, candidiasis, and ectodermal dystrophy; APS, autoimmune polyglandular syndrome; AR-HIES, autosomal recessive hyperimmunoglobulin syndrome; AT, ataxia-telangiectasia; ATLD, ataxia-telangiectasia–like disorder; ATM, ataxia-telangiectasia mutated; BCG, bacillus Calmette-Guérin; *BLM*, the causative gene of Bloom syndrome; BS, Bloom syndrome; BTK, Bruton tyrosine kinase; C, complement; CARD, caspase recruitment domain-containing protein; CD40L, CD40 ligand; CHARGE, coloboma of the eye, heart defects, atresia of the nasal choanae, retardation of growth and/or development, genital and/or urinary abnormalities, and ear abnormalities and deafness; CID, combined immune deficiency; CMC, chronic mucocutaneous candidiasis; CMV, cytomegalovirus; CSR, class switch recombination; CTL, cytotoxic T lymphocyte; CTLA-4, cytotoxic T-lymphocyte antigen-4; CTPS1, cytidine 5-triphosphate synthase 1; CVID, common variable immunodeficiency; D, diversity; DC, dendritic cell; DGS, DiGeorge syndrome; DOCK8, dedicator of cytokinesis 8; EBV, Epstein-Barr virus; FHL, familial hemophagocytic lymphohistiocytosis; G-CSF, granulocyte colony-stimulating factor; GM-CSF, granulocyte-macrophage colony-stimulating factor; GS2, Griscelli syndrome type 2; HIES, hyperimmunoglobulin E syndrome; HLA, human leukocyte antigen; HLH, hemophagocytic lymphohistiocytosis; HPV, human papillomavirus; HSCT, hematopoietic stem cell transplantation; HSE, herpes simplex virus encephalitis; HSV, herpes simplex virus; IBD, inflammatory bowel disease; ICF, immunodeficiency with centromere instability and facial anomalies; IFN, interferon; Ig, immunoglobulin; IGF-1, insulin-like growth factor 1; IGHM, immunoglobulin heavy constant mu; IGLL1, immunoglobulin lambda-like polypeptide 1; IKK, IκB kinase; IL, interleukin; IL-7R, IL-7 receptor; iNKT, invariant natural killer T cell; IPEX, immune dysregulation, polyendocrinopathy, enteropathy, X-linked; IRAK, IL-1 receptor-associated kinase; IRF8, interferon-regulated factor 8; ISG15, interferon-stimulated gene 15; ITCH, itchy E3 ubiquitin protein ligase; ITK, interleukin-2–inducible T-cell kinase; IVIG, intravenous immunoglobulin; J, joining; JAK3, Janus-associated tyrosine kinase 3; LCK, lymphocyte-specific protein tyrosine kinase; LGL, large granular lymphocytic leukemia; LIG4, DNA ligase IV; LRBA, lipopolysaccharide responsive beige-like anchor; LYST, lysosomal trafficking regulator; MAGT1, magnesium transporter 1; MHC, major histocompatibility complex; MMF, mycophenolate mofetil; MonoMAC, monocytopenia, B-cell and NK-cell lymphopenia associated with mycobacterial, fungal, and viral infections; MSMD, mendelian susceptibility to mycobacterial disease; MyD88, myeloid differentiation factor 88; NBS, Nijmegen breakage syndrome; NEMO, nuclear factor-κB essential modulator; NF, nuclear factor; NK, natural killer; NKT, natural killer T cell; ORAI1, calcium release-activated calcium channel protein 1; PI3K, phosphatidylinositol 3-kinase; PIDD, primary immune deficiency disease; PLDN, pallidin; PMS2, postmeiotic segregation increased 2 *(Saccharomyces cerevisiae)*; PNP, purine nucleoside phosphorylase; *RAG1/2*, recombination activating gene 1/2; RMRP, ribonuclease mitochondrial RNA processing complex; SAP, signaling lymphocyte activation molecule (SLAM)-associated protein; SCID, severe combined immune deficiency; SHM, somatic hypermutation; SLAM, signaling lymphocyte activation molecule; SMARCAL1, switch/sucrose nonfermentable (SWI/SNF)-related matrix-associated actin-dependent regulator of chromatin subfamily A–like protein 1; SNP, single nucleotide polymorphism; STIM1, stromal interaction molecule 1; TAP-1/2, transport-associated protein 1/2; TCR, T-cell receptor; T$_{EMRA}$, T memory; TLR, toll-like receptor; TNF, tumor necrosis factor; TRAF, TRIF-related adaptor molecule; TREC, T-cell–receptor excision circle; TRIF, toll-interleukin 1 receptor domain-containing adaptor-inducing IFN-β; TYK2, tyrosine kinase 2; UNG, uracil N-glycosylase; V, variable; VODI, venoocclusive disease with immunodeficiency; WAS, Wiskott-Aldrich syndrome; WASp, Wiskott-Aldrich syndrome protein; WHIM, warts, hypogammaglobulinemia, infections, myelokathexis; WIP, WASp-interacting protein; WRN, Werner syndrome, RecQ helicase-like; XHIGM, X-linked hyperimmunoglobulin M; XLA, X-linked agammaglobulinemia; XLP1 and XLP2, X-linked lymphoproliferative syndrome types 1 and 2; XLT, X-linked thrombocytopenia; ZAP-70, zeta-associated protein of 70 kDa.

The clinical presentation and the results of these screening evaluations may prompt additional laboratory testing. For instance, patients with a profound hypogammaglobulinemia and a history of recurrent infections should be tested for the presence of circulating B lymphocytes (CD19+ or CD20+ cells), which are absent or markedly reduced in X-linked agammaglobulinemia. On the other hand, early presentation with severe and/or opportunistic infections, especially if associated with lymphopenia, should prompt enumeration of lymphocyte subsets. A severe reduction of circulating CD3+ T cells is typically observed in severe combined immune deficiency, and may be associated with defects of B and/or natural killer cells. Deep bacterial infections, or infections sustained by *Aspergillus*, require evaluation of neutrophil count and function, to identify patients with congenital neutropenia and chronic granulomatous disease, respectively. Invasive recurrent infections sustained by *Neisseria* species are an indication for assessing complement levels and function. The complement component deficiencies may also lead to systemic lupus erythematosus-like features or other autoimmune disorders. Laboratory results should be compared to age-matched control values, as white blood cell counts, lymphocyte subsets, complement components, immunoglobulin levels, and antibody production (especially to polysaccharide antigens) undergo significant changes and progressive maturation in the first years of life. It is important to rule out secondary forms of immunodeficiency, such as human immunodeficiency virus infection, protein loss, and immunodeficiency secondary to use of immunosuppressive drugs, as well as anatomical and/or functional problems (e.g., asplenia) that may lead to increased susceptibility to infections.

Recognition of PIDDs is essential to start optimal therapies at an early age. These include immunoglobulin substitution for patients with antibody deficiency; allogeneic hematopoietic stem cell transplantation for patients with severe combined immune deficiency; and in some cases, gene therapy or enzyme replacement therapy may be considered. Antimicrobial prophylaxis and aggressive treatment of infections is necessary in most cases of PIDD. Some patients with significant immune dysregulation may benefit from immunosuppressive therapy.

This chapter focuses on defects that primarily affect T and B lymphocytes, the complement system, and innate immunity. It discusses specific immunodeficiency syndromes, reviews etiology and pathogenesis, clinical and laboratory features, treatment, and prognosis. Chapters 65 and 66 discuss in detail disorders of neutrophil number and function.

● PREDOMINANT ANTIBODY DEFICIENCIES

X-LINKED AND AUTOSOMAL RECESSIVE AGAMMAGLOBULINEMIA

Definition and Genetic Features

X-linked agammaglobulinemia (XLA) is the prototypic antibody deficiency characterized by profound hypogammaglobulinemia caused by a maturation defect in B-cell development.[1,2] XLA, originally described in 1953, is one of the first primary immunodeficiencies in which the underlying defect, a mutation of Bruton tyrosine kinase (BTK) was identified. Autosomal recessive agammaglobulinemia, a variant form of agammaglobulinemia, has been reported in patients with a clinical phenotype resembling XLA including very low B-cell numbers and severe

bacterial infections but normal BTK.[2] Several responsible gene mutations have been identified, including those involving the B-cell receptor complex μ heavy chain (immunoglobulin heavy constant mu [IGHM]), the surrogate light chain component λ5 (immunoglobulin lambda-like polypeptide 1 [IGLL1]), the signal transducer complex of the pre–B-cell receptors immunoglobulin (Ig) α (CD79a), Igβ (CD79b), and mutations in the B-cell adaptor molecule BLINK, the p85α subunit of phosphatidylinositol 3-kinase (PI3K)[3] and a dominant negative E47 mutation causing autosomal dominant agammaglobulinemia.[4]

Clinical Features

Because IgG is actively transported across the placenta, infants born with XLA have normal levels of IgG at birth and are frequently asymptomatic for the first few months of life. Following metabolism of the maternal antibodies, affected boys begin to develop recurrent infections usually between 4 and 12 months of age. In a review of 96 XLA patients, 20 percent experienced initial clinical symptoms after their first birthday and approximately 10 percent after 18 months of age.[5] In an Italian study of 73 patients with mutation-verified XLA, the mean age of onset of symptoms was 2 years.[6] The presenting symptoms vary greatly and may be mild or severe (Table 80–1). Otitis media and chronic sinusitis, pneumonia, pyoderma, and diarrhea are frequent clinical presentations. Serious complications include septicemia, meningitis, septic arthritis, and osteomyelitis. In young children with XLA, acute infections are often associated with neutropenia. Pyogenic bacteria, such as *Haemophilus influenzae*, *Streptococcus pneumoniae*, and *Staphylococcus aureus* are the most common pathogens observed in XLA. Opportunistic infections, such as *Pneumocystis jirovecii*, are rarely observed. Infections with *Ureaplasma urealyticum* have been reported in XLA patients with mycoplasma arthritis.[7] Although resistance to viral infections is generally intact, XLA patients are unusually susceptible to enteroviruses such as echovirus, coxsackievirus, and poliovirus. Poliomyelitis after live-attenuated (Sabin) poliovirus vaccine, especially if given at a time when maternal antibodies had disappeared, is associated with high morbidity and mortality.[5] Before the introduction of intravenous immunoglobulin (IVIG), XLA patients frequently developed chronic, disseminated echovirus and coxsackievirus infections presenting as meningoencephalitis, dermatomyositis/fasciitis, and hepatitis.[8] Gastroenteritis caused by *Giardia lamblia*, *Campylobacter* species, or rotavirus is not uncommon and may be associated with malabsorption. Chronic intestinal inflammation resembling Crohn disease may develop in children and adults with XLA. Interestingly, an increased incidence of rectosigmoid cancer with high mortality has been reported.[9] Pyoderma gangrenosum-like ulcers of the lower extremities have been observed to be caused by *Helicobacter* species.[10]

Laboratory Features

Most patients have markedly reduced levels of all classes of immunoglobulins; circulating B cells are less than 1 percent of total lymphocytes and tonsils are absent. Because of the maturation arrest at the pre–B-cell stage, very few B cells undergo differentiation into plasma cells. As a result, lymph nodes, lymphoid follicles, germinal centers, and intestinal mucosal biopsies lack plasma cells. As expected, specific antibodies to microorganisms or vaccines are markedly reduced or undetectable (Table 80–2).

BTK, a cytoplasmic protein tyrosine kinase known to interact with other cytoplasmic proteins, plays an important role in the pre–B-cell expansion and the survival of mature B cells by facilitating signaling through the B-cell antigen receptor. BTK is present in all hematopoietic cells except T cells, natural killer (NK) cells, and plasma cells. The presence of BTK in normal monocytes and platelets allows assessment of BTK in most XLA patients with low or absent

TABLE 80–1. Principal Clinical Features of Primary Immunodeficiency Disorders

Neutrophil Numerical or Functional Defects (See Chaps. 65, 66)	Antibody Deficiencies	Combined Immune Deficiencies	Complement Deficiencies
Severe bacterial and fungal infections	Recurrent bacterial infections after 4 to 6 months of age	Early onset respiratory and gut infections (bacterial, viral, fungal)	Recurrent or severe infections sustained by encapsulated pathogens
Skin or deep bacterial and fungal abscesses	Intestinal Giardia lamblia infection	Opportunistic infections	Recurrent Neisseria meningitidis infections
Infections sustained by unusual bacteria and fungi		Persistent candidiasis	
	Enteroviral meningoencephalitis	Erythroderma	Autoimmune manifestations (systemic lupus erythematosus-like)
Colitis		Growth failure	
			Atypical hemolyticuremic syndrome
			Recurrent angioedema (C1-INH deficiency)

BTK levels using flow cytometry, and to identify carrier females.[11] Sequence analysis of the *BTK* gene confirms the diagnosis of XLA and allows prenatal diagnosis. Autosomal recessive (and dominant) forms of agammaglobulinemia are rare and require sequence analysis of the genes listed above.

Treatment

Intravenous or subcutaneous IgG infusions at a dose of 400 to 600 mg/kg every 3 to 4 weeks are highly effective in preventing chronic infections in agammaglobulinemic patients. Prophylactic antibiotics are indicated in those with chronic lung disease. Adequate IVIG replacement has markedly reduced the incidence of enteroviral infections, but other complications, such as Crohn-like disease, are difficult to prevent, and progressive neurodegeneration has been observed in a small number of XLA patients without identification of an infectious agent.[12]

HYPERIMMUNOGLOBULIN M SYNDROMES

Definition and Genetic Abnormalities

Hyper-IgM syndromes are characterized by recurrent infections associated with low serum levels of IgG, IgA, and IgE, but normal or increased levels of IgM (see Table 80–2). They are the direct result of mutations affecting genes involved in B-cell activation, class switch recombination (CSR), and somatic hypermutation (SHM). Mutations in the genes encoding CD40 ligand (CD40L) or CD40 interfere with the triggering of events that lead to CSR and SHM. Mutations in the B-cell intrinsic enzymes, activation-induced cytosine deaminase (AID) and uracil N-glycosylase (UNG), directly affect CSR and SHM. Mutations in the *NEMO* gene (nuclear factor [NF]-κB essential modulator), a protein crucial for NF-κB activation, cause clinical features of anhydrotic ectodermal dysplasia with associated immune deficiency in males and incontinentia pigmenti in females.[13] A novel B-cell–intrinsic CSR deficiency characterized by susceptibility to malignancies was found to be associated with mutations in the gene encoding the postmeiotic segregation increased 2 (*Saccharomyces cerevisiae*) (PMS2) component of the mismatch repair machinery.[14] A subset of patients with ataxia telangiectasia present with elevated serum IgM and CSR deficiency.[15]

X-Linked Hyperimmunoglobulin M as a Result of CD40 Ligand Deficiency

Clinical Features In addition to recurrent bacterial infections, affected infants with X-linked hyperimmunoglobulin M (XHIGM) often present with interstitial pneumonia caused by *P. jirovecii* approximately 50 percent of affected males will develop neutropenia.[16] Patients with XHIGM are at high risk of developing chronic *Cryptosporidium* infections complicated by ascending cholangiolitis and chronic liver disease. Progressive neurodegeneration in XHIGM patients similar to those with XLA has been reported.[12] Abortive germinal center formation and severe depletion of follicular dendritic cells of lymph nodes occurs. Affected patients are at risk to develop neoplasms, most often lymphomas, but also tumors of the biliary and gastrointestinal tract,[17] which are rarely observed in other primary immunodeficiencies.

Laboratory Features Circulating lymphocyte subsets are present in normal numbers but B cells are predominantly naïve and few are of the switched memory B-cell subtype (IgD−, IgM− CD27+).[18] Lymphocyte proliferation in response to mitogens is normal, but responses to specific antigens are often reduced.[19] XHIGM is caused by mutations in CD40L, a surface protein expressed by activated CD4+ lymphocytes. CD40L interacts with the CD40 membrane protein constitutively expressed by B cells, macrophages, and dendritic cells (DCs). The interaction of CD40L/CD40 sets in motion a signaling event that results in the expression of AID and UNG, and induces CSR and SHM. Mutations in CD40L are distributed throughout the gene and may result in nonfunctional or absent protein.[16] Several patients with mild cases of XHIGM not treated with IVIG have developed chronic pure red cell aplasia as a result of persistent parvovirus B19 infection.[20]

Treatment Prophylactic treatment with trimethoprim-sulfamethoxazole is indicated during infancy and childhood to prevent *P. jirovecii* pneumonia. Intravenous or subcutaneous immunoglobulin at doses similar to patients with XLA is used to prevent chronic infections, including parvovirus B19. Exposure to *Cryptosporidium* should be prevented by avoiding the use of potentially contaminated water. Because of the high incidence of serious complications and the unfavorable long-term outcome,[21] allogeneic stem cell transplantation should be considered if an optimal donor can be identified. Severe and persistent neutropenia may

TABLE 80–2. Common Adaptive Immunodeficiencies: Laboratory and Clinical Features*

	Lymphocytes*			Cellular Immunity	Humoral Immunity Serum Immunoglobulins (Ig)				Antibody Responses	Common Infections
	B	T	NK		M	G	A	E		
Predominantly antibody deficiencies										
X-linked agammaglobulinemia BTK deficiency	−	+	+	+	↓	↓	↓	↓	−	Bacteria, *Giardia lamblia*
Autosomal recessive agammaglobulinemia										
λ5, Igα, Igβ, BLNK, p85α, E47 deficiency	−	+	+	+	↓	↓	↓	↓	−	Bacteria
Transient hypogamma-globulinemia of infancy	+	+	+	+	N/↓	N/↓	N/↓	N/↓	+/−	Bacteria
Selective IgA deficiency	+	+	+	+	N	N	↓	N	+/−	Bacteria, *G. lamblia*
Common variable immune deficiency (CVID)	+	+	+	+	N/↓	↓	↓	↓	−	Bacteria, *G. lamblia*
Hyper-IgM syndromes										
CD40 ligand deficiency (X-linked)	+	+	+	+/−	N/↑	↓	↓	↓	+/−	Bacteria, viruses, fungi
CD40 deficiency	+	+	+	+	N/↑	↓	↓	↓	+/−	Bacteria, viruses, fungi
Activation-induced cytidine deaminase deficiency (AID)	+	+	+	+	N/↑	↓	↓	↓	+/−	Bacteria
Uracil-DNA glycosylase deficiency (UNG)	+	+	+	+	N/↑	↓	↓	↓	+/−	Bacteria
X-linked NF-κB Essential Modulator (NEMO) deficiency, due to mutations in *IKBKG*	+	+	+	+	N/↑	↓	↓	↓	+/−	Bacteria, viruses, fungi
Severe combined immunodeficiencies (SCID)										
Interleukin receptor γ-chain deficiency (X-linked SCID)	+	−	−	−	N	↓	↓	↓	−	Bacteria, viruses, fungi
Janus-associated kinase 3 (JAK3) deficiency	+	−	−	−	N	↓	↓	↓	−	Bacteria, viruses, fungi
Interleukin-7 receptor α-chain deficiency	+	−	+	−	N	↓	↓	↓	−	Bacteria, viruses, fungi
ZAP-70 tyrosine kinase deficiency	+	+/−	+	−	N	N/↓	N/↓	N/↓	+/−	Bacteria, viruses, fungi
Adenosine deaminase (ADA) deficiency	−	−	−	−	↓	↓	↓	↓	−	Bacteria, viruses, fungi
Purine nucleotide phosphorylase (PNP) deficiency	+	−	+	−	N	↓	↓	↓	+/−	Bacteria, viruses, fungi
Recombinase activating genes (RAG 1/2) deficiency	−	−	+	−	↓	↓	↓	↓	−	Bacteria, viruses, fungi
Artemis deficiency	−	−	+	−	↓	↓	↓	↓	−	Bacteria, viruses, fungi
Reticular dysgenesis (AK2 deficiency)	−	−	−	−	↓	↓	↓	↓	−	Bacteria, viruses, fungi
Primary T-cell deficiencies										
Congenital thymic aplasia (DiGeorge syndrome)	+	−	+	+/−	N	N	N	N	+/−	Bacteria, viruses, fungi

(Continued)

TABLE 80-2. Common Adaptive Immunodeficiencies: Laboratory and Clinical Features* (Continued)

| | Lymphocytes* | | | | Humoral Immunity | | | | | |
| | | | | Cellular Immunity | Serum Immunoglobulins (Ig) | | | | Antibody Responses | Common Infections |
	B	T	NK		M	G	A	E		
MHC class II deficiency	+	+/−	+	+	N/↓	↓	N/↓	↓	+/−	Bacteria, viruses, fungi
TAP-1, TAP-2 deficiency (MHC class I deficiency)	+	+/−	+/−	+/−	N	N	N	N	+/−	Bacteria, viruses, fungi
Other well-defined immunodeficiency syndromes										
Ataxia-telangiectasia	+	+	+	+/−	N/↑	N/↓	N/↓	↓	+/−	Bacteria
Wiskott-Aldrich syndrome	+	+/−	+	+/−	↓	N	↑	↑	+/−	Bacteria
Hyper IgE Syndromes										
STAT3 deficiency (AD)	+/−	+	+	+/−	N	N	N	↑↑	+/−	Staph, Candida
DOCK8 deficiency (AR)	+/−	+/−	+/−	+/−	↓	N	N	↑↑	+/−	Candida, viruses, fungi
GATA 2 deficiency (AD)	−	+	−	+/−	N	N	N	N	+/−	Atypical mycobacteria, viruses, fungi
IPEX, IPEX-like	+	(lack of Tregs)	+	+	N	N	↑	↑	+	Autoimmunity, Staph, Candida, CMV

*Natural killer lymphocytes (NK), T cells (T), B cells (B).

Normal levels (+), reduced or absent levels (−); normal (N), elevated (↑), or reduced (↓) serum immunoglobulins.

require treatment with granulocyte colony-stimulating factor (G-CSF), at least on a temporary basis.

Autosomal Recessive Hyperimmunoglobulin M with CD40 Mutations

Autosomal recessive hyperimmunoglobulin M caused by mutations in CD40 have been reported, mostly in consanguineous families.[16,22] Affected members have similar clinical and laboratory findings as those with CD40L mutations. Treatment and prognosis of CD40 deficiency is similar to XHIGM.

Autosomal Recessive Hyperimmunoglobulin M Syndrome Caused by an Intrinsic B-Cell Defect

Definition AID is expressed only in B cells undergoing CSR or SHM and is thought to affect DNA editing.[23] Because of milder symptoms, the diagnosis of AID deficiency is often established later in life.

Clinical Features AID-deficient patients present with recurrent bacterial infections, mostly affecting the upper and lower respiratory tract. In contrast to patients with XHIGM, AID-deficient individuals have an excellent long-term prognosis, especially if given IVIG prophylaxis. Most affected individuals present with striking lymphoid hyperplasia involving tonsils and lymph nodes as a result of marked follicular hyperplasia. The number of circulating T- and B-cell subsets are normal, including normal proportion of memory B cells; however, all CD27+ memory B cells fail to isotype switch and only express IgM and IgD. Mutations of *AID* affect the entire gene and include missense, nonsense mutations, and small deletions.

UNG is expressed in proliferating cells, including B cells undergoing CSR. Following AID-induced deamination of cytosine into uracil residues on single-stranded DNA, UNG deglycosylates and removes uracil residues, thus leading to a single-stranded DNA break. The repair of the DNA nick leads to successful CSR and SHM. Because AID and UNG are functionally closely linked, lack of UNG results in a clinical phenotype similar to AID deficiency. The three UNG deficient patients reported to date have a history of frequent bacterial infections, lymphadenopathy, and an excellent response to IVIG therapy.[23]

X-Linked Anhydrotic Ectodermal Dysplasia with Immunodeficiency Caused by Mutations in Nuclear Factor-κB Essential Modulator

Definition Anhydrotic (or hypohidrotic) ectodermal dysplasia is a rare syndrome with partial or complete absence of sweat glands, sparse hair growth, and abnormal dentition. A subset of these patients has an X-linked mode of inheritance and immunodeficiency characterized by low-serum IgG levels, variably elevated IgM levels, and decreased antibody responses. This syndrome results from mutations in the *IKBKG* gene encoding NEMO, a key subunit of I-κB kinase that regulates NF-κB dimerization and nuclear transfer.[24] Most affected boys have a hypomorphic NEMO mutation that allows some function, and present with bacterial (*S. pneumoniae, S. aureus*) and often atypical mycobacterial infections. Loss-of-function mutations cause the X-linked dominant condition of incontinentia pigmenti in females and are embryonically lethal in males. A similar phenotype with autosomal dominant inheritance is caused by gain-of-function mutations in *IKBA*.[25]

Clinical Features A review of 72 individuals with NEMO mutations has demonstrated a wide spectrum of clinical phenotypes.[26] Thirty-two different mutations of NEMO were identified, with 70 percent being associated with ectodermal dysplasia, 86 percent with serious pyogenic infections, 39 percent with mycobacterial infections, 19 percent with serious viral infections, and 21 percent with inflammatory bowel disease. One-third of this cohort of NEMO patients died prematurely (mean age: 6.4 years).

Treatment Treatment with IVIG is useful but does not prevent the occurrence of serious complications. Symptomatic treatment depends on those complications.

COMMON VARIABLE IMMUNODEFICIENCY AND SELECTIVE IMMUNOGLOBULIN A DEFICIENCY

Definition

Common variable immunodeficiency (CVID) is a clinically and molecularly heterogeneous disorder, presenting at any age, but most often during adulthood. CVID is characterized by recurrent bacterial infections, hypogammaglobulinemia, and impaired antibody responses. Together with selective IgA deficiency, CVID is the most common primary immune deficiency, with an incidence of 1 in 10,000 individuals. Familial inheritance is observed in approximately 20 percent of cases and CVID and IgA deficiency may be present in the same families. In rare instances, patients with selective IgA deficiency may progress to CVID. Attempts have been made to associate CVID and IgA deficiency with genes located within the major histocompatibility complex (MHC) region on chromosome 6; however, no specific genes within this region have been identified. A small proportion of patients with CVID have been molecularly defined as having mutations in several genes involved directly or indirectly with B-cell differentiation, including *ICOS*, *TACI*, *BAFF*-receptor, CD19, CD20, CD21, and CD81.[27] The recent discovery of CVID-like phenotypes resulting from heterozygous mutations in NF-κB2[28,29] and gain-of-function mutations in PI3Kδ,[30] and CVID with autosomal recessive inheritance as a result of mutations in protein kinase Cδ[31] further support the idea that CVID is a heterogeneous primary immune deficiency disease (PIDD) with strong genetic roots. In addition, patients with mutations in BTK, CD40L, and SH2D1A have been mistakenly diagnosed as CVID.

Clinical Features and Treatment of Common Variable Immunodeficiency

The majority of CVID patients present with recurring sinopulmonary infections, most often bacterial pneumonia.[27,32] If the diagnosis is delayed or if treatment is inadequate, bronchiectasis and chronic lung disease may develop. Gastrointestinal complaints are frequent and may be caused by chronic *G. lamblia* or *Campylobacter* infections, resembling chronic inflammatory bowel disease. Lymphoid hyperplasia of the small bowel is a frequent finding. Autoimmune disorders are common and may resemble rheumatoid arthritis, dermatomyositis, or scleroderma. In addition, CVID patients may develop autoimmune hemolytic anemia, autoimmune thrombocytopenia, autoimmune neutropenia, pernicious anemia, and chronic active hepatitis. Lymphadenopathy and splenomegaly are common, the result of follicular hyperplasia. Caseating granulomas of the lung, spleen, liver, skin, and other tissues may develop at any age, and a condition resembling sarcoidosis has been described. The cause of this devastating granuloma formation is unknown. A high incidence of lymphoma and gastrointestinal malignancies have been reported in older CVID patients,[33] with a 438-fold increase in the risk of lymphomas in affected women during the fifth and sixth decades.[34] Despite normal numbers of blood B lymphocytes and the presence of lymphoid cortical follicles, CVID patients have hypogammaglobulinemia that may be as profound as in XLA (see Table 80–2). Antibody responses to recall and to neoantigens are diminished and some CVID patients have decreased numbers of memory B cells, especially of switched memory B cells. A subset of CVID patients have a substantial T-cell deficiency characterized by decreased expression of CD40L by activated CD4+ T cells (without a mutation of CD40L) and by reversed CD4:CD8 ratio. Treatment with IVIG substitution and prophylactic antibiotics is beneficial but often insufficient to prevent serious complications. Allogeneic hematopoietic stem cell transplantation (HSCT) is generally not recommended, except in patients with lymphoid malignancies. There is a rare association between immune

deficiency and thymoma, which is estimated to be present in 4 percent of patients with hypogammaglobulinemia.[35]

Clinical Features and Treatment of Selective Immunoglobulin A Deficiency

The incidence of selective IgA deficiency, defined as IgA less than 5 to 10 mg/dL, differs greatly between ethnic groups, being highest in Scandinavia (1 in 396 in a Finnish study)[36] and lowest in Asian populations (1 in 14,000 in Japan).[37] Because secretory IgA is considered to be most important in protecting mucus surfaces, it is surprising that most IgA-deficient patients remain healthy. Other defense systems, for example, noncirculatory IgM or neutrophils, may compensate for this deficiency. Symptomatic individuals are not only IgA deficient, but often have deficient antibody responses to specific antigens. IgA deficiency may be associated with IgG$_2$ and IgG$_3$ deficiency and poor responses to polysaccharide antigens.[38] Selective IgA deficiency, if associated with symptoms, often leads to recurrent sinopulmonary infections and atopic symptoms including allergic conjunctivitis, rhinitis, and eczema. Food allergy may be more common in IgA-deficient patients and asthma associated with IgA deficiency appears to be more refractory to therapy. Gastrointestinal tract disorders include chronic giardiasis, malabsorption, celiac disease, primary biliary cirrhosis, pernicious anemia, and nodular lymphoid hyperplasia. A number of autoimmune diseases are associated with selective IgA deficiency, including rheumatoid arthritis, systemic lupus erythematous, thyroiditis, myasthenia gravis, and ulcerative colitis.

A significant proportion of IgA-deficient individuals has anti-IgA antibodies in their serum and may react to blood products containing IgA, including IVIG preparations with low IgA content. However, patients with selective IgA deficiency who make normal IgG antibody do not need IVIG therapy.

The fundamental defect in selective IgA deficiency is the failure of IgA-bearing B lymphocytes to mature into IgA-secreting plasma cells. There is no specific treatment that would correct this problem. Intermittent or continuous prophylactic antibiotics may be helpful in patients with recurrent respiratory tract infections, who develop chronic symptoms of lung disease. On the other hand, if IgA deficiency is associated with poor antibody responses to selected antigens, for example, to polysaccharides, an attempt with IVIG substitution should be made.

LIPOPOLYSACCHARIDE RESPONSIVE BEIGE-LIKE ANCHOR DEFICIENCY

Lipopolysaccharide responsive beige-like anchor (LRBA) is a broadly expressed, cytosolic protein involved in endocytosis of ligand-activated receptors. LRBA deficiency is inherited as an autosomal recessive trait and is characterized by recurrent bacterial and viral infections, and prominent autoimmune manifestations, cytopenias, and inflammatory bowel disease, in particular.[39,40] Hypothyroidism and myasthenia gravis have been also reported. Immunologic abnormalities include progressive hypogammaglobulinemia, impaired activation and decreased survival of T and B lymphocytes, reduced number of marginal zone-like and switched memory B cells, and defective autophagy.

● SEVERE COMBINED IMMUNODEFICIENCIES

DEFINITION AND HISTORY

The first description of severe combined immunodeficiencies (SCIDs) dates back to 1950, when Glanzmann and Riniker described infants

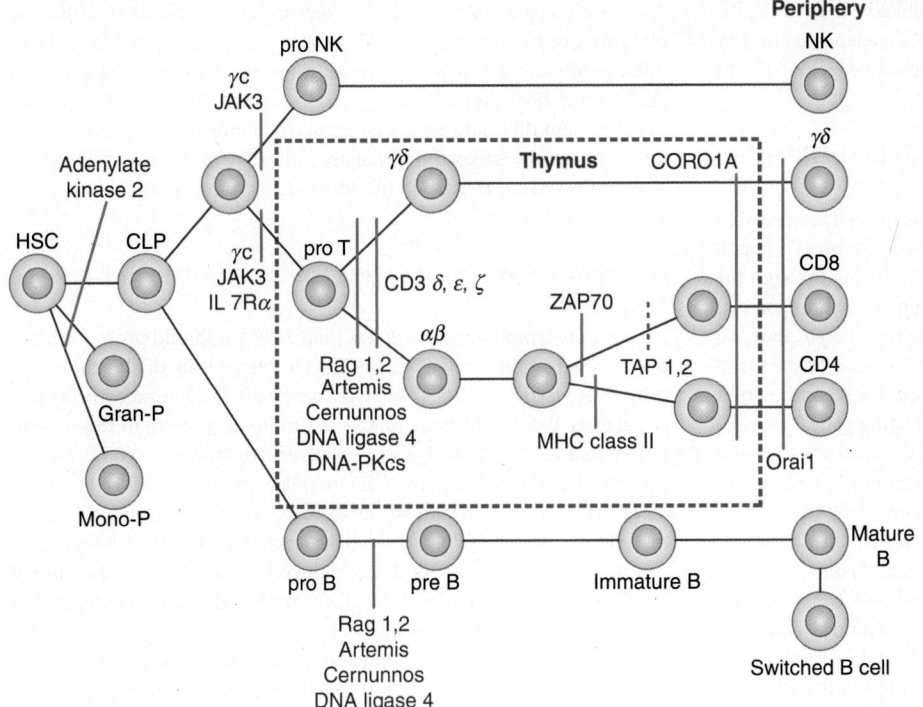

Figure 80–1. Disruption of the normal T-cell development by mutations of genes known to cause a severe combined immunodeficiency disease phenotype. B, B lymphocyte; CLP, common lymphocyte progenitor; γc, common gamma; Gran-P, granulocyte progenitor; HSC, hematopoietic stem cell; JAK3, Janus-associated tyrosine kinase 3; MHC, major histocompatibility complex; Mono-P, monocyte progenitor; NK, natural kill lymphocyte; ORAI1, calcium release-activated calcium channel protein 1; T, T lymphocyte; TAP-1/2, transport-associated protein 1/2; ZAP70, zeta-associated protein of 70 kDa.

who died with overwhelming infections, intractable diarrhea, thrush, and profound lymphophenia.[41] The SCID phenotype represents a heterogeneous group of genetic disorders that are characterized by a severe impairment of T-lymphocyte development and function (Fig. 80–1).[42–44] Depending on whether the development of B and/or NK lymphocytes is also affected, SCID can be classified into four distinct immunologic phenotypes: (1) T⁻B⁺NK⁻ SCID (the most common variant); (2) T⁻B⁺NK⁺ SCID; (3) T⁻B⁻NK⁺ SCID; or (4) T⁻B⁻NK⁻ SCID (see Table 80–2). The term *combined immune deficiency* (CID) is used to define disorders with residual development and/or function of T lymphocytes. Unless treated by allogeneic HSCT or, in selected cases, by gene therapy or enzyme replacement therapy, SCID is inevitably fatal.

MOLECULAR DEFECTS AND PATHOGENESIS OF SEVERE COMBINED IMMUNE DEFICIENCY

SCIDs are mendelian disorders, and their overall prevalence is estimated to be approximately 1 in 50,000 births. In Western countries, the most common form of SCID is inherited as an X-linked trait; however, a variety of autosomal recessive forms are also known. SCID can be grouped in different categories that illustrate the various pathogenetic mechanisms involved in T-cell development.

Severe Combined Immune Deficiency as a Result of Increased Apoptosis of Lymphocyte Precursors

Adenosine Deaminase Deficiency Approximately 5 to 10 percent of infants with SCID have a deficiency of adenosine deaminase (ADA), the enzyme that converts adenosine and deoxyadenosine into inosine and deoxyinosine, respectively.[45] In the absence of ADA, high intracellular levels of adenosine, deoxyadenosine, and their toxic phosphorylated metabolites cause apoptosis of lymphoid precursors, and hence result in the virtual absence of T lymphocytes, that is usually associated with marked reduction of B and NK lymphocytes (T⁻B⁻NK⁻SCID).[46] ADA-SCID is inherited as an autosomal recessive trait, and its clinical manifestations extend beyond the immune system, reflecting the fact that ADA is a general housekeeping enzyme.

Purine Nucleoside Phosphorylase Deficiency Purine nucleoside phosphorylase (PNP) is another enzyme of the purine salvage pathway. PNP catalyzes the phosphorylation of inosine, guanosine, and deoxyguanosine.[45] In the absence of PNP, high intracellular levels of deoxyguanosine triphosphatase cause lymphoid and neuronal toxicity. Immature thymocytes are particularly susceptible to PNP deficiency. Accordingly, the immunologic phenotype of PNP deficiency is characterized by decreased T-cell counts, whereas B and NK lymphocytes are often unaffected.[47] PNP deficiency accounts for 1 to 2 percent of all forms of SCID, and is inherited as an autosomal recessive trait.

Adenylate Kinase 2 Deficiency Another rare variant of autosomal recessive SCID, reticular dysgenesis, is characterized by extreme lymphopenia, absence of neutrophils, and sensorineural deafness.[48] The disease is caused by mutations of adenylate kinase 2 that result in apoptosis of myeloid precursors of neutrophils, and of lymphoid progenitor cells.[49,50]

Severe Combined Immune Deficiency as a Result of Defects of Cytokine-Mediated Signaling

Thymic T-cell progenitors depend on interleukin (IL)-7 for cell proliferation. The IL-7 receptor (IL-7R) is composed of an α chain (encoded by the *IL7R* gene) and a common γ chain (γc), that is shared also by IL-2R, IL-4R, IL-9R, IL-15R, and IL-21R,[51] and is encoded by the *IL2RG* gene, located on the X chromosome. Cytokine-mediated signaling through γc—containing receptors involves activation of Janus-associated tyrosine kinase 3 (JAK3).[51] In humans, defects of IL-7–mediated signaling abrogate T-cell development, whereas impaired signaling through IL-15R affects development of NK cells.[51] X-linked SCID, caused by *IL2RG* mutations,[52] represents approximately 30 percent of all cases of SCID, and is characterized by lack of T and NK lymphocytes but normal development of B cells (T⁻B⁺NK⁻ SCID). B-lymphocyte function, however, is severely compromised by both the lack of T-cell help and nonfunctional γc. JAK3 deficiency is inherited as an autosomal recessive trait, and its phenotype is identical to that of X-linked SCID (T⁻B⁺NK⁻ SCID).[53,54] In contrast, autosomal recessive IL-7R deficiency caused by mutation of the α chain is characterized by the selective lack of T cells (T⁻B⁺NK⁺ SCID).[55]

Severe Combined Immune Deficiency as a Result of Defective Signaling Through the T-Cell Receptor

One of the distinctive features of developing thymocytes is the expression of the pre–T-cell receptor (TCR), that is composed of a pre-Tα chain, a TCRβ chain, and the CD3 γ, δ, ε, and ζ chains. Signaling through the pre-TCR permits rearrangement of the TCRα chain and expression of a mature TCRαβ. Alternatively, thymocytes may express the γδ chains of the TCR. Rearrangement of the TCR loci is accomplished by means of the V(D)J recombination, whereby the lymphoid specific recombination activating gene 1 (*RAG1*) and recombination activating gene 2 (*RAG2*) proteins mediate DNA cleavage at the variable (V), diversity (D), and joining (J) elements of the TCR loci. The DNA double-strand break of the coding ends is initially sealed as a hairpin, followed by nonhomologous endjoining via the nuclease Artemis (encoded by the *DCLRE1C* gene). Eventually, joining of coding (and signal) elements is mediated by a series of proteins, that include the Ku70/80 heterodimer, XRCC4, DNA ligase IV (LIG4), DNA-protein kinase catalytic subunit, and Cernunnos/ XLF. Defects in V(D)J recombination affect both T- and B-cell development and hence cause T⁻B⁻NK⁺ SCID, because this process is also essential to mediate rearrangement of the immunoglobulin genes, a key step in B-cell development. RAG1 or RAG2 deficiencies account for 3 to 20 percent of all SCID cases in different series.[42,56] Artemis (*DCLRE1C*),[57] DNA-protein kinase catalytic subunit,[58] LIG4,[59,60] and Cernunnos/ XLF[61] deficiencies are less frequent and their cellular and clinical phenotypes extend beyond impaired T- and B-cell development, because enzymes that mediate DNA double-strand break repair are ubiquitously expressed, and their deficiency results in increased cellular radiosensitivity.[57–61] The phenotype of LIG4 deficiency can be extremely variable, from T⁻B⁻NK⁺ SCID to mild or no immunodeficiency, whereas Cernunnos/XLF deficiency is characterized by significant T-cell lymphopenia and progressive decrease in the number of B cells.

Defects of the CD3 δ, ε, or ζ chains affect signaling through the pre-TCR and the TCR and hence cause autosomal recessive T⁻B⁺NK⁺ SCID.[62–64] In contrast, CD3γ deficiency is associated with mild T-cell lymphopenia and a variable clinical phenotype.[65,66]

Mutations of the TCRα constant (*TCRA*) gene cause impaired differentiation of T cells expressing TCRαβ.[67]

Mutations of CD45, a pan-leukocyte tyrosine phosphatase that has been implicated in signaling through the TCR and the B-cell receptor, have been reported in few patients with T⁻B⁺NK⁺ SCID.[68,69]

Clinical Features of Severe Combined Immunodeficiency Syndrome

Despite genetic heterogeneity, SCID is characterized by a consistent clinical phenotype. Interstitial pneumonia, often sustained by *P. jirovecii*, cytomegalovirus (CMV), adenovirus, parainfluenza 3 virus, respiratory syncytial virus, chronic diarrhea, failure to thrive, and persistent candidiasis are common features (see Table 80–1). Typically, infections develop in the first months of life. Skin manifestations (maculopapular rash, erythroderma, alopecia) are also common, especially in infants with maternal T-cell engraftment. Hypoplastic lymphoid tissue (tonsils, lymph nodes), and absence of a thymic shadow on chest radiography are characteristic.[70]

Because of the inability to control replication of live microorganisms, administration of live-attenuated vaccines often leads to severe, life-threatening complications in infants with SCID.[71]

T-cell engraftment derived from maternal cells that cross the placenta occurs in more than 50 percent of infants with SCID. Most often asymptomatic, it may cause skin rash or, less frequently, typical graft-versus-host disease with generalized rash, liver disease, profuse diarrhea, jaundice, and severe hematologic abnormalities (thrombocytopenia, anemia, leukopenia) that are indicative of marrow damage.[72,73] Transfusion of un-irradiated blood products often leads to fatal graft-versus-host disease.

Laboratory Features of Severe Combined Immunodeficiency Syndrome

An absolute lymphocyte count less than 2000/μL should prompt immediate investigation for SCID, regardless of the severity of clinical symptoms.[42] Typically, infants with SCID have markedly reduced or absent circulating T cells which are unable to proliferate *in vitro* in response to mitogens and specific antigens.[74] However, T lymphocyte count may be preserved, at least in part, in SCID infants with maternal T-cell engraftment, with "leaky" variants of the disease,[74] or with somatic reversions that allow for some autologous T-cell development.[75] Finally, T-lymphocyte count can be normal or modestly reduced in patients with functional T-cell immunodeficiencies (see other combined immunodeficiencies; defective thymic development).

Maternal T-cell engraftment and "leaky" SCID with residual development of autologous T cells are characterized by the expression of the CD45R0 memory/activation antigen on the surface of circulating T lymphocytes (whereas most T cells in normal infants have a naïve CD45RA⁺ phenotype).

TCR excision circles, consisting of circularized signal joints, are a byproduct of V(D)J recombination and are exported to the blood by recent thymic emigrants. Levels of TCR excision circles in circulating lymphocytes are particularly high in newborns and infants, and progressively decline with age. Because TCR excision circles cannot be detected in infants with SCID, assessment of TCR excision circle levels by polymerase chain reaction has been successfully introduced for newborn screening for SCID.[76]

Although the number of circulating B lymphocytes can vary depending on the nature of the genetic defect, serum immunoglobulin levels are low in infants with SCID (see Table 80–2). Normal serum IgG levels early in life reflect transplacental passage of maternal immunoglobulins. Antibody response to immunization antigens is abolished.

Eosinophilia may be observed in SCID, and IgE serum levels may be elevated in spite of hypogammaglobulinemia. Cytopenias, caused by infections or marrow damage, may also be present. Autoimmune hemolytic anemia is frequent in PNP deficiency.[47] Marrow abnormalities (dysplasia or aplasia) can be observed in ADA,[77] PNP,[78] Cernunnos/ XLF,[79,80] and LIG4[81] deficiencies.

The diagnosis of ADA and PNP deficiency is facilitated by the demonstration of increased levels of deoxyadenosine triphosphate and deoxyguanosine triphosphate, respectively, in red blood cells.

Differential diagnosis of SCID includes secondary forms of immunodeficiencies, especially HIV infection, congenital rubella, and CMV infections, severe malnutrition, marrow failure syndromes,[82] and defects of vitamin B₁₂ and folate metabolism.[83,84]

Therapy, Course, and Prognosis of Severe Combined Immunodeficiency Syndrome

SCID is a medical emergency and is inevitably fatal if untreated. Confirmation of diagnosis by appropriate laboratory assays, referral to a tertiary care center, and aggressive treatment of infections should be immediately initiated in infants with possible SCID. High-dose intravenous sulfamethoxazole-trimethoprim (20 mg/kg) is effective in treating

P. jirovecii pneumonia. CMV should be treated with ganciclovir and adenoviral infections should be treated with cidofovir. Infants who have received bacillus Calmette-Guérin (BCG) vaccination at birth should receive isoniazid and rifampicin, regardless of the presence of overt signs of mycobacteriosis. Administration of IVIG and antimicrobial prophylaxis are necessary to reduce the risk of infections. Parenteral nutrition may be necessary, especially if chronic diarrhea and failure to thrive are present.

Survival, however, is ultimately dependent on immune reconstitution. Allogeneic HSCT was first performed in 1968 in an infant with X-linked SCID,[85] and is the treatment of choice. A multiinstitutional analysis of outcome of HSCT for SCID performed in North America in the period 2000 to 2009 demonstrates that survival following HSCT from a human leukocyte antigen (HLA)-identical sibling is as high as 97 percent.[86] T-cell–depleted transplantation from haploidentical donors results in a 79 percent 5-year-survival rate if no conditioning regimen is used. Importantly, survival is as high as 94 percent, regardless of donor type, if the transplant is performed within the first 3.5 months of age.[86] Moreover, 90 percent survival rate has been reported for older infants who received HSCT and did not have a prior history of infection.[86] For patients who do not have a matched sibling donor, use of pretransplantation conditioning regimen increases the chance of achieving more robust B-cell reconstitution, but this benefit must be balanced against toxicity of chemotherapy.[86] By contrast, HSCT from unrelated cord blood is associated with a lower survival rate (58 percent).[86]

Failure to achieve sufficient T- and B-cell reconstitution is associated with prolonged morbidity after transplantation, but most patients with SCID enjoy good quality of life after transplantation.[56] However, neurologic complications and developmental problems after transplantation are more common in patients with SCID associated with increased radiosensitivity and in patients with defects of purine metabolism.[56,87–89]

Enzyme replacement therapy offers rapid normalization of the toxic metabolites in ADA deficiency in those who do not have a matched donor, and may result in immune reconstitution and significant clinical improvement in patients with ADA deficiency, although T-cell counts often remain low.[45]

Gene therapy is an attractive form of therapy for SCID patients who lack fully matched donors. Transplantation of gene-modified autologous hematopoietic stem cells (aHSCs) may lead to immune reconstitution without the risk of graft-versus-host disease. More than 40 patients with ADA deficiency have received gene therapy using nonmyeloablative conditioning regimen and transfusion of aHSCs transduced with ADA-encoding retroviral vectors. All of these patients are alive, and approximately 75 percent of them have attained sufficient immune reconstitution.[90–92]

Twenty patients with X-linked SCID received gene therapy with retroviral vectors in Paris and London, without conditioning regimen. Seventeen of them are alive (as of this writing) with robust T-cell immune reconstitution, but variable B-cell function.[93,94] However, five patients developed leukemia as the result of insertional mutagenesis.[95,96] This prompted development of novel, hopefully safer, vectors. A new multiinstitutional trial of gene therapy for X-linked SCID with a self-inactivating γ-retroviral vector is being conducted as of this writing. Of nine patients treated, eight are surviving, and seven have attained good T-cell reconstitution. No leukemic proliferations have been observed.[97] Variable, but often poor, B-cell reconstitution has been reported after gene therapy for X-linked SCID without conditioning. To overcome this problem, a new trial based on use of a self-inactivating lentiviral trial and reduced intensity conditioning is under way at the National Institutes of Health as of this writing.

OTHER COMBINED IMMUNODEFICIENCIES

In some cases, significant impairment of T-cell immunity is associated with residual development and/or function of T lymphocytes. These conditions are also known as CID to distinguish them from SCID, in which both T-cell development and function are abrogated. The clinical features of CID overlap with SCID, but also include autoimmunity and/or inflammatory manifestations reflecting unbalanced immune homeostasis. CID is caused by two main mechanisms: (1) hypomorphic mutations in SCID-causing genes that allow for some T-cell development; and (2) genetic defects that affect late stages in T-cell development or peripheral T-cell function.

OMENN SYNDROME

Definition
Originally described in 1965, Omenn syndrome is characterized by severe infections, associated with early onset diffuse rash or generalized erythroderma, alopecia, eosinophilia, lymphadenopathy, hepatosplenomegaly, hypoproteinemia with edema, and oligoclonal expansion of activated autologous T lymphocytes that infiltrate and damage target tissues.[98,99]

Genetic Abnormalities
Various gene defects can cause this syndrome. Hypomorphic mutations in the *RAG1* and *RAG2* genes are most common,[100] but virtually any gene defect that severely impairs, but does not abolish, T-cell development may cause the disease.[101]

Pathophysiology
Defects of immunologic tolerance have been implied in the pathophysiology of Omenn syndrome. Thymic expression of AIRE (autoimmune regulator), a transcription factor involved in presentation of self-antigens and negative selection of autoreactive thymocytes, is reduced.[102] Impaired generation of natural regulatory T cells, and homeostatic proliferation of T lymphocytes in a lymphopenic environment, may also play a critical role in the pathophysiology of the disease.[103]

Laboratory Features
Laboratory investigations demonstrate that leukocytosis with eosinophilia and hypogammaglobulinemia are common findings, and that serum IgE is often elevated. The number of circulating T lymphocytes may vary, but they have a characteristic activated/memory (CD45R0+) phenotype. T cells have a restricted repertoire, and the distribution of CD4 and CD8 subsets is generally skewed. There is also a skewing to a T-helper (Th) type 2 (Th2) profile, with increased production of IL-4 and IL-5. The *in vitro* lymphocyte response to antigens is abrogated; responses to mitogens are variable, but in general are reduced.[74,104] The number of circulating B and NK lymphocytes may vary, depending on the nature of the underlying genetic defect. Absence of invariant NK T cells has been reported in RAG-deficient Omenn syndrome.[105]

Differential Diagnosis
Differential diagnosis includes maternal T-cell engraftment in patients with SCID, complete atypical DiGeorge syndrome, CHARGE syndrome (coloboma of the eye, heart defects, atresia of the nasal choanae, retardation of growth and/or development, genital and/or urinary abnormalities, and ear abnormalities and deafness), immune dysregulation-polyendocrinopathy-enteropathy-X-linked (IPEX) syndrome

and other conditions of neonatal erythroderma.[106–109] Male infants with NEMO deficiency can also present with severe skin manifestations resembling Omenn syndrome.

Treatment

In preparation for allogeneic HSCT, the only curative treatment available,[56] patients require aggressive nutritional support, correction of hypoproteinemia, and treatment or prevention of infections with antibiotics, antifungals, and immunoglobulin replacement therapy. Immune suppression with steroids or cyclosporine is beneficial in controlling T-cell–mediated tissue damage.

DEFECTS OF T-CELL–RECEPTOR SIGNALING

Definition

TCR ligation promotes activation of the p56Lck kinase, which mediates phosphorylation of components of the CD3 complex. This allows recruitment and phosphorylation of the zeta-associated protein of 70 kDa (ZAP-70), activation of downstream signaling molecules, release of Ca^{2+} from intracellular endoplasmic reticulum stores, and initiation of Ca^{2+} influx. Mutations of lymphocyte-specific protein tyrosine kinase (LCK), ZAP-70, and of other TCR-associated signaling molecules (RHOH, MST1, IL-2–inducible T-cell kinase [ITK]) result in various forms of CID with dysfunctional T cells.[110–115] Finally, PI3K, composed of a p110δ and a p85 subunit, is involved in generation of phosphatidylinositol 4,5-triphosphate (PIP_3) and activation of mammalian target of rapamycin (mTOR) and AKT. Activating mutations of the PI3KD gene (encoding for the PI3K subunit p110δ) results in increased activation-induced cell death of T lymphocytes, and consequently immunodeficiency.[29,30]

Clinical and Laboratory Features

Patients with these disorders present with early onset and severe infections. Warts, molluscum contagiosum, infections caused by herpes viruses, and a high risk of Epstein-Barr virus (EBV)-driven lymphoproliferative disease have been reported in patients with LCK, RHOH, and MST1 deficiency, and with activating PI3KD mutations.[29,30,110,113,114] Moreover, autoimmunity and lung granulomatous disease may also occur. From a laboratory standpoint, selective loss of CD8+ lymphocytes is observed in patients with ZAP-70 deficiency, and although the number of CD4+ lymphocytes is preserved, in vitro response to mitogens is markedly reduced, consistent with a signaling defect.[111,112] Patients with LCK, RHOH, MST1, and ITK deficiency and with gain-of-function PI3KD mutations have a reduced number of naïve CD4+ T cells. Oligoclonality of the T-cell repertoire and an increased proportion of exhausted CD8+ T memory (T_{EMRA}) cells have been reported in these patients.[29,30,107,113–115]

Differential Diagnosis

Differential diagnosis of ZAP-70 deficiency includes MHC class I deficiency and CD8α deficiency, two conditions characterized by a severe reduction of CD8+ lymphocytes. Patients with CD8α deficiency have an unusual population of CD3+ TCR αβ+ CD4- CD8- cells that have normal proliferative responses and usually survive to adulthood, although a late death from infections has been reported.[116,117] The other defects of TCR signaling have an overlapping phenotype. Ultimately, biochemical and molecular tests are needed to define the diagnosis.

Treatment

The only curative treatment of this group of disorders is allogeneic HSCT. Treatment with rapamycin (an mTOR inhibitor) or phosphoinositide

3-kinase inhibitor may reduce lymphoproliferation and hepatosplenomegaly in patients with activating PI3KD mutations.[29,30]

T-CELL IMMUNODEFICIENCIES WITH IMPAIRED NUCLEAR FACTOR-κB ACTIVATION

Following TCR signaling, the complex composed of MALT1, BCL-10, and caspase recruitment domain-containing protein (CARD)-11 proteins is activated, resulting in recruitment of TRIF-related adaptor molecule (TRAF) 6 and activation of IKK, permitting nuclear translocation of the p50 and p65 subunits of NF-κB and consequently induction of activation of NF-κB–dependent genes. Mutations of MALT1,[118] CARD11,[119,120] and IKBKB[121] (encoding for the IKKβ component of the IKK complex) genes are associated with increased susceptibility to bacterial, viral and fungal infections. Although the number of circulating T lymphocytes is normal, generation of memory T cells is impaired and proliferative responses to CD3 stimulation are decreased. Patients with CARD11 mutations have a block in B-cell development at the transitional stage,[119,120] and virtual absence of class-switched memory B cells is observed in patients with IKBKB mutations.[121]

As reported above, mutations of the IKBKG/NEMO gene are responsible for X-linked immunodeficiency with ectodermal dysplasia, whose clinical manifestations may also include opportunistic infections, resembling CID. Finally, gain-of-functions mutations of the IKBA gene, that prevent phosphorylation and degradation of the IKB-α subunit of the IKB complex, cause T-cell immunodeficiency with ectodermal dystrophy. The immunologic phenotype includes deficiency of memory T cells, impaired in vitro proliferation of naïve T cells to TCR/CD3 stimulation, and hypogammaglobulinemia with inability to mount specific antibody responses.[122] In addition to TCR signaling, activation of toll-like receptor (TLR) and tumor necrosis factor (TNF) pathways can also be compromised, causing increased susceptibility to a broad range of pathogens (pyogenic bacteria, mycobacteria, Candida, other opportunistic pathogens).[123]

CORONIN-1A DEFICIENCY

Coronin-1A is an actin regulator that is predominantly expressed in hematopoietic cells, plays a key role in regulating T-cell survival and migration. Mutations affecting both alleles of the CORO1A gene have been reported in patients with CID and an increased risk of severe varicella and EBV lymphoproliferative disease.[124,125] The immunologic phenotype includes naïve T-cell lymphopenia with normal numbers of B and NK cells, oligoclonal T-cell repertoire and reduced number of circulating invariant NKT (iNKT) cells and mucosa associated invariant T (MAIT) lymphocytes. Immunoglobulin serum levels are low, and antibody responses to antigens are absent. The disease can be treated by allogeneic HSCT.[124]

CD27 DEFICIENCY

The CD27 costimulatory molecule regulates survival and activation of T, B, and NK cells. CD27 deficiency is a CID with risk of EBV lymphoproliferative disease. In vitro T-cell proliferation to mitogens and antigens is reduced.[126] Immunoglobulin serum levels may be initially high, but patients eventually become hypogammaglobulinemic.

CTPS1 DEFICIENCY

Cytidine 5-triphosphate synthase 1 (CTPS1) is involved in de novo synthesis of cytidine 5-triphosphate (CTP), a nucleotide required for DNA and RNA metabolism. Impaired de novo synthesis of CTP causes a proliferation defect in both T and B lymphocytes. CTPS1 mutations have been identified in several infants from Northwestern England. The disease is characterized by severe bacterial and viral infections since early in life, and an increased risk of EBV-driven non-Hodgkin lymphoma. There are no extra-immune manifestations. Variable degrees of lymphopenia (especially of CD4+ cells), increased proportion of effector memory T cells and reduced *in vitro* proliferation to mitogens and antigens have been reported. Immunoglobulin levels may be normal, but specific antibody titers are reduced, and there is a low number of memory B cells.[127]

MAJOR HISTOCOMPATIBILITY COMPLEX CLASS I DEFICIENCY

Definition
MHC class I deficiency is characterized by reduced expression of MHC class I molecules at the cell surface. The disease is inherited as an autosomal recessive trait, and may be caused by defects in the *TAP1*,[128] *TAP2*,[129] or *Tapasin*[130] genes. These defects interfere with intracellular transport of peptide antigens and their loading onto MHC class I molecules, and cell-surface expression of the complex.

Clinical and Laboratory Features
MHC class I deficiency manifests with recurrent respiratory infections in childhood, and chronic inflammatory lung disease and skin lesions, mimicking Wegener granulomatosis in patients with transporter-associated with antigen-processing (TAP)-1 and TAP-2 deficiencies.[131,132] Chronic lung disease is a prominent cause of death. Glomerulonephritis and herpes zoster infections have been reported in Tapasin deficiency.[130]

The number of circulating CD8+ T cells is reduced, because positive selection of CD8+ lymphocytes in the thymus depends on the recognition of MHC class I molecules. *In vitro* T-cell function is normal, which facilitates differential diagnosis with ZAP-70 deficiency in patients who have significantly reduced CD8+ cells. The NK cytolytic activity is usually significantly reduced (see Table 80–2). Serum immunoglobulin levels are variable.

Treatment
Prophylactic measures, similar to those used in cystic fibrosis, may be beneficial. Treatment of the granulomatous lesions is based on use of topical antiseptics; immunosuppressive drugs may worsen symptoms and should be avoided.

MAJOR HISTOCOMPATIBILITY COMPLEX CLASS II DEFICIENCY

Definition
MHC class II deficiency is defined by the lack of MHC class II expression and autosomal recessive inheritance. There is a higher prevalence in populations of North African origin. MHC class II deficiency is caused by mutations of transcription factors that bind to the proximal promoters of the MHC class II gene. Four different gene defects are known and include mutations of the *CIITA*, *RFXANK*, *RFX5*, and *RFXAP* genes.[133]

Clinical and Laboratory Features
Typically, patients present early in life with increased susceptibility to bacterial, viral, and opportunistic infections. Severe lung infections, chronic diarrhea, and sclerosing cholangitis, often secondary to *Cryptosporidium* or CMV infection, are frequently observed. Less-severe presentations and survival into adulthood have been reported.[133]

The number of circulating CD4+ T cells is markedly reduced, reflecting an impairment of positive selection in the thymus.

Delayed-type hypersensitivity responses are absent, but *in vitro* proliferative responses to mitogens are preserved. Hypogammaglobulinemia is common and poor antibody response to immunization antigens is consistently observed (see Table 80–2).[133] The diagnosis is based on demonstrating lack of MHC class II expression on monocytes, B lymphocytes and *in vitro* activated T cells. Differential diagnoses include HIV infection and idiopathic CD4 lymphopenia; however, in these conditions expression of MHC class II molecules is preserved.

Treatment and Course
MHC class II deficiency has a poor prognosis. If untreated, most patients die in infancy or childhood. Respiratory infections are the predominant cause of death. Liver failure is observed in patients who develop sclerosing cholangitis. Antibiotic prophylaxis and immunoglobulin replacement therapy, with adequate nutritional support, are required. HSCT is the only curative approach, but survival rate is lower than in other forms of CID and graft-versus-host disease is common, especially in patients with preexisting viral infections.[133]

DEFECTS OF STORE-OPERATED CA²⁺ ENTRY

Calcium mobilization is a key event in the activation process of lymphocytes and nonimmune cells. Two molecules, calcium release-activated calcium channel protein 1 (ORAI1) and stromal interaction molecule 1 (STIM1), mediate the function of Ca²⁺ entry channels. ORAI1 is a ubiquitously expressed protein that constitutes the pore-forming subunits of the Ca²⁺ release-activated channels located in the cell membrane. STIM1 senses the Ca²⁺ concentration in the endoplasmic reticulum and activates Ca²⁺ release-activated channels. Mutations of both the *ORAI1* and *STIM1* genes in humans result in an autosomal recessive immunodeficiency with increased susceptibility to severe infections, especially from herpesviruses infections, associated with nonprogressive myopathy and ectodermal dysplasia. Manifestations of immune dysregulation (autoimmune cytopenias, hepatosplenomegaly) are common, especially in STIM1 deficiency.[134,135] Although T-cell development is unaffected, *in vitro* proliferation of circulating T cells to mitogens and to a combination of phorbol ester and ionomycin is drastically reduced, and the Ca²⁺ influx following T-cell activation is absent. Lack of natural killer T (NKT) cells and functional defects of NK lymphocytes have been reported. In spite of hypergammaglobulinemia, specific antibody responses are typically absent. Allogeneic HSCT has been used in some patients to correct the defect.[135]

DEFECTS OF MAGNESIUM TRANSPORTER 1

Mg²⁺ is an important second messenger in the immune system. Mutations of the X-linked magnesium transporter 1 (*MAGT1*) gene, that encodes for a protein that permits transport of Mg²⁺ across the cell membrane, cause immunodeficiency with increased susceptibility to bacterial and viral infections, and a high risk of EBV-driven lymphoproliferative disease.[136] Patients have CD4 lymphopenia, defective lymphocyte proliferation *in vitro* and impaired NK cytolytic function.[137]

DEDICATOR OF CYTOKINESIS 8 DEFICIENCY

Dedicator of cytokinesis 8 (DOCK8) is an atypical guanosine triphosphatase (GTPase) that regulates cytoskeleton reorganization and intracellular signaling. Although it is broadly expressed, it plays a critical role in T, B, and NK lymphocytes. DOCK8 deficiency is inherited as an autosomal recessive trait, and is characterized by recurrent and severe bacterial, fungal, and viral infections, eczema and other manifestations of immune dysregulation, including autoimmune cytopenias. Cutaneous viral infections (warts, molluscum contagiosum, herpes simplex) are especially common, but systemic viral disease (varicella, CMV, EBV) has been also reported. Cutaneous infections frequently evolve into squamous cell carcinoma. Vascular thrombosis in the central nervous system has been described in several patients.[138,139] Multiple immunologic abnormalities have been reported,[138–142] including a variable degree of lymphopenia that affects especially naïve T cells, increased proportion of CD8+ T_{EMRA} cells, decreased *in vitro* proliferation to CD3 stimulation, impaired generation of Th17 cells, and defects of NK cytolytic function. Immunoglobulin levels are variable, but IgM serum levels are often low. B-cell response to TLR9 stimulation is defective, and specific antibody responses are blunted. Large, intragenic deletion of the gene has been frequently reported in affected patients,[139] and lack of DOCK8 protein expression can be demonstrated by flow cytometry.[143] The disease has a poor prognosis, but can be cured by allogeneic HSCT.[144] Good results have been reported in the treatment of severe herpetic infections with interferon (IFN)-α (see also "The Hyperimmunoglobulin E Syndromes" below).[145]

COMBINED IMMUNODEFICIENCY WITH MULTIPLE INTESTINAL ATRESIA

Multiple intestinal atresia is a congenital disease characterized by atresias that may affect the gastrointestinal tract, from stomach to anus.[146–149] In many cases, CID is associated, with reduced number of T (and in some patients, B) lymphocytes, impaired *in vitro* proliferation to mitogens, and profound hypogammaglobulinemia. A high risk of sepsis because of Gram-negative bacteria has been reported, but viral, fungal, and opportunistic infections are also common. The disease is inherited as an autosomal recessive trait and is caused by mutations of the tetratricopeptide repeat domain 7A *(TTC7A)* gene,[146,147] which plays an important role in intestinal and immune homeostasis by maintaining cell polarity and regulation of cell survival, proliferation, adhesion, and migration.[148,149] In the thymus, TTC7A is expressed both by thymic epithelial cells and by thymocytes.[147,148] Multiple surgeries are often required to establish canalization of the gastrointestinal tract. Total parenteral nutrition often leads to severe liver disease, and combined small bowel and liver transplantation may be needed.[150] Most patients die early in life. Partial immune reconstitution has been reported in a few cases following HSCT.[147]

VENOOCCLUSIVE DISEASE WITH IMMUNODEFICIENCY

Venoocclusive disease with immunodeficiency (VODI) is a congenital disorder characterized by liver abnormalities and immunodeficiency, with onset in the first months of life.[151] Liver abnormalities include venoocclusive disease, fibrosis, hepatomegaly, and hepatic failure. Patients are prone to recurrent infections, sustained by viruses, bacteria, and opportunistic pathogens (*P. jirovecii*, *Candida*, CMV). Thrombocytopenia is frequent. Infections may precede development of liver abnormalities. Immunologic defects include low number of memory T and B lymphocytes, defective B-cell differentiation *in vitro* into antibody-secreting cells, and hypogammaglobulinemia.[151] The disease is more common in the Lebanese population. It is inherited as an autosomal recessive trait and is caused by mutations of the *SP110* gene,[152] which encodes for a nuclear body protein that acts as a transcription factor driving expression of genes with a retinoic acid response element. Treatment is based on immunoglobulin replacement therapy, prophylactic antibiotics, prompt treatment of infections, and ursodiol; however, the prognosis remains dismal. HSCT is the only curative approach, but the outcome is often problematic because of liver toxicity as a result of conditioning regimen.[153]

● DEFECTIVE THYMIC DEVELOPMENT

DIGEORGE SYNDROME (22q 11.2 DELETION SYNDROME)

Definition

The DiGeorge syndrome (DGS) is a developmental disorder caused by abnormal cephalic neural crest cell migration and differentiation in the third and fourth pharyngeal arches during early embryonic development.[154] The vast majority of patients with DGS have partial monosomy of human chromosome 22q11.2. However, a significant fraction (10 to 45 percent) of patients with DGS do not have a chromosome 22q11.2 deletion and some 2 percent have small deletions in chromosome 10p.

Clinical and Laboratory Features

The clinical phenotype of DGS consists of the triad congenital cardiac defects, hypocalcemia as a result of parathyroid insufficiency, and immune deficiency as a consequence of aplasia or hypoplasia of the thymus.[154] However, there is significant phenotypic variability. Cardiac defects (especially interrupted aortic arch type B and truncus arteriosus) occur in 50 to 80 percent of patients with 22q11.2 deletion. Hypocalcemia is observed in 50 to 60 percent, and may cause neonatal seizures. Facial dysmorphisms include micrognathia, hypertelorism, antimongoloid slant of the eyes, and ear malformations. A third of DGS patients have velopharyngeal incompetence, leading to feeding difficulties and speech delay; 10 percent have a cleft palate. As young adults, many develop social, behavioral, and psychiatric problems.

There is also significant variability of the severity of immunologic phenotype. Most patients have residual thymic tissue and hence mild to moderate T-cell lymphopenia (see Table 80–2). Approximately 1 percent of DGS patients lack T cells completely, resembling SCID (complete DGS). In some cases, generation of oligoclonal T cells that infiltrate target tissues is associated with generalized skin rash and lymphadenopathy, resembling Omenn syndrome. This phenotype is known as atypical complete DGS.[155] As in other cellular immunodeficiencies, patients with DGS have a high incidence of autoimmune diseases such as cytopenia and thyroiditis. A retrospective analysis of TCR excision circle (TREC) levels at birth in patients with DGS has shown that approximately 20 percent of them had low TRECs; these infants had lower CD8+ T-cell count and were more prone to viral infections than DGS infants with normal TREC levels at birth.[156]

Treatment

Cardiovascular anomalies require prompt attention and hypocalcemia appropriate medical treatment. Depending on the extent of the immune deficiency, patients may require antibiotic prophylaxis or IVIG therapy. However, patients with complete DGS (including complete atypical phenotype) require more aggressive treatment. Allogenic thymic transplantation may restore T-cell development and function in approximately 75 percent of these patients.[155] Unmanipulated marrow from matched donors can also lead to immune reconstitution by providing mature T lymphocytes contained in the graft.[157]

COLOBOMA, HEART DEFECTS, ATRESIA OF THE CHOANAE, RETARDED GROWTH, GENITAL HYPOPLASIA AND EAR ANOMALIES SYNDROME

A syndrome with a severe T-cell defect, CHARGE is caused by heterozygous *de novo* mutations in the *CHD7* gene.[158] Circulating T lymphocytes are decreased in most CHARGE patients and respond poorly to mitogens.

CONGENITAL ALOPECIA AND ABSENCE OF THYMUS

Mutations of the *FOXN1* gene, encoding for a transcription factor that plays a critical role in development of thymic epithelial cells, causes thymic aplasia, associated with congenital alopecia, nail dystrophy, and a severe neural tube defect.[159] This phenotype is the equivalent of the mouse nude/SCID phenotype. Successful outcome has been reported after thymic transplantation.[160]

● PRIMARY IMMUNODEFICIENCY DISORDERS PRESENTING AS AUTOIMMUNE DISEASES

The concept of a link between immune dysregulation and autoimmunity has been strengthened by the discovery of distinct single-gene defects resulting in unusual susceptibility to autoimmune diseases. The three representative syndromes in this category include (1) IPEX, (2) autoimmune polyendocrinopathy, candidiasis, and ectodermal dystrophy (APECED), and (3) the autoimmune lymphoproliferative syndrome (ALPS).

IMMUNE DYSREGULATION, POLYENDOCRINOPATHY, ENTEROPATHY, X-LINKED SYNDROME

Clinical Findings

The most prominent IPEX symptoms include early onset diarrhea secondary to autoimmune enteropathy, eczematous dermatitis, multiple endocrinopathies including early onset insulin-dependent type 1 diabetes mellitus, thyroiditis, and, rarely, adrenal insufficiency. Autoimmune hemolytic anemia, thrombocytopenia, and neutropenia are common complications. Eczema is the most frequent pathology of the skin, but erythematous, psoriasiform dermatitis, and *alopecia universalis* have been reported. Autoimmune hepatitis is present in 20 percent of IPEX patients. Lymphadenopathy and hepatosplenomegaly are less common.[108] Loss of small bowel villi and lymphocytic infiltrates in the intestinal mucosa, the pancreas, thyroid, lung, and liver are commonly observed. Immunologic abnormalities include elevated serum IgA and IgE concentrations and the absence of CD4+CD25+ FOXP3+ regulatory T cells.

IPEX is caused by mutations in the *FOXP3* gene located in the centromeric region of the X chromosome.[161] The transcription factor FOXP3 binds to more than 700 promotors and acts as a transcriptional repressor of the IL-2, IL-4, and IFN-γ promoters by interfering with the cytokine regulator, NFAT (nuclear factor of activated T cells).[162] FOXP3 plays a crucial role in the generation of T-regulatory cells (Tregs) in the thymus.

Treatment

Immunosuppressive drugs such as cyclosporine, tacrolimus, sirolimus, and glucocorticoids provide temporary remission. Allogeneic HSCT can cure this disease.[163]

IMMUNE DYSREGULATION, POLYENDOCRINOPATHY, ENTEROPATHY, X-LINKED–LIKE SYNDROMES

An IPEX-like phenotype has been associated with mutations in a number of genes, including *CD25*, *STAT5B*, *STAT1* (gain-of-function mutations) *STAT3* (gain-of-function) and ITCH/AIP4.

Cd25 Deficiency

CD25 (IL-2 receptor α chain) was found to be deficient in three infants from two unrelated families. Clinical features resemble those of both IPEX and SCID. CD25-deficient infants presented with severe chronic diarrhea, villous atrophy and autoimmune hepatitis at an early age.[164,165] Early onset insulin-dependent diabetes was observed in one patient; all presented with eczema and developed autoantibodies, hepatosplenomegaly, lymphadenopathy, and lymphocytic infiltrates in the lung, gut, and liver.[165] However, CD25-deficient patients suffered from infectious complications more commonly observed in patients with SCID, including recurrent CMV pneumonitis, persistent thrush, and EBV infection. One patient was treated successfully with HSCT.[164]

STAT5B Deficiency

The transcription factor STAT5B is activated/phosphorylated in response to growth hormone and the cytokines IL-2, IL-7, IL-15 and IFN-γ, and promotes the transcription of nonimmune and immune genes. STAT5B plays a crucial role in the transcription of insulin-like growth factor 1 (IGF-1), which is required for *in utero* and postnatal growth. In addition, STAT5B is required for the transcription of IL-2Rα, a crucial component of the IL-2 receptor necessary for induction of FOXP3, which programs the development of Tregs in the thymus. The clinical phenotype of homozygous STAT5B deficiency reflects these molecular observations. Affected patients suffer from intrauterine and postnatal growth failure from lack of IGF-1 resulting in growth hormone insensitivity.[166] Moderate T and NK cell lymphopenia may be the cause of susceptibility to viral infections.[167] Importantly, STAT5B-deficient patients have reduced numbers of Tregs with low FOXP3 expression, and decreased suppressor function.[168] As a result of abnormal Treg homeostasis, STAT5B-deficient patients have immune dysfunction and multiple autoimmune problems, including arthritis, lymphocytic interstitial pneumonia, severe eczema, autoimmune thyroiditis, and idiopathic thrombocytopenic purpura.[169]

STAT1 Gain-of-Function Mutations

Heterozygous mutations in STAT1 were recently identified in patients with chronic mucocutaneous candidiasis.[170] These mutations were within the coiled-coil and DNA-binding domains, leading to hyperphosphorylation of STAT1 in response to cytokines such as IFN-γ. Screening of a cohort of patients with IPEX-like symptoms who also had mucocutaneous fungal infections revealed heterozygous STAT1 gain of function mutations. The clinical characteristics included enteropathy with villous atrophy, type I diabetes, thyroiditis, eczema, short stature, vascular aneurysms and viral infections. FOXP3+ Treg numbers were within the normal range, and showed normal suppressive function.[171] It has been hypothesized that effector cells may be less responsive to suppression as a result of excessive STAT1 activity.

STAT3 Gain-of-Function Mutations

A Finnish-British consortium discovered heterozygous gain-of-function mutations in several patients with short stature, polyendocrinopathy including type 1 diabetes starting at a very young age (*in utero* or before 3 weeks of age). The clinical phenotype included the presence of multiple autoantibodies, celiac disease or autoimmune enteropathy, eczema, thyroiditis, arthritis, autoimmune cytopenias and large granular lymphocytic (LGL) leukemia in one in five patients.[172] Except for eczema, none of the patients with STAT3 gain-of-function mutations had the clinical features of autosomal dominant (AD) hyperimmunoglobulin E syndrome (HIES) as a result of heterozygous dominant negative STAT3 mutations, although the mutations, all missense, were located in the same domains (DNA binding, SH3 [Src homology 3], and transactivation) as those observed in AD-HIES. When studied for STAT3 activity using a luciferase reporter assay gain-of-function mutations showed an increase, whereas those with heterozygous loss of function mutations causing AD-HIES had decreased activity.

Cytotoxic T-Lymphocyte Antigen-4 Haploinsufficiency

Cytotoxic T-lymphocyte antigen-4 (CTLA-4) is an inhibitory receptor expressed by T lymphocytes including Tregs, and by B cells. While CD28 transmits a stimulatory signal to lymphocytes, CTLA-4 provides an inhibitory signal.[173] CTLA-4 can also affect signaling in B cells by competing with CD28 for CD80/86 binding.

In a recent report, heterozygous mutations in the *CTLA4* gene were observed in members of four unrelated families suffering from multiple autoimmune diseases, recurrent infections, and lymphocytic infiltrates in a number of target organs.[174] Affected patients developed hypogammaglobulinemia, CD4 lymphopenia, progressive loss of circulating B cells and defective/dysregulated Treg cells. Reduced CTLA-4 expression in T cells, B cells, and Tregs, and increased T- and B-cell apoptosis are characteristic findings and may contribute to the clinical phenotype.

ITCH E3 Ubiquitin Protein Ligase Deficiency

The clinical features of ITCH E3 ubiquitin protein ligase (ITCH) deficiency caused by mutations in E3 ubiquitin ligase *(ITCH/AIP4)* include dysmorphic facial features, failure to thrive and developmental delay. In addition, immune dysregulation that is characterized by chronic interstitial pneumonitis, thyroiditis, type I diabetes, enteropathy, and hepatitis were common.[175] This is a rare syndrome observed in a single large Amish kindred with 10 affected family members. ITCH can affect T-cell anergy in mice because of defective FOXP3 expression.[176]

AUTOIMMUNE POLYENDOCRINOPATHY, CANDIDIASIS, AND ECTODERMAL DYSTROPHY SYNDROME

APECED is a rare autosomal recessive disorder, also known as autoimmune polyglandular syndrome (APS) type I. The incidence is high in certain isolated populations, for example, Finns, Iranian Jews, and Sardinians. Most patients with APECED present with chronic mucocutaneous candidiasis and endocrinopathies predominantly involving the parathyroid and adrenal glands, less frequently the thyroid and the pancreas. The syndrome is often associated with ectodermal manifestations such as dystrophic dental enamel and fingernails.[177] APECED results from mutations in the *AIRE* gene. AIRE expression is limited to medullary thymic epithelial cells which express MHC class II and the costimulatory molecule CD80. These cells are endowed with the remarkable ability to "promiscuously" express a wide variety of tissue-restricted antigens derived from nearly all organs in the body.[178] Expression of these organ specific proteins allows for the negative selection of autoreactive T cells or the generation of immunoregulatory FOXP3+ T cells in the thymus. A lack of AIRE function causes decreased expression of tissue-restricted antigens in the thymus, resulting in the escape of autoreactive T-cell clones into the periphery.[179] Autoantibodies against type 1 interferons,[180] and against IL-17A, IL-17F and/or IL-22,[181] were detected at high titers in most patients. Treatment for APECED is largely supportive.

AUTOIMMUNE LYMPHOPROLIFERATIVE SYNDROME

Definition, Clinical Features, and Pathogenesis

ALPS is caused by defective apoptosis of lymphocytes, resulting in nonmalignant lymphadenopathy, hepatosplenomegaly, and autoimmune disorders, which most commonly include Coombs-positive autoimmune hemolytic anemia, thrombocytopenia, and neutropenia. The incidence of lymphoma is estimated to be 9 percent in the National Institutes of Health cohort of 79 probands[182] and consist of both Hodgkin and non-Hodgkin lymphoma. Both lymph nodes and spleen show pronounced hyperplasia and contain a CD3+ lymphocyte population of which a large proportion consists of TCR$\alpha\beta$+ CD4-CD8- cells. This phenomenon is also observed in blood lymphocytes from ALPS patients in which the proportion of double-negative T cells is typically between 5 and 20 percent (range: 1.5 to 68 percent).[182] Many of these cells express MHC class II and secrete high levels of IL-4, IL-5, and IL-10.

The FAS-mediated apoptosis pathway is important for the downregulation of antigen-induced immune responses and the elimination of autoreactive lymphocytes. ALPS patients have mutations in genes required for "programmed cell death." The most common defect involves heterozygous (dominant) mutations in the gene encoding the T-cell surface molecule FAS, also known as CD95 or TNFRSF6 (ALPS-FAS, formerly ALPS type Ia); rare patients with compound heterozygous or homozygous FAS-mutations (ALPS-FAS or type 0) have been reported. In some patients, somatic mutations of FAS have been identified in double-negative T cells (ALPS-sFAS or type 1m). A few families have been identified with mutations affecting the FAS ligand (CD95L; TNFSF6) which is responsible for ALPS-FASL or ALPS type Ib. Approximately 3 percent of ALPS patients have mutations in caspase 10 (ALPS-CASP10 or ALPS type II). Ten to 20 percent of patients with the ALPS phenotype do not have mutations in FAS, FASL, or caspases and are classified as ALPS-U or ALPS type III.[182] Because three Fas molecules form a trimeric complex to interact with a FasL trimer, most families with ALPS have AD inheritance (dominant negative effect) with variable penetrance (mutations in caspase 8 and 10 are autosomal recessive).

Treatment

Immunosuppressive therapy including steroids, mycophenolate mofetil (MMF), and rituximab, has been used with variable success to treat autoimmune symptoms.[182] A recent clinical trial with sirolimus achieved complete or near complete resolution of autoimmune cytopenia, colitis, lymphadenopathy, and splenomegaly and all patients had a reduction in double-negative T cells.[183] Splenectomy is recommended only in patients with excessively large spleens or splenic rupture and requires lifetime antibiotic prophylaxis. The long-term prognosis is guarded, but patients can achieve a normal life span.

● OTHER WELL-DEFINED IMMUNODEFICIENCY SYNDROMES

WISKOTT-ALDRICH SYNDROME

Definition

The Wiskott-Aldrich syndrome (WAS) is a rare X-linked disorder characterized by thrombocytopenia (Chap. 117) and small platelets, eczema, recurrent infections, immunodeficiency, and a high incidence of autoimmune diseases and malignancies.[184] A classic WAS phenotype is generally associated with null-mutations of the gene that encode the WAS protein (WASp). WASp is the key regulator of actin polymerization in hematopoietic cells and has well-defined domains that are involved in cytoplasmic signaling, cell locomotion, and immunologic synapse formation. A milder phenotype, X-linked thrombocytopenia (XLT), is often associated with mutations that result in expression of mutated protein. XLT patients have either no or very mild eczema and few problems, if any, with infections, autoimmunity, and malignancy.[185] Amino acid substitutions within the GTPase-binding domain of WASp interfere with the intramolecular autoinhibitory mechanism, resulting in gain-of-function–impaired actin polymerization, causing X-linked neutropenia (Chap. 65).[186]

Clinical and Laboratory Features

By definition, WAS and XLT patients have congenital thrombocytopenia in the range of 20,000 to 60,000/μL and microplatelets, but normal numbers of megakaryocytes. Hemorrhagic problems may be mild, consisting of bruises and petechiae, or serious, including gastrointestinal and central nervous system hemorrhages. Patients with classic WAS are susceptible to bacterial, fungal, and viral infections.

Treatment

Patients may require antibiotic prophylaxis and IVIG replacement therapy. Immunosuppressive therapy may be needed if autoimmune symptoms occur. Splenectomy ameliorates the bleeding tendency by increasing the number of blood platelets. However, splenectomy substantially increases the risk of septicemia, sometimes in spite of antibiotic prophylaxis, and often results in fatal bacterial infections. Because of the poor long-term outcome of WAS, early allogeneic HSCT is the treatment of choice. The outcome is excellent if a matched-related or matched-unrelated donor can be identified, or if a partially matched cord blood unit is available.[187] Haploidentical transplantation is not recommended. Patients with XLT have an excellent prognosis, but may develop complications including serious bleeding, autoimmune diseases, and malignancies.[144,185] Therefore, allogeneic HSCT for XLT may be considered if an appropriate donor is available. Because complete myeloid and lymphoid engraftment is required to correct all aspects of WAS/XLT, standard-conditioning using myeloablative protocols (busulfan, cyclophosphamide, with or without antithymocyte globulin) are required. A European followup study of WAS patients who received HSCT reports a strong association of autoimmunity with mixed chimerism, clearly demonstrating that reduced intensity conditioning is not sufficient.[188]

WASp-INTERACTING PROTEIN DEFICIENCY

A syndrome exhibiting symptoms and laboratory abnormalities typical for classic WAS has been observed in a female infant with a homozygous nonsense mutation in *WIPF1* that encodes WASp-interacting protein (WIP). The patient presented at 11 days of age with eczema, thrombocytopenia (but normal platelet size) and infections.[189] Both WIP and WASp were absent in patient leukocytes, demonstrating that WIP is required for stabilization of WASp. The patient was successfully transplanted at age 4.5 months.

THE HYPERIMMUNOGLOBULIN E SYNDROMES

Autosomal Dominant Hyperimmunoglobulin E Syndrome

HIES (or Job syndrome) is a rare AD or sporadic multisystem immunodeficiency characterized by eczema, *S. aureus*-induced skin abscesses, recurrent pneumonia with abscess and pneumatocele formation, *Candida* infections, and skeletal and connective tissue abnormalities.[190] In 1966, two girls suffering from eczema, recurrent respiratory tract infections, and "cold" staphylococcus skin abscesses were described as having Job syndrome because of the phenotypic similarity to the biblical figure Job, who had been "smitten with sore boils from the soles of his feet unto his crown."[191] Subsequently, patients with similar clinical findings were reported to have very-high serum IgE concentrations[192] and additional characteristic abnormalities were recognized, including distinct facial features, often described as "coarse," hyperextensive joints, pathologic bone fractures, scoliosis, craniosynostosis, and retained primary teeth.[193,194] Serum IgE levels of greater than 2000 IU/mL have been used as arbitrary diagnostic values, but often are greater than 10,000 IU/mL.

Other abnormal laboratory tests include eosinophilia, abnormal B-cell maturation and defective antibody responses to neoantigens,[195] chemotactic defects of neutrophils, and reduced lymphocyte proliferation to specific antigens.

Most patients with HIES were noted to arise sporadically from unaffected, healthy parents. With the advent of improved antibiotic therapy, patients survived into adulthood and had affected children, suggesting AD inheritance.[193] This observation was validated by the finding that heterozygous mutations of the gene encoding the transcription factor STAT3 are the cause of AD-HIES. All STAT3 mutations identified to date in patients with AD-HIES are either amino acid substitutions or in-frame deletions strongly supporting the concept that coexpression of wild-type and mutant STAT3 protein is required to cause the syndrome. The notable lack of nonsense or frameshift mutations strengthens the notion that AD-HIES is a result of a dominant-negative effect.[196–198] The molecular analysis of a large cohort of patients (n = 38) with "classic" HIES and a score of greater than 40 points using the National Institutes of Health clinical scoring system, identified STAT3 mutations in all but one individual. The mutations clustered in three domains of the STAT3 protein known to have distinct functional characteristics, the DNA-binding, and the SH2 and the transactivation domains. This finding suggests that more than one molecular mechanism causes the AD-HIES phenotype. This notion is supported by the observation that mutations in the SH2 domain, but not those in the DNA-binding domain, affect tyrosine phosphorylation of STAT3, whereas mutations in the DNA-binding domain interfere with nuclear import and DNA-binding.[198] Because STAT3 plays a key role in the development of IL-17 producing Th17 cells, AD-HIES patients have a marked decrease in circulating Th17 cells.[199] Given that IL-17 plays an important role in host defense against extracellular bacteria and fungi and upregulates production of β defensins and S100 proteins by neutrophils,[200] the absence of Th17 cells may directly affect susceptibility to *S. aureus* and *Candida albicans*.

Treatment

To prevent progressive lung destruction, prophylactic antibiotic therapy to decrease the frequency of *S. aureus* infections is important. Antifungal therapy is indicated to prevent recurrent *Candida* infections. A surgical approach to treating chronic lung disease should be avoided, if possible. Allogeneic HSCT has been performed in a few patients with variable benefits.[201,202]

Autosomal Recessive Hyperimmunoglobulin E Syndromes

In 2004, a cohort of 13 patients from consanguineous families were reported to have marked eosinophilia, elevated serum IgE levels, eczema, skin abscesses, recurrent bacterial, fungal, and viral infections including herpes simplex, therapy-resistant molluscum contagiosum, and recurrent varicella zoster. Lymphopenia and decreased lymphocyte proliferation suggested a significant T-cell defect. In contrast to HIES caused by STAT3 mutations, autosomal recessive hyper-IgE syndrome (AR-HIES) patients frequently present with neurologic complications but do not develop skeletal abnormalities or postpneumonia pneumatoceles. Most have large deletions in the *DOCK8* gene, resulting in absent DOCK8 protein.[138,139] (See DOCK8 deficiency in "Other Combined Immunodeficiencies" above.) Because of a high incidence of malignancies and early death, HSCT is recommended.[203] A single adult patient with eczema; moderately elevated serum IgE; a history of bacterial (BCG complications, salmonellosis), fungal, and viral infections, including molluscum contagiosum; and a mild T-cell deficiency was found to have a mutation in tyrosine kinase 2 (TYK2), a receptor-associated cytoplasmatic tyrosine kinase that plays an important role in multiple cytokine signaling of T cells.[204]

IMMUNOOSSEOUS DYSPLASIAS

Cartilage Hair Hypoplasia

Cartilage hair hypoplasia is an autosomal recessive condition characterized by short-limbed dwarfism and light-colored, hypoplastic hair.[205] Patients may also present with marrow cell dysplasia, increased susceptibility to malignancies, Hirschsprung disease, defects of spermatogenesis, and a variable degree of immune deficiency (resembling SCID, Omenn syndrome, partial T-cell deficiency) or may have normal immune function.[206] The rare disorder is more common in certain populations, such as the Amish and Finns, and is caused by mutations in the gene encoding for untranslated RNA component of the ribonuclease mitochondrial RNA processing (*RMRP*) complex, which is involved in cleavage of ribosomal RNA, processing of mitochondrial RNA, and cell-cycle control.[207] Decreased numbers of T lymphocytes, especially of CD8+ cells, and impaired *in vitro* proliferative responses to mitogens have been reported and may be from reduced thymic output, cell-cycle abnormalities, and increased apoptosis.[208,209] Impairment of cellular immunity may cause increased susceptibility to severe varicella or other viral diseases, and administration of live-attenuated viral vaccines should be avoided. Defects of humoral immunity are less frequent, and may contribute to recurrent infections. Autoimmune manifestations (hemolytic anemia, neutropenia, and thrombocytopenia) may also occur. Similar to what has been observed in other disorders of ribosomal biogenesis (Diamond-Blackfan anemia, Shwachman-Diamond syndrome), disturbances of hematopoiesis, such as anemia, leukopenia, thrombocytopenia, and marrow dysplasia, are frequent manifestations of cartilage hair hypoplasia. Allogeneic HSCT has been successfully used to correct those forms of cartilage hair hypoplasia presenting with a SCID or Omenn syndrome phenotype.[210]

Schimke Syndrome

Schimke syndrome is an autosomal recessive condition characterized by dwarfism with short neck and trunk because of spondyloepiphyseal dysplasia, progressive renal impairment evolving to renal failure, facial dysmorphisms, lentigines, immunodeficiency (ranging from T-cell lymphopenia to SCID), and increased occurrence of marrow failure and of early onset arteriosclerosis associated with cerebral infarcts.[211] Microcephaly and cognitive, motor, or social abnormalities have been reported in a significant proportion of the patients.[212] The disease is caused by mutations of the switch/sucrose nonfermentable (SWI/SNF)-related matrix-associated actin-dependent regulator of chromatin subfamily A-like protein 1 (*SMARCAL1*) gene that encodes for a chromatin remodeling protein.[211] Recurrent infections of bacterial, viral, and fungal origin, and opportunistic infections (*P. jirovecii* pneumonia) are seen in half of the patients. Severe presentations lead to death in the first decade of life, and development of renal failure is common among those who survive. Combined HSCT and renal transplantation has been used to correct immune deficiency and renal problems.[213]

WHIM SYNDROME

Warts, hypogammaglobulinemia, infections, and myelokathexis (WHIM) syndrome[214] is an AD disorder, caused by heterozygous mutations in the *CXCR4* gene that encodes for the receptor for the CXCL12 chemokine, involved in leukocyte trafficking.[215] The term *myelokathexis* indicates retention of mature neutrophils in the marrow. WHIM mutations result in truncation or structural abnormalities in the intracytoplasmic tail of CXCR4 that interfere with ligand-induced internalization and ultimately cause increased cellular responsiveness to CXCL12.[214]

Patients with WHIM syndrome may present with early onset recurrent bacterial infections, but the clinical phenotype may vary greatly.[216] Warts, caused by human papillomavirus (HPV), tend to develop in the second decade of life. Severe neutropenia contrasts with accumulation of mature neutrophils in the marrow. Spontaneous apoptosis of neutrophils has been reported.[217] Lymphopenia, including low B-cell numbers, is a frequent finding. Hypogammaglobulinemia of variable degree can be observed, and immunizations result in short-lived antibody responses and impaired class switch.[218] EBV-positive B-cell lymphoma can occur.

Immunoglobulin replacement therapy and antibiotic prophylaxis may reduce the incidence of infections. Recombinant G-CSF has been used to increase the absolute neutrophil count. Warts are resistant to local therapy and need to be monitored for neoplastic transformation.

● CHROMOSOMAL INSTABILITY SYNDROMES ASSOCIATED WITH IMMUNODEFICIENCY

Chromosomal instability syndromes have in common increased spontaneous or induced DNA breaks, susceptibility to infections secondary to immune deficiency, and an increased risk of malignancies. Disease-specific abnormalities involving growth and development, the central nervous system, and the skin provide useful diagnostic clues. The classic chromosomal instability syndromes include ataxia-telangiectasia (AT), Nijmegen breakage syndrome (NBS), Bloom syndrome (BS), and AT-like disorder (ATLD). The genes responsible for these syndromes protect human genome integrity by contributing to the complex task of double-strand break repair. Together with the proteins associated with Fanconi anemia, the gene products of the chromosomal instability syndromes form or regulate a large protein complex that is active in the surveillance and maintenance of genomic integrity.[219] The triad of immunodeficiency, neoplasia, and infertility is the direct consequence of defective double-strand break repair, and involves nonhomologous end-joining or homologous rejoining. Because nonhomologous end-joining is crucial for the generation of TCR diversity and polyclonal immunoglobulins, any interruption of this process will predictably result in defective adaptive immunity. Tumor development and infertility may be a direct consequence of defective DNA repair during miotic recombination of lymphocytes, other somatic cells, or germ cells, respectively.

ATAXIA-TELANGIECTASIA

AT is a multisystem disorder, characterized by immunodeficiency, progressive neurologic impairment, and ocular and cutaneous telangiectasia.[220]

The immune deficiency in AT is highly variable, involving both cellular and humoral immunity. Respiratory infections are common and often result in chronic lung disease. Opportunistic infections are rare. The majority of AT patients have low or absent IgA and IgE, often combined with IgG_2 and IgG_4 deficiency.[221] Specific antibody responses may be depressed or normal. The number of circulating lymphocytes is often reduced, and proliferation in response to mitogens is variably depressed. Spontaneous cytogenetic abnormalities include chromosomal breaks, translocations, rearrangements, and inversions; these defects increase following *in vitro* exposure to radiation. The thymus is often small, showing marked paucity of thymocytes and absence of Hassall corpuscles. The most consistent laboratory abnormality, an elevation of serum α-fetoprotein, is diagnostic in adults and children older than age 8 months as it is not observed in the other chromosomal instability syndromes.

Cancer is the second most common cause of death, after infections.[220] Most malignancies are non-Hodgkin lymphomas (40 percent), leukemias (25 percent), and solid tumors (25 percent); 10 percent are Hodgkin lymphoma. In contrast to other immune deficiency syndromes with increased incidence of malignancies, the leukemias and lymphomas observed in AT are predominantly of T-cell origin. The solid tumors in AT patients include adenocarcinoma, dysgerminoma, gonadoblastoma, and medulloblastoma.

Cerebellar ataxia is the earliest clinical manifestation of AT and becomes evident when a child begins to walk at the end of the first year of life. The ataxic gait persists, and most patients never develop normal speech. Eventually, involuntary movements become a major handicap and the child may require a wheelchair by the end of the first decade of life. Cortical cerebellar degeneration involves primarily Purkinje and granular cells; progressive changes to the central nervous system also occur.

A variety of other features have been reported. Growth retardation is present in 30 percent of the patients. Female hypogonadism is common and associated with hypoplasia of the ovaries. Hypogonadism is also observed in male AT patients.

The AT gene *(AT mutated [ATM])* encodes a large transcript that predicts a protein of 3056 amino acids.[222] ATM is a predominantly nuclear protein with a strong serine-threonine kinase activity. Its major function is to rapidly respond to the induction of double-stranded breaks in DNA. The activation of ATM leads to phosphorylation of an extensive array of target proteins, each of which plays a key role in a unique damage response pathway. Specifically, ATM is involved in cell-cycle checkpoint control and delays the passage of cells through the various phases of the cell cycle, allowing time for DNA damage repair. Additionally, ATM is functionally linked to telomere maintenance, a process crucial to aging and cancer.[223] The more than 400 unique mutations of ATM described to date are distributed throughout the gene with a majority predicted to cause premature termination resulting in unstable truncated proteins.

AT patients should avoid X-radiation and chemotherapeutic agents. Treatment is symptomatic and includes prophylactic antibiotics for those with recurrent pulmonary infections and IVIG for those with antibody deficiency.

ATAXIA-TELANGIECTASIA–LIKE DISORDER

ATLD[224] has many features of AT and is the result of mutations in the Mre11 protein, which is part of the DNA-repair complex (Mre11/Rad50/Nbs1).[225] Affected patients have progressive ataxia, but show less-severe neurodegeneration and may be ambulatory until their early twenties. They do not develop telangiectasia and α-fetoprotein levels are normal. However, similar to AT, ATLD patients have increased spontaneous chromosomal abnormalities in blood lymphocytes and show increased radiation sensitivity.

NIJMEGEN BREAKAGE SYNDROME

NBS is characterized by short stature, microcephaly, a bird-like face, immunodeficiency, chromosomal instability, increased radiosensitivity, and a high incidence of malignancies.[226] Although NBS shares many characteristics with AT and ATLD, it can be distinguished from these disorders by an absence of neurodegeneration, impressive microcephaly with mild to moderate mental retardation, and absence of telangiectasia.

Most NBS patients develop respiratory tract infections, including recurrent pneumonia that may result in bronchiectasis and premature death from respiratory failure. Both humoral and cellular immunity are defective and include hypogammaglobulinemia, except for normal or elevated IgM, abnormal antibody responses to protein and polysaccharide antigens, suggesting a defect in CSR, reduced numbers of T lymphocytes, and abnormal lymphoproliferation to mitogens and specific antigens.[226]

NBS lymphocytes show the typical features of chromosomal instability syndromes characterized by increased chromatid and chromosome breaks, rearrangement/translocations of chromosome 7 and 14, telomere fusions, radioresistant DNA synthesis, and hypersensitivity to ionizing radiation and radiomimetic agents.[226]

The extensive immunodeficiency and the chromosomal instability explain the high incidence of lymphoid malignancies, including non-Hodgkin lymphoma (both of B- and T-cell origin), lymphoblastic leukemia/lymphoma, and, less frequently, Hodgkin lymphoma and acute myeloblastic leukemia. Solid tumors are less frequent and include medulloblastoma and rhabdomyosarcoma. Because of hypersensitivity to radiation and radiomimetic/alkylating agents, tumor therapy is limited. Magnetic resonance imaging and ultrasound examinations are the preferred imaging techniques, rather than x-ray and CT scan. Prophylactic therapy with antibiotics and IVIG is indicated in patients with recurrent infections. Several patients have been successfully treated with allogeneic HSCT.[227]

BLOOM SYNDROME

BS is characterized by short stature, hypersensitivity to sunlight, increased susceptibility to infections, and a predisposition to early development of a variety of cancers.[219] Susceptibility to bacterial infections, affecting mainly the upper and lower respiratory tract, is associated with hypogammaglobulinemia and variable T-cell deficiency. Most affected patients have decreased fertility and some may develop early onset type II diabetes mellitus. By age 25 years, approximately half of the patients with BS will have developed one or more malignancies. Leukemia and non-Hodgkin lymphoma predominate during the first two decades; later, carcinoma affecting the colon, skin, and breast are common. The diagnosis of BS can be confirmed by demonstrating excessive numbers of sister-chromatid exchanges, increased chromatid gaps and breaks, and the presence of quadriradial configuration composed of two homologous chromosomes. The causative gene, *BLM*, encodes a 1417-amino-acid protein with homology to the RecQ family of helicases. This family of helicases includes the Werner syndrome, RecQ helicase-like (WRN) protein, which is mutated in Werner syndrome. BLM is a member of a group of proteins that associate with BRCA1 to form a large complex that co-localizes to large nuclear foci if cells are treated with agents that interfere with DNA synthesis. As part of this complex, BLM plays a role in sensing DNA damage and contributes to the maintenance and genomic integrity during the process of DNA replication and repair. More than 60 unique mutations in the *BLM* gene have been identified. The most common mutation is a 6-bp deletion/7-bp insertion in exon 10, which is the homozygous mutation causing BS in Ashkenazi Jews.

BS patients with significant antibody deficiency may benefit from antibiotic prophylaxis and IVIG therapy. Because of increased radiation sensitivity, exposure to any form of irradiation should be restricted.

RARE SYNDROMES WITH CHROMOSOMAL INSTABILITY

NBS-like phenotypes have been linked to mutations in *LIG4, RAD50,* and nonhomologous end-joining factor 1 *(NHEJ1).*[219] Other syndromes with chromosomal instability include Werner syndrome, Riddle syndrome and immunodeficiency with centromere instability and facial anomalies (ICF) syndrome.

● CYTOTOXICITY DISORDERS

Defense against viruses is primarily dependent on cell-mediated cytotoxicity. Cytotoxic T lymphocytes (CTLs) and NK cells are capable of killing virus-infected target cells using pore-forming perforin and cytolytic granzymes A and B. Different genetic defects can affect various steps in the formation, intracellular transport, and delivery of cytolytic granules,[228,229] and result in different defects of cell-mediated cytotoxicity, that include various forms of familial hemophagocytic lymphohistiocytosis (FHL), Chédiak-Higashi syndrome, Griscelli syndrome type II, and Hermansky-Pudlak syndrome type II. Overall, these disorders are characterized by increased susceptibility to severe viral infections that in some cases is associated with defects of hair and skin pigmentation, and neurologic problems. Dysregulation in CTL and NK homeostasis, with increased production of inflammatory cytokines and accumulation of activated lymphocytes, characterizes the two genetic variants of X-linked lymphoproliferative syndrome (XLP1 and XLP2).

FAMILIAL HEMOPHAGOCYTIC LYMPHOHISTIOCYTOSIS

FHL includes a group of genetically heterogeneous conditions that are characterized by the uncontrolled proliferation of activated lymphocytes and histiocytes that secrete large amounts of proinflammatory cytokines. This results in life-threatening manifestations, characterized by fever, hepatosplenomegaly, marrow infiltration and pancytopenia, and severe neurologic manifestations (Chap. 71).

There are at least five different forms of FHL, four of which have been defined at the molecular level. FHL2 is caused by mutations of the *PRF1* gene, which encodes perforin.[230] FHL3 is caused by mutations in *UNC13D*, also known as Munc13–4.[231] FHL4 is caused by defects of the *STX11* gene, that encodes syntaxin 11,[232] whereas FHL5 is a result of mutations of the *STXBP2* gene, that encodes for Munc18–2, a protein that interacts with STX11.[233] Each of these defects interferes with a specific step of the cytolytic machinery, and ultimately causes inefficient pathogen clearance, uncontrolled activation of CTLs, and release of IFN-γ and other inflammatory cytokines, resulting in recruitment and activation of macrophages, and inhibition of hematopoiesis.

Clinical and Laboratory Features

In approximately 85 percent of the cases, FHL becomes clinically evident within the first year of life,[234] but late presentations may occur in patients with hypomorphic mutations.[235–237] High fever, severe hepatosplenomegaly, lymphadenopathy, hemorrhagic manifestations as a result of thrombocytopenia, and edema are common. Neurologic symptoms, including seizures and decreased level of consciousness, may lead to long-term disability.[238]

The FHL diagnostic guidelines were updated in 2007.[239] Anemia and thrombocytopenia are early signs followed by increased serum levels of triglycerides, bilirubin, liver enzymes, ferritin, and coagulation abnormalities. Hemophagocytosis can be observed in the marrow, lymph nodes, and cerebrospinal fluid, which often shows abundant mononuclear cells and increased proteins, even in the absence of overt neurologic symptoms. Immunologic findings include persistently impaired cytolytic activity of NK cells and elevated levels of inflammatory cytokines (IFN-γ, IL-1, IL-6, TNF-γ) in the blood. Monitoring circulating soluble CD25 (IL-2Rα) is also useful as a measure of increased cellular activation.

Flow-cytometry enables analysis of perforin expression, which is absent except for hypomorphic mutations, and may thus facilitate diagnosis of FHL2. The diagnosis of FHL forms that are characterized by reduced NK cell degranulation (such as *UNC13D* and *STX11* defects) may be facilitated by the analysis of membrane expression of the lysosomal marker CD107a.[240]

Treatment and Prognosis

Without treatment, FHL is usually rapidly fatal. Treatment of active disease should focus on controlling or eliminating possible triggers (infections in particular), blocking T-cell activation, and stopping the hyperinflammatory cytokine response. To this purpose, antimicrobials, etoposide, immune suppression (antithymocyte globulin), cyclosporine, and dexamethasone are commonly used.[239,241] Alemtuzumab has shown some efficacy in controlling etoposide-resistant forms.[242] However, relapses are common in FHL. Patients should be monitored carefully for reactivation of the disease, especially in the central nervous system. Administration of anti–IFN-γ monoclonal antibody has given interesting results in animal model of the disease,[243] and is currently being tested in a clinical trial. Permanent cure for FHL can be only provided by allogeneic HSCT. A higher success rate is obtained when HLA-matched related or unrelated donors are available. Use of myeloablative conditioning regimen is associated with high transplantation-related mortality. Considering that partial chimerism is enough to achieve disease control,[244] reduced intensity conditioning is being increasingly used, with promising results.[245] Outcome of HSCT is worse if the disease is not in remission at the time of transplantation.

X-LINKED LYMPHOPROLIFERATIVE DISEASE

Definition and History

In 1975, Purtilo described a family in which numerous males in multiple generations presented with fulminant infectious mononucleosis, lymphoma, or hypogammaglobulinemia after primary EBV infection.[246] XLP1 is caused by mutations in the *SH2D1A* gene[247,248] that encodes an adaptor protein (SLAM [signaling lymphocyte activation molecule]-associated protein [SAP]) involved in T- and NK-cell signaling.[249] Thus, defects of SAP drastically affect both T- and NK-mediated cytotoxicity.[250–252] SAP also plays an important role in germinal center formation and antibody production by modulating development and function of follicular helper T cells.[253] Finally, SAP is required for the development of iNKT cells, which are immunoregulatory cells that are involved in the responses to pathogens and cancer cells.[254] In the absence of SAP, EBV and other virus infections result in dysregulated immune responses, because of persistent antigenic stimulation that leads to hyperactive cytotoxic T lymphocytes and macrophages, with increased production of IFN-γ.

However, not all males with X-linked lymphoproliferative syndrome (XLP) features have mutations in *SH2D1A* and mutations in another X-chromosome–associated gene (*XIAP*; X-linked inhibitor of apoptosis, also known as *BIRC4*) have been identified,[255] resulting in XLP2.

Clinical and Laboratory Features

Although lymphoproliferative disease is observed in both XLP1 and XLP2, there are some important differences in the disease phenotype. Most often, XLP1 becomes clinically manifest following EBV infection in childhood, although later presentations are possible. Fulminant infectious mononucleosis has been observed in 50 to 60 percent of cases, and EBV-related lymphoma in 30 percent of the cases. Most lymphomas are of B-cell origin, and approximately half are of the Burkitt type. Persistent dysgammaglobulinemia, with low IgG and low to increased levels of IgM, is common among survivors. Other clinical manifestations of XLP1 include vasculitis, marrow aplasia secondary to hemophagocytic lymphohistiocytosis, and lymphoid granulomatosis.

Although less frequently encountered, other viral infections (CMV, other herpes viruses) may unmask the clinical phenotype of XLP1.[256]

Fulminant infectious mononucleosis is marked by a rapid increase of liver enzymes, followed by impaired coagulation, hepatic encephalopathy, and signs of hemophagocytic lymphohistiocytosis (HLH), associated with a high EBV viral load in the blood and other tissues. B-cell lymphomas carry monoclonal immunoglobulin gene rearrangements. Patients who develop dysgammaglobulinemia show impaired antibody responses. Antibody levels to the EBV nuclear antigen usually remain undetectable, even in patients who survive the acute EBV infection. In contrast, antibodies to the EBV viral capsid antigen can be low to elevated. During clinical manifestations of XLP, the proportion of CD8+ T cells carrying activation markers is increased and the number of memory (CD27+), and specifically switched memory (CD27+IgD−) B cells, is reduced. NK cell cytotoxicity is usually normal, when measured in a conventional K562 killing assay. However, NK cytolytic activity is markedly reduced in XLP1, when costimulation through CD244 is provided.[250] Flow cytometry can be used to detect a lack of SAP protein expression in circulating T and NK lymphocytes in patients with XLP1.[257]

XLP2 often manifests with HLH, and EBV is a common trigger.[258] However, some important differences exist in the phenotype of XLP2 versus XLP1. In particular, recurrent splenomegaly often associated with cytopenia and fever is preferentially observed in XLP2, and may represent an attenuated manifestation of HLH. By contrast, lymphoma, a common complication of XLP1, is not frequently observed in XLP2. Importantly, severe inflammatory bowel disease (IBD) has been reported in a significant proportion of patients with XLP2,[258,259] and in some cases may represent the dominant clinical phenotype.[259] Moreover, XLP2 may also manifest as delayed-onset Crohn disease.[260] The occurrence of IBD in XLP2 may reflect the notion that the RING domain of XIAP is required for NOD2 signaling.[261]

A flow-cytometry-based assay can be used to facilitate differential diagnosis of XLP1 and XLP2.[262]

Treatment and Prognosis

If untreated, approximately 70 percent of XLP1 patients die within 10 years of onset. The mortality rate is particularly high (96 percent) in patients who present with fulminant infectious mononucleosis.[263] Allogeneic HSCT is the treatment of choice, yielding the best results when the transplant is performed early in life, prior to EBV infection. However, transplantation using reduced-intensity conditioning may permit correction of the disease in EBV-positive patients with severe organ toxicity.[264] The use of anti-CD20 monoclonal antibody can reduce viral load and improve the clinical status, and anti–TNF-α therapy or etoposide may be beneficial in patients with active EBV infection and severe systemic inflammatory response.[265-267] Administration of immunoglobulin may reduce the risk of infections, but does not prevent or attenuate the symptoms of primary EBV infection.

Similar survival rates have been reported in XLP2 and in XLP1.[258] However, this figure does not take into account forms of XLP2 that may present with features other than HLH, and IBD in particular. Sulfasalazine, glucocorticoids, 5-amino salicylic acid, and anti-TNF medications have been used in the treatment of IBD in patients with XLP2, however the only curative approach is allogeneic HSCT. Use of myeloablative conditioning is associated with high mortality and toxicity rate, but good results have been reported with reduced intensity conditioning.[268]

CYTOTOXICITY DEFECTS ASSOCIATED WITH PIGMENTARY DILUTION DISORDERS

Chédiak-Higashi Syndrome

Chédiak-Higashi syndrome is an autosomal recessive disorder characterized by immune dysregulation with impaired cellular cytotoxicity, partial oculocutaneous albinism, platelet functional abnormalities, and neurologic involvement.[269] The disease is caused by mutations in the *lysosomal trafficking regulator (LYST)* gene.[270] LYST plays an important role in sorting of lysosomal proteins, and in docking and fusion of lysosomal vesicles.[228]

Patients are susceptible to recurrent pyogenic and viral infections. Bruises are common and reflect deficiency of the platelet specific granules responsible for secondary aggregation (Chap. 120). Both bacterial and viral infections may trigger the life-threatening "accelerated phase" of the disease, characterized by high fever, hepatosplenomegaly, coagulation abnormalities, increase of liver enzymes and bilirubin (with possible jaundice), edema, and neurologic symptoms, with seizures, ataxia, cranial nerve palsies, and peripheral neuropathy.[269]

Abnormally large granules in lymphocytes, neutrophils, platelets, melanocytes, and neurons represent a morphologic hallmark of the disease. Light microscopy examination of hair reveals large and evenly distributed granules of melanin. Reduced NK cytotoxic activity and prolonged bleeding time are typical findings.

Treatment requires control of infections, and immunosuppressive intervention during the accelerated phase. Allogeneic HSCT, best performed during remission, is the only permanent cure of the immunohematologic problems.[271] However, HSCT does not seem to prevent progressive neurologic involvement.[272]

Griscelli Syndrome Type 2

Griscelli syndrome type 2 (GS2) is an autosomal recessive syndrome characterized by immunodeficiency and hypopigmentation, and a variable degree of neurologic involvement.[269] The presence of immune deficiency distinguishes GS2 from Griscelli syndrome type 1 (GS1; marked by the association of partial albinism and neurologic involvement) and Griscelli syndrome type 3 (GS3; with isolated hypopigmentation). GS2 is caused by mutations of the *RAB27A* gene,[273] which encodes for a GTPase involved in intracellular transport of granules.

GS2 patients are highly susceptible to recurrent pyogenic infections and to episodes of "accelerated phase" of the disease, with typical features of HLH. Prominent hypopigmentation is a result of large clumps of melanin in the hair shafts. NK cytotoxicity is defective and CD107 expression at the cell membrane of NK lymphocytes is impaired upon coculture with target cells. Treatment is based on allogeneic HSCT, and promising results have been reported with reduced intensity conditioning.[274]

Hermansky-Pudlak Syndrome Type 2

This autosomal recessive disease is characterized by oculocutaneous albinism, bleeding tendency, recurrent infections, and moderate to severe neutropenia (Chap. 120).[269] Bone anomalies (with dysplastic acetabula), facial dysmorphisms and development of pulmonary fibrosis are also part of the clinical phenotype. Hermansky-Pudlak type 2 is caused by mutations of the *AP3B1* gene that encode for the β_1 subunit of the AP-3 endosomal protein, which is required for sorting of lysosomal membrane proteins to the granules.[275] Missorting of tyrosinase in melanocytes accounts for oculocutaneous albinism. Reduced platelet-dense granules and impaired platelet degranulation are responsible for increased susceptibility to bleeding. Absence of AP-3 leads to low intracellular content of neutrophil elastase in myeloid progenitors causing neutropenia. Even though CTL and NK cell cytolytic activity is defective,[276] the risk of progression to HLH is lower than in Chediak-Higashi syndrome or GS2.[277] Consequently, preemptive use of HSCT is not justified.

Hermansky-Pudlak syndrome type 9 is caused by mutations of the pallidin (*PLDN*) gene, and is characterized by recurrent infections, partial albinism and nystagmus.[278] NK cell cytolytic activity is impaired.[279]

● IMMUNODEFICIENCIES WITH SELECTIVE SUSCEPTIBILITY TO PATHOGENS

Although classical forms of PIDD are characterized by susceptibility to a broad range of pathogens, several disorders have been identified with selective susceptibility to certain microorganisms. Some of these diseases (e.g., mendelian susceptibility to herpes simplex virus encephalitis [HSE] or to pyogenic infections, especially *S. pneumoniae*) are the result of defects of innate immunity, in particular TLR signaling. Others (mendelian susceptibility to mycobacterial disease) involve defects of the IL-12/IFN-γ axis at the interface of innate and adaptive immunity. Susceptibility to recurrent meningitis caused by *Neisseria meningitidis* is discussed in "Genetically Determined Deficiencies of the Complement System" below.

IMMUNODEFICIENCIES WITH IMPAIRED SIGNALING THROUGH TOLL-LIKE RECEPTORS

TLRs are transmembrane proteins (Chap. 17) expressed on a variety of cell types that recognize pathogen-associated molecular patterns, such as lipopolysaccharide derived from Gram-negative bacteria, lipopeptide, double-stranded RNA that is generated during viral replication, viral single-stranded RNA, viral cytosine phosphate guanine DNA moieties, and flagellin. Although most TLRs are expressed at the cell surface, TLRs 7, 8, and 9 are expressed on the membrane of endosomal vesicles.[280]

The recognition of pathogen-associated molecular patterns by TLRs induces characteristic intracellular signaling.[280] The classical pathway of TLR activation involves the adaptor molecules MyD88 (myeloid differentiation factor 88) and toll–IL-1R domain-containing adaptor protein (TIRAP), and the intracellular kinases IL-1R–associated kinase (IRAK)-4 and IRAK-1, ultimately resulting in the nuclear transfer of NF-κB and the production of inflammatory cytokines (IL-1, IL-6, TNF-α, IL-12). TLRs 3, 7, 8, and 9 activate an alternative pathway that involves other adaptor molecules, such as TRIF, TRAF3, and the UNC-93B protein, and ultimately results in the induction of type 1 interferons (IFN-α/β). Deficiencies of IRAK-4, MyD88, TLR3, and UNC-93B have been identified in humans, and are associated with two distinct phenotypes.

Toll-Like Receptor Signaling Defects with Increased Susceptibility to Herpes Simplex Virus Encephalitis

Selective susceptibility to HSE is associated with monogenic disorders that affect TLR3,[281,282] or components of the TLR3 signaling pathway, including UNC-93B,[283] TRAF3,[284] TRIF,[285] and TBK1.[286] The disease reflects a CNS-intrinsic defect of neurons and oligodendrocytes to produce type 1 IFN in response to herpes simplex virus (HSV).[287]

Because TLR3 recognizes double-stranded RNA and is normally expressed in CNS-resident cells, mutations of TLR3 or other components of the TLR3-dependent signaling pathway impair the response of these cells to actively replicating HSV-1. Because cellular responsiveness to type 1 IFN is intact in both UNC-93B–deficient and TLR3-deficient patients, the use of IFN-α along with acyclovir should be considered to treat HSE in these patients.[281,287]

HSE may also be a result of null mutations of STAT1, a transcription factor that is activated upon interaction of type 1 IFN with their receptors, and is critical for the induction of IFN-responsive genes. However, these patients are also prone to other severe viral infections. Furthermore, because STAT1 is also involved in the response to IFN-γ,

patients with null *STAT1* mutations are also at risk for mycobacterial disease.[288]

Other Immunodeficiencies with Increased Susceptibility to Viral Infections

Mutations of STAT2, leading to impaired response to IFN-α and IFN-β predispose to severe viral infections, including disseminated vaccine-strain measles.[289]

Skin warts caused by HPV infection are the hallmark of epidermodysplasia verruciformis. This disease is caused by mutations of the *EVER1* and *EVER2* genes.[290] There is an increased risk of squamous cell carcinoma.

Toll-Like Receptor Signaling Defects with Increased Susceptibility to Pyogenic Infections

IRAK-4 and MyD88 deficiencies are characterized by recurrent and invasive pyogenic bacterial infections, particularly from *S. pneumoniae* and *S. aureus*.[123,291,292] These infections are common especially during the first years of life (when lethality rate can be as high as 50 percent), but their frequency tends to decline with age.[293] Fever and systemic inflammatory responses are absent or unusually modest, reflecting poor induction of inflammatory cytokines and reduced response through the IL-1R.

Use of antimicrobic prophylaxis is important to prevent invasive pyogenic infections, especially in childhood. Substitution therapy with immunoglobulins may be beneficial in patients with impaired antibody responses.

Defects Involving Other Pattern-Recognition Signaling Pathways with Increased Susceptibility to Fungal Infections

Several inborn errors of immunity have unraveled key mechanisms of defense against *Candida*. Chronic mucocutaneous candidiasis (CMC) is a common complication affecting patients with APECED; it results from a mutation in the transcription factor AIRE.[177] CMC also affects those with AD-HIES; in this case, it is a result of mutations in the transcription factor STAT3.[190] Autoantibodies to IL-17 are a common feature of APECED,[181,294] and Th17 differentiation is impaired in HIES because of *STAT3* mutations. The Th17 cytokines IL-17A, IL-17F, and IL-22 induce the synthesis of chemokines that recruit neutrophils, and promote production of antimicrobial peptides from epithelial cells, thereby playing a key role in mucocutaneous resistance to *Candida* spp. Heterozygous, dominant negative mutations in *IL17F* gene, and biallelic loss-of-function mutations in the *IL-17RA* gene (encoding for the α chain of IL-17 receptor) have been linked with CMC.[305] Furthermore, mutations of the *ACT1* gene[296] (that encodes for an adaptor molecule that interacts with IL-17R) and gain-of-function *STAT1* mutations impairing Th17 immunity[170] are associated with CMC.

Mutations of the *CARD9* gene have been identified in patients with CMC or disseminated candidiasis, including infection of the brain.[297] CARD9 is recruited by Dectin-1, a transmembrane pattern-recognition receptor that senses the β-glucan component of fungal cell walls, and together with other cytoplasmic proteins, forms an intracellular signaling complex that leads to the nuclear import of NF-κB and the induction of key cytokines including IL-1, IL-6, IL-23, and the generation of IL-17 cells, which are required to control antifungal immune responses. However, invasive fungal infections in CARD9 deficiency are not restricted to *Candida*, but also include other species, such as *Exophiala*, an environmental black yeast with low virulence.[298] Granulocyte macrophage-colony stimulating factor (GM-CSF) therapy resulting in complete clinical remission has been reported in one CARD9-deficient patient with relapsing albicans meningoencephalitis.[299]

MENDELIAN SUSCEPTIBILITY TO MYCOBACTERIAL DISEASE

The IL-12/IFN-γ axis is essential for controlling mycobacterial infections. Following phagocytosis of mycobacteria, macrophages secrete IL-12, a heterodimer composed of IL-12p40 and IL-12p70. IL-12 binds to the heterodimeric IL-12R (composed of IL12Rβ_1 and IL-12Rβ_2 chains) expressed by Th1 and NK cells. This results in activation of the JAK-STAT4 pathway, and ultimately in the production of IFN-γ, which binds to its receptor (comprising IFN-γR1 and IFN-γR2 chains) on the surface of macrophages, triggering a signaling cascade that involves the transcription factor STAT1 and induction of IFN-γ-responsive genes that are essential to contain the infection and kill the mycobacteria. A variety of defects along this pathway have been shown to account for mendelian susceptibility to mycobacterial disease (MSMD) in humans.[300] The basis for increased susceptibility to mycobacterial disease in patients with NEMO deficiency was discussed in "X-Linked Anhydrotic Ectodermal Dysplasia with Immunodeficiency Caused by Mutations in Nuclear Factor-κB Essential Modulator" above.

IL-12p40 Deficiency

Affected patients are at increased risk of childhood infections because of BCG and *Salmonella*; *Candida* infections have also been reported. Recurrence of *Salmonella* infection is common.[301] IL-12p40 can associate with IL-12p70 to form the IL-12 heterodimer, or with IL-23p19 subunit to form IL-23. Consequently, patients with IL-12p40 deficiency have defects in both IL-12 and in IL-23–dependent immunity, with the latter causing a Th17 deficiency. The clinical course is variable, with some genetically affected siblings being asymptomatic, but approximately 32 percent of symptomatic IL-12p40–deficient patients die prematurely of infections.[301] Treatment with antimicrobial drugs and IFN-γ has been tried with variable results.

IL-12Rβ_1 Deficiency

Autosomal recessive IL-12Rβ_1 deficiency is characterized by infections with mycobacteria of low virulence and *Salmonella* species.[302] However, infections with *Mycobacterium tuberculosis*, *Cryptococcus*, and disseminated coccidioidomycosis have also been reported.[302-304] Unlike salmonellosis, mycobacterial infections tend not to recur and the overall prognosis is good. In most cases, IL-12Rβ_1 expression on the cell surface is absent, and *in vitro* IFN-γ production in response to IL-12 is abrogated. Treatment with appropriate antibiotics and IFN-γ is effective.

IFN-γR1 and IFN-γR2 Deficiencies

The genetic and biochemical pathophysiology of IFN-γR1 and IFN-γR2 deficiencies are remarkably complex. Autosomal recessive forms are most often associated with mutations that abrogate cell surface expression of IFN-γR1 or result in the expression of receptors that do not bind IFN-γ. Partial autosomal recessive deficiency is the result of hypomorphic mutations, with residual IFN-γ binding and signaling.[305] Dominant partial forms reflect the presence of heterozygous mutations in the cytoplasmic tail of IFN-γR1, allowing the expression of mutant molecules on the cell surface (often in increased density because of defective receptor shedding) which are unable to mediate signal transduction.[306]

The severity of the clinical features reflects the nature of the biochemical defect.[307] Patients with complete deficiency develop severe infections with environmental mycobacteria infections early in life, with lack of granuloma formation. Osteomyelitis caused by BCG or by environmental mycobacteria has been reported in several patients with dominant partial IFN-γR1 deficiency.

Treatment of partial deficiency should be based on careful identification and typing of the mycobacterial strains and appropriate antimicrobial therapy; addition of IFN-γ may be useful in patients with AD mutations in IFN-γR1 who are able to express reduced amounts of normal IFN-γR1 on the cell surface. Recessive forms are resistant to medical treatment. Although allogeneic HSCT may be curative, a high rate of graft failure has been observed[308] as a consequence of the inhibitory effect of high levels of circulating IFN-γ.[309]

GATA2

The syndrome of monocytopenia, B-cell and NK-cell lymphopenia associated with mycobacterial, fungal and viral infections, also called MonoMAC syndrome or familial myelodysplasia/leukemia with lymphedema (Emberger) syndrome was first described in 2010.[310] One year later, heterozygous mutations in *GATA2* resulting in haploinsufficiency were identified as the molecular defect causing MonoMAC[311] and Emberger syndrome.[312,313]

GATA2 plays a role in the early development of lymphatics and their valves,[314] explaining the connection with Emberger syndrome. The transcription of GATA2 occurs in early and undifferentiated hematopoietic cells, but also in somatic cells. Because of its progression to myelodysplastic syndrome or acute myeloid leukemia, mortality can be as high as 28 percent.[310] HSCT has successfully reversed clinical symptoms.[315]

STAT1 Deficiency

Complete STAT1 deficiency causes increased susceptibility to viral infections and to mycobacterial disease with a severe clinical course and early death.[288]

Dominant partial STAT1 deficiency is caused by a heterozygous mutation that allows formation of the IFN-α/β-dependent ISGF3 transcription factor, but abrogates expression of the γ-activating factor, which is composed of STAT1 homodimers. Affected individuals have either a mild clinical course, characterized by selective susceptibility to mycobacterial infections, or are asymptomatic.[316]

Partial autosomal recessive STAT1 deficiency is associated with impaired, but not abrogated, IFN-α/β and IFN-γ signaling, and occurrence of severe, but curable, intracellular bacterial and viral infections.[317]

Heterozygous STAT1 gain-of-function mutations result in susceptibility to mycobacterial infections, candidiasis, and IPEX-like phenotype (see "Immune Dysregulation, Polyendocrinopathy, Enteropathy, X-Linked–Like Syndromes" above).[171]

Other Genetic Disorders with Mendelian Susceptibility to Mycobacterial Disease

Interferon-regulated factor 8 (IRF8) is a transcription factor that regulates the differentiation of granulocytes and macrophages, and the development of DCs. IRF8 mutations in humans cause MSMD.[318] Two variants of the disease have been described: an autosomal recessive form characterized by extreme leukocytosis (up to 98×10^9/L cells), marked expansion of lymphocytes and granulocytes, and absence of monocytes, myeloid DCs, and plasmacytoid DCs; and an AD variant, in which monocytes and DCs are present, but there is selective loss of IL-12–producing CD1c$^+$ DCs. The clinical phenotype of autosomal recessive IRF8 deficiency is more severe, with early onset, failure to thrive, and disseminated BCG. HSCT is curative. The AD variant of the disease is characterized by disseminated but curable BCG infection.

The interferon stimulated gene 15 (ISG15) protein is an IFN-α/β-inducible, ubiquitin-like protein involved in ISGylation, but can be also secreted by granulocytes and act upon T and NK lymphocytes, inducing IFN-γ production. Inherited ISG15 deficiency causes severe MSMD, with disseminated BCG infection, which is responsive to antimycobacterial treatment.[319]

● GENETICALLY DETERMINED DEFICIENCIES OF THE COMPLEMENT SYSTEM

The complement (C) system[320] consists of the classical and alternative pathways and the membrane attack complex, and is composed of a series of plasma proteins that play an important role in host defense, inflammation, clearance of immune complexes and apoptotic cells, and induction of a normal humoral immune response (Chap. 19). Mutations in the classical pathway (C1q, C1r/C1s, C4, C2, and C3) result in pyogenic infections and autoimmune diseases. Mutations affecting the alternative pathway (factors B, D, properidin) result in meningococcal and pneumococcal sepsis. Mutations in the terminal components (C5–C9) are associated with an increased susceptibility to *Neisseria* species, especially meningococcal sepsis and meningitis. C1 inhibitor deficiency, an AD disorder, is the cause of hereditary angioedema. All other complement-component deficiencies have an autosomal recessive mode of inheritance with the exception of properidin deficiency, which is X-linked.

The most important screening tests for complement deficiencies are those using the assessment of the hemolytic function of both the classic and alternative pathways, CH50 and AH50, respectively. If both tests are normal, a complement deficiency is unlikely. If CH50 is absent and AH50 normal, a defect of C1, C4, or C2 is likely. Normal CH50 but absent AH50 suggests a defect of properdin or factor D. If both tests are abnormal, the defect most likely affects C3 to C8. Deficiency of C9 results usually in a CH50 value that is approximately half of normal. To pinpoint the specific complement component deficiency, immunochemical tests using component specific antibodies or functional assays using *in vitro* reconstitution of the hemolytic function are recommended. Mutations and single nucleotide polymorphisms (SNPs) in the complement regulatory proteins factor H and factor I are implicated in atypical hemolytic uremic syndrome and age-related macular degeneration.[320,321] Treatment of complement-component deficiencies depends on the defect and may include frequent immunizations using the appropriate vaccines, antibiotic prophylaxis, and workup for sepsis if the clinical symptoms suggest bacterial infections. Autoimmune disorders are treated symptomatically, using the same immunosuppressive agents and antiinflammatory medications as those used in the general population. Management of angioedema has been revolutionized by C1 esterase inhibitor concentrate (Cinryze, Berinert), which is most effective for the treatment of acute attacks and by the kallikrein inhibitor Kalbitor (Dyax) and the bradykinin receptor antagonist Firazyr (Shire).

REFERENCES

1. Winkelstein JA, Marino MC, Lederman HM, et al: X-linked agammaglobulinemia: Report on a United States registry of 201 patients. *Medicine (Baltimore)* 85:193–202, 2006.
2. Conley ME, Dobbs AK, Farmer DM, et al: Primary B cell immunodeficiencies: Comparisons and contrasts. *Annu Rev Immunol* 27:199–227, 2009.
3. Conley ME, Dobbs AK, Quintana AM, et al: Agammaglobulinemia and absent B lineage cells in a patient lacking the p85alpha subunit of PI3K. *J Exp Med* 209:463–470, 2012.
4. Boisson B, Wang YD, Bosompem A, et al: A recurrent dominant negative E47 mutation causes agammaglobulinemia and BCR(−) B cells. *J Clin Invest* 123:4781–4785, 2013.
5. Lederman HM, Winkelstein JA: X-linked agammaglobulinemia: An analysis of 96 patients. *Medicine (Baltimore)* 64:145–156, 1985.
6. Plebani A, Soresina A, Rondelli R, et al: Clinical, immunological, and molecular analysis in a large cohort of patients with X-linked agammaglobulinemia: An Italian multicenter study. *Clin Immunol* 104:221–230, 2002.
7. Franz A, Webster AD, Furr PM, et al: Mycoplasmal arthritis in patients with primary immunoglobulin deficiency: Clinical features and outcome in 18 patients. *Br J Rheumatol* 36:661–668, 1997.
8. McKinney RE Jr, Katz SL, Wilfert CM: Chronic enteroviral meningoencephalitis in agammaglobulinemic patients. *Rev Infect Dis* 9:334–356, 1987.
9. van der Meer JW, Weening RS, Schellekens PT, et al: Colorectal cancer in patients with X-linked agammaglobulinaemia. *Lancet* 341:1439–1440, 1993.
10. Murray PR, Jain A, Uzel G, et al: Pyoderma gangrenosum-like ulcer in a patient with X-linked agammaglobulinemia: Identification of Helicobacter bilis by mass spectrometry analysis. *Arch Dermatol* 146:523–526, 2010.
11. Futatani T, Watanabe C, Baba Y, et al: Bruton's tyrosine kinase is present in normal platelets and its absence identifies patients with X-linked agammaglobulinaemia and carrier females. *Br J Haematol* 114:141–149, 2001.
12. Ziegner UH, Kobayashi RH, Cunningham-Rundles C, et al: Progressive neurodegeneration in patients with primary immunodeficiency disease on IVIG treatment. *Clin Immunol* 102:19–24, 2002.
13. Jain A, Ma CA, Liu S, et al: Specific missense mutations in NEMO result in hyper-IgM syndrome with hypohydrotic ectodermal dysplasia. *Nat Immunol* 2:223–228, 2001.
14. Peron S, Metin A, Gardes P, et al: Human PMS2 deficiency is associated with impaired immunoglobulin class switch recombination. *J Exp Med* 205:2465–2472, 2008.
15. Etzioni A, Ben-Barak A, Peron S, et al: Ataxia-telangiectasia in twins presenting as autosomal recessive hyper-immunoglobulin M syndrome. *Isr Med Assoc J* 9:406–407, 2007.
16. Notarangelo LD, Gilani S, Pleabani A: CD40 and CD40 ligand deficiencies, in *Primary Immunodeficiency Diseases, A Molecular and Genetic Approach*, 3rd ed, edited by Ochs HD, Smith CIE, Puck JM, p 324. Oxford University Press, New York, 2014.
17. Hayward AR, Levy J, Facchetti F, et al: Cholangiopathy and tumors of the pancreas, liver, and biliary tree in boys with X-linked immunodeficiency with hyper-IgM. *J Immunol* 158:977–983, 1997.
18. Agematsu K, Nagumo H, Shinozaki K, et al: Absence of IgD-CD27(+) memory B cell population in X-linked hyper-IgM syndrome. *J Clin Invest* 102:853–860, 1998.
19. Ameratunga R, Lederman HM, Sullivan KE, et al: Defective antigen-induced lymphocyte proliferation in the X-linked hyper-IgM syndrome. *J Pediatr* 131:147–150, 1997.
20. Seyama K, Kobayashi R, Hasle H, et al: Parvovirus B19-induced anemia as the presenting manifestation of X-linked hyper-IgM syndrome. *J Infect Dis* 178:318–324, 1998.
21. Levy J, Espanol-Boren T, Thomas C, et al: Clinical spectrum of X-linked hyper-IgM syndrome. *J Pediatr* 131:47–54, 1997.
22. Al-Saud BK, Al-Sum Z, Alassiri H, et al: Clinical, immunological, and molecular characterization of hyper-IgM syndrome due to CD40 deficiency in eleven patients. *J Clin Immunol* 33:1325–1335, 2013.
23. Durandy A, Kracker S, Fischer A: Autosomal IgCSR deficiencies caused by an intrinsic B-cell defect, in *Primary Immunodeficiency Diseases, A Molecular and Genetic Approach*, 3rd ed, edited by Ochs HD, Smith CIE, Puck JM, p 343. Oxford University Press, New York, 2014.
24. Picard C, Orange JS, Puel A, et al: Inborn errors of NF-KB immunity, in *Primary Immunodeficiency Diseases, A Molecular and Genetic Approach*, 3rd ed, edited by Ochs HD, Smith CIE, Puck JM, p 467. Oxford University Press, New York, 2014.
25. Schimke LF, Rieber N, Rylaarsdam S, et al: A novel gain-of-function IKBA mutation underlies ectodermal dysplasia with immunodeficiency and polyendocrinopathy. *J Clin Immunol* 33:1088–1099, 2013.
26. Hanson EP, Monaco-Shawver L, Solt LA, et al: Hypomorphic nuclear factor-kappaB essential modulator mutation database and reconstitution system identifies phenotypic and immunologic diversity. *J Allergy Clin Immunol* 122:1169–1177 e16, 2008.
27. Salzer U, Warnatz K, Peter HH: Common variable immunodeficiency—An update. *Arthritis Res Ther* 14:223, 2012.
28. Chen K, Coonrod EM, Kumanovics A, et al: Germline mutations in NFKB2 implicate the noncanonical NF-kappaB pathway in the pathogenesis of common variable immunodeficiency. *Am J Hum Genet* 93:812–824, 2013.
29. Lucas CL, Kuehn HS, Zhao F, et al: Dominant-activating germline mutations in the gene encoding the PI(3)K catalytic subunit p110delta result in T cell senescence and human immunodeficiency. *Nat Immunol* 15:88–97, 2014.
30. Angulo I, Vadas O, Garcon F, et al: Phosphoinositide 3-kinase delta gene mutation predisposes to respiratory infection and airway damage. *Science* 342:866–871, 2013.
31. Salzer E, Santos-Valente E, Klaver S, et al: B-cell deficiency and severe autoimmunity caused by deficiency of protein kinase C delta. *Blood* 121:3112–3116, 2013.
32. Resnick ES, Moshier EL, Godbold JH, et al: Morbidity and mortality in common variable immune deficiency over 4 decades. *Blood* 119:1650–1657, 2012.
33. Cunningham-Rundles C, Siegal FP, Cunningham-Rundles S, et al: Incidence of cancer in 98 patients with common varied immunodeficiency. *J Clin Immunol* 7:294–299, 1987.
34. Cunningham-Rundles C, Cooper DL, Duffy TP, et al: Lymphomas of mucosal-associated lymphoid tissue in common variable immunodeficiency. *Am J Hematol* 69:171–178, 2002.
35. Van der Hilst JC, Smits BW, van der Meer JW: Hypogammaglobulinaemia: Cumulative experience in 49 patients in a tertiary care institution. *Neth J Med* 60:140–147, 2002.
36. Koistinen J: Selective IgA deficiency in blood donors. *Vox Sang* 29:192–202, 1975.
37. Kanoh T, Mizumoto T, Yasuda N, et al: Selective IgA deficiency in Japanese blood donors: Frequency and statistical analysis. *Vox Sang* 50:81–86, 1986.
38. Oxelius VA, Laurell AB, Lindquist B, et al: IgG subclasses in selective IgA deficiency: Importance of IgG2-IgA deficiency. *N Engl J Med* 304:1476–1477, 1981.
39. Lopez-Herrera G, Tampella G, Pan-Hammarstrom Q, et al: Deleterious mutations in LRBA are associated with a syndrome of immune deficiency and autoimmunity. *Am J Hum Genet* 90:986–1001, 2012.
40. Alangari A, Alsultan A, Adly N, et al: LPS-responsive beige-like anchor (LRBA) gene mutation in a family with inflammatory bowel disease and combined immunodeficiency. *J Allergy Clin Immunol* 130:481–488 e2, 2012.

41. Glanzman ERP: Essentielle lymphocytophtise. Ein neues Krankheitsbild aus der Sauglingspathologie. *Ann Paediatr* 175, 1950.

42. Buckley RH: Molecular defects in human severe combined immunodeficiency and approaches to immune reconstitution. *Annu Rev Immunol* 22:625–655, 2004.

43. Fischer A, Le Deist F, Hacein-Bey-Abina S, et al: Severe combined immunodeficiency. A model disease for molecular immunology and therapy. *Immunol Rev* 203:98–109, 2005.

44. Al-Herz W, Bousfiha A, Casanova JL, et al: Primary immunodeficiency diseases: An update on the classification from the international union of immunological societies expert committee for primary immunodeficiency. *Front Immunol* 5:162, 2014.

45. Grunebaum E, Cohen A, Roifman CM: Recent advances in understanding and managing adenosine deaminase and purine nucleoside phosphorylase deficiencies. *Curr Opin Allergy Clin Immunol* 13:630–638, 2013.

46. Cassani B, Mirolo M, Cattaneo F, et al: Altered intracellular and extracellular signaling leads to impaired T-cell functions in ADA-SCID patients. *Blood* 111:4209–4219, 2008.

47. Cohen AGE, Arpaia E, Roifman CM: Immunodeficiency caused by purine nucleoside phosphorylase deficiency. *Immunol Allergy Clin North Am* 20 (1):143–159, 2000.

48. Small TN, Wall DA, Kurtzberg J, et al: Association of reticular dysgenesis (thymic alymphoplasia and congenital aleukocytosis) with bilateral sensorineural deafness. *J Pediatr* 135:387–389, 1999.

49. Pannicke U, Honig M, Hess I, et al: Reticular dysgenesis (aleukocytosis) is caused by mutations in the gene encoding mitochondrial adenylate kinase 2. *Nat Genet* 41:101–105, 2009.

50. Lagresle-Peyrou C, Six EM, Picard C, et al: Human adenylate kinase 2 deficiency causes a profound hematopoietic defect associated with sensorineural deafness. *Nat Genet* 41:106–111, 2009.

51. Rochman Y, Spolski R, Leonard WJ: New insights into the regulation of T cells by gamma(c) family cytokines. *Nat Rev Immunol* 9:480–490, 2009.

52. Noguchi M, Yi H, Rosenblatt HM, et al: Interleukin-2 receptor gamma chain mutation results in X-linked severe combined immunodeficiency in humans. *Cell* 73:147–157, 1993.

53. Macchi P, Villa A, Giliani S, et al: Mutations of Jak-3 gene in patients with autosomal severe combined immune deficiency (SCID). *Nature* 377:65–68, 1995.

54. Russell SM, Tayebi N, Nakajima H, et al: Mutation of Jak3 in a patient with SCID: Essential role of Jak3 in lymphoid development. *Science* 270:797–800, 1995.

55. Puel A, Ziegler SF, Buckley RH, et al: Defective IL7R expression in T(-)B(+)NK(+) severe combined immunodeficiency. *Nat Genet* 20:394–397, 1998.

56. Neven B, Leroy S, Decaluwe H, et al: Long-term outcome after hematopoietic stem cell transplantation of a single-center cohort of 90 patients with severe combined immunodeficiency. *Blood* 113:4114–4124, 2009.

57. Moshous D, Callebaut I, de Chasseval R, et al: Artemis, a novel DNA double-strand break repair/V(D)J recombination protein, is mutated in human severe combined immune deficiency. *Cell* 105:177–186, 2001.

58. van der Burg M, Ijspeert H, Verkaik NS, et al: A DNA-PKcs mutation in a radiosensitive T-B- SCID patient inhibits Artemis activation and nonhomologous end-joining. *J Clin Invest* 119:91–98, 2009.

59. Buck D, Moshous D, de Chasseval R, et al: Severe combined immunodeficiency and microcephaly in siblings with hypomorphic mutations in DNA ligase IV. *Eur J Immunol* 36:224–235, 2006.

60. van der Burg M, van Veelen LR, Verkaik NS, et al: A new type of radiosensitive T-B-NK+ severe combined immunodeficiency caused by a LIG4 mutation. *J Clin Invest* 116:137–145, 2006.

61. Ahnesorg P, Smith P, Jackson SP: XLF interacts with the XRCC4-DNA ligase IV complex to promote DNA nonhomologous end-joining. *Cell* 124:301–313, 2006.

62. Dadi HK, Simon AJ, Roifman CM: Effect of CD3delta deficiency on maturation of alpha/beta and gamma/delta T-cell lineages in severe combined immunodeficiency. *N Engl J Med* 349:1821–1828, 2003.

63. de Saint Basile G, Geissmann F, Flori E, et al: Severe combined immunodeficiency caused by deficiency in either the delta or the epsilon subunit of CD3. *J Clin Invest* 114:1512–1517, 2004.

64. Rieux-Laucat F, Hivroz C, Lim A, et al: Inherited and somatic CD3zeta mutations in a patient with T-cell deficiency. *N Engl J Med* 354:1913–1921, 2006.

65. Arnaiz-Villena A, Timon M, Corell A, et al: Brief report: Primary immunodeficiency caused by mutations in the gene encoding the CD3-gamma subunit of the T-lymphocyte receptor. *N Engl J Med* 327:529–533, 1992.

66. Recio MJ, Moreno-Pelayo MA, Kilic SS, et al: Differential biological role of CD3 chains revealed by human immunodeficiencies. *J Immunol* 178:2556–2564, 2007.

67. Morgan NV, Goddard S, Cardno TS, et al: Mutation in the TCRalpha subunit constant gene (TRAC) leads to a human immunodeficiency disorder characterized by a lack of TCRalphabeta+ T cells. *J Clin Invest* 121:695–702, 2011.

68. Kung C, Pingel JT, Heikinheimo M, et al: Mutations in the tyrosine phosphatase CD45 gene in a child with severe combined immunodeficiency disease. *Nat Med* 6:343–345, 2000.

69. Tchilian EZ, Wallace DL, Wells RS, et al: A deletion in the gene encoding the CD45 antigen in a patient with SCID. *J Immunol* 166:1308–1313, 2001.

70. Buckley RH, Schiff RI, Schiff SE, et al: Human severe combined immunodeficiency: Genetic, phenotypic, and functional diversity in one hundred eight infants. *J Pediatr* 130:378–387, 1997.

71. Yeganeh M, Heidarzade M, Pourpak Z, et al: Severe combined immunodeficiency: A cohort of 40 patients. *Pediatr Allergy Immunol* 19:303–306, 2008.

72. Muller SM, Ege M, Pottharst A, et al: Transplacentally acquired maternal T lymphocytes in severe combined immunodeficiency: A study of 121 patients. *Blood* 98:1847–1851, 2001.

73. Palmer K, Green TD, Roberts JL, et al: Unusual clinical and immunologic manifestations of transplacentally acquired maternal T cells in severe combined immunodeficiency. *J Allergy Clin Immunol* 120:423–428, 2007.

74. Shearer WT, Dunn E, Notarangelo LD, et al: Establishing diagnostic criteria for severe combined immunodeficiency disease (SCID), leaky SCID, and Omenn syndrome: The Primary Immune Deficiency Treatment Consortium experience. *J Allergy Clin Immunol* 133:1092–1098, 2014.

75. Hirschhorn R: In vivo reversion to normal of inherited mutations in humans. *J Med Genet* 40:721–728, 2003.

76. Kwan A, Abraham RS, Currier R, et al: Newborn screening for severe combined immunodeficiency in 11 screening programs in the United States. *JAMA* 312:729–738, 2014.

77. Engel BC, Podsakoff GM, Ireland JL, et al: Prolonged pancytopenia in a gene therapy patient with ADA-deficient SCID and trisomy 8 mosaicism: A case report. *Blood* 109:503–506, 2007.

78. Dror Y, Grunebaum E, Hitzler J, et al: Purine nucleoside phosphorylase deficiency associated with a dysplastic marrow morphology. *Pediatr Res* 55:472–477, 2004.

79. Buck D, Malivert L, de Chasseval R, et al: Cernunnos, a novel nonhomologous end-joining factor, is mutated in human immunodeficiency with microcephaly. *Cell* 124:287–299, 2006.

80. Faraci M, Lanino E, Micalizzi C, et al: Unrelated hematopoietic stem cell transplantation for Cernunnos-XLF deficiency. *Pediatr Transplant* 13:785–789, 2009.

81. Gruhn B, Seidel J, Zintl F, et al: Successful bone marrow transplantation in a patient with DNA ligase IV deficiency and bone marrow failure. *Orphanet J Rare Dis* 2:5, 2007.

82. Cossu F, Vulliamy TJ, Marrone A, et al: A novel DKC1 mutation, severe combined immunodeficiency (T+B-NK- SCID) and bone marrow transplantation in an infant with Hoyeraal-Hreidarsson syndrome. *Br J Haematol* 119:765–768, 2002.

83. Hitzig WH, Kenny AB: The role of vitamin B12 and its transport globulins in the production of antibodies. *Clin Exp Immunol* 20:105–111, 1975.

84. Wong SN, Low LC, Lau YL, et al: Immunodeficiency in methylmalonic acidaemia. *J Paediatr Child Health* 28:180–183, 1992.

85. Gatti RA, Meuwissen HJ, Allen HD, et al: Immunological reconstitution of sex-linked lymphopenic immunological deficiency. *Lancet* 2:1366–1369, 1968.

86. Pai SY, Logan BR, Griffith LM, et al: Transplantation outcomes for severe combined immunodeficiency, 2000–2009. *N Engl J Med* 371:434–446, 2014.

87. Honig M, Albert MH, Schulz A, et al: Patients with adenosine deaminase deficiency surviving after hematopoietic stem cell transplantation are at high risk of CNS complications. *Blood* 109:3595–3602, 2007.

88. Titman P, Pink E, Skucek E, et al: Cognitive and behavioral abnormalities in children after hematopoietic stem cell transplantation for severe congenital immunodeficiencies. *Blood* 112:3907–3913, 2008.

89. Schuetz C, Neven B, Dvorak CC, et al: SCID patients with ARTEMIS vs RAG deficiencies following HCT: Increased risk of late toxicity in ARTEMIS-deficient SCID. *Blood* 123:281–289, 2014.

90. Aiuti A, Cattaneo F, Galimberti S, et al: Gene therapy for immunodeficiency due to adenosine deaminase deficiency. *N Engl J Med* 360:447–458, 2009.

91. Gaspar HB, Cooray S, Gilmour KC, et al: Hematopoietic stem cell gene therapy for adenosine deaminase-deficient severe combined immunodeficiency leads to long-term immunological recovery and metabolic correction. *Sci Transl Med* 3:97ra80, 2011.

92. Candotti F, Shaw KL, Muul L, et al: Gene therapy for adenosine deaminase-deficient severe combined immune deficiency: Clinical comparison of retroviral vectors and treatment plans. *Blood* 120:3635–3646, 2012.

93. Hacein-Bey-Abina S, Hauer J, Lim A, et al: Efficacy of gene therapy for X-linked severe combined immunodeficiency. *N Engl J Med* 363:355–364, 2010.

94. Gaspar HB, Cooray S, Gilmour KC, et al: Long-term persistence of a polyclonal T cell repertoire after gene therapy for X-linked severe combined immunodeficiency. *Sci Transl Med* 3:97ra79, 2011.

95. Hacein-Bey-Abina S, Garrigue A, Wang GP, et al: Insertional oncogenesis in 4 patients after retrovirus-mediated gene therapy of SCID-X1. *J Clin Invest* 118:3132–3142, 2008.

96. Howe SJ, Mansour MR, Schwarzwaelder K, et al: Insertional mutagenesis combined with acquired somatic mutations causes leukemogenesis following gene therapy of SCID-X1 patients. *J Clin Invest* 118:3143–3150, 2008.

97. Hacein-Bey-Abina S, Pai SY, Gaspar HB: Improved gene therapy for X-linked severe combined immunodeficiency. *N Engl J Med* 371:1407–1417, 2014.

98. Omenn GS: Familial reticuloendotheliosis with eosinophilia. *N Engl J Med* 273:427–432, 1965.

99. Signorini S, Imberti L, Pirovano S, et al: Intrathymic restriction and peripheral expansion of the T-cell repertoire in Omenn syndrome. *Blood* 94:3468–3478, 1999.

100. Villa A, Santagata S, Bozzi F, et al: Partial V(D)J recombination activity leads to Omenn syndrome. *Cell* 93:885–896, 1998.

101. Marrella V, Maina V, Villa A: Omenn syndrome does not live by V(D)J recombination alone. *Curr Opin Allergy Clin Immunol* 11:525–531, 2011.

102. Cavadini P, Vermi W, Facchetti F, et al: AIRE deficiency in thymus of 2 patients with Omenn syndrome. *J Clin Invest* 115:728–732, 2005.

103. Villa A, Marrella V, Rucci F, et al: Genetically determined lymphopenia and autoimmune manifestations. *Curr Opin Immunol* 20:318–324, 2008.

104. Villa A, Notarangelo LD, Roifman CM: Omenn syndrome: Inflammation in leaky severe combined immunodeficiency. *J Allergy Clin Immunol* 122:1082–1086, 2008.

105. Matangkasombut P, Pichavant M, Saez DE, et al: Lack of iNKT cells in patients with combined immune deficiency due to hypomorphic RAG mutations. *Blood* 111:271–274, 2008.

106. Markert ML, Alexieff MJ, Li J, et al: Complete DiGeorge syndrome: Development of rash, lymphadenopathy, and oligoclonal T cells in 5 cases. *J Allergy Clin Immunol* 113:734–741, 2004.

107. Gennery AR, Slatter MA, Rice J, et al: Mutations in CHD7 in patients with CHARGE syndrome cause T-B + natural killer cell + severe combined immune deficiency and may cause Omenn-like syndrome. *Clin Exp Immunol* 153:75–80, 2008.

108. Torgerson TR, Gambineri E, Ochs HD: Immune dysregulation, polyendocrinopathy, enteropathy, and X-linked inheritance, in *Primary Immunodeficiency Diseases, A Molecular and Genetic Approach*, 3rd ed, edited by Ochs HD, Smith CIE, Puck JM, pp 395–413. Oxford University Press, New York, 2014.

109. Fraitag S, Bodemer C: Neonatal erythroderma. *Curr Opin Pediatr* 22:438–444, 2010.

110. Hauck F, Randriamampita C, Martin E, et al: Primary T-cell immunodeficiency with immunodysregulation caused by autosomal recessive LCK deficiency. *J Allergy Clin Immunol* 130:1144–1152 e11, 2012.

111. Chan AC, Kadlecek TA, Elder ME, et al: ZAP-70 deficiency in an autosomal recessive form of severe combined immunodeficiency. *Science* 264:1599–1601, 1994.

112. Elder ME, Lin D, Clever J, et al: Human severe combined immunodeficiency due to a defect in ZAP-70, a T cell tyrosine kinase. *Science* 264:1596–1599, 1994.

113. Crequer A, Troeger A, Patin E, et al: Human RHOH deficiency causes T cell defects and susceptibility to EV-HPV infections. *J Clin Invest* 122:3239–3247, 2012.

114. Nehme NT, Pachlopnik Schmid J, Debeurme F, et al: MST1 mutations in autosomal recessive primary immunodeficiency characterized by defective naive T-cell survival. *Blood* 119:3458–3468, 2012.

115. Abdollahpour H, Appaswamy G, Kotlarz D, et al: The phenotype of human STK4 deficiency. *Blood* 119:3450–3457, 2012.

116. de la Calle-Martin O, Hernandez M, Ordi J, et al: Familial CD8 deficiency due to a mutation in the CD8 alpha gene. *J Clin Invest* 108:117–123, 2001.

117. Mancebo E, Moreno-Pelayo MA, Mencia A, et al: Gly111Ser mutation in CD8A gene causing CD8 immunodeficiency is found in Spanish Gypsies. *Mol Immunol* 45:479–484, 2008.

118. Jabara HH, Ohsumi T, Chou J, et al: A homozygous mucosa-associated lymphoid tissue 1 (MALT1) mutation in a family with combined immunodeficiency. *J Allergy Clin Immunol* 132:151–158, 2013.

119. Stepensky P, Keller B, Buchta M, et al: Deficiency of caspase recruitment domain family, member 11 (CARD11), causes profound combined immunodeficiency in human subjects. *J Allergy Clin Immunol* 131:477–85 e1, 2013.

120. Greil J, Rausch T, Giese T, et al: Whole-exome sequencing links caspase recruitment domain 11 (CARD11) inactivation to severe combined immunodeficiency. *J Allergy Clin Immunol* 131:1376–1383 e3, 2013.

121. Pannicke U, Baumann B, Fuchs S, et al: Deficiency of innate and acquired immunity caused by an IKBKB mutation. *N Engl J Med* 369:2504–2514, 2013.

122. Courtois G, Smahi A, Reichenbach J, et al: A hypermorphic IkappaBalpha mutation is associated with autosomal dominant anhidrotic ectodermal dysplasia and T cell immunodeficiency. *J Clin Invest* 112:1108–1115, 2003.

123. Picard C, Casanova JL, Puel A: Infectious diseases in patients with IRAK-4, MyD88, NEMO, or IkappaBalpha deficiency. *Clin Microbiol Rev* 24:490–497, 2011.

124. Shiow LR, Roadcap DW, Paris K, et al: The actin regulator coronin 1A is mutant in a thymic egress-deficient mouse strain and in a patient with severe combined immunodeficiency. *Nat Immunol* 9:1307–1315, 2008.

125. Moshous D, Martin E, Carpentier W, et al: Whole-exome sequencing identifies Coronin-1A deficiency in 3 siblings with immunodeficiency and EBV-associated B-cell lymphoproliferation. *J Allergy Clin Immunol* 131:1594–1603, 2013.

126. van Montfrans JM, Hoepelman AI, Otto S, et al: CD27 deficiency is associated with combined immunodeficiency and persistent symptomatic EBV viremia. *J Allergy Clin Immunol* 129:787–793 e6, 2012.

127. Martin E, Palmic N, Sanquer S, et al: CTP synthase 1 deficiency in humans reveals its central role in lymphocyte proliferation. *Nature* 510:288–292, 2014.

128. de la Salle H, Zimmer J, Fricker D, et al: HLA class I deficiencies due to mutations in subunit 1 of the peptide transporter TAP1. *J Clin Invest* 103:R9–R13, 1999.

129. de la Salle H, Hanau D, Fricker D, et al: Homozygous human TAP peptide transporter mutation in HLA class I deficiency. *Science* 265:237–241, 1994.

130. Yabe T, Kawamura S, Sato M, et al: A subject with a novel type I bare lymphocyte syndrome has tapasin deficiency due to deletion of 4 exons by Alu-mediated recombination. *Blood* 100:1496–1498, 2002.

131. Gadola SD, Moins-Teisserenc HT, Trowsdale J, et al: TAP deficiency syndrome. *Clin Exp Immunol* 121:173–178, 2000.

132. Zimmer J, Andres E, Donato L, et al: Clinical and immunological aspects of HLA class I deficiency. *QJM* 98:719–727, 2005.

133. Picard C, Fischer A: Hematopoietic stem cell transplantation and other management strategies for MHC class II deficiency. *Immunol Allergy Clin North Am* 30:173–178, 2010.

134. Feske S, Gwack Y, Prakriya M, et al: A mutation in Orai1 causes immune deficiency by abrogating CRAC channel function. *Nature* 441:179–185, 2006.

135. Picard C, McCarl CA, Papolos A, et al: STIM1 mutation associated with a syndrome of immunodeficiency and autoimmunity. *N Engl J Med* 360:1971–1980, 2009.

136. Li FY, Chaigne-Delalande B, Kanellopoulou C, et al: Second messenger role for Mg2+ revealed by human T-cell immunodeficiency. *Nature* 475:471–476, 2011.

137. Chaigne-Delalande B, Li FY, O'Connor GM, et al: Mg2+ regulates cytotoxic functions of NK and CD8 T cells in chronic EBV infection through NKG2D. *Science* 341:186–191, 2013.

138. Zhang Q, Davis JC, Lamborn IT, et al: Combined immunodeficiency associated with DOCK8 mutations. *N Engl J Med* 361:2046–2055, 2009.

139. Engelhardt KR, McGhee S, Winkler S, et al: Large deletions and point mutations involving the dedicator of cytokinesis 8 (DOCK8) in the autosomal-recessive form of hyper-IgE syndrome. *J Allergy Clin Immunol* 124:1289–1302 e4, 2009.

140. Randall KL, Chan SS, Ma CS, et al: DOCK8 deficiency impairs CD8 T cell survival and function in humans and mice. *J Exp Med* 208:2305–2320, 2011.

141. Mizesko MC, Banerjee PP, Monaco-Shawver L, et al: Defective actin accumulation impairs human natural killer cell function in patients with dedicator of cytokinesis 8 deficiency. *J Allergy Clin Immunol* 131:840–848, 2013.

142. Jabara HH, McDonald DR, Janssen E, et al: DOCK8 functions as an adaptor that links TLR-MyD88 signaling to B cell activation. *Nat Immunol* 13:612–620, 2012.

143. Pai SY, de Boer H, Massaad MJ, et al: Flow cytometry diagnosis of dedicator of cytokinesis 8 (DOCK8) deficiency. *J Allergy Clin Immunol* 134:221–223 e7, 2014.

144. Barlogis V, Galambrun C, Chambost H, et al: Successful allogeneic hematopoietic stem cell transplantation for DOCK8 deficiency. *J Allergy Clin Immunol* 128:420–422 e2, 2011.

145. Keles S, Jabara HH, Reisli I, et al: Plasmacytoid dendritic cell depletion in DOCK8 deficiency: Rescue of severe herpetic infections with IFN-alpha 2b therapy. *J Allergy Clin Immunol* 133:1753–1755 e3, 2014.

146. Samuels ME, Majewski J, Alirezaie N, et al: Exome sequencing identifies mutations in the gene TTC7A in French-Canadian cases with hereditary multiple intestinal atresia. *J Med Genet* 50:324–329, 2013.

147. Chen R, Giliani S, Lanzi G, et al: Whole-exome sequencing identifies tetratricopeptide repeat domain 7A (TTC7A) mutations for combined immunodeficiency with intestinal atresias. *J Allergy Clin Immunol* 132:656–664 e17, 2013.

148. Bigorgne AE, Farin HF, Lemoine R, et al: TTC7A mutations disrupt intestinal epithelial apicobasal polarity. *J Clin Invest* 124:328–337, 2014.

149. Avitzur Y, Guo C, Mastropaolo LA, et al: Mutations in tetratricopeptide repeat domain 7A result in a severe form of very early onset inflammatory bowel disease. *Gastroenterology* 146:1028–1039, 2014.

150. Fischer RT, Friend B, Talmon GA, et al: Intestinal transplantation in children with multiple intestinal atresias and immunodeficiency. *Pediatr Transplant* 18:190–196, 2014.

151. Cliffe ST, Bloch DB, Suryani S, et al: Clinical, molecular, and cellular immunologic findings in patients with SP110-associated veno-occlusive disease with immunodeficiency syndrome. *J Allergy Clin Immunol* 130:735–742 e6, 2012.

152. Roscioli T, Cliffe ST, Bloch DB, et al: Mutations in the gene encoding the PML nuclear body protein Sp110 are associated with immunodeficiency and hepatic veno-occlusive disease. *Nat Genet* 38:620–622, 2006.

153. Ganaiem H, Eisenstein EM, Tenenbaum A, et al: The role of hematopoietic stem cell transplantation in SP110 associated veno-occlusive disease with immunodeficiency syndrome. *Pediatr Allergy Immunol* 24:250–256, 2013.

154. Kobrynski LJ, Sullivan KE: Velocardiofacial syndrome, DiGeorge syndrome: The chromosome 22q11.2 deletion syndromes. *Lancet* 370:1443–1452, 2007.

155. Markert ML, Devlin BH, Alexieff MJ, et al: Review of 54 patients with complete DiGeorge anomaly enrolled in protocols for thymus transplantation: Outcome of 44 consecutive transplants. *Blood* 109:4539–4547, 2007.

156. Lingman Framme J, Borte S, von Dobeln U, et al: Retrospective analysis of TREC based newborn screening results and clinical phenotypes in infants with the 22q11 deletion syndrome. *J Clin Immunol* 34:514–519, 2014.

157. Land MH, Garcia-Lloret MI, Borzy MS, et al: Long-term results of bone marrow transplantation in complete DiGeorge syndrome. *J Allergy Clin Immunol* 120:908–915, 2007.

158. Jongmans MC, Admiraal RJ, van der Donk KP, et al: CHARGE syndrome: The phenotypic spectrum of mutations in the CHD7 gene. *J Med Genet* 43:306–314, 2006.

159. Pignata C, Fiore M, Guzzetta V, et al: Congenital Alopecia and nail dystrophy associated with severe functional T-cell immunodeficiency in two sibs. *Am J Med Genet* 65:167–170, 1996.

160. Markert ML, Marques JG, Neven B, et al: First use of thymus transplantation therapy for FOXN1 deficiency (nude/SCID): A report of 2 cases. *Blood* 117:688–696, 2011.

161. Bennett CL, Christie J, Ramsdell F, et al: The immune dysregulation, polyendocrinopathy, enteropathy, X-linked syndrome (IPEX) is caused by mutations of FOXP3. *Nat Genet* 27:20–21, 2001.

162. Torgerson TR, Genin A, Chen C, et al: FOXP3 inhibits activation-induced NFAT2 expression in T cells thereby limiting effector cytokine expression. *J Immunol* 183:907–915, 2009.

163. Burroughs LM, Torgerson TR, Storb R, et al: Stable hematopoietic cell engraftment after low-intensity nonmyeloablative conditioning in patients with immune dysregulation, polyendocrinopathy, enteropathy, X-linked syndrome. *J Allergy Clin Immunol* 126:1000–1005, 2010.

164. Aoki CA, Roifman CM, Lian ZX, et al: IL-2 receptor alpha deficiency and features of primary biliary cirrhosis. *J Autoimmun* 27:50–53, 2006.

165. Caudy AA, Reddy ST, Chatila T, et al: CD25 deficiency causes an immune dysregulation, polyendocrinopathy, enteropathy, X-linked-like syndrome, and defective IL-10 expression from CD4 lymphocytes. *J Allergy Clin Immunol* 119:482–487, 2007.

166. Kofoed EM, Hwa V, Little B, et al: Growth hormone insensitivity associated with a STAT5b mutation. *N Engl J Med* 349:1139–1147, 2003.

167. Nadeau K, Hwa V, Rosenfeld RG: STAT5b deficiency: An unsuspected cause of growth failure, immunodeficiency, and severe pulmonary disease. *J Pediatr* 158:701–708, 2011.

168. Cohen AC, Nadeau KC, Tu W, et al: Cutting edge: Decreased accumulation and regulatory function of CD4+ CD25(high) T cells in human STAT5b deficiency. *J Immunol* 177:2770–2774, 2006.

169. Hwa V, Nadeau K, Wit JM, et al: STAT5b deficiency: Lessons from STAT5b gene mutations. *Best Pract Res Clin Endocrinol Metab* 25:61–75, 2011.

170. Liu L, Okada S, Kong XF, et al: Gain-of-function human STAT1 mutations impair IL-17 immunity and underlie chronic mucocutaneous candidiasis. *J Exp Med* 208:1635–1648, 2011.

171. Uzel G, Sampaio EP, Lawrence MG, et al: Dominant gain-of-function STAT1 mutations in FOXP3 wild-type immune dysregulation-polyendocrinopathy-enteropathy-X-linked-like syndrome. *J Allergy Clin Immunol* 131:1611–1623, 2013.

172. Flanagan SE, Haapaniemi E, Russell MA, et al: Activating germline mutations in STAT3 cause early-onset multi-organ autoimmune disease. *Nat Genet* 46:812–814, 2014.

173. Krummel MF, Allison JP: CD28 and CTLA-4 have opposing effects on the response of T cells to stimulation. *J Exp Med* 182:459–465, 1995.

174. Kuehn HS, Ouyang W, Lo B, et al: Immune dysregulation in human subjects with heterozygous germline mutations in CTLA4. *Science* 345:1623–1627, 2014.

175. Lohr NJ, Molleston JP, Strauss KA, et al: Human ITCH E3 ubiquitin ligase deficiency causes syndromic multisystem autoimmune disease. *Am J Hum Genet* 86:447–453, 2010.

176. Venuprasad K: Cbl-b and itch: Key regulators of peripheral T-cell tolerance. *Cancer Res* 70:3009–3012, 2010.

177. Ahonen P, Myllarniemi S, Sipila I, et al: Clinical variation of autoimmune polyendocrinopathy-candidiasis-ectodermal dystrophy (APECED) in a series of 68 patients. *N Engl J Med* 322:1829–1836, 1990.

178. Anderson MS, Venanzi ES, Klein L, et al: Projection of an immunological self shadow within the thymus by the aire protein. *Science* 298:1395–1401, 2002.

179. Kont V, Laan M, Kisand K, et al: Modulation of Aire regulates the expression of tissue-restricted antigens. *Mol Immunol* 45:25–33, 2008.

180. Meager A, Visvalingam K, Peterson P, et al: Anti-interferon autoantibodies in autoimmune polyendocrinopathy syndrome type 1. *PLoS Med* 3:e289, 2006.

181. Puel A, Doffinger R, Natividad A, et al: Autoantibodies against IL-17A, IL-17F, and IL-22 in patients with chronic mucocutaneous candidiasis and autoimmune polyendocrine syndrome type I. *J Exp Med* 207:291–297, 2010.

182. Fleisher TA, Rieux-Laucat F, Puck JM: Autoimmune lymphoproliferative syndrome, in *Primary Immunodeficiency Diseases, A Molecular and Genetic Approach*, 3rd ed, edited by Ochs HD, Smith CIE, Puck JM, p 368. Oxford University Press, New York, 2014.

183. Teachey DT, Greiner R, Seif A, et al: Treatment with sirolimus results in complete responses in patients with autoimmune lymphoproliferative syndrome. *Br J Haematol* 145:101–106, 2009.

184. Ochs HD, Notarangelo L: Wiskott-Aldrich syndrome, in *Primary Immunodeficiency Diseases, A Molecular and Genetic Approach*, 3rd ed, edited by Ochs HD, Smith CIE, Puck JM, p 454. Oxford University Press, New York, 2014.

185. Albert MH, Bittner TC, Nonoyama S, et al: X-linked thrombocytopenia (XLT) due to WAS mutations: Clinical characteristics, long-term outcome, and treatment options. *Blood* 115:3231–3238, 2010.

186. Ancliff PJ, Blundell MP, Cory GO, et al: Two novel activating mutations in the Wiskott-Aldrich syndrome protein result in congenital neutropenia. *Blood* 108:2182–2189, 2006.

187. Moratto D, Giliani S, Bonfim C, et al: Long-term outcome and lineage-specific chimerism in 194 patients with Wiskott-Aldrich syndrome treated by hematopoietic cell transplantation in the period 1980–2009: An international collaborative study. *Blood* 118:1675–1684, 2011.

188. Ozsahin H, Cavazzana-Calvo M, Notarangelo LD, et al: Long-term outcome following hematopoietic stem-cell transplantation in Wiskott-Aldrich syndrome: Collaborative study of the European Society for Immunodeficiencies and European Group for Blood and Marrow Transplantation. *Blood* 111:439–445, 2008.

189. Lanzi G, Moratto D, Vairo D, et al: A novel primary human immunodeficiency due to deficiency in the WASP-interacting protein WIP. *J Exp Med* 209:29–34, 2012.

190. Grimbacher B, Holland SM, Gallin JI, et al: Hyper-IgE syndrome with recurrent infections—An autosomal dominant multisystem disorder. *N Engl J Med* 340:692–702, 1999.

191. Davis SD, Schaller J, Wedgwood RJ: Job's syndrome. Recurrent, "cold," staphylococcal abscesses. *Lancet* 1:1013–1015, 1966.

192. Buckley RH, Wray BB, Belmaker EZ: Extreme hyperimmunoglobulinemia E and undue susceptibility to infection. *Pediatrics* 49:59–70, 1972.

193. Grimbacher B, Schaffer AA, Holland SM, et al: Genetic linkage of hyper-IgE syndrome to chromosome 4. *Am J Hum Genet* 65:735–744, 1999.

194. Borges WG, Hensley T, Carey JC, et al: The face of Job. *J Pediatr* 133:303–305, 1998.

195. Meyer-Bahlburg A, Renner ED, Rylaarsdam S, et al: Heterozygous signal transducer and activator of transcription 3 mutations in hyper-IgE syndrome result in altered B-cell maturation. *J Allergy Clin Immunol* 129:559–562, 562 e1–e2, 2012.

196. Renner ED, Torgerson TR, Rylaarsdam S, et al: STAT3 mutation in the original patient with Job's syndrome. *N Engl J Med* 357:1667–1668, 2007.

197. Holland SM, DeLeo FR, Elloumi HZ, et al: STAT3 mutations in the hyper-IgE syndrome. *N Engl J Med* 357:1608–1619, 2007.

198. Minegishi Y, Saito M, Tsuchiya S, et al: Dominant-negative mutations in the DNA-binding domain of STAT3 cause hyper-IgE syndrome. *Nature* 448:1058–1062, 2007.

199. Renner ED, Rylaarsdam S, Anover-Sombke S, et al: Novel signal transducer and activator of transcription 3 (STAT3) mutations, reduced T(H)17 cell numbers, and variably defective STAT3 phosphorylation in hyper-IgE syndrome. *J Allergy Clin Immunol* 122:181–187, 2008.

200. Huang W, Na L, Fidel PL, et al: Requirement of interleukin-17A for systemic anti-Candida albicans host defense in mice. *J Infect Dis* 190:624–631, 2004.

201. Gennery AR, Flood TJ, Abinun M, et al: Bone marrow transplantation does not correct the hyper IgE syndrome. *Bone Marrow Transplant* 25:1303–1305, 2000.

202. Goussetis E, Peristeri I, Kitra V, et al: Successful long-term immunologic reconstitution by allogeneic hematopoietic stem cell transplantation cures patients with autosomal dominant hyper-IgE syndrome. *J Allergy Clin Immunol* 126:392–394, 2010.

203. Bittner TC, Pannicke U, Renner ED, et al: Successful long-term correction of autosomal recessive hyper-IgE syndrome due to DOCK8 deficiency by hematopoietic stem cell transplantation. *Klin Padiatr* 222:351–355, 2010.

204. Minegishi Y, Saito M, Morio T, et al: Human tyrosine kinase 2 deficiency reveals its requisite roles in multiple cytokine signals involved in innate and acquired immunity. *Immunity* 25:745–755, 2006.

205. McKusick VA, Eldridge R, Hostetler JA, et al: Dwarfism in the Amish. II. Cartilage-hair hypoplasia. *Bull Johns Hopkins Hosp* 116:285–326, 1965.

206. Notarangelo LD, Roifman CM, Giliani S: Cartilage-hair hypoplasia: Molecular basis and heterogeneity of the immunological phenotype. *Curr Opin Allergy Clin Immunol* 8:534–539, 2008.

207. Ridanpaa M, van Eenennaam H, Pelin K, et al: Mutations in the RNA component of RNase MRP cause a pleiotropic human disease, cartilage-hair hypoplasia. *Cell* 104:195–203, 2001.

208. de la Fuente MA, Recher M, Rider NL, et al: Reduced thymic output, cell cycle abnormalities, and increased apoptosis of T lymphocytes in patients with cartilage-hair hypoplasia. *J Allergy Clin Immunol* 128:139–146, 2011.

209. Kavadas FD, Giliani S, Gu Y, et al: Variability of clinical and laboratory features among patients with ribonuclease mitochondrial RNA processing endoribonuclease gene mutations. *J Allergy Clin Immunol* 122:1178–1184, 2008.

210. Guggenheim R, Somech R, Grunebaum E, et al: Bone marrow transplantation for cartilage-hair-hypoplasia. *Bone Marrow Transplant* 38:751–756, 2006.

211. Boerkoel CF, Takashima H, John J, et al: Mutant chromatin remodeling protein SMAR-CAL1 causes Schimke immuno-osseous dysplasia. *Nat Genet* 30:215–220, 2002.

212. Deguchi K, Clewing JM, Elizondo LI, et al: Neurologic phenotype of Schimke immuno-osseous dysplasia and neurodevelopmental expression of SMARCAL1. *J Neuropathol Exp Neurol* 67:565–577, 2008.

213. Boerkoel CF, O'Neill S, Andre JL, et al: Manifestations and treatment of Schimke immuno-osseous dysplasia: 14 new cases and a review of the literature. *Eur J Pediatr* 159:1–7, 2000.

214. Gorlin RJ, Gelb B, Diaz GA, et al: WHIM syndrome, an autosomal dominant disorder: Clinical, hematological, and molecular studies. *Am J Med Genet* 91:368–376, 2000.

215. Hernandez PA, Gorlin RJ, Lukens JN, et al: Mutations in the chemokine receptor gene CXCR4 are associated with WHIM syndrome, a combined immunodeficiency disease. *Nat Genet* 34:70–74, 2003.

216. Tassone L, Notarangelo LD, Bonomi V, et al: Clinical and genetic diagnosis of warts, hypogammaglobulinemia, infections, and myelokathexis syndrome in 10 patients. *J Allergy Clin Immunol* 123:1170–1173, 1173 e1–e3, 2009.

217. Sanmun D, Garwicz D, Smith CI, et al: Stromal-derived factor-1 abolishes constitutive apoptosis of WHIM syndrome neutrophils harbouring a truncating CXCR4 mutation. *Br J Haematol* 134:640–644, 2006.

218. Mc Guire PJ, Cunningham-Rundles C, Ochs H, et al: Oligoclonality, impaired class switch and B-cell memory responses in WHIM syndrome. *Clin Immunol* 135:412–421, 2010.

219. Wegner R-D, German JJ, Chrzanowska KH, et al: Chromosomal instability syndromes other than ataxia-telangiectasia, in *Primary Immunodeficiency Diseases, A Molecular and Genetic Approach*, 3rd ed, edited by Ochs HD, Smith CIE, Puck JM, p 632. Oxford University Press, New York, 2014.

220. Yel L, Lavin MF, Shiloh Y: Ataxia-telangiectasia, in *Primary Immunodeficiency Diseases, A Molecular and Genetic Approach*, 3rd ed, edited by Ochs HD, Smith CIE, Puck JM, p 602. Oxford University Press, New York, 2014.

221. Nowak-Wegrzyn A, Crawford TO, Winkelstein JA, et al: Immunodeficiency and infections in ataxia-telangiectasia. *J Pediatr* 144:505–511, 2004.

222. Savitsky K, Bar-Shira A, Gilad S, et al: A single ataxia telangiectasia gene with a product similar to PI-3 kinase. *Science* 268:1749–1753, 1995.

223. Pandita TK: The role of ATM in telomere structure and function. *Radiat Res* 156:642–647, 2001.

224. Klein C, Wenning GK, Quinn NP, et al: Ataxia without telangiectasia masquerading as benign hereditary chorea. *Mov Disord* 11:217–220, 1996.

225. Stewart GS, Maser RS, Stankovic T, et al: The DNA double-strand break repair gene hMRE11 is mutated in individuals with an ataxia-telangiectasia-like disorder. *Cell* 99:577–587, 1999.

226. Chrzanowska KH, Gregorek H, Dembowska-Baginska B, et al: Nijmegen breakage syndrome (NBS). *Orphanet J Rare Dis* 7:13, 2012.

227. Albert MH, Gennery AR, Greil J, et al: Successful SCT for Nijmegen breakage syndrome. *Bone Marrow Transplant* 45:622–626, 2010.

228. de Saint Basile G, Menasche G, Fischer A: Molecular mechanisms of biogenesis and exocytosis of cytotoxic granules. *Nat Rev Immunol* 10:568–579, 2010.

229. Chandrakasan S, Filipovich AH: Hemophagocytic lymphohistiocytosis: Advances in pathophysiology, diagnosis, and treatment. *J Pediatr* 163:1253–1259, 2013.

230. Stepp SE, Dufourcq-Lagelouse R, Le Deist F, et al: Perforin gene defects in familial hemophagocytic lymphohistiocytosis. *Science* 286:1957–1959, 1999.

231. Feldmann J, Callebaut I, Raposo G, et al: Munc13-4 is essential for cytolytic granules fusion and is mutated in a form of familial hemophagocytic lymphohistiocytosis (FHL3). *Cell* 115:461–473, 2003.

232. zur Stadt U, Schmidt S, Kasper B, et al: Linkage of familial hemophagocytic lymphohistiocytosis (FHL) type-4 to chromosome 6q24 and identification of mutations in syntaxin 11. *Hum Mol Genet* 14:827–834, 2005.

233. Cote M, Menager MM, Burgess A, et al: Munc18–2 deficiency causes familial hemophagocytic lymphohistiocytosis type 5 and impairs cytotoxic granule exocytosis in patient NK cells. *J Clin Invest* 119:3765–3773, 2009.

234. Janka GE: Hemophagocytic syndromes. *Blood Rev* 21:245–253, 2007.

235. Trizzino A, zur Stadt U, Ueda I, et al: Genotype-phenotype study of familial haemophagocytic lymphohistiocytosis due to perforin mutations. *J Med Genet* 45:15–21, 2008.

236. Ueda I, Kurokawa Y, Koike K, et al: Late-onset cases of familial hemophagocytic lymphohistiocytosis with missense perforin gene mutations. *Am J Hematol* 82:427–432, 2007.

237. Rudd E, Bryceson YT, Zheng C, et al: Spectrum, and clinical and functional implications of UNC13D mutations in familial haemophagocytic lymphohistiocytosis. *J Med Genet* 45:134–141, 2008.

238. Horne A, Trottestam H, Arico M, et al: Frequency and spectrum of central nervous system involvement in 193 children with haemophagocytic lymphohistiocytosis. *Br J Haematol* 140:327–335, 2008.

239. Henter JI, Horne A, Arico M, et al: HLH-2004: Diagnostic and therapeutic guidelines for hemophagocytic lymphohistiocytosis. *Pediatr Blood Cancer* 48:124–131, 2007.

240. Marcenaro S, Gallo F, Martini S, et al: Analysis of natural killer-cell function in familial hemophagocytic lymphohistiocytosis (FHL): Defective CD107a surface expression heralds Munc13–4 defect and discriminates between genetic subtypes of the disease. *Blood* 108:2316–2323, 2006.

241. Mahlaoui N, Ouachee-Chardin M, de Saint Basile G, et al: Immunotherapy of familial hemophagocytic lymphohistiocytosis with antithymocyte globulins: A single-center retrospective report of 38 patients. *Pediatrics* 120:e622–e628, 2007.

242. Marsh RA, Allen CE, McClain KL, et al: Salvage therapy of refractory hemophagocytic lymphohistiocytosis with alemtuzumab. *Pediatr Blood Cancer* 60:101–109, 2013.

243. Pachlopnik Schmid J, Ho CH, Chretien F, et al: Neutralization of IFNgamma defeats haemophagocytosis in LCMV-infected perforin- and Rab27a-deficient mice. *EMBO Mol Med* 1:112–124, 2009.

244. Ouachee-Chardin M, Elie C, de Saint Basile G, et al: Hematopoietic stem cell transplantation in hemophagocytic lymphohistiocytosis: A single-center report of 48 patients. *Pediatrics* 117:e743–50, 2006.

245. Marsh RA, Vaughn G, Kim MO, et al: Reduced-intensity conditioning significantly improves survival of patients with hemophagocytic lymphohistiocytosis undergoing allogeneic hematopoietic cell transplantation. *Blood* 116:5824–5831, 2010.

246. Purtilo DT, Cassel CK, Yang JP, et al: X-linked recessive progressive combined variable immunodeficiency (Duncan's disease). *Lancet* 1:935–940, 1975.

247. Coffey AJ, Brooksbank RA, Brandau O, et al: Host response to EBV infection in X-linked lymphoproliferative disease results from mutations in an SH2-domain encoding gene. *Nat Genet* 20:129–135, 1998.

248. Sayos J, Wu C, Morra M, et al: The X-linked lymphoproliferative-disease gene product SAP regulates signals induced through the co-receptor SLAM. *Nature* 395:462–469, 1998.

249. Calpe S, Wang N, Romero X, et al: The SLAM and SAP gene families control innate and adaptive immune responses. *Adv Immunol* 97:177–250, 2008.

250. Parolini S, Bottino C, Falco M, et al: X-linked lymphoproliferative disease. 2B4 molecules displaying inhibitory rather than activating function are responsible for the inability of natural killer cells to kill Epstein-Barr virus-infected cells. *J Exp Med* 192:337–346, 2000.

251. Bottino C, Falco M, Parolini S, et al: NTB-A [correction of GNTB-A], a novel SH2D1A-associated surface molecule contributing to the inability of natural killer cells to kill Epstein-Barr virus-infected B cells in X-linked lymphoproliferative disease. *J Exp Med* 194:235–246, 2001.

252. Dupre L, Andolfi G, Tangye SG, et al: SAP controls the cytolytic activity of CD8+ T cells against EBV-infected cells. *Blood* 105:4383–4389, 2005.

253. Qi H, Cannons JL, Klauschen F, et al: SAP-controlled T-B cell interactions underlie germinal centre formation. *Nature* 455:764–769, 2008.

254. Pasquier B, Yin L, Fondaneche MC, et al: Defective NKT cell development in mice and humans lacking the adapter SAP, the X-linked lymphoproliferative syndrome gene product. *J Exp Med* 201:695–701, 2005.

255. Rigaud S, Fondaneche MC, Lambert N, et al: XIAP deficiency in humans causes an X-linked lymphoproliferative syndrome. *Nature* 444:110–114, 2006.

256. Sumegi J, Huang D, Lanyi A, et al: Correlation of mutations of the SH2D1A gene and epstein-barr virus infection with clinical phenotype and outcome in X-linked lymphoproliferative disease. *Blood* 96:3118–3125, 2000.

257. Tabata Y, Villanueva J, Lee SM, et al: Rapid detection of intracellular SH2D1A protein in cytotoxic lymphocytes from patients with X-linked lymphoproliferative disease and their family members. *Blood* 105:3066–3071, 2005.

258. Pachlopnik Schmid J, Canioni D, Moshous D, et al: Clinical similarities and differences of patients with X-linked lymphoproliferative syndrome type 1 (XLP-1/SAP deficiency) versus type 2 (XLP-2/XIAP deficiency). *Blood* 117:1522–1529, 2011.

259. Speckmann C, Lehmberg K, Albert MH, et al: X-linked inhibitor of apoptosis (XIAP) deficiency: The spectrum of presenting manifestations beyond hemophagocytic lymphohistiocytosis. *Clin Immunol* 149:133–141, 2013.

260. Speckmann C, Ehl S: XIAP deficiency is a mendelian cause of late-onset IBD. *Gut* 63:1031–1032, 2014.

261. Damgaard RB, Nachbur U, Yabal M, et al: The ubiquitin ligase XIAP recruits LUBAC for NOD2 signaling in inflammation and innate immunity. *Mol Cell* 46:746–758, 2012.

262. Gifford CE, Weingartner E, Villanueva J, et al: Clinical flow cytometric screening of SAP and XIAP expression accurately identifies patients with SH2D1A and XIAP/BIRC4 mutations. *Cytometry B Clin Cytom* 86:263–271, 2014.

263. Seemayer TA, Gross TG, Egeler RM, et al: X-linked lymphoproliferative disease: Twenty-five years after the discovery. *Pediatr Res* 38:471–478, 1995.

264. Lankester AC, Visser LF, Hartwig NG, et al: Allogeneic stem cell transplantation in X-linked lymphoproliferative disease: Two cases in one family and review of the literature. *Bone Marrow Transplant* 36:99–105, 2005.

265. Milone MC, Tsai DE, Hodinka RL, et al: Treatment of primary Epstein-Barr virus infection in patients with X-linked lymphoproliferative disease using B-cell-directed therapy. *Blood* 105:994–996, 2005.

266. Mischler M, Fleming GM, Shanley TP, et al: Epstein-Barr virus-induced hemophagocytic lymphoproliferative disease: A mimicker of sepsis in the pediatric intensive care unit. *Pediatrics* 119:e1212–e1218, 2007.

267. Migliorati R, Castaldo A, Russo S, et al: Treatment of EBV-induced lymphoproliferative disorder with epipodophyllotoxin VP16–213. *Acta Paediatr* 83:1322–1325, 1994.

268. Marsh RA, Rao K, Satwani P, et al: Allogeneic hematopoietic cell transplantation for XIAP deficiency: An international survey reveals poor outcomes. *Blood* 121:877–883, 2013.

269. Dotta L, Parolini S, Prandini A, et al: Clinical, laboratory and molecular signs of immunodeficiency in patients with partial oculo-cutaneous albinism. *Orphanet J Rare Dis* 8:168, 2013.

270. Nagle DL, Karim MA, Woolf EA, et al: Identification and mutation analysis of the complete gene for Chediak-Higashi syndrome. *Nat Genet* 14:307–311, 1996.

271. Eapen M, DeLaat CA, Baker KS, et al: Hematopoietic cell transplantation for Chediak-Higashi syndrome. *Bone Marrow Transplant* 39:411–415, 2007.

272. Tardieu M, Lacroix C, Neven B, et al: Progressive neurologic dysfunctions 20 years after allogeneic bone marrow transplantation for Chediak-Higashi syndrome. *Blood* 106:40–42, 2005.

273. Menasche G, Pastural E, Feldmann J, et al: Mutations in RAB27A cause Griscelli syndrome associated with haemophagocytic syndrome. *Nat Genet* 25:173–176, 2000.

274. Hamidieh AA, Pourpak Z, Yari K, et al: Hematopoietic stem cell transplantation with a reduced-intensity conditioning regimen in pediatric patients with Griscelli syndrome type 2. *Pediatr Transplant* 17:487–491, 2013.

275. Dell'Angelica EC, Shotelersuk V, Aguilar RC, et al: Altered trafficking of lysosomal proteins in Hermansky-Pudlak syndrome due to mutations in the beta 3A subunit of the AP-3 adaptor. *Mol Cell* 3:11–21, 1999.

276. Fontana S, Parolini S, Vermi W, et al: Innate immunity defects in Hermansky-Pudlak type 2 syndrome. *Blood* 107:4857–4864, 2006.

277. Jessen B, Bode SF, Ammann S, et al: The risk of hemophagocytic lymphohistiocytosis in Hermansky-Pudlak syndrome type 2. *Blood* 121:2943–2951, 2013.

278. Cullinane AR, Curry JA, Carmona-Rivera C, et al: A BLOC-1 mutation screen reveals that PLDN is mutated in Hermansky-Pudlak Syndrome type 9. *Am J Hum Genet* 88:778–787, 2011.

279. Badolato R, Prandini A, Caracciolo S, et al: Exome sequencing reveals a pallidin mutation in a Hermansky-Pudlak-like primary immunodeficiency syndrome. *Blood* 119:3185–3187, 2012.

280. Kawai T, Akira S: Toll-like receptors and their crosstalk with other innate receptors in infection and immunity. *Immunity* 34:637–650, 2011.

281. Zhang SY, Jouanguy E, Ugolini S, et al: TLR3 deficiency in patients with herpes simplex encephalitis. *Science* 317:1522–1527, 2007.

282. Guo Y, Audry M, Ciancanelli M, et al: Herpes simplex virus encephalitis in a patient with complete TLR3 deficiency: TLR3 is otherwise redundant in protective immunity. *J Exp Med* 208:2083–2098, 2011.

283. Casrouge A, Zhang SY, Eidenschenk C, et al: Herpes simplex virus encephalitis in human UNC-93B deficiency. *Science* 314:308–312, 2006.

284. Perez de Diego R, Sancho-Shimizu V, Lorenzo L, et al: Human TRAF3 adaptor molecule deficiency leads to impaired Toll-like receptor 3 response and susceptibility to herpes simplex encephalitis. *Immunity* 33:400–411, 2010.

285. Sancho-Shimizu V, Perez de Diego R, Lorenzo L, et al: Herpes simplex encephalitis in children with autosomal recessive and dominant TRIF deficiency. *J Clin Invest* 121:4889–4902, 2011.

286. Herman M, Ciancanelli M, Ou YH, et al: Heterozygous TBK1 mutations impair TLR3 immunity and underlie herpes simplex encephalitis of childhood. *J Exp Med* 209:1567–1582, 2012.

287. Lafaille FG, Pessach IM, Zhang SY, et al: Impaired intrinsic immunity to HSV-1 in human iPSC-derived TLR3-deficient CNS cells. *Nature* 491:769–773, 2012.

288. Dupuis S, Jouanguy E, Al-Hajjar S, et al: Impaired response to interferon-alpha/beta and lethal viral disease in human STAT1 deficiency. *Nat Genet* 33:388–391, 2003.

289. Hambleton S, Goodbourn S, Young DF, et al: STAT2 deficiency and susceptibility to viral illness in humans. *Proc Natl Acad Sci U S A* 110:3053–3058, 2013.

290. Ramoz N, Rueda LA, Bouadjar B, et al: Mutations in two adjacent novel genes are associated with epidermodysplasia verruciformis. *Nat Genet* 32:579–581, 2002.

291. Picard C, Puel A, Bonnet M, et al: Pyogenic bacterial infections in humans with IRAK-4 deficiency. *Science* 299:2076–2079, 2003.

292. von Bernuth H, Picard C, Jin Z, et al: Pyogenic bacterial infections in humans with MyD88 deficiency. *Science* 321:691–696, 2008.

293. Ku CL, von Bernuth H, Picard C, et al: Selective predisposition to bacterial infections in IRAK-4-deficient children: IRAK-4-dependent TLRs are otherwise redundant in protective immunity. *J Exp Med* 204:2407–2422, 2007.

294. Kisand K, Boe Wolff AS, Podkrajsek KT, et al: Chronic mucocutaneous candidiasis in APECED or thymoma patients correlates with autoimmunity to Th17-associated cytokines. *J Exp Med* 207:299–308, 2010.

295. Puel A, Cypowyj S, Bustamante J, et al: Chronic mucocutaneous candidiasis in humans with inborn errors of interleukin-17 immunity. *Science* 332:65–68, 2011.

296. Boisson B, Wang C, Pedergnana V, et al: An ACT1 mutation selectively abolishes interleukin-17 responses in humans with chronic mucocutaneous candidiasis. *Immunity* 39:676–686, 2013.

297. Glocker EO, Hennigs A, Nabavi M, et al: A homozygous CARD9 mutation in a family with susceptibility to fungal infections. *N Engl J Med* 361:1727–1735, 2009.

298. Lanternier F, Barbati E, Meinzer U, et al: Inherited CARD9 deficiency in 2 unrelated patients with invasive exophiala infection. *J Infect Dis* 211(8):1241–50, 2015.

299. Gavino C, Cotter A, Lichtenstein D, et al: CARD9 deficiency and spontaneous central nervous system candidiasis: Complete clinical remission with GM-CSF therapy. *Clin Infect Dis* 59:81–84, 2014.

300. Al-Muhsen S, Casanova JL: The genetic heterogeneity of mendelian susceptibility to mycobacterial diseases. *J Allergy Clin Immunol* 122:1043–1051; quiz 52–53, 2008.

301. Prando C, Samarina A, Bustamante J, et al: Inherited IL-12p40 deficiency: Genetic, immunologic, and clinical features of 49 patients from 30 kindreds. *Medicine (Baltimore)* 92:109–122, 2013.

302. Altare F, Durandy A, Lammas D, et al: Impairment of mycobacterial immunity in human interleukin-12 receptor deficiency. *Science* 280:1432–1435, 1998.

303. Jirapongsananuruk O, Luangwedchakarn V, Niemela JE, et al: Cryptococcal osteomyelitis in a child with a novel compound mutation of the IL12RB1 gene. *Asian Pac J Allergy Immunol* 30:79–82, 2012.

304. Vinh DC, Schwartz B, Hsu AP, et al: Interleukin-12 receptor beta1 deficiency predisposing to disseminated Coccidioidomycosis. *Clin Infect Dis* 52:e99–e102, 2011.

305. Sologuren I, Boisson-Dupuis S, Pestano J, et al: Partial recessive IFN-gammaR1 deficiency: Genetic, immunological and clinical features of 14 patients from 11 kindreds. *Hum Mol Genet* 20:1509–1523, 2011.

306. Jouanguy E, Lamhamedi-Cherradi S, Lammas D, et al: A human IFNGR1 small deletion hotspot associated with dominant susceptibility to mycobacterial infection. *Nat Genet* 21:370–378, 1999.

307. Dorman SE, Picard C, Lammas D, et al: Clinical features of dominant and recessive interferon gamma receptor 1 deficiencies. *Lancet* 364:2113–2121, 2004.

308. Roesler J, Horwitz ME, Picard C, et al: Hematopoietic stem cell transplantation for complete IFN-gamma receptor 1 deficiency: A multi-institutional survey. *J Pediatr* 145:806–812, 2004.

309. Rottman M, Soudais C, Vogt G, et al: IFN-gamma mediates the rejection of haematopoietic stem cells in IFN-gammaR1-deficient hosts. *PLoS Med* 5:e26, 2008.

310. Vinh DC, Patel SY, Uzel G, et al: Autosomal dominant and sporadic monocytopenia with susceptibility to mycobacteria, fungi, papillomaviruses, and myelodysplasia. *Blood* 115:1519–1529, 2010.

311. Hsu AP, Sampaio EP, Khan J, et al: Mutations in GATA2 are associated with the autosomal dominant and sporadic monocytopenia and mycobacterial infection (MonoMAC) syndrome. *Blood* 118:2653–2655, 2011.

312. Hahn CN, Chong CE, Carmichael CL, et al: Heritable GATA2 mutations associated with familial myelodysplastic syndrome and acute myeloid leukemia. *Nat Genet* 43:1012–1017, 2011.

313. Ostergaard P, Simpson MA, Connell FC, et al: Mutations in GATA2 cause primary lymphedema associated with a predisposition to acute myeloid leukemia (Emberger syndrome). *Nat Genet* 43:929–931, 2011.

314. Kazenwadel J, Secker GA, Liu YJ, et al: Loss-of-function germline GATA2 mutations in patients with MDS/AML or MonoMAC syndrome and primary lymphedema reveal a key role for GATA2 in the lymphatic vasculature. *Blood* 119:1283–1291, 2012.

315. Cuellar-Rodriguez J, Gea-Banacloche J, Freeman AF, et al: Successful allogeneic hematopoietic stem cell transplantation for GATA2 deficiency. *Blood* 118:3715–3720, 2011.

316. Dupuis S, Dargemont C, Fieschi C, et al: Impairment of mycobacterial but not viral immunity by a germline human STAT1 mutation. *Science* 293:300–303, 2001.

317. Chapgier A, Kong XF, Boisson-Dupuis S, et al: A partial form of recessive STAT1 deficiency in humans. *J Clin Invest* 119:1502–1514, 2009.

318. Hambleton S, Salem S, Bustamante J, et al: IRF8 mutations and human dendritic-cell immunodeficiency. *N Engl J Med* 365:127–138, 2011.

319. Bogunovic D, Byun M, Durfee LA, et al: Mycobacterial disease and impaired IFN-gamma immunity in humans with inherited ISG15 deficiency. *Science* 337:1684–1688, 2012.

320. Sullivan KE, Winkelstein JA: Genetically determined deficiencies of the complement components, in *Primary Immunodeficiency Diseases, A Molecular and Genetic Approach*, 3rd ed, edited by Ochs HD, Smith CIE, Puck JM, p 757. Oxford University Press, New York, 2014.

321. Donoso LA, Vrabec T, Kuivaniemi H: The role of complement factor H in age-related macular degeneration: A review. *Surv Ophthalmol* 55:227–246, 2010.

CHAPTER 81
HEMATOLOGIC MANIFESTATIONS OF ACQUIRED IMMUNODEFICIENCY SYNDROME

Virginia C. Broudy and Robert D. Harrington

SUMMARY

The prevalence of HIV in the United States continues to rise as a result of the combined effects of a declining HIV death rate, and a sustained rate of new infections. Furthermore, HIV-infected patients on antiretroviral therapy can expect to live nearly as long as uninfected persons (within 5 years) providing ample time for individuals to develop AIDS-associated and non–AIDS-associated hematologic and oncologic conditions. HIV-infected individuals remain at increased risk of AIDS-defining malignancies such as Kaposi sarcoma, aggressive non-Hodgkin lymphoma, primary central nervous system lymphoma, and invasive cervical cancer and a number of non–AIDS-defining malignancies, including Hodgkin lymphoma, as well as anemia and thrombocytopenia. When individuals present with any of these hematologic or malignant illnesses it should be the standard of care to obtain HIV testing so as to provide optimal treatment to both the presenting illness and the HIV.

Acronyms and Abbreviations: ABVD, Adriamycin, bleomycin, vinblastine, dacarbazine; ADAMTS 13, a disintegrin and metalloproteinase with a thrombospondin type 1 motif, member 13; AMC, AIDS Malignancy Consortium; ART, antiretroviral therapy; AVD, Adriamycin, vinblastine, dacarbazine; BEACOPP, bleomycin, etoposide, Adriamycin, cyclophosphamide, vincristine, procarbazine, prednisone; BFU-E, burst-forming unit–erythroid; CFU-GM, granulocyte-macrophage colony-forming unit; CFU-GEMM, granulocyte-erythrocyte-monocyte and megakaryocyte colony-forming unit; CHOP, cyclophosphamide, doxorubicin, vincristine, prednisone; CHORUS, Collaboration in HIV Outcomes Research/U.S. study; CMV, cytomegalovirus; CODOX-M/IVAC, cyclophosphamide, vincristine, doxorubicin, methotrexate/ifosfamide, mesna, etoposide, cytarabine; CRF, circulating recombinant form; CSF, cerebrospinal fluid; CTL, cytotoxic T-lymphocyte; DHHS, Department of Health and Human Services; EBV, Epstein-Barr virus; ECOG, Eastern Cooperative Oncology Group; EPOCH, etoposide, prednisone, vincristine, cyclophosphamide, doxorubicin; ESHAP, etoposide, methylprednisolone, high-dose cytarabine, cisplatin; G6PD, glucose-6-phosphate dehydrogenase; HHV8, human herpesvirus-8; HPV, human papillomavirus; HSV, herpes simplex virus; HUS, hemolytic-uremic syndrome; hyperCVAD, cyclophosphamide, vincristine, doxorubicin, dexamethasone; IL, interleukin; IRIS, immune reconstitution inflammatory syndrome; ITP, idiopathic thrombocytopenic purpura; KICS, KSHV-associated inflammatory cytokine syndrome; KSHV, Kaposi sarcoma-associated herpesvirus; LDH, lactate dehydrogenase; LPS, lipopolysaccharide; MRI, magnetic resonance imaging; NHL, non-Hodgkin lymphoma; nnRTI, nonnucleoside reverse transcriptase inhibitor; nRTI, nucleoside reverse transcriptase inhibitor; PCR, polymerase chain reaction; PET-CT, positron emission tomography–computed tomography; PrEP, preexposure prophylaxis; R-CHOP, rituximab plus CHOP; R-EPOCH, rituximab plus EPOCH; R-ICE, rituximab plus ifosfamide, carboplatin, etoposide; SEER, Surveillance, Epidemiology, and End Results Program; SIV, simian immunodeficiency virus; TTP, thrombotic thrombocytopenic purpura.

HISTORY AND HUMAN IMMUNODEFICIENCY VIRUS

HIV, the virus that causes AIDS, is a lentivirus that originated as a simian immunodeficiency virus (SIV) in chimpanzees and entered the human population in the early 20th century in equatorial Africa.[1,2] First isolated in 1983,[3,4] HIV-1 actually comprises four distinct viruses (types M, N, O, and P) that represent four separate transmission events that occurred between chimpanzees and humans, likely the result of predation of monkeys by humans and mucosal or nonintact skin contact with infected fluids. Group M, the viral type responsible for the HIV-1 pandemic, was detected in a tissue sample from 1959 and probably entered the human population in or around Kinshasa, Democratic Republic of Congo (then Leopoldville, Belgium Congo) between 1910 and 1930 based on phylogenetic analysis.[2] HIV-2 originated in West Africa, the result of cross-species transmission of SIV from sooty mangabeys to humans. Patients infected with HIV-2 progress more slowly and have lower plasma viral loads (often nondetectable) than those with HIV-1, reflective of the different virology and adaptation to humans of this SIV.[5] Because of lower rates of replication and transmission, HIV-2 prevalence is declining and is being replaced by HIV-1 in countries where both viruses are endemic.[5,6] Among those infected with HIV-1, group M is the globally predominant viral strain and is further divided into nine subtypes and many more recombinant viruses (circulating recombinant forms [CRFs]) with some geographic localization. Subtypes A and D predominate in East Africa; subtype C in South Africa, India, and Asia; subtype B in the Caribbean, the Americas, and Western Europe; and CRF01 in Southeast Asia.[1]

EPIDEMIOLOGY, TRANSMISSION

The development of *Pneumocystis jiroveci* (*Pneumocystis carinii*) pneumonia and Kaposi sarcoma in previously healthy men who have sex with men on both coasts of the United States in 1981 represented the first clinical manifestations of HIV and the onset of the HIV-1 pandemic.[7–9] Subsequent reports of similar illnesses in the sexual partners of index cases, injection drug users, patients with hemophilia and other transfusion recipients, infants born to infected mothers, and Haitian immigrants[10–17] helped identify the routes of transmission as bloodborne, sexual, or vertical. With the discovery of HIV in 1983 and the subsequent development of serologic testing, more systematic detection of HIV infections became possible providing an understanding of the regional and global HIV epidemiology. While sexual contact between men was responsible for most infections in the United States, Northern Europe, Australia, and parts of Central and South America, heterosexual spread predominated in sub-Saharan Africa and injection drug use followed by sexual transmission was responsible for most infections in Southern and Eastern Europe and Southeast Asia.[18] Transmission rates between individuals per incident/act is dictated by the viral load in the HIV-infected person,[19] the presence of modifying factors such as concurrent ulcerative sexually transmitted diseases and the type of exposure.[20] Rates vary between 93 percent for blood transfusion from an infected person to less than 0.04 percent for oral sex. Estimated rates for mother-to-child transmission (in the absence of antiretroviral therapy [ART] prophylaxis) are 23 percent, for needle sharing 0.63 percent, for needle stick 0.23 percent, for receptive anal intercourse 1.38 percent, for insertive anal intercourse 0.11 percent, for receptive vaginal intercourse 0.08 percent, and for insertive vaginal intercourse 0.04 percent.[20] In 2012 there were an estimated 35.3 million people living with HIV, including 2.3 million newly infected persons.[21] Although the global incidence of HIV is thought to have peaked in 1997, the prevalence of HIV is increasing because of ongoing new infections and the shrinking death rate of those already infected and on ART (2.3 million deaths in 2005 versus 1.6 million deaths in 2012). The majority of HIV-infected persons (approximately 23 million) now live in sub-Saharan Africa with 4 million in Asia and Southeast Asia and roughly 3 million in the Americas and Caribbean.

● PATHOGENESIS

Eighty percent of HIV infections occur via mucosal transmission during sex[22] when cell-free and cell-associated virions transverse the epithelium to gain access to macrophages, Langerhans cells, dendritic cells, and CD4-expressing T lymphocytes.[23] To infect most cells HIV must bind to CD4 and one of two major coreceptors (CCR5 or CXCR4); in most cases, CCR5-utilizing viral strains are those that are transmitted and predominate early in disease. Rare individuals who do not express CCR5 (homozygote for a 32 bp deletion mutation in the CCR5 gene) are highly resistant to HIV infection although they can be infected with isolates utilizing CXCR4. After transmission, low-level replication of HIV in tissue macrophages and dendritic cells can occur, but the key role these cells play is in trapping and trafficking virions and presenting them to CD4+ T lymphocytes within regional lymphatics (e.g., gut-associated lymphoid tissue and lymph nodes where the infection is amplified).[24] High-level viral replication proceeds within these local tissues leading to profound CD4+ T-cell depletion, establishment of a reservoir of latently infected memory T cells and eventually to high plasma levels of virus that are the hallmark of acute infection. The immune response to HIV is brisk but ineffective and may, in fact, fuel the infection because the expression of inflammatory cytokines[25] and migration of activated CD4+ T cells to the site of HIV-1 concentration provides additional activated cells that the virus coopts for its own replication.[26] The initial antibody response to HIV does not contain neutralizing antibodies; these develop only later, months after chronic infection is established. Furthermore, HIV escapes these antibodies by mutations within N-glycosylation sites that prevent antibody binding.[27] The CD8+ cytotoxic T-lymphocyte (CTL) cell response to HIV controls high-level viral replication during primary infection and establishes the viral "setpoint" or plasma level of HIV RNA in chronic infection. Evidence for the controlling anti-HIV effect of CD8+ T cells includes their detection immediately prior to peak viremia, the development of viral escape mutations[28–30] and the requirement for CD8+ T cells to control SIV infection in Rhesus macaques.[31] The rate of viral escape mutations slows during chronic infection[32,33] and is not associated with further declines in viral load, reaching a stalemate where viral replication continues under the pressure of a slowly evolving CTL response leading to viral strains with reduced replication capacity.[34–36] As important as the direct cytolytic effect of HIV on CD4+ T cells, the virus induces a state of chronic immune activation of both the adaptive and innate immune systems that is central to disease pathogenesis.[37–41] Because the immune response to HIV is defective and does not clear the virus, the immune system remains continually activated with high rates of T-cell turnover that eventually leads to T-cell exhaustion and depletion. This is particularly evident in gut-associated lymphoid tissue where early T-cell losses alter the integrity of the mucosal border leading to microbial translocation and leakage of lipopolysaccharide (LPS) into the blood which, in turn, amplifies the state of immune activation.[42] This persistent,

systemic inflammatory state leads to tissue fibrosis over time[43,44] that is partly responsible for immune failure and the increased frequency of nonimmune, nontraditional chronic diseases that now plague an aging HIV population.[45]

● CLINICAL FEATURES AND DISEASE PROGRESSION

Primary HIV infection that comes to medical attention presents as a febrile illness that may include headache, pharyngitis, lymphadenopathy, gastrointestinal symptoms, and rash and may be mistaken for mononucleosis or other nonspecific viral infections. Key to making the diagnosis is taking a history for HIV risk factors and obtaining appropriate laboratory testing (combined HIV Ag/Ab assays and plasma HIV RNA testing). However, in most cases, primary infection goes undiagnosed and patients are later identified in the chronic, asymptomatic phase of infection by routine screening or later still, after the development of symptoms that are often caused by opportunistic infections. Typically, the asymptomatic phase of chronic infection will last for 8 to 10 years, although there is great interindividual variation dictated by the effectiveness of the immune response in controlling HIV replication (the viral "setpoint," see above). Long-term nonprogressors (those who maintain CD4+ T-cell counts >500 for 5 years without therapy) and elite controllers (those with low or nondetectable plasma HIV RNA without treatment) can live for decades with limited or no disease progression, while others with high viral setpoints in the range of 100,000 to >1,000,000 copies/mL can develop AIDS-defining illnesses quickly after primary infection. In untreated individuals CD4+ T-cell counts (typically at CD4 counts) typically decline by 50 to 100 cells/µL per year, taking 8 to 10 years before counts are in the range where symptoms develop (typically at CD4 count <500 cells/µL) or AIDS-defining illnesses occur (typically at CD4 count <200 cells/µL). Historically, opportunistic infections provided the first evidence for the existence of HIV and remain the most visible manifestation of infection in countries with limited access to ART and in individuals who are diagnosed late in the course of their disease. The development of opportunistic infections and AIDS-defining conditions is dependent on the virulence properties of the organism and the degree of host immune suppression. Pathogens with high virulence potential (e.g., *Mycobacterium tuberculosis*, *Salmonella* sp., the bacterial agents of community-acquired pneumonia) cause disease in patients without HIV and do so in HIV-infected persons regardless of CD4 count (although more severe and prolonged illness occurs with more profound immunodeficiency). Agents with more limited pathogenic potential typically cause disease at lower CD4 counts, for example, *P. jiroveci* at CD4 counts below 200 cells/µL, while those that rarely cause disease in immunocompetent persons, such as disseminated *Mycobacterium avium* complex, *Toxoplasma gondii* encephalitis, and JC virus (the agent of progressive multifocal leukoencephalopathy), typically occur only in those with very advanced HIV disease and CD4 counts less than 100 cells/µL or less than 50 cells/µL, respectively (Table 81–1 lists HIV staging; Table 81–2

TABLE 81–1. HIV Staging

HIV Stage	Description
0	Infection within the previous 6 months
1	CD4 count ≥500 cells/µL (or ≥26%)
2	CD4 count 200–499 cells/µL (or 14–25%)
3	AIDS-defining condition or CD4 count <200 cells/µL (or <14%)
Unknown	If none of the above apply

TABLE 81-2. Aids-Defining Conditions

Bacterial infections, multiple or recurrent*

Candidiasis of bronchi, trachea, or lungs

Candidiasis of esophagus†

Cervical cancer, invasive§

Coccidioidomycosis, disseminated or extrapulmonary

Cryptococcosis, extrapulmonary

Cryptosporidiosis, chronic intestinal (>1 month's duration)

Cytomegalovirus disease (other than liver, spleen, or nodes), onset at age >1 month

Cytomegalovirus retinitis (with loss of vision)†

Encephalopathy, HIV related

Herpes simplex: chronic ulcers (>1 month's duration) or bronchitis, pneumonitis, or esophagitis (onset at age >1 month)

Histoplasmosis, disseminated or extrapulmonary

Isosporiasis, chronic intestinal (>1 month's duration)

Kaposi sarcoma†

Lymphoid interstitial pneumonia or pulmonary lymphoid hyperplasia complex*†

Lymphoma, Burkitt (or equivalent term)

Lymphoma, immunoblastic (or equivalent term)

Lymphoma, primary, of brain

Mycobacterium avium complex or *Mycobacterium kansasii*, disseminated or extrapulmonary†

Mycobacterium tuberculosis of any site, pulmonary,†§ disseminated,† or extrapulmonary†

Mycobacterium, other species or unidentified species, disseminated† or extrapulmonary†

Pneumocystis jiroveci pneumonia†

Pneumonia, recurrent†§

Progressive multifocal leukoencephalopathy

Salmonella septicemia, recurrent

Toxoplasmosis of brain, onset at age >1 month†

Wasting syndrome attributed to HIV

*Only among children younger than age 13 years. (*Centers for Disease Control and Prevention (CDC). 1994 Revised classification system for human immunodeficiency virus infection in children less than 13 years of age. MMWR Morb Mortal Wkly Rep 1994;43(RR-12). Available at: http://www.cdc.gov/mmwr/PDF/rr/rr4312.pdf)*

†Condition that might be diagnosed presumptively.

§Only among adults and adolescents older than age 13 years. (*Centers for Disease Control and Prevention (CDC). 1993 Revised classification system for HIV infection and expanded surveillance case definition for AIDS among adolescents and adults. MMWR Morb Mortal Wkly Rep 41(RR-17):1–19, 1992.)*

Data from Centers for Disease Control and Prevention (CDC): 1994 Revised classification system for human immunodeficiency virus infection in children less than 13 years of age. *MMWR Morb Mortal Wkly Rep* 1994;43(RR-12) (available at: http://www.cdc.gov/mmwr/PDF/rr/rr4312.pdf), and Centers for Disease Control and Prevention (CDC): 1993 Revised classification system for HIV infection and expanded surveillance case definition for AIDS among adolescents and adults. *MMWR Morb Mortal Wkly Rep* 41(RR-17):1–19, 1992.

TABLE 81-3. Examples of Common Opportunistic Infections By CD4 Count

CD4 Count	Opportunistic Infection or Condition
>500 cells/μL	Any condition that can occur in HIV-uninfected persons, e.g., bacterial pneumonia, tuberculosis, varicella-zoster, herpes simplex virus
350–499 cells/μL	Thrush, seborrheic dermatitis, oral hairy leucoplakia, molluscum contagiosum
200–349 cells/μL	Kaposi sarcoma, lymphoma
100–199 cells/μL	Pneumocystis pneumonia, *Candida* esophagitis, cryptococcal meningitis
<100 cells/μL	*Toxoplasma* encephalitis, disseminated *Mycobacterium avium* complex, progressive multifocal leukoencephalopathy, cytomegalovirus retinitis, primary central nervous system lymphoma, microsporidia

lists AIDS-defining conditions; and Table 81–3 lists common HIV-associated conditions by CD4 count). Prophylaxis against the development of these infections is provided when the infection is common and significant and when the prophylaxis is effective, inexpensive and well tolerated. (Table 81–4 lists the organisms and medications used for primary prophylaxis.) Tumors classified as AIDS-defining malignancies are Kaposi sarcoma, Burkitt lymphoma, immunoblastic lymphoma, primary CNS lymphoma and cervical cancer, as these were first identified at high rates among infected persons early in the epidemic. Many other cancers also occur at increased rates among HIV-infected patients because of a higher rate of traditional cancer risk factors and the long-term effects of immune dysregulation leading to decreased tumor surveillance and chronic systemic inflammation. Outside of the immune defects levied by HIV, the virus can directly or indirectly cause specific organ or tissue damage including the nervous system (causing cognitive impairment, dementia and peripheral neuropathy), cardiovascular system (HIV cardiomyopathy), kidney (HIV nephropathy), gastrointestinal system (HIV enteropathy and cholangiopathy), and can accelerate disease progression as a result of other infections, such as hepatitides

TABLE 81-4. Primary Prophylaxis

Infection	Criteria	Treatment
Pneumocystis pneumonia	CD4 <200 cells/μL or <14% or oral candidiasis or an AIDS-defining illness	Trimethoprim-sulfamethoxazole or dapsone or aerosolized pentamidine
Tuberculosis	Purified protein derivative >5 mm or + Interferon-γ release assay	Isoniazid (INH) + pyridoxine
Toxoplasmosis	Immunoglobulin G+ and CD4 <100 cells/μL	Trimethoprim-sulfamethoxazole or dapsone+ pyrimethamine+ leucovorin
Mycobacterium avium complex	CD4 <50 cells/μL	Azithromycin or clarithromycin

B and C.[46,47] Finally, the long-term effects of chronic immune activation and persistent inflammation is likely a factor in the development of coronary artery disease,[45] chronic liver disease,[47,48] and a hypercoagulable state[49-51] that is only partly corrected by the initiation of ART. These "aging effects" of HIV are likely to dominate the health issues for infected persons now that opportunistic infections are readily treated or avoided altogether through a combination of prophylaxis and ART.

THERAPY

The story of ART from the first reports that zidovudine had activity against HIV to the current formulary of drugs, including single-tablet, fixed-dose, once-daily formulations, is one of the great achievements in medicine. Early studies of zidovudine monotherapy demonstrated a delay to the development of AIDS and short-term mortality benefits but no long-term effect on survival; zidovudine also carried significant toxicity.[52-57] Combination therapy with other nucleoside reverse transcriptase inhibitors (nRTIs) proved slightly more effective than zidovudine alone, but not until combination nRTI was used with a third drug from another class, first nonnucleoside reverse transcriptase inhibitors (nnRTIs)[58] and then protease inhibitors,[59-62] were sustained viral suppression and substantive, dramatic improvements in survival realized.[63] The recommended time to initiate ART has evolved in response to studies demonstrating benefits of ART at high CD4 counts and improvements in drug tolerability and formulation. Current Department of Health and Human Services (DHHS) guidelines suggest that all HIV-infected persons be offered ART regardless of CD4 count, although the strength of evidence supporting this recommendation varies by CD4 count (Table 81–5 lists the criteria for initiating ART), while the World Health Organization sets a CD4 count threshold of 350 cells/μL for initiating ART in more resource-limited countries. The rationale for these expanded ART recommendations include the recognition that newer therapies are more convenient, have fewer adverse effects and are associated with lower rates of drug resistance. Furthermore, in addition to

improved all-cause survival, ART preserves renal function in those with HIV-associated nephropathy,[64] slows the progression of hepatic fibrosis in those coinfected with hepatitis C,[65-68] decreases (but does not normalize) markers of chronic inflammation[69] and may be associated with reduced cardiovascular disease,[70] prevents the development of HIV-associated dementia,[71,72] and is highly effective in reducing mother-to-child[73,74] and sexual transmission.[19,22,75] Adverse effects related to ART do occur but are less common with current regimens and can usually be effectively managed with corrective treatments and by substitution of the offending drug with an alternative medication.[76,77] Similarly, the presence or development of drug resistance can usually be overcome by the use of secondary or salvage ART regimens that are fully suppressive. At the current time, only rare patients who are fully adherent to ART fail to control HIV replication. Treatment of early and primary infection provides a unique opportunity to intervene and possibly alter the course of HIV infection. Several studies have demonstrated that treatment in early or primary HIV lowers the rate of disease progression if treatment is subsequently interrupted[78-83] and may also limit the size of the latent HIV reservoir,[84-87] the impediment to curing patients. One interesting group of 14 patients initiated ART during primary infection and stayed on treatment for a median of 3 years and then controlled HIV replication for a median of 7 years after ART interruption.[88] Finally, given the high viral loads typical of primary HIV, these patients are thought to be highly infectious; therefore identifying them and initiating treatment should prevent transmission to their uninfected partners. One consequence of initiating ART in the setting of a known or occult infection is the development of an acute inflammatory reaction as a result of reconstitution of the immune system in the presence of organisms or foreign antigens.[89-93] The immune reconstitution inflammatory syndrome (IRIS) occurs in between 8 and 30 percent of patients who start ART, depending on the opportunistic infection and the timing of ART.[94] Risk factors for the development of IRIS include a low baseline CD4 count, more-severe disease and a short interval between treatment of the opportunistic infection and initiation of ART. The treatment of IRIS should include treatment of the underlying infection or condition, continued ART, and antiinflammatory medication, such as corticosteroids, depending on the severity of the reaction.[95]

PREVENTION AND CURE

The future of the HIV epidemic will differ by region and be dictated by local public health responses, HIV testing rates, sociobehavioral prevention interventions, and access to ART. Expanded HIV testing is an essential element of any prevention campaign as an estimated 50 percent of all new infections originate from individuals unaware of their HIV status.[96] Behavioral interventions can have some preventative effect[97-99] but biomedical methods have emerged as the most effective means to prevent new infections. Male circumcision can reduce female-to-male sexual transmission by 51 percent[100] and is being implemented on a population level in some African countries. ART administered peripartum will prevent most mother-to-child transmissions[101,102] and fully suppressive ART provided throughout pregnancy essentially eliminates all infant infections.[73,74] A prospective randomized trial of HIV-discordant couples demonstrated that ART provided to the HIV-infected partner was almost 100 percent effective in preventing transmission[22] and other studies have shown that elements of ART given to HIV-negative but at-risk persons (preexposure prophylaxis [PrEP]) can prevent HIV acquisition when subjects are adherent to treatment.[103-105] These studies point the way to the best strategies and interventions to curtail the HIV epidemic until an effective HIV vaccine is available.

The persistence of replication-competent but transcriptionally silent HIV proviral DNA in long-lived resting cells (the HIV latent

TABLE 81–5. Criteria for Initiating Antiretroviral Therapy

CD4 Count	Recommendation
<350 cells/μL	Start antiretroviral therapy (ART) (AI)
350–500 cells/μL	Start ART (AII)
>500 cells/μL	Start ART (BIII)

Clinical conditions favoring initiation of therapy regardless of CD4 count.

- History of AIDS-defining illness (AI)
- Pregnancy (AI)
- HIV-associated nephropathy (AII)
- Hepatitis B coinfection (AII)
- Patients at risk of transmitting HIV to sexual partners (AI, heterosexuals; AIII, others)
- Hepatitis C coinfection (BII)
- Patients older than 50 years of age (BIII)

A, strong recommendation; B, moderate recommendation; C, optional recommendation; I, one or more randomized trials with clinical outcomes and/or validated laboratory end points; II, one or more well-designed, nonrandomized trials or observational cohort studies with long-term clinical outcomes; III, expert opinion.

Adapted from Department of Health and Human Services Guidelines. http://aidsinfo.nih.gov/guidelines.

reservoir) is the impediment to cure for nearly all HIV-infected people.[87,106-109] Although combination ART is highly effective at controlling HIV replication in activated cells, it has no effect on the latent HIV reservoir, which will persist as long as the cells harboring HIV survive. Because most HIV genomes reside in central and effector memory T cells that decay at a negligible rate, there is no possibility of cure with ART alone. The only individual cured of *chronic* HIV infection (Timothy Brown, the Berlin patient) developed acute myelogenous leukemia that was treated with high-dose conditioning and transplantation of HIV-resistant (CCR5D32/D32) allogeneic blood stem cells.[109] While this case provides proof-of-principle that the latent HIV reservoir can be eliminated by allogeneic hematopoietic cell transplantation, the approach is impractical for widespread application because of the high toxicity associated with this procedure, the morbidity of graft-versus-host disease, and the scarcity of CCR5D32/D32 donors. To date, most HIV cure efforts have focused on the strategy of reversing latency with the notion that once resting cells begin producing HIV they will be targeted by the immune system or die from apoptosis. However, early studies suggest that activating latent cells to express HIV does not reliably lead to their death and additional treatments including vaccination to boost cytotoxic responses will be needed.[109A] Gene therapy is also being pursued as a means to control or cure HIV; specifically, DNA editing enzymes that disrupt CCR5 have been used to eliminate CCR5 expression in cells that are then expanded *ex vivo* and reinfused into patients, creating a population of HIV-resistant CD4+ T cells.[110,111]

● HUMAN IMMUNODEFICIENCY VIRUS–ASSOCIATED MALIGNANCIES

When AIDS was first identified as a clinical syndrome it was quickly appreciated that these patients were at greatly increased risk for certain types of malignancies, including Kaposi sarcoma, various types of non-Hodgkin lymphoma (NHL), and invasive cervical cancer. Each of these AIDS-defining cancers is frequently associated with an oncogenic virus (Table 81–6). As effective ART was developed and patients began living into their 50s, 60s, and 70s,[112,113] it became apparent that many non–AIDS-defining malignancies were also more common in this population compared to HIV-uninfected patients. Anal cancer is 120-fold more common in people living with HIV, particularly among men who have sex with men. Hodgkin lymphoma incidence is increased approximately 20-fold, hepatocellular cancer fivefold, and the risk of lung cancer is increased twofold. In contrast, the risks of other common cancers, including breast cancer, prostate cancer, and colon cancer, are not increased in comparison to HIV-negative people.[114] In the ART era, non–AIDS-defining malignancies comprise approximately half of the cancers in people living with HIV, and overall cancer causes approximately 25 to 33 percent of all deaths in HIV-infected

TABLE 81–6. AIDS-Defining Malignancies and Oncogenic Viruses

AIDS-Defining Malignancy	Oncogenic Virus
Kaposi sarcoma	HHV8
Aggressive non-Hodgkin lymphoma	EBV, HHV8
Primary central nervous system lymphoma	EBV
Invasive cervical cancer	HPV

EBV, Epstein-Barr virus; HHV, human herpesvirus; HPV, human papillomavirus.

patients, supporting the importance of age-appropriate standard cancer screening.[115]

The Centers for Disease Control estimates that 20 percent of HIV+ people in the United States do not know that they are HIV+,[116] and HIV testing is strongly recommended in all patients who present to the hematologist with NHL, Hodgkin lymphoma, or idiopathic thrombocytopenic purpura (ITP), or other malignancies.[117] This recommendation is made because approximately 5 percent of those with diffuse large B-cell lymphoma and 22 percent of patients with Burkitt lymphoma in the United States are HIV+ (Fig. 81–1). These proportions vary substantially by demographic group[118]: among men, 10 percent of those with diffuse large B-cell lymphoma are HIV+, in contrast to 1 percent of women, and approximately 40 percent of those 30 to 59 years old with Burkitt lymphoma are HIV+. It is important to diagnose HIV infection when present, as effective treatment of HIV is essential for successful treatment of the malignancy or ITP.

HUMAN IMMUNODEFICIENCY VIRUS–ASSOCIATED DIFFUSE LARGE B-CELL LYMPHOMA

Among HIV+ patients in the United States, diffuse large B-cell lymphoma is now more common than Kaposi sarcoma, although Kaposi sarcoma remains the most common malignancy in people living with HIV worldwide.[118] The pathophysiology of diffuse large B-cell lymphoma in HIV has been reviewed.[119,120] In a recent case series, HIV+ patients presented with diffuse large B-cell lymphoma at a median age of 43 years, 2 decades younger than HIV– patients.[121] Patients often present with a rapidly growing lymph node or extranodal mass, and frequently have B symptoms (drenching night sweats, fever, or loss of 10 percent of body weight). Involvement of extranodal sites, including the gastrointestinal tract, liver, CNS, lung, and other sites is common.[121,122] Diagnosis is most commonly made by excisional lymph node biopsy. Evaluation should include careful examination of all lymph nodes sites, and the oral cavity. Standard staging with positron emission tomography–computed tomography (PET-CT), marrow evaluation, and lumbar puncture for cerebrospinal fluid cytology and flow cytometry[123] should be performed. Patients should be evaluated for hepatitis B prior to initiation of chemotherapy. If active hepatitis B is found (hepatitis B DNA+), it must be managed in the context of the HIV treatment, as several commonly used medications for hepatitis B are also active against HIV. Although initial studies in the pre-ART era focused on low-dose chemotherapy,[124] it is now appreciated that full-dose multiagent systemic chemotherapy with appropriate supportive care using filgrastim or peg-filgrastim and prophylaxis against infectious complications, offers the best chance for permanent cure. Cohort studies show that the 5-year overall survival in the ART era is far better than the pre-ART era.[125] A National Cancer Institute study using six cycles of dose-adjusted etoposide, prednisone, vincristine, cyclophosphamide, and doxorubicin (EPOCH), in which the initial cyclophosphamide dose was adjusted based on the CD4 count, and subsequent cycles cyclophosphamide dosing was adjusted based on the neutrophil nadir, showed an overall survival of 60 percent at 53 months (39 patients, 79 percent had diffuse large B-cell lymphoma, 18 percent had Burkitt lymphoma, and none were on ART during chemotherapy).[126] CD4 counts dropped by 190 cells/μL during chemotherapy, but recovered to baseline by 6 to 12 months following chemotherapy. All patients received *P. jiroveci* prophylaxis, and if CD4 counts were less than 100 cells/μL, *M. avium* complex prophylaxis. All patients also received filgrastim following each cycle of chemotherapy. This key study demonstrated that EPOCH is safe and effective in HIV+ patients with aggressive lymphoma. Outcomes differed markedly depending on the initial CD4 count: patients with an

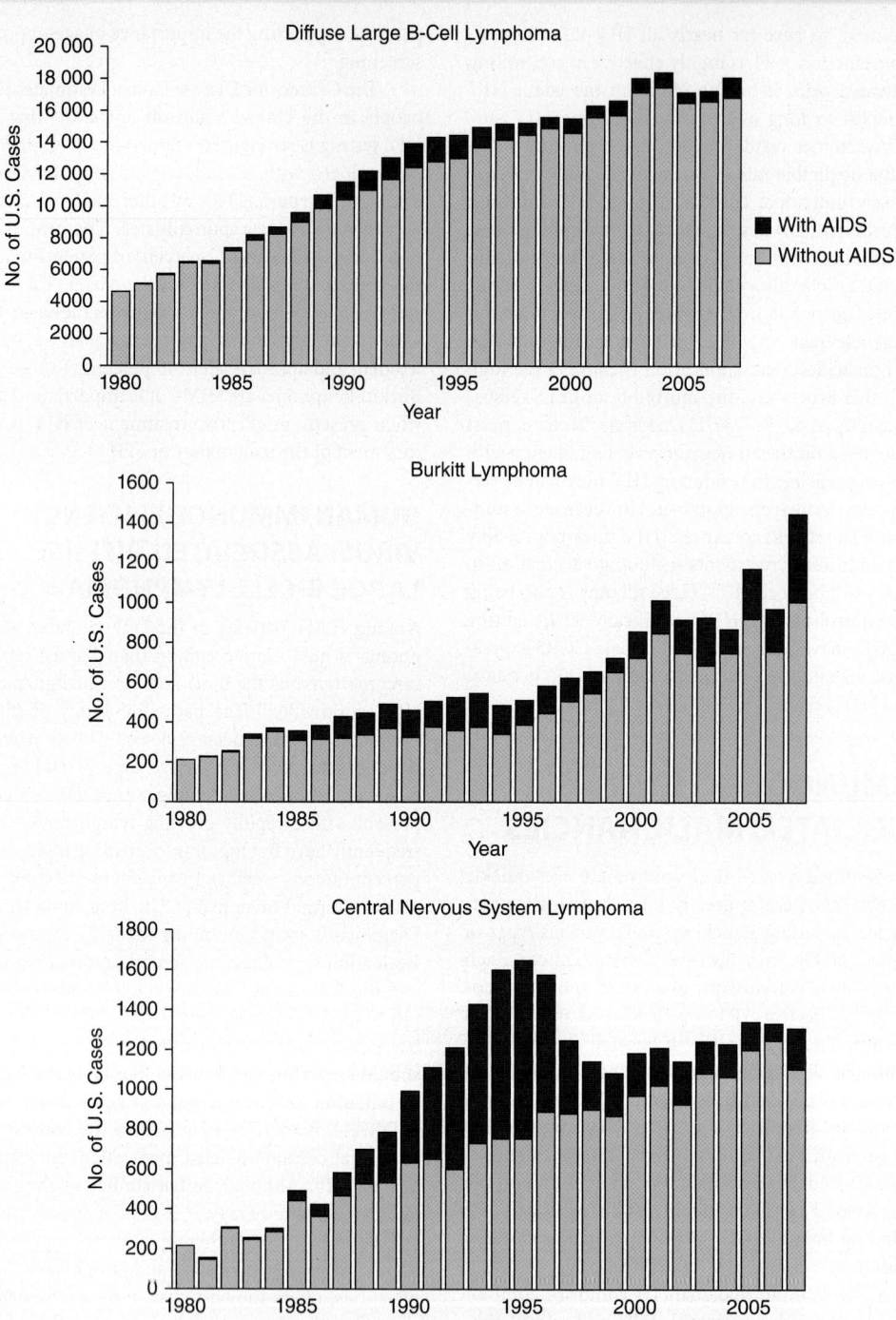

Figure 81–1. Number of AIDS-defining cancer cases in the United States in persons with and without AIDS by calendar year. *(Reproduced with permission from Shiels MS, Pfeiffer RM, Hall HI, et al.: Proportions of Kaposi sarcoma, selected non-Hodgkin lymphomas, and cervical cancer in the United States occurring in persons with AIDS, 1980-2007. JAMA 13;305(14):1450–1459, 2011.)*

initial CD4 count greater than 100 cells/μL had an 87 percent overall survival at 53 months, whereas those with CD counts of less than 100 cells/μL had a 16 percent overall survival at 53 months.[126] A larger multiinstitution study done by the AIDS Malignancy Consortium (AMC-034) randomized patients to receive EPOCH with concurrent rituximab versus EPOCH with sequential rituximab (given weekly for 6 weeks following completion of EPOCH) in 101 patients with HIV-associated NHL (approximately 75 percent of the patients had diffuse large B-cell

lymphoma and 25 percent had mainly Burkitt lymphoma).[127] Administration of EPOCH with concurrent rituximab resulted in a high complete response rate (73 percent) in comparison to EPOCH with sequential rituximab (55 percent complete response rate). The National Cancer Institute evaluated short-course EPOCH with dose-dense rituximab (rituximab day 1 and day 5 of each cycle of EPOCH), and achieved an overall survival of 68 percent at 5 years in 33 patients with diffuse large B-cell lymphoma.[128] In this study, the initial cyclophosphamide dose was 750 mg/m^2 (even in those patients with a low CD4 count) and was dose adjusted, depending on the neutrophil nadir, in subsequent cycles of EPOCH. Patients were treated to complete response plus one additional cycle. The majority (79 percent) of patients received three cycles of short-course EPOCH with dose-dense rituximab, and ART was suspended during chemotherapy because of concern about alteration in the pharmacokinetics or pharmacodynamics of the chemotherapy agents or overlapping toxicity. CD4 counts dropped a median of 64 cells/μL, and recovered to baseline by 6 to 12 months. Consistent with other studies, patients with initial CD4 counts of 100 cells/μL or greater had a much better 5-year overall survival (90 percent) than did the patients with a CD4 count of less than 100 cells/μL (20 percent). Cyclophosphamide, doxorubicin, vincristine, prednisone (CHOP) has also been studied in HIV+ patients with diffuse large B-cell lymphoma. In an AMC phase III multiinstitution clinical trial (AMC 010), patients with HIV-associated NHL (diffuse large B-cell lymphoma in 80 percent, Burkitt lymphoma in 9 percent) were randomized to six cycles of CHOP (n = 50) versus rituximab plus CHOP (R-CHOP) (n = 99), with all patients on ART.[129] The R-CHOP group also received three monthly doses of rituximab following completion of chemotherapy. Of note, the median CD4 count at enrollment was 133 cells/μL and 24 percent of the patients had advanced HIV with CD4 counts less than 50 cells/μL, so this was a fairly immunocompromised group of patients. Overall survival was identical with CHOP or R-CHOP, unlike HIV-negative patients in whom the addition of rituximab significantly improves outcome. In the AMC 010 clinical trial, there were significantly more deaths from infection in the R-CHOP arm in comparison to the CHOP arm, which offset the trend toward better control of lymphoma with R-CHOP. The majority of these infectious deaths occurred in patients with a CD4 count of less than 50 cells/μL, suggesting that rituximab should be used cautiously in immunologically vulnerable patients. As in studies of EPOCH, patients with a CD4 count greater than 100 cells/μL had a better overall survival than those with a lower CD4 count. Other reports suggest that R-CHOP treatment in HIV+ patients with diffuse large B-cell lymphoma is safe and effective,[121,130] including in those with a low CD4 count.[131] In a phase II study of modified R-CHOP in 40 patients with diffuse large B-cell lymphoma, pegylated liposomal doxorubicin was substituted for doxorubicin[132] and the complete response rate was 48 percent, lower than what is reported with rituximab plus EPOCH (R-EPOCH) or R-CHOP. At the time of this writing, there are no phase III data comparing R-EPOCH to R-CHOP in HIV+ patients. Pooled analysis of two sequential AMC clinical trials, AMC 010 (99 patients on the R-CHOP arm) and AMC 034 (51 patients on the concurrent R-EPOCH arm) showed that the 2-year overall survival was approximately 50 percent with R-CHOP and approximately 65 percent with R-EPOCH (p <0.01), suggesting superiority of R-EPOCH.[133] Similarly, a pooled analysis of 1546 patients enrolled in 19 prospective clinical trials, concluded that EPOCH was associated with a better overall survival than CHOP in patients with HIV-associated diffuse large B-cell lymphoma (hazard ratio 0.33, p = 0.03).[134] However these observations require validation in prospective randomized studies. For patients with relapsed or refractory HIV-associated diffuse large B-cell lymphoma, salvage regimens such as gemcitabine/dexamethasone/cisplatin[135] or etoposide, methylprednisolone, high-dose cytarabine, cisplatin (ESHAP)[136] can provide response rates of approximately 50 percent.

HUMAN IMMUNODEFICIENCY VIRUS–ASSOCIATED BURKITT LYMPHOMA

HIV-associated Burkitt lymphoma is approximately one-third as common as HIV-associated diffuse large B-cell lymphoma in the Western world, and occurs at a higher CD4 count.[137] In a Surveillance,

Epidemiology, and End Results (SEER) Registry–based study, there was an increase in the number of cases of Burkitt lymphoma in the United States in the late 1980s that is maintained to the present time (see Fig. 81-1), particularly in men, and is thought to be attributable to the HIV epidemic.[138] The pathogenesis of HIV-associated Burkitt lymphoma is similar to that of Burkitt lymphoma in HIV– people, and involves translocation of the *Myc* gene on chromosome 8 with one of the immunoglobulin genes on chromosomes, 2, 14, or 22, resulting in overexpression of Myc.[139] HIV-associated Burkitt lymphoma is an aggressive malignancy, and it is important to act decisively in these often very ill patients. More than 80 percent of patients with HIV-associated Burkitt lymphoma present with stage IV disease[140] and extranodal sites are often involved. Marrow, liver, gastrointestinal tract, kidney, and CNS involvement are common, with cranial nerve palsies a common feature of CNS involvement.[141] The serum lactate dehydrogenase (LDH) is elevated in more than 80 percent of patients, often to high levels (greater than five-fold normal). A number of chemotherapy regimens have been studied in HIV+ patients with Burkitt lymphoma. As in the HIV– setting, CHOP is not adequate treatment for Burkitt lymphoma,[140,142] and should not be used. Recent data show excellent outcomes with a variant of the R-EPOCH regimen.[143] In this single-institution, small prospective clinical trial, a total of 30 patients with Burkitt lymphoma were treated, including 11 who were HIV+ with a median CD4 count of 322 cells/μL. The short-course EPOCH-RR used in this clinical trial included two doses of rituximab per cycle of EPOCH, and a total of three or four cycles of EPOCH (to complete response plus one additional cycle), and included prophylactic intrathecal methotrexate. With a median follow up of 6 years, the overall survival of the HIV+ patients was 90 percent. The major toxicity was neutropenia in 31 percent of cycles of EPOCH-RR, and hospital admission for febrile neutropenia was required in 10 percent of cycles. This study showed that low-intensity therapy administered primarily in the outpatient setting can be effective for HIV-associated Burkitt lymphoma. Other studies of R-EPOCH that included a subset of patients with HIV-associated Burkitt lymphoma also report excellent outcomes with R-EPOCH.[127] Other regimens reported in patients with HIV-associated Burkitt lymphoma include cyclophosphamide, vincristine, doxorubicin, and dexamethasone (HyperCVAD) alternating with high-dose methotrexate plus cytarabine.[144] In this study, patients were very immunocompromised with a median CD4 count of 77 cells/μL; nevertheless, complete remission was achieved in more than 90 percent of patients, with 48 percent of patients alive at 2 years. Severe myelosuppression was universal, but infectious complications were similar to HIV– patients. In this small study, those on ART had a better outcome than those not on ART. Cyclophosphamide, vincristine, doxorubicin, methotrexate/ifosfamide, mesna, etoposide, cytarabine (CODOX-M/IVAC) has also been employed to treat HIV-associated Burkitt lymphoma,[145–147] with 3-year overall survival of approximately 50 percent.[146] A retrospective review compared eight HIV+ patients who received CODOX-M/IVAC to 24 HIV– patients with Burkitt lymphoma[145]: Patients had similar rates of myelosuppression, infection, and complete response regardless of HIV status. The LMB86 protocol (including high-dose methotrexate plus cytarabine) was used to treat HIV-related Burkitt lymphoma[141] in a prospective single center study of 63 patients on ART. The complete response rate was 70 percent and the estimated disease-free survival at 2 years was 67 percent. This regimen was characterized by severe marrow toxicity, and more than 10 percent of patients died of regimen-related toxicity. Poor prognostic factors included a CD4 count of less than 200 cells/μL and an Eastern Cooperative Oncology Group (ECOG) performance status of greater than 2. Other intensive regimens have also been used, with 4-year overall survival of 70 percent, but with death in 11 percent from regimen-related toxicity.[148]

HUMAN IMMUNODEFICIENCY VIRUS–ASSOCIATED PRIMARY CENTRAL NERVOUS SYSTEM LYMPHOMA

Primary CNS lymphoma in HIV+ patients is an Epstein-Barr virus (EBV)–related diffuse large B-cell lymphoma occurring in the brain, typically in patients with very advanced HIV: These patients usually have a CD4 count of less than 50 cells/μL, and often of less than 20 cells/μL.[137,149–151] The epidemiology of primary CNS lymphoma illustrates the concept of specific types of lymphoma occurring at different levels of immunodepletion. The incidence of primary CNS lymphoma has declined markedly since the availability of ART (see Fig. 81–1).[150,152] The pathophysiology of HIV-associated primary CNS lymphoma is related to EBV which is detectable in virtually all cases.[139] Primary CNS lymphoma should be considered in an HIV+ patient who presents with neurologic symptoms (confusion, cognitive decline, memory loss), headache, seizures, or ataxia. In one series, the most common symptom was headache, followed by memory loss, ataxia, and seizure.[153] Characteristic features on magnetic resonance imaging (MRI) of the brain include a single to several mass lesions in the subcortical white matter.[154] Anatomic sites commonly involved are predominantly the cerebral cortex and periventricular area, but the basal ganglia can be involved in up to one-third of cases. Cerebellar or brain stem involvement is rare.[150] A thorough physical exam for signs of systemic lymphoma is key, including a testicular exam as testicular lymphoma frequently involves the CNS. A slit-lamp exam to assess for vitreous disease should be done; this may assist in diagnoses of primary CNS lymphoma and may affect therapy. Evaluation with a chest, abdomen, and pelvic CT and a marrow aspirate and biopsy should be performed. If a lumbar puncture can be safely done, cerebrospinal fluid (CSF) should be sent for cytology and flow cytometry to evaluate for leptomeningeal involvement with lymphoma, and also for polymerase chain reaction (PCR) for EBV. Detection of EBV in the CSF supports, but does not confirm, the diagnosis of primary CNS lymphoma in these patients.[155] PET-CT of the brain can also help distinguish primary CNS lymphoma from other common causes of focal brain lesions in profoundly immunosuppressed patients with HIV, namely, cerebral toxoplasmosis and other infections.[156,157] Evaluation of HIV+ patients with CNS mass lesions should include blood serology for toxoplasmosis, although a small percentage of patients with CNS toxoplasmosis will have negative serologies. Stereotactic brain biopsy should be performed if possible, but some lesions are not readily accessible to biopsy; in these cases, the diagnosis of primary CNS lymphoma may rest on CSF cytology, detection of EBV in the CSF, and the results of PET-CT. Because of the rarity of primary CNS lymphoma in the ART era, there are no large prospective clinical trial data to define optimal therapy. Case reports document long-term responses to initiation of ART as a sole intervention in a small number of patients who refused other therapy. All HIV+ patients with primary CNS lymphoma should be on effective ART. Systemic glucocorticoid treatment can temporarily ameliorate symptoms. Small retrospective series report that whole-brain radiation therapy can result in improved survival,[149] but approximately one-third of these patients had detectable leukoencephalopathy on followup. A large retrospective study found that treatment with whole-brain radiation therapy and/or chemotherapy was associated with a decreased risk of death,[151] but this analysis is confounded by lack of information on performance status. Small numbers of patients have been treated with multiple cycles of high-dose methotrexate with leucovorin rescue, without radiation therapy, with prolonged survival and no cognitive dysfunction,[158,159] and this may be a reasonable option in patients with good performance status. In the pre-ART era, median survival of the HIV+ patient with primary CNS lymphoma was approximately 2 months. The outcome has improved in the present era, but remains inferior to that of patients without HIV.[153] The Center for AIDS Research database for 1996 to 2010 shows that the 2-year survival of HIV+ patients with primary CNS lymphoma was 24 percent, inferior to other major types of HIV-associated lymphoma (diffuse large B-cell lymphoma, Burkitt lymphoma, Hodgkin lymphoma).[137] Prior CNS opportunistic infection[151] and poor performance status[149,150] confer an increased risk of death.

HUMAN IMMUNODEFICIENCY VIRUS–ASSOCIATED PLASMABLASTIC LYMPHOMA

Described in 1997,[160] plasmablastic lymphoma is a rare and very aggressive B-cell NHL with plasmacytic differentiation that often involves the oral cavity, typically the gingiva and the palate. In the original report, 15 of the 16 cases were HIV+, and subsequent studies showed that plasmablastic lymphoma comprises approximately 2 to 3 percent of NHL in people living with HIV.[161] A review of 112 cases of HIV-associated plasmablastic lymphoma showed that the median age of presentation was approximately 40 years, and the median CD4 count was approximately 180 cells/μL. Of the 112 patients, 58 percent had primary oral involvement. Other common sites of involvement were the gastrointestinal track, the lymph nodes and skin, among other sites.[162] In a recent series of 50 cases of plasmablastic lymphoma,[163] approximately 25 percent of the patients had oral cavity involvement, and extraoral involvement was common. Diagnosis requires biopsy. The pathology shows a monomorphic diffuse lymphoid infiltrate with cells resembling plasmablasts. The cells have a high proliferative rate with a Ki-67 often exceeding 90 percent, and are positive for plasma cell markers. CD20 is expressed in 2 percent or fewer of the cases and the majority of the cases (>80 percent) are EBV+. The differential diagnosis of an oral cavity lesion in a person with HIV includes odontogenic infection, squamous carcinoma, Kaposi sarcoma, and diffuse large B-cell lymphoma or Burkitt lymphoma.

Many of the patients with plasmablastic lymphoma have been treated with CHOP or with EPOCH, with poor outcome. In one retrospective series,[163] median overall survival was 11 months with no difference in outcome between CHOP versus more intensive chemotherapy (EPOCH, hyperCVAD, or other regimens). Data from the German AIDS Related Lymphoma Cohort Study in the ART era confirmed the poor outcome of these patients, with a median survival of 5 months.[164] There are no prospective clinical trials to define optimal treatment for patients with HIV-associated plasmablastic lymphoma. Case reports of individual patients suggest that bortezomib may have activity in these patients, and this should be explored in future clinical trials.[165,166]

HUMAN IMMUNODEFICIENCY VIRUS–ASSOCIATED PRIMARY EFFUSION LYMPHOMA

Primary effusion lymphoma is an aggressive B-cell lymphoma characterized by lymphomatous effusions in body cavities, most commonly pleural effusion,[167,168] followed by ascites and pericardial effusion or multiple body cavities; lymph nodes, marrow, and skin can also be involved. A solid variant of primary effusion lymphoma presents without effusion, but with lymph node, gastrointestinal, skin, or liver involvement has been reported.[169] Primary effusion lymphoma comprises approximately 4 percent of HIV-associated NHL[170] and occurs much more frequently in men than in women (10:1 ratio), usually associated with low CD4 counts (50 to 200 cells/μL).[171] Of primary effusion lymphoma cases, 100 percent are human herpesvirus-8+ (HHV8+), and approximately 80 percent are EBV+. HHV8 plays a key pathophysiologic role, possibly by elaboration of a viral homologue of FLICE inhibitory protein and a viral homologue of interleukin (IL)-6.[120] Other HHV8-related disorders include Castleman disease and Kaposi sarcoma, both of which may coexist with primary effusion lymphoma in a substantial proportion of patients.[168] Patients may present with dyspnea from pleural effusions or new-onset ascites. A high index of suspicion for lymphoma is needed so that appropriate samples are sent to Hematopathology for analysis. Primary effusion lymphoma cells have an immunoblastic, plasmablastic, or anaplastic appearance and are CD45+ and CD30+; CD20 is expressed less than 5 percent of the time. The malignant cells are latently infected with HHV8, which is detectable by immunocytochemistry. There are no large prospective studies of treatment of primary effusion lymphoma, a consequence of its rarity, and the majority of the available information is derived from retrospective case series. There are a few case reports of complete remission following initiation of ART without chemotherapy, and ART should be a component of the treatment plan. Patients have been treated with CHOP, EPOCH, and other regimens. Approximately 50 percent of patients with primary effusion lymphoma achieve a complete response, but relapse within the next few months is common, and the median survival is approximately 6 months, with most deaths a result of progressive lymphoma. In one series, poor prognostic features included an ECOG performance status greater than 2 and ART noncompliance. Promising preclinical data show that treatment with the anti-CD30 agent brentuximab vedotin[172] or bortezomib with or without vorinostat[173] can decrease growth of primary effusion lymphoma cell lines and prolong survival in a mouse xenograft model.

Prognosis

As ART improves, the prognosis for patients with HIV-associated NHL is defined mainly by lymphoma-related features, and less by HIV.[121] A retrospective review of patients with HIV-associated diffuse large B-cell lymphoma diagnosed in the pre-ART era (120 patients), and in the ART era (72 patients) showed a median survival of 8 months in the pre-ART era and 43 months in the ART era; this held true for each of the different International Prognostic Index groups.[125] Pooled data for 1546 patients with HIV-associated diffuse large B-cell lymphoma or Burkitt lymphoma who had been enrolled in phase II or phase III clinical trials was evaluated to identify treatment-related factors associated with overall survival. The use of rituximab was significantly associated with improved overall survival (hazard ratio 0.55, p <0.001) for patients with a CD4 count of greater than 50 cells/μL but not for those patients with CD4 counts of less than 50 cells/μL. A focus on the 1059 patients with diffuse large B-cell lymphoma suggested that treatment with EPOCH resulted in a better overall survival (hazard ratio 0.33, p = 0.031) than treatment with CHOP. On multivariant analysis of R-EPOCH versus R-CHOP, the hazard ratio for overall survival was 0.34 favoring R-EPOCH, although this did not achieve statistical significance. An enhanced internal prognostic index based on 650 adults with *de novo* diffuse large B-cell lymphoma treated at seven National Comprehensive Cancer Network Cancer Centers in the rituximab era included a small portion of HIV+ patients.[174] Patients were risk stratified on an 8-point scale. Patients with a low score (0 to 1 points) had a 5-year overall survival of 96 percent; patients with a low intermediate score (2 to 3 points) had a 5-year overall survival of 82 percent; patients with a high intermediate score (4 to 5 points) had a 5-year overall survival of 64 percent, and patients with high risk (6 to 8 points) had an overall 5-year survival of 33 percent. This scale offered better risk stratification than the original International Prognostic Index, which was developed in the prerituximab era. It is recommended that this enhanced International Prognostic Index be used as a guide, in addition to the very robust data that patients with CD4 counts of less than 100 cells/μL at the time of diagnosis of lymphoma have a much worse outcome than those with higher CD4 counts.

HUMAN IMMUNODEFICIENCY VIRUS–ASSOCIATED HODGKIN LYMPHOMA

Hodgkin lymphoma tends to occur at moderate levels immunosuppression in HIV+ patients, unlike NHL, where the risk increases as the CD4 count decreases.[175] A retrospective cohort study from the Veterans Administration Clinical Case Registry from 1985 to 2010 showed that Hodgkin lymphoma was most common in patients with CD4 counts of 200 to 350 cells/μL. The risk was highest in the first year after starting ART, and was lower in people with a greater percent of time with an undetectable viral load.[176] Data from 14 U.S. Cancer Registries representing 25 percent of the U.S. population was used to compare the clinical features of HIV+ and HIV– patients with Hodgkin lymphoma in the ART era.[177] In this study, Hodgkin lymphoma occurring in HIV+ people was shown to be a clinically aggressive disease. Of the 22,355 patients with Hodgkin lymphoma, 3.8 percent were HIV+. However this percentage varied depending on sex, ethnicity, and age. Prevalent HIV infection was higher in men (6 percent) than in women (1.2 percent), and among men in the 40- to 59-year-old age group, those newly diagnosed with Hodgkin lymphoma had a 14.2 percent chance of being HIV+. Non-Hispanic blacks with newly diagnosed Hodgkin lymphoma had a 16.9 percent chance of being HIV+ and Hispanics with newly diagnosed Hodgkin lymphoma had a 9.9 percent chance of being HIV+. Unlike NHL, the incidence of Hodgkin lymphoma is comparable in the pre- and post-ART era. The pathology of Hodgkin lymphoma in HIV+ cases differs from that of HIV– cases, with a higher percent of HIV+ patients having a more aggressive histology (mixed cellularity or lymphocyte depleted; Table 81–7). An HIV-AIDS cancer match study that linked HIV and cancer registry data found that an even higher percent of patients with HIV-associated Hodgkin lymphoma had mixed cellularity on biopsy (53.7 percent).[175] The Ann Arbor stage at diagnosis is higher in HIV+ Hodgkin patients than in HIV– cases, with 41.5 percent of those with HIV+ Hodgkin lymphoma having stage IV disease at presentation, compared to 17 percent of those with HIV– Hodgkin lymphoma (Table 81–7). B symptoms (drenching night sweats, fever, or loss of 10 percent of body weight) are also more common in HIV+ patients with Hodgkin lymphoma (Table 81–7).[177]

A retrospective study of Adriamycin, bleomycin, vinblastine, and dacarbazine (ABVD) chemotherapy in 62 HIV+ patients newly diagnosed with advanced-stage Hodgkin lymphoma showed that ABVD and ART could be given safely together.[178] In this study, the median CD4 count at diagnosis was 129 cells/μL, and all patients had stage III or stage IV Hodgkin lymphoma. Patients received ABVD with filgrastim support, as well as trimethoprim-sulfamethoxazole or pentamidine for *P. jiroveci* prophylaxis. The overall survival was 76 percent at 5 years, with treatment-related mortality of 10 percent. In a large retrospective study[179] of 93 HIV+ patients and 131 HIV– patients with Hodgkin lymphoma who were treated with ABVD, (HIV+ patients also received concomitant ART), those with stage I or II nonbulky disease received four cycles of ABVD plus involved field radiation therapy; the rest received six cycles of ABVD with involved field radiation therapy if bulky disease was present. All patients received prophylaxis for opportunistic infections. The HIV+ patients had more advanced-stage Hodgkin lymphoma and a worse International Prognostic Score[180]; despite this the 5-year overall survival was 81 percent for the HIV+ patients compared to 88 percent for the HIV– patients, a nonsignificant difference. This retrospective case series demonstrated comparable overall survival in HIV+ and HIV– patients with Hodgkin lymphoma, and that ART could be given safely with ABVD chemotherapy.

The German HIV Related Lymphoma Study Group[181] conducted a prospective multicenter study in which HIV+ patients with early stage favorable Hodgkin lymphoma were treated with two to four cycles of

TABLE 81–7. Characteristics of Hodgkin Lymphoma in HIV+ and HIV– Populations

	HIV+	HIV–
Number of individuals	848	21,507
Percent (%) men	86.2	53.7
HISTOLOGY		
Lymphocyte rich	1.9%	3.2%
Nodular lymphocyte predominant	0.9%	4.4%
Nodular sclerosis	30.7%	59.6%
Mixed cellularity	25.0%	12.2%
Lymphocyte depleted	3.7%	1.3%
Classical Hodgkin lymphoma NOS	37.9%	19.3%
ANN ARBOR STAGE		
I	14.3%	18.4%
II	17.6%	39.5%
III	22.4%	19.1%
IV	41.5%	17.0%
unknown	4.3%	6.0%
B SYMPTOMS		
Present	57.4%	34.2%
Absent	28.9%	43.9%
Unknown	13.7%	21.9%

Adapted with permission from Shiels MS, Koritzinsky EH, Clarke CA, et al: Prevalence of HIV Infection among U.S. Hodgkin lymphoma cases. *Cancer Epidemiol Biomarkers Prev* 23(2):274–281, 2014.

ABVD plus 30 Gy of involved field radiation therapy, while patients with early stage unfavorable Hodgkin lymphoma received four cycles of bleomycin, etoposide, Adriamycin, cyclophosphamide, vincristine, procarbazine, and prednisone (BEACOPP) baseline or four cycles of ABVD plus 30 Gy of involved field radiation therapy. More advanced-stage Hodgkin lymphoma patients received six to eight cycles of BEA-COPP. Patients with advanced HIV infection (defined as two of the following: CD4 count <50 cells/μL, prior AIDS-defining opportunistic infection, performance status >2) were treated with six to eight cycles of ABVD. ART was used with chemotherapy. CD4 count decreased with chemotherapy, but recovered over the subsequent 6 to 9 months and treatment-related mortality was 5.6 percent, mainly from sepsis. Using this risk-adapted approach, the 2-year overall survival was 90.7 percent, comparable to HIV– patients with Hodgkin lymphoma.

Areas of controversy in treatment of Hodgkin lymphoma in HIV– patients include whether BEACOPP escalated is better than ABVD for advanced Hodgkin lymphoma.[182–184] Until this controversy is settled, most authorities recommend using ABVD for patients with HIV-associated Hodgkin lymphoma. Brentuximab vedotin, an antibody-drug conjugate that targets CD30, has been combined with Adriamycin, vinblastine, and dacarbazine (AVD) to treat HIV- patients with Hodgkin lymphoma.[185] Whether brentuximab vedotin plus AVD will be effective for HIV+ patients with Hodgkin lymphoma is being addressed in a prospective phase II clinical trial being done by the AMC (AMC 085).

In the ART era, HIV+ patients with Hodgkin lymphoma have similar excellent outcomes with systemic chemotherapy as do HIV– patients. This is corroborated by the SEER Study[177] in which the 5-year risk of death from Hodgkin lymphoma was 6.2 percent in the HIV+ patients and 9 percent in the HIV– patients. However, this interpretation is confounded by competing risks of death: the overall risk of death was higher in the HIV+ cohort, and the majority of the deaths were from HIV. Many[179] but not all[181] studies conclude that the International Prognostic Score has predictive value for HIV+ patients with Hodgkin lymphoma.

Stem Cell Transplant

There is more than a decade of experience in high-dose therapy followed by autologous blood stem cell transplantation showing that this technique is feasible, safe, and effective in patients with HIV and NHL or Hodgkin lymphoma.[186,187] Adequate numbers of blood stem cells can be mobilized in the majority of patients with HIV-associated NHL or Hodgkin lymphoma. A retrospective study of 155 patients with either NHL or Hodgkin lymphoma in the ART era showed that mobilization of greater than 2×10^6 CD34+ cells/kg was achieved in 73 percent of patients and greater than 5×10^6 CD34+ cells/kg was achieved in 48 percent. Factors reducing the chance of optimal mobilization included a low platelet count, a low CD4 count, and use of filgrastim alone, rather than chemotherapy plus filgrastim, to mobilize blood stem cells.[188]

Studies of autologous blood stem cell transplantation in HIV+ patients with NHL (mainly diffuse large B-cell lymphoma) or Hodgkin lymphoma show that outcomes are similar to those reported for patients without HIV infection.[189,190] The median time to neutrophil and platelet engraftment is 11 and 14 days, respectively. The risk for nonrelapse mortality is in the 5 to 8 percent range and the overall survival at 3 to 4 years after transplantation is approximately 50 percent.[191–193] These patients were supported throughout the transplantation with ART, as well as with antibacterial, antifungal, and antiviral prophylaxis. The European group for Blood and Marrow Transplant performed a case-control study that included 53 HIV+ patients with either NHL (two-thirds of patients) or Hodgkin lymphoma (one-third of patients) that matched patients on the basis of histology, Ann Arbor stage, International Prognostic Index and disease status. The overall survival, progression-free survival, and relapse rates were similar in the HIV+ and the HIV– groups across all histologies and disease states. Nonrelapse mortality at 1 year was 8 percent in the HIV+ group and 2 percent in the HIV– group; the difference mainly was a result of early bacterial infections. Overall survival at 30 months was 59 percent for both HIV+ and HIV– patients with NHL, and the main cause of death in both HIV+ and HIV– patients was relapse. A single-institution matched case-control study of HIV+ and HIV– NHL patients showed nonrelapse mortality of 11 percent in the HIV+ group, and 4 percent in the HIV– group. Overall survival at 2 years was 75 percent for both the HIV+ and HIV– groups.[190] Thus, HIV status did not affect the outcome of autologous transplantation for NHL although there were more viral opportunistic infections, particularly cytomegalovirus (CMV), adenovirus, and varicella in the HIV+ population. The main cause of death was relapse and the major predictor of outcome in both groups was disease status at time of transplantation. Together these data suggest that long-term outcomes are similar in the HIV+ and HIV– patients who undergo autologous blood stem cell transplant in the setting of NHL or Hodgkin lymphoma and the reconstitution of neutrophils and platelets are similar in both groups.[194] Experience with allogeneic stem cell transplantation HIV+ patients is less extensive.[195–197] This remains an area of intensive research, in part because of the report of cure of HIV in a patient who underwent allogeneic transplant to treat acute myeloid leukemia and received a donor graft that was homozygous for a deletion mutation eliminating the chemokine and HIV coreceptor CCR5.[109]

Antiretroviral Therapy and Chemotherapy

Controversy persists regarding whether ART should be initiated or continued during multiagent systemic chemotherapy. In the pre-ART era, the outcomes for treatment of lymphoma in HIV+ patients were markedly inferior to the present era.[125] Some clinical trial groups stop or do not initiate ART during systemic chemotherapy,[198] whereas others continue ART or initiate ART after the first cycle of chemotherapy in those patients not on ART at time of lymphoma diagnosis.[199,200] Certain classes of ART medications, notably protease inhibitors and nnRTIs can alter the metabolism of other medications primarily though inhibition or induction of the cytochrome P450 enzymes, potentially leading to higher or lower concentrations of other drugs (including chemotherapy agents).[201] Unfortunately, there are limited pharmacokinetic data from clinical trials to elucidate these potential drug interactions and their effects on drug levels. Chemotherapy agents eliminated by non-P450 routes are less likely to be affected by ART. A study of 154 HIV+ patients with a broad range of malignancies (many with hematologic malignancies) treated at the MD Anderson Cancer Center showed that clinically relevant drug interactions between ART and chemotherapy drugs were rare (4 percent of cases) and confined to the protease inhibitor class.[202] The nnRTIs and the integrase strand-transfer inhibitors had a better safety profile when combined with chemotherapy than did the protease inhibitors, in this retrospective series. Others have also found that protease inhibitors may exacerbate chemotherapy-induced neutropenia,[203] although this is controversial.[204,205] A retrospective review of 34 patients with diffuse large B-cell lymphoma showed similar complete response rates and toxicities in those receiving CHOP while also on an HIV protease inhibitor as those who were receiving a nonprotease inhibitor ART regimen.[206] In another study of HIV+ patients with Hodgkin lymphoma receiving ABVD chemotherapy, the use of the protease inhibitor ritonavir appeared to increase the risk of peripheral neuropathy.[207] More accurate information regarding drug interactions between ART and chemotherapy agents will become available through the AMC, which is currently conducting clinical trials in which patients are stratified by the type of ART and its potential for inducing or inhibiting cytochrome P450 enzymes, and obtaining detailed pharmacokinetic data. With the growing number of available ART agents, including integrase strand-transfer inhibitors, it is usually possible to adjust an ART regimen that minimizes potential drug interactions but still suppresses HIV replication throughout the course of chemotherapy.

A second issue is overlapping toxic effects between ART and chemotherapy drugs. Zidovudine causes marrow suppression, and should be avoided in patients receiving myelosuppressive chemotherapy. Didanosine and stavudine (older, infrequently used agents) cause peripheral neuropathy, and their use should be reconsidered in patients who will receive potentially neurotoxic chemotherapy. Atazanavir, a commonly prescribed protease inhibitor, causes unconjugated hyperbilirubinemia similar to Gilbert syndrome and can complicate the administration of some chemotherapy agents. However, if there is no other evidence of hepatotoxicity, chemotherapy can be given at standard doses. Earlier studies suggested some ART drugs (saquinavir, efavirenz, nelfinavir) might cause cardiac conduction abnormalities (prolongation of the electrocardiographic "QTc interval"), but this has not been confirmed in subsequent studies. If the patient is stable on ART with excellent HIV virologic control, a reasonable approach is to consult the infectious diseases physician who is managing the patient and also the chemotherapy pharmacist to identify potential drug interactions between ART and the planned chemotherapy, to adjust ART as necessary, and then proceed with chemotherapy with concurrent ART. If the patient is not on ART, it is reasonable to give one cycle of chemotherapy and then start ART with the second cycle of chemotherapy following

multidisciplinary consultation with the pharmacist and infectious diseases physician.

HUMAN IMMUNODEFICIENCY VIRUS–ASSOCIATED CASTLEMAN DISEASE

Castleman disease is a rare polyclonal lymphoproliferative disorder characterized by periodic flares (an inflammatory illness accompanied by lymphadenopathy and splenomegaly), and a high risk of progression to lymphoma.[208] Castleman disease occurs with higher frequency in people living with HIV.[209] The pathophysiology of Castleman disease is related to IL-6 (reviewed in Ref. 210). Virtually all patients with HIV-associated Castleman disease are infected with HHV8, whose viral genome encodes a viral homologue of IL-6. Sequential analysis of human IL-6, viral IL-6, and a variety of other cytokines in patients with HIV-associated Castleman disease during and after flares showed that either human IL-6, viral IL-6, or both were elevated during the flare and diminished during remission.[211] IL-6 is a proinflammatory cytokine and stimulates polyclonal proliferation of B lymphocytes. Serologic evidence of HHV8 infection is present in 7 percent of healthy U.S. blood donors,[212] but few healthy adults or HIV+ patients without Castleman disease, Kaposi sarcoma, or primary effusion lymphoma have detectable HHV8 virus in the blood. More than 80 percent of HIV+ patients with symptomatic multicentric Castleman disease have detectable HHV8 viremia, often at a high level.[209] A retrospective analysis of 52 HIV+ patients with multicentric Castleman disease at time of presentation[213] showed that more than 50 percent of the patients had a prior diagnosis of Kaposi sarcoma, and 80 percent were on ART. The mean CD4 count at time of diagnosis of Castleman disease was 287 cells/μL, indicating that Castleman disease occurs in moderately immunocompromised patients. Symptoms at presentation included fever, lymphadenopathy, and splenomegaly in 98 to 100 percent, pulmonary symptoms in 60 percent, and edema in 40 percent of patients. A single-institution study of 113 patients with Castleman disease[214] also reported that approximately half of the patients had a prior diagnosis of Kaposi sarcoma. The median CD4 count in this study was 188 cells/μL. The ECOG performance status at diagnosis of Castleman disease was greater than 2 in 45 percent of patients, 36 percent had hemophagocytosis, and 30 percent required an ICU stay, illustrating how ill these patients often are. During a Castleman disease flare, patients may rapidly develop cytopenias: half the patients in this series had a hemoglobin of less than 8 g/dL and 29 percent had a platelet count of less than 150,000/μL. High C-reactive protein (often 10-fold higher than normal) and plasma HHV8 levels (median 30,000 copies/mL, range: 60 to 1 million copies/mL) are found during a flare,[215,216] and these values can be helpful. Diagnosis requires a lymph node biopsy that is consistent with Castleman disease, ideally an excisional biopsy rather than a needle biopsy. The morphology of multicentric Castleman disease in HIV+ patients shows plasmablastic cells in the mantle zone of the follicles; HHV8 is detectable in the plasmablasts.[217] Often, lymph nodes diagnostic of Castleman disease also contain malignant appearing spindle cells characteristic of Kaposi sarcoma.

Castleman disease is rare, and treatment recommendations are largely based on case series and small clinical trials. Several clinical trials show that the anti-CD20 monoclonal antibody rituximab is very effective for treatment of Castleman disease. Prospective studies[213,218,219] demonstrate that 375 mg/m² of rituximab administered intravenously weekly for 4 doses resulted in rapid symptomatic improvement, and 90 percent of patients achieved a response that lasted for more than 6 months. Clinical improvement with rituximab may begin within hours to days and is associated with diminished levels of serum IL-6.[220] In one series of 113 HIV+ patients with multicentric Castleman disease, some of whom received rituximab, the overall median survival was longer than 12 years with therapy; this is much improved in comparison to 20 years ago when Castleman disease was rapidly fatal.

Incipient flares of Castleman disease may be heralded by cytopenias, increased C-reactive protein, or by increased levels of HHV8 in the blood.[216] Serial studies of 52 HIV+ patients with multicentric Castleman disease showed that approximately 75 percent had elevated C-reactive protein and 90 percent had detectable plasma HHV8 during a flare, with a median HHV8 viral load of 27,000 copies/mL. HHV8 was detectable in 38 percent of patients during remission. If relapse occurs, patients can safely be retreated with rituximab.[221] Up to 20 percent of HIV+ patients with Castleman disease will develop lymphoma,[208,214] often primary effusion lymphoma, plasmablastic lymphoma, or diffuse large B-cell lymphoma, but occasionally Hodgkin lymphoma, so it is important to consider this during followup. Use of rituximab to treat Castleman disease may decrease the risk of subsequent NHL.[214] In HIV+ patients with both Castleman disease and Kaposi sarcoma, Kaposi sarcoma may progress following treatment with rituximab.[218,219,222] When Kaposi sarcoma involves a key clinical location such as the lungs, where progression might result in significant respiratory compromise, a regimen of rituximab plus liposomal doxorubicin can be considered to address both the Castleman disease flare and Kaposi sarcoma.[223] R-CHOP or other multiagent systemic chemotherapy has also been used to treat Castleman disease, but given the excellent response to rituximab alone, R-CHOP is usually not necessary. An alternative therapeutic approach focuses on the central role of IL-6. A multiinstitution, randomized, placebo-controlled clinical trial of an anti–IL-6 monoclonal antibody siltuximab in 79 HIV– patients with Castleman disease showed a 34 percent response rate.[224] Siltuximab was given IV every 3 weeks and can be administered long-term (up to 60 months).[225] Siltuximab is FDA-approved for treatment of Castleman disease in HIV– patients but not in HIV+ patients. Tocilizumab, an anti–IL-6 receptor monoclonal antibody has been FDA-approved for use in rheumatoid arthritis. Tocilizumab had short-term effects in two HIV+ patients with Castleman disease, but both patients relapsed within 6 months and required subsequent treatment with rituximab.[226] Tocilizumab is not FDA-approved for treatment of Castleman disease. Another approach to treatment of Castleman disease is to use antiviral therapy, such as ganciclovir, valganciclovir, foscarnet, cidofovir, or zidovudine, to suppress HHV8 replication.[227,228] When 14 HIV+ patients with Castleman disease were treated with high-dose zidovudine plus valganciclovir, the C-reactive protein level, human IL-6 levels and HHV8 viral load improved. The median progression-free period was 6 months and the major toxicity was marrow suppression. However, until additional information is available from clinical trials, the data at this time most strongly support the use of rituximab as the backbone of treatment of Castleman disease.

KAPOSI SARCOMA–ASSOCIATED HERPESVIRUS–ASSOCIATED INFLAMMATORY CYTOKINE SYNDROME

A new syndrome termed Kaposi sarcoma-associated herpesvirus (KSHV)-associated inflammatory cytokine syndrome (KICS) is characterized by an inflammatory illness similar to a flare of Castleman disease, but without the pathologic diagnosis of Castleman disease.[229–231] Patients present with fever, sweating, anorexia, leukopenia, anemia, thrombocytopenia, hypoalbuminemia, and hyponatremia, and may also have dyspnea or abdominal pain. Four of the six patients in the original report also had severe manifestations of Kaposi sarcoma. Patients with KICS have a very high HHV8 viral load, similar to that seen in patients during a flare of multicentric Castleman disease. Levels of other cytokines, including human IL-6, viral IL-6, and IL-10, are similar in KICS

and multicentric Castleman disease patients, and much higher than in patients with isolated Kaposi sarcoma. Whether KICS represents a *form fruste* of multicentric Castleman disease, part of the clinical spectrum of Castleman disease, or a distinct clinical syndrome requires more investigation. There is scant information on treatment of KICS.

HUMAN IMMUNODEFICIENCY VIRUS–ASSOCIATED HEMOPHAGOCYTIC SYNDROME

Hemophagocytic syndrome is a rare and potentially fatal disorder characterized by excess immune activation that occurs with increased frequency in people living with HIV. An autopsy study in the pre-ART era identified hemophagocytosis in 20 percent of 56 patients who died of AIDS.[232] The pathogenesis of the hemophagocytic syndrome results from failure to regulate the immune response, resulting in excess activation of T lymphocytes, increased cytokine secretion, and hyperactivation of macrophages. There are primary and secondary forms of hemophagocytic syndrome. Secondary forms can occur in the setting of infection, hematologic malignancy, or autoimmune disease.[233] In HIV+ patients, the hemophagocytic syndrome is usually secondary to a viral infection, either HIV itself or, more commonly, a member of the herpes virus family (EBV, CMV, HHV8), but can also occur in patients with Hodgkin lymphoma, NHL, or Castleman disease.[234] A study of 58 HIV+ patients with hemophagocytic syndrome performed in the ART era[234] showed that the median duration of HIV at the time of diagnosis was 4 years. Most patients were on ART, and the median CD4 count was 91 cells/μL, demonstrating advanced HIV disease. Patients with hemophagocytic syndrome are typically very ill: greater than 40 percent of the patients in this series required ICU care and 31 percent died within a year of diagnosis. The clinical features of hemophagocytic syndrome in HIV+ patients include fever, hepatosplenomegaly, and cytopenias. Patients often have a markedly elevated ferritin (greater than 10-fold the upper range of normal), coagulopathy, and increased triglycerides.[234]

The differential diagnosis of hemophagocytic syndrome in HIV+ patients includes a Castleman disease flare or KICS, and the clinical features of these syndromes may overlap. Table 81–8 shows the diagnostic criteria for hemophagocytic syndrome . If an underlying trigger for the hemophagocytic syndrome is identified, specific therapy should be directed at the trigger. Treatment for hemophagocytic syndrome is standardized using the Histiocytosis Society 1994 protocol[235] or the

TABLE 81–8. Diagnostic Criteria for Secondary Hemophagocytic Syndrome*

1. Fever ≥38.5°C
2. Splenomegaly
3. Cytopenias in at least 2 of 3 lineages (hemoglobin <9 g/dL, platelets <100,000/μL, neutrophils <1000/μL)
4. Hypertriglyceridemia (fasting >265 mg/dL) and/or low fibrinogen (<150 mg/dL)
5. Hemophagocytosis found on biopsy of the marrow, spleen, lymph nodes, or liver
6. Low or absent natural killer cell activity
7. Ferritin >500 mg/mL
8. Elevated soluble CD25

*Presence of 5 of these 8 criteria is required for diagnosis of hemophagocytic syndrome.

Adapted with permission from Henter JI, Horne A, Arico M, et al: HLH-2004: Diagnostic and therapeutic guidelines for hemophagocytic lymphohistiocytosis. *Pediatr Blood Cancer* 48(2):124–131, 2007.

Histiocytosis Society 2004 protocol[236] (Chapter 71). Caution regarding interaction of cyclosporine with specific ART medications is warranted.

ANEMIA AND HUMAN IMMUNODEFICIENCY VIRUS

Anemia is common in people living with HIV. The multisite Adult and Adolescent Spectrum of HIV Disease Surveillance Project[237] included approximately 32,000 HIV+ people living in the United States in the pre-ART era, 1990 to 1996. In this study, the first hemoglobin measured was less than 10 g/dL in 37 percent of men and 43 percent of women with clinical AIDS (an AIDS-defining illness). Even patients with a CD4 count of greater than 200 cells/μL and no AIDS-defining illness had a high prevalence of anemia: 28 percent of men and 31 percent of women had anemia defined as hemoglobin less than 14 g/dL for men or less than 12 g/dL for women. At the 1-year followup, the incidence of anemia was 3.2 percent for HIV+ people without immunologic or clinical AIDS, 12.1 percent for those with immunologic AIDS, and 36.9 percent for those with clinical AIDS. Notably, anemia was associated with a 1.5- to 2.5-fold increased risk of death during followup.[237] One prospective study showed a moderate correlation between the hemoglobin and CD4 count at entry into the cohort, and found that initiation of ART could increase the hemoglobin value.[238] Similarly, interruption of ART increased the risk of anemia.[239] An investigation of 2056 HIV+ women at six sites in the United States showed that use of ART for as little as 6 months was associated with improvement of anemia,[240] while several factors, including CD4 count less than 200 cells/μL, HIV viral load greater than 50,000 copies/mL, and mean corpuscular volume less than 80 fL were associated with decreased ability to correct the anemia. Anemia was identified as a key prognostic factor in large European and South African HIV+ cohorts.[241,242] The Veterans Aging Cohort Study evaluated HIV+ patients who had been on ART for 1 year, to identify factors predictive of mortality.[243] This study identified age, CD4 count, HIV viral load, hemoglobin, glomerular filtration rate, presence or absence of hepatitis C, and a composite measure of liver function as predictive factors for mortality. Even a mild decrease in the hemoglobin contributed significantly to mortality in this index. The Veterans Aging Cohort Study Index was subsequently validated in an independent cohort.[244] Thus, even in the ART era, anemia is associated with a worse prognosis, independent of the traditional risk markers such as the CD4 count and the HIV viral load.

Pathophysiology of Anemia in Human Immunodeficiency Virus

There are many pathophysiologic causes of anemia in HIV+ people (Table 81–9), and often anemia in an individual is multifactorial in origin. Unique to HIV are the effects of the virus on hematopoiesis, including direct infection of hematopoietic progenitor cells (impairing their survival, proliferation, differentiation, and maturation), infection of marrow stromal cells (affecting their ability to support hematopoiesis in the marrow microenvironment[245]), and alterations in hematopoietic growth factor production or function. Additionally, HIV infection is associated with a chronic inflammatory state[38] that may also contribute to ineffective erythropoiesis. Markers of inflammation, including IL-6, are higher in HIV+ individuals than in their HIV– counterparts, and this holds true even for those on ART with an undetectable viral load.[69] Inflammation, in part mediated by IL-6, upregulates hepcidin, a key regulator of iron trafficking, and serum hepcidin levels are inversely correlated with CD4 counts.[246,247]

Attempts to infect normal hematopoietic progenitor cells *in vitro* with HIV and studies of hematopoietic progenitor cells obtained from HIV+ patients initially suggested that HIV infection of hematopoietic

TABLE 81–9. Causes of Anemia in Human Immunodeficiency Virus

DECREASED PRODUCTION
HIV effect on hematopoiesis
Marrow infiltration (e.g., *Mycobacterium avium* complex, histoplasmosis, non-Hodgkin lymphoma, Hodgkin lymphoma)
Pure red cell aplasia (Parvovirus B19)
Drug suppression of hematopoiesis (e.g., Zidovudine)
Nutritional deficiency (e.g., vitamin B$_{12}$, folate, iron)
Inflammation
INCREASED DESTRUCTION
Thrombotic thrombocytopenic purpura
Immunohemolytic anemia
Glucose-6-phosphate dehydrogenase deficiency (e.g., dapsone, trimethoprim-sulfamethoxazole)
Hemophagocytic syndrome
LOSS
Gastrointestinal bleeding (e.g., Kaposi sarcoma in gastrointestinal tract)

progenitor cells was an infrequent event. However, subsequent studies of HIV subgroup C (the subtype that predominates in African populations) showed that a proportion of burst-forming unit–erythroid (BFU-E), granulocyte-macrophage colony-forming units (CFU-GM), and granulocyte-erythrocyte-monocyte and megakaryocyte colony-forming units (CFU-GEMM) can be infected with HIV *in vitro*.[248] The proportion of hematopoietic progenitor cells that could be infected with HIV subtype B (the predominant subtype in the United States and in Europe) was smaller (in the 1 percent range). Proviral HIV was detected by PCR in a small fraction of isolated CD34+ cells from some but not all HIV+ patients on ART with an undetectable viral load,[249] suggesting that HIV can latently infect hematopoietic progenitor cells *in vivo*; similar results were obtained using CD133+ sorted marrow cells.[250] Recent studies using a specific strain of humanized mice showed that some human CD34+, CD38+ intermediate progenitor cells could be infected with HIV *in vivo*, and that these progenitor cells when cultured *in vitro* had impaired growth, particularly in the erythroid and megakaryocytic lineages.[251]

The normal response of the kidneys to a decline in hemoglobin is to produce more erythropoietin. However in HIV+ people, the incremental increase in erythropoietin is blunted.[252,253] Additionally, antierythropoietin antibodies can be detected in a portion of HIV+ patients and are associated with increased risk of anemia.[254] The antierythropoietin antibodies recognize a peptide that is needed for erythropoietin binding to the erythropoietin receptor. This peptide has sequence homology to an HIV protein, suggesting molecular mimicry as a potential mechanism for development of the antierythropoietin antibodies.[255]

A cross-sectional study of 200 HIV+ patients in San Francisco during the ART era suggested an association between low testosterone levels and anemia in men living with HIV.[256] Hypogonadism is associated with weight loss, osteoporosis, and AIDS wasting syndrome, but whether testosterone treatment can correct anemia in these patients awaits further study.

Another, occasionally dramatic, cause of anemia in those living with HIV is pure red cell aplasia caused by parvovirus B19. Parvovirus

B19 is a small DNA virus that infects and lyses late human erythroid precursor cells,[257] causing transient reticulocytopenia in immunocompetent patients. The clinical spectrum of parvovirus B19–related disease includes "slapped cheek rash" in children and arthralgias in adults, but most immunocompetent patients are asymptomatic. Patients with hemolytic anemia who depend on high production of reticulocytes may develop transient aplastic crisis following infection with parvovirus B19. Immunoincompetent individuals may not be able to mount an adequate antibody response to clear parvovirus B19 from the blood and marrow, resulting in sustained infection with reticulocytopenia and anemia. In a series of HIV+ patients with parvovirus B19–related anemia, the median CD4 count was 42 cells/μL, indicating that parvovirus B19–associated pure red cell aplasia is associated with advanced immunodeficiency.[258] Characteristically, these patients have a normocytic anemia with virtual absence of reticulocytes, but normal white blood cells and platelets. Parvovirus immunoglobulin (Ig) G and IgM levels are generally not helpful in making the diagnosis, but PCR to detect parvovirus in the blood can be a reliable diagnostic test.[259] Marrow evaluation may show characteristic giant proerythroblasts and markedly diminished late erythroid precursor cells, with full maturation of the myeloid and megakaryocytic lineages. Some patients respond to initiation of ART in addition to transfusion support, but the majority of patients require additional therapy. A high prevalence of antibodies to B19 parvovirus exists in the general population; therefore, pooled human IgG preparations are a rich source of antiparvovirus antibody. Infusion of human IgG results in clearance of parvovirus B19 from the blood and improved reticulocyte production and resolution of anemia in HIV+ patients with parvovirus B19–induced pure red cell aplasia.[259,260] However, patients with a CD4 count of less than 80 cells/μL are prone to relapse within 6 months and may require retreatment.

Medications and Anemia

An important cause of anemia in people living with HIV is medications; both ART and medications used for prophylaxis against infections are implicated. Zidovudine can cause macrocytic anemia and leukopenia, and is not commonly used at present because of its toxicity. Stavudine is associated with anemia, although at lower rates than zidovudine.[261] Dapsone or trimethoprim-sulfamethoxazole, used for *P. jiroveci* prophylaxis, can cause hemolytic anemia in patients with glucose-6-phosphate dehydrogenase (G6PD) deficiency. Ganciclovir or valganciclovir, used to treat herpes simplex virus (HSV), Varicella-zoster, CMV, and sometimes HHV8, often cause pancytopenia. Trimethoprim-sulfamethoxazole can also cause myelosuppression and pancytopenia.

Treatment of Anemia

Initiation of ART is the optimal treatment for HIV-associated anemia. If a specific cause of anemia is identified, such as parvovirus B19, specific treatment can be provided. Early clinical trials demonstrated that erythropoietin treatment in anemic HIV+ patients taking zidovudine can improve the hemoglobin and decrease red blood cell transfusion requirements,[262] although responses were confined to patients with an endogenous erythropoietin level of 500 mU/mL or less.[262,263] Since zidovudine is no longer commonly used as a component of ART, the use of erythropoietin has declined. Nevertheless, treatment of anemia caused by zidovudine in patients with HIV and an erythropoietin level of 500 mU/mL or less is an FDA-approved indication for erythropoietin. However, a Cochrane analysis[264] that included six studies and more than 500 anemic HIV+ patients treated with erythropoietin or placebo concluded that erythropoietin did not reduce the risk of death and did not have a clear effect on quality of life. Additionally, erythropoietin has side effects including the potential to exacerbate hypertension, increased risk of thrombosis, a very rare risk of pure red cell aplasia, and increased risk of tumor progression or recurrence in specific types of cancer, as well as high cost.

HUMAN IMMUNODEFICIENCY VIRUS–ASSOCIATED THROMBOTIC MICROANGIOPATHY

Early in the HIV epidemic, it was reported that HIV+ people are at increased risk of thrombotic microangiopathy, either thrombotic thrombocytopenic purpura (TTP) or hemolytic-uremic syndrome (HUS). In a retrospective survey of 1223 patients with clinical AIDS in the pre-ART era, 1.4 percent met criteria for thrombotic microangiopathy. However, a prospective cohort of 347 patients followed from 1997 to 2000 identified no patients with thrombotic microangiopathy, suggesting that the incidence may have declined as a result of effective ART.[265] In support of this, a study done in the ART era followed 6022 HIV+ patients and found that 0.3 percent of patients developed thrombotic microangiopathy.[266] The group with thrombotic microangiopathy had a lower mean CD4 count, a higher plasma viral load, and a higher incidence of clinical AIDS than did HIV+ patients without microangiopathy. Registries of patients with TTP have been used to investigate what fraction of the patients are HIV+; of 362 patients in the Oklahoma TTP/HUS registry from 1989 to 2007, 1.84 percent were HIV+ while the prevalence of HIV in the local community was 0.3 percent.[267] In this study, several of the HIV+ patients were thought to have alternative causes of their microangiopathic hemolytic anemia, reinforcing the importance of a thorough consideration of the full spectrum of illnesses causing thrombotic microangiopathy, which may, in turn, affect the decision to use plasmapheresis/plasma exchange.[267] One series of 24 HIV+ patients with TTP reported that these patients presented with a mean hemoglobin of 6.8 g/dL, a mean platelet count of 20,000/μL, a mean LDH of 4.5-fold normal, and a mean CD4 count of 236 cells/μL, and the majority had an HIV viral load of greater than 10,000 copies/mL. Patients were treated with prompt plasma exchange (mean of 13 treatments) and initiation of ART and achieved excellent outcomes comparable to HIV– patients with TTP, with death occurring in a single patient. However six of the 24 patients suffered relapse of TTP, often in the setting of increased viral load, and required retreatment.[268] A study of patients enrolled in the French thrombotic microangiopathy (TMA) network revealed that 29 of 236 patients were HIV+. Of the HIV+ patients who had a disintegrin and metalloproteinase with a thrombospondin type 1 motif, member 13 (ADAMTS 13) activity of less than 5 percent, outcome was very similar to HIV– patients with a low ADAMTS 13 activity. However the HIV+ patients with an ADAMTS 13 activity of greater than 5 percent tended to have far advanced HIV with a median CD4 count of 30 cells/μL, more infectious complications present at the diagnoses of thrombotic microangiopathy, multiple AIDS-associated complications, and a high mortality.[269] Thus the outcome of TTP in HIV+ patients can be excellent in patients without advanced HIV when treated promptly with plasmapheresis/plasma exchange and ART.

HUMAN IMMUNODEFICIENCY VIRUS–ASSOCIATED THROMBOCYTOPENIA

In the pre-ART era, approximately 10 to 30 percent of people living with HIV had thrombocytopenia, defined as a platelet count of less than 150,000/μL, and thrombocytopenia was the initial manifestation of HIV in approximately 10 percent of patients. Those whose risk factor for HIV was intravenous drug abuse had a higher incidence of thrombocytopenia, attributed to increased coinfection with hepatitis C and hepatic cirrhosis. A British study evaluated selective testing for HIV in patients who presented with specific medical conditions, including thrombocytopenia. They found an increased rate of HIV infection in patients presenting with thrombocytopenia,[270] providing a rationale for including HIV testing in the evaluation of patients presenting with isolated thrombocytopenia. In the ART era, 26 percent of 5290 patients followed at the British Columbia Center for Excellence in HIV/AIDS had at least one platelet count less than 100,000/μL, and 3 percent had at least one platelet count less than 20,000/μL.[271] A study of the frequency and severity of thrombocytopenia in a large cohort of patients in the Collaboration in HIV Outcomes Research/U.S. study (CHORUS) included 6300 HIV+ people from 1997 to 2006[272] and found a prevalence of thrombocytopenia (platelet count <150,000/μL) of 14 percent. However, this cohort excluded patients who had hepatitis C or hepatitis B infection, so the prevalence of thrombocytopenia would likely be higher if these patients had been included.[272] In this study, 3.1 percent of patients had a platelet count of 50,000/μL or less, and 1.7 percent of patients had a platelet count of 30,000/μL or less. The majority of patients with severe thrombocytopenia who had not started ART had a CD4 count greater than 200 cells/μL, demonstrating that thrombocytopenia can occur prior to severe immunodepletion. These data are consistent with the findings of the British Columbia Center for Excellence in AIDS/HIV study, in which the CD4 count at diagnosis of ITP was 200 or greater in 72 percent of patients.[271]

Mild thrombocytopenia also occurs during primary HIV infection, a time of unfettered HIV replication and intense immune activation. In one study of 957 patients evaluated during primary HIV infection, 9.7 percent had a platelet count of less than 150,000/μL, 2.3 percent had a platelet count of less than 100,000/μL, and none had a platelet count of less than 50,000/μL.[273] Of those who started ART, the time to platelet recovery was approximately 1 month. Of those who did not start ART, the time to platelet recovery was just under 2 months. Those who developed thrombocytopenia during acute HIV infection had a threefold higher incidence of developing a low platelet count in the next 3 years (13.3 percent) in comparison to those who maintained a normal platelet count throughout. Thus, most patients who develop thrombocytopenia during primary HIV infection recover quickly, even if ART is not started immediately. A study to evaluate the risk factors for HIV-associated thrombocytopenia included 73 HIV+ people with a platelet count of less than 100,000/μL for 3 months matched to 73 nonthrombocytopenic controls. Identified risk factors were an HIV viral load of greater than 400 copies/mL, hepatitis C coinfection, and cirrhosis.[274] The platelet count correlated inversely with the viral load in a study of 207 patients naïve to ART.[275]

Platelet kinetic studies demonstrate shortened platelet survival in HIV+ patients not on ART (92 hours) compared to HIV– healthy volunteers (198 hours).[276] Even HIV+ patients with normal platelet counts had modestly diminished platelet survival in these studies as well as decreased platelet production in comparison to HIV– normal volunteers. As discussed above, some human hematopoietic progenitor cells can be infected with HIV *in vivo*, and these cells demonstrate impaired megakaryopoiesis *in vitro*.[251] Additionally megakaryocytes can be infected with HIV[277] and these observations may contribute to the decreased production of platelets in the marrow of HIV+ individuals. The more frequent and severe thrombocytopenia seen in patients with HIV and hepatitis C coinfection can be explained by the increased risk of cirrhosis in people coinfected with HIV and hepatitis C. The combined effects of diminished production of thrombopoietin, the major thrombopoietic growth factor, together with portal hypertension, splenomegaly, and sequestration of platelets in the enlarged spleen can result in severe thrombocytopenia. Patients with severe liver failure

TABLE 81–10. Pancytopenia in Human Immunodeficiency Virus

- Advanced HIV with high viral load
- Medication side effect
- Malignancy in the marrow
  - Non-Hodgkin lymphoma, Hodgkin lymphoma
- Infection in the marrow
  - *Mycobacterium avium* complex, histoplasmosis, cytomegalovirus, *Mycobacterium tuberculosis*
- Castleman disease
- Hemophagocytic syndrome
- Alcohol abuse
- Vitamin B$_{12}$ or folate deficiency

may also have a component of low-grade disseminated intravascular coagulation.

Evaluation of thrombocytopenia in HIV+ patients is similar to HIV– patients and should include a thorough history and physical exam looking for symptoms and signs of platelet-type bleeding, to assess the clinical severity of the thrombocytopenia. The blood film should be reviewed to confirm that the patient does have low platelets, rather than platelet clumping, and to evaluate for abnormalities in red blood cell and white blood cell numbers and morphology. If not already done, the patient should be tested for hepatitis C. The HIV viral load and CD4 count should be determined, as noncompliance or development of resistance to the current ART regimen can exacerbate HIV-associated thrombocytopenia. The patient should be asked what percent of the patient's HIV medications are taken, or alternatively how many missed doses the patient has had in the past month. The medication list, including nonprescription medications, naturopathic medications, and dietary supplements, should be thoroughly reviewed. The differential diagnosis for isolated thrombocytopenia includes HIV-associated ITP, hepatitis C-associated ITP, *Helicobacter pylori*–associated ITP, medication side effect, or antiphospholipid antibody syndrome. If the patient also has anemia, immunohemolytic anemia with ITP (Evans syndrome) or TTP should be considered. In a febrile and ill patient who has additional cytopenias, Castleman disease and hemophagocytic syndrome should be included in the differential diagnosis (Table 81–10).

Treatment of Human Immunodeficiency Virus–Associated Idiopathic Thrombocytopenic Purpura

ART improves the platelet count in patients with HIV-associated ITP over a period of approximately 3 months in the majority of patients.[278–280] The primary treatment of HIV-associated ITP is initiation of ART if the patient is not on ART, and assessment of the effectiveness of ART if the patient is taking ART. Reasons for failure of ART include suboptimal compliance with the medications, as the ability of ART to control the HIV viral load is related to adherence.[281] Alternatively, the patient's HIV may have developed ART resistance which can be detected by resistance testing. Close communication between the hematologist and the infectious disease/HIV physician is essential for optimal management of these issues.

Because ART typically takes 3 months to improve the platelet count, additional interventions are needed if the patient is experiencing severe thrombocytopenia (platelets <20,000/μL) or has platelet-type bleeding. If the patient is Rh+ and has an intact spleen, intravenous anti-D can be very effective.[282] In a study that included both HIV+ and

HIV– patients, treatment with intravenous anti-D increased the platelet count by an average of 45,000/μL in adults in both groups. In the majority of patients, the platelet increment lasted more than 21 days. The major side effect of anti-D treatment was a drop in the hemoglobin (average decrease in hemoglobin of 1 g/dL). Another approach is to use intravenous immunoglobulin although one study of immunoglobulin treatment reported a smaller increase in the platelet count (average of 29,000/μL), and a shorter duration of response (19 days) than was obtained with intravenous anti-D.[283] Furthermore, intravenous anti-D may be less expensive than intravenous immunoglobulin. However, anti-D has the potential to cause significant hemolysis and has a "Black Box" warning because of this rare complication. Alternative approaches include the use of standard doses of prednisone or pulse dexamethasone, as in HIV– patients. Steroids are less attractive in HIV+ patients because of the potential to decrease CD4 counts, increase the risk of infection, and increase risk of Kaposi sarcoma progression. Splenectomy can be effective in HIV+ patients,[284] but is rarely required. Case reports document the use of romiplostim or eltrombopag in HIV+ patients.[285,286]

HIV+ patients with ITP should be counseled not to take aspirin or nonsteroidal antiinflammatory drugs or fish oil while severely thrombocytopenic, and educated on the symptoms of relapse of ITP (spontaneous nose bleeds, spontaneous large bruises, bleeding gums), and encouraged to report promptly for medical care should any of these occur. Most patients with HIV-associated ITP can be started on ART and treated with 1 or 2 doses of anti-D at 3-week intervals and will subsequently experience sustained platelet count response with effective control of HIV.

HUMAN IMMUNODEFICIENCY VIRUS–ASSOCIATED NEUTROPENIA

The prevalence of neutropenia (defined as a neutrophil count <1300/μL) in patients naïve to ART in Africa, Asia, the Americas, and the Caribbean was 14.3 percent,[287] with the U.S. cohort having a slightly higher prevalence of approximately 16 percent. A multicenter prospective study of HIV+ women in the United States followed 1729 women[288] and found that 7 percent had a pre-ART absolute neutrophil count of less than 1000/μL, and during 7.5 years of follow up 31 percent had an absolute neutrophil count of less than 1000/μL. Low CD4 count and high viral load were significant risk factors for development of neutropenia whereas initiation of ART correlated with resolution of neutropenia. Patients living with HIV may have neutropenia for a variety of reasons and neutropenia may be a component of pancytopenia (see Table 81–10) or occur as an isolated finding. As discussed in the section "Pathophysiology of Anemia in HIV" above, HIV has a multitude of effects on hematopoiesis, and the effects on progenitor cell survival, growth and differentiation and on the marrow microenvironment pertain to myelopoiesis as well as erythropoiesis and megakaryopoiesis. A study of 87 consecutive patients attending an HIV clinic who developed an absolute neutrophil count of less than 1000/μL showed that the vast majority were receiving at least one known myelosuppressive medication, and 59 of the 87 patients were receiving three or more myelosuppressive drugs. Many other medications are rare causes of neutropenia,[289] illustrating the importance of drug-induced neutropenia in this population of patients.

Other causes of neutropenia reported in HIV+ patients include deficiency of vitamins such as folate or vitamin B$_{12}$, hepatitis C-associated autoimmune neutropenia, alcohol toxicity, and levamisole-adulterated cocaine, which can cause severe neutropenia (neutrophil counts as low as 0). Patients should be specifically asked about cocaine use if they are found to have severe neutropenia with normal hemoglobin and platelet count.[290]

REFERENCES

1. Sharp PM, Hahn BH: Origins of HIV and the AIDS pandemic. *Cold Spring Harb Perspect Med* 1:a006841, 2011.
2. Worobey M, Gemmel M, Teuwen DE, et al: Direct evidence of extensive diversity of HIV-1 in Kinshasa by 1960. *Nature* 455:661–664, 2008.
3. Gallo RC, Sarin PS, Gelmann EP, et al: Isolation of human T-cell leukemia virus in acquired immune deficiency syndrome (AIDS). *Science* 220:865–867, 1983.
4. Barre-Sinoussi F, Chermann JC, Rey F, et al: Isolation of a T-lymphotropic retrovirus from a patient at risk for acquired immune deficiency syndrome (AIDS). *Science* 220:868–871, 1983.
5. de Silva TI, Cotten M, Rowland-Jones SL: HIV-2: The forgotten AIDS virus. *Trends Microbiol* 16:588–595, 2008.
6. de Silva TI, van Tienen C, Onyango C, et al: Population dynamics of HIV-2 in rural West Africa: Comparison with HIV-1 and ongoing transmission at the heart of the epidemic. *AIDS* 27:125–134, 2013.
7. Centers for Disease Control (CDC): Follow-up on Kaposi's sarcoma and *Pneumocystis* pneumonia. *MMWR Morb Mortal Wkly Rep* 30:409–410, 1981.
8. Centers for Disease Control (CDC): Kaposi's sarcoma and *Pneumocystis* pneumonia among homosexual men—New York City and California. *MMWR Morb Mortal Wkly Rep* 30:305–308, 1981.
9. Centers for Disease Control (CDC): *Pneumocystis* pneumonia—Los Angeles. *MMWR Morb Mortal Wkly Rep* 30:250–252, 1981.
10. Jaffe HW, Bregman DJ, Selik RM: Acquired immune deficiency syndrome in the United States: The first 1,000 cases. *J Infect Dis* 148:339–345, 1983.
11. Centers for Disease Control (CDC): *Pneumocystis carinii* pneumonia among persons with hemophilia A. *MMWR Morb Mortal Wkly Rep* 31:365–367, 1982.
12. Centers for Disease Control (CDC): Possible transfusion-associated acquired immune deficiency syndrome (AIDS)—California. *MMWR Morb Mortal Wkly Rep* 31:652–654, 1982.
13. Leads from the MMWR. Prevention of acquired immune deficiency syndrome (AIDS): Report of inter-agency recommendations. *JAMA* 249:1544–1545, 1983.
14. Centers for Disease Control (CDC): Immunodeficiency among female sexual partners of males with acquired immune deficiency syndrome (AIDS)—New York. *MMWR Morb Mortal Wkly Rep* 31:697–698, 1983.
15. Centers for Disease Control (CDC): Update: Acquired immunodeficiency syndrome (AIDS) among patients with hemophilia—United States. *MMWR Morb Mortal Wkly Rep* 32:613–615, 1983.
16. Pape JW, Liautaud B, Thomas F, et al: The acquired immunodeficiency syndrome in Haiti. *Ann Intern Med* 103:674–678, 1985.
17. Pape JW, Liautaud B, Thomas F, et al: Characteristics of the acquired immunodeficiency syndrome (AIDS) in Haiti. *N Engl J Med* 309:945–950, 1983.
18. De Cock KM, Jaffe HW, Curran JW: The evolving epidemiology of HIV/AIDS. *AIDS* 26:1205–1213, 2012.
19. Quinn TC, Wawer MJ, Sewankambo N, et al: Viral load and heterosexual transmission of human immunodeficiency virus type 1. Rakai Project Study Group. *N Engl J Med* 342:921–929, 2000.
20. Patel P, Borkowf CB, Brooks JT, et al: Estimating per-act HIV transmission risk: A systematic review. *AIDS* 28:1509–1519, 2014.
21. Bar M, Wyman SK, Fritz BR, et al: MicroRNA discovery and profiling in human embryonic stem cells by deep sequencing of small RNA libraries. *Stem Cells* 26:2496–2505, 2008.
22. Cohen MS, Chen YQ, McCauley M, et al: Prevention of HIV-1 infection with early antiretroviral therapy. *N Engl J Med* 365:493–505, 2011.
23. Hladik F, McElrath MJ: Setting the stage: Host invasion by HIV. *Nat Rev Immunol* 8:447–457, 2008.
24. Hu Q, Frank I, Williams V, et al: Blockade of attachment and fusion receptors inhibits HIV-1 infection of human cervical tissue. *J Exp Med* 199:1065–1075, 2004.
25. Borrow P: Innate immunity in acute HIV-1 infection. *Curr Opin HIV AIDS* 6:353–363, 2011.
26. Cohen MS, Shaw GM, McMichael AJ, et al: Acute HIV-1 Infection. *N Engl J Med* 364:1943–1954, 2011.
27. Wei X, Decker JM, Wang S, et al: Antibody neutralization and escape by HIV-1. *Nature* 422:307–312, 2003.
28. Borrow P, Lewicki H, Hahn BH, et al: Virus-specific CD8+ cytotoxic T-lymphocyte activity associated with control of viremia in primary human immunodeficiency virus type 1 infection. *J Virol* 68:6103–6110, 1994.
29. Borrow P, Lewicki H, Wei X, et al: Antiviral pressure exerted by HIV-1-specific cytotoxic T lymphocytes (CTLs) during primary infection demonstrated by rapid selection of CTL escape virus. *Nat Med* 3:205–211, 1997.
30. Cao J, McNevin J, Malhotra U, et al: Evolution of CD8+ T cell immunity and viral escape following acute HIV-1 infection. *J Immunol* 171:3837–3846, 2003.
31. Schmitz JE, Kuroda MJ, Santra S, et al: Control of viremia in simian immunodeficiency virus infection by CD8+ lymphocytes. *Science* 283:857–860, 1999.
32. Ganusov VV, Goonetilleke N, Liu MK, et al: Fitness costs and diversity of the cytotoxic T lymphocyte (CTL) response determine the rate of CTL escape during acute and chronic phases of HIV infection. *J Virol* 85:10518–10528, 2011.
33. Goonetilleke N, Liu MK, Salazar-Gonzalez JF, et al: The first T cell response to transmitted/founder virus contributes to the control of acute viremia in HIV-1 infection. *J Exp Med* 206:1253–1272, 2009.

34. Allen BJ, Raja C, Rizvi S, et al: Intralesional targeted alpha therapy for metastatic melanoma. *Cancer Biol Ther* 4:1318–1324, 2005.

35. Allen TM, Altfeld M, Yu XG, et al: Selection, transmission, and reversion of an antigen-processing cytotoxic T-lymphocyte escape mutation in human immunodeficiency virus type 1 infection. *J Virol* 78:7069–7078, 2004.

36. Allen TM, Altfeld M, Geer SC, et al: Selective escape from CD8+ T-cell responses represents a major driving force of human immunodeficiency virus type 1 (HIV-1) sequence diversity and reveals constraints on HIV-1 evolution. *J Virol* 79:13239–13249, 2005.

37. Deeks SG, Kitchen CM, Liu L, et al: Immune activation set point during early HIV infection predicts subsequent CD4+ T-cell changes independent of viral load. *Blood* 104:942–947, 2004.

38. Deeks SG, Tracy R, Douek DC: Systemic effects of inflammation on health during chronic HIV infection. *Immunity* 39:633–645, 2013.

39. Douek DC, Roederer M, Koup RA: Emerging concepts in the immunopathogenesis of AIDS. *Annu Rev Med* 60:471–484, 2009.

40. Giorgi JV, Hultin LE, McKeating JA, et al: Shorter survival in advanced human immunodeficiency virus type 1 infection is more closely associated with T lymphocyte activation than with plasma virus burden or virus chemokine coreceptor usage. *J Infect Dis* 179:859–870, 1999.

41. Liu Z, Cumberland WG, Hultin LE, et al: Elevated CD38 antigen expression on CD8+ T cells is a stronger marker for the risk of chronic HIV disease progression to AIDS and death in the Multicenter AIDS Cohort Study than CD4+ cell count, soluble immune activation markers, or combinations of HLA-DR and CD38 expression. *J Acquir Immune Defic Syndr Hum Retrovirol* 16:83–92, 1997.

42. Brenchley JM, Price DA, Schacker TW, et al: Microbial translocation is a cause of systemic immune activation in chronic HIV infection. *Nat Med* 12:1365–1371, 2006.

43. Zeng M, Smith AJ, Wietgrefe SW, et al: Cumulative mechanisms of lymphoid tissue fibrosis and T cell depletion in HIV-1 and SIV infections. *J Clin Invest* 121:998–1008, 2011.

44. Zeng M, Southern PJ, Reilly CS, et al: Lymphoid tissue damage in HIV-1 infection depletes naive T cells and limits T cell reconstitution after antiretroviral therapy. *PLoS Pathog* 8:e1002437, 2012.

45. Freiberg MS, Chang CC, Kuller LH, et al: HIV infection and the risk of acute myocardial infarction. *JAMA Intern Med* 173:614–622, 2013.

46. Weber R, Sabin CA, Friis-Moller N, et al: Liver-related deaths in persons infected with the human immunodeficiency virus: The D:A:D study. *Arch Intern Med* 166:1632–1641, 2006.

47. Balagopal A, Ray SC, De Oca RM, et al: Kupffer cells are depleted with HIV immunodeficiency and partially recovered with antiretroviral immune reconstitution. *AIDS* 23:2397–2404, 2009.

48. Peters L, Neuhaus J, Mocroft A, et al: Hyaluronic acid levels predict increased risk of non-AIDS death in hepatitis-coinfected persons interrupting antiretroviral therapy in the SMART Study. *Antivir Ther* 16:667–675, 2011.

49. Duprez DA, Neuhaus J, Kuller LH, et al: Inflammation, coagulation and cardiovascular disease in HIV-infected individuals. *PLoS One* 7:e44454, 2012.

50. Shen YM, Frenkel EP: Thrombosis and a hypercoagulable state in HIV-infected patients. *Clin Appl Thromb Hemost* 10:277–280, 2004.

51. Lijfering WM, Sprenger HG, Georg RR, et al: Relationship between progression to AIDS and thrombophilic abnormalities in HIV infection. *Clin Chem* 54:1226–1233, 2008.

52. Fischl MA, Richman DD, Grieco MH, et al: The efficacy of azidothymidine (AZT) in the treatment of patients with AIDS and AIDS-related complex. A double-blind, placebo-controlled trial. *N Engl J Med* 317:185–191, 1987.

53. Fischl MA, Richman DD, Hansen N, et al: The safety and efficacy of zidovudine (AZT) in the treatment of subjects with mildly symptomatic human immunodeficiency virus type 1 (HIV) infection. A double-blind, placebo-controlled trial. The AIDS Clinical Trials Group. *Ann Intern Med* 112:727–737, 1990.

54. Lundgren JD, Phillips AN, Pedersen C, et al: Comparison of long-term prognosis of patients with AIDS treated and not treated with zidovudine. AIDS in Europe Study Group. *JAMA* 271:1088–1092, 1994.

55. Richman DD, Fischl MA, Grieco MH, et al: The toxicity of azidothymidine (AZT) in the treatment of patients with AIDS and AIDS-related complex. A double-blind, placebo-controlled trial. *N Engl J Med* 317:192–197, 1987.

56. Volberding PA, Lagakos SW, Grimes JM, et al: A comparison of immediate with deferred zidovudine therapy for asymptomatic HIV-infected adults with CD4 cell counts of 500 or more per cubic millimeter. AIDS Clinical Trials Group. *N Engl J Med* 333:401–407, 1995.

57. Volberding PA, Lagakos SW, Koch MA, et al: Zidovudine in asymptomatic human immunodeficiency virus infection. A controlled trial in persons with fewer than 500 CD4-positive cells per cubic millimeter. The AIDS Clinical Trials Group of the National Institute of Allergy and Infectious Diseases. *N Engl J Med* 322:941–949, 1990.

58. Montaner JS, Reiss P, Cooper D, et al: A randomized, double-blind trial comparing combinations of nevirapine, didanosine, and zidovudine for HIV-infected patients: The INCAS Trial. Italy, The Netherlands, Canada and Australia Study. *JAMA* 279:930–937, 1998.

59. Cameron DW, Japour AJ, Xu Y, et al: Ritonavir and saquinavir combination therapy for the treatment of HIV infection. *AIDS* 13:213–224, 1999.

60. Gulick RM, Mellors JW, Havlir D, et al: 3-year suppression of HIV viremia with indinavir, zidovudine, and lamivudine. *Ann Intern Med* 133:35–39, 2000.

61. Hammer SM, Squires KE, Hughes MD, et al: A controlled trial of two nucleoside analogues plus indinavir in persons with human immunodeficiency virus infection and CD4 cell counts of 200 per cubic millimeter or less. AIDS Clinical Trials Group 320 Study Team. *N Engl J Med* 337:725–733, 1997.

62. Walmsley S, Bernstein B, King M, et al: Lopinavir-ritonavir versus nelfinavir for the initial treatment of HIV infection. *N Engl J Med* 346:2039–2046, 2002.

63. Palella FJ Jr, Delaney KM, Moorman AC, et al: Declining morbidity and mortality among patients with advanced human immunodeficiency virus infection. HIV Outpatient Study Investigators. *N Engl J Med* 338:853–860, 1998.

64. Kalayjian RC, Franceschini N, Gupta SK, et al: Suppression of HIV-1 replication by antiretroviral therapy improves renal function in persons with low CD4 cell counts and chronic kidney disease. *AIDS* 22:481–487, 2008.

65. Brau N, Salvatore M, Rios-Bedoya CF, et al: Slower fibrosis progression in HIV/HCV-coinfected patients with successful HIV suppression using antiretroviral therapy. *J Hepatol* 44:47–55, 2006.

66. Loko MA, Bani-Sadr F, Valantin MA, et al: Antiretroviral therapy and sustained virological response to HCV therapy are associated with slower liver fibrosis progression in HIV-HCV-coinfected patients: Study from the ANRS CO 13 HEPAVIH cohort. *Antivir Ther* 17:1335–1343, 2012.

67. Thorpe J, Saeed S, Moodie EE, et al: Antiretroviral treatment interruption leads to progression of liver fibrosis in HIV-hepatitis C virus co-infection. *AIDS* 25:967–975, 2011.

68. Limketkai BN, Mehta SH, Sutcliffe CG, et al: Relationship of liver disease stage and antiviral therapy with liver-related events and death in adults coinfected with HIV/HCV. *JAMA* 308:370–378, 2012.

69. Neuhaus J, Jacobs DR, Jr., Baker JV, et al: Markers of inflammation, coagulation, and renal function are elevated in adults with HIV infection. *J Infect Dis* 201:1788–1795, 2010.

70. El-Sadr WM, Lundgren J, Neaton JD, et al: CD4+ count-guided interruption of antiretroviral treatment. *N Engl J Med* 355:2283–2296, 2006.

71. Bhaskaran K, Mussini C, Antinori A, et al: Changes in the incidence and predictors of human immunodeficiency virus-associated dementia in the era of highly active antiretroviral therapy. *Ann Neurol* 63:213–221, 2008.

72. d'Arminio Monforte A, Cinque P, Mocroft A, et al: Changing incidence of central nervous system diseases in the EuroSIDA cohort. *Ann Neurol* 55:320–328, 2004.

73. Townsend CL, Cortina-Borja M, Peckham CS, et al: Low rates of mother-to-child transmission of HIV following effective pregnancy interventions in the United Kingdom and Ireland, 2000–2006. *AIDS* 22:973–981, 2008.

74. Tubiana R, Le Chenadec J, Rouzioux C, et al: Factors associated with mother-to-child transmission of HIV-1 despite a maternal viral load <500 copies/ml at delivery: A case-control study nested in the French perinatal cohort (EPF-ANRS CO1). *Clin Infect Dis* 50:585–596, 2010.

75. Coombs RW, Reichelderfer PS, Landay AL: Recent observations on HIV type-1 infection in the genital tract of men and women. *AIDS* 17:455–480, 2003.

76. Keiser O, Fellay J, Opravil M, et al: Adverse events to antiretrovirals in the Swiss HIV Cohort Study: Effect on mortality and treatment modification. *Antivir Ther* 12:1157–1164, 2007.

77. O'Brien ME, Clark RA, Besch CL, et al: Patterns and correlates of discontinuation of the initial HAART regimen in an urban outpatient cohort. *J Acquir Immune Defic Syndr* 34:407–414, 2003.

78. Fidler S, Porter K, Ewings F, et al: Short-course antiretroviral therapy in primary HIV infection. *N Engl J Med* 368:207–217, 2013.

79. Grijsen ML, Steingrover R, Wit FW, et al: No treatment versus 24 or 60 weeks of antiretroviral treatment during primary HIV infection: The randomized Primo-SHM trial. *PLoS Med* 9:e1001196, 2012.

80. Hogan CM, Degruttola V, Sun X, et al: The setpoint study (ACTG A5217): Effect of immediate versus deferred antiretroviral therapy on virologic set point in recently HIV-1-infected individuals. *J Infect Dis* 205:87–96, 2012.

81. Timing of HAART initiation and clinical outcomes in human immunodeficiency virus type 1 seroconverters. *Arch Intern Med* 171:1560–1569, 2011.

82. Hocqueloux L, Prazuck T, Avettand-Fenoel V, et al: Long-term immunovirologic control following antiretroviral therapy interruption in patients treated at the time of primary HIV-1 infection. *AIDS* 24:1598–1601, 2010.

83. Le T, Wright EJ, Smith DM, et al: Enhanced CD4+ T-cell recovery with earlier HIV-1 antiretroviral therapy. *N Engl J Med* 368:218–230, 2013.

84. Strain MC, Little SJ, Daar ES, et al: Effect of treatment, during primary infection, on establishment and clearance of cellular reservoirs of HIV-1. *J Infect Dis* 191:1410–1418, 2005.

85. Ananworanich J, Schuetz A, Vandergeeten C, et al: Impact of multi-targeted antiretroviral treatment on gut T cell depletion and HIV reservoir seeding during acute HIV infection. *PLoS One* 7:e33948, 2012.

86. Archin NM, Vaidya NK, Kuruc JD, et al: Immediate antiviral therapy appears to restrict resting CD4+ cell HIV-1 infection without accelerating the decay of latent infection. *Proc Natl Acad Sci U S A* 109:9523–9528, 2012.

87. Chun TW, Justement JS, Moir S, et al: Decay of the HIV reservoir in patients receiving antiretroviral therapy for extended periods: Implications for eradication of virus. *J Infect Dis* 195:1762–1764, 2007.

88. Saez-Cirion A, Bacchus C, Hocqueloux L, et al: Post-treatment HIV-1 controllers with a long-term virological remission after the interruption of early initiated antiretroviral therapy ANRS VISCONTI Study. *PLoS Pathog* 9:e1003211, 2013.

89. French MA: HIV/AIDS: Immune reconstitution inflammatory syndrome: A reappraisal. *Clin Infect Dis* 48:101–107, 2009.

90. Grant PM, Komarow L, Andersen J, et al: Risk factor analyses for immune reconstitution inflammatory syndrome in a randomized study of early vs. deferred ART during an opportunistic infection. *PLoS One* 5:e11416, 2010.

91. Lawn SD, Myer L, Bekker LG, et al: Tuberculosis-associated immune reconstitution disease: Incidence, risk factors and impact in an antiretroviral treatment service in South Africa. *AIDS* 21:335–341, 2007.

92. Muller M, Wandel S, Colebunders R, et al: Immune reconstitution inflammatory syndrome in patients starting antiretroviral therapy for HIV infection: A systematic review and meta-analysis. *Lancet Infect Dis* 10:251–261, 2010.

93. Robertson J, Meier M, Wall J, et al: Immune reconstitution syndrome in HIV: Validating a case definition and identifying clinical predictors in persons initiating antiretroviral therapy. *Clin Infect Dis* 42:1639–1646, 2006.

94. Achenbach CJ, Harrington RD, Dhanireddy S, et al: Paradoxical immune reconstitution inflammatory syndrome in HIV-infected patients treated with combination antiretroviral therapy after AIDS-defining opportunistic infection. *Clin Infect Dis* 54:424–433, 2012.

95. Meintjes G, Wilkinson RJ, Morroni C, et al: Randomized placebo-controlled trial of prednisone for paradoxical tuberculosis-associated immune reconstitution inflammatory syndrome. *AIDS* 24:2381–2390, 2010.

96. Hall HI, Song R, Rhodes P, et al: Estimation of HIV incidence in the United States. *JAMA* 300:520–529, 2008.

97. Marks G, Crepaz N, Senterfitt JW, et al: Meta-analysis of high-risk sexual behavior in persons aware and unaware they are infected with HIV in the United States: Implications for HIV prevention programs. *J Acquir Immune Defic Syndr* 39:446–453, 2005.

98. Crepaz N, Lyles CM, Wolitski RJ, et al: Do prevention interventions reduce HIV risk behaviours among people living with HIV? A meta-analytic review of controlled trials. *AIDS* 20:143–157, 2006.

99. Lyles CM, Kay LS, Crepaz N, et al: Best-evidence interventions: Findings from a systematic review of HIV behavioral interventions for US populations at high risk, 2000–2004. *Am J Public Health* 97:133–143, 2007.

100. Gray RH, Kigozi G, Serwadda D, et al: Male circumcision for HIV prevention in men in Rakai, Uganda: A randomised trial. *Lancet* 369:657–666, 2007.

101. Connor EM, Sperling RS, Gelber R, et al: Reduction of maternal-infant transmission of human immunodeficiency virus type 1 with zidovudine treatment. Pediatric AIDS Clinical Trials Group Protocol 076 Study Group. *N Engl J Med* 331:1173–1180, 1994.

102. Guay LA, Musoke P, Fleming T, et al: Intrapartum and neonatal single-dose nevirapine compared with zidovudine for prevention of mother-to-child transmission of HIV-1 in Kampala, Uganda: HIVNET 012 randomised trial. *Lancet* 354:795–802, 1999.

103. Baeten JM, Donnell D, Ndase P, et al: Antiretroviral prophylaxis for HIV prevention in heterosexual men and women. *N Engl J Med* 367:399–410, 2012.

104. Abdool Karim Q, Abdool Karim SS, Frohlich JA, et al: Effectiveness and safety of tenofovir gel, an antiretroviral microbicide, for the prevention of HIV infection in women. *Science* 329:1168–1174, 2010.

105. Karim SS, Kashuba AD, Werner L, et al: Drug concentrations after topical and oral antiretroviral pre-exposure prophylaxis: Implications for HIV prevention in women. *Lancet* 378:279–281, 2011.

106. Chun TW, Carruth L, Finzi D, et al: Quantification of latent tissue reservoirs and total body viral load in HIV-1 infection. *Nature* 387:183–188, 1997.

107. Finzi D, Blankson J, Siliciano JD, et al: Latent infection of CD4+ T cells provides a mechanism for lifelong persistence of HIV-1, even in patients on effective combination therapy. *Nat Med* 5:512–517, 1999.

108. Siliciano JD, Kajdas J, Finzi D, et al: Long-term follow-up studies confirm the stability of the latent reservoir for HIV-1 in resting CD4+ T cells. *Nat Med* 9:727–728, 2003.

109. Hutter G, Nowak D, Mossner M, et al: Long-term control of HIV by CCR5 Delta32/Delta32 stem-cell transplantation. *N Engl J Med* 360:692–698, 2009.

109A. Shan L, Deng K, Shroff Neeta S, et al: Stimulation of HIV-1-Specific Cytolytic T Lymphocytes Facilitates Elimination of Latent Viral Reservoir after Virus Reactivation. *Immunity* 36(3):491-501, 2012.

110. Tebas P, Stein D, Binder-Scholl G, et al: Antiviral effects of autologous CD4 T cells genetically modified with a conditionally replicating lentiviral vector expressing long antisense to HIV. *Blood* 121:1524–1533, 2013.

111. Tebas P, Stein D, Tang WW, et al: Gene editing of CCR5 in autologous CD4 T cells of persons infected with HIV. *N Engl J Med* 370:901–910, 2014.

112. Work Group for HIV and Aging Consensus Project: Summary report from the Human Immunodeficiency Virus and Aging Consensus Project: Treatment strategies for clinicians managing older individuals with the human immunodeficiency virus. *J Am Geriatr Soc* 60:974, 2012.

113. Deeks SG, Lewin SR, Havlir DV: The end of AIDS: HIV infection as a chronic disease. *Lancet* 382:1525–1533, 2013.

114. Powles T, Robinson D, Stebbing J, et al: Highly active antiretroviral therapy and the incidence of non-AIDS-defining cancers in people with HIV infection. *J Clin Oncol* 27:884–890, 2009.

115. Causes of death in HIV-1-infected patients treated with antiretroviral therapy, 1996–2006: Collaborative analysis of 13 HIV cohort studies. *Clin Infect Dis* 50:1387–1396, 2010.

116. Campsmith ML, Rhodes PH, Hall HI, et al: Undiagnosed HIV prevalence among adults and adolescents in the United States at the end of 2006. *J Acquir Immune Defic Syndr* 53:619–624, 2010.

117. Chiao EY, Dezube BJ, Krown SE, et al: Time for oncologists to opt in for routine opt-out HIV testing? *JAMA* 304:334–339, 2010.

118. Shiels MS, Pfeiffer RM, Hall HI, et al: Proportions of Kaposi sarcoma, selected non-Hodgkin lymphomas, and cervical cancer in the United States occurring in persons with AIDS, 1980–2007. *JAMA* 305:1450–1459, 2011.

119. Liapis K, Clear A, Owen A, et al: The microenvironment of AIDS-related diffuse large B-cell lymphoma provides insight into the pathophysiology and indicates possible therapeutic strategies. *Blood* 122:424–433, 2013.

120. Gloghini A, Dolcetti R, Carbone A: Lymphomas occurring specifically in HIV-infected patients: From pathogenesis to pathology. *Semin Cancer Biol* 23:457–467, 2013.

121. Coutinho R, Pria AD, Gandhi S, et al: HIV status does not impair the outcome of patients diagnosed with diffuse large B-cell lymphoma treated with R-CHOP in the cART era. *AIDS* 28:689–697, 2013.

122. Tirelli U, Spina M, Gaidano G, et al: Epidemiological, biological and clinical features of HIV-related lymphomas in the era of highly active antiretroviral therapy. *AIDS* 14:1675–1688, 2000.

123. Hegde U, Filie A, Little RF, et al: High incidence of occult leptomeningeal disease detected by flow cytometry in newly diagnosed aggressive B-cell lymphomas at risk for central nervous system involvement: The role of flow cytometry versus cytology. *Blood* 105:496–502, 2005.

124. Kaplan LD, Straus DJ, Testa MA, et al: Low-dose compared with standard-dose m-BACOD chemotherapy for non-Hodgkin's lymphoma associated with human immunodeficiency virus infection. National Institute of Allergy and Infectious Diseases AIDS Clinical Trials Group. *N Engl J Med* 336:1641–1648, 1997.

125. Lim ST, Karim R, Tulpule A, et al: Prognostic factors in HIV-related diffuse large-cell lymphoma: Before versus after highly active antiretroviral therapy. *J Clin Oncol* 23:8477–8482, 2005.

126. Little RF, Pittaluga S, Grant N, et al: Highly effective treatment of acquired immunodeficiency syndrome-related lymphoma with dose-adjusted EPOCH: Impact of antiretroviral therapy suspension and tumor biology. *Blood* 101:4653–4659, 2003.

127. Sparano JA, Lee JY, Kaplan LD, et al: Rituximab plus concurrent infusional EPOCH chemotherapy is highly effective in HIV-associated B-cell non-Hodgkin lymphoma. *Blood* 115:3008–3016, 2010.

128. Dunleavy K, Little RF, Pittaluga S, et al: The role of tumor histogenesis, FDG-PET, and short-course EPOCH with dose-dense rituximab (SC-EPOCH-RR) in HIV-associated diffuse large B-cell lymphoma. *Blood* 115:3017–3024, 2010.

129. Kaplan LD, Lee JY, Ambinder RF, et al: Rituximab does not improve clinical outcome in a randomized phase 3 trial of CHOP with or without rituximab in patients with HIV-associated non-Hodgkin lymphoma: AIDS-Malignancies Consortium Trial 010. *Blood* 106:1538–1543, 2005.

130. Ribera JM, Oriol A, Morgades M, et al: Safety and efficacy of cyclophosphamide, Adriamycin, vincristine, prednisone and rituximab in patients with human immunodeficiency virus-associated diffuse large B-cell lymphoma: Results of a phase II trial. *Br J Haematol* 140:411–419, 2008.

131. Wyen C, Jensen B, Hentrich M, et al: Treatment of AIDS-related lymphomas: Rituximab is beneficial even in severely immunosuppressed patients. *AIDS* 26:457–464, 2012.

132. Levine AM, Noy A, Lee JY, et al: Pegylated liposomal doxorubicin, rituximab, cyclophosphamide, vincristine, and prednisone in AIDS-related lymphoma: AIDS Malignancy Consortium Study 047. *J Clin Oncol* 31:58–64, 2013.

133. Barta SK, Lee JY, Kaplan LD, et al: Pooled analysis of AIDS malignancy consortium trials evaluating rituximab plus CHOP or infusional EPOCH chemotherapy in HIV-associated non-Hodgkin lymphoma. *Cancer* 118:3977–3983, 2012.

134. Barta SK, Xue X, Wang D, et al: Treatment factors affecting outcomes in HIV-associated non-Hodgkin lymphomas: A pooled analysis of 1546 patients. *Blood* 122:3251–3262, 2013.

135. Zhong DT, Shi CM, Chen Q, et al: Study on effectiveness of gemcitabine, dexamethasone, and cisplatin (GDP) for relapsed or refractory AIDS-related non-Hodgkin's lymphoma. *Ann Hematol* 91:1757–1763, 2012.

136. Bi J, Espina BM, Tulpule A, et al: High-dose cytosine-arabinoside and cisplatin regimens as salvage therapy for refractory or relapsed AIDS-related non-Hodgkin's lymphoma. *J Acquir Immune Defic Syndr* 28:416–421, 2001.

137. Gopal S, Patel MR, Yanik EL, et al: Temporal trends in presentation and survival for HIV-associated lymphoma in the antiretroviral therapy era. *J Natl Cancer Inst* 105:1221–1229, 2013.

138. Costa LJ, Xavier AC, Wahlquist AE, et al: Trends in survival of patients with Burkitt lymphoma/leukemia in the USA: An analysis of 3691 cases. *Blood* 121:4861–4866, 2013.

139. Dolcetti R, Dal Col J, Martorelli D, et al: Interplay among viral antigens, cellular pathways and tumor microenvironment in the pathogenesis of EBV-driven lymphomas. *Semin Cancer Biol* 23:441–456, 2013.

140. Lim ST, Karim R, Nathwani BN, et al: AIDS-related Burkitt's lymphoma versus diffuse large-cell lymphoma in the pre-highly active antiretroviral therapy (HAART) and HAART eras: Significant differences in survival with standard chemotherapy. *J Clin Oncol* 23:4430–4438, 2005.

141. Galicier L, Fieschi C, Borie R, et al: Intensive chemotherapy regimen (LMB86) for St Jude stage IV AIDS-related Burkitt lymphoma/leukemia: A prospective study. *Blood* 110:2846–2854, 2007.

142. Xicoy B, Ribera JM, Miralles P, et al: Comparison of CHOP treatment with specific short-intensive chemotherapy in AIDS-related Burkitt's lymphoma or leukemia. *Med Clin (Barc)* 136:323–328, 2011.

143. Dunleavy K, Pittaluga S, Shovlin M, et al: Low-intensity therapy in adults with Burkitt's lymphoma. *N Engl J Med* 369:1915–1925, 2013.

144. Cortes J, Thomas D, Rios A, et al: Hyperfractionated cyclophosphamide, vincristine, doxorubicin, and dexamethasone and highly active antiretroviral therapy for patients with acquired immunodeficiency syndrome-related Burkitt lymphoma/leukemia. *Cancer* 94:1492–1499, 2002.

145. Wang ES, Straus DJ, Teruya-Feldstein J, et al: Intensive chemotherapy with cyclophosphamide, doxorubicin, high-dose methotrexate/ifosfamide, etoposide, and high-dose cytarabine (CODOX-M/IVAC) for human immunodeficiency virus-associated Burkitt lymphoma. *Cancer* 98:1196–1205, 2003.

146. Montoto S, Wilson J, Shaw K, et al: Excellent immunological recovery following CODOX-M/IVAC, an effective intensive chemotherapy for HIV-associated Burkitt's lymphoma. *AIDS* 24:851–856, 2010.

147. Rodrigo JA, Hicks LK, Cheung MC, et al: HIV-Associated Burkitt Lymphoma: Good Efficacy and Tolerance of Intensive Chemotherapy Including CODOX-M/IVAC with or without Rituximab in the HAART Era. *Adv Hematol* 2012:735392, 2012.

148. Xicoy B, Ribera JM, Muller M, et al: Dose-intensive chemotherapy including rituximab is highly effective but toxic in human immunodeficiency virus-infected patients with Burkitt lymphoma/leukemia: Parallel study of 81 patients. *Leuk Lymphoma* 55:2341–2348, 2014.

149. Nagai H, Odawara T, Ajisawa A, et al: Whole brain radiation alone produces favourable outcomes for AIDS-related primary central nervous system lymphoma in the HAART era. *Eur J Haematol* 84:499–505, 2010.

150. Newell ME, Hoy JF, Cooper SG, et al: Human immunodeficiency virus-related primary central nervous system lymphoma: Factors influencing survival in 111 patients. *Cancer* 100:2627–2636, 2004.

151. Uldrick TS, Pipkin S, Scheer S, et al: Factors associated with survival among patients with AIDS-related primary central nervous system lymphoma. *AIDS* 28:397–405, 2014.

152. Ammassari A, Cingolani A, Pezzotti P, et al: AIDS-related focal brain lesions in the era of highly active antiretroviral therapy. *Neurology* 55:1194–1200, 2000.

153. Bayraktar S, Bayraktar UD, Ramos JC, et al: Primary CNS lymphoma in HIV positive and negative patients: Comparison of clinical characteristics, outcome and prognostic factors. *J Neurooncol* 101:257–265, 2011.

154. Erdag N, Bhorade RM, Alberico RA, et al: Primary lymphoma of the central nervous system: Typical and atypical CT and MR imaging appearances. *AJR Am J Roentgenol* 176:1319–1326, 2001.

155. Antinori A, De Rossi G, Ammassari A, et al: Value of combined approach with thallium-201 single-photon emission computed tomography and Epstein-Barr virus DNA polymerase chain reaction in CSF for the diagnosis of AIDS-related primary CNS lymphoma. *J Clin Oncol* 17:554–560, 1999.

156. Lewitschnig S, Gedela K, Toby M, et al: ^{18}F-FDG PET/CT in HIV-related central nervous system pathology. *Eur J Nucl Med Mol Imaging* 40:1420–1427, 2013.

157. Westwood TD, Hogan C, Julyan PJ, et al: Utility of FDG-PET CT and magnetic resonance spectroscopy in differentiating between cerebral lymphoma and non-malignant CNS lesions in HIV-infected patients. *Eur J Radiol* 82:e374–e379, 2013.

158. Jacomet C, Girard PM, Lebrette MG, et al: Intravenous methotrexate for primary central nervous system non-Hodgkin's lymphoma in AIDS. *AIDS* 11:1725–1730, 1997.

159. Rubenstein JL, Gupta NK, Mannis GN, et al: How I treat CNS lymphomas. *Blood* 122:2318–2330, 2013.

160. Delecluse HJ, Anagnostopoulos I, Dallenbach F, et al: Plasmablastic lymphomas of the oral cavity: A new entity associated with the human immunodeficiency virus infection. *Blood* 89:1413–1420, 1997.

161. Carbone A, Gloghini A, Canzonieri V, et al: AIDS-related extranodal non-Hodgkin's lymphomas with plasma cell differentiation. *Blood* 90:1337–1338, 1997.

162. Castillo J, Pantanowitz L, Dezube BJ: HIV-associated plasmablastic lymphoma: Lessons learned from 112 published cases. *Am J Hematol* 83:804–809, 2008.

163. Castillo JJ, Furman M, Beltran BE, et al: Human immunodeficiency virus-associated plasmablastic lymphoma: Poor prognosis in the era of highly active antiretroviral therapy. *Cancer* 118:5270–5277, 2012.

164. Schommers P, Wyen C, Hentrich M, et al: Poor outcome of HIV-infected patients with plasmablastic lymphoma: Results from the German AIDS-related lymphoma cohort study. *AIDS* 27:842–845, 2013.

165. Bibas M, Grisetti S, Alba L, et al: Patient with HIV-associated plasmablastic lymphoma responding to bortezomib alone and in combination with dexamethasone, gemcitabine, oxaliplatin, cytarabine, and pegfilgrastim chemotherapy and lenalidomide alone. *J Clin Oncol* 28:e704–e708, 2010.

166. Saba NS, Dang D, Saba J, et al: Bortezomib in plasmablastic lymphoma: A case report and review of the literature. *Onkologie* 36:287–291, 2013.

167. Ammari ZA, Mollberg NM, Abdelhady K, et al: Diagnosis and management of primary effusion lymphoma in the immunocompetent and immunocompromised hosts. *Thorac Cardiovasc Surg* 61:343–349, 2013.

168. Boulanger E, Gerard L, Gabarre J, et al: Prognostic factors and outcome of human herpesvirus 8-associated primary effusion lymphoma in patients with AIDS. *J Clin Oncol* 23:4372–4380, 2005.

169. Pan ZG, Zhang QY, Lu ZB, et al: Extracavitary KSHV-associated large B-Cell lymphoma: A distinct entity or a subtype of primary effusion lymphoma? Study of 9 cases and review of an additional 43 cases. *Am J Surg Pathol* 36:1129–1140, 2012.

170. Simonelli C, Spina M, Cinelli R, et al: Clinical features and outcome of primary effusion lymphoma in HIV-infected patients: A single-institution study. *J Clin Oncol* 21:3948–3954, 2003.

171. Chen YB, Rahemtullah A, Hochberg E: Primary effusion lymphoma. *Oncologist* 12:569–576, 2007.

172. Bhatt S, Ashlock BM, Natkunam Y, et al: CD30 targeting with brentuximab vedotin: A novel therapeutic approach to primary effusion lymphoma. *Blood* 122:1233–1242, 2013.

173. Bhatt S, Ashlock BM, Toomey NL, et al: Efficacious proteasome/HDAC inhibitor combination therapy for primary effusion lymphoma. *J Clin Invest* 123:2616–2628, 2013.

174. Zhou Z, Sehn LH, Rademaker AW, et al: An enhanced International Prognostic Index (NCCN-IPI) for patients with diffuse large B-cell lymphoma treated in the rituximab era. *Blood* 123:837–842, 2014.

175. Biggar RJ, Jaffe ES, Goedert JJ, et al: Hodgkin lymphoma and immunodeficiency in persons with HIV/AIDS. *Blood* 108:3786–3791, 2006.

176. Kowalkowski MA, Mims MP, Amiran ES, et al: Effect of immune reconstitution on the incidence of HIV-related Hodgkin lymphoma. *PLoS One* 8:e77409, 2013.

177. Shiels MS, Koritzinsky EH, Clarke CA, et al: Prevalence of HIV Infection among U.S. Hodgkin lymphoma cases. *Cancer Epidemiol Biomarkers Prev* 23:274–281, 2014.

178. Xicoy B, Ribera JM, Miralles P, et al: Results of treatment with doxorubicin, bleomycin, vinblastine and dacarbazine and highly active antiretroviral therapy in advanced stage, human immunodeficiency virus-related Hodgkin's lymphoma. *Haematologica* 92:191–198, 2007.

179. Montoto S, Shaw K, Okosun J, et al: HIV status does not influence outcome in patients with classical Hodgkin lymphoma treated with chemotherapy using doxorubicin, bleomycin, vinblastine, and dacarbazine in the highly active antiretroviral therapy era. *J Clin Oncol* 30:4111–4116, 2012.

180. Hasenclever D, Diehl V: A prognostic score for advanced Hodgkin's disease. International Prognostic Factors Project on Advanced Hodgkin's Disease. *N Engl J Med* 339:1506–1514, 1998.

181. Hentrich M, Berger M, Wyen C, et al: Stage-adapted treatment of HIV-associated Hodgkin lymphoma: Results of a prospective multicenter study. *J Clin Oncol* 30:4117–4123, 2012.

182. Borchmann P, Skoetz N, Trelle S: BEACOPP or no BEACOPP?—Authors' reply. *Lancet Oncol* 14:e488–e489, 2013.

183. Federico M, Bellei M, Cheson BD: BEACOPP or no BEACOPP? *Lancet Oncol* 14:e487–e488, 2013.

184. Skoetz N, Trelle S, Rancea M, et al: Effect of initial treatment strategy on survival of patients with advanced-stage Hodgkin's lymphoma: A systematic review and network meta-analysis. *Lancet Oncol* 14:943–952, 2013.

185. Younes A, Connors JM, Park SI, et al: Brentuximab vedotin combined with ABVD or AVD for patients with newly diagnosed Hodgkin's lymphoma: A phase 1, open-label, dose-escalation study. *Lancet Oncol* 14:1348–1356, 2013.

186. Re A, Cattaneo C, Michieli M, et al: High-dose therapy and autologous peripheral-blood stem-cell transplantation as salvage treatment for HIV-associated lymphoma in patients receiving highly active antiretroviral therapy. *J Clin Oncol* 21:4423–4427, 2003.

187. Krishnan A, Molina A, Zaia J, et al: Durable remissions with autologous stem cell transplantation for high-risk HIV-associated lymphomas. *Blood* 105:874–878, 2005.

188. Re A, Cattaneo C, Skert c, et al: Stem cell mobilization in HIV seropositive patients with lymphoma. *Haematologica* 98:1762–1768, 2013.

189. Diez-Martin JL, Balsalobre P, Re A, et al: Comparable survival between HIV+ and HIV-non-Hodgkin and Hodgkin lymphoma patients undergoing autologous peripheral blood stem cell transplantation. *Blood* 113:6011–6014, 2009.

190. Krishnan A, Palmer JM, Zaia JA, et al: HIV status does not affect the outcome of autologous stem cell transplantation (ASCT) for non-Hodgkin lymphoma (NHL). *Biol Blood Marrow Transplant* 16:1302–1308, 2010.

191. Balsalobre P, Diez-Martin JL, Re A, et al: Autologous stem-cell transplantation in patients with HIV-related lymphoma. *J Clin Oncol* 27:2192–2198, 2009.

192. Re A, Michieli M, Casari S, et al: High-dose therapy and autologous peripheral blood stem cell transplantation as salvage treatment for AIDS-related lymphoma: Long-term results of the Italian Cooperative Group on AIDS and Tumors (GICAT) study with analysis of prognostic factors. *Blood* 114:1306–1313, 2009.

193. Spitzer TR, Ambinder RF, Lee JY, et al: Dose-reduced busulfan, cyclophosphamide, and autologous stem cell transplantation for human immunodeficiency virus-associated lymphoma: AIDS Malignancy Consortium study 020. *Biol Blood Marrow Transplant* 14:59–66, 2008.

194. Michieli M, Mazzucato M, Tirelli U, et al: Stem cell transplantation for lymphoma patients with HIV infection. *Cell Transplant* 20:351–370, 2011.

195. Henrich TJ, Hu Z, Li JZ, et al: Long-term reduction in peripheral blood HIV type 1 reservoirs following reduced-intensity conditioning allogeneic stem cell transplantation. *J Infect Dis* 207:1694–1702, 2013.

196. Hutter G, Zaia JA: Allogeneic haematopoietic stem cell transplantation in patients with human immunodeficiency virus: The experiences of more than 25 years. *Clin Exp Immunol* 163:284–295, 2011.

197. Serrano D, Miralles P, Balsalobre P, et al: Graft-versus-tumor effect after allogeneic stem cell transplantation in HIV-positive patients with high-risk hematologic malignancies. *AIDS Res Hum Retroviruses* 29:1340–1345, 2013.

198. Dunleavy K, Wilson WH: How I treat HIV-associated lymphoma. *Blood* 119:3245–3255, 2012.

199. Bower M, Collins S, Cottrill C, et al: British HIV Association guidelines for HIV-associated malignancies 2008. *HIV Med* 9:336–388, 2008.

200. Hentrich M, Hoffmann C, Mosthaf F, et al: Therapy of HIV-associated lymphoma-recommendations of the oncology working group of the German Study Group of

Physicians in Private Practice Treating HIV-Infected Patients (DAGNA), in cooperation with the German AIDS Society (DAIG). *Ann Hematol* 93:913–921, 2014.

201. Rudek MA, Flexner C, Ambinder RF: Use of antineoplastic agents in patients with cancer who have HIV/AIDS. *Lancet Oncol* 12:905–912, 2011.

202. Torres HA, Rallapalli V, Saxena A, et al: Efficacy and safety of antiretrovirals in HIV-infected patients with cancer. *Clin Microbiol Infect* 20:O672–O679, 2014.

203. Bower M, McCall-Peat N, Ryan N, et al: Protease inhibitors potentiate chemotherapy-induced neutropenia. *Blood* 104:2943–2946, 2004.

204. Bower M, Powles T, Stebbing J, et al: Potential antiretroviral drug interactions with cyclophosphamide, doxorubicin, and etoposide. *J Clin Oncol* 23:1328–1329; author reply 1329–1330, 2005.

205. Sparano JA, Lee S, Chen MG, et al: Phase II trial of infusional cyclophosphamide, doxorubicin, and etoposide in patients with HIV-associated non-Hodgkin's lymphoma: An Eastern Cooperative Oncology Group Trial (E1494). *J Clin Oncol* 22:1491–1500, 2004.

206. Wong AY, Marcotte S, Laroche M, et al: Safety and efficacy of CHOP for treatment of diffuse large B-cell lymphoma with different combination antiretroviral therapy regimens: SCULPT study. *Antivir Ther* 18:699–707, 2013.

207. Ezzat HM, Cheung MC, Hicks LK, et al: Incidence, predictors and significance of severe toxicity in patients with human immunodeficiency virus-associated Hodgkin lymphoma. *Leuk Lymphoma* 53:2390–2396, 2012.

208. Oksenhendler E, Boulanger E, Galicier L, et al: High incidence of Kaposi sarcoma-associated herpesvirus-related non-Hodgkin lymphoma in patients with HIV infection and multicentric Castleman disease. *Blood* 99:2331–2336, 2002.

209. Powles T, Stebbing J, Bazeos A, et al: The role of immune suppression and HHV-8 in the increasing incidence of HIV-associated multicentric Castleman's disease. *Ann Oncol* 20:775–779, 2009.

210. Carbone A, De Paoli P, Gloghini A, et al: KSHV-associated multicentric Castleman disease: A tangle of different entities requiring multitarget treatment strategies. *Int J Cancer* 137:251–261, 2015.

211. Polizzotto MN, Uldrick TS, Wang V, et al: Human and viral interleukin-6 and other cytokines in Kaposi sarcoma herpesvirus-associated multicentric Castleman disease. *Blood* 122:4189–4198, 2013.

212. Qu L, Jenkins F, Triulzi DJ: Human herpesvirus 8 genomes and seroprevalence in United States blood donors. *Transfusion* 50:1050–1056, 2010.

213. Hoffmann C, Schmid H, Muller M, et al: Improved outcome with rituximab in patients with HIV-associated multicentric Castleman disease. *Blood* 118:3499–3503, 2011.

214. Gerard L, Michot JM, Burcheri S, et al: Rituximab decreases the risk of lymphoma in patients with HIV-associated multicentric Castleman disease. *Blood* 119:2228–2233, 2012.

215. Oksenhendler E, Carcelain G, Aoki Y, et al: High levels of human herpesvirus 8 viral load, human interleukin-6, interleukin-10, and C reactive protein correlate with exacerbation of multicentric Castleman disease in HIV-infected patients. *Blood* 96:2069–2073, 2000.

216. Stebbing J, Adams C, Sanitt A, et al: Plasma HHV8 DNA predicts relapse in individuals with HIV-associated multicentric Castleman disease. *Blood* 118:271–275, 2011.

217. Bower M: How I treat HIV-associated multicentric Castleman disease. *Blood* 116:4415–4421, 2010.

218. Bower M, Powles T, Williams S, et al: Brief communication: Rituximab in HIV-associated multicentric Castleman disease. *Ann Intern Med* 147:836–839, 2007.

219. Gerard L, Berezne A, Galicier L, et al: Prospective study of rituximab in chemotherapy-dependent human immunodeficiency virus associated multicentric Castleman's disease: ANRS 117 CastlemaB Trial. *J Clin Oncol* 25:3350–3356, 2007.

220. Bower M, Veraitch O, Szydlo R, et al: Cytokine changes during rituximab therapy in HIV-associated multicentric Castleman disease. *Blood* 113:4521–4524, 2009.

221. Powles T, Stebbing J, Montoto S, et al: Rituximab as retreatment for rituximab pretreated HIV-associated multicentric Castleman disease. *Blood* 110:4132–4133, 2007.

222. Marcelin AG, Aaron L, Mateus C, et al: Rituximab therapy for HIV-associated Castleman disease. *Blood* 102:2786–2788, 2003.

223. Uldrick TS, Polizzotto MN, Aleman K, et al: Rituximab plus liposomal doxorubicin in HIV-infected patients with KSHV-associated multicentric Castleman disease. *Blood* 124:3544–3552, 2014.

224. van Rhee F, Wong RS, Munshi N, et al: Siltuximab for multicentric Castleman's disease: A randomised, double-blind, placebo-controlled trial. *Lancet Oncol* 15:966–974, 2014.

225. Kurzrock R, Voorhees PM, Casper C, et al: A phase I, open-label study of siltuximab, an anti-IL-6 monoclonal antibody, in patients with B-cell non-Hodgkin lymphoma, multiple myeloma, or Castleman disease. *Clin Cancer Res* 19:3659–3670, 2013.

226. Nagao A, Nakazawa S, Hanabusa H: Short-term efficacy of the IL6 receptor antibody tocilizumab in patients with HIV-associated multicentric Castleman disease: Report of two cases. *J Hematol Oncol* 7:10, 2014.

227. Casper C, Nichols WG, Huang ML, et al: Remission of HHV-8 and HIV-associated multicentric Castleman disease with ganciclovir treatment. *Blood* 103:1632–1634, 2004.

228. Uldrick TS, Polizzotto MN, Aleman K, et al: High-dose zidovudine plus valganciclovir for Kaposi sarcoma herpesvirus-associated multicentric Castleman disease: A pilot study of virus-activated cytotoxic therapy. *Blood* 117:6977–6986, 2011.

229. Polizzotto MN, Uldrick TS, Hu D, et al: Clinical manifestations of Kaposi sarcoma herpesvirus lytic activation: Multicentric Castleman disease (KSHV-MCD) and the KSHV inflammatory cytokine syndrome. *Front Microbiol* 3:73, 2012.

230. Ray A, Marshall V, Uldrick T, et al: Sequence analysis of Kaposi sarcoma-associated herpesvirus (KSHV) microRNAs in patients with multicentric Castleman disease and KSHV-associated inflammatory cytokine syndrome. *J Infect Dis* 205:1665–1676, 2012.

231. Uldrick TS, Wang V, O'Mahony D, et al: An interleukin-6-related systemic inflammatory syndrome in patients co-infected with Kaposi sarcoma-associated herpesvirus and HIV but without Multicentric Castleman disease. *Clin Infect Dis* 51:350–358, 2010.

232. Niedt GW, Schinella RA: Acquired immunodeficiency syndrome. Clinicopathologic study of 56 autopsies. *Arch Pathol Lab Med* 109:727–734, 1985.

233. Jordan MB, Allen CE, Weitzman S, et al: How I treat hemophagocytic lymphohistiocytosis. *Blood* 118:4041–4052, 2011.

234. Fardet L, Lambotte O, Meynard JL, et al: Reactive haemophagocytic syndrome in 58 HIV-1-infected patients: Clinical features, underlying diseases and prognosis. *AIDS* 24:1299–1306, 2010.

235. Trottestam H, Horne A, Arico M, et al: Chemoimmunotherapy for hemophagocytic lymphohistiocytosis: Long-term results of the HLH-94 treatment protocol. *Blood* 118:4577–4584, 2011.

236. Henter JI, Horne A, Arico M, et al: HLH-2004: Diagnostic and therapeutic guidelines for hemophagocytic lymphohistiocytosis. *Pediatr Blood Cancer* 48:124–131, 2007.

237. Sullivan PS, Hanson DL, Chu SY, et al: Epidemiology of anemia in human immunodeficiency virus (HIV)-infected persons: Results from the multistate adult and adolescent spectrum of HIV disease surveillance project. *Blood* 91:301–308, 1998.

238. Mocroft A, Kirk O, Barton SE, et al: Anaemia is an independent predictive marker for clinical prognosis in HIV-infected patients from across Europe. EuroSIDA study group. *AIDS* 13:943–950, 1999.

239. Mocroft A, Lifson AR, Touloumi G, et al: Haemoglobin and anaemia in the SMART study. *Antivir Ther* 16:329–337, 2011.

240. Berhane K, Karim R, Cohen MH, et al: Impact of highly active antiretroviral therapy on anemia and relationship between anemia and survival in a large cohort of HIV-infected women: Women's Interagency HIV Study. *J Acquir Immune Defic Syndr* 37:1245–1252, 2004.

241. Hoffmann CJ, Fielding KL, Johnston V, et al: Changing predictors of mortality over time from cART start: Implications for care. *J Acquir Immune Defic Syndr* 58:269–276, 2011.

242. Mocroft A, Ledergerber B, Zilmer K, et al: Short-term clinical disease progression in HIV-1-positive patients taking combination antiretroviral therapy: The EuroSIDA risk-score. *AIDS* 21:1867–1875, 2007.

243. Tate JP, Justice AC, Hughes MD, et al: An internationally generalizable risk index for mortality after one year of antiretroviral therapy. *AIDS* 27:563–572, 2013.

244. Justice AC, Modur SP, Tate JP, et al: Predictive accuracy of the Veterans Aging Cohort Study index for mortality with HIV infection: A North American cross cohort analysis. *J Acquir Immune Defic Syndr* 62:149–163, 2013.

245. Moses AV, Williams S, Heneveld ML, et al: Human immunodeficiency virus infection of bone marrow endothelium reduces induction of stromal hematopoietic growth factors. *Blood* 87:919–925, 1996.

246. Drakesmith H, Prentice AM: Hepcidin and the iron-infection axis. *Science* 338:768–772, 2012.

247. Wisaksana R, de Mast Q, Alisjahbana B, et al: Inverse relationship of serum hepcidin levels with CD4 cell counts in HIV-infected patients selected from an Indonesian prospective cohort study. *PLoS One* 8:e79904, 2013.

248. Redd AD, Avalos A, Essex M: Infection of hematopoietic progenitor cells by HIV-1 subtype C, and its association with anemia in southern Africa. *Blood* 110:3143–3149, 2007.

249. Carter CC, Onafuwa-Nuga A, McNamara LA, et al: HIV-1 infects multipotent progenitor cells causing cell death and establishing latent cellular reservoirs. *Nat Med* 16:446–451, 2010.

250. McNamara LA, Onafuwa-Nuga A, Sebastian NT, et al: CD133+ hematopoietic progenitor cells harbor HIV genomes in a subset of optimally treated people with long term viral suppression. *J Infect Dis* 207:1807–1816, 2013.

251. Nixon CC, Vatakis DN, Reichelderfer SN, et al: HIV-1 infection of hematopoietic progenitor cells *in vivo* in humanized mice. *Blood* 122:2195–2204, 2013.

252. Camacho J, Poveda F, Zamorano AF, et al: Serum erythropoietin levels in anaemic patients with advanced human immunodeficiency virus infection. *Br J Haematol* 82:608–614, 1992.

253. Spivak JL, Barnes DC, Fuchs E, et al: Serum immunoreactive erythropoietin in HIV-infected patients. *JAMA* 261:3104–3107, 1989.

254. Tsiakalos A, Kordossis T, Ziakas PD, et al: Circulating antibodies to endogenous erythropoietin and risk for HIV-1-related anemia. *J Infect* 60:238–243, 2010.

255. Tsiakalos A, Routsias JG, Kordossis T, et al: Fine epitope specificity of anti-erythropoietin antibodies reveals molecular mimicry with HIV-1 p17 protein: A pathogenetic mechanism for HIV-1-related anemia. *J Infect Dis* 204:902–911, 2011.

256. Behler C, Shade S, Gregory K, et al: Anemia and HIV in the antiretroviral era: Potential significance of testosterone. *AIDS Res Hum Retroviruses* 21:200–206, 2005.

257. Young NS, Brown KE: Parvovirus B19. *N Engl J Med* 350:586–597, 2004.

258. Koduri PR: Parvovirus B19-related anemia in HIV-infected patients. *AIDS Patient Care STDS* 14:7–11, 2000.

259. Abkowitz JL, Brown KE, Wood RW, et al: Clinical relevance of parvovirus B19 as a cause of anemia in patients with human immunodeficiency virus infection. *J Infect Dis* 176:269–273, 1997.

260. Koduri PR, Kumapley R, Valladares J, et al: Chronic pure red cell aplasia caused by parvovirus B19 in AIDS: Use of intravenous immunoglobulin—A report of eight patients. *Am J Hematol* 61:16–20, 1999.

261. Moyle G, Sawyer W, Law M, et al: Changes in hematologic parameters and efficacy of thymidine analogue-based, highly active antiretroviral therapy: A meta-analysis of six prospective, randomized, comparative studies. *Clin Ther* 26:92–97, 2004.

262. Fischl M, Galpin JE, Levine JD, et al: Recombinant human erythropoietin for patients with AIDS treated with zidovudine. *N Engl J Med* 322:1488–1493, 1990.

263. Henry DH, Beall GN, Benson CA, et al: Recombinant human erythropoietin in the treatment of anemia associated with human immunodeficiency virus (HIV) infection and zidovudine therapy. Overview of four clinical trials. *Ann Intern Med* 117:739–748, 1992.

264. Marti-Carvajal AJ, Sola I, Pena-Marti GE, et al: Treatment for anemia in people with AIDS. *Cochrane Database Syst Rev* (10):CD004776, 2011.

265. Gervasoni C, Ridolfo AL, Vaccarezza M, et al: Thrombotic microangiopathy in patients with acquired immunodeficiency syndrome before and during the era of introduction of highly active antiretroviral therapy. *Clin Infect Dis* 35:1534–1540, 2002.

266. Becker S, Fusco G, Fusco J, et al: HIV-associated thrombotic microangiopathy in the era of highly active antiretroviral therapy: An observational study. *Clin Infect Dis* 39 Suppl 5:S267–S275, 2004.

267. Benjamin M, Terrell DR, Vesely SK, et al: Frequency and significance of HIV infection among patients diagnosed with thrombotic thrombocytopenic purpura. *Clin Infect Dis* 48:1129–1137, 2009.

268. Hart D, Sayer R, Miller R, et al: Human immunodeficiency virus associated thrombotic thrombocytopenic purpura—Favourable outcome with plasma exchange and prompt initiation of highly active antiretroviral therapy. *Br J Haematol* 153:515–519, 2011.

269. Malak S, Wolf M, Millot GA, et al: Human immunodeficiency virus-associated thrombotic microangiopathies: Clinical characteristics and outcome according to ADAMTS13 activity. *Scand J Immunol* 68:337–344, 2008.

270. Sogaard OS, Lohse N, Ostergaard L, et al: Morbidity and risk of subsequent diagnosis of HIV: A population based case control study identifying indicator diseases for HIV infection. *PLoS One* 7:e32538, 2012.

271. Ambler KL, Vickars LM, Leger CS, et al: Clinical Features, Treatment, and Outcome of HIV-Associated Immune Thrombocytopenia in the HAART Era. *Adv Hematol* 2012:910954, 2012.

272. Vannappagari V, Nkhoma ET, Atashili J, et al: Prevalence, severity, and duration of thrombocytopenia among HIV patients in the era of highly active antiretroviral therapy. *Platelets* 22:611–618, 2011.

273. Ghosn J, Persoz A, Zitoun Y, et al: Thrombocytopenia during primary HIV-1 infection predicts the risk of recurrence during chronic infection. *J Acquir Immune Defic Syndr* 60:e112–e114, 2012.

274. Marks KM, Clarke RM, Bussel JB, et al: Risk factors for thrombocytopenia in HIV-infected persons in the era of potent antiretroviral therapy. *J Acquir Immune Defic Syndr* 52:595–599, 2009.

275. Servais J, Nkoghe D, Schmit JC, et al: HIV-associated hematologic disorders are correlated with plasma viral load and improve under highly active antiretroviral therapy. *J Acquir Immune Defic Syndr* 28:221–225, 2001.

276. Ballem PJ, Belzberg A, Devine DV, et al: Kinetic studies of the mechanism of thrombocytopenia in patients with human immunodeficiency virus infection. *N Engl J Med* 327:1779–1784, 1992.

277. Zucker-Franklin D, Cao YZ: Megakaryocytes of human immunodeficiency virus-infected individuals express viral RNA. *Proc Natl Acad Sci U S A* 86:5595–5599, 1989.

278. Zidovudine for the treatment of thrombocytopenia associated with human immunodeficiency virus (HIV). A prospective study. The Swiss Group for Clinical Studies on the Acquired Immunodeficiency Syndrome (AIDS). *Ann Intern Med* 109:718–721, 1988.

279. Arranz Caso JA, Sanchez Mingo C, Garcia Tena J: Effect of highly active antiretroviral therapy on thrombocytopenia in patients with HIV infection. *N Engl J Med* 341:1239–1240, 1999.

280. Carbonara S, Fiorentino G, Serio G, et al: Response of severe HIV-associated thrombocytopenia to highly active antiretroviral therapy including protease inhibitors. *J Infect* 42:251–256, 2001.

281. Rosenblum M, Deeks SG, van der Laan M, et al: The risk of virologic failure decreases with duration of HIV suppression, at greater than 50% adherence to antiretroviral therapy. *PLoS One* 4:e7196, 2009.

282. Scaradavou A, Woo B, Woloski BM, et al: Intravenous anti-D treatment of immune thrombocytopenic purpura: Experience in 272 patients. *Blood* 89:2689–2700, 1997.

283. Scaradavou A, Cunningham-Rundles S, Ho JL, et al: Superior effect of intravenous anti-D compared with IV gammaglobulin in the treatment of HIV-thrombocytopenia: Results of a small, randomized prospective comparison. *Am J Hematol* 82:335–341, 2007.

284. Oksenhendler E, Bierling P, Chevret S, et al: Splenectomy is safe and effective in human immunodeficiency virus-related immune thrombocytopenia. *Blood* 82:29–32, 1993.

285. Aslam MI, Cardile AP, Crawford GE: Use of peptide thrombopoietin receptor agonist romiplostim (Nplate) in a case of primary HIV-associated thrombocytopenia. *J Int Assoc Provid AIDS Care* 13:22–23, 2014.

286. Quach H, Lee LY, Smith B, et al: Successful use of eltrombopag without splenectomy in refractory HIV-related immune reconstitution thrombocytopenia. *AIDS* 26:1977–1979, 2012.

287. Firnhaber C, Smeaton L, Saukila N, et al: Comparisons of anemia, thrombocytopenia, and neutropenia at initiation of HIV antiretroviral therapy in Africa, Asia, and the Americas. *Int J Infect Dis* 14:e1088–e1092, 2010.

288. Levine AM, Karim R, Mack W, et al: Neutropenia in human immunodeficiency virus infection: Data from the women's interagency HIV study. *Arch Intern Med* 166:405–410, 2006.

289. Moore DA, Benepal T, Portsmouth S, et al: Etiology and natural history of neutropenia in human immunodeficiency virus disease: A prospective study. *Clin Infect Dis* 32:469–475, 2001.

290. Zhu NY, Legatt DF, Turner AR: Agranulocytosis after consumption of cocaine adulterated with levamisole. *Ann Intern Med* 150:287–289, 2009.

CHAPTER 82
MONONUCLEOSIS SYNDROMES

Robert F. Betts

SUMMARY

The defining clinical features of a mononucleosis syndrome are fever and reactive lymphocytes in the blood. The two most common causes of mononucleosis are Epstein-Barr virus (EBV) and cytomegalovirus (CMV) infection. The clinical manifestations of EBV and CMV mononucleosis depend on a vigorous host response to the viral infection. Patients who become infected without a host response develop antibodies to the virus but no or minimal clinical manifestations. Several clinical similarities exist between EBV and CMV mononucleosis. Both infections have a febrile prodrome before the mononucleosis phase develops. Both infections can induce fever, an enlarged spleen, and an erythematous skin rash—the mononucleosis phase. The disease is self-limited in the vast majority of patients, although resolution may take several weeks, especially in older individuals. In both viral infections, lymphocytes represent greater than 50 percent of blood cells, and at least 10 percent are reactive lymphocytes. Differences in clinical and laboratory findings are observed. Severe pharyngitis and tender lymph node enlargement, often in several lymph node groups, occur in infection with EBV and perhaps with some unknown agents, but not to the same degree in infections with CMV. The majority of cases of EBV mononucleosis occur in teenagers and young adults, whereas CMV-induced disease occurs most commonly in adults in their 30s to 60s. A much larger percentage of adults have unrecognized primary infection with CMV than with EBV. EBV results in the development of heterophile antibodies, active against sheep and horse red cells among others, but this development does not occur in CMV. The pathway leading to lymphocytosis and reactive lymphocytes differs between the two agents. The B cell is infected in EBV infection which eventually may lead to hematologic malignancy, whereas the macrophage is infected in CMV. This may explain its important role after allogeneic transplantation. In both infections, the T lymphocyte is the reactive cell. Other agents, including *Toxoplasma gondii*, human immune deficiency virus type 1, and several other viruses, can cause a mononucleosis-like syndrome with reactive lymphocytes in the blood.

DEFINITION AND HISTORY

The first clinical description of what was probably infectious mononucleosis was published in 1885 when Pfeiffer[1] described a disorder termed *Drüsenfieber* (glandular fever). In 1920, Sprunt and Evans[2] introduced the term *infectious mononucleosis* for an acute, self-limited syndrome

Acronyms and Abbreviations: CMV, cytomegalovirus; EA, early antigen; EBNA, Epstein-Barr nuclear antigen; EBV, Epstein-Barr virus; NK, natural killer; PCR, polymerase chain reaction; PTLD, posttransplantation lymphoproliferative disease; VCA, virus capsid antigen.

of mononuclear leukocytosis in febrile patients. In 1932, Paul and Bunnell[3] showed that the sera from patients with infectious mononucleosis agglutinated red cells from sheep and horses, a reaction that was termed the *heterophile antibody test*. Paul was investigating heterophile antibodies in human sera that reacted with sheep red blood cells. These antibodies were unrelated by phylogenetic features to the antigen with which they reacted, the so-called Forssman antigen. He found that the highest titer had developed in the serum of an individual recovering from infectious mononucleosis. Davidson showed that serum, after absorption by guinea pig kidney cells, no longer reacted with sheep or horse cells. This absorption of these antibodies made this test very specific for Epstein Barr virus (EBV) infection.[4] In 1964, Epstein, Ashong, and Barr reported the isolation of a virus from the cells of a patient with African Burkitt lymphoma and hence the derivation of its name, EBV. The etiologic role of EBV in infectious mononucleosis was discovered serendipitously in the laboratory of Gertrude and Werner Henle.[5] A technician in their laboratory whose serum had been negative for EBV antibodies and was used as a seronegative control was discovered to be EBV antibody-positive after she recovered from infectious mononucleosis. The association later was confirmed in seroepidemiologic studies of college students.[6-9]

Much of the clinical nature and the incubation period of mononucleosis were documented by Hoagland[10] in studies of cadets at West Point. He established that oral transmission was the principal route of viral transmission, which led to mononucleosis being dubbed the "kissing disease." He also noted that cadets developed the disease approximately 6 weeks after they returned from their vacation.[11]

Although EBV is the most common cause of infectious mononucleosis, other agents produce a febrile syndrome with a blood lymphocytosis that mimics some aspects of EBV mononucleosis.

ETIOLOGY AND PATHOGENESIS

The infectious mononucleosis syndrome is most commonly caused by one of two members of the herpes virus family: EBV or cytomegalovirus (CMV). Occasionally the HIV and, less commonly, the parasite *Toxoplasma gondii* produce a febrile illness with lymphocytosis. Other viral agents produce a febrile syndrome with a blood lymphocytosis, but only infrequently (Table 82–1). For both EBV and CMV mononucleosis, the T-lymphocyte response to the infected target cell, resulting in reactive lymphocytosis, is a hallmark of the disease. The difference is that for EBV, the B lymphocyte is the cell that becomes infected and thus the target of the responding T lymphocyte, whereas it is the macrophage/monocyte lineage that is infected by CMV, which engenders the T-lymphocyte response.[13,14]

EPIDEMIOLOGY OF EPSTEIN-BARR VIRUS AND CYTOMEGALOVIRUS

Some similar and several distinct epidemiologic and clinical differences exist between EBV and CMV infection. Both EBV and CMV infect young children.[15] Those who develop EBV infection at a very young age (1 to 5 years) have an illness similar to other illnesses occurring during their youth. CMV infection presents similarly, but in the young patients there is low-grade fever, mild elevation in liver function, and, quite often, lymphadenopathy. The latter seldom occurs in older people with primary CMV infection.

If an individual escaped EBV infection when he or she was young, it is very common for the individual to develop infection during the teen and young adult years, that is, between the ages of 12 and 25 years.[8] By contrast, CMV infection is uncommon in that age range but begins

TABLE 82–1. Etiologic Agents Associated with a Mononucleosis Syndrome

Epstein-Barr virus
Cytomegalovirus
Human immunodeficiency virus
Human herpes virus-6
Metapneumovirus
Rubella
Hepatitis A
Adenovirus
Toxoplasma gondii
Bartonella henselae
Brucella abortus

to increase in frequency after the age of 25 years.[16,17] Primary CMV infection is also far more common than EBV in those older than 50 years of age.[16] Between the ages of 12 and 25 years, the classic mononucleosis illness develops in the majority of those with primary EBV infection.[8] In the few older individuals in whom EBV occurs, clinical illness that develops resembles the clinical illness that occurs in those with new CMV infection.[18] Congenital infection with EBV occurs,[19] but it occurs only in babies of mothers who were infected with EBV during pregnancy and it is very uncommon. By contrast, it is estimated that 1 to 2 percent of all livebirths have CMV congenital infection. Furthermore, it occurs associated with primary infection in mothers; it also occurs in babies of mothers who were seropositive preconception.[20] CMV infection of the monocyte/macrophage[21] helps explain its role in disease following solid-organ transplant. Because latent CMV is present in all solid organs of those with previous CMV infection, when immunosuppression is administered latent CMV is reactivated. EBV infection posttransplantation occurs only in those recipients who have not been infected before transplantation and, as with CMV, the EBV is reactivated in the donor organ.[22]

● EPSTEIN-BARR VIRUS MONONUCLEOSIS

VIROLOGY AND PATHOGENESIS

EBV is a DNA virus of the Gammaherpesvirinae subfamily. The virus is estimated to infect 90 percent of the world's population. In the process of this infection, the EBV intercalates itself primarily into the long-lived memory B cell, not the naïve B cell,[23] and thereafter establishes lifelong residence in its host. Early after infection, the virus is continuously shed into oral secretions. The virus then usually undergoes latency, but it may be reactivated periodically.[24]

Following primary infection, varying severity of disease ensues. Infection occurs via virus attachment to the cell surface CD21 glycoprotein, a 140-kDa complement receptor type 2. Infection induces polyclonal proliferation of infected B cells in the nodes in the pharynx. There is increasing evidence that host genetic factors predict the severity and duration of disease following primary EBV infection.[25,26] Specifically, the interferon (IFN)-γ +874T/A or the interleukin (IL)-10 –592C/A polymorphisms are the important genetic factors. Using measures of severity of illness such as fatigue, myalgia, and height of fever, individuals who have the IFN-γ +874TT (high interferon production) allele have a striking increase in the risk of experiencing these severe manifestations compared to those with IFN-γ +874 A and IL-10 –592.[24] When a subject's blood monocytes are tested in vitro, the high-risk group has

a higher production of IFN-γ in stimulated cells.[27] Other factors in host response, which include the height of the virus load in the blood, the number of CD 8+ cells, and the T-cell granzyme expression in the CD8+ cell also have been described as contributing to disease severity.[28] As a corollary to this, variability in the symptoms, signs, physical findings, and laboratory abnormalities occurs in primary infection.[28,29] At the time serology confirms evidence of primary infection, some, but not all individuals with primary infection, have classic symptomatic disease.[28,29] In those who develop the classical syndrome, T lymphocytes recognize viral replicative antigens on the infected B cell as foreign, and an exuberant polyclonal cytotoxic T-cell response ensues. The proliferative rate of CD8+ T cells is estimated to be approximately 50 percent of this population of cells proliferating per day. This translates into a population doubling time of 1.5 days so that 5×10^9 CD8+ T cells per day appear in the blood. The later rate of appearance is two orders of magnitude greater than normal.[30] The surface activation marker SLAM (signaling lymphocyte activation molecule)-associated protein (SAP) on T lymphocytes stimulates cell activation in response to a signal from CD244 and CD150 (SLAM) on the T-cell surface.[31] In the healthy individual, this process subsides over days to weeks. In parallel, the signs and symptoms of the infection subside, although fatigue may persist for a longer period of time.

EPIDEMIOLOGY

There is an apparent seasonal pattern with its peak incidence in the summer. Close person-to-person contact is required for transmission to a susceptible individual.[29] Subclinical primary infection[28] or frequent asymptomatic reactivation of EBV in the previously infected individual provides an opportunity for transmission at all ages. Although, transmission from breast milk or from the cervix occurs, it is very uncommon.[32] Nonetheless, nearly everyone in the developing world is infected by age 5 years and mononucleosis is rarely seen. Similar rates of infection occur in the lower socioeconomic class in the developed world. In the upper socioeconomic strata of the developed world, the majority of persons avoid infection when they are young. However, between the ages of 12 and 25, infection is very common. Characteristically, primary infection occurs in an individual a few months after the individual develops a relationship with someone who has latent infection.[24,28] Transmission occurs from a virus-positive asymptomatic individual who transmits his or her virus to a previously uninfected person. Individuals who are raised in more protected environments may reach their 30s before they are infected. If both individuals in an initial relationship are seronegative, years may pass before they become infected. Individuals who are seropositive usually do not develop clinical disease upon reexposure, although a second infection with a different strain may occur.[33,35]

CLINICAL MANIFESTATIONS

Clinical manifestations vary by age.[15,18,36–41] When young children acquire illness they develop a typical childhood illness of upper respiratory infection (43 percent), otitis media (29 percent) pharyngitis (21 percent), gastroenteritis (7 percent), or typical mononucleosis (<10 percent). Rashes and/or periorbital swelling occur more frequently in younger children than in the teens. In the age group 12 to 25 years, many, but not all, present with the classical presentation of infectious mononucleosis. However, there are a substantial proportion of newly infected individuals who have minimal or very mild disease.[28,29] Furthermore, evidence of virus in the blood may be present for several days before disease appears.[28] For those who present with the classical disease of infectious mononucleosis, the earliest manifestations of disease develop 35 to 42 days after the individual develops infection (Table 82–2). Infection occurs via virus attachment to the cell-surface CD21 glycoprotein, a 140-kDa complement receptor type 2. Infection

TABLE 82–2. Signs and Symptoms of Epstein-Barr Virus and Cytomegalovirus Mononucleosis: Effect of Age (Percent of Patients)

Signs and Symptoms	EBV (Age 14–35 Years*)	EBV (Age 40–72 Years†)	CMV (Age 30–70 Years‡)
Fever	95	94	85
Pharyngitis	95	46	15
Lymphadenopathy	98	49	24
Splenomegaly	65	33	3
Hepatomegaly	23	42	N/A
Jaundice	8	27	24

CMV, cytomegalovirus; EBV, Epstein-Barr virus.

*Data from RJ Hoagland.[10]

†Data from Hoagland RJ: The clinical manifestations of infectious mononucleosis: A report of 200 cases. *Am J Med* Sci 240:55, 1960; Schmader KE, van der Horst CM, Klotman ME: Epstein-Barr virus and the elderly host. *Rev Infect Dis* 11:64–73, 1989; Axelrod P, Finestone AJ: Infectious mononucleosis in older adults. *Am Fam Physician* 42:1599, 1990; Hurwitz CA, Henle W, Henle G, et al: Infectious mononucleosis in patients aged 40 to 72 years: Report of 27 cases, including 3 without heterophile-antibody responses. *Medicine* 62:256, 1983.

‡Data from reference Just-Nubling, G. Korn, S. Ludwig, B. et.al: Primary cytomegalovirus infection in an outpatient setting–laboratory markers and clinical aspects. *Infection* 31:318, 2003.

induces polyclonal proliferation of infected B cells in the nodes in the pharynx. Initial symptoms are lassitude and fever with no evidence of lymphocytosis or pharyngitis. Fever results from infection and proliferation of the B lymphocytes. From the nodes in the pharynx, the infected cells make their way into the circulating lymphocyte pool.[42,43] Although the duration of virus in the blood is much shorter than it is in the secretions, it is the movement into the blood that leads to the manifestation of the disease. Subsequent, massive T-cell response to the neoantigens on the infected B lymphocyte is evident by the lymphocytosis with reactive blood lymphocytes and other disease manifestations. The pharyngitis that develops is a result of the T-cell response to the infected B cells that are found in Waldeyer ring in the tonsils. Sometimes enlargement of the tonsils occurs to the extent that they touch each other in the midline. Blood lymphocytosis occurs in response to the virus in the blood. Periorbital swelling, which occurs in mononucleosis, is an important clue to the diagnosis, even in young adults. Other manifestations include lymphadenopathy, hepatitis and splenic enlargement. (Table 82–2).[8,28] Although the liver is not an organ rich in lymphocytes and hepatocytes are not damaged by the infection, CD4+ and CD8+ lymphocytes are trapped in that organ and their release of cytokines contributes to the inflammation in the liver and the changes in liver function that occur.[44] However, hyperbilirubinemia is very uncommon. The frequency of each clinical finding of the typical syndrome in newly infected patients is variable (Table 82–3).[28,29] The disease abates with the occurrence of a T-cell–mediated counterresponse to the virus-induced initial polyclonal B-cell proliferation. During this time, dramatic clinical improvement can occur in 24 to 48 hours. Subsequently, EBV remains in the patient's B cells throughout life, but expresses only Epstein-Barr nuclear antigen-1 (EBNA-1), which does not elicit a T-cell response because of a glycine-alanine repeat that inhibits its processing.[45]

Group A streptococcus is found in the pharynx occasionally (3 to 4 percent of cases) in concert with an EBV primary infection. Although treatment of the streptococcus eradicates the organism, the severe pharyngitis changes little, and the disease follows its usual course. Thus, treatment should be administered only if the test result for β-streptococcus is positive. If a penicillin congener is used, quite often, but not always, a rash develops[46,47] and the patient is labeled "penicillin allergic." The patient should be reevaluated after the mononucleosis resolves to determine if the patient has a true allergy.

There are exceptions to the usual situation of most people becoming infected by age 25 years. The first is found in a woman who is protected by her family from intimate male contact. She avoids infection until she is married at which time she may become infected from her husband. The second situation occurs when a long-term relationship is established when a couple is young. If they are both seronegative, infection does not occur. When they reach parenting age or older, they become infected by a child or a grandchild. When that occurs, the presentation is less likely to include lymphadenopathy and pharyngitis (see Table 82–3).[18,40,41] Fever almost always occurs and abdominal pain, hepatomegaly, and abnormal liver function develops in most. Older adults are less likely to develop lymphocytosis, they have fewer reactive lymphocytes, and splenomegaly is less evident. This leads to the clinical impression of infiltrative hepatic disease or cholecystitis. The illness at this age may be very protracted.

TABLE 82–3. Complications of Epstein-Barr Virus and Cytomegalovirus Mononucleosis

Complication	Epstein-Barr Virus	Cytomegalovirus
Hemolytic anemia	++	+
Thrombocytopenia	+	+
Aplastic anemia	+	−
Splenic rupture	+	−
Jaundice (age >25 years)	++	++
Guillain-Barré syndrome	+	++
Encephalitis*	++	+/−
Pneumonitis*	+/−	+
Myocarditis*	+	−
B-cell lymphoma	+	−
Agammaglobulinemia	+	−

++, Common; +, less common; +/−, uncommon; −, not observed.

*Can occur without the mononucleosis syndrome.

LABORATORY FINDINGS

Antibody Responses

By week three of a mononucleosis caused by primary EBV infection, an heterophile antibody response will occur in approximately 85 percent of patients. The test is called the monospot test and may be falsely negative, especially in young children.[36,48]

The infection of B cells results in their production of a variety of antibodies against uninvolved infectious agents. The B-cell clones expanded, non-specifically, result in antibodies against *Chlamydia*, *Borrelia burgdorferi*, the yellow fever virus, and many other infectious agents. If the patient's febrile illness is considered a fever of unknown origin, diagnostic conclusions may be misleading. A variety of other antibodies against antigens that are not those of infectious agents also are produced because of polyclonal B-cell activation. These include antiplatelet, anti–red cell (anti-i cold agglutinin), and antinuclear antibodies.

At the time clinical disease is evident, both immunoglobulin (Ig) G and IgM antibodies to Epstein-Barr virus capsid antigen (VCA) usually are detectable. Later, antibody to early antigen (EA) develops. A small proportion of individuals will also have developed antibody to EBNA-1 on presentation. However, usually EBNA-1 antibody does not appear until the recovery phase of the illness. For those patients suspected of having infectious mononucleosis but who do not develop heterophile antibody, detection of IgG and IgM antibody to VCA with the absence of EBNA-1 antibody leads to the diagnosis.[49] A real-time positive polymerase chain reaction (PCR) is sometimes useful.[50]

Reactive Lymphocytosis

Expansion of cytotoxic T lymphocytes produces lymphocytosis. Reactive lymphocytes are larger than the lymphocytes normally found in the blood (Fig. 82–1). They may have a vacuolated cytoplasm, lobulated and eccentrically placed nucleus, and a cell membrane that often is indented by neighboring erythrocytes. A more darkly staining peripheral cytoplasm, called "skirting," occurs. Reactive lymphocytes are a hematologic hallmark of infectious mononucleosis, but they are not always found[29] and are not pathognomonic. They also are found in CMV infection, roseola (caused by human herpes virus-6), viral hepatitis, toxoplasmosis, rubella, mumps, and drug reactions.

Sheets of lymphocytes are noted on a stained slide preparation of tonsillar exudate. The immunophenotype of lymphocytes in mononucleosis syndromes assessed by multiparametric flow cytometry has confirmed that lymphocytosis results from CD8+ T cells. CD4+ T

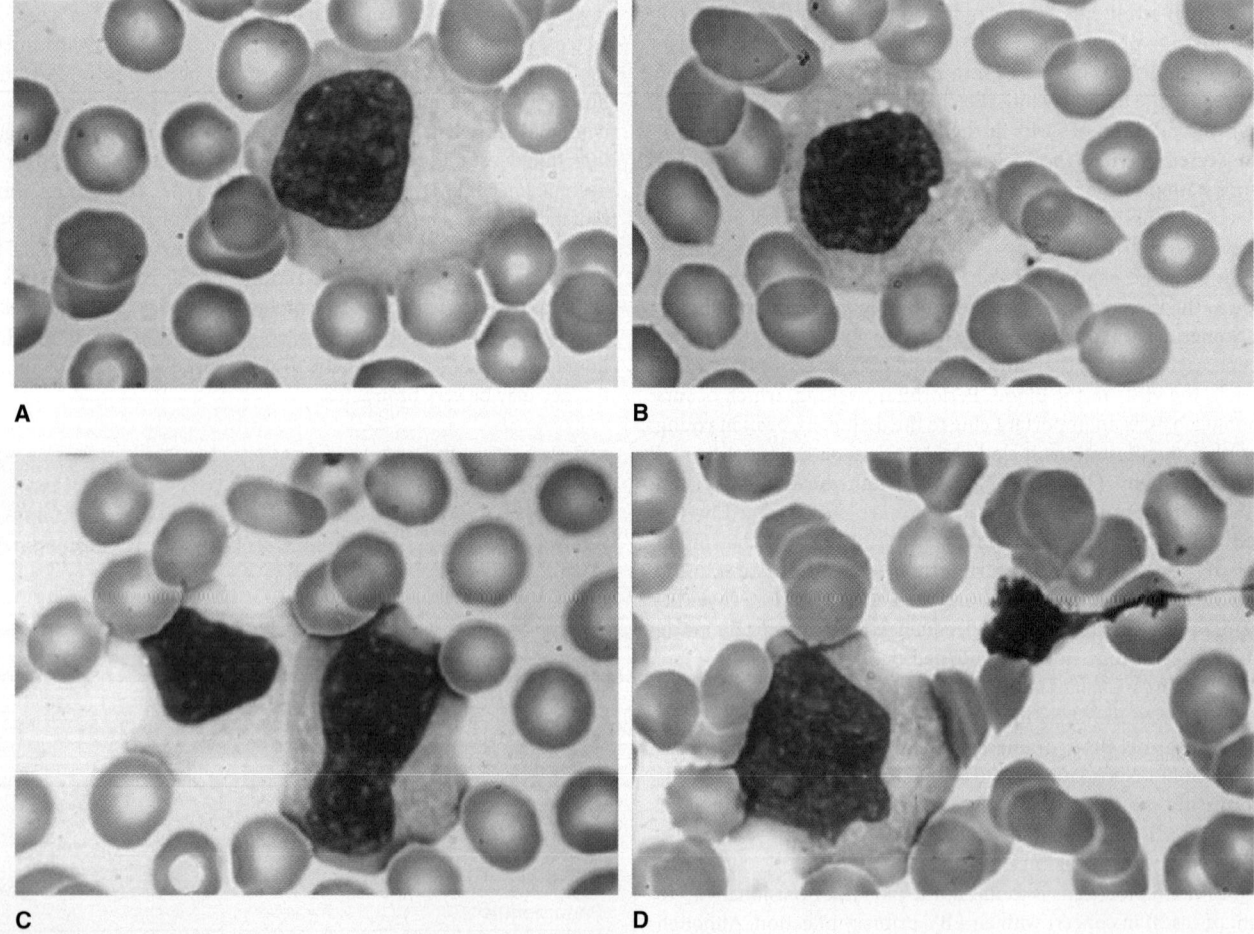

A **B** **C** **D**

Figure 82–1. A-D. Blood films from patients with Epstein-Barr virus–induced mononucleosis. These reactive lymphocytes exhibit the characteristic changes seen in patients with infectious mononucleosis: large lymphocytes with abundant cytoplasm. The cytoplasmic margin often spreads around (is indented by) neighboring red cells and the margin may take on a densely basophilic coloration (skirting). This type of reactive T lymphocyte may be seen in a variety of diseases and is not a specific change but is characteristic and helpful in pointing to the diagnosis in concert with other characteristic clinical findings. (*Reproduced with permission from Lichtman's Atlas of Hematology, www.accessmedicine.com.*)

cells and B cells are not increased. In EBV mononucleosis, the notable populations increased are CD8+CD57− and CD3+γδ+ T cells.[51] If β-streptococcal infection accompanies the EBV infection segmented neutrophils may be present in the tonsillar exudate.

Other Blood Test Abnormalities

Liver function abnormalities are common, especially elevated serum alkaline phosphatase and γ-aminotransferase. There is no or only slight elevation of bilirubin. Studies in Israel have found a higher frequency of hyperbilirubinemia (15 percent), a lower incidence of leukocytosis (46 percent), and elevated liver enzymes (58 percent) than previously reported. The differences may be geographical or genetic.[29]

COURSE AND PROGNOSIS

Complications of Epstein-Barr Virus Mononucleosis

Hematologic Virtually all subjects with acute mononucleosis develop a mildly decreased platelet count (see Table 82–2). More-severe hematologic complications occur infrequently, but include severe immune thrombocytopenia with petechiae, immune hemolytic anemia, immune-mediated granulocytopenia, and aplastic anemia.[52–60] Uncommonly, the splenomegaly that accompanies the lymphoid proliferation accentuates an underlying, previously undiagnosed, hereditary spherocytosis.[60] Splenic rupture is estimated to occur in 1 to 5 per 1000 cases. It is the leading cause of death from EBV mononucleosis.[61,62] Avoidance of athletic activities is prudent until the signs of the disease have disappeared and the spleen has returned to normal size.[62]

Neurologic Neurologic complication include Guillain-Barré syndrome, acute encephalitis, acute disseminated encephalomyelitis (Alice-in-Wonderland syndrome), acute cerebellar ataxia, viral meningitis, transverse myelitis, and cranial nerve palsies.[57,58,63–65] There is evidence that antibody to gangliosides plays a role in the pathogenesis of Guillain-Barré syndrome Neurologic complications may occur in the absence of clinical mononucleosis. Diagnosis of EBV-induced neurologic disease requires obtaining specific antibodies to EBV (see "Antibody Responses" above) and a positive PCR for EBV in the cerebrospinal fluid.[63] Neurologic disease can be associated with primary infection, reactivated infection or chronic EBV infection.[63] Table 82–2 lists other complications.

Chronic Fatigue Fatigue is a very prominent feature of acute infectious mononucleosis. Most recover from this fatigue fairly quickly but a few remain fatigued for a very long period of time. The source of this fatigue is not certain but there is evidence that dysfunction of the midbrain plays a role.[68,69] Furthermore, there are genetic factors that are present in those who remain fatigued. Limited information suggests improvement in some with antiviral treatment.[69]

Multiple Sclerosis There are reports indicating that EBV infection is linked to the development of multiple sclerosis.[70,71] Further studies to clarify which molecular mechanisms link the immune response to a natural infection of humans with EBV to the subsequent development of chronic inflammatory damage to the CNS are required to explain this relationship

Systemic Lupus Erythematosus and Rheumatoid Arthritis There are epidemiologic links between previous infection with EBV and development of systemic lupus erythematosus (SLE).[72] Not unexpectedly, virtually everyone with SLE has had previous infection with EBV. Therefore, the link may be fortuitous. Alternatively, a history of infection with EBV might lead to induction of autoimmunity.[73,74] There has also been a suggested relationship between increased viral load in rheumatoid arthritis leading to expansion of CD8+ cells and its consequences.[75]

Chronic Progressive Epstein-Barr Virus Infections, T-Cell or Natural Killer–Cell Lymphoproliferation, Lymphoma, and Hemophagocytic Syndrome Chronic EBV infection is a rare outcome of primary EBV infection, notable in persons with an immunodeficiency state.[76,77] In chronic EBV infection, fever, marrow hypoplasia, interstitial pneumonia, hepatosplenomegaly, persistent hepatitis often to the point of hepatic failure, lymphadenitis, and uveitis are frequent clinical manifestations. These findings may persist for months or years and eventuate in a high fatality rate.[75] EBV antibodies may be very elevated (VCA in excess of 1:5120, anti-EA greater than 1:640) but with no detectable EBNA-1 antibody. A persistently elevated blood PCR for EBV is a feature. The more-severe form of this manifestation may evolve into a natural killer (NK)- or T-cell lymphoproliferative disease that ranges from chronic to fulminant.[78] Alternatively, EBV hemophagocytic syndrome may develop. The latter is a severe multiorgan, inflammatory disease provoked by massive cytokine elaboration. In some case, clonal proliferation induced by EBV develops (Chap. 71).[78–81]

OTHER EPSTEIN-BARR VIRUS–ASSOCIATED DISEASE PROCESSES

Neoplastic Potential of Epstein-Barr Virus

EBV was the first human tumor virus identified[82] from the cultured cells of a patient with African Burkitt lymphoma. EBV can confer unlimited proliferative potential of infected B lymphocytes in culture.[83] EBV has since been associated with tumors other than Burkitt lymphoma, including some patients with Hodgkin lymphoma (Chap. 97). Although proof of causality still eludes investigators, there is an intriguing relationship between EBV and Hodgkin lymphoma.[84–87] EBV is detectable in the neoplastic B cells (Reed-Sternberg cells) of a significant percent of patients with Hodgkin lymphoma. The etiologic role of EBV in this setting is unknown.[84–87]

There is also a relationship between EBV and lymphoma in immune-deficient individuals including the posttransplantation lymphoproliferative disease (PTLD).[88] Recipient PTLD is a more serious problem than donor PTLD[89] and investigators avoid certain immunosuppressive programs if there is a risk of PTLD.[90] Use of positron emission tomography helps determine who of those at risk for PTLD have evidence for disease.[91] X-chromosome–linked lymphoproliferative disease,[92] T-cell and NK-cell lymphomas that follow chronic EBV infection,[93–95] nasopharyngeal carcinoma in patients in the Far East,[96] the latter disease generating efforts to develop a vaccine,[97] leiomyoma and leiomyosarcoma in patients with HIV infection or immunodeficiency posttransplantation,[98] and a small fraction of cases of gastric carcinoma[99] are each associated with EBV infection (Table 82–4). In three types of lymphomas, Burkitt, Hodgkin, and PTLD, the cell that mutates to produce the clonal disease is a germinal center B cell with a circular viral genome in the tumor cells that expresses the EBV-encoded latent genes.[100]

In the case of PTLD, the most characteristic clinical setting involves an EBV seronegative person receiving an organ from an EBV seropositive donor.[89] EBV is latent in the B lymphocytes of the transplanted marrow or solid organ. Immunosuppression allows reactivation of the latent virus. Because basiliximab, calcineurin inhibitor, sirolimus, and glucocorticoids seem to increase the frequency of PTLD, that regimen is avoided where the potential for PTLD is present.[90] Because the recipient is not immune, there is no T-cell response and the B cells may proliferate unchecked, sometimes eventuating in PTLD. In the EBV-seronegative recipient who develops PTLD posttransplantation, this disease usually develops within the first posttransplantation year

TABLE 82–4. Special Problems with Epstein-Barr Virus or Cytomegalovirus Infection

Epstein-Barr Virus	Cytomegalovirus
Rare congenital infection[129,130]	Congenital infection[110]
Chronic progressive mononucleosis[65–67,72–74]	Posttransplant primary infection[114,115]
Hemophagocytic syndrome[77,78]	Graft-versus-host disease association[143]
XX-linked B cell lymphoma[92]	Transfusion-related infection[144]
Posttransplant lymphoprolifera-tive disease[88–91]	*Aspergillus* and/or *Pneumocystis* infection[122,123]
T or NK lymphoproliferative disease[94,95]	
African Burkitt lymphoma[5]	
Approximately 20% of Burkitt lymphoma in the United States[5]	
Approximately 35% of Hodgkin lymphoma[84–87]	
Nasopharyngeal carcinoma[96,97]	
Approximately 5% of gastric carcinoma[99]	
Leiomyoma and leiomyosar-coma in HIV or immunosup-pressed patients[98]	
Oral hairy leukoplakia[102]	

and often within the first few months. The abnormally proliferating cell almost always is a B cell and the process at an early stage may be monoclonal. In the initial states, the disease may respond to lowering of immunosuppressive medications. Although administration of anti-viral prophylaxis seems to lower the frequency of development of the disease, once the disease develops, antiviral agents are ineffective.[101] When disease develops, in addition to reduction in immunosuppression, administration of anti-CD20 therapy with rituximab is used. Occasionally, PTLD occurs in a person who is EBV antibody-positive pretransplantation. When this occurs, the onset is usually greater than 1 year posttransplantation.

In young males with an X-linked lymphoproliferative syndrome, primary EBV infection leads to unabated B-cell proliferation and evolution into a frank B-cell lymphoma, the so-called Duncan syndrome.[92] These young males do not develop a T-cell response and hence do not develop mononucleosis. Although control of this effect of EBV infection by treatment with antiviral agents and/or chemotherapy has been attempted, the Duncan syndrome usually is fatal.

Oral hairy leukoplakia, a characteristic white lingual lesion with hairy projections, occurs in patients with HIV infection. It is caused by EBV infection of the lingual epithelium.[102]

FUTURE THERAPEUTIC APPROACHES TO EPSTEIN-BARR VIRUS INFECTION AND NEOPLASIA

Because of the severe consequences of EBV infection, several approaches to preventing or treating these disorders are underway, such as an EBV vaccine,[103] adoptive transfer of activated cytotoxic T cells,[104] and the development of peptides that inhibit viral replication.[105]

● CYTOMEGALOVIRUS MONONUCLEOSIS

HISTORY

The early description of CMV-related disease was that of an uncommon congenital syndrome with abnormal liver function and thrombocytopenia leading to petechiae.[106] Subsequently, it was recognized that previously healthy young children with a primary infection with CMV[107] had prolonged abnormal liver function, hepatosplenomegaly, lymphocytosis, and thrombocytopenia. Later, primary CMV infection was linked to a febrile mononucleosis syndrome.[108]

EPIDEMIOLOGY

In the developing world, CMV infects the majority of individuals by the age of 5 or 6 years. Three factors contribute to this. In those societies, mothers are still in their teen years when they deliver their children. These young women have active CMV virus in their cervix that has persisted since they were younger. The cervical virus is aspirated by the child during the birthing process. Transmission to the newborn also occurs through breast milk. In addition, all of these young children play together when they are young and virus is transmitted readily to those who have avoided earlier infection. Infection at the time of birth from the cervical virus or shortly after birth from breast milk or another child does not lead to any known consequences. However, congenital infection occurs in all populations. For less-than-clear reasons, a seropositive mother may deliver a child who has become infected in utero.[109] In the developing world, most often it occurs in the babies whose mothers are seropositive before they become pregnant and the disease in the new born is not clinically obvious at birth.[109] These children, who have asymptomatic congenital infection, may develop unilateral or bilateral hearing deficits later. Congenital CMV infection in the babies of seropositive women and may account for a significant number of people with hearing loss.[109]

In the developed world, first children often have parents who have not had CMV infection. If primary infection occurs in the mother at or near the time of impregnation in anticipation of the second child, severe congenital infection may develop.[110] It is not clear which of the several possible factors contribute to why that child acquires congenital CMV infection and more study is required to lead to intelligent management decisions.

Presence of CMV in oral secretions and in urine in children living together in families where there is known CMV has been recognized for many years.[107] The source of the virus is not entirely clear. It is not always certain whether these children acquired infection at birth or from breast milk and they continue to have active infection or whether it is resulting from transmission among children. The latter is suspected but not proven.

It is strongly suspected that when a CMV-infected child comes in contact with a CMV-seronegative grandparent, primary infection in that grandparent may occur. This can be associated with CMV disease in the older person, although the development of disease associated with the infection is uncommon.[18] Very little is known about the risk of CMV-infected semen in those undergoing heterosexual intercourse. However, there is a very high frequency of CMV infection in young homosexual males. Almost all active homosexual young men are seropositive to CMV by age 20 years, which contrasts to only 20 percent of heterosexual young men. Presumably that 20 percent of heterosexual men were infected as children.

CLINICAL MANIFESTATIONS

In most cases, the new infection with CMV is clinically silent. However, some newly infected individuals will develop high fever (40°C often), weight loss, and associated malaise and myalgia.[111] Abnormal liver function and a palpable spleen similar to that seen with EBV occur. A left shift in the differential white count may occur initially, evidenced by a higher proportion of band neutrophils. The incidence of lymphadenopathy is much higher in the young then in the older person with primary CMV. Infection occurs in the older individual because they have not been infected during their younger years (Tables 82–2 and 82–3 list additional clinical and laboratory findings). Because no classic manifestation, such as severe exudative pharyngitis, develops, CMV is not considered in the differential diagnosis. Instead, it is assumed that the patient has a bacterial infection and antibiotics are administered. How frequently this occurs is uncertain but administration of a β-lactam antibiotic may be associated with development of a rash and the mistaken impression that the recipient is allergic to penicillin. Because the disease occurs in the older population, including those older than age 50 years, the causes of fever of unknown origin often are pursued in an expensive evaluation prior to the diagnosis. A number of the laboratory and physical findings raise many diagnostic possibilities. Development of antinuclear factor and thrombocytopenia (Table 82–5) often erroneously leads to the diagnosis of a collagen vascular disease. The presence of splenomegaly raises the question of lymphoma.

LABORATORY FINDINGS

The cell that becomes infected initially is not the B lymphocyte but a cell in the monocyte–macrophage lineage and it is that cell or cells to which the T-lymphocyte responds.[112,113] Lymphocytosis that develops is indistinguishable from that of EBV-induced disease. In some patients, neutrophilia with band forms occurs early in the infection. In addition, because the incubation period is 30 to 40 days, IgG and IgM antibodies to CMV have already developed when the disease first becomes manifest. The PCR of a blood sample for CMV usually is positive, and CMV can be isolated from specimens of urine or saliva. Liver function abnormalities (see Tables 82–2 and 82–3) include bilirubin elevation. Jaundice may occur in up to 25 percent of these ill patients.[18] Prolonged illness and severe fatigue is quite common in this subset of ill individuals.

TABLE 82–5. Laboratory Findings in Mononucleosis

Complication	Epstein-Barr Virus	Cytomegalovirus
Heterophile antibody	+++	–
Lymphocytosis	+++	++
Reactive lymphocytes	+++	++
Abnormal liver function	++	++
Antinuclear factor	+	+
Cold agglutinins	+	+
Cryoglobulins	+	+
Decreased platelets	++	+

+++, Characteristic; ++, common; +, occurs.

COMPLICATIONS

Hemolytic anemia and thrombocytopenia occur in primary CMV infection and are other findings that may lead the clinician initially to consider a diagnosis of lymphoma. There are a variety of pathogenic factors, which explain these hematologic changes. The most prominent neurologic complication is Guillain-Barré syndrome and, less commonly, transverse myelitis and aseptic meningitis (see Table 82–3). Antibody that develops to CMV-infected cells cross reacts with GM_2 antigen that may explain the development of Guillain-Barré syndrome.[66,67] This antibody can be absorbed with CMV-infected fibroblasts but not by uninfected fibroblasts.

Because it is not the B cell that is the target of infection, but the monocyte–macrophage lineage,[112,113] evolution to unrestrained B-cell replication, lymphoma, and PTLD do not occur.

CYTOMEGALOVIRUS IN TRANSPLANTATION

CMV does not predispose to hematologic malignancy. However, it plays a critical role in all of the transplantation settings, with some very similar findings in lung and allogeneic hematopoietic stem cell transplants. It is rare in autologous hematopoietic stem cell transplantations, but can occur and be a serious infection (Chap. 23 discusses CMV infection in allogeneic hematopoietic stem cell transplantation).

In all solid-organ transplantations, there are three potential types of infection that can occur because of CMV.[114-116] The monocyte-macrophage cells in all solid organs, for example, heart, kidney, pancreas, and liver of CMV-seropositive individuals, harbor CMV that can be reactivated. The CMV-seronegative recipient who receives an organ from a CMV-positive donor can develop a primary infection when the CMV reactivates from the donor organ. Because this occurs when the recipient is receiving immunosuppression, this is the most serious clinical problem.[115,116] The classic situation occurs when a parent, who is older and has developed infection in the past, donates a kidney or a segment of their liver containing CMV to their child.[116] A second possibility is that the CMV in the seropositive recipient, even when the donor is CMV-seronegative, can be reactivated. Because it is the recipient's own latent CMV that is reactivated, the clinical manifestations of infection usually are mild or absent.[116] The third occurs when both the donor and the recipient are both CMV-seropositive. Clinical disease can sometimes occur, but its severity is difficult to predict. Clinical disease consists of fever, liver function abnormalities, and inflammatory bowel changes. Prior to the availability of antiviral agents, most patients who developed primary CMV infection did well.[116] In solid-organ transplantation patients, in the majority of situations, immunosuppressive therapy starts with the transplantation and then is maintained for prolonged periods.

CMV pulmonary problems occur mainly in lung and allogeneic hematopoietic stem cell transplantations. One contributing factor is that an ideal *in vitro* growth system for CMV is pulmonary macrophages obtained by bronchoalveolar lavage (BAL) from humans.[117] That raises the question, does the CMV grow well in the pulmonary macrophage *in vivo*? Does latency in the macrophage–monocyte cellular system from which it reactivates play an important role in lung and allogeneic hematopoietic stem cell transplant patient populations?[118-120] It is in that setting that the infected macrophage is either occurring in a foreign tissue, the lung transplant, or is being seen as foreign by the allogeneic hematopoietic stem cell cellular derivatives.

In patients receiving an allogeneic hematopoietic stem cell transplant, the immunosuppressive regimen is of relatively short duration, unless the patient develops graft-versus-host disease compared to that for solid-organ recipients. If both the recipient and the donor are CMV-seronegative, posttransplantation, CMV infection does not develop.[121] In the allogeneic hematopoietic stem cell transplantation setting, if the recipient is CMV-seronegative and the donor is positive for CMV, infection occurs often, but not in everyone. Although pulmonary involvement is most common, the retina and gastrointestinal tract also can be involved. Because the donor cells are not exposed to immunosuppressive medication, other factors need to come into play for CMV infection to become manifest. The other possible matches with respect to CMV are that the recipient is CMV-seropositive and the donor is negative, or both the recipient and the donor are seropositive. If the recipient is seropositive and has been repeatedly exposed to therapeutic regimens in the process of treatment for the recipient's underlying disease, reactivation of CMV could occur before the recipient undergoes transplantation. It would be a "self-vaccination" process for some. One needs to consider whether serious infection with CMV is a major problem in allogeneic hematopoietic stem cell transplantations, or whether it is the interaction between the virus, the pulmonary macrophage, and the host.[117-120] CMV continues to be a problem, but there are now preliminary studies of a CMV DNA vaccine that are promising.

Two approaches have been taken to manage CMV infection for solid-organ recipients. The first is to provide anti-CMV antiviral agents when the donor, the recipient, or both are CMV-seropositive. Antiviral prophylaxis is initiated at transplantation and continued for up to 120 days thereafter. The second is to provide CMV antiviral prophylaxis only for those situations where the donor is seropositive and the recipient is seronegative. For other situations, weekly monitoring for CMV by PCR is done. If that result is positive, the subject is treated for approximately 1 month. In those who undergo specific monitoring, fewer people receive anti-CMV antiviral drugs and for those who do, the duration is shorter. It also makes the best sense as those recipients who were seropositive pre-solid-organ transplantation have a very low frequency of disease.[116]

For solid-organ transplantations, clinical illness caused by CMV and rejection of the transplanted organ are difficult to differentiate. Fever develops in the recipient when they begin to mount an immune response. Because the cells in the transplanted organ are now "more foreign" than they were prior to virus reactivation, an immune response occurs directed at the infected monocyte. Although both hepatic and gastrointestinal changes occur, mononucleosis usually does not. There is the potential for rejection of the donated organ. Reactivation of one's own latent CMV in a solid-organ recipient does not lead to a problem.[116] On occasion, reactivation of CMV in the donor organ in a previously seropositive recipient can lead to illness.

Other infectious problems develop in solid-organ recipients. It is proposed that reactivation of the CMV in the macrophage system inhibits the protective function of that system. In the lung where inhalation of potentially infectious agents occurs continuously, new infection can develop because of impairment of the protective action of the macrophages or the neutrophils.[122,123] In addition, a number of organisms can, in the case of renal transplantation, be transplanted with the kidney. Besides the viruses discussed above, these can include bacteria, yeast, and parasites, such as *Strongyloides* sp.

When fever develops there is a tendency for the transplantation physician to increase immunosuppression under the assumption that rejection is occurring. If the fever is a result of development of primary infection with CMV, the immunosuppressive therapy leads to permanent interference with development of posttransplantation immunity to the CMV. That, in turn, leads to life-long continued problems with CMV infection.

One of the other confusing features for the transplantation physician has stemmed from the common practice to provide ganciclovir prophylaxis to prevent CMV infection posttransplantation to everyone (see above). Those who are seronegative, receive an organ from a seropositive donor, and receive ganciclovir that suppresses reactivation

from that organ. When the ganciclovir is discontinued, CMV sometimes reactivates from that organ and primary infection can develop several months later. When this happens, patients present with fever and diarrhea and often have a negative blood CMV by PCR. CMV-induced bowel disease develops because the colonic mucosal cells, as noted previously, are targets for primary infection and virus replication. However, because the blood PCR for CMV is negative, the diagnosis eludes the transplant clinician until colonoscopy and biopsy are carried out.

There are other clinical settings where CMV may play a role. There are hints that HIV patients with pneumocystis pneumonia who also have CMV secretions do less well than those who simply have pneumocystis pneumonia.[124] In the intensive care unit, CMV reactivation may occur in the very ill nonimmunosuppressed patient. It is uncertain what role the virus plays in this setting.

● PRIMARY HIV INFECTION MONONUCLEOSIS

An acute syndrome develops very frequently at the time of development of primary infection with HIV.[124-127] The frequency with which the HIV mononucleosis syndrome develops is uncertain, but for this discussion the difference in features is more important. The acute retroviral syndrome must be recognized for both the patient's health and the public health. Fever is sudden in onset, followed by sore throat, lymphadenopathy, tonsillar hypertrophy, painful oral ulcerations, conjunctivitis, and rash. Nausea, vomiting, and diarrhea also occur. Leucopenia, thrombocytopenia, a relative increase in band neutrophils, and a small proportion of reactive lymphocytes usually can be identified on the blood film. Although absolute lymphocytosis is uncommon, the syndrome is referred to as *HIV mononucleosis*. Uncommonly, patients may also develop a heterophile antibody.[126] Among a group of 563 heterophile antibody-positive patient samples retrospectively tested for HIV-1 RNA and p24 antigen, approximately 1 percent had evidence of primary HIV-1 infection.[126] In another study, none of 132 cases was positive.[127] Because in this situation, anti-HIV antibody response has not yet developed, HIV load in the blood should be measured by PCR to make a diagnosis of HIV infection. Usually, viral load is very high (greater than 50,000 viral particles per milliliter of blood). Early treatment may reduce the incidence of HIV-1 complications (Chap. 81). Acute HIV-1 infection may be particularly contagious.[128] Discussion of the findings with the patient may prevent transmission to a sexual partner.[124,128]

● OTHER AGENTS LINKED TO A MONONUCLEOSIS SYNDROME

Human herpes virus-6 occasionally has been associated with a mononucleosis-type syndrome as has metapneumonia virus (see Table 82–1).[129,130] Hepatitis A and rubella virus infection have produced the typical blood lymphocytic changes. Pharyngitis is not a prominent feature in patients infected with *T. gondii*. Lymphocytosis is mild, and liver functions are normal even when the liver is enlarged. Usually, toxoplasmosis presents as posterior cervical lymphadenopathy. In the United States, exposure to oocysts from cat feces is the primary route of infection. In other countries, ingestion of partially cooked meat, especially from sheep, is a route of infection. The IgM immunofluorescent antibody test for *T. gondii* is useful in diagnosing the disease.

Cat scratch disease, *Corynebacterium diphtheriae* pharyngitis, infection with brucellosis, or lymphoma can be mistaken for mononucleosis. Other, as yet unidentified, agents probably produce the classic syndrome as laboratory studies for all of the known infectious agents, including EBV and CMV, are negative in a small percentage of typical mononucleosis cases.

DIFFERENTIAL DIAGNOSIS OF MONONUCLEOSIS SYNDROMES

At a very young age, EBV and CMV mimic each other. They present as one of the many febrile illnesses in young children.[15] The difference here is that the children with CMV present with abnormal liver function tests.[107] The importance of documenting primary CMV is that with this information, one can develop a strategy to prevent transmission to a pregnant woman when she might not be immune. By so doing, a severe congenital CMV infection may be avoided.[110] The latter possibility is much more likely in the developed world, because only 20 to 30 percent of women have been infected with CMV before they reach reproductive age. In the older teenage child, both EBV and CMV may cause the mononucleosis syndrome but EBV is far more common. If exudative pharyngitis or lymphadenopathy is present then it is most likely to be EBV. If the patient has intraoral ulcers tests for HIV should be done.

In the sexually active teen, both EBV and HIV testing should be done but CMV remains a possibility.[108] Simultaneous infection with EBV and HIV has occurred, although this, too, is very uncommon. Presence of heterophile antibody strongly supports EBV, although these have been reported in HIV.[127] In adults in their 30s or 40s, mononucleosis more likely results from infection with CMV than EBV because almost all individuals have been infected with EBV by age 25 years. Furthermore, absence of exudative pharyngitis points to CMV, but HIV also should be considered in this age group. Patients infected with either CMV or HIV can present with blood neutrophilia with an increased proportion of band neutrophils. Rash or aseptic meningitis is more common in patients infected with HIV than CMV. In the middle-aged patient, primary CMV infection is by far the most important possibility, although the unusual individual who has escaped infection with EBV earlier in life may present with EBV with clinical manifestations similar to patients with primary CMV infection at that age.[18,40,41]

THERAPY

For the majority of patients with primary CMV or EBV infection, treatment is supportive. Salicylates or other analgesics are appropriate for control of fever, headache, and sore throat. Contact sports should be avoided until the spleen has returned to normal size because splenic rupture can occur in the first few weeks after diagnosis. The vast majority of subjects improve and have resolution of most symptoms. Almost half of patients recovering from EBV mononucleosis still feel fatigued at 60 days and a small percent at 6 months. Severe fatigue can persist after CMV mononucleosis as well.

Antiviral therapy may be considered in special settings for treatment of EBV mononucleosis. The nucleoside analogue acyclovir blocks EBV replication by inhibition of viral DNA polymerase and can prevent viral shedding from the oropharynx.[131,132] However, acyclovir has little if any effect on the course of mononucleosis, presumably because the disease at that point results from the immunopathologic process and not viral proliferation. Antiviral therapy may be useful in chronic aggressive EBV infection and in EBV infection posttransplantation.

Glucocorticoids have been used for management of specific complications. Their specific benefit is difficult to determine because glucocorticoids often are started late in the clinical course, when immunologic reaction to infection is leading to improvement. One carefully controlled trial showed little benefit from glucocorticoids in EBV mononucleosis, and the treated group did less well at 30 days than the

placebo group.[133] Nevertheless, treatment with glucocorticoid is reasonable when the tonsils are touching in the midline when airway obstruction is imminent. Prednisone 40 to 60 mg/day is given for 7 to 10 days, then rapidly tapered once a clinical response is achieved. Urgent tonsillectomy and adenoidectomy may be required.[134,135] The same prednisone regimen is used for severe immune hemolytic anemia, severe symptomatic immune thrombocytopenia, neurologic complications, pancreatitis, and myocarditis.

The same dose of glucocorticoid has been used for the hematologic or neurologic complications of CMV mononucleosis. Results of ganciclovir 5 mg/kg/day given intravenously for 14 days for severe CMV mononucleosis occasionally have been dramatic. However, ganciclovir is seldom used because of the potential long-term risk to spermatogenesis (aspermia) or potentially on female fertility. Thus, when the disease appears to be self-limited, many physicians do not treat it. Therapy that already was started is stopped after a few weeks. Antiretroviral therapy has been suggested for severe HIV primary disease.

Acyclovir use for other manifestations of EBV infection not resulting from host response but from a high titer of EBV replication, such as oral hairy leukoplakia of AIDS, rapidly resolves lingual lesions.[136] However, treatment with acyclovir does not appear to be effective for the carrier state.[137]

MONONUCLEOSIS IN PREGNANCY

CYTOMEGALOVIRUS AND EPSTEIN-BARR VIRUS INFECTION

For CMV, immunity does not necessarily protect against congenital infection.[109] CMV viruria at birth occurs in babies of mothers known to be seropositive before they became pregnant. Some viruric children whose mother is seropositive at conception go on to develop unilateral or bilateral hearing loss. The reason for the susceptibility to this type of infection in the apparently immune mother is not clear. If primary CMV infection occurs during gestation the baby can have very severe disease. Microcephaly, mental retardation, cataracts, hepatosplenomegaly, and fetal loss or postnatal death have can occur.[110] When EBV mononucleosis occurs during pregnancy, severe abnormalities similar to those as described for CMV have occurred (see Table 82–4).[138,139] Ganciclovir for congenital CMV infection in a very young child is being studied for those who are viruric at birth. Antiviral therapy with famciclovir or valacyclovir has been used for EBV primary infection during pregnancy, but the number of patients treated is too small to draw conclusions.

HIV INFECTION

Primary infection with HIV during pregnancy may not be recognized because HIV antibody is absent early in infection and the antibody screening process is performed at the first prenatal visit. If suspicion of HIV infection is raised during pregnancy and the antibody test for HIV is negative, then viral load should be measured. If positive, antiretroviral therapy for the mother to prevent HIV transmission to the fetus or newborn is indicated.[140]

TOXOPLASMA INFECTION

T. gondii producing primary infection during pregnancy can lead to congenital abnormalities. Although no controlled trials are available, treatment of the mother with pyrimethamine plus sulfonamides or spiramycin may eradicate parasites from the infant and the placenta.[141,142]

REFERENCES

1. Pfeiffer E: Drüsenfieber. *Jahrbuch für Kinderheilkunde* 23:257, 1885.
2. Sprunt TP, Evans FA: Mononucleosis in reaction to acute infections ("infectious mononucleosis"). *Johns Hopkins Bull* 31:410, 1920.
3. Paul JR, Bunnell WW: The presence of heterophile antibodies in infectious mononucleosis. *Am J Med Sci* 183:91, 1932.
4. Davidson I, Walker PH: The nature of the heterophile antibodies in infectious mononucleosis. *Am J Clin Pathol* 5:455, 1935.
5. Henle G, Henle W, Diehl V: Relation of Burkitt's tumor associated herpes type virus to infectious mononucleosis. *Proc Natl Acad Sci U S A* 59:94, 1968.
6. Niederman JC, McCollum RW, Henle G, et al: Infectious mononucleosis: Clinical manifestations in relation to EB virus antibodies. *JAMA* 203:205, 1968.
7. Evans AS, Niederman JC, McCollum RW: Seroepidemiologic studies of infectious mononucleosis with EB virus. *N Engl J Med* 279:1121, 1968.
8. Sawyer RN, Evans AS, Niederman JC, et al: Prospective studies of a group of Yale University freshman: I. Occurrence of infectious mononucleosis. *J Infect Dis* 123:263, 1971.
9. Infectious mononucleosis and its relationship to EB virus antibody. A joint investigation by university health physicians and P.H.L.S. laboratories. *Br Med J* 4:643, 1971.
10. Hoagland RJ: The clinical manifestations of infectious mononucleosis: A report of 200 cases. *Am J Med Sci* 240:55, 1960.
11. Hoagland RJ: The incubation period of infectious mononucleosis. *Am J Public Health* 54:1699, 1964.
12. Tanner J, Weis J, Fearon D, et al: Epstein-Barr virus gp350/220 binding to the B lymphocyte C3d receptor mediates adsorption, capping, and endocytosis. *Cell* 50:203, 1987.
13. Söderberg-Nauclér C, Fish KN, Nelson JA: Reactivation of latent human cytomegalovirus by allogeneic stimulation of blood cells from healthy donors. *Cell* 91:119, 1997.
14. Tomkinson BE, Wagner DK, Nelson DL, Sullivan JL: Activated lymphocytes during acute Epstein-Barr virus infection. *J Immunol* 139:3802, 1987.
15. Lajo A, Borque C, Del Castillo F, Martin-Ancel A: Mononucleosis caused by Epstein-Barr virus and Cytomegalovirus in children: A comparative study of 124 cases. *Pediatr Infect Dis J* 13:56, 1994.
16. Porter DP, Wimberly I, Benyesh-Melnick M: Prevalence of antibodies to EB virus and other herpes viruses. *JAMA* 209:1675, 1969.
17. Ross SA, Arora N, Novak Z, et al: Cytomegalovirus reinfections in healthy seroimmune women. *J Infect Dis* 201:386, 2010.
18. Schmader KE, van der Horst CM, Klotman ME: Epstein-Barr virus and the elderly host. *Rev Infect Dis* 11:64, 1989.
19. Fleisher G, Bolognese R: Epstein-Barr virus infections in pregnancy: A prospective study. *J Pediatr* 104:374, 1984.
20. Istas AS, Demmler GJ, Dobbins JG, Stewart JA: Surveillance for congenital cytomegalovirus disease: A report from the National Congenital Cytomegalovirus Disease Registry. *Clin Infect Dis* 20:665, 1995.
21. Senechal B, Boruchov AM, Reagan JL, et al: Infection of mature monocyte-derived dendritic cells with human cytomegalovirus inhibits stimulation of T-cell proliferation via the release of soluble CD83. *Blood* 103:420, 2004.
22. Hussein K, Tiede C, Maecker-Kolhoff B, Kreipe H: Posttransplant lymphoproliferative disorder in pediatric patients. *Pathobiology* 80:289, 2013.
23. Hochberg D, Souza T, Catalina M, et al: Acute infection with Epstein-Barr virus targets and overwhelms peripheral memory B-cell compartment with resting, latently infected cells. *J Virol* 78:5194, 2004.
24. Hadinoto V, Shapiro M, Greenough TC, et al: On the dynamics of acute EBV infection and the pathogenesis of infectious mononucleosis. *Blood* 111:1420, 2008.
25. McAulay KA, Higgins CD, Macsween KF, et al: HLA class I polymorphisms are associated with development of infectious mononucleosis upon primary EBV infection. *J Clin Invest* 117:3042, 2007.
26. Vollmer-Conner U, Piraino B, Cameron B, et al: Cytokine polymorphisms have a synergistic effect on the acute sickness response to infection. *Clin Infect Dis* 47:1418, 2008.
27. Scherrenburg J, Piriou ER, Nanlohy NM, van Baarle D: Detailed analysis of Epstein-Barr virus specific CD4+ and CD8+ T cell response during infectious mononucleosis. *Clin Exp Immunol* 153:231, 2008.
28. Balfour HH Jr, Odumade OA, Schmeling DO, et al: Behavioral, virologic, and immunologic factors associated with acquisition and severity of primary Epstein-Barr virus infection in university students. *J Infect Dis* 207:80, 2013.
29. Grotto I, Mimouni D, Huerta M, et al: Clinical and laboratory presentation of EBV positive infectious mononucleosis in young adults. *Epidemiol Infect* 131:683, 2003.
30. Macallan DC, Wallace DL, Irvine AJ, et al: Rapid turnover of T cells in acute infectious mononucleosis. *Eur J Immunol* 33:2655, 2003.
31. Williams H, Macsween K, McAulay K, et al: Analysis of immune activation and clinical events in acute infectious mononucleosis. *J Infect Dis* 190:63, 2004.
32. Kusuhara K, Takabayashi A, Ueda K, et al: Breast milk is not a significant source of early Epstein-Barr virus or human herpes 6 infections in infants. A sero-epidemiologic study in two 2 areas of human T cell lymphotropic virus type 1 in Japan. *Microbiol Immunol* 41:309, 1997.
33. Sixbey JW, Shirley P, Chesney PJ, et al: Detection of a second widespread strain of Epstein-Barr virus. *Lancet* 2:76, 1989.
34. Yao QY, Croom-Carter DSG, Tierney RJ, et al: Epidemiology of infection with Epstein-Barr virus types 1 and 2: Lessons from the study of a T cell immunocompromised hemophiliac cohort. *J Virol* 72:4352, 1998.
35. Pichler R, Berg J, Hengtschlager A, et al: Recurrent infectious mononucleosis caused by Epstein-Barr virus with persistent splenomegaly. *Mil Med* 166:733, 2001.
36. Sumaya CV, Ench Y: Epstein-Barr virus infectious mononucleosis. I. Clinical and general laboratory findings. *Pediatrics* 75:1003, 1985.
37. Sumaya CV, Ench Y: Epstein-Barr virus infectious mononucleosis. II. Heterophil antibody and viral-specific responses. *Pediatrics* 75:1011, 1985.
38. Fleisher G, Henle W, Henle G, et al: Primary infection with Epstein-Barr virus in the United States: Clinical and serologic observations. *J Infect Dis* 139:553, 1979.
39. Hickey SM, Strasburger VC: What every pediatrician should know about infectious mononucleosis in adolescents. *Pediatr Clin North Am* 44:1541, 1997.
40. Axelrod P, Finestone AJ: Infectious mononucleosis in older adults. *Am Fam Physician* 42:1599, 1990.
41. Hurwitz CA, Henle W, Henle G, et al: Infectious mononucleosis in patients aged 40 to 72 years: Report of 27 cases, including 3 without heterophile-antibody responses. *Medicine (Baltimore)* 62:256, 1983.
42. Karajannis MA, Hummel M, Anagnostopoulos I, Stein H: Strict lymphotropism of Epstein-Barr virus during acute infectious mononucleosis in non-immunocompromised individuals. *Blood* 89:2856, 1997.
43. Yefenof E, Bakacs T, Einhorn L, et al: Epstein-Barr virus (EBV) receptors, complement receptors and EBV infectibility of different lymphocyte fractions of human peripheral blood: I. Complement receptor distribution and complement binding by separated lymphocyte subpopulations. *Cell Immunol* 35:34, 1978.
44. Drebber U, Kasper HU, Krupacz J: et al: The role of Epstein-Barr virus in acute and chronic hepatitis. *J Hepatol* 44:879, 2006.
45. Levitskaya K, Coram M, Levitsky V, et al: Inhibition of antigen processing by the internal repeat region of the Epstein-Barr Nuclear antigen-1. *Nature* 375:685, 1995.
46. Renn CN, Straff W, Dorfmuller A, et al: Amoxicillin-induced exanthema in young adults with infectious mononucleosis: Demonstration of drug-specific lymphocyte reactivity. *Br J Dermatol* 147:1166, 2002.
47. Haverkos HW, Amsel Z, Drotman DP: Adverse virus-drug interactions. *Rev Infect Dis* 13:697, 1991.
48. Linderholm M, Boman J, Juto P, Linde A: Comparative evaluation of nine kits for rapid diagnosis of infectious mononucleosis and Epstein-Barr virus-specific serology. *J Clin Microbiol* 32:259, 1994.
49. Rea TD, Ashley TL, Russo JE, Buchwald DS: A systematic study of Epstein-Barr virus serologic assays following acute infection. *Am J Clin Pathol* 117:156, 2002.
50. Pitetti RD, Laus S, Wadowsky RM: Clinical evaluation of a quantitative real time polymerase chain reaction assay for diagnosis of primary Epstein-Barr virus infection in children. *Pediatr Infect Dis J* 22:736, 2003.
51. Hudnall SD, Patel JU, Schwab H, Martinez J: Comparative immunophenotypic features of EBV-positive and EBV-negative atypical lymphocytosis. *Cytometry* 55B:22, 2003.
52. Matsukawa Y, Okano M, Ishikawa N, Imasi S: Severe thrombocytopenic purpura associated with primary Epstein-Barr virus infection. *J Infect* 29:107, 1994.
53. Whitelaw F, Brook MG, Kennedy N, Weir WR: Haemolytic anemia complicating Epstein-Barr virus infection. *Br J Clin Pract* 49:212, 1995.
54. Lazarus KH, Baehner RL: Aplastic anemia complicating infectious mononucleosis: A case report and review of the literature. *Pediatrics* 67:907, 1981.
55. Auvin S, Dalle JH, Ganga-Zandzou PS, Ythier H: Is agranulocytosis following infectious mononucleosis caused by autoimmunity? *Pediatr Hematol Oncol* 20:611, 2003.
56. Tanaka M, Kamijo T, Koike T, et al: Specific auto antibodies to platelet glycoprotein in Epstein-Barr virus-associated immune thrombocytopenia. *Int J Hematol* 78:168, 2003.
57. Evans AS: Infectious mononucleosis and related syndromes. *Am J Med Sci* 276:325, 1978.
58. Jones JF: A perspective on Epstein-Barr virus diseases. *Adv Pediatr* 36:307, 1989.
59. Bhaskaran J, Harkness DR: Hereditary spherocytosis unmasked by infectious mononucleosis with autoimmune hemolytic anemia. *J Fla Med Assoc* 67:483, 1980.
60. Taylor JJ: Haemolysis in infectious mononucleosis: Inapparent congenital spherocytosis. *Br Med J* 4:525, 1973.
61. Asgari MM, Begos DG: Spontaneous splenic rupture in infectious mononucleosis: A review. *Yale J Biol Med* 70:175, 1997.
62. Kinderknecht JJ: Infectious mononucleosis and the spleen. *Curr Sports Med Rep* 1:116, 2002.
63. Fujimoto H, Asaoka K, Imaaizumi T, et al: Epstein-Barr virus infections of the central nervous system. *Intern Med* 42:33, 2003.
64. Connelly KP, DeWitt LD: Neurologic complications of infectious mononucleosis. *Pediatr Neurol* 10:181, 1994.
65. Jacobs BC, Rothbarth PH, van der Meche, et al: The spectrum of antecedent infections in Guillain-Barré syndrome. *Neurology* 51:1110, 1998.
66. Hughes RA, Hadden RD, Gregson NA, Smith KJ: Pathogenesis of Guillain-Barré syndrome. *J Neuroimmunol* 100:74, 1999.
67. Ang CW, Lang BC, Laman JD: The Guillain-Barré syndrome, a true case of molecular mimicry. *Trends Immunol* 25:561, 2004.
68. Cameron B, Galbraith S, Zhang Y, et al: Gene expression correlates of post fatigue syndrome after infectious mononucleosis. *J Infect Dis* 196:56, 2007.
69. Lerner AM, Benquai SM, Deeter RG, Fitzgerald JT: Valacyclovir treatment in Epstein-Barr virus subset of chronic fatigue syndrome-36 month follow up. *In Vivo* 21:707, 2007.
70. Thacker EL, Mirzaei F, Ascherio A: Infectious mononucleosis and risk of multiple sclerosis: A meta-analysis. *Ann Neurol* 59:499, 2006.

71. Zaadstra BM, Chorus AM, van Buuren S, et al: Selective association of multiple sclerosis with infectious mononucleosis. *Mult Scler* 14:307, 2008.

72. James JA, Neas BR, Moser KL, et al: Systemic lupus in adults associated with previous Epstein-Barr virus exposure. *Arthritis Rheum* 44:1122, 2001.

73. Harley JB, Harley IT, Guthridge JM, James JA: The curiously suspicious: A role of Epstein-Barr virus in lupus. *Lupus* 15:768, 2006.

74. Lunemann JD, Frey O, Eidner T, et al: Increased frequency of EBV specific effector memory CD 8+ T cells correlates with higher viral load in rheumatoid arthritis. *J Immunol* 181:991, 2008.

75. Kawano Y, Iwata S, Kawada J, et al: Plasma viral microRNA profiles reveal potential biomarkers for chronic active Epstein-Barr virus infection. *J Infect Dis* 208:771, 2013.

76. Buchwald DS, Rea TD, Katon WJ, et al: Acute infectious mononucleosis: Characteristics of patients who report failure to recover. *Am J Med* 109:531, 2000.

77. Okano M: Overview and problematic standpoints of severe chronic active Epstein-Barr virus infection syndrome. *Crit Rev Oncol Hematol* 44:273, 2002.

78. Suzuki K, Ohshima K, Karube K, et al: Clinicopathological states of Epstein-Barr virus-associated T/NK cell proliferative disorders (severe chronic active EBV infection) of children and young adults. *Int J Oncol* 24:1165, 2004.

79. Chen CJ, Huang YC, Jaing TH, et al: Hemophagocytic syndrome: A review of 18 pediatric cases. *J Microbiol Immunol Infect* 37:157, 2004.

80. Imashuku S, Kuriyama K, Sakai R, et al: Treatment of Epstein-Barr virus-associated hemophagocytic lymphohistiocytosis (EBV-HLH) in young adults: A report from HLH study center. *Med Pediatr Oncol* 41:103, 2003.

81. Imashuku S, Teramura T, Tauchi H, et al: Longitudinal follow-up of patients with Epstein-Barr virus-associated hemophagocytic lymphohistiocytosis. *Haematologica* 89:183, 2004.

82. Pagano JS: Epstein-Barr virus. The first human tumor virus and its role in cancer. *Proc Assoc Am Physicians* 111:573, 1999.

83. Endo R, Kikuta H, Ebihara T, et al: Possible involvement in oncogenesis of a single base mutation in internal ribosome entry site of Epstein-Barr nuclear antigen 1 mRNA. *J Med Virol* 72:630, 2004.

84. Flavell KJ, Murray PG: Hodgkin disease and Epstein-Barr virus. *Mol Pathol* 53:262, 2000.

85. Hjalgrim H, Askling J, Rostgaard K, et al: Characteristics of Hodgkin's lymphoma after infectious mononucleosis. *N Engl J Med* 349:1324, 2003.

86. Hjalgrim H, Rostgaard K, Johnson PC, et al: HLA-A alleles and infectious mononucleosis suggest a critical role for cytotoxic T-cell response in EBV-related Hodgkin lymphoma. *Proc Natl Acad Sci U S A* 107:6400, 2010.

87. Kanakry JA, Li H, Gellert LL, et al: Plasma Epstein-Barr virus DNA predicts outcome in advanced Hodgkin lymphoma: Correlative analysis from a large North American cooperative group trial. *Blood* 121:3547, 2013.

88. Gao SZ, Chapparro SV, Perlroth M, et al: Post-transplant lymphoproliferative disease in heart and heart-lung transplant recipients: 30 year experience at Stanford University. *J Heart Lung Transplant* 22:505, 2003.

89. Ballen KK, Cutler C, Yeap BY, et al: Donor-derived second hematologic malignancies after cord blood transplantation. *Biol Blood Marrow Transplant* 16:1025, 2010.

90. McDonald RA, Smith JM, Ho M, et al: Incidence of PTLD in pediatric renal transplant recipients receiving basiliximab, calcineurin inhibitor, sirolimus and steroids. *Am J Transplant* 8:984, 2008.

91. Dierickx D, Tousseyn T, Requilé A, et al: The accuracy of positron emission tomography in the detection of post-transplant lymphoproliferative disorder. *Haematologica* 98:771, 2013.

92. MacGinnitie AJ, Geha R: X-linked lymphoproliferative disease: Genetic lesions and clinical consequences. *Curr Allergy Asthma Rep* 2:361, 2002.

93. Cohen JI: Benign and malignant Epstein-Barr virus-associated B-cell lymphoproliferative diseases. *Semin Hematol* 40:116, 2003.

94. Yachie A, Kanegane H, Kasahara Y: Epstein-Barr virus associated T-/natural killer cell lymphoproliferative diseases. *Semin Hematol* 40:124, 2003.

95. Kawa K, Okamura T, Yasui M, et al: Allogeneic hematopoietic stem cell transplantation for Epstein-Barr virus-associated T/NK-cell lymphoproliferative disease. *Crit Rev Oncol Hematol* 44:251, 2002.

96. Cheng WM, Chan KH, Chen HL, et al: Assessing the risk of nasopharyngeal cancer on the basis of EBV antibody spectrum. *Int J Cancer* 97:489, 2002.

97. Moss DJ, Khanna R, Bharadwaj M: Will a vaccine to nasopharyngeal carcinoma retain orphan status? *Dev Biol* 110:67, 2002.

98. Lee ES, Locker J, Nalesnik M, et al: The association of Epstein-Barr virus with smooth muscle tumors occurring after organ transplantation. *N Engl J Med* 332:19, 1995.

99. Oda K, Koda K, Takiguchi N, et al: Detection of Epstein-Barr virus in gastric carcinoma cells and surrounding lymphocytes. *Gastric Cancer* 6:173, 2003.

100. Murray PG, Young LS: Epstein-Barr virus infection: Basis of malignancy and potential for therapy. *Expert Rev Mol Med* 15:2001, 2001.

101. Malouf MA, Chajed PN, Hopkins P, et al: Anti-viral prophylaxis reduces the incidence of lymphoproliferative disease in lung transplant recipients. *J Heart Lung Transplant* 21:547, 2002.

102. Greenspan JS, Greenspan D, Lennette ET: Replication of Epstein-Barr virus within epithelial cells of hairy oral leukoplakia an AIDS associated lesion. *N Engl J Med* 332:19, 1986.

103. Sokal EM, Hoppenbrouwers K, Vandermeulen C, et al: Recombinant gp350 vaccine for infectious mononucleosis. A phase 2 randomized, double blind, placebo controlled trial to evaluate the safety, immunogenicity, efficacy of Epstein-Barr virus vaccine in healthy young adults. *J Infect Dis* 196:1749, 2007.

104. Davis JE, Moss DJ: Treatment options for post-transplant lymphoproliferative disorder and other Epstein-Barr virus associated malignancies. *Tissue Antigens* 63:285, 2004.

105. Farrell CJ, Lee JM, Shin EC, et al: Inhibition of Epstein-Barr virus–induced growth proliferation by nuclear antigen EBNA-2 peptide. *Proc Natl Acad Sci U S A* 101:4625, 2004.

106. Weller TH, Hanshaw JB: Virologic and clinical observations in cytomegalic inclusion disease. *N Engl J Med* 266:1233, 1962.

107. Hanshaw, JB, Betts RF, Simon G, Boynton RC: Acquired cytomegalovirus infection. *N Engl J Med* 272:602, 1965.

108. Klemola E, Von Essen R, Henle G, et al: Infectious mononucleosis like disease with negative heterophile agglutinin test. Clinical features in relation to Epstein-Barr virus and cytomegalic virus antibodies. *J Infect Dis* 121:808, 1970.

109. de Vries JJ, van Zwet EW, Dekker FW, et al: The apparent paradox of maternal seropositivity as a risk factor for congenital cytomegalovirus infection: A population-based prediction model. *Rev Med Virol* 23:241, 2013.

110. Stagno S, Pass RF, Dworsky ME, et al: Congenital cytomegalovirus infection: The relative importance of primary or recurrent maternal infection. *N Engl J Med* 306:945, 1982.

111. Just-Nubling G, Korn S, Ludwig B, et al: Primary cytomegalovirus infection in an outpatient setting—Laboratory markers and clinical aspects. *Infection* 31:318, 2003.

112. Söderberg-Nauclér C, Fish KN, Nelson JA: Reactivation of latent human cytomegalovirus by allogeneic stimulation of blood cells from healthy donors. *Cell* 91:119, 1997.

113. Smith MS, Bentz GL, Alexander JS, Yurochko AD: Human cytomegalovirus induces monocyte differentiation and migration as a strategy for dissemination and persistence. *J Virol* 78:4444, 2004.

114. Betts RF, Freeman RB, Douglas RG Jr, et al: Transmission of cytomegalovirus with the renal allograft. *Kidney Int* 8:385, 1975.

115. Ho M, Suwansirkul S, Dowling JN, et al: The transplanted kidney is a source of cytomegalovirus infection. *N Engl J Med* 293:1109, 1975.

116. Betts RF, Freeman RB, Douglas RG Jr, Talley TE: Clinical manifestations of renal allograft derived primary cytomegalovirus infection. *Am J Dis Child* 131:759, 1977.

117. Drew WL, Mintz L, Hoo R, Finley TN: Growth of herpes simplex and cytomegalovirus in cultured human alveolar macrophages. *Am Rev Respir Dis* 119:287, 1979.

118. Chien J, Chan CK, Chamberlain D, et al: Cytomegalovirus pneumonia in allogeneic bone marrow transplantation. An immunopathologic process? *Chest* 98:1034, 1990.

119. Huisman C, van der Straaten HM, Canninga-van Dijk MR, et al: Pulmonary complications after T-cell-depleted allogeneic stem cell transplantation: Low incidence and strong association with acute graft-versus-host disease. *Bone Marrow Transplant* 38:561, 2006.

120. Snyder LD, Finlen-Copeland CA, Turbyfill WJ: Cytomegalovirus pneumonitis is a risk for bronchiolitis obliterans syndrome in lung transplantation. *Am J Respir Crit Care Med* 181:1391, 2010.

121. Ljungman P: Cytomegalovirus infections in transplant patients. *Scand J Infect Dis Suppl* 100:59, 1996.

122. Schooley RT, Hirsch MS, Colvin RB, et al: Association of herpes virus infections with T-lymphocyte subset alterations, glomerulopathy, and opportunistic infections after renal transplantation. *N Engl J Med* 308:307, 1983.

123. George MJ, Snydman DR, Werner BG, et al: The independent role of cytomegalovirus for invasive fungal infections in orthotopic liver transplant recipients. Boston Center for Liver Transplantation CMVIG-Study Group. Cytogam, MedImmune, Inc. Gaithersburg, Maryland. *Am J Med* 103:106, 1997.

124. Tindall B, Cooper DA, Donovan B, Penny R: Primary human immunodeficiency infection. Clinical and serologic aspects. *Infect Dis Clin North Am* 2:329, 1988.

125. Vanhems P, Allard R, Cooper DA, et al: Acute human immunodeficiency virus type 1 disease as a mononucleosis-like illness: Is the diagnosis too restrictive? *Clin Infect Dis* 24:965, 1997.

126. Rosenberg ES, Caliendo AM, Walker BD: Acute HIV among patients tested for mononucleosis [letter]. *N Engl J Med* 340:969, 1999.

127. Walensky RP, Rosenberg ES, Ferraro MJ, et al: Investigation of primary human immunodeficiency virus infection in patients who test positive for heterophile antibody. *Clin Infect Dis* 33:570, 2001.

128. Dalman J, Puertas MC, Azuara M, et al: Contribution of immunologic and virological factors to the extremely severe primary HIV type 1 infection. *Clin Infect Dis* 48:229, 2009.

129. Steeper TA, Horwitz CA, Ablashi DV, et al: The spectrum of clinical and laboratory findings resulting from human Herpesvirus-6 (HHV-6) in patients with mononucleosis-like illness not resulting from Epstein-Barr virus or cytomegalovirus. *Am J Clin Pathol* 93:776, 1990.

130. Li IW, To KK, Tang BS, et al: Human metapneumonia virus infections in a human immunocompetent adult presenting as mononucleosis-like illness. *J Infect* 56:389, 2008.

131. Andersson J, Britton S, Ernberg I, et al: Effect of acyclovir on infectious mononucleosis: A double-blinded, placebo-controlled study. *J Infect Dis* 153:283, 1986.

132. Torre D, Tambini R: Acyclovir for treatment of infectious mononucleosis: A meta-analysis. *Scand J Infect Dis* 31:543, 1999.

133. Collins M, Fleisher G, Kreisberg J, Fager S: Role of steroids in the treatment of infectious mononucleosis in the ambulatory college student. *J Am Coll Health* 33:101, 1984.

134. Chan SC, Dawes PJ: The management of severe infectious mononucleosis tonsillitis and upper airway obstruction. *J Laryngol Otol* 115:973; 2001.

135. Peter J, Ray GG: Infectious mononucleosis. *Pediatr Rev* 19:276, 1998.

136. Walling DM, Flaitz CM, Nichols CM: Epstein-Barr virus replication in oral hairy leukoplakia: Response, persistence, and resistance to treatment with valacyclovir. *J Infect Dis* 188:883, 2003.

137. Yao QY, Ogan P, Rowe M, et al: Epstein-Barr virus-infected B cells persist in the circulation of acyclovir-treated virus carriers. *Int J Cancer* 43:67, 1989.

138. Goldberg GN, Fulginiti VA, Ray CG, et al: In utero Epstein-Barr virus (infectious mononucleosis) infection. *JAMA* 246:1579, 1981.

139. Avgil M, Diav-Citrin O, Shechtman S, et al: Epstein-Barr virus in pregnancy: A prospective controlled study. *Reprod Toxicol* 25:468, 2008.

140. Connor EM, Sperling RS, Gelber R, et al: Reduction of maternal-infant transmission of human immunodeficiency virus type 1 with zidovudine treatment. Pediatrics AIDS Clinical Trials Group Protocol 076 Study Group. *N Engl J Med* 331:1173, 1994.

141. Cengir SD, Ortac F, Soylemez F: Treatment and results of chronic toxoplasmosis. Analysis of 33 cases. *Gynecol Obstet Invest* 33:105, 1992.

142. Stray-Pedersen B: Treatment of toxoplasmosis in the pregnant mother and newborn child. *Scand J Infect Dis* 84:23, 1992.

143. Nichols WG, Price TH, Gooley T, et al: Transfusion-transmitted cytomegalovirus infection after receipt of leukoreduced blood products. *Blood* 101:4195, 2003.

144. Meyers JD: Prevention and treatment of cytomegalovirus infection after marrow transplantation. *Bone Marrow Transplant* 3:95, 1988.

Part X Malignant Myeloid Diseases

83. Classification and Clinical Manifestations of the Clonal Myeloid Disorders..... 1275

84. Polycythemia Vera...................1291

85. Essential Thrombocythemia 1307

86. Primary Myelofibrosis 1319

87. Myelodysplastic Syndromes 1341

88. Acute Myelogenous Leukemia.......1373

89. Chronic Myelogenous Leukemia and Related Disorders 1437

CHAPTER 83

CLASSIFICATION AND CLINICAL MANIFESTATIONS OF THE CLONAL MYELOID DISORDERS

Marshall A. Lichtman

SUMMARY

The clonal myeloid neoplasms result from acquired driver and cooperating mutations within a multipotential marrow cell, or sometimes, perhaps, a stem cell. Translocations, inversions, duplications (e.g., trisomy, tetrasomy), and deletions of chromosomes can result in (1) the expression of fusion genes that encode oncogenic fusion proteins or (2) the overexpression or underexpression of genes that encode molecules critical to the control of cell growth, programmed cell death, cell differentiation and maturation, or other regulatory pathways. Gene sequencing has also identified relevant somatic mutations in cases without an overt cytogenetic abnormality. The different mutations may result in phenotypes that range from mild impairment of the steady-state levels of blood cells, insignificant functional impairment of cells, and a modest effect on longevity to severe cytopenias and death in days, if the disorder is untreated. The somatically mutated multipotential cell from which the clonal expansion of neoplastic hematopoietic cells derives acquires the features of a stem cell and retains the ability, with varying degrees of imperfection, to differentiate and mature into each blood cell lineage. A particular disease in this spectrum of phenotypes may have altered blood cell concentrations and cell structural and functional abnormalities, and these may range from minimal to severe, involving several blood cell lineages. The effect on any one lineage occurs in an unpredictable way, even in subjects within the same category of disease. The resulting phenotypes are, therefore, innumerable and varied. In polycythemia vera or essential thrombocythemia, differentiation and subsequent maturation of unipotential progenitor cells results in blood cells nearly normal in appearance and function, but their level in the blood is excessive. Moreover, overlapping features are common, such as thrombocytosis as a feature of polycythemia vera, essential thrombocythemia, primary myelofibrosis, and chronic myelogenous leukemia. The clonal (refractory) anemias may be accompanied by functionally insignificant or very severe neutropenia or thrombocytopenia or sometimes thrombocytosis. These findings reflect the unpredictable expression of the mutant multipotential hematopoietic cell's differentiation and maturation capabilities for which the genetic explanations are not well defined. The mutant cell of origin takes on the features of a (leukemic) stem cell, responsible for sustaining the disease process. Tight relationships between the genetic alteration and phenotype occur in only a few circumstances, and even these are imperfect, for example, t(9;22)(q34;q11)(BCR-ABL1; p210) with chronic myelogenous leukemia and t(15;17)(q22;q21) (PML-RARα) with acute promyelocytic leukemia. However, most patients can be grouped into a classic diagnostic designations listed in Table 83–1. The mutant stem cells that maintain the clone may undergo further somatic mutations over time resulting in a more aggressive phenotype, notably acute leukemia, usually of the myeloid type. An important feature of the clonal myeloid diseases is the potentially reversible suppression of normal (polyclonal) stem cells by the clonally expanded neoplastic cells. The coexistence of normal polyclonal stem cells and their competition with the neoplastic clone forms the basis for the remission-relapse pattern seen in acute myelogenous leukemia after intensive chemotherapy and the reappearance of polyclonal, normal hematopoiesis in patients with chronic myelogenous leukemia after tyrosine kinase BCR-ABL inhibitor therapy. This reciprocal relationship between the leukemic clonal and polyclonal normal stem cells may be mediated by the effects of the mass of neoplastic cells (inhibitory cytokine elaboration) and/or to the effect of the neoplastic clone on the stem cell niche and the resulting disturbance of stromal cell support for normal stem cell function.

Acronyms and Abbreviations: ABL1, Abelson murine leukemia viral oncogene homologue 1; ALL, acute lymphocytic leukemia; AML, acute myelogenous leukemia; BCR, breakpoint cluster gene; CALR, calreticulin gene; CD, cluster of differentiation; CEPBA, CCAAT/enhancer-binding protein a gene; CML, chronic myelogenous leukemia; FGFR, fibroblast growth factor receptor; FLT-3, FMS-like tyrosine kinase 3; G-banding, Giemsa banding; GPI, glycosylphosphatidylinositol; inv, inversion; JAK2, Janus kinase 2; miRNA, microribonucleic acid; MPL, myeloproliferative leukemia virus gene; NPM1, nucleophosmin 1 gene; PDGFR, platelet-derived growth factor receptor; PNH, paroxysmal nocturnal hemoglobinuria; t, translocation; WHO, World Health Organization.

A wide array of clonal (neoplastic) syndromes or diseases can result from somatic mutations in a multipotential hematopoietic progenitor cell (Table 83–1). This mutated neoplastic cell behaves like a hematopoietic stem cell (albeit, a cancer or leukemia stem cell), in that it is self-replicating, can differentiate, and feed progenitor cells into the various hematopoietic lineages. These leukemic, unipotential progenitors can undergo varying degrees of maturation to phenocopies of mature blood cells. Strong circumstantial evidence has existed for a myelogenous leukemia stem cell for approximately 60 years. This concept has been buttressed by experimental verification of such cells by transplantation of the human disease into immunodeficient mice[1] and by techniques to isolate and characterize their stem cell phenotype.[2,3] Although most attention has been given to the leukemic stem cell in acute myelogenous leukemia (AML) and chronic myelogenous leukemia (CML), it is very likely that a similar cell underlies (initiates and sustains) each of the phenotypically distinctive clonal myeloid diseases.

The clonal myeloid diseases can be grouped, somewhat arbitrarily, by their degree of malignancy, using the classic terminology of experimental carcinogenesis, which considers the degree of loss of differentiation and maturation potential and the rate of progression of the disease. Thus, myeloid malignancies can be viewed in the spectrum of minimally to severely deviated neoplasms (leukemias). The term *deviation* refers to the relationship of the disease in question to normal cellular differentiation and maturation and the regulation of cell population homeostasis (birth and death rates). This terminology has been used here to array the diagnostic categories of clonal hematopoietic diseases into a

TABLE 83–1. Neoplastic (Clonal) Myeloid Disorders

I. Minimal-deviation neoplasms (no increase in blast cells [<2%] are evident in marrow)

  A. Underproduction of mature cells is prominent

    1. Clonal (refractory sideroblastic or non-sideroblastic) anemia[a] (Chap. 87)

    2. Clonal bi- or tricytopenia[a] (Chap. 87)

    3. Paroxysmal nocturnal hemoglobinuria (Chap. 40)

  B. Overproduction of mature cells is prominent

    1. Polycythemia vera[b] (Chap. 84)

    2. Essential thrombocythemia[b] (Chap. 85)

II. Moderate-deviation neoplasms (very small proportions of leukemic blast cells present in marrow)

  A. Chronic myelogenous leukemia (Chap. 89)

    1. Philadelphia (Ph) chromosome-positive, *BCR* rearrangement positive (~90%)

    2. Ph chromosome-negative, *BCR* rearrangement positive (~6%)

    3. Ph chromosome-negative, *BCR* rearrangement negative (~4%)

  B. Primary myelofibrosis[b] (chronic megakaryocytic leukemia) (Chap. 86)

  C. Chronic eosinophilic leukemia (Chaps. 62 and 89)

    1. *PDGFR* rearrangement-positive

    2. *FGFR1* rearrangement-positive

  D. Chronic neutrophilic leukemia (Chap. 89)

    1. *CSF3R*-rearrangement-positive

    2. *CSF3R* and *SETBP1*-rearrangement positive

    3. *JAK2*^{V617F}-rearrangement positive

  E. Chronic basophilic leukemia (Chap. 89)

  F. Systemic mastocytosis (chronic mast cell leukemia) (Chap. 63)

    1. *KITD*^{816V} mutation-positive (~90%)

    2. *KITV*^{560G} mutation-positive (rare)

    3. *FILIPI-PDGFRα*

III. Moderately severe-deviation neoplasms (moderate concentration of leukemic blast cells present in marrow)

  A. Oligoblastic myelogenous leukemia (refractory anemia with excess blasts)[a] (Chap. 87)

  B. Chronic myelomonocytic leukemia (Chap. 89)

    1. *PDGFR* rearrangement positive (rare)

  C. Atypical myeloproliferative disease (syn. atypical chronic myelogenous leukemia)

  D. Juvenile myelomonocytic leukemia (Chap. 89)

IV. Severe-deviation neoplasms (leukemic blast or early progenitor cells frequent in the marrow and blood)

  A. Phenotypic variants of acute myelogenous leukemia (Chap. 88)

    1. Myeloblastic (granuloblastic)

    2. Myelomonocytic (granulomonoblastic)

    3. Promyelocytic

    4. Erythroid

    5. Monocytic

    6. Megakaryocytic

    7. Eosinophilic[c]

    8. Basophilic[d]

    9. Mastocytic[e]

    10. Histiocytic or dendritic[f]

  B. High-frequency genotypic variants of acute myelogenous leukemia [t(8;21), Inv16 or t(16;16), t(15;17), or (11q23)][g]

  C. Myeloid sarcoma

  D. Acute biphenotypic (myeloid and lymphoid markers) leukemia[h]

  E. Acute leukemia with lymphoid markers evolving from a prior clonal myeloid disease

[a]The World Health Organization includes these disorders under the rubric of the "Myelodysplastic Syndromes," the classification of which is discussed in Chap. 87.

[b]The World Health Organization includes these three disorders under the rubric of the "Myeloproliferative Syndromes."

[c]Acute eosinophilic leukemia is rare. Most cases are subacute or chronic and formerly were included in the category of the hypereosinophilic syndromes.

[d]Rare cases of acute basophilic leukemia are *BCR*-rearrangement-negative and are variants of acute myelogenous leukemia. Most cases have the *BCR* rearrangement and evolve from chronic myelogenous leukemia (Chaps. 63, 88, and 89).

[e]See Chap. 63.

[f]See Chap. 71.

[g]The World Health Organization has designated these subtypes as separate entities. They also have phenotypes listed under phenotypic variants.[1] For example, approximately 90 percent of cases of t(8;21) AML are of the phenotype acute myelogenous leukemia with maturation. Occasional cases are of the phenotypes acute myeloblastic leukemia (no evidence of maturation) or acute myelomonocytic leukemia. Inv(16) is usually an acute myelomonocytic leukemia but can be of other phenotypes, and t(15;17) invariably manifests itself as an acute promyelocytic leukemia.

[h]Approximately 10 percent of cases of acute myeloblastic leukemia may be biphenotypic (myeloid and lymphoid CD markers on individual cells) when studied with antimyeloid and antilymphoid monoclonal antibodies (Chap. 88).

framework related to their pathogenesis for the reader. This approach is an effort to encourage thinking about these somewhat arbitrary diagnostic categories in pathobiologic terms and not just as a list of conditions or by epiphenomena such as disturbed morphology of blood cells that is shared to varying degrees in all categories of these disease (e.g., the dysmorphia of primary myelofibrosis is as dramatic as that of clonal cytopenias or oligoblastic myelogenous leukemia, so-called myelodysplastic syndromes.)

MINIMAL-DEVIATION CLONAL MYELOID DISORDERS

The neoplasms in this category in Table 83–1 retain a higher degree of differentiation and maturation capability and permit median life spans measured in decades without treatment or with minimally toxic treatment approaches.[4] Use of the term *minimal-deviation* should not be construed as indicating these conditions do not have morbidity, shorten life, and have other consequences to the patient. The term is used relative to AML, in which differentiation and maturation and regulation of cell proliferation and cell death are profoundly disturbed, and in which expected life span is measured in days to weeks, if untreated. The minimal-deviation clonal myeloid diseases include one group in which late precursor apoptosis (ineffective myeloproliferation) is characteristic (the clonal cytopenias) and one group in which proliferation is exaggerated and cellular maturation approximates normal (effective myeloproliferation).

PRECURSOR APOPTOSIS PROMINENT

The clonal (refractory) anemias and bi- and tricytopenias are characteristic of this category. Cytopenias resulting from exaggerated apoptosis of marrow late precursors (referred to as "ineffective hematopoiesis") are a principal feature of this subgroup of clonal hematopoietic multipotential cell diseases. A common additional characteristic is variable dysmorphogenesis of blood cells. The blood cell abnormalities, characteristic of the clonal anemias, bicytopenias, or pancytopenia, include abnormalities of (1) red cell size (macrocytosis, anisocytosis), shape (poikilocytosis), and cytoplasm (basophilic stippling), (2) neutrophil nuclear or organelle structure (cytoplasmic hypogranulation, nuclear hypolobulation or hyperlobulation and condensation), and (3) platelet variation in size (megathrombocytes) and granulation (hypogranulation or abnormal granulation). These structural changes are the result of neoplasia. Abnormal maturation of blood cells may also leads to biochemical and functional alterations of the cells, such as disturbed hemostasis, despite adequate platelet numbers, and dysfunctional phagocytes. Dysmorphic changes in marrow precursors are evident, also (Chap. 87). Ineffective erythropoiesis, the intramedullary, apoptotic death of late erythroblasts before they reach full maturation and release, is a common feature, a major factor in development of anemia. Ineffective granulopoiesis and thrombopoiesis also occur, resulting in varying degrees of neutropenia and thrombocytopenia, despite a cellular marrow.

There is no clinical distinction in the presenting manifestation or the course of clonal anemia with less than 15 or equal to or greater than 15 percent pathologic sideroblasts in the marrow,[5] not surprisingly, as there is no pathobiologic basis for this arbitrary boundary. Therefore, this distinction nonsideroblastic vis-à-vis sideroblastic clonal (refractory) anemia has no nosologic or clinical utility, although the World Health Organization (WHO) has retained it.[6] Indeed, the clonal anemias frequently have some degree of pathologic sideroblasts in the marrow, and, thus, usually have some degree of sideroblastic erythropoiesis. Another important feature of these syndromes is that there is

no quantitative evidence of leukemic blast cells in marrow or blood. If marrow blasts are elevated above the normal upper limit of 2 percent, the disorder should be considered oligoblastic myelogenous leukemia (synonym: *refractory anemia with excess blasts*; see "Moderately Severe-Deviation Disorders" below).

The WHO has defined "AML" as having equal to or greater than 20 percent leukemic blast cells in marrow; whereas, a marrow with fewer blasts (5 to 20 percent) is referred to as refractory anemia with excess blasts (e.g., one of the myelodysplastic syndromes). The use of an arbitrary boundary of 20 percent blasts has no pathobiologic basis.[7,8] In addition, the use of less than 5 percent of blasts as a threshold to distinguish clonal anemia (refractory anemia) from oligoblastic myelogenous leukemia (refractory anemia with excess blasts) is an anachronism that dates back approximately 60 years to a time when supportive care was inadequate for children undergoing newly developed multidrug chemotherapy for acute lymphoblastic leukemia (ALL). At that time, the mid-1950s, there was no accessibility to platelet transfusions. There were very limited antibiotic options and no antifungal agents. There were no venous access devices. The risk of death during prolonged posttherapy marrow aplasia was substantial and it was not yet evident that intensive antileukemic therapy would produce a net benefit to the children so treated. In children with ALL, there were often occasional residual atypical lymphoid cells in the marrow after treatment. To deal with these circumstances an arbitrary threshold of less than 5 percent atypical lymphoid cells (suspected blasts) was used as a measure of successful induction therapy to avoid an unnecessarily long period of posttreatment–induced aplasia.[7] That boundary, however, was not intended to be a threshold to be used at the time of diagnosis. The normal myeloblast percentage is a very tightly regulated variable (mean: 1.0; SD: 0.4). In severe inflammatory states with leukemoid reactions, the marrow myeloblast percent is usually decreased because in this circumstance precursor cell expansion in the postblast cell myelocyte pool is greater. Three or 4 percent blast cells in the marrow at the time of presentation or suspected relapse should not be considered "normal" and is usually evidence of leukemic hematopoiesis. Indeed, in the presence of an established clonal myeloid disorder (e.g., clonal anemia), any percentage of blast cells, no matter how low the percentage is presumably part of the clone and thus "leukemic." Not surprisingly, sophisticated multicolor flow analysis has found immunophenotypic abnormalities in such blast cells indicating that they are not "normal" blasts.[9]

In no other cancer is the diagnosis defined by the proportion of cancer cells in histologic or cytologic examinations. Thus, using equal to or greater than 20 percent blasts as the basis for diagnosis of AML versus myelodysplasia represents an aberration in cancer diagnosis and has no pathophysiologic basis.[7,8] Indeed, studies have shown that there are no differences in the presenting hematologic findings or a series of prognostic genetic markers, for example, the FMS-like tyrosine kinase 3 *(FLT-3)* gene mutation in patients with 10 to 19 percent versus 20 to 30 percent marrow leukemic myeloblasts at the time of diagnosis.[7] The patient's disease features are the same regardless of whether they have 10 or 30 percent blast cells in the marrow at diagnosis; prognosis was correlated with patient age at diagnosis and the cytogenetic risk category and not the blast count. Moreover, several phenotypes of AML may have less than 20 percent blasts at diagnosis (e.g., acute promyelocytic leukemia, acute monocytic leukemia, acute myelomonocytic leukemia, and others).

The term *hematopoietic dysplasia*, later simplified to *myelodysplasia*, has become ensconced as the category into which clonal anemia, clonal multicytopenia, and oligoblastic myelogenous leukemia (refractory anemia with excess blasts) have been grouped. In strict pathologic terms, a dysplasia is a polyclonal, and thus nonmalignant, change in the cells of a tissue.[8,10] These myeloid syndromes are clonal, often have aneuploid or pseudodiploid cells in the clone, are the result of the expansion of a somatically mutated cell, and can be associated with significant morbidity and premature death; thus, they are neoplasias not dysplasias. They demonstrate clonal (genomic) instability, and each has a propensity to evolve into AML at a rate that far exceeds the incidence of the disease in the general population. The term *myelodysplasia* was proposed at a conference in Paris in 1976 at a time when prominent dysmorphogenesis and cytopenias were thought to be the singular abnormalities and arguments existed as to whether some of these syndromes without increased blast cell percentages represented a preneoplastic (preleukemic) condition.[11] They have long been established as neoplastic (a spectrum of minimal-deviation to severe-deviation leukemias)—indeed, those with overt leukemic hematopoiesis (quantitatively increased leukemic blast cell counts), which made up approximately 50 percent of cases, were known at the time to be neoplasms—but the terminology has not been rectified.

OVERPRODUCTION OF CELLS PROMINENT

Polycythemia vera (Chap. 84) and essential thrombocythemia (Chap. 85) are clonal myeloid disorders so named because of the overaccumulation of red cells, and often neutrophils, and platelets in the blood in polycythemia, and of platelets, and to a lesser extent neutrophils, in thrombocythemia.[12] Each cell lineage is affected in each disorder, reflecting a multipotential hematopoietic cell origin, but the magnitude of the effect on each lineage differs. The decrease in red cell production in essential thrombocythemia usually is slight to mild. Polycythemia vera and essential thrombocythemia do not show morphologic evidence of leukemic hematopoiesis; the proportion of blast cells in the marrow is never increased above normal, and blast cells are never present in the blood. Hematopoietic differentiation and maturation are maintained. These are minimal-deviation neoplasms. These disorders do not have a specific cytogenetic abnormality, but approximately 95 percent of cases of polycythemia and approximately 50 percent of cases of essential thrombocythemia have an acquired mutation in the Janus kinase 2 *(JAK2)* gene. In thrombocythemia, 25 percent of patients have wild-type *JAK2* genes and mutations in the calreticulin *(CALR)* gene. A few percent of patients with thrombocythemia have nonmutated *JAK2* and *CALR* but a mutation in the myeloproliferative leukemia virus gene *(MPL;* Chaps. 84 and 85).[13,14] Several studies of comparative survival of the chronic myeloproliferative neoplasms have been reported.[4,15–18,18a] In the most comprehensive study of survival as of this writing, patients with essential thrombocythemia have only slightly decreased survival than expected over 10 years of observation, but this widens somewhat over longer periods. The difference in survival of patients with primary myelofibrosis is dramatically less than expected for age- and gender-matched unaffected persons and the survival of patients with polycythemia vera is intermediate (Table 83–2).[18a]

MODERATE-DEVIATION CLONAL MYELOID DISORDERS

Primary myelofibrosis (Chap. 86) and CML (Chap. 89) classically share the features of overproduction of granulocytes and platelets and impaired production of red cells. In contrast to the minimally deviated clonal myeloid neoplasms, CML and primary myelofibrosis may have a small to moderate proportion of leukemic blast cells in marrow and blood. The most constant feature in primary myelofibrosis is the abundance of neoplastic, dysmorphic megakaryocytes and the resultant predisposition to marrow reticulin and collagen fibrosis, osteosclerosis, extramedullary fibrohematopoietic tumors, splenomegaly, and teardrop-shaped red cells (dacryocytes) in every oil immersion field on the blood film. The megakaryocytic abnormalities are so dominant and consistent in this disorder that it could be considered chronic megakaryocytic leukemia.[19] The cells in this disorder have no specific cytogenetic change, but approximately 50 percent of cases carry a mutation in the *JAK2* gene and approximately one-third have wild-type *JAK2* but a mutation in the *CALR* gene (Chap. 86).[13,14] These two mutations give primary myelofibrosis a genetic kinship with polycythemia vera and essential thrombocytosis. They are often referred to as "the myeloproliferative neoplasms," but virtually all clonal myeloid diseases are fundamentally myeloproliferative as the term refers, principally, to marrow hematopoiesis. The clinical behavior of primary myelofibrosis is, in most cases of a progressive neoplasm with morphologic evidence, of lower-level leukemic hematopoiesis and with a median survival significantly less than polycythemia vera or essential thrombocythemia. Primary myelofibrosis is another misnomer perpetuated in the WHO classification. The fibrosis is secondary to cytokines released by neoplastic (leukemic) megakaryocytes (an epiphenomenon) and it is the only cancer in the medical lexicon named after connective tissue fibers and not the cells in which the cancer arises.[19]

In contrast to primary myelofibrosis, CML has a rearrangement of the breakpoint cluster *(BCR)* gene on chromosome 22. The shortening of the long arm of chromosome 22 gives it the designation of the Philadelphia chromosome, now called the Ph chromosome. It can be identified by Giemsa (G)-banding cytogenetic studies in approximately 90 percent of patients with CML. This mutation is caused by and is a reflection of the translocation t(9;22)(q34;q11)(*BCR-ABL1* [Abelson murine leukemia viral oncogene homologue 1]). The *BCR-ABL1* fusion in CML cells can be found in virtually all cases studied by fluorescence *in situ* hybridization or the polymerase chain reaction. Only approximately 4 percent of patients with a phenotype indistinguishable from *BCR*-rearrangement–positive CML do not have the rearrangement (see Table 83–1 and Chap. 89). An unrelenting increase in the white cell (granulocyte) count, anemia, splenomegaly, and a progressive course are common features of CML. Blast cells are very slightly increased in marrow

TABLE 83–2. Comparative Survival Among Persons with Myeloproliferative Neoplasms

Years of Survival	Percent (%) of Cohort Alive			
	Expected	Essential Thrombocythemia	Polycythemia Vera	Primary Myelofibrosis
5	90	90	85	55
10	85	80	70	30
15	75	70	45	30
20	65	50	30	15
25	55	40	20	10

Data from Tefferi A, Guglielmelli P, Larson DR, et al: Long-term survival and blast transformation in molecularly annotated essential thrombocythemia, polycythemia vera, and myelofibrosis. *Blood* 2014 Oct 16;124(16):2507–2513.

and in the blood in patients with these two disorders, although this is a function of time of diagnosis in relation to the time of onset. CML, if untreated, has a very high propensity to progress through clonal evolution to acute leukemia.

Primary myelofibrosis terminates in acute leukemia in approximately 15 percent of patients. Median life span in these disorders is measured in years, but is significantly decreased compared to age- and gender-matched unaffected cohorts. Therapy is required in all cases of CML, and in most, but not all, cases of primary myelofibrosis at the time of diagnosis. Both diseases can be cured by allogeneic hematopoietic stem cell transplantation. Median life span is projected to be increased by decades in CML as a result of the introduction of tyrosine kinase inhibitors, which results in involution of the malignant clone, restoration of polyclonal normal hematopoiesis, and a reduction in the risk of transformation to an accelerated phase of the disease and to acute leukemia in many patients (Chap. 89).[20] A significant median prolongation of life (e.g., approximately median 2 years) result from JAK inhibitors in poor-prognosis primary myelofibrosis (Chap. 86).

Chronic neutrophilic leukemia, chronic eosinophilic leukemia, systemic mastocytosis, and chronic basophilic leukemia are included in this category. Chronic basophilic leukemia is a rare disease (Chap 89).[21] Chronic neutrophilic leukemia is uncommon but well described and defined (Chap. 89). Chronic neutrophilic leukemia is associated with a mutation in the colony-stimulating factor 3 receptor gene *(CSF3R)* alone (approximately 30 percent of cases), or a combination of mutated *CSF3R* and a SET binding protein gene *(SETBP1)* mutation (approximately 60 percent of cases) or the $JAK2^{V617F}$ mutation alone (approximately 10 percent of cases). Chronic eosinophilic leukemia represents cases previously called hypereosinophilic syndrome with evidence of clonal hematopoiesis involving eosinopoiesis. Some cases are associated with a rearrangement of the platelet-derived growth factor receptor-β *(PDGFR-β)* gene (these are indicted in Table 83–1) because they are specifically responsive to the tyrosine kinase inhibitor imatinib mesylate or to a congener (Chaps. 62 and 89). Chronic clonal eosinophilia also may be associated with a *PDGFR-α* gene rearrangement, but histopathologic examination of the marrow also may be consistent with systemic mastocytosis with eosinophilia, with sheets of spindle-shaped mast cells and intense eosinophilia in blood and marrow. This rearrangement is usually the result of a *FIP1L1–PDGFR-α* fusion gene. Identification of this fusion gene in cases of mastocytosis with eosinophilia is important because of the sensitivity of the gene product to imatinib mesylate (or a congener). The mutation is inferred by a deletion in the *CHIC2* gene found using fluorescence *in situ* hybridization, which narrowly separates *FIP1L1* and *PDGFR-α* at chromosome 4q band 12. The cryptic deletion involving *CHIC2* is too small to be seen on standard G-banding. A clonal myeloid syndrome that includes eosinophilia and a translocation between 8p11, at the site of the tyrosine kinase domain of the fibroblast growth factor receptor-1 *(FGFR1)* gene, and several different partner chromosomes, is not responsive to imatinib mesylate. Systemic mastocytosis may have several types of *KIT* gene mutation; KIT^{V560G} is sensitive to imatinib mesylate and KIT^{D816V} is insensitive to imatinib but may be responsive to second-generation tyrosine kinase inhibitors. *PDGFR-α* mutations also may be present in the cells of patients with systemic mastocytosis and be responsive to imatinib mesylate (or a congener).[22]

MODERATELY SEVERE-DEVIATION CLONAL MYELOID DISORDERS

These disorders fall into a group that progresses less rapidly than acute leukemia and more rapidly than CML.[23,24] They have a predisposition

to develop with a granulocytic and monocytic phenotype, either morphologically or cytochemically. These diseases include oligoblastic myelogenous leukemia (refractory anemia with excess blasts), chronic myelomonocytic leukemia, and juvenile myelomonocytic leukemia. Occasional patients have an atypical or unclassifiable syndrome. The "unclassifiable syndrome" designation is used for uncommon cases that do not fall into a classical or easily classifiable designation and usually are seen in patients older than age 70 years.

The subacute syndromes produce more morbidity than do the chronic syndromes, and patients have a shorter life expectancy. These are leukemic states that have low or moderate concentrations of leukemic blast cells in marrow and often blood, anemia, often thrombocytopenia, and usually prominent monocytic maturation of cells (Chap. 88). The oligoblastic myelogenous leukemias compose approximately 50 percent of the cases that have been grouped under the title *myelodysplastic syndromes*. In all other malignancies, the presence of tumor cells determines the diagnosis, such as carcinoma of the colon or the uterine cervix, whether *in situ*, invasive, or metastatic. Use of the percentage of tumor (leukemic blast) cells as a threshold for the diagnosis of leukemia versus "dysplasia" is not consistent with usual practice; hence, the preference for oligoblastic myelogenous leukemia rather than myelodysplasia for patients with a quantitative increase in blast cells (>2 percent blasts), cytopenias, and dysmorphic cell maturation.[8] Moreover, CML, chronic neutrophilic leukemia, chronic myelomonocytic leukemia, acute promyelocytic leukemia, and several other subtypes of AML invariably have fewer than 20 percent blasts in the marrow. Thus, the criteria used in the WHO classification system for clonal myeloid diseases have internal inconsistencies that can be dealt with by experts but are confusing to the less experienced and are not unifying.

A group of clonal myeloid diseases are referred to as atypical myeloproliferative disease or atypical CML (aCML) in the WHO classification. They are usually seen in older patients (>65 years), have a relatively low myeloblast percentage in marrow (<5 percent) and blood, and have an elevated white cell count ranging between 15 and 100×10^9/L, but which may be higher. They have anemia and thrombocytopenia and often splenomegaly. The blood and marrow usually have a progressively increasing proportion of promyelocytes and myelocytes as well as neutrophils, superficially simulating the appearance of CML, hence the use of the designation "aCML." These cases never have a rearrangement in the *BCR* gene, are not responsive to tyrosine kinase inhibitors, and have a poor prognosis with a median survival of approximately 15 to 20 months. Because the granulocytic series often has some dysmorphia (e.g., acquired Pelger-Huët nuclear anomaly), the WHO seems reluctant to call it an atypical myeloproliferative disorder, which should be done as aCML is an inadvisable term. Their inconsistency is evident in the classification of primary myelofibrosis as a myeloproliferative disorder despite florid dysmorphia of all three major lineages. Dysmorphia is a feature of most neoplastic cells, of considerable diagnostic utility, of interest cytologically, but an epiphenomenon not central to the pathobiology of the neoplasm. Atypical myeloproliferative disease (aCML) has a relatively high frequency of *CSF3R* gene mutations, akin to chronic neutrophilic leukemia. Because the mutant gene is thought to cause dysregulation evidenced by *myeloproliferation* and exaggerated neutrophil counts, it underlines the preferred terminology.

SEVERE-DEVIATION CLONAL MYELOID DISORDERS

Morphologic, histochemical, immunocytologic, and cytogenetic characteristics of cells in the blood and marrow provide the major basis for the diagnosis and classification of AML and its subtypes

(Chaps. 11 and 88). Correlation among observers and between the morphologic method of classification and the monoclonal antibody reactivity-dependent classification of AML is imperfect.[25-27] The approach that uses morphology, immunocytochemistry, and the immunophenotype is the most inclusive because virtually all cases can be placed into a morphologic subtype. Because immunophenotyping is a standard procedure in most clinical hematopathology laboratories, the results are readily available. Classification by cytogenetics is more limited because approximately 45 percent of cases of AML do not have a discernible cytogenetic abnormality by G-banding and many cases have different infrequent abnormalities, making this approach complex. Hundreds of unique patterns of cytogenetic abnormalities have been reported in cells of patients with AML, including unbalanced structural abnormalities, such as loss of part or all of chromosome 5 or 7, numerical abnormalities, such as an additional chromosome 8 (e.g., trisomy 8), or unbalanced and balanced structural abnormalities, such as translocation between chromosomes 8 and 21 or 15 and 17, or between chromosome 11 and many chromosome partners, or any one of numerous other abnormalities involving other chromosomes.[28] Despite this heterogeneity, knowing the cytogenetic alteration is useful for estimating the probability of entering a sustained remission (risk category). For example, AML patients whose cells contain t(8;21), t(15;17), t(16;16), or inv(16) (approximately 20 percent of cases considering all age groups) are more likely to enter a prolonged remission or be cured with therapy. The cytogenetic findings may influence the drugs used for remission-induction therapy. Notably, patients with t(15;17) AML (approximately 7 percent of all new AML cases in the United States and twice that frequency in China) uniquely require use of all-*trans*-retinoic acid and arsenic trioxide to result in the best long-term outcome and, in many cases, a cure. Thus, combining light microscopy of blood and marrow with immunocytochemistry and cell-flow analysis immunophenotyping to designate the phenotypic subtype, supplemented by cytogenetics or molecular diagnostic methods, currently is the best approach to categorization of the AML subtype. The polymerase chain reaction may be particularly useful for determining subclinical (minimal) residual disease and monitoring therapy in cases in which an appropriate genetic marker is available, such as the t(8;21) or t(15;17) (Chaps. 88 and 89).

Gene expression profiling using chips containing tens, hundreds, or thousands of relevant genes can be used to further genotype and subclassify AML into prognostic groups.[29,30] One would predict, based on cytogenetics, a large and diverse group of gene expression profiles for cases of AML. In one study of 200 cases of AML, some of 270 mutated genes among nine genes families (i.e., transcription factor, tumor-suppressor, signaling pathway, nucleophosmin encoder, DNA-methylation–related, chromatin-modifying, myeloid transcription factor, cohesion complex, and spliceosome-complex genes) were found in at least two cases.[31] Genetic analysis is currently most useful in analyzing cases with prior stratification by some relevant variable. For example, a study of patients with AML who have normal karyotypes by standard cytogenetic methods (e.g., G-banding) has identified two groups by hierarchical gene clustering with significantly different survival after current therapy.[32] Patients with AML whose cells contain a *FLT-3* internal tandem duplication also can be stratified into more discriminating prognostic groups using hierarchical gene cluster analysis.[33] Gene expression profiling can identify groups of patients with AML who have covert gene abnormalities, such as a mutation in the DNA methyltransferase gene (*DNMT3A*) or the nucleophosmin 1 (*NPM1*) gene. The former gene encodes one of a family of enzymes that catalyze the transfer of a methyl group to DNA, using *S*-adenosyl methionine as the methyl donor; and, the latter gene encodes a protein that shuttles between the nucleus and cytoplasm. Gene expression studies in AML are important because they (1) identify genes that cooperate or interact to result in a fully malignant

phenotype, (2) provide potential new targets for therapy, (3) help identify patients who might benefit from early hematopoietic stem cell transplantation, (4) may be used to measure minimal residual disease,[34] and (5) may permit analysis of the mutational evolution from the earliest neoplastic cell without malignant potential to cells with additional mutations capable of developing lethal clones.[35]

Another molecular technique applied to understanding the molecular pathology of AML and to defining prognostic groups is the leukemic cell microribonucleic acid (miRNA) signature.[36,37] The miRNAs are small (19 to 25 nucleotides), noncoding RNAs that regulate messenger RNA stability and its translation into protein. miRNA signatures can be analyzed by polymerase chain reaction technology of RNA samples from leukemic cells and compared to normal or compared among different categories of AML cases. For example, miRNA analysis can distinguish among cytogenetically normal cases of AML as to their expression of different genes that influence prognosis, such as *NPM1* and the CCAAT/enhancer binding protein α gene (*CEPBA*). Specific microribonucleic acids (miRNAs) may regulate lineage differentiation of stem cells, indicating critical roles for these molecules in the regulation of hematopoiesis and in leukemogenesis.[38] Prognostic group stratification of AML, at the moment, has value principally in assessing the utility of using allogeneic hematopoietic stem cell transplantation as an early therapy. It also may inform the therapist about considering a clinical trial of new therapeutic combinations, if the prognostic indicators suggest use of cytarabine and an anthracycline regimen, as the backbone of therapy, is unlikely to be successful and the patient is not a candidate for allogeneic hematopoietic stem cell transplantation (Chap. 88).

TRANSITIONS AMONG CLONAL MYELOID DISEASES

Patients with minimal-, moderate-, and moderately severe-deviation clonal myeloid disorders have an increased likelihood of progressing to florid (polyblastic) AML, with a frequency ranging from approximately less than 1 percent of patients with paroxysmal nocturnal hemoglobinuria, approximately 10 percent of patients with clonal anemia, approximately 35 percent of patients with clonal bi- or tricytopenia, and as many as 66 percent of patients with oligoblastic myelogenous leukemia.[39] Approximately 30 percent of patients within the spectrum of clonal cytopenia to oligoblastic myelogenous leukemia (myelodysplastic syndromes) develop AML when the WHO boundary of equal to or greater than 20 percent blast cells is applied.[39] Approximately 15 percent of patients with polycythemia vera evolve to a syndrome indistinguishable from primary myelofibrosis and the same evolution can occur in patients with essential thrombocythemia.[40,41] Occasional cases of apparent essential thrombocythemia or rare cases of primary myelofibrosis can evolve into polycythemia vera. Apparent essential thrombocythemia with cells containing the *BCR-ABL1* fusion gene may progress to CML or acute blast crisis of CML.

Approximately 5 percent of patients with essential thrombocythemia develop AML over 20 years of observation, but this rises to 10 percent over 25 years.[18a] Approximately 12 percent of patients with polycythemia vera evolve to AML over 20 years of observation.[18a] Approximately 20 percent of patients with primary myelofibrosis progress to overt AML over 10 years of observation.[18a] Virtually all patients with CML have the potential to progress to acute leukemia of any subtype, including in about a quarter of cases to lymphoid phenotypes, although in some cases the patient enters an accelerated phase that behaves like oligoblastic leukemia before it progresses to acute leukemia. The accelerated phase of CML is associated with inadequate response to therapy, progressive anemia, bone pain, enlarging spleen, thrombocytopenia, among other changes (Chap. 89). The progression from chronic to accelerated phase or blast phase of CML, however, has been delayed in the majority of patients by the application of tyrosine kinase inhibitor therapy during the chronic phase of the disease. Determining the frequency of evolution to AML in those patients with CML who enter a complete molecular remission with tyrosine kinase inhibitors must await observations over the next decade.

This process of clonal evolution is an intrinsic feature of the genomic instability of clonal myeloid diseases. The practice of calling the result of this process "secondary AML" is obfuscating. This choice of terms is notable in the case of myelodysplastic syndrome, which is "leukemia" at the time of diagnosis. (Leukemia is defined as the neoplastic transformation of a primitive multipotential hematopoietic [myeloid] cell.) The neoplastic transformation has occurred and the progression to a more advanced myeloid neoplasm is a process quite different from the secondary AML that occurs as a result of recent chemotherapy for a lymphoma or an unrelated cancer (e.g., breast cancer). When there is progression to AML from a previously diagnosed clonal myeloid disease, it should be designated as clonally evolved AML (ceAML). This distinction is important because an effort to develop methods to prevent clonal evolution is very likely to be different from methods to prevent true secondary leukemia.

PATHOGENESIS OF CLONAL MYELOID DISEASES

In AML, a sequence of mutations in a single multipotential cell results in a clone that is severely defective and contains precursor cells that are largely unable to mature.[42,43] Proliferation of primitive progenitors is excessive when considered in absolute terms, that is, the total number of blast cells proliferating. AML is a clinical disease with many forms of morphologic expression. This variation of phenotype is consistent with the large number of genetic lesions identified and the behavior of the leukemic stem cell, which is capable of differentiation into all the blood cell lineages (Fig. 83–1). Hence, the asymmetrical and uncoordinated differentiation and maturation of leukemic progenitor cells may allow one or another cell type to predominate.[44] The different morphologic or cytogenetic variants of AML are each rapidly progressive, however, if not treated successfully (Chap. 88).

Important epiphenomena are related to certain morphologic types of AML, such as tissue infiltration, including into the central nervous system in monocytic leukemia, disseminated intravascular coagulation, fibrinolysis, and hemorrhage in promyelocytic leukemia, and to a lesser extent in monocytic leukemia, hepatosplenomegaly (eosinophilic

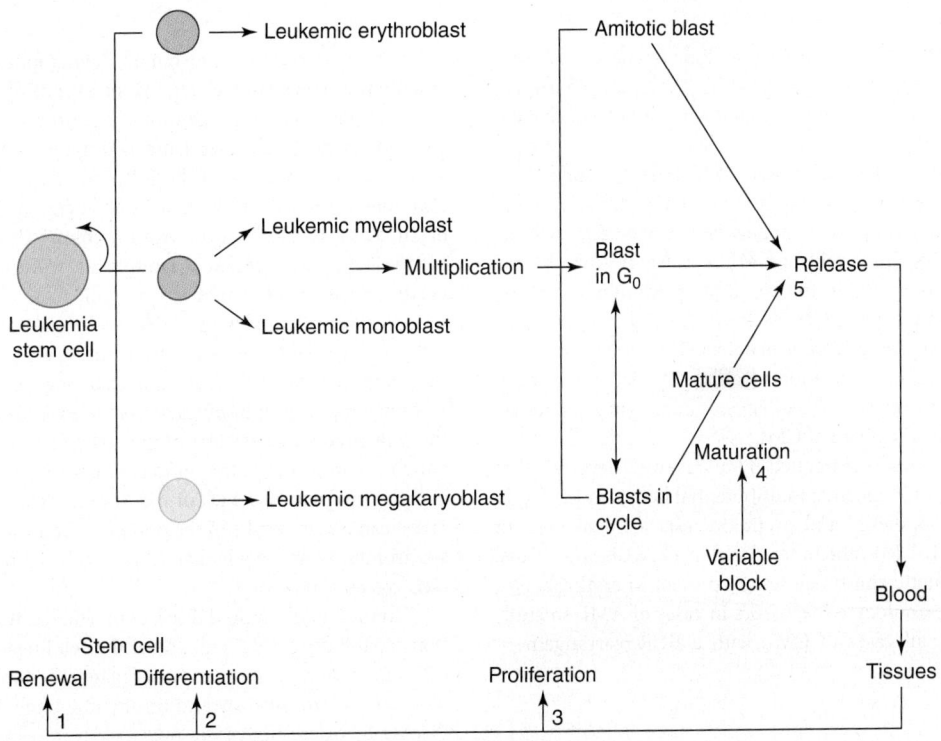

Figure 83–1. Leukemic hematopoiesis in acute myelogenous leukemia. The malignant process evolves from a single mutant multipotential cell. This cell on the basis of a sequence of somatic mutations becomes a leukemia stem cell with a growth advantage in relationship to normal pluripotential stem cells. This cell originates at either level 1 or level 2 or level 3 in Fig. 83–2. Whether all cases of acute myelogenous leukemia originate in the pluripotential stem cell pool is still under study (see text). This cell is capable of multivariate commitment to leukemic erythroid, granulocytic, monocytic, and megakaryocytic progenitors. In most cases, granulocytic and monocytic commitment predominates, and myeloblasts and promonocytes or their immediate derivatives are the dominant cell types. Leukemic blast cells accumulate in the marrow. The leukemic blast cells may become amitotic (sterile) and undergo programmed cell death, may stop dividing for prolonged periods (blasts in G_0) but have the potential to reenter the mitotic cycle, or may divide and then undergo varying degrees of maturation. Maturation may lead to mature cells, such as red cells, segmented neutrophils, monocytes, or platelets. A severe block in maturation is characteristic of AML, whereas a high proportion of leukemic primitive multipotential cells mature into terminally differentiated cells of all lineages in patients with CML. The disturbance in differentiation and maturation in myelogenous leukemia is quantitative, thus many patterns are possible. At least five major steps in hematopoiesis are regulated: (1) stem cell self-renewal, (2) differentiation into hematopoietic cell lineages (e.g., red cells, granulocytes, monocytes, platelets), (3) proliferation (cell multiplication), (4) maturation of progenitor and precursor cells, and (5) release of mature cells into the blood. These control points are defective in acute myelogenous leukemia. Premature or delayed apoptosis of cells may be another key abnormality contributing to premature cell death or cell accumulation.

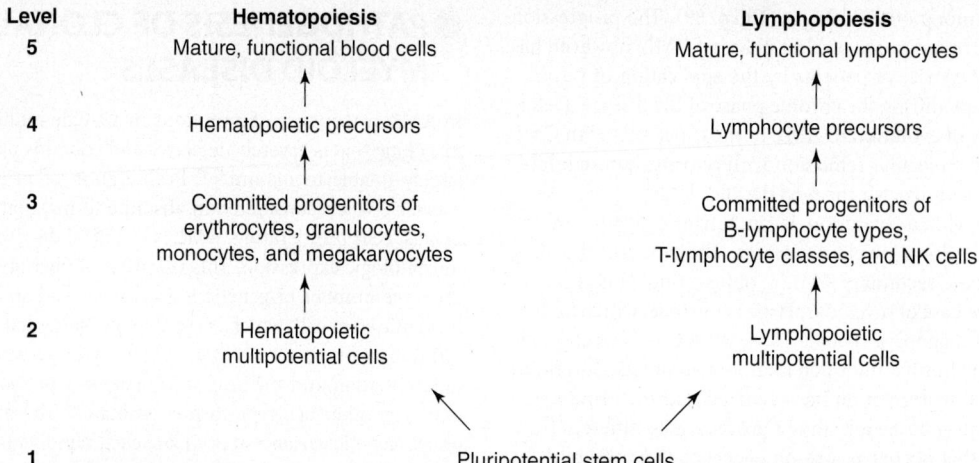

Level	Hematopoiesis	Lymphopoiesis

Figure 83–2. Differentiation and maturation of hematopoietic stem cells. The functioning stem cell pool is thought to be at *level 1*, the pluripotential (lymphohematopoietic) stem cells. In healthy humans, two multipotential progenitor cell pools are operative *(level 2)*. The multipotential progenitors differentiate further to unipotential progenitors, which are sensitive to specific cytokines *(level 3)*. The committed progenitor cells are referred to as colony-forming units or colony-forming cells because they form clonal colonies of cells in semisolid medium in the presence of the appropriate growth factors. These growth factors are capable of inducing proliferation and maturation of the committed progenitor cells so that they achieve *level 4*, at which the first morphologically identifiable marrow precursors have developed, such as myeloblasts, proerythroblasts, promonocytes, megakaryocytes and, ultimately, *level 5*, the mature, functional blood cells. NK, natural killer.

leukemia), mediator-release syndromes (basophilic or mast cell leukemia), predisposition to myeloid sarcomas (AML with t[8;21] or inv[16] cytogenetic abnormalities), and intense marrow fibrosis (megakaryocytic leukemia) (Chap. 88).

In CML, injury to a single cell results in a clone in which there is an enormous expansion of progenitors for granulocytic and, often, megakaryocytic cells. Erythropoiesis is effective but decreased. Unlike AML, maturation of progenitor cells in CML is nearly normal; hence, the predominant leukemic cells in the blood are postmitotic, mature, or partially matured cells, such as late myelocytes and segmented neutrophils, monocytes, erythrocytes, and platelets. This process of multilineage differentiation and maturation to cells with virtually normal function accounts for the relative infrequency of hemorrhage or recurrent infection in the chronic phase of CML.

Because hematopoiesis is generated by a leukemic stem cell that has functional analogies to a normal multipotential hematopoietic cell, erythropoiesis, thrombopoiesis, and granulopoiesis are leukemic in most patients with AML, CML, and other clonal myeloid diseases. Thus, identical clonal cytogenetic abnormalities are present in erythroblasts, megakaryocytes, and granulocyte precursors in cases of AML so studied (Chap. 88) and in all cases of CML with a BCR-rearrangement (Chap. 89).

PHENOTYPE OF MYELOID CLONAL DISEASES AS A RESULT OF THE MATRIX OF DIFFERENTIATION AND MATURATION

The phenotype of clonal myeloid diseases is a reflection of a neoplastic stem cell's capability to differentiate into abnormal committed progenitor cells and the ability of those progenitor cells to mature into identifiable cells of the erythroid, granulocytic (neutrophilic, basophilic, mastocytic, eosinophilic), monocytic, dendritic, and megakaryocytic cell lineages (Fig. 83–3).[42,45,46]

Under normal circumstances, hematopoietic differentiation represents the irreversible change from a multipotential cell to multiple, unipotential lineage progenitors. Maturation represents the physical and chemical changes from a unipotential progenitor through a sequence of precursors to the fully mature and functional blood cell, including progression from a burst-forming unit–erythroid to proerythroblast to erythrocyte; from a colony-forming unit–granulocyte to myeloblast to segmented neutrophil; from a colony-forming unit-eosinophil to a segmented eosinophil; from a colony-forming unit-basophil to a mature basophil; from a colony-forming unit–mast cell to a mature mast cell; from a colony-forming unit–monocyte-macrophage to promonocyte to monocyte to macrophage or dendritic cell; and from a colony-forming unit–megakaryocyte to a diploid megakaryoblast to the polyploidy, platelet-forming megakaryocyte (Chap. 18). A matrix, which is composed of the options of commitment to different lineages and the progressive stages of maturation at which partial or complete arrest can occur, results in the potential for a wide array of morphologic syndromes by which a leukemic stem cell can dominate hematopoiesis (see Fig. 83–2).

In the clonal myeloid diseases in which differentiation and maturation capability are retained, one of the cell lines—for example, erythrocytes, granulocytes, monocytes, or platelets—tends to accumulate in the blood more prominently and results in a phenotypic expression of the disease that determines the nosology (e.g., exaggerated blood platelet accumulation and essential thrombocythemia). In AML, the phenotypic expression may be predominantly myeloblastic (granuloblastic), erythroid, monocytic, megakaryocytic, or combinations thereof. Certain patterns are favored. In AML, myelocytic leukemia, monocytic leukemia, or a mosaic of the two cell types (myelomonocytic leukemia) are more common than erythroid or megakaryocytic leukemia. Eosinophilic, basophilic, and dendritic cell leukemias are rare. However, AML usually has a disturbance in all cell lines. In myeloblastic or myelomonocytic leukemia, overt, qualitative abnormalities of erythroblasts and megakaryocytes may occur. The prevalence of the abnormalities in the latter two lineages may not be great enough or evident enough for the observer to designate a case as erythroid or megakaryocytic leukemia. In the latter two cases, identification of markers unique for erythroid

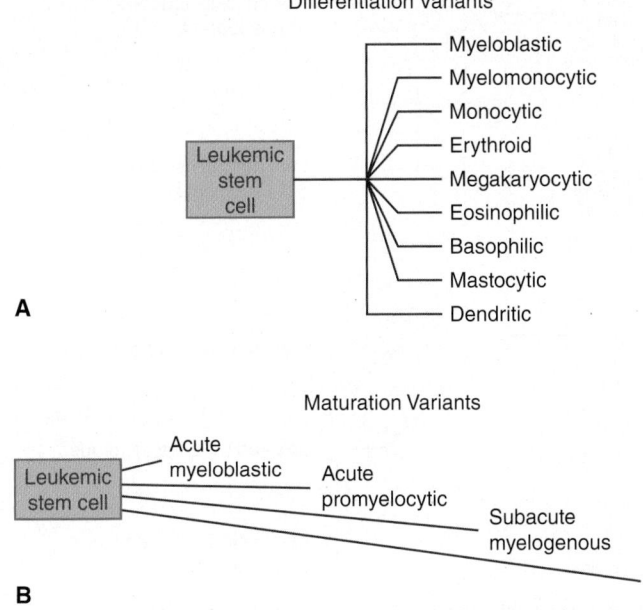

Differentiation Variants

Maturation Variants

Figure 83–3. Phenotypic subtypes of acute myelogenous leukemia. Acute myelogenous leukemia has variable morphologic expression and a variable degree of maturation of leukemic cells into recognizable precursors of each blood cell type. This phenotypic variation results because the leukemic lesion resides in a multipotential cell normally capable of all the hematopoietic lineage commitment decisions. **A.** Morphologic variants of AML can be considered differentiation variants in which the cells derived from one of the options of commitment accumulate prominently (e.g., leukemic erythroblasts, leukemic monocytes, leukemic megakaryocytes). **B.** Acute myeloblastic leukemia, promyelocytic leukemia, subacute myelogenous leukemia, and chronic myelogenous leukemia can be considered maturation variants in which blocks at different levels of maturation may be present or do not exist (e.g., CML).

(e.g., cluster of differentiation [CD] 71) or megakaryocytic cells (e.g., CD41, CD42, or CD61), rather than reliance solely on light microscopy, has increased the frequency of identification of these variants.

The continuum of maturation can be completely or partially blocked at various levels, leading to morphologic variants such as acute myeloblastic, acute promyelocytic, AML with maturation, and CML.

PLURIPOTENTIAL STEM CELL POOL AS SITE OF THE NEOPLASTIC EVENTS

Evidence points to a lesion in the multipotential hematopoietic cell pool in most of the clonal myeloid diseases, explaining the involvement of erythropoiesis, granulopoiesis, monopoiesis, and thrombopoiesis. Debate continues whether the cell of origin is a pluripotential (lymphohematopoietic) stem cell or a somewhat more differentiated multipotential cell.[47,48] (Chapter 88 provides a more detailed discussion of this topic.) In CML patients, the mutation is thought to be in the pluripotential stem cell; in other syndromes, evidence for involvement of B, T, and natural killer (NK) lymphocytes is variable. B lymphocytes are derived from the clone in some cases. Evidence that affected T lymphocytes undergo apoptosis before entering the blood in patients with CML may explain the absence of clonal markers in T lymphocytes in some cases of CML and other clonal myeloid disorders.[49]

PROGENITOR CELL LEUKEMIA

Analysis of cases of AML in informative girls (young women) and older women who were heterozygous for X chromosome-linked gene products isotypes A and B of the enzyme glucose-6-phosphate dehydrogenase indicated that the AML clone in the young women was restricted to the granulocyte–monocyte pathway, whereas monoclonality was expressed in all hematopoietic cell lines in the older women. This approach had been validated in prior studies of CML and AML, using enzymes or chromosome markers.[50,51] These findings supported the possibility that a leukemic transformation in young patients can occur in progenitor cells (e.g., colony-forming unit—granulocyte-monocyte; level 3 in Fig. 83–2) and result in a true acute "granulocytic"

leukemia. If progenitor cell myelogenous leukemia is common in younger patients, this pattern might explain their better response to treatment. In a subset of patients with acute monocytic leukemia,[52] t(8;21) AML,[53] and t(15;17) AML,[54] studies indicated that the leukemia derives from the neoplastic transformation of a more differentiated progenitor cell not the pluripotential lymphohematopoietic stem cell. The acute transformation of CML also appears to occur in a granulocyte-monocyte progenitor (Chap. 89).

More sophisticated approaches to the site of the lesion in mouse models of AML have indicated that disorders like acute promyelocytic leukemia for which there is evidence in humans that it may originate in a more differentiated progenitor, such as the granulocyte-monocyte colony-forming cell,[54] places the neoplastic event(s) in a much earlier multipotential (?stem) cell.[55] Indeed, some experts have concluded that all clonal myeloid neoplasms originate in a mutated lymphohematopoietic stem cell, whereas others do not feel the evidence is either consistent or conclusive and that either a stem cell or an early multipotential progenitor cell could be the site of the transformation.

QUANTITATIVENESS OF CLONAL MYELOID DISEASES

The mutational lesions of the primitive hematopoietic multipotential cell compartment are qualitative in the sense that a distinct alteration from normal is seen in the function of that cell pool. The alteration reflects an acquired change in the genome of one primitive hematopoietic cell. This qualitative change, however, is such that the mutant multipotential cell can express all or some of the normal differentiation and maturation options. This expression can mimic closely the differentiation (commitment) and maturation expected of normal hematopoietic cells, as occurs in CML, essential thrombocythemia, and polycythemia vera. Most cases tend to conform to readily recognized patterns, but the opportunity for a large number of variations on the most common themes is possible. Thus, some mixed and "in-between" syndromes occur in which features of ineffective hematopoiesis and myeloproliferation of different cell lineages are present. For example, extreme thrombocytosis, usually confined to essential thrombocythemia, may accompany CML, primary myelofibrosis, or clonal bicytopenia with thrombocytosis. Erythrocytosis may rarely accompany CML. Atypical myeloproliferative syndromes or other clonal myeloid diseases may have mixtures of anemia, granulocytopenia, and thrombocytosis or of anemia, granulocytosis, and thrombocytopenia rather than pancytopenia. Qualitative abnormalities of red cell, granulocyte, or platelet structure or function may be more or less prominent in a given patient. For example, qualitative abnormalities of erythroblast development may result in acquired α-thalassemia (acquired hemoglobin H disease), especially in patients with primary myelofibrosis, or occasionally other clonal myeloid diseases. In AML, unusual patterns of phenotypic expression occur frequently. For example, prominent leukemic erythroblasts and monocytes or eosinophils and monocytes may be seen in patients. So much opportunity for variation in disease expression exists among patients with AML that observation of patients in whom the phenotype of their leukemic cells is identical to the phenotype of other patients is unusual. Choice of treatment is little affected by these variations. Decisions about whether to treat and which drugs to use are greatly influenced by whether a patient has a chronic, subacute, or acute clonal myeloid disease; by the rate of progression of the disease; by the extent of the leukemic blast cell infiltrate; by the cytogenetic findings; and by the severity of the cytopenias. The experienced diagnostician and therapist usually can identify variants as a clonal myeloid disorder and can manage the disorder as dictated by their manifestations regardless of their precise subclassification.

INTERPLAY OF CLONAL AND POLYCLONAL HEMATOPOIESIS

Although potentially curative chemotherapy of myelogenous leukemia was introduced in the mid-20th century to kill "the last leukemic cell," two important factors were not explicitly appreciated. The first was whether residual normal stem cells coexisted in marrow to restore polyclonal (normal) hematopoiesis if ablation of the leukemia was accomplished. The second was whether, given the estimates of 1 trillion leukemic cells in a patient, the therapist had to eliminate all the leukemic cells to achieve a cure. A corollary of the latter was whether the disease was the result of a leukemic stem cell and, if so, was the undifferentiated replicates of the leukemic stem cell the only cells that mattered, ultimately, in the eradication process. We know that remissions result from sufficient suppression of the leukemic population by intensive chemotherapy to permit restitution of polyclonal hematopoiesis by normal stem cells (Fig. 83–4).[56] Why monoclonal leukemic hematopoiesis is so difficult to subdue, even temporarily, with intensive chemotherapy (pre–tyrosine kinase therapy) in the chronic myeloid neoplasms (e.g., CML) compared to the acute myeloid neoplasms (AML) is unclear. Prolonged remission (longer than 3 years) may occur in some cases of AML with late relapse occurring from the same clone, suggesting a new symbiotic relationship occurs after intensive therapy that suppresses the growth potential of leukemic cells for an extended period of time. A role for the patient's immune system in such protracted remissions has been hypothesized and forms the basis for attempts to manipulate cellular and innate immunity in an attempt to improve therapeutic results.

CLINICAL MANIFESTATIONS

DEFICIENCY, EXCESS, OR DYSFUNCTION OF BLOOD CELLS

Alterations in blood cell concentration are the primary manifestations of clonal hematopoietic disorders. The clinical manifestations of deficiencies or excesses of individual blood cell types are described in the chapters

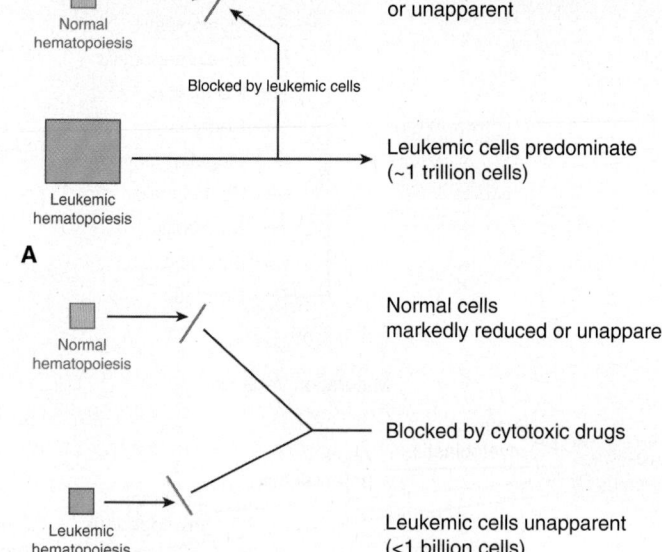

A

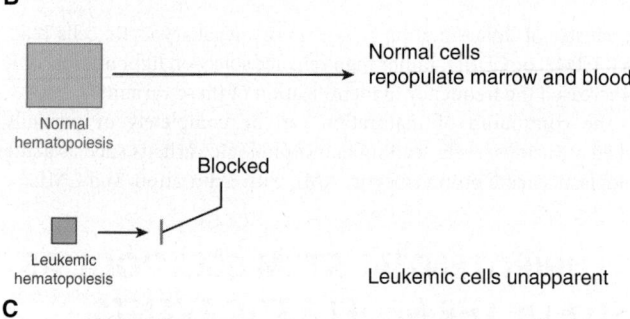

B

C

Figure 83–4. Remission–relapse pattern of acute myelogenous leukemia. **A.** Acute myelogenous leukemia at diagnosis or in relapse. Monoclonal leukemic hematopoiesis predominates. Normal polyclonal stem cell function is suppressed. **B.** Following effective cytotoxic treatment leukemic cells are unapparent in marrow and blood. Severe pancytopenia exists as a result of cytotoxic therapy. The reduction in leukemic cells can release inhibition of normal polyclonal stem cell function. **C.** If reconstitution of normal hematopoiesis ensues, a remission is established and blood cells return to near normal as a result of the recovery of polyclonal hematopoiesis. This relapse–remission pattern has not been seen, generally, in the subacute and chronic myeloid leukemias treated with similar chemotherapy. Either it has not been possible to minimize the leukemic cell population with cytotoxic therapy to a point at which polyclonal hematopoiesis is restored or some other factors inhibit normal stem cell recovery. The principal exception is the effect of BCR-ABL1 inhibitor therapy in which suppression of BCR-ABL1–positive cells in CML can be achieved with return of polyclonal hematopoiesis. Uncommon examples of tyrosine kinase inhibitor responses in myeloid neoplasms with *PDGFR* or certain *KIT* mutations may also show this pattern. In a proportion of cases, BCR-ABL1 transcripts (minimal residual disease) can be detectable along with normal, polyclonal hematopoiesis (mosaic hematopoiesis). *(Reproduced with permission from Lichtman MA: Interrupting the inhibiton of normal hematopoiesis in myelogenous leukemia: A hypothetical approach to therapy. Stem Cells 18(5):304–306, 2000.)*

on clinical manifestations of disorders of erythrocytes (Chap. 34), granulocytes (Chap. 64), monocytes (Chap. 69), and platelets (Chap. 116).

Several clonal hematopoietic diseases frequently manifest as qualitative abnormalities of blood cells. Abnormal red cell shapes, red cell or granulocyte enzyme deficiencies, abnormal neutrophil granules, bizarre nuclear configurations, disorders of neutrophil chemotaxis, phagocytosis or microbial killing, giant platelets, abnormal platelet granules, and disturbed platelet function can occur in some patients with oligoblastic myelogenous leukemia and primary myelofibrosis. In oligoblastic myelogenous leukemia, the effects of severe cytopenia usually dominate. In primary myelofibrosis and essential thrombocythemia, functional platelet abnormalities may contribute to the hemorrhagic diathesis, especially if surgery or injury occurs. Paroxysmal nocturnal hemoglobinuria is a hematopoietic multipotential cell disease resulting from a somatic mutation of the *PIG-A* gene on the active X chromosome. The mutation causes a highly specific alteration in blood cell membranes, a deficiency in the glycosylphosphatidylinositol (GPI) anchor, with decreased cell-surface CD59, rendering the blood cells exquisitely sensitive to complement lysis. In its classic form, chronic hemolytic anemia is coupled with mild decreases in neutrophil and platelet counts but depressions in hematopoiesis often occur (hypoplastic marrow; Chap. 40). Patients with CML or polycythemia vera usually do not have clinically significant functional abnormalities of cells, although in polycythemia vera, neutrophils often are activated with heightened metabolic rates and enhanced phagocytosis.

Secondary clinical manifestations occur as a result of the proliferation and accumulation of the malignant (leukemic) cells.

EFFECTS OF LEUKEMIC BLAST CELLS

Extramedullary Tumors

Myeloid (granulocytic) sarcomas (also called *chloromas* or *myeloblastomas*) are discrete tumors of leukemic cells that form in skin and soft tissues, breast, periosteum and bone, lymph nodes, mediastinum, lung, pleura, gastrointestinal tract, gonads, urinary tract, uterus, central nervous system, and virtually any other site (Chap. 88).[57-59] They can develop in patients with AML or the accelerated phase of CML and, occasionally, may be the first manifestation of AML, preceding morphologic evidence of the disease in marrow and blood by months or, sometimes, years. AML with the t(8;21) and inv(16) has a predisposition to form myeloid sarcomas, although other AML types may also. Myeloid sarcomas can be mistaken for large cell lymphomas because of the similarity of the histopathology in biopsy specimens from soft tissues. In the past, approximately 50 percent of cases that occur in the absence of blood and marrow involvement initially were misdiagnosed, usually as lymphoma.[57] The presence of eosinophils or other granulocytes in the mass may arouse suspicion of a myeloid sarcoma; however, immunohistochemistry should be used on such lesions to identify myeloperoxidase, lysozyme, CD117, CD61, CD68/KP1, and other relevant CD markers of myeloid cells. One of four histopathologic patterns usually is evident by immunocytochemistry: myeloblastic, monoblastic, myelomonoblastic, or megakaryoblastic.

More diffuse collections of leukemic promonocytes or monoblasts can invade the skin, gingiva, anal canal, lymph nodes, central nervous system, or other tissues of patients with AML of the monocytic subtype and may form tumors in those locations. Leukemic monocytes tend to mature to the point at which they develop many of the cytoplasmic and membrane features required for motility and tissue entry.[60-62] Moreover, leukemic monocytes proliferate and survive in tissues for long periods. Consequently, this AML phenotype has a higher frequency of overt infiltrative tissue lesions than do other forms of AML.

Extramedullary tumors may usher in the accelerated phase of CML. These tumors may be composed of myeloblasts or lymphoblasts, although in each case the Ph chromosome or the *BCR-ABL1* fusion is present in the cells, indicating the extramedullary Ph-positive

lymphoblastomas are the tissue variant of the predisposition of CML to transform into a terminal deoxynucleotidyl transferase-positive lymphoblastic leukemia in approximately 30 percent of patients who enter blast crisis (Chap. 89).

Release of Procoagulants and Fibrinolytic Activators

Microvascular thrombosis is a feature of AML of the promyelocytic type, although thrombosis can occur in other forms of acute leukemia, especially in cases with elevated white cell counts or monocytic phenotypes.[63,64] The leukemic promyelocytes liberate tissue factor and other procoagulants, giving rise to disseminated intravascular coagulation, and annexin II, which augments conversion of plasminogen to plasmin and contributes to the activation of fibrinolysis (Chaps. 88, 129, and 135). Each mechanism contributes to hypofibrinogenemia and hemorrhage. Thrombin generation may mediate the microvascular thrombotic aspect of this process, which can occur in acute promyelocytic, acute monocytic, or acute myelomonocytic leukemia, either before or after cytotoxic treatment.[65,66] The increased fibrinolytic activity further complicates coagulopathy in patients with promyelocytic leukemia.

Large-vessel arterial thrombosis is very rare as a presenting feature or complication of leukemia but has occurred in the setting of hyperleukocytosis and as a presenting feature of acute promyelocytic leukemia.[67,68]

The plasma levels of protein C antigen, functional protein C, free protein S, and antithrombin are decreased in some patients with AML. Although these changes are particularly notable in acute promyelocytic leukemia, they occur occasionally in other morphologic variants of AML. The changes are not related to liver disease or white cell count.[69,70]

Hyperleukocytic Syndromes

A proportion of patients with AML (5 to 15 percent) and CML (10 to 20 percent) manifest extraordinarily high blood leukocyte counts.[71-75] These patients present special problems because of the effects of blast cells in the microcirculation of the lung, brain, eye, ear, and penis, and the metabolic effects that result when massive numbers of leukemic cells in blood, marrow, and tissues are simultaneously killed by cytotoxic drugs. Cell concentrations greater than $100,000/\mu L$ (100×10^9/L) in AML and greater than $300,000/\mu L$ (300×10^9/L) in CML usually are required to produce such problems. In CML, the manifestations of hyperleukocytosis are usually reversed by cytoreduction and may not portend a poor outcome with anti–tyrosine kinase therapy. In AML, intracerebral hemorrhage and the impairment of pulmonary function are the most serious manifestations in predicting early death.[74,75] A respiratory distress syndrome attributed to pulmonary leukostasis occurs in some patients with acute promyelocytic leukemia after all-*trans*-retinoic acid therapy.[76] The syndrome is usually, but not always, associated with prominent neutrophilia.

The viscosity of blood is related to the total cytocrit and usually is not increased in hyperleukocytic leukemias because the reduced hematocrit compensates for increased leukocrit. This compensatory change is invariably present in AML. In CML there is a very close negative correlation of hematocrit with leukocrit, preventing an increase in bulk viscosity.[71] Occasional patients with hyperleukocytic CML who are transfused initially with red cells may have a blood viscosity increased above normal.

Pathologic studies of patients who have died with hyperleukocytosis have identified leukoocclusion and vascular invasion in small vessels of the lung, brain, or other sites. Because viscosity in the microcirculation is a function of the plasma viscosity and the deformability of individual cells in capillaries, leukocytes should transiently raise the viscosity in such small channels. Flow in microvascular channels decreases if poorly deformable blast cells enter capillary channels.[77]

TABLE 83–3. Clinical Features of the Hyperleukocytic Syndrome

I. Pulmonary circulation
   A. Tachypnea, dyspnea, cyanosis
   B. Alveolar–capillary block
   C. Pulmonary infiltrates
   D. Postchemotherapy respiratory dysfunction
II. Predisposition to tumor lysis syndrome
III. Central nervous system circulation
   A. Dizziness, slurred speech, delirium, stupor
   B. Intracranial (cerebral) hemorrhage
IV. Special sensory organ circulation
   A. Visual blurring
   B. Papilledema
   C. Diplopia
   D. Tinnitus, impaired hearing
   E. Retinal vein distention, retinal hemorrhages
V. Penile circulation
   A. Priapism
VI. Spurious laboratory results
   A. Decreased blood partial pressure of oxygen (P_{O_2}); increased serum potassium
   B. Decreased plasma glucose; increased mean corpuscular volume, red cell count, hemoglobin, and hematocrit

With high leukocyte counts, chronically reduced flow may reduce oxygen transport to tissues because the probability of leukocytes being in microchannels should increase as a function of white cell count. Moreover, trapped leukemic cells have an oxygen consumption rate that contributes to deleterious effects in the microcirculation. Leukocyte aggregation, leukocyte microthrombi, release of toxic products from leukocytes, endothelial cell damage, and microvascular invasion can contribute to vascular injury and flow impedance. Adhesive interactions between leukemic blast cells and endothelium may also be involved but have not been defined.

High leukemic blast cell counts in AML and CML may be associated with pulmonary, central nervous system, special sensory, or penile circulatory impairment (Table 83–3). Sudden death can occur in patients with hyperleukocytic acute leukemia as a result of intracranial hemorrhage.[74,75] Hyperleukocytosis can be treated initially with hydration, leukapheresis, and/or cytotoxic therapy, usually hydroxyurea (Chaps. 88 and 89). In patients with CML, leukapheresis reverses the hyperleukocytic syndrome and can reduce the extent of cytolysis-induced hyperuricemia, hyperkalemia, and hyperphosphatemia by reducing tumor cell mass before hydroxyurea therapy. Hydroxyurea may follow as, or soon after, the tumor cell burden is decreased. Unfortunately, the specific effect of leukapheresis, hydroxyurea therapy, or cranial irradiation in patients with hyperleukocytic AML on duration of survival appears to be negligible.[73–75]

THROMBOCYTHEMIC SYNDROMES: HEMORRHAGE AND THROMBOPHILIA

Hemorrhagic or thrombotic episodes can develop during the course of essential thrombocythemia or thrombocythemia associated with other clonal myeloid diseases.[76–78] Arterial vascular insufficiency and venous thromboses are the major vascular manifestations of thrombocythemia.

Peripheral vascular insufficiency with gangrene and cerebral vascular thrombi can develop. Thrombosis of superficial or deep veins of the extremities occurs frequently.[79] Mesenteric, hepatic, portal, splenic, or penile venous thrombosis can ensue. Patients with essential thrombocythemia who have the *CALR* mutation have a significantly lower risk of thrombotic disease than those with a *JAK2* or *MPL* mutation.[80] Hemorrhage is an occasional manifestation of thrombocythemia and can occur concomitantly with thrombotic episodes. Gastrointestinal hemorrhage and cutaneous hemorrhage, the latter especially after trauma, happen most frequently, but bleeding from other sites also can result (Chap. 85).

Procoagulant factors, such as the content of platelet tissue factor and blood platelet neutrophil aggregates, are more frequent in patients with essential thrombocythemia than normal subjects and are more frequent among patients with the *JAK2*[V617F] mutation than patients with the wild-type gene.[79,81]

Thrombotic complications occur in approximately 40 percent of patients with polycythemia vera.[79,82] The presence of homozygosity for the *JAK2* mutation as a result of uniparental disomy in as many as one-third of patients with polycythemia vera increases the risk of thrombosis. Erythrocytosis and thrombocytosis may interact and cause hypercoagulability, especially in the abdominal venous circulation. A syndrome of splanchnic venous thrombosis associated with endogenous erythroid colony growth, the latter characteristic of polycythemia vera, but without blood cell count changes indicative of a myeloproliferative disease, has accounted for a high proportion of patients with apparent idiopathic hepatic or portal vein thrombosis.[83,84] These cases may have blood cells with the *JAK2* gene mutation without a clinically apparent myeloproliferative phenotype.[85]

Nearly half of patients with paroxysmal nocturnal hemoglobinuria have thrombosis, especially in the venous system. Thrombosis of the veins of the abdomen, liver, and other organs, characteristic complications of paroxysmal nocturnal hemoglobinuria, may result from a complex thrombophilic state related to nitric oxide depletion, formation of prothrombotic platelet microvesicles, the dysfunction of tissue factor pathway inhibitor, and other factors.[86,87] Thrombosis is more common in paroxysmal nocturnal hemoglobinuria (PNH) patients with the classical hemolytic syndrome than in those with the PNH-aplastic anemia hybrid (Chap. 40).

SYSTEMIC SYMPTOMS

Fever, weight loss, and malaise occur as early manifestations of AML. At the time of diagnosis, low-grade fever is present in nearly 50 percent of patients.[88] Although minor infections may be present, severe systemic infections are relatively uncommon at the time of AML diagnosis.[89] However, fever during cytotoxic therapy, when neutrophil counts are extremely low, nearly always is a sign of infection. Fever also may be a manifestation of the acute leukemic transformation of CML and can occur in patients with oligoblastic myelogenous leukemia (refractory anemia with excess blasts).

Weight loss occurs in nearly 20 percent of patients with AML.[89] Loss of well-being and intolerance to exertion may be disproportionate to the extent of anemia and may not be corrected by red cell transfusions. The pathogenesis of these effects is unknown.

METABOLIC SIGNS

Hyperuricemia and hyperuricosuria are common manifestations of AML and CML. Acute gouty arthritis and hyperuricosuric nephropathy are less common. If therapy is instituted without a reduction in plasma uric acid and without adequate hydration, saturation of the urine with uric acid can lead to precipitation of urate (gravel) and obstructive uropathy. If the uropathy is severe, urine flow can be obliterated, and renal failure ensues. Hyponatremia can occur in AML, and in some cases results from inappropriate antidiuretic hormone secretion. Hyponatremia also can result from an osmotic diuresis of urea, creatinine, urate, and other substances released from blast cells and wasting muscles. Hypernatremia is rare but may be seen in cases with central diabetes insipidus. Hypokalemia is commonly seen in AML[89–91] and is thought to be caused by injury to the kidney by increased plasma and urine lysozyme and subsequent kaliuresis. Hypokalemia is related to excessive urinary potassium loss, but the correlation with lysozymuria is imperfect. Other mechanisms probably are responsible in most cases, including osmotic diuresis and tubular dysfunction. Kaliuretic antibiotics, often administered to patients with AML, may accentuate the hypokalemia. Hyperkalemia is very unusual, but may be seen with tumor lysis syndrome. Hypercalcemia occurs in occasional patients with AML. Several causes have been proposed, including bone resorption as a result of leukemic infiltration. This explanation is in keeping with the normal serum inorganic phosphate in most patients. Occasional patients with hypercalcemia, and hypophosphatemia can have ectopic parathyroid hormone secretion by leukemic blast cells. Hypophosphatemia also can occur because of rapid utilization of plasma inorganic phosphate in some cases of myelogenous leukemia with a high blood blast cell count and a high fraction of proliferative cells. Hyperphosphatemia is uncommon, except as a reflection of the tumor lysis syndrome. Approximately 10 percent of persons with AML show varying degrees of tumor lysis syndrome in the week after onset of therapy, reflected in at least doubling of baseline creatinine, and increases in serum phosphate (>1.6 mmol/L [>5 mg/dL]), uric acid (>416 mmol/L [>7mg/dL]), or potassium (>5 mmol/L [>5 mEq/L]).[92] Hypomagnesemia is common as a result of low intake coupled with gastrointestinal loss and a shift of magnesium to the intracellular compartment.

Acid–base disturbances occur in approximately 25 percent of patients, the majority having respiratory or metabolic alkalosis.[91] The latter may be secondary to volume depletion, upper gastrointestinal fluid loss, and hypokalemia. Lactic acidosis also has been observed in association with AML, although the mechanism is obscure. True hypoxia can result from the hyperleukocytic syndrome as a consequence of pulmonary vascular leukostasis (see also "Factitious Laboratory Results" below).

Increased serum concentrations of lipoprotein (a) and decreased concentrations of both low-density and high-density lipoproteins have been observed in a high proportion of patients with AML.[93] The increased level of lipoprotein (a), which returns to normal after successful treatment, correlates with the presence of leukemic blast cells. Serum prolactin also is increased in some patients with AML.[94] Leukemic blast cells may be an ectopic source of this hormone.[94]

Colony-stimulating factor-1 is elevated in a variety of lymphoid and hemopoietic malignancies, including AML and CML.[95] The malignant cells have been proposed as the source of excess cytokine.

FACTITIOUS LABORATORY RESULTS

Elevations of serum potassium levels have resulted from the release of potassium from platelets or, less often, leukocytes in patients with myeloproliferative diseases and extreme elevations in those blood cell concentrations. If blood is collected in a tube that contains an anticoagulant and the plasma is removed after high-speed centrifugation, the potassium concentration is normal. Glucose can be falsely decreased, especially because autoanalyzer techniques call for omission of glycolytic inhibitors such as sodium fluoride in collection tubes. Blood with high leukocyte counts, if it stands prior to separation of the plasma, may have a significant amount of glucose metabolism by leukocytes. Factitious hypoglycemia also can occur as a result of red cell utilization

of glucose, especially in polycythemic patients. True hypoglycemia has been observed rarely in patients with leukemia. Arterial blood oxygen content also can be lowered spuriously as a result of *in vitro* utilization by large numbers of leukocytes, while the anticoagulated blood awaits measurement.

SPECIFIC ORGAN INVOLVEMENT

Clonal myeloid diseases lead to disturbances principally in marrow, blood, and spleen. Although clusters of cells may be found in all organs, major infiltrates and organ dysfunction are unusual. In AML and the acute blastic phase of CML, clinically significant infiltration of the larynx, central nervous system, heart, lungs, bone, joints, gastrointestinal tract, genitourinary tract, skin, or virtually any other organ can occur.

Splenomegaly

In AML, palpable splenomegaly is present in approximately one-third of cases, but usually is slight in extent. In the chronic myeloproliferative diseases, palpable splenomegaly is present in a high proportion of cases (polycythemia vera ~80 percent, CML ~90 percent, primary myelofibrosis ~100 percent). In essential thrombocythemia, splenic enlargement is present in approximately 30 percent of patients. A predisposition to silent splenic vascular thrombi, infarction, and subsequent splenic atrophy, analogous to that occurring in sickle cell anemia, is postulated as the cause of the lower frequency of splenic enlargement in essential thrombocythemia. Early satiety, left-upper-quadrant discomfort, splenic infarctions with painful perisplenitis, diaphragmatic pleuritis, and referred shoulder pain may occur in patients with splenomegaly, especially in the acute phase of CML and in primary myelofibrosis. In primary myelofibrosis, the spleen can become enormous, occupying the left hemiabdomen. Blood flow through the splenic vein can be so great as to lead to portal hypertension and gastroesophageal varices. Usually, reduced hepatic venous compliance also is present (Chap. 86). Bleeding and, occasionally, encephalopathy can result from portal–systemic venous shunts.

Marrow Necrosis

Extensive marrow necrosis, an uncommon event, can occur in any clonal myeloid disease, especially AML, and less often, primary myelofibrosis, CML, essential thrombocythemia, and polycythemia vera. Bone pain and fever are the most common initial findings. Anemia and thrombocytopenia are very common, as are nucleated red cells and myelocytes in the blood (leukoerythroblastic reaction).[96,97] Marrow aspiration does not result in a useful sample but biopsy early in the process usually shows hypocellularity with loss of marrow cell structural definition (blurred staining of residual cells), evidence of cell necrosis, gelatinous transformation of marrow, and, often, an amorphous eosinophilic material throughout. The mechanism is thought to be microvascular dysfunction. Restitution of marrow and repopulation of hematopoietic tissue often may follow. The prognosis is a function of the underlying disease.

REFERENCES

1. Dick JE, Lapidot T: Biology of normal and acute myeloid leukemia stem cells. *Int J Hematol* 82:389, 2005.
2. Eppert K, Takenaka K, Lechman ER, et al: Stem cell gene expression programs influence clinical outcome in human leukemia. *Nat Med* 17:1086, 2011.
3. Pei S, Jordan CT: How close are we to targeting the leukemia stem cell? *Best Pract Res Clin Haematol* 25:415, 2012.
4. Rozman CGM, Feliu E, Rubio D, et al: Life expectancy of patients with chronic nonleukemic myeloproliferative disorders. *Cancer* 67:2658, 1991.

5. Bacher U, Kern W, Alpermann T et al: Prognoses of MDS subtypes RARS, RCMD and RCMD-RS are comparable but cytogenetics separates a subgroup with inferior clinical course. *Leuk Res* 36:826, 2012.

6. Jaffe ES, Harris NL, Stein H, Vardiman JW: *World Health Organization Classification of Tumours: Pathology and Genetics of Tumours of Haematopoietic and Lymphoid Tissues.* IARC Press, Lyon, 2008.

7. Bacher U, Kern W, Alpermann T, et al: Prognosis in patients with MDS or AML and bone marrow blasts between 10% and 30% is not associated with blast counts but depends on cytogenetic and molecular genetic characteristics. *Leukemia* 25:1361, 2011.

8. Lichtman MA: Does a diagnosis of myelogenous leukemia require 20% marrow myeloblasts, and does <5% marrow myeloblasts represent a remission? The history and ambiguity of arbitrary diagnostic boundaries in the understanding of myelodysplasia. *Oncologist* 18:973, 2013.

9. van de Loosdrecht AA, Westers TM: Cutting edge: Flow cytometry in myelodysplastic syndromes. *J Natl Compr Canc Netw* 11:892, 2013.

10. Lichtman MA: Myelodysplasia or myeloneoplasia: Thoughts on the nosology of clonal myeloid diseases. *Blood Cells Mol Dis* 26:572, 2000.

11. Bessis M, Bernard J: Hematopoietic dysplasias (preleukemic states). *Blood Cells* 2:5, 1976.

12. Spivak JL, Silver RT: The revised World Health Organization diagnostic criteria for polycythemia vera, essential thrombocytosis, and primary myelofibrosis: An alternative proposal. *Blood* 112:231, 2008.

13. Nangalia J, Massie CE, Baxter EJ, et al: Somatic CALR mutations in myeloproliferative neoplasms with non-mutated JAK2. *N Engl J Med* 369:2391, 2013.

14. Klampfl T, Gisslinger H, Harutyunyan AS, et al: Somatic mutations of calreticulin in myeloproliferative neoplasms. *N Engl J Med* 369:2379, 2013.

15. Kiladjian JJ, Gardin C, Renoux M, et al: Long-term outcomes of polycythemia vera patients treated with pipobroman as initial therapy. *Hematol J* 4:198, 2003.

16. Tefferi A, Fonesca R, Pereira DL, Hoagland HC: A long-term retrospective study of young women with essential thrombocythemia. *Mayo Clin Proc* 76:22, 2001.

17. Passamonti F, Malabarba L, Orlandi E, et al: Polycythemia in young patients: A study on the long-term risk of thrombosis, myelofibrosis and leukemia. *Haematologica* 88:13, 2003.

18. Stein BL, Saraf S, Sobol U, et al: Age-related differences in disease characteristics and clinical outcomes in polycythemia vera. *Leuk Lymphoma* 54:1989, 2013.

18a. Tefferi A, Guglielmelli P, Larson DR, et al: Long-term survival and blast transformation in molecularly annotated essential thrombocythemia, polycythemia vera, and myelofibrosis. *Blood* 124:2507, 2014.

19. Lichtman MA: Is it chronic idiopathic myelofibrosis, myelofibrosis with myeloid metaplasia, chronic megakaryocytic-granulocytic myelosis, or chronic megakaryocytic leukemia? Further thoughts on the nosology of the clonal myeloid disorders. *Leukemia* 19:1139, 2005.

20. Simon W, Segel GB, Lichtman MA: Early allogeneic stem cell transplantation for chronic myelogenous leukemia in the imatinib era: A preliminary assessment. *Blood Cells Mol Dis* 37:116, 2006.

21. Tefferi A, Elliott MA, Pardanani A: Atypical myeloproliferative disorders: Diagnosis and management. *Mayo Clin Proc* 81:553, 2006.

22. Tefferi A, Vardiman JW: Classification and diagnosis of myeloproliferative neoplasms: The 2008 World Health Organization criteria and point-of-care diagnostic algorithms. *Leukemia* 22:14, 2008.

23. Breccia M, Cannella L, Frustaci A, et al: Chronic myelomonocytic leukemia with antecedent refractory anemia with excess blasts: Further evidence for the arbitrary nature of current classification systems. *Leuk Lymphoma* 49:1292, 2008.

24. Breccia M, Latagliata R, Cannella L, et al: Analysis of prognostic factors in patients with refractory anemia with excess of blasts (RAEB) reclassified according to WHO proposal. *Leuk Res* 33:391, 2009.

25. Barnard DR, Kalousek DK, Wiersma SR, et al: Morphologic, immunologic, and cytogenetic classification of acute myeloid leukemia and myelodysplastic syndrome in childhood. *Leukemia* 10:5, 1996.

26. Bene MC, Castoldi G, Knapp W, et al: Proposals for the immunological classification of acute leukemias. *Leukemia* 9:1783, 1995.

27. Jennings CD, Foon KA: Recent advances in flow cytometry: Application to the diagnosis of hematologic malignancy. *Blood* 90:2863, 1997.

28. Cancer Genome Anatomy Project: *Mitelman Database of Chromosome Aberrations and Gene Fusions in Cancer.* Available at: http://cgap.nci.nih.gov/Chromosomes/Mitelman (accessed August 2008).

29. Oyan AM, Bø TH, Jonassen I, et al: Global gene expression in classification, pathogenetic understanding and identification of therapeutic targets in acute myeloid leukemia. *Curr Pharm Biotechnol* 8:344, 2007.

30. Verhaak RG, Valk PJ: Genes predictive of outcome and novel molecular classification schemes in adult acute myeloid leukemia. *Cancer Treat Res* 145:67, 2010.

31. Cancer Genome Atlas Research Network. Genomic and epigenomic landscapes of adult de novo acute myeloid leukemia. *N Engl J Med* 368:2059, 2013.

32. Valk PJM, Verhaak RGW, Beijen A, et al: Prognostically useful gene expression profiles in acute myeloid leukemia. *N Engl J Med* 350:1617, 2004.

33. Bullinger L, Döhner K, Kranz R, et al: An FLT3 gene-expression signature predicts clinical outcome in normal karyotype AML. *Blood* 111:4490, 2008.

34. Welch JS, Ley TJ, Link DC, et al: The origin and evolution of mutations in acute myeloid leukemia. *Cell* 150:264, 2012.

35. Shlush LI, Zandi S, Mitchell A, et al: Identification of pre-leukaemic haematopoietic stem cells in acute leukaemia. *Nature* 506:328, 2014.

36. Jongen-Lavrencic M, Sun SM, Dijkstra MK, et al: MicroRNA expression profiling in relation to the genetic heterogeneity of acute myeloid leukemia. *Blood* 111:5078, 2008.

37. Garzon R, Croce CM: MicroRNAs in normal and malignant hematopoiesis. *Curr Opin Hematol* 15:352 2008.

38. Mills KI: Gene expression profiling for the diagnosis and prognosis of acute myeloid leukemia. *Front Biosci* 13:4605, 2008.

39. Shukron O, Vainstein V, Kündgen A, et al: Analyzing transformation of myelodysplastic syndrome to secondary acute myeloid leukemia using a large patient database. *Am J Hematol* 87:853, 2012.

40. Andrieux J, Demory JL, Caulier MT, et al: Karyotype abnormalities in myelofibrosis following polycythemia vera. *Cancer Genet Cytogenet* 140:118, 2003.

41. Finazzi G, Caruso V, Marchioli R, et al: Acute leukemia in polycythemia vera: An analysis of 1638 patients enrolled in a prospective observational study. *Blood* 105:2664, 2005.

42. Lichtman MA: The stem cell in the pathogenesis and treatment of myelogenous leukemia: A perspective. *Leukemia* 15:1489, 2001.

43. Gilliland DG: Molecular genetics of human leukemias: New insights into therapy. *Semin Hematol* 39:6, 2002.

44. Lichtman MA, Segel GB: Uncommon phenotypes of acute myelogenous leukemia: Basophilic, mast cell, eosinophilic, and myeloid dendritic cell subtypes: A review. *Blood Cells Mol Dis* 35:370, 2005.

45. Ploemacher RE: Characterization and biology of normal human haematopoietic stem cells. *Haematologica* 84 Suppl EHA-4:4, 1999.

46. Bonnet D, Dick J: Human acute myeloid leukemia is organized as a hierarchy that originates from a primitive hematopoietic cell. *Nat Med* 3:730, 1997.

47. Sarry JE, Murphy K, Perry R, et al: Human acute myelogenous leukemia stem cells are rare and heterogeneous when assayed in NOD/SCID/IL2Rγc-deficient mice. *J Clin Invest* 121:384, 2011.

48. Corces-Zimmerman MR, Majeti R: Pre-leukemic evolution of hematopoietic stem cells: the importance of early mutations in leukemogenesis. *Leukemia* 28:2276, 2014.

49. Takahashi N, Maura I, Saitoh K, Miura AB: Lineage involvement of stem cells bearing the Philadelphia chromosome in chronic myeloid leukemia in the chronic phase as shown by combination of fluorescence-activated cell sorting and fluorescence in situ hybridization. *Blood* 92:4758, 1998.

50. Fialkow PJ, Singer JW, Adamson JW, et al: Acute nonlymphocytic leukemia: Expression in cells restricted to granulocytic and monocytic differentiation. *N Engl J Med* 301:1, 1979.

51. Fialkow PJ, Singer JW, Adamson JW, et al: Acute nonlymphocytic leukemia: Heterogeneity of stem cell origin. *Blood* 57:1068, 1981.

52. Ferraris AM, Broccia G, Meloni T, et al: Clonal origin of cells restricted to monocytic differentiation in acute nonlymphocytic leukemia. *Blood* 64:817, 1984.

53. Van Lom K, Hagenmaijer A, Vandekerckhove F, et al: Clonality analysis of hematopoietic cell lineages in acute myeloid leukemia and trans-location (8;21): Only myeloid cells are part of the malignant clone. *Leukemia* 11:202, 1997.

54. Grimwade D, Enver T: Acute promyelocytic leukemia: Where does it stem from? *Leukemia* 18:375, 2004.

55. Wartman LD, Welch JS, Uy GL, et al: Expression and function of PML-RARA in the hematopoietic progenitor cells of CTGS-PML-RARA mice. *PLoS One* 7:e46529, 2012.

56. Lichtman MA: Interrupting the inhibition of normal hematopoiesis in myelogenous leukemia: A hypothetical approach to therapy. *Stem Cells* 18(5):304, 2000.

57. Menasce LP, Banerjee SS, Becket E, Harris M: Extramedullary myeloid tumor (granulocytic sarcoma) is often misdiagnosed. A study of 26 cases. *Histopathology* 34:391, 1999.

58. Pileri SA, Ascani S, Cox MC, et al: Myeloid sarcoma: Clinico-pathologic, phenotypic and cytogenetic analysis of 92 adult patients. *Leukemia* 21:340, 2007.

59. Tsimberidou AM, Kantarjian HM, Wen S, et al: Myeloid sarcoma is associated with superior event-free survival and overall survival compared with acute myeloid leukemia. *Cancer* 113:1370, 2008.

60. Lichtman MA, Weed RI: Peripheral cytoplasmic characteristics of leukemia cells in monocytic leukemia: Relationship to clinical manifestations. *Blood* 40:52, 1972.

61. Peterson L, Dekner LP, Brunning RD: Extramedullary masses as presenting features of acute monoblastic leukemia. *Am J Clin Pathol* 75:140, 1981.

62. Tobelem G, Jacquillat C, Chastang C, et al: Acute monoblastic leukemia: A clinical and biologic study of 74 cases. *Blood* 55:71, 1980.

63. Weltermann A, Pabinger I, Geissler K, et al: Hypofibrinogenemia in non-M3 acute myeloid leukemia. Incidence, clinical and laboratory characteristics and prognosis. *Leukemia* 12:1182, 1998.

64. Uchiumi H, Matsushima T, Yamane A, et al: Prevalence and clinical characteristics of acute myeloid leukemia associated with disseminated intravascular coagulation. *Int J Hematol* 86:137, 2007.

65. Falanga A, Rickles FR: Pathogenesis and management of the bleeding diathesis in acute promyelocytic leukaemia. *Best Pract Res Clin Haematol* 16:463, 2003.

66. Tallman MS, Abutalib SA, Altman JK: The double hazard of thrombophilia and bleeding in acute promyelocytic leukemia. *Semin Thromb Hemost* 33:330, 2007.

67. Kalk E, Goede A, Rose P: Acute arterial thrombosis in acute promyelocytic leukaemia. *Clin Lab Haematol* 25:267, 2003.

68. Reisch N, Roehnisch T, Sadeghi M, et al: AML M1 presenting with recurrent acute large arterial vessel thromboembolism. *Leuk Res* 31:869, 2007.

69. Troy K, Essex D, Rand J, et al: Protein C and S levels in acute leukemia. *Am J Hematol* 37:159, 1991.

70. Dixit A, Kannan M, Mahapatra M, et al: Roles of protein C, protein S, and antithrombin III in acute leukemia. *Am J Hematol* 81:171, 2006.

71. Lichtman MA, Heal J, Rowe JM: Hyperleukocytic leukaemia: Rheological and clinical features and management. *Baillieres Clin Haematol* 1:725, 1987.

72. Rowe JM, Lichtman MA: Hyperleukocytosis and leukostasis: Common features of childhood chronic myelogenous leukemia. *Blood* 63:1230, 1984.

73. Porcu P, Cripe LD, Ng EW, et al: Hyperleukocytic leukemias and leukostasis: A review of pathophysiology, clinical presentation and management. *Leuk Lymphoma* 39:1, 2000.

74. Marbello L, Ricci F, Nosari AM: Outcome of hyperleukocytic adult acute myeloid leukaemia: A single-center retrospective study and review of literature. *Leuk Res* 32:1221, 2008.

75. Chang MC, Chen TY, Tang JL, et al: Leukapheresis and cranial irradiation in patients with hyperleukocytic acute myeloid leukemia: No impact on early mortality and intracranial hemorrhage. *Am J Hematol* 82:976, 2007.

76. Patatanian E, Thompson DF: Retinoic acid syndrome: A review. *J Clin Pharm Ther* 33:331, 2008.

77. Östergren J, Fagrell B, Björkholm M: Hyperleukocytic effects on skin capillary circulation in patients with leukaemia. *J Intern Med* 231:19, 1992.

78. Cortelazzo S, Vicero P, Finazzi G, et al: Incidence and risk factors for thrombotic complications in a historical cohort of 100 patients with thrombocythemia. *J Clin Oncol* 8:556, 1990.

79. Falanga A, Barbui T, Rickles FR: Hypercoagulability and tissue factor gene upregulation in hematologic malignancies. *Semin Thromb Hemost* 34:204, 2008.

80. Rotunno G, Mannarelli C, Guglielmelli P, et al: Impact of calreticulin mutations on clinical and hematological phenotype and outcome in essential thrombocythemia. *Blood* 123:1552, 2014.

81. Dahabreh IJ, Zoi K, Giannouli S, et al: Is JAK2 V617F mutation more than a diagnostic index? A meta-analysis of clinical outcomes in essential thrombocythemia. *Leuk Res* 33:67, 2009.

82. Landolfi R: Bleeding and thrombosis in myeloproliferative disorders. *Curr Opin Hematol* 5:327, 1998.

83. Anger B, Haugh U, Seidler R, Heimpel H: Polycythemia vera: A clinical study of 141 patients. *Blut* 59:493, 1989.

84. Teofili L, De Stefano V, Leone G, et al: Hematologic causes of venous thrombosis in young people: High incidence of myeloproliferative disorder as underlying disease in patients with splanchnic venous thrombosis. *Thromb Haemost* 67:297, 1992.

85. Colaizzo D, Amitrano L, Tiscia GL, et al: Occurrence of the JAK2 V617F mutation in the Budd-Chiari syndrome. *Blood Coagul Fibrinolysis* 19:459, 2008.

86. Peffault de Latour R, Mary JY, Salanoubat C, et al: Paroxysmal nocturnal hemoglobinuria: Natural history of disease subcategories. *Blood* 112:3099, 2008.

87. Brodsky RA: Advances in the diagnosis and therapy of paroxysmal nocturnal hemoglobinuria. *Blood Rev* 22:65, 2008.

88. Burke PJ, Braine HG, Rathbun HK, Owens AH Jr: The clinical significance of fever in acute myelocytic leukemia. *Johns Hopkins Med J* 139:1, 1976.

89. Burns CP, Armitage JO, Frey AL, et al: Analysis of the presenting features of adult acute leukemia. *Cancer* 47:2460, 1981.

90. Mir MA, Delamore JW: Metabolic disorders in acute myeloid leukaemia. *Br J Haematol* 40:79, 1978.

91. Filippatos TD, Milionis HJ, Elisaf MS: Alterations in electrolyte equilibrium in patients with acute leukemia. *Eur J Haematol* 75:449, 2005.

92. Mato AR, Riccio BE, Qin L, et al: A predictive model for the detection of tumor lysis syndrome during AML induction therapy. *Leuk Lymphoma* 47:877, 2006.

93. Niendorf A, Stang A, Beisiegel U, et al: Elevated lipoprotein (a) levels in patients with acute myeloblastic leukaemia decrease after successful chemotherapeutic treatment. *Clin Investig* 70:683, 1990.

94. Hatfill SJ, Kirby R, Hanley M, et al: Hyperprolactinemia in acute myeloid leukemia and indication of ectopic expression of human prolactin in blast cells of a patient of subtype M4. *Leuk Res* 14:57, 1990.

95. Janowska-Wieczarek A, Belch AR, Jacobs A, et al: Increased circulating colony-stimulating factor-1 in patients with preleukemia, leukemia and lymphoid malignancies. *Blood* 77:1796, 1991.

96. Janssens AM, Offner FC, Van Hove WZ: Bone marrow necrosis. *Cancer* 88:1769, 2000.

97. Paydas S, Ergin M, Baslamisli F, et al: Bone marrow necrosis: Clinicopathologic analysis of 20 cases and review of the literature. *Am J Hematol* 70:300, 2002.

CHAPTER 84
POLYCYTHEMIA VERA

Jaroslav F. Prchal and Josef T. Prchal

SUMMARY

Polycythemia vera (PV) is classified in the group of Philadelphia chromosome–negative myeloproliferative neoplasms (MPNs) that also includes essential thrombocythemia (ET) and primary myelofibrosis (PMF). Chronic myelogenous leukemia was historically classified as a MPN, but is now considered a separate entity. PV is an acquired primary clonal polycythemic disorder. Primary polycythemias result from abnormal intrinsic properties of erythroid progenitors that proliferate independently or excessively in response to extrinsic regulators; low serum erythropoietin is their hallmark. PV is the most common primary polycythemia. It arises from mutation(s) of a pluripotent hematopoietic stem cell, which results in excess production of erythrocytes and variable overproduction of granulocytes and platelets. It is often accompanied by splenomegaly. Most patients with PV have a somatic mutation of the Janus-type tyrosine kinase-2 gene (JAK2) that is detectable in blood myeloid cells. The mutation results in constitutive hyperactivity of JAK2 kinase stemming from loss-of-function of its negative regulatory domain. The most common mutation is $JAK2^{V617F}$, which is present in virtually all cases of PV; a small minority of PV patients have a mutation in other parts of JAK2 (exon 12). The $JAK2^{V617F}$ mutation is also found in many patients with ET and myelofibrosis (MF), albeit at lower frequency (55 percent in ET and 65 percent in MF). As with other clonal hematologic disorders, PV can undergo a clonal evolution to PMF ($JAK2^{V617F}$-positive) or acute leukemia (either $JAK2^{V617F}$-negative or positive). In virtually all $JAK2^{V617F}$-positive PV patients, at least some progenitors exist that become homozygous for the $JAK2^{V617F}$ mutation by uniparental disomy-acquired mitotic recombination. The majority of these progenitors account for the erythropoietin-independent erythroid colonies detected in vitro by clonogenic burst-forming unit–erythroid assay. The $JAK2^{V617F}$ mutation is often not the initial cause of clonal proliferation, but may be preceded by other germline and somatic mutation(s) (e.g., TET2).

Arterial and venous thromboses are a major cause of morbidity and mortality in PV, and a small proportion of patients develop secondary myelofibrosis (sometimes called the *spent phase*) and/or an invariably fatal acute leukemic transformation. Myelosuppressive therapy has been an effective mode of therapy, with drugs such as hydroxyurea, busulfan, pipobroman, and radioactive phosphorus useful in controlling proliferation of all blood cell lineages. However, while myelosuppressive therapy controls the cellular proliferation and decreases the incidence of thrombotic complications, many of these drugs have leukemogenic potential. In contrast, pegylated interferon-*a* may lead to complete hematologic remission and restoration of polyclonal hematopoiesis and avoid the leukemogenic complications. Targeted therapy with JAK2 kinase inhibitors is currently being evaluated in clinical trials and, thus far, have been found effective in decreasing the need for phlebotomies, decreasing the number of white cells and splenomegaly, and improving the patient's quality of life.

DEFINITION AND HISTORY

The term *polycythemia*, denoting an increased amount of blood, has traditionally been applied to those conditions in which the mass of erythrocytes is increased. In polycythemia vera (PV), an increase in the erythroid mass is frequently accompanied by an increase in neutrophils and platelets. For a classification of the polycythemias, see Chap. 57 and Chap. 34, Table 34–2. Although several clinical stages of PV are recognized (masked PV, plethoric phase, stable phase, transformation, spent phase, and acute leukemia), it is not clear whether these stages represent a sequential progression of the disease or whether all patients progress through all stages.

PV, the sole clonal form of primary polycythemia, was first described in 1892 by Vaquez.[1] In 1903, Osler reviewed four of his own PV cases and an additional five cases from the literature and wrote, "The condition is characterized by chronic cyanosis, polycythemia, and variable moderate enlargement of the spleen. The chief symptoms have been weakness, prostration, constipation, headache, and vertigo."[2] The increased proliferation of granulocyte precursors and megakaryocytes was first described by Türk in 1904.[3]

EPIDEMIOLOGY

A recent analysis of 20 studies of PV patients from around the world revealed an annual incidence rate of 0.84 cases per 100,000 people, with no bias for gender.[4,5] The true incidence may be higher, as many cases are asymptomatic and thus not diagnosed. Testing for the Janus-type tyrosine kinase 2 $(JAK2)^{V617F}$ mutation can uncover hidden cases of PV among subjects with thrombosis or concomitant iron deficiency. The incidence of PV may be higher among Ashkenazi Jews.[6,7]

Although most patients with PV do not have a history of polycythemia in the family, familial incidence of the disorder is known to occur[8–10] and is very likely underreported. In a large Swedish study of more than 25,000 first-degree relatives of 11,000 myeloproliferative neoplasm (MPN) patients, the incidence of MPNs were five to seven times higher in relatives than in controls.[11] In familial cases of PV, an inherited predisposition, perhaps in the form of a germline mutation, presumably facilitates the acquired somatic mutation(s) necessary for disease onset.[9,12]

ETIOLOGY AND PATHOGENESIS

PV arises from the neoplastic transformation of a single normal hematopoietic pluripotent cell, which acquires a selective proliferative and survival advantage, resulting in the development of a variable degree

Acronyms and Abbreviations: AML, acute myelogenous leukemia; BFU-E, burst-forming unit–erythroid; ECLAP, European Collaboration on Low-Dose Aspirin in Polycythemia Vera; EEC, endogenous erythroid colony; ELN, European Leukemia Net; ET, essential thrombocytosis; HDAC, histone deacetylase; HU, hydroxyurea; IFN-*a*, interferon-*a*; IWG-MRT, International Working Group for Myeloproliferative Neoplasms Research and Treatment; JAK2, Janus-type tyrosine kinase 2; MDS, myelodysplastic syndrome; MF, myelofibrosis; MPN, myeloproliferative neoplasm; PCR, polymerase chain reaction; PEG-IFN, pegylated interferon; PFCP, primary familial and congenital polycythemia; PMF, primary myelofibrosis; PV, polycythemia vera; SNP, single nucleotide polymorphism; UPD, uniparental disomy; TET2, a homologue of chromosome 10-11 translocation; WHO, World Health Organization.

of clonal hematopoiesis. Once large enough, the clone then suppresses and replaces normal polyclonal hematopoiesis. The clonal origin of PV has been demonstrated in women heterozygous for a polymorphic X-chromosome marker such as, glucose-6-phosphate dehydrogenase[13] as well as by more modern clonality assays (Chap. 10).[14] In both cases, all hematopoietic cell lineages[9] express either one isoform of the enzyme, or some polymorphic allele encoded by the maternal or paternal X chromosome, whereas T lymphocytes and nonhematopoietic cells are a mosaic of both enzyme types.

In vitro marrow- or blood-derived erythroid colonies of PV patients arise from both normal burst-forming unit–erythroid (BFU-E) precursors and BFU-E precursors that are erythropoietin-independent. Erythropoietin-independent BFU-E precursors form so-called endogenous erythroid colonies (EECs),[15–18] a characteristic feature of PV. The fibroblasts that accumulate in the marrow of patients with PV as the disease progresses are not part of the abnormal PV clone. Rather, they seem to accumulate in response to cytokines released by megakaryocytes and other cells (Chap. 86).[19]

Other abnormalities that have been described include decreased levels of a platelet thrombopoietin receptor,[20] deregulation of bcl-x, an inhibitor of apoptosis,[21] increased expression of protein tyrosine phosphatase activity by red cell precursors,[22] and acquired loss-of-heterozygosity of chromosome 9p as a result of uniparental disomy (UPD).[9] This last observation was one of two routes that led to the discovery of the *JAK2* 2343G > T mutation encoding the V617F mutation located on chromosome 9p,[12,23] which has improved our understanding of disease pathogenesis, improved the specificity of diagnosis, and led to an explosion of research in MPN (see "*JAK2*^V617F Mutation" below).

There are no specific karyotypic markers occurring with high frequency in PV. Fewer than 25 percent of patients have karyotypic abnormalities at diagnosis,[24–29] but the incidence rises with the increasing duration of the disease,[25,30] suggesting that karyotypic abnormalities represent secondary genetic events.[31] Cytogenetic abnormalities may potentially herald transformation from PV to myelofibrosis, acute myeloid leukemia, or a myelodysplastic syndrome, but as of now, these associations are weak.[29]

JAK2^V617F MUTATION

JAK2 kinase is present in all hematopoietic cells and is essential for proliferative intracellular signaling in response to a variety of hematopoietic growth factors (Chaps. 34 and 57). The V617F mutation was first identified in PV in 2004,[23] and was simultaneously reported by several laboratories.[32–34] The V617F mutation is present in virtually all patients with PV and in more than 50 percent of patients with essential thrombocytosis (ET; Chap. 85) and myelofibrosis (MF; Chap. 86); rarely is it found in the minority of patients with other myeloproliferative disorders.[35,36] In PV (unlike in ET), it is often in its associated homozygous form as a result of UPD, at least in some of the progenitors.[26,37] Patients bearing homozygous *JAK2*^V617F tend to have a longer duration of disease,[33] higher hemoglobin levels, and increased incidence of pruritus[38] and are more likely to transform to post-PV MF (Chap. 86).[39] The *JAK2*^V617F allele burden in PV may also be correlated with increased spleen volume, increased leukocytosis, and severity of MF.[39–42] It should be noted, however, that PV patients can achieve a complete hematologic remission without a significant molecular response (i.e., a decrease in *JAK2*^V617F allele burden).[43] In some of the rare PV patients who are *JAK2*^V617F-negative, a different *JAK2* mutation is present in exon 12.[44] Several different *JAK2* exon 12 mutations, including missense mutations, insertions, and deletions, have been described. Patients with exon 12 mutations may present with different clinical manifestations from those with the classic *JAK2*^V617F mutation: erythrocytosis only, higher

hemoglobin, and differences in marrow morphology.[45] Disease course and clinical outcome, however, are similar.[46]

Studies of families of MPN patients, in which several different MPNs occur in a single pedigree,[47] indicate that *JAK2* mutations may not be solely responsible for the disease phenotype and may not even represent the disease-initiating event. A number of compelling lines of evidence support this conclusion. First, in familial PV, there is no clear linkage between the disease and chromosome 9p, the genetic site of *JAK2*, suggesting an independent germline predisposition to PV.[12] Second, in familial PV, affected members can be either *JAK2*^V617F-positive or -negative.[48] Third, acquisition of the *JAK2*^V617F mutation may be a late genetic event.[49] Fourth, in sporadic PV, only a proportion of clonal PV cells are *JAK2*^V617F-positive.[37] And fifth, acute leukemic transformation of any *JAK2*-positive MPN, including PV, is frequently negative for the *JAK2*^V617F mutation.[35,50] These diverse observations strongly suggest that the somatic mutation of the *JAK2* gene is not the initiating or sole pathogenic process in PV, but in most patients is essential for the clinical phenotype of PV. The pathways leading to acquisition of the *JAK2*^V617F mutation, homozygosity of *JAK2*^V617F, and participation of many other genes in the 9p UPD region may have phenotypic and prognostic significance.[51,52] Additional prognostic significance can be ascertained by analysis for clustering of specific genes.[53]

A genomic chromosome 9p functional variant might also be relevant to the pathogenesis of *JAK2*^V617F. Independent occurrence of the *JAK2*^V617F mutation on different haplotypes was found, although a specific constitutional inherited *JAK2* haplotype (GGCC, 46/1), associated with the *JAK2*^V617F somatic mutation, was found in most *JAK2*^V617F-positive individuals.[54] The risk of acquiring a *JAK2*^V617F-positive MPN is three to four fold higher in patients with the *JAK2* GGCC (46/1) haplotype.[54–57] This *GGCC* haplotype of *JAK2* also confers susceptibility to *JAK2* exon 12 mutation-positive PV.[55] These studies suggest that pre-JAK2 hypermutability events exist and that germline genetics play an important role in the early pathogenesis of MPNs.

OTHER MUTATIONS

In addition to the important role of *JAK2*^V617F and other *JAK2* mutations in the etiology of PV and other MPNs, mutations in other genes may be important to the full genesis of these disorders.

TET2 is a homologue of the gene originally discovered at the chromosome ten-eleven translocation (TET) site in a subset of patients with acute leukemia. *TET2* mutations were found in hematopoietic cells from a significant proportion of patients with PV and other MPNs.[58,59] It has been established that *TET2* loss-of-function mutations originate in pluripotent hematopoietic stem cells but seem to favor myeloid rather than lymphoid proliferation, and that in many patients both *TET2* alleles were affected. However, studies in familial PV demonstrated that the *TET2* mutation is often not disease-initiating, as the *TET2* mutations differ among affected relatives and, in some instances, the *TET2* mutations followed, rather than preceded, the appearance of *JAK2*^V617F.[60] Additionally, recurrent *TET2* mutations have been reported in elderly patients with clonal hematopoiesis but no evidence of hematological malignancy.[61] Several additional genes commonly bear mutations in PV patients, including *ASXL1*, *DNMT3A*, and *IDH1/2*.[62,63] The quantitative proportion of clones carrying different mutations may change during disease progression.[64]

AUTOIMMUNITY AND CHRONIC INFLAMMATION

Although JAK2 kinase is clearly involved in the pathogenesis of PV, immune dysfunction and chronic inflammation may also be implicated. A history of any autoimmune disorder is associated with a 20 percent increased risk of developing an MPN,[65] and chronic inflammation is suggested to contribute to mutagenesis and clonal evolution in PV.[66–68] A recent molecular profiling study found that a number of immune and inflammatory genes were either up- or downregulated in PV patients, among them interleukin-10, interleukin-4, complement 5, short pentraxin C-reactive protein, fibrinogen, orosomucoid, and transforming growth factor-β_1.[69] The dysregulation of immune and inflammatory genes in PV may represent an additional avenue for future therapeutic development.

CLINICAL FEATURES

SIGNS AND SYMPTOMS

PV usually has an insidious onset, most commonly during the sixth decade of life, although onset may occur from childhood to old age.[70] Presenting signs and symptoms may include headache, plethora, pruritus, thrombosis, and gastrointestinal bleeding, but many patients are diagnosed because elevated hemoglobin, and sometimes other cell counts, are found on a periodic medical examination. Others cases may be uncovered during investigation for blood loss, iron-deficiency anemia, or thrombosis. Symptoms are reported by at least 30 percent of patients at the time of diagnosis; other patients may admit to symptoms on direct questioning. The most common symptoms, in decreasing order of frequency, are headache, fatigue, weakness, pruritus, dizziness, and night sweats, but these symptoms are more likely in those PV patients transforming to MF (Chap. 86).[70]

PV generally occurs in older patients, a population who may already have an elevated rate of vascular abnormalities (e.g., coronary artery disease). Development of PV represents an additional increase in the risk of vascular events.

Thrombosis and Hemorrhage

Thrombotic episodes are the most common and most important complication of PV,[71–73] occurring in approximately one-third of PV patients.[74] From one-half to three-quarters of these events are arterial[75]; ischemic strokes and transient ischemic attacks account for the majority of arterial complications. In some studies, 40 to 60 percent of patients develop at least one thrombotic event over a period of 10 years, the annual incidence being approximately equal throughout this period.[76] However, in prospective studies, thrombosis was most common just prior to and during the first few years after diagnosis.[74,77,78] The most common serious complication is a cerebrovascular accident, which accounts for approximately one-third of thrombotic events, followed in frequency by myocardial infarction, deep vein thrombosis, and pulmonary embolism.[76] The allelic burden of the $JAK2^{V617F}$ mutation has been correlated with activation of thrombotic pathways in PV patients,[79,80] although this idea is not universally accepted.[39]

Bleeding and bruising is a common complication of PV, occurring in approximately one-quarter of patients in some series.[74] Although such episodes are usually minor (e.g., gingival bleeding, nose bleeding, easy bruising), serious gastrointestinal and other hemorrhagic complications with a fatal outcome can also occur.[31,75,81,82]

Hepatic Vein Thrombosis (Budd-Chiari Syndrome) Budd-Chiari syndrome is a catastrophic and often fatal complication of PV. In one series, it occurred in 10 percent of 140 PV patients,[83] but was less common in a European collaborative study.[75] Budd-Chiari syndrome is caused by a thrombosis in the hepatic venous outflow, leading to ischemia from reduced perfusion through hepatic arterioles and necrosis of hepatocytes. Budd-Chiari syndrome may present as ascites with or without right-upper-quadrant abdominal pain, hepatosplenomegaly, and jaundice.

Budd-Chiari syndrome may be the first clinical manifestation of PV; endogenous erythroid colony formation and $JAK2^{V617F}$ mutation have been described in many of these patients before any clinical evidence of polycythemia.[84,85] PV is the most frequent underlying disease associated with Budd-Chiari syndrome. The association of Budd-Chiari syndrome and PV is so strong that many experts advocate screening for PV with $JAK2^{V617F}$ mutation analysis in all patients who present with hepatic vein thrombosis.[86,87] Budd-Chiari syndrome is a serious condition, often requiring a liver transplant for treatment.[85,88,89]

Cutaneous Findings

Pruritus occurs in approximately 40 percent of PV patients.[90] It is usually aggravated by bathing or showering (aquagenic pruritus), and may be so severe it markedly compromises the quality of life of the patient.[82,91] It has been attributed to increased numbers of mast cells in the skin[92] and to elevated histamine levels,[93] although these associations were not found in other studies.[94]

Several PV patients have developed the dermatologic disorder, acute febrile neutrophilic dermatosis (i.e., Sweet syndrome).[95,96]

Erythromelalgia

Erythromelalgia is a syndrome characterized by warmth of the extremities; painful, reddened digits; a burning sensation; and erythema of the fingers, hands, and feet (Fig. 84–1) that is associated with thrombocytosis. It characteristically responds rapidly to low-dose aspirin therapy. In severe cases, it results in ischemic necrosis of the digits and may lead to their amputation. This syndrome occurs in less than 5 percent of PV patients.[75,81] It is not specific to PV or other MPNs, and in one series of 168 patients with erythromelalgia, less than 10 percent had PV.[97] A causative role for transient microvascular occlusion by platelet aggregates has been proposed (Chap. 112).[98,99]

Abdominal Findings

Portal hypertension, varices, and abdominal pain are not uncommon,[100] and are often caused by unrecognized splenic or hepatic vein thromboses. The occurrence of Budd-Chiari syndrome is noted above (see "Hepatic Vein Thrombosis [Budd-Chiari Syndrome]" above). The incidence of peptic ulcer is four to five times greater than in the general population.[101] Gastrointestinal bleeding may be the first presenting symptom of PV, with iron deficiency caused by gastrointestinal blood loss frequently masking erythrocytosis.[87]

Cardiovascular Findings

Cardiovascular complications include angina, myocardial infarction, and congestive heart failure, related to a predisposition to thrombosis in the coronary circulation.[31,75,77]

Pulmonary Hypertension

Pulmonary hypertension occurs in a higher than expected frequency in patients with PV. The suggested etiologies include smooth muscle hyperplasia induced by the release of platelet-derived growth factor from activated platelets, obstruction of pulmonary circulation by megakaryocytes, extramedullary hematopoiesis, and unrecognized recurrent thrombotic events.[102,103] None of these etiologies are clearly established.

Neurologic Findings

Neurologic symptoms such as dizziness and headache are very common in PV.[31,75,77,81,104] Spinal cord compression secondary to extramedullary hematopoiesis has been documented.[105]

Findings in Other Organ Systems

The increased nucleic acid turnover that results from the excessive proliferation of marrow cells often leads to an increase in blood uric acid concentration; gout can be exacerbated in some patients.[31]

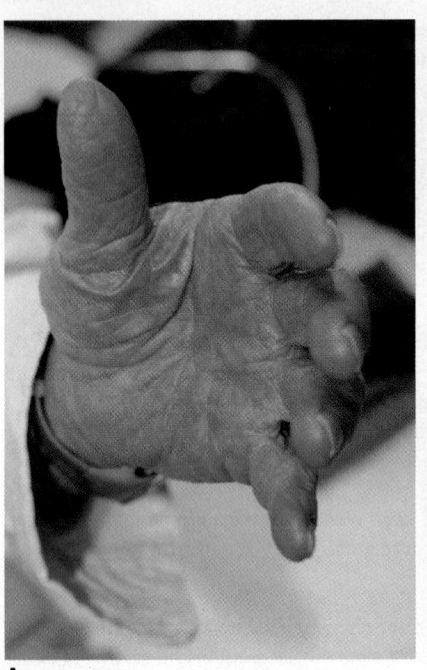

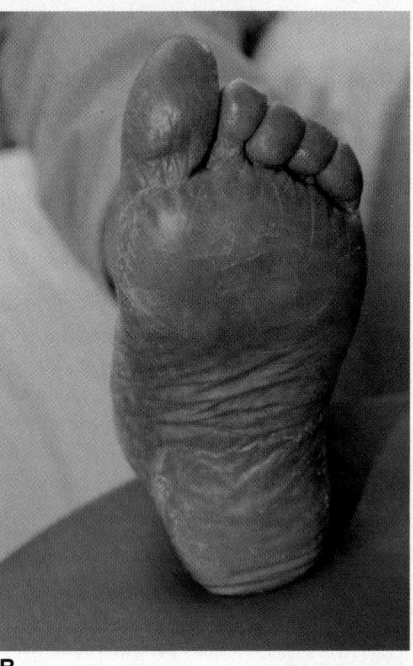

Figure 84–1. A. Patient with erythromelalgia of hand and fingers. **B.** Erythromelalgia of feet and toes that progressed to necrosis and amputation of the toes. *(Used with permission of Steven Fruchtman, MD, Allos Therapeutics, Princeton, New Jersey.)*

A   **B**

SPECIAL CONSIDERATIONS

Surgery

More than 75 percent of patients with uncontrolled PV develop complications during or after major surgery because both bleeding and thromboses are common.[82,106] Thus, it is advised to normalize blood counts and blood volume before surgical interventions, which may lower the frequency of intraoperative and postoperative complications.

Pregnancy

Chapter 8 discusses the complications of PV in pregnancy.

SPENT PHASE OF POLYCYTHEMIA VERA

The spent phase of PV, also referred to as post-PV MF, is a frequent and often terminal complication of the disease.[75,78,107] It is characterized by a combination of anemia (non–iron deficiency), progressive increase of splenic size (Fig. 84–2), and marrow fibrosis (Chap. 86). The spent phase may first be noticed when phlebotomy requirements decrease. Thrombocytosis and granulocytosis (often with immature myeloid cells) are common. In a minority of cases, thrombocytopenia and granulocytopenia may occur. Affected individuals are frequently symptomatic with anemia, bleeding, splenic enlargement with early satiety, and/

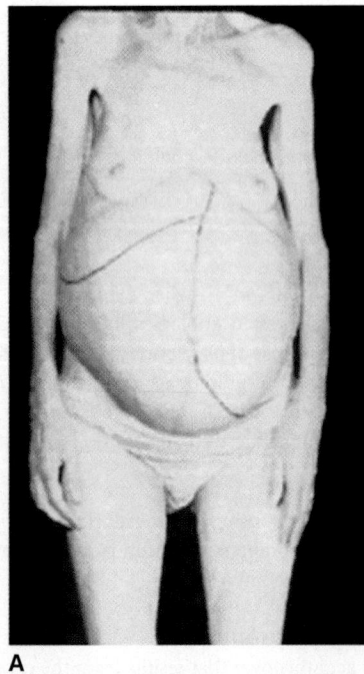

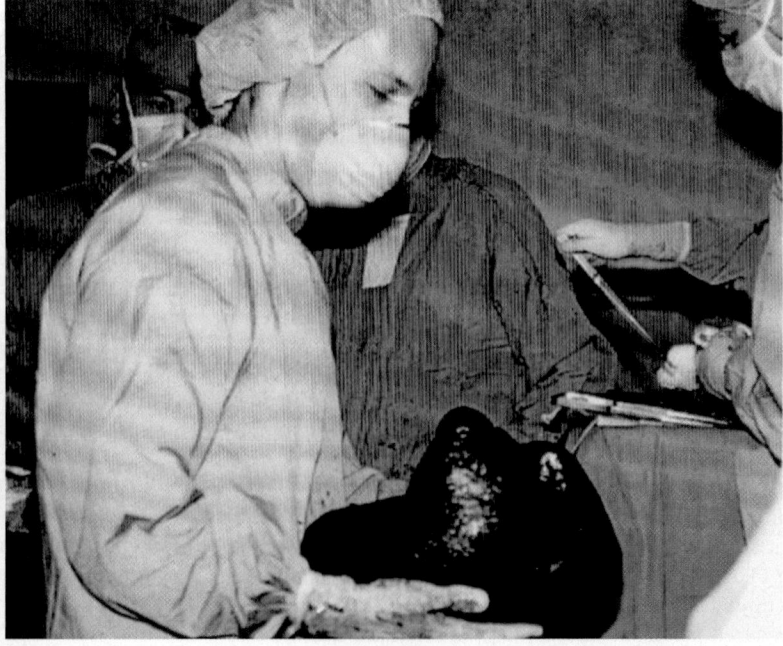

A   **B**

Figure 84–2. Patient with spent phase of PV with a massive increase of splenic size **(A)** and surgically removed spleen **(B)**. *(Used with permission of Steven Fruchtman, MD, Allos Therapeutics, Princeton, New Jersey.)*

or upper abdominal pain secondary to splenic infarcts. Most patients become dependent on transfusions or erythropoietin therapy.[31,75,77,81,107] Development of the spent phase is associated with an increased risk of leukemic transformation[31,108]; in the PV Study Group-01 study, the incidence of acute leukemia was 24 percent in PV patients with MF, compared to 7 percent in those without MF, although it should be noted that a sizable number of the patients in this study had been treated with alkylating agents or ^{32}P.[78] Therapy, including use of JAK2 inhibitors, is described in Chap. 86.

LEUKEMIC AND MYELODYSPLASTIC TRANSFORMATION OF POLYCYTHEMIA VERA

Patients with PV have an increased risk of developing leukemia.[71,82] This contrasts with other nonclonal polycythemic disorders, wherein progression to leukemia is not part of the disease process. Acute leukemia, usually myelogenous, is an invariably fatal complication of PV. A European multicenter observational study of 1638 patients reported a 6.3 percent relative risk of developing leukemia within 10 years after the diagnosis of PV.[75] Different treatments can also influence the risk of transformation from PV to leukemia. In the PV Study Group-01 randomized trial, the incidence of acute leukemia at 18 years of followup was 1.5 percent on the phlebotomy-only treatment arm, 10 percent on the ^{32}P treatment arm, and 13 percent on the chlorambucil treatment arm.[81] In a more recent study of 1638 patients, the risk of transformation to acute myelogenous leukemia (AML) or a myelodysplastic syndrome (MDS) in PV patients also varied by treatment. Treatment-specific risk of transformation, ordered by increasing risk, was: phlebotomy (hazard ratio [HR]: 0.91), hydroxyurea (HR: 1.09), interferon (INF)-α (HR: 1.24), busulfan (HR: 8.64), pipobroman (HR: 4.32), and ^{32}P (HR: 8.96).[109] Leukemic transformation was not significantly different between phlebotomy, hydroxyurea, and INF-α treatments.[109]

Acute leukemia as the terminal PV event may arise from either the *JAK2*[V617F]-positive clone or, more frequently, from a hematopoietic cell that does not carry the *JAK2* mutation.[35,47,50]

● LABORATORY FEATURES

BLOOD FINDINGS

Erythrocytes

The hemoglobin concentration, erythrocyte count, and hematocrit are usually increased, and the mean cell volume is usually low-normal or low in untreated patients, and low in patients who have undergone phlebotomies or had gastrointestinal bleeding episodes. Red cells are hypochromic and microcytic, with morphology characteristic of iron deficiency. Although increased hemoglobin is generally a diagnostic feature of PV, at times the hemoglobin level may be low, normal, or borderline, a condition termed "masked" PV.[110–112]

The appearance of significant aniso- and poikilocytosis and teardrop cells (dacryocytes; Chap. 31) heralds the onset of the spent phase and post-PV MF (Chap. 86).

Red Cell Mass Determination

The Polycythemia Vera Study Group employed the direct determination of red cell mass as the *sine qua non* of the diagnosis of PV for all patients entered into their studies.[76] Some believe that even in the routine clinical setting, this procedure should be performed on all patients to establish a diagnosis of PV.[76,113] Unfortunately, the determination of red cell mass is expensive, requires the use of radioactive isotopes in patients, and, when performed by the inexperienced, is often inaccurate.[114] Red cell mass determination is not useful in distinguishing PV

from secondary polycythemia because the red cell mass is increased in both disorders. The principal value of red cell mass determination is to distinguish apparent or spurious polycythemia from PV and secondary polycythemia.[110,111] It could also be useful in distinguishing cases of masked PV from ET.[115] The availability of the JAK2 assay has made red cell mass determination only rarely important.

Leukocytes

Absolute neutrophilia occurs in approximately two-thirds of PV patients.[70] Occasional myelocytes and metamyelocytes are present in the blood, and considerable degrees of cell immaturity are present in patients with longstanding, advanced disease. Again, these abnormalities herald the onset of the spent phase (Chap. 86). Basophilia occurs in approximately two-thirds of patients with uncontrolled disease.[31,81,116] In PV, the proportion of activated neutrophils is increased,[117] and it is possible that neutrophils may be an important factor in PV-associated thrombosis.[118]

The leukocyte alkaline phosphatase level is elevated in approximately 70 percent of patients with PV,[70] but this assay has now become largely obsolete.

Platelets

The platelet count is increased in approximately 50 percent of PV patients at the time of diagnosis, and in approximately 10 percent of patients it is greater than 1000×10^9/L.[70] There are no consistent abnormalities of thrombopoietin levels in PV patients.[119] A significant proportion of PV patients first present with isolated thrombocytosis without elevated hemoglobin, especially if the patient has a reason for iron deficiency, and are sometimes misdiagnosed with essential thrombocythemia.[120]

Qualitative platelet abnormalities have been described which may play a role in the pathogenesis of thrombotic and hemorrhagic events. *In vitro* spontaneous platelet aggregation is accelerated. On the other hand, patients with MPNs often display a nearly pathognomonic defect in the primary wave of platelet aggregation induced by epinephrine (Chaps. 112 and 121).[121]

There are a number of additional platelet abnormalities associated with PV, including increased platelet thromboxane A_2 generation[122] and increased excretion of thromboxane metabolites.[123] Platelet factor-4 levels are elevated.[124] Platelet survival may be shortened.[124,125] Fibrinogen binding after stimulation with a platelet-activating factor is diminished,[126] and there is reduced expression of the thrombopoietin receptor.[20] However, none of these changes are specific for PV. In a prospective study, a Pl^{A2} polymorphism of the platelet glycoprotein IIIa was associated with an increased risk of arterial thrombosis in PV patients,[127] although this conclusion remains controversial.

Platelet counts greater than 1000 to 1500×10^9/L are associated with progressive decrease of von Willebrand factor (an acquired, type 2 von Willebrand disease) and increased risk of bleeding, but not of thrombosis.[128]

Plasma

Serum lysozyme levels are slightly increased in some patients,[129] and because of increased leukocyte turnover and increased levels of B$_{12}$ binding protein, serum B$_{12}$ determination is usually increased.[130] Hyperuricemia, a consequence of hyperproliferative myelopoiesis, is frequently encountered.[31]

JAK2[V617F] AND EXON 12 MUTATIONS

JAK2 G1849T Creating V617F

Mutations within the *JAK2* gene cause deregulation of the hematopoietic process, which is expressed in a wide spectrum of disorders involving the expansion of erythrocytes, granulocytes, or leukocytes. The primary lesion associated with these disorders was discovered in exon 14: A single nucleotide change *JAK2* G1849T resulting in the amino acid substitution V617F. Detection of the *JAK2*[V617F] mutation provides a qualitative diagnostic marker for the identification of the Philadelphia-chromosome-negative subgroup of MPNs, and differentiates them from congenital and acquired reactive hematopoietic disorders. In general, the *JAK2*[V617F] allele burden is lower in ET patients than in either PV or primary myelofibrosis (PMF).[131,132] In many, but not all, *JAK2*[V617F]-positive PV patients, at least some progenitors exist that became homozygous for the *JAK2*[V617F] mutation by UPD acquired by mitotic recombination.[37,133]

Allele-specific polymerase chain reaction (PCR) is widely used for single nucleotide polymorphism (SNP) genotyping; the technique is based on amplification of DNA by an allele-specific primer matching the polymorphism at the 3′ position. This approach is directly applicable to analysis of *JAK2*[V617F] because the mutation *(G1849T)* is analogous to a SNP. To improve the specificity, sensitivity, and reliability for quantitating the *JAK2*[V617F] allele burden, two modifications of technique were incorporated: Inclusion of a second mismatch at the –1 position, and substitution of a modified locked nucleic acid at the –2 position. A study comparing 11 different techniques was undertaken and carried out in 16 laboratories using various testing platforms.[134] Although five of the 11 techniques were similarly reliable for quantification of *JAK2*[V617F] loads that were equal to or greater than 1 percent of total *JAK2*[V617F], the allele-specific quantitative PCR technique could detect 0.2 percent of *JAK2*[V617F].

The majority of laboratories analyze quantitative assays of *JAK2*[V617F] allele burden from (clonal) granulocytes; nonquantitative analyses use total leukocytes, whole blood, or marrow for screening. A proportion of *JAK2*[V617F]-negative assays are positive using sensitive quantitative analyses.[134] Plasma has been used for detection of the *JAK2*[V617F] DNA and mRNA mutation and zygosity state,[135,136] but plasma analysis is not reliable.[137]

JAK2 Exon 12 Mutations

Although the most common *JAK2* mutation is a single SNP in exon 14, many MPN cases negative for the exon 14 *JAK2*[V617F] mutation may carry one of a number of mutations in exon 12. Almost 40 different mutations in exon 12 have been identified within codons 536 to 547, including substitutions, deletions, and duplications.[45,138–142] In addition to the various mutations observed in this region, the proportion of mutations within a given sample may be small and therefore difficult to detect in the high background of a normal sequence.[45] *JAK2* exon 12 mutations have been observed primarily in younger patients and in patients with isolated erythrocytosis, and thus may represent a somewhat different phenotype from *JAK2*[V617F]-positive PV.

ERYTHROPOIETIN LEVELS

PV is distinguished by the fact that erythroid cells proliferate even in the absence of normal levels of erythropoietin; thus, one would expect that at high hematocrit levels, the production of erythropoietin would be inhibited and serum levels consequently reduced. Indeed, several studies have documented serum erythropoietin levels below the normal reference range in patients with PV.[143–145]

Patients with secondary polycythemia usually have normal to elevated erythropoietin levels, although considerable overlap exists in the range of erythropoietin levels between patients with PV and those with secondary polycythemia rendering the test of marginal value in distinguishing between diagnostic possibilties.[144,146] An elevated erythropoietin level generally excludes the diagnosis of PV, but a low erythropoietin

level is not pathognomonic of PV; patients with primary familial and congenital polycythemia (PFCP) have levels of erythropoietin that are as low or lower than in PV,[147] and instances of normal erythropoietin levels occur in PV patients without apparent explanation. The latter is more likely to occur in PV patients with exon 12 *JAK2* mutations.[44]

ERYTHROID COLONY CULTURES

In vitro assays of erythroid progenitor cells permit the study of their responsiveness to erythropoietin. In PV patient samples, erythroid BFU-E progenitors grow in culture without added erythropoietin,[17] forming colonies that are termed EECs. Detection of EECs in cultures of blood or marrow had previously been the most specific test for PV.[12,14,148] In one study, all patients with PV, but none with secondary or other causes of polycythemia, formed EECs *in vitro*.[149] Rare EECs may, at times, be observed in PFCP and in congenital disorders of hypoxia sensing, but unlike EECs in PV, these are abrogated by pretreatment with erythropoietin and erythropoietin receptor-blocking antibodies.[150,151]

In experienced hands, the EEC assay is a specific and sensitive means for detecting PV. It may be useful in diagnosing patients with unusual presentations of PV, such as Budd-Chiari syndrome,[85,89,152,153] isolated thrombocytosis, or the rare *JAK2*[V617F]-negative PV patient. It has not been fully standardized, however, and is expensive and laborious, so it is now used primarily in a research setting where it remains informative.

MARROW FINDINGS

In PV, the marrow is characteristically hypercellular, with an increase in erythroid and granulocytic precursor cells and megakaryocytes. Whereas marrow morphology is part of the World Health Organization (WHO) diagnostic criteria of PV,[154] the morphologic features have not yet been validated and may be subject to inter- and intraobserver variation. Marrow morphology in patients with *JAK2* exon 12 mutations may be subtly different, with subtle or no megakaryocytic clustering and a lack of panmyelosis.[45,155] Absent or decreased iron stores are seen in the marrow of most PV patients. Various cytogenetic findings have been reported,[156] but they are not sufficiently specific to be of diagnostic utility (Chap. 13).

CLONALITY IN FEMALE SUBJECTS USING ASSAYS EMPLOYING X-CHROMOSOME–BASED POLYMORPHISM

PV results from an acquired mutation in a pluripotent hematopoietic stem cell. Clonality studies based on the phenomenon of X-chromosome inactivation[157] show that red cells, granulocytes, platelets, monocytes, and B lymphocytes are all part of the neoplastic clone.[13,158] The majority of T lymphocytes and natural killer cells are polyclonal, but a small proportion of these cells are also derived from the PV clone[9]; this is presumed to be the result of the presence of long-lived, normal T cells that preceded the development of the clone and younger, clonal cells. Unfortunately, the applicability of X-chromosome inactivation for the differential diagnosis of PV is hampered by the many methodologic and conceptual differences that have drawn conflicting conclusions.[159] Some of these discrepancies result from using two different approaches[160] to distinguish the active from inactive X-chromosomes (Chap. 10).[161–164] In a study of approximately 100 female PV patients, their reticulocytes, platelets, and granulocytes were always clonal, with the exception of a few patients who converted to polyclonal hematopoiesis after therapy with IFN-α.[14]

DIFFERENTIAL DIAGNOSIS

Also refer to Chap. 34, Table 34–2, and Chap. 57, Fig. 57–6.

PV has to be differentiated from spurious polycythemia, secondary polycythemias, congenital disorders of hypoxia sensing, and primary congenital polycythemias. The differential diagnostic task has been facilitated by the discovery of the $JAK2^{V617F}$ mutation that is present in 95 percent or more of all PV patients.[165,166] Thus, the majority of PV patients can be diagnosed with a complete blood count repeated twice and molecular studies to confirm the presence of the $JAK2^{V617F}$ mutation.

For the remainder of polycythemic patients, additional diagnostic measures need to be undertaken. These may include measuring serum erythropoietin level, measuring venous oxygen saturation to calculate hemoglobin P50, measuring arterial oxygen saturation (less than 92 percent suggests cardiac or pulmonary etiologies), abdominal CT scan (to exclude renal, hepatic, and cerebral tumors), brain magnetic resonance imaging (to rule out a cerebellar hemangioblastoma), and detailed family studies.

If a diagnosis at this point has not yet been made, the patient could be referred to a specialized center for further testing. These studies may include measuring changes in serum erythropoietin levels after phlebotomies, red blood cell and plasma volume studies (to diagnose spurious polycythemia or masked PV), genomic sequencing studies, testing for $JAK2$ exon 12 mutations, and in vitro studies for EECs. The latter two are used to diagnose $JAK2^{V617F}$-negative PV patients (<5 percent of all PVs).

Distinguishing between PV and other polycythemic disorders may, at times, be challenging. Although the diagnosis of PV may be straightforward if patients have the classic features of PV as defined by the most recent WHO guidelines,[154] patients often present with an incomplete phenotype. Some of the clinical and laboratory features that can be helpful for differential diagnosis are summarized in Chap. 34, Table 34–2 and Chap. 57, Fig. 57–6. While the current WHO diagnostic criteria (presented in Table 84–1)[154] represent an improvement over previous guidelines, they do not necessarily discriminate between individual MPNs,[167] and are still a matter of some debate.[168,169] Children with PV are especially unlikely to fit the most recent WHO criteria.[170] Most importantly, often laborious and time-consuming efforts to rule out congenital polycythemia should always be undertaken in patients with atypical presentations; however, the presence of polycythemia in other relatives does not rule out PV.

TABLE 84–1. World Health Organization Criteria for the Diagnosis of Polycythemia Vera, 2008

MAJOR CRITERIA	
1	Hgb >18.5 g/dL (men), >16.5 g/dL (women)
	or
	Hgb >17 g/dL (men), >15 g/dL (women)
	if associated with a sustained increase of ≥2 g/dL from baseline that cannot be attributed to correction of iron deficiency
2	Presence of $JAK2^{V617F}$ or similar mutation

MINOR CRITERIA	
1	Marrow trilineage myeloproliferation
2	Subnormal serum EPO level
3	EEC growth

EEC, endogenous erythroid colony; EPO, erythropoietin; Hgb, hemoglobin.

A diagnosis of PV requires the presence of both major criteria and one minor criterion, or the first major criterion and two minor criteria.

TREATMENT

The major causes of morbidity and mortality in PV are an increased incidence of vascular complications (i.e., thrombosis and/or hemorrhage), and progression to MF or acute leukemia/myelodysplasia. In the first randomized trial of PV patients, a history of previous thrombosis, age, treatment with phlebotomies, and rate of phlebotomies contributed to the increased risk of thrombosis.[76] Presently, the age of the patient (>60 years) and previous thrombotic events are universally acknowledged major risk factors for major vascular complications in PV.[71]

Thus, PV patients are classified as low risk or high risk, with age greater than 60 years and previous thrombotic events (including transient ischemic attacks) defining the high-risk category. The assigned risk classification has a major impact on therapeutic decisions, as high-risk patients are treated with cytoreductive therapies. Other risk factors may also play a role in the pathogenesis of thrombosis, such as hypertension, diabetes, or smoking,[171] as well as leukocytosis[172–176] and $JAK2^{V617F}$ mutational allele burden.[80,177] There is a need for prospective clinical studies with stratification of patients according to these criteria, but until such evidence is available, patients with high leukocyte levels and/or high $JAK2^{V617F}$ mutational allele burden should be managed according to conventional criteria.

An elevated platelet count does not increase the risk of thrombosis, but it may increase the risk of hemorrhage.[128] Bleeding is more frequent in patients with platelet counts in excess of 1500×10^9/L, thought to be the result of an acquired type 2 von Willebrand disease.

Treatment of PV depends on risk evaluation at diagnosis and evolution of the disease over time. Treatment should be given both to alleviate symptoms and prevent complications. Updated consensus-based guidelines for the management of PV and other major MPNs were published by a panel of experts formed by European LeukemiaNet (ELN).[178] Response criteria by which new therapies are evaluated were also updated to facilitate direct comparison of therapeutic efficacy across clinical trials (Table 84–2).[179] This joint effort between ELN and the International Working Group for Myeloproliferative Neoplasms Research and Treatment (IWG-MRT) provides updated guidelines incorporating assessment of clinical, hematologic, and histologic response, as well as symptoms, disease progression, and vascular events.[179]

It is useful to consider treatment for the plethoric and spent phases separately. In the plethoric phase, the mainstay of therapy remains nonspecific myelosuppression, which many practitioners supplement with phlebotomies.[82,178,180] Additional measures prevent thrombotic events (i.e., aspirin) and relieve symptoms. Promising therapies include pegylated interferon (PEG-IFN) preparations and JAK2 inhibitors; these are, at the time of this writing, being evaluated by prospective randomized trials. A minority of patients (i.e., low-risk patients) can be treated with phlebotomies and low-dose aspirin alone. PV patients in the spent phase may be treated with a number of therapies (Chap. 86), which may include hydroxyurea, transfusion, erythropoiesis-stimulating drugs, JAK2 inhibitors, splenectomy, or allogeneic stem cell transplantation; only JAK2 inhibitors have been proven to be beneficial in prospective trials.[235]

THE PLETHORIC PHASE

Treatment of PV patients in the plethoric phase of the disease is aimed at reducing marrow proliferation and blood counts, thereby ameliorating symptoms and decreasing the risk of thrombosis and bleeding.[180,181] This

TABLE 84–2. Response Criteria for Polycythemia Vera[179]

A. CLINICAL RESPONSE

Response	Criteria
Complete remission	
A	Durable* resolution of disease-related signs including palpable hepatosplenomegaly, large improvement in symptoms,[†] AND
B	Durable* blood count remission, defined as hematocrit lower than 45% without phlebotomies; platelet count ≤400 × 10^9/L, white blood cell count <10 × 10^9/L, AND
C	Without progressive disease, and absence of any hemorrhagic or thrombotic event, AND
D	Marrow histologic remission defined as the presence of age-adjusted normocellularity and disappearance of trilinear hyperplasia, and absence of > grade 1 reticulin fibrosis.
Partial remission	
A	Durable* resolution of disease-related signs including palpable hepatosplenomegaly, large improvement in symptoms,[†] AND
B	Durable* blood count remission, defined as hematocrit lower than 45% without phlebotomies; platelet count ≤400 × 10^9/L, white blood cell count <10 × 10^9/L, AND
C	Without progressive disease, and absence of any hemorrhagic or thrombotic event, AND
D	Without marrow histologic remission defined as persistence of trilinear hyperplasia.
No response	Any response that does not satisfy partial remission.
Progressive disease	Transformation into post-PV myelofibrosis, myelodysplastic syndrome or acute leukemia.

B. MOLECULAR RESPONSE[‡]

Response	Criteria
Complete response	Eradication of a preexisting abnormality
Partial response	≥50% decrease in allele burden, in patients with >20% allele burden at baseline

*Lasting at least 12 weeks.

[†]Large improvement in symptoms (≥10-point decrease) in MPN Symptom Assessment Form total assessment score.

[‡]Evaluation requires analysis in blood granulocytes. Molecular response is not required for assignment as complete response or partial response.

is best accomplished by myelosuppressive drugs and, in some patients, combination therapy consisting of myelosuppression, phlebotomies, and platelet-reducing agents and/or IFN-α. Table 84–3 summarizes the advantages and disadvantages of various forms of therapy for PV.

Myelosuppression

Myelosuppression decreases blood counts, decreases the risk of vascular events, and ameliorates symptoms, thus increasing an overall sense of well-being. Although there may be an impression that it increases patients' long-term survival, there are no long-term clinical studies to document this.

TABLE 84–3. Treatment of Polycythemia Vera

Treatment	Advantages	Disadvantages
Phlebotomy	Low Risk. Simple to perform.	Does not control thrombocytosis or leukocytosis.
Hydroxyurea	Controls leukocytosis and thrombocytosis as well as erythrocytosis.	Continuous therapy required. Long-term leukemogenic potential is not completely known.
Busulfan	Easy to administer. Prolonged remissions.	Overdose produces prolonged marrow suppression. Risks of leukemogenesis, long-term pulmonary and cutaneous toxicity.
^{32}P	Patient compliance not required. Long-term control of thrombocytosis, leukocytosis, and erythrocytosis.	Expensive and relatively inconvenient to administer. Likely leukemogenic risk.
Chlorambucil	Easy to administer. Good control of thrombocytosis and leukocytosis.	High risk of leukemogenesis.
Interferon	Low leukemogenic potential. Beneficial effect on pruritus. Potential deep suppression of the polycythemic clone.	Inconvenient to administer (injectable), costly, and adverse effects are common.
Anagrelide	Selective effect on platelets.	Selective effect on platelets.
JAK2 Inhibitors	Decreased need for phlebotomy. Improvement in quality of life.	Clinical trials experience only. Long-term benefits are unknown.

Hydroxyurea Hydroxyurea (HU) is the most common myelosuppressive agent used in the treatment of PV.[182,183] HU is an effective therapy for controlling erythrocyte, leukocyte, and platelet counts, and it decreases the risk of thrombosis during the first few years of therapy when compared to an historical cohort treated with phlebotomy alone.[78] Because its suppressive effect is of short duration, continuous rather than intermittent therapy is required. Because it is short acting, it is relatively safe to use even when excessive marrow suppression occurs, as blood counts rise within a few days of decreasing the dose or stopping the drug. Several groups have investigated the effects of HU on $JAK2^{V617F}$ allele burden, and as of yet, the results have been conflicting.[184–187] Interestingly, it has been suggested that the $JAK2^{V617F}$ allele burden in PV may be a reliable predictor of response to HU, and of the HU dose necessary to control the disease.[188]

The leukemogenic risk of HU has been an ongoing debate for many years. Because HU is not an alkylating agent, it has less potential to cause acute leukemic transformation than other myelosuppressive agents, but its leukemogenicity was questioned in some historical studies. A large meta-analysis of patients with sickle cell disease did not find an increased risk of the development of acute leukemia following HU treatment.[189] Two large studies in PV have also suggested a similar low risk associated with HU; analysis of 1638 PV patients enrolled in a prospective observational study[109] and 1545 patients followed under IWG-MRT[190] did not find an increased incidence of leukemic or myelodysplastic transformation with HU treatment.

Unfortunately, despite its safety and effectiveness, approximately 10 percent of PV patients develop HU resistance or intolerance (i.e., skin ulcers or gastrointestinal intolerance).[191-193] Resistance to HU is correlated with decreased survival and a higher rate of transformation to AML or MF.[191] Effective alternative treatments are available.

Busulfan Busulfan is a useful second-line agent in patients whose disease is difficult to control or who have adverse reactions to HU. The administration of busulfan is a convenient and effective means for treating PV. The marrow suppression produced by this drug is long-lasting and, as a consequence, it can be given intermittently at a dose of 2 to 8 mg daily for a period not exceeding several weeks; blood counts continue to fall for several weeks after drug administration is discontinued. The disease is usually controlled for many months or even years. In one large study, the median first remission duration of busulfan-treated patients was 4 years.[194] The prolonged depression of marrow activity brought about by busulfan is its major advantage in the treatment of PV, but it also poses a hazard of long-term pancytopenia. The incidence of transformation to leukemia may be increased with busulfan treatment. In a large study of 1638 PV patients, busulfan was one of the agents which was associated with an increased rate of transformation to AML/MDS.[109] When tested as a second-line therapy, busulfan robustly reduces the $JAK2^{V617F}$ allelic burden and causes a complete hematologic response in the majority of patients,[195,196] but also has a higher rate of transformation to leukemia compared to first-line busulfan treatment.[196]

Radioactive Phosphorus ^{32}P therapy was one of the first effective modes of treatment used in PV. Extensive investigations of the long-term outcome of treatment with ^{32}P have been documented.[76,197] Satisfactory control of the disease usually can be achieved with initial doses of 2 to 4 mCi. It is rarely used at present, but it may be the treatment of choice for older patients and patients who may be difficult to follow.[198,199]

Interferon Since the pioneering work of Silver,[200] IFN-α treatment has been confirmed to result in clinical and hematologic remission in PV in more than a dozen studies.[201-204] Although these studies have many design similarities, they do not lend themselves to accurate meta-analysis; various formulations of IFN were used (INF-α2a and -α2b, PEG-INF-α2a, and -α2b, human leukocyte IFN), and heterogeneous criteria were employed to measure response. Nevertheless, it is clear that IFN-α effectively decreases many PV symptoms, including pruritus, results in a hematologic response in approximately 80 percent of patients, and decreases the need for phlebotomies in approximately 60 percent of patients.[201-204]

In addition to clinical and hematologic responses, administration of IFN-α has led to a decrease in $JAK2^{V617F}$ allelic burden[43,205,206] and conversion from clonal to polyclonal hematopoiesis[14] in the small number of patients studied thus far. Two comparisons of IFN-α2b and HU suggest that IFN-α2b may cause a greater molecular and hematologic response than HU in PV patients.[207,208]

However, IFN-α has significant adverse effects. Approximately 25 percent of patients with PV and ET given IFN-α discontinue treatment, half of them within the first year. The hematologic toxicities include anemia, thrombocytopenia, and neutropenia. Other potential untoward effects of IFN-α include depression, mood changes, disabling fatigue, skin toxicity, hair loss, nausea, diarrhea, weight loss, liver function abnormalities, and cardiac and neurologic toxicity. Immunologic abnormalities in the form of autoimmune processes (e.g., hypothyroidism, autoimmune hemolytic anemia, polyarthritis, glomerulonephritis, connective tissue diseases, and asymptomatic antinuclear antibodies) may be consequences of IFN therapy.[209] Conceivably, the development

of IFN-induced autoimmune processes reflects the immunomodulatory activity of the drug, through which at least part of its antitumor activity is mediated.

A pegylated version of IFN-α (PEG-IFN-α) is better tolerated than standard IFN-α and requires less frequent administration.[210] A number of phase II trials have shown that PEG-IFN-α2a induces a complete hematologic response in the vast majority of patients and a reduction in $JAK2^{V617F}$ allelic burden in some.[211-215] Using $JAK2^{V617F}$ as a molecular marker, a French group studied 40 PV patients treated with PEG-IFN-α2a; 95 percent of evaluable patients had a complete hematologic remission, 90 percent had a decrease in $JAK2^{V617F}$ allelic burden, and in 20 percent the $JAK2^{V617F}$ allelic burden became undetectable.[214] However, the experience of the authors of this chapter is that we have not seen any true molecular remission in our therapy of more than 50 PV subjects and always detect a small level of $JAK2$ mutant in those considered in "molecular remission," albeit it at times at levels of less than 0.2 percent.

Although IFN-α and PEG-IFN-α can be used as first-line therapy in PV, they are more often used as second-line treatments.[193] PEG-IFN-α is the drug of choice in pregnant patients (Chap. 8).

Phlebotomy

Often, the initial treatment for patients with uncomplicated PV is phlebotomy.[31,197] Together with low-dose aspirin, it is at present the recommended therapy for low-risk PV cases.

When phlebotomy is instituted, the hemoglobin may be reduced to normal or near-normal values by the removal of 450 mL of blood at one time every 2 to 4 days; smaller amounts should be removed from patients who weigh less than 50 kg. Patients with impaired cardiovascular function are better treated with smaller phlebotomies at more frequent intervals.

Phlebotomy is an effective way by which to lower or normalize the elevated blood viscosity of patients with PV. The reduction of hemoglobin levels may result in improvement of symptoms such as headaches or feeling of increased pressure. However, it does not reduce the leukocyte or platelet count, nor does it affect pruritus or gout. Iron deficiency and resulting microcytosis are usual consequences of repeated phlebotomies. An iron-deficient state may help control hemoglobin concentration in the long run, but it may increase platelet counts and fatigue in some patients. Judicious use of oral iron replacement therapy may improve the fatigue associated with iron deficiency without significantly increasing hematocrit.

A randomized study[76,216] of a small number of PV patients comparing phlebotomy to other treatments indicated that the survival of patients treated only with phlebotomy was slightly better than for patients treated with chlorambucil, and no worse than those given ^{32}P. Patients undergoing phlebotomy did suffer more thrombotic episodes than patients treated with myelosuppressive therapy, although this risk seemed limited to the first 3 years of therapy.[78] This documented increased risk of thrombosis associated with phlebotomy was balanced by a lower incidence of acute leukemia late in the patient's course. There was no correlation between platelet count and development of thrombotic complications.[216]

The rationale for phlebotomy in patients with PV is based on a widely quoted study that suggested the risk of thrombosis in PV was proportional to the elevation in hematocrit.[217] Although the underlying mechanisms causing thrombosis in PV are not fully understood, hematocrit is unlikely to be the only, or even a major risk factor, as the risk of thrombosis is not elevated in patients with non-PV polycythemia or in patients with secondary polycythemia caused by chronic exposure to high altitude, Eisenmenger syndrome,[218] or other cyanotic heart diseases.[219,220] In patients with Chuvash polycythemia, the risk of stroke is similar regardless of whether hematocrit is controlled by phlebotomies (Chap. 37). Furthermore, the European Collaboration on Low-Dose

Aspirin in the Polycythemia Vera study (ECLAP), which included 1638 patients from 12 countries and 94 centers, found no difference in thrombotic complications for patients with hematocrits in the range of 40 to 55 percent.[221] An important attempt to clarify this issue was a prospective study of the effect of hematocrit in PV patients, as evaluated by univariate analysis, which reported that patients treated with phlebotomies had a decreased rate of thrombosis.[222] However, patients in the high-hematocrit group received less HU than those in the low-hematocrit group and had higher levels of leukocytes, both independent correlates of thrombotic risk.[223]

Anagrelide

Anagrelide can be used in PV for thrombocytosis, as an adjunct to other treatments. Among 113 PV patients with thrombocytosis, the administration of anagrelide produced a platelet response in 85 cases (75 percent).[224] The starting dose was 0.5 or 1.0 mg given four times daily, and a response was noted in most patients within 1 week. The average dose required to control the platelet count was 2.4 mg per day. Adverse events included headache, palpitations, diarrhea, and fluid retention, and were occasionally sufficiently severe to require discontinuation of the treatment.[225] In patients with ET (Chap. 85), a randomized trial in the United Kingdom indicated superior results for HU plus aspirin compared to anagrelide plus aspirin for control of elevated platelet count, MF, and hemorrhagic complications.[26] However, a later randomized trial showed a noninferiority of anagrelide to HU.[226]

Symptomatic Therapy for Pruritus

Although some symptoms of PV can be controlled using phlebotomy, control of pruritus is at times achieved using myelosuppression. Pruritus is a major symptom of PV and, in some patients, it is nearly intolerable. When marrow proliferation is well controlled, pruritus becomes milder or disappears entirely. Because bathing or showering usually intensifies the itching, the term *aquagenic pruritus* is often used. Some level of control of pruritus may be achieved by moisturization of the skin. Photochemotherapy with psoralens and ultraviolet light can be helpful.[227] Antihistamines are often given, but are usually not very effective, and neither is aspirin.[228] Both IFN-α[229-231] and the JAK2 inhibitors provide a generally effective treatment modality to alleviate pruritus.[232,233]

Aspirin

Because thromboembolic episodes represent a major source of morbidity and mortality in patients with polycythemia, aspirin is an important drug in the arsenal of treatment modalities for PV.

The results of early trials using 300 mg of aspirin daily showed an increase in the incidence of bleeding without a measurable impact on the incidence of thrombotic episodes.[234] Subsequently, several studies showed positive benefits of aspirin use in PV. A pilot-controlled trial found that low-dose aspirin was well tolerated by PV patients and fully inhibited synthesis of the platelet aggregating compound thromboxane, but not the endothelial cell protectant prostacyclin.[235] An ECLAP study showed that daily low-dose aspirin decreased arterial and venous thromboses, albeit incompletely.[75] Because thrombotic complications were not completely prevented, this study suggested that only a minor fraction of thromboses are attributable to platelets, and additional pathogenetic pathways in PV should be investigated. The increased risk of bleeding with high platelet counts and associated acquired von Willebrand disease is discussed in the preceding section entitled Platelets; aspirin should not be used when the platelet count exceeds 1000 to 1500 × 10⁹/L.

JAK2 Inhibitors

JAK2 inhibitors represent a promising new therapeutic avenue that arose with the discovery of abnormal JAK-STAT signaling in MPNs.[236]

Currently available JAK2 inhibitors target the catalytic site of the enzyme and therefore inhibit both wild-type and mutant forms of JAK2, as well as variable inhibition of JAK1, JAK3, and other kinases. A number of JAK2 inhibitors are in clinical testing for PV,[236,237] including ruxolitinib (INCB018424), which is effective and FDA approved for use in patients with PMF.[238-241] Ruxolitinib is an oral JAK1/JAK2 inhibitor that has been shown effective in preclinical testing with PV primary cultures[242] and in phase II trials in HU-intolerant or refractory PV patients,[233,243,244] ruxolitinib effectively reduced PV-associated symptoms, such as night sweats, pruritus, and bone pain, within 4 weeks, decreased spleen size to nonpalpable in 44 percent of patients by week 24, induced a complete hematologic response in 59 percent of patients, and reduced the *JAK2*^V617F allelic burden by equal to or greater than 50 percent within the first 3 years of treatment in 24 percent of patients.[233] Phase III trial showed that patients with HU-intolerant or refractory PV treated with ruxolitinib have a decreased requirement for phlebotomy, decreased spleen size, and improvement in other PV-associated symptoms.[232]

Despite the encouraging advances with JAK2 inhibitors, modulation of the JAK2 pathways may not be the sole optimal treatment for PV and other MPNs. *JAK2*^V617F may not be the disease-initiating step in patients with MPNs,[37,245] and additional mutations may require specific therapeutic targeting. Additionally, disease progression is characterized by clonal heterogeneity and genetic instability.[246] Better characterization of the pathogenesis of PV is needed to facilitate further therapeutic developments.

Epigenetic Modulation

A high incidence of mutation in genes involved in epigenetic modification in MPNs (i.e., *TET2, DNMT3A, IDH1/2, PRC2, ASXL1*) provides potential targets for therapy.[247,248] One currently used approach in cancer treatment is interference of histone acetylation, as the acetylation status of histones can alter DNA-protein and protein-protein interactions.[249] The expression levels of histone deacetylases (HDAC) were found to be altered in all three major MPNs,[250] which has made HDAC inhibitors a new therapy of interest in PV. For instance, Givinostat is an HDAC inhibitor which specifically inhibits the proliferation of *JAK2*^V617F-positive cells compared to normal cells[251] by inhibiting hematopoietic transcription factors NFE2 and c-MYB.[252] It has been found to reduce splenomegaly and pruritus in Phase II trials with PV patients.[253,254]

Summary of Therapeutic Approach

The current approach for the management of the majority of PV patients (i.e., high risk) who are not participating in a clinical trial is a combination of therapeutic and preventative approaches:

1. Myelosuppression with HU daily, both as initial therapy (1500 mg qd) and long-term treatment (500 to 2000 mg qd), aiming to maintain neutrophil counts at low-normal levels. In addition, some patients will require the use of phlebotomies and/or anagrelide to maintain hemoglobin and platelet levels in normal ranges. Myelosuppression can also be achieved by other agents such as IFN-α or PEG-IFN-α. PEG-IFN-α is better tolerated than IFN-α and is the most effective therapy, but it is not as well tolerated as HU.

2. Low-dose aspirin at 80 mg qd (or 100 mg outside of North America) is given to all patients without history of major bleeding or gastric intolerance, or those with platelets over 1000 to 1500 × 10⁹/L.

3. Medication to control pruritus and gout may be added if required.

4. Judicious use of phlebotomies in patients with hematocrits greater than 45 to 55 percent and in patients who find phlebotomy relieves their symptoms, such as headaches, difficulty concentrating, and fatigue.

THE SPENT PHASE

Sometimes after only a few years and usually after 15 years or more, erythrocytosis in patients with PV gradually abates in the absence of iron deficiency, phlebotomy requirements decrease and cease, and anemia develops. During this "spent" phase of the disease, marrow fibrosis becomes more marked and the spleen often becomes greatly enlarged (see Fig. 84–2A). Instead of phlebotomies, transfusions or erythropoietin may be required in such patients.[255] The platelet count may remain high or may decline, even to pronounced thrombocytopenic levels. Marked leukopenia or leukocytosis may occur, and immature granulocytes may appear in the blood. At this point, the disease closely mimics PMF (Chap. 86) and is termed post-PV MF. Treatment of this phase of the disease is difficult and requires the judicious use of a combination of therapeutic approaches, including HU, erythropoiesis-stimulating drugs, transfusions, JAK2 inhibitors, and/or allogeneic stem cell transplantation.

Splenectomy

Splenectomy may be warranted (see Fig. 84–2B), particularly in patients with severe fatigue and cytopenias, and in those where a greatly enlarged spleen produces physical discomfort and postprandial fullness.[256] However, a large Mayo Clinic series reported significant morbidity and mortality associated with splenectomy at this stage of the disease.[257]

Hematopoietic Stem Cell Transplantation

Nonmyeloablative allogeneic stem cell transplantation should be considered for otherwise healthy PV patients in the spent phase, even in the seventh decade of life (Chap. 23).[255,258,259] Transplantation is the treatment of choice in patients with early signs of MDS/AML transformation, and the only treatment offering the possibility of a cure.[260] The rate of relapse and nonrelapse mortality following allogeneic stem cell transplantation is negatively associated with increased age, a matched but unrelated donor, and a diagnosis of AML.[260]

● COURSE AND PROGNOSIS

PV is a chronic disease that runs a course over many years. Thrombotic complications, discussed in the preceding sections, are the dominant cause of morbidity and mortality in patients with PV. In contrast to other polycythemic disorders, PV has an increased risk and increased mortality resulting from development of acute leukemia.

The Polycythemia Vera Study Group[76] found that the median survival from the beginning of treatment was 13.9 years for those treated by phlebotomy alone, 11.8 years for ^{32}P-treated patients, and 8.9 years for chlorambucil-treated patients. Thrombosis was the most common cause of death, accounting for 31 percent of fatalities. Nineteen percent of patients died of acute leukemia, 15 percent from other neoplasms, and approximately 5 percent each from hemorrhage or development of the spent phase.

There is excess mortality attributable to thrombotic complications and acute leukemia transformation as a direct consequence of PV.[75] Acute leukemia occurs even in patients who have been treated only by phlebotomy, although its incidence is increased by the various forms of cytotoxic therapy employed. While AML is most common, acute lymphoid leukemia[261] and chronic neutrophilic leukemia[262] have occurred as well. The IWG-MRT reported a rate of transformation to leukemia of 2.3 percent at 10 years and 5.5 percent at 15 years,[190] but a unified scoring system that predicts the likelihood of transformation is yet to be developed.[263,264]

Although it has been suggested that the overall survival of PV patients is near normal,[265,266] a number of other studies have found

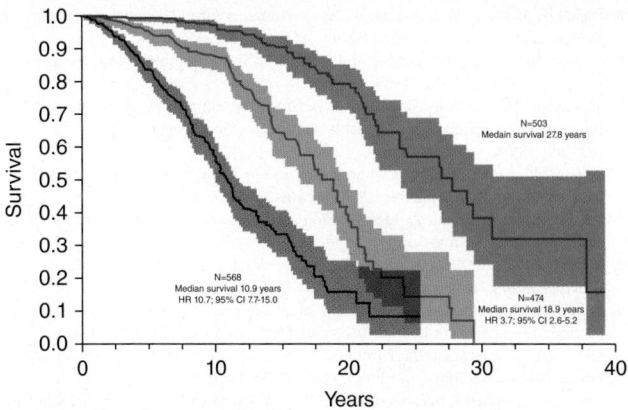

Figure 84–3. Survival of PV patients stratified by prognostic low-risk *(blue)*, intermediate-risk *(green)*, and high-risk *(red)* groups. Patients are scored based on three risk criteria: venous thrombosis (1 point), a leukocyte count $\geq 15 \times 10^9$/L (1 point), and age (≥ 67 years: 5 points, 57–66 years: 2 points). The sum of these points classifies patients as prognostic low risk (0 points), intermediate risk (1–2 points) or high risk (≥ 3 points). *(Reproduced with permission from Tefferi A, Rumi E, Finazzi G, et al: Survival and prognosis among 1545 patients with contemporary polycythemia vera: An international study.* Leukemia 27(9):1874–1881, 2013.)

reduced survival of PV patients compared to controls.[4] A recent study of 1545 patients by the IWG-MRT found that survival for PV patients was negatively correlated to leukocytosis, older age, venous thrombosis, and atypical karyotype. The median overall survival ranged from 10.9 and 27.8 years for different PV prognostic risk groups (Fig. 84–3).[190]

REFERENCES

1. Vaquez MH: Sue une forme spéciale de cyanose s'accompagnant d'hyperglobulie excessive et persistante. *CR Soc Biol* 44:384, 1892.
2. Osler W: Chronic cyanosis, with polycythemia and enlarged spleen: A new clinical entity. *Am J Med Sci* 126:187, 1903.
3. Türk W: Beitrage zur Kenntnis des Symptomenbildes Polycythamie mit Milztumor und Zyanose. *Wien Klin Wochenschr* 17:153, 1904.
4. Anderson LA, McMullin MF: Epidemiology of MPN: What do we know? *Curr Hematol Malig Rep* 2014.
5. Titmarsh GJ, Duncombe AS, McMullin MF, et al: How common are myeloproliferative neoplasms? A systematic review and meta-analysis. *Am J Hematol* 89(6):581–587, 2014.
6. Chaiter Y, Brenner B, Aghai E, et al: High incidence of myeloproliferative disorders in Ashkenazi Jews in northern Israel. *Leuk Lymphoma* 7(3):251–255, 1992.
7. Modan B, Kallner H, Zemer D, et al: A note on the increased risk of polycythemia vera in Jews. *Blood* 37(2):172–176, 1971.
8. Bellanne-Chantelot C, Chaumarel I, Labopin M, et al: Genetic and clinical implications of the Val617Phe JAK2 mutation in 72 families with myeloproliferative disorders. *Blood* 108(1):346–352, 2006.
9. Kralovics R, Stockton DW, Prchal JT: Clonal hematopoiesis in familial polycythemia vera suggests the involvement of multiple mutational events in the early pathogenesis of the disease. *Blood* 102(10):3793–3796, 2003.
10. Ranjan A, Penninga E, Jelsig AM, et al: Inheritance of the chronic myeloproliferative neoplasms. A systematic review. *Clin Genet* 83(2):99–107, 2013.
11. Landgren O, Goldin LR, Kristinsson SY, et al: Increased risks of polycythemia vera, essential thrombocythemia, and myelofibrosis among 24,577 first-degree relatives of 11,039 patients with myeloproliferative neoplasms in Sweden. *Blood* 112(6):2199–2204, 2008.
12. Kralovics R, Guan Y, Prchal JT: Acquired uniparental disomy of chromosome 9p is a frequent stem cell defect in polycythemia vera. *Exp Hematol* 30(3):229–236, 2002.
13. Adamson JW, Fialkow PJ, Murphy S, et al: Polycythemia vera: Stem-cell and probable clonal origin of the disease. *N Engl J Med* 295(17):913–916, 1976.
14. Liu E, Jelinek J, Pastore YD, et al: Discrimination of polycythemias and thrombocytoses by novel, simple, accurate clonality assays and comparison with PRV-1 expression and BFU-E response to erythropoietin. *Blood* 101(8):3294–3301, 2003.
15. Eaves CJ, Eaves AC: Erythropoietin (Ep) dose-response curves for three classes of erythroid progenitors in normal human marrow and in patients with polycythemia vera. *Blood* 52(6):1196–1210, 1978.
16. Prchal JF, Adamson JW, Murphy S, et al: Polycythemia vera. The *in vitro* response of normal and abnormal stem cell lines to erythropoietin. *J Clin Invest* 61(4):1044–1047, 1978.
17. Prchal JF, Axelrad AA: Bone-marrow responses in polycythemia vera [letter]. *N Engl J Med* 290(24):1382, 1974.

18. Prchal JF, Adamson JW, Steinmann L, et al: Human erythroid colony formation *in vitro*: Evidence for clonal origin. *J Cell Physiol* 89(3):489–492, 1976.

19. Groopman JE: The pathogenesis of myelofibrosis in myeloproliferative disorders. *Ann Intern Med* 92(6):857–858, 1980.

20. Moliterno AR, Hankins WD, Spivak JL: Impaired expression of the thrombopoietin receptor by platelets from patients with polycythemia vera. *N Engl J Med* 338(9):572–580, 1998.

21. Silva M, Richard C, Benito A, et al: Expression of Bcl-x in erythroid precursors from patients with polycythemia vera. *N Engl J Med* 338(9):564–571, 1998.

22. Sui X, Krantz SB, Zhao Z: Identification of increased protein tyrosine phosphatase activity in polycythemia vera erythroid progenitor cells. *Blood* 90(2):651–657, 1997.

23. James C, Ugo V, Le Couedic JP, et al: A unique clonal JAK2 mutation leading to constitutive signalling causes polycythaemia vera. *Nature* 434(7037):1144–1148, 2005.

24. Bench AJ, Nacheva EP, Champion KM, et al: Molecular genetics and cytogenetics of myeloproliferative disorders. *Baillieres Clin Haematol* 11(4):819–848, 1998.

25. Diez-Martin JL, Graham DL, Petitt RM, et al: Chromosome studies in 104 patients with polycythemia vera. *Mayo Clin Proc* 66(3):287–299, 1991.

26. Green A, Campbell P, Buck G, et al: The Medical Research Council PT1 Trial in Essential Thrombocythemia. *Blood* 104(Suppl 1):5a, 2004.

27. Najfeld V, Montella L, Scalise A, et al: Exploring polycythaemia vera with fluorescence in situ hybridization: Additional cryptic 9p is the most frequent abnormality detected. *Br J Haematol* 119(2):558–566, 2002.

28. Wurster-Hill D, Whang-Peng J, McIntyre OR, et al: Cytogenetic studies in polycythemia vera. *Semin Hematol* 13(1):13–32, 1976.

29. Sever M, Quintas-Cardama A, Pierce S, et al: Significance of cytogenetic abnormalities in patients with polycythemia vera. *Leuk Lymphoma* 54(12):2667–2670, 2013.

30. Swolin B, Weinfeld A, Westin J: A prospective long-term cytogenetic study in polycythemia vera in relation to treatment and clinical course. *Blood* 72(2):386–395, 1988.

31. Spivak JL: Polycythemia vera: Myths, mechanisms, and management. *Blood* 100(13):4272–4290, 2002.

32. Baxter EJ, Scott LM, Campbell PJ, et al: Acquired mutation of the tyrosine kinase JAK2 in human myeloproliferative disorders. *Lancet* 365(9464):1054–1061, 2005.

33. Kralovics R, Passamonti F, Buser AS, et al: A gain-of-function mutation of JAK2 in myeloproliferative disorders. *N Engl J Med* 352(17):1779–1790, 2005.

34. Levine RL, Wadleigh M, Cools J, et al: Activating mutation in the tyrosine kinase JAK2 in polycythemia vera, essential thrombocythemia, and myeloid metaplasia with myelofibrosis. *Cancer Cell* 7(4):387–397, 2005.

35. Jelinek J, Oki Y, Gharibyan V, et al: JAK2 mutation 1849G>T is rare in acute leukemias but can be found in CMML, Philadelphia chromosome-negative CML, and megakaryocytic leukemia. *Blood* 106(10):3370–3373, 2005.

36. Jones AV, Kreil S, Zoi K, et al: Widespread occurrence of the JAK2 V617F mutation in chronic myeloproliferative disorders. *Blood* 106(6):2162–2168, 2005.

37. Nussenzveig RH, Swierczek SI, Jelinek J, et al: Polycythemia vera is not initiated by JAK2V617F mutation. *Exp Hematol* 35(1):32–38, 2007.

38. Tefferi A, Lasho TL, Schwager SM, et al: The clinical phenotype of wild-type, heterozygous, and homozygous JAK2V617F in polycythemia vera. *Cancer* 106(3):631–635, 2006.

39. Passamonti F, Rumi E, Pietra D, et al: A prospective study of 338 patients with polycythemia vera: The impact of JAK2 (V617F) allele burden and leukocytosis on fibrotic or leukemic disease transformation and vascular complications. *Leukemia* 24(9):1574–1579, 2010.

40. Silver RT, Vandris K, Wang YL, et al: JAK2(V617F) allele burden in polycythemia vera correlates with grade of myelofibrosis, but is not substantially affected by therapy. *Leuk Res* 35(2):177–182, 2011.

41. Alvarez-Larran A, Bellosillo B, Pereira A, et al: JAK2V617F monitoring in polycythemia vera and essential thrombocythemia: Clinical usefulness for predicting myelofibrotic transformation and thrombotic events. *Am J Hematol* 89(5):517–523, 2014.

42. Koren-Michowitz M, Landman J, Cohen Y, et al: JAK2V617F allele burden is associated with transformation to myelofibrosis. *Leuk Lymphoma* 53(11):2210–2213, 2012.

43. Kuriakose E, Vandris K, Wang YL, et al: Decrease in JAK2 V617F allele burden is not a prerequisite to clinical response in patients with polycythemia vera. *Haematologica* 97(4):538–542, 2012.

44. Scott LM, Tong W, Levine RL, et al: JAK2 exon 12 mutations in polycythemia vera and idiopathic erythrocytosis. *N Engl J Med* 356(5):459–468, 2007.

45. Scott LM: The JAK2 exon 12 mutations: A comprehensive review. *Am J Hematol* 86(8):668–676, 2011.

46. Passamonti F, Elena C, Schnittger S, et al: Molecular and clinical features of the myeloproliferative neoplasm associated with JAK2 exon 12 mutations. *Blood* 117(10):2813–2816, 2011.

47. Skoda R, Prchal JT: Lessons from familial myeloproliferative disorders. *Semin Hematol* 42(4):266–273, 2005.

48. Cario H, Schwarz K, Herter JM, et al: Clinical and molecular characterisation of a prospectively collected cohort of children and adolescents with polycythemia vera. *Br J Haematol* 142(4):622–626, 2008.

49. Kralovics R, Teo SS, Buser AS, et al: Altered gene expression in myeloproliferative disorders correlates with activation of signaling by the V617F mutation of Jak2. *Blood* 106(10):3374–3376, 2005.

50. Theocharides A, Boissinot M, Girodon F, et al: Leukemic blasts in transformed JAK2-V617F-positive myeloproliferative disorders are frequently negative for the JAK2-V617F mutation. *Blood* 110(1):375–379, 2007.

51. Wang L, Swierczek SI, Drummond J: Whole-exome sequencing of polycythemia vera revealed novel driver genes and somatic mutation shared by T cells and granulocytes. 28(4):935–938, 2014.

52. Wang L, Swierczek SI, Lanikova L, et al: The relationship of JAK2(V617F) and acquired UPD at chromosome 9p in polycythemia vera. *Leukemia* 28(4):938–941, 2014.

53. Spivak JL, Considine M, Williams DM, et al: Two clinical phenotypes in polycythemia vera. *N Engl J Med* 371(9):808–817, 2014.

54. Olcaydu D, Harutyunyan A, Jager R, et al: A common JAK2 haplotype confers susceptibility to myeloproliferative neoplasms. *Nat Genet* 41(4):450–454, 2009.

55. Olcaydu D, Skoda RC, Looser R, et al: The "GGCC" haplotype of JAK2 confers susceptibility to JAK2 exon 12 mutation-positive polycythemia vera. *Leukemia* 23(10):1924–1926, 2009.

56. Kilpivaara O, Mukherjee S, Schram AM, et al: A germline JAK2 SNP is associated with predisposition to the development of JAK2(V617F)-positive myeloproliferative neoplasms. *Nat Genet* 41(4):455–459, 2009.

57. Jones AV, Chase A, Silver RT, et al: JAK2 haplotype is a major risk factor for the development of myeloproliferative neoplasms. *Nat Genet* 41(4):446–449, 2009.

58. Delhommeau F, Dupont S, Della Valle V, et al: Mutation in TET2 in myeloid cancers. *N Engl J Med* 360(22):2289–2301, 2009.

59. Tefferi A, Pardanani A, Lim KH, et al: TET2 mutations and their clinical correlates in polycythemia vera, essential thrombocythemia and myelofibrosis. *Leukemia* 23(5):905–911, 2009.

60. Saint-Martin C, Leroy G, Delhommeau F, et al: Analysis of the ten-eleven translocation 2 (TET2) gene in familial myeloproliferative neoplasms. *Blood* 114(8):1628–1632, 2009.

61. Busque L, Patel JP, Figueroa ME, et al: Recurrent somatic TET2 mutations in normal elderly individuals with clonal hematopoiesis. *Nat Genet* 44(11):1179–1181, 2012.

62. Cazzola M, Kralovics R: From Janus kinase 2 to calreticulin: The clinically relevant genomic landscape of myeloproliferative neoplasms. *Blood* 123(24):3714–3719, 2014.

63. Wang L, Swierczek SI, Drummond J, et al: Whole-exome sequencing of polycythemia vera revealed novel driver genes and somatic mutation shared by T cells and granulocytes. *Leukemia* 28(4):935–938, 2014.

64. Li S, Kralovics R, De Libero G, et al: Clonal heterogeneity in polycythemia vera patients with JAK2 exon12 and JAK2-V617F mutations. *Blood* 111(7):3863–3866, 2008.

65. Kristinsson SY, Landgren O, Samuelsson J, et al: Autoimmunity and the risk of myeloproliferative neoplasms. *Haematologica* 95(7):1216–1220, 2010.

66. Hasselbalch HC: Perspectives on chronic inflammation in essential thrombocythemia, polycythemia vera, and myelofibrosis: Is chronic inflammation a trigger and driver of clonal evolution and development of accelerated atherosclerosis and second cancer? *Blood* 119(14):3219–3225, 2012.

67. Hasselbalch HC: Chronic inflammation as a promotor of mutagenesis in essential thrombocythemia, polycythemia vera and myelofibrosis. A human inflammation model for cancer development? *Leuk Res* 37(2):214–220, 2013.

68. Hasselbalch HC: A role of NF-E2 in chronic inflammation and clonal evolution in essential thrombocythemia, polycythemia vera and myelofibrosis? *Leuk Res* 38(2):263–266, 2014.

69. Skov V, Larsen TS, Thomassen M, et al: Molecular profiling of peripheral blood cells from patients with polycythemia vera and related neoplasms: Identification of deregulated genes of significance for inflammation and immune surveillance. *Leuk Res* 36(11):1387–1392, 2012.

70. Berlin NI: Diagnosis and classification of the polycythemias. *Semin Hematol* 12(4):339–351, 1975.

71. Marchioli R, Finazzi G, Landolfi R, et al: Vascular and neoplastic risk in a large cohort of patients with polycythemia vera. *J Clin Oncol* 23(10):2224–2232, 2005.

72. Falanga A, Marchetti M: Thrombotic disease in the myeloproliferative neoplasms. *Hematology Am Soc Hematol Educ Program* 2012:571–581, 2012.

73. Falanga A, Marchetti M: Thrombosis in myeloproliferative neoplasms. *Semin Thromb Hemost* 40(3):348–358, 2014.

74. Wehmeier A, Daum I, Jamin H, et al: Incidence and clinical risk factors for bleeding and thrombotic complications in myeloproliferative disorders. A retrospective analysis of 260 patients. *Ann Hematol* 63(2):101–106, 1991.

75. Landolfi R, Marchioli R, Kutti J, et al: Efficacy and safety of low-dose aspirin in polycythemia vera. *N Engl J Med* 350(2):114–124, 2004.

76. Berk PD, Goldberg JD, Donovan PB, et al: Therapeutic recommendations in polycythemia vera based on Polycythemia Vera Study Group protocols. *Semin Hematol* 23(2):132–143, 1986.

77. Polycythemia vera: The natural history of 1213 patients followed for 20 years. Gruppo Italiano Studio Policitemia. *Ann Intern Med* 123(9):656–664, 1995.

78. Berk P, Wasserman L, Fruchtman S: Treatment of polycythemia vera. A summary of clinical trials conducted by the Polycythemia Study Group, in *Polycythemia Vera and the Myeloproliferative Disorders*, edited by Wasserman L, Berk P, Berlin N. WB Saunders, Philadelphia, 1995.

79. Coucelo M, Caetano G, Sevivas T, et al: JAK2V617F allele burden is associated with thrombotic mechanisms activation in polycythemia vera and essential thrombocythemia patients. *Int J Hematol* 99(1):32–40, 2014.

80. Carobbio A, Finazzi G, Antonioli E, et al: JAK2V617F allele burden and thrombosis: A direct comparison in essential thrombocythemia and polycythemia vera. *Exp Hematol* 37(9):1016–1021, 2009.

81. Spivak JL, Barosi G, Tognoni G, et al: Chronic myeloproliferative disorders. *Hematology Am Soc Hematol Educ Program* 200–224, 2003.

82. Barbui T, Finazzi G: Special issues in myeloproliferative neoplasms. *Curr Hematol Malig Rep* 6(1):28–35, 2011.

83. Anger BR, Seifried E, Scheppach J, et al: Budd-Chiari syndrome and thrombosis of other abdominal vessels in the chronic myeloproliferative diseases. *Klin Wochenschr* 67(16):818–825, 1989.

84. De Stefano V, Fiorini A, Rossi E, et al: Incidence of the JAK2 V617F mutation among patients with splanchnic or cerebral venous thrombosis and without overt chronic myeloproliferative disorders. *J Thromb Haemost* 5(4):708–714, 2007.

85. De Stefano V, Teofili L, Leone G, et al: Spontaneous erythroid colony formation as the clue to an underlying myeloproliferative disorder in patients with Budd-Chiari syndrome or portal vein thrombosis. *Semin Thromb Hemost* 23(5):411–418, 1997.

86. Colaizzo D, Amitrano L, Tiscia GL, et al: The JAK2 V617F mutation frequently occurs in patients with portal and mesenteric venous thrombosis. *J Thromb Haemost* 5(1):55–61, 2007.

87. Reikvam H, Tiu RV: Venous thromboembolism in patients with essential thrombocythemia and polycythemia vera. *Leukemia* 26(4):563–571, 2012.

88. Srinivasan P, Rela M, Prachalias A, et al: Liver transplantation for Budd-Chiari syndrome. *Transplantation* 73(6):973–977, 2002.

89. Valla D, Casadevall N, Lacombe C, et al: Primary myeloproliferative disorder and hepatic vein thrombosis. A prospective study of erythroid colony formation in vitro in 20 patients with Budd-Chiari syndrome. *Ann Intern Med* 103(3):329–334, 1985.

90. Murphy S: Polycythemia vera. *Dis Mon* 38(3):153–212, 1992.

91. Siegel FP, Tauscher J, Petrides PE: Aquagenic pruritus in polycythemia vera: Characteristics and influence on quality of life in 441 patients. *Am J Hematol* 88(8):665–669, 2013.

92. Jackson N, Burt D, Crocker J, et al: Skin mast cells in polycythemia vera: Relationship to the pathogenesis and treatment of pruritus. *Br J Dermatol* 116(1):21–29, 1987.

93. Steinman HK, Kobza-Black A, Lotti TM, et al: Polycythaemia rubra vera and water-induced pruritus: Blood histamine levels and cutaneous fibrinolytic activity before and after water challenge. *Br J Dermatol* 116(3):329–333, 1987.

94. Buchanan JG, Ameratunga RV, Hawkins RC: Polycythemia vera and water-induced pruritus: Evidence against mast cell involvement. *Pathology* 26(1):43–45, 1994.

95. Cox NH, Leggat H: Sweet's syndrome associated with polycythemia rubra vera. *J Am Acad Dermatol* 23(6 Pt 1):1171–1172, 1990.

96. Furukawa T, Takahashi M, Shimada H, et al: Polycythaemia vera with Sweet's syndrome. *Clin Lab Haematol* 11(1):67–70, 1989.

97. Davis MD, O'Fallon WM, Rogers RS, 3rd, et al: Natural history of erythromelalgia: Presentation and outcome in 168 patients. *Arch Dermatol* 136(3):330–336, 2000.

98. van Genderen PJ, Lucas IS, van Strik R, et al: Erythromelalgia in essential thrombocythemia is characterized by platelet activation and endothelial cell damage but not by thrombin generation. *Thromb Haemost* 76(3):333–338, 1996.

99. van Genderen PJ, Michiels JJ: Erythromelalgia: A pathognomonic microvascular thrombotic complication in essential thrombocythemia and polycythemia vera. *Semin Thromb Hemost* 23(4):357–363, 1997.

100. Wanless IR, Peterson P, Das A, et al: Hepatic vascular disease and portal hypertension in polycythemia vera and agnogenic myeloid metaplasia: A clinicopathological study of 145 patients examined at autopsy. *Hepatology* 12(5):1166–1174, 1990.

101. Tinney WS, Hall BE, Giffin HZ: Polycythemia vera and peptic ulcer. *Mayo Clin Proc* 18:24, 1943.

102. Dingli D, Utz JP, Krowka MJ, et al: Unexplained pulmonary hypertension in chronic myeloproliferative disorders. *Chest* 120(3):801–808, 2001.

103. Garcia-Manero G, Schuster SJ, Patrick H, et al: Pulmonary hypertension in patients with myelofibrosis secondary to myeloproliferative diseases. *Am J Hematol* 60(2):130–135, 1999.

104. Newton LK: Neurologic complications of polycythemia and their impact on therapy. *Oncology (Williston Park)* 4(3):59–64; discussion 64–66, 1990.

105. Jackson A, Burton IE: Retroperitoneal mass and spinal cord compression due to extramedullary haemopoiesis in polycythaemia rubra vera. *Br J Radiol* 62(742):944–947, 1989.

106. Wasserman LR, Gilbert HS: Surgical bleeding in polycythemia vera. *Ann N Y Acad Sci* 115:122–138, 1964.

107. Gilbert HS: Modern treatment strategies in polycythemia vera. *Semin Hematol* 40(1 Suppl 1):26–29, 2003.

108. Thiele J, Kvasnicka HM: Diagnostic impact of bone marrow histopathology in polycythemia vera (PV). *Histol Histopathol* 20(1):317–328, 2005.

109. Finazzi G, Caruso V, Marchioli R, et al: Acute leukemia in polycythemia vera: An analysis of 1638 patients enrolled in a prospective observational study. *Blood* 105(7):2664–2670, 2005.

110. Cassinat B, Laguillier C, Gardin C, et al: Classification of myeloproliferative disorders in the JAK2 era: Is there a role for red cell mass? *Leukemia* 22(2):452–453, 2008.

111. Johansson PL, Safai-Kutti S, Kutti J: An elevated venous haemoglobin concentration cannot be used as a surrogate marker for absolute erythrocytosis: A study of patients with polycythaemia vera and apparent polycythaemia. *Br J Haematol* 129(5):701–705, 2005.

112. Barbui T, Thiele J, Gisslinger H, et al: Masked polycythemia vera (mPV): Results of an international study. *Am J Hematol* 89(1):52–54, 2014.

113. Spivak JL: Diagnosis of the myeloproliferative disorders: Resolving phenotypic mimicry. *Semin Hematol* 40(1 Suppl 1):1–5, 2003.

114. Beutler E: Polycythemia. *Med Grand Rounds* 3:142, 1984.

115. Spivak JL, Silver RT: The revised World Health Organization diagnostic criteria for polycythemia vera, essential thrombocytosis, and primary myelofibrosis: An alternative proposal. *Blood* 112(2):231–239, 2008.

116. Gilbert HS, Warner RR, Wasserman LR: A study of histamine in myeloproliferative disease. *Blood* 28(6):795–806, 1966.

117. Falanga A, Marchetti M, Evangelista V, et al: Polymorphonuclear leukocyte activation and hemostasis in patients with essential thrombocythemia and polycythemia vera. *Blood* 96(13):4261–4266, 2000.

118. Vannucchi AM: Insights into the pathogenesis and management of thrombosis in polycythemia vera and essential thrombocythemia. *Intern Emerg Med* 5(3):177–184, 2010.

119. Cerutti A, Custodi P, Duranti M, et al: Thrombopoietin levels in patients with primary and reactive thrombocytosis. *Br J Haematol* 99(2):281–284, 1997.

120. Shih LY, Lee CT: Identification of masked polycythemia vera from patients with idiopathic marked thrombocytosis by endogenous erythroid colony assay. *Blood* 83(3):744–748, 1994.

121. Yamamoto K, Sekiguchi E, Takatani O: Abnormalities of epinephrine-induced platelet aggregation and adenine nucleotides in myeloproliferative disorders. *Thromb Haemost* 52(3):292–296, 1984.

122. Mehta P, Mehta J, Ross M, et al: Decreased platelet aggregation but increased thromboxane A2 generation in polycythemia vera. *Arch Intern Med* 145(7):1225–1227, 1985.

123. Landolfi R, Ciabattoni G, Patrignani P, et al: Increased thromboxane biosynthesis in patients with polycythemia vera: Evidence for aspirin-suppressible platelet activation in vivo. *Blood* 80(8):1965–1971, 1992.

124. Berild D, Hasselbalch H, Knudsen JB: Platelet survival, platelet factor-4 and bleeding time in myeloproliferative disorders. *Scand J Clin Lab Invest* 47(5):497–501, 1987.

125. Kutti J, Weinfeld A: Platelet survival in active polycythaemia vera with reference to the haematocrit level. An experimental study before and after phlebotomy. *Scand J Haematol* 8(5):405–414, 1971.

126. Le Blanc K, Lindahl T, Rosendahl K, et al: Impaired platelet binding of fibrinogen due to a lower number of GPIIB/IIIA receptors in polycythemia vera. *Thromb Res* 91(6):287–295, 1998.

127. Afshar-Kharghan V, Lopez JA, Gray LA, et al: Hemostatic gene polymorphisms and the prevalence of thrombotic complications in polycythemia vera and essential thrombocythemia. *Blood Coagul Fibrinolysis* 15(1):21–24, 2004.

128. Landolfi R, Cipriani MC, Novarese L: Thrombosis and bleeding in polycythemia vera and essential thrombocythemia: Pathogenetic mechanisms and prevention. *Best Pract Res Clin Haematol* 19(3):617–633, 2006.

129. Binder RA, Gilbert HS: Muramidase in polycythemia vera. *Blood* 36(2):228–232, 1970.

130. Gilbert HS, Krauss S, Pasternack B, et al: Serum vitamin B12 content and unsaturated vitamin B12-binding capacity in myeloproliferative disease. Value in differential diagnosis and as indicators of disease activity. *Ann Intern Med* 71(4):719–729, 1969.

131. Moliterno AR, Williams DM, Rogers O, et al: Molecular mimicry in the chronic myeloproliferative disorders: Reciprocity between quantitative JAK2 V617F and Mpl expression. *Blood* 108(12):3913–3915, 2006.

132. Antonioli E, Guglielmelli P, Poli G, et al: Influence of JAK2V617F allele burden on phenotype in essential thrombocythemia. *Haematologica* 93(1):41–48, 2008.

133. Wang L, Swierczek SI, Lanikova L, et al: The relationship of JAK2(V617F) and acquired UPD at chromosome 9p in polycythemia vera. *Leukemia* 28(4):938–941, 2014.

134. Lippert E, Girodon F, Hammond E, et al: Concordance of assays designed for the quantification of JAK2V617F: A multicenter study. *Haematologica* 94(1):38–45, 2009.

135. Ma W, Kantarjian H, Zhang X, et al: Higher detection rate of JAK2 mutation using plasma. *Blood* 111(7):3906–3907, 2008.

136. Ma W, Kantarjian H, Verstovsek S, et al: Hemizygous/homozygous and heterozygous JAK2 mutation detected in plasma of patients with myeloproliferative diseases: Correlation with clinical behaviour. *Br J Haematol* 134(3):341–343, 2006.

137. Salama ME, Swierczek SI, Hickman K, et al: Plasma quantitation of JAK2 mutation is not suitable as a clinical test: An artifact of storage. *Blood* 114(1):223–224; author reply 224, 2009.

138. Jones AV, Cross NC, White HE, et al: Rapid identification of JAK2 exon 12 mutations using high resolution melting analysis. *Haematologica* 93(10):1560–1564, 2008.

139. Percy MJ, Scott LM, Erber WN, et al: The frequency of JAK2 exon 12 mutations in idiopathic erythrocytosis patients with low serum erythropoietin levels. *Haematologica* 92(12):1607–1614, 2007.

140. Pietra D, Li S, Brisci A, et al: Somatic mutations of JAK2 exon 12 in patients with JAK2 (V617F)-negative myeloproliferative disorders. *Blood* 111(3):1686–1689, 2008.

141. Rapado I, Grande S, Albizua E, et al: High resolution melting analysis for JAK2 Exon 14 and Exon 12 mutations: A diagnostic tool for myeloproliferative neoplasms. *J Mol Diagn* 11(2):155–161, 2009.

142. Schnittger S, Bacher U, Haferlach C, et al: Detection of JAK2 exon 12 mutations in 15 patients with JAK2V617F negative polycythemia vera. *Haematologica* 94(3):414–418, 2009.

143. Birgegard G, Wide L: Serum erythropoietin in the diagnosis of polycythaemia and after phlebotomy treatment. *Br J Haematol* 81(4):603–606, 1992.

144. Messinezy M, Westwood NB, El-Hemaidi I, et al: Serum erythropoietin values in erythrocytoses and in primary thrombocythaemia. *Br J Haematol* 117(1):47–53, 2002.

145. Mossuz P, Girodon F, Donnard M, et al: Diagnostic value of serum erythropoietin level in patients with absolute erythrocytosis. *Haematologica* 89(10):1194–1198, 2004.

146. Remacha AF, Montserrat I, Santamaria A, et al: Serum erythropoietin in the diagnosis of polycythemia vera. A follow-up study. *Haematologica* 82(4):406–410, 1997.

147. Prchal JT: Classification and molecular biology of polycythemias (erythrocytoses) and thrombocytosis. *Hematol Oncol Clin North Am* 17(5):1151–1158, vi, 2003.

148. Weinberg RS: *In vitro* erythropoiesis in polycythemia vera and other myeloproliferative disorders. *Semin Hematol* 34(1):64–69, 1997.

149. Shih LY, Lee CT, See LC, et al: *In vitro* culture growth of erythroid progenitors and serum erythropoietin assay in the differential diagnosis of polycythaemia. *Eur J Clin Invest* 28(7):569–576, 1998.

150. Fisher MJ, Prchal JF, Prchal JT, et al: Anti-erythropoietin (EPO) receptor monoclonal antibodies distinguish EPO-dependent and EPO-independent erythroid progenitors in polycythemia vera. *Blood* 84(6):1982–1991, 1994.

151. Kralovics R, Sokol L, Prchal JT: Absence of polycythemia in a child with a unique erythropoietin receptor mutation in a family with autosomal dominant primary polycythemia. *J Clin Invest* 102(1):124–129, 1998.

152. Acharya J, Westwood NB, Sawyer BM, et al: Identification of latent myeloproliferative disease in patients with Budd-Chiari syndrome using X-chromosome inactivation patterns and in vitro erythroid colony formation. *Eur J Haematol* 55(5):315–321, 1995.

153. Pagliuca A, Mufti GJ, Janossa-Tahernia M, et al: In vitro colony culture and chromosomal studies in hepatic and portal vein thrombosis—Possible evidence of an occult myeloproliferative state. *Q J Med* 76(281):981–989, 1990.

154. Tefferi A, Thiele J, Vardiman JW: The 2008 World Health Organization classification system for myeloproliferative neoplasms: Order out of chaos. *Cancer* 115(17):3842–3847, 2009.

155. Lakey MA, Pardanani A, Hoyer JD, et al: Bone marrow morphologic features in polycythemia vera with JAK2 exon 12 mutations. *Am J Clin Pathol* 133(6):942–948, 2010.

156. Wang X, LeBlanc A, Gruenstein S, et al: Clonal analyses define the relationships between chromosomal abnormalities and JAK2V617F in patients with Ph-negative myeloproliferative neoplasms. *Exp Hematol* 37(10):1194–1200, 2009.

157. Beutler E, Yeh M, Fairbanks VF: The normal human female as a mosaic of X-chromosome activity: Studies using the gene for C-6-PD-deficiency as a marker. *Proc Natl Acad Sci U S A* 48:9–16, 1962.

158. Prchal JT: Pathogenetic mechanisms of polycythemia vera and congenital polycythemic disorders. *Semin Hematol* 38(1 Suppl 2):10–20, 2001.

159. Swierczek SI, Piterkova L, Jelinek J, et al: Methylation of AR locus does not always reflect X chromosome inactivation state. *Blood* 119:e100–e109, 2012.

160. Swierczek SI, Agarwal N, Nussenzveig RH, et al: Hematopoiesis is not clonal in healthy elderly women. *Blood* 112(8):3186–3193, 2008.

161. Vogelstein B, Fearon ER, Hamilton SR, et al: Use of restriction fragment length polymorphisms to determine the clonal origin of human tumors. *Science* 227(4687):642–645, 1985.

162. Allen RC, Zoghbi HY, Moseley AB, et al: Methylation of HpaII and HhaI sites near the polymorphic CAG repeat in the human androgen-receptor gene correlates with X chromosome inactivation. *Am J Hum Genet* 51(6):1229–1239, 1992.

163. Curnutte JT, Hopkins PJ, Kuhl W, et al: Studying X inactivation. *Lancet* 339(8795):749, 1992.

164. Prchal JT, Guan YL, Prchal JF, et al: Transcriptional analysis of the active X-chromosome in normal and clonal hematopoiesis. *Blood* 81(1):269–271, 1993.

165. McMullin MF, Reilly JT, Campbell P, et al: Amendment to the guideline for diagnosis and investigation of polycythaemia/erythrocytosis. *Br J Haematol* 138(6):821–822, 2007.

166. Bench AJ, White HE, Foroni L, et al: Molecular diagnosis of the myeloproliferative neoplasms: UK guidelines for the detection of JAK2 V617F and other relevant mutations. *Br J Haematol* 160(1):25–34, 2013.

167. Samuelson SJ, Parker CJ, Prchal JT: Revised criteria for the myeloproliferative disorders: Too much too soon? *Blood* 111(3):1741; author reply 1742, 2008.

168. Barbui T, Thiele J, Vannucchi AM, et al: Rethinking the diagnostic criteria of polycythemia vera. *Leukemia* 28(6):1191–1195, 2014.

169. Silver RT, Chow W, Orazi A, et al: Evaluation of WHO criteria for diagnosis of polycythemia vera: A prospective analysis. *Blood* 122(11):1881–1886, 2013.

170. Teofili L, Giona F, Martini M, et al: The revised WHO diagnostic criteria for Ph-negative myeloproliferative diseases are not appropriate for the diagnostic screening of childhood polycythemia vera and essential thrombocythemia. *Blood* 110(9):3384–3386, 2007.

171. Finazzi G, Barbui T: Evidence and expertise in the management of polycythemia vera and essential thrombocythemia. *Leukemia* 22(8):1494–1502, 2008.

172. Barbui T, Carobbio A, Rambaldi A, et al: Perspectives on thrombosis in essential thrombocythemia and polycythemia vera: Is leukocytosis a causative factor? *Blood* 114(4):759–763, 2009.

173. Caramazza D, Caracciolo C, Barone R, et al: Correlation between leukocytosis and thrombosis in Philadelphia-negative chronic myeloproliferative neoplasms. *Ann Hematol* 88(10):967–971, 2009.

174. Landolfi R, Di Gennaro L, Barbui T, et al: Leukocytosis as a major thrombotic risk factor in patients with polycythemia vera. *Blood* 109(6):2446–2452, 2007.

175. Gangat N, Strand J, Li CY, et al: Leucocytosis in polycythaemia vera predicts both inferior survival and leukaemic transformation. *Br J Haematol* 138(3):354–358, 2007.

176. De Stefano V, Za T, Rossi E, et al: Leukocytosis is a risk factor for recurrent arterial thrombosis in young patients with polycythemia vera and essential thrombocythemia. *Am J Hematol* 85(2):97–100, 2010.

177. Vannucchi AM, Antonioli E, Guglielmelli P, et al: Clinical correlates of JAK2V617F presence or allele burden in myeloproliferative neoplasms: A critical reappraisal. *Leukemia* 22(7):1299–1307, 2008.

178. Barbui T, Barosi G, Birgegard G, et al: Philadelphia-negative classical myeloproliferative neoplasms: Critical concepts and management recommendations from European LeukemiaNet. *J Clin Oncol* 29(6):761–770, 2011.

179. Barosi G, Mesa R, Finazzi G, et al: Revised response criteria for polycythemia vera and essential thrombocythemia: An ELN and IWG-MRT consensus project. *Blood* 121(23):4778–4781, 2013.

180. Harrison C: Rethinking disease definitions and therapeutic strategies in essential thrombocythemia and polycythemia vera. *Hematology Am Soc Hematol Educ Program* 2010:129–134, 2010.

181. Tefferi A: Polycythemia vera and essential thrombocythemia: 2013 Update on diagnosis, risk-stratification, and management. *Am J Hematol* 88(6):507–516, 2013.

182. Dingli D, Tefferi A: Hydroxyurea: The drug of choice for polycythemia vera and essential thrombocythemia. *Curr Hematol Malig Rep* 1(2):69–74, 2006.

183. Barbui T, Finazzi G: Evidence-based management of polycythemia vera. *Best Pract Res Clin Haematol* 19(3):483–493, 2006.

184. Antonioli E, Carobbio A, Pieri L, et al: Hydroxyurea does not appreciably reduce JAK2 V617F allele burden in patients with polycythemia vera or essential thrombocythemia. *Haematologica* 95(8):1435–1438, 2010.

185. Ricksten A, Palmqvist L, Johansson P, et al: Rapid decline of JAK2V617F levels during hydroxyurea treatment in patients with polycythemia vera and essential thrombocythemia. *Haematologica* 93(8):1260–1261, 2008.

186. Spanoudakis E, Bazdiara I, Kotsianidis I, et al: Hydroxyurea (HU) is effective in reducing JAK2V617F mutated clone size in the peripheral blood of essential thrombocythemia (ET) and polycythemia vera (PV) patients. *Ann Hematol* 88(7):629–632, 2009.

187. Zalcberg IR, Ayres-Silva J, de Azevedo AM, et al: Hydroxyurea dose impacts hematologic parameters in polycythemia vera and essential thrombocythemia but does not appreciably affect JAK2-V617F allele burden. *Haematologica* 96(3):e18–e20, 2011.

188. Sirhan S, Lasho TL, Hanson CA, et al: The presence of JAK2V617F in primary myelofibrosis or its allele burden in polycythemia vera predicts chemosensitivity to hydroxyurea. *Am J Hematol* 83(5):363–365, 2008.

189. Lanzkron S, Strouse JJ, Wilson R, et al: Systematic review: Hydroxyurea for the treatment of adults with sickle cell disease. *Ann Intern Med* 148(12):939–955, 2008.

190. Tefferi A, Rumi E, Finazzi G, et al: Survival and prognosis among 1545 patients with contemporary polycythemia vera: An international study. *Leukemia* 27(9):1874–1881, 2013.

191. Alvarez-Larran A, Pereira A, Cervantes F, et al: Assessment and prognostic value of the European LeukemiaNet criteria for clinicohematologic response, resistance, and intolerance to hydroxyurea in polycythemia vera. *Blood* 119(6):1363–1369, 2012.

192. Barosi G, Birgegard G, Finazzi G, et al: A unified definition of clinical resistance and intolerance to hydroxycarbamide in polycythaemia vera and primary myelofibrosis: Results of a European LeukemiaNet (ELN) consensus process. *Br J Haematol* 148(6):961–963, 2010.

193. Sever M, Newberry KJ, Verstovsek S: Therapeutic options for patients with polycythemia vera and essential thrombocythemia refractory/resistant to hydroxyurea. *Leuk Lymphoma* 55(12):2685–2690, 2014.

194. Treatment of polycythaemia vera by radiophosphorus or busulphan: A randomized trial. "Leukemia and Hematosarcoma" Cooperative Group, European Organization for Research on Treatment of Cancer (E.O.R.T.C.). *Br J Cancer* 44(1):75–80, 1981.

195. Kuriakose ET, Gjoni S, Wang YL, et al: JAK2V617F allele burden is reduced by busulfan therapy: A new observation using an old drug. *Haematologica* 98(11):e135–e137, 2013.

196. Alvarez-Larrán A, Martínez-Avilés L, Hernández-Boluda JC, et al: Busulfan in patients with polycythemia vera or essential thrombocythemia refractory or intolerant to hydroxyurea. *Ann Hematol* 93(12):2037–2043, 2014.

197. Tefferi A: Polycythemia vera: A comprehensive review and clinical recommendations. *Mayo Clin Proc* 78(2):174–194, 2003.

198. Balan KK, Critchley M: Outcome of 259 patients with primary proliferative polycythaemia (PPP) and idiopathic thrombocythaemia (IT) treated in a regional nuclear medicine department with phosphorus-32—A 15 year review. *Br J Radiol* 70(839):1169–1173, 1997.

199. Roberts BE, Smith AH: Use of radioactive phosphorus in haematology. *Blood Rev* 11(3):146–153, 1997.

200. Silver RT: Recombinant interferon-alpha for treatment of polycythaemia vera. *Lancet* 2(8607):403, 1988.

201. Hasselbalch HC: A new era for IFN-alpha in the treatment of Philadelphia-negative chronic myeloproliferative neoplasms. *Expert Rev Hematol* 4(6):637–655, 2011.

202. Hasselbalch HC, Larsen TS, Riley CH, et al: Interferon-alpha in the treatment of Philadelphia-negative chronic myeloproliferative neoplasms. Status and perspectives. *Curr Drug Targets* 12(3):392–419, 2011.

203. Silver RT, Kiladjian JJ, Hasselbalch HC: Interferon and the treatment of polycythemia vera, essential thrombocythemia and myelofibrosis. *Expert Rev Hematol* 6(1):49–58, 2013.

204. Kiladjian JJ, Mesa RA, Hoffman R: The renaissance of interferon therapy for the treatment of myeloid malignancies. *Blood* 117(18):4706–4715, 2011.

205. Jones AV, Silver RT, Waghorn K, et al: Minimal molecular response in polycythemia vera patients treated with imatinib or interferon alpha. *Blood* 107(8):3339–3341, 2006.

206. Larsen TS, Moller MB, de Stricker K, et al: Minimal residual disease and normalization of the bone marrow after long-term treatment with alpha-interferon2b in polycythemia vera. A report on molecular response patterns in seven patients in sustained complete hematological remission. *Hematology* 14(6):331–334, 2009.

207. Zhang ZR, Duan YC: Interferon apha 2b for treating patients with JAK2V617F positive polycythemia vera and essential thrombocytosis. *Asian Pac J Cancer Prev* 15(4):1681–1684, 2014.

208. Huang BT, Zeng QC, Zhao WH, et al: Interferon alpha-2b gains high sustained response therapy for advanced essential thrombocythemia and polycythemia vera with JAK2V617F positive mutation. *Leuk Res* 38(10):1177–1183, 2014.

209. Steegmann JL, Requena MJ, Martin-Regueira P, et al: High incidence of autoimmune alterations in chronic myeloid leukemia patients treated with interferon-alpha. *Am J Hematol* 72(3):170–176, 2003.

210. Quintas-Cardama A, Kantarjian HM, Giles F, et al: Pegylated interferon therapy for patients with Philadelphia chromosome-negative myeloproliferative disorders. *Semin Thromb Hemost* 32(4 Pt 2):409–416, 2006.

211. Jabbour E, Kantarjian H, Cortes J, et al: PEG-IFN-alpha-2b therapy in BCR-ABL-negative myeloproliferative disorders: Final result of a phase 2 study. *Cancer* 110(9):2012–2018, 2007.

212. Samuelsson J, Hasselbalch H, Bruserud O, et al: A phase II trial of pegylated interferon alpha-2b therapy for polycythemia vera and essential thrombocythemia: Feasibility, clinical and biologic effects, and impact on quality of life. *Cancer* 106(11):2397–2405, 2006.

213. Samuelsson J, Mutschler M, Birgegard G, et al: Limited effects on JAK2 mutational status after pegylated interferon alpha-2b therapy in polycythemia vera and essential thrombocythemia. *Haematologica* 91(9):1281–1282, 2006.

214. Kiladjian JJ, Cassinat B, Chevret S, et al: Pegylated interferon-alfa-2a induces complete hematologic and molecular responses with low toxicity in polycythemia vera. *Blood* 112(8):3065–3072, 2008.

215. Kiladjian JJ, Cassinat B, Turlure P, et al: High molecular response rate of polycythemia vera patients treated with pegylated interferon alpha-2a. *Blood* 108(6):2037–2040, 2006.

216. Berlin NI, Wasserman LR: Polycythemia vera: A retrospective and reprise. *J Lab Clin Med* 130(4):365–373, 1997.

217. Pearson TC, Wetherley-Mein G: Vascular occlusive episodes and venous haematocrit in primary proliferative polycythaemia. *Lancet* 2(8102):1219–1222, 1978.

218. Vongpatanasin W, Brickner ME, Hillis LD, et al: The Eisenmenger syndrome in adults. *Ann Intern Med* 128(9):745–755, 1998.

219. Thorne SA: Management of polycythaemia in adults with cyanotic congenital heart disease. *Heart* 79(4):315–316, 1998.

220. Perloff JK, Marelli AJ, Miner PD: Risk of stroke in adults with cyanotic congenital heart disease. *Circulation* 87(6):1954–1959, 1993.

221. Di Nisio M, Barbui T, Di Gennaro L, et al: The haematocrit and platelet target in polycythemia vera. *Br J Haematol* 136(2):249–259, 2007.

222. Marchioli R, Finazzi G, Specchia G, et al: Cardiovascular events and intensity of treatment in polycythemia vera. *N Engl J Med* 368(1):22–33, 2013.

223. Prchal JT, Gordeuk VR: Treatment target in polycythemia vera. *N Engl J Med* 368(16):1555–1556, 2013.

224. Petitt RM, Silverstein MN, Petrone ME: Anagrelide for control of thrombocythemia in polycythemia and other myeloproliferative disorders. *Semin Hematol* 34(1):51–54, 1997.

225. Storen EC, Tefferi A: Long-term use of anagrelide in young patients with essential thrombocythemia. *Blood* 97(4):863–866, 2001.

226. Gisslinger H, Gotic M, Holowiecki J, et al: Anagrelide compared with hydroxyurea in WHO-classified essential thrombocythemia: The ANAHYDRET Study, a randomized controlled trial. *Blood* 121(10):1720–1728, 2013.

227. Swerlick RA: Photochemotherapy treatment of pruritus associated with polycythemia vera. *J Am Acad Dermatol* 13(4):675–677, 1985.

228. Bircher AJ: Water-induced itching. *Dermatologica* 181(2):83–87, 1990.

229. de Wolf JT, Hendriks DW, Egger RC, et al: Alpha-interferon for intractable pruritus in polycythaemia vera. *Lancet* 337(8735):241, 1991.

230. Foa P, Massaro P, Caldera S, et al: Long-term therapeutic efficacy and toxicity of recombinant interferon-alpha 2a in polycythaemia vera. *Eur J Haematol* 60(5):273–277, 1998.

231. Ozturk A, Gunay A, Uskent N: Therapeutic efficacy of recombinant interferon-alpha in polycythaemia vera. *Acta Haematol* 99(2):89–91, 1998.

232. Verstovsek S, Kiladjian JJ, Grieshammer M, et al: *Results of a Prospective, Randomized, Open-Label Phase 3 Study of Ruxolitinib (RUX) in Polycythemia Vera (PV) Patients Resistant to or Intolerant of Hydroxyurea (HU): The RESPONSE Trial*, abstract #7026. American Society of Clinical Oncology (ASCO), Chicago, 2014.

233. Verstovsek S, Passamonti F, Rambaldi A, et al: A phase 2 study of ruxolitinib, an oral JAK1 and JAK2 Inhibitor, in patients with advanced polycythemia vera who are refractory or intolerant to hydroxyurea. *Cancer* 120(4):513–520, 2014.

234. Tartaglia AP, Goldberg JD, Berk PD, et al: Adverse effects of antiaggregating platelet therapy in the treatment of polycythemia vera. *Semin Hematol* 23(3):172–176, 1986.

235. Landolfi R, Marchioli R: European Collaboration on Low-dose Aspirin in Polycythemia Vera (ECLAP): A randomized trial. *Semin Thromb Hemost* 23(5):473–478, 1997.

236. Mascarenhas JO, Cross NC, Mesa RA: The future of JAK inhibition in myelofibrosis and beyond. *Blood Rev* 28(5):189–196, 2014.

237. Scherber R, Mesa RA: Future therapies for the myeloproliferative neoplasms. *Curr Hematol Malig Rep* 6(1):22–27, 2011.

238. Harrison C, Kiladjian JJ, Al-Ali HK, et al: JAK inhibition with ruxolitinib versus best available therapy for myelofibrosis. *N Engl J Med* 366(9):787–798, 2012.

239. Santos FP, Verstovsek S: Efficacy of ruxolitinib for myelofibrosis. *Expert Opin Pharmacother* 15(10):1465–1473, 2014.

240. Verstovsek S, Kantarjian H, Mesa RA, et al: Safety and efficacy of INCB018424, a JAK1 and JAK2 inhibitor, in myelofibrosis. *N Engl J Med* 363(12):1117–1127, 2010.

241. Verstovsek S, Mesa RA, Gotlib J, et al: A double-blind, placebo-controlled trial of ruxolitinib for myelofibrosis. *N Engl J Med* 366(9):799–807, 2012.

242. Quintas-Cardama A, Vaddi K, Liu P, et al: Preclinical characterization of the selective JAK1/2 inhibitor INCB018424: Therapeutic implications for the treatment of myeloproliferative neoplasms. *Blood* 115(15):3109–3117, 2010.

243. Garber K: JAK2 inhibitors: Not the next imatinib but researchers see other possibilities. *J Natl Cancer Inst* 101(14):980–982, 2009.

244. Mesa RA, Tefferi A: Emerging drugs for the therapy of primary and post essential thrombocytemia, post polycythemia vera myelofibrosis. *Expert Opin Emerg Drugs* 14(3):471–479, 2009.

245. Kralovics R, Teo SS, Li S, et al: Acquisition of the V617F mutation of JAK2 is a late genetic event in a subset of patients with myeloproliferative disorders. *Blood* 108(4):1377–1380, 2006.

246. Plo I, Nakatake M, Malivert L, et al: JAK2 stimulates homologous recombination and genetic instability: Potential implication in the heterogeneity of myeloproliferative disorders. *Blood* 112(4):1402–1412, 2008.

247. Nguyen HM, Gotlib J: Insights into the molecular genetics of myeloproliferative neoplasms. *Am Soc Clin Oncol Educ Book* 411–418, 2012.

248. Reuther GW: Recurring mutations in myeloproliferative neoplasms alter epigenetic regulation of gene expression. *Am J Cancer Res* 1(6):752–762, 2011.

249. Mascarenhas J, Roper N, Chaurasia P, et al: Epigenetic abnormalities in myeloproliferative neoplasms: A target for novel therapeutic strategies. *Clin Epigenetics* 2(2):197–212, 2011.

250. Skov V, Larsen TS, Thomassen M, et al: Increased gene expression of histone deacetylases in patients with Philadelphia-negative chronic myeloproliferative neoplasms. *Leuk Lymphoma* 53(1):123–129, 2012.

251. Guerini V, Barbui V, Spinelli O, et al: The histone deacetylase inhibitor ITF2357 selectively targets cells bearing mutated JAK2(V617F). *Leukemia* 22(4):740–747, 2008.

252. Amaru Calzada A, Todoerti K, Donadoni L, et al: The HDAC inhibitor Givinostat modulates the hematopoietic transcription factors NFE2 and C-MYB in JAK2(V617F) myeloproliferative neoplasm cells. *Exp Hematol* 40(8):634–645 e10, 2012.

253. Andersen CL, McMullin MF, Ejerblad E, et al: A phase II study of vorinostat (MK-0683) in patients with polycythaemia vera and essential thrombocythaemia. *Br J Haematol* 162(4):498–508, 2013.

254. Rambaldi A, Dellacasa CM, Finazzi G, et al: A pilot study of the histone-deacetylase inhibitor Givinostat in patients with JAK2V617F positive chronic myeloproliferative neoplasms. *Br J Haematol* 150(4):446–455, 2010.

255. Hoffman R, Prchal JT, Samuelson S, et al: Philadelphia chromosome-negative myeloproliferative disorders: Biology and treatment. *Biol Blood Marrow Transplant* 13(1 Suppl 1):64–72, 2007.

256. Rosenthal DS: Clinical aspects of chronic myeloproliferative diseases. *Am J Med Sci* 304(2):109–124, 1992.

257. Tefferi A, Mesa RA, Nagorney DM, et al: Splenectomy in myelofibrosis with myeloid metaplasia: A single-institution experience with 223 patients. *Blood* 95(7):2226–2233, 2000.

258. Devine SM, Hoffman R, Verma A, et al: Allogeneic blood cell transplantation following reduced-intensity conditioning is effective therapy for older patients with myelofibrosis with myeloid metaplasia. *Blood* 99(6):2255–2258, 2002.

259. Anderson JE, Sale G, Appelbaum FR, et al: Allogeneic marrow transplantation for primary myelofibrosis and myelofibrosis secondary to polycythaemia vera or essential thrombocytosis. *Br J Haematol* 98(4):1010–1016, 1997.

260. Lussana F, Rambaldi A, Finazzi MC, et al: Allogeneic hematopoietic stem cell transplantation in patients with polycythemia vera or essential thrombocythemia transformed to myelofibrosis or acute myeloid leukemia: A report from the MPN Subcommittee of the Chronic Malignancies Working Party of the European Group for Blood and Marrow Transplantation. *Haematologica* 99(5):916–921, 2014.

261. Camos M, Cervantes F, Montoto S, et al: Acute lymphoid leukemia following polycythemia vera. *Leuk Lymphoma* 32(3–4):395–398, 1999.

262. Higuchi T, Oba R, Endo M, et al: Transition of polycythemia vera to chronic neutrophilic leukemia. *Leuk Lymphoma* 33(1–2):203–206, 1999.

263. Shariff F, Harrison C: Polycythemia vera: Can we do better? *Expert Opin Pharmacother* 14(6):687–689, 2013.

264. Hensley B, Geyer H, Mesa R: Polycythemia vera: Current pharmacotherapy and future directions. *Expert Opin Pharmacother* 14(5):609–617, 2013.

265. Passamonti F, Malabarba L, Orlandi E, et al: Polycythemia vera in young patients: A study on the long-term risk of thrombosis, myelofibrosis and leukemia. *Haematologica* 88(1):13–18, 2003.

266. Rozman C, Giralt M, Feliu E, et al: Life expectancy of patients with chronic nonleukemic myeloproliferative disorders. *Cancer* 67(10):2658–2663, 1991.

CHAPTER 85
ESSENTIAL THROMBOCYTHEMIA

Philip A. Beer and Anthony R. Green

SUMMARY

Essential thrombocythemia is a clonal stem cell disorder characterized by an overproduction of platelets and associated with mutations in the *JAK2, CALR,* or *MPL* gene. Complications include thrombosis (predominantly arterial), hemorrhage, and progression to myelofibrosis or acute myeloid leukemia. Diagnosis requires exclusion of reactive thrombocytosis and other myeloid malignancies associated with a raised platelet count. Therapy is aimed at reducing thrombotic complications and includes modification of known cardiovascular risk factors and antiplatelet therapy for the majority of patients. Those at high risk of thrombosis are also considered for cytoreductive therapy with agents such as hydroxyurea, anagrelide or interferon-*a*. Although the majority of patients can expect to live for many years, mortality rates are increased compared to the general population as a consequence of disease complications.

DEFINITION AND HISTORY

Essential thrombocythemia (ET), one of the myeloproliferative neoplasms (MPNs), is a clonal hematopoietic stem cell disorder characterized by thrombocytosis and associated with thrombotic and hemorrhagic complications. First recognized as a specific disease entity in 1934[1] and as a clonal disorder in 1981,[2] ET shares clinical and pathologic similarities with other MPNs, particularly polycythemia vera (PV) and primary myelofibrosis (PMF).

EPIDEMIOLOGY

The annual incidence of ET is in the order of 1 to 2.5 per 100,000 per population and appears slightly more common in females.[3,4] Patients may present at any age, although ET is largely a disorder of later life with a peak incidence between the ages of 50 and 70 years. Presentation in childhood is rare but well recognized.

ETIOLOGY

Little is known about the precise etiology of this disorder, although environmental factors such as exposure to radiation have been implicated in the genesis of other MPNs.[5] Both registry data and kindred

studies suggest a familial tendency to develop MPNs, including ET.[6,7] This predisposition appears to be explained in part by inheritance of a specific haplotype that contains the Janus family of tyrosine kinases type 2 *(JAK2)* gene.[8]

PATHOGENESIS

ET is characterized by hyperactive cytokine signaling which in 50 to 60 percent of cases is the result of somatic mutations targeting components of signaling pathways, including the *JAK2* gene or the thrombopoietin receptor gene *(MPL)*. Mutations in calreticulin gene *(CALR)* are present in the majority of *JAK2/MPL*–wild-type patients, leaving approximately 10 percent of ET patients without a mutation in any of these genes (*JAK2/MPL/CALR*–wild-type or "triple-negative" patients). A minority of ET patients also harbor mutations in transcriptional regulation pathways (Fig. 85–1).

A *JAK2*[V617F] mutation is found in approximately 50 percent of patients with ET.[9] JAK2, a cytoplasmic tyrosine kinase, forms a complex with and is essential for signaling by the erythropoietin and thrombopoietin receptors[10,11]; JAK2 also contributes to signaling by the granulocyte colony-stimulating factor, granulocyte-macrophage colony-stimulating factor, and interferon-*γ* receptors.[12] Cytokine binding leads to a conformational change in the JAK2-receptor complex, with consequent activation of JAK2 kinase activity and recruitment of downstream signaling pathways.[10,13,14] The *JAK2*[V617F] mutation alters a critical residue within the autoinhibitory pseudokinase (JH2) domain, resulting in increased JAK2 basal kinase and downstream signaling activity.[15] The cellular consequences of mutant *JAK2* expression include increased proliferation, cytokine hypersensitivity, cytokine-independent differentiation, and inhibition of apoptosis.[9] The central role of JAK2 in erythropoiesis is highlighted by a *JAK2* knockout mouse, which dies in midgestation from severe anemia.[12] In addition, mice engineered to express the *JAK2*[V617F] allele recapitulate features of human ET or PV.[16]

Acquired mutations in *MPL* are found in 4 percent of ET patients, the majority of whom are *JAK2*–wild-type, and a similar proportion of those with PMF, but not in patients with PV.[17,18] These mutations alter residues in the juxtamembrane (*MPL*[W515]) or transmembrane (*MPL*[S505N]) regions and lead to constitutive activation of the receptor complex.[19,20] Expression of the *MPL*[W515L] allele in a mouse model recapitulated features of human ET and PMF.[21] Occasional patients with ET, as well as PV and PMF, harbor loss of function mutations in *SH2B3* which encodes LNK, an important negative regulator of JAK/STAT (signal transducer and activator of transcription) signaling.[22]

The majority of ET patients without a signaling pathway mutation harbor a somatic mutation in *CALR* (encoding calreticulin). *CALR* mutations are found in 15 to 35 percent of ET patients and a similar proportion of those with PMF but not in PV. Calreticulin is a key endoplasmic reticulum protein with calcium buffering and protein chaperone activity.[23] Although *CALR*-mutant patients generally lack mutations in *JAK2* or *MPL*, they nonetheless show signaling pathway activation, suggesting an as yet undetermined role for CALR in cytokine signaling.[24–26]

Mutations targeting pathways implicated in the control of gene transcription are found in a minority of patients with ET, as well as those with PV, PMF and other myeloid neoplasms (see Fig. 85–1B). These mutations, which may coexist with mutations in *JAK2, MPL,* or *CALR,* target genes involved in DNA methylation (*TET2, IDH1/2, DNMT3A*), histone modification (*EZH2*) or RNA splicing (*SF3B1*).[27] In addition to its roles in cytokine signaling, JAK2 has also been shown to translocate to the nucleus where it acts as a mediator of gene transcription through the direct modification of histone proteins. Whereas nuclear translocation of wild-type JAK2 appears to be activation-dependent,

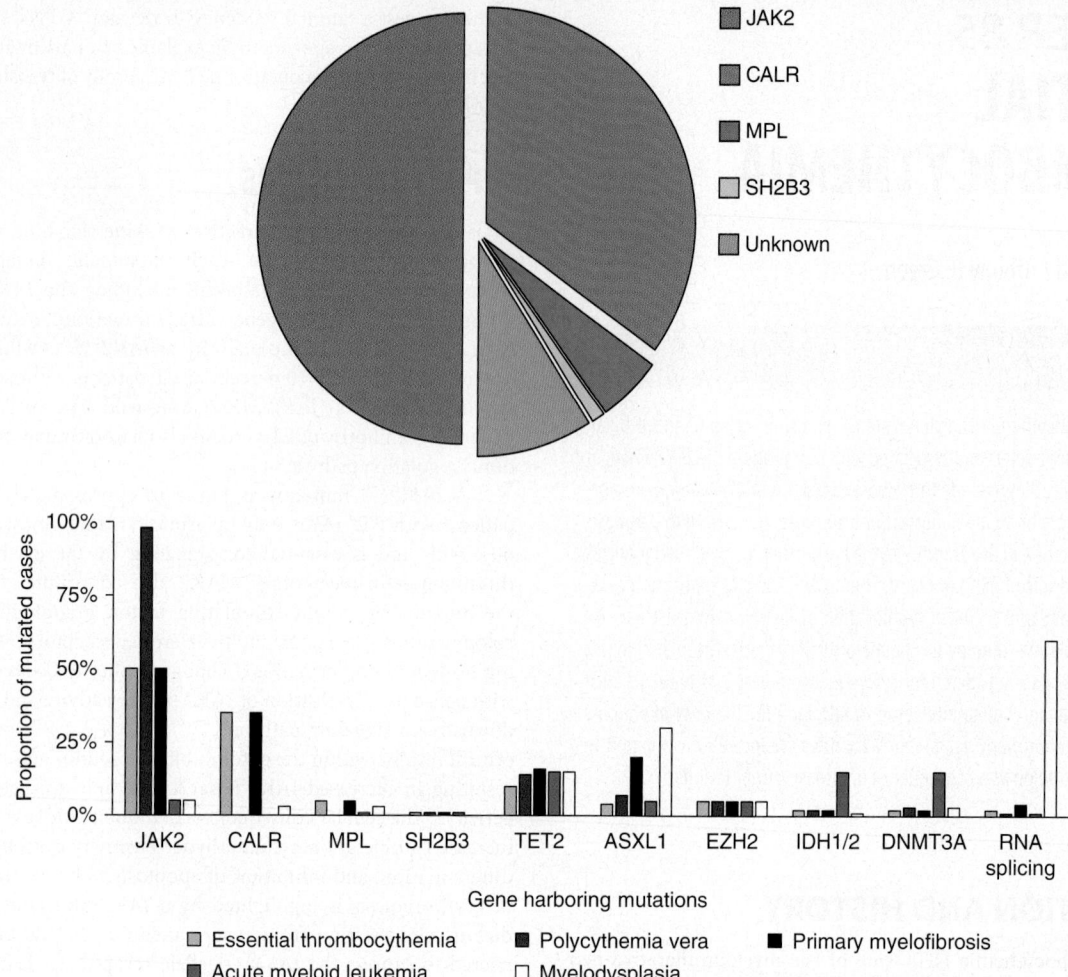

Figure 85–1. The spectrum and frequency of somatic mutations in myeloid neoplasms. **A.** Frequency of mutations in essential thrombocythemia associated with activated cytokine signaling pathways. **B.** Comparison of mutation frequencies in ET, related myeloproliferative neoplasms and other myeloid malignancies.

JAK2 harboring a V617F substitution shows nuclear localization in the absence of cytokine stimulation.[28,29]

CLINICAL FEATURES

SYMPTOMS AND SIGNS

ET is often diagnosed following the incidental finding of a high platelet count, although a proportion of patients present with thrombotic or hemorrhage complications. A detailed clinical history and physical examination are necessary to exclude causes for a reactive thrombocytosis. Approximately 10 percent of ET patients have a mild degree of palpable splenomegaly at diagnosis,[30] although significant splenic enlargement should raise the possibility of another MPN such as PMF or chronic myeloid leukemia (CML).

THROMBOSIS

Thrombotic complications are the major source of morbidity and mortality in ET, with a prospective study indicating a cumulative incidence of 24 percent over 27 months for untreated high-risk patients.[31] Arterial thrombosis predominates, affecting the central nervous system (stroke, transient ischemic attack) and cardiovascular system (myocardial infarction, unstable angina, peripheral arterial occlusion).[30,31]

Erythromelalgia, a distinct clinicopathologic syndrome caused by occlusion of small blood vessels, is manifest by discomfort and burning sensations in the fingers or toes, sometimes accompanied by mottling or discoloration of the skin.[32] Venous events mainly comprise deep vein thrombosis and pulmonary embolism. Involvement of unusual sites such as hepatic, portal or mesenteric veins also occurs and may precede the onset of clinically overt ET (Fig. 85–2A). In one series, half of all patients presenting with hepatic vein thrombosis and a normal blood count tested positive for the JAK2[V617F] mutation, and a quarter of these subsequently developed a clinically overt MPN, most commonly ET.[33]

The strongest predictive factors for thrombotic complications are older than 60 years of age or a history of previous thrombosis.[34] The platelet count and leucocyte count at diagnosis are poor predictors of thrombotic risk.[35] Meta-analysis confirmed detection of a JAK2[V617F] mutation as a risk factor for both arterial and venous thrombosis.[36,37] Other reported risk factors include predisposition to cardiovascular disease or increased marrow fibrosis at diagnosis.[38]

HEMORRHAGE

Serious bleeding is less common than thrombosis and mainly affects the nasal and buccal mucosa and the gastrointestinal tract, although central nervous system hemorrhage may occur.[30,31] ET patients often demonstrate prolongation of the bleeding time and various abnormalities of

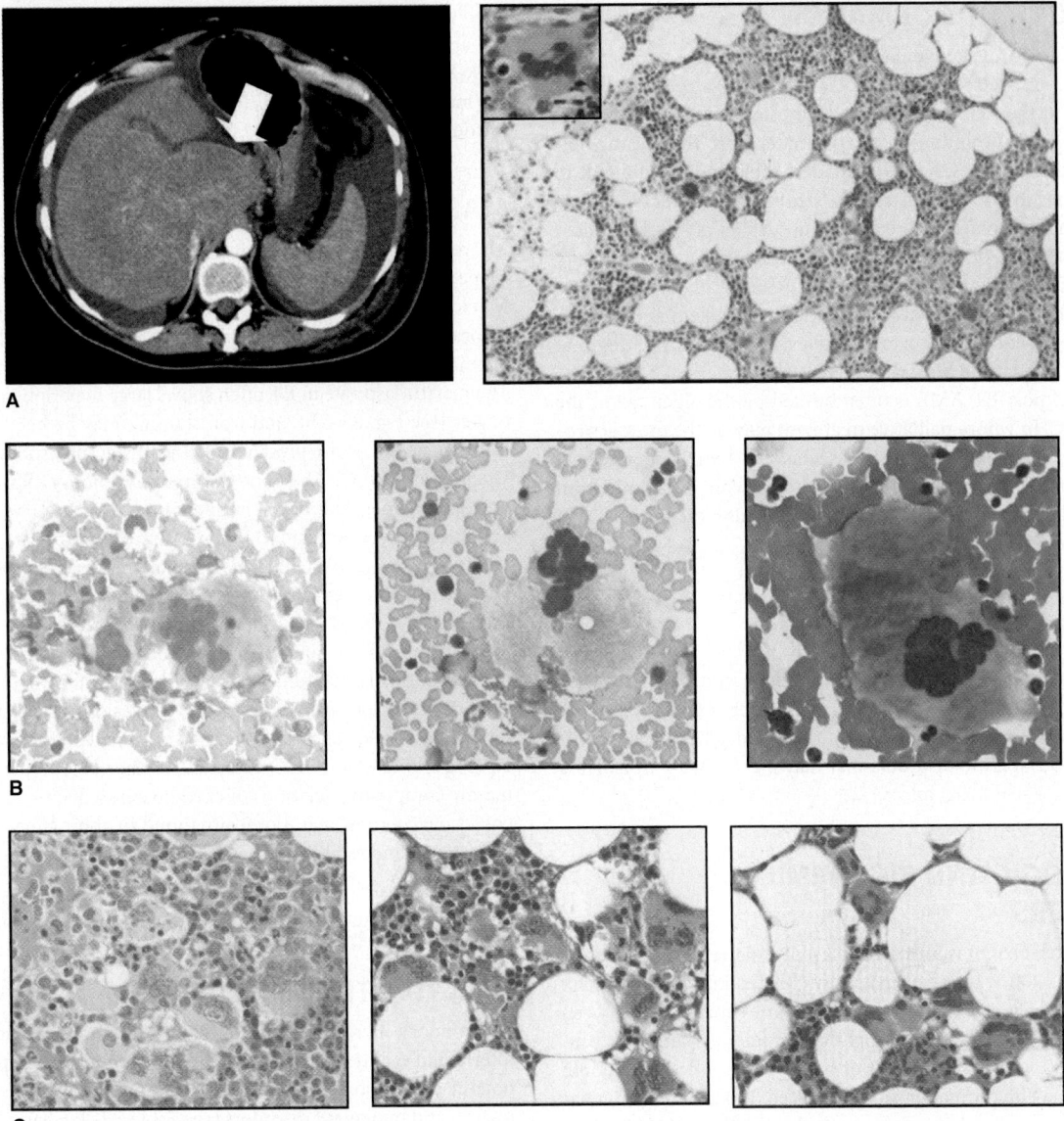

Figure 85–2. Morphologic features of essential thrombocythemia. **A.** Contrast-enhanced abdominal computed tomography (CT) scan showing features of established hepatic vein thrombosis in a 53-year-old female, including hypertrophy of the caudate lobe *(arrow)* with atrophy of the remaining liver and surrounding ascites; the spleen is of normal size. Hematoxylin and eosin (H&E)-stained marrow trephine biopsy showing normal cellularity and increased megakaryocytes with occasional hyperlobulated forms *(inset)*. Although the patient was *JAK2*[V617F]-positive, other investigations performed at this time, including blood count, red cell mass and cytogenetic analysis, were normal. **B.** Marrow aspirate from a *JAK2*[V617F]-positive essential thrombocythemia (ET) patient showing large, hyperlobulated megakaryocytes (slide stained with Wright-Giemsa). **C.** Marrow trephine biopsy samples from patients with ET (slide stained with H&E).

in vitro coagulation studies, including abnormal platelet aggregation or loss of large von Willebrand factor multimers; however, the relationship of these findings to episodes of clinical bleeding is unclear.[39] In a prospective study, rates of major hemorrhage were increased in patients with increased marrow fibrosis at diagnosis[38] and in those with an increased platelet or leucocyte count during followup.[35]

MYELOFIBROTIC TRANSFORMATION

Evolution to myelofibrosis is seen in a proportion of ET patients, although the reported prevalence varies widely, reflecting differences in study design, therapeutic intervention and diagnostic criteria for post-ET myelofibrosis (Chap. 86). Retrospective studies suggest that disease duration is a major predictor of progressive disease, with rates of myelofibrosis in the first decade after diagnosis of 3 to 10 percent rising to 6 to 30 percent in the second decade.[34,40] The presence of marrow fibrosis at diagnosis also appears to presage progression to myelofibrosis,[38] although the predictive value of other histologic features of early stage PMF, such as megakaryocyte dysplasia, remains controversial.[41] Mutations in *JAK2*,[42,43] *MPL*,[17,18] or *CALR*[44,45] appear to lack prognostic significance. A prospective study of high-risk ET patients indicated increased progression to myelofibrosis with anagrelide therapy, with a 5-year cumulative incidence of 7 percent for anagrelide plus aspirin versus 2 percent for hydroxyurea plus aspirin-treated patients.[30] The clinical consequences of post-ET myelofibrosis are similar to *de novo* myelofibrosis, and the conditions are managed in the same way.

LEUKEMIC TRANSFORMATION

Progression to acute myeloid leukemia (AML) occurs in a small minority of patients, with retrospective studies suggesting a prevalence of 1 to 2.5 percent in the first decade after diagnosis, 5 to 8 percent in the second decade, and continuing to rise thereafter.[34,40,46] Therapeutic heterogeneity in these studies, however, renders their findings difficult to interpret. Studies in PV demonstrated a significantly increased risk of AML in patients receiving genotoxic agents such as radioactive phosphorus, chlorambucil, or busulphan.[47,48] The potential leukemogenicity of hydroxyurea remains controversial (see "Choice of Cytoreductive Agent" below). Importantly, transformation to leukemia has been reported in the absence of any cytoreductive therapy,[49,50] indicating that AML is part of the natural history of this disorder.

Therapy of post-ET AML is often limited by the older age of the affected patients, in whom palliative treatment may be the most appropriate strategy. Overall the prognosis of secondary AML is poor (Chap. 88). Younger patients who do achieve remission with AML induction therapy may be considered for allogeneic hematopoietic stem cell transplantation.

● LABORATORY FEATURES

An unexplained and persistently raised platelet count generally warrants further investigation (Fig. 85–3). Establishing a diagnosis of ET requires exclusion of both reactive conditions and other myeloproliferative or myelodysplastic disorders that may present with an isolated thrombocytosis (Tables 85–1 and 85–2).

HEMATOLOGIC AND BIOCHEMICAL PARAMETERS

An elevated platelet count is invariably present and may be only slightly increased (e.g., $\geq 400 \times 10^9$/L) or massively elevated into the millions $\times 10^9$/L. Thus, the degree of thrombocytosis varies markedly between patients. The white count may be slightly to mildly elevated but usually not above 20×10^9/L as a result of neutrophilia. The hemoglobin concentration may be normal or mildly reduced. If occult bleeding has been present, the hemoglobin may be further decreased and indications of iron deficiency may be evident in the red cells (microcytosis and hypochromia; see "Differential Diagnosis" below). Examination of the blood film often reveals large platelets which may stain poorly, and is useful in excluding features of PMF such as teardrop cells (dacryocytes) or circulating immature granulocyte precursors.

SERUM CHEMICAL FINDINGS

Levels of thrombopoietin are normal or slightly elevated in ET and have no diagnostic utility. ET patients may show a spurious increase in serum potassium level as a result of *in vitro* activation of platelets and leukocytes during processing of serum; this phenomenon can be circumvented by using a plasma sample for biochemical analysis.

MOLECULAR TESTING

Molecular testing for genetic mutations has become the investigation of choice for patients with an unexplained and persistent increase in platelet count (see Fig. 85–3). A reasonable approach is to screen all patients for the $JAK2^{V617F}$ mutation, following by screening for mutations in *CALR* and uncommon *MPL* in negative cases. Suitable techniques include allele-specific or real-time polymerase chain reaction (PCR) for $JAK2^{V617F}$, pyrosequencing or high-resolution melt curve

analysis for *MPL*, and fragment length analysis for *CALR* exon 9.[25,51] In the absence of marrow cytogenetic analysis, molecular testing for the *BCR-ABL1* fusion gene is also recommended to exclude CML. Screening for additional mutations (e.g., *TET2*) is currently of uncertain utility in routine clinical practice.

MARROW STUDIES

Marrow aspiration and trephine biopsy is particularly recommended in suspected cases of ET that are negative for a relevant somatic mutation. Marrow studies may also be useful in cases showing atypical clinical or laboratory features (for example, palpable splenomegaly, unexplained anemia or blood film abnormalities) or in the context of a clinical study. The marrow aspirate in ET often shows large hyperlobulated megakaryocytes (see Fig. 85–2B), and iron staining may be helpful in excluding iron deficiency or the presence of ringed sideroblasts (see "Differential Diagnosis" below). The marrow trephine biopsy typically shows an increase in megakaryocyte frequency with megakaryocyte clustering and nuclear hyperlobulation in the absence of significant reticulin fibrosis (see Fig. 85–2C). Cellularity is usually normal or slightly increased, but occasional cases may show a hypocellular marrow, for example, a proportion of those with mutations in *MPL*.[17,18]

Chromosomal analysis, by G-banding or *in situ* fluorescent hybridization, is helpful in suspected cases of ET lacking a relevant somatic mutation, primarily to exclude lesions associated with other myeloid disorders such as t(9;22) (CML) or deletions of chromosome 5q ("5q-minus syndrome"; Chap. 87). Other karyotypic abnormalities, mainly comprising deletions of chromosomes 20q or 13q or additional copies of chromosomes 8 or 9, are found in approximately 5 percent of ET patients and establish the existence of clonal hematopoiesis.

● DIFFERENTIAL DIAGNOSIS

REACTIVE THROMBOCYTOSIS

A secondary increase in platelet count, initiated by cytokines such as interleukin-6 and directly driven by the induction of hepatic thrombopoietin production is associated with a number of infectious, inflammatory and malignant disorders (see Table 85–2; Chap. 119). In reports of unselected patients attending various hospital departments, an increased platelet count was attributable to reactive causes in more than 80 percent of cases; the degree of thrombocytosis did not permit distinction between a clonal versus a reactive pathogenesis.[52,53]

FAMILIAL THROMBOCYTOSIS

Familial thrombocytosis is a rare disorder caused by mutations in the thrombopoietin gene, *MPL*, or other unknown genes. Changes in the 5′-untranslated region or splice donor/acceptor sites of the thrombopoietin gene are associated with increased translation of thrombopoietin and consequent thrombocytosis.[54] These alleles are dominantly inherited and have not been seen in clonal MPNs.[55] A dominantly inherited, activating *MPL* allele (MPL^{S505N}) has been reported in Japanese and Italian kindreds.[54] Of interest, this allele has also been reported as a somatic mutation in patients with a clonal MPN.[17] Several different inherited *JAK2* alleles have been reported in families with autosomal dominant thrombocytosis (including $JAK2^{R564Q}$, $JAK2^{V617I}$, $JAK2^{R867Q}$, and $JAK2^{S755R/R938Q}$).[56,57] Although complicated by occasional thrombotic or bleeding episodes, the clinical phenotype of familial thrombocytosis is relatively mild, although exceptions occur.[54] The genetic cause underlying a subset of familial cases remains to be elucidated.

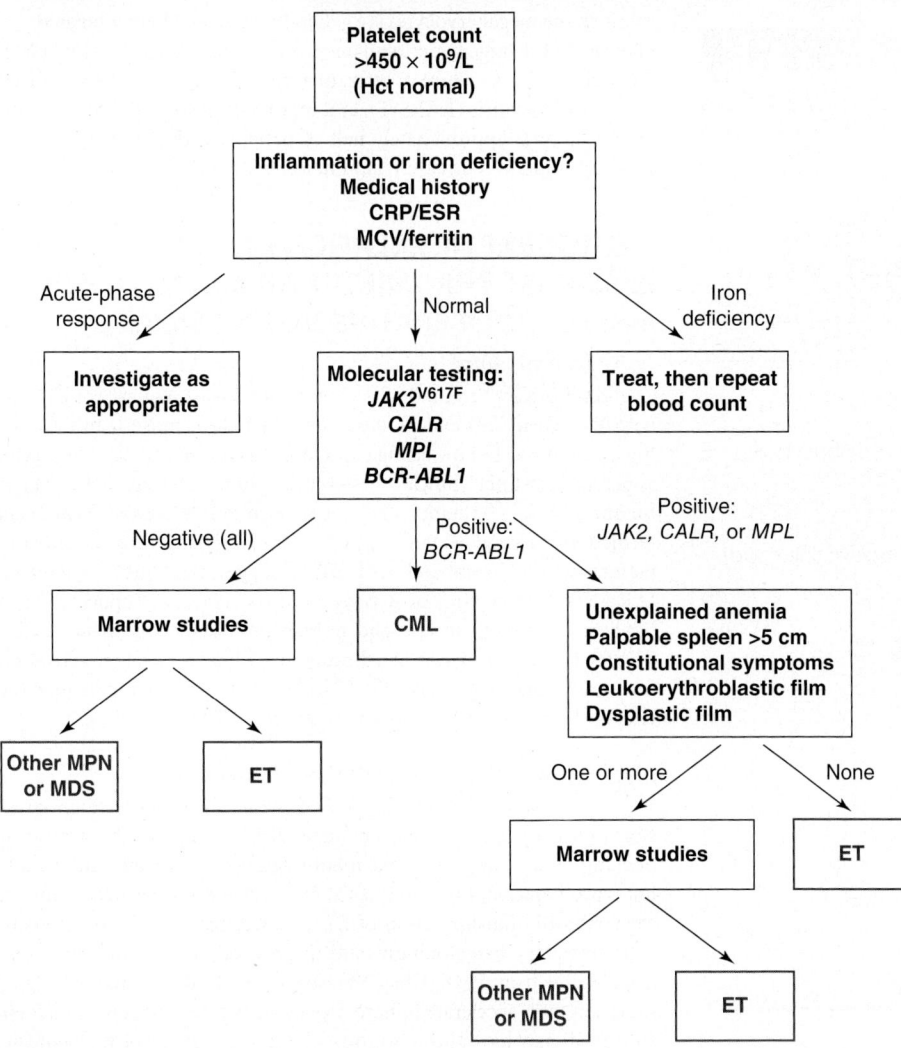

Figure 85–3. Investigation of patients with thrombocythemia. Algorithm outlining the investigation of a patient with an unexplained and persistently raised platelet count.

POLYCYTHEMIA VERA

PV (Chap. 84) is often associated with thrombocytosis, and may present with a normal hemoglobin level in the presence of iron depletion, mimicking ET, although in such cases the mean corpuscular volume is usually decreased. In addition, ET and PV form a phenotypic spectrum, resulting in diagnostic difficulties in a subset of patients. There are inherent limitations to the utility of continuous variables, such as hematocrit, to make this distinction, as the group of patients with intermediate values

will inevitably include both disorders (Fig. 85–4). Controversy persists over how to best distinguish these two conditions.[58]

PRIMARY MYELOFIBROSIS

PMF may present with an isolated thrombocytosis, but palpable splenomegaly, circulating teardrop red cells and progenitor cells, and marrow fibrosis are usually present (Chap. 86). An area of ongoing controversy relates to the 15 to 20 percent of ET patients who harbor distinct marrow morphology, coined *prefibrotic PMF*, at diagnosis in the absence of other features to indicate PMF. Although such patients have higher rates of myelofibrotic transformation, thrombosis, and hemorrhage, their overall survival is not different from other patients with ET.[59] A second area of controversy relates to the suggestion that marrow trephine appearances can distinguish ET and prefibrotic PMF from the early stages of PMF[60]; however, the reproducibility and clinical utility of this distinction is unclear.[41,58]

CHRONIC MYELOID LEUKEMIA

Occasional patients with CML present with an isolated thrombocytosis. Such cases are predominantly female with absent or minimal splenomegaly and a normal or marginally elevated white cell count, often without basophilia or circulating myeloid progenitors.[61] Marrow studies, however, are usually informative, showing small hypolobulated megakaryocytes typical of CML, and not the large hyperlobulated forms observed

TABLE 85–1. Diagnostic Criteria for Essential Thrombocythemia

Diagnosis requires A1 to A3 or A1 + A3 to A5

A1 Sustained platelet count >450 × 10⁹/L

A2 Presence of an acquired pathogenic mutation (e.g., in *JAK2*, *CALR*, or *MPL*)

A3 No other myeloid malignancy, especially polycythemia vera, primary myelofibrosis, chronic myeloid leukemia, or myelodysplastic syndrome

A4 No reactive cause for thrombocytosis and normal iron stores

A5 Marrow studies showing increased megakaryocytes displaying a spectrum of morphology with prominent large hyperlobulated forms; reticulin is generally not increased

TABLE 85–2. Causes of Thrombocytosis

CLONAL THROMBOCYTOSIS

Essential thrombocythemia

Polycythemia vera

Primary myelofibrosis

Chronic myeloid leukemia

Refractory anemia with ringed sideroblasts and thrombocytosis

5q-minus syndrome

REACTIVE (SECONDARY) THROMBOCYTOSIS

Transient thrombocytosis

    Acute blood loss

    Recovery from thrombocytopenia (rebound thrombocytosis)

    Acute infection or inflammation

    Response to exercise

    Response to drugs (vincristine, epinephrine, all-*trans*-retinoic acid)

Sustained thrombocytosis

    Iron deficiency

    Splenectomy or congenital absence of spleen

    Malignancy

    Chronic infection or inflammation

    Hemolytic anemia

FAMILIAL THROMBOCYTOSIS

SPURIOUS THROMBOCYTOSIS

Cryoglobulinemia

Cytoplasmic fragmentation in acute leukemia

Red cell fragmentation

Bacteremia

in ET. Given the significant impact of tyrosine kinase inhibitors on the prognosis of CML, it is important that this unusual presentation is not overlooked. It is therefore recommended that suspected cases of ET that are negative for a relevant somatic mutation undergo molecular analysis of blood for the BCR-ABL1 fusion gene. Marrow aspiration, biopsy and G-banding cytogenetic analysis, may be useful in a specific case.

MYELODYSPLASIA

Thrombocytosis, usually in association with anemia, may be seen in the myelodysplastic disorder associated with an isolated deletion of chromosome 5q ("5q-minus syndrome"). Although often increased in

number, the megakaryocytes are generally small and hypolobulated,[60] in contrast to the large hyperlobulated forms typical of ET. A raised platelet count is also a feature of refractory anemia with ringed sideroblasts and thrombocytosis (RARS-T), and may be associated with thrombotic complications. Approximately half of patients with RARS-T harbor a $JAK2^{V617F}$ mutation or, rarely, a mutation in *MPL*.

PATHOGENETIC RELATIONSHIP OF ESSENTIAL THROMBOCYTHEMIA TO OTHER MYELOPROLIFERATIVE NEOPLASMS

Polycythemia Vera

The same $JAK2^{V617F}$ mutation is present in the vast majority of patients with PV (Chap. 84) and in approximately half of those with ET, raising questions as to how a single mutation is commonly associated with apparently distinct clinical phenotypes. Clones that are homozygous for the $JAK2^{V617F}$ mutation (arising by a mitotic recombination event termed *uniparental disomy*; Fig. 85–5) are larger and more frequent in patients with PV compared with ET,[62,63] suggesting a role for increased JAK2-STAT5 signaling in driving erythrocytosis. In support of this hypothesis, in both mouse and human model systems strong JAK2-STAT5 activation drives erythropoiesis whereas weaker activation favors a megakaryopoiesis.[16,64,65] Other contributing factors include the effects of patient gender[63] and modulation of STAT1 signaling.[66]

Myelofibrosis and Accelerated Phase Disease

A proportion of patients diagnosed with ET experience progression to an accelerated phase characterized by increasingly disordered hematopoiesis. The phenotypic manifestations are variable and include hyperproliferation, myelodysplasia, or, most commonly, myelofibrosis. Myelofibrotic transformation of ET, characterized by marrow fibrosis, extramedullary hematopoiesis and marrow failure, is clinically indistinguishable from PMF (Chap. 86), suggesting PMF may represent presentation with accelerated phase disease. Consistent with this, patients with PMF may have thrombocytosis for many years prior to diagnosis, suggestive of undiagnosed ET.[58]

The prevalence of mutations in *JAK2, CALR,* or *MPL* is similar in ET compared to myelofibrosis; however, karyotypic abnormalities are present in up to 50 percent of myelofibrosis patients (Chap. 86) compared to only approximately 5 percent of patients in ET, indicating a greater degree of genetic instability. In addition, mutations in genes implicated in transcriptional regulation (including *ASXL1, IDH1/2,* and *EZH2*) appear more common in patients with PMF compared with ET. Together, these findings suggest that progression to advanced phase disease arises through a process of clonal evolution driven by the acquisition of additional genetic events or epigenetic alterations; to date, however, no combination of genetic events has been shown to reliably

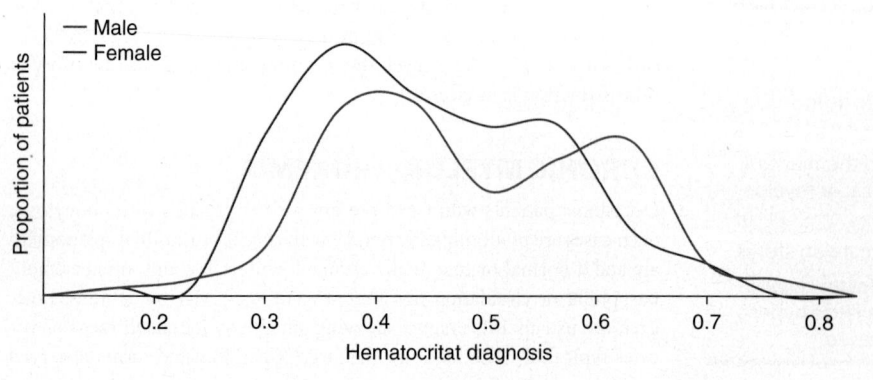

Figure 85–4. Distribution of diagnostic hematocrit levels in a cohort of 243 patients with $JAK2^{V617F}$-positive disease (essential thrombocythemia or polycythemia vera).

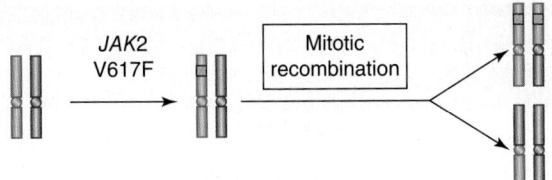

Figure 85–5. Mitotic recombination leads to duplication of the $JAK2^{V617F}$ mutation, resulting in a V617F-homozygous subclone.

TABLE 85–3. Risk Stratification for Patients with Essential Thrombocythemia

| High Risk | No High-Risk Features | |
	Low Risk	Intermediate Risk
Age >60 years	Age <40 years	Age 40–60 years
Prior thrombosis		
Platelets >1500 × 10⁹/L		

distinguish ET from PMF. Constitutive activation of JAK2 has been implicated as a driver of clonal progression, as expression of mutant JAK2 leads to the accumulation of reactive oxygen species, increased DNA damage, and aberrant DNA repair.[67–70]

Blastic Phase Disease

For a minority of patients with ET, their disease terminates in AML, also referred to as blastic phase. In some patients, the disease phenotype shows a stepwise transition from ET to PMF to AML, thus mimicking the triphasic disease pattern of CML observed in the preimatinib era (Chap. 89). In other cases, AML arises directly following ET.[71]

The mutational profile of blastic phase disease shares some similarities with *de novo* AML. Mutations in transcriptional control pathways (including *TET2, ASXL1, EZH2,* and *IDH1*) are more common in blastic phase than in the early disease phases. In addition, mutations are seen in DNA repair and cellular differentiation pathways (including *TP53, RUNX1,* and *IKZF1*) which are rarely mutated in early stage MPNs. In contrast to *de novo* AML, balanced chromosomal translocations are rare in post-MPN AML.[72–74] Of note, patients with $JAK2^{V617F}$-positive ET may develop AML that is negative for the *JAK2* mutation.[49,71]

●THERAPY

MODIFICATION OF CARDIOVASCULAR RISK FACTORS

Established risk factors for cardiovascular disease, such as hypertension, diabetes, smoking, hypercholesterolemia, and obesity, should be identified and treated appropriately. The broad efficacy of the cholesterol-lowering statin drugs in the prevention of atherosclerotic disease has raised the possibility that such agents may be useful in ET, although this has yet to be tested in a prospective study.

ANTIPLATELET THERAPY

A large randomized trial in PV demonstrated a reduction in thrombotic events in those taking low-dose aspirin (100 mg daily) without a concomitant increase in the risk of hemorrhage.[75] Although retrospective studies have suggested a similar protective effect in ET,[32] prospective trials have not been performed. Based on current evidence, aspirin is recommended for all ET patients unless contraindicated. Although there are few data concerning the use of newer antiplatelet agents such as clopidogrel in ET, their proven track record in preventing complications of atherosclerotic disease suggests they may be appropriate for patients unable to tolerate aspirin.

CYTOREDUCTIVE THERAPY

Indications to Treat

A prospective randomized trial demonstrated a clear role for cytoreductive therapy with hydroxyurea in reducing thrombotic events in high-risk ET patients (age >60 years or history of prior thrombosis), approximately 70 percent of whom were also receiving antiplatelet

agents.[31] Although retrospective studies suggest that thrombotic complications in those younger than 60 years of age without additional risk factors may be no higher than controls, prospective data are lacking. Patients with ET are currently stratified on the basis of their risk of thrombotic complications (Table 85–3), with cytoreductive therapy likely to benefit high-risk patients. Patients without high-risk features can be divided into low risk (age less than 40 years) and intermediate risk (age 40 to 60 years). Cytoreductive therapy is unlikely to offer a significant protective effect for those with low-risk disease, in whom the *a priori* risk of thrombosis is small. There is currently little evidence available to guide treatment decisions in the intermediate-risk group. The ongoing PT-1 trials (http://www.haem.cam.ac.uk/primary-thrombocy-thaemia/), comprising a randomized trial of hydroxyurea and aspirin versus aspirin alone for intermediate-risk patients and an observational study of low-risk patients treated with aspirin alone, will provide prospective data to help clarify therapeutic decisions for these patients. Although the degree of thrombocytosis is not a reliable indicator of thrombotic risk, many physicians consider cytoreductive therapy in patients with a very high platelet count (e.g., greater than 1500 × 10⁹/L).

Once cytoreductive therapy is instituted, dose adjustment is recommended to keep the platelet and leucocyte counts within the normal range.[35]

Choice of Cytoreductive Agent (Table 85–4)

Choices of first and second line therapies for patients with ET are summarized in Table 85–4). Hydroxyurea, a ribonucleotide reductase inhibitor also known as hydroxycarbamide, is widely regarded as first-line therapy for patients requiring treatment, and is the only cytoreductive agent proven to reduce thrombotic events in a randomized controlled trial.[31] Major complications of this drug include reversible myelosuppression and ulceration of the buccal mucosa or lower leg. Although hydroxyurea appears nonleukemogenic when used to treat sickle cell

TABLE 85–4. Choice of Cytoreductive Agent in Essential Thrombocythemia

Age Group	First Line	Second Line
<40 years old	Interferon-α	Hydroxyurea Anagrelide
40–60 years	Interferon-α Hydroxyurea	Anagrelide
>60 years	Hydroxyurea	Anagrelide Pipobroman* Busulphan* Radioactive phosphorus*

*These agents increase the frequency of transformation to acute leukemia in PV studies and their use is only recommended in patients older than 75 years of age after careful consideration on a case-by-case basis.

disease,[76] controversy remains about potential leukemogenicity in the MPNs. Some studies suggest an increased risk of acute leukemia in hydroxyurea-treated ET patients,[77,78] but others have failed to observe this association.[79,80] Problems with these studies include small patient numbers, inclusion of patients who have received multiple cytotoxic agents, lack of proper controls, retrospective data collection, and relatively short followup. Of note, analysis of blood cells from sickle cell and MPN patients receiving hydroxyurea showed equivalent rates of DNA mutations to normal controls, suggesting that the mutagenic potential of hydroxyurea is low.[81] At present it is not clear whether hydroxyurea used as a single agent is associated with an increased risk of acute leukemia; however, any increased risk is likely to be small and should be balanced against the reduction in thrombotic complications.

Anagrelide, a quinazoline derivative, reduces the platelet count by inhibition of megakaryocyte differentiation. Although the white cell count is unaffected, anemia is common and often progressive.[38] Up to a third of patients cannot tolerate anagrelide because of side effects, many of which result from its vasodilatory and positive inotropic actions including palpitations and arrhythmias, fluid retention, heart failure and headaches. Use of this drug requires particular caution in elderly patients or those with preexisting cardiac disease. Although anagrelide is not cytotoxic, and therefore unlikely to be leukemogenic, the PT-1 randomized trial demonstrated that anagrelide plus aspirin was inferior to hydroxyurea plus aspirin in high-risk ET patients. In this study, anagrelide-treated patients experienced reduced event-free survival (p = 0.03) with higher rates of arterial thrombosis (p = 0.004), major hemorrhage (p = 0.008) and progression to myelofibrosis (p = 0.01), despite equivalent control of the platelet count, although rates of venous thrombosis were decreased (p = 0.006).[30] In contrast to hydroxyurea, anagrelide therapy was also associated with an increase in marrow reticulin over time.[38] Comparison of patients in the PT-1 (comparison of hydroxyurea versus anagrelide) and Italian (comparison of hydroxyurea versus no cytoreductive therapy) prospective studies suggests that anagrelide does provide partial protection from thrombosis,[82] and therefore may be suitable as second-line therapy for patients in whom hydroxyurea therapy is inadequate or not tolerated. It has been suggested that the results of the ANAHYDRET trial (comparing hydroxyurea to anagrelide) show that anagrelide is not inferior to hydroxyurea in the treatment of ET.[83] However, the number of patients enrolled, duration of followup, and primary end points recorded were relatively small (Table 85–5) and as such this trial was not powered to see the differences observed in the PT-1 study. In addition, the ethical basis for performing noninferiority trials may be questioned.[84]

Recombinant interferon-α is effective at controlling the platelet count in ET, although there is little direct evidence of efficacy in prevention of thrombosis. Treatment is often associated with significant side effects, including flu-like symptoms and psychiatric disturbance that may mandate cessation of therapy. As this agent is free from leukemogenic or teratogenic effects,[85] interferon-α is often used for younger patients or during conception and pregnancy. The adverse side-effect profile, however, means that it is generally avoided in older patients. Pegylated interferon-α, for which less-frequent administration is required, may be more convenient but the side-effect profile appears similar to the native compound.

Radioactive phosphorus and alkylating agents such as busulphan are effective at controlling the platelet count, but are associated with an increased risk of progression to acute leukemia, particularly when used sequentially with hydroxyurea, and thus should be avoided in younger patients. Both radioactive phosphorus and busulphan can be given intermittently with long intervals between doses, and may be useful in treating older patients who are unable to attend the clinic on a regular basis. Pipobroman, a piperazine derivative, is effective at reducing

TABLE 85–5. ANAHYDRET and PT-1 Randomized Controlled Trials of Anagrelide versus Hydroxyurea for the Treatment of Essential Thrombocythemia

	ANAHYDRET Trial[83]	PT-1 Trial[30]
Diagnosis	WHO criteria (2001)	PVSG criteria
	Central review of histology*	Diagnosis by treating physician
Patients	High risk	High risk
	Treatment naïve	Treated or untreated
Median age: AN/HU	58/56	61/62
Patient number: AN/HU	122/131	405/404
Followup	730 patient-years	2653 patient-years
Total events:		
Arterial thrombosis	15	54
Venous thrombosis	8	17
Hemorrhage	7	30
Transformation to MF	3	21

AN, anagrelide; HU, hydroxyurea; MF, myelofibrosis; WHO, World Health Organization.

*82.2 percent of patients met WHO 2001 diagnostic criteria for ET.

the platelet count in ET, although there is little direct evidence for efficacy in thrombosis prevention. However, studies of patients with PV have indicated that long-term use of this agent is associated with an increased risk of developing leukemia.[80,86]

The identification of mutations in *JAK2* and studies highlighting a central role for increased JAK2 activity in the pathogenesis of the MPNs have driven the rapid development of targeted JAK2 inhibitors (e.g., ruxolitinib). Randomized trials indicate a role for these agents in relieving symptoms and possibly prolonging survival in patients with PMF.[87,88] Although early phase clinical trials have demonstrated efficacy in reducing the platelet count in patients with ET, their place in routine management has yet to be defined.

SPECIAL CONSIDERATIONS

Conception and Pregnancy

First trimester fetal loss complicates up to 50 percent of pregnancies in ET patients, with other complications such as intrauterine growth retardation, stillbirth, and preeclampsia also occurring more frequently. Such complications occur irrespective of the platelet count prior to conception but may be more prominent in those with *JAK2*[V617F]-positive disease. Whether the use of aspirin or cytoreductive agents can improve pregnancy outcome is uncertain, with studies reporting contradictory results.[89] However, a large meta-analysis of preeclampsia patients without ET suggested that aspirin use in pregnancy is safe for both mother and fetus,[90] and it therefore seems reasonable to consider its use for all pregnant ET patients. Although hydroxyurea has been used during pregnancy, usually without adverse effects for mother or fetus, it is teratogenic in various non-human mammals[91] and should be avoided if possible. Anagrelide can cross the placenta with unknown effects on fetal development and should also be avoided. Interferon-α is nonteratogenic[85] and is the agent of choice for patients with high-risk disease

TABLE 85–6. Risk Factors for Complications in Essential Thrombocythemia

Thrombosis	Hemorrhage	Myelofibrotic Transformation	Acute Myeloid Leukemia
Age >60 years	Marrow fibrosis[‡]	Disease duration	Disease duration
Prior thrombosis	Thrombocytosis[†]	Anagrelide therapy[¶]	Genotoxic therapy
Cardiovascular risk*	Leucocytosis[†]	Marrow fibrosis[‡]	Use of >1 cytoreductive agent
Leukocytosis[†]			
Marrow fibrosis[‡]			
JAK2[V617F] mutation[§]			

*Diabetes, hypertension, hypercholesterolemia or tobacco use.
[†]During followup.
[‡]At diagnosis.
[§]Venous and arterial thrombosis.
[¶]Compared with hydroxyurea.

should cytoreductive therapy be required during pregnancy. Although studies in ET patients are lacking, thromboprophylaxis appears safe in pregnancy (e.g., with low doses of low-molecular-weight heparin),[92] and may be considered for patients with a history of thrombosis or pregnancy loss; in those with prior thrombosis, treatment should be continued for 6 weeks postpartum. Pregnant ET patients should ideally be managed in a center where regular fetal monitoring can be performed, with good communication between the obstetric, hematology, and anesthetic departments. Pregnancy does not appear to affect the natural history of the disease, although the platelet count often falls during gestation. In animal studies, hydroxyurea is associated with reduced spermatogenesis and genetic damage to spermatogonia.[91] Male patients requiring cytoreductive treatment should therefore consider interferon-α therapy prior to attempted conception.

Surgery

Although thrombotic and bleeding complications appear increased in ET patients undergoing surgical procedures, it is not clear whether these risks can be ameliorated by specific therapeutic interventions. In general, antiplatelet agents should be stopped 7 to 10 days prior to major surgery or surgery to critical sites, and recommended as soon as the surgeon is confident of secure hemostasis. Postoperative thromboprophylaxis should be administered according to local protocols. For patients receiving cytoreductive therapy, control of blood counts should be optimized preoperatively and interruptions in therapy kept to a minimum. For patients not receiving treatment, temporary cytoreductive therapy may be considered on a case-by-case basis, taking into account the individual's thrombotic risk profile, the degree of thrombocytosis, and the nature of the surgery.

Splenectomy in ET patients generally results in an increase in the platelet count and also in increased thrombotic and hemorrhagic complications. Normalization of the platelet count is therefore advisable for all ET patients prior to elective splenectomy. Thromboprophylaxis and daily monitoring of bloods counts is recommended during the postoperative period.

● COURSE AND PROGNOSIS

There is a lack of good quality prospective data concerning long-term survival in ET. Data from cancer registries and retrospective studies indicate that overall survival is reduced compared with population controls.[93–95] This excess mortality results from disease complications such as thrombosis and transformation to PMF or AML. However,

management paradigms have changed significantly over the last 10 to 20 years, including more aggressive intervention to prevent thrombosis and decreasing use of leukemogenic agents. These changes, which may be related to observed improvements in patient outcomes in recent years,[94] render some long-term followup studies difficult to interpret.

A number of predictive factors for thrombotic complications have been identified (Table 85–6), the best established of which are age older than 60 years or a history of previous thrombosis. Factors independently associated with decreased overall survival in ET include history of prior thrombosis, anemia and leukocytosis,[93] the latter two factors likely representing markers of more advanced disease. Additional factors associated with an increased risk of thrombosis include predisposition to atherosclerotic disease (diabetes, hypertension, hypercholesterolemia, or tobacco use), presence of a JAK2[V617F] mutation or increased marrow fibrosis at diagnosis (see section "Thrombosis"). At the present time, age older than 60 years or history of previous thrombosis are generally considered to mandate cytoreductive therapy in ET patients. Whether additional factors, such as presence of a JAK2 mutation, can be used to improve patient stratification is yet to be tested formally in a clinical trial.

In contrast to thrombotic complications, there are few identifiable factors that predict for progression to PMF or acute leukemia. The incidence of both complications increases progressively with disease duration. Choice of therapy also plays a role, with anagrelide increasing the risk of myelofibrotic transformation compared to hydroxyurea[30] and genotoxic agents increasing the risk of leukemia, especially when used sequentially with hydroxyurea. Marrow fibrosis at diagnosis was associated with an increased risk of subsequent PMF in a prospective study,[38] but other markers, including the presence of different somatic mutations, have failed to show a consistent association with either myelofibrotic or leukemic transformation.

REFERENCES

1. Epstein E, Geoedel A: Hemorrhagic thrombocythemia with cascular, sclerotic spleen. *Virchows Archiv A Pathol Anat Histopathol* 293:233, 1934.
2. Fialkow PJ, Faguet GB, Jacobson RJ, et al: Evidence that essential thrombocythemia is a clonal disorder with origin in a multipotent stem cell. *Blood* 58:916, 1981.
3. McNally RJ, Rowland D, Roman E, Cartwright RA: Age and sex distributions of hematological malignancies in the U.K. *Hematol Oncol* 15:173, 1997.
4. Mesa RA, Silverstein MN, Jacobsen SJ, et al: Population-based incidence and survival figures in essential thrombocythemia and agnogenic myeloid metaplasia: An Olmsted County Study, 1976-1995. *Am J Hematol* 61:10, 1999.
5. Anderson RE, Hoshino T, Yamamoto T: Myelofibrosis with myeloid metaplasia in survivors of the atomic bomb in Hiroshima. *Ann Intern Med* 60:1, 1964.
6. Kralovics R, Stockton DW, Prchal JT: Clonal hematopoiesis in familial polycythemia vera suggests the involvement of multiple mutational events in the early pathogenesis of the disease. *Blood* 102:3793, 2003.

7. Landgren O, Goldin LR, Kristinsson SY, et al: Increased risks of polycythemia vera, essential thrombocythemia, and myelofibrosis among 24,577 first-degree relatives of 11,039 patients with myeloproliferative neoplasms in Sweden. *Blood* 112:2199, 2008.

8. Cross NCP: Genetic and epigenetic complexity in myeloproliferative neoplasms. *Hematology Am Soc Hematol Educ Program* 2011:208, 2011.

9. Levine RL, Pardanani A, Tefferi A, Gilliland DG: Role of JAK2 in the pathogenesis and therapy of myeloproliferative disorders. *Nat Rev Cancer* 7:673, 2007.

10. Witthuhn BA, Quelle FW, Silvennoinen O, et al: JAK2 associates with the erythropoietin receptor and is tyrosine phosphorylated and activated following stimulation with erythropoietin. *Cell* 74:227, 1993.

11. Drachman JG, Millett KM, Kaushansky K: Thrombopoietin signal transduction requires functional JAK2, not TYK2. *J Biol Chem* 274:13480, 1999.

12. Parganas E, Wang D, Stravopodis D, et al: Jak2 is essential for signaling through a variety of cytokine receptors. *Cell* 93:385, 1998.

13. Remy I, Wilson IA, Michnick SW: Erythropoietin receptor activation by a ligand-induced conformation change. *Science* 283:990, 1999.

14. Brooks AJ, Dai W, O'Mara ML, et al: Mechanism of activation of protein kinase JAK2 by the growth hormone receptor. *Science* 344:1249783, 2014.

15. Bandaranayake RM, Ungureanu D, Shan Y, et al: Crystal structures of the JAK2 pseudokinase domain and the pathogenic mutant V617F. *Nat Struct Mol Biol* 19:754, 2012.

16. Li J, Kent DG, Chen E, Green AR: Mouse models of myeloproliferative neoplasms: JAK of all grades. *Dis Model Mech* 4:311, 2011.

17. Beer PA, Campbell PJ, Scott LM, et al: MPL mutations in myeloproliferative disorders: Analysis of the PT-1 cohort. *Blood* 112:141, 2008.

18. Vannucchi AM, Antonioli E, Guglielmelli P, et al: Characteristics and clinical correlates of MPL 515W>L/K mutation in essential thrombocythemia. *Blood* 112:844, 2008.

19. Staerk J, Lacout C, Sato T, et al: An amphipathic motif at the transmembrane-cytoplasmic junction prevents autonomous activation of the thrombopoietin receptor. *Blood* 107:1864, 2006.

20. Ding J, Komatsu H, Iida S, et al: The Asn505 mutation of c-MPL gene, which causes familial essential thrombocythemia, induces autonomous homodimerization of the c-Mpl protein due to strong amino acid polarity. *Blood* 114:3325, 2009.

21. Pikman Y, Lee BH, Mercher T, et al: MPLW515L is a novel somatic activating mutation in myelofibrosis with myeloid metaplasia. *PLoS Med* 3:e270, 2006.

22. Oh ST, Simonds EF, Jones C, et al: Novel mutations in the inhibitory adaptor protein LNK drive JAK-STAT signaling in patients with myeloproliferative neoplasms. *Blood* 116:988, 2010.

23. Wang WA, Groenendyk J, Michalak M: Calreticulin signaling in health and disease. *Int J Biochem Cell Biol* 44:842, 2012.

24. Nangalia J, Massie CE, Baxter EJ, et al: Somatic CALR mutations in myeloproliferative neoplasms with nonmutated JAK2. *N Engl J Med* 369:2391, 2013.

25. Klampfl T, Gisslinger H, Harutyunyan AS, et al: Somatic mutations of calreticulin in myeloproliferative neoplasms. *N Engl J Med* 369:2379, 2013.

26. Rampal R, Al-Shahrour F, Abdel-Wahab O, et al: Integrated genomic analysis illustrates the central role of JAK-STAT pathway activation in myeloproliferative neoplasm pathogenesis. *Blood* 123:e123, 2014.

27. Kim E, Abdel-Wahab O: Focus on the epigenome in the myeloproliferative neoplasms. *Hematology Am Soc Hematol Educ Program* 2013:538, 2013.

28. Dawson MA, Bannister AJ, Gottgens B, et al: JAK2 phosphorylates histone H3Y41 and excludes HP1alpha from chromatin. *Nature* 461:819, 2009.

29. Rinaldi CR, Rinaldi P, Alagia A, et al: Preferential nuclear accumulation of JAK2V617F in CD34+ but not in granulocytic, megakaryocytic, or erythroid cells of patients with Philadelphia-negative myeloproliferative neoplasia. *Blood* 116:6023, 2010.

30. Harrison CN, Campbell PJ, Buck G, et al: Hydroxyurea compared with anagrelide in high-risk essential thrombocythemia. *N Engl J Med* 353:33, 2005.

31. Cortelazzo S, Finazzi G, Ruggeri M, et al: Hydroxyurea for patients with essential thrombocythemia and a high risk of thrombosis. *N Engl J Med* 332:1132, 1995.

32. Michiels JJ, van Genderen PJ, Lindemans J, van Vliet HH: Erythromelalgic, thrombotic and hemorrhagic manifestations in 50 cases of thrombocythemia. *Leuk Lymphoma* 22 Suppl 1:47, 1996.

33. Patel RK, Lea NC, Heneghan MA, et al: Prevalence of the activating JAK2 tyrosine kinase mutation V617F in the Budd-Chiari syndrome. *Gastroenterology* 130:2031, 2006.

34. Passamonti F, Rumi E, Arcaini L, et al: Prognostic factors for thrombosis, myelofibrosis, and leukemia in essential thrombocythemia: A study of 605 patients. *Haematologica* 93:1645, 2008.

35. Campbell PJ, MacLean C, Beer PA, et al: Correlation of blood counts with vascular complications in essential thrombocythemia: Analysis of the prospective PT1 cohort. *Blood* 120:1409, 2012.

36. Dahabreh IJ, Zoi K, Giannouli S, et al: Is JAK2 V617F mutation more than a diagnostic index? A meta-analysis of clinical outcomes in essential thrombocythemia. *Leuk Res* 33:67, 2009.

37. Lussana F, Caberlon S, Pagani C, et al: Association of V617F Jak2 mutation with the risk of thrombosis among patients with essential thrombocythaemia or idiopathic myelofibrosis: A systematic review. *Thromb Res* 124:409, 2009.

38. Campbell PJ, Bareford D, Erber WN, et al: Reticulin accumulation in essential thrombocythemia: Prognostic significance and relationship to therapy. *J Clin Oncol* 27:2991, 2009.

39. Elliott MA, Tefferi A: Thrombosis and haemorrhage in polycythaemia vera and essential thrombocythaemia. *Br J Haematol* 128:275, 2005.

40. Wolanskyj AP, Schwager SM, McClure RF, et al: Essential thrombocythemia beyond the first decade: Life expectancy, long-term complication rates, and prognostic factors. *Mayo Clin Proc* 81:159, 2006.

41. Wilkins BS, Erber WN, Bareford D, et al: Bone marrow pathology in essential thrombocythemia: Interobserver reliability and utility for identifying disease subtypes. *Blood* 111:60, 2008.

42. Campbell PJ, Scott LM, Buck G, et al: Definition of subtypes of essential thrombocythaemia and relation to polycythaemia vera based on JAK2 V617F mutation status: A prospective study. *Lancet* 366:1945, 2005.

43. Vannucchi AM, Antonioli E, Guglielmelli P, et al: Clinical correlates of JAK2V617F presence or allele burden in myeloproliferative neoplasms: A critical reappraisal. *Leukemia* 22:1299, 2008.

44. Rotunno G, Mannarelli C, Guglielmelli P, et al: Impact of calreticulin mutations on clinical and hematological phenotype and outcome in essential thrombocythemia. *Blood* 123:1552, 2014.

45. Rumi E, Pietra D, Ferretti V, et al: JAK2 or CALR mutation status defines subtypes of essential thrombocythemia with substantially different clinical course and outcomes. *Blood* 123:1544, 2014.

46. Kiladjian JJ, Rain JD, Bernard JF, et al: Long-term incidence of hematological evolution in three French prospective studies of hydroxyurea and pipobroman in polycythemia vera and essential thrombocythemia. *Semin Thromb Hemost* 32:417, 2006.

47. Finazzi G, Caruso V, Marchioli R, et al: Acute leukemia in polycythemia vera: An analysis of 1638 patients enrolled in a prospective observational study. *Blood* 105:2664, 2005.

48. Berk PD, Goldberg JD, Silverstein MN, et al: Increased incidence of acute leukemia in polycythemia vera associated with chlorambucil therapy. *N Engl J Med* 304:441, 1981.

49. Theocharides A, Boissinot M, Girodon F, et al: Leukemic blasts in transformed JAK2-V617F-positive myeloproliferative disorders are frequently negative for the JAK2-V617F mutation. *Blood* 110:375, 2007.

50. Andersson PO, Ridell B, Wadenvik H, Kutti J: Leukemic transformation of essential thrombocythemia without previous cytoreductive treatment. *Ann Hematol* 79:40, 2000.

51. Bench AJ, White HE, Foroni L, et al: Molecular diagnosis of the myeloproliferative neoplasms: UK guidelines for the detection of JAK2 V617F and other relevant mutations. *Br J Haematol* 160:25, 2013.

52. Griesshammer M, Bangerter M, Sauer T, et al: Aetiology and clinical significance of thrombocytosis: Analysis of 732 patients with an elevated platelet count. *J Intern Med* 245:295, 1999.

53. Buss DH, Cashell AW, O'Connor ML, et al: Occurrence, etiology, and clinical significance of extreme thrombocytosis: A study of 280 cases. *Am J Med* 96:247, 1994.

54. Skoda R: The genetic basis of myeloproliferative disorders. *Hematology Am Soc Hematol Educ Program* 2007:1, 2007.

55. Harrison CN, Gale RE, Wiestner AC, et al: The activating splice mutation in intron 3 of the thrombopoietin gene is not found in patients with non-familial essential thrombocythaemia. *Br J Haematol* 102:1341, 1998.

56. Mead AJ, Rugless MJ, Jacobsen SE, Schuh A: Germline JAK2 mutation in a family with hereditary thrombocytosis. *N Engl J Med* 366:967, 2012.

57. Marty C, Saint-Martin C, Pecquet C, et al: Germ-line JAK2 mutations in the kinase domain are responsible for hereditary thrombocytosis and are resistant to JAK2 and HSP90 inhibitors. *Blood* 123:1372, 2014.

58. Beer PA, Erber WN, Campbell PJ, Green AR: How I treat essential thrombocythemia. *Blood* 117:1472, 2010.

59. Campbell PJ, Bareford D, Erber WN, et al: Reticulin accumulation in essential thrombocythemia: Prognostic significance and relationship to therapy. *J Clin Oncol* 27:2991, 2009.

60. Swerdlow SH, Campo E, Harris NL, et al: *WHO Classification of Tumours of Haematopoietic and Lymphoid Tissues.* IARC Press, Lyon, 2008.

61. Michiels JJ, Berneman Z, Schroyens W, et al: Philadelphia (Ph) chromosome-positive thrombocythemia without features of chronic myeloid leukemia in peripheral blood: Natural history and diagnostic differentiation from Ph-negative essential thrombocythemia. *Ann Hematol* 83:504, 2004.

62. Godfrey AL, Chen E, Pagano F, et al: JAK2V617F homozygosity arises commonly and recurrently in PV and ET, but PV is characterized by expansion of a dominant homozygous subclone. *Blood* 120:2704, 2012.

63. Godfrey AL, Chen E, Pagano F, et al: Clonal analyses reveal associations of JAK2V617F homozygosity with hematologic features, age and gender in polycythemia vera and essential thrombocythemia. *Haematologica* 98:718, 2013.

64. Olthof SG, Fatrai S, Drayer AL, et al: Downregulation of signal transducer and activator of transcription 5 (STAT5) in CD34+ cells promotes megakaryocytic development, whereas activation of STAT5 drives erythropoiesis. *Stem Cells* 26:1732, 2008.

65. Li J, Kent DG, Godfrey AL, et al: JAK2V617F homozygosity drives a phenotypic switch in myeloproliferative neoplasms, but is insufficient to sustain disease. *Blood* 123:3139, 2014.

66. Chen E, Beer PA, Godfrey AL, et al: Distinct clinical phenotypes associated with JAK2V617F reflect differential STAT1 signaling. *Cancer Cell* 18:524, 2010.

67. Plo I, Nakatake M, Malivert L, et al: JAK2 stimulates homologous recombination and genetic instability: Potential implication in the heterogeneity of myeloproliferative disorders. *Blood* 112:1402, 2008.

68. Zhao R, Follows GA, Beer PA, et al: Inhibition of the Bcl-xL deamidation pathway in myeloproliferative disorders. *N Engl J Med* 359:2778, 2008.

69. Marty C, Lacout C, Droin N, et al: A role for reactive oxygen species in JAK2 V617F myeloproliferative neoplasm progression. *Leukemia* 27:2187, 2013.

70. Nieborowska-Skorska M, Kopinski PK, Ray R, et al: Rac2-MRC-cIII-generated ROS cause genomic instability in chronic myeloid leukemia stem cells and primitive progenitors. *Blood* 119:4253, 2012.

71. Beer PA, Delhommeau F, Lecouedic JP, et al: Two routes to leukemic transformation following a JAK2 mutation-positive myeloproliferative neoplasm. *Blood* 115:2891, 2010.

72. Abdel-Wahab O, Manshouri T, Patel J, et al: Genetic analysis of transforming events that convert chronic myeloproliferative neoplasms to leukemias. *Cancer Res* 70:447, 2010.

73. Jager R, Gisslinger H, Passamonti F, et al: Deletions of the transcription factor Ikaros in myeloproliferative neoplasms. *Leukemia* 24:1290, 2010.

74. Milosevic JD, Puda A, Malcovati L, et al: Clinical significance of genetic aberrations in secondary acute myeloid leukemia. *Am J Hematol* 87:1010, 2012.

75. Landolfi R, Marchioli R, Kutti J, et al: Efficacy and safety of low-dose aspirin in polycythemia vera. *N Engl J Med* 350:114, 2004.

76. Lanzkron S, Strouse JJ, Wilson R, et al: Systematic review: Hydroxyurea for the treatment of adults with sickle cell disease. *Ann Intern Med* 148:939, 2008.

77. Sterkers Y, Preudhomme C, Lai JL, et al: Acute myeloid leukemia and myelodysplastic syndromes following essential thrombocythemia treated with hydroxyurea: High proportion of cases with 17p deletion. *Blood* 91:616, 1998.

78. Weinfeld A, Swolin B, Westin J: Acute leukaemia after hydroxyurea therapy in polycythaemia vera and allied disorders: Prospective study of efficacy and leukaemogenicity with therapeutic implications. *Eur J Haematol* 52:134, 1994.

79. Bjorkholm M, Derolf AR, Hultcrantz M, et al: Treatment-related risk factors for transformation to acute myeloid leukemia and myelodysplastic syndromes in myeloproliferative neoplasms. *J Clin Oncol* 29:2410, 2011.

80. Tefferi A, Rumi E, Finazzi G, et al: Survival and prognosis among 1545 patients with contemporary polycythemia vera: An international study. *Leukemia* 27:1874, 2013.

81. Hanft VN, Fruchtman SR, Pickens CV, et al: Acquired DNA mutations associated with in vivo hydroxyurea exposure. *Blood* 95:3589, 2000.

82. Campbell PJ, Green AR: Management of polycythemia vera and essential thrombocythemia. *Hematology* 2005:201, 2005.

83. Gisslinger H, Gotic M, Holowiecki J, et al: Anagrelide compared with hydroxyurea in WHO-classified essential thrombocythemia: The ANAHYDRET Study, a randomized controlled trial. *Blood* 121:1720, 2013.

84. Garattini S, Bertele V: Non-inferiority trials are unethical because they disregard patients' interests. *Lancet* 370:1875, 2007.

85. Yazdani Brojeni P, Matok I, Garcia Bournissen F, Koren G: A systematic review of the fetal safety of interferon alpha. *Reprod Toxicol* 33:265, 2012.

86. Kiladjian JJ, Chevret S, Dosquet C, et al: Treatment of polycythemia vera with hydroxyurea and pipobroman: Final results of a randomized trial initiated in 1980. *J Clin Oncol* 29:3907, 2011.

87. Verstovsek S, Kantarjian H, Mesa RA, et al: Safety and efficacy of INCB018424, a JAK1 and JAK2 inhibitor, in myelofibrosis. *N Engl J Med* 363:1117, 2010.

88. Cervantes F, Vannucchi AM, Kiladjian JJ, et al: Three-year efficacy, safety, and survival findings from COMFORT-II, a phase 3 study comparing ruxolitinib with best available therapy for myelofibrosis. *Blood* 122:4047, 2013.

89. Harrison C: Pregnancy and its management in the Philadelphia negative myeloproliferative diseases. *Br J Haematol* 129:293, 2005.

90. Askie LM, Duley L, Henderson-Smart DJ, Stewart LA: Antiplatelet agents for prevention of pre-eclampsia: A meta-analysis of individual patient data. *Lancet* 369:1791, 2007.

91. Liebelt EL, Balk SJ, Faber W, et al: NTP-CERHR expert panel report on the reproductive and developmental toxicity of hydroxyurea. *Birth Defects Res B Dev Reprod Toxicol* 80:259, 2007.

92. Patel JP, Hunt BJ: Where do we go now with low molecular weight heparin use in obstetric care? *J Thromb Haemost* 6:1461, 2008.

93. Montanaro M, Latagliata R, Cedrone M, et al: Thrombosis and survival in essential thrombocythemia: A regional study of 1,144 patients. *Am J Hematol* 89:542, 2014.

94. Hultcrantz M, Kristinsson SY, Andersson TM, et al: Patterns of survival among patients with myeloproliferative neoplasms diagnosed in Sweden from 1973 to 2008: A population-based study. *J Clin Oncol* 30:2995, 2012.

95. Price GL, Davis KL, Karve S, et al: Survival patterns in United States (US) medicare enrollees with non-CML myeloproliferative neoplasms (MPN). *PLoS One* 9:e90299, 2014.

CHAPTER 86
PRIMARY MYELOFIBROSIS

Marshall A. Lichtman and Josef T. Prchal

SUMMARY

Primary myelofibrosis is one of several disorders in the spectrum of clonal myeloid diseases, malignant diseases that originate in the clonal expansion of a single hematopoietic multipotential cell reprogrammed by several somatic mutations. It is one of the eight neoplasms, including polycythemia vera and essential thrombocythemia, classified as a myeloproliferative disease by the World Health Organization. Approximately 90 percent of cases have a mutation in the Janus kinase 2 *(JAK2)* gene (~50 percent), the calreticulin *(CALR)* gene (~35 percent), or the thrombopoietin receptor *(MPL)* gene (~4 percent). The disease is characterized, classically, by anemia, mild neutrophilia, thrombocytosis, and splenomegaly. Occasional cases may present with bi- or tricytopenias (~15 percent). Immature myeloid and nucleated red cells, teardrop-shaped erythrocytes, and large platelets (megakaryocyte cytoplasmic fragments) are characteristic features of the blood film. The marrow contains an increased number of neoplastic dysmorphic megakaryocytes and increased reticulin fibers and, often later, collagen fibrosis. This reactive, polyclonal fibroplasia is the result of cytokines (e.g., transforming growth factor-β) released locally by the numerous neoplastic megakaryocytes. Osteosclerosis, also, may be present. The disease may be complicated by (1) portal hypertension and gastroesophageal varices as a result of a very large splenic blood flow and loss of compliance of hepatic vessels, (2) extramedullary fibrohematopoietic tumors that can develop in any tissue and lead to symptoms by compression of vital structures, and (3) abdominal vein thrombosis (Budd-Chiari syndrome). Newly developed JAK2 inhibitors are now first-line therapy for splenomegaly and constitutional symptoms (fever, night sweats, and weight loss). Other treatment has included hydroxyurea for thrombocytosis and massive splenomegaly, androgens, erythropoietin, or red cell transfusions for severe anemia, local irradiation of fibrohematopoietic tumors or of a massive, symptomatic spleen, or splenectomy for severe cytopenias, if splenic effects are not controlled by JAK2 inhibitors. Portosystemic shunt surgery may be required for gastroesophageal variceal bleeding. In younger patients, allogeneic hematopoietic stem cell transplantation can be curative and nonmyeloablative transplantation has been successful, at least up to age 60 years. The disease may remain indolent for years or may progress rapidly by further deterioration in hematopoiesis, by massive splenic enlargement and its sequelae, or by transformation to acute myelogenous leukemia.

Acronyms and Abbreviations: AML, acute myelogenous leukemia; bFGF, basic fibroblast growth factor; bp, base pair; *CALR*, calreticulin gene; CD, cluster of differentiation; CML, chronic myelogenous leukemia; FISH, fluorescence *in situ* hybridization; G6PD, glucose-6-phosphate dehydrogenase; G-CSF, granulocyte colony-stimulating factor; IL, interleukin; *JAK2*, Janus kinase 2 gene; *MPL*, thrombopoietin receptor gene; MRI, magnetic resonance imaging; PDGF, platelet-derived growth factor; TGF, transforming growth factor; TNFR, tumor necrosis factor receptor.

● DEFINITION AND HISTORY

Primary myelofibrosis is a chronic clonal myeloid neoplasm characterized by (1) anemia; (2) neutrophilia and thrombocytosis or, in a minority, thrombocytopenia and leukopenia; (3) splenomegaly; (4) immature granulocytes, increased cluster of differentiation (CD) 34+ cells, erythroblasts, and teardrop-shaped red cells in the blood; (5) marrow fibrosis; and (6) osteosclerosis. The disorder originally was described by Heuck[1] in 1879 under the title "Two Cases of Leukemia and Peculiar Blood and Bone Marrow Findings." In his monograph, Silverstein traced the history of the concepts set forth during the first half of the 20th century to explain the pathogenesis of this disease, including its origin in the marrow, the appearance of extramedullary hematopoiesis, and the relationship of fibrosis to hematopoietic changes.[2] The disease occurs, often, *de novo* but can develop as a later phase of polycythemia vera (Chap. 84), essential thrombocythemia (Chap. 85), or, rarely, chronic myelogenous leukemia (Chap. 89), or an atypical myeloproliferative disease (Chap. 89). It may be preceded by a prefibrotic phase (see "Special Clinical Features: Prefibrotic Primary Myelofibrosis" below). Numerous designations for the disease have been proposed or used, and different names were preferred in different countries.[3] *Primary myelofibrosis* has been designated the most recent "official" name of the disease by a working group on classification of the World Health Organization.[3] This compromise selection is unfortunate as the fibrosis is secondary, not primary, and the choice omits focusing on the central pathologic change: a clonal myeloid disease with the singular finding of neoplastic (dysmorphic) megakaryocytopoiesis.[4] It is a disease of cells, not fibers, and is the only cancer in the medical lexicon not so designated; rather, it is named for an epiphenomenon in the extracellular matrix.

The discovery that the mutated Janus kinase 2 *(JAK2)* gene mutation can play a role in the causation and behavior of several myeloproliferative diseases[5] and that approximately 50 percent of cases of primary myelofibrosis have a mutation of the *JAK2* gene[6] or, far less commonly, thrombopoietin receptor *(MPL)* gene has led to better understanding of the pathogenesis of the disease and its relationship to other myeloproliferative diseases. The JAK signaling pathways also represent an important new target for therapy. The subsequent observation of mutations of the calreticulin *(CALR)* gene in approximately 70 percent of patients without a *JAK2* or *MPL* mutation has provided deeper insights into the pathogenesis of myelofibrosis, the opportunity to examine interactions among somatic mutations in the cells of patents, and the opportunity for new therapeutic approaches (see "Etiology and Pathogenesis" below).[7]

● EPIDEMIOLOGY

INCIDENCE

Age and Sex

Primary myelofibrosis characteristically occurs after age 50 years.[2,8–16] The median age at diagnosis is approximately 65 to 70 years,[8,12–14,17] but the disease also can occur in neonates and children.[2,12,14,18–20] In infants, the disorder can mimic the classic disease or show certain features but not others, such as absence of hepatosplenomegaly.[19] Familial infantile myelofibrosis mimics the adult disease and in some cases is transmitted by autosomal recessive inheritance.[20–23] The occurrence of primary myelofibrosis in children usually is in the first 3 years of life.[20,24,25] In young children, girls are afflicted with the disease twice as frequently as boys.[19] In young and middle-age adults, the disease is similar to that in older subjects, although the proportion of indolent cases may be higher.[18,20,26] In adults, the disease occurs with about equal frequency in men and women.[8,12–16] Like virtually all clonal myeloid diseases,[27] primary myelofibrosis can cluster in families, suggesting transmission of an unidentified predisposition gene.[28-30] A large Swedish study found a significant relative risk (five- to sevenfold) for a familial occurrence of another myeloproliferative disease neoplasm, although not specifically primary myelofibrosis. The latter finding may relate to the small number of cases of primary myelofibrosis in that study.[17] The incidence of the disease is approximately 0.5 cases per 100,000 population per year in northern European countries.[31-34] A survey in Olmstead County, Minnesota reported an incidence of 1.5 case per 100,000 population per year and a median age of onset of 67 years,[35] similar to other studies (see above in this section).

● ETIOLOGY AND PATHOGENESIS

EXOGENOUS FACTORS

Exposure to high concentrations of benzene[36-38] or very-high-dose ionizing radiation[39] preceded the development of primary myelofibrosis in a very small number of cases in the past. Epidemiologic studies have not determined a relative risk of myelofibrosis after high-dose benzene exposure. Lower-level benzene exposure was not found to be associated with the risk of myeloproliferative disease in a comprehensive study.[40] Thus, the few case reports must be viewed with caution in assessing causation. Benzene in exposures greater than 40 to 200 ppm-years is associated with an increased relative risk of acute myelogenous leukemia (AML),[41,42] but not of chronic myelogenous leukemias (CMLs; Chap. 89) These levels of exposures are far above the current levels permitted by the Occupational Safety and Health Administration.

IMMUNE MECHANISMS

Reports of myelofibrosis in patients with lupus erythematosus, have suggested the possibility of immunologic-mediated hyperplasia of marrow connective tissue (see "Immune and Inflammatory Manifestations" below).[2] These forms of myelofibrosis are different from the monoclonal multipotential hematopoietic cell disease, which is the principal type considered in this chapter.

CLONAL MYELOID DISEASE, ANIMAL MODELS, AND ACTIVATING MUTATIONS

The disease arises from the neoplastic transformation of a single hematopoietic multipotential cell, a conclusion derived from the presence of clonal cytogenetic abnormalities in patients with an identifiable chromosomal abnormality and in studies in women with primary myelofibrosis who also were heterozygous for isotypes A and B of glucose-6-phosphate dehydrogenase (G6PD).[43,44] Although the nonhematopoietic tissues of these patients expressed both isotypes, each patient had blood cells with only one G6PD isotype. The findings strongly imply the blood cells of each patient arose from only one transformed stem cell. Furthermore, chromosome studies of colonies of hematopoietic progenitor cells in primary myelofibrosis established that the same clonal cytogenetic abnormality is present in erythroblasts, neutrophils, macrophages, basophils, and megakaryocytes.[45] These studies were confirmed by (1) examining X-linked restriction fragment length polymorphisms in women with primary myelofibrosis with heterozygosity for X chromosome-linked genes[46,47] and (2) verifying the presence of a mutation of codon 12 of the N-RAS gene in five blood cell lineages of a patient with the disease.[48,49] Lymphocyte derivation from the clone has been noted using mutation in codon 12 of the RAS gene as the marker.[48] Using fluorescence in situ hybridization (FISH) analysis, T and B lymphocytes were found to be derived from clonal expansion of a multipotential hematopoietic cell in three of four patients with primary myelofibrosis with a 13q– or 20q– clonal cytogenetic abnormality.[50] Primary myelofibrosis

can be distinguished from secondary myelofibrosis in women by clonality studies.[51] The discovery of the $JAK2^{V617F}$ mutation has permitted this marker to be used in assessing clonality (as will mutations in CALR and MPL as their determination reaches the clinic). Mutated JAK2-containing cells were identified in all blood lineages of patients with primary myelofibrosis and in the common multipotential hematopoietic cell.[52]

The neoplastic hematopoietic stem cells in primary myelofibrosis containing the $JAK2^{V617F}$ mutation behave differently from the same cell population in polycythemia vera when studied in nonobese, diabetic, severe combined immunodeficient mice. Although studied in a nonhuman environment, the findings are consistent with the presence of $JAK2^{V617F}$ mutations in three phenotypically different myeloproliferative diseases: polycythemia vera, essential thrombocythemia, and primary myelofibrosis.[53]

Animal models allowed the derivation of the murine myeloproliferative leukemia (mpl) virus, carrying the oncogene v-mpl, which in mice produced a syndrome having features of a mixed idiopathic myelofibrotic–polycythemic disorder (Chap. 111).[54] The availability of v-mpl led to the isolation of the thrombopoietin receptor and its ligand thrombopoietin.[55] Later models of myelofibrosis and osteosclerosis, mimicking some of the important features of human primary myelofibrosis, were induced in mice by retroviral-mediated overexpression of thrombopoietin.[56,57] The concomitant high levels of fibroblastic factors (transforming growth factor [TGF]-β_1 and platelet-derived growth factor [PDGF]) resulted in intense fibrosis.[58] In this model, increased osteoprotegerin was thought to be the principal cause of osteosclerosis.[59] The disease was cured by murine hematopoietic stem cell transplantation.[56] These findings were extended and led to the discovery of the human analogue of v-mpl, c-MPL that encodes the human thrombopoietin receptor. Two gain-of-function somatic mutations, MPL^{W515L} and MPL^{W515K}, were found to be associated with primary myelofibrosis and essential thrombocythemia.[60,61] These gain-of-function mutations may also be germline and in such a case are associated with familial (hereditary) thrombocytosis.[62]

A syndrome in mice that results from the GATA-1 (low) mutation also leads to a phenotype that closely simulates human myelofibrosis. The mice gradually develop anemia, teardrop poikilocytes, myeloid immaturity, marrow fibrosis, extramedullary hematopoiesis, and overexpression of profibrotic cytokines in marrow.[63] GATA-1 is a transcription factor required for normal megakaryocyte development. GATA-1 deficiency in mice leads to increased megakaryocytic proliferation, followed by myelofibrosis and osteosclerosis, as a result of exaggerated elaboration of fibroblast-inducing and osteoblast-stimulating factors.[64,65]

The discovery in 2005 that an activating somatic G→T point mutation (V617F) in JAK2 was associated with the three major myeloproliferative diseases—polycythemia vera, essential thrombocythemia, and primary myelofibrosis—has rapidly led to a fuller understanding of the pathogenesis of these diseases.[48,66] A dominant, gain-of-function mutation in the gene JAK2 residing on chromosome 9p24, which encodes the JAK2 tyrosine kinase, is present in approximately 50 percent of patients with primary myelofibrosis, in approximately 95 percent of patients with polycythemia vera (Chap. 84), and in approximately 60 percent of patients with essential thrombocythemia (Chap. 85), but is absent in healthy individuals.[67,68] In confirmation, the expression of the mutated human JAK2 gene transferred into mice can induce a myeloproliferative disease with features characteristic of the human disorders.[69-74] Homozygosity results from allelic duplication as a result of uniparental disomy of chromosome 9p, not loss of the normal allele corresponding to the mutation.[72]

It is not yet precisely known how $JAK2^{V617F}$, the most prevalent mutation, links the three diseases and what modifiers explain the dramatically different phenotype and expected survival of the patients with polycythemia and primary myelofibrosis. At least four other modifying factors have been proposed to account for the different phenotypes and the apparent absence of the mutation in a high proportion of patients with primary myelofibrosis: (1) gene dosage, (2) germline modifiers, (3) predisposition alleles, and (4) additional somatic mutations.[66,68,73] An example of each influence follows. There is an increasing $JAK2^{V617F}$ allele burden from essential thrombocythemia, to polycythemia vera, to primary myelofibrosis.[74] For example, the $JAK2^{V617F}$ allele burden may be a key determinant of the degree of myeloproliferation and myeloid metaplasia reflected by significantly higher levels of white blood cell counts, CD34+ cell counts, lower platelet counts, and a higher frequency of splenomegaly in homozygous polycythemia vera patients compared to their heterozygous counterparts. These findings are consistent with $JAK2^{V617F}$-positive chronic myeloproliferative disorders as a biologic continuum with phenotypic presentation in part influenced by $JAK2^{V617F}$ mutational load.[74] Myeloproliferative neoplasm predisposition alleles could provide a selective advantage for the development of mutations in the $JAK2$ signaling pathway. A number of pre-$JAK2$ alleles, which arise in cells prior to $JAK2$ mutation, may contribute to the phenotype displayed.[68]

A mutation in the thrombopoietin receptor gene, MPL, ($MPL^{515L/K}$) has been found in some mutant $JAK2$-negative patients with primary myelofibrosis. The finding of an activating $JAK2$ (~50 percent of patients) or MPL (~4 percent of patients) mutation, which employs JAK2 for signaling, reinforces the critical role of unregulated activation of the JAK-STAT (signal transducer and activator of transcription) signaling pathway in the pathogenesis of primary myelofibrosis.[75–77] Using next-generation gene whole-exome sequencing, primary myelofibrosis patients who did not have mutated $JAK2$ or MPL genes (approximately half of all patients) were only found to have an occasional somatic mutation.[78]

It came as a surprise that nearly a decade after the description of the $JAK2$ mutation in primary myelofibrosis and related myeloproliferative diseases, two groups reported, simultaneously, the presence of $CALR$ mutations in approximately 70 percent of patients with primary myelofibrosis who did not carry the $JAK2$ or MPL mutations (35 percent of total population).[79,80] The $CALR$ mutations were either from deletions or insertions, explaining the failure to identify them by Sanger sequencing technology. The 52-bp deletion (type 1 mutation) or 5-bp insertion (type 2 mutation) are the most frequent types, accounting for approximately 85 percent of the $CALR$ mutations. The $CALR$ mutations are missense for the gene's final domain, encoding the calcium binding site.

Patients with primary myelofibrosis and $JAK2$, $CALR$, or MPL mutations may have an additional two to four somatic mutations. Some of the principal genes mutated are $TET2$, $ASXL1$, $DNMT3A$, $EZH2$, and $IDH1$, which are implicated in epigenetic regulation, and $TP53$ and CBL.[7] As many as five somatic mutations could be identified in 3 percent of patients, whereas 12 percent of patients with primary myelofibrosis did not have an identifiable somatically mutated gene, using targeted next-generation whole-exome gene sequencing.[7] However, the proportion of these additional somatic mutations was less that that detected by similar studies in polycythemia vera,[81] suggesting that these sequencing technologies, capable of uncovering only approximately 1 percent of the genome, may leave unidentified additional somatic and germline mutations present in a much greater proportion of primary myelofibrosis patients.

Isolated genetic findings in individual patients have included (13q14) deletions, mutation or overexpression of the retinoblastoma gene,[82,83] $NF1$ (17q11) deletions,[84] RAS mutations in approximately one in 20 patients studied, and occasional patients with mutations in KIT.[71] Uniparental disomy has been found on chromosomes 9p (site of $JAK2$, creating a second allele of V617F) and 1p.[83]

$HMGA2$, a gene on chromosome 12, normally is not expressed in humans and is implicated in mesenchymal tumors. $HMGA2$ was expressed in 12 of 12 patients with idiopathic myelofibrosis studied, implying that, if confirmed, expression of this gene in myeloid cells may play a role in the disease.[87]

CENTRALITY OF CD34+ CELL EGRESS AND NEOPLASTIC MEGAKARYOCYTOPOIESIS

Neoplastic megakaryopoiesis is the most prominent alteration in this clonal myeloid disease and is responsible for most of its major manifestations. Constitutive mobilization and circulation of CD34+ cells are prominent features of the clonal expansion. This phenomenon, probably, is the result of epigenetic methylation of the CXCR4 promotor, a resultant decrease in CXCR4 mRNA, decreased expression of CXCR4 on CD34+ cells, and their resultant enhanced migration into the blood in primary myelofibrosis patients.[85]

Circulating CD34+ cells in patients with primary myelofibrosis generate about 24-fold the number of megakaryocytes in culture than do CD34+ cells from normal subjects, express increased levels of BCL-XL, and have delayed apoptosis.[86,87] Media conditioned with CD61+ cells (presumptive megakaryocytes) elaborated greater quantities of growth factors and proteases, including TGF-β and metalloprotease-9, than did CD61+ cells generated from normal CD34+ cells.

Circulating CD34+ cells in patients with primary myelofibrosis also had a higher expression of eight genes ($CD9$, $GAS2$, $DLK1$, $CDH1$, $WT1$, $NFE2$, $HMGA2$, and $CXCR4$) than did normal CD34+ cells. These genes or subsets of them are likely related to disease pathogenesis and were shown to be related to specific manifestations in patients (e.g., increased expression of $CD9$ and $DLK1$ with platelet count and $WT1$ with severity score).[88]

ENHANCED ANGIOGENESIS AND SPLENIC ENDOTHELIAL CELLS

Microvessel density and marrow blood flow are increased in patients with myelofibrosis. These changes may be related to an increase in circulating endothelial cell progenitors.[89] The endothelial cells examined by laser microdissection, cell sorting, or cell culture from spleen capillaries and splenic vein contained the $JAK2^{V617F}$ mutation in 12 of 18 patients studied who had the mutation in their granulocytes. A definitive explanation for this finding has not been established.[90]

DYSFUNCTION OF HEMATOPOIESIS

Neoplastic myeloproliferation usually is the dominant marrow abnormality in the granulocytic and megakaryocytic lineages resulting in intensely cellular marrows and mild to moderate blood granulocytosis and thrombocytosis. Hypocellular hematopoiesis, resulting from exaggerated apoptosis of very early precursors, can be present initially or emerge later, leading to granulocytopenia and/or thrombocytopenia. Anemia is a frequent finding and results from a combination of decreased erythropoiesis, shortened red cell survival, and the effects of splenomegaly on the distribution of red cells in the circulation. Hemolysis can be a prominent factor in some cases. Neoplastic megakaryocyte expansion and intense dysmorphogenesis of megakaryocytes are constant features of the disease. Even in intensely fibrotic marrows with severe decreases in erythroid and granulocytic precursors, clusters of megakaryocytes are easily found interspersed between collagen bundles. The term *megakaryocytic myelosis*, one of the many synonymous terms for the disease, exemplifies the constancy of this finding. The dominance of megakaryopoiesis may relate to the average fivefold overexpression of *FKBP51* in megakaryocytes in primary myelofibrosis and the marked predisposition of CD34+ cells to differentiate into megakaryocytes (see "Centrality of CD34+ Cell Egress and Neoplastic Megakaryocytopoiesis" above). *FKBP51* increases resistance to apoptosis, possibly by an effect through the calcineurin pathway.[91] Thus, the designation "chronic megakaryocytic leukemia" would be a more accurate designation for primary myelofibrosis, if one used an internally consistent classification.[7] Although elevated levels of thrombopoietin (and interleukin [IL]-6 and IL-11) are found in the serum of patients with primary myelofibrosis, their etiologic role in the human disease is unresolved.[92] A marked increase in the thrombopoietin receptor MPL is observed on the platelets and megakaryocytes of a proportion of patients with primary myelofibrosis.[93] Despite the animal models of thrombopoietin-induced myeloproliferation and osteomyelofibrosis and the apparent abnormality of MPL receptor sites on human megakaryocytes, autonomous megakaryocyte growth, characteristic of human primary myelofibrosis marrow in culture, has not been associated with either an autocrine effect of MPL ligand (thrombopoietin) or of a mutation in *MPL*.

FIBROPLASIA

Four of the five major types of collagen[94] are present in normal marrow: type I in bone, type III in blood vessels, and types IV and V in basement membranes. The fine reticulin fibers that appear after silver impregnation of marrow are principally type III collagen. They do not stain with trichrome dyes. The thicker collagen fibers are principally type I collagen and stain with trichrome dyes, but do not impregnate with silver. The amount of the very fine fibrous network barely perceptible in normal marrow that is stained by silver impregnation techniques[95] increases in the marrow of patients with primary myelofibrosis (Table 86–1 and Fig. 86-1C).[96] The fibrous network contains collagen and occasionally progresses to include thick collagen bands that are evident with trichrome stains. Collagen types I, III, IV, and V are increased in myelofibrosis, but type III collagen is increased uniformly and preferentially.[97-104] The latter occurrence accounts for the increased plasma concentration of procollagen III aminoterminal peptide, a component of collagen type III, which is cleaved during collagen biosynthesis.[96,101,102] Serum prolyl-hydroxylase and marrow and plasma fibronectin also increase in patients with idiopathic myelofibrosis or myelofibrosis from other causes.[98,99] Several other matrix materials are increased in marrow or plasma (Tables 86–1 and 86–2).[105-119]

Marrow fibrosis in primary myelofibrosis is most closely correlated with increased neoplastic and dysmorphic megakaryocytes in the marrow. Even densely fibrotic marrow with little residual granulopoiesis or erythropoiesis usually has numerous megakaryocytes scattered throughout the fibrotic areas.[96,120] The increased pathologic emperipolesis (the entry of neutrophils and other marrow cells into the canalicular system of megakaryocytes), evident in human primary myelofibrosis and in mouse models, suggests this may be an additional mechanism of α-granule injury and release of TGF-β and PDGF.[121] Animal models also indicate that marrow monocytes and macrophages may play a subsidiary role in the induction of fibrosis.[121-123] Secretion of PDGF, basic fibroblast growth factor (bFGF), and TGF-β from monocytes that are part of the clone have the potential to act as myeloproliferative growth factors and profibrotic cytokines.[114]

The increased content of marrow collagen types I and III results from release of fibroblast growth factors, which include PDGF,[123,124] epidermal growth factor,[126] endothelial cell growth factor,[126] TGF-β,[114,127,128] and bFGF,[114,129] each of which is present in megakaryocyte α granules. Other factors, such as tumor necrosis factor α, IL-1α, IL-1β, and lysyl oxidase, which can be released from marrow cells, also can stimulate

TABLE 86–1. Fibroplasia in Primary Myelofibrosis
I.   Marrow stroma
A. *Increased amount of*
1. Total collagen (hydroxyproline)[97,101]
2. Type I collagen[97-99,103]
3. Type III collagen[97-99,103]
4. Type III procollagen[98,101,103,104]
5. Type IV collagen[98,105,106]
6. Matrix metalloproteinase-14[107]
7. Bone morphogenetic protein[108]
8. Laminin[98,105,109]
9. Fibronectin[110,111]
10. Tenascin[112]
11. Vitronectin[113]
12. Microenvironment transforming growth factor-β,[114] basic fibroblast growth factor,[114] and substance P[115]
B. *Decreased amount of*
1. Collagenase[107]
II. Plasma
A. *Increased concentration of*
1. Prolylhydroxylase[116]
2. C-terminal peptide of procollagen type I[100]
3. N-terminal peptide of procollagen type III[99,101,117,118]
4. Type IV collagen[99,109]
5. Laminin[99,109]
6. Fibronectin[110,111]
7. Hyaluronan[119]

fibroblasts.[130-132] Platelet factor 4, also derived from megakaryocytes, inhibits collagenase and could contribute to collagen accumulation,[120] although studies showing a poor correlation between plasma platelet factor 4 concentration and marrow fibrosis have dampened enthusiasm for the role of this factor.[133] Substance P, a peptide that acts as a neurotransmitter and a modulator of immune and hematopoietic functions, is increased in the fibrotic marrow and colocalizes with fibronectin. It is angiogenic and is a fibroblast mitogen.[115] Its precise role in the complex interactions among fibroblasts, cytokines, and matrix protein deposition is not clear. The high urinary excretion of platelet-derived calmodulin, a putative fibroblast growth factor, in patients with myelofibrosis has added this compound to the array of factors that may contribute to the fibroplasia.[130] The plasma level of matrix metalloprotein III is decreased and the level of tissue inhibitor of metalloproteinase is increased in patients with idiopathic myelofibrosis.[134] The expression of matrix metalloproteinase-14 in marrow increases by nearly two orders of magnitude as fibroplasia progresses during the course of the disease; and, megakaryocytes and endothelial cells are the major sources of this protein.[107] Neutrophil collagenase (matrix metalloproteinase-8) content is decreased early in the disease.[107] Bone morphogenetic proteins (BMPs) also are implicated as a contributory factor in fibroplasia. BMP1, BMP6, BMP7, and BMP-receptor 2 are increased in marrow in myelofibrosis as a result of release from megakaryocytes and stromal cells. These proteins are activators of latent TGF-β₁ and processors of collagen precursors. In addition, TGF-β₁ induces release of BMP6.[108]

This complex combination of alterations contributes to matrix deposition. The pathogenetic role of released growth factors in

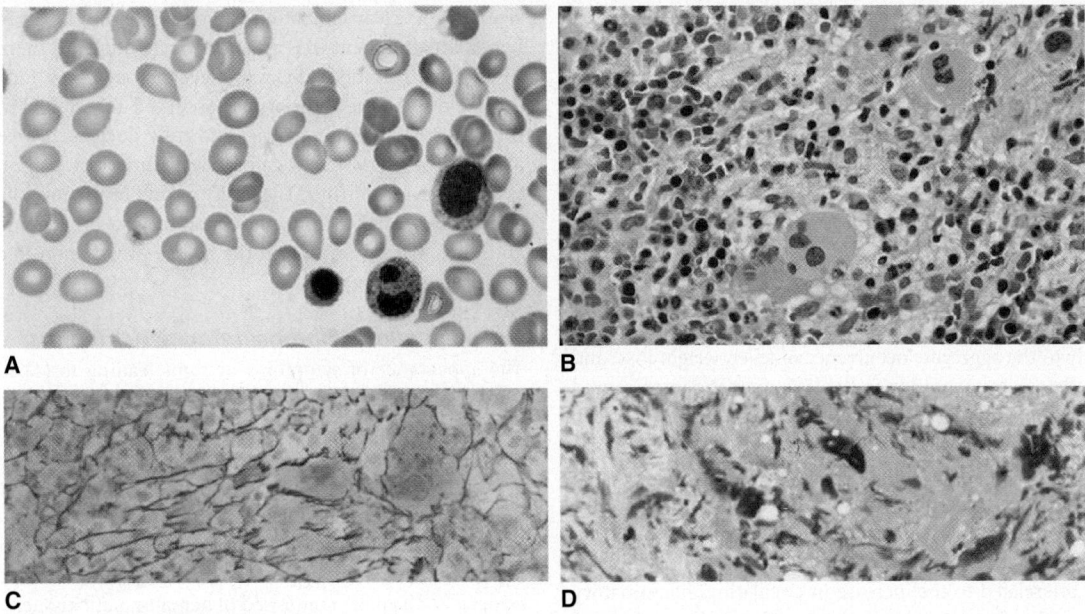

Figure 86–1. Blood film and marrow sections from patients with primary myelofibrosis. **A.** Blood film. Characteristic teardrop poikilocytes, a nucleated red cell, and a segmented neutrophil with a dysmorphic nucleus are evident. **B.** Marrow section. Low power. Hypercellular marrow with increased number of hypolobular megakaryocytes. **C.** Marrow section. Silver impregnation stain. Marked increase in argentophilic fibers representing collagen type III (reticulin). **D.** Marrow section. Collagen fibrosis with extensive replacement of marrow with swirls of collagen fibers. (*Reproduced with permission from* Lichtman's Atlas of Hematology, *www.accessmedicine.com.*)

TABLE 86–2. Diagnostic Findings in Primary Myelofibrosis

PREFIBROTIC STAGE

Anemia may be absent or mild

Leukocytosis may be absent or slight

Thrombocythemia is invariable

BCR-ABL fusion gene absent

Presence of *JAK2, CALR, or MPL* mutations indicative of diagnosis of myeloproliferative disease (one of these mutations present in ~90% of patients)

Cellular marrow with mild increase in granulopoiesis; increased megakaryocytes, clusters of very dysmorphic megakaryocytes and megakaryocytic nuclei; no to very slight increase in reticular fibers on silver stain

Palpable splenomegaly infrequent

Absent or slight anisopoikilocytosis including teardrop red cells

FULLY DEVELOPED STAGE

Marrow reticulin fibrosis plus or minus collagen fibrosis

BCR-ABL fusion gene absent

JAK2, CALR, or MPL mutation in approximately 90% of patients

Splenomegaly

Anisopoikilocytosis with teardrop red cells in virtually every oil immersion field

Immature myeloid cells in blood

Increased CD34+ cells in blood

Nucleated red cells in blood

Marrow usually hypercellular but invariably has increased megakaryocytes, clusters of highly dysmorphic megakaryocytes, and megakaryocyte bare nuclei regardless of overall marrow cellularity

fibroplasia is not completely understood. Generalizations from *in vitro* experiments or correlation between two variables provide only a limited perspective. For example, TGF-β can stimulate or inhibit fibroblast growth, depending on the repertoire of other growth factors in the environment.[127,128]

Fibroplasia is associated with an increase in the number and size of marrow sinuses,[111] the number of endothelial cells,[135] an increase in vascular volume in the marrow,[106] and an increase in blood flow through the marrow.[136,137] These processes are responsible for the increase in marrow collagen types IV and V and laminin synthesized by endothelial cells in the marrow of patients.[126]

The fibroblastic proliferation in marrow is not an intrinsic part of the abnormal clonal expansion of hematopoiesis.[138] In cases of primary myelofibrosis in which G6PD isoenzyme studies or chromosome karyotyping establish monoclonal growth of hematopoietic cells, marrow fibroblasts contain both G6PD isoenzymes and do not share the clonal chromosome abnormality.[139] The findings strongly imply that the fibroblasts differentiate from a primordial cell different from the neoplastic hematopoietic stem cell in primary myelofibrosis and that fibroblast proliferation and enhanced collagen synthesis are secondary results of abnormal hematopoiesis.

EXTRAMEDULLARY HEMATOPOIESIS

Extramedullary hemopoiesis is almost always present in liver and spleen, where it contributes to organ enlargement.[8-10] Escape of progenitor cells from marrow and their lodgment in other organs contributes to extramedullary blood cell formation. Reversion of the liver and spleen to their fetal hematopoietic functions (metaplasia) is not a major factor in extramedullary hematopoiesis, and quantitatively significant, effective hematopoiesis does not occur outside of the marrow (see also "Extramedullary (Fibrohematopoietic) Tumors" below).

CLINICAL FEATURES

PRESENTING SYMPTOMS

Some patients are asymptomatic at the time of diagnosis; in which case the disease is detected by medical examination for an unrelated reason. In symptomatic patients, fatigue, weakness, shortness of breath, pruritus, and palpitations are nonspecific but frequent complaints.[9-13] Fatigue is the most frequent self-reported complaint and is disproportionate to the degree of anemia. Weight loss is common, but anorexia is less so, and fever and night sweats may occur. The term *constitutional symptoms*, often used in studies of the response to treatment of myelofibrosis, refers specifically to the aggregate occurrence of fever, weight loss, and night sweats.[140] A dragging sensation in the left upper abdomen caused by an enlarged spleen or early satiety from encroachment of the spleen on the stomach may occur. Severe left upper quadrant or left shoulder pain can occur from splenic infarction and perisplenitis. Patients may report unexpected bleeding. Occasionally, bone pain is prominent, especially in the lower extremities. Fever, weight loss, cachexia, night sweats, and bone pain are more frequent later in the course of the disease and are related to the increase in circulating inflammatory cytokines that are a key feature of the disease (see "Immune and Inflammatory Manifestations" below).

PRESENTING SIGNS

Hepatomegaly is detectable in two-thirds of patients, and splenomegaly is present on palpation or imaging studies in almost all patients at the time of diagnosis.[8-12] The spleen is mildly enlarged in one-fourth, moderately enlarged in half, and massively enlarged in approximately one-fourth of patients. Muscle wasting, peripheral edema, and purpura are present infrequently. Bone tenderness may be present. The latter signs may develop in a larger proportion of patients over the course of the disease.

Neutrophilic dermatosis, a syndrome that closely mimics the raised and tender plaques of Sweet syndrome, may occur.[141-143] It can be the presenting or a significant complicating feature, and can progress to bullae or pyoderma gangrenosum.[141,144] The dermatopathology of neutrophilic dermatosis is different from leukemia cutis and is unrelated to infection or vasculitis. The predominant histologic lesion is an intense polymorphonuclear neutrophilic infiltrate.

Skin infiltrates related to hematopoietic cells (leukemia cutis) are uncommon.[145] These cutaneous lesions may have myeloid cells with giant cells carrying CD61 markers characteristic of megakaryocytes.[146,147] Skin lesions representing cutaneous fibrohematopoietic tumors may occur.

SPECIAL CLINICAL FEATURES

Prefibrotic Primary Myelofibrosis

The presenting findings of the clonal myeloid diseases are changing because of more and earlier access to healthcare in industrialized countries (see Table 86–2). A subset of patients, perhaps as many as 25 percent, with primary myelofibrosis present without overt reticulin fibrosis in the marrow.[148,149] Blood hemoglobin may be normal and white cell count mildly elevated. The classic findings of frequent teardrop red cells, myelocytes, and nucleated red cells in the blood film and palpable splenomegaly often are absent. Thrombocytosis is a constant finding. Essential thrombocythemia is closely simulated, but observation eventually shows evolution to primary myelofibrosis. The most important distinction with essential thrombocythemia is the nature of the megakaryocytic expansion.[150] In primary myelofibrosis, bizarre changes are evident with wide variation in megakaryocyte size, from very small to giant

size cells. Nuclear lobulation is abnormal, with bulky multilobulation, hypolobulation, and free megakaryocyte nuclei in the marrow spaces. In essential thrombocythemia, megakaryocytes are increased but they do not display the dysmorphia observed in myelofibrosis. The prefibrotic disease usually evolves into fully developed myelofibrosis over a period of years. Investigators, evaluating histopathology in a blind fashion, have confirmed the entity of prefibrotic myelofibrosis and this abnormality predicts for progression to an overt primary myelofibrosis and, thus, has an impact on the risk of progression to acute leukemia and prognosis in general.[151]

Extramedullary (Fibrohematopoietic) Tumors

The appearance of symptoms or signs leading to (1) identification of a mass on imaging regardless of location, (2) appearance of signs or symptoms of an effusion in the thorax or abdomen, (3) unexpected neurologic signs, or (4) another finding that appears unexpected in a patient with primary myelofibrosis should be considered a fibrohematopoietic (extramedullary) tumor(s) until proven otherwise. Foci of hematopoiesis may become clinically apparent as fibrohematopoietic tumors in the adrenal glands,[152,153] renal parenchyma,[154-156] and lymph nodes.[157-159] Tumors composed of hematopoietic tissue, sometimes with intense fibrosis, can develop in the bowel,[160-163] breast,[164-166] liver,[167,168] lungs,[169-171] mediastinum,[172] pleura and mesentery,[169,171,173] skin,[174,175] synovium,[176] thymus,[169] thyroid,[177] thorax,[178] prostate,[179] spleen,[180] or urinary tract.[178,181-184]

Extramedullary hematopoiesis in the intracranial or intraspinal epidural space can lead to serious neurologic complications, including subdural hemorrhage,[185] delirium,[185,186] increased intracranial pressure,[187] orbital apex syndrome,[188] papilledema,[189] cerebral tumor,[190] coma,[191] motor and sensory impairment,[192,193] spinal cord compression,[194,195] and limb paralysis.[195,196] Intraspinal myelography,[193-199] computed axial tomography,[185,187,191-197,199] positron emission tomography after ^{52}Fe infusion,[186] and magnetic resonance imaging (MRI)[198,199] each has been used to define the location and nature of the masses.

Hematopoietic foci on serosal surfaces can produce effusions, sometimes massive, in the thorax,[178,180] abdomen,[172,173,201,202] and pericardial space.[203-206] The effusion fluid often contains megakaryocytes, immature granulocytes, and, occasionally, erythroblasts.[207-209] Splenectomy is sometimes followed by extramedullary hematopoietic tumors in soft tissues,[210] in body cavities, or on serosal surfaces,[209] perhaps as a result of an increase in circulating hematopoietic progenitors[211] and loss of the filtration function of the spleen. In rare cases, extramedullary soft-tissue megakaryoblastic tumors simulate the myeloid sarcoma (synonyms: chloroma, granulocytic sarcoma) of other types of myelogenous leukemia.[212,213]

Portal Hypertension and Varices and Pulmonary Arterial Hypertension

In patients with primary myelofibrosis, there can be a massive increase in splenoportal blood flow and a decrease in hepatic vascular compliance or the presence of hepatic vein thrombosis, either of which can result in severe portal hypertension, ascites, esophageal and gastric varices, intraluminal gastrointestinal bleeding, and hepatic encephalopathy.[214-216] The hepatic venous pressure gradient, normally less than 6 torr, is markedly elevated.[217]

Perisinusoidal fibrosis,[218-220] collagen bundles in the spaces of Disse,[219] perisinusoidal fibroplasia,[218-221] and foci of hematopoietic cells[219,222] appear to contribute to the decreased sinusoidal compliance. Portal vein thrombosis is a complication of primary myelofibrosis and occasionally precedes disease onset.[223]

Rarely, portal hypertension is accompanied by pulmonary hypertension and may result from pulmonary fibrosis[171] or hydrodynamic factors.[224] Pulmonary arterial hypertension, also, may be the principal problem.[225,226] Although as many as one-third of patients with primary myelofibrosis have an elevated systolic pulmonary artery pressures (>35 torr), the fraction that is symptomatic is very small. Elevated vascular endothelial growth factor (VEGF) levels, elevated circulating endothelial cells, and elevated marrow microvessel density in patients suggest that proangiogenic factors may contribute to the hypertension.[227] Contrariwise, secondary myelofibrosis with polyclonal hematopoiesis and normal blood CD34 cell concentrations frequently occurs in patients with primary pulmonary hypertension.[228]

Immune and Inflammatory Manifestations

Abnormalities of humoral immune mechanisms have been observed in up to half of patients with primary myelofibrosis.[229-234] The array of immune products and events reported includes anti–red cell antibodies,[233-237] antiplatelet antibodies,[238,239] antinuclear antibodies,[229,230,234] elevated plasma-soluble IL-2 receptor,[240] anti-Gal (galactoside determinants) antibodies,[241] anti-γ-globulins,[229,230,234] antiphospholipid antibodies,[234,242] antitissue or organ-specific antibodies,[231,233] and circulating immune complexes,[234,243-245] as well as complement activation,[234,246] immune complex deposition,[231] interstitial immunoglobulin deposition,[231] increased numbers of marrow plasmacytoid lymphocytes,[231,243] and development of amyloidosis.[244-247]

Inflammatory cytokines, including IL-1β, IL-6, IL-8, tumor necrosis factor (TNF)-α, TNF receptor II (TNFRII), and C-reactive protein also are markedly elevated and play a role in the constitutional symptoms seen in patients with progressive disease,[248] which explains the often rapid, symptomatic improvement in patients treated with JAK2 inhibitors before splenic size is reduced.

Occasional reports of nonclonal secondary myelofibrosis associated with lupus erythematosus,[249-254] vasculitis,[255] polyarteritis nodosa,[234,255] ulcerative colitis,[256] scleroderma,[257] biliary cirrhosis,[237,258,259] Sjögren syndrome,[260] and acute reversible myelofibrosis responsive to glucocorticoids,[261] although fundamentally different processes from primary myelofibrosis, have raised the possibility that immune mechanisms play a role in the development of marrow fibrosis in some circumstances.

Bone Changes

A large proportion of patients have osteosclerosis at diagnosis or develop osteosclerosis during the course of the disease,[11-15,262-265] as reflected by increased bone density on imaging studies and histomorphometric analysis of a bone biopsy (Table 86–3).[263-268] The proximal femur and humerus, pelvis, vertebrae, ribs, and skull may be involved. MRI can uncover evidence of new bone formation and periosteal thickening. Lumbar spine dual-energy x-ray absorption studies and quantitative computed tomography provide evidence for increased bone formation, bone thickening, and higher proportions of cancellous and of woven bone.[268,269] Osteolytic lesions are rare[270] and may reflect a myeloid sarcoma.[271] Periostitis, although infrequent, can lead to debilitating bone pain.[272]

Thrombosis

The risk of arterial and venous thrombosis is elevated in patients with primary myelofibrosis, although not to the degree seen in polycythemia vera or essential thrombocythemia.[273] Approximately 10 percent of patients with myelofibrosis will develop a significant thrombotic event during the first 4 years of the disease. The two principal risk factors are an elevated leukocyte count and age, but not platelet count.[274] In a large multicenter study of 707 patients with primary myelofibrosis, thromboses occurred in 7.2 percent of patients over the period of observation, or 1.8 percent patient-years. The combination of the JAK2 mutation, leukocytosis, and age predicted the highest incidence of thrombosis.[275]

TABLE 86–3. Serum, Urine, and Bone Changes Reflecting Osteosclerosis[243,244]

- Increased serum alkaline phosphatase
- Increased serum bone GLA-protein
- Increased serum carboxytelopeptidase
- Increased urinary deoxypyridinoline
- Increased bone density by dual-energy x-ray absorption
- Increased bone density by quantitative computed tomography
- Histomorphometry
  - Increased percentage of cancellous bone volume to tissue volume
  - Increased bone formation and resorption (high turnover)
  - Increased trabecular plate thickness
  - Increased percentage of woven bone volume
  - Increased percentage of fibrous area
- No evidence of mineralization defect

The cardiovascular risk factor, such as hypertension, hypercholesterolemia, or smoking, further increase thrombotic risk. Multiple thrombotic episodes may occur; and, the thrombotic event may occur at or just before diagnosis.

Noncirrhotic splanchnic vein thrombosis includes hepatic vein thrombosis (Budd-Chiari syndrome) and portal vein thrombosis, which may occur with minimal evidence of a clonal myeloproliferative disease. In the past marrow examination or evidence of erythropoietin-independent colony growth was used to determine if an occult or incipient myeloproliferative disease may underlie the thrombosis. Now JAK2 mutational analysis can be done and is positive in 35 percent of seemingly idiopathic hepatic vein thrombosis and 25 percent seemingly idiopathic portal vein thrombosis.[276] Presumably, future use of CALR gene mutational analysis will increase the proportion of cases of hepatic vein thrombosis indicative of an underlying occult myeloproliferative disease.

● LABORATORY FEATURES

BLOOD CELL COUNTS AND MORPHOLOGY

The range of values for blood cell counts at the time of diagnosis is very broad. Normocytic–normochromic anemia is present in most, but not all, patients (see Table 86–2).[8-10,273-280] Mean hemoglobin concentration in a series of patients at diagnosis was approximately 9 to 12 g/dL (range: 4–20 g/dL).[8-16,279,280] Anisocytosis and poikilocytosis are a constant finding. In all cases, teardrop-shaped red cells (dacryocytes) are present in sufficient number to be found in every oil immersion field (see Fig. 86–1). Nucleated red cells are present in the blood film of most patients and average 2 percent of nucleated cells (range: 0 to 30 percent). The percentage of reticulocytes is mildly increased but may vary widely in a given case. A decreased blood hemoglobin may be attributed in part to the expansion of plasma volume and a higher than normal proportion of the red cell volume in an enlarged spleen. Ineffective erythropoiesis can result in a decrease in red cell mass.[277] Erythroid hypoplasia is present in many patients.[281,282] In some patients, hemolysis may be prominent, and polychromatophilia and very elevated reticulocyte counts can occur.[278,279] The antiglobulin (Coombs) test usually is negative, but red cell autoantibodies can develop and lead to immune-mediated hemolysis,[234-236,283] which rarely has been a presenting finding of the disease.[236] Occasional patients have had a positive acid hemolysis and sucrose hemolysis test, reflecting a concurrent clone of cells consistent with paroxysmal nocturnal hemoglobinuria.[284] Acquired hemoglobin H disease, coincident with typical white cells and platelet changes of myelofibrosis, can occur[285] and results in hemolysis, hypochromic–microcytic red cells, marked poikilocytosis, and hemoglobin H inclusions that stain with brilliant cresyl blue. Red cell aplasia, in association with primary myelofibrosis, has been observed.[280,286]

The total white cell count usually is usually moderately elevated as a result of granulocytosis.[8-16] The mean total blood white cell count was 10,000 to 14,000/µL (10 to 14 × 10⁹/L) in four large studies. Neutropenia, however, is present in approximately 20 percent of patients at the time of diagnosis.[8-16] The range of white cell counts was 400 to 237,000/µL (0.4 to 237.0 × 10⁹/L) at the time of diagnosis.[8-15,278,279] Myelocytes and promyelocytes are present in small proportions in the blood film in most patients, and a low proportion of blast cells (0.5 to 2.0 percent) may be found in the blood film. The blood blast cells range from 0 to 20 percent at the time of diagnosis. In patients with blast counts at the high end, which is unusual at presentation, the disease merges with or may progress rapidly to AML. Hypersegmentation, hyposegmentation (acquired Pelger-Huët anomaly), and abnormal granulation of neutrophils may be present.[8-16] Neutrophil alkaline phosphatase scores may be elevated (25 percent of patients) or decreased (25 percent of patients).[287] The percentage of basophils may be slightly increased.[279] The mean platelet count in patient series ranges from 175,000 to 580,000/µL (175 to 580 × 10⁹/L) at the time of diagnosis. Individual platelet counts can range from 15,000 to 3,215,000/µL (15 to 3215 × 10⁹/L).[8-16,278,279] The platelet count is elevated above the normal upper limit in approximately 40 percent of patients.[279] Mild to moderate thrombocytopenia is present in approximately one-third of patients at the time of diagnosis, particularly if splenomegaly is massive. Giant platelets and abnormal platelet granulation in the blood film are characteristic features of the disease.

Approximately 10 percent of patients present with pancytopenia because of severe impairment of hematopoiesis affecting each cell lineage, coupled with sequestration in a massively enlarged spleen. Pancytopenia usually is associated with intense marrow fibrosis.

Increased concentrations of multipotential,[288,289] granulocytic,[290,291] monocytic,[291] erythroid,[292] and megakaryocytic[293] progenitor cells are present in the blood of patients, as measured by clonogenic assays in semisolid cultures. The frequency of hematopoietic progenitor cells in the blood is correlated with the extent of marrow reticular fiber density.[293] Megakaryocytes also are present in the systemic venous blood.[294] An increase in blood CD34+ cells is very characteristic of primary myelofibrosis, and the concentration of these cells lends weight to the diagnosis. The height of the CD34+ cell count is correlated with the extent of disease and disease progression. Greater than 15 × 10⁶/L blood CD34+ cells is virtually diagnostic of primary myelofibrosis, and patients with greater than 300 × 10⁶/L CD34+ cells have more rapid progression of disease than patients with fewer CD34+ cells.[289]

Endothelial progenitor cells (CD34+CD133+ and VEGF receptor 2–positive cells) are significantly higher in the blood of primary myelofibrosis patients than of normal subjects.[89]

Mild lymphocytopenia resulting from decreased CD3+, CD4+, CD8+, and CD3–/CD56+ T cells is the rule.[295]

FUNCTIONAL ABNORMALITIES OF BLOOD CELLS

The neutrophils of some patients have impaired phagocytosis, oxygen consumption, nitroblue tetrazolium reduction, and hydrogen peroxide generation, and decreased myeloperoxidase[296,297] and glutathione reductase activities.[297] CD34+ cells have impaired *in vitro* differentiation to

natural killer cells, which appears to be related to a dysregulation in control of IL-15.[298]

Bleeding time can be prolonged disproportionately to the platelet count.[299,300] Platelet abnormalities include impaired aggregation in response to epinephrine, depletion of dense granule adenosine diphosphate content,[301] decreased platelet lipoxygenase pathway activity,[302] and others.[303,304] The correlation of bleeding or thrombosis with platelet functional abnormalities is weak.[303,304] The lupus anticoagulant has been present, rarely.[242]

MARROW EXAMINATION

Morphology

In the fibrotic phase, marrow aspiration often is unsuccessful because of the fibrosis.[8-16,96,97] The marrow biopsy specimen usually is cellular and shows granulocytic and megakaryocytic hyperplasia (see Fig. 86–1).[8-16,288,289] Erythroid cells may be decreased, normal, or increased in number. Silver stain usually shows an increase in reticular fibers, and in half of patients a striking increase in reticular fibers is seen.[289] Hematoxylin and eosin stains of the biopsy specimen may show mild collagen fibrosis; occasionally the fibrosis is extreme (see Fig. 86–1). Collagen fibrosis may be more evident using a Gomori trichrome stain with which collagen characteristically stains green. In intensely fibrotic marrows, cellularity may be markedly decreased but megakaryocytes usually remain evident.[289] Giant megakaryocytes and micromegakaryocytes, abnormal nuclear lobulation, and naked megakaryocyte nuclei are present.[8-16,305] Thrombopoietin receptors are decreased on megakaryocytes and platelets.[93] Granulocytes may show hyperlobulation and hypolobulation of the nucleus, acquired Pelger-Huët anomaly, nuclear blebs, and nuclear–cytoplasmic maturation asynchrony.[306] Clusters of blasts and CD34+ cells are often present. Dilated marrow sinusoids are common. Intrasinusoidal, immature hematopoietic cells, and megakaryocytes are present.[98] As a reflection of the high blood flow to marrow-bearing bone and the widened sinusoidal system, microvessel density is significantly increased in approximately 70 percent of patients.[306,307] Histomorphometric analysis of marrow biopsies permit detection of osteosclerosis.[263,265,266] Grading of the degree of myelofibrosis has used the Bauermeister scale,[308] which assesses fibrosis on a scale of 0 to 4, and the revised European grading scale of 0 to 3.[309] Digital imaging may be used for less subjective, quantitative grading of fibrosis or osteosclerosis, if its utility is confirmed in additional studies.[310]

The marrow in the prefibrotic stage usually has no or slight reticular fibrosis. The marrow is cellular and there is often an increase proportion of late neutrophil precursors (myelocytes, metamyelocytes, bands). Myeloblasts and CD34+ cells are inconspicuous. Erythropoiesis may be slightly decreased. Increased and abnormal megakaryocytopoiesis is the hallmark of this phase. Clusters of megakaryocytes are present. Megakaryocytes are large and admixed with small megakaryocytes. Nuclei are often ballooned and have scalloped margins. Bare megakaryocyte nuclei are present. Megakaryocyte involvement is facilitated by staining the marrow with a megakaryocyte marker such as CD61.

Cytogenetic Findings

Chromosome abnormalities of hematopoietic cells are evident in approximately 40 percent of patients at the time of diagnosis.[311-316] The most frequent findings are partial trisomy 1q, interstitial deletion of a segment of the long arm of chromosome 13, del(13)(q12–22), which bears the retinoblastoma gene,[312-314,317] del 20q, and trisomy 8.[318] Involvement of chromosome 5, 6, 7, 9, 13, 20, or 21 occurs with heightened frequency.[318] The 5q– abnormality is more prevalent in primary myelofibrosis than any other chronic myeloproliferative disorder. Abnormality of chromosome 12 resulting from several translocations or deletion or inversion occurs in approximately 3 percent of patients.[301] The del(13) and der(6)t(1;6)(q21–23;p21.3) are associated with myelofibrosis but are not exclusively seen in patients with primary myelofibrosis.[320] Aneuploidy as a result of monosomy or trisomy is common. Pseudodiploidy, manifested by partial deletions and translocations, occurs. Patients with the clinical features of typical primary myelofibrosis very rarely have the Philadelphia (Ph) chromosome in their marrow cells.[321] Approximately 15 percent of patients present with unfavorable karyotypes, including three or more abnormalities, +9, –7/7q–, 5/5q–, i(17q), inv(3), 12p–, or 11q23. An unfavorable karyotype is associated with a sixfold greater risk of acute leukemic transformation than a favorable karyotype.[322] With increasing knowledge of the chromosomes commonly affected, interphase FISH of blood cells is used to look for prevalent abnormalities, compensating for the technical difficulties of harvesting cell suspensions, given the intense marrow fibrosis.[314] Clonal chromosomal abnormalities found in hematopoietic cells have not been observed in marrow fibroblasts.[139]

Magnetic Resonance Imaging

Marrow fibrosis alters the hyperintensity of T1-weighted images that normally results from marrow fat. As cellularity and fibrosis progress, hypointensity of T1-weighted and T2-weighted images develops. MRI does not distinguish between primary myelofibrosis and secondary causes of fibrosis,[264,323,324] but the clinical distinctions usually are very evident from the results of prior physical, blood, and marrow examinations and the evidence for mutations in *JAK2*, *CALR*, or *MPL*. Patchy or diffuse osteosclerosis is a common finding, as are "sandwich vertebrae," so called because of marked radiodensity of superior and inferior margins of the vertebral body. MRI can identify the uncommon periosteal reactions that usually occur in the distal femur, proximal tibia, or ankle. The reactions represent expansion of marrow cellularity into normally inactive regions of long bones or extramedullary space-occupying lesions of fibrohematopoietic tissue.[264] The findings of sodium fluoride (^{18}F) positron emission tomography can be virtually specific for osteosclerosis of primary myelofibrosis.[325]

PLASMA AND URINE CHEMICAL CHANGES

Serum levels of uric acid, lactic dehydrogenase, bilirubin, alkaline phosphatase, and high-density lipoprotein frequently are elevated.[8–16] Serum cholesterol is often decreased and is a negative prognostic factor.[326–328] Serum levels of albumin and cholesterol frequently are decreased.[329] Hypocalcemia[330] or hypercalcemia[331] may occur. Plasma levels of thrombopoietin and IL-6 are elevated but do not correlate with either platelet or megakaryocyte mass.[332,333] Elevated thrombopoietin is not explained by increased marrow hematopoietic or stromal cell production.[334] Serum-soluble IL-2 receptor[335] and serum VEGF[336] levels are increased. Urinary excretion of calmodulin is approximately three times normal.[130] The serum contains evidence of increased collagen (see Table 86–1) and bone (see Table 86–2) synthesis.

● DIFFERENTIAL DIAGNOSIS

CML (Chap. 89) should be considered in the differential diagnosis of primary myelofibrosis. In CML, the white cell count is usually greater than 30,000/μL (30 × 10^9/L) in almost all patients and greater than 100,000/μL (100 × 10^9/L) in half of patients. In myelofibrosis, the white cell count usually is less than 30,000/μL (30 × 10^9/L) at the time of diagnosis. In CML, red cell shape usually is normal or slightly perturbed. In myelofibrosis, teardrop poikilocytes are present in every oil immersion field and exaggerated anisocytosis and anisochromia are often prominent. The marrow in CML shows intense granulocytic hyperplasia, with

almost 100 percent cellularity and usually no or very slight fibrosis.[337] In myelofibrosis, the marrow has mildly increased cellularity or is hypocellular, with moderate to marked reticulin fibrosis. Occasionally, patients with CML develop intense marrow fibrosis and dysmorphic blood cell changes that make distinction between the two diseases difficult on merely morphological grounds.[319] However, the Ph chromosome or the *BCR-ABL* fusion gene is present in CML and is absent in primary myelofibrosis; whereas, the *JAK2*^{V617F} or the *CALR*, or the *MPL* mutation is present in approximately 90 percent of cases of primary myelofibrosis and absent in CML. Most cases are readily separable based on the aforementioned distinctions.

Patients with primary myelofibrosis may have pancytopenia or bicytopenia and in that respect mimic patients with oligoblastic myelogenous leukemia (myelodysplasia [MDS]; Chap. 87). Contrariwise, patients with oligoblastic leukemia rarely have intense fibrosis.[338] Prominent splenomegaly is expected in patients with primary myelofibrosis but not in patients with oligoblastic myelogenous leukemia, which helps to distinguish the former from the latter patients. The absence of a high frequency of teardrop-shaped red cells, nucleated red cells, and striking anisopoikilocytosis in the blood film mitigates against primary myelofibrosis.

Because some patients with primary myelofibrosis have platelet counts greater than 450,000/μL (450 × 10^9/L), the diagnosis of primary thrombocythemia may be considered. Moreover, some patients may be in transition from thrombocythemia to myelofibrosis. The anisopoikilocytosis, nucleated red cells, and myeloid immaturity in the blood film characteristic of myelofibrosis are not present in patients with thrombocythemia. Marrow fibrosis usually is insignificant in thrombocythemia, and splenic enlargement often is absent or slight. For these reasons, a clear distinction usually exists between the two disorders.[279,339] The prefibrotic phase of primary myelofibrosis may mimic essential thrombocythemia, but the more prominent splenomegaly and the more disordered and characteristic dysmorphic megakaryopoiesis in primary myelofibrosis can be used to distinguish the two entities by an experienced hematopathologist.[340] Careful observation of disease evolution is, also, important.[341]

Hairy cell leukemia (Chap. 93), when associated with shape abnormalities of red cells, pancytopenia, splenomegaly, and fibrotic marrow, can closely mimic primary myelofibrosis.[336,342] Usually, careful scrutiny of the blood and marrow by microscopy, histochemistry, and cell immunophenotype shows evidence of the abnormal mononuclear (hairy) cells characteristic of the disease.

Hepatic disease can be associated with cytopenias and splenomegaly, although the specific blood and marrow findings usually make the distinction with primary myelofibrosis obvious. In a review of 170 cases of splenomegaly in a county hospital, hepatic disease was the second most common cause of massive splenomegaly after primary myelofibrosis.[343]

Primary autoimmune myelofibrosis is characterized by intense marrow fibrosis and an increase in marrow polyclonal T and B lymphocytes.[344,345] Serologic or clinical evidence of lupus erythematosus or other connective tissue diseases is absent, giving primary autoimmune myelofibrosis a definitive diagnostic niche. Cytopenias that occur may be immune mediated (e.g., immune hemolytic disease), and the blood cell findings (anisopoikilocytosis, nucleated red cells, myeloid immaturity) characteristic of primary myelofibrosis usually are absent. The marrow may be cellular with increased megakaryocytes, but strikingly dysmorphic megakaryocytopoiesis is absent. Splenomegaly, a nearly constant feature of primary myelofibrosis, usually is absent. Polyclonal hyperglobulinemia may be present.

Patients with sporadic idiopathic or familial pulmonary hypertension have significant marrow fibrosis. They can be distinguished from patients with primary myelofibrosis with pulmonary hypertension by the latter's high-circulating CD34+ cell count, the presence of clonal platelets and granulocytes, a high frequency of dacryocytes in the blood film, and a *JAK2*[V617F] mutation.[346]

Metastatic carcinoma, especially derived from carcinoma of breast or prostate[347-352] or disseminated mycobacterial infection,[353,354] can induce reactive marrow fibrosis and occasionally simulate primary myelofibrosis. Demonstration of metastatic carcinoma cells or mycobacteria in the marrow indicates the etiology. Other disorders reported with secondary myelofibrosis include mastocytosis,[355-358] angioimmunoblastic lymphadenopathy,[359] angiosarcoma,[360] lymphoma,[361-363] multiple myeloma,[364-366] renal osteodystrophy,[367] hypertrophic osteoarthropathy,[368] gray platelet syndrome,[369] systemic lupus erythematosus,[251-254] polyarteritis nodosa,[256] hypereosinophilic syndrome,[370,371] kala azar,[372] primary thrombocytopenic purpura,[373] thrombotic thrombocytopenic purpura,[374] tretinoin administration,[375] neuroblastoma,[376] giant lymph node hyperplasia,[377] vitamin D-deficiency rickets,[378-381] Langerhans cell histiocytosis,[382] acute promyelocytic leukemia,[383,384] and malignant histiocytosis.[385] Correction or amelioration of the primary disorder can lead to disappearance of the marrow fibrosis.

Lymphoma,[386,387] chronic lymphocytic leukemia,[388,389] hairy cell leukemia,[342,390] systemic mastocytosis,[391] macroglobulinemia,[392] amyloidosis,[244,245] myeloma,[393,394] malignant teratoma,[395] and essential monoclonal gammopathy[396] can coincide with primary myelofibrosis.

● TRANSITIONS TO AND FROM MYELOFIBROSIS AMONG CLONAL HEMOPATHIES

All clonal hematopoietic diseases (AML, CML, oligoblastic myelogenous leukemia [MDS], lymphomas) may have increased marrow reticulin fibers but only infrequently have collagen fibrosis.[397] Acute megakaryoblastic leukemia is accompanied by intense marrow fibrosis (Chap. 88). Approximately 15 percent of patients with polycythemia vera, whether treated by phlebotomy, alkylating agents, or ^{32}P, develop a clinical state indistinguishable from primary myelofibrosis during 20 years of observation (Chap. 84).[398-400] Essential thrombocythemia may evolve into a myelofibrotic stage, estimated to occur in approximately 7 percent of cases (Chap. 85). This estimate is complicated by the question of whether some cases of essential thrombocythemia actually were distinguished as early (prefibrotic) primary myelofibrosis.[340,341] Sideroblastic anemia has progressed to primary myelofibrosis.[401] Rarely, primary myelofibrosis reverts to polycythemia vera, with disappearance of marrow fibrosis.[402,403] Even more rarely, primary myelofibrosis, carrying the *JAK2* mutation, has undergone clonal evolution to BCR-ABL–positive CML or vice versa.[404,405]

● THERAPY

DECISION TO TREAT

A proportion of asymptomatic patients remains stable for years and they do not require specific treatment. Constitutional symptoms, anemia, thrombocytopenia, and splenomegaly are the principal initial reasons for therapy. A hemoglobin less than 10 g/dL,[12,14,20] a white count less than 4000/μL (4.0 × 10[9]/L) or greater than 30,000/μL (30.0 × 10[9]/L),[13] a platelet count under 100,000/μL (100 × 10[9]/L), and blood blasts above 1 percent of total leukocytes[12,20,406] predict more rapid progression of disease. In addition, patients may have a loss of sense of well-being, fatigue, night sweats, loss of weight, low-grade fever, and loss of functionality as a result of the accompanying elaboration of inflammatory cytokines.

Staging protocols may be useful in comparing concurrent and sequential clinical trial results (see "Course and Prognosis" below). In an individual patient under the care of a clinician experienced in the disease, following the disease for evidence of progression is a very important additional factor in determining the timing of treatment, even in patients deemed at higher risk by formulaic techniques, especially before introducing allogeneic stem cell transplantation with its morbidity and potential mortality in this age group.

RED CELL TRANSFUSION

Patients with severe anemia or with moderate but symptomatic anemia may require periodic red cell transfusions (Chap. 138). Alternative mechanisms for raising the blood hemoglobin concentration include use of recombinant erythropoietin and androgen therapy.

RECOMBINANT HUMAN ERYTHROPOIETIN FOR ANEMIA

Serum erythropoietin levels usually are appropriate to the severity of anemia in patients with myelofibrosis.[407] Thus, use of erythropoietin for anemia is, usually, disappointing. In some studies, patients selected by their inappropriately low serum erythropoietin levels (<125 U/L) for the degree of anemia, beneficial effects can result.[408,409]

ANDROGENS AND GLUCOCORTICOIDS FOR ANEMIA

Severe anemia may improve with androgen therapy in some patients.[410] Testosterone, oxymetholone, and fluoxymesterone have been used but have virilizing effects. In addition, they have the potential for hepatic injury and other side effects. Danazol, 600 to 800 mg/day orally for up to 6 months, can be used. The drug is tapered to the minimum effective dose or discontinued if no significant response occurs. Improvement may be limited to a decreased frequency of red cell transfusion. Androgens often are used after splenectomy if anemia returns and requires transfusion of red cells. They are more effective in splenectomized patients or those with less splenic enlargement. Patients undergoing androgen therapy should have periodic assessment of liver size by physical examination, measurement of liver function tests, and, if appropriate, ultrasonographic imaging to detect liver injury (e.g., peliosis) or tumors.[411] Evaluation of male patients for prostatic enlargement or cancer is prudent before starting androgen therapy. Patients with significant hemolytic anemia may benefit from glucocorticoid therapy. Prednisone 25 mg/m[2] per day orally can be tried. If tolerated, the dose can be continued for 1 to 2 months and then tapered gradually. In children, high-dose glucocorticoid therapy can ameliorate marrow fibrosis and improves hematopoiesis.[412,413]

DRUG THERAPY FOR MYELOPROLIFERATION, SPLENOMEGALY, OR CYTOPENIAS

A variety of drugs have been used for treatment of massive splenomegaly, thrombocytosis, or constitutional symptoms.

JAK2[V617F] *Kinase Inhibitors*

Because *JAK2* mutations and the resulting effects on JAK-STAT signaling are thought to be a key factor in the clonal expansion leading to primary myelofibrosis in at least 50 percent of patients, an effort to synthesize and test inhibitors of the mutant JAK2 protein product were conducted.[414] Early studies of the JAK2 kinase inhibitor TG101209, an oral, bioavailable small molecule, and a potent inhibitor of JAK2 kinase, showed its ability to inhibit *JAK2*[V617F]-dependent phosphorylation of

STAT3 and STAT5, inhibit colony growth of cells harboring *JAK2* and *MPL* mutations, and to have therapeutic effects in a nude mouse model of *JAK2*[V617F]-induced myeloproliferative disease.[415] The effects of several JAK2 inhibitors have been described.[416–418] Although their effects are somewhat different, the most striking and consistent effect with each agent is a decrease in spleen size and reversal of constitutional symptoms. They often suppress blood cell counts, and thrombocytopenia can be dose-limiting. At least initially, the anemia worsens although this laboratory deterioration may be transient, lasting only for few months. Typically, in spite of progression of anemia, most treated patients report decreased fatigue. The reduction in large spleen size and the improvement in the quality of life of many patients have been dramatic and were similar in those with and without a *JAK2* mutation. This effect may be explained by the drug's ability to inhibit JAK1 and JAK2 isoforms, the former having a role in cytokine elaboration. These agents may decrease morbidity and mortality, prolonging survival (see "Course and Prognosis" below).[419–423]

In 2011, ruxolitinib, an oral JAK2 inhibitor, was approved by the FDA for use in patients with intermediate or high-risk myelofibrosis. It decreases spleen size, fatigue, night sweats, pruritus, and red cell transfusion requirements, and can result in weight gain in a significant proportion of patients. The principal dose-limiting side effect is a decreased platelet count. Although some patients may have worsened anemia or neutropenia, the net effect often was beneficial, with improvement in fatigue and other symptoms. Headache, dizziness, and diarrhea also may occur but are usually manageable without discontinuing the drug. After 6 months of treatment approximately 40 percent of treated patients have a significant decrease in spleen size and constitutional symptoms. The initial drug trials were limited to patients with a platelet count at the initiation of ruxolitinib therapy of 100×10^9/L; however, newer studies using lower starting doses of ruxolitinib and gradually incrementing those doses have indicated that patients with platelet counts of between 50 and 100×10^9/L may receive similar benefits from carefully incremented drug doses. Table 86–4 shows a suggested approach to initial dosage. Of all available therapeutic modalities for primary myelofibrosis, ruxolitinib is the only therapy that has shown benefit in clinical trials that included a comparison group given a placebo.

Hydroxyurea

Hydroxyurea is a commonly used agent for exaggerated accumulation of platelets, occasional very high leukocyte counts, troublesome areas of extramedullary hematopoiesis, and symptomatic splenomegaly.[424–426]

Hydroxyurea can, inconsistently, decrease the size of the spleen and liver, decrease or eliminate constitutional symptoms of night sweats or weight loss, and occasionally lead to an increase in hemoglobin concentration, a decrease of platelet counts, and a decrease in the degree of marrow fibrosis. Patients with myelofibrosis often do not have the marrow tolerance to chemotherapy of patients with other chronic myeloproliferative diseases. Hydroxyurea can be administered in doses of 0.5 to 1.0 g/day or 1 to 2 g orally two to three times per week, depending on the level of pretreatment blood cell counts. Patients should be evaluated for dose adjustment at least every week for 1 month and, if appropriate, eventually extended to evaluation every 3 months. Although alkylating agents, especially busulfan and other cytotoxic agents, have been used successfully, they have largely been replaced by hydroxyurea. Use of alkylating agents has resurfaced with the suggestion that melphalan or busulfan may be useful as therapy.[427,428]

Thalidomide and Lenalidomide

Thalidomide is poorly tolerated at optimal doses of approximately 800 mg/day. Most patients receive about half that amount and are tapered to the lowest effective dose. One study of 14 patients found the drug was not beneficial and had high toxicity rates.[429] Other studies found some decrease in spleen size and improvement in blood hemoglobin and platelet counts in a minority of patients receiving up to 600 mg/day.[430,431] In subsequent studies, lower doses of thalidomide (50 mg/day) coupled with prednisone were more tolerable and resulted in improvement of anemia and thrombocytopenia in about half of patients, with sustained improvement in some patients after treatment was stopped.[432] The thalidomide congener lenalidomide may supersede thalidomide use. Lenalidomide has provided responses in a significant minority of patients.[433–436] The drug can result in marked improvement in hemoglobin concentration or avoidance of a requirement for transfusion (22 percent of patients treated), improvement in platelet count (50 percent of patients treated), and decrease in spleen size (33 percent of patients treated). Neutropenia and thrombocytopenia were the most troubling side effects.[433] The drug has also been useful in patients with primary myelofibrosis who have a 5q– cytogenetic abnormality.[435,436] Another thalidomide congener, pomalidomide, has completed a phase 3 trial and has not been shown to decrease transfusion requirements.[437]

Cyclosporine, Etanercept, Imatinib Mesylate, and Tipifarnib

Cyclosporine has been used to achieve a serum level of 100 to 200 ng/mL in severely anemic patients with evidence of immune abnormalities (positive Coombs test, antinuclear antibodies).[438] Three of six patients responded with an increased hemoglobin concentration. Cyclosporine has been used with apparent success in a single patient with myelofibrosis and red cell aplasia.[439]

TNF-α has been proposed as a target to inhibit its possible effects in the pathogenesis of primary myelofibrosis.[440] Of 20 patients treated with soluble TNF-α receptor (etanercept), 12 had improvement in constitutional symptoms (fever, night sweats, fatigue, weight loss), and four had improved blood counts and decreased spleen size.[441,442]

Imatinib mesylate for treatment of myelofibrosis has been examined on empirical grounds and has been largely ineffective in influencing the disease course.[442,443] Modest doses have not been well tolerated, and responses have been infrequent and insubstantial.

The farnesyl transferase inhibitor tipifarnib is not well tolerated.[444] Although it may decrease spleen size, it has shown no advantages over hydroxyurea.

Interferons

Interferon-α and interferon-γ act synergistically to inhibit myeloproliferation.[445] Interferon-α has been used extensively for treatment of CML

TABLE 86–4. Guideline for Initial Oral Ruxolitinib Dose in Primary Myelofibrosis

Platelet Count	Dose
>200 × 10⁹/L	20 mg twice daily
100–200 × 10⁹/L	15 mg twice daily
50–100 × 10⁹/L	5 mg twice daily (increasing each month by 5 mg daily until maximal splenic size reduction, only if platelet count stays above 40 × 10⁹/L)*

*Drug not FDA approved for starting platelet counts of 50 to 100 × 10⁹/L.

If platelet count decreases while on ruxolitinib therapy, dose reduction should be made in relation to level of platelet count. The drug should not be administered if platelet counts falls to less than 50 × 10⁹/L. Therapists should consult more detailed guidelines, *Prescribing Information*, published by Incyte, for use of ruxolitinib (Jakafi) (revised November 2011).

prior to the availability of mutant tyrosine kinase (BCR-ABL) inhibitors (Chap. 89). Interferon-α has not been used extensively in primary myelofibrosis, but has been useful for treatment of splenic enlargement, bone pain, and thrombocytosis in select patients.[446] Trials comparing interferon therapy with hydroxyurea or other therapy have not been reported.[447] Hydroxyurea is easier to use (oral versus parenteral) and has less-frequent and less-severe side effects than interferon, especially in older patients. A polyethylene glycol conjugated interferon-α preparation may prove more practical and tolerable for use in patients with myelofibrosis. Although largely ineffective in later stages of myelofibrosis, it has shown efficacy in the early myeloproliferative stage of primary myelofibrosis with mild to moderate marrow fibrosis.[448–451]

Serosal Implants

Cytarabine Ascites resulting from peritoneal hematopoietic implants has been treated with intraperitoneal cytarabine.[452] Intrasplenic cytarabine administered via a splenic artery catheter has resulted in significant improvement in a patient (see also "Radiotherapy" below).[453]

IMMUNE-RELATED FIBROSIS

Intravenous Immunoglobulin

Although autoimmune or systemic lupus erythematosus-related myelofibrosis has responded to glucocorticoids or intravenous immune globulin[251,254] and a variety of other fibrotic disorders occasionally respond,[454] primary myelofibrosis does not have a sustained response to such therapy because the fundamental lesion is the hematopoietic multipotential cell neoplasm, neoplastic megakaryocytosis, severe megakaryocytic dysmorphia, and cytokine release with resultant fibrogenesis and, sometimes, osteogenesis.

BISPHOSPHONATES FOR BONE DISEASE

Debilitating bone pain can be a vexing problem in some patients with osteosclerosis and periostitis. Dramatic improvement in bone pain and hematopoiesis after etidronate 6 mg/kg per day on alternate months[455] or clodronate 30 mg/kg per day for several months, during which marked improvement was still present 33 months later,[456] highlight the potential usefulness of this family of drugs for bone symptoms.[457]

RADIOTHERAPY

Radiotherapy can be useful for patients with primary myelofibrosis in several situations. For example, in the presence of severe splenic pain (splenic infarctions) or massive splenic enlargement with contraindication to splenectomy (e.g., thrombocytosis), repeated doses of 0.5 to 2.0 Gy to the spleen can ameliorate the pain.[458] Splenic radiation can result in further cytopenias or worsening cytopenias, especially thrombocytopenia, referred to as an abscopal effect on marrow production, perhaps because of the circulation of large numbers of CD34+ cells exposed in the spleen. Other situations in which radiation may be useful are ascites resulting from myeloid metaplasia of the peritoneum,[459] focal areas of severe bone pain (periostitis or the osteolysis of a myeloid sarcoma),[272,458,460] and extramedullary fibrohematopoietic tumors,[157,458] especially of the epidural space.[191] Low-dose radiation to the liver for symptomatic hepatomegaly and ascites provides only short-term relief.[458,461] Low-dose radiotherapy to the lung has been used successfully to palliate the effects of pulmonary hypertension thought to result from extensive extramedullary hematopoiesis in the organ. Low-dose radiotherapy has relieved signs of respiratory insufficiency, especially hypoxemia,[226] but in several unreported instances known to the authors, this approach has led to deterioration of pulmonary function.

SPLENECTOMY

Splenectomy has been important in the management of primary myelofibrosis.[462] The major indications for splenectomy include (1) painful enlarged spleen (~50 percent of patients), (2) excessive transfusion requirements or refractory hemolytic anemia (~25 percent of patients), (3) portal hypertension (~15 percent of patients), and (4) severe thrombocytopenia (~10 percent of patients).

Patients who have a prolonged bleeding time or coagulation times are at serious risk for hemorrhage with surgery and should not undergo the procedure unless the abnormalities can be corrected by platelet transfusion and factor replacement therapy. Evidence of low-grade intravascular coagulation, such as elevated D-dimer levels, may require prophylactic heparin therapy and platelet transfusion should excessive bleeding occur.

Removal of the spleen in patients with primary myelofibrosis may be difficult. Usually the spleen is adherent to neighboring serosal surfaces and structures (e.g., inferior surface of left hemidiaphragm) and has numerous collateral vessels and very dilated splenoportal arteries and veins. Immediate postoperative mortality is a function of surgical experience and skill and of the rapidity of recognition of postoperative complications. In experienced hands, perioperative mortality is approximately 10 percent. Postoperative morbidity from hemorrhage, subphrenic hematoma, subphrenic abscess, injury to the tail of the pancreas, pancreatic fistulas, or portal vein stump or mesenteric vessel thrombosis occurs in approximately 30 percent of patients. Infection, especially, pneumonia occurs in approximately 10 percent of patients. Later postoperative changes include liver enlargement (sometimes massive), extramedullary hematopoietic tumors, thrombocytosis, and a decrease in teardrop-shaped red cells. Leukemic blast transformation occurs in approximately 15 percent of patients after splenectomy. Hydroxyurea or aspirin and anagrelide may be useful for exaggerated thrombocytosis (Chap. 85). The morbidity and mortality from splenectomy and the modest extension of life have led to increasing conservatism regarding its use. However, splenectomy can improve the condition for which it was performed in approximately 50 percent of patients. Median survival after splenectomy has been approximately 18 months.

PORTAL-SYSTEMIC VASCULAR SHUNT SURGERY

Circulatory dynamic studies are performed at the time of surgery in patients undergoing operation for portal hypertension and bleeding varices or refractory ascites. In patients in whom the hepatic wedge pressure elevations result from markedly increased blood flow from the spleen to the liver, the preferred treatment procedure for portal hypertension is splenectomy. In patients who have portal hypertension resulting from intrahepatic block or hepatic vein thrombosis and who have a hepatic venous pressure gradient well above the upper limits of normal (6 torr), a splenorenal shunt can be performed[463] or, to avoid abdominal surgery, a transjugular intrahepatic portosystemic shunt can be used.[464,465] Variceal sclerotherapy or variceal ligation has been used to treat bleeding varices resulting from portal hypertension.

HEMATOPOIETIC STEM CELL TRANSPLANTATION

Marrow transplantation is the only curative approach to primary myelofibrosis. Marrow transplantation therapy has been used increasingly in younger patients with a poor prognosis (e.g., severe anemia and leukopenia or exaggerated leukocytosis) who have a histocompatible sibling.[466–473] The median age in most studies is approximately 50 years, whereas the median age of all patients is approximately 70 years.[322]

Patients engraft at a rate similar to the rate of patients with hematologic diseases without marrow fibrosis (Chap. 23). The decision to use full-conditioning allogeneic transplantation is a function of the patient's age (<50 years), the severity of the blood cell and marrow abnormalities, and the likelihood of a protracted indolent course without transplantation. Younger patients, especially those younger than age 50 years, with a DNA-based matched sibling donor, progressive disease, and poor prognostic findings, such as hemoglobin less than 10 g/dL, blast cells greater than 1 percent of blood cells, unfavorable cytogenetics (e.g., abnormalities involving chromosome 5, 7, or 17, or cells with three or more abnormalities) are usually considered for transplantation. Although a large spleen may slightly delay the expression of donor granulopoiesis, on average the results in patients with a spleen is the same as those who had prior splenectomy.[471,474] In addition, the latter procedure incurs significant risk of morbidity or mortality.

Patients younger than age 50 years who are transplanted with stem cells from a matched sibling donor have a lower posttransplantation mortality and have better outcomes than those older than age 50 years.[460] Transplant-related mortality using full-conditioning regimens is approximately 35 to 40 percent and 5-year survival is approximately 50 percent in patients younger than 50 years of age.

Donor lymphocyte infusion in patients who have lost donor dominance of hematopoiesis and a return of myelofibrosis can result in regression of fibrosis and return to normal hematopoiesis for at least 6 and 20 months at the time of reporting.[475,476]

In $JAK2^{V617F}$-positive patients, real-time polymerase chain reaction analysis can permit a sensitive determination of residual $JAK2^{V617F}$-positive cells after transplantation. In a study of patients receiving low-intensity conditioning, 17 of 21 patients became $JAK2^{V617F}$-negative, and in one case donor lymphocyte infusion eliminated $JAK2^{V617F}$-positive cells.[477]

The option of nonmyeloablative transplantation in older patients is gaining favor.[470,471,478–482] Several reports of lower posttransplantation mortality and salutary outcomes have led some to consider this approach as the preferred approach in patients older than 50 years of age, and perhaps in younger patients as well. One study showed that the outcome of nonmyeloablative transplantation was dramatically better than myeloablative transplant.[470] The study compared 17 patients receiving a myeloablative conditioning regimen and 10 receiving nonmyeloablative conditioning. The median age was 50 years (age range: 5 to 63 years) at transplantation. After a median followup of 55 months, 20 patients were alive. The transplantation-related mortality was 10 percent in the nonmyeloablative group and 30 percent in the myeloablative group. There was no difference in survival for high- or low-risk patients or between sibling and unrelated donor transplantations. This study confirmed prior smaller comparisons of myeloablative and nonmyeloablative stem cell transplantation.[483]

A large cooperative study of reduced conditioning transplantation found the most favorable results in transplants using matched-related donors and in intermediate stage disease.[482]

Autologous blood stem cells mobilized with granulocyte colony-stimulating factor (G-CSF) and administered after busulfan conditioning produced clinical benefit, including improved erythropoiesis, improved platelet counts, and decreased splenic size, in a plurality of 21 patients with primary myelofibrosis whose age range was 45 to 75 years. The 2-year actuarial survival rate was 61 percent.[484]

● COURSE AND PROGNOSIS

The rate of disease progression is associated with at least 16 variables measured at the time of diagnosis, namely: (1) older age; (2) severity of anemia; (3) exaggerated leukocytosis (>25 × 10⁹/L) or leukopenia (<4.0 × 10⁹/L); (4) constitutional symptoms of fever, sweating, or weight loss at the time of diagnosis; (5) proportion of blast cells in the blood (≥1 percent); (6) male gender; (7) severity of thrombocytopenia; (8) proportion of CD34+ cells in the blood; (9) the presence of the V617F mutation in *JAK2*; (10) monocytosis; (11) a decreased proliferating cell nuclear antigen index and a decreased apoptotic index by *in situ* end labeling; (12) degree of liver enlargement; (13) extent of marrow fibrosis; (14) postsplenectomy spleen histology; (15) *WT1* expression in CD34+ cells; and (16) certain clonal cytogenetic abnormalities, especially involving chromosome 5, 7, or 17, or with three or more abnormalities. Abnormalities such as 13q or 20q did not affect patient survival compared to those patients without cytogenetic alterations.

Each retrospective study has found a different subset of these factors to be significant prognostic factors. The most consistent predictive variables appear to be advanced age, severity of anemia, and higher-risk clonal cytogenetic abnormality at the time of diagnosis, each of which represents a poor prognostic indicator.[8,12,14,16,312,314,485–490]

In a study of more than 1000 consecutive cases of myelofibrosis at seven centers, among which the median survival was 69 months, variables (1) through (5) (listed above) proved to be the most useful in dividing patients into four risk-factor categories. Shorter survival was observed in patients who were older than age 65 years, had a hemoglobin concentration less than 10 g/dL, a leukocyte count greater than 25 × 10⁹/L (25,000/µL), a blood blast cell count equal to or greater than 1 percent, and constitutional symptoms. The patients were assigned to a risk group based on the number of risk factors present. If no risk factors were present, risk was low; if one factor was present, risk was low-intermediate; if two risk factors were present, risk was high-intermediate; and if three or more risk factors were present, risk was high. The application of these variables could distinguish among patients with low risk with a survival of 135 months, low-intermediate risk with a survival of 95 months, high-intermediate risk with a survival of 48 months, and high risk with a survival of 27 months.[491] Overall, the 5-year survival of patients with primary myelofibrosis is approximately 40 percent of the survival expected for healthy age- and sex-matched controls.[492]

Some data suggest that the use of JAK2 inhibitors in the treatment of primary fibrosis may not only decrease symptomatology and spleen size, but may prolong survival.[493,494] An analysis of 100 patients receiving ruxolitinib compared to 350 carefully matched patients who did not receive ruxolitinib showed a median 18-month prolongation in survival in patients with poorer prognosis disease. At the upper range some patients had a 4- to 5-year prolongation of life.[494] In addition, the clinical improvement in vitality and functionality can be dramatic.

The major causes of death are infection, hemorrhage, postsplenectomy mortality, and acute leukemic transformation.[495–499] Acute leukemia occasionally is preceded by the development of myeloid sarcomas.[35,460,499,500] Evolution of the disease to acute lymphocytic leukemia or lymphoma may occur.[501,502] An increased risk of progression to leukemia has been reported in splenectomized patients.[503] Progression to acute leukemia is associated with a blast count greater than 3 percent and a platelet count less than 100,000/µL (100 × 10⁹/L) at the time of diagnosis. Treatment with erythropoietin or androgens is associated with increased risk of progression to acute leukemia, as well.[504] The administration of JAK2 inhibitors may provide improved efficacy for the treatment of AML evolving in patients with primary myelofibrosis. Rare spontaneous remissions of apparent primary myelofibrosis are documented.[505,506]

A variety of gene mutations have been associated with prognosis in patients with primary myelofibrosis, either overall survival or risk of conversion to acute myelogenous leukemia. These include the following gene mutations: *IDH, EZH, ASXLI,* and *SRSF2*.[507,508] The A3669G (rs6198) single nucleotide polymorphism of the glucocorticoid receptor contributes to the erythrocytosis in polycythemia and contributes to the risk of evolution to AML.[509] About 5 to 10 percent of patients with primary myelofibrosis do not have a mutation in *JAK2, CALR,* or *MPL.* These so-called "triple-negative" patients with myelofibrosis appear to have a less favorable prognosis as do those whose neoplastic cells have wild type CALR and an ASXL1 mutation.[509A]

Primary myelofibrosis in infants and children has a more varied pathobiology than in adults. Patients have been followed for decades without requiring significant treatment,[510] and spontaneous remission has been described.[511] Because of its variable course, conservative management may be appropriate while the course of the disease is followed.

REFERENCES

1. Heuck G: Zwei Fälle von Leukämie mit eigenthümlichem Blut-resp Knochenmarksbe-fund. *Virchows Arch Pathol Anat Physiol Klin Med* 78:475, 1879.
2. Silverstein MN: *Agnogenic Myeloid Metaplasia.* Publishing Science, Boston, 1975.
3. Mesa RA, Verstovsek S, Cervantes F, et al: Primary myelofibrosis (PMF), post poly-cythemia vera myelofibrosis (post-PV MF), post essential thrombocythemia myelofi-brosis (post-ET MF), blast phase PMF (PMF-BP): Consensus on terminology by the international working group for myelofibrosis research and treatment (IWG-MRT). *Leuk Res* 31:737, 2007.
4. Lichtman MA: Is it chronic idiopathic myelofibrosis, myelofibrosis with myeloid meta-plasia, chronic megakaryocytic-granulocytic myelosis, or chronic megakaryocytic leu-kemia? Further thoughts on the nosology of the clonal myeloid disorders. *Leukemia* 19:1139, 2005.
5. James C, Ugo V, Le Couédic JP, et al: A unique clonal JAK2 mutation leading to consti-tutive signalling causes polycythaemia vera. *Nature* 434:1144, 2005.
6. Baxter EJ, Scott LM, Campbell PJ, et al: Acquired mutation of the tyrosine kinase JAK2 in human myeloproliferative disorders. *Lancet* 365:1054, 2005.
7. Lundberg P, Karow A, Nienhold R, et al: Clonal evolution and clinical correlates of somatic mutations in myeloproliferative neoplasms. *Blood* 123:2220, 2014.
8. Barosi G: Myelofibrosis with myeloid metaplasia. *Hematol Oncol Clin North Am* 17:1211, 2003.
9. Ward HP, Block MH: The natural history of agnogenic myeloid metaplasia (AMM) and a critical evaluation of its relationship with myeloproliferative syndrome. *Medicine (Baltimore)* 50:357, 1971.
10. Varki A, Lottenberg R, Griffith R, et al: The syndrome of idiopathic myelofibrosis. *Medicine (Baltimore)* 62:353, 1983.
11. Barosi G: Myelofibrosis with myeloid metaplasia. *Hematol Oncol Clin North Am* 17:1211, 2003.
12. Okamura T, Kinukawa N, Niho Y, Mizoguichi H: Primary chronic myelofibrosis: Clin-ical and prognostic evaluation in 336 Japanese patients. *Int J Hematol* 73:194, 2001.
13. Cervantes F, Pereira A, Esteve J, et al: Idiopathic myelofibrosis: Initial features, evolution-ary pattern and survival in a series of 106 patients. *Med Clin North Am* 109:651, 1997.
14. Dupriez B, Morel P, Demory JL, et al: Prognostic factors in agnogenic myeloid metapla-sia: A report on 195 cases with a new scoring system. *Blood* 88:1013, 1996.
15. Rupoli S, DaLio L, Sisti S, et al: Primary myelofibrosis: A detailed analysis of the clini-copathologic variables influencing survival. *Ann Hematol* 68:205, 1994.
16. Ozen S, Ferhanoglu B, Senocak M, Tüzüner N: Idiopathic myelofibrosis (agnogenic myeloid metaplasia). *Leuk Res* 21:125, 1997.
17. Landgren O, Goldin LR, Kristinsson SY, et al: Increased risks of polycythemia vera, essential thrombocythemia, and myelofibrosis among 24,577 first-degree relatives of 11,039 patients with myeloproliferative neoplasms in Sweden. *Blood* 112:2199, 2008.
18. Shalev O, Goldfarb A, Ariel I, et al: Myelofibrosis in young adults. *Acta Haematol* 70:396, 1983.
19. Sekhar M, Prentice HG, Poyat U, et al: Idiopathic myelofibrosis in children. *Br J Haematol* 93:394, 1996.
20. Cervantes F, Barosi G, Demory JL, et al: Myelofibrosis with myeloid metaplasia in young individuals: Disease characteristics, prognostic factors and identification of risk groups. *Br J Haematol* 102:684, 1998.
21. Sieff CA, Malleson P: Familial myelofibrosis. *Arch Dis Child* 55:888, 1980.
22. Sheikha A: Fatal familial infantile myelofibrosis. *J Pediatr Hematol Oncol* 26:164, 2004.
23. Rossbach HC: Familial infantile myelofibrosis as an autosomal recessive disorder: Pre-ponderance among children from Saudi Arabia. *Pediatr Hematol Oncol* 23:453, 2006.
24. Cohn SL, Cohn RA, Chou P, et al: Infantile myelofibrosis with nephromegaly secondary to myeloid metaplasia. *Clin Pediatr (Phila)* 30:59, 1991.
25. Mallouh AA, Sa'di AR: Agnogenic myeloid metaplasia in children. *Am J Dis Child* 146:965, 1992.
26. Cervantes F, Barosi G, Hernández-Boluda J-C, et al: Myelofibrosis with myeloid meta-plasia in adult individuals 30 years old or younger: Presenting features, evolution and survival. *Eur J Haematol* 66:324, 2001.
27. Segel GB, Lichtman MA: Familial (inherited) leukemia, lymphoma, and myeloma. *Blood Cells Mol Dis* 32:246, 2004.
28. Rumi E: Familial chronic myeloproliferative disorders: The state of the art. *Hematol Oncol* 26:131, 2008.
29. Kaufman S, Briere J, Bernard J: Familial myeloproliferative syndromes: Study of 6 fam-ilies and review of literature. *Nouv Rev Fr Hematol* 20:1, 1978.
30. Péres-Encinas M, Bello JL, Perez-Crespo S, et al: Familial myeloproliferative syndrome. *Am J Hematol* 46:225, 1994.
31. Kutty J, Ridell B: Epidemiology of the myeloproliferative disorders: Essential thrombo-cythaemia, polycythemia vera, and idiopathic myelofibrosis. *Pathol Biol* 49:164, 2001.
32. McNally RJ, Rowland D, Roman E, Cartwright RA: Age and sex distributions of haema-tological malignancies in the U.K. *Hematol Oncol* 15:173, 1997.
33. Ridell B, Carneskog J, Wedel H, et al: Incidence of chronic myeloproliferative disorders in the city of Gotesborg, Sweden 1983–1992. *Eur J Haematol* 65:267, 2000.
34. Phekoo KJ, Richards MA, Møller H, Schey SA: The incidence and outcome of mye-loid malignancies in 2,112 adult patients in southeast England. *Haematologica* 91:1400, 2006.
35. Mesa RA, Silverstein MN, Jacobsen SJ, et al: Population-based incidence and survival figures in essential thrombocythemia and agnogenic myeloid metaplasia: An Olmstead County Study 1976–1995. *Am J Hematol* 61:10, 1999.
36. Aksoy M, Erdem S, Dincol G: Two rare complications of chronic benzene poisoning: Myeloid metaplasia and paroxysmal nocturnal hemoglobinuria. *Blut* 30:255, 1975.
37. Hu H: Benzene-associated myelofibrosis. *Ann Intern Med* 106:171, 1987.
38. Tondel M, Perrson B, Carstensen J: Myelofibrosis and benzene exposure. *Occup Med* 45:31, 1995.
39. Anderson RE, Hoshino T, Yamamoto T: Myelofibrosis with myeloid metaplasia in sur-vivors of the atomic bomb in Hiroshima. *Ann Intern Med* 60:1, 1964.
40. Glass DC, Schnatter AR, Tang G, et al: Risk of myeloproliferative disease and chronic myeloid leukaemia following exposure to low-level benzene in a nested case-control study of petroleum workers. *Occup Environ Med* 71:266, 2014.
41. Rinsky RA, Smith AB, Hornung R, et al: Benzene and leukemia. An epidemiologic risk assessment. *N Engl J Med* 316:1044, 1987.
42. Johnson ES, Harbison SC, McCluskey JD, Harbison RD: Characterization of cancer risk from airborne benzene exposure. *Regul Toxicol Pharmacol* 55:361, 2009.
43. Jacobson RS, Salo A, Fialkow PS: Agnogenic myeloid metaplasia: A clonal proliferation of hematopoietic stem cells with secondary myelofibrosis. *Blood* 51:189, 1978.
44. Kahn A, Bernard JF, Cottreau D, et al: A deficient G-6-PD variant with hemizygous expression in blood cells of a woman with primary myelofibrosis. *Humangenetik* 30:41, 1975.
45. Sato Y, Suda T, Suda J, et al: Multilineage expression of haemopoietic precursors with an abnormal clone in idiopathic myelofibrosis. *Br J Haematol* 64:657, 1986.
46. Kreipe H, Jaquet K, Falgner J, et al: Clonal granulocytes and bone marrow cells in the cellular phase of agnogenic myeloid metaplasia. *Blood* 78:1814, 1991.
47. Tsukamoto N, Morita K, Maehara T, et al: Clonality in chronic myeloproliferative dis-orders defined by X-chromosome linked probes. *Br J Haematol* 86:253, 1994.
48. Buschle M, Janssen JWG, Drexler H, et al: Evidence for pluripotent stem cell origin of idiopathic myelofibrosis: Clonal analysis of a case characterized by a N-*ras* gene muta-tion. *Leukemia* 2:658, 1988.
49. Lebowitz P, Papac R, Ghosh PK: Impaired retinoblastoma susceptibility (Rb) gene expression in agnogenic myeloid metaplasia. *Blood* 76(Suppl 1):236A, 1990.
50. Reeder TL, Bailey RJ, Dewald GW, Tefferi A: Both B and T lymphocytes may be clonally involved in myelofibrosis with myeloid metaplasia. *Blood* 101:1981, 2003.
51. Popat U, Frost A, Liu E, et al: High levels of circulating CD34 cells, dacryocytes, clonal hematopoiesis, and JAK2 mutation differentiate myelofibrosis with myeloid meta-plasia from secondary myelofibrosis associated with pulmonary hypertension. *Blood* 107:3486, 2006.
52. Delhommeau F, Dupont S, Tonetti C, et al: Evidence that the JAK2 G1849T (V617F) mutation occurs in a lymphomyeloid progenitor in polycythemia vera and idiopathic myelofibrosis. *Blood* 109:71, 2007.
53. James C, Mazurier F, Dupont S, et al: The hematopoietic stem cell compartment of JAK2V617F-positive myeloproliferative disorders is a reflection of disease heterogene-ity. *Blood* 112:2429, 2008.
54. Wendling F, Varlet P, Charon M, Tambourin P: MPLV: A retrovirus complex inducing an acute myeloproliferative leukemic disorder in adult mice. *Virology* 149:242, 1986.
55. Kaushansky K: Thrombopoietin. *N Engl J Med* 339:746, 1998.
56. Yan X-Q, Lacey D, Hill D, et al: A model of myelofibrosis and osteosclerosis in mice induced by overexpressing thrombopoietin (mpl ligand). *Blood* 88:402, 1996.
57. Villeval JL, Cohen-Solal K, Tuliez M, et al: High thrombopoietin production by hematopoietic cells induces a fatal myeloproliferative syndrome in mice. *Blood* 90:4396, 1997.
58. Chagraoui H, Komura E, Tulliez M, et al: Prominent role of TGF-beta 1 in thrombopoietin-induced myelofibrosis in mice. *Blood* 100:3495, 2002.
59. Chagraoui H, Tulliez M, Smayra T, et al: Stimulation of osteoprotegerin production is responsible for osteosclerosis in mice overexpressing TPO. *Blood* 101:2983, 2003.
60. Pikman Y, Lee BH, Mercher T, et al: MPLW515L is a novel somatic activating mutation in myelofibrosis with myeloid metaplasia. *PLoS Med* 3:e270, 2006.
61. Vannucchi AM, Lasho TL, Guglielmelli P, et al: Mutations and prognosis in primary myelofibrosis. *Leukemia* 27:1861, 2013.
62. Cazzola M, Kralovics R: From Janus kinase 2 to calreticulin: The clinically relevant genomic landscape of myeloproliferative neoplasms. *Blood* 123:3714, 2014.
63. Vannucchi AM, Bianchi L, Cellai C, et al: Development of myelofibrosis in mice genet-ically impaired for GATA-1 expression (GATA-1(low) mice). *Blood* 100:1123, 2002.
64. Vannucchi AM, Migliaccio AR, Paoletti F, et al: Pathogenesis of myelofibrosis with mye-loid metaplasia: Lessons from mouse models of the disease. *Semin Oncol* 32:365, 2005.

65. Garimella R, Kacena MA, Tague SE, et al: Expression of bone morphogenetic proteins and their receptors in the bone marrow megakaryocytes of GATA-1(low) mice: A possible role in osteosclerosis. *J Histochem Cytochem* 55:745, 2007.

66. Levine RL, Gilliland DG: Myeloproliferative disorders. *Blood* 112:2190, 2008.

67. Levine RL, Wadleigh M, Cools J, et al: Activating mutation in the tyrosine kinase JAK2 in polycythemia vera, essential thrombocythemia, and myeloid metaplasia with myelofibrosis. *Cancer Cell* 7:387, 2005.

68. Kilpivaara O, Levine RL: JAK2 and MPL mutations in myeloproliferative neoplasms: Discovery and science. *Leukemia* 22:1813, 2008.

69. Wernig G, Mercher T, Okabe R, et al: Expression of Jak2V617F causes a polycythemia vera-like disease with associated myelofibrosis in a murine bone marrow transplant model. *Blood* 107:4274, 2006.

70. Lacout C, Pisani DF, Tulliez M, et al: JAK2V617F expression in murine hematopoietic cells leads to MPD mimicking human PV with secondary myelofibrosis. *Blood* 108:1652, 2006.

71. Zaleskas VM, Krause DS, Lazarides K, et al: Molecular pathogenesis and therapy of polycythemia induced in mice by JAK2 V617F. *PLoS One* 1:e18, 2006.

72. Kralovics R, Guan Y, Prchal JT: Acquired uniparental disomy of chromosome 9p is a frequent stem cell defect in polycythemia vera. *Exp Hematol* 30:229, 2002.

73. Tiedt R, Hao-Shen H, Sobas MA, et al: Ratio of mutant JAK2-V617F to wild-type Jak2 determines the MPD phenotypes in transgenic mice. *Blood* 111:3931, 2008.

74. Larsen TS, Pallisgaard N, Møller MB, Hasselbalch HC: The JAK2 V617F allele burden in essential thrombocythemia, polycythemia vera and primary myelofibrosis—Impact on disease phenotype. *Eur J Haematol* 79:508, 2007.

75. Pikman Y, Lee BH, Mercher T, et al: MPLW515L is a novel somatic activating mutation in myelofibrosis with myeloid metaplasia. *PLoS Med* 3:e270, 2006.

76. Pardanani AD, Levine RL, Lasho T, et al: MPL515 mutations in myeloproliferative and other myeloid disorders: A study of 1182 patients. *Blood* 108:3472, 2006.

77. Tefferi A: JAK and MPL mutations in myeloid malignancies. *Leuk Lymphoma* 49:388, 2008.

78. Tefferi A: Primary myelofibrosis: 2013 update on diagnosis, risk-stratification, and management. *Am J Hematol* 88:141, 2013.

79. Klampfl T, Gisslinger H, Harutyunyan AS, et al: Somatic mutations of calreticulin in myeloproliferative neoplasms. *N Engl J Med* 369:2379, 2013.

80. Nangalia J, Massie CE, Baxter EJ, et al: Somatic CALR mutations in myeloproliferative neoplasms with nonmutated JAK2. *N Engl J Med* 369:2391, 2013.

81. Wang L, Swierczek SI, Drummond J, et al: Whole-exome sequencing of polycythemia vera revealed novel driver genes and somatic mutation shared by T-cells and granulocytes. *Leukemia* 28:935, 2014.

82. Abu-Duhier FM, Goodeve AC, Care RS, et al: Mutational analysis of class III receptor tyrosine kinases (C-KIT, C-FMS, FLT3) in idiopathic myelofibrosis. *Br J Haematol* 120:464, 2003.

83. Kawamata N, Ogawa S, Yamamoto G, et al: Genetic profiling of myeloproliferative disorders by single-nucleotide polymorphism oligonucleotide microarray. *Exp Hematol* 36(11):1477, 2008.

84. Andrieux J, Demory JL, Dupriez B, et al: Dysregulation and overexpression of HMGA2 in myelofibrosis with myeloid metaplasia. *Genes Chromosomes Cancer* 39:82, 2004.

85. Bogani C, Ponziani V, Guglielmelli P, et al: Myeloproliferative Disorders Research Consortium. Hypermethylation of CXCR4 promoter in CD34+ cells from patients with primary myelofibrosis. *Stem Cells* 26:1920, 2008.

86. Rosti V, Massa M, Vannucchi AM, et al: The expression of CXCR4 is down-regulated on the CD34+ cells of patients with myelofibrosis with myeloid metaplasia. *Blood Cells Mol Dis* 38:280, 2007.

87. Ciurea SO, Merchant D, Mahmud N, et al: Pivotal contributions of megakaryocytes to the biology of idiopathic myelofibrosis. *Blood* 110:986, 2007.

88. Guglielmelli P, Zini R, Bogani C, et al: Molecular profiling of CD34+ cells in idiopathic myelofibrosis identifies a set of disease-associated genes and reveals the clinical significance of Wilms' tumor gene 1 (WT1). *Stem Cells* 25:165, 2007.

89. Massa M, Rosti V, Ramajoli I, et al: Circulating CD34+, CD133+, and vascular endothelial growth factor receptor 2-positive endothelial progenitor cells in myelofibrosis with myeloid metaplasia. *J Clin Oncol* 23:5688, 2005.

90. Rosti V, Villani L, Riboni R, et al: Spleen endothelial cells from patients with myelofibrosis harbor the JAK2V617F mutation. *Blood* 121:360, 2013.

91. Giraudier S, Chagraoui H, Komura E, et al: Overexpression of FKBP51 in idiopathic myelofibrosis regulates the growth factor independence of megakaryocyte progenitors. *Blood* 100:2932, 2002.

92. Wang JC, Chen C, Lou LH, et al: Blood thrombopoietin, IL-6, and IL-11 levels in patients with agnogenic myeloid metaplasia. *Leukemia* 11:1827, 1997.

93. Moliterno AR, Hankins WD, Spivak JL: Impaired expression of the thrombopoietin receptor by patients with polycythemia vera. *N Engl J Med* 338:572, 1998.

94. Prockop DJ, Kivirikko KI, Tuderman L, et al: The biosynthesis of collagen and its disorders. *N Engl J Med* 301:13, 1979.

95. Bauermeister DE: Quantitation of bone marrow reticulin: A normal range. *Am J Clin Pathol* 56:24, 1971.

96. Ivànyi JL, Mahunka M, Papp A, Telek B: Prognostic significance of bone marrow reticulum fibers in idiopathic myelofibrosis: Evolution of clinicopathological parameters in a scoring system. *Haematologica* 26:75, 1994.

97. McCarthy DM: Annotation: Fibrosis of the bone marrow: Content and causes. *Br J Haematol* 59:1, 1985.

98. Apaja-Sarkkinen M, Autio-Harmainen H, Alavaikko M, et al: Immunohistochemical study of basement membrane proteins and type III procollagen in myelofibrosis. *Br J Haematol* 63:571, 1986.

99. Hasselbalch H, Junker P, Lisse I, et al: Serum markers for type IV collagen and type III procollagen in the myelofibrosis-osteomyelosclerosis syndrome and other chronic myeloproliferative disorders. *Am J Hematol* 23:101, 1986.

100. Reilly JT: Pathogenesis of idiopathic myelofibrosis: Role of growth factors. *J Clin Pathol* 45:461, 1992.

101. Charron D, Robert L, Couty MC, Binet JL: Biochemical and histological analysis of bone marrow collagen in myelofibrosis. *Br J Haematol* 41:151, 1979.

102. Podolak-Dawidziak M, Wróbel T, Jelen M: Serum concentration of the amino terminal peptide of type III procollagen (PIIINP) in patients with myeloproliferative disorders (MPD). *Pol Arch Med Wewn* 99:24, 1998.

103. Gay S, Gay RE, Prohal JT: Immunohistological studies of bone marrow collagen, in *Myelofibrosis and the Biology of Connective Tissue*, edited by Berk P, Castro-Malaspina H, Wasserman LR, p 291. Alan R. Liss, New York, 1984.

104. Hasselbalch H, Junker P, Horslev-Patersen K, et al: Procollagen type III amino-terminal peptide in serum in idiopathic myelofibrosis and allied conditions. *Am J Hematol* 33:18, 1990.

105. Reilly JT, Nash JRG, Mackie MJ, McVerry BA: Endothelial cell proliferation in myelofibrosis. *Br J Haematol* 60:625, 1985.

106. Baglin TP, Crocker MA, Timmins A, et al: Bone marrow hypervascularity in patients with myelofibrosis identified by infrared thermography. *Clin Lab Haematol* 13:341, 1991.

107. Bock O, Neuse J, Hussein K, et al: Aberrant collagenase expression in chronic idiopathic myelofibrosis is related to the stage of disease but not to the JAK2 mutation status. *Am J Pathol* 169:471, 2006.

108. Bock O, Höftmann J, Theophile K, et al: Bone morphogenetic proteins are overexpressed in the bone marrow of primary myelofibrosis and are apparently induced by fibrogenic cytokines. *Am J Pathol* 172:951, 2008.

109. Dolan G, Forrest P, Eastham J, et al: Serum laminin, procollagen terminal peptide III and thrombocyte platelet derived growth factor concentrations in idiopathic myelofibrosis. *Br J Haematol* 77(Suppl 1):73, 1991.

110. Reilly JT, Nash JRG, Mackie MJ, McVerry BA: Immunoenzymatic detection of fibronectin in normal and pathological haemopoietic tissue. *Br J Haematol* 59:497, 1985.

111. Hasselbalch H, Clemmensen I: Plasma fibronectin in idiopathic myelofibrosis and related chronic myeloproliferative disorders. *Scand J Clin Lab Invest* 47:429, 1987.

112. Soini Y, Kamel D, Apaja-Sarkkinen M, et al: Tenascin immunoreactivity in normal and pathological bone marrow. *J Clin Pathol* 46:218, 1993.

113. Reilly JT, Nash JRG: Vitronectin (serum spreading factor): Its localization in normal and fibrotic tissue. *J Clin Pathol* 41:1269, 1988.

114. Le Bousse-Kerdilès MC, Martyré MC, et al: Involvement of the fibrogenic cytokines, TGF-β and bFGF, in the pathogenesis of idiopathic myelofibrosis. *Pathol Biol* 49:153, 2001.

115. Rameshwar P, Oh HS, Yook C, Chang VT: Substance P-fibronectin cytokine interactions in myeloproliferative disorders with bone marrow fibrosis. *Acta Haematol* 109:1, 2003.

116. Wang JC, Wong C, Kao WW: Immunoreactive prolylhydroxylase in patients with primary and secondary myelofibrosis. *Br J Haematol* 65:171, 1987.

117. Barosi G, Costa A, Liberato LN, et al: Serum procollagen III peptide level correlates with disease activity in myelofibrosis with myeloid metaplasia. *Br J Haematol* 72:16, 1989.

118. Hochweiss S, Fruchtman S, Hahn EG, et al: Increased serum procollagen III amino-terminal peptide in myelofibrosis. *Am J Hematol* 15:343, 1983.

119. Hasselbalch H, Junker P, Lisse I, et al: Circulating hyaluronan in the myelofibrosis/osteomyelosclerosis syndrome and other myeloproliferative disorders. *Am J Hematol* 36:1, 1991.

120. Thiele J, Kvasnicka HM, Fischer R, Diehl V: Clinicopathological impact of the interactivity between megakaryocytes and myeloid stroma in chronic myeloproliferative disorders: A concise update. *Leuk Lymphoma* 24:463, 1997.

121. Schmitt A, Drouin A, Masse J-M, et al: Polymorphonuclear neutrophil and megakaryocyte mutual involvement in myelofibrosis pathogenesis. *Leuk Lymphoma* 43:719, 2002.

122. Frey BM, Rafii S, Teterson M, et al: Adenovector-mediated expression of human thrombopoietin cDNA in immune-compromised mice: Insights into the pathophysiology of osteomyelosclerosis. *J Immunol* 160:691, 1998.

123. Rameshwar P, Chang VT, Thacker UF, Gascón P: Systemic transforming growth factor-beta in patients with bone marrow fibrosis-pathophysiological implications. *Am J Hematol* 59:133, 1998.

124. Rosenfeld M, Keating A, Bowen-Pope BF, et al: Responsiveness of the *in vitro* hematopoietic microenvironment to platelet-derived growth factor. *Leuk Res* 9:427, 1985.

125. Bernabei PA, Arcangeli A, Casini M, et al: Platelet-derived growth factor(s) mitogenic activity in patients with myeloproliferative disease. *Br J Haematol* 63:353, 1986.

126. Thiele J, Rompick V, Wagner S, Fischer R: Vascular architecture and collagen type IV in primary myelofibrosis and polycythemia vera. *Br J Haematol* 80:227, 1992.

127. Johnston JB, Dalal BI, Israels SJ, et al: Deposition of transforming growth factor-β in the marrow in myelofibrosis, and the intracellular localization and secretion of TGF-β by leukemic cells. *Am J Clin Pathol* 103:574, 1995.

128. Martré M-C: TGF-β and megakaryocytes in the pathogenesis of myelofibrosis in myeloproliferative disorders. *Leuk Lymphoma* 20:39, 1995.

129. Martré M-C, LeBousse-Kerdiles M-C, Romquin N, et al: Elevated levels of basic fibroblast growth factor in megakaryocytes and platelets from patients with idiopathic myelofibrosis. *Br J Haematol* 97:441, 1997.

130. Dalley A, Smith JM, Reilly JT, MacNeil S: Investigation of calmodulin and basic fibroblast growth factor (bFGF) in idiopathic myelofibrosis: Evidence for a role of extracellular calmodulin in fibroblast proliferation. *Br J Haematol* 93:856, 1996.

131. Nathan C: Secretory products of macrophages. *J Clin Invest* 79:319, 1987.

132. Papadantonakis N, Matsuura S, Ravid K: Megakaryocyte pathology and bone marrow fibrosis: The lysyl oxidase connection. *Blood* 120:1774, 2012.

133. Burstein SA, Malpass TW, Yee E, et al: Platelet factor-4 excretion in myeloproliferative disease: Implication for the aetiology of myelofibrosis. *Br J Haematol* 57:383, 1984.

134. Wang JC, Novetsky A, Chen C, et al: Plasm matrix metalloproteinase and tissue inhibitor of metalloproteinase in patients with agnogenic myeloid metaplasia or idiopathic primary myelofibrosis. *Br J Haematol* 119:709, 2002.

135. Reilly JT, Nash JR, Mackie MJ, et al: Endothelial cell proliferation in myelofibrosis. *Br J Haematol* 60:625, 1985.

136. Charbord P: Increased vascularity of bone marrow in myelofibrosis. *Br J Haematol* 62:595, 1986.

137. VanDyke D, Anger HO, Parker H, et al: Markedly increased bone blood flow in myelofibrosis. *J Nucl Med* 12:506, 1971.

138. Hotta T, Utsumi M, Katoh T, et al: Granulocytic and stromal progenitors in the bone marrow of patient with primary myelofibrosis. *Scand J Haematol* 34:251, 1985.

139. Greenberg BR, Woo L, Veomett JC, et al: Cytogenetics of bone marrow fibroblastic cells in idiopathic chronic myelofibrosis. *Br J Haematol* 66:487, 1987.

140. Mesa RA, Shields A, Hare T, et al: Progressive burden of myelofibrosis in untreated patients: Assessment of patient-reported outcomes in patients randomized to placebo in the COMFORT-I study. *Leuk Res* 37:911, 2013.

141. Caughman W, Stern R, Haynes H: Neutrophilic dermatosis of myeloproliferative disorders: Atypical forms of pyoderma gangrenosum and Sweet's syndrome associated with myeloproliferative disorders. *J Am Acad Dermatol* 9:751, 1983.

142. Gibson LE, Dicken CH, Flach DB: Neutrophilic dermatoses and myeloproliferative disease: Report of two cases. *Mayo Clin Proc* 60:735, 1985.

143. Su WPD, Alegre VA, White WL: Myelofibrosis discovered after diagnosis of Sweet's syndrome. *Int J Dermatol* 29:201, 1990.

144. Kanel KT, Kroboth FJ, Swartz WM: Pyoderma gangrenosum with myelofibrosis. *Am J Med* 82:1031, 1987.

145. Loewy G, Matthew A, Distenfeld A: Skin manifestations of agnogenic myeloid metaplasia. *Am J Hematol* 45:167, 1994.

146. Patel BM, Perniciaro C, Gertz MA: Cutaneous extramedullary hematopoiesis. *J Am Acad Dermatol* 32:805, 1995.

147. Rogalski C, Paasch U, Friedrich T, et al: Cutaneous extramedullary hematopoiesis in idiopathic myelofibrosis. *Int J Dermatol* 41:883, 2002.

148. Thiele J, Kvasnicka HM, Zankovich R, Diehl V: Early-stage idiopathic (primary) myelofibrosis—Current issues of diagnostic features. *Leuk Lymphoma* 43:1035, 2002.

149. Buhr T, Büsche G, Choritz H, et al: Evolution of myelofibrosis in chronic idiopathic myelofibrosis as evidenced in sequential bone marrow biopsy specimens. *Am J Clin Pathol* 119:152, 2003.

150. Thiele J, Kvasnicka HM: Chronic myeloproliferative disorders with thrombocythemia comparative study of two classification systems (PSSG, WHO) on 839 patients. *Ann Hematol* 82:148, 2003.

151. Barbui T, Thiele J, Passamonti F, et al: Survival and disease progression in essential thrombocythemia are significantly influenced by accurate morphologic diagnosis: An international study. *J Clin Oncol* 29:3179, 2011.

152. King BF, Kopecky KK, Baker MK, et al: Extramedullary hematopoiesis in the adrenal glands: CT characteristics. *J Comput Assist Tomogr* 11:342, 1987.

153. Wat NM, Tse KK, Chan FL, Lam KS: Adrenal extramedullary hematopoiesis. *Br J Haematol* 100:725, 1998.

154. Gibbins J, Pankhurst T, Murray J, et al: Extramedullary haematopoiesis in the kidney: A case report and review of literature. *Clin Lab Haematol* 27:391, 2005.

155. Schunuelle P, Waldherr R, Lehmann KJ, et al: Idiopathic myelofibrosis with extramedullary hematopoiesis in the kidneys. *Clin Nephrol* 52:256, 1999.

156. Ablett MJ, Vosylius P: Perirenal extramedullary haematopoiesis in myelofibrosis demonstrated on computed tomography. *Br J Haematol* 124:406, 2004.

157. Shaver RW, Clore FC: Extramedullary hemopoiesis in myeloid metaplasia. *AJR Am J Roentgenol* 137:874, 1981.

158. Williams ME, Innes DJ, Hutchison WT, et al: Extramedullary hematopoiesis: A cause of severe generalized lymphadenopathy in agnogenic myeloid metaplasia. *Arch Intern Med* 145:1308, 1985.

159. La Fianza A, Alberici E, Toretta L: The irreplaceable image: Rapidly growing extramedullary hematopoiesis in lymph nodes: Unusual findings of long-standing idiopathic myelofibrosis. *Haematologica* 86:784, 2001.

160. Sharma BK, Pounder RE, Cruse JP, et al: Extramedullary haematopoiesis in the small bowel. *Gut* 27:873, 1986.

161. MacKinnon S, McNicol AM, Lee FD, et al: Myelofibrosis complicated by intestinal extramedullary haematopoiesis and acute small bowel obstruction. *J Clin Pathol* 39:677, 1986.

162. Soloman D, Goodman H, Jacobs P: Rectal stenosis due to extramedullary hematopoiesis. *Clin Radiol* 49:726, 1994.

163. Sunderland K, Barratt J, Pidcock M: Extramedullary hemopoiesis arising in the gut mimicking carcinoma of the cecum. *Pathology* 26:62, 1994.

164. Brooks JJ, Krugman DT, Danjanor I: Myeloid metaplasia presenting as a breast mass. *Am J Surg Pathol* 4:281, 1980.

165. Martinelli G, Santini D, Bazzocchi F, et al: Myeloid metaplasia of the breast: A lesion which clinically mimics carcinoma. *Virchows Arch* 401:203, 1983.

166. Zonderland HM, Michiels JJ, Ten Kate FJW: Mammographic and sonographic demonstration of extramedullary hematopoiesis of the breast. *Clin Radiol* 44:64, 1991.

167. Navarro M, Crespo C, Pérez L, et al: Massive intrahepatic extramedullary hematopoiesis in myelofibrosis. *Abdom Imaging* 25:184, 2000.

168. Lee IJ, Kim SH, Kim DS, et al: Intrahepatic extramedullary hematopoiesis mimicking a hypervascular hepatic neoplasm on dynamic- and SPIO-enhanced MRI. *Korean J Radiol* 9(Suppl):S34, 2008.

169. Yusen RD, Kollef MH: Acute respiratory failure due to extramedullary hematopoiesis. *Chest* 108:1170, 1995.

170. Schwarz C, Bittner R, Kirsch A, et al: A 62-year-old woman with bilateral pleural effusions and pulmonary infiltrates caused by extramedullary hematopoiesis. *Respiration* 78:110, 2009.

171. García-Manero G, Schuster S, Patrick H, Martinez J: Pulmonary hypertension in patients with myelofibrosis secondary to myeloproliferative diseases. *Am J Hematol* 60:130, 1999.

172. Yang X, Bhuiya T, Esposito M: Sclerosing extramedullary tumor. *Ann Diagn Pathol* 6:183, 2002.

173. Oren I, Goldman A, Haddad N, et al: Ascites and pleural effusion a secondary to extramedullary hematopoiesis. *Am J Med Sci* 318:286, 1999.

174. Miyata T, Masuzawa M, Katsuoka K, Higashihara M: Cutaneous extramedullary hematopoiesis in a patient with idiopathic myelofibrosis. *J Dermatol* 35:456, 2008.

175. Mizoguchi M, Kawa Y, Minami T, et al: Cutaneous extramedullary hematopoiesis in myelofibrosis. *J Am Acad Dermatol* 22:351, 1990.

176. Heinicke MH, Zarrabi MH, Gorevic PD: Arthritis due to synovial involvement by extramedullary haematopoiesis in myelofibrosis with myeloid metaplasia. *Ann Rheum Dis* 42:196, 1983.

177. Leoni F, Fabbri R, Pascarella A, et al: Extramedullary hematopoiesis in thyroid multinodular goiter preceding clinical evidence of agnogenic myeloid metaplasia. *Histopathology* 28:559, 1996.

178. Kwak H-S, Lee J-M: CT findings of extramedullary hematopoiesis in the thorax, liver, and kidneys in a patient with myelofibrosis. *J Korean Med Sci* 15:460, 2000.

179. Humphrey PA, Vollmer RT: Extramedullary hematopoiesis in the prostate. *Am J Surg Pathol* 15:486, 1991.

180. Macumber C, Young GAR, Selby WS: Myelofibrosis presenting as splenic tumor. *Dig Dis Sci* 44:1817, 1999.

181. Balogh K, O'Hara CJ: Myeloid metaplasia masquerading as a urethral caruncle. *J Urol* 135:789, 1986.

182. Oesterling JE, Keating JP, Leroy AJ, et al: Idiopathic myelofibrosis with myeloid metaplasia involving the renal pelvis, ureters and bladder. *J Urol* 147:1360, 1992.

183. La Fianza A, Torretta L, Spinazzola A: Extramedullary hematopoiesis in chronic myelofibrosis encasing the pelvicaliceal system and perirenal spaces: CT findings. *Urol Int* 75:281, 2005.

184. Perazella MA, Buller GK: Nephrotic syndrome associated with agnogenic myeloid metaplasia. *Am J Nephrol* 14:223, 1994.

185. Brown JA, Gomez-Leon G: Subdural hemorrhage secondary to extramedullary hematopoiesis in postpolycythemic myeloid metaplasia. *Neurosurgery* 14:588, 1984.

186. Cornfield DB, Shipkin P, Alluvia A, et al: Intracranial myeloid metaplasia: Diagnosis by CT and Fe52 scans and treatment by cranial irradiation. *Am J Hematol* 15:273, 1983.

187. Lundh B, Brandt L, Cronqvist S, et al: Intracranial myeloid metaplasia in myelofibrosis. *Scand J Haematol* 28:91, 1982.

188. Pless M, Rizzo JF III, Shang J: Orbital apex syndrome: A rare presentation of extramedullary hematopoiesis. *J Neurooncol* 57:37, 2002.

189. Cameron WR, Ronnert M, Brun A: Extramedullary hematopoiesis of CNS in postpolycythemic myeloid metaplasia. *N Engl J Med* 305:765, 1981.

190. Chan SW, Datta NN, Thomas TM, Chan KW: Intracranial chloroma in myelofibrosis. *Surg Neurol* 59:55, 2003.

191. Haidar S, Ortiz-Neira C, Shroff M, et al: Intracranial involvement in extramedullary hematopoiesis: Case report and review of the literature. *Pediatr Radiol* 35:630, 2005.

192. Goh DH, Lee SH, Cho DC, et al: Chronic idiopathic myelofibrosis presenting as cauda equina compression due to extramedullary hematopoiesis: A case report. *J Korean Med Sci* 22:1090, 2007.

193. Cook G, Sharp RA: Spinal cord compression due to extramedullary haemopoiesis in myelofibrosis. *J Clin Pathol* 47:464, 1994.

194. Horwood E, Dowson H, Gupta R, et al: Myelofibrosis presenting as spinal cord compression. *J Clin Pathol* 56:154, 2003.

195. Scott IC, Poynton CH: Polycythaemia rubra vera and myelofibrosis with spinal cord compression. *J Clin Pathol* 61:681, 2008.

196. Ohtsubo M, Hayaski K, Fukushima T, et al: Intracranial extramedullary haematopoiesis in postpolycythemia myelofibrosis. *Br J Radiol* 67:299, 1994.

197. Urman M, O'Sullivan RA, Nugent RA, Lentle BC: Intracranial extramedullary hematopoiesis. *Clin Nucl Med* 16:431, 1991.

198. Lanir A, Aghai E, Simon JS, et al: MR imaging in myelofibrosis. *J Comput Assist Tomogr* 10:634, 1986.

199. Koch BL, Bisset GS, Bisset RR, Zimmer MB: Intracranial extramedullary hematopoiesis: MR findings with pathologic correlation. *AJR Am J Roentgenol* 162:1419, 1994.

200. Bartlett RP, Greipp PR, Tefferi A, et al: Extramedullary hematopoiesis manifesting as a symptomatic pleural effusion. *Mayo Clin Proc* 70:1165, 1995.
201. Oren I, Goldman A, Haddad N, et al: Ascites and pleural effusion secondary to extramedullary hematopoiesis. *Am J Med Sci* 318:286, 1999.
202. Lioté F, Yeni P, Teillet-Thiebaud F, et al: Ascites revealing peritoneal and hepatic extramedullary hematopoiesis with peliosis in agnogenic myeloid metaplasia. *Am J Med* 90:111, 1991.
203. Vilaseca J, Arnau JM, Tallada N, et al: Agnogenic myeloid metaplasia presenting as massive pericardial effusion due to extramedullary hematopoiesis. *Acta Haematol* 73:239, 1985.
204. Haedersdal C, Hasselbalch H, Devantier A, et al: Pericardial haematopoiesis with tamponade in myelofibrosis. *Scand J Haematol* 34:270, 1985.
205. Imam TH, Doll DC: Acute cardiac tamponade associated with pericardial extramedullary hematopoieses in agnogenic myeloid metaplasia. *Acta Haematol* 98:42, 1997.
206. Nagler A, Brenner B, Argov S, et al: Postsplenectomy pericardial effusion in two patients with myeloid metaplasia. *Arch Intern Med* 146:600, 1986.
207. Pedio G, Krause M, Jansova I: Megakaryocytes in ascitic fluid in a case of agnogenic myeloid metaplasia [letter]. *Acta Cytol* 29:89, 1985.
208. Silverman JF: Extramedullary hematopoietic ascitic fluid cytology in myelofibrosis. *Am J Clin Pathol* 84:125, 1985.
209. Stephenson RW, Britt DA, Schumann GB: Primary cytodiagnosis of peritoneal extramedullary hematopoiesis. *Diagn Cytopathol* 2:241, 1986.
210. Hocking WG, Lazar GS, Lipsett JA, et al: Cutaneous extramedullary hematopoiesis following splenectomy for idiopathic myelofibrosis. *Am J Med* 76:956, 1984.
211. Partanen S, Ruutu T, Jubonen E, et al: Effect of splenectomy on circulating haematopoietic progenitors in myelofibrosis. *Scand J Haematol* 37:87, 1986.
212. Hirose Y, Masaki Y, Shimoyama K, et al: Granulocytic sarcoma of megakaryoblastic differentiation in the lymph nodes terminating as acute megakaryocytic leukemia in a case of chronic idiopathic myelofibrosis persisting 16 years. *Eur J Haematol* 67:194, 2001.
213. Chan ACL, Kwong Y-L, Lam CCK: Granulocytic sarcoma megakaryoblastic differentiation complicating chronic idiopathic myelofibrosis. *Hum Pathol* 27:417, 1996.
214. Oishi N, Swisher SN, Stormont JM, et al: Portal hypertension in myeloid metaplasia. *Arch Surg* 81:80, 1960.
215. Rosenbaum DL, Murphy GW, Swisher SN: Hemodynamic studies of the portal circulation in myeloid metaplasia. *Am J Med* 41:360, 1966.
216. Jacobs P, Maze S, Tayob F, et al: Myelofibrosis, splenomegaly, and portal hypertension. *Acta Haematol* 74:45, 1985.
217. Dubois A, Dauzat M, Pignodel C, et al: Portal hypertension in lymphoproliferative and myeloproliferative disorders: Hemodynamic and histological correlations. *Hepatology* 17:246, 1993.
218. Degott C, Capron JP, Bettan L, et al: Myeloid metaplasia, perisinusoidal fibrosis, and nodular regenerative hyperplasia of the liver. *Liver* 5:276, 1985.
219. Bioulac-Sage P, Roux D, Quinton A, et al: Ultrastructure of sinusoids in patients with agnogenic myeloid metaplasia. *J Submicrosc Cytol* 18:815, 1986.
220. Roux D, Merlio JP, Quinton A, et al: Agnogenic myeloid metaplasia, portal hypertension and sinusoidal abnormalities. *Gastroenterology* 92:1067, 1987.
221. Tsao MS: Hepatic sinusoidal fibrosis in agnogenic myeloid metaplasia. *Am J Clin Pathol* 91:302, 1989.
222. Pereira A, Bruguera M, Cervantes F, Rozman C: Liver involvement at diagnosis of primary myelofibrosis: A clinicopathological study of twenty-two cases. *Eur J Haematol* 40:355, 1988.
223. Valla D, Casadevall N, Huisse MG, et al: Etiology of portal vein thrombosis in adults. *Gastroenterology* 94:1063, 1988.
224. Lee W-C, Lin H-C, Tsay S-H, et al: Esophageal variceal ligation for esophageal variceal hemorrhage in a patient with portal and primary pulmonary hypertension complicating myelofibrosis. *Dig Dis Sci* 46:915, 2001.
225. Yusen RD, Kollef MH: Acute respiratory failure due to extramedullary hematopoiesis. *Chest* 108:1170, 1995.
226. Steensma DP, Hook CC, Stafford SL, Tefferi A: Low-dose, single fraction, whole-lung radiotherapy for pulmonary hypertension associated with myelofibrosis and myeloid metaplasia. *Br J Haematol* 118:813, 2002.
227. Cortelezzi A, Gritti G, et al: Pulmonary arterial hypertension in primary myelofibrosis is common and associated with an altered angiogenic status. *Leukemia* 22:646, 2008.
228. Popat U, Frost A, Liu E, et al: New onset of myelofibrosis in association with pulmonary arterial hypertension. *Ann Intern Med* 143:466, 2005.
229. Boivin P, Bernard JF, Hakim J, Woroclans M: Anomalies immunitaires au cours de splenomegalies myeloides myelosclerose. *Acta Haematol* 51:91, 1974.
230. Lang JM, Oberling F, Mayer S, et al: Autoimmunity in primary myelofibrosis. *Biomedicine* 25:39, 1976.
231. Barge J, Slabodshy-Brousse N, Bernard JF: Histoimmunology of myelofibrosis: A study of 100 cases. *Biomedicine* 29:73, 1978.
232. Vellenga E, Mulder NH, The TH, Nieweg HO: A study of the cellular and humoral immune response in patients with myelofibrosis. *Clin Lab Haematol* 4:239, 1982.
233. Rondeau E, Solal-Celigny P, Dhermy D, et al: Immune disorders in agnogenic myeloid metaplasia: Relations to myelofibrosis. *Br J Haematol* 53:467, 1983.
234. Gordon B: Immunological abnormalities in myelofibrosis. *Prog Clin Biol Res* 154:455, 1984.
235. Khumbananda M, Horowitz HI, Eyster ME: Coombs' positive hemolytic anemia in myelofibrosis with myeloid metaplasia. *Am J Med Sci* 258:89, 1969.
236. Mohite U, Pathare A, Al Kindi S, et al: Autoimmune haemolytic anemia as the presenting manifestation of agnogenic myeloid metaplasia. *Haematologica* 32:495, 2002.
237. Kornblihtt LI, Vassalllu PS, Heller PG, et al: Primary myelofibrosis in a patient who developed primary biliary cirrhosis, autoimmune hemolytic anemia and fibrillary glomerulonephritis. *Ann Hematol* 87:1019, 2008.
238. Schreiber ZA: Immune thrombocytopenia in postpolythemic myelofibrosis. *Am J Hematol* 54:146, 1997.
239. Seelen MA, de Meijer PH, Posthuma EF, Meinders AE: Myelofibrosis and thrombocytopenic purpura. *Ann Hematol* 75:129, 1997.
240. Wang JC, Wang A: Plasma soluble interleukin-2 receptor in patients with primary myelofibrosis. *Br J Haematol* 86:380, 1994.
241. Leoni P, Rupoli S, Salvi A, et al: Antibodies against terminal galactosyl alpha(1–3) galactose epitopes in patients with idiopathic myelofibrosis. *Br J Haematol* 85:313, 1993.
242. Bernhardt B, Valleta M: Lupus anticoagulant in myelofibrosis. *Am J Med Sci* 272:229, 1976.
243. Cappio FC, Vigliani R, Novarino A, et al: Idiopathic myelofibrosis: A possible role for immune-complexes in the pathogenesis of bone marrow fibrosis. *Br J Haematol* 49:17, 1981.
244. Akikusa B, Komatsu T, Kondo Y, et al: Amyloidosis complicating idiopathic myelofibrosis. *Arch Pathol Lab Med* 111:525, 1987.
245. Hasselbalch H, Nielsen H, Berild D, et al: Circulating immune complexes in myelofibrosis. *Scand J Haematol* 34:177, 1985.
246. Gordon BR, Coleman M, Kohen P, et al: Immunologic abnormalities in myelofibrosis with activation of the complement system. *Blood* 58:904, 1981.
247. Ferhanoğlu B, Erzin Y, Başlar Z, Tüzüner HA: Secondary amyloidosis in the course of idiopathic myelofibrosis. *Leuk Res* 21:897, 1997.
248. Tefferi A, Kantarjian HM, Pardanani AD, et al: The clinical phenotype of myelofibrosis encompasses a chronic inflammatory state that is favorably altered by INCB018424, a selective inhibitor of JAK1/2. *Blood* 112:968, 2008.
249. el Mouzan MI, Ahmad MA, al Fadel Saleh M, et al: Myelofibrosis and pancytopenia in systemic lupus erythematosus. *Am J Med* 81:935, 1986.
250. Matsouka CH, Lioouris J, Andrianakis A: Systemic lupus erythematosus and myelofibrosis. *Clin Rheumatol* 8:402, 1989.
251. Paquette RL, Meshkinpour A, Rosen PJ: Autoimmune myelofibrosis. A steroid-responsive cause of bone marrow fibrosis associated with systemic lupus erythematosus. *Medicine (Baltimore)* 73:145, 1994.
252. Ramakrishna R, Kyle PW, Day PJ, Mansharan A: Evan's syndrome, myelofibrosis and systemic lupus erythematosus: Role of procollagens in myelofibrosis. *Pathology* 27:255, 1995.
253. Kiss E, Gál I, Simkovics E, et al: Myelofibrosis in systemic lupus erythematosus. *Leuk Lymphoma* 39:661, 2000.
254. Aharon A, Levy Y, Bar-Dayan Y, et al: Successful treatment of early secondary myelofibrosis in SLE with IVIG. *Lupus* 6:408, 1997.
255. von Knorring J, Selroos O, Wasastjerna C, Wegelius O: Myeloid metaplasia in disseminated vascular disease. *Acta Med Scand* 195:137, 1974.
256. Connelly TJ, Abruzzo JL, Schwab RH: Agnogenic myeloid metaplasia with polyarteritis. *J Rheumatol* 9:954, 1982.
257. Arellano-Rodrigo E, Esteve J, Giné E, et al: Idiopathic myelofibrosis associated with ulcerative colitis. *Leuk Lymphoma* 43:1481, 2002.
258. Ben-Chetrit E, Gross DJ, Ikon E, et al: The association between auto-immunity and agnogenic myeloid metaplasia. *Scand J Haematol* 31:410, 1983.
259. Hernández-Beluda JC, Jiménez M, Rosiñol L, Cervantes F: Idiopathic myelofibrosis associated with primary biliary cirrhosis. *Leuk Lymphoma* 43:673, 2002.
260. Marie I, Levesque H, Cailleux N, et al: An uncommon association: Sjögren syndrome and autoimmune myelofibrosis. *Rheumatology* 38:370, 1999.
261. Hasselbalch H, Jans H, Nielsen PL: A distinct subtype of idiopathic myelofibrosis with bone marrow features mimicking hairy cell leukemia: Evidence of an autoimmune pathogenesis. *Am J Hematol* 25:225, 1987.
262. Thiele J, Chen Y-S, Kvasnicka H-M, et al: Evolution of fibro-osteosclerotic bone marrow lesions in primary (idiopathic) osteomyelosclerosis—A histomorphometric study on sequential trephine biopsies. *Leuk Lymphoma* 14:163, 1994.
263. Thiele J, Hoeppner B, Zankovich R, Fischer R: Histomorphometry of bone marrow biopsies in primary osteomyelofibrosis-sclerosis (agnogenic myeloid metaplasia): Correlation between clinical and morphological features. *Virchows Arch* 415:191, 1989.
264. Guermazi A, de Kerviler E, Cazals-Hatem D, et al: Imaging findings in myelofibrosis. *Eur J Radiol* 9:1366, 1999.
265. Thiele J, Kvasnicka HM, Fischer R: Histochemistry and morphometry on bone marrow biopsies in chronic myeloproliferative disorders: Aids to diagnosis and classification. *Ann Hematol* 78:496, 1999.
266. Poulsen LW, Melsen F, Bendix K: Histomorphometric study of haematologic disorders with respect to marrow fibrosis and osteosclerosis. *Acta Pathol Microbiol Immunol Scand* 106:495, 1998.
267. Coindre JM, Reiffers J, Goussot JF, et al: Histomorphometric analysis of sclerotic bone from idiopathic myeloid metaplasia. *J Pathol* 144:163, 1984.
268. Diamond T, Smith A, Schnier R, Manoharan A: Syndrome of myelofibrosis and osteosclerosis: A series of case reports and review of the literature. *Bone* 3:498, 2002.
269. Parfitt AM, Drezner MK, Glorieux FH, et al: Bone histomorphometry: Standardization of nomenclature, symbols, and units. *J Bone Miner Res* 2:595, 1987.
270. Cassi E, DePaoli A, Tosi A, et al: Pure osteolytic lesions in myelofibrosis: Report of 2 cases. *Haematologica* 70:178, 1985.

271. Fayemi AO, Gerber MA, Cohen I, et al: Myeloid sarcoma. *Cancer* 32:253, 1973.

272. Yu JS, Greenway G, Resnick D: Myelofibrosis associated with prominent periosteal bone apposition. *Clin Imaging* 18:89, 1994.

273. Cervantes F, Alvarez-Larrán A, Arellano-Rodrigo E, et al: Frequency and risk factors for thrombosis in idiopathic myelofibrosis: Analysis in a series of 155 patients from a single institution. *Leukemia* 20:55, 2006.

274. Buxhofer-Ausch V, Gisslinger H, Thiele J, et al: Leukocytosis as an important risk factor for arterial thrombosis in WHO-defined early/prefibrotic myelofibrosis: An international study of 264 patients. *Am J Hematol* 87:669, 2012.

275. Barbui T, Carobbio A, Cervantes F, et al: Thrombosis in primary myelofibrosis: Incidence and risk factors. *Blood* 115:778, 2010.

276. Smalberg JH, Arends LR, Valla DC, et al: Myeloproliferative neoplasms in Budd-Chiari syndrome and portal vein thrombosis: A meta-analysis. *Blood* 120:4921, 2012.

277. Barosi G, Cazzoli M, Frassoni F: Erythropoiesis in myelofibrosis with myeloid metaplasia: Recognition of different classes of patients by erythrokinetics. *Br J Haematol* 48:263, 1981.

278. Barosi G, Berzuinic C, Liberato LN, et al: A prognostic classification of myelofibrosis with myeloid metaplasia. *Br J Haematol* 70:397, 1988.

279. Thiele J, Kvasnicka H-M, Werden C, et al: Idiopathic primary osteomyelofibrosis. *Leuk Lymphoma* 22:303, 1996.

280. Njoku OS, Lewis SM, Catovsky D, et al: Anaemia in myelofibrosis: Its value in prognosis. *Br J Haematol* 54:79, 1983.

281. Howarth JE, Waters HM, Hyde K, Geary CG: Detection of erythroid hypoplasia in myelofibrosis using erythrokinetic studies. *J Clin Pathol* 42:1250, 1989.

282. Thiele J, Windecker R, Kvasnicka HM, et al: Erythropoiesis in primary (idiopathic) osteomyelofibrosis. *Am J Hematol* 46:36, 1994.

283. Bird GW, Wingham J, Richardson SG: Myelofibrosis, autoimmune haemolytic anaemia and Tn-polyagglutinability. *Haematologica* 18:99, 1985.

284. Kuo CY, VanVoolen GA, Morrison AN: Primary and secondary myelofibrosis: Its relationship to the PNH-like defect. *Blood* 40:875, 1972.

285. Veer A, Kosciolek BA, Bauman AW, et al: Acquired hemoglobin H disease in idiopathic myelofibrosis. *Am J Hematol* 6:199, 1979.

286. Barosi G, Baraldi A, Cassola M, et al: Red cell aplasia in myelofibrosis with myeloid metaplasia. *Cancer* 52:1290, 1983.

287. Silverstein MN, Elveback LR: Leukocyte alkaline phosphatase in agnogenic myeloid metaplasia. *Am J Clin Pathol* 61:307, 1974.

288. Douer D, Fabian I, Cline MJ: Circulation pluripotent haemopoietic cells in patients with myeloproliferative disorders. *Br J Haematol* 54:373, 1983.

289. Barosi G, Viarengo G, Pecci A, et al: Diagnostic and clinical relevance of the number of circulating CD34+ cells in myelofibrosis with myeloid metaplasia. *Blood* 98:3249, 2001.

290. Partanen S, Ruutu T, Vuopio P: Circulating haematopoietic progenitors in myelofibrosis. *Scand J Haematol* 29:325, 1982.

291. Wang JC, Cheung CP, Ahmed F, et al: Circulating granulocyte and macrophage progenitor cells in primary and secondary myelofibrosis. *Br J Haematol* 54:301, 1983.

292. Kornberg A, Fibach E, Treves A, et al: Circulating erythroid progenitors in patients with "spent" polycythaemia vera and myelofibrosis with myeloid metaplasia. *Br J Haematol* 52:573, 1982.

293. Colovi MD, Wiernik PH, Jankovi GM, et al: Circulating haematopoietic progenitor cells in primary and secondary myelofibrosis: Relation to collagen and reticulin fibrosis. *Eur J Haematol* 62:155, 1999.

294. Tinggaard-Pedersen N, Laursen B: Megakaryocytes in cubital venous blood in patients with chronic myeloproliferative diseases. *Scand J Haematol* 30:50, 1983.

295. Cervantes F, Hernandez-Boluda JC, Villamor N, et al: Assessment of peripheral blood lymphocyte subsets in idiopathic myelofibrosis. *Eur J Haematol* 65:104, 2000.

296. Marquetty C, Labro-Bryskier MT, Perianin A, et al: Impaired metabolic activity of phagocytosis neutrophils in agnogenic osteomyelofibrosis with splenomegaly. *Am J Med* 16:243, 1984.

297. Perianin A, Labro-Bryskier MT, Marquetty C, et al: Glutathione reductase and nitroblue tetrazolium reduction deficiencies in neutrophils of patients with primary idiopathic myelofibrosis. *Clin Exp Immunol* 57:244, 1984.

298. Briard D, Brouty-Boyé D, Giron-Michel J, et al: Impaired NK cell differentiation of blood-derived CD34+ progenitors from patients with myeloid metaplasia with myelofibrosis. *Clin Immunol* 106:201, 2003.

299. Murphy S, Davis JL, Walsh PN: Template bleeding time and clinical hemorrhage in myeloproliferative disease. *Arch Intern Med* 138:1251, 1978.

300. Malpass TW, Savage B, Hanson SR, et al: Correlation between bleeding time and depletion of platelet dense granule ADP in patients with myelodysplastic and myeloproliferative disorders. *J Lab Clin Med* 103:894, 1984.

301. Cunietti E, Gandini R, Marcaro G, et al: Defective platelet aggregation and increased platelet turnover in patients with myelofibrosis and other myeloproliferative diseases. *Scand J Haematol* 26:339, 1981.

302. Schafer AL: Deficiency of platelet lipoxygenase activity in myeloproliferative disorders. *N Engl J Med* 306:381, 1982.

303. Shafer AL: Bleeding and thrombosis in the myeloproliferative disorders. *Blood* 64:1, 1984.

304. Barbui T, Cortelazzo S, Viero P, et al: Thrombohaemorrhagic complications in 101 cases of myeloproliferative disorders: Relationship to platelet number and function. *Eur J Cancer Clin Oncol* 19:1593, 1983.

305. Thiele J, Lorenzen J, Manich B, et al: Apoptosis (programmed cell death) in idiopathic (primary) osteo-/myelofibrosis. *Acta Haematol* 97:137, 1997.

306. Thiele J, Holgado S, Choritz H, et al: Chronic megakaryocyte-granulocytic myelosis—An electron microscope study including freeze-fracture. *Virchows Arch A Pathol Anat Histol* 375:129, 1977.

307. Mesa RA, Hanson CA, Rajkumar SV, et al: Evaluation and clinical correlations of bone marrow angiogenesis in myelofibrosis with myeloid metaplasia. *Blood* 15:3374, 2000.

308. Bauermeister DE. Quantitation of bone marrow reticulin—a normal range. *Am J Clin Pathol* 56:24, 1971.

309. Thiele J, Kvasnicka HM: Myelofibrosis—What's in a name? Consensus on definition and EUMNET grading. *Pathobiology* 74:89, 2007.

310. Teman CJ, Wilson AR, Perkins SL, et al: Quantification of fibrosis and osteosclerosis in myeloproliferative neoplasms: A computer-assisted image study. *Leuk Res* 34:871, 2010.

311. Hussein K, Van Dyke DL, Tefferi A: Conventional cytogenetics in myelofibrosis: Literature review and discussion. *Eur J Haematol* 82:329, 2009.

312. Tam CS, Abruzzo LV, Lin KI, et al: The role of cytogenetic abnormalities as a prognostic marker in primary myelofibrosis: Applicability at the time of diagnosis and later during disease course. *Blood* 30:113, 2009.

313. Nakamura H, Sadamori N, Mine M, et al: Effects of short-term liquid culture of peripheral blood mononuclear cells with recombinant human granulocyte or granulocyte-macrophage colony-stimulating factor in cytogenetic studies of myelofibrosis with myeloid metaplasia. *Leukemia* 6:853, 1992.

314. Reilly JT, Snowden JA, Spearing RL, et al: Cytogenetic abnormalities and their prognostic significance in idiopathic myelofibrosis. *Br J Haematol* 98:96, 1997.

315. Tefferi A, Mesa RA, Schroeder G, et al: Cytogenetic findings and their clinical relevance in myelofibrosis with myeloid metaplasia. *Br J Haematol* 113:763, 2001.

316. Tefferi A, Meyer RG, Wyatt WA, et al: Comparison of peripheral blood interphase cytogenetics with bone marrow karyotype analysis in myelofibrosis with myeloid metaplasia. *Br J Haematol* 115:316, 2001.

317. Sinclair EJ, Forrest EC, Reilly JT, et al: Fluorescence *in situ* hybridization analysis of 25 cases of idiopathic myelofibrosis and two cases of secondary idiopathic: Monoallelic loss of RB1, D13S319 and D13S25 loci associated with cytogenetic deletion and translocation involving 13q14. *Br J Haematol* 113:365, 2001.

318. Reilly JT: Cytogenetic and molecular genetic aspects of idiopathic myelofibrosis. *Acta Haematol* 108:113, 2002.

319. Andrieux J, Demory JL, Morel P, et al: Frequency of structural abnormalities of the long arm of chromosome 12 in myelofibrosis with myeloid metaplasia. *Cancer Genet Cytogenet* 137:68, 2002.

320. Dingli D, Grand FH, Mahaffey V, et al: Der(6)t(1;6)(q21–23;p21.3): A specific cytogenetic abnormality in myelofibrosis with myeloid metaplasia. *Br J Haematol* 130:229, 2005.

321. Forrester RH, Louro JM: Philadelphia chromosome abnormality in agnogenic myeloid metaplasia. *Ann Intern Med* 64:622, 1966.

322. Gupta V, Hari P, Hoffman R. Allogeneic hematopoietic cell transplantation for myelofibrosis in the era of JAK inhibitors. *Blood* 120:1367, 2012.

323. Weda F, Takashima T, Suzuki M, Kadoya M: MR diagnosis of myelofibrosis. *Radiat Med* 12:135, 1994.

324. Amano Y, Onda M, Amano M, Kumazaki T: Magnetic resonance imaging of myelofibrosis. STIR and gadolinium-enhanced MR images. *Clin Imaging* 21:264, 1997.

325. Schirrmeister H, Bommer M, Buck A, Reske SN: The bone scan ion osteosclerosis. *J Bone Miner Res* 16:2361, 2001.

326. Spanos G, Narasimhan P, Rosner F. Hypocholesterolemia in myelofibrosis. *JAMA* 245:235, 1981.

327. Cervantes F, Pereira A, Esteve J, et al: Identification of "short-lived" and "long-lived" patients at presentation of idiopathic myelofibrosis. *Br J Haematol* 97:635, 1997.

328. Barosi G, Rosti V, Bonetti E, et al: Evidence that prefibrotic myelofibrosis is aligned along a clinical and biological continuum featuring primary myelofibrosis. *PLoS One* 7:e35631, 2012.

329. Gilbert HS, Ginsberg H, Fagerstrom R, Brown WV: Characterization of hypocholesterolemia in myeloproliferative diseases. *Am J Med* 71:595, 1981.

330. Naggar L, Jaeger P, Burckhardt P, et al: Hypocalcemia and myelofibrosis: An unrecognized association. *Schweiz Med Wochenschr* 116:1771, 1986.

331. Voss A, Schmidt K, Haesselbalch H, Junker P: Hypercalcemia in idiopathic myelofibrosis. *Am J Hematol* 39:231, 1992.

332. Wang JC, Chen C, Lou LH, Mora M: Blood thrombopoietin, IL-6 and IL-11 levels in patients with agnogenic myeloid metaplasia. *Leukemia* 11:1827, 1997.

333. Elliott MA, Yoon SY, Kao P, et al: Simultaneous measurement of serum thrombopoietin and expression of megakaryocyte c-MPL with clinical and laboratory correlates for myelofibrosis with myeloid metaplasia. *Eur J Haematol* 68:175, 2002.

334. Wang JC, Hashmi G: Elevated thrombopoietin levels in patients with myelofibrosis may not be due to enhanced production of thrombopoietin by bone marrow. *Leuk Res* 27:13, 2003.

335. Wang J, Wang A: Plasma soluble interleukin-2 receptor in patients with primary myelofibrosis. *Br J Haematol* 86:180, 1994.

336. Di Raimondo F, Azzaro MP, Palumbo GA, et al: Elevated vascular endothelial growth factor (VEGF) serum levels in idiopathic myelofibrosis. *Leukemia* 15:976, 2001.

337. Dekmezian R, Kantarjian HM, Heating MJ, et al: The relevance of reticulin stain-measured fibrosis at diagnosis in chronic myelogenous leukemia. *Cancer* 59:1739, 1987.

338. Steensma DP, Hanson C, Letendre L, Teffari A: Myelodysplasia with fibrosis: A distinct entity? *Leuk Res* 25:829, 2001.

339. Thiele J, Zankovich R, Steinberg T, et al: Primary (essential) thrombocythemia versus initial hyperplastic stages of agnogenic myeloid metaplasia with thrombocytosis. *Acta Haematol* 81:192, 1989.

340. Barbui T, Thiele J, Passamonti F, et al: Survival and disease progression in essential thrombocythemia are significantly influenced by accurate morphologic diagnosis: An international study. *J Clin Oncol* 29:3179, 2011.

341. Thiele J, Kvasnicka HM, Zankovich R, Diehl V: Relevance of bone marrow features in the differential diagnosis between essential thrombocythemia and early stage idiopathic myelofibrosis. *Haematologica* 85:1126, 2000.

342. Hasselbach H, Jans H, Nielsen PL: A distinct subtype of idiopathic myelofibrosis with bone marrow features mimicking hairy cell leukemia. Evidence of an autoimmune pathogenesis. *Am J Hematol* 25:225, 1979.

343. O'Reilly RA: Splenomegaly at a United States County Hospital: Diagnostic evaluation of 170 patients. *Am J Med Sci* 312:160, 1996.

344. Pullarkat V, Bass RD, Gong JZ, et al: Primary autoimmune myelofibrosis: Definition of a distinct clinicopathologic syndrome. *Am J Hematol* 72:8, 2003.

345. Harrison JS, Corcoran KE, Joshi D, et al: Peripheral monocytes and CD4+ cells are potential sources for increased circulating levels of TGF-beta and substance P in autoimmune myelofibrosis. *Am J Hematol* 81:51, 2006.

346. Popat U, Frost A, Liu E, et al: High levels of circulating CD34 cells, dacryocytes, clonal hematopoiesis, and JAK2 mutation differentiate myelofibrosis with myeloid metaplasia from secondary myelofibrosis associated with pulmonary hypertension. *Blood* 107:3486, 2006.

347. Fortunato A, Mazzone A, Ricevuti G: Myelofibrosis caused by cancer: Presentation of a clinical case with a very difficult diagnosis. *Minerva Med* 76:1051, 1985.

348. Yablonski-Peretz T, Sulkes A, Polliack A, et al: Secondary myelofibrosis with metastatic breast cancer simulating agnogenic myeloid metaplasia: Report of a case and review of the literature. *Med Pediatr Oncol* 13:92, 1985.

349. Ishimura J, Fukushi M: Scintigraphic evaluation of secondary myelofibrosis associated with prostatic cancer before hormonal therapy. *Clin Nucl Med* 15:330, 1990.

350. Smart HE, Canney PA, Kerr DJ: Myelofibrosis associated with metastatic seminoma. *Clin Oncol* 4:132, 1992.

351. Takahashi T, Akihama T, Yamaguchi A, et al: Lysozyme secreting tumor: A case of gastric cancer associated with myelofibrosis due to disseminated bone marrow metastasis. *Jpn J Med* 26:58, 1987.

352. Rubins JM: The role of myelofibrosis in malignant leukoerythroblastosis. *Cancer* 51:308, 1983.

353. Hashim MSK, Kordofani AYA, El Dabi MA: Tuberculosis and myelofibrosis in children. *Ann Trop Paediatr* 17:61, 1997.

354. Viallard J-F, Parrens M, Boiron J-M, et al: Reversible myelofibrosis induced by tuberculosis. *Clin Infect Dis* 34:1641, 2002.

355. Sawers AH, Davson J, Braganza J, et al: Systemic mastocytosis, myelofibrosis and portal hypertension. *J Clin Pathol* 35:617, 1982.

356. Reisberg IR, Oyakawa S: Mastocytosis with malabsorption, myelofibrosis, and massive ascites. *Am J Gastroenterol* 82:54, 1987.

357. Kanbe N, Kurosawa M, Nagata H, et al: Production of fibrogenic cytokines by cord blood-derived cultured human mast cells. *J Allergy Clin Immunol* 106:S85, 2000.

358. Berton A, Levi-Schaffer F, Emonard H, et al: Activation of fibroblasts in collagen lattices by mast cell extracts: A model of fibrosis. *Clin Exp Allergy* 30:485, 2000.

359. Brenner B, Green J, Rosenbaum H, et al: Severe pancytopenia due to marked marrow fibrosis associated with angioimmunoblastic lymphadenopathy. *Acta Haematol* 74:43, 1985.

360. Varma N, Vaiphei K, Varma S: Angiosarcoma presenting with leucoerythroblastic anaemia bone marrow fibrosis and massive splenomegaly. *Br J Haematol* 110:503, 2000.

361. Meckenstock G, Wehmeier A, Schaefer HE, et al: Lymphoid myelofibrosis associated with high grade B cell lymphoma of the liver. *Leuk Lymphoma* 26:197, 1997.

362. Abe Y, Ohshima K, Shiratsuchi M, et al: Cytotoxic T-cell lymphoma presenting as secondary myelofibrosis with high levels of PDGF and TGF-β. *Eur J Haematol* 66:210, 2001.

363. Weirich G, Sandherr M, Fellbaum C, et al: Molecular evidence of bone marrow involvement in advanced case of Tgammadelta lymphoma with secondary myelofibrosis. *Hum Pathol* 29:761, 1998.

364. Subramanian R, Basu D, Dutta TK: Significance of bone marrow fibrosis in multiple myeloma. *Pathology* 39:512, 2007.

365. Schmidt U, Ruwe M, Leder LD: Multiple myeloma with bone marrow biopsy features simulating concomitant chronic idiopathic myelofibrosis. *Nouv Rev Fr Hematol* 37:159, 1995.

366. Abildgaard N, Bendix-Hansen K, Kristensen JE, et al: Bone marrow fibrosis and disease activity in multiple myeloma monitored by the aminoterminal propeptide of procollagen III in serum. *Br J Haematol* 99:641, 1997.

367. Kim CD, Kim SH, Kim YL, et al: Bone marrow immunoscintigraphy (BMIS): A new and important tool for the assessment of marrow fibrosis in renal osteodystrophy? *Adv Perit Dial* 14:183, 1998.

368. Bachmeyer C, Blum L, Cadranel JF, Delfraissy JF: Myelofibrosis in a patient with pachydermoperiostosis. *Clin Exp Dermatol* 30:646, 2005.

369. Nurden AT, Nurden P: The gray platelet syndrome: Clinical spectrum of the disease. *Blood Rev* 21:21, 2007.

370. Sadoun A, Lacotte L, Delwail V, et al: Allogeneic bone marrow transplantation for hypereosinophilic syndrome with advanced myelofibrosis. *Bone Marrow Transplant* 19:741, 1997.

371. Vasquez L, Caballero D, Del Cañizo C, et al: Allogeneic peripheral blood cell transplantation for hypereosinophilic syndrome with myelofibrosis. *Bone Marrow Transplant* 25:217, 2000.

372. Filho FDR, Ferreira VDA, Mendes FDO, et al: Bone marrow fibrosis (pseudo-myelofibrosis) in kala-azar. *Rev Soc Bras Med Trop* 33:363, 2000.

373. Seelen MA, de Meijer PH, Posthuma EF, Meinders AE: Myelofibrosis and idiopathic thrombocytopenic purpura. *Ann Hematol* 75:129, 1997.

374. Chang JC, Naqvi T: Thrombotic thrombocytopenic purpura associated with bone marrow metastasis and secondary myelofibrosis in cancer. *Oncologist* 8:375, 2003.

375. Hatake K, Ohtsuki T, Uwai M, et al: Tretinoin induces bone marrow collagenous fibrosis in acute promyelocytic leukemia. *Br J Haematol* 93:646, 1996.

376. Labotka RJ, Morgan RR: Myelofibrosis with neuroblastoma. *Med Pediatr Oncol* 10:21, 1982.

377. Karcher DS, Pearson CE, Butler WM, et al: Giant lymph node hyperplasia involving the thymus with associated nephrotic syndrome and myelofibrosis. *Am J Clin Pathol* 77:100, 1982.

378. Kamien B, Harris L: Twin troubles—Rickets causing myelofibrosis. *J Paediatr Child Health* 43:573, 2007.

379. Stéphan JL, Galambrun C, Dutour A, Freycon F: Myelofibrosis: An unusual presentation of vitamin D-deficient rickets. *Eur J Pediatr* 158:828, 1999.

380. Gruner BA, DeNapoli TS, Elshihabi S, et al: Anemia and hepatosplenomegaly as presenting features in a child with rickets and secondary myelofibrosis. *J Pediatr Hematol Oncol* 25:813, 2003.

381. Razali NN, Hwu TT, Thilakavathy K: Phosphate homeostasis and genetic mutations of familial hypophosphatemic rickets. *J Pediatr Endocrinol Metab* 2015. [Epub ahead of print]

382. Sartoris DJ, Resnick D: Myelofibrosis arising in treated histiocytosis X. *Eur J Pediatr* 144:200, 1985.

383. Fukuno K, Tsurumi H, Yoshikawa T, et al: A variant of acute promyelocytic leukemia with marked myelofibrosis. *Int J Hematol* 74:322, 2001.

384. Mori A, Wada H, Okada M, et al: Acute promyelocytic leukemia with marrow fibrosis at initial presentation. Possible involvement of transforming growth factor-beta(1). *Acta Haematol* 103:220, 2000.

385. Shah-Reddy I, Subramanian L, Narang S: Myelofibrosis and true histiocytic lymphoma. *Tumori* 71:509, 1985.

386. Jennings WH, Li CY, Kiely JM: Concomitant myelofibrosis with agnogenic myeloid metaplasia and malignant lymphoma. *Mayo Clin Proc* 58:617, 1983.

387. Epstein RJ, Joshua DE, Kronenberg H: Idiopathic myelofibrosis complicated by lymphoma: Report of two cases. *Acta Haematol* 73:40, 1985.

388. Kaufman S, Iuclea S, Reif R: Idiopathic myelofibrosis complicated by chronic lymphatic leukaemia. *Clin Lab Haematol* 9:81, 1987.

389. Nieto LH, Raya Sánchez JM, Arguelles HA, et al: A case of chronic lymphocytic leukemia overwhelmed by rapidly progressive idiopathic myelofibrosis. *Haematologica* 85:973, 2000.

390. Subramanian VP, Gomez GA, Han T, et al: Coexistence of myeloid metaplasia with myelofibrosis and hairy-cell leukemia. *Arch Intern Med* 145:164, 1985.

391. Sotlar K, Bache A, Stellmacher F, et al: Systemic mastocytosis associated with chronic idiopathic myelofibrosis: A distinct subtype of systemic mastocytosis associated with a clonal hematological non-mast cell lineage disorder carrying the activating point mutations KITD816V and JAK2V617F. *J Mol Diagn* 10:58, 2008.

392. Ji SQ, Zhu M, Wang YZ: Primary macroglobulinemia with myelofibrosis: Report of a case. *Chin Med J* 100:83, 1987.

393. Humphrey CA, Morris TC: The intimate relationship of myelofibrosis and myeloma: Effect of therapy. *Br J Haematol* 73:269, 1989.

394. Meerkin D, Ashkenazi Y, Gottschalk-Sabag S, Hershko C: Plasma cell dyscrasia with myelofibrosis. A reversible syndrome mimicking agnogenic myeloid metaplasia. *Cancer* 73:625, 1994.

395. Kakkar N, Vashishta RK, Banerjee AK, et al: Primary pulmonary malignant teratoma with yolk sac element associated with hematologic neoplasia. *Respiration* 63:52, 1996.

396. Berner Y, Berrebi A: Myeloproliferative disorders and nonmyelomatous paraprotein: A study of five patients and review of the literature. *Isr J Med Sci* 22:109, 1986.

397. Ellis JT, Peterson P: Myelofibrosis in the myeloproliferative disorders. *Prog Clin Biol Res* 154:19, 1984.

398. Najean Y, Rain JD, Dresch C, et al: Risk of leukaemia, carcinoma and myelofibrosis in ^{32}P- or chemotherapy-treated patients with polycythaemia vera. *Leuk Lymphoma* 22(Suppl 1):111, 1996.

399. Najean Y, Rain JD: Treatment of polycythemia vera: Use of ^{32}P alone or in combination with maintenance therapy using hydroxyurea in 461 patients greater than 65 years of age. *Blood* 89:2319, 1997.

400. Randi ML, Barbone E, Fabris F, et al: Post-polycythemia myeloid metaplasia. *J Med* 25:363, 1994.

401. Lukowicz DF, Myers TJ, Grasso JA, et al: Sideroblastic anemia terminating in myelofibrosis. *Am J Hematol* 13:253, 1982.

402. Talarico L, Wolf BC, Kumar A, Weintraub LR: Reversal of bone marrow fibrosis and subsequent development of polycythemia vera in patients with myeloproliferative disorders. *Am J Hematol* 30:248, 1989.

403. Butler MJ, Roda PI, Dorion P: Molecular characterization of a transformation from primary myelofibrosis into polycythemia vera: A case report. *Blood* 122:297, 2013.

404. Jallades L, Hayette S, Tigaud I, et al: Emergence of therapy-unrelated CML on a background of BCR-ABL-negative JAK2V617F-positive chronic idiopathic myelofibrosis. *Leuk Res* 32:1608, 2008.

405. Hussein K, Bock O, Seegers A, et al: Myelofibrosis evolving during imatinib treatment of a chronic myeloproliferative disease with coexisting BCR-ABL translocation and JAK2 V617F mutation. *Blood* 109:4106, 2007.

406. Cervantes F, Dupriez B, Pereira A, et al: New prognostic scoring system for primary myelofibrosis based on a study of the International Working Group for Myelofibrosis Research and Treatment. *Blood* 113:2895, 2009.

407. Barois G, Liberato LN, Guarnone R: Serum erythropoietin in patients with myeloid metaplasia. *Br J Haematol* 83:365, 1993.

408. Cervantes F, Alvarez-Larrán A, Hernández-Boluda JC, et al: Erythropoietin treatment of the anaemia of myelofibrosis with myeloid metaplasia: Results in 20 patients and review of the literature. *Br J Haematol* 127:399, 2004.

409. Cervantes F, Alvarez-Larrán A, Hernández-Boluda JC, et al: Darbepoetin-alpha for the anaemia of myelofibrosis with myeloid metaplasia. *Br J Haematol* 134:184, 2006.

410. Cervantes F, Alvarez-Larrán A, Domingo A, et al: Efficacy and tolerability of danazol as a treatment for the anaemia of myelofibrosis with myeloid metaplasia: Long-term results in 30 patients. *Br J Haematol* 129:771, 2005.

411. Makdisi WJ, Cherian R, Vanveldhuizen PJ, et al: Fatal peliosis of the liver and spleen in a patient with agnogenic myeloid metaplasia treated with danazol. *Am J Gastroenterol* 90:317, 1995.

412. Ozsoylu S, Ruacan S: High-dose intravenous corticosteroid treatment in childhood idiopathic myelofibrosis. *Acta Haematol* 75:49, 1986.

413. Cetingül N, Yener E, Oztop S, et al: Agnogenic myeloid metaplasia in childhood: A report of two cases and efficiency of intravenous high dose methylprednisolone treatment. *Acta Paediatr Jpn* 36:697, 1994.

414. Wilks AF: The JAK kinases: Not just another kinase drug discovery target. *Semin Cell Dev Biol* 19:319, 2008.

415. Pardanani A, Hood J, Lasho T, et al: TG101209, a small molecule JAK2-selective kinase inhibitor potently inhibits myeloproliferative disorder-associated JAK2V617F and MPLW515L/K mutations. *Leukemia* 21:1658, 2007.

416. Verstovsek S, Kantarjian HM, Pardanani AD, et al: The JAK inhibitor, INCB018424, demonstrates durable and marked clinical responses in primary myelofibrosis (PMF) and post-polycythemia/essential thrombocythemia myelofibrosis (PV/ET-MF). *Blood* 112:622, 2008.

417. Pardanani AD, Gotlib J, Jamieson C, et al: A phase I study of TG101348, an orally bioavailable JAK-2 selective inhibitor, in patients with myelofibrosis. *Blood* 112:43, 2008.

418. Shah, NP, Olszynski P, Sokol, L, et al: A phase I study of XL019, a selective JAK2 inhibitor, in patients with primary myelofibrosis polycythemia vera, or post-essential thrombocythemia myelofibrosis. *Blood* 112:441, 2008.

419. Harrison C, Kiladjian JJ, Al-Ali HK, et al: JAK inhibition with ruxolitinib versus best available therapy for myelofibrosis. *N Engl J Med* 366:787, 2012.

420. Verstovsek S, Mesa RA, Gotlib J, et al: The clinical benefit of ruxolitinib across patient subgroups: Analysis of a placebo-controlled, phase III study in patients with myelofibrosis. *Br J Haematol* 161:508, 2013.

421. Mesa RA, Gotlib J, Gupta V, et al: Effect of ruxolitinib therapy on myelofibrosis-related symptoms and other patient-reported outcomes in COMFORT-I: A randomized, double-blind, placebo-controlled trial. *J Clin Oncol* 31:1285, 2013.

422. Mesa RA, Kiladjian JJ, Verstovsek S, et al: Comparison of placebo and best available therapy for the treatment of myelofibrosis in the phase 3 COMFORT studies. *Haematologica* 99:292, 2014.

423. Talpaz M, Paquette R, Afrin L, et al: Interim analysis of safety and efficacy of ruxolitinib in patients with myelofibrosis and low platelet counts. *J Hematol Oncol* 6:81, 2013.

424. Lofvenberg E, Wahlin A: Management of polycythaemia vera, essential thrombocythaemia and myelofibrosis with hydroxyurea. *Eur J Haematol* 41:375, 1988.

425. Lofvenberg E, Wahlin A, Roos G, Ost A: Reversal of myelofibrosis by hydroxyurea. *Eur J Haematol* 44:33, 1990.

426. Manoharan A: Management of myelofibrosis with intermittent hydroxyurea. *Br J Haematol* 71:252, 1991.

427. Petti MC, Latagliata R, Spadea T, et al: Melphalan treatment in patients with myelofibrosis with myeloid metaplasia. *Br J Haematol* 116:576, 2002.

428. Tefferi A: Polycythemia vera and essential thrombocythemia: 2013 Update on diagnosis, risk-stratification, and management. *Am J Hematol* 88:507, 2013.

429. Merup M, Kutti J, Birgerård G, et al: Negligible clinical effects of thalidomide in patient with myelofibrosis with myeloid metaplasia. *Med Oncol* 19:79, 2002.

430. Piccaluga PP, Visani G, Pileri SA, et al: Clinical efficacy and antiangiogenic activity of thalidomide in myelofibrosis with myeloid metaplasia. A pilot study. *Leukemia* 16:1609, 2002.

431. Strupp C, Germing U, Scherer A, et al: Thalidomide for treatment of idiopathic myelofibrosis. *Eur J Haematol* 72:52, 2004.

432. Mesa RA, Lliott MA, Schroeder G, Tefferi A: Durable responses to thalidomide-based drug therapy for myelofibrosis with myeloid metaplasia. *Mayo Clin Proc* 79:883, 2004.

433. Tefferi A, Cortes J, Verstovsek S, et al: Lenalidomide therapy in myelofibrosis with myeloid metaplasia. *Blood* 108:1158, 2006.

434. Santana-Davila R, Tefferi A, Holtan SG, et al: Primary myelofibrosis is the most frequent myeloproliferative neoplasm associated with del(5q): Clinicopathologic comparison of del(5q)-positive and -negative cases. *Leuk Res* 32:1927, 2008.

435. Tefferi A, Lasho TL, Mesa RA, et al: Lenalidomide therapy in del(5)(q31)-associated myelofibrosis: Cytogenetic and JAK2V617F molecular remissions. *Leukemia* 21:1827, 2007.

436. Cervantes F, Mesa R, Barosi G: New and old treatment modalities in primary myelofibrosis. *Cancer J* 13:377, 2007.

437. Begna KH, Pardanani A, Mesa R, et al: Long-term outcome of pomalidomide therapy in myelofibrosis. *Am J Hematol* 87:66, 2012.

438. Centanara E, Guarone R, Ippoliti G, Barosi G: Cyclosporine-A in severe refractory anemia of myelofibrosis with myeloid metaplasia: A preliminary report. *Haematologica* 83:622, 1998.

439. Nemoto Y, Tsutani H, Imamura S, et al: Successful treatment of acquired myelofibrosis with pure red cell aplasia. *Br J Haematol* 104:420, 1999.

440. Tsimberidou AM, Giles FJ: TNF-α targeted therapeutic approaches in patients with hematologic malignancies. *Expert Rev Anticancer Ther* 2:277, 2002.

441. Steensma DP, Mesa RA, Li CY, et al: Etanercept, a soluble tumor necrosis factor receptor, palliates constitutional symptoms in patients with myelofibrosis with myeloid metaplasia: Results of a pilot study. *Blood* 99:2252, 2002.

442. Mesa RA: The therapy of myelofibrosis: Targeting pathogenesis. *Int J Hematol* 76 Suppl 2:296, 2002.

443. Tefferi A, Mesa RA, Gray LA, et al: Phase 2 trial of imatinib mesylate in myelofibrosis with myeloid metaplasia. *Blood* 99:3854, 2002.

444. Mesa RA, Camoriano JK, Geyer SM, et al: A phase II trial of tipifarnib in myelofibrosis: Primary, post-polycythemia vera and post-essential thrombocythemia. *Leukemia* 21:1964, 2007.

445. Carlo-Stella C, Cazzola M, Gasner A, et al: Effects of recombinant alpha and gamma interferons on the *in vitro* growth of circulating hematopoietic progenitors from patients with myelofibrosis and myeloid metaplasia. *Blood* 70:1014, 1987.

446. Sacchi S: The role of alpha-interferon in essential thrombocythaemia, polycythaemia vera and myelofibrosis with myeloid metaplasia (MMM): A concise update. *Leuk Lymphoma* 19:13, 1995.

447. Bachleitner-Hofmann T, Gisslinger H: The role of interferon-alpha in the treatment of idiopathic myelofibrosis. *Ann Hematol* 78:533, 1999.

448. Heis-Vahidi-Fard N, Forberg E, Eichinger S, et al: Ineffectiveness of interferon-gamma in the treatment of idiopathic myelofibrosis: A pilot study. *Ann Hematol* 80:79, 2001.

449. Gowin K, Thapaliya P, Samuelson J, et al: Experience with pegylated interferon α-2a in advanced myeloproliferative neoplasms in an international cohort of 118 patients. *Haematologica* 97:1570, 2012.

450. Ianotto JC, Boyer-Perrard F, Gyan E, et al: Efficacy and safety of pegylated-interferon α-2a in myelofibrosis: A study by the FIM and GEM French cooperative groups. *Br J Haematol* 162:783, 2013.

451. Silver RT, Vandris K, Goldman JJ: Recombinant interferon-α may retard progression of early primary myelofibrosis: A preliminary report. *Blood* 117:6669, 2011.

452. Stahl RL, Hoppstein L, Davidson TG: Intraperitoneal chemotherapy with cytosine arabinoside in agnogenic myelofibrosis with myeloid metaplasia and ascites due to peritoneal extramedullary hematopoiesis. *Am J Hematol* 43:156, 1993.

453. Camba L, Aldrighetti L, Ciceri F, et al: Locoregional intrasplenic chemotherapy for hypersplenism in myelofibrosis. *Br J Haematol* 114:638, 2001.

454. Amital H, Rewald E, Levy Y, et al: Fibrosis regression induced by intravenous gamma-globulin treatment. *Ann Rheum Dis* 62:175, 2003.

455. Sivera P, Cesano L, Guerrasio A, et al: Clinical and hematological improvement induced by etidronate in a patient with idiopathic myelofibrosis and osteosclerosis. *Br J Haematol* 86:397, 1994.

456. Froom P, Elmalah I, Braester A, et al: Clodronate in myelofibrosis: A case report. *Am J Med Sci* 323:115, 2002.

457. Assous N, Foltz V, Fautrel B, et al: Bone involvement in myelofibrosis: Effectiveness of bisphosphonates. *Joint Bone Spine* 72:591, 2005.

458. Elliott MA, Tefferi A: Splenic irradiation in myelofibrosis with myeloid metaplasia: A review. *Blood Rev* 13:163, 1999.

459. Jacobs P, Wood L, Robson S: Refractory ascites in the chronic myeloproliferative syndrome. *Am J Hematol* 37:128, 1991.

460. Jacobs P, Sellars S: Granulocytic sarcoma preceding leukaemic transformation in myelofibrosis. *Postgrad Med J* 61:1069, 1985.

461. Teffari A, Jimenez T, Gray LA, et al: Radiation therapy for symptomatic hepatomegaly in myelofibrosis with myeloid metaplasia. *Eur J Haematol* 66:37, 2001.

462. Mesa RA, Nagorney DS, Schwager S, et al: Palliative goals, patient selection, and perioperative platelet management: Outcomes and lessons from 3 decades of splenectomy for myelofibrosis with myeloid metaplasia at the Mayo Clinic. *Cancer* 107:361, 2006.

463. Tefferi A, Barrett SM, Silverstein NM, Nagorney DM: Outcome of portal-systemic shunt surgery for portal hypertension associated with intrahepatic obstruction in patients with agnogenic myeloid metaplasia. *Am J Hematol* 46:325, 1994.

464. Angermayr B, Cejna M, Schoder M, et al: Transjugular intrahepatic portosystemic shunt for treatment of portal hypertension due to extramedullary hematopoiesis in idiopathic myelofibrosis. *Blood* 99:4246, 2002.

465. Belohlavek J, Schwarz J, Jirásek A, et al: Idiopathic myelofibrosis complicated by portal hypertension treated with a transjugular intrahepatic portosystemic shunt (TIPS). *Wien Klin Wochenschr* 113:208, 2001.

466. Guardiola P, Anderson JE, Bandini G, et al: Allogeneic stem cell transplantation for agnogenic myeloid metaplasia: A European Group for Blood and Marrow Transplantation, Société Française de Greffe de Moelle, Gruppo Italiano per il Trapianto Midollo Osseo, and Fred Hutchinson Cancer Center Collaborative Study. *Blood* 93:2831, 1999.

467. Deeg HJ, Appelbaum FR: Stem-cell transplantation for myelofibrosis. *N Engl J Med* 334:775, 2001.

468. McCarty JM: Transplant strategies for idiopathic myelofibrosis. *Semin Hematol* 41(Suppl 3):23, 2004.

469. Mittal P, Saliba RM, Giralt SA, et al: Allogeneic transplantation: A therapeutic option for myelofibrosis, chronic myelomonocytic leukemia, and Philadelphia-negative BCR-ABL-negative chronic myelogenous leukemia. *Bone Marrow Transplant* 33:1005, 2004.

470. Papageorgiou SG, Castleton A, Bloor A, Kottaridis PD: Allogeneic stem cell transplantation as treatment for myelofibrosis. *Bone Marrow Transplant* 38:721, 2006.

471. Barosi G, Bacigalupo A: Allogeneic hematopoietic stem cell transplantation for myelofibrosis. *Curr Opin Hematol* 13:74, 2006.

472. Kerbauy DM, Gooley TA, Sale GE, et al: Hematopoietic cell transplantation as curative therapy for idiopathic myelofibrosis, advanced polycythemia vera, and essential thrombocythemia. *Biol Blood Marrow Transplant* 13:355, 2007.

473. Rondelli D: Allogeneic hematopoietic stem cell transplantation for myelofibrosis. *Haematologica* 93:1449, 2008.

474. Li Z, Deeg HJ: Pros and cons of splenectomy in patients with myelofibrosis undergoing stem cell transplantation. *Leukemia* 15:465, 2001.

475. Byrne JL, Beshti H, Clark D, et al: Induction of remission after donor leucocyte infusion for the treatment of relapsed chronic idiopathic myelofibrosis following allogeneic transplantation: Evidence for a "graft vs. myelofibrosis" effect. *Br J Haematol* 108:430, 2000.

476. Cervantes F, Rovira M, Urbano-Ispizua A, et al: Complete remission of idiopathic myelofibrosis following donor lymphocyte infusion after failure of allogeneic transplantation: Demonstration of a graft-versus-myelofibrosis effect. *Bone Marrow Transplant* 26:697, 2000.

477. Kröger N, Badbaran A, Holler E, et al: Monitoring of the JAK2-V617F mutation by highly sensitive quantitative real-time PCR after allogeneic stem cell transplantation in patients with myelofibrosis. *Blood* 109:1316, 2007.

478. Devine SM, Hoffman R, Verma A, et al: Allogeneic blood cell transplantation following reduced-intensity conditioning is effective therapy for older patients with myelofibrosis with myeloid metaplasia. *Blood* 99:2255, 2002.

479. Hessling J, Kroger N, Werner M, et al: Dose-reduced conditioning regimen followed by allogeneic stem cell transplantation in patients with myelofibrosis with myeloid metaplasia. *Br J Haematol* 119:769, 2002.

480. Merup M, Lazarevic V, Nahi H, et al: Different outcome of allogeneic transplantation in myelofibrosis using conventional or reduced-intensity conditioning regimens. *Br J Haematol* 135:367, 2006.

481. Greyz N, Miller WE, Andrey J, Masson J: Long-term remission of myelofibrosis following nonmyeloablative allogenic peripheral blood progenitor cell transplantation in older age. *Bone Marrow Transplant* 34:833, 2004.

482. Gupta V, Malone AK, Hari PN, et al: Reduced-intensity hematopoietic cell transplantation for patients with primary myelofibrosis: A cohort analysis from the center for international blood and marrow transplant research. *Biol Blood Marrow Transplant* 20:89, 2014.

483. Hoffman R, Prchal JT, Samuelson S, et al: Philadelphia chromosome-negative myeloproliferative disorders: Biology and treatment. *Biol Blood Marrow Transplant* 13(Suppl 1):64, 2007.

484. Anderson JE, Tefferi A, Craig F, et al: Myeloablation and autologous peripheral blood stem cell rescue results in hematologic and clinical responses in patients with myeloid metaplasia with myelofibrosis. *Blood* 98:586, 2001.

485. Visini G, Finelli C, Castelli U, et al: Myelofibrosis with myeloid metaplasia: Clinical and haematological parameters predicting survival in a series of 133 patients. *Br J Haematol* 75:4, 1990.

486. Cervantes F: Prognostic and current practice in treatment of myelofibrosis and myeloid metaplasia: An update anno 2000. *Pathol Biol (Paris)* 49:148, 2001.

487. Mesa RA, Li C-Y, Schroeder G, Tefferi A: Clinical correlates of splenic histology and splenic karyotype in myelofibrosis with myeloid metaplasia. *Blood* 97:3665, 2001.

488. Kvasnicka HM, Thiele J, Regn C, et al: Prognostic impact of apoptosis and proliferation in idiopathic (primary) myelofibrosis. *Ann Hematol* 78:65, 1999.

489. Elliott MA, Verstovsek S, Dingli D, et al: Monocytosis is an adverse prognostic factor for survival in younger patients with primary myelofibrosis. *Leuk Res* 31:1503, 2007.

490. Campbell PJ, Griesshammer M, Döhner K, et al: V617F mutation in JAK2 is associated with poorer survival in idiopathic myelofibrosis. *Blood* 107:2098, 2006.

491. Cervantes F, Dupriez B, Pereira A, et al: A new prognostic scoring system for primary myelofibrosis based on a study of the International Working Group for Myelofibrosis Research and Treatment. *Blood* 113:2895, 2009.

492. Rozman C, Giralt M, Feliu E, et al: Life expectancy of patients with chronic nonleukemic myeloproliferative disorders. *Cancer* 67:2658, 1991.

493. Mascarenhas J, Hoffman R: A comprehensive review and analysis of the effect of ruxolitinib therapy on the survival of patients with myelofibrosis. *Blood* 121:4832, 2013.

494. Passamonti F, Maffioli M, Cervantes F, et al: Impact of ruxolitinib on the natural history of primary myelofibrosis: A comparison of the DIPSS and the COMFORT-2 cohorts. *Blood* 123:1833, 2014.

495. Silverstein MN, Brown AL, Linman JW: Idiopathic myeloid metaplasia, its evolution into acute leukemia. *Arch Intern Med* 132:709, 1973.

496. Marcus RE, Hibbin JA, Matutes E, et al: Megakaryoblastic transformation of myelofibrosis with expression of the c-*sis* oncogene. *Am J Hematol* 36:186, 1986.

497. Hernandez JM, SanMiguel JF, Gonzalez M, et al: Development of acute leukaemia after idiopathic myelofibrosis. *J Clin Pathol* 45:427, 1992.

498. Palphilon DH, Creamer P, Keeling DH, et al: Restoration of active haemopoiesis in a patient with myelofibrosis and subsequent termination in acute myeloblastic leukaemia: Case report and review of the literature. *Eur J Haematol* 38:279, 1987.

499. Chan ACL, Kwong Y-L, Lam CCK: Granulocytic sarcoma of megakaryoblastic differentiation complicating chronic idiopathic myelofibrosis. *Hum Pathol* 27:417, 1996.

500. Barnes HM, Prchal JT, Scott CW: Extramedullary blast transformation in the central nervous system in idiopathic myelofibrosis. *Am J Hematol* 11:305, 1981.

501. Polliack A, Prokocimer M, Matzner Y, et al: Lymphoblastic leukemic transformation (lymphoblastic crisis) in myelofibrosis and myeloid metaplasia. *Am J Hematol* 9:211, 1980.

502. Yinon A, Kopolovic J, Dollberg L, Hershko C: Evolution of malignant lymphoma in agnogenic myeloid metaplasia. *Oncology* 45:373, 1988.

503. Barosi G, Ambrosetti A, Centra A: Splenectomy and risk of blast transformation in myelofibrosis with myeloid metaplasia. *Blood* 91:3630, 1998.

504. Huang J, Li CY, Mesa RA, et al: Risk factors for leukemic transformation in patients with primary myelofibrosis. *Cancer* 112:2726, 2008.

505. Shreiner DP: Spontaneous hematologic remission in agnogenic myeloid metaplasia. *Am J Med* 60:1014, 1976.

506. Rani MV, Shreiner DP: Spontaneous "remission" of agnogenic myeloid metaplasia and termination in acute myeloid leukemia. *Arch Intern Med* 141:1481, 1981.

507. Vannucchi AM, Lasho TL, Guglielmelli P, et al: Mutations and prognosis in primary myelofibrosis. *Leukemia* 27:1861, 2013.

508. Guglielmelli P, Lasho TL, Rotunno G, et al: The number of prognostically detrimental mutations and prognosis in primary myelofibrosis: An international study of 797 patients. *Leukemia* 28:1804, 2014.

509. Poletto V, Rosti V, Villani L, et al: A3669G polymorphism of glucocorticoid receptor is a susceptibility allele for primary myelofibrosis and contributes to phenotypic diversity and blast transformation. *Blood* 120:3112, 2012.

509A. Tefferi A, Lasho TL, Finke CM, et al: CALR vs JAK2 vs MPL-mutated or triple-negative myelofibrosis: clinical, cytogenetic and molecular comparisons. Leukemia 28:1472, 2014.

510. Altura RA, Headv DR, Wang WC: Long-term survival of infants with idiopathic myelofibrosis. *Br J Haematol* 109:459, 2000.

511. Sah A, Minford A, Parapia LA: Spontaneous remission of juvenile idiopathic myelofibrosis. *Br J Haematol* 112:1083, 2001.

CHAPTER 87
MYELODYSPLASTIC SYNDROMES

Rafael Bejar and David P. Steensma*

SUMMARY

Myelodysplastic syndromes (MDS) are a heterogenous group of clonal hematopoietic neoplasms defined by morphologic dysmorphia, one or more blood cytopenias, and an increased risk of clonal evolution to acute myelogenous leukemia (AML). These disorders can occur at any age but have an incidence that rises exponentially after age 40 years with a median age at diagnosis of 72 years. Most cases are acquired *de novo* through the accumulation of somatic mutations, although a small fraction arises after exposure to DNA damaging agents, such as chemotherapy and radiation. A minority of cases are the result of inherited mutations that predispose to the development of MDS and related myeloid disorders. Subtypes of MDS are largely defined by clinical features and range from refractory cytopenias (typically including anemia) to oligoblastic myelogenous leukemia with an increase in marrow myeloblasts (5 to 19 percent). Cases with 20 percent or more myeloblasts in the marrow (an arbitrary boundary) or specific chromosomal translocations are defined as AML. The diagnostic criteria for MDS include dysmorphogenesis in one or more blood cell lineages, often resulting in exaggerated apoptosis during later stages of maturation. Poikilocytosis, anisocytosis, anisochromia, and basophilic stippling are features of the abnormal red cells. The marrow usually contains increased erythroid precursors with dysmorphic features, including nuclear distortions and scanty, poorly hemoglobinized cytoplasm or macroerythroblasts. Pathologic ring sideroblasts are a common feature used to define particular subtypes of MDS. Neutrophils may have bilobed or hypersegmented nuclei and hypogranulated cytoplasm in association with increased marrow granulocyte precursors. Giant and microcytic platelets, sometimes with abnormal or absent granulation, in the blood are associated with megakaryocytic hyperplasia and atypical lobulation of the nucleus, megakaryocyte clustering, and decreased marrow megakaryocyte size. Clonal cytogenetic abnormalities occur in approximately 50 percent of patients, typically as recurrent deletions of entire chromosomes or chromosomal segments. Trisomy 8 is the only frequent copy number gain and recurrent translocations are rare. Various prognostic models for MDS incorporate cytogenetic abnormalities along with marrow blast proportion and blood cytopenias to predict the mortality and risk of clonal evolution to AML. The selection and timing of therapy for MDS is largely driven by risk stratification. Newer prognostic scoring systems have begun to consider somatic mutations as markers of disease-associated risk as pathogenic driver mutations can be identified in almost all cases of MDS and several lesions have a prognostic significance that is independent of other known risk factors. As detectable somatic events, driver mutations are markers of clonal hematopoiesis and could help establish the diagnosis in some cases. Recurrent somatic mutations identify the heterogenous molecular pathways frequently disordered in MDS. These include mutations in multiple components of the RNA splicing machinery, several epigenetic regulators of DNA methylation and histone modifications, various hematopoietic transcription factors, and growth factor signaling pathway members among others. Certain mutations are tightly associated with clinical features including ring sideroblasts, chromosomal instability, and severe cytopenias. Current treatment guidelines for MDS are based on clinical risk assessments and generally do not consider genetic abnormalities. The exception are cases with del(5q) and noncomplex karyotypes that have a high rate of deep and sustained responses to the immunomodulator drug lenalidomide. Many patients with lower-risk MDS may not require treatment. Others may benefit from hematopoietic growth factor support or immune suppression with antithymocyte globulin and a calcineurin inhibitor, depending on specific clinical features. Higher-risk MDS is typically treated with one of the hypomethylating agents, azacitidine or decitabine, and eligible patients are evaluated for hematopoietic allogeneic hematopoietic stem cell transplantation, the only potentially curative treatment for MDS. Despite these treatment options, outcomes for persons with MDS remain poor overall. Novel therapies targeting recently identified molecular pathways have been developed and are being pursued in clinical trials.

Acronyms and Abbreviations: AHSCT, allogeneic hematopoietic stem cell transplantation; ALIP, abnormal localized immature precursor; ALL, acute lymphocytic leukemia; AML, acute myelogenous leukemia; ATG, antithymocyte globulin; ATRA, all-*trans*-retinoic acid; aUPD, acquired uniparental disomy; CALGB, Cancer and Leukemia Group B; CDR, commonly deleted region; CLL, chronic lymphocytic leukemia; CMML, chronic myelomonocytic leukemia; ESA, erythropoiesis-stimulating agent; FAB, French-American-British; FPD, familial platelet disorder; G-CSF, granulocyte colony-stimulating factor; GM-CSF, granulocyte-macrophage colony-stimulating factor; HLA, human leukocyte antigens; IDH, isocitrate dehydrogenase; IL, interleukin; IPSS, International Prognosis Scoring System; IPSS-R, International Prognosis Scoring System Revised; LGL, large granular lymphocyte; MAP, mitogen-activated protein; M-CSF, monocyte colony-stimulating factor; MDS, myelodysplastic syndrome; MDS/MPN, myelodysplastic syndrome/myeloproliferative neoplasm; miRNA, microRNA; NCI, National Cancer Institute; NK, natural killer; PLK, polo-like kinase; PRC, protein-repressive complex; RA, refractory anemia; RAEB, refractory anemia with excess blasts; RAEB-t, refractory anemia with excess blasts in transformation; RARS, refractory anemia with ring sideroblasts; RARS-t, refractory anemia with ring sideroblasts and thrombocytosis; RBC, red blood cell; SEER, Surveillance, Epidemiology and End Results; snRNP, small nuclear riboprotein complex; TET, ten-eleven translocation; TGF, transforming growth factor; TNF, tumor necrosis factor; WT, Wilms tumor; WHO, World Health Organization.

*We acknowledge Drs. Marshall Lichtman and Jane Liesveld who wrote this chapter in previous editions of this text. We have retained sections of their previous chapter.

DEFINITION

Myelodysplastic syndromes (MDS) represent a collection of hemapoietic neoplasms characterized by abnormal differentiation, dysmorphology, and resultant blood cytopenias. The hallmarks of these clonal disorders include exaggerated apoptosis of hematopoietic precursors in the marrow, common chromosomal abnormalities, frequent somatic gene mutations, and a variable predilection to undergo clonal evolution to acute myelogenous leukemia (AML). The clinical course of patients with MDS is variable and ranges from relatively indolent clonal cytopenias (e.g., refractory anemia) with a low rate of AML transformation, to more aggressive disease defined by an increased proportion of marrow myeloblasts, oligoblastic myelogenous leukemia (refractory anemia with excess blasts), and a greater risk of progression to AML.

Despite their phenotypic variability, MDS share a common pathophysiology. They are neoplasms derived from the clonal expansion of a somatically mutated, multipotent hematopoietic progenitor cell. A wide range of genetic aberrations can contribute to the development and progression of MDS and these somatic mutations can exist in an even greater variety of combinations. The specific profile of genetic lesions present in a given case contributes to the eventual disease phenotype.

MDS are closely related to other myeloid neoplasms such as AML and some myeloproliferative neoplasms. The *dysmorphia of neoplasia* (commonly referred to as *dysplasia* in describing MDS) refers to the abnormal morphology than can be observed in neoplastic mature blood cells and maturing marrow erythroid, granulocytic, and megakaryocytic precursor cells, and is one of the distinguishing characteristics of MDS. The dysmorphia is essential in diagnosis, but is an epiphenomenon. The essential abnormality is the neoplastic transformation of a primitive multipotential myeloid cell. A lower fraction of myeloblasts in the marrow is a reflection of its being at the less-severe end of the spectrum of myelogenous leukemia and is a feature of the diagnosis, creating an arbitrary division between MDS and AML. The diagnostic criteria that separate various myeloid neoplasms (and MDS subtypes) from each other are somewhat ambiguous because they are so closely related. This is evident at the molecular level where no particular genetic abnormality or mutation profile is entirely unique to MDS. Both somatic mutations and chromosomal abnormalities found in MDS are observed in related disorders, albeit often with different frequency. RNA splicing factors and epigenetic regulators are the most common classes of genes affected by mutations in MDS followed by mutations in transcription factors, tyrosine kinase signaling genes, and *TP53*. MDS should be thought of as a minimal to moderately deviated neoplasm in the spectrum of myelogenous leukemias (Chap. 83).

A minority of MDS cases are attributable to prior exposure to DNA-damaging agents, including chemotherapy, high-dose ionizing radiation, and benzene-containing compounds. The latter external factor requires an exposure of sufficient duration and magnitude to be considered causal, rare now in countries with regulations regarding the content of benzene in products such as paints and solvents. Cigarette smoking is considered a risk factor for AML by the U.S. Public Health Service and, presumably, this should apply to MDS, although it has not been studied as extensively. Other chemical exposures have not been established as causative agents by the International Agency for Research on Cancer. A small number of patients come from families with a high penetrance of MDS and related myeloid disorders or have an inherited or congenital syndrome predisposing to MDS. Although rare, identification of the genetic abnormalities in many of these cases has informed our understanding of the molecular pathophysiology of MDS in general. Yet, the vast majority of MDS cases are age-related without a clear precipitating factor. Although MDS can occur at any age, including rare pediatric forms, its incidence increases exponentially after 40 years of age, making it one of the most common myeloid neoplasms of older adults. This pattern is related to the evidence that somatic mutations in primitive hematopoietic cells increase significantly with age.[1]

● HISTORY

MDS have historically been subject to confusing and shifting terminology and definitions related to incomplete biologic understanding of disease.[2,3] With the advent of routine molecular analysis of primary patient samples and increasing insight into disease pathobiology, classification of MDS is likely to evolve from the current systems based on cytologic morphology and enumeration of marrow and blood cell subsets to nosology based on DNA mutation patterns, clonal architecture, and predicted evolution to AML.[4]

Although anemia had been recognized since the early 19th century as a specific deficiency of red cells (also known as "colored corpuscles," a term that distinguished these cells from leukocytes in the era before histological stains), marrow biopsies were not regularly performed on living patients until after the 1920s.[5] Therefore, conditions such as MDS that are associated with and defined by specific marrow findings could not be described as distinct syndromes until the first half of the 20th century. Still, early suggestive reports can be found in the medical literature: a 1907 report by Luzzatto of megaloblastic "pseudo-aplastic anemia,"[6] for example, could have included MDS cases.

In the mid-1920s, Di Guglielmo in Naples described a group of marrow disorders associated with bizarrely shaped erythrocytes and cytopenias, which in some cases ultimately proved fatal.[7] For many years thereafter, a heterogeneous group of marrow disorders associated with anemia and erythroid dysmorphology were called "Di Guglielmo syndrome" by hematologists, a term that was used variably and is still employed occasionally as an eponymous description of erythroleukemia (AML M6). Some cases of Di Guglielmo syndrome would be called MDS today.

The first MDS-specific term familiar to contemporary hematologists, "refractory anemia," was coined in the 1930s to describe patients who had unexplained anemia as a consequence of marrow underproduction and who failed to respond to treatment with the available hematinics: iron salts and the liver extract found by Minot and Murphy in the early 1920s to cure pernicious anemia.[8,9] It is not clear how many of the 100 cases of refractory anemia in the classic 1938 series of Rhoads and Barker in New York City actually had MDS—many appear to have had anemia of chronic disease from infections or associated malignancies, such as Hodgkin lymphoma—but this term and its cognate, "refractory cytopenias," are still used today to describe some of the lower-risk forms of MDS with blast proportions less than 5 percent.[9,10]

In 1942, Chevallier and colleagues in France discussed syndromes they labeled as "odo-leukemias."[11] The French investigators chose the Greek word *odo*, meaning threshold, to highlight disorders on the threshold of leukemia, and proposed *leucoses* as a generic term for the leukemias so that marked variations in white cell counts and other highly variable presenting features would not engender inappropriate terminology. However, this proposal was neglected, in part because the paper was published in French and there was no international network of hematologists with which to discuss such concepts in the 1940s.

Despite such provincialism, the idea that what would later be known as MDS could precede and terminate in AML soon made its way in the English medical literature. In 1949, Hamilton-Paterson in London used the term *preleukaemic anemia* to describe patients with refractory anemia antecedent to AML.[12] In 1953, Block and coworkers in Chicago expanded the concept to include cytopenias of all lineages and described cases that closely fit with our current concepts of a clonal myeloid hemopathy prior to evolution to overt AML.[13] In 1956, Björkman in Malmö, Sweden described four cases of idiopathic refractory sideroblastic anemia, one of which terminated in AML.[14] Descriptive terms, such as *herald state of leukemia, refractory anemia, sideroachrestic anemia, pancytopenia with hyperplastic marrow*, and others, were coined to describe the various hematopoietic derangements that preceded the onset of florid AML. By the 1970s, the relationship of acquired idiopathic cytopenias to the subsequent onset of AML had become broadly appreciated, although such cases were still thought to be rare. In a 1973 review, Saarni and Linman found only 143 cases of "preleukemic anemia" in the medical literature.[15]

In 1970, Dreyfus proposed the designation "les anémies réfractaires avec excès de myéloblastes" (i.e., refractory anemia with excess myeloblasts) and in 1976 he and colleagues proposed a preliminary classification of these syndromes. Dreyfus published a paper in which refractory anemia with an excess of myeloblasts was amplified, parenthetically, as smoldering acute leukemia.[16,17] The synonym, *oligoblastic leukemias*, had been used also to describe those cases with low proportions of leukemic myeloblasts and relatively protracted courses.[18,19]

In 1975, at a conference held in Paris, Bessis and Bernard used the term *hematopoietic dysplasia*, later shortened to *myelodysplasia*, for the group of disorders having a more indolent course than AML. The concept that neoplasia is a tissue abnormality defined by its origin in the mutation(s) within a single cell (monoclonality) and that dysplasia is a polyclonal tissue change, not neoplasia, was ignored and took a back seat to the participants' primary interest in the dysmorphia of cells that characterized most of these syndromes, hence the application of the term *dysplasia*, which has become entrenched.

In the year following the Paris conference, a group of seven hematopathologists from France, the United States, and England—the "French-American-British (FAB) Co-Operative Group"—instituted the classification of acute leukemia,[19] developed by Dalton and Dacie, and called it the FAB classification.[20] In the FAB classification, acute leukemia was defined by the presence of 30 percent blasts in the marrow; the original report also included two preleukemic syndromes that should be distinguished from acute leukemia, refractory anemia with excess blasts (RAEB), and chronic myelomonocytic leukemia (CMML), defined by greater than 1000/µL of blood monocytes. Because most patients with preleukemia do not go on to develop leukemia, the FAB group proposed the term "dysmyelopoietic syndrome" as an alternative to preleukemia.[20] A few years later, "dysmyelopoietic syndrome" was revised to become the "myelodysplastic syndrome(s)" still used today.

The 1976 FAB classification included only two subtypes of dysmyelopoietic syndromes, but in 1982 the FAB proposed a specific MDS classification that included five entities: refractory anemia (RA), refractory anemia with ring sideroblasts (RARS), RAEB (defined by 5 to 19 percent marrow blasts), refractory anemia with excess blasts in transformation (RAEB-t, defined by 20 to 29 percent marrow blasts), and CMML.[21] The 1982 FAB classification, while not without limitations, proved influential and was the basis of subsequent classifications of MDS and related disorders by the World Health Organization (WHO). Subsequent developments in prognostic scoring systems and biologic understanding of MDS are described below.

● CLASSIFICATION

A classification of MDS and related disorders was defined by the WHO in 2001 and revised in 2008. It includes six major subtypes of disease distinguished by the type and number of dysplastic lineages, the proportion of marrow blasts, and in one subtype, the presence of a specific chromosomal abnormality, del(5q). These subtypes include (1) refractory cytopenia with unilineage dysplasia (RCUD), which is typically RA, (2) RARS, (3) RA with ringed sideroblasts and thrombocytosis (RARS-t), (4) MDS with isolated del(5q), (5) refractory cytopenia with multilineage dysplasia, (6) RAEB (type 1 or type 2 depending in the proportion of marrow or blood blasts), and (7) unclassifiable MDS (Table 87–1). MDS patients with 20 to 29 percent marrow blasts, previously defined as RAEB-t, are considered to have AML in the WHO classification. However, this sharp cutoff is arbitrarily defined. In practice, patients with blast proportions in this range have comparable outcomes to patients with RAEB-2, including similar rates of benefit from MDS-directed therapy.

The boundaries between subtypes involving percentages of myeloblasts or ring sideroblasts are also arbitrarily defined. Patients may see their disease classification change over time as a result of clinical

TABLE 87–1. World Health Organization Classification of the Myelodysplastic Syndromes

1. Refractory cytopenia with unilineage dysplasia (RCUD)

   Dysplasia in ≥10% of cells from a single myeloid lineage

   <5% marrow blasts, <1% blood blasts, and no Auer rods

   <15% of erythroid precursors are ring sideroblasts

   Most often is refractory anemia (RA) but can be refractory neutropenia (RN) or refractory thrombocytopenia (RT) in rare cases

2. Refractory anemia with ring sideroblasts (RARS)

   Isolated erythroid dysplasia

   <5% marrow blasts, <1% blood blasts, and no Auer rods

   ≥15% of erythroid precursors are ring sideroblasts

   The cutoff for ring sideroblasts is arbitrary and does not reflect the clinical behavior of this subtype as accurately as the frequently associated mutations of SF3B1

3. Myelodysplastic syndromes (MDS) associated with isolated del(5q)

   5q31 deletion as the sole chromosomal abnormality

   Normal to increased megakaryocytes with hypolobated nuclei

   Normal to increase platelet count

   <5% marrow blasts, <1% blood blasts, and no Auer rods

   This subtype overlaps with, but is not entirely synonymous with the "5q-minus syndrome" recognized prior to the establishment of the WHO classification system for MDS

4. Refractory cytopenia with multilineage dysplasia (RCMD)

   Dysplasia in ≥10% of cells from two or more myeloid lineages

   <5% marrow blasts, <1% blood blasts, and no Auer rods

   Blood monocyte count <1 × 10⁹/L

5. Refractory anemia with excess blasts (RAEB)

   Type 1: 5–9% marrow blasts, <5% blood blasts, *and* no Auer rods

   Type 2: 10–19% marrow blasts, 5–19% blood blasts, *or* Auer rods

   Blood monocyte count <1 × 10⁹/L

6. Unclassifiable MDS (MDS-U)

   Minimal dysplasia in the presence of a clonal cytogenetic lesion considered presumptive evidence of MDS

   <5% marrow blasts, <1% blood blasts, and no Auer rods

NOTE: Other acute and chronic clonal myeloid diseases are categorized in Chap. 83, Table 83–1.

progression or response to therapy. Clonal cytopenias with dysmorphia may also be present in patients with myeloproliferative features such as thrombocytosis or monocytosis. CMML, for example, was previously considered an MDS subtype in the FAB classification, but is now recognized as a myelodysplastic/myeloproliferative neoplasm (MDS/MPN) overlap syndrome. Some patients diagnosed with MDS may have their diagnosis change to CMML once their monocyte count exceeds 1 × 10⁹/L. Similarly, RARS may be reclassified as RARS-t, if the platelet count rises above 450 × 10⁹/L. CMML, RARS-t, and related MDS/MPN subtypes are discussed separately in Chap. 89 with the chronic myelogenous leukemias.

Classification systems for MDS have descriptive merit, but do not capture many disease variables with clinical significance. The WHO subtypes of MDS identify patients with similar prognoses because patients with multilineage dysplasia and increasing blast percentages are at higher risk of AML transformation and death. However, dedicated prognostic models that include features not considered by the WHO classification system are better suited for the estimation of disease risk. Similarly, WHO-defined subtypes do not necessarily share common pathogenic elements or identify groups of patients most likely to respond to particular therapies. Our greater understanding about the underlying molecular abnormalities that occur in MDS demonstrate how clinically defined subtypes are genetically very heterogenous. It is likely that future classification systems will consider somatic mutations in MDS driver genes, genes responsible for the clonal outgrowth and the eventual development of disease, as a basis for defining disease subtypes.

EPIDEMIOLOGY

INCIDENCE BY AGE, SEX, AND OCCUPATION

The incidence and prevalence of MDS have been difficult to establish, in part because patients are not consistently reported to central cancer registries.[22-24] Only since 2001 has the United States (U.S.) National Cancer Institute (NCI) Surveillance, Epidemiology and End Results (SEER) database included MDS cases (Fig. 87–1).[25] In 2003, approximately 10,000 new cases were reported to NCI SEER, most "unclassified" (i.e., not distinguished as lower- or higher-risk).[25] Improved methods of case ascertainment using claims-based data suggest a high rate of unreported cases and also indicate that MDS is one of the most common hematological malignancies.[26]

Claims-based data suggest that conservatively, at least 30,000 new cases annually are diagnosed in the United States.[27] It is likely that many additional elderly patients with unexplained cytopenias have MDS, but are incompletely evaluated because of severe comorbid conditions limiting life expectancy, clinician oversight of blood test results, or a sense of nihilism. Rates of MDS are similar in Western Europe and the United States.[28]

In certain Asian countries and Eastern Europe, MDS is diagnosed at a younger age on average than in the United States and Western Europe.[29-31] The subtypes of MDS that are diagnosed in different regions of the world are also distinct[32,33]; for instance, for unclear reasons RARS is rare in Japan compared to the West.[34] Exposure to ionizing radiation from the 1945 Hiroshima and Nagasaki atomic bomb explosions continues to be associated with an increased MDS risk among exposed Japanese more than 50 years after the events.[35]

The median age at MDS diagnosis in the United States is approximately 71 years.[36] Onset of MDS before the age of 50 years is uncommon, except in cases preceded by irradiation or cytotoxic chemotherapy given for another malignancy.[37-39] MDS, as defined by the WHO classification, occurs in children ages 5 months to 15 years at a rate of approximately one per 1 million children per year. In contrast to adults, most pediatric cases are oligoblastic myelogenous leukemia (RAEB); clonal sideroblastic anemia is rare.[40,41] A proportion of childhood cases evolve from inherited predisposing diseases, such as Down syndrome and Fanconi anemia, or are associated with germline *GATA2* or *RUNX1* mutations.[42-44] Some cases of Fanconi anemia first present in adulthood as MDS, often in the absence of typical dysmorphology.[45] Dyskeratosis congenita and other telomeropathies can also end in MDS, but many

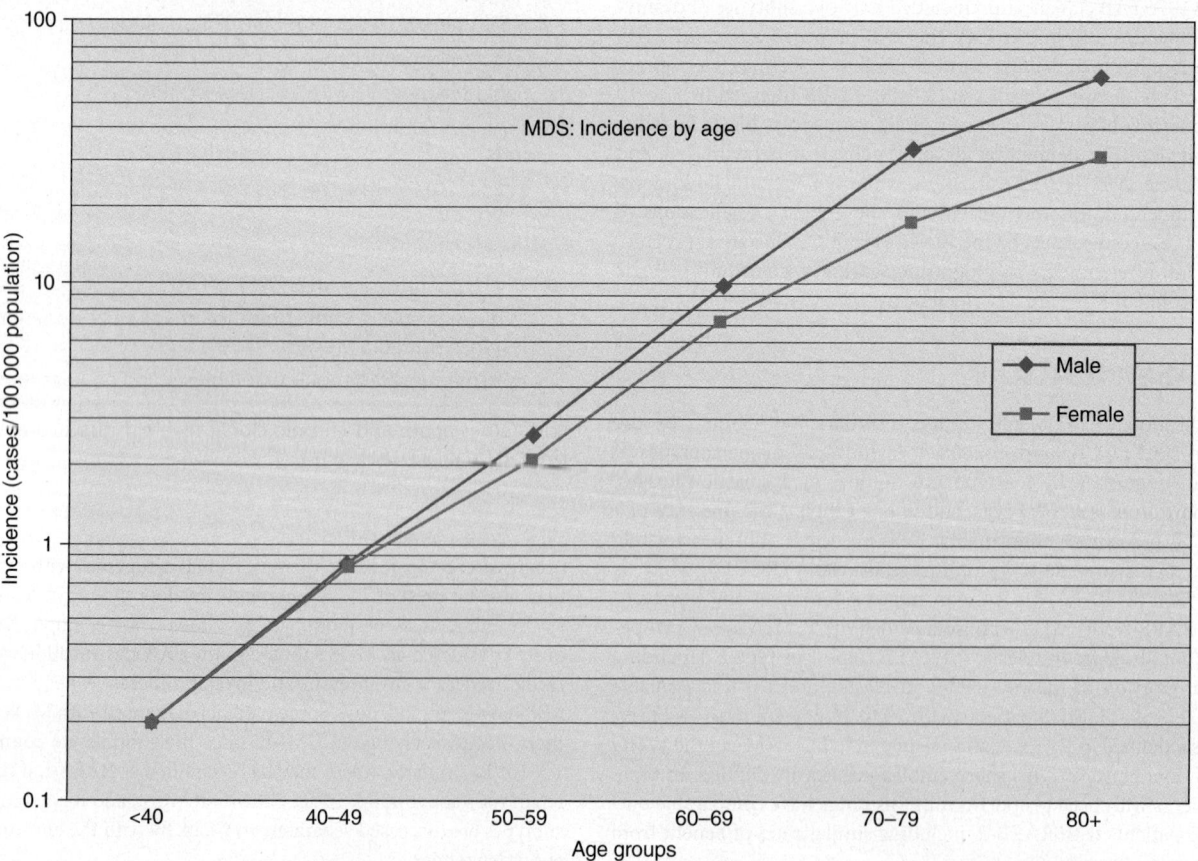

Figure 87–1. The annual incidence of myelodysplastic syndrome shown by age. There is an exponential (approximately linear on semilogarithmic plot) increase in incidence from age 40 years on. In persons younger than age 40 years, the incidence is so low that it is aggregated as <40 years. (*Data from the United States National Cancer Institute, Surveillance, Epidemiology, and End-Results Program.*)

congenital marrow failure syndromes such as Diamond-Blackfan anemia or Shwachman-Diamond syndrome do not carry an increased MDS risk.[46]

With the exception of the 5q-minus syndrome, males are affected with MDS up to 1.5 times as often as females.[47] Case-control studies of possible occupational or environmental associations have provided many possible candidates as contributors to MDS, but none other than benzene (exposure of ≥40 parts per million [ppm]-years) has been observed consistently.[48-51] Cigarette smoking, and a family history of hematologic malignancy also seem plausible risk factors.[52] Chemicals other than benzene have not been established as causative factors by epidemiologic studies that fully meet the guidelines proposed by Bradford Hill for causation by an external factor. Moreover, given the requirement for biologic plausibility, such chemicals should be shown to induce the specific driver mutations required to cause MDS.

● ETIOLOGY AND PATHOGENESIS

ETIOLOGY

The etiologic factors that increase the incidence of MDS are similar to the factors affecting the incidence of AML (Chap. 88). Exposure to prolonged or high levels of benzene,[34,35] chemotherapeutic agents, particularly alkylating agents and topoisomerase inhibitors,[36-43] and radiation[44,45] increases the risk of these clonal hemopathies. These agents may cause DNA damage, impair DNA repair enzymes, and induce loss of chromosome integrity. Most cases of secondary or posttreatment MDS occur in patients treated for a lymphoma or a solid tumor. Increasing reports of MDS as a complication of treatment of myeloid diseases, such as acute promyelocytic leukemia, may reflect a second clonal myeloid disease from another primitive hematopoietic cell injured during therapy.[43] The increased life span of patients with acute promyelocytic leukemia and other cancers after effective therapy may make these events more common. More common environmental exposures, such as cigarette smoke, may contribute to the likelihood of developing MDS.

Inherited diseases, such as Fanconi anemia, known to predispose to AML development occasionally evolve instead into a clonal myeloid hemopathy (see Chap. 88, Table 88–1).[46] Other syndromes, of either a familial (inherited) or spontaneous nature, have been associated with a high risk of developing myeloid neoplasms. Germline mutations of the hematopoietic transcription factor *RUNX1* are associated with a familial platelet disorder with predisposition at AML (FPD-AML). Affected individuals often have qualitative and quantitative platelet abnormalities that precede the development of a more aggressive myeloid neoplasm such as MDS or AML. Transformation typically occurs in the third decade of life, but penetrance is variable between individuals and kinships. The long latency prior to progression suggests that the acquisition of additional cooperating mutations is required for transformation. Somatic *RUNX1* mutations are also common in *de novo* and therapy-related MDS cases highlighting the oncogenic driver nature of these abnormalities. In contrast, somatic mutations of Fanconi anemia genes are extremely rare in MDS. Congenital *FANC* mutations may instead cause DNA damage and accelerated exhaustion of normal stem cells allowing mutant clones to expand more readily. Similarly, inherited CCAAT/enhancer binding protein alpha (*C/EBPA*) mutations, often associated with eosinophilia, typically predispose to AML without an MDS-like clinical phase and are only rarely found as somatic mutations in MDS.

Congenital mutations of another hematopoietic transcription factor, *GATA2*, have been linked to familial MDS.[53] The syndromic manifestations of germline *GATA2* mutations are highly varied and can include lymphedema, cutaneous warts, sensorineural hearing loss, pulmonary alveolar proteinosis, and disseminated nontuberculous mycobacterial infections.[54,55] Several distinct clinical syndromes that include subsets of these features are now known to be caused by germline *GATA2* mutations. These include Emberger syndrome comprising MDS, verrucae, and congenital lymphedema, as well as the MonoMAC syndrome comprising monocytopenia and nontuberculous mycobacterial infections.[55-58] Not all patients show overt syndromic features prior to developing MDS, even as adults, and several pediatric marrow failure syndromes can be associated with germlinel *GATA2* mutation in the absence of syndromic features.[59]

The combined incidence of familial (<2 percent) and therapy-related MDS (~5 to 10 percent) pales in comparison to the frequency of *de novo* MDS that has age as its dominant predisposing factor. This may be simply a matter of probability, with aged stem cells being more likely to have acquired somatic driver mutations. It may also reflect age-related changes in the microenvironment or stem cell epigenetic state as hematopoietic stem cells from elderly persons without disease are known to have an exaggerated myeloid differentiation bias.[60] In concert, age-related drop out of normal hematopoietic stem cells could lead to oligoclonal, or even monoclonal, hematopoiesis derived from stem cells with weakly selective abnormalities that then serve as fertile ground for cooperating MDS-related somatic mutations.[61]

PATHOGENESIS

MDS arise from the clonal expansion of a mutated multipotential hematopoietic cell. For patients without excess blasts, the cell of origin is presumed to be a lymphohematopoietic pluripotential stem cell based on the presence of disease-associated driver mutations in cells that share the surface protein immunophenotype of functionally defined stem cells.[62] Subsequent evolution measured by the acquisition of additional mutations takes place in this cellular compartment and can occur in more differentiated progenitors, if they confer the capacity for sustained self-renewal. Evidence for the clonal nature of MDS is supported by studies of skewed X-chromosome inactivation in female patients heterozygous for glucose-6-phosphate dehydrogenase isoenzymes. The hematopoietic progenitors,[63,64] and sometimes B lymphocytes,[65] of such patients had only one isoenzyme present, supporting the concept of clonal expansion of a neoplastic early progenitor cell. Subsequent studies confirm the presence of acquired chromosomal abnormalities and somatic mutations in hematopoietic progenitors as well as in B and T lymphocytes in some, but not all, cases.[62,66-72]

This process of clonal expansion takes place in the context of the marrow microenvironment and host immune response (Chap. 5). These features extrinsic to the cells in the neoplastic clone generate the selection pressures that drive disease evolution and can significantly influence the clinical manifestations of MDS.

The hallmark of clonal hematopoiesis is the presence of a somatic genetic abnormality. Approximately 50 percent of patients with MDS will have a grossly abnormal karyotype, typically in the form of a partial or total chromosomal deletion. A fraction of the remaining cases with a "normal" karyotype will have cryptic cytogenetic abnormalities that can include small microdeletions and areas of copy number neutral loss of heterozygosity. This latter phenomenon occurs by mitotic recombination during cell division and results in acquired uniparental disomy (aUPD) where both copies of a large chromosomal segment appear to be derived from a single parent. The most common somatic genetic lesions in MDS are mutations of individual genes. More than 50 recurrently mutated genes have been identified with nearly all patients harboring one or more such mutations (Table 87–2).

The recurrent nature of many of these genetic events has helped identify molecular mechanisms associated with the development and

TABLE 87–2. Recurrently Mutated Myelodysplastic Syndrome Genes

	Mutated Gene	Frequency in MDS (%)	Prognostic Value	Additional Information
Splicing	SF3B1	20–30	Favorable	Strongly associated with ring sideroblasts
	SRSF2	10–15	Adverse	More frequent in CMML
	U2AF1	8–12	Adverse	Associated with del(20q)
	ZRSR2	5–10	?	
Epigenetic regulators	TET2	20–25	Neutral	More frequent in CMML
	DNMT3A	12–18	Adverse	
	IDH1/IDH2	<5	?	
	ASXL1	15–25	Adverse	More frequent in CMML
	EZH2	5–10	Adverse	More frequent in CMML
	ATRX	<2	?	Associated with ATMDS
	KMD6A	<2	?	
Transcription	RUNX1	10–15	Adverse	Familial in rare cases
	GATA2	<2	?	Commonly familial, rarely somatic
	ETV6	<5	Adverse	Rarely translocated in MDS
	PHF6	<2	?	
	TP53	8–12	Adverse	Associated with complex karyotypes
Cohesins	STAG2	5–10	?	
	RAD21	<5	?	
	SMC3	<2	?	
	SMC1A	<2	?	
Signaling	NRAS/KRAS	5–10	Adverse	More frequent in CMML
	JAK2	<5	Neutral	Enriched in RARS-t
	CBL/CBLB	<5	Adverse	More frequent in CMML
	PTPN11	<2	Adverse	More frequent in JMML, can be germline
Others	GNAS/GNB1	<2	?	G-protein signalling pathway
	BRCC3	<2	?	DNA repair pathway
	PIGA	<2	?	Cause of PNH clones
	TERT/TERC	<2	?	Can be germline
	FANC genes	<2	?	Typically germline

ATMDS, acquired thalassemia and myelodysplastic syndrome; CMML, chronic myelomonocytic leukemia; JMML, juvenile myelomonocytic leukemia; MDS, myelodysplastic syndrome; PNH, paroxysmal nocturnal hemoglobinuria; RARS-t, refractory anemia with ringed sideroblasts and thrombocytosis.

progression of MDS. Many of these lesions are associated with particular clinical phenotypes, including differences in disease manifestation, response to therapy, risk of AML transformation and overall survival. However, the use of genetic features to classify disease subtypes or personalize the care of individual patients is still rudimentary.

Cytogenetics

Chromosomal amplifications and translocations are relatively rare events in MDS compared with other hematologic malignancies. The most frequent chromosomal abnormalities seen in MDS, present in nearly half of all cases, are deletions of chromosomal segments or loss of entire chromosomes (monosomies). Several such lesions are recurrent and typically involve commonly deleted regions that are presumed to harbor one or more tumor-suppressor genes. Identifying individual gene drivers from these regions has been challenging because of the large amount of genomic territory that they encompass and the

likelihood that multiple gene losses cooperate to generate a disease-related phenotype.[73] However, MDS-related chromosomal abnormalities do have important clinical significance. For example, they can establish the presence of clonal hematopoiesis and in the appropriate context, can serve as presumptive evidence of MDS. Chromosomal abnormalities are key elements in the determination of prognosis and in the case of del(5q), can predict response to a particular treatment.

Del(5q) Deletion of the long arm of chromosome 5 is the most common karyotypic abnormality observed in MDS, occurring in 15 percent of cases, half of which have several other karyotype abnormalities. Studies examining the breakpoints of deletions across multiple patients have identified two commonly deleted regions (CDRs), one on 5q31.1 and the other at 5q32–33.3. Patients with del(5q) often have deletions that encompass both CDRs and can include proximal and distal chromosomal regions as well. Larger deletions that include more proximal genes, like *APC*, and more distal genes, like *NPM1*, are much more

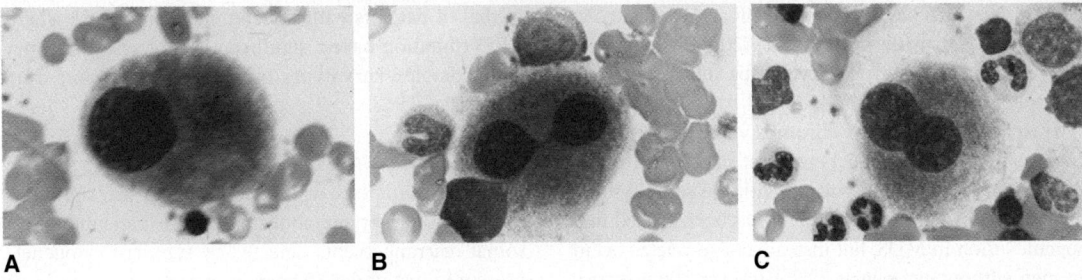

Figure 87–2. Composite from marrow films of patient with the 5q– syndrome. Characteristic hypolobulated megakaryocytes. **A.** Monolobed megakaryocyte. **B.** Bilobed megakaryocyte. Lobes connected by a nuclear bridge. **C.** Bilobed megakaryocyte. *(Reproduced with permission from Lichtman's Atlas of Hematology, www.accessmedicine.com.)*

common in higher-risk MDS and AML where del(5q) is considered an adverse cytogenetic abnormality.[74] In MDS, smaller deletions that include the 5q32–33.3 region are associated with a more favorable prognosis and a marked sensitivity to treatment with lenalidomide. Such patients with a sole del(5q) abnormality and no excess blasts represent the only genetically defined MDS subtype in the WHO classification system. Some of these patients have characteristics of the "5q-minus syndrome," which is characterized by dyserythropoietic anemia, micromegakaryocytes with a preserved or elevated platelet count, female predominance, and lower risk of transformation to AML (Fig. 87–2).

The pathogenic mechanisms associated with del(5q) are not completely understood. Patients with del(5q) do not routinely carry point mutations on the remaining intact 5q arm, suggesting that the inactivation of classic tumor-suppressor genes is not responsible for the selective advantage associated with this lesion.[75] Instead, haploinsufficiency of genes lost in the deleted regions of chromosome 5q is largely responsible for the disease phenotype. For example, deletion of the ribosomal subunit gene *RPS14* creates dyserythropoiesis mediated by TP53 activation in differentiating erythroid cells analogous to that seen in congenital haploinsufficient ribosomopathies such as Diamond-Blackfan anemia.[76–79] Isolated mutations or deletions of *RPS14* are not known to occur in MDS, suggesting that loss of this gene may influence the clinical presentation of MDS, but is not directly responsible for its development. Instead, codeleted genes must be drivers of transformation and several candidates have been proposed. These include microRNA (miRNA) genes 145 and 146a involved in the regulation of innate immune signaling and megakaryocyte differentiation,[80–82] a mitochondrial heat shock protein *HSPA9*,[83,84] and the zinc finger transcription factor *EGR1*.[85,86] Several other genes, both in and out of the CDRs, have been implicated in the pathogenesis of MDS, including *MAML1*, a coactivator of the Notch signaling pathway, and the casein kinase gene, *CSNK1A1*.[74,87]

A del(5q) is frequently found as one of several chromosomal abnormalities in patients with complex disease karyotypes (defined as three or more chromosomal abnormalities).[88] In this context, it is associated with an adverse prognosis, a poor response to lenalidomide, and frequently cooccurs with mutations of *TP53* or abnormalities of 17p where *TP53* resides.[89–92] The association between del(5q) and *TP53* lesions occur more often than predicted by their independent incidences alone, suggesting pathogenic cooperation between these abnormalities.[86] Even in cases of isolated del(5q), small subclonal *TP53* mutations can be found in 15 to 20 percent of cases. These patients appear to have a greater than predicted risk of AML transformation and inferior responses to treatment with lenalidomide.[93–95]

Monosomy 7 and Del(7q) Abnormalities of chromosome 7 are prognostically adverse lesions found in approximately 5 percent of MDS patients, often as part of a complex karyotype. Studies indicate that isolated monosomy 7 is a more adverse abnormality than isolated del(7q),

and both occur more frequently (~50 percent) in patients with prior exposure to alkylating agents.[88,89,96] Several distinct CDRs have been reported, including regions 7q22, 7q32–34, and 7q36.[97–99] The relative pathogenic contribution of deletions in each of these regions is not well understood.

Several recurrently mutated genes reside on chromosome 7q. The histone methyltransferase gene, *EZH2*, is located on 7q36 and is mutated in approximately 6 percent of MDS cases.[100–102] In some patients, an *EZH2* mutation is accompanied by aUPD of 7q, but most *EZH2* mutant patients do not have –7 or del(7q) and most patients with these chromosomal lesions do not harbor *EZH2* mutations. In AML, the *MLL3* gene, also located at 7q36, has been proposed as a haploinsufficient driven of disease.[103] More proximal lies *CUX1*, a 7q22 gene implicated in MDS pathogenesis, which, like *EZH2*, is associated with a poor prognosis when mutated.[104] Inactivating mutations of *CUX1* tend to be heterozygous, suggesting that haploinsufficiency of this gene found in 7q22 might be a disease driver.[104] However, deletion in mice of the region syngeneic to 7q22 produced no discernable phenotype.[105]

Trisomy 8 This is the only large-scale amplification frequently encountered in MDS, present in approximately 5 percent of cases. It is also highly nonspecific as it can occur in patients with myeloproliferative neoplasms, acute myeloid leukemia, and even aplastic anemia. Trisomy 8 is associated with an intermediate prognosis and is often acquired late in the disease course.[106] In some cases, it may be acquired in myeloid progenitors as opposed to more pluripotential CD34+CD38–CD90+ stem cells where the MDS-initiating clone is presumed to have developed.[107] How trisomy 8 leads to a selective growth advantage is not well understood. Progenitor cells with trisomy 8 express high levels of apoptosis-related genes and demonstrate dysregulation of immune response genes. Patients can harbor T cells that preferentially suppress trisomy 8 progenitor cells, particularly in response to overexpression of Wilms tumor 1 (WT1), which is upregulated in trisomy 8 cells.[108,109] These findings may indicate selective pressure from the immune system on the disease clone with potential for collateral autoimmune suppression of normal hematopoiesis. Patients with trisomy 8 may benefit from immune suppression even if the aneuploid clone expands after response to treatment.[110] Other autoimmune phenomena, such as Behçet disease, have been associated with trisomy 8 MDS.[111–113]

Del(20q) This abnormality is another nonspecific, yet recurrent, chromosomal abnormality found in approximately 2 percent of MDS cases. As an isolated lesion it is associated with disease risk comparable to that of MDS patients with normal karyotypes.[114,115] However, del(20q) may be acquired late in the course of disease, indicating clonal progression and a more adverse prognosis.[116] A CDR on 20q has been defined, but no single gene has been identified as the pathogenic driver responsible for the recurrent selection of del(20q) clones in MDS.[117,118] Candidate disease genes on 20q include *MYBL2*,[119,120] which lies within the CDR, and *ASXL1*,[121,122] which lies outside the CDR and is mutated in a large fraction of MDS patients with or without del(20q). Patients with del(20q) appear more likely to have thrombocytopenia and are enriched in mutations of the splicing factor gene *U2AF1*.[123,124]

Loss of Y The isolated loss of the Y chromosome is a rare recurrent abnormality observed in just over 2 percent of males with MDS. Like the del(20q) abnormality, –Y is associated with the same cytogenetic risk as patients with normal karyotypes.[114] It has been argued that –Y is not a pathogenic lesion in MDS, but instead an age-related event that can occur in men without cytopenias.[125,126] However, the presence of –Y as a somatic change is indicative of oligoclonal, if not monoclonal hematopoiesis and is therefore consistent with the diagnosis of MDS in a cytopenic patient. The larger the –Y clone, the more likely that evidence of an underlying neoplasm like MDS will be found.[127] Other genetic abnormalities, including mutations in ten-eleven translocation 2 (*TET2*) and *DNMT3A* have also been identified in elderly patients without cytopenias or other evidence of hematologic disease, yet these are considered pathogenic lesions in MDS. It is unclear if cytopenic patients with these markers of clonality, such as –Y, and insufficient evidence for an MDS diagnosis have comparable prognoses to patients with MDS.

Chromosome 17 Abnormalities Including del(17p) A small fraction of MDS patients will have an abnormality of chromosome 17, typically in the context of a complex karyotype. The *TP53* gene is located on 17p13.1 in a region that is recurrently deleted in those rare patients with either del(17p) or monosomy 17. One copy of 17p is typically retained in these cases suggesting that total loss of this region is not tolerated. However, the *TP53* gene on the remaining chromosome is often mutated leaving no wild-type protein. Patients with chromosome 17 abnormalities typically have a poor prognosis, particularly in the presence of a *TP53* mutation. The 17p region can be effectively lost in patients with an isochromosome 17p abnormality [i(17q)], occurring in just under 1 percent of cases. While these lesions predict a high rate of leukemic transformation, they are rarely associated with a coexisting TP53 mutation.[128] Instead, they are often found to cooccur with mutations of *SETBP1*, abnormalities that are found more often in patients with both dysplastic and proliferative disease features.[129]

Complex and Monosomal Karyotypes MDS karyotypes can be defined by the number of abnormalities present instead of focusing on the specific regions involved. Complex karyotypes are defined as having three or more cytogenetic abnormalities of any sort and are strongly associated with an adverse prognosis. In the International Prognosis Scoring System-Revised (IPSS-R), complex karyotypes are further separated in those with exactly three abnormalities and those with four or more, with the latter group having the highest associated disease risk. Monosomal karyotypes are defined as the loss of two or more entire chromosomes or the deletion of a single chromosome and the presence of another structural cytogenetic abnormality. Monosomal karyotypes are not necessarily complex and complex karyotypes are not necessarily monosomal, but in practice, there is substantial overlap between the two. The most frequent abnormalities seen in both monosomal and complex karyotypes involve chromosomes 5 and 7. The IPSS-R considers complex, but not monosomal karyotype as an independent risk factor and there has been ambiguity about whether complex versus monosomal karyotypes are better predictors of disease risk.[130–133]

Approximately 50 percent of patients with complex karyotypes have a concomitant *TP53* mutation and account for the majority of patients with mutations of this gene.[134] The incidence of *TP53* mutation is particularly high when the complex karyotype includes del(5q) as an associated abnormality.[90,92,135] The adverse prognostic significance associated with complex karyotypes may be largely driven by their frequent association with *TP53* mutations.[134,136] Complex karyotype MDS patients with intact *TP53* have a median overall survival comparable

to that of patients with noncomplex karyotypes, whereas those with a *TP53* mutation have a significantly shorter overall survival.[134] Patients with complex karyotypes on average have fewer mutations in genes other than *TP53*.

Somatic Mutations

Acquired mutations of individual genes are significantly more common than karyotypic abnormalities in patients with MDS. Chromosomal rearrangements detected by standard cytogenetic techniqes are present in just under 50 percent of cases and more sensitive techniques with greater resolution can uncover small scale or copy number neutral abnormalities in an additional 25 percent. However, recurrent mutations of single genes can be identified in more than 80 percent of patients with MDS using targeted sequencing techniques and are likely to be found in all cases studied with whole-genome approaches. Unlike most chromosomal abnormalities that span large regions of the genome containing many candidate disease genes, most recurrent mutations affect the coding sequence of single genes, identifying them and their associated molecular pathways as pathogenic drivers. As of this writing, there are more than 50 genes known to be recurrently mutated in patients with MDS. A handful of these genes are mutated in a significant fraction of cases (10 to 35 percent) with several others in the 5 to 10 percent range. But the majority of recurrently mutated genes are found only rarely, encompassing fewer than 5 percent and, generally, less than 1 percent of cases. In some instances, these rare mutations occur in genes, like the splicing factors *U2AF2* or *SF1* that are in the same family as more commonly mutated genes. In other cases, the infrequently mutated genes, like *GNAS* and *GNB1*, represent their own molecular pathways suggesting that clonal myelodysplasia is a phenotypic manifestation that can be caused by a variety of pathogenic mechanisms. The large number of potentially mutated genes and multitude of ways in which they can be combined result in a staggering number of possible genetic profiles. The apparent cooperativity between some lesions and the mutual exclusivity of other limits this variability to some extent, but still allows for tremendous complexity at the genetic level. As a determinant of disease phenotypes, this variation likely explains much of the clinical heterogeneity seen in patients with MDS.[137]

Not all somatic mutations have equal pathogenic or clinical significance. Any patient with clonal hematopoiesis will harbor a large number of acquired mutations throughout their genome. The vast majority of these are incidental mutations acquired over the lifetime of the particular stem cell that eventually grew to clonally dominate hematopoiesis, most of which occurred prior to its expansion. These preceding mutations are not related to the development of disease and are distributed randomly, typically in noncoding and nonconserved areas of the genome, suggesting that they have no positive or negative selective significance. Collectively, these nonrecurrent mutations without pathogenic significance are described as *passenger mutations* because their presence in the expanded clone is only because they happen to coexist with much rarer *driver mutations*, responsible for the clonal outgrowth and the eventual development of disease. Driver mutations are typically recurrent and predicted to have pathogenic consequences like the alteration of a protein coding sequence or changes in the expression of one or more disease-related genes. Driver mutations can be early transformative events, in which case they would be found in every subsequent disease cell derived from that clone, or they can be late events, often associated with progressive disease. Some genes, like splicing factors, are predominantly mutated early and are typically found as part of the dominant disease clone. Other genes, like *NRAS* and *SETBP1*, are typically secondary mutations acquired later in the disease course and are often found as emergent subclones that may expand in size during progression.[90,138,139]

Somatic mutations can have important clinical implications for patients with MDS and the physicians who treat them, but their interpretation can be challenging. Several factors may influence the clinical significance or recurrent gene mutations. These include the type of mutation present (e.g., missense, nonsense, splicing, or frameshift), the configuration of the mutations (e.g., homozygous, heterozygous, hemizygous, or compound heterozygous), the fraction of disease cells that contain the mutations (i.e., presence in the dominant clone versus a subclone), the mutations that coexist in that patient and if these mutations are in the same clone or a sister clone, and whether mutations add information above and beyond what can be learned by looking at more readily accessible clinical variables like age, blast proportion, and blood counts. Despite these complexities, there are several scenarios in which specific gene mutations can inform the clinical care of patients with clonal cytopenias like MDS.

Splicing Factors The most frequently mutated class of genes in patients with MDS encode splicing factor proteins involved in the excision of introns and the ligation of exons from maturing pre-mRNA strands. There are at least eight recurrently mutated splicing factor genes identified in MDS and nearly two-thirds of patients will carry at mutation of a member of this gene family.[140] Splicing factor mutations are largely mutually exclusive. Patients with one splicing factor mutation rarely have a mutation in another suggesting that these lesions are either not tolerated in combination or, more likely, have a common mechanism of action. Thus, a disease stem cell that acquires a second splicing factor mutation would gain no selective advantage and may well develop a selective disadvantage as a consequence of that second mutation. Despite a presumed common pathogenic role, patients with mutations in different splicing factor genes often have very disparate clinical phenotypes.[137] This is partially because disease manifestations are often determined by the effect of driver mutations in the differentiating progeny of disease stem cells. Some may induce profound dysplasia while others promote lineage-specific proliferation, for example. Different splicing factor mutations may also be associated with certain clinical phenotypes because of their distinct patterns of comutation with other MDS-related genes.[90,135,141] These comutations may, for example, drive the disease manifestations or prognosis. If there is a common mechanism by which splicing factor mutations drive the development of MDS, it is not yet well understood. These mutations are not unique to MDS as they can be found in other malignancies, including some solid tumors, where they occur at low frequency. Several studies have identified changes in splicing efficiency and gene expression associated with splicing factor mutations, but these effects are subtle and do not readily identify a downstream pathogenic mechanism.

SF3B1 is the most frequently mutated splicing factor gene and encodes the U2 small nuclear riboprotein complex (snRNP) subunit responsible for branch site recognition. Mutations of *SF3B1* are present in 20 to 30 percent of patients and are the only somatic mutations associated with a favorable prognosis. The pattern of mutation of *SF3B1* suggests an oncogenic gain or change of function for its encoded protein. Mutations are always heterozygous to an intact wild-type allele and are relatively conservative missense substitutions at very specific hotspots.[142] These mutations occur in the middle of several consecutive HEAT protein domains of which the K700E substitution is the most common, accounting for more than half of all mutations of *SF3B1*. Clinically, mutations of *SF3B1* are very tightly associated with the presence of ring sideroblasts (Fig. 87–3). More than 85 percent of patients with RARS or RARS-t will have an *SF3B1* mutation. These mutations are common in patients with other subtypes of MDS, like refractory cytopenia with multilineage dysplasia, when ring sideroblasts are present. *SF3B1* mutations have been associated with a more favorable prognosis but it is unclear if it is independent of other known risk factors.

For example, *SF3B1* mutant patients are less likely to have cytogenetic abnormalities, including complex karyotypes, and are less likely to have other mutations in genes associated with a poor prognosis. Only mutations in *DNMT3A* cooccur with *SF3B1* mutations more often than would be predicted by chance alone, suggesting a cooperative interaction between these lesions.[90,141] *SF3B1*-mutant MDS may represent its own nosologic entity based on its common clinical features and patterns of comutation regardless of WHO subtype.[137] Mutation of *SF3B1* is also common in chronic lymphocytic leukemia (CLL) where it occurs in 15 to 20 percent of cases (Chap. 92). However, in contrast with MDS, these mutations in CLL are often subclonal or acquired after initial diagnosis and are associated with treatment resistance and a poor prognosis.[143] *SF3B1* hotspot mutations are enriched in uveal melanoma and can be found in various other solid tumors at lower frequency, demonstrating that it is not a tissue-specific oncogene.[144,145]

SRSF2 is the second most frequently mutated splicing factor, present in 10 to 15 percent of MDS and 40 percent of CMML cases. It encodes a serine-arginine–rich protein that interacts with the U2 and U1 components of the spliceosome. The predominant mutation in this gene is a missense substitution of the proline at codon 95, although small insertions and deletions at this position that conserve the reading frame have also been reported. As with *SF3B1*, mutations are heterozygous to a wild-type allele suggesting a very specific gain or change of function. *SRSF2* mutations cooccur with mutations of several other genes, such as *TET2, ASXL1, CUX1, IDH2,* and *STAG2,* many of which are also enriched in patients with CMML.[90] *SRSF2* mutations are generally associated with an inferior prognosis.

U2AF1 is the third frequently mutated splicing factor, present in approximately 12 percent of patients. Like *SF3B1* and *SRSF2*, mutations are heterozygous to a wild-type allele and occur as missense mutations at fixed hotspots. The affected amino acids at codons 34 and 157 are in the zinc finger DNA-binding regions of the protein.[140,146] *U2AF1* encodes an auxiliary factor in the U2 spliceosome responsible for the recognition of the AG splice acceptor dinucleotide at the 3′ end of introns. *U2AF1* mutations appear to affect splicing in reporter assays and transgenic mouse models, but how these changes confer a selective advantage to mutant cells is not well understood.[140,147] Clinically, *U2AF1* mutations are associated with shorter overall survival and increased risk of transformation to acute leukemia.[148] Patient with del(20q) may be enriched or *U2AF1* mutations.[123] Several additional splicing factors can be mutated in MDS, including *ZRSR2, SF1,* and *U2AF2.*[140] Most of these appear to harbor loss-of-function mutations, but remain largely exclusive of mutations in other splicing factors, suggesting a shared pathogenic mechanism.

Epigenetic Regulators

Epigenetic changes, defined as heritable covalent modifications of chromatin that do not alter the DNA base sequence, play a role in the development of MDS and other malignancies. Methylation of cytosine residues in DNA represents one form epigenetic modification that can be dysregulated in MDS. Specifically, patients may have global DNA hypomethylation, but will demonstrate hypermethylation in specific regions such as the CpG islands (areas rich in CG dinucleotides) found at or near gene promoters. These epigenetic marks have been associated with a closed chromatin configuration and relative silencing of nearby genes. The simplistic explanation is that aberrant DNA methylation leads to the pathogenic silencing of critical tumor-suppressor genes and is, therefore, oncogenic. Hypomethylating agents, which are inhibitors of the DNA methyltransferases that catalyze cytosine methylation, have been presumed to undo the silencing of these tumor-suppressor genes leading to therapeutic benefit. However, it is not certain that hypomethylating agents work in this way. It is known that several genes involved

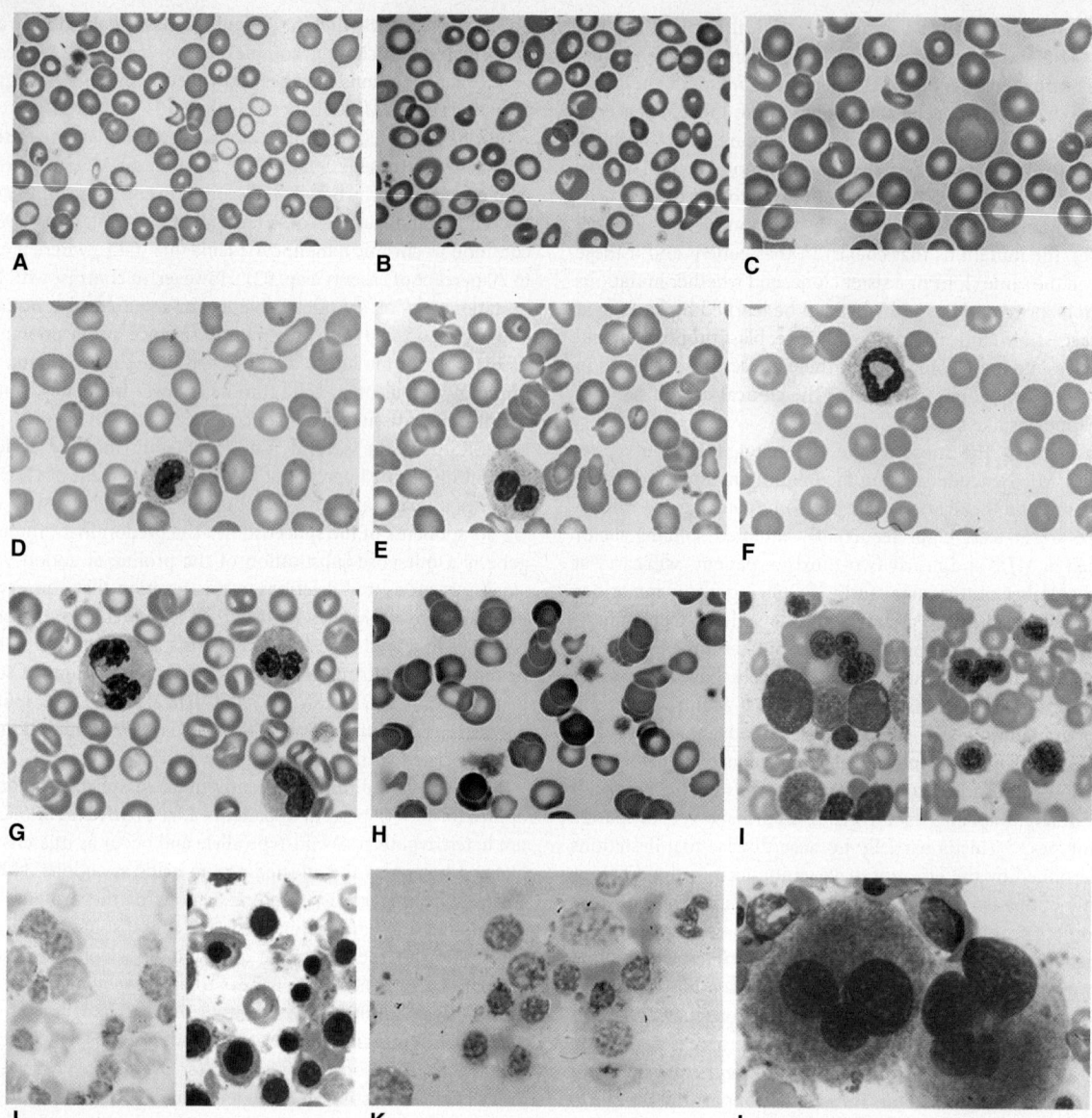

Figure 87–3. Blood and marrow films from patients with clonal cytopenias (myelodysplastic syndromes). **A.** Blood film. Anisocytosis. Poikilocytosis with occasional fragmented cells. Marked anisochromia with marked hypochromia, mild hypochromia and normochromic cells. **B.** Blood film. Marked anisocytosis. Mild anisochromia. Poikilocytes with occasional fragmented cells and oval and elliptical cells. Two polychromatophilic macrocytes. **C.** Blood film. Striking anisocytosis with giant macrocytes and microcytes. Poikilocytes with tiny red cell fragment and elliptocyte. **D.** Blood film. Mild anisocytosis. Ovalocytes and elliptocytes. Dacryocyte. Hyposegmented neutrophil with poor granulation. **E.** Blood film. Marked anisocytosis (macrocytes and microcytes). Ovalocytes and elliptocytes. Acquired Pelger-Hüet nuclear anomaly (classic pince-nez shape) in neutrophil. **F.** Blood film. Mild anisocytosis. Abnormal neutrophil with ring nucleus. **G.** Blood film. Anisochromia. Stomatocytes. Abnormal neutrophil nuclei with hyperlobulation and hyperchromatic staining. Note abnormal elongated nuclear bridge in neutrophil on left. **H.** Blood film. Atypical platelets. Two macrothrombocytes with excess cytoplasm and atypical central granules. Anisocytosis (conspicuous microcytes). Anisochromia (conspicuous hypochromic cells). Poikilocytosis with occasional fragmented red cells. **I.** Marrow film. Wright stain. Trilobed megakaryocyte. Wright stain. Macroerythroblasts. **J.** Marrow films. Prussian blue stain. Ring sideroblasts. Wright stain. Erythroid hyperplasia with macroerythroblasts. **K.** Marrow film. Prussian blue stain. Ring sideroblasts. **L.** Marrow film. Wright stain. Trilobed megakaryocytes. *(Reproduced with permission from* Lichtman's Atlas of Hematology, *www. accessmedicine.com.)*

in the regulation of DNA methylation are mutated in a large proportion of patients with MDS as are genes involved in the regulation of DNA-associated histone modifications. Together these epigenetic regulators form the second largest class of genes mutated in MDS. Unlike the splicing factors, most mutated epigenetic regulator genes are not exclusive of each other and frequently coexist.

DNMT3A This gene encodes a *de novo* DNA methyltransferase and is the only DNA methyltransferase gene frequently mutated in MDS. It

is mutated in approximately 15 percent of cases in a pattern that suggests a resultant loss of function.[149,150] Mutations can include frameshifts and premature stop codons, as well as missense mutations spread throughout the length of the gene. The one exception is a high frequency of missense mutations at the hotspot codon 882, which have been shown to impair catalytic activity.[151] As with nearly all of the genes mutated in MDS, *DNMT3A* mutations are not unique to these disorders and can be found in AML, myeloproliferative neoplasms (MPNs), and even lymphoid malignancies. Mouse models of *Dnmt3a* loss demonstrate hematopoietic stem cell expansion with impaired differentiation. Dysplasia and leukemic transformation do not occur in this mouse model, suggesting that *DNMT3A* loss is sufficient to provide a stem cell growth advantage, but insufficient to cause an MDS or AML disease phenotype. This is consistent with the finding that somatic *DNMT3A* mutations can be found in persons without cytopenias or other elements of disease.[152] Therefore, cooperating mutations or microenvironmental changes are likely necessary determinants of disease. Mutations of *DNMT3A* are found most often in patients with normal karyotypes and cooccur with *SF3B1* mutations more often than expected by chance.[90,153] *DNMT3A* mutations in MDS patients appear to confer a poor prognosis.[150,154]

TET2 The second member of the ten-eleven translocation gene family, *TET2*, is among the most frequently mutated MDS genes present in 20 to 30 percent of cases, and in more than 40 percent of patients with CMML. It encodes a methylcytosine oxygenase that converts 5-methylcytosine (5-mC) in to 5-hydroxymethylcytosine (5-hmC) using iron and α-ketoglutarate (αKG) as cofactors.[155] The TET2 enzyme can further oxidize 5-hmC into 5-formyl- and 5-carobxycytosine (5-fC and 5-caC, respectively).[156] This may represent a mechanism for the active demethylation of cytosines as 5-caC can be decarboxylated to form cytosine or treated as a mismatched nucleotide by the base excision DNA repair pathway. Mutations in *TET2* are typically truncating or clustered in regions that encode catalytic domains indicating an associated loss of function. Mutations are often compound heterozygous or in areas of aUPD on chromosome 4q, resulting in no viable wild-type allele.[157] Patients with *TET2* mutations demonstrate increased global DNA methylation, lower levels of 5-hmC and are more likely to have an elevated monocyte count.[158,159] Mouse models of *Tet2* loss show a similar phenotype with increased stem cell and progenitor numbers, impaired differentiation, and myeloid skewing of hematopoiesis.[160-163] As with *DNMT3A*, *TET2* mutations can also be found in various myeloid and lymphoid malignancies, as well as in persons with clonal hematopoiesis and no hematologic disesase.[152] Clinically, *TET2* mutations are not likely drivers of MDS prognosis and have variably been associated with favorable, neutral, or poor outcomes.[134,164,165]

IDH1 and IDH2 Only mutations in the isocitrate dehydrogenase genes 1 and 2 (*IDH1* and *IDH2*, respectively) are exclusive of *TET2* mutations, suggesting that they share a common pathogenic mechanism. Mutations of these *IDH* genes are common in AML and gliomas, but relatively rare in MDS, comprising approximately 5 percent of cases. Oncogenic *IDH* mutations are always heterozygous missense mutations of specific codons that result in an important change of enzyme function. Instead of converting isocitrate to αKG while generating an nicotinamide adenine dinucleotide phosphate (NADPH) from nicotinamide adenine dinucleotide phosphate–positive (NADP⁺), the mutant forms of *IDH1* and *IDH2* catalyze the conversion of αKG to 2-hydroxyglutarate (2-HG) while oxidizing NADPH to NADP⁺.[166] The 2-HG produced is considered an *oncometabolite,* which can interfere with the activity of αKG-dependent oxygenases, including the *TET* family of genes, prolyl hydroxylases, collagen synthesis enzymes, and various histone demethylases.[167-171] Mouse models of leukemic *IDH* mutations in the hematopoietic system share several features with *Tet2*-null mice, including global DNA hypermethylation and increased proportions of early progenitor cells.[172] In MDS, the clinical significance of IDH mutations is mixed and may depend on the nature of the mutation.[173] Inhibitors of the neomorphic activity of mutant IDH enzymes represent promising therapies as the effects of 2-HG exposure appear to be reversible.[174]

EZH2 and Other Rare Mutations Several regulators of histone modifications are recurrently mutated in MDS and MDS/MPN disorders. These include the histone methylase *EZH2*, which encodes the catalytic subunit of the protein-repressive complex 2 (PRC2) responsible

for methylating lysine 27 on histone 3 (H3K27). The H3K27 methyl mark is associated with closed chromatic and reduced expression of neighboring genes. Loss-of-function mutations in *EZH2*, present in 6 percent of MDS, are associated with a poor prognosis in a manner that is independent of common prognostic scoring systems.[100,102,134] This is largely because *EZH2* mutations are not strongly associated with adverse clinical features such as increased proportions of blasts, complex karyotypes, or severe cytopenias.[141] Other members of the PRC2, *EED* and *SUZ12*, can also be mutated in very rare cases of MDS.[175] Loss of PRC2 activity may, in part, promote the development and progression of MDS through derepression of HOX genes, which are often upregulated or aberrantly expressed in self-renewing leukemic cells.[176]

ASXL1 *ASXL1* is a frequently mutated MDS gene believed to be an epigenetic "reader" capable of binding to specific histone marks through its highly conserved PHD domain. Mutations of *ASXL1*, present in 20 percent of MDS and 40 percent of CMML, are largely heterozygous truncating mutations in its terminal exon. These lesions are associated with a poorer prognosis than predicted by common clinical assessments alone.[134,177,178] *ASXL1* interacts directly with the PRC2, directing the activity of *EZH2* to specific genomic regions. Loss of *ASXL1* is associated with absent H3K27 trimethylation at the *HOXA* gene cluster.[179] *ASXL1* mutations may cooperate with mutations in various other genes such as *SRSF2*, *U2AF1*, *TET2*, and *NRAS*, as mutations of these genes cooccur more often than predicted by chance alone.[90] In patients with germline mutations of the transcription factor *GATA2*, somatic *ASXL1* mutation appears to be a common concurrent event at the time of MDS or AML development.[180,181]

Mutated Transcription Factor Genes Mutations of hematopoietic transcription factors in MDS are typically somatic events, but can be present in the germline either as inherited or spontaneous congenital events in rare cases. *RUNX1* is the most frequently mutated transcription factor in MDS. This gene, previously known as *AML1*, encodes the alpha core binding transcription factor subunit and is altered in many myeloid and lymphoid malignancies. In the acute leukemias, *RUNX1* is a frequent translocation partner with other genes such as *RUNX1T1* (previously known as *ETO*) as part of t(8;21) in AML and with *ETV6* in (previously known as *TEL*) as part of t(12;21) in acute lymphocytic leukemia (ALL). *RUNX1* is mutated in 10 to 15 percent of MDS where it is associated with a poor prognosis, increased rates of leukemic progression, and thrombocytopenia.[134,135] Mutations can affect one or both alleles and often involve the DNA-binding RUNT domain or truncate the more distal protein interaction domain.[182-184] Persons with congenital mutations of *RUNX1* can have an autosomal dominant FPD-AML characterized by numerical and functional platelet abnormalities that precede transformation to AML by many years. Penetrance of FPD-AML is variable and the long latency to transform indicates the need to acquire cooperating mutations.[43,185,186] Mutations of *C/EBPA* can also cause familial propensity for AML in an autosomal dominant fashion, but are very rare mutations in MDS as somatic or inherited abnormalities.[187]

ETV6 The ets-like transcription factor 6, *ETV6*, is frequently rearranged, deleted, or mutated in hematologic malignancies. In MDS, *ETV6* mutations are present in approximately 5 percent of cases, where they are independently associated with shorter overall survival and progressive disease.[134,188]

GATA2 Germline *GATA2* mutations are responsible for several different congenital syndromes with overlapping features including a predisposition to marrow failure, MDS, and AML.[53,58,189,190] Familial *GATA2* mutations can manifest as the monoMAC syndrome, characterized by monocytopenia and mycobacterial infections; Emberger syndrome, characterized by congenital lymphedema and risk of developing MDS; or as a deficiency in monocytes, B and natural killer (NK) lymphocytes, and dendritic cells.[191] Patients can also have sensorineural hearing loss, alveolar proteinosis, and dermatologic abnormalities. Penetrance is variable and patients with one syndrome often will have features of the others. Several cases of congenital neutropenia or apparently de novo MDS in childhood have been ascribed to germline *GATA2* mutations in the absence of other syndromic features.[56] However, unlike *RUNX1* and *ETV6* mutations, mutations of *GATA2* are only very rarely somatic events.

TP53 *TP53* mutations are present in approximately 10 percent of MDS cases and are strongly associated with a poor prognosis independent of other risk factors.[134] Most patients with mutations of *TP53* will have a complex karyotype and tend to have fewer point mutations in other typical MDS genes. Patients with del(5q) are more likely to have a *TP53* mutation, particularly in the context of a complex karyotype, suggesting pathologic synergy between these abnormalities.[90,135] Unfortunately, treatment with either hypomethylating agents or allogeneic hematopoietic stem cell transplantation (AHSCT) fails to rescue the adverse outcomes associated with mutations of *TP53*.[192–194]

Mutations of Growth Factor Signaling Pathway Genes Mutations of receptor tyrosine kinase genes are common in proliferative myeloid disorders, such as *FLT3* in AML, *KIT* in mast cell neoplasms, and of the receptor gene *MPL* in MPN, but only rarely present in MDS. Instead, several genes encoding downstream signaling proteins are more frequently mutated in MDS. Many of these mutations are associated with proliferative features and often presage more advance disease or progression to secondary AML. Signaling pathway mutations are typically mutually exclusive, indicating some redundancy in function and are more common in CMML where monocytic proliferation is a defining feature. In MDS, these mutations are frequently present in minor disease subclones demonstrating that they were acquired later in the course of disease. Despite their small abundance, signaling pathway mutations are often predictive of transformation and shorter overall survival.[195,196]

Activating *NRAS* mutations are the most common in this category, but found in only 5 to 10 percent of cases. These lesions are associated with excess blasts and thrombocytopenia.[134] The E3-ubiquitin ligase CBL regulates tyrosine kinase receptors by marking them for degradation.[197] *CBL* mutations that impair this function are found in 3 to 5 percent of MDS cases and are associated with monocytosis.[198,199] Somatic mutations of the tyrosine phosphatase encoded by *PTPN11* are seen in very rare cases of MDS and CMML, but are more common in juvenile myelomonocytic leukemia where mutations are often germline lesions and part of a congenital syndrome.[200,201] Other genes that are very rarely but recurrently mutated in this pathway include *KRAS, BRAF, KIT*, and *CBLB*.

The V617F mutation in *JAK2* is found in 3 to 5 percent of patients with MDS and is exclusive of other signaling pathway mutations. However, it does not appear to have prognostic significance and is not associated with an increased red cell mass as it is in polycythemia vera.[134] This is likely because *JAK2* mutations in MDS are often late events and coexist with other genetic lesions that result in dysplasia, limiting the production of mature red cells. *JAK2* mutations are enriched in patients with RARS-t, and MDS/MPN overlap disease.[202] Half of these patients will carry a *JAK2*[V617F] mutation. This is roughly the same proportion observed in patients with essential thrombocythemia (ET); leading to the speculation that RARS-t is a "frustrated" form of ET with dysplasia caused by the other mutations like those in *SF3B1* associated with ring sideroblasts.[203] Approximately 5 percent of RARS-t patients will instead have a mutation in *MPL*, which is similar to the rate at which it occurs in ET as well (Chap. 85).

Cohesin Genes *RAD21, STAG2, SMC3*, and *SMC1A* are recurrently mutated members of the cohesin gene family. Collectively, they are mutated in approximately 10 percent of MDS cases, where they may

be associated with a poor prognosis.[204,205] Cohesins bind to chromatin in a large complex believed to protect chromatid structure and shepherd chromosomes through mitosis. However, mutations of this complex are not associated with chromosomal instability in MDS. Instead, they identify patients more likely to have multilineage dysplasia.[137] The pathogenic mechanism of cohesin mutations in myeloid disorders remains poorly understood.

Other Classes of Mutated Genes Several other classes of genes are recurrently mutated in MDS, including DNA repair enzymes, RNA helicases, and members of the G-protein signaling pathway. The long tail of recurrent, but rarely mutated genes in MDS suggest that dysplasia is common final phenotype that can be caused by a variety of different pathogenic abnormalities, each with their own degree of severity, risk of progression, and variation in clinical presentation.

Microenvironmental Changes

Not all abnormalities identified in the marrow of patients with MDS are intrinsic to the clonal cells that give rise to the disease. There are many microenvironmental alterations that contribute to the distorted hematopoiesis that is characteristic of MDS. Marrow cytokine levels are altered in many cases. Circulating monocyte colony-stimulating factor (M-CSF) is increased in some patients with MDS, AML, and other hematologic malignancies.[206] Interleukin (IL)-1α and granulocyte-macrophage colony-stimulating factor (GM-CSF) levels have been undetectable in most patients. IL-6, granulocyte colony-stimulating factor (G-CSF), and erythropoietin concentrations have been variable. Tumor necrosis factor (TNF) concentrations has been inversely related to hematocrit.[207] Stem cell factor, a multilineage hematopoietin, can be decreased in some patients.[208]

The neoplastic clone may induce activation of the innate immune system. Loss of miRNAs 145 and 146a from the CDR of chromosome 5q lead upregulation of toll-interleukin receptor adaptor protein (TIRAP) and tumor receptor-associated factor (TRAF) 6, members of the innate immune signaling pathway downstream of toll-like receptors.[80] Toll-like receptors may also be targets of somatic mutations leading to nuclear factor (NF)-κB activation.[209] Myeloid-derived suppressor cells, distinct from the clonal disease cells, may contribute to the altered cytokine microenvironment and promote disordered hematopoiesis.[210]

Dysregulation of the adaptive immune system has also been described. CD40 expression on monocytes is increased, as is CD40L on T lymphocytes, and has been postulated as being a contributing factor to hematopoietic failure in some patients with less-advanced disease.[86] Many patients with MDS will demonstrate oligoclonal T-cell expansion with skewing of Vβ-subunits of the T-cell receptor similar to that seen in aplastic anemia.[211] In patients that respond to immunosuppressive therapy, this oligoclonality of T cells may be normalized.[212] There likely exists substantial pathogenic overlap between aplastic anemia and hypoplastic MDS. Immunosuppression can improve hematopoiesis in both disorders, both can exhibit paroxysmal nocturnal hemoglobinuria (PNH) clones, and both can have somatic mutations typical of MDS (Chap. 35).[213] Large granular lymphocyte (LGL) leukemia can cause immune cytopenias and LGL cells are present in some cases of both MDS and aplastic anemia. These lymphocytes can carry somatic mutations of *STAT3* indicating their clonal nature, distinct from the MDS clone.[214]

● CLINICAL FEATURES

SYMPTOMS AND SIGNS

Patients can be asymptomatic or, if anemia is more severe, can have pallor, weakness, loss of a sense of well-being, and exertional dyspnea.[215] Fatigue is a major complaint that is not necessarily related to degree of anemia.[216] A small proportion of patients have infections related to severe neutropenia or neutrophil dysfunction, or hemorrhage related to severe thrombocytopenia or platelet dysfunction at the time of diagnosis. Patients with severe depressions of neutrophil and platelet counts at diagnosis usually have more advanced disease. Rarely, patients have fever unrelated to infection. Arthralgia is the initial complaint in some patients. The presentation, infrequently, can mimic a rheumatologic disease. Hepatomegaly or splenomegaly occurs in approximately 5 or 10 percent of patients, respectively.

LABORATORY FEATURES

BLOOD

Red Cells
Anemia is present in greater than 85 percent of patients.[217–219] In approximately 4 percent of patients, the anemia results from erythroid aplasia.[220] Mean cell volume often is increased. Red cell shape abnormalities include oval, elliptical, teardrop, spherical, and fragmented cells. Red cell findings occur in a spectrum. Some patients have only slight anisocytosis. Elliptical red cells sometimes dominate. Basophilic stippling of red cells occurs (see Fig. 87–3). Nucleated red cells are seen in the blood film in approximately 10 percent of cases. Reticulocyte counts are low for the degree of anemia. Other abnormalities of red cells occur, such as an increased proportion of hemoglobin F[221] and decreased red cell enzyme activities, especially acquired pyruvate kinase deficiency.[222] Hemolysis has occurred in some patients with the latter deficiency. Enhanced sensitivity of membranes to complement[223] and modification of red cell blood group antigens may be observed.[224] Acquired hemoglobin H disease, a rare superimposition, results in red cell morphology similar to thalassemia (microcytosis, anisocytosis, basophilic stippling, poikilocytosis with target cells, fragmented cells, and teardrop cells). Intracellular precipitates of β-chain tetramers (identified by crystal violet stain) reflect an acquired decrease in the rate of α-chain synthesis in erythroblasts.[225–227] The decrease in α-globin–chain synthesis is profound, involves each of the four α-chain loci, and results from a transcription abnormality. No gross alterations in genes (e.g., insertions, deletions) are seen in these cases.[227] Acquired hemoglobin H disease in this setting has been dubbed the α-thalassemia–myelodysplastic syndrome and is the consequence of acquired mutations in *ATRX*, the gene associated with the X-linked α-thalassemia/mental retardation (ATR-X) syndrome.[225]

Granulocytes and Monocytes
Neutropenia is present in approximately 50 percent of patients at the time of diagnosis.[228] The proportion of monocytes often is increased, and monocytosis per se can be the dominant manifestation of the hematopoietic abnormality for months or years.[229–231] Morphologic abnormalities of neutrophils can occur, sometimes resulting in the acquired Pelger-Huët anomaly (see Fig. 87–3E). In this condition, neutrophils have very condensed chromatin and unilobed or bilobed nuclei that often have a pince-nez shape. The neutrophils may be in the process of apoptosis.[232] Ring-shaped nuclei also can occur in neutrophils (see Fig. 87–3F).[233] Neutrophil alkaline phosphatase activity is decreased in some patients.[234] Expression of normal surface antigens on neutrophils and monocytes is decreased, and abnormal surface antigen expression occurs in some cases.[235] Defective primary granules of abnormal size and shape with decreased myeloperoxidase content can be present.[236] Specific neutrophil granules are often decreased in number, producing hypogranular cells.[237] Neutrophil granule membranes frequently are deficient in glycoproteins.[238] Chemotactic, phagocytic,

and bactericidal capability may be impaired.[239–241] Formyl-leucyl-methionyl-phenylamine receptor signaling and actin polymerization can be abnormal.[242,243] Muramidase (lysozyme) activity in blood and urine may be increased, reflecting granulocytic hyperplasia, heightened monocytopoiesis, and monocyte turnover.

Platelets
Approximately 25 to 50 percent of patients have mild to moderate thrombocytopenia at the time of diagnosis.[228,234] Mild thrombocytosis also can occur.[228,234] Platelets may be abnormally large, have poor granulation, or have large, fused central granules (see Fig. 87–3H).[244,245] Abnormal platelet function can contribute to a prolonged closure time, easy bruising, or exaggerated bleeding. Decreased platelet aggregation in response to collagen or epinephrine is a frequent functional abnormality.[246]

Lymphocytes
Patients with clonal hemopathies may have immunologic deficiencies, such as a decrease in NK cells in the blood but no decrease in LGLs,[247–250] a decrease in helper T lymphocytes,[248] and a decrease in Epstein-Barr virus receptors on B lymphocytes.[248–251] Antibody-dependent cellular cytotoxicity is normal.[248] Thymidine incorporation after mitogenic stimulation[252,253] and colony growth of T lymphocytes are decreased.[248] Lymphocytes may have an increased sensitivity to irradiation.[253] The defects in lymphoid cells could reflect the level of the somatic mutation in a primitive multipotential cell in different cases. Intrinsic, rather than secondary, alterations in lymphocytes are determined by whether no lymphocytes are generated from the clone, B cells are part of the clone, or B and T cells are part of the clone.[254] Clonally derived, CD8+CD57+CD244+CD28–CD62L– T lymphocytes are present in marrow and to a lesser extent in blood in approximately 50 percent of patients, independent of type of MDS, age, and sex of the patient,[255,256] as are NK and B cells (see "Pathogenesis" above).[256]

PLASMA ABNORMALITIES
Serum iron, transferrin, and ferritin levels may be elevated as a result of anemia and the shift of erythron iron to plasma and storage compartments. Lactic dehydrogenase and uric acid concentrations can be increased as a result of ineffective hematopoiesis and a high death fraction of maturing marrow precursors. Monoclonal gammopathy, polyclonal hypergammaglobulinemia, and hypogammaglobulinemia each occur with increased frequency.[257,258] The frequency of autoantibodies was increased in one report[240] but not in another.[258] β_2-Microglobulin serum levels are increased in proportion to the prognostic category of the disease.[259]

MARROW

Cellularity
Marrow cellularity usually is normal or increased.[234,260,261] Cellularity is decreased in approximately 15 percent of cases[260] and may simulate hypoplastic or aplastic anemia.[262] However, islands of dysmorphic cells, especially atypical megakaryocytes, usually are present (see Fig. 87–3L). An increased proportion of blast cells in this setting suggests hypoplastic myelogenous leukemia (Chap. 88).

Erythropoiesis
Erythroid hyperplasia is frequent. Very large or small erythroblasts, nuclear fragmentation, stippled erythroblasts, and poor hemoglobinization may be seen.[234,260,261] Proerythroblasts may be present in excess, and the marrow may lack normal clusters or islets of erythroblasts.

Erythroblasts may resemble megaloblasts that have nuclear-cytoplasmic maturation asynchrony, nuclear fragmentation, or cytoplasmic nuclear remnants. The asynchrony is manifest morphologically by nuclear immaturity with prominent euchromatin in cells with more advanced cytoplasmic maturation. This pattern is referred to as *megaloblastoid erythropoiesis* (see Fig. 87–3*I*). Erythroid aplasia seen in occasional cases results in a hypocellular marrow.[220]

Pathologic sideroblasts may be identified when the marrow is stained with Prussian blue stain (see Fig. 87–3*J* and *K*). The sideroblasts include erythroblasts with an increased number and size of siderosomes (cytoplasmic ferritin-containing vacuoles), referred to as *intermediate sideroblasts*, or erythroblasts with mitochondrial iron aggregates that take the form of a partial or complete circumnuclear ring of iron globules, referred to as *ring sideroblasts*. Macrophage iron often is increased. Ring sideroblasts are uncommon or present only in very low proportions in clonal myeloid disorders other than RA.

Granulopoiesis

Granulocytic hyperplasia is frequent.[228,234,260,261] Marrow monocytes may be increased in number. Abnormalities of granulocytes include hypogranulation, a monocytoid appearance of neutrophilic granulocytes, and the acquired Pelger-Huët nuclear abnormality of neutrophils.[232,263] Progranulocytes and myelocytes may be increased. The proportion of blast cells is not increased in clonal hemopathies that are categorized as RA (defined as <5 percent); although, a blast percentage of greater than 2 percent should be considered oligoblastic leukemia and is recognized as having prognostic risk. Marrow biopsy may show abnormal localized immature precursors (ALIPs),[264,265] which are clusters of immature myeloid, CD34+ cells[266] located centrally rather than subjacent to the endosteum. These clusters of atypical cells are present in almost all cases of oligoblastic leukemia where blast cells compose 3 percent or more of nucleated marrow cells (RAEBs) and in approximately one-third of patients with RA, suggesting these patients have a disorder closely approaching oligoblastic leukemia. Patients with this abnormality are more prone to develop overt AML. Vascular endothelial growth factor and its receptor are expressed on cells forming ALIP clusters and have been proposed as providing an autocrine loop to promote leukemia progenitor cell formation.[267] The number of plasma cells may be slightly increased. Marrow basophilia or eosinophilia occurs in approximately one in seven patients and is associated with a higher probability of evolution to AML.[268]

Thrombopoiesis

Megakaryocytes are present in normal or increased numbers.[234,260,261] Micromegakaryocytes (dwarf megakaryocytes) may occur.[261,269,270] Megakaryocytes with unilobed or bilobed nuclei may be increased, and hypersegmented and hyposegmented megakaryocytes may be present (see Fig. 87–3*L*). Clusters of megakaryocytes may be seen. Megakaryocytes may be distributed laterally from their usual parasinusoidal location.[271]

Fibrosis and Angiogenesis

An increase in reticulin and collagen fibers of varying degree is common (approximately 15 percent of cases), especially in oligoblastic myelogenous leukemia.[266] When fibrosis is prominent, the disorder can resemble primary myelofibrosis, although, in contrast to the latter, splenomegaly usually is not marked and mutations of *CALR*, *JAK2*, or *MPL*, genes frequently truncated in primary myelofibrosis and ET, are extremely rare.[272] Because primary myelofibrosis is an oligoblastic leukemia with striking dysmorphogenesis of cells, some confusion in classification with other fibrotic clonal myeloid disorders may occur.[273] Marrow fibrosis is correlated with higher blast counts and poor-risk cytogenetics.[266] Some physicians have proposed a category of myelofibrotic myelodysplasia,

but all clonal myeloid diseases, including AML, chronic myelogenous leukemia, and CMML may have within their spectrum of expression occasional cases with intense myelofibrosis. Like numerous other epiphenomena that occur in the expression of hematopoietic stem cell diseases, extending the general classifications is not warranted.

Increased angiogenesis is a feature of MDS. Microvessel density increases with more advanced stages of the disease.[274] Mast cell frequency and mast cell tryptase activity are highly correlated with microvessel density.[275] Circulating endothelial cells are also increased in concentration in patients with MDS and their concentration is correlated with marrow neoangiogenesis (microvessel density).[276]

● THERAPY-RELATED MYELODYSPLASTIC SYNDROMES

Therapy-related MDS are increasing in frequency as the use of intensive chemotherapy and radiation increases in other solid tumors and lymphoma.[277–284] These cases have a poor prognosis and are not included in either the original IPSS or the revised IPSS-R. Cellular abnormalities of chromosomes 5, 7, and 8 are common in these cases.[285] MDS following breast cancer is associated with older age, presence of other cancers, and multiple first-degree relatives with cancer.[286] As compared to patients with myeloma or germ cell tumors, patients with lymphoma undergoing autologous stem cell transplantation have a higher incidence of treatment-related MDS. In this group, pretransplantation therapy, total-body irradiation, and other transplantation-related factors play a role, as do inherited polymorphisms in genes governing drug metabolism and DNA repair.[287] Therapy-related MDS has been reported after high-dose melphalan for myeloma treatment, particularly in patients treated with lenalidomide.[288]

Accelerated telomere shortening precedes development of therapy-related myelodysplasia after autologous transplantation for lymphoma.[289] Treatment-related MDS is managed as are *de novo* cases of MDS, but are very refractory to treatment. AHSCT can result in long-term disease-free survival, but most patients with therapy-related MDS are not candidates because of advanced age, comorbidities, or the inability to control the primary cancer.[290]

● DIAGNOSTIC CRITERIA FOR MYELODYSPLASTIC SYNDROMES

The current diagnostic criteria for MDS are well defined, but can be difficult to apply in practice. Many diagnostic elements, such as the extent of dysplasia in the marrow and the quantification of blasts, are subjective measures associated with high rates of interobserver variability.[291,292] Current guidelines require a blast proportion of 5 percent or greater in the marrow as definitive evidence for MDS absent other criteria and this threshold distinguishes RAEB from other MDS subtypes. However, more than 2 percent marrow blasts is abnormal and likely evidence of oligoblastic leukemia. This lower threshold is recognized as prognostically adverse in the IPSS-R. Even when dysplasia is clearly present, benign and potentially reversible causes of morphologic abnormalities must be excluded (Table 87–3). The presence of acquired chromosomal abnormalities is indicative of clonal hematopoiesis and can aid in the diagnostic evaluation. Specific karyotypes found more commonly in patients with MDS serve as presumptive evidence of the disorder in patients with clinically meaningful cytopenias and insufficient dysplasia to meet the morphologic criteria for diagnosis. Somatic mutations, which are more frequent than chromosomal abnormalities may soon be formally used in this manner to aid the diagnosis of MDS.

TABLE 87–3. Diagnostic Criteria for Myelodysplastic Syndromes[577]

Presence of one or more otherwise unexplained cytopenias*
Hemoglobin <11 g/dL
Absolute neutrophil count <1500/μL
Platelet count <100,000/μL
Presence of one or more myelodysplastic syndrome (MDS) decisive criteria
>10% dysplastic cells in erythroid, myeloid, and/or megakaryocyte lineages
5 to 19% marrow blasts

Evidence of a cytogenetic abnormality typical for MDS[†]:

–7 or del(7q)	del(12p) or t(12p)	t(1;3)(p36.3;q21.1)
–5 or del(5q)	del(9q)	t(2;11)(p21;q23)
i(17q) or t(17p)	idic(X)(q13)	inv(3)(q21q26.2)
–13 or del(13q)	t(11;16)(q23;p13.3)	t(6;9)(p23;q34)
del(11q)	t(3;21)(q26.2;q22.1)	

Exclusion of alternative diagnosis that explain blood and marrow findings
No AML-defining criteria (e.g., t[8;11], i[16], t[16;16], t[15;17], or erythroleukemia)
No other hematologic disorders (e.g., acute lymphocytic leukemia, aplastic anemia, or various lymphomas)

Not explained by
- HIV or other viral infection
- Deficiencies of iron or copper
- B$_{12}$, folate, or other vitamin deficiency
- Medications (e.g., methotrexate, azathioprine, or chemotherapy)
- Alcohol abuse (typically heavy and prolonged usage)
- Autoimmune conditions (e.g., immune thrombocytopenia purpura, immune hemolytic anemia, Evans syndrome, Felty syndrome, or systemic lupus erythematosus)
- Congenital disorders (e.g., Fanconi anemia, Diamond-Blackfan anemia, and Shwachman-Diamond syndrome, etc…)

*Present for 6 months or longer, if there is no typical cytogenetic abnormality identified.

†The list of cytogenetic abnormalities shown in this Table was taken from reference 578 and reiterated here.

CLINICAL PROGNOSTIC SCORING SYSTEMS

The estimation of prognosis is an integral element in the care for patients with MDS. It sets expectations for patients about their disease and helps physicians weigh the risks and benefits of specific treatments versus observation alone. Historically, they have been used to describe participants with MDS in clinical trials, which has allowed for comparison among studies. The most prevalent prognostic model in clinical use is the IPSS, first published in 1997. This model was created by examining 816 MDS patients at the time of their diagnosis. Patients with therapy-related MDS, proliferative CMML, and those who received disease-modifying therapy, such as AHSCT, were excluded. The IPSS considered three major risk markers: the percentage of blasts in the marrow, the presence of specific cytogenetic abnormalities, and the number of cytopenias present in the blood. These elements were weighted as shown in Table 87–4 to assign patients to one of four IPSS risk groups

TABLE 87–4. International Prognostic Scoring System for Myelodysplastic Syndromes[579]

Score Value	0	0.5	1.0	1.5
Prognostic Variables				
Marrow Blasts (%)	<5	5–10		11–20
Karyotype	Good	Intermediate	Poor	
Cytopenias	0, 1	2, 3		

Risk groups: Low, 0; intermediate-1, 0.5–1.0; intermediate-2, 1.5–2.0; high, ≥2.5. Survival for each risk group is displayed in Table 87–5.

Karyotype: Good score, –Y, del(5q); poor score, complex abnormalities and chromosome 7 abnormalities; intermediate score, all other abnormalities. See "Marrow: Cytogenetics" in text above for further details.

Cytopenias: anemia, hemoglobin <10 g/dL; neutropenia, absolute neutrophil count <1.8 × 10^9/L; thrombocytopenia, platelet count <100 × 10^9/L.

with significant differences in overall survival and risk of clonal evolution to AML (Table 87–5). The IPSS was an extremely useful tool that gained wide acceptance in clinical practice and is incorporated into clinical practice guidelines published by the National Comprehensive Cancer Network and European LeukemiaNet.[293,294] However, the IPSS has several limitations that include consideration of blast proportions that were later redefined by the WHO classification system as AML and a propensity to underestimate risk in patients with severe cytopenias. Several subsequent prognostic models that improve upon the IPSS have been published and validated, but have generally not been widely adopted in routine clinical practice.[295–297]

The IPSS-R, published in 2012, addresses most of the limitations of the IPSS and provides improved prognostic accuracy over the IPSS and subsequent models.[298–300] The IPSS-R examined clinical data from 7012 MDS patients at the time of their diagnosis (Table 87–6). Like the IPSS, the IPSS-R excluded patients with proliferative CMML or therapy-related disease and censored patients if and when they received disease-modifying therapy. The IPSS-R differs from the IPSS in that it includes a much broader range of cytogenetic abnormalities which are given greater weight in the overall risk calculation. The IPSS-R refines the marrow blast percentages to exclude patients with 20 percent or greater blasts and considers each type of cytopenia as an independent risk factor weighted by severity. Based on the total risk score, patients are assigned to one of five risk groups instead of the four used by the IPSS. The risk score can be adjusted for age to take this variable into account. Patients assigned to the "very low" and "low risk" groups are considered to have lower-risk MDS whereas those in the "high" or "very high" groups have higher-risk disease. Patients in the intermediate category may be treated as lower or higher risk based on other prognostic factors such as serum ferritin and serum lactate dehydrogenase (LDH) which are not formally considered in the model.

The IPSS-R has been validated and shown to apply in contexts for which it was not originally defined. This includes risk stratification at times other than diagnosis, use in patients who go on to receive disease-modifying treatment, and use in patients undergoing AHSCT.[299,301–303] It is important to note that the median overall survival for patients stratified by the IPSS and IPSS-R represent estimates based on patients who did not receive disease-modifying therapy. Patients who respond to active treatments may, in fact, have a greater expected median survival than predicted by these scoring systems. Currently, somatic mutations are not considered by any prognostic scoring system in widespread

TABLE 87–5. Survival of Patients Based on the International Prognostic Scoring System

IPSS Group at Diagnosis	No. of Patients	2-Year Survival	5-Year Survival	10-Year Survival	15-Year Survival
Low	267	85%	55%	28%	20%
Intermediate-1	314	70%	35%	17%	12%
Intermediate-2	179	30%	8%	0	–
High	56	5%	0	–	–

IPSS, International Prognostic Scoring System.

clinic use even though these lesions have been shown to have independent prognostic significance. Future prognostic models are likely to combine clinical and molecular information to refine the prediction of prognosis in MDS.

TREATMENT OF MYELODYSPLASTIC SYNDROMES BASED ON PROGNOSTIC SCORE

Therapeutic decisions in patients with MDS patients can be based on the predicted evolution of disease, as measured by prognostic tools such as the IPSS and IPSS-R.[304] Lower-risk patients are commonly treated with lower-intensity therapies such as hematopoietic growth factors or immunomodulatory agents, while use of hypomethylating agents, cytotoxic agents, or AHSCT is typically reserved for higher-risk patients.[305–307] In addition, two biomarkers—the presence of del(5q) in lower-risk patients with anemia, and the serum erythropoietin level in anemic patients—are strong enough predictors of treatment response as to permit selection or avoidance of individual drugs (i.e., the use of lenalidomide[308] or erythropoiesis-stimulating agents,[309] respectively). While other predictive biomarkers in MDS have been proposed, such as *TET2* and *DNMT3A* mutation status as predictors of the likelihood of response to hypomethylating agents[194,310,311]; patient age, marrow hypocellularity or human leukocyte antigen (HLA) DR-B15 status and response to immunosuppressive therapy[312]; serum thrombopoietin and intensity of platelet transfusion requirements and response to thrombopoietin agonist romiplostim[313]; or flow cytometry patterns and response to erythropoiesis-stimulating agents[314], these are not strong enough predictors of response to specific therapies to influence management

TABLE 87–6. Revised International Prognostic Scoring System for Myelodysplastic Syndromes[8]

Cytogenetic Groups	IPSS-R Karyotype Abnormalities				
Very good	del(11q), –Y				
Good	Normal, del(20q), del(5q) alone or with 1 other anomaly, del(12p)				
Intermediate	+8, del(7q), i(17q), +19, +21, any single or double abnormality not listed, or two or more independent clones				
Poor	der(3q), –7, double with del(7q), complex with 3 abnormalities				
Very poor	Complex with >3 abnormalities				

IPSS-R Parameter	Categories and Associated Scores				
	Very Good	**Good**	**Intermediate**	**Poor**	**Very Poor**
Cytogenetic Risk Group	0	1	2	3	4
Marrow blast %	≤2	>2–<5	5–10	>10	
	0	1	2	3	
Hemoglobin (g/dL)	≥10	8–<10	<8		
	0	1	1.5		
Platelet count (× 10⁹/L)	≥100	50–<100	<50		
	0	0.5	1		
Neutrophil count (× 10⁹/L)	≥0.8	<0.8			
	0	0.5			

IPSS-R Risk Group	Total Score	% of Patients	Median Survival, Years	25% with AML, at Years
Very low	≤1.5	19	8.8	NR
Low	>1.5–3	38	5.3	10.8
Intermediate	>3–4.5	20	3	3.2
High	>4.5–6	13	1.6	1.4
Very high	>6	10	0.8	0.73

AML, acute myelogenous leukemia; IPSS-R, International Prognostic Scoring System–Revised; NR, not reached.
These data were found in Ref 298 and reiterated in this table.

decisions. Patients with *TP53* mutations may comprise a special group, as they have such a poor outlook with conventional therapies that either clinical trial enrollment or palliative care may be most appropriate for individuals with a *TP53* mutant genotype.[315,316]

The calculated prognostic score should not be the sole guide to treatment of a patient, as many patients deviate from the average expectation of disease behavior. The prognostic scores are based on the average behavior of large numbers of patients without confidence intervals to show the degree of variation, which is substantial. Unexpected progression or evolution of disease may also necessitate changes in treatment approach, and patients' comorbid conditions may preclude use of specific therapies (e.g., renal failure requires dose adjustment or avoidance of lenalidomide). There is also uncertainty among clinical investigators about the optimal therapeutic approach in many situations, such as for IPSS lower-risk patients with severe cytopenias other than anemia, anemic IPSS lower-risk patients without del(5q) and with a serum erythropoietin level greater than 500 U/L, and IPSS higher-risk patients who are not transplant candidates and for whom azacitidine and decitabine have failed.[317]

Measurement of treatment response in a clinical trial usually involves comparison to the 2006 International Working Group (IWG) response criteria.[318] Although IWG response criteria focus on improvements in specific measurable and objective variables such as hemoglobin level, the number of abnormal metaphases on karyotyping, and marrow blast proportion, surveys have shown that what matters most to patients is decreased symptoms,[319,320] improved quality of life,[321–323] avoidance of hospitalization and extended survival, which overlap with but are not identical to numerical disease measurements. Economic considerations also determine clinical care patterns, and the high cost of MDS care is a burden for many patients.[324]

THERAPEUTIC APPROACHES TO PATIENTS WITH LOWER-RISK DISEASE

All patients, regardless of risk score, deserve "best supportive care." Supportive care consists of improving quality of life by treatment of cytopenias or their complications (e.g., dyspnea, bleeding, infection) and providing ongoing psychosocial support, while monitoring the patient's clinical status at intervals.[325] The inclusion of palliative care can be very helpful to many patients, especially those at higher-risk and does not imply the cessation of treatment. Counseling by experienced palliative care physicians can provide patients with important support in their understanding of the best ways to manage their disabilities and to make therapeutic decisions.

Red Cell Transfusion

Red blood cell (RBC) transfusions should be administered for symptomatic anemia. Often patients will tolerate hemoglobin levels lower than 8 g/dL, but the level at which symptoms develop varies from patient to patient. Higher thresholds have been suggested to prevent cardiac consequences of prolonged anemia,[326,327] while lower thresholds have been recommended based on superior outcomes with restrictive RBC transfusion strategies in inpatient populations[328–330] and the need to preserve the blood supply. Patients with MDS may receive hundreds of units of RBCs over the course of their illness.[331,332]

Platelet Transfusion

Thrombocytopenia is common in MDS and has a higher prevalence in higher-risk IPSS categories.[333] Furthermore, many therapies used in MDS may worsen thrombocytopenia. Hemorrhage is the second most common cause of death in patients with MDS.[333] Platelet transfusions may be required if the platelet count falls below 10×10^9 cells/L or at

higher levels if the patient is actively bleeding. Antifibrinolytic agents, such as aminocaproic acid or tranexamic acid, can be used in patients who have mucosal bleeding despite platelet transfusion or to decrease the need of platelet transfusions.[93] This strategy is especially effective in patients with urinary bleeding or bleeding from arteriovenous malformations of the gut.

Antimicrobial Agents

Febrile events are common in higher-risk syndromes because of the frequency of moderately severe neutropenia and functional disorders of neutrophils and monocytes. Also, chemotherapy is more likely to be used in these situations, inducing severe neutropenia. Appropriate cultures and use of broad-spectrum antibiotics until and if a specific organism is found is important, with subsequent therapy tailored to microbiologic data. Chapter 24 discusses an approach to febrile neutropenia. The use of prophylactic antimicrobial agents in neutropenic patients is of uncertain usefulness in MDS, but may help prevent infections in those who have had previous problems with recurrent infection.[334] In this setting, levofloxacin and acyclovir are the best studied.[335] Prophylactic antifungal agents are used more frequently in AML patients, and some guidelines recommend posaconazole or voriconazole in MDS patients who have prolonged neutropenia and are at increased risk for fungal infections or who are undergoing induction chemotherapy.[336–339]

Erythropoiesis-Stimulating Agents

RBC transfusion dependency negatively influences clinical outcomes in MDS.[340] RBC transfusion dependence is a marker of more severe marrow failure, increased risk of transformation to AML, and increased iron overload from repetitive transfusions. Less-well-defined immunomodulatory effects of transfusions may contribute to poor outcomes.[341] In contrast, some studies found that neither the serum ferritin nor the number of RBC transfusions were associated with survival in clonal sideroblastic anemia.[342,343]

Erythropoiesis-stimulating agents (ESAs), such as recombinant human erythropoietin analogues, can be used to treat anemia in patients who are transfusion-dependent, if the serum erythropoietin level is lower than optimal for the hemoglobin level. Responses are best in patients with low serum erythropoietin levels,[309] normal blast counts, lower IPSS scores,[344] normal cytogenetics,[345] lower levels of inflammatory cytokines,[346] absence of aberrant marker expression by flow cytometry,[314] and in patients who do not require regular RBC transfusions.[309,347] Hemolysis and deficiencies of iron, vitamin B_{12}, or folate should be excluded as a cause of anemia before ESA therapy is started. Iron stores should be kept replete during ESA therapy.[348,349]

Epoetin alfa at a dose of 150 to 300 U/kg per day three times per week or single weekly doses of 40,000 to 60,000 U are effective.[350–362] There is no increase in response with doses exceeding 60,000 U weekly.[358] In clinical practice, weekly epoetin is more commonly administered than three times per week, a dosing schedule that was developed in the hemodialysis setting. Darbepoetin alfa in various schedules of administration (e.g., 500 mcg fixed dose once every 3 weeks) has also been found effective in increasing hemoglobin levels and in enhancing quality of life.[363,364] Meta-analysis has confirmed erythropoietic response rates are similar for those treated either with epoetin alfa or with the longer-acting darbepoetin alfa.[365]

The probability of a response to ESA therapy increases modestly with duration of therapy, but from a practical standpoint it is difficult to obtain reimbursement to continue patients on ESA treatment beyond 12 weeks in the absence of an objective response.[366] Unlike in patients with solid tumors or renal failure, there is no evidence that ESAs increase thromboembolic disease or accelerate progress to leukemia, but followup in studies to date have been short.[367] Several series have reported increased survival in ESA-treated patients compared to controls.[344,368] There is evidence that marrow erythroid cells of MDS patients who respond to erythropoietin have a different gene expression pattern than do those of nonresponders.[369]

Filgrastim (G-CSF) combined with erythropoietin may produce a response more frequently than with an ESA alone, perhaps as a result of lineage crosstalk of growth factors at the progenitor cell level.[360,370] This combination does not appear to affect the risk of leukemic transformation and may have a positive impact on survival in those with low transfusion needs.[371]

Granulocyte-Stimulating Factors

Infection is the major cause of mortality in MDS.[372] Both neutropenia and granulocyte dysfunction contribute to the risk of infection.[373,374] Granulocyte transfusions are of little utility,[375] and, unfortunately, randomized, double-blind studies have not shown that any cytokine prolongs survival or reduces morbidity in MDS.[376] Treatment with GM-CSF (sargramostim) or G-CSF (filgrastim) increases neutrophil counts and function in some patients, but this is inconsistent.[360,377,378] G-CSF receptor expression on hematopoietic progenitor cells may be low in some patients with MDS and prevents response to endogenous or exogenously administered G-CSF.[379] Rare remissions have been reported in hypoplastic AML/MDS with G-CSF alone.[380]

The most common adverse effects of G-CSF and GM-CSF include bone pain, low-grade fevers, and soreness at the injection site. Rare serious complications such as splenic rupture, have been reported with use of G-CSF.[381] Pegfilgrastim may allow less-frequent dosing than filgrastim, but is poorly studied in MDS, in which leukemoid reactions and splenic ruptures have been described.[376,382,383] G-CSF is not generally recommended for those with intermediate-2 risk or high-risk IPSS scores because of the risk of leukemoid reactions.[384] In one review, 22 of 83 reported cases of MDS treated with G-CSF or GM-CSF had an increase in marrow blast percentage, and AML evolved in 12 of 69 patients. An increased percentage of abnormal macrophages has been reported during G-CSF therapy.[385] Use of these agents without chemotherapy in oligoblastic leukemias carries a risk of promoting expansion of leukemic blast cells.[386] Combinations of growth factors alone with maturing agents (so-called differentiating therapy) such as retinoic acid have not significantly improved response or survival rates.[387,388]

Platelet and Megakaryocyte Growth Factors

Low-dose IL-11 (oprelvekin), a megakaryocyte growth factor, was studied in patients with symptomatic thrombocytopenia associated with marrow failure syndromes including MDS, but efficacy was low and adverse effects such as fluid retention and atrial dysrhythmias were common.[389,390] Although this drug is approved by the FDA, it is rarely used and uncommonly reimbursed by third-party payers.

Initial development of thrombopoietin analogues was halted in the 1990s,[391] but newer thrombopoietin-receptor agonists have shown efficacy in MDS. Romiplostim (formerly AMG-531), a peptibody that stimulates the thrombopoietin receptor (c-Mpl), can decrease thrombocytopenia and reduce platelet transfusion needs and clinically significant bleeding events in patients with MDS and severe thrombocytopenia, including both those who are receiving no treatment and those who are receiving therapy with azacitidine, lenalidomide or decitabine.[392-395] The optimal MDS romiplostim dose determined by early clinical studies, 750 mcg subcutaneously once weekly, is higher than that required for immune thrombocytopenia. Eltrombopag, an orally administered small molecule c-Mpl agonist, has also shown efficacy in early phase MDS studies.[376,396-400]

Although there was initially concern about AML progression with romiplostim therapy as some leukemic blasts express functional

c-Mpl, a randomized study comparing romiplostim to placebo in lower-risk patients showed no increase in AML progression in patients receiving active treatment, although this study was stopped early by its Data Safety Monitoring Committee because of concern about such progression.[401] Another theoretical risk based on thrombopoietin-overexpressing murine models, marrow reticulin formation, appears to be uncommon in immune thrombocytopenia (ITP), but has not been systematically investigated in romiplostim-treated patients with MDS.[402] A model to predict response to romiplostim based on platelet transfusion need and serum thrombopoietin (TPO) level that parallels the similar model for ESAs based on RBC transfusion and serum erythropoietin (EPO) level has recently been developed.[313] The pathophysiology of ITP overlaps that of MDS, and other treatments for ITP such as rituximab or γ-globulin may be beneficial in cases of lower-risk MDS where the degree of thrombocytopenia is disproportionate to other cytopenias.

Iron-Chelation Therapy

The magnitude of risk from iron overload in patients with receiving frequent RBC transfusions compared to the risk of death intrinsic to the disease and the utility of chelation therapy is one of the most controversial areas in MDS clinical management.[403-406] Claims-based data suggest increased risk of complications in transfused patients with MDS, but correlation does not prove causation and patients at higher risk of complications may have been more likely to be transfused (e.g., diabetic patients might have had more renal insufficiency and insufficient EPO production, rather than repeated transfusion causing pancreatic islet injury via hemosiderosis and inducing diabetes mellitus).[407,408] Retrospective comparisons suggest superior outcomes in chelated patients compared to unchelated patients, but are subject to confounding by patient selection bias.[409-412]

Despite the absence of high-quality evidence from prospective trials, numerous consensus guidelines have been published regarding the treatment of iron overload in MDS.[413] These guidelines make general recommendations about iron monitoring and chelation in RBC transfusion-requiring patients, but emphasize that there is no prospectively validated threshold for either the number of units of transfused blood or the level of serum ferritin that should trigger iron chelation, as patients accumulate iron at different rates and serum ferritin is sensitive to other influences such as inflammation. Most guidelines take into account the patient's candidacy for AHSCT,[414] life expectancy, and evidence of iron-related organ damage.[415,416] Several guidelines use a serum ferritin greater than 1000 mcg/L and a transfusion history of 20 to 30 RBC units as a threshold for starting iron-chelation therapy, but this strategy is not validated. The use of $T2^*/R2^*$ magnetic resonance imaging techniques may allow noninvasive assessment of organ iron deposition,[331,332,417] but it is not clear whether labile plasma iron levels or total-body iron burden poses a greater risk.[418,419]

Both deferoxamine given subcutaneously or intravenously and deferasirox given orally are available for chelation therapy in MDS patients. Deferasirox rapidly reduces labile plasma iron and mobilizes iron stores and is more convenient than deferoxamine, but in both U.S. and European studies, one-half of patients discontinued deferasirox therapy within a year of study enrollment because of disease progression or adverse effects (renal insufficiency, rash, and gastroenterologic distress).[418,420] There are several reports of improved hematopoiesis in chelated patients.[421,422]

Low-Dose Cytarabine

Since the early 1980s,[423-425] low-dose cytarabine at doses of 5 to 20 mg/m^2 per day by subcutaneous injection every 12 hours for 8 to 16 weeks or by continuous intravenous infusion has been used in MDS in lieu of intensive chemotherapy.[426-429] Although this approach leads to remission in approximately 10 to 20 percent of patients with MDS, the median duration of remission is less than 1 year, and survival has not been prolonged nor has AML progression been delayed compared with supportive care alone.[430] Moreover, low-dose cytosine arabinoside usually is cytotoxic, inducing marrow hypoplasia and worsening cytopenias. Although occasional reports of remission following low-dose cytarabine have been consistent with an effect on leukemia cell maturation, most patients experience suppression of the malignant cell clone, leading to marrow repopulation with polyclonal hemopoiesis. This treatment approach is used less often since the advent of other FDA-approved agents for MDS, especially as azacitidine treatment is associated with superior overall survival compared to cytarabine,[431] but may still have a role in some patients.[432]

Immunosuppressive Therapy: Cyclosporine and Antithymocyte Globulin

In some patients with MDS, autoreactive T-lymphocyte–mediated inhibition of hematopoiesis occurs and contributes to cytopenias.[433] In such patients, cytopenias may be ameliorated by treatment with immunosuppressive agents directed at T cells such as antithymocyte globulin (ATG) or calcineurin inhibitors.[212] In patients who recover effective hematopoiesis after immunosuppressive treatment, the $V\beta$ (T-cell receptor-β) spectra-type representative of clonal or oligoclonal T-cell populations typically reverts to normal patterns. In one older study, a nonclonal X-chromosome inactivation pattern in the marrow, as assessed by the human androgen receptor gene assay and the phosphoglycerated kinase-1 assay, was associated with a response to ATG.[434] This finding was attributed to incomplete clonal expansion, with ATG improving normal hematopoiesis by relieving the immunologic pressure on the remaining normal progenitors. Other investigators have postulated that responses may result from suppression of interferon-γ secretion by CD4+ T cells regardless of clonality.[435]

Some series in MDS have reported response rates to ATG of 15 to 60 percent and longer survival times in patients who respond.[436–438] The mortality with ATG-based therapy is higher in MDS patients than in aplastic anemia.[439] With cyclosporine alone, responses seem to be less common than with ATG-based regimens and mostly consist of minor hematologic improvements.[440,441] There are case reports of responses to tacrolimus.[442]

HLA-DR15 (DR2) is overrepresented in MDS and predicts a response to immunosuppressive therapy.[312,443] In one series of 60 patients who were treated with ATG and cyclosporine, 60 percent had hematologic improvement, and more responders had good karyotype or HLA-DRB1 1501.[3123] Most of the patients in this series had RA and an IPSS score of intermediate-1. In a series of 129 patients who were treated with immunosuppressive therapy at a single institution, 30 percent had either a complete or partial response; younger patient age and intermediate-1 or low-risk IPSS score favored survival.[110]

In some series a hypocellular marrow has predicted a higher likelihood of response, analogous to the response to immunosuppressive therapy in aplastic anemia, but this has not been consistent.[439,441,444] Younger age, normal karyotype or trisomy 8, lack of transfusion dependence, and the presence of either a PNH clone[445] or HLA-DR15 have predicted response to immunosuppressive therapy, but none is a robust biomarker.[312]

Not all groups have seen success with immunosuppressive therapy approaches. One study of ATG was stopped early because of lack of efficacy and development of adverse reactions.[446] Other studies also have reported lack of efficacy of single-agent cyclosporine.[447]

Among highly selected patients seen at the National Institutes of Health, the anti-CD52 monoclonal antibody alemtuzumab was associated with a response rate exceeding 90 percent in IPSS Intermediate-1 risk patients.[448] However, these patients were 20 years younger than the median age for MDS diagnosis (median age of approximately 50 years) and most were women with a normal karyotype, suggesting that they were not representative of the typical MDS patient seen in most clinics.

Immunomodulatory Agents: Thalidomide and Lenalidomide

The immunomodulatory drug (IMiD) thalidomide induced hematopoietic responses in 20 to 25 percent of patients with MDS at doses ranging from 50 to 800 mg per day, but thalidomide is difficult to tolerate (especially at higher doses) because of neuropathy, rashes, and constipation; in addition, risk of teratogenicity limited distribution of the drug.[449,450] Although thalidomide was initially promoted as an angiogenesis inhibitor following a vogue for such therapies in the 1990s, more recent data indicate that thalidomide's effects depend on modulation of the activity of cereblon, a component of an E3 ubiquitin ligase complex.[451] Alteration of ubiquitination by IMiD therapy has pleiotropic effects, such as alteration of transcription factors, and downstream effects on levels of cytokines and immune cell subsets.[452–455]

Lenalidomide, a thalidomide analogue with a more favorable risk-to-benefit ratio than the parent compound, induces improvement in approximately 85 percent of patients with lower-risk MDS associated with deletion of chromosome 5q, and results in RBC transfusion independence in almost 70 percent of patients.[308,456] The median hemoglobin increment in responding patients is 5.4 g/dL and responses last a median of more than 2 years. A randomized trial of a starting dose of 5 mg/day versus 10 mg/day showed a higher cytogenetic response rate with the higher dose; in that study, there was no increase in AML risk compared to placebo.[457] Most responses occur in the first 8 weeks. Neutropenia and thrombocytopenia can be adverse effects of lenalidomide, but treatment-emergent cytopenias correlate with response.[458] Pretreatment thrombocytopenia, in contrast, is associated with lower response rate.

The results with lenalidomide therapy are less favorable if chromosome 5q is absent; patients with normal karyotype and lower-risk MDS have approximately a 25 percent response rate with a median response duration of less than 1 year.[459] Case reports suggest patients with trisomy 13 may respond favorably.[460] Another thalidomide derivative, pomalidomide, has activity in primary myelofibrosis but has not yet been studied in MDS.

Antitumor Necrosis Factor Therapy

Patients with MDS overlap with the anemia of chronic inflammation in that they often have elevated levels of inflammatory cytokines such as TNF-α, which inhibit hematopoiesis. Whereas both thalidomide and lenalidomide indirectly lower TNF levels, strategies more directly inhibiting TNF also have been pursued. The soluble TNF receptor fusion protein etanercept (p75 TNFR:Fc), FDA approved for rheumatoid arthritis, has produced mixed results in MDS. In one pilot series, moderate improvement in cytopenias was noted,[461] whereas in another trial, no responses were noted in 10 patients.[462] In another pilot study of 3 months duration, one of 16 enrolled patients became transfusion-independent temporarily.[463] There is a report of two patients who had sustained erythroid responses during treatment with the chimeric anti–TNF-α monoclonal antibody infliximab, which also decreased the percentage of apoptotic cells in the marrow.[464] Etanercept has been combined with ATG[465] and with azacitidine,[466] but the independent contribution of etanercept to the responses observed is unclear.

Other Treatment Options in Low- or Intermediate-1–Risk Patients

A number of miscellaneous therapies have been tried for lower-risk patients with MDS by analogy with other diseases such as inflammatory anemias or promyelocytic leukemia, or based on theoretical constructs.

There are anecdotes of hematopoietic responses to vitamin K$_2$ (menatetrenone), for unclear reasons.[467,468] Glucocorticoids, vitamin A analogues (retinoids), vitamin D analogues such as dihydroxyvitamin D$_3$, the polar-planar solvent hexamethylene bisacetamide, the antioxidant amifostine, and interferon are among other agents that can induce *in vitro* maturation of mouse and human leukemic cells but have limited clinical activity.[469–471] Glucocorticoids can induce neutrophil increment via demargination, but this does not prevent infections and there is at least some reason for concern about increased risk of fungal infections.[472,473] Use of *cis*-retinoic acid, isotretinoin, or all-*trans*-retinoic acid (ATRA) has produced only slight, transient (few weeks) improvement in a very small proportion of patients with oligoblastic leukemia.[474,475]

Arsenic trioxide, used as a single agent or in combination with other therapies, results in responses in up to 20 percent of cases.[472,476–478] Lower-risk MDS patients were most likely to show benefit in one arsenic study.[479] The mechanism of action of arsenic in MDS is unclear.

Bortezomib, a proteasome inhibitor that indirectly targets NF-κB, has limited activity in MDS as a single agent but might be useful in combination.[480–482] The AKT/mTOR (mammalian target of rapamycin) pathway is active in MDS, but there are no data on treatment with mTOR inhibitors.[483,484]

For those patients who are unlikely to respond to the therapies described above or for those for whom such treatments have been attempted and failed, treatments more commonly used for higher-risk MDS such as azacitidine or decitabine can be used. In those not responding to these approved agents, AHSCT or other investigational options can be considered (see below).

A number of novel agents are currently undergoing clinical trials for patients with lower risk MDS for whom ESAs and other agents have failed. For instance, a multicenter trial of sotatercept, a soluble activin receptor type 2A immunoglobulin (Ig) G-Fc fusion protein that acts as a ligand trap for members of the transforming growth factor beta (TGF-β) superfamily, is ongoing in MDS.[485] The dual p38 mitogen-activated protein (MAP) kinase/Tie2 kinase inhibitor Arry-614 was associated with hematologic improvements in patients for whom hypomethylating agents have failed yet who still meet IPSS criteria for lower-risk disease.[486] Although activating kinase mutations are rare in MDS and kinase inhibitors such as imatinib have not shown efficacy in MDS with the exception of the rare CMML-like syndrome associated with t(5;12) and translocation of a gene encoding platelet-derived growth factor,[487,488] several other kinase inhibitors besides Arry-614 are also being studied. The glutathione analogue TLK199 (ezatiostat hydrochloride [Telintra]) had some activity in lower-risk MDS and restored sensitivity to lenalidomide in some patients who had lost response, but development of this agent appears to have been abandoned.[489–491]

THERAPY FOR PATIENTS WITH HIGHER-RISK DISEASE

Hypomethylating Agents (DNA Methyltransferase Inhibitors): Azacitidine and Decitabine

Recognition of the high prevalence of DNA cytosine methylation abnormalities in MDS, including hypermethylation and consequent silencing of expression of tumor-suppressor genes, contributed to clinical development of DNA hypomethylating agents.[492,493] Another factor in development of these agents was the detection *in vitro* of the potential for DNA hypomethylating agents to induce differentiation of immature hematopoietic cells, including neoplastically transformed cells.[388,494,495]

5-Azacytidine (azacitidine) is an azo-substituted pyrimidine analogue that is primarily incorporated into RNA. It can be converted to a deoxynucleotide by ribonucleotide reductase and incorporated into DNA where it binds to and irreversibly inhibits the enzyme DNA methyltransferase 1, reduces cytosine methylation, and induces maturation of some leukemic cell lines. In addition to epigenetic changes, azacitidine also is an antiproliferative drug, alters NF-κB and other signaling pathways, alters expression of cell-surface antigenic epitopes that can stimulate a regulatory T-cell immunologic response, and retains some cytotoxic activity akin to low-dose cytarabine as measured by induction of γH2AX (a marker of DNA strand breaks).[496–499] Administration of the drug and its congener decitabine has resulted in improvement of some patient's MDS, and these agents are also active in AML.[500–502]

Azacitidine is typically administered at a dose of 75 mg/m^2 once per day given subcutaneously for 7 consecutive days each month. In a cooperative group randomized study conducted in the 1990s (Cancer and Leukemia Group B [CALGB] 9221), azacitidine was superior to supportive care in terms of hematopoietic improvement and AML progression.[503] Quality of life was also enhanced.[323,503] Complete responses were seen in approximately 15 percent of azacitidine-treated patients, and nearly 50 percent of patients had hematologic improvement, reduction of blasts, decrease in abnormal metaphases on cytogenetic analysis, or some combination of those changes.[504] Ninety percent of responses were seen by cycle six of therapy, although a few patients responded to further cycles beyond six.[505] In another series, subclasses of MDS did not predict for response to azacitidine therapy.[506] Consequently, azacitidine was approved by the FDA in 2004 for treatment of all FAB subtypes of MDS.

In a randomized multicenter study of higher-risk MDS patients where azacitidine was compared to the physician's choice of one of three conventional care regimens that included supportive care, low-dose cytarabine treatment, or intensive induction chemotherapy, azacitidine increased survival by a median of 9 months compared to standard care regimens (24 vs. 15 months).[507] This was the first agent shown in a randomized fashion to extend survival in MDS.

Treatment with azacitidine can usually be accomplished on an outpatient basis, and the efficacy of intravenous administration seems to be similar to that with subcutaneous drug delivery.[508] An oral formulation of azacitidine is being studied.[509] Other schedules of administration to accommodate outpatient therapy have been reported to have benefit but have not been directly compared to the 75 mg/m^2 daily dose for 7 days every 4 weeks.[510] Adverse events associated with azacitidine include treatment-emergent cytopenias, skin rash, injection site soreness (which may respond to evening primrose oil[511]), mucositis, renal insufficiency (uncommon), and gastrointestinal upset.

5-Aza-2′-deoxycytidine (decitabine) is also FDA approved for all MDS risk categories. Although also a 5-azo–substituted pyrimidine nucleoside analogue that inhibits DNA methyltransferase, decitabine differs from azacitidine in that it is primarily incorporated into DNA, has a distinct profile of sensitive cell lines among the NCI-60 panel compared to azacitidine (more similar to cytarabine), and may work faster.[512] In one study, 90 percent of patients had responded by the end of cycle four of decitabine therapy, compared to cycle six with azacitidine, but this was a cross-study comparison and not randomization.[513] Seventeen percent of patients in one series had a major cytogenetic response on an intention-to-treat basis after a median of three courses.[514] The median duration of cytogenetic response was 7.5 months in all IPSS groups.[515] Patients who responded had improved survival compared with patients in whom the cytogenetically abnormal clone persisted. While decitabine was initially developed using a 3-day, nine-dose inpatient schedule, a 5-day intravenous administration schedule for outpatient use was found to be optimal in one series, which compared several doses and schedules; examination of optimal doses and schedules continues.[516–518] Decitabine also has cytotoxic activity like cytarabine, but may work at least partly through demethylation, as it has resulted in demethylation of a hypermethylated *INK4B* gene in patients.[519] Treatment-emergent demethylation is associated with clinical responses, although it is unclear whether the same cells are being compared pre- and posttreatment, and clonal shift could account for these results.[520] Adverse events associated with decitabine are similar to those observed with azacitidine. Oligodeoxynucleotide antisense approaches to DNA methyltransferase-1 inhibition are also being explored in MDS.[521]

Therapy with demethylating agents in patients who are not suitable candidates for AHSCT usually continues for as long as it seems like the patient is deriving benefit and as long as the drug is well tolerated. For patients who are going to AHSCT, these agents may be helpful as a bridge to transplant, and retrospective studies show that pretransplant treatment with azacitidine is at least as effective as treatment with induction chemotherapy.[522]

Histone Deacetylase Inhibitors

Inhibitors of histone deacetylation exhibit *in vitro* synergy with hypomethylating agents and have clinical activity in MDS, albeit limited, when they are used as single agents. This class of drugs is under active investigation at many centers.[523,524] Numerous agents are being studied and include valproic acid,[525,526] vorinostat (SAHA), mocetinostat (MGCD0103),[527] panobinostat (LBH589),[528] pracinostat and others. Belinostat had no activity.[529] Randomized trials combining histone deacetylation inhibitors with DNA methyltransferase inhibitors are ongoing, such as the U.S.–Canadian Intergroup study S1117, which compares azacitidine monotherapy to azacitidine plus lenalidomide[530] and azacitidine plus vorinostat.[531,532] In a randomized cooperative group trial of azacitidine with or without entinostat (MS-275), the combination arm was not associated with an increase in response rate but was associated with more adverse events, including fatigue and thrombocytopenia.[533]

Failure of Hypomethylating Agents

In higher-risk patients whom azacitidine or decitabine has failed, overall life expectancy is less than 6 months and patients who receive only supportive/palliative care have a life expectancy of only 3 to 4 months.[534,535] Novel approaches are needed for this group of patients. A randomized trial of rigosertib, an injectable phosphatidylinositol-4,5-bisphosphate 3-kinase (PI3K) kinase/polo-like kinase 1 (PLK-1) inhibitor, in higher-risk patients for whom azacitidine or decitabine had failed showed no survival benefit of the active agent compared with low-dose cytarabine or supportive care controls.[536] An oral formulation of rigosertib is being studied in lower-risk patients.[537]

A new dinucleotide decitabine-guanosine hypomethylating agent with increased resistance to cytidine deaminase degradation, SGI-110, has activity in relapsed/refractory patients.[538,539] The quinolone derivative vosaroxin, the nucleoside analogue sapacitabine, and inhibitors of PLK-1, such as volasertib, are also undergoing clinical trials in this setting.

Intensive Chemotherapy Similar to That Used for Acute Myelogenous Leukemia

Intensive chemotherapeutic regimens containing standard doses of cytarabine, an anthracycline, with or without etoposide (Chap. 88) result in remission in fewer than 20 percent of patients with high-risk MDS, primarily because of incomplete hematopoietic recovery or recovery with dysplastic/leukemia cells, and are no longer commonly used. The advanced age of many patients with MDS and the high frequency of cardiac, renal, immunologic, and other organ system impairment in most patients are thought to be largely responsible for the poor outcome. In a randomized trial of patients with WHO-defined AML and up to 30 percent blasts (oligoblastic leukemia), azacitidine was superior to a daunorubicin and cytarabine induction regimen.[540]

Patients who are younger than age 60 years have higher remission rates with AML-like regimens—rates up to 50 percent[541]—and can be considered for intensive therapy, but this is usually only done as a bridge to AHSCT. Patients older than age 60 years have a median survival of only 9.5 months with this approach and the survival is reduced to 4 months in those with unfavorable karyotypes, indicating a lack of benefit in this group.[542] In addition to the standard combination of anthracycline and cytarabine, other regimens, such as liposomal daunorubicin and topotecan with or without thalidomide, did not result in clinical benefit in patients with AML or high-risk MDS.[543] The so-called FLAG-Ida regimen (fludarabine, cytarabine, idarubicin, and G-CSF) resulted in 53 percent complete remissions and 11 percent improvement in 45 patients with high-risk myeloid malignancies, 13 of whom had MDS.[544] CPX-351, a liposomal nanoparticle with cytarabine and daunorubicin in a fixed 5:1 ratio is currently being studied in patients with AML arising from MDS and may be more effective than standard anthracycline-based regimens.

Allogeneic Hematopoietic Stem Cell Transplantation

AHSCT has been used to treat various types of MDS in patients ranging in age from 1 month to older than 70 years.[545,546] AHSCT remains the only treatment that can cure patients with the disease. Conditioning regimens have consisted of cyclophosphamide plus irradiation, fludarabine and busulfan, fludarabine and melphalan, or busulfan plus cyclophosphamide. Most patients have received transplants from histocompatible sibling donors, but the use of unrelated donors and of cord blood and haploidentical donors has increased. Patients with higher-risk karyotypes and more advanced disease do more poorly with transplantation, as do those with certain higher-risk genotypes such as a *TP53* mutation. Despite the increased age of donors and recipients and increased use of unrelated donors, transplantation outcomes in MDS are improving, in part as a result of molecular tissue typing and better supportive care.[547] Numerous factors such as disease stage, patient age, comorbidities, prior therapies, type of donor, and source of stem cells need to be considered when recommending AHSCT to MDS patients.

AHSCT for MDS should be performed before the disease progresses to AML, but modeling of data from the International Bone Marrow Transplant Registry suggests that patients (age 60 to 70 years) with lower-risk disease have net loss of life whether fully myeloablative conditioning or reduced-intensity conditioning is used.[548,549] When T-cell depletion is used to prevent graft-versus-host disease, the best outcomes occur in those who are transplanted while in remission, because T-cell depletion diminishes the graft-versus-leukemia effect.[550]

Poor-risk cytogenetic patterns may increase risk of relapse but not of nonrelapse mortality, but elevated pretransplant serum ferritin is correlated with less-favorable outcomes.[414,551] In one retrospective series, blast percentage less than 5 percent at time of transplantation was the best predictor of improved disease-free survival, and myeloablative conditioning was associated with lower relapse risk but could not overcome the unfavorable effect of increased disease burden.[552] Patients with secondary MDS have comparable outcomes after AHSCT as those with *de novo* MDS when high-risk cytogenetics are considered.[553,554] Pretransplantation neutropenia is also associated with inferior outcomes as a result of infection-related mortality.[555] Prior therapy with demethylating agents does not appear to increase the toxicity of transplantation and whether it will improve outcomes by decreasing disease burden has yet to be studied systematically.[556,557] Posttransplantation therapy with azacitidine and decitabine is also being explored, either as maintenance therapy, in an attempt to augment graft-versus-leukemia effect, or in an attempt to stave off imminent relapse.[496,558]

The morbidity and mortality of various transplantation approaches for MDS remain high—at least 20 percent of patients—and currently most patients are not candidates for any form of transplantation because of advanced age or comorbid conditions. Outcomes are similar for those treated with myeloablative and reduced-intensity conditioning.[559] For those patients who relapse after AHSCT, outcomes are grim. Salvage therapy with donor lymphocyte infusions, second transplantations, or other immunologic manipulations may be feasible, but less than 10 percent of patients will experience prolonged disease-free survival.[560,561]

Autologous Stem Cell Infusion

Patients with oligoblastic leukemia have been infused with their own stem cells after intensive chemotherapy.[562–564] This strategy is rarely used in the present era. In MDS, autologous transplantation is limited by contamination of the stem cell product with a repopulating leukemic cell and the absence of a graft-versus-leukemia effect. In selected patients, peritransplantation mortality with intensive therapy and stem cell rescue has been approximately 10 percent, and approximately 50 percent of selected patients had extended survivals.[565] The more advanced the disease at the time of treatment, the worse the outcome. With the increasing use of reduced-intensity AHSCT, autologous stem cell transplantation has been used less often. An antecedent diagnosis of RAEB had no influence on mobilization of blood stem cells and hematopoietic recovery after autologous stem cell transplantation for acute myeloid leukemia.[566]

Other Cytotoxic Drugs

Hydroxyurea and low-dose etoposide are useful in controlling leukemic cell proliferation but usually produce only partial responses in higher-risk MDS and do not influence survival duration.[567,568] Occasional patients have achieved remissions with etoposide (50 mg as a 2-hour infusion, two to seven times weekly for 4 weeks; or 100 mg/day orally for 3 days and then 50 mg twice weekly).[568] Low-dose melphalan,[569] gemcitabine,[570] irinotecan (CPT-11), a DNA topoisomerase I inhibitor,[571] troxacitabine, an enantiomer of cytarabine,[572,573] and weekly doses of oral idarubicin[574] have each resulted in responses in some patients. Clofarabine, a purine nucleoside analogue, also has activity in MDS, although renal insufficiency and hepatotoxicity limit its use to patients who require cytoreduction prior to transplant.[575]

Future Approaches

The FDA has not approved any new drugs for MDS therapy since 2006, and currently available therapies will lose effectiveness in the majority of patients within 2 to 3 years after treatment initiation. Unfortunately, targetable constitutively activating kinase mutations are rare in MDS, and for many MDS-associated mutations summarized above, including those that alter transcriptional regulation or pre-mRNA splicing, it is not clear how best to develop targeted therapy. In addition, clonal heterogeneity and the clonal architecture of MDS mean that currently it is often not known which mutations are early initiating events and which are later events important only for survival of a subclone.[576] The advent of high-throughput techniques for genetic analysis and improved understanding of disease biology may lead to development of new, more effective approaches in the future.

REFERENCES

1. Welch JS, Ley TJ, Link DC, et al: The origin and evolution of mutations in acute myeloid leukemia. *Cell* 150(2):264–278, 2012.
2. Steensma DP: Historical perspectives on myelodysplastic syndromes. *Leuk Res* 36(12):1441–1452, 2012.
3. Layton DM, Mufti GJ: Myelodysplastic syndromes: Their history, evolution and relation to acute myeloid leukaemia. *Blut* 53(6):423–436, 1986.
4. Lichtman MA: Does a diagnosis of myelogenous leukemia require 20% marrow myeloblasts, and does <5% marrow myeloblasts represent a remission? The history and ambiguity of arbitrary diagnostic boundaries in the understanding of myelodysplasia. *Oncologist* 18(9):973–980, 2013.
5. Parapia LA: Trepanning or trephines: A history of bone marrow biopsy. *Br J Haematol* 139(1):14–19, 2007.
6. Luzzatto AM: Sull' anemia grave megaloblastica senza reporto ematologico corrispondente (anemia pseudoaplastica). *Riv veneta di sc med Venezia* 47:193–212, 1907.
7. di Guglielmo G: Eritremie acute. *Boll Soc Med Chir* 1:665–673, 1926.
8. Minot GR, Murphy WP: Treatment of pernicious anemia by a special diet. *J Am Med Assoc* 87:470–476, 1926.
9. Rhoads CP, Barker WH: Refractory anemia: Analysis of 100 cases. *JAMA* 110:794–796, 1938.
10. Rosati S, Mick R, Xu F, et al: Refractory cytopenia with multilineage dysplasia: Further characterization of an "unclassifiable" myelodysplastic syndrome. *Leukemia* 10(1):20–26, 1996.
11. Chevallier P: Sur la terminologie des leucoses et les affections-frontieres: Les odoleucoses. *Sangre (Barc)* 15:587–593, 1942–1943.
12. Hamilton-Paterson JL: Pre-leukaemic anaemia. *Acta Haematol* 2:309–316, 1949.
13. Block M, Jacobson LO, Bethard WF: Preleukemic acute human leukemia. *JAMA* 152:1018–1028, 1953.
14. Bjorkman SE: Chronic refractory anemia with sideroblastic bone marrow: A study of four cases. *Blood* 11:250–259, 1956.
15. Saarni MI, Linman JW: Preleukemia. The hematologic syndrome preceding acute leukemia. *Am J Med* 55(1):38–48, 1973.
16. Dreyfus B, Rochant H, Sultan C, et al: [Refractory anemia with excess myeloblasts in the bone marrow. Study of 11 cases]. *Presse Med* 78(8):359–364, 1970.
17. Dreyfus B: Preleukemic states. I. Definition and classification. II. Refractory anemia with an excess of myeloblasts in the bone marrow (smoldering acute leukemia). *Nouv Rev Fr Hematol Blood Cells* 17(1–2):33–55, 1976.
18. Izrael V, Jacquillat C, Chastang C, et al: [New data about oligoblastic leukemias. Apropos of an analysis of 120 cases]. *Nouv Presse Med* 4(13):947–952, 1975.
19. Bennett JM, Catovsky D, Daniel MT, et al: Proposals for the classification of the acute leukaemias. French-American-British (FAB) co-operative group. *Br J Haematol* 33(4):451–458, 1976.
20. Galton DAG, Dacie, JV: Classification of the acute leukemias. *Blood Cells* 1:17–24, 1975.
21. Bennett JM, Catovsky D, Daniel MT, et al: Proposals for the classification of the myelodysplastic syndromes. *Br J Haematol* 51(2):189–199, 1982.
22. Ma X: Epidemiology of myelodysplastic syndromes. *Am J Med* 125(7 Suppl):S2–S5, 2012.
23. Sekeres MA: The epidemiology of myelodysplastic syndromes. *Hematol Oncol Clin North Am* 24(2):287–294, 2010.
24. Craig BM, Rollison DE, List AF, Cogle CR: Underreporting of myeloid malignancies by United States cancer registries. *Cancer Epidemiol Biomarkers Prev* 21(3):474–481, 2012.
25. Ma X, Does M, Raza A, Mayne ST: Myelodysplastic syndromes: Incidence and survival in the United States. *Cancer* 109(8):1536–1542, 2007.
26. Cogle CR, Iannacone MR, Yu D, et al: High rate of uncaptured myelodysplastic syndrome cases and an improved method of case ascertainment. *Leuk Res* 38(1):71–75, 2014.
27. Cogle CR, Craig BM, Rollison DE, List AF: Incidence of the myelodysplastic syndromes using a novel claims-based algorithm: High number of uncaptured cases by cancer registries. *Blood* 117(26):7121–7125, 2011.
28. Visser O, Trama A, Maynadie M, et al: Incidence, survival and prevalence of myeloid malignancies in Europe. *Eur J Cancer* 48(17):3257–3266, 2012.
29. Gologan R: Epidemiological data on myelodysplastic syndrome patients under 50 years in a single center of Romania. *Leuk Res* 34(11):1442–1446, 2010.
30. Chen B, Zhao WL, Jin J, et al: Clinical and cytogenetic features of 508 Chinese patients with myelodysplastic syndrome and comparison with those in Western countries. *Leukemia* 19(5):767–775, 2005.
31. Chatterjee T, Dixit A, Mohapatra M, et al: Clinical, haematological and histomorphological profile of adult myelodysplastic syndrome. Study of 96 cases in a single institute. *Eur J Haematol* 73(2):93–97, 2004.
32. Kuendgen A, Matsuda A, Germing U: Differences in epidemiology of MDS between Western and Eastern countries: Ethnic differences or environmental influence? *Leuk Res* 31(1):103–104, 2007.
33. Matsuda A, Germing U, Jinnai I, et al: Differences in the distribution of subtypes according to the WHO classification 2008 between Japanese and German patients with refractory anemia according to the FAB classification in myelodysplastic syndromes. *Leuk Res* 34(8):974–980, 2010.
34. Ohba R, Furuyama K, Yoshida K, et al: Clinical and genetic characteristics of congenital sideroblastic anemia: Comparison with myelodysplastic syndrome with ring sideroblast (MDS-RS). *Ann Hematol* 92(1):1–9, 2013.
35. Iwanaga M, Hsu WL, Soda M, et al: Risk of myelodysplastic syndromes in people exposed to ionizing radiation: A retrospective cohort study of Nagasaki atomic bomb survivors. *J Clin Oncol* 29(4):428–434, 2011.
36. Sekeres MA, Schoonen WM, Kantarjian H, et al: Characteristics of US patients with myelodysplastic syndromes: Results of six cross-sectional physician surveys. *J Natl Cancer Inst* 100(21):1542–1551, 2008.
37. Breccia M, Mengarelli A, Mancini M, et al: Myelodysplastic syndromes in patients under 50 years old: A single institution experience. *Leuk Res* 29(7):749–754, 2005.
38. Stary J, Baumann I, Creutzig U, et al: Getting the numbers straight in pediatric MDS: Distribution of subtypes after exclusion of down syndrome. *Pediatr Blood Cancer* 50(2):435–436, 2008.
39. Niemeyer CM, Kratz CP, Hasle H: Pediatric myelodysplastic syndromes. *Curr Treat Options Oncol* 6(3):209–214, 2005.

40. Hasle H, Niemeyer CM, Chessells JM, et al: A pediatric approach to the WHO classification of myelodysplastic and myeloproliferative diseases. *Leukemia* 17(2):277–282, 2003.

41. Sasaki H, Manabe A, Kojima S, et al: Myelodysplastic syndrome in childhood: A retrospective study of 189 patients in Japan. *Leukemia* 15(11):1713–1720, 2001.

42. Hyde RK, Liu PP: GATA2 mutations lead to MDS and AML. *Nat Genet* 43(10):926–927, 2011.

43. Owen CJ, Toze CL, Koochin A, et al: Five new pedigrees with inherited RUNX1 mutations causing familial platelet disorder with propensity to myeloid malignancy. *Blood* 112(12):4639–4645, 2008.

44. Song WJ, Sullivan MG, Legare RD, et al: Haploinsufficiency of CBFA2 causes familial thrombocytopenia with propensity to develop acute myelogenous leukaemia. *Nat Genet* 23(2):166–175, 1999.

45. Bagby GC, Lipton JM, Sloand EM, Schiffer CA: Marrow failure. *Hematology Am Soc Hematol Educ Program* 318–336, 2004.

46. Alter BP, Giri N, Savage SA, et al: Malignancies and survival patterns in the National Cancer Institute inherited bone marrow failure syndromes cohort study. *Br J Haematol* 150(2):179–188, 2010.

47. Kelaidi C, Stamatoullas A, Beyne-Rauzy O, et al: Daily practice management of myelodysplastic syndromes in France: Data from 907 patients in a one-week cross-sectional study by the Groupe Francophone des Myélodysplasies. *Haematologica* 95(6):892–899, 2010.

48. Nisse C, Haguenoer JM, Grandbastien B, et al: Occupational and environmental risk factors of the myelodysplastic syndromes in the North of France. *Br J Haematol* 112(4):927–935, 2001.

49. Yin SN, Hayes RB, Linet MS, et al: A cohort study of cancer among benzene-exposed workers in China: Overall results. *Am J Ind Med* 29(3):227–235, 1996.

50. Lv L, Lin G, Gao X, et al: Case-control study of risk factors of myelodysplastic syndromes according to World Health Organization classification in a Chinese population. *Am J Hematol* 86(2):163–169, 2011.

51. Rushton L, Schnatter AR, Tang G, Glass DC: Acute myeloid and chronic lymphoid leukaemias and exposure to low-level benzene among petroleum workers. *Br J Cancer* 110(3):783–787, 2014.

52. Strom SS, Gu Y, Gruschkus SK, et al: Risk factors of myelodysplastic syndromes: A case-control study. *Leukemia* 19(11):1912–1918, 2005.

53. Hahn CN, Chong CE, Carmichael CL, et al: Heritable GATA2 mutations associated with familial myelodysplastic syndrome and acute myeloid leukemia. *Nat Genet* 43(10):1012–1017, 2011.

54. Horwitz MS: GATA2 deficiency: Flesh and blood. *Blood* 123(6):799–800, 2014.

55. Holme H, Hossain U, Kirwan M, et al: Marked genetic heterogeneity in familial myelodysplasia/acute myeloid leukaemia. *Br J Haematol* 158(2):242–248, 2012.

56. Pasquet M, Bellanne-Chantelot C, Tavitian S, et al: High frequency of GATA2 mutations in patients with mild chronic neutropenia evolving to MonoMac syndrome, myelodysplasia, and acute myeloid leukemia. *Blood* 121(5):822–829, 2013.

57. Kazenwadel J, Secker GA, Liu YJ, et al: Loss-of-function germline GATA2 mutations in patients with MDS/AML or MonoMAC syndrome and primary lymphedema reveal a key role for GATA2 in the lymphatic vasculature. *Blood* 119(5):1283–1291, 2012.

58. Hsu AP, Sampaio EP, Khan J, et al: Mutations in GATA2 are associated with the autosomal dominant and sporadic monocytopenia and mycobacterial infection (MonoMAC) syndrome. *Blood* 118(10):2653–2655, 2011.

59. Hirabayashi S, Strahm B, Urbaniak S, et al: Unexpected high frequency of GATA2 mutations in children with non-familial MDS and monosomy 7. *ASH Annu Meet Abstr* 120(21): Abstract no. 1699, 2012.

60. Vas V, Senger K, Dorr K, et al: Aging of the microenvironment influences clonality in hematopoiesis. *PLoS One* 7(8):e42080, 2012.

61. Henry CJ, Marusyk A, DeGregori J: Aging-associated changes in hematopoiesis and leukemogenesis: What's the connection? *Aging (Albany NY)* 3(6):643–656, 2011.

62. Woll PS, Kjallquist U, Chowdhury O, et al: Myelodysplastic syndromes are propagated by rare and distinct human cancer stem cells *in vivo*. *Cancer Cell* 25(6):794–808, 2014.

63. Raskind WH, Tirumali N, Jacobson R, Singer J, Fialkow PJ: Evidence for a multistep pathogenesis of a myelodysplastic syndrome. *Blood* 63(6):1318–1323, 1984.

64. Abkowitz JL, Fialkow PJ, Niebrugge DJ, et al: Pancytopenia as a clonal disorder of a multipotent hematopoietic stem-cell. *J Clin Invest* 73(1):258–261, 1984.

65. Mongkonsritragoon W, Letendre L, Li CY: Multiple lymphoid nodules in bone marrow have the same clonality as underlying myelodysplastic syndrome recognized with fluorescent in situ hybridization technique. *Am J Hematol* 59(3):252–257, 1998.

66. Tehranchi R, Woll PS, Anderson K, et al: Persistent malignant stem cells in del(5q) myelodysplasia in remission. *N Engl J Med* 363(11):1025–1037, 2010.

67. Damm F, Fontenay M, Bernard OA: Point mutations in myelodysplastic syndromes. *N Engl J Med* 365(12):1154–1155, 2011.

68. Vercauteren SM, Starczynowski DT, Sung S, et al: T cells of patients with myelodysplastic syndrome are frequently derived from the malignant clone. *Br J Haematol* 156(3):409–412, 2012.

69. Nilsson L, Astrand-Grundstrom I, Arvidsson I, et al: Isolation and characterization of hematopoietic progenitor/stem cells in 5q-deleted myelodysplastic syndromes: Evidence for involvement at the hematopoietic stem cell level. *Blood* 96(6):2012–2021, 2000.

70. van Lom K, Hagemeijer A, Smit E, et al: Cytogenetic clonality analysis in myelodysplastic syndrome: Monosomy 7 can be demonstrated in the myeloid and in the lymphoid lineage. *Leukemia* 9(11):1818–1821, 1995.

71. Anastasi J, Feng J, Le Beau MM, et al: Cytogenetic clonality in myelodysplastic syndromes studied with fluorescence in situ hybridization: Lineage, response to growth factor therapy, and clone expansion. *Blood* 81(6):1580–1585, 1993.

72. Gerritsen WR, Donohue J, Bauman J, et al: Clonal analysis of myelodysplastic syndrome-monosomy-7 is expressed in the myeloid lineage, but not in the lymphoid lineage as detected by fluorescent *in situ* hybridization. *Blood* 80(1):217–224, 1992.

73. Will B, Steidl U: Combinatorial haplo-deficient tumor suppression in 7q-deficient myelodysplastic syndrome and acute myeloid leukemia. *Cancer Cell* 25(5):555–557, 2014.

74. Jerez A, Gondek LP, Jankowska AM, et al: Topography, clinical, and genomic correlates of 5q myeloid malignancies revisited. *J Clin Oncol* 30(12):1343–1349, 2012.

75. Graubert TA, Payton MA, Shao J, et al: Integrated genomic analysis implicates haploinsufficiency of multiple chromosome 5q31.2 genes in de novo myelodysplastic syndromes pathogenesis. *PLoS One* 4(2):e4583, 2009.

76. Ebert BL, Pretz J, Bosco J, et al: Identification of RPS14 as a 5q- syndrome gene by RNA interference screen. *Nature* 451(7176):335–339, 2008.

77. Dutt S, Narla A, Lin K, et al: Haploinsufficiency for ribosomal protein genes causes selective activation of p53 in human erythroid progenitor cells. *Blood* 117(9):2567–2576, 2011.

78. Boultwood J, Pellagatti A, Wainscoat JS: Haploinsufficiency of ribosomal proteins and p53 activation in anemia: Diamond-Blackfan anemia and the 5q- syndrome. *Adv Biol Regul* 52(1):196–203, 2012.

79. Caceres G, McGraw K, Yip BH, et al: TP53 suppression promotes erythropoiesis in del(5q) MDS, suggesting a targeted therapeutic strategy in lenalidomide-resistant patients. *Proc Natl Acad Sci U S A* 110(40):16127–16132, 2013.

80. Starczynowski DT, Kuchenbauer F, Argiropoulos B, et al: Identification of miR-145 and miR-146a as mediators of the 5q- syndrome phenotype. *Nat Med* 16(1):49–58, 2010.

81. Kumar MS, Narla A, Nonami A, et al: Coordinate loss of a microRNA and protein-coding gene cooperate in the pathogenesis of 5q- syndrome. *Blood* 118(17):4666–4673, 2011.

82. Starczynowski DT, Kuchenbauer F, Wegrzyn J, et al: MicroRNA-146a disrupts hematopoietic differentiation and survival. *Exp Hematol* 39(2):167–178 e164, 2011.

83. Chen TH, Kambal A, Krysiak K, et al: Knockdown of Hspa9, a del(5q31.2) gene, results in a decrease in hematopoietic progenitors in mice. *Blood* 117(5):1530–1539, 2011.

84. Craven SE, French D, Ye W, et al: Loss of Hspa9b in zebrafish recapitulates the ineffective hematopoiesis of the myelodysplastic syndrome. *Blood* 105(9):3528–3534, 2005.

85. Joslin JM, Fernald AA, Tennant TR, et al: Haploinsufficiency of EGR1, a candidate gene in the del(5q), leads to the development of myeloid disorders. *Blood* 110(2):719–726, 2007.

86. Stoddart A, Fernald AA, Wang J, et al: Haploinsufficiency of del(5q) genes, Egr1 and Apc, cooperate with Tp53 loss to induce acute myeloid leukemia in mice. *Blood* 123(7):1069–1078, 2014.

87. Jaras M, Miller PG, Chu LP, et al: Csnk1a1 inhibition has p53-dependent therapeutic efficacy in acute myeloid leukemia. *J Exp Med* 211(4):605–612, 2014.

88. Schanz J, Steidl C, Fonatsch C, et al: Coalesced multicentric analysis of 2,351 patients with myelodysplastic syndromes indicates an underestimation of poor-risk cytogenetics of myelodysplastic syndromes in the international prognostic scoring system. *J Clin Oncol* 29(15):1963–1970, 2011.

89. Andersen MK, Christiansen DH, Pedersen-Bjergaard J: Centromeric breakage and highly rearranged chromosome derivatives associated with mutations of TP53 are common in therapy-related MDS and AML after therapy with alkylating agents: An M-FISH study. *Genes Chromosomes Cancer* 42(4):358–371, 2005.

90. Papaemmanuil E, Gerstung M, Malcovati L, et al: Clinical and biological implications of driver mutations in myelodysplastic syndromes. *Blood* 122(22):3616–3627, 2013.

91. Volkert S, Kohlmann A, Schnittger S, et al: Association of the type of 5q loss with complex karyotype, clonal evolution, TP53 mutation status, and prognosis in acute myeloid leukemia and myelodysplastic syndrome. *Genes Chromosomes Cancer* 3(10):22151, 2014.

92. Christiansen DH, Andersen MK, Pedersen-Bjergaard J: Mutations with loss of heterozygosity of p53 are common in therapy-related myelodysplasia and acute myeloid leukemia after exposure to alkylating agents and significantly associated with deletion or loss of 5q, a complex karyotype, and a poor prognosis. *J Clin Oncol* 19(5):1405–1413, 2001.

93. Jadersten M, Saft L, Smith A, et al: TP53 mutations in low-risk myelodysplastic syndromes with del(5q) predict disease progression. *J Clin Oncol* 29(15):1971–1979, 2011.

94. Jadersten M, Saft L, Pellagatti A, et al: Clonal heterogeneity in the 5q- syndrome: P53 expressing progenitors prevail during lenalidomide treatment and expand at disease progression. *Haematologica* 94(12):1762–1766, 2009.

95. Saft L, Karimi M, Ghaderi M, et al: P53 protein expression independently predicts outcome in patients with lower-risk myelodysplastic syndromes with del(5q). *Haematologica* 99(6):1041–1049, 2014.

96. Cordoba I, Gonzalez-Porras JR, Nomdedeu B, et al: Better prognosis for patients with del(7q) than for patients with monosomy 7 in myelodysplastic syndrome. *Cancer* 118(1):127–133, 2012.

97. Tosi S, Scherer SW, Giudici G, et al: Delineation of multiple deleted regions in 7q in myeloid disorders. *Genes Chromosomes Cancer* 25(4):384–392, 1999.

98. Le Beau MM, Espinosa R 3rd, Davis EM, et al: Cytogenetic and molecular delineation of a region of chromosome 7 commonly deleted in malignant myeloid diseases. *Blood* 88(6):1930–1935, 1996.

99. Lewis S, Abrahamson G, Boultwood J, et al: Molecular characterization of the 7q deletion in myeloid disorders. *Br J Haematol* 93(1):75–80, 1996.

100. Ernst T, Chase AJ, Score J, et al: Inactivating mutations of the histone methyltransferase gene EZH2 in myeloid disorders. *Nat Genet* 42(8):722–726, 2010.

101. Makishima H, Jankowska AM, Tiu RV, et al: Novel homo- and hemizygous mutations in EZH2 in myeloid malignancies. *Leukemia* 24(10):1799–1804, 2010.

102. Nikoloski G, Langemeijer SM, Kuiper RP, et al: Somatic mutations of the histone methyltransferase gene EZH2 in myelodysplastic syndromes. *Nat Genet* 42(8):665–667, 2010.

103. Chen C, Liu Y, Rappaport AR, et al: MLL3 is a haploinsufficient 7q tumor suppressor in acute myeloid leukemia. *Cancer Cell* 25(5):652–665, 2014.

104. Wong CC, Martincorena I, Rust AG, et al: Inactivating CUX1 mutations promote tumorigenesis. *Nat Genet* 46(1):33–38, 2014.

105. Wong JC, Zhang Y, Lieuw KH, et al: Use of chromosome engineering to model a segmental deletion of chromosome band 7q22 found in myeloid malignancies. *Blood* 115(22):4524–4532, 2010.

106. Saumell S, Florensa L, Luno E, et al: Prognostic value of trisomy 8 as a single anomaly and the influence of additional cytogenetic aberrations in primary myelodysplastic syndromes. *Br J Haematol* 159(3):311–321, 2012.

107. Nilsson L, Astrand-Grundstrom I, Anderson K, et al: Involvement and functional impairment of the CD34(+)CD38(−)Thy-1(+) hematopoietic stem cell pool in myelodysplastic syndromes with trisomy 8. *Blood* 100(1):259–267, 2002.

108. Sloand EM, Mainwaring L, Fuhrer M, et al: Preferential suppression of trisomy 8 compared with normal hematopoietic cell growth by autologous lymphocytes in patients with trisomy 8 myelodysplastic syndrome. *Blood* 106(3):841–851, 2005.

109. Sloand EM, Melenhorst JJ, Tucker ZC, et al: T-cell immune responses to Wilms tumor 1 protein in myelodysplasia responsive to immunosuppressive therapy. *Blood* 117(9):2691–2699, 2011.

110. Sloand EM, Wu CO, Greenberg P, Young N, Barrett J: Factors affecting response and survival in patients with myelodysplasia treated with immunosuppressive therapy. *J Clin Oncol* 26(15):2505–2511, 2008.

111. Handa T, Nakatsue T, Baba M, et al: Clinical features of three cases with pulmonary alveolar proteinosis secondary to myelodysplastic syndrome developed during the course of Behcet's disease. *Respir Investig* 52(1):75–79, 2014.

112. Kawabata H, Sawaki T, Kawanami T, et al: Myelodysplastic syndrome complicated with inflammatory intestinal ulcers: Significance of trisomy 8. *Intern Med* 45(22):1309–1314, 2006.

113. Toyonaga T, Nakase H, Matsuura M, et al: Refractoriness of intestinal Behcet's disease with myelodysplastic syndrome involving trisomy 8 to medical therapies—Our case experience and review of the literature. *Digestion* 88(4):217–221, 2013.

114. Schanz J, Tuchler H, Sole F, et al: New comprehensive cytogenetic scoring system for primary myelodysplastic syndromes (MDS) and oligoblastic acute myeloid leukemia after MDS derived from an international database merge. *J Clin Oncol* 30(8):820–829, 2012.

115. Braun T, de Botton S, Taksin AL, et al: Characteristics and outcome of myelodysplastic syndromes (MDS) with isolated 20q deletion: A report on 62 cases. *Leuk Res* 35(7):863–867, 2011.

116. Liu YC, Ito Y, Hsiao HH, et al: Risk factor analysis in myelodysplastic syndrome patients with del(20q): Prognosis revisited. *Cancer Genet Cytogenet* 171(1):9–16, 2006.

117. Wang PW, Eisenbart JD, Espinosa R 3rd, et al: Refinement of the smallest commonly deleted segment of chromosome 20 in malignant myeloid diseases and development of a PAC-based physical and transcription map. *Genomics* 67(1):28–39, 2000.

118. Huh J, Tiu RV, Gondek LP, et al: Characterization of chromosome arm 20q abnormalities in myeloid malignancies using genome-wide single nucleotide polymorphism array analysis. *Genes Chromosomes Cancer* 49(4):390–399, 2010.

119. Clarke M, Dumon S, Ward C, et al: MYBL2 haploinsufficiency increases susceptibility to age-related haematopoietic neoplasia. *Leukemia* 27(3):661–670, 2013.

120. Heinrichs S, Conover LF, Bueso-Ramos CE, et al: MYBL2 is a sub-haploinsufficient tumor suppressor gene in myeloid malignancy. *Elife* 2(2):00825, 2013.

121. Gelsi-Boyer V, Trouplin V, Adelaide J, et al: Mutations of polycomb-associated gene ASXL1 in myelodysplastic syndromes and chronic myelomonocytic leukaemia. *Br J Haematol* 145(6):788–800, 2009.

122. Abdel-Wahab O, Gao J, Adli M, et al: Deletion of Asxl1 results in myelodysplasia and severe developmental defects in vivo. *J Exp Med* 210(12):2641–2659, 2013.

123. Bacher U, Haferlach T, Schnittger S, et al: Investigation of 305 patients with myelodysplastic syndromes and 20q deletion for associated cytogenetic and molecular genetic lesions and their prognostic impact. *Br J Haematol* 164(6):822–833, 2014.

124. Gupta R, Soupir CP, Johari V, Hasserjian RP: Myelodysplastic syndrome with isolated deletion of chromosome 20q: An indolent disease with minimal morphological dysplasia and frequent thrombocytopenic presentation. *Br J Haematol* 139(2):265–268, 2007.

125. Abeliovich D, Yehuda O, Ben-Neriah S, Or R: Loss of Y chromosome. An age-related event or a cytogenetic marker of a malignant clone? *Cancer Genet Cytogenet* 76(1):70–71, 1994.

126. Wong AK, Fang B, Zhang L, et al: Loss of the Y chromosome: An age-related or clonal phenomenon in acute myelogenous leukemia/myelodysplastic syndrome? *Arch Pathol Lab Med* 132(8):1329–1332, 2008.

127. Wiktor A, Rybicki BA, Piao ZS, et al: Clinical significance of Y chromosome loss in hematologic cancer. *Genes Chromosomes Cancer* 27(1):11–16, 2000.

128. Kanagal-Shamanna R, Bueso-Ramos CE, Barkoh B, et al: Myeloid neoplasms with isolated isochromosome 17q represent a clinicopathologic entity associated with myelodysplastic/myeloproliferative features, a high risk of leukemic transformation, and wild-type TP53. *Cancer* 118(11):2879–2888, 2012.

129. Meggendorfer M, Bacher U, Alpermann T, et al: SETBP1 mutations occur in 9% of MDS/MPN and in 4% of MPN cases and are strongly associated with atypical CML, monosomy 7, isochromosome i(17)(q10), ASXL1 and CBL mutations. *Leukemia* 27(9):1852–1860, 2013.

130. Valcarcel D, Adema V, Sole F, et al: Complex, not monosomal, karyotype is the cytogenetic marker of poorest prognosis in patients with primary myelodysplastic syndrome. *J Clin Oncol* 31(7):916–922, 2013.

131. Schanz J, Tuchler H, Sole F, et al: Monosomal karyotype in MDS: Explaining the poor prognosis? *Leukemia* 27(10):1988–1995, 2013.

132. Cluzeau T, Mounier N, Karsenti JM, et al: Monosomal karyotype improves IPSS-R stratification in MDS and AML patients treated with azacitidine. *Am J Hematol* 88(9):780–783, 2013.

133. Patnaik MM, Hanson CA, Hodnefield JM, et al: Monosomal karyotype in myelodysplastic syndromes, with or without monosomy 7 or 5, is prognostically worse than an otherwise complex karyotype. *Leukemia* 25(2):266–270, 2011.

134. Bejar R, Stevenson K, Abdel-Wahab O, et al: Clinical effect of point mutations in myelodysplastic syndromes. *N Engl J Med* 364(26):2496–2506, 2011.

135. Haferlach T, Nagata Y, Grossmann V, et al: Landscape of genetic lesions in 944 patients with myelodysplastic syndromes. *Leukemia* 28(2):241–247, 2014.

136. Bejar R: Clinical and genetic predictors of prognosis in myelodysplastic syndromes. *Haematologica* 99(6):956–964, 2014.

137. Malcovati L, Papaemmanuil E, Ambaglio I, et al: Driver somatic mutations identify distinct disease entities within myeloid neoplasms with myelodysplasia. *Blood* 26:2014–2003, 2014.

138. Walter MJ, Shen D, Ding L, et al: Clonal architecture of secondary acute myeloid leukemia. *N Engl J Med* 366(12):1090–1098, 2012.

139. Walter MJ, Shen D, Shao J, et al: Clonal diversity of recurrently mutated genes in myelodysplastic syndromes. *Leukemia* 27(6):1275–1282, 2013.

140. Yoshida K, Sanada M, Shiraishi Y, et al: Frequent pathway mutations of splicing machinery in myelodysplasia. *Nature* 478(7367):64–69, 2011.

141. Bejar R, Stevenson KE, Caughey BA, et al: Validation of a prognostic model and the impact of mutations in patients with lower-risk myelodysplastic syndromes. *J Clin Oncol* 30(27):3376–3382, 2012.

142. Papaemmanuil E, Cazzola M, Boultwood J, et al: Somatic SF3B1 mutation in myelodysplasia with ring sideroblasts. *N Engl J Med* 365(15):1384–1395, 2011.

143. Baliakas P, Hadzidimitriou A, Sutton LA, et al: Recurrent mutations refine prognosis in chronic lymphocytic leukemia. *Leukemia* 19(10):196, 2014.

144. Scott LM, Rebel VI: Acquired mutations that affect pre-mRNA splicing in hematologic malignancies and solid tumors. *J Natl Cancer Inst* 105(20):1540–1549, 2013.

145. Furney SJ, Pedersen M, Gentien D, et al: SF3B1 mutations are associated with alternative splicing in uveal melanoma. *Cancer Discov* 3(10):1122–1129, 2013.

146. Graubert TA, Shen D, Ding L, et al: Recurrent mutations in the U2AF1 splicing factor in myelodysplastic syndromes. *Nat Genet* 44(1):53–57, 2011.

147. Przychodzen B, Jerez A, Guinta K, et al: Patterns of missplicing due to somatic U2AF1 mutations in myeloid neoplasms. *Blood* 122(6):999–1006, 2013.

148. Patnaik MM, Lasho TL, Finke CM, et al: Spliceosome mutations involving SRSF2, SF3B1, and U2AF35 in chronic myelomonocytic leukemia: Prevalence, clinical correlates, and prognostic relevance. *Am J Hematol* 88(3):201–206, 2013.

149. Ley TJ, Ding L, Walter MJ, et al: DNMT3A mutations in acute myeloid leukemia. *N Engl J Med* 363(25):2424–2433, 2010.

150. Walter MJ, Ding L, Shen D, et al: Recurrent DNMT3A mutations in patients with myelodysplastic syndromes. *Leukemia* 25(7):1153–1158, 2011.

151. Kim SJ, Zhao H, Hardikar S, et al: A DNMT3A mutation common in AML exhibits dominant-negative effects in murine ES cells. *Blood* 122(25):4086–4089, 2013.

152. Busque L, Patel JP, Figueroa ME, et al: Recurrent somatic TET2 mutations in normal elderly individuals with clonal hematopoiesis. *Nat Genet* 44(11):1179–1181, 2012.

153. Bejar R, Stevenson KE, Caughey BA, et al: Validation of a prognostic model and the impact of mutations in patients with lower-risk myelodysplastic syndromes. *J Clin Oncol* 30(27):3376–3382, 2012.

154. Thol F, Winschel C, Ludeking A, et al: Rare occurrence of DNMT3A mutations in myelodysplastic syndromes. *Haematologica* 96(12):1870–1873, 2011.

155. Tahiliani M, Koh KP, Shen Y, et al: Conversion of 5-methylcytosine to 5-hydroxymethylcytosine in mammalian DNA by MLL partner TET1. *Science* 324(5929):930–935, 2009.

156. Ito S, Shen L, Dai Q, et al: Tet proteins can convert 5-methylcytosine to 5-formylcytosine and 5-carboxylcytosine. *Science* 333(6047):1300–1303, 2011.

157. Jankowska AM, Szpurka H, Tiu RV, et al: Loss of heterozygosity 4q24 and TET2 mutations associated with myelodysplastic/myeloproliferative neoplasms. *Blood* 113(25):6403–6410, 2009.

158. Ko M, Huang Y, Jankowska AM, et al: Impaired hydroxylation of 5-methylcytosine in myeloid cancers with mutant TET2. *Nature* 468(7325):839–843, 2010.

159. Yamazaki J, Taby R, Vasanthakumar A, et al: Effects of TET2 mutations on DNA methylation in chronic myelomonocytic leukemia. *Epigenetics* 7(2):201–207, 2012.

160. Ko M, Bandukwala HS, An J, et al: Ten-eleven-translocation 2 (TET2) negatively regulates homeostasis and differentiation of hematopoietic stem cells in mice. *Proc Natl Acad Sci U S A* 108(35):14566–14571, 2011.

161. Moran-Crusio K, Reavie L, Shih A, et al: Tet2 loss leads to increased hematopoietic stem cell self-renewal and myeloid transformation. *Cancer Cell* 20(1):11–24, 2011.

162. Quivoron C, Couronne L, Della Valle V, et al: TET2 inactivation results in pleiotropic hematopoietic abnormalities in mouse and is a recurrent event during human lymphomagenesis. *Cancer Cell* 20(1):25–38, 2011.

163. Li Z, Cai X, Cai CL, et al: Deletion of Tet2 in mice leads to dysregulated hematopoietic stem cells and subsequent development of myeloid malignancies. *Blood* 118(17): 4509–4518, 2011.

164. Kosmider O, Gelsi-Boyer V, Cheok M, et al: TET2 mutation is an independent favorable prognostic factor in myelodysplastic syndromes (MDS). *Blood* 114(15):3285–3291, 2009.

165. Kosmider O, Gelsi-Boyer V, Ciudad M, et al: TET2 gene mutation is a frequent and adverse event in chronic myelomonocytic leukemia. *Haematologica* 94(12):1676–1681, 2009.

166. Ward PS, Patel J, Wise DR, et al: The common feature of leukemia-associated IDH1 and IDH2 mutations is a neomorphic enzyme activity converting alpha-ketoglutarate to 2-hydroxyglutarate. *Cancer Cell* 17(3):225–234, 2010.

167. Figueroa ME, Abdel-Wahab O, Lu C, et al: Leukemic IDH1 and IDH2 mutations result in a hypermethylation phenotype, disrupt TET2 function, and impair hematopoietic differentiation. *Cancer Cell* 18(6):553–567, 2010.

168. Koivunen P, Lee S, Duncan CG, et al: Transformation by the (R)-enantiomer of 2-hydroxyglutarate linked to EGLN activation. *Nature* 483(7390):484–488, 2012.

169. Cairns RA, Mak TW: Oncogenic isocitrate dehydrogenase mutations: Mechanisms, models, and clinical opportunities. *Cancer Discov* 3(7):730–741, 2013.

170. Xu W, Yang H, Liu Y, et al: Oncometabolite 2-hydroxyglutarate is a competitive inhibitor of alpha-ketoglutarate-dependent dioxygenases. *Cancer Cell* 19(1):17–30, 2011.

171. Lu C, Ward PS, Kapoor GS, et al: IDH mutation impairs histone demethylation and results in a block to cell differentiation. *Nature* 483(7390):474–478, 2012.

172. Sasaki M, Knobbe CB, Munger JC, et al: IDH1(R132H) mutation increases murine haematopoietic progenitors and alters epigenetics. *Nature* 488(7413):656–659, 2012.

173. Patnaik MM, Hanson CA, Hodnefield JM, et al: Differential prognostic effect of IDH1 versus IDH2 mutations in myelodysplastic syndromes: A Mayo Clinic study of 277 patients. *Leukemia* 26(1):101–105, 2012.

174. Losman JA, Looper RE, Koivunen P, et al: (R)-2-hydroxyglutarate is sufficient to promote leukemogenesis and its effects are reversible. *Science* 339(6127):1621–1625, 2013.

175. Score J, Hidalgo-Curtis C, Jones AV, et al: Inactivation of polycomb repressive complex 2 components in myeloproliferative and myelodysplastic/myeloproliferative neoplasms. *Blood* 119(5):1208–1213, 2012.

176. Khan SN, Jankowska AM, Mahfouz R, et al: Multiple mechanisms deregulate EZH2 and histone H3 lysine 27 epigenetic changes in myeloid malignancies. *Leukemia* 27(6):1301–1309, 2013.

177. Itzykson R, Kosmider O, Renneville A, et al: Prognostic score including gene mutations in chronic myelomonocytic leukemia. *J Clin Oncol* 31(19):2428–2436, 2013.

178. Thol F, Friesen I, Damm F, et al: Prognostic significance of ASXL1 mutations in patients with myelodysplastic syndromes. *J Clin Oncol* 29(18):2499–2506, 2011.

179. Abdel-Wahab O, Adli M, LaFave Lindsay M, et al: ASXL1 mutations promote myeloid transformation through loss of PRC2-mediated gene repression. *Cancer Cell* 22(2): 180–193, 2012.

180. Micol JB, Abdel-Wahab O: Collaborating constitutive and somatic genetic events in myeloid malignancies: ASXL1 mutations in patients with germline GATA2 mutations. *Haematologica* 99(2):201–203, 2014.

181. West RR, Hsu AP, Holland SM, Cuellar-Rodriguez J, Hickstein DD: Acquired ASXL1 mutations are common in patients with inherited GATA2 mutations and correlate with myeloid transformation. *Haematologica* 99(2):276–281, 2014.

182. Harada H, Harada Y, Niimi H, et al: High incidence of somatic mutations in the AML1/RUNX1 gene in myelodysplastic syndrome and low blast percentage myeloid leukemia with myelodysplasia. *Blood* 103(6):2316–2324, 2004.

183. Harada Y, Harada H: Molecular pathways mediating MDS/AML with focus on AML1/RUNX1 point mutations. *J Cell Physiol* 220(1):16–20, 2009.

184. Kuo MC, Liang DC, Huang CF, et al: RUNX1 mutations are frequent in chronic myelomonocytic leukemia and mutations at the C-terminal region might predict acute myeloid leukemia transformation. *Leukemia* 23(8):1426–1431, 2009.

185. Preudhomme C, Renneville A, Bourdon V, et al: High frequency of RUNX1 biallelic alteration in acute myeloid leukemia secondary to familial platelet disorder. *Blood* 113(22):5583–5587, 2009.

186. Owen C: Insights into familial platelet disorder with propensity to myeloid malignancy (FPD/AML). *Leuk Res* 34(2):141–142, 2010.

187. Smith ML, Cavenagh JD, Lister TA, Fitzgibbon J: Mutation of CEBPA in familial acute myeloid leukemia. *N Engl J Med* 351(23):2403–2407, 2004.

188. Padron E, Yoder S, Kunigal S, et al: ETV6 and signaling gene mutations are associated with secondary transformation of myelodysplastic syndromes to chronic myelomonocytic leukemia. *Blood* 123(23):3675–3677, 2014.

189. Ostergaard P, Simpson MA, Connell FC, et al: Mutations in GATA2 cause primary lymphedema associated with a predisposition to acute myeloid leukemia (Emberger syndrome). *Nat Genet* 43(10):929–931, 2011.

190. Dickinson RE, Griffin H, Bigley V, et al: Exome sequencing identifies GATA-2 mutation as the cause of dendritic cell, monocyte, B and NK lymphoid deficiency. *Blood* 118(10):2656–2658, 2011.

191. Dickinson RE, Milne P, Jardine L, et al: The evolution of cellular deficiency in GATA2 mutation. *Blood* 123(6):863–874, 2014.

192. Bejar R, Stevenson KE, Caughey B, et al: Somatic mutations predict poor outcome in patients with myelodysplastic syndrome after hematopoietic stem-cell transplantation. *J Clin Oncol* 32(25):2691–2698, 2014.

193. Bally C, Ades L, Renneville A, et al: Prognostic value of TP53 gene mutations in myelodysplastic syndromes and acute myeloid leukemia treated with azacitidine. *Leuk Res* 38(7):751–755, 2014.

194. Bejar R, Lord A, Stevenson K, et al: TET2 mutations predict response to hypomethylating agents in myelodysplastic syndrome patients. *Blood* 15:2014–2006, 2014.

195. Murphy DM, Bejar R, Stevenson K, et al: NRAS mutations with low allele burden have independent prognostic significance for patients with lower risk myelodysplastic syndromes. *Leukemia* 27(10):2077–2081, 2013.

196. Takahashi K, Jabbour E, Wang X, et al: Dynamic acquisition of FLT3 or RAS alterations drive a subset of patients with lower risk MDS to secondary AML. *Leukemia* 27(10):2081–2083, 2013.

197. Saur SJ, Sangkhae V, Geddis AE, et al: Ubiquitination and degradation of the thrombopoietin receptor c-Mpl. *Blood* 115(6):1254–1263, 2010.

198. Sanada M, Suzuki T, Shih LY, et al: Gain-of-function of mutated C-CBL tumour suppressor in myeloid neoplasms. *Nature* 460(7257):904–908, 2009.

199. Makishima H, Cazzolli H, Szpurka H, et al: Mutations of e3 ubiquitin ligase cbl family members constitute a novel common pathogenic lesion in myeloid malignancies. *J Clin Oncol* 27(36):6109–6116, 2009.

200. Loh ML, Martinelli S, Corddeu V, et al: Acquired PTPN11 mutations occur rarely in adult patients with myelodysplastic syndromes and chronic myelomonocytic leukemia. *Leuk Res* 29(4):459–462, 2005.

201. Sakaguchi H, Okuno Y, Muramatsu H, et al: Exome sequencing identifies secondary mutations of SETBP1 and JAK3 in juvenile myelomonocytic leukemia. *Nat Genet* 45(8):937–941, 2013.

202. Broseus J, Alpermann T, Wulfert M, et al: Age, JAK2(V617F) and SF3B1 mutations are the main predicting factors for survival in refractory anaemia with ring sideroblasts and marked thrombocytosis. *Leukemia* 27(9):1826–1831, 2013.

203. Hellstrom-Lindberg E, Cazzola M: The role of JAK2 mutations in RARS and other MDS. *Hematology Am Soc Hematol Educ Program* 52–59, 2008.

204. Kon A, Shih LY, Minamino M, et al: Recurrent mutations in multiple components of the cohesin complex in myeloid neoplasms. *Nat Genet* 45(10):1232–1237, 2013.

205. Thota S, Viny AD, Makishima H, et al: Genetic alterations of the cohesin complex genes in myeloid malignancies. *Blood* 8:2014–2004, 2014.

206. Janowska-Wieczorek A, Belch AR, Jacobs A, et al: Increased circulating colony-stimulating factor-1 in patients with preleukemia, leukemia, and lymphoid malignancies. *Blood* 77(8):1796–1803, 1991.

207. Verhoef GE, De Schouwer P, Ceuppens JL, et al: Measurement of serum cytokine levels in patients with myelodysplastic syndromes. *Leukemia* 6(12):1268–1272, 1992.

208. Bowen D, Yancik S, Bennett L, et al: Serum stem cell factor concentration in patients with myelodysplastic syndromes. *Br J Haematol* 85(1):63–66, 1993.

209. Wei Y, Dimicoli S, Bueso-Ramos C, et al: Toll-like receptor alterations in myelodysplastic syndrome. *Leukemia* 27(9):1832–1840, 2013.

210. Chen X, Eksioglu EA, Zhou J, et al: Induction of myelodysplasia by myeloid-derived suppressor cells. *J Clin Invest* 123(11):4595–4611, 2013.

211. Epperson DE, Nakamura R, Saunthararajah Y, et al: Oligoclonal T cell expansion in myelodysplastic syndrome: Evidence for an autoimmune process. *Leuk Res* 25(12):1075–1083, 2001.

212. Kochenderfer JN, Kobayashi S, Wieder ED, et al: Loss of T-lymphocyte clonal dominance in patients with myelodysplastic syndrome responsive to immunosuppression. *Blood* 100(10):3639–3645, 2002.

213. Kulasekararaj AG, Jiang J, Smith AE, et al: Somatic mutations identify a sub-group of aplastic anemia patients that progress to myelodysplastic syndrome. *Blood* 18: 2014–2005, 2014.

214. Jerez A, Clemente MJ, Makishima H, et al: STAT3 mutations indicate the presence of subclinical T-cell clones in a subset of aplastic anemia and myelodysplastic syndrome patients. *Blood* 122(14):2453–2459, 2013.

215. Steensma DP, Bennett JM: The myelodysplastic syndromes: Diagnosis and treatment. *Mayo Clin Proc* 81(1):104–130, 2006.

216. Steensma DP, Heptinstall KV, Johnson VM, et al: Common troublesome symptoms and their impact on quality of life in patients with myelodysplastic syndromes (MDS): Results of a large internet-based survey. *Leuk Res* 32(5):691–698, 2008.

217. Linman JW, Bagby GC Jr: The preleukemic syndrome (hemopoietic dysplasia). *Cancer* 42(2 Suppl):854–864, 1978.

218. Bagby GC: The preleukemic syndrome (hematopoietic dysplasia). *Blood Rev* 2(3): 194–205, 1988.

219. Noel P, Solberg LA Jr: Myelodysplastic syndromes. Pathogenesis, diagnosis and treatment. *Crit Rev Oncol Hematol* 12(3):193–215, 1992.

220. Park S, Merlat A, Guesnu M, et al: Pure red cell aplasia associated with myelodysplastic syndromes. *Leukemia* 14(9):1709–1710, 2000.

221. Choi JW, Kim Y, Fujino M, Ito M: Significance of fetal hemoglobin-containing erythroblasts (F blasts) and the F blast/F cell ratio in myelodysplastic syndromes. *Leukemia* 16(8):1478–1483, 2002.

222. Kornberg A, Goldfarb A: Preleukemia manifested by hemolytic anemia with pyruvate-kinase deficiency. *Arch Intern Med* 146(4):785–786, 1986.

223. Harris JW, Koscick R, Lazarus HM, et al: Leukemia arising out of paroxysmal nocturnal hemoglobinuria. *Leuk Lymphoma* 32(5–6):401–426, 1999.

224. Lopez M, Bonnetgajdos M, Reviron M, et al: An acute-leukemia augured before clinical signs by blood-group antigen abnormalities and low-levels of A-blood and H-blood group transferase activities in erythrocytes. *Br J Haematol* 63(3):535–539, 1986.

225. Steensma DP, Higgs DR, Fisher CA, Gibbons RJ: Acquired somatic ATRX mutations in myelodysplastic syndrome associated with alpha thalassemia (ATMDS) convey a more severe hematologic phenotype than germline ATRX mutations. *Blood* 103(6): 2019–2026, 2004.

226. Helder J, Deisseroth A: S1 nuclease analysis of alpha-globin gene expression in preleukemic patients with acquired hemoglobin H disease after transfer to mouse erythroleukemia cells. *Proc Natl Acad Sci U S A* 84(8):2387–2390, 1987.

227. Anagnou NP, Ley TJ, Chesbro B, et al: Acquired alpha-thalassemia in preleukemia is due to decreased expression of all four alpha-globin genes. *Proc Natl Acad Sci U S A* 80(19):6051–6055, 1983.

228. French registry of acute leukemia and myelodysplastic syndromes. Age distribution and hemogram analysis of the 4496 cases recorded during 1982–1983 and classified according to FAB criteria. Groupe Francais de Morphologie Hematologique. *Cancer* 60(6):1385–1394, 1987.

229. Friedland ML, Ward H, Wittels EG, Arlin ZA: A monocytic leukemoid reaction: A manifestation of preleukemia. *R I Med J* 68(4):173–174, 1985.

230. Jaworkowsky LI, Solovey DY, Rhausova LY, Udris OY: Monocytosis as a sign of subsequent leukemia in patients with cytopenias (preleukemia). *Folia Haematol Int Mag Klin Morphol Blutforsch* 110(3):395–401, 1983.

231. Economopoulos T, Stathakis N, Maragoyannis Z, et al: Myelodysplastic syndrome. Clinical and prognostic significance of monocyte count, degree of blastic infiltration, and ring sideroblasts. *Acta Haematol* 65(2):97–102, 1981.

232. Shetty VT, Mundle SD, Raza A: Pseudo Pelger-Huet anomaly in myelodysplastic syndrome: Hyposegmented apoptotic neutrophil? *Blood* 98(4):1273–1275, 2001.

233. Langenhuijsen MM: Neutrophils with ring-shaped nuclei in myeloproliferative disease. *Br J Haematol* 58(2):227–230, 1984.

234. Linman JW, Bagby C Jr: The preleukemic syndrome: Clinical and laboratory features, natural course, and management. *Nouv Rev Fr Hematol Blood Cells* 17(1–2):11–31, 1976.

235. Clark RE, Smith SA, Jacobs A: Myeloid surface antigen abnormalities in myelodysplasia: Relation to prognosis and modification by 13-cis retinoic acid. *J Clin Pathol* 40(6):652–656, 1987.

236. Cech P, Markert M, Perrin LH: Partial myeloperoxidase deficiency in preleukemia. *Blut* 47(1):21–30, 1983.

237. Schofield KP, Stone PC, Kelsey P, et al: Quantitative cytochemistry of blood neutrophils in myelodysplastic syndromes and chronic granulocytic leukaemia. *Cell Biochem Funct* 1(2):92–96, 1983.

238. Elghetany MT, Peterson B, MacCallum J, et al: Deficiency of neutrophilic granule membrane glycoproteins in the myelodysplastic syndromes: A common deficiency in 216 patients studied by the Cancer and Leukemia Group B. *Leuk Res* 21(9):801–806, 1997.

239. Prodan M, Tulissi P, Perticarari S, et al: Flow cytometric assay for the evaluation of phagocytosis and oxidative burst of polymorphonuclear leukocytes and monocytes in myelodysplastic disorders. *Haematologica* 80(3):212–218, 1995.

240. Piva E, De Toni S, Caenazzo A, et al: Neutrophil NADPH oxidase activity in chronic myeloproliferative and myelodysplastic diseases by microscopic and photometric assays. *Acta Haematol* 94(1):16–22, 1995.

241. Ruutu P: Granulocyte function in myelodysplastic syndromes. *Scand J Haematol Suppl* 45:66–70, 1986.

242. Carulli G, Sbrana S, Minnucci S, et al: Actin polymerization in neutrophils from patients affected by myelodysplastic syndromes—A flow cytometric study. *Leuk Res* 21(6):513–518, 1997.

243. Nakaseko C, Asai T, Wakita H, et al: Signalling defect in FMLP-induced neutrophil respiratory burst in myelodysplastic syndromes. *Br J Haematol* 95(3):482–488, 1996.

244. Payne CM, Glasser L: An ultrastructural morphometric analysis of platelet giant and fusion granules. *Blood* 67(2):299–309, 1986.

245. Pamphilon DH, Aparicio SR, Roberts BE, et al: The myelodysplastic syndromes—A study of haemostatic function and platelet ultrastructure. *Scand J Haematol* 33(5):486–491, 1984.

246. Rasi V, Lintula R: Platelet function in the myelodysplastic syndromes. *Scand J Haematol Suppl* 45:71–73, 1986.

247. Hamblin TJ: Immunological abnormalities in myelodysplastic syndromes. *Semin Hematol* 33(2):150–162, 1996.

248. Anderson RW, Volsky DJ, Greenberg B, et al: Lymphocyte abnormalities in preleukemia—I. Decreased NK activity, anomalous immunoregulatory cell subsets and deficient EBV receptors. *Leuk Res* 7(3):389–395, 1983.

249. Kerndrup G, Meyer K, Ellegaard J, Hokland P: Natural killer (NK)-cell activity and antibody-dependent cellular cytotoxicity (ADCC) in primary preleukemic syndrome. *Leuk Res* 8(2):239–247, 1984.

250. Takagi S, Kitagawa S, Takeda A, et al: Natural killer-interferon system in patients with preleukemic states. *Br J Haematol* 58(1):71–81, 1984.

251. Volsky DJ, Anderson RW: Deficiency in Epstein-Barr virus receptors on B-lymphocytes of preleukemia patients. *Cancer Res* 43(8):3923–3926, 1983.

252. Baumann MA, Milson TJ, Patrick CW, et al: Immunoregulatory abnormalities in myelodysplastic disorders. *Am J Hematol* 22(1):17–26, 1986.

253. Knox SJ, Greenberg BR, Anderson RW, Rosenblatt LS: Studies of T-lymphocytes in preleukemic disorders and acute nonlymphocytic leukemia: In vitro radiosensitivity, mitogenic responsiveness, colony formation, and enumeration of lymphocytic subpopulations. *Blood* 61(3):449–455, 1983.

254. Lawrence HJ, Broudy VC, Magenis RE, et al: Cytogenetic evidence for involvement of B lymphocytes in acquired idiopathic sideroblastic anemias. *Blood* 70(4):1003–1005, 1987.

255. Meers S, Vandenberghe P, Boogaerts M, et al: The clinical significance of activated lymphocytes in patients with myelodysplastic syndromes: A single centre study of 131 patients. *Leuk Res* 32(7):1026–1035, 2008.

256. Epling-Burnette PK, Painter JS, Rollison DE, et al: Prevalence and clinical association of clonal T-cell expansions in myelodysplastic syndrome. *Leukemia* 21(4):659–667, 2007.

257. Mufti GJ, Figes A, Hamblin TJ, et al: Immunological abnormalities in myelodysplastic syndromes. I. Serum immunoglobulins and autoantibodies. *Br J Haematol* 63(1):143–147, 1986.

258. Economopoulos T, Economidou J, Giannopoulos G, et al: Immune abnormalities in myelodysplastic syndromes. *J Clin Pathol* 38(8):908–911, 1985.

259. Gatto S, Ball G, Onida F, et al: Contribution of beta-2 microglobulin levels to the prognostic stratification of survival in patients with myelodysplastic syndrome (MDS). *Blood* 102(5):1622–1625, 2003.

260. Yue G, Hao S, Fadare O, et al: Hypocellularity in myelodysplastic syndrome is an independent factor which predicts a favorable outcome. *Leuk Res* 32(4):553–558, 2008.

261. Delacretaz F, Schmidt PM, Piguet D, et al: Histopathology of myelodysplastic syndromes. The FAB classification (proposals) applied to bone marrow biopsy. *Am J Clin Pathol* 87(2):180–186, 1987.

262. Fohlmeister I, Fischer R, Modder B, et al: Aplastic anaemia and the hypocellular myelodysplastic syndrome: Histomorphological, diagnostic, and prognostic features. *J Clin Pathol* 38(11):1218–1224, 1985.

263. Kuriyama K, Tomonaga M, Matsuo T, et al: Diagnostic significance of detecting pseudo-Pelger-Huet anomalies and micro-megakaryocytes in myelodysplastic syndrome. *Br J Haematol* 63(4):665–669, 1986.

264. Mangi MH, Mufti GJ: Primary myelodysplastic syndromes: Diagnostic and prognostic significance of immunohistochemical assessment of bone marrow biopsies. *Blood* 79(1):198–205, 1992.

265. Tricot G, De Wolf-Peeters C, Vlietinck R, Verwilghen RL: Bone marrow histology in myelodysplastic syndromes. II. Prognostic value of abnormal localization of immature precursors in MDS. *Br J Haematol* 58(2):217–225, 1984.

266. Della Porta MG, Malcovati L, Boveri E, et al: Clinical relevance of bone marrow fibrosis and CD34-positive cell clusters in primary myelodysplastic syndromes. *J Clin Oncol* 27(5):754–762, 2009.

267. Bellamy WT, Richter L, Sirjani D, et al: Vascular endothelial cell growth factor is an autocrine promoter of abnormal localized immature myeloid precursors and leukemia progenitor formation in myelodysplastic syndromes. *Blood* 97(5):1427–1434, 2001.

268. Matsushima T, Handa H, Yokohama A, et al: Prevalence and clinical characteristics of myelodysplastic syndrome with bone marrow eosinophilia or basophilia. *Blood* 101(9):3386–3390, 2003.

269. Queisser W, Queisser U, Ansmann M, et al: Megakaryocyte polyploidization in acute leukaemia and preleukaemia. *Br J Haematol* 28(2):261–270, 1974.

270. Smith WB, Ablin A, Goodman JR, Brecher G: Atypical megakaryocytes in preleukemic phase of acute myeloid leukemia. *Blood* 42(4):535–540, 1973.

271. Bartl R, Frisch B, Baumgart R: Morphological classification of the myelodysplastic syndromes (MDS): Combined utilization of bone marrow aspirates and trephine biopsies. *Leuk Res* 16(1):15–33, 1992.

272. Della Porta MG, Travaglino E, Boveri E, et al: Minimal morphological criteria for defining bone marrow dysplasia: A basis for clinical implementation of WHO classification of myelodysplastic syndromes. *Leukemia* 20(10):161, 2014.

273. Maschek H, Georgii A, Kaloutsi V, et al: Myelofibrosis in primary myelodysplastic syndromes: A retrospective study of 352 patients. *Eur J Haematol* 48(4):208–214, 1992.

274. Moehler TM, Ho AD, Goldschmidt H, Barlogie B: Angiogenesis in hematologic malignancies. *Crit Rev Oncol Hematol* 45(3):227–244, 2003.

275. Ribatti D, Polimeno G, Vacca A, et al: Correlation of bone marrow angiogenesis and mast cells with tryptase activity in myelodysplastic syndromes. *Leukemia* 16(9):1680–1684, 2002.

276. Della Porta MG, Malcovati L, Rigolin GM, et al: Immunophenotypic, cytogenetic and functional characterization of circulating endothelial cells in myelodysplastic syndromes. *Leukemia* 22(3):530–537, 2008.

277. Lobe I, Rigal-Huguet F, Vekhoff A, et al: Myelodysplastic syndrome after acute promyelocytic leukemia: The European APL group experience. *Leukemia* 17(8):1600–1604, 2003.

278. Smith SM, Le Beau MM, Huo D, et al: Clinical-cytogenetic associations in 306 patients with therapy-related myelodysplasia and myeloid leukemia: The University of Chicago series. *Blood* 102(1):43–52, 2003.

279. Krishnan A, Bhatia S, Slovak ML, et al: Predictors of therapy-related leukemia and myelodysplasia following autologous transplantation for lymphoma: An assessment of risk factors. *Blood* 95(5):1588–1593, 2000.

280. Abruzzese E, Radford JE, Miller JS, et al: Detection of abnormal pretransplant clones in progenitor cells of patients who developed myelodysplasia after autologous transplantation. *Blood* 94(5):1814–1819, 1999.

281. Van Den Neste E, Louviaux I, Michaux JL, et al: Myelodysplastic syndrome with monosomy 5 and/or 7 following therapy with 2-chloro-2′-deoxyadenosine. *Br J Haematol* 105(1):268–270, 1999.

282. Rigolin GM, Cuneo A, Roberti MG, et al: Exposure to myelotoxic agents and myelodysplasia: Case-control study and correlation with clinicobiological findings. *Br J Haematol* 103(1):189–197, 1998.

283. Sterkers Y, Preudhomme C, Lai JL, et al: Acute myeloid leukemia and myelodysplastic syndromes following essential thrombocythemia treated with hydroxyurea: High proportion of cases with 17p deletion. *Blood* 91(2):616–622, 1998.

284. Park DJ, Koeffler HP: Therapy-related myelodysplastic syndromes. *Semin Hematol* 33(3):256–273, 1996.

285. Karp JE, Sarkodee-Adoo CB: Therapy-related acute leukemia. *Clin Lab Med* 20(1):71–81, ix, 2000.

286. Padmanabhan A, Baker JA, Zirpoli G, et al: Acute myeloid leukemia and myelodysplastic syndrome following breast cancer: Increased frequency of other cancers and of cancers in multiple family members. *Leuk Res* 2008;32(12):1820–1823, 2000.

287. Hake CR, Graubert TA, Fenske TS: Does autologous transplantation directly increase the risk of secondary leukemia in lymphoma patients? *Bone Marrow Transplant* 39(2):59–70, 2007.

288. Palumbo A, Bringhen S, Kumar SK, et al: Second primary malignancies with lenalidomide therapy for newly diagnosed myeloma: A meta-analysis of individual patient data. *Lancet Oncol* 15(3):333–342, 2014.

289. Chakraborty S, Sun CL, Francisco L, et al: Accelerated telomere shortening precedes development of therapy-related myelodysplasia or acute myelogenous leukemia after autologous transplantation for lymphoma. *J Clin Oncol* 27(5):791–798, 2009.

290. Fukumoto JS, Greenberg PL: Management of patients with higher risk myelodysplastic syndromes. *Crit Rev Oncol Hematol* 56(2):179–192, 2005.

291. Senent L, Arenillas L, Luno E, Ruiz JC, Sanz G, Florensa L: Reproducibility of the World Health Organization 2008 criteria for myelodysplastic syndromes. *Haematologica* 98(4):568–575, 2013.

292. Font P, Loscertales J, Benavente C, et al: Inter-observer variance with the diagnosis of myelodysplastic syndromes (MDS) following the 2008 WHO classification. *Ann Hematol* 92(1):19–24, 2013.

293. Greenberg PL, Attar E, Bennett JM, et al: Myelodysplastic syndromes: Clinical practice guidelines in oncology. *J Natl Compr Canc Netw* 11(7):838–874, 2013.

294. Malcovati L, Hellstrom-Lindberg E, Bowen D, et al: Diagnosis and treatment of primary myelodysplastic syndromes in adults: Recommendations from the European LeukemiaNet. *Blood* 122(17):2943–2964, 2013.

295. Garcia-Manero G, Shan J, Faderl S, et al: A prognostic score for patients with lower risk myelodysplastic syndrome. *Leukemia* 22(3):538–543, 2008.

296. Kantarjian H, O'Brien S, Ravandi F, et al: Proposal for a new risk model in myelodysplastic syndrome that accounts for events not considered in the original International Prognostic Scoring System. *Cancer* 113(6):1351–1361, 2008.

297. Malcovati L, Della Porta MG, Strupp C, et al: Impact of the degree of anemia on the outcome of patients with myelodysplastic syndrome and its integration into the WHO classification-based Prognostic Scoring System (WPSS). *Haematologica* 96(10):1433–1440, 2011.

298. Greenberg PL, Tuechler H, Schanz J, et al: Revised international prognostic scoring system for myelodysplastic syndromes. *Blood* 120(12):2454–2465, 2012.

299. Neukirchen J, Lauseker M, Blum S, et al: Validation of the revised International Prognostic Scoring System (IPSS-R) in patients with myelodysplastic syndrome: A multi-center study. *Leuk Res* 38(1):57–64, 2014.

300. Voso MT, Fenu S, Latagliata R, et al: Revised International Prognostic Scoring System (IPSS) predicts survival and leukemic evolution of myelodysplastic syndromes significantly better than IPSS and WHO Prognostic Scoring System: Validation by the Gruppo Romano Mielodisplasie Italian Regional Database. *J Clin Oncol* 31(21):2671–2677, 2013.

301. Zeidan AM, Lee JW, Prebet T, et al: Comparison of the prognostic utility of the revised International Prognostic Scoring System and the French Prognostic Scoring System in azacitidine-treated patients with myelodysplastic syndromes. *Br J Haematol* 166(3):352–359, 2014.

302. Sekeres MA, Swern AS, Fenaux P, et al: Validation of the IPSS-R in lenalidomide-treated, lower-risk myelodysplastic syndrome patients with del(5q). *Blood Cancer J* 4(4):e242, 2014.

303. Della Porta MG, Alessandrino EP, Bacigalupo A, et al: Predictive factors for the outcome of allogeneic transplantation in patients with MDS stratified according to the revised IPSS-R. *Blood* 123(15):2333–2342, 2014.

304. Steensma DP, Tefferi A: Risk-based management of myelodysplastic syndrome. *Oncology (Williston Park)* 21(1):43–54; discussion 57–58, 62, 2007.

305. Sekeres MA: How to manage lower-risk myelodysplastic syndromes. *Leukemia* 26(3):390–394, 2012.

306. Sekeres MA, Cutler C: How we treat higher-risk myelodysplastic syndromes. *Blood* 123(6):829–836, 2014.

307. Fenaux P, Ades L: How we treat lower-risk myelodysplastic syndromes. *Blood* 121(21):4280–4286, 2013.

308. List A, Dewald G, Bennett J, et al: Lenalidomide in the myelodysplastic syndrome with chromosome 5q deletion. *N Engl J Med* 355(14):1456–1465, 2006.

309. Hellstrom-Lindberg E, Gulbrandsen N, Lindberg G, et al: A validated decision model for treating the anaemia of myelodysplastic syndromes with erythropoietin + granulocyte colony-stimulating factor: Significant effects on quality of life. *Br J Haematol* 120(6):1037–1046, 2003.

310. Traina F, Visconte V, Elson P, et al: Impact of molecular mutations on treatment response to DNMT inhibitors in myelodysplasia and related neoplasms. *Leukemia* 28(1):78–87, 2014.

311. Itzykson R, Kosmider O, Cluzeau T, et al: Impact of TET2 mutations on response rate to azacitidine in myelodysplastic syndromes and low blast count acute myeloid leukemias. *Leukemia* 25(7):1147–1152, 2011.

312. Saunthararajah Y, Nakamura R, Wesley R, et al: A simple method to predict response to immunosuppressive therapy in patients with myelodysplastic syndrome. *Blood* 102(8):3025–3027, 2003.

313. Sekeres MA, Giagounidis A, Kantarjian H, et al: Development and validation of a model to predict platelet response to romiplostim in patients with lower-risk myelodysplastic syndromes. *Br J Haematol* 167(3):337–345, 2014.

314. Westers TM, Alhan C, Chamuleau ME, et al: Aberrant immunophenotype of blasts in myelodysplastic syndromes is a clinically relevant biomarker in predicting response to growth factor treatment. *Blood* 115(9):1779–1784, 2010.

315. Saft L, Karimi M, Ghaderi M, et al: P53 protein expression independently predicts outcome in patients with lower-risk myelodysplastic syndromes with del(5q). *Haematologica* 99(6):1041–1049, 2014.

316. Bejar R, Stevenson K, Abdel-Wahab O, et al: Clinical effect of point mutations in myelodysplastic syndromes. *N Engl J Med* 364(26):2496–2506, 2011.

317. Greenberg PL, Attar E, Bennett JM, et al: Myelodysplastic syndromes: Clinical practice guidelines in oncology. *J Natl Compr Canc Netw* 11(7):838–874, 2013.

318. Cheson BD, Greenberg PL, Bennett JM, et al: Clinical application and proposal for modification of the International Working Group (IWG) response criteria in myelodysplasia. *Blood* 108(2):419–425, 2006.

319. Steensma DP, Heptinstall KV, Johnson VM, et al: Common troublesome symptoms and their impact on quality of life in patients with myelodysplastic syndromes (MDS): Results of a large internet-based survey. *Leuk Res* 32(5):691–698, 2008.

320. Sekeres MA, Maciejewski JP, List AF, et al: Perceptions of disease state, treatment outcomes, and prognosis among patients with myelodysplastic syndromes: Results from an internet-based survey. *Oncologist* 16(6):904–911, 2011.

321. Abel GA, Klaassen R, Lee SJ, et al: Patient-reported outcomes for the myelodysplastic syndromes: A new MDS-specific measure of quality of life. *Blood* 123(3):451–452, 2014.

322. Jansen AJ, Essink-Bot ML, Beckers EA, et al: Quality of life measurement in patients with transfusion-dependent myelodysplastic syndromes. *Br J Haematol* 121(2):270–274, 2003.

323. Kornblith AB, Herndon JE 2nd, Silverman LR, et al: Impact of azacytidine on the quality of life of patients with myelodysplastic syndrome treated in a randomized phase III trial: A Cancer and Leukemia Group B study. *J Clin Oncol* 20(10):2441–2452, 2002.

324. Lindquist KJ, Danese MD, Mikhael J, et al: Health care utilization and mortality among elderly patients with myelodysplastic syndromes. *Ann Oncol* 22(5):1181–1188, 2011.

325. Hellstrom-Lindberg E, Malcovati L: Supportive care and use of hematopoietic growth factors in myelodysplastic syndromes. *Semin Hematol* 45(1):14–22, 2008.

326. Oliva EN, Schey C, Hutchings AS: A review of anemia as a cardiovascular risk factor in patients with myelodysplastic syndromes. *Am J Blood Res* 1(2):160–166, 2011.

327. Fakhry SM, Fata P: How low is too low? Cardiac risks with anemia. *Crit Care* 8 Suppl 2:S11–S14, 2004.

328. Hajjar LA, Vincent JL, Galas FR, et al: Transfusion requirements after cardiac surgery: The TRACS randomized controlled trial. *JAMA* 304(14):1559–1567, 2010.

329. Hebert PC, Wells G, Blajchman MA, et al: A multicenter, randomized, controlled clinical trial of transfusion requirements in critical care. Transfusion Requirements in Critical Care Investigators, Canadian Critical Care Trials Group. *N Engl J Med* 340(6):409–417, 1999.

330. Hogshire L, Carson JL: Red blood cell transfusion: What is the evidence when to transfuse? *Curr Opin Hematol* 20(6):546–551, 2013.

331. Pascal L, Beyne-Rauzy O, Brechignac S, et al: Cardiac iron overload assessed by T2* magnetic resonance imaging and cardiac function in regularly transfused myelodysplastic syndrome patients. *Br J Haematol* 162(3):413–415, 2013.

332. Chacko J, Pennell DJ, Tanner MA, et al: Myocardial iron loading by magnetic resonance imaging T2* in good prognostic myelodysplastic syndrome patients on long-term blood transfusions. *Br J Haematol* 138(5):587–593, 2007.

333. Kantarjian H, Giles F, List A, et al: The incidence and impact of thrombocytopenia in myelodysplastic syndromes. *Cancer* 109(7):1705–1714, 2007.

334. Cullen M, Baijal S: Prevention of febrile neutropenia: Use of prophylactic antibiotics. *Br J Cancer* 101 Suppl 1:S11–S14, 2009.

335. Bergmann OJ, Mogensen SC, Ellermann-Eriksen S, Ellegaard J: Acyclovir prophylaxis and fever during remission-induction therapy of patients with acute myeloid leukemia: A randomized, double-blind, placebo-controlled trial. *J Clin Oncol* 15(6):2269–2274, 1997.

336. Cornely OA, Maertens J, Winston DJ, et al: Posaconazole vs. fluconazole or itraconazole prophylaxis in patients with neutropenia. *N Engl J Med* 356(4):348–359, 2007.

337. Steensma DP, Stone RM: Practical recommendations for hypomethylating agent therapy of patients with myelodysplastic syndromes. *Hematol Oncol Clin North Am* 24(2):389–406, 2010.

338. Cornely OA, Bohme A, Buchheidt D, et al: Primary prophylaxis of invasive fungal infections in patients with hematologic malignancies. Recommendations of the Infectious Diseases Working Party of the German Society for Haematology and Oncology. *Haematologica* 94(1):113–122, 2009.

339. Mattiuzzi GN, Kantarjian H, Faderl S, et al: Amphotericin B lipid complex as prophylaxis of invasive fungal infections in patients with acute myelogenous leukemia and myelodysplastic syndrome undergoing induction chemotherapy. *Cancer* 100(3):581–589, 2004.

340. Cazzola M, Malcovati L: Myelodysplastic syndromes—Coping with ineffective hematopoiesis. *N Engl J Med* 352(6):536–538, 2005.

341. Malcovati L: Impact of transfusion dependency and secondary iron overload on the survival of patients with myelodysplastic syndromes. *Leuk Res* 31 (Suppl 3):S2–S6, 2007.

342. Chee CE, Steensma DP, Wu W, et al: Neither serum ferritin nor the number of red blood cell transfusions affect overall survival in refractory anemia with ringed sideroblasts. *Am J Hematol* 83(8):611–613, 2008.

343. Leitch HA, Chan C, Leger CS, et al: Improved survival with iron chelation therapy for red blood cell transfusion dependent lower IPSS risk MDS may be more significant in patients with a non-RARS diagnosis. *Leuk Res* 36(11):1380–1386, 2012.

344. Park S, Grabar S, Kelaidi C, et al: Predictive factors of response and survival in myelodysplastic syndrome treated with erythropoietin and G-CSF: The GFM experience. *Blood* 111(2):574–582, 2008.

345. Rigolin GM, Porta MD, Ciccone M, et al: In patients with myelodysplastic syndromes response to rHuEPO and G-CSF treatment is related to an increase of cytogenetically normal CD34 cells. *Br J Haematol* 126(4):501–507, 2004.

346. Musto P, Matera R, Minervini MM, et al: Low serum levels of tumor necrosis factor and interleukin-1 beta in myelodysplastic syndromes responsive to recombinant erythropoietin. *Haematologica* 79(3):265–268, 1994.

347. Wallvik J, Stenke L, Bernell P, et al: Serum erythropoietin (EPO) levels correlate with survival and independently predict response to EPO treatment in patients with myelodysplastic syndromes. *Eur J Haematol* 68(3):180–185, 2002.

348. Auerbach M, Ballard H: Clinical use of intravenous iron: Administration, efficacy, and safety. *Hematology Am Soc Hematol Educ Program* 2010:338–347, 2010.

349. Rizzo JD, Brouwers M, Hurley P, et al: American Society of Hematology/American Society of Clinical Oncology clinical practice guideline update on the use of epoetin and darbepoetin in adult patients with cancer. *Blood* 116(20):4045–4059, 2010.

350. Rose EH, Abels RI, Nelson RA, et al: The use of r-HuEpo in the treatment of anaemia related to myelodysplasia (MDS). *Br J Haematol* 89(4):831–837, 1995.

351. Negrin RS, Stein R, Vardiman J, et al: Treatment of the anemia of myelodysplastic syndromes using recombinant human granulocyte colony-stimulating factor in combination with erythropoietin. *Blood* 82(3):737–743, 1993.

352. Bessho M, Jinnai I, Matsuda A, et al: Improvement of anemia by recombinant erythropoietin in patients with myelodysplastic syndromes and aplastic anemia. *Int J Cell Cloning* 8(6):445–458, 1990.

353. Stebler C, Tichelli A, Dazzi H, et al: High-dose recombinant human erythropoietin for treatment of anemia in myelodysplastic syndromes and paroxysmal nocturnal hemoglobinuria: A pilot study. *Exp Hematol* 18(11):1204–1208, 1990.

354. Bowen D, Culligan D, Jacobs A: The treatment of anaemia in the myelodysplastic syndromes with recombinant human erythropoietin. *Br J Haematol* 77(3):419–423, 1991.

355. Hellstrom E, Birgegard G, Lockner D, et al: Treatment of myelodysplastic syndromes with recombinant human erythropoietin. *Eur J Haematol* 47(5):355–360, 1991.

356. Schouten HC, Vellenga E, van Rhenen DJ, et al: Recombinant human erythropoietin in patients with myelodysplastic syndromes. *Leukemia* 5(5):432–436, 1991.

357. Stein RS, Abels RI, Krantz SB: Pharmacologic doses of recombinant human erythropoietin in the treatment of myelodysplastic syndromes. *Blood* 78(7):1658–1663, 1991.

358. Goy A, Belanger C, Casadevall N, et al: High doses of intravenous recombinant erythropoietin for the treatment of anaemia in myelodysplastic syndrome. *Br J Haematol* 84(2):232–237, 1993.

359. A randomized double-blind placebo-controlled study with subcutaneous recombinant human erythropoietin in patients with low-risk myelodysplastic syndromes. Italian Cooperative Study Group for rHuEpo in Myelodysplastic Syndromes. *Br J Haematol* 103(4):1070–1074, 1998.

360. Thompson JA, Gilliland DG, Prchal JT, et al: Effect of recombinant human erythropoietin combined with granulocyte/macrophage colony-stimulating factor in the treatment of patients with myelodysplastic syndrome. GM/EPO MDS Study Group. *Blood* 95(4):1175–1179, 2000.

361. Spiriti MA, Latagliata R, Niscola P, et al: Impact of a new dosing regimen of epoetin alfa on quality of life and anemia in patients with low-risk myelodysplastic syndrome. *Ann Hematol* 84(3):167–176, 2005.

362. Stone RM, Bernstein SH, Demetri G, et al: Therapy with recombinant human erythropoietin in patients with myelodysplastic syndromes. *Leuk Res* 18(10):769–776, 1994.

363. Gabrilove J, Paquette R, Lyons RM, et al: Phase 2, single-arm trial to evaluate the effectiveness of darbepoetin alfa for correcting anaemia in patients with myelodysplastic syndromes. *Br J Haematol* 142(3):379–393, 2008.

364. Stasi R, Abruzzese E, Lanzetta G, et al: Darbepoetin alfa for the treatment of anemic patients with low- and intermediate-1-risk myelodysplastic syndromes. *Ann Oncol* 16(12):1921–1927, 2005.

365. Moyo V, Lefebvre P, Duh MS, et al: Erythropoiesis-stimulating agents in the treatment of anemia in myelodysplastic syndromes: A meta-analysis. *Ann Hematol* 87(7):527–536, 2008.

366. Terpos E, Mougiou A, Kouraklis A, et al: Prolonged administration of erythropoietin increases erythroid response rate in myelodysplastic syndromes: A phase II trial in 281 patients. *Br J Haematol* 118(1):174–180, 2002.

367. Bohlius J, Schmidlin K, Brillant C, et al: Recombinant human erythropoiesis-stimulating agents and mortality in patients with cancer: A meta-analysis of randomised trials. *Lancet* 373(9674):1532–1542, 2009.

368. Jadersten M, Malcovati L, Dybedal I, et al: Erythropoietin and granulocyte-colony stimulating factor treatment associated with improved survival in myelodysplastic syndrome. *J Clin Oncol* 26(21):3607–3613, 2008.

369. Cortelezzi A, Colombo G, Pellegrini C, et al: Bone marrow glycophorin-positive erythroid cells of myelodysplastic patients responding to high-dose rHuEPO therapy have a different gene expression pattern from those of nonresponders. *Am J Hematol* 83(7):531–539, 2008.

370. Negrin RS, Stein R, Doherty K, et al: Maintenance treatment of the anemia of myelodysplastic syndromes with recombinant human granulocyte colony-stimulating factor and erythropoietin: Evidence for *in vivo* synergy. *Blood* 87(10):4076–4081, 1996.

371. Mundle S, Lefebvre P, Vekeman F, et al: An assessment of erythroid response to epoetin alpha as a single agent versus in combination with granulocyte- or granulocyte-macrophage-colony-stimulating factor in myelodysplastic syndromes using a meta-analysis approach. *Cancer* 115(4):706–715, 2009.

372. Pomeroy C, Oken MM, Rydell RE, Filice GA: Infection in the myelodysplastic syndromes. *Am J Med* 90(3):338–344, 1991.

373. Boogaerts MA, Nelissen V, Roelant C, Goossens W: Blood neutrophil function in primary myelodysplastic syndromes. *Br J Haematol* 55(2):217–227, 1983.

374. Davey FR, Erber WN, Gatter KC, Mason DY: Abnormal neutrophils in acute myeloid leukemia and myelodysplastic syndrome. *Hum Pathol* 19(4):454–459, 1988.

375. Engelfriet CP, k HW, Klein HG, et al: International forum: Granulocyte transfusions. *Vox Sang* 79(1):59–66, 2000.

376. Steensma DP: Hematopoietic growth factors in myelodysplastic syndromes. *Semin Oncol* 38(5):635–647, 2011.

377. Vadhan-Raj S, Keating M, LeMaistre A, et al: Effects of recombinant human granulocyte-macrophage colony-stimulating factor in patients with myelodysplastic syndromes. *N Engl J Med* 317(25):1545–1552, 1987.

378. Chuncharunee S, Intragumtornchai T, Chaimongkol B, et al: Treatment of myelodysplastic syndrome with low-dose human granulocyte colony-stimulating factor: A multicenter study. *Int J Hematol* 74(2):144–146, 2001.

379. Sultana TA, Harada H, Ito K, et al: Expression and functional analysis of granulocyte colony-stimulating factor receptors on CD34++ cells in patients with myelodysplastic syndrome (MDS) and MDS-acute myeloid leukaemia. *Br J Haematol* 121(1):63–75, 2003.

380. Nimubona S, Grulois I, Bernard M, et al: Complete remission in hypoplastic acute myeloid leukemia induced by G-CSF without chemotherapy: Report on three cases. *Leukemia* 16(9):1871–1873, 2002.

381. O'Malley DP, Whalen M, Banks PM: Spontaneous splenic rupture with fatal outcome following G-CSF administration for myelodysplastic syndrome. *Am J Hematol* 73(4):294–295, 2003.

382. Arshad M, Seiter K, Bilaniuk J, et al: Side effects related to cancer treatment: CASE 2. Splenic rupture following pegfilgrastim. *J Clin Oncol* 23(33):8533–8534, 2005.

383. Jakob A, Hirsch FW, Engelhardt M: Successful treatment of a patient with myelodysplastic syndrome (RAEB) with Darbepoetin-alfa in combination with Pegfilgrastim. *Ann Hematol* 84(10):694–695, 2005.

384. Jadersten M, Montgomery SM, Dybedal I, et al: Long-term outcome of treatment of anemia in MDS with erythropoietin and G-CSF. *Blood* 106(3):803–811, 2005.

385. Verhoef G, Van den Berghe H, Boogaerts M: Cytogenetic effects on cells derived from patients with myelodysplastic syndromes during treatment with hemopoietic growth factors. *Leukemia* 6(8):766–769, 1992.

386. Tohyama K, Ohmori S, Michishita M, et al: Effects of recombinant G-CSF and GM-CSF on in vitro differentiation of the blast cells of RAEB and RAEB-T. *Eur J Haematol* 42(4):348–353, 1989.

387. Ferrero D, Bruno B, Pregno P, et al: Combined differentiating therapy for myelodysplastic syndromes: A phase II study. *Leuk Res* 20(10):867–876, 1996.

388. Hofmann WK, Koeffler HP: Differentiation therapy for myelodysplastic syndrome. *Clin Cancer Res* 8(4):939–941, 2002.

389. Kurzrock R, Cortes J, Thomas DA, et al: Pilot study of low-dose interleukin-11 in patients with bone marrow failure. *J Clin Oncol* 19(21):4165–4172, 2001.

390. Tsimberidou AM, Giles FJ, Khouri I, et al: Low-dose interleukin-11 in patients with bone marrow failure: Update of the M. D. Anderson Cancer Center experience. *Ann Oncol* 16(1):139–145, 2005.

391. Kuter DJ, Begley CG: Recombinant human thrombopoietin: Basic biology and evaluation of clinical studies. *Blood* 100(10):3457–3469, 2002.

392. Greenberg PL, Garcia-Manero G, Moore M, et al: A randomized controlled trial of romiplostim in patients with low- or intermediate-risk myelodysplastic syndrome receiving decitabine. *Leuk Lymphoma* 54(2):321–328, 2013.

393. Kantarjian H, Fenaux P, Sekeres MA, et al: Safety and efficacy of romiplostim in patients with lower-risk myelodysplastic syndrome and thrombocytopenia. *J Clin Oncol* 28(3):437–444, 2010.

394. Kantarjian IIM, Giles FJ, Greenberg PL, et al: Phase 2 study of romiplostim in patients with low- or intermediate-risk myelodysplastic syndrome receiving azacitidine therapy. *Blood* 116(17):3163–3170, 2010.

395. Sekeres MA, Kantarjian H, Fenaux P, et al: Subcutaneous or intravenous administration of romiplostim in thrombocytopenic patients with lower risk myelodysplastic syndromes. *Cancer* 117(5):992–1000, 2011.

396. Wroblewski S, Shi W, Mudd P Jr, Aivado M: Eltrombopag in thrombocytopenic patients with advanced myelodysplastic syndromes (MDS) or secondary acute myeloid leukemia after MDS: A phase I/II study. *J Clin Oncol.* 28:15s [abstract], 2010 (available at http://meetinglibrary.asco.org/content/53792-74).

397. Mavroudi I, Pyrovolaki K, Pavlaki K, et al: Effect of the nonpeptide thrombopoietin receptor agonist eltrombopag on megakaryopoiesis of patients with lower risk myelodysplastic syndrome. *Leuk Res* 2011;35(3):323–328, 2010.

398. Svensson T, Chowdhury O, Garelius H, et al: A pilot phase I dose finding safety study of the thrombopoietin-receptor agonist, eltrombopag, in patients with myelodysplastic syndrome treated with azacitidine. *Eur J Haematol* 93(5):439–445, 2014.

399. Tamari R, Schinke C, Bhagat T, et al: Eltrombopag can overcome the anti-megakaryopoietic effects of lenalidomide without increasing proliferation of the malignant myelodysplastic syndrome/acute myelogenous leukemia clone. *Leuk Lymphoma* 55(12):2901–2906, 2014.

400. Will B, Kawahara M, Luciano JP, et al: Effect of the nonpeptide thrombopoietin receptor agonist Eltrombopag on bone marrow cells from patients with acute myeloid leukemia and myelodysplastic syndrome. *Blood* 114(18):3899–3908, 2009.

401. Giagounidis A, Mufti GJ, Fenaux P, et al: Results of a randomized, double-blind study of romiplostim versus placebo in patients with low/intermediate-1-risk myelodysplastic syndrome and thrombocytopenia. *Cancer* 120(12):1838–1846, 2014.

402. Kuter DJ, Mufti GJ, Bain BJ, et al: Evaluation of bone marrow reticulin formation in chronic immune thrombocytopenia patients treated with romiplostim. *Blood* 114(18):3748–3756, 2009.

403. Steensma DP, Gattermann N: When is iron overload deleterious, and when and how should iron chelation therapy be administered in myelodysplastic syndromes? *Best Pract Res Clin Haematol* 26(4):431–444, 2013.

404. Steensma DP: The role of iron chelation therapy for patients with myelodysplastic syndromes. *J Natl Compr Canc Netw* 9(1):65–75, 2011.

405. Steensma DP: The relevance of iron overload and the appropriateness of iron chelation therapy for patients with myelodysplastic syndromes: A dialogue and debate. *Curr Hematol Malig Rep* 6(2):136–144, 2011.

406. Leitch HA: Controversies surrounding iron chelation therapy for MDS. *Blood Rev* 25(1):17–31, 2011.

407. Goldberg SL, Chen E, Sasane M, et al: Economic impact on US Medicare of a new diagnosis of myelodysplastic syndromes and the incremental costs associated with blood transfusion need. *Transfusion* 52(10):2131–2138, 2012.

408. Goldberg SL, Chen E, Corral M, et al: Incidence and clinical complications of myelodysplastic syndromes among United States Medicare beneficiaries. *J Clin Oncol* 28(17):2847–2852, 2010.

409. Leitch HA: Improving clinical outcome in patients with myelodysplastic syndrome and iron overload using iron chelation therapy. *Leuk Res* 31 Suppl 3:S7–S9, 2007.

410. Lyons RM, Marek BJ, Paley C, et al: Comparison of 24-month outcomes in chelated and non-chelated lower-risk patients with myelodysplastic syndromes in a prospective registry. *Leuk Res* 38(2):149–154, 2014.

411. Rose C, Brechignac S, Vassilief D, et al: Does iron chelation therapy improve survival in regularly transfused lower risk MDS patients? A multicenter study by the GFM (Groupe Francophone des Myelodysplasies). *Leuk Res* 34(7):864–870, 2010.

412. Neukirchen J, Fox F, Kundgen A, et al: Improved survival in MDS patients receiving iron chelation therapy-a matched pair analysis of 188 patients from the Dusseldorf MDS registry. *Leuk Res* 36(8):1067–1070, 2012.

413. Gattermann N: Overview of guidelines on iron chelation therapy in patients with myelodysplastic syndromes and transfusional iron overload. *Int J Hematol* 88(1):24–29, 2008.

414. Armand P, Kim HT, Cutler CS, et al: Prognostic impact of elevated pretransplantation serum ferritin in patients undergoing myeloablative stem cell transplantation. *Blood* 109(10):4586–4588, 2007.

415. Bennett JM; MDS Foundation's Working Group on Transfusional Iron Overload: Consensus statement on iron overload in myelodysplastic syndromes. *Am J Hematol* 83(11):858–861, 2008.

416. Wells RA, Leber B, Buckstein R, et al: Iron overload in myelodysplastic syndromes: A Canadian consensus guideline. *Leuk Res* 32(9):1338–1353, 2008.

417. Di Tucci AA, Matta G, Deplano S, et al: Myocardial iron overload assessment by T2* magnetic resonance imaging in adult transfusion dependent patients with acquired anemias. *Haematologica* 93(9):1385–1388, 2008.

418. List AF, Baer MR, Steensma DP, et al: Deferasirox reduces serum ferritin and labile plasma iron in RBC transfusion-dependent patients with myelodysplastic syndrome. *J Clin Oncol* 30(17):2134–2139, 2012.

419. Pullarkat V: Objectives of iron chelation therapy in myelodysplastic syndromes: More than meets the eye? *Blood* 114(26):5251–5255, 2009.

420. Cappellini MD, Porter J, El-Beshlawy A, et al: Tailoring iron chelation by iron intake and serum ferritin: The prospective EPIC study of deferasirox in 1744 patients with transfusion-dependent anemias. *Haematologica* 95(4):557–566, 2010.

421. Guariglia R, Martorelli MC, Villani O, et al: Positive effects on hematopoiesis in patients with myelodysplastic syndrome receiving deferasirox as oral iron chelation therapy: A brief review. *Leuk Res* 35(5):566–570, 2011.

422. Jensen PD, Heickendorff L, Pedersen B, et al: The effect of iron chelation on haemopoiesis in MDS patients with transfusional iron overload. *Br J Haematol* 94(2):288–299, 1996.

423. Wisch JS, Griffin JD, Kufe DW: Response of preleukemic syndromes to continuous infusion of low-dose cytarabine. *N Engl J Med* 309(26):1599–1602, 1983.

424. Mufti GJ, Oscier DG, Hamblin TJ, Bell AJ: Low doses of cytarabine in the treatment of myelodysplastic syndrome and acute myeloid leukemia. *N Engl J Med* 309(26):1653–1654, 1983.

425. Manoharan A: Low-dose cytarabine therapy in hypoplastic acute leukemia. *N Engl J Med* 309(26):1652–1653, 1983.

426. Hellstrom-Lindberg E, Robert KH, Gahrton G, et al: A predictive model for the clinical response to low dose ara-C: A study of 102 patients with myelodysplastic syndromes or acute leukaemia. *Br J Haematol* 81(4):503–511, 1992.

427. Ganser A, Seipelt G, Eder M, et al: Treatment of myelodysplastic syndromes with cytokines and cytotoxic drugs. *Semin Oncol* 19(2 Suppl 4):95–101, 1992.

428. Gerhartz HH, Marcus R, Delmer A, et al: A randomized phase II study of low-dose cytosine arabinoside (LD-AraC) plus granulocyte-macrophage colony-stimulating factor (rhGM-CSF) in myelodysplastic syndromes (MDS) with a high risk of developing leukemia. EORTC Leukemia Cooperative Group. *Leukemia* 8(1):16–23, 1994.

429. Aul C, Gattermann N: The role of low-dose chemotherapy in myelodysplastic syndromes. *Leuk Res* 16(3):207–215, 1992.

430. Miller KB, Kim K, Morrison FS, et al: The evaluation of low-dose cytarabine in the treatment of myelodysplastic syndromes: A phase-III intergroup study. *Ann Hematol* 65(4):162–168, 1992.

431. Fenaux P, Gattermann N, Seymour JF, et al: Prolonged survival with improved tolerability in higher-risk myelodysplastic syndromes: Azacitidine compared with low dose ara-C. *Br J Haematol* 149(2):244–249, 2010.

432. Visani G, Malagola M, Piccaluga PP, Isidori A: Low dose Ara-C for myelodysplastic syndromes: Is it still a current therapy? *Leuk Lymphoma* 45(8):1531–1538, 2004.

433. Sloand EM, Rezvani K: The role of the immune system in myelodysplasia: Implications for therapy. *Semin Hematol* 45(1):39–48, 2008.

434. Aivado M, Rong A, Stadler M, et al: Favourable response to antithymocyte or antilymphocyte globulin in low-risk myelodysplastic syndrome patients with a "non-clonal" pattern of X-chromosome inactivation in bone marrow cells. *Eur J Haematol* 68(4):210–216, 2002.

435. Selleri C, Maciejewski JP, Catalano L, et al: Effects of cyclosporine on hematopoietic and immune functions in patients with hypoplastic myelodysplasia: *In vitro* and *in vivo* studies. *Cancer* 95(9):1911–1922, 2002.

436. Yazji S, Giles FJ, Tsimberidou AM, et al: Antithymocyte globulin (ATG)-based therapy in patients with myelodysplastic syndromes. *Leukemia* 17(11):2101–2106, 2003.

437. Killick SB, Mufti G, Cavenagh JD, et al: A pilot study of antithymocyte globulin (ATG) in the treatment of patients with "low-risk" myelodysplasia. *Br J Haematol* 120(4):679–684, 2003.

438. Molldrem JJ, Caples M, Mavroudis D, et al: Antithymocyte globulin for patients with myelodysplastic syndrome. *Br J Haematol* 99(3):699–705, 1997.

439. Kadia TM, Borthakur G, Garcia-Manero G, et al: Final results of the phase II study of rabbit anti-thymocyte globulin, ciclosporin, methylprednisone, and granulocyte colony-stimulating factor in patients with aplastic anaemia and myelodysplastic syndrome. *Br J Haematol* 157(3):312–320, 2012.

440. Dixit A, Chatterjee T, Mishra P, et al: Cyclosporin A in myelodysplastic syndrome: A preliminary report. *Ann Hematol* 84(9):565–568, 2005.

441. Shimamoto T, Tohyama K, Okamoto T, et al: Cyclosporin A therapy for patients with myelodysplastic syndrome: Multicenter pilot studies in Japan. *Leuk Res* 27(9):783–788, 2003.

442. Nozaki Y, Nagare Y, Kinoshita K, et al: Successful treatment using tacrolimus plus corticosteroid in a patient with RA associated with MDS. *Rheumatol Int* 28(5):487–490, 2008.

443. Saunthararajah Y, Nakamura R, Nam JM, et al: HLA-DR15 (DR2) is overrepresented in myelodysplastic syndrome and aplastic anemia and predicts a response to immunosuppression in myelodysplastic syndrome. *Blood* 100(5):1570–1574, 2002.

444. Lim ZY, Killick S, Germing U, et al: Low IPSS score and bone marrow hypocellularity in MDS patients predict hematological responses to antithymocyte globulin. *Leukemia* 21(7):1436–1441, 2007.

445. Wang H, Chuhjo T, Yasue S, et al: Clinical significance of a minor population of paroxysmal nocturnal hemoglobinuria-type cells in bone marrow failure syndrome. *Blood* 100(12):3897–3902, 2002.

446. Steensma DP, Dispenzieri A, Moore SB, et al: Antithymocyte globulin has limited efficacy and substantial toxicity in unselected anemic patients with myelodysplastic syndrome. *Blood* 101(6):2156–2158, 2003.

447. Atoyebi W, Bywater L, Rawlings L, et al: Treatment of myelodysplasia with oral cyclosporin. *Clin Lab Haematol* 24(4):211–214, 2002.

448. Sloand EM, Olnes MJ, Shenoy A, et al: Alemtuzumab treatment of intermediate-1 myelodysplasia patients is associated with sustained improvement in blood counts and cytogenetic remissions. *J Clin Oncol* 28(35):5166–5173, 2010.

449. Moreno-Aspitia A, Geyer S, Li C, et al: N998B: Multicenter phase II trial of thalidomide (Thal) in adult patients with myelodysplastic syndromes (MDS). *Blood* 100:96a, 2002.

450. Zorat F, Shetty V, Dutt D, et al: The clinical and biological effects of thalidomide in patients with myelodysplastic syndromes. *Br J Haematol* 115(4):881–894, 2001.

451. Ito T, Ando H, Suzuki T, et al: Identification of a primary target of thalidomide teratogenicity. *Science* 327(5971):1345–1350, 2010.

452. Kronke J, Udeshi ND, Narla A, et al: Lenalidomide causes selective degradation of IKZF1 and IKZF3 in multiple myeloma cells. *Science* 343(6168):301–305, 2014.

453. Lu G, Middleton RE, Sun H, et al: The myeloma drug lenalidomide promotes the cereblon-dependent destruction of Ikaros proteins. *Science* 343(6168):305–309, 2014.

454. Zhu YX, Braggio E, Shi CX, et al: Identification of cereblon-binding proteins and relationship with response and survival after IMiDs in multiple myeloma. *Blood* 124(4):536–545, 2014.

455. Kotla V, Goel S, Nischal S, et al: Mechanism of action of lenalidomide in hematological malignancies. *J Hematol Oncol* 2:36, 2009.

456. List A, Kurtin S, Roe DJ, et al: Efficacy of lenalidomide in myelodysplastic syndromes. *N Engl J Med* 352(6):549–557, 2005.

457. Fenaux P, Giagounidis A, Selleslag D, et al: A randomized phase 3 study of lenalidomide versus placebo in RBC transfusion-dependent patients with Low-/Intermediate-1-risk myelodysplastic syndromes with del5q. *Blood* 118(14):3765–3776, 2011.

458. Sekeres MA, Maciejewski JP, Giagounidis AA, et al: Relationship of treatment-related cytopenias and response to lenalidomide in patients with lower-risk myelodysplastic syndromes. *J Clin Oncol* 26(36):5943–5949, 2008.

459. Raza A, Reeves JA, Feldman EJ, et al: Phase 2 study of lenalidomide in transfusion-dependent, low-risk, and intermediate-1 risk myelodysplastic syndromes with karyotypes other than deletion 5q. *Blood* 111(1):86–93, 2008.

460. Fehniger TA, Byrd JC, Marcucci G, et al: Single-agent lenalidomide induces complete remission of acute myeloid leukemia in patients with isolated trisomy 13. *Blood* 113(5):1002–1005, 2009.

461. Deeg HJ, Gotlib J, Beckham C, et al: Soluble TNF receptor fusion protein (etanercept) for the treatment of myelodysplastic syndrome: A pilot study. *Leukemia* 16(2):162–164, 2002.

462. Rosenfeld C, Bedell C: Pilot study of recombinant human soluble tumor necrosis factor receptor (TNFR:Fc) in patients with low risk myelodysplastic syndrome. *Leuk Res* 26(8):721–724, 2002.

463. Maciejewski JP, Risitano AM, Sloand EM, et al: A pilot study of the recombinant soluble human tumour necrosis factor receptor (p75)-Fc fusion protein in patients with myelodysplastic syndrome. *Br J Haematol* 117(1):119–126, 2002.

464. Stasi R, Amadori S: Infliximab chimaeric anti-tumour necrosis factor alpha monoclonal antibody treatment for patients with myelodysplastic syndromes. *Br J Haematol* 116(2):334–337, 2002.

465. Scott BL, Ramakrishnan A, Fosdal M, et al: Anti-thymocyte globulin plus etanercept as therapy for myelodysplastic syndromes (MDS): A phase II study. *Br J Haematol* 149(5):706–710, 2010.

466. Scott BL, Ramakrishnan A, Storer B, et al: Prolonged responses in patients with MDS and CMML treated with azacitidine and etanercept. *Br J Haematol* 148(6):944–947, 2010.

467. Yaguchi M, Miyazawa K, Katagiri T, et al: Vitamin K2 and its derivatives induce apoptosis in leukemia cells and enhance the effect of all-*trans* retinoic acid. *Leukemia* 11(6):779–787, 1997.

468. Takami A, Nakao S, Ontachi Y, et al: Successful therapy of myelodysplastic syndrome with menatetrenone, a vitamin K2 analog. *Int J Hematol* 69(1):24–26, 1999.

469. Nagler A, Rikilis I, Tatarsky I, Fabian I: Effect of 1,25-dihydroxyvitamin D3 and 13-*cis*-retinoic acid on *in vitro* hematopoiesis in the myelodysplastic syndromes. *J Lab Clin Med* 110(2):237–244, 1987.

470. Rowinsky EK, Conley BA, Jones RJ, et al: Hexamethylene bisacetamide in myelodysplastic syndrome: Effect of five-day exposure to maximal therapeutic concentrations. *Leukemia* 6(6):526–534, 1992.

471. Tefferi A, Elliott MA, Steensma DP, et al: Amifostine alone and in combination with erythropoietin for the treatment of favorable myelodysplastic syndrome. *Leuk Res* 25(2):183–185, 2001.

472. Raza A, Qawi H, Lisak L, et al: Patients with myelodysplastic syndromes benefit from palliative therapy with amifostine, pentoxifylline, and ciprofloxacin with or without dexamethasone. *Blood* 95(5):1580–1587, 2000.

473. Jantunen E, Ruutu P, Niskanen L, et al: Incidence and risk factors for invasive fungal infections in allogeneic BMT recipients. *Bone Marrow Transplant* 19(8):801–808, 1997.

474. Hast R, Axdorph S, Lauren L, Reizenstein P: Absent clinical effects of retinoic acid and isoretinoin treatment in the myelodysplastic syndrome. *Hematol Oncol* 7(4):297–301, 1989.

475. Ohno R, Naoe T, Hirano M, et al: Treatment of myelodysplastic syndromes with all-*trans* retinoic acid. Leukemia Study Group of the Ministry of Health and Welfare. *Blood* 81(5):1152–1154, 1993.

476. List A, Beran M, DiPersio J, et al: Opportunities for Trisenox (arsenic trioxide) in the treatment of myelodysplastic syndromes. *Leukemia* 17(8):1499–1507, 2003.

477. Sekeres MA, Maciejewski JP, Erba HP, et al: A Phase 2 study of combination therapy with arsenic trioxide and gemtuzumab ozogamicin in patients with myelodysplastic syndromes or secondary acute myeloid leukemia. *Cancer* 117(6):1253–1261, 2011.

478. Bejanyan N, Tiu RV, Raza A, et al: A phase 2 trial of combination therapy with thalidomide, arsenic trioxide, dexamethasone, and ascorbic acid (TADA) in patients with overlap myelodysplastic/myeloproliferative neoplasms (MDS/MPN) or primary myelofibrosis (PMF). *Cancer* 118(16):3968–3976, 2011.

479. Schiller GJ, Slack J, Hainsworth JD, et al: Phase II multicenter study of arsenic trioxide in patients with myelodysplastic syndromes. *J Clin Oncol* 24(16):2456–2464, 2006.

480. Terpos E, Verrou E, Banti A, et al: Bortezomib is an effective agent for MDS/MPD syndrome with 5q– anomaly and thrombocytosis. *Leuk Res* 31(4):559–562, 2007.

481. Braun T, Carvalho G, Coquelle A, et al: NF-kappaB constitutes a potential therapeutic target in high-risk myelodysplastic syndrome. *Blood* 107(3):1156–1165, 2006.

482. Attar EC, Amrein PC, Fraser JW, et al: Phase I dose escalation study of bortezomib in combination with lenalidomide in patients with myelodysplastic syndromes (MDS) and acute myeloid leukemia (AML). *Leuk Res* 37(9):1016–1020, 2013.

483. Maeda Y, Yamaguchi T, Hijikata Y, et al: Possible molecular target therapy with rapamycin in MDS. *Leuk Lymphoma* 47(5):907–911, 2006.

484. Follo MY, Mongiorgi S, Bosi C, et al: The Akt/mammalian target of rapamycin signal transduction pathway is activated in high-risk myelodysplastic syndromes and influences cell survival and proliferation. *Cancer Res* 67(9):4287–4294, 2007.

485. Carrancio S, Markovics J, Wong P, et al: An activin receptor IIA ligand trap promotes erythropoiesis resulting in a rapid induction of red blood cells and haemoglobin. *Br J Haematol* 165(6):870–882, 2014.

486. Bachegowda L, Gligich O, Mantzaris I, et al: Signal transduction inhibitors in treatment of myelodysplastic syndromes. *J Hematol Oncol* 6:50, 2013.

487. Cortes J, Giles F, O'Brien S, et al: Results of imatinib mesylate therapy in patients with refractory or recurrent acute myeloid leukemia, high-risk myelodysplastic syndrome, and myeloproliferative disorders. *Cancer* 97(11):2760–2766, 2003.

488. Gunby RH, Cazzaniga G, Tassi E, et al: Sensitivity to imatinib but low frequency of the TEL/PDGFRbeta fusion protein in chronic myelomonocytic leukemia. *Haematologica* 88(4):408–415, 2003.

489. Raza A, Galili N, Smith S, et al: Phase 1 multicenter dose-escalation study of ezatiostat hydrochloride (TLK199 tablets), a novel glutathione analog prodrug, in patients with myelodysplastic syndrome. *Blood* 113(26):6533–6540, 2009.

490. Raza A, Galili N, Mulford D, et al: Phase 1 dose-ranging study of ezatiostat hydrochloride in combination with lenalidomide in patients with non-deletion (5q) low to intermediate-1 risk myelodysplastic syndrome (MDS). *J Hematol Oncol* 5:18, 2012.

491. Raza A, Galili N, Callander N, et al: Phase 1–2a multicenter dose-escalation study of ezatiostat hydrochloride liposomes for injection (Telintra, TLK199), a novel glutathione analog prodrug in patients with myelodysplastic syndrome. *J Hematol Oncol* 2:20, 2009.

492. Leone G, Teofili L, Voso MT, Lubbert M: DNA methylation and demethylating drugs in myelodysplastic syndromes and secondary leukemias. *Haematologica* 87(12):1324–1341, 2002.

493. Quesnel B, Fenaux P: P15INK4b gene methylation and myelodysplastic syndromes. *Leuk Lymphoma* 35(5–6):437–443, 1999.

494. Silverman LR: Targeting hypomethylation of DNA to achieve cellular differentiation in myelodysplastic syndromes (MDS). *Oncologist* 6 (Suppl 5):8–14, 2001.

495. Saunthararajah Y, Hillery CA, Lavelle D, et al: Effects of 5-aza-2′-deoxycytidine on fetal hemoglobin levels, red cell adhesion, and hematopoietic differentiation in patients with sickle cell disease. *Blood* 102(12):3865–3870, 2003.

496. Goodyear OC, Dennis M, Jilani NY, et al: Azacitidine augments expansion of regulatory T cells after allogeneic stem cell transplantation in patients with acute myeloid leukemia (AML). *Blood* 119(14):3361–3369, 2012.

497. de Vos D: Epigenetic drugs: A longstanding story. *Semin Oncol* 32(5):437–442, 2005.

498. Palii SS, Van Emburgh BO, Sankpal UT, et al: DNA methylation inhibitor 5-Aza-2′-deoxycytidine induces reversible genome-wide DNA damage that is distinctly influenced by DNA methyltransferases 1 and 3B. *Mol Cell Biol* 28(2):752–771, 2008.

499. Fabre C, Grosjean J, Tailler M, et al: A novel effect of DNA methyltransferase and histone deacetylase inhibitors: NFkappaB inhibition in malignant myeloblasts. *Cell Cycle* 7(14):2139–2145, 2008.

500. Itzykson R, Fenaux P: Optimizing hypomethylating agents in myelodysplastic syndromes. *Curr Opin Hematol* 19(2):65–70, 2012.

501. Baer MR, Gojo I: Novel agents for the treatment of acute myeloid leukemia in the older patient. *J Natl Compr Canc Netw* 9(3):331–335, 2011.

502. Garcia-Manero G. Demethylating agents in myeloid malignancies. *Curr Opin Oncol* 20(6):705–710, 2008.

503. Silverman LR, Demakos EP, Peterson BL, et al: Randomized controlled trial of azacitidine in patients with the myelodysplastic syndrome: A study of the cancer and leukemia group B. *J Clin Oncol* 20(10):2429–2440, 2002.

504. Silverman LR, McKenzie DR, Peterson BL, et al: Further analysis of trials with azacitidine in patients with myelodysplastic syndrome: Studies 8421, 8921, and 9221 by the Cancer and Leukemia Group B. *J Clin Oncol* 24(24):3895–3903, 2006.

505. Silverman LR, Fenaux P, Mufti GJ, et al: The effects of continued azacitidine treatment cycles on response in higher risk patients with myelodysplastic syndromes: An update. *Ecancermedicalscience* 2:118, 2008.

506. Gryn J, Zeigler ZR, Shadduck RK, et al: Treatment of myelodysplastic syndromes with 5-azacytidine. *Leuk Res* 26(10):893–897, 2002.

507. Fenaux P, Mufti GJ, Hellstrom-Lindberg E, et al: Efficacy of azacitidine compared with that of conventional care regimens in the treatment of higher-risk myelodysplastic syndromes: A randomised, open-label, phase III study. *Lancet Oncol* 10(3):223–232, 2009.

508. Sekeres MA, Maciejewski JP, Donley DW, et al: A study comparing dosing regimens and efficacy of subcutaneous to intravenous azacitidine (AZA) for the treatment of myelodysplastic syndromes (MDS). *ASH Annu Meet Abstr* 114(22):3797, 2009.

509. Garcia-Manero G, Stoltz ML, Ward MR, et al: A pilot pharmacokinetic study of oral azacitidine. *Leukemia* 22(9):1680–1684, 2008.

510. Lyons RM, Cosgriff TM, Modi SS, et al: Hematologic response to three alternative dosing schedules of azacitidine in patients with myelodysplastic syndromes. *J Clin Oncol* 27(11):1850–1856, 2009.

511. Platzbecker U, Aul C, Ehninger G, Giagounidis A: Reduction of 5-azacitidine induced skin reactions in MDS patients with evening primrose oil. *Ann Hematol* 89(4):427–428, 2010.

512. Qin T, Castoro R, El Ahdab S, et al: Mechanisms of resistance to decitabine in the myelodysplastic syndrome. *PLoS One* 6(8):e23372, 2011.

513. Steensma DP, Baer MR, Slack JL, et al: Multicenter study of decitabine administered daily for 5 days every 4 weeks to adults with myelodysplastic syndromes: The alternative dosing for outpatient treatment (ADOPT) trial. *J Clin Oncol* 27(23):3842–3848, 2009.

514. Kantarjian H, Issa JP, Rosenfeld CS, et al: Decitabine improves patient outcomes in myelodysplastic syndromes: Results of a phase III randomized study. *Cancer* 106(8):1794–1803, 2006.

515. Lubbert M, Wijermans P, Kunzmann R, et al: Cytogenetic responses in high-risk myelodysplastic syndrome following low-dose treatment with the DNA methylation inhibitor 5-aza-2′-deoxycytidine. *Br J Haematol* 114(2):349–357, 2001.

516. Kantarjian H, Oki Y, Garcia-Manero G, et al: Results of a randomized study of 3 schedules of low-dose decitabine in higher-risk myelodysplastic syndrome and chronic myelomonocytic leukemia. *Blood* 109(1):52–57, 2007.

517. Blum W, Garzon R, Klisovic RB, et al: Clinical response and miR-29b predictive significance in older AML patients treated with a 10-day schedule of decitabine. *Proc Natl Acad Sci U S A* 107(16):7473–7478, 2010.

518. Blum W: How much? How frequent? How long? A clinical guide to new therapies in myelodysplastic syndromes. *Hematology Am Soc Hematol Educ Program* 2010:314–321, 2010.

519. Daskalakis M, Nguyen TT, Nguyen C, et al: Demethylation of a hypermethylated P15/INK4B gene in patients with myelodysplastic syndrome by 5-Aza-2′-deoxycytidine (decitabine) treatment. *Blood* 100(8):2957–2964, 2002.

520. Shen L, Kantarjian H, Guo Y, et al: DNA methylation predicts survival and response to therapy in patients with myelodysplastic syndromes. *J Clin Oncol* 28(4):605–613, 2010.

521. Klisovic RB, Stock W, Cataland S, et al: A phase I biological study of MG98, an oligodeoxynucleotide antisense to DNA methyltransferase 1, in patients with high-risk myelodysplasia and acute myeloid leukemia. *Clin Cancer Res* 14(8):2444–2449, 2008.

522. Gerds AT, Gooley TA, Estey EH, et al: Pretransplantation therapy with azacitidine vs. induction chemotherapy and posttransplantation outcome in patients with MDS. *Biol Blood Marrow Transplant* 18(8):1211–1218, 2012.

523. Quintas-Cardama A, Santos FP, Garcia-Manero G. Histone deacetylase inhibitors for the treatment of myelodysplastic syndrome and acute myeloid leukemia. *Leukemia* 25(2):226–235, 2011.

524. Prebet T, Vey N: Vorinostat in acute myeloid leukemia and myelodysplastic syndromes. *Expert Opin Investig Drugs* 20(2):287–295, 2011.

525. Kuendgen A, Bug G, Ottmann OG, et al: Treatment of poor-risk myelodysplastic syndromes and acute myeloid leukemia with a combination of 5-azacytidine and valproic acid. *Clin Epigenetics* 2(2):389–399, 2011.

526. Voso MT, Santini V, Finelli C, et al: Valproic acid at therapeutic plasma levels may increase 5-azacytidine efficacy in higher risk myelodysplastic syndromes. *Clin Cancer Res* 15(15):5002–5007, 2009.

527. Garcia-Manero G, Assouline S, Cortes J, et al: Phase 1 study of the oral isotype specific histone deacetylase inhibitor MGCD0103 in leukemia. *Blood* 112(4):981–989, 2008.

528. Ottmann OG, DeAngelo DJ, Garcia-Manero G, et al: Determination of a phase II dose of panobinostat in combination with 5-azacitidine in patients with myelodysplastic syndromes, chronic myelomonocytic leukemia, or acute myeloid leukemia. *Blood (ASH Annu Meet Abstr)* 118:459, 2011.

529. Cashen A, Juckett M, Jumonville A, et al: Phase II study of the histone deacetylase inhibitor belinostat (PXD101) for the treatment of myelodysplastic syndrome (MDS). *Ann Hematol* 91(1):33–38, 2012.

530. Sekeres MA, O'Keefe C, List AF, et al: Demonstration of additional benefit in adding lenalidomide to azacitidine in patients with higher-risk myelodysplastic syndromes. *Am J Hematol* 86(1):102–103, 2011.

531. Silverman LR, Verma A, Odchimar-Reissig R, et al: Abstract #386: A phase II trial of epigenetic modulators vorinostat in combination with azacitidine (azaC) in patients with the myelodysplastic syndrome (MDS): Initial results of study 6898 of the New York Cancer Consortium. *Blood (ASH Annu Meet Abstr)* 122(11a).

532. Garcia-Manero G, Estey E, Jabbour E, et al: Final report of a phase II study of 5-azacitidine and vorinostat in patients with newly diagnosed myelodysplastic syndrome or acute myelogenous leukemia not eligible for clinical trials because poor performance and presence of other comorbidities. *Blood (ASH Annu Meet Abstr)* 118:608, 2011.

533. Prebet T, Gore SD, Sun Z, et al: Prolonged administration of azacitidine with or without entinostat increases rate of hematologic normalization for myelodysplastic syndrome and acute myeloid leukemia with myelodysplasia-related changes: Results of the US Leukemia Intergroup Trial E1905. *J Clin Oncol.* 20;32(12):1242-8, 2014.

534. Prebet T, Gore SD, Esterni B, et al: Outcome of high-risk myelodysplastic syndrome after azacitidine treatment failure. *J Clin Oncol* 29(24):3322–3327, 2011.

535. Jabbour E, Garcia-Manero G, Batty N, et al: Outcome of patients with myelodysplastic syndrome after failure of decitabine therapy. *Cancer* 116(16):3830–3834, 2010.

536. Guillermo Garcia-Manero, Pierre Fenaux, Aref Al-Kali, et al: Overall survival and subgroup analysis from a randomized phase III study of intravenous rigosertib versus best supportive care (BSC) in patients (pts) with higher-risk myelodysplastic ssyndrome (HR-MDS) after failure of hypomethylating agents (HMAs). *Blood (ASH Annu Meet Abstr)* 163(124).

537. Komrokji RS, Raza A, Lancet JE, et al: Phase I clinical trial of oral rigosertib in patients with myelodysplastic syndromes. *Br J Haematol* 162(4):517–524, 2013.

538. Singh V, Sharma P, Capalash N: DNA methyltransferase-1 inhibitors as epigenetic therapy for cancer. *Curr Cancer Drug Targets* 13(4):379–399, 2013.

539. Coral S, Parisi G, Nicolay HJ, et al: Immunomodulatory activity of SGI-110, a 5-aza-2′-deoxycytidine-containing demethylating dinucleotide. *Cancer Immunol Immunother* 62(3):605–614, 2013.

540. Fenaux P, Mufti GJ, Hellstrom-Lindberg E, et al: Azacitidine prolongs overall survival compared with conventional care regimens in elderly patients with low bone marrow blast count acute myeloid leukemia. *J Clin Oncol* 28(4):562–569, 2010.

541. Beran M, Shen Y, Kantarjian H, et al: High-dose chemotherapy in high-risk myelodysplastic syndrome: Covariate-adjusted comparison of five regimens. *Cancer* 92(8):1999–2015, 2001.

542. Knipp S, Hildebrand B, Kundgen A, et al: Intensive chemotherapy is not recommended for patients aged >60 years who have myelodysplastic syndromes or acute myeloid leukemia with high-risk karyotypes. *Cancer* 110(2):345–352, 2007.

543. Cortes J, Kantarjian H, Albitar M, et al: A randomized trial of liposomal daunorubicin and cytarabine versus liposomal daunorubicin and topotecan with or without thalidomide as initial therapy for patients with poor prognosis acute myelogenous leukemia or myelodysplastic syndrome. *Cancer* 97(5):1234–1241, 2003.

544. de la Rubia J, Regadera A, Martin G, et al: FLAG-IDA regimen (fludarabine, cytarabine, idarubicin, and G-CSF) in the treatment of patients with high-risk myeloid malignancies. *Leuk Res* 26(8):725–730, 2002.

545. Marcondes M, Deeg HJ: Hematopoietic cell transplantation for patients with myelodysplastic syndromes (MDS): When, how and for whom? *Best Pract Res Clin Haematol* 21(1):67–77, 2008.

546. Oliansky DM, Antin JH, Bennett JM, et al: The role of cytotoxic therapy with hematopoietic stem cell transplantation in the therapy of myelodysplastic syndromes: An evidence-based review. *Biol Blood Marrow Transplant* 15(2):137–172, 2009.

547. Hahn T, McCarthy PL Jr, Hassebroek A, et al: Significant improvement in survival after allogeneic hematopoietic cell transplantation during a period of significantly increased use, older recipient age, and use of unrelated donors. *J Clin Oncol* 31(19):2437–2449, 2013.

548. Cutler CS, Lee SJ, Greenberg P, et al: A decision analysis of allogeneic bone marrow transplantation for the myelodysplastic syndromes: Delayed transplantation for low-risk myelodysplasia is associated with improved outcome. *Blood* 104(2):579–585, 2004.

549. Koreth J, Pidala J, Perez WS, et al: Role of reduced-intensity conditioning allogeneic hematopoietic stem-cell transplantation in older patients with *de novo* myelodysplastic syndromes: An international collaborative decision analysis. *J Clin Oncol* 31(21):2662–2670, 2013.

550. Castro-Malaspina H, Harris RE, Gajewski J, et al: Unrelated donor marrow transplantation for myelodysplastic syndromes: Outcome analysis in 510 transplants facilitated by the National Marrow Donor Program. *Blood* 99(6):1943–1951, 2002.

551. Armand P, Kim HT, DeAngelo DJ, et al: Impact of cytogenetics on outcome of *de novo* and therapy-related AML and MDS after allogeneic transplantation. *Biol Blood Marrow Transplant* 13(6):655–664, 2007.

552. Warlick ED, Cioc A, Defor T, et al: Allogeneic stem cell transplantation for adults with myelodysplastic syndromes: Importance of pretransplant disease burden. *Biol Blood Marrow Transplant* 15(1):30–38, 2009.

553. Chang C, Storer BE, Scott BL, et al: Hematopoietic cell transplantation in patients with myelodysplastic syndrome or acute myeloid leukemia arising from myelodysplastic syndrome: Similar outcomes in patients with de novo disease and disease following prior therapy or antecedent hematologic disorders. *Blood* 110(4):1379–1387, 2007.

554. Kroger N, Brand R, van Biezen A, et al: Risk factors for therapy-related myelodysplastic syndrome and acute myeloid leukemia treated with allogeneic stem cell transplantation. *Haematologica* 94(4):542–549, 2009.

555. Scott BL, Park JY, Deeg HJ, et al: Pretransplant neutropenia is associated with poor-risk cytogenetic features and increased infection-related mortality in patients with myelodysplastic syndromes. *Biol Blood Marrow Transplant* 14(7):799–806, 2008.

556. Platzbecker U, Schetelig J, Finke J, et al: Allogeneic hematopoietic cell transplantation in patients aged 60–70 years with *de novo* high-risk myelodysplastic syndrome or secondary acute myelogenous leukemia: Comparison with patients lacking donors who received azacitidine. *Biol Blood Marrow Transplant* 18(9):1415–1421, 2012.

557. Kim DY, Lee JH, Park YH, et al: Feasibility of hypomethylating agents followed by allogeneic hematopoietic cell transplantation in patients with myelodysplastic syndrome. *Bone Marrow Transplant* 47(3):374–379, 2012.

558. Platzbecker U, Wermke M, Radke J, et al: Azacitidine for treatment of imminent relapse in MDS or AML patients after allogeneic HSCT: Results of the RELAZA trial. *Leukemia* 26(3):381–389, 2012.

559. Luger SM, Ringden O, Zhang MJ, et al: Similar outcomes using myeloablative vs reduced-intensity allogeneic transplant preparative regimens for AML or MDS. *Bone Marrow Transplant* 47(2):203–211, 2012.

560. Pollyea DA, Artz AS, Stock W, et al: Outcomes of patients with AML and MDS who relapse or progress after reduced intensity allogeneic hematopoietic cell transplantation. *Bone Marrow Transplant* 40(11):1027–1032, 2007.

561. Campregher PV, Gooley T, Scott BL, et al: Results of donor lymphocyte infusions for relapsed myelodysplastic syndrome after hematopoietic cell transplantation. *Bone Marrow Transplant* 40(10):965–971, 2007.

562. de Witte T, Oosterveld M, Muus P: Autologous and allogeneic stem cell transplantation for myelodysplastic syndrome. *Blood Rev* 21(1):49–59, 2007.

563. de Witte T, Suciu S, Brand R, et al: Autologous stem cell transplantation in myelodysplastic syndromes. *Semin Hematol* 44(4):274–277, 2007.

564. de Witte T, Van Biezen A, Hermans J, et al: Autologous bone marrow transplantation for patients with myelodysplastic syndrome (MDS) or acute myeloid leukemia following MDS. Chronic and Acute Leukemia Working Parties of the European Group for Blood and Marrow Transplantation. *Blood* 90(10):3853–3857, 1997.

565. Wattel E, Solary E, Leleu X, et al: A prospective study of autologous bone marrow or peripheral blood stem cell transplantation after intensive chemotherapy in myelodysplastic syndromes. Groupe Francais des Myelodysplasies. Group Ouest-Est d'etude des Leucemies aigues myeloides. *Leukemia* 13(4):524–529, 1999.

566. Viola A, Falco C, D'Elia R, et al: An antecedent diagnosis of refractory anemia with excess blasts has no influence on mobilization of peripheral blood stem cells and hematopoietic recovery after autologous stem cell transplantation in acute myeloid leukemia. *Eur J Haematol* 78(1):41–47, 2007.

567. Burnett AK, Milligan D, Prentice AG, et al: A comparison of low-dose cytarabine and hydroxyurea with or without all-*trans* retinoic acid for acute myeloid leukemia and high-risk myelodysplastic syndrome in patients not considered fit for intensive treatment. *Cancer* 109(6):1114–1124, 2007.

568. Ogata K, Nomura T: Application of low-dose etoposide therapy for myelodysplastic syndromes. *Leuk Lymphoma* 12(1–2):35–39, 1993.

569. Robak T, Szmigielska-Kaplon A, Urbanska-Rys H, et al: Efficacy and toxicity of low-dose melphalan in myelodysplastic syndromes and acute myeloid leukemia with multi-lineage dysplasia. *Neoplasma* 50(3):172–175, 2003.

570. Mario AD, Pagano L, Mele L, et al: Use of gemcitabine (GEM) in advanced myelodysplastic syndromes. *Ann Oncol* 12(10):1494, 2001.

571. Ribrag V, Suzan F, Ravoet C, et al: Phase II trial of CPT-11 in myelodysplastic syndromes with excess of marrow blasts. *Leukemia* 17(2):319–322, 2003.

572. Giles FJ, Faderl S, Thomas DA, et al: Randomized phase I/II study of troxacitabine combined with cytarabine, idarubicin, or topotecan in patients with refractory myeloid leukemias. *J Clin Oncol* 21(6):1050–1056, 2003.

573. Giles FJ, Garcia-Manero G, Cortes JE, et al: Phase II study of troxacitabine, a novel dioxolane nucleoside analog, in patients with refractory leukemia. *J Clin Oncol* 20(3):656–664, 2002.

574. Bouabdallah R, Lefrere F, Rose C, et al: A phase II trial of induction and consolidation therapy of acute myeloid leukemia with weekly oral idarubicin alone in poor risk elderly patients. *Leukemia* 13(10):1491–1496, 1999.

575. Bryan J, Kantarjian H, Prescott H, Jabbour E: Clofarabine in the treatment of myelodysplastic syndromes. *Expert Opin Investig Drugs* 23(2):255–263, 2014.

576. Walter MJ, Shen D, Ding L, et al: Clonal architecture of secondary acute myeloid leukemia. *N Engl J Med* 366(12):1090–1098, 2012.

577. Steensma DP: Dysplasia has a differential diagnosis: Distinguishing genuine myelodysplastic syndromes (MDS) from mimics, imitators, copycats and impostors. *Curr Hematol Malig Rep* 7(4):310–320, 2012.

578. Vardiman JW, Thiele J, Arber DA, et al: The 2008 revision of the World Health Organization (WHO) classification of myeloid neoplasms and acute leukemia: Rationale and important changes. *Blood* 114(5):937–951, 2009.

579. Greenberg P, Cox C, LeBeau MM, et al: International scoring system for evaluating prognosis in myelodysplastic syndromes. *Blood* 89(6):2079–2088, 1997.

CHAPTER 88
ACUTE MYELOGENOUS LEUKEMIA

Jane L. Liesveld and Marshall A. Lichtman

SUMMARY

Acute myelogenous leukemia (AML) is the result of a sequence of somatic mutations in a primitive multipotential hematopoietic cell. Exposure to radiation, chronic exposure to high doses of benzene, and chronic inhalation of tobacco smoke increase the incidence of the disease. Obesity has been found to be an endogenous risk factor. A small but increasing proportion of cases develop after a patient with lymphoma, a nonhematologic cancer, or an autoimmune disorder is exposed to intensive chemotherapy, especially with alkylating agents or topoisomerase II inhibitors. The mutant (leukemic) hematopoietic cell acquires the features of a leukemic stem cell capable of self-renewal and desultory differentiation and maturation. It gains a growth and survival advantage in relationship to the normal polyclonal pool of hematopoietic stem cells. As the progeny of this mutant, now leukemic, multipotential cell proliferates to form approximately 10 to 100 billion or more cells, normal hematopoiesis is inhibited, and normal red cell, neutrophil, and platelet blood levels fall. The resultant anemia leads to weakness, exertional limitations, and pallor; the thrombocytopenia to spontaneous hemorrhage, usually in the skin and mucous membranes; and the neutropenia and monocytopenia to poor wound healing and minor infections. Severe infection usually does not occur at diagnosis, but often does if the disease progresses because of lack of treatment or if chemotherapy intensifies the decrease of blood neutrophil and monocyte levels. The diagnosis is made by measurement of blood cell counts and examination of blood and marrow cells and is based on identification of leukemic blast cells in the blood and marrow. The diagnosis of the myelogenous form of acute leukemia is confirmed specifically by identification of myeloperoxidase activity in blast cells or by identifying characteristic cluster of differentiation (CD) antigens on the blast cells (e.g., CD13, CD33). Because the leukemic stem cell is capable of imperfect differentiation and maturation, the clone may contain cells that have the morphologic or immunophenotypic features of erythroblasts, megakaryocytes, monocytes, eosinophils, or, rarely, basophils or mast cells, in addition to myeloblasts or promyelocytes. When one cell line is sufficiently dominant, the leukemia may be referred to by that lineage: for example, acute erythroid, acute megakaryocytic, acute monocytic leukemia, and so on. Certain cytogenetic alterations are more frequent; these abnormalities include t(8;21), t(15;17), inversion 16 or t(16;16), trisomy 8, and deletions of all or part of chromosome 5 or 7. A translocation involving chromosome 17 at the site of the retinoic acid receptor–a (RAR-a) gene is uniquely associated with acute promyelocytic leukemia. AML usually is treated with cytarabine and an anthracycline antibiotic, although other drugs may be added or substituted in poor-prognosis, older, refractory, or relapsed patients. The exception to this approach is the treatment of acute promyelocytic leukemia with all-trans-retinoic acid, arsenic trioxide, and sometimes an anthracycline antibiotic. High-dose chemotherapy and either autologous stem cell infusion or allogeneic hematopoietic stem cell transplantation may be used in an effort to treat relapse or patients at high risk to relapse after chemotherapy treatment. The probability of remission in acute myelogenous leukemia ranges from approximately 80 percent in children to less than 25 percent in octogenarians. The probability for cure decreases from approximately 50 percent in children to virtually zero in octogenarians.

● DEFINITION AND HISTORY

Acute myelogenous leukemia (AML) is a clonal, malignant disease of hematopoietic tissues that is characterized by (1) accumulation of abnormal (leukemic) blast cells, principally in the marrow, and (2) impaired production of normal blood cells. Thus, the leukemic cell infiltration in marrow is accompanied, nearly invariably, by anemia and thrombocytopenia. The absolute neutrophil count may be low or normal, depending on the total white cell count.

The first well-documented case of acute leukemia is attributed to Friedreich,[1] but Ebstein[2] was the first to use the term *acute leukämie* in 1889. This work led to the general appreciation of the clinical distinctions between AML and chronic myelogenous leukemia (CML).[3] In 1878, Neumann,[4] who proposed that marrow was the site of blood cell production, first suggested that leukemia originated in the marrow and used the term *myelogene* (myelogenous) leukemia. The availability of polychromatic stains, as a result of the work of Ehrlich,[5] the description of the myeloblast and myelocyte by Naegeli,[6] and the earliest appreciation of the common origin of red cells and leukocytes by Hirschfield[7] laid the foundation for our current understanding of the disease.

Although Theodor Boveri proposed a critical role for chromosomal abnormalities in the development of cancer in 1914, a series of technical developments in the 1950s was needed to permit informed examination of the chromosomes of human cancer cells. Thereafter, the discovery that a G group chromosome consistently had a foreshortened long arm in the cells of patients with CML (Philadelphia chromosome) supported the concept that chromosome abnormalities may be specifically linked to a cancer phenotype. This finding was followed by the introduction of banding of chromosomes, which enhanced the specific identification of individual chromosomes and the point at which they break in the formation of a translocation, inversion, or deletion. This technologic advance unleashed the power of cancer cytogenetics and initiated an era of leukemia study based not solely on the appearance of cells under the microscope (phenotype) but also by their chromosomal or genetic abnormality (genotype).[8] The completion of the human genome project further enhanced the specificity of the identification of gene alterations.[9] These advances permitted (1) more precise understanding of the molecular pathology of specific leukemia subtypes, (2) improvement of diagnostic and prognostic methods for the study of AML, and (3) identification of molecular targets for therapy.

The introduction to the clinic by Holland, Ellison, and colleagues[10] of arabinosyl cytosine (cytarabine) in the late 1960s as the first potent drug for treatment of AML, followed by their introduction of the combination of 7 days of cytosine arabinoside and 3 days of daunorubicin in the early 1970s (the "7 plus 3 regimen")[11] opened the era of effective therapy for AML. This drug combination or its congeners remains the mainstay of treatment over 4 decades later.[12] The description of allogeneic marrow (stem cell) transplantation as a curative therapy for AML by Thomas and colleagues[13] in 1977 ushered in the era of hematopoietic stem cell (HSC) transplantation as a modality to cure eligible patients with AML.

ETIOLOGY AND PATHOGENESIS

ENVIRONMENTAL FACTORS

Table 88-1 lists the major conditions that predispose to development of AML. Only four environmental factors are established causal agents: high-dose radiation exposure,[14,15] chronic, high-dose benzene exposure (≥40 parts per million [ppm]-years),[16-18] chronic tobacco smoking,[19] and chemotherapeutic (DNA-damaging) agents.[20-22] Most patients have not been exposed to an antecedent causative factor. Exposure to high-linear energy transfer radiation from α-emitting radioisotopes such as thorium dioxide increases the risk of AML.[23] Case-control studies have sometimes found a relationship between AML and organic solvents, petroleum products, radon exposure, pesticides, and herbicides, but these data have been inconsistent, have shown no association in other studies, and have not reached a level comparable to the strong association that exists for high-dose benzene, high-dose external irradiation, and certain chemotherapeutic agents. There is a significant association between tobacco smoking and AML with a relative risk of about 1.5 to 2.0.[24,25] Although formaldehyde has been suspected of being a leukemogen, detailed analysis has not supported this contention.[26,27]

An endogenous factor that increases risk is obesity. Studies in North America show an increased risk of AML in men and women with elevated body mass index, and this is particularly notable for acute promyelocytic leukemia. The precise mechanisms are still unclear but may be related, in part, to elevated leptin levels, decreased adiponectin levels, shortened telomeres, and as yet unknown factors in obese subjects.[28]

EVOLUTION FROM A CHRONIC MYELOID NEOPLASM

AML may develop from the progression of other clonal disorders of a multipotential hematopoietic cell, including CML, chronic myelomonocytic leukemia, chronic neutrophilic leukemia (CNL), polycythemia vera, primary myelofibrosis, essential thrombocythemia, and clonal cytopenia or oligoblastic myelogenous leukemia. The latter two are considered forms of myelodysplastic syndrome (MDS) (see Table 88-1). Clonal progression occurs as a result of genomic instability and the acquisition of additional mutations, although with a different

TABLE 88–1. Conditions Predisposing to Development of Acute Myelogenous Leukemia

Environmental factors
  Radiation[14,15]
  Benzene[16-18]
  Alkylating agents, topoisomerase II inhibitors, and other cytotoxic drugs[20-22]
  Tobacco smoke[19,24,25]
Acquired diseases
  Clonal myeloid diseases
    Chronic myelogenous leukemias (CML, CMML, CNL, etc.) (Chap. 89)
    Primary myelofibrosis (Chap. 86)
    Essential thrombocythemia (Chap. 85)
    Polycythemia vera (Chap. 84)
    Clonal cytopenias (Chap. 87)
    Oligoblastic myelogenous leukemia (Chap.87)
    Paroxysmal nocturnal hemoglobinuria (Chap. 40)
Other hematopoietic disorders
  Aplastic anemia (Chap. 35)
  Eosinophilic fasciitis (Chap. 87)
  Myeloma (Chap. 107)[31,32]
Other disorders
  Human immunodeficiency virus infection[32]
  Langerhans cell histiocytosis[33,34]
  Thyroid disorders[35]
  Polyendocrine disorders[36]
Inherited or congenital conditions
  Sibling with AML[37-39]
  Amegakaryocytic thrombocytopenia, congenital[40,41]
  Ataxia-pancytopenia[42,43]
  Bloom syndrome[44,45]
  Congenital agranulocytosis (Kostmann syndrome)[46-49]
  Chronic thrombocytopenia with chromosome 21q 22.12 microdeletion[50]
  Diamond-Blackfan syndrome[51,52]
  Down syndrome[53,54]
  Dubowitz syndrome[55]
  Dyskeratosis congenita[56,57]
  Familial (pure, nonsyndromic) AML[58]
  Familial platelet disorder[59,60]
  Fanconi anemia[61,62]
  MonoMAC and Emberger syndromes (*GATA2* mutations)[63]
  Naxos syndrome[64]
  Neurofibromatosis 1[65,66]
  Noonan syndrome[67,68]
  Poland syndrome[69]
  Rothmund-Thomson syndrome[70,71]
  Seckel syndrome[72]
  Shwachman syndrome[73-75]
  Werner syndrome (progeria)[76-78]
  Wolf-Hirschhorn syndrome[79]
  WT syndrome[80]

AML, acute myelogenous leukemia; CML, chronic myelogenous leukemia; CMML, chronic myelomonocytic leukemia; CNL, chronic neutrophilic leukemia; MonoMAC, monocytopenia and mycobacterial infections.

probability of occurrence in each chronic myeloid neoplasm (Chap. 83). The frequency of clonal progression to AML is enhanced by radiation or chemotherapy in patients with polycythemia vera (Chap. 84) or essential thrombocythemia (Chap. 85).[29] Although some refer to this as secondary AML, it should be called clonally evolved AML (ceAML) to distinguish it from secondary AML that results from radiation or chemotherapy given to patients who do not have a precedent clonal myeloid disease. In the population of patients with preceding clonal myeloid neoplasms, a myeloid leukemic clone already exists and is not induced secondarily. Evolution to AML represents the natural history of the neoplasm, albeit sometimes accelerated by various external mutagens.

AGING AND ACUTE MYELOGENOUS LEUKEMIA–RELEVANT SOMATIC MUTATIONS

Very low copy number gene mutations characteristic of leukemia or lymphoma have been detected in the blood of healthy individuals. An analysis of blood cell DNA sequence data has identified 77 blood cell–specific mutations in cancer-associated genes, the majority being associated with advanced age. A large majority of these mutations were from 19 leukemia and/or lymphoma-associated genes, and nine were recurrently mutated (*DNMT3A*, *TET2*, *JAK2*, *ASXL1*, *TP53*, *GNAS*, *PPM1D*, *BCORL1*, and *SF3B1*). Additional mutations were found in a very small fraction of blood cells. Comparison of these findings to mutations in hematologic malignancies identified other recurrently mutated genes.

The blood cells of more than 2 percent of individuals (5 to 6 percent of people older than 70 years) contain mutations that may represent premalignant events that can cause clonal hematopoietic expansion. These events may, in part, explain the age-dependent incidence of AML (Fig. 88–1).[29a]

PREDISPOSING DISEASES

Patients who develop AML may have an antecedent predisposing nonmyeloid disease, such as aplastic anemia (poly- or oligoclonal T-cell disorder), myeloma (monoclonal B-cell disorder),[30,31] or, rarely, AIDS (HIV-induced polyclonal T-cell disorder).[32] An association between Langerhans cell histiocytosis, immune thyroid diseases, and familial polyendocrine disorder and AML has been reported.[33-36] A number of inherited conditions carry an increased risk of AML (see Table 88–1).[37-80] In the inherited syndromes, at least several pathogenetic types of gene alterations are represented: (1) DNA repair defects, for example, Fanconi anemia; (2) susceptibility genes favoring a second mutation, for example, familial platelet syndrome; (3) tumor-suppressor defects, for example, dyskeratosis congenita; and (4) unknown mechanisms, for example, ataxia-pancytopenia (See Tables 35-8 and 35-9 in Chap. 35 for further details of each pathogenetic process). There is evidence from central registry studies that any disorder that results in chronic immune stimulation, such as infection or autoimmune diseases may be associated with AML and MDS.[81] The prevalence of essential monoclonal gammopathy is not increased in AML patients.[82]

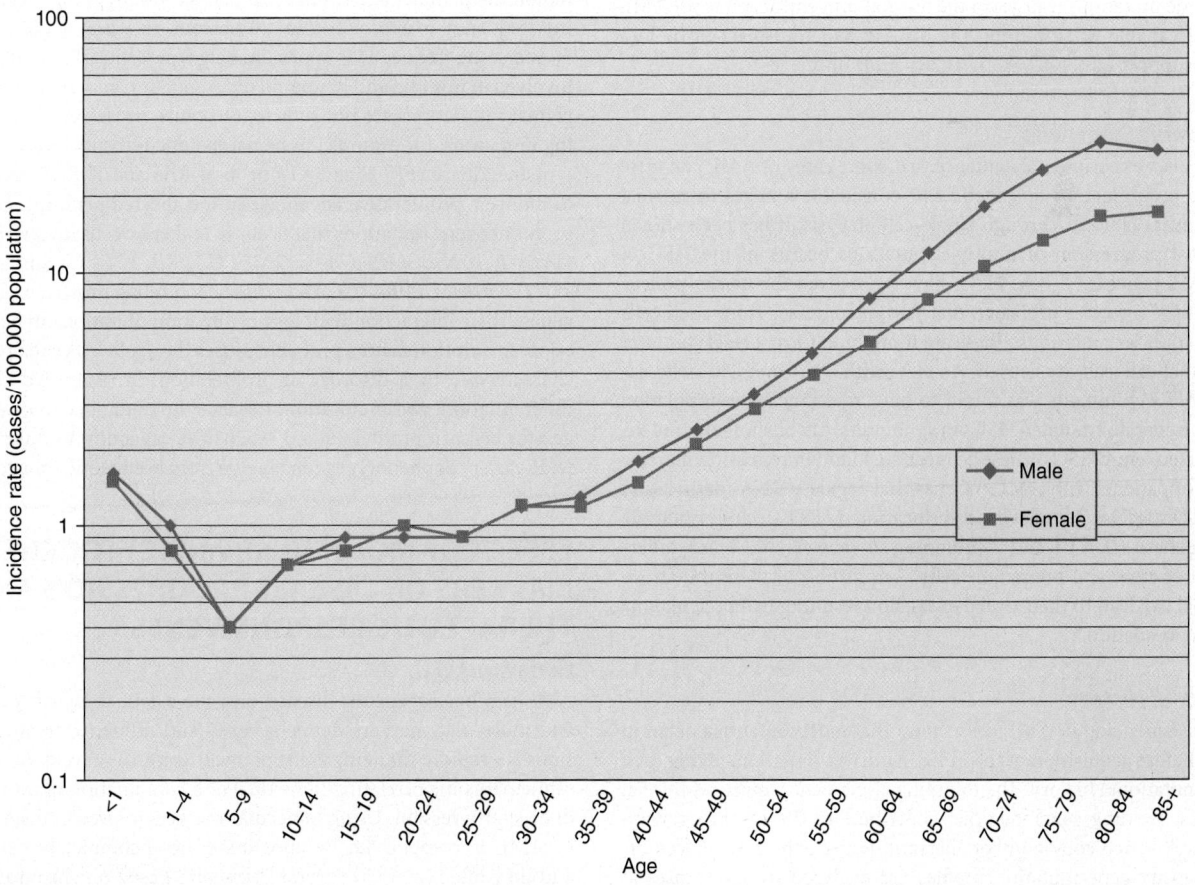

Figure 88–1. The annual incidence of acute myelogenous leukemia as a function of age. There is a relatively small increase to approximately 1.5 cases per 100,000 persons in the first year of life, representing congenital, neonatal, and infant AML. The incidence falls to a nadir of 0.4 new cases per 100,000 persons over the first 10 years of life and then rises again to 1 case per 100,000 in the second decade of life. From approximately 25 years of age, the incidence increases exponentially (log-linear) to approximately 25 cases per 100,000 population in octogenarians.

MOLECULAR PATHOGENESIS

The Leukemia Stem Cell

AML results from a series of somatic mutations in a primitive hematopoietic multipotential progenitor cell or, very occasionally, a more differentiated, more lineage-restricted progenitor cell.[83,84] Some cases of monocytic leukemia, promyelocytic leukemia, and AML in younger individuals may arise in a progenitor cell with lineage restrictions (progenitor cell leukemia).[85–87] Other morphologic phenotypes and older patients likely have a disease that originates in a primitive multipotential cell. In the latter case, all myeloid blood cell lineages can be derived from the leukemic stem cell because it retains the ability for some degree of differentiation and maturation (Chap. 83). Because the T lymphocytes, B lymphocytes, and natural killer cells in cases of AML, often, have not carried a cytogenetic abnormality as did the myeloid cells, claims of origin in the pluripotential lymphohematopoietic cell have been ambiguous. The most compelling data indicate that the bulk of AML cases arise from one of two predominant CD34+ cell populations: CD34+CD45RA+CD38–CD90– (multipotential myeloid progenitor) or CD34+CD38+CD45RA+CD110+ (granulocyte-monocyte progenitor). Both of these cell populations correspond to normal hematopoietic progenitor cells and not the normal pluripotential lymphohematopoietic stem cell.[86,88] This finding was confirmed by showing that the two leukemic cell populations were more similar to the corresponding normal progenitor populations than to pluripotential lymphohematopoietic stem cells by microarray gene expression analysis.[88] The AML stem cell arises from somatic mutations in one of these populations in most, but not all, cases of AML. Because progenitor cells are not self-renewing, the somatic mutations transform the normal progenitor cell to an AML stem cell capable of sustaining the disease and transplanting it into immunosuppressed (NOD/SCID/IL2Rγ null) mice.

Preleukemic Stem Cells

There is, also, experimental evidence that some cases of AML can arise from the accumulation of genetic and epigenetic changes in normal pluripotential HSCs.[89] Through single-cell analysis, it has been shown that clonal progression of multiple mutations occurs in the HSC of some AML patients.[90] These HSCs have been given the name "preleukemic HSCs" and it is proposed that AML progresses from such cells carrying founder mutations. These are thought to form a reservoir after therapy that can lead to relapse.[89] An HSC with DNA methyltransferase 3A (DNMT3A) mutants was found to have multilineage repopulation advantage over nonmutated HSCs in xenografts, establishing their identity as preleukemic HSCs. These cells can be found in remission marrow samples of patients with AML.[91] Genes that regulate DNA methylation such as DNMT3A, ten-eleven translocation (TET) 2, and isocitrate dehydrogenase (IDH) 1 and 2 promote self-renewal and block differentiation of stem and progenitor cells. Acquisition of these mutations in an HSC can lead to their clonal expansion resulting in a preleukemia stem cell population.[92]

Mutational History

Genome sequencing in AML cells shows that most mutations occur at random before acquisition of the initiating driver mutation, giving each clone a mutational history. The founding clone may acquire additional mutations, yielding subclones that contribute to disease progression or relapse.[93] When copy number aberrations and copy-neutral loss-of-heterozygosity gene mutation profiles are analyzed in AML cases at diagnosis and at relapse, the relapsed leukemia always reflects reemergence of the founder clone. In persistent AML cases, sometimes two coexisting dominant clones can be seen, one chemotherapy-sensitive and one chemotherapy-resistant, suggesting that refractory or relapsed

AML cases represent incomplete eradication of founder clones and not emergence of unrelated clones.[94]

Role of Telomeres

AML with multiple chromosome aberrations is always characterized by critically short telomeres. Age-related critical telomere shortening may have a role in generating chromosome instability in AML pathogenesis.[95] Leukemic cells show variable reduction in length of telomeric DNA, and telomere length in blood cells during remission is greater.[96]

Somatic Mutations

Somatic mutation results from a chromosomal translocation in a large fraction of patients.[97] The translocation results in rearrangement of a critical region of a protooncogene. Fusion of portions of two genes often does not prevent the processes of transcription and translation; thus, the fusion oncogene encodes a fusion protein that, because of its abnormal structure, disrupts a normal cell pathway and predisposes to a malignant transformation of the cell. The mutant protein product often is a transcription factor or an element in the transcription pathway that disrupts the regulatory sequences controlling growth rate or survival of blood cell progenitors and their differentiation and maturation.[97–99] Examples of genes often mutated are core binding factor (CBF), retinoic acid receptor-α (RAR-α), HOX family, mixed-lineage leukemia (MLL), and others. CBF has two subunits: CBF-β and runt-related transcription factor 1(RUNX1, formerly AML1). Approximately 10 percent of AML cases have translocations involving one or the other of these latter two genes (CBF-β and RUNX1), although the percentage varies depending on the patient's age at onset. In patients younger than age 50 years, the frequency is approximately 20 percent. In patients older than age 50 years, the frequency is approximately 6 percent. CBF activates genes involved in myeloid and lymphoid differentiation and maturation. These primary mutations are not sufficient to cause AML. Additional activating mutations, for example, in hematopoietic tyrosine kinases Fms-like tyrosine kinase (FLT)3 and KIT or in N-RAS and K-RAS, are required to induce a proliferative advantage in the affected primitive cell. Other protooncogene mutations that occur in leukemic cells involve FES, FOS, GATA-1, JUN B, MPL, MYC, p53, PU.1, RB, WT1 (Wilms tumor 1), WNT, NPM1, CEPBA (CCAAT-enhancer binding protein A), and other genes. Their interaction with loss-of-function mutations in hematopoietic transcription factors probably causes the acute leukemia phenotype characterized by a disorder of proliferation, programmed cell death, differentiation, and maturation. Because the mutant stem or early progenitor cell can proliferate and retains the capability to differentiate, a wide variety of phenotypes can emerge from a leukemic transformation.

EFFECT OF MOLECULAR AND CYTOGENETIC MARKERS ON DISEASE PROGRESSION AND THERAPEUTIC RESPONSIVENESS

Gene Markers

AML is a heterogeneous disease, and the extent to which cytogenetic and molecular markers define severity and influence treatment decisions is a rapidly changing arena of investigation as a result of continued refinements in correlating individual or a combination of mutations on disease progression. Using molecular markers to predict disease course in AML is complicated because these are incompletely determined, and they often interact. Several risk scores based on chromosome and molecular markers have integrated factors such as age and white blood cell (WBC) count into the scoring systems.[100,101] Others have identified common gene signatures that can be independent predictors of disease progression or therapeutic response and provide a structure for risk stratification. Some of these signatures have 24 genes,[102] and some have a seven gene-epigene score.[103] Some have relied on genetic profiling,[104] some on expression of a subset of molecular mutations,[105] and some have combined epigenetic and genetic markers.[106] Prognostic models of AML based solely on molecular markers have been proposed. In one, *PML-RARa* or *CEPBA* double mutations were very favorable (overall survival [OS] at 3 years of 83 percent), *RUNX1-RUNX1T1*, *CFB-B-MYH11*, or *NPM1* (nucleophosmin-1 mutation) without *FLT3-ITD* (OS of 62.6 percent), intermediate with no mutation allowing assignment to other groups (OS of 44 percent), *MLL-PTD* or *RUNX1*, or *ASXL1* mutation (OS of 22 percent), and very unfavorable, *TP53* mutation (OS at 3 years, 0 percent).

Chromosome Markers

In general, those patients with changes involving CBF, that is, t(8/21), inv(16), t(16;16), or t(15;17), a feature of acute promyelocytic leukemia (APL), are considered predictors of a more favorable outcome. Those with complex karyotype, 11q23, t(6;9), abnormalities of chromosome 5 or 7 or inv3 (t3;3) are associated with a poor outcome. The remainder of cytogenetic abnormalities and those patients with a normal karyotype are considered of intermediate risk.[107] These are determined by the behavior of the average of very large groups of patients and confidence intervals are not calculated. Patients with favorable cytogenetic patterns may have poor outcomes and those with less favorable patterns may do better than anticipated.

Deletions of all or part of a chromosome (e.g., chromosome 5, 7, or 9) or additional chromosomes (such as trisomy 4, 8, or 13) are common cytogenetic abnormalities (Chap. 11), although the specific causative oncogenes or tumor-suppressor genes in these latter circumstances have not been defined. Deletions in chromosomes 5 and 7 and complex cytogenetic abnormalities are associated with a worse prognosis and are increased in frequency in older patients and cases of AML following cytotoxic therapy compared to *de novo* cases.[108] Because the genes residing on the undeleted homologous segment of chromosome 5 are not mutated, an epigenetic lesion, such as hypermethylation of a gene allelic to one on the deleted segment on chromosome 5, may contribute to the leukemogenic event.

In APL, *PML-RAR-α* fusion protein represses retinoic acid-inducible genes, which prevent appropriate maturation of promyelocytes. The induced disruption, which involves corepressor–histone deacetylase complexes, results in the leukemic phenotype (see "Acute Promyelocytic Leukemia" below).[109,110]

Patients with CBF leukemias are younger on average and in addition to t(8;21) or inv(16)/t(16;16) may have *RUNX1/RUNX1T1* and *CBFB/MYH11* oncogenes.[111] The cure rate in these so-called good-risk patients is only approximately 55 percent, however. Patients with CBF leukemias expressing *KIT* have a worse prognosis.[112] In the case of inv(16)/t(16;16), different fusion transcripts can be formed, and these may have associated with *KIT* mutations and other abnormal chromosomal associations with differing prognosis, possibly from activation of caspase activity.[113] Secondary genetic changes in inv(16) or t(16;16) cases may have an impact on prognosis. *RAS*, *KIT*, *FLT3*-internal tandem duplication (ITD), and *FLT3-TKD* each affect prognosis. *FLT3-TKD*, trisomy 8, age, and therapy-related AML were associated with worse prognosis.[114] In t(8;21) leukemias, epigenetic silencing of *microR-NA-193a* activates the PTEN/PI3K signaling pathway,[115] and wild-type *RUNX1* can attenuate nuclear factor-kappaB (NF-κB) signaling, events not present in the t(8;21) translocation leukemias.[116]

3q Abnormalities EVI1 and *MDS1/EVI1* expression in AML is associated with poor prognosis and is a distinct entity. These chromosome 3 abnormalities are found in only approximately 4 percent of AML cases. These include inv(3) or t(3;3), t(3q26), t(3q21), and other miscellaneous 3q abnormalities.[117] These generally have an unfavorable prognosis.[118]

Monosomal Karyotype A monosomy has been associated with decreased chance of achieving remission or of survival, especially when combined with *TP53* mutations.[119,120]

OTHER ACQUIRED MUTATIONS

Approximately 45 percent of AML cases have a normal karyotype. Sequencing has shown that mutations in *NPM1, DNMT1, FLT3, KIT, CEBPA, TET2,* and others may have diagnostic and prognostic implications. When genomes of APL with a known founder event (*PML-RARa*) are sequenced and compared with normal karyotype AML and exomes of HSCs from normal donors, most mutations in AML genomes are random events that occurred in HSC before the initiating mutation occurred. As the clone expands, one or two additional, cooperating mutations may result in development of a leukemia, and these clones may acquire additional mutations, leading to subclones.[121] DNA sequences of leukemia cell and normal skin cell genomes of a patient with AML showed 12 acquired mutations within coding sequences of genes and 532 somatic point mutations in conserved or regulatory portions of the genome.[122] When whole-genome or whole-exome sequencing was performed in 200 AML cases, it was found that an average of only 13 mutations occurred in the genes. Only a total of 23 genes were mutated. There were nine categories of genes thought relevant for pathogenesis: (1) transcription-factor fusions, (2) nucleophosmin, tumor-suppressor, (3) DNA methylation-related, (4) signaling, chromatin-modifying, (5) transcription-factor, (6) cohesion-complex, and (7) spliceosome-complex genes. Many of these genes had patterns of cooperation and mutual exclusivity.[123] Table 88–2 lists commonly mutated genes in cytogenetically normal AML in order of decreasing frequency.

Nucleophosmin-1 Mutations *NPM1* mutations are the most frequent genetic alterations in AML, found in approximately half of patients with a normal karyotype.[124,125] The mutation in exon 12 results in loss of the residue that requires its binding to nucleoli such that the NPM1 protein is abnormally localized to the cytoplasm.[126] Studies show that mutant *NPM1* without *FLT3-ITD* represents a favorable prognostic marker.[127] NPM1 mutations also have a favorable prognostic impact in older patients.[128] Mutated regions of *NPM1* elicit T-cell responses which might indicate that immunotherapy could have a role in these mutated cases.[129]

FLT3 Mutations *FLT3* encodes a tyrosine kinase receptor in normal myeloid and lymphoid progenitors. ITD of *FLT3* on chromosome 13 occurs in approximately 25 percent of adult AML cases, but occurs more frequently in cases of AML with normal cytogenetic patterns, monocytic phenotype, and *PML-RAR-α* or *DEK-CAN* translocations.[124,125,130] The *FLT3-ITD* mutation confers a poor prognosis if the ratio of mutant to wild-type expression is high.[130–132] FLT3-ITD expression is often higher at relapse.[133] *FLT3-ITD* upregulates *MCL-1* to promote survival of AML stem cells through signal transducer and activator of transcription (STAT) 5 activation.[134] *FLT3-ITD* adversely affects the outcome of an allogeneic stem cell transplant, but more than half of patients harboring this mutation who receive transplants can survive leukemia free for 2 or more years.[135] Point mutations in the tyrosine kinase domain (TKD) of *FLT3* (*FLT3-TKD*) mutations occur in approximately 6 percent of AML cases and have little impact on outcomes.[136]

DNMT3A Mutations The *DNMT3A* gene encodes a DNA methyltransferase isoform. The process of DNA methylation involves the addition of a methyl group on a cytosine residue at a C-G site. If this methylation happens in the promoter region of a coding gene, the gene will be silenced. The DNMT enzymes contribute to leukemogenesis by mediating tumor suppressor gene silencing.[137] *DNMT3A* mutations have been found in approximately 20 percent of AML patients with normal

TABLE 88–2. Commonly Mutated Genes In Cytogenetically Normal Acute Myelogenous Leukemia

Mutated Gene	Approximate Frequency in AML with Normal Karyotype (%)	Implication	Comments	References
NPM1	50	More-favorable outcomes	Most frequently mutated gene in AML. Allogenic transplantation not needed in first remission if this mutation occurs in absence of mutated FLT3-ITD	124–129
FLT3 ITD	40	Less-favorable outcomes		124, 125, 130–137
DNMT3A	20	Less-favorable outcomes	Seen more often in AML patients with normal cytogenetics. Mutant NPM1, FLT3-ITD, and IDH1 have been found more frequently in AML patients with DNMT3A mutations compared to those with wild-type DNMT3A	137–143
RUNX1	15	Less-favorable outcomes		144–149
TET2	15	Less-favorable outcomes	Coincidence of mutated TET2 with NPM1 mutation in the absence of FLT3-ITD mutation predicts a less-favorable outcome	150–153
CEBPA	15	More-favorable outcomes	Only cases with double mutations associated with favorable outcomes	124, 154–157
NRAS	10	Little effect on prognosis		144
IDH1 or IDH2	10	Little effect on outcomes	More frequent in AML patients with normal cytogenetics. Frequently associated with NPM1. Adverse prognostic factor if present with mutated NPM1 without FLT3-ITD. Serum 2-hydroxyglutarate levels indicate high probability of IDH mutation	138, 158, 159–164
MLL-PTD	8	Less-favorable outcomes		144
WT1	6	Less-favorable outcomes	More frequent in females than in males (6.6 vs. 4.7%; P = 0.014) and in patients <60 than in patients >60 years (P <0.001)	166, 167
FLT3-TKD	6	Little effect on outcomes	May appear after use of FLT3-ITD inhibitor	132, 136

Gene frequencies are approximations with some variation from study to study. Outcome statement does not reflect effect of interacting mutations unless otherwise noted in comments. Outcome statements are based on consensus and vary from one study to another.

AML, acute myelogenous leukemia; CEPBa, CCAAT/enhancer binding protein alpha; DNMT3A, DNA methyltransferase 3A; FLT, FMS-like tyrosine kinase; IDH, isocitrate dehydrogenase; ITD, internal tandem duplication; MLL, myeloid-lymphoid (mixed-lineage) leukemia; NPM, nucleophosmin; PTD, partial tandem deletion; RAS, rat sarcoma; RUNX, Runt-related transcription factor; TET, ten-eleven translocation; TKD, tyrosine kinase domain; WT, Wilms tumor.

cytogenetic patterns.[138] These cases more frequently had mutations in NPM1, FLT3, and IDH1 genes as well.[139] DNMT3A mutations are associated with a poorer prognosis[139–142] and their significance appears to be age-dependent.[143] The R882 mutation was associated with adverse prognosis in older patients, and non-R882 mutations with adverse prognosis in younger patients.

RUNX1 Mutations The RUNX1 gene is located on chromosome 21q22 and is involved in hematopoiesis at all stages through its interaction with CBFβ. It acts as an activator or repressor of numerous genes, including transcription factors.[144,145] In de novo AML, RUNX1 mutations were found with normal and noncomplex karyotypes. They were sometimes associated with MLL-PTD (partial tandem duplication [PTD]) and FLT3-ITD, and they were associated with a poor prognosis independent of other molecular mutations.[146] Another group found these mutations in 5.6 percent of cases, associated with cytogenetically normal AML and an association with MLL-PTD mutations, refractory disease, and, as an independent risk factor, an inferior relapse-free survival and overall survival. The use of allogeneic HSC transplant did have a

favorable impact in such cases.[147] Another series found RUNX1 mutations to be twice as common in older than younger patients with normal cytogenetics, and to have an adverse outcome effect in both age groups. Mutated blasts had molecular signatures suggesting origin in a primitive hematopoietic cell.[148] RUNX1 mutations have been found to cooperate with granulocyte colony-stimulating factor receptor (CSFR) mutations in congenital neutropenia to lead to acute leukemia or MDS.[149]

TET2 Mutations The TET2 protein inactivation may occur through a loss of function mutation, deletion, or through IDH1/2 mutations. It is a member of a family of dioxygenases that catalyze conversion of 5-methyl-cytosine to 5-hydroxymethyl-cytosine and promote DNA demethylation. TET2 has many roles in normal hematopoiesis, and knockout mice show that it is a tumor suppressor, which haploinsufficiency initiates myeloid transformations.[150] TET2 mutations are found in approximately 25 percent of patients and in those who have mutated CEBPα and/or mutated NPM1 without a FLT3/ITD mutation.[151,152] Patients with AML and a TET2 mutation had a shorter event-free and overall survival compared with patients who were TET2 wild-type. They did not predict for outcomes in those with cytogenetically normal AML and with wild-type *CEBPα*, *NPM1,* and/or *FLT3/ITD*.[153] Whether these patients would benefit from alternate therapies, such as hypomethylating agents or HSC transplantation, has not been determined.

CEBPα Mutation CEBPα is a leucine zipper transcription factor involved in myeloid differentiation. Mutations have been described in approximately 10 percent of AML patients.[124] Single or double mutations can occur, and these rarely are associated with *FLT3/ITD* or with *NPM1* mutations. *CEBPα*-double, but not *CEBPα*-single, mutation patients had a significantly better overall survival at 8 years than wild-type, *CEBPα*-single, or *CEBPα*-double and *FLT3/ITD*-positive patients.[154] A multivariate analysis found that only double-mutant *CEBPα* was associated with a favorable event-free, relapse-free, and overall survival. Double-mutant cases were also associated with a unique gene signature as compared with single-mutant cases.[155,156] Some AML patients with *CEBPα*-double mutations harbor *TET2* and *GATA2* mutations, which can affect prognostic outlook unfavorably with *TET2* or favorably with *GATA2* mutations.[157]

IDH1 and IDH2 Mutations The IDHs catalyze oxidative decarboxylation of isocitrate into α-hemoglutarate. The nicotinamide adenine dinucleotide phosphate–dependent IDH1 enzyme is encoded by the *IDH1* gene on chromosome 2q33.3, and the nicotinamide adenine dinucleotide phosphate–dependent-dependent IDH2 enzyme is encoded by the *IDH2* gene on chromosome 15q26.1.[158] Mutations in *IDH1* (R132) or *IDH2* (R172) occur in 10 percent of AML patients.[158,159] Both were found to adversely impact relapse-free survival and overall survival. Multivariate analysis showed that *IDH* mutation conferred an adverse impact in those patients with an *NPM1* mutation without *FLT3-ITD*. Favorable genotype cytogenetically normal AML is therefore defined as *NPM1* or *CEBPα* mutation with neither a *FLT3-ITD* nor an *IDH1* mutation. An *IDH1* mutation was also associated with a higher relapse rate and shorter overall survival.[160] Another group found a higher frequency of *IDH1* and *IDH2* mutations in cytogenetically normal AML. Both were found to have an unfavorable impact on outcome.[161] *IDH1* was exclusive of other mutations. Serum 2-hydroxyglutarate production has been found to predict for the presence of *IDH1/2* mutations.[162,163] A level of 700 mg/mL was found to discriminate mutated from nonmutated cases, and those with levels greater than 20 ng/mL at the time of remission had shorter overall survival.[163] Mutant *IDH1* has been found to accelerate cell-cycle transition and to activate mitogen-activated protein kinase signaling. Mutant *IDH1* can be inhibited, suggesting this may be a therapeutic target.[164]

WT1 Mutations Mutations of the *WT1* gene have been reported in approximately 5 to 10 percent of cytogenetically normal patients with AML.[165] Some studies suggest association with a poor prognosis, but others have not. *WT1* SNP rs 16754 was associated with a favorable risk, but acquired mutations did not affect the development of complete remission, relapse-free survival, or overall survival.[166] A study of *WT1* mutations in older patients with cytogenetically normal AML also showed poor treatment response across all age-groups and association with a distinct gene expression signature.[167]

Prognostic Impact of Other Molecular Abnormalities

Other methodologies to evaluate genomic aberrations have been reported to have prognostic importance beyond the impact of the individual mutations described above and in Table 88–2. Abnormal genome-wide single nucleotide polymorphisms have adverse prognosis in patients with AML and a normal karyotype.[168] Expression signatures of cytokines and chemokines have an independent prognostic impact in AML.[169] Profiling transcriptional pathways may have prognostic importance in AML as well.[170]

There is also interplay among molecular aberrancies in AML. These include: (1) gene interaction with a microRNA; for example,

BAALC and *miR-3151* in cytogenetically normal AML,[171] (2) distinct patterns of dual or multiple gene mutation patterns that have prognostic impact,[172] and (3) concurrence of somatic mutations and transcriptional regulators such as interaction between *ERG* expression and a heptad of transcriptional factors[173] that maintains a stem cell-like signature. Furthermore, interactions between genetic and epigenetic changes (DNA methylation, histone acetylation, histone methylation, and others) are anticipated to have prognostic impact.[174,175]

DEREGULATED SIGNALING PATHWAYS

The mutations in AML result in deregulation of any of several signal transduction pathways, which disrupt pathways that ensure the normal behavior of (1) differentiation and maturation, (2) proliferation, and (3) survival signals in hematopoietic cells. The pathways involved are myriad, but several represent the majority of cases such as the (1) PI3K-AKT, (2) RAS-RAF-MEK-ERK, and (3) STAT3 signaling sequences.[176] The expectation is that a relative small number of downstream signaling pathways mediate the leukemogenic effect of gene mutations, making the potential targets for therapy less diffuse than suggested by the number of gene mutations involved in AML.

MODE OF INHERITANCE

In most cases, little evidence is seen for a strong influence of inherited factors. The identical twin of a child with acute leukemia has a heightened risk of developing the disease. However, the risk appears to be related to intraplacental metastasis and thus falls to the risk of a nonidentical sibling after the first few years of life.[177,178] The risk of AML in a nonidentical sibling in the United States is elevated, perhaps twofold to threefold, compared to the risk of AML in unrelated American children of European descent younger than age 15 years.[177,179] A registry study in Sweden showed no significant aggregation in relatives of patients with AML. An increased risk of AML/MDS was found among relatives of patients diagnosed at younger than age 21 years (relative risk 6.5).[180] Clusters of AML cases in families have been documented, but their frequency is low.[58] Clusters of AML in unrelated persons in a community are uncommon and, when investigated, usually prove to be a chance occurrence. Heritable *GATA2* mutations may be associated with familial MDS and AML,[181] and loss-of-function germline *GATA2* mutations (the MonoMAC [monocytopenia and mycobacterial infections] syndrome) may be associated with primary lymphedema and a predisposition to AML (Emberger syndrome).[182–184] Mutations of *CEBPα* have been found in familial AML.[185] In one study of 27 families with familial MDS/AML, genetic characterization could be shown in 10 (four with *GATA2* mutations, five with telomerase mutations, and one with mutated *RUNX1*).[186] Mutations in telomerase RNA *(TERC)* or telomerase reverse transcriptase component *(TERT)* are also associated with familial AML.[185,187]

EPIDEMIOLOGY

AML is the predominant form of leukemia during the neonatal period but represents a small proportion of cases during childhood and adolescence. Approximately 20,000 new cases of AML occur annually, representing approximately 35 percent of the new cases of leukemia in the United States each year. Approximately 12,000 patients with AML in the United States die each year as a result of the disease. The incidence rate of AML is approximately 1.5 per 100,000 in infants younger than 1 year of age, decreases to approximately 0.4 per 100,000 children ages 5 to 9 years, increases gradually to approximately 1.0 persons per 100,000 population until age 25 years, and thereafter increases exponentially until the rate reaches approximately 25 per 100,000 persons in octogenarians (see Fig. 88–1). The exception to this exponential age-related increase in incidence is APL, which does not change greatly in incidence with age.[188]

AML accounts for 15 to 20 percent of the acute leukemias in children and 80 percent of the acute leukemias in adults. It is slightly more common in males. Little difference in incidence is seen between individuals of African or European descent at any age. A somewhat lower incidence is seen in persons of Asian descent.[189] An increase in the frequency of AML is seen in Jews, especially those of Eastern European descent. The acute promyelocytic variant of AML is somewhat more common in Latinos.[190,191] In a large population study of 426,068 patients treated with chemotherapy for malignancy, 301 AML cases occurred, 4.7 times the number expected. Over time (1975 to 2008), the risks increased for non-Hodgkin lymphoma, declined for ovarian cancer and myeloma, and were heterogeneous for breast and Hodgkin lymphoma, reflecting changing treatment patterns.[192]

CLASSIFICATION

Variants of AML can be identified by morphologic features of blood films using polychromatic stains and histochemical reactions,[193] monoclonal antibodies against surface markers,[194] or by the presence of specific chromosome translocations or other molecular changes as discussed above.[104,105] The epitopes on the progenitor cells of several phenotypic variants overlap, and several monoclonal antibodies are required to make specific distinctions among cell types (Table 88–3; see also "Morphologic Variants of Acute Myelogenous Leukemia" below). Correlation between morphologic and immunologic phenotyping of AML is poor. However, poor correlation is expected because morphologic phenotyping is more subjective, given to observer variation, and is based on qualitative factors, whereas the immunologic phenotyping, which characterizes surface molecular features, is more accurate and reproducible. The correlation is improved only somewhat if morphology and histochemistry are coupled.[195] Gene-expression profiling is early in its use as a classification technique for AML but will be more specific and informative than current methods.[104,105] The outcome will depend on the simplification and automation of such techniques, and the availability of drugs that make such distinctions in the prognostic category of practical utility. Chapter 83 contains the classification of morphologic

TABLE 88–3. Immunologic Phenotypes of Acute Myelogenous Leukemia

Phenotype	Usually Positive
Myeloblastic	CD11b, CD13, CD15, CD33, CD117, HLA-DR
Myelomonocytic	CD11b, CD13, CD14, CD15, CD32, CD33, HLA-DR
Erythroid	Glycophorin, spectrin, ABH antigens, carbonic anhydrase I, HLA-DR, CD71 (transferrin receptor)
Promyelocytic	CD13, CD33
Monocytic	CD11b, 11c, CD13, CD14, CD33, CD65, HLA-DR
Megakaryoblastic	CD34, CD41, CD42, CD61, anti–von Willebrand factor
Basophilic	CD11b, CD13, CD33, CD123, CD203c
Mast cell	CD13, CD33, CD117

variants of AML (see Chap. 83, Table 83–1 and Fig. 83–3). A cogent argument has been made that, for practical purposes, a classification that initially considers morphologic phenotype and immunophenotype is advisable. Cytogenetics, molecular genetics, gene-expression profiling, and other considerations can, and should, be layered on as available and useful in influencing therapy, and these features are starting to be incorporated into the World Health Organization (WHO) Classification of AML.[196] It is anticipated that molecular classifications will continue to evolve and dominate clinical decision making in the future.[105]

CLINICAL FEATURES

SIGNS AND SYMPTOMS

General
Signs and symptoms that signal the onset of AML include pallor, fatigue, weakness, palpitations, and dyspnea on exertion. The signs and symptoms reflect the development of anemia; however, weakness, loss of sense of well-being, and fatigue on exertion can be disproportionate to the severity of anemia.[197–201]

Easy bruising, petechiae, epistaxis, gingival bleeding, conjunctival hemorrhages, and prolonged bleeding from skin injuries reflect thrombocytopenia and are frequent early manifestations of the disease. Very infrequently, gastrointestinal, genitourinary, bronchopulmonary, or CNS bleeding occurs at the onset of disease.

Pustules or other minor pyogenic infections of the skin and of minor cuts or wounds are most common. Major infections, such as sinusitis, pneumonia, pyelonephritis, and meningitis, are uncommon presenting features of the disease, partly because absolute neutrophil counts less than 0.5×10^9/L are uncommon until chemotherapy starts. With intensification of neutropenia and monocytopenia after chemotherapy, major bacterial, fungal, or viral infections become more frequent. Anorexia and weight loss are frequent findings. Fever is present in many patients at the time of diagnosis.[200,202–204] Palpable splenomegaly or hepatomegaly occurs in approximately one-quarter of patients.[197,198,201] Lymphadenopathy is extremely uncommon,[201,205,206] except in the monocytic variant of AML.[207]

SPECIFIC ORGAN SYSTEM INVOLVEMENT
Leukemic blast cells circulate and enter most tissues in small numbers. Occasionally, biopsy (or autopsy) uncovers marked aggregates or infiltrates of leukemic cells. Collections of such cells may cause functional disturbances. Extramedullary involvement is most common in monocytic or myelomonocytic leukemia.[208,209]

Skin involvement may be of three types: nonspecific lesions, leukemia cutis, or granulocytic (myeloid) sarcoma of skin and subcutis.[210–213] Nonspecific lesions include macules, papules, vesicles, pyoderma gangrenosum, vasculitis,[214–216] neutrophilic dermatitis (Sweet syndrome),[217] cutis vertices gyrata,[218] and erythema multiforme or nodosum.[211,212] Skin involvement preceding marrow and blood involvement or relapse occurs, but is rare.[219–222]

Sensory organ involvement is very unusual, but retinal, choroidal, iridial, and optic nerve infiltration can occur.[223] Otitis externa and interna, inner ear hemorrhage, and mastoid tumors with seventh nerve involvement may be presenting signs.[224–226]

The *gastrointestinal tract* may be involved at any point, but functional disturbances are unusual.[227,228] The mouth, colon, and anal canal are sites of involvement that most commonly lead to symptoms. Oral manifestations may prompt the patient to visit the dentist. Gingival or periodontal infiltration and dental abscesses may lead to an extraction, followed by prolonged bleeding of an infected tooth socket.[229] Ileotyphlitis (enterocolitis), a necrotizing inflammatory lesion involving the terminal ileum, cecum, and ascending colon, can be a presenting syndrome or occur during treatment.[230–233] Fever, abdominal pain, bloody diarrhea, or ileus may be present and occasionally mimic appendicitis. Intestinal perforation, an inflammatory mass, and associated infection with enteric gram-negative bacilli or clostridial species often are associated with a fatal outcome. Isolated involvement of the gastrointestinal tract is rare.[234,235] Proctitis, especially common in the monocytic variant of AML, can be a presenting sign or a vexing problem during periods of severe granulocytopenia and diarrhea.[227]

The *respiratory tract* can be involved by infiltrates or tumors, leading to laryngeal obstruction, parenchymal infiltrates, alveolar septal infiltration, or pleural seeding. Each of these events can result in severe symptoms and radiologic findings.[236–240]

Cardiac involvement is frequent but rarely causes symptoms. Symptomatic pericardial infiltrates, transmural ventricular infiltrates with hemorrhage, and endocardial foci with associated intracavitary thrombi can occasionally cause heart failure, arrhythmia, and death.[241] Infiltration of the conducting system or valve leaflets or myocardial infarction has occurred.[242]

The *urogenital system* can be affected. The kidneys are infiltrated with leukemic cells in a high proportion of cases, but functional abnormalities are rare. Hemorrhage in the pelvis or collecting system is frequent.[243,244] Cases of vulvar, bladder neck, prostatic, and testicular involvement have been described.[245–247]

Osteoarticular symptoms may occur. Bone pain, joint pain, and bone necrosis can occur, and, rarely, arthritis with effusion is present.[248] Crystal-induced arthritis of either calcium pyrophosphate dihydrate (pseudogout) or monosodium urate (gout) may be responsible for the synovitis in some cases.[249]

Central or peripheral *nervous system* involvement by infiltration of leukemic cells is very uncommon, although meningeal involvement is an important consideration in the treatment of the monocytic type of AML.[250,251] An association of CNS involvement and diabetes insipidus in AML with monosomy 7[252] and inversion of chromosome 16[253,254] has been reported.

MYELOID (GRANULOCYTIC) SARCOMA

Myeloid sarcoma (synonyms: granulocytic sarcoma, chloroma, myeloblastoma, monocytoma) is a tumor composed of myeloblasts, monoblasts, or megakaryocyes.[255–260] The tumor may occur as an extramedullary mass without evidence of leukemia in blood or marrow, so-called nonleukemic myeloid sarcomas, or in association with AML. When the tumor appears as an isolated lesion, it initially may be misdiagnosed as extranodal lymphoma because they look like lymphoid cells on biopsy.[257] They may be found in virtually any location, including the skin; orbit; paranasal sinuses; bone; chest wall; breast; heart; gastrointestinal, respiratory, or genitourinary tract; central or peripheral nervous system; or lymph nodes and spleen. The tumors originally were called *chloromas* because of the green color imparted by the high concentration of the enzyme myeloperoxidase present in myelogenous leukemic cells. Biopsy specimens are positive for chloracetate esterase, lysozyme, myeloperoxidase, and cluster of differentiation (CD) markers of myeloid cells. When myeloid sarcomas are the initial manifestation of AML, the appearance of the disease in the blood and marrow may follow weeks or months later. Abnormalities in chromosome 8 are the most frequent cytogenetic disturbance in myeloid sarcomas.[258] Systemic chemotherapy, rather than local therapy, should be used for treatment, although the long-term outcome in such cases usually is poor.[260–262] Patients having AML with t(8;21) or inv16 have a propensity to develop extramedullary leukemia,[263–266] and such patients with myeloid sarcomas have a poorer outcome after treatment than those who do not have extramedullary lesions.[263,265]

● LABORATORY FEATURES

BLOOD CELL FINDINGS

Anemia is an almost constant feature.[197–201] Red cell life span may be mildly shortened, but the principal cause of anemia is inadequate production of red cells. The reticulocyte count usually is between 0.5 and 2.0 percent. Occasionally patients have rapid destruction of autologous and transfused red cells as a result of an unknown mechanism, referred to as milieu hemolysis. The presence of red cell autoantibodies (positive direct antiglobulin test) is very uncommon and may be nonspecific (anti-C_3), perhaps related to circulating immune complexes. Red cell morphology is mildly abnormal, with exaggerated variation in cell size and occasional poikilocytes. Nucleated red cells or stippled erythrocytes may be present. Less often, extreme abnormalities of red cell size, shape, and hemoglobin content occur (AML with trilineage dysmorphia), but these changes are seen more often in oligoblastic myelogenous leukemia (Chap. 87).

Thrombocytopenia is nearly always present at the time of diagnosis. The mechanism of thrombocytopenia is a combination of inadequate production and decreased survival of platelets. More than half of patients have a platelet count less than 50×10^9/L at the time of diagnosis.[267] Giant platelets and poorly granulated platelets with functional abnormalities can occur.[268] Defects in platelet aggregation and 5-hydroxytryptamine release are frequent.[268]

The total leukocyte count is less than 5×10^9/L in approximately half of patients at the time of diagnosis.[197–201] The absolute neutrophil count is less than 1×10^9/L in more than half of cases at diagnosis.[97–201] Patients with very elevated total leukocyte counts have a low proportion of mature neutrophils but may have a normal absolute neutrophil count. Hypersegmented, hyposegmented, and hypogranular mature neutrophils may be present. Cytochemical abnormalities of blood neutrophils include low or absent myeloperoxidase or low alkaline phosphatase activity.[269] Defects in phagocytosis or microbial killing are common.[270,270A]

Myeloblasts almost always are present in the blood but may be infrequent in severely leukopenic patients. Diligent search may uncover the myeloblasts, or examination of a white cell concentrate (buffy coat) may permit their identification. Classic leukemic blast cells are agranular, but mixtures of immature cells, including agranular and slightly granular cells ranging up to overt progranulocytes, can occur. Auer rods are elliptical cytoplasmic inclusions approximately 1.0 to 1.5 μm long and 0.5 μm wide that derive from azurophilic granules (Fig. 88–2B). The inclusions are present in the blast cells of approximately 15 percent of cases. When present, the inclusions are found in only a small percentage of blast cells when examined with polychrome stains.[193] An exception is APL, in which a higher proportion of cells have Auer rods and some have multiple (bundles) of rods (faggot cells). This finding can be dramatic if peroxidase stain is used to highlight the Auer rods.

MARROW FINDINGS

Morphology

The marrow always contains leukemic blast cells. From 3 to 95 percent of marrow cells are blasts at the time of diagnosis or relapse (see Fig. 88–2A). The WHO has invoked an arbitrary threshold of 20 percent of marrow nucleated cells being blast cells to distinguish polyblastic AML (≥20 percent blasts) from oligoblastic myelogenous leukemia (<20 percent blasts).[197–201] The latter situation is referred to as refractory anemia with excess blasts, a MDS (Chap. 87). The WHO choice of ≥20 percent blasts is an arbitrary standard as acute monocytic leukemia, APL, acute erythroid leukemia, and other variants often have less than 20 percent blast cells at the time of diagnosis,[271] and if any blasts are found with a case of AML in which the cells have a t(8;21) or other CBF inversions or

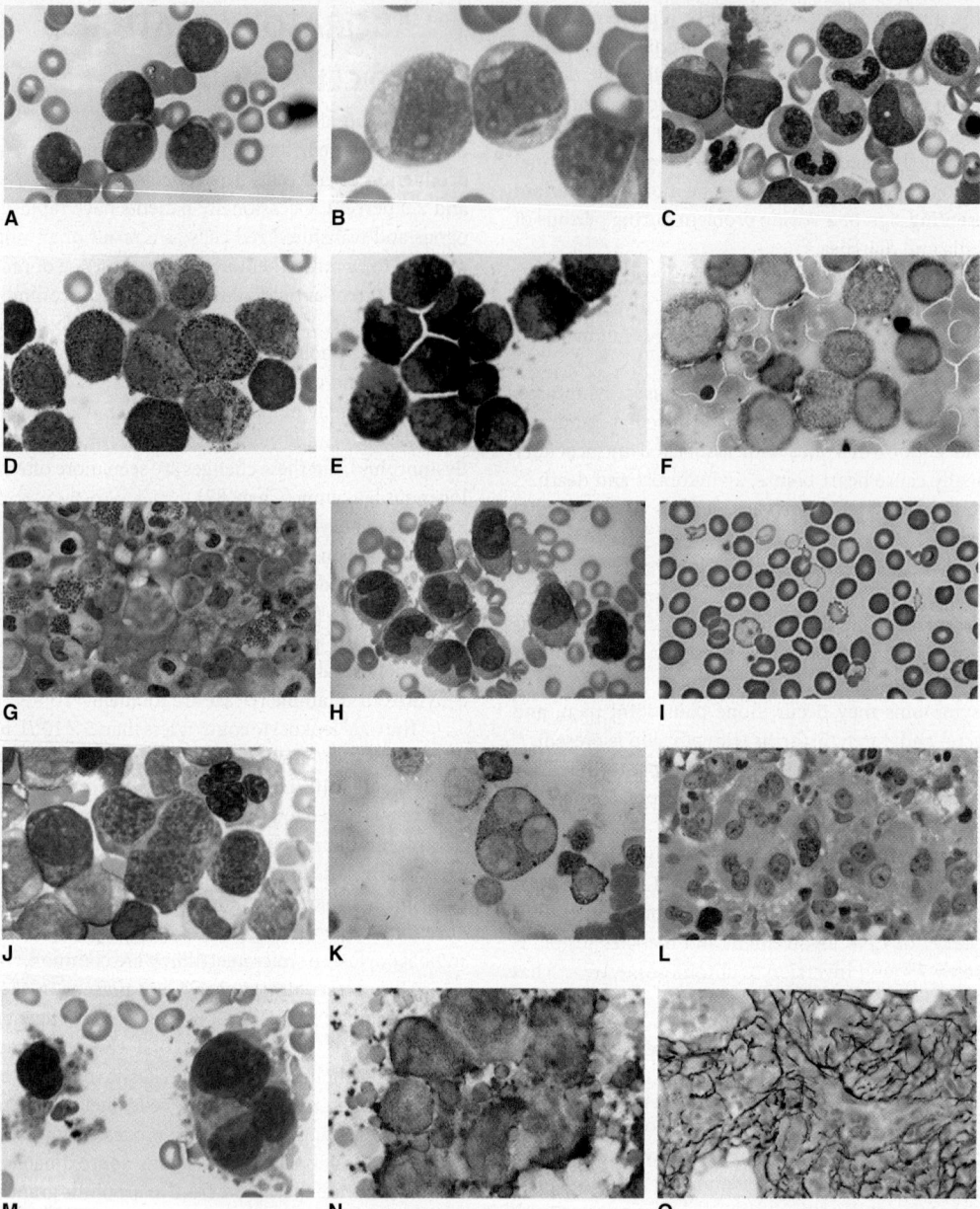

Figure 88–2. Blood and marrow images of major subtypes of acute myelogenous leukemia. **A.** Blood film of acute myelogenous leukemia (AML) without maturation (acute myeloblastic leukemia). Five myeloblasts are evident. High nuclear-to-cytoplasmic ratio. Agranular cells. Nucleoli in each cell. **B.** Blood film. AML without maturation (acute myeloblastic leukemia). Three myeloblasts, one containing an Auer rod. **C.** Marrow film. AML with maturation. Three leukemic myeloblasts admixed with myelocytes, bands, and segmented neutrophils. **D.** Blood film. Acute promyelocytic leukemia. Majority of cells are heavily granulated leukemic promyelocytes. **E.** Blood film. Acute promyelocytic leukemia. Myeloperoxidase stain. Intensely positive. Numerous stained (black) granules in cytoplasm of leukemic progranulocytes. **F.** Blood film. Acute myelomonocytic leukemia. Double esterase stain. Leukemic monocytic cells stained dark blue and leukemic neutrophil precursors stained reddish-brown. **G.** Marrow film. AML with inv16. Note high proportion of eosinophils in field. Note myeloblasts with very large nucleoli at upper right. Also, intermediate leukemic granulocytic forms. **H.** Blood film. Acute monocytic leukemia. Leukemic cells have characteristics of monocytes with agranular gray cytoplasm and reniform or folded nuclei with characteristic chromatin staining. This case had hyperleukocytosis as evident by leukemic monocyte frequency in the blood film. **I.** Blood film. Acute erythroid leukemia. Note population of extremely hypochromic cells with scattered bizarre-shaped poikilocytes admixed with normal-appearing red cells. **J.** Marrow film. Acute erythroid leukemia. Giant erythroblasts with multilobulated nuclei. **K.** Marrow film. Acute erythroid leukemia. Note giant trinucleate erythroblast and other leukemic erythroblasts with periodic acid–Schiff–positive cytoplasmic staining (reddish granules). **L.** Marrow section. Acute megakaryoblastic leukemia. Marrow replaced with atypical two- and three-lobed leukemic megakaryocytes with bold nucleoli. **M.** Marrow film. Acute megakaryoblastic leukemia. Marrow replaced with atypical megakaryocytes and megakaryoblasts with cytoplasmic disorganization, fragmentation, and budding. **N.** Marrow film. Acute megakaryoblastic leukemia. Marrow replaced with atypical megakaryocytes and megakaryoblasts staining for platelet glycoprotein IIIA (reddish-brown). Platelets in background also stained. **O.** Marrow section. Acute megakaryoblastic leukemia. Argentophilic (silver) stain shows marked increase in collagen, type III fibrils (marrow reticulin fibrosis), characteristic of this AML subtype. (*Reproduced with permission from* Lichtman's Atlas of Hematology, *www.accessmedicine.com.*)

translocations, AML is the diagnosis. Moreover, relapse of AML can be identified at any increase in blast count >2 percent. In addition, patients with oligoblastic leukemia with 10 to 19 percent marrow leukemic blast cells are identical in all other phenotypic findings and survival to those with 20 to 29 percent marrow blast cells. Any distinctions between the two groups in survival are a function of age, cytogenetic risk category, and molecular features, not the blast count.[272] This arbitrary boundary prevents patients, otherwise suitable, to enter clinical trials.

Myeloblasts are distinguished from lymphoblasts by any of three pathognomonic features: reactivity with specific histochemical stains; Auer rods in the cells (see Fig. 88–2B); or reactivity with a panel of monoclonal antibodies against epitopes present on myeloblasts (e.g., CD13, CD33, CD117) (see Table 88–3). Leukemic myeloblasts give positive histochemical reactions for myeloperoxidase, Sudan black B, or naphthyl AS-D-chloroacetate esterase stains. Auer rods can be found in the marrow blast cells in approximately one-sixth of cases. Blast cells may express granulocytic (CD15, CD65) or monocytic (CD11b, CD11c, CD14, CD64) surface antigens. They typically do not express either lymphoid surface markers or membrane or cytoplasmic immunoglobulin. No immunoglobulin gene rearrangement or T-lymphocyte receptor gene rearrangement is evident with molecular probes (see "Hybrid and Mixed Leukemias" below). In a proportion of otherwise typical cases of AML, the cells may contain terminal deoxynucleotidyl transferase (TdT).[273,274] Variations in marrow findings are discussed below in "Morphologic Variants of Acute Myelogenous Leukemia." Normal erythropoiesis, megakaryocytopoiesis, and granulopoiesis are decreased or absent in the marrow aspirate. The biopsy may contain residual islands of erythroblasts or megakaryocytes. Dysmorphic changes in hematopoietic cells, including very small or large erythroblasts with nuclear fragmentation or binucleation or delayed nuclear condensation; small or monolobed megakaryocytes; or hypogranulated, bilobed, or monolobed neutrophils, may occur in 30 to 50 percent of patients with de novo AML.[275] Marrow reticulin fibrosis is common but usually is slight to moderate except in cases of megakaryoblastic leukemia, in which intense fibrosis is the rule.[276] Increased blood vessel density (angiogenesis) is present in the marrow of patients with AML compared to normal subjects.[277,278] Various angiogenic factors, including vascular endothelial growth factor (VEGF), basic fibroblast growth factor, angiogenin, and angiopoietin-1, are increased. VEGF detected histochemically in human marrow is closely correlated with the prevalence of leukemic myeloblasts in the various AML subtypes.[279] AML cytogenetic variants may result in marrow basophilia (usually t(6;9))[280] or marrow eosinophilia (usually inv16 or t(16;16)).[281]

Cytogenetic and Genic Features

An abnormal number (aneuploidy) or structure (pseudodiploidy) of chromosomes or both are evident in approximately 55 percent of cases.[282–285] The most prevalent abnormalities are trisomy 8, monosomy 7, monosomy 21, trisomy 21, and loss of an X or Y chromosome. However, any chromosome can be rearranged, added, or lost (Chap. 13). In cases of AML following chemotherapy or radiotherapy, loss of part or all of chromosomes 5 and 7 are a common features,[286–288] as are the cytogenetic findings noted above for AML, occurring de novo. Table 88–4 lists the most frequent abnormalities and translocations seen in AML.[282,283,286–308] The t(8;21) and inv(16) confer a more favorable outcome on average. t(15;17) confers a highly favorable prognosis. Deletion of all or part of chromosomes 5 and 7 or the presence of complex changes (greater than 3 abnormalities) confers an unfavorable prognosis. Other findings (e.g., normal karyotype, +8, 11q23) generally confer an intermediate prognosis (Chap. 13 has further details and discussion regarding impact of specific translocations).[282–284]

Approximately 45 percent of cases of AML contain cells that are cytogenetically normal. When five genes—NPM1, FLT3, CEPBA, MLL, and NRAS—were examined in 872 adults who were younger than 60 years of age with a normal karyotype, approximately 85 percent had a mutation in at least one of these genes. Mutations in NPM1 or CEPBA were associated with more favorable outcomes, analogous to the category of favorable cytogenetics noted above. The microarray expression signature in patients with AML younger than age 60 years who have cytogenetically normal cells but high-risk molecular features, especially FLT3-ITD and/or wild-type NMP1 expression, is correlated with outcome of therapy (see "Effect of Molecular and Cytogenetic Markers on Disease Progression and Therapeutic Responsiveness" above and Table 88–2). MicroRNAs regulate gene expression and the downregulation of the microRNA-181 family predicts a poor outcome. The microRNAs studied also revealed several important gene families that appear to be involved in the pathogenesis of AML, including genes involved in innate immunity (e.g., toll-like receptors and interleukin-1β expression and regulation).[309] (Chapters 13 and 83 provide further discussion of gene-array profiling and microRNA analysis and the section "Other Acquired Mutations" on molecular pathogenesis has a more detailed discussion of specific molecular markers.) Microarray-based gene-expression profiling is anticipated to become more important in precise diagnosis and subclassification of AML in the future.[310]

PLASMA CHEMICAL FINDINGS

Prior to treatment, mild to moderate increases in serum uric acid and lactic dehydrogenase levels are frequent. Both levels are higher in myelomonocytic and monocytic AML than in other AML phenotypes.[200,201] Occasional patients have very elevated uric acid levels, which usually occur after chemotherapy if proper precautions are not taken (e.g., hypouricemic agents and hydration therapy).[311] Abnormalities of sodium, potassium, calcium, or hydrogen ion concentration are infrequent and usually mild.[312,313] Severe hyponatremia associated with inappropriate antidiuretic hormone secretion has occurred at presentation.[312,313] Severe hypernatremia as a consequence of diabetes insipidus can be an initial event.[314] Hypokalemia is a more frequent finding at presentation and is related to kaliuresis, although the reason for the proximal renal tubular dysfunction is unclear.[312,313,315] The hypokalemia can be severe and often is worsened by the effects of treatment, especially use of kaliuretic antibiotics.[315] Factitious elevations in serum potassium levels have been reported in patients with hyperleukocytosis as a result of leakage from white cells in vitro.[316,317] Factitious hypoglycemia and spurious hypoxia from the effects of high blast cell counts in blood can occur.[314,318]

The presence of hypercalcemia is multifactorial,[319] but cases with increased ectopic parathormone-like activity in the plasma have been described.[320] Severe lactic acidosis prior to treatment has been reported.[312,321,322] Hypophosphatemia as a result of phosphate uptake by leukemic cells can occur.[323] Ectopic adrenocorticotropic hormone secretion,[324] circulating immune complexes,[325] and abnormal concentrations of coagulation factors or their inhibitors[326] may be present.

Although prothrombin and partial thromboplastin times usually are normal or near normal, abnormal concentrations of coagulation factors are frequent. Elevations of platelet factor 4 and thromboxane B_2 occur often.[327] Decreases in α_2-antiplasmin, protein C, and antithrombin III levels are frequent[327] and may be associated with venous thrombosis.[328] APL and acute monocytic leukemia are associated with hypofibrinogenemia and other indicators of activation of coagulation or fibrinolysis (see "Morphologic Variants of Acute Myelogenous Leukemia" below).[329]

TABLE 88–4. Clinical Correlates of Frequent Cytogenetic Abnormalities Observed in Acute Myelogenous Leukemia

Chromosome Abnormality	Genes Affected	Clinical Correlation
Loss or gain of chromosome		
Deletions of part or all of chromosome 5 or 7	Not defined	Frequent in patients with acute myelogenous leukemia (AML) occurring *de novo* and in patients with history of chemical, drug, or radiation exposure and/or previous hematologic disease.[282,283,286,287]
Trisomy 8	Not defined	Very common abnormality in acute myeloblastic leukemia. Poor prognosis, often a secondary change.[283,289]
Translocation		
t(8;21) (q22;q22)	*RUNX1(AML1)– RUNX1T1(ETO)*	Present in ~8% of patients <50 years old and in 3% of patients >50 years old with AML.[288] Approximately 75% of cases have additional cytogenetic abnormalities, including loss of Y in males or X in females. Secondary cooperative mutations of *KRAS, NRAS, KIT* common. Present in ~40% of myelomonocytic phenotype. Higher frequency of myeloid sarcomas.[263–266]
t(15;17) (q31; q22)	*PML-RAR-α*	Represents ~6% of cases of AML.[288] Translocation involving chromosome 17, t(15;17), t(11;17), or t(5;17) is present in most cases of promyelocytic leukemia.[290,291]
t(9;11); (p22; q23)	*MLL (especially MLLT3)*	Present in ~7% of cases of AML. Associated with monocytic leukemia.[292,293] 11q23 translocations in 60% of infants with AML and carries poor prognosis. Rearranges *MLL* gene.[292–296] Many translocation partners for 11q23 translocation.[295–298] *MLL1, MLL4, MLL10* may also result in AML phenotype.
t(9;22) (q34; q22)	*BCR-ABL1*	Present in ~2% of patients with AML.[299,300]
t(1;22)(p13;q13)	*RBMIS-MKL1*	<1% of cases of AML. Admixture of myeloblasts, megakaryoblasts, micromegakaryocytes with cytoplasmic blebbing, dysmorphic megakaryocytes. Reticulin fibrosis common.[301]
t(10;11) (p12-13;q14-21)	*PICALM-MLLT10*	Outcome similar to that of intermediate prognosis group; more extramedullary disease and CD7 expression.[302]
Inversion		
Inv(16) (p13.1;q22) or t(16;16) (p13.1;q22)	*CBF-β MYH11*	Present in ~8% of patients <50 years of age and in ~3% of patients >50 years of age with AML[288]; often acute myelomonocytic phenotype; associated with increased marrow eosinophils; predisposition to cervical lymphadenopathy,[303] better response to therapy.[304–307] Predisposed to myeloid sarcoma.
Inv(3) (q21q26.2)	*RPN1-EVI1*	~1% of cases of AML. Approximately 85% of cases with normal or increased platelet count. Marrow has increased dysmorphic, hypolobulated megakaryocytes. Hepatosplenomegaly more frequent than usual in AML.[308]

SPECIAL CLINICAL FEATURES

Hyperleukocytosis

Leukocyte count is an independent prognostic factor in the outcome of AML treatment.[330] Approximately 5 percent of patients with AML develop signs or symptoms attributable to a markedly elevated blood blast cell count, usually greater than 100×10^9/L (Chap. 83).[331] Several subsets of AML are associated with a greater likelihood of presenting with hyperleukocytosis. These include acute myelomonocytic, acute monocytic, the microgranular variant of APL, and AML with inv16,11q23 rearrangements, or FLT3-ITD. The circulations of the CNS, lungs, and penis are most sensitive to the effects of leukostasis. Intracerebral hemorrhage from vascular occlusion, invasion, and disruption, sometimes complicated by thrombocytopenia and vascular insufficiency are the most virulent manifestations of the syndrome.[332–336] Dizziness, stupor, dyspnea, and priapism may occur. Diabetes insipidus is another association.[337,338] Other severe organ involvement also may occur infrequently. A high early mortality in patients with AML correlates with hyperleukocytosis greater than 100×10^9/L.[334,335,339,340] Chemotherapy in hyperleukocytic patients may lead to a pulmonary leukostatic syndrome, presumably from the effects of rigid, effete blast cells, or the discharge of large amounts of cell contents and resultant cell aggregation or other effects.[341–343] Larger-vessel vascular occlusion as a result of white thrombi or masses of leukemic cells is rare.[344,348] The upregulation of endothelial cell intercellular adhesion molecule-1 and of leukemic blast cell lymphocyte function-associated antigen-1 may mediate the vessel wall interaction contributing to leukostasis.[349]

Hypoplastic Leukemia

Approximately 10 percent of patients with AML present with a syndrome that includes pancytopenia, often with inapparent blood blast cells, and absence of hepatic, splenic, or lymph nodal enlargement.[350–352] If one corrects for the decrease in marrow cellularity with age, hypoplastic AML occurs in approximately 2 percent of cases.[353] Approximately 75 percent of these patients are men older than 50 years of age. Marrow biopsy is hypocellular, which is the unusual feature of the syndrome, but leukemic blast cells are evident and present in a proportion of 10 to 90 percent of marrow cells. Response to intensive chemotherapeutic treatment, often with low-dose cytarabine because of the patients' very advanced age, has been relatively good, and 3-year survival rates are approximately the same as the rates of other age-matched patients.[354]

Oligoblastic Myelogenous (Subacute, Smoldering, Low-Infiltrate, Pauciblastic) Leukemia

Not infrequently, usually in patients older than 50 years of age, myelogenous leukemia is manifested by anemia and often thrombocytopenia. The leukocyte count may be low, normal, or increased, and a small proportion of blast cells are present in the blood (0 to 15 percent) and marrow (3 to 19 percent). Such cases have been referred to as *oligoblastic myelogenous leukemia, subacute,* or *smoldering leukemia,*[355] or classified as a MDS, particularly refractory anemia with excess blasts. The clinical course of the untreated disease can be protracted. The disease has a high morbidity and mortality from infection and hemorrhage and can evolve into overt (polyblastic) AML. The smoldering or oligoblastic leukemias (refractory anemia with excess blasts) historically have been grouped along with the clonal cytopenias as composing MDS; and, the diagnosis and treatment of these variants are discussed in Chap. 87. Biologically and clinically, the disorders in this subset of the MDS with blast cell proportions in the marrow above normal are leukemias, not dysplasias, but they have a slower rate of progression than polyblastic myelogenous leukemia. Dysmorphogenesis of red cells, neutrophils, and platelets is more frequent and more striking than in the average case of polyblastic AML (Chap. 87), but such dysmorphogenesis also occurs in polyblastic leukemia, so-called AML with trilineage dysmorphia.[275] A discussion of the spectrum of myelogenous leukemias, ranging from minimal to severe deviation neoplasms, can be found in Chap. 83.

Philadelphia Chromosome–Positive Acute Myelogenous Leukemia

Approximately 2 percent of patients with AML have the Philadelphia (Ph) chromosome t(9;22)(q34;q11) in a significant proportion (10 to 100 percent) of leukemic blast cells.[356–358] The blast cells have surface antigens, such as CD13 and CD33, characteristic of myeloid leukemias.[359,360] One interpretation of the concurrence of AML with t(9;22) is that it represents CML presenting in myeloid blast crisis.[361–363] The arguments in favor of this proposal are as follows: (1) Blast crisis may occur within days after diagnosis of Ph chromosome–positive CML. (2) Cases can present with additional cytogenetic changes comparable to CML in blast crisis.[361,363] (3) Marked hepatosplenomegaly, uncharacteristic of AML, may be present.[362,363] (4) Platelet counts may be normal, and basophils can be increased.[361,363] (5) A long prodromal period of weakness and weight loss may occur, and some features of CML, such as granulocytosis, can appear after treatment with chemotherapy.[364] (6) Ph chromosome–positive AML has a poor prognosis, as in myeloid blast crisis of CML. (7) The breakpoint on chromosome 22 in the M-bcr may be typical of CML, and the product of the fusion *BCR-ABL* gene is a p210 tyrosine kinase identical to that of classic CML.[360,363–368] (8) Occasional cases express p210 and p190 tyrosine kinases, now known to be features of CML.[368] (9) Some patients enter a remission by converting to a phenotype analogous to chronic phase CML. An alternative view has been promulgated because (1) cases of Ph chromosome–positive AML can be a mosaic (normal and abnormal karyotypes)[360]; (2) the Ph chromosome may appear later in the course of the disease[369]; (3) additional chromosomal abnormalities often are different from those seen in the myeloblastic crisis of CML[360,370,371]; and (4) in some cases, the *BCR-ABL* gene is not encoding a p210 but a p190 mutant tyrosine kinase,[357,365,368,372] the former being most characteristic of CML. Moreover, Ph chromosome–positive AML has developed following Ph chromosome–negative oligoblastic myelogenous leukemia.[357,373,374] Many cases of Ph chromosome–positive acute leukemia are myeloid-lymphoid hybrids.[364,368,370,375] Thus, Ph chromosome–positive AML comes in two varieties: one with a break in M-BCR of chromosome 22 with a p210 product, which could be considered analogous to acute blast crisis of CML, and one with a molecular pathology resulting in the oncogene product being a p190 protein (m-BCR) that could be considered a *de novo* case.

Marrow Necrosis

Necrosis of the marrow is an uncommon event and can be seen in a wide variety of malignant and nonmalignant clinical disorders, but approximately two-thirds of cases are associated with lymphoid or myeloid malignancies and about one-quarter of cases occur in patients with AML.[376] Bone pain (approximately 80 percent of patients) and fever (approximately 70 percent of patients) are the two most common symptoms or signs. Anemia and thrombocytopenia, if not already present, results. White cell counts may be low or high. The blood may contain nucleated red cells and myeloid immaturity (approximately 50 percent of cases). Lactic dehydrogenase and alkaline phosphatase are elevated in approximately 50 percent of cases. The marrow aspirate is often watery and serosanguineous. An amorphous extracellular eosinophilic background with disintegrating cells that have lost their staining characteristics with indistinct margins and varying degrees of pyknosis and karyorrhexis is characteristic. Rare cases have been described in which the marrow contained Charcot-Leyden crystals without an increase in eosinophils or basophils.[377] Bony spicules may also show evidence of necrosis. Destruction of spicule architecture with loss of osteocytes, osteoblasts, and osteocytes may be seen. It is important not to identify these changes as artifact. Usually more than 50 percent of the biopsy is involved. Careful search may identify the underlying hematologic disorder in small islands of intact cells. Technetium-99m sulfur colloid scans show little or no uptake. Magnetic resonance imaging (MRI) may not be diagnostic but can show the extent of the necrosis by changes in signal intensity signifying an increase in water content in relation to fat. Both technetium scanning and MRI can point to areas of intact marrow that may be used to make a diagnosis of the underlying disease, if it is unknown. The pathophysiology is uncertain but is thought to be related to marrow vascular injury and or thrombosis secondary to inflammatory or immune factors and cytokines. The prognosis of marrow necrosis is largely related to the underlying disease. Repair of marrow can occur, if the patient enters remission.

NEONATAL MYELOPROLIFERATION AND LEUKEMIA

Four myeloproliferative syndromes related to AML have been identified in the neonate: transient myeloproliferative disorder, transient leukemia, congenital leukemia, and neonatal leukemia. Transient myeloproliferative disorder and transient leukemia are considered to represent the same phenomenon.

Transient myeloproliferative disease (TMD) can be present at birth or occur shortly thereafter in approximately 10 percent of infants with Down syndrome.[378–384] The leukocyte count is markedly elevated, blast cells are present in the blood and marrow, and anemia and thrombocytopenia may be present, but the latter are not constant findings. The liver and spleen may be enlarged. Results of cytogenetic studies and marrow cell culture studies are normal, except for trisomy 21, which is characteristic of Down syndrome. The blast cells usually have the immunophenotype of megakaryocytes. In contrast to congenital leukemia, the elevated white cell and blast cell counts disappear in most patients (approximately 80 percent) over a period of weeks to months. In approximately 20 percent of patients, severe and potentially lethal complications of hydrops fetalis, hepatic fibrosis, or cardiorespiratory failure may occur.

In some cases, an additional cytogenetic abnormality is present, which disappears after regression of the myeloproliferative syndrome, suggesting a reversible clonal disorder (transient leukemia) that is replaced by normal hematopoiesis. The presence of a trisomy of chromosome 21 is essential for the disease as judged by three observations: the trisomy occurs in (1) the TMD clone of patients with constitutional trisomy 21, (2) the TMD clone in patients with Down syndrome with a cell mosaic pattern of trisomy 21, and (3) in the TMD clone of phenotypically normal infants without a constitutional trisomy 21, but with TMD. In the last case, trisomy 21 disappears with resolution of the myeloproliferation.[385] Candidate oncogenes on chromosome 21 responsible for the phenomenon include *FPDMM, RUNX1 (CBF-β),* and *IFNAR,* among others.[385] *GATA-1* mutations have been found in nearly all patients with TMD and in acute megakaryocytic leukemia in Down patients.[386] The TMD syndrome may disappear, only to be followed shortly thereafter by acute leukemia, predominantly AML, but occasionally acute lymphocytic leukemia (ALL).

One hypothesis for TMD is that the disorder originates in a primitive cell of fetal hepatic hematopoiesis. The cell involutes and is replaced with marrow stem cells. Approximately 25 percent of newborns with Down syndrome and transient leukemia develop acute megakaryocytic leukemia in the first 4 years of life.[387–389]

Very-low-dose cytarabine has been suggested for those patients with severe hepatic fibrosis, very high white cell counts, or hydrops fetalis.[385] TMD cells in these infants are very sensitive to cytarabine.[390,391]

Children with Down syndrome have a 150-fold risk of AML and about a 40-fold risk of ALL by age 5 years. A slightly increased risk of acute leukemia persists into older age. Myelogenous leukemia in patients with Down syndrome often has a megakaryoblastic or erythroid phenotype and may have an interstitial deletion of chromosome 21.[380,381,392–395] This requires mutation in the *GATA1* gene in addition to trisomy 21, and sequential epigenetic changes occur as well in the evolution of acute megakaryoblastic leukemia.[395,396] The response rate of infants with Down syndrome and AML to chemotherapy is very high over prolonged followup and better than the response of patients without Down syndrome.[387,391,397,398] The response to adjusted-dose anthracycline antibiotic and cytarabine in Down syndrome children with AML is approximately 90 percent and the event-free 5-year survival is approximately 80 percent.[394] In those cases with relapsed or refractory disease, outcomes are poor even with allogeneic HSC transplantation.[399] ALL may occur, and the response to therapy is similar to the response of patients without Down syndrome of the same age. Most solid tumors occur less frequently in Down syndrome patients.[390]

Congenital or neonatal leukemia, a rare syndrome, occurs 10 times more frequently in newborns with Down syndrome than in newborns without trisomy 21.[392,393] Leukocytosis, blood and marrow blast cells, hepatosplenomegaly, thrombocytopenia, purpura, anemia, and skin infiltrates are usual. The disease has been diagnosed prenatally. Cytogenetic abnormalities can occur and mark the leukemic clone.[393,400,401] Monocytic leukemia and t(4;11) are the most common phenotype and karyotype.[401–403] A case of vertical (transplacental) transmission of acute monocytic leukemia from mother to son has been reported.[404]

Infants who are normal at birth but develop AML in the first few weeks of life (neonatal leukemia) often display pallor, inadequate food intake, insufficient weight gain, diarrhea, and lethargy. The presence of a cytogenetic abnormality on band q23 of chromosome 11 is a very poor prognostic sign. Most infants with congenital or neonatal leukemia do not survive for more than a few weeks or months. Because treatment has been largely ineffective, observation to ascertain if TMD or a transient leukemia is present has been recommended if the clinical picture is unclear.[405]

HYBRID AND MIXED LEUKEMIAS

Hybrid Leukemias

Although coincidental myeloid and lymphoid clonal diseases have been reported for more than 60 years, the availability of techniques to identify surface antigens with monoclonal antibodies, immunoglobulin gene, and T-lymphocyte receptor gene rearrangements with molecular methods, and chromosome translocations by chromosome banding cytogenetic techniques has led to the appreciation of several types of hybrid acute leukemia.[406–411]

In bilineal (interlineal) acute leukemias, a proportion of cells (>10 percent) have lymphoid and myeloid markers; *interlineal* here refers to lymphopoietic and myeloid gene expression. Bilineal (biphenotypic) leukemias are heterogeneous. Some patients have cells with both lymphoid and myeloid markers (chimeric), whereas other patients have cells with either lymphoid or myeloid markers but evidence that all the cells are part of the same malignant clone (mosaic). The bilineal leukemias may be synchronous (lymphoid and myeloid cells are present simultaneously) or asynchronous (in which lymphoid cells are succeeded by myeloid cells or vice versa), but evidence exists for their origin from the same clone.

Cases of biphenotypic leukemia that are morphologically or cytochemically indicative of myelogenous leukemia have been referred to as LY+AML; the cases that are more indicative of lymphocytic leukemia are referred to as MY+ALL. As a group, interlineal hybrid leukemias treated with current regimens respond to therapy at approximately the same rate as AML cases without lymphoid markers.[406] Some observers suggest altering drug regimens, depending on the balance between lymphoid and myeloid biochemical (drug-response) patterns.[412]

Acute leukemias may be intralineal hybrids in that the blast cells have markers for two or more myeloid lineages (e.g., erythroid, granulocytic, and megakaryocytic) or, in the case of lymphocytic leukemias, both immunoglobulin gene rearrangement (B-lymphocyte type) and T-cell receptor gene rearrangement (T-lymphocyte type).

Myeloid–Natural Killer Cell Hybrids and t(8;13) Myeloid–Lymphoid Leukemias

Although most hybrid leukemias share myeloid and either B- or T-lymphocyte markers, two notable syndromes are associated with hybrid leukemias: (1) the myeloid leukemia and natural killer cell hybrid (CD56+, CD7+, CD13+, CD33+)[413–419] and (2) the lymphoma, eosinophilia, and t(8;13) myeloid leukemia hybrid.[420,421] Signs of lymphoma, such as mediastinal or other lymphadenopathy and extranodal lymphoid tumor, are mixed with findings compatible with AML in both syndromes. The morphology of the myeloid–natural killer cell leukemia often simulates APL, with hypergranular cytoplasm present but abnormality of chromosome 17 absent. The hybrids can appear *de novo* or after relapse of a lymphoma, T-cell leukemia, or blast crisis of CML. The hybrid leukemias usually have a poor prognosis. Myeloid antigens may not be evident at diagnosis in the natural killer cell hybrid but appear later in the course.[422] Hematopoietic stem cell transplantation should be considered in an eligible patient.[423]

Hybrid leukemias may result from either lineage infidelity caused by genetic misprogramming[413] or promiscuous gene expression, which occurs transiently in the differentiation of normal pluripotential HSCs. In the case of promiscuity, persistence of the transient normal event is thought to be present because of the block in differentiation that occurs.[408] Genetic misprogramming (infidelity) could result from rearrangements of the DNA sequences that control the transcription of genes designating differentiation antigens.[424]

Mixed Leukemias

In these cases, lymphoid and myeloid cells are present simultaneously but are derived from separate clones, or sequential myeloid and lymphoid leukemia are present but the two lineages are derived from separate clones.

MEDIASTINAL GERM CELL TUMORS AND ACUTE MYELOGENOUS LEUKEMIA

An unusual but significant concordance has been reported between nonseminomatous mediastinal germ cell tumors and AML, especially the megakaryoblastic variant.[425–430] Mediastinal tumors are rare variants of germ cell tumors. The latter ordinarily occur as testicular teratomas and seminomas in men or as ovarian teratomas in women. They are thought to be derived from yolk sac cells that failed to migrate.[428,429] AML is a HSC tumor derived from a cell type that is present in the yolk sac. Cytogenetic studies are compatible with a clonal relationship (identity) of mediastinal germ cells and myelogenous leukemia cells.[426,427] Apparently, hematopoietic lineage genes are predisposed to expression in extragonadal (mediastinal) germ cell tumors. Use of etoposide, platinum, and related cytotoxic drugs for treatment of mediastinal germ cell tumors may induce secondary AML in a predisposed cell population.[431]

GASTROINTESTINAL TUMORS AND ACUTE MYELOGENOUS LEUKEMIA

A study of 1892 patients with KIT-positive mesenchymal gastrointestinal stromal tumors found a significant subsequent incidence of AML (nine patients). The standardized incidence ratio was approximately 3.0 (confidence interval: 1.1 to 5.8). The patients had not received prior chemotherapy or radiotherapy and the median duration of gastrointestinal stromal tumors before onset of AML was 6 years.[432]

● MORPHOLOGIC VARIANTS OF ACUTE MYELOGENOUS LEUKEMIA

Morphologic variants of AML (Table 88–5) may occur *de novo* or may be the manifestation of clonal evolution from essential thrombocythemia, idiopathic myelofibrosis, CML, or other chronic clonal myeloid disorders. For example, every phenotypic variant of AML can occur as the blast crisis of CML (Chap. 89).

ACUTE MYELOBLASTIC LEUKEMIA

The designation *acute myeloblastic leukemia* came into existence in the second decade of the 20th century,[4] following the specific description of the myeloblast.[6] Approximately 25 percent of AML cases have the features of acute myeloblastic leukemia, a variant in which the leukemic myeloblast is the predominant cell in the marrow. Acute myeloblastic leukemia was divided into two forms, designated *M0* and *M1* in the French-American-British (FAB) Classification. In either type, little evidence of maturation of myeloblasts exists, and the marrow is replaced by a monotonous population of blasts. In acute myeloblastic leukemia (M0), the patient's age distribution, presenting white cell count, and cytogenetic abnormalities are not distinctive. The blasts are nonreactive when stained for myeloperoxidase activity, and Auer rods are not seen. The blasts react with antibodies to myeloperoxidase and antibodies to CD13, CD33, and CD34. Human leukocyte antigen (HLA)-DR is positive in most patients. Occasional cases require *in situ* hybridization to identify the myeloperoxidase gene[433] or genomic profiling for early myeloid-associated genes.[434] Abnormal and unfavorable karyotypes (e.g., 5q–,7q–) and expression of the multidrug resistance (MDR) glycoprotein (p170) are more frequent. This phenotypic variant has a poor prognosis.[435–438] In the other type of myeloblastic leukemia, designated *M1*, myeloblasts are present in the blood and make up more than 70 percent of marrow cells. Less than 15 percent of marrow cells are promyelocytes and myelocytes. Auer rods may be present in occasional blasts, but azurophilic granules are not evident in the blasts by light microscopy. At least 3 percent, but usually a much higher percentage, of the blast cells, have a positive reaction when stained for peroxidase or with Sudan black or react with monoclonal antibodies specific to myeloblasts, such as CD33. This morphologic subtype is denoted as M1 in

the FAB classification. The WHO has divided acute myeloblastic leukemia into three types: AML without differentiation, AML without maturation, and AML with maturation. There is no evidence of a clinical distinction in response to therapy or in prognosis within these rarified designations.

In many cases of myeloblastic leukemia, more prominent granulocytic maturation is evident (FAB type *M2* or WHO designation AML with maturation). This variant is present in approximately 15 percent of AML cases; thus, approximately 45 percent of cases of AML are myeloblastic leukemia with or without maturation. Blasts usually constitute at least 20 percent of the marrow cells. Auer rods may be present in blast cells. Promyelocytes, myelocytes, and segmented neutrophils, the latter often with the acquired Pelger-Huët anomaly, may constitute 20 to 60 percent of marrow granulocytes. The anomaly is reflected in bilobed or monolobed neutrophils. Histochemical and surface markers of blast cells are typical of myeloblastic leukemia, and monocytic markers are absent or infrequent. Monocytes represent less than 10 percent of cells. A translocation between chromosomes 8 and 21 t(8;21)(q22; q22), often accompanied by loss of the Y chromosome in men or loss of an X chromosome in women, is associated with the phenotype and occurs in younger patients (average age approximately 30 years).[439–441] Patients whose cells contain t(8;21) are more prone to develop myeloid sarcoma.[263,266]

ACUTE MYELOMONOCYTIC LEUKEMIA

The ability of AML to express cells of the monocytic and granulocytic lineages was first highlighted in the early 1900s by Naegeli. Later, Hal Downey, a leading hematologist of the day, proposed the eponym *Naegeli type* for myelomonocytic leukemia.[442] Approximately 15 percent of patients with AML present with this variant, and they are more likely to have extramedullary infiltrates in gingiva, skin, or CNS than are patients with acute myeloblastic leukemia (see "Myeloid [Granulocytic] Sarcoma" above).[443] A mixture of myeloblasts and monoblasts is found in the blood and marrow. More than 30 percent of marrow cells are a mixed population of myeloblasts, which react with peroxidase or chloracetate esterase, and monoblasts or promonocytes, which react with fluoride-inhibitable nonspecific esterase (see Fig. 88–2F). More than 20 percent of cells are monoblasts or promonocytes in blood and marrow. In some cases, individual cells react with monocytic and granulocytic histochemical stains.[444] Serum and urinary lysozyme levels are increased in most cases. This variant of AML is referred to as *M4* in the FAB classification and as acute myelomonocytic leukemia in the WHO classification. Translocations involving chromosome 3 are associated with this phenotype.[445]

The proportion of marrow eosinophils[446] or basophils[447] may be increased. A particular variant of myelomonocytic leukemia has increased numbers of marrow eosinophils (10 to 50 percent), Auer rods in blast cells, and inversion or rearrangement of chromosome 16 (see Fig. 88–2G).[304–307] The eosinophils are abnormally large, and the eosinophilic myelocytes contain large basophilic granules. Macrophages with ingested Charcot-Leyden crystals may be present. This phenotypic variant of AML has been designated *M4Eo* in the FAB classification. Although this variant has an increased risk of CNS involvement, it carries a more favorable prognosis than the average case of AML. Fluorescence *in situ* hybridization (FISH) is a more accurate method for detection of cryptic 16q22 gene rearrangements and is useful in conjunction with conventional cytogenetics for patients with M4Eo AML. AML with t(6;9)(p23;q34) is an uncommon variant, occurring in approximately 1 percent of cases, and may express itself as acute myelomonocytic or acute myeloblastic leukemia. Anemia, thrombocytopenia, a variable white cell count, and increased myeloblasts are frequent.

TABLE 88–5. Morphologic Variants of Acute Myelogenous Leukemia

Variant	Cytologic Features	Special Clinical Features	Special Laboratory Features
Acute myeloblastic leukemia (M0, M1, M2)	1. Myeloblasts range from 20–90% of marrow cells. Cytoplasm occasionally contains Auer bodies. Nucleus shows fine reticular pattern and distinct nucleolus (1 or 2 usually). 2. Blast cells are sudanophilic. They are positive for myeloperoxidase and chloroacetate esterase, negative for nonspecific esterase, and negative or diffusely positive for PAS (no clumps or blocks). 3. Electron microscopy shows cytoplasmic primary granules.	1. Most common in adults, and most frequent variety in infants. 2. Three morphologic-cytochemical types (M0, M1, M2)	1. Chromosomes +8, –5, –7, del(11q), and complex abnormalities common. *RUNX1(AML1)* and *FLT3* mutations occur in approximately 20–25% of cases. 2. M0 type blast cells positive with antibody to myeloperoxidase and CD34 and CD13 or CD33 coexpression. *AML1* mutations in ~25%. 3. M1 expresses CD13 and CD33. Positive for myeloperoxidase by cytochemistry. 4. M2 AML with maturation often associated with t(8;21) karyotype. 5. M2 AML with t(6;9)(p23;q34), an uncommon variant, is associated with marrow basophilia, a high blast count, a high frequency of *FLT3*-ITD, and a poor outcome.
Acute promyelocytic leukemia (M3, M3v)	1. Leukemic cells resemble promyelocytes. They have large atypical primary granules and a kidney-shaped nucleus. Branched or adherent Auer rods are common. 2. Peroxidase stain intensely positive. 3. A variant has microgranules (M3v), otherwise the same course and prognosis.	1. Usually in adults. 2. Hypofibrinogenemia and hemorrhage common. 3. Leukemic cells mature in response to all-*trans*-retinoic acid.	1. Cells contain t(15;17) in >95% of cases or another rearrangement involving the *RAR-α* gene on chromosome 17. 2. Cells are HLA-DR–negative.
Acute myelomonocytic leukemia (M4, M4Eo)	1. Both myeloblastic and monoblastic leukemic cells in blood and marrow. 2. Peroxidase-, Sudan-, chloroacetate esterase-, and nonspecific esterase-positive cells. 3. M4Eo variant has marrow eosinophilia.	1. Similar to myeloblastic leukemia but with more frequent extramedullary disease. 2. Mildly elevated serum and urine lysozyme.	1. Leukemic cells in eosinophilic variant (M4Eo) usually have inversion or translocation of chromosome 16.
Acute monocytic leukemia (M5)	1. Leukemia cells are large; nuclear cytoplasmic ratio lower than myeloblast. Cytoplasm contains fine granules. Auer rods are rare. Nucleus is convoluted and cell simulates promonocytes (M5a) or may simulate monoblasts (M5b) and contain large nucleoli. 2. Nonspecific esterase-positive inhibited by NaF; Sudan-, peroxidase-, and chloroacetate esterase-negative. PAS occurs in granules, blocks.	1. Seen in children or young adults. 2. Gum, CNS, lymph node, and extramedullary infiltrations are common. 3. DIC occurs. 4. Plasma and urine lysozyme elevated. 5. Hyperleukocytosis common.	1. t(4;11) common in infants. 2. Rearrangement of q11;q23 very frequent.

(continued)

TABLE 88–5. Morphologic Variants of Acute Myelogenous Leukemia (Continued)

Variant	Cytologic Features	Special Clinical Features	Special Laboratory Features
Acute erythroid leukemia (M6)	1. Abnormal erythroblasts are in abundance initially in marrow and often in blood. Later the morphologic findings may be indistinguishable from those of AML.	1. Pancytopenia common at diagnosis.	1. Cells reactive with antihemoglobin antibody. Erythroblasts usually are strongly PAS and CD71-positive, express ABH blood group antigens, and react with antihemoglobin antibody. 2. Cells reactive with anti–Rc-84 (antihuman erythroleukemia cell-line antigen).
Acute megakaryocytic leukemia (M7)	1. Small blasts with pale agranular cytoplasm and cytoplasmic blebs. May mimic lymphoblasts of medium to larger size. 2. Leukemic cells with megakaryocytic morphology may coexist with megakaryoblasts.	1. Usually presents with pancytopenia. 2. Markedly elevated serum lactic dehydrogenase levels. 3. Marrow aspirates are usually "dry taps" because of the invariable presence of myelofibrosis. 4. Common phenotype in the AML of Down syndrome.	1. Antigens of von Willebrand factor, and glycoprotein Ib (CD42), IIb/IIIa (CD41), IIIa (CD61) on blast cells. 2. Platelet peroxidase positive.
Acute eosinophilic leukemia	1. Mixture of blasts and cells with dysmorphic eosinophilic granules (smaller and less refractile).	1. Hepatomegaly, splenomegaly, lymphadenopathy may be prominent. 2. Absence of neurologic, respiratory, or cardiac signs or symptoms characteristic of chronic eosinophilic leukemia (clonal hypereosinophilic syndrome).	1. Cyanide-resistant peroxidase stains eosinophilic granules. TEM shows eosinophilic granules to be smaller and missing central crystalloid. 2. Biopsy may show Charcot-Leyden crystals in skin, marrow, or other sites of eosinophil accumulation.
Acute basophilic leukemia	Mixture of blast cells and cells with basophilic granules in blood and marrow.	1. Often has hepatomegaly and or splenomegaly; symptoms often present. 2. Rash with urticaria, headaches, prominent gastrointestinal symptoms.	1. CD9-, CD11b-, CD25-, CD123-positive cells are usually present. 2. Toluidine blue-positive cells. 3. Hyperhistaminemia and hyperhistaminuria. 4. Cells negative for tryptase but positive for histidine decarboxylase.
Acute mast cell leukemia	1. Mast cells in blood and marrow. Most contain granules but some are agranular and may simulate monocytes.	1. Fever, headache, flushing of face and trunk, pruritus may be present. 2. Abdominal pain, peptic ulcer, bone pain, diarrhea more common than other AML subtypes. 3. Hepatomegaly, splenomegaly common. 4. Hemorrhagic diathesis may be evident.	1. CD13, CD33, CD68, CD117 often positive. 2. Cells positive for tryptase staining and serum tryptase elevated. 3. Hyperhistaminemia and hyperhistaminuria.

AML, acute myelogenous leukemia; DIC, disseminated intravascular coagulation; HLA-DR, human leukocyte antigen-D related; NaF, sodium fluoride; PAS, periodic acid–Schiff; RAR, retinoic acid receptor; TEM, transmission electron microscopy.

NOTE: Parentheses indicate French-American-British (FAB) classification designations M0 through M7.

The myeloblasts often contain Auer rods. Marrow basophilia is present in about half the cases.[208,280,448] The variant occurs at a younger age, has a poor prognosis, and has a tendency to trilineage dysmorphia and ringed sideroblasts.[449]

ACUTE ERYTHROID LEUKEMIA

Prominence of erythroid cell proliferation in AML cases was noted by Copelli[450] and DiGuglielmo[451] in the early 20th century. Moeschlin[452] used the term *erythroleukemia*. Dameshek[453] suggested the name *DiGuglielmo syndrome* and dissected the disorder into three phases, depending on the decreasing prevalence of dysmorphic erythroblasts and the reciprocal increasing prevalence of myeloblasts. Erythroid leukemia makes up approximately 5 percent of AML cases and is referred to as *M6* in the FAB classification.[454] Familial erythroleukemia has been described.[455,456] Erythroid leukemia is arbitrarily divided into three degrees of severity: (1) *erythroleukemia* in which more than 50 percent of the marrow cells are dysmorphic; (2) erythroblasts admixed with myeloblasts, the latter composing approximately 20 percent of non-erythroid cells or approximately 5 to 10 percent of total marrow cells; and (3) a form in which dysmorphic erythroblasts dominate the marrow, *pure erythroid leukemia*, in which more than 80 percent of marrow cells are dysmorphic erythroblasts with a trivial granulocytic proportion of cells and very few if any myeloblasts. This last form of the disease may start in as a milder variant, formerly called *erythremic myelosis*, in which granulopoiesis, and thrombopoiesis may be only mildly abnormal. This phase, dominated morphologically by bizarre dysmorphia of erythroblasts, can be protracted but eventually evolves into a dimorphic phase in which myeloblasts are more prominent, severe neutropenia and thrombocytopenia develop, and the patient progresses to erythroid leukemia. The disease may evolve further into polyblastic AML.[457–460] In the erythremic myelosis variant, erythropoiesis is ineffective. However, some normal regulation may remain because hypertransfusion decreases both erythropoietin levels and the amount of abnormal erythropoiesis.[461] Spontaneous growth of leukemic erythroid clonogenic cells is a feature of the disease.[462] Periodic acid–Schiff (PAS)-positive erythroblasts are evident in almost all cases.[457,460]

The erythroid leukemias are characterized by a striking population of dysmorphic erythroblasts in marrow and red cells in blood (see Fig. 88–2I, J, and K). Anemia and thrombocytopenia are present in nearly all cases. Some patients may have elevated total leukocyte counts. The red cells show marked anisocytosis, poikilocytosis, anisochromia, and basophilic stippling. Nucleated red cells are present in the blood. The marrow erythroblasts are extremely abnormal, with giant multinucleate forms, nuclear budding, and nuclear fragmentation. Cytogenetic abnormalities are present in approximately 70 percent of patients and complex cytogenetic abnormalities are frequent. The frequency of erythroid leukemia is increased if methods for detecting erythroid differentiation more sensitive than light microscopy are used. These cell features include glycophorin A, spectrin, carbonic anhydrase I, ABH blood group antigens, and other antigens that occur on early erythroid progenitors, such as the transferrin receptor (CD71).[463–465] Antihemoglobin antibody and antihuman erythroleukemic cell line antibody often are positive.[458]

Erythremic myelosis can have an indolent course and may be managed for a time without intensive chemotherapy. Treatment is warranted in patients with erythroleukemia and acute erythroid leukemia, and the results are approximately the same as with other phenotypes in patients of similar age.[460] The more predominant the erythroid component and the lower the proportion of myeloblasts, the better the response to therapy.[403]

ACUTE PROMYELOCYTIC LEUKEMIA

The association of an exaggerated hemorrhagic syndrome with certain leukemias was described by French hematologists in 1949.[466] In 1957, Hillstad[467] bestowed the appellation *promyelocytic leukemia* upon this morphologic-clinical subtype of AML. This variant, which is called *M3* in the FAB classification and APL in the WHO classification, occurs at any age and constitutes approximately 7 percent of AML cases.[290,291,468,469] APL occurs with greater frequency among Latinos from Europe and South and Central America.[190,191] APL represents 19 percent of AML cases in the Chinese[189] as compared to 8 percent among persons of European descent. APL is also increased among persons with an increased body mass index.[470–472] Unlike all other major variants of AML, which increase in incidence logarithmically with age, the incidence of APL is constant over the human life span.[188] Hemorrhagic manifestations are prominent including hemoptysis, hematuria, vaginal bleeding, melena, hematemesis, and pulmonary and intracranial bleeding, as well as the more typical skin and mucous membrane bleeding. In severely leukopenic patients, blasts may not be evident in the blood. Moderately severe thrombocytopenia ($<50 \times 10^9/L$) is present in most cases. The marrow contains few agranular blast cells and some blast-like cells with scant granules. The dominant cells are promyelocytes, which comprise 30 to 90 percent of marrow cells (see Fig. 88–2D and E). Auer rods and cells with multiple Auer rods (1 to 10 percent) are present in nearly every case. Promyelocytes with multiple Auer rods have been referred to as *faggot cells*. Leukemic promyelocytes stain intensely with myeloperoxidase and Sudan black and express CD 9, CD13, and CD33, but not CD34 or HLA-DR.[290,291,468,469]

A variant type of promyelocytic leukemia is referred to as *microgranular* (*M3v* in the FAB nomenclature).[473–476] Microgranular cases represent approximately 20 percent of patients with promyelocytic leukemia. The leukemic cells may mimic promonocytes with convoluted or lobulated nuclei. Auer rods may be present but are less evident. The majority of the leukemic cells contain azurophilic granules that are so small they are not visible by light microscopy, but the peroxidase stain usually is strongly positive. Typical hypergranulated promyelocytes usually are present on careful inspection. The total white cell count often is highly elevated, and severe coagulopathy is prominent in microgranular cases.[474] Rarely, the cells contain eosinophilic or basophilic granules, but t(15;17) is present, and the response to all-*trans* retinoic acid (ATRA) persists,[477–479] although the basophilic variant can be virulent.[480]

A translocation between chromosome 17(q21), which rearranges the *RAR-α* gene at band q21, and another chromosome is present in all cases of APL and in the acute promyelocytic transformation of CML; it is not found in other AML variants. The t(15;17)(q22;q21) is the most frequent cytogenetic abnormality (>95 percent), but variant translocations between chromosome 3, 5, or 11 and chromosome 17 or isochromosome 17, and other even less common variants have been described.[290,468,481–483] In some cases, cytogenetic analysis is inadequate and Southern blot analysis is required to identify the rearrangement of the *RAR-α* gene. A functional distinction is that the t(15;17), *PML–RAR-α* fusion, the t(5;17), *NPM–RAR-α* fusion, and the t(3;17), *TBLR1–RAR-α* fusion confer retinoid therapy responsiveness, whereas t(11;17), *PLZF–RAR-α* fusion, usually is retinoid resistant. In cells with the t(11;17), Auer rods are absent and CD56 expression usually is present, offering some clinical variables to provoke special molecular investigations.[484] The retinoid resistance may not always be present.[485]

The breakpoint on chromosome 17 is within the gene encoding the RAR-α, and the breakpoint on chromosome 15 is within the locus of a gene originally referred to as *MYL* and renamed *PML* (to indicate its relationship to promyelocytic leukemia).[290,486] The gene encodes a unique transcription factor. The translocation results in two new chimeric or fusion genes: *RAR-α–PML,* which is actively transcribed in APL, and *PML–RAR-α,* which also is transcribed and may account for the aberrancy in hematopoiesis. The *PML–RAR-α* gene has two isoforms that produce a short- and a long-type fusion messenger RNA, respectively.[487] Patients with the short isoform may have a worse outcome than those with the longer form. Polymerase chain reaction (PCR) for the mRNA of the fusion gene can be used to identify residual cells during remission and may predict relapse. The *PML–RAR-α* transgene can reproduce the disease in mice,[488] although in some models a superimposed *FLT3* mutation is required to express the disease. *FLT3* mutations are frequently found in human disease, especially in the hypogranular variant.[157]

A propensity to hemorrhage is a striking feature of this subtype. The prothrombin and partial thromboplastin times are prolonged, and the plasma fibrinogen level is decreased in most cases. The disturbance in coagulation first was thought to principally result from intravascular coagulation initiated by procoagulant released from the granules of the leukemic promyelocytes. Elevated thrombin–antithrombin complexes, prothrombin fragment 1+2, and fibrinopeptide A plasma levels support that supposition. Increased levels of fibrinogen–fibrin degradation products, D-dimer, and evidence of plasminogen activation indicate fibrinolysis.[489–491] Furthermore, decreased levels of plasminogen, increased expression of annexin II on the leukemic cells,[492] and reports of responses to tranexamic acid support a role for fibrinolysis in the bleeding in APL.[493] Release of nonspecific proteases may further contribute to fibrinogenolysis. Thus, the coagulopathy is now considered tripartite.[494]

Although APL responded to chemotherapy regimens for AML, especially those containing an anthracycline antibiotic,[495] the cytologic pattern of response in the marrow often was paradoxical.[496–499] Persistence of leukemic promyelocytes preceded remission in the absence of further therapy, whereas induction of marrow cell hypoplasia was classically considered a requirement for remission in patients with AML. Generally, if leukemic blast cells persist after therapy for AML, relapse ensues unless hypoplasia is induced by more cytotoxic therapy. The unusual pattern of response in APL was put into context by reports of successful treatment with isomers of retinoic acid, an agent that leads to maturation of leukemic promyelocytes *in vitro.*[499] In 1988, the success of ATRA in remission induction was reported[500,501] and confirmed.[290,291] Relapse occurs invariably, however, so chemotherapy regimens or addition of arsenic trioxide also were required. Use of ATRA has decreased the risk of early hemorrhagic complications and death and has enhanced the long-term response to chemotherapy. Despite the improvement in therapy, approximately 5 to 10 percent of patients die during remission induction, most of hemorrhage, often into the brain. The prolonged remissions of patients with promyelocytic leukemia has been interrupted in approximately 3 percent of cases by the later appearance of oligoblastic myelogenous leukemia with deletions of all or part of chromosome 5 or 7 and no evidence of involvement of chromosome 17, compatible with a myelogenous leukemia secondary to cytotoxic chemotherapy.[501–503] The responsiveness to arsenic trioxide has provided additional treatment approaches that are discussed in the "Therapy" section below.

ACUTE MONOCYTIC LEUKEMIA

Monocytic leukemia was first reported by Reschad and Schilling-Torgau[504] in 1913. Approximately 8 percent of patients with AML present with monocytic leukemia, which is referred to as *M5* in the FAB classification. Patients with monocytic leukemia have a higher prevalence (50 percent) of extramedullary tumors in the skin, gingiva, eyes, larynx, lung, rectum and anal canal, bladder, lymph nodes, meninges, CNS, and other sites than do other phenotypes (<5 percent).

Hepatomegaly, splenomegaly, and lymphadenopathy are more frequent in monocytic leukemia.[207,505–507]

The proportion of monocytic cells is usually greater than 75 percent. The total leukocyte count is higher in a larger proportion of patients, and hyperleukocytosis occurs more frequently (approximately 35 percent) than in other variants.[508–510] The marrow and blood cells may be largely monoblasts (acute monoblastic leukemia) or more mature-appearing promonocytes and monocytes (acute monocytic leukemia) (see Fig. 88–2*H*). When the blood contains more mature-appearing monocytic cells, the marrow contains a lower proportion of blast cells, approximately 15 to 50 percent. When the blood monocytes are largely blast cells, the marrow contains approximately 50 to 90 percent blasts. In nearly all cases, 10 to 90 percent of monocytic cells react for nonspecific esterase stains, *α*-naphthyl acetate esterase, and naphthol AS-D-chloroacetate esterase; in a cytochemical or chemoluminescence assay; or with monoclonal antibodies against monocyte surface antigens, especially CD14. Immunoreactivity of cells for lysozyme is characteristic. Serum and urine lysozyme levels are elevated in most patients. Serum lactic dehydrogenase and β_2-microglobulin concentrations are increased in greater than 80 percent of patients.[511] Plasminogen activator inhibitor-2 is present in the plasma and the cells of a high proportion of patients.[512] Auer rods are absent when monoblasts dominate but may be present in cases where promonocytes and monocytes are prevalent in blood and marrow. Leukemic monocytes have Fc receptors and can ingest and kill microorganisms in some cases.[513,514]

There is an association between translocations involving chromosome 11, especially region 11q23, and monocytic leukemia.[292–294] In particular, t(9;11) is found in leukemic monocytes.[295,296,507,508] In t(9;11) the β_1-interferon gene is translocated to chromosome 11, and the protooncogene *ETS*-1 is translocated to chromosome 9 adjacent to the *α*-interferon gene. The latter juxtaposition may be important in the pathogenesis of monocytic leukemia.[515]

The expression of *FOS* is closely correlated with monocytic maturation of cells in myelomonocytic and monocytic leukemia and in normal monocytopoiesis.[516,517] Absence or markedly decreased expression of the retinoblastoma gene growth-suppressor product (p105) is present in approximately half of patients with monocytic leukemia. Patients express a more dramatic phenotype.[518] A variant of acute monocytic leukemia in which the leukemic cells have monocytoid features and are positive for early and late monocytic lineage antigens and for TdT activity often occurs after prior radiotherapy or chemotherapy and is relatively resistant to treatment.[519] A syndrome of acute monoblastic leukemia with t(8;16), resulting in *MOZ-CBP* fusion gene, is characterized by mildly granular promonocytes (simulating hypogranular promyelocytes), intense phagocytosis of red cells, erythroblasts, and sometimes neutrophils and platelets in blood and marrow, simulating macrophagic hemophagocytic syndrome, intravascular coagulation or primary fibrinolysis, and a high frequency of extramedullary disease.[520]

The management of monocytic leukemia is complicated by a greater incidence of CNS or meningeal disease either at the time of diagnosis or as a form of relapse during remission. Thus, examination of cerebrospinal fluid is often recommended, even in the absence of symptoms, when remission has been achieved.[208,507,508] Some therapists recommend prophylactic intrathecal therapy with methotrexate or cytosine arabinoside for patients who enter remission after having presented with hyperleukocytic acute monocytic leukemia because of the risk of subclinical meningeal involvement. Others posit that high-dose cytarabine with CNS penetration potential used in consolidation chemotherapy suffices for this purpose. There are few data for guidance in this matter.

Rare cases of dendritic cell or Langerhans cell phenotype have been described (Chap. 71).[521,522] Uncommon cases of histiocytic sarcoma are the tissue or extramedullary variant of monocytic leukemia (Chap. 71).[523,524] The outcome of treatment, once thought to be less favorable than with other forms of AML, is comparable to the outcome of other subtypes.[525]

ACUTE MEGAKARYOBLASTIC (MEGAKARYOCYTIC) LEUKEMIA

In 1963, Szur and Lewis[526] reported patients with pancytopenia, low percentages of blast cells, and intense myelofibrosis but an absence of teardrop red cells, splenomegaly, leukocytosis, and thrombocytosis, the usual features of primary myelofibrosis. They designated the syndrome *malignant myelosclerosis*.[526] Reports of similar cases ensued, with some investigators referring to the syndrome as *acute myelofibrosis*.[527] The development of methods to phenotype megakaryoblasts indicated the cases were variants of AML rather than of primary myelofibrosis and have been designated *acute megakaryocytic* or *acute megakaryoblastic leukemia*.[391,528,529] This leukemia is referred to as M7 in the FAB classification. The prevalence of this phenotype is approximately 5 percent of all AML cases if appropriate cell markers are used in the diagnosis, and is at least twice that frequency in childhood AML.[530,531] The syndrome is an especially prevalent variant of AML that develops in patients with Down syndrome[398,532] or in patients with mediastinal germ cell tumors and coincident AML.[425–429]

Leukemic megakaryoblasts and promegakaryocytes can be difficult to identify by light microscopy using polychrome staining. However, with experience, heightened suspicion can be engendered by blasts in the blood with abundant budding cytoplasm or blasts having a lymphoid appearance, especially if the marrow cannot be aspirated because of intense myelofibrosis, the latter evident on the marrow biopsy. Initially high-resolution histochemistry for platelet peroxidase and identification of the demarcation membrane system using transmission electron microscopy were required for diagnosis. Now antibodies to von Willebrand factor or to platelet glycoprotein Ib (CD42), IIb/IIIa (CD41), or IIIa (CD61) can be used to identify very primitive megakaryocytic cells.[528,529] A small proportion of megakaryoblasts may be present in other cases of AML, but in megakaryocytic leukemia they are the prominent or the dominant leukemic cells (see Fig. 88–2*L* through *O*). Moreover, the other key features of the syndrome usually are present, especially severe myelofibrosis.[530]

Patients usually present with pallor, weakness, excessive bleeding and anemia, and leukopenia. Lymphadenopathy or hepatosplenomegaly is uncommon at the time of diagnosis. High leukocyte and blood blast cell counts may be present initially or may develop later. The platelet count may be normal or elevated in many patients at the time of presentation. Abnormal platelets or megakaryocytic cytoplasmic fragments may be found in the blood. Marrow aspiration often is unsuccessful ("dry tap") because of extensive marrow fibrosis in most cases, although not all. The marrow biopsy contains small blast cells, large blast cells, or a combination of both. The former have a high nuclear-to-cytoplasmic ratio, have dense chromatin with distinct nucleoli, and resemble lymphoblasts. Cases have been mistaken for ALL. The larger blasts may have some features of maturing megakaryocytes with agranular cytoplasm with cytoplasmic protrusions, clusters of platelet-like structures, or shedding of cytoplasmic blebs. The blast cells are peroxidase negative and tend to aggregate. Confirmation of their megakaryoblastic maturation requires immunocytologic studies for the presence of von Willebrand factor and the immunoreactivity to CD41, CD42, or CD61. The more mature megakaryocytes, which often coexist in the marrow, stain with PAS reagent, contain sodium fluoride–inhibitable nonspecific esterase, and fail to react for α-naphthylbutyrate

esterase or myeloperoxidase. The thrombopoietin receptor gene (*MPL*) is expressed in megakaryocytes (CD116) and exhibits the gain-of-function point mutation W515K/L in approximately 25 percent of cases of acute megakaryoblastic leukemia.[533]

The serum lactic acid dehydrogenase level frequently is strikingly increased and has an isomorphic pattern unlike that seen with other acute leukemias. Complex chromosome aberrations are common.[534] An association of megakaryoblastic leukemia in infants with t(1;22)(p13;q13) has been reported.[534–537] Abnormalities of chromosome 3 have been linked to clonal hemopathies expressing a prominent megakaryocytic phenotype.[538,539] Progression of primary myelofibrosis or essential thrombocythemia to AML may have the phenotype of acute megakaryocytic leukemia. Paradoxically, in children with Down syndrome the disease can be treated with modified doses of chemotherapy, with a very high remission rate and long-term event-free survival.[540–542] The result is thought to be related to the exquisite sensitivity of the leukemic cells to drug-induced apoptosis,[475] whereas the long-term remission rate as a result of chemotherapy in children without Down syndrome or in adults are not as good.[543,544]

ACUTE EOSINOPHILIC LEUKEMIA

Acute eosinophilic leukemia is rare. Increased eosinophils in the marrow but not in the blood is a variant of acute myelomonocytic leukemia and inversion 16 or other abnormalities of chromosome 16 but is not considered an acute eosinophilic leukemia.[303–306] First described in 1912,[545] acute eosinophilic leukemia is a distinct entity that can arise *de novo* as AML, with 50 to 80 percent of eosinophilic cells in the blood and marrow.[546–549] Anemia, thrombocytopenia, and blast cells in blood and marrow are present. There is apparent eosinophilic differentiation in striking proportions. The eosinophilic cells are dysmorphic and the cytoplasm hypogranulated with smaller than normal eosinophilic granules. The granules stain less intensely and are less refractile with polychrome stains. These findings are the result of the loss of the central crystalloid in the eosinophilic granules that can be identified with electron microscopic analysis. Biopsy of skin, marrow, or other sites of eosinophil accumulation often shows Charcot-Leyden crystals. A specific histochemical reaction, cyanide-resistant peroxidase, permits identification of leukemic cells with eosinophilic differentiation and diagnosis of acute eosinoblastic leukemia in some cases of AML with fewer identifiable eosinophils in blood or marrow.[550] Eosinophilia, not part of the malignant clone, may be a feature of occasional patients with AML, an uncommon reactive phenomenon. In many cases, idiopathic eosinophilia (hypereosinophilic syndrome) is a monoclonal disorder representing a spectrum of more indolent chronic or subacute eosinophilic leukemia to more progressive acute leukemia (Chaps. 62 and 89).[551] Acute eosinophilic leukemia may develop in patients having the chronic form of a hypereosinophilic syndrome. Overexpression of *WT* gene expression has been proposed as a means of distinguishing acute eosinophilic leukemia from a polyclonal, reactive eosinophilia.[552]

Patients with acute eosinophilic leukemia do not usually develop bronchospastic signs, neurologic signs, and heart failure from endomyocardial fibrosis as is seen in chronic eosinophilic leukemia, probably because those tissue changes are the result of release of toxins in the granule crystalloid, absent in most eosinophils in acute eosinophilic leukemia and because of the shorter duration of survival in acute eosinophilic leukemia. Hepatomegaly, splenomegaly, and lymphadenopathy are more common than in other variants of AML. The treatment approach is similar to other types of AML. A combination of cytarabine and an anthracycline antibiotic is an appropriate choice for treatment. Response to treatment is approximately the same as in other types of AML.[550]

ACUTE BASOPHILIC AND MAST CELL LEUKEMIA

First described in 1906,[553] basophilic differentiation as a feature of AML is an uncommon event, occurring in approximately one in 100 cases of AML.[549] Most cases of acute basophilic leukemia evolve from the chronic phase of CML,[554] but de novo acute basophilic leukemia, in which the cells do not contain the Ph chromosome, does occur.[549,535–560] The cells stain with toluidine blue, and the basophilic granules can be most striking in myelocytes. In some cases of acute myelomonocytic leukemia associated with t(6;9)(p23;q34), basophils may be increased in the marrow but not in the blood. Because CML with t(9;22)(q34;q11) has the same breakpoint (q34) on chromosome 9 as AML with t(6;9) and both diseases are strongly associated with marrow basophilia, a gene(s) at the breakpoint on chromosome 9 may influence basophilopoiesis.[448]

Anemia, thrombocytopenia, and blast cells in the blood are present at the time of diagnosis. The blood leukocyte count usually is elevated, and proportions of the cells are basophils. The marrow is cellular with a high proportion of blasts and early and late basophilic myelocytes. Special staining with toluidine blue or Astra blue often is necessary to distinguish basophilic from neutrophilic promyelocytes and myelocytes. Immunophenotyping may show myeloid markers (CD33, CD13) that are not specific. Presence of CD9, CD25, or both is characteristic of basophilic differentiation. Cells may have granules with ultrastructural features of basophils and mast cells.[558] Electron microscopy can be useful in identifying basophilic granules in cases where no granules are evident by light microscopy and the phenotype simulates M0.[558] Basophilic leukemia can be confused with promyelocytic leukemia if the basophilic early myelocytes are mistaken for promyelocytes.[561] On the contrary, promyelocytic leukemia may have basophilic maturation and can be mistaken for basophilic leukemia. However, if the cells contain t(15;17), the disease should respond to ATRA and an anthracycline antibiotic.[474,477,478] Prolonged clotting time, intravascular coagulation, and hemorrhage are uncommon presenting features in patients with basophilic leukemia, but are common in patients with promyelocytic leukemia. Coagulopathy can occur after chemotherapy. Cluster headaches, skin rashes, often with an urticarial component, and gastrointestinal symptoms may be present. Elevated blood and urine histamine and urinary methylhistamine levels are characteristic features. Rare cases of a chronic course in *BCR-ABL*–negative basophilic leukemia preceding the onset of rapid progression have occurred.[562] Treatment for acute (Ph-negative) basophilic leukemia is similar to that for other variants of AML.

Mast cell leukemia is a rare manifestation of systemic mast cell disease (Chap. 63).[549,563] It can be related to a mutation of the *KIT* gene.[507] The leukemic mast cells are KIT (CD117) positive, naphthol AS-D-chloracetate esterase positive, tryptase positive, myeloperoxidase negative, and CD25-negative.[564,565] Plasma tryptase is elevated. In some cases, electron microscopy of the granule-containing cells, which demonstrates the characteristic scroll-like granules of mast cells, may aid in distinguishing basophils from mast cells (Chap. 63). Extensive, apparently reactive, mast cell tissue infiltrations may be provoked by cytokines during the course of AML.[566,567]

The key laboratory distinctions between acute basophilic leukemia and acute mast cell leukemia are that the cells in the former are naphthol AS-D-chloracetate esterase negative, CD11b positive, CD117 negative or weakly positive, CD123 positive, have no increase in cell or plasma tryptase, and have basophilic-like granules on electron microscopy; whereas, the cells in mast cell leukemia are naphthol AS-D-chloracetate esterase positive, CD11b-negative, CD117-positive, CD123-negative, have an increase in cell and plasma tryptase, and have mast cell-like granules on electron microscopy.[549]

HISTIOCYTIC AND ACUTE MYELOID DENDRITIC CELL LEUKEMIA

Chapter 71 discusses histiocytic and myeloid dendritic cell leukemia.

● DIFFERENTIAL DIAGNOSIS

Acute leukemia in infants with Down syndrome should be differentiated from TMD (see "Neonatal Myeloproliferation and Leukemia" above). In adults, the term *pseudoleukemia* has been applied to circumstances that mimic the marrow appearance of promyelocytic leukemia. Recovery from drug-induced or *Pseudomonas aeruginosa*–induced agranulocytosis is characterized by a striking cohort of promyelocytes in the marrow, which upon inspection of the marrow aspirate or biopsy mimics promyelocytic leukemia.[568–570]

In pseudoleukemia, the platelet count may be normal; the degree of leukopenia often is more profound ($<1.0 \times 10^9$/L) than usually seen in AML[511,512]; promyelocytes contain a prominent paranuclear clear (Golgi) zone not covered with granules; and promyelocytes do not have Auer rods.[570–572] Similar reactions have been reported after granulocyte colony-stimulating factor (G-CSF) administration.[573] In patients suspected of having pseudoleukemia, observation for a few days usually clarifies the significance of the marrow appearance, because progressive maturation to segmented neutrophils normalizes the marrow and leads to an increased blood neutrophil count.

In patients with hypoplastic marrows, careful examination of specimens is required to distinguish among aplastic anemia, hypoplastic acute leukemia,[350–352] and hypoplastic oligoblastic myelogenous leukemia (MDS).[574] Leukemic blast cells are evident in the marrow in hypoplastic leukemia, and islands of dysmorphic cells, especially megakaryocytes, are present in hypoplastic oligoblastic leukemia.

Leukemoid reactions and nonleukemic pancytopenias can be distinguished from AML by the absence of leukemic blast cells in the blood or marrow.[575] In older children and adults, myeloblasts usually do not constitute more than 2 percent of marrow cells except in patients with a myeloid neoplasm, and the proportion of blast cells usually decreases in the marrow as a result of exaggerated expansion of the myelocyte compartment with neutrophilic leukemoid reactions.

● THERAPY

OVERVIEW OF TREATMENT PLAN

The usual treatment of AML includes an initial program termed the *induction* phase. Induction may involve the simultaneous use of multiple agents or a planned sequence of therapy called *timed sequential treatment*. Once a remission is obtained, further treatment is indicated to preserve the remission state. Remission is defined as elimination of the leukemic cell population in marrow as judged by microscopy and flow cytometry and the restitution of marrow hematopoiesis resulting in a normal or virtually normal white cell, hemoglobin, and platelet concentrations in the blood. The postinduction treatment can consist of cytotoxic chemotherapy, HSC transplantation, or low-dose maintenance chemotherapy, depending upon patient performance status and risk factors. If relapse occurs, treatment options may include different chemotherapy regimens, allogeneic HSC transplantation, or other investigational regimens, often as part of a clinical trial.

DECISION TO TREAT

Most patients with AML should be advised to undergo treatment promptly after diagnosis. Patients younger than 60 years of age have a poorer outcome as the time from diagnosis to treatment lengthens.[576] Although remission rates are lower in older patients, a significant proportion enter remission. Occasionally, very elderly patients refuse treatment or are so ill from unrelated illnesses that treatment may be unreasonable. Age per se is not a contraindication to treatment, and septuagenarians and octogenarians who are fit can enter remissions. Treatment can be tailored to the decreased tolerance of older patients, some of whom have a smoldering course (see "Treatment of Older Patients" below). Associated problems, such as hemorrhagic manifestations, severe anemia, or infections, should be treated in parallel.

PREPARATION OF THE PATIENT

Orientation of the patient and the family should provide them with an understanding of the disease, the treatment planned, and the adverse effects of treatment, as well as information about long-term prognosis to the extent this can be provided while awaiting cytogenetic and molecular markers. Socioeconomic status and distance from the treatment center have minimal effects on survival in AML,[577] but impaired Karnofsky performance status and instrumental activities of daily living score do impact outcomes.[578]

Pretreatment laboratory examination should include blood cell counts, cytochemistry analysis and immunophenotyping of leukemic cells from blood or marrow, marrow examination including cytogenetic and molecular analyses to include *FLT3* ITD, *NPM-1*, *CEBPα*, and *KIT* mutation status in CBF leukemias, if available. If these are not available, they can performed later as required based on AML subtype from a cryopreserved specimen. Blood chemistry studies, chest radiography, electrocardiogram, and determination of partial thromboplastin time, prothrombin time, and fibrinogen level should be obtained. More extensive evaluation of coagulation factors should be made if (1) clotting times are abnormal, (2) bleeding is exaggerated for the level of the platelet count, or (3) APL or acute monocytic leukemia is the phenotype. Early HLA typing is useful so that compatible platelet products can be provided if alloimmunization (Chap. 139) occurs and for patients who will become marrow transplantation candidates (Chap. 23). *Herpes simplex* virus and cytomegalovirus serotyping may be helpful, especially if transplantation is a consideration. HIV and hepatitis serology is indicated in patients with appropriate risk factors, and patients should have a baseline cardiac scan to determine ejection fraction prior to administration of an anthracycline antibiotic.

A peripherally inserted central catheter or a tunneled central venous catheter should be placed. This access to the circulation facilitates administration of chemotherapy, blood components, antibiotics, and other intravenous fluids and medications. It also permits sampling blood for analysis without patient discomfort or concern about venous access. Meticulous skin care at the catheter exit site is required to minimize tunnel infections. Central venous catheters have become a major source of infection during neutropenia, especially with Gram-positive organisms.[579] In some patients with severe coagulopathy such as those with APL, a tunneled catheter may be best deferred to avoid significant bleeding or vessel activation during insertion. In those with neurologic symptoms, a head computed tomographic study or MRI followed by a lumbar puncture should be obtained. Before procedures, adequate platelet counts and control of coagulopathy should be achieved, if possible.

Therapy for hyperuricemia is required if (1) the pretreatment uric acid level is greater than 7 mg/dL (0.4 mmol/L), (2) the marrow is packed with blast cells, or (3) the blood blast cell count is moderately or markedly elevated. Allopurinol 300 mg/day orally should be given. Allopurinol can cause allergic dermatitis and should not be used if the uric acid level is less than 7 mg/dL and the total white cell count is less

than approximately 20×10^9/L, as long as hydration is adequate and urine flow is high (>150 mL/h). The dermatitis may appear when antibiotics are instituted. This concurrence may confound the decision to continue antibiotics. Thus, allopurinol should be discontinued after the risk of acute hyperuricosuria or tumor lysis has passed (usually 4 to 7 days). Recombinant urate oxidase (rasburicase) can be used to prevent urate-induced nephropathy. This preparation, although costly, can reduce plasma urate levels by approximately 80 percent within 4 hours of the first drug dose. It is well tolerated, and the recommended dose of rasburicase is 0.2 mg/kg daily for 5 to 7 days intravenously, although shorter courses are usually effective.[580]

Attention to decreasing pathogen exposure by assiduous hand washing and meticulous care of catheter and intravenous sites is important, especially when the total neutrophil count is less than 0.5×10^9/L. Care of the patient in *a single room* is advisable to provide privacy during periods of intensive care and to help decrease the risk of exogenously acquired infection until the neutrophil count recovers.

REMISSION-INDUCTION THERAPY

Principles

The cytotoxic therapy of AML rests on two tenets: (1) two competing populations of cells are present in marrow—a normal polyclonal and a leukemic monoclonal population; and (2) profound suppression of the leukemic cells to the point they are inapparent in the marrow aspirate and biopsy is required to permit restoration of polyclonal hematopoiesis.[581,582] Although these two principles hold in most cases, two deviations from these guidelines are (1) the predisposition of patients with APL to enter remission despite cellular posttherapy marrow[583] and (2) the rare presence of monoclonal hematopoiesis in some cases of AML during remission (see "Results of Treatment" below). AML is a heterogeneous disease, and subgroups with different prognosis can be identified. In the future, incorporation of knowledge about the biology of the particular AML subtype may be utilized for adapted therapies, but at present, all subtypes of AML classified by cytogenetics or molecular changes with the exception of APL are approached similarly during induction, and often induction therapy must be started before knowledge of cytogenetic and molecular factors is available.[584]

The goal of induction therapy in AML is achievement of complete remission (<2 percent blasts in the marrow), a neutrophil count greater than 1000/μL, and a platelet count greater than 100,000/μL. An International Working Group for Diagnosis, Standardization of Response Criteria, Treatment Outcomes, and Reporting Standards has redefined outcomes in an effort to standardize reporting and comparison of data (see "Course and Prognosis: Results of Treatment: Definition of Remission" below).[585] Other treatment guidelines have been published.[586,587] The majority of adults enter remission with standard induction therapy, but for patients with high-risk disease, consideration can be given to an experimental approach, and complete remission rates do not reach 100 percent, so clinical trial participation can be considered during induction chemotherapy. How durable a complete remission will be attained in an individual patient often is difficult to predict at diagnosis. Gene-expression profiling can separate some patients into prognostic groups that may indicate patients with a high risk of not responding to standard approaches.[105]

Cytotoxic Regimens

Anthracycline Antibiotic or Anthraquinone and Cytarabine Current standard induction treatment for non-APL AML involves drug regimens with two or more agents that include an anthracycline antibiotic

TABLE 88–6. Remission Induction for Acute Myelogenous Leukemia: Examples of Cytosine Arabinoside and Anthracycline Antibiotic Combinations

Cytarabine	Anthracycline Antibiotic ± Another Agent	No. of Patients	Age Range in Years (Median)	Complete Remissions (%)	Year of Report	Reference
100 mg/m², days 1–7	DNR 50 mg/m² days 1–5	407	15–64 (47)	77.5	2011	596
100 mg/m², days 1–7	IDA 12 mg/m² days 1–3	525	15–64 (47)	78.2	2011	596
100 mg/m², days 1–7	DNR 45 mg/m², days 1–3	330	17–60 (47)	57	2009	593
100 mg/m², days 1–7	DNR 90 mg/m², days 1–3	327	18–60 (48)	71	2009	593
200 mg/m², days 1–7	DNR 60 mg/m², days 1–3	200	16–60 (45)	72	2004	611
200 mg/m², days 1–7	DNR 60 mg/m², days 1–3 Cladribine 5 mg/m², days 1–5	200	16–60 (45)	69	2004	611
200 mg/m² twice per day for 10 days (some in this report received FLAG-IDA vs. H-DAT)	DNR 50 mg/m², days 1, 3, 5 Thioguanine 100 mg/m² twice per day, days 10–20 Gemtuzumab ozogamicin 3 mg/m², day 1	64	18–59 (46.5)	91	2003	609
3 g/m² every 12 h for 8 doses	60 mg/m² DNR daily for 2 days	122	Adults	80	2000	603
100 mg/m² daily for 7 days (2 courses always given)	IDA 12 mg/m² daily for 3 days	153	NR	63	2000	589
500 mg/m² by continuous infusion, days 1–3, 8–10	Mitoxantrone 12 mg/m² for 3 days Etoposide 200 mg/m² days 8–10	133	15–70 (43)	60	1996	606
100 mg/m² daily for 7 days	DNR 45 mg/m² for 3 days	113	NR (55)	59	1992	588
100 mg/m² daily for 7 days	IDA 13 mg/m² for 3 days	101	NR (56)	70	1992	588

DNR, daunorubicin; FLAG, fludarabine, cytarabine, and granulocyte colony-stimulating factor; H-DAT, hydroxydaunorubicin, cytarabine, and thioguanine; IDA, idarubicin; NR, not reported.

All drugs are administered intravenously, except for thioguanine, which is administered orally. The reader is advised to consult the original reports for details of induction, consolidation or continuation therapy, and ancillary therapy.

or an anthraquinone and cytarabine (see "Special Therapeutic Considerations: Acute Promyelocytic Leukemia" below for therapy of APL).[588–617] Remission rates in the studies cited range from approximately 55 to 90 percent in adult subjects, depending on the composition of the population treated (Table 88–6). The two most important variables are the age of the patients and the proportion of patients with therapy-induced leukemia or an antecedent clonal myeloid disease. In the studies listed in Table 88–6, the median age of the patient populations was much younger (approximately 50 years) than the median age of the population of AML patients at large (approximately 70 years); thus the results cannot be generalized (see "Treatment of Older Patients" below). A combination of anthracycline and cytarabine has been the standard induction therapy since 1973.[11,12] A now classic standard induction regimen is cytarabine 100 mg/m² daily by continuous infusion on days 1 through 7 and daunorubicin at 45 to 90 mg/m² on days 1 through 3, the "7 plus 3" regimen. Dose or schedule modulation of the anthracycline or cytarabine, addition of other agents such as etoposide, in various schedules of administration, represent attempts to improve upon results obtained with "7 plus 3" therapy.

Choice of Anthracycline Development of drug resistance is reduced with idarubicin relative to other anthracyclines. Idarubicin does not induce P-glycoprotein expression, but daunorubicin, doxorubicin, and epirubicin do.[590] Idarubicin 12 mg/m² gives better complete remission rates in younger adults than does daunorubicin 45 mg/m², each given for 3 days. Amsacrine, aclarubicin, and mitoxantrone give improved results over standard-dose daunorubicin. In older adults, mitoxantrone may reduce cardiotoxicity, but this is controversial.[591] In two randomized studies, high-dose daunorubicin (90 mg/m²) for 3 days resulted in superior complete remission rates as compared to 45 mg/m² for 3 days when combined with cytarabine.[592,593] When idarubicin 12 mg/m² was compared to daunorubicin 80 mg/m² for 3 days in patients 50 to 70 years of age, the remission rate with idarubicin was 83 percent compared to 40 percent with daunorubicin.[594] Another analysis of idarubicin compared with high-dose daunorubicin in patients with AML showed idarubicin to result in a higher remission rate but not overall survival.[595] In contrast, a randomized study showed no difference in remission and long-term efficacy between idarubicin 12 mg/m² daily for 3 days as compared to daunorubicin, 50 mg/m² daily for

5 days.[596] In light of these studies, many therapists, when using dauno-rubicin, use the 90 mg/m² dose for 3 days in younger patients, and this is in keeping with the current National Comprehensive Cancer Network (NCCN) guidelines.[597] This benefit of higher dose applies only to younger and favorable or intermediate-risk patients.[593] Dexrazoxane may be given during induction to reduce the risk of cardiotoxicity in patients at higher than usual risk because of a history of coronary artery disease or congestive heart failure, but this is rarely used in adults.[598] Other regimens that incorporate fludarabine with cytarabine can be used in those patients for which an anthracycline would not be ideal.

High-Dose versus Standard-Dose Cytarabine High-Dose cytarabine does not increase complete remission rates and increases toxicity compared to conventional doses, especially in older patients (for doses of these regimens, see "Intensive Consolidation Therapy" below). Patients receiving high-dose cytarabine have more leukopenia, thrombocytopenia, gastrointestinal problems, and eye toxicity. Disease-free survival and overall survival may be better than that achieved with standard therapy, leading some investigators to suggest use of high-dose therapy for induction in patients younger than age 50 years, but this approach is not a standard one, and these studies do not take into account the role of high-dose cytarabine in postremission therapy.[599] Some studies show that marrow blast clearance is higher after an induction with high-dose cytarabine and that there is an improvement in disease-free survival for patients 50 years of age or younger.[600] When high-dose cytarabine was compared to intermediate doses in induction therapy, no improvement in outcome was noted, and higher incidences of grades 3 and 4 toxic effects were noted.[600] A trial in younger patients with multiple arms; fludarabine, high-dose cytarabine, and G-CSF (FLAG regimen) with idarubicin resulted in a higher remission rate than did standard daunorubicin plus cytarabine with or without etoposide. Relapse rates were also less with the high-dose cytarabine induction (38 vs. 55 percent).[601] A superior remission rate and survival was achieved in younger patients (<46 years) induced with a regimen containing high-dose cytarabine, 82 versus 76 percent rate of remission and a 52 versus 43 percent rate of overall survival. These differences were also seen in secondary AML cases and in those with *FLT3-ITD* mutations.[602] Also, complete remission rates of greater than 60 percent have been noted with high-dose cytarabine in patients with poor-risk cytogenetics.[603,604]

Timed Sequential Therapy and Other Drugs Timed sequential therapy, which uses agents in a scheduled sequence rather than concurrently, may prolong remission duration.[605-607] Timed sequential chemotherapy combining mitoxantrone intravenously (IV) on days 1 to 3, etoposide IV on days 8 to 10, and cytarabine IV on days 1 to 3 and 8 to 10 resulted in a complete remission in 60 percent of patients, but treatment-related death in 9 percent of patients. Median disease-free survival was 9 months.[605]

Adding ATRA,[608] gemtuzumab ozogamicin,[609] fludarabine,[610] cladribine or topotecan[611,612] to induction regimens has not improved results significantly. A recent randomized study showed that the addition of the purine analogue cladribine, but not fludarabine, to daunorubicin and cytarabine improved the remission rate and prolonged survival in patients younger than 60 years of age.[613] The addition of bortezomib to daunorubicin and cytarabine in those 60 to 75 years of age resulted in a remission rate of 65 percent. This was a single-arm trial with dose escalation of bortezomib.[614] There are preliminary reports suggesting that the addition of gemtuzumab ozogamicin to standard induction chemotherapy may increase disease-free survival in patients with low- and standard-risk cytogenetic abnormalities,[615] and inhibitors of FLT3 ITD are now being examined, but no data are available regarding utility of this approach.[616] A recent prospective comparison of five different treatment strategies, adjusted for differences in prognostic

characteristics, did not show clinically relevant differences in outcome when compared to a standard cytarabine and anthracycline containing arm.[617] Thus, the standard practice guideline for AML, other than promyelocytic leukemia, recommends standard-dose cytarabine plus an anthracycline antibiotic as treatment.[587]

Hematopoietic Cytokines to Enhance Chemotherapy G-CSF and granulocyte-monocyte colony-stimulating factor (GM-CSF), when used in untreated leukemia, can increase the percentage of leukemic cells in the DNA synthetic phase, resulting in blast population expansion during short-term administration. This process could render the cells more sensitive to simultaneous chemotherapy, but clinical benefit from growth-factor priming has not been observed[618,619] despite an increased ratio of intracellular cytosine arabinoside triphosphate to deoxycytidine-5′-triphosphate and enhanced cytarabine incorporation into the DNA of AML blasts.[619] Remission rates or overall survival did not differ among adult patients who received cytarabine plus idarubicin or cytarabine plus amsacrine with or without G-CSF given concurrently, but relapse rates decreased in patients who received G-CSF.[620] GM-CSF priming in a younger patient group treated with timed-sequential therapy increased complete remission rates but did not impact overall survival.[621] Thus, these growth factors are not generally considered useful as enhancers of chemotherapy. A study did, however, suggest that an improved event-free survival and overall survival was noted in patients treated with high-dose cytarabine during remission induction,[622] and complete remissions have occurred in hypoplastic AML after G-CSF treatment without chemotherapy.[623]

Reinduction Therapy Patients who have persistent leukemia after the first course of induction chemotherapy generally are given the same regimen a second time. The effect is usually assessed by marrow aspirate and biopsy 7 to 10 days after completion of chemotherapy (the "14-day marrow" examination). For those with hypocellular marrow and no evidence of residual leukemic blasts, recovery of normal counts is awaited, and for those with a hypocellular marrow and a small number of residual blasts, additional therapy may be delayed until count recovery or until another marrow assessment. For those with significant amounts of leukemic cells remaining, repeating the original induction therapy or use of a high-dose cytarabine regimen can be considered. The patient's long-term outcome is worse if two courses of treatment are required, even if a complete remission is achieved. Approximately 40 percent of patients with persistent AML after one course of induction therapy have a complete remission after a second course,[624] and disease-free survival at 5 years is approximately 10 percent. In some European centers, two courses of induction chemotherapy are given routinely, but the impact on remission rates or overall survival is uncertain.[625] The longer the time to remission after the first induction therapy, the shorter the duration of disease-free survival.[626] High-risk cytogenetic abnormalities, antecedent hematologic disorders, and other poor prognostic factors can be used to assign nonresponders to an experimental chemotherapy regimen designed to treat refractory disease, rather than repeating induction therapy. In one study, overall response to reinduction was 53 percent. Those patients with poor risk cytogenetics and those with a marrow blast percentage of 60 percent or greater following the 7-plus-3 regimen induction treatment were found to have a low probability of achieving a complete remission with reinduction.[627] Mortality during induction therapy correlates with age[628] and, perhaps, leukocyte count.[629]

Special Considerations during Induction Therapy

Hyperleukocytosis Patients with blast counts greater than 100×10^9/L require prompt treatment to prevent the most serious complications of hyperleukocytosis: intracranial hemorrhage or pulmonary insufficiency. Hydration should be administered promptly to maintain urine flow greater than 100 mL/h/m². Cytoreduction therapy can be initiated with hydroxyurea 1.5 to 2.5 g orally every 6 hours (total dose 6 to 10 g/day) for approximately 36 hours. Appropriate remission-induction therapy should be initiated as soon as possible after the leukocyte count has been decreased significantly. Simultaneous leukapheresis can decrease blast cell concentration by approximately 30 percent within several hours[331,630,631] without contributing to uric acid or cellular phosphate release. Leukapheresis may improve acute disturbances resulting from the vascular effects of blast cells, but the procedure may not alter the long-term outcome with current therapeutic programs.[339,340,630] Inhaled nitric oxide may improve the hypoxemia related to hyperleukocytosis.[631]

Antibiotic Therapy Pancytopenia is worsened or induced shortly after treatment is instituted. Absolute neutrophil counts less than 100/μL (0.1 × 10⁹/L) are expected and are a sign of effective drug action. The patient usually becomes febrile (>38°C), often with associated rigors. Cultures of urine, blood, nasopharynx, and, if available, sputum should be obtained. Because the inflammatory response is blunted by severe neutropenia and monocytopenia, evidence of exudates on physical examination or imaging studies may be minimal or absent. Antibiotics should be started immediately after cultures are obtained.[632] Chapter 24 describes antibiotic usage in the setting of intensive chemotherapy. Infections remain a major cause of therapy-associated morbidity and mortality.[633,634] Gram-positive bacterial isolates now outnumber Gram-negative organisms.[634] Cultures are often negative, but if fever and other signs are present, antibiotic therapy should be continued until neutrophil recovery.

Some centers use prophylactic antibacterial, antifungal, and/or antiviral antibiotics, whereas other centers do not. Antifungal prophylaxis can consist of low-dose amphotericin or azoles such as fluconazole, itraconazole, posaconazole, or voriconazole.[635,636] In a randomized study in patients undergoing induction therapy, posaconazole was more effective in preventing invasive fungal infections than fluconazole or itraconazole.[637] Voriconazole was not included in the comparison. Acyclovir, valacyclovir, or famciclovir prophylaxis during remission-induction therapy of patients with AML does not affect the duration of fever or the need for antibiotics. The incidence of bacteremia is not reduced, but acute oral infections are less severe.[638] Liposomal amphotericin, the caspofungins and azoles are available for treatment of established fungal infections.[639] Some centers use outpatient supportive therapy, including oral antimicrobials, immediately after induction therapy administration in adult AML.[640]

Hematopoietic Growth Factors to Treat Cytopenias Cytokine therapy as an adjunctive treatment for AML remains controversial.[641] GM-CSF and G-CSF accelerate neutrophil recovery; neither GM-CSF nor G-CSF reproducibly decreases major morbidity or mortality. However, one study has shown decreased mortality from fungal infections in older patients.[642] Use of cytokines during periods of cytopenia following induction therapy is safe, and nearly all trials have shown a modestly reduced duration of severe neutropenia with a variable effect on the incidence of severe infections, antibiotic usage, and duration of hospital stays. Although no increase in relapse has been noted when growth factors are started after completion of chemotherapy, no consistent enhancement of remission, event-free survival, or overall survival has been noted.[643] Therefore, the cost-effectiveness and clinical effectiveness of growth factor usage is doubtful. Also, growth factor usage can cloud marrow interpretation when used during induction.

Component Transfusion Therapy Red cell transfusions should be used to keep the hemoglobin level greater than 7.0 g/dL, or higher in special cases (e.g., symptomatic coronary artery disease; Chap. 138). Platelet transfusions should be used for hemorrhagic manifestations related to thrombocytopenia and prophylactically if necessary to maintain the platelet count between 5 × 10⁹/L and 10 × 10⁹/L.[644] Patients

without coagulation abnormalities, anticoagulant use, sepsis, or other complications usually can maintain hemostasis with platelet counts of 5 to 10 × 10⁹/L. Initially, random donor platelets can be used, although single-donor platelets or HLA-matched platelets may be preferable products and should be tried if random-donor platelets do not raise the platelet count significantly A no-prophylaxis platelet-transfusion strategy for blood cancers has been examined, but data support the need for prophylactic platelet transfusions.[645] Family members may be effective donors, if allogeneic HSC transplantation is not being considered (Chap. 139). There are data that fever should result in increasing the platelet count used as a transfusion threshold, and there is some suggestion that higher hemoglobin values protect against bleeding related to thrombocytopenia.[646]

All red cell and platelet products should be depleted of leukocytes, and all products, including granulocytes for transfusions, should be irradiated to prevent transfusion-associated graft-versus-host disease (GVHD) in this immunosuppressed population (Chaps. 138 and 139).

Granulocyte transfusion should not be used prophylactically for neutropenia but may be used in patients with high fever, rigors, and bacteremia unresponsive to antibiotics, with blood fungal infections, or with septic shock. G-CSF administration to a volunteer donor increases neutrophil yield fourfold and results in posttransfusion blood neutrophil increments for more than 24 hours after transfusion.[647] There is still ambiguity about the usefulness of this approach. GM-CSF administration may be warranted for treatment of major fungal infections (Chap. 24).

Jehovah's Witnesses and others who refuse blood product support can survive tailored chemotherapy.[648] In general, phlebotomy is minimized, and antifibrinolytics, hematinics, and growth factors are used to support such patients during severe cytopenias.

Therapy for Hypofibrinogenemic Hemorrhage Patients with evidence of intravascular coagulation (Chap. 129) or exaggerated primary fibrinolysis (Chap. 135) should be considered for platelet and fresh-frozen plasma administration before antileukemic therapy is started. Infusion of cryoprecipitate can be used for fibrinogen levels under approximately 125 mg/dL. If the findings are equivocal, patients should be monitored closely with measurements of fibrinogen levels, fibrin(ogen) degradation products, D-dimer assay, and coagulation times. Intravascular coagulation or primary fibrinolysis may occur in patients with APL and acute monocytic leukemia, but also may occur in occasional patients with other AML subtypes.

Management of Central Nervous System Disease CNS disease occurs in approximately one in 50 cases at presentation.[649] Prophylactic therapy usually is not indicated, but examination of the spinal fluid after remission should be considered in (1) monocytic subtypes,[508] (2) cases with extramedullary disease, (3) cases with inversion 16[254] and t(8;21)[263,266] cytogenetics, (4) CD7- and CD56-positive (neural-cell adhesion molecule) immunophenotypes,[650] and (5) patients who present with very high blood blast cell counts. In these situations, the risk of meningeal leukemia or a brain myeloid sarcoma is heightened, but prophylactic intrathecal chemotherapy is not recommended if high-dose cytarabine is used for consolidation. Patients who present with neurologic symptoms should have a head computed tomogram or MRI to rule out hemorrhage or mass effect. If negative, a lumbar puncture should be performed. Treatment of meningeal leukemia can include high-dose intravenous cytarabine (which penetrates the blood–brain barrier), intrathecal methotrexate, intrathecal cytarabine, cranial radiation, or chemotherapy and radiation in combination.[649] If CNS leukemia is present, intrathecal therapy is often given twice per week until blasts are cleared, and then once per week for 4 to 6 weeks. This therapy can be accomplished via the lumbar puncture route or through placement of an Ommaya reservoir. If there is a mass present, radiation or high-dose cytarabine with glucocorticoids can be considered.[651] Systemic relapse commonly follows relapse in the meninges, and concurrent systemic treatment usually is indicated. Long-term success is unusual unless allogeneic HSC transplantation is possible. Unless the patient has neurologic symptoms, lumbar puncture generally is deferred until blood blast cells have cleared. No consensus exists on a trigger for platelet transfusion in adults with AML undergoing lumbar puncture, but a platelet count less than 20×10^9/L has been proposed as such a trigger,[652] but many therapists use a higher platelet count (e.g., 50×10^9/L) as a safety threshold for lumbar puncture.

Management of Nonleukemic Myeloid Sarcoma Some patients present with myeloid (granulocytic) sarcomas without evidence of leukemia in the blood or marrow (see "Myeloid [Granulocytic] Sarcoma" earlier). Myeloid sarcoma may be the presenting finding in approximately 1 percent of patients with AML. Such patients should receive intensive AML induction therapy.[262] Intensive therapy results in a longer nonleukemic period than patients who have undergone surgical resection or resection followed by local irradiation.[250] Whether such patients should undergo allogeneic HSC transplantation in first remission irrespective of other factors has not been determined.[653,654] Median relapse-free survival is approximately 12 months after AML-type chemotherapy.[262] Patients with trisomy 8 have poorer survival rates.[260]

POSTREMISSION THERAPY

Cytotoxic Therapy

General Considerations Postremission therapy is intended to prolong remission duration and overall survival, but no consensus exists regarding the best approach. Postremission chemotherapy that does not produce profound prolonged cytopenias, closely simulating intensive induction therapy, has produced on average only slight prolongation of remission or life. Regimens that fall between these intensities have been used, with equivocal results. Intensive consolidation therapy after remission results in a somewhat longer remission duration and, more significantly, a subset of patients who have a remission of more than 3 years. The issue of postremission therapy and its impact is complicated by the large proportion of patients with AML who are older than 60 years of age and have limited tolerance for intensive therapy. In addition, a very small pool of leukemic stem cells may sustain the process, and elimination of these cells may require approaches other than intensive chemotherapy, especially in adults.

Several randomized trials have studied whether AML patients in first remission should receive consolidation chemotherapy alone, autologous transplantation, or allogeneic HSC transplantation, without reaching a consensus. Allogeneic transplantation was compared to autologous transplantation using unpurged marrow and two courses of intensive chemotherapy in 623 patients who had a complete remission after induction chemotherapy.[655] Disease-free survival was 53 percent at 4 years for those receiving allogeneic transplantation, 48 percent for those receiving autologous transplantation, and 30 percent for patients receiving intensive chemotherapy. Overall survival after complete remission was similar in all three groups because patients who relapsed after chemotherapy could be rescued with allogeneic HSC transplantation. No significant difference in the 4-year disease-free survival between allogeneic HSC transplantation (42 percent) and other types of intensive postremission therapy (40 percent) has been found.[656] In another study, only patients younger than 35 years of age with poor-risk cytogenetics had improved disease-free survival if they had a sibling donor and underwent allogeneic transplantation (43.5 percent vs. 18.5 percent at 4 years).[657] Thus, in several studies, the early mortality after allogeneic HSC transplantation and the chemotherapy-induced remissions in patients who relapse following autologous transplantation or

chemotherapy have led to comparable overall survival rates. However, leukemia-free survival was greater after allogeneic transplantation.[658] In the last decade, treatment-related mortality from transplantation has declined and matched unrelated donor transplantations are as effective as those from a matched sibling donor, so currently, transplantation is recommended for all but good-prognosis patients (CBF leukemias or those with *NPM1* mutation without a *FLT3* mutation).[659] A Markov decision analysis has shown that patients treated with allogeneic HSC transplantation have a longer life expectancy compared with those treated with chemotherapy among patients with an intermediate- or unfavorable-risk prognosis.[660] A prospective matched-pairs analysis has also concluded that allogeneic HSC transplantation is the most effective postremission therapy for AML, especially for those 45 to 59 years of age and/or with high-risk cytogenetics.[661] When quality of life was measured for patients in complete remission for 1 to 7 years, those treated with chemotherapy had the highest quality of life, whereas those who underwent allogeneic HSC transplantation had the lowest.[662]

The decision to utilize autologous or allogeneic HSC transplantation or high-dose cytarabine alone for consolidation should be individualized, based on the patient's age and other prognostic factors, such as high-risk cytogenetic findings and antecedent hematologic disease. Patients with good-risk cytogenetics should receive up to four cycles of high-dose cytarabine. Patients with poor-risk cytogenetics should be considered for allogeneic HSC transplantation as soon as feasible. A meta-analysis has also shown that compared with nonallogeneic therapies, allogeneic HSC transplantation has superior relapse-free survival and overall survival for cases of AML classified intermediate and poor-risk, but not for cases considered good-risk AML in first remission.[663]

Intensive Consolidation Therapy For patients who do not receive high-dose chemotherapy with autologous or allogeneic transplantation in first remission, consolidation chemotherapy regimens containing high-dose cytarabine provide better results than intermediate-dose cytarabine,[664,665] but these regimens are not universally accepted.[666] Patients who are to have allogeneic HSC transplantation do not require four cycles of high-dose cytarabine, and may not benefit from even one, if a donor is readily available.[667] *RAS* mutations are associated with benefit from high-dose cytarabine therapy.[668] Patients with CBF leukemias such as t(8;21) also have particularly favorable responses to repetitive cycles of high-dose cytarabine. In patients who received three or more cycles, a relapse rate of 19 percent was reported.[669]

Other regimens, such as those containing gemtuzumab ozogamicin and fludarabine, have been used in postremission therapy, but whether they provide benefit over use of high-dose cytarabine has not been studied.[670] Long-term disease-free survival at 5 years generally is approximately 30 percent when two to four cytarabine-containing regimens are administered.[671,672] Adding mitoxantrone or amsacrine to high-doses cytarabine has not improved treatment outcomes in consolidation,[673] and timed sequential chemotherapy used in consolidation did not improve outcome as compared with high-dose cytarabine.[674] Most centers use four cycles of therapy. A cycle is 3 g/m² twice daily on days 1, 3, and 5, providing six doses per cycle, with cycle durations dependent on normal blood count recovery. The optimal number of cycles for this therapy is not known.[675] High-dose cytarabine can be administered at a dose of 3 g/m² in a 1- to 3-hour intravenous infusion every 12 hours for up to 6 days (12 doses), but this schedule is almost never used because of its toxicity. There is some evidence that two cycles of intermediate-dose cytarabine (1 g/m² every 12 hours for 6 days) may be a viable alternative to the 3 g/m² for six doses schedules.[676] When 36 g/m² total dosing was compared with 12 g/m² dosing in the first consolidation, there was no improvement in treatment outcomes.[677] High-dose cytarabine frequently causes conjunctivitis and photophobia, and glucocorticoid eye drops are usually used every 6 hours until 24 hours after the last dose of the drug.[678] Cerebellar function abnormalities also may occur, and these require cessation of drug administration. A 1-hour duration infusion of high-dose or reduced-dose (e.g., 2 g/m^2) cytarabine may decrease the likelihood of severe cerebellar toxicity.[678] Older patients and patients with renal insufficiency require dose attenuation (i.e., to 1 to 2 g/m^2).[679]

Additional Maintenance Therapy

Various forms of less-intensive maintenance chemotherapy have been attempted after completion of intensive consolidation chemotherapy. Many of the regimens consist of monthly chemotherapy, for example, low-dose 6-thioguanine or cytarabine. Although improved disease-free survival was noted in some studies, no improvement in overall survival has been demonstrated in most studies.[680] Some groups are examining the role of demethylating agents (e.g., 5-azacytidine or decitabine) as maintenance therapy.[681]

Autologous Stem Cell Infusion after Myeloablative Chemotherapy or Chemoradiotherapy for Consolidation Removal and cryopreservation of postremission marrow or collection of mobilized blood stem cells from patients with AML and reinfusion of these products following intensive chemotherapy and/or radiotherapy is a form of postremission therapy (Chap. 23).[682] This approach is loosely referred to as autologous transplantation but does not cross transplantation barriers. Autologous marrow or blood stem cell rescue can be used in patients with AML who achieve a remission, do not have a compatible stem cell donor, and are as old as 70 years. With the availability of high-resolution HLA-matched unrelated donors, cord blood and haploidentical donors, the number of autologous stem cell transplants used in AML has diminished.

Various treatment regimens for autologous transplantation in AML have been used,[683] such as busulfan-cyclophosphamide, busulfan-etoposide-cytarabine, high-dose cytarabine-mitoxantrone plus total-body irradiation, melphalan plus total-body irradiation, and cyclophosphamide plus total-body irradiation. A disease-free survival rate of approximately 40 percent at 3 years is average after such regimens in the age-range treated.[684,685] Long-term disease-free survival can occur in patients who undergo this treatment for AML in second remission.[686] Patients older than age 50 years have inferior outcomes, but no strict upper-age limit for this procedure has been determined.[687] Administration of two or more courses of consolidation chemotherapy prior to harvest and transplant is associated with decreased relapse rates and improved disease-free survival. A marrow nucleated cell dose greater than 2×10^8/kg improves disease-free survival.[688] Chemotherapy agents such as 4-hydroperoxycyclophosphamide have been used for purging residual leukemic cells in marrow before infusion,[689,690] and antisense agents reportedly diminish leukemic cell contamination.[691] Use of marrow grafts purged of residual leukemia cells has not significantly improved the results obtained with unpurged marrow in many studies, suggesting that low proportions of leukemic stem cells may not transplant easily or that they do not survive the freeze–thaw cycle to which autologous marrow is subjected as well as do normal HSCs.[692] In addition, residual leukemia in the patient may contribute to relapse. For these reasons, marrow purging is rarely used in AML autografting (Chap. 23). In long-term cultures from patients newly diagnosed with AML, normal progenitors can be detected, and their numbers are increased by *in vitro* culture with cytokines.[693] In oligoblastic myelogenous leukemia (high-risk myelodysplasia), secondary AML, and therapy-related AML, leukapheresis products obtained after chemotherapy and growth factor treatment contain normal progenitors,[694] indicating mobilized stem cells may be relatively free of leukemic counterparts even in the absence of *ex vivo* purging.[695] Early mortality may be decreased using blood stem cells because they engraft more rapidly, but relapse rates may be higher.[696] Mobilized stem cells can be collected

after high-dose cytarabine plus G-CSF or after G-CSF alone.[697] There is a plateau in the survival curve after autologous stem cell transplantation at about 2.2 years,[698] and there is evidence that autologous transplantation improves disease-free survival but not overall survival.[699] The total number of CD34+ cells infused influences early engraftment, but durable engraftment is associated more closely with the CD34+/CD38– subset of cells in the graft.[700]

Chemoradiotherapy Plus Allogeneic Hematopoietic Stem Cell Transplantation for Consolidation Therapy

General Considerations Utilization of allogeneic HSC transplantation for AML is increasing in Europe and the United States.[701] No strict upper-age limit for transplantation exists,[702] but many centers use age 60 or 65 years for transplantations following ablation of hematopoiesis and 70 to 75 years for transplantations not preceded by ablation of hematopoiesis (nonmyeloablative or reduced-intensity transplants). Decisions to proceed to allogeneic transplantation should be individualized, and feasibility depends on (1) the availability of a suitable donor, (2) the recipient's age and health status, and (3) whether AML is in remission.

For full-intensity transplantations, the patient is prepared with a regimen that includes total-body irradiation and/or high-dose chemotherapy, after which the donor stem cells are infused by vein. Patients given allogeneic blood stem cells have more rapid hematopoietic reconstitution than patients given marrow stem cells, but they may have more chronic GVHD and comparable risk of relapse.[703,704] Chapter 23 describes the indications, procedure, and preparative regimens for allogeneic stem cell transplantation. In general, no single preparative regimen is superior for patients with AML in first remission.[705] In one study, cyclophosphamide and total-body irradiation lowered relapse risk, but overall results were comparable to conditioning with chemotherapy alone.[706] Another retrospective study showed outcomes with intravenous busulfan and cyclophosphamide were not different from those with cyclophosphamide and total-body irradiation in AML in remission.[707] A retrospective registry analysis showed that leukemia-free and overall survivals were better with busulfan and cyclophosphamide, as compared with total body irradiation in AML in first remission.[708] Postremission consolidation with cytarabine before allogeneic transplantation for AML in first remission does not improve outcome compared with immediate transplant after successful induction.[709] It is unclear that this result will also hold in the setting of reduced-intensity transplants or for transplants performed beyond first remission.[710]

Related Donors When matched-sibling transplantation is performed for AML in first remission, approximately half of patients have a disease-free survival of 4 years. Small series using T-cell depletion have reported 4-year disease-free survival of 65 percent.[711] Leukemia relapses occur in approximately 20 percent of patients who receive an allogeneic transplant. Patients who are alive with good performance status 3 years after transplantation have excellent prospects of long-term survival.[711] In the posttransplantation period, approximately one-third of patients die of severe GVHD, opportunistic infection, or interstitial pneumonitis. The outlook for long-term survival is improved if (1) the AML is in remission prior to transplantation, (2) grades III to IV acute GVHD does not occur, and (3) chronic GVHD is low grade.[712,713] For patients with unfavorable cytogenetics, an allogeneic sibling transplantation in first remission is often recommended.[714] Patients with FLT3/ITD-positive AML may also benefit from allogeneic HSC transplantation in first remission.[715,716] When AML patients in first remission were compared on a donor versus no donor basis, and more than 80 percent of patients with a donor went on to transplantation, patients with a donor had a significantly better disease-free survival, although treatment-related mortality was higher.[717] For patients with intermediate-risk cytogenetics, where the decision is made to delay transplantation until first relapse and second remission, physicians should identify a source of a HSC graft and ensure that careful monitoring of the patient occurs so that transplantation can be instituted as quickly as possible.[718]

In an attempt to decrease the relapse rate after stem cell transplantation for advanced acute leukemia,[202] I-labeled anti-CD45 antibody to deliver radiation to leukemic cells, followed by a standard transplant preparative regimen, has been used. With this regimen, more radiation can be delivered to hematopoietic tissues compared with liver, lung, or kidney, which may improve the efficacy of the transplant.[719]

Unrelated Donors Approximately 70 percent of all patients with AML are older than 50 years of age, and the current mean family size in the United States is slightly more than two children per family. Thus, only approximately 10 to 15 percent of subjects with AML are within the age-range and have a sibling donor for marrow transplantation. The ability to extend the proportion of patients who can be transplanted has led to histocompatible, unrelated donors or HLA type-mismatched sibling or parent (haploidentical) donor transplants.[720] More than 70 percent of patients of European descent can find a suitable unrelated -matched donor in the available donor registries,[721] and another study showed that the majority of patients with AML in first remission for whom transplantation is recommended are able to undergo the procedure; the main barriers to transplantation are relapse of disease while awaiting a donor and poor performance status.[722] Molecular matching of classes I and II HLA alleles adds to the clinical success of unrelated donor transplantations, but makes finding a donor more difficult.[723] Using such typing, studies have demonstrated that use of matched-unrelated donors as compared with matched-related donors result in similar survival times in AML.[724] Transplantation benefits younger adults in first remission, but no difference in outcome between matched-related donors and matched unrelated donors.[725] HLA-matched or HLA-mismatched cord blood stem cells can be used in adults with acute leukemia but generally not for patients in first remission.[726,727] In adults, the numbers of stem cells available in a single cord product may not result in engraftment, which has led to the use of two-cord blood units for grafting (Chap. 23).[728]

Reduced-Intensity and Nonmyeloablative Transplantation Patients who, based upon comorbidities or performance status, are deemed too old or too ill to undergo a full-intensity (myeloablative) allogeneic stem cell transplantation may be offered a reduced-intensity transplantation procedure or a nonmyeloablative conditioning regimen, provided a suitable donor is available. Reduced-intensity transplant results in some degree of myeloablation but in non-ablative transplants, autologous stem cell recovery would occur in the case of graft failure.[729,730] This type of transplantation for AML and closely related hematologic malignancies relies upon the graft-versus-leukemia effect as primary therapy.[731-733] These regimens have moderate hematologic and nonhematologic toxicity, and often can be performed on an outpatient basis. Engraftment and establishment of complete donor chimerism are successful in most patients. GVHD rates have been variable, and the ultimate risk of acute and chronic GVHD with these regimens is unclear. A variety of low-intensity regimens have been proposed.[734] In AML in first remission, the 1-year progression-free survival is approximately 55 percent.[735,736] The role of this approach in the treatment of AML remains to be defined, and comparative trials with longer followup are needed. Nonmyeloablative conditioning with unrelated donors has been used successfully.[737,738] Although randomized trials of ablative versus reduced dose-intensity conditioning regimens for transplantation of AML patients in first remission have not been done, there is evidence that reduced dose intensity is an inferior option for disease control, but that disadvantage is offset by the decreased treatment-related mortality.[739] One study found that reduced-intensity conditioning compared with myeloablative conditioning using unrelated

donors in AML gave similar rates of leukemia-free survival.[740] In a multivariate analysis, active disease at transplant and development of grades II to IV GVHD after transplantation had a negative impact on survival in reduced-dose-intensity transplantations.[741] Reduced-intensity transplantations are feasible in elderly patients with both fludarabine and low-dose total-body irradiation[742] and with fludarabine and IV busulfan[743] but donor availability and coexisting medical problems often limit its use.[744]

Use of Transplantation in Relapsed Patients Some form of allograft usually is recommended for patients in early first relapse or second remission, because long-term survival with chemotherapy alone is improbable, whereas histocompatible sibling transplants in these situations have a 25 percent survival rate. For patients who lack a sibling donor, matched-unrelated donor transplantations can be effective, but treatment-related mortality is high, suggesting that patients with unfavorable cytogenetics should undergo a matched-unrelated donor transplantation in first complete remission, if an acceptable donor can be found.[745] However, when transplantation was compared to chemotherapy for AML in second remission, the 3-year probability of event-free survival was 17 percent with chemotherapy and 16 percent with transplantation. Patients younger than 30 years of age who were in remission for at least 1 year fared best.[746] Development of chronic GVHD, an unrelated donor, a young age of donor, and blast cell count less than 30 percent at transplantation were found in another series to be favorable predictors of survival for transplantations performed in leukemia relapse.[747] Another study found that those with a remission duration of less than 6 months, circulating blasts, donor other than an HLA-matched sibling, poor-performance status, and poor-risk cytogenetics were adverse pretransplantation variables for those in relapse or primary induction failure.[748] Patients with extramedullary sites of leukemia are more likely to relapse after allogeneic transplantation.[749]

Patients with AML who relapse after allogeneic stem cell transplantation can have a long-term remission, if they undergo retransplantation.[750] A second stem cell transplantation can induce 2-year overall survival in approximately 25 percent of patients and is effective after either related or unrelated donor transplantations. A clear advantage of changing the donor for the second transplantation has not been demonstrated.[751]

The mechanism of benefit of allogeneic stem cell transplantation was thought to result from high-dose ablative chemoradiotherapy followed by marrow "rescue." The increased relapse rate of AML in patients transplanted with marrow from identical twins, compared to nonidentical siblings, or transplanted with T-lymphocyte–depleted marrow has indicated that an immunologic effect of donor lymphocytes may determine the results of transplantation. This immunologic response, referred to as *graft-versus-leukemia effect*, may play a role in preventing leukemia relapses.[752]

Donor Leukocyte Infusion In an attempt to enhance graft-versus-leukemia effects, adoptive immunotherapy with donor mononuclear cell infusions is sometimes used to treat relapse of leukemia after allografting.[753,754] These infusions have been successful in only a minority of patients with AML, but given the high mortality associated with alternative procedures such as a second transplantation, the infusions are a reasonable approach for patients who relapse after allogeneic transplantation.[755] GVHD and marrow aplasia are the major complications of this form of treatment.[756] The graft-versus-leukemia reaction is thought to be directed against minor histocompatibility antigens on the cell surface of hematopoietic cells, but reactions against leukemia-specific antigens are possible. Relapses after donor leukocyte infusions for recurring acute leukemia have a higher probability of being extramedullary.[757] Donor lymphocyte infusions are most effective in early relapses and in the absence of extensive of chronic GVHD.[758] Some patients also enter a new remission upon withdrawal of immune suppression. Patients who enter remission by donor lymphocyte infusion or cessation of immunosuppressive agents have a better survival than those who entered remission with chemotherapy alone or after a second transplantation.[759] Unrelated donor-leukocyte infusions can be used to treat relapsed leukemia after unrelated donor stem cell transplantation.[760] Approximately 40 percent of AML patients enter remission with this treatment. G-CSF has been used as an alternative to donor leukocyte infusions after AML relapse posttransplantation.[761] Donor blood stem cells can be combined with chemotherapy for early relapse of AML after allogeneic stem cell transplantation.[762] Strategies with donor leukocyte infusions are anticipated to become more effective once the effector cells are identified and the tumor target antigens better understood.[763]

Other Modalities to Decrease or Treat Relapse after Transplant. Killer-cell immunoglobulin-like receptor (KIR) genes among HLA-matched potential donors can point to donors with donor KIR genotype that are associated with enhanced disease-free survival.[764] Early cytomegalovirus replication after transplantation is also associated with decreased relapse risk, possibly because of a virus-versus-leukemia effect in AML.[765] Hypomethylating agents have been used for the treatment of relapse after allogeneic transplantation with some success and with induction of T-regulatory cells.[766,767] Extramedullary sites of relapse are more common after transplant.[767]

Recurrent Leukemia in Donor Cells or New Leukemia in Recipient Cells Recurrence of AML in donor cells has been reported in patients who received transplants from healthy siblings. These recurrences in donor cells occurred in approximately one in 18 relapsed patients who received marrow from a donor of the opposite sex.[768] A similar frequency of relapsed AML is observed in recipient cells but with a different clonal cytogenetic abnormality, suggesting a "new" leukemia.[768] The frequencies are dependent on the sensitivity and specificity of cytogenetic techniques, which have been challenged. AML developing in a stem cell recipient but of donor cell origin long after transplantation has been documented in rare cases.[768,769]

Summary of Postremission Therapy In younger patients with favorable cytogenetics (CBF with no mutation of *KIT*) or with *NPM1* or double *CEBPα* mutations in the absence of a *FLT3* mutation, there is no advantage to do an allograft in first remission and four cycles of high-dose cytarabine is appropriate treatment. Another option would be two cycles of high-dose cytarabine followed by autografting, an approach often favored in Europe. In those with intermediate-risk cytogenetics, an allograft should be considered as consolidation, and three to four cycles of high-dose cytarabine could be offered if a transplant donor cannot be found. Those with poor-risk cytogenetics or a *FLT3-ITD* mutation should be considered for an allograft in first complete remission. These recommendations may change as transplant mortality improves and subclasses of the "normal" cytogenetics group are better defined such that targeted agents might have an impact on relapse rates. After patients complete consolidation therapy, they are generally followed with blood counts every 3 months for 2 years, and then every 3 to 6 months for 5 years. Marrow examination is done to confirm continued remission after consolidation is completed but is rarely pursued regularly thereafter unless blood counts change.

TREATMENT OF RELAPSED OR REFRACTORY PATIENTS

Chemotherapy

Patients who relapse after remission-induction and postinduction therapy have a decreased probability of entering a subsequent remission, and the duration of any remission that occurs is usually shorter. In

patients who relapse more than 1 year after the first remission, the original remission-induction regimen can be readministered or a combination salvage chemotherapy regimen can be administered. At relapse, cell lineage trees suggest that the leukemic cell sustaining the relapse resembles the leukemic stem cell of origin.[770] When primary tumor and relapse genomes are compared, two primary patterns of relapse are discerned: gain of mutations in a founding clone that evolved into the relapse clone or a subclone of the founding clone that survived induction, gained mutations, and gained ascendancy to become the dominant clone at relapse.[771]

Refractory leukemia is defined as leukemia that does not respond to initial induction chemotherapy with cytarabine and an anthracycline antibiotic or anthraquinone. Patients with refractory disease are more likely to have disease with adverse cytogenetic findings, a history of antecedent clonal myeloid disease, adverse immunophenotypic features, and expression of MDR.[772]

Relapsed leukemia is leukemia that recurs following a remission. The duration of remission greatly affects the patient's prognosis and response to additional treatment. The wide range of response rates may not only reflect the regimen used but may also reflect variability in patient selection, age, and other prognostic factors.[772,773]

Chemotherapy regimens can be divided into cytarabine-based, noncytarabine-based, and timed sequential therapy with growth factors and cytotoxic drugs. Table 88–6 lists regimens and their response rates; the duration of response usually is measured in months, and, therefore, clinical trials are also recommended for this patient group. The duration of response is difficult to define because many patients go on to other therapies, including allogeneic stem cell transplantation.

In a large patient cohort treated on successive Medical Research Council trials, of those patients who relapsed after first remission, 55 percent entered a second remission. For those with favorable cytogenetics, 5-year survival was 32 percent; for those with intermediate cytogenetics, 5-year survival was 17 percent; and for those with adverse cytogenetic patterns, 5-year survival was 7 percent. In those in a second remission who underwent transplant, 42 as compared to 16 percent survived 5 years.[774] Results from therapy were better in younger patients, and in those with longer first remissions, longer durations since last chemotherapy, and better general health. The probability of a second remission is approximately 40 percent in younger (ages 15 to 60 years) and approximately 25 percent in older (ages 60 to 80 years) patients, but the duration of remission is nearly always much shorter than the first remission. An eventual fatal outcome is nearly certain unless allogeneic HSC transplantation can be performed. Rare patients may have a third (or more) relapse followed by a remission when treated with cytotoxic drugs, but each remission is shorter than the preceding one and usually is measured in weeks. For those who have favorable or normal karyotype, long second remission, and no previous stem cell transplantation, intensive chemotherapy can be useful.[775] In one study, 21 (approximately 17 percent) of 124 patients had a second remission duration at least 2 months longer than the first remission.[776] In patients in relapse treated with the sequential high-dose cytosine arabinoside and mitoxantrone (S-HAM) regimen, the duration of the first remission was the only factor associated with a successful outcome, and unfavorable karyotype was the only factor related to duration of survival.[777] Patients who relapse less than 1 year from remission should be treated with investigational agents, whereas patients who relapse more than 1 year later may benefit from standard reinduction therapy.[778] No standard chemotherapy regimen provides a durable remission of AML patients who relapse (Table 88–7),[779–789] and all such patients should be considered for clinical trials if available. For patients not fit for intensive salvage regimens, low-dose cytarabine, hypomethylating agents, or supportive or palliative care can be offered.

TABLE 88–7. Examples of Chemotherapy Regimens Used for Relapsed or Refractory Patients

Regimen	No. of Patients	Percent of Patients Entering a Complete Remission (Median Duration)	Year	Reference
Clofarabine 40 mg/m², IV, days 1–5	163	35.2 (6.6 months)	2012	789
Cytarabine 1 g/m², IV, days 1-5	163	17.8 (6.3 months)	2012	789
Clofarabine 25 mg/m², IV, daily for 5 days Cytarabine 2 g/m², IV, daily for 5 days G-CSF 5 mcg/kg per day subcutaneously daily until ANC ≥2,000/μL	50	46 (9 months)	2011	787
Gemtuzumab ozogamicin 6 mg/m², IV, days 1 and 13 Idarubicin 12 mg/m², IV, days 2–4 Cytarabine 1.5 g/m², IV, days 2–5	15	21 (27 weeks)	2003	780
Mitoxantrone 12 mg/m², IV, days 1–3 Cytarabine 500 mg/m², IV, days 1–3 Followed (at blood count recovery) by: Etoposide 200 mg/m², IV, days 1–3 Cytarabine 500 mg/m², IV, days 1–3	66	36 (5 months)	2003	781
Cladribine 5 mg/m², IV, days 1–5 Cytarabine 2 g/m², IV, days 1–5, 2 h after cladribine G-CSF 10 mcg/kg subcutaneously, each day, days 1–5	58	50 (29% disease-free at 1 year)	2003	782
Fludarabine 30 mg/m², IV, days 1–5 Cytarabine 2 g/m², IV, days 1–5 Idarubicin 10/m², IV, days 1–3 G-CSF 5 mcg/kg subcutaneously each day, up to 6 doses until neutrophil recovery	46	52 (13 months)	2003	783
Gemtuzumab ozogamicin 9 mg/m², IV, days 1 and 15	43	9	2002	784
Mitoxantrone 4 mg/m², IV, days 1–3 Etoposide 40 mg/m², IV, days 1–3 Cytarabine 1 g/m², IV, days 1–3, ± valspodar (PSC-833)	37	32	1999	785
Fludarabine 30 mg/m², IV, days 1–5 Cytarabine 2 g/m², IV, days 1–5± Idarubicin 12 mg/m², IV, days 1–3 G-CSF 400 mcg/m², subcutaneously, daily until complete remission	85	66	1995	786

ANC, absolute neutrophil count; G-CSF, granulocyte-colony-stimulating factor.

NOTE: The reader is advised to consult the original reference for details of chemotherapy regimen administration.

Allogeneic Hematopoietic Stem Cell Transplantation

Allogeneic stem cell transplantation may be the only means to induce a sustained remission in patients with AML who do not enter remission with cytotoxic drug therapy or who relapse after a first remission. Approximately 25 percent of patients with refractory or relapsed AML have a sustained remission of at least 3 years.[790] Transplant-related mortality at 3 years is approximately 50 percent. Relapse rates are higher after sibling than matched-unrelated transplantation.[791,792] If a histocompatible donor is available and the patient is younger than age 50 years, allogeneic stem cell transplantation can be as successful, if it is performed when the patient is in early relapse compared with in second remission, but this is often done in the context of a clinical trial.[793]

Relapse after Stem Cell Transplantation For patients who relapse after allogeneic stem cell transplantation, the prognosis is extremely poor and available chemotherapy, donor leukocyte infusions,

or second transplants do not result in consistent durable remissions.[794] For patients who relapse after reduced-intensity allogeneic transplantations, median overall survival after relapse was found to be 6 months, and no advantage was found for donor leukocyte infusions or second transplantations as compared with chemotherapy.[795] Patients who relapse after autologous stem cell transplantation can sometimes be salvaged with reduced-intensity allogeneic transplantation or with full-intensity allogeneic transplantations with high treatment-related mortality rates even in younger patients.

OTHER TREATMENT MODALITIES

Chemotherapy

Several newer chemotherapeutic agents are being examined for treatment of AML. For example, liposomal preparations of fixed ratios of daunorubicin and cytarabine have entered trials.[796] This has shown some responses in older adults with secondary leukemia.

Epigenetic Modulation

Methylation of DNA at critical sites can cause transcriptional inactivation of genes or chromosomal instability. In AML, aberrant methylation, especially preferential methylation of chromosome 11, has been described.[797] Epigenetic gene silencing caused by DNA methylation is a target for presumptive demethylating agents such as 5-azacytidine or decitabine, and silencing mediated by histone deacetylation is a target for histone deacetylases.[798] Decitabine, a potent agent, can cause maturation and growth arrest of AML cells.[799–801] 5-Azacytidine also has activity in AML, and it is being studied in an oral formulation.[802] These agents, singly or in combination, have resulted in response rates of 25 to 60 percent.[803] Methylome analysis may be useful as a pharmacodynamic end point in those treated with decitabine,[804] and higher levels of *miR-29b* are associated with responses to decitabine.[805] Histone deacetylase inhibitors can restore retinoic acid-dependent transcriptional activation and maturation in AML blasts.[806] Depsipeptide can promote histone acetylation and gene transcription in RUNX1/ETO-positive leukemic cells.[807] Depsipeptide (romidepsin),[808] LBH589,[809] vorinostat (suberoylanilide hydroxamic acid [SAHA]),[810] and MGCD0103[811] have each been studied in early phase trials in leukemia. Combination therapy of these agents with other targeted therapies is being explored,[812] and combination therapy with hypomethylating agents and histone deacetylase inhibitors has been reported.[813]

Inhibitors of DOT1L, Isocitric Dehydrogenase, and MDM2

The histone methyltransferase DOT1L is necessary for sustaining *MLL*-rearranged, AML. EPZ-5676, an aminonucleoside inhibitor of DOT1L histone methyltransferase activity is under clinical investigation in *MLL*-rearranged leukemias.[814] Other DOLT1L inhibitors are being explored in IDH1/2 mutated AML.[815] AGI-6780 has been identified as an IDH2 R140Q inhibitor with potential for differentiation.[816] Inhibitors of MDM2, a regulator of p53 and p53-specific E3 ubiquitin ligase have also entered trials.[817]

Antibodies to CD33

The CD33 antigen is expressed on approximately 90 percent of AML blasts and is a target for antibody-mediated destruction. Gemtuzumab ozogamicin is a recombinant humanized anti-CD33 monoclonal immunoglobulin G$_4$ antibody conjugated to the cytotoxin calicheamicin.[818] The conjugated antibody is rapidly internalized and causes subsequent cell apoptosis.[819] Hyperbilirubinemia and transaminase elevations can occur. Although it results in similar survival rates as standard chemotherapy reinduction, its use was associated with fewer days of hospitalization.[820] In patients who relapsed between 3 and 11 months, gemtuzumab ozogamicin resulted in higher remission rates compared to regimens containing high-dose cytarabine in different trials. However, in patients who had prolonged first remissions of greater than 19 months, cytarabine resulted in superior remission rates.[821] Prior gemtuzumab ozogamicin exposure may increase the risk of venoocclusive disease in patients who later undergo myeloablative allogeneic HSC transplantation procedures.[822] Gemtuzumab ozogamicin was approved by the FDA in 2000, but withdrawn from the market in 2010. Studies in Europe are examining its role in induction treatment coupled with standard chemotherapy, in postremission therapy, and in the treatment of APL.[823–825] In those studies, it did not alter remission rates but appeared to decrease relapse rate or improve relapse-free survival.

Therapies Targeted to Signal Transduction Mediators

Tyrosine Kinase Inhibitors: *FLT3* Inhibitors Constitutively activating FLT3 receptor mutations have been found in approximately 30 percent of patients with AML. Several small-molecule *FLT3* tyrosine kinase inhibitors have been formulated, but none have yet received regulatory approval.[826–831] Myeloblast differentiation may occur, including a syndrome with neutrophilic dermatosis wherein the neutrophils are *FLT3*-positive.[832] *FLT3*-mutant allelic burden may predict response to such inhibitors.[833] These agents are in phase I and phase II trials, in which they have induced a decline in blood blast cells, but rarely result in complete remissions.[834,835] Newer-generation *FLT3* inhibitors have been developed in an attempt to improve their effects.[836] Crenolanib may inhibit both ITD and TKD mutations.[837] Quizartinib (previously AC220) showed activity in a phase I study in relapsed/refractory AML, especially in patients with *FLT3-ITD* mutations.[838] Trials are now under way to examine inhibitors such as midostaurin (PKC412)[839] and sorafenib[840] in combination with cytostatic drugs for AML.

Kit Tyrosine Kinase Inhibitors: Imatinib Mesylate Activation of the KIT tyrosine kinase by somatic mutation has been documented in a small minority of AML cases. Paracrine or autocrine activation of *KIT* may occur in AML cells.[841] Imatinib mesylate has induced a complete remission in refractory secondary AML,[842] but this is a very uncommon result of its use.[843] Dasatinib has been studied in CBF leukemias with a *KIT* mutation in conjunction with chemotherapy, but final results of studies are awaited.[844]

Nuclear Factor-Kappa B Inhibitors AML leukemia stem cells have activated NF-κB, unlike normal HSCs.[845] Proteasome inhibitors such as bortezomib inhibit NF-κB and have been examined in AML. They have been found to increase sensitivity to chemotherapy agents in *NPM1*-mutated AML.[846] Bortezomib is also being combined with chemotherapy agents in AML patients.[847] Other inhibitors more specific to the NF-κB family have been proposed for study in AML.[848]

Other Signal Transduction and Tyrosine Kinase Inhibitors Numerous inhibitors of activated tyrosine kinases have been examined for AML therapy.[849,850] These include mammalian target of rapamycin (mTOR) inhibitors,[851,852] phosphoinositol 3′-kinase inhibitors,[853,854] AKT inhibitors, such as perifosine,[855] small-molecule mitogen-activated protein kinase (MEK) kinase inhibitors,[856] Aurora kinase inhibitors,[857] and heat-shock protein inhibitors.[858] None of these agents have had an impact on AML survival as single agents, but using a combination of agents that target multiple pathways or using multitargeted tyrosine kinase inhibitors may hold promise for incremental improvements in AML therapy.[859] There is some indication that extramedullary disease may increase in incidence in cases treated with signal transduction agents alone.[860]

Other Inhibitors of Signal Transduction and Apoptosis Pathways Many malignancies overexpress antiapoptotic proteins, such as BCL-2 and BCL-x$_L$.[861] Small-molecule BCL-2 homology domain-3 (BH3) mimetics such as ABT-737[862] and GX15–070 (obatoclax)[863] inhibit BCL-2. CDDO-Me, a triterpenoid, studied *in vitro* induces apoptosis and differentiation in AML cells through activation of caspase-8 and caspase-3 and induction of mitochondrial cytochrome *c* release.[864]

Prenylation Inhibitors: Farnesyltransferase inhibitors (FTIs)[865–868] and geranylgeranyltransferase-1 inhibitors (GTIs), such as statins, have been examined as therapy in AML. Examples of responses of AML to lovastatin have been reported.[869] Simvastatin adds to the effect of cytarabine's inhibition of AML cell lines.[870] Other studies suggest that the statins may mediate antileukemic effects independent of Ras/Rho prenylation through blockade of cholesterol responses to cellular injury.[871] Effectiveness of either FTIs or GTIs as single agents has been minimal in untreated AML patients.[865–868]

Maturation Therapies Several analogues of vitamin D inhibit AML cells by inducing inhibition of cyclin-dependent kinases.[872] In general, AML cells have not responded to retinoids. Single-strand conformational polymorphism analysis and DNA sequencing of leukemic cells from AML, other than APL, have not found mutations of *RAR-α*.[873] Nevertheless, combinations of retinoids, growth factors, and chemotherapeutic agents are being examined for therapeutic potential in AML.[874] Leukemias with 11q, −5, and −7 chromosome abnormalities have high telomerase activity, which can be inhibited by maturation-inducing agents.[875] In one study, addition of ATRA to chemotherapy did not improve patient outcome but did result in a 25 percent increase in apoptosis in AML marrow cells *in vitro*.[876] ATRA has induced a complete remission in a patient with acute myelomonocytic leukemia.[877,878] Arsenic trioxide induces apoptosis and cytotoxic effects in blasts from patients with AML other than APL, and it is not influenced by permeability glycoprotein (P-gp) expression.[879,880]

Antiangiogenesis Agents and Agents That Inhibit Microenvironmental Interactions

Targeting the increased vascular density of marrow noted in AML or cytokines secreted by marrow endothelium has been examined as means to inhibit AML cell growth. Amifostine,[881] thalidomide,[880] sunitinib,[881] and other agents that target VEGF and interleukin (IL)-8,[882] as well as of the angiopoietin signaling pathway,[883] are potential antiangiogenic agents in the treatment of AML. Lenalidomide, which also has antiangiogenic properties, is used to treat deletion 5q− AML.[884] Antagonists of the chemokine receptor CXCR4, which plays a role in retention of hematopoietic cells in marrow and of integrins or selectins, have been proposed as therapeutic agents to overcome stromal-mediated resistance and to enhance chemotherapy-induced cell death.[885,886]

Modulation of Drug Resistance

Numerous mechanisms of drug resistance occur in AML,[887] and several attempts to overcome this resistance have been instituted, but none of the agents used, such as cyclosporine or PSC-833, have had a significant impact on AML outcomes to date. P-gp, MDR protein-1 (MRP-1), and breast cancer resistance protein (BCRP) expression all have been found in AML.[888]

Other Immunotherapy and Antisense DNA Approaches

Culture of AML blasts upregulates costimulatory molecules, and the role of dendritic cells in antileukemia therapy is being examined.[889–891] Other approaches to generating autologous T-cell antileukemic activity include vaccination with AML-specific peptides, immunization with AML blasts exhibiting dendritic cell phenotype and function,[892,893] and pulsing normal dendritic cells with AML-specific peptide sequences.[894] Natural killer cells may mediate antileukemia effects.[895] Low doses of IL-2 have been used in the maintenance phase of AML, and some patients have remained on this regimen for 10 or more years without significant side effects.[896] However, low-dose IL-2 does not improve outcomes when used as maintenance treatment in older AML patients.[897] The WT gene *WT1* is expressed on AML blasts, and a *WT1* vaccine may elicit cytotoxic T-cell responses against this protein.[898] Peptides derived from the mutated nucleophosmin I gene can elicit *in vitro* CD4 and CD8 T-cell responses.[129] Other proteins against which such humoral responses have been elicited include minor HLA antigens and proteinase-3.[899] Coinhibitory molecule signaling can hamper benefit of immune therapies, so efforts to modulate coinhibitory networks are underway in leukemias.[900] Small interfering RNA (siRNA) targeting of transcription factors[901] and GTI-2040, an antisense to ribonucleotide reductase, have been used in AML therapy.[902] In addition to CD33, CD45, CD66, and CD38 have been examined as targets for immunotherapy of AML.[903,904] Immunotoxin conjugates are being examined in AML as well to increase potency of naked monoclonal antibodies.[905] Alloreactive haploidentical KIR ligand-mismatched natural killer cells are also being examined in high-risk elderly AML cases.[906]

The immunomodulatory drug lenalidomide has also been examined in AML and has some activity in high doses in relapsed or refractory AML.[907,908]

The IL-3 receptor α (CD123) is overexpressed in AML as compared with normal HSCs, so it has been proposed as a target for chimeric antigen receptors (CARS) as a bridge to allogeneic HSC transplantation.[909,910]

SPECIAL THERAPEUTIC CONSIDERATIONS

Acute Promyelocytic Leukemia

General Consideration in Therapy Because of the early induction mortality in APL, patients who are suspected based on morphology and presence of coagulopathy should begin ATRA without waiting for definitive FISH or molecular confirmation. There is now an International Consortium on APL, the goal is to improve outcomes through education and guidelines formulaton.[911] While many trials with variations in the induction, consolidation, and maintenance phases are published, the clinician is urged to consider clinical trials and to follow one protocol plan through all the phases of therapy.

Induction Treatment ATRA has become a standard component of induction therapy for APL. Used alone, ATRA can induce a short-term remission in at least 80 percent of patients.[912] However, ATRA should be combined with an anthracycline such as idarubicin or with arsenic trioxide during induction treatment for most benefit and to prevent drug resistance.[913] Idarubicin by itself can induce remission in approximately 75 percent of patients.[914] A typical induction regimen for APL is ATRA 45 mg/m² daily in divided doses with idarubicin at standard induction doses (e.g., 12 mg/m² on days 1 to 3).[915,916] Although cytarabine has been largely abandoned as part of induction, some studies show a high degree of efficacy of high-dose cytarabine combined with ATRA.[917] There is evidence that in patients who present with a white cell count of 10×10^9/L or greater, the complete remission rate and overall survival may be superior when cytarabine is added to induction or consolidation regimens, especially if arsenic trioxide is not part of the induction regimen.[918,919] The addition of arsenic trioxide to ATRA and idarubicin in induction regimens results in approximately 95 percent complete remission rates. This approach allows reduction in anthracycline usage and excellent overall survival (93 percent).[920] In low- to intermediate-risk APL (WBC $<10 \times 10^9$/L), the combination of ATRA and arsenic trioxide was found equal to, or possibly superior to, an ATRA plus chemotherapy regimen.[921,922] Also, there was less hematologic toxicity and fewer infections with that combination of drugs. Older patients generally tolerate a combination of ATRA and an anthracycline.[923] Combinations that include gemtuzumab ozogamicin are being examined for their effectiveness in APL induction therapy, but this antibody is no longer marketed in the United States.[924] The combination of ATRA and arsenic trioxide results in more rapid remissions and lower PML-RAR-α transcript levels than either agent alone.[925] Despite the high remission rates and frequency of long-term event-free survival achieved in this disease, controversies remain regarding therapy because of the 5 to 10 percent of patients who die as a result of fatal intracranial hemorrhage.[926] This relatively high early death rate (17.3 percent) persisted despite use of ATRA in induction therapy.[927] Thus, there are several induction regimens that can be chosen to treat APL based on WBC at diagnosis and, to a lesser extent, patient age and ability to tolerate anthracyclines. For those with low-risk disease, a combination of ATRA plus arsenic trioxide, ATRA plus idarubicin alone, or ATRA plus daunorubicin plus cytarabine can be used. In high-risk patients, ATRA plus daunorubicin and cytarabine, ATRA plus idarubicin, or ATRA and arsenic trioxide with idarubicin (dose-adjusted based on age) can be used.[928] Table 88–8 lists APL induction regimens.

All-*Trans* Retinoic Acid: Dose and Mechanism of Action ATRA, an analogue of vitamin A, has been used to initiate the therapy of APL

TABLE 88–8. Examples of Treatment Protocols for Acute Promyelocytic Leukemia

Induction	Consolidation	Reference
HIGH-RISK PATIENT		
ATRA 45 mg/m² PO in divided doses Daunorubicin 60 mg/m² IV for 3 days Cytarabine 200 mg/m² IV for 7 days	1st Cycle: Daunorubicin 60 mg/m² IV for 3 days; Cytarabine 200 mg/m² IV for 7 days 2nd Cycle: Cytarabine 2 g/m² (or 1.5 g/m² in older patients) IV, every 12 hours for 5 days plus daunorubicin 45 mg/m² IV for 3 days	922
ATRA 45 mg/m² PO (days 1–36 in divided doses) Idarubicin (6–12 mg/m² based on age) IV on days 2, 4, 6, and 8 Arsenic trioxide 0.15 mg/kg IV (days 9–26)	1st Cycle: ATRA 45 mg/m² PO in divided doses for 28 days; arsenic trioxide 0.15 mg/kg IV per day for 28 days 2nd Cycle: ATRA 45 mg/m² PO for 7 days every 2 weeks × 3. Arsenic trioxide 0.15 mg/kg per day × 5 days IV for 5 weeks	928
LOW-RISK PATIENT		
ATRA 45 mg/m² PO in divided doses daily until remission; arsenic trioxide 0.15 mg/kg IV daily until remission	Arsenic trioxide 0.15 mg/kg IV per day, 5 days per week for 4 weeks every 8 weeks for 4 cycles ATRA 45 mg/m² PO per day for 2 weeks every 4 weeks for 7 cycles	921
ATRA 45 mg/m² PO in divided doses until clinical remission; Idarubicin 12 mg/m² IV on days 2, 4, 6, and 8	1st Cycle: ATRA 45 mg/m² PO for 15 days; idarubicin 5 mg/m² IV for 4 days 2nd Cycle: ATRA 45 mg/m² PO for 15 days; mitoxantrone 10 mg/m² IV for 5 days 3rd Cycle: ATRA 45 mg/m² PO for 15 days; idarubicin 12 mg/m² IV for 1 dose	919

NOTE: The reader is advised to consult the original reference for details of the administration of the chemotherapy regimens. "High risk" is defined as a white cell count at diagnosis ≥10 × 10⁹/L. "Low risk" is defined as a white cell count at diagnosis <10 × 10⁹/L.

since 1987 in the United States. ATRA induces complete remissions in approximately 80 percent of previously untreated patients.[929] *In vitro*, ATRA is 10 times more potent in inducing maturation of leukemic promyelocytes to neutrophils than 13-*cis* retinoic acid, the other naturally occurring isomer.[930] ATRA induces maturation of the leukemic cells and their apoptosis results in the reappearance of normal polyclonal hematopoiesis and a remission in most cases.[931] ATRA may induce synthesis of a protein that selectively degrades PML-RAR-α. ATRA can overcome the recruitment of histone deacetylase activity by the *PML-RAR-α* fusion gene through interference with a nuclear corepressor.[932] STAT1 is induced and activated by ATRA. Promyelocytic leukemia cells with PML-RAR-α break-fusion sites in *PML* exon 6 have decreased *in*

vitro responsiveness to ATRA.[933] The t(11;17) variant of APL, in which the promyelocytic leukemia zinc finger *(PLZF)* gene is fused to *RAR-α*, does not respond to ATRA.[934] Other nonpromyelocytic leukemia subtypes of AML have not responded to ATRA therapy. ATRA is beneficial in APL during the induction and maintenance phases of disease,[935] and improved outcome with ATRA is reflected in the 5-year survival rates of 75 to 80 percent.[936] Additional cytogenetic changes do not influence treatment outcomes with ATRA plus an anthracycline.[937] ATRA induction therapy can result in favorable results without blood product support.[938]

Toxic Effects of All-*Trans* Retinoic Acid ATRA therapy is associated with dryness of the skin and lips, occasionally leading to mild exfoliation, nausea, headache, arthralgia, and bone pain. The white cell count may rise dramatically in the first week or two of therapy. Serum glutamic-pyruvate transaminase and triglyceride concentrations often increase. Leukemic promyelocytes disappear from the blood in 2 to 4 weeks, and a normal marrow aspirate may be obtained in 4 to 10 weeks. Anemia improves gradually. The majority of patients become PML-RAR-α–negative by PCR after the second consolidation therapy in conjunction with ATRA.[939] ATRA has been used successfully to treat APL diagnosed during pregnancy.[940] ATRA has been used from week 3 of gestation, but may result in fetal malformations when it is used during the first trimester.[941]

Differentiation Syndrome A rapid increase in the total blood leukocyte count to as high as 80 × 10⁹/L in the first several weeks of therapy, referred to as the *differentiation syndrome* (previously called the *retinoic acid syndrome*), is a potential cause of early death during therapy.[942-944] The median time of onset is 11 days, but the syndrome has occurred up to 47 days after therapy starts.[944] Two approaches to treatment of this phenomenon have been suggested: early use of cytotoxic chemotherapy[945,946] and glucocorticoid administration.[947,948] The syndrome consists of fever, weight gain, dependent edema, pleural or pericardial effusion, and bouts of hypotension. Respiratory distress is the key feature. In fatal cases, pulmonary interstitial infiltration with maturing granulocytes is prominent. Once respiratory distress is evident, the patient should receive dexamethasone 10 mg IV every 12 hours for several days. Because the syndrome may occur at relatively low total white cell counts and its onset is unpredictable, high-dose glucocorticoid therapy should be instituted if respiratory symptoms develop even in the absence of pulmonary infiltrates or an elevated white cell count.[942,946] ATRA can be continued or resumed with glucocorticoids or with concurrent cytotoxic chemotherapy, but the syndrome may recur.[942] This syndrome is not observed during maintenance therapy. It may also occur with arsenic trioxide therapy, and some recommend prophylactic glucocorticoids in those with a WBC greater than 10 × 10⁹/L or in those receiving both ATRA and arsenic trioxide.[943]

Treatment of Coagulopathy Reducing the risk of early death from hemorrhage as a result of the coagulopathy accompanying APL requires use of fresh-frozen plasma, platelet replacement, and fibrinogen replacement.[489,490,949] Targeted levels for platelet counts are usually 30 to 50 × 10⁹/L[928] and for fibrinogen levels 1.5 g/L or higher, but these levels are often difficult to achieve in patients with active hemorrhage.[950] Heparin treatment was used during induction chemotherapy in the past to prevent onset of disseminated intravascular coagulopathy during treatment, but rarely is used now.[951] ATRA may have some corrective effect on coagulation disorders in APL.[952] However, a reduction of 5 to 10 percent of fatal hemorrhages has not been significant with ATRA used early during treatment. Paradoxically, hypercoagulable clotting tendency may occur in patients during the first months of ATRA therapy.[931] In the coagulopathy of APL, the blasts overexpress annexin II, and there is evidence that the effects of annexin II can be reversed by L-methionine administration.[953]

Chemotherapy Induction of remission with ATRA alone is followed by relapse in weeks to months unless intensive chemotherapy is used concomitantly.[954] At relapse, cells show high levels of a cytosolic retinoic-acid-binding protein not detected prior to ATRA therapy.[932] The mechanism of retinoid resistance in leukemic cells may involve cytochrome P450 and P-gp because of induction of various enzymes that may alter ATRA metabolism.[955] ATRA, whether administered as part of induction therapy or as maintenance therapy, confers a disease-free survival advantage. More than 70 percent of patients receiving ATRA at any point were in continuous remission at 2.5 years versus less than 20 percent of patients who never received ATRA.[936] The acquired *in vivo* resistance that occurs rapidly to ATRA as a single agent requires consolidation of ATRA-induced complete remission with intensive chemotherapy using an anthracycline antibiotic. Customary treatment today involves simultaneous administration of ATRA and an anthracycline and/or arsenic trioxide. Some therapists have returned to combining an anthracycline antibiotic with cytarabine in an effort to decrease CNS relapse, especially in patients younger than 60 years of age with white counts greater than 10×10^9/L at presentation.[956] Maintenance therapy with ATRA alone or in combination with mercaptopurine or methotrexate has been recommended. This additional therapy has not been examined in a randomized trial of ATRA dosing and scheduling, but ATRA usually is given in an interrupted fashion. Intensified maintenance therapy may have a negative impact on those patients who have become negative for the PML-RAR-α fusion transcript after induction plus consolidation therapy.[957] Some therapists have proposed that elderly patients can be treated with ATRA and arsenic trioxide without chemotherapy and with addition of gemtuzumab ozogamicin in the event of an elevated white count at the time of diagnosis.[958]

Arsenic Trioxide Arsenic trioxide can trigger apoptosis of APL cells at high concentrations and maturation at low concentrations. The presence of PML-RAR-α is important for the response. Apoptosis may occur through induction of activation of caspase-1 and caspase-3 after changes in the mitochondrial membrane potential with increase in H_2O_2.[959,960] It also may function through NF-κB inhibition.[961] Death-associated protein 5 also contributes to arsenic trioxide–induced apoptosis in APL.[962] Arsenic trioxide given at 0.06 to 0.12 mg/kg body weight per day until leukemic cells were eliminated from the marrow induced remission within 12 to 89 days in 11 of 12 patients.[963] Suppression of hematopoiesis did not occur. Rash, light-headedness, fatigue, and musculoskeletal pain were the main side effects. Arsenic trioxide can be combined with idarubicin in relapsed patients; it also has been used with ATRA.[921,964,965] A retinoic acid–like syndrome (see "All-*Trans*-Retinoic Acid: Dose and Mechanism of Action" above) has been described in patients with APL treated with arsenic trioxide.[966] Torsade de pointes, an uncommon variant of ventricular tachycardia in which the underlying etiology and management are different from those of the usual variety of ventricular tachycardia, has been described with arsenic trioxide use,[967] and monitoring of electrocardiographic QTc intervals and electrolyte levels during therapy is recommended.[968]

Consolidation Therapy Consolidation therapy is required in APL to achieve a durable molecular remission. Consolidation typically consists of anthracycline plus ATRA, but in high-risk patients, the addition of cytarabine or use of arsenic trioxide can be used to diminish the rate of relapse. Almost every induction regimen described in APL has a distinct consolidation regimen attached to it, dependent on disease stratification. To achieve uniformly good responses, it is recommended that one follow a given protocol's induction, consolidation, and maintenance regimen. Table 88–8 provides examples of paired induction and consolidation regimens. Excellent results can be achieved with all of these regimens, if treatment plans are executed faithfully.

Maintenance Therapy After consolidation phases of therapy are complete, patients should be in a molecular remission, that is, PCR-negative for PML-RAR-α. ATRA maintenance with chemotherapy is recommended based on the APL 93 trial, which showed that relapse-free survival was superior with ATRA versus no ATRA, and that the best results were achieved when ATRA was combined with 6-mercaptopurine and methotrexate.[969] The 10-year cumulative relapse rates were 43 percent with no maintenance, 33 percent with ATRA alone, 23 percent with chemotherapy alone, and 13 percent with ATRA and chemotherapy.[970] Maintenance is usually recommended for 2 years, and studies to examine whether maintenance is beneficial in low-risk disease are ongoing.[928] During maintenance, PCR monitoring on blood samples is recommended.[928] If the PCR is positive in blood, a marrow examination should be done.

Treatment for Relapsed Acute Promyelocytic Leukemia Conventional chemotherapy can be effective after relapse. Arsenic trioxide has been used in those who do not achieve molecular remission at completion of consolidation or who subsequently demonstrate molecular relapse and can generate high molecular remission rates in more than 80 percent of patients alone or when combined with chemotherapy.[971] It is still uncertain whether ATRA has benefit in patients previously exposed to ATRA. Patients younger than age 70 years should be considered for allogeneic or autologous HSC transplantation after they have achieved a second remission or for allogeneic transplantation if a second remission cannot be induced.[972] Other treatments for patients in relapse include the combination of ATRA, arsenic trioxide, and gemtuzumab ozogamicin. This combination has resulted in durable remissions.[973] Transplantation generally is not recommended for patients with APL in first remission given the prolonged remissions after standard treatments. Allogeneic stem cell transplant is best used in advanced APL, especially in patients with persistent disease by PCR.[974] The outcome of autologous stem cell transplantation in second complete remission is excellent if the stem cells used are negative for PML-RAR-α.[941] High-dose cytarabine can be used for stem cell mobilization which will also treat CNS relapse, and when a second molecular remission is followed by an autograft, the 5-year disease-free survival is approximately 75 percent. This result is superior to survival after allografting, but a direct comparison of autologous transplantation, allogeneic transplantation, and arsenic trioxide or ATRA with standard chemotherapy has not been made in patients with APL in a second remission after relapse.[975] For patients in a second remission who are not candidates for allogeneic stem cell transplant, up to six cycles of arsenic can be used.

Many cases of extramedullary relapse in APL have been reported.[976] Many of the relapses occur in patients who received ATRA and who initially were diagnosed with hyperleukocytosis,[977] and many of the patients are in marrow remission. Relapses occurring more than 5 years after diagnosis have been reported, some at extramedullary sites such as in the mastoid bone.[978] Early detection of relapse is important as those with molecular relapse before hematologic relapse has occurred fare best.[979] Patients should be monitored with PCR every 3 months for 2 years after remission induction, especially those with intermediate- or high-risk disease.[928]

MDS can occur in patients in remission with APL, usually 24 months or more after diagnosis. The complication results from a second (drug-induced) clonal disease in long-term responders.[980–992] Cases of therapy-related APL have been described.[983] Patients with APL who are FLT3-ITD–positive generally have worse overall outcomes than do those persons who present with elevated white cell counts and older age.[984] There is also evidence that mutations in the ATRA-targeted ligand binding domain of *PML-RAR-α* and additional chromosome abnormalities may be associated with reduced postrelapse survival in those on

ATRA.[985] Oral arsenic trioxide and tamibarotene, a synthetic retinoid, are being examined in relapsed APL.[986,987] Children older than 4 years and adolescents have outcomes with ATRA-treated APL equivalent to that of adults, but younger children have more frequent relapses.[988]

SECONDARY ACUTE MYELOGENOUS LEUKEMIA

Secondary leukemias arise after treatment of another malignancy or an autoimmune disease with cytotoxic chemotherapy or radiation. Secondary AML responds more poorly to chemotherapy and allogeneic stem cell transplantation than does *de novo* AML. Secondary AML accounts for approximately 5 to 10 percent of all AML cases, although this percentage is increasing.[980,990] The leukemogenic risk of treatment regimens depends on the agents used. Future development of agents with lower risk of inducing AML is an important goal.[991]

Effect of Topoisomerase II Inhibitors

Exposure to topoisomerase II inhibitors (e.g., etoposide, mitoxantrone, amsacrine) can lead to AML with *MLL* gene rearrangements on chromosome 11q32.[992] Inversion 16 is an uncommon aberration in secondary AML and, like balanced translocations of chromosome bands 11q32, 21q22, and t(15;17), is associated with prior chemotherapy with topoisomerase II inhibitors when seen in the setting of treatment-induced leukemias. The site of breakpoints within the *MYH*11 gene involved in inversion 16 may vary between therapy-induced AML and AML occurring *de novo*.[993] The latency period for development of AML after topoisomerase II inhibitors is approximately 2 years. No relationship with higher cumulative dose has been identified. Studies of single nucleotide polymorphisms to ascertain genetic predisposition are ongoing.[994] Polymorphisms in detoxification genes and in genes involved in DNA repair pathways might be involved.[995] Even the use of low-dose or oral etoposide can be associated with development of secondary AML.

Effect of Alkylating Agents and Cisplatin

Alkylating agents cause secondary AML, often preceded by myelodysplasia. The mean latency period after onset of treatment is approximately 6 years. Deletions of all or part of chromosome 5 or 7 are the most common cytogenetic changes. The risk is related to cumulative alkylating agent dose. Germline aberrancies of *NFI* and *p53* may increase the risk of AML. Cisplatin used for treatment of ovarian cancer also increases the risk of secondary leukemia.[996]

Other Cytotoxic Agents

Other drugs that may increase the risk of secondary leukemias include low-dose weekly methotrexate for rheumatoid arthritis,[997] etanercept therapy,[998] temozolamide,[999] growth hormone administration,[1000] and G-CSF given to patients with congenital, but not idiopathic or cyclic neutropenia.[1001] In the latter cases, a cause-and-effect relationship between MDS/AML and G-CSF therapy has not been established. Improved survival duration with G-CSF may allow expression of an underlying leukemic predisposition.

Other Settings for Secondary Leukemia

Patients with APL in remission may develop a new MDS (oligoblastic leukemia), presumably secondary to therapy.[1002] Series of children with treatment-related myelodysplasia or AML have the same latency period as do adults treated with alkylating agents or topoisomerase II inhibitors for AML.[1003] Breast cancer patients receiving doxorubicin and cyclophosphamide regimens of such intensity that they required G-CSF support had increased rates of posttherapy AML. Breast and prostate radiotherapy are associated with an increased risk of AML.[1004,1005] In patients with non-Hodgkin lymphoma, up to 10 percent of patients treated with either conventional chemotherapy or high-dose therapy developed secondary AML within 10 years.[1006] Secondary leukemia is seen after autologous marrow or blood stem cell transplants involving high-dose chemotherapy and/or radiotherapy. In a study of 83 patients after autografting, 12 had nonclonal cytogenetic abnormalities and 10 had clonal abnormalities, five of whom developed secondary AML. Onset occurred 12 to 48 months after autografting. The relative contribution of the underlying disease and the conditioning therapy is uncertain.[1007] Clonality analysis using an X chromosome gene, based on methylation of the human androgen receptor locus in cell samples in patients with lymphoma, found a clonal marrow cell population 6 months after autologous transplantation at a time when no morphologic or clinical evidence of AML was present. AML appeared later in some patients.[1008] More than 10 percent of patients with non-Hodgkin lymphoma who underwent stem cell rescue after total body irradiation and cyclophosphamide developed AML at a median followup of 6 years.[1009] Using a triple FISH assay to detect loss of chromosomal material from 5q31, 7q22, or 13q14, abnormal cells were detected before high-dose therapy was given to non-Hodgkin lymphoma patients.[1010] Thus, some patients are at increased risk for developing secondary AML based on pretreatment chromosome studies.

Treatment of Secondary Leukemia

Secondary leukemia generally is treated similarly to *de novo* leukemia. However, given the lower response rates and remission durations of secondary leukemia, patients can be treated in clinical trials examining new therapies or treated initially with chemotherapy regimens used for refractory disease.[1011] Some patients may benefit from early allogeneic HSC transplantation.[1012] Autologous transplant can be successful if stem cells are harvested prior to the development of secondary AML.[1013] In those who have low blood blast counts, allogeneic stem cell transplantation as initial therapy may be superior to induction chemotherapy followed by transplantation, but this remains an area of controversy.[1014] Although patients may have a response rate of approximately 50 percent to standard induction chemotherapy, most soon relapse, and long-term survival is approximately 10 percent.[1015] Secondary AML more often has unfavorable cytogenetic features compared to *de novo* leukemia.[1016]

TREATMENT OF Ph CHROMOSOME–POSITIVE AML

This cytogenetic variant of acute leukemia is characterized by extraordinary drug resistance. Imatinib mesylate in doses of 600 to 800 mg/day may produce a hematologic remission in a small proportion of patients with Ph chromosome–positive AML, based on the response in patients with CML who go on to a myeloid blast crisis. No formal studies of the response to imatinib mesylate of *de novo* Ph chromosome–positive AML have been performed. In myeloid blast crisis of CML, the uncommon full hematologic response (blood and marrow) usually is short lived, measured in weeks or a few months. This outcome also seems to be the case when therapy with other drugs (e.g., cytarabine, etoposide, anthracycline antibiotics) is included. Occasional cases in which chemotherapy has induced remission in Ph chromosome–positive AML and imatinib mesylate has appeared to help induce and sustain the remission have been reported.[1017] Thus, in Ph chromosome–positive AML, a matched-related or matched-unrelated donor stem cell transplant should be considered if the patient is younger than age 50 years. This approach may have the highest probability of a long-term remission. There is little information about the use of second generation *BCR-ABL* inhibitors in this setting.

TREATMENT OF OLDER PATIENTS

Biologic Features

Approximately 65 percent of patients with AML are older than age 60 years at the time of diagnosis.[1018] The disease in this age group is less responsive to therapy, and this age group has a higher proportion of patients who have oligoblastic myelogenous leukemia (MDS); an antecedent clonal myeloid disease; prior chemotherapy for cancer of another site; and comorbid conditions that decrease the tolerance to intensive chemotherapy programs.[1019–1022] The AML cells of elderly patients often have more CD34 expression, suggesting origin from a more primitive multipotential (? stem) cell. This finding is thought to contribute to longer duration of postchemotherapy aplasia and to the increased risk of induction deaths in this age group.[1023] Patients older than age 60 years also have a high frequency of unfavorable cytogenetic findings (32 percent) and higher *MDR1* expression (71 percent) and functional drug efflux (58 percent).[1024,1025]

Chemotherapy

The therapist and patient determine whether a standard regimen, a standard regimen with dose reductions, or a special regimen is used.[1026,1027] Decisions based on chronologic age should be supplanted by measurements of cognitive, neurologic, and physical fitness used by geriatricians to evaluate the wisdom of considering intensive treatment.[1028] These are often not well-validated in geriatric AML populations, but there is evidence that assessments focused on cognition and objective measures of physical function may predict for overall survival in those older than age 60 years who undergo standard induction chemotherapy.[1029] In patients older than age 60 years who are fit and otherwise are considered good candidates, standard two-drug therapy can be used: cytarabine and an anthracycline antibiotic, and on some occasions the addition of a third drug, etoposide. Remission rates of approximately 35 to 45 percent can be achieved. Based on case studies, those who are able to receive induction chemotherapy may have a median survival slightly better than those who receive supportive care alone,[1030,1031] but there are no randomized trials that address this issue.[1032] Patients older than 70 years (median: 74; range: 70 to 88) may not have much benefit from intensive chemotherapy with an 8-week mortality of greater than 30 percent and a median survival of less than 6 months.[1033] Some investigators have proposed waiting for cytogenetic information before therapy decisions are made in older patients. Those with unfavorable cytogenetics and two or more other criteria including age older than 75 years, poor performance status, and WBC greater than 50×10^9/L were found not to benefit from chemotherapy.[1034] Chemotherapy has been combined with growth factor support to accelerate neutrophil recovery in older patients.[1035] In a study in which patients older than age 55 years were randomized to receive either placebo or G-CSF after induction therapy, no reduction in the duration of hospitalization, survival prolongation, or cost of supportive care was noted.[1036] In previously untreated elderly patients with AML, mitoxantrone induction therapy produces a slightly higher remission rate than did daunorubicin, but had no significant effect on remission duration and survival.[1037] Oral idarubicin alone has been used with success.[1038]

Attenuated standard regimens can be used in older patients. An example of an attenuated regimen is cytarabine 100 mg/m² subcutaneously every 12 hours for 10 doses on days 1 through 5 and daunorubicin 30 mg/m² IV on days 1 through 3 of treatment. One induction regimen is not superior to another in older patients. Outcomes achieved with cytarabine and daunorubicin are comparable to results with mitoxantrone and etoposide.[1039] Other regimens for older patients include lower total doses of idarubicin, etoposide, and cytarabine (DIVA regimen)[1040] and a combination of continuous infusion low-dose

cytarabine with etoposide and G-CSF.[1041] Temozolomide has been used in this age group,[1042] and clofarabine is also being tested in patients age 60 years and older.[1043] In one study of clofarabine in older patients who were deemed unfit for 7-plus-3 chemotherapy, a 5-day clofarabine regimen resulted in a 48 percent response rate, and 18 percent died within 30 days.[1044] Another study in those older than 60 years showed a response rate of 46 percent and an overall median survival of 41 weeks and a 30-day all-cause mortality of approximately 10 percent.[1045] Several investigational therapies, including 5-azacytidine, decitabine, cloretazine, and depsipeptide, are also being studied. There are also several reports concerning addition of other agents to standard chemotherapy to improve responses. These include bevacizumab,[1046] sorafenib,[1047] and gemtuzumab ozogamicin.[1048,1049] Thus far, none of these drugs have resulted in improvement in overall survival.

Autologous Stem Cell Infusion or Nonmyeloablative Allogeneic Transplantation

Autologous stem cell transplantation has been used in fit patients older than age 60 years.[1050] The incidence of relapse is lower when marrow stem cells are used compared to blood stem cells. Some patients older than age 60 years may be eligible for reduced-intensity allogeneic stem cell transplantation from related or unrelated donors, but more data regarding outcomes are needed.[1051] In a large registry study, examining reduced-intensity allogeneic HSC transplantation for older patients with AML and MDS in first remission, older age was not found to affect 2-year nonrelapse mortality, disease-free or overall survival.[1052]

Postremission Therapy in Older Patients

No consensus exists regarding the best regimen or the number of treatment cycles for postremission therapy in older adults. Regardless of the consolidation regimen, the duration of the leukemia-free survival is longer with high-dose cytarabine and autologous stem cell transplantation, just as it is in younger patients,[1042] but fewer older patients can tolerate this degree of therapeutic intensity. Higher-dose cytarabine can be used in older adults with AML, but usually at a reduced dose.[1053] Older patients treated with attenuated high-dose cytarabine at 750 mg/m² intravenously for 12 doses and then consolidated with four to six doses had an approximately 50 percent remission rate with a median duration of remission of 326 days.[1054] Fifty-one percent of 110 patients older than 60 years of age had a 9-month median remission duration when consolidated with high-dose cytarabine.[1055] Older patients are at higher risk for relapse despite successfully completing intensive consolidation therapy, regardless of whether other adverse prognostic features are present. Cytarabine as maintenance therapy may prolong disease-free survival but does not improve overall survival.[1056] Decitabine and 5-azacytidine are also being examined for maintenance therapy. In one randomized study, those receiving consolidation therapies had more hospitalizations and more transfusion requirements.[1057]

Patients older than 80 years of age do not tolerate treatments well. Remission rates are approximately 30 percent, but the median survival of treated patients is approximately 1 month. Less than 10 percent of patients survive for 1 year.[1058]

Unlike the case in younger patients, the treatment outcomes for older patients have not improved over the last two decades.[1059] Treatment options in older patients include (1) no treatment, (2) supportive care, (3) palliative low-dose chemotherapy, (4) attenuated induction chemotherapy, or (5) high-dose chemotherapy regimens. Investigative agents should also be given strong consideration in this population.[1060] Comorbidities are independent predictors of complete remission and should be taken into account during decision making,[1061] as should performance status.[1062] Some argue that the approximately 15 percent rate of death in those older than 60 years of age in the first month after standard induction chemotherapy is unacceptable given the less than 1 year median survival expected.[1063] Lower-dose regimens can also be toxic and can lead to severe cytopenias. Use of colony-stimulating factor permits older patients to tolerate full-dose induction therapy. The Medical Research Council of the United Kingdom observed remission rates of 80 percent in children, 70 percent in adults younger than 50 years of age, 68 percent in adults 50 to 59 years old, 53 percent in adults 60 to 69 years old, 39 percent in adults 70 to 75 years old, and 22 percent in adults older than 75 years of age.[1064] In one study of patients older than 60 years of age, the 2-, 5-, and 10-year survivals were 22, 11, and 8 percent, respectively.[1065,1066] The older patients who remain free of leukemia beyond 1 year have a reasonable quality of life.[1067,1068] The National Cancer Institute 5-year relative survival rates for patients with AML are 11 percent for adults ages 65 to 74 years and 1.8 percent for adults ages 75 years and older.[1069]

Even though t(8;21) and inversion 16 are rare in older AML patients, remission rates are high with these favorable prognostic chromosome changes, so induction chemotherapy is often recommended, although rates of relapse remain high.[1070] In parallel, elderly patients with unfavorable cytogenetics have a dismal prognosis, and those who have a monosomal karyotype have low complete remission and overall survival rates; 37 versus 64 percent and 8 versus 28 percent, respectively, in those with and without monosomal karyotype.[1071]

TREATMENT OF PREGNANT PATIENTS

Leukemia (AML, ALL, CML) is the second most common malignancy of women in the childbearing age group and is expected to occur in approximately 1 in 75,000 to 100,000 pregnancies.[1072,1073] No systematic studies of the (1) effects of leukemia on pregnancy or delivery, (2) effects of the leukemia or its treatment on the fetus, or (3) postnatal development of the offspring exposed to maternal chemotherapy *in utero* have been performed. A recent literature review led to the conclusion that treatment during the second and third trimesters resulted in fewer complications to the fetus, but delaying treatment adversely affected the outcome of mothers. Remission rates were comparable to that of nonpregnant patients.[1074] Folic acid inhibitors, purine, pyrimidine, or retinoid analogues given during the first trimester of pregnancy increase the probability of major congenital malformations. In a French study of 37 patients with acute leukemia during pregnancy, 34 patients achieved remission, and disease-free survival appeared equivalent to that of patients who were not treated during pregnancy.[1075] In another study from Saudi Arabia, of 21 pregnant patients with acute leukemia, 10 were given chemotherapy with seven livebirths and three spontaneous abortions without any teratogenetic or congenital malformations. In the 11 not given chemotherapy until after 34 weeks of gestation, three had normal births and eight had an abortion before starting chemotherapy.[1076]

If the pregnancy is not terminated, leukapheresis might be useful in the first trimester, when chemotherapy poses a high risk to the embryo. Intensive chemotherapy given to women in the second and third trimesters of pregnancy does not present an inordinate risk to fetal or neonatal development,[1077,1078] although an increased frequency of premature delivery, higher perinatal mortality, and lower birthweight for gestational age are observed, especially if the fetus is exposed to chemotherapy.

Cytarabine is highly teratogenic in animal models and malformations have been described in women who were treated in the first trimester of pregnancy. Doxorubicin is the preferred anthracycline antibiotic to treat pregnant women as it has lower transplacental transfer. Doxorubicin is considered relatively safe when used in pregnant women.[1079] Newborn infants may be transiently cytopenic if the mother receives chemotherapy near the time of delivery. Development of the

newborn usually is normal after intensive chemotherapy for AML during pregnancy, if therapy is started after the first trimester.[1072,1077,1078] Vaginal delivery should be used whenever possible. Pregnant women with AML who enter remission have little difficulty with childbirth or postparturition. The remission rates of AML are approximately the rates expected for the age group, and long-term remissions can occur with current therapy. Leukemic infiltrates can be found on the maternal side of the placenta, but usually not in the villi. One case of maternal-to-fetal transmission of AML has been documented.[1080] Transmission of AML from one identical twin to another through a shared placental circulation accounts for the dual occurrence in twins in the first several years of life.[177] There are reports of the use of ATRA for APL treatment during pregnancy, but use during the first trimester is discouraged, and data are sparse.[941,1081,1082]

TREATMENT OF CHILDREN

AML represents approximately 15 percent of the acute leukemias in children (younger than 20 years of age) in the United States. APL is treated as in adults, with ATRA and an anthracycline antibiotic. In other phenotypes of AML, intensive treatment—including initial therapy with cytarabine and daunomycin or doxorubicin and a third drug such as mitoxantrone or 6-thioguanine, followed by intensive multidrug consolidation therapy including additional agents such as etoposide, and intrathecal cytarabine—has resulted in remission in approximately 80 percent of children and 5-year relapse-free remissions in approximately 50 percent of treated children.[1083–1086] Most of the children in long-term remission are considered cured.

Monocytic leukemia and hyperleukocytic (>100 × 10^9/L) myelogenous leukemia are unfavorable phenotypes. In children, *FLT3-ITD* mutations are approximately half as common (15 percent) as in adults (30 percent), but are a very poor prognostic indicator.[1087] Therapy can be adjusted for children based on the presence of poor prognostic variables, which include age younger than 2 years or older than 10 years; abnormalities of chromosome 3, 5, or 7, complex karyotypes, *FLT3* mutations, elevated white cell count of 50 × 10^9/L or greater, male gender; and, perhaps, most importantly, because it reflects the effect of all factors, the presence of greater than 15 percent blast cells in the marrow examined 14 days after onset of treatment.[1088,1089] The presence of residual blast cells detected by flow cytometry after induction therapy is a very poor prognostic finding.[1090] The duration of first remission predicts the subsequent remission rate and long-term survival in children with relapse.

Translocations 8;21, 15;17, or inv16 are good prognostic markers. Loss of a sex chromosome in the t(8;21) group is especially favorable. Monosomy 7 and abnormalities of chromosomes 3 or 5 are poor prognostic features.[1091] Pediatric AML with t(8;16)(p11;p13) has been found to be a distinct clinical entity, and in a subset of neonatal cases, spontaneous remissions can occur.[1092] In childhood 11p23/*MLL* AML, there are large differences in outcome based on translocation partners that are independent prognostic markers as assessed in a large international study.[1093] When gene mutations were examined in childhood leukemia, *FLT3-ITD* was most frequent, and 29 percent had more than one gene mutation. Mutated epigenetic regulators were less than in adults, but were often seen with other mutations.[1094]

In the United Kingdom Medical Research Council Trial 12, completed in 2002, using daunorubicin, mitoxantrone cytarabine, etoposide, and asparaginase in different combinations, approximately 90 percent of children with AML had a remission, 60 percent of children had a 5-year disease-free survival, and most were considered cured.[1091] Approximately 4 percent of children are drug resistant with this program and approximately 4 percent die during induction and intensification therapy. Studies are under way to examine the effects of using fludarabine in the regimen (Medical Research Council 15 Trial).

Autologous stem cell transplantation has not improved outcome compared to current intensive chemotherapy treatment regimens.[1095] Allogeneic stem cell transplantation from a histocompatible sibling should be considered in children in first remission with a donor and poor prognostic indicators or in children who relapse.[1095] Trials have shown good results of allogeneic transplantation in first remission; event-free survival was better in childhood AML with those allografted than with those who underwent autografting.[1096] Children younger than age 2 years previously had a very poor prognosis. They tend to present with myelomonocytic or monocytic leukemia with high blast counts and CNS involvement. The t(9;11) abnormality has a more favorable prognosis. Intensive multidrug regimens have resulted in 3-year survivals approaching 70 percent of all infants treated. Thus, most infants can be successfully treated with intensive chemotherapy or allogeneic stem cell transplantation.[1097,1098] Cord blood may be a suitable allograft option for children with AML who lack an acceptably matched unrelated marrow donor.[1099]

Growth failure, neurocognitive abnormalities, endocrine deficiencies, and cardiac abnormalities are found in children treated at a young age.[1100] The occurrence of a second malignancy in cured children is approximately 10-fold greater than expected in a matched population by age.[1101] Indefinite followup of children in remission or believed to be cured is important to assess developmental and intellectual progress and to evaluate long-term adverse events.

NONHEMATOPOIETIC ADVERSE EFFECTS OF TREATMENT

Skin Rashes

More than 50 percent of patients with AML develop skin lesions during remission-induction or remission-consolidation therapy. The rash may be on the trunk and extremities. The rash usually is maculopapular initially but can become hemorrhagic in patients who have thrombocytopenia. Allopurinol, trimethoprim-sulfamethoxazole, and other β-lactam antibiotics are commonly implicated causes. Use of multiple drugs enhances the probability of skin reactivity of patients.[1102] Cytostatic therapy coupled with the effects of leukemia predisposes patients to an increased frequency of allergic dermatitis.

Cardiac Toxicity

Alterations in cardiac function, especially left ventricular and intraventricular septal diastolic wall motion abnormalities, occur frequently in patients after they are exposed to the anthracycline antibiotics, daunorubicin, or doxorubicin.[1103] The risk of serious cardiac effects is correlated with increasing dose of anthracycline antibiotic, increasing patient age, and presence of underlying heart disease. Adverse effects include electrocardiographic changes, such as prolonged QT interval, myocarditis, pericarditis, myocardial infarction, and congestive heart failure. The incidence of congestive heart failure is dose related and ranges from approximately 5 percent at doses of 550 mg/m^2 to greater than 30 percent at doses of 600 mg/m^2.[1104] The frequency and long-term sequelae increase as anthracycline dose increases. However, even lower doses of these agents exert negative effects on cardiac myocytes. Measurement of heart wall behavior, valvular competence, and ejection fraction by ultrasonography can assist in assessing the risk of proceeding with anthracycline treatment in patients with or without pretreatment heart disease.[1105,1106] In younger patients, transient abnormalities, although frequent, often improve after therapy is completed. Increased long-term remissions in children and younger adults have led to an increase

in serious ventricular and valvular disturbances years after therapy in some patients. Periodic evaluation of cardiac status by ultrasonography should be undertaken in long-term survivors.[1106] Cardiomyopathy and heart failure can occur 10 to 15 years after therapy. Two approaches that may ameliorate the cardiomyopathic effect of anthracycline antibiotics are the use of these agents in liposome encapsulated preparations[1107] and the use of dexrazoxane. Either approach may reduce the cardiotoxicity of anthracycline antibiotics.[1108]

Hepatitis

Hepatitis may occur in multiply transfused patients and usually is mild, but persistent hepatitis can develop, although hepatitis viruses A and B infection are not increased above the expected incidence in the general population. Hepatitis caused by type A virus is nearly nonexistent early in the course of AML. Cases of type B hepatitis can occur infrequently in patients who are carriers of the B virus and in whom chemotherapy and transient immunosuppression reactivate the virus.[1109–1111] These rare cases of fibrosing cholestatic hepatitis can be fulminant. Screening blood products for hepatitis virus C has markedly decreased the risk of hepatitis C.[1112] Reactivation of carriers of the C virus after chemotherapy is unusual.[1113] Medication induced chemical hepatitis or cholestasis can occur but is usually reversible. Iron overload in the multiply transfused survival may lead to later liver abnormalities.

Systemic Candidiasis Syndrome

The syndrome is manifested by fever, abdominal pain, and hepatomegaly. Increased serum alkaline phosphatase activity often is noted. Blood cultures are often negative. Abdominal ultrasonography, computed tomography, and MRI show characteristic hepatic lesions: circular areas of decreased attenuation of liver and often spleen, kidney, lung, or paraspinal muscles by imaging.[1114] Ultrasonography reveals multiple hypoechogenic areas with a bull's-eye appearance. Laparoscopic-guided liver biopsy reveals yellow nodules on the liver surface, which on microscopic examination are large granulomas with *Candida* and pseudohyphae. Cure of this infection is possible with long-term (2 to 10 months) antifungals. Hepatosplenic candidiasis is seen much less frequently when azoles are used for fungal prophylaxis.

Neutropenic Enterocolitis

Necrotizing inflammation of the cecum with secondary infection can occur in patients with acute leukemia on intensive chemotherapy.[233] Bacteremia may occur. Right lower abdominal pain and fever can simulate appendicitis. The diagnosis can be confirmed by sonography or computerized tomographic scanning in which a characteristic mucosal thickening and polypoid appearance are evident.[1115,1116] Management includes bowel rest, nasogastric suction, fluids, and antibiotics. Parenteral alimentation is sometimes used but is generally not helpful.[1117] Restoration of the neutrophil count after chemotherapy is an important feature of resolution. In the absence of resolution, right hemicolectomy should be considered but is a last resort in neutropenic patients, usually imposed if hemodynamic stability is lost.[233]

Thromboembolic Disease

Although bleeding is associated with AML, thrombotic complications can also occur; up to 10 percent in APL and up to 3 percent in other AML subtypes.[1118] Management can be difficult because of thrombocytopenia. Central lines may contribute to this incidence.[1119] Thrombotic thrombocytopenic purpura has also been reported in patients in remission of AML during consolidation chemotherapy.[1120] Patients with AML undergoing allogeneic stem cell transplantation also may develop posttransplantation thrombotic thrombocytopenic purpura, which rarely responds to plasmapheresis.

Fertility and Gonadal Function

Patients treated for AML, especially patients undergoing conditioning for allogeneic stem cell transplantation, have decreased gonadal function.[1121–1123] Men may develop oligospermia. Women may develop ovarian dysfunction and very high gonadotropin levels.[1124] Men recover gonadal function more often and sooner than do women. Recovery of ovarian function in women is partly dependent on a younger age at the time of treatment. In survivors of childhood AML treated only with chemotherapy and not transplantation, normal pubertal development and fertility are found, but antimüllerian hormone was low in some women.[1125] Women in remission following treatment for AML with allogeneic transplantation can become pregnant and deliver healthy infants[1126,1127]; however, this preservation of fertility is rare.[1128] Histologic studies of the testes show marked suppression of spermatogenesis as a function of duration of treatment for AML and not of the specific agents used or the patient's age. Residual spermatogenesis in intensively treated patients enables recovery of reproductive function in males.[1129] Males receiving intensive daunorubicin, cytosine arabinoside, or 6-thioguanine treatment for AML have conceived children during therapy.[1130] Banking of sperm should be offered, and cryopreservation of ova can be attempted prior to institution of cytotoxic therapy, but often neither is logistically possible or successful in patients with AML who are acutely ill at presentation and require urgent chemotherapy.[1121] Banking of sperm or ova-ovarian tissue should be considered before myeloablative conditioning regimens for transplantation are administered. Many AML survivors report they were not, or not fully, informed about fertility-related issues.[1131]

● COURSE AND PROGNOSIS

RESULTS OF TREATMENT

Definition of Remission

Complete remission (CR) after AML therapy is defined as neutrophil count greater than $1000/\mu L$ and platelet count greater than $100,000/\mu L$[1132] with less than 5 percent blasts morphologically in marrow and the absence of extramedullary AML, although this definition has been called into question.[1133] Remission with incomplete platelet recovery $CR_{platelets}$ (CRp) has all these requirements but the platelet count does not reach $100 \times 10^9/L$. In a large cooperative group study, at least 94 percent of patients receiving cytarabine-based therapy who survived more than 3 or 5 years achieved a remission. Three- and 5-year survivals with CRp were less frequent.[1134] With residual leukemic cell detection now possible by flow cytometry, cytogenetic, and molecular methodologies, definitions of remission may change. Persistence of

cytogenetic abnormalities at morphologic remission after induction therapy predicts for a significantly shorter relapse-free survival and overall survival, for example.[1135]

Rates of Remission

Remission rates have improved dramatically in the last 60 years, but remission, relative 5-year survival, and cure rates are most dependent on the patient's age when AML occurs.[1136,1137] Initial remission rates now approach 90 percent in children, 70 percent in young adults, 60 percent in middle-aged patients, and 40 percent in older patients. Within age groups, remission is related to other variables such as cytogenetic risk category and expression of *MDR* genes in leukemic cells, but these variables also are correlated with age at onset. For example, the more favorable cytogenetic patterns t(8;21), t(15;17), inv16, or t(16;16) are present in approximately 30 percent of patients between 10 and 39 years old, 15 percent of patients between 40 and 59 years old, and 5 percent of patients 60 to 90 years old (Table 88–9).[1137] Other factors, such as AML evolving from a prior clonal myeloid disease or developing as a result of cytotoxic treatment for another cancer or immune disorder, can decrease the expected remission and survival rates for the age group. In one study, treatment-related AML was an adverse prognostic factor for death in remission for younger patients and for relapse in remission in older patients.[1138] Age-related comorbid conditions may limit the appropriateness or tolerance of intensive therapy, decreasing the opportunity for remission. The expected increase in the proportion of old and old-old individuals in the population may decrease remission rates and their duration unless counteracting improvements in treatment approaches are developed. In one study of 1069 consecutive AML patients in first CR treated between 1991 and 2003, the yearly risk of treatment failure was 69.1 in the first year, 37.7 in the second year, 17 in the third year, 7.6 in the fourth year, and 6.6 in the fifth year. The effects of cytogenetics remained constant during the first 3 years, but the effect of age increased with time. The probability of relapse-free survival at 6 years was 84 percent for those in remission at 3 years, but for the group older than 60 years old, it was only 56 percent, suggesting that different variables contribute differently over time to overall outcomes.[1139]

Early death can occur during induction chemotherapy, and performance status and age are the most important predictors of treatment related mortality. Age may be primarily a surrogate for other factors which also predict treatment related mortality.[1140]

Clonal Remissions

A small proportion of patients who enter remission have apparently normal hematopoiesis supported by a single clone rather than the expected polyclonal hematopoiesis. Evidence points to this clone being

TABLE 88–9. Frequency of Cytogenetic Findings with a More Favorable Prognosis by Age Group

Age (Years)	No. of Cases Studied	t(8;21) (No. of Cases)	t(15;17) (No. of Cases)	Inv16/t(16;16) (No. of Cases)	Total (No. of Cases)	Favorable Karyotypes (% of All Cases)
10–39	307	27	38	33	98	32
40–59	584	36	28	28	92	16
60–69	579	18	24	21	63	11
70–79	381	5	7	5	17	4.5
>80	45	1	2	0	3	6.6
Total	1896	87	99	87	273	22

These observations were made in Germany by Claudia Schoch and colleagues and kindly provided to the authors. (See also Schoch C, Kern W, Krawitz P, et al: Dependence of age-specific incidence of acute myeloid leukemia on karyotype. *Blood* 98:3500, 2001.)

a preleukemic cell rather than a normal stem cell.[1141-1144] This finding is in keeping with previous hypotheses about the possible patterns of remission and relapse in AML[1145-1148] and has implications for minimal residual disease detection.

Spontaneous Remissions

Spontaneous disappearance of AML has been reported for more than 100 years; however, most cases reported before 1960 had poor documentation of the diagnosis. Bona fide cases of AML patients who entered CR, usually after or concurrent with an infection, occur but are very rare.[1148-1151] The occurrence of spontaneous remission with infection is consistent with the observation that the antibody response to *Pseudomonas* vaccine[1152] correlates with improved probability of chemotherapy-induced remission. Spontaneous remissions often are short lived but have lasted up to 3 years in adults and more than 9 years in children.[1153] A particularly notable case of remission for more than 60 years has been documented following "treatment" prior to the introduction of chemotherapeutic drugs. The regimen included arsenic.[1154]

LONG-TERM SURVIVAL

Prior to the introduction of chemotherapy for AML 60 years ago, the median survival of patients was approximately 6 weeks,[1155] the 1-year survival was approximately 3 percent, and longer survival occurred in less than 1 percent of patients. Five-year relative survival rates of patients in the United States from 2004 to 2010, based on the Surveillance, Epidemiology, and End Results Program of the National Cancer Institute, are 56 percent for patients younger than age 45 years, 39 percent for patients 45 to 54 years old, 27 percent for patients 55 to 64 years old, 11 percent for patients 65 to 74 years old, and 1.8 percent for patients older than age 75 years at the time of diagnosis (Table 88-10).[1069] Considering that the median age at disease onset is approximately 70 years and that 75 percent of patients are older than 45 years, the overall median survival is approximately 12 months. A study of the cost of care of older AML patients using Medicare data found that in adults older than age 65 years who were diagnosed between 1991 and 1996, the median survival was 2 months and the 2-year survival was 6 percent.[1156] Very similar results were found in a study of nearly 10,000 patients in Sweden.[1157] Better survival has been reported for younger patients who have received allogeneic stem cell transplantation in first remission, but the confidence limits for remission duration and survival are overlapping for drug-treated and drug- and transplantation-treated

TABLE 88–10. Acute Myelogenous Leukemia: Five-Year Percent Relative Survival Rates (2004–2010)

Age (Years)	Acute Myelogenous Leukemia*
<45	56
45–54	39
55–64	27
65–74	11
>75	1.8
<65	43
>65	6.0

*Percent rounded to nearest integer.

Data from SEER Cancer Statistics. Table 13.6. National Cancer Institute, Washington, DC. Available at: http://seer.cancer.gov/csr/1975_2011/browse_csr.php?sectionSEL=13&pageSEL=sect_13_table.16.html

groups, and the proportion of AML patients receiving transplantation is very small.[1136,1158-1161] Abnormalities of chromosomes 17p and –5/5q– have negative impact on outcomes after allogeneic transplant.[1162,1163]

In contrast to other AML subtypes, APL has had an increased incidence as well as improved survival since the introduction of ATRA. In one large study, relative survival rates were 0.18 for the period 1975 to 1990, with increase to 0.64 from 2000 to 2008. Age did remain an important predictor of survival; 0.38 in those older than age 60 years and 0.73 for those 20 to 29 years old.[1164]

Relapse (or a new leukemic event) in long-term survivors occurring as late as 8 years after remission has been reported in adults[1153,1154] and after more than 16 years in children.[1153,1154] Relapse in long-term survivors nearly always occurs in the marrow in adults and usually in the marrow in children, with occasional childhood cases of CNS or gonadal relapses occurring initially, followed by relapse in the marrow.[1159] Studies of long-term survivors of AML show that most can return to work and that, at a median followup of 9 years, no increased risk of secondary invasive cancer or secondary AML had occurred.[1160,1161] An exception to this finding is the occasional report of myelodysplasia or presumably secondary AML in long-term survivors of APL. Health-related quality of life in long-term survivors appears to recover completely as related to physical, psychological, and emotional well-being, but continued sexual dysfunction has been reported.[1165] The quality of life at the time of diagnosis and during the course of therapy usually is poor.[1165,1166]

FEATURES INFLUENCING OUTCOME OF THERAPY IN ACUTE MYELOGENOUS LEUKEMIA

Numerous features are related to outcome of AML treatment. Older age and less-favorable cytogenetic risk group are the two most compelling determinants of a poor outcome. Even with multivariate analysis, dissecting which other features are themselves important or are associations that segregate with another prognostic factor is difficult (Table 88-11).[1167-1264] As noted previously, prognostic models of AML that rely solely on molecular mutations have been proposed.[105]

Determining useful prognostic variables in patients with AML is imprecise because negative prognostic factors may be eliminated by better treatment protocols. Moreover, several prognostic factors are significant only when AML is stratified by age or by morphologic phenotype. Conflicting findings are common among studies. In addition, although a prognostic variable may be correlated significantly with a favorable outcome, the lack of a very strong statistical correlation with the outcome of treatment makes the variable's presence or absence of little prognostic value in an individual patient. If a stem cell donor is available, unfavorable prognostic factors could influence the therapist to use allogeneic stem cell transplantation as a means of remission maintenance in patients entering remission. The impact of prognostic factors may change in patients treated with allogeneic stem cell transplantation compared with conventional cytotoxic treatment.[1265,1266]

DETECTION OF MINIMAL RESIDUAL DISEASE

General Considerations

The tumor cell burden in acute leukemia at presentation is approximately one trillion (10^{12}) cells. Apparent marrow aplasia followed by restitution of normal hematopoiesis can occur with at least a three-log reduction in leukemic cell numbers, which represents a residual tumor cell burden of approximately one billion cells. Intensification therapy is intended to decrease further the residual cell numbers. With the advent of specific monoclonal antibodies for leukemic cell antigens and FISH coupled with flow cytometry and DNA amplification by PCR, residual leukemic cell populations at or below the level of one billion cells,

TABLE 88–11. Prognostic Factors in Acute Myelogenous Leukemia

Better prognosis than average of all patients

Early blast clearance during remission induction therapy[1167,1168]

Leukemic cells contain t(8;21), t(15;17), inv(16) t(16;16), trisomy 21[282,284,1169]

CEBPA mutations in cytogenetically normal AML[1170]

Absence of exaggerated dysmyelopoiesis[1170]

Residual normal metaphases admixed with clonal cytogenetic abnormalities[1172]

High telomerase activity levels[1173]

Low levels of TdT expression by flow cytometry (<5%)[1172]

High BAX expression[1175] and high BAX/BCL-2 ratios[1176]

High expression of integrin CD11b[1177]

Absence of VLA-4 expression on AML blast cells[1178]

High levels of soluble VCAM-1 binding to AML blast cells[1179]

High levels of caspase-3[1180]

Mutant CEBPA expression[1181]

NPM1 gene expression in adults or children (usually present in cytogenetically normal cases)[1182]

Higher neutrophil and higher platelet counts at time of complete remission[1183]

<5% blasts on day 14 marrow predicts for complete remission but not for overall survival[1184]

MiR-181a expression in NK AML[1185]

High methylation levels of polycomb group genes[1186]

Poorer prognosis than average of all patients

Older age: Age at the time of diagnosis has the greatest impact on the probability of remission and on duration of survival. Children in the first 15 years of life, exclusive of the neonatal period, have the highest rate of remission and longest relapse-free remission; patients older than age 60 years have only half the chance of a young adult to enter remission and less likelihood of a long relapse-free remission.[1137] There is a gradient of poor response to treatment through adulthood, with the largest decrease after the sixth decade of life

Unfavorable karyotypes: The cytogenetic pattern of leukemic blast cells influences outcome, but the relationship is complex.[212–284] The presence of –5, –7, 5q–, 7q–, or of exaggerated hyperdiploidy (>47 chromosomes), trisomy 8, t(6;9), trisomy 11, and multiple chromosomal abnormalities in leukemic cells are poor prognostic signs.

Multidrug resistance phenotype: Leukemic cells expressing P-glycoprotein, a unidirectional drug efflux pump, encoded by the MDR1.[1187] Expression of this gene product can result in decreased accumulation of anthracyclines, amsacrine, mitoxantrone, and etoposide. Expression of P-glycoprotein does not influence outcome of treatment, but if rhodamine-123 efflux also is increased, relapse is more common.[1188–1191] Frequently observed in AML cells after relapse. Associated with CD34 expression and chromosome 7 abnormalities.[1190] Alternative non–MDR1-mediated drug efflux mechanisms are important also.[1191–1194] MDR1 expression is low in favorable prognosis subtypes of AML[1195]

Presence of mutated KIT with t(8;21): Associated with higher relapse risk and poorer overall survival[1196]

Prior clonal hemopathy: Chemotherapy or radiotherapy remission rates are one-third to one-half that of de novo AML in the same age group. Remission duration is shorter with remissions >3 years very uncommon.[1197–1198] AML developing from the clonal

hemopathy may relapse as a smoldering leukemia. It then reverts to AML but can be treated with remissions lasting several years[1199–1203]

Higher white cell count: Count >30 × 10^9/L or a blast cell count >15 × 10^9/L[1204–1206]

Very low platelet count (<30 × 10^9/L)[1205]

High serum lactic dehydrogenase[1207]

High stem cell mobilizing capacity during complete remission predicts for relapse risk[1208]

Another medical disorder: extreme obesity, diabetes mellitus, chronic renal disease.

Low serum albumin or prealbumin

Need for intubation or ventilator support during induction therapy[1209]

Autonomous clonal growth of leukemic blast cells[1210]

High BCL-2 expression[1211,1212]

High MCL-1 expression: Elevated at the time of leukemic relapse. Suggests prognostic importance or that chemotherapeutic regimen selects for leukemia cells with elevated levels of apoptosis inhibitors[1213]

Low expression of retinoblastoma gene[1214]

High levels of WAF/Cip1 protein: This is a regulator at the G_1 checkpoint of cell cycle[1215]

High CD34 expression: High CD34 antigen expression often in AML subtypes M0, M1, and M4.[1216] Remission rate of 61% vs. to 88% in AML not expressing CD34. Correlation is stronger between high-intensity expression of CD34 and lower remission rate.[1216–1217] CD34 expression in APL[1218]

GATA-1 expression[1219]

Neural cell adhesion molecule (CD56) expression[1220]

Elevated soluble L-selectin: Seen especially in extramedullary disease[1221]

Higher expression of interleukin (IL)-1β gene[1222]

Low FMS expression[1222]

Expression of the thrombopoietin receptor (c-MPL) mRNA[1223]

FLT3 mutations[1224,1225]

Increased angiogenesis/vascular endothelial growth factor levels[1226]

High β_2-microglobulin levels in adults younger than 60 years old[1227]

MN1 (meningioma 1) gene overexpression in AML patients with normal cytogenetics[1228]

Young adults with the genotype WT1(mutation)/FLT3-ITD(positive) have a lower complete remission rate and an inferior relapse-free and overall survival compared to those with the genotype WT1(mutation)/FLT3-ITD(negative)[1229]

WT1 gene mutations in patients with AML and a normal karyotype[1230,1231]

Patients with AML with a large number of AML stem cells

Elevated expression of IL-3Rα[1232]

MLL tandem duplications[1233] and 11p23/MLL abnormalities[1234]

CD56 expression in APL.[1235] High incidence of CNS involvement, especially with CD7 expression.[1236] Also contributes to poorer outcomes in t(8;21) cases[1237]

P15 methylation[1238]

(continued)

TABLE 88–11. Prognostic Factors in Acute Myelogenous Leukemia (Continued)

Microsatellite instability[1239] (may not be independent of age and t-AML)	High Nrf2 and high ROS expression[1254,1255]
AC133 expression (shorter remissions and disease-free survival)[1240]	Overexpression of IL-1 receptor accessory protein[1256]
Constitutive activity of signal transducer and activator of transcription 3 protein (shorter disease-free survival)[1241]	Survivin expression in CD34+CD38– cells[1257]
	High TRAIL-R3 (tumor necrosis factor [TNF]-related apoptosis-inducing ligand) expression[1258]
BAALC gene expression[1242]	PICALM-MLLT10 fusion gene expression[302]
High S-phase activity in cells surviving after 7 days of induction[1243]	**Factors with no or uncertain prognostic findings**
High EVI1 expression[1244,1245]	Complex karyotype or secondary aberrations in patients with t(8;21), inv(16) t(16;16), or t(9;11)[1259]
Overexpression of CXCR4[1246]	Myeloid antigens: CD11b expression may be predictive of shorter survival[1260]
Increased marrow angiogenesis as measured by magnetic resonance imaging[1247]	Detection of the WT1 (Wilms tumor) transcript[1261]
The presence of the CTLA4 CT60 A/G genotype adult patients with AML[1248]	FLT3-ITD or Asp835 mutations in APL[1262]
miR 155 upregulaation[1249]	Levels of initiator caspase[1263]
ERG expression[1250]	Persistent thrombocytopenia after remission induction[1264]
EVI1 expression in MLL_rearranged AML[1251]	Lung resistance protein: Functional test is needed to assess activity.[1265] Expression may predict poor outcome in de novo AML[1193,1266]
Clonal heterogeneity by metaphase karyotyping[1252]	
Abnormal expression of FLI1 protein[1253]	

which are undetectable by light microscopy of stained marrow films, can be quantified.[1267] When real-time PCR is used to quantify PML-RAR-α, RUNX1/ETO, or CBF-β/MYH11, risk for treatment failure can be determined by the levels of the fusion gene at diagnosis and after the first 3 to 4 months of therapy.[1268] Sampling remains an important problem because marrow aspiration contains approximately 1/10,000 of the marrow cell population, and variation among sites of aspiration is well documented. In addition, the markers of the leukemic cell used for detection can change during the course of the disease. For example, persistence of circulating cells containing t(8;21) in patients with AML despite long-term remission has been established using PCR.[1269]

There are many other pitfalls when interpreting these studies, including timing of sampling in relationship to therapy, sensitivity of the PCR reaction for target genes, interlaboratory standardization, selection of patients, and retrospective or prospective design of the study.[1270] There is emerging evidence, however, that detection of minimal residual disease (MRD) by multiparameter flow cytometry has prognostic relevance in older patients,[1271] in children with de novo AML,[1272] and in adults younger than age 60 years.[1273] Pretransplantation, detection of MRD by flow cytometry has negative impact on outcome in patients with AML in either first or second remission. Even MRD levels less than 0.1 percent have an adverse correlation with outcome.[1274] Detection of MRD in the after allogeneic stem cell transplantation is also important. Sensitive chimerism assays have been developed using PCR-based technology to detect short tandem-repeat polymorphisms. Whether these will have impact on management of posttransplantation relapses is still undetermined.[1275,1276]

Marrow examinations are not needed in the majority of AML patients in first CR.[1277] Because of increased myeloid precursors in regenerating marrow, detection of residual disease may be difficult early after a given therapeutic modality.[1278] Cytogenetic followup usually is not helpful. Emergence of a karyotypically unrelated clone of AML cells, especially containing chromosome 7, can occur. Studies using multiparameter flow cytometry to identify leukemic cells by aberrant antigen expression have a high positive predictive value in identifying relapse.[1279] Detection of residual disease in AML patients using double immunologic marker analysis for TdT and myeloid CD antigens can

be useful because these two markers are expressed on leukemic cells in the majority of AML patients and these markers are rare in normal marrow cells.[1280,1281] In other cases, aberrant combinations of surface antigens[1280,1282] or increased expression of various surface antigens, such as CD34, are seen.[1283] Immunophenotype may change at relapse and has implications for MRD detection.[1284] Five-color staining has been reported to improve the percentage of AML cases in which a leukemia-associated aberrant immunophenotype can be identified.[1285] Various markers, such as CLL-1 (C-type lectin-like molecule-1) and other lineage markers and marker combinations, have been found aberrantly expressed on leukemic CD34+CD38–, cells allowing residual disease detection at the stem cell level.[1286] Other methods for detecting MRD include MRI; fluorescence DNA in FISH[1287,1288]; reverse transcriptase (RT)-PCR to detect amplification of abnormal fusion genes, such as t(15;17), t(8;21), inversion 16, and 11q23; and DNA PCR for mutations in the RAS coding regions.[1267] Quantitative assessment of WT1 expression[1289] or presence of a FLT3 mutation[1290] can also be evaluated for MDR monitoring. Real-time quantitative PCR can be used to quantitate MDR more precisely than other methods, but this test requires standardized criteria and is not widely available clinically.[1291]

Multiparameter flow cytometry is applicable to most AML cases, whereas real-time quantitative PCR is applicable in just above half the cases when NPM1 and FLT3 mutations are examined in addition to fusion oncogenes.[1292] Gene profiling of CD34+CD38– cells, a fraction that contains both normal and leukemic stem cells, might be important in MRD measurement, but 34 percent of genes modulated in AML stem cells are shared with normal stem cells.[1293]

Detecting Inversion 16

Minimal residual disease in acute myelomonocytic leukemia with inversion 16 can be detected by nested PCR with allele-specific amplifications (CBF-β on 16q and MYH11 on 16p).[1294,1295] This fusion transcript occurs not only in the majority of cases of acute myelomonocytic leukemia with marrow eosinophilia (M4Eo), but also in 10 percent of acute myelomonocytic leukemia M4 without eosinophilic abnormalities, a much higher incidence than suggested by the sporadic reports of chromosome 16 abnormalities in AML. Following completion of chemotherapy (induction and consolidation), patients who had a CBF-β/MYH11 fusion transcript copy number greater than 10 had a shorter remission duration and higher risk for relapse than did patients with a copy number less than 10.[1295] Evidence indicates transcript ratios of samples may have utility in establishing thresholds for curability and for relapse risk in standard clinical CR states in the future.[1296]

Detecting t(8;21)

Translocation 8;21 is one of the most common translocations in AML, especially in younger patients (see Table 88–9). This translocation fuses the *RUNX1* gene on chromosome 21p to RUNXIT1 (ETO) on chromosome 8p to produce the fusion gene.[1297,1298] The fusion has been detected in the majority of patients in remission. One study found its persistence in all patients with t(8;21) after chemotherapy or autologous marrow transplantation.[1299–1301] Quantitation of the amount of the fusion transcript during remission may be more predictive of cure or relapse than a simple qualitative assessment.[1302,1303] Real-time quantitative RT-PCR can be used for this purpose.

In general, CBF leukemias lend themselves to MRD monitoring by quantitative RT-PCR. In a trial from the Medical Research Council, in 163 patients with t(8;21) and 115 with inv(16), quantitative PCR transcripts at end of induction and end of consolidation course three were informative for relapse. Rising MRD levels in blood also predicted relapse.[1304] Another study showed that a three-log reduction in MRD after one consolidation had prognostic value whereas expression of *KIT* and *FLT3* mutations did not.[1305]

Detecting t(15;17)

Unlike AML with the fusion transcript t(8;21), in APL the t(15;17) fusion transcript usually disappears after intensive therapy.[1306] At least one in 100,000 cells with the *PML-RAR-α* transcript can be detected by RT-PCR.[1306] FISH also can be used.[1307] Molecular monitoring has shown treatment is capable of achieving a molecular remission (negative RT-PCR).[1308] Nested PCR can be used to determine the need for additional treatment at the end of consolidation, to determine the advisability of autologous stem cell transplantation in second remission, and to predict relapse after transplantation.[1309] Real-time quantitative RT-PCR may improve the predictive value of MDR assessment and aid in laboratory standardization.[1310]

Detecting NPM-1 and FLT3 Mutations

In AML patients who have normal cytogenetics, mutational status of *NPM1, FLT3, CEPBA, MLL,* and *RAS* have implications for treatment outcomes and prognosis.[1311] Whether detection of these mutations as a reflection of MRD will have implications for relapse and therapy remains undetermined. Cumulative incidence of relapse is higher in those who remain positive using real-time quantitative PCR consolidation.[1312] There is evidence in *NPM1*-mutated cases, relapse was accompanied by an increase of mutant gene copy numbers; it has been concluded that quantitative PCR monitoring may have prognostic impact in such patients.[1313]

The technology to detect MRD has increased in sensitivity and availability. Detection of MRD to determine a patient's treatment or prognosis remains an evolving area of investigation. The role that proteomic[1314,1315] and microRNA profiles[1316–1319] will play in MRD detection is under study.

Marshall A. Lichtman has been an expert witness on behalf of defendants in toxic tort cases involving occupational exposure to chemicals, including benzene.

REFERENCES

1. Friedreich N: Ein neuer Fall von Leukämie. *Arch Pathol* 12:37, 1857.
2. Ebstein W: Ueber die acute Leukämie und Pseudoleukämie. *Dtsch Arch Klin Med* 44:343, 1889.
3. Fraenkel A: Ueber acute Leukämie. *Dtsch Med Wochenschr* 21:639, 1895.
4. Neumann E: Ueber myelogene leukäemie. *Berl Klin Wochenschr* 15:69, 1878.
5. Ehrlich P: *Farbenanolytische Untersuchungen zur Histologie und Klinik des Blutes.* Hirschwald, Berlin, 1891.
6. Naegeli O: Ueber rothes Knochenmark und Myeloblasten. *Dtsch Med Wochenschr* 26:287, 1900.
7. Hirschfield H: Zur Kenntnis der Histogenese der granulirten Knochenmarkzellen. *Arch Pathol* 153:335, 1898.
8. Hsu TC: *Human and Mammalian Cytogenetics: An Historical Perspective.* Springer-Verlag, New York, 1979.
9. Subramanian G, Adams MD, Venter JC, Broder S: Implications of the human genome for understanding human biology and medicine. *JAMA* 286:2296, 2001.
10. Ellison RR, Holland JF, Weil M, et al: Arabinosyl cytosine: A useful agent in the treatment of acute leukemia in adults. *Blood* 33:507, 1968.
11. Yates JW, Wallace HJ, Ellison RR, Holland JF: Cytosine arabinoside and daunorubicin therapy in acute non-lymphocytic leukemia. *Cancer Chemother Rep* 52:485, 1973.
12. Lichtman MA: A historical perspective on the development of the cytarabine (7 days) and daunorubicin (3 days) treatment regimen for acute myelogenous leukemia: 2013 the 40th anniversary of 7+3. *Blood Cells Mol Dis* 50:119, 2013.
13. Thomas ED, Buckner CD, Banaji M, et al: One hundred patients with acute leukemia treated by chemotherapy, total body irradiation, and allogeneic bone marrow transplantation. *Blood* 49:511, 1977.
14. Preston DL, Kusumi S, Tomonaga M, et al: Cancer incidence in atomic bomb survivors. Part III. Leukemia, lymphoma and multiple myeloma, 1950–1987. *Radiat Res* 137(2 Suppl):S68, 1994.
15. Tsushima H, Iwanaga M, Miyazaki Y. Late effect of atomic bomb radiation on myeloid disorders: Leukemia and myelodysplastic syndromes. *Int J Hematol* 95:232, 2012.
16. Rinsky RA, Smith AB, Hornung R, et al: Benzene and leukemia. An epidemiologic risk assessment. *N Engl J Med* 316:1044, 1987.
17. Johnson GT, Harbison SC, McCluskey JD, Harbison RD: Characterization of cancer risk from airborne benzene exposure. *Regul Toxicol Pharmacol* 55:361, 2009.
18. Pyatt D: Benzene and hematopoietic malignancies. *Clin Occup Environ Med* 4:529, 2004.
19. Lichtman MA: Cigarette smoking, cytogenetic abnormalities, and acute myelogenous leukemia. *Leukemia* 21:1137, 2007.
20. Rund D, Ben-Yehuda D: Therapy-related leukemia and myelodysplasia: Evolving concepts of pathogenesis and treatment. *Hematology* 9:179, 2004.
21. Larson RA, Le Beau MM: Therapy-related myeloid leukaemia: A model for leukemogenesis in humans. *Chem Biol Interact* 153–154:187, 2005.
22. Yeasmin S, Nakayama K, Ishibashi M, et al: Therapy-related myelodysplasia and acute myeloid leukemia following paclitaxel- and carboplatin-based chemotherapy in an ovarian cancer patient: A case report and literature review. *Int J Gynecol Cancer* 18:1371, 2008.
23. Visfeldt J, Anderson M: Pathoanatomical aspects of malignant haematological disorders among Danish patients exposed to thorium dioxide. *APMIS* 103:29, 1995.
24. Brownson RC, Novotny TE, Perry MC: Cigarette smoking and adult leukemia: A meta-analysis. *Arch Intern Med* 153:469, 1993.
25. Stewart SL, Cardinez CJ, Richardson LC, et al: Surveillance for cancers associated with tobacco use—United States, 1999–2004. *MMWR Surveill Summ* 57:1, 2008.
26. Rhomberg LR, Bailey LA, Goodman JE, et al: Is exposure to formaldehyde in air causally associated with leukemia?—A hypothesis-based weight-of-evidence analysis. *Crit Rev Toxicol* 41:555, 2011.
27. Checkoway H, Boffetta P, Mundt DJ, et al: Critical review and synthesis of the epidemiologic evidence on formaldehyde exposure and risk of leukemia and other lymphohematopoietic malignancies. *Cancer Causes Control* 23:1747, 2012.
28. Lichtman MA: Obesity and the risk for a hematological malignancy: Leukemia, lymphoma, or myeloma. *Oncologist* 15:1083, 2010.
29. Swolin B, Rödjer S, Westin J: Therapy-related patterns of cytogenetic abnormalities in acute myeloid leukemia and myelodysplastic syndrome post polycythemia vera: Single center experience and review of literature. *Ann Hematol* 87:467, 2008.
29a. Xie M, Lu C, Wang J, et al: Age-related mutations associated with clonal hematopoietic expansion and malignancies. *Nat Med* 20:1472, 2014.
30. Wiernik P: Leukemias and plasma cell myeloma. *Cancer Chemother Biol Response Modif* 17:390, 1997.
31. Luca DC, Almanaseer IY: Simultaneous presentation of multiple myeloma and acute monocytic leukemia. *Arch Pathol Lab Med* 127:1506, 2003.
32. Pulik M, Genet P, Jary L, et al: Acute myeloid leukemias, multiple myelomas, and chronic leukemias in the setting of HIV infection. *AIDS Patient Care STDS* 12:913, 1998.
33. Yohe SL, Chenault CB, Torlakovic EE, et al: Langerhans cell histiocytosis in acute leukemias of ambiguous or myeloid lineage in adult patients: Support for a possible clonal relationship. *Mod Pathol* 27:651, 2014.
34. Edelbroek JR, Vermeer MH, Jansen P, et al: Langerhans cell histiocytosis first presenting in the skin in adults: Frequent association with a second haematological malignancy. *Br J Dermatol Dermatology* 167:1287, 2012.
35. Moskowitz C, Dutcher JP, Wiernik PH: Association of thyroid disease with acute leukemia. *Am J Hematol* 39:102, 1992.

36. Willems E, Valdes-Socin H, Betea D, et al: Association of acute leukemia and autoimmune polyendocrine syndrome in two kindreds. *Leukemia* 17:1912, 2003.

37. Lichtenstein P, Holm NV, Verkasalo PK, et al: Environmental and hereditable factors in causation of cancer—Analyses of cohorts of twins from Sweden, Denmark, and Finland. *N Engl J Med* 343:78, 2000.

38. Risch N: The genetic epidemiology of cancer. Interpreting family and twin studies and their implications for molecular genetic approaches. *Cancer Epidemiol Biomarkers Prev* 10:733, 2001.

39. Hemminki K, Vaittinen P, Dong C, Easton D: Sibling risks in cancer: Clues to recessive or X-linked genes? *Br J Cancer* 84:388, 2001.

40. Germeshausen M, Ballmaier M, Welte K: Implications of mutations in hematopoietic growth factor receptor genes in congenital cytopenias. *Ann N Y Acad Sci* 938:305, 2001.

41. Tonelli R, Scardovi AL, Pession A, et al: Compound heterozygosity for two different amino-acid substitution mutations in the thrombopoietin receptor (c-mpl gene) in congenital amegakaryocytic thrombocytopenia (CAMT). *Hum Genet* 107:225, 2000.

42. Li FP, Hecht F, Kaiser-McCaw B, et al: Ataxia-pancytopenia: Syndrome of cerebellar ataxia, hypoplastic anemia, monosomy 7, and acute myelogenous leukemia. *Cancer Genet Cytogenet* 4:189, 1981.

43. Gonzales-del Angel A, Cervera M, Gomez L, et al: Ataxia-pancytopenia syndrome. *Am J Med Genet* 90:252, 2000.

44. German J: Bloom's syndrome: Incidence, age of onset, and types of leukemia in the Bloom's syndrome registry, in *Genetics in Hematologic Disorders*, edited by Bartsocas CS, Loukopoulos D, p 241. Hemisphere, Washington, 1992.

45. Poppe B, Van Limbergen H, Van Roy N, et al: Chromosomal aberrations in Bloom syndrome patients with myeloid malignancies. *Cancer Genet Cytogenet* 128:39, 2001.

46. Freedman MH, Alter BP: Risk of myelodysplastic syndrome and acute myeloid leukemia in congenital neutropenia. *Semin Hematol* 39:128, 2002.

47. Aprikyan AA, Kutyavin T, Stein S, et al: Cellular and molecular abnormalities in severe congenital neutropenia predisposing to leukemia. *Exp Hematol* 31:372, 2003.

48. Rosenberg PS, Alter BP, Link DC, et al: Neutrophil elastase mutations and risk of leukaemia in severe congenital neutropenia. *Br J Haematol* 140:210, 2008.

49. Link DC, Kunter G, Kasai Y, et al: Distinct patterns of mutations occurring in *de novo* AML versus AML arising in the setting of severe congenital neutropenia. *Blood* 110:1648, 2007.

50. Shinawi M, Erez A, Shardy DL, et al: Syndromic thrombocytopenia and predisposition to acute myelogenous leukemia caused by constitutional microdeletions on chromosome 21q. *Blood* 112:1042, 2008.

51. Janov AJ, Leong T, Nathan DG, Guinan EC: Diamond-Blackfan anemia: Natural history and sequelae of treatment. *Medicine (Baltimore)* 75:77, 1996.

52. Vlachos A, Klein G, Lipton J: The Blackfan-Diamond anemia registry: Tool for investigating the epidemiology and biology of Diamond-Blackfan anemia. *Pediatr Hematol Oncol* 23:377, 2001.

53. Forestier E, Izraeli S, Beverloo B, et al: Cytogenetic features of acute lymphoblastic and myeloid leukemias in pediatric patients with Down syndrome: An iBFM-SG study. *Blood* 111:1575, 2008.

54. Puumala SE, Ross JA, Olshan AF, et al: Reproductive history, infertility treatment, and the risk of acute leukemia in children with down syndrome: A report from the Children's Oncology Group. *Cancer* 110:2067, 2007.

55. Andrade-Machado R, Machado-Rojas A, de la Torre-Santos ME: Dubowitz syndrome, polymyositis, and aleucemic myeloblastic leukemia. A new association. *Rev Neurol* 35:500, 2001.

56. Savage SA, Alter BP: The role of telomere biology in bone marrow failure and other disorders. *Mech Ageing Dev* 129:35, 2008.

57. Röth A, Baerlocher GM: Dyskeratosis congenita. *Br J Haematol* 141:412, 2008.

58. Segel GB, Lichtman MA: Familial (inherited) leukemia, lymphoma, and myeloma. *Blood Cells Mol Dis* 32:246, 2004.

59. Owen CJ, Toze CL, Koochin A, et al: Five new pedigrees with inherited RUNX1 mutations causing familial platelet disorder with propensity to myeloid malignancy (FPD/AML). *Blood* 112:4639, 2008.

60. Minelli A, Maserati E, Rossi G, et al: Familial platelet disorder with propensity to acute myelogenous leukemia: Genetic heterogeneity and progression to leukemia via acquisition of clonal chromosome anomalies. *Genes Chromosomes Cancer* 40:165, 2004.

61. Rosenberg PS, Greene MH, Alter BP: Cancer incidence in persons with Fanconi anemia. *Blood* 101:822, 2003.

62. Rosenberg PS, Alter BP, Ebell W: Cancer risks in Fanconi anemia: Findings from the German Fanconi Anemia Registry. *Haematologica* 93:511, 2008.

63. Dickinson RE, Milne P, Jardine L, et al: The evolution of cellular deficiency in GATA2 mutation. *Blood* 123:863, 2014.

64. Polychronopoulou S, Tsatsopoulou A, Papadhimitriou SI, et al: Myelodysplasia and Naxos disease: A novel pathogenetic association? *Leukemia* 16:2335, 2002.

65. Kratz CP, Antonietti L, Shannon KM, et al: Acute myeloid leukemia associated with t(8;21) or trisomy 8 in children with neurofibromatosis type 1. *Pediatr Hematol Oncol* 25:343, 2003.

66. Lurgaespada DA, Brannan CI, Shaughnessy JD, et al: The neurofibromatosis type 1 (NF1) tumor suppressor gene and myeloid leukemia. *Curr Top Microbiol Immunol* 211:233, 1996.

67. Bader-Meunier B, Tchernia G, Miélot F, et al: Occurrence of myeloproliferative disorder in patients with Noonan syndrome. *J Pediatr* 130:885, 1997.

68. Bentires-Alj M, Paez JG, David FS, et al: Activating mutations of the Noonan syndrome-associated SHP2/PTPN11 gene in human solid tumors and adult acute myelogenous leukemia. *Cancer Res* 64:8816,2004.

69. Fokin AA, Robicsek F: Poland's syndrome revisited. *Ann Thorac Surg* 74:2218, 2002.

70. Pianigiani E, DeAloe G, Andreassi A, et al: Rothmund-Thomson syndrome (Thomson type) and myelodysplasia. *Pediatr Dermatol* 18:422, 2001.

71. Duker NJ: Chromosome breakage syndromes and cancer. *Am J Med Genet* 115:125, 2002.

72. Hayani A, Suarez CR, Molnar Z, et al: Acute myeloid leukemia in a patient with Seckel syndrome. *J Med Genet* 31:148, 1994.

73. Boocock GR, Morrison JA, Popovic M, et al: Mutations in SBDS are associated with Shwachman-Diamond syndrome. *Nat Genet* 33:97, 2003.

74. Rujkijyanont P, Beyene J, Wei K, et al: Leukaemia-related gene expression in bone marrow cells from patients with the preleukaemic disorder Shwachman-Diamond syndrome. *Br J Haematol* 137:537, 2007.

75. Mitsui T, Kawakami T, Sendo D, et al: Successful unrelated donor bone marrow transplantation for Shwachman-Diamond syndrome with leukemia. *Int J Hematol* 79:189, 2004.

76. Yamada T, Tsurumi H, Murakami N, et al: Werner's syndrome developing acute megakaryoblastic leukemia with der(1;7). *Rinsho Ketsueki* 38:28, 1997.

77. Tao LC, Stecker E, Gardner HA: Werner's syndrome and acute myeloid leukemia. *CMAJ* 105:951, 1971.

78. Muftuoglu M, Oshima J, von Kobbe C, et al: The clinical characteristics of Werner syndrome: Molecular and biochemical diagnosis. *Hum Genet* 124:369, 2008.

79. Sharathkumar A, Kirby M, Freedman M, et al: Malignant hematological disorders in children with Wolf-Hirschhorn syndrome. *Am J Med Genet* 119A:194, 2003.

80. Gonzalez CH, Durkin-Stamm MV, Geimer NF, et al: The WT syndrome—A "new" autosomal dominant pleiotropic trait of radial/ulnar hypoplasia with high risk of bone marrow failure and/or leukemia. *Birth Defects Orig Artic Ser* 13:31, 1977.

81. Kristinsson SY, Bjorkholm M, Hultcrantz M, et al: Chronic immune stimulation might act as a trigger for the development of acute myeloid leukemia or myelodysplastic syndromes. *J Clin Oncol* 29: 2897, 2011.

82. Wu SP, Costello R, Hofmann JN, et al: MGUS prevalence in a cohort of AML patients. *Blood* 122:294, 2013.

83. Fialkow PH, Singer JW, Adamson JW, et al: Acute nonlymphocytic leukemia. Heterogeneity of stem cell origin. *Blood* 57:1068, 1991.

84. Ferraris AM, Broccia G, Meloni T, et al: Clonal origin of cells restricted to monocytic differentiation in acute nonlymphocytic leukemia. *Blood* 64:817, 1984.

85. Turhan AG, Lemoire FB, Debert C, et al: Highly purified primitive hematopoietic stem cells are PML-RARA negative and generate nonclonal progenitors in acute promyelocytic leukemia. *Blood* 85:2154, 1995.

86. Van Lom K, Hagemeijer A, Vandekerckhove F, et al: Clonality analysis of hematopoietic cell lineages in acute myeloid leukemia and translocation (8;21): Only myeloid cells are part of malignant clone. *Leukemia* 11:202, 1997.

87. Goardon N, Marchi E, Atzberger A, et al: Coexistence of LMPP-like and GMP-like leukemia stem cells in acute myeloid leukemia. *Cancer Cell* 19:138, 2011.

88. Majeti R, Weissman IL: Human acute myelogenous leukemia stem cells revisited: There's more than meets the eye. *Cancer Cell* 19:9, 2011.

89. Pandolfi A, Barreyro L, Steidl U: Concise review: Preleukemic stem cells: Molecular biology and clinical implications of the precursors to leukemia stem cells. *Stem Cells Transl Med* 2:143, 2013.

90. Jan M, Snyder TM, Ryan M, et al: Clonal evolution of preleukemic hematopoietic stem cells precedes human acute myeloid leukemia. *Sci Transl Med* 149:149ra118, 2012.

91. Shlush LI, Zandi S, Mitchell A, et al: Identification of pre-leukaemic haematopoietic stem cells in acute leukaemia. *Nature* 506:328, 2014.

92. Chan SM, Majeti R: Role of DNMT3A, TET2, and IDH-1/2 mutations in pre-leukemic stem cells in acute myeloid leukemia. *Int J Hematol* 98:648, 2013.

93. Welch JS, Ley TJ, Link DC, et al: The origin and evolution of mutations in acute myeloid leukemia. *Cell* 150:264, 2012.

94. Parkin B, Ouillette P, Li Y, et al: Clonal evolution and devolution after chemotherapy in adult acute myelogenous leukemia. *Blood* 121:369, 2013.

95. Swiggers SJJ, Kuijpers MA, de Cort MJM, et al: Critically short telomeres in acute myeloid leukemia with loss or gain of parts of chromosomes. *Genes Chromosomes Cancer* 45:247, 2006.

96. Yamada O, Oshimi K, Motoji, et al: Telomeric DNA in normal and leukemic blood cells. *J Clin Invest* 95:1117, 1995.

97. Look AT: Oncogene transcription factors in human acute leukemias. *Science* 278:1059, 1997.

98. Pabst T, Mueller BU: Transcriptional dysregulation during myeloid transformation in AML. *Oncogene* 26:6829, 2007.

99. Kelly LM, Gilliland DG: Genetics of myeloid leukemias. *Annu Rev Genomics Hum Genet* 3:179, 2002.

100. Damm F, Heuser M, Morgan M, et al: Integrative prognostic risk score in acute myeloid leukemia with normal karyotype. *Blood* 117:4561, 2011.

101. Pastore F, Duforu A, Benthaus T, et al: Combined molecular and clinical prognostic index for relapse and survival in cytogenetically normal acute myeloid leukemia. *J Clin Oncol* 32:1586, 2014.

102. Li Z, Herold T, He C, et al: Identification of a 24-gene prognostic signature that improves the European Leukemia Net risk classification of acute myeloid leukemia: An international collaborative study. *J Clin Oncol* 31:1172, 2013.

103. Marcucci G, Yan P, Maharry K, et al: Epigenetics meets genetics in acute myeloid leukemia: Clinical impact of a novel seven-gene score. *J Clin Oncol* 32:548, 2013.

104. Patel JP, Gonen M, Figueroa MF, et al: Prognostic relevance of integrated genetic profiling in acute myeloid leukemia. *N Engl J Med* 266:1079, 2012.

105. Grossmann V, Schnittger S, Kohlmann A, et al: A novel hierarchical prognostic model of AML solely based on molecular mutations. *Blood* 120:2963, 2012.

106. Abdel-Wahab O, Levine RL: Mutations in epigenetic modifiers in the pathogenesis and therapy of acute myeloid leukemia. *Blood* 121:3563, 2013.

107. Grimwade D, Hills RK, Moorman AV, et al: Refinement of cytogenetic classification in acute myeloid leukemia: Determination of prognostic significance or rare recurring chromosomal abnormalities amongst 5,875 younger adult patients treated in the UK Medical Research Council trials. *Blood* 116: 354, 2010.

108. Mauritzson N, Albin M, Rylander L, et al: Pooled analysis of clinical and cytogenetic features in treatment-related and de novo adult acute myeloid leukemia and myelodysplastic syndromes based on consecutive series of 761 patients analyzed 1976–1993 and on 5098 unselected cases reported in the literature 1974–2001. *Leukemia* 16:2366, 2002.

109. Grimwade D, Enver T: Acute promyelocytic leukemia: Where does it stem from? *Leukemia* 18:375, 2004.

110. Zeisig BB, Kwok C, Zelent A, et al: Recruitment of RXR by homotetrameric RARalpha fusion proteins is essential for Transformation. *Cancer Cell* 12:36, 2007.

111. Cox MC, Panetta P, Venditti A, et al: Comparison between conventional banding analysis and FISH screening with an AML-specific set of probes in 260 patients. *Hematol J* 24:263, 2003.

112. Paschka P, Marcucci G, l Ruppert AS, et al: Adverse prognostic significance of KIT mutations in adult acute myeloid leukemia with inv(16 and t(8;21): A Cancer and Leukemia Group B Study. *J Clin Oncol* 24:3904, 2006.

113. Schwind S, Edward CG, Nicolet D, et al: Inv (16)/t(16;16) acute myeloid leukemia with non-type A (CBFB-MYH11) fusions associate with distinct clinical and genetic features and lack KIT mutations. *Blood* 212:385, 2013.

114. Paschka P, Du J, Schlenk FR, et al: Secondary genetic lesions in acute myeloid leukemia with Inv(16) or t(16;16): A study of the German-Austrian AML study group (AMLSG), *Blood* 121:170, 2013.

115. Li Y, Gao L, Luo X, et al: Epigenetic silencing of *microRNA-193a* contributes to leukemogenesis in t(8;21) acute myeloid leukemia by activating the *PTEN*/PI3K signal pathway. *Blood* 121:499, 2013.

116. Nakagawa M, Shimabe M, Watanabe-Okochi N, et al: AML1/RUNX1 functions as a cytoplasmic attenuator of NF-κB signaling in the repression of myeloid tumors. *Blood* 118:6626, 2011.

117. Lughart S, Groschel S, Beverloo HB, et al: Clinical, molecular, and prognostic significance of WHO type inv(3)(q21q26.2)/t(3;3)(q21;q26.2) and various other 3q abnormalities in acute myeloid leukemia. *J Clin Oncol* 28:3890, 2010.

118. Weisser M, Haferlach C, Haferlach T, et al: Advanced age and high initial WBC influence the outcome of inv(3)(q21q26)/t(3;3)(q21;q26) positive AML. *Leuk Lymphoma* 48:2145, 2007.

119. Kayser S, Zucknick M, Dohner K, et al: Monosomal karyotype in adult acute myeloid leukemia: Prognostic impact and outcome after different treatment strategies. *Blood* 119:551, 2012.

120. Rucker FG, Schlenk RF, Bulolinger L, et al: TP53 alterations in acute myeloid leukemia with complex karyotype correlate with specific copy number alterations, monosomal karyotype, and dismal outcome. *Blood* 119:214, 2012.

121. Welch JS, Ley TJ, Link DC, et al: The origin and evolution of mutations in acute myeloid leukemia. *Cell* 150:264, 2012.

122. Mardi ER, Ding L, Dooling DJ, et al: Recurring mutations found by sequencing an acute myeloid leukemia genome. *N Engl J Med* 361:1058, 2009.

123. The Cancer Genome Atlas Research Network. Genomic and epigenomic landscapes of adult de novo acute myeloid leukemia. *N Engl J Med* 268:2059, 2013.

124. Port M, Bottcher M, Thol F, et al: Prognostic significance of FLT3 internal tandem duplication, nucleophosmin1, and CEBPA gene mutations for acute myeloid leukemia patients with normal karyotype and younger than 60 years: A systematic review and meta-analysis. *Ann Hematol* 93:1279, 2014.

125. Hirsch P, Qassa G, Marzac C, et al: Acute myeloid leukemia in patients older than 75: Prognostic impact of FLT3-ITD and NPM1 mutations. *Leuk Lymphoma* 16:1, 2014.

126. Falni B, Mecucci C, Tiacci E, et al: GIMEMA acute leukemia working party. Cytoplasmic nucleophosmin in acute myelogenous leukemia with a normal karyotype. *N Engl J Med* 352:254, 2005.

127. Schlenk RE, Dohner K, Krauter J, et al: Mutations and treatment outcome in cytogenetically normal acute myeloid leukemia. *N Engl J Med* 358, 1909, 2008.

128. Becker H, Marcucci G, Maharry K, et al: Favorable prognostic impact of NPM1 mutations in older pateints with cytogenetically normal de novo acute myeloid leukemia and associated gene-and microRNA-expression signatures: A Cancer and Leukemia Group B Study. *J Clin Oncol* 28:596, 2009.

129. Greiner J, Ono Y, Hofmann S, et al: Mutated regions of nucleophosmin 1 elicit both CD4+ and CD8+ T cell responses in patients with acute myeloid leukemia. *Blood* 120: 1282, 2012.

130. Renneville A, Roumier C, Biggio V, et al: Cooperating gene mutations in acute myeloid leukemia: A review of the literature. *Leukemia* 22:915, 2008.

131. Small D: Targeting FLT3 for the treatment of leukemia. *Semin Hematol* 45(3 Suppl 2): S17, 2008.

132. Janke H, Pastore F, Schumacher D, et al: Activating FLT3 mutants show distinct gain-of-function phenotypes *in vitro* and a characteristic signaling pathway profile associated with prognosis in acute myeloid leukemia. *PLoS One* 9:e89560, 2014.

133. Levis M: FLT3/ITD AML and the law of unintended consequences. *Blood* 117:6987, 2011.

134. Yoshimoto G, Miyamoto T, Jabbarzadeh-Tabrizi S, et al: FLT3-ITD up-regulates MCL-1 to promote survival of stem cell sin acute myeloid leukemia via FLT3-ITD-specific STAT5 activation. *Blood* 114:5034, 2009.

135. Brunet S, Labopin M, Esteve J, et al: Impact of FLT3 internal tandem duplication on the outcome of related and unrelated hematopoietic transplantation for adult myeloid leukemia in the first remission: A retrospective analysis. *J Clin Oncol* 30:735, 2012.

136. Yamamoto Y, Kiyoi H, Nakano Y, et al: Activating mutation of D835 within the activation loop of FLT3 in human hematologic malignancies. *Blood* 97:2434, 2001.

137. Mizuno S, Chijiwa T, Okamura T, et al: Expression of DNA methyltransferases DNMT1, D1, and 3B in normal hematopoiesis and in acute and chronic myelogenous leukemia. *Blood* 97:1172, 2001.

138. Im AP, Sehgal AR, Carroll MP et al: DNMT3A and IDH mutations in acute myeloid leukemia and other myeloid malignancies: Associations with prognosis and potential treatment strategies. *Leukemia* 28:1774, 2014.

139. Thol P, Damm F, Ludeking A, et al: Incidence and prognostic influence of DNMT3A mutations in acute myeloid leukemia. *J Clin Oncol* 29:2889, 2011.

140. Ley TJ, Ding L, Walther MJ, et al: DNMT3A mutations in acute myeloid leukemia *N Engl J Med* 363:2424, 2010.

141. Marcucci G, Metzeler KH, Schwind S, et al: Age-related prognostic impact of different types of DNMT3A mutations in adults with primary cytogenetically normal acute myeloid leukemia. *J Clin Oncol* 80:742, 2012.

142. Shivarov V, Gueroguieva R, Stoimenov A, et al: *DNMT3A* mutation is a poor prognosis biomarker in AML: Results of a meta-analysis of 4500 AML patients. *Leuk Res* 37:1445, 2013.

143. Gaidzik VI, Schlenk RF, Paschka P, et al: Clinical impact of DNMT3A mutations in younger adult patients with acute myeloid leukemia: Results of the AML study group (AMLSG). *Blood* 121:4769, 2013.

144. Kihara R, Nagata Y, Kiyoi H, et al: Comprehensive analysis of genetic alterations and their prognosis impacts in adult acute myeloid leukemia patients. *Leukemia* 28:1586, 2014.

145. Ito Y: Oncogenic potential of the RUNX gene family: "Overview." *Oncogene* 23:4198, 2004.

146. Schnittger S, Dicker F, Kern W, et al: RUNX1 mutations are frequent in de novo AML with noncomplex karyotype and confer an unfavorable prognosis. *Blood* 117:2348, 2011.

147. Gaidzik VI, Bullinger L, Schlenk RF, et al: RUNX1 mutations in acute myeloid leukemia: Results from a comprehensive genetic and clinical analysis from the AML study group. *J Clin Oncol* 29:1364, 2011.

148. Mendler JH, Maharry K, Radmacher MD, et al: RUNX1 mutations are associated with poor outcome in younger and older patients with cytogenetically normal acute myeloid leukemia and with distinct gene and microRNA expression signatures. *J Clin Oncol* 30:3109, 2012.

149. Skokowa J, Stenemann D, Katsman-Kuipers JE, et al: Cooperativity of RUNX1 and CSF3R mutations in severe congenital neutropenia: A unique pathway in myeloid leukemogenesis. *Blood* 123:2229, 2014.

150. Solary E, Bernard OA, Terfferi A, et al: The Ten-Eleven Translocation (TET2) gene in hematopoiesis and hematopoietic diseases. *Leukemia* 38:485, 2014.

151. Tian X, Yu Y, Yin J, et al: TET2 gene mutation is unfavorable prognostic factor in cytogenetically normal acute myeloid leukemia patient with NPM1+ and FLT3-ITD- mutations. *Int J Hematol* 100:96, 2014.

152. Aslanyan MG, Kroeze LI, Langemeijer SM, et al: Clinical and biological impact of TET2 mutations and expression in younger adult AML patients treated within the EORTC/GIMEMA AML-12 clinical trial. *Ann Hematol* 92:1401, 2014.

153. Metzeler KH, Maharry K, Radmacher MD, et al: TET2 mutations improve the new European LeukemiaNet risk classification of acute myeloid leukemia: A Cancer and Leukemia Group B study. *J Clin Oncol* 29:1373, 2011.

154. Green CL, Koo KK, Hills FR, et al: Prognostic significance of CEBPA mutations in a large cohort of younger adult patients with acute myeloid leukemia: Impact of double CEBPA mutations and the interaction with FLT3 and NPM1 mutations. *J Clin Oncol* 28:2739, 2010.

155. Taskesen E, Bullinger L, Corbacioglu A, et al: Prognostic impact, concurrent genetic mutations, and gene expression features of AML with CEBPA mutations in a cohort of 1183 cytogenetically normal AML patients: Further evidence of CEBPA double mutant AML as a distinctive disease entity. *Blood* 1107:2469, 2011.

156. Fasan A, Haferlach C, Alpermann T, et al: The role of different genetic subtypes of *CEBPA* mutated AML. *Leukemia* 28:791, 2013.

157. Grossman V, Haferlach C, Nadarajah N, et al: *CEBPA* double-mutated acute myeloid leukaemia harbours concomitant molecular mutations in 76.8% of cases with TET2 and GATGA2 alterations impacting prognosis. *Br J Haematol* 161:642, 2013.

158. Paschka P, Schlenk RF, Gaidzik VI, et al: IDH1 and IDH2 mutations are frequent genetic alterations in acute myeloid leukemia and confer adverse prognosis in cytogenetically normal acute myeloid leukemia with NPM1 mutation without FLT3 internal tandem duplication. *J Clin Oncol* 28:3636, 2010.

159. Guan L, Gao L, Wang L, et al: The frequency and clinical significance of IDH1 mutations in Chinese acute myeloid leukemia patients. *PLoS One* 8:e83334, 2013.

160. Boissel N, Nibourel O, Renneville A, et al: Prognostic impact of isocitrate dehydrogenase enzyme isoforms 1 and 2 mutations in acute myeloid leukemia: A study by the acute leukemia French association group. *J Clin Oncol* 28:3717, 2010.

161. Marcucci G, Maharry K, Wu Y-Z, et al: IDH1 and IDH2 gene mutations identify novel molecular subsets within de novo cytogenetically normal acute myeloid leukemia: A Cancer and Leukemia Group B study. *J Clin Oncol* 28:2348, 2010.

162. Janin M, Mylonas E, Saada V, et al: Serum-2-hydroxyglutarate production in IDH1- and IDH2-mutated de novo acute myeloid leukemia: A study by the Acute Leukemia French Association Group. *J Clin Oncol* 32:297, 2013.

163. Dinardo CD, Propert KJ, Loren AW, et al: Serum 2-hydroxyglutarate levels predict isocitrate dehydrogenase mutations and clinical outcome in acute myeloid leukemia. *Blood* 121;4917, 2013.

164. Chaturvedi A, Cruz MMA, Jyotsana N, et al: Mutant IDH1 promotes leukemogenesis in vivo and can be specifically targeted in human AML. *Blood* 122;2877, 2013.

165. Krauth MT, Alpermann T, Bacher U, et al: WT1 mutations are secondary events in AML, show varying frequencies and impact on prognosis between genetic subgroups. *Leukemia* 29:660, 2015.

166. Damm F, Heuser M, Morgan M, et al: Single nucleotide polymorphism in the mutational hotspot of WT1 predicts a favorable outcome in patients with cytogenetically normal acute myeloid leukemia. *J Clin Oncol* 28:473, 2009.

167. Becker H, Marcucci G, Maharry K, et al: Mutations of the Wilms tumor 1 gene (WT1) in older patients with primary cytogenetically normal acute myeloid leukemia: A Cancer and Leukemia Group B study. *Blood* 116;788, 2010.

168. Yi JH, Huh J, Kin H-J, et al: Adverse prognostic impact of abnormal lesions detected by genome-wide single nucleotide polymorphism array-based karyotyping analysis in acute myeloid leukemia with normal karyotype. *J Clin Oncol* 29:4702, 2011.

169. Kornblau SM, McCue D, Singh N, et al;, Recurrent expression signatures of cytokines and chemokines are present and are independently prognostic in acute myelogenous leukemia and myelodysplasia. *Blood* 116:4251, 2010.

170. Rapin N, Bagger FO, Jendholm J, et al: Comparing cancer vs normal gene expression profiles identifies new disease entities and common transcriptional programs in AML patients. *Blood* 123:894, 2014.

171. Eisfled A-K, Marcucci G, Maharry K, et al: *mIR-3151* interplays with its host gene BAALC and independently affects outcome of patients with cytogenetically normal acute myeloid leukemia. *Blood* 120:249, 2012.

172. Shen Y, Zhyu Y-M, Fan X, et al: Gene mutation patterns and their prognostic impact in a cohort of 1185 patients with acute myeloid leukemia. *Blood* 118:5593, 2011.

173. Diffner E, Beck D, Gudgin E, et al: Activity of a heptad of transcription factors is associated with stem cell programs and clinical outcome in acute myeloid leukemia. *Blood* 121:2289, 2013.

174. Gutierrez SE, Romero-Oliva FA. Epigenetic changes: A common theme in acute myelogenous leukemogenesis. *J Hematol Oncol* 6:57, 2013.

175. Schoofs T, Berdel WE, Muller-Tidow C: Origins of aberrant DNA methylation in acute myeloid leukemia. *Leukemia* 28:1, 2014.

176. Scholl C, Gilliland DG, Fröhling S: Deregulation of signaling pathways in acute myeloid leukemia. *Semin Oncol* 35:336, 2008.

177. Greaves MF, Maia AT, Wiemels JL, Ford AM: Leukemia in twins: Lessons in natural history. *Blood* 102:2321, 2003.

178. Wiemels JL, Xiao Z, Buffler PA, et al: *In utero* origin of t(8;21) AML1-ETO translocation in childhood acute leukemia. *Blood* 99:3801, 2002.

179. Groves FD, Linet MS, Devesa SS: Epidemiology of leukemia, in *Leukemia*, ed 6, edited by Henderson ES, Lister TA, Greaves MF, p 145. WB Saunders, New York, 1986.

180. Goldin LR, Kristinsson SY, Liang XS, et al: Familial aggregation of acute myeloid leukemia and myelodysplastic syndromes. *J Clin Oncol* 30:179, 2011.

181. Hahn CN, Chong C-E, Carmichael CL, et al: Heritable GATA2 mutations associated with familial myelodysplastic syndrome and acute myeloid leukemia. *Nat Genet* 43:1012, 2012.

182. Ostergaard P, Simpson MA, Connell FC, et al: Mutations in GATA2 cause primary lymphedema associated with a predisposition to acute myeloid leukemia (Emberger syndrome). *Nat Genet* 43:929, 2011.

183. Calvo KR, Vihn DC, Maric I, et al: Myelodysplasia in autosomal dominant and sporadic monocytopenia immunodeficiency syndrome: Diagnostic features and clinical implications. *Haematologica* 96:1221, 2010.

184. Kazenwadel J, Secker GA, Liu YJ, et al: Loss-of-function germline GATA2 mutations in patients with MDS/AML or MonoMAC syndrome and primary lymphedema reveal a key role for GATA2 in the lymphatic vasculature. *Blood* 119:1283, 2012.

185. Smith ML, Cavenagh JD, Lister A, Fitzgibbon J: Mutation of CEBPA in familial acute myeloid leukemia. *N Engl J Med* 351:2403, 2004.

186. Holme H, Hossain U, Kirwan M, et al: Marked genetic heterogeneity in familial myelodysplasia/acute myeloid leukaemia. *Br J Haematol* 158:242, 2012.

187. Kirwan M, Vuillamy T, Marrone A, et al: Defining the pathogenic role of telomerase mutations in myelodysplastic syndrome and acute myeloid leukemia. *Hum Mutat* 30:1567, 2009.

188. Vickers M, Jackson G, Taylor P: The incidence of acute promyelocytic leukemia appears constant over most of a human life span, implying only one rate limiting mutation. *Leukemia* 14:727, 2000.

189. Chongli Y, Xiaobo Z: Incidence survey of leukemia in China. *Chinese J Med Sci* 6:65, 1991.

190. Douer D, Santillana S, Ramezani L, et al: Acute promyelocytic leukaemia in patients originating in Latin America is associated with an increased frequency of the bcr1 subtype of the PML/RARalpha fusion gene. *Br J Haematol* 122:563, 2003.

191. Otero JC, Santillana S, Fereyros G: High frequency of acute promyelocytic leukemia among Latinos with acute myeloid leukemias. *Blood* 88:377, 1996.

192. Morton LM, Dores GM, Tucker MA, et al: Evolving risk of therapy-related acute myeloid leukemia following cancer chemotherapy among adults in the United States, 1975–2008. *Blood* 121:2996, 2013.

193. Stanley M, McKenna RW, Ellinger G, Brunning RD: Classification of 358 cases of acute myeloid leukemia by FAB criteria: Analysis of clinical and morphologic features, in *Chronic and Acute Leukemias in Adults*, edited by Bloomfield CD, p 147. Martinus Nijhoff, Boston, 1985.

194. Paietta E: Classification of acute leukemias: Proposals for the immunological classification of acute leukemias. *Leukemia* 9:2147, 1995.

195. Kheiri SA, MacKerrell T, Bonagura VR, et al: Flow cytometry with or without cytochemistry for the diagnosis of acute leukemias? *Cytometry* 34:82, 1998.

196. Arber B, Brunning R, LeBeau M, et al: Acute myeloid leukemia with recurrent genetic abnormalities, in *WHO Classification of Tumors of Hematopoietic and Lymphoid Tissues*, ed 4, edited by Swerdlow S, Compo E, Harris NL, p 110. World Health Organization, Geneva, 2008.

197. Boggs DR, Wintrobe MM, Cartwright GE: The acute leukemias. Analysis of 322 cases and review of the literature. *Medicine (Baltimore)* 41:163, 1962.

198. Roath S, Isräels MCG, Wilkinson JF: The acute leukemias: A study of 580 patients. *Q J Med* 33:256, 1964.

199. Choi SI, Simone JV: Acute nonlymphocytic leukemia in 171 children. *Med Pediatr Oncol* 2:119, 1976.

200. Chessels JM, O'Calloghan U, Hardisty RM: Acute myeloid leukaemia in childhood: Clinical features and prognosis. *Br J Haematol* 63:555, 1986.

201. Burns CP, Armitage JO, Frey AL, et al: Analysis of presenting features of adult leukemia. *Cancer* 47:2460, 1981.

202. Goodall PT, Vosti KL: Fever in acute myelogenous leukemia. *Arch Intern Med* 135:1197, 1975.

203. Burke PJ, Braine HG, Rothbun HK, Owens AH: The clinical significance and management of fever in acute myelocytic leukemia. *Johns Hopkins Med J* 139:1, 1976.

204. Chang JC: How to differentiate neoplastic fever from infectious fever in patients with cancer. Usefulness of the naproxen test. *Heart Lung* 16:122, 1987.

205. Gollard RP, Robbins BA, Piro L, Saven A: Acute myelogenous leukemia presenting with bulky lymphadenopathy. *Acta Haematol* 95:129, 1996.

206. Davey DD, Fourcar K, Burns CP, Goekin JA: Acute myelocytic leukemia manifested by prominent generalized lymphadenopathy. *Am J Hematol* 21:89, 1986.

207. Tobelem G, Jacquillat C, Chastang C, et al: Acute monoblastic leukemia: A clinical and biologic study of 74 cases. *Blood* 55:71, 1980.

208. Sepp N, Radaszkiewicz T, Meijer CJ, et al: Specific skin manifestations in acute leukemia with monocytic differentiation. *Cancer* 71:124, 1993.

209. Hejmadi RK, Thompson D, Shah F, Naresh KN: Cutaneous presentation of aleukemic monoblastic leukemia cutis—A case report and review of literature with focus on immunohistochemistry. *J Cutan Pathol* 35:46, 2008.

210. Cibull TL, Thomas AB, O'Malley DP, Billings SD: Myeloid leukemia cutis: A histologic and immunohistochemical review. *J Cutan Pathol* 35:180, 2008.

211. Kaiserling E, Horny H-P, Geerts M-L, Schmid U: Skin involvement in myelogenous leukemia. Morphologic and immunophenotypic heterogeneity of skin infiltrates. *Mod Pathol* 7:771, 1994.

212. Longacre TA, Smoller BR: Leukemia cutis: Analysis of 50 biopsy-proven cases with an emphasis on occurrences in myelodysplastic syndromes. *Am J Clin Pathol* 100:276, 1993.

213. Cho-Vega JH, Medeiros LJ, Prieto VG, Vega F: Leukemia cutis. *Am J Clin Pathol* 129:130, 2008.

214. Bourantas K, Malamou-Mitsi V, Christou L, et al: Cutaneous vasculitis as the initial manifestation in acute myelomonocytic leukemia. *Ann Intern Med* 121:942, 1994.

215. Sheps M, Shapero H, Ramsay C: Bullous pyoderma gangrenosum and acute leukemia. *Arch Dermatol* 114:1842, 1978.

216. Lewis SJ, Poh-Fitzpatrick MB, Walther RR: A typical pyoderma gangrenosum with leukemia. *JAMA* 239:935, 1978.

217. Cohen PR: Sweet's syndrome—A comprehensive review of an acute febrile neutrophilic dermatosis. *Orphanet J Rare Dis* 26(2):34, 2007.

218. Cheson BD, Christensen RM: Cutis verticis gyrata: Unusual chloromatous disease in acute myelogenous leukemia. *Am J Hematol* 8:415, 1980.

219. Stern M, Halter J, Buser A, et al: Leukemia cutis preceding systemic relapse of acute myeloid leukemia. *Int J Hematol* 87:108, 2008.

220. Markowski TR, Martin DB, Kao GF, et al: Leukemia cutis: A presenting sign in acute promyelocytic leukemia. *Arch Dermatol* 143:1220, 2007.

221. Long JC, Mihm MC: Multiple granulocytic tumors of the skin: Report of six cases of myelogenous leukemia with initial manifestations in the skin. *Cancer* 39:2004, 1977.

222. Rallis E, Stavropoulou E, Michalakeas I, et al: Monoblastic sarcoma cutis preceding acute monoblastic leukemia. *Am J Hematol* 84:590, 2008.

223. Kincaid MC, Green WR: Ocular and orbital involvement in leukemia. *Surv Ophthalmol* 27:211, 1983.

224. Paparella MM, Berlinger NT, Oda M: Otological manifestations of leukemia. *Laryngoscope* 83:1510, 1973.

225. Bertrand Y, Lefrère JJ, Leverger G, et al: Acute myeloblastic leukemia presenting as apparent acute otitis media. *Am J Hematol* 27:136, 1988.

226. Shiknecht HF, Igarashi M, Chasin WD: Inner ear hemorrhage in leukemia. *Laryngoscope* 75:662, 1965.

227. Dewar GJ, Lim CN, Michalyshyn B, Akabutu J: Gastrointestinal complications in patients with acute and chronic leukemia. *Can J Surg* 24:67, 1981.

228. Hunter TB, Bjelland JC: Gastrointestinal complications of leukemia and its treatment. *AJR Am J Roentgenol* 142:513, 1984.

229. Duffy JH, Driscoll EJ: Oral manifestations of leukemia. *Oral Surg Oral Med Oral Pathol* 11:484, 1958.

230. Ahsan N, Schen-Chih, JS, John DD: Acute ileotyphlitis as presenting manifestation of acute myelogenous leukemia. *Am J Clin Pathol* 89:407, 1988.

231. Rodgers B, Seibert JJ: Unusual combination of an appendicolith in a leukemic patient with typhlitis-ultrasound diagnosis. *J Clin Ultrasound* 18:141, 1990.

232. Abramson SJ, Berdon WE, Baker DH: Childhood typhlitis: Its increasing association with acute myelogenous leukemia. *Radiology* 146:61, 1983.

233. Bagnoli P, Castagna L, Cozzaglio L, et al: Neutropenic enterocolitis: Is there a right timing for surgery? Assessment of a clinical case. *Tumori* 93:608, 2007.

234. Roy J, Vercellotti G, Fenderson M, et al: Isolated relapse of acute myelogenous leukemia presenting as a gastric ulcer. *Am J Hematol* 37:270, 1991.

235. Thompson BC, Feczko PJ, Mezwa DG: Dysphagia caused by acute leukemia infiltration of the esophagus. *AJR Am J Roentgenol* 155:654, 1990.

236. Ti M, Villafuerte R, Chase PH, Dosik H: Acute leukemia presenting as laryngeal obstruction. *Cancer* 34:427, 1974.

237. Bodey GP, Powell RD, Hersh EM, et al: Pulmonary complications of acute leukemia. *Cancer* 19:781, 1966.

238. Maile CW, Moore AV, Ulreich S, Putnam CE: Chest radiographic pathologic correlation in adult leukemia patients. *Invest Radiol* 18:495, 1983.

239. Armstrong P, Dyer R, Alford BA, O'Hara M: Leukemic pulmonary infiltrates. Rapid development mimicking pulmonary edema. *AJR Am J Roentgenol* 135:373, 1980.

240. Wu KK, Burns CP: Leukemic pleural infiltrates during bone marrow remission of acute myelocytic leukemia. *Cancer* 33:1179, 1974.

241. Roberts WC, Bodey GP, Wertlake PT: The heart in acute leukemia. A study of 420 autopsy cases. *Am J Cardiol* 21:388, 1968.

242. Lisker SA, Finkelstein D, Brody JI, Beizer LH: Myocardial infarction in acute leukemia. *Arch Intern Med* 119:332, 1967.

243. Norris NH, Weiner J: The renal lesions in leukemia. *Am J Med Sci* 241:512, 1961.

244. Uno Y: Histopathological study of leukemic cell infiltration in the kidney. *Med J Osaka Univ* 18:185, 1967.

245. Russo A, Basquez E, Russo G, Schilvio G: Testicular relapse in acute myelogenous leukemia after 3 1/2 years of complete remission. *Acta Haematol* 65:131, 1981.

246. Quien ET, Wallach B, Sandhaus L, et al: Primary extramedullary leukemia of the prostate. *Am J Hematol* 53:267, 1996.

247. Vanden Broecke R, Van Droogenbroek J, Dhont M: Vulvovaginal manifestations of acute myeloblastic leukemia. *Obstet Gynecol* 88:735, 1996.

248. Marsh WL, Byland DJ, Heath VC, Anderson MJ: Osteoarticular and pulmonary manifestations of acute leukemia. *Cancer* 57:385, 1986.

249. Weinberger A, Schumacher R, Schimmer BM, et al: Arthritis in acute leukemia. *Arch Intern Med* 141:1183, 1981.

250. Pavlovsky S, Eppinger-Helft M, Murill FS: Factors that influence the appearance of central nervous system leukemia. *Blood* 42:935, 1973.

251. Meyer RJ, Ferreira PP, Cuttner J, et al: Central nervous system involvement at presentation in acute granulocytic leukemia. *Am J Med* 68:691, 1980.

252. Castagnola C, Morra E, Bernasconi P, et al: Acute myeloid leukemia and diabetes insipidus: Results in five patients. *Acta Haematol* 93:1, 1995.

253. Holmes R, Keating MJ, Cork A, et al: A unique pattern of central nervous system leukemia in acute myelomonocytic leukemia associated with inv (16) (p13;q32). *Blood* 65:1071, 1985.

254. Glass JP, VanTassel P, Keating MJ, et al: Central nervous system complications of a newly recognized subtype of leukemia: AMML with a pencentric inversion of chromosome 16. *Neurology* 38:639, 1987.

255. Neiman RS, Barcos M, Berard C, et al: Granulocytic sarcoma: A clinicopathologic study of 61 biopsied cases. *Cancer* 48:426, 1981.

256. Byrd JC, Edenfield WJ, Shields DJ, Dawson NA: Extramedullary myeloid cell tumors in acute nonlymphocytic leukemia. A clinical review. *J Clin Oncol* 13:1800, 1995.

257. Menasce LP, Banerjee SS, Becket E, Harris M: Extramedullary myeloid tumor (granulocytic sarcoma) is often misdiagnosed. A study of 26 cases. *Histopathology* 34:391, 1999.

258. Audouin J, Comperat E, Le Tourneau A, et al: Myeloid sarcoma: Clinical and morphologic criteria useful for diagnosis. *Int J Surg Pathol* 11:271, 2003.

259. Hernandez JA, Navarro JT, Rozman M, et al: Primary myeloid sarcoma of the gynecologic tract: A report of two cases progressing to acute leukemia. *Leuk Lymphoma* 43:2151, 2002.

260. Tsimberidou AM, Kantarjian HM, Estey E, et al: Outcome in patients with nonleukemic granulocytic sarcoma treated with chemotherapy with or without radiotherapy. *Leukemia* 17:1100, 2003.

261. Yamauchi K, Yasuda M: Comparison of nonleukenic granulocytic sarcoma. *Cancer* 94:1739, 2002.

262. Tsimberidou AM, Kantarjian HM, Wen S, et al: Myeloid sarcoma is associated with superior event-free survival and overall survival compared with acute myeloid leukemia. *Cancer* 113:1370, 2008.

263. Byrd JC, Weiss RB, Arthur DC, et al: Extramedullary leukemia adversely affects hematologic complete remission rate and overall survival in patients with t(8;21)(q22;q22): Results from Cancer and Leukemia Group B 8461. *J Clin Oncol* 15:466, 1997.

264. Andrieu V, Radford-Weill I, Troussand X, et al: Molecular detection of t(8;21)/AML1-ETO in AML M1/M2: Correlation with cytogenetics, morphology and immunophenotype. *Br J Haematol* 92:855, 1996.

265. Rege K, Swansbury GJ, Atra AA, et al: Disease features in acute myeloid leukemia with t(8;21)(q22;q22). Influence of age, secondary karyotypic abnormalities, CD19 status, and extramedullary leukemia. *Leuk Lymphoma* 40:67, 2000.

266. Nguyen S, Leblanc T, Fenaux P, et al: A white blood cell index as the main prognostic factor in t(8;21) acute myeloid leukemia (AML): A survey of 161 cases from the French AML intergroup. *Blood* 99:3517, 2002.

267. Rowe JM: Clinical and laboratory features of the myeloid and lymphoid leukemias. *Am J Med Technol* 49:103, 1983.

268. Woodcock BE, Cooper PC, Brown PR, et al: The platelet defect in acute myeloid leukemia. *J Clin Pathol* 37:1339, 1984.

269. Hofmann WK, Stauch M, Höffken K: Impaired granulocytic function in patients with acute leukaemia: Only partial normalization after successful remission-inducing treatment. *J Clin Res Clin Oncol* 124:113, 1998.

270. Suda T, Onai T, Maekawa T: Studies on abnormal polymorphonuclear neutrophils in acute myelogenous leukemia. *Am J Hematol* 15:45, 1983.

270a. Glick AD, Paniker K, Flexner JM, et al: Acute leukemia of adults: Ultrastructural, cytochemical, and histological observations in 100 cases. *Am J Pathol* 73:459, 1980.

271. Lichtman MA: Does a diagnosis of myelogenous leukemia require 20% marrow myeloblasts, and does <5% marrow myeloblasts represent a remission? The history and ambiguity of arbitrary diagnostic boundaries in the understanding of myelodysplasia. *Oncologist* 18:973, 2013.

272. Bacher U, Kern W, Alpermann T, et al: Prognosis in patients with MDS or AML and bone marrow blasts between 10% and 30% is not associated with blast counts but depends on cytogenetic and molecular genetic characteristics. *Leukemia* 25:1361, 2011.

273. San Miguel JF, Conzalez M, Canizo MC, et al: TdT activity in acute myeloid leukemias defined by monoclonal antibodies. *Am J Hematol* 23:9, 1986.

274. Kaplan SS, Penchansky L, Krause JR, et al: Simultaneous evaluation of terminal deoxynucleotidyl transferase and myeloperoxidase in acute leukemias using an immunocytochemical method. *Am J Clin Pathol* 87:732, 1987.

275. Kahl C, Florschü tz A, Müller G, et al: Prognostic significance of dysplastic features of hematopoiesis in patients with de novo acute myelogenous leukemia. *Ann Hematol* 75:91, 1997.

276. Manoharan A, Horsley R, Pitney WR: The reticulin content of bone marrow in acute leukemia in adults. *Br J Haematol* 43:185, 1979.

277. Moehler TM, Ho AD, Goldschmidt H, Barlogie B: Angiogenesis in hematologic malignancies. *Crit Rev Oncol Hematol* 45:227, 2003.

278. Albitar M: Angiogenesis in acute myeloid leukemia and myelodysplastic syndrome. *Acta Haematol* 106:170, 2001.

279. Ghannadan M, Wimazal F, Simonitsch I, et al: Immunohistochemical detection of VEGF in the bone marrow of patients with acute myeloid leukemia. Correlation between VEGF expression and the FAB category. *Am J Clin Pathol* 119:663, 2003.

280. Chi Y, Lindgren V, Quigley S, Gaitonde S: Acute myelogenous leukemia with t(6;9)(p23;q34) and marrow basophilia: An overview. *Arch Pathol Lab Med* 132:1835, 2008.

281. Seiter K: Diagnosis and management of core-binding factor leukemias. *Curr Hematol Rep* 2:78, 2003.

282. Mrózek K, Heinonen K, De la Chapelle A, Bloomfield C: Clinical significance of cytogenetics in acute myeloid leukemia. *Semin Oncol* 24:17, 1997.

283. Schoch C, Haferlach T, Haase D, et al: Patients with de novo acute myeloid leukaemia and complex karyotype aberrations show a poor prognosis despite intensive treatment: A study of 90 patients. *Br J Haematol* 112:118, 2001.

284. Weltermann A, Fonatsch C, Haas OA, et al: Impact of cytogenetics on the prognosis of adults with de novo AML in first relapse. *Leukemia* 18:293, 2004.

285. Martinez-Climent JA, Lane NJ, Rubin CM, et al: Clinical and prognostic significance of chromosomal abnormalities in childhood acute myeloid leukemia de novo. *Leukemia* 9:95, 1995.

286. Pedersen-Bjergaard J, Philip P: Chromosome characteristics of therapy-related acute nonlymphocytic leukemia and preleukemia: Possible implications for pathogenesis of the disease. *Leuk Res* 11:315, 1987.

287. Zaccarea A, Alimena G, Baccarani M, et al: Cytogenetic analyses in 89 patients with secondary hematologic disorders: Results of a cooperative study. *Cancer Genet Cytogenet* 26:65, 1987.

288. Schoch C, Kern W, Krawitz P, et al: Dependence of age-specific incidence of acute myeloid leukemia on karyotype. *Blood* 98:3500, 2002.

289. Byrd JC, Lawrence D, Arthur DC, et al: Patients with isolated trisomy 8 in acute myeloid leukemia are not cured with cytarabine-based chemotherapy: Results from Cancer and Leukemia Group B 8461. *Clin Cancer Res* 4:1235, 1998.

290. Melnick A, Licht J: Deconstructing a disease, RARalpha, its fusion partners, and their roles in the pathogenesis of acute promyelocytic leukemia. *Blood* 93:3167, 1999.

291. LoCoco F, Diverio D, Falini B, et al: Genetic diagnosis and molecular monitoring in the management of acute promyelocytic leukemia. *Blood* 94:12, 1999.

292. Poirel H, Rack K, Dalbesse E, et al: Incidence and characterization of MLL gene (11q23) rearrangements in acute myeloid leukemia M1 and M5. *Blood* 87:2496, 1996.

293. Schoch C, Schnittger S, Klaus M, et al: AML with 11q23/MLL abnormalities as defined by the WHO classification: Incidence, partner chromosomes, FAB subtype, age distribution, and prognostic impact in an unselected series of 1897 cytogenetically analyzed AML cases. *Blood* 102:2395, 2003.

294. Mrózek K, Heinonen K, Lawrence D, et al: Adult patients with *de novo* acute myeloid leukemia and t(9;11) (p22;q23) have a superior outcome to patients with other translocations involving band 11q23: A Cancer and Leukemia Group B study. *Blood* 90:4532, 1997.

295. Swansbury GJ, Slater R, Bain BJ, et al: Hematologic malignancies with t(9;11) (p21–22; q23)—A laboratory and clinical study of 125 cases. *Leukemia* 12:792, 1998.

296. Huret JL, Dessen P, Bernheim A: An atlas of chromosomes in hematological malignancies. Example: 11q23 and MLL partners. *Leukemia* 15:987, 2001.

297. Scholl C, Breitinger H, Schlenk RF, et al: Development of a real-time RT-PCR assay for the quantification of the most frequent MLL/AF9 fusion types resulting from translocation t(9;11)(p22;q23) in acute myeloid leukemia. *Genes Chromosomes Cancer* 38:274, 2003.

298. Meyer C, Schneider B, Jakob S, et al: The MLL recombinome of acute leukemias. *Leukemia* 20:777, 2006.

299. Soupir CP, Vergilio JA, Dal Cin P, et al: Philadelphia chromosome-positive acute myeloid leukemia: A rare aggressive leukemia with clinicopathologic features distinct from chronic myeloid leukemia in myeloid blast crisis. *Am J Clin Pathol* 127:642, 2007.

300. Tien HF, Wang CH, Chuang SM, et al: Characterization of Philadelphia-chromosome-positive acute leukemia by clinical, cytochemical, and gene analysis. *Leukemia* 6:907, 1992.

301. Duchayne E, Fenneteau O, Pages MP, et al: Acute megakaryoblastic leukaemia: A national clinical and biological study of 53 adult and childhood cases by the Groupe Français d'Hématologie Cellulaire (GFHC). *Leuk Lymphoma* 44:49, 2003.

302. Borel C, Dastugue N, Cances-Lauwers V, et al: PICALM-MLLT10 acute myeloid leukemia: A French cohort of 18 patients. *Leuk Res* 36:1365, 2012.

303. Billstrom R, Ahlgren T, Bekassy AN, et al: Acute myeloid leukemia with inv(16) (p13q22): Involvement of cervical lymph nodes and tonsils is common and may be a negative prognostic sign. *Am J Hematol* 71:15, 2002.

304. Speck NA, Gilliland DG: Core-binding factors in haematopoiesis and leukaemia. *Nat Rev Cancer* 2:502, 2002.

305. Delauney J, Ve3y N, Leblanc T, et al: Prognosis of Inv 16/t(16;16) acute myeloid leukemia (AML): A survey of 110 cases from the French AML Intergroup. *Blood* 102:462, 2003.

306. Poirel H, Radford-Weiss I, Rack K, et al: Detection of the chromosome 16 CBFβ-MYH11 fusion transcript in myelomonocytic leukemias. *Blood* 85:1313, 1995.

307. Haferlach T, Winkemann M, Löffler H, et al: The abnormal eosinophils are part of the leukemic cell population in acute myelomonocytic leukemia with abnormal eosinophils (AML M4 Eo) and carry pericentric inversion 16: A combination of May-Grünwald-Giemsa a staining and fluorescence *in situ* hybridization. *Blood* 87:2459, 1996.

308. Secker-Walker LM, Mehta A, Bain B: Abnormalities of 3q21 and 3q26 in myeloid malignancy: A United Kingdom Cancer Cytogenetic Group study. *Br J Haematol* 91:490, 1995.

309. Marcucci G, Radmacher MD, Maharry K, et al: MicroRNA expression in cytogenetically normal acute myeloid leukemia. *N Engl J Med* 358:1919, 2008.

310. Haferlach T, Kohlmann A, Wieczorek L, et al: Clinical utility of microarray-based gene expression profiling in the diagnosis and subclassification of leukemia: Report from the international microarray innovations in leukemia study group. *J Clin Oncol* 28:2529, 2010.

311. Kjellstrand CM, Campbell DC, Von Hartitzsch B, Buselmeier TJ: Hyperuricemic acute renal failure. *Arch Intern Med* 133:349, 1974.

312. O'Regan S, Carson S, Chesney RW, Drummond KN: Electrolyte and acid–base disturbances in the management of leukemia. *Blood* 49:345, 1977.

313. Mir MA, Delamore IW: Metabolic disorders in acute myeloid leukaemia. *Br J Haematol* 40:79, 1978.

314. Bergman GE, Baluarte HJ, Naiman JL: Diabetes insipidus as a presenting manifestation of acute myelogenous leukemia. *J Pediatr* 88:355, 1976.

315. Mir MA, Brabin B, Tang OT, et al: Hypokalemia in acute myeloid leukaemia. *Ann Intern Med* 82:54, 1975.

316. Salomon J: Spurious hypoglycemia and hyperkalemia in myelomonocytic leukemia. *Am J Med Sci* 267:359, 1974.

317. Bellevue R, Disik H, Speigel G, Gussoff BD: Pseudohyperkalemia and extreme leukocytosis. *J Lab Clin Med* 85:660, 1975.

318. Fox MJ, Brody JS, Weintraub LR, et al: Leukocyte larceny: A cause of spurious hypoxia. *Am J Med* 67:742, 1979.

319. Palva IP, Salokannel SJ: Hypercalcemia in acute leukemia. *Blut* 24:209, 1972.

320. Zidar BL, Shadduck RK, Winkelstein A, et al: Acute myeloblastic leukemia and hypercalcemia. *N Engl J Med* 295:692, 1976.

321. Roth GJ, Poite D: Chronic lactic acidosis and acute leukemia. *Arch Intern Med* 125:317, 1970.

322. Wainer RA, Wiernik PH, Thompson WL: Metabolic and therapeutic studies of a patient with acute leukemia and severe lactic acidosis of prolonged duration. *Am J Med* 55:255, 1973.

323. Zamkoff KW, Kirshner JJ: Marked hypophosphatemia associated with acute myelomonocytic leukemia. *Arch Intern Med* 140:1523, 1980.

324. Pflüger K-H, Gramse M, Gropp C, Havemann K: Ectopic ACTH production with autoantibody formation in a patient with acute myeloblastic leukemia. *N Engl J Med* 305:1632, 1981.

325. Carpenter NA, Fiere DM, Schuh D, et al: Circulating immune complexes and the prognosis of acute myeloid leukemia. *N Engl J Med* 307:1174, 1982.

326. Bratt G, Bromback M, Paul C, et al: Factors and inhibitors of blood coagulation and fibrinolysis in acute nonlymphoblastic leukaemia. *Scand J Haematol* 34:332, 1985.

327. Reddy VB, Kowal-Vern A, Hoppensteadt DA, et al: Global and molecular hemostatic markers in acute myeloid leukemia. *Am J Clin Pathol* 94:397, 1990.

328. Tsumita Y, Matsushima T, Uchiumi H, et al: Acute myeloid leukemia accompanied by multiple thrombophlebitis. *Intern Med* 36:595, 1997.

329. Weltermann A, Pabinger I, Geiseler K, et al: Hypofibrinogenemia in non-M3 acute myeloid leukemia. Incidence, clinical and laboratory characteristics and prognosis. *Leukemia* 12:1182, 1998.

330. Greenwood MJ, Seftel MD, Richardson C, et al: Leukocyte count as a predictor of death during remission induction in acute myeloid leukemia. *Leuk Lymphoma* 47: 1245, 2006.

331. Lichtman MA, Heal J, Rowe JM: Hyperleukocytic leukaemia: Rheological and clinical features and management. *Baillieres Clin Haematol* 1:725, 1987.

332. Nowacki P, Zdziarska B, Fryze C, Urasinski I: Co-existence of thrombocytopenia and hyperleukocytosis ("critical period") as a risk factor of haemorrhage into the central nervous system in patients with acute leukaemias. *Haematologia (Budap)* 31:347, 2002.

333. Wurthner JU, Kohler G, Behringer D, et al: Leukostasis followed by hemorrhage complicating the initiation of chemotherapy in patients with acute myeloid leukemia and hyperleukocytosis: A clinicopathologic report of four cases. *Cancer* 85:368, 1999.

334. Ventura GJ, Hester JP, Smith TL, Keating MJ: Acute myeloblastic leukemia with hyperleukocytosis: Risk factors for early mortality in induction. *Am J Hematol* 27:34, 1988.

335. Dutcher J, Schiffer CA, Wiernik PH: Hyperleukocytosis in adult acute nonlymphocytic leukemia: Impact on remission rate, duration, and survival. *J Clin Oncol* 5:1364, 1987.

336. VanBuchem MA, Te Velde J, Willemze R, Spaander PJ: Leucostasis, an underestimated cause of death in leukaemia. *Blut* 56:39, 1988.

337. Dilek I, Uysal A, Demirer T, et al: Acute myeloblastic leukemia associated with hyperleukocytosis and diabetes insipidus. *Leuk Lymphoma* 30:657, 1998.

338. Lavabre-Bertrand T, Bourquard P, Chiesa J, et al: Diabetes insipidus revealing acute myelogenous leukaemia with a high platelet count, monosomy 7 and abnormalities of chromosome 3: A new entity? *Eur J Haematol* 66:66, 2001.

339. Inaba H, Fan Y, Pounds S, et al: Clinical and biologic features and treatment outcome of children with newly diagnosed acute myeloid leukemia and hyperleukocytosis. *Cancer* 113:522, 2008.

340. Bug G, Anargyrou K, Tonn T, et al: Impact of leukapheresis on early death rate in adult acute myeloid leukemia presenting with hyperleukocytosis. *Transfusion* 47:1843, 2007.

341. Nagler A, Brenner B, Zuckerman E, et al: Acute respiratory failure in hyperleukocytic acute myeloid leukemia. *Am J Hematol* 27:65, 1988.

342. Von Eyben FE, Siddiqui MZ, Spanosi G: High-voltage irradiation and hydroxyurea for pulmonary leukostasis in acute myelomonocytic leukemia. *Acta Haematol* 77:180, 1987.

343. Azoulay E, Fieux F, Moreau D, et al: Acute monocytic leukemia presenting as respiratory failure. *Am J Respir Crit Care Med* 167:1329, 2003.

344. Koote AMM, Thompson J, Bruijn JA: Acute myelocytic leukemia with acute aortic occlusion as presenting symptoms. *Acta Haematol* 75:120, 1986.

345. Foss R, Haddad M, Zaizov R, et al: Recurrent peripheral arterial occlusion by leukemic cells sedimentation in acute promyelocytic leukemia. *J Pediatr Surg* 27:665, 1992.

346. Mataix R, Gómez-Casares MT, Campo C, et al: Acute leg ischaemia as a presentation of hyperleukocytosis syndrome in acute myeloid leukaemia. *Am J Hematol* 51:250, 1996.

347. Murray JC, Dorfman SR, Brandt ML, Dreyer ZE: Renal venous thrombosis complicating acute myeloid leukemia in the hyperleukocytosis. *J Pediatr Hematol Oncol* 18:327, 1996.

348. Cohen Y, Amir G, Da'as N, et al: Acute myocardial infarction as the presenting symptom of acute myeloblastic leukemia with extreme hyperleukocytosis. *Am J Hematol* 71:47, 2002.

349. Zhang W, Zhang X, Fan X, et al: Effect of ICAM-1 and LFA-1 in hyperleukocytic acute myeloid leukaemia. *Clin Lab Haematol* 28:177, 2006.

350. Berdeaux DH, Glosser L, Serokman R: Hypoplastic acute leukemia. Review of 70 cases with multivariate regression analysis. *Hematol Oncol* 4:291, 1986.

351. Tuzuner N, Cox C, Rowe JM, Bennett JM: Hypocellular acute leukemia. *Hematol Pathol* 9:195, 1995.

352. Nagai K, Kohno T, Chen Y-X, et al: Diagnostic criteria for hypocellular acute leukemia. *Leuk Res* 7:563, 1996.

353. Bennett JM, Orazi A: Diagnostic criteria to distinguish hypocellular acute myeloid leukemia from hypocellular myelodysplastic syndromes and aplastic anemia: Recommendations for a standardized approach. *Haematologica* 94:264, 2009.

354. Iwakiri R, Ohta M, Mikoshiba M, et al: Prognosis of elderly patients with acute myelogenous leukemia: Analysis of 126 AML cases. *Int J Hematol* 75:45, 2002.

355. Niissler V, Sauer H, Pelka-Fleischer R, et al: Clinical, biochemical and cytokinetic parameters for distinguishing smouldering and rapidly proliferating variants of acute leukaemia. *Eur J Haematol* 45:19, 1990.

356. Paietta E, Racevskis J, Bennett JM, et al: Biologic heterogeneity in Philadelphia chromosome-positive acute leukemia with myeloid morphology. *Leukemia* 12:1881, 1998.

357. Keung YK, Beaty M, Powell BL, et al: Philadelphia chromosome positive myelodysplastic syndrome and acute myeloid leukemia—Retrospective study and review of literature. *Leuk Res* 28:579, 2004.

358. Saikevych IA, Kerrigan DP, McConnell TS, et al: Multiparameter analysis of acute mixed lineage leukemia: Correlation of a B/myeloid immunophenotype and immunoglobulin and T-cell receptor gene rearrangements with the presence of the Philadelphia chromosome translocation in acute leukemias with myeloid morphology. *Leukemia* 5:373, 1991.

359. Neuman MP, deSolas I, Parkin JL, et al: Monoclonal antibody study of Philadelphia chromosome-positive blastic leukemias using the alkaline phosphatase anti-alkaline phosphatase (APAAP) technique. *Am J Clin Pathol* 85:564, 1986.

360. Cuneo A, Ferrant A, Michaux JL, et al: Philadelphia chromosome-positive acute myeloid leukemia: Cytoimmunologic and cytogenetic features. *Haematologica* 81:423, 1996.

361. Bornstein RS, Nesbit M, Kennedy BJ: Chronic myelogenous leukemia presenting in blast crisis. *Cancer* 30:939, 1972.

362. Peterson LC, Bloomfield CD, Brunning RD: Blast crisis as an initial or terminal manifestation of chronic myeloid leukemia. *Am J Med* 60:209, 1976.

363. Worm AM, Pedersen-Bjergaard J: Chronic myelocytic leukemia presenting in blast transformation. *Scand J Haematol* 18:288, 1977.

364. Kantarjian HM, Talpaz M, Chingra K, et al: Significance of the p210 versus p190 molecular abnormalities in adults with Philadelphia chromosome-positive acute leukemia. *Blood* 78:2411, 1991.

365. Chen SJ, Flandrin G, Daniel M-T, et al: Philadelphia-positive acute leukemia: Lineage promiscuity and inconsistently rearranged breakpoint cluster region. *Leukemia* 2:261, 1988.

366. Price CM, Rassool F, Shivji MK, et al: Rearrangement of the breakpoint cluster region and expression of p210 BCR-ABL in a "masked" Philadelphia chromosome-positive acute myeloid leukemia. *Blood* 72:1829, 1988.

367. Westbrook CA, Hooberman AL, Spino C, et al: Clinical significance of the BCR-ABL fusion gene in adult acute lymphoblastic leukemia: A Cancer and Leukemia Group B study. *Blood* 80:2983, 1992.

368. Lim LC, Heng KK, Vellupillai M, et al: Molecular and phenotypic spectrum of de novo Philadelphia positive acute leukemia. *Int J Mol Med* 4:665, 1999.

369. Vandenberghe E, Martiat P, Baens M, et al: Megakaryoblastic leukemia with an N-ras mutation and late acquisition of a Philadelphia chromosome. *Leukemia* 5:683, 1991.

370. Helenglass G, Testa JR, Schiffer CA: Philadelphia chromosome-positive acute leukemia. *Am J Hematol* 25:311, 1987.

371. Mecucci C, Noens L, Aventin A, et al: Philadelphia-positive acute myelomonocytic leukemia with inversion of chromosome 16 and eosinobasophils. *Am J Hematol* 27:69, 1988.

372. Kurzrock R, Shtalrid M, Talpaz M, et al: Expression of c-abl in Philadelphia-positive acute myelogenous leukemia. *Blood* 70:1584, 1987.

373. Smadja N, Krulik M, DeGramont A, et al: Acquisition of Philadelphia chromosome concomitant with transformation of a refractory anemia into acute leukemia. *Cancer* 55:1477, 1985.

374. Primo D, Tabernero MD, Rasillo A, et al: Patterns of BCR/ABL gene rearrangements by interphase fluorescence *in situ* hybridization (FISH) in BCR/ABL+ leukemia: Incidence and underlying genetic abnormalities. *Leukemia* 17:1124, 2003.

375. Lo Coco F, Basso G, di Celle PF, et al: Molecular characterization of Ph´ + hybrid acute leukemia. *Leuk Res* 13:1061, 1989.

376. Janssens AM, Offner FC, Van Hove WZ: Bone marrow necrosis. *Cancer* 88:1769, 2000.

377. Vermeersch P, Zachee P, Brusselmans C: Acute myeloid leukemia with bone marrow necrosis and Charcot Leyden crystals. *Am J Hematol* 82:1029, 2007.

378. Yumura-Yagi K, Hara J, Talva A, Kawa-Ha K: Phenotypic characteristics of acute megakaryocytic leukemia and transient myelopoiesis. *Leuk Lymphoma* 13:393, 1994.

379. Bhatt S, Schreck R, Graham JM, et al: Transient leukemia with trisomy 21. *Am J Med Genet* 58:310, 1995.

380. Litz CE, Davies S, Brunning RD, et al: Acute leukemia and the transient myeloproliferative disorder associated with Down syndrome: Morphologic immunophenotypic and cytogenetic manifestations. *Leukemia* 9:1432, 1999.

381. Ito E, Kasai M, Hayashi Y, et al: Expression of erythroid-specific genes in acute megakaryoblastic leukaemia and transient myeloproliferative disorder in Down syndrome. *Br J Haematol* 90:607, 1995.

382. Kurukashi H, Junichi H, Keiko Y, et al: Monoclonal nature of transient abnormal myelopoiesis in Down's syndrome. *Blood* 77:1161, 1991.

383. Apollonsky N, Shende A, Ouansafi I, et al: Transient myeloproliferative disorder in neonates with and without Down syndrome: A tale of 2 syndromes. *J Pediatr Hematol Oncol* 30:860, 2008.

384. Muramatsu H, Kato K, Watanabe N, et al: Risk factors for early death in neonates with Down syndrome and transient leukaemia. *Br J Haematol* 142:610, 2008.

385. Gamis AS, Hilden J: Transient myeloproliferative disorder. *J Pediatr Hematol Oncol* 241:2, 2002.

386. Gurbuxani S, Vyas P, Crispino JD: Recent insights into the mechanism of myeloid leukemogenesis in Down syndrome. *Blood* 103:399, 2004.

387. Zipursky A, Poon A, Doyle J: Leukemia in Down syndrome: A review. *Pediatr Hematol Oncol* 9:139, 1992.

388. Creutzig U, Ritter J, Vormoor J, et al: Myelodysplasia and acute myelogenous leukemia in Down's syndrome. *Leukemia* 10:1677, 1996.

389. Avet-Loiseau H, Mechinaud F, Harousseau J-L: Clonal hematologic disorders in Down syndrome. *J Pediatr Hematol Oncol* 17:19, 1995.

390. Taub J, Huang X, Ge Y, et al: Cystathionine-beta-synthase cDNA transfection alters sensitivity and metabolism of 1-beta-D-arabinofuranosylcytosine in CCRF-CEM leukemic cells *in vitro* and *in vivo*: A model of leukemia in Down syndrome. *Cancer Res* 60:6421, 2000.

391. Lange BJ, Kobrinsky N, Barnard DR, et al: Distinctive demography, biology, and outcome of acute myeloid leukemia and myelodysplastic syndrome in children with Down syndrome: Children's Cancer Group Studies 2861 and 2891. *Blood* 91:608, 1998.

392. McCoy JP Jr, Overton WR: Immunophenotyping of congenital leukemia. *Cytometry* 22:85, 1995.

393. Kempski HM, Chessells JM, Reeves BR: Deletions of chromosome 21 restricted to the leukemia cells of children with Down syndrome and leukemia. *Leukemia* 11:1973, 1997.

394. Hama A, Yagasaki H, Takahashi Y, et al: Acute megakaryoblastic leukaemia (AMKL) in children: A comparison of AMKL with and without Down syndrome. *Br J Haematol* 140:552, 2008.

395. Hasle H, Abrahamsson J, Arola M, et al: Myeloid leukemia in children 4 years or older with Down syndrome often lacks GATA1 mutation and cytogenetics and risk of relapse are more akin to sporadic AML. *Leukemia* 22:1428, 2008.

396. Malinge S, Chlon T, Dore LC, et al: Development of acute megakaryoblastic leukemia in Down syndrome is associated with sequential epigenetic changes. *Blood* 122:e33, 2013.

397. Ravindranath Y, Abella E, Kruscher JP, et al: Acute myeloid leukemia (AML) in Down's syndrome is highly responsive to chemotherapy: Experience on Pediatric Oncology Group AML Study 8498. *Blood* 80:2210, 1992.

398. Pui C-H, Kane JR, Crist WM: Biology and treatment of infant leukemias. *Leukemia* 9:762, 1995.

399. Taga T, Salto AM, Kudo K, et al: Clinical characteristics and outcome of refractory/relapsed myeloid leukemia in children with Down syndrome. *Blood* 120:1810, 2012.

400. Lampert F, Harbott J, Ritterbach J: Cytogenetic findings in acute leukaemias of infants. *Br J Cancer Suppl* 18:S20, 1992.

401. Nagasaka M, Maeda S, Maeda H, et al: Four cases of t(4;11) acute leukemia and its myelomonocytic nature in infants. *Blood* 61:1174, 1983.

402. Hunger SP, Cleary ML: What significance should we attribute to the detection of MLL fusion transcripts? *Blood* 92:709, 1998.

403. Bresters D, Reus AC, Veerman AJ, et al: Congenital leukaemia: The Dutch experience and review of the literature. *Br J Haematol* 7:513, 2002.

404. Osada S, Horibe K, Oiwa K, et al: A case of infantile acute monocytic leukemia caused by vertical transmission of the mother's leukemic cells. *Cancer* 65:1146, 1990.

405. Lampkin BC, Peipon JJ, Price JK, et al: Spontaneous remission of presumed congenital acute nonlymphoblastic leukemia (ANLL) in a karyotypically normal neonate. *Am J Pediatr Hematol Oncol* 7:346, 1985.

406. Lauria F, Raspadori D, Ventura MA, et al: The presence of lymphoid-associated antigens in adult acute myeloid leukemia is devoid of prognostic relevance. *Stem Cells* 13:428, 1995.

407. Carbonell F, Swansbury J, Min T, et al: Cytogenetic findings in acute biphenotypic leukaemia. *Leukemia* 10:1283, 1996.

408. Greaves MF, Chan LC, Furley AJ, et al: Lineage promiscuity in hemopoietic differentiation and leukemia. *Blood* 67:1, 1986.

409. Neame PB, Soamboonsrup P, Browman G, et al: Simultaneous or sequential expression of lymphoid and myeloid phenotypes in acute leukemia. *Blood* 65:142, 1985.

410. Scott CS, Vulliamy T, Catovsky D, et al: DNA genotypic conservation during phenotypic switch from T-cell acute lymphoblastic leukaemia to acute myeloblastic leukaemia. *Leuk Lymphoma* 1:21, 1989.

411. Jensen AW, Hokland M, Jorgensen H, et al: Solitary expression of CD 7 among T-cell antigens in acute myeloid leukemia. *Blood* 78:1291, 1991.

412. Ferra F, DelVecchio L: Clinical relevance of acute mixed-lineage leukemia. *Blood* 79:2799, 1992.

413. Miwa H, Nakase K, Kita K: Biological characteristics of CD7(+) acute leukemia. *Leuk Lymphoma* 21:239, 1996.

414. Suzuki R, Yamamoto K, Seto M, et al: CD7+ and CD56+ myeloid/natural killer cell precursor acute leukemia: A distinct hematolymphoid disease entity. *Blood* 90:2417, 1997.

415. Scott AA, Head DR, Kropecky KJ, et al: HLA-DR–, CD33+, CD56+, CD16– myeloid/natural killer cell acute leukemia. *Blood* 84:244, 1994.

416. Paietta E, Gallagher RE, Wiernik PH: Myeloid/natural killer cell acute leukemia. *Blood* 84:2824, 1994.

417. Lee PS, Lin CN, Liu C, et al: Acute leukemia with myeloid, B-, and natural killer cell differentiation. *Arch Pathol Lab Med* 127:E93, 2003.

418. Handa H, Motohashi S, Isozumi K, et al: CD7+ and CD56+ myeloid/natural killer cell precursor acute leukemia treated with idarubicin and cytosine arabinoside. *Acta Haematol* 108:47, 2001.

419. Oshimi K: Progress in understanding and managing natural killer-cell malignancies. *Br J Haematol* 139:532, 2007.

420. Inhorn RC, Aster JC, Roach SA, et al: A syndrome of lymphoblastic lymphoma, eosinophilia, and myeloid hyperplasia malignancy associated with t(8;13) (p11;q11): Description of a distinctive clinical entity. *Blood* 85:1881, 1995.

421. Still IH, Chernova O, Hurd D, et al: Molecular characterization of the t(8;13) (p11;q12) translocation associated with an atypical myeloproliferative disorder: Evidence for three discrete loci involved in myeloid leukemias on 8 p11. *Blood* 90:3136, 1997.

422. Ogura K, Kimura F, Kobayashi S, et al: Myeloid/NK cell precursor acute leukemia lost both CD13 and CD33 at first diagnosis. *Leuk Res* 30:761, 2006.

423. Suzuki R, Suzumiya J, Nakamura S, et al: NK-cell Tumor Study Group. Hematopoietic stem cell transplantation for natural killer-cell lineage neoplasms. *Bone Marrow Transplant* 37:425, 2006.

424. Mirro J, Kitchingman GR, Williams DL, Murphy SB: Mixed lineage leukemia: The implication for hemopoietic differentiation [letter]. *Blood* 68:597, 1986.

425. Ladanyi M, Samaniego F, Reuter VE, et al: Cytogenetic and immunohistochemical evidence for the germ cell origin of a subset of acute leukemias associated with mediastinal germ cell tumors. *J Natl Cancer Inst* 82:221, 1990.

426. DeMent, CR, Roth BJ, Heerema N, et al: Hematologic neoplasia associated with primary mediastinal germ-cell tumors. *Hum Pathol* 21:699, 1990.

427. Nichols CR, Roth BJ, Heerema N, et al: Hematologic neoplasia associated with primary mediastinal germ-cell tumors. *N Engl J Med* 322:1425, 1990.

428. Kiffer JD, Sandeman TF: Primary malignant mediastinal germ cell tumors: A study of eleven cases and a review of the literature. *Int J Radiat Oncol Biol Phys* 17:835, 1990.

429. Nichols CR: Mediastinal germ cell tumors: Clinical features and biologic correlates. *Chest* 99:472, 1991.

430. Brahmanday GR, Gheorghe G, Jaiyesimi IA, et al: Primary mediastinal germ cell tumor evolving into an extramedullary acute megakaryoblastic leukemia causing cord compression. *J Clin Oncol* 26:4686, 2008.

431. Kollmannsberger C, Beyer J, Droz JP, et al: Secondary leukemia following high cumulative doses of etoposide in patients treated for advanced germ cell tumors. *J Clin Oncol* 16:3386, 1998.

432. Miettinen M, Kraszewska E, Sobin LH, Lasota J: A nonrandom association between gastrointestinal stromal tumors and myeloid leukemia. *Cancer* 112:645, 2008.

433. Miyazato H, Sono H, Nasiki Y, et al: Detection of myeloperoxidase gene expression by in situ hybridization in a case of granulocytic sarcoma associated with AML-M0. *Leukemia* 14:1797, 2001.

434. Testa U, Torelli GF, Riccioni R, et al: Human acute stem cell leukemia with multilineage differentiation potential via cascade activation of growth factor receptors. *Blood* 99:4534, 2002.

435. Cuneo A, Ferrant A, Michaux JL, et al: Cytogenetic profile of minimally differentiated (FAB M0) acute myeloid leukemia: Correlation with clinicobiologic findings. *Blood* 85:3688, 1995.

436. Venditti A, Del Poeta G, Buccisano F, et al: Minimally differentiated acute myeloid leukemia (AML M0): Comparison of 25 cases with other French-American-British subtypes. *Blood* 89:621, 1997.

437. Villamor N, Zarco M-A, Rozman M, et al: Acute myeloblastic leukemia with minimal myeloid differentiation: Phenotypical and ultrastructural characteristics. *Leukemia* 12:1071, 1998.

438. Roumier C, Eclache V, Imbert M, et al: M0 AML, clinical and biologic features of the disease, including *AML1* gene mutations. *Blood* 101:1277, 2003.

439. Maruyami F, Stass SA, Estey EH, et al: Detection of AML1/ETO fusion transcript as a tool for diagnosing t(8;21) positive acute myelogenous leukemia. *Leukemia* 8:40, 1994.

440. Schoch C, Haase D, Haferlach T, et al: Fifty-one patients with acute myeloid leukemia and translocation t(8;21) (q22; q22): An additional deletion in 9q is an adverse prognostic factor. *Leukemia* 10:1288, 1996.

441. Wang J, Wang M, Liu JM: Transformation properties of the ETO gene, fusion partner in t(8;21) leukemias. *Cancer Res* 57:2951, 1997.

442. Watkins CH, Hall BE: Monocytic leukemia of the Naegeli and Schilling types. *Am J Clin Pathol* 10:387, 1940.

443. Huhn D, Twardzik L: Acute myelomonocytic leukemia and the French-American-British classification. *Acta Haematol* 69:36, 1983.

444. Scott CS, Morgan M, Limbert HJ, et al: Cytochemical, immunological and ANAE-isoenzyme studies in acute myelomonocytic leukaemia: A study of 39 cases. *Scand J Haematol* 35:284, 1985.

445. Bloomfield CD, Garson OM, Violin L, et al: t(1;3)(p36; q21) in acute nonlymphocytic leukemia: A new cytogenetic-clinicopathologic association. *Blood* 66:1409, 1985.

446. Creictzig U, Niederbiermann G, Kitter J, et al: Prognostic significance of eosinophilia in acute myelomonocytic leukemia in relation to induction treatment. *Haematol Blood Transfus* 33:226, 1990.

447. Hoyle CF, Sherrington PD, Fischer P, Hayhoe FGT: Basophils in acute leukemia. *J Clin Pathol* 42:785, 1989.

448. Pearson MG, Vardiman JW, LeBeau MM, et al: Increased numbers of marrow basophils may be associated with t(6;9) in ANLL. *Am J Hematol* 18:393, 1985.

449. Alsabeh R, Byrnes RK, Slovak ML, Arber DA: Acute myeloid leukemia with t(6;9) (p23;q34): Association with myelodysplasia, basophilia, and initial CD34 negative phenotype. *Am J Clin Pathol* 107:430, 1997.

450. Copelli M: Di una emopatia sistemizzata rappresentata da una iperplasia eritroblastica (eritromatosi). *Path Riv Quindicin* 4:460, 1912.

451. DiGuglielmo G: Richerche di hematologia: I. Una casa di eritroleucemia. *Folia Med* 13:386, 1917.

452. Moeschlin S: Erythroblastosen, erythroleukemien und erythroblastamien. *Folia Haematol (Frankf)* 64:262, 1940.

453. Dameshek W: The Di Guglielmo syndrome. *Blood* 13:192, 1940.

454. Fouillard L, Labopin M, Gorin N-C, et al: Hematopoietic stem cell transplantation for de novo erythroleukemia: A study of the European Group for Blood and Marrow Transplantation (EBMT). *Blood* 100:3135, 2002.

455. Novick Y, Marino P, Makower DF, Wiernik PH: Familial erythroleukemia: A distinct clinical and genetic type of familial leukemia. *Leuk Lymphoma* 80:395, 1998.

456. Lee EJ, Schiffer CA, Misawa S, Testa JR: Clinical and cytogenetic features of familial erythroleukaemia. *Br J Haematol* 65:313, 1987.

457. Cuneo A, VanOrshoven A, Michaux JL, et al: Morphologic, immunologic and cytogenetic studies in erythroleukemia: Evidence for multilineage involvement and identification of two distinct cytogenetic clinicopathologic types. *Br J Haematol* 75:346, 1990.

458. Goldberg SL, Noel P, Klumpp TR, Dewald GW: The erythroid leukemias. *Am J Clin Oncol* 21:42, 1998.

459. Olopade OI, Thangavelu M, Larson RA, et al: Clinical, morphologic, and cytogenetic characteristics of 26 patients with acute erythroblastic leukemia. *Blood* 80:2873, 1992.

460. Davey FR, Abraham N Jr, Bronetto VL, et al: Morphologic characteristics of erythroleukemia (Acute myeloid leukemia; FAB-M6): A CALGB study. *Am J Hematol* 49:29, 1995.

461. Adamson JW, Finch CA: Erythropoietin and the regulation of erythropoiesis in di Guglielmo's syndrome. *Blood* 36:590, 1970.

462. Mitjavila MT, Villeval JL, Cramer P, et al: Effects of granulocyte-macrophage colony-stimulating factor and erythropoietin on leukemic erythroid colony formation in human early erythroblastic leukemia. *Blood* 70:965, 1987.

463. Mazella FM, Kowel-Vern A, Shrit MA, et al: Acute erythroleukemia evaluation of 48 cases with reference to classification, cell proliferation, cytogenetics, and prognosis. *Am J Clin Pathol* 110:590, 1998.

464. Breton-Gorius J: Phenotypes of blasts in acute erythroblastic and megakaryoblastic leukemia—A review. *Keio J Med* 36:23, 1987.

465. Peterson BA, Levine EG: Uncommon subtypes of acute nonlymphocytic leukemia: Clinical features and management of FAB M5, M6 and M7. *Semin Oncol* 14:425, 1987.

466. Croizat P, Favre-Gilly J: Les aspects du syndrome hémorrhagiue des leucémies. *Sang* 20:417, 1949.

467. Hillstad LK: Acute promyelocytic leukemia. *Acta Med Scand* 159:189, 1957.

468. LoCoco F, Nervi C, Avvisati G, Mandelli F: Acute promyelocytic leukemia: A curable disease. *Leukemia* 12:1866, 1998.

469. Avvisati G, Lo Coco F, Mandelli F: Acute promyelocytic leukemia: Clinical and morphological features and prognostic factors. *Semin Hematol* 38:4, 2001.

470. Estey E, Thall P, Kantarjian H, et al: Association between increased body mass index and a diagnosis of acute promyelocytic leukemia in patients with acute myeloid leukemia. *Leukemia* 11:1661, 1997.

471. Wong O, Harris F, Yiying W, Hua F: A hospital-based case-control study of acute myeloid leukemia in Shanghai: Analysis of personal characteristics, lifestyle and environmental risk factors by subtypes of the WHO classification. *Regul Toxicol Pharmacol* 55:340, 2009

472. Elliott MA(1), Letendre L, Tefferi A, et al: Therapy-related acute promyelocytic leukemia: Observations relating to APL pathogenesis and therapy. *Eur J Haematol* 88:237, 2012.

473. Golomb HM, Rowley JD, Vardiman J, et al: "Microgranular" acute promyelocytic leukemia: A distinct clinical, ultrastructural, and cyto-genetic entity. *Blood* 55:253, 1980.

474. McKenna RW, Parkin J, Bloomfield C, et al: Acute promyelocytic leukaemia: A study of 39 cases with identification of a hyperbasophilic microgranular variant. *Br J Haematol* 50:201, 1982.

475. Rovelli A, Biondi A, Rajnoldi AC, et al: Microgranular variant of acute promyelocytic leukemia in children. *J Clin Oncol* 10:1413, 1992.

476. Castoldi GL, Liso V, Speechia G, Thomasi P: Acute promyelocytic leukemia: Morphological aspects. *Leukemia* 8(Suppl 2):S27, 1994.

477. Umeda M, Nojima Z, Yamaguchi R, et al: Two cases of acute promyelocytic leukemia with marked basophilia—A variant type of APL with the capability of differentiating into basophils. *Rinsho Ketsueki* 28:2004, 1987.

478. Gotoh H, Murakani S, Oku N, et al: Translocation t(15;17) and t(9;14) (q34;q22) in a case of acute promyelocytic leukemia with increased number of basophils. *Cancer Genet Cytogenet* 36:103, 1988.

479. Yu RQ, Huang W, Chen SJ, et al: A case of acute eosinophilic granulocytic leukemia with PML-RAR alpha fusion gene expression and response to all-*trans* retinoic acid. *Leukemia* 11:609, 1997.

480. Invernizzi R, Iannone AM, Bernuzzi S, et al: Acute promyelocytic leukemia toluidine blue subtype. *Leuk Lymphoma* 18(Suppl 1):57, 1995.

481. Rowley JD, Golomb HM, Dogherty C: 15/17 translocation, a consistent chromosomal change in acute promyelocytic leukaemia. *Lancet* 1:549, 1977.

482. Lavau C, Dejean A: The t(15;17) translocation in acute promyelocytic leukemia. *Leukemia* 8:1615, 1994.

483. Chen Y, Li S, Zhou C, et al: TBLR1 fuses to retinoid acid receptor α in a variant t(3;17) (q26;q21) translocation of acute promyelocytic leukemia. *Blood* 124:936, 2014.

484. Sainty D, Liso V, Cantu-Rajnoldi A, et al: A new morphologic classification system for acute promyelocytic leukemia distinguishes cases with underlying PLZF/RARA gene rearrangements. *Blood* 96:1287, 2000.

485. Petti MC, Fazi F, Gentile M, et al: Complete remission through blast cell differentiation in PLZF/RARα-positive acute promyelocytic leukemia: In vitro and in vivo studies. *Blood* 100:1065, 2002.

486. de Thé H, Chomienne C, Lanotte M, et al: The t(15;17) translocation of acute promyelocytic leukaemia fuses the retinoic acid receptor alpha gene to a novel transcribed locus. *Nature* 347:558, 1990.

487. Huang W, Sun GL, Li XS, et al: Acute promyelocytic leukemia: Clinical relevance of two major PML-RAR alpha isoforms and detection of minimal residual disease by retrotranscriptase/polymerase chain reaction to predict relapse. *Blood* 82:1264, 1993.

488. Rego EM, Pandolfi PP: Analysis of molecular genetics of acute promyelocytic leukemia in mouse models. *Semin Hematol* 38:54, 2001.

489. Dombret H, Scrobohaci ML, Ghorra P, et al: Coagulation disorder associated with acute promyelocytic leukemia: Correct effect of all-*trans* retinoic acid. *Leukemia* 7:2, 1993.

490. Tallman MS, Kwaan HC: Reassessing the hemostatic disorder associated with acute promyelocytic leukemia. *Blood* 79:543, 1992.

491. Barbui T, Finazzi G, Falanga A: The impact of all-*trans* retinoic acid on the coagulopathy of acute promyelocytic leukemia. *Blood* 91:3093, 1998.

492. Menell JS, Cesarman GM, Jacovina AT, et al: Annexin II and bleeding in acute promyelocytic leukemia. *N Engl J Med* 340:994, 1999.

493. Avvisati G, Ten Cate JW, Büller H, Mandelli F: Tranexamic acid for control of haemorrhage in patients with acute promyelocyte leukaemia. *Lancet* 2:122, 1989.

494. Tallman MS, Abutalib SA, Altman JK: The double hazard of thrombophilia and bleeding in acute promyelocytic leukemia. *Semin Thromb Hemost* 33:330, 2007.

495. Fenaux P, Tertian G, Castaigne S, et al: A randomized trial of amsacrine and rubidazone on 39 patients with acute promyelocytic leukemia. *J Clin Oncol* 9:1556, 1991.

496. Craddock CG, Crandall BF, Como R: Restoration of effective hemopoiesis preceding suppression of leukemia clone in myeloblastic leukemia. *Am J Med* 59:737, 1975.

497. Amato R, Kantarjian H, Walter R, Keating M: Rebound peripheral blastosis with subsequent remission during induction in a patient with acute promyelocytic leukemia. *Cancer* 61:650, 1988.

498. Stone RM, Maguire M, Goldberg MA, et al: Complete remission in acute promyelocytic leukemia despite persistence of abnormal marrow promyelocytes during induction therapy: Experience in 34 patients. *Blood* 71:690, 1988.

499. Breitman TR, Collins SJ, Keene BR: Terminal differentiation of human promyelocytic leukemic cells in primary culture in response to retinoic acid. *Blood* 57:1000, 1981.

500. Huang ME, Ye YC, Chen SR, et al: Use of all-*trans* retinoic acid in the treatment of acute promyelocytic leukemia. *Blood* 72:567, 1988.

501. Wu X, Wang X, Qen X, et al: Four years' experience with treatment of all-*trans* retinoic acid in acute promyelocytic leukemia. *Am J Hematol* 43:183, 1993.

502. Lobe I, Regal-Huguet FR, Vekhoff A, et al: Myelodysplastic syndrome after acute promyelocytic leukemia: The European APLK group experience. *Leukemia* 17:1600, 2003.

503. Garcia-Manero G, Kantarjian HM, Kornblau S, Estey E: Therapy-related myelodysplastic syndrome or acute myelogenous leukemia in patients with acute promyelocytic leukemia. *Leukemia* 17:1888, 2002.

504. Reschad H, Schilling-Torgau V: Ueber eine neue Leukämie durch echte Uebergangsformen (Splenozyten-leukämie) und ihre Bedeutung für die Selbstständigkeit dieser Zellen. *Munch Med Wochenschr* 60:1981, 1913.

505. Straus DJ, Mertelsmann R, Koziner B, et al: The acute monocytic leukemias. *Medicine (Baltimore)* 59:409, 1980.

506. Janvier M, Tobelem G, Daniel MT, et al: Acute monoblastic leukaemia. Clinical, biological data and survival in 45 cases. *Scand J Haematol* 32:385, 1984.

507. Finaux P, Vanhaesbroucke C, Estienne MH, et al: Acute monocytic leukaemia in adults: Treatment and prognosis in 99 cases. *Br J Haematol* 75:41, 1990.

508. Fung H, Shepard JD, Naiman SC, et al: Acute monocytic leukemia: A single institution experience. *Leuk Lymphoma* 19:259, 1995.

509. Cuttner J, Conjalka MS, Reilly M, et al: Association of monocyte leukemia in patients with extreme leukocytosis. *Am J Med* 69:555, 1980.

510. Jourdan E, Dombret H, Glaisner S, et al: Unexpected high incidence of intracranial subdural haematoma during intensive chemotherapy for acute myeloid leukaemia with a monoblastic component. *Br J Haematol* 89:527, 1995.

511. Scott CS, Stark AN, Limbert HJ, et al: Diagnostic and prognostic factors in acute monocytic leukemia: An analysis of 51 cases. *Br J Haematol* 69:247, 1988.

512. Scherrer A, Kruithof EK, Grob JP: Plasminogen activator inhibitor-2 in patients with monocytic leukemia. *Leukemia* 5:479, 1991.

513. van Furth R, van Zwet TL: Cytochemical, functional, and proliferative characteristics of promonocytes and monocytes from patients with monocytic leukemia. *Blood* 62:298, 1983.

514. van Furth R, Leijh PCJ, van Zwet TL, van den Barselaar MT: Phagocytic and intracellular killing by peripheral blood monocytes of patients with monocytic leukemia. *Blood* 59:1234, 1982.

515. Diaz MO, LeBeau MM, Pitha P, Rowley JD: Interferon and *c-est*-1 genes in the translocation (9;11)(p22;q23) in human acute monocytic leukemia. *Science* 231:265, 1986.

516. Mavilo F, Testa U, Sposi NM, et al: Selective expression of *fos* protooncogene in human acute myelomonocytic and monocytic leukemias: A molecular marker of terminal differentiation. *Blood* 69:160, 1987.

517. Pinto A, Colletta G, DeVecchio L, et al: *C-fos* oncogene expression in human hemopoietic malignancies is restricted to acute leukemias with monocytic phenotype and to subsets of B cell leukemias. *Blood* 70:1450, 1987.

518. Weide R, Parviz B, Pflüger K-H, Haveman K: Altered expression of the human retinoblastoma gene in monocytic leukaemias. *Br J Haematol* 83:428, 1993.

519. Cuttner J, Seremetis S, Najfield V, et al: TdT-positive acute leukemia with monocytoid characteristics: Clinical, cytochemical, cytogenetic, and immunologic findings. *Blood* 64:237, 1984.

520. Sun T, Wu E: Acute monoblastic leukemia with t(8;16): A distinct clinicopathologic entity. *Am J Hematol* 66:207, 2001.

521. Santiago-Schwarz F, Coppock DL, Hindenburg A, Kern J: Identification of a malignant counterpart of the monocytic-dendritic cell progenitor in acute myeloid leukemia. *Blood* 84:3054, 1994.

522. Pileri SA, Grogan TM, Harris NL, et al: Tumors of histiocytes and accessory dendritic cells: An immunohistochemical approach to classification from the International Lymphoma Study Group based on 61 cases. *Histopathology* 41:1, 2002.

523. Elghetany MT: True histiocytic lymphoma: Is it an entity? *Leukemia* 11:762, 1997.

524. Esteve J, Rozman M, Campo E, et al: Leukemia after true histiocytic lymphoma: Another type of acute monocytic leukemia with histiocytic differentiation (AML-M5c). *Leukemia* 9:1389, 1995.

525. Tallman MS, Kim HT, Paietta E, et al: Acute monocytic leukemia (French-American-British classification M5) does not have a worse prognosis than other subtypes of acute myeloid leukemia: Report from the Eastern Cooperative Group. *J Clin Oncol* 22:1276, 2004.

526. Lewis SM, Szur L: Malignant myelosclerosis. *Br Med J* 2:472, 1963.

527. Bergsman KL, VanSlyck EJ: Acute myelofibrosis. *Ann Intern Med* 74:232, 1971.

528. Huang MJ, Li CY, Nichols WL, et al: Acute leukemia with megakaryocytic differentiation. A study of twelve cases identified immunocytochemically. *Blood* 64:427, 1984.

529. Gassman W, Löffler H: Acute megakaryoblastic leukemia. *Leuk Lymphoma* 18:69, 1995.

530. Cripe LD, Hromas R: Malignant disorders of megakaryocytes. *Semin Hematol* 35:200, 1998.

531. Paredes-Aguilera R, Romero-Guzman L, Lopez-Santiago N, Trejo RA: Biological, clinical, and hematological features of acute megakaryoblastic leukemia in children. *Am J Hematol* 73:71, 2003.

532. Zipursky A, Brown E, Christensen H, et al: Leukemia and/or myeloproliferative syndrome in neonates with Down syndrome. *Semin Perinatol* 21:97, 1997.

533. Hussein K, Bock O, Theophile K, et al: MPL(W515L) mutation in acute megakaryoblastic leukaemia. *Leukemia* 23:852, 2009.

534. Dastugue N, Lafage-Pochitaloff M, Pages MP, et al: Cytogenetic profile of childhood and adult megakaryoblastic leukemia (M7): A study of the Groupe Francais de Cytogenetique Hematologique (GFCH). *Blood* 100:618, 2002.

535. Carroll A, Civin C, Schneider N, et al: The t(1;22)(p13;q13) is non-random and restricted to infants with acute megakaryoblastic leukemia: A pediatric oncology group study. *Blood* 78:748, 1991.

536. Duchayne F, Fenneteau O, Pages MP, et al: Acute megakaryoblastic leukaemia: A national clinical and biological study of adult and childhood cases by the Group Francais d'Hematologie Cellulaire (GFHC). *Leuk Lymphoma* 44:49, 2003.

537. Bernstein J, Dastugue N, Haas OA, et al: Nineteen cases of the t(1;22)(p13;q13) acute megakaryoblastic leukaemia of infants/children and a review of 39 cases: Report from a t(1;22) study group. *Leukemia* 14:216, 2000.

538. Cuneo A, Mecucci C, Kerim S, et al: Multipotent stem cell involvement in megakaryoblastic leukemia: Cytologic and cytogenetic evidence in 15 patients. *Blood* 74:1781, 1989.

539. Dhyashiki K, Ohyashiki JH, Hojo H, et al: Cytogenetic findings in adult acute leukemia in myeloproliferative disorders with an involvement of megakaryocytic lineage. *Cancer* 65:940, 1990.

540. Kojima S, Sako M, Kato K, et al: An effective chemotherapeutic regimen for acute myeloid leukemia and myelodysplastic syndrome in children with Down's syndrome. *Leukemia* 14:786, 2000.

541. Athale UH, Razzouk BI, Raimondi SC, et al: Biology and outcome of childhood acute megakaryoblastic leukemia: A single institution's experience. *Blood* 97:3727, 2001.

542. Yamada S, Hongo T, Okada S, et al: Distinctive multidrug sensitivity and outcome of acute erythroblastic and megakaryoblastic leukemia in children with Down syndrome. *Int J Hematol* 74:428, 2001.

543. Tallman MS, Neuberg D, Bennett JM, et al: Acute megakaryocytic leukemia: The Eastern Cooperative Group experience. *Blood* 96:2405, 2000.

544. Pagano L, Pulsoni A, Vignetti M, et al: Acute megakaryoblastic leukemia: Experience of GIMEMA trial. *Leukemia* 16:1622, 2002.

545. Stillman RG: A case of myeloid leukemia with predominance of eosinophilic cells. *Med Rec* 81:594, 1912.

546. Harrington DS, Peterson C, Ness M, et al: Acute myelogenous leukemia with eosinophilic differentiation. *Am J Clin Pathol* 90:464, 1988.

547. Kueck BD, Smith RE, Parkin J, et al: Eosinophilic leukemia: A myeloproliferative disorder distinct from the hypereosinophilic syndrome. *Hematol Pathol* 5:195, 1991.

548. Sanada I, Asou N, Kajima S, et al: Acute myelogenous leukemia (FABM1) associated with t(5;16) and eosinophilia. *Cancer Genet Cytogenet* 43:139, 1989.

549. Lichtman MA, Segel GB: Uncommon phenotypes of acute myelogenous leukemia: Basophilic, mast cell, eosinophilic, and myeloid dendritic cell subtypes: A review. *Blood Cells Mol Dis* 35:370, 2005.

550. Gabbas AG, Li CF: Acute non-lymphocytic leukemia with eosinophilic differentiation. *Am J Hematol* 21:29, 1986.

551. Brito-Babapulle F: Clonal eosinophilic disorders and the hypereosinophilic syndrome. *Blood Rev* 11:129, 1997.

552. Menssen HD, Renkl H-J, Rieder H, et al: Distinction of eosinophilic leukemia from idiopathic hypereosinophilic syndrome by analysis of Wilms tumor gene expression. *Br J Haematol* 101:325, 1998.

553. Joachim G: Über mastzellenleukämien. *Dtsch Arch Klin Med* 87:437, 1906.

554. Goh KO, Anderson FW: Cytogenetic studies in basophilic chronic myelocytic leukemia. *Arch Pathol Lab Med* 193:288, 1979.

555. Shvidel L, Shaft D, Stark B, et al: Acute basophilic leukaemia: Eight unsuspected new cases diagnosed by electron microscopy. *Br J Haematol* 120:774, 2003.

556. Yokohama A, Tsukamoto N, Hatsumi N, et al: Acute basophilic leukemia lacking basophil-specific antigens: The importance of cytokine receptor expression in differential diagnosis. *Int J Hematol* 75:309, 2002.

557. Kubota M, Akiyama Y, Tabata Y, et al: Acute nonlymphocytic leukemia with basophilic differentiation and t(9;11)(p22;q23) in a child. *Am J Hematol* 31:133, 1989.

558. Mezger J, Permanetter W, Gerhartz H, et al: Philadelphia chromosome–negative acute hematopoietic malignancy: Ultrastructural, cytochemical, and immunocytochemical evidence of mast cell and basophil differentiation. *Leuk Res* 14:169, 1990.

559. Duchayne E, Demur C, Rubie H, et al: Diagnosis of acute basophilic leukemia. *Leuk Lymphoma* 32:269, 1999.

560. Petersen LC, Parkin JL, Arthur DC, Brunning RD: Acute basophilic leukemia. A clinical, morphologic, and cytogenetic study of eight cases. *Am J Clin Pathol* 96:160, 1991.

561. Kubonishi I, Fijishita M, Niiya K, et al: Basophilic differentiation in acute promyelocytic leukaemia. *Nippon Ketsueki Gakkai Zasshi* 48:1390, 1985.

562. Pardanani AD, Morice WG, Hoyer JD, Tefferi A: Chronic basophilic leukemia: A distinct clinico-pathologic entity. *Eur J Haematol* 71:18, 2003.

563. Travis WD, Li C-Y, Hoaglan HC, et al: Mast cell leukemia. Report of a case and review of the literature. *Mayo Clin Proc* 61:957, 1986.

564. Beghini A, Cairoli R, Morra E, Larizza L: *In vivo* differentiation of mast cells from acute myeloid leukemia blasts carrying a novel activating ligand-independent c-Kit mutation. *Blood Cells Mol Dis* 24:262, 1998.

565. Sperr WR, Horny HP, Lechner K, Valent P: Clinical and biological diversity of leukemias occurring in patients with mastocytosis. *Leuk Lymphoma* 37:473, 2000.

566. Fukuda T, Kakihara T, Kamishima T, et al: Leukemic cell membrane from acute myelogenous leukemias with massive mast cell infiltration has a mast celldifferentiation activity under culture condition containing interleukin 3. *Leuk Res* 18:749, 1994.

567. Valent P, Sperr WR, Samorapoompichit P, et al: Myelomastocytic overlap syndromes: Biology, criteria, and relationship to mastocytosis. *Leuk Res* 25:595, 2001.

568. Levine PH, Weintraub LR: Pseudoleukemia during recovery from dapsone-induced agranulocytosis. *Ann Intern Med* 68:1060, 1968.

569. Sanal SM, Campbell EW, Bowdler AJ, Brat PJ: Pseudoleukemia. *Postgrad Med* 65:143, 1979.

570. Dreskin SC, Iberti TJ, Watson-Williams EJ: Pseudoleukemia due to infection. *J Med* 14:147, 1983.

571. Lanham GR, Dahl GV, Billings FT, Stass SA: *Pseudomonas aeruginosa* infection with marrow suppression simulating acute promyelocytic leukemia. *Am J Clin Pathol* 80:404, 1983.

572. Orchard PJ, Moffet HL, Hafez R, Sondel PM: Pseudomonas sepsis simulating acute promyelocytic leukemia. *Pediatr Infect Dis J* 7:66, 1988.

573. Reykdal S, Sham R, Phatak P, Kouides P: Pseudoleukemia following the use of G-CSF. *Am J Hematol* 49:258, 1995.

574. Innes DJ, Hess CE, Bertholf MF, Wade P: Promyelocyte morphology: Differentiation of acute promyelocytic leukemia from benign myeloid proliferations. *Am J Clin Pathol* 88:725, 1987.

575. Ahmed MA: Promyelocytic leukaemoid reaction: An atypical presentation of mycobacterial infection. *Acta Haematol* 85:143, 1991.

576. Sekeres MA, Elson P, Kalaycio ME: Time from diagnosis to treatment initiation predicts survival in younger, but not older, acute myeloid leukemia patients. *Blood* 113:28, 2009.

577. Rodriguez CP, Baz R, Jawde RA, et al: Impact of socioeconomic status and distance from treatment center on survival in patients receiving remission induction therapy for newly diagnosed acute myeloid leukemia. *Leuk Res* 32:413, 2008.

578. Wedding U, Röhrig B, Klippstein A, et al: Impairment in functional status and survival in patients with acute myeloid leukaemia. *J Cancer Res Clin Oncol* 132:665, 2006.

579. Karthaus M, Doellmann T, Klimasch T, et al: Central venous catheter infections in patients with acute leukemia. *Chemotherapy* 48:154, 2002.

580. Hummel M, Duchheidt D, Reiter S, et al: Successful treatment of hyperuricemia with low doses of recombinant urate oxidase in four patients with hematologic malignancy and tumor lysis syndrome. *Leukemia* 17:2542, 2003.

581. Lo Coco F, Pelicci PG, D'Adamo F, et al: Polyclonal hematopoietic reconstitution in leukemia patients in remission after suppression of specific gene rearrangements. *Blood* 82:606, 1993.

582. Lichtman MA: The stem cell in the pathogenesis and treatment of myelogenous leukemia. *Leukemia* 15:1489, 2001.

583. Sanz MA, Jarque I, Martin G, et al: Acute promyelocytic leukemia. *Cancer* 6:7, 1988.

584. Hiddemann W, Spiekermann K, Buske C, et al: Towards a pathogenesis-oriented therapy of acute myeloid leukemia. *Crit Rev Oncol Hematol* 56:235, 2005.

585. Cheson BD, Bennett JM, Kopecky KJ, et al: Revised recommendations of the International Working Group for Diagnosis, Standards for Therapeutic Trials in Acute Myeloid Leukemia. *J Clin Oncol* 21:4642, 2003.

586. Fey M, Dreyling M: ESMO Guidelines Working Group: Acute myeloblastic leukemia in adult patients: ESMO clinical recommendations for diagnosis, treatment and follow-up. *Ann Oncol* 19 Suppl 2:ii58, 2008.

587. O'Donnell MR, Abboud CN, Altman J, et al: Acute myeloid leukemia. *J Natl Compr Canc Netw* 10:984, 1012, 2012.

588. Wiernik PH, Banks PLC, Case DC Jr, et al: Cytarabine plus idarubicin or daunorubicin as induction and consolidation therapy for previously untreated adult patients with acute myeloid leukemia. *Blood* 79:313, 1992.

589. Flasshove M, Meusers P, Schutte J, et al: Long-term survival after induction therapy with idarubicin and cytosine arabinoside for de novo acute myeloid leukemia. *Ann Hematol* 79:533, 2000.

590. Hargrave RM, Davey MW, Davey RA, Kidman AD: Development of drug resistance in reduced idarubicin relative to other anthracyclines. *Anticancer Drugs* 6:432, 1995.

591. Feldman EJ: High-dose mitoxantrone in acute leukaemia: New York Medical College experience. *Eur J Cancer Care (Engl)* 6:27, 1997.

592. Fernandez HF, Sun Z, Yao X, et al: Anthracycline dose intensification in acute myeloid leukemia. *N Engl J Med* 361:1249, 2009.

593. Lowenberg B, Ossenkoppele GJ, van Putten W, et al: High-dose daunorubicin in older patients with acute myeloid leukemia. *N Engl J Med* 361:1235, 2009.

594. Kern W, Estey EH: High-dose cytosine arabinoside in the treatment of acute myeloid leukemia: Review of three randomized trials. *Cancer* 107:116, 2006.

595. Gardin C, Chevret S, Pautas C, et al: Superior long-term outcome with idarubicin compared with high-dose daunorubicin in patients with acute myeloid leukemia age 50 years and older. *J Clin Oncol* 31:321, 2012.

596. Ohtake S, Miyawaki S, Fujita H, et al: Randomized study of induction therapy comparing standard-dose idarubicin with high-dose daunorubicin in adult patients with previously untreated acute myeloid leukemia: The JALSG AML201 study. *Blood* 117:358, 2011.

597. NCCN Guidelines Version 2.2014 Acute Myeloid Leukemia. http://www.nccn.org/professionals/physician_gls/f_guidelines.asp. Last accessed July 2015.

598. Woodlock TJ, Lifton R, DiSalle M: Coincident acute myelogenous leukemia and ischemic heart disease: Use of the cardioprotectant dexrazoxane during induction chemotherapy. *Am J Hematol* 59:246, 1998.

599. Kern W, Estey EH: High-dose cytosine arabinoside in the treatment of acute myeloid leukemia: Review of three randomized trials. *Cancer* 107:116, 2006.

600. Lowenberg B, Pabst T, Vellenga E, et al: Cytarabine dose for acute myeloid leukemia. *N Engl J Med* 264:1027, 2011.

601. Burnett AK, Russell NH, Hills RK, et al: Optimization of chemotherapy for younger patients with acute myeloid leukemia: Results of the medial research council AML15 trial. *J Clin Oncol* 31:3360, 2013.

602. Willemze R, Suciu S, Meloni G, et al: High-dose cytarabine in induction treatment improves the outcome of adult patients younger than age 46 years with acute myeloid leukemia: Results of the EORTC-GIMEMA AML-12 trial. *J Clin Oncol* 32:219, 2013.

603. Stein AS, O'Donnell MR, Slovak ML, et al: High-dose cytosine arabinoside and daunorubicin induction therapy for adult patients with de novo non M3 acute myelogenous leukemia: Impact of cytogenetics on achieving a complete remission. *Leukemia* 14:1191, 2000.

604. Mehta J, Powles R, Treleaven J, et al: The impact of karyotype on remission rates in adult patients with de novo acute myeloid leukemia receiving high-dose cytarabine-based induction chemotherapy. *Leuk Lymphoma* 34:553, 1999.

605. Archimbaud E, Thomas X, Leblond V, et al: Timed sequential chemotherapy for previously treated patients with acute myeloid leukemia: Long-term follow-up of the etoposide, mitoxantrone, and cytarabine-86 trial. *J Clin Oncol* 13:11, 1995.

606. Archimbaud E, Leblond V, Fenaux P, et al: Timed sequential chemotherapy for advanced acute myeloid leukemia. *Hematol Cell Ther* 38:161, 1996.

607. Thomas X, Dombret H: Timed-sequential chemotherapy as induction and/or consolidation regimen for younger adults with acute myelogenous leukemia. *Hematology* 12:15, 2007.

608. Bolanos-Meade J, Karp JE, Guo C, et al: Timed sequential therapy of acute myelogenous leukemia in adults: A phase II study of retinoids in combination with the sequential administration of cytosine arabinoside, idarubicin and etoposide. *Leuk Res* 27:313, 2003.

609. Kell WJ, Burnett AK, Chopra R, et al: A feasibility study of simultaneous administration of gemtuzumab ozogamicin with intensive chemotherapy in induction and consolidation in younger patients with acute myeloid leukemia. *Blood* 102:4277, 2003.

610. Borthakur G, Kantarjian H, Wang X, et al: Treatment of core-binding-factor in acute myelogenous leukemia with fludarabine, cytarabine, and granulocyte colony-stimulating factor results in improved event-free survival. *Cancer* 113:3181, 2008.

611. Holowiecki J, Grosicki S, Robak T, et al: Addition of cladribine to daunomycin and cytarabine increases remission rate after a single course of induction treatment in acute myeloid leukemia. Multicenter phase III study. *Leukemia* 18:989, 2004.

612. Estey EH, Thall PF, Cortes JE, et al: Comparison of idarubicin + ara-C, and topotecan + ara-C-, and topotecan + ara-C-based regimens in treatment of newly diagnosed acute myeloid leukemia, refractory anemia with excess blasts in transformation, or refractory anemia with excess blasts. *Blood* 98:3575, 2001.

613. Holowiecki J, Grosicki S, Giebel S et al: Cladribine, but not fludarabine, added to daunorubicin and cytarabine during induction prolongs survival of patients with acute myeloid leukemia: A multicenter, randomized phase II study. *J Clin Oncol* 30:2441, 2012.

614. Attar EC, Johnson JL, Amrein PC, et al: Bortezomib added to daunorubicin and cytarabine during induction therapy and to intermediate-dose cytarabine for consolidation in patients with previously untreated acute myeloid leukemia age 60 to 75 years: CALGB (Alliance) study 10502. *J Clin Oncol* 31:923, 2012,

615. Giles F: Gemtuzumab ozogamicin: A component of induction therapy in AML? *Leuk Res* 29:1, 2005.

616. Tallman M: Existing and emerging therapeutic options for the treatment of acute myeloid leukemia. *Clin Adv Hematol Oncol* 6:3, 2008.

617. Buchner T, Schlenk RF, Schaich M, et al: Acute myeloid leukemia (AML): Different treatment strategies versus a common standard arm—Combined prospective analysis by the German AML intergroup. *J Clin Oncol* 30:3604, 2012.

618. Rowe JM, Neuberg D, Friedenberg W, et al: A phase 3 study of three induction regimens and of priming with GM-CSF in older adults with acute myeloid leukemia: A trial by the Eastern Cooperative Oncology Group. *Blood* 103:479, 2004.

619. Ganser A, Heil G: Use of hematopoietic growth factors in the treatment of acute myelogenous leukemia. *Curr Opin Hematol* 4:191, 1997.

620. Lowenberg B, Van Putten W, Theobald M, et al: Effect of priming with granulocyte colony-stimulating factor on the outcome of chemotherapy for acute myeloid leukemia. *N Engl J Med* 348:743, 2003.

621. Thomas X, Raffoux E, Botton S, et al: Effect of priming with granulocyte-macrophage colony-stimulating factor in younger adults with newly diagnosed acute myeloid leukemia: A trial by the Acute Leukemia French Association (ALFA) Group. *Leukemia* 21:453, 2007.

622. Pabst T, Vellenga E, van Putten W, et al: Favorable effect of priming with granulocyte colony-stimulating factor in remission induction of acute myeloid leukemia restricted to dose escalation of cytarabine. *Blood* 119:5367, 2012.

623. Nimubona S, Grulois I, Bernard M, et al: Complete remission in hypoplastic acute myeloid leukemia induced by G-CSF without chemotherapy: Report on three cases. *Leukemia* 16:1872, 2002.

624. Schlenk RF, Benner A, Hartmann F, et al: Risk-adapted postremission therapy in acute myeloid leukemia: Results of the German multicenter AML HD93 treatment trial. *Leuk Res* 17:1521, 2003.

625. Anderlini P, Ghaddar HM, Smith TL, et al: Factors predicting complete remission and subsequent disease-free survival after a second course of induction therapy in patients with acute myelogenous leukemia resistant to the first. *Leukemia* 10:964, 1996.

626. Estey EH, Shen Yu, Thall PF: Effect of time to complete remission on subsequent survival and disease-free survival time in AML, RAEB-t, and RAEB. *Blood* 95:72, 2000.

627. Brandwein JM, Gupta V, Schuh AC, et al: Predictors of response to reinduction chemotherapy for patients with acute myeloid leukemia who do not achieve complete remission with frontline induction chemotherapy. *Am J Hematol* 83:54, 2008.

628. Tsimberidou AM, Estey E: Induction mortality risk in adult acute myeloid leukemia. *Leuk Lymphoma* 47:1199, 2006.

629. Greenwood MJ, Seftel MD, Richardson C, et al: Leukocyte count as a predictor of death during remission induction in acute myeloid leukemia. *Leuk Lymphoma* 47:1245, 2006.

630. Blum W, Porcu P: Therapeutic apheresis in hyperleukocytosis and hyperviscosity syndrome. *Semin Thromb Hemost* 33:350, 2007.

631. Schmidt JE, Tamburro RF, Sillos EM, et al: Pathophysiology-directed therapy for acute hypoxemic respiratory failure in acute myeloid leukemia with hyperleukocytosis. *J Pediatr Hematol Oncol* 25:569, 2003.

632. Hughes WT, Armstrong D, Bodey GP, et al: 1997 Guidelines for the use of antimicrobial agents in neutropenic patients with unexplained fever. Infectious Diseases Society of America. *Clin Infect Dis* 25:551, 1997.

633. Lehrenbecher T, Varig D, Kaiser J, et al: Infectious complications in pediatric acute myeloid leukemia: Analysis of the prospective multi-institutional clinical trial AML-BFM 93. *Leukemia* 18:72, 2004.

634. Jagarlamidi R, Kumar L, Kochupillai V, et al: Infections in acute leukemia: An analysis of 240 febrile episodes. *Med Oncol* 17:111, 2000.

635. Uzun O, Anaissie EJ: Antifungal prophylaxis in patients with hematologic malignancies: A reappraisal. *Blood* 86:2063, 1995.

636. Glasmacher A, Molitor E, Hahn C, et al: Antifungal prophylaxis with itraconazole in neutropenic patients with acute leukaemia. *Leukemia* 12:1338, 1998.

637. Cornely OA, Maertens J, Winston DJ et al: Posaconazole vs fluconazole or itraconazole prophylaxis in patients with neutropenia. *N Engl J Med* 356:348, 2007.

638. Bergmann OJ, Mogensen SC, Ellermann-Eriksen S, Ellegaard J: Acyclovir prophylaxis and fever during remission-induction therapy of patients with acute myeloid leukemia: A randomized, double-blind, placebo-controlled trial. *J Clin Oncol* 15:2269, 1997.

639. Marr KA: New approaches to invasive fungal infections. *Curr Opin Hematol* 10:445, 2003.

640. Walter RB, Taylor LR, Gardner KM, et al: Outpatient management following intensive induction or salvage chemotherapy for acute myeloid leukemia. *Clin Adv Hematol Oncol* 9: 571, 2013.

641. Ravandi F: Role of cytokines in the treatment of acute leukemias: A review. *Leukemia* 20:563, 2006.

642. Rowe J, Anderson JW, Mazza JJ, et al: A randomized placebo-controlled phase III study of granulocyte-macrophage colony-stimulating factor in adult patients (>55 to 70 years of age) with acute myelogenous leukemia: A study of the Eastern Cooperative Oncology Group (E1490). *Blood* 86:457, 1995.

643. Hoelzer D, Seipelt G: Granulocyte colony-stimulating factor and granulocyte-macrophage colony-stimulating factor in the treatment of myeloid leukemia. *Curr Opin Hematol* 2:196, 1995.

644. Beutler E: Platelet transfusions: The 20,000/microL trigger. *Blood* 81:1441, 1993.

645. Stanworth SJ, Estcourt LJ, Powder G, et al: A no-prophylaxis platelet-transfusion strategy for hematologic cancers. *N Engl J Med* 368:1771, 2013.

646. Webert K, Cook RJ, Sigouin CS, et al: The risk of bleeding in thrombocytopenic patients with acute myeloid leukemia. *Haematologica* 91:1530, 2006.

647. Schiffer CA: Granulocyte transfusion therapy. *Curr Opin Hematol* 6:3, 1999.

648. Cullis JO, Duncombe AS, Dudley JM, et al: Acute leukaemia in Jehovah's Witnesses. *Br J Haematol* 100:664, 1998.

649. Castagnola C, Nozza A, Corso A, Bernasconi C: The value of combination therapy in adult acute myeloid leukemia with central nervous system involvement. *Haematologia (Budap)* 82:577, 1997.

650. Hatano Y, Miura I, Horiuchi T, et al: Cerebellar myeloblastoma formation in CD7-positive, neural cell adhesion molecule (CD56)-positive acute myelogenous leukemia (M1). *Ann Hematol* 75:125, 1997.

651. Zuckerman T, Ganzel C, Tallman MS, et al: How I treat hematologic emergencies in adults with acute leukemia. *Blood* 120:1993, 2012.

652. Vavricka SR, Walter RB, Irani S, et al: Safety of lumbar puncture for adults with acute leukemia and restrictive prophylactic platelet trans-fusion. *Ann Hematol* 82:570, 2003.

653. Slomowitz SJ, Shami PJ: Management of extramedullary leukemia as a presentation of acute myeloid leukemia. *J Natl Compr Canc Netw* 10:1165, 2012.

654. Breccia M, Mandelli F, Petti MC, et al: Clinico-pathological characteristics of myeloid sarcoma at diagnosis and during follow-up: Report of 12 cases from a single institution. *Leuk Res* 28:1165, 2014

655. Zittoun RA, Madelli F, Willemze R, et al: Autologous or allogeneic bone marrow transplantation compared with intensive chemotherapy in acute myelogenous leukemia. European Organization for Research and Treatment of Cancer (EORTC) and the Gruppo Italiano Malattie Ematologiche Maligne dell-Adulto (GIMEMA) Leukemia Cooperative Groups. *N Engl J Med* 332:217, 1995.

656. Harousseau JL, Cahn JY, Pignon B, et al: Comparison of autologous bone marrow transplantation and intensive chemotherapy as postremission therapy in adult acute myeloid leukemia. The Group Ouest Est Leucemies Aigues Myeloblastiques (GOELAM). *Blood* 90:2978, 1997.

657. Suciu S, Mandelli F, De Witte T, et al: Allogeneic compared with autologous stem cell transplantation in the treatment of patients younger than 46 years with acute myeloid leukemia (AML) in first complete remission (CR1): An intention-to-treat analysis of the EORTC/GIMEMAAML-10 trial. *Blood* 102:1232, 2003.

658. Bassara N, Schulze A, Wedding U, et al: Early related or unrelated haematopoietic cell transplantation results in higher overall survival and leukaemia-free survival compared with conventional chemotherapy in high-risk acute myeloid leukaemia patients in first complete remission. *Leukemia* 23:635, 2009.

659. Stone RM: Acute myeloid leukemia in first remission: To choose transplantation or not? *J Clin Oncol* 31:1262, 2013.

660. Kurosawa S, Yamaguchi T, Miyawski S, et al: A Markov decision analysis of allogeneic hematopoietic cell transplantation versus chemotherapy in patient with acute myeloid leukemia in first remission. *Blood* 117:2113, 2011.

661. Stelljes M, Krug U, Beelen DW, et al: Allogeneic transplantation versus chemotherapy as postremission therapy for acute myeloid leukemia: A prospective matched pairs analysis. *J Clin Oncol* 32:388, 2013.

662. Messerer D, Engel J, Hasford J, et al: Impact of different post-remission strategies on quality of life in patients with acute myeloid leukemia. *Haematologica* 93:826, 2008.

663. Koreth J, Schlenk R, Kopecky KJ, et al: Allogeneic stem cell transplantation for acute myeloid leukemia in first complete remission: Systematic review and meta-analysis of prospective clinical trials. *JAMA* 301:2349, 2009.

664. Shpilberg O, Haddad N, Sofer O, et al: Postremission therapy with two different dose regimens of cytarabine in adults with acute myelogenous leukemia. *Leuk Res* 19:893, 1995.

665. Heil G, Mitrou PS, Hoeizer D, et al: High-dose cytosine arabinoside and daunorubicin postremission therapy in adults with *de novo* acute myeloid leukemia. Long-term follow-up of a prospective multicenter trial. *Ann Hematol* 71:219, 1995.

666. Rowe JM: Uncertainties in the standard care of acute myelogenous leukemia. *Leukemia* 15:677, 2001.

667. Cahn JY, Labopin M, Sierra J, et al: No impact of high-dose cytarabine on the outcome of patients transplanted for acute myeloblastic leukemia in first remission. Acute Leukemia Working Party of the European Group for Blood and Marrow Transplantation (EBMT). *Br J Haematol* 110:308, 2000.

668. Neubauer A, Maharry K, Mrózek K, et al: Patients with acute myeloid leukemia and RAS mutations benefit most from postremission high-dose cytarabine: A Cancer and Leukemia Group B study. *J Clin Oncol* 26:4603, 2008.

669. Byrd JC, Dodge RK, Carroll A, et al: Patients with t(8;21) (q22) and acute myeloid leukemia have superior failure-free and overall survival when repetitive cycles of high-dose cytarabine are administered. *J Clin Oncol* 17:3767, 1999.

670. Tsimberidou AM, Estey E, Cortes JE, et al: Mylotarg, fludarabine, cytarabine (ara-C), and cyclosporine (MFAC) regimen as post-remission therapy in acute myelogenous leukemia. *Cancer Chemother Pharmacol* 52:449, 2003.

671. Schiller G: Dose-intensive treatment of acute myelogenous leukemia: Improved survival [letter, comment]. *J Clin Oncol* 13:1828, 1995.

672. Mayer RJ, Davis RB, Schiffer CA, et al: Intensive postremission chemotherapy in adults with acute myeloid leukemia. Cancer and Leukemia Group B. *N Engl J Med* 331:896, 1994.

673. Schaich M, Parmentier S, Kramer M, et al: High-dose cytarabine consolidation with or without additional amsacrine and mitoxantrone in acute myeloid leukemia: Results of the prospective randomized AML2003 trial. *J Clin Oncol* 31:2094, 2013.

674. Thomas X, Elhamri M, Ralfoux E, et al: Comparison of high-dose cytarabine and timed-sequential chemotherapy as consolidation for younger adults with AML in first remission: The ALFA-9802 study. *Blood* 118:1754, 2011.

675. Elonen E, Almqvist A, Hanninen A, et al: Comparison between four and eight cycles of intensive chemotherapy in adult acute myeloid leukemia: A randomized trial of the Finnish Leukemia Group. *Leukemia* 12:1041, 1998.

676. Lowenberg B: Sense and nonsense of high-dose cytarabine for acute myeloid leukemia. *Blood* 121:26, 2013.
677. Schaich M, Rollig C, Soucek S, et al: Cytarabine dose of 36 g/m² compared with 12 g/m² within first consolidation in acute myeloid leukemia: Results of patients enrolled onto the prospective randomized AML96 study. *J Clin Oncol* 29:2696, 2011.
678. Graves T, Hooks MA: Drug-induced toxicities associated with high-dose cytosine arabinoside infusions. *Pharmacotherapy* 9:23, 1989.
679. Smith GA, Damon LE, Rugo HS, et al: High-dose cytarabine dose modification reduces the incidence of neurotoxicity in patients with renal insufficiency. *J Clin Oncol* 15:833, 1997.
680. Hewlett J, Kopecky KJ, Head D, et al: A prospective evaluation of the roles of allogeneic marrow transplantation and low-dose monthly maintenance chemotherapy in the treatment of adult acute myelogenous leukemia (AML): A Southwest Oncology Group study. *Leukemia* 9:562, 1995.
681. Laille E, Savona MR, Scott BL, et al: Pharmacokinetics of different formulations of oral azacitidine (CC-486) and the effect of food and modified gastric pH on pharmacokinetics in subjects with hematologic malignancies *J Clin Pharmacol* 54:630, 2014.
682. Breems DA, Löwenberg B: Autologous stem cell transplantation in the treatment of adults with acute myeloid leukaemia. *Br J Haematol* 130:825, 2005.
683. Gorin NC: Autologous stem cell transplantation in acute myelocytic leukemia. *Blood* 92:1073, 1998.
684. Schiller G, Lee M, Miller T, et al: Transplantation of autologous peripheral blood progenitor cells procured after high-dose cytarabine-based consolidation chemotherapy for adults with acute myelogenous leukemia in first remission. *Leukemia* 11:1533, 1997.
685. Gondo H, Harada M, Miyamoto T, et al: Autologous peripheral blood stem cell transplantation for acute myelogenous leukemia. *Bone Marrow Transplant* 20:821, 1997.
686. Meloni G, Vignetti M, Avvisati G, et al: BAVC regimen and autograft for acute myelogenous leukemia in second complete remission. *Bone Marrow Transplant* 18:693, 1996.
687. Kusnierz-Glaz CR, Schlegel PG, Wong RM, et al: Influence of age on the outcome of 500 autologous bone marrow transplant procedures for hematologic malignancies. *J Clin Oncol* 15:18, 1997.
688. Mehta J, Powles R, Singhal S, et al: Autologous bone marrow transplantation for acute myeloid leukemia in first remission: Identification of modifiable prognostic factors. *Bone Marrow Transplant* 16:499, 1995.
689. Miller CB, Rowlings PA, Zhang MJ, et al: The effect of graft purging with 4-hydroperoxycyclophosphamie in autologous bone marrow transplantation or acute myelogenous leukemia. *Exp Hematol* 29:1336, 2001.
690. Abdallah A, Egerer G, Weberf-Nordt RM, et al: Long-term outcome in acute myelogenous leukemia autografted with mafosfamide-purged marrow in a single institution: Adverse events and incidence of secondary myelodysplasia. *Bone Marrow Transplant* 30:15, 2002.
691. Bishop MR, Jackson JD, Tarantolo SR, et al: *Ex vivo* treatment of bone marrow with phosphorothioate oligonucleotide OL(l) p53 for autologous transplantation in acute myelogenous leukemia and myelodysplastic syndrome. *J Hematother* 6:441, 1997.
692. To LB, Haylock DN, Thorp D, et al: The optimization of collection of peripheral blood stem cells for autotransplantation in acute myeloid leukaemia. *Bone Marrow Transplant* 4:41, 1989.
693. Hogge DE, Ailles LE, Gerhard B: Cytokine responsiveness of primitive progenitors in acute myelogenous leukemia. *Leukemia* 11:2220, 1997.
694. Carella AM, Dejana A, Lerma E, et al: *In vivo* mobilization of karyotypically normal peripheral blood progenitor cells in high-risk MDS, secondary or therapy-related acute myelogenous leukaemia. *Br J Haematol* 95:127, 1996.
695. Mehta J, Powles R, Horton C, et al: Factors affecting engraftment and hematopoietic recovery after unpurged autografting in acute leukemia. *Bone Marrow Transplant* 18:319, 1996.
696. Gorin NC, Labopin M, Blaise D, et al: Higher incidence of relapse with peripheral blood rather than marrow as a source of stem cells in adults with acute myelocytic leukemia autografted in their first remission. *J Clin Oncol* 27:3987, 2009.
697. Voog E, Le QH, Philip I, et al: Autologous transplantation in acute myeloid leukemia: Peripheral blood stem cell harvest after mobilization in steady state by granulocyte colony-stimulating factor alone. *Ann Hematol* 80:584, 2001.
698. Ganguly S, Singh J, Divine CL, et al: Is there a plateau in the survival curve after autologous transplantation in patients with intermediate and high-risk acute myeloid leukemia? A 20-year single institution experience. *Leuk Res* 31:1253, 2007.
699. Chauncey TR: Autologous bone marrow transplantation improves disease-free survival but not overall survival in people with acute myeloid leukaemia. *Cancer Treat Rev* 30:483, 2004.
700. Specchia G, Pastore D, Mestice A, et al: Early and long-term engraftment after autologous peripheral stem cell transplantation in acute myeloid leukemia patients. *Acta Haematol* 116:229, 2006.
701. Gupta V, Tallman MS, Weisdorf DJ: Allogeneic hematopoietic cell transplantation for adults with acute myeloid leukemia: Myths, controversies, and unknowns. *Blood* 117:2307, 2011.
702. Popplewell LL, Forman SJ: Is there an upper age limit for bone marrow transplantation? *Bone Marrow Transplant* 29:277, 2002.
703. Lemoli RM, Bandini G, Leopardi G, et al: Allogeneic peripheral blood stem cell transplantation in patients with early-phase hematologic malignancy: A retrospective comparison of short-term outcome with bone marrow transplantation. *Haematologica* 83:48, 1998.
704. Anasetti C, Logan BR, Lee SJ, et al: Peripheral-blood stem cells versus bone marrow from unrelated donors. *N Engl J Med* 367:1487, 2012.
705. Applebaum FR: Is there a best transplant conditioning regimen for acute myeloid leukemia? *Leukemia* 14:497, 2000.
706. Litzow MR, Perez WS, Klein JP, et al: Comparison of outcome following allogeneic bone marrow transplantation with cyclophosphamide-total body irradiation versus busulphan-cyclophosphamide conditioning regimens for acute myelogenous leukaemia in first remission. *Br J Haematol* 119:1115, 2002.
707. Nagler A, Racha V, Labopin M, et al: Allogeneic hematopoietic stem cell transplantation for acute myeloid leukemia in remission: Comparison of intravenous busulfan plus cyclophosphamide (Cy) versus total-body irradiation plus Cy as conditioning regimen—A report from the acute leukemia working party of the European group for blood and marrow transplantation. *J Clin Oncol* 31:3549, 2013.
708. Copelan EA, Hamilton BK, Avalos B, et al: Better leukemia-free and overall survival in AML in first remission following cyclophosphamide in combination with busulfan compared with TBI. *Blood* 122;3863, 2013.
709. Tallman MS, Rowlings PA, Milone G, et al: Effect of postremission chemotherapy before human leukocyte antigen-identical sibling transplantation for acute myelogenous leukemia in first complete remission. *Blood* 96:1254, 2000.
710. Rowe JM: Is there a role for consolidation therapy pre-transplantation? *Best Pract Res Clin Haematol* 19:301, 2006.
711. Mehta J, Powles R, Treleaven J, et al: Long-term follow-up of patients undergoing allogeneic bone marrow transplantation for acute myeloid leukemia in first complete remission after cyclophosphamide-total body irradiation and cyclosporine. *Bone Marrow Transplant* 18:741, 1996.
712. Robin M, Guardiola P, Dombret H, et al: Allogeneic bone marrow transplantation for acute myeloblastic leukaemic in remission: Risk factors for long-term morbidity and mortality. *Bone Marrow Transplant* 31:877, 2003.
713. Greinex HT, Nachbaur D, Krieger O, et al: Factors affecting long-term outcome after allogeneic haematopoietic stem cell transplantation for acute myelogenous leukaemia: A retrospective study of 172 adult patients reported to the Austrian Stem Cell Transplant Registry. *Br J Haematol* 117:914, 2002.
714. Mathews V, DiPersio JF: Stem cell transplantation in acute myelogenous leukemia in first remission: What are the options? *Curr Hematol Rep* 3:235, 2004.
715. Bornhäuser M, Illmer T, Schaich M, et al: Improved outcome after stem-cell transplantation in FLT3/ITD-positive AML. *Blood* 109:2264, 2007.
716. DeZern AE, Sung A, Kim S, et al: Role of allogeneic transplantation for FLT3/ITD actue myeloid leukemia: Outcomes from 133 consecutive newly diagnosed patients from a single institution. *Biol Blood Marrow Transplant* 17:1404, 2011.
717. Cornelissen JJ, van Putten WL, Verdonck LF, et al: Results of a HOVON/SAKK donor versus no-donor analysis of myeloablative HLA-identical sibling stem cell transplantation in first remission acute myeloid leukemia in young and middle-aged adults: Benefits for whom? *Blood* 109:3658, 2007.
718. Appelbaum FR, Pearce SF: Hematopoietic cell transplantation in first complete remission versus early relapse. *Best Pract Res Clin Haematol* 19:333, 2006.
719. Matthews DC, Appelbaum FR, Eary JF, et al: Development of a marrow transplant regimen for acute leukemia using targeted hematopoietic irradiation delivered by ¹³¹I-labeled anti-CD45 antibody, combined with cyclophosphamide and total body irradiation. *Blood* 85:1122, 1995.
720. Zuckerman T, Rowe JM: Alternative donor transplantation in acute myeloid leukemia: Which source and when? *Curr Opin Hematol* 14:152, 2007.
721. Gragert L, Eapen M, Williams E, et al: HLA match likelihoods for hematopoietic stem-cell grafts in the U. S. registry. *N Engl J Med* 371:339, 2014.
722. Mawad B, Gooley TA, Sandhu V, et al: Frequency of allogeneic hematopoietic cell transplantation among patients with high- or intermediate-risk acute myeloid leukemia in first complete remission. *J Clin Oncol* 31:3883, 2013.
723. Sasazuki T, Juji T, Morishima Y, et al: Effect of matching of class I HLA alleles on clinical outcome after transplantation of hematopoietic stem cells from an unrelated donor. Japan Marrow Donor Program. *N Engl J Med* 339:1177, 1998.
724. Saber W, Opie S, Rizzo JD, et al: Outcomes after matched unrelated donor versus identical sibling hematopoietic cell transplantation in adults with acute myelogenous leukemia. *Blood* 119: 3908, 2012.
725. Schlenk RF, Dohner K, Mack S, et al: Prospective evaluation of allogeneic hematopoietic stem cell transplantation from matched related and matched unrelated donors in younger adults with high-risk acute myeloid leukemia: German-Austrian trial AMLHD98A. *J Clin Oncol* 28:4642, 2010.
726. Ooi J, Iseki T, Takahashi S, et al: Unrelated cord blood transplantation for adult patients with de novo acute myeloid leukemia. *Blood* 103:489, 2004.
727. Michel G, Rocha V, Chevret S, et al: Unrelated cord blood transplantation for childhood acute myeloid leukemia: A Eurocord Group Analysis. *Blood* 102:4290, 2003.
728. Haspel RL, Ballen KK: Double cord blood transplants: Filling a niche? *Stem Cell Rev* 2:81, 2006.
729. Bacigalupo A, Ballen K, Rizzo D, et al: Defining the intensity of conditioning regimens: Working definitions. *Biol Blood Marrow Transplant* 15:1628, 2009.
730. Giralt S, Ballen K, Rizzo D, et al: Reduced-intensity conditioning regimen workshop: Defining the dose spectrum. Report of a workshop convened by the center for international blood and marrow transplant research. *Biol Blood Marrow Transplant* 15:367, 2009.
731. Storb R: Mixed allogeneic chimerism and graft-versus-leukemia effects in acute myeloid leukemia. *Leukemia* 16:753, 2002.

732. Lekakis L, de Lima M: Reduced-intensity conditioning and allogeneic hematopoietic stem cell transplantation for acute myeloid leukemia. *Expert Rev Anticancer Ther* 8:785, 2008.

733. Blaise D, Vey N, Faucher C, Mohty M: Current status of reduced-intensity-conditioning allogeneic stem cell transplantation for acute myeloid leukemia. *Haematologica* 92:533, 2007.

734. Schlenk RF, Hartmann F, Hensel M, et al: Less intense conditioning with fludarabine, cyclophosphamide, idarubicin and etoposide (FCIE) followed by allogeneic unselected peripheral blood stem cell transplantation in elderly patients with leukemia. *Leukemia* 16:581, 2002.

735. Massenkeil G, Nagy M, Lawang M, et al: Reduced intensity conditioning and prophylactic DLI can cure patients with high-risk acute leukaemia if complete donor chimerism can be achieved. *Bone Marrow Transplant* 31:339, 2003.

736. Giralt S, Anagnostopoulos A, Shahjahan M, Champlin R: Nonablative stem cell transplantation for older patients with acute leukemias and myelodysplastic syndromes. *Semin Hematol* 39:57, 2002.

737. Maris MB, Niederwieser D, Sandmaier BM, et al: HLA-matched unrelated donor hematopoietic cell transplantation after nonmyeloablative conditioning for patients with hematologic malignancies. *Blood* 102:2021, 2003.

738. Chakraverty R, Peggs K, Chopra R, et al: Limiting transplantation-related mortality following unrelated donor stem cell transplantation by using a nonmyeloablative conditioning regimen. *Blood* 99:1071, 2002.

739. Alyea EP, Kim HT, Ho V, et al: Impact of conditioning regimen intensity on outcome of allogeneic hematopoietic cell transplantation for advanced acute myelogenous leukemia and myelodysplastic syndrome. *Biol Blood Marrow Transplant* 12:1047, 2006.

740. Ringdén O, Labopin M, Ehninger G, et al: Reduced intensity conditioning compared with myeloablative conditioning using unrelated donor transplants in patients with acute myeloid leukemia. *J Clin Oncol* 27:4570, 2009.

741. Oran B, Giralt S, Saliba R, et al: Allogeneic hematopoietic stem cell transplantation for the treatment of high-risk acute myelogenous leukemia and myelodysplastic syndrome using reduced-intensity conditioning with fludarabine and melphalan. *Biol Blood Marrow Transplant* 13:454, 2007.

742. Gyurkocza B, Storb, R, Storer BE, et al: Nonmyeloablative allogeneic hematopoietic cell transplantation in patients with acute myeloid leukemia. *J Clin Oncol* 38:2859, 2010.

743. Alatrash G, de Lima M, Hamerschlak N, et al: Myeloablative reduced-toxicity i.v. busulfan-fludarabine and allogeneic hematopoietic stem cell transplant for patients with acute myeloid leukemia or myelodysplastic syndrome in the sixth through eighth decades of life. *Biol Blood Marrow Transplant* 17:1490, 2011.

744. Estey E, de Lima M, Tibes R, et al: Prospective feasibility analysis of reduced-intensity conditioning (RIC) regimens for hematopoietic stem cell transplantation (HSCT) in elderly patients with acute myeloid leukemia (AML) and high-risk myelodysplastic syndrome (MDS). *Blood* 109:1395, 2007.

745. Tallman MS, Dewald GW, Gandham S, et al: Impact of cytogenetics on outcome of matched unrelated donor hematopoietic stem cell transplantation for acute myeloid leukemia in first or second complete remission. *Blood* 110:409, 2007.

746. Gale RP, Horowitz MM, Rees JK, et al: Chemotherapy versus transplants for acute myelogenous leukemia in second remission. *Leukemia* 10:13, 1996.

747. Bacigalupo A, Lamparelli T, Gualandi F, et al: Allogeneic hemopoietic stem cell transplants for patients with relapsed acute leukemia: Long-term outcome. *Bone Marrow Transplant* 39:341, 2007.

748. Duval M, Klein JP, He W, et al: Hematopoietic stem-cell transplantation for acute leukemia in relapse or primary induction failure. *J Clin Oncol* 28:3730, 2010.

749. Michel G, Boulad F, Small TN, et al: Risk of extramedullary relapse following allogeneic bone marrow transplantation for acute myelogenous leukemia with leukemia cutis. *Bone Marrow Transplant* 20:107, 1997.

750. Blau IW, Basara N, Bischoff M, et al: Second allogeneic hematopoietic stem cell transplantation as treatment for leukemia relapsing following a first transplant. *Bone Marrow Transplant* 25:41, 2000.

751. Christopeit M, Kuss O, Finke J, et al: Second allograft for hematologic relapse of acute leukemia after first allogeneic stem-cell transplantation from related and unrelated donors: The role of donor change. *J Clin Oncol* 31:3259, 2013.

752. Shlomchik WD, Emerson SG: The immunobiology of T cell therapies for leukemias. *Acta Haematol* 96:189, 1996.

753. Porter DL, Roth MS, Lee SJ, et al: Adoptive immunotherapy with donor mononuclear cell infusions to treat relapse of acute leukemia or myelodysplasia after allogeneic bone marrow transplantation. *Bone Marrow Transplant* 18:975, 1996.

754. Porter DL: Donor leukocyte infusions in acute myelogenous leukemia. *Leukemia* 17:1035, 2003.

755. Greinix NT: DLI or second transplant. *Ann Hematol* 81:S34, 2002.

756. van Rhee F, Kolb HJ: Donor leukocyte transfusions for leukemic relapse. *Curr Opin Hematol* 2:423, 1995.

757. Berthou C, Leglise MC, Herry A, et al: Extramedullary relapse after favorable molecular response to donor leukocyte infusions for recurring acute leukemia. *Leukemia* 12:1676, 1998.

758. Carlens S, Remberger M, Aschan J, Ringden O: The role of disease stage in the response to donor lymphocyte infusions as treatment for leukemic relapse. *Biol Blood Marrow Transplant* 7:31, 2001.

759. Keil F, Prinz E, Kalhs P, et al: Treatment of leukemic relapse after allogeneic stem cell transplantation with cytoreductive chemotherapy and/or second transplants. *Leukemia* 15:355, 2001.

760. Porter DL, Collins RH, Hardy C, et al: Treatment of relapsed leukemia after unrelated donor marrow transplantation with unrelated donor leukocyte infusions. *Blood* 95:1214, 2000.

761. Bishop MR, Tarantolo SR, Pavletic ZS, et al: Filgrastim as an alternative to donor leukocyte infusion for relapse after allogeneic stem-cell transplantation. *J Clin Oncol* 18:2269, 2000.

762. Trenschel R, Bernier M, Stryckmans P, et al: Complete remission following donor PBSC after low-dose cytarabine chemotherapy for early relapse of acute myelogenous leukemia after allogeneic stem cell transplantation. *Bone Marrow Transplant* 19:381, 1997.

763. Porter DL, Antin JH: Donor leukocyte infusions in myeloid malignancies: New strategies. *Best Pract Res Clin Haematol* 19:737, 2006.

764. Cooley S, Weisdorf DJ, Guethlein LA, et al: Donor selection for natural killer cell receptor genes leads to superior survival after unrelated transplantation for acute myelogenous leukemia. *Blood* 116:2411, 2010.

765. Elmaagacli A, Steckel NK, Koldehoff M, et al: Early human cytomegalovirus replication after transplantation is associated with a decreased relapse risk: Evidence for a putative virus-versus-leukemia effect in acute myelogenous leukemia patients. *Blood* 118:1402, 2011.

766. Czibere A, Bruns I, Kröger N, et al: 5-Azacytidine for the treatment of patients with acute myeloid leukemia or myelodysplastic syndrome who relapse after allo-SCT: A retrospective analysis. *Bone Marrow Transplant* 45:872, 2010.

767. Cunningham I: Extramedullary sites of leukemia relapse after transplant. *Leuk Lymphoma* 45:1754, 2006.

768. Murata M, Ishikawa Y, Ohashi H, et al: Donor cell leukemia after allogeneic peripheral blood stem cell transplantation: A case report and literature review. *Int J Hematol* 88:111, 2008.

769. Reichard KK, Zhang QY, Sanchez L, et al: Acute myeloid leukemia of donor origin after allogeneic bone marrow transplantation for precursor T-cell acute lymphoblastic leukemia: Case report and review of the literature. *Am J Hematol* 81:178, 2006.

770. Shlush LI, Ilani NC, Ader R, et al: Cell lineage analysis of acute leukemia relapse uncovers the role of replication-rate heterogeneity and microsatellite instability. *Blood* 120:603, 2012.

771. Ding L, Ley TJ, Larson DE, et al: Clonal evolution in relapsed acute myeloid leukaemia revealed by whole-genome sequencing. *Nature* 481:506, 2012.

772. Estey E: Treatment of refractory AML. *Leukemia* 10:932, 1996.

773. Estey E, Kornblau S, Pierce S, et al: A stratification system for evaluating and selecting therapies in patients with relapsed or primary refractory acute myelogenous leukemia. *Blood* 88:756, 1996.

774. Burnett AK, Goldstone A, Hills RK, et al: Curability of patients with acute myeloid leukemia who did not undergo transplantation in first remission. *J Clin Oncol* 31:1293, 2013.

775. Stoiser B, Knöbl P, Fonatsch C, et al: Prognosis of patients with second relapse of acute myeloid leukemia. *Leukemia* 14:2059, 2000.

776. Lee S, Tallman MS, Oken MM, et al: Duration of second complete remission compared with first complete remission in patients with acute myeloid leukemia. *Leukemia* 14:1345, 2000.

777. Kern W, Schoch C, Haferlach T, et al: Multivariate analysis of prognostic factors in patients with refractory and relapsed acute myeloid leukemia undergoing sequential high-dose cytosine arabinoside and mitoxantrone (S-HAM) salvage therapy: Relevance of cytogenetic abnormalities. *Leukemia* 14:226, 2000.

778. Estey EH: Treatment of relapsed and refractory acute myelogenous leukemia. *Leukemia* 14:476, 2000.

779. Leopold LH, Willemze R: The treatment of acute myeloid leukemia in first relapse: A comprehensive review of the literature. *Leuk Lymphoma* 43:1715, 2002.

780. Alvarado Y, Tsimberidou A, Kantarjian H, et al: Pilot study of Mylotarg, idarubicin and cytarabine combination regimen in patients with primary resistant or relapsed acute myeloid leukemia. *Cancer Chemother Pharmacol* 51:87, 2003.

781. Revesz D, Chelghoum Y, Le QH, et al: Salvage by timed sequential chemotherapy in primary resistant acute myeloid leukemia: Analysis of prognostic factors. *Ann Hematol* 82:684, 2003.

782. Wrzesień-Kuś A, Robak T, Lech-Marańda E, et al: A multicenter, open, non-comparative, phase II study of the combination of cladribine (2-chlorodeoxyadenosine), cytarabine, and G-CSF as induction therapy in refractory acute myeloid leukemia: A report of the Polish Adult Leukemia Group (PALG). *Eur J Haematol* 71:155, 2003.

783. Pastore D, Specchia G, Carluccio P, et al: FLAG-IDA in the treatment of refractory/relapsed acute myeloid leukemia: Single-center experience. *Ann Hematol* 82:231, 2003.

784. Roboz GJ, Knovich MA, Bayer RL, et al: Efficacy and safety of gemtuzumab ozogamicin in patients with poor-prognosis acute myeloid leukemia. *Leuk Lymphoma* 43:1951, 2002.

785. Advani R, Saba HI, Tallman MS, et al: Treatment of refractory and relapsed acute myelogenous leukemia with combination chemotherapy plus the multidrug resistance modulator PSC 833 (Valspodar). *Blood* 93:787, 1999.

786. Estey EH, Kantarjian HM, O'Brien S, et al: High remission rate, short remission duration in patients with refractory anemia with excess blasts (RAEB) in transformation (RAEB-t) given acute myelogenous leukemia (AML)-type chemotherapy in combination with granulocyte-CSF (G-CSF). *Cytokines Mol Ther* 1:21, 1995.

787. Becker PS, Kantarjain HM, Appelbaum FR, et al: Clofarabine with high dose cytarabine and granulocyte colony-stimulaing factor (G-CSF) priming for relapsed and refractory acute myeloid leukemia. *Br J Haematol* 155:182, 2011.

788. Faderl S, Ferrajoli A, Wierda W, et al: Clofarabine combinations as acute myeloid leukemia salvage therapy. *Cancer* 113:2090, 2008.

789. Faderl S, Wetzler M, Roizzieri D, et al: Clofarabine plus cytarabine compared with cytarabine alone in older patients with relapsed or refractory acute myelogenous leukemia: Results from the CLASSIC 1 Trial. *J Clin Oncol* 30:2492, 2012.

790. Greinix HT, Keil F, Brugger SA, et al: Long-term leukemia-free survival after allogeneic marrow transplantation in patients with acute myelogenous leukemia. *Ann Hematol* 72:53, 1996.

791. Appelbaum FR: Hematopoietic cell transplantation beyond first remission. *Leukemia* 16:157, 2002.

792. Singhal S, Powles R, Henslee-Downey PJ, et al: Allogeneic transplantation from HLA-matched sibling or partially HLA-mismatched related donors for primary refractory acute leukemia. *Bone Marrow Transplant* 29:291, 2002.

793. Biggs JC, Horowitz MM, Gale RP, et al: Bone marrow transplants may cure patients with acute leukemia never achieving remission with chemotherapy. *Blood* 80:1090, 1992.

794. Arellano ML, Langston A, Winton E, et al: Treatment of relapsed acute leukemia after allogeneic transplantation: A single center experience. *Biol Blood Marrow Transplant* 13:116, 2007.

795. Pollyea DA, Artz AS, Stock W, et al: Outcomes of patients with AML and MDS who relapse or progress after reduced intensity allogeneic hematopoietic cell transplantation. *Bone Marrow Transplant* 40:1027, 2007.

796. Lancet JE, Cortes JE, Hogge DE, et al: Phase 2 trial of CPX-351, a fixed 5:1 molar ration of cytarabine/daunorubicin, vs cytarabine/daunorubicin in older adults with untreated AML. *Blood* 123:3238, 2014.

797. Rush LJ, Dai Z, Smiraglia DJ, et al: Novel methylation targets in *de novo* acute myeloid leukemia with prevalence of chromosome 11 loci. *Blood* 97:3226, 2001.

798. Blum W, Marcucci G: Targeting epigenetic changes in acute myeloid leukemia. *Clin Adv Hematol Oncol* 3:855, 2005.

799. Lübbert M, Minden M: Decitabine in acute myeloid leukemia. *Semin Hematol* 42(Suppl 2):S38, 2005.

800. Kihslinger JE, Godley LA: The use of hypomethylating agents in the treatment of hematologic malignancies. *Leuk Lymphoma* 48:1676, 2007.

801. Plimack ER, Kantarjian HM, Issa JP, et al: Decitabine and its role in the treatment of hematopoietic malignancies. *Leuk Lymphoma* 48:1472, 2007.

802. Garcia-Manero G, Stoltz ML, Ward MR, et al: A pilot pharmacokinetic study of oral azacitidine. *Leukemia* 22:1680, 2008.

803. Kantarjian HM, O'Brien SM, Estey E, et al: Decitabine studies in chronic and acute myelogenous leukemia. *Leukemia* 11(Suppl 1):S35, 1997.

804. Yan P, Frankhouser D, Murphy M, et al: Genome-wide methylation profiling in decitabine-treated patients with acute myeloid leukemia. *Blood* 120:2466, 2012.

805. Blum W, Garzon R, Kilisovic RB, et al: Clinical response and miR-29B predictive significance in older patients treated with a 10-day schedule of decitabine. *Proc Natl Acad Sci U S A* 107:7473, 2010.

806. Ferrara EF, Fazi F, Bianchini A, et al: Histone deacetylase-targeted treatment restores retinoic acid signaling and differentiation in acute myeloid leukemia. *Cancer Res* 61:2, 2001.

807. Klisovic MI, Maghraby EA, Parthun MR, et al: Depsipeptide (FR 901228) promotes histone acetylation, gene transcription, apoptosis and its activity is enhanced by DNA methyltransferase inhibitors in AML1/ETO-positive leukemic cells. *Leukemia* 17:350, 2003.

808. Klimek VM, Fircanis S, Maslak P, et al: Tolerability, pharmacodynamics, and pharmacokinetics studies of depsipeptide (romidepsin) in patients with acute myelogenous leukemia or advanced myelodysplastic syndromes. *Clin Cancer Res* 14:826, 2008.

809. Giles F, Fischer T, Cortes J, et al: A phase I study of intravenous LBH589, a novel cinnamic hydroxamic acid analogue histone deacetylase inhibitor, in patients with refractory hematologic malignancies. *Clin Cancer Res* 12:4628, 2006.

810. Garcia-Manero G, Yang H, Bueso-Ramos C, et al: Phase 1 study of the histone deacetylase inhibitor vorinostat (suberoylanilide hydroxamic acid [SAHA]) in patients with advanced leukemias and myelodysplastic syndromes. *Blood* 111:1060, 2008.

811. Garcia-Manero G, Assouline S, Cortes J, et al: Phase 1 study of the oral isotype specific histone deacetylase inhibitor MGCD0103 in leukemia. *Blood* 112:981, 2008.

812. Gore SD: Combination therapy with DNA methyltransferase inhibitors in hematologic malignancies. *Nat Clin Pract Oncol* 2 Suppl 1:S30, 2005.

813. Blum W, Klisovic RB, Hackanson B, et al: Phase I study of decitabine alone or in combination with valproic acid in acute myeloid leukemia. *J Clin Oncol* 25:3884, 2007.

814. Daigle SR, Oihava EJ, Therkeisen CA, et al: Potent inhibition of DOT1L as treatment of MLL-fusion leukemia. *Blood* 122:1017, 2013.

815. Sarkaria SM, Christopher MJ, Klco JM, Ley TJ: Primary acute myeloid leukemia cells with *IDH1* or *IDH2* mutations respond to a DOT1L inhibitor *in vitro*. *Leukemia* 28:2403, 2014.

816. Lee WY, Chen KC, Chen HY, Chen CY: Potential mitochondrial isocitrate dehydrogenase R140Q mutant inhibitor from traditional Chinese medicine against cancers. *Biomed Res Int* 2014:364625, 2014.

817. Lu M, Xia L, Li Y, et al: The orally bioavailable MDM2 antagonist RG7112 and pegylated interferon α 2a target JAK2V617F-positive progenitor and stem cells. *Blood* 124:771, 2014.

818. Larson RA: Current use and future development of gemtuzumab ozogamicin. *Semin Hematol* 38:24, 2001.

819. van Der Velden VH, te Marvelde JG, Hoogeveen PG, et al: Targeting of the CD33-calicheamicin immunoconjugate Mylotarg (CMA-676) in acute myeloid leukemia: *In vivo* and *in vitro* saturation and internalization by leukemic and normal myeloid cells. *Blood* 97:3197, 2001.

820. Lang K, Menzin J, Earle CC, Mallick R: Outcomes in patients treated with gemtuzumab ozogamicin for relapsed acute myelogenous leukemia. *Am J Health Syst Pharm* 59:941, 2002.

821. Leopold LH, Berger MS, Cheng SC, et al: Comparative efficacy and safety of Gemtuzumab ozogamicin monotherapy and high-dose cytarabine combination therapy in patients with acute myeloid leukemia in first relapse. *Clin Adv Hematol Oncol* 1:220, 2003.

822. Wadleigh M, Richardson PG, Zahrieh D, et al: Prior gemtuzumab ozogamicin exposure significantly increases the risk of veno-occlusive disease in patients who undergo myeloablative allogeneic stem cell transplantation. *Blood* 102:1578, 2003.

823. Stasi R, Evangelista ML, Buccisano F, et al: Gemtuzumab ozogamicin in the treatment of acute myeloid leukemia. *Cancer Treat Rev* 34:49, 2008.

824. Burnett AK, Russell NH, Hills RK, et al: Addition of gemtuzumab ozogamicin in induction chemotherapy improves survival in older patients with acute myeloid leukemia. *J Clin Oncol* 30:3924, 2012.

825. Castaigne S, Pautas C, Terré C, et al: Effect of gemtuzumab ozogamicin on survival of adult patients with *de-novo* acute myeloid leukaemia (ALFA-07010). A randomized, open-label, phase 3 study. *Lancet* 379:1508, 2012.

826. Weisberg E, Boulton C, Kelly LM, et al: Inhibition of mutant FLT3 receptors in leukemia cells by the small molecule tyrosine kinase inhibitor PKC412. *Cancer Cell* 1:433, 2002.

827. Kelly LM, Yu JC, Boulton CL, et al: CT53518, a novel selective FLT3 antagonist for the treatment of acute myelogenous leukemia (AML). *Cancer Cell* 1:421, 2002.

828. Levis M, Allebach J, Tse KF, et al: A FLT3-targeted tyrosine kinase inhibitor is cytotoxic to leukemia cells *in vitro* and *in vivo*. *Blood* 99:3885, 2002.

829. Spiekermann K, Dirschinger RJ, Schwab R, et al: The protein tyrosine kinase inhibitor SU5614 inhibits FLT3 and induces growth arrest and apoptosis in AML-derived cell lines expressing a constitutively activated FLT3. *Blood* 101:1494, 2003.

830. DeAngelo DJ, Stone RM, Heaney ML, et al: Phase 1 clinical results with tandutinib (MLN518), a novel FLT3 antagonist, in patients with acute myelogenous leukemia or high-risk myelodysplastic syndrome: Safety, pharmacokinetics, and pharmacodynamics. *Blood* 108:3674, 2006.

831. Tickenbrock L, Müller-Tidow C, Berdel WE, Serve H: Emerging Flt3 kinase inhibitors in the treatment of leukaemia. *Expert Opin Emerg Drugs* 11:153, 2006.

832. Fathi AT, Le L, Hasserjian RP: FLT3 inhibitor-induced neutrophilic dermatosis. *Blood* 122:239, 2013.

833. Pratz KW, Sato T, Murphy KM, et al: FLT3-mutant allelic burden and clinical status are predictive of response to FLT3 inhibitors in AML. *Blood* 115:1425, 2010.

834. Stone RM, De Angelo DJ, Klimek V, et al: Patients with acute myeloid leukemia and an activating mutation in FLT3 respond to a small molecule FLT3 tyrosine kinase inhibitor. *Blood* 105:54, 2005.

835. Knapper S, Burnett AK, Littlewood T, et al: A phase 2 trial of the FLT3 inhibitor lestaurtinib (CEP701) as first-line treatment for older patients with acute myeloid leukemia not considered fit for intensive chemotherapy. *Blood* 108:3262, 2006.

836. Kindler T, Lipka DB, Fischer T: FLT3 as a therapeutic target in AML: Still challenging after all these years. *Blood* 116:5089, 2010.

837. Zimmerman EI, Turner DC, Buaboonnam J, et al: Crenolanib is active against models of drug-resistant FLT3-ITD–positive acute myeloid leukemia. *Blood* 122:3607, 2013.

838. Cortes JE, Kantarjian H, Foran JM, et al: Phase I study of quizartinib administered daily to patients with relapsed or refractory acute myeloid leukemia irrespective of FMS-like tyrosine kinase 3-internal tandem duplication status. *J Clin Oncol* 31:3681, 2013.

839. Fischer T, Stone RM, DeAngelo DJ, et al: Phase IIB trial of oral midostaurin (PKC412), the FMS-like tyrosine kinase 3 receptor (FLT3) and multi-targeted kinase inhibitor, in patients with acute myeloid leukemia and high-risk myelodysplastic syndrome with either wild-type of mutated FLT3. *J Clin Oncol* 28:4339, 2010.

840. Ravandi F, Cortes JE, Jones D, et al: Phase I/II study of combination therapy with sorafenib, idarubicin, and decitabine in younger patients with acute myeloid leukemia. *J Clin Oncol* 28:1856, 2010.

841. Heinrich MC, Blanke CD, Druker BJ, Corless CL: Inhibition of KIT tyrosine kinase activity: A novel molecular approach to the treatment of KIT-positive malignancies. *J Clin Oncol* 20:1692, 2002.

842. Kindler T, Breitenbuecher F, Marx A, et al: Sustained complete hematologic remission after administration of the tyrosine kinase inhibitor imatinib mesylate in a patient with refractory, secondary AML. *Blood* 101:2960, 2003.

843. Kindler T, Breitenbuecher F, Marx A, et al: Efficacy and safety of imatinib in adult patients with C-kit-positive acute myeloid leukemia. *Blood* 103:3644, 2004.

844. Marcucci G, Geyer S, Zhao J, et al: Adding the KIT inhibitor Dasatinib (DAS) to standard induction and consolidation therapy for newly diagnosed patients (pts) with core binding factor (CBF) acute myeloid leukemia (AML): Initial results of the CALGB 10801 (Alliance) study [abstract]. *Blood* 122:2013.

845. Guzman ML, Jordan CT: Considerations for targeting malignant stem cells in leukemia. *Cancer Control* 11:97, 2004.

846. Cilloni D, Messa F, Rosso V, et al: Increase sensitivity to chemotherapeutical agents and cytoplasmatic interaction between NPM leukemic mutant and NF-kappaB in AML carrying NPM1 mutations. *Leukemia* 22:1234, 2008.

847. Minderman H, Zhou Y, O'Loughlin KL, Baer MR: Bortezomib activity and *in vitro* interactions with anthracyclines and cytarabine in acute myeloid leukemia cells are independent of multidrug resistance mechanisms and p53 status. *Cancer Chemother Pharmacol* 60:245, 2007.

848. Frelin C, Imbert V, Griessinger E, et al: Targeting NF-kappaB activation via pharmacologic inhibition of IKK2-induced apoptosis of human acute myeloid leukemia cells. *Blood* 105: 804, 2005.

849. Stone RM: Novel therapeutic agents in acute myeloid leukemia. *Exp Hematol* 35(Suppl 1):163, 2007.

850. Chalandon Y, Schwaller J: Targeting mutated protein tyrosine kinases and their signaling pathways in hematologic malignancies. *Haematologica* 90:949, 2005.

851. Tamburini J, Chapuis N, Bardet V, et al: Mammalian target of rapamycin (mTOR) inhibition activates phosphatidylinositol 3-kinase/Akt by up-regulating insulin-like growth factor-1 receptor signaling in acute myeloid leukemia: Rationale for therapeutic inhibition of both pathways. *Blood* 111:379, 2008.

852. Wei G, Twomey D, Lamb J, et al: Gene expression-based chemical genomics identifies rapamycin as a modulator of MCL1 and glucocorticoid resistance. *Cancer Cell* 10:331, 2006.

853. Kojima K, Shimanuki M, Shikami M, et al: The dual PI3 kinase/mTOR inhibitor PI-103 prevents p53 induction by Mdm2 inhibition but enhances p53-mediated mitochondrial apoptosis in p53 wild-type AML. *Leukemia* 22:1728, 2008.

854. Martelli AM, Nyåkern M, Tabellini G, et al: Phosphoinositide 3-kinase/Akt signaling pathway and its therapeutical implications for human acute myeloid leukemia. *Leukemia* 20:911, 2006.

855. Papa V, Tazzari PL, Chiarini F, et al: Proapoptotic activity and chemosensitizing effect of the novel Akt inhibitor perifosine in acute myelogenous leukemia cells. *Leukemia* 22:147, 2008.

856. Milella M, Kornblau SM, Estrov Z, et al: Therapeutic targeting of the MEK/MAPK signal transduction module in acute myeloid leukemia. *J Clin Invest* 108:851, 2001.

857. Ikezoe T, Yang J, Nishioka C, et al: A novel treatment strategy targeting Aurora kinases in acute Myelogenous leukemia. *Mol Cancer Ther* 6:1851, 2007.

858. Thomas X, Campos L, Le QH, Guyotat D: Heat shock proteins and acute leukemias. *Hematology* 10:225, 2005.

859. Hu S, Niu H, Minkin P, et al: Comparison of antitumor effects of multitargeted tyrosine kinase inhibitors in acute myelogenous leukemia. *Mol Cancer Ther* 7:1110, 2008.

860. Raanani P, Shpilberg O, Ben-Bassat I, et al: Extramedullary disease and targeted therapies for hematological malignancies—Is the association real? *Ann Oncol* 18:7, 2007.

861. Shangary S, Johnson DE: Recent advances in the development of anticancer agents targeting cell death inhibitors in the Bcl-2 protein family. *Leukemia* 17:1470, 2003.

862. Konopleva M, Contractor R, Tsao T, et al: Mechanisms of apoptosis sensitivity and resistance to the BH3 mimetic ABT-737 in acute myeloid leukemia. *Cancer Cell* 10:375, 2006.

863. Konopleva M, Watt J, Contractor R, et al: Mechanisms of antileukemic activity of the novel Bcl-2 homology domain-3 mimetic GX15–070 (obatoclax). *Cancer Res* 68:3413, 2008.

864. Konopleva M, Tsao T, Ruvolo P, et al: Novel triterpenoid CDDO-Me is a potent inducer of apoptosis and differentiation in acute myelogenous leukemia. *Blood* 99:326, 2002.

865. Morgan MA, Ganser A, Reuter CWM: Therapeutic efficacy of prenylation inhibitors in the treatment of myeloid leukemia. *Leukemia* 17:1482, 2003.

866. Kurzrock R, Cortes J, Kantarjian H: Clinical development of farnesyltransferase inhibitors in leukemias and myelodysplastic syndrome. *Semin Hematol* 39:20, 2002.

867. Brunner TB, Hahn SM, Gupta AK, et al: Farnesyltransferase inhibitors: An overview of the results of preclinical and clinical investigations. *Cancer Res* 63:5656, 2003.

868. Karp JE, Lancet JE, Kaufmann SH, et al: Clinical and biologic activity of the farnesyltransferase inhibitor R115777 in adults with refractory and relapsed acute leukemias: A phase 1 clinical-laboratory correlative trial. *Blood* 97:3361, 2001.

869. Minden MD, Dimitroulakos J, Nohynek D, Penn LZ: Lovastatin induced control of blast cell growth in an elderly patient with acute myeloblastic leukemia. *Leuk Lymphoma* 40:659, 2001.

870. Lishner M, Bar-Sef A, Elis A, Fabian I: Effect of simvastatin alone and in combination with cytosine arabinoside on the proliferation of myeloid leukemia cell lines. *J Investig Med* 49:319, 2001.

871. Li HY, Appelbaum FR, Willman CL, et al: Cholesterol-modulating agents kill acute myeloid leukemia cells and sensitize them to therapeutics by blocking adaptive cholesterol responses. *Blood* 101:3628, 2003.

872. Munker R, Kobayashi T, Eistner E, et al: A new series of vitamin D analogs is highly active for clonal inhibition, differentiation, and induction of WAF1 in myeloid leukemia. *Blood* 88:2201, 1996.

873. Morosetti R, Grignani F, Liberatore C, et al: Infrequent alterations of the RAR alpha gene in acute myelogenous leukemias, retinoic acid-resistant acute promyelocytic leukemias, myelodysplastic syndromes, and cell lines. *Blood* 87:4399, 1996.

874. Usuki K, Kitazume K, Endo M, et al: Combination therapy with granulocyte colony-stimulating factor, all-*trans* retinoic acid, and low-dose cytotoxic drugs for acute myelogenous leukemia. *Intern Med* 34:1186, 1995.

875. Zhang W, Piatyszek MA, Kobayashi T, et al: Telomerase activity in human acute myelogenous leukemia: Inhibition of telomerase activity by differentiation-inducing agents. *Clin Cancer Res* 2:799, 1996.

876. Seiter K, Feldman EJ, Dorota Halicka H, et al: Clinical and laboratory evaluation of all-trans retinoic acid modulation of chemotherapy in patients with acute myelogenous leukaemia. *Br J Haematol* 108:40, 2000.

877. Chen Z, Wang Y, Wang W, et al: All-*trans* retinoic acid as a single agent induces complete remission in a patient with acute leukemia of M2a subtype. *Chin Med J* 115:58, 2002.

878. Lehman S, Bengtzen S, Paul A, et al: Effects of arsenic trioxide (As$_2$O$_3$) on leukemic cells from patients with non-M3 acute myelogenous leukemia: Studies of cytotoxicity, apoptosis and the pattern of resistance. *Eur J Haematol* 66:357, 2001.

879. Ozturk A, Orhan B, Turken O, et al: Acute myeloblastic leukemia achieving complete remission with amifostine alone. *Leuk Lymphoma* 43:451, 2002.

880. Steins MB, Padro T, Bieker R, et al: Efficacy and safety of thalidomide in patients with acute myeloid leukemia. *Blood* 99:834, 2002.

881. Cabebe E, Wakelee H: Sunitinib: A newly approved small-molecule inhibitor of angiogenesis. *Drugs Today (Barc)* 42:387, 2006.

882. Hatfield KJ, Olsnes AM, Gjertsen BT, Bruserud Ø: Antiangiogenic therapy in acute myelogenous leukaemia: Targeting of vascular endothelial growth factor and interleukin 8 as possible antileukemic strategies. *Curr Cancer Drug Targets* 5:229, 2005.

883. Kitagawa M: The angiopoietin signaling pathway as a promising target for the treatment of acute myeloid leukemia. *Haematologica* 91:1155B, 2006.

884. Lancet JE, List AF, Moscinski LC, et al: Treatment of deletion 5q acute myeloid leukemia with lenalidomide. *Leukemia* 21:586, 2007.

885. Burger JA, Bürkle A: The CXCR4 chemokine receptor in acute and chronic leukaemia: A marrow homing receptor and potential therapeutic target. *Br J Haematol* 137:288, 2007.

886. Zeng Z, Samudio IJ, Munsell M, et al: Inhibition of CXCR4 with the novel RCP168 peptide overcomes stroma-mediated chemoresistance in chronic and acute leukemias. *Mol Cancer Ther* 5:3113, 2006.

887. Andreeff M, Konopleva M: Mechanisms of drug resistance in AML. *Cancer Treat Res* 112:237, 2002.

888. Van der Kolk DM, De Vries EG, Muller M, Vellenga E: The role of drug efflux pumps in acute myeloid leukemia. *Leuk Lymphoma* 43:685, 2002.

889. Claxton D, Choudhury A: Potential for therapy with AML-derived dendritic cells. *Leukemia* 15:668, 2001.

890. Rosenblatt J, Avigan D: Can leukemia-derived dendritic cells generate antileukemia immunity? *Expert Rev Vaccines* 5:467, 2006.

891. Panoskaltsis N: Dendritic cells in MDS and AML—Cause, effect or solution to the immune pathogenesis of disease? *Leukemia* 19:354, 2005.

892. Woiciechowsky A, Regn S, Kolb H-J, Roskrow M: Leukemic dendritic cells generated in the presence of FLT3 ligand have the capacity to stimulate an autologous leukemia-specific cytotoxic T cell response from patients with acute myeloid leukemia. *Leukemia* 15:246, 2001.

893. Stripecke R, Levine AM, Pullarkat V, Cardoso AA: Immunotherapy with acute leukemia cells modified into antigen-presenting cells: *Ex vivo* culture and gene transfer methods. *Leukemia* 16:1974, 2002.

894. Galea-Lauri J, Darling D, Mufti G, et al: Eliciting cytotoxic T lymphocytes against acute myeloid leukemia-derived antigens: Evaluation of dendritic cell-leukemia cell hybrids and other antigen-loading strategies for dendritic cell-based vaccination. *Cancer Immunol Immunother* 51:299, 2002.

895. Cooper MA, Caligiuri MA: Immunologic manipulation in AML: From bench to bedside. *Leukemia* 16:736, 2002.

896. Meloni G, Trisolini SM, Capria S, et al: How long can we give interleukin-2? Clinical and immunological evaluation of AML patients after 10 or more years of IL2 administration. *Leukemia* 16:2016, 2002.

897. Baer MR, George SL, Caligiuri MA, et al: Low-dose interleukin-2 immunotherapy does not improve outcome of patients age 60 years and older with acute myeloid leukemia in first complete remission: Cancer and Leukemia Group B Study 9720. *J Clin Oncol* 26:4934, 2008.

898. Elisseeva OA, Oka Y, Tsuboi A, et al: Humoral immune responses against Wilms tumor gene WT1 product in patients with hematopoietic malignancies. *Blood* 99:3272, 2002.

899. Molldrem J: Immune therapy of AML. *Cytotherapy* 4:437, 2002.

900. Norde WJ, Hobo W, van der Voort R, et al: Coinhibitory molecules in hematologic malignancies: Targets for therapeutic intervention. *Blood* 120:728, 2012.

901. Choo A, Palladinetti P, Holmes T, et al: SiRNA targeting the IRF2 transcription factor inhibits leukaemic cell growth. *Int J Oncol* 33:175, 2008.

902. Klisovic RB, Blum W, Wei X, et al: Phase I study of GTI-2040, an antisense to ribonucleotide reductase, in combination with high-dose cytarabine in patients with acute myeloid leukemia. *Clin Cancer Res* 14:3889, 2008.

903. Stevenson GT: CD38 as a therapeutic target. *Mol Med* 12:345, 2006.

904. Abutalib SA, Tallman MS: Monoclonal antibodies for the treatment of acute myeloid leukemia. *Curr Pharm Biotechnol* 7:343, 2006.

905. Wayne AS, FitzGerald DJ, Kreitman RJ, et al: Immunotoxins for leukemia. *Blood* 123:2470, 2014.

906. Curti A, Ruggeri L, D'Addio A, et al: Successful transfer of alloreactive haploidentical KIR ligand-mismatched natural killer cells after infusion in elderly after high risk acute myeloid leukemia patients. *Blood* 11:3273, 2011.

907. Sekeres MA, Gundacker H, Lancet J, et al: A phase 2 study of lenalidomide monotherapy in patients with 5q acute myeloid leukemia: Southwest Oncology Group Study S0605. *Blood* 118: 523, 2011.

908. Blum W, Klisovic RB, Becker H, et al: Dose escalation of lenalidomide in relapsed or refractory acute leukemias. *J Clin Oncol* 28:4919, 2010.

909. Mardiors A, Dos Santos C, McDonald T, et al: T cells expressing CD123=specific chimeric antigen receptors exhibit specific cytolytic effector functions and antitumor effects against human acute myeloid leukemia. *Blood* 122:3138, 2013.

910. Tettamanti S, Biondi A, Biagl E, et al: CD123 AML targeting by chimeric antigen receptors. *Oncoimmunology* 3:e28835, 2014.

911. Rego EM, Kim HT, Ruiz-Arguelles GJ, et al: Improving acute promyelocytic leukemia (APL) outcome in developing countries through networking, results of the International consortium on APL. *Blood* 121:1935, 2013.

912. Sanz MA, Martin G, Gonzalez M, et al: Risk-adapted treatment of acute promyelocytic leukemia with all-trans-retinoic acid and anthracycline monochemotherapy: A multicenter study by the PETHEMA. *Blood* 103:1237, 2004.

913. Avvisati G, Petti MC, Lo-Coco F, et al: Induction therapy with idarubicin alone significantly influences event-free survival duration in patients with newly diagnosed hypergranular acute promyelocytic leukemia: Final results of the GIMEMA randomized study LAP 0389 with 7 years of minimal follow-up. *Blood* 100:3141, 2002.

914. Sanz MA, Tallman MS, Lo-Coco F, et al: Practice points, consensus, and controversial issues in the management of patients with newly diagnosed acute promyelocytic leukemia. *Oncologist* 10:806, 2005.

915. Sanz MA, Lo-Coco F: Standard practice and controversial issues in front-line therapy of acute promyelocytic leukemia. *Haematologica* 90:840, 2005.

916. Sanz MA, Grimwade D, Tallman MS, et al: Management of acute promyelocytic leukemia: Recommendations from an expert panel on behalf of the European LeukemiaNet. *Blood* 113:1875, 2009.

917. Lengfelder E, Reichert A, Schoch C, et al: Double induction strategy including high dose cytarabine in combination with all-trans retinoic acid: Effects in patients with newly diagnosed acute promyelocytic leukemia. German AML Cooperative Group. *Leukemia* 14:1362, 2000.

918. Adès L, Sanz MA, Chevret S, et al: Treatment of newly diagnosed acute promyelocytic leukemia (APL): A comparison of French-Belgian-Swiss and PETHEMA results. *Blood* 111:1078, 2008.

919. Sanz MA, Montesions P, Rayon C, et al: Risk-adapted treatment of acute promyelocytic leukemia based on all-trans retinoic acid and anthracycline with addition of cytarabine in consolidation therapy for high-risk patients; further improvements in treatment outcome. *Blood* 115:5137, 2010.

920. Iland HJ, Bradstock K, Supple SG, et al: All-trans-retinoic acid, idarubicin and IV arsenic trioxide as initial therapy in acute promyelocytic leukemia (APML4). *Blood* 120:1570, 2012.

921. Lo-Coco F, Avvisati G, Vignetti M, et al: Retinoic acid and arsenic trioxide for acute promyelocytic leukemia. *N Engl J Med* 369:111, 2013.

922. Lallemand-Breittenbach V, de The H: Retinoic acid plus arsenic trioxide, the ultimate panacea for acute promyelocytic leukemia? *Blood* 122:2008, 2013.

923. Mandelli F, Latagliata R, Avvisati G, et al: Treatment of elderly patients (> or = 60 years) with newly diagnosed acute promyelocytic leukemia. Results of the Italian multicenter group GIMEMA with ATRA and idarubicin (AIDA) protocols. *Leukemia* 17:1085, 2003.

924. Estey EH, Giles FJ, Beran M, et al: Experience with gemtuzumab ozogamicin ("Mylotarg") and all-trans retinoic acid in untreated acute promyelocytic leukemia. *Blood* 99:4222, 2002.

925. Shen ZX, Shi ZZ, Fang J, et al: All-trans retinoic acid/As_2O_3 combination yields a high quality remission and survival in newly diagnosed acute promyelocytic leukemia. *Proc Natl Acad Sci U S A* 10:1073, 2004.

926. Tallman MS, Rowe JM: Long-term follow-up and potential for cure in acute promyelocytic leukaemia. *Best Pract Res Clin Haematol* 16:535, 2003.

927. Park JH, Qiao B, Panageas KS, et al: Early death rate in acute promyelocytic leukemia remains high despite all-trans retinoic acid. *Blood* 118:1248, 2011.

928. Tallman MS, Altman JK: How I treat acute promyelocytic leukemia. *Blood* 114:5126, 2009.

929. Tallman MS, Andersen JW, Schiffer CA, et al: All-trans-retinoic acid in acute promyelocytic leukemia. *N Engl J Med* 337:1021, 1997.

930. Chomienne C, Ballerini P, Balitrand N, et al: All-trans retinoic acid in acute promyelocytic leukemia: II. In vitro studies: Structure–function relationship. *Blood* 76:1710, 1990.

931. Degos L: Is acute promyelocytic leukemia a curable disease? Treatment strategy for a long-term survival. *Leukemia* 8:911, 1994.

932. Degos L, Dombret H, Chomienne C, et al: All-trans-retinoic acid as a differentiating agent in the treatment of acute promyelocytic leukemia. *Blood* 85:2643, 1995.

933. Gallagher RE, Li YP, Rao S, et al: Characterization of acute promyelocytic leukemia cases with PML-RAR alpha break/fusion sites in PML exon 6: Identification of a subgroup with decreased in vitro responsiveness to all-trans retinoic acid. *Blood* 86:1540, 1995.

934. Licht JD, Chomienne C, Goy A, et al: Clinical and molecular characterization of a rare syndrome of acute promyelocytic leukemia associated with translocation (11;17). *Blood* 85:1083, 1995.

935. Jansen JH, De Ridder MC, Geertsma WM, et al: Complete remission of t(11;17) positive acute promyelocytic leukemia induced by all-trans retinoic acid and granulocyte colony-stimulating factor. *Blood* 94:39, 1999.

936. Tallman MS, Andersen JW, Schiffer CA, et al: All-trans retinoic acid in acute promyelocytic leukemia: Long-term outcome and prognostic factor analysis from the North American Intergroup protocol. *Blood* 100:4298, 2002.

937. Hernandez JM, Martin G, Gutierrez MC, et al: Additional cytogenetic changes do not influence the outcome of patients with newly diagnosed acute promyelocytic leukemia treated with an ATRA plus anthracycline based protocol. A report of the Spanish group PETHEMA. *Haematologica* 86:807, 2001.

938. Kennedy GA, Marlton P, Cobcroft R, Gill D: Molecular remission without blood product support using all-trans retinoic acid (ATRA) induction and combined arsenic trioxide/ATRA consolidation in a Jehovah's Witness with de novo acute promyelocytic leukemia. *Br J Haematol* 111:1103, 2000.

939. Martinelli G, Ottaviani E, Testoni N, et al: Disappearance of PML/RAR alpha acute promyelocytic leukemia associated transcript during consolidation chemotherapy. *Haematologica* 83:985, 1998.

940. Fadilah SA, Hatta AZ, Keng CS, et al: Successful treatment of acute promyelocytic leukemia in pregnancy with all-trans retinoic acid. *Leukemia* 15:1665, 2001.

941. Carridice D, Austin N, Bayston K, Ganly PS: Successful treatment of acute promyelocytic leukaemia during pregnancy. *Clin Lab Haematol* 24:307, 2002.

942. Tallman MS, Andersen JW, Schiffer CA, et al: Clinical description of 44 patients with acute promyelocytic leukemia who developed the retinoic acid syndrome. *Blood* 95:90, 2000.

943. Sanz MA, Montesinos P: How we prevent and treat differentiation syndrome in patients with acute promyelocytic leukemia. *Blood* 123:2777, 2014.

944. Larsen RS, Tallman MS: Retinoic acid syndrome: Manifestations, pathogenesis, and treatment. *Best Pract Res Clin Haematol* 16:453, 2003.

945. Frankel SR, Eardley A, Lauwers G, et al: The "retinoic acid syndrome" in acute promyelocytic leukemia. *Ann Intern Med* 117:292, 1992.

946. De Botton S, Dombret H, Sanz M, et al: Incidence, clinical features, and outcome of all trans-retinoic acid syndrome in 413 cases of newly diagnosed acute promyelocytic leukemia. The European APL Group. *Blood* 92:2712, 1998.

947. Azlin ZA, Ahmed T: Cure in acute promyelocytic leukemia—Now more readily achievable with less toxic therapy. *Blood* 79:2492, 1992.

948. Tallman MS: Retinoic acid syndrome: A problem of the past? *Leukemia* 16:160, 2002.

949. Falanga A, Barbui T: Coagulopathy of acute promyelocytic leukemia. *Acta Haematol* 106:43, 2001.

950. Yanada M, Matsushita T, Asou N, et al: Severe hemorrhagic complications during remission induction therapy for acute promyelocytic leukemia: Incidence, risk factors, and influence on outcome. *Eur J Haematol* 78:213, 2007.

951. Goldberg MA, Ginsburg D, Mayer RJ, et al: Is heparin administration necessary during induction chemotherapy for patients with acute promyelocytic leukemia? *Blood* 69:187, 1987.

952. Visani G, Gugliotta L, Tosi P, et al: All-trans retinoic acid significantly reduces the incidence of early hemorrhagic death during induction therapy of acute promyelocytic leukemia. *Eur J Haematol* 64:139, 2000.

953. Jacomo RH, Santana-Lemos BA, Lima ASG, et al: Methionine-induced hyperhomocysteinemia reverses fibrinolytic pathway activation in a murine model of actue promyelocytic leukemia. *Blood* 120:207, 2012.

954. Petti MC, Avvisati G, Amadori S, et al: Acute promyelocytic leukaemia: Clinical aspects and results of treatment in 62 patients. *Haematologica* 72:151, 1987.

955. Kizaki M, Ueno H, Yamazoe Y, et al: Mechanisms of retinoid resistance in leukemic cells: Possible role of cytochrome P450 and P-glycoprotein. *Blood* 87:725, 1996.

956. Adès L, Chevret S, Raffoux E, et al: Is cytarabine useful in the treatment of acute promyelocytic leukemia? Results of a randomized trial from the European Acute Promyelocytic Leukemia Group. *J Clin Oncol* 24:5703, 2006.

957. Asou N, Kishimoto Y, Kiyoi H, et al: A randomized study with or without intensified maintenance chemotherapy in patients with acute promyelocytic leukemia who have become negative for PML-RARalpha transcript after consolidation therapy: The Japan Adult Leukemia Study Group (JALSG) APL97 study. *Blood* 110:59, 2007.

958. Tsimberidou AM, Kantarjian H, Keating MJ, Estey E: Optimizing treatment for elderly patients with acute promyelocytic leukemia: Is it time to replace chemotherapy with all-trans retinoic acid and arsenic trioxide? *Leuk Lymphoma* 47:2282, 2006.

959. Chen GQ, Shi XG, Tang W, et al: Use of arsenic trioxide (As_2O_3) in the treatment of acute promyelocytic leukemia (APL): 1. As_2O_3 exerts dose-dependent dual effects on APL cells. *Blood* 89:3345, 1997.

960. Jing Y, Dai J, Chalmers-Redman RME, et al: Arsenic trioxide selectively induces acute promyelocytic leukemia cell apoptosis via a hydrogen peroxide-dependent pathway. *Blood* 94:2102, 1999.

961. Mathas S, Lietz A, Janz M, et al: Inhibition of NF-kappaB essentially contributes to arsenic-induced apoptosis. *Blood* 102:1028, 2003.

962. Ozpolat B, Akar U, Zorrilla-Calancha I, et al: Death-associated protein 5 (DAP5/p97/NAT1) contributes to retinoic acid-induced granulocytic differentiation and arsenic trioxide-induced apoptosis in acute promyelocytic leukemia. *Apoptosis* 13:915, 2008.

963. Soignet SL, Maslak P, Wang ZG, et al: Complete remission after treatment of acute promyelocytic leukemia with arsenic trioxide. *N Engl J Med* 339:1341, 1998.

964. Kwong YL, Au WY, Chim CS, et al: Arsenic trioxide- and idarubicin-induced remissions in relapsed acute promyelocytic leukaemia: Clinicopathological and molecular features of a pilot study. *Am J Hematol* 66:274, 2001.

965. Raffoux E, Rousselot P, Poupon J, et al: Combined treatment with arsenic trioxide and all-trans-retinoic acid in patients with relapsed acute promyelocytic leukemia. *J Clin Oncol* 21:2326, 2003.

966. Comacho LH, Soignet SL, Chanel S, et al: Leukocytosis and the retinoic acid syndrome in patients with acute promyelocytic leukemia treated with arsenic trioxide. *J Clin Oncol* 18:2620, 2000.

967. Unnikrishnan D, Dutcher JP, Varshneya N, et al: Torsades de pointes in 3 patients with leukemia treated with arsenic trioxide. *Blood* 97:1514, 2001.

968. Zhou J, Meng R, Li X, et al: The effect of arsenic trioxide on QT interval prolongation during APL therapy. *Chin Med J* 116:1764, 2003.

969. Fenaux P, Chastang C, Chevret S, et al: A randomized comparison of all-*trans* retinoic acid (ATRA) followed by chemotherapy and ATRA plus chemotherapy and the role of maintenance therapy in newly diagnosed acute promyelocytic leukemia. The European APL Group. *Blood* 94:1192, 1999.

970. Ades L, Guerci A, Raffoux E, et al: Very long-term outcome of acute promyelocytic leukemia after treatment with all-*trans* retinoic acid and chemotherapy: The European APL Group experience. *Blood* 115:1690, 2010.

971. Thirugnanam R, George B, Chendamarai E, et al: Comparison of clinical outcomes of patients with relapsed acute promyelocytic leukemia induced with arsenic trioxide and consolidated with either an autologous stem cel transplant or an arsenic trioxide-based regimen. *Biol Blood Marrow Transplant* 15:1479, 2009.

972. de Bottom S, Fawaz A, Chevret S, et al: Autologous and allogeneic stem-cell transplantation as salvage treatment of acute promyelocytic leukemia initially treated with all-trans-retinoic acid: A retrospective analysis of the European acute promyelocytic leukemia groups. *J Clin Oncol* 23:120, 2005.

973. Aribi A, Kantarjian HM, Estey EH, et al: Combination therapy with arsenic trioxide, all-trans retinoic acid, and gemtuzumab ozogamicin in recurrent acute promyelocytic leukemia. *Cancer* 109:1355, 2007.

974. Lo-Coco F, Romano A, Mengarelli A, et al: Allogeneic stem cell transplantation for advanced acute promyelocytic leukemia: Results in patients treated in second molecular remission or with molecularly persistent disease. *Leukemia* 17:1930, 2003.

975. Nabhan C, Mehta J, Tallman MS: The role of bone marrow transplantation in acute promyelocytic leukemia. *Bone Marrow Transplant* 28:219, 2001.

976. Colvic N, Bogdanovic A, Miljic P, et al: Central nervous system relapse in acute promyelocytic leukemia. *Am J Hematol* 71:60, 2002.

977. Sanz MA, Larrea L, Sanz G, et al: Cutaneous promyelocytic sarcoma at sites of vascular access and marrow aspiration. A characteristic localization of chloromas in acute promyelocytic leukemia? *Haematologica* 85:758, 2000.

978. Latagliata R, Carmosino I, Breccia M, et al: Late relapses in acute promyelocytic leukaemia. *Acta Haematol* 117:106, 2007.

979. Esteve J, Escoda L, Martín G, et al: Outcome of patients with acute promyelocytic leukemia failing to front-line treatment with all-*trans* retinoic acid and anthracycline-based chemotherapy (PETHEMA protocols LPA96 and LPA99): Benefit of an early intervention. *Leukemia* 21:446, 2007.

980. Latagliata R, Petti MC, Fenu S, et al: Therapy-related myelodysplastic syndrome-acute myelogenous leukemia in patients treated for acute promyelocytic leukemia: An emerging problem. *Blood* 99:822, 2002.

981. Lobe I, Rigal-Huguet F, Vekhoff A, et al: Myelodysplastic syndrome after acute promyelocytic leukemia: The European APL group. *Leukemia* 17:1600, 2003.

982. Garcia-Manero G, Kantarjian HM, Kornblau S, Estey E: Therapy-related myelodysplastic syndrome or acute myelogenous leukemia in patients with acute promyelocytic leukemia (APL). *Leukemia* 16:1888, 2002.

983. Jantunen E, Heinonen K, Mahlamäki E, et al: Secondary acute promyelocytic leukemia: An increasingly common entity. *Leuk Lymphoma* 48:190, 2007.

984. Yoo SJ, Park CJ, Jang S, et al: Inferior prognostic outcome in acute promyelocytic leukemia with alterations of FLT3 gene. *Leuk Lymphoma* 47:1788, 2006.

985. Gallagher RE, Moser BK, Racevskis J, et al: Treatment-influenced associations of PML-RARα mutations, FLT3 mutations, and additional chromosome abnormalities in relapsed acute promyelocytic leukemia. *Blood* 120: 2098, 2012.

986. Lu DP, Qiui JY, Jiang B, et al: Tetra-arsenic tetra-sulfide for the treatment of acute promyelocytic leukemia: A pilot report. *Blood* 99:2136, 2002.

987. Takeuchi M, Yano T, Omoto E, et al: Relapsed acute promyelocytic leukemia previously treated with all-*trans* retinoic acid: Clinical experience with a new synthetic retinoid, Am-80. *Leuk Lymphoma* 31:441, 1998.

988. Bally C, FadallahJ, Leverger G, et al: Outcome of acute promyelocytic leukemia (APL) in children and adolescents: An analysis in two consecutive trials of the European APL group. *J Clin Oncol* 30:1641, 2012.

989. Smith MA, McCaffrey RP, Karp JE: The secondary leukemias: Challenges and research directions. *J Natl Cancer Inst* 88:407, 1996.

990. Smith MA, Rubinstein L, Anderson JR, et al: Secondary leukemia or myelodysplastic syndrome after treatment with epipodophyllotoxins. *J Clin Oncol* 17:569, 1999.

991. Ng A, Taylor GM, Eden OB: Treatment-related leukaemia: A clinical and scientific challenge. *Cancer Treat Rev* 26:377, 2000.

992. Super HJ, McCabe NR, Thirman MJ, et al: Rearrangements of the MLL gene in therapy-related acute myeloid leukemia in patients previously treated with agents targeting DNA-topoisomerase 11. *Blood* 82:3705, 1993.

993. Dissing M, Le Beau MM, Pedersen-Bjergaard J: Inversion of chromosome 16 and uncommon rearrangements of the CBFB and MYHI1 genes in therapy-related acute myeloid leukemia: Rare events related to DNA-topoisomerase II inhibitors? *J Clin Oncol* 16:1890, 1998.

994. Gondek LP, Tiu R, O'Keefe CL, et al: Chromosomal lesions and uniparental disomy detected by SNP arrays in MDS, MDS/MPD, and MDS-derived AML. *Blood* 111:1534, 2008.

995. Seedhouse C, Russell N: Advances in the understanding of susceptibility to treatment-related acute myeloid leukaemia. *Br J Haematol* 137:513, 2007.

996. Pogliani EM, Pioltelli P, Russini F, et al: Acute leukemia following cisplatin for ovarian cancer [letter]. *Haematologica* 72:184, 1987.

997. Kolte B, Baer AN, Sait SN, et al: Acute myeloid leukemia in the setting of low dose weekly methotrexate therapy for rheumatoid arthritis. *Leuk Lymphoma* 42:371, 2001.

998. Bakland G, Nossent H: Acute myelogenous leukemia following etanercept therapy. *Rheumatology (Oxford)* 42:900, 2003.

999. Noronha V, Berliner N, Ballen KK, et al: Treatment-related myelodysplasia/AML in a patient with a history of breast cancer and an oligodendroglioma treated with temozolomide: Case study and review of the literature. *Neuro Oncol* 8:280, 2006.

1000. Aktan M, Tanakol R, Nalcaci M, Dincol G: Leukemia in a patient treated with growth hormone. *Endocr J* 47:471, 2000.

1001. Freedman MH, Bonilla MA, Fier C, et al: Myelodysplasia syndrome and acute myeloid leukemia in patients with congenital neutropenia receiving G-CSF therapy. *Blood* 96:429, 2000.

1002. Andersen MK, Pedersen-Bjergaard J: Therapy-related MDS and AML in acute promyelocytic leukemia. *Blood* 100:1928, 2002.

1003. Barnard DR, Lange B, Alonzo TA, et al: Acute myeloid leukemia and myelodysplastic syndrome in children treated for cancer: Comparison with primary presentation. *Blood* 100:427, 2002.

1004. Smith RE, Bryant J, DeCillis A, et al: Acute myeloid leukemia and myelodysplastic syndrome after doxorubicin-cyclophosphamide adjuvant therapy for operable breast cancer: The National Surgical Adjuvant Breast and Bowel Project Experience. *J Clin Oncol* 21:1195, 2003.

1005. Gershkevitsh E, Rosenberg I, Dearnaley DP, Trott KR: Bone marrow doses and leukemia risk in radiotherapy of prostate cancer. *Radiother Oncol* 53:189, 1999.

1006. Armitage JO, Carbone PP, Connors JM, et al: Treatment-related myelodysplasia and acute leukemia in non-Hodgkin's lymphoma. *J Clin Oncol* 21:897, 2003.

1007. Lambertenghi Deliliers G, Annaloro C, Pozzoli E, et al: Cytogenetic and myelodysplastic alterations after autologous hemopoietic stem cell transplantation. *Leuk Res* 23:291, 1999.

1008. Legare RD, Gribben JG, Maragh M, et al: Prediction of therapy-related acute myelogenous leukemia (AML) and myelodysplastic syndrome (MDS) after autologous bone marrow transplant (ABMT) for lymphoma. *Am J Hematol* 56:45, 1997.

1009. Micallef IN, Lillington DM, Apostolidis J, et al: Therapy-related myelodysplasia and secondary acute myelogenous leukemia after high-dose therapy with autologous hematopoietic progenitor-cell support for lymphoid malignancies. *J Clin Oncol* 18:847, 2000.

1010. Lillington DM, Micallef IN, Carpenter E, et al: Detection of chromosome abnormalities pre-high-dose treatment in patients developing therapy-related myelodysplasia and secondary acute myelogenous leukemia after treatment for non-Hodgkin's lymphoma. *J Clin Oncol* 19:2472, 2001.

1011. Estey EH: Treatment of acute myelogenous leukemia and myelodys-plastic syndromes. *Semin Hematol* 32:132, 1995.

1012. Witherspoon RP, Deeg HJ, Storer B, et al: Hematopoietic stem-cell transplantation for treatment-related leukemia or myelodysplasia. *J Clin Oncol* 19:2134, 2001.

1013. Costa LJ, Rodriguez V, Porrata LF, et al: Autologous HSC transplant in t-MDS/AML using cells harvested prior to the development of the secondary malignancy. *Bone Marrow Transplant* 42:497, 2008.

1014. Anderson JE, Gooley TA, Schoch G, et al: Stem cell transplantation for secondary acute myeloid leukemia: Evaluation of transplantation as initial therapy or following induction chemotherapy. *Blood* 89:2578, 1997.

1015. Rowe JM: Therapy of secondary leukemia. *Leukemia* 16:748, 2002.

1016. Rosenfield C, Kantarjian H: Is myelodysplastic related acute myelogenous leukemia a distinct entity from *de novo* acute myelogenous leukemia? Potential for targeted therapies. *Leuk Lymphoma* 41:493, 2001.

1017. Viniou NA, Vassilakopoulos TP, Giakoumi X, et al: Ida-FLAG plus imatinib mesylate-induced remission with chemoresistant Ph1+ acute myeloid leukemia. *Eur J Haematol* 72:58, 2004.

1018. Brincker H: Estimate of overall treatment results in acute nonlymphocytic leukemia based on age-specific rates of incidence and complete remission. *Cancer Treat Rep* 69:5, 1985.

1019. Büchner T, Berdel WE, Haferlach C, et al: Age-related risk profile and chemotherapy dose response in acute myeloid leukemia: A study by the German Acute Myeloid Leukemia Cooperative Group. *J Clin Oncol* 27:61, 2009.

1020. Kuendgen A, Germing U: Emerging treatment strategies for acute myeloid leukemia (AML) in the elderly. *Cancer Treat Rev* 35:97, 2009.

1021. Dombret H, Raffoux E, Gardin C: Acute myeloid leukemia in the elderly. *Semin Oncol* 35:430, 2008.

1022. Ferrara F, Pinto A: Acute myeloid leukemia in the elderly: Current therapeutic results and perspectives for clinical research. *Rev Recent Clin Trials* 2:33, 2007.

1023. Pinto A, Zulian GB, Archimbaud E: Acute myelogenous leukaemia. *Crit Rev Oncol Hematol* 27:161, 1998.

1024. Leith CP, Kopecky KJ, Godwin J, et al: Acute myeloid leukemia in the elderly: Assessment of multidrug resistance (MDR1) and cytogenetics distinguishes biologic subgroups with remarkably distinct responses to standard chemotherapy. A Southwest Oncology Group study. *Blood* 89:3323, 1997.

1025. Bacher U, Kern W, Schnittger S, et al: Population-based age-specific incidences of cytogenetic subgroups of acute myeloid leukemia. *Haematologica* 90:1502, 2005.

1026. Ballester O, Moscinski LC, Morris D, Balducci L: Acute myelogenous leukemia in the elderly. *J Am Geriatr Soc* 40:277, 1992.

1027. Klepin HD, Rao AV, Pardee TS: Acute myeloid leukemia and myelodysplastic syndromes in older adults. *J Clin Oncol* 23:2541, 2014.

1028. Klepin H, Balducci L: Acute myelogenous leukemia in older adults, *Oncologist* 13:222, 2009.

1029. Klepin HD, Geiger AM, Tooze JA, et al: Geriatric assessment predicts survival for older adults receiving induction chemotherapy for acute myelogenous leukemia. *Blood* 121:4287, 2013.

1030. Baz R, Rodriguez C, Fu AZ, et al: Impact of remission induction chemotherapy on survival in older adults with acute myeloid leukemia. *Cancer* 110:1752, 2007.

1031. Juliusson G, Antunovic P, Derolf A, et al: Age and acute myeloid leukemia: Real world data on decision to treat and outcomes from the Swedish Acute Leukemia Registry. *Blood* 113:4179, 2009.

1032. Deschler B, de Witte T, Mertelsmann R, Lübbert M: Treatment decision-making for older patients with high-risk myelodysplastic syndrome or acute myeloid leukemia: Problems and approaches. *Haematologica* 91:1513, 2006.

1033. Kantarjian H, Ravandi F, O'Brien S, et al: Intensive chemotherapy does not benefit most older patients (age 70 year or older) with acute myeloid leukemia. *Blood* 116:4422, 2010.

1034. Malfusion J-V, Etienne A, Turlure P, et al: Risk factors and decision criteria for intensive chemotherapy in older patients with acute myeloid leukemia. *Haematologica* 93:1806, 2008.

1035. Kalaycio M, Pohlman B, Elson P, et al: Chemotherapy for acute myelogenous leukemia in the elderly with cytarabine, mitoxantrone, and granulocyte-macrophage colony-stimulating factor. *Am J Clin Oncol* 24:58, 2001.

1036. Bennett CL, Hynes D, Godwin J, et al: Economic analysis of granulocyte colony stimulating factor as adjunct therapy for older patients with acute myelogenous leukemia (AML): Estimates from a Southwest Oncology Group clinical trial. *Cancer Invest* 19:603, 2001.

1037. Löwenberg B, Suciu S, Archimbaud E, et al: Mitoxantrone versus daunorubicin in induction-consolidation chemotherapy—The value of low-dose cytarabine for maintenance of remission, and an assessment of prognostic factors in acute myeloid leukemia in the elderly: Final report. European Organization for the Research and Treatment of Cancer and the Dutch-Belgian Hemato-Oncology Cooperative Hovon Group. *J Clin Oncol* 16:872, 1998.

1038. Harousseau JL, Rigal-Huguet F, Hurteloup P, et al: Treatment of acute myeloid leukemia in elderly patients with oral idarubicin as a single agent. *Eur J Haematol* 42:182, 1989.

1039. Anderson JE, Kopecky KJ, Willman CL, et al: Outcome after induction chemotherapy for older patients with acute myeloid leukemia is not improved with mitoxantrone and etoposide compared to cytarabine and daunorubicin: A Southwest Oncology Group study. *Blood* 100:3869, 2002.

1040. Hartman F, Jacobs G, Gotto H, et al: Cytosine arabinoside, idarubicin and divided dose etoposide for the treatment of acute myeloid leukemia in elderly patients. *Leuk Lymphoma* 42:347, 2001.

1041. Kanemura N, Tsurumi H, Kasahara S, et al: Continuous drip infusion of low dose cytarabine and etoposide with granulocyte colony-stimulating factor for elderly patients with acute myeloid leukaemia ineligible for intensive chemotherapy. *Hematol Oncol* 26:33, 2008.

1042. Brandwein JM, Yang L, Schimmer AD, et al: A phase II study of temozolomide therapy for poor-risk patients aged > or = 60 years with acute myeloid leukemia: Low levels of MGMT predict for response. *Leukemia* 21:821, 2007.

1043. Faderl S, Ravandi F, Huang X, et al: A randomized study of clofarabine versus clofarabine plus low-dose cytarabine as front-line therapy for patients aged 60 years and older with acute myeloid leukemia and high-risk myelodysplastic syndrome. *Blood* 112:1638, 2008.

1044. Burnett AK, Russell NH, Kell J, et al: European development of clofarabine as treatment for older patients with acute myeloid leukemia considered unsuitable for intensive chemotherapy. *J Clin Oncol* 28:2389, 2010.

1045. Kantarjian HM, Erba HP, Claxton D, et al: Phase II study of clofarabine monotherapy in previously untreated older adults with acute myeloid leukemia and unfavorable prognostic factors. *J Clin Oncol* 28:549, 2009.

1046. Ossenkoppele GJ, Stussi G, Maertens J, et al: Addition of bevacizumab to chemotherapy in acute myeloid leukemia at older age: A randomized phase 2 trial of the Dutch-Belgian Cooperative Trial Group for Hemato-Oncology (HOVON) and the Swiss Group for Cancer Research (SAKK). *Blood* 120:4706, 2012.

1047. Serve H, Krug U, Wagner R, et al: Sorafenib in combination with intensive chemotherapy in elderly patients with acute myeloid leukemia: Results from a randomized, placebo-controlled trial. *J Clin Oncol* 31:3110, 2013.

1048. Burnett AK, Hills RK, Hunter AE, et al: The addition of gemtuzumab ozogamicin to low-dose Ara-C improves remission rate but does not significantly prolong survival in older patients with acute myeloid leukaemia: Results from the LFR AML14 and NCRI AML16 pick-a-winner comparison. *Leukemia* 27:75, 2013.

1049. Amadori S, Suciu S, Stasi R, et al: Sequential combination of gemtuzumab ozogamicin and standard chemotherapy in older patients with newly diagnosed acute myeloid leukemia; results of a randomized phase III trial by the EORTC and GIMEMA consortium (AML-17). *J Clin Oncol* 31:4424, 2013.

1050. Schiller GJ: Postremission therapy of acute myeloid leukemia in older adults. *Leukemia* 10(Suppl 1):S18, 1996.

1051. Kiss TL, Sabry W, Lazarus HM, Lipton JH: Blood and marrow transplantation in elderly acute myeloid leukaemia patients—Older certainly is not better. *Bone Marrow Transplant* 40:405, 2007.

1052. McClune BL, Weisdorf DJ, Pedersen TI, et al: Effect of age on outcome of reduced-intensity hematopoietic cell transplantation for older patients with acute myeloid leukemia in first complete remission or with myelodysplastic syndrome. *J Clin Oncol* 28:1878, 2010.

1053. Herzig RH: High-dose ara-C in older adults with acute leukemia. *Leukemia* 10(Suppl 1): S10, 1996.

1054. Letendre L, Noel P, Litzow MR, et al: Treatment of acute myelogenous leukemia in the older patient with attenuated high-dose ara-C. *Am J Clin Oncol* 21:142, 1998.

1055. Schiller G, Lee M: Long-term outcome of high-dose cytarabine-based consolidation chemotherapy for older patients with acute myelogenous leukemia. *Leuk Lymphoma* 25:111, 1997.

1056. Löwenberg B: Post-remission treatment of acute myelogenous leukemia. *N Engl J Med* 332:260, 1995.

1057. Gardin C, Turlure P, Fagot T, et al: Postremission treatment of elderly patients with acute myeloid leukemia in first complete remission after intensive induction chemotherapy: Results of the multicenter randomized Acute Leukemia French Association (ALFA) 9803 trial. *Blood* 109:5129, 2007.

1058. DeLima M, Ghaddar H, Pierce S, Estey E: Treatment of newly-diagnosed acute myelogenous leukaemia in patients aged 80 years and above. *Br J Haematol* 93:89, 1996.

1059. Burnett AK, Mohite U: Treatment of older patients with acute myeloid leukemia—New agents. *Semin Hematol* 43:96, 2006.

1060. Estey EH: Older adults: Should the paradigm shift from standard therapy? *Best Pract Res Clin Haematol* 21:61, 2008.

1061. Etienne A, Esterni B, Charbonnier A, et al: Comorbidity is an independent predictor of complete remission in elderly patients receiving induction chemotherapy for acute myeloid leukemia. *Cancer* 109:1376, 2007.

1062. Gupta V, Xu W, Keng C, et al: The outcome of intensive induction therapy in patients > or = 70 years with acute myeloid leukemia. *Leukemia* 21:1321, 2007.

1063. Estey EH: General approach to, and perspectives on clinical research in, older patients with newly diagnosed acute myeloid leukemia. *Semin Hematol* 43:89, 2006.

1064. Johnson PR, Yin JA: Prognostic factors in elderly patients with acute myeloid leukaemia. *Leuk Lymphoma* 16:51, 1994.

1065. Oberg G, Killander A, Björeman M, et al: Long-term follow-up of patients > or = 60 yr old with acute myeloid leukaemia. *Eur J Haematol* 68:376, 2002.

1066. Stone RM: The difficult problem of acute myeloid leukemia in the older adult. *CA Cancer J Clin* 52:363, 2002.

1067. Alibhai SM, Leach M, Kermalli H, et al: The impact of acute myeloid leukemia and its treatment on quality of life and functional status in older adults. *Crit Rev Oncol Hematol* 64:19, 2007.

1068. Büchner T, Berdel WE, Wörmann B, et al: Treatment of older patients with AML. *Crit Rev Oncol Hematol* 56:247, 2005.

1069. Surveillance, Epidemiology, and End Results (SEER): Myeloid leukemia: 5-Year relative and period survival by race, sex, diagnosis year and age, 1975-2011. Available at: http://seer.cancer.gov/csr/1975_2011/browse_csr.php?sectionSEL=13&pageSEL=sect_13_table.16.html

1070. Prebet T, Boissel N, Reutenauer S, et al: Acute myeloid leukemia with translocation (8;21) or inversion (16) in elderly patients treated with conventional chemotherapy: A collaborative study of the French CBF-AML intergroup. *J Clin Oncol* 27:4747, 2009.

1071. Perrot A, Luquet I, Pigneux A, et al: Dismal prognostic value of monosomal karyotype in elderly patients with acute myeloid leukemia: A GOELAMS study of 186 patients with unfavorable cytogenetic abnormalities. *Blood* 118:679, 2011.

1072. Renosos EE, Shepard FA, Messner HA, et al: Acute leukemia during pregnancy: The Toronto Leukemia Study Group Experience with long-term follow-up of children exposed in utero to chemotherapeutic agents. *J Clin Oncol* 5:1098, 1987.

1073. Caligiuri MA, Mayer RJ: Pregnancy and leukemia. *Semin Oncol* 16:388, 1989.

1074. Chang A, Patel S: Treatment of acute myeloid leukemia during pregnancy: A systematic review of the literature. *Ann Pharmacother* 49:48, 2015.

1075. Chelghoum Y, Vey N, Raffoux E, et al: Acute leukemia during pregnancy: A report on 37 patients and a review of the literature. *Cancer* 104:110, 2005.

1076. Salah AJ, Alhejazi A, Ahmed SO, et al: Leukemia during pregnancy: Long term follow up of 32 cases form a single institution. *Hematol Oncol Stem Cell Ther* 7:63, 2014.

1077. Aviles A, Neri N: Hematological malignancies and pregnancy: A final report of 84 children who received chemotherapy *in utero*. *Clin Lymphoma* 2:173, 2001.

1078. Greenlund LJ, Letendre L, Tefferi A: Acute leukemia during pregnancy: A single institutional experience with 17 cases. *Leuk Lymphoma* 41:571, 2001.

1079. Shapira T, Pereg D, Lishner M: How I treat acute and chronic leukemia in pregnancy. *Blood Rev* 22:247, 2008.

1080. Osada S, Horibe K, Oiwa K, et al: A case of infantile acute monocytic leukemia caused by vertical transmission of the mother's leukemic cells. *Cancer* 65:1146, 1990.

1081. Lipovsky MM, Biesma DH, Christiaens GC, Petersen EJ: Successful treatment of acute promyelocytic leukemia with all-*trans* retinoic acid during late pregnancy. *Br J Haematol* 94:669, 1996.

1082. Valappil S, Kurkar M, Howell R, et al: Outcome of pregnancy in women treated with all-trans retinoic acid; a case report and review of literature. *Hematology* 12:415, 2007.

1083. Gregory J, Arceci R: Acute myeloid leukemia in children: A review of risk factors and recent trials. *Cancer Invest* 20:1027, 2002.

1084. Clark JJ, Smith FO, Arceci RJ: Update in childhood myeloid leukemia: Recent developments in the molecular basis of disease and novel therapies. *Curr Opin Hematol* 10:31, 2002.

1085. Arceci RJ: Progress and controversies in the treatment of pediatric acute myelogenous leukemia. *Curr Opin Hematol* 9:353, 2002.

1086. Webb DKH, Harrison G, Stevens RF, et al: Relationships between age at diagnosis, clinical features, and outcome of therapy in children in the Medical Research Council AML 10 and 12 trials for acute myeloid leukemia. *Blood* 98:1714, 2001.

1087. Zwaan CM, Meshinchi S, Radich JP, et al: FLT3 internal tandem duplication in 234 children with acute myeloid leukemia: Prognostic significance and relation to cellular drug resistance. *Blood* 102:2387, 2002.

1088. Wheatley K, Burnett AK, Goldstone AH, et al: A simple robust, validated and highly predictive index for the determination of risk-directed therapy in acute myeloid leukaemia derived from the MRC AML 10 trial. *Br J Haematol* 107:69, 1999.

1089. Wells RJ, Arthur DC, Srivastava A, et al: Prognostic variables in newly diagnosed children and adolescents with acute myeloid leukemia. *Leukemia* 16:601, 2002.

1090. Sievers EL, Lange BJ, Alonzo TA, et al: Immunophenotypic evidence of leukemia after induction therapy predicts relapse: Results from a prospective Children's Cancer Group study of 252 patients with acute myeloid leukemia. *Blood* 101:3398, 2003.

1091. Hann IM, Webb DK, Gibson BE, Harrison CJ: MRC trials in childhood acute myeloid leukaemia. *Ann Hematol* 83 (Suppl 1):S108, 2004.

1092. Coenen EV, Zwaan CM, Reinhardt D, et al: Pediatric acute myeloid leukemia with t(8;16)(p11;p13), a distinct clinical and biological entity: A collaborative study by the International-Berlin-Frankfurt-Munster AML study group. *Blood* 122:2702, 2013.

1093. Balgobind BV, Raimondi SC, Harbott J, et al: Novel prognostic subgroups in childhood 11p23/MLL-rearranged acute myeloid leukemia: Results of an international retrospective study. *Blood* 114:2489, 2009.

1094. Liang DC, Liu HC, Yang CP, et al: Cooperating gene mutations in childhood acute myeloid leukemia with special reference on mutations of ASXL1, TET2, IDH1, IDH2, and DNMT3A. *Blood* 121:2988, 2013.

1095. Woods WG, Neudorf S, Gold S, et al: A comparison of allogeneic bone marrow transplantation, autologous bone marrow transplantation, and aggressive chemotherapy in children with acute myeloid leukemia in remission: A report from the Children's Cancer Group. *Blood* 97:56, 2001.

1096. Pession A, Masetti R, Rizzari C, et al: Results of the AIEOP AML 2002/01 multicenter prospective trial for the treatment of children with acute myeloid leukemia. *Blood* 122:170, 2013.

1097. Kawasaki H, Isoyama K, Eguchi M, et al: Superior outcome of infant acute myeloid leukemia with intensive chemotherapy: Results of the Japan Infant Leukemia Study Group. *Blood* 98:3589, 2001.

1098. Chessels JM, Harrison CJ, Kempski H, et al: Clinical features, cytogenetics, and outcome in acute lymphoblastic and myeloid leukemia of infancy: Report from the MRC Childhood Leukemia working party. *Leukemia* 16:776, 2002.

1099. Rocha V, Cornish J, Sievers EL, et al: Comparison of outcomes of unrelated bone marrow and umbilical cord blood transplants in children with acute leukemia. *Blood* 97:2962, 2001.

1100. Leung W, Hudson MM, Strickland DK, et al: Late effects of treatment in survivors of childhood acute myeloid leukemia. *J Clin Oncol* 18:3273, 2000.

1101. Leung W, Ribiero RC, Hudson MM, et al: Second malignancy after treatment of childhood acute myeloid leukemia. *Leukemia* 15:41, 2001.

1102. Verhagen C, Stalpers LJ, dePauw BE, Haanen C: Drug-induced skin reactions in patients with acute non-lymphocytic leukaemia. *Eur J Haematol* 38:225, 1987.

1103. Kapusta L, Groot-Loonen J, Thijssen JM, et al: Regional cardiac wall motion abnormalities during and shortly after anthracyclines therapy. *Med Pediatr Oncol* 41:426, 2003.

1104. Sawyer DB: Anthracyclines and heart failure. *N Engl J Med* 368:1154, 2013.

1105. Benvenuto GM, Ometto R, Fontanelli A, et al: Chemotherapy-related cardiotoxicity: New diagnostic and preventive strategies. *Ital Heart J* 4:655, 2003.

1106. Dietz B, van der Hem KG: Late-onset cardiotoxicity of chemotherapy and radiotherapy. *Neth J Med* 61:228, 2003.

1107. Theodoulou M, Hudis C: Cardiac profiles of liposomal anthracyclines: Greater cardiac safety versus conventional doxorubicin? *Cancer* 100:2052, 2004.

1108. Swain SM, Vici P: The current and future role of dexrazoxane as a cardioprotectant in anthracycline treatment: Expert panel review. *J Cancer Res Clin Oncol* 130:1, 2004.

1109. Anderson LA, Pfeiffer R, Warren JL, et al: Hematopoietic malignancies associated with viral and alcoholic hepatitis. *Cancer Epidemiol Biomarkers Prev* 17:3069, 2008.

1110. Kojima H, Abei M, Takei N, et al: Fatal reactivation of hepatitis B virus following cytotoxic chemotherapy for acute myelogenous leukemia: Fibrosing cholestatic hepatitis. *Eur J Haematol* 69:101, 2002.

1111. Ishiga K, Kawatani T, Suou T, et al: Fulminant hepatitis type B after chemotherapy in a serologically negative hepatitis B virus carrier with acute myelogenous leukemia. *Int J Hematol* 73:115, 2001.

1112. Bianco E, Marcucci F, Mele A, et al: Prevalence of hepatitis C virus infection in lymphoproliferative diseases other than B-cell non-Hodgkin's lymphoma, and in myeloproliferative diseases: An Italian Multi-Center case-control study. *Haematologica* 89:70, 2004.

1113. Zuckerman E, Zuckerman T, Douer D, et al: Liver dysfunction in patients infected with hepatitis C virus undergoing chemotherapy for hematologic malignancies. *Cancer* 15:1224, 1998.

1114. Colovic M, Lazarevic V, Colovic R, et al: Hepatosplenic candidiasis after neutropenic phase of acute leukaemia. *Med Oncol* 16:139, 1999.

1115. Teefey SA, Montana MA, Goldfogel GA, Shuman WP: Sonographic diagnosis of neutropenic typhlitis. *AJR Am J Roentgenol* 149:731, 1987.

1116. Keidan RD, Fanning J, Gatenby RA, Weese JL: Recurrent typhlitis. A disease resulting from aggressive chemotherapy. *Dis Colon Rectum* 32:206, 1989.

1117. Zuckerman T, Ganzel C, Tallman MS, et al: How I treat hematologic emergencies in adults with acute leukemia. *Blood* 120:1993, 2012.

1118. De Stefano V, Sora F, Rossi E, et al: The risk of thrombosis in patients with acute leukemia: Occurrence of thrombosis at diagnosis and during treatment. *J Thromb Haemost* 3:1985, 2004.

1119. Kwann HC, Huyck T: Thromboembolic and bleeding complication in acute leukemia. *Expert Rev Hematol* 3:719, 2010.

1120. Byrnes JJ, Baqueiro H, Gonzalez M, Henseley GT: Thrombotic thrombocytopenic purpura subsequent to acute myelogenous leukemia chemotherapy. *Am J Hematol* 21:299, 1986.

1121. Blumenfeld Z, Avivi I, Ritter M, Rowe JM: Preservation of fertility and ovarian function and minimizing chemotherapy-induced gonadotoxicity in young women. *J Soc Gynecol Investig* 6:229, 1999.

1122. Lopez Andreu JA, Fernandez PJ, Ferrisi Tortajada J, et al: Persistent altered spermatogenesis in long-term childhood cancer survivors. *Pediatr Hematol Oncol* 17:21, 2000.

1123. Relander T, Cavallin-Stahl E, Garwicz S, et al: Gonadal and sexual function in men treated for childhood cancer. *Med Pediatr Oncol* 35:52, 2000.

1124. Rossi BV, Missmer S, Correia KF, et al: Ovarian reserve in women treated for acute lymphocytic leukemia or acute myeloid leukemia with chemotherapy, but not stem cell transplantation. *ISRN Oncol* 2012:956190, 2012.

1125. Molgaard-Hansen L, Skou AS, Juul A, et al: Pubertal development and fertility in survivors of childhood acute myeloid leukemia treated with chemotherapy only: A NOPHO-AML study. *Pediatr Blood Cancer* 60:1988, 2013.

1126. Hinterberger-Fischer M, Kier P, Kalhs P, et al: Fertility, pregnancies and offspring complications after bone marrow transplantation. *Bone Marrow Transplant* 7:5, 1991.

1127. Giri N, Vowels MR, Barr AL, Mameghan H: Successful pregnancy after total body irradiation and bone marrow transplantation for acute leukaemia. *Bone Marrow Transplant* 10:93, 1992.

1128. Lemez P, Urbánek V: Chemotherapy for acute myeloid leukemias with cytosine arabinoside, daunorubicin, etoposide, and mitoxantrone may cause permanent oligoasthenozoospermia or amenorrhea in middle-aged patients. *Neoplasma* 52:398, 2005.

1129. Maguire LC, Dick FR, Sherman BM: The effects of anti-leukemic therapy on gonadal histology in adult males. *Cancer* 48:1967, 1981.

1130. Matthews JH, Wood JK: Male fertility during chemotherapy for acute leukemia. *N Engl J Med* 303:1235, 1980.

1131. Branvall E, Derolf AR, Johansson E, et al: Self-reported fertility in long-term survivors of acute myeloid leukemia. *Ann Hematol* 93:1491, 2014.

1132. Cheson BD, Bennett J, Kopecky KJ, et al: Revised recommendations of the International Working Group for Diagnosis, Standardization of Response Criteria, Treatment Outcomes, and Reporting Standards for Therapeutic Trials in Acute Myeloid Leukemia. *J Clin Oncol* 21:4642, 2003.

1133. Lichtman MA: Does a diagnosis of myelogenous leukemia require 20% marrow myeloblasts, and does <5% marrow myeloblasts represent a remission? The history and ambiguity of arbitrary diagnostic boundaries in the understanding of myelodysplasia. *Oncologist* 18:973, 2013.

1134. Walter RB, Kantarjian HM, Hunag X, et al: Effect of complete remission and responses less than complete remission on survival in acute myeloid leukemia: A combined Eastern Cooperative Oncology Group, Southwest Oncology Group, and M. D. Anderson Cancer Center study. *J Clin Oncol* 28:1766, 2010.

1135. Chen Y, Cortes J, Estrov Z, et al: Persistence of cytogenetic abnormalities at complete remission after induction in patients with acute myeloid leukemia: Prognostic significance and the potential role of allogeneic stem-cell transplantation. *J Clin Oncol* 29:2507, 2011.

1136. Wahlin A, Markevarn B, Gololeva I, et al: Improved outcome in adult acute myeloid leukemia is almost entirely restricted to young patients and associated stem cell transplantation. *Eur J Haematol* 68:54, 2002.

1137. Lichtman MA, Rowe JM: The relationship of patient age to the pathobiology of the clonal myeloid disease. *Semin Oncol* 31:185, 2004.

1138. Kayser S, Dohen K, Krauter, et al: The impact of therapy-related acute myeloid leukemia (AML) on outcome in 2853 adult patients with newly diagnosed AML. *Blood* 117:2137, 2011.

1139. Yanada M, Garcia-Manero G, Borthakur G, et al: Potential cure of acute myeloid leukemia: Analysis of 1069 consecutive patients in first complete remission. *Cancer* 110:2756, 2007.

1140. Walter RB, Othus M, Borthakur G, et al: Prediction of early death after induction therapy for newly diagnosed acute myeloid leukemia with pretreatment risk scores: A novel paradigm for treatment assignment. *J Clin Oncol* 29:4417, 2011.

1141. Fialkow PJ, Singer JW, Roskind WH, et al: Clonal development, stem cell differentiation and the nature of clinical remissions in acute nonlymphocytic leukemia: Studies of patients heterozygous for glucose-6-phosphate dehydrogenase. *N Engl J Med* 317:468, 1987.

1142. Bartram CR, Ludwig W-D, Hiddemann W, et al: Acute myeloid leukemia: Analysis of ras gene mutations and clonality defined by polymorphic X-linked loci. *Leukemia* 3:247, 1989.

1143. Fialkow PJ, Janssen JWG, Bartram CR: Clonal remissions in acute nonlymphocytic leukemia: Evidence for a multistep pathogenesis of the malignancy. *Blood* 77:1415, 1991.

1144. Busque L, Gilliland DG: Clonal evolution in acute myeloid leukemia. *Blood* 82:337, 1993.

1145. Gale RE, Wheadon H, Goldstone AH, et al: Frequency of clonal remission in acute myeloid leukaemia. *Lancet* 341:138, 1993.

1146. Killman SA: Acute leukemia: Development, remission/relapse pattern, relationship between normal and leukaemic haemopoiesis, and the "sleeper-to-feeder" stem cell hypothesis. *Baillieres Clin Haematol* 4:577, 1991.

1147. Kudoh S, Asou H, Kyo T, et al: Emergence of karyotypically unrelated clone in remission of de novo acute myeloblastic leukaemias. Br J Haematol 89:531, 1995.

1148. Jinnai I, Nagai K, Yoshida S, et al: Incidence and characteristics of clonal hematopoiesis in remission of acute myeloid leukemia in relation to morphological dysplasia. Leukemia 9:1756, 1995.

1149. Robert EE: Spontaneous complete remission in acute promyelocytic leukemia. N Y State J Med 86:662, 1985.

1150. Takue Y, Culbert SJ, Van Eys J, et al: Spontaneous cure of end-stage acute nonlymphocytic leukemia complicated with chloroma (granulocytic sarcoma). Cancer 58:1101, 1986.

1151. Jehn UW, Mempel MA: Spontaneous remission of acute myeloid leukemia. Blut 52:165, 1986.

1152. Passe S, Miké V, Mertelsmann R, et al: Acute nonlymphoblastic leukemia: Prognostic factors in adults with long-term follow-up. Cancer 50:1462, 1982.

1153. Evansen SA, Stavem P: Long-term survival in acute leukemia. Acta Med Scand 219:79, 1986.

1154. Grunwald HW: The cure of acute myeloblastic leukemia in adults. JAMA 247:1698, 1982.

1155. MacMahon B, Forman D: Variations in the duration of survival of patients with acute leukemia. Blood 12:683, 1957.

1156. Menzin J, Lang K, Earle C, et al: The outcomes and costs of acute myeloid leukemia among the elderly. Arch Intern Med 162:1597, 2002.

1157. Derolf AR, Kristinsson SY, Andersson TM, et al: Improved patient survival for acute myeloid leukemia: A population-based study of 9,729 patients diagnosed in Sweden 1973–2005. Blood 113:3666, 2009.

1158. Burnett AK: Transplantation in first remission of acute myeloid leukemia. N Engl J Med 339:1698, 1998.

1159. Burnett AK, Goldstone AH, Stevens RM, et al: Randomised comparison of addition of autologous bone-marrow transplantation to intensive chemotherapy for acute myeloid leukaemia in first remission: Results of MRC AML 10 trial. U.K. Medical Research Council Adult and Children's Leukaemia Working Parties. Lancet 351:700, 1998.

1160. Clift RA, Buckner CD: Marrow transplantation for acute myeloid leukemia. Cancer Invest 16:53, 1998.

1161. Gale RP, Butturini A: Transplants for acute myelogenous leukemia. Cancer Invest 16:66, 1998.

1162. Middeke JM, Beelen D, Stadler M, et al: Outcome of high-risk acute myeloid leukemia after allogeneic hematopoietic cell transplantation: Negative impact of abnl(17p) and −5/5q−. Blood 120:2521, 2012.

1163. Middeke JM, Fang M, Cornelissen JJ, et al: Outcome of patients with abnl(1p) acute myeloid leukemia after allogeneic hematopoietic stem cell transplantation. Blood 123:2960, 2014.

1164. Chen Y, Kantarjian H, Wang H, et al: Acute promyelocytic leukemia: A population-based study on incidence and survival in the United States, 1975–2008. Cancer 118:5811, 2012.

1165. Redaelli A, Stephens JM, Brandt S, et al: Short- and long-term effects of acute myeloid leukemia on patient health-related quality of life. Cancer Treat Rev 30:103, 2004.

1166. Hsu C, Wang JD, Hwang JS, et al: Survival-weighted health profile for long-term survivors of acute myelogenous leukemia. Qual Life Res 12:519, 2003.

1167. Kern W, Haferlach T, Schoch C, et al: Early blast clearance by remission induction therapy is a major independent prognostic factor for both achievement of complete remission and long-term outcome in acute myeloid leukemia: Data from the German AML Cooperative Group (AMLCG) 1992 Trial. Blood 101:64, 2003.

1168. Elliott MA, Litzow MR, Letendre LL, et al: Early peripheral blood blast clearance during induction chemotherapy for acute myeloid leukemia predicts superior relapse-free survival. Blood 110:4172, 2007.

1169. Cortes JE, Kantarjian H, O'Brien S, et al: Clinical and prognostic significance of trisomy 21 in adult patients with acute myelogenous leukemia and myelodysplastic syndromes. Leukemia 9:115, 1995.

1170. Marcucci G, Maharry K, Radmacher MD, et al: Prognostic significance of, and gene and microRNA expression signatures associated with, CEBPA mutations in cytogenetically normal acute myeloid leukemia with high-risk molecular features: A Cancer and Leukemia Group B Study. J Clin Oncol 26:5078, 2008.

1171. Buchner T, Heinecke A: The role of prognostic factors in acute myeloid leukemia. Leukemia 10(Suppl 1):S28, 1996.

1172. Ghaddar HM, Pierce S, Reed P, Estey EH: Prognostic value of residual normal metaphases in acute myelogenous leukemia patients presenting with abnormal karyotype. Leukemia 9:779, 1995.

1173. Seol JG, Kim ES, Park WH, et al: Telomerase activity in acute myelogenous leukaemia: Clinical and biological implications. Br J Haematol 100:156, 1998.

1174. Huh Y, Smith TL, Collins P, et al: Terminal deoxynucleotidyl transferase expression in acute myelogenous leukemia and myelodysplasia as determined by flow cytometry. Leuk Lymphoma 37:319, 2000.

1175. Del Poeta G, Venditti A, Del Principe MI, et al: Amount of spontaneous apoptosis detected by Bax/Bcl-2 ratio predicts outcome in acute myeloid leukemia (AML). Blood 101:2125, 2003.

1176. Ong YL, McMullin MF, Bailie KE, et al: High bax expression is a good prognostic indicator in acute myeloid leukaemia. Br J Haematol 111:182, 2000.

1177. Amirghofran Z, Zakerinia M, Shamseddin A: Significant association between expression of the CD11b surface molecule and favorable outcome for patients with acute myeloblastic leukemia. Int J Hematol 73:502, 2001.

1178. Matsunaga T, Takemoto N, Sato T, et al: Interaction between leukemic-cell VLA-4 and stromal fibronectin is a decisive factor for minimal residual disease of acute myelogenous leukemia. Nat Med 9:1158, 2003.

1179. Becker PS, Kopecky KJ, Wilks AN, et al: Very late antigen-4 (VLA-4) function of myeloblasts correlates with improved overall survival for patients with acute myeloid leukemia. Blood 113:866, 2009.

1180. Estrov Z, Thall PF, Talpaz M, et al: Caspase 2 and caspase 3 protein levels as predictors of survival in acute myelogenous leukemia. Blood 92:3090, 1998.

1181. Frehling S, Schlenk RF, Stolze I, et al: CEBPA mutation in younger adults with acute myeloid leukemia and normal cytogenetics: Prognostic relevance and analysis of cooperating mutations. J Clin Oncol 22:624, 2004.

1182. Hollink IH, Zwaan CM, Zimmermann M, et al: Favorable prognostic impact of NPM1 gene mutations in childhood acute myeloid leukemia, with emphasis on cytogenetically normal AML. Leukemia 23:262, 2009.

1183. Yanada M, Borthakur G, Garcia-Manero G, et al: Blood counts at time of complete remission provide additional independent prognostic information in acute myeloid leukemia. Leuk Res 32:1505, 2008.

1184. Hussein K, Jahagirdar B, Gupta P, et al: Day 14 bone marrow biopsy in predicting complete remission and survival in acute myeloid leukemia. Am J Hematol 83:446, 2008.

1185. Schwind S, Maharry K, Radmacher MD, et al: Prognostic significance of expression of a single microRNA, miR-181a, in cytogenetically normal acute myeloid leukemia: A Cancer and Leukemia Group B study. J Clin Oncol 28:5257, 2010.

1186. Deneberg S, Guardiola P, Lennartsson A, et al: Prognostic DNA methylation patterns in cytogenetically normal acute myeloid leukemia are predefined by stem cell chromatin marks. Blood 118:5573, 2011.

1187. Paietta E: Classical multidrug resistance in acute myeloid leukaemia. Med Oncol 14:53, 1997.

1188. Ino T, Miyazaki H, Isogai M, et al: Expression of P-glycoprotein in de novo acute myelogenous leukemia at initial diagnosis: Results of molecular and functional assays and correlation with treatment outcome. Leukemia 8:1492, 1994.

1189. Hart SM, Ganeshaguru K, Hoffbrand AV: Expression of the multidrug resistance-associated protein (MRP) in acute leukaemia. Leukemia 8:2163, 1994.

1190. Guerci A, Merlin JL, Missoum N, et al: Predictive value for treatment outcome in acute myeloid leukemia of cellular daunorubicin accumulation and P-glycoprotein expression simultaneously determined by flow cytometry. Blood 85:2147, 1995.

1191. Leith CP, Chen IM, Kopecky KJ, et al: Correlation of multidrug resistance (MDR1) protein expression with functional dye/drug efflux in acute myeloid leukemia by multiparameter flow cytometry: Identification of discordant MDR/efflux+ and MDR1+/efflux− cases. Blood 86:2329, 1995.

1192. Kohler T, Eller J, Leiblein S, et al: Mechanisms responsible for therapy resistance of acute myelogenous leukemia (AML). Int J Clin Pharmacol Ther 36:97, 1998.

1193. Filipits M, Stranzl T, Pohl G, et al: Drug resistance factors in acute myeloid leukemia: A comparative analysis. Leukemia 14:68, 2000.

1194. Massaad-Massade L, Ribrag V, Marie JP, et al: Glutathione system, topoisomerase II level and multidrug resistance phenotype in acute myelogenous leukemia before treatment and at relapse. Anticancer Res 17:4647, 1997.

1195. Drach D, Zhao S, Drach J, Andreeff M: Low incidence of MDR1 expression in acute promyelocytic leukaemia. Br J Haematol 90:369, 1995.

1196. Paschka P, Marcucci G, Ruppert AS, et al: Adverse prognostic significance of KIT mutations in adult acute myeloid leukemia with inv(16) and t(8;21): A Cancer and Leukemia Group B Study. J Clin Oncol 24:3904, 2006.

1197. Hoyle CF, DeBastos M, Wheatley K, et al: AML associated with previous cytotoxic therapy, MDS or myeloproliferative disorders: Results from the MRC's 9th AML trial. Br J Haematol 72:45, 1989.

1198. DeWitte T, Muus P, DePauw B, Haanen C: Intensive antileukemic treatment of patients younger than 65 years with myelodysplastic syndromes and secondary acute myelogenous leukemia. Cancer 66:831, 1990.

1199. Brito-Babapulle F, Catovsky D, Galton DAG: Clinical and laboratory features of de novo acute myeloid leukaemia with trilineage myelodysplasia. Br J Haematol 66:445, 1987.

1200. Brito-Babapulle F, Catovsky D, Galton DAG: Myelodysplastic relapse of de novo acute myeloid leukaemia with trilineage myelodysplasia. Br J Haematol 66:411, 1988.

1201. Rosenthal NS, Farhi DC: Dysmegakaryopoiesis resembling acute megakaryoblastic leukemia in treated acute myeloid leukemia. Am J Clin Pathol 95:556, 1991.

1202. Layton DM, Ireland RM, Mufti GJ, Bellingham AJ: Myelodysplastic relapse of de novo AML: A heterogenous entity. Leuk Res 11:1055, 1987.

1203. Jowitt SN, Yin JAL, Saunders MJ: Relapsed myelodysplastic clone differs from acute onset clone as shown by X-linked DNA polymorphism patterns in a patient with acute myeloid leukemia. Blood 82:613, 1993.

1204. O'Brien S, Kantarjian HM, Keating M, et al: Association of granulocytosis with poor prognosis in patients with acute myelogenous leukemia and translocation of chromosomes 8 and 21. J Clin Oncol 7:1081, 1989.

1205. Krykowski E, Polkowska-Kulesza E, Robak T, et al: Analysis of prognostic factors in acute leukemias in adults. Haematol Blood Transfus 30:369, 1987.

1206. Greenwood MJ, Seftel MD, Richardson C, et al: Leukocyte count as a predictor of death during remission induction in acute myeloid leukemia. Leuk Lymphoma 47:1245, 2006.

1207. Bernard P, Reiffers J, LaComb F, et al: A stage classification for prognosis in adult acute myelogenous leukaemia based upon patient's age, bone marrow karyotype, and clinical features. Scand J Haematol 32:429, 1984.

1208. Keating S, Suciu S, De Witte T, et al: The stem cell mobilizing capacity of patients with acute myeloid leukemia in complete remission correlates with relapse risk: Results of the EORTC-GIMEMA AML-10 trial. *Leukemia* 17:60, 2003.

1209. Tremblay LN, Hyland RH, Schouten BD, Hanly PJ: Survival of acute myelogenous leukemia patients requiring intubation/ventilatory support. *Clin Invest Med* 18:19, 1995.

1210. Hunter AE, Rogers SY, Roberts IAG, et al: Autonomous growth of blast cells is associated with reduced survival in acute myeloblastic leukemia. *Blood* 82:399, 1993.

1211. Campos L, Rouault JP, Sabido O, et al: High expression of bcl-2 protein in acute myeloid leukemia cells is associated with poor response to chemotherapy. *Blood* 81:3091, 1993.

1212. Sharawat SK, Bakhshi R, Vishnubhatla S, Bakhshi S: High receptor tyrosine kinase (FLT3, KIT) transcript versus anti-apoptotic (BCL2) transcript ratio independently predicts inferior outcome in pediatric acute myeloid leukemia. *Blood Cells Mol Dis* 54:56, 2015.

1213. Kaufmann SH, Karp JE, Svingen PA, et al: Elevated expression of the apoptotic regulator Mcl-1 at the time of leukemic relapse. *Blood* 91:991, 1998.

1214. Zhang W, Xu HJ, Kornblau SM, et al: Growth-factor stimulation reveals two mechanisms of retinoblastoma gene inactivation in human myelogenous leukemia cells. *Leuk Lymphoma* 16:191, 1995.

1215. Zhang W, Kornblau SM, Kobayashi T, et al: High levels of constitutive WAFl/Cipl protein are associated with chemoresistance in acute myelogenous leukemia. *Clin Cancer Res* 1:1051, 1995.

1216. Raspadori D, Lauria F, Ventura MA, et al: Incidence and prognostic relevance of CD34 expression in acute myeloblastic leukemia: Analysis of 141 cases. *Leuk Res* 21:603, 1997.

1217. Dalal Bi, Wu V, Barnett MJ, et al: Induction failure in de novo acute myelogenous leukemia is associated with expression of high levels of CD34 antigen by the leukemic blasts. *Leuk Lymphoma* 26:299, 1997.

1218. Lee JJ, Cho D, Chung IJ, et al: CD34 expression is associated with poor clinical outcome in patients with acute promyelocytic leukemia. *Am J Hematol* 73:149, 2003.

1219. Shimamoto T, Ohyashiki K, Ohyashiki JH, et al: The expression pattern of erythrocyte/megakaryocyte-related transcription factors GATA-1 and the stem cell leukemia gene correlates with hematopoietic differentiation and is associated with outcome of acute myeloid leukemia. *Blood* 86:3173, 1995.

1220. Baer MR, Stewart CC, Lawrence D, et al: Expression of the neural cell adhesion molecule CD56 is associated with short remission duration and survival in acute myeloid leukemia with t(8;21)(q22;q22). *Blood* 90:1643, 1997.

1221. Extermann M, Bacchi M, Monai N, et al: Relationship between cleaved L-selectin levels and the outcome of acute myeloid leukemia. *Blood* 92:3115, 1998.

1222. Raza A, Preisler HD, Li YQ, et al: Biologic characteristics of newly diagnosed poor prognosis acute myelogenous leukemia. *Am J Hematol* 42:359, 1993.

1223. Wetzler M, Baer MR, Bernstein SH, et al: Expression of c-mpl MRNA, the receptor for thrombopoietin, in acute myeloid leukemia blasts identifies a group of patients with poor response to intensive chemotherapy. *J Clin Oncol* 15:2262, 1997.

1224. Small D: Targeting FLT3 for the treatment of leukemia. *Semin Hematol* 45(3 Suppl 2):S17, 2008.

1225. Libura M, Asnafi V, Delabesse E, et al: *FLT3* and *MLL* intragenic abnormalities in AML reflect a common category of genotoxic stress. *Blood* 1902:2198, 2003.

1226. Kim DH, Lee NY, Lee MH, et al: Vascular endothelial growth factor (VEGF) gene (VEGFA) polymorphism can predict the prognosis in acute myeloid leukaemia patients. *Br J Haematol* 140:71, 2008.

1227. Tsimberidou AM, Kantarjian HM, Wen S, et al: The prognostic significance of serum beta2 microglobulin levels in acute myeloid leukemia and prognostic scores predicting survival: Analysis of 1,180 patients. *Clin Cancer Res* 14:721, 2008.

1228. Heuser M, Beutel G, Krauter J, et al: High meningioma 1 (MN1) expression as a predictor for poor outcome in acute myeloid leukemia with normal cytogenetics. *Blood* 108:3898, 2006.

1229. Gaidzik VI, Schlenk RF, Moschny S, et al: Prognostic impact of WT1 mutations in cytogenetically normal acute myeloid leukemia (AML): A study of the German-Austrian AML Study Group (AMLSG). *Blood* 113:4505, 2009.

1230. Virappane P, Gale R, Hills R, et al: Mutation of the Wilms' tumor 1 gene is poor prognostic factor associated with chemotherapy resistance in normal karyotype acute myeloid leukemia: The United Kingdom Medical Research Council Adult Leukemia Working Party. *J Clin Oncol* 26:5429, 2008.

1231. Paschka P, Marcucci G, Ruppert AS, et al: Wilms' tumor 1 gene mutations independently predict poor outcome in adults with cytogenetically normal acute myeloid leukemia: A cancer and leukemia group B study. *J Clin Oncol* 26:4595, 2008.

1232. Testa U, Riccioni R, Militi S, et al: Elevated expression of IL-3Ralpha in acute myelogenous leukemia is associated with enhanced blast proliferation, increased cellularity, and poor prognosis. *Blood* 100:2980, 2002.

1233. Schnittger S, Kinkelin U, Schoch C, et al: Screening for MLL tandem duplication in 387 unselected patients with AML identify a prognostically unfavorable subset of AML. *Leukemia* 14:796, 2000.

1234. Schoch C, Schnittger S, Klaus M, et al: AML with 11q23/MLL abnormalities as defined by the WHO classification: Incidence, partner chromosomes, FAB subtype, age distribution, and prognostic impact in an unselected series of 1897 cytogenetically analyzed AML cases. *Blood* 102:2395, 2003.

1235. Di Bono E, Sartori R, Zambello R, et al: Prognostic significance of CD56 antigen expression in acute myeloid leukemia. *Haematologica* 87:250, 2002.

1236. Kahl C, Florschutz A, Jentsch-Ullrich K, et al: Primary intracranial manifestation of CD7/CD56-positive acute myelogenous leukemia. *Onkologie* 23:580, 2000.

1237. Yang DH, Lee JJ, Mun YC, et al: Predictable prognostic factor of CD56 expression in patients with acute myeloid leukemia with t(8;21) after high dose cytarabine or allogeneic hematopoietic stem cell transplantation. *Am J Hematol* 82:1, 2007.

1238. Chim CS, Liang R, Tam CY, Kwong YL: Methylation of p15 and p16 genes in acute promyelocytic leukemia: Potential diagnostic and prognostic significance. *J Clin Oncol* 19:2033, 2001.

1239. Das-Gupta EP, Seedhouse CH, Russell NH: Microsatellite instability occurs in defined subsets of patients with acute myeloblastic leukaemia. *Br J Haematol* 114:307, 2001.

1240. Lee ST, Jang JH, Min YH, et al: AC133 antigen as a prognostic factor in acute leukemia. *Leuk Res* 25:757, 2001.

1241. Benekle M, Xia Z, Donohue KA, et al: Constitutive activity of signal transducer and activator of transcription 3 protein in acute myeloid leukemia blasts is associated with short disease-free survival. *Blood* 99:252, 2002.

1242. Baldus CD, Tanner SM, Ruppert AS, et al: *BAALC* expression predicts clinical outcome of de novo acute myeloid leukemia patients with normal cytogenetics. *Blood* 102:1613, 2003.

1243. Smith MA, Luxton RW, Pallister CJ, Smith JG: A novel predictive model of outcome in de novo AML based on S-phase activity and proliferative response of blast cells to haemopoietic growth factors. *Leuk Res* 26:345, 2002.

1244. Barjesteh van Waalwijk van Doorn-Khosrovani S, Erpelinck C, van Putten WL, et al: High *EVI1* expression predicts poor survival in acute myeloid leukemia: A study of 319 de novo AML patients. *Blood* 101:837, 2003.

1245. Lugthart S, van Drunen E, van Norden Y, et al: High EVI1 levels predict adverse outcome in acute myeloid leukemia: Prevalence of EVI1 overexpression and chromosome 3q26 abnormalities underestimated. *Blood* 111:4329, 2008.

1246. Konoplev S, Rassidakis GZ, Estey E, et al: Overexpression of CXCR4 predicts adverse overall and event-free survival in patients with unmutated FLT3 acute myeloid leukemia with normal karyotype. *Cancer* 109:1152, 2007.

1247. Shih TT, Hou HA, Liu CY, et al: Bone marrow angiogenesis magnetic resonance imaging in patients with acute myeloid leukemia: Peak enhancement ratio is an independent predictor for overall survival. *Blood* 113:3161, 2009.

1248. Pérez-García A, Brunet S, Berlanga JJ, et al: CTLA-4 genotype and relapse incidence in patients with acute myeloid leukemia in first complete remission after induction chemotherapy. *Leukemia* 23:486, 2009.

1249. Marcucci G, Maharry KS, Metzeler KH, et al: Clinical role of microRNAs in cytogenetically normal acute myeloid leukemia: *MiR-155* upregulation independently identifies high-risk patients. *J Clin Oncol* 31:2086, 2013.

1250. Metzeler KH, Dufour A, Benthaus T, et al: *ERG* expression is an independent prognostic factor and allows refined risk stratification in cytogenetically normal acute myeloid leukemia: A comprehensive analysis of Erg, MN1, and BAALC transcript levels using oligonucleotide microarrays. *J Clin Oncol* 27:5031, 2009.

1251. Groschel S, Schlenk RF, Engelmann J, et al: Deregulated expression of *EVI1* defines a poor prognostic subset of *MLL*-rearranged acute myeloid leukemias: A study of the German-Austrian acute myeloid leukemia study group and the Dutch-Belgian-Swiss HOVON/SAKK cooperative group. *J Clin Oncol* 31:95, 2012.

1252. Bochtler T, Stolzel F, Heilig CE, et al: Clonal heterogeneity as detected by metaphase karyotyping is an indicator of poor prognosis in acute myeloid leukemia. *J Clin Oncol* 31:2898, 2013.

1253. Kornblau SM, Qui YH, Zhang N, et al: Abnormal expression of FLI1 protein is an adverse prognostic factor in acute myeloid leukemia. *Blood* 118:5604, 2011.

1254. Rushworth SA, Zaitseva L, Murray MY, et al: The high Nrf2 expression in human acute myeloid leukemia is driven by NF-κB and underlies its chemoresistance. *Blood* 120:5188, 2012.

1255. Hole PS, Darley RL, Tonks A: Do reactive oxygen species play a role in myeloid leukemias? *Blood* 117:5816, 2011.

1256. Barreyro L, Will B, Bartholdy B, et al: Overexpression of IL-1 receptor accessory protein in stem and progenitor cells and outcome correlation in AML and MDS. *Blood* 120:1290, 2012.

1257. Carter BZ, Qiu Y, Huang X, et al: Survivin is highly expressed in CD34(+)38(–) leukemic stem/progenitor cells and predicts poor clinical outcomes in AML. *Blood* 120:173, 2012.

1258. Chamuleau ME, Ossenkoppele GJ, van Rhenen A, et al: High TRAIL-R3 expression on leukemic blasts is associated with poor outcome and induces apoptosis-resistance which can be overcome by targeting TRAIL-R2. *Leuk Res* 35:741, 2011.

1259. Byrd JC, Mrozek K, Dodge RK, et al: Pretreatment cytogenetic abnormalities are predictive of induction success, cumulative incidence of relapse, and overall survival in adult patients with de novo acute myeloid leukemia: Results from Cancer and Leukemia Group B (CALGB 8461). *Blood* 100:4325, 2002.

1260. Bradstock K, Matthews J, Benson E, et al: Prognostic value of immunophenotyping in acute myeloid leukemia. Australian Leukaemia Study Group. *Blood* 84:1220, 1994.

1261. Gaiger A, Schmid D, Heinze G, et al: Detection of the WT1 transcript by RT-PCR in complete remission has no prognostic relevance in de novo acute myeloid leukemia. *Leukemia* 12:1886, 1998.

1262. Shih LY, Kuo MC, Liang DC, et al: Internal tandem duplication and Asp835 mutations of the FMS-like tyrosine kinase 3 (FLT3) gene in acute promyelocytic leukemia. *Cancer* 98:1206, 2003.

1263. Svingen PA, Karp JE, Krajewski S, et al: Evaluation of Apaf-1 and procaspases-2, -3, -7, -8, and -9 as potential prognostic markers in acute leukemia. *Blood* 96:3922, 2000.

1264. Heckman KD, Weiner GJ, Burns CP: Persistent thrombocytopenia during remission in acute leukemia does not preclude long-term disease-free survival. *Am J Hematol* 71:236, 2002.

1265. Legrand O, Simonin G, Zittoun R, Marie JP: Lung resistance protein (LRP) gene expression in adult acute myeloid leukemia: A critical evaluation by three techniques. *Leukemia* 12:1367, 1998.

1266. Filipits M, Pohl G, Stranzl T, et al: Expression of the lung resistance protein predicts poor outcome in *de novo* acute myeloid leukemia. *Blood* 91:1508, 1998.

1267. Gale RP, Horowitz MM, Weiner RS, et al: Impact of cytogenetic abnormalities on outcome of bone marrow transplants in acute myelogenous leukemia in first remission. *Bone Marrow Transplant* 16:203, 1995.

1268. Zapatero A, Martin de Vidales C, Pinar B, et al: Prognostic factors affecting leukemia relapse after allogeneic BMT conditioned with cyclophosphamide and fractionated TBI. *Bone Marrow Transplant* 18:591, 1996.

1269. Sievers EL, Loken MR: Detection of minimal residual disease in acute myelogenous leukemia. *J Pediatr Hematol Oncol* 17:123, 1995.

1270. Schnittger S, Weisser M, Schoch C, et al: New score predicting for prognosis in PML-RARA+, AML1-ETO+, or CBFBMYH11+ acute myeloid leukemia based on quantification of fusion transcripts. *Blood* 102:2746, 2003.

1271. Nucifora G, Larson RA, Rowley JD: Persistence of the 8;21 translocation in patients with acute myeloid leukemia type M2 in long-term remission. *Blood* 82:712, 1993.

1272. Cazzaniga G, Gaipa G, Rossi V, Biondi A: Monitoring of minimal residual disease in leukemia, advantages and pitfalls. *Ann Med* 38:512, 2006.

1273. Freeman SD, Virgo P, Couzens S, et al: Prognostic relevance of treatment response measured by flow cytometric residual disease detection in older patients with acute myeloid leukemia. *J Clin Oncol* 31:4123, 2013.

1274. Loken MR, Alonzzo TA, Pardo L, et al: Residual disease detected by multidimensional flow cytometry signifies high relapse risk in patients with *de novo* acute myeloid leukemia: A report from Children's Oncology Group. *Blood* 120:1561, 2012.

1275. Terwijn M, van Putten WI, Kelder A, et al: High prognostic impact of flow cytometric minimal residual disease detection in acute myeloid leukemia: Data from the HOVON/SAKK AML 42A study. *J Clin Oncol* 31:3889, 2013.

1276. Walter RB, Buckley SA, Pagel JM, et al: Significance of minimal residual disease before myeloablative allogeneic hematopoietic cell transplantation for AML in first and second complete remission. *Blood* 122:1813, 2013.

1277. Bacher U, Zander AR, Haferlach T, et al: Minimal residual disease diagnostics in myeloid malignancies in the post transplant period. *Bone Marrow Transplant* 42:145, 2008.

1278. Huisman C, de Weger RA, de Vries L, et al: Chimerism analysis within 6 months of allogeneic stem cell transplantation predicts relapse in acute myeloid leukemia. *Bone Marrow Transplant* 39:285, 2007.

1279. Estey E, Pierce S: Routine bone marrow exam during first remission of acute myeloid leukemia. *Blood* 87:3899, 1996.

1280. Zeleznikova T, Stevulova L, Kovarikova A, Babusikova O: Increased myeloid precursors in regenerating bone marrow; implications for detection of minimal residual disease in acute myeloid leukemia. *Neoplasma* 54:471, 2007.

1281. Campana D, Coustan-Smith E: Detection of minimal residual disease in acute leukemia by flow cytometry. *Cytometry* 38:139, 1999.

1282. Adriaansen HJ, Jacobs BC, Kappers-Klunne MC, et al: Detection of residual disease in AML patients by use of double immunological marker analysis for terminal deoxynucleotidyl transferase and myeloid markers. *Leukemia* 7:472, 1993.

1283. Reading CL, Estey EH, Huh YO, et al: Expression of unusual immunophenotype combinations in acute myelogenous leukemia. *Blood* 81:3083, 1993.

1284. Kita K, Miwa H, Nakase K, et al: Clinical importance of CD7 expression in acute myelocytic leukemia. The Japan Cooperative Group of Leukemia/Lymphoma. *Blood* 81:2399, 1993.

1285. Porwit-MacDonald A, Janossy G, Ivory K, et al: Leukemia-associated changes identified by quantitative flow cytometry: IV. CD34 overexpression in acute myelogenous leukemia M2 with t(8;21). *Blood* 87:1162, 1996.

1286. Baer MR, Stewart CC, Dodge RK, et al: High frequency of immunophenotype changes in acute myeloid leukemia at relapse: Implications for residual disease detection (Cancer and Leukemia Group B Study 8361). *Blood* 97:3574, 2001.

1287. Voskova D, Schnittger S, Schoch C, et al: Use of five-color staining improves the sensitivity of multiparameter flow cytometric assessment of minimal residual disease in patients with acute myeloid leukemia. *Leuk Lymphoma* 48:80, 2007.

1288. van Rhenen A, Moshaver B, Kelder A, et al: Aberrant marker expression patterns on the CD34+CD38− stem cell compartment in acute myeloid leukemia allows to distinguish the malignant from the normal stem cell compartment both at diagnosis and in remission. *Leukemia* 21:1700, 2007.

1289. Arkesteijn GJ, Erpelinck SL, Martens AC, et al: The use of FISH with chromosome specific repetitive DNA probes for the follow-up of leukemia patients. Correlations and discrepancies with bone marrow cytology. *Cancer Genet Cytogenet* 88:69;1996.

1290. Engel H, Drach J, Keyhani A, et al: Quantitation of minimal residual disease in acute myelogenous leukemia and myelodysplastic syndromes in complete remission by molecular cytogenetics of progenitor cells. *Leukemia* 13:568, 1999.

1291. Cilloni D, Gottardi E, De Micheli D, et al: Quantitative assessment of WT1 expression by real time quantitative PCR may be a useful tool for monitoring minimal residual disease in acute leukemia patients. *Leukemia* 16:2115, 2002.

1292. Elmaagacli AH: Molecular methods used for detection of minimal residual disease following hematopoietic stem cell transplantation in myeloid disorders. *Methods Mol Med* 134:161, 2007.

1293. van der Velden VH, Hochhaus A, Cazzaniga G, et al: Detection of minimal residual disease in hematologic malignancies by real-time quantitative PCR: Principles, approaches, and laboratory aspects. *Leukemia* 17:1013, 2003.

1294. Kern W, Haferlach C, Haferlach T, Schnittger S: Monitoring of minimal residual disease in acute myeloid leukemia. *Cancer* 112:4, 2008.

1295. Gal H, Amariglio N, Trakhtenbrot L, et al: Gene expression profiles of AML derived stem cells; similarity to hematopoietic stem cells. *Leukemia* 20:2147, 2006.

1296. Laczika K, Novak M, Hilgarth B, et al: Competitive CBFbeta/MYH11 reverse-transcriptase polymerase chain reaction for quantitative assessment of minimal residual disease during postremission therapy in acute myeloid leukemia with inversion(16): A pilot study. *J Clin Oncol* 16:1519, 1998.

1297. Marucci G, Caligiuri MA, Dohner H, et al: Quantification of CBFbeta/MYH11 fusion transcript by real time RT-PCR in patients with INV(16) acute myeloid leukemia. *Leukemia* 15:1072, 2001.

1298. Buonamici S, Ottaviani E, Testoni N, et al: Real-time quantitation of minimal residual disease in inv(16)-positive acute myeloid leukemia may indicate risk for clinical relapse and may identify patients in a curable state. *Blood* 99:443, 2002.

1299. Nucifora G, Birn DJ, Erickson P, et al: Detection of DNA rearrangements in the AML1 and ETO loci and of an AML 1/ETO fusion mRNA in patients with t(8;21) acute myeloid leukemia. *Blood* 81:1573, 1993.

1300. Maseki N, Miyoshi H, Shimuzu K, et al: The 8;21 chromosome trans-location in acute myeloid leukemia is always detectable by molecular analysis using AML 1. *Blood* 81:1573, 1993.

1301. Kusec R, Laczika K, Knobl P, et al: AML1/ETO fusion mRNA can be detected in remission blood samples of all patients with t(8;21) acute myeloid leukemia after chemotherapy or autologous bone marrow transplantation. *Leukemia* 8:735, 1994.

1302. Marcucci G, Livak KJ, Bi W, et al: Detection of minimal residual disease in patients with AML1/ETO-associated acute myeloid leukemia using a novel quantitative reverse transcription polymerase chain reaction assay. *Leukemia* 12:1482, 1998.

1303. Miyamoto T, Nagafuji K, Akashi K, et al: Persistence of multipotent progenitors expressing AML1/ETO transcripts in long-term remission patients with t(8;21) acute myelogenous leukemia. *Blood* 87:4789, 1996.

1304. Miyamoto T, Nagafuji K, Harada M, et al: Quantitative analysis of AML1/ETO transcripts in peripheral blood stem cell harvests from patients with t(8;21) acute myelogenous leukaemia. *Br J Haematol* 91:132, 1995.

1305. Miyamoto T, Nagafuji K, Harada M, Niho Y: Significance of quantitative analysis of AML1/ETO transcripts in peripheral blood stem cells from t(8;21) acute myelogenous leukemia. *Leuk Lymphoma* 25:69, 1997.

1306. Yin JAL, O'Brien MA, Hills RK, et al: Minimal residual disease monitoring by quantitative RT-PCR in core binding factor AML allows risk stratification and predicts relapse: Results of the United Kingdom MRC AML-15 trial. *Blood* 120:2826, 2012.

1307. Jourdan E, Boisle N, Chevret S, et al: Prospective evaluation of gene mutations and minimal residual disease in patients with core binding factor acute myeloid leukemia. *Blood* 121:2213, 2013.

1308. Takatsuki H, Umemura T, Sadamura S, et al: Detection of minimal residual disease by reverse transcriptase polymerase chain reaction for the PML/RAR alpha fusion MRNA: A study in patients with acute promyelocytic leukemia following peripheral stem cell transplantation. *Leukemia* 9:889, 1995.

1309. Zhao L, Chang KS, Estey EH, et al: Detection of residual leukemic cells in patients with acute promyelocytic leukemia by the fluorescence *in situ* hybridization method: Potential for predicting relapse. *Blood* 85:495, 1995.

1310. Grimwade D, Lo-Coco F: Acute promyelocytic leukemia: A model for the role of molecular diagnosis and residual disease monitoring in a directing treatment approach in acute myeloid leukemia. *Leukemia* 16:1959, 2002.

1311. Lo-Coco F, Breccia M, Diverio D: The importance of molecular monitoring in acute promyelocytic leukaemia. *Best Pract Res Clin Haematol* 16:503, 2003.

1312. Tobal K, Moore H, Macheta M, Liu Yin JA: Monitoring minimal residual disease and predicting relapse in APL by quantitating *PML-RARalpha* transcripts with a sensitive competitive RT-PCR method. *Leukemia* 15:1060, 2001.

1313. Schlenk RF, Döhner K, Krauter J, et al: Mutations and treatment outcome in cytogenetically normal acute myeloid leukemia. *N Engl J Med* 358:1909, 2008.

1314. Kronke J, Schlenk RF, Jensen KO, et al: Monitoring of minimal residual disease in NPM1-mutated acute myeloid leukemia; a study from the German-Austrian Acute myeloid leukemia study group. *J Clin Oncol* 29:2709, 2011.

1315. Chou WC, Tang JL, Wu SJ, et al: Clinical implications of minimal residual disease monitoring by quantitative polymerase chain reaction in acute myeloid leukemia patients bearing nucleophosmin (NPM1) mutations. *Leukemia* 21:998, 2007.

1316. Sjøholt G, Anensen N, Wergeland L, et al: Proteomics in acute myelogenous leukaemia (AML): Methodological strategies and identification of protein targets for novel antileukaemic therapy. *Curr Drug Targets* 6:631, 2005.

1317. Czibere A, Grall F, Aivado M: Perspectives of proteomics in acute myeloid leukemia. *Expert Rev Anticancer Ther* 6:1663, 2006.

1318. Wang XS, Zhang JW: The microRNAs involved in human myeloid differentiation and myelogenous/myeloblastic leukemia. *J Cell Mol Med* 12:1445, 2008.

1319. Garzon R, Volinia S, Liu CG, et al: MicroRNA signatures associated with cytogenetics and prognosis in acute myeloid leukemia. *Blood* 111:3183, 2008.

CHAPTER 89
CHRONIC MYELOGENOUS LEUKEMIA AND RELATED DISORDERS

Jane L. Liesveld and Marshall A. Lichtman

SUMMARY

The chronic myelogenous leukemias (CMLs) include *BCR* rearrangement-positive CML, chronic myelomonocytic leukemia, juvenile myelomonocytic leukemia, chronic neutrophilic leukemia, chronic eosinophilic leukemia, and chronic basophilic leukemia. The term *chronic*, in contrast to *acute*, once had prognostic implications. However, although the terms remain useful for nosology, they no longer reflect an invariable difference in prognosis. For example, acute myelogenous leukemia in children and young adults has higher remission and cure rates than juvenile or chronic myelomonocytic leukemia in children or adults, respectively. *BCR* rearrangement-positive CML presents with anemia, exaggerated granulocytosis, a large proportion of myelocytes and mature neutrophils, absolute basophilia, normal or elevated platelet counts, and, frequently, splenomegaly. The marrow is intensely hypercellular, and marrow cells contain the Philadelphia (Ph) chromosome in approximately 90 percent of cases by cytogenetic analysis. A rearrangement of the *BCR* gene on chromosome 22 is present by molecular diagnostic analysis in approximately 96 percent of cases that have a classic morphologic appearance. The BCR-rearranged form of the

Acronyms and Abbreviations: ALL, acute lymphocytic leukemia; BCR, breakpoint cluster region; CCyR, complete cytogenetic response; CFU-GM, colony-forming unit–granulocyte-monocyte; CHR, complete hematologic response; CLL, chronic lymphocytic leukemia; CML, chronic myelogenous leukemia; CMML, chronic myelomonocytic leukemia; CMR, complete molecular response; DLI, donor lymphocyte infusion; FISH, fluorescence *in situ* hybridization; G-CSF, granulocyte colony-stimulating factor; GM-CSF, granulocyte-monocyte colony-stimulating factor; GRB2, growth factor receptor–bound protein-2; GTP, guanosine triphosphate; GTPase, guanosine triphosphatase; GVHD, graft-versus-host disease; HLA, human leukocyte antigen; HPRT, hypoxanthine phosphoribosyltransferase; hsp, heat shock protein; HUMARA, human androgen receptor assay; IFN, interferon; IL, interleukin; IRIS, International Randomized Study of Interferon; JAK, Janus-associated kinase; LTC-IC, long-term culture–initiating cell; MCP, monocyte chemotactic protein; MCyR, major cytogenetic response; MDS, myelodysplastic syndrome; MIP, macrophage inflammatory protein; MMR, major molecular response; NF-κB, nuclear factor-κB; *NF1*, neurofibromatosis tumor-suppressor gene; NK, natural killer; NOD, nonobese diabetic; OCT-1, organic cation transporter 1; PCR, polymerase chain reaction; PCyR, partial cytogenetic response; PDGFR, platelet-derived growth factor receptor; Ph, Philadelphia chromosome; PI3K, phosphatidylinositol 3′-kinase; Rb, retinoblastoma; RT-PCR, reverse transcriptase polymerase chain reaction; SCID, severe combined immunodeficiency; STAT, signal transducer and activator of transcription; TBI, total-body irradiation; TdT, terminal deoxynucleotidyl transferase; TGF, transforming growth factor; TKI, tyrosine kinase inhibitor; VEGF, vascular endothelial growth factor; WT, Wilms tumor.

disease usually responds to a tyrosine kinase inhibitor, and median survival has been extended significantly. Allogeneic hematopoietic stem cell transplantation can cure the disease, especially if the transplantation is applied early in the chronic phase, although this approach is now uncommon as a result of the effect of tyrosine kinase inhibitor therapy. The effect of stem cell transplantation is related in part to a robust graft-versus-leukemia effect, engendered by donor T lymphocytes. The natural history of the chronic phase is to evolve into an accelerated phase that often terminates in acute leukemia (blast crisis), but the frequency of this progression has been markedly decreased by the advent of tyrosine kinase inhibitors. Blast crisis results in a myelogenous leukemic phenotype in 75 percent of cases and a lymphoblastic leukemic phenotype in approximately 25 percent of cases. Ph chromosome–positive acute myeloblastic leukemia (AML) may appear *de novo* in approximately 1 percent of cases of AML, and Ph chromosome–positive acute lymphocytic leukemia (ALL) may occur *de novo* in approximately 20 percent of cases of adult ALL and approximately 5 percent of childhood ALL cases. In Ph chromosome–positive ALL, the translocation between chromosomes 9 and 22 results in the fusion gene encoding a mutant tyrosine kinase oncoprotein that may be identical in size to that in classic CML (210 kDa) in approximately one-third of cases. A smaller mutant tyrosine kinase (190 kDa) is encoded in approximately two-thirds of cases. In children, the cells in approximately 90 percent of cases contain a 190-kDa mutant tyrosine kinase. These acute leukemias may reflect (1) the presentation of CML in acute blastic transformation without a preceding chronic phase or (2) *de novo* cases resulting from a *BCR-ABL1* mutation occurring in a different early hematopoietic cell from the event in CML or with as yet unidentified modifying gene alterations. Chronic myelomonocytic leukemia has variable presenting features. Anemia may be accompanied by mildly or moderately elevated leukocyte counts; an elevated total monocyte count; a low, normal, or elevated platelet count; and sometimes splenomegaly. Although cytogenetic abnormalities may be present, there is no specific genetic marker of the disease. In a very small proportion of cases, a translocation involving the platelet-derived growth factor receptor (PDGFR)-β gene is associated with eosinophilia and is responsive to a tyrosine kinase inhibitor. Juvenile myelomonocytic leukemia occurs in infancy or very early childhood. Anemia, thrombocytopenia, and leukocytosis with monocytosis are usual. The disease is refractory to treatment and, even with current maximal therapy and stem cell rescue, cures are uncommon. Chronic neutrophilic leukemia presents with mild anemia and exaggerated neutrophilia, with very few immature cells in the blood. Splenomegaly is common. The disease usually occurs after age 60 years. Chronic and juvenile myelomonocytic leukemia and chronic neutrophilic leukemia have a propensity to evolve into acute myelogenous leukemia. Prior to that evolution, morbidity and mortality are related to infection, hemorrhage, and complicating medical conditions. Chronic eosinophilic leukemia represents the major subset of the hypereosinophilic syndrome. It is a clonal disorder with a striking absolute eosinophilia, often neurologic and cardiac manifestations secondary to toxic effects of eosinophil granules, and sometimes a translocation involving the PDGFR-*a* gene that encodes a mutant tyrosine kinase, imparting sensitivity to a tyrosine kinase inhibitor.

● DEFINITION AND HISTORY

Chronic myelogenous leukemia (CML) is a multipotential hematopoietic stem cell disease characterized by anemia, extreme blood granulocytosis and granulocytic immaturity, basophilia, often thrombocytosis, and splenomegaly. The hematopoietic cells contain a reciprocal translocation between chromosomes 9 and 22 in more than

95 percent of patients with classic morphologic findings, which leads to an overtly foreshortened long arm of one of the pair of chromosome 22 (i.e., 22,22q−), referred to as the *Philadelphia (Ph) chromosome*. A rearrangement of the breakpoint cluster region gene *(BCR)* on the long arm of chromosome 22 defines this form of CML and is present even in the 10 percent of patients without an overt 22q abnormality by Giemsa chromosome banding. The natural history of the disease is to undergo clonal evolution into an accelerated phase and/or a rapidly progressive blast phase, an acute leukemia, highly refractory to therapy, which had been a frequent event prior to the introduction of tyrosine kinase inhibitors (TKIs) in 2001.

In 1845, Bennett[1] in Scotland and Virchow[2] in Germany described patients with splenic enlargement, severe anemia, and enormous concentrations of leukocytes in their blood at autopsy. Bennett initially favored an extreme pyemia as the explanation, but Virchow argued against suppuration as a cause. Additional cases were reported by Craige[3] and others, and in 1847 Virchow[4] introduced the designation *weisses Blut* and *leukämie* (leukemia). In 1878, Neumann[5] proposed that the marrow not only was the site of normal blood cell production, but also was the site from which leukemia originated and used the term *myelogene* (myelogenous) leukemia. Subsequent observations amplified the clinical and laboratory features of the disease, but few fundamental insights were gained until the discovery by Nowell and Hungerford,[6] who reported in 1960 that two patients with the disease had an apparent loss of the long arm of chromosome 21 or 22, an abnormality that was quickly confirmed[7-9] and designated the Ph chromosome.[7] Advanced cytogenetic techniques confirmed that it was chromosome 22. This observation led to a new approach to diagnosis, a marker to study the pathogenesis of the disease, and a focus for future studies of the molecular pathology of the disease. The availability of banding techniques to define the fine structure of chromosomes[10,11] led to the discovery by Rowley[12] that the apparent lost chromosomal material on chromosome 22 was part of a reciprocal translocation between chromosomes 9 and 22. The discovery that the cellular oncogene *ABL1* on chromosome 9 and a segment of chromosome 22, the BCR, fuse as a result of the translocation provided a basis for the study of the molecular cause of the disease.[13,14] The appreciation that the fusion gene encoded a constitutively active tyrosine kinase (BCR-ABL1) that was capable of inducing the disease in mice established the fusion gene product as the proximate cause of the malignant transformation. The search for, identification of, and clinical development of a small molecule inhibitor of the mutant tyrosine kinase provided a specific agent, imatinib mesylate, with which to inhibit the molecule that incites the disease.[15] Several more potent congeners have also been synthesized (see "Etiology and Pathogenesis" below). Thomas and colleagues established that allogeneic hematopoietic stem cell transplantation could cure the disease.[16] An engaging monograph on the discoveries and the scientists involved from the identification of the Ph chromosome to the development of imatinib has been published.[17]

EPIDEMIOLOGY

CML accounts for approximately 15 percent of all cases of leukemia, or approximately 6500 new cases in the United States in 2015. The age-adjusted incidence rate in the United States is approximately 2.3 per 100,000 persons for men and approximately 1.2 per 100,000 persons for women. The incidence around the world varies by a factor of approximately twofold. The lowest incidence is in Sweden and China (approximately 0.7 per 100,000 persons), and the highest incidence is in Switzerland and the United States (approximately 1.5 per 100,000 persons).[18] The age-specific incidence rate for CML in the United States increases logarithmically with age, from approximately 0.2 per 100,000

per year in persons younger than 20 years to a rate of approximately 10.0 per 100,000 in octogenarians (Fig. 89–1). Although CML occurs in children and adolescents, less than 10 percent of all cases occur in persons between 1 and 20 years old. CML represents approximately 3 percent of all childhood leukemias. Multiple occurrences of CML in families are rare. There is no concordance of the disease between identical twins. There is no analytical epidemiologic evidence for a familial predisposition to CML in Swedish databases.[19] There is some evidence that overweightness and obesity can increase the incidence of CML.[20]

ETIOLOGY AND PATHOGENESIS

ENVIRONMENTAL LEUKEMOGENS

Exposure to very high doses of ionizing radiation can increase the occurrence of CML above the expected frequency in comparable populations. Three major populations—the Japanese exposed to the radiation released by the atomic bomb detonations at Nagasaki and Hiroshima,[21] British patients with ankylosing spondylitis treated with spine irradiation,[22] and women with uterine cervical carcinoma who received radiation therapy[23]—had a frequency of CML (as well as acute leukemia) significantly above the frequency expected in comparable unexposed groups. The median latent period was approximately 4 years in irradiated spondylitics, among whom approximately 20 percent of the leukemia cases were CML; 9 years in the uterine cervical cancer patients, of whom approximately 30 percent had CML; and 11 years in the Japanese survivors of the atomic bombs, of whom approximately 30 percent of the leukemia patients had CML.[24] Chemical leukemogens, such as benzene and alkylating agents, are not causative agents of CML, presumably because of their inability to induce the specific chromosome translocation required to cause the disease.[25-27]

ORIGIN FROM A MUTANT HEMATOPOIETIC STEM CELL

CML results from the malignant transformation of a single hematopoietic stem cell. The disease is acquired (somatic mutation), given that the identical twin of patients with CML and the offspring of mothers with the disease neither carry the Ph chromosome nor develop the disease.[28] The origin of CML from a single hematopoietic stem cell is supported by the following lines of evidence:

1. Involvement of erythropoiesis, neutrophilopoiesis, eosinophilopoiesis, basophilopoiesis, monocytopoiesis, and thrombopoiesis in chronic phase CML.[29]
2. Presence of the Ph chromosome (22q−) in erythroblasts; neutrophilic, eosinophilic, and basophilic granulocytes; macrophages; and megakaryocytes.[30]
3. Presence of a single glucose-6-phosphate dehydrogenase isoenzyme in red cells, neutrophils, eosinophils, basophils, monocytes, and platelets, but not in fibroblasts or other somatic cells in women with CML who are heterozygotes for isoenzymes A and B.[31-33]
4. Presence of the Ph translocation only on a structurally anomalous chromosome 9 or 22 of each chromosome pair in every cell analyzed in occasional patients with a structurally dissimilar 9 or 22 chromosome within the pair.[34-36]
5. Presence of the Ph chromosome in one, but not the other, cell lineage of patients who are a mosaic for sex chromosomes, as in Turner syndrome (45X/46XX)[37] and Klinefelter syndrome (46XY/47XXY).[38]
6. Molecular studies showing variation in the breakpoint of chromosome 22 among different patients with CML but precisely the same breakpoint among cells within a single patient with CML.[39,40]

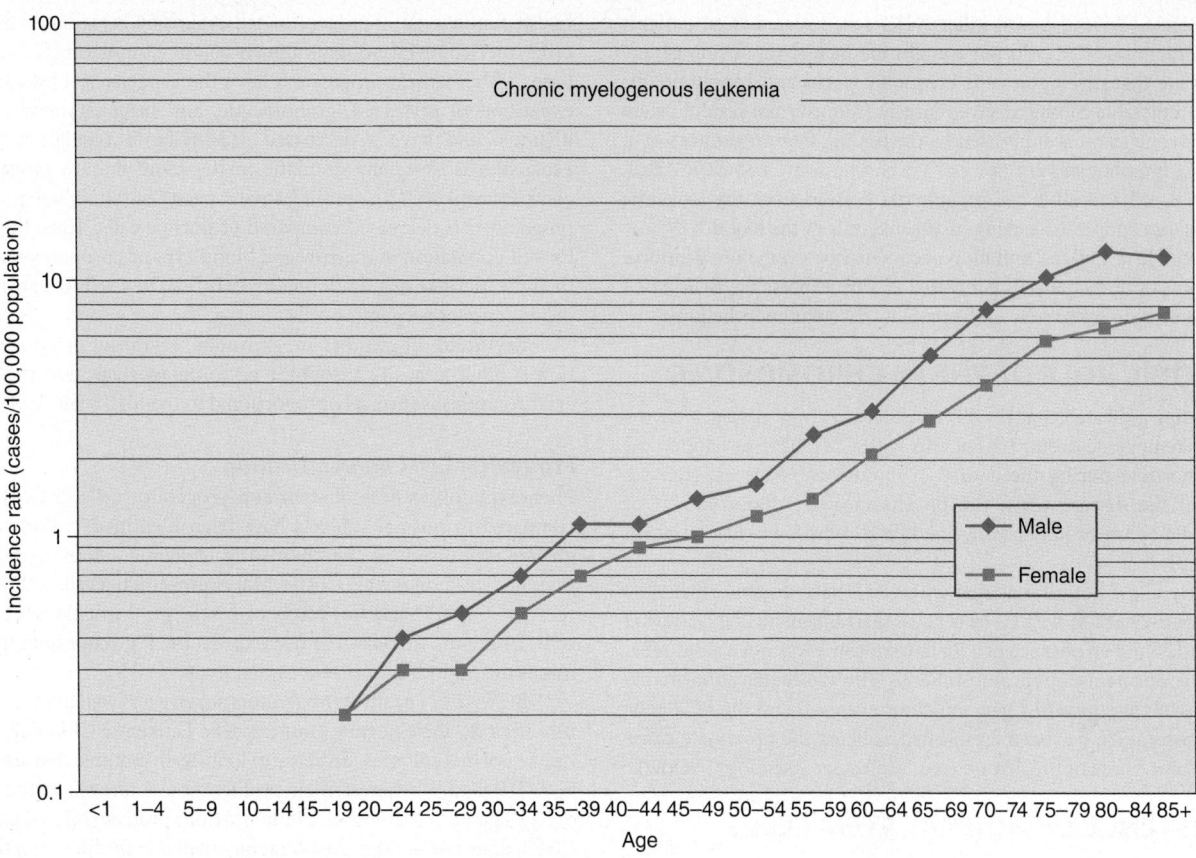

Figure 89–1. Incidence of chronic myelogenous leukemia by age. Note the exponential increase in incidence with age from about teenagers to octogenarians. Rare cases occur in younger children but too few to generate an incidence rate.

7. Combined DNA hybridization-methylation analysis of women who have restriction fragment length polymorphisms at the X-linked locus for hypoxanthine phosphoribosyltransferase (HPRT), which enables distinction of the two alleles of the HPRT gene in heterozygous females, coupled with methylation-sensitive restriction-enzyme cleavage patterns, which permits delineation of whether cells contain either the maternally derived or the paternally derived copy of the gene.[41]

The foregoing observations place the parent cell of the clone at least at the level of the hematopoietic multipotential cell.

THE CHRONIC MYELOGENOUS LEUKEMIA STEM CELL

Acquisition of the *BCR-ABL1* fusion gene as a result of the t(9;22) (q34;q11.2) in a single primitive multipotential hematopoietic cell (possibly the pluripotential stem cell) results in the CML stem cell, necessary for the initiation and maintenance of the chronic phase of CML.[42,43] The phenotype of the CML stem cell is not fully defined but they are among the CD34+CD33–Lin–Thy1+ KIT– fraction of CML cells.[43] A proportion of CML stem cells is in the G_0 phase of the cell cycle and is resistant to therapy with *BCR-ABL1* inhibitors. These cells represent a pool for the regrowth of the tumor in most patients, if suppressive therapy is interrupted. The leukemia stem cell is resistant to TKI therapy, but a pan-BCL2 inhibitor has been found to sensitize marrow leukemia stem cells to tyrosine kinase inhibition.[44] N-cadherin and WNT-β-catenin signaling are also thought to mediate microenvironmental protection of CML stem cells from TKIs.[45] The acquisition of genetic and epigenetic

events in a derivative *BCR-ABL1*–positive cell can result in evolution to accelerated phase and blastic transformation[46] (see "Accelerated Phase and Blast Crisis of Chronic Myelogenous Leukemia" below).

PLURIPOTENTIAL STEM CELL LESION

Some patients in chronic phase CML have lymphocytes that are derived from the primordial malignant cell. Evidence for this finding includes the following: A single isoenzyme for glucose-6-phosphate dehydrogenase has been found in some T and B lymphocytes in women with CML who are heterozygous for isoenzymes A and B[47]; blood cells from patients with CML induced to proliferate with Epstein-Barr virus (presumptive B lymphocytes) are of the same glucose-6-phosphate dehydrogenase isoenzyme type, have cytoplasmic immunoglobulin heavy and light chains, and contain the Ph chromosome[48]; blood lymphocytes stimulated with B lymphocyte mitogens contain the Ph chromosome[49,50]; purified B lymphocytes from the blood in chronic phase CML contain an abnormal, elongated phosphoprotein coded for by the chimeric gene resulting from the t(9;22)[51]; and fluorescence *in situ* hybridization (FISH) has detected the *BCR-ABL1* fusion gene in approximately 25 percent of B lymphocytes in some, but not all, patients in chronic phase.[52,53] These findings suggest that B lymphocytes are derived from the malignant clone, placing the lesion closer to, if not in, the pluripotential lymphohematopoietic stem cell.[47–51] Previous studies have found that the B lymphocyte pool is a mosaic, containing both Ph chromosome– and *BCR-ABL1*–positive cells and Ph chromosome– or *BCR-ABL1*–negative cells. Results of studies examining the derivation of T lymphocytes from the malignant clone are more ambiguous but indicate that T lymphocytes are derived from the malignant clone in some patients.[47,49,54–63] Natural killer (NK) cells isolated from patients with chronic phase CML do not contain the *BCR-ABL1* fusion gene.[64] It is possible that myelopoiesis is invariably clonal and lymphopoiesis is an unpredictable mosaic derived largely from normal residual stem cells. This conclusion is supported by the finding that progenitors of T, B, and NK lymphocytes contain the Ph chromosome and *BCR-ABL1*, but most B-cell and all T-cell progenitors derived from the leukemic clone undergo apoptosis, leaving unaffected cells in the blood.[65–68]

The cell in which the mutation occurs may be even more primitive in that some endothelial cells generated *in vitro* express the *BCR-ABL1* fusion gene, as do some cells in the patient's vascular endothelium.[69]

ETIOLOGIC ROLE OF THE Ph CHROMOSOME

Early studies indicated that the Ph chromosome may appear after the initial leukemogenic event.[70–73] Patients with CML have developed the Ph chromosome during the course of the disease, have experienced periods of the disease when the Ph chromosome disappeared,[74] or have had Ph chromosome–positive and Ph chromosome–negative cells concurrently.[75–79]

Nearly all, if not all, patients with CML have an abnormality of chromosome 22 at a molecular level (*BCR* rearrangement). Thus, earlier studies indicating an absence of a Ph chromosome was not a valid measure of the normality of chromosome 22. The molecular abnormality in CML involving the *ABL1* gene on chromosome 9 and the *BCR* gene on chromosome 22 has been established as being the proximate cause of the chronic phase of the disease (see "Molecular Pathology" below).

COEXISTENCE OF NORMAL STEM CELLS

Most, if not all, patients with CML have hematopoietic stem cells that, after treatment[80–82] or culture *in vitro*,[83–85] use of special cell isolation techniques,[81,82] or use of cell transfer to nonobese diabetic (NOD)/severe combined immunodeficiency (SCID) mice[88] do not have the Ph chromosome[89,90] or the *BCR-ABL1* fusion gene.[91–95] The switch to Ph chromosome–negative cells *in vitro* is associated with a loss of monoclonal glucose-6-phosphate dehydrogenase isoenzyme patterns, indicating the persistence and reemergence of normal polyclonal hematopoiesis rather than reversion to a Ph chromosome–negative clone.[96] In confirmation, *BCR-ABL1*+, CD34+, human leukocyte antigen (HLA)-DR– cells isolated from women with early phase CML are polyclonal using the human androgen receptor assay (HUMARA) to assess X chromosome inactivation patterns.[97] Very primitive hematopoietic cells, the long-term culture–initiating cells (LTC-ICs), are present in Ph chromosome–negative cytapheresis samples collected during early recovery after chemotherapy for CML.[98] These LTC-ICs are most commonly present when samples are collected within 3 months of diagnosis.[99] Variable levels of *BCR-ABL1*–negative progenitors are found in the CD34+DR– population, but low levels are found in the CD34+CD38– population.[95,100] Preprogenitors for the CD34+DR– cells are predominantly *BCR-ABL1*–negative in both marrow and blood at diagnosis.[101] However, some cells with surface marker characteristics of very primitive normal hematopoietic cells do express the *BCR-ABL1* gene.[102] Both normal and leukemic SCID-repopulating cells coexist in the marrow and blood from CML patients in chronic phase, whereas only leukemic SCID-repopulating cells are detected in blast crisis.[103,104]

PROGENITOR CELL CHARACTERISTICS

Progenitor Cell Dysfunction

The leukemic transformation resulting from the *BCR-ABL1* fusion oncogene is maintained by a relatively small number of BCR-ABL1 stem cells that favor differentiation over self-renewal.[105] This predisposition to differentiation and progenitor cell expansion is mediated by an autocrine interleukin (IL)-3–granulocyte colony-stimulating factor (G-CSF) loop.[105] The earliest progenitors have the capacity to undergo marked expansion of erythroid, granulocytic, and megakaryocytic cell populations, and have a decreased sensitivity to regulation.[105–107] This expansion is especially dramatic in the more mature progenitor cell compartment.[105,108] The proliferative capacity of individual granulocytic progenitors is decreased compared to normal cells. Thus, the progenitor cell population in marrow and blood expands proportionately more than the increase in granulopoiesis.[109] BCR-ABL1 reduces growth factor dependence of progenitor cells.

Erythroid progenitors are expanded, erythroid precursor maturation is blocked at the basophilic erythroblast stage, and the extent of erythropoiesis is inversely proportional to the total white cell count.[110]

Progenitor Cell Characterization

Phenotypic differences of stem and progenitor cells in CML patients compared to normal subjects have been identified.[111] For example, a greater proportion of the circulating leukemic colony-forming unit–granulocyte-monocytes (CFU-GMs) express high levels of the adhesion receptor CD44[112] and low levels of L-selectin[113] in contrast to normal cells. Leukemic CD34+ cells overexpress the P glycoprotein that determines the multidrug resistance phenotype.[114]

BCR-ABL1–positive progenitors survive less well in long-term culture than do their normal counterparts. Leukemic CFU-GM colonies, unlike normal colonies, decrease in long-term cultures that are deficient in KIT ligand,[115] whereas their proliferation is favored in the presence of KIT ligand.[116] Macrophage inflammatory protein (MIP)-1α, renamed CCL3, does not inhibit growth factor-mediated proliferation of CD34+ cells from CML patients, as it does CD34+ cells from normal subjects, even though the CCL3 receptor is expressed.[117] Another chemokine, monocyte chemotactic protein (MCP)-1 or CCL2, unlike CCL3, is an endogenous chemokine that cooperates with transforming growth factor beta (TGF-β) to inhibit the cycling of primitive normal, but not CML, progenitors in long-term human marrow cultures.[118] Leukemic progenitors are less sensitive than normal progenitors to the antiproliferative effects of TGF-β.[119]

Effects of BCR-ABL1 on Cell Adhesion

Primitive progenitors and blast colony-forming cells from patients with CML have decreased adherence to marrow stromal cells.[120] This defect is normalized if stromal cells are treated with interferon (IFN)-α.[121] As a result, *BCR-ABL1*–negative progenitors are enriched in the adherent fraction of circulating CD34+ cells in chronic phase CML patients. The most primitive *BCR-ABL1*–positive cells in the blood of patients with CML differ from their normal counterparts. They are increased in frequency and are activated, such that signals that block cell mitosis are bypassed.[122]

Ph chromosome–positive colony-forming cells adhere less to fibronectin (and to marrow stroma) than do their normal counterparts. Adhesion is fostered as a result of restoration of cooperation between activated β_1 integrins and the altered epitopes of CD44.[123,124] CML granulocytes have reduced and altered binding to P-selectin because of modification in the CD15 antigens.[125] *BCR-ABL1*–induced defects in integrin function may underlie the abnormal circulation and proliferation of progenitors[126,127] because growth signaling can occur through the fibronectin receptor.[128] IFN-α restores normal integrin-mediated inhibition of hematopoietic progenitor proliferation by the marrow microenvironment.[129] There are conflicting data regarding the effects of TKI effects on adhesion of CML cells to stroma.[130,131]

BCR-ABL1–encoded fusion protein p210[BCR-ABL] binds to actin, and several cytoskeletal proteins are thereby phosphorylated. The p210[BCR-ABL] interacts with actin filaments through an actin-binding domain. *BCR-ABL1* transfection is associated with increased spontaneous motility, membrane ruffling, formation of long actin extensions (filopodia), and accelerated rate of protrusion and retraction of pseudopodia on fibronectin-coated surfaces. IFN-α treatment slowly converts the abnormal motility phenotype of *BCR-ABL1*–transformed cells toward normal.[132] Integrins regulate the c-*ABL*–encoded tyrosine kinase activity and its cytoplasmic nuclear transport.[133] The p210[BCR-ABL] abrogates the anchorage requirement but not the growth factor requirement for proliferation.[134]

In normal cells exposed to IL-3, paxillin tyrosine residues are phosphorylated. In cells transformed by p210[BCR-ABL], the tyrosines of paxillin, vinculin, p125[FAK], talin, and tensin are constitutively phosphorylated. Pseudopodia enriched in focal adhesion proteins[134,135] are present in cells expressing p210[BCR-ABL].

The sum of evidence suggests that defects in adhesion (contact and anchoring) of CML primitive cells remove them from their controlling signals normally received from microenvironmental cells via cytokine messages. These signals retain the balance among cell survival, cell death, cell proliferation, and cell differentiation. Inappropriate phosphorylation of cytoskeletal proteins, possibly independent of the mutant tyrosine kinase, is thought to be the key factor in disturbed integrin function of CML cells.

MOLECULAR PATHOLOGY

Ph Chromosome

The genetic disturbance became evident with the knowledge that CML was derived from a primitive cell containing a 22q– abnormality.[6,11] The abnormal chromosome contained only 60 percent of the DNA in other G-group chromosomes.[136] Cytogenetic analysis indicated the G-group chromosome involved was different from the extra G-group chromosome in Down syndrome, which had been assigned number 21. Thus, the former was assigned number 22—even though it proved to be slightly longer than the chromosome involved in Down syndrome.[11,137] The Paris Conference on Nomenclature decided not to undo the concept that Down syndrome is trisomy 21 and assigned the Ph

chromosome and its normal counterpart, 22.[138] Using quinacrine (Q) and Giemsa (G) banding, Rowley[12] reported in 1973 that the material missing from chromosome 22 was not lost (deleted) from the cell, but was translocated to the distal portion of the long arm of chromosome 9. The amount of material translocated to chromosome 9 was approximately equivalent to that lost from chromosome 22, and the translocation was predicted to be balanced.[12] Moreover, the breaks were localized to band 34 on the long arm of chromosome 9 and band 11 on the long arm of chromosome 22. Therefore, the classic Ph chromosome is t(9;22) (q34;q11), abbreviated t(Ph) (Fig. 89–2). The Ph chromosome can develop on either the maternal or the paternal member of the pair.[139]

Mutation of ABL1 and BCR Genes

Mutations of the *ABL1* gene on chromosome 9 and of the *BCR* gene on chromosome 22 are central to the development of CML (Fig. 89–3).[140–142]

In 1982, the human cellular homologue *ABL1* of the transforming sequence of the Abelson murine leukemia virus was localized to human chromosome 9.[143] In 1983, *ABL1* was shown to be on the segment of chromosome 9 that is translocated to chromosome 22[144] by demonstrating reaction to hybridization probes for *ABL1* only in somatic cell hybrids of human CML cells containing 22q– but not those containing 9q+. v-*abl* is the viral oncogenic homologue of the normal cellular *ABL1* gene. This gene (v-*abl*) can induce malignant transformation of cells in culture and can induce leukemia in susceptible mice.[145]

The *ABL1* gene is rearranged and amplified in cell lines from patients with CML.[146] Cell lines and fresh isolates of CML cells contain an abnormal, elongated 8-kb RNA transcript,[147–150] which is transcribed from the new chimeric gene produced by the fusion of the 5′ portion of the *BCR* gene left on chromosome 22 with the 3′ portion of the *ABL1* gene translocated from chromosome 9 (Fig. 89–4).[144] The fusion mRNA leads to the translation of a unique tyrosine phosphoprotein kinase of 210 kDa (p210[BCR-ABL]), which can phosphorylate tyrosine residues on cellular proteins similar to the action of the v-*abl* protein product.[151–155] The *ABL1* locus contains at least two alleles, one having a 500-bp deletion.[157] In normal cells, the *ABL1* protooncogene codes for a tyrosine kinase of molecular weight 145,000, which is translated only in trace quantities and lacks any *in vitro* kinase activity.[152] The fusion product

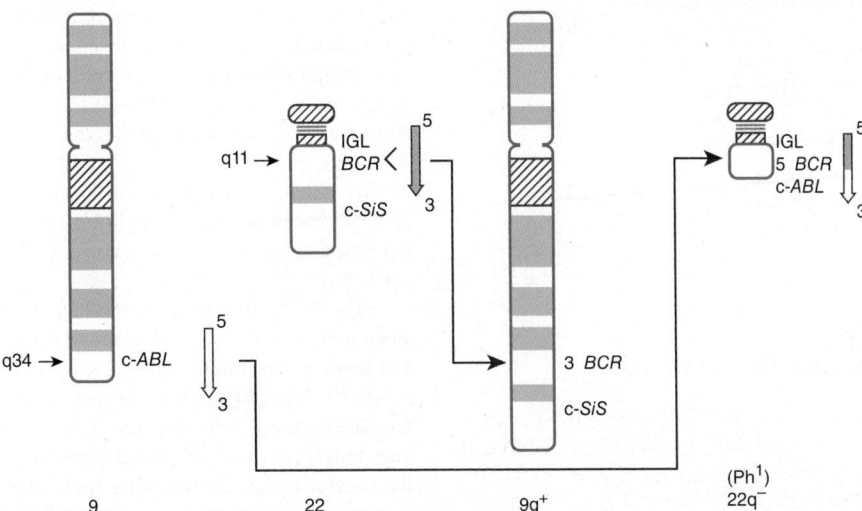

Figure 89–2. Schematic of normal chromosome 9 showing the *ABL* gene between bands q34 and qter of chromosome 22, which has the *BCR* and *SIS* genes between bands q11 and qter. The t(9;22) is shown on the *right*. The *ABL* from chromosome 9 is transposed to the chromosome 22 M-*bcr* sequences, and the terminal portion of chromosome 22 is transposed to the long arm of chromosome 9. The 22q– is the Ph chromosome. bcr, breakpoint cluster region; c-SiS, cellular homologue of the viral simian sarcoma virus-transforming gene; IGL, gene for immunoglobulin light chains. *(Reproduced with permission from De Klein A: Oncogene activation by chromosomal rearrangement in chronic myelocytic leukemia. Mutat Res 1987 Sep;186(2):161–172.)*

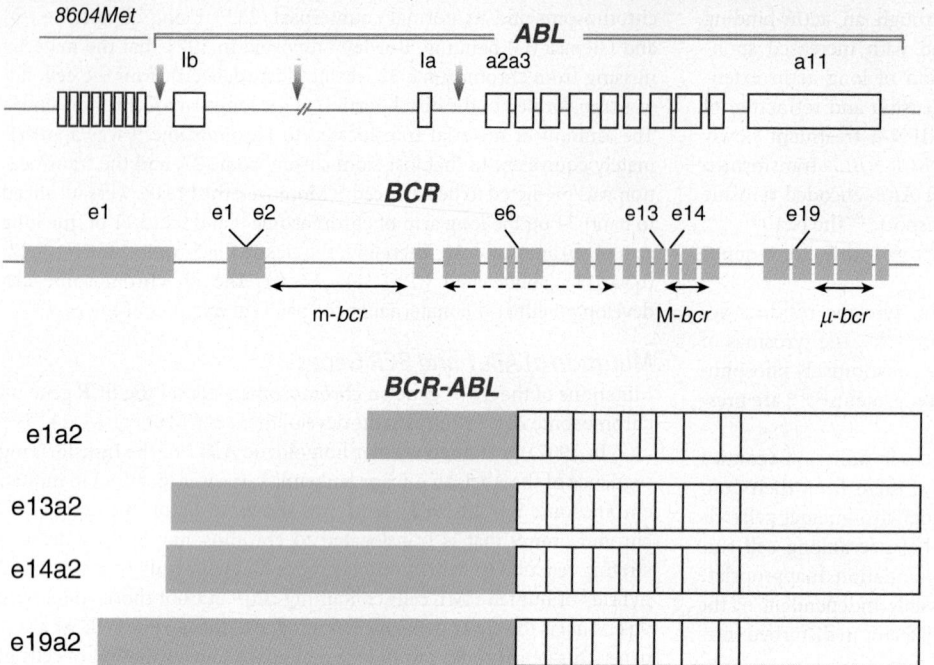

Figure 89–3. Schematic of the normal *ABL* and *BCR* genes and of the *BCR-ABL* fusion transcripts. In the *upper panel* of the diagram, the possible breakpoint positions in *ABL* are marked by *vertical arrows*. Note the position immediately upstream of the *ABL* locus of the *8604Met* gene. The *BCR* gene contains 25 exons, including first (e1) and second (e2) exons. The positions of the three breakpoint cluster regions, m-*bcr*, M-*bcr*, and μ-*bcr*, are shown. The *lower panel* of the figure shows the structure of the *BCR-ABL* messenger RNA fusion transcripts. Breakpoints in μ-*bcr* result in *BCR-ABL* transcripts with an e19a2 junction. The associated number designates the exon (location) at which the break occurs in each gene.

expressed by the *BCR-ABL1* gene is hypothesized to lead to malignant transformation because of the abnormally regulated enzymatic activity of the chimeric tyrosine protein kinase.[153,154,158,159] Construction of *BCR-ABL1* fusion genes indicated that *BCR* sequences could also activate a microfilament-binding function, but the tyrosine kinase and microfilament-binding functions were not linked. Nevertheless, tyrosine kinase modification of actin filament function has been proposed as a step in leukemogenesis.[160]

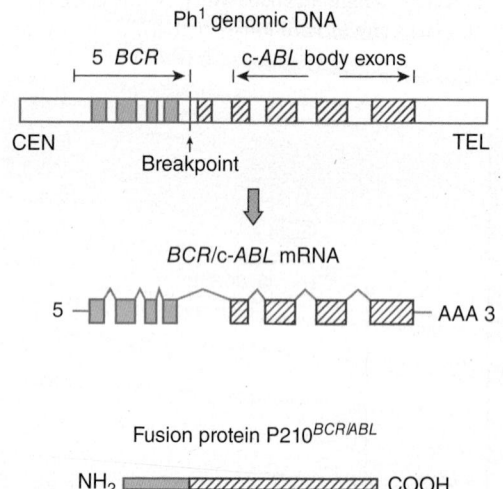

Figure 89–4. Molecular effects of the Ph chromosome translocation t(9;22)(q34;q11). The *upper panel* shows the physically joined 5′ *BCR* and the 3′ *ABL* regions on chromosome 22. The exons are *solid* (from chromosome 22, *BCR*) and *hatched* (from chromosome 9, *ABL*). The *middle panel* depicts transcription of chimeric messenger RNA. The *lower panel* shows the translated fusion protein with the aminoterminus derived from the *BCR* of chromosome 22 and the carboxy-terminus from the *ABL* of chromosome 9. *(Reproduced with permission from De Klein A: Oncogene activation by chromosomal rearrangement in chronic myelocytic leukemia. Mutat Res 1987 Sep;186(2):161–172.)*

p210^BCR-ABL *Fusion Protein*

The breakpoints on chromosome 9 are not narrowly clustered, ranging from approximately 15 to more than 40 kb upstream from the most proximate region (first exon) of the *ABL1* gene.[143,144,161] The breakpoints on chromosome 22 occur over a very short, approximately 5 to 6 kb, stretch of DNA referred to as the breakpoint cluster region (M-*bcr*),[162,163] which is part of a much longer *BCR*[164,165] gene (see Fig. 89–4). Three main BCRs have been characterized on chromosome 22: major (M-*bcr*), minor (m-*bcr*), and micro (μ-*bcr*). The three different breakpoints result in a p210, p190, and p230 fusion protein, respectively (see Fig. 89–3). The overwhelming majority of CML patients have a *BCR-ABL1* fusion gene that encodes a fusion protein of 210 kDa (p210^BCR-ABL1), for which mRNA transcripts have e14a2 or a e13a2 fusion junction (see Fig. 89–3).[166] The "e" represents the *BCR* exon and "a" the *ABL1* exon sites involved in the translocation. A *BCR-ABL1* with an e1a2 type of junction has been identified in approximately 50 percent of the Ph chromosome–positive acute lymphoblastic leukemia cases and results in the production of a *BCR-ABL1* protein of 190 kDa (p190^BCR-ABL). Almost all CML cases at diagnosis that encode a p210^BCR-ABL also express *BCR-ABL* transcripts for p190.[167] The biologic or clinical significance of these dual transcripts is not known. Transgenic mice expressing p210^BCR-ABL develop acute lymphoblastic leukemia in the founder mice, but all transgenic progeny have a myeloproliferative disorder resembling CML.[168]

The *BCR* gene encodes a 160-kDa serine-threonine kinase, which, when it oligomerizes, autophosphorylates and transphosphorylates several protein substrates.[169] Aberrant methylation of the M-*bcr* in CML occurs.[166] The first exon sequences of the *BCR* gene potentiate the tyrosine kinase of *ABL* when they fuse as a result of the translocation.[170] The central portion of *BCR* has homology to *DBL*, a gene involved in the control of cell division after the S phase of the cell cycle. The C-terminus of *BCR* has a guanosine triphosphatase (GTPase)-activating protein for p21^rac, a member of the *RAS* family of guanosine triphosphate (GTP)-binding proteins.[171] A reciprocal hybrid gene *ABL-BCR1* is formed on chromosome 9q+ when *BCR-ABL1* fuses on chromosome 22. The *ABL-BCR1* fusion gene actively transcribes in most patients with CML.[172]

Variations in breakpoints involving smaller stretches of chromosome 9 and rearrangements outside the M-bcr of chromosome 22 can occur.[37] In a few cases of CML with no evident elongation of chromosome 9, molecular probes have shown that *ABL1* still is translocated to chromosome 22.[173] In occasional patients with Ph chromosome–positive CML, the break in chromosome 22 is outside the M-bcr, and transcription of a fusion RNA of the usual type fails or a fusion RNA is transcribed that does not hybridize with the classic M-bcr complementary DNA (cDNA) probe.[174]

In cases in which the Ph chromosome is not found, *BCR-ABL1* still may be located on chromosome 9 (a masked Ph chromosome).[175] The *BCR* gene can recombine with genomically distinct sites on band 11q13 in complex translocations in a region rich in Alu repeat elements.[176] *ETV6/ABL1* fusion genes have also been found in *BCR-ABL1*–negative CML.[177]

The *BCR* breakpoint site has been examined as a factor in disease prognosis. Some studies have shown no correlation between CML chronicity and breakpoint site, although thrombocytosis may be more common with 3′ breakpoint sites and basophilia with 5′ breakpoint sites.[178] No difference in response to IFN-α therapy was noted, and survival was not significantly different, although patients with 3′ deletions tended to have shorter survival.[179] Others have observed a better response to IFN-α in patients with a 3′ rearrangement, which is being examined with imatinib mesylate therapy.[180]

CML patients with m-bcr breakpoints develop a blast crisis with monocytosis and an absence of splenomegaly and basophilia.[181] The p230 (e19a2 RNA junction) encoded by μ-bcr is rarely expressed but has been associated with neutrophilic CML or thrombocytosis (see "Special Clinical Features" below). Other rare breakpoints have been described.[182] For example, a case with a 12-bp insert between BCR and ABL1 resulted in a *BCR-ABL1*–negative (false-negative), Ph chromosome–positive CML with thrombocythemia.[183] Another novel *BCR-ABL1* fusion gene (e6a2) in a patient with Ph chromosome–negative CML encoded an oncoprotein of 185 kDa.[184] Typical CML also has been associated with an e19a2 junction *BCR-ABL1* transcript.[185]

Experimental support for the hypothesis that p210[BCR-ABL1] tyrosine phosphoprotein kinase is transforming is provided by a retroviral gene transfer system that permits expression of the protein. Mouse marrow cells transfected with *BCR-ABL1* develop clonal outgrowths of immature cells expressing the p210[BCR-ABL1] tyrosine kinase. Some clones progress to a malignant phenotype, can be transplanted, and can induce tumors in syngeneic mice.[186] Similar studies suggest that the p210[BCR-ABL] can transform 3T3 murine fibroblasts if the *gag* gene sequence from a helper virus cooperates.[187] The *BCR-ABL1* gene from a retroviral vector has been expressed in an IL-3–dependent cell line. Clones derived from the infected line transform over months to IL-3 independency, are capable of increased proliferation, and develop chromosomal abnormalities.[188]

A series of mouse models in which the *BCR-ABL1* was used to induce leukemogenesis have been described.[189–197] Lethally irradiated mice have been reconstituted with marrow enriched for cycling stem cells infected with a *BCR-ABL1*–bearing retrovirus. Fatal diseases with abnormal accumulations of macrophagic, erythroid, mast, and lymphoid cells develop.[188] Classic CML did not occur, and complete transformation was not documented. The cell lines from spleen and marrow from mice with a *BCR-ABL1* retrovirus infection were predominantly mast cells; however, in some cases these cell lines spontaneously switched to either erythroid and megakaryocytic, erythroid, or granulocytic lineages displaying maturation. They were transplantable (transformed) and contained the same proviral inserts as the original mast cell line.[198] Murine marrow also has been infected with a retrovirus encoding p210[BCR-ABL] and transplanted into irradiated syngeneic recipients.[189] Although several types of hematologic malignancies developed,

a syndrome mimicking human CML also occurred. Mice transgenic for a p190[BCR-ABL] develop an acute lymphocytic leukemia (ALL) lymphoma syndrome[190] that resembles human Ph chromosome–positive ALL. When a p210[BCR-ABL] transcript is introduced into a mouse germline (one-cell fertilized eggs), the p210 founder and progeny transgenic animals developed leukemia of B or T lymphoid or of myeloid origin after a relatively long latency period. In contrast, p190 transgenic mice exclusively developed leukemia of B-cell origin, with a relatively short period of latency. This finding was believed to be consistent with the apparent indolent nature of human CML during the chronic phase.[191] When transgenic mice express p210[BCR-ABL], the transgenes develop ALL, whereas the progeny develop a myeloproliferative disorder.[192]

Mouse models remain important for exploring the pathogenesis of the acute and chronic BCR-ABL1–mediated leukemias *in vivo* and in examining the potential effects of new drugs targeted at BCR-ABL1.[199]

BCR-ABL IN HEALTHY SUBJECTS

BCR-ABL1 fusion genes can be found in the leukocytes of some normal individuals using a two-step reverse transcriptase polymerase chain reaction assay. Thus, although *BCR-ABL1* may be expressed relatively frequently at very low levels in hematopoietic cells, only infrequently do the cells acquire the additional changes necessary to produce leukemia. This may be a dosage effect.[200]

BCR-ABL1 AND SIGNAL TRANSDUCTION

The tyrosine phosphoprotein kinase activity of p210[BCR-ABL1] has been causally linked to the development of Ph chromosome–positive leukemia in man.[201–212] p210[BCR-ABL1] is, unlike the ABL1 protein that is located principally in the nucleus, located in the cytoplasm making it accessible to a large number of interactions, especially components of signal transduction pathways.[205,206,213] It binds and/or phosphorylates more than 20 cellular proteins in its role as an oncoprotein.[206] A subunit of phosphatidylinositol 3′-kinase (PI3K) associates with p210[BCR-ABL]; this interaction is required for the proliferation of *BCR-ABL1*–dependent cell lines and primary CML cells. Wortmannin, a nonspecific inhibitor of the p110 subunit of the kinase, inhibits growth of these cells.[207]

The pathways and interactions invoked by BCR-ABL1 acting on mitogen-activated protein kinases are multiple and complex.[214,215] A RAF-encoded serine-threonine kinase activity is regulated by p210[BCR-ABL]. Downregulation of RAF expression inhibits both *BCR-ABL1*–dependent growth of CML cells and growth factor–dependent proliferation of normal hematopoietic progenitors.[208] The efficiency of cell transformation by *BCR-ABL1* is affected by an adaptor protein that can relate tyrosine kinase signals to RAS. This involves growth factor receptor–bound protein-2 (GRB2). p210[BCR-ABL] also activates multiple alternative pathways of RAS.[209] PI3K is constitutively activated by BCR-ABL1, generates inositol lipids, and is dysregulated through the downregulation by BCR-ABL1 of polyinositol phosphate tumor suppressors, such as PTEN and SHIP1.[213] Figure 89–5 demonstrates interaction of p210[BCR-ABL] with various mediators of signal transduction.

Reactive oxygen species are increased in BCR-ABL1–transformed cells and may act as a second messenger to modulate enzymes regulated by the reduction-oxidation (redox) equilibrium. An increase in these reactive oxygen products is postulated to play a role in the acquisition of additional mutations as a result of production of reactive oxygen species through the chronic phase, contributing to the progression to accelerated phase.[213,216]

The adaptor molecule CRKL is a major *in vivo* substrate for p210[BCR-ABL], and it acts to relate p210[BCR-ABL] to downstream effectors. CRKL is a linker protein that has homology to the *v-crk* oncogene

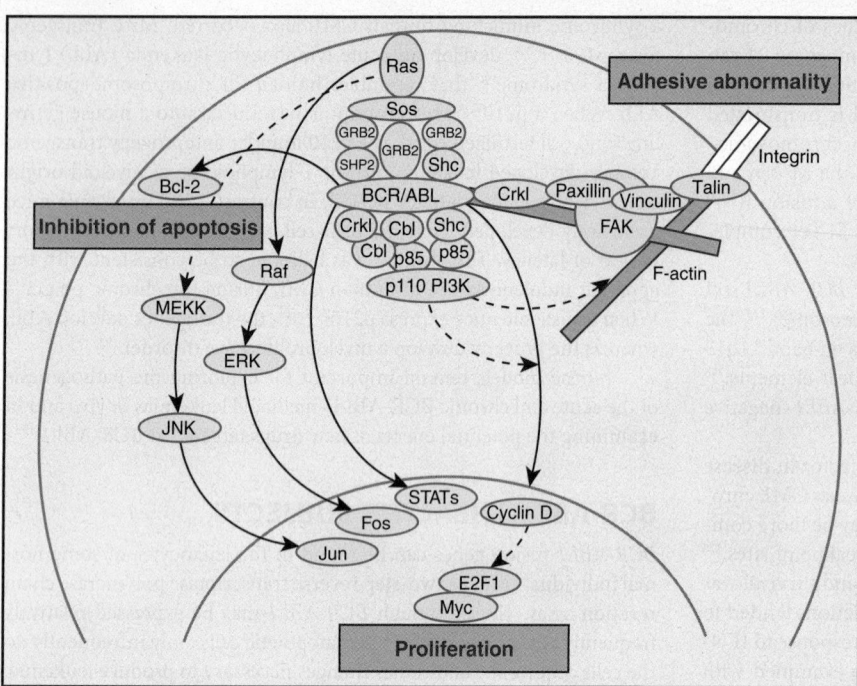

Figure 89–5. Major intracellular signaling events associated with *BCR/ABL*. Constitutive activation of ABL protein tyrosine kinase (PTK) induces phosphorylation of the tyrosine moiety of various substrates, including autophosphorylation of *BCR/ABL* and complex formation of *BCR/ABL* with adaptor proteins. This process subsequently activates multiple intracellular signaling pathways, including *RAS* activation and phosphatidylinositol 3′-kinase (PI3K) activation pathways. *BCR/ABL* also activates the c-MYC pathway, which involves *ABL*-SH2 domain. *BCR/ABL* inhibits apoptosis, possibly in part through upregulation of Bcl-2, and alters cellular adhesive properties, possibly by interacting with focal adhesion proteins and the actin cytomatrix. *Broken lines* indicate hypothetical pathways. ERK, extracellular signal-regulated kinase; FAK, focal adhesion kinase; JNK, Jun N-terminal kinase; MEKK, MEK kinase; Sos, Son-of-sevenless; STAT, signal transducer and activator of transcription. *(Reproduced with permission from Gotoh A, Broxmeyer HE: The function of BCR/ABL and related proto-oncogenes.* Curr Opin Hematol *4(1):3–11, 1997.)*

product. Antibodies to CRKL can immunoprecipitate paxillin. Paxillin is a focal adhesion protein[210] that is phosphorylated by p210[BCR-ABL]. The p210[BCR-ABL] may be physically linked to paxillin by CRKL. CRKL binds to CBL, an oncogene product that induces B cell and myeloid leukemias in mice.[211] The Src homology 3 domains of CRKL do not bind to CBL, but they do bind *BCR-ABL*. Therefore, CRKL mediates the oncogenic signal of *BCR-ABL* to CBL. The p120[CBL] and the adaptor proteins CRKL and c-CRK also link c-abl, p190[BCR-ABL], and p210[BCR-ABL] to the PI3K pathway.[212] The p120[CBL] also coprecipitates with the p85 subunit of PI3K, CRKL, and c-CRK. The p210[BCR-ABL] may, therefore, induce the formation of multimeric complexes of signaling proteins.[217] These complexes contain paxillin and talin and may explain some of the adhesive defects of CML cells.[218]

Hef2 also binds to CRKL in leukemic tissues of p190[BCR-ABL] transgenic mice. Hef2 is involved in the integrin signaling pathway[219] and encodes a protein that accelerates GTP hydrolysis of RAS-encoded proteins and neurofibromin. The latter negatively regulates granulocyte-monocyte colony-stimulating factor (GM-CSF) signaling through RAS in hematopoietic cells.[220] p62[DOK], a constitutively tyrosine-phosphorylated, p120[RAS] GAP-associated protein, which is rapidly tyrosine phosphorylated upon activation of the c-kit receptor,[221] is also associated with ABL1.[222]

Nuclear factor (NF)-κB activation is also required for p210[BCR-ABL]-mediated transformation.[223] Expression of p210[BCR-ABL] leads to activation of NF-κB–dependent transcription via nuclear translocation.[224]

Cell lines that express p210[BCR-ABL] also demonstrate constitutive activation of Janus kinases (JAKs) and signal transducers and activators of transcription (STATs), usually STAT5.[225] STAT5 is also activated in primary mouse marrow cells acutely transformed by the *BCR-ABL1*[226]; p210[BCR-ABL1] coimmunoprecipitates with and constitutively phosphorylates the common β subunit of the IL-3 and GM-CSF receptors and JAK2.[227] Both ABL1 and BCR are also multifunctional regulators of the GTP-binding protein family Rho[228,229] and the growth factor-binding protein GRB2, which links tyrosine kinases to RAS and forms a complex with *BCR-ABL1* and the nucleotide exchange factor Sos that leads to activation of RAS.[230]

The p210[BCR-ABL1] also activates Jun kinase and requires Jun for transformation.[231] In some CML cell lines, p210[BCR-ABL1] is associated with the retinoblastoma (Rb) protein.[232] Loss of the neurofibromatosis (*NF1*) tumor-suppressor gene, a RAS GTPase-activating protein, also is sufficient to produce a myeloproliferative neoplasm in mice akin to human CML resulting from RAS-mediated hypersensitivity to GM-CSF.[233]

EFFECTS OF BCR-ABL ON APOPTOSIS

Whether p210[BCR-ABL1] influences the expansion of the malignant clone in CML by inhibiting apoptosis is uncertain. In one study, the survival of normal and CML progenitors was the same after *in vitro* incubation in serum-deprived conditions and after treatment with X-irradiation or glucocorticoids.[234] p210[BCR-ABL1] inhibits apoptosis by delaying the G2/M transition of the cell cycle after DNA damage.[235] The p210[BCR-ABL1] also may exert an antiapoptotic effect in factor-dependent hematopoietic cells.[236,237]

p210[BCR-ABL1] does not prevent apoptotic death induced by human NK or lymphokine-activated killer cells directed against CML or normal cells.[238] In accelerated and blast phases, apoptosis rates were lower in CML neutrophils. G-CSF and GM-CSF considerably decreased the rate of apoptosis in CML neutrophils.[239]

TELOMERE LENGTH

Patients with CML present with a somewhat shortened mean telomere length in granulocytic cells but not blood T lymphocytes at diagnosis, but considerable overlap exists in the distribution of telomere length with healthy individuals.[240–242] The rate of shortening of telomere length during the chronic phase is correlated with a more rapid onset of accelerated phase.[240,242] Telomerase reverse transcriptase (TERT) is the catalytic subunit, expression of which is closely correlated with telomerase activity. In CML CD34+ cells containing BCR-ABL1, the expression of TERT is significantly lower than in normal CD34+ cells, consistent with accelerated shortening of telomeres in CML cells.[243] A further significant decrease in telomere length occurs in the accelerated phase of

CML. Telomerase activity is increased in the accelerated phase.[244] When therapy permits restoration of Ph chromosome–negative cells in the blood, these cells have telomere length comparable to that in matched healthy controls.[245]

CLINICAL FEATURES

SIGNS AND SYMPTOMS

In the 70 percent of patients who are symptomatic at diagnosis, the most frequent complaints include easy fatigability, loss of sense of well-being, decreased tolerance to exertion, anorexia, abdominal discomfort, early satiety (related to splenic enlargement), weight loss, and excessive sweating.[246-248] The symptoms are vague, nonspecific, and gradual in onset (weeks to months). A physical examination may detect pallor and splenomegaly. The latter was present in approximately 90 percent of patients at diagnosis, but with medical care being sought earlier, the presence of splenomegaly at the time of diagnosis is decreasing in frequency.[247] Sternal tenderness, especially the lower portion, is common; occasionally, patients notice it themselves.

Uncommon presenting symptoms include those of dramatic hypermetabolism (night sweats, heat intolerance, weight loss) simulating thyrotoxicosis; acute gouty arthritis, presumably related in part to hyperuricemia; priapism, tinnitus, or stupor from the leukostasis associated with greatly exaggerated blood leukocyte count elevations[249-251]; left upper quadrant and left shoulder pain as a consequence of splenic infarction and perisplenitis; vasopressin-responsive diabetes insipidus[252,253]; and acne urticata associated with hyperhistaminemia.[254] Acute febrile neutrophilic dermatosis (Sweet syndrome), a perivascular infiltrate of neutrophils in the dermis, can occur. In the latter situation, fever accompanied by painful maculonodular violaceous lesions on the trunk, arms, legs, and face are characteristic.[255,256] Spontaneous rupture of the spleen is a rare event.[257,258] Digital necrosis has been reported as a rare paraneoplastic event.[259,260]

In an increasing proportion of patients, the disease is discovered, coincidentally, when blood cell counts are measured at a periodic medical examination.

CHILDHOOD PRESENTATION

Hyperleukocytosis and symptoms or signs therefrom are a more common feature in patients who present with CML before the age of 20 years. The white cell counts at diagnosis are on average more than twice that in adults, the fraction of blood blasts, promyelocytes, and myelocytes is significantly higher, and clinical manifestations of hyperleukocytosis are far more frequent in children than adults.[250]

LABORATORY FINDINGS

Blood

The presumptive diagnosis of CML can be made from the results of the blood cell counts and examination of the blood film.[26,246,247] The blood hemoglobin concentration is decreased in most patients at the time of diagnosis. Red cells usually are only slightly altered, with an increase in variation from small to large size and only occasional misshapen (elliptical or irregular) erythrocytes. Small numbers of nucleated red cells are commonly present. The reticulocyte count is normal or slightly elevated, but clinically significant hemolysis is rare.[246,261,262] Rare cases of mild erythrocytosis[263,264] or erythroid aplasia[265,266] have been documented.

The total leukocyte count is always elevated at the time of diagnosis and is nearly always greater than 25×10^9/L; at least half the patients have total white counts greater than 100×10^9/L (Fig. 89–6).[26,246,247] The total leukocyte count rises progressively in untreated patients. Rare patients

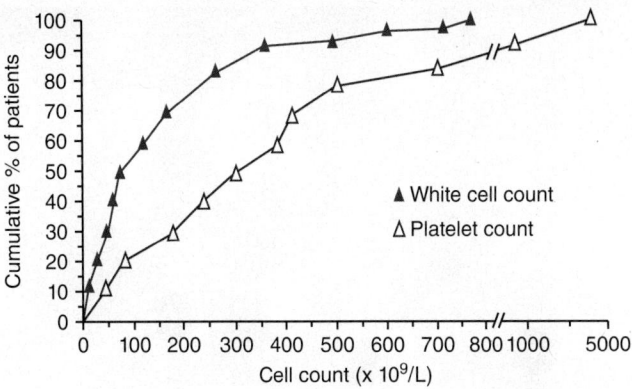

Figure 89–6. Total white cell count and platelet count of 90 patients with CML at the time of diagnosis. The cumulative percent of patients is on the *ordinate,* and the cell count is on the *abscissa.* Fifty percent of patients had a white cell count greater than 100×10^9/L and a platelet count greater than approximately 300×10^9/L at the time of diagnosis.

may have dramatic cyclic variations in white cell counts as much as an order of magnitude with cycle intervals of approximately 60 days.[267,268] Granulocytes at all stages of development are present in the blood and are generally normal in appearance (Fig. 89–7). In this series, the mean blast cell prevalence was approximately 3 percent but can range from 0 to 10 percent; progranulocyte prevalence was approximately 4 percent; myelocytes, metamyelocytes, and bands accounted for approximately 40 percent; and segmented neutrophils accounted for approximately 35 percent of total leukocytes (Table 89–1). Often, there is a "myelocyte bulge" in which the differential count shows an exaggerated proportion of myelocytes compared to the proportion observed in normal persons. Hypersegmented neutrophils are commonly present.

Neutrophil alkaline phosphatase activity is low or absent in more than 90 percent of patients with CML.[269-271] The mRNA for alkaline phosphatase is undetectable in neutrophils of patients with CML.[272] The activity increases toward or to normal in the presence of intense inflammation or infection and when the total leukocytic count is decreased to or near normal with treatment.[271,273] CML neutrophils regain alkaline phosphatase activity after infusion into leukopenic recipients, suggesting the effect of regulators or factors extrinsic to the neutrophils. With the availability of specific markers, *BCR-ABL1* in CML and *JAK2* mutations in polycythemia, leukocyte alkaline phosphatase is no longer used for diagnostic purposes.

The proportion of eosinophils usually is not increased, but the absolute eosinophil count nearly always is increased. Rarely, eosinophils are so prominent that they dominate the granulocytic cells and lead to the designation *Ph chromosome–positive eosinophilic CML.* An absolute increase in the basophil concentration is present in almost all patients, and this finding can be useful in preliminary consideration of the differential diagnosis.[26,278] Basophilic progenitor cells are increased in the blood.[279] The proportion of basophils usually is not greater than 10 to 15 percent during the chronic phase but may, in rare patients, represent 30 to 80 percent of the total leukocyte count during chronic phase and lead to the designation of Ph chromosome–positive basophilic CML.[280] Flow cytometry using anti-CD203c provides very accurate assessment of the basophil frequency. Basophils may be hypogranulated or have an immature phenotype and may be left uncounted in an optical differential white cell count. Anti-CD203c recognizes these cells as basophils.[281] Granules of basophils in patients with CML, unlike normal basophils, contain mast cell α-tryptase.[281,282] Granulocytes containing both eosinophilic and basophilic granules (mixed granulation) are commonly present.[283]

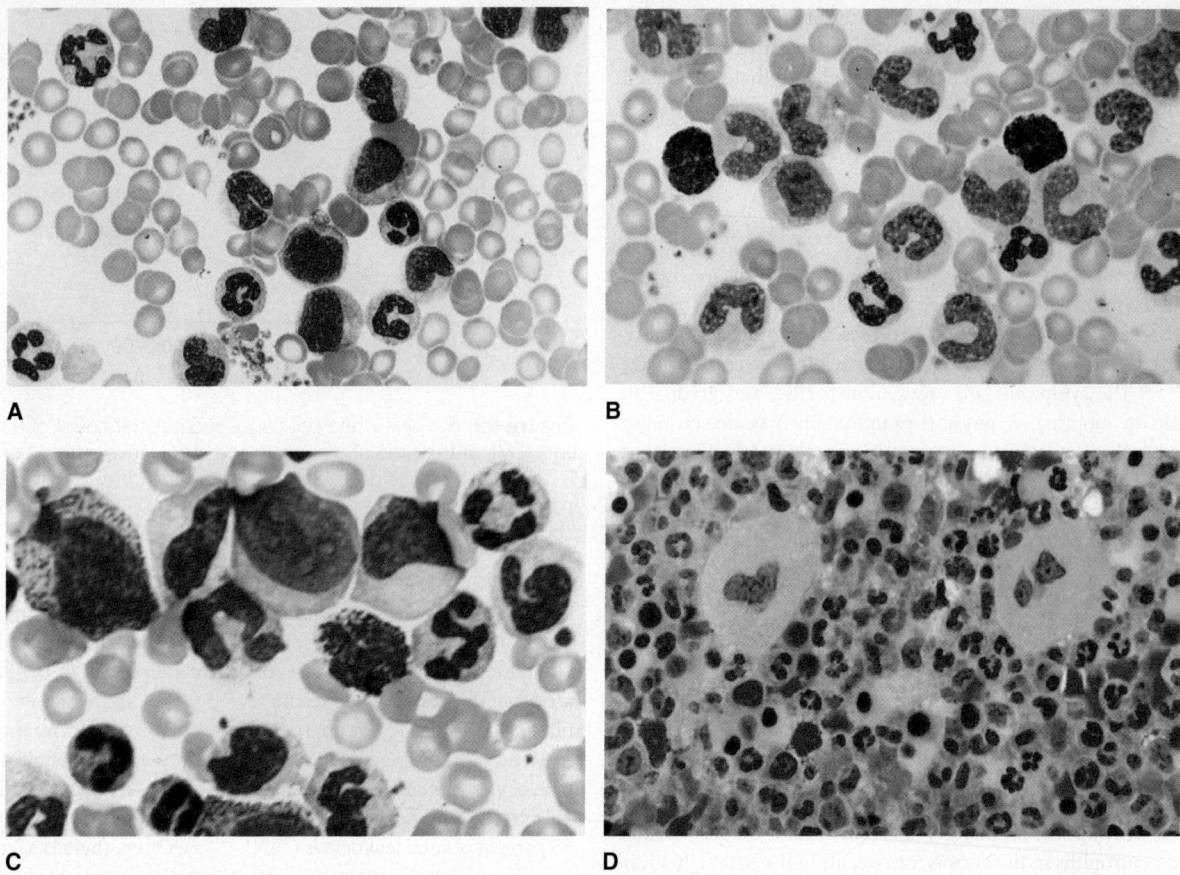

Figure 89–7. Blood and marrow cells characteristic of chronic myelogenous leukemia. **A.** Blood film. Elevated leukocyte count. Elevated platelet count (aggregates). Characteristic array of immature (myelocytes, metamyelocytes, band forms) and mature neutrophils. **B.** Blood film. Elevated leukocyte count. Characteristic array of immature (myelocytes, metamyelocytes, band forms) and mature neutrophils. Two basophils in the field. Absolute basophilia is a constant finding in CML. **C.** Blood film. Elevated leukocyte count. Characteristic array of immature (promyelocytes, myelocytes, metamyelocytes, band forms) and mature neutrophils. Basophil in the field. Two myeloblasts in upper center. Note multiple nucleoli (abnormal) and agranular cytoplasm. **D.** Marrow section. Hypercellular. Replacement of fatty tissue (normally approximately 60 percent of marrow volume in adults of this patient's age) with hematopoietic cells. Intense granulopoiesis and evident megakaryocytopoiesis. Decreased erythropoiesis. *(Reproduced with permission Lichtman's Atlas of Hematology, www.accessmedicine.com.)*

The total absolute lymphocyte count is increased (mean: approximately 15×10^9/L) in patients with CML at the time of diagnosis[284] as a result of the balanced increase in T-helper and T-suppressor cells.[285] B lymphocytes are not increased.[288] T lymphocytes also are increased in the spleen.[286] NK cell activity is defective in CML patients as a result of decreased maturation of these cells *in vivo*[287,288] and a decrease in the absolute number of circulating NK cells in patients with CML. The latter change can perhaps be related to increased apoptosis.[289] The CD56 bright subset of NK cells is particularly decreased. These cells are reduced more as CML progresses, and they respond less to stimuli that recruit clonogenic NK cells compared to NK cells from normal subjects.[290]

The platelet count is elevated in approximately 50 percent of patients at the time of diagnosis and is normal in most of the rest.[291] The median value in patients at diagnosis is approximately 400×10^9 cells/L. The platelet count may increase during the course of the chronic phase. Platelet counts greater than 1000×10^9/L are not unusual, and platelet counts as high as 5000 to 7000×10^9/L have occurred. Thrombohemorrhagic complications of thrombocytosis are infrequent. Occasionally, the platelet count may be below normal at the time of diagnosis, but this finding usually signals an impending progression to the accelerated phase of the disease (see "Accelerated Phase and Blast Crisis of Chronic

Myelogenous Leukemia" below) and may also occur in with massive splenomegaly.

Functional abnormalities of neutrophils (adhesion, emigration, phagocytosis) are mild; are compensated for by high neutrophil concentrations; and do not predispose patients in chronic phase to infections by either usual or opportunistic organisms.[292–294] Platelet dysfunction can occur but is not associated with spontaneous or exaggerated bleeding. A decrease in the second wave of epinephrine-induced platelet aggregation is the most common abnormality and is associated with a deficiency of adenine nucleotides in the storage pool.[295,296]

Marrow

Morphology The marrow is markedly hypercellular, and hematopoietic tissue takes up 75 to 90 percent of the marrow volume, with fat markedly reduced (see Fig. 89–7).[297,298] Granulopoiesis is dominant, with a granulocytic-to-erythroid ratio between 10:1 and 30:1, rather than the normal 2:1 to 4:1. Erythropoiesis usually is decreased, and megakaryocytes are normal or increased in number. Eosinophils and basophils may be increased, usually in proportion to their increase in the blood. Mitotic figures are increased in number. Mast cells are often seen, and uncommonly a juxtamembrane domain mutant of *KIT* coincides with *BCR-ABL1* in CML.[299] Rare reports of marrow mastocytosis

TABLE 89–1. White Blood Cell Differential Count at the Time of Diagnosis in 90 Cases of Ph Chromosome–Positive Chronic Myelogenous Leukemia

	Percent of Total Leukocytes (Mean Values)
Myeloblasts	3
Promyelocytes	4
Myelocytes	12
Metamyelocytes	7
Band forms	14
Segmented forms	38
Basophils	3
Eosinophils	2
Nucleated red cells	0.5
Monocytes	8
Lymphocytes	8

In these 90 patients, the mean hematocrit was 31 mL/dL, mean total white cell count was 160 × 10⁹/L, and mean platelet count was 442 × 10⁹/L at the time of diagnosis.
Data from Hematology Unit, University of Rochester Medical Center.

have been explained by a *KIT* mutation as an additional genetic abnormality or by dual clones in the marrow.[300,301] Macrophages that mimic Gaucher cells in appearance are sometimes seen. This finding is a result of the inability of normal cellular glucocerebrosidase activity to degrade the increased glucocerebroside load associated with markedly increased cell turnover.[302] Macrophages also can become engorged with lipids, which, when oxidized and polymerized, yield ceroid pigment. This pigment imparts a granular and bluish cast to the cells after polychrome staining; such cells have been referred to as *sea-blue histiocytes*.[302]

Collagen type III (reticulin fibrosis), which takes the silver impregnation stain, is commonly increased at the time of diagnosis in nearly half the patients,[303] and is correlated with the proportion of megakaryocytes in the marrow.[304,305] Increased fibrosis also is correlated with larger spleen size, more severe anemia, and a higher proportion of marrow and blood blast cells.

The marrows of CML patients have a mean doubling of microvessel density compared to healthy controls and have more angiogenesis in marrow than other forms of leukemia.[306–308] This increased marrow vascularity decreases to normal after treatment.[309]

Progenitor Cell Growth Cells that form colonies of neutrophils and macrophages or eosinophils (CFUs) are increased in the marrow and blood. The increase in CFUs in marrow is approximately 20-fold normal and in blood approximately 500-fold normal. The CFUs are of lighter buoyant density than those in normal marrow.[100] More primitive progenitors that can initiate long-term cultures of hematopoiesis also are markedly increased.[311] Spontaneous blood-derived granulocyte-macrophage colony growth is common, although CFUs also respond to growth factor stimulation.

Cytogenetics The marrow and nucleated blood cells of more than 90 percent of patients with clinical and laboratory signs that fall within the criteria for the diagnosis of CML contain the Ph chromosome (22q–) as measured by G-banding, and virtually all patients have the t(9;22)(q34;q11)(*BCR-ABL1*) by FISH. The Ph chromosome is present in all blood cell lineages (erythroblasts, granulocytes, monocytes,

megakaryocytes, T- and B-cell progenitors) but is not present in the majority of blood B lymphocytes or in most T lymphocytes.[54,56] Approximately 70 percent of patients in the chronic phase have the classic Ph chromosome in their cells.[312] The remaining 20 percent also have a missing Y chromosome [t(Ph),–Y]; an additional C-group chromosome, usually number 8 [t(Ph),+8]; an additional chromosome 22q– but without the 9q+ [t(Ph), 22q–]; or t(Ph) plus either another stable translocation or another minor clone. These variations have not been shown to affect the duration of the chronic phase. Deletion of the Y chromosome occurs in approximately 10 percent of healthy men older than 60 years.[313,314]

Variant Ph chromosome translocations occur in approximately 5 percent of subjects with CML and involve complex rearrangements (three chromosomes), and every chromosome except the Y chromosome can be involved.[315–319] The Ph chromosome, that is, 22q–, is present, but the gross exchange of chromosomal material involves a chromosome other than 9 (simple variant) or involves exchange of material among chromosomes 9 and 22 and a third or more chromosomes (complex variant; Fig. 89–8). High-resolution techniques have indicated that 9q34-qter is transposed to 22q11 in simple and in complex translocations.[320,321] Thus, the fusion of 9q34 with 22q11 seems to occur in the cells of most patients with CML.[323] Complex translocations involving chromosome 3 have been notable.[322–324] In rare cases, a reciprocal translocation with a chromosome other than 9 to chromosome 22 is larger than usual, and the posttranslocation shortening of the long arms of 22 is not apparent. This circumstance has been referred to as a *masked Ph chromosome* or *masked translocation* because the 22q– is not evident by microscopic examination,[325,326] although t(9;22) may occur as judged by banding techniques or molecular probes.[327]

Approximately 10 percent of patients have a deletion of the derivative 9 chromosome adjacent to the chromosome breakpoint. Although this deletion is thought to be an important factor in resistance to drug effects with IFN therapy, it does not appear to be significant with the use of imatinib.[214]

Molecular Probes In a small proportion of patients with a clinical disease analogous to CML, cytogenetic studies do not disclose a classic, variant, or masked Ph chromosome. In these cases, use of a panel of restriction enzymes and Southern blot analyses with a molecular probe for the breakpoint cluster region on chromosome 22 nearly always detects rearrangement of fragments. This finding has led to the conclusion that almost all cases of CML have an abnormality of the long arm of chromosome number 22 (*BCR* rearrangement).[328–332] Ph chromosome-negative CML cells with *BCR* rearrangement can express p210^BCR-ABL1, and such patients have a clinical course similar to Ph chromosome-positive CML.[328,333–336]

The ability to identify the molecular consequences of the t(9;22), that is, *BCR* rearrangement, mRNA transcripts of the mutant fusion gene, and p210^BCR-ABL1, has resulted in diagnostic tests supplementary to cytogenetic analysis.[332] These tests include Southern blot analysis of *BCR* rearrangement,[334–338] polymerase chain reaction (PCR) amplification of the abnormal mRNA,[339] and a less complex variation on the latter, a hybridization protection assay.[340]

PCR can achieve a sensitivity of one positive cell in approximately 500,000 to one million cells. This extreme sensitivity requires special care in analysis and the inclusion of negative controls.[341–344] Fusions e13a3, e14a3, and e19a2 are not detectable with standard PCR primers.[344A]

A multicolor FISH method to detect the *BCR-ABL1* fusion in patients with CML is a rapid and sensitive alternative to Southern blot and PCR-dependent methods.[345] For diagnostic purposes, FISH is simple, accurate, and sensitive, and can detect the various molecular fusions (e.g., e13a2, e14a2, e1a2).[346–350] Interphase FISH is faster and more sensitive than cytogenetics in identifying the Ph chromosome. If

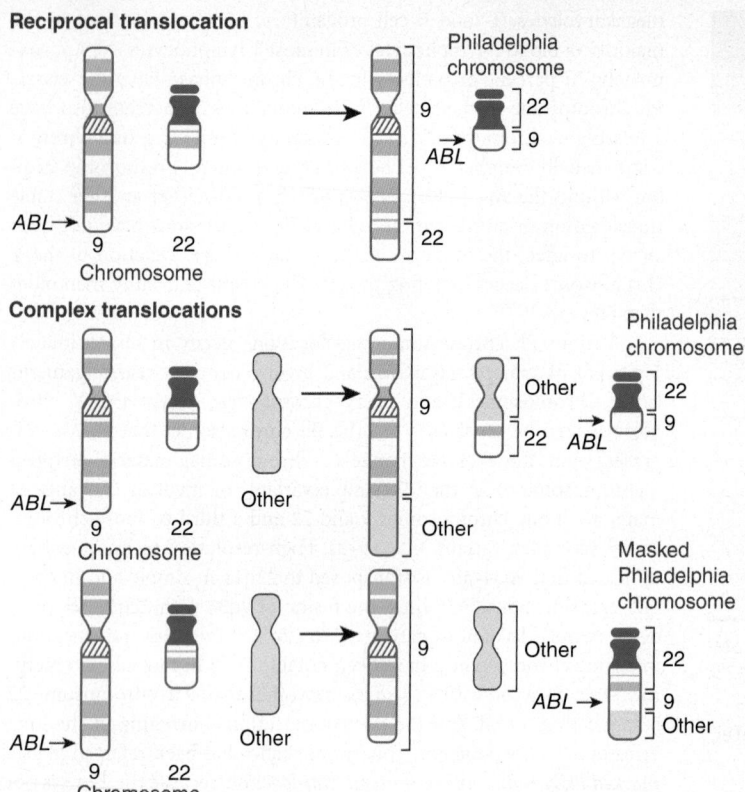

Reciprocal translocation

Complex translocations

Figure 89–8. Translocations involved in chronic myelogenous leukemia. The positions of the *ABL* gene in each of the chromosomes before and after the translocation are noted. The origin of the chromosomal segments in each of the translocated chromosomes is indicated by a *bracket* on the side of the chromosome. (*Reproduced with permission from Rosson D, Reddy EP: Activation of the abl oncogene and its involvement in chromosomal translocations in human leukemia. Mutat Res 1988 May;195(3):231–243.*)

the concentration of CML cells is very low, interphase FISH may not detect *BCR-ABL1*, so it has limited use for detecting minimal residual disease.[351] Hypermetaphase FISH allows analysis of up to 500 metaphases per sample in 1 day. Several factors influence the false-positive and false-negative rates of FISH identification of *BCR-ABL1*, including definition of a fusion signal, nuclear size, and the genomic position of the *ABL1* breakpoint.[352] Double BCR-ABL fusion signals (double-fusion [D]-FISH) have been proposed as being more accurate than the fusion signal used in dual color (single-fusion) S-FISH, because in the latter case a small percentage of the normal *BCR* and *ABL1* signals overlap.[353]

The frequency of cytogenetic analysis can be reduced if patients are monitored by molecular methods such as competitive reverse transcriptase (RT)-PCR. Molecular analyses can be performed on blood samples and therefore are much easier to use than cytogenetic analysis of marrow cell metaphases. Quantitative RT-PCR is the method of choice for monitoring patients for residual disease or reappearance of disease after marrow transplantation and for following response to TKIs once routine cytogenetics and FISH are negative for the Ph chromosome. Competitive PCR can detect reappearance of or increasing levels of *BCR-ABL1* RNA transcripts prior to clinical relapse in patients after transplantation.[354–356]

Chemical Abnormalities

Uric Acid An increased production of uric acid with hyperuricemia and hyperuricosuria occurs in untreated CML.[357] Uric acid excretion often is two to three times normal in patients with CML. If aggressive therapy leads to rapid cell lysis, excretion of the additional purine load may produce urinary tract blockage from uric acid precipitates. Formation of urinary urate stones is common in patients with CML, and some patients with latent gout may develop acute gouty arthritis or uric acid nephropathy.[358] The likelihood of complications from urate overproduction is greatly increased by starvation, acidosis, renal disease, or diuretic drug therapy.

Serum Vitamin B_{12}–Binding Proteins and Vitamin B_{12} Neutrophils contain vitamin B_{12}–binding proteins, including transcobalamins I and III (synonym: R-type B_{12}-binding protein or cobalophilin).[359–362] Patients with myeloproliferative neoplasms have an increased serum level of vitamin B_{12}–binding capacity, and the source of the protein is principally mature neutrophilic granulocytes.[359,360] The increase in transcobalamin level and the resultant increase in vitamin B_{12} concentration are particularly notable in CML, although any increase in the number of neutrophilic granulocytes, as in leukemoid reactions, can be accompanied by an increase in serum vitamin B_{12}–binding protein levels and vitamin B_{12} concentration.[362] The serum vitamin B_{12} level in CML patients is increased on average to more than 10 times normal.[363] The increase is proportional to the total leukocyte count in untreated patients and falls toward normal levels with treatment, although increased vitamin B_{12} levels commonly persist even after the white cell count is lowered to near normal with therapy.

Pernicious anemia and CML may rarely coexist. In this situation, the tissues are vitamin B_{12} deficient, but the serum vitamin B_{12} level may be normal because of the elevated level of transcobalamin I, a binder with a very high affinity for vitamin B_{12}.[363]

Whole Blood Histamine Mean histamine levels are markedly increased in patients in chronic phase (median: approximately 5000 ng/mL) compared to healthy individuals (median: approximately 50 ng/mL); and, this elevation is correlated with the blood basophil count.[364] Cases of exaggerated basophilia and disabling pruritus, urticaria, and gastric hyperacidity have occurred, associated with enormous increases (several hundredfold) of blood histamine concentration.[365,366]

Serum Lactic Dehydrogenase, Potassium, Calcium, and Cholesterol The level of serum lactic acid dehydrogenase (LDH) is elevated in CML.[367] Pseudohyperkalemia resulting from the release of potassium from white cells during clotting[368] and spurious hypoxemia or pseudohypoglycemia from *in vitro* utilization of oxygen or glucose by granulocytes can occur. Hypercalcemia[369] or hypokalemia[370] has occurred during the chronic phase of the disease, but such complications are very rare until the disorder transforms to acute leukemia. Elevated serum and urinary lysozyme levels are features of leukemia with greater monocytic components and are not features of CML.[371] Serum cholesterol is decreased in patients with CML.[372,373]

Serum Angiogenic Factors Angiogenin, endoglin (CD105), vascular endothelial growth factor (VEGF), β-fibroblast growth factor, and hepatocyte growth factor are increased strikingly in the serum of CML patients.[307,308,374,375]

SPECIAL CLINICAL FEATURES

BCR-ABL1–POSITIVE THROMBOCYTHEMIA

Either of two syndromes—thrombocythemia with the Ph chromosome and BCR-ABL1 rearrangement or thrombocythemia without a Ph chromosome but with the BCR-ABL1 rearrangement—may precede the overt signs of CML or its accelerated phase.[376–379] In general, the disease closely mimics classic essential thrombocythemia initially: marked platelet elevation, extreme megakaryocytic hyperplasia, normal or mildly elevated white cell count, no or very slight myeloid immaturity in the blood, and minimal anemia. Minor bleeding, such as epistaxis, erythromelalgia, or signs of thrombosis, such as cerebral or limb ischemia, are occasionally present. In some cases, the absolute basophil count is mildly elevated. Approximately 5 percent of patients with apparent essential thrombocythemia have a Ph chromosome.[376] In another study, two of 121 patients with essential thrombocythemia had BCR-ABL1 transcripts, and one of these patients also had a Ph chromosome in the marrow cells, whereas in a different study, four of 32 patients with thrombocythemia had low levels of BCR-ABL1 transcripts in blood cells. Approximately one in 20 patients with CML present with the features of essential thrombocythemia.[377,378] Evolution to blast crisis may occur.[380,381]

NEUTROPHILIC CHRONIC MYELOGENOUS LEUKEMIA

A rare variant of BCR-ABL1–positive CML has been described in which the elevated white cell count is composed principally of mature neutrophils.[382,383] The white cell count is lower (on average: 30 to 50 × 10^9/L) at the time of diagnosis than is the case with classic CML (median: 100 to 150 × 10^9/L). Moreover, patients with neutrophilic CML usually do not have basophilia, notable myeloid immaturity in the blood, prominent splenomegaly, or low leukocyte alkaline phosphatase scores. The cells of these patients have the Ph chromosome but have an unusual BCR-ABL1 fusion gene in that the breakpoint in the BCR gene is between exons 19 and 20. This breakpoint location results in fusion of most of the BCR gene with ABL1 (e19a2 type BCR-ABL1), which leads to a larger fusion protein (230 kDa) compared to the fusion protein in classic CML (210 kDa; see Fig. 89–3). This correlation between genotype and phenotype has not been observed in all cases.[384] This variant usually has an indolent course, which may be the result of very low levels of mRNA for p230 and the undetectable or barely detectable p230 protein in cells.[385]

MINOR-BCR BREAKPOINT–POSITIVE CHRONIC MYELOGENOUS LEUKEMIA

A small portion of patients with BCR-ABL1–positive CML have the breakpoint on the BCR gene in the first intron (m-bcr), resulting in a 190-kDa fusion protein instead of the classic 210-kDa protein observed in most patients with CML (see Fig. 89–3). The m-bcr molecular lesion is similar to that observed in approximately 60 percent of patients with BCR rearrangement-positive ALL. In patients with m-bcr CML, monocytes are more prominent, the white cell count is lower on average, and basophilia and splenomegaly are less prominent than in disease with classic BCR breakpoint (M-bcr). The few reported cases had a short interval before either myeloid or lymphoid blast transformation developed.[386,387]

HYPERLEUKOCYTOSIS

Approximately 15 percent of patients present with symptoms or signs referable to leukostasis as a result of the intravascular flow-impeding effects of white cell counts greater than 300 × 10^9/L.[249] Hyperleukocytosis is more prevalent in children with Ph chromosome–positive CML.[250] The effects of total leukocyte counts from 300 to 800 × 10^9/L include impaired circulation of the lung, central nervous system, special sensory organs, and penis, resulting in some combination of tachypnea, dyspnea, cyanosis, dizziness, slurred speech, delirium, stupor, visual blurring, diplopia, retinal vein distention, retinal hemorrhages, papilledema, tinnitus, impaired hearing, and priapism.[251] In asymptomatic patients with hyperleukocytosis, initial treatment with hydration and hydroxyurea usually can be used to decrease the white cell count. Hydroxyurea treatment should be designed to accomplish a gradual decrease in white cell count over a few days so as to avoid the tumor lysis syndrome. If signs of hyperleukocytosis are present, hydration, leukapheresis, and hydroxyurea can be used simultaneously; hydroxyurea dose should be selected to avoid exaggerated tumor lysis.

CONCURRENCE OF LYMPHOID MALIGNANCIES

CML may emerge in patients with established chronic lymphocytic leukemia (CLL).[388–390] A few patients have presented with simultaneous occurrence of the two diseases.[391,392] A single case of lymphocytic leukemoid reaction simulating CLL that regressed as CML emerged has been reported.[393] In some cases, the CLL lymphocytes did not contain the Ph chromosome, whereas the CML cells did, suggesting the presence of two independent clonal disorders.[388,389,393,394] In other cases, the Ph chromosome was present in the myeloid and lymphoid cells, indicating a common origin.[392] Patients may present with Ph chromosome–positive acute lymphoblastic leukemia and, following chemotherapy-induced remission, develop the features of typical CML.[395]

DIFFERENTIAL DIAGNOSIS

DISEASES MIMICKING CHRONIC MYELOGENOUS LEUKEMIA

The diagnosis of CML is made based on the characteristic granulocytosis, white cell differential count, increased absolute basophil count, and splenomegaly coupled with the presence of the Ph chromosome or its variants (90 percent of patients) or a BCR rearrangement on chromosome 22 (>95 percent of patients).

Patients with other chronic hematopoietic stem cell diseases, such as polycythemia vera, essential thrombocythemia, or primary myelofibrosis, only occasionally have closely overlapping features. For example, the total white cell count is greater than 30 × 10^9/L in more than 90 percent of patients with CML and increases inexorably over weeks or months of observation, whereas the total white cell count is less than 30 × 10^9/L in more than 90 percent of patients with the three other classic chronic clonal myeloid diseases and usually does not change significantly over months to years. Polycythemia vera is associated with increased red cell mass and hemoglobin concentration and displays clinical signs of plethora; CML does not have these features. Patients with primary myelofibrosis invariably have marked teardrop poikilocytes and other severe red cell shape, size, and chromicity changes, as well as prominent nucleated red cells in the blood; CML rarely has these features. Patients with essential thrombocythemia have a platelet count greater than 450×10^9/L and usually only mild neutrophilia ($<20 \times 10^9$/L); the slight neutrophilia distinguishes it from the proportion (approximately 25 percent) of CML patients with platelet counts greater than 450×10^9/L, who at the time of diagnosis have white cell counts above 25×10^9/L. In addition, patients with the clinical features of polycythemia vera or primary myelofibrosis do not have the Ph chromosome or *BCR* rearrangement in their blood and marrow cells, except in extremely rare cases. A very small proportion of patients with apparent essential thrombocythemia has BCR-ABL1 transcripts in their marrow and blood cells, and occasionally a Ph chromosome and may represent an atypical initial phase of CML (see "*BCR-ABL1*–Positive Thrombocythemia" above). The presence of a mutation in the *JAK2* gene in more than 95 percent of patients with polycythemia vera is an important distinguishing feature (Chap. 84). The blood cells of approximately 50 percent of patients with primary myelofibrosis or essential thrombocythemia carry the *JAK2* gene mutation and in those with primary myelofibrosis who do not, a significant proportion have a mutation in the calreticulin or the *c-MPL* gene (Chap. 86).

Increased awareness of the features of related disorders, such as chronic myelomonocytic leukemia (CMML) and chronic neutrophilic leukemia, and an appreciation that older patients are prone to atypical clonal myeloid diseases, have minimized the inappropriate diagnosis of Ph chromosome–negative CML, which should be avoided unless the clinical features are characteristic of classic CML and a masked Ph chromosome or *BCR* rearrangement is not found.

Reactive leukocytosis can occur with absolute neutrophil counts of 30 to 100×10^9/L. Usually these leukemoid reactions occur in the setting of an overt inflammatory disease (e.g., pancreatitis), cancer (e.g., lung), or infection (e.g., pneumococcal pneumonia). If the incitant is not apparent, the absence of granulocytic immaturity, basophilia, or splenomegaly, and the absence of *BCR/ABL1* in blood cells virtually eliminates classic CML as a consideration.

The precise diagnosis of CML is helpful in estimating the patient's prognosis, identifying the utility of TKIs, and assessing the timing of special therapies, such as allogeneic hematopoietic stem cell transplantation.

Ph CHROMOSOME–POSITIVE CLONAL MYELOID DISEASES AND APLASTIC ANEMIA

The Ph chromosome has been found rarely in patients with apparent polycythemia vera,[396] polycythemia vera that later evolves into Ph chromosome–positive CML,[397-399] primary myelofibrosis,[400,401] and myelodysplastic syndrome (MDS).[402,403] Molecular studies to determine the presence of the *BCR-ABL1* were not performed in cases reported before 1985. Essential thrombocythemia with a Ph chromosome and/or *BCR-ABL1* rearrangement in blood cells was discussed earlier (see "Special Clinical Features" above). Rare cases of aplastic anemia have presented with *BCR-ABL1*–positive cells or have evolved into BCR-ABL1 CML.[404,405]

●THERAPY

HYPERURICEMIA

Hyperuricemia and hyperuricosuria are frequent features of CML at diagnosis or in relapse.[406] The need for treatment of hyperuricemia is a function of the elevated pretreatment serum uric acid concentration,

blood white cell concentration, spleen size, and dose of cytolytic therapy planned. If these variables suggest a high risk for a significant amount of cell lysis, allopurinol 300 mg/day orally and adequate hydration to maintain a good urine flow should be instituted prior to therapy. Allopurinol is associated with a high frequency of allergic skin reactions and should be discontinued after the blood leukocyte count and spleen size have decreased and the risk of exaggerated cell lysis has passed. If hyperuricemia is extreme, usually over 9 mg/dL, rasburicase can be administered.[407] Rasburicase is a recombinant urate oxidase that converts uric acid to allantoin. Rasburicase, unlike allopurinol, reduces the uric acid pool very rapidly, does not result in the accumulation of xanthine or hypoxanthine, and does not require alkalinization of urine facilitating phosphate excretion.[408] Although the manufacturer recommends a dose every day for 5 days, several reports have indicated that one injection will produce a rapid and sustained decrease in serum uric acid, significantly decreasing the cost of therapy.[409] Another alternative is to use allopurinol for a few days after one injection of rasburicase. A dose of 0.2 mg/kg of ideal body weight of rasburicase intravenously has been used.[410]

INITIAL CYTOREDUCTION THERAPY

A TKI is now used as initial therapy in patients with CML. In cases where the white cell count is markedly elevated, hydroxyurea can be used prior to or in conjunction with a TKI. If rapid cytoreduction is required because of signs of the hyperleukocytic syndrome, leukapheresis and hydroxyurea often are combined.

Leukapheresis

Leukapheresis can control CML only temporarily. For this reason, it is rarely used in chronic phase CML and is useful in only two types of patients: the hyperleukocytic patient in whom rapid cytoreduction can reverse symptoms and signs of leukostasis (e.g., stupor, hypoxia, tinnitus, papilledema, priapism),[249-251] and in the pregnant patient with CML who can be controlled by leukapheresis treatment without other therapy either during the early months of pregnancy when therapy poses a higher risk to the fetus or, in some cases, throughout the pregnancy.[411,412] Because of the large body burden of leukocytes in marrow, blood, and spleen, and the high proliferative rate in CML, leukocyte reduction by apheresis is less efficient than in other types of leukemia.[249,251] Leukapheresis reduces the burden of tumor cells subject to chemotherapeutically induced cytolysis and thus the production and the excretion of uric acid. In hyperleukocytic nonpregnant patients, leukapheresis is best used in conjunction with hydroxyurea to ensure rapid and optimal reduction in white cell count.

Hydroxyurea

Hydroxyurea 1 to 6 g/day orally, depending on the height of the white cell count, can be used to initiate elective therapy.[413] Urgent treatment of extraordinary total white cell counts may require higher doses. The dose of hydroxyurea should be decreased as the total white cell count decreases and usually is given at 1 to 2 g/day when the total white cell count reaches 20×10^9/L. The drug should be temporarily discontinued if the white cell count drops below 5×10^9/L. If hydroxyurea is being used in combination with a TKI, it is usually tapered and discontinued once a hematologic response to the TKI is observed.

Anagrelide

Anagrelide can be used for platelet reduction in patients who present with elevated platelet counts. This agent acts directly to decrease megakaryocyte mass, and it can lead to a precipitous fall in platelet counts. In occasional patients who still have significant thrombocythemia after a

TKI is initiated, combination with anagrelide is associated with a normalization of platelet counts.[414]

INITIAL THERAPY WITH A TYROSINE KINASE INHIBITOR

Imatinib mesylate (imatinib) was the first TKI developed, and it was approved by the FDA for initial therapy of CML in 2002. Subsequently, two second-generation TKIs, nilotinib and dasatinib, were approved for initial therapy in 2010. This approval was based upon superior cytogenetic and molecular response rates with nilotinib and dasatinib at benchmark time points and lower rates of conversion to accelerated or blast phase as compared with imatinib. Thus far, an overall survival advantage of dasatinib or nilotinib compared with imatinib has not been shown.[415] Third-generation TKIs, bosutinib and ponatinib, are under study. Table 89–2 compares these inhibitors.

Imatinib Patients with newly diagnosed, chronic phase CML can be started on imatinib, 400 mg/day by mouth. The goal of imatinib therapy is to decrease the cells bearing the t(9;22) translocation (leukemic cells) to the lowest levels possible, during which process normal (polyclonal) hematopoiesis is restored. The efficacy of imatinib is judged by measuring three benchmarks: hematologic response, cytogenetic response, and molecular response as defined in Table 89–3.[416,417] These benchmarks are used to determine its maximal therapeutic effect. The time to achieve

TABLE 89–2. Comparison of Tyrosine Kinase Inhibitors				
	Imatinib (Gleevec)	**Nilotinib (Tasigna)**	**Dasatinib (Sprycel)**	**Bosutinib (Bosulif)**	**Ponatinib (Iclusig)**
Indications	First-line therapy (CP, AP, BP); relapsed/refractory Ph+ ALL	First-line therapy (CP), resistance or intolerance to imatinib (CP and AP)	First-line therapy (CP), resistance or intolerance to other TKIs (CP, AP, or BP); Ph+ ALL with resistance or intolerance to prior therapy	Second-line therapy (CP, AP, BP with resistance or intolerance)	Resistance or intolerance to prior TKI or Ph+ ALL resistant or intolerant to all other TKIs; all T315I + casesl
Usual dosing	CP 400 mg/day AP/BP/progression 600–800 mg/day	CP 300 mg BID AP/BP 400 mg BID	CP 100 mg/day AP/BP 140 mg/day	500 mg/day	45 mg/day
Common toxicities (nonhematologic)	GI disturbance, edema (including periorbital), muscle cramps, arthralgias, Hypophosphatemia, rash	Rash, GI disturbances, elevated lipase, hyperglycemia, low phosphorus, increased LFTs	Edema, pleural effusions, GI symptoms, rash, low phosphorus	GI (diarrhea), rash, edema, fatigue, low phosphorus, elevated LFTs	HBP, rash, GI, fatigue, headache
Other significant toxicities	Elevated LFTs (usually appear in first month); rare cardiac toxicity reported	Peripheral vascular disease, PT prolongation, pancreatitis	Pulmonary arterial hypertension, QTc prolongation		Arterial and venous thrombosis, pancreatitis, liver failure, ocular toxicity, cardiac failure
Drug–drug interactions	CYP3A4 inducers decrease levels CYP3A4 inhibitors may increase levels It is an inhibitor of CYP3A4 and CYP2D6 Pgp substrate	CYP3A4 inhibitors increase levels CYP3A4 inducers may decrease levels Inhibitor of CYP3A4, CYP2C8, CYP2C9, CYP2D6 Induces CYP2B6, CYP2C8, and CYP2C9	CYP3A4 inhibitors increase levels CYP3A4 inducer decrease levels Antacids decrease levels H₂ antagonists/proton pump inhibitors decrease levels	CYP3A inhibitors and inducers may alter levels Acid-reducing medication may lower levels	Strong CYP3A inhibitors increased serum levels
Administration considerations	Taken with food	Taken on empty stomach; avoid food 2 hours before and 2 hours after dose	Can be taken with or without a meal	Taken with food	Taken with and without food
Black box warnings	None	QT prolongation and sudden death	None	None	Arterial thrombosis; hepatotoxicity
Other considerations	Approved in pediatric patients (340 mg/m²/day) in CP	Keep potassium, Mg, calcium, phosphorus repleted	Ascites and pericardial effusion can also occur; has CSF penetration		Has activity with T315I mutations; Available in U.S. through ARIAD PASS program

ALL, acute lymphocytic leukemia; AP, accelerated phase; BP, blast phase; CP, chronic phase; CSF, cerebrospinal fluid; CYP, cytochrome P450; GI, gastrointestinal; HBP, high blood pressure; LFT, liver function tests; Pgp, P-glycoprotein; PT, prothrombin time; TKI, tyrosine kinase inhibitor.

All information is from the commercial package insert of the TKIs as listed.

TABLE 89–3. Definition of a Treatment Response to a Tyrosine Kinase Inhibitor

Complete hematologic response (CHR)	White cell count <10 × 10⁹/L, platelet count <450 × 10⁹/L, no immature myeloid cells in the blood, and disappearance of all signs and symptoms related to leukemia (including palpable splenomegaly) lasting for at least 4 weeks.
Minor cytogenetic response (mCyR)	>35% of cell metaphases are Philadelphia (Ph) chromosome–positive by cytogenetic analysis of marrow cells.
Partial cytogenetic response (pCyR)	1–35% of cell metaphases are Ph chromosome–positive by cytogenetic analysis of marrow cells.
Major cytogenetic response (MCyR)	<35% of cell metaphases contain the Ph chromosome by cytogenetic analysis of marrow cells.
Complete cytogenetic response (CCyR)	No cells containing the Ph chromosome by cytogenetic analysis of marrow cells.
Major molecular response (MMR)	*BCR-ABL1/ABL1* ratio <0.1% or a 3-log reduction in quantitative polymerase chain reaction (qPCR) signal from mean pretreatment baseline value, if International Standard (IS)-based PCR not available.
Complete molecular response (CMR)	*BCR-ABL1* mRNA levels undetectable by qPCR with assay sensitivity at least 4.5 logs below baseline (IS).

a maximal effect is variable, but as long as a patient is having a continued reduction in the size of the leukemic clone as judged by cytogenetic or PCR measurements, and has met response benchmarks, the drug is continued at 400 mg/day. If the patient stops responding before a complete cytogenetic remission or complete molecular remission is achieved, the dose can be increased to 600 mg/day or to 800 mg/day (400 mg every 12 hours), if tolerated. Alternatively, another TKI can be used. About two-thirds of patients who do not have a significant hematologic response or who relapse while receiving imatinib at a dose of 400 mg/day achieve a complete or partial hematologic response with higher doses, but few cytogenetic responses occur.[418] Some patients without a cytogenetic response can enter a partial or complete cytogenetic response(CCyR) with higher doses of imatinib. Unfortunately, the responses to higher doses of imatinib in patients lacking a hematologic or cytogenetic response at 400 mg/day usually are transient.[419,420]

Several studies have examined use of imatinib at doses higher than 400 mg/day. Patients with newly diagnosed chronic phase CML treated with imatinib, 800 mg/day, administered in two 400-mg doses, every 12 hours, had a frequency of 90 percent CCyR, and 96 percent had at least a major cytogenetic response (MCyR). At a median of 15 months, no patients had progressed and 63 percent showed blood *BCR-ABL1/ABL1* percentage ratios of less than 0.05 percent. Twenty-eight percent

of patients had undetectable *BCR-ABL1* blood levels.[421] In one trial, major molecular remission (MMR) at 12 and 24 months was higher in those receiving doses of imatinib greater than 600 mg/day.[422] In another trial, patients receiving 400 mg twice per day had a MCyR of 90 and 96 percent at 12 and 18 months, respectively. MMR rates were 48 percent and 54 percent at 6 and 12 months, respectively. These results compared favorably to historical data in the IRIS (International Randomized Study of Interferon) trial studying 400 mg/day of imatinib, but myelosuppression, rash, fatigue, and musculoskeletal symptoms were greater with these higher doses. Responses were, also, more rapid with the higher doses. More edema, gastrointestinal symptoms, rash, and myelosuppression occurred at the higher doses.[423] Despite these reports the current starting dose is customarily 400 mg/day, balancing both effectiveness and tolerability in newly diagnosed patients. Moreover, the more rapid response with higher doses of imatinib may not translate into better long-term results.[424,425] For example, in another trial, MMR and CCyR at 12 months were not significantly different between standard and high-dose patients, although patients in higher-risk categories based on Sokal scores, fared better with high-dose imatinib.[424] (See "Course and Prognosis" below for an explanation of the Sokal Score.)

Doses of imatinib lower than 400 mg/day result in fewer CCyR and a shorter duration of that response. Patients who are older and who have lower body weight may only tolerate a lower dose, but they are less likely to achieve a CCyR.[426] If however, a patient is on a lower dose (e.g., 300 mg/day) for a special reason (body size or tolerance level) and achieves a complete hematologic response (CHR) and CCyR within 12 months of onset of therapy, acceptable outcomes without excess toxicity can result.[427]

Some patients have been followed for up to 8 years on imatinib in the IRIS trial (IFN vs. STI571).[428] With median followup of 60 months, the best observed MCyR and CCyR rates were 89 percent and 82 percent, respectively. Only 7 percent had progressed to accelerated or blast phase, and overall survival rate was 89 percent. The best MMR rate was 86 percent during the 8-year followup. No patient with an MMR at 12 months progressed to accelerated or blast phase. By 8 years of follow up on the IRIS trial, 22 percent of patients had discontinued imatinib treatment because of an unsatisfactory response or toxicity, and only 55 percent remained on study. The 5-year probability of remaining in MCyR while receiving imatinib was approximately 60 percent. Achieving a CCyR correlated with progression-free survival, but achieving a MMR conferred no further survival benefit.[429]

Use of Imatinib in Patients with Variant Chromosomal Translocations or Breakpoints

Patients with variant Ph chromosome translocations have a similar prognosis to that of patients with classic Ph chromosome translocations who are treated with imatinib.[430] (See Fig. 89–3 for a diagram of breakpoints.) Patients with the e13a2, p210*BCR-ABL* translocation respond well to imatinib, with similar rates of complete cytogenetic remission.[431] The e13a2 transcript may be more sensitive to imatinib than the e14a2 transcript.[432] In a patient with both e1a2 and e14a2 fusion transcripts, only the p210 e14a2 transcript disappeared, whereas the e1a2 transcript persisted during progression to blast phase. No mutation in the kinase domain of *ABL1* was found.[433] Thus, different clones in a patient may have a different sensitivity to imatinib. Deletions of the derivative chromosome 9 do not influence the response and outcomes in CML chronic phase when using imatinib.[434]

Response to Imatinib in Children and Older Patients

More than 80 percent of children with chronic phase CML who are treated with imatinib, 260 to 570 mg/m², enter a complete cytogenetic remission. Imatinib is now approved for use in pediatric patients.

Weight gain is the most common side effect of imatinib.[435] In patients who were older than age 60 years, similar cytogenetic response rates and survival rates were noted as in younger patients in the late chronic phase who were treated concurrently, suggesting that age is not usually a factor in response.[436,437]

Side Effects and Special Treatment Considerations

Imatinib is usually tolerated. Most adverse effects are manageable and seldom require permanent cessation of therapy. Reduction to subtherapeutic doses is not recommended; it is better to interrupt therapy for a time.[438]

Myelosuppression is common, especially at treatment onset when the CML clone accounts for most of the blood cells. Dose reduction to less than 300 mg/day is not advisable for myelosuppression. The drug should be stopped until blood counts recover. G-CSF or GM-CSF can prevent or treat neutropenia.[439,440] Platelet transfusion may be used for severe thrombocytopenia. Patients with imatinib-induced chronic cytopenias have inferior responses.[441] Myelosuppression is an independent adverse factor for achieving cytogenetic responses with imatinib.[442] Erythropoiesis-stimulating agents may be used to raise hemoglobin levels, and their use does not appear to affect CML outcomes, but may increase the risk of thrombosis.[443] Severe irreversible marrow aplasias after imatinib exposure can occur.[444]

The main side effects noted with imatinib include fatigue, edema, nausea, diarrhea, muscle cramps, and rash.[445] Elevated hepatic transaminases can occur. Mild transaminase elevations often respond to glucocorticoid use.[446] Hepatotoxicity is uncommon, occurring in approximately 3 percent of patients, usually within 6 months of onset of imatinib use. Acute liver failure has been described.[447] The severe periorbital edema occasionally observed is postulated to be a drug effect on the function of platelet-derived growth factor receptor (PDGFR) and KIT expressed by dermal dendrocytes. Surgical decompression of severe edema rarely has been required.[448] Although no effects on spermatogenesis have been reported, women of childbearing age are at risk of teratogenic effects on their fetus.[448]

Weight gain is associated with imatinib use.[449] Patients with renal impairment require lower doses of imatinib.[450] Hypophosphatemia[451] and altered bone and mineral metabolism have occurred.[452,453] Cutaneous reactions with imatinib therapy occur in approximately 15 percent of patients.[454] Except for severe reactions (approximately 5 percent of patients), such as Stevens-Johnson syndrome, exfoliative dermatitis, and erythema multiforme, cutaneous reactions rarely require permanent discontinuation of therapy. With milder reactions, concomitant glucocorticoid therapy or brief discontinuation of imatinib with gradual reintroduction at a lower dose and then a gradual increase in dose can be accomplished.[456,457] With very mild cases, concurrent treatment with antihistamine or other symptomatic therapy may be successful. Oral desensitization regimens have been described that allow some patients to continue imatinib therapy. Hair depigmentation[458] and hypopigmentation of the skin,[459] probably related to the inhibition of the KIT receptor tyrosine kinase by imatinib, have been reported.

Other Effects of Imatinib

Imatinib has been found to cause regression of marrow fibrosis.[460] One study found that the extent of marrow fibrosis in CML is not a prognostic factor with imatinib therapy,[461] whereas another study observed that although imatinib reverses marrow fibrosis in patients with CML, it does not change the unfavorable prognosis associated with fibrosis.[462] Imatinib reverses exaggerated VEGF secretion in patients with CML,[463] and it may reverse exaggerated marrow angiogenesis.[464] It can reduce marrow cellularity and normalize morphologic features regardless of cytogenetic response. *BCR-ABL1*–positive cells persist in patients despite prolonged treatment responses with imatinib.[465]

Pharmacokinetic Considerations During Imatinib Therapy

Mean plasma trough concentration of imatinib and its metabolite, CGP74588, obtained at about 1 month (presumptive steady-state) was 979 ± 530 ng/mL. The rate of CCyR and MMR was higher within the highest quartiles of imatinib trough levels.[466] Some therapists suggest that imatinib plasma levels be checked in cases of suboptimal response in order to adjust the dose, but access to this monitoring is not routinely available.[467] Comedications and population covariates, such as body weight and white cell count, had no, or minimal, effect on imatinib clearance.[468] Patients with CML on hemodialysis have been successfully treated with imatinib.[469] Therapy interruptions and nonadherence with oral imatinib usage are common, and patient education and close monitoring are important to ensure compliance.[470]

Initiation of Therapy with Newer Tyrosine Kinase Inhibitors

Dasatinib Dasatinib is a second-generation oral BCR-ABL1 inhibitor with dual inhibition of ABL1 and SRC.[471] It can bind to both the active and inactive conformation of the *ABL1* kinase domain, so it may be affected by mutations resulting in resistance.[471]

Dasatinib was first studied for use in initial therapy in a phase II trial that accrued 62 patients. Ninety-eight percent achieved a CCyR, and the median time to CCyR was 3 months. The MMR rate was 82 percent. Responses were durable, and the recommended treatment schedule based on a safety profile was 100 mg, once daily.[472] A randomized, phase III trial compared the efficacy of dasatinib to imatinib.[473] In this study, 259 patients received dasatinib, 100 mg/day, and 260 received imatinib, 400 mg/day. After 12 months of followup, the rates of CCyR by 3, 6, and 9 months were 54, 73, and 78 percent, respectively, for patients on dasatinib as compared to 31, 59, and 67 percent, respectively, for those on imatinib. The 24-month CCyR was 80 percent for patients using dasatinib, as compared to 74 percent for those on imatinib. The MMR showed a similar trend, and the median time to MMR was 15 months for those using dasatinib, compared to 36 months for those using imatinib.

Long-term followup data have confirmed faster and deeper responses to dasatinib as compared to imatinib.[474] At 4 years, 76 percent of dasatinib-treated patients had attained a MMR (*BCR/ABL1* <0.1 percent) as compared to 63 percent using imatinib. At 3, 6, and 12 months, more patients achieved molecular responses using dasatinib than those using imatinib. There were fewer patients who progressed to accelerated or blast phase using dasatinib as compared to imatinib. To date, there is no difference in progression-free survival or overall survival between the two groups.[474] In a randomized study, with a minimal followup of 3 years, the proportion of patients with *BCR-ABL1* transcript levels less than 10 percent was higher in those using dasatinib as compared to those using imatinib.[475] Better responses were observed at 3, 6, and 12 months in the patients using dasatinib. The achievement of an early molecular response was predictive of improved progression-free and overall survival.[476]

Toxicity of Dasatinib Most grade 3 or 4 adverse events with dasatinib are hematologic and all cell lines can be affected. Some patients may have bleeding from inhibition of platelet aggregation.[477] Adverse events noted less frequently with dasatinib than imatinib include nausea, vomiting, myalgia, rash, and fluid retention, including superficial edema. Pleural effusions can be seen with dasatinib use. In one trial, 14 percent of patients had grade 1 or 2 pleural effusions at 24 months, but grade 3 or 4 effusions occurred in only 2 patients. This toxicity did not affect drug efficacy. Dasatinib may also increase the risk of pulmonary arterial hypertension at any time, and this is an indication to discontinue dasatinib.[478] Dasatinib may prolong the QTc interval, and it should be used with caution in those who have long QT syndrome or those taking drugs that may lengthen the QT interval.[474] Hypophosphatemia was found in 7 percent of cases.[474]

Dasatinib is metabolized primarily by hepatic cytochrome P450 (CYP) 3A4 enzymes, so inducers of this enzyme may decrease the effective dose, and inhibitors may increase the effective dose. Increases or decreases in administered dose may be needed to compensate for these effects. Antacids can also reduce dasatinib effects.[479] Lymphocytosis from the clonal expansion of NK/T cells has occurred during dasatinib treatment.[480] In a population of dasatinib-treated patients with large granular lymphocyte expansion, 90 percent had T-cell receptor delta rearrangements, the functional significance of which is unknown.[481] Lymph node follicular hyperplasia has been noted on dasatinib therapy.[482] Unlike the case with imatinib, dasatinib cellular uptake is not affected by octamer-binding protein-1 (OCT-1) activity, which is a substrate of the efflux proteins, ABCB1 and ABCG2. Resistance to dasatinib is often found with point mutations in *ABL1* at residue 315 or 317.

Nilotinib Unlike dasatinib, nilotinib is a selective, orally bioavailable, ATP-competitive inhibitor of BCR-ABL1 which is 20 to 50 times more potent than imatinib *in vitro*.[483] Like imatinib, it does not induce apoptosis in CD34+ CML cells.[484] As with dasatinib, nilotinib was first tested as initial therapy in phase II trials,[485] which were followed by a randomized phase III trial. In one phase II trial, 51 patients received nilotinib 400 mg, twice a day, and 98 percent entered CCyR and 76 percent had a MMR by 6 months.[486] The phase III trial compared nilotinib, 300 mg twice daily, 400 mg twice daily, and imatinib 400 mg daily.[487] At 12 months, the MMR which had been chosen as the primary end point, was 44 percent (nilotinib 300 mg dose), 43 percent (nilotinib 400 mg dose), and 22 percent (imatinib 400 mg daily). The CCyR rates were 15 percent higher with nilotinib than imatinib. The rate of progression to accelerated or blast phase was 4 percent at 1 year with imatinib and less than 1 percent with nilotinib. These improvements were observed in each prognostic group based on Sokal risk groups. The patients using either 300 or 400 mg doses had minimal differences, so in 2010, nilotinib was approved at a dose of 300 mg twice daily for initial CML therapy. At 4 years of followup, more patients using either dose of nilotinib achieved a MMR than those using imatinib (73 and 70 percent vs. 53 percent).[488] The rates of progression to accelerated and blast phase were also lower for nilotinib than imatinib. The 4-year freedom-from-progression and overall-survival rates were not different between the two groups. MMR rates at 3 years were higher for those patients using nilotinib, 300 mg, twice per day, in the three risk groups of Sokal (low risk, 79 percent; intermediate risk, 76 percent; and high risk, 52 percent progression as compared to those using imatinib (65, 55, and 30 percent progression, respectively).[488] There was a reduced incidence of *BCR-ABL1* mutations in in patients using nilotinib compared to those using imatinib. Nilotinib use led to fewer (less than half as many) treatment-emergent *BCR-ABL1* mutations than did imatinib treatment, and to reduced rates of progression to accelerated phase and blast crisis in patients with these mutations.[489]

Toxicity of Nilotinib Nilotinib is rarely associated with edema or muscle cramps. Grades 3 and 4 cytopenias were seen in 29 percent of cases in one trial.[487] Grade 3 or 4 elevations in lipase, bilirubin, and hyperglycemia were observed in 17, 8, and 12 percent of patients, and hypophosphatemia was seen in 16 percent. QTc prolongation can occur, so one should monitor the electrocardiogram (EKG) readings for 7 days after starting therapy and with dose changes.[483] Electrolyte abnormalities should be corrected at outset of treatment. Nilotinib may be associated with an increased risk of peripheral vascular disease, which may be arterial or venous.[490] If thrombosis occurs, it should no longer be used for therapy.

Bosutinib and Ponatinib These TKIs are not approved for use in initial therapy. In the one trial, which compared efficacy for bosutinib, 500 mg once daily, with imatinib, 400 mg daily in newly diagnosed chronic phase patients, the primary end point of CCyR at 12 months

was 70 percent for bosutinib and 63 percent for imatinib.[491,492] Results from followup of MMR rates, transformation rates, and durability of remission are not yet available.

Summary of Tyrosine Kinase Inhibitor Selection for Initial Therapy of Chronic Phase Chronic Myelogenous Leukemia

The goal of initial TKI therapy is to achieve a CCyR within 12 months or no later than 18 months of therapy, and to prevent progression to the accelerated or blast phase. How best to achieve these goals remains controversial. Hence, the National Comprehensive Cancer Network (NCCN) guidelines list imatinib, nilotinib, and dasatinib as all being acceptable TKIs for initial treatment of CML.[492] Many clinicians would choose a second-generation TKI, given the rapidity and depth of response and the lower rates of transformation to advanced phases of the disease, but others use imatinib because of the lack of proof of prolongation of survival with nilotinib or dasatinib. In those with intermediate- or high-risk disease as assessed by the Sokal and Hasford models (see "Course and Prognosis" below for details of these scores), nilotinib or dasatinib may be preferred over imatinib to achieve rapid, better responses—the "hit hard, hit early" approach.[493] Thus, until survival data are available, any one of the three approved TKIs may be used for initial therapy. Choice of agent may be dependent upon cost considerations, ease of administration, patient risk scores or perceived risk,[494] and the drug's side-effect profile (see Table 89–2).

Defining a Response to Tyrosine Kinase Inhibitors

Table 89–3 contains definitions of hematologic, cytogenetic, and molecular responses. The guidelines for periodic monitoring patients who are in chronic phase and receiving TKI therapy are shown in Table 89–4. The median *BCR-ABL1* levels for imatinib-treated patients can decrease over at least 5 years. Table 89–5[495] lists the milestones at 3, 6, 12, and 18 months expected of patients as indicators of an appropriate response in patients treated initially with a TKI.[434] There is variation in an individual patient's time to maximal response. Consequently, if a patient has not met those precise milestones but shows a continued decrease in the proportion of Ph chromosome–positive cells on cytogenetic examination of marrow, or if in a CCyR, a continued decrease in the level of the PCR signal for *BCR-ABL1* and is near the benchmark, the treatment can be continued. Only (1) failure to meet the benchmarks at 3, 6, or 12 months or (2) loss of response as defined as loss of a CHR or CCyR, (3) development of new cytogenetic abnormalities, (4) acquisition of a *BCR-ABL1* mutation, or (5) an increase in the *BCR-ABL1/ABL1* ratio of 1-log or more on serial RT-PCR testing or into the range associated with reappearance of the Ph chromosome on G-banding should generate a change in treatment to limit the risk of progression of the disease. Because of the variability in PCR testing, those changes should be confirmed within 1 month. Patients who have 100 percent Ph chromosome–positive cells after 6 months of therapy have a minimal chance of achieving a MCyR or CCyR and may be offered allogeneic stem cell transplantation, if applicable.[417,496]

Achieving a cytogenetic response is associated with progression-free survival in patients treated with imatinib and is an important goal of therapy (97 percent in those with a CCyR vs. 81 percent in those without a MCyR).[497] At 5 years of followup, of those patients who achieved CCyR on imatinib in the IRIS study, only 3 percent had progressed to accelerated or blast phase during treatment.[428] A CCyR at 1 year may be the major predictor for overall survival and progression-free survival.[498] In patients in chronic phase treated with imatinib, nilotinib, or dasatinib, early responses (at 3 months) in *BCR-ABL1* transcript reduction or decrease of Ph chromosome frequency predicted for better outcomes as measured by event-free or overall survival. For example, patients with less than 10 percent *BCR-ABL1*

TABLE 89–4. Guidelines for Monitoring of Patients in Chronic Phase Who are Undergoing Tyrosine Kinase Inhibitor Therapy

1. At diagnosis, before starting therapy, obtain Giemsa-banding cytogenetics and measure *BCR-ABL1* transcript numbers by qPCR using marrow cells. If marrow cannot be obtained, use FISH on a blood specimen to confirm the diagnosis.

2. At 3, 6, 9, and 12 months after initiating therapy, measure qPCR for *BCR-ABL1* transcripts. (If qPCR using the International Standard is not available, perform marrow cytogenetics.) If there is a rising level of *BCR-ABL1* transcript or 1 log increase after MMR achieved, qPCR should be repeated in 1 to 3 months.

3. At 12 months obtain marrow cytogenetics for cells with Ph chromosome if no CCyR or MMR.

4. Once CCyR is obtained, monitor qPCR on blood cells every 3 months for 3 years and then every 4 to 6 months, thereafter. If there is a rising level of *BCR/ABL1* transcripts (1 log increase after MMR achieved), repeat quantitative PCR in 1 to 2 months for confirmation.

5. These guidelines presume continued response to a TKI until CCyR achieved. If this does not occur see text for approach.

6. Mutation analysis should be performed with loss of chronic phase, loss of any previous level of response, inadequate initial response (*BCR/ABL1* transcripts >10%) at 3 or 6 months or no CCyR at 12 or 18 months, and a 1-log increase in BCR/ABL after MMR once achieved.

CCyR, complete cytogenetic response; CP, chronic phase; FISH, fluorescence *in situ* hybridization; MMR, major molecular response; Ph, Philadelphia; qPCR, quantitative polymerase chain reaction; TKI, tyrosine kinase inhibitor.

Data from http://www.nccn.org/professionals/physicians_gls/PDF/cml.pdf.

TABLE 89–5. Milestones for Assessing Response to Tyrosine Kinase Inhibitors[417,495]

Time of Observation (months)	Disease Response		
	Unsatisfactory	Suboptimal Response/ Warning	Optimal Response
3	No CHR and/or Ph+ >95%	*BCR/ABL1* >10% and/or Ph+ 36–95%	*BCR/ABL1* ≤10% and/or MCyR
6	*BCR/ABL1* >10% and/or no MCyR	*BCR–ABL1* 1–10% and/or MCyR	*BCR/ABL1* <1% and/or CCyR
12	*BCR/ABL1* >1% and/or no CCyR	*BCR–ABL1* <0.1–1%	*BCR/ABL1* <0.1%
18	No CCyR	CCyR if no MMR	CCyR or MMR

CHR, complete hematologic response; CCyR, complete cytogenetic response; MCyR, major cytogenetic response; MMR, major molecular response.

Response is defined in Table 89–3. These data were derived from studies with imatinib but are applicable to therapy with any tyrosine kinase inhibitor (TKI) as initial therapy in chronic phase. "Unsatisfactory" implies the need to consider change in treatment approach, as appropriate for that patient. Usually this change is an increase in the dose of imatinib, a shift to an alternative TKI, or allogeneic hematopoietic stem cell transplantation, if eligible. These guidelines are approximate in that a patient showing continued response to a TKI can be continued on that therapy until a response plateau has been reached, at which time the response can be evaluated using the milestones described. The suboptimal category indicates at least closer monitoring is recommended. See text for further details.

transcripts at 3 months had a 3-year event-free survival of 95 percent or greater, whereas those with greater than 10 percent transcript level at 3 months had a 61 percent event-free survival.[499]

Molecular response is determined by the decrease in *BCR-ABL1* mRNA by PCR. This is the only means to measure the depth of the response once a CCyR is attained. The achievement of MMR after treatment with imatinib is associated with durable long-term CCyR and a lower rate of disease progression. Only 5 percent of patients achieving a MMR with imatinib lost a CCyR compared to 37 percent who did not achieve that degree of response.[500] Also, the 5-year followup of the IRIS trial showed that no patient with a CCyR and MMR at 12 months had progressed to a more advanced phase of the disease.[497] The IRIS study 7-year followup also showed that in those with a MMR at that point in time, progression was rare. The estimated event-free survival was 95 percent for those with MMR at 18 months compared with 86 percent in those without a MMR.[501] To date, there is no evidence that a change of therapy would improve survival in those with CCyR but not a MMR. In those with stable CCyR after treatment with a second-generation TKI, achievement of MMR may not have significance as a predictor of survival.[499]

The time taken to achieve MMR is also thought to have prognostic significance. In the IRIS study, the chance of disease progression was higher in those who failed to achieve a 1-log reduction in *BCR/ABL1* transcripts by 3 months or a 2-log reduction by 6 months.[502] A *BCR-ABL1* transcript level greater than 10 percent after 3 months is a significant predictor for long-term outcomes.[503] In another analysis, chronic phase patients treated with imatinib 400 mg/day who had

BCR-ABL1 transcripts of 9.84 percent or less at 3 months had better overall, progression-free, and event-free survival at 8 years than did those with values of 9.84 percent or greater.[503] Also, there is evidence that early molecular response to initial therapy with dasatinib or nilotinib in patients with CML is a predictor of overall response. In one trial with dasatinib, patients with *BCR-ABL1* transcripts of 10 percent or less at 3 months had significantly better 5-year progression-free (92 vs. 67 percent) and 4-year overall survival than did those with greater than 10 percent transcripts (95 vs. 83 percent).[504] In another study with nilotinib, patients with *BCR-ABL1* of 10 percent or less at 3 months also had improved 4-year progression-free survival compared to those with *BCR-ABL1* greater than 10 percent at 3 months (95 vs. 85 percent).[505] Progression was defined as transformation to accelerated or blast phase.

Rising *BCR-ABL1* Transcript Levels Rising *BCR-ABL1* transcripts can indicate a new mutation or cytogenetic relapse. A significant change has been defined as either a twofold increase, serially increasing levels, or a 1-log increase.[492,495] There are no current recommendations for therapy changes based on an increase in *BCR-ABL1* transcripts. Serial increases or increases of 1-log or more should trigger *ABL* mutational analysis and frequent monitoring of *BCR-ABL1* transcripts.

Suboptimal Therapeutic Responses The initial European Leukemia Network guidelines defined suboptimal response as no cytogenetic response at 3 months, less than a partial cytogenetic response (PCyR) at 6 months, a PCyR at 12 months, and less than a MMR at 18 months.[495,506] The significance of a suboptimal response is dependent on the cause; for example, this may be insignificant if the result of drug intolerance or noncompliance as opposed to drug resistance (see

"Acquired Resistance" below). The significance also depends on time of suboptimal response with earlier time points indicating a worse prognosis. Currently, CCyR and PCyR at 3 months are considered optimal and suboptimal responses. Suboptimal responses are labeled as a "warning" response in the Network guidelines.[495] These response levels may trigger *ABL* mutation analysis or closer monitoring.

Secondary Chromosomal Changes with Tyrosine Kinase Inhibitors

Because of its earlier development, most of these data are obtained with imatinib treatment. Clonal abnormalities in cells lacking a detectable Ph chromosome or *BCR-ABL1* rearrangements have been detected in patients undergoing imatinib therapy who previously were treated with IFN-α.[507,508] These cytogenetic changes were noted in seven patients at a median of 13 months of imatinib therapy, and trisomy 8 was the most frequent abnormality. All of these patients had MCyRs to imatinib.[507] The presence of additional chromosomal abnormalities is considered to be a feature of the accelerated phase of CML. In some patients, clonal evolution may be related to imatinib resistance.[509] Clonal abnormalities may be present in up to 10 percent of patients taking imatinib.[510] Some of these cases may be associated with a MDS, especially in those patients with previous exposure to cytarabine and idarubicin. The antiproliferative effect of imatinib allows restoration of polyclonal hematopoiesis in CCyR, which could permit the manifestation of a Ph chromosome–negative disorder.[511] Some investigators have found that, with the possible exception of +8, +Ph, and i(17), additional chromosomal abnormalities at diagnosis are not associated with an inferior outcome to imatinib therapy.[512,513] In contrast, another group found that development of trisomy 8 in patients taking imatinib, while associated with pancytopenia, did not result in signs of disease progression. In a series of 34 CML patients who developed Ph chromosome–negative clones while taking imatinib, the most common abnormalities were trisomy 8 and monosomy 7. In 11 of these patients, no archival evidence of these clones was present before imatinib therapy was initiated, and none of the patients developed myelodysplasia.[514] In patients treated at diagnosis with imatinib, 9 percent developed chromosomal abnormalities in Ph chromosome-negative metaphases. These appeared at a median of 18 months, and the most common abnormalities were −Y and +8. Most were temporary and disappeared within 5 months. Only one patient with −7 progressed to acute myelogenous leukemia (AML).[515] Cytogenetic clonal evolution may not be an important impediment to achieving a MCyR or CCyR with imatinib, but it is an independent poor prognostic factor for survival of patients in chronic and accelerated phases of CML.[516] Imatinib therapy may overcome the poor prognostic significance of derivative chromosome 9 in CML.[517]

Adherence to Tyrosine Kinase Inhibitor Therapy

Noncompliance with therapy is associated with poorer outcomes. In one trial, patients with a suboptimal response had higher nonadherence (23 percent) than did those with optimal responses (7 percent).[518] In another study, adherence was the only independent predictor for achieving a complete molecular response (CMR) on imatinib. Patients with an adherence rate of 85 percent or less had a greater chance of losing their CCyR at 2 years (27 percent) than did those with better adherence (1.5 percent). They, also, had a lower chance of remaining on imatinib.[519] Adherence has also been correlated with level of molecular response. In patients using a TKI for about 5 years, median adherence was 98 percent (range: 24 to 100 percent). If adherence was greater than 90 percent, there was a higher probability for a 3-log reduction in *BCR/ABL1* transcripts and a CMR. If adherence was less than 80 percent, no MMRs occurred.[520] The poor adherence to second-generation TKIs has not been studied for a sufficient duration to determine its impact.

Management of side effects is of importance in maintaining a high rate of adherence.

Development of Tyrosine Kinase Inhibitor Resistance

The development of resistance to imatinib is not surprising.[521,522] Its specificity and "snug fit" into the *ABL1*-kinase pocket provide the ideal circumstance for resistance.[523] Some cases demonstrate primary resistance to imatinib, and gene profiling has demonstrated differential expression of about 46 genes in responders compared to nonresponders.[524] Even in patients with CCyR, malignant progenitors at the LTC-IC stage persist. Chronic phase CML stem cells are resistant to imatinib and are genetically unstable.[525] These cells have a high level of *BCR-ABL1* transcription, and they are thought to express transporter proteins that result in abnormal imatinib flux.[526] Mathematical models suggest that imatinib rapidly eliminates leukemic progenitors, but does not deplete CML stem cells. Such models predict the probability of developing resistant mutations and can estimate the time that resistance will emerge.[527] Several potential mechanisms of resistance include *BCR-ABL1* amplification in the presence of imatinib, P-glycoprotein–mediated drug efflux, altered drug metabolism, acquisition of BCR-ABL1–independent signaling characteristics, and point mutations in the *ABL1* kinase domain that decrease imatinib binding. Each of these mechanisms of resistance may have clinical relevance.

Primary Resistance Primary resistance to imatinib is defined as lack of CHR at 6 months or failure to achieve any level of cytogenetic response at 6 months, a MCyR at 12 months, or a CCyR at 18 months. This may occur in 15 to 25 percent of patients. Primary resistance may often be the result of inadequate plasma concentration because of binding of the drug to proteins, such as albumin or α_1-acid glycoprotein. In an analysis of the IRIS study, plasma levels of imatinib following the first month of treatment proved to be a significant predictor for clinical response. Plasma levels are not available for clinical use, however, so these have minimal influence on treatment decisions when responses are not as expected. Only one gene, prostaglandin-endoperoxide synthase 1/cyclooxygenase1 (*PTGS1/COX1*) was found to differentiate primary imatinib resistance. Eleven genes were associated with secondary resistance after imatinib therapy in those without an *ABL1* kinase domain mutation.[528] Expression of the OCT-1, which mediates drug influx, is thought to be important for imatinib but not dasatinib effectiveness.[529,530] Many CML patients who have a suboptimal response to imatinib have low OCT-1 activity, but this can be overcome with higher doses of imatinib or use of dasatinib, which uptake is not dependent on OCT-1 expression.[530] OCT-1 expression is associated with MMR at 12 and 24 months, and it is a predictor of the long-term risk of resistance and of transformation in patients treated with imatinib.[531] CML CD34+ cells overexpress the drug transporter ABCG2, and imatinib, dasatinib, and nilotinib are substrates for ABCB1 and ABCG2. Overexpression of MDR1 has been associated with decreased intracellular concentration of imatinib.[532]

Acquired Resistance Acquired resistance is that which occurs after exposure to TKIs or other treatments. Amplified gene expression and increased BCR-ABL1 protein expression are often reported in resistant patients. Duplication of the Ph chromosome and isodicentric chromosomes are a possible mechanism of resistance to imatinib.[533,534]

Mutations in the *ABL1* kinase domain are a frequent mechanism of resistance. Kinase domain mutations were the only independent predictor for the loss of CCyR and progression when compared to those without a mutation.[535] Mutations in the *ABL1* kinase domain may predate imatinib treatment,[536] and several *BCR-ABL1* kinase domain mutants associated with imatinib resistance remain sensitive to the drug, suggesting a need for characterization before a resistant phenotype can be attributed to the given mutation.[537] The mutant clone does not always have a proliferative advantage.[538] Some of these mutations may lie outside the kinase domain, and more than 40 such mutations have been described. Screening early phase CML patients for mutations before the start of imatinib therapy is not cost-effective because of their low incidence, but in patients with evidence of an increase in CML cells while on imatinib, mutation searches are indicated.[539] *BCR-ABL1* kinase domain point mutations are rare in those who have had good cytogenetic responses to imatinib, and when detected in that setting, their presence does not always predict relapse.[540] Mutations in the *ABL1* portion of the *BCR-ABL1* oncogene are present in approximately 40 percent of patients who do not achieve a CHR or CCyR to imatinib. *ABL1* mutations were found in those patients with both primary and acquired resistance. Amino acid substitutions in seven residues accounted for 85 percent of all mutations associated with resistance.[541] The mutations most associated with resistance are Thr315ILe, Gly250Glu, Glu255Lys, and Thr253His substitutions. Few of the described mutations directly affect imatinib binding.[542] Mutations in the *ABL1*–ATP phosphate-binding loop (P-loop) are most closely associated with a poor prognosis,[543] and these P-loop mutations predict for disease progression. Overall survival is worse for P-loop and for T315I mutations, but not significantly different when other mutations are present.[544]

Ultra-deep sequencing approaches have shown that routine Sanger sequencing underestimates *BCR-ABL1* mutation in 55 percent of samples where the missed mutations had low abundance.[545] Mass spectrometry can detect a 0.05 to 0.5 percent level of mutations, as well.[546] For many mutations, the concentration that inhibits 50 percent (IC_{50}) of various TKIs and response have not been documented.[547]

Second-generation BCR-ABL1 inhibitors (see "Dasatinib and Nilotinib" below) are able to overcome imatinib-resistant mutants, with the exception of the T315I mutations (Table 89–6). Mutations F317L and V299L are resistant to dasatinib and mutations Y253H, E255K, and F359I are resistant to nilotinib. Ponatinib was active against T315I and against other BCR-ABL1 mutations resistant to dasatinib or nilotinib.[548] Ponatinib may be effective against individual *ABL1* point mutations but may not overcome some compound mutations, which are two or more mutations in the same BCR/ABL1 molecule. Some mutations may be polyclonal as well.[549] The T315I mutation results in steric hindrance, which precludes access of some TKIs to the ATP-binding pocket of the *ABL1 kinase* domain.[550] In a series of 27 patients with T315I mutation, survival was dependent on stage of disease, with many of the chronic phase patients described as having an indolent course.[551] In addition to ponatinib, agents such as IFN-α and homoharringtonine have also been proposed as therapy for those with the T315I mutation.[552]

In some cases of resistance associated with imatinib, other signal pathways independent of BCR-ABL1 may become important in cell proliferation.[553] These include heat shock protein (hsp) 70,[554] survivin,[555] LYN kinase,[556] SRC,[557] and GRB2, among others.[558]

Dose escalation, combination therapy, and treatment interruption have been proposed as means to overcome drug resistance.[559] Combination therapy from the outset[560] also has been proposed to prevent development of resistance. Treatment interruption to stop clonal selection of resistant cells has been proposed.[557] Gene-expression profiles may be useful to predict the clinical effectiveness of imatinib for CML treatment, thereby allowing individualized therapy from the outset.[560] In patients with relapse or resistance, alternative approaches include increasing the dose of imatinib or switching to dasatinib or nilotinib.[561] Allogeneic hematopoietic stem cell transplantation is not recommended unless patients have inadequate response or intolerance to multiple TKIs or have the T315I mutation. Mutational analysis is not recommended at diagnosis but is of help in selecting TKI therapy for patients with an inadequate initial response or loss of response to TKI therapy. Mutation type may dictate choice of the next TKI.[562]

Management of Resistance

Dose Escalation If the patient is on imatinib, 400 mg/day, dose escalation to 800 mg/day can be tried. This may be most efficacious in patients with cytogenetic relapse who had achieved a cytogenetic response with the initial dose of imatinib, but is not likely to benefit those who have not had a cytogenetic response with imatinib at 400 mg/day.

Second-Generation Tyrosine Kinase Inhibitor Therapy Several TKIs are approved for use in the case of imatinib resistance or intolerance. In general, outcome with each is comparable, so the choice of agent often depends on its side-effect profile or in some cases on mutation type (see Tables 89–2 and 89–6).[562]

The 3-month molecular response after initiation of a second TKI is also a predictor of overall and event-free survival for those patients in chronic phase when switched from imatinib to another TKI.[505] A *BCR-ABL1* level of 10 percent or less at 3 months is desirable. In patients treated with nilotinib after imatinib resistance or intolerance, the 4-year progression-free and overall survival was 85 and 95 percent, respectively, if *BCR-ABL1* transcripts were 10 percent or less as compared to 42 and 71 percent for those with *BCR-ABL1* transcripts greater than 10 percent at 3 months.[563]

Either dasatinib or nilotinib can be used in cases of imatinib resistance or intolerance. Dasatinib is 325-fold more potent than imatinib; and, as a dual inhibitor of SRC and ABL1 kinases, dasatinib is able to bind to *BCR-ABL1* with less-stringent conformational requirements.[564] In patients resistant to imatinib, dasatinib, 140 mg/day (70 mg q12h), resulted in a higher proportion of MCyR, CCyR, and MMR than did 800 mg/day (400 mg q12h) of imatinib. Treatment failure was decreased and progression-free survival was improved with dasatinib.[565] Unlike imatinib, dasatinib penetrates the blood–brain barrier.[566] In long-term followup of 670 patients with imatinib-resistant or intolerant CML, treated with various doses of dasatinib, 28 percent of patients remained on study treatment at 6 years. Survival was in the range of 76 to 83 percent and a MMR was achieved in 45 percent on a dose of 100 mg daily. Molecular and cytogenetic responses at 3 and 6 months were predictive of survival. For those with *BCR-ABL1* transcripts less than 10 percent at 3 months, progression-free survival was 68 percent, whereas it was only 26 percent for those with *BCR-ABL1* transcripts greater than 10 percent.[567] Nilotinib in a dose of 400 mg every 12 hours induced approximately 40 percent of patients who were resistant to or intolerant of imatinib into a MCyR, and approximately 30 percent into a CCyR. Nilotinib, 400 mg BID, is the recommended dose for those intolerant or resistant to imatinib.

Bosutinib and Ponatinib In addition to dasatinib and nilotinib, bosutinib and ponatinib, third-generation TKIs, are active against many of the imatinib-resistant *BCR-ABL1* kinase domain mutations and are

Mutation	Treatment Recommendation
T315I	Ponatinib or stem cell transplant
V299L, T315A, F317L/V/I/C	Consider nilotinib over dasatinib; bosutinib and ponatinib may be effective
F359V/C/I	Consider dasatinib rather than imatinib; bosutinib and ponatinib may be effective
Others	Any tyrosine kinase inhibitor not previously used or high-dose imatinib

TABLE 89–6. Prevalent *ABL1* Mutations Conferring Resistance to a Tyrosine Kinase Inhibitor

The reader is referred to the text, which includes references describing listings of known sensitivities of reported mutations.

effective treatment options for CML resistant to standard-dose imatinib. Both were FDA approved for this indication in 2012. Bosutinib is active with F317L, Y253H, and F359C/I/V mutations. Ponatinib is also effective against many mutations resistant to nilotinib or dasatinib and has activity in cases with a T315I mutation (see Table 89–6).

Bosutinib is a dual SRC-ABL1 TKI that resulted in a CCyR in 24 percent and CHR in 73 percent of patients who had used two prior TKIs.[568] All mutations except T315I were responsive. It is approved for chronic phase, accelerated phase, or blast phase in those resistant or intolerant to prior TKI therapy. The dose is 500 mg/day, orally, with food. Diarrhea, nausea, decreased platelet count, other gastrointestinal complaints, rash, and anemia were the most common adverse events, and most of these were of low-grade. Bosutinib is not yet approved for use as an initial agent in CML, as it did not demonstrate significant improvement in CCyR rates at 1 year compared to imatinib. It was, however, associated with higher 1-year MMR rates, faster time to response, and less disease progression.[491]

Ponatinib blocks native and mutated *BCR-ABL1* including the gatekeeper mutation T315I. In a phase I dose escalation study, pancreatitis, rash, and myelosuppression were major toxicities. In 12 patients with T315I mutations, 92 percent had a MCyR. In those with accelerated or blast phase, or Ph chromosome–positive ALL, 36 percent had a major hematologic response and 32 percent had a MCyRs. Arterial thrombotic events occurred, however.[548] Retrospective analyses of these incidents led to temporary withdrawal of this medication, which is now used primarily in cases of T315I mutation or failure of several other TKIs. If vascular occlusion occurs, therapy should be halted immediately.[569] Ponatinib has a black box warning for vascular occlusion, heart failure, and hepatotoxicity.

A third-line TKI should be considered in patients who have failed two prior generations of TKI therapy, but responses tend to be infrequent and are usually not durable, so clinical trials, other agents, or allogeneic hematopoietic stem cell transplantation should be considered. A prior CCyR on either imatinib or subsequent nilotinib or dasatinib therapy was the only predictor of a cytogenetic remission on a third-line therapy.[570]

Non–Tyrosine Kinase Inhibitor Therapies

Omacetaxine Omacetaxine (homoharringtonine) is a *Cephalotaxus* alkaloid that has activity against the T315I mutation. Omacetaxine was approved on the basis of a study that recruited patients who had already been on two or more TKIs. In those enrolled in chronic phase, 67 percent had a CHR; a MCyR or a CCyR was achieved in 22 and 4 percent, respectively. Median overall survival was 30 months.[570] In those with T315I mutations enrolled on a separate study, MMR was achieved in 17 percent of patients and the T315I clone was reduced in 61 percent of patients.[571] The most common side effects with this medication are cytopenias. This agent also has activity in accelerated phase CML, but little in blast phase. It was approved by the FDA in October 2012 for chronic and accelerated phase patients intolerant of other therapy or in cases not responding to two or more TKIs.

Several inhibitors of signal transduction mediators involved in the downstream effects of BCR-ABL have been proposed for use in imatinib-resistant CML. These inhibitors include the JAK2 inhibitor AG490,[572] SRC kinase inhibitors, mTOR (mammalian target of rapamycin) inhibitors, such as rapamycin,[573] the proteasome inhibitor bortezomib,[574,575] histone deacetylators,[576,577] PI3K or MEK (mitogen-activated kinase) inhibitors and inhibitors of the WNT/β-catenin pathway thought to be active in CML stem cells. Imatinib resistance often is associated with restored activation of the BCR-ABL1 signal transduction pathway, suggesting that BCR-ABL1 remains a valid target to overcome resistance in these cases.[578] *BCR-ABL1* point mutations isolated from patients with

imatinib-resistant CML are sensitive to inhibitors of the BCR-ABL1 chaperone hsp90, such as geldanamycin.[579] Many of these agents have not yet entered clinical trials, but some are in early phase trials, such as inhibitors of the hedgehog pathway, which is activated in CML but not normal hematopoietic stem cells.[580] Some are being used in conjunction with imatinib in resistant cases.

Combined Therapy Agents that have been proposed for use in combination to improve response rates or to overcome resistance to imatinib have included IFN-α, cytarabine, omacetaxine multiagent chemotherapy, arsenic trioxide, and decitabine, with some supporting *in vitro* data.[581–586] Combining imatinib with chemotherapeutic agents is more myelosuppressive, and final effects on response rates and survival have yet to be determined. This approach is rarely used in chronic phase CML, but is used in accelerated or blast phase or in Ph chromosome–positive acute lymphoblastic leukemia.[587]

Disease Prognosis and Monitoring During Tyrosine Kinase Inhibitor Therapy

Treatment failure should lead to alterations in therapeutic strategy.[588] For patients treated initially with imatinib, BCR-ABL1 expression in cytogenetic responders and nonresponders was similar. BCR-ABL1 expression became significantly different 3 months after treatment and became increasingly different between responders and nonresponders with continued therapy at 6, 9, and 12 months.[589]

One mode of monitoring patients undergoing TKI therapy is to measure blood counts at least once per month and to obtain marrow samples every 6 months until a complete cytogenetic remission is obtained.[590] Thereafter, marrow samples are obtained no more often than yearly to monitor for other clonal abnormalities. Quantitative RT-PCR is performed every 3 months on blood or marrow. A 1-log increase in the level of *BCR-ABL1* reactivity, confirmed on a repeat sample at least 1 month later, suggests a loss of response to treatment. In patients who do not have a CHR at 3 months, or a MCyR after 6 to 12 months, other therapeutic options are considered.[591] The molecular response after 2 to 3 months of therapy is a strong predictor of clinical and cytogenetic response.[592] Sequencing the *BCR-ABL1* kinase domain can reveal emergence of resistant clones and is useful if there is an insufficient initial response to imatinib or a second-generation TKI (see Table 89–5) or any sign of loss of response, such as relapse to Ph chromosome–positive status, a 1-log increase in BCR/ABL1 transcript ratio, or loss of a MMR.[417]

In patients receiving second-generation TKIs as second-line therapy, those who have no cytogenetic response at 3 to 6 months should be considered for allogeneic transplantation or switched to an alternative therapy in a clinical trial. After CCyR is attained, molecular monitoring is recommended every 3 months for 3 years and every 4 to 6 months thereafter.[492] After 12 months, those with a MCyR had a significant survival advantage over those with lesser responses.[593] Those with *BCR-ABL1* transcripts greater than 10 percent following initial imatinib treatment should be switched to dasatinib, nilotinib, or bosutinib. If this is not an option because of cost or availability, high-dose imatinib can be considered, but it also unlikely to have benefit for more than a few months. For those already on a second-generation TKI, a clinical trial or alternative TKI could be tried or patients may continue on the same TKI with very careful followup, as the impact of this benchmark on overall survival is not yet known.[492] The 6-month evaluation should identify patients with a poor outcome. For those who have MCyR or *BCR-ABL1* of less than 10 percent at 6 months, overall survival was 100 percent as compared to 79 percent for those with no response.[594] At 12 and 18 months, CCyR is the optimal response.[417] In those who have achieved CCyR, MMR may not be of prognostic significance.[595]

Rising BCR-ABL1 levels may be associated with an *ABL1* mutation or relapse of disease. Those with more than a twofold rise in BCR-ABL1 are more likely to have a mutation.[596] A serial rise in the BCR-ABL1 level may also indicate loss of response to therapy.[415]

OTHER AGENTS USED IN TREATMENT OF CHRONIC PHASE

Interferon-α

IFN-α, formerly the most effective agent, is rarely used in the treatment of CML. A CCyR with IFN-α was uncommon (13 percent), but 10-year survival rates in responders were approximately 70 percent.[597] CCyRs to IFN-α were stable and durable.[598] Approximately 50 percent of complete responders become long-term survivors. Common toxicities of IFN-α use include fatigue, low-grade fever, weight loss, liver function test abnormalities, hematologic changes, and neuropsychiatric symptoms. Overall survival is improved in imatinib-treated patients compared with patients treated with IFN-α or IFN-α plus cytarabine.[599] Nevertheless, among all patients who attained a major or CCyR at 12 months, the survival rate was comparable in either case. IFN-α has also been proposed as an immune stimulant to consolidate imatinib remissions because additive effects have been noted.[600,601] Conversely, those treated initially with INF-α who achieve a CCyR have an improved molecular response with imatinib.[602,603] Some patients intolerant to a TKI may be treated successfully with INF-α.

Use of Other Chemotherapeutic Agents in Chronic Phase

Hydroxyurea The major side effect of hydroxyurea is an extension of its pharmacologic effect, that is, reversible suppression of hematopoiesis, often with megaloblastic erythropoiesis. The median survival of patients with CML treated with hydroxyurea alone is approximately 5 years. Studies with high-dose hydroxyurea indicate that marrow metaphase cells in some patients lose the Ph chromosome either partially or completely after such therapy.[604] Hydroxyurea often is used for initial cytoreduction, but it has few other indications in the TKI era of CML therapeutics. Chronic use of hydroxyurea is associated with leg ulcers.[605]

Cytarabine IFN-α$_{2b}$ combined with cytarabine (20 mg/m² per day for 10 days per month) in the chronic phase was associated with a greater proportion of MCyRs at 12 months and with greater survival prolongation than was IFN alone.[606] Toxicities with these drug combinations were greater, and this combination has been replaced by TKI therapy and is rarely used.

Busulfan Once the mainstay of treatment for the chronic phase, busulfan usage now is rare.[607] It is used primarily as part of the preparative regimen for allografting or autografting. It may be used occasionally in older patients who do not tolerate TKIs.

Other Cytotoxic Agents Intensive multidrug regimens have been used in an attempt to eradicate the Ph chromosome–positive clone and, occasionally, have led to prolongation of remission or cure of the disease. This approach did not significantly increase population survival.[608]

Other Potential Therapeutic Agents in Chronic Phase Chronic Myelogenous Leukemia The farnesyltransferase inhibitors lonafarnib and tipifarnib have been combined with imatinib and have activity after imatinib failure.[609,610] The hypomethylation agent decitabine has activity in imatinib refractory CML. INNO-406, a dual BCR-ABL/LYN inhibitor, suppresses the growth of CML cells in the central nervous system.[611] MicroRNA approaches may eventually play a role in CML treatment,[612] and synthetic *BCR-ABL1* small interfering ribonucleic acid (siRNA) has been used in a patient with resistant CML, postallografting with inhibition of *BCR-ABL1* noted.[613] Ribozymes targeting *BCR-ABL1* mRNA have been used as CML treatment,[614,615] and these approaches probably will have the most utility for *in vitro* purging of CML marrow cells before autotransplantation.[616,617]

RADIOTHERAPY

Palliative splenic irradiation may be useful occasionally in subjects who have entered the accelerated or advanced chronic phase and are troubled with extreme splenomegaly with splenic pain, perisplenitis, and encroachment of the spleen on the gastrointestinal tract.[618] Splenic irradiation may palliate symptoms for a short time.[619] Spleen size associated with chronic phase disease usually is decreased with TKI therapy.

Palliative radiotherapy may be useful for extramedullary myeloid sarcomas, which may occur occasionally in bone or soft tissue during the late chronic or accelerated phase.

SPLENECTOMY

Splenectomy does not prolong the chronic phase of CML, delay the onset of the accelerated phase, enhance sensitivity to TKIs or chemotherapy, or prolong survival of patients.[620] In carefully selected patients with symptomatic thrombocytopenia unresponsive to therapy, mechanical discomfort, hypercatabolic symptoms, and portal hypertension, splenectomy may be useful. Postoperative morbidity from infection, thrombosis, or hemorrhage has been high, with mortality rates up to 10 percent reported.[621] Splenectomy performed before allografting has not been found to influence the severity of graft-versus-host disease (GVHD) or survival after allogeneic hematopoietic stem cell transplantation.[622]

TREATMENT OF CHRONIC PHASE CHRONIC MYELOGENOUS LEUKEMIA DURING PREGNANCY

Treatment of chronic phase CML during pregnancy is sometimes needed to prevent placental insufficiency from hyperleukocytosis. Imatinib may be teratogenic. Normal newborns have been delivered by patients who conceived and ingested imatinib during early pregnancy.[623–626] In 125 women exposed to imatinib during pregnancy, 50 percent delivered normal infants, and 25 percent underwent elective terminations, three of the latter following the identification of fetal abnormalities. Twelve other infants had abnormalities.[627] The majority of patients who discontinue imatinib during pregnancy lose their complete hematologic remission and their cytogenetic responses.[628] One fetal fatality during pregnancy as a result of a meningocele has been reported. Males treated with imatinib have fathered healthy infants.[629] Current recommendations are to practice contraception during treatment with any TKI, or, if pregnant, at the onset of the disease, to consider IFN treatment until delivery.[626,630] Imatinib does appear in breast milk.[631]

IFN can be used during pregnancy with minimum risk of teratogenicity. Eight patients treated with IFN from the first trimester have been described, and each of these pregnancies resulted in normal infants, except for one with mild neonatal thrombocytopenia. All infants had normal growth patterns.[632] Hydroxyurea may be useful during the second and third trimester but should be avoided in the first trimester.[626,633] Leukapheresis in the first trimester (or longer) also can be used to avoid fetal drug exposure early in pregnancy (see "Leukapheresis" above). It is important to use a TKI after delivery to achieve the best outcome. Further observation may show it to be safe later in pregnancy. Although controversial, stopping and later restarting TKI therapy may not result in as favorable an outcome of therapy as use of IFN or other approaches, initially.[626] If conception is desired, attaining a MMR before the TKI therapy is discontinued and a 3-month washout period are recommended.[415] The patient should be made aware of the risk for CML progression during the pregnancy.

DISCONTINUATION OF TYROSINE KINASE INHIBITOR THERAPY

Patients responding to TKI therapy are likely to maintain their response. TKIs are associated with a significant symptom burden, however,[634] and one-third have persistent moderate to severe symptoms. Persistent CMR is seen in only a minority of patients, and the vast majority of patients on TKIs have minimal residual disease even if their *BCR-ABL1* transcripts are undetectable, and this may lead to relapse if the drug is stopped. Thus, in the absence of a clinical trial, life-long therapy with a TKI is recommended.

Some patients in a CMR for 2 years or more have been able to discontinue imatinib without relapse.[635,636] Discontinuation of imatinib in 12 patients who had undetectable disease for at least 2 years resulted in six patients having a molecular relapse within 1 to 5 months (imatinib was reintroduced with a response) and six others remaining in CMR for a median of 18 months.[637] There are numerous anecdotes of patients relapsing when imatinib was stopped. In patients with intolerable side effects on imatinib, the dose may be reduced in some cases without the loss of a CMR.[638] In occasional patients in whom imatinib is stopped, a cytogenetic response of up to 15 months has persisted.[639–642] In a study of 100 patients with a CMR (>5-log reduction in *BCR/ABL1* transcripts) for at least 2 years who stopped imatinib, 69 patients had at least 12 months of followup. Of these, 39 percent were stable and 61 percent relapsed, most within the first 6 months. The outcome of stopping was better for those with a lower Sokal risk score at diagnosis.[636] In another study, 40 patients were evaluated, and treatment-free remission at 24 months was 47.1 percent for all patients and was higher if patients had prior IFN treatment.[635] Female sex and early molecular response predict stable undetectable *BCR-ABL1* transcripts in chronic phase CML, the criteria for early stopping.[643] In a series of 423 CML patients treated with imatinib, the rate of undetectable *BCR/ABL1* transcripts and stable MMR (4.5-log decrease) was 36.5 percent.[643] A model to analyze the risk of molecular relapse after cessation of TKIs has been developed.[644] Reports of discontinuations, reappearance of the clone, treatment with a second prolonged course of imatinib, discontinuation with retention of MMR at 32 months followup, and retention of CMR in 12.5 percent have been described.[645]

Discontinuation of nilotinib or dasatinib has not been reported in a significant series, and larger prospective studies will be needed to determine in which patients stopping treatment can be safely attempted. Because early, quiescent Ph chromosome–positive cells (CD34+Lin−) are insensitive to imatinib *in vitro*,[546] at present it is advisable to maintain treatment indefinitely until the criteria for cessation, if any, can be established in clinical trials. Intermittent imatinib dosing has been explored in selected elderly patients with CML without adverse impact on overall and progression-free survival.[647]

HIGH-DOSE CHEMOTHERAPY WITH AUTOLOGOUS STEM CELL INFUSION

Since the availability of imatinib, autografting in CML is rarely used.[648] Ph chromosome–negative stem cells are present in most patients with CML at the time of diagnosis. Techniques that use these cells to reconstitute hematopoiesis after high-dose therapy have been developed.[649] Ph chromosome–negative progenitors can be mobilized with G-CSF and collected from the blood of patients who have responded to prior treatment with a TKI.[650] Such cells also can be collected after recovery from chemotherapy regimens, such as after idarubicin and cytarabine,

followed by G-CSF stimulation.[649] G-CSF was used for at least 4 days while imatinib treatment was continued for stem cell mobilization in 58 patients with a CCyR. The cells were collected in two cytapheresis procedures in 74 percent of patients, and the cells of 84 percent of those cytapheresis products were negative for the Ph chromosome.[651]

In another series, stem cells were mobilized in 32 patients in complete cytogenetic remission after imatinib, with uninterrupted imatinib therapy in 50 percent of patients and with imatinib temporarily withheld in approximately 50 percent. Blood levels of *BCR-ABL1* transcripts were not changed by the use of G-CSF.[652] In yet another series, 13 of 15 patients were successfully mobilized with G-CSF while receiving imatinib, and 28 percent of stem cell harvests were negative for *BCR-ABL* mRNA. No change in blood *BCR-ABL1* transcript level was noted after stem cell mobilization as assessed by RT-PCR.[653] No series of patients autografted with cells mobilized while they were receiving imatinib have been reported.[654] Autografting might find a role in cases of imatinib resistance,[655] or to reduce the level of residual disease in cases without a molecular response.[656] Imatinib can be effective and safe in chronic phase CML patients who have previously undergone autografting,[657] although there is an increased frequency of hematologic toxicity.

ALLOGENEIC HEMATOPOIETIC STEM CELL TRANSPLANTATION

Until imatinib became available in 2001, allogeneic transplantation was used in most new patients with CML who were younger than 65 years of age and who had a suitable donor. The advent of imatinib treatment and the projected survival of patients with a complete cytogenetic remission has changed the indications for transplantation in CML.[658,659] There has been a marked reduction in number of transplants performed for CML worldwide and a decline in the proportion performed in first chronic phase.[660,661] Although no randomized trials of imatinib versus transplantation have been or are likely to be conducted, there is circumstantial evidence that survival is superior for populations of patients treated with drugs who have a CCyR as compared to transplantation.[662] Allografting continues to play a role in the treatment of patients, who are refractory or intolerant to serial TKIs, and remains the optimal therapy in those who progress to accelerated or blast crisis in the face of treatment with a series of TKIs.

Patients in the chronic phase of CML who are younger than approximately 70 years and who have an identical twin,[663] or a histocompatible sibling,[664,665] or access to a histocompatible unrelated donor,[666] can be transplanted after intensive therapy, usually with cyclophosphamide and fractionated total-body irradiation (TBI) or a combination of busulfan and cyclophosphamide. Busulfan can be administered as an intravenous preparation and as a single daily dose.[667] When targeted steady-state busulfan levels are used, a 3-year survival rate of 86 percent and a disease-free survival rate of 78 percent with no age effect is achieved.[668] With nonmyeloablative or "reduced-intensity" conditioning regimens, older patients and those with comorbidities can undergo successful allografting.[669] With the success of TKI therapy, allogeneic stem cell transplantation is no longer recommended as a treatment option in chronic phase CML responding to any sequence of TKIs.[670] Allogeneic transplant should be considered for patients with disease progression to accelerated or blast phase on TKI therapy. In these cases, TKIs to which the patient has not been previously exposed and for which they do not possess a resistant mutation can be used to bridge or prepare for the transplant.[671] Allogeneic transplant can be used in those rare patients who present with blast crisis and in those with T315I mutations who do not respond to ponatinib.[672,673] In those who do not respond to their first TKI exposure and are switched to a second TKI, transplantation in chronic phase would be indicated for those patients with *BCR-ABL1* transcripts greater than 10 percent or less than a PCyR at 3 and 6 months, minor or no cytogenetic response at 12 months, and only a PCyR at 18 months or cytogenetic relapse at 12 or 18 months.[417]

Myeloablative Allogeneic Transplants

Stem cell transplantation from HLA-compatible siblings results in engraftment and an actual or projected long-term survival in 45 to 85 percent of recipients.[674-676] In patients older than age 50 years, survival rates are slightly less at 5 years. The risk of CML relapse is approximately 20 percent, with a plateau of relapse at 5 to 7 years. Transplanted T lymphocytes, especially if activated by a (mild) GVHD, may be an important factor in preventing leukemic relapse. This phenomenon, referred to as *graft-versus-leukemia reaction*, is thought to suppress the leukemic process through T-cell–mediated cytotoxicity.[634] The relative benefit of marrow compared to mobilized blood stem cells as the source of the allograft has not been established.[677,678] Mobilized blood stem cells engraft more rapidly but may be associated with more chronic GVHD. The majority of survivors have no evidence of residual leukemia.[679]

For younger patients who do not have a histocompatible sibling, an unrelated donor or a mismatched family member as a source of stem cells is feasible. When class I HLA genes are typed with molecular methods, an improvement in matching and better outcomes using unrelated donors have been demonstrated and are comparable to those transplanted with a matched-sibling donor. When matched-unrelated donor and sibling donor transplants were compared, unrelated donor transplants had increased risk of graft failure and acute GVHD, but only a slightly poorer survival and disease-free survival. For patients who survived to 1 year, only a slightly inferior disease-free survival was observed.[680] The rate of extensive chronic GVHD is up to 60 percent with unrelated donor transplants, but 63 percent disease-free survival in younger CML chronic phase patients has been reported. Cord blood stem cell transplantation from an unrelated donor has also been used in adults with CML.[681]

Pretransplantation imatinib is not associated with increased transplant-related morbidity or decreased survival, but those who are transplanted with suboptimal response to imatinib or loss of response to imatinib fare worse, probably related to a higher disease burden at the time of transplantation and more aggressive disease.[682,683] Second-generation TKIs do not increase transplant-related toxicity.[684] Disease status after allografting can be monitored with cytogenetic studies, PCR, or FISH analysis. A positive PCR assay 3 months after allogeneic transplantation has not been found to correlate with an increased risk of relapse compared with PCR-negative patients. A positive assay at 6 months and beyond is associated with subsequent relapse. In one series, 42 percent of patients with a positive PCR assay at 6 to 12 months relapsed versus 3 percent with a negative assay.[685] Paradoxically, patients who remain *BCR-ABL1* positive more than 36 months after transplantation have little propensity for relapse.[685] Serial quantitative RT-PCR analysis of blood specimens has been proposed to distinguish patients destined to relapse.[686] Patients who remain in remission have undetectable, low, or falling *BCR-ABL1* levels on sequential analysis. After 6 to 9 months, these levels are undetectable in most cases. Recognition of relapse at the molecular level may allow for early therapeutic intervention.

Killer immunoglobulin-like receptors (KIRs) are expressed by NK cells and subpopulations of T cells. NK clones from a single individual can vary substantially in the type of KIR molecules they express. The ligands for several of the inhibitory KIR have been shown to be subsets of HLA class I molecules. Missing KIR ligands in recipients lead to less relapse and increased GVHD based on NK alloreactivity.[687] KIR ligand mismatch has also been found to be an important prognostic factor in achieving molecular responses after transplantation for CML.[688] Increased frequency of regulatory T cells characterized as CD4+,

CD25-high are associated with higher rates of relapse after allografting in CML.[689]

Nonmyeloablative Allogeneic Transplants

Nonablative regimens have been developed in an attempt to expand the indication for allogeneic transplantation to older patients. These regimens rely on immunosuppressive therapy to allow engraftment of cells that potentially will generate a graft-versus-leukemia effect. These procedures in general are associated with acceptable degrees of engraftment, less mortality, similar rates of GVHD, and possible durable effects on persistent or recurrent disease.[690] Approximately 60 percent of patients, mostly in initial chronic phase (median age: 50 years) and transplanted with reduced-intensity conditioning regimens, had a 3-year survival and about one-third had a 3-year progression-free survival.[691] Patients no longer in first chronic phase do not fare as well.[712] Conditioning regimens include fludarabine and busulfan,[693,694] low-dose TBI and fludarabine, and low-dose TBI and cyclophosphamide, but no prospective randomized trials comparing regimens or comparing ablative and nonmyeloablative transplant approaches have been conducted.[693,695,696] In one case, imatinib given concurrently with nonmyeloablative stem cell transplantation did not compromise engraftment and resulted in a cytogenetic remission in a patient with CML in blast crisis.[697] Whereas nonmyeloablative or reduced intensity regimens are still considered investigational, they can achieve molecular remissions.

USE OF TYROSINE KINASE INHIBITORS AFTER STEM CELL TRANSPLANT

In patients treated with stem cell transplantation before the wide availability of imatinib, complete cytogenetic remissions with imatinib treatment can occur if treated at relapse after allografting and after donor lymphocyte infusion (DLI) fails to give a response. Such remissions may include a molecular response.[698] Complete responses after imatinib therapy have been noted in accelerated or blast phase CML persisting after stem cell transplantation.[699] In another series, 45 percent of relapsed patients had a CCyR of up to 28 months and without significant GVHD.[700] In a series of 28 adults with relapse after allogeneic stem cell transplantation who then received imatinib, the response rate was 74 percent, and the complete cytogenetic remission rate was 35 percent. Five patients had recurrence of GVHD, and 13 had received previous DLI infusions.[698] In one series, imatinib was able to generate complete molecular remissions in 26 percent of chronic phase patients after allografting, with full donor chimerism usually observed.[701] One study found that more relapsed patients had a molecular remission with DLI at 5 years than with imatinib alone. Most of these patients had cytogenetic relapses only.[702] In a retrospective comparison of 37 patients with hematologic or molecular relapse of CML who received imatinib, DLI, or a combination of both in concurrent or sequential regimens, the overall survival was 100, 89, and 54 percent for both modalities, imatinib, alone, and DLI alone, respectively.[703] There are few studies examining use of nilotinib or dasatinib for posttransplantation relapses.[704]

Prophylactic administration of imatinib after transplantation has been used for patients at high risk of relapse.[705] Posttransplantation imatinib may also postpone the requirement for DLI with its attendant risks of GVHD and marrow aplasia.[706] Some have found that DLI are superior to imatinib therapy in preventing relapse and increasing leukemia-free survival. Posttransplantation imatinib is usually well-tolerated; pancytopenia is the principal toxicity. The cytopenias resolve with doses adjustments or temporary drug discontinuation. Many questions remain regarding the use of posttransplantation TKIs. When should they be started? Which drug is superior? For how long should the drugs be used? Should they only be started in cases of molecular relapse? How can they be best combined with DLI in cases of relapse?

IMMUNOTHERAPY: ADOPTIVE CELL THERAPY FOR POSTTRANSPLANTATION RELAPSE

Substantial evidence indicates that the effectiveness of allografting in CML does not result solely from the eradication of the leukemic clone with high-dose chemoradiotherapy conditioning regimens, but also from adoptive immunotherapy provided by lymphocytes in the allograft, the graft-versus-leukemia effect (see "Myeloablative Allogeneic Transplants" above).[707] This phenomenon has been recreated to produce a therapeutic response by infusing the lymphocytes from the stem cell donor after a relapse following allogeneic stem cell transplantation.[708,709] The overall response rate to DLI is approximately 75 percent. The response rate is higher when this approach is used early after detecting a relapse by PCR,[710] compared to use after a hematologic or cytogenetic relapse. Patients with a short interval between transplantation and DLI have a higher probability of response than patients with longer intervals. Responses are the same with related versus unrelated donors.[711] Some patients show a very rapid decline of *BCR-ABL1* transcript levels (<6 months after DLI), whereas other patients demonstrate PCR negativity only over a longer period.[712] The responses to DLI can be durable.[713] Molecular responses can occur in up to two-thirds of patients.[714]

The main toxicities of DLI have been the induction of GVHD and myelosuppression. Chronic GVHD can occur in up to 60 percent of cases.[715] Attempts to diminish these toxicities have included use of CD8-depleted DLIs and infusion of smaller numbers of T cells.[716,717] Lower initial cell dose is associated with less myelosuppression, the same response rate, better survival, and less DLI-related mortality, leading to suggestions that the initial dose should not exceed 0.2×10^8 mononuclear cells/kg.[718] The initial doses should be lower when matched unrelated donors are used. Immune suppression should first be tapered before DLIs are administered. As noted above, imatinib may synergize with DLI to foster rapid molecular responses after relapse.[719]

● COURSE AND PROGNOSIS

Imatinib was first used experimentally for CML treatment in June 1998. Although it has completely altered the treatment approach to CML, its use has raised several questions. Studies require long-term followup of survival, but the degree of cytogenetic response, and degree of molecular response can be used as surrogate end points. The durability of cytogenetic and molecular responses in the face of persistent minimal residual disease during imatinib therapy require longer followup of larger numbers of patients, as more than 95 percent of cases have molecular evidence of disease at 2 years.

With the advent of TKI treatment, median survival in chronic phase CML is estimated to be 25 to 30 years. The prevalence of CML in the TKI era is estimated to reach a plateau 35 times the annual incidence with plateau estimated to occur in 2050. Therefore, the prevalence of CML is predicted to increase by a factor of 10.[720] Using the Swedish Cancer Registry over a 36-year period, relative survival rates compared with the total population for CML improved from 0.21 in 1973 to 1979 to 0.80 for 2001 to 2008; imatinib was introduced in Sweden in 2001.[721] Another study from the Swedish CML registry of 779 patients showed that the mean survival ratio at 5 years was close to 1.0 for those younger than 60 years old and 0.9 for those 60 to 80 years old. Only 3 percent had progressed to accelerated or blast phase at 12 months.[722] Resistance rates decline with each passing year, and adverse effects have not emerged over time.[723] Those who require 1 year or more of imatinib therapy to attain a complete cytogenetic remission have comparable rates of

TABLE 89–7. Chronic Myelogenous Leukemia: 5-Year Period Relative Survival Rates (2004–2012) by Age at Diagnosis

Age (years)	Percent of Patients*
<45	86
45–54	82
55–64	70
65–74	51
<75	27

*Percent rounded to nearest whole number.

Data from Surveillance, Epidemiology, End Results Cancer Statistics: *5-Year Survival Rates, Table 13.6, All Races and Sexes.* National Cancer Institute, Washington, DC. Available at http://www.seer.cancer.gov.

molecular response, progression-free, and overall survival to those who achieve a cytogenetic remission sooner.[724] In patients with failure to respond or intolerance to imatinib the estimated 3-year survival rate was approximately 70 percent for patients in chronic phase. Survival in chronic phase was better when subsequent therapy was nilotinib or dasatinib as compared to allogeneic hematopoietic stem cell transplantation or to others agents. This result was at a median followup of 2 years.[725] Older patients have lower response rates when treated in late chronic phase, but if they attain a CCyR, no difference was found in the level of molecular response.[724] Table 89–7 shows the most recent 5-year relative survival data by age at diagnosis in the United States.

The introduction of imatinib has minimized the impact of prognostic factors at diagnosis of chronic phase CML.[726] Several prognostic scales have been proposed in CML, including the Sokal and Hasford systems for patients at the time of diagnosis (Table 89–8). The European Bone Marrow Transplantation Consortium Risk Score was introduced

TABLE 89–8. The Variables Used to Calculate the Risk Group (High, Intermediate, Low) at Diagnosis in Patients with Chronic Phase Chronic Myelogenous Leukemia to Estimate Prognosis

The Sokal score, which is a hazard ratio, is calculated using the following formula based on age, spleen size, platelet count, and blood percent blast cells: exp (0.0116 × (age [years]–43.4)) + (0.0345 × (spleen size [cm] – 7.51) + (0.188 × ((platelets [10^9/L]/700)^2 – 0.563)) + (0.0887 × (blasts [%] – 2.10)). There are three risk groups: low-risk (Sokal score <0.8), intermediate-risk (Sokal score 0.8–1.2), and high-risk (Sokal score >1.2).

The Hasford score (or Euro score) is calculated using the following formula based on the four Sokal variables plus percent eosinophils and basophils in the blood: (0.6666 × age [0 when age <50 years; 1 otherwise]) + (0.0420 × spleen size [cm]) + (0.0584 × blasts [%]) + (0.0413 × eosinophils [%]) + (0.2039 × basophils [0 when basophils <3%; 1 otherwise]) + (1.0956 × platelet count [0 when platelets <1500 × 10^9/L; 1 otherwise]) × 1000). Three risk groups are: low-risk (score ≤780, 40.6% of patients), intermediate-risk (score 781–1480, 44.7% of patients), and high-risk (score ≥1481, 14.6% of patients).

These scores may be calculated electronically by insertion of the individual variables, such as age, spleen size, blood blast percentage, etc. at the following website. http://bloodref.com/myeloid/cml/sokal-hasford.

for patients undergoing allogeneic hematopoietic stem cell transplantation,[727] in which performance status is added to five variables (age, spleen size, blood blast cell count, basophil and eosinophil count, and platelet count [Hasford score]), and has been validated with good discrimination for survival.[728] The Sokal score based on age, spleen size, platelet count, and percent blasts was developed much earlier during the busulfan era of treatment and was less accurate in patients treated with IFN. The European Treatment and Outcome Study (EUTOS) score uses basophils and spleen size but has not been well-validated. A simple prognostic scale that includes donor type, stage of disease at time of transplantation, age of recipient, sex of donor and recipient, and interval between diagnosis and transplantation has been proposed to predict outcome of allogeneic hematopoietic stem cell transplantation.[729] These prognostic scales require revalidation given the dramatic impact of conversion to TKI therapy. There is evidence that a patient with chronic phase CML and a favorable Sokal Score at the time of diagnosis has a higher proportion of CHR and CCyR than other patients.[730] Cytogenetic response and molecular response as a surrogate marker for survival is useful in patients undergoing TKI therapy.[731] The score of a patient may be calculated, easily, using an online website (Table 89–8). Studies suggest that in certain healthcare systems, healthcare setting may influence survival time, especially for those in advanced phases of the disease.[732]

Outcomes after allogenic hematopoietic stem cell transplantation have also improved in the imatinib era, but those in chronic phase have better 3-year survival rates than those in advanced phases (91 percent vs. 59 percent, respectively).[733] There is favorable long-term survival after 5 years free of relapse after allogeneic hematopoietic stem cell transplantation.[734] Prognostic factors in the TKI era for allogeneic transplantation are also being defined, and in addition to disease phase, donor-match, age, sex, and calculated comorbidity indices are of importance.[735]

DETECTION OF MINIMAL RESIDUAL DISEASE

Detection of minimal residual disease by molecular probes makes possible the identification of approximately one cell in 1,000,000 that is derived from the CML clone.[736] Techniques used to monitor residual disease have been reviewed.[737,738] PCR permits observation of regression or persistence of subclinical disease following therapy and of progression of subclinical disease prior to the disease becoming overt, and it is therefore critical for monitoring responses to CML treatment.[739,740] The stable persistence of subclinical disease does not invariably predict early relapse.[741,742]

Efforts are underway to standardize the technique for measuring and reporting real-time RT-PCR,[743] and serial measurements are required for treatment decisions based on increases in transcript numbers.[744] Some studies show that marrow values tend to be higher than blood in real-time RT-PCR assays, but both follow a similar trend during treatment.[745] Interchanging these may lead to misinterpretation of disease status.[745] In patients on imatinib, who have MMR, confirmed by real-time quantitative PCR, no marrow cell cytogenetic abnormalities were found, indicating that patients with MMR do not require regular marrow examinations for cytogenetics. The International Standard uses baseline diagnosis levels in the IRIS study as 100 percent and fixes a 3-log reduction from a standardized baseline (MMR) at 0.1 percent. Widespread use of the International Standard will require laboratories to send in specimens for analysis,[743,746] but is a priority in order to ascertain response to therapy accurately and to be able to analyze responses among treatment centers.

Patients who achieve a MMR (expressed as a 3-log reduction from median baseline value) at the time of achieving a CCyR have been found to have longer cytogenetic remissions than those without this magnitude of molecular response.[749] The achievement of a 2-log molecular

response at the time of a CCyR or a 3-log response anytime thereafter is an independent prognostic marker of progression-free survival.[748] Other studies, however, show that patients who achieve CCyR do not derive additional benefit from a CMR.[749] The treatment response, to imatinib, nilotinib, or dasatinib showed the 3-year event-free survival was 95 percent for those with BCR-ABL1 transcripts of 1 percent or less at 3 months, 98 percent for greater than 1 percent to 10 percent, and 61 percent for greater than 10 percent. These 3-month responses translated into overall survival of 98, 96, and 92 percent, respectively.[750]

Interphase FISH is not standardized, but a large number of cells can be rapidly analyzed (100 to 500). Fixation, specimen preparation, and hybridization conditions may account for differing false-positive ranges and scoring criteria.[751] In CML patients treated with imatinib, FISH for BCR-ABL1 on interphase blood neutrophils, but not unselected white cells, correlates with marrow cytogenetics.[752] FISH and RT-PCR can be useful complementary techniques,[753] but FISH is generally not suitable for monitoring minimal residual disease.[754]

For patients who are undergoing allogeneic hematopoietic stem cell transplantation, the kinetics of minimal residual disease in either standard or nonmyeloablative transplants differ. BCR-ABL1/ABL1 ratios were 0.2 percent with reduced-intensity transplants versus 0.01 percent in transplantation patients with traditional conditioning regimens in the first 3 months. By 12 months, however, 20 percent of patients who received standard transplants and 50 percent of patients who received reduced-intensity transplants had reached a level less than 0.01 percent, supporting the concept of different kinetics of disease eradication between the two transplantation modalities.[755] Patients who relapse after allografting have reappearance and/or rising levels of BCR-ABL1 transcripts.[756] Use of quantitative RT-PCR early (3 to 5 months) after stem cell transplantation can project long-term outcomes.[757] When RT-PCR was negative, the 3-year risk of relapse was 16.7 percent; when RT-PCR was positive at a ratio of less than 0.02 percent, the relapse rate was 42.9 percent; and when RT-PCR was positive at a level greater than 0.02 percent, the relapse rate was 86.5 percent. Another group found that detection of blood BCR-ABL1 at 18 or more months after transplantation was associated with a highly significant risk of relapse and that patients who had a positive test result but failed to relapse generally had only one positive test result at a low copy number.[758] Performance of quantitative PCR (qPCR) at regular intervals after allogeneic transplant (every 2 to 4 months in the first year and every 6 months thereafter) is appropriate. If the PCR results are persistently positive or become positive, qPCR should be performed at monthly or shorter intervals. Molecular relapse is defined as a 10-fold increase of PCR positivity without any signs of cytogenetic relapse.[759] Detection of increasing recipient chimerism by FISH for the male chromosome in sex-mismatched donor–recipient pairs or variable number of tandem repeats after allogeneic transplantation or after DLI infusion also is usually associated with a relapse.[760]

In an imatinib-treated patient, the absence of BCR-ABL1 transcripts should not be interpreted as an absence of the leukemic clone.[761] In terms of response to second-generation TKIs, there was no difference in event-free survival and CCyR duration between patients with CCyR with and without MMR up to 18 months with followup at 3-month intervals.[762] One study examined 116 patients with durable cytogenetic responses on imatinib who had increased PCR levels on at least two occasions. Only 9 percent of those had CML progression. Ten patients had lost MMR or had never had it, and all of these had more than 1-log increase in qPCR.[763] With second-generation TKI, the BCR-ABL1 transcript levels at 3 months are also correlated with CCyR and MMR by 24 months, with levels less than 10 percent at 3 months being optimal.[764] The European Leukemia Net criteria for failure or suboptimal response may also identify CML in early chronic phase treated with imatinib where the eventual outcome will be poor. These landmarks at 3, 6, 12, and 18 months are associated with poorer overall survival and cytogenetic responses.[505] Only 60 percent of patients on the IRIS trial were in CCyR on imatinib after 6 years of therapy, indicating the need for close monitoring and for alternative therapies.[765] There is also evidence that the *BCR-ABL1* transcript doubling-time more reliably assesses CML relapse as compared to the fold rise in *BCR-ABL1* transcripts. A short doubling-time for a patient in chronic phase should raise suspicion of nonadherence.[766]

ACCELERATED PHASE AND BLAST CRISIS OF CHRONIC MYELOGENOUS LEUKEMIA

DEFINITION

In all patients with chronic phase CML, the disease has the potential to evolve into a more aggressive, more symptomatic, and troublesome phase, which is poorly responsive to the therapy that formerly controlled the chronic phase. The failure of therapy to restore or maintain near-normal red cell and white cell counts, increased spleen size, increased numbers of marrow blasts and blood basophils, loss of the sense of well-being, and appearance of extramedullary tumors are the most consistent clinical hallmarks of the metamorphosis of the chronic to the accelerated phase of CML. The most objective findings are a blood blast percentage greater than 10, a platelet count less than 100×10^9/L, blood basophils greater than 20 percent, and new clonal cytogenetic abnormalities accompanying the Ph chromosome.[767]

Several criteria have been published to define accelerated phase and blast crisis.[768–770] The terminology used has included *accelerated phase, acute phase, acute transformation*, or, in its most dramatic expression, *blast crisis*, but the metamorphosis, which can be acute, often is more gradual, hence the preference for *transformation* or *accelerated phase* to describe this transition from a controllable to a poorly controlled malignancy. Blast phase is the most severe manifestation of the accelerated phase and can occur abruptly or after a period of worsening disease. Blast crisis is in effect the evolution to overt acute leukemia, either myeloid or lymphoid.

PATHOGENESIS

Effect of Tyrosine Kinase Inhibitors in Rate of Progression

The advent of TKI therapy for CML has resulted in a marked increase in the duration of a subclinical chronic phase, with normal blood counts and spleen size, often with the loss of identifiable Ph chromosome-bearing cells in blood and marrow, and sometimes with the loss of laboratory evidence of the *BCR-ABL1* oncogene as judged by PCR. This therapeutic advance has greatly delayed the evolution to accelerated phase and blast crisis, but the risk for such a conversion exists since under experimental conditions CML stem cells do not undergo apoptosis when exposed to BCR-ABL1 TKIs and *BCR-ABL1*–positive cells return in virtually all patients if tyrosine kinase therapy is interrupted. There is evidence that genomic instability may derive from an imatinib-refractory CML stem cell.[771]

Blast Crisis Stem Cells

The onset of accelerated phase is thought to occur in a *BCR-ABL1*–bearing granulocyte-monocyte progenitor. Experimental[772,773] and theoretical[774] evidence supports this concept. This progenitor for clonal evolution also could explain the reversion to chronic phase in some patients in whom the suppression of the advanced phase of the disease is achieved.

Molecular and Genetic Alterations

The transformation of chronic phase CML to accelerated and then blast crisis or directly to blast crisis is thought to be the result of seven molecular processes: (1) maturation arrest, (2) failure of genome surveillance, (3) failure of adequate DNA repair, (4) development of a mutator phenotype, (5) telomere shortening, (6) loss of tumor-suppressor function, and (7) unknown factors.[775,776]

Progression of chronic phase to accelerated phase is marked by an increase in *BCR-ABL1* expression.[777,778] Superimposed on the increased transcription of mRNA[BCR-ABL1] are additional cytogenetic abnormalities that are added to the persistent Ph chromosome in approximately 50 to 65 percent of patients.[779–781] In lymphoid blast crisis, in which the blast cells have a lymphocytic phenotype, acquisition of mutations in tumor suppressor genes, such as p16/*ARF*, occurs in approximately 50 percent of cases, and *RB* gene mutations occurs in approximately 20 percent of cases. In myeloid blast crisis, in which blast cells have a myeloid phenotype, approximately 25 percent of cases have cells containing a p53 mutation.[782] The possible role of loss of p53 function in fostering transformation of a human chronic phase CML clone has been demonstrated in transgenic mice in which p53 function was abrogated.[783,784] Progression of the clone to a more malignant clone is reflected in a more disordered growth and maturation pattern of progenitor cells in culture, ultimately mimicking the growth failure of acute leukemia,[779] and in increased morphologic and functional abnormalities of blood cells,[785,786] eventuating in a block in maturation and replacement of blood and marrow by blast cells.

Approximately 65 percent of patients have cytogenetic abnormalities in addition to the Ph chromosome. A double Ph chromosome, trisomy 8, and isochromosome 17p are the secondary changes most commonly seen.[782,787] Because the frequency of trisomy 8 was greater after treatment with busulfan compared to hydroxyurea, the frequency of secondary chromosomal changes may be quite different after imatinib therapy.[782] Clonal instability has also been found in cases of lymphoid blast crisis. Clones distinct from those identified later may be detected before overt lymphoid transformation. Identification of these abortive clones suggests clonal instability before the onset of transformation, which might have prognostic value.[788] FISH has been used to determine which cells have secondary cytogenetic abnormalities, and these cells often are not the blast cells. This finding suggests that some chromosomal abnormalities merely denote genomic instability.[789] The abnormal mRNA and protein product p210[BCR-ABL1] are present in the marrow and blood cells of patients who have transformed to acute leukemia.[790–792]

Although the breakpoint site on M-*bcr* was thought to be correlated with the time of the onset of the accelerated phase,[793] subsequent studies have not indicated a correlation between length of chronic phase and the specific site of the *BCR-ABL1* fusion.[794] Rare cases have displayed deletion of the *BCR-ABL1* fusion gene, loss of transcription of the message, and loss of expression of the p210 tyrosine kinase after transformation, the latter finding indicating the abnormal protein kinase may not always play a unique role in sustaining the acute state.[795] In contrast, the frequent response, albeit temporary, to imatinib suggests that the *mutant BCR-ABL1* product usually plays a role at this stage of the disease.

Numerous molecular changes identified in the cells of patients with acute transformation that might contribute to the increased malignant behavior of the CML clone, include activation of the *N-RAS* gene,[796,797] rearrangement of the p53 gene,[797–800] hypermethylation of the calcitonin gene,[801] and methylation of the *ABL1* gene.[802] One report described p53 mutations in 17 percent of blast crisis patients. An association between the failure of CML cells to express the *RB1* gene product and acute blast crisis with a megakaryoblastic phenotype has been reported.[802] Homozygous deletions of the *p16* gene are associated with lymphoid transformation of CML,[804] but such deletions are not seen in the chronic phase and in myeloid blast crisis. p16 is also known as the *cyclin-dependent kinase 4 inhibitor gene* and is located on chromosome 9p21.[805,806] This gene inhibits the kinase CDK-4, which regulates a cell-cycle checkpoint prior to commitment to DNA synthesis. The Wilms tumor *(WT)* gene on chromosome 11p13 encodes a zinc finger motif-containing transcription factor found in CML patients only after progression to blast crisis.[807] Overexpression of the *EVI-1* gene has also been found in CML blast crisis.[808,809] Microsatellite instability has not been found to be involved with progression to blast crisis.[810] *BCL-2, c-MYC, RUNX1, IKZF1, ASXL1, WT1, TET2, IDH1, NRAS, KRAS, CBL,* and various other genes have also been implicated in the evolution of CML.[811–815]

Approximately 50 genes have been identified that could play a role in the progression to accelerated phase or blast crisis,[775] including genes identified by expression profiling that are dysregulated in accelerated phase compared to chronic phase.[816,817] These include the WNT-β-catenin and JunB pathways.

CLINICAL FEATURES

Signs and Symptoms

The features that might signal the conversion of the chronic to the accelerated phase include unexplained fever, bone pain, weakness, night sweats, weight loss, loss of sense of well-being, arthralgia, and left upper quadrant pain related to splenic enlargement or infarcts. These features may occur weeks in advance of laboratory evidence of the accelerated phase. Localized or diffuse lymphadenopathy or enlarging masses in extralymphatic and extramedullary sites containing *BCR-ABL1*–positive myeloblasts or lymphoblasts may develop. A poor response of blood cell counts and splenic enlargement despite previously effective therapy may be evident.[767,782,818–820] Symptoms caused by histamine excess in basophilic crisis can be present.[821]

Several of these changes may occur in series or in parallel. The time of onset of transformation and the appearance of a blast crisis and its clinical expression are unpredictable.

LABORATORY FEATURES

Blood Findings[782,818–820]

Anemia may worsen and be associated with increasing poikilocytosis, anisocytosis, and anisochromia. The number of nucleated red cells in the blood may increase. These red cell changes may be accentuated further if advancing marrow fibrosis is a feature of the disease.

The total leukocyte count may fall without treatment. The proportion of blasts increases to greater than 10 percent in blood and marrow in the accelerated phase and when blast crisis ensues represents 20 to 90 percent of the cells. The morphology of the blast cells may be lymphoid or myeloid. Myelocytes decrease in number. Hyposegmented neutrophils (Pelger-Huët cells) and other dysmorphic changes may become evident. Basophils increase and often represent 20 to 80 percent of the total blood leukocytes. A decrease of the platelet count to less than 100×10^9/L develops. Giant platelets, micromegakaryocytes, and megakaryocyte fragments may enter the blood. Decreased progenitor cell growth in culture is present, akin to that in acute leukemia.

Marrow Findings[782,818–820]

The marrow findings are widely variable. Marked dysmorphic changes in one, two, or three of the major cell lineages; an increase in blast count to greater than 10 percent; marrow morphology simulating subacute myelomonocytic leukemia; or, in the extreme, florid blastic transformation with blast counts greater than 30 percent can occur. Reticulin fibers may increase in prominence, and occasionally severe reticulin

and collagen fibrosis develop. Additional clonal cytogenetic abnormalities develop in as many as half the patients in accelerated phase (see "Cytogenetic Studies" below).

EXTRAMEDULLARY BLAST CRISIS

A variety of symptoms or signs may occur as a result of the specific effects of new extramedullary blastic tumors, referred to as *extramedullary blast crisis*.[821–824] Extramedullary blast crisis is the first manifestation of accelerated phase in approximately 10 percent of patients with CML. Lymph nodes,[822–824] serosal surfaces,[825,826] skin and soft tissue,[821–824] breast,[824,827] gastrointestinal or genitourinary tract,[822,824] bone,[822,824,824–831] and central nervous system[822,832–836] are among the principal areas involved. Isolated or diffuse lymphadenopathy may occur. Bone involvement may lead to severe pain, tenderness, and pathologic fracture, and may be evident on imaging of the involved area. Central nervous system involvement usually is meningeal and may be preceded by headache, vomiting, stupor, cranial nerve palsies, and papilledema and is associated with an increase in cells, protein, and the presence of blasts in the spinal fluid.[824,832–834]

Appropriate histochemical and immunologic tests are required to determine if the extramedullary disease is composed of phenotypic myeloblasts or lymphoblasts. Because the tumor cells may have features of lymphoma cells, the terms *myeloid* or *granulocytic sarcoma, chloroma,* and *myeloblastoma* can be misnomers, and the term *extramedullary blast crisis* is used for this circumstance in CML.[833,835–837] The lymphoblasts, like the myeloblasts, are Ph chromosome–positive. A combination of morphology, histochemistry (e.g., peroxidase, lysozyme), terminal deoxynucleotidyl transferase assay, and monoclonal antibodies specific for lymphoid or myeloid cells can be used to classify the extramedullary blast cells.

MARROW BLAST CRISIS

Approximately half of patients with CML enter the accelerated phase by developing acute leukemia. The onset of blast crisis can develop from days[838–840] to decades after diagnosis of CML. The signs and symptoms may include fever, hemorrhage, bone pain, and lymphadenopathy.[776,838–840] The morphology of the acute leukemia usually is myeloblastic or myelomonocytic.[776,841] A substantial proportion of myeloid leukemia in this setting may not have myeloperoxidase demonstrable by cytochemistry.[842] The proportion of cases classified as erythroblastic leukemia is approximately 10 percent, based on morphologic features,[843] but may be as high as 20 percent if expression of glycophorin-A is used as the determinant.[844] Occasional cases have megakaryoblastic transformation.[803,845] These cases may be difficult to identify by light microscopy because the megakaryoblasts may be mistaken for lymphoid cells or undifferentiated blasts. Myelofibrosis is a feature of this variant. Antiplatelet glycoprotein antibodies and other monoclonal antiplatelet antibodies now are available as reagents to identify megakaryoblasts without the need for ultrastructural studies.[845] Promyelocytic[846–848] and eosinophilic[849] blast crises also can occur. Basophilic leukemia is a known variant of CML.[850] Patients with promyelocytic crisis often have t(15;17) in addition to the Ph chromosome, and some have presented with disseminated intravascular coagulation.[851]

CML may transform into acute lymphoblastic leukemia in approximately 30 percent of blastic crisis cases.[767,852–856] The lymphoid cells generally express terminal deoxynucleotidyl transferase (TdT)[852,853] and are of the B-cell lineage,[856–878] as judged by antiimmunoglobulin staining. TdT is a DNA polymerase that adds deoxynucleoside monophosphates from triphosphate substrates to single-stranded DNA by end addition, differing in the latter respect from replicative polymerases.[859]

The enzyme is present in normal immature thymocytes and in the blast cells of nearly all patients with acute lymphoblastic leukemia. Rare patients have blasts with a T-lymphocyte phenotype.[835,836,860-862] Some cases are biphenotypic; the blasts have both lymphoid and myeloid markers.[841,863-865] Some cases may have myeloperoxidase activity in blast cells and express CD33 or CD13. Myeloid to lymphoid clonal succession following autologous transplantation in the second chronic phase has been described.[866] Patients with lymphoid blast crisis seldom have an intermediate accelerated phase, have less splenomegaly and basophilia, and usually have a higher degree of marrow blast infiltration. With non-TKI therapy, remission rate and survival were somewhat longer in cases of lymphoid than in myeloid blast crisis.[867]

CYTOGENETIC STUDIES

Most large studies have shown seven recurrent changes in patients' cells prior to, or during, the accelerated phase: trisomy 8 (33 percent of cases), additional 22q– (30 percent of cases), isochromosome 17 (20 percent of cases), trisomy 19 (12 percent of cases), loss of Y chromosome (8 percent of males), trisomy 21 (7 percent of cases), and monosomy 7 (5 percent of cases).[867-870] In addition, a large number of other chromosome abnormalities have been described.[871-875] In one study, 46 (63 percent) of 73 blast crisis patients had secondary cytogenetic abnormalities. These abnormalities were more common in myeloid blast crisis and were associated with shorter remission.[788] The changes may be features of myeloid blast crisis compared to lymphoid crisis.[869,874] Some abnormalities, such as inv16, are associated with early transformation to AML.[870,874-877] A significant proportion (50 percent) of patients in the accelerated phase or blast crisis have no additional cytogenetic abnormalities beyond t(9;22)(q34;q11) after banding and multicolor FISH analysis.[876] In cases where the blastic transformation is in extramedullary sites, such as lymph nodes or spleen, the additional cytogenetic abnormalities may be in the cells at those sites but not in cells in the blood or marrow.[878]

TREATMENT

Optimal treatment is allogeneic stem cell transplantation if the patient is eligible based upon patient's age and donor availability. The role of stem cell transplantation is also evolving as TKI use in these phases of diseases becomes better defined. Thus far, treatment with TKIs has improved survival only modestly in blast crisis, and most long-term survivors have been transplanted. At present, it is recommended that patients in blast crisis be treated with TKIs with or without chemotherapy to a second chronic phase and proceed to stem cell transplant as soon as possible once a donor is identified. One of the major goals of treatment of chronic phase CML is the prevention of evolution to accelerated or blast phases of the disease.

Tyrosine Kinase Inhibitors in Accelerated and Blast Crisis

The initial dose of imatinib in accelerated phase is 600 mg/day.[879] Imatinib, dasatinib 140 mg/day, and nilotinib 400 mg BID, bosutinib 500 mg daily, and ponatinib 45 mg/day have been used as bridging therapies to permit allogeneic stem cell transplantation in accelerated phase.[880] Dasatinib and nilotinib can achieve a better molecular response, and thus the role for and timing of transplantation in accelerated phase CML is being redefined. Imatinib can be combined with an anthracycline plus cytarabine for patients in myeloid blast crisis.[881] Imatinib has produced complete hematologic remissions in approximately 20 percent of patients.[882,883] However, CCyRs are uncommon. Central nervous system and other extramedullary blast crisis can occur during imatinib therapy for accelerated phase disease,[884,885] and all types of blast crisis,

including promyelocytic blast crisis,[886] can occur during imatinib therapy. Compared to historical controls in which various combinations of chemotherapy were utilized, imatinib used alone results in comparable outcomes (6-month median survival of patients in blast crisis).[887] Although dasatinib therapy can result in CCyRs in 29 percent of blast crisis CML, and nilotinib can result in CCyRs in 27 percent of myeloid blast crisis and in 43 percent of lymphoid blast crisis, these responses are rarely durable, so in a patient of appropriate age with an acceptable donor, transplantation options should be considered with the second-line TKIs used as a bridge to transplantation therapy.[888,889] The choice of TKI in accelerated phase is based on prior therapy and/or mutational status. If response to TKI therapy is inadequate in accelerated phase, allogeneic hematopoietic stem cell transplantation should be considered. In lymphoid or myeloid blast phase, allogeneic hematopoietic stem cell transplantation is recommended if there is a suitable donor.[417] Omacetaxine has shown activity in patients with disease progression to accelerated phase CML after prior TKI use.[890]

Chemotherapy

The treatment approach is predicated on the phenotype of the blast cells in CML patients with blast crisis and is rarely used in accelerated phase. In patients with myeloid phenotypes, the approach has been similar to that used for AML: combinations of an anthracycline antibiotic, such as idarubicin or daunorubicin, with cytosine arabinoside and sometimes etoposide.[891] Because this approach produces few remissions that are of short duration (median survival approximately 6 months), a variety of other drug combinations have been used, but with no significant improvement in outcome.[887] Complete hematologic response is observed in only a quarter to a third of patients with this approach.

In patients with lymphoid phenotypes, vincristine sulfate 1.4 mg/m^2 (not to exceed 2 mg/dose) given intravenously once per week and prednisone 60 mg/m^2 per day given orally are the mainstay of treatment. A minimum of two cycles of treatment (2 weeks) should be given to judge responsivity. Other more intense ALL-type regimens, such as Hyper-CVAD (cyclophosphamide, vincristine, doxorubicin, and dexamethasone),[892] have also been used. Approximately one-third of patients with lymphoid blast transformation reenter the chronic phase after such treatment. However, because only about one-third of patients have lymphoid blasts, this number represents a remission rate of only approximately 10 percent of patients who enter blast crisis using this approach. The benefit of intensive chemotherapy has been small because remission durations have been modest. TdT-positive, CD10 (CALLA)-positive lymphoblasts may be the lymphoblast phenotype most responsive to vincristine and prednisone.[855] mTOR inhibitors may be useful in lymphoid blast crisis.[897]

Use of Chemotherapy with Tyrosine Kinase Inhibitors in Accelerated Phase or Blast Crisis

Imatinib has been successfully combined with decitabine, low-dose cytarabine, and standard anthracycline plus cytarabine ("7 + 3") where complete remission can be as high as 75 percent. Median time to relapse and overall survival are brief, however.[815] Imatinib and dasatinib have been combined with HyperCVAD in lymphoid blast crisis.[892,893]

Allogeneic Hematopoietic Stem Cell Transplantation

Stem cell transplantation from an appropriately HLA-matched donor has been used in some patients after entry into the blastic crisis. Occasional patients have had long-term survival. The 3-year survival rate is approximately 15 to 20 percent,[894-896] unlike transplantation in the chronic phase, in which the 3-year survival rate is 50 to 60 percent. However, for patients who present in blast crisis, who develop blast crisis in the first year of the chronic phase, or who delay transplantation for other reasons, transplantation remains the best hope for long-term survival if a histocompatible donor is available.[832,833] Relapse of accelerated phase after allogeneic stem cell transplantation has responded to infusion of donor cytotoxic T lymphocytes.[897] The use of TKIs before allogeneic stem cell transplantation for patients in advanced phases of disease may favorably improve transplantation outcomes, especially when MCyR occurs before transplantation.[898]

Autologous Hematopoietic Stem Cell Transplantation

Autografting in the accelerated phase or blast crisis, either with stem cells collected during chronic phase or with mobilized Ph chromosome–negative progenitor cells collected upon cell rebound after intensive chemotherapy, has resulted in apparent prolonged remission in some patients, but this procedure is rarely used in advanced disease because of the high rate of relapse.[899] Whether Ph chromosome–negative cells collected during imatinib therapy have the same potential is unknown.

Splenectomy

Splenectomy may be performed for palliation of painful splenic infarctions or hemorrhage. However, the complication rates are high, and the procedure performed in this setting should be avoided if possible.[900]

COURSE AND PROGNOSIS

The accelerated phase of CML generally is very poorly responsive or refractory to treatment and is a morbid state that can be fatal in weeks to months in all but a few patients who undergo a successful stem cell transplant from a histocompatible donor. Patients with myeloid blast crisis have a median survival of approximately 6 months, whereas patients with lymphoid blast crisis have a median survival of approximately 12 months.[887–901] In the earliest study of imatinib in blast crisis, patients with myeloblastic crisis had a slightly longer median survival (approximately 5 months) than patients with lymphoid blast crisis plus Ph chromosome–positive ALL (3 months). The results are poor in either case. A worse survival was seen with abnormalities of chromosome 17, other superimposed translocations, or a high percentage of abnormal metaphases.[902] Severe cytopenias from repeated courses of cytotoxic therapy contribute to infections, hemorrhage, and organ dysfunction, especially liver and kidney dysfunction. Opportunistic infections with herpes viruses, cytomegalovirus, or fungi often supervene. The addition of imatinib or other TKI therapies has made only a small difference in long-term outcome, although formal studies of combinations of chemotherapy and imatinib at a higher dose (600 mg/day) have not been completed, and the results of trials with second-generation TKIs are anticipated.

● RELATED CLONAL MYELOID DISEASES WITHOUT THE BCR REARRANGEMENT

In addition to classic CML with the *BCR-ABL1* fusion gene, there are several other chronic myeloid leukemias which are listed in Table 89–9.

CHRONIC MYELOMONOCYTIC LEUKEMIA

This leukemia is part of the spectrum of clonal myeloid diseases that may have findings that simulate CML. In the past, when rigorous criteria for the diagnosis of CML were not applied, CMML was among a heterogenous group of related diseases that sometimes were referred to as *Ph chromosome–negative CML*. These diseases share the feature of originating in the clonal expansion of a primitive multipotential hematopoietic cell.[903]

Epidemiology

Most patients with CMML are older than age 50 years, the median age is approximately 72 years, and approximately 90 percent of patients are older than age 60 years at the time of diagnosis.[904] Occasional cases have been reported in older children and younger adults. Men are affected more frequently than women (approximately 2:1).[904–906] An evaluation of exogenous factors that might increase the incidence of CMML, did not find an association with benzene or other occupational or nonoccupational risk factors.[907]

The disease may occur following therapy for an unrelated malignancy, most commonly lymphoma, breast, or prostate cancer. The prior therapy was radiation, combined radiation and chemotherapy, or chemotherapy, alone. The median time of onset of CMML was 6 years.[908]

Clinical Findings

Signs and Symptoms The onset usually is insidious, and weakness, infection, or exaggerated bleeding may bring patients to medical attention.[905,906] Hepatomegaly and splenomegaly occur in approximately 50 percent of patients. Leukemia cutis occurs in a small proportion of patients and the skin cellular infiltrate is usually has a monocytic phenotype: CD45, CD68, and lysozyme positive by immunostaining. Immune manifestations, such as vasculitis, pyoderma gangrenosum, immune cytopenias, and connective tissue diseases, may occur in coincidence with CMML.[909]

Blood and Marrow Findings The disease is characterized by anemia and blood monocytosis greater than 1×10^9/L.[910] The white cell count may be decreased, normal, or moderately elevated. In one study of 275 patients, the range in 247 informative patients was 0.9 to 160×10^9/L.[904] Occasional patients, however, may have hyperleukocytosis with total white cell counts of 250 to 300×10^9/L associated with respiratory insufficiency resulting from pulmonary leukostasis.[911] Promonocytes and monocytes are present in blood and may have dysmorphic features. Immature granulocytes (promyelocytes and myelocytes) may be present in the blood. Blood myeloblasts are absent in approximately 75 percent of patients or, when present, usually do not exceed 10 percent of total white cells. Most patients have thrombocytopenia, but normal or elevated platelet counts may occur (range: 3.0 to 1385×10^9/L among 227 patients in one series).[904] Eosinophilia may be so prominent in occasional cases that the designation *chronic eosinophilic leukemia* may be appropriate.[905,906,912]

The marrow is hypercellular as a result of granulomonocytic hyperplasia; the dominant cells are early myelocytes. Blasts cells are 1 to 4 percent in about two-thirds of patients and are from 5 to 19 percent in one-third of cases.[904] The proportion of promyelocytes is increased. Promonocytes and monocytes also are increased in number. Distinction between poorly granulated myelocytes and promonocytes with primary granules can be difficult. Macronormoblasts and hypersegmented or hyposegmented, often bilobed (acquired Pelger-Huët anomaly), neutrophils may be evident but are more frequent in cases with lower white cell counts. Despite thrombocytopenia, megakaryocytes usually are present in the marrow. Microvessel density is increased in the marrow, and myelomonocytic cells contain cytoplasmic mRNA for VEGF and membrane VEGF receptors.[912,913] *In vitro* colony studies suggest that autocrine stimulation of cell growth by VEGF may occur. "Spontaneous" cluster/colony growth of granulocyte-monocyte colony-forming cells occurs *in vitro*. The spontaneous growth may result from autocrine or paracrine production of GM-CSF, based on anti–GM-CSF inhibition of colony growth.[914]

Cytogenetic and Genetic Findings Patients with CMML have an approximately 35 percent frequency of chromosomal abnormalities. Trisomy 8 and, to a lesser extent, monosomy 7 and –Y are the most prevalent findings. A low–risk karyotype is either a normal pattern or

TABLE 89–9. Types of Chronic Myelogenous Leukemia

Type of Chronic Myelogenous Leukemia	Molecular Genetics	Major Clinical Features	Further Details
BCR rearrangement-positive chronic myelogenous leukemia	>95% p210$^{BCR-ABL}$; <5% p190 or p230	Splenomegaly in 80% of cases; WBC >25 × 10⁹/L; blood blasts <5%; absolute basophilia in virtually all cases. Ph chromosome in 90% of cases; BCR gene rearrangement in 100% of cases	Pages 1437–1467
Chronic myelomonocytic leukemia	>40% mutation in SRSF2 gene and 90% have a mutation in 1 of 9 genes.[1032] Various cytogenetic abnormalities	Anemia, monocytosis >1.0 × 10⁹/L; blood blasts <10%; increased plasma and urine lysozyme; BCR rearrangement absent; rare cases with PDGFR-β mutation respond to imatinib	Page 1467
Chronic eosinophilic leukemia	Various cytogenetic abnormalities; PDGFR-α mutations in some cases.	Blood eosinophil count >1.5 × 10⁹/L; cardiac and neurologic manifestations common; a proportion of cases have PDGFR-α mutations and are responsive to imatinib mesylate	Page 1469
Chronic basophilic leukemia	Various cytogenetic abnormalities	Only 5 cases reported; hemoglobin 6–13 g/dL; basophilia of 3.4–41 × 10⁹/L; 2 of 5 cases with splenomegaly; very cellular marrow (>90%) in each case with mild increase in type III collagen, and megakaryocytic dysmorphia; increase in marrow mast cells in 3 of 5 cases	Page 1470
Juvenile myelomonocytic leukemia	RAS pathway mutations (PTPN11, NF1, NRAS, KRAS and CBL) in 89% of cases.[1033] Various cytogenetic changes	Infants and children <4 years; eczematoid or maculopapular rash; anemia and thrombocytopenia; increased Hgb F in 70% of cases; neurofibromatosis in 10% of cases; abnormality of chromosome 7 (e.g., del 7, del 7q, etc.) in approximately 20% of patients; BCR rearrangement absent	Page 1470
Chronic neutrophilic leukemia	Colony-stimulating factor 3 receptor gene (CSF3R) alone (~30% of cases); a combination of mutated CSF3R and a SET binding protein gene (SETBP1) mutation (~60% of cases); the JAK2^{V617F} mutation alone (~10% of cases)[990–992]	Segmented neutrophilia >20,000/μL; splenomegaly >90% of cases; no blood blasts; platelets >100 × 10⁹/L; 75% of cases have normal cytogenetics; BCR rearrangement absent	Page 1471
BCR rearrangement-negative chronic myelogenous leukemia	Various cytogenetic changes	Clinical findings indistinguishable from BCR rearrangement-positive CML; Ph chromosome and BCR-ABL fusion gene absent	Page 1472
Atypical myeloproliferative disease	Various cytogenetic changes	Usually older patient (>65 years); variable blood cell changes: anemia, granulocytosis, normal or decreased platelet counts; hypercellular marrow, marrow blasts <10%; dysmorphia of blood and marrow cells common (e.g., Pelger-Huët neutrophils, dyserythropoiesis, and megakaryopoiesis; often splenomegaly)	Page 1473

Hgb, hemoglobin; PDGFR, platelet-derived growth factor receptor; Ph, Philadelphia; WBC, white blood cells.

isolated –Y, an intermediate-risk is any other abnormality, and high-risk is trisomy 8 or complex karyotypes (more than three abnormalities). Approximately 35 percent of patients have point mutations of the K-RAS or N-RAS gene.[904] The RAS gene also may be involved in the transforming events. Abnormal methylation of p15^{INK4B} is a common finding in CMML.[915] Translocation between the gene PDGFR-β on chromosome 5(q33) and four partner genes—TEL at 12(p13), HIP-1 at 7(q11.2), H4 at 10(q22), and Rabaptin-5 at 17(p13)—occur in a very small proportion of patients (approximately 3 to 4 percent).[905,916–919] This mutation juxtaposes the gene encoding the PDGFR-β with a partner gene, which results in the encoding of a mutant tyrosine kinase that is constitutively activated and sensitive to inhibition by imatinib or a congener[920] (see "Treatment" below). The cases with PDGFR-β translocations are more likely to be accompanied by eosinophilia than are cases with other cytogenetic abnormalities. Other gene mutations identified

in the leukemic cells of patients with CMML include RUNX1, IDH1/2, CBL, JAK2, TET2, DNMT3A, ASXL1, UTX, EZH2. The gene SRSF2 (serine/arginine-rich splicing factor 2), was found to be the most frequently mutated gene in patients with CMML, 28 percent of patients studied. In an effort to determine the frequency of the mutation in a large sample of patients and to look for coincident mutations with SRSF2 in CMML patient's cells, eight other genes known to be mutated in some patients with CMML were studied among 275 patients with the disease.[904] SRSF2 was mutated in 47 percent of patients in this large series, and had a significantly increased coincidence with EZH2 and TET2. Ninety-three percent of patients had at least one mutated gene.

Serum and Urine Findings Plasma and urine lysozyme concentrations nearly always are elevated. Plasma levels of VEGF, hepatocyte growth factor, and tumor necrosis factor alpha are elevated. Serum vitamin B$_{12}$, β_2-microglobulin, and LDH levels often are elevated.[905,906]

Treatment

Treatment of most patients with CMML has been unsatisfactory, and remissions of any duration are uncommon. The age and performance status of the patient are considered in determining the intensity of treatment. Cytarabine, either standard or low-dose, etoposide, hydroxyurea, and other approaches used for the oligoblastic myelogenous leukemias have been attempted, but with little success (Chap. 88). Decitabine and 5-azacytidine have been useful in a small proportion of patients.[905,906] One study of azacytidine treatment reported a complete response in 11 percent, a partial response in 3 percent, and hematologic improvement in 25 percent. The median survival of responders was 15 months compared to 12 months among nonresponders, a modest result.[921] Unfortunately, although a particular approach may confer significant benefit in a small proportion of cases, determining which patients will respond is not possible, except by trial and error. An exception is the patient with a translocation involving PDGFR-β, which itself occurs in only a small percentage of patients. In the case of PDGFR-β fusion genes with several of the partner genes, imatinib 400 mg/day has resulted in normal blood counts, cytogenetic remissions, and, occasionally, molecular remission.[915–917,922,923] These fortunate patients probably will benefit from this treatment, as evidenced by prolonged remissions and survival, compared to other drug options, but the number of patients and duration of followup do not permit quantitative estimates at this point. Allogeneic stem cell transplantation is an option for the small proportion of younger patients with an appropriate matched-related or unrelated donor.[924]

Course and Prognosis

Median survival in CMML is approximately 12 months, with a range from approximately 1 to more than 60 months. Approximately 20 percent of patients progress to frank AML. Arbitrary stratification of CMML into types 1 (<5 percent blood myeloblasts) and 2 (5 to 20 percent blood myeloblasts) based on the height of the blast count has been proposed, but distinguishing patients by whether, for example, they have 4 (type 1) or 8 percent blasts (type 2) on a marrow examination is of little use for care of an individual patient. Blast percentage may be a significant correlate with outcome in any large group of patients with a clonal myeloid disease, and this factor among several others should guide therapy. Clusters of prognostic variables have been used to stratify patients into risk groups for survival duration. In general, the severity of the anemia, the cytogenetic risk category, and the height of the blast percentage are the most important. Other variables that may confer a shorter life expectancy are height of the absolute lymphocyte count, high spontaneous rates of myelomonocytic colony growth, higher total leukocyte counts, higher LDH level, and larger spleen size.[925–927] These risk factors for progression are validated in large groups of patients but the confidence intervals are not shown. In an individual patient the variability in outcome is great based on such variables; careful clinical observation for progression is most important. Unfortunately, at this time, unless the patient is a candidate for imatinib therapy or allogeneic stem cell transplantation, long-term salutary therapeutic effects are uncommon.

CHRONIC EOSINOPHILIC LEUKEMIA

History and Definition

The recognition of eosinophilic lineage prominence in myelogenous leukemia dates to a case published in 1912.[928] In 1968, the term *hypereosinophilic syndrome* was introduced to encompass a group of disorders with (1) prolonged exaggerated eosinophilia without an apparent cause, (2) frequent cardiac and neurologic tissue damage, (3) a poor or transient response to therapy, and (4) a progressive course and a high fatality rate. Shortly thereafter, Benvenisti and Ultmann[929] presented five cases of eosinophilic leukemia and reviewed the literature regarding that phenotypic designation. In 1975, Chusid and colleagues[930] described 14 cases of hypereosinophilic syndrome, highlighted the frequency of secondary cardiac and neurologic disorders, and suggested the existence of a continuum of manifestations. Because some cases had clonal cytogenetic abnormalities and hematologic findings compatible with a clonal myeloid disease, the presence of eosinophilic leukemia was suspected in this apparently heterogeneous group of patients.

The relationship of blood eosinophilia to clonal myeloid diseases is complex because the former can be reactive or represent acute eosinophilic leukemia, chronic eosinophilic leukemia, or eosinophilia associated with a different category of disease, such as BCR-ABL1–positive CML, primary myelofibrosis, oligoblastic leukemia (MDS), or mastocytosis.[931] Chronic eosinophilic leukemia is a BCR-ABL1–negative, clonal myeloid disease with a striking eosinophilia in the blood and marrow, often with clonal cytogenetic abnormalities that have features including, when present, cytogenetic findings that usually distinguish chronic eosinophilic leukemia from other clonal myeloid diseases that may have an associated eosinophilia, such as CMML. The phenotype of the eosinophilic variant of CMML overlaps somewhat with that of chronic eosinophilic leukemia. However, the fusion gene associated with CMML involves the PDGFR-β (see "Chronic Myelomonocytic Leukemia" above), whereas in chronic eosinophilic leukemia the cytogenetic findings are different and in some cases involve PDGFR-α. This definition of chronic eosinophilic leukemia recognizes that, at the margins, classification may be arbitrary. Studies in cases with the FIP1L1–PDGFR-α translocation were consistent with multilineage involvement, consistent with an origin in a pluripotent lymphohematopoietic cell.[932] Another report found multilineage involvement but with a presumptive lesion in a multipotent, not pluripotent, hematopoietic cell.[933]

Signs and Symptoms

Fever, cough, weakness, easy fatigability, dyspnea, abdominal pain, maculopapular rash, cardiac symptoms and signs of heart failure, and a variety of neurologic manifestations ranging from peripheral neuropathy to cerebral encephalomalacia may occur, ranging from mild to severe in expression. Splenomegaly often is evident.

Laboratory Findings

Eosinophilia is a constant finding (see Chap. 62, Fig. 62–3). Anemia usually but not always is present at the time of presentation. The leukocyte count may be high-normal or more often elevated. Platelet counts often are normal or mildly decreased. The marrow shows myelocytic and eosinophilic hyperplasia and, occasionally, Charcot-Leyden crystals. Mast cells, often spindle-shaped, may be increased. In the FIP1L1–PDGFR-α type of chronic eosinophilic leukemia, which may make up approximately 14 percent of cases of primary eosinophilia not found to be reactive to another disease, marrow aggregates of spindle-shaped mast cells are invariably found (see "Cytogenetic Findings" below).[933,934] Megakaryocytes usually are present but may appear dysmorphic. Reticulin fibrosis is common. Immunophenotyping and PCR do not show evidence of either a clonal T-cell population or T-cell–receptor rearrangement. Pulmonary function studies may provide evidence of fibrotic (restrictive) lung disease. Echocardiography may detect mural thrombi, thickening (fibrosis) of the ventricular wall, valvular dysfunction from papillary muscle, and chordae fibrosis. Magnetic resonance imaging can detect subendocardial fibrosis, thickening of ventricles, and markedly reduced ventricular lumen volume. Serum immunoglobulin (Ig) E, vitamin B_{12}, and tryptase levels usually are elevated. Skin biopsy of lesions uncovers intense eosinophilic infiltrates. Neural or brain biopsy may disclose eosinophilic infiltrates, often perivascular, with microthrombi, axonal degeneration, and gliosis.

Cytogenetic Findings A wide array of cytogenetic findings have been reported in cases of chronic eosinophilic leukemia.[935] Notable translocations include a high frequency of translocations involving chromosome 5, t(1;5), t(2;5), t(5;12), t(6;11), 8p11, trisomy 8, and numerous others, infrequently. Chromosome 5 often is translocated at the site of the *PDGFR-β* gene, and the phenotype usually is more compatible with CMML with eosinophilia. Chromosome 5 from band q31–35 contains several genes relevant to eosinophilopoiesis, including those encoding IL-5, IL-3, GM-CSF, and PDGFR-β. A cryptic interstitial *CHIC2* deletion on chromosome 4 (q12;q12) results in the fusion gene *FIL1L1–PDGFR-α*, normally separated by the *CHIC2* gene, and in a phenotype that can be considered a form of chronic eosinophilic leukemia, virtually always associated with marrow mastocytosis, which is of particular note because, like the *PDGFR-β* mutations in CMML with eosinophilia, of a near-universal response to treatment with imatinib.[935–937]

Serum Tryptase Level Elevation Versus Normal Levels

The elevation of serum tryptase level (>11.5 ng/mL) has been used to distinguish a subset of patients who (1) are male, (2) have marrows that are intensely hypercellular with a higher proportion of immature eosinophils and with dysmorphic mast cells with a CD117−CD25+CD2− genotype and phenotype (distinguishing these cells from classic mastocytosis, which are CD117+CD25+CD2+), (3) have dramatically higher serum vitamin B_{12} and IgE levels, (4) are more prone to restrictive pulmonary disease and endomyocardial fibrosis, (5) have the *FIP1L1–PDGFR-α* fusion gene, and (6) are responsive to imatinib.[869] Patients with normal serum tryptase levels are more prone to obstructive pulmonary restrictive disease, eosinophilic dermatitis, and gastrointestinal complaints.

Differential Diagnosis

Eosinophilia can occur for many reasons (Chap. 62). The first step is to identify signs that may point to a clonal myeloid disease. These signs include anemia, thrombocytopenia, splenomegaly, immature eosinophils in the marrow examination, evidence of dysmorphic cells in blood or marrow, for example, atypical megakaryocytes or dysmorphic mast cells, cardiac or pulmonary manifestations, which may occur secondary to chronic eosinophilic leukemia, and markedly elevated serum tryptase or vitamin B_{12} level. The former signs, especially in the aggregate, are highly suggestive, but the presence of a cytogenetic abnormality in myeloid cells is diagnostic of a clonal myeloid disease (leukemia). If the latter is not evident, PCR and/or flow cytometry to search for a clonal T lymphocyte abnormality should be performed. Whether the eosinophilic leukemia is typical or represents an eosinophilia with idiopathic myelofibrosis, CMML, or MDS is less important than if it has a mutation that is imatinib sensitive (e.g., *PDGFR* mutation).

Therapy

Patients (nearly always men) whose cells display a *FIP1L1–PDGFR-α* have a very high probability of responding to imatinib at a dose of 100 to 400 mg/day.[936–940] The tyrosine kinase activity of this fusion protein is two orders of magnitude more sensitive to imatinib than that of BCR-ABL1. However, because not all patients taking 400 mg/day achieve a molecular remission, and that goal may be more likely to result in long-term remission, initial therapy remains at 400 mg/day or an equivalent dose of another TKI, such as dasatinib or nilotinib, and PCR monitoring is appropriate. Dose adjustment upward if molecular remission is not achieved can be considered. Unlike the case in CML, patients with chronic eosinophilic leukemia with significant side effects when taking imatinib, 400 mg/day, have a reasonable probability of having a good response at lower doses.[950] Dasatinib and nilotinib are also active.[941]

In patients with eosinophilic leukemia without an imatinib-sensitive mutation or in patients who become resistant to imatinib and unresponsive to a second-generation TKI (e.g., dasatinib or nilotinib) and who are progressing, ablative or nonablative allogeneic stem cell transplantation can be considered if they are in an acceptable age range and have access to a matched-related or matched-unrelated donor.[942,943]

In TKI-insensitive patients without the option of transplantation, empirical treatment with glucocorticoids, hydroxyurea, or anti–IL-5[944,945] to decrease eosinophil counts and mute the progress of eosinophil-mediated cutaneous, cardiac, pulmonary, and neurologic tissue damage should be considered. These approaches may relieve symptoms for a time, but are temporizing if therapy with drugs that might be effective in inhibiting clonal expansion or evolution is not effective (e.g., cytarabine, anthracycline antibiotic, etoposide).

Course and Prognosis

If chronic eosinophilic leukemia is not TKI-sensitive, the long-term outlook is one of probable progressive cardiac and neurologic disability. Transformation to acute eosinophilic or myelogenous leukemia can occur. Allogeneic stem cell transplantation is potentially curative. In tyrosine kinase sensitive cases, hematologic normalization, reversal of marrow fibrosis and mastocytosis, resolution of skin lesions, normalization of spleen size, and restoration of well-being occurs in the great preponderance of cases. Cardiac, neurologic, and pulmonary changes usually cannot be reversed but should be stabilized. The long-term outlook with tyrosine kinase therapy is uncertain. However, it likely will decisively and dramatically improve survival compared to other prior therapy and should greatly improve the prognosis of patients with a molecular target for the drug.

CHRONIC BASOPHILIC LEUKEMIA

This type of clinical disorder, in which the patient has marrow and blood basophilia and other findings compatible with a clonal myeloid disease without evidence of the *BCR-ABL1* translocation, is rare. Two reports of such a syndrome occurring in five patients have been published.[946,947] The marrow was intensely hypercellular in the three major lineages. Dysmorphic megakaryocytes were evident. Basophilia in marrow and blood was striking, although eosinophilia also was evident in two patients and increased mast cells in three patients. The clinical effects of basophilic mediator release were evident in two patients. One patient evolved to AML; another recovered after allogeneic transplantation. The cases had similar findings, leading to the suggestion they represented Ph chromosome–negative chronic basophilic leukemia. In one case, a *PRKG2–PDGFR-β* fusion gene was evident and the patient responded to imatinib.

JUVENILE MYELOMONOCYTIC LEUKEMIA

Epidemiology

Ph chromosome–positive, adult-type CML occurring in children younger than age 15 years makes up approximately 3 percent of childhood leukemias and approximately 10 percent of all cases of CML.[948] Although CML occurs in children of all ages, it is rare in children younger than age 5 years. With the exception of a propensity to present with higher total leukocyte counts and with leukostatic signs or symptoms, CML in children has the typical manifestations and course of the disorder seen in adults.

A disorder different from adult-type CML, designated *juvenile myelomonocytic leukemia*, represents approximately 1.5 percent of childhood leukemias. It occurs most often in infants and children younger than age 4 years and is similar in some respects to adult subacute or

CMML because the two diseases share a prominent monocytic component in the leukemic cell population.[949–952]

Pathogenesis

This disorder is a clonal myeloid disease that originates in an early hematopoietic multipotential cell. Evidence indicates this cell may be pluripotential (myeloid-lymphoid) in some cases and myeloid in others.[953–956] Patient-derived induced pluripotential stem cells recapitulated the growth patterns *in vitro* of the human disease and drug inhibition of MEK kinase reduced their GM-CSF growth potential.[957] *RAS* mutations in hematopoietic cells are present in approximately 20 percent of patients.[958] Approximately one in 10 patients with juvenile myelomonocytic leukemia have mutations of *NF1* and manifest type 1 neurofibromatosis. This frequency is approximately 400 times the expected occurrence in a comparable pediatric population.[959–961] The linkage between neurofibromin, the protein encoded by the *NF1* gene, GTPase activity proteins, and the activation state of *RAS*-encoded proteins has led to a postulated sequence of events that may be triggered by the extraordinarily heightened sensitivity of the colony-forming cells in the marrow and blood of infants with the disease to the proliferative effects of GM-CSF. The latter initiates signal transduction from the cell membrane to the nucleus via *RAS* protein activation.[961,962] Mutations in the *PTPN11* gene have been found in approximately one-third of children with juvenile myelomonocytic leukemia, and the mutations in *NF1*, *RAS*, and *PTPN11* usually do not coincide.[1025,1026] However, they each may act through a common pathway. *PTPN11* encodes SHP-2, a phosphatase, which is an upstream regulator of RAS; thus, all three mutations can contribute to deregulation of RAS signaling. As an aside, children with Noonan syndrome, which is characterized by short stature, dysmorphic facies, skeletal abnormalities, and cardiac defects, have a germ-cell mutation of *PTPN1*. These children may have a transient disorder that closely mimics juvenile myelomonocytic leukemia.[963]

Clinical Findings

Symptoms and Signs Infants present with failure to thrive, and children present with malaise, fever, persistent infections, and exaggerated skin, oral, or nasal bleeding. Hepatomegaly can occur. Splenomegaly, sometimes massive, is present in almost all cases. Lymphadenopathy is frequent.[949–952] More than half of the patients have eczematoid or maculopapular skin lesions[964] and xanthomatous lesions, and multiple *café-au-lait* spots (neurofibromatosis type 1) may occur.[950] The xanthomas may be the earliest signs of neurofibromatosis.[950,951] Noonan syndrome (dysmorphic facies, short stature, heart disease, mental retardation, cryptorchidism, webbed neck, chest deformities, and bleeding diathesis) may coexist.[951]

Laboratory Findings Anemia, thrombocytopenia, and mild to moderate leukocytosis are common. The leukocyte count usually is greater than 10×10^9/L with a median leukocyte count at diagnosis of approximately 35×10^9/L. The blood has an increased monocyte concentration of 1 to 100×10^9/L, immature granulocytes including a small percentage of blast cells, and nucleated red cells. Fetal hemoglobin concentration is increased in approximately two-thirds of the patients. The marrow aspirate is hypercellular as a result of granulocytic hyperplasia; the number of erythroblasts and megakaryocytes usually are decreased. Monocytic cells are increased but may not be as striking as in the blood. Leukemic blast cells are present in modest proportions (<20 percent).

Cell culture of blood and marrow shows a striking preponderance of monocytic progenitors, even in the absence of overt monocytosis in the marrow.[965,966] Granulocyte-monocyte colony-forming cells show a marked tendency to spontaneous growth if adherent (monocytic) cells are not depleted from culture.[966] The effect is mediated by a release of large quantities of GM-CSF by monocytes in culture.[967]

Although clonal chromosome abnormalities have been found in some cases,[968] the cytogenetic abnormalities have no consistent pattern, and more than half of the patients have normal karyotypes. The *BCR-ABL1* fusion gene is not present.[968–970] The phenotype of monosomy 7 syndrome overlaps with juvenile myelomonocytic leukemia, and an abnormality of chromosome 7 (del 7, del 7q, others) is present in approximately one-fifth of patients.[949]

Course, Prognosis, and Treatment

The median survival of patients with juvenile myelomonocytic leukemia has been less than 2 years.[949,950] Children younger than 2 years are more likely to have a protracted course.[882] The disease has been refractory to most chemotherapy. In a study of nine patients, four of whom were treated with a five- or six-drug intensive regimen, remissions were 11 months to more than 27 months, compared with untreated or lightly treated patients, four of whom died within 7 months.[971] Even in the treated patients, complete suppression of the disease did not occur, and treatment protocols to induce and sustain remissions were lacking.[966] A program of cytosine arabinoside, etoposide, vincristine, and isotretinoin resulted in a highly favorable response in five children treated. Three patients relapsed and were treated with cytarabine by infusion and subcutaneously and with etoposide. All patients were alive, and the range of survival at the time of publication was 8 to 89 months, with a median survival of 27 months. The resistance of these cells to currently available therapy is distressingly highlighted by the sense of success in prolonging the life of infants and young children by a few years. Intensive therapy can control disease, but curative chemotherapy has been elusive.[972] The inclusion of isotretinoin was based on a prior report of responsiveness to the drug used alone; however, this observation has not been confirmed.[973] The GM-CSF antagonist E21R, inhibitors of *RAF-1* gene expression, blockers of RAS protein farnesylation, and angiogenesis inhibitors are among other drug approaches to the disease being studied.[952,974]

Allogeneic stem cell transplantation is an important approach to therapy and may provide the best chance of long-term survival in selected children.[975–977] Hence, a rapid search for a matched-unrelated donor, including cord blood sources, is important in patients without matched sibling donors. Transplantation from a histocompatible sibling or matched-unrelated donor resulted in an event-free survival at 5 years of approximately 50 percent, and from matched-cord blood stem cells of approximately 45 percent, unless monosomy 7 was present, which lowers 5-year survival to approximately 25 percent.[977] Children transplanted before age 1 year had better results (approximately 50 percent) than did older children (approximately 30 percent).[977] DLI has placed a posttransplantation patient in relapse into remission,[978] but, in general, this procedure is ineffective in patients who relapse after transplantation.

A minority of patients have a smoldering course for 2 to 4 years. Thereafter, the disease usually rapidly progresses, and patients die of infection or hemorrhage. Occasional patients have a very long survival (>10 years) despite persistence of abnormal blood counts and splenomegaly, independent of the type or intensity of therapy. Some children convert to a full-blown AML with a rapidly fatal outcome. Cases of juvenile myelomonocytic leukemia may be associated with transformation to acute lymphoblastic leukemia.[979]

CHRONIC NEUTROPHILIC LEUKEMIA

History, Pathogenesis, and Epidemiology

In 1920, Tuohey[980] described the first recorded case of an unusual sustained neutrophilia with splenomegaly without fever, inflammation, cancer, or other cause of a leukemoid reaction. Use of X-chromosome-linked polymorphic genes in blood cells and FISH of chromosome abnormalities have been indicative of a clonal myeloid disorder.[981-983] Some cases may arise in the hematopoietic multipotential cell, others in a neutrophil progenitor cell (Chap. 85).[981-985] Evidence points to defective apoptotic signals accounting, in part, for the striking accumulation of segmented neutrophils in the blood.[986] The median age at onset is approximately age 65 years. Younger patients may be affected.[987] As in most clonal myeloid diseases, men are affected more frequently than are women.

Clinical Features

Symptoms and Signs Patients may complain of weakness, anorexia, weight loss, abdominal pain, and easy bruising. Symptoms and signs of gouty arthritis occur in approximately one-third of cases. The spleen is enlarged in almost all cases, and the liver frequently is enlarged. Lymphadenopathy is very infrequent.[985] A hemorrhagic tendency is present in some patients.

Laboratory Findings Although some patients have a normal hemoglobin concentration at the time of presentation, most have mild to moderate anemia on presentation. The reticulocyte count usually is between 0.5 and 3.0 percent. The platelet count rarely is less than 125×10^9/L and usually is normal. Coagulation times are normal. The total leukocyte count usually is between 25 and 100×10^9/L in most cases, and only rarely is less than 20×10^9/L or exceeds 100×10^9/L. Neutrophils compose 85 to 95 percent of the white cells. Although segmented cells usually dominate, occasional cases have a high proportion of band forms. Very infrequently, metamyelocytes, myelocytes, and nucleated red cells may be present in patients. Basophil and eosinophil counts are not increased. Blasts nearly always are absent from the blood. Neutrophil alkaline phosphatase activity is increased in almost all cases.

The marrow invariably shows granulocytic hyperplasia with myeloid-to-erythroid ratios as high as 10:1. Myeloblasts are not overtly increased in number (0.5 to 3.0 percent). Megakaryocytes are either normal or slightly increased in number and have normal distribution and morphology. Erythropoiesis usually is mildly decreased. Unlike CML, reticulin fibrosis is unusual. A few cases with dysmorphic features in the marrow (acquired Pelger-Hüet anomaly, erythroid, dysplasia, micromegakaryocytes) have been reported. Serum vitamin B_{12}-binding protein and vitamin B_{12} levels both are markedly increased above normal. Serum uric acid concentration is increased, and serum LDH activity may be increased.

Almost every case examined postmortem had liver and splenic enlargement. Portal hepatic and splenic red pulp infiltrates of neutrophils or islands of extramedullary hematopoiesis with immature myeloid cells and megakaryocytes are characteristic.

Cytogenetic and Genetic Findings By definition, the Ph chromosome, *BCR* gene rearrangements, and *BCR-ABL1* transcripts are absent.[987-990] Most patients have normal karyotypes, but approximately 25 percent of patients have nonrandom abnormalities of chromosomes.[990] Deletions of chromosome 20q and trisomy 21 or 9 are the most common abnormalities. The disease has been shown to be associated with a mutation in the colony-stimulating factor 3 receptor gene (*CSF3R*) alone (approximately 30 percent of cases), or a combination of mutated *CSF3R* and a SET binding protein gene (*SETBP1*) mutation (approximately 60 percent of cases) or the *JAK2*[V617F] mutation alone (approximately 10 percent of cases).[991,992] Two principal mutations were observed in *CSF3R*: membrane proximal *CSF3R*[S783fs] mutation and truncated *CSF3R*[T618I] mutation. The former results in deregulation of the JAK family kinases and may respond to JAK inhibitors, whereas the later deregulates SRC family-TNK2 kinases and confers sensitivity to dasatinib.[991] Four of five prior reports of *JAK2* mutations in a single patient with chronic neutrophilic leukemia were cited. In the fifth report, six patients with the disease were studied and one had a *JAK2*[V617F] mutation.

Differential Diagnosis

Most leukemoid reactions are associated with an obvious underlying cause, such as pancreatitis, carcinoma, connective tissue disease, smoker's neutrophilia, and chronic bacterial or fungal infection. The leukocyte alkaline phosphatase level usually is markedly elevated in chronic neutrophilic leukemia and markedly decreased in CML. More to the point, molecular studies identifying *BCR* gene rearrangement or the presence of *BCR-ABL1* transcripts should distinguish chronic neutrophilic leukemia (*BCR-ABL1*–negative) from neutrophilic CML (*BCR-ABL1*–positive; see "Special Clinical Features" above). In the latter case, more than half of the patients have thrombocytosis and megakaryocytic hyperplasia, which are uncharacteristic of chronic neutrophilic leukemia. The presence of a *CSF3R* or *JAK2* mutation with a classical clinical picture would be strong diagnostic evidence for the disease.

Treatment

No systematic studies of treatment have been reported. Although hydroxyurea, IFN-α, or cytarabine may decrease the white count and spleen size, long-term benefit is unusual.[987-990] Intensive therapy has led to early posttreatment deaths. With identification of a specific genetic mutation, either a JAK2 inhibitor (e.g., ruxolitinib) (for the *CSF3R*[T618I] mutation) or dasatinib (for the *CSF3R*[S783fs] mutation) should be considered. The disease is rare and clinical trials would be difficult. *In vitro* studies of cell sensitivity and reports of individual responses may have to be relied upon.[991-993] Allogeneic stem cell transplantation in eligible patients may be curative.[994]

Course and Prognosis

The disease is fatal, with a median survival of approximately 2.5 years and a range of 0.5 to 6 years.[987-990] A case of spontaneous remission has been reported. The prognosis is considerably worse than the prognosis for CML despite the prevalence of mature neutrophils and the paucity of blasts. Newer approaches with dasatinib or ruxolitinib for the appropriate genetic mutations (see "Treatment" above) may provide better outcomes. Causes of death have included (1) intracranial hemorrhage, sometimes in the presence of adequate platelet counts and coagulation times, suggesting a vascular infiltrative process; (2) severe infection; (3) transformation to AML; and (4) the toxic effects of intensive therapy. The disease usually afflicts older persons, and cardiac, pulmonary, and vascular diseases contribute to a fatal outcome.

A remarkable frequency of concordant essential monoclonal gammopathy or myeloma has been described.[983,995-1003] In two cases, the extreme neutrophilia proved to be a polyclonal response to a plasma cell disorder.[983,1004] Chronic neutrophilic leukemia has evolved from polycythemia vera or oligoblastic leukemia,[1005-1009] supporting its relationship to the clonal hemopathies.[983,1010,1011]

BCR REARRANGEMENT-NEGATIVE PHENOTYPICALLY TYPICAL CHRONIC MYELOGENOUS LEUKEMIA

A very small proportion of patients (approximately 4 percent) with clinical manifestations within the limits usually applied to the diagnosis of CML have neither a Ph chromosome (classic, variant, or masked) nor evidence of rearrangement of *BCR* on chromosome 22. This circumstance represents *BCR*-negative CML. The literature describing Ph chromosome–negative CML prior to 1987 is difficult to evaluate because many cases were not studied carefully for masked or variant translocations and for the *BCR* gene rearrangement. Ph chromosome–negative CML is a clonal disease[903] that has the propensity for lymphoid and myeloid transformation.[1012,1013] Although most cases of *BCR* rearrangement–negative CML are closer in manifestations to

CMML,[903,927,1014-1016] some cases are indistinguishable from classic CML but without the *BCR-ABL1* after exhaustive molecular diagnostic evaluation.[1017-1021] In a report of 76 such patients, the median age was 66 years (range: 24 to 88), splenomegaly was present in 50 percent of cases, the median white cell count was 38,000 cells/μL (38 × 10⁹ cells/L; range: 11 to 296), and the median hemoglobin was 11 g/dL (range: 7 to 16), with classical morphologic features in blood and marrow.[1021] As the disease progressed, patients developed severe cytopenias.[1018] Median survival was 24 months and only 7 percent survived for more than 5 years. Myeloid blast phase occurred in one-third of those followed until their death. Occasional patients had extended complete remissions with IFN-γ therapy.[1020] Hydroxyurea can be useful as palliative therapy.

Some patients have transposition of *ABL1* to chromosome 22 but not the classic translocation. In such cases, including *TEL-ABL1* translocations, transient responses to imatinib have been observed.[1022]

Uncommon cases of coexisting BCR-negative and BCR-positive clones have been described, and the basis for such cases is in dispute.[1023] One proposed explanation is that this case is an example of "field carcinogenesis" in which multiple clones coexist.[1023] An alternative explanation is that these cases represent the dual progeny of a single unstable clone.[1024] The long-term survival of patients with CML may permit the emergence of a drug-induced or spontaneous second malignancy, and in the former it may be notably associated with imatinib (see "Secondary Chromosomal Changes with Tyrosine Kinase Inhibitors above).[1025-1027]

ATYPICAL MYELOPROLIFERATIVE DISEASE

Definition

There is a small but measurable frequency of patients who do not fit the diagnostic criteria of the other chronic myeloproliferative diseases, yet their findings represent the manifestations of a clonal myeloid neoplasm.[1028-1031] A neoplasm of a hematopoietic stem cell has many variations in expression (Chap. 83), and it is surprising that nearly all can be pigeonholed into a generally agreed upon phenotype. These cases are among those that do not fit a standard diagnostic pattern. These cases have been classified by the WHO as atypical CML (aCML) or alternatively myelodysplastic-myeloproliferative syndrome, which category excludes BCR-rearrangement–positive CML, CMML, chronic neutrophilic leukemia, refractory sideroblastic anemia with thrombocytosis, and other classical syndromes, as judged phenotypically and genotypically. An attempt at teasing apart these syndromes into specific classifications proved how difficult that was, even when very arbitrary criteria were applied.[1031] Until a genetic basis is more clearly defined and specific therapy becomes available, we prefer to use the term atypical myeloproliferative disease for this category of hematopoietic multipotential (stem) cell disorder because, when starting with a single patient, the clinical features do not allow clear distinctions among patients and therapy is based on the manifestations in a given case, the consensus between patient and physician about the desirability and likely utility of therapy, and the rate of progression of the disease in that patient.

Clinical Features These patients are principally in the 60 to 90 year-old age range, but atypical expression of a multipotential hematopoietic cell neoplasm can occur at any age. Hepatomegaly and (or) splenomegaly are present in a minority of patients. Anemia and nearly always granulocytosis (granulocytes, notably neutrophils, and granulocytic precursors), sometimes with neutrophilic dysmorphia (e.g., acquired Pelger-Huët neutrophils) are characteristic. Neutrophilic precursors represent less than 15 percent of blood cells. The blast cell count in blood and marrow is low, usually less than 10 percent. Monocytes are not increased and eosinophils or basophils are usually not increased but may be as high as 10 percent of total leukocytes.

Laboratory Features The LDH is often elevated. The marrow is hypercellular with variable evidence of dysmorphic granulopoiesis and dysmorphic megakaryocytopoiesis. Mild marrow reticular fibrosis may be evident. Clonal cytogenetic abnormalities may occur but do not include translocations characteristic of classical chronic myeloid neoplasms, such as a BCR-ABL1 or translocations involving PDGFR-α, PDGFR-β, or FGFR1 seen in chronic eosinophilic leukemia with or without mastocytosis. Common myeloid-related cytogenetic abnormalities may occur, such as trisomy 8, del(20q), and others.

Therapy This type of neoplasm has no specific treatment and is usually treated "symptomatically" with red cell or platelet transfusion and an agent to reduce the white cell count, if that is a problem (e.g., hydroxyurea, 5-azacytidine, low-dose cytarabine, numerous others).[1031] Appropriate patients may be considered for allogeneic hematopoietic stem cell transplantation, if a suitable donor is available, but this approach is problematic in an older population because they would be transplanted during active disease and with a higher-risk of GVHD. Nonmyeloablative allogeneic stem cell transplantation has also been used.

Course and Prognosis This patient population has a median survival of approximately 18 months, but the upper range is approximately 5 years. The disease may undergo clonal evolution to AML.

REFERENCES

1. Bennett JH: Case of hypertrophy of the spleen and liver, in which death took place from suppuration of the blood. *Edinburgh Med Surg J* 64:313, 1845.
2. Virchow R: Weisses blut. *Froieps Notizen* 36:151, 1845.
3. Craige D: Case of disease of the spleen in which death took place in consequence of the presence of purulent matter in the blood. *Edinburgh Med Surg J* 64:400, 1845.
4. Virchow R: *Die Leukaemie in Gesammelte Abhandlungen zur Wissen-Schaftlichen Medizin.* Meidinger, Frankfort, 1865.
5. Neumann E: Ueber myelogene leukämie. *Berl Klin Wochenschr* 15:69, 1878.
6. Nowell PC, Hungerford DA: A minute chromosome in human chronic granulocytic leukemia. *J Natl Cancer Inst* 25:85, 1960.
7. Baike AG, Court Brown WM, Buckton KE, et al: A possible specific chromosome abnormality in human chronic myeloid leukemia. *Nature* 188:1165, 1960.
8. Nowell PC, Hungerford DA: Chromosome studies in human leukemia: II. Chronic granulocytic leukemia. *J Natl Cancer Inst* 27:1013, 1961.
9. Tough IM, Court Brown WM, Buckton KE, et al: Cytogenetic studies in chronic leukemia and acute leukemia associated with mongolism. *Lancet* 1:411, 1961.
10. Caspersson T, Zech L, Johansson C, Modest EJ: Identification of human chromosomes by DNA binding fluorescent agents. *Chromosoma* 30:215, 1970.
11. Caspersson T, Gahrton G, Lindsten J, Zech L: Identification of the Philadelphia chromosome as a number 22 by quinacrine mustard fluorescence analysis. *Exp Cell Res* 63:238, 1970.
12. Rowley JD: A new consistent abnormality in chronic myelogenous leukemia identified by quinacrine fluorescence and Giemsa staining. *Nature* 243:290, 1973.
13. de Klein A, Van Kessel AG, Grosveld G, et al: A cellular oncogene is translocated to the Philadelphia chromosome in chronic myelocytic leukemia. *Nature* 300:765, 1982.
14. Bartram CR, de Klein A, Hagemeijer A, et al: Translocation of c-abl oncogene correlates with the presence of a Philadelphia chromosome in chronic myelocytic leukemia. *Nature* 306:277, 1983.
15. Drucker BJ, Tamura S, Buchdunger E, et al: Effects of a selective inhibitor of the ABL tyrosine kinase in the growth of BCR-ABL positive cells. *Nat Med* 2:561, 1996.
16. Thomas ED, Clift RA, Fefer A, et al: Marrow transplantation for the treatment of chronic myelogenous leukemia. *Ann Intern Med* 104:155, 1986.
17. Wapner J: *The Philadelphia Chromosome. A mutant gene and the quest to cure cancer at the molecular level.* The Experiment, New York, NY, 2013.
18. Redaelli A, Bell C, Casagrande J, et al: Clinical and epidemiologic burden of chronic myelogenous leukemia. *Expert Rev Anticancer Ther* 4:85, 2004.
19. Björkholm M: No familial aggregation in chronic myeloid leukemia. *Blood* 122:460, 2013.
20. Lichtman MA: Obesity and the risk of chronic myelogenous leukemia: Is this another example of the neoplastic effects of increased body fat? *Leukemia* 26:183, 2012.
21. Ichimaru M, Ichimaru T, Belsky JL: Incidence of leukemia in atomic bomb survivors belonging to a fixed cohort in Hiroshima and Nagasaki 1950–1971. *J Radiat Res (Tokyo)* 19:262, 1978.
22. Court Brown WM, Doll R: Adult leukemia. *Br Med J* 1:1753, 1960.
23. Boice JD Jr, Day NE, Anderson A, et al: Second cancers following radiation treatment for cervical cancer. *J Natl Cancer Inst* 74:955, 1985.
24. Maloney WC: Radiation leukemia revisited. *Blood* 70:905, 1987.

25. Lichtman MA: Is there an entity of chemically induced BCR-ABL-positive chronic myelogenous leukemia? *Oncologist* 13:645, 2008.

26. Lamm SH, Engel A, Joshi KP, et al: Chronic myelogenous leukemia and benzene exposure: A systematic review and meta-analysis of the case-control literature. *Chem Biol Interact* 182:93, 2009.

27. Khalade A, Jaakkola MS, Pukkala E, Jaakkola JJ: Exposure to benzene at work and the risk of leukemia: A systematic review and meta-analysis. *Environ Health* 9:31, 2010.

28. Whang-Peng J, Knutsen T: Chromosomal abnormalities, in *Chronic Granulocytic Leukaemia*, edited by Shaw MT, p 49. Praeger, East Sussex, UK, 1982.

29. Spiers ASD, Bain BJ, Turner JE: The peripheral blood in chronic granulocytic leukemia: A study of 50 untreated Philadelphia positive cases. *Scand J Haematol* 18:25, 1977.

30. Sandberg AA: The leukemias: The Philadelphia chromosome, in *The Chromosomes in Human Cancer and Leukemia*, 2nd ed, p 183. Elsevier, New York, 1990.

31. Fialkow PJ, Garther SM, Yoshida A: Clonal origin of chronic myelocytic leukemia in men. *Proc Natl Acad Sci U S A* 58:1468, 1967.

32. Fialkow PJ, Jacobsen RJ, Papayannopoulou T: Chronic myelocytic leukemia: Clonal origin in a stem cell common to granulocyte, erythrocyte, platelet, and monocyte/macrophage. *Am J Med* 63:125, 1977.

33. Koeffler HP, Levine AM, Sparkes LM, Sparkes RS: Chronic myelocytic leukemia: Eosinophils involved in the malignant clone. *Blood* 55:1063, 1980.

34. Hayata I, Kakati S, Sandberg AA: On the monoclonal origin of chronic myelocytic leukemia. *Proc Jpn Acad* 30:351, 1974.

35. Lawler SD, O'Malley F, Lobb DS: Chromosome banding studies in Philadelphia chromosome positive myeloid leukemia. *Scand J Haematol* 17:17, 1976.

36. Harrison CJ, Chang J, Johnson D, et al: Chromosomal evidence of a common stem cell in acute lymphoblastic leukemia and chronic granulocytic leukemia. *Cancer Genet Cytogenet* 13:331, 1984.

37. Chaganti RS, Bailey RB, Jhanwar SC, et al: Chronic myelogenous leukemia in the monosomic cell line of a fertile Turner syndrome mosaic (45, X/46, XX). *Cancer Genet Cytogenet* 5:215, 1982.

38. Fitzgerald PH, Pickering AF, Eiby JR: Clonal origin of the Philadelphia chromosome and chronic leukemia. *Br J Haematol* 21:473, 1971.

39. Groffen J, Stephenson JR, Heisterkamp N, et al: Philadelphia chromosomal breakpoints are clustered within a limited region, bcr, on chromosome 22. *Cell* 36:93, 1984.

40. Leibowitz D, Schaefer-Rego K, Popenoe DW, et al: Variable breakpoints on the Philadelphia chromosome in chronic myelogenous leukemia. *Blood* 66:243, 1985.

41. Yoffe G, Chinault AG, Talpaz M, et al: Clonal nature of Philadelphia chromosome positive and negative chronic myelogenous leukemia by DNA hybridization analysis. *Exp Hematol* 15:725, 1987.

42. Savona M, Talpaz M: Getting to the stem of chronic myeloid leukaemia. *Nat Rev Cancer* 8:341, 2008.

43. Janssen JJ, Schuurhuis GJ, Terwijn M, Ossenkoppele GJ: Towards cure of CML: Why we need to know more about CML stem cells? *Curr Stem Cell Res Ther* 4:224, 2009.

44. Goff DJ, Recart AC, Sadarangani A, et al: A pan-BCL1 inhibitor renders bone marrow resident human leukemia stem cells sensitive to tyrosine kinase inhibition. *Cell Stem Cell* 12:316, 2013.

45. Zhang B, Li M, McDonald T, et al: Microenvironmental protection of CML stem and progenitor cells from tyrosine kinase inhibitors through N-cadherin and Wnt-β-catenin signaling. *Blood* 121:1824, 2013.

46. Radich JP, Dai H, Mao M, et al: Gene expression changes associated with progression and response in chronic myeloid leukemia. *Proc Natl Acad Sci U S A* 103:2794, 2006.

47. Fialkow PJ, Denman AM, Jacobsen RJ, Lowenthal MN: Chronic myelocytic leukemia. Origin of some lymphocytes from leukemic stem cells. *J Clin Invest* 62:815, 1978.

48. Martin PJ, Najfeld V, Hansen JA, et al: Involvement of the B-lymphoid system in chronic myelogenous leukemia. *Nature* 287:49, 1980.

49. Boggs DR: Hematopoietic stem cell theory in relation to possible lymphoblastic conversion in chronic myeloid leukemia. *Blood* 44:449, 1974.

50. Bernheim A, Berger R, Preud'homme JL, et al: Philadelphia chromosome positive blood B lymphocytes in chronic myelocytic leukemia. *Leuk Res* 5:331, 1981.

51. Collins S, Coleman H, Groudine M: Expression of bcr and bcr-abl fusion transcripts in normal and leukemic cells. *Mol Cell Biol* 7:2870, 1987.

52. Al-Amin A, Lennartz K, Runde V, et al: Frequency of clonal B lymphocytes in chronic myelogenous leukemia evaluated by fluorescence in situ hybridization. *Cancer Genet Cytogenet* 104:45, 1998.

53. Torlakovic E, Litz CE, McClure JS, Brunning RD: Direct detection of the Philadelphia chromosome in CD20-positive lymphocytes in chronic myelogenous leukemia by tricolor immunophenotyping/FISH. *Leukemia* 8:1940, 1994.

54. Kearney L, Orchard KH, Hibbin JA, Goldman JM: T-cell cytogenetics in chronic granulocytic leukaemia. *Lancet* 1:858, 1981.

55. Nogueira-Costa R, Spitzer G, Cock A, Trijillo JM: E rosette-positive agar colonies containing the Philadelphia chromosome in chronic myeloid leukemia. *Scand J Haematol* 34:184, 1985.

56. Bartram CR, Raghavachar A, Anger B, et al: T lymphocytes lack rearrangement of the bcr gene in Philadelphia chromosome-positive chronic myelogenous leukemia. *Blood* 69:1682, 1985.

57. Fauser AA, Kanz L, Bross KJ, et al: T cells and probably B cells arise from the malignant clone in chronic myelogenous leukemia. *J Clin Invest* 75:1080, 1985.

58. Nitta M, Kato Y, Strife A, et al: Incidence of the B and T lymphocyte lineages in chronic myelogenous leukemia. *Blood* 66:1053, 1985.

59. Ariad S, Dajee D, Willem P, Bezwoda WR: Lack of involvement of T-lymphocytes in the leukaemic population during prolonged chronic phase of Philadelphia chromosome positive chronic myeloid leukaemia. *Leuk Lymphoma* 10:217, 1993.

60. Tsukamoto N, Karasawa M, Maehara T, et al: The majority of T lymphocytes are polyclonal during the chronic phase of chronic myelogenous leukemia. *Ann Hematol* 72:61, 1996.

61. Garicochea B, Chase A, Lazaridou A, Goldman JM: T lymphocytes in chronic myelogenous leukaemia (CML). *Leukemia* 8:1197, 1994.

62. Jonas D, Lubbert M, Kawasaki ES, et al: Clonal analysis of bcr-abl rearrangement in T lymphocytes from patients in the chronic myelogenous leukemia. *Blood* 79:1017, 1992.

63. Haferlach T, Winkemann M, Nickening C, et al: Which components are involved in Philadelphia-chromosome-positive chronic leukemia? *Br J Haematol* 97:99, 1997.

64. Verfaillie C, Miller W, Kay N, McClave P: Adherent lymphokine-activated killer cells in chronic myelogenous leukemia: A benign cell population with potent cytotoxic activity. *Blood* 74:793, 1989.

65. Takahashi N, Miura I, Saitoh K, Miura AB: Lineage involvement of stem cells bearing the Philadelphia chromosome in chronic myeloid leukemia in the chronic phase as shown by a combination of fluorescence-activated cell sorting and fluorescence in situ hybridization. *Blood* 92:4758, 1998.

66. Muñoz L, Bellido M, Sierra J, Nomdedéu JF: Flow cytometric detection of B cell abnormal maturation in chronic myeloid leukemia. *Leukemia* 14:339, 2000.

67. Miura A: Progress in laboratory medicine in chronic myeloid leukemia. *Rinsho Byori* 46:1226, 1998.

68. Kovacic B, Hoelbl A, Litos G, et al: Diverging fates of cells of origin in acute and chronic leukaemia. *EMBO Mol Med* 4:283, 2012.

69. Gunsilius E, Duba H-C, Petzer AL, et al: Evidence from a leukaemia model for maintenance of vascular endothelium by bone-marrow-derived endothelial cells. *Lancet* 355:1688, 2000.

70. Fialkow PJ, Martin PJ, Najfeld V, et al: Evidence for a multistep pathogenesis of chronic myelogenous leukemia. *Blood* 58:158, 1981.

71. Lisker R, Casas L, Mutchinick O, et al: Late-appearing Philadelphia chromosome in two patients with chronic myelogenous leukemia. *Blood* 56:812, 1980.

72. Kamada N, Uchino H: Chronologic sequence in appearance of clinical and laboratory findings characteristic of chronic myelogenous leukemia. *Blood* 51:843, 1978.

73. Smadja N, Krulik M, DeGramont A, et al: Acquisition of a Philadelphia chromosome concomitant with transformation of a refractory anemia into an acute leukemia. *Cancer* 55:1477, 1985.

74. Fegan C, Morgan G, Whittaker JA: Spontaneous remission in a patient with chronic myeloid leukaemia. *Br J Haematol* 72:594, 1989.

75. Brandt L, Mitelman F, Panani A, Lenner HC: Extremely long duration of chronic myeloid leukaemia with Ph1 negative and Ph1 positive bone marrow cells. *Scand J Haematol* 16:321, 1976.

76. Hagemeijer A, Smith EME, Lowenberg B, Abels J: Chronic myeloid leukemia with permanent disappearance of the Ph1 chromosome and development of new clonal subpopulations. *Blood* 53:1, 1979.

77. Singer JN, Arlin ZA, Najfeld V, et al: Restoration of nonclonal hematopoiesis in chronic myelogenous leukemia (CML) following a chemotherapy induced loss of the Ph1 chromosome. *Blood* 56:356, 1980.

78. Sokal JE: Significance of Ph1-negative marrow cells in Ph1-positive chronic granulocytic leukemia. *Blood* 56:1072, 1980.

79. Smadja N, Krulik M, Audebert AA, et al: Spontaneous regression of cytogenetic and haematologic anomalies in Ph1-positive chronic myelogenous leukaemia. *Br J Haematol* 63:257, 1986.

80. Goldman JM, Kearney L, Pittman S, et al: Hemopoietic stem cell grafting for chronic granulocytic leukemia. *Exp Hematol* 10:76, 1982.

81. Reiffers J, Vezon G, David B, et al: Philadelphia negative cells in a patient treated with autografting for Ph1 positive chronic granulocytic leukaemia in transformation. *Br J Haematol* 55:382, 1983.

82. Reiffers J, Broustet A, Goldman JM: Philadelphia chromosome-negative progenitors in chronic granulocytic leukemia. *N Engl J Med* 309:1460, 1983.

83. Coulombel L, Kalousek DK, Eaves CJ, et al: Long-term marrow culture reveals chromosomally normal hemopoietic progenitor cells in patients with Philadelphia chromosome-positive chronic myelogenous leukemia. *N Engl J Med* 308:1493, 1983.

84. Degliantoni G, Mangori L, Rizzoli V: *In vitro* restoration of polyclonal hematopoiesis in a chronic myelogenous leukemia after *in vitro* treatment with 4-hydroperoxy-cyclophosphamide. *Blood* 65:753, 1985.

85. Barnett MJ, Eaves CJ, Phillips GL, et al: Successful autografting in chronic myeloid leukemia after maintenance of marrow in culture. *Bone Marrow Transplant* 4:345, 1989.

86. Verfaillie CM, Miller WJ, Boylan K, McGlave PB: Selection of benign primitive hematopoietic progenitors in chronic myelogenous leukemia on the basis of HLA-DR antigen expression. *Blood* 79:1003, 1992.

87. Leemhuis T, Leibowitz D, Cox G, et al: Identification of BCR/ABL-negative primitive hematopoietic progenitor cells within chronic myeloid leukemia marrow. *Blood* 81:801, 1993.

88. Wang JCY, Lapidot T, Cashman JD, et al: High level engraftment of NOD/SCID mice by primitive normal and leukemic hemopoietic cells from patients with chronic myeloid leukemia in chronic phase. *Blood* 91:2406, 1998.

89. Dunbar CE, Stewart FM: Separating the wheat from the chaff: Selection of benign hematopoietic cells in chronic myeloid leukemia. *Blood* 79:1107, 1992.

90. Strife A, Clarkson B: Biology of chronic myelogenous leukemia: Is discordant maturation the primary defect? *Semin Hematol* 25:1, 1988.

91. Heinzinger M, Waller CF, Rosentiel A, et al: Quality of IL-3 and G-CSF-mobilized peripheral blood stem cells in patients with early chronic phase CML. *Leukemia* 12:333, 1998.

92. Verfaillie CM, Bhatia R, Miller W, et al: BCR/ABL-negative primitive progenitors suitable for transplantation can be selected from the marrow of most early-chronic phase but not accelerated-phase chronic myelogenous leukemia patients. *Blood* 87:4770, 1996.

93. Grand FH, Marley SB, Chase A, et al: BCR/ABL-negative progenitors are enriched in the adherent fraction of CD34+ cells circulating in the blood of chronic phase chronic myeloid leukemia patients. *Leukemia* 11:1486, 1997.

94. Carella AM, Podesta M, Frassoni R, et al: Collection of "normal" blood repopulating cells during early hemopoietic recovery after intensive conventional chemotherapy in chronic myelogenous leukemia. *Bone Marrow Transplant* 12:267, 1993.

95. Guyootat D, Wahabi K, Viallet A, et al: Selection of BCR/ABL-negative stem cells from marrow or blood of patients with chronic myeloid leukemia. *Leukemia* 13:991, 1999.

96. Hogge DE, Coulumbel L, Kalousek D, et al: Nonclonal hemopoietic progenitors in a G6PD heterozygote with chronic myelogenous leukemia revealed after long-term marrow culture. *Am J Hematol* 24:389, 1987.

97. Delforge M, Boogaerts MA, McGlave PB, Verfaillie CM: BCR/ABL-CD34+HLA-DR− progenitor cells in early phase, but not in more advanced phases, of chronic myelogenous leukemia are polyclonal. *Blood* 93:284, 1999.

98. Van den Berg D, Wessman M, Murray L, et al: Leukemic burden in subpopulations of CD34+ cells isolated from the mobilized peripheral blood of alpha-interferon-resistant or -intolerant patients with chronic myeloid leukemia. *Blood* 87:4348, 1996.

99. Podesta M, Piaggio G, Frassoni F, et al: Very primitive hemopoietic cells (LTC-IC) are present in Philadelphia negative cytaphereses collected during early recovery after chemotherapy for chronic myeloid leukemia (CML). *Bone Marrow Transplant* 16:549, 1995.

100. Kirk JA, Reems JA, Roecklein BA, et al: Benign marrow progenitors are enriched in the CD34+/HLA-DRlo population but not in the CD34+/CD38lo population in chronic myeloid leukemia: An analysis using interphase fluorescence *in situ* hybridization. *Blood* 86:737, 1995.

101. Lewis ID, Haylock DN, Moore S, et al: Peripheral blood is a source of BCR-ABL–negative pre-progenitors in early chronic phase chronic myeloid leukemia. *Leukemia* 11:581, 1997.

102. Maguer-Satta V, Petzer AL, Eaves AC, Eaves CJ: BCR-ABL expression in different subpopulations of functionally characterized Ph+ CD34+ cells from patients with chronic myeloid leukemia. *Blood* 88:1796, 1996.

103. Sirard C, Lapidot T, Vormoor J, et al: Normal and leukemia SCID-repopulating cells (SRC) coexist in the bone marrow and peripheral blood from CML patients in chronic phase, whereas leukemic SRC are detected in blast crisis. *Blood* 87:1539, 1996.

104. Dazzi F, Capelli D, Hasserjian R, et al: The kinetics and extent of engraftment of chronic myelogenous leukemia cells in nonobese diabetic/severe combined immunodeficiency mice reflect the phase of the donor's disease: An *in vivo* model for chronic myelogenous leukemia biology. *Blood* 92:1390, 1998.

105. Holyoake TL, Jiang X, Drummond MW, et al: Elucidating critical mechanisms of deregulated stem cell turnover in the chronic phase of chronic myelogenous leukemia. *Leukemia* 16:549, 2002.

106. Eaves C, Cashman J, Eaves A: Defective regulation of leukemic hematopoiesis in chronic myeloid leukemia. *Leuk Res* 22:1085, 1998.

107. Clarkson BD, Strife A, Wisniewski D, et al: New understanding of the pathogenesis of CML: A prototype of early neoplasia. *Leukemia* 11:1404, 1997.

108. Bedi A, Zehnbauer BA, Collector MI, et al: BCR-ABL gene rearrangement and expression of primitive hematopoietic progenitors in chronic myeloid leukemia. *Blood* 81:2898, 1993.

109. Moore MA: *In vitro* culture studies in chronic granulocytic leukaemia. *Clin Haematol* 6:97, 1977.

110. Sjögren U, Brandt L: Composition and mitotic activity of the erythropoietic part of the bone marrow in chronic myeloid leukaemia. *Scand J Haematol* 12:18, 1974.

111. Verfaillie CM: Stem cells in chronic myelogenous leukemia. *Hematol Oncol Clin North Am* 11:1079, 1997.

112. Ghaffari S, Dougherty GJ, Lansdorp PM, et al: Differentiation-associated changes in CD44 isoform expression during normal hematopoiesis and their alteration in chronic myeloid leukemia. *Blood* 86:2976, 1995.

113. Kawaishi K, Kimura A, Katch O, et al: Decreased L-selectin expression in CD34-positive cells from patients with chronic myelocytic leukaemia. *Br J Haematol* 93:367, 1996.

114. Turkina AG, Baryshnikov AY, Sedyakhina NP, et al: Studies of P-glycoprotein in chronic myeloid leukaemia patients: Expression, activity and correlations with CD34 antigen. *Br J Haematol* 92:88, 1996.

115. Agarwal R, Doren S, Hicks B, Dunbar CE: Long-term culture of chronic myelogenous leukemia marrow cells on stem cell factor-deficient stroma favors benign progenitors. *Blood* 85:1306, 1995.

116. Moore S, Haylock DN, Lévesque JP, et al: Stem cell factor as a single agent induces selective proliferation of the Philadelphia chromosome positive fraction of chronic myeloid leukemia CD34+ cells. *Blood* 92:2461, 1998.

117. Chasty RC, Lucas GS, Owen-Lynch PJ, et al: Macrophage inflammatory protein-1 alpha receptors are present on cells enriched for CD34 expression from patients with chronic myeloid leukemia. *Blood* 86:4270, 1995.

118. Cashman JD, Eaves CJ, Sarris AH, Eaves AC: MCP-1, not MIP-1α, is the endogenous chemokine that cooperates with TGF-β to inhibit the cycling of primitive normal but not leukemic (CML) progenitors in long-term human marrow cultures. *Blood* 92:2338, 1998.

119. Murohashi I, Endho K, Nishida S, et al: Differential effects of TGF-beta 1 on normal and leukemic human hematopoietic cell proliferation. *Exp Hematol* 23:970, 1995.

120. Gordon MY, Dowding C, Riley G, et al: Altered adhesive interactions with marrow stroma of haematopoietic progenitor cells in chronic myeloid leukaemia. *Nature* 328:342, 1987.

121. Bhatia R, Wayner EA, McGlave PB, Verfaillie CM: Interferon-α restores normal adhesion of chronic myelogenous leukemia hematopoietic progenitors to bone marrow stroma by correcting impaired β1 integrin receptor function. *J Clin Invest* 94:384, 1994.

122. Verfaillie CM: Stem cells in chronic myelogenous leukemia. *Hematol Oncol Clin North Am* 11:1079, 1997.

123. Bhatia R, Munthe HA, Verfaillie CM: Tyrphostin AG957, a tyrosine kinase inhibitor with anti-BCR/ABL tyrosine activity restores β₁ integrin-mediated adhesion and inhibiting signaling in chronic myelogenous leukemia hematopoietic progenitors. *Leukemia* 12:1708, 1998.

124. Lundell BI, McCarthy JB, Kovach NL, Verfaillie CM: Activation of beta 1 integrins on CML progenitors reveals cooperation between beta1 integrins and CD44 in the regulation of adhesion and proliferation. *Leukemia* 11:822, 1997.

125. Vijayan KV, Advani SH, Zingde SM: Chronic myeloid leukemic granulocytes exhibit reduced and altered binding to P-selectin; modification in the CD15 antigens and sialylation. *Leuk Res* 21:59, 1997.

126. Deininger MW, Vieira S, Mendiola R, et al: BCR-ABL tyrosine kinase activity regulates the expression of multiple genes implicated in the pathogenesis of chronic myeloid leukemia. *Cancer Res* 60:2049, 2000.

127. Verfaillie CM, Hurley R, Lundell BI, et al: Integrin-mediated regulation of hematopoiesis: Do BCR/ABL-induced defects in integrin function underlie the abnormal circulation and proliferation of CML progenitors? *Acta Haematol* 29:40, 1997.

128. Symington BE: Growth signalling through the alpha 5 beta 1 fibronectin receptor. *Biochem Biophys Res Commun* 208:126, 1995.

129. Bhatia R, McCarthy JB, Verfaillie CM: Interferon-alpha restores normal beta 1 integrin-mediated inhibition of hematopoietic progenitor proliferation by the marrow microenvironment in chronic myelogenous leukemia. *Blood* 87:3883, 1996.

130. Wertheim JA, Forsythe K, Druker BJ, et al: BCR-ABL-induced adhesion defects are tyrosine kinase-independent. *Blood* 99:4122, 2002.

131. Fruehauf S, Topaly J, Schad M, Paschka P, et al: Imatinib restores expression of CD62L in BCR-ABL-positive cells. *J Leukoc Biol* 73:600, 2003.

132. Salgia R, Li JL, Ewaniuk DS, et al: BCR/ABL induces multiple abnormalities of cytoskeletal function. *J Clin Invest* 100:46, 1997.

133. Lewis JM, Baskaran R, Taagepera S, et al: Integrin regulation of c-ABL tyrosine kinase activity and cytoplasmic-nuclear transport. *Proc Natl Acad Sci U S A* 93:15174, 1996.

134. Renshaw MW, McWhirter JR, Wang JY: The human leukemia oncogene bcr-abl abrogates the anchorage requirement but not the growth factor requirement for proliferation. *Mol Cell Biol* 15:1286, 1995.

135. Salgia R, Brunkhorst B, Pisick E, et al: Increased tyrosine phosphorylation of focal adhesion proteins in myeloid cell lines expressing p210BCR/ABL. *Oncogene* 11:1149, 1995.

136. Rudkin GT, Hungerford DA, Nowell PC: DNA content of chromosome Ph1 and chromosome 21 in human chronic granulocytic leukemia. *Science* 144:1229, 1964.

137. O'Riordan ML, Robinson JA, Buckton KE, Evans HJ: Distinguishing between the chromosome involved in Down's syndrome (trisomy 21) and chronic myeloid leukaemia (Ph1) by fluorescence. *Nature* 230:167, 1971.

138. Lawler SD: The cytogenetics of chronic granulocytic leukaemia. *Clin Haematol* 6:55, 1977.

139. Melo JV, Yan XH, Diamond J, Goldman JM: Balanced parental contribution to the ABL component of the BCR-ABL gene in chronic myeloid leukemia. *Leukemia* 9:734, 1995.

140. Chissoe SL, Bodenteich A, Wang YF, et al: Sequence and analysis of the human ABL gene, the BCR gene, and regions involved in the Philadelphia chromosomal translocation. *Genomics* 27:67, 1995.

141. Melo JV, Deininger MW: Biology of chronic myelogenous leukemia-signaling pathways of initiation and transformation. *Hematol Oncol Clin North Am* 18:545, 2004.

142. Daley GQ, Ben-Neriah Y: Implicating the bcr/abl gene in the pathogenesis of Philadelphia chromosome-positive human leukemia. *Adv Cancer Res* 57:151, 1991.

143. Heisterkamp N, Groffen J, Stephenson JR, et al: Chromosomal localization of human cellular homologues of two viral oncogenes. *Nature* 299:747, 1982.

144. Heisterkamp N, Stephenson JR, Groffen J, et al: Localization of the c-abl oncogene adjacent to a translocation breakpoint in chronic myelocytic leukemia. *Nature* 306:239, 1983.

145. Konopka JB, Witte ON: Activation of the abl oncogene in murine and human leukemias. *Biochim Biophys Acta* 823:1, 1985.

146. Collins SJ, Groudine MT: Rearrangements and amplification of c-abl sequences in the human chronic myelogenous leukemia cell line K562. *Proc Natl Acad Sci U S A* 80:4813, 1983.

147. Canaani E, Gale RP, Steiner-Seltz D, et al: Altered transcription of an oncogene in chronic myelocytic leukemia. *Lancet* 1:593, 1984.

148. Gale RP, Canaani E: An 8 kilobase abl RNA transcript in chronic myelogenous leukemia. *Proc Natl Acad Sci U S A* 81:5648, 1984.

149. Collins SJ, Kubonishi I, Miyoshi I, Groudine MT: Altered transcription of the c-abl oncogene in K562 and other chronic myelogenous leukemia cells. *Science* 225:72, 1984.

150. Leibowitz D, Cubbon RM, Bank A: Increased expression of a novel c-abl related RNA in K562 cells. *Blood* 65:526, 1985.

151. Konopka JB, Watanabe SM, Witte ON: An alteration of the human c-abl protein in K562 leukemia cells unmasks associated tyrosine kinase activity. *Cell* 37:1035, 1984.

152. Konopka JB, Watanabe SM, Singer JW, et al: Cell lines and clinical isolates derived from Ph1-positive chronic myelogenous leukemia patients express c-abl proteins with a common structural alteration. *Proc Natl Acad Sci U S A* 82:1810, 1985.

153. Stam K, Heisterkamp N, Grosveld G, et al: Evidence of a new chimeric bcr/c-abl mRNA in patients with chronic myelocytic leukemia and the Philadelphia chromosome. *N Engl J Med* 313:1429, 1985.

154. Ben-Neriah Y, Daley GQ, Mes-Masson AM, et al: The chronic myelogenous leukemia-specific P210 protein is the product of the bcr/abl hybrid gene. *Science* 233:212, 1985.

155. Maxwell SA, Kurzrock R, Parson SJ, et al: Analysis of P210bcr/abl tyrosine protein kinase activity in various subtypes of Philadelphia chromosome-positive cells from chronic myelogenous leukemia patients. *Cancer Res* 47:1731, 1987.

157. Xu DQ, Galibert F: Restriction fragment length polymorphism caused by a deletion within the human c-abl gene (ABL). *Proc Natl Acad Sci U S A* 83:3447, 1986.

158. Popenoe DW, Schaefer-Rego K, Mears JC, et al: Frequent and extensive deletion during the 9,22 translocation in CML. *Blood* 68:1123, 1986.

159. Shtivelman E, Gale RP, Dreazen O, et al: Bcr-abl RNA in patients with chronic granulocytic leukemia. *Blood* 69:971, 1987.

160. McWhirter JR, Wang JJ: Activation of tyrosine kinase and microfilament-binding functions of *c-abl* by *bcr* sequences in *bcr/abl* fusion proteins. *Mol Cell Biol* 11:1553, 1991.

161. Bernards A, Rubin CM, Westbrook CA, et al: The first intron in the human c-abl gene is at least 200 kilobases long and is the target for translocations in chronic myelogenous leukemia. *Mol Cell Biol* 7:3231, 1987.

162. Eisenberg A, Silver R, Soper L, et al: The location of breakpoints within the breakpoint cluster region (bcr) of chromosome 22 in chronic myeloid leukemia. *Leukemia* 2:642, 1988.

163. Collins SJ: Breakpoints on chromosomes 9 and 22 in Philadelphia chromosome-positive chronic myelogenous leukemia. *J Clin Invest* 78:1392, 1986.

164. Heisterkamp N, Stam K, Groffen J, et al: Structural organization of the bcr gene and its role in the Ph1 translocation. *Nature* 315:758, 1985.

165. Gao LM, Goldman J: Long-range mapping of the normal BCR gene. *Leukemia* 5:555, 1991.

166. Melo JV: BCR-ABL gene variants. *Baillieres Clin Haematol* 10:203, 1997.

167. Saglio G, Pane F, Gottardi E, et al: Consistent amounts of acute leukemia-associated P190BCR/ABL transcripts are expressed by chronic myelogenous leukemia patients at diagnosis. *Blood* 87:1075, 1996.

168. Honda H, Oda H, Suzuki T, et al: Development of acute lymphoblastic leukemia and myeloproliferative disorder in transgenic mice expressing p210bcr/abl: A novel transgenic model for human Ph1-positive leukemias. *Blood* 91:2067, 1998.

169. Maru Y, Witte ON: The BCR gene encodes a novel serine/threonine kinase activity within a single exon. *Cell* 67:459, 1991.

170. Muller AJ, Young JC, Pendergast A-M, et al: BCR first exon sequences specifically activate the BCR/ABL tyrosine kinase oncogene of Philadelphia chromosome-positive human leukemia. *Mol Cell Biol* 11:1785, 1991.

171. Diekmann D, Brill S, Garrett MD, et al: BCR encodes a GTPase-activating protein for p21rac. *Nature* 351:400, 1991.

172. Melo JV, Gordon DE, Goldman JM: The ABL-BCR fusion gene is expressed in chronic myeloid leukemia. *Blood* 81:158, 1993.

173. Bartram CR, de Klein A, Hagemeijer A, et al: Translocation of the human c-abl oncogene correlates with the presence of a Philadelphia chromosome in chronic myelocytic leukaemia. *Nature* 306;277, 1983.

174. Selleri L, Narni F, Emilia G, et al: Philadelphia-positive chronic myeloid leukemia with a chromosome 22 breakpoint outside the breakpoint cluster region. *Blood* 70:1659, 1987.

175. Mohamed AN, Koppitch F, Varterasian M, et al: BCR/ABL fusion located on chromosome 9 in chronic myeloid leukemia with a masked Ph chromosome. *Genes Chromosomes Cancer* 13:133, 1995.

176. Morris C, Jeffs A, Smith T, et al: BCR gene recombines with genomically distinct sites on band 11Q13 in complex BCR-ABL translocations of chronic myeloid leukemia. *Oncogene* 12:677, 1996.

177. Andreasson P, Johansson B, Carlsson M, et al: BCR/ABL-negative chronic myeloid leukemia with ETV6/ABL fusion. *Genes Chromosomes Cancer* 20:299, 1997.

178. Rozman C, Urbano-Ispizua A, Cervantes F, et al: Analysis of the clinical relevance of the breakpoint location within M-BCR and the type of chimeric mRNA in chronic myelogenous leukemia. *Leukemia* 9:1104, 1995.

179. Verschraegen CF, Kantarjian HM, Hirsch-Ginsberg C, et al: The breakpoint cluster region site in patients with Philadelphia chromosome-positive chronic myelogenous leukemia. Clinical, laboratory, and prognostic correlations. *Cancer* 76:992, 1995.

180. Zaccaria A, Martinelli G, Testoni N, et al: Does the type of BCR/ABL junction predict the survival of patients with Ph1-positive chronic myeloid leukemia? *Leuk Lymphoma* 16:231, 1995.

181. Ohno T, Hada S, Sugiyama T, et al: Chronic myeloid leukemia with minor bcr breakpoint developed hybrid type of blast crisis. *Am J Hematol* 57:320, 1998.

182. Melo JV: The diversity of BCR-ABL fusion proteins and their relationship to leukemia phenotype. *Blood* 88:2375, 1996.

183. Rubinstein R, Purves LR: A novel BCR-ABL rearrangement in a Philadelphia chromosome-positive chronic myelogenous leukaemia variant with thrombocythaemia. *Leukemia* 12:230, 1998.

184. Hochhaus A, Reither A, Skladny H, et al: A novel BCR-ABL fusion gene (e6a2) in a patient with Philadelphia chromosome-negative chronic myelogenous leukemia. *Blood* 88:2236, 1996.

185. Briz M, Vilches C, Cabrera R, et al: Typical chronic myelogenous leukemia with e19a2 junction BCR/ABL transcript. *Blood* 90:5024, 1997.

186. McLaughlin J, Chianese E, Witte ON: *In vitro* transformation of immature hemopoietic cells by P210 bcr/abl oncogene product of the Philadelphia chromosome. *Proc Natl Acad Sci U S A* 84:6558, 1987.

187. Daley GQ, McLaughlin J, Witte ON, Baltimore D: The CML-specific P210 bcr/abl protein, unlike v-abl, does not transform NIH/3T3 fibroblasts. *Science* 237:532, 1987.

188. Elefanty AG, Hariharan IK, Cory S: Bcr-abl, the hallmark of chronic myeloid leukaemia in man, induces multiple haemopoietic neoplasms in mice. *EMBO J* 9:1069, 1990.

189. Daley GQ, Van Etten RA, Baltimore D: Induction of chronic myelogenous leukemia in mice by the p210bcr/abl gene of the Philadelphia chromosome. *Science* 247:824, 1990.

190. Voncken JW, Morris C, Pattengale P, et al: Clonal development and karyotype evolution during leukemogenesis of BCR/ABL transgenic mice. *Blood* 79:1029, 1992.

191. Gishizky ML, Johnson-White J, Witte O: Efficient transplantation of BCR-ABL-induced chronic myelogenous leukemia-like syndrome in mice. *Proc Natl Acad Sci U S A* 90:3755, 1993.

192. Daley GQ: Animal models of BCR/ABL-induced leukemias. *Leuk Lymphoma* 11:57, 1993.

193. Voncken JW, Kaartinen V, Pattengale PK, et al: BCR/ABL P210 and P190 cause distinct leukemia in transgenic mice. *Blood* 86:4603, 1995.

194. Honda H, Oda H, Suzuki T, et al: Development of acute lymphoblastic leukemia and myeloproliferative disorder in transgenic mice expressing p210bcr/abl: A novel transgenic model for human Ph 1-positive leukemias. *Blood* 91:2067, 1998.

195. Pear WS, Miller JP, Xu L, et al: Efficient and rapid induction of a chronic myelogenous leukemia-like myeloproliferative disease in mice receiving P210 bcr/abl-transduced bone marrow. *Blood* 92:3780, 1998.

196. Honda M, Ohno S, Takahashi T, et al: Establishment, characterization, and chromosomal analysis of new leukemic cell lines derived from MT/p210/bcr/abl transgenic mice. *Exp Hematol* 26:188, 1998.

197. Zhang X, Ren R: Bcr-Abl efficiency induces in a myeloproliferative disease and production of excess interleukin-3 and granulocyte-macrophage colony-stimulating factor in mice: A novel model for chronic myelogenous leukemia. *Blood* 92:3829, 1998.

198. Elefanty AG, Corsy S: Bcr-abl-induced cell lines can switch from mast cell to erythroid or myeloid differentiation *in vitro*. *Blood* 79:1271, 1992.

199. Van Etten RA: Pathogenesis and treatment of Ph+ leukemia: Recent insights from mouse models. *Curr Opin Hematol* 8:224, 2001.

200. Bose S, Deininger M, Goora-Tybor J, et al: The presence of typical and atypical BCR-ABL fusion genes in leukocytes of normal individuals: Biological significance and implications for the assessment of minimal residual disease. *Blood* 92:3362, 1998.

201. Hirai HS, Tanaka M, Azuma Y, et al: Transforming genes in human leukemia cells. *Blood* 66:1371, 1985.

202. Clarkson BD, Strife A, Wisniewski D, et al: New understanding of the pathogenesis of CML: A prototype of early neoplasia. *Leukemia* 11:1404, 1997.

203. Verfaillie CM: Chronic myelogenous leukemia: From pathogenesis to therapy. *J Hematother* 8:3, 1999.

204. Pasternak G, Hochhaus A, Schultheis B, Hehlmann R: Chronic myelogenous leukemia: Molecular and cellular aspects. *J Cancer Res Clin Oncol* 124:643, 1998.

205. Gotoh A, Broxmeyer HE: The function of BCR/ABL and related protooncogenes. *Curr Opin Hematol* 4:3, 1997.

206. Sattler M, Salgia R: Activation of hematopoietic growth factor signal transduction pathways by the human oncogene BCR/ABL. *Cytokine Growth Factor Rev* 8:63, 1997.

207. Skorski T, Kanakaraj P, Nieborowska-Skorska M, et al: Phosphatidylinositol-3 kinase activity is regulated by BCR/ABL and is required for the growth of Philadelphia chromosome-positive cells. *Blood* 86:726, 1995.

208. Skorski T, Nieborowska-Skorska M, Szczylik C, et al: C-RAF-1 serine/threonine kinase is required in BCR/ABL-dependent and normal hematopoiesis. *Cancer Res* 55:2275, 1995.

209. Goga A, McLaughlin J, Afar DE, et al: Alternative signals to RAS for hematopoietic transformation by the BCR-ABL oncogene. *Cell* 82:981, 1995.

210. Salgia R, Uemura N, Okuda K, et al: CRKL links p210BCR/ABL with paxillin in chronic myelogenous leukemia cells. *J Biol Chem* 270:29145, 1995.

211. De Jong R, ten Hoeve J, Heisterkamp N, Groffen J: Crkl is complexed with tyrosine-phosphorylated Cbl in Ph-positive leukemia. *J Biol Chem* 270:21468, 1995.

212. Salgia R, Pisick E, Sattler M, et al: P130CAS forms a signalling complex with the adapter protein CRKL in hematopoietic cells transformed by the BCR/ABL oncogene. *J Biol Chem* 271:25198, 1996.

213. Sattler M, Griffin JD: Molecular mechanisms of transformation by the *BCR-ABL* oncogene. *Semin Hematol* 40:4, 2003.

214. Melo JV, Deininger MW: Biology of chronic myelogenous-signaling pathways of initiation and transformation. *Hematol Oncol Clin North Am* 18:545, 2004.

215. Wong S, Witte ON: The BCR-ABL story: Bench to bedside and back. *Annu Rev Immunol* 22:247, 2004.

216. Sattler M, Verma S, Shrinkhande G, et al: The BCR/ABL tyrosine kinase induces production of reactive species in hematopoietic cells. *J Biol Chem* 275:24273, 2000.
217. Sattler M, Salgia R, Okuda K, et al: The proto-oncogene product p120CBL and the adaptor proteins CRKL and c-CR link c-ABL, p190BCR/ABL and p210BCR/ABL to the phosphatidylinositol-3; kinase pathway. *Oncogene* 12:832, 1996.
218. Salgia R, Sattler M, Pisick E, et al: P210BCR/ABL induces formation of complexes containing focal adhesion proteins and the protooncogene product p120c-CBL. *Exp Hematol* 24:310, 1996.
219. De Jong R, van Wijk A, Haataja L, et al: BCR/ABL-induced leukemogenesis causes phosphorylation of Hef2 and its association with Crkl. *J Biol Chem* 272:32649, 1997.
220. Bollag G, Clapp DW, Shih S, et al: Loss of NF1 results in activation of the Ras signaling pathway and leads to aberrant growth in haematopoietic cells. *Nat Genet* 12:144, 1996.
221. Carpino N, Wisniewski D, Strife A, et al: P62dok: A constitutively tyrosine-phosphorylated, GAP-associated protein in chronic myelogenous leukemia progenitor cells. *Cell* 88:197, 1997.
222. Yamanashi Y, Baltimore D: Identification of the Abl- and ras GAP-associated 62 kDa protein as a docking protein, Dok. *Cell* 88:205, 1997.
223. Reuther JY, Reuther GW, Cortez D, et al: A requirement for NFkappaB activation in BCR/ABL-mediated transformation. *Genes Dev* 1:12:968, 1998.
224. LaMontagne KR, Flint AJ, Franza BR, et al: Protein tyrosine phosphatase 1B antagonizes signalling by oncoprotein tyrosine kinase p210 bcr/abl *in vivo*. *Mol Cell Biol* 18:2965, 1998.
225. Chai SK, Nichols GL, Rothman P: Constitutive activation of JAKs and STATs in BCR-abl-expressing cell lines and peripheral blood cells derived from leukemic patients. *J Immunol* 159:4720, 1997.
226. Shuai K, Halpern J, ten Hoeve J, et al: Constitutive activation of STAT5 by the BCR-ABL oncogene in chronic myelogenous leukemia. *Oncogene* 13:247, 1996.
227. Wilson-Rawls J, Xie S, Liu J, et al: P210 Bcr-Abl interacts with the interleukin 3 receptor beta (c) subunit and constitutively induces its tyrosine phosphorylation. *Cancer Res* 56:3426, 1996.
228. Chuang TH, Xu X, Kaartinen V, et al: Abl and Bcr are multifunctional regulators of the Rho GTP-binding protein family. *Proc Natl Acad Sci U S A* 92:10282, 1995.
229. Afar DE, Witte O: Characterization of breakpoint cluster region kinase and SH2-binding activities. *Methods Enzymol* 256:125, 1995.
230. Gishizky ML, Cortez D, Pendergast AM: Mutant forms of growth factor-binding protein-2 reverse BCR-ABL-induced transformation. *Proc Natl Acad Sci U S A* 92:10889, 1995.
231. Raitano AB, Halpern JR, Hambuch TM, Sawyers CL: The Bcr-Abl leukemia oncogene activates Jun kinase and requires Jun for transformation. *Proc Natl Acad Sci U S A* 92:11746, 1995.
232. Miyamura T, Nishimura J, Yufu Y, Nawata H: Interaction of BCR-ABL with the retinoblastoma protein in Philadelphia chromosome-positive cell lines. *Int J Hematol* 67:115, 1997.
233. Largaespada DA, Brannan CI, Jenkins NA, Copeland NG: NF1 deficiency causes Ras-mediated granulocyte/macrophage colony stimulating factor hypersensitivity and chronic myeloid leukaemia. *Nat Genet* 12:137, 1996.
234. Amos TA, Lewis JL, Grand FH, et al: Apoptosis in chronic myeloid leukaemia: Normal responses by progenitor cells to growth factor deprivation, X-irradiation and glucocorticoids. *Br J Haematol* 91:387, 1995.
235. Bedi A, Barber JP, Bedi GC, et al: BCR-ABL-mediated inhibition of apoptosis with delay of G2/M transition after DNA damage: A mechanism of resistance to multiple anticancer agents. *Blood* 86:1148, 1995.
236. Amarante-Mendes GP, Naekyung KC, Liu L, et al: Bcr-Abl exerts its antiapoptotic effect against diverse apoptotic stimuli through blockage of mitochondrial release of cytochrome C and activation of caspase-3. *Blood* 92:1700, 1998.
237. Maguer-Satta V, Burl S, Liu L, et al: BCR-ABL accelerates C2-ceramide-induced apoptosis. *Oncogene* 16:237, 1998.
238. Pierson BA, Miller JS: CD56+bright and CD56+dim natural killer cells in patients with chronic myelogenous leukemia progressively decrease in number, respond less to stimuli that recruit clonogenic natural killer cells, and exhibit decreased proliferation on a per cell basis. *Blood* 88:2279, 1996.
239. Gissinger H, Kurzrock R, Wetzler M, et al: Apoptosis in chronic myelogenous leukemia: Studies of stage-specific differences. *Leuk Lymphoma* 25:121, 1997.
240. Boultwood J, Peniket A, Watkins F, et al: Telomere length shortening in chronic myelogenous leukemia is associated with reduced time to accelerated phase. *Blood* 96:358, 2000.
241. Terasaki Y, Okamura H, Ohtake S, Nakao S: Accelerated telomere length shortening in granulocytes: A diagnostic marker for myeloproliferative diseases. *Exp Hematol* 30:1399, 2002.
242. Drummond MW, Lennard A, Brummendorf TH, Holyoake TL: Telomere shortening correlates with prognostic score at diagnosis and proceeds rapidly during progression of chronic myeloid leukemia. *Leuk Lymphoma* 45:1775, 2004.
243. Campbell LJ, Fidler C, Eagleton H, et al: HTERT, the catalytic component of telomerase, is downregulated in the haematopoietic stem cells of patients with chronic myeloid leukaemia. *Leukemia* 20:671, 2006.
244. Ohyashiki K, Ohyashiki JH, Iwama H, et al: Telomerase activity and cytogenetic changes in chronic myeloid leukemia with disease progression. *Leukemia* 11:190, 1997.
245. Brümmendorf TH, Ersöz I, Hartmann U, et al: Telomere length in peripheral blood granulocytes reflects response to treatment with imatinib in patients with chronic myeloid leukemia. *Blood* 101:375, 2003.
246. Thompson RB, Stainsby D: The clinical and haematological features of chronic granulocytic leukaemia in the chronic phase, in *Chronic Granulocytic Leukaemia*, edited by Shaw MT, p 137. Praeger, East Sussex, UK, 1982.
247. Cortes JE, Talpaz M, Kantarkian H: Chronic myelogenous leukemia: A review. *Am J Med* 100:555, 1996.
248. Goldman JM: Chronic myeloid leukaemia. *Curr Opin Hematol* 4:277, 1997.
249. Lichtman MA, Rowe JM: Hyperleukocytic leukemias: Rheological, clinical and therapeutic considerations. *Blood* 60:279, 1982.
250. Rowe JM, Lichtman MA: Hyperleukocytosis and leukostasis: Common features of childhood chronic myelogenous leukemia. *Blood* 63:1230, 1984.
251. Lichtman MA, Heal J, Rowe JM: Hyperleukocytic leukaemia. *Baillieres Clin Haematol* 1:725, 1987.
252. Ungaro PC, Gonzalez JJ, Werk EE, MacKay JC: Chronic myelogenous leukemia presenting clinically as diabetes insipidus. *N C Med J* 45:640, 1984.
253. Juan D, Hsu SD, Hunter J: Case report of vasopressin-responsive diabetes insipidus associated with chronic myelogenous leukemia. *Cancer* 56:1468, 1985.
254. Brydon J, Lucky PA, Duffy T: Acne urticaria associated with chronic myelogenous leukemia. *Cancer* 56:2083, 1985.
255. Cohen PR, Talpaz M, Kurzrock R: Malignancy-associated Sweet's syndrome: A review of the world's literature. *J Clin Oncol* 6:1887, 1988.
256. López JLB, Fonseca E, Mauso F: Sweet's syndrome during the chronic phase of chronic myeloid leukemia. *Acta Haematol* 84:207, 1990.
257. Nestok BR, Goldstein JD, Lipkovic P: Splenic rupture as a cause of sudden death in undiagnosed chronic myelogenous leukemia. *Am J Forensic Med Pathol* 9:241, 1988.
258. Giagounidis AAN, Burk M, Meckenstock G, et al: Pathological rupture of the spleen in hematologic malignancies. *Ann Hematol* 73:297, 1996.
259. Hild DH, Myers TJ: Hyperviscosity in chronic granulocytic leukemia. *Cancer* 46:1418, 1980.
260. D'Hondt L, Guillaume TH, Hemblit Y, Symann M: Digital necrosis associated with chronic myeloid leukemia. *Acta Clin Belg* 52:49, 1997.
261. Arbaje YM, Betran G: Chronic myelogenous leukemia complicated by autoimmune hemolytic anemia. *Am J Med* 88:197, 1990.
262. Steegmann JL, Pinilla I, Requena MJ, et al: The direct antiglobulin test is frequently positive in chronic myeloid leukemia patients treated with interferon-alpha. *Transfusion* 37:446, 1997.
263. Hoppin EC, Lewis JP: Polycythemia rubra vera progressing to Ph1-positive chronic myelogenous leukemia. *Ann Intern Med* 83:820, 1975.
264. Shenkenberg TD, Waddell CC, Rice L: Erythrocytosis and marked leukocytosis in overlapping myeloproliferative diseases. *South Med J* 75:868, 1982.
265. Haas O, Hinterberger W, Morz R: Pure red cell aplasia as possible early manifestation of chronic myeloid leukemia. *Am J Hematol* 27:20, 1986.
266. Mijovic A, Rolovic Z, Novak A, et al: Chronic myeloid leukemia associated with pure red cell aplasia and terminating in promyelocytic transformation. *Am J Hematol* 31:128, 1989.
267. Inbal A, Akstein E, Barak I, et al: Cyclic leukocytosis and long survival in chronic myeloid leukemia. *Acta Haematol* 69:353, 1983.
268. Umemura T, Hirata J, Kaneko S, et al: Periodic appearance of erythropoietin-independent erythropoiesis in chronic myelogenous leukemia with cyclic oscillation. *Acta Haematol* 76:230, 1986.
269. Mitus WJ, Kiossoglou KA: Leukocyte alkaline phosphatase in myeloproliferative syndrome. *Ann N Y Acad Sci* 155:976, 1968.
270. DePalma L, Delgado P, Werner M: Diagnostic discrimination and cost-effective assay strategy for leukocyte alkaline phosphate. *Clin Chim Acta* 6:83, 1996.
271. Pedersen F: Functional and biochemical phenotype in relation to cellular age of differentiated neutrophils in chronic myeloid leukemia. *Br J Haematol* 51:339, 1982.
272. Rambaldi A, Terao M, Bettoni S, et al: Differences in the expression of alkaline phosphatase in mRNA in chronic myelogenous leukemia and paroxysmal nocturnal hemoglobinuria polymorphonuclear leukocytes. *Blood* 73:1113, 1989.
273. Perillie PE: Studies of the changes in leukocyte alkaline phosphatase following pyrogen stimulation in chronic granulocytic leukemia. *Blood* 29:401, 1967.
278. Kamada N, Uchino H: Chronologic sequence in appearance of clinical and laboratory findings characteristic of chronic myelocytic leukemia. *Blood* 51:843, 1978.
279. Denburg JA, Wilson WE, Goodacre R, Bienenstock J: Chronic myeloid leukemia: Evidence for basophil differentiation and histamine synthesis from cultured peripheral blood cells. *Br J Haematol* 45:1, 1980.
280. Goh KO, Anderson FW: Cytogenetic studies in basophilic chronic myelocytic leukemia. *Arch Pathol Lab Med* 103:288, 1979.
281. Valent P, Agis H, Sperr W, et al: Diagnostic and prognostic value of new biochemical and immunohistochemical parameters in chronic myeloid leukemia. *Leuk Lymphoma* 49:635, 2008.
282. Samorapoompichit P, Kiener HP, Schernthaner GH, et al: Detection of tryptase in cytoplasmic granules of basophils in patients with chronic myeloid leukemia and other myeloid neoplasms. *Blood* 98:2580, 2001.
283. Weil SC, Hrisinko MA: A hybrid eosinophilic-basophilic granulocyte in chronic granulocytic leukemia. *Am J Clin Pathol* 87:66, 1987.
284. Velardi A, Rambotti P, Cernetti C, et al: Monoclonal antibody defined T-cell phenotypes and phytohemagglutinin reactivity of E-rosette forming circulating lymphocytes from untreated chronic myelocyte leukemia patients. *Cancer* 53:913, 1984.
285. Dowding C, Th'ng KH, Goldman JM, Galton DA: Increased T-lymphocyte numbers in chronic granulocytic leukemia before treatment. *Exp Hematol* 12:811, 1984.

286. Kaur J, Catovsky D, Spiers AS, Galton DA: Increase of T-lymphocytes in the spleen in chronic granulocytic leukaemia. *Lancet* 1:834, 1974.
287. Fujimiya Y, Bakke A, Chang WC, et al: Natural killer-cell immunodeficiency in patients with chronic myelogenous leukemia. *Int J Cancer* 37:639, 1986.
288. Fujimiya Y, Chang WC, Bakke A, et al: Natural killer cell immunodeficiency in patients with chronic myelogenous leukemia. *Cancer Immunol Immunother* 24:213, 1987.
289. Mellqvist UH, Hansson M, Brune M, et al: Natural killer cell dysfunction and apoptosis induced by chronic myelogenous leukemia cells: Role of reactive oxygen species and regulation by histamine. *Blood* 96:1961, 2000.
290. Pierson BA, Miller JS: The role of autologous natural killer cells in chronic myelogenous leukemia. *Leukemia* 11:1404, 1997.
291. Mason JE, DeVita VT, Canellos GP: Thrombocytosis in chronic granulocytic leukemia: Incidence and clinical significance. *Blood* 44:483, 1974.
292. Pederson B: Kinetics and cell function, in *Chronic Granulocytic Leukaemia*, edited by Shaw MT, p 93. Praeger, East Sussex, UK, 1982.
293. Radhika V, Thennarasu S, Naik NR, et al: Granulocytes from chronic myeloid leukemia (CML) patients show differential response to different chemoattractants. *Am J Hematol* 52:155, 1996.
294. Kasimir-Bauer S, Ottinger H, Brittinger G, König W: Philadelphia chromosome-positive chronic myelogenous leukemia: Functional defects in circulating mature neutrophils of untreated and interferon-α-treated patients. *Exp Hematol* 22:426, 1994.
295. Adams T, Schultz L, Goldberg L: Platelet function abnormalities in the myeloproliferative disorders. *Scand J Haematol* 13:215, 1974.
296. Gerrard JM, Stoddard SF, Shapiro RS, et al: Platelet storage pool deficiency and prostaglandin synthesis in chronic granulocytic leukaemia. *Br J Haematol* 40:597, 1978.
297. Knox WF, Bhavani M, Davson J, Geary CG: Histological classification of chronic granulocytic leukemia. *Clin Lab Haematol* 6:171, 1984.
298. Lorand-Metze I, Vassalo J, Souza CA: Histological and cytological heterogeneity of bone marrow in Philadelphia-positive chronic myelogenous leukaemia at diagnosis. *Br J Haematol* 67:45, 1987.
299. Inokuchi K, Yamaguchi H, Tarusawa M, et al: Abnormality of c-kit oncoprotein in certain patients with chronic myelogenous leukaemia—Potential clinical significance. *Leukemia* 16:170, 2002.
300. Cairoli R, Grillo G, Beghini A, et al: Chronic myelogenous leukemia with acquired c-kit activating mutation and transient bone marrow mastocytosis. *Hematol J* 5:273, 2004.
301. Agis H, Sotlar K, Valent P, Horny HP: Ph-chromosome-positive chronic myeloid leukemia with associated bone marrow mastocytosis. *Leuk Res* 29:1227, 2005.
302. Kelsey PR, Geary CG: Sea-blue histiocytes and Gaucher's cells in bone marrow of patients with chronic myeloid leukaemia. *J Clin Pathol* 41:960, 1988.
303. Dekmezian R, Kantarjian HM, Keating MJ, et al: The relevance of reticulin stain-measured fibrosis at diagnosis in chronic myelogenous leukemia. *Cancer* 59:1739, 1987.
304. Ghosh K, Varma N, Varma S, Dash S: Cellular composition and reticulin fibrosis in chronic myeloid leukaemia. *Indian J Cancer* 25:128, 1988.
305. Buhr T, Choritz H, Georgii A: The impact of megakaryocyte proliferation for the evolution of myelofibrosis. *Virchows Arch* 420:473, 1992.
306. Korkolopoulou P, Viniou N, Kavantzas N, et al: Clinicopathologic correlations of bone marrow angiogenesis in chronic myeloid leukemia: A morphometric study. *Leukemia* 17:89, 2003.
307. Aguayo A, Kantarjian H, Manshouri T, et al: Angiogenesis in acute and chronic leukemias and myelodysplastic syndromes. *Blood* 96:2240, 2000.
308. Zhelyazkova AG, Tonchev AB, Kolova P, et al: Prognostic significance of hepatocyte growth factor and microvessel bone marrow density in patients with chronic myeloid leukaemia. *Scand J Clin Lab Invest* 18:1, 2008.
309. Rumpel M, Friedrich T, Deininger MW: Imatinib normalizes bone marrow vascularity in patients with chronic myeloid leukemia in first chronic phase. *Blood* 101:4641, 2003.
311. Udomsakdi C, Eaves CJ, Lansdorp PM, Eaves AC: Phenotypic heterogeneity of primitive leukemic hematopoietic cells in patients with chronic myeloid leukemia. *Blood* 80:2522, 1992.
312. Huret JL: Complex translocations, simple variant translocation and Ph-negative cases in chronic myelogenous leukaemia. *Hum Genet* 85:565, 1990.
313. Sakurai M, Sandberg AA: The chromosomes and causation of human cancer and leukemia: XVIII. The missing Y in acute myeloblastic leukemia (AML) and Ph1-positive chronic myelocytic leukemia. *Cancer* 38:762, 1976.
314. Berger R, Bernheim A: Y chromosome loss in leukemias. *Cancer Genet Cytogenet* 1:1, 1979.
315. Ishihara T, Sasaki M, Oshimura M, et al: A summary of cytogenetic studies on 534 cases of chronic myelogenous leukemia in Japan. *Cancer Genet Cytogenet* 9:81, 1983.
316. Mitelman F: Catalogue of chromosomal aberrations in cancer. *Cytogenet Cell Genet* 36:9, 1983.
317. Heim S, Billstrom R, Kristoffersson U, et al: Variant Ph translocations in chronic myeloid leukemia. *Cancer Genet Cytogenet* 18:215, 1985.
318. Bartram CR, Anger B, Carbonell F, Kleihauer E: Involvement of chromosome 9 in variant Ph1 translocation. *Leuk Res* 9:1133, 1985.
319. Morris CM, Rosman I, Archer SA, et al: A cytogenetic and molecular analysis of five variant Philadelphia translocations in chronic myeloid leukemia. *Cancer Genet Cytogenet* 35:179, 1988.
320. Teyssier JR, Bartram CR, DeVille J, et al: C-abl oncogene and chromosome 22 "bcr" juxtaposition in chronic myelogenous leukemia. *N Engl J Med* 312:1393, 1985.

321. Hagemeijer A, Bartram CR, Smith EME, et al: Is the chromosomal region 9q34 always involved in variants of the Ph1 translocation? *Cancer Genet Cytogenet* 13:1, 1984.
322. De Braekeleer M, Chui HM, Fiser J, Gardner HA: A further case of Philadelphia chromosome-positive chronic myeloid leukemia with t(3;9;22). *Cancer Genet Cytogenet* 35:279, 1988.
323. Lafage-Pochitaloff-Huvalé M1, Sainty D, Adriaanssen HJ, et al: Translocation (3;21) in Philadelphia positive chronic myeloid leukemia. *Leukemia* 3:554, 1989.
324. Thompson PW, Whittaker JA: Translocation 3;21 in Philadelphia chromosome positive chronic myeloid leukemia at diagnosis. *Cancer* 39:143, 1989.
325. Engel E, McGee BJ, Flexner JM, et al: Philadelphia chromosome (Ph1) translocation in an apparently Ph1 negative, minus G22, case of chronic myeloid leukemia. *N Engl J Med* 291:154, 1974.
326. Verma RS, Dosik H: "Masked" Ph1 chromosome in chronic myelogenous leukaemia (CML). *Blut* 50:129, 1985.
327. Hagemeijer A, de Klein A, Godde-Salz E, et al: Translocation of c-abl to "masked" Ph in chronic myeloid leukemia. *Cancer Genet Cytogenet* 18:95, 1985.
328. Melo JV: The diversity of BCR-ABL fusion proteins and their relationship to leukemic phenotype. *Blood* 88:2375, 1996.
329. O'Brien S, Thall PR, Siciliano MJ: Cytogenetics of chronic myeloid leukemia. *Baillieres Clin Haematol* 10:259, 1997.
330. Bartram CR, Carbonell F: Bcr rearrangement in Ph-negative CML. *Cancer Genet Cytogenet* 21:183, 1986.
331. Bartram CR: Rearrangement of bcr and c-abl sequences in Ph-positive acute leukemias and Ph-negative CML—An update. *Curr Stud Hematol Blood Transfus* 31:160, 1987.
332. Ganesan TS, Rassool F, Guo A-P, et al: Rearrangement of the bcr gene in Philadelphia-chromosome negative chronic myeloid leukemia. *Curr Stud Hematol Blood Transfus* 31:153, 1987.
333. Wiedemann LM, Karhi K, Chan LC: Similar molecular alterations occur in related leukemias with and without the Philadelphia chromosome. *Curr Stud Hematol Blood Transfus* 31:149, 1987.
334. Benn P, Loper L, Eisenberg A, et al: Utility of molecular genetic analysis of bcr rearrangement in the diagnosis of chronic myeloid leukemia. *Cancer Genet Cytogenet* 29:1, 1987.
335. Epner DE, Koeffler AP: Molecular genetic advances in chronic myelogenous leukemia. *Ann Intern Med* 113:3, 1990.
336. Dubé I, Dixon J, Beckett T, et al: Location of breakpoints within the major breakpoint cluster region (bcr) in 33 patients with *bcr* rearrangement-positive chronic myeloid leukemia with complex or absent Philadelphia chromosomes. *Genes Chromosomes Cancer* 1:106, 1989.
337. Morris C, Heisterkamp N, Kennedy MA, et al: Ph-negative chronic myeloid leukemia: Molecular analysis of ABL insertion into M-BCR on chromosome 22. *Blood* 76:1812, 1990.
338. Blennerhassett GT, Furth ME, Anderson A, et al: Clinical evaluation of DNA probe assay for the Philadelphia (Ph1) translocation in chronic myelogenous leukemia. *Leukemia* 2:648, 1988.
339. Lange W, Snyder DS, Castro R, et al: Detection by enzymatic amplification of bcr-abl mRNA in peripheral blood and bone marrow cells of patients with chronic myelogenous leukemia. *Blood* 73:1735, 1989.
340. Dhingra K, Talpaz M, Riggs MC, et al: Hybridization protection assay: A rapid, sensitive, and specific method for detection of Philadelphia chromosome-positive leukemias. *Blood* 77:238, 1991.
341. Stock W, Westbrook CA, Peterson B, et al: Value of molecular monitoring during the treatment of chronic myeloid leukemia: A Cancer and Leukemia Group B study. *J Clin Oncol* 15:26, 1997.
342. Frenoy N, Chabli A, Sol D, et al: Application of a new protocol for nested PCR to the detection of minimal residual bcr/abl transcripts. *Leukemia* 8:1411, 1994.
343. Melo JV, Yan XH, Diamond J, et al: Reverse transcription/polymerase chain reaction (RT/PCR) amplification of very small numbers of transcripts: The risk in misinterpreting negative results. *Leukemia* 10:1217, 1996.
344. Lin F, Chase A, Bunget J, et al: Correlation between the proportion of Philadelphia chromosome-positive metaphase cells and levels of BCR-ABL mRNA in chronic myeloid leukaemia. *Genes Chromosomes Cancer* 13:110, 1995.
344A. Cortes J and Kantarjian H: How I treat newly diagnosed chronic phase CML. *Blood* 120:1390, 2012.
345. Dewald GW, Schad CR, Christensen ER, et al: The application of in situ fluorescent hybridization to detect M bcr/abl fusion in variant Ph chromosomes in CML and ALL. *Cancer Genet Cytogenet* 71:7, 1993.
346. Cox MC, Maffei L, Buffolino S, et al: A comparative analysis of FISH, RT-PCR, and cytogenetics for the diagnosis of bcr-abl-positive leukemias. *Am J Clin Pathol* 109:24, 1998.
347. Sinclair PB, Green AR, Grace C, Nacheva EP: Improved sensitivity of BCR-ABL detection: A triple-probe three-color fluorescence in situ hybridization system. *Blood* 90:1395, 1997.
348. Acar H, Stewart J, Boyd E, Connor MJ: Identification of variant translocations in chronic myeloid leukemia by fluorescence in situ hybridization. *Cancer Genet Cytogenet* 93:115, 1997.
349. Schoch C, Schnittger S, Bursch S, et al: Comparison of chromosome banding analysis, interphase- and hypermetaphase-FISH, qualitative and quantitative PCR for

diagnosis and for follow-up in chronic myeloid leukemia: A study of 350 cases. *Leukemia* 16:53, 2002.

350. Yanagi M, Shinjo K, Takeshita A, et al: Simple and reliably sensitive diagnosis and monitoring of Philadelphia chromosome-positive cells in chronic myeloid leukemia by interphase fluorescence in situ hybridization of peripheral blood cells. *Leukemia* 13:542, 1999.

351. Werner M, Ewig M, Nasarek A, et al: Value of fluorescence in situ hybridization for detecting the bcr/abl gene fusion in interphase cells of routine bone marrow specimens. *Diagn Mol Pathol* 6:282, 1997.

352. Chase A, Grand F, Zhang JG, et al: Factors influencing the false positive and negative rates of BCR-ABL fluorescence in situ hybridization. *Genes Chromosomes Cancer* 18:246, 1997.

353. Pelz AF, Kroning H, Franke A, Wieacker P: High reliability and sensitivity of the BCR/ABL1 D-FISH test for the detection of BCR/ABL rearrangements. *Ann Hematol* 81:147, 2002.

354. Hochhaus A, Reiter A, Skladny H, et al: Molecular monitoring of residual disease in chronic myelogenous leukemia patients after therapy. *Recent Results Cancer Res* 144:36, 1998.

355. Wells SJ, Phillips CN, Winton EF, Farhi DC: Reverse transcriptase polymerase chain reaction for bcr-abl fusion in chronic myelogenous leukemia. *Am J Clin Pathol* 105:756, 1996.

356. Cox MC, Maffei L, Buffolino S, et al: A comparative analysis of FISH, RT-PCR, and cytogenetics for the diagnosis of bcr-abl-positive leukemias. *Am J Clin Pathol* 109:24, 1998.

357. Krackoff IH: Studies of uric acid biosynthesis in the chronic leukemias. *Arthritis Rheum* 8:772, 1965.

358. Vogler WR, Bain JA, Huguley CM Jr, et al: Metabolic and therapeutic effects of allopurinol in patients with leukemia and gout. *Am J Med* 40:548, 1966.

359. Zittoun J, Marquet J, Zittoun R: The intracellular content of the three cobalamins at various stages of normal and leukaemic myeloid cell development. *Br J Haematol* 31:299, 1975.

360. Zittoun J, Zittoun R, Marquet J, Sultan C: The three transcobalamins in myeloproliferative disorders and acute leukaemia. *Br J Haematol* 31:287, 1975.

361. Rosner F, Schreiber ZA: Serum vitamin B12 and vitamin B12 binding capacity in chronic myelogenous leukemia and other disorders. *Am J Med Sci* 263:473, 1972.

362. Sternman U-H: Intrinsic factor and the B12 binding proteins. *Clin Haematol* 5:473, 1976.

363. Corcino JJ, Zalusky R, Greenberg M, Herbert V: Coexistence of pernicious anaemia and chronic myeloid leukaemia: An experiment of nature involving vitamin B12 metabolism. *Br J Haematol* 20:511, 1971.

364. Agis H, Sperr WR, Herndlhofer S, et al: Clinical and prognostic significance of histamine monitoring in patients with CML during treatment with imatinib (STI571). *Ann Oncol* 18:1834, 2007.

365. Youman JD, Taddeini L, Cooper T: Histamine excess symptoms in basophilic chronic granulocytic leukemia. *Arch Intern Med* 131:560, 1973.

366. Rosenthal S, Schwartz JH, Canellos GP: Basophilic chronic granulocytic leukemia with hyperhistaminemia. *Br J Haematol* 36:367, 1977.

367. Gomez GA, Sokal JE, Walsh D: Prognostic features at diagnosis of chronic myelocytic leukemia. *Cancer* 47:2470, 1981.

368. Bellevue R, Dosik H, Spergel G, Gussoff BD: Pseudohyperkalemia and extreme leukocytosis. *J Lab Clin Med* 85:660, 1975.

369. Ballard HS, Marcus AJ: Hypercalcemia in chronic myelogenous leukemia. *N Engl J Med* 282:663, 1970.

370. Evans JJ, Bozdech MJ: Hypokalemia in nonblastic chronic myelogenous leukemia. *Arch Intern Med* 141:786, 1981.

371. Perillie PE, Finch SC: Muramidase studies in Philadelphia-chromosome-positive and chromosome-negative chronic granulocytic leukemia. *N Engl J Med* 283:456, 1970.

372. Gilbert HS, Ginsberg H: Hypocholesterolemia as a manifestation of disease activity in chronic myeloid leukemia. *Cancer* 51:1428, 1983.

373. Muller CP, Wagner AN, Maucher C, Steinke B: Hypocholesterolemia, an unfavorable feature of prognostic value in chronic myeloid leukemia. *Eur J Haematol* 43:235, 1989.

374. Musolino C, Alonci A, Bellomo G, et al: Levels of soluble angiogenin in chronic myeloid malignancies. *Eur J Haematol* 72:416, 2004.

375. Calabro L, Fonsatti E, Bellomo G, et al: Differential levels of soluble endoglin (CD105) in myeloid malignancies. *J Cell Physiol* 194:171, 2003.

376. Sessarego M, Defferrari R, Dejana AM, et al: Cytogenetic analysis in essential thrombocythemia at diagnosis and at transformation. *Cancer Genet Cytogenet* 43:57, 1989.

377. Pajor L, Kereskai L, Zsdral K, et al: Philadelphia chromosome and/or bcr-abl mRNA-positive primary thrombocytosis: Morphometric evidence for the transition from essential thrombocythemia to chronic myeloid leukaemia type myeloproliferation. *Histopathology* 42:53, 2003.

378. Blickstein D, Aviram A, Luboshitz J, et al: BCR-ABL transcripts in bone marrow aspirates of Philadelphia-negative essential thrombocythemia patients: Clinical presentation. *Blood* 90:2768, 1997.

379. Cervantes F, Colomer D, Vives-Corrons JL, et al: Chronic myeloid leukemia of thrombocythemic onset: A CML subtype with distinct hematological and molecular features. *Leukemia* 10:1241, 1996.

380. Paietta E, Rosen N, Roberts M, et al: Philadelphia chromosome positive essential thrombocythemia evolving into lymphoid blast crisis. *Cancer Genet Cytogenet* 25:227, 1987.

381. Michiels JJ, Prins ME, Hagermeijer A, et al: Philadelphia chromosome-positive thrombocythemia and megakaryoblast leukemia. *Am J Clin Pathol* 88:645, 1987.

382. Sanadi I, Yamamoto S, Ogata M, et al: Detection of the Philadelphia chromosome in chronic neutrophilic leukemia. *Jpn J Clin Oncol* 15:553, 1985.

383. Christopoulos C, Kottoris K, Mikraki V, Anevlavis E: Presence of bcr/abl rearrangement in a patient with chronic neutrophilic leukaemia. *J Clin Pathol* 49:1013, 1996.

384. Pane F, Frigeri F, Sindina M, et al: Neutrophilic-chronic myeloid leukemia: A distinct disease with a specific molecular marker (BCR/ABL with C3/A2 junction). *Blood* 88:2410, 1996.

385. Verstovsek S, Lin H, Kantarjian H, et al: Neutrophilic-chronic myeloid leukemia: Low levels of p 230 BCR/ABL mRNA and undetectable BCR/ABL protein may predict an indolent course. *Cancer* 94:2416, 2002.

386. Ohsaka A, Shiina S, Kobayashi M, et al: Philadelphia chromosome-positive chronic myeloid leukemia expressing p190(BCR-ABL). *Intern Med* 41:1183, 2002.

387. Barnes DJ, Melo JV: Cytogenetic and molecular genetic aspects of chronic myeloid leukaemia. *Acta Haematol* 108:180, 2002.

388. Whang-Peng J, Gralnick HR, Johnson RE, et al: Chronic granulocytic leukemia (CGL) during the course of chronic lymphocytic leukemia (CLL): Correlation of blood, marrow, and spleen morphology and cytogenetics. *Blood* 43:333, 1974.

389. Schrieber ZA, Axelrod MR, Abebe LS: Coexistence of chronic myelogenous leukemia and chronic myelocytic leukemia. *Cancer* 54:697, 1984.

390. Specchia G, Buquicchio C, Albano F, et al: Non-treatment-related chronic myeloid leukemia as a second malignancy. *Leuk Res* 28:115, 2004.

391. Esteve J, Cervantes F, Rives S, et al: Simultaneous occurrence of B-cell chronic lymphocytic leukemia and chronic myeloid leukemia with further evolution to lymphoid blast status. *Haematologica* 82:596, 1997.

392. Leoni F, Ferrini PR, Castoldi GL, et al: Simultaneous occurrence of chronic granulocytic leukemia and chronic lymphoid leukemia. *Haematologica* 72:253, 1987.

393. Crescenzi B, Sacchi S, Marasca R, et al: Distinct genomic events in the myeloid and lymphoid lineages in simultaneous presentation of chronic myeloid leukemia and B-chronic lymphocytic leukemia. *Leukemia* 16:955, 2002.

394. Mansat-De Mas V, Rigal-Huguet F, Cassar G, et al: Chronic myeloid leukemia associated with B-cell chronic lymphocytic leukemia: Evidence of two separate clones as shown by combined cell-sorting and fluorescence *in situ* hybridization. *Leuk Lymphoma* 44:867, 2003.

395. Faguet GB, Little T, Agee JF, Garver FA: Chronic lymphatic leukemia evolving into chronic myelocytic leukemia. *Cancer* 52:1647, 1983.

396. Jantunen E, Nousiainen T: Ph-positive chronic myelogenous leukemia evolving after polycythemia vera. *Am J Hematol* 37:212, 1991.

397. Hoppen EC, Lewis JP: Polycythemia rubra vera progressing to Ph-positive chronic myelogenous leukemia. *Ann Intern Med* 83:820, 1975.

398. Haq AU: Transformation of polycythemia vera to Ph-positive chronic myelogenous leukemia. *Am J Hematol* 356:110, 1990.

399. Roth AD, Oral A, Przepiorka D, et al: Chronic myelogenous leukemia and acute lymphoblastic leukemia occurring in the course of polycythemia vera. *Am J Hematol* 43:123, 1993.

400. Foviester RH, Louro JM: Philadelphia chromosome abnormality in angiogenic myeloid metaplasia. *Ann Intern Med* 64:622, 1966.

401. Nowell PC, Kant JA, Finan JB, et al: Marrow fibrosis associated with a Philadelphia chromosome. *Cancer Genet Cytogenet* 59:89, 1992.

402. Roth DG, Richman CM, Rowley JD: Chronic myelodysplastic syndrome (preleukemia) with the Philadelphia chromosome. *Blood* 56:262, 1980.

403. Berrebi A, Bruck R, Shtalrid M, Chemke J: Philadelphia chromosome in idiopathic acquired sideroblastic anemia. *Acta Haematol* 72:343, 1984.

404. Suzan F, Terré C, Garcia I, et al: Three cases of typical aplastic anaemia associated with a Philadelphia chromosome. *Br J Haematol* 112:385, 2001.

405. Sica S, Chiusolo P, Zollino M, et al: The association of severe aplastic anaemia with the Philadelphia chromosome and the bcr/abl transcript. *Br J Haematol* 114:961, 2001.

406. Hande K: Hyperuricemia, uric acid nephropathy and the tumor lysis syndrome, in *Renal Complications of Neoplasia*, edited by McKinney TD, p 134. Praeger, New York, 1986.

407. Navolanic PM, Pui CH, Larson RA, et al: Elitek-rasburicase: An effective means to prevent and treat hyperuricemia associated with tumor lysis syndrome, a Meeting Report, Dallas, TX, January, 2002. *Leukemia* 17:499, 2003.

408. Jeha S, Pui CH: Recombinant urate oxidase (rasburicase) in the prophylaxis and treatment of tumor lysis syndrome. *Contrib Nephrol* 147:69, 2005.

409. Liu CY, Sims-McCallum RP, Schiffer CA: A single dose of rasburicase is sufficient for the treatment of hyperuricemia in patients receiving chemotherapy. *Leuk Res* 29:463, 2005.

410. Arnold TM, Reuter JP, Delman BS, Shanholtz CB: Use of single-dose rasburicase in an obese female. *Ann Pharmacother* 38:1428, 2004.

411. Bazarbashi MS, Smith MR, Karanes C, et al: Successful management of Ph chromosome chronic myelogenous leukemia with leukapheresis during pregnancy. *Am J Hematol* 38:235, 1991.

412. Strobl FJ, Voelkerding KY, Smith EP: Management of chronic myeloid leukemia during pregnancy with leukapheresis. *J Clin Apher* 14:42, 1999.

413. Kennedy BJ: The evolution of hydroxyurea therapy in chronic myelogenous leukemia. *Semin Oncol* 19(Suppl 9):21, 1992.

414. Tsimberidou AM, Colburn DE, Welch MA, et al: Anagrelide and imatinib mesylate combination therapy in patients with chronic myeloproliferative disorders. *Cancer Chemother Pharmacol* 52:229, 2003.

415. Cortes J, Kantarjian H: How I treat newly diagnosed chronic phase CML. *Blood* 120:1390, 2012.

416. Baccarani M, Saglio G, Goldman J, et al: Evolving concepts in the management of chronic myeloid leukemia. Recommendations from an expert panel of behalf of the European LeukemiaNet. *Blood* 108:1809, 2006.

417. *NCCN Practice Guidelines in Oncology.* v.3.2014. Available at: http://www.nccn.org/professionsals/physician_gls/.

418. Kantarjian HM, Talpaz M, O'Brien S, et al: Dose escalation of imatinib mesylate can overcome resistance to standard-dose therapy in patients with chronic myeloid leukemia. *Blood* 101:473, 2003.

419. Marin D, Goldman JM, Olavarria E, Apperley JF: Transient benefit only from increasing the imatinib dose in CML patients who do not achieve complete cytogenetic remissions on conventional doses. *Blood* 102:2702, 2003.

420. Zonder JA, Pemberton P, Brandt H, et al: The effect of dose increase of imatinib mesylate in patients with chronic or accelerated phase chronic myelogenous leukemia with inadequate hematologic or cytogenetic response to initial treatment. *Clin Cancer Res* 9:2092, 2003.

421. Kantarjian H, Talpaz M, O'Brien S, et al: High-dose imatinib mesylate therapy in newly diagnosed Philadelphia chromosome-positive chronic phase chronic myeloid leukemia. *Blood* 103:2873, 2004.

422. Hughes T, Branford S, White D, et al: Impact of early dose intensity on cytogenetic and molecular responses in chronic-phase CML patients receiving 600 mg/day of imatinib as initial therapy. *Blood* 112:3967, 2008.

423. Cortes JE, Kantarjian HM, Goldberg SL, et al: High-dose imatinib in newly diagnosed chronic-phase chronic myeloid leukemia: High rates of rapid cytogenetic and molecular responses. *J Clin Oncol* 27:4754, 2009.

424. Hehlmann R, Lauseker M, Jung-Munkwitz S, et al: Tolerability-adapted imatinib 800 mg/d versus 400 mg/d versus 400 gm/d plus interferon-α in newly diagnosed chronic myeloid leukemia. *J Clin Oncol* 29:1634, 2011.

425. Castagnetti F, Palandri F, Amabile M, et al: Results of high-dose imatinib mesylate in intermediate Sokal risk chronic myeloid leukemia patients in early chronic phase: A phase 2 trial of the GIMEMA CML Working Party. *Blood* 113:4497, 2009.

426. Kanda Y, Okamoto S, Tauchi T, et al: Multicenter prospective trial evaluating the tolerability of imatinib for Japanese patients with chronic myelogenous leukemia in the chronic phase: Does body weight matter? *Am J Hematol* 83:835, 2008.

427. Kobayashi S, Kimura F, Kobayashi A, et al: Efficacy of low-dose imatinib in chronic-phase chronic myelogenous leukemia patients. *Ann Hematol* 88:311, 2009.

428. Deininger M, O'Brien SG, Ghilhot F, et al: International randomized study of interferon vs STI571 (IRIS) 8 year follow up: Sustained survival and low risk for progression or events in patients with newly diagnosed chronic myeloid leukemia in chronic phase (CML-CP) treated with imatinib. *Blood* 14: Abstract 1126, 2009.

429. de Lavallade H, Apperley JF, Khorashad JS, et al: Imatinib for newly diagnosed patients with chronic myeloid leukemia: Incidence of sustained responses in an intention-to-treat analysis. *J Clin Oncol* 26:3358, 2008.

430. El-Zimaity MM, Kantarjian H, Talpaz M, et al: Results of imatinib mesylate therapy in chronic myelogenous leukaemia with variant Philadelphia chromosome. *Br J Haematol* 125:187, 2004.

431. Synder DS, McMahon R, Cohen SR, Slovak ML: Chronic myeloid leukemia with an e13a3 BCR-ABL fusion: Benign course responsive to imatinib with an RT-PCR advisory. *Am J Hematol* 75:92, 2004.

432. de Lemos JA, de Oliveira CM, Scerni AC, et al: Differential molecular response of the transcripts B2A2 and B3A2 to imatinib mesylate in chronic myeloid leukemia. *Genet Mol Res* 4:803, 2005.

433. Agirre X, Román-Gómez J, Vázquez I, et al: Coexistence of different clonal populations harboring the b3a2 (p210) and e1a2 (p190) BCR-ABL1 fusion transcripts in chronic myelogenous leukemia resistant to imatinib. *Cancer Genet Cytogenet* 160:22, 2005.

434. Castagnetti F, Testoni N, Luati S, et al: Deletions of the derivative chromosome 9 do not influence the response and the outcome of chronic myeloid leukemia in early chronic phase treated with inmatinib mesylate: GIMEMA CML working party analysis. *J Clin Oncol* 28:2743, 2010.

435. Champagne MA, Capdeville R, Krailo M, et al: Imatinib mesylate (STI571) for treatment of children with Philadelphia chromosome-positive leukemia: Results from a Children's Oncology Group phase I study. *Blood* 104:2655, 2004.

436. Cortes J, Talpaz M, O'Brien S, et al: Effects of age on prognosis with imatinib mesylate therapy for patients with Philadelphia chromosome-positive chronic myelogenous leukemia. *Cancer* 98:1105, 2003.

437. Latagliata R, Breccia M, Carmosino I, et al: Elderly patients with Ph+ chronic myelogenous leukemia (CML): Results of imatinib mesylate treatment. *Leuk Res* 29:287, 2005.

438. Guilhot F: Indications for imatinib mesylate therapy and clinical management. *Oncologist* 9:271, 2004.

439. Marin D, Marktel S, Foot N, et al: Granulocyte colony-stimulating factor reverses cytopenia and may permit cytogenetic responses in patients with chronic myeloid leukemia treated with imatinib mesylate. *Haematologica* 88:227, 2003.

440. Quintas-Cardama A, Kantarjian H, O'Brien S, et al: Granulocyte-colony-stimulating factor (filgrastim) may overcome imatinib-induced neutropenia in patients with chronic-phase chronic myelogenous leukemia. *Cancer* 100:2592, 2004.

441. van Deventer HW, Hall MD, Orlowski RZ, et al: Clinical course of thrombocytopenia in patients treated with imatinib mesylate for accelerated phase chronic myelogenous leukemia. *Am J Hematol* 71:184, 2002.

442. Sneed TB, Kantarjian HM, Talpaz M, et al: The significance of myelosuppression during therapy with imatinib mesylate in patients with chronic myelogenous leukemia in chronic phase. *Cancer* 100:116, 2004.

443. Santos FP, Alvarado Y, Kantarjian H, et al: Long-term prognostic impact of the use of erythropoietic-stimulating agents in patients with chronic myeloid leukemia in chronic phase treated with imatinib. *Cancer* 117:982, 2011.

444. Lokeshwar N, Kumar L, Kumari M: Severe bone marrow aplasia following imatinib mesylate in a patient with chronic myelogenous leukemia. *Leuk Lymphoma* 46:781, 2005.

445. Hensley ML, Ford JM: Imatinib treatment: Specific issues related to safety, fertility, and pregnancy. *Semin Hematol* 40:21, 2003.

446. Ferrero D, Pogliani EM, Rege-Cambrin G, et al: Corticosteroids can reverse severe imatinib-induced hepatotoxicity. *Haematologica* 91(6 Suppl):ECR27, 2006.

447. Cross TJ, Bagot C, Portmann B, et al: Imatinib mesylate as a cause of acute liver failure. *Am J Hematol* 83:189, 2006.

448. Esmaeli B, Prieto VG, Butler CE, et al: Severe periorbital edema secondary to STI571 (Gleevec). *Cancer* 95:881, 2002.

449. Aduwa E, Szydlo R, Marin D, et al: Significant weight gain in patients with chronic myeloid leukemia after imatinib therapy. *Blood* 120:5087, 2012.

450. Pappas P, Karavasilis V, Briasoulis E, et al: Pharmacokinetics of imatinib mesylate in end stage renal disease. A case study. *Cancer Chemother Pharmacol* 56:358, 2005.

451. Osorio S, Noblejas AG, Durán A, Steegmann JL: Imatinib mesylate induces hypophosphatemia in patients with chronic myeloid leukemia in late chronic phase, and this effect is associated with response. *Am J Hematol* 82:394, 2007.

452. Fitter S, Dewar AL, Kostakis P, et al: Long-term imatinib therapy promotes bone formation in CML patients. *Blood* 111:2538, 2008.

453. Berman E, Nicolaides M, Maki RG, et al: Altered bone and mineral metabolism in patients receiving imatinib mesylate. *N Engl J Med* 354:2006, 2006.

454. Sanchez-Gonzalez B, Pascual-Ramirez JC, Fernandez-Abellan P, et al: Severe skin reaction to imatinib in a case of Philadelphia-positive acute lymphoblastic leukemia. *Blood* 101:2446, 2003.

455. Pascual JC, Matarredona J, Miralles J, et al: Oral and cutaneous lichenoid reaction secondary to imatinib: Report of two cases. *Int J Dermatol* 45:1471, 2006.

456. Drummond A, Micallef-Eynaud P, Douglas WS, et al: A spectrum of skin reactions caused by the tyrosine kinase inhibitor imatinib mesylate (STI 571, Glivec). *Br J Haematol* 120:911, 2003.

457. Rule SAJ, O'Brien SG, Crossman LC: Managing cutaneous reactions to imatinib therapy. *Blood* 100:3434, 2002.

458. Etienne G, Cony-Makhoul P, Mahon FX: Imatinib mesylate and gray hair. *N Engl J Med* 346:645, 2002.

459. Tjao AS, Kantarjian H, Cortes J, et al: Imatinib mesylate causes hypopigmentation in the skin. *Cancer* 98:2483, 2003.

460. Beham-Schmid C, Apfelbeck U, Sill H, et al: Treatment of chronic myelogenous leukemia with the tyrosine kinase inhibitor STI571 results in marked regression of bone marrow fibrosis. *Blood* 99:381, 2002.

461. Kantarjian HM, Bueso-Ramos CE, Talpaz M, et al: The degree of bone marrow fibrosis in chronic myelogenous leukemia is not a prognostic factor with imatinib mesylate therapy. *Leuk Lymphoma* 46:993, 2005.

462. Buesche G, Ganser A, Schlegelberger B, et al: Marrow fibrosis and its relevance during imatinib treatment of chronic myeloid leukemia. *Leukemia* 21:2420, 2007.

463. Ebos JM, Tran J, Master Z, et al: Imatinib mesylate (STI-571) reduces the Bcr-Abl-mediated vascular endothelial growth factor secretion in chronic myelogenous leukemia. *Mol Cancer Res* 1:89, 2002.

464. Kvasnicka HM, Thiele J, Staib P, et al: Reversal of bone marrow angiogenesis in chronic myeloid leukemia following imatinib mesylate (STI571) therapy. *Blood* 103:3549, 2004.

465. Chu S, McDonald T, Lin A, et al: Persistence of leukemia stem cells in chronic myelogenous leukemia patients in prolonged remission with imatinib treatment. *Blood* 118:5065, 2011.

466. Larson RA, Druker BJ, Guilhot F, et al: Imatinib pharmacokinetics and its correlation with response and safety in chronic-phase chronic myeloid leukemia: A subanalysis of the IRIS study. *Blood* 111:4022, 2008.

467. Picard S, Titier K, Etienne G, et al: Trough imatinib plasma levels are associated with both cytogenetic and molecular responses to standard-dose imatinib in chronic myeloid leukemia. *Blood* 109:3496, 2007.

468. Schmidli H, Peng B, Riviere GJ, et al: Population pharmacokinetics of imatinib mesylate in patients with chronic-phase chronic myeloid leukaemia: Results of a phase III study. *Br J Clin Pharmacol* 60:35, 2005.

469. Ozdemir E, Koc Y, Kansu E: Successful treatment of chronic myeloid leukemia with imatinib mesylate in a patient with chronic renal failure on hemodialysis. *Am J Hematol* 81:474, 2006.

470. Darkow T, Henk HJ, Thomas SK, et al: Treatment interruptions and non-adherence with imatinib and associated healthcare costs: A retrospective analysis among managed care patients with chronic myelogenous leukaemia. *Pharmacoeconomics* 25:481, 2007.

471. Shah P, Tran C, Lee FY, et al: Overriding imatinib resistance with a novel ABL kinase inhibitor. *Science* 305:399, 2004.

472. Cortes JE, Jones D, O'Brien S, et al: Results of dasatinib therapy in patients with early chronic-phase chronic myeloid leukemia. *J Clin Oncol* 28:398, 2010.

473. Kantarjian H, Shah NP, Hochhaus A, et al: Dasatinib versus imatinib in newly diagnosed chronic-phase chronic myeloid leukemia. *N Engl J Med* 362:2260, 2010.

474. Quintás-Cardama A, Choi S, Kantarjian H, et al: Predicting outcomes in patients with chronic myeloid leukemia at any time during tyrosine kinase inhibitor therapy. *Clin Lymph Myeloma Leuk* 14:327, 2014.

475. Jabbour E, Kantarjian HM, Saglio G, et al: Early response with dasatinib or imatinib in chronic myeloid leukemia: 3-year follow-up from a randomized phase 3 trial (DASISION). *Blood* 123:494, 2013.

476. Radich JP, Kopecky KJ, Appelbaum FR, et al: A randomized trial of dasatinib 100 mg versus imatinib 400 mg in newly diagnosed chronic-phase chronic myeloid leukemia. *Blood* 120:3898, 2012.

477. Quintas-Cardama A, Han X, Kantarjian H, Cortes J, Tyrosine kinase inhibitor-induced platelet dysfunction in patients with chronic myeloid leukemia. *Blood* 114: 261, 2009.

478. Montani D, Bergot E, Gunther S, et al: Pulmonary arterial hypertension in patients treated by dasatinib. *Circulation* 125:2128, 2012.

479. Ault P: Dasatinib in the first-line treatment of chronic myeloid leukemia. *Community Oncol* 9:336, 2012.

480. Schiffer CA, Cortes JE, Saglio G, et al: Lymphocytosis following first-line treatment for CML in chronic phase with dasatinib is associated with improved responses: A comparison with imatinib. *Blood* 116: Abstract 358, 2010.

481. Kreutzman A, Juvonen V, Karisto V, et al: Mono/oligoclonal T and NK cells are common in chronic myeloid leukemia patients at diagnosis and expand during dasatinib therapy. *Blood* 116:772, 2010.

482. Roux C, Nicolini F-E, Rea D, et al: Reversible lymph node follicular hyperplasia associated with dasatinib treatment of chronic myeloid leukemia in chronic phase. *Blood* 122:3082, 2013.

483. Weisberg E, Manley P, Mestan J, et al: AMN107 (nilotinib): A novel and selective inhibitor of BCR-ABL. *Br J Cancer* 94:1765, 2006.

484. Jørgensen HG, Allan EK, Jordanides NE, et al: Nilotinib exerts equipotent antiproliferative effects to imatinib and does not induce apoptosis in CD34+ CML cells. *Blood* 109:4016, 2007.

485. Rosti G, Palandri F, Castagnetti F, et al: Nilotinib for the frontline treatment of Ph+_ chronic myeloid leukemia. *Blood* 114:4933, 2009.

486. Cortes JE, Jones D, O'Brien S, et al: Nilotinib as front-line treatment for patients with chronic myeloid leukemia in early chronic phase. *J Clin Oncol* 28:392, 2009.

487. Saglio G, Kim DW, Issaragrisil S, et al: Nilotinib versus imatinib for newly diagnosed chronic myeloid leukemia. *N Engl J Med* 362:2251, 2010.

488. Larson RA, Hochhaus A, Hughes TP, et al: Nilotinib vs imatinib in patients with newly diagnosed Philadelphia chromosome-positive chronic myeloid leukemia in chronic phase: ENESTnd 3-year follow-up. *Leukemia* 26:2197, 2012.

489. Hochhuas A, Saglio G, Larson RA, et al: Nilotinib is associated with a reduced incidence of BCR-ABL mutations vs imatinib in patients with newly diagnosed chronic myeloid leukemia in chronic phase. *Blood* 121:3703, 2013.

490. Giles FJ, Mauro MJ, Hong F, et al: Rates of peripheral arterial occlusive disease in patients with chronic myeloid leukemia in the chronic phase treated with imatinib, nilotinib, or non-tyrosine kinase therapy: A retrospective cohort analysis. *Leukemia* 27:1310, 2013.

491. Stenger MS: Bosutinib in previously treated CML and in first-line comparison with imatinib. *Community Oncol* 10:105, 2013.

492. Cortes JE, Kim DW, Kantarjian HM, et al: Bosutinib versus imatinib in newly diagnosed chronic-phase chronic myeloid leukemia: Results from the BELA trail. *J Clin Oncol* 30:3486, 2012.

493. Akard LP, Albitar M, Hill CE, Pinilla-Ibarz J: The "hit hard and hit early" approach to the treatment of chronic myeloid leukemia: Implications of the updated national comprehensive cancer network clinical practice guidelines for routine practice. *Clin Adv Hematol Oncol* 11:421, 2013.

494. Goldman JM, Marin D: Is imatinib still an acceptable first-line treatment for CML in chronic phase? *Oncology (Williston Park)* 26:901, 2012.

495. Baccarani M, Deininger MW, Rosli G, et al: European LeukemiaNet recommendations for the management of chronic myeloid leukemia: 2013. *Blood* 122:872, 2013.

496. Kantarjian H, Talpaz M, O'Brien S, et al: Prediction of initial cytogenetic response for subsequent major and complete cytogenetic response to imatinib mesylate therapy in patients with Philadelphia chromosome-positive chronic myelogenous leukemia. *Cancer* 98:1776, 2003.

497. Druker BJ, Guilhot F, O'Brien SG, et al: Five-year follow-up of patients receiving imatinib for chronic myeloid leukemia. *N Engl J Med* 355:2408, 2006.

498. de Lavallade H, Apperley JF, Khorashad JS, et al: Imatinib for newly diagnosed patients with chronic myeloid leukemia: Incidence of sustained response in an intention-to-treat analysis. *J Clin Oncol* 26:3358, 2008.

499. Jabbour E, Kantarjian H, O'Brien S, et al: The achievement of an early complete cytogenetic response is a major determinant for outcome in patients with early chronic phase chronic myeloid leukemia treated with tyrosine kinase inhibitors. *Blood* 118:4541, 2011.

500. Cortes J, Talpaz M, O'Brien S, et al: Molecular response in patients with chronic myelogenous leukemia in chronic phase treated with imatinib mesylate. *Clin Cancer Res* 22:3425, 2005.

501. Hughes T, Hochhaus A, Branford S, et al: Long-term prognostic significance of early molecular response to imatinib in newly diagnosed chronic myeloid leukemia: An analysis from the International Randomized Study of Interferon and STI571 (IRIS). *Blood* 116:3758, 2010.

502. Quintas-Cardama A, Kantarjian H, Jones D, et al: Delayed achievement of cytogenetic and molecular response is associated with increased risk of progression among patients with chronic myeloid leukemia in early chronic phase receiving high-dose of standard-dose imatinib therapy. *Blood* 113:6315, 2009.

503. Marin D, Ibrahim AR, Lucas C, et al: Assessment of BCR-ABL1 transcript levels at 3 months is the only requirement for predicting outcome for patients with chronic myeloid leukemia treated with tyrosine kinase inhibitors. *J Clin Oncol* 30:232, 2012.

504. Saglio G, Kantarjian HM, Shah N, et al: Early response (molecular and cytogenetic) and long-term outcomes in newly diagnosed chronic myeloid leukemia in chronic phase (CML-CP): Exploratory analysis of DASISION 3-year data. *Blood* 12: Abstract 1675, 2012.

505. Saglio G, Hughes TP, Larson RA, et al: Impact of early molecular response to nilotinib (NIL) or imatinib (IM) on the long-term outcomes of newly diagnosed patients (pts) with chronic myeloid leukemia in chronic phase (CML-CP): Landmark analysis of 4=year (y) data form ENESTnd. *J Clin Oncol* 31: Abstract 7054, 2013.

506. Marin D, Milojkovic D, Olavarria E, et al: European LeukemiaNet criteria for failure or suboptimal response reliably identify patients with CML in early chronic phase treated with imatinib whose eventual outcome is poor. *Blood* 112:4437, 2008.

507. O'Dwyer ME, Gatter KM, Loriaux M, et al: Demonstration of Philadelphia chromosome negative abnormal clones in patients with chronic myelogenous leukemia during major cytogenetic responses induced by imatinib mesylate. *Leukemia* 17:481, 2003.

508. Guilbert-Douet N, Morel F, LeBris M-J, et al: Clonal chromosomal abnormalities in the Philadelphia chromosome negative cells of chronic myeloid leukemia patients treated with imatinib. *Leukemia* 18:1140, 2004.

509. Deininger MW: Cytogenetic studies in patients on imatinib. *Semin Hematol* 40:50, 2003.

510. Bumm T, Muller C, Al-Ali K, et al: Emergence of clonal cytogenetic abnormalities in Ph-cells in some CML patients in cytogenetic remission to imatinib but restoration of polyclonal hematopoiesis in the majority. *Blood* 101:1941, 2003.

511. Goldberg SL, Medan RA, Rowley SD, et al: Myelodysplastic subclones in chronic myeloid leukemia: Implications for imatinib mesylate therapy. *Blood* 101:781, 2003.

512. Farag SS, Ruppert AS, Mrozek K, et al: Prognostic significance of additional cytogenetic abnormalities in newly diagnosed patients with Philadelphia chromosome-positive chronic myelogenous leukemia treated with interferon-alpha: A Cancer and Leukemia Group B study. *Int J Oncol* 25:143, 2004.

513. Andersen MK, Pedersen-Bjergaard J, Kjeldsen L, et al: Clonal Ph-negative hematopoiesis in CML after therapy with imatinib mesylate is frequently characterized by trisomy 8. *Leukemia* 16:1390, 2002.

514. Terre C, Eclache V, Rousselot P, et al: Report of 34 patients with clonal chromosomal abnormalities in Philadelphia-negative cells during imatinib treatment of Philadelphia-positive chronic myeloid leukemia. *Leukemia* 18:1340, 2004.

515. Jabbour E, Kantarjian HM, Abruzzo LV, et al: Chromosomal abnormalities in Philadelphia chromosome negative metaphases appearing during imatinib mesylate therapy in patients with newly diagnosed chronic myeloid leukemia in chronic phase. *Blood* 110:2991, 2007.

516. Cortes JE, Talpaz M, Giles F, et al: Prognostic significance of cytogenetic clonal evolution in patients with chronic myelogenous leukemia on imatinib mesylate therapy. *Blood* 101:3794, 2003.

517. Chee YL, Vickers MA, Stevenson D, et al: Fatal myelodysplastic syndrome developing during therapy with imatinib mesylate and characterised by the emergence of complex Philadelphia negative clones. *Leukemia* 17:634, 2003.

518. Noens L, van Lierde MA, De Bock R, et al: Prevalence, determinants, and outcomes of nonadherence ot imatinib therapy in patients with chronic myeloid leukemia: The ADAGIO study. *Blood* 113:5401, 2009.

519. Ibrahim AR, Eliasson L, Apperley JF, et al: Poor adherence is the main reason for loss of CCyR and imatinib failure for chronic myeloid leukemia patients on long-term therapy. *Blood* 1176:3722, 2011.

520. Marin D, Bazeos A, Mahon F-X, et al: Adherence is the critical factor for achieving molecular responses in patients with chronic myeloid leukemia who achieve complete cytogenetic responses on imatinib. *J Clin Oncol* 28:2381, 2010.

521. Hochhaus A, La Rosse P: Imatinib therapy in chronic myelogenous leukemia: Strategies to avoid and overcome resistance. *Leukemia* 18:1320, 2004.

522. Cowan-Jacob SW, Guez V, Fendrich G, et al: Imatinib (STI571) resistance in chronic myelogenous leukemia: Molecular basis of the underlying mechanism and potential strategies for treatment. *Mini Rev Med Chem* 4:285, 2004.

523. Melo JV: Resistance to imatinib mesylate in CML: All BCR-ABL mutations "are created equal but some are more equal than others." *Blood* 101:4231, 2003.

524. Villuendas R, Steegmann JL, Pollán M, et al: Identification of genes involved in imatinib resistance in CML: A gene-expression profiling approach. *Leukemia* 20:1047, 2006.

525. Jiang X, Zhao Y, Forrest D, et al: Stem cell biomarkers in chronic myeloid leukemia. *Dis Markers* 24:201, 2008.

526. Barnes DJ, Melo JV: Primitive, quiescent and difficult to kill: The role of non-proliferating stem cells in chronic myeloid leukemia. *Cell Cycle* 5:2862, 2006.

527. Michor F, Hughes TP, Iwasa Y, et al: Dynamics of chronic myeloid leukaemia. *Nature* 435:1267, 2005.

528. Zhang WW, Cortes JE, Yao H, et al: Predictors of primary imatinib resistance in chronic myelogenous leukemia are distinct from those in secondary imatinib resistance. *J Clin Oncol* 27:3642, 2009.

529. White DL, Saunders VA, Dang P, et al: OCT-1-mediated influx is a key determinant of the intracellular uptake of imatinib but not nilotinib (AMN107): Reduced OCT-1 activity is the cause of low in vitro sensitivity to imatinib. *Blood* 108:697, 2006.

530. Hiwase DK, Saunders V, Hewett D, et al: Dasatinib cellular uptake and efflux in chronic myeloid leukemia cells: Therapeutic implications. *Clin Cancer Res* 14:3881, 2008.

531. White DL, Dang P, Engler J, et al: Functional activity of the OCT-1 protein is predictive of long-term outcome in patients with chronic-phase chronic myeloid leukemia treated with imatinib. *J Clin Oncol* 28:2761, 2010.

532. Jordanides NE, Jorgensen HG, Holyoake TL, et al: Functional ABCG2 is overexpressed on primary CML CD34+ cells and is inhibited by imatinib mesylate. *Blood* 108:1370, 2006.

533. Ossard-Receveur A, Bernheim A, Clausse B, et al: Duplication of the Ph-chromosome as a possible mechanism of resistance to imatinib mesylate in patients with chronic myelogenous leukemia. *Cancer Genet Cytogenet* 163:189, 2005.

534. Szych CM, Liesveld JL, Iqbal MA, et al: Isodicentric Philadelphia chromosomes in imatinib mesylate (Gleevec)-resistant patients. *Cancer Genet Cytogenet* 174:132, 2007.

535. Khorashad JS, Kelley TW, Szankasi P, et al: BCR-ABL1 Compound mutations in tyrosine kinase inhibitor-resistant CML: Frequency and clonal relationships. *Blood* 121:489, 2013.

536. Roche-Lestienne C, Preudhomme C: Mutations in the ABL kinase domain pre-exist the onset of imatinib treatment. *Semin Hematol* 21:80, 2003.

537. Corbin AS, La Rosee P, Stoffregen EP, et al: Several Bcr-Abl kinase domain mutants associated with imatinib mesylate resistance remain sensitive to imatinib. *Blood* 101:4611, 2003.

538. Khorashad JS, Anand M, Marin D, et al: The presence of a BCR-ABL mutant allele in CML does not always explain clinical resistance to imatinib. *Leukemia* 20:658, 2006.

539. Wei Y, Hardling M, Olsson B, et al: Not all imatinib resistance in CML are BCR-ABL kinase domain mutations. *Ann Hematol* 85:841, 2006.

540. Soverini S, Colarossi S, Gnani A, et al: Contribution of ABL kinase domain mutations to imatinib resistance in different subsets of Philadelphia-positive patients: By the GIMEMA Working Party on Chronic Myeloid Leukemia. *Clin Cancer Res* 12:7374, 2006.

541. Sherbenou DW, Wong MJ, Humayun A, et al: Mutations of the BCR-ABL-kinase domain occur in a minority of patients with stable complete cytogenetic response to imatinib. *Leukemia* 21:489, 2007.

542. Miething C, Mugler C, Grundler R, et al: Phosphorylation of tyrosine 393 in the kinase domain of Bcr-Abl influences the sensitivity towards imatinib in vivo. *Leukemia* 17:1695, 2003.

543. Branford S, Rudzki Z, Walsh S, et al: Detection of BRC-ABL mutations in patients with CML treated with imatinib is virtually always accompanied by clinical resistance, and mutations in the ATP phosphate-binding loop (P-loop) are associated with a poor prognosis. *Blood* 102:276, 2003.

544. Nicolini FE, Corm S, Lê QH, et al: Mutation status and clinical outcome of 89 imatinib mesylate-resistant chronic myelogenous leukemia patients: A retrospective analysis from the French intergroup of CML (Fi(phi)-LMC GROUP). *Leukemia* 20:1061, 2006.

545. Soverini S, De Benedittis C, Machova Polakova K, et al: Unraveling the complexity of tyrosine kinase inhibitor-resistant populations by ultra-deep sequencing of the BCR-ABL kinase domain. *Blood* 122:1634, 2013.

546. Parker WT, Lawrence RM, Ho M, et al: Sensitive detection of BDR-ABL! Mutations in patients with chronic myeloid leukemia after imatinib resistance is predictive of outcome during subsequent therapy. *J Clin Oncol* 29:4250, 2011.

547. Vainstein V, Eide CA, O'Hare T, et al: Integrating in vitro sensitivity and dose-response slope is predictive of clinical response to ABL kinase inhibitors in chronic myeloid leukemia. *Blood* 122:3331, 2013.

548. Cortes JE, Kim DW, Pinilla-Ibarz J, et al: A phase 2 trial of ponatinib in Philadelphia chromosome-positive leukemias. *N Engl J Med* 369:1783, 2013.

549. Khorashad JS, Kelley TW, Szankasi P, et al: BCR-ABL1 compound mutations in tyrosine kinase inhibitor-resistant CML: Frequency and clonal relationships. *Blood* 121:489, 2013.

550. Quintás-Cardama A, Cortes J: Therapeutic options against BCR-ABL1 T315I-positive chronic myelogenous leukemia. *Clin Cancer Res* 14:4392, 2008.

551. Jabbour E, Kantarjian H, Jones D, et al: Characteristics and outcomes of patients with chronic myeloid leukemia and T315I mutation following failure of imatinib mesylate therapy. *Blood* 112:53, 2008.

552. de Lavallade H, Khorashad JS, Davis HP, et al: Interferon-alpha or homoharringtonine as salvage treatment for chronic myeloid leukemia patients who acquire the T315I BCR-ABL mutation. *Blood* 110:2779, 2007.

553. Jilani I, Kantarjian H, Gorre M, et al: Phosphorylation levels of BCR-ABL, CrkL, AKT and STAT5 in imatinib-resistant chronic myeloid leukemia cells implicate alternative pathway usage as a survival strategy. *Leuk Res* 32:643, 2008.

554. Pocaly M, Lagarde V, Etienne G, et al: Overexpression of the heat-shock protein 70 is associated to imatinib resistance in chronic myeloid leukemia. *Leukemia* 21:93, 2007.

555. Carter BZ, Mak DH, Schober WD, et al: Regulation of survivin expression through Bcr-Abl/MAPK cascade: Targeting survivin overcomes imatinib resistance and increases imatinib sensitivity in imatinib-responsive CML cells. *Blood* 107:1555, 2006.

556. Wu J, Meng F, Kong LY, et al: Association between imatinib-resistant BCR-ABL mutation-negative leukemia and persistent activation of LYN kinase. *J Natl Cancer Inst* 100:926, 2008.

557. Hochhaus A, Erben P, Ernst T, Mueller MC: Resistance to targeted therapy in chronic myelogenous leukemia. *Semin Hematol* 44:S15, 2007.

558. Feller SM, Tuchscherer G, Voss J: High affinity molecular disruption of GRB2 protein complexes as a therapeutic strategy for chronic myelogenous leukemia. *Leuk Lymphoma* 44:411, 2003.

559. Hochhaus A: Cytogenetic and molecular mechanisms of resistance to imatinib. *Semin Hematol* 40:69, 2003.

560. Ohno R, Nakamura Y: Prediction of response to imatinib by cDNA microarray analysis. *Semin Hematol* 40:42, 2003.

561. Cortes J, Kantarjian H: Beyond dose escalation: Clinical options for relapse or resistance in chronic myelogenous leukemia. *J Natl Compr Canc Netw* 6 Suppl 2:S22, 2008.

562. Soverini S, Hochhaus A, Nicolini FE, et al: BCR-ABL kinase domain mutation analysis in chronic myeloid leukemia patients treated with tyrosine kinase inhibitors: Recommendations from an expert panel on behalf of European LeukemiaNet. *Blood* 118:1208, 2011.

563. Jabbour E, Kantarjian HM, Saglio G, et al: Early response with dasatinib or imatinib in chronic myeloid leukemia: 3-year follow-up from a randomized phase 3 trial (DASISION). *Blood* 123:494, 2014.

564. Martinelli G, Soverini S, Rosti G, Baccarani M: Dual tyrosine kinase inhibitors in chronic myeloid leukemia. *Leukemia* 19:1872, 2005.

565. Kantarjian H, Pasquini R, Hamerschlak N, et al: Dasatinib or high-dose imatinib for chronic-phase chronic myeloid leukemia after failure of first-line imatinib: A randomized phase 2 trial. *Blood* 109:5143, 2007.

566. Porkka K, Koskenvesa P, Lundán T, et al: Dasatinib crosses the blood–brain barrier and is an efficient therapy for central nervous system Philadelphia chromosome-positive leukemia. *Blood* 112:1005, 2008.

567. Shah NP, Guilhot F, Cortes JE, et al: Long-term outcome with dasatinib after imatinib failure in chronic-phase chronic myeloid leukemia: Follow-up of a phase 3 study. *Blood* 123:2317, 2014.

568. Khoury HJ, Cortes JE, Kantarjian HM, et al: Bosutinib is active in chronic phase chronic myeloid leukemia after imatinib and dasatinib and/or nilotinib therapy failure. *Blood* 119:343, 2012.

569. Ibrahim AR, Pallompeis C, Bua M, et al: Efficacy of tyrosine kinase inhibitors (TKIs) as third-line therapy in patients with chronic myeloid leukemia in chronic phase who have failed 2 prior lines of TKI therapy. *Blood* 116:5497, 2010.

570. Cortes JE, Nicolini FE, Wetzler M, et al: Subcutaneous omacetaxine mepesuccinate in patients with chronic-phase chronic myeloid leukemia previously treated with 2 or more tyrosine kinase inhibitors including Imatinib. *Clin Lymphoma Myeloma Leuk* 13:584, 2013.

571. Cortes J, Digumatri R, Parikh PM, et al: Phase 2 study of subcutaneous omacetaxine mepesuccinate for chronic-phase chronic myeloid leukemia patients resistant to or intolerant of tyrosine kinase inhibitors. *Am J Hematol* 88:350, 2013.

572. Sun X, Layton JE, Elefanty A, Lieschke GJ: Comparison of effects of the tyrosine kinase inhibitors AG957, AG490, and STI571 on BCR-ABL-expressing cells, demonstrating synergy between AG490 and STI571. *Blood* 97:2008, 2001.

573. Mohi MG, Boulton C, Gu TL, et al: Combination of rapamycin and protein tyrosine kinase (PTK) inhibitors for the treatment of leukemias caused by oncogenic PTKs. *Proc Natl Acad Sci U S A* 101:3130, 2004.

574. Gatto S, Scappini B, Pham L, et al: The proteasome inhibitor PS-341 inhibits growth and induces apoptosis in Bcr/Abl-positive cell lines sensitive and resistant to imatinib mesylate. *Haematologica* 88:853, 2003.

575. Dai Y, Rahmani M, Pei XY, et al: Bortezomib and flavopiridol interact synergistically to induce apoptosis in chronic myeloid leukemia cells resistant to imatinib mesylate through both Bcr/Abl-dependent and -independent mechanisms. *Blood* 104:509, 2004.

576. Yu C, Rahmani M, Conrad D, et al: The proteasome inhibitor bortezomib interacts synergistically with histone deacetylase inhibitors to induce apoptosis in Bcr/Abl+ cells sensitive and resistant to STI571. *Blood* 102:3765, 2003.

577. Fiskus W, Pranpat M, Bali P, et al: Combined effects of novel tyrosine kinase inhibitor AMN107 and histone deacetylase inhibitor LBH589 against Bcr-Abl-expressing human leukemia cells. *Blood* 108:645, 2006.

578. Sawyers CL, Hochhaus A, Feldman E, et al: Imatinib induces hematologic and cytogenetic responses in patients with chronic myelogenous leukemia in myeloid blast crisis: Results of a phase II study. *Blood* 99:3530, 2002.

579. Gorre ME, Ellwood-Yen K, Chiosis G, et al: BCR-ABL point mutants isolated from patients with imatinib mesylate-resistant chronic myeloid leukemia remain sensitive to inhibitors of the BCR-ABL chaperone heat shock protein 90. *Blood* 100:3041, 2002.

580. Zhao C, Chen A, Jamieson CH, et al: Hedgehog signaling is essential for maintenance of cancer stem cells in myeloid leukaemia. *Nature* 458:776, 2009.

581. Tipping AJ, Mahon FX, Zafirides G, et al: Drug responses of imatinib mesylate-resistant cells: Synergism of imatinib with other chemotherapeutic drugs. *Leukemia* 16:2349, 2002.

582. Tipping AJ, Melo JV: Imatinib mesylate in combination with other chemotherapeutic drugs: In vitro studies. *Semin Hematol* 40:83, 2003.

583. Kantarjian HM, Talpaz M, Smith TL, et al: Homoharringtonine and low-dose cytarabine in the management of late chronic-phase chronic myelogenous leukemia. *J Clin Oncol* 18:3513, 2000.

584. O'Dwyer ME, La Rosee P, Nimmanapalli R, et al: Recent advances in Philadelphia chromosome-positive malignancies: The potential role of arsenic trioxide. *Semin Hematol* 39:18, 2002.

585. Kantarjian HM, O'Brien S, Corteo J, et al: Results of decitabine (5-aza-2′-deoxycytidine) therapy in 130 patients with chronic myelogenous leukemia. *Cancer* 98:522, 2003.

586. Issa JP, Garcia-Manero G, Giles FJ, et al: Phase 1 study of low-dose prolonged exposure schedules of the hypomethylating agent 5-aza-2′-deoxycytidine (decitabine) in hematopoietic malignancies. *Blood* 103:1635, 2004.

587. Chand M, Thakuri M, Keung YK: Imatinib mesylate associated with delayed hematopoietic recovery after concomitant chemotherapy. *Leukemia* 18:886, 2004.

588. Deininger M: Resistance and relapse with imatinib in CML: Causes and consequences. *J Natl Compr Canc Netw* 6 Suppl 2:S11, 2008.

589. Wu CJ, Neuberg D, Chillemi A, et al: Quantitative monitoring of BCR/ABL transcript during STI-571 therapy. *Leuk Lymphoma* 43:2281, 2002.

590. Druker BJ: Imatinib as a paradigm of targeted therapies. *J Clin Oncol* 21:239, 2003.

591. Druker BJ: STI571 (Gleevec) as a paradigm for cancer therapy. *Trends Mol Med* 8:S14, 2002.

592. Merx K, Muller MC, Kreil S, et al: Early reduction of BCR-ABL mRNA transcript levels predicts cytogenetic response in chronic phase CML patients treated with imatinib after failure of interferon alpha. *Leukemia* 16:1579, 2002.

593. Tam CS, Kantarjian H, Garcia-Manero G, et al: Failure to achieve a major cytogenetic response by 12 months defines inadequate response in patients receiving nilotinib or dasatinib as second or subsequent line therapy for chronic myeloid leukemia. *Blood* 112:516, 2008.

594. Nzha A, Kantarjian HM, Jain P, et al: Disease patterns for patients (pts) with chronic myeloid leukemia (CML) that have BCR0ABL transcript level >10% at 3 months of therapy with tyrosine kinase inhibitors (TKIs). *Blood* 12: Abstract 3757, 2012.

595. Kantarjian HM, Shan J, Jones D, et al: Significance of increasing levels of minimal residual disease in patients with Philadelphia chromosome-positive chronic myelogenous leukemia in complete cytogenetic response. *J Clin Oncol* 27:3659, 2009.

596. Branford S, Rudzki Z, Parkinson I, et al: Real-time quantitative PCR analysis can be used as a primary screen to identify patient with CML treated with imatinib who have BCR-ABL kinase domain mutations. *Blood* 104:2926, 2014.

597. Bonifazi F, Bandini G, Rondelli D, et al: Reduced incidence of GVHD without increase in relapse with low-dose rabbit ATG in the preparative regimen for unrelated bone marrow transplants in CML. *Bone Marrow Transplant* 32:237, 2003.

598. Baccarani M, Russo D, Rosti G, Martinelli G: Interferon-alpha for chronic myeloid leukemia. *Semin Hematol* 40:22, 2003.

599. Roy L, Guilhot J, Krahnke T, et al: Survival advantage from imatinib compared with the combination interferon-alpha plus cytarabine in chronic-phase chronic myelogenous leukemia: Historical comparison between two phase 3 trials. *Blood* 108:1478, 2006.

600. Talpaz M: Interferon-alfa-based treatment of chronic myeloid leukemia and implications of signal transduction inhibition. *Semin Hematol* 38:22, 2001.

601. Kujawski LA, Talpaz M: The role of interferon-alpha in the treatment of chronic myeloid leukemia. *Cytokine Growth Factor Rev* 18:459, 2007.

602. Alimena G, Breccia M, Luciano L, et al: Imatinib mesylate therapy in chronic myeloid leukemia patients in stable complete cytogenic response after interferon-alpha results in a very high complete molecular response rate. *Leuk Res* 32:255, 2008.

603. Branford S, Hughes T, Milner A, et al: Efficacy and safety of imatinib in patients with chronic myeloid leukemia and complete or near-complete cytogenetic response to interferon-alpha. *Cancer* 110:801, 2007.

604. Kolitz JE, Kempin SF, Schluger A, et al: A phase II trial of high-dose hydroxyurea in chronic myelogenous leukemia. *Semin Oncol* 19:27, 1992.

605. Abhyankar D, Shende C, Saikia T, Advani SH: Hydroxyurea induced leg ulcers. *J Assoc Physicians India* 48:926, 2000.

606. Guilhot F, Chastang C, Michallet M, et al: Interferon alfa-2b combined with cytarabine versus interferon alone in chronic myelogenous leukemia. *N Engl J Med* 337:223, 1997.

607. Hehlmann R, Heimpel H, Hasford J, et al: Randomized comparison of busulfan and hydroxyurea in chronic myelogenous leukemia: Prolongation of survival by hydroxyurea. *Blood* 82:398, 1993.

608. Clarkson B: Chronic myelogenous leukemia: Is aggressive treatment indicated? *J Clin Oncol* 3:135, 1985.

609. Cortes J, Jabbour E, Daley GQ, et al: Phase 1 study of lonafarnib (SCH 66336) and imatinib mesylate in patients with chronic myeloid leukemia who have failed prior single-agent therapy with imatinib. *Cancer* 110:1295, 2007.

610. Cortes J, Quintás-Cardama A, Garcia-Manero G, et al: Phase 1 study of tipifarnib in combination with imatinib for patients with chronic myelogenous leukemia in chronic phase after imatinib failure. *Cancer* 110:2000, 2007.

611. Carew JS, Nawrocki ST, Kahue CN, et al: Targeting autophagy augments the anticancer activity of the histone deacetylase inhibitor SAHA to overcome Bcr-Abl-mediated drug resistance. *Blood* 110:313, 2007.

612. Barbarotto E, Calin GA: Potential therapeutic applications of miRNA-based technology in hematological malignancies. *Curr Pharm Des* 14:2040, 2008.

613. Koldehoff M, Steckel NK, Beelen DW, Elmaagacli AH: Therapeutic application of small interfering RNA directed against bcr-abl transcripts to a patient with imatinib-resistant chronic myeloid leukaemia. *Clin Exp Med* 7:47, 2007.

614. James HA: The potential application of ribozymes for the treatment of hematological disorders. *J Leukoc Biol* 66:361, 1999.

615. Mendoza-Maldonado R, Zentilin L, Fanin R, Giacca M: Purging of chronic myelogenous leukemia cells by retrovirally expressed anti-bcrabl ribozymes with specific cellular compartmentalization. *Cancer Gene Ther* 9:71, 2002.

616. Cotter FE: Antisense oligonucleotides for haematological malignancies. *Haematologica* 84:19, 1999.

617. Verfaillie CM, McIvor S, Zhao RCH: Gene therapy for chronic myelogenous leukemia. *Mol Med Today* 5:359, 1999.

618. Wagner H, McKeough PG, Desforges J, Madoc-Jones H: Splenic irradiation in the treatment of patients with chronic myelogenous leukemia or myelofibrosis and myeloid metaplasia. *Cancer* 58:1204, 1986.

619. McFarland JT, Kuzma C, Millard FE, Johnstone PA: Palliative irradiation of the spleen. *Am J Clin Oncol* 26:178, 2003.

620. The Italian Cooperative Study Group on Chronic Myeloid Leukemia: Results of a prospective randomized trial of early splenectomy in chronic myeloid leukemia. *Cancer* 54:333, 1984.

621. Mesa RA, Elliott MA, Tefferi A: Splenectomy in chronic myeloid leukemia and myelofibrosis with myeloid metaplasia. *Blood Rev* 14:121, 2000.

622. Kalhs P, Schwarzinger I, Anderson G, et al: A retrospective analysis of the long-term effect of splenectomy on late infections, graft-versus-host disease, relapse, and survival after allogeneic marrow transplantation for chronic myelogenous leukemia. *Blood* 86:2028, 1995.

623. Meera V, Jijina F, Shrikande M, et al: Twin pregnancy in a patient of chronic myeloid leukemia on imatinib therapy. *Leuk Res* 32:1620, 2008.

624. Skoumalova I, Vondrakova J, Rohon P, et al: Successful childbirth in a patient with chronic myelogenous leukemia treated with imatinib during early pregnancy. *Biomed Pap Med Fac Univ Palacky Olomouc Czech Repub* 152:121, 2008.

625. Ali R, Ozkalemkas F, Ozçelik T, et al: Pregnancy under treatment of imatinib and successful labor in a patient with chronic myelogenous leukemia (CML). Outcome of discontinuation of imatinib therapy after achieving a molecular remission. *Leuk Res* 29:971, 2005.

626. Shapira T, Pereg D, Lishner M: How I treat acute and chronic leukemia in pregnancy. *Blood Rev* 22:247, 2008.

627. Pye SM, Cortes J, Ault P, Hatfield A, et al: The effects of imatinib on pregnancy outcome. *Blood* 111:5505, 2008.

628. Ault P, Kantarjian H, O'Brien S, et al: Pregnancy among patients with chronic myeloid leukemia treated with imatinib. *J Clin Oncol* 24:1204, 2006.

629. Ramasamy K, Hayden J, Lim Z, et al: Successful pregnancies involving men with chronic myeloid leukaemia on imatinib therapy. *Br J Haematol* 137:374, 2007.

630. Breccia M, Cannella L, Montefusco E, et al: Male patients with chronic myeloid leukemia treated with imatinib involved in healthy pregnancies: Report of five cases. *Leuk Res* 32:519, 2008.

631. Gambacorti-Passerini CB, Tornaghi L, Marangon E, et al: Imatinib concentrations in human milk. *Blood* 109:1790, 2007.

632. Mubarek AA, Kakil IR, Al-Homsi U, et al: Normal outcome of pregnancy in chronic myeloid leukemia treated with interferon-alpha in 1st trimester: Report of 3 cases and review of the literature. *Am J Hematol* 69:115, 2002.

633. Fadilah SA, Ahmad-Zailani R, Soon-Keng C, Norlaila M: Successful treatment of chronic myeloid leukemia during pregnancy with hydroxyurea. *Leukemia* 16:1202, 2002.

634. Williams LA Garcia Gonzalez AG, Ault P, et al: Measuring the symptom burden associated with the treatment of chronic myeloid leukemia. *Blood* 122:641, 2013.

635. Ross DM, Branford S, Seymour JF, et al: Safety and efficacy of imatinib cessation for CML patients with stable undetectable minimal residual disease: Results from the TWISTER study. *Blood* 122:515, 2013.

636. Mahon F-X, Rea D, Guilhot J, et al: Discontinuation of imatinib in patients with chronic myeloid leukaemia who have maintained complete molecular remission for at least 2 years: The prospective, multicenter Stop Imatinib (STIM) trial. *Lancet Oncol* 11:1029, 2010.

637. Rousselot P, Huguet F, Rea D, et al: Imatinib mesylate discontinuation in patients with chronic myelogenous leukemia in complete molecular remission for more than 2 years. *Blood* 109:58, 2007.

638. Carella AM, Lerma E: Durable responses in chronic myeloid leukemia patients maintained with lower doses of imatinib mesylate after achieving molecular remission. *Ann Hematol* 86:749, 2007.

639. Ghanima W, Kahrs J, Dahl TG 3rd, Tjonnfjord GE: Sustained cytogenetic response after discontinuation of imatinib mesylate in a patient with chronic myeloid leukaemia. *Eur J Haematol* 72:441, 2004.

640. Cortes J, O'Brien S, Kantarjian H: Discontinuation of imatinib therapy after achieving a molecular response. *Blood* 104:2204, 2004.

641. Okabe S, Tauchi T, Ishii Y, et al: Sustained complete cytogenetic remission in a patient with chronic myeloid leukemia after discontinuation of imatinib mesylate therapy. *Int J Hematol* 85:173, 2007.

642. Merante S, Orlandi E, Bernasconi P, et al: Outcome of four patients with chronic myeloid leukemia after imatinib mesylate discontinuation. *Haematologica* 90:979, 2005.

643. Branford S, Yeung DT, Ross DM, et al: Early molecular response and female sex strongly predict stable undetectable BCR-abl1, the criteria for imatinib discontinuation in patients with CML. *Blood* 121:3818, 2013.

644. Horn M, Glauche I, Muller MC, et al: Model-based decision rules reduce the risk of molecular relapse after cessation of tyrosine kinase inhibitor therapy in chronic myeloid leukemia. *Blood* 121:378, 2013.

645. Legros L, Rousselot P, Giraudier S, et al: Second attempt to discontinue imatinib in CP-CML patients with a second sustained complete molecular response. *Blood* 120:1959, 2012.

646. Graham SM, Jørgensen HG, Allan E, et al: Primitive, quiescent, Philadelphia-positive stem cells from patients with chronic myeloid leukemia are insensitive to STI571 *in vitro. Blood* 99:319, 2002.

647. Russo D, Martinelli G, Malagola M, et al: Effects and outcome of a policy of intermittent imatinib treatment in elderly patients with chronic myeloid leukemia. *Blood* 121:5138, 2013.

648. CML Autograft Trials Collaboration: Autologous stem cell transplantation in chronic myeloid leukaemia: A meta-analysis of six randomized trials. *Cancer Treat Rev* 33:39, 2007.

649. Goldman J: Autologous stem-cell transplantation for chronic myelogenous leukemia. *Semin Hematol* 30:53, 1993.

650. Talpaz M, Kantarjian H, Liang J, et al: Percentage of Philadelphia chromosome (Ph)-negative and Ph-positive cells found after autologous transplantation for chronic myelogenous leukemia depends on percentage of diploid cells induced by conventional dose chemotherapy before collection of autologous cells. *Blood* 85:3257, 1995.

651. Drummond MW, Marin D, Clark RE, et al: Mobilization of Ph chromosome-negative peripheral blood stem cells in chronic myeloid leukemia patients with imatinib mesylate-induced complete cytogenetic remission. *Br J Haematol* 123:479, 2003.

652. Hui CH, Goh KY, White D, et al: Successful peripheral blood stem cell mobilisation with filgrastim in patients with chronic myeloid leukaemia achieving complete cytogenetic response with imatinib, without increasing disease burden as measured by quantitative real-time PCR. *Leukemia* 17:821, 2003.

653. Kreuzer KA, Kluhs C, Baskaynak G, et al: Filgrastim-induced stem cell mobilization in chronic myeloid leukaemia patients during imatinib therapy: Safety, feasibility and evidence for an efficient in vivo purging. *Br J Haematol* 124:195, 2004.

654. Gordon MK, Sher D, Karrison T, et al: Successful autologous stem cell collection in patients with chronic myeloid leukemia in complete cytogenetic response, with quantitative measurement of BCR-ABL expression in blood, marrow, and apheresis products. *Leuk Lymphoma* 49:531, 2008.

655. Olavarria E: Autologous stem cell transplantation in chronic myeloid leukemia. *Semin Hematol* 44:252, 2007.

656. Perseghin P, Gambacorti-Passerini C, Tornaghi L, et al: Peripheral blood progenitor cell collection in chronic myeloid leukemia patients with complete cytogenetic response after treatment with imatinib mesylate. *Transfusion* 45:1214, 2005.

657. Cervantes F, Hernandez-Boluda JC, Odriozola J, et al: Imatinib mesylate (STI571) treatment in patients with chronic-phase chronic myelogenous leukaemia previously submitted to autologous stem cell transplantation. *Br J Haematol* 120:500, 2003.

658. Simon W, Segel GB, Lichtman MA: Early allogeneic stem cell transplantation for chronic myelogenous leukemia in the imatinib era: A preliminary assessment. *Blood Cells Mol Dis* 37:116, 2006.

659. Goldman J: Allogeneic stem cell transplantation for chronic myeloid leukemia—Status in 2007. *Bone Marrow Transplant* 42:S11, 2008.

660. Giralt SA, Arora M, Goldman JM, et al: Chronic Leukemia Working Committee, Center for International Blood and Marrow Transplant Research: Impact of imatinib therapy on the use of allogeneic haematopoietic progenitor cell transplantation for the treatment of chronic myeloid leukaemia. *Br J Haematol* 137:461, 2007.

661. Maziarz RT: Who with chronic myelogenous leukemia to transplant in the era of tyrosine kinase inhibitors? *Curr Opin Hematol* 15:127, 2008.

662. Hehlmann R, Berger U, Pfirrmann M, et al: Drug treatment is superior to allografting as first-line therapy in chronic myeloid leukemia. *Blood* 109:4686, 2007.

663. Thomas ED, Clift RA, Fefer A, et al: Marrow transplantation for the treatment of chronic myelogenous leukemia. *Ann Intern Med* 104:155, 1986.

664. Apperley JF: Hematopoietic stem cell transplantation in chronic myeloid leukemia. *Curr Opin Hematol* 5:445, 1998.

665. Cooperative Study Group on Chromosomes in Transplanted Patients: Cytogenetic follow-up of 100 patients submitted to bone marrow transplantation for Philadelphia chromosome-positive chronic myeloid leukemia. *Eur J Haematol* 40:50, 1988.

666. McGlave P, Bartoch G, Anasetti C, et al: Unrelated donor marrow transplantation therapy for chronic myelogenous leukemia. *Blood* 81:543, 1993.

667. Fernandez HF, Tran HT, Albrecht F, et al: Evaluation of safety and pharmacokinetics of administering intravenous busulfan in a twice-daily or daily schedule to patients with advanced hematologic malignant disease undergoing stem cell transplantation. *Biol Blood Marrow Transplant* 8:486, 2002.

668. Radich JP, Gooley T, Bensinger W, et al: HLA-matched related hematopoietic cell transplantation for chronic-phase CML using a targeted busulfan and cyclophosphamide preparative regimen. *Blood* 102:31, 2003.

669. Warlick E, Ahn KW, Pedersen TL, et al: Reduced intensity conditioning is superior to nonmyeloablative conditioning for older chronic myelogenous leukemia patients undergoing hematopoietic cell transplant during the tyrosine kinase inhibitor era. *Blood* 119:4083, 2012.

670. Radich J: Stem cell transplant for chronic myeloid leukemia in the imatinib era. *Semin Hematol* 47:354, 2010.

671. Jabbour E, Cortes J, Santos FP, et al: Results of allogeneic hematopoietic stem cell transplantation for chronic myelogenous leukemia patients who failed tyrosine kinase inhibitors after developing BCR-ABL1 kinase domain mutations. *Blood* 117:3641, 2011.

672. Velev N, Cortes J, Champlin R, et al: Stem cell transplantation for patients with chronic myeloid leukemia resistant to tyrosine kinase inhibitors with BCR-ALB kinase domain mutation T315I. *Cancer* 116:3631, 1010.

673. Nicolini FE, Basak GW, Soverini S, et al: Allogeneic stem cell transplantation for patients harboring T315I BCR-ABL mutated leukemias. *Blood* 118:5697, 2011.

674. Goldman J: Implications of imatinib mesylate for hematopoietic stem cell transplantation. *Semin Hematol* 38:28, 2001.

675. Barrett J: Allogeneic stem cell transplantation for chronic myeloid leukemia. *Semin Hematol* 40:59, 2003.

676. Messner HA, Curtis JE, Lipton JL, et al: Three decades of allogeneic bone marrow transplants at the Princess Margaret Hospital. *Clin Transplant* 289, 1999.

677. Byrne JL, Stainer C, Hyde H, et al: Low incidence of acute graft-versus-host disease and recurrent leukemia in patients undergoing allogeneic haemopoietic stem cell transplantation from sibling donors with methotrexate and dose-monitored cyclosporin A prophylaxis. *Bone Marrow Transplant* 22:541, 1988.

678. Goldman J, Apperley J, Kanfer E, et al: Imatinib or transplant for chronic myeloid leukemia? *Lancet* 362:172, 2003.

679. Van Rhee F, Szydlo RM, Hermans J, et al: Long-term results after allogeneic bone marrow transplantation for chronic myelogenous leukemia in chronic phase: A report from the Chronic Leukemia Working Party of the European Groups for Blood and Marrow Transplantation. *Bone Marrow Transplant* 20:553, 1997.

680. Weisdorf DJ, Anasetti C, Antin JH, et al: Allogeneic bone marrow transplantation for chronic myelogenous leukemia: Comparative analysis of unrelated versus matched sibling donor transplantation. *Blood* 99:1971, 2002.

681. Laporte JP, Gorin NC, Rubinstein P, et al: Cord-blood transplantation from an unrelated donor in an adult with chronic myelogenous leukemia. *N Engl J Med* 335:167, 1997.

682. Oehler VG, Gooley T, Snyder DS, et al: The effects of imatinib mesylate treatment before allogeneic transplantation for chronic myeloid leukemia. *Blood* 109:1782, 2007.

683. Weisser M, Schmid C, Schoch C, et al: Resistance to pretransplant imatinib therapy may adversely affect the outcome of allogeneic stem cell transplantation in CML. *Bone Marrow Transplant* 36:1017, 2005.

684. Jabbour E, Cortes J, Kantarjian H, et al: Novel tyrosine kinase inhibitor therapy before allogeneic stem cell transplantation in patients with chronic myeloid leukemia: No evidence for increased transplant-related toxicity. *Cancer* 110:340, 2007.

685. Radich JP, Gehly G, Gooley T, et al: Polymerase chain reaction detection of the BCR-ABL fusion transcript after allogeneic marrow transplantation for chronic myeloid leukemia: Results and implications in 346 patients. *Blood* 85:2632, 1995.

686. Goldman JM: Therapeutic strategies for chronic myeloid leukemia in chronic (stable) phase. *Semin Hematol* 40:10, 2003.

687. Miller JS, Cooley S, Parham P, et al: Missing KIR ligands are associated with less relapse and increased graft-versus-host disease (GVHD) following unrelated donor allogeneic HCT. *Blood* 109:5058, 2007.

688. Elmaagacli AH, Ottinger H, Koldehoff M, et al: Reduced risk for molecular disease in patients with chronic myeloid leukemia after transplantation from a KIR-mismatched donor. *Transplantation* 79:1741, 2005.

689. Nadal E, Garin M, Kaeda J, et al: Increased frequencies of CD4(+)CD25(high) T(regs) correlate with disease relapse after allogeneic stem cell transplantation for chronic myeloid leukemia. *Leukemia* 21:472, 2007.

690. Crawley C, Szydlo R, Lalancette M, et al: Outcomes of reduced-intensity transplantation for chronic myeloid leukemia: An analysis of prognostic factors from the Chronic Leukemia Working Party of the EBMT. *Blood* 106:2969, 2005.

691. Kebriaei P, Detry MA, Giralt S: Long-term follow-up of allogeneic hematopoietic stem-cell transplantation with reduced-intensity conditioning for patients with chronic myeloid leukemia. *Blood* 110:3456, 2007.

692. Uzunel M, Mattsson J, Brune M, et al: Kinetics of minimal residual disease and chimerism in patients with chronic myeloid leukemia after nonmyeloablative conditioning and allogeneic stem cell transplantation. *Blood* 101:469, 2003.

693. Or R, Shapira MY, Resnick I, et al: Nonmyeloablative allogeneic stem cell transplantation for the treatment of chronic myeloid leukemia in first chronic phase. *Blood* 101:441, 2003.

694. Bornhauser M, Kiehl M, Siegert W, et al: Dose-reduced conditioning for allografting in 44 patients with chronic myeloid leukaemia: A retrospective analysis. *Br J Haematol* 115:119, 2001.

695. Das M, Saikia TK, Advani SH, et al: Use of a reduced-intensity conditioning regimen for allogeneic transplantation in patients with chronic myeloid leukemia. *Bone Marrow Transplant* 32:125, 2003.

696. Feinstein L, Storb R: Reducing transplant toxicity. *Curr Opin Hematol* 8:342, 2001.

697. Koh LP, Hwang WY, Chuah CT, et al: Imatinib mesylate (STI-571) given concurrently with nonmyeloablative stem cell transplantation did not compromise engraftment and resulted in cytogenetic remission in a patient with chronic myeloid leukemia in blast crisis. *Bone Marrow Transplant* 31:305, 2003.

698. McCann SR: Molecular response to imatinib mesylate following relapse after allogeneic SCT for CML. *Blood* 101:1200, 2003.

699. Vandenberghe P, Boeckx N, Ronsyn E, et al: Imatinib mesylate induces durable complete remission of advanced CML persisting after allogeneic bone marrow transplantation. *Leukemia* 17:458, 2003.

700. Ullmann AJ, Hess G, Kolbe K, et al: Current results on the use of imatinib mesylate in patients with relapsed Philadelphia chromosome positive leukemia after allogeneic or syngeneic hematopoietic stem cell transplantation. *Keio J Med* 52:182, 2003.
701. Olavarria E, Craddock C, Dazzi F, et al: Imatinib mesylate (STI571) in the treatment of relapse of chronic myeloid leukemia after allogeneic stem cell transplantation. *Blood* 99:3861, 2002.
702. Weisser M, Tischer J, Schnittger S, et al: A comparison of donor lymphocyte infusions or imatinib mesylate for patients with chronic myelogenous leukemia who have relapsed after allogeneic stem cell transplantation. *Haematologica* 91:663, 2006
703. Savani BN, Montero A, Kurlander R, et al: Imatinib synergizes with donor lymphocyte infusions to achieve rapid molecular remission of CML relapsing after allogeneic stem stem cell transplantation. *Bone Marrow Transplant* 36;1009, 2005.
704. Bar M, Radich J: Maintenance therapy with tyrosine kinase inhibitors after transplant in patients with chronic myeloid leukemia. *J Natl Compr Canc Netw* 11:308, 2013.
705. Carpenter PA, Snyder DS, Flowers ME, et al: Prophylactic administration of imatinib after hematopoietic cell transplantation for high-risk Philadelphia chromosome-positive leukemia. *Blood* 109:2791, 2007.
706. Olavarria E, Siddique S, Griffiths MJ, et al: Posttransplantation imatinib as a strategy to postpone the requirement for immunotherapy in patients undergoing reduced-intensity allografts for chronic myeloid leukemia. *Blood* 110:4614, 2007.
707. Sullivan KM: Marrow transplantation for disorders of hematopoiesis. *Leukemia* 7:1098, 1993.
708. Kolb HJ, Mittermuller J, Clemm CH, et al: Donor leukocyte transfusions for treatment of recurrent chronic myelogenous leukemia in marrow transplant patients. *Blood* 76:2462, 1990.
709. Dazzi F, Szydlo RM, Goldman JM: Donor lymphocyte infusion for relapse of chronic myeloid leukemia after allogeneic stem cell transplant: Where we now stand. *Exp Hematol* 27:1477, 1999.
710. Van Rhee F, Lin F, Cullis JO, et al: Relapse of chronic myeloid leukemia after allogeneic bone marrow transplant: The case of giving donor leukocyte transfusions before the onset of hematologic relapse. *Blood* 83:3377, 1994.
711. Leis J, Porter DL: Unrelated donor leukocyte infusions to treat relapse after unrelated donor bone marrow transplantation. *Leuk Lymphoma* 43:9, 2002.
712. Dazzi F, Goldman J: Donor lymphocyte infusions. *Curr Opin Hematol* 6:394, 1999.
713. Dazzi F, Szydlo RM, Cross NCP, et al: Durability of responses following donor lymphocyte infusions for patients who relapse after allogeneic stem cell transplantation for chronic myeloid leukemia. *Blood* 96:2712, 2000.
714. Dazzi F: Monitoring of minimal residual disease after allografting: A requirement to guide DLI treatment. *Ann Hematol* 81 Suppl 2:S29, 2002.
715. Porter D, Levine JE: Graft-versus-host disease and graft-versus-leukemia after donor leukocyte infusion. *Semin Hematol* 43:53, 2006.
716. MacKinnon S: Donor leukocyte infusions. *Baillieres Clin Haematol* 10:357, 1997.
717. Giralt S, Hester J, Huh T, et al: CD8-depleted donor lymphocyte infusion as treatment for relapsed chronic myelogenous leukemia after allogeneic bone marrow transplantation. *Blood* 86:4337, 1995.
718. Guglielma C, Arcese W, Dazzi F, et al: Donor lymphocyte infusion for relapsed chronic myelogenous leukemia: Prognostic relevance of the initial cell dose. *Blood* 100:397, 2002.
719. Savani BN, Montero A, Kurlander R, et al: Imatinib synergizes with donor lymphocyte infusions to achieve rapid molecular remission of CML relapsing after allogeneic stem cell transplantation. *Bone Marrow Transplant* 36:1009, 2005.
720. Huang X, Cortes J, Kantarjian H: Estimations of the increasing prevalence and plateau prevalence of chronic myeloid leukemia in the era of tyrosine kinase inhibitor therapy. *Cancer* 118:3123, 2012.
721. Bjorkholm M, Ohm L, Eloranta S, et al: Success of targeted therapy in chronic myeloid leukemia: A population-based study of patients diagnosed in Sweden from 1973 to 2008. *J Clin Oncol* 29:2514, 2011.
722. Höglund M, Sandin F, Hellström K, et al: Tyrosine kinase inhibitor usage, treatment, outcome, and prognostic scores in CML: Report from the population-based Swedish CML registry. *Blood* 122:1284, 2013.
723. Druker BJ, Guilhot F, O'Brien SG, et al: Five-year follow-up of patients receiving imatinib for chronic myeloid leukemia. *N Engl J Med* 355:2408, 2006.
724. Rosti G, Iacobucci I, Bassi S, et al: Impact of age on the outcome of patients with chronic myeloid leukemia in late chronic phase: Results of a phase II study of the GIMEMA CML Working Party. *Haematologica* 92:101, 2007.
725. Kantarjian H, O'Brien S, Talpaz M, et al: Outcome of patients with Philadelphia chromosome-positive chronic myelogenous leukemia post-imatinib mesylate failure. *Cancer* 109:1556, 2007.
726. Kantarjian H, O'Brien S, Jabbour E, et al: Improved survival in chronic myeloid leukemia since the introduction of imatinib therapy: A single-institution historical experience. *Blood* 119:1981, 2012.
727. Passweg JR, Walker I, Sobocinski KA, et al: Validation and extension of the EBMT Risk Score for patients with chronic myeloid leukemia (CML) receiving allogeneic haematopoietic stem cell transplants. *Br J Haematol* 125:613, 2004.
728. Hasford J, Pfirrmann M, Hehlmann R, et al: Prognosis and prognostic factors for patients with chronic myeloid leukemia: Nontransplant therapy. *Semin Hematol* 40:4, 2003.
729. Qazilbash MH, Devetten MP, Abraham J, et al: Utility of a prognostic scoring system for allogeneic stem cell transplantation in patients with chronic myeloid leukemia. *Acta Haematol* 109:119, 2003.
730. Usman M, Syed NN, Kakepoto GN, et al: Chronic phase chronic myeloid leukemia: Response of imatinib mesylate and significance of Sokal score, age and disease duration in predicting the hematological and cytogenetic response. *J Assoc Physicians India* 55:103, 2007.
731. Rosti G, Martinelli G, Bassi S, et al: Molecular response to imatinib in late chronic-phase chronic myeloid leukemia. *Blood* 103:2284, 2004.
732. Lauseker M, Hasford J, Pfirmann M, et al: The impact of health care settings on survival time of patients with chronic phase myeloid leukemia. *Blood* 123:2494, 2014.
733. Boehm A, Walcherberger B, Sperr WR, et al: Improved outcome in patients with chronic myeloid leukemia after allogeneic hematopoietic stem cell transplantation over the past 25 years: A single center experience. *Biol Blood Marrow Transplant* 17:133, 2011.
734. Goldman JM, Majhail NS, Klein JP, et al: Relapse and late mortality in 5-year survivors of myeloablative allogeneic hematopoietic cell transplantation for chronic myeloid leukemia in first chronic phase. *J Clin Oncol* 28:1888, 2010.
735. Khoury HJ, Kukreja M, Goldman JM, et al: Prognostic factors for outcomes in allogeneic transplantation (allo SCT) for chronic myeloid leukemia in the imatinib era: Evaluation of its impact within a subgroup of the randomized German CMLA Study IV. *Blood* 115:1880, 2010.
736. Yee K, Anglin P, Keating A: Molecular approaches to the detection and monitoring of chronic myeloid leukemia: Theory and practice. *Blood Rev* 13:105, 1999.
737. Hughes T, Branford S: Molecular monitoring of chronic myeloid leukemia. *Semin Hematol* 40:62, 2003.
738. Kantarjian H, Schiffer C, Jones D, Cortes J: Monitoring the response and course of chronic myeloid leukemia in the modern era of BCR-ABL tyrosine kinase inhibitors: Practical advice on the use and interpretation of monitoring methods. *Blood* 111(4):1774, 2008.
739. Lowenberg B: Minimal residual disease in chronic myeloid leukemia. *N Engl J Med* 349:1399, 2003.
740. Gabert J: Detection of recurrent translocations using real time PCR; assessment of the technique for diagnosis and detection of minimal residual disease. *Haematologica* 84:107, 1999.
741. Negrin RS, Blume KG: The use of polymerase chain reaction for the detection of minimal residual malignant disease. *Blood* 78:255, 1991.
742. Lee MS, Kantarjian H, Talpaz M, et al: Detection of minimal residual disease by polymerase chain reaction in Philadelphia chromosome-positive chronic myelogenous leukemia following interferon therapy. *Blood* 79:1920, 1992.
743. Branford S, Fletcher L, Cross NC, et al: Desirable performance characteristics for BCR-ABL measurement on an international reporting scale to allow consistent interpretation of individual patient response and comparison of response rates between clinical trials. *Blood* 112:3330, 2008.
744. Sahay T, Schiffer CA: Monitoring minimal residual disease in patients with chronic myeloid leukemia after treatment with tyrosine kinase inhibitors. *Curr Opin Hematol* 15:134, 2008.
745. Stock W, Yu D, Karrison T, et al: Quantitative real-time RT-PCR monitoring of BCR-ABL in chronic Myelogenous leukemia shows lack of agreement in blood and bone marrow samples. *Int J Oncol* 28:1099, 2006
746. Hughes T, Deininger M, Hochhaus A, et al: CML patients responding to treatment with tyrosine kinase inhibitors: Review and recommendations for harmonizing current methodology for detecting BCR-ABL transcripts and kinase domain mutations and for expressing results. *Blood* 108:28, 2006.
747. Iacobucci I, Saglio G, Rosti G, et al: Achieving a major molecular response at the time of a complete cytogenetic response (CCgR) predicts a better duration of CCgR in imatinib-treated chronic myeloid leukemia patients. *Clin Cancer Res* 12:3037, 2006.
748. Press RD, Love Z, Tronnes AA, et al: BCR-ABL mRNA levels at and after the time of a complete cytogenetic response (CCR) predict the duration of CCR in imatinib mesylate-treated patients with CML. *Blood* 107:4250, 2006.
749. Jabbour E, Cortes JE, Kantarjian HM: Molecular monitoring in chronic myeloid leukemia: Response to tyrosine kinase inhibitors and prognostic implications. *Cancer* 112:2112, 2008.
750. Jain P, Kantarjian H, Nazha A, et al: Early responses predict better outcomes in patients with newly diagnosed chronic myeloid leukemia; results with four tyrosine kinase inhibitor modalities. *Blood* 121:4867, 2013.
751. Cohen N, Novikov I, Hardan I, et al: Standardization criteria for the detection of BCR/ABL fusion in interphase nuclei of chronic myelogenous leukemia patients by fluorescence in situ hybridization. *Cancer Genet Cytogenet* 123:102, 2000.
752. Rheinhold U, Hennig E, Leiblein S, et al: FISH for BCR-ABL on interphases of peripheral blood neutrophils but not of unselected white cells correlates with bone marrow cytogenetics in CML patients treated with imatinib. *Leukemia* 17:1925, 2003.
753. Kim YJ, Kim DW, Lee S, et al: Comprehensive comparison of FISH, RT-PCR, and RQ-PCR for monitoring the BCR-ABL gene after hematopoietic stem cell transplantation in CML. *Eur J Haematol* 68:272, 2002.
754. Bao F, Munker R, Lowery C, et al: Comparison of FISH and quantitative RT-PCR for the diagnosis and follow-up of BCR-ABL-positive leukemias. *Mol Diagn Ther* 11:239, 2007.
755. Uzunel M, Mattsson J, Brune M, et al: Kinetics of minimal residual disease and chimerism in patients with chronic myeloid leukemia after nonmyeloablative conditioning and allogeneic stem cell transplantation. *Blood* 101:469, 2003.
756. Hochhaus A, Weisser A, LaRosee P, et al: Detection and quantification of residual disease in chronic myelogenous leukemia. *Leukemia* 14:998, 2000.

757. Olavarria E, Kanfer E, Szydlo R, et al: Early detection of *BCR-ABL* transcripts by quantitative reverse transcriptase-polymerase chain reaction predicts outcome after allogeneic stem cell transplantation for chronic myeloid leukemia. *Blood* 97:1560, 2001.

758. Radich JP, Gooley T, Bryant E, et al: The significance of *bcr-abl* molecular detection in chronic myeloid leukemia patients "late" 18 months or more after transplantation. *Blood* 98:1701, 2001.

759. Lion T: Minimal residual disease. *Curr Opin Hematol* 6:406, 1999.

760. Thiele J, Wickenhauser C, Kvasnicka HM, et al: Mixed chimerism of bone marrow CD34+ progenitor cells (genotyping, bcr/abl analysis) after allogeneic transplantation for chronic myelogenous leukemia. *Transplantation* 74:982, 2002.

761. Sobrinho-Simões M, Wilczek V, Score J, et al: In search of the original leukemic clone in chronic myeloid leukemia paients in complete molecular remission after stem cell transplantation or imatinib. *Blood* 116:1329, 2010.

762. Jabbour E, Kantarjian HM, O'Brien S, et al: Front-line therapy with second-generation tyrosine kinase inhibitors in patients with early chronic phase chronic myeloid leukemia: What is the optimal response? *J Clin Oncol* 29:4260, 2011.

763. Kantarjian HM, Shan J, Jones D et al: Significance of increasing levels of minimal residual disease in patients with Philadelphia chromosome-positive chronic myelogenous leukemia in complete cytogenetic response. *J Clin Oncol* 27:3659, 2009.

764. Branford S, Kim DW, Soverini S, et al: Initial molecular response at 3 months may predict both response and event-free survival at 24 months in imatinib-resistant or -intolerant patients with Philadelphia chromosome-positive chronic myeloid leukemia in chronic phase treated with nilotinib. *J Clin Oncol* 30:4323, 2012.

765. Radich JP: How I monitor residual disease in chronic myeloid leukemia. *Blood* 114:3376, 2009.

766. Branford S, Yeung DT, Prime JA, et al: *BCR-ABL1* doubling times more reliably assess the dynamics of CML relapse compared with the *BCR-ABL1* fold rise: Implications for monitoring and management. *Blood* 119:4264, 2012.

767. Giles FJ, Cortes JE, Kantarjian HM, O'Brien S: Accelerated and blastic phase of chronic myelogenous leukemia. *Hematol Oncol Clin North Am* 18:753, 2004.

768. Kantarjian HM, Deisseroth A, Kurzrock R, et al: Chronic myelogenous leukemia: A concise update. *Blood* 82:691, 1993.

769. Swerdlow SH, Campo E, Harris NL, et al: *World Health Organization Classification of Tumours of Haematopoieitc and Lymphoid Tissues*. IARC Press, Lyon, 2008.

770. Druker BJ: Chronic myelogenous leukemia, in *Principles & Practice of Oncology*, vol 2, ed 8, edited by DeVita VT, Lawrence TS, Rosenburg SA, p 2267. Lippincott, Williams and Wilkins, Baltimore, MD, 2007.

771. Bolton-Gillespie E, Schemionek M, Klein HU, et al: Genomic instability may originate from imatinib-refractory chronic myeloid leukemia stem cells. *Blood* 121:4175, 2013.

772. Jamieson CH, Ailles LE, Dylla SJ, et al: Granulocyte-macrophage progenitors as candidate leukemic stem cells in blast-crisis CML. *N Engl J Med* 351:657, 2004.

773. Michor F: Chronic myeloid leukemia blast crisis arises from progenitors. *Stem Cells* 25:1114, 2007.

774. Wodarz D: Stem cell regulation and the development of blast crisis in chronic myeloid leukemia: Implications for the outcome of Imatinib treatment and discontinuation. *Med Hypotheses* 70:128, 2008.

775. Melo JV, Barnes DJ: Chronic myeloid leukaemia as a model of disease evolution in human cancer. *Nat Rev Cancer* 7:441, 2007.

776. Brazma D, Grace C, Howard J, et al: Genomic profile of chronic myelogenous leukemia: Imbalances associated with disease progression. *Genes Chromosomes Cancer* 46:1039, 2007.

777. Gaiger A, Henn T, Horth E, et al: Increase of bcr/abl chimeric mRNA expression in tumor cells of patients with chronic myeloid leukemia precedes disease progression. *Blood* 86:2371, 1995.

778. Elmaaglacli AH, Beelen DW, Opalka B, et al: The amount of BCR/ABL fusion transcripts detected by real time quantitative polymerase chain reaction method in patients with Philadelphia chromosome positive chronic myeloid leukemia disease stages correlates with the disease stages. *Ann Hematol* 79:424, 2000.

779. Lowenberg B, Hagemeijer A, Swart K, Abels J: Serial follow-up of patients with chronic myeloid leukemia (CML) with combined cytogenetic and colony culture methods. *Exp Hematol* 10:123, 1982.

780. Haas OA, Schwarzmeier JD, Nachera E, et al: Investigations on karyotype evolution in patients with chronic myeloid leukemia (CML). *Blut* 48:33, 1984.

781. Swolin B, Weinfeld A, Westin J, et al: Karyotypic evolution in Ph-positive chronic myeloid leukemia in relation to management and disease progression. *Cancer Genet Cytogenet* 18:65, 1985.

782. Cortes J, O'Dwyer ME: Clonal evolution in chronic myelogenous leukemia. *Hematol Oncol Clin North Am* 18:671, 2004.

783. Honda H, Ushijima K, Oda H, et al: Acquired loss of p53 induces blast transformation in p210bcr/abl-expressing hematopoietic cells: A transgenic study for blast crisis in human CML. *Blood* 95:1144, 2000.

784. Yamaguchi H, Inokuchi K, Sakuma Y, Dan K: Mutation of p51/p63 gene is associated with blast crisis in chronic myelogenous leukemia. *Leukemia* 15:1729, 2001.

785. Coiffier B, Byron PA, Flere D, et al: Chronic granulocytic leukemia: Early detection of metamorphosis with "in vitro" culture of granulocytic progenitors. *Biomedicine* 33:96, 1980.

786. Todd MB, Waldron JA, Jennings TA, et al: Loss of myeloid differentiation antigens precedes blastic transformation in chronic myelogenous leukemia. *Blood* 70:122, 1987.

787. Griesshammer M, Heinze B, Bangerter M, et al: Karyotype abnormalities and their clinical significance in blast crisis of chronic myeloid leukemia. *J Mol Med* 75:8836, 1997.

788. Spencer A, Vulliamy T, Kaeda J, et al: Clonal instability preceding lymphoid blastic transformation of chronic myeloid leukemia. *Leukemia* 11:195, 1997.

789. Anastasi J, Feng J, LeBeau MM, et al: The relationship between secondary chromosomal abnormalities and blast transformation in chronic myelogenous leukemia. *Leukemia* 9:628, 1995.

790. Bartram CR, de Klein A, Hagemeijer A, et al: Additional C-abl/bcr rearrangements in a CML patient exhibiting two Ph1 chromosomes during blast crisis. *Leuk Res* 10:221, 1986.

791. Collins SJ, Grudine MT: Chronic myelogenous leukemia: Amplification of a rearranged c-abl oncogene in both chronic phase and blast crisis. *Blood* 69:893, 1987.

792. Mughal TI, Goldman JM: Chronic myeloid leukemia: Why does it evolve from chronic phase to blast transformation? *Front Biosci* 11:198, 2006.

793. Schaefer-Rego K, Dudek H, Popenoe D, et al: CML patients in blast crisis have breakpoints localized to a specific region of the bcr. *Blood* 70:448, 1987.

794. Mills KI, Benn P, Birnie GD: Does the breakpoint within the major breakpoint region (M-bcr) influence the duration of the chronic phase in chronic myeloid leukemia? An analytical comparison of current literature. *Blood* 78:1155, 1991.

795. Bartram CR, Janssen JWG, Becher R, et al: Persistence of chronic myelocytic leukemia despite deletion of rearranged bcr/c-abl sequences in blast crisis. *J Exp Med* 164:1389, 1986.

796. Okabe M, Matsushima S: Philadelphia chromosome-positive leukemia: Molecular analysis of *bcr* and *abl* genes and transforming genes. *Nippon Ketsueki Gakkai Zasshi* 51:1471, 1988.

797. Ahuja H, Bar-Eli M, Arlin Z, et al: The spectrum of molecular alterations in the evolution of chronic myelocytic leukemia. *J Clin Invest* 87:2042, 1991.

798. Kelman Z, Prokocimer M, Peller S, et al: Rearrangements in the p53 gene in Philadelphia chromosome positive chronic myelogenous leukemia. *Blood* 74:2318, 1989.

799. Mashal R, Shtalrid M, Talpaz M, et al: Rearrangement and expression of p53 in the chronic phase and blast crisis of chronic myelocytic leukemia. *Blood* 75:180, 1990.

800. Guinn BA, Mello KI: P53 mutations, methylation and genomic instability in the progression of chronic myeloid leukemia. *Leuk Lymphoma* 26:241, 1997.

801. Malinen T, Palotie A, Pakkala S, et al: Acceleration of chronic myeloid leukemia correlates with calcitonin gene methylation. *Blood* 77:2435, 1991.

802. Asimakopoolos FA, Shteper PJ, Krichevsky S, et al: *ABL1* methylation is a distinct molecular event associated with clonal evolution of chronic myeloid leukemia. *Blood* 94:2452, 1999.

803. Towatari M, Adachi K, Kato H, Saito H: Absence of the human retinoblastoma gene product in the megakaryoblastic crisis of chronic myelogenous leukemia. *Blood* 78:2178, 1991.

804. Sill H, Goldman JM, Cross NC: Homozygous deletions of the p16 tumor-suppressor gene are associated with lymphoid transformation of chronic myeloid leukemia. *Blood* 85:2013, 1995.

805. Hernandez-Boluda JC, Cervantes F, Colomer D, et al: Genomic p16 abnormalities in the progression of chronic myeloid leukemia into blast crisis. *Exp Hematol* 31:204, 2003.

806. Serra A, Gottardi E, Della Ragione F, et al: Involvement at the cyclin-dependent kinase-4 inhibitor (CDKN2) gene in the pathogenesis of lymphoid blast crisis of chronic myelogenous leukaemia. *Br J Haematol* 91:625, 1995.

807. Menssen HD, Renkl HJ, Rodeck U, et al: Presence of Wilms' tumor gene (wt1) transcripts and the WT1 nuclear protein in the majority of human acute leukemias. *Leukemia* 9:1060, 1995.

808. Mitarri K, Ogawa S, Tanaka T, et al: Generation of the AML1-EVI-1 fusion gene in the t(3;21) (q26;q22) causes blastic crisis in chronic myelocytic leukemia. *EMBO J* 13:504, 1994.

809. Carapeti M, Goldman JM, Cross NC: Overexpression of EV-l in blast crisis of chronic myeloid leukemia. *Leukemia* 10:1561, 1996.

810. Mori N, Takeuchi S, Tasaka T, et al: Absence of microsatellite instability during the progression of chronic myelocytic leukemia. *Leukemia* 11:151, 1997.

811. Handa H, Hegde UP, Kuteninikov VM, et al: Bcl-2 and c-myc expressions, cell cycle kinetics and apoptosis during the progression of chronic myelogenous leukemia from diagnosis to blastic phase. *Leuk Res* 21:479, 1997.

812. Daheron L, Salmeron S, Patri S, et al: Identification of several genes differentially expressed during progression of chronic myelogenous leukemia. *Leukemia* 12:326, 1998.

813. Foti A, Ahuja HG, Allen SL, et al: Correlation between molecular and clinical events in the evolution of chronic myelocytic leukemia to blast crisis. *Blood* 77:2441, 1991.

814. Mori N, Morosetti R, Loe S, et al: Allelotype analysis in the evolution of chronic myelocytic leukemia. *Blood* 90:2010, 1997.

815. Hehlmann R: How I treat CML blast crisis. *Blood* 120:737, 2012.

816. Radich JP, Dai H, Mao M, et al: Gene expression changes associated with progression and response in chronic myeloid leukemia. *Proc Natl Acad Sci U S A* 103:2794, 2006.

817. Yong AS, Szydlo RM, Goldman JM, et al: Molecular profiling of CD34+ cells identifies low expression of CD7, along with high expression of proteinase 3 or elastase, as predictors of longer survival in patients with CML. *Blood* 107:205, 2006.

818. Spiers ASD: Metamorphosis of chronic granulocytic leukemia: Diagnosis, classification and management. *Br J Haematol* 49:1, 1979.

819. Grignani F: Chronic myelogenous leukemia. *Crit Rev Oncol Hematol* 4:31, 1985.

820. Matsuo T, Tomonaga M, Kuriyama K, et al: Prognostic significance of the morphological dysplastic changes in chronic myelogenous leukemia. *Leuk Res* 10:331, 1986.

821. Specchia G, Palumbo G, Pastore D, et al: Extramedullary blast crisis in chronic myeloid leukemia. *Leuk Res* 20:905, 1996.

822. Inveradi D, Lazzarino M, Morra E, et al: Extramedullary disease in Ph-positive chronic myelogenous leukemia: Frequency, clinical features, prognostic significance. *Haematologica* 75:146, 1990.

823. Jacknow J, Fizzera G, Gajl-Peczalska K, et al: Extramedullary presentation of the blast crisis of chronic myelogenous leukemia. *Br J Haematol* 61:225, 1985.

824. Terjanian T, Kantarjian H, Keating M, et al: Clinical and prognostic features of patients with Philadelphia chromosome-positive chronic myelogenous leukemia and extramedullary disease. *Cancer* 59:297, 1987.

825. Miksanek T, Reyes CV, Semkuo Z, Molnar ZJ: Granulocytic sarcoma of the peritoneum. *CA Cancer J Clin* 33:40, 1983.

826. Jones TI: Pleural blast crisis in chronic myelogenous leukemia. *Am J Hematol* 44:75, 1993.

827. Pascoe HR: Tumors composed of immature granulocytes occurring in the breast in chronic granulocytic leukemia. *Cancer* 25:697, 1970.

828. Chabner BA, Haskell CM, Canellos GP: Destructive bone lesions in chronic granulocytic leukemia. *Medicine (Baltimore)* 48:401, 1969.

829. Licht A, Many N, Rachmilewitz EA: Myelofibrosis, osteolytic bone lesions and hypercalcemia in chronic myeloid leukemia. *Acta Haematol* 49:182, 1973.

830. Lee CH, Morris TCM: Bone marrow necrosis and extramedullary myeloid tumor necrosis in aggressive chronic myeloid leukemia. *Pathology* 11:551, 1979.

831. Asarro S, Sato N, Ueshima Y, et al: Localized blastoma preceding blastic transformation in Ph1-positive chronic myelogenous leukemia. *Scand J Haematol* 25:251, 1980.

832. Ohyashiki K, Ito H: Characterization of extramedullary tumors in a case of Ph-positive chronic myelogenous leukemia. *Cancer Genet Cytogenet* 15:119, 1985.

833. Sun T, Susin M, Koduru P, et al: Extramedullary blast crisis in chronic myelogenous leukemia. *Cancer* 68:605, 1991.

834. Saikia TK, Dhabhar B, Iyer RS, et al: High incidence of meningeal leukemia in lymphoid blast crisis of chronic myelogenous leukemia. *Am J Hematol* 43:10, 1993.

835. Falini B, Tabilio A, Pelicci PG, et al: T-cell receptor B-chain gene rearrangement in a case of Ph1-positive chronic myeloid leukaemia blast crisis. *Br J Haematol* 62:776, 1986.

836. Giannone L, Whitlock JA, Kinney MC, et al: Use of the BCR probe to demonstrate extramedullary recurrence of CML with a T cell lymphoid phenotype following bone marrow transplantation. *Bone Marrow Transplant* 3:631, 1988.

837. Ohyashiki J, Ohyashiki K, Shimizu H, et al: Testicular tumor as the first manifestation of B-lymphoid blastic crisis in a case of Ph-positive chronic myelogenous leukemia. *Am J Hematol* 29:164, 1988.

838. Rosenthal S, Canellos GP, DeVita VT Jr, Gralnick HR: Characteristics of blast crisis in chronic granulocytic leukemia. *Blood* 49:705, 1977.

839. Barton JC, Conrad ME: Current status of blastic transformation in chronic myelogenous leukemia. *Am J Hematol* 4:281, 1978.

840. Peterson LC, Bloomfield CD, Brunning RD: Blast crisis as an initial or terminal manifestation of chronic myeloid leukemia. *Am J Med* 60:209, 1976.

841. Bettelheim P, Lutz D, Majdic O, et al: Cell lineage heterogeneity in blast crisis of chronic myeloid leukaemia. *Br J Haematol* 59:395, 1985.

842. Nair C, Chopra M, Shinde S, et al: Immunophenotype and ultrastructural studies in blast crisis of chronic myeloid leukemia. *Leuk Lymphoma* 19:309, 1995.

843. Rosenthal S, Canellos GP, Gralnick HR: Erythroblastic transformation of chronic granulocytic leukemia. *Am J Med* 63:116, 1977.

844. Ekblom M, Borgstrom G, von Willebrand E, et al: Erythroid blast crisis in chronic myelogenous leukemia. *Blood* 62:591, 1983.

845. Lingg G, Schmalzl F, Breton-Gorius J, et al: Megakaryoblastic micro-megakaryocytic crisis in chronic myeloid leukemia. *Blut* 51:275, 1985.

846. Castaigne S, Berger R, Jolly V, et al: Promyelocytic blast crisis of chronic myelocytic leukemia with both t(9;22) and t(15;17) in M3 cells. *Cancer* 54:2409, 1984.

847. Berger R, Bernheim A, Daniel MT, Flandrin G: T(15;17) in a promyelocytic form of chronic myeloid leukemia blastic crisis. *Cancer Genet Cytogenet* 8:149, 1983.

848. Misawa S, Lee E, Schiffer CA, et al: Association of translocation (15;17) with malignant proliferation of promyelocytes in acute leukemia and chronic myelogenous leukemia in blast crisis. *Blood* 67:270, 1986.

849. Marinone G, Rossi G, Verzura P: Eosinophilic blast crisis in a case of chronic myeloid leukaemia. *Br J Haematol* 55:251, 1983.

850. Goh KO, Anderson FW: Cytogenetic studies in basophilic chronic myelocytic leukemia. *Arch Pathol Lab Med* 103:288, 1979.

851. Rosenthal NS, Knapp D, Farhi DC: Promyelocytic blast crisis of chronic myelogenous leukemia. A rare subtype associated with disseminated intravascular coagulation. *Am J Clin Pathol* 103:185, 1995.

852. Lemes A, Gomez Casares MT, de la Iglesia S, et al: P190 BCR-ABL rearrangement in chronic myeloid leukemia and acute lymphoblastic leukemia. *Cancer Genet Cytogenet* 113:100, 1999.

853. Bertazzoni U, Brusamolino E, Isernia P, et al: Diagnostic significance of terminal transferase and adenosine deaminase in acute and chronic myeloid leukemia. *Blood* 60:685, 1982.

854. Schuh AC, Sutherland DR, Horsfall W, et al: Chronic myeloid leukemia arising in a progenitor common to T cells and myeloid cells. *Leukemia* 4:631, 1990.

855. Uike N, Takeichi N, Kimura N, et al: Dual arrangement of immunoglobulin and T-cell receptor genes in blast crisis of CML. *Eur J Haematol* 42:460, 1989.

856. Greaves MF, Verbi W, Reeves BR, et al: "Pre-B" phenotypes in blast crisis of Ph1 positive CML: Evidence for a pluripotential stem cell "target." *Leuk Res* 3:181, 1979.

857. Bakhshi A, Minowada J, Arnold A, et al: Lymphoid blast crisis of chronic myelogenous leukemia represents stages in the development of B-cell precursors. *N Engl J Med* 309:826, 1983.

858. Griffin JD, Todd RF, Ritz J, et al: Differentiation patterns in the blastic phase of chronic myeloid leukemia. *Blood* 61:85, 1983.

859. Bollum FJ: Terminal deoxynucleotidyl transferase, in *The Enzymes*, edited by Boyer RD, p 145. Academic, New York, 1974.

860. Dorfman DM, Longtine JA, Fox EA, et al: T-cell blast crisis in chronic myelogenous leukemia. *Am J Clin Pathol* 107:168, 1997.

861. Allouche M, Bourinbaiar A, Georgoulias V, et al: T-cell lineage involvement in lymphoid blast crisis of chronic myeloid leukemia. *Blood* 66:1155, 1985.

862. Gramatzki M, Bartram CR, Muller D, et al: Early T-cell differentiated chronic myeloid leukemia blast crisis with rearrangement of the breakpoint cluster region but not of the T-cell receptor beta chain genes. *Blood* 69:1082, 1987.

863. Dastugue N, Kuhlein E, Duchayne E, et al: T(14;14)(q11;q32) in biphenotypic blastic phase of chronic myeloid leukemia. *Blood* 68:949, 1986.

864. Kuriyama K, Tomonaga M, Yao E, et al: Dual expression of lymphoid/basophil markers on single blast cells transformed from chronic myeloid leukemia. *Leuk Res* 10:1015, 1986.

865. Yasukawa M, Iwamasa K, Kawamura S, et al: Phenotypic and genotypic analysis of chronic myelogenous leukaemia with T lymphoblastic and megakaryoblastic mixed crisis. *Br J Haematol* 66:331, 1987.

866. Spencer A, Vulliamy T, Chase A, et al: Myeloid to lymphoid clonal suppression following autologous transplantation in second chronic phase of chronic myeloid leukemia. *Leukemia* 9:2138, 1995.

867. Cervantes F, Villamor N, Esteve J, et al: "Lymphoid" blast crisis of chronic myeloid leukaemia is associated with distinct clinicohaematological features. *Br J Haematol* 100:123, 1998.

868. Stoll C, Oberline F: Non-random clonal evolution in 45 cases of chronic myeloid leukemia. *Leuk Res* 46:61, 1980.

869. Sandberg AA: The cytogenetics of chronic myelocytic leukemia (CML): Chronic phase and blast crisis. *Cancer Genet Cytogenet* 1:1980.

870. Myint H, Ross FM, Hall JL, et al: Early transformation to acute myeloblastic leukaemia with the acquisition of inv(16) in Ph positive chronic granulocytic leukaemia. *Leuk Res* 21:473, 1997.

871. Johansson B, Fioretos T, Mitelman F: Cytogenetic and molecular genetic evolution of chronic myeloid leukemia. *Acta Haematol* 107:76, 2002.

872. Sandberg AA: Chronic myelocytic leukemia, in *The Chromosomes in Human Cancer and Leukemia*, 2nd ed, p 465. Elsevier North Holland, New York, 1990.

873. Mitani K, Miyazono K, Urabe A, Takaku F: Karyotypic changes during the course of blastic crisis of chronic myelogenous leukemia. *Cancer Genet Cytogenet* 39:299, 1989.

874. Diez-Martin JL, DeWald GW, Pierre RV, et al: Possible cytogenetic distinction between lymphoid and myeloid blast crisis in chronic granulocytic leukemia. *Am J Hematol* 27:194, 1988.

875. Feinstein E, Cimino G, Gale RP, Canaani E: Initiation and progression of chronic myelogenous leukemia. *Leukemia* 6(Suppl 1):37, 1992.

876. Brizard F, Cividin M, Villalva C, et al: Comparison of M-FISH and conventional cytogenetic analysis in accelerated and acute phases of CML. *Leuk Res* 28:345, 2004.

877. Heim S, Christensen EB, Fioretos T, et al: Acute myelomonocytic leukemia with inv(16) (p13q22) complicating Philadelphia chromosome positive chronic myeloid leukemia. *Cancer Genet Cytogenet* 59:35, 1992.

878. Hogge DE, Misawa S, Testa JR, et al: Unusual karyotypic changes and B-cell involvement in a case of lymph node blast crisis of chronic myelogenous leukemia. *Blood* 64:123, 1984.

879. Kantarjian H, Talpaz M, O'Brien S, et al: Survival benefit with imatinib mesylate therapy in patients with accelerated-phase chronic myelogenous leukemia—Comparison with historic experience. *Cancer* 103:2099, 2005.

880. Shah NP: Advanced CML: Therapeutic options for patients in accelerated and blast phases. *J Natl Compr Canc Netw* 6 Suppl 2:S31, 2008.

881. Fruehauf S, Topaly J, Buss EC, et al: Imatinib combined with mitoxantrone/etoposide and cytarabine is an effective induction therapy for patients with chronic myeloid leukemia in myeloid blast crisis. *Cancer* 109:1543, 2007.

882. Cortes J, Kantarjian H: Advanced-phase chronic myeloid leukemia. *Semin Hematol* 40:79, 2003.

883. Druker BJ, Sawyers CL, Kantarjian H, et al: Activity of a specific inhibitor of the BCR-ABL tyrosine kinase in the blast crisis of chronic myeloid leukemia and acute lymphoblastic leukemia with the Philadelphia chromosome. *N Engl J Med* 344:1038, 2001.

884. Altintas A, Cil T, Kilinc I, et al: Central nervous system blastic crisis in chronic myeloid leukemia on imatinib mesylate therapy: A case report. *J Neurooncol* 84:103, 2007.

885. Simpson E, O'Brien SG, Reilly JT: Extramedullary blast crises in CML patients in complete hematological remission treated with imatinib mesylate. *Clin Lab Haematol* 28:215, 2006.

886. Gozzetti A, Bocchia M, Calabrese S, et al: Promyelocytic blast crisis of chronic myelogenous leukemia during imatinib treatment. *Acta Haematol* 117:236, 2007.

887. Kantarjian HM, Cortes J, O'Brien S, et al: Imatinib mesylate (STI571) therapy for Philadelphia chromosome–positive chronic myelogenous leukemia in blast phase. *Blood* 99:3547, 2002.

888. Giles FJ, Larson RA, Kantarjian HM, et al: Nilotinib in patients with Philadelphia chromosome-positive chronic myelogenous leukemia in blast crisis (CML-BC) who are resistant or intolerant to imatinib. *J Clin Oncol* 26:376, 2008.

889. Cortes J, Rousselot P, Kin DW, et al: Dasatinib induces complete hematologic and cytogenetic responses in patients with imatinib-resistant or intolerant chronic myeloid leukemia in blast crisis. *Blood* 109:3207, 2007.

890. Nicolini FE, Khoury HJ, Akard L, et al: Omacetaxine mepesuccinate for patients with accelerated phase chronic myeloid leukemia with resistance or intolerance to two or more tyrosine kinase inhibitors. *Haematologica* 29:e78, 2013.

891. Barone S, Baer MR, Sait SNJ, et al: High-dose cytosine arabinoside and idarubicin treatment of chronic myeloid leukemia in myeloid blast crisis. *Am J Hematol* 67:119, 2001.

892. Thomas DA, O'Brien SM, Faderl S, et al: Long-term outcome after hyper-CVAD and imatinib (IM) for de novo or minimally treated Philadelphia chromosome-positive acute lymphoblastic leukemia (Ph-ALL) *J Clin Oncol* 28: Abstract 6506, 2010.

893. Benjamini O, Dumlao TL, Kantarjian H, O'Brien S, et al: Phase II trial of hyper CVAD and dasatinib in patients with relapsed Philadelphia chromosome positive acute lymphoblastic leukemia or blast phase chronic myeloid leukemia. *Am J Hematol* 89:282, 2014.

894. Champlain R, Ho W, Arenson E, Gale RP: Allogeneic bone marrow transplantation for chronic myelogenous leukemia in chronic or accelerated phase. *Blood* 60:1038, 1982.

895. McGlave PB, Kim TH, Hard DD, et al: Successful allogeneic bone-marrow transplantation for patients in the accelerated phase of chronic granulocytic leukaemia. *Lancet* 2:625, 1982.

896. Martin PJ, Clift RA, Fisher LD, et al: HLA-identical marrow transplantation during accelerated-phase chronic myelogenous leukemia: Analysis of survival and remission duration. *Blood* 77:1978, 1988.

897. Falkenberg JHF, Wafelman AR, Joosten P, et al: Complete remission of accelerated phase chronic myeloid leukemia by treatment with leukemia-reactive cytotoxic T lymphocytes. *Blood* 94:1201, 1999.

898. Weisser M, Schleuning M, Haferlach C, et al: Allogeneic stem-cell transplantation provides excellent results in advanced stage chronic myeloid leukemia with major cytogenetic response to pre-transplant imatinib therapy. *Leuk Lymphoma* 48:295, 2007.

899. Carella AM, Gaozza E, Raffo MR, et al: Therapy of acute phase chronic myelogenous leukemia with intensive chemotherapy, blood cell autotransplant and cyclosporin A. *Leukemia* 5:517, 1991.

900. Bouvet M, Babiera GV, Termuhlen PM, et al: Splenectomy in the accelerated or blastic phase of chronic myelogenous leukemia: A single-institution 25-year experience. *Surgery* 122:20, 1997.

901. Wadhwa J, Szydio RM, Apperley J, et al: Factors affecting duration of survival after onset of blastic transformation of chronic myeloid leukemia. *Blood* 99:2304, 2002.

902. Majiis A, Smith TL, Talpaz M, et al: Significance of cytogenetic clonal evolution in chronic myelogenous leukemia. *J Clin Oncol* 14:196, 1996.

903. Fialkow PJ, Jacobsen RJ, Singer JW, et al: Philadelphia chromosome (Ph1)-negative chronic myelogenous leukemia (CML): A clonal disease with origin in a multipotent stem cell. *Blood* 56:70, 1980.

904. Such E, Germing U, Malcovati L, et al: Development and validation of a prognostic scoring system for patients with chronic myelomonocytic leukemia. *Blood* 121:3005, 2013.

905. Cortes J: CMML: A biologically distinct disease. *Curr Hematol Rep* 2:202, 2003.

906. Onida F, Beran M: Chronic myelomonocytic leukemia: Myeloproliferative variant. *Curr Hematol Rep* 3:218, 2004.

907. Gross SA, Irons RD, Scott PK, et al: A case-control study of chronic myelomonocytic leukemia (CMML) in Shanghai, China: Evaluation of risk factors for CMML, with special focus on benzene. *Arch Environ Occup Health* 67:206, 2012.

908. Takahashi K, Pemmaraju N, Strati P, et al: Clinical characteristics and outcomes of therapy-related chronic myelomonocytic leukemia. *Blood* 122:2807, 2013.

909. Saif MW, Hopkins JL, Gore SD: Autoimmune phenomena in patients with myelodysplastic syndromes and chronic myelomonocytic leukemia. *Leuk Lymphoma* 43:2083, 2002.

910. Cambier N, Baruchel A, Schlageter MH, et al: Chronic myelomonocytic leukemia: From biology to therapy. *Hematol Cell Ther* 39:41, 1997.

911. Stemmler J, Wittman GW, Hacker U, Heinemann V: Leukapheresis in chronic myelomonocytic leukemia with leukostasis syndrome: Elevated serum lactate levels as an early sign of microcirculation failure. *Leuk Lymphoma* 43:1427, 2002.

912. Bain BJ: Hypereosinophilia. *Curr Opin Hematol* 7:21, 2000.

913. Aguayo A, Kantarjian H, Manshouri T, et al: Angiogenesis in acute and chronic leukemias and myelodysplastic syndromes. *Blood* 96:2240, 2000.

914. Ramshaw HS, Bardy PG, Lee MA, Lopez AQF: Chronic myelomonocytic leukemia requires granulocytic-macrophage colony-stimulating factor for growth *in vitro* and *in vivo*. *Exp Hematol* 30:1124, 2002.

915. Tessema M, Länger F, Dingemann J, et al: Aberrant methylation and impaired expression of the p14INK4B cell cycle regulatory gene in chronic myelomonocytic leukemia (CMML). *Leukemia* 17:910, 2003.

916. Magnusson MK, Meade KE, Nakamura R, et al: Activity of STI571 in chronic myelomonocytic leukemia with a platelet-derived growth factor B receptor fusion oncogene. *Blood* 100:1088, 2002.

917. Apperley JF, Gardembas M, Melo JV, et al: Response to imatinib mesylate in patients with chronic myeloproliferative diseases with rearrangements of the platelet-derived growth factor receptor beta. *N Engl J Med* 347:481, 2002.

918. Wessels JW, Fibbe WE, van der Keur D, et al: T(5;12)(q31;p12): A clinical entity with features of both myeloid leukemia and chronic myelomonocytic leukemia. *Cancer Genet Cytogenet* 65:7, 1993.

919. Golub TR, Barker GF, Lovett HM, Gilliland DG: Fusion of PDGF receptor beta to a novel *ets*-like gen, *tel*, in chronic myelomonocytic leukemia with t(5;12) chromosomal translocation. *Cell* 77:307, 1994.

920. Cross NCP, Reiter A: Tyrosine kinase genes in chronic myeloproliferative diseases. *Leukemia* 16:1207, 2002.

921. Costa R, Abdulhaq H, Haq B, et al: Activity of azacitidine in chronic myelomonocytic leukemia. *Cancer* 117:2690, 2011.

922. Gunby RH, Cazzaniga G, Tassi E, et al: Sensitivity to imatinib but low frequency of the TEL/PDGFRbeta fusion protein in chronic myelomonocytic leukemia. *Haematologica* 88:408, 2003.

923. Pitini V, Arrigo C, Teti D, et al: Response to STI571 in chronic myelomonocytic leukemia with platelet derived growth factor beta receptor involvement: A new case report. *Haematologica* 88:ECR18, 2003.

924. Kröger N, Zabelina T, Guardiola P, et al: Allogeneic stem cell transplantation of adult chronic myelomonocytic leukemia. *Br J Haematol* 118:67, 2002.

925. Onida F, Kantarjian HM, Smith TL, et al: Prognostic factors and scoring systems in chronic myelomonocytic leukemia: A prospective analysis of 213 patients. *Blood* 99:840, 2002.

926. Germing U, Strupp C, Alvado M, Gattermann N: New prognostic parameters for chronic myelomonocytic leukemia? *Blood* 100:731, 2002.

927. Sagaster V, Ohler L, Berer A, et al: High spontaneous colony growth in chronic myelomonocytic leukemia correlates with increased disease activity and is a novel prognostic factor for predicting short survival. *Ann Hematol* 83:9, 2004.

928. Stillman RG: A case of myeloid leukemia with predominance of eosinophil cells. *Med Rec* 81:594, 1912.

929. Benvenisti DS, Ultmann JE: Eosinophilic leukemia. *Ann Intern Med* 71:731, 1969.

930. Chusid MJ, Dale D, West BG, Wolff SM: The hypereosinophilic syndrome: Analysis of fourteen cases with a review of the literature. *Medicine (Baltimore)* 54:1, 1975.

931. Brito-Babapulle F: The eosinophilias: Including the idiopathic hypereosinophilic syndrome. *Br J Haematol* 121:203, 2003.

932. Robyn J, Lemery S, McCoy JP, et al: Multilineage involvement of the fusion gene in patients with FIP1L1/PDGFRA-positive hypereosinophilic syndrome. *Br J Haematol* 132:286, 2006.

933. Crescenzi B, Chase A, Starza RL, et al: FIP1L1-PDGFRA in chronic eosinophilic leukemia and BCR-ABL1 in chronic myeloid leukemia affect different leukemic cells. *Leukemia* 21:397, 2007.

934. Pardanani A, Brockman SR, Paternoster SF, et al: FIP1L1-PDGFRA fusion: Prevalence and clinicopathologic correlates in 89 consecutive patients with moderate to severe eosinophilia. *Blood* 104:3038, 2004.

935. Bain BJ: Cytogenetic and molecular genetic aspects of eosinophilic leukemia. *Br J Haematol* 122:173, 2003.

936. Gotlib J, Cools J, Malone JM III, et al: The FIP1L1-PDGFRA fusion tyrosine kinase in hypereosinophilic syndrome and chronic eosinophilic leukemia: Implications for diagnosis, classification, and management. *Blood* 103:2879, 2004.

937. Vandenberghe P, Wlodarska I, Michaux L, et al: Clinical and molecular features of FIP1L1-PDFGRA (+) chronic eosinophilic leukemia. *Leukemia* 18:734, 2004.

938. Klion AD, Noel P, Akin C, et al: Elevated serum tryptase levels identify a subset of patients with a myeloproliferative variant of idiopathic hypereosinophilic syndrome associated with tissue fibrosis, poor prognosis, and imatinib responsiveness. *Blood* 101:4660, 2003.

939. Florian S, Esterbauer H, Binder T, et al: Systemic mastocytosis (SM) associated with chronic eosinophilic leukemia (SM-CEL): Detection of FIP1L1/PDGFRalpha, classification by WHO criteria, and response to therapy with imatinib. *Leuk Res* 30:1201, 2006.

940. Klion AD, Robyn J, Maric I, et al: Relapse following discontinuation of imatinib mesylate therapy for FIP1L1/PDGFRA-positive chronic eosinophilic leukemia: Implications for optimal dosing. *Blood* 110:3552, 2007.

941. Verstovsek S, Tefferi A, Cortes J, et al: Phase II study of dasatinib in Philadelphia chromosome-negative acute and chronic myeloid disease, including systemic mastocytosis. *Clin Cancer Res* 14:3906, 2008.

942. Esteva-Lorenzo FJ, Meehan KR, Spitzer TR, Mazumder A: Allogeneic bone marrow transplantation in a patient with hypereosinophilic syndrome. *Am J Hematol* 51:164, 1996.

943. Juvonen E, Volin L, Koponen A, Ruutu T: Allogeneic blood stem cell transplantation following non-myeloablative conditioning for hypereosinophilic syndrome. *Bone Marrow Transplant* 29:457, 2002.

944. Plotz SG, Simon HU, Darsow U, et al: Use of anti-interleukin-5 antibody in the hypereosinophilic syndrome with eosinophilic dermatitis. *N Engl J Med* 349:2334, 2003.

945. Klion AD, Law MA, Noel P, et al: Safety and efficacy of the monoclonal anti-interleukin-5 antibody SCH55700 in the treatment of patients with hypereosinophilic syndrome. *Blood* 103:2939, 2004.

946. Ardanani AD, Morice WG, Hoyer JD, Tefferi A: Chronic basophilic leukemia: A distinct clinical entity. *Eur J Haematol* 71:18, 2003.

947. Lahortiga I, Akin C, Cools J, et al: Activity of imatinib in systemic mastocytosis with chronic basophilic leukemia and a PRKG2-PDGFRB fusion. *Haematologica* 93:49, 2008.

948. Castro-Malaspina H, Schaison G, Brier J, et al: Philadelphia chromosome positive chronic myelocytic leukemia in children: Survival and prognostic factors. *Cancer* 51:721, 1983.

949. Arico M, Biondi A, Pui C-H: Juvenile myelomonocytic leukemia. *Blood* 90:479, 1997.

950. Neimeyer CM, Arico M, Basso A, et al: Chronic myelomonocytic leukemia in childhood. *Blood* 89:3535, 1997.

951. Emanuel PD: Juvenile myelomonocytic leukemia and chronic myelomonocytic leukemia. *Leukemia* 22:1335, 2008.

952. Niemeyer CM, Kratz C: Juvenile myelomonocytic leukemia. *Curr Oncol Rep* 5:510, 2003.

953. Busque L, Gilliland DG, Prchal JT, et al: Clonality in juvenile chronic myelogenous leukemia. *Blood* 85:21, 1995.

954. Cooper LJN, Shannon KM, Loken MR, et al: Evidence that juvenile chronic myelomonocytic leukemia can arise from a pluripotential stem cell. *Blood* 96:2310, 2000.

955. Emanuel PD: RAS pathway mutations in juvenile myelomonocytic leukemia. *Acta Haematol* 119:207, 2008.

956. Guilbert-Douet N, Morel F, Le Bris M-J, et al: Somatic *PTPN11* mutation with a heterogeneous clonal origin in children with juvenile myelomonocytic leukemia. *Leukemia* 18:1142, 2004.

957. Gandre-Babbe S, Paluru P, Aribeana C, Chou ST, et al: Patient-derived induced pluripotent stem cells recapitulate hematopoietic abnormalities of juvenile myelomonocytic leukemia. *Blood* 121:4925, 2013.

958. Miyauchi J, Asada M, Sasaki M, et al: Mutations of the N-*ras* gene in juvenile chronic myelogenous leukemia. *Blood* 83:2248, 1994.

959. Bader JL, Miller RW: Neurofibromatosis and childhood leukemia. *J Pediatr* 92:925, 1978.

960. Brodeur GM: The NF1 gene in myelopoiesis and childhood myelodysplastic syndrome. *N Engl J Med* 330:637, 1994.

961. Shannon KM: Loss of normal NF1 allele from the bone marrow of children with type 1 neurofibromatosis and malignant myeloid disorders. *N Engl J Med* 330:597, 1994.

962. Bollag G: Loss of NF1 results in activation of RAS signaling pathway and leads to aberrant growth in haematopoietic cells. *Nat Genet* 12:137, 1996.

963. Tartaglia M, Niemeyer CM, Fragale A, et al: Somatic mutations in PTPN11 in juvenile myelomonocytic leukemia, myelodysplastic syndrome and acute myeloid leukemia. *Nat Genet* 34:148, 2003.

964. Owen G, Lewis IJ, Morgan M, et al: Prognostic factors in juvenile chronic granulocytic leukaemia. *Br J Cancer Suppl* 18:S68, 1992.

965. Estrov Z, Grunberger T, Chan HS, Freedman MH: Juvenile chronic myelogenous leukemia. Characterization of the disease using cell cultures. *Blood* 67:1382, 1986.

966. Estrov Z, Dube ID, Chan HS, Freedman MH: Residual juvenile chronic myelogenous leukemia cells detected in peripheral blood during clinical remission. *Blood* 70:1466, 1987.

967. Emanuel PD, Bates LJ, Zhu SW, et al: The role of monocyte-derived hemopoietic growth factors in the regulation of myeloproliferation in juvenile chronic myelogenous leukemia. *Exp Hematol* 19:1017, 1991.

968. Morerio C, Acquila M, Rosanda C, et al: HCMOGT-1 is a novel fusion partner to *PDGFRB* in juvenile myelomonocytic leukemia with t(5;17)(q33;p11.2). *Cancer Res* 64:2649, 2004.

969. Inoue S, Ravindranath Y, Thompson RI, et al: Cytogenetics of juvenile type chronic granulocytic leukemia. *Cancer* 39:2017, 1977.

970. Brodeur GM, Dow LW, Williams DL: Cytogenetic features of juvenile chronic myelogenous leukemia. *Blood* 53:812, 1979.

971. Chan HS, Estrov Z, Weitzman SS, Freedman MH: The value of intensive combination chemotherapy for juvenile chronic myelogenous leukemia. *J Clin Oncol* 5:1960, 1987.

972. Kang HJ, Shin HY, Choi HS, Ahn HS: Novel regimen for the treatment of juvenile myelomonocytic leukemia (JMML). *Leuk Res* 28:167, 2004.

973. Pui CH, Arico M: Isotretinoin for juvenile chronic myelogenous leukemia. *N Engl J Med* 332:1520, 1995.

974. Bernard F, Thomas C, Emile JF, et al: Transient hematologic and clinical effects of E21R in a child with end-stage juvenile myelomonocytic leukemia. *Blood* 99:2615, 2002.

975. Locatelli F, Niemeyer C, Angelucci E, et al: Allogeneic bone marrow transplantation for chronic myelogenous leukemia in childhood. *J Clin Oncol* 15:556, 1997.

976. Manabe A, Okamura J, Yumura-Yagi K, et al: Allogeneic hematopoietic stem cell transplantation for 27 children with juvenile myelomonocytic leukemia diagnosed based on the criteria of the International JMML Working Group. *Leukemia* 16:645, 2002.

977. Locatelli F, Crotta A, Ruggeri A, et al: Analysis of risk factors influencing outcomes after cord blood transplantation in children with juvenile myelomonocytic leukemia: A EUROCORD, EBMT, EWOG-MDS, CIBMTR study. *Blood* 122:2135, 2013.

978. Worth A, Rao K, Webb D, et al: Successful treatment of juvenile myelomonocytic leukemia relapsing after stem cell transplantation using donor lymphocyte infusion. *Blood* 101:1713, 2003.

979. Scrideli CA, Baruffi MR, Rogatto SR, et al: B lineage acute lymphoblastic leukemia transformation in a child with juvenile myelomonocytic leukemia, type 1 neurofibromatosis and monosomy of chromosome 7. Possible implications in the leukemogenesis. *Leuk Res* 27:371, 2003.

980. Tuohey EL: A case of splenomegaly with polymorphonuclear neutrophil hyperleukocytosis. *Am J Med Sci* 160:18, 1920.

981. Froberg MK, Brunning RD, Dorion P, et al: Demonstration of clonality in neutrophils using FISH in a case of chronic neutrophilic leukemia. *Leukemia* 12:623, 1998.

982. Böhm J, Schaefer HE: Chronic neutrophilic leukemia:14 new cases of an uncommon myeloproliferative disorder. *J Clin Pathol* 55:862, 2002.

983. Standen GR, Steers FJ, Jones L: Clonality in chronic neutrophilic leukemia associated with myeloma: Analysis using the X-linked probe M27 beta. *J Clin Pathol* 46:297, 1993.

984. Bohm J, Kock S, Schaefer HE, Fisch P: Evidence of clonality in chronic neutrophilic leukaemia. *J Clin Pathol* 56:292, 2003.

985. Yanagisawa K, Ohminami H, Sato M, et al: Neoplastic involvement of granulocytic lineage, not granulocytic-monocytic, monocytic, or erythrocytic lineage, in a patient with chronic neutrophilic leukemia. *Am J Hematol* 57:221, 1998.

986. Hasegawa T, Suzuki K, Sakamoto C, et al: Expression of the inhibitor of apoptosis (IAP) family members in human neutrophils: Up-regulation of cIAP2 in chronic neutrophilic leukemia. *Blood* 101:1164, 2003.

987. Hasle H, Olesen G, Kerndrup G, et al: Chronic neutrophilic leukaemia in adolescence and young adulthood. *Br J Haematol* 94:628, 1996.

988. Elliott MA, Dewald GW, Tefferi A, Hanson CA: Chronic neutrophilic leukemia (CNL): A clinical and pathological entity. *Leukemia* 15:35, 2001.

989. Reilly JT: Chronic neutrophilic leukaemia: A distinct clinical entity? *Br J Haematol* 116:10, 2002.

990. Elliott MA: Chronic neutrophilic leukemia. *Curr Hematol Rep* 3:210, 2004.

991. Gotlib J, Maxson JE, George TI, Tyner JW. The new genetics of chronic neutrophilic leukemia and atypical CML: Implications for diagnosis and treatment. *Blood* 122:1707, 2013.

992. Ortiz-Cruz K, Amog-Jones G, Salvatore JR: Chronic neutrophilic leukemia with JAK2 gene mutation. *Clin Commun Oncol* 9:127, 2012.

993. Fleischman AG, Maxson JE, Luty SB et al: The CSF3R T618I mutation causes a lethal neutrophilic neoplasia in mice that is responsive to therapeutic JAK inhibition. *Blood* 122:3628, 2013.

994. Piliotis E, Kutas G, Lipton JH: Allogeneic bone marrow transplantation in the management of chronic neutrophilic leukemia. *Leuk Lymphoma* 43:2051, 2002.

995. Ito T, Kojima H, Otani K, et al: Chronic neutrophilic leukemia associated with monoclonal gammopathy of undetermined significance. *Acta Haematol* 95:140, 1996.

996. Vorobiof DA, Benjamin J, Kaplan H, Dvilansky A: Chronic granulocytic leukemia, neutrophilic type with paraproteinemia (IgA type K). *Acta Haematol* 60:316, 1978.

997. Carcassonne Y, Gastaut JA, Sebahoun G, Gratecos N: Découverte simultanée chez un même malade d'un myélome, d'une leucémie granuleuse (à polynucléaires neutrophils) et d'une maladie de Paget. *Nouv Rev Fr Hematol* 18:240, 1977.

998. Franchi F, Seminara P, Gruinchi G: Chronic neutrophilic leukemia and myeloma. Report on long survival. *Tumori* 70:105, 1984.

999. Lewis MJ, Oelbaum MH, Coleman M, Allen S: An association between chronic neutrophilic leukaemia and multiple myeloma with a study of cobalamin-binding proteins. *Br J Haematol* 63:173, 1986.

1000. Rovira M, Cervantes F, Namdedeu B, Rozman C: Chronic neutrophilic leukaemia preceding for seven years the development of multiple myeloma. *Acta Haematol* 3:94, 1990.

1001. Standen GR, Jasani B, Wagstaff M, Wardrop CAJ: Chronic neutrophilic leukemia and multiple myeloma. *Cancer* 66:162, 1990.

1002. Nagai M, Oda S, Iwamoto M, et al: Granulocyte-colony stimulating factor concentrates in a patient with plasma cell dyscrasia and clinical features of chronic neutrophilic leukaemia. *J Clin Pathol* 49:858, 1996.

1003. Dinçol G, Nalçaci M, Dogan O, et al: Coexistence of chronic neutrophilic leukemia with multiple myeloma. *Leuk Lymphoma* 43:649, 2002.

1004. Masini L, Salvarani C, Macchioni P, et al: Chronic neutrophilic leukemia (CNL) with karyotype abnormalities associated with plasma cell dyscrasia. *Haematologica* 77:277, 1992.

1005. Pascucci M, Dorion P, Makary A, Froberg MK: Chronic neutrophilic leukemia evolving from the myelodysplastic syndrome. *Acta Haematol* 98:163, 1997.

1006. Takamatsu Y, Kondo S, Inoue M, Tamura K: Chronic neutrophilic leukemia with dysplastic features mimicking myelodysplastic syndrome. *Int J Hematol* 63:65, 1996.

1007. Higuchi T, Oba R, Endo M, et al: Transition of polycythemia vera to chronic neutrophilic leukemia. *Leuk Lymphoma* 33:203, 1999.

1008. Billio A, Venturi R, Morello E, et al: Chronic neutrophilic leukemia evolving from polycythemia vera along with multiple chromosome rearrangements: A case report. *Haematologica* 86:1225, 2001.

1009. Foa P, Iurlo A, Saglio G, et al: Chronic neutrophilic leukemia associated with polycythemia vera. *Br J Haematol* 78:286, 1991.

1010. Higuchi T, Oba R, Endo M, et al: Transition of polycythemia vera to chronic neutrophilic leukemia. *Leuk Lymphoma* 33:203, 1999.

1011. Iurlo A, Foa P, Mailo AT, et al: Polycythemia vera terminating in chronic neutrophilic leukemia. *Am J Hematol* 35:139, 1990.

1012. Soda H, Kuriyama K, Tomonaga M, et al: Lymphoid crisis with T-cell phenotypes in a patient with Philadelphia chromosome negative chronic myeloid leukemia. *Br J Haematol* 59:671, 1985.

1013. Kessler JF, Grogan TM, Greenberg BR: Philadelphia-chromosome-negative chronic myelogenous leukemia with lymphoid stem cell blastic transformation. *Am J Hematol* 18:201, 1985.

1014. Martiat P, Michaux JL, Rodhain J, et al: Philadelphia-negative (Ph−) chronic myeloid leukemia (CML): Comparison with Ph+ CML and chronic myelomonocytic leukemia. *Blood* 78:205, 1991.

1015. van der Plas DC, Grosveld G, Hagemeijer A: Review of clinical, cytogenetic, and molecular aspects of Ph-negative CML. *Cancer Genet Cytogenet* 52:143, 1991.

1016. Galton DA: Haematological differences between chronic granulocytic leukemia, atypical chronic myeloid leukaemia and chronic myelomonocytic leukaemia. *Leuk Lymphoma* 7:343, 1992.

1017. Kato Y, Sawada H, Tashima M et al: Heterogeneous features of Ph-negative CML—Possible existence of Ph-negative, bcr-rearrangement-negative CML. *Acta Haematol* 52:1004, 1989.

1018. Selleri L, Emilia G, Luppi M, et al: Chronic myelogenous leukemia with typical clinical and morphological features can be Philadelphia chromosome negative and "bcr negative." *Hematol Pathol* 4:67, 1990.

1019. Costello R, Sainty D, Lafage-Pochitaloff M, Gabert J: Clinical and biological aspects of Philadelphia-negative/BCR-negative chronic myeloid leukemia. *Leuk Lymphoma* 25:225, 1997.

1020. Kurzrock R, Bueso-Ramos CE, Kantarjian H, et al: BCR rearrangement-negative chronic myelogenous leukemia revisited. *J Clin Oncol* 19:2915, 2001.

1021. Onida F, Ball G, Kantarjian HM, et al: Characteristics and outcome of patients with Philadelphia chromosome negative, bcr/abl negative chronic myelogenous leukemia. *Cancer* 95:1673, 2002.

1022. O'Brien SG, Viera SA, Connors S, et al: Transient response to imatinib mesylate (STI571) in a patient with ETV6-ABL t(9;12) translocation. *Blood* 99:3465, 2002.

1023. Mauro MJ, Loriaux M, Deininger MW: Ph-positive and -negative myeloproliferative syndromes may coexist. *Leukemia* 18:1305, 2004.

1024. Raskind WH, Ferraris AM, Najfeld V, et al: Further evidence for the existence of a clonal Ph-negative stage in some cases of Ph-positive chronic myelocytic leukemia. *Leukemia* 18:1305, 2004.

1025. Chee YL, Vickers MA, Stevenson D, et al: Fatal myelodysplastic syndrome developing during therapy with imatinib mesylate and characterized by the emergence of complex Philadelphia negative clones. *Leukemia* 17:634, 2003.

1026. Meeus P, Demuynck H, Martiat P, et al: Sustained clonal karyotype abnormalities in the Philadelphia chromosome negative cells of CML patients successfully treated with imatinib. *Leukemia* 17:465, 2003.

1027. Bumm T, Muller C, Al Ali HK, et al: Emergence of clonal cytogenetic abnormalities in Ph-cells in some CML patients in cytogenetic remission to imatinib but restoration of polyclonal hematopoiesis in the majority. *Blood* 101:1941, 2001.

1028. Galton DA: Haematological differences between chronic granulocytic leukaemia, atypical chronic myeloid leukaemia, and chronic myelomonocytic leukaemia. *Leuk Lymphoma* 7:343, 1992.

1029. Breccia M, Biondo F, Latagliata R, et al: Identification of risk factors in atypical chronic myeloid leukemia. *Haematologica* 91:1566, 2006.

1030. Dinardo CD, Daver N, Jain N, et al: Myelodysplastic/myeloproliferative neoplasms, unclassifiable (MDS/MPN, U): Natural history and clinical outcome by treatment strategy. *Leukemia* 28:958, 2014.

1031. Wang SA, Hasserjian RP, Fox PS, et al: Atypical chronic myeloid leukemia is clinically distinct from unclassifiable myelodysplastic/myeloproliferative neoplasms. *Blood* 123:2645, 2014.

1032. Meggendorfer M, Roller A, Haferlach T, et al: SRSF2 mutations in 275 cases with chronic myelomonocytic leukemia (CMML). *Blood* 120:3080, 2012.

1033. Sakaguchi H(1), Okuno Y, Muramatsu H, et al: Exome sequencing identifies secondary mutations of SETBP1 and JAK3 in juvenile myelomonocytic leukemia. *Nat Genet* 45:937, 2013.

Part XI **Malignant Lymphoid Diseases**

90. Classification of Malignant Lymphoid Disorders 1493

91. Acute Lymphocytic Leukemia 1505

92. Chronic Lymphocytic Leukemia 1527

93. Hairy Cell Leukemia 1553

94. Large Granular Lymphocytic Leukemia 1563

95. General Considerations for Lymphomas: Epidemiology, Etiology, Heterogeneity, and Primary Extranodal Disease 1569

96. Pathology of Lymphomas 1587

97. Hodgkin Lymphoma 1603

98. Diffuse Large B-Cell Lymphoma and Related Diseases 1625

99. Follicular Lymphoma................... 1641

100. Mantle Cell Lymphoma................. 1653

101. Marginal Zone B-Cell Lymphomas 1663

102. Burkitt Lymphoma 1671

103. Cutaneous T-Cell Lymphoma (Mycosis Fungoides and Sézary Syndrome) 1679

104. Mature T-Cell and Natural Killer Cell Lymphomas 1693

105. Plasma Cell Neoplasms: General Considerations........................ 1707

106. Essential Monoclonal Gammopathy 1721

107. Myeloma 1733

108. Immunoglobulin Light-Chain Amyloidosis 1773

109. Macroglobulinemia 1785

110. Heavy-Chain Disease.................. 1803

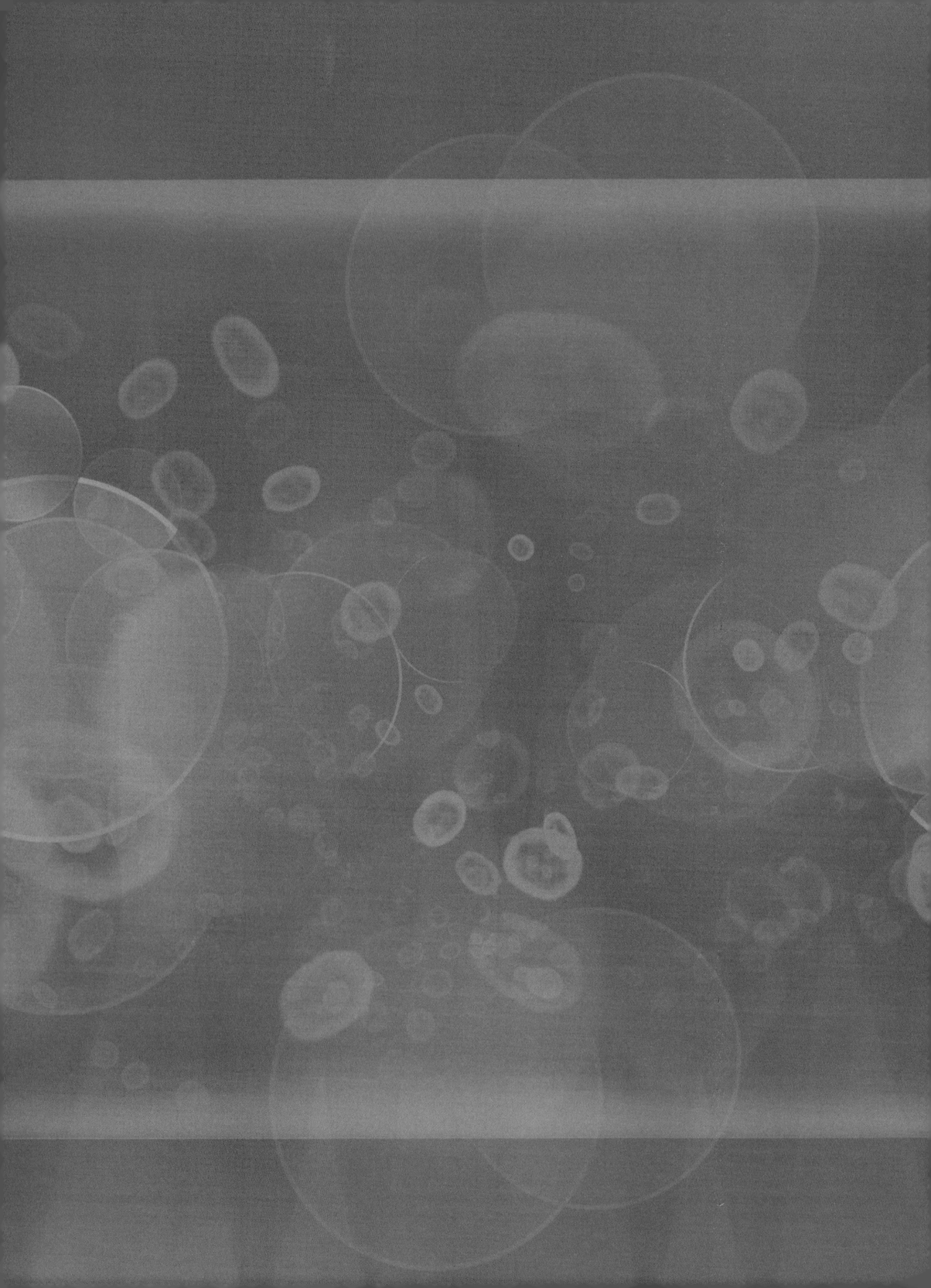

CHAPTER 90
CLASSIFICATION OF MALIGNANT LYMPHOID DISORDERS

Robert A. Baiocchi

SUMMARY

This chapter outlines the category of preneoplastic and neoplastic lymphocyte and plasma cell disorders. It introduces a framework for evaluating neoplastic lymphocyte and plasma cell disorders, outlines clinical syndromes associated with such disorders, and guides the reader to the chapters in the text that discuss each of these disorders in greater detail. Chapter 78 outlines the diseases caused by nonneoplastic disorders of lymphocytes and plasma cells.

CLASSIFICATION

Lymphocyte and plasma cell malignancies present a broad spectrum of different morphologic features and clinical syndromes (Table 90–1). Lymphocyte neoplasms can originate from cells that are at a stage prior to T- and B-lymphocyte differentiation from a primitive stem cell or from cells at stages of maturation after stem cell differentiation. Thus, acute lymphoblastic leukemias arise from an early lymphoid progenitor cell that may give rise to cells with either B- or T-cell phenotypes (Chap. 91). On the other hand, chronic lymphocytic leukemia arises from a more mature B-lymphocyte progenitor (Chap. 92) and myeloma from progenitors at even later stages of B-lymphocyte maturation (Chap. 107). Disorders of lymphoid progenitors may result in a broad spectrum of lymphocytic diseases such as B or T cell lymphomas (Chaps. 98 and 104), hairy cell leukemia

Acronyms and Abbreviations: a/β TCR, T-cell-receptor genes encoding the a and β chains of the T-cell receptor (Chap. 76); ALK, gene encoding anaplastic lymphoma kinase; BCL2, gene encoding B-cell chronic lymphocytic leukemia (CLL)/lymphoma 2; BCL6, gene encoding B-cell chronic lymphocytic leukemia (CLL)/lymphoma 6; clg, cytoplasmic immunoglobulin; EBER, Epstein-Barr-virus-encoded RNA; EBV, Epstein-Barr virus; γ/δ TCR, T-cell-receptor genes encoding the γ and δ chains of the T-cell receptor (Chap. 76); HL, Hodgkin lymphoma; HLA, human leukocyte antigen; HTLV-1, human T-cell leukemia virus type 1; HHV8, human herpes virus 8; Ig, immunoglobulin; IgR, immunoglobulin gene rearrangement (Chap. 75); IL, interleukin; MALT, mucosa-associated lymphoid tissue; MUM1, gene encoding multiple myeloma oncogene 1; neg., negative; NK cell, natural killer cell; NOS, not otherwise specified; NPM, gene encoding nucleophosmin; PAX5, paired box gene 5; POEMS, polyneuropathy, organomegaly, endocrinopathy, monoclonal gammopathy, and skin changes; REAL, revised European-American lymphoma; R-S, Reed-Sternberg; slg, surface immunoglobulin (Chap. 75); slgD, surface immunoglobulin D; slgM, surface immunoglobulin M; TAL1, gene encoding T-cell acute leukemia-1; TCR, T-cell receptor; TdT, terminal deoxynucleotidyl transferase; Th2, T-helper type 2; WHO, World Health Organization.

(Chap. 93), prolymphocytic leukemia (Chap. 92), natural killer cell large granular lymphocytic leukemia (Chap. 94),[1] myeloma, and plasmacytoma (Chap. 107). Hodgkin lymphoma also is derived from a neoplastic B cell that has highly mutated immunoglobulin genes that are no longer expressed as protein (Chap. 97).

To provide a unified international basis for clinical and investigative work in this field, the International Lymphoma Study Group proposed a classification termed the *revised European-American Lymphoma* (REAL) classification (Chap. 95),[2] which was modified in 2001 and again in 2008 by the World Health Organization (WHO).[3,4] The REAL/WHO classification scheme makes use of the pathologic, immunophenotypic, genetic, and clinical features of a given lymphocyte tumor to delineate them into separate disease entities (see Table 90–1 and Chap. 96).[5] For some of these entities, the neoplastic lymphocytes have distinctive cytogenetic abnormalities, which can be identified using molecular techniques that increasingly are being used in clinical pathology laboratories.[6,7]

The REAL/WHO classification recognizes a basic distinction between nodular lymphocyte-predominant Hodgkin lymphoma and classic Hodgkin lymphoma, reflecting the differences in clinical presentation and behavior, morphology, phenotype, and molecular features (Chap. 97).[3] Studies have identified features that can be used to distinguish classical Hodgkin lymphoma from anaplastic large cell lymphoma and, to a lesser extent, between nodular lymphocyte-predominant Hodgkin lymphoma and T-cell/histiocyte-rich large B-cell lymphoma.

The updated WHO classification (summarized in Ref. 4) provided several revised guidelines for defining diseases such as chronic lymphocytic leukemia (CLL),[8] Waldenström macroglobulinemia,[9] plasma cell neoplasms,[10] and diffuse large B-cell lymphoma (DLBCL).[11-14] The classification of several T-cell lymphomas were also refined including enteropathy-associated T-cell lymphoma, anaplastic large cell lymphoma (ALK-positive and ALK-negative), and subcutaneous panniculitis-like T-cell lymphoma.[4] This chapter has summarized these new distinctions in Table 90–1.

CLINICAL BEHAVIOR

Lymphomas of similar histology can have widely different spectra of associated clinical symptoms and clinical aggressiveness, making the categorization of lymphoid tumors impossible using a generic grading system based on morphology alone. For example, the neoplastic cells in mantle cell lymphoma appear smaller and more differentiated than those of anaplastic large cell lymphomas. However, the validation studies for the REAL classification revealed that patients with mantle cell lymphoma or anaplastic large cell lymphomas have a 5-year survival rate of approximately 30 percent and approximately 80 percent, respectively.[15,16] Generally, T-cell lymphomas/leukemias have a more aggressive clinical behavior than B-cell lymphomas of comparable histology. The tendency for more aggressive disease also applies to lymphoid tumors derived from natural killer cells. A helpful distinction is to divide the lymphoid tumors into one of two categories, namely, indolent lymphomas versus aggressive lymphomas, based upon on the characteristics of the disease at the time of presentation and the patients' life expectancy if the disease is left untreated.[17,18] Clinical studies have verified that the different disease categories defined in the REAL/WHO classification each can be segregated into one or the other of these two major categories (Tables 90–2 and 90–3).[15] Analyses of gene-expression patterns using microarray technology (Chaps. 11 and 12) have enabled identification of subcategories within some of the disease categories defined by the REAL/WHO classification that have different tendencies for disease progression, survival, and/or response rates to standard therapies (Chap. 96).[19-25] An example of how gene-expression profiling has had a major impact on refining lymphoma diagnoses can be found

TABLE 90–1. Classification of Lymphoma and Lymphoid Leukemia by World Health Organization

Neoplasm	Morphology	Phenotype*	Genotype†
B-CELL NEOPLASMS			
Immature B-Cell Neoplasms			
Lymphoblastic leukemia/ lymphoma not otherwise specified (NOS) (Chap. 91)	Medium to large cells with finely stippled chromatin and scant cytoplasm	TdT+, sIg–, CD10+, CD13+/–, CD19+, CD20–, CD22+, CD24+, CD34+/–, CD33+/–, CD45+/–, CD79a+, PAX5+	Clonal DJ rearrangement of *IGH* gene T(17;19), *E2A-HLF*, *AML1* iAMP21 associated with poor prognosis
Lymphoblastic leukemia/ lymphoma with recurrent genetic abnormalities (Chap. 91)	See above	See above. B-ALL with t(9;22) with CD25 and more frequent myeloid antigens CD13, CD33	See individual genetic features in B-ALL subtypes below
B-ALL with t(v;11q23); *MLL* rearranged	See above	CD19+, CD10–, CD24–, CD15+	Multiple MLL (11q23) fusion partners including *AF4* (4q21), *AF9* (9p22), and *ENL* (19p13). B-ALL with MLL translocations over express *FLT-3*. Poor prognosis
B-ALL with t(12;21) (p13;q22); *TEL-AML1* (*ETV6-RUNX1*)	See above	CD19+, CD10+, CD34+. Characteristically negative for CD9, CD20, and CD66c	t(12;21)(p13;q22) *ETV6-RUNX* translocation
B-ALL with hyperdiploidy	See above	CD19+, CD10+, CD45–, CD34+	Numerical increase in chromosomes without structural abnormalities. Most frequent chromosomes +21, X, 14 and 4. +1,2, 3 rarely seen. Favorable prognosis
B-ALL with hypodiploidy	See above	See above	Loss of at least one or more chromosomes (range from 45 chromosomes to near haploid). Rare chromosome abnormalities. Poor prognosis
B-ALL with t(5;14) (q31;q32); *IL3-IGH*	See above with increase in reactive eosinophilia	See above. Even rare blasts with B-ALL immunophenotype with eosinophilia strongly suggestive of this subtype of B-ALL	t(5;14)(q31;q32); *IL3-IGH* leading to overexpression of IL3. Unclear prognosis
B-ALL with t(1;19) (q23;p13.3); *E2A-PBX1*	See above	CD10+, CD19+, cytoplasmic μ heavy chain. CD9+, CD34–	t(1;19)(q23;p13.3); leads to overexpression of *E2A-PBX1* fusion gene product interfering with normal transcription factor activity of E2A and PBX1
Mature B-Cell Neoplasms			
Leukemias			
Chronic lymphocytic leukemia/small lymphocytic lymphoma (Chap. 92)	Small cells with round, dense nuclei	sIg+(dim), CD5+, CD10–, CD19+, CD20+(dim), CD22+(dim), CD23+, CD38+/–, CD45+, FMC-7–	IgR+, trisomy 12 (~30%), del at 13q14 (~50%), 11q22–23, 17p13, and *IGHV* mutated status associated with poor prognosis
Prolymphocytic leukemia (Chap. 92)	≥55% prolymphocytes	sIg+(bright), CD5+/–, CD10–, CD19+, CD22+, CD23+/–, CD45+, CD79a+, FMC7+	del13q.14(~30%); del17p (50%), IgR+
Hairy cell leukemia (Chap. 93)	Small cells with cytoplasmic projections	sIg+(bright), CD5–, CD10–, CD11c+(bright), CD19+, CD20+, CD25+, CD45+, CD103+, Annexin A+	BRAF mutations (~100%), IgR+
Lymphomas			
Lymphoplasmacytic lymphoma (Chap. 109)	Small cells with plasmacytoid differentiation	cIg+, CD5–, CD10–, CD19+, CD20+/– Plasma cell population: CD38+, CD138+, cIgM+	IgR, 6q- in 50% of marrow-based cases [the t(9;14) was proved to be wrong], +4 (20%)
Mantle cell lymphoma (Chap. 100)	Small to medium cells	sIgM+, sIgD+, CD5+, CD10–, CD19+, CD20+, CD23–, Cyclin D1+, FMC-7+, SOX11+ in nearly 100% of cases	IgR, t(11;14)(q13;q32) (~100% by FISH), involving *BCL1* and IgH. Highly proliferative variants often show TP53 mutation, deletion of *INK4a/ART* and *p18INK4c*

(Continued)

TABLE 90–1. Classification of Lymphoma and Lymphoid Leukemia by World Health Organization (Continued)

Neoplasm	Morphology	Phenotype*	Genotype†
Follicular lymphoma (follicle center lymphoma; Chap. 99)	Small, medium, or large cells with cleaved nuclei	sIg, CD5−, CD10+, CD19+, CD20+(bright), CD23−/+, CD38+, CD45+	IgR, t(14;18)(q32;q21) (~85%) involving *BCL2* and IgH. Mutated 3q27 (5–15%, *BCL6*)
Nodal marginal zone B-cell lymphoma (Chap. 101)	Small or large monocytoid cells	sIgM+, sIgD−, cIg+ (~50%), CD5-, CD10−, CD11c+/−, CD19+, CD20+, CD23−, CD43+/−	IgR, commonly with trisomies 3, 7, and 18
Extranodal marginal zone lymphoma of mucosa-associated lymphoid tissue (MALT) type (Chap. 101)	See above	See above	t(11;18)(q21;q21) involving *API2*, *MLT1*, or t(1;14)(p22;q32) involving *BCL10*
Splenic B-cell marginal zone lymphoma	Small round lymphocytes replaces reactive germinal centers and/or villous lymphocytes in blood	sIgM+, sIgD−, CD5+/−, CD19+, CD20+, CD23−, CD103−	IgR, allelic loss of chromosome 7q31–32 (40%)
Splenic B-cell lymphoma, unclassifiable			
Splenic diffuse red pulp small B-cell lymphoma	Blood: villous lymphocytes similar to SMZL. Marrow: intrasinusoidal infiltration. Spleen: monomorphous small to medium lymphocytes with round nuclei, vesicular chromatin, occasional small nucleoli	CD20+, DBA.44+, IgG+/IgD−, CD25−, CD5−, CD103−, CD123−	T(9;14)(p13;q32) involving *PAX5* and *IGH*
Hairy cell leukemia variant	Hybrid features of prolymphocytic leukemia and classic hairy cell leukemia	sIg+(bright), CD5−, CD10−, CD11c+(bright), CD19+, CD20+, CD25−, CD45+, CD103+, FMC7+, CD123−, Annexin A1−, TRAP−	BRAF mutation negative
Diffuse large B-cell lymphoma (DLBCL, Chap. 98)			
DLBCL NOS			
Common Morphologic Variants:			
Centroblastic	Medium to large lymphoid cells with vesicular nuclei containing fine chromatin. Multiple nucleoli	sIgM+, sIgD+/−, CD5-, CD10−/+, CD19+, CD20+, CD22+, CD79a+, CD45+, PAX5+	IgR, 3q27 abnormalities and/or t(3;14)(q27;q32) involving *BCL6* (~30%) or t(14;18)(q32;q21) (~25%) involving *BCL2*
Immunoblastic	>90% of cells are immunoblasts with central nucleolus	See above. May express CD30+	See above
Anaplastic	Very large round, oval, or polygonal cells with bizarre pleomorphic nuclei resembling R-S cells	See above. Often CD30+	See above
Molecular Subgroups			
Germinal center B cell like (GCB)	See above	See above	See above
Activated B-cell–like (ABC)	See above. Often with more immunoblastic morphology	See above	T(14;18) (35%), 12q12 (20%), IG mutation, BCL2 rearrangement (20–25%), Rel amplification (15%). Amplification of microRNA-17-92 cluster
Immunohistochemical Subgroups			Gain of 3q (26%), 9p (6%), 12q12 (5%), NF-κB activation
CD5-positive DLBCL	See above	See above. CD5+	t(11;14) and t(14;18) negative. +3 and gain on chromosome 16/16p and 18/18q common. Deletion p16/INK4a

(Continued)

TABLE 90–1. Classification of Lymphoma and Lymphoid Leukemia by World Health Organization (Continued)

Neoplasm	Morphology	Phenotype*	Genotype†
Nongerminal center B-cell–like (non-GCB)	See above	See above	See above. Uniform FOXP1 expression with IRF4/MUM1 and BCL6 expression
Primary mediastinal (thymic) large B-cell lymphoma (Chap. 98)	Variable from case to case. Medium to large cells often with pleomorphic nuclei (R-S–like cells)	sIg–, CD5–, CD10–/+, CD15–, CD19+, CD20+, CD22+, CD23+, CD30+ (80%), CD45+, CD79a+, IRF4/MUM1 (75%). Variable BCL2 (50–80%) and BCL6 (45–100%) expression	IgR+, Gain of 9q24 (75%), gain 2p15 (50%) Amplification of *REL, BCL11A, JAK2, PDL1, PDL2*. Transcriptome similar to CHL
Intravascular large B-cell lymphoma	Neoplastic cells infiltrated within small to intermediate vessels of all organs	CD19+, CD20+, CD5 (38%), CD10 (13%). Lack of CD29 (β1 integrin) and CD54 (ICAM1) may account for intravascular growth pattern	IgR+, otherwise poorly characterized
ALK-positive large B-cell lymphoma	Sinusoidal growth pattern, monomorphic large immunoblast-like cells	Strongly positive for ALK, CD138+, VS38+, cytoplasmic IgA or IgG	IgR+, t(2;17) *ALK/CLTC*
Plasmablastic lymphoma	Diffuse proliferation of immunoblasts with plasmacytic differentiation, frequent mitotic figures, monomorphic morphology common in HIV+ patients. Frequently extranodal, EBV+	CD138+, CD38+, VS38C, IRF4/MUM1+, high Ki67, CD79a+ CD30+ in most cases. Negative for CD45, CD20, PAX5. Cytoplasmic Ig (50–70%). CD56 negative (if positive, suspect plasma cell myeloma)	IgR+, frequently Epstein-Barr virus-encoded RNA (EBER)+ (60–70%) but most cases negative for LMP1. HHV8+ status consistent with large B-cell lymphoma from MCD (below)
Large B-cell lymphoma arising from multicentric, HHV8+ Castleman disease (MCD)	HHV8 MCD: B cell follicles with involution and hyalinization of germinal centers with prominent mantle zones. Large plasmablastic cells within mantle zone HHV8 plasmablastic lymphoma. Confluent sheets of HHV8+ LANA1+ cells effacing lymph node architecture. Extranodal involvement common	HHV8+, LANA1+, viral IL6+, cytoplasmic IgM, CD20+/–, Negative for CD79a, CD138, and EBV (EBER)	Polyclonal IgM. IgVH unmutated. IL6R pathway activation. Cytogenetics poorly characterized
Primary effusion lymphoma	Range of infiltrating cells with highly abnormal morphology including immunoblastic, plasmablastic, anaplastic. Large nuclei with prominent nucleoli	CD45+, Lack expression of CD19, CD20, CD79a, sIg	IgR+ and hypermutated. No recurrent chromosomal anomalies
Burkitt lymphoma (Chap. 98)	Medium cells arranged in diffuse, monotonous pattern. Basophilic cytoplasm, high proliferative index with frequent mitotic figures. "Starry sky" pattern present	Positive for CD19, CD20, CD10, BCL6, CD38, CD77, and CD43. Negative for BCL2 and TdT. Ki67+ in nearly 100% of tumor cells	t(8;14)(q24;q32), t(2;8)(q11;q24), or t(8;22)(q24;q11), involving Ig loci and *C-MYC* at 8q24
B-cell lymphoma unclassifiable, features intermediate between DLBCL and Burkitt lymphoma (BL) (Chap. 102)	Medium, round cells with abundant cytoplasm. More variation in nuclear size and contour compared to BL. Commonly >90% Ki67+. Unlike BL, can show strong BCL2 expression	Same as above except sIg–, cIg+/–, and CD10–	Same as above except more typically expresses high levels of *BCL2* and ~30% have *BCL2* rearrangements (double-hit type)

(Continued)

TABLE 90–1. Classification of Lymphoma and Lymphoid Leukemia by World Health Organization (Continued)

Neoplasm	Morphology	Phenotype*	Genotype†
B-cell lymphoma unclassifiable, features intermediate between DLBCL and classical Hodgkin lymphoma (HL)	Confluent, diffuse, sheet-like growth of pleomorphic cells within a fibrotic stroma. Pleomorphic cells resembling HL R-S–like cells and lacunar cells. Necrosis frequent	In contrast to HL, CD45+. Positive for CD30 and CD15	Poorly characterized
Plasma Cell Neoplasms			
Monoclonal gammopathy of undetermined significance (MGUS)	Marrow infiltrate with mature plasma cells comprising 1–9% of cellularity	M-protein <30 g/L, marrow <10% plasma cells, no end-organ damage. CD138+. Often difficult to demonstrate LC restriction because of small numbers of plasma cells	Abnormal cytogenetics rarely encountered in MGUS. FISH studies involving *IgH* occur in ~50% of cases: t(11;14), t(4;14). Del13q. Hyperdiploidy 40%
Plasma cell myeloma	Myeloma plasma cells seen in marrow arranged in interstitial clusters	sIg+, CD5–, CD10–, CD19–, CD20–, CD38+(bright), CD45+/–, CD56+, CD117+(bright), CD138+(bright)	IgR, commonly with complex karyotypes and or t(6;14)(p25;q32) involving *MUM1*. t(11;14) seen in 15–25% cases
Extraosseous plasmacytoma	Plasma cells in extraosseous organs must be distinguished from other lymphoproliferative disorders (i.e., MALT type)	Same as plasma cell myeloma	Same as above
Solitary plasmacytoma of bone	Plasma cells	Same as plasma cell myeloma	Same as above
Monoclonal immunoglobulin deposition disease	Prominent organ (kidney most common, occasionally liver, heart, nerve, blood vessels involved) deposits of nonamyloid, nonfibrillary, amorphous eosinophilic material that does not stain with congo red. Heavy chain (HCDD) and light chain (LCDD)	LCDD is κ light chain predominant. HCDD shows λ chain predominance. Marrow may show abnormal κ/λ ratio	HCDD with VλVI overrepresentation. LCDD with VκIV variable region
Hodgkin Lymphoma (Hl)			
Nodular lymphocyte predominant HL (Chap. 97)	"Popcorn cells" with nuclei resembling those of centroblasts	BCL6+, CD19+, CD20+, CD22+, CD45+, CD79a+, CD15–, and rarely CD30+/–, Bob1+, Oct2+, PAX5+	IgR, with high-level expression of *BCL6*
Classic Hl (Chap. 97)			
Nodular sclerosis HL	R-S cells and lacunar cells dispersed in reactive lymphoid nodules	R-S cells typically are CD15+, CD20–/+, CD30+, CD45–, CD79a–, PAX5+(dim)	R-S cells generally express *PAX5* and *MUM1*, variable expression of *BCL6*, and have IgR without functional Ig
Lymphocyte-rich HL	Few R-S cells with occasional "popcorn" appearance dispersed in lymphoid nodules	Same as above	Same as above
Mixed cellularity HL	R-S cells dispersed among plasma cells, epithelioid histiocytes, eosinophils, and T cells	R-S cells typically are CD15+, CD20–/+, CD30+, CD45–, CD79a–	R-S cells generally express *PAX5* and *MUM1*, variable expression of *BCL6*, and have IgR without functional Ig
Lymphocyte-depleted HL	Prominent numbers of R-S cells with effacement of the nodal structure	Same as above	Same as above

(Continued)

TABLE 90–1. Classification of Lymphoma and Lymphoid Leukemia by World Health Organization (Continued)

Neoplasm	Morphology	Phenotype*	Genotype†
T-CELL NEOPLASMS			
Immature T-cell neoplasms			
Lymphoblastic leukemia (Chap. 91)	Medium to large cells with finely stippled chromatin and scant cytoplasm	TdT+, CD2+/−, cytoplasmic CD3+, CD1a+/−, CD5+/−, CD7+, CD10−/+, CD4+/CD8+ or CD4−/CD8−, CD34+/−	Abnormalities in *TCR* loci at 14q11 (TCR-α), 7q34 (TCR-β), or 7p15 (TCR-γ), and/or t(1;14)(p32-34; q11) involving *TAL1*
Lymphoblastic lymphoma (Chap. 91)	Same as above	Same as above	Same as above
Mature T and NK cell neoplasms			
Leukemias			
T-cell prolymphocytic leukemia (Chap. 104)	Small to medium cells with cytoplasmic protrusions or blebs	TdT−, CD2+, CD3+, CD5+, CD7+, CD4+ and CD8− is more common than CD4− and CD8+, but can be CD4+ and CD8+	α/β TCR rearrangement, inv14(q11;q32)(~75%). Inv14 in ~80% of cases. Translocations frequently involve *TCL1A* and *TCL1B* genes. +8q seen in ~75% cases. del 11q23 and abnormalities with chromosome 6 (33%) and 17P (26%) seen
T-cell large granular lymphocytic leukemia (Chap. 94)	Abundant cytoplasm and sparse azurophilic granules	CD2+, CD3+, CD4 −/+, CD5+, CD7+, CD8+/−, CD16+/−, CD56−, CD57+/−	α/β TCR rearrangement, γ/δ rearrangement can be seen
Lymphomas/Lymphoproliferative Disorders			
Extranodal T/NK-cell lymphoma, nasal type ("angiocentric lymphoma"; Chaps. 94 and 104)	Angiocentric and angiodestructive growth	CD2+, cytoplasmic CD3+, CD4−, CD5−/+, CD7+, CD8−, CD56+, EBV+	TCR rearrangements usually neg., EBV present by *in situ* hybridization
Cutaneous T-cell lymphoma (mycosis fungoides; Chap. 103)	Small to large cells with cerebriform nuclei	CD2+, CD3+, CD4+, CD5+, CD7+/−, CD8−, CD25−, CD26+	α/β TCR rearrangements, complex karyotype common. STAT3 activation
Sézary syndrome (Chap. 103)	Same as above	Same as above	Same as above
Angioimmunoblastic T-cell lymphoma[34]	Small to medium immunoblasts with clear to pale cytoplasm around follicles and high endothelial venules	CD3+/−, CD4+, CD10+, CXCL13+, PD-1+ (60–100%), EBV+	α/β TCR rearrangement (75–90%), IgR (25–30%), trisomy 3 or 5 noted
Peripheral T-cell lymphoma (not otherwise unspecified; Chap. 104)	Highly variable	CD2+, CD3+, CD5+, CD7−, CD4+CD8− more often than CD4−CD8+, which is more often than CD4+CD8+	α/β TCR rearrangement
Subcutaneous panniculitis-like T-cell lymphoma[35]	Variably sized atypical cells with hyperchromasia infiltrating fat lobule	CD2+, CD3+, CD4−, CD5+, CD7−, CD8+, and cytoxic molecules (perforin, granzyme B, and TIA1)	α/β TCR rearrangement
Enteropathy associated T cell lymphoma	Medium to large cells with prominent nucleoli, abundant pale cytoplasm invading mucosal membranes of the small intestine	CD3+, CD5−, CD7+, CD8+/−, CD4−, CD103+, TCRβ+/−. CD30+ (most cases)	*TRB, TRG* clonally rearranged. >90% *HLADQA1*0501, DQB1*0201*
Hepatosplenic T-cell lymphoma[37–39]	Small to medium cells with condensed chromatin and round nuclei	CD2+, CD3+, CD4−, CD5−, CD7+/−, CD8+/−	γ/δ TCR rearrangement, rarely α/β TCR rearrangement, isochromosome 7q
Adult T-cell leukemia/lymphoma (Chap. 91)	Highly pleomorphic with multilobed nuclei	CD2+, CD3+, CD5+, CD7−, CD25+, CD4+CD8− more often than CD4−CD8+	α/β TCR rearrangement, integrated HTLV-1

(Continued)

TABLE 90–1. Classification of Lymphoma and Lymphoid Leukemia by World Health Organization (Continued)

Neoplasm	Morphology	Phenotype*	Genotype†
Anaplastic large cell lymphoma ALK-positive	Large pleomorphic cells with "horseshoe"-shaped nuclei, prominent nucleoli, and abundant cytoplasm	TdT–, ALK1+, CD2+/–, CD3–/+, CD4–/+, CD5–/+, CD7+/–, CD8–/+, CD13–/+, CD25+/–, CD30+, CD33–/+, CD45+, HLA-DR+, TIA+/–	TCR rearrangement, t(2;5)(p23;q35) resulting in nucleophosmin—anaplastic lymphoma kinase fusion protein (NPM/ALK); other translocations involving 2p23 are also seen
Anaplastic large cell lymphoma ALK-negative	Similar morphologic spectrum to that seen in ALK+ ALCL. No small cell variant seen in ALK–	TdT–, ALK1–, CD2+/–, CD3–/+, CD4–/+, CD5–/+, CD7+/–, CD8–/+, CD13–/+, CD25+/–, CD30+, CD33–/+, CD45+, HLA-DR+, TIA+/–	TCR rearrangement, no recurrent cytogenetic features seen
Primary cutaneous CD30+ anaplastic large cell lymphoma[43,44]	Anaplastic large cells as above in cutaneous nodules	TdT–, CD2–/+, CD3+/–, CD4+, CD5–/+, CD7+/–, CD25+/–, CD30+, CD45+	TCR rearrangement but without t(2;5)(p23;q35)
Lymphomatoid papulosis	Three histologic subtypes (A, B, C). Type A: scattered clusters of large R-S–like cells admixed with histiocyte rich infiltrate. Type B: rarely seen, epidermotropic infiltrate of small atypical cells with cerebriform nuclei (MF-like). Type C: monotonous large CD30+ T cells with few inflammatory cells	Type A and C have similar phenotype to C-ALCL. Type B phenotype CD3+, CD4+, CD8–, CD30–	TCR rearrangement in 60% cases. No t(2;5)(p23;135)
Primary cutaneous peripheral T cell lymphomas, rare subtypes:			
Primary cutaneous γ/δ T-cell lymphoma	Epidermotropic, dermal and subcutaneous histologic patterns. Neoplastic cells medium to large with coarse chromatin, frequent apoptosis/necrosis	CD3+, CD2+, CD5–, CD7+/–, CD56+. Most cases CD4–, CD8–	TCRG, TCRD clonal rearrangement. EBV negative
Primary cutaneous CD8+ aggressive epidermotropic cytotoxic T-cell lymphoma	Variable histology ranging from lichenoid epidermotropism to deeper nodular infiltrates. Tumor cells small to medium with pleomorphic or blastic nuclei	CD3+, CD8+, granzyme B+, perforin+, TIA1+, CD45RA+/–, CD45RO–, CD2+/–, CD4–, CD5–, CD7+/–	Clonal TCR rearrangement. EBV negative
Primary cutaneous CD4+ small/medium T-cell lymphoma	Dense, diffuse, dermal infiltrates. Predominance of small/medium pleomorphic cells	CD3+, CD4+, CD8–, CD30–. No cytotoxic proteins expressed	Clonal TCR rearrangement. EBV negative
EBV+ T-cell lymphoproliferative diseases of childhood	Infiltrating T cells are EBV+, but lack cytologic atypia. Erythrophagocytosis and histiocytosis seen frequently	CD2+, CD3+, CD56–, CD8+, EBER+	Clonal TCR rearrangement. EBV+ with LMP1 expression
Hydroa vacciniforme-like lymphoma	Cutaneous presentation, small to medium cells without clear cytology atypical	CD3+, CD8+, CD56+	Clonal TCR rearrangement. EBV+ without LMP1

NATURAL KILLER (NK) CELL NEOPLASMS

Neoplasm	Morphology	Phenotype*	Genotype†
Large granular lymphocytic leukemia (Chap. 94)	Abundant cytoplasm and sparse azurophilic granules	TdT–, CD2+, CD3–, CD4–, CD5–/+, CD7+, CD8–/+, CD11b+, CD16+, CD56+, CD57+/–	No TCR rearrangement
Aggressive NK-cell leukemia[1]	Same as above	Same as above	No TCR rearrangement, EBV present

(Continued)

TABLE 90–1. Classification of Lymphoma and Lymphoid Leukemia by World Health Organization (Continued)

Neoplasm	Morphology	Phenotype*	Genotype†
Extranodal NK-cell lymphoma, nasal-type ("angiocentric lymphoma")[1,45,46]	Angiocentric and angiodestructive growth	CD2+, cytoplasmic CD3ε +, CD4–, CD5–/+, CD7+, CD8–, CD56+	No TCR rearrangement, EBV present
Immunodeficiency-associated lymphoproliferative disorders			
Lymphoproliferative disorders associated with primary immune disorders	Range of morphology from reactive hyperplasia, polymorphous lymphoid infiltrate, to high-grade lymphomas. Lymphoma and HL morphology is similar to that seen in immune competent patients	Immunophenotype similar to that seen in immune competent patients with corresponding malignancy	FAS mutation seen in *ALPS*. Mutations in *SAP/SLAM* in XLP. *ATM* mutations in AT
Lymphomas associated with HIV infection	Similar to above. Typical histologic features seen in Burkitt lymphoma, HL, DLBCL. Lymphomas seen more frequently in HIV setting include primary effusion, plasmablastic, lymphomas, multicentric Castleman disease	Similar to above	*MYC* and *BCL2* translocations seen in DLBCL
Posttransplant lymphoproliferative disorders (PTLDs)			
Early lesions: plasmacytic hyperplasia (PH) and infectious mononucleosis (IM)-like	PH: numerous plasma cells, lymphocytes, and immunoblasts. IM: numerous immunoblasts on a background of T cells	Similar to above	EBV+ in both IM and PH. Oligoclonal polyclonal IgH rearrangement. EBV+
Polymorphic PTLD	Effacement of tissue architecture with infiltrate showing full range of B-cell maturation	Similar to above with exception that R-S cells in HLs often express CD30+, CD20+ but frequently are CD15–	Clonal *IG* rearrangement. EBV+ by EBER ISH. Mutated IgH in 75% of cases
Monomorphic PTLD	Similar to DLBCL, Burkitt lymphoma or plasmacytoma morphology	Similar to above	EBV+/–. Clonal B cell or T cells. Cytogenetics frequently with *TP53, RAS* mutations, *BCL6* translocations
Other iatrogenic immunodeficiency-associated lymphoproliferative disorders	Increased frequency of HL and lymphoproliferation with Hodgkin-like features. Histologic features can otherwise resemble the range of features seen in other immune deficiency-related LPDs	HL-like show CD20+, CD30+, CD15– or CD20–, CD30+, CD15+ staining. EBV is variably positive	Same as above

FISH, fluorescence *in situ* hybridization; IgR, immunoglobulin gene rearrangement; IgVH, immunoglobulin variable heavy chain; MCD, multicentric castleman's disease; neg., negative; NF-κB, nuclear factor-κB; NK, natural killer; R-S, Reed-Sternberg; SMZL, splenic marginal zone lymphoma; STAT, signal transducer and activator of transcription; TCR, T-cell receptor. Also see acronyms and abbreviations at the beginning of this chapter.

*The immunophenotype revealed by immunohistochemistry and/or flow cytometry of surface antigens that typically are found for neoplastic cells of a given disorder are listed. If a CD antigen is indicated, then most of the neoplastic cells express that particular surface protein that is expressed by most tumor cells. CD antigens that have a minus (–) sign suffix are characteristically not expressed by the neoplastic cells of that disease entity. CD antigens that have a +/– sign suffix are not expressed by the neoplastic cells of all patients with that entity or are expressed at low or variable levels on the tumor cells. Antigens that have a –/+ sign suffix are expressed at very low levels or by the tumor cells of a minority of patients.

†The common genetic features associated with a given type of neoplasm are indicated. The numbers in parentheses provide the approximate proportion of cases that have the defined phenotype or genetic abnormality.

TABLE 90–2. Indolent Lymphomas

Disseminated lymphomas/leukemias

   Chronic lymphocytic leukemia

   Hairy cell leukemia

   Lymphoplasmacytic lymphoma

   Splenic marginal zone B-cell lymphoma (with or without villous lymphocytes)

   Plasma cell myeloma/plasmacytoma

Nodal lymphomas

   Follicular lymphoma

   Nodal marginal zone B-cell lymphoma (with or without mono-cytoid B cells)

   Small lymphocytic lymphoma

Extranodal lymphomas

   Extranodal marginal zone B-cell lymphoma of mucosa-associated lymphoid tissue (MALT) type

with two newly defined working categories as "gray zone" lymphomas between Hodgkin lymphoma and primary mediastinal large B-cell lymphoma[12,26] and between Burkitt and DLBCL.[13,14] These new intermediate groups make clear distinctions between biologic and clinical features of conventional DLBCL and HL.

TABLE 90–3. Aggressive Lymphomas

Immature B-cell neoplasms

   B-lymphoblastic leukemia/lymphoma

Mature B-cell neoplasms

   Burkitt lymphoma/Burkitt cell leukemia

   Diffuse large B-cell lymphoma

   Follicular lymphoma grade III

   Mantle cell lymphoma

Immature T-cell neoplasms

   T-lymphoblastic lymphoma/leukemia

Peripheral T- and natural killer (NK) cell neoplasms

   T-cell prolymphocytic leukemia/lymphoma

   Aggressive NK cell leukemia/lymphoma

   Adult T-cell lymphoma/leukemia (associated with HTLV-1 [human T-cell leukemia virus type 1])

   Extranodal NK/T-cell lymphoma

   Enteropathy-associated T-cell lymphoma

   Hepatosplenic T-cell lymphoma

   Subcutaneous panniculitis-like T-cell lymphoma

   Peripheral T-cell lymphomas, not otherwise specified

   Angioimmunoblastic T-cell lymphoma

   Anaplastic large cell lymphoma, primary, systemic

   Immune deficiency-associated lymphoproliferative disorders

● ASSOCIATED CLINICAL SYNDROMES

EARLY PRECURSOR LESIONS IN LYMPHOID NEOPLASMS

The 2008 WHO classification highlights several clinical, histologic, and immunophenotypic observations supporting the notion that lymphoid neoplasms arise from clonal expansion and ultimately, malignant transformation of precursor lesions. Monoclonal B-cell lymphocytosis (MBL) can be found in first-degree relatives of patients with CLL and in 5 to 15 percent of adults older than 60 years of age who present with lymphocytosis.[27,28] The documented rate of progression to CLL of 1 to 2 percent/year and immunophenotypic evidence of evolving CLL-like clones with cytogenetic anomalies suggest that mantle cell lymphoma may represent a potential precursor to CLL.[29] Other potential precursor lesions for follicular lymphoma and mantle cell lymphoma are currently under investigation.[4]

ABNORMAL PRODUCTION OF IMMUNOGLOBULIN

When B lymphocytes undergo neoplastic transformation and clonal proliferation, they can secrete monoclonal proteins inappropriately (Chaps. 105 and 106). If the monoclonal protein is immunoglobulin (Ig) M, IgA, or a member of certain subclasses of IgG (e.g., IgG$_3$), its presence may increase the viscosity of the blood, impairing blood flow through the microcirculation (Chaps. 107 and 109). This process may be impeded further by the associated homotypic erythrocyte aggregation (pathologic rouleaux) that often occurs in blood with a high concentration of immunoglobulin protein. Collectively, this situation may result in the hyperviscosity syndrome, manifested clinically by headache, dizziness, diplopia, stupor, retinal venous engorgement, or frank coma (Chap. 109).[30,31]

Monoclonal immunoglobulin proteins also can interact with cell surfaces and impair granulocyte or platelet function, or they can interact with coagulation proteins to impair their function in hemostasis (Chap. 120). Excessive excretion of immunoglobulin light chains can lead to several types of renal tubular dysfunction and renal insufficiency (Chaps. 106 and 107). IgM deposited in glomerular tufts also can lead to renal disease (Chap. 109). Cryoglobulins (immunoglobulins that precipitate at temperatures below 37°C) can result in Raynaud syndrome, skin ulcerations, purpura, digital infarction, and gangrene (Chap. 54). These manifestations result from immune complex formation, complement activation, and precipitation of cryoglobulins in cutaneous blood vessels. Excessive production of monoclonal immunoglobulin or immunoglobulin fragments in myeloma (Chap. 107) or in heavy-chain disease (Chap. 110) may lead to formation of amyloid, resulting in primary amyloidosis (Chap. 108).

Production of autoreactive antibodies spontaneously or in relationship to a B-lymphocyte neoplasm may lead to autoimmune hemolytic anemia (Chap. 54), autoimmune thrombocytopenia (Chap. 117), or, rarely, autoimmune neutropenia (Chap. 65). Autoantibodies directed against tissues are implicated in the pathogenesis of diseases such as autoimmune thyroiditis, adrenalitis, encephalitis, and conditions with other organ involvement. Peripheral neuropathies as a result of demyelinization can occur in patients with monoclonal immunoglobulin (Chaps. 106, 107, and 109). The neural injury often is related to antibody activity against myelin-associated glycoproteins or absorption by nerve tissue.[31] Rarely, the polyneuropathy is part of the polyneuropathy, organomegaly, endocrinopathy, monoclonal protein, and skin changes (POEMS) syndrome (Chap. 107).[32]

MARROW AND OTHER TISSUE INFILTRATION

Well-differentiated malignant B lymphocytes, such as those found in the early stages of CLL or Waldrenstrom's macroglobulinemia, may infiltrate the marrow extensively, causing impairment of hemopoiesis. Eventually, however, massive infiltration of marrow by malignant B lymphocytes can suppress normal hemopoiesis, resulting in varying combinations of anemia, neutropenia, and/or thrombocytopenia (Chap. 92). Malignant B-lymphocyte proliferation or infiltration may result in any combination of splenomegaly and lymphadenopathy of either superficial or deep lymph nodes. Diffuse large B cell lymphomas tend to involve isolated lymph node groups (Chaps. 97 and 98), whereas low-grade lymphomas (follicular lymphoma) and lymphoproliferative disorders (CLL) tend to present with more diffuse lymphadenopathy and splenic involvement (Chaps. 92 to 94). Prolymphocytic leukemia and hairy cell leukemia, two uncommon B-lymphocyte malignancies, are prone to infiltrate the marrow and spleen, sometimes causing bone marrow fibrosis and massive splenomegaly (Chaps. 92 and 93).

LYMPHOKINE-INDUCED DISORDERS

In addition to the consequences of monoclonal immunoglobulin and tumor proliferation, some lymphoid malignancies may produce cytokines that contribute to the disease morbidity. Recent work has identified several immune activation syndromes, mediated in large part as a result of unchecked inflammatory cytokines (interleukin [IL]-1, IL-6) and defects in perforin/granzyme pathways are associated with lymphomas and infection with oncogenic herpes viruses. Hemophagocytic lymphohistiocytosis and macrophage activating syndrome are two distinct complications arising from dysregulated effector lymphocyte-tumor interaction at the immunologic synapse and can lead to life-threatening complications if not rapidly diagnosed and treated with immunochemotherapy.[33] Patients with cutaneous T-cell lymphomas have elevated plasma levels of T-helper type 2 (Th2)-associated cytokines, which may account for the relatively high incidence of eosinophilia (Chap. 103) and eosinophilic pneumonia observed in patients with this disease.[34] In addition, the neoplastic plasma cells in myeloma may secrete various cytokines and osteoclast activating factors that stimulate osteoclast proliferation and activity leading to extensive osteolysis, severe bone pain, and pathologic fractures (Chap. 107).[35] Dysregulated extrarenal production of calcitriol, the active metabolite of vitamin D, appears to underlie the hypercalcemia associated with Hodgkin lymphoma and other lymphomas (Chaps. 95 and 97).[36]

SYSTEMIC SYMPTOMS

Large cell lymphoma, poorly differentiated lymphoma, and Hodgkin lymphoma frequently are associated with fever, night sweats, weight loss, and anorexia-cachexia (Chaps. 95, 97, and 98). Patients with lymphomas or Hodgkin lymphoma have an increased incidence of localized or disseminated herpes zoster,[37] and 10 percent or more of these patients may be affected at some time during the course of their illness. Pruritus is common in Hodgkin lymphoma,[38] and its severity parallels disease activity (Chap. 97). Systemic symptoms may be present in Hodgkin lymphoma in the absence of obvious, bulky lymph node or splenic tumors, whereas in well-differentiated small cell lymphomas, such as CLL or Waldenström macroglobulinemia, fever, night sweats, and significant weight loss are uncommon despite generalized lymphadenopathy and splenomegaly. Rather, fever in patients with CLL or

macroglobulinemia usually is secondary to infectious disease (Chaps. 92 and 109).

METABOLIC SIGNS

Lymphoid malignancies are associated with several dramatic metabolic disturbances associated with cancers (Chap. 95). Some lymphomas and lymphocytic leukemias may have a high proliferative rate, a high death fraction of cells, and, therefore, an enormous turnover of nucleoproteins, sometimes causing hyperuricemia and extreme hyperuricosuria. Highly proliferative neoplasms like Burkitt lymphoma or lymphoblastic lymphoma are particularly likely to cause an extreme degree of hyperuricemia, sometimes leading to renal failure complicating initiation of cytotoxic therapy (Chaps. 91 and 102). Also, because these and other lymphocytic malignancies are sensitive to cytotoxic drugs and glucocorticoids, cytotoxic therapy may cause a *tumor lysis syndrome*, characterized by extreme hyperuricemia, hyperuricosuria, hyperkalemia, and/or hyperphosphatemia.[39,40] Precipitation of uric acid in the renal tubules and collecting system can lead to acute obstructive nephropathy and renal failure unless precautions are taken, such as pretreatment with allopurinol, hydration, and alkalization of the urine.[41] For extreme cases, or in cases in which allopurinol cannot be administered (e.g., drug allergy), the drug rasburicase may be required for treatment of hyperuricemia (Chap. 102).[42]

Hypercalcemia and calciuria are common complications of myeloma because of osteolysis. Hypercalcemia also may occur during the course of lymphomas (Chap. 94) or myeloma (Chap. 107). This situation may be caused by several mechanisms, including tumor cell production of IL-1, ectopic parathyroid hormone elaboration, excessive bone resorption, and impaired bone formation.[43]

EXTRANODAL INVOLVEMENT

T-cell leukemias and lymphomas, in addition to causing lymph node and spleen enlargement, may involve the skin, mediastinum, or CNS. As the name implies, cutaneous T-cell lymphomas have malignant cells that home to the skin,[44] sometimes producing a severe desquamating erythroderma, as in Sézary syndrome, or small (<2 cm) subcutaneous nodules, as in primary cutaneous CD30-positive T-cell lymphoproliferative disease or anaplastic large cell lymphoma,[45] or a variety of nodular infiltrative lesions, as in mycosis fungoides or adult T-cell leukemia/lymphoma associated with human T-cell leukemia virus type 1 (HTLV-1; Chap. 103).[46] T-cell acute lymphoblastic leukemia and lymphoblastic lymphoma frequently cause mediastinal enlargement (Chap. 91). These diseases frequently involve testicles and the leptomeninges and other structures that are transverse to the subarachnoid space, such as the cranial and peripheral nerves.

B-cell lymphomas frequently may involve the salivary glands, endocrine glands, joints, heart, lung, kidney, bowel, bone, or, less frequently, other extranodal sites such as the CNS and testes (Chap. 95). These diseases may begin as an extranodal tumor, or the tumor may develop during the course of the disease. Aggressive lymphomas, such as Burkitt lymphoma,[47] primary testicular lymphoma,[47,48] and double-hit DLBCLs (Chap. 98),[49] frequently involve the CNS and require upfront assessment during diagnosis and treatment with either intrathecal chemotherapy or regimens capable of crossing blood–brain barrier that contain high-dose methotrexate. Marginal zone B-cell lymphoma of the mucosa-associated lymphoid tissue (MALT) type frequently involves the stomach and salivary glands, although the disease may be encountered in any extranodal site distinguished by the presence of a columnar or cuboidal epithelium.

REFERENCES

1. Liang X, Graham DK: Natural killer cell neoplasms. *Cancer* 112:1425–1436, 2008.
2. Harris NL, Jaffe ES, Stein H, et al: A revised European-American classification of lymphoid neoplasms: A proposal from the International Lymphoma Study Group. *Blood* 84:1361–1392, 1994.
3. Chan JK: The new World Health Organization classification of lymphomas: The past, the present and the future. *Hematol Oncol* 19:129–150, 2001.
4. Campo E, Swerdlow SH, Harris NL, et al: The 2008 WHO classification of lymphoid neoplasms and beyond: Evolving concepts and practical applications. *Blood* 117:5019–5032, 2011.
5. Segal GH, Kjeldsberg CR: Practical lymphoma diagnosis: An approach to using the information organized in the REAL proposal. Revised European-American Lymphoid Neoplasm. *Anat Pathol* 3:147–168, 1998.
6. Spagnolo DV, Ellis DW, Juneja S, et al: The role of molecular studies in lymphoma diagnosis: A review. *Pathology* 36:19–44, 2004.
7. Strauchen JA: Immunophenotypic and molecular studies in the diagnosis and classification of malignant lymphoma. *Cancer Invest* 22:138–148, 2004.
8. Hallek M, Cheson BD, Catovsky D, et al: Guidelines for the diagnosis and treatment of chronic lymphocytic leukemia: A report from the International Workshop on Chronic Lymphocytic Leukemia updating the National Cancer Institute-Working Group 1996 guidelines. *Blood* 111:5446–5456, 2008.
9. Owen RG, Treon SP, Al-Katib A, et al: Clinicopathological definition of Waldenström's macroglobulinemia: Consensus panel recommendations from the Second International Workshop on Waldenström's Macroglobulinemia. *Semin Oncol* 30:110–115, 2003.
10. International Myeloma Working Group: Criteria for the classification of monoclonal gammopathies, multiple myeloma and related disorders: A report of the International Myeloma Working Group. *Br J Haematol* 121:749–757, 2003.
11. Calvo KR, Traverse-Glehen A, Pittaluga S, et al: Molecular profiling provides evidence of primary mediastinal large B-cell lymphoma as a distinct entity related to classic Hodgkin lymphoma: Implications for mediastinal gray zone lymphomas as an intermediate form of B-cell lymphoma. *Adv Anat Pathol* 11:227–238, 2004.
12. Traverse-Glehen A, Pittaluga S, Gaulard P, et al: Mediastinal gray zone lymphoma: The missing link between classic Hodgkin's lymphoma and mediastinal large B-cell lymphoma. *Am J Surg Pathol* 29:1411–1421, 2005.
13. Salaverria I, Zettl A, Bea S, et al: Chromosomal alterations detected by comparative genomic hybridization in subgroups of gene expression-defined Burkitt's lymphoma. *Haematologica* 93:1327–1334, 2008.
14. Hummel M, Bentink S, Berger H, et al: A biologic definition of Burkitt's lymphoma from transcriptional and genomic profiling. *N Engl J Med* 354:2419–2430, 2006.
15. A clinical evaluation of the International Lymphoma Study Group classification of non-Hodgkin's lymphoma. The Non-Hodgkin's Lymphoma Classification Project. *Blood* 89:3909–3918, 1997.
16. Fisher RI, Miller TP, Grogan TM: New REAL clinical entities. *Cancer J Sci Am* 4 (Suppl 2):S5–S12, 1998.
17. Pileri SA, Ascani S, Sabattini E, et al: The pathologist's view point. Part II—Aggressive lymphomas. *Haematologica* 85:1308–1321, 2000.
18. Pileri SA, Ascani S, Sabattini E, et al: The pathologist's view point. Part I—Indolent lymphomas. *Haematologica* 85:1291–1307, 2000.
19. Alizadeh AA, Eisen MB, Davis RE, et al: Distinct types of diffuse large B-cell lymphoma identified by gene expression profiling. *Nature* 403:503–511, 2000.
20. Rosenwald A, Alizadeh AA, Widhopf G, et al: Relation of gene expression phenotype to immunoglobulin mutation genotype in B cell chronic lymphocytic leukemia. *J Exp Med* 194:1639–1647, 2001.
21. Davis RE, Staudt LM: Molecular diagnosis of lymphoid malignancies by gene expression profiling. *Curr Opin Hematol* 9:333–338, 2002.
22. Pileri SA, Ascani S, Leoncini L, et al: Hodgkin's lymphoma: The pathologist's viewpoint. *J Clin Pathol* 55:162–176, 2002.
23. Copur MS, Ledakis P, Bolton M: Molecular profiling of lymphoma. *N Engl J Med* 347:1376–1377, 2002.
24. Lossos IS, Czerwinski DK, Alizadeh AA, et al: Prediction of survival in diffuse large-B-cell lymphoma based on the expression of six genes. *N Engl J Med* 350:1828–1837, 2004.
25. Ramaswamy S: Translating cancer genomics into clinical oncology. *N Engl J Med* 350:1814–1816, 2004.
26. Garcia JF, Mollejo M, Fraga M, et al: Large B-cell lymphoma with Hodgkin's features. *Histopathology* 47:101–110, 2005.
27. Shanafelt TD, Ghia P, Lanasa MC, et al: Monoclonal B-cell lymphocytosis (MBL): Biology, natural history and clinical management. *Leukemia* 24:512–520, 2010.
28. Rawstron AC, Bennett FL, O'Connor SJ, et al: Monoclonal B-cell lymphocytosis and chronic lymphocytic leukemia. *N Engl J Med* 359:575–583, 2008.
29. Nieto WG, Almeida J, Romero A, et al: Increased frequency (12%) of circulating chronic lymphocytic leukemia-like B-cell clones in healthy subjects using a highly sensitive multicolor flow cytometry approach. *Blood* 114:33–37, 2009.
30. Stone MJ: Waldenström's macroglobulinemia: Hyperviscosity syndrome and cryoglobulinemia. *Clin Lymphoma Myeloma* 9:97–99, 2009.
31. Decaux O, Laurat E, Perlat A, et al: Systemic manifestations of monoclonal gammopathy. *Eur J Intern Med* 20:457–461, 2009.
32. Silberman J, Lonial S: Review of peripheral neuropathy in plasma cell disorders. *Hematol Oncol* 26:55–65, 2008.
33. Jordan MB, Allen CE, Weitzman S, et al: How I treat hemophagocytic lymphohistiocytosis. *Blood* 118:4041–4052, 2011.
34. Lee CH, Mamelak AJ, Vonderheid EC: Erythrodermic cutaneous T cell lymphoma with hypereosinophilic syndrome: Treatment with interferon alfa and extracorporeal photopheresis. *Int J Dermatol* 46:1198–1204, 2007.
35. Roodman GD: Pathogenesis of myeloma bone disease. *Leukemia* 23:435–441, 2009.
36. Gupta R, Neal JM: Hypercalcemia due to vitamin D-secreting Hodgkin's lymphoma exacerbated by oral calcium supplementation. *Endocr Pract* 12:227–229, 2006.
37. Johnson RW, Wasner G, Saddier P, et al: Herpes zoster and postherpetic neuralgia optimizing management in the elderly patient. *Drugs Aging* 25:991–1006, 2008.
38. Hiramanek N: Itch: A symptom of occult disease. *Aust Fam Physician* 33:495–499, 2004.
39. Tiu RV, Mountantonakis SE, Dunbar AJ, et al: Tumor lysis syndrome. *Semin Thromb Hemost* 33:397–407, 2007.
40. Cheson BD: Etiology and management of tumor lysis syndrome in patients with chronic lymphocytic leukemia. *Clin Adv Hematol Oncol* 7:263–271, 2009.
41. Tosi P, Barosi G, Lazzaro C, et al: Consensus conference on the management of tumor lysis syndrome. *Haematologica* 93:1877–1885, 2008.
42. Cammalleri L, Malaguarnera M: Rasburicase represents a new tool for hyperuricemia in tumor lysis syndrome and in gout. *Int J Med Sci* 4:83–93, 2007.
43. Roodman GD: Mechanisms of bone lesions in multiple myeloma and lymphoma. *Cancer* 80:1557–1563, 1997.
44. Lansigan F, Choi J, Foss FM: Cutaneous T-cell lymphoma. *Hematol Oncol Clin North Am* 22:979–996, x, 2008.
45. Chuang SS, Hsieh YC, Ye H, et al: Lymphohistiocytic anaplastic large cell lymphoma involving skin: A diagnostic challenge. *Pathol Res Pract* 205:283–287, 2009.
46. Hwang ST, Janik JE, Jaffe ES, et al: Mycosis fungoides and Sézary syndrome. *Lancet* 371:945–957, 2008.
47. Blum KA, Lozanski G, Byrd JC: Adult Burkitt leukemia and lymphoma. *Blood* 104:3009–3020, 2004.
48. Cheah CY, Wirth A, Seymour JF: Primary testicular lymphoma. *Blood* 123:486–493, 2014.
49. Aukema SM, Siebert R, Schuuring E, et al: Double-hit B-cell lymphomas. *Blood* 117:2319–2331, 2011.

CHAPTER 91
ACUTE LYMPHOBLASTIC LEUKEMIA

Richard A. Larson

SUMMARY

Acute lymphoblastic leukemia (ALL) is a malignant disorder that originates in a single B- or T-lymphocyte progenitor. Proliferation and accumulation of clonal blast cells in the marrow result in suppression of hematopoiesis and, thereafter, anemia, thrombocytopenia, and neutropenia. Lymphoblasts can accumulate in various extramedullary sites, especially the meninges, gonads, thymus, liver, spleen, and lymph nodes. The disease is most common in children but can be seen in individuals of any age. ALL has many subtypes and can be classified by immunologic, cytogenetic, and molecular genetic methods. These methods can identify clinically important, biologic subtypes, requiring treatment approaches that differ in their use of specific drugs or drug combinations, dosages of drug, or duration of treatment required to achieve optimal results. For example, cases of childhood ALL having a hyperdiploid karyotype respond well to extended treatment with methotrexate and mercaptopurine, whereas adults whose leukemic cells contain the Philadelphia chromosome and *BCR-ABL1* fusion benefit from intensive treatment that includes a tyrosine kinase inhibitor and transplantation of allogeneic hematopoietic stem cells. The relative lack of therapeutic success in adult ALL is partly related to a high frequency of cases having unfavorable genetic abnormalities and partly related to poor tolerance for intensive treatment. Nearly 90 percent of children and 40 percent of adults can expect long-term, leukemia-free survival—and probable cure—with contemporary treatment. Novel immunotherapeutic approaches are under development. Currently, emphasis is placed not only on improving the cure rate but also on improving quality of life by preventing acute and late treatment-related complications, such as second malignancies, cardiotoxicity, and endocrinopathy.

DEFINITION AND HISTORY

Acute lymphoblastic leukemia (ALL) is a neoplastic disease that results from multistep somatic mutations in a single lymphoid progenitor cell at one of several discrete stages of development. The immunophenotype of leukemic cells at diagnosis reflects the level of differentiation achieved by the dominant clone. The clonal origin of ALL has been established by cytogenetic analysis, by analysis of restriction fragments in female patients who are heterozygous for polymorphic X chromosome-linked genes, and by analysis of rearrangements of T-cell receptor or immunoglobulin genes. Leukemic cells divide more slowly and require more time to synthesize DNA than do normal hematopoietic counterparts. However, leukemic cells accumulate relentlessly because of their altered response to growth and death signals.[1,2] They compete successfully with normal hematopoietic cells, resulting in anemia, thrombocytopenia, and neutropenia. At diagnosis, leukemic cells not only have replaced normal marrow cells but also have disseminated to various extramedullary sites.

Velpeau[3] is generally credited with the earliest report of leukemia in 1827. Virchow,[4] Bennett,[5] and Craigie[6] recognized the condition as a distinct entity by 1845. In 1847, Virchow coined the term "weisses blut" and, later, "leucaemie," applying it to two distinct types of the disease— splenic and lymphatic—that could be distinguished from each other based on splenomegaly and enlarged lymph nodes and on the morphologic similarities of the leukemic cells to those normally found in these organs.[7] Ehrlich's introduction of staining methods in 1891 allowed further distinction of leukemia subtypes.[8] By 1913, leukemia could be classified as acute or chronic, and as lymphatic or myelogenous.[9] The greater prevalence of ALL in children, especially those ages 1 to 5 years, was recognized in 1917.[10]

Shortly after leukemia was recognized as a discrete disease entity, physicians began using chemicals as palliative therapy. The first advance was the use of a 4-amino analogue of folic acid (aminopterin), prompted by Farber's observation that folic acid appeared to accelerate the proliferation of leukemic cells. Strikingly, for the first time, complete clinical and hematologic remissions that lasted for several months were seen in children.[11] A year after the report of aminopterin-induced clinical remissions, a newly isolated adrenocorticotrophic hormone was reported to induce prompt, though brief, remissions in patients with leukemia.[12] Almost concurrently, Elion and colleagues synthesized antimetabolites that interfere with synthesis of purines and pyrimidines.[13] Their findings led to the introduction of mercaptopurine, 6-thioguanine, and allopurinol into clinical use. From 1950 to 1960, many new antileukemic agents were introduced, and occasional cures were seen. Pinkel and colleagues at St. Jude Children's Research Hospital, in 1962, devised a "total therapy" approach, consisting of four treatment phases: remission induction; intensification or consolidation; therapy for subclinical CNS leukemia (or preventive meningeal treatment); and prolonged continuation therapy.[14] By the early 1970s, as many as 50 percent of children achieved long-term event-free survival (EFS) using this innovative strategy. During the same period, a better understanding of the genetics of human histocompatibility and wider use of human leukocyte antigen (HLA) typing culminated in the successful use of hematopoietic stem cell transplantation for treatment of patients in whom leukemia relapsed. In the early 1980s, Riehm and coworkers introduced a so-called reinduction or delayed intensification treatment during early continuation therapy, consisting mainly of repetition of the initial remission induction and early intensification phases, and further improved the EFS to approximately 70 percent.[15] Parallel to advances in treatment has been the improved understanding of the biology of ALL. The recognition of ALL as a heterogeneous group of diseases—clinically, immunologically, and genetically[16]—set the stage for risk-directed therapy.[16a]

Treatment of ALL has progressed incrementally, beginning with the development of effective therapy for CNS disease, followed by intensification of early treatment, especially for patients at high risk of relapse. The current cure rates of nearly 90 percent for children (Fig. 91–1) and 40 percent for adults attest to the steady progress made in treating this disease.[17,18] Rapid evolution and convergence of multiple genome-wide platforms to identify the total complement of genetic and

Acronyms and Abbreviations: ALL, acute lymphoblastic leukemia; ARID5B, AT-rich interactive domain 5b; *ATM*, ataxia-telangiectasia mutated gene; CD, cluster of differentiation; CNAs, copy number abnormalities; CSF, cerebrospinal fluid; EFS, event-free survival; FISH, fluorescence *in situ* hybridization; HLA, human leukocyte antigen; MRI, magnetic resonance imaging; PCR, polymerase chain reaction; RT-PCR, reverse transcriptase polymerase chain reaction; SEER, Surveillance, Epidemiology, and End Results; SNP, single nucleotide polymorphism.

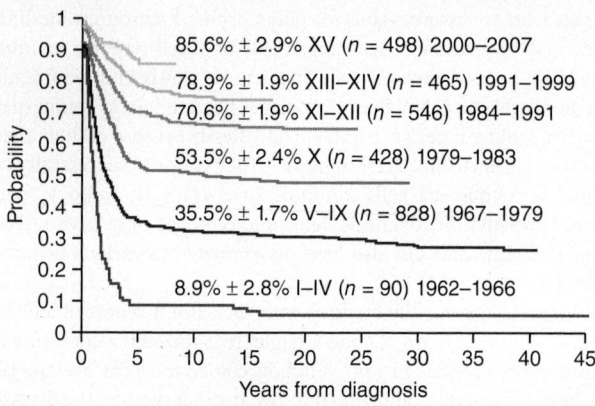

Figure 91–1. Kaplan-Meier analysis of event-free survival for 2855 children with ALL treated in 15 consecutive total-therapy studies at St. Jude Children's Research Hospital. Early intensification of systemic and intrathecal chemotherapy with a risk assignment based on sequential measurements of minimal residual disease in the 2000s has boosted the event-free survival estimate to 85.6 percent ± 2.9 percent (SE). *(Data from CH Pui and is unpublished.)*

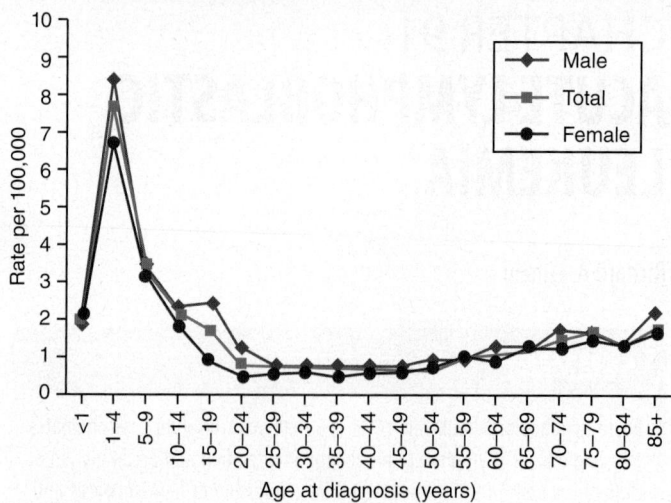

Figure 91–2. Age-specific incidence rates for acute lymphoblastic leukemia by sex. *(Data from SEER Cancer Statistics Review, 1975–2010, National Cancer Institute. Bethesda, MD, http://seer.cancer.gov/csr/1975_2010. Accessed July 4, 2014.)*

epigenetic alterations almost certainly will lead to the identification of new targets for specific treatment.[19,20] A clear advance was the development of imatinib mesylate and dasatinib, which target leukemias with the *BCR-ABL1* fusion.[21]

● ETIOLOGY AND PATHOGENESIS

Initiation and progression of ALL are driven by successive mutations that alter cellular functions, including an enhanced ability of self-renewal, a subversion of control of normal proliferation, a block in differentiation, and an increased resistance to death signals (apoptosis).[1,2] Familial disorders of DNA repair may play a role. Environmental agents, such as ionizing radiation and chemical mutagens, have been implicated in the induction of ALL in some patients. However, in most cases, no etiologic factors are discernible. In the favored theory, leukemogenesis reflects the interaction between host pharmacogenetics (susceptibility) and environmental factors, a model that requires confirmation in well-designed population and molecular epidemiologic studies.

INCIDENCE

The American Cancer Society has estimated that in the United States there will be approximately 6020 new cases of ALL in 2014 (3140 in males and 2880 in females) and approximately 1440 deaths from ALL (810 in males and 630 in females).[22] Most cases of ALL occur in children, but most deaths from ALL (approximately four of five) occur in adults.

The age-adjusted incidence rate of ALL was 1.6 per 100,000 males and 1.2 for females per year in the United States, based on cases diagnosed in 1975 to 2010 from 17 Surveillance, Epidemiology, and End Results (SEER) geographic areas.[23] The risk for developing ALL is highest in children younger than 5 years of age. The risk then declines slowly until the mid-20s, and begins to rise again slowly after age 50. The incidence is 7.9 per 100,000 children 1 to 4 years old and 1.2 for those older than age 60 years. Only 20 percent of adult acute leukemias are ALL, but about one-third of ALL cases are in adults. The average person's lifetime risk of developing ALL is less than one in 750. The risk is slightly higher in males than in females, and higher in whites than in African Americans (Fig. 91–2).[23] The median age at diagnosis for ALL is 13 years and approximately 61 percent are diagnosed before the age of 20 years,

however, because of the bimodal peak in incidence, the age of 13 years is mathematically correct but medically nearly useless. ALL is the most common malignancy diagnosed in patients younger than age 15 years, accounting for 23 percent of all cancers and 76 percent of all leukemias in this age group.

The sharp incidence peak of ALL during early childhood has been observed only since the 1930s in the United Kingdom and the United States.[24] In the United States, the peak first appeared in children of European descent, and subsequently was seen in children of African descent in the 1960s. The age peak is absent in many developing or underdeveloped countries, suggesting a leukemogenic contribution from factors associated with industrialization. Except for a slight predominance for females in infancy, ALL affects males of European descent more often than females in all age groups (see Fig. 91–2). The frequency distribution is similar among those of African descent. In most age groups, the incidence of ALL is higher in those of European descent than in those of African descent, especially among children ages 2 to 3 years.

The incidence of ALL differs substantially in different geographic areas. Rates are higher among populations in northern and western Europe, North America, and Oceania, with lower rates in Asian and African populations.[25] In Europe, the highest rates of ALL among males are found in Spain and the highest rates among females in Denmark. In the United States, the highest rates for both sexes are among Latinos in Los Angeles.

RISK FACTORS

Genetic Syndromes

The precise pathogenetic events leading to the development of ALL are unknown. Only a minority (5 percent) of cases are associated with inherited, predisposing genetic syndromes. Children with Down syndrome have a 10 to 30 times greater risk of leukemia; acute megakaryoblastic leukemia predominates in those patients younger than age 3 years, and ALL is predominant in older age groups. ALL in patients with Down syndrome is a heterogeneous disorder, comprising subtypes with the same well-recognized genetic abnormalities found in the general population, such as hyperdiploidy greater than 50 and t(12;21)[*ETV6-RUNX1*], plus those more commonly associated with Down syndrome such as +X, del(9), and *CEBPD* rearrangement.[26,27] Studies show that *P2RY8-CRLF2* fusion and activating *JAK* mutations together contribute to leukemogenesis in approximately half of the cases of Down syndrome patients with ALL.[28,29] Almost all ALL patients with Down syndrome have a deletion of IKZF1.[30] Autosomal recessive genetic diseases associated with increased chromosomal fragility and a predisposition to ALL include ataxia-telangiectasia, Nijmegen breakage syndrome, and Bloom syndrome.[31] Patients with ataxia-telangiectasia have a 70 times greater risk of leukemia and a 250 times greater risk of lymphoma, particularly of the T-cell phenotype.[32] The causative gene, termed *ATM* (ataxia-telangiectasia mutated), encodes a protein involved in DNA repair, regulation of cell proliferation, and apoptosis. Laboratory studies supporting the diagnosis of ataxia-telangiectasia include an elevated serum concentration of α-fetoprotein, presence of characteristic chromosomal aberrations, absent or reduced intranuclear serine protein kinase ATM, and increased *in vitro* radiosensitivity. A high prevalence of germline truncating and missense *ATM* gene alterations in children with sporadic T-cell ALL suggests a pathogenetic role of *ATM* in lymphoid malignancies. Although impaired immune surveillance contributes to the increased risk of Epstein-Barr virus-related malignancies in patients with acquired immunodeficiencies, no compelling evidence indicates defective immunity contributes to the predisposition to ALL in patients with ataxia-telangiectasia or other congenital immunodeficiency syndromes. Genome-wide association studies have identified common allelic variants in four genes (*IKZF1, ARID5B, CEBPE,* and *CDKN2a*) that are consistently associated with childhood ALL.[33-35] These genes are key regulators of blood cell development, and acquired mutations of each are also detected in ALL cases. Thus, the risk of childhood ALL may be influenced by coinheritance of multiple low-risk variants. Inherited allelic variation may also affect response to treatment.[36]

Environmental Factors

In utero (but not postnatal) exposure to diagnostic x-rays confers a slightly increased risk of ALL, which correlates positively with the number of exposures.[37] The evidence is weak for an association between the development of ALL and nuclear fallout; exposure to occupational, natural terrestrial, or cosmic ionizing radiation exposure; or paternal radiation exposure prior to conception. There has been concern that exposure to low-energy electromagnetic fields produced by a residential power supply may be associated with the development of childhood ALL. Case-control studies suggested a slightly increased risk of leukemia at very high levels of exposure; assuming the association is real, only approximately 1 percent of leukemias could be attributed to the exposure.[38,39] Pesticide exposure (occupational or home use) and parental cigarette smoking before or during pregnancy, administration of vitamin K to neonates, maternal alcohol consumption during pregnancy, and increased consumption of dietary nitrites have each been suggested causes. However, each of these associations is controversial, and most have been refuted after careful, controlled investigation. High birth weight is associated with an increased risk of leukemia before the age of 5 years with fair consistency,[40] and the birth weight is likely a marker for an endogenous factor, such as insulin-like growth factor.

Host Pharmacogenetics

Subtle genetic polymorphisms of xenobiotic-metabolizing enzymes, DNA repair pathways, and cell-cycle checkpoint functions might interact with environmental, dietary, maternal, and other external factors to affect the development of ALL.[2,41] Although the number of investigations and sample sizes are limited, data exist to support a causal role for polymorphisms in genes encoding detoxifying enzymes (e.g., glutathione *S*-transferase, nicotinamide adenine dinucleotide phosphate [NAD(P)H]:quinone oxidoreductase), folate-metabolizing enzymes (serine hydroxymethyltransferase and thymidylate synthase), cytochrome P450, methylenetetrahydrofolate reductase, and cell-cycle

inhibitors in the development of adult and childhood ALL.[42,43] However, all these associations must be confirmed by larger studies with careful attention to ethnic and geographic diversity in the frequency of polymorphisms. Using genome-wide analysis, germline single-nucleotide polymorphisms (SNPs) of AT-rich interactive domain 5b (*ARID5B*) gene have been associated with childhood hyperdiploid B-cell precursor ALL,[44] a clear example of host genetic variations affecting the susceptibility to the development of childhood ALL.

Development of Acute Lymphoblastic Leukemia in Utero

Retrospective identification of leukemia-specific fusion genes (e.g., *KMT2A/AFF1* [also known as *MLL-AF4*] and *ETV6-RUNX1* [also known as *TEL-AML1*]), hyperdiploidy, or clonotypic rearrangements of immunoglobulin or T-cell receptor loci in archived neonatal blood spots (Guthrie cards), and development of concordant leukemia in identical twins clearly indicate some leukemias have a prenatal origin.[45,46] In identical twins with the t(4;11)/*KMT2A/AFF1*, the concordance rate is nearly 100 percent, and the latency in the time of occurrence in the two twins is short (a few weeks to a few months). These findings suggest this fusion gene alone either is leukemogenic or requires only a small number of cooperative mutations to cause leukemia. By contrast, the lower concordance rate in twins with the *ETV6-RUNX1* fusion or T-cell phenotype and the longer postnatal latency period suggest additional postnatal events are required for leukemic transformation in these subtypes.[45] This theory is supported by the identification of rare cells expressing *ETV6-RUNX1* fusion transcripts in approximately 1 percent of cord blood samples from newborns, a frequency 100 times higher than the incidence of ALL defined by this fusion transcript.[45] The presence of a preleukemic clone with the *ETV6-RUNX1* has been established.[47] Hyperdiploid ALL, another common subtype of childhood ALL, also appears to arise before birth but requires postnatal events for full malignant transformation.[46] The observations of a peak age of development of childhood ALL of 2 to 5 years, an association of industrialization and modern or affluent societies with increased prevalence of ALL, and the occasional clustering of childhood leukemia cases have fueled two parallel infection-based hypotheses to account for postnatal events. The "delayed-infection" hypothesis suggests that some susceptible individuals with a prenatally acquired preleukemic clone had low or no exposure to common infections early in life because they lived in an affluent hygienic environments.[45] Such infectious insulation predisposes the immune system of these individuals to aberrant or pathologic responses after subsequent or delayed exposure to common infections at an age commensurate with increased lymphoid cell proliferation. The "population-mixing" hypothesis predicts that clusters of childhood ALL result from exposure of susceptible (nonimmune) individuals to common but fairly nonpathologic infections after population mixing with carriers.[48] However, clearly not all childhood cases develop *in utero*. For example, t(1;19)/*TCF3-PBX1* (also known as *E2A-PBX1*) ALL appears to have a postnatal origin in most cases.[49] Cases of adult ALL most certainly arise over a protracted time.

ACQUIRED GENETIC CHANGES

Acquired genetic abnormalities are a hallmark of ALL; 80 percent of all cases have recurring cytogenetic or molecular lesions with prognostic and therapeutic relevance (Table 91–1).[2,19,41] Chromosomal changes include abnormalities in the number (ploidy) and structure of chromosomes.[50-52] The latter comprise translocations (the most frequent abnormality), inversions, deletions, point mutations, and amplifications. Although the frequency of particular genetic subtypes differs between childhood and adult cases, the general mechanisms underlying the induction are similar. Mechanisms include aberrant expression of oncoproteins, loss of

TABLE 91–1. Frequencies of Common Genetic Aberrations in Childhood and Adult Acute Lymphoblastic Leukemia

Abnormality	Children (%)	Adults (%)
Hyperdiploidy (>50 chromosomes)	23–29	6–7
Hypodiploidy (<45 chromosomes)	1	2
t(1;19)(q23;p13.3) [TCF3-PBX1]	4 in white, 12 in black	2–3
t(9;22)(q34;q11.2) [BCR-ABL1]	2–3	25–30
t(4;11)(q21;q23) [MLL-AF4]	2	3–7
t(8;14)(q23;q32.3)	2	4
t(12;21)(p13;q22) [ETV6-RUNX1]	20–25	0–3
NOTCH1 mutations*	7	15
HOX11L2 overexpression*	20	13
LYL1 overexpression*	9	15
TAL1 overexpression*	15	3
HOX11 overexpression*	7	30
MLL-ENL fusion	2	3
Abnormal 9p	7–11	6–30
Abnormal 12p	7–9	4–6
del(7p)/del(7q)/monosomy 7	4	6–11
+8	2	10–12
Intrachromosomal amplification of chromosome 21 (iAMP21)	2	?

*Abnormalities found in T-cell acute lymphoblastic leukemia (ALL).

tumor-suppressor genes, and chromosomal translocations that generate fusion genes encoding transcription factors or active kinases.

Primary genetic rearrangement by itself is insufficient to induce overt leukemia. Cooperative mutations are necessary for leukemic transformation and include genetic and epigenetic changes in key growth regulatory pathways.[19,20] The candidate gene approach has identified deletion of the CDKN2A/CDKN2B tumor-suppressor locus[53] and mutations of NOTCH1 in T-cell ALL.[54] Current searches applying genome-wide microarray and high-throughput sequencing methodologies have identified a high frequency of common genetic alterations in both B-cell precursor ALL and T-cell ALL. Using SNP microarray, a mean of 6.46 DNA copy number abnormalities (CNAs) per case was identified, suggesting that gross genomic instability is not a feature for most ALL cases.[55] There was a wide variation in the number of CNAs across leukemic subtypes. Interestingly, infant ALL cases with MLL rearrangement had less than one CNA per case, suggesting that few additional genetic lesions are required for leukemogenesis in these cases. By contrast, ETV6-RUNX1 and BCR-ABL1 cases had more than six CNAs per case, with some having more than 20 lesions, a finding consistent with the concept that, although the initiating events may occur early in childhood, additional lesions are required for subsequent development of ALL. More than 40 percent of B-cell precursor ALL cases had mutations in genes encoding regulators of normal lymphoid development.[55] The most frequent target was the lymphoid transcription factor PAX5 (mutated in approximately 32 percent of cases), which encode a paired-domain protein required for the pro–B-cell to pre–B-cell transition and B-lineage fidelity. The second most frequently involved gene was IKZF1 (mutated in almost 28 percent of the cases), encoding the

IKAROS zinc finger DNA-binding protein that is required for the earliest lymphoid differentiation. IKZF1 was deleted in the vast majority of cases of BCR-ABL1 ALL cases as well as chronic myeloid leukemia in lymphoid blast crisis (but not chronic phase).[56] Approximately half of BCR-ABL1 ALL cases also had deletions of CDKN2A/B and PAX5. This finding further supports the concept that multiple signaling pathways need to be disrupted to induce leukemia. A subgroup of ALL with very poor outcome was strongly associated with the presence of IKZF1 deletions.[57,58] Together, these findings suggest that IKZF1 directly contributes to treatment resistance in ALL.

BCR-ABL1–like B-cell ALL lacks the BCR-ABL1 fusion or t(9;22) by cytogenetic, fluorescence in situ hybridization (FISH), or molecular analyses, but it shares the same gene-expression profile with typical BCR-ABL1–positive ALL.[59] In half of these cases, the CRLF2 gene is involved in a cryptic translocation with the IGH gene or is fused to the P2RY8 gene; both rearrangements lead to overexpression of CRLF2.[29,60] Mutations in JAK2 or JAK1 are detected in 30 to 40 percent of these cases, and many of the remaining have activating mutations in cytokine receptor and kinase signaling pathways.[30] Microarrays and genomic DNA sequencing identified monoallelic deletion of the PAX5 gene at chromosome band 9p13.2 in 28 percent of ALL patients with cryptic or larger deletions on 9p.[55]

Gene-expression profiling with DNA microarrays allows nearly all T-cell cases to be grouped according to multistep oncogenic pathways.[61] Gene-expression studies also show that overexpression of FLT3, a receptor tyrosine kinase important for development of hematopoietic stem cells, is a secondary event in almost all cases with either MLL rearrangements or hyperdiploidy.[62] The finding has provided an impetus for clinical testing of FLT3 inhibitors in ALL. Other genome-wide interrogations of both leukemia cells and germline tissues have identified other genetic variations with prognostic or therapeutic relevance and may lead to the development of specific treatment.[17,36]

Epigenetic changes, including hypermethylation and silencing of tumor-suppressor genes and hypomethylation of oncogenes and abnormalities in posttranscriptional control mechanisms, such as those involving microRNA, are common findings in cancer. These changes are reversible and do not alter the DNA sequence, yet they can alter gene expression in subtle ways that encourage malignant transformation and progression. The analysis of epigenetic alterations has begun to apply to the development of new biomarkers for risk assignment or disease monitoring, and to the design of alternative treatment in ALL.[63] Evidence indicates that the methylation of multiple genes in ALL is associated with a worse outcome. Surprisingly, methylation of genes was as prominent in childhood as in adult ALL. The differences in the response of children and adults appear not to be related to quantitative methylation but to the specific genes and the specific pathways deactivated. Preliminary studies of hypomethylating agents (e.g., azacitidine and decitabine) are being tested in patients refractory or resistant to current drug programs.[64]

CLINICAL FEATURES

SIGNS AND SYMPTOMS

The clinical presentation of ALL is highly variable. Symptoms may appear insidiously or acutely. The presenting features generally reflect the degree of marrow failure and the extent of extramedullary spread (Table 91–2).[18,65–67] Approximately half of patients present with fever, which can be caused by either neutropenia-induced infection or leukemia-released cytokines (e.g., interleukin-1, interleukin-6, and tumor necrosis factor) released from leukemia cells. In these patients, fever resolves within 72 hours after the start of antileukemia therapy.

TABLE 91–2. Presenting Clinical Features in Children and Adults with Acute Lymphoblastic Leukemia

Feature	Children (%)	Adult (%)
Age (years)		
<1	2	—
1–9	72–78	—
10–19	20–26	—
20–39	—	40
40–59	—	40
≥60	—	20
Male	56–57	62
Symptoms		
Fever	57	33–56
Fatigue	50	Common
Bleeding	43	33
Bone or joint pain	25	25
Lymphadenopathy		
None	30	51
Marked (>3 cm)	15	11
Hepatomegaly		
None	34	65
Marked (below umbilicus)	17	Rare
Splenomegaly		
None	41	56
Marked (below umbilicus)	17	Uncommon
Mediastinal mass	8–10	15
CNS leukemia	3	8
Testicular leukemia	1	0.3

Data from Pui CH: *Acute lymphoblastic leukemia, in Childhood Leukemias,* 2nd ed, edited by CH Pui, p 439. Cambridge University Press, New York, 2006 and Larson RA, Dodge RK, Burns CP, et al: A five-drug remission induction regimen with intensive consolidation for adults with acute lymphoblastic leukemia: Cancer and Leukemia Group B study 8811. *Blood* 85:2025, 1995.

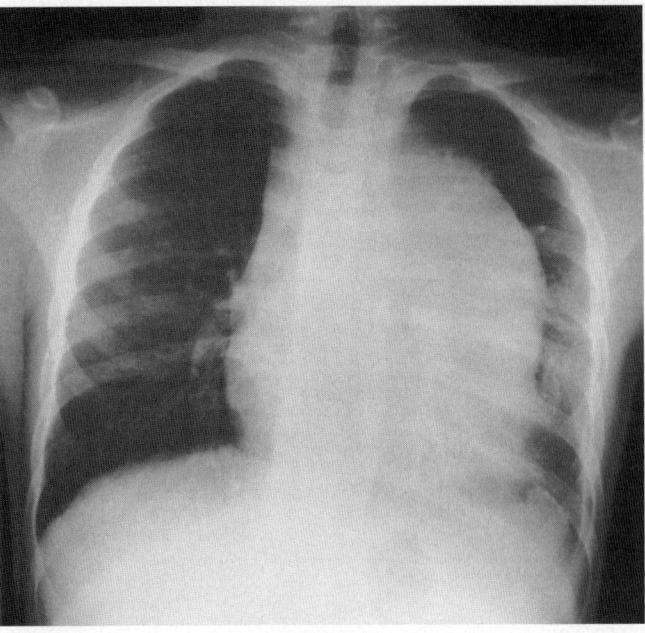

Figure 91–3. Chest radiograph of a 12-year-old black male with T-cell acute lymphoblastic leukemia (ALL) and an anterior mediastinal mass.

PHYSICAL FINDINGS

Among frequent findings are pallor, petechiae, and ecchymosis in the skin and mucous membranes, and bone tenderness as a result of leukemic infiltration or hemorrhage that stretches the periosteum. Liver, spleen, and lymph nodes are the most common sites of extramedullary involvement, and the degree of organomegaly is more pronounced in children than in adults. An anterior mediastinal (thymic) mass is present in 8 to 10 percent of childhood cases and in 15 percent of adult cases (Fig. 91–3). A bulky, anterior mediastinal mass can compress the great vessels and trachea and possibly lead to the superior vena cava syndrome. Patients with this syndrome present with cough, dyspnea, orthopnea, stridor, cyanosis, dysphagia, facial edema, increased intracranial pressure, and sometimes syncope. Painless enlargement of the scrotum can be a sign of testicular leukemia cell infiltration or hydrocele, the latter resulting from lymphatic obstruction. Both conditions can be readily diagnosed by ultrasonography. Overt testicular disease is relatively rare, is generally seen in infants or adolescents with T-cell leukemia and/or hyperleukocytosis, and does not require radiation therapy.[71] Other uncommon presenting features include ocular involvement (leukemic infiltration of the orbit, optic nerve, retina, iris, cornea, or conjunctiva), subcutaneous nodules (leukemia cutis), enlarged salivary glands (Mikulicz syndrome), cranial nerve palsy, and priapism (resulting from leukostasis of the corpora cavernosa and dorsal veins or sacral nerve involvement). Epidural spinal cord compression at presentation is a rare but serious finding that requires immediate treatment to prevent permanent paraparesis or paraplegia. In some pediatric patients, infiltration of tonsils, adenoids, appendix, or mesenteric lymph nodes leads to surgical intervention before leukemia is diagnosed.

● LABORATORY FEATURES

Anemia, neutropenia, and thrombocytopenia are common in patients with newly diagnosed ALL. The severity reflects the degree of marrow replacement by leukemic lymphoblasts (Table 91–3).[18,65–67] Presenting leukocyte counts range widely, from 0.1 to 1500 × 10⁹/L (median:

Fatigue and lethargy are common manifestations of anemia in patients with ALL. In older patients, anemia-related dyspnea and lightheadedness may be the dominant presenting features. More than 25 percent of patients, especially young children, may have a limp from bone pain or arthralgia, or an unwillingness to walk because of leukemic infiltration of the periosteum, bone, or joint or because of expansion of the marrow cavity by leukemia cells. Children with prominent bone pain often have nearly normal blood counts, which can contribute to delayed diagnosis. In a small proportion of patients, marrow necrosis can result in severe bone pain and tenderness, fever, and a very high level of serum lactate dehydrogenase.[68,69] Arthralgia and bone pain are less severe in adults. Less common signs and symptoms include headache, vomiting, altered mental function, oliguria, and anuria. Occasionally, patients present with a life-threatening infection or bleeding (e.g., intracranial hematoma). Intracranial hemorrhage occurs mainly in patients with an initial leukocyte count greater than 400 × 10⁹/L.[70] Very rarely, ALL produces no signs or symptoms and is detected during routine examination.

TABLE 91–3. Presenting Laboratory Features in Children and Adults with Acute Lymphoblastic Leukemia

Feature	Percent of Total	
	Children, White/ Black (%)	Adults (%)
Cell lineage		
T cell	15/24	25
B-cell precursor	85/76	75
Leukocyte count (× 10⁹/L)		
<10	47–49/34	41
10–49	28–31/29	31
50–99	8–12/14	12
>100	11–13/23	16
Hemoglobin concentration (g/dL)		
<8	48/58	28
8–10	24/22	26
>10	28/20	46
Platelet count (× 10⁹/L)		
<50	46/40	52
50–100	23/20	22
>100	31/40	26
CNS status*		
CNS1	67–79/60	92–95
CNS2	5–24/27	?
CNS3	3/3	5–8
Traumatic lumbar puncture with blasts	6–7/10	?
Leukemic blasts in marrow (%)		
<90	33/46	29
>90	67/54	71
Leukemic blasts in blood		
Present	87/90	92
Absent	13/10	8

*CNS1, no blast cells in cerebrospinal fluid sample; CNS2, <5 leukocytes/µL with blast cells in a nontraumatic sample; CNS3, ≥5 leukocytes/µL with blast cells in a nontraumatic sample or the presence of a cranial nerve palsy; and traumatic lumbar puncture with blasts (≥10 erythrocytes/µL with blasts). Data on CNS2 and traumatic lumbar puncture with blasts are not available in adults.

Data from Pui CH: *Acute lymphoblastic leukemia, in Childhood Leukemias*, 2nd ed, edited by CH Pui, p 439. Cambridge University Press, New York, 2006 and Larson RA, Dodge RK, Burns CP, et al: A five-drug remission induction regimen with intensive consolidation for adults with acute lymphoblastic leukemia: Cancer and Leukemia Group B study 8811. *Blood* 85:2025, 1995.

10–12 × 10⁹/L). Hyperleukocytosis (>100 × 10⁹ white cells/L) occurs in 11 to 13 percent of white children, but occurs more often in black children (23 percent) and in adults (16 percent) because they are more likely to have T-cell ALL. Profound neutropenia (<0.5 × 10⁹/L) is found in 20 to 40 percent of patients, elevating their risk for infection. Approximately 90 percent of patients have circulating leukemic blast cells at diagnosis. Hypereosinophilia, generally reactive, may precede the diagnosis of ALL by several months. Some patients, mostly male, have ALL with the t(5;14)(q31;q32) chromosomal abnormality and a hypereosinophilic syndrome (pulmonary infiltration, cardiomegaly, and congestive heart failure). These patients often do not have circulating leukemic blasts or other cytopenias and have a relatively low percentage of blasts in the marrow.[72] Activation of the interleukin-3 gene on chromosome

5 by the enhancer element of the immunoglobulin heavy-chain gene on chromosome 14 is thought to contribute to leukemogenesis and the associated eosinophilia in these cases.[72] In patients with anemia, hemoglobin levels are lower in younger children. Occasionally, a child with ALL has a hemoglobin level as low as 1 g/dL.

Decreased platelet counts are common at diagnosis (median: 48–52 × 10⁹/L). Severe bleeding is uncommon, even when platelet counts are as low as 20 × 10⁹/L, provided infection and fever are absent.[73,74] Occasional patients, principally male, present with thrombocytosis (>400 × 10⁹/L). Pancytopenia followed by a period of spontaneous hematopoietic recovery may precede the diagnosis of ALL in rare cases.[75] Coagulopathy, usually mild, can be seen in 3 to 5 percent of patients, most of whom have T-cell ALL, and is only rarely associated with clinical bleeding.[76] The level of serum lactate dehydrogenase is increased in most patients with ALL and is well correlated with tumor burden. Increased levels of serum uric acid are common in patients with a large leukemia cell burden, reflecting an increased rate of purine catabolism. Leukemic infiltration of the kidneys can lead to increased levels of creatinine, urea nitrogen, uric acid, and phosphorus. Rarely, patients present with hypercalcemia resulting from release of parathyroid hormone-like protein from lymphoblasts and leukemic infiltration of bone. The t(17;19)(q22;p13.3) with *E2A-HLF* fusion, found in 0.5 percent of B-cell precursor ALL, is associated with adolescent age group, disseminated coagulopathy, hypercalcemia, and dismal prognosis.[77] Liver dysfunction as a result of leukemic infiltration occurs in 10 to 20 percent of patients and is usually mild. However, recognition of carriers of hepatitis B virus is important because prompt lamivudine therapy can prevent serious complications from virus reactivation during immunosuppressive treatment.[78]

Chest radiography is needed to detect enlargement of the thymus or mediastinal nodes and pleural effusions (see Fig. 91–3). Although bony abnormalities, such as metaphyseal banding, periosteal reactions, osteolysis, osteosclerosis, and osteopenia, can be found in 50 percent of patients, especially children with low leukocyte counts at presentation, skeletal films are not necessary for management. Magnetic resonance imaging (MRI) is useful in patients with suspected vertebral collapse or meningeal or nerve root involvement.

Examination of the cerebrospinal fluid (CSF) is an essential diagnostic procedure. Leukemic blasts can be identified in as many as one-third of pediatric patients and approximately 5 percent of adult patients at diagnosis of ALL; most of these patients lack neurologic symptoms.[79,80] Traditionally, CNS leukemia is defined by the presence of at least 5 leukocytes/µL of CSF (with leukemic blast cells apparent in a cytocentrifuged sample) or by the presence of cranial nerve palsies. However, with the omission of prophylactic cranial irradiation in contemporary clinical trials, the presence of any leukemic blast cells in the CSF is associated with increased risk of CNS relapse and is an indication to intensify intrathecal therapy.[80] Different opinions exist regarding when the first lumbar puncture should be performed. Most protocols now require the procedure at diagnosis and instill the first dose of chemotherapeutic agents intrathecally. Contamination of the CSF by leukemia cells as a result of traumatic lumbar puncture at diagnosis is associated with an inferior treatment outcome in children with ALL.[81] The risk of traumatic lumbar puncture can be decreased by administering platelet transfusions to thrombocytopenic patients and by having the most experienced clinician perform the procedure.

DIAGNOSIS AND CELL CLASSIFICATION

Examination of a marrow aspirate is recommended for diagnosis of ALL because as many as 10 percent of patients lack circulating blasts at the time of diagnosis and because high concentrations of marrow cells are better than blood cells for genetic studies. Fibrosis or tightly packed marrow can lead to difficulties with marrow aspiration that necessitate biopsy. In patients with marrow necrosis, multiple marrow aspirations are sometimes needed to obtain diagnostic tissue.

Morphologic and Cytochemical Analysis

Diagnosis of ALL begins with morphologic analysis of Romanowsky-stained (Wright-Giemsa or May-Grünwald-Giemsa) marrow films. Lymphoblasts tend to be relatively small (ranging from the same size to twice the size of small lymphocytes) with scanty, often light-blue cytoplasm; a round or slightly indented nucleus; fine to slightly coarse and clumped chromatin; and inconspicuous nucleoli (Fig. 91–4A). In some cases, the lymphoblasts are large, with prominent nucleoli, moderate amounts of cytoplasm, admixed with smaller blasts (Fig. 91–4B). Cytoplasmic granules are found in the lymphoblasts of some patients with ALL (Fig. 91–4C). The granules usually are amphophilic (and stain fuchsia), readily distinguishable from primary myeloid granules (which stain deep purple), and demonstrated to be mitochondria by electron microscopy. B-cell blasts in Burkitt-type ALL are characterized by intensely basophilic cytoplasm, prominent nucleoli, and cytoplasmic vacuolation (Fig. 91–4D).

Cytochemical stains (Sudan black stain and the stains for myeloperoxidase and the nonspecific esterases) distinguish ALL from acute myeloid leukemia but are now less commonly used for diagnosis than immunophenotyping.

Immunologic Classification

Immunophenotyping is an essential part of the diagnostic evaluation. Antibodies distinguish clusters of differentiation (CD) groups, but most leukocyte antigens lack specificity. Hence, a panel of antibodies is needed to establish the diagnosis and to distinguish among the different immunologic subclasses of leukemic cells. Typical panels include antibodies to at least one highly sensitive marker (CD19 for B-cell lineage, CD7 for T-cell lineage, and CD13 or CD33 for myeloid cells) and antibodies to a highly specific marker (cytoplasmic CD79a and CD22 for B-cell lineage, cytoplasmic CD3 for T-cell lineage, and cytoplasmic myeloperoxidase for myeloid cells).[17] Although ALL can be further subclassified according to the recognized steps of normal maturation within the B-cell lineage (pro-B, early pre-B, pre-B, transitional pre-B, and mature B cells) or T-cell lineage (pre-T, mid-, and late thymocyte) pathways, the only distinctions of therapeutic importance at present are those between T-cell, mature B, and other B-cell lineage (B-cell precursor type) immunophenotypes (Table 91–4).[17] A distinct subset of T-cell

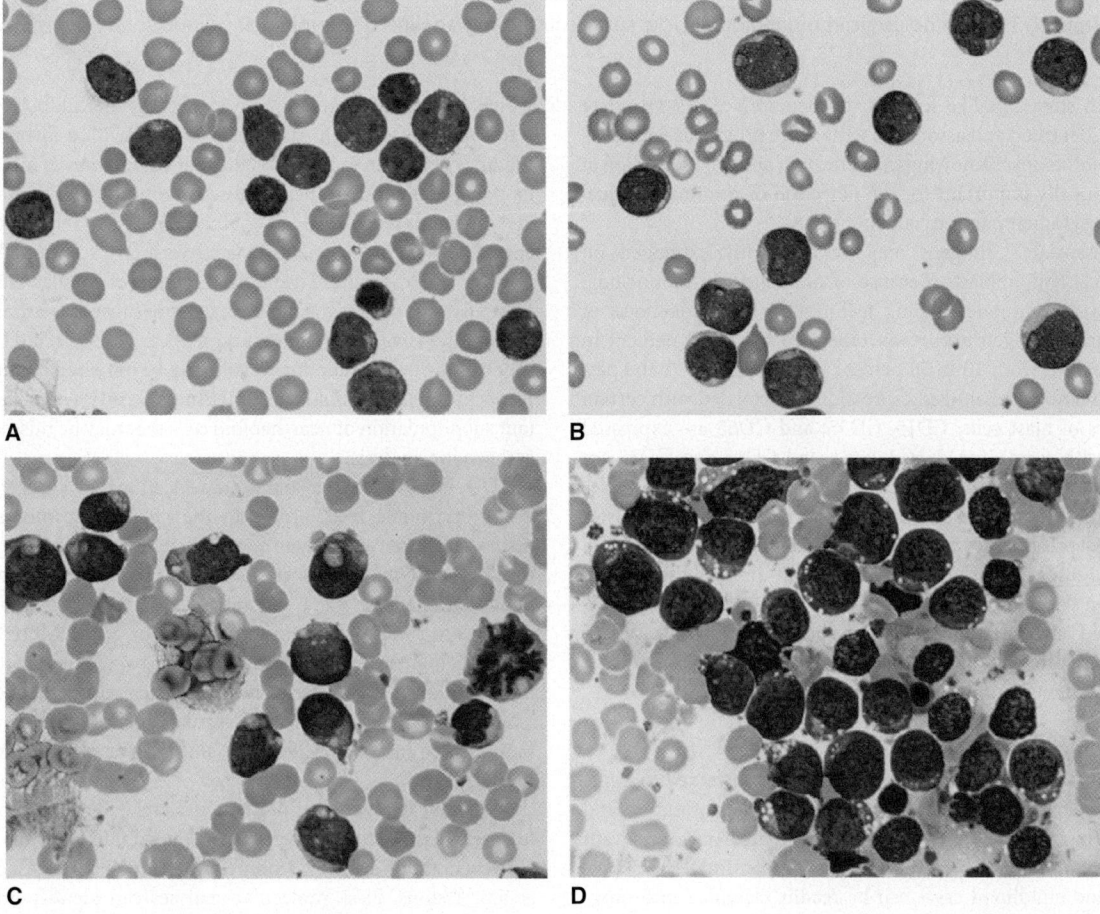

A   B

C   D

Figure 91–4. A. Typical lymphoblasts with scanty cytoplasm, regular nuclear shape, fine chromatin, and indistinct nucleoli. **B.** Acute lymphoblastic leukemia (ALL) with large blasts showing prominent nucleoli, moderate amounts of cytoplasm, and an admixture of smaller blasts. **C.** ALL with cytoplasmic granules. Fuchsia granules are present in the cytoplasm of many blasts. Such granules may lead to a misdiagnosis of acute myeloid leukemia; however, the granules are negative for myeloperoxidase and myeloid-pattern Sudan black B staining. **D.** B-cell ALL lymphoblasts. The blasts in this phenotype are characterized by intensely basophilic cytoplasm, regular cellular features, and cytoplasmic vacuolation. (Images **A** to **D,** Wright-Giemsa stain; original magnification ×1000.)

TABLE 91–4. Presenting Features of Acute Lymphoblastic Leukemia According to Immunologic Subtype

Subtype	Typical Markers	Childhood (%)	Adult (%)	Associated Features
B-cell precursor	CD19+, CD22+, CD79a+, cIg+/–, sIgμ–, HLA-DR+			
Pro-B	CD10–	5	11	Infants and adult age group, high leukocyte count, initial CNS leukemia, pseudodiploidy, *MLL* rearrangement, unfavorable prognosis
Early pre-B	CD10+	63	52	Favorable age group (1–9 years), low leukocyte count, hyperdiploidy (>50 chromosomes)
Pre-B	CD10+/–, cIg+	16	9	High leukocyte count, black race, pseudodiploidy
Mature B cell (Burkitt)	CD19+, CD22+, CD79a+, cIg+, sIg+ (kappa or lambda+)	3	4	Male predominance, initial CNS leukemia, abdominal masses, often renal involvement
T lineage	CD7+, cCD3+			
T cell	CD2+, CD1+/–, CD4+/–, CD8+/–, HLA-DR–, TdT+/–	10	18	Male predominance, hyperleukocytosis, extramedullary disease
Pre-T	CD2–, CD1–, CD4–, CD8–, HLA-DR+/–, TdT+	1	6	Male predominance, hyperleukocytosis, extramedullary disease, unfavorable prognosis
Early T-cell precursor	CD1–, CD8–, CD5[weak], CD13+, CD33+, CD11b+, CD117+, CD65+, HLA-DR+	2	?	Male predominance, age >10 years, poor prognosis

cCD3, cytoplasmic CD3; cIg, cytoplasmic immunoglobulin; sIg, surface immunoglobulin; TdT, terminal deoxynucleotidyl transferase.

ALL that retain stem cell–like features, termed *early T-cell precursor ALL*, has been identified and associated with a dire prognosis with conventional chemotherapy.[82] Knowing the pattern of antigen expression at diagnosis is critically important for the detection of minimal residual disease by flow cytometry after treatment.[83]

Myeloid-associated antigens may be aberrantly expressed on otherwise typical lymphoblasts. Because of differences in monoclonal antibodies and immunophenotyping techniques, the frequencies of myeloid-associated antigen expression range from 5 to 30 percent in childhood cases and from 10 to 50 percent in adult cases.[67,84] The pattern of myeloid-associated antigen expression is correlated with certain genetic features of blast cells. CD15, CD33, and CD65 are expressed in ALL cases with a rearranged *MLL* gene, and CD13 and CD33 are expressed in cases with the *ETV6-RUNX1*.[84] There is a subset of cases that coexpress both lymphoid and myeloid markers but do not cluster with T-cell, B-cell precursor, or acute myeloid leukemia in gene-expression profiling. These cases may not respond to myeloid-directed therapy but attain remission with ALL-directed induction treatment.[85,86] The presence of myeloid-associated antigens lacks prognostic significance in contemporary treatment programs but can be useful in immunologic monitoring of patients for minimal residual leukemia.[67,83]

Genetic Classification

ALL arises from a lymphoid progenitor cell that has sustained multiple specific genetic alterations that lead to malignant transformation and proliferation. Thus, genetic classification of ALL yields more relevant biologic information than any other means. Approximately 75 percent of adult and childhood cases can be readily classified into prognostically or therapeutically relevant subgroups based on the modal chromosome number (or DNA content estimated by flow cytometry), specific chromosomal rearrangements, and molecular genetic changes.[1,2,17–20,41,54–56,87–89] Table 91–5 summarizes the prominent clinical and biologic features of cases with the most common genetic abnormalities.

Two ploidy groups (hyperdiploidy >50 chromosomes and hypodiploidy <44 chromosomes) have clinical relevance. Hyperdiploidy, which is seen in approximately 25 percent of childhood cases and in 6 to 7 percent of adult cases, is associated with a favorable prognosis that may reflect an increased cellular accumulation of methotrexate and its polyglutamates, an increased sensitivity to therapeutic antimetabolites, and a marked propensity of these cells to undergo apoptosis.[90,91] By contrast, hypodiploidy is associated with an exceptionally poor prognosis.[88,89,92] Flow cytometric determination of cellular DNA content is a useful adjunct to cytogenetic analysis because it is automated, rapid, and inexpensive, and its measurements are not affected by the mitotic index of the cell population; results can be obtained in almost all cases. Flow cytometric studies can sometimes identify a small but drug-resistant subpopulation of near-haploid cells that may be missed by standard cytogenetic analysis.

Reciprocal chromosomal translocations in cases of B-cell and T-cell ALL arise from errors in the normal recombination mechanisms that generate antigen receptor genes. Such rearrangements can fuse the promoter/enhancer element of the immunoglobulin heavy- or light-chain gene or the T-cell antigen receptor β/γ or α/δ gene to sites adjacent to a variety of transcription factor genes. More often, genetic rearrangements result from the fusion of two genes encoding different transcription factors. These chimeric genes encode active kinases and altered transcription factors that regulate genes involved in the differentiation, self-renewal, proliferation, and drug resistance of hematopoietic stem cells.

Specific cytogenetic findings are correlated with presenting clinical features, blast-cell phenotypes, and clinical outcome (see Table 91–5). However, there are now compelling reasons to focus on molecular genetic lesions. First, molecular analyses can identify important submicroscopic genetic alterations not visible by standard karyotyping, such as the *ETV6-RUNX1* fusion, intrachromosomal amplification of chromosome 21, deletions of tumor-suppressor genes, and mutations of protooncogenes.[1,2,87,93–95] Second, cases with clinically important genetic rearrangements can be missed because of technical errors (e.g., karyotyping residual normal metaphase cells rather than leukemic metaphase cells). Hence, FISH and reverse transcriptase polymerase chain reaction

TABLE 91-5. Clinical and Biologic Features Associated with the Most Common Genetic Subtypes of Acute Lymphoblastic Leukemia

Subtype	Associated Features	Estimated Event-Free Survival (%)	
		Children	Adults
Hyperdiploidy (>50 chromosomes)	Predominant precursor B-cell phenotype; low leukocyte count; favorable age group (1–9 years) and prognosis in children	80–90 at 5 years	30–50 at 5 years
Hypodiploidy (<45 chromosomes)	Predominant precursor B-cell phenotype; increased leukocyte count; poor prognosis	30–40 at 3 years	10–20 at 3 years
t(12;21)(p13;q22) [ETV6-RUNX1]	CD13+/–CD33+/– precursor B-cell phenotype; pseudodiploidy; age 1–9 years; favorable prognosis	90–95 at 5 years	Unknown
t(1;19)(q23;p13.3) [TCF3-PBX1]	CD10+/–CD20–CD34– pre-B phenotype; pseudodiploidy; increased leukocyte count; black race; CNS leukemia; prognosis depends on treatment	82–90 at 5 years	20–40 at 3 years
t(9;22)(q34;q11.2) [BCR-ABL1]	Predominant precursor B-cell phenotype; older age; increased leukocyte count; myeloid antigens; improved early outcome with tyrosine kinase inhibitor treatment	80–90 at 3 years	~60 at 1 year
t(4;11)(q21;23) with MLL-AF4 fusion	CD10+/–CD15+/–CD33+/–CD65+/– precursor B-cell phenotype; infant and older adult age groups; hyperleukocytosis; CNS leukemia; poor outcome	32–40 at 5 years	10–20 at 3 years
t(8;14)(q24;q32.3)	Mature B-cell phenotype; L3 morphology; male predominance; bulky extramedullary disease; favorable prognosis with short-term intensive chemotherapy including high-dose methotrexate, cytarabine, and cyclophosphamide/ifosfamide	75–85 at 5 years	70–80 at 4 years
NOTCH 1 mutations	T-cell phenotype; favorable prognosis	90 at 5 years	50 at 4 years
HOX11 overexpression	CD10+ T-cell phenotype; favorable prognosis with chemotherapy alone	90 at 5 years	80 at 3 years
Intrachromosomal amplification of chromosome 21	Precursor B-cell phenotype; low white blood cell count; intensified treatment required to avert a poor prognosis	30 at 5 years	?

Data from Pui CH, Robison LL, Look AT: Acute lymphoblastic leukemia. *Lancet* 371:1030, 2008; Schultz KR, Bowman WP, Aledo A, et al: Improved early event free survival with imatinib in Philadelphia chromosome-positive acute lymphoblastic leukemia: A Children's Oncology Group Study. *J Clin Oncol* 27:5715, 2009; Larson RA, Dodge RK, Burns CP, et al: A five-drug remission induction regimen with intensive consolidation for adults with acute lymphoblastic leukemia: Cancer and Leukemia Group B study 8811. *Blood* 85:2025, 1995; Rizzieri DA, Johnson JL, Byrd JC, et al; Alliance for Clinical Trials In Oncology (ACTION). Improved efficacy using rituximab and brief duration, high intensity chemotherapy with filgrastim support for Burkitt or aggressive lymphomas: Cancer and Leukemia Group B study 10002. *Br J Haematol* 165(1):102-111, 2014.

(RT-PCR) assays are increasingly used. The application of microarray-based genome-wide analysis of gene expression and DNA copy number, complemented by transcriptional profiling, resequencing and epigenetic approaches, and next-generation sequencing have identified specific genetic alterations with biologic and therapeutic implications.

● DIFFERENTIAL DIAGNOSIS

The initial manifestations of ALL can mimic a variety of disorders. The acute onset of petechiae, ecchymoses, and bleeding can suggest idiopathic thrombocytopenic purpura. The latter disorder often is associated with a recent viral infection, large platelets in blood films, normal hemoglobin concentration, and absence of leukocyte abnormalities in blood or marrow. Patients with ALL, or promyelocytic leukemia, or aplastic anemia can present with pancytopenia and complications associated with marrow failure. However, in aplastic anemia, hepatosplenomegaly and lymphadenopathy are rare, and the skeletal pain associated with ALL is absent. The results of marrow aspiration or biopsy usually distinguish between these diseases, although the diagnosis can be difficult in a patient who has hypocellular marrow that is later replaced by lymphoblasts. In one study, transient pancytopenia preceded ALL in 2 percent of all pediatric cases.[75] During the preleukemic phase in these patients,

polymerase chain reaction (PCR) analysis demonstrated monoclonality, suggesting inhibition of normal hematopoiesis by leukemia cells.[96] ALL should be considered in the differential diagnosis of patients with hypereosinophilia, which can be a presenting feature of leukemia or can precede its diagnosis by several months. Occasionally, hematogones in a regenerative marrow may mimic leukemic blast cells; flow cytometry with optimal combinations of antibodies may be required to distinguish them.[97]

Infectious mononucleosis and other viral infections, especially those associated with thrombocytopenia or hemolytic anemia, can be confused with leukemia. Detection of reactive lymphocytes or serologic evidence of Epstein-Barr virus infection helps establish the diagnosis. Patients with acute infectious lymphocytosis, pertussis, or parapertussis can have marked lymphocytosis. However, even when leukocyte counts are as high as 50×10^9/L, the affected cells are mature lymphocytes rather than lymphoblasts. Bone pain, arthralgia, and occasionally arthritis mimic juvenile rheumatoid arthritis, rheumatic fever, other collagen diseases, or osteomyelitis. The marrow should be examined if glucocorticoid treatment is planned for presumed rheumatoid diseases.

In children, ALL should be distinguished from small, round cell tumors involving the marrow, including neuroblastoma, rhabdomyosarcoma, and retinoblastoma. Generally, in patients with solid tumors, a primary lesion will be found by standard diagnostic studies. Disseminated tumor cells often present in characteristic aggregates, and immunophenotypic characteristics of lymphoblasts are absent.

●THERAPY

SUPPORTIVE CARE

Optimal management of patients with ALL requires careful attention to supportive care, including immediate treatment or prevention of metabolic and infectious complications (Chap. 24) and rational use of blood products (Chaps. 138 and 139). Other important supportive care measures, such as use of indwelling catheters, amelioration of nausea and vomiting, pain control, and continuous psychosocial support for the patient and family, are essential.

Metabolic Complications

Hyperuricemia and hyperphosphatemia with secondary hypocalcemia are frequently encountered at diagnosis, even before chemotherapy is initiated, especially in patients with B-cell or T-cell ALL or precursor B-cell leukemia with high leukemic cell burden.[98] Patients should be given intravenous fluids; allopurinol or rasburicase (recombinant urate oxidase) to treat hyperuricemia; and a phosphate binder, such as aluminum hydroxide, calcium carbonate (if the serum calcium concentration is low), lanthanum carbonate, or sevelamer to treat hyperphosphatemia. Allopurinol, a relatively inexpensive drug, is usually used if the uric acid is less than 7 mg/dL. Allergic skin reactions occur in approximately 10 percent, and allopurinol should be stopped as soon as the risk of hyperuricemia from the destruction of a large leukemic cell burden has passed. By inhibiting *de novo* purine synthesis in leukemic blast cells, allopurinol can reduce the peripheral blast-cell count before chemotherapy.[99] Allopurinol can decrease both the anabolism and catabolism of mercaptopurine by depleting intracellular phosphoribosyl pyrophosphate and by inhibiting xanthine oxidase. If mercaptopurine and allopurinol are given together orally, the dosage of mercaptopurine must be reduced.

Rasburicase works very rapidly and is extremely effective, especially for very elevated uric acid levels (>7 mg/dL), often with one infusion (a far smaller dose than the manufacturer recommends). Rasburicase breaks down uric acid to allantoin, a readily excreted metabolite that is five to 10 times more soluble than uric acid. Rasburicase is more effective than allopurinol, and it facilitates phosphorus excretion, partly because of rasburicase's potent uricolytic effect (which obviates the need to alkalinize urine) and partly because of improved renal function with its use.[100] However, rasburicase is contraindicated in patients with glucose-6-dehydrogenase deficiency because hydrogen peroxide, a by-product of uric acid breakdown, can cause methemoglobinemia or hemolytic anemia.

Hyperleukocytosis

For patients with extreme leukocytosis (leukocyte count >400 × 10⁹/L), either leukapheresis or exchange transfusion (in small children) can be used to reduce the burden of leukemic cells. In theory, either treatment should reduce the complications associated with leukostasis, but the short- and long-term benefits of the procedures are questionable.[70] Emergency cranial irradiation, once advocated by some leukemia therapists, probably has no role in the treatment of these patients. Preinduction therapy with low-dose glucocorticoids, with addition of vincristine and cyclophosphamide in cases of B-cell ALL, is a favored means of ameliorating hyperleukocytosis. This method, when used in conjunction with urate oxidase, has largely eliminated tumor lysis syndrome and the need for hemodialysis in patients with mature B-cell ALL.

Infection Control

Infections are common in febrile patients with newly diagnosed ALL. Therefore, any patient presenting with fever, especially a patient with neutropenia, should be given broad-spectrum antibiotics until infection is excluded. Remission induction therapy can increase susceptibility to infection by exacerbating myelosuppression, immunosuppression, and mucosal breakdown. At least 50 percent of patients undergoing induction therapy experience infections. Special precautions should be taken to reduce the risk of infection during this critical phase of treatment, including protective contact isolation and air filtration; elimination of contact with people with infections; refraining from eating certain food products, such as raw cheese, uncooked vegetables, or unpeeled fruits; and use of antiseptic mouthwash or sitz baths, especially for patients with mucositis. Good hand washing practices and the use of alcohol-based cleansers are important. Administration of granulocyte colony-stimulating factor can hasten recovery from neutropenia and reduce the complications of intensive chemotherapy, but does not improve the EFS rate for children or adults.[101,102] One study suggested growth factor increased the risk of therapy-related acute myeloid leukemia in the context of epipodophyllotoxin-based therapy.[103] Intensified remission induction regimens, especially in combination with high-dose glucocorticoids, have resulted in an increased risk of disseminated fungal infection and death. Antifungal prophylaxis is commonly given.

All nonallergic patients with ALL are given trimethoprim-sulfamethoxazole, 2 to 3 days per week, as prophylactic therapy for *Pneumocystis carinii (Pneumocystis jiroveci)* pneumonia. Prophylaxis is started after 2 weeks of remission induction and continues for several months after completion of all chemotherapy. Alternative treatments for patients who cannot tolerate trimethoprim-sulfamethoxazole include aerosolized pentamidine, dapsone, and atovaquone.[104] Live-virus vaccines should not be administered during immunosuppressive therapy. Siblings and other children who have frequent contact with patients can receive routine immunizations, including inactivated poliomyelitis vaccine. Susceptible patients exposed to varicella virus should receive zoster immunoglobulin within 96 hours of exposure together with acyclovir. Such treatment usually prevents or mitigates the clinical manifestations of varicella.

Hematologic Support

ALL and its treatment leads to pancytopenia. Hemorrhagic manifestations are common but usually are limited to the skin and mucous membranes. Although rare, bleeding in the CNS, lungs, or gastrointestinal tract can be life-threatening. Patients with extremely high leukocyte counts (>400 × 10⁹/L) at diagnosis are more likely to develop such complications.[70] Coagulopathy attributable to disseminated intravascular coagulation, hepatic dysfunction, or chemotherapy is usually mild.[76] Patients receiving L-asparaginase and a glucocorticoid have a hypercoagulable state. Platelet transfusions should be given therapeutically for overt bleeding and may be used prophylactically when platelet counts are less than 10 × 10⁹/L.[105] Anticoagulants and antiplatelet agents such as aspirin must be avoided. Children generally do not have active bleeding during remission induction therapy with prednisone, vincristine, and L-asparaginase, even when platelet counts are less than 10 × 10⁹/L. A higher threshold for prophylactic platelet transfusions should be considered for active toddlers and patients with fever or infection. Transfusion of packed leukocyte-poor red cells is indicated in patients with anemia and marrow suppression but should be delayed until the leukocyte count is reduced in patients with extreme hyperleukocytosis. Transfusions should be given slowly in patients with profound but chronic anemia to prevent development of congestive heart failure. Granulocyte transfusions are rarely needed, but should be considered for patients with absolute neutropenia and documented Gram-negative septicemia or disseminated fungal infection that is responding poorly to antimicrobial treatment alone. All blood products should be irradiated to prevent transfusion-related graft-versus-host disease.

ANTILEUKEMIC THERAPY

Because ALL is a heterogeneous disease with many distinct subtypes, there is no uniform approach to therapy. Increasingly, treatment is targeted to biologically distinct subgroups. The best results have been reported from experienced treatment centers using well-designed and rigorously applied protocols.[106–109] No consensus exists on the risk criteria and the terminology for defining prognostic subgroups. Usually, childhood ALL cases are divided into standard-risk, high- (intermediate- or average-) risk, and very-high-risk groups, although the United States' Children's Oncology Group advocates four categories, including low risk, to accommodate patients with a very low risk of relapse. Adult cases are generally divided into two risk groups. Often infant and elderly ALL are considered special subgroups of ALL that require different treatment, primarily related to intolerance. One study showed improved outcome for infant ALL, using a hybrid treatment protocol with elements to treat both ALL and acute myeloid leukemia, and reducing dose intensity in the very young infants.[110] Few studies have been performed in those older than 60 years of age and their management remains a therapeutic challenge.[111,112] Some successes have been achieved with the use of dose-reduced regimens and the addition of imatinib or dasatinib for patients with Philadelphia chromosome–positive ALL.[113,114] Because cure is not common in patients older than age 70 years, maintenance of a good quality of life is a major goal for this age group.

Mature B-Cell Acute Lymphoblastic Leukemia (Burkitt-Type)

The most effective contemporary treatment regimens for mature B-cell (Burkitt-type) ALL are drug combinations that include cyclophosphamide and/or ifosfamide given over a relatively short time (3 to 6 months). The first major breakthrough in this disease was reported by French investigators, who achieved a 68 percent EFS rate in their LMB84 study featuring high-dose cyclophosphamide, high-dose methotrexate, vincristine, doxorubicin, and conventional doses of cytarabine. In the LMB89 study, the same group reported a cure rate of 87 percent, which was achieved by using increased doses of methotrexate (to 8 g/m² per dose) and cytarabine (3 g/m² per dose) and by adding etoposide for patients with a large leukemia cell burden.[115] This excellent result has been confirmed in a randomized international study.[116] Successful treatments also have been developed by the Berlin-Frankfurt-Münster consortium, which uses a multiagent regimen that incorporates cyclophosphamide, high-dose methotrexate (1 g/m² per dose), etoposide, ifosfamide, doxorubicin, dexamethasone, and cytarabine (3 g/m² per dose).[117] These intensive pediatric protocols have been translated into adult treatment regimens that are completed in as little as 18 weeks.[118–120] Because of its demonstrated efficacy in B-cell lymphoma, rituximab (anti-CD20) has been incorporated in frontline clinical trials for adults with B-cell ALL.[118,120] Maintenance or continuation therapy is not needed. The remission rate is very high, and most remissions are durable. B-cell ALL rarely, if ever, reoccur after the first year.

Effective CNS therapy is an essential component of successful regimens for B-cell ALL and generally consists of methotrexate and cytarabine administered both systematically and intrathecally. Cranial irradiation does not appear to be necessary even for patients presenting with CNS leukemia.[116,120]

Precursor B-Cell and T-Cell Acute Lymphoblastic Leukemia

Treatment for leukemias affecting the precursor B-cell and T-cell lineages consists of three standard phases: remission induction, intensification (consolidation), and prolonged continuation (maintenance)

therapy.[121] CNS-directed therapy, which overlaps other treatments, is started early and is given for different lengths of time, depending on the patient's risk of relapse and the intensity of the primary systemic regimen.

Remission Induction The first goal of therapy is inducing a complete remission and restoring normal hematopoiesis. The induction regimen typically includes a glucocorticoid (prednisone, prednisolone, or dexamethasone), vincristine, and L-asparaginase for children or an anthracycline for adults.[17,67,106–108] Children with high- or very-high-risk ALL, and nearly all young adults with ALL, receive four or more drugs (daunorubicin, vincristine, glucocorticoid, and L-asparaginase) during remission induction in contemporary clinical trials. Improvements in chemotherapy and supportive care have resulted in complete remission rates of approximately 98 percent for children and 85 to 90 percent for adults. When a complete clinical remission is induced, patients have various degrees of residual leukemia.[122] Because the extent of residual disease is well correlated with long-term outcome,[83,123–129] the concept of a "molecular" or "immunologic" remission, defined as leukemia less than 0.01 percent of nucleated marrow cells,[122] is beginning to supplant the traditional perception of remission, which is based solely on microscopic criteria.[129] Prospective trials are needed to demonstrate that outcomes will improve when interventions to change therapy are based on measurements of residual disease.

Attempts have been made to intensify induction therapy based on the premise that more rapid and complete reduction of the leukemia cell burden forestalls the development of drug resistance. However, several studies have suggested intensive induction therapy is unnecessary for children with standard-risk ALL, provided patients receive postinduction intensification therapy.[107] Intensive induction can lead to increased early morbidity and mortality. More intensive induction regimens with additional cyclophosphamide, high-dose cytarabine, or high-dose anthracycline also have been tested in adults with ALL and have yielded no clear benefit, partly because of the low tolerance of adults to drug toxicity.[130,131] However, in one study, the use of high-dose dexamethasone (10 mg/m² per day) instead of prednisone (60 mg/m² per day) during remission induction significantly improved treatment outcome for children with ALL, especially those with T-cell ALL and good prednisone response, despite a higher induction death rate.[121,132] Conceivably, intensified remission induction with other relatively nonmyelosuppressive drugs can also improve treatment outcome. Dexamethasone provided better control of systemic and CNS disease than did prednisone in two randomized studies of childhood ALL.[133,134]

The pharmacodynamics of asparaginase differ by formulation and three forms are available: one derived from *Erwinia chrysanthemi*, another prepared from *Escherichia coli*, and a third made of a polyethylene glycol form of the *E. coli* product (pegaspargase).[135,136] In terms of leukemic control, the dose intensity and duration of asparaginase treatment (i.e., the amount of asparagine depletion) are far more important than the type of asparaginase used. The dosages of the three preparations are based on their half-lives. Pegaspargase, which has the longest half-life, usually is administered at 2500 IU/m² every other week for one to two doses in cases of newly diagnosed ALL. By contrast, the *Erwinia* preparation, which has the shortest half-life, is administered at 20,000 IU/m² three times per week for 6 to 12 doses. The doses of *E. coli* L-asparaginase range from 5000 to 10,000 IU/m², administered two to three times per week for 6 to 12 doses. Because of lower immunogenicity, improved efficacy, and less-frequent administration, pegaspargase has replaced the native product as the first-line treatment for children and adults in the United States, and is also increasingly used in other ALL trials around the world.[137–140] None of the various anthracyclines (daunorubicin, doxorubicin, idarubicin, and mitoxantrone) given to adults with ALL has proven superior to any other; daunorubicin is used most commonly.

Intensification (Consolidation) Therapy After normal hematopoiesis is restored, patients in remission become candidates for intensification therapy. Such treatment, administered shortly after remission induction, refers to readministration of the induction regimen or to high doses of multiple agents not used during the induction phase. Although there is no dispute on the importance of this treatment in childhood ALL, there is no consensus on the best regimen and duration of treatment. More commonly used regimens for childhood ALL include high-dose methotrexate with or without mercaptopurine, high-dose L-asparaginase given for an extended period, or a combination of dexamethasone, vincristine, L-asparaginase, and doxorubicin, followed by thioguanine, cytarabine, and cyclophosphamide.[107,108,121,137,141,142] This phase of therapy has improved outcomes, even for patients with low-risk ALL.[143] Patients with *ETV6-RUNX1* have an especially good outcome in clinical trials featuring intensive postremission treatment with glucocorticoids, vincristine, and asparaginase.[144,145] A very high dose of methotrexate (5 g/m^2) appears to improve the treatment outcome of patients with T-cell ALL.[141,146] This finding is consistent with data indicating T-cell blasts accumulate methotrexate polyglutamates (active metabolites of the parent compound) less avidly than do B-cell precursors; consequently, higher serum levels of the drug are needed for an adequate therapeutic effect.[147,148] The conventional dose of methotrexate (1 g/m^2) may be too low for many patients with B-cell precursor ALL. Among B-lineage ALL, blasts with either *ETV6-RUNX1* or *TCF3-PBX1* gene fusion accumulate significantly lower methotrexate polyglutamates compared to those with hyperdiploidy or other genetic abnormalities.[149] This finding suggested that patients with *ETV6-RUNX1* or *TCF3-PBX1* gene fusion would also benefit from a higher dose of methotrexate.

Based on pediatric studies, intensive consolidation therapy has become a standard in the treatment of adult ALL even though early studies failed to show the benefit of this phase of treatment. Various drugs have been used for intensification, including high-dose methotrexate, high-dose cytarabine, cyclophosphamide, and asparaginase.[67,102,150–153] Increasingly, intensification treatment is risk-adapted and subtype specific. In the German 06/93 study, high-dose methotrexate was used for patients with standard-risk B-cell precursor ALL, high-dose methotrexate and high-dose cytarabine for high-risk B-cell precursor ALL, and cyclophosphamide for T-cell ALL. The hyper-CVAD (cyclophosphamide, vincristine, Adriamycin, dexamethasone) regimen of the MD Anderson Cancer Center alternates the combination of cyclophosphamide, vincristine, doxorubicin (Adriamycin), and dexamethasone, with high-dose methotrexate and high-dose cytarabine for four courses each. More recently, rituximab has been added for patients with CD20 expression on lymphoblasts.[150,151] In adults, methotrexate dose should probably be limited to 1.5 to 2.0 g/m^2 because higher doses may lead to excessive toxicities, delayed subsequent treatment, and reduced compliance. In a Cancer and Leukemia Group B study, a five-drug remission induction was followed by early and late intensification courses with eight drugs.[67] These studies and others suggested the benefit of early intensive consolidation therapy, especially in young adults. In adult T-cell ALL, benefit is derived from cyclophosphamide and cytarabine.[67,102] In other adult cases of standard-risk and high-risk ALL, the benefit is derived from high-dose cytarabine. Two German multicenter trials using high-dose cytarabine, mitoxantrone, and allogeneic hematopoietic stem cell transplantation showed markedly improved results in cases bearing the t(4;11), which generally confers an adverse prognosis.[154] Several ongoing trials are testing the efficacy of asparaginase during intensification in young adult ALL[137] because this drug clearly improves outcome in childhood ALL and is better tolerated during consolidation treatment than during remission induction.

Patients diagnosed with ALL between the ages of 16 and 39, often considered together as adolescents and young adults, are commonly treated by either adult or pediatric hematologists. Several retrospective comparative analyses have reported that adolescents and young adults with ALL treated on pediatric protocols have had superior event-free and overall survival rates when compared with similar patients enrolled on adult ALL trials. Preliminary data suggest that these patients have better outcomes when treated with pediatric-inspired regimens, and that excess toxicity is not observed.[153,155–162]

Continuation Therapy Although unnecessary for cure of mature B-cell leukemia, continuation therapy for 2 to 3 years is an integral part of pediatric and adult ALL regimens. Attempts to shorten the duration of treatment have led to inferior outcomes in both childhood and adult ALL,[163] although as many as two-thirds of childhood cases might be cured with only 12 months of treatment.[164] However, which subgroups of childhood ALL can be cured with abbreviated therapy is unclear. In a meta-analysis of 42 trials, a third year of continuation therapy reduced the likelihood of relapse during the third year, but no advantage to prolonging treatment beyond 3 years was observed.[165] Early studies demonstrated that the third year of continuation therapy benefits boys but not girls.[166,167] Hence, most studies discontinue all therapy for girls after 2 to 2.5 years of treatment. It is uncertain whether with improved contemporary treatment boys still require prolonged continuation treatment. Whether adults with ALL benefit from prolonged continuation therapy is also unclear. In most adult trials, continuation therapy is given for 2 years from diagnosis.

Methotrexate administered weekly and mercaptopurine administered daily constitute the usual continuation regimen for ALL. Accumulation of higher intracellular concentrations of the active metabolites of methotrexate and mercaptopurine and administration of this combination to the limits of tolerance (as indicated by low leukocyte counts) have been associated with improved clinical outcome.[168,169] Many investigators advocate that drug dosage be adjusted to maintain leukocyte counts below 3×10^9/L and neutrophil counts between 0.5 and 1.5×10^9/L to ensure adequate dose intensity during the continuation treatment in childhood ALL.[2] In one study, the dose intensity of mercaptopurine was the most important pharmacologic factor influencing treatment outcome.[170] Mercaptopurine is most effective when it is given orally on a daily basis. However, overzealous use of mercaptopurine is counterproductive, as such use results in neutropenia and interruption of chemotherapy, reducing overall dose intensity. The effect of mercaptopurine is better when the drug is administered in the evening.[171] Mercaptopurine should not be given with milk or milk products containing xanthine oxidase, which can degrade the drug.[172] Antimetabolite treatment should not be withheld because of isolated increases of liver enzymes since such liver function abnormalities are tolerable and reversible.[173]

A few patients (one in 300) have an inherited homozygous deficiency of thiopurine *S*-methyltransferase, the enzyme that catalyzes the *S*-methylation (inactivation) of mercaptopurine. In these patients, standard doses of mercaptopurine have potentially fatal hematologic side effects. The drug should be given in much smaller doses (e.g., 10-fold reduction).[174] Approximately 10 percent of patients are heterozygous for the enzyme deficiency and have intermediate levels of thiopurine methyltransferase.[175] This subgroup can be treated safely with only moderate reductions in mercaptopurine dosage and appears to have better clinical outcomes than do patients with the homozygous wild-type phenotype. Importantly, patients with this enzyme deficiency are at risk for therapy-related myeloid leukemia and radiation-related brain tumors.[176–178] Identification of this autosomal codominant trait has been enabled by molecular diagnosis and led to increased emphasis on inherited differences in drug metabolism and disposition resulting from genetic polymorphisms in drug-metabolizing enzymes and in drug transporters, receptors, and targets.[1,179,180] Ultimately, therapy can be designed according to the genetic constitution of both the host and the host's leukemia cells.

Because thioguanine is more potent than mercaptopurine in model systems and leads to higher concentrations of thioguanine nucleotides in cells and cytotoxic concentrations in CSF,[181] randomized trials have been performed in children to compare the effectiveness of these two drugs.[182] Thioguanine, given at a daily dose of 40 mg/m^2 or more, produced superior antileukemic responses to mercaptopurine, but was associated with profound thrombocytopenia, an increased risk of death, and unacceptable rate of hepatic venoocclusive disease.[182] Consequently, mercaptopurine, remains the drug of choice for ALL, although thioguanine is still used in short-term courses during the intensification phase of therapy.

Intermittent pulses of vincristine and a glucocorticoid improved the efficacy of antimetabolite-based continuation regimens and have been widely adopted for both childhood and adult ALL.[165,183] In older children and adults, prolonged glucocorticoid therapy may lead to increased risk of osteonecrosis.[184] Another integral component of many protocols is reinduction therapy introduced relatively soon after the first remission. This treatment, which relies on the same drugs used during the initial phase of induction therapy, has improved outcomes for children and adults with ALL.[67,106–108] A second reinduction phase during continuation treatment may further improve the outcome of patients with standard- or high-risk ALL.[142,185] The benefit of such a double-delayed intensification may result from either the increased dose intensity of other agents such as asparaginase or anthracycline or the timing or scheduling of the intensification regimen.

Therapy of the Central Nervous System The CNS is a common sanctuary for leukemic cells and requires prophylactic or presymptomatic therapy. In the 1970s, the cornerstone of ALL therapy was cranial irradiation (2400 cGy) plus methotrexate administered intrathecally after complete remission was induced. Concerns that cranial irradiation could cause second cancer, late neurocognitive deficits, and endocrinopathy stimulated efforts to replace cranial irradiation with early intensification by intrathecal and systemic chemotherapy. Two early clinical trials tested the feasibility of complete omission of prophylactic cranial irradiation in the treatment of childhood ALL.[186–188] Although the cumulative risk of an isolated CNS relapse was relatively low (3 to 4 percent), the EFS rates in the two studies were only 68.4 percent and 60.7 percent.[186–188] In another study, prophylactic cranial irradiation appeared to improve outcome in T-cell ALL with leukocyte counts >100 × 10^9/L.[189] Thus, until recently, virtually all childhood study groups continued to rely on prophylactic cranial irradiation for up to 20 percent of patients.[80] A radiation dose of 1200 cGy appeared to provide adequate protection against CNS relapse, even in high-risk patients (e.g., those with T-cell ALL and leukocyte counts >100 × 10^9/L).[141] More recently, a study at St. Jude Children's Research Hospital again tested the feasibility of total omission of prophylactic cranial irradiation in the context of risk-adapted intrathecal and systemic chemotherapy.[190] The 5-year survival rate for the 498 patients enrolled was 93.5 percent and the cumulative risk of an isolated CNS relapse rate was only 2.7 percent, a promising result, suggesting that prophylactic cranial irradiation can be safely omitted in the context of the effective intrathecal and systemic chemotherapy. Another study by the Dutch Childhood Oncology Group also showed that prophylactic cranial irradiation can be safely omitted from children with ALL.[191] Preliminary data from additional trials also indicate that prophylactic cranial irradiation is not necessary.

Systemic treatment including high-dose methotrexate, intensive asparaginase, and dexamethasone, as well as optimal intrathecal therapy, is important to control CNS leukemia.[80,192] Triple intrathecal therapy with methotrexate, cytarabine, and hydrocortisone is more effective than intrathecal methotrexate in preventing CNS relapse.[193] Because the presence of ALL blasts in the CSF, even from traumatic lumbar puncture, is associated with an increased risk of CNS relapse and poor EFS,[80,81] intrathecal therapy should be intensified in patients with this feature. With CNS prophylaxis and high-dose systemic therapy most adults with ALL remain free of CNS disease. CNS disease at the time of leukemia relapse in adults occurs in approximately 10 percent of cases. The frequency of CNS recurrence is about the same whether CNS radiation therapy (12 to 24 Gy) is used or whether only intrathecal cytotoxic therapy is used. Systemic high-dose methotrexate and cytarabine add to the CNS therapy. The outcome after CNS relapse is poor. Survival after CNS relapse is usually less than 1 year in adults. Treatment of CNS relapse requires cranial irradiation, intrathecal chemotherapy, typically via an Ommaya shunt, plus reinduction and reconsolidation systemic therapy.

Stem Cell Transplantation Hematopoietic stem cell transplantation during first remission remains controversial.[194] In adult ALL, long-term disease-free survival rates range from 35 to 50 percent with chemotherapy alone and from 45 to 60 percent with allogeneic transplantation.[195,196] However, interpretation of these results is difficult because of the lack of true randomization. Even so, results from both adult and pediatric studies suggest allogeneic transplantation benefits some high-risk patients.[194,196,197] Because of their unfavorable prognosis, patients with the Philadelphia chromosome–positive ALL and those with a poor initial response to induction therapy have been recommended to undergo allogeneic stem cell transplantation during the first remission.[194–196,198] However, the advent of improved chemotherapy has diminished the survival advantage from transplantation in children with Philadelphia chromosome–positive ALL.[199] The use of a tyrosine kinase inhibitor has further improved the early treatment results,[200] casting doubt on the benefit from transplantation in first remission in childhood cases.[201] Allogeneic transplantation appears to improve the outcome of adults with the t(4;11),[154] but not that of children or infants with the same genotype.[202]

Allogeneic transplantation has not been compared to chemotherapy alone in a true randomized trial, and thus the results of comparative studies are biased by availability of appropriate donors and other factors.[194,203–205] The more potent antileukemia activity of allogeneic transplantation is balanced against the considerable nonrelapse mortality and long-term consequences of graft-versus-host disease. A meta-analysis involving 3157 patients supports matched sibling donor allogeneic transplantation as the optimal postremission therapy for adults with ALL with a significant reduction in relapses and a significant increase in treatment related mortality. Results may differ depending upon stem cell source, that is, related or unrelated donors or umbilical cord stem cells. A retrospective study of 421 adults who underwent allogeneic cord blood transplantation reported 2-year leukemia-free survival of 39 percent for patients in first complete remission and 31 percent for second remission. In multivariate analysis, factors associated with poor outcomes were age older than 35 years, myeloablative conditioning, and more advanced disease. Reduced intensity-conditioning allografting has yielded lower nonrelapse mortality and higher relapse rates than myeloablative conditioning with no significant differences in leukemia-free survival.[206,207] The indications for allogeneic transplantation in first remission should be reevaluated as chemotherapy and transplantation continue to improve. Autologous transplantation failed to improve outcome in adult ALL overall, mainly because of a high rate of relapse.[195] Several small studies indicate that autologous stem cell transplantation is feasible and beneficial for adults with Philadelphia chromosome–positive ALL who achieve a molecular remission after combined chemotherapy and imatinib.[208,209]

Targeted Therapies The best example of targeted therapy is the use of the tyrosine kinase inhibitors imatinib or dasatinib in Philadelphia chromosome–positive ALL.[21,113,114,210] Used as single agents or with a glucocorticoid, they can induce complete remission in older patients where this subset of ALL is more common.[114,210,211] In combination with chemotherapy, they not only induce a higher complete remission rate but also a high rate of molecular remission in children and adults.[200,201,212–216] The duration of these remissions is uncertain, but some have been quite long after additional chemotherapy. Although the need for early transplantation in childhood cases is uncertain, this treatment modality is still a standard for adult cases.[206,217] The use of imatinib or dasatinib yields a higher proportion of adult cases suitable for transplantation. The outcome depends on minimal residual disease before and after transplantation.[218] In patients with residual disease after transplantation, rapid response to imatinib was associated with a superior survival.[219] It is uncertain whether and when to discontinue imatinib or dasatinib after the patient is treated with chemotherapy or transplantation.

Surface expression of CD20 by leukemia cells is associated with an inferior outcome in adult,[220] but not childhood, ALL.[221] Chemotherapy trials incorporating rituximab, an anti-CD20 antibody, have yielded promising results in adults with CD20-positive B-cell precursor ALL.[150,222] Other monoclonal antibodies that bind CD22 and CD19 are in late-stage clinical development.[223] Nelarabine is an approved antimetabolite drug that has shown considerable activity in T-cell ALL, both alone and in combination with other chemotherapy.[224–226]

COURSE AND PROGNOSIS

RELAPSE

Relapse is defined as the reappearance of leukemia cells at any site in the body. Most relapses occur during treatment or within the first 2 years after its completion, although initial relapses have been observed 10 or more years after diagnosis.[227] Molecular studies suggest that in some cases, especially those with the *ETV6-RUNX1* fusion, subsequent mutations of the residual preleukemic clone that were not eradicated during initial treatment account for the "late relapse."[228] The marrow remains the most common site of relapse in ALL. Anemia, leukocytosis or leukopenia, thrombocytopenia, enlargement of the liver or spleen, bone pain, fever, or a sudden decrease in tolerance to continuation chemotherapy may signal the onset of marrow relapse. In contemporary treatment programs for childhood ALL, the rates of CNS and testicular relapse have decreased to 3 percent or less.[190,192] Leukemic relapse occasionally occurs at other extramedullary sites, including the eye, ear, ovary, uterus, bone, muscle, tonsil, kidney, mediastinum, pleura, and paranasal sinus.

For ALL patients who have received a modern, intensive multiagent treatment regimen, with delayed intensification and prolonged continuation therapy, a relapse of disease portends a very poor survival. Although some individuals can be rescued with additional chemotherapy alone, in general, only allogeneic hematopoietic stem cell transplantation offers a reasonable chance for cure and long-term survival. Thus, treatment for relapse is often considered as "a bridge to transplant." Two new drugs, clofarabine and liposomal vincristine, were approved as single agents in large part based upon their ability to enable patients with relapsed ALL to proceed to a transplant.[229,230] Because the outcome of allogeneic transplantation is poor in the presence of overt ALL, reinduction therapy aims for rapid cytoreduction of lymphoblasts while efforts proceed concurrently to identify an HLA-matched donor. The optimal pretransplant conditioning regimen then depends largely on the age and medical condition of the patient.

Marrow relapse, with or without extramedullary involvement, portends a poor outcome for most patients.[231,232] Factors indicating an especially poor prognosis include relapse while on therapy or after a short initial remission, T-cell immunophenotype, the presence of the Philadelphia chromosome, and an isolated hematologic relapse.[232–234] Prolonged second remissions (>3 years) can be achieved with chemotherapy in as many as half of patients with late relapses (i.e., >6 months after cessation of therapy) but in only approximately 10 percent of those with early relapse. The persistence of minimal residual disease after reinduction treatment also portends a very poor prognosis.[235] In patients who develop hematologic relapse while on therapy or shortly thereafter, and in those with residual disease after remission induction for relapse, allogeneic hematopoietic stem cell transplantation is the treatment of choice.[236] Autologous transplantation as postinduction treatment offers no substantial advantage over chemotherapy.[190,192,237] For patients without histocompatible related donors, transplantation of stem cells from cord blood or marrow from matched unrelated donors is recommended.[201,238–241] For patients with ALL that has relapsed after allogeneic transplantation, a second transplant or donor T-lymphocyte infusion occasionally results in sustained remission.[242]

Central Nervous System Relapse

Although extramedullary relapse is frequently an isolated clinical finding, many occurrences are associated with recurrent disease detectable in the marrow. CNS relapses are associated with higher level of minimal residual disease in the marrow than testicular relapses.[243] Submicroscopic marrow involvement at a level of 10^{-4} or higher at the time of overt extramedullary relapse confers a very poor outcome.[243] Hence, patients with extramedullary relapse and detectable disease in marrow require intensive systemic treatment to prevent subsequent hematologic relapse. The efficacy of salvage therapy in children with an isolated CNS relapse depends partly on duration of first complete remission and partly on whether CNS irradiation was previously performed. The strategy of delaying cranial or craniospinal irradiation for 6 to 12 months to allow initial intensification with systemic chemotherapy has yielded long-term second EFS of 70 to 80 percent in children with isolated CNS relapse.[244,245] In one study, 12 months of intensive systemic chemotherapy and reduced-dose cranial irradiation (18 Gy) resulted in an excellent 4-year EFS rate among children with precursor B-cell ALL who had not received cranial irradiation during initial treatment and who had an initial remission duration of 18 months or more.[246] Notably, in this study, a favorable age group of 1 to 9.9 years plus a low presenting leukocyte count (<50 × 10⁹/L) at diagnosis of ALL was an independent favorable prognostic factor. For patients, especially those with T-cell ALL, in whom relapse develops during therapy and who had previously undergone cranial irradiation, the remission rate generally does not exceed 30 percent.[244,245] Adults with isolated CNS relapse fare much more poorly than children. However, the recommended treatment strategy remains the same–combining CNS-directed treatment with additional systemic chemotherapy.

Testicular Relapse

One-third of patients with early testicular relapse and two-thirds of patients with late testicular recurrence became long-term survivors after salvage chemotherapy and testicular irradiation.[232,247,248] In one study, some patients with late isolated testicular relapses were successfully treated with chemotherapy that included very high-dose methotrexate, without the addition of radiation therapy.[249] The optimal treatment and prognosis for patients with relapse at unusual extramedullary sites are unclear. However, the same principles that apply to the clinical management of CNS or testicular relapse probably apply to this subgroup.

TREATMENT SEQUELAE

Despite the increasing intensity of curative treatment for childhood ALL, judicious use of supportive care reduced the rate of early death from 8 percent in the early 1970s to less than 2 percent in the 1990s.[16,17] Currently, the induction mortality ranges between 2 percent and 11 percent in adult ALL, with increasing age associated with higher death rate.[66,67,150–153] Most deaths are caused by bacterial or fungal infections. The death rate among older patients receiving remission induction therapy can be as high as 30 percent because of increased hematologic and nonhematologic toxicities (e.g., hepatotoxicity and cardiotoxicity).[111,112] This poor tolerance for chemotherapy and consequent reduction of dose intensity largely account for the poor clinical outcome in older patients.

Patients previously treated for ALL are best monitored in dedicated cancer survivorship clinics where both early and late complications can be identified and managed. Table 91–6 summarizes common side effects associated with antileukemia therapy. Hyperglycemia develops in 10 to 20 percent of children during induction therapy with prednisone, vincristine, and L-asparaginase but has no long-term consequence nor prognostic implication; in some cases, short-term insulin treatment is required.[250] Adolescent and older adult age, obesity, a family history of diabetes mellitus, and Down syndrome are associated with increased susceptibility to hyperglycemia.[250,251] This induction regimen causes a hypercoagulable state leading to cerebral thrombosis, peripheral vein thrombosis, or both, in as many as 5 percent of patients. Cerebral thrombosis should be distinguished from transient ischemic lesions (posterior reversible encephalopathy syndrome) which are associated with acute hypertension and severe constipation.[252] These lesions are located at the watershed areas between the major cerebral arteries and

TABLE 91–6. Side Effects Associated with Antileukemic Therapy

Treatment	Acute Complications	Late Complications
Prednisone (or prednisolone)	Hyperglycemia, hypertension, changes in mood or behavior, acne, increased appetite, weight gain, peptic ulcer, hepatomegaly, myopathy	Avascular necrosis of bone, osteopenia, growth retardation
Dexamethasone	Same as prednisone, except for increased changes in mood or behavior and myopathy, but less salt retention	Same as prednisone
Vincristine	Peripheral neuropathy, constipation, chemical cellulitis, jaw pain, seizures, hair loss	
Daunorubicin, idarubicin, doxorubicin, or epirubicin	Nausea and vomiting, hair loss, mucositis, marrow suppression, chemical cellulitis, increased skin pigmentation	Cardiomyopathy (after high cumulative dose)
L-Asparaginase	Nausea and vomiting, allergic reactions (manifested as rashes, bronchospasm, severe pain at intramuscular injection site), hyperglycemia, pancreatitis, liver dysfunction, large vein thrombosis, encephalopathy	None
Mercaptopurine	Nausea and vomiting, mucositis, marrow suppression, solar dermatitis, liver dysfunction: increased hematologic toxicity in persons lacking thiopurine methyltransferase	Osteoporosis (long-term use), acute myeloid leukemia in persons with thiopurine methyltransferase deficiency
Methotrexate	Nausea and vomiting, liver dysfunction, marrow suppression, mucositis (resulting from high-dose treatment), solar dermatitis	Leukoencephalopathy, osteopenia (resulting from long-term use)
Etoposide, teniposide	Nausea and vomiting, hair loss, mucositis, marrow suppression, allergic reactions (bronchospasm, urticaria, angioedema, hypotension)	Acute myeloid leukemia
Cytarabine	Nausea and vomiting, fever, skin rashes, mucositis, marrow suppression, liver dysfunction, conjunctivitis (from high-dose treatment)	Decreased fertility (with high cumulative dose)
Cyclophosphamide	Nausea and vomiting, hemorrhagic cystitis, marrow suppression, syndrome of inappropriate secretion of antidiuretic hormone, hair loss	Bladder cancer or acute myeloid leukemia (rare), decreased fertility (with high cumulative dose)
Rituximab	Infusion reactions, mucocutaneous reactions, lymphopenia, pulmonary infiltrates	Reactivation of virus infections (hepatitis B), progressive multifocal leukoencephalopathy from JC virus infection
Intrathecal methotrexate	Headache, fever, seizure, marrow suppression, mucositis (in patients with renal dysfunction)	Encephalopathy or myelopathy (with high cumulative dose)
Brain irradiation	Hair loss, postirradiation somnolence syndrome (6–10 weeks after treatment)	Seizure, mineralizing microangiopathy, growth hormone deficiency, thyroid dysfunction, obesity, osteopenia, brain tumors, basal cell carcinoma, parotid gland carcinoma, hair loss, cataract (rare), dental abnormalities

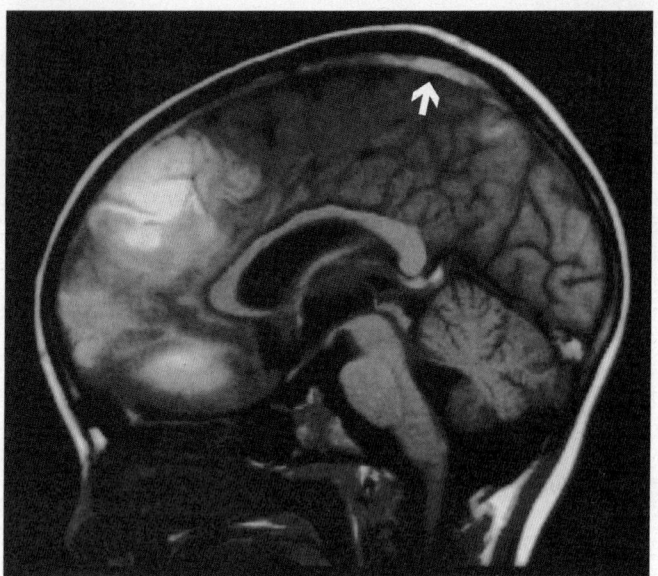

Figure 91–5. T1-weighted magnetic resonance image without contrast demonstrates a clot in the superior sagittal sinus *(arrow)* and several frontal lobe hematomas.

generally are reversible. Cerebral thrombosis can be readily distinguished from transient ischemic lesions by magnetic resonance imaging or computed tomography (Fig. 91–5). Occasionally, cerebral thrombosis may not be apparent by diagnostic imaging until a few days after the onset of symptoms and signs. Thrombotic complications (especially in leg veins or inferior vena cava) are also common in adults receiving asparaginase.[136–140]

Emphasis on the intensive use of vincristine, methotrexate and glucocorticoids has led to an increased frequency of neurotoxicity,[252,253] and of osteonecrosis.[254] Many long-term survivors of childhood ALL, especially those who received high cumulative doses of glucocorticoid, methotrexate, or cranial irradiation, have developed severe osteoporosis.[254–257] Early identification of bone lesions and the introduction of therapy to prevent fractures is recommended. Treatment with anthracyclines can produce severe cardiomyopathy, especially when anthracyclines are given in high cumulative and peak doses to children, and particularly young girls.[258–260] Prolonged infusion did not appear to reduce late cardiotoxicity compared to bolus administration.[261] The existence of a safe cumulative dose of anthracycline is controversial. Cardiac abnormalities are persistent and progressive years after anthracycline therapy.[262] In one study, dexrazoxane prevented or reduced anthracycline-induced cardiotoxicity without interfering with antileukemic activity.[263,264] In current pediatric trials, limited doses of anthracyclines are used, even for high-risk cases, to decrease the risk of subsequent cardiomyopathy. Most regimens for adult ALL restrict cumulative anthracycline dosage to levels associated with less than 5 percent risk of congestive heart failure.

Cranial irradiation has been implicated as the cause of numerous late sequelae in children, including second cancer, neurocognitive deficits, and endocrine abnormalities that can lead to obesity, short stature, precocious puberty, and osteoporosis.[265–269] In general, these complications are seen in girls more often than in boys and in young children more often than in older children or adults. Long-term followup studies of survivors of childhood ALL reveal a greater than 10 percent cumulative risk of second neoplasms after 30 years of observation, and a higher-than-average mortality rate among patients who had received cranial irradiation.[266,267] Patients who had been irradiated also had a high unemployment rate and, among

women, a low marital rate. Many children with profound deficiencies of growth hormone receive hormone replacement therapy, which permits attainment of acceptable final heights without an increased chance of relapse.[270]

The most devastating complication is the development of brain tumors and therapy-related myeloid leukemia.[271,272] Children who undergo cranial irradiation at age 6 years or younger are most susceptible to development of brain tumors.[273] Intensive use of antimetabolites before and during cranial irradiation also increases the risk of brain tumor.[177] The median latency period for high-grade brain tumors is 9 years; it is 20 years for low-grade tumors (e.g., meningioma).[266,273]

Therapy-related myeloid leukemia has been linked to intensive treatment with epipodophyllotoxins (teniposide and etoposide). The risk of disease depends on treatment schedule, concomitant use of other agents (e.g., L-asparaginase, alkylating agents, perhaps antimetabolites), and host pharmacogenetics.[176,274] The long-term survival rate for patients with this complication is very low, even when the patients undergo allogeneic stem cell transplantation. No evidence indicates an increased incidence of cancer or birth defects among the offspring of adult survivors of childhood ALL.[275,276]

PROGNOSTIC FACTORS

The cornerstone of the modern therapeutic approach to childhood ALL has been careful assessment of the risk of relapse so that only high-risk or very-high-risk patients are treated with intensive therapy.[277,278] Less-toxic treatments (usually antimetabolites) are reserved for low-risk or standard-risk patients. By contrast, almost all adult patients are candidates for intensive therapy. Of the many variables that influence prognosis, treatment is the most important. Some of the factors that emerged as useful prognostic indicators in the past have disappeared as treatment has improved; others have shown predictive strength in one or several trials, but not in others. For example, T-cell ALL, once associated with a poor prognosis, now has long-term response rates of 70 to 85 percent in children[2,17,190] and 50 to 60 percent in adults[66,67,279] as a result of effective intensive chemotherapy. Outcomes for mature B-cell ALL, also a poor prognostic subset in the past, have improved in both children and adults and 80 percent or more are cured with short but intensive chemotherapy treatments.[280]

Age and leukocyte count continue to be used for risk classification in almost every pediatric clinical trial involving precursor B-cell ALL. In a workshop sponsored by the National Cancer Institute, participants agreed on a presenting age of between 1 and 9 years and a leukocyte count of less than 50×10^9/L as the minimum criteria for low-risk ALL. These criteria apply only to precursor B-cell ALL and not to T-cell ALL. Among adults, the outcome of therapy worsens with increasing age and leukocyte count. Age younger than 35 years and leukocyte count less than 30×10^9/L are considered favorable prognostic indicators (Table 91–7).[67,150,152] In general, age younger than 60 years is considered a practical guide for selecting candidates who might benefit from intensive therapy, including allogeneic transplantation. Any decision to begin aggressive treatment in patients older than age 60 years must be weighed against the risk of increased morbidity and mortality.[111,112]

Male sex has long been recognized as an adverse prognostic factor in childhood ALL but has less influence in adult ALL. Its prognostic significance was abolished in a number of childhood studies in which overall outcome was improved. Black race conferred a poor outcome in the national clinical trials,[281,282] but in a single-institution study with equal access to effective treatment regimens, race had no prognostic significance.[283]

Primary genetic abnormalities have important prognostic significance. Hyperdiploidy (>50 chromosomes) and *ETV6-RUNX1*

TABLE 91–7. Adverse Prognostic Factors in Adult Acute Lymphoblastic Leukemia

Factors	Precursor B Cell	Precursor T Cell
Age (years)*	>35	>35
Leukocyte count (×10⁹/L)	>30	>100
Immunophenotype	Pro-B (CD10–)	Pre-T
Genetics	t(9;22) [BCR-ABL1]	HOX11L2 expression?
	t(4;11) [MLL-AF4]	ERG expression?
	Hypodiploidy?	
Treatment response	Delayed remission (>4 weeks)	Delayed remission (>4 weeks)
	Minimal residual disease >10⁻⁴ after induction	Minimal residual disease >10⁻⁴ after induction

*Continuous factor with increasing age associated with progressively worse outcome.

TABLE 91–8. Risk Classification System Used in St. Jude Total Therapy Study XVI

Risk Group	Feature
Standard	Precursor B-cell phenotype in patients ages 1–9 years with a presenting leukocyte count <50 × 10⁹/L, ETV6-RUNX1 fusion, or hyperdiploidy (>50 chromosomes or DNA index >1.16)
	Must not have CNS3 status, testicular leukemia, t(9;22), t(1;19), rearranged MLL gene, hypodiploidy, or ≥0.01% leukemia cells in marrow after 6-week remission induction
High	T-cell acute lymphoblastic leukemia (ALL) and all cases of B-cell precursor ALL that do not meet the criteria for standard or very-high-risk ALL
Very high	Early T-cell precursor, initial induction failure, or ≥1% leukemic cells in marrow after 6-week remission induction

fusion—seen primarily in children ages 1 to 9 years but very rarely in adults—are associated with a favorable prognosis.[2,17] MLL rearrangements, which occur in 70 to 80 percent of infants younger than age 1 year and in 10 percent of adults, and Philadelphia chromosome with BCR-ABL1 fusion, which is found in 3 percent of children but in 25 to 30 percent of adult patients, historically confer a poor outcome.[1,2,17,199] Interestingly, there is a marked influence of age on the prognosis of genetic subtypes of ALL. For example, Philadelphia chromosome–positive ALL is associated with a poor outcome in adolescents but a relatively favorable outcome in children ages 1 to 9 years old who have a low leukocyte count at presentation.[198] Once associated with a dismal outcome, the early treatment outcome of Philadelphia chromosome–positive ALL in both children and adults has improved substantially with the advent of BCR/ABL1 tyrosine kinase inhibitors.[113,114,200,201,210–216] Among patients with MLL-rearranged ALL, infants younger than age 1 year fare considerably worse than older children.[202] The basis of these differences may be related to some combination of secondary genetic events, the developmental stage of the target cell undergoing malignant transformation, and the pharmacogenetics or pharmacokinetic features of the patient. In T-cell ALL, NOTCH1 or FBXW7 mutation identifies a subgroup of childhood or adult cases with a favorable outcome.[284–286]

A useful adjunct in risk assessment is the response to early treatment, as measured by the rate of clearance of leukemia cells from the blood or marrow with the use of flow cytometric detection of aberrant immunophenotype or analysis by PCR of clonal antigen receptor gene rearrangements.[83,123–129,190,287,288] This measure reflects the drug sensitivity or resistance of leukemia cells and the pharmacodynamics of the drugs, which is affected by the pharmacogenetics of the host. Current techniques allow measurement of minimal residual disease in all patients, and it has become the most important prognostic factor (Table 91–8). The expectation is that alteration of treatment intensity according to the level of minimal residual disease at early time points will improve the long-term outcome of patients with ALL. The level of measureable residual leukemia is also a strong predictor of treatment outcome before allogeneic stem cell transplantation for relapsed leukemia.[235,289] Pediatric trials have shown better outcomes when treatment decisions have been based in part on measurable levels of residual disease. However, similar benefit remains to be shown convincingly in adults.

REFERENCES

1. Pui CH, Relling MV, Downing JR: Acute lymphoblastic leukemia. N Engl J Med 350:1535, 2004.
2. Pui CH, Robison LL, Look AT: Acute lymphoblastic leukemia. Lancet 371:1030, 2008.
3. Velpeau A: Sur la resorption du pus et sur l'alteration du sang dans les maladies, Clinique de persection nenemant. Premier observation. Rev Med 26:216, 1827.
4. Virchow R: Weisses blut. Notiz Geg Natur Heilk 36:152, 1845.
5. Bennett JH: Case of hypertrophy of the spleen and liver in which death took place from suppuration of the blood. Edinburgh Med Surg J 64:413, 1845.
6. Craigie D: Case of disease of the spleen, in which death took place in consequence of the presence of purulent matter in the blood. Edinburgh Med Surg J 64:400, 1845.
7. Virchow R: Weisses Blut und Milztumoren. Part II. Med Z, 1847, 16, 9. Virchows Arch Path Anat Physiol 1:565, 1847.
8. Ehrlich P: Farbenanalytische untersuchungen zur histologie und klinick des blutes. Berl Hirschwald 137, 1891.
9. Reschad H, Schilling-Torgau V: Ueber eine neue Leukämie durch echte Uebergangsformen (Splenozytenleuämie) und ihre bedeutung für dies, selbständigkeit dieser Zellen. Munchener Med Wochenschr 60:1981, 1913.
10. Ward G: The infective theory of acute leukemia. Br J Child Dis 14:10, 1917.
11. Farber S, Diamond LK, Mercer RD, et al: Temporary remissions in acute leukemia in children produced by folic acid antagonist, 4-aminopteroylglumatic acid (aminopterin). N Engl J Med 238:787, 1948.
12. Farber S: The effect of ACTH in acute leukemia in childhood, in Proceedings of the First Clinical Conference on the Use of ACTH, edited by Mote JR, p 325. Blakiston, Philadelphia, 1950.
13. Elion GB, Hitchings GH, Vanderwerff H: Antagonists of nucleic acid derivatives. VI. Purines. J Biol Chem 192:505, 1951.
14. Pinkel D, Hernandez K, Borella L, et al: Drug dosage and remission duration in childhood lymphocytic leukemia. Cancer 27:247, 1971.
15. Riehm H, Gadner H, Henze G, et al: The Berlin childhood acute lymphoblastic leukemia therapy study, 1970–1976. Am J Pediatr Hematol Oncol 2:299, 1980.
16. Pui CH, Evans WE: A 50-year journey to cure childhood acute lymphoblastic leukemia. Semin Hematol 50:185, 2013.
16a. Laszlo J: The Cure of Childhood Leukemia: Into the Age of Miracles. Rutgers University Press, New Brunswick, NJ, 1995.
17. Pui CH, Evans WE: Treatment of acute lymphoblastic leukemia. N Engl J Med 354:166, 2006.
18. Bassan R, Hoelzer D: Modern therapy of acute lymphoblastic leukemia. J Clin Oncol 29:532, 2011.
19. Mulligan CG: The molecular genetic makeup of acute lymphoblastic leukemia. Hematology Am Soc Hematol Educ Program 2012:389, 2012.
20. Mulligan CG: Genomic characterization of childhood acute lymphoblastic leukemia. Semin Hematol 50:314, 2013.
21. Lee HJ, Thompson JE, Wang ES, Wetzler M: Philadelphia chromosome-positive acute lymphoblastic leukemia: Current treatment and future perspectives. Cancer 117:1583, 2011.
22. American Cancer Society: Cancer Facts and Figures 2014. http://www.cancer.org. Accessed July 4, 2014.

23. SEER Cancer Statistics Review, 1975–2010, National Cancer Institute. Bethesda, MD, http://seer.cancer.gov/csr/1975_2010. Accessed July 4, 2014.

24. Sandler DP, Ross JA: Epidemiology of acute leukemia in children and adults. *Semin Oncol* 24:3, 1997.

25. Ferlay J, Shin HR, Bray F, et al: Estimates of worldwide burden of cancer in 2008: GLOBOCAN 2008. *Int J Cancer* 127:2893, 2010.

26. Forestier E, Izraeli S, Beverloo B, et al: Cytogenetic features of acute lymphoblastic and myeloid leukemias in pediatric patients with Down syndrome: An iBFM-SG study. *Blood* 111:1575, 2008.

27. Izraeli S, Vora A, Zwaan CM, Whitlock J: How I treat ALL in Down's syndrome: Pathobiology and management. *Blood* 123:35, 2014.

28. Mullighan CG, Zhang J, Harvey RC, et al: JAK mutations in high-risk childhood acute lymphoblastic leukemia. *Proc Natl Acad Sci U S A* 106:9414, 2009.

29. Mullighan CG, Collins-Underwood JR, Phillips LA, et al: Rearrangement of CRLF2 in B-progenitor- and Down syndrome-associated acute lymphoblastic leukemia. *Nat Genet* 41:1243, 2009.

30. Hertzberg L, Vendramini E, Ganmore I, et al: Down syndrome acute lymphoblastic leukemia, a highly heterogeneous disease in which aberrant expression of CRLF2 is associated with mutated JAK2: A report from the International BFM Study Group. *Blood* 115:1006, 2010.

31. Vanasse GJ, Concannon P, Willerford DM: Regulated genomic instability and neoplasia in the lymphoid lineage. *Blood* 94:3997, 1999.

32. Liberzon E, Avigad S, Stark B, et al: Germ-line ATM gene alterations are associated with susceptibility to sporadic T-cell acute lymphoblastic leukemia in children. *Genes Chromosomes Cancer* 39:161, 2004.

33. Papaemmanuil E, Hosking FJ, Vijayakrishnan J, et al: Loci on 7p12.2, 10q21.2 and 14q11.2 are associated with risk of childhood acute lymphoblastic leukemia. *Nat Genet* 41:1006–1010, 2009.

34. Trevino LR, Yang W, French D, et al: Germline genomic variants associated with childhood acute lymphoblastic leukemia. *Nat Genet* 41:1001, 2009.

35. Sherborne AL, Hosking FJ, Prasad RB, et al: Variation in CDKN2A at 9p21.3 influences childhood acute lymphoblastic leukemia risk. *Nat Genet* 42:492, 2010.

36. Yang JJ, Cheng C, Yang W, et al: Genome-wide interrogation of germline genetic variation associated with treatment response in childhood acute lymphoblastic leukemia. *JAMA* 301:393, 2009.

37. Doll R, Wakeford R: Risk of childhood cancer from fetal irradiation. *Br J Radiol* 70:130, 1997.

38. Draper G, Vincent T, Kroll ME, Swanson J: Childhood cancer in relation to distance from high voltage power lines in England and Wales: A case-control study. *BMJ* 330:1290, 2005.

39. Sermage-Faure C, Demoury C, Rudant J, et al: Childhood leukaemia close to high-voltage power lines—The Geocap study, 2002–2007. *Br J Cancer* 108:1899, 2013.

40. Hjalgrim LL, Rostgaard K, Hjalgrim H, et al: Birth weight and risk for childhood leukemia in Denmark, Sweden, Norway, and Iceland. *J Natl Cancer Inst* 96:1549, 2004.

41. Inaba H, Greaves M, Mullighan CG: Acute lymphoblastic leukaemia. *Lancet* 381:1943, 2013.

42. Li C, Zhou Y: Association between NQO1 C609T polymorphism and acute lymphoblastic leukemia risk: Evidence from an updated meta-analysis based on 17 case-control studies. *J Cancer Res Clin Oncol* 140:873, 2014.

43. Sherborne AL, Hemminki K, Kumar R, et al: Rationale for an international consortium to study inherited genetic susceptibility to childhood acute lymphoblastic leukaemia. *Haematologica* 96:1049, 2011.

44. Trevino LR, Yang W, French D, et al: Germline genomic variants associated with childhood acute lymphoblastic leukemia. *Nat Genet* 41:1001, 2009.

45. Greaves M: Infection, immune responses and the aetiology of childhood leukaemia. *Nat Rev Cancer* 6:193, 2006.

46. Maia AT, Tussiwand R, Cazzaniga G, et al: Identification of preleukemic precursors of hyperdiploid acute lymphoblastic leukemia in cord blood. *Genes Chromosomes Cancer* 40:38, 2004.

47. Hong D, Gupta R, Ancliff P, et al: Initiating and cancer-propagating cells in TEL-AML1-associated childhood leukemia. *Science* 319:336, 2008.

48. Kinlen LJ: Infection, immune factors in cancer: The role of epidemiology. *Oncogene* 23:6341, 2004.

49. Wiemels JL, Leonard BC, Wang Y, et al: Site-specific translocation and evidence of postnatal origin of the t(1;19) E2A-PBX1 fusion in childhood acute lymphoblastic leukemia. *Proc Natl Acad Sci U S A* 99:15101, 2002.

50. Moorman AV, Chilton L, Wilkinson J, et al: A population-based cytogenetic study of adults with acute lymphoblastic leukemia. *Blood* 115:206, 2010.

51. Mrózek K, Harper DP, Aplan PD: Cytogenetics and molecular genetics of acute lymphoblastic leukemia. *Hematol Oncol Clin North Am* 23:991, 2009.

52. Harrison CJ: Cytogenetics of paediatric and adolescent acute lymphoblastic leukaemia. *Br J Haematol* 144:147, 2009.

53. Sherr CJ: The INK4a/ARF network in tumour suppression. *Nat Rev Mol Cell Biol* 2:731, 2001.

54. Weng P, Ferrando AA, Lee W, et al: Activating mutations of NOTCH1 in human T cell acute lymphoblastic leukemia. *Science* 306:269, 2004.

55. Mullighan CG, Goorha S, Radtke I, et al: Genome-wide analysis of genetic alterations in acute lymphoblastic leukemia. *Nature* 446:758, 2007.

56. Mullighan CG, Miller CB, Radtke I, et al: BCR-ABL1 lymphoblastic leukemia is characterized by the deletion of Ikaros. *Nature* 453:110, 2008.

57. Mullighan CG, Su X, Zhang J, et al: Deletion of IKZF1 and prognosis in acute lymphoblastic leukemia. *N Engl J Med* 360:470, 2009.

58. Den Boer ML, van Slegtenhorst M, De Menezes RX, et al: A subtype of childhood acute lymphoblastic leukemia with poor treatment outcome: A genome-wide classification study. *Lancet Oncol* 10:125, 2009.

59. Harvey RC, Mullighan CG, Wang X, et al: Identification of novel cluster groups in pediatric high-risk B-precursor acute lymphoblastic leukemia with gene expression profiling: Correlation with genome-wide DNA copy number alterations, clinical characteristics, and outcome. *Blood* 116; 4874, 2010.

60. Mullighan CG, Collins-Underwood JR, Phillips LA, et al: Rearrangement of CRLF2 in B-progenitor- and Down syndrome-associated acute lymphoblastic leukemia. *Nat Genet* 41:1243, 2009.

61. Ferrando AA, Look AT: Gene expression profiling in T-cell acute lymphoblastic leukemia. *Semin Hematol* 40:274, 2003.

62. Armstrong SA, Kung AL, Mabon ME, et al: Inhibition of FLT3 in MLL: Validation of a therapeutic target identified by gene expression based classification. *Cancer Cell* 3:173, 2003.

63. Garcia-Manero G, Yang H, Kuang SQ, et al: Epigenetics of acute lymphoblastic leukemia. *Semin Hematol* 46:24, 2009.

64. Geng H, Brennan S, Milne TA, et al: Integrative epigenomic analysis identifies biomarkers and therapeutic targets in adult B-acute lymphoblastic leukemia. *Cancer Discov* 2:1004, 2012.

65. Pui CH: Acute lymphoblastic leukemia, in *Childhood Leukemias*, ed 2, edited by Pui CH, p 439. Cambridge University Press, New York, 2006.

66. Freedman AS, Aster JC: Clinical manifestations, pathologic features, and diagnosis of precursor B-cell acute lymphoblastic leukemia/lymphoma, in *UpToDate*, edited by Post TW. UpToDate, Waltham, MA. http://www.uptodate.com/contents/clinical-manifestations-pathologic-features-and-diagnosis-of-precursor-b-cell-acute-lymphoblastic-leukemia-lymphoma. (Accessed on August 07, 2015.)

67. Larson RA, Dodge RK, Burns CP, et al: A five-drug remission induction regimen with intensive consolidation for adults with acute lymphoblastic leukemia: Cancer and Leukemia Group B study 8811. *Blood* 85:2025, 1995.

68. Pui C-H, Stass S, Green A: Bone marrow necrosis in children with malignant disease. *Cancer* 56:1522, 1985.

69. Shah NR, Landi DB, Kreissman SG, et al: Presentation and outcomes for children with bone marrow necrosis and acute lymphoblastic leukemia: A literature review. *J Pediatr Hematol Oncol* 33:e316, 2011.

70. Lowe EJ, Pui CH, Hancock ML, et al: Early complications in children with acute lymphoblastic leukemia presenting with hyperleukocytosis. *Pediatr Blood Cancer* 45:10, 2005.

71. Hijiya N, Liu W, Sandlund JT, et al: Overt testicular disease at diagnosis of childhood acute lymphoblastic leukemia: Lack of therapeutic role of local irradiation. *Leukemia* 19:1399, 2005.

72. Huang MS, Hasserjian RP: Case 19-2004: A 12-year-old boy with fatigue and eosinophilia. *N Engl J Med* 350:2604, 2004.

73. Beutler E: Platelet transfusions: The 20,000/microL trigger. *Blood* 81:1411, 1993.

74. Slichter SJ: Evidence-based platelet transfusion guidelines. *Hematology Am Soc Hematol Educ Program* 2007:172, 2007.

75. Hasle H, Heim S, Schroeder H, et al: Transient pancytopenia preceding acute lymphoblastic leukemia (pre-ALL). *Leukemia* 9:605, 1995.

76. Ribeiro RC, Pui CH: The clinical and biological correlates of coagulopathy in children with acute leukemia. *J Clin Oncol* 4:1212, 1986.

77. Inukai T, Hirose K, Inaba T, et al: Hypercalcemia in childhood acute lymphoblastic leukemia: Frequent implication of parathyroid hormone-related peptide and E2A-HLF from translocation 17;19. *Leukemia* 21:288, 2007.

78. Liang R: How I treat and monitor viral hepatitis B infection in patients receiving intensive immunosuppressive therapies or undergoing hematopoietic stem cell transplantation. *Blood* 113:3147, 2009.

79. Pui CH, Mahmoud HH, Rivera GK, et al: Early intensification of intrathecal chemotherapy virtually eliminates central nervous system relapse in children with acute lymphoblastic leukemia. *Blood* 92:411, 1998.

80. Pui CH, Howard SC: Current management and challenges of malignant disease in the CNS in paediatric leukaemia. *Lancet Oncol* 9:257, 2008.

81. Bürger B, Zimmermann M, Mann G, et al: Diagnostic cerebrospinal fluid examination in children with acute lymphoblastic leukemia: Significance of low leukocyte counts with blasts or traumatic lumbar puncture. *J Clin Oncol* 21:184, 2003.

82. Coustan-Smith E, Mullighan CG, Onciu M, et al: Early T-cell precursor leukaemia: A subtype of very high-risk acute lymphoblastic leukaemia. *Lancet Oncol* 10:147, 2009.

83. Campana D: Minimal residual disease in acute lymphoblastic leukemia. *Semin Hematol* 46:100, 2009.

84. Pui CH, Rubnitz JE, Hancock ML, et al: Reappraisal of the clinical and biologic significance of myeloid-associated antigen expression in childhood acute lymphoblastic leukemia. *J Clin Oncol* 16:3768, 1998.

85. Rubnitz JE, Onciu M, Pounds S, et al: Acute mixed lineage leukemia in children: The experience of St. Jude Children's Research Hospital. *Blood* 113:5083, 2009.

86. Neff T, Armstrong SA: Recent progress toward epigenetic therapies: The example of mixed lineage leukemia. *Blood* 121:4847, 2013.

87. Meijerink JP, Den Boer ML, Pieters R: New genetic abnormalities and treatment response in acute lymphoblastic leukemia. *Semin Hematol* 46:16, 2009.

88. Moorman AV, Harrison CJ, Buck GA, et al: Karyotype is an independent prognostic factor in adult acute lymphoblastic leukemia (ALL): Analysis of cytogenetic data from patients treated on the Medical Research Council (MRC) UKALLXII/Eastern Cooperative Oncology Group (ECOG) 2993 trial. *Blood* 109:3189, 2007.

89. Pullarkat V, Slovak ML, Kopecky KJ, et al: Impact of cytogenetics on the outcome of adult acute lymphoblastic leukemia: Results of Southwest Oncology Group 9400 study. *Blood* 111:2563, 2008.

90. Ito C, Kumagai M, Manabe A, et al: Hyperdiploid acute lymphoblastic leukemia with 51 to 65 chromosomes: A distinct biological entity with a marked propensity to undergo apoptosis. *Blood* 93:315, 1999.

91. Dastugue N, Suciu S, Plat G, et al: Hyperdiploidy with 58-66 chromosomes in childhood B-acute lymphoblastic leukemia is highly curable: 58951 CLG-EORTC results. *Blood* 121:2415, 2013.

92. Nachman JB, Heerema NA, Sather H, et al: Outcome of treatment in children with hypodiploid acute lymphoblastic leukemia. *Blood* 110:1112, 2007.

93. Moorman AV, Richards SM, Robinson HM, et al: Prognosis of children with acute lymphoblastic leukemia (ALL) and intrachromosomal amplification of chromosome 21 (iAMP21). *Blood* 109:2327, 2007.

94. Harrison CJ, Moorman AV, Schwab C, et al: An international study of intrachromosomal amplification of chromosome 21 (iAMP21): Cytogenetic characterization and outcome. *Leukemia* 28:1015, 2014.

95. Paulsson K, Horvat A, Strömbeck B, et al: Mutations in FLT3, NRAS, KRAS, and PTPN11 are frequent and possibly mutually exclusive in high hyperdiploid childhood acute lymphoblastic leukemia. *Genes Chromosomes Cancer* 47:26, 2008.

96. Morely AA, Brisco MJ, Rice M, et al: Leukaemia presenting as marrow hypoplasia: Molecular detection of the leukaemic clone at the time of initial presentation. *Br J Haematol* 98:940, 1997.

97. McKenna RW, Washington LT, Aquino DB, et al: Immunophenotypic analysis of hematogones (B-lymphocyte precursors) in 662 consecutive bone marrow specimens by 4-color flow cytometry. *Blood* 98:2498, 2001.

98. Coiffier B, Altman A, Pui CH, et al: Guidelines for the management of pediatric and adult tumor lysis syndrome: An evidence-based review. *J Clin Oncol* 26:2767, 2008.

99. Masson E, Synold TW, Relling MV, et al: Allopurinol inhibits de novo purine synthesis in lymphoblasts of children with acute lymphoblastic leukemia. *Leukemia* 10:56, 1996.

100. Cairo MS, Coiffier B, Reiter A, Younes A; TLS Expert Panel: Recommendations for the evaluation of risk and prophylaxis of tumour lysis syndrome (TLS) in adults and children with malignant diseases: An expert TLS panel consensus. *Br J Haematol* 149:578, 2010.

101. Pui CH, Boyett JM, Hughes WT, et al: Human granulocyte colony-stimulating factor after induction chemotherapy in children with acute lymphoblastic leukemia. *N Engl J Med* 336:1781, 1997.

102. Larson RA, Dodge RK, Linker CA, et al: A randomized controlled trial of filgrastim during remission induction and consolidation chemotherapy for adults with acute lymphoblastic leukemia: CALGB study 9111. *Blood* 92:1556, 1998.

103. Relling MV, Boyett JM, Blanco JG, et al: Granulocyte-colony stimulating factor and the risk of secondary myeloid malignancy. *Blood* 101:3862, 2003.

104. Madden RM, Pui CH, Hughes WT, et al: Prophylaxis of *Pneumocystis carinii* pneumonia with atovaquone in children with leukemia. *Cancer* 109:1654, 2007.

105. Heckman KD, Weiner GJ, Davis CS, et al: Randomized study of prophylactic platelet transfusion threshold during induction therapy for adult acute leukemia: 10,000/microL versus 20,000/microL. *J Clin Oncol* 15:1143, 1997.

106. Pieters R, Carroll WL: Biology and treatment of acute lymphoblastic leukemia. *Hematol Oncol Clin North Am* 24:1, 2010.

107. Hunger, SP, Lu X, Devidas M, et al: Improved survival for children and adolescents with acute lymphoblastic leukemia between 1990 and 2005: A report from the Children's Oncology Group. *J Clin Oncol* 29:551, 2011.

108. Pui CH, Carroll WL, Meshinchi S, Arceci RJ: Biology, risk stratification, and therapy of pediatric acute leukemias: An update. *J Clin Oncol* 29:551, 2011.

109. Harrison CJ: Targeting signaling pathways in acute lymphoblastic leukemia: New insights. *Hematology Am Soc Hematol Educ Program* 2013:118, 2013.

110. Mann G, Attarbaschi A, Schrappe M, et al; Interfant-99 Study Group: Improved outcome with hematopoietic stem cell transplantation in a poor prognostic subgroup of infants with mixed-lineage-leukemia (MLL)-rearranged acute lymphoblastic leukemia: Results from the Interfant-99 Study. *Blood* 116:2644, 2010.

111. Larson RA: Management of acute lymphoblastic leukemia in older patients. *Semin Hematol* 43:126, 2006.

112. Gokbuget N: How I treat older patients with ALL. *Blood* 122:1366, 2013.

113. Fielding AK: How I treat Philadelphia chromosome-positive acute lymphoblastic leukemia. *Blood* 116:3409, 2010.

114. Foa R, Vitale A, Vignetti M, et al; GIMEMA Acute Leukemia Working Party: Dasatinib as first-line treatment for adult patients with Philadelphia chromosome-positive acute lymphoblastic leukemia. *Blood* 118:6521, 2011.

115. Patte C, Auperin A, Michon J, et al: The Société Francaise d'Oncologie Pédiatrique LMB89 protocol: Highly effective multiagent chemotherapy tailored to the tumor burden and initial response in 561 unselected children with B-cell lymphomas and L3 leukemia. *Blood* 97:3370, 2001.

116. Cairo MS, Gerrard M, Sposto R, et al: Results of a randomized international study of high-risk central nervous system B non-Hodgkin lymphoma and B acute lymphoblastic leukemia in children and adolescents. *Blood* 109:2736, 2007.

117. Woessmann W, Seidemann K, Mann G, et al: The impact of the methotrexate administration schedule and dose in the treatment of children and adolescents with B-cell neoplasms: A report of the BFM Group Study NHL-BFM95. *Blood* 105:948, 2005.

118. Thomas DA, Faderl S, O'Brien S, et al: Chemoimmunotherapy with hyper-CVAD plus rituximab for the treatment of adult Burkitt and Burkitt-type lymphoma or acute lymphoblastic leukemia. *Cancer* 106:1569, 2006.

119. Mead GM, Barrans SL, Qian W, et al. for the UK National Cancer Research Institute Lymphoma Clinical Studies Group, Australasian Leukaemia and Lymphoma Group: A prospective clinicopathologic study of dose-modified CODOX-M/IVAC in patients with sporadic Burkitt lymphoma defined using cytogenetic and immunophenotypic criteria (MRC/NCRI LY10 trial). *Blood* 112:2248, 2008.

120. Rizzieri DA, Johnson JL, Byrd JC, et al; Alliance for Clinical Trials In Oncology (ACTION): Improved efficacy using rituximab and brief duration, high intensity chemotherapy with filgrastim support for Burkitt or aggressive lymphomas: Cancer and Leukemia Group B study 10002. *Br J Haematol* 165:102, 2014.

121. Schrappe M, Möricke A, Reiter A, et al: Key treatment questions in childhood acute lymphoblastic leukemia: Results in 5 consecutive trials performed by the ALL-BFM study group from 1981 to 2000. *Klin Padiatr* 225 Suppl 1:S62, 2013.

122. Pui CH, Campana D: New definition of remission in childhood acute lymphoblastic leukemia. *Leukemia* 14:783, 2000.

123. Borowitz MJ, Devidas M, Hunger S, et al: Clinical significance of minimal residual disease in childhood acute lymphoblastic leukemia and its relationship to other prognostic factors: A Children's Oncology Group study. *Blood* 111:5477, 2008.

124. Bruggemann M, Schrauder A, Raff R, et al; European Working Group for Adult Acute Lymphoblastic Leukemia (EWALL) and the International Berlin-Frankfurt-Munster Study Group (I-BFM-SG), Standardized MRD quantification in European ALL trials: Proceedings of the Second International Symposium on MRD assessment in Kiel, Germany, 18-20 September 2008. *Leukemia* 24:521, 2010.

125. Schrappe M: Minimal residual disease: Optimal methods, timing, and clinical relevance for an individual patient. *Hematology Am Soc Hematol Educ Program* 2012:137, 2012.

126. Gaipa G, Basso G, Biondi A, Campana D: Detection of minimal residual disease in pediatric acute lymphoblastic leukemia. *Cytometry B Clin Cytom* 84:359, 2013.

127. Bassan R, Spinelli O, Oldani E, et al: Improved risk classification for risk-specific therapy based on the molecular study of minimal residual disease (MRD) in adult acute lymphoblastic leukemia (ALL). *Blood* 113:4153, 2009.

128. Patel B, Rai L, Buck, et al: Minimal residual disease is a significant predictor of treatment failure in non T-lineage adult acute lymphoblastic leukemia: Final results of the international trial UKALL XII/ECOG 2993. *Br J Haematol* 148:80, 2010.

129. Beldjord K, Chevret S, Aasnafi V, et al; Group for Research on Adult Acute Lymphoblastic Leukemia (GRAALL): Oncogenetics and minimal residual disease are independent outcome predictors in adult patients with acute lymphoblastic leukemia. *Blood* 123:3739, 2014.

130. Annino L, Vegna ML, Camera A, et al: Treatment of adult acute lymphoblastic leukemia (ALL): Long-term follow-up of the GIMEMA ALL 0288 randomized study. *Blood* 99:863, 2002.

131. Stock W, Johnson JL, Stone RM, et al: Dose intensification of daunorubicin and cytarabine during treatment of adult acute lymphoblastic leukemia: Results of Cancer and Leukemia Group B Study 19802. *Cancer* 119:90, 2013.

132. Conter V, Bartram CR, Valsecchi MG, et al: Molecular response to treatment redefines all prognostic factors in children and adolescents with B-cell precursor acute lymphoblastic leukemia: Results in 3184 patients of the AIEOP-BFM ALL 2000 study. *Blood* 115:3206, 2010.

133. Bostrom BC, Sensel MR, Sather HN, et al: Dexamethasone versus prednisone and daily oral versus weekly intravenous mercaptopurine for patients with standard-risk acute lymphoblastic leukemia: A report from the Children's Cancer Group. *Blood* 101:3809, 2003.

134. Mitchell CD, Richards SM, Kinsey SE, et al: Benefit of dexamethasone compared with prednisolone for childhood acute lymphoblastic leukaemia: Results of the UK Medical Research Council ALL97 randomized trial. *Br J Haematol* 129:734, 2005.

135. Asselin BL, Whitin JC, Coppola DJ, et al: Comparative pharmacokinetic studies of three asparaginase preparations. *J Clin Oncol* 11:1780, 1993.

136. Douer D, Yampolsky H, Cohen LJ, et al: Pharmacodynamics and safety of intravenous pegaspargase during remission induction in adults aged 55 years or younger with newly diagnosed acute lymphoblastic leukemia. *Blood* 109:2744, 2007.

137. Vrooman LM, Stevenson KE, Supko JG, et al: Postinduction dexamethasone and individualized dosing of Escherichia coli L-asparaginase each improve outcome of children and adolescents with newly diagnosed acute lymphoblastic leukemia: Results from a randomized study—Dana-Farber Cancer Institute ALL Consortium Protocol 00-01. *J Clin Oncol* 31:1202, 2013.

138. Wetzler M, Sanford BL, Kurtzberg J, et al: Effective asparagine depletion with pegylated asparaginase results in improved outcomes in adult acute lymphoblastic leukemia: Cancer and Leukemia Group B Study 9511. *Blood* 109:4164, 2007.

139. Douer D, Aldoss I, Lunning MA, et al: Pharmacokinetics-based integration of multiple doses of intravenous pegaspargase in a pediatric regimen for adults with newly diagnosed acute lymphoblastic leukemia. *J Clin Oncol* 32:905, 2014.

140. Stock W, Douer D, DeAngelo DJ, et al: Prevention and management of asparaginase/pegasparaginase-associated toxicities in adults and older adolescents: Recommendations of an expert panel. *Leuk Lymphoma* 52:2237, 2011.

141. Schrappe M, Reiter A, Ludwig WD, et al: Improved outcome in childhood acute lymphoblastic leukemia despite reduced use of anthracyclines and cranial radiotherapy: Results of trial ALL-BFM 90. German-Austrian-Swiss ALL-BFM Study Group. *Blood* 95:3310, 2000.

142. Nachman JB, Sather HN, Sensel MG, et al: Augmented post-induction therapy for children with high-risk acute lymphoblastic leukemia and a slow response to initial therapy. *N Engl J Med* 338:1663, 1998.

143. Chessells JM, Bailey C, Richards SM: Intensification of treatment and survival in all children with lymphoblastic leukaemia: Results of UK Medical Research Council Trial

UKALL X. Medical Research Council Working Party on Childhood Leukaemia. *Lancet* 345:143, 1995.

144. Pui CH, Sandlund JT, Pei D, et al: Improved outcome for children with acute lymphoblastic leukemia: Results of Total Therapy Study XIIIB at St. Jude Children's Research Hospital. *Blood* 104:2690, 2004.

145. Loh ML, Goldwasser MA, Silverman LB, et al: Prospective analysis of TEL/AML1-positive patients treated on Dana-Farber Cancer Institute Consortium Protocol 95-01. *Blood* 107:4508, 2006.

146. Asselin BL, Devida M, Wang C, et al: Effectiveness of high-dose methotrexate in T-cell lymphoblastic leukemia and advanced-stage lymphoblastic lymphoma: A randomized study by the Children's Oncology Group (POG 9404). *Blood* 118:874, 2011.

147. Galpin AJ, Schuetz JD, Masson E, et al: Differences in folylpolyglutamate synthetase and dihydrofolate reductase expression in human B-lineage versus T-lineage leukemic lymphoblasts: Mechanisms for lineage differences in methotrexate polyglutamylation and cytotoxicity. *Mol Pharmacol* 52:155, 1997.

148. Mikkelsen TS, Sparreboom A, Cheng C, et al: Shortening infusion time for high-dose methotrexate alters antileukemic effects: A randomized prospective clinical trial. *J Clin Oncol* 29:1771, 2011.

149. Kager L, Cheok M, Yang W, et al: Folate pathway gene expression differs in subtypes of acute lymphoblastic leukemia and influences methotrexate pharmacodynamics. *J Clin Invest* 115:110, 2005.

150. Hoelzer D, Gökbuget N: Chemoimmunotherapy in acute lymphoblastic leukemia. *Blood Rev* 26:25, 2012.

151. Thomas DA, O'Brien S, Faderl S, et al: Chemoimmunotherapy with a modified hyper-CVAD and rituximab regimen improves outcome in de novo Philadelphia chromosome-negative precursor B-lineage acute lymphoblastic leukemia. *J Clin Oncol* 28:3880, 2010.

152. Rowe JM, Buck G, Burnett AK, et al. for the ECOG and the MRC/NCRI Adult Leukemia Working Party: Induction therapy for adults with acute lymphoblastic leukemia: Results of more than 1500 patients from the international ALL trial: MRC UKALL XII/ECOG E2993. *Blood* 106:3760, 2005.

153. Huguet F, Leguay T, Raffoux E, et al: Pediatric-inspired therapy in adults with Philadelphia chromosome-negative acute lymphoblastic leukemia: The GRAALL-2003 study. *J Clin Oncol* 27:911, 2009.

154. Ludwig WD, Rieder H, Bartram CR, et al: Immunophenotypic and genotypic features, clinical characteristics, and treatment outcome of adult pro-B acute lymphoblastic leukemia: Results of the German multicenter trials GMALL 03/87 and 04/89. *Blood* 92:1898, 1998.

155. Nakano TA, Hunger SP: Blood consult: Therapeutic strategy and complications in the adolescent and young adult with acute lymphoblastic leukemia. *Blood* 119:4372, 2012.

156. Stock W, La M, Sanford B, et al: What determines the outcomes for adolescents and young adults with acute lymphoblastic leukemia treated on cooperative group protocols? A comparison of Children's Cancer Group and Cancer and Leukemia Group B studies. *Blood* 112:1646, 2008.

157. Boissel N, Auclerc MF, Lhéritier V, et al: Should adolescents with acute lymphoblastic leukemia be treated as old children or young adults? Comparison of the French FRALLE-93 and LALA-94 trials. *J Clin Oncol* 21:774, 2003.

158. Ribera JM, Oriol A, Sanz MA, et al: Comparison of the results of the treatment of adolescents and young adults with standard-risk acute lymphoblastic leukemia with the Programa Espanol de Tratamiento en Hematologia Pediatric-based protocol 96. *J Clin Oncol* 26:1843, 2008.

159. Nachman JB, La MK, Hunger SP, et al: Young adults with acute lymphoblastic leukemia have an excellent outcome with chemotherapy alone and benefit from intensive postinduction treatment: A report from the Children's Oncology Group. *J Clin Oncol* 27:5189, 2009.

160. Pui CH, Pei D, Campana D, et al: Improved prognosis for older adolescents with acute lymphoblastic leukemia. *J Clin Oncol* 29:386, 2011.

161. Schafer ES, Hunger SP: Optimal therapy for acute lymphoblastic leukemia in adolescents and young adults. *Nat Rev Clin Oncol* 8:417, 2011.

162. Deangelo DJ, Stevenson KE, Dahlberg SE, et al: Long-term outcome of a pediatric-inspired regimen used for adults ages 18 to 50 with newly diagnosed acute lymphoblastic leukemia. *Leukemia* 29:526, 2015.

163. Riehm H, Gadner H, Henze G, et al: Results and significance of six randomized trials in four consecutive ALL-BFM studies. *Haematol Blood Transfus* 33:439, 1990.

164. Toyoda Y, Manabe A, Tsuchida M, et al: Six months of maintenance chemotherapy after intensified treatment for acute lymphoblastic leukemia of childhood. *J Clin Oncol* 18:1508, 2000.

165. Childhood ALL Collaborative Group: Duration and intensity of maintenance chemotherapy in acute lymphoblastic leukaemia: Overview of 42 trials involving 12,000 randomised children. *Lancet* 347:1783, 1996.

166. Sather H, Miller D, Nesbit M, et al: Differences in prognosis for boys and girls with acute lymphoblastic leukaemia. *Lancet* 1:739, 1981.

167. The Medical Research Council's Working Party on Leukaemia in Childhood: Duration of chemotherapy-in-childhood acute lymphoblastic leukaemia. *Med Pediatr Oncol* 10:511, 1982.

168. Schmiegelow K, Schroder H, Gustafsson G, et al: Risk of relapse in childhood acute lymphoblastic leukaemia is related to RBC methotrexate and mercaptopurine metabolites during maintenance chemotherapy. Nordic Society for Pediatric Hematology and Oncology. *J Clin Oncol* 13:345, 1995.

169. Chessells JM, Harrison G, Lilleyman JS, et al: Continuing (maintenance) therapy in lymphoblastic leukaemia: Lessons from MRC UKALL X. Medical Research Council Working Party in Childhood Leukaemia. *Br J Haematol* 98:945, 1997.

170. Relling MV, Hancock ML, Boyett JM, et al: Prognostic importance of 6-mercaptopurine dose intensity in acute lymphoblastic leukemia. *Blood* 93:2817, 1999.

171. Schmiegelow K, Glomstein A, Kristinsson J, et al: Impact of morning versus evening schedule for oral methotrexate and 6-mercaptopurine on relapse risk for children with acute lymphoblastic leukemia. Nordic Society for Pediatric Hematology and Oncology (NOPHO). *J Pediatr Hematol Oncol* 19:102, 1997.

172. Rivard GE, Lin KT, Leclerc JM, David M: Milk could decrease the bioavailability of 6-mercaptopurine. *Am J Pediatr Hematol Oncol* 11:402, 1989.

173. Farrow AC, Buchanan GR, Zwiener RJ, et al: Serum aminotransferase elevation during and following treatment of childhood acute lymphoblastic leukemia. *J Clin Oncol* 15:1560, 1997.

174. Evans WE, Horner M, Chu YQ, et al: Altered mercaptopurine metabolism, toxic effects, and dosage requirement in a thiopurine methyltransferase-deficient child with acute lymphocytic leukemia. *J Pediatr* 119:985, 1991.

175. Relling MV, Hancock ML, Rivera GK, et al: Mercaptopurine therapy intolerance and heterozygosity at the thiopurine S-methyltransferase gene locus. *J Natl Cancer Inst* 91:2001, 1999.

176. Pui CH, Relling MV: Topoisomerase II inhibitor-related acute myeloid leukaemia. *Br J Haematol* 109:13, 2000.

177. Schmiegelow K, Al-Modhwahi I, Andersen MK, et al: Methotrexate/6-mercaptopurine maintenance therapy influences the risk of a second malignant neoplasm after childhood acute lymphoblastic leukemia: Results from the NOPHOALL-92 study. *Blood* 113:6077, 2009.

178. Relling MV, Rubnitz JE, Rivera GK, et al: High incidence of secondary brain tumours after radiotherapy and antimetabolites. *Lancet* 354:34, 1999.

179. Cheok MH, Pottier N, Kager L, Evans WE: Pharmacogenetics in acute lymphoblastic leukemia. *Semin Hematol* 46:39, 2009.

180. Relling MV, Ramsey LB: Pharmacogenomics of acute lymphoid leukemia: New insights into treatment toxicity and efficacy. *Hematology Am Soc Hematol Educ Program* 2013:126, 2013.

181. Jacobs SS, Stork LC, Bostrom BC, et al: Substitution of oral and intravenous thioguanine for mercaptopurine in a treatment regimen for children with standard risk acute lymphoblastic leukemia: A collaborative Children's Oncology Group/National Cancer Institute pilot trial (CCG-1942). *Pediatr Blood Cancer* 49:250, 2007.

182. Vora A, Mitchell CD, Lennard L, et al: Toxicity and efficacy of 6-thioguanine versus 6-mercaptopurine in childhood lymphoblastic leukaemia: A randomised trial. *Lancet* 368:1339, 2006.

183. Eden T, Pieters R, Richards S; Childhood Acute Lymphoblastic Leukaemia Collaborative Group (CALLCG): Systematic review of the addition of vincristine plus steroid pulses in maintenance treatment for childhood acute lymphoblastic leukaemia—An individual patient data meta-analysis involving 5,659 children. *Br J Haematol* 149:722, 2010.

184. Mattano LA Jr, Devidas M, Nachman JB, et al. for the Children's Oncology Group: Effect of alternate-week versus continuous dexamethasone scheduling on the risk of osteonecrosis in paediatric patients with acute lymphoblastic leukaemia: Results from the CCG-1961 randomised cohort trial. *Lancet Oncol* 13:906, 2012.

185. Lange BJ, Bostrom BC, Cherlow JM, et al: Double-delayed intensification improves event-free survival for children with intermediate-risk acute lymphoblastic leukemia: A report from the Children's Cancer Group. *Blood* 99:825, 2002.

186. Pui CH, Thiel E: Central nervous system disease in hematologic malignancies: Historical perspective and practical applications. *Semin Oncol* 36(4 Suppl 2):S2, 2009.

187. Vilmer E, Suciu S, Ferster A, et al: Long-term results of three randomized trials (58831, 58832, 58881) in childhood acute lymphoblastic leukemia: A CLCG-EORTC report. *Leukemia* 14:2257, 2000.

188. Manera R, Ramirez I, Mullins J, Pinkel D: Pilot studies of species-specific chemotherapy of childhood acute lymphoblastic leukemia using genotype and immunophenotype. *Leukemia* 14:1354, 2000.

189. Conter V, Schrappe M, Aric M, et al: Role of cranial radiotherapy for childhood T-cell acute lymphoblastic leukemia with high WBC count and good response to prednisone. Associazione Italiana Ematalogia Oncologia Pediatrica and the Berlin-Frankfurt-Munster groups. *J Clin Oncol* 15:2786, 1997.

190. Pui CH, Campana D, Pei D, et al: Treating childhood acute lymphoblastic leukemia without prophylactic cranial irradiation. *N Engl J Med* 360:2730, 2009.

191. Veerman AJ, Kamps WA, ven den Berg H, et al: Dexamethasone-based therapy for childhood acute lymphoblastic leukaemia: Results of the prospective Dutch Childhood Oncology Group (DCOG) protocol ALL-9 (1997–2004). *Lancet Oncol* 10:957, 2009.

192. Richards S, Pui CH, Gayon P; Childhood Acute Lymphoblastic Leukemia Collaborative Group (CALLCG): Systematic review and meta-analysis of randomized trials of central nervous system directed therapy for childhood acute lymphoblastic leukemia. *Pediatr Blood Cancer* 60:185, 2013.

193. Matloub Y, Lindemulder S, Gaynon PS, et al: Intrathecal triple therapy decreases central nervous system relapse but fails to improve event-free survival when compared to intrathecal methotrexate: Results of the Children's Cancer Group (CCG) 1952 study for standard-risk acute lymphoblastic leukemia. A report from the Children's Oncology Group. *Blood* 108:1165, 2006.

194. Oliansky DM, Larson RA, Weisdorf D, et al: The role of cytotoxic therapy with hematopoietic stem cell transplantation in the treatment of adult acute lymphoblastic leukemia: Update of the 2006 evidence-based review. *Biol Blood Marrow Transplant* 18:18, 2012.

195. Goldstone AH, Richards SM, Lazarus HM, et al: In adults with standard-risk acute lymphoblastic leukemia, the greatest benefit is achieved from a matched sibling allogeneic transplantation in first complete remission, and an autologous transplantation is less effective than conventional consolidation/maintenance chemotherapy in all patients: Final results of the International ALL Trial (MRC UKALL XII/ECOG E2993). *Blood* 111:1827, 2008.

196. Gupta V, Richards S, Rowe J, Acute Leukemia Stem Cell Transplantation Trialists' Collaborative Group: Allogeneic, but not autologous, hematopoietic cell transplantation improves survival only among younger adults with acute lymphoblastic leukemia in first remission: An individual patient data meta-analysis. *Blood* 121:339, 2013.

197. Mark DJ, Perez WS, He W, et al: Unrelated donor transplants in adults with Philadelphia-negative acute lymphoblastic leukemia in first complete remission. *Blood* 112:426, 2008.

198. Aricò M, Valsecchi MG, Camitta B, et al: Outcome of treatment in children with Philadelphia chromosome-positive acute lymphoblastic leukemia. *N Engl J Med* 342:998, 2000.

199. Arico M, Schrappe M, Hunger SP, et al: Clinical outcome of children with newly diagnosed Philadelphia chromosome-positive acute lymphoblastic leukemia treated between 1995 and 2005. *J Clin Oncol* 28:4755, 2010.

200. Schultz KR, Bowman WP, Aledo A, et al: Improved early event free survival with imatinib in Philadelphia chromosome-positive acute lymphoblastic leukemia: A Children's Oncology Group Study. *J Clin Oncol* 27:5715, 2009.

201. Schultz KR, Carroll A, Heerema NA, et al: Long-term follow-up of imatinib in pediatric Philadelphia chromosome-positive acute lymphoblastic leukemia: Children's Oncology Group Study AALL0031. *Leukemia* 28:1467, 2014.

202. Pui CH, Gaynon PS, Boyett JM, et al: Outcome of treatment in childhood acute lymphoblastic leukaemia with rearrangements of the 11q23 chromosomal region. *Lancet* 359:1909, 2002.

203. Rowe JM: Interpreting data on transplant selection outcome in adult acute lymphoblastic leukemia (ALL). *Biol Blood Marrow Transplant* 17:S76, 2011.

204. Pidala J, Djulbegovic B, Anasetti C, et al: Allogeneic hematopoietic cell transplantation for adult acute lymphoblastic leukemia (ALL) in first complete remission. *Cochrane Database Syst Rev* (10):CD008818, 2011.

205. Tucunduva L, Ruggeri A, Sanz G, et al: Risk factors for outcomes after unrelated cord blood transplantation for adults with acute lymphoblastic leukemia: A report on behalf of Eurocord and the Acute Leukemia Working party of the European Group for Blood and Marrow Transplantation. *Bone Marrow Transplant* 49:887, 2014.

206. Bachanova V, Verneris MR, DeFor T, et al: Prolonged survival in adults with acute lymphoblastic leukemia after reduced-intensity conditioning with cord blood or sibling donor transplantation. *Blood* 113:2902, 2009.

207. Mohty M, Labopin M, Volin L, et al: Reduced-intensity versus conventional myeloablative conditioning allogeneic stem cell transplantation for patients with acute lymphoblastic leukemia: A retrospective study from the European Group for Blood and Marrow Transplantation. *Blood* 116:4439, 2010.

208. Wetzler M, Watson D, Stock W, et al: Autologous transplantation for Philadelphia chromosome-positive acute lymphoblastic leukemia achieves outcomes similar to allogeneic transplantation: Results of CALGB Study 10001 (Alliance). *Haematologica* 99:111, 2014.

209. Giebel S, Labopin M, Gorin NC, et al: Improving results of autologous stem cell transplantation for Philadelphia-positive acute lymphoblastic leukaemia in the era of tyrosine kinase inhibitors: A report from the Acute Leukaemia Working Party of the European Group for Blood and Marrow Transplantation. *Eur J Cancer* 50:411, 2014.

210. Ottmann OG, Wassmann B, Pfeifer H, et al: Imatinib compared with chemotherapy as front-line treatment of elderly patients with Philadelphia chromosome-positive acute lymphoblastic leukemia (Ph+ALL). *Cancer* 109:2068, 2007.

211. Vignetti M, Fazi P, Cimino G, et al: Imatinib plus steroids induces complete remissions and prolonged survival in elderly Philadelphia chromosome-positive acute lymphoblastic leukemia patients without additional chemotherapy: Results of the GIMEMA LAL0201-B protocol. *Blood* 109:3676, 2007.

212. Thomas DA, Faderl S, Cortes J, et al: Treatment of Philadelphia chromosome-positive acute lymphocytic leukemia with hyper-CVAD and imatinib mesylate. *Blood* 103:4396, 2004.

213. Fielding AK, Rowe JM, Buck G, et al: UKALL XII/ECOG 2993: Addition of imatinib to a standard treatment regimen enhances long-term outcomes in Philadelphia positive acute lymphoblastic leukemia. *Blood* 123:843, 2014.

214. Ravandi F, O'Brien S, Thomas D, et al: First report of phase 2 study of dasatinib with hyper-CVAD for the frontline treatment of patients with Philadelphia chromosome-positive (Ph+) acute lymphoblastic leukemia. *Blood* 116:2070, 2010.

215. Zwaan CM, Rizzari C, Mechinaud F, et al: Dasatinib in children and adolescents with relapsed or refractory leukemia: Results of the CA180-018 phase I dose-escalation study of the Innovative Therapies for Children with Cancer Consortium. *J Clin Oncol* 31:2460, 2013.

216. Biondi A, Schrappe M, De Lorenzo P, et al: Imatinib after induction for treatment of children and adolescents with Philadelphia-chromosome-positive acute lymphoblastic leukaemia (EsPhALL): A randomised, open-label, intergroup study. *Lancet Oncol* 13:936, 2012.

217. Bachanova V, Marks DI, Zhang MJ, et al: Ph+ ALL patients in first complete remission have similar survival after reduced intensity and myeloablative allogeneic transplantation: Impact of tyrosine kinase inhibitor and minimal residual disease. *Leukemia* 28:658, 2014.

218. Campana D, Leung W: Clinical significance of minimal residual disease in patients with acute leukaemia undergoing haematopoietic stem cell transplantation. *Br J Haematol* 162:147, 2013.

219. Wassermann B, Pfeifer H, Stadler M, et al: Early molecular response to posttransplantation imatinib determines outcome in MRD+ Philadelphia-positive acute lymphoblastic leukemia (PH+ALL). *Blood* 106:458, 2005.

220. Thomas DA, O'Brien S, Jorgensen JL, et al: Prognostic significance of CD20 expression in adults with de novo precursor B-lineage acute lymphoblastic leukemia. *Blood* 113:6330, 2009.

221. Jeha S, Behm F, Pei D, et al: Prognostic significance of CD20 expression in childhood B-cell precursor acute lymphoblastic leukemia. *Blood* 108:3302, 2006.

222. Thomas DA, O'Brien S, Faderl S, et al: Chemoimmunotherapy with a modified hyper-CVAD and rituximab regimen improves outcome in de novo Philadelphia chromosome-negative precursor B-lineage acute lymphoblastic leukemia. *J Clin Oncol* 28:3880, 2010.

223. Advani AS: New immune strategies for the treatment of acute lymphoblastic leukemia: Antibodies and chimeric antigen receptors. *Hematology Am Soc Hematol Educ Program* 2013:131, 2013.

224. DeAngelo DJ, Yu D, Johnson JL, et al: Nelarabine induces complete remissions in adults with relapsed or refractory T-lineage acute lymphoblastic leukemia or lymphoblastic lymphoma: Cancer and Leukemia Group B study 19801. *Blood* 109:5136, 2007.

225. Cohen MH, Johnson JR, Justice R, Pazdur R: FDA drug approval summary: Nelarabine (Arranon) for the treatment of T-cell lymphoblastic leukemia/lymphoma. *Oncologist* 13:709, 2008.

226. Dunsmore KP, Devidas M, Linda SB, et al: Pilot study of nelarabine in combination with intensive chemotherapy in high-risk T-cell acute lymphoblastic leukemia: A report from the Children's Oncology Group. *J Clin Oncol* 30:2753, 2012.

227. Bhojwani D, Pui CH: Relapsed childhood acute lymphoblastic leukaemia. *Lancet Oncol* 14:e205, 2013.

228. Mullighan GC, Phillips LA, Su X, et al: Genomic analysis of the clonal origins of relapsed acute lymphoblastic leukemia. *Science* 322:1377, 2008.

229. O'Brien S, Schiller G, Lister J, et al: High-dose vincristine sulphate liposome injection for advanced, relapsed, and refractory adult Philadelphia chromosome-negative acute lymphoblastic leukemia. *J Clin Oncol* 31:676, 2013.

230. Huguet F, Leguay T, Raffoux E, et al: Clofarabine for the treatment of adult acute lymphoid leukemia: A review article by the GRAALL intergroup. *Leuk Lymphoma* 4:1, 2014.

231. Locatelli F, Schrappe M, Bernardo ME, Rutella S: How I treat relapsed childhood acute lymphoblastic leukemia. *Blood* 120:2807, 2012.

232. Nguyen K, Devidas M, Cheng SC, et al: Factors influencing survival after relapse from acute lymphoblastic leukemia: A Children's Oncology Group study. *Leukemia* 22:2142, 2008.

233. Bhatla T, Jones CL, Meyer JA, et al: The biology of relapsed acute lymphoblastic leukemia: Opportunities for therapeutic interventions. *J Pediatr Hematol Oncol* 36:413, 2014.

234. Freyer DR, Devidas M, La M, et al: Postrelapse survival in childhood acute lymphoblastic leukemia is independent of initial treatment intensity: A report from the Children's Oncology Group. *Blood* 117:3010, 2011.

235. Paganin M, Zecca M, Fabbri G, et al: Minimal residual disease is an important predictive factor of outcome in children with relapsed "high-risk" acute lymphoblastic leukemia. *Leukemia* 22:2193, 2008.

236. Doney K, Hagglund H, Leisenring W, et al: Predictive factors for outcome of allogeneic hematopoietic cell transplantation for adult acute lymphoblastic leukemia. *Biol Blood Marrow Transplant* 9:472, 2003.

237. Borgmann A, Schmid H, Hartmann R, et al: Autologous bone-marrow transplants compared with chemotherapy for children with acute lymphoblastic leukaemia in a second remission: A matched-pair analysis. The Berlin-Frankfurt-Munster Study Group. *Lancet* 346:873, 1995.

238. Smith AR, Baker KS, Defor TE, et al: Hematopoietic cell transplantation for children with acute lymphoblastic leukemia in second complete remission: Similar outcomes in recipients of unrelated marrow and umbilical cord blood versus marrow from HLA matched sibling donors. *Biol Blood Marrow Transplant* 15:1086, 2009.

239. Marks DI, Woo KA, Zhong X, et al: Unrelated umbilical cord blood transplant for adult acute lymphoblastic leukemia in first and second complete remission: A comparison with allografts from adult unrelated donors. *Haematologica* 99:322, 2014.

240. Doney K, Gooley TA, Deeg HJ, et al: Allogeneic hematopoietic cell transplantation with full-intensity conditioning for adult acute lymphoblastic leukemia: Results from a single center, 1998-2006. *Biol Blood Marrow Transplant* 17:1187, 2011.

241. Borgmann A, von Stackelberg A, Hartmann R, et al: Unrelated donor stem cell transplantation compared with chemotherapy for children with acute lymphoblastic leukemia in a second remission: A matched-pair analysis. *Blood* 101:3835, 2003.

242. Spyridonidis A, Labopin M, Schmid C, et al: Outcomes and prognostic factors of adults with acute lymphoblastic leukemia who relapse after allogeneic hematopoietic cell transplantation. An analysis on behalf of the Acute Leukemia Working Party of EBMT. *Leukemia* 26:1211, 2012.

243. Hagedorn N, Acquaviva C, Fronkova E, et al: Submicroscopic bone marrow involvement in isolated extramedullary relapses in childhood acute lymphoblastic leukemia: A more precise definition of "isolated" and its possible clinical implications, a collaborative study of the Resistant Disease Committee of the international BFM study group. *Blood* 110:4022, 2007.

244. Ribeiro RC, Rivera GK, Hudson M, et al: An intensive re-treatment protocol for children with an isolated CNS relapse of acute lymphoblastic leukemia. *J Clin Oncol* 13:333, 1995.

245. Ritchey AK, Pollock BH, Lauer SJ, et al: Improved survival of children with isolated CNS relapse of acute lymphoblastic leukemia: A Pediatric Oncology Group study. *J Clin Oncol* 17:3745, 1999.

246. Barredo J, Devidas M, Lauer SJ, et al: Isolated CNS relapse of acute lymphoblastic leukemia treated with intensive systemic chemotherapy and delayed CNS radiation: A Pediatric Oncology Group study. *J Clin Oncol* 24:3142, 2006.

247. Wofford MM, Smith SD, Shuster JJ, et al: Treatment of occult or late overt testicular relapse in children with acute lymphoblastic leukemia: A Pediatric Oncology Group study. *J Clin Oncol* 10:624, 1992.

248. Finklestein JZ, Miller DR, Feusner J, et al: Treatment of overt isolated testicular relapse in children on therapy for acute lymphoblastic leukemia. A report from the Children's Cancer Group. *Cancer* 73:219, 1994.

249. van den Berg H, Langeveld NE, Veenhof CH, Behrendt H: Treatment of isolated testicular recurrence of acute lymphoblastic leukemia without radiotherapy. Report from the Dutch Late Effects Study Group. *Cancer* 79:2257, 1997.

250. Roberson JR, Raju S, Shelso J, et al: Diabetic ketoacidosis during therapy for childhood acute lymphoblastic leukemia. *Pediatr Blood Cancer* 50:1207, 2008.

251. Pui CH, Burghen GA, Bowman WP, Aur RJ: Risk factors for hyperglycemia in children with leukemia receiving l-asparaginase and prednisone. *J Pediatr* 99:46, 1981.

252. Laningham FH, Kun LE, Reddick, et al: Childhood central nervous system leukemia: Historical perspectives, current therapy, and acute neurological sequelae. *Neuroradiology* 49:873, 2007.

253. Bhojwani D, Sabin ND, Pei D, et al: Methotrexate-induced neurotoxicity and leukoencephalopathy in childhood acute lymphoblastic leukemia. *J Clin Oncol* 32:949, 2014.

254. Kadan-Lottick NS, Dinu I, Wasilewski-Masker K, et al: Osteonecrosis in adult survivors of childhood cancer: A report from the childhood cancer survivor study. *J Clin Oncol* 26:3038, 2008.

255. Rai SN, Hudson MM, McCammon E, et al: Implementing an intervention to improve bone mineral density in survivors of childhood acute lymphoblastic leukemia: BONEII, a prospective placebo-controlled double-blind randomized interventional longitudinal study design. *Contemp Clin Trials* 29:711, 2008.

256. Thomas IH, Donohue JE, Ness KK, et al: Bone mineral density in your adult survivors of acute lymphoblastic leukemia. *Cancer* 113:3248, 2008.

257. Te Winkel ML, Pieters R, Wind EJ, et al: Management and treatment of osteonecrosis in children and adolescents with acute lymphoblastic leukemia. *Haematologica* 99:430, 2014.

258. Grenier MA, Lipshultz SE: Epidemiology of anthracycline cardiotoxicity in children and adults. *Semin Oncol* 25:72, 1998.

259. Childhood Acute Lymphoblastic Leukaemia Collaborative Group (CALLCG): Beneficial and harmful effects of anthracyclines in the treatment of childhood acute lymphoblastic leukaemia: A systematic review and meta-analysis. *Br J Haematol* 145:376, 2009.

260. Zerra P, Cochran TR, Franco VI, Lipshultz SE: An expert opinion on pharmacologic approaches to reducing the cardiotoxicity of childhood acute lymphoblastic leukemia therapies. *Expert Opin Pharmacother* 14:1497, 2013.

261. Levitt GA, Dorup I, Sorensen K, Sullivan I: Does anthracycline administration by infusion in children affect late cardiotoxicity? *Br J Haematol* 124:463, 2004.

262. Lipshultz S, Lipsitz SR, Sallan SE, et al: Chronic progressive cardiac dysfunction years after doxorubicin therapy for acute lymphoblastic leukemia. *J Clin Oncol* 23:2629, 2005.

263. Lipshultz SE, Rifai N, Dalton VM, et al: The effect of dexrazoxane on myocardial injury in doxorubicin-treated children with acute lymphoblastic leukemia. *N Engl J Med* 351:145, 2004.

264. Sieswerda E, van Dalen EC, Postma A, et al: Medical interventions for treating anthracycline-induced symptomatic and asymptomatic cardiotoxicity during and after treatment for childhood cancer. *Cochrane Database Syst Rev* (9):CD008011, 2011.

265. Oeffinger KC, Mertesn AC, Sklar CA, et al: Chronic health conditions in adult survivors of childhood cancer. *N Engl J Med* 355:1572, 2006.

266. Pui CH, Cheng C, Leung W, et al: Extended follow-up of long-term survivors of childhood acute lymphoblastic leukemia. *N Engl J Med* 349:640, 2003.

267. Hijiya N, Hudson MM, Lensing S, et al: Cumulative incidence of secondary neoplasms as a first event after childhood acute lymphoblastic leukemia. *JAMA* 297:1207, 2007.

268. Geenen MM, Cardous-Ubbink MC, Kremer LCM, et al: Medical assessment of adverse health outcomes in long-term survivors of childhood cancer. *JAMA* 297:2705, 2007.

269. Waber DP, Turek J, Catania L, et al: Neuropsychological outcomes from a randomized trial of triple intrathecal chemotherapy compared with 18 Gy cranial radiation as CNS treatment in acute lymphoblastic leukemia: Findings from Dana-Farber Cancer Institute ALL Consortium Protocol 95–01. *J Clin Oncol* 25:4914, 2007.

270. Leung W, Rose SR, Zhou Y, et al: Outcomes of growth hormone replacement therapy in survivors of childhood acute lymphoblastic leukemia. *J Clin Oncol* 20:2959, 2002.

271. Perkins SM, Dewees T, Shinohara ET, et al: Risk of subsequent malignancies in survivors of childhood leukemia. *J Cancer Surviv* 7:544, 2013.

272. Schmiegelow K, Levinsen MF, Attarbaschi A, et al: Second malignant neoplasms after treatment of childhood acute lymphoblastic leukemia. *J Clin Oncol* 31:2469, 2013.

273. Walter AW, Hancock ML, Pui CH, et al: Secondary brain tumors in children treated for acute lymphoblastic leukemia at St. Jude Children's Research Hospital. *J Clin Oncol* 16:3761, 1998.

274. Pui CH, Ribeiro RC, Hancock ML, et al: Acute myeloid leukemia in children treated with epipodophyllotoxins for acute lymphoblastic leukemia. *N Engl J Med* 325:1682, 1991.

275. Kenney LB, Nicholson HS, Brasseux C, et al: Birth defects in offspring of adult survivors of childhood acute lymphoblastic leukemia. A Children's Cancer Group/National Institutes of Health Report. *Cancer* 78:169, 1996.

276. Sankila R, Olsen JH, Anderson H, et al: Risk of cancer among offspring of childhood-cancer survivors. Association of the Nordic Cancer Registries and the Nordic Society of Paediatric Haematology and Oncology. *N Engl J Med* 338:1339, 1998.

277. Pui CH, Mullighan CG, Evans WE, Relling MV: Pediatric acute lymphoblastic leukemia: Where are we going and how do we get there? *Blood* 120:1165, 2012.

278. Creutzig U1, van den Heuvel-Eibrink MM, Gibson B,, et al; AML Committee of the International BFM Study Group: Diagnosis and management of acute myeloid leukemia in children and adolescents: Recommendations from an international expert panel. *Blood* 120:3187, 2012.

279. Fielding AK, Banerjee L, Marks DI: Recent developments in the management of T-cell precursor acute lymphoblastic leukemia/lymphoma. *Curr Hematol Malig Rep* 7:160, 2012.

280. Freedman AS, Friedberg JW: Treatment of Burkitt leukemia/lymphoma in adults, in *UpToDate*, edited by Post TW TW. UpToDate, Waltham, MA. http://www.uptodate.com/contents/treatment-of-burkitt-leukemia-lymphoma-in-adults. (Accessed on August 07, 2015.)

281. Bhatia S, Sather HN, Heerema NA, et al: Racial and ethnic differences in survival of children with acute lymphoblastic leukemia. *Blood* 100:1957, 2002.

282. Kadan-Lottick NS, Ness KK, Bhatia S, Gurney JG: Survival variability by race and ethnicity in childhood acute lymphoblastic leukemia. *JAMA* 290:2008, 2003.

283. Pui CH, Sandlund JT, Pei D, et al: Results of therapy for acute lymphoblastic leukemia in black and white children. *JAMA* 290:2001, 2003.

284. Breit S, Stanulla M, Flohr T, et al: Activating NOTCH1 mutations predict favorable early treatment response and long-term outcome in childhood precursor T-cell lymphoblastic leukemia. *Blood* 108:1151, 2009.

285. Asnafi V, Buzyn A, Le NS, et al: NOTCH1/FBXW7 mutation identifies a large subgroup with favorable outcome in adult T-cell acute lymphoblastic leukemia (T-ALL): A Group for Research on Adult Acute Lymphoblastic Leukemia (GRAALL) study. *Blood* 113:3918, 2009.

286. Abdelali RB, Asnafi V, Leguay T, et al: Pediatric-inspired intensified therapy of adult T-ALL reveals the favourable outcome of NOTCH/FBXW7 mutations, but not of low ERG/BAALC expression: A GRAALL study. *Blood* 118:5099, 2011.

287. Raff T, Gokbuget N, Luschen S, et al: Molecular relapse in adult standard-risk ALL patients detected by prospective MRD monitoring during and after maintenance treatment: Data from the GMALL 06/99 and 07/03 trials. *Blood* 109:910, 2007.

288. Coustan-Smith E, Sancho J, Hancock ML, et al: Use of peripheral blood instead of bone marrow to monitor residual disease in children with acute lymphoblastic leukemia. *Blood* 100:2399, 2002.

289. Bader P, Kreyenberg H, Henze GHR, et al: Prognostic value of minimal residual disease quantification before allogeneic stem-cell transplantation in relapsed childhood acute lymphoblastic leukemia: The ALL-REZ BFM Study Group. *J Clin Oncol* 27:377, 2008.

290. Gokbuget N, Stanze D, Beck J, et al: Outcome of relapsed adult lymphoblastic leukemia depends on response to salvage chemotherapy, prognostic factors, and performance of stem cell transplantation. *Blood* 120:2032, 2012.

CHAPTER 92
CHRONIC LYMPHOCYTIC LEUKEMIA

Farrukh T. Awan and John C. Byrd

SUMMARY

Chronic lymphocytic leukemia is a malignancy of mature B cells characterized by progressive lymphocytosis, lymphadenopathy, splenomegaly, and cytopenias. The progressive accumulation of leukemic B cells is a consequence of defective apoptosis and survival signals derived from the microenvironment. Progressive disease results in dysregulation of the cellular and humoral components of the effector immune system with a resultant increase in the incidence of infectious complications, which constitutes the leading cause of morbidity and mortality in this disease. Significant therapeutic advances have been realized in recent years, especially with the development of well-tolerated targeted antibodies and kinase inhibitors. Although not curative, these therapies have resulted in significant improvements in patient outcomes with substantial increases in progression-free and overall survival intervals. Multiple novel agents are also in development with the potential to alter the treatment paradigms for this disease and ultimately to affect a cure.

● DEFINITION AND EPIDEMIOLOGY

Chronic lymphocytic leukemia (CLL) is one of the most common leukemias in the Western hemisphere. CLL is a malignant lymphoid neoplasm that is characterized by the accumulation of a population of small mature B cells. The diagnosis of CLL requires the presence of at least 5000 circulating B cells/μL with clonality demonstrated by flow cytometry according to International Workshop on Chronic Lymphocytic Leukemia (IWCLL) criteria.[1] Over the last 2 centuries, significant strides have been made in the understanding of the disease pathophysiology, clinical features, and complications arising from CLL. CLL was initially described by Virchow in the 1840s when he described patients with lymph node enlargement and leukocytosis. Subsequent studies revealed the involvement of the spleen and marrow and led to the introduction of the term "lymphosarcoma." Ensuing natural history studies established the malignant and clonal nature of the disease and categorized patients based on clinical presentation. Surveillance, Epidemiology, and End Results Program (SEER) data from 2013 estimate the prevalence of CLL in the United States at 126,553 patients, of whom 72,569 are males. The American Cancer Society estimates 15,720 new cases of CLL in 2014 with a median age of diagnosis of 72 years. This cancer is more common in men,[2] uncommon in patients younger than the age of 40 years, and extremely rare in children. The risk also increases progressively with age[3] and decreases with increasing parity in women.[4] It is also relatively uncommon in Asians,[5] even in Asian immigrants to the Western hemisphere,[6] suggesting a possibility of a genetic predisposition. In the last few years there has been a tremendous growth in the understanding of the disease biology, which has resulted in the development of numerous new therapeutic options with resultant transformation in the management of this illness. Despite the significant improvement in the prognosis of this disease, cure currently remains elusive.

Acronyms and Abbreviations: ABC, activated B cell; ABVD, Adriamycin, bleomycin, vinblastine, and dacarbazine; ADCC, antibody-dependent cell-mediated cytotoxicity; ADP, adenosine diphosphate; AIHA, autoimmune hemolytic anemia; ALL, acute lymphoblastic lymphoma; ARLTS1, ADP-ribosylation factor-like tumor-suppressor gene 1; ATM, ataxia-telangiectasia mutated; BAK, Bcl-2 homologous antagonist/killer; BCL-2, B-cell lymphoma-2; BCR, B-cell receptor; BiTE, Bi-specific T-cell engaging; BR, bendamustine and rituximab; BTK, Bruton tyrosine kinase; CALGB, Cancer and Leukemia Group B; CAP, cyclophosphamide, doxorubicin, and prednisone; CAR-T, chimeric antigen receptor T cell; CD, cluster of differentiation; CDC, complement-dependent cytotoxicity; CDK, cyclin-dependent kinase; CHOP, cyclophosphamide, doxorubicin, vincristine, and prednisone; CIRS, cumulative illness rating scale; CLL, chronic lymphocytic leukemia; CMP, cyclophosphamide, melphalan, and prednisone; CMV, cytomegalovirus; CR, complete response; CRi, complete response with incomplete count recovery; CT, computed tomography; CVP, cyclophosphamide, vincristine, and prednisone; CXCR4, C-X-C chemokine receptor type 4; DAPK, death-associated protein kinase; ERK1, extracellular signal-regulated kinase 1; FC, fludarabine and cyclophosphamide; FCR, fludarabine, cyclophosphamide, and rituximab; FDG-PET, fluorodeoxyglucose positron emission tomography; FISH, fluorescent *in situ* hybridization; FR, fludarabine and rituximab; G-CSF, granulocyte colony-stimulating factor; GM-CSF, granulocyte-macrophage colony-stimulating factor; GVL, graft-versus-leukemia; HCL, hairy cell leukemia; HLA, human leukocyte antigen; Ig, immunoglobulin; IGH, immunoglobulin heavy chain; IGHV, immunoglobulin heavy-chain variable region; IL, interleukin; ITK, IL-2–inducible T-cell kinase; ITP, immune thrombocytopenia; IVIG, intravenous immunoglobulins; IWCLL, International Workshop on Chronic Lymphocytic Leukemia; KLHL6, Kelch-like protein-6; LDH, lactate dehydrogenase; LYN, Lck/Yes novel; MBL, monoclonal B-cell lymphocytosis; MCL-1, myeloid cell leukemia-1; MHC, major histocompatibility complex; miRNA, microRNA; MMP, matrix metalloproteinase; MMR, measles, mumps, and rubella; MRD, minimal residual disease; MYD88, myeloid differentiation primary response gene 88; NAD, nicotinic acid adenine; NCCN, National Comprehensive Cancer Network; NFAT, nuclear factor of activated T cells; NF-κB, nuclear factor kappa B; NK, natural killer; NOTCH1, Notch homologue 1, translocation-associated; NRM, nonrelapse mortality; OFAR, oxaliplatin, fludarabine, and rituximab; ORR, overall response rate; OS, overall survival; PCR, pentostatin, cyclophosphamide, and rituximab; PCV-13, pneumococcal 13-valent conjugate vaccine; PFS, progression-free survival; PI3K, phosphatidylinositol-4,5-bisphosphate 3-kinase; PLCγ_2, phospholipase C-gamma-2; PLL, prolymphocytic leukemia; PR, partial response; PR+L, partial response with lymphocytosis; PRCA, pure red cell aplasia; RB, retinoblastoma; R-CHOP, rituximab, cyclophosphamide, doxorubicin, vincristine, and prednisone; R-EPOCH, rituximab, etoposide, prednisone, vincristine, cyclophosphamide, and doxorubicin; R-hyperCVXD, fractionated cyclophosphamide, vincristine, liposomal daunorubicin, and dexamethasone; RS, Richter syndrome; SCT, stem cell transplantation; SDF-1, stromal cell–derived factor-1; SF3B1, splicing factor 3B subunit 1; SLL, small lymphocytic B-cell lymphoma; SNP, single nucleotide polymorphism; STAT3, signal transducer and activator of transcription 3; SUV, standardized uptake value; SYK, spleen tyrosine kinase; TCL1, T-cell leukemia/lymphoma protein 1A; TGF-β, transforming growth factor-β; T-LGL, T-cell large granular lymphoma; TNF-α, tumor necrosis factor-α; TP53, tumor protein p53; T-PLL, T-cell prolymphocytic lymphoma; TRAP, tartrate-resistant acid phosphatase; TRM, transplant-related mortality; VCAM, vascular cell adhesion molecule; XIAP, X-linked inhibitor of apoptosis protein; XPO1, gene encoding exportin-1; ZAP-70, zeta-chain–associated protein kinase of 70 kDa.

ENVIRONMENTAL FACTORS

Multiple studies have been conducted in an attempt to identify environmental factors that predispose people to the development of CLL. These studies have consistently identified a family history of hematologic malignancies as a strong predictive factor for the development of CLL.[7,8] In the reported International Lymphoma Epidemiology Consortium (InterLymph) Non-Hodgkin Lymphoma Subtypes Project,[9] detailed correlative studies were performed on a large cohort of white patients with CLL as compared to normal controls. The Inter-Lymph study identified multiple factors that were associated with the presence of CLL, including: (1) family history of a first-degree relative with hematologic malignancy including lymphomas, leukemias, and myeloma; (2) a history of working or living on a farm; (3) hairdressers; and (4) a history of hepatitis C infection. Factors that were found to be protective include a history of allergies, blood transfusions, sun exposure, and smoking. CLL is also recognized as a service-connected illness among Vietnam War veterans who were exposed to Agent Orange.[10] Limited data suggests a possible risk of CLL in individuals chronically exposed to electromagnetic fields.[11,12] Radiation exposure, however, has not been shown to correlate with the development of CLL as revealed by population-based studies on survivors of the Hiroshima atomic bomb and studies on nuclear reactor workers.[13,14] A smaller study conducted on survivors of the Chernobyl nuclear power plant accident did, however, suggest a slightly higher incidence of CLL in these people.[15]

HEREDITARY FACTORS

CLL has a strong familial predisposition with up to 10 percent of patients with a first- or second-degree relative with CLL and an even higher percentage when also considering individuals with monoclonal B-cell lymphocytosis.[16,17] Risk of acquiring CLL is also potentially increased in patients with first-degree relatives with other indolent non-Hodgkin lymphomas including lymphoplasmacytic lymphomas.[18] Death-associated protein kinase (DAPK) and CD57 (LEU7) germline mutations have been linked to familial predisposition in a single CLL family.[19] Association studies have identified multiple putative genes, polymorphisms, and genetic factors including CD5,[20] CD38,[21] tumor necrosis factor (TNF)-α,[22] and human leukocyte antigen (HLA) haplotypes,[23] among others,[24] but definite mechanistic studies demonstrating clear contribution to pathogenesis are lacking.

DISEASE BIOLOGY

CLL has varied presentations and complex biology that is the focus of ongoing studies of particular relevance to the practicing oncologist. CLL cells are derived from the B-lymphocyte lineage as demonstrated by their expression of the pan–B-cell surface markers including CD19, and a weaker expression of CD20.[25,26] Furthermore, CLL B cells express the memory B-cell marker CD27,[27] and also exhibit similar microarray profiles, suggesting a potential relationship to the normal memory B cell.[28,29] Most CLL B cells also express κ and λ immunoglobulin light chains on their surface, along with M and D immunoglobulin heavy chains.[30,31] These immunoglobulins are often reactive toward self-antigens and polyreactive,[32,33] and may play a role in the survival and expansion of the leukemia cell clone.

CLL is characterized by gradual accumulation of leukemic cells primarily from defective apoptosis that is partly contributed by microenvironment interaction. Overexpression of multiple antiapoptotic proteins like BCL-2 (B-cell lymphoma-2), MCL-1 (myeloid cell leukemia-1),[34,35] BAK (Bcl-2 homologous antagonist/killer), and XIAP

(X-linked inhibitor of apoptosis protein) along with transcription factors like NF-κB (nuclear factor kappa B), NFAT (nuclear factor of activated T cells), and STAT3 (signal transducer and activator of transcription 3) have been clearly demonstrated in CLL.[36] Additional survival signals are provided by the microenvironment and include cellular factors like nurse-like cells,[37] and various chemokines like CXCR4 (C-X-C chemokine receptor type 4) and SDF-1 (stromal cell–derived factor-1).[38] A combination of these factors results in providing the CLL cells with a survival and proliferative advantage. CLL B cells exhibit differential proliferation in the various disease compartments, including the blood, spleen, and marrow.[39,40] CLL B cells isolated from the blood of patients lack proliferative potential *in vitro* and are restricted to the resting phase of the cell cycle.[41,42] These cells also undergo spontaneous apoptosis in routine culture conditions. Their survival can be extended when these cells are cultured on stromal cells or nurse like cells that are generally found in the secondary lymphoid organs.[43,44] These secondary lymphoid organs are generally diffusely infiltrated by the B cells and are potentially the sites of cell division and proliferation.[45] *In vivo*, the leukemic cell clones increase by 0.1 to 1 percent per day despite a stable blood lymphocyte count as assessed by elegant heavy water studies.[46]

IMMUNE DYSREGULATION

CLL is characterized by progressive immune dysregulation both in the cellular and humoral compartments.[47] Progression of CLL is associated with an early increase in the absolute number of circulating T cells and specifically an increase in the immunosuppressive T-regulatory cells.[48,49] Functional studies on T cells from patients with CLL have also shown the T cells to be anergic and with impaired proliferative potential, but with a retained capacity to produce cytokines.[50] Functional defects have also been observed in granulocytes.[51] The leukemic B cells are responsible for initiating and propagating the immune dysregulation observed in the disease by producing immunosuppressive cytokines like transforming growth factor-β (TGF-β) or by downregulating critical surface molecules required for development of a functional immune system such as CD154 and CD80.[52–54] Moreover, the microenvironment is potentially responsible for developing an immunosuppressive niche in the lymph nodes and marrow that allow for active immune evasion of the leukemic B-cells.[55] Collectively, these cellular defects predispose patients to recurrent opportunistic infections especially with herpes zoster virus and cytomegalovirus (CMV).[56,57] Defects in class switching of immunoglobulins and normal B-cell function also result in progressive hypogammaglobulinemia that predisposes patients to recurrent infections with encapsulated organisms.[58] This may in part be related to the downregulation of CD154 on CLL B-cells or through CD95 interaction with its ligand.[59,60] Understanding of these putative pathways has resulted in development of mechanistically relevant targeted therapy.[61]

ROLE OF THE B-CELL RECEPTOR PATHWAY

The B-cell receptor (BCR) plays an integral part in the development and maturation of B cells. Constitutive activation of the BCR is one of the most important survival signals for the propagation of CLL B cells.[62] The surface immunoglobulin heterodimer that forms an integral part of the BCR, is critical for both antigen-dependent and antigen-independent signaling through the BCR.[63–65] This signal is transduced through a variety of kinases including LYN (Lck/Yes novel), PI3K (phosphatidylinositol-4,5-bisphosphate 3-kinase), SYK (spleen tyrosine kinase), and BTK (Bruton tyrosine kinase).[64] Their activation results in phosphorylation of phospholipase C-gamma-2 (PLCγ₂) and induction of downstream second messengers that further modulate cell-survival regulators.[35,63] Targeting the various kinases involved in the BCR pathway has resulted in significant improvements in the therapeutic options for this disease. Early results from studies done with BTK, PI3K, and SYK inhibitors have all shown excellent efficacy and tolerability, and these agents are currently being used in various combinations to improve disease outcomes.

BTK was initially characterized as a deficient kinase in patients with X-linked agammaglobulinemia, a disease characterized by a severe immunodeficient state.[66] Specific mutations in BTK results in severe impairments in B-cell development and humoral immunity.[66] Activating mutations of BTK have not been identified in CLL or other cancers. However, CLL B cells tend to have higher levels of BTK that can be induced through the BCR signaling pathway.[67] Efficient targeting of BTK with the irreversible inhibitor ibrutinib results in significant abrogation of downstream survival signaling transduced through this pathway and results in the inhibition of cell survival and proliferation.[67] Moreover, ibrutinib irreversibly targets interleukin (IL)-2–inducible T-cell kinase (ITK) in T cells, thus potentiating T-helper type 1 (Th1)–driven immune responses and reversing tumor-induced T-cell anergy.[68]

Similar to BTK, both SYK and PI3K can be induced by both the autonomous and antigen-dependent BCR activation and result in providing the critical signals that result in leukemic cell survival and proliferation.[69,70] Similar to ibrutinib, the PI3K isoform delta inhibitor idelalisib antagonizes internal and external survival signals to the CLL cells and results in significant clinical response. Idelalisib is currently approved for the treatment of relapsed CLL.[71] Similar results are observed with SYK inhibitors that are currently in early phase clinical trials.[72]

GENETICS OF CHRONIC LYMPHOCYTIC LEUKEMIA

Improved understanding of the genetics of CLL has resulted in significant improvements in our ability to determine the prognosis of this disease and to tailor therapy for our patients. Initial efforts to study the cytogenetic abnormalities in CLL were hindered by the inability of the tumor cells to proliferate *in vitro* for standard metaphase analyses. Improvements in our ability to stimulate the CLL B cells *in vitro* and the development of interphase fluorescent *in situ* hybridization techniques (FISH) have significantly improved and refined the study of cytogenetic abnormalities in this disease.[73] Using these methods, del 13q14 was identified as the most common abnormality in patients with CLL, being present in approximately 50 percent of all patients, followed by trisomy 12, which is present in approximately 15 to 20 percent of patients, and del 11q22.3, which is present in approximately 10 to 15 percent of patients. Other abnormalities that were identified in significant numbers include del 6q21 and del 17p13.1. These abnormalities impart differential prognostic impact on disease outcomes.[74]

Functional studies have been performed to determine the association of these cytogenetic abnormalities to disease physiology. Specifically, deletion in the long arm of chromosome 13 results in a loss of the tumor-suppressor gene ARLTS1 with potential physiologic impact.[75] Moreover, this region also includes genes encoding microRNA (miRNA) including miRNA-15 and miRNA-16.[76] These abundant and evolutionarily conserved short, noncoding miRNA, that range in size from 21 to 25 nucleotides, have the potential to regulate the expression of a number of different genes at the posttranscriptional level significantly impacting cell signaling. They are also known to modulate the expression of various pro- and antiapoptotic proteins of significant relevance to CLL B-cell proliferation, including BCL-2 (miRNA-15 and miRNA-16), MCL-1 (miRNA-29), and TCL1 (miRNA-29 and miRNA-181).[76–78] Recent studies have identified miRNA-150 as potentially the most abundantly expressed miRNA in patients with CLL and may be involved in the regulation of BCR signaling and subsequent survival signals.[79] Multiple studies are currently underway to further define the full impact of the role of miRNAs in the pathogenesis of CLL and to develop strategies to modulate their expression and function for therapeutic benefit.

With regards to other cytogenetic abnormalities, trisomy 12 is often found in patients with progressive or relapsed disease or Richter transformation.[80] Numerous genes are affected as a result of the trisomy and B cells obtained from patients with this abnormality tend to have higher surface expression of CD19, CD20, CD38, and immunoglobulins when compared to patients without this abnormality.[80–82] Multiple genetic alterations have also been described in patients with del 11q22.3, but most importantly, it may involve the loss of the ataxia-telangiectasia mutated *(ATM)* gene, which normally activates p53 and results in either apoptosis or cellular repair in response to cytotoxic stimuli.[83] Moreover, there is a decrease in the expression of miRNA-29 and miRNA-181, which are involved in the down regulation of the T-cell leukemia/lymphoma protein 1A *(TCL1)* oncogene.[84] Patients with del 11q22.3 tend to have more aggressive disease with bulky lymphadenopathy[85]; historically have had a worse prognosis with disease poorly responsive to conventional nucleoside analogue-based therapy; and have specifically required the addition of alkylating agents like cyclophosphamide to overcome the poor prognostic impact.[86,87]

The del 17p13.1 is present in less than 10 percent of patients with CLL and frequently involves the deletion of the tumor protein p53 *(TP53)* gene that encodes the p53 protein which, as noted above, is critical for cellular apoptosis or repair specifically in response to cytotoxic stimuli.[88] Patients with this abnormality have rapidly progressive disease with significantly inferior survival outcomes and poor response to therapy.[89] This mutation also confers chemoresistance; consequently, responses to conventional chemotherapy-based regimens have been dismal.[90] These patients also have higher risk of Richter transformation to more aggressive lymphomas over the course of their disease.[89] The inferior outcomes observed in patients with del 11q or del 17p appears to persist in the era of treatment with kinase inhibitors, with patients experiencing a shorter progression-free interval, but are significantly better as compared to historic controls.[91,92]

Multiple other cytogenetic abnormalities have been reported from patients with CLL, including del 6q21, those involving the immunoglobulin heavy chain (IGH) locus on chromosome 14q32, and those involving the *BCL-2* gene located on chromosome 18q21.[93,94] These are generally associated with progressive, relapsed, and aggressive disease and frequently observed in patients with an unmutated immunoglobulin heavy-chain variable region (IGHV).[93,95]

Other recurring abnormalities in CLL involving *SF3B1* (splicing factor 3B subunit 1), *NOTCH1* (Notch homologue 1, translocation-associated), *MYD88* (myeloid differentiation primary response gene 88), *XPO1* (gene encoding exportin-1), *KLHL6* (Kelch-like protein-6), and *ERK1* (extracellular signal-regulated kinase 1) have been described using whole-exon and whole-genome sequencing with potential prognostic impact.[96–98] With the advent of single nucleotide polymorphism (SNP) arrays, comparative genomic hybridization techniques, and determination of acquired copy number aberrations, more detailed studies can be performed assessing the mechanistic significance and impact of these genetic mutations on prognosis and customizing therapy.

CLINICAL PRESENTATION OF CHRONIC LYMPHOCYTIC LEUKEMIA

CLL is a disease of the elderly with the median age at diagnosis being 72 years. Most patients are asymptomatic at diagnosis and are diagnosed as a result of incidental finding of lymphadenopathy and lymphocytosis of uncertain etiology as part of an evaluation unrelated to CLL. A vast majority of patients may not have any significant symptoms related to the disease but some patients may experience mild fatigue or minor limitations in their activities of daily living. A subset of patients may present with recurring infectious complications, especially upper respiratory tract infections. Patients with advanced disease can uncommonly present with drenching night sweats, fevers, and weight loss (B symptoms), and signs and symptoms related to anemia, thrombocytopenia, and lymphadenopathy. The lymphadenopathy typically observed in patients with CLL is generally not fixed or tender and very rarely causes symptoms of organ dysfunction or resulting dependent-limb lymphedema. Patients can have exacerbations of their lymphadenopathy during an acute infectious episode, but this typically returns to baseline upon resolution of the underlying infectious complication.[99] Splenomegaly is seen commonly in patients with CLL with resultant hypersplenism and thrombocytopenia. Significant hepatomegaly because of leukemic infiltration is unusual. CLL infiltration of multiple organs has been described but these are typically seen in patients with advanced disease and will occasionally cause symptoms. Pulmonary involvement has been observed in patients with high lymphocyte count and typically presents as an interstitial infiltrate on chest radiography. Chylous and hemorrhagic pleural effusions have also been reported.[100-102] Similarly, leukemic infiltration of the gastrointestinal tract may result in chronic diarrhea or iron-deficiency anemia secondary to chronic bleeding or malabsorption. However, this mucosal infiltration is more commonly seen in patients with mantle cell lymphoma. CLL involvement of the central nervous system is rare and may result in headaches, confusion, meningismus, or cranial nerve palsies.[103] More commonly, these patients are at higher risk for opportunistic infections of the central nervous system because of their deficient immune system. Patients with CLL are also known to have insect bite hypersensitivity.[104,105] Patient's typically present with recurrent, erythematous, painful eruptions usually on the exposed part of the extremities. Evaluation of skin biopsies from these patients reveal a mixed infiltrating population of T cells, B cells, and eosinophils. These resolve over time and can be effectively treated with a short course of glucocorticoid.

EVALUATION OF THE PATIENT WITH CHRONIC LYMPHOCYTIC LEUKEMIA

According to the IWCLL-2008 criteria, the diagnosis of CLL requires a sustained monoclonal lymphocytosis of greater than 5000 cells/μL of monoclonal B cells.[1] This requires blood flow cytometry for immunophenotyping the B cells, which additionally reveals the cells to be positive for CD19, dim CD20, dim surface immunoglobulin, and negative for CD10, CD79b, and FMC7. A similar disease presentation with no evidence of hematopoietic involvement and with only lymph node involvement by cells of comparable morphology will be classified as small lymphocytic lymphoma. These patients are essentially managed similar to patients with CLL. CLL cells appear as small blue lymphocytes with scant cytoplasm on the Wright-Giemsa staining commonly used for evaluating blood films (Fig. 92–1). Smudge cells are also commonly observed on the blood film and this results from the mechanical disruption of the cells during the slide preparation process (Fig. 92–2). For an improved evaluation of the cellular morphology on the blood

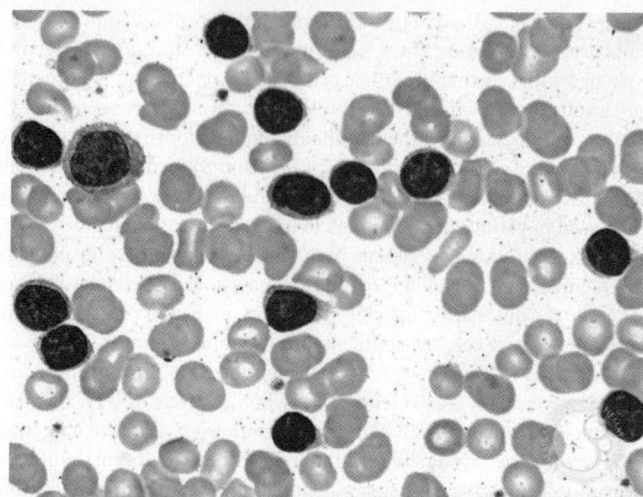

Figure 92–1. Typical chronic lymphocytic leukemia blood film. *(Reproduced with permission from Ash Image Bank, Peter Maslak, 2013, © the American Society of Hematology.)*

film, an albumin preparation is sometimes required. Patients can also have large prolymphocytes with prominent nucleoli in the blood but these lymphocytes must be less than 55 percent of the total lymphocyte population. The anemia is typically normocytic and normochromic and platelet morphology is typically preserved. A marrow aspirate and biopsy is not required for the vast majority of patients with CLL at initial presentation to establish a diagnosis. However, we do recommend performing a marrow aspirate and biopsy in patients with anemia and thrombocytopenia to evaluate the presence of autoimmune hemolytic anemia and/or immune thrombocytopenia. Marrow biopsy typically shows diffuse marrow involvement with a monotypic population of small lymphocytes. Variability of marrow involvement has been historically used as a potential marker for prognosis but has limited applicability given the availability of more specific and sensitive prognostic markers.[106,107] The red cell precursors and megakaryocytes usually display an unremarkable morphology but do diminish in numbers with

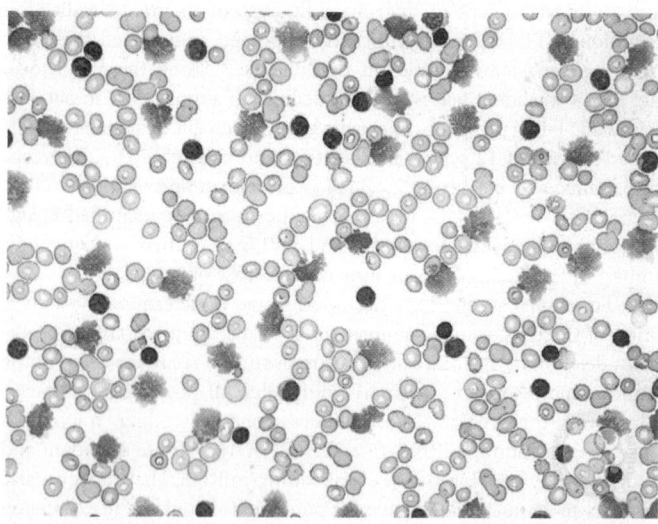

Figure 92–2. Typical chronic lymphocytic leukemia blood film with smudge cells. *(Reproduced with permission from ASH image bank, Peter Maslak, 2010. © the American Society of Hematology.)*

progressive disease. Conventional stimulated karyotype analysis and interphase FISH cytogenetic study, to evaluate for abnormalities commonly seen in patients with CLL, should be performed on all patients at the time of diagnosis and every time the disease changes character in order to determine the extent of a clonal evolution. Patients with atypical presentations, especially those with absent or low CD23 expression should have a negative FISH study for t(11;14) to exclude mantle cell lymphoma. Lymph node biopsy is not typically required for further establishing the diagnosis of CLL. Lymph nodes typically show architectural effacement by diffuse infiltration by cells of a similar morphology as observed in the peripheral circulation.

When anemia is present from CLL, patients typically will have normocytic and normochromic anemia, often with thrombocytopenia and lymphocytosis. Patients with a macrocytic anemia or an isolated anemia should have a Coombs test, haptoglobin test, and reticulocyte count performed to rule out autoimmune hemolytic anemia. These patients should also be evaluated for vitamin B_{12} and folic acid deficiencies, and malabsorption or gastrointestinal bleeding from CLL involvement should be ruled out.

Patients with CLL will frequently have hypogammaglobulinemia with decrease in the serum concentration of immunoglobulin (Ig) G, IgA, and IgM. The degree of hypogammaglobulinemia correlates with progressive disease and predisposes patients to recurrent sinopulmonary infections with encapsulated organisms. T-cell defects, which increase the risks of viral infections, have also been described; however, this is not routinely assessed at the time of initial presentation. A small percentage of patients also have monoclonal gammopathy with IgM or IgG or light-chain monoclonal paraproteinemia, which can be detected on serum protein electrophoresis and immunofixation. Excessively high heavy-chain paraproteinemia can result in symptoms related to hyperviscosity as seen in patients with Waldenström macroglobulinemia and should be managed as such.[108-110] The presence of a monoclonal paraproteinemia and/or hypogammaglobulinemia may be related to inferior survival outcomes in patients with advanced disease stage, but not necessarily in patients with early stage disease.[111,112]

● PROGNOSTIC MARKERS

CYTOGENETICS AND FLUORESCENCE *IN SITU* HYBRIDIZATION

All patients must undergo a comprehensive prognostic evaluation at the time of initial presentation. This allows the clinician to explain the specific disease characteristic to the patient and also helps the patient with the emotional adjustment process that they have to go through when initially diagnosed with this disease. All patients should undergo conventional karyotype analysis and stimulated interphase FISH either on blood or marrow aspirate. The minimum FISH panel should include assessment for del 17p13, del 11q23, trisomy 12, and del 13q14, and for t(11;14) in selected patients suspected of having mantle cell lymphoma. Conventional stimulated karyotype analysis is helpful in identifying the global structural abnormalities in chromosomes, especially of chromosomes 14, 3, and 6, that cannot be routinely detected on FISH analysis.[113] Together, these assays have strong prognostic significance with regards to treatment-free and overall survival (Table 92–1).[114] Patients with CLL acquire additional cytogenetic abnormalities, as detected by stimulated karyotyping and FISH analysis, with disease progression and especially after chemotherapy. This "clonal evolution" is predominantly observed in patients with unmutated IGHV and portends poor survival and inferior response to therapy.[115] We therefore recommend repeating the stimulated karyotyping and FISH studies prior to initiation of a new line of treatment.

TABLE 92–1. Survival Outcomes and Time to First Treatment Based on FISH Cytogenetics and IGHV Status

	Prognostic Variables	Median Survival (Months)	Median Time to First Treatment
Interphase FISH cytogenetics	13q– (sole)	133	92 months
	Trisomy 12	114	33 months
	Normal	111	49 months
	11q–	79	13 months
	17p–	32	9 months
IGHV mutational status	Unmutated (≥98 percent)	89	3.5 years
	Mutated (<98 percent)	>152	9.2 years

FISH, fluorescence *in situ* hybridization; IGHV, immunoglobulin heavy-chain variable region.

IMMUNOGLOBULIN HEAVY-CHAIN VARIABLE REGION MUTATION ANALYSIS

The assessment of IGHV somatic mutation by a polymerase chain reaction–based assay has been shown to be an extremely reliable and important prognostic tool for patients with CLL. Patients with less than 2 percent homology in their nucleotide sequence as compared to consensus germline sequence are considered unmutated.[116] Patients with a mutated IGHV, which is present in approximately 60 percent of patients with CLL, have a significantly prolonged treatment-free interval, longer remission durations, and overall survival (OS).[117] These patients also have a very low incidence of clonal evolution or transformation to an aggressive histology.[114,118] The IGHV mutation status does not vary over time and does serve as a reliable marker for predicting long-term disease outcomes.[119] The only known exception to the mutation rule currently is the presence of IGHV 3–21 somatic mutation, which may confer an aggressive phenotype similar to leukemic cells from patients with unmutated IGHV at least in a subset of patients.[120,121]

ZETA-CHAIN–ASSOCIATED PROTEIN KINASE OF 70 kDa AND ITS METHYLATION STATUS

Zeta-chain–associated protein kinase of 70 kDa (ZAP-70) is an intracellular tyrosine kinase that is typically associated with T-cell development and T-cell receptor (TCR) signaling. Expression of ZAP-70 in CLL B cells provides a survival advantage through intrinsic and extrinsic signals mediated through the BCR.[122] Cytoplasmic assessment of ZAP-70 in CLL B cells by flow cytometry correlates strongly with IGHV mutational status and clinical outcomes, with an expression of 20 percent or more predictive of poor outcomes.[123] The assessment of ZAP-70 by flow cytometric testing has been plagued with several issues, including lack of reproducibility and reliability of the reagents. Consequently, the National Comprehensive Cancer Network (NCCN) guidelines do not recommend the routine use of ZAP-70 as a prognostic marker outside of clinical trials. Given the stability of DNA and epigenetic modification by methylation, investigators have also sought to assess ZAP-70 expression by the absence of promoter methylation.[124] Methylation analysis of select proximal 5′ regions of the ZAP-70 gene correlates very strongly with expression of ZAP-70 and has been established as an important and reliable prognostic marker with regards to predicting time to treatment and OS.[125,126] This assay can be done by pyrosequencing with significant reproducibility among different laboratories.[126]

CD38 EXPRESSION

CD38 is a 45-kDa transmembrane glycoprotein that can be detected on the surface of CLL B cells by flow cytometry; a level of expression greater than 30 percent correlates strongly with progression-free survival (PFS).[118] Newer reports, however, suggest that an even lower level of CD38 expression might also have a prognostic impact.[127,128] CD38 appears to be involved in cellular metabolism by synthesizing cyclic adenosine diphosphate (cADP)-ribose from nicotinic acid adenine (NAD),[129] and its activity and expression correlates with proliferation of the lymphocytes and progressive disease as demonstrated by their high Ki-67 proliferation index.[130] CD38 expression also changes with disease progression and the assessment of the extent of expression of CD38 is based on nonstandardized, subjective parameters.[131]

CD49d EXPRESSION

CD49d can also be used as a reliable predictive marker. CD49d is a surface subunit of the integrin heterodimer that is involved in promoting survival of the CLL cells through growth signals derived from the microenvironment.[132,133] Patients with 30 percent or greater cells expressing CD49d by flow cytometry are considered to be positive and constitute a group of patients with an aggressive disease course and inferior survival.[134]

OTHER PROGNOSTIC MARKERS

Serum lactate dehydrogenase (LDH) and β_2-microglobulin are readily available, validated markers of disease aggressiveness and prognosis. Specifically, β_2-microglobulin is an independent prognostic marker for remission duration, PFS, and OS, and a higher level is observed in patients with advanced and extensive disease.[135–137] Elevated LDH is associated with more-aggressive disease and with Richter syndrome. Lymphocyte doubling time could also be used as a tool to determine the prognosis of CLL. Patients with a lymphocyte doubling time of 12 months or less have worse OS and treatment-free survival.[138] Other reasons for transient elevation in lymphocyte count should be ruled out before making the determination of lymphocyte doubling time. Thymidine kinase is an important intracellular enzyme; the soluble form can be detected in patients with CLL and predicts for advanced stage and progressive disease. However, the assay is not widely available and the test is rarely used in routine clinic care.[139–141] Over the years, various other serum proteins have been found to be associated with various measures of disease outcomes, including soluble factors like CD23,[142] CD44,[143] vascular cell adhesion molecule (VCAM)-1,[144] CD27,[144] and matrix metalloproteinase (MMP)-9,[145] IL-6,[146] and IL-8.[147] However, none of these is routinely used for clinical decision making (Table 92–2).

Various miRNAs have also been validated as useful prognostic markers. miRNAs are noncoding RNAs that are 19 to 25 nucleotides in length and modulate mRNA translation and synthesis of various proteins. miRNA-15a and miRNA-16–1 were the first ones to be identified as underexpressed in CLL patient B cells.[76] Genes for these miRNAs are located in the deleted region of chromosome 13q14 and modulate the expression of the antiapoptotic bcl-2 protein, which is overexpressed in patients with CLL and other B-cell lymphoproliferative disorders.[148] Similarly, miRNA-34c is involved in patients with del 11q23 and regulates the expression of ZAP-70 and other proteins involved in the TP53 pathway.[149] Using mass array methods, miRNA profiles have also been found to be predictive for disease progression, fludarabine resistance, and clinical outcomes.[150,151]

TABLE 92–2. Outcomes of Selected Prognostic Factors

	Favorable Outcome	Unfavorable Outcome
Lactate dehydrogenase	Low or normal	Elevated
Lymphocyte doubling time	>12 months	≤12 months
Thymidine kinase activity	Low or normal	Elevated
β_2-microglobulin	Low or normal	Elevated
Soluble CD23 levels	Low or normal	Elevated
CD38 expression	<30 percent	>30 percent
Interphase FISH cytogenetics	Normal	11q–
	Trisomy 12	17p–
	13q– (sole)	
IGHV mutational status	Mutated (<98 percent)	Unmutated (≥98 percent)
CD49d expression	<30 percent	>30 percent

FISH, fluorescence *in situ* hybridization; IGHV, immunoglobulin heavy-chain variable region.

● STAGING FOR CHRONIC LYMPHOCYTIC LEUKEMIA

The Rai[152] and Binet[153] staging systems have been used for a long time for patients with CLL (Tables 92–3 and 92–4). These easy-to-use staging systems are based on assessment of disease burden as determined by lymphadenopathy and splenomegaly demonstrated on physical examination and the presence of cytopenias. Further modifications and development of the Binet system established low-risk (stage 0: lymphocytosis only), intermediate-risk (stages 1–2: lymphocytosis with lymphadenopathy and hepatosplenomegaly), and high-risk groups of patients with CLL (stages 3–4: lymphocytosis with anemia and thrombocytopenia).[153] These classification systems provided an estimate of median OS of 150, 90, and 19 months, respectively, and helped classify patients for subsequent therapeutic intervention. The staging systems still remain relevant and complementary to molecular testing in the modern era.[154]

Marrow aspirate and biopsy is not routinely required for the initial diagnosis and management of the patient with CLL. Marrow biopsy is especially helpful in determining the etiology of thrombocytopenia and anemia, which can frequently be related to concomitant autoimmune processes. It may also be helpful in determining the extent of involvement by large prolymphocytes and in establishing the diagnosis of prolymphocytic leukemia. A diffuse pattern of involvement of the biopsy specimen by characteristic small lymphocytes is also associated with a worse prognosis than interstitial or nodular involvement.[106,155] Ideally, a marrow biopsy is performed at the start of therapy to document the disease extent and to detect any atypical features.

Computed tomography (CT) scans are generally not required for the routine initial evaluation of patients with CLL and conventional staging systems rely on physical examination findings. Similarly, routine CT scans for the serial evaluation of disease extent have no role in patients with CLL. CT scans should be performed in patients with symptomatic disease and prior to starting therapy. Similarly, a positron emission tomography (PET) scan has no role in the routine management of patients with CLL. CLL lymph nodes are fluorodeoxyglucose

TABLE 92–3. Modified Rai Clinical Staging System

Stage at Diagnosis	Risk Level	Rai Stage at Diagnosis	Patients Never Requiring Therapy (%)	Median Survival (Months)
0	Low	Lymphocytosis >5 × 10⁹/L only	59	150
1	Intermediate	Lymphocytosis + lymph node (LN) enlargement	21	101
2		Lymphocytosis + spleen/liver (S/L) enlargement ± LN	23	71
3	High	Lymphocytosis + anemia (with hemoglobin <11 g/dL) ± LN or S/L	5	19
4		Lymphocytosis + thrombocytopenia (< 100 × 10¹²/L ± LN) or S/L	0	19

(FDG) nonavid; however, FDG-PET scanning can be used for the identification of patients with Richter transformation with a high sensitivity and negative predictive value.[156,157]

Based on disease extent, characteristics and prognostic markers, various nomograms have been developed and validated for use in patients with CLL. These nomograms provide a robust predictive tool for outcomes and incorporates various aspects of the CLL patient and disease and can be used for standardized risk assessment.[136,137,158]

●TREATMENT OF CHRONIC LYMPHOCYTIC LEUKEMIA

Treatment of patients with CLL is initiated at the time of symptomatic progressive disease. The specific criteria for initiating therapy have been detailed in the IWCLL-2008 guidelines.[1] This recommendation is primarily based on older studies that failed to demonstrate a survival advantage in patients treated early in the course of disease.[159,160] These results were validated by a large study of fludarabine treatment in patients with early stage disease conducted by the German CLL study group, which failed to show a survival advantage with early treatment using conventional chemotherapeutic agents.[161] Trials are currently underway with kinase inhibitors to determine if early intervention can alter the natural history of the disease. We recommend initiating treatment when patients fulfill the IWCLL-2008 criteria for treatment, regardless of the prognostic factors.

Patients with autoimmune complications of CLL can be managed accordingly with steroids and immunosuppressive therapies prior to proceeding with definitive therapy for the underlying disease. Patients with CLL rarely exhibit evidence of leukostasis resulting from profound leukocytosis, therefore, an elevated white cell count should not be used as a sole criteria for initiating treatment. Similarly, hypogammaglobulinemia should not be used as a reason to treat the disease. Periodic intravenous immunoglobulin infusions can be used in patients with hypogammaglobulinemia and recurrent life-threatening infections with encapsulated organisms. The IWCLL-2008 criteria should also be used when determining the timing of therapy for patients with relapsed disease.

One of the most important factors to consider prior to initiating treatment is the functional state of the patient. Historically, age cutoff has been successfully used in developing specific therapies. Because the median age of diagnosis for CLL is 72 years, the vast majority of patients treated in the community are older and with multiple comorbid conditions. Unfortunately, there is limited data available in this patient population and until recently they had very limited options for therapy. Most of the clinical trial participants have been younger patients who are in their 50s and 60s. The gradual functional decline, decrease in organ function, especially renal and hepatic function, and an increase in the comorbid conditions in the majority of patients older than age 65 years significantly increases the risks and toxicities of conventional chemotherapeutic regimens especially nucleoside analogues. To address these issues, different approaches are being used to treat patients older than 65 years versus younger patients. A cumulative illness rating scale (CIRS) has been proposed and used primarily by the German CLL study group. It allows patients to be stratified based on an aggregate score derived from multiple factors including age, comorbid conditions and organ function.[162]

TABLE 92–4. Binet Clinical Staging System

Stage at Diagnosis	Equivalent Rai staging	Rai Stage at Diagnosis	Proportion of Patients (%)	Median Survival (Years)
A	0–2	Lymphocytosis >5 × 10⁹/L only with <3 enlarged nodal areas*; no anemia, no thrombocytopenia	15	12+
B	1–2	Lymphocytosis >5 × 10⁹/L + ≥3 enlarged nodal areas*; no anemia, no thrombocytopenia	30	7
C	3–4	Lymphocytosis >5 × 10⁹/L + anemia (hemoglobin <10 g/dL) or thrombocytopenia (<100 × 10¹²/L) regardless of the number of enlarged nodal areas*	55	2

*Nodal areas counted as one each of the following: axillary, cervical, inguinal lymph nodes, whether unilateral or bilateral, spleen, and liver.

DEVELOPMENT OF CHEMOTHERAPY FOR THE TREATMENT OF CHRONIC LYMPHOCYTIC LEUKEMIA

Alkylating Agents

Chlorambucil has been used as the prominent alkylating agent for the treatment of CLL for the last 60 years. Chlorambucil is taken orally and is generally well-tolerated but does have multiple side effects, including nausea, vomiting, and cytopenias. Various doses and schedules have been used with different responses and tolerability profiles. Older studies compared chlorambucil to conventional high-grade lymphoma therapy, including cyclophosphamide, vincristine, and prednisone (CVP) and cyclophosphamide, doxorubicin, vincristine, and prednisone (CHOP), and found no improvement in survival outcomes with the use of high-grade lymphoma-like therapies.[159] Multiple doses of chlorambucil have been evaluated in various clinical trials with differing but similarly modest overall response rate (ORR) and PFS. No single-dosing regimen has been shown to be superior to another. One dosing regimen that has been used in cooperative group studies is 40 mg/m^2 oral dose every 28 days for 12 cycles.[163] An argument, however, can be made that escalating the dose of chlorambucil in younger patients might result in a higher response rate.[164] Despite its ease of use and reasonable tolerability, chlorambucil is not very commonly used today because of the availability of better and potentially safer alternatives. Moreover, responses observed with chlorambucil are modest and not durable.[165] Nevertheless, chlorambucil is potentially an option for treatment of elderly patients with multiple comorbidities and limited other options for treatment. It should, however, not be used for asymptomatic patients with early stage disease.[160]

Cyclophosphamide is also approved for the use in patients with CLL and has moderate efficacy and reasonable tolerability. Care should be taken to avoid nighttime dosing and aggressive hydration should encouraged to avoid hemorrhagic cystitis.[166] Low-dose etoposide, either as a single agent or in combination with cladribine, also shows modest responses in patients with relapsed and refractory disease. Treatment with etoposide is associated with significant myelosuppression and resultant infectious complications.[167,168]

Bendamustine was approved for the treatment of patients with CLL in 2008. This was based on a phase III trial that demonstrated the superior efficacy of bendamustine as compared to chlorambucil with regards to response rate and PFS.[169] Structurally, bendamustine has features common with alkylating agents and purine analogues, but its activity is primarily derived from the alkylating agent moiety.[170] Bendamustine appears to be generally better tolerated than fludarabine but causes significant myelosuppression, requiring dose reductions, especially in elderly and infirm. Tolerability is better in patients with impaired renal function since excretion is primarily through the feces.[171]

Nucleoside Analogues

Nucleoside analogues have also been used for the treatment of patients with CLL for the last 25 to 30 years. Fludarabine has been the most commonly used agent from this class of drugs. Fludarabine has moderate activity especially in the younger patients with good nutritional status and with untreated, early stage disease.[172] After demonstrating promising activity as a single agent in early phase clinical trials, fludarabine was compared to chlorambucil in a randomized phase III study for the initial treatment of patients with CLL. Patients treated with fludarabine demonstrated improvement in PFS and OS compared to chlorambucil, albeit with a higher rate of infectious complications; however, all patients ultimately had recurrent disease.[163] Similar to chlorambucil, fludarabine was also more effective compared to combination chemotherapy regimens like cyclophosphamide, doxorubicin, and prednisone (CAP).[173]

However, PFS and OS advantage was not shown in another randomized trial of elderly patients older than age 70 years treated with fludarabine on chlorambucil despite the higher overall and complete response (CR) rate in the fludarabine-treated patients.[174]

The use of fludarabine and similar nucleoside analogues is associated with significant hematologic and immunologic toxicities. Patients can experience prolonged cytopenias and especially neutropenia, which can result in a significant increase in the risk of infectious complications. These drugs are also exquisitely toxic to T cells, especially to CD4+ T cells. This effect may last for an extended period of time and predisposes patients to acquiring opportunistic infections.[175,176] Neurologic toxicities have also been observed in patients receiving the usual dose of fludarabine.[177] Patients treated with fludarabine occasionally develop autoimmune hemolytic anemia. In this situation, further use of fludarabine is contraindicated.[178–180] Fludarabine is also poorly tolerated in patients with compromised renal function as a significant percentage of the metabolites are cleared via the renal system. Hemodialysis is a useful tool to limit fludarabine toxicity in patients who develop acute renal failure while receiving treatment.[181] Moreover, fludarabine treatment in patients older than age 65 years was poorly tolerated and did not result in improvements in PFS and resulted in a trend toward inferior OS outcome when compared to chlorambucil.[174]

Other nucleoside analogues used in the treatment CLL include cladribine and pentostatin which have similar outcomes and toxicities as fludarabine.[182–185] A phase III trial comparing fludarabine, cladribine, and chlorambucil showed similar ORR and CR rate with all three agents, but median PFS was superior with cladribine (25 months) versus 10 and 9 months with fludarabine and chlorambucil, respectively.[186] No advantages, however, were observed in OS. Cytarabine has also shown modest activity, especially in combination with oxaliplatin, fludarabine, and rituximab (OFAR regimen) in patients with refractory disease and patients with Richter transformation.[187,188]

COMBINATION CHEMOTHERAPY

Multiple chemotherapeutic combinations have been studied in patients with CLL. One of the earlier combinations to be used was chlorambucil and prednisone with ORR of approximately 80 percent with CR rates of approximately 10 to 15 percent.[165,189] This regimen was also found to be as effective as other combination regimens like CVP, cyclophosphamide, melphalan, and prednisone (CMP), CAP, or CHOP.[159,190–192] A meta-analysis comparing lymphoma-like combination therapies found no improvements in survival outcomes over chlorambucil alone.[159] High-dose combination therapies like CAP, CHOP, and CVP have no role in the routine management of patients with CLL.

Given the improvement in outcomes with single-agent fludarabine as compared to chlorambucil, multiple combinations were developed with fludarabine to improve on its efficacy. Both the combination of fludarabine and chlorambucil and fludarabine and prednisone were found to be similar to fludarabine and not developed further.[172,193,194] Fludarabine was combined with cyclophosphamide (FC) and resulted in encouraging responses even in patients with heavily pretreated disease.[195] Multiple phase III trials were subsequently conducted in predominantly younger patients, comparing fludarabine with FC and revealed an ORR of 74 to 94 percent with CR rates of 23 to 38 percent and median PFS of 33 to 48 months, all significantly better with the combination.[87,196,197] Early toxicities were mostly related to cytopenias secondary to myelosuppression and the resultant increase in infectious complications resulted in a slight dose adjustment and a dose of fludarabine 25 to 30 mg/m^2 for 3 days and cyclophosphamide 250 mg/m^2 for 3 days every 28 days for six cycles was used for subsequent studies. Notably, the combination of FC was the first regimen that was able to overcome the adverse prognostic impact of del 11q.[86]

Similarly, other combinations of alkylating agents with nucleoside agents have been tested with varying success. These include cladribine and prednisone, which combination was shown to be better than chlorambucil and prednisone in terms of responses, but without improvements in OS and with a higher incidence of infectious complications in the cladribine-treated arm.[198,199] Similarly, the addition of cyclophosphamide and prednisone to cladribine resulted in higher responses but more myelosuppression and related complications.[200–202] Pentostatin was also combined with cyclophosphamide and resulted in ORR of 74 percent and CR rates of 17 percent in patients with fludarabine refractory disease.[203] Pentostatin in combination with chlorambucil and prednisone also resulted in promising responses but was extremely immunosuppressive and resulted in an unacceptably high incidence of infectious complications.[204]

Fludarabine was also combined with mitoxantrone without significant improvements in outcome. Although mitoxantrone appeared to improve outcomes when added to cladribine, it came at the cost of significant toxicity.[205,206] Likewise, the combination of fludarabine, cyclophosphamide, and mitoxantrone resulted in an ORR of 78 percent and CR rates of 50 percent in patients with relapsed disease and an ORR of 90 percent with a CR rate of 38 percent in patients with previously untreated disease. The major toxicity was myelosuppression.[206,207]

ANTIBODY THERAPY

The advent of antibodies for the treatment of patients with CLL has been a major advance in the management of this disease with the first true consistent evidence of improving survival. Numerous antibodies targeting different receptors have been developed and are at various stages of development. Four antibodies are currently approved for routine management. Unfortunately, one of these (alemtuzumab) is no longer actively marketed for this indication.

Alemtuzumab

Alemtuzumab is a CD52-targeting, humanized, monoclonal antibody that mediates its efficacy through direct cytotoxicity, complement-dependent cytotoxicity (CDC) and antibody-dependent cell-mediated cytotoxicity (ADCC). CD52 is ubiquitously expressed on lymphocytes (including B and T cells) and monocytes and this explains the efficacy and toxicity of the antibody. Alemtuzumab is extremely effective in clearing the blood and marrow of disease and is also active in patients with del 17p disease which is generally refractory to conventional chemotherapy.[208] However, alemtuzumab has limited efficacy in patients with bulky lymphadenopathy, especially in patients with lymph nodes that are greater than 5 cm in diameter.[209–211] Alemtuzumab was initially approved in 2001 by the FDA for the treatment of patients who had failed prior therapy with nucleoside analogues. This was primarily based on small trials that administered alemtuzumab intravenously three times a week for 12 weeks and showed modest response rates of approximately 30 to 40 percent and CRs in less than 5 percent of patients.[209–211] Responses were short-lived in this cohort of patients and the median response duration was approximately 9 months. Treatment was also complicated by infusion-related toxicities in the vast majority of patients. To minimize these reactions, alemtuzumab is started at a dose of 3 mg and escalated to 10 mg for the second dose and 30 mg for the third dose, as tolerated. Another major toxicity was immunosuppression that resulted in multiple recurrent infections especially with opportunistic organisms that are commonly seen in patients with chronic immunocompromised states like HIV/AIDS such as CMV, pneumocystis, or varicella zoster.[209–211] Patients also experienced prolonged cytopenias, especially of natural killer (NK) and T cells, which can persist for more than 9 months following therapy.[212] Consequently, antiviral and antimicrobial prophylaxis therapy should be initiated in all patients receiving alemtuzumab and should be continued for at least 6 months after completing therapy.

A subsequent large phase III (CAM307) clinical trial was performed that compared alemtuzumab to chlorambucil as first-line therapy.[213] Two hundred ninety-seven patients were randomized to chlorambucil 40 mg/m² every 4 weeks for 12 cycles or alemtuzumab 30 mg intravenous infusion three times per week for 12 weeks. Overall response with alemtuzumab was 83 percent, with 24 percent CRs and with time to next treatment of 23 months. This was significantly better than the results observed with chlorambucil, which resulted in an ORR of 55 percent with 2 percent CRs and time to next treatment of 14 months. Moreover, approximately one-third of patients treated with alemtuzumab achieved a minimal residual disease (MRD)-negative CR that was later shown to correlate with OS. Both agents were well-tolerated but alemtuzumab resulted in a higher incidence of CMV infections. This trial resulted in the approval of alemtuzumab as initial therapy for CLL in 2007.

Infusion reactions and infectious complications are the major issues observed with the use of alemtuzumab. Infusion reactions can be diminished with a subcutaneous administration which appears to be equally efficacious but with similar toxicity profiles.[214,215] Despite the encouraging results and approvals by the FDA, alemtuzumab never gained mass popularity and was not used by practicing physicians very often. It is no longer being marketed by the company for CLL but (as of 2015) can be obtained upon written request at no cost. The limited future prospects of alemtuzumab precludes exhaustive discussion. Alemtuzumab has been studied in combination with chemotherapy and as consolidative therapy after chemotherapy and has shown some benefit, but is generally associated with significant serious infectious morbidity.[216–219]

CD20 Targeting Antibodies

Rituximab Rituximab is a chimeric, murine, CD20-targeting, monoclonal antibody that has been extensively used for the treatment of patients with CD20+ lymphoid malignancies. CD20 is a calcium channel that interacts with BCR complex and is ubiquitously expressed on B-cell non-Hodgkin lymphomas and has a weak expression on CLL cells. Rituximab exerts its efficacy through direct CDC and ADCC.[220–222]

The dose and schedule of treatment with rituximab was determined empirically and has since been modified repeatedly. Initial trials were performed with four weekly infusions at 375 mg/m² and showed limited efficacy in patients with CLL.[223,224] Responses were higher when higher doses (up to 2250 mg/m²) or dose-dense regimens (375 mg/m² three times a week) were used but was primarily limited to the blood and nodal areas.[225,226] Nonetheless, these studies established the efficacy of rituximab and supported combination trials with chemoimmunotherapy where their impact has been most impactful.

Rituximab is generally tolerated very well with the most common toxicity being infusion reactions that are predominantly observed primarily with the first dose. These are generally mild fevers or chills, but occasionally may result in serious reactions that mimic severe allergic or anaphylactic reactions or cytokine release syndrome. The infusion reactions can be minimized with the routine use of prophylactic acetaminophen, antihistamine, and corticosteroids, glucocorticoid, and by slowing the infusion rate. Patients may also experience transient, severe thrombocytopenia, the mechanism of which is poorly understood. Therefore, rituximab should be used with caution in patients with a preexisting thrombocytopenia. Another important and potentially severe toxicity is tumor lysis syndrome, which is generally observed in patients with a high circulating peripheral lymphocyte count. These patients should be monitored closely and should receive prophylactic hydration, allopurinol, and electrolyte monitoring during and after the infusion. Other uncommon toxicities include delayed neutropenia, hepatitis B reactivation, interstitial pneumonitis, rash, and serum sickness. Patients with a prior history of hepatitis B infection should receive monitoring for reactivation while being treated with rituximab or similar agents, with rapid implementation of antiviral therapy if reactivation is observed. Fatal cases of progressive multifocal leukoencephalopathy from JC polyomavirus infection has also been reported with the use of rituximab and similar monoclonal antibodies. These infections typically occur during treatment or soon after, with virtually all cases observed during the first year posttherapy.[227,228]

Ofatumumab Ofatumumab is a fully human, type 1, IgG₁, CD20-targeting, monoclonal antibody that binds more effectively to a different epitope of CD20 than rituximab.[229] *In vitro* it was shown to have improved CDC and ADCC as compared to rituximab.[230,231] Ofatumumab is given as a test dose of 300 mg followed by eight weekly intravenous infusions of 2000 mg, after which patients can go on a maintenance schedule of four monthly infusions of 2000 mg. The half-life of ofatumumab is 21 days, but the B-cell–depleting effects may last for up to 7 months after the last infusion.[232]

Early results with ofatumumab as a single agent in patients who were refractory to alemtuzumab and/or fludarabine showed encouraging ORR of 58 percent in the double refractory group and 47 percent in the fludarabine refractory cohort with bulky disease. Responses were all partial except for one CR in the fludarabine refractory group. Response was also short lived and the median duration of response was 7 months in the fludarabine refractory group and 5.6 months in the double refractory group with most patients progressing during treatment.[233] These results led to the approval of ofatumumab in patients with relapsed disease refractory to alemtuzumab and/or fludarabine in 2009. Subsequent studies compared ofatumumab (300 mg on day 1 followed by eight weekly infusions of 1000 mg, followed by 1000 mg on day 1 of subsequent 28-day cycles, for a maximum of 12 cycles) given in combination with oral chlorambucil (10 mg/m² on days 1 to 7 of each 28-day cycle) versus chlorambucil alone, in patients with previously untreated CLL who required treatment and were not considered candidates for conventional chemoimmunotherapy. The combination resulted in an ORR of 82 percent versus 68 percent with chlorambucil alone. However, CR rates were 12 percent versus 1 percent and median duration of response was 22 months versus 13 months in the combination versus chlorambucil arms, respectively.[234] Based on these results, the combination of ofatumumab and chlorambucil was granted approval in 2014 for the treatment of previously untreated patients with CLL for whom fludarabine-based therapy is considered inappropriate.

Ofatumumab has also been studied in the upfront setting in combination with FC in smaller phase II studies of a relatively young patient population (median age: 56 years). This study revealed an ORR of 75 percent with 41 percent CRs.[235] The combination of ofatumumab with pentostatin and cyclophosphamide resulted in a 96 percent ORR with 46 percent complete remission rate.[236,237] This compares favorably to the results seen with the combination of rituximab and chemotherapy, but large multiinstitution randomized trials are lacking.

Ofatumumab is generally well-tolerated, with the most common reaction being an infusion-related reaction that typically occurs with the first infusion and includes fevers, rash, fatigue, chills, and diaphoresis. These reactions tend to get better with subsequent infusions. Infectious complications are similar to those reported with other CD20 monoclonal antibodies.

Obinutuzumab Obinutuzumab is a CD20-targeting antibody that was approved in combination with chlorambucil for the initial treatment of patients with CLL in 2014. Obinutuzumab is a fully humanized, type II, IgG₁ antibody[238] with additional structural modifications that explain its enhanced activity. It binds selectively to the extracellular domain of CD20 with reduced internalization. This persistence of the antibody on the cell surface along with a fucosylation in its Fc region allow for enhanced ADCC through robust engagement of Fc-gamma receptor type III on effector cells. Another modification in the hinge region allows for more potent direct cytotoxicity.[239–241] Together, these modifications translate into a higher efficacy as compared with rituximab in both preclinical and clinical studies.[239–243]

Obinutuzumab in combination with chlorambucil was compared to rituximab and chlorambucil and chlorambucil alone in patients with untreated CLL in the CLL-11 trial conducted by the German CLL study group.[244] Patients had a median age of 73 years, which is closer to the median age of 72 years at diagnosis for CLL patients, and significantly higher than the median ages of 58 to 62 years which have historically been the population that has been enrolled in chemotherapy-based clinical trials for CLL. More importantly, these patients had clinically meaningful comorbid conditions. Treatment of this patient population has historically been challenging and no prior chemotherapeutic option, including fludarabine, has improved survival outcomes as compared to chlorambucil alone.[174] The combination of obinutuzumab and chlorambucil improved ORRs (77.3 percent [obinutuzumab and chlorambucil] vs. 65.7 percent [rituximab and chlorambucil] vs. 31.4 percent [chlorambucil]), CR rates (22.3 percent [obinutuzumab and chlorambucil] vs. 7.3 percent [rituximab and chlorambucil] vs. 0 percent [chlorambucil]) and median PFS (26.7 months [obinutuzumab and chlorambucil] vs. 16.3 months [rituximab and chlorambucil] vs. 11.1 months [chlorambucil]). Obinutuzumab with chlorambucil also prolonged OS over that which was observed with chlorambucil. Notably, the combination also resulted in significant improvement in the rate of MRD-negative status in both marrow (19.5 percent vs. 2.6 percent) and blood (37.7 percent vs. 3.3 percent) as compared to rituximab and chlorambucil.

Obinutuzumab is generally well-tolerated, but has a high incidence of infusion reactions that are seen primarily with the first infusion. Unlike rituximab or ofatumumab where infusion events occur 1 to 2 hours into therapy, those with obinutuzumab typically occur within the first 5 to 10 minutes of starting therapy. These may be minimized by a test dose, slower infusion rate, and prophylactic steroids, acetaminophen, and antihistamines. Tumor lysis is also seen in a small number of patients, reflecting the higher efficacy of obinutuzumab. Hematologic toxicities, like neutropenia and thrombocytopenia, are also observed. All CD20-targeting antibodies increase the risk of hepatitis B virus reactivation and progressive multifocal leukoencephalopathy.

The activity of obinutuzumab in patients with untreated CLL is very exciting and this antibody is being combined with other novel agents and chemotherapy to further improve outcomes in patients with CLL.

Other Antibodies and Antibody-Like Compounds

Multiple antibodies targeting various antigens like CD19 and CD37 are at various stages of development for the treatment of CLL.[245–247] Advances in antibody manufacturing technology are enabling us to synthesize more potent and bispecific antibodies like blinatumomab, which has already shown promising activity in patients with acute lymphoblastic lymphoma (ALL) and CLL.[248]

GLUCOCORTICOIDS

Glucocorticoids are effective agents in the management of patients with relapsed CLL and especially patients with del 17p and fludarabine refractory disease. High-dose methylprednisolone, either as a single agent or in combination with multiple other chemotherapeutic agents, produced sustained responses in the majority of patients with refractory and high-risk disease.[249] High-dose methylprednisolone at 1 g/m for 5 days with weekly rituximab for three cycles induces response rates as high as 93 percent with a CR of 36 percent.[250] Therapy, however, is complicated by significant hyperglycemia, fluid retention, and immune suppression resulting in increased incidence of opportunistic infections requiring close followup and aggressive supportive care with prophylactic anti-biotics. The addition of weekly rituximab and decreasing the duration of methylprednisone dose to 3 days resulted in similar responses and reduction in the incidence of adverse events.[250,251] Similar results were observed when methylprednisolone was substituted for dexamethasone 40 mg weekly or every 2 weeks for 4 days.[252] Glucocorticoids at lower doses are also very useful in the management of patients with autoimmune complications as a result of their CLL.

CHEMOIMMUNOTHERAPY

The combining of chemotherapy with targeted antibodies has been a major advance in the management of patients with CLL. Multiple thera-peutic combinations have been developed and validated for use and are summarized below.

Fludarabine and Rituximab

The impact of sequential or concurrent administration of rituximab with fludarabine (FR) was assessed in the Cancer and Leukemia Group B (CALGB) 9712 randomized study of 104 previously untreated CLL patients.[253] Fludarabine was given at 25 mg/m² days 1 to 5 every 4 weeks for six cycles, with or without concurrent rituximab 375 mg/m² on day 1 of each cycle, and an additional dose on day 4 of cycle 1. Patients in both arms received rituximab 375 mg/m² weekly for four doses beginning 2 months after completion of fludarabine; thus, patients in the concur-rent arm received 11 total doses of rituximab, compared to four in the sequential arm. ORR was 90 percent versus 77 percent and CR rates were 47 percent versus 28 percent in the concurrent versus sequential arm, respectively. A retrospective comparison to a fludarabine-only treatment (CALGB 9011) demonstrated improved PFS and OS with the use of FR.[254] This regimen had limited efficacy in patients with del 17p and del 11q. The median PFS was 42 months and 27 percent were progression free at 5 years. Notably, there were no cases of treatment-related-myeloid neoplasms occurring before disease relapse.[255]

Fludarabine, Cyclophosphamide, and Rituximab

Fludarabine, cyclophosphamide, and rituximab (FCR) chemotherapy has been studied extensively in patients with previously treated and untreated CLL.[256–259] Fludarabine was administered at 25 mg/m², cyclo-phosphamide at 250 mg/m² on days 2 to 4 of cycle 1 and on days 1 to 3 of cycles 2 to 6, and rituximab at 375 mg/m² on day 1 of cycle 1 and 500 mg/m² on day 1 of cycles 2 to 6. In the initial single institution, phase II experience of 300 untreated CLL patients, this combination resulted in exciting ORR of 95 percent with CR rate of 72 percent with median time to progression of 80 months in patients with untreated CLL.[259] However, despite a younger patient population with a median age of 57 years, FCR resulted in significant and sustained myelosuppres-sion, with 35 percent of patients experiencing cytopenias 3 months after completing therapy.[260] Notably, therapy-related myeloid neoplasms/myelodysplastic syndromes occurred in 5.1 percent of patients and Richter transformation in 9 percent.[261] FCR was subsequently compared to FC in a large multicenter trial of 817 young patients (median age: 61 years) with previously untreated CLL.[262] The responses observed with FCR were more modest in larger phase III trials. Patients treated

with FCR had a significantly higher ORR of 90 percent with a CR rate of 44 percent as compared to FC, which resulted in an ORR of 80 percent and a CR rate of 22 percent. More importantly, this study established the improvement in OS with the addition of rituximab to chemother-apy. As a result, rituximab was approved for the treatment of patients with CLL in combination with chemotherapy in 2010. The use of FCR was also associated with a significantly higher risk of cytopenias that did not result in a higher incidence of serious infectious complications which were similar in both arms as was the treatment-related mortality. All genomic groups appear to benefit from the addition of FCR, except for those without any common interphase cytogenetic abnormalities and those with del 17p.[263] Long-term followup of FCR by both the MD Anderson group and the German CLL Study Group suggests that the patients benefiting most from FCR may be those with IGHV mutated disease where prolonged complete remissions can be obtained. For patients with IGHV unmutated disease there does not appear to be any evidence of sustained stable remission, with all eventually relapsing and requiring additional therapy.[263,264]

Given the poor tolerability and increased toxicity observed with the use of FCR in elderly patients and patients with compromised renal function and to enhance efficacy of FCR, multiple variations of the reg-imen were tested with similar results in small cohorts of patients.[265,266] None of these regimens are commonly used and the advent of alterna-tive agents have made these regimens of limited utility.

Bendamustine and Rituximab

The combination of bendamustine and rituximab (BR) has been tested both in patients with relapsed and in patients with untreated CLL. In the first BR study with relapsed CLL bendamustine was administered to 78 patients at a dose of 70 mg/m² on days 1 and 2 with rituximab 375 mg/m² on day 0 of cycle 1 and 500 mg/m² on day 1 of cycles 2 to 6. The ORR was 59 percent with a CR rate of 9 percent and a median PFS of 14.7 months. Minimal activity was observed in patients with del 17p.[267] In the subsequent followup study, 117 patients with previously untreated CLL were treated at the same schedule but with a higher dose of bendamustine at 90 mg/m² on days 1 and 2 and resulted in ORR of 91 percent with CR rate of 33 percent.[268] In the large, multicenter, CLL10 trial, 564 patients with previously untreated CLL, good performance status, and low comor-bidity burden were randomized to FCR or BR.[269] ORR was similar in both arms at 97 percent but CR rates were higher in the FCR arm at 40 percent versus 31 percent with BR. MRD rates were also higher with FCR (74 per-cent vs. 62 percent). Median PFS was 53 months in the FCR arm and 43 months in the BR arm. FCR was more toxic and severe neutropenia was more often observed in the FCR arm (87 percent vs. 67 percent) as were severe infections (39 percent vs. 25 percent). Treatment-related mortality was 3.9 percent with FCR and 2.1 percent with BR. Given these results, FCR appears to be the more effective therapeutic option for younger patients and patients without significant comorbid conditions, and BR can be used for older and unfit patients.

Other Chemoimmunotherapeutic Regimens

Pentostatin and rituximab and pentostatin, cyclophosphamide, and rituximab (PCR) both resulted in promising ORR (91 percent vs. 76 percent) and CR rates (41 percent vs. 27 percent).[237,270] Importantly, the PCR regimen appeared to be generally well-tolerated in young and older patients and in patients with high-risk genetic features. Levels of Mcl-1, an antiapoptotic protein, were also shown to be predictive of response and OS.[34] The most common toxicity was neutropenia and thrombo-cytopenia. Similarly, cladribine and cladribine plus cyclophosphamide were also combined with rituximab and resulted in predictable efficacy and toxicity.[271–273]

KINASE INHIBITORS

The introduction of BCR kinase inhibitors has significantly improved the management options for patients with CLL and represents a group of agents that very likely will change the natural history of this disease. Early results with these agents including ibrutinib and idelalisib that target BTK and PI3K, respectively, have shown promising efficacy and excellent tolerability but long-term data is limited to 4 years of followup and decision rules need to be developed that allow for eventual treatment discontinuation.[72] Much of what was learned from the transition of chemoimmunotherapy management of chronic myeloid leukemia will likely become relevant to CLL as additional follow up develops with the use of BCR antagonists in this disease.

Ibrutinib

Ibrutinib is a first-in-class, irreversible inhibitor of BTK and covalently binds to Cys-481 near the ATP binding domain of the BTK molecule, and abrogates enzyme activity and BCR-mediated survival signals. Ibrutinib also has the ability to irreversibly target ITK in T cells and other Tec family of kinases.[274]

A 420-mg daily oral dose of ibrutinib has been used in the treatment of patients with relapsed CLL and demonstrated an ORR of 71 percent with an additional 20 percent of patients experiencing partial response (PR) with lymphocytosis (PR+L), which, interestingly, does not appear to predict for inferior PFS.[275] The responses observed with ibrutinib are sustained and resulted in PFS of 75 percent at 26 months.[92] Patients with del 17p had an ORR of 55.9 percent with a median duration of response of 25 months.[276] Historical comparisons reveal a significantly improved response rate and PFS when ibrutinib was compared to either cyclin-dependent kinase (CDK) inhibitors or other conventional therapies used in the past for patients with del 17p.[91] Similar exciting results were reported in elderly, treatment-naïve patients treated with ibrutinib with ORR of 71 percent and 13 percent PR+L. These responses also appear to be sustained over time with PFS of 96.1 percent at 2 years.[277] Ibrutinib in general is well-tolerated, with the most common side effects being mild diarrhea, nausea, and fatigue. A randomized study comparing ibrutinib to ofatumumab in relapsed CLL confirmed the benefits of ibrutinib with improved response rate, PFS, and OS.[278] However, this study also demonstrated a higher incidence of both minor bleeding and atrial fibrillation with ibrutinib. The bleeding diathesis observed with ibrutinib is possibly caused by a collagen-mediated platelet aggregation defect.[278,279] Caution should be taken to avoid the use of ibrutinib in patients on concurrent anticoagulation with warfarin and treatment should be held 3 to 7 days before and after surgical procedures. The pathophysiologic reason for increased risk of atrial fibrillation with ibrutinib is uncertain. Ibrutinib treatment also results in a progressive decline in the incidence of infectious complications with ongoing therapy, primarily as a result of disease control.[92] Most patients do not require routine antimicrobial prophylaxis commonly used with chemoimmunotherapy. Moreover, improvements are also observed in stress, depressive symptoms, fatigue, and quality-of-life in patients treated with ibrutinib.[280] Based on these exciting data, ibrutinib was approved in 2014 for the treatment of all patients with relapsed CLL and for the treatment of all patients with del 17p CLL regardless of prior therapy.

Treatment with ibrutinib does not result in CRs in most patients and discontinuing this treatment in heavily pretreated patients often results in patients experiencing rapid disease progression. Therefore, we currently recommend that ibrutinib be continued in responding patients until disease progression or unacceptable toxicity. However, this chronic exposure to kinase inhibitors might result in the emergence of resistant malignant cell clones, although this has been quite rare.[72] Data derived from whole-exome sequencing of paired samples at baseline and at the time of relapse while being treated with ibrutinib identified a cysteine-to-serine mutation in BTK at the binding site of ibrutinib and three distinct mutations in PLCγ_2.[281] Functional analysis revealed that the C481S mutation of BTK results in a protein that is only reversibly inhibited by ibrutinib. The R665W and L845F mutations in PLCγ_2 are both potentially gain-of-function mutations that lead to autonomous BCR activity. Interestingly, these mutations were not found in any of the patients with prolonged lymphocytosis who were taking ibrutinib, suggesting an alternative and as yet unidentified mechanism for the persistence of lymphocytosis in those patients. Furthermore, the clinical impact of this persistent lymphocytosis was not demonstrated, with individuals having persistent lymphocytosis actually having similar outcome to those patients with PRs or better.

Ibrutinib is being combined with various other agents to improve the depth of response and outcomes. The combination of ibrutinib and rituximab in patients with high-risk CLL was generally well-tolerated and resulted in an ORR of 95 percent and a PFS of 78 percent at 18 months.[282] PFS was 72 percent at 18 months in patients with del 17p. Multiple trials are ongoing with ibrutinib in the frontline setting and in comparison to chemoimmunotherapy. These trials and the development of newer BTK inhibitors have the potential to change the treatment paradigms for CLL.

Idelalisib

Idelalisib is an orally bioavailable, first-in-class isoform selective PI3K-δ inhibitor that promoted apoptosis of CLL B cells *ex vivo*, along with abrogating the survival signals provided by the microenvironment.[283] The PI3K family of enzymes are involved in an extraordinarily diverse group of cellular functions, including cell growth, proliferation, differentiation, motility, survival, and intracellular trafficking.[284] Many of these functions relate to the ability of class I PI3Ks to activate the PI3K/AKT/mTOR (mammalian target of rapamycin) pathway.[285] The p110δ isoform regulates different aspects of cellular proliferation and survival and is constitutively overexpressed in CLL B cells[286]; consequently, targeting it with specific inhibitors has become a useful therapeutic option.[72]

In a phase I trial of 54 patients, with relapsed/refractory high-risk CLL patients, idelalisib resulted in an ORR of 72 percent (including PR+L).[71] The median PFS was 15.8 months. Therapy was generally well-tolerated with the most commonly observed grade 3 or greater adverse events being pneumonia (20 percent), neutropenic fever (11 percent), and diarrhea (6 percent). The combination of idelalisib and rituximab was also compared to rituximab and placebo in a phase III trial and resulted in an ORR of 81 percent versus 13 percent and PFS at 1 year in excess of 90 percent versus 5.5 months in the rituximab and placebo arms, respectively.[287] Serious toxicities observed with idelalisib included transaminase elevations, diarrhea with colitis, and pneumonitis that were primarily observed after continued drug exposure. Based on these results, idelalisib was approved in 2014 in combination with rituximab for the treatment of patients with relapsed CLL with significant comorbid conditions that would make them ineligible for treatment with standard chemotherapy.

Lenalidomide

Lenalidomide is an immunomodulatory analogue of thalidomide and is approved for the treatment of multiple myeloma and myelodysplastic syndrome.[288] Lenalidomide has also shown exciting efficacy in patients with previously treated and untreated CLL in multiple studies.[289-293] Multiple dose levels and schedules have been tested in CLL with varying responses. From compilation of all the data it appears that 5 mg daily continuous dose of lenalidomide appears to be the best-tolerated dose in the vast majority of patients with CLL.[294] The responses observed with CLL are mostly PRs in 40 to 60 percent of patients, with approximately 10 percent of the patients experiencing a CR. However, response improves with ongoing therapy. Cytopenias are the most common, and dose-limiting, side effect. Patients can also experience tumor flare and tumor lysis, especially at the start of therapy. Care should be taken to minimize these reactions with the early use of steroids and aggressive hydration and uricosuric agents. In a recent phase III study, lenalidomide was shown to increase mortality in patients older than 80 years of age and thus is not recommended for the elderly. Combination of lenalidomide with monoclonal antibodies has also resulted in improved sustained responses.[295–297] Despite the advent of kinase inhibitors, lenalidomide continues to be an exciting agent for the treatment of CLL as it is one of the only agents that appears to have the potential to reverse the immune dysfunction associated with CLL; it also appears to have efficacy in patients with del 17p disease.[49,298–301]

CHIMERIC ANTIGEN RECEPTOR T CELLS

Chimeric antigen receptor T (CAR-T) cells are engineered autologous lentiviral modified T cells that contain an altered TCR targeting a surface antigen (e.g., CD19) on the surface of CLL B cells. The modified TCR has a higher affinity and specificity toward the target antigen and is not major histocompatibility complex (MHC) restricted. Multiple CAR-T cells have been developed and tested in clinical trials with exciting results.[302,303] These modified T cells persisted *in vivo* for an extended period and were able to induce prolonged clinical responses in the majority of patients.[304] The treatment is associated with severe cytokine release syndrome and macrophage activation syndrome that require aggressive and intensive supportive care and anti–IL-6–directed therapy. These modified CAR-T cells also result in the sustained elimination of normal B cells and subsequent sustained hypogammaglobulinemia that require ongoing supportive care and infection prophylaxis to limit the incidence of infectious complications in these patients.[303] Development of these agents on a larger scale is ongoing to allow for larger studies to confirm their promising effect.

OTHER AGENTS

Venetoclax (ABT-199) is an oral Bcl-2–targeting agent that has shown impressive activity with deep remissions in patients with relapsed and refractory CLL, including those who have del 17p.[305] Bcl-2 is an antiapoptotic protein overexpressed in CLL and causes disruption of apoptosis in CLL cells. Early efforts with the first-generation compound navitoclax, demonstrated single-agent activity, but also resulted in profound thrombocytopenia as a result of off-target effects on Bcl-xl expressed in platelets. Venetoclax is significantly more potent and more specific to Bcl-2 with limited off-target effects.[306] Combination studies are already underway with kinase inhibitors and monoclonal antibodies to improve outcomes. Therapy with venetoclax has been complicated by fulminant tumor lysis syndrome, especially in patients with a high burden of disease that has greatly slowed down clinical development of this agent.

Blinatumomab is an engineered bi-specific T-cell engaging (BiTE) antibody that has shown promising activity in CD19+ B-cell malignancies, including CLL and ALL.[248] It was approved in 2014 for the treatment of relapsed ALL. Blinatumomab engages the CD19+ cell and brings it in close proximity to a CD3+ T-cell that is also activated upon binding to the bi-specific antibody. The resultant interaction leads to the apoptosis of the CD19+ B cells. The antibody has shown promising and durable responses and is currently in clinical trials for CLL. Therapy is complicated by hypogammaglobulinemia, cytokine release and neurologic symptoms.[307]

CDK inhibitors like flavopiridol and dinaciclib have also demonstrated promising activity in patients with CLL, and are able to induce durable remissions even in patients with high-risk del 17p disease with or without concomitant chemotherapy.[308–311] Therapy with CDK inhibitors is complicated by fulminant hyperacute tumor lysis that requires aggressive supportive care including hemodialysis. Diarrhea and fatigue are also seen as off target effects.

STEM CELL TRANSPLANTATION IN PATIENTS WITH CHRONIC LYMPHOCYTIC LEUKEMIA

With the advent of effective therapy for patients with relapsed and refractory disease and even for patients with high-risk disease, the role of stem cell transplantation (SCT) for the routine management of patients with CLL is diminishing. Autologous transplantation has the ability to induce deeper and more frequent remissions that may result in longer disease-free remission, but does not translate into an OS advantage and is associated with significantly higher morbidity and mortality and secondary cancers, including therapy-related myeloid neoplasms that may impact long-term survival.[312–314] Moreover, autologous transplantation, which is essentially high-dose chemotherapy, is unable to overcome the chemoresistance conferred by del 17p or TP53 mutation. Consequently, autologous transplantation has no role in the routine management of patients with CLL.

Allogeneic SCT potentially offers a curative approach for patients with CLL, but its utility and timing is currently under considerable debate given the availability of multiple novel agents. Myeloablative conditioning prior to allogeneic SCT is associated with an unacceptably high transplant-related mortality (TRM) in excess of 30 percent and is not generally recommended.[314–316] Nonmyeloablative conditioning regimens afford the opportunity to reduce TRM without impacting the graft-versus-leukemia (GVL) effect. Long-term disease-free survival is generally in the 30 to 45 percent range. However, nonrelapse mortality (NRM) is still in the 15 to 30 percent range, but decreasing with improvements in supportive care techniques. Moreover, chronic graft-versus-host disease still impacts long-term quality-of-life after nonmyeloablative allogeneic SCT in approximately 25 percent of survivors.[317–320] Various patient-, disease-, and transplant-specific factors at the time of transplantation impact SCT outcomes.[321] In particular, the number of prior treatments and the presence of a complex karyotype contribute to success and also toxicity observed after transplantation.[322–324] Studies have identified that implementation of an effective quality management system and experience of the transplantation center are associated with a significant decrease in NRM.[325–327] Patients who relapse after SCT can sometimes be effectively salvaged with the use of currently approved novel therapeutic agents. Given the availability of kinase inhibitors such as ibrutinib, we recommend that patients be offered therapy with these novel agents and nonmyeloablative SCT evaluation should be reserved for those failing ibrutinib unless no other cytoreductive therapy is available after receipt of this agent. Moreover, we recommend that patients who progress after treatment with kinase inhibitors be referred to a treatment center with established expertise for treating CLL, as this can significantly impact their therapeutic options and outcomes.[325–327]

SPLENECTOMY

Splenectomy is rarely used today given the availability of effective therapeutic agents to treat CLL. It can be an effective option for ameliorating refractory autoimmune hemolytic anemia and thrombocytopenia for which medical management has been unsuccessful.[328] It can also be used to provide relief to patients with symptomatic splenomegaly secondary to refractory disease.[329–331]

RADIATION

Involved field radiation therapy is an extremely useful treatment modality for the management of locally symptomatic lymphadenopathy and isolated Richter transformation. Splenic irradiation can be used in patients with symptomatic splenomegaly, but its efficacy is limited and short-lived with significant and sometimes prolonged myelosuppression.[332-334] Systemic radiation or extracorporeal photopheresis has no role in the routine management of patients with CLL.[335-337]

LEUKAPHERESIS

Patients with CLL will very rarely experience hyperviscosity-related signs and symptoms secondary to hyperleukocytosis. However, this modality can be used for the occasional patient who becomes symptomatic from hyperleukocytosis. When this is initiated, it should be performed in conjunction conventional therapy, to cytoreduce the CLL. Leukapheresis has been used in the past for patients with refractory disease as a therapeutic option, but it results in modest and transient benefits.[338-340] With the advent of modern therapeutic options, the role of leukapheresis is limited in the management of routine CLL patients with hyperleukocytosis. While the BCR signaling agents can cause profound hyperleukocytosis in some patients, it virtually never results in symptoms mandating leukapheresis.

● ASSESSMENT OF RESPONSE

Patients who complete therapy should be assessed for response. This involves performing a detailed history for any disease-related symptoms, physical examination for any palpable lymphadenopathy, and laboratory studies to evaluate for persistent cytopenias or leukocytosis. Outside of a clinical trial, if the patient fails to have a CR on routine history, physical evaluation, and blood counts, then a CT scan and a marrow biopsy have limited utility. However, if the patient does achieve a CR on clinical and laboratory evaluation, we recommend proceeding with a CT scan of the chest, abdomen, and pelvis with contrast, along with a marrow aspirate and biopsy in the event that the CT scan is negative. These patients should undergo evaluation for MRD assessment on the marrow aspirate. Formal response criteria for disease evaluation were revised with the advent of kinase inhibitors. Conventionally, patients with no evidence of disease on CT scan and marrow biopsy with complete hematologic count recovery would be classified as a complete remission. Patients with a CR but with persistent cytopenias that are related to drug toxicity are classified as having CR with incomplete count recovery (CRi). These are also detailed in the IWCLL-2008 criteria.[1] Evaluation of the marrow aspirate and biopsy is also useful in assessing the etiology of cytopenias that can be seen frequently after chemotherapy use. We recommend waiting until count recovery or 3 to 6 months after chemotherapy to repeat a marrow biopsy for persistent cytopenias. Occasionally, patients will have no evidence of disease on flow cytometry of the aspirate or on the biopsy specimen but may have nodular lymphoid aggregates. If these aggregates are confirmed to be consistent with a collection of CLL cells by immunohistochemical studies, then these patients should be classified as having a nodular PR. Given the advent of kinase inhibitors, the response criteria are undergoing significant modifications especially because most patients will not experience traditional responses as observed with chemotherapy use despite having similar or even better outcomes.[341] This is especially evident in patients with PR+L after kinase inhibitor therapy with ibrutinib who demonstrate significant and sustained improvement in clinical signs and symptoms related to CLL and in lymphadenopathy and organomegaly and potentially may have a longer progression-free interval as compared to people with a more conventional partial remission.[275]

● EVALUATION FOR MINIMAL RESIDUAL DISEASE

CLL is currently considered incurable, but a subset of patients who achieve a complete remission will have undetectable disease even after using highly sensitive techniques. The evaluation for MRD is now fairly well established and can be performed by either flow cytometry or allele-specific oligonucleotide polymerase chain reaction–based methods.[342-345] Both these tests have excellent comparable sensitivity and are able to identify one leukemia cell in 10,000 leukocytes.[343] These tests can be performed on blood but sensitivity is higher when performed on marrow aspirate, especially with the current use of monoclonal antibodies that are able to effectively clear the circulating blood of the disease but are not equally effective in eliminating disease from the marrow or lymph nodes. Patients with MRD-negative disease at the completion of therapy experience longer treatment-free and OS periods.[346,347] This advantage in outcomes has been shown both for chemotherapy-based regimens and for regimens based primarily on antibodies.[262,347] The utility of MRD assessment in the era of kinase inhibitors is currently under discussion as kinase inhibitors are not typically able to induce deep remissions as monotherapy in the majority of patients with short followup. MRD assessment, however, can be used as a surrogate for survival outcomes and to potentially develop a stopping rule for kinase inhibitor-based combination approaches.

● RECOMMENDATIONS FOR TREATMENT OF PATIENTS WITH UNTREATED DISEASE

All patients should be offered therapy on a clinical trial whenever possible. This is increasingly important as therapy for CLL is evolving rapidly and clinical trials are required to answer the multiple questions regarding the best possible therapeutic option. For patients being treated off-trial, we recommend discussion of the potential risks and benefits of chemoimmunotherapy with FCR, particularly when low-risk disease is present (e.g., IGHV mutated disease) that might result in prolonged remission. For those with IGHV unmutated disease, chemoimmunotherapy with FCR or alternative non–chemotherapy-based regimens are considered. For patients older than age 65 years and those with multiple comorbid conditions or renal insufficiency, we recommend therapy with either obinutuzumab or ofatumumab with chlorambucil. Younger and healthier patients can be treated with chemoimmunotherapy. Patients with del 17p should be treated with ibrutinib in the first-line setting.

● RECOMMENDATIONS FOR TREATMENT OF PATIENTS WITH RELAPSED DISEASE

Patients who relapse after conventional chemoimmunotherapy-based approaches should, in most cases, be treated with ibrutinib unless a need for chronic anticoagulation with warfarin (Coumadin) is required. In such settings, treatment with idelalisib with or without rituximab should be considered. With both ibrutinib and idelalisib, the benefit of adding rituximab at this time is not known. Repeating a different chemoimmunotherapy regimen is also an option in younger and otherwise healthy patients, but is associated with higher toxicity and risk of secondary neoplasms. Patients who relapse after one kinase inhibitor should be treated with the other and referred to a specialized center for clinical trial participation on subsequent relapses.

SECONDARY CANCER RISK WITH CHRONIC LYMPHOCYTIC LEUKEMIA

Patients with CLL have a significantly higher risk of developing a secondary malignancy. This includes cancers of the skin, connective tissue and peripheral nerves, eye, lip and oral cavity, lung, kidney, colorectal, prostate, breast, and genitourinary cancers.[348] Skin cancer is one of the most common cancers seen in patients with CLL.[349–351] This includes basal cell carcinoma, squamous cell carcinoma, cutaneous melanoma, and Merkel cell carcinoma. Patients with skin cancers also appear to have a worse prognosis from their melanoma and Merkel cell cancer if they also have a concomitant CLL history.[348,352] This is also true for solid tumors, as patients with breast, colorectal, prostate, lung, and kidney cancers have an inferior prognosis if they have a preexisting diagnosis of CLL.[353] We therefore recommend an annual mammogram and pap smear for female patients and annual prostate evaluation in male patients and annual dermatologic evaluation and screening colonoscopy every 5 years for all patients with CLL. Multiple myeloma also occurs at a higher frequency in patients with CLL, but appears to arise from a separate B-cell clone.[354–356] Non-Hodgkin lymphomas are typically not associated with CLL and appearance of a large cell lymphoma is considered to be Richter transformation.[357]

MANAGEMENT OF INFECTIOUS COMPLICATIONS

Infectious complications constitute the leading cause of morbidity and mortality in patients with CLL. Patients with CLL develop progressive hypogammaglobulinemia with progressive disease that results in a higher incidence of infections with encapsulated organisms like *Streptococcus pneumoniae* and *Haemophilus influenzae*.[358] This has historically been further compounded by the effect of cytotoxic chemotherapeutics like fludarabine or antibodies like alemtuzumab that cause profound T-cell depletion along with worsening normal B-cell depletion and resultant hypogammaglobulinemia.[359] This combined effect of disease and therapy results in a higher incidence of opportunistic bacterial and viral infections with herpes simplex virus, CMV, herpes zoster virus, and *Listeria monocytogenes*. Fungal infections with *Cryptococcus neoformans* and *Pneumocystis jiroveci* are also seen in these patients and patients treated with high-dose glucocorticoids.[359–361] Patients respond to appropriate antibiotics early in their disease course, but might require prolonged and repeated courses of antibiotics later in their disease course and after therapy with chemotherapeutic agents. Prophylaxis for herpes zoster infections with acyclovir and for *P. jiroveci* with trimethoprim-sulfamethoxazole is routinely used for patients with prior therapy with nucleoside analogues.[362] Fungal prophylaxis is also employed with voriconazole or posaconazole for the prevention of invasive aspergillosis in patients on high-dose steroids. Patients treated with ibrutinib experience a lower incidence of infection, possibly because of effective disease control and despite a significant improvement in immunoglobulin levels.[92]

Hypogammaglobulinemia is universally present in patients with CLL and progressively worsens with advancing stage of the disease. Intravenous immunoglobulin (IVIG) at doses of 250 to 600 mg/kg administered every 4 to 6 weeks may result in a significant reduction of major infections requiring intensive supportive care and a modest reduction in the incidence of clinically significant infections. However, there is no significant improvement in survival.[363–365] Consequently, we recommend the judicious use of IVIG in patients at high risk of developing infectious complications.

Along with the disease-related immune defects, patients with CLL also respond poorly to routine prophylactic vaccinations. Response to protein-conjugated vaccines can be modestly augmented with concomitant use of antihistamine (H$_2$) blockers.[366–369] Protein-conjugated vaccines also appear to be more immunogenic than polysaccharide vaccines. In the absence of definitive data of the use of vaccines in CLL we recommend following the adult immunization schedule for immunocompromised adults for 2014, recommended by the Advisory Committee on Immunization Practices. This includes annual influenza vaccine and pneumococcal 13-valent conjugate (PCV-13) vaccine.[370–372] Vaccination with live virus vaccines including the zoster, varicella and measles, mumps, and rubella (MMR) vaccine are contraindicated in patients with CLL.[372]

The routine of use of granulocyte colony-stimulating factor (G-CSF) for patients with CLL is not recommended. G-CSF and granulocyte-macrophage colony-stimulating factor (GM-CSF) can be used to treat therapy-related neutropenia and for patients with febrile neutropenia to shorten the duration and severity of illness. Also, please see Chap. 24.

MANAGEMENT OF AUTOIMMUNE COMPLICATIONS OF CHRONIC LYMPHOCYTIC LEUKEMIA

Patients with CLL have a greater risk of developing autoimmune complications including autoimmune hemolytic anemia (AIHA; Chap. 54), immune thrombocytopenia (ITP; Chap. 117), and pure red cell aplasia (PRCA; Chap. 36). In the majority of patients, the nonmalignant B-cell clone produces the autoantibody, reflecting a dysregulation of humoral immune tolerance.[373,374] Patients who present with autoimmune cytopenias may not have a worse prognosis than patients in whom cytopenias develop because of extensive marrow infiltration by the disease.[328,375–377] AIHA can present in up to a third of patients with CLL at some time during the course of their disease and in a small proportion of patients (10 to 15 percent) at the time of diagnosis.[328] Patients present with signs and symptoms of acute onset of anemia with weakness, fatigue, lethargy, and shortness of breath on exertion. Physical examination reveals pallor, jaundice, lymphadenopathy, and hepatosplenomegaly. Laboratory evaluation reveals anemia, elevated LDH, hyperbilirubinemia, positive direct Coombs test, and decreased serum haptoglobin. Not all patients who have a positive Coombs test, however, develop hemolysis. Most patients have warm reactive antibodies, but some patients may develop cold agglutinin disease.[373] Occasionally, patients may develop concomitant ITP with AIHA or Evans syndrome. Certain miRNAs have been correlated with the development of AIHA but their mechanistic explanation in the pathogenesis of AIHA is lacking.[378]

ITP results in development of sudden profound thrombocytopenia with associated bleeding diathesis. Accurate diagnosis requires a marrow aspirate and biopsy to evaluate the extent of CLL in the marrow and the presence of adequate or increased numbers of megakaryocytes.

Patients often require periodic red cell transfusions for symptomatic anemia and platelet transfusions may be employed in patients with severe thrombocytopenias with bleeding complications. Glucocorticoids have been the mainstay of treatment for AIHA and ITP, However, steroids need to be dosed at 0.5 to 1.0 mg/kg/day for 2 to 3 weeks followed by a slow taper over several weeks. Unfortunately, a large number of patients relapse after discontinuation of the steroids and may need subsequent therapy with IVIG or rituximab. The early use of IVIG and weekly rituximab for four doses may allow for better disease control and rapid glucocorticoid withdrawal. Other immunosuppressive agents that have been used include cyclosporine, the dose of which can be titrated to stable hemoglobin or platelet levels or serum trough levels between 100 and 150 ng/mL.[331] Erythropoiesis-stimulating agents have been used and may decrease the frequency of packed red cell transfusions; however, their use can be complicated by polycythemia and thromboembolic disease.[379,380] Thrombopoietin agonists can also be considered in refractory patients, but conclusive data is currently lacking.[381] Refractory cases may require definitive treatment with therapeutic agents for the underlying CLL. Initiating nucleoside analogue-based chemotherapy in patients with preexisting AIHA or ITP is not contraindicated, but their use is contraindicated if these complications arise while patients are on these agents. In general for patients presenting with both active CLL and autoimmune manifestations, our approach is to first treat the autoimmune complication and then the CLL if symptoms persist.

PRCA is a rare complication of CLL that can arise spontaneously. PRCA needs to be differentiated from other forms of anemia, including AIHA and anemia resulting from extensive marrow infiltration. PRCA is characterized by a decrease in red cell precursors.[382] Additionally, select infections, such as parvovirus, can cause PRCA in CLL. The etiology of disease-related PRCA is believed to be related to the cytotoxic effect of a T-cell large granular lymphoma (T-LGL) clone on erythroid progenitor cells (Chap. 94). These CD3-, CD8-, and CD57-positive cells slowly accumulate in the marrow of patients with PRCA. Occasional cases have been observed after parvovirus B19 infection.[383] Treatment with immunosuppressive agents like glucocorticoids, cyclophosphamide, and/or cyclosporine result in reticulocytosis and slow correction of the anemia over several weeks.[384] IVIG, rituximab, and antithymocyte globulin have also been used in refractory cases.[385–388]

● RICHTER SYNDROME

Richter syndrome (RS) is defined as a transformation of CLL into an aggressive, high-grade, large B-cell non-Hodgkin lymphoma. The large cell lymphoma is typically of the activated B-cell (ABC) subtype by immunohistochemistry.[389] Incidence estimates vary from 2 to 10 percent.[390] Transformation typically occurs in patients with unmutated IGHV genes, but occasionally may be seen in patients with mutated IGHV genes who have been heavily pretreated.[391] The development of transformation may be related to the evolution of an alternate clone of malignant B cells distinct from the original CLL clone in a subset of patients.[392] Transformation appears to occur independent of disease stage, duration of disease, type of therapy, or response to therapy. However, the presence of bulky and advanced stage disease, IGHV unmutated disease, especially with involvement of 4 to 39 loci, high CD38 expression, absence of del 13q, presence of del 17p or del 2p and trisomy 12, typically in combination with NOTCH1 mutations, may predict the development of RS.[393–396] The syndrome is characterized by rapid development of B symptoms and rapidly progressive lymphadenopathy. Cytopenias may worsen rapidly because of transformation in the marrow. LDH is also increased in the majority of patients. Patients typically have complex karyotype and involvement of TP53, ATM, RB (retinoblastoma), and c-myc genes.[397] PET scans have generally no role in the routine management of patients with CLL but can be very useful in the diagnosis of transformation. A standardized uptake value (SUV) of 5 or less on a lymph node by PET scan has a high negative predictive value and patients with a higher SUV require an excisional biopsy for definitive diagnosis.[156,398,399] Prognosis of RS is related to the clonality of the malignant clone in that patients with clones unrelated to the CLL tend to have a much better prognosis than patients with a clonally related RS.[389] Additionally, patients who present with RS prior to treatment for their CLL often have a better outcome. Treatment of patients with RS has historically been treated with regimens similar to those used for the treatment of patients with large cell lymphoma with mixed results. These include R-CHOP (rituximab, cyclophosphamide, doxorubicin, vincristine, and prednisone) or R-EPOCH (rituximab, etoposide, prednisone,

vincristine, cyclophosphamide, and doxorubicin) and R-hyperCVXD (rituximab, fractionated cyclophosphamide, vincristine, liposomal daunorubicin, and dexamethasone). However, the use of hyperCVXD is associated unacceptably high treatment-related mortality and its use is not recommended.[400,401] The OFAR combination also has modest but short-lived responses with significant toxicities.[400] The use of dose-adjusted R-EPOCH is our preferred regimen to debulk patients before we proceed with more definitive therapy, including allogeneic SCT.

Along with large B-cell transformation, patients can also experience prolymphocytic leukemia (PLL) transformation, characterized by the presence of more than 55 percent prolymphocytes in the marrow, or Hodgkin lymphoma.[402–404] Unlike large cell transformation, patients with Hodgkin lymphoma have a similar outcome to *de novo* disease when matched by stage and can be treated with adriamycin, bleomycin, vinblastine, and dacarbazine (ABVD) based therapy (Chap. 97).[405]

The prolymphocytic transformation is similar to the distinct entity of B-cell PLL which is characterized by subacute accumulation of prolymphocytes in a predominantly older, male population with presence of chromosome 14q abnormalities and del 17p.[406–408] Gene-expression profiling suggests subgroups of patients with PLL that are similar to CLL and others that are similar to mantle cell lymphoma.[409] Patients present with B symptoms, massive splenomegaly, and palpable lymphadenopathy. Occasionally, patients may have organ infiltration and extralymphatic invasion, including neurologic involvement and leukostasis from hyperleukocytosis.[410,411] Prolymphocytes have variable expression of CD5 and are negative for CD23. Indications and therapeutic options for patients with PLL are similar to those used for CLL.[412–414]

T-cell prolymphocytic lymphoma (T-PLL) is a distinct clinical entity that was previously classified as T-CLL. These patients typically present with B symptoms and paraneoplastic phenomenon associated with rapid splenomegaly and lymphadenopathy with leukocytosis. Evaluation results in the demonstration of prolymphocytes on tissue biopsy with markers typical for T-cell disorders, including CD3, CD5, CD4, CD7, and CD8. TCR gene rearrangements are also observed. These features help distinguish them from B-cell CLL. The most effective treatment for this entity is alemtuzumab, although regimens for aggressive T-cell lymphomas have also been used.[412,415–419] In general, all patients relapse from these therapies, making consolidation allogeneic transplantation a viable consideration for these patients if a donor is available and patient comorbid features allow.

● MONOCLONAL B-CELL LYMPHOCYTOSIS

Monoclonal B-cell lymphocytosis (MBL) can be characterized as a precursor state of CLL. Patients who have greater than 5000 B-lymphocytes/μL in their blood, in the absence of B symptoms, lymphadenopathy, organomegaly, or cytopenias, are classified as having monoclonal B-cell lymphocytosis. Presence of a lymphoid aggregate or infiltration of lymph node or marrow by cells with a characteristic CLL phenotype establishes the diagnosis of CLL regardless of blood lymphocytosis. The prevalence of MBL varies from 3.5 percent in normal healthy people[420] with normal counts to 13.5 percent to 17 percent in normal healthy people with a family history of CLL,[16,421] which suggests a familial predisposition to the development of CLL. The vast majority of patients with MBL have clonal populations with a characteristic CLL phenotype on sensitive flow cytometry assay that is positive for CD5 and CD23, negative for CD10, and dim positive for CD20. Other phenotypes that have been observed are the atypical CLL phenotype with positive CD5, CD23, and bright CD20, and the non-CLL phenotype that is negative for CD5 and CD23 and appears to be more consistent with low-grade lymphoproliferative disorders like marginal zone lymphoma or lymphoplasmacytic lymphoma.[422] MBL is more prevalent in men and increases in incidence with age. The cumulative annual risk of patients with MBL who require CLL-specific therapy is approximately 1 percent.[16,17,420] Retrospective analysis of samples collected on longitudinal, prospective studies have also demonstrated that the development of overt CLL is almost always preceded by MBL.[423] Management of patients with MBL is similar to patients with early stage CLL and the vast majority of these patients can be followed with watchful waiting. Like early stage CLL, these patients are predisposed to a higher frequency of infections and also secondary malignancies mandating follow up similar to that recommended for CLL. Our own practice is to see MBL patients yearly with exams and complete blood count assessment.

SMALL LYMPHOCYTIC LYMPHOMA

Small lymphocytic B-cell lymphoma (SLL) is closely related to CLL and mimics it with regards to clinical course and outcomes. The malignant B cells have similar immunophenotypic features and prognostic markers on lymph node assessment but without the presence of malignant monoclonal B-cell lymphocytosis on blood or marrow assessment. Treatment and outcomes of these patients are similar to those for patients with CLL and as such this disorder should be considered analogous to CLL.[1,45,424,425]

DIFFERENTIAL DIAGNOSES

Multiple low-grade lymphoid malignancies can mimic the presentation and laboratory evidence of CLL and are discussed in detail in the chapters on non-Hodgkin lymphomas (Chaps. 95, 96, 99–101). The most common entities mimicking CLL are briefly discussed below.

MANTLE CELL LYMPHOMA

Mantle cell lymphoma frequently mimics the clinical presentation and laboratory findings observed in patients with CLL (Chap. 100). However, the malignant lymphocytes observed in mantle cell lymphoma express CD5 without coexpression of CD23 and have a higher level of expression of CD79. Cases of CD23-negative CLL and CD23-positive mantle cell lymphoma have been described. An important discriminating feature between the two disorders is the presence of t(11;14) in mantle cell lymphoma, which results in the bcl-1-IGH translocation and the overexpression of cyclin D1. Therapy for mantle cell lymphoma employs some of the agents used for CLL but is covered in detail elsewhere.[426–429]

HAIRY CELL LEUKEMIA

Hairy cell leukemia (HCL) presents with B symptoms, splenomegaly and the presence of typical villous "hairy" projections from the surface of its cells (Chap. 93). The cells are also strongly positive for tartrate-resistant acid phosphatase (TRAP) and express CD11c, CD25, and CD103. With the discovery of the BRAF[V600E] in HCL, significant improvements have been made in the availability of therapeutic agents for the management of these patients.[430–433]

OTHER LYMPHOID MALIGNANCIES

Various low-grade lymphoid malignancies can mimic the clinical and laboratory presentation of CLL and include marginal zone lymphomas and lymphoplasmacytic lymphomas. However, pathologic evaluation results in the identification of surface markers CD19 and CD20 without coexpression of CD5 or CD23. Therapy is directed at the specific lymphoid malignancy identified.[434–436] B-cell ALL is also included in the list of differential diagnoses, but it is an aggressive malignancy involving immature B cells with distinct molecular features and outcomes (Chap. 91). Transformation of CLL into ALL has been reported and managed with regimens suitable for ALL.[437–439]

REFERENCES

1. Hallek M, Cheson BD, Catovsky D, et al: Guidelines for the diagnosis and treatment of chronic lymphocytic leukemia: A report from the International Workshop on Chronic Lymphocytic Leukemia updating the National Cancer Institute-Working Group 1996 guidelines. *Blood* 111:5446–5456, 2008.
2. Cartwright RA, Gurney KA, Moorman AV: Sex ratios and the risks of haematological malignancies. *Br J Haematol* 118:1071–1077, 2002.
3. Diehl LF, Karnell LH, Menck HR: The American College of Surgeons Commission on Cancer and the American Cancer Society. The National Cancer Data Base report on age, gender, treatment, and outcomes of patients with chronic lymphocytic leukemia. *Cancer* 86:2684–2692, 1999.
4. Adami HO, Tsaih S, Lambe M, et al: Pregnancy and risk of non-Hodgkin's lymphoma: A prospective study. *Int J Cancer* 70:155–158, 1997.
5. Ahn YO, Koo HH, Park BJ, et al: Incidence estimation of leukemia among Koreans. *J Korean Med Sci* 6:299–307, 1991.
6. Haenszel W, Kurihara M: Studies of Japanese migrants. I. Mortality from cancer and other diseases among Japanese in the United States. *J Natl Cancer Inst* 40:43–68, 1968.
7. Goldin LR, Bjorkholm M, Kristinsson SY, et al: Elevated risk of chronic lymphocytic leukemia and other indolent non-Hodgkin's lymphomas among relatives of patients with chronic lymphocytic leukemia. *Haematologica* 94:647–653, 2009.
8. Wang SS, Slager SL, Brennan P, et al: Family history of hematopoietic malignancies and risk of non-Hodgkin lymphoma (NHL): A pooled analysis of 10,211 cases and 11,905 controls from the International Lymphoma Epidemiology Consortium (InterLymph). *Blood* 109:3479–3488, 2007.
9. Slager SL, Benavente Y, Blair A, et al: Medical history, lifestyle, family history, and occupational risk factors for chronic lymphocytic leukemia/small lymphocytic lymphoma: The InterLymph Non-Hodgkin Lymphoma Subtypes Project. *J Natl Cancer Inst Monogr* 2014:41–51, 2014.
10. Marwick C: Link found between Agent Orange and chronic lymphocytic leukaemia. *BMJ* 326:242, 2003.
11. Floderus B, Persson T, Stenlund C, et al: Occupational exposure to electromagnetic fields in relation to leukemia and brain tumors: A case-control study in Sweden. *Cancer Causes Control* 4:465–476, 1993.
12. Feychting M, Forssen U, Floderus B: Occupational and residential magnetic field exposure and leukemia and central nervous system tumors. *Epidemiology* 8:384–389, 1997.
13. Vrijheid M, Cardis E, Ashmore P, et al: Ionizing radiation and risk of chronic lymphocytic leukemia in the 15-country study of nuclear industry workers. *Radiat Res* 170:661–665, 2008.
14. Richardson DB, Wing S, Schroeder J, et al: Ionizing radiation and chronic lymphocytic leukemia. *Environ Health Perspect* 113:1–5, 2005.
15. Abramenko I, Bilous N, Chumak A, et al: Chronic lymphocytic leukemia patients exposed to ionizing radiation due to the Chernobyl NPP accident—With focus on immunoglobulin heavy chain gene analysis. *Leuk Res* 32:535–545, 2008.
16. Rawstron AC, Yuille MR, Fuller J, et al: Inherited predisposition to CLL is detectable as subclinical monoclonal B-lymphocyte expansion. *Blood* 100:2289–2290, 2002.
17. Rawstron AC, Bennett FL, O'Connor SJ, et al: Monoclonal B-cell lymphocytosis and chronic lymphocytic leukemia. *N Engl J Med* 359:575–583, 2008.
18. Kristinsson SY, Bjorkholm M, Goldin LR, et al: Risk of lymphoproliferative disorders among first-degree relatives of lymphoplasmacytic lymphoma/Waldenstrom macroglobulinemia patients: A population-based study in Sweden. *Blood* 112:3052–3056, 2008.
19. Raval A, Tanner SM, Byrd JC, et al: Downregulation of death-associated protein kinase 1 (DAPK1) in chronic lymphocytic leukemia. *Cell* 129:879–890, 2007.
20. Perez-Chacon G, Contreras-Martin B, Cuni S, et al: Polymorphism in the CD5 gene promoter in B-cell chronic lymphocytic leukemia and mantle cell lymphoma. *Am J Clin Pathol* 123:646–650, 2005.
21. Aydin S, Rossi D, Bergui L, et al: CD38 gene polymorphism and chronic lymphocytic leukemia: A role in transformation to Richter syndrome? *Blood* 111:5646–5653, 2008.
22. Jevtovic-Stoimenov T, Kocic G, Pavlovic D, et al: Polymorphisms of tumor-necrosis factor-alpha -308 and lymphotoxin-alpha + 250: Possible modulation of susceptibility to apoptosis in chronic lymphocytic leukemia and non-Hodgkin lymphoma mononuclear cells. *Leuk Lymphoma* 49:2163–2169, 2008.
23. Sellick GS, Goldin LR, Wild RW, et al: A high-density SNP genome-wide linkage search of 206 families identifies susceptibility loci for chronic lymphocytic leukemia. *Blood* 110:3326–3333, 2007.
24. Di Bernardo MC, Crowther-Swanepoel D, Broderick P, et al: A genome-wide association study identifies six susceptibility loci for chronic lymphocytic leukemia. *Nat Genet* 40:1204–1210, 2008.
25. Marti GE, Faguet G, Bertin P, et al: CD20 and CD5 expression in B-chronic lymphocytic leukemia. *Ann N Y Acad Sci* 651:480–483, 1992.
26. Almasri NM, Duque RE, Iturraspe J, et al: Reduced expression of CD20 antigen as a characteristic marker for chronic lymphocytic leukemia. *Am J Hematol* 40:259–263, 1992.

27. Ranheim EA, Cantwell MJ, Kipps TJ: Expression of CD27 and its ligand, CD70, on chronic lymphocytic leukemia B cells. *Blood* 85:3556–3565, 1995.

28. Klein U, Dalla-Favera R: New insights into the phenotype and cell derivation of B cell chronic lymphocytic leukemia. *Curr Top Microbiol Immunol* 294:31–49, 2005.

29. Klein U, Tu Y, Stolovitzky GA, et al: Gene expression profiling of B cell chronic lymphocytic leukemia reveals a homogeneous phenotype related to memory B cells. *J Exp Med* 194:1625–1638, 2001.

30. Geisler CH, Larsen JK, Hansen NE, et al: Prognostic importance of flow cytometric immunophenotyping of 540 consecutive patients with B-cell chronic lymphocytic leukemia. *Blood* 78:1795–1802, 1991.

31. Vilpo J, Tobin G, Hulkkonen J, et al: Surface antigen expression and correlation with variable heavy-chain gene mutation status in chronic lymphocytic leukemia. *Eur J Haematol* 70:53–59, 2003.

32. Caligaris-Cappio F: B-chronic lymphocytic leukemia: A malignancy of anti-self B cells. *Blood* 87:2615–2620, 1996.

33. Wardemann H, Yurasov S, Schaefer A, et al: Predominant autoantibody production by early human B cell precursors. *Science* 301:1374–1377, 2003.

34. Awan FT, Kay NE, Davis ME, et al: Mcl-1 expression predicts progression-free survival in chronic lymphocytic leukemia patients treated with pentostatin, cyclophosphamide, and rituximab. *Blood* 113:535–537, 2009.

35. Petlickovski A, Laurenti L, Li X, et al: Sustained signaling through the B-cell receptor induces Mcl-1 and promotes survival of chronic lymphocytic leukemia B cells. *Blood* 105:4820–4827, 2005.

36. Liu Z, Hazan-Halevy I, Harris DM, et al: STAT-3 activates NF-kappaB in chronic lymphocytic leukemia cells. *Mol Cancer Res* 9:507–515, 2011.

37. Burger JA, Tsukada N, Burger M, et al: Blood-derived nurse-like cells protect chronic lymphocytic leukemia B cells from spontaneous apoptosis through stromal cell-derived factor-1. *Blood* 96:2655–2663, 2000.

38. Burger JA, Burger M, Kipps TJ: Chronic lymphocytic leukemia B cells express functional CXCR4 chemokine receptors that mediate spontaneous migration beneath bone marrow stromal cells. *Blood* 94:3658–3667, 1999.

39. Herishanu Y, Perez-Galan P, Liu D, et al: The lymph node microenvironment promotes B-cell receptor signaling, NF-kappaB activation, and tumor proliferation in chronic lymphocytic leukemia. *Blood* 117:563–574, 2011.

40. Herishanu Y, Katz BZ, Lipsky A, et al: Biology of chronic lymphocytic leukemia in different microenvironments: Clinical and therapeutic implications. *Hematol Oncol Clin North Am* 27:173–206, 2013.

41. Zimmerman TS, Godwin HA, Perry S: Studies of leukocyte kinetics in chronic lymphocytic leukemia. *Blood* 31:277–291, 1968.

42. Andreeff M, Darzynkiewicz Z, Sharpless TK, et al: Discrimination of human leukemia subtypes by flow cytometric analysis of cellular DNA and RNA. *Blood* 55:282–293, 1980.

43. Panayiotidis P, Jones D, Ganeshaguru K, et al: Human bone marrow stromal cells prevent apoptosis and support the survival of chronic lymphocytic leukaemia cells *in vitro*. *Br J Haematol* 92:97–103, 1996.

44. Lagneaux L, Delforge A, Bron D, et al: Chronic lymphocytic leukemic B cells but not normal B cells are rescued from apoptosis by contact with normal bone marrow stromal cells. *Blood* 91:2387–2396, 1998.

45. Ben-Ezra J, Burke JS, Swartz WG, et al: Small lymphocytic lymphoma: A clinicopathologic analysis of 268 cases. *Blood* 73:579–587, 1989.

46. Messmer BT, Messmer D, Allen SL, et al: In vivo measurements document the dynamic cellular kinetics of chronic lymphocytic leukemia B cells. *J Clin Invest* 115:755–764, 2005.

47. Riches JC, Gribben JG: Immunomodulation and immune reconstitution in chronic lymphocytic leukemia. *Semin Hematol* 51:228–234, 2014.

48. D'Arena G, D'Auria F, Simeon V, et al: A shorter time to the first treatment may be predicted by the absolute number of regulatory T-cells in patients with Rai stage 0 chronic lymphocytic leukemia. *Am J Hematol* 87:628–631, 2012.

49. Huergo-Zapico L, Acebes-Huerta A, Gonzalez-Rodriguez AP, et al: Expansion of NK cells and reduction of NKG2D expression in chronic lymphocytic leukemia. Correlation with progressive disease. *PLoS One* 9:e108326, 2014.

50. Riches JC, Davies JK, McClanahan F, et al: T cells from CLL patients exhibit features of T-cell exhaustion but retain capacity for cytokine production. *Blood* 121:1612–1621, 2013.

51. Itala M, Vainio O, Remes K: Functional abnormalities in granulocytes predict susceptibility to bacterial infections in chronic lymphocytic leukaemia. *Eur J Haematol* 57:46–53, 1996.

52. Cantwell M, Hua T, Pappas J, et al: Acquired CD40-ligand deficiency in chronic lymphocytic leukemia. *Nat Med* 3:984–989, 1997.

53. Lagneaux L, Delforge A, Bron D, et al: Heterogenous response of B lymphocytes to transforming growth factor-beta in B-cell chronic lymphocytic leukaemia: Correlation with the expression of TGF-beta receptors. *Br J Haematol* 97:612–620, 1997.

54. Romano C, De Fanis U, Sellitto A, et al: Effects of preactivated autologous T lymphocytes on CD80, CD86 and CD95 expression by chronic lymphocytic leukemia B cells. *Leuk Lymphoma* 44:1963–1971, 2003.

55. Jitschin R, Braun M, Buttner M, et al: CLL-cells induce IDOhi CD14+HLA-DRlo myeloid-derived suppressor cells that inhibit T-cell responses and promote TRegs. *Blood* 124:750–760, 2014.

56. Hermouet S, Sutton CA, Rose TM, et al: Qualitative and quantitative analysis of human herpesviruses in chronic and acute B cell lymphocytic leukemia and in multiple myeloma. *Leukemia* 17:185–195, 2003.

57. Laurenti L, Piccioni P, Cattani P, et al: Cytomegalovirus reactivation during alemtuzumab therapy for chronic lymphocytic leukemia: Incidence and treatment with oral ganciclovir. *Haematologica* 89:1248–1252, 2004.

58. Hersey P, Wotherspoon J, Reid G, et al: Hypogammaglobulinaemia associated with abnormalities of both B and T lymphocytes in patients with chronic lymphatic leukaemia. *Clin Exp Immunol* 39:698–707, 1980.

59. Lacombe C, Gombert J, Dreyfus B, et al: Heterogeneity of serum IgG subclass deficiencies in B chronic lymphocytic leukemia. *Clin Immunol* 90:128–132, 1999.

60. Sampalo A, Navas G, Medina F, et al: Chronic lymphocytic leukemia B cells inhibit spontaneous Ig production by autologous bone marrow cells: Role of CD95-CD95L interaction. *Blood* 96:3168–3174, 2000.

61. Herman SE, Mustafa RZ, Gyamfi JA, et al: Ibrutinib inhibits BCR and NF-kappaB signaling and reduces tumor proliferation in tissue-resident cells of patients with CLL. *Blood* 123:3286–3295, 2014.

62. Duhren-von Minden M, Ubelhart R, Schneider D, et al: Chronic lymphocytic leukaemia is driven by antigen-independent cell-autonomous signalling. *Nature* 489:309–312, 2012.

63. Pierce SK, Liu W: The tipping points in the initiation of B cell signalling: How small changes make big differences. *Nat Rev Immunol* 10:767–777, 2010.

64. Stevenson FK, Krysov S, Davies AJ, et al: B-cell receptor signaling in chronic lymphocytic leukemia. *Blood* 118:4313–4320, 2011.

65. Chiorazzi N, Efremov DG: Chronic lymphocytic leukemia: A tale of one or two signals? *Cell Res* 23:182–185, 2013.

66. Buckley RH: Primary immunodeficiency diseases due to defects in lymphocytes. *N Engl J Med* 343:1313–1324, 2000.

67. Herman SE, Gordon AL, Hertlein E, et al: Bruton tyrosine kinase represents a promising therapeutic target for treatment of chronic lymphocytic leukemia and is effectively targeted by PCI-32765. *Blood* 117:6287–6296, 2011.

68. Dubovsky JA, Beckwith KA, Natarajan G, et al: Ibrutinib is an irreversible molecular inhibitor of ITK driving a Th1-selective pressure in T lymphocytes. *Blood* 122:2539–2549, 2013.

69. Pogue SL, Kurosaki T, Bolen J, et al: B cell antigen receptor-induced activation of Akt promotes B cell survival and is dependent on Syk kinase. *J Immunol* 165:1300–1306, 2000.

70. Srinivasan L, Sasaki Y, Calado DP, et al: PI3 kinase signals BCR-dependent mature B cell survival. *Cell* 139:573–586, 2009.

71. Brown JR, Byrd JC, Coutre SE, et al: Idelalisib, an inhibitor of phosphatidylinositol 3-kinase p110delta, for relapsed/refractory chronic lymphocytic leukemia. *Blood* 123:3390–3397, 2014.

72. Awan FT, Byrd JC: New strategies in chronic lymphocytic leukemia: Shifting treatment paradigms. *Clin Cancer Res* 20:5869–5874, 2014.

73. Garcia-Marco JA, Price CM, Catovsky D: Interphase cytogenetics in chronic lymphocytic leukemia. *Cancer Genet Cytogenet* 94:52–58, 1997.

74. Malek S: Molecular biomarkers in chronic lymphocytic leukemia. *Adv Exp Med Biol* 792:193–214, 2013.

75. Bullrich F, Fujii H, Calin G, et al: Characterization of the 13q14 tumor suppressor locus in CLL: Identification of ALT1, an alternative splice variant of the LEU2 gene. *Cancer Res* 61:6640–6648, 2001.

76. Calin GA, Dumitru CD, Shimizu M, et al: Frequent deletions and down-regulation of micro- RNA genes miR15 and miR16 at 13q14 in chronic lymphocytic leukemia. *Proc Natl Acad Sci U S A* 99:15524–15529, 2002.

77. Mott JL, Kobayashi S, Bronk SF, et al: Mir-29 regulates Mcl-1 protein expression and apoptosis. *Oncogene* 26:6133–6140, 2007.

78. Pekarsky Y, Santanam U, Cimmino A, et al: Tcl1 expression in chronic lymphocytic leukemia is regulated by miR-29 and miR-181. *Cancer Res* 66:11590–11593, 2006.

79. Mraz M, Chen L, Rassenti LZ, et al: MiR-150 influences B-cell receptor signaling in chronic lymphocytic leukemia by regulating expression of GAB1 and FOXP1. *Blood* 124:84–95, 2014.

80. Quijano S, Lopez A, Rasillo A, et al: Association between the proliferative rate of neoplastic B cells, their maturation stage, and underlying cytogenetic abnormalities in B-cell chronic lymphoproliferative disorders: Analysis of a series of 432 patients. *Blood* 111:5130–5141, 2008.

81. Hjalmar V, Hast R, Kimby E: Cell surface expression of CD25, CD54, and CD95 on B- and T-cells in chronic lymphocytic leukaemia in relation to trisomy 12, atypical morphology and clinical course. *Eur J Haematol* 68:127–134, 2002.

82. Quijano S, Lopez A, Rasillo A, et al: Impact of trisomy 12, del(13q), del(17p), and del(11q) on the immunophenotype, DNA ploidy status, and proliferative rate of leukemic B-cells in chronic lymphocytic leukemia. *Cytometry B Clin Cytom* 74:139–149, 2008.

83. Bullrich F, Rasio D, Kitada S, et al: ATM mutations in B-cell chronic lymphocytic leukemia. *Cancer Res* 59:24–27, 1999.

84. Dohner H, Stilgenbauer S, James MR, et al: 11q deletions identify a new subset of B-cell chronic lymphocytic leukemia characterized by extensive nodal involvement and inferior prognosis. *Blood* 89:2516–2522, 1997.

85. Starostik P, Manshouri T, O'Brien S, et al: Deficiency of the ATM protein expression defines an aggressive subgroup of B-cell chronic lymphocytic leukemia. *Cancer Res* 58:4552–4557, 1998.

86. Grever MR, Lucas DM, Dewald GW, et al: Comprehensive assessment of genetic and molecular features predicting outcome in patients with chronic lymphocytic leukemia: Results from the US Intergroup Phase III Trial E2997. *J Clin Oncol* 25:799–804, 2007.

87. Flinn IW, Neuberg DS, Grever MR, et al: Phase III trial of fludarabine plus cyclophosphamide compared with fludarabine for patients with previously untreated chronic lymphocytic leukemia: US Intergroup Trial E2997. *J Clin Oncol* 25:793–798, 2007.

88. Bixby D, Kujawski L, Wang S, et al: The pre-clinical development of MDM2 inhibitors in chronic lymphocytic leukemia uncovers a central role for p53 status in sensitivity to MDM2 inhibitor-mediated apoptosis. *Cell Cycle* 7:971–979, 2008.

89. Cordone I, Masi S, Mauro FR, et al: P53 expression in B-cell chronic lymphocytic leukemia: A marker of disease progression and poor prognosis. *Blood* 91:4342–4349, 1998.

90. el Rouby S, Thomas A, Costin D, et al: P53 gene mutation in B-cell chronic lymphocytic leukemia is associated with drug resistance and is independent of MDR1/MDR3 gene expression. *Blood* 82:3452–3459, 1993.

91. Stephens DM, Ruppert AS, Jones JA, et al: Impact of targeted therapy on outcome of chronic lymphocytic leukemia patients with relapsed del(17p13.1) karyotype at a single center. *Leukemia* 28:1365–1368, 2014.

92. Byrd JC, Furman RR, Coutre SE, et al: Targeting BTK with ibrutinib in relapsed chronic lymphocytic leukemia. *N Engl J Med* 369:32–42, 2013.

93. Berkova A, Pavlistova L, Babicka L, et al: Combined molecular biological and molecular cytogenetic analysis of genomic changes in 146 patients with B-cell chronic lymphocytic leukemia. *Neoplasma* 55:400–408, 2008.

94. Rechavi G, Katzir N, Brok-Simoni F, et al: A search for bcl1, bcl2, and c-myc oncogene rearrangements in chronic lymphocytic leukemia. *Leukemia* 3:57–60, 1989.

95. Cuneo A, Rigolin GM, Bigoni R, et al: Chronic lymphocytic leukemia with 6q- shows distinct hematological features and intermediate prognosis. *Leukemia* 18:476–483, 2004.

96. Puente XS, Pinyol M, Quesada V, et al: Whole-genome sequencing identifies recurrent mutations in chronic lymphocytic leukaemia. *Nature* 475:101–105, 2011.

97. Jeromin S, Weissmann S, Haferlach C, et al: SF3B1 mutations correlated to cytogenetics and mutations in NOTCH1, FBXW7, MYD88, XPO1 and TP53 in 1160 untreated CLL patients. *Leukemia* 28:108–117, 2014.

98. Quesada V, Conde L, Villamor N, et al: Exome sequencing identifies recurrent mutations of the splicing factor SF3B1 gene in chronic lymphocytic leukemia. *Nat Genet* 44:47–52, 2012.

99. Higgins JP, Warnke RA: Herpes lymphadenitis in association with chronic lymphocytic leukemia. *Cancer* 86:1210–1215, 1999.

100. Sivakumaran M, Qureshi H, Chapman CS: Chylous effusions in CLL. *Leuk Lymphoma* 18:365–366, 1995.

101. Zeidman A, Yarmolovsky A, Djaldetti M, et al: Hemorrhagic pleural effusion as a complication of chronic lymphocytic leukemia. *Haematologia (Budap)* 26:173–175, 1995.

102. Dhodapkar M, Yale SH, Hoagland HC: Hemorrhagic pleural effusion and pleural thickening as a complication of chronic lymphocytic leukemia. *Am J Hematol* 42:221–224, 1993.

103. Elliott MA, Letendre L, Li CY, et al: Chronic lymphocytic leukaemia with symptomatic diffuse central nervous system infiltration responding to therapy with systemic fludarabine. *Br J Haematol* 104:689–694, 1999.

104. Asakura K, Kizaki M, Ikeda Y: Exaggerated cutaneous response to mosquito bites in a patient with chronic lymphocytic leukemia. *Int J Hematol* 80:59–61, 2004.

105. Weed RI: Exaggerated delayed hypersensitivity to mosquito bites in chronic lymphocytic leukemia. *Blood* 26:257–268, 1965.

106. Pangalis GA, Roussou PA, Kittas C, et al: Patterns of bone marrow involvement in chronic lymphocytic leukemia and small lymphocytic (well differentiated) non-Hodgkin's lymphoma. Its clinical significance in relation to their differential diagnosis and prognosis. *Cancer* 54:702–708, 1984.

107. Pangalis GA, Roussou PA, Kittas C, et al: B-chronic lymphocytic leukemia. Prognostic implication of bone marrow histology in 120 patients experience from a single hematology unit. *Cancer* 59:767–771, 1987.

108. Deegan MJ, Abraham JP, Sawdyk M, et al: High incidence of monoclonal proteins in the serum and urine of chronic lymphocytic leukemia patients. *Blood* 64:1207–1211, 1984.

109. Sinclair D, Dagg JH, Dewar AE, et al: The incidence, clonal origin and secretory nature of serum paraproteins in chronic lymphocytic leukaemia. *Br J Haematol* 64:725–735, 1986.

110. Pangalis GA, Moutsopoulos HM, Papadopoulos NM, et al: Monoclonal and oligoclonal immunoglobulins in the serum of patients with B-chronic lymphocytic leukemia. *Acta Haematol* 80:23–27, 1988.

111. Bernstein ZP, Fitzpatrick JE, O'Donnell A, et al: Clinical significance of monoclonal proteins in chronic lymphocytic leukemia. *Leukemia* 6:1243–1245, 1992.

112. Shvidel L, Tadmor T, Braester A, et al: Serum immunoglobulin levels at diagnosis have no prognostic significance in stage A chronic lymphocytic leukemia: A study of 1113 cases from the Israeli CLL Study Group. *Eur J Haematol* 93:29–33, 2014.

113. Mayr C, Speicher MR, Kofler DM, et al: Chromosomal translocations are associated with poor prognosis in chronic lymphocytic leukemia. *Blood* 107:742–751, 2006.

114. Dohner H, Stilgenbauer S, Benner A, et al: Genomic aberrations and survival in chronic lymphocytic leukemia. *N Engl J Med* 343:1910–1916, 2000.

115. Stilgenbauer S, Sander S, Bullinger L, et al: Clonal evolution in chronic lymphocytic leukemia: Acquisition of high-risk genomic aberrations associated with unmutated VH, resistance to therapy, and short survival. *Haematologica* 92:1242–1245, 2007.

116. Kipps TJ, Tomhave E, Chen PP, et al: Autoantibody-associated kappa light chain variable region gene expressed in chronic lymphocytic leukemia with little or no somatic mutation. Implications for etiology and immunotherapy. *J Exp Med* 167:840–852, 1988.

117. Lin KI, Tam CS, Keating MJ, et al: Relevance of the immunoglobulin VH somatic mutation status in patients with chronic lymphocytic leukemia treated with fludarabine, cyclophosphamide, and rituximab (FCR) or related chemoimmunotherapy regimens. *Blood* 113:3168–3171, 2009.

118. Damle RN, Wasil T, Fais F, et al: Ig V gene mutation status and CD38 expression as novel prognostic indicators in chronic lymphocytic leukemia. *Blood* 94:1840–1847, 1999.

119. Byrd JC, Stilgenbauer S, Flinn IW: Chronic lymphocytic leukemia. *Hematology Am Soc Hematol Educ Program* 163–183, 2004.

120. Ghia EM, Jain S, Widhopf GF, 2nd, et al: Use of IGHV3–21 in chronic lymphocytic leukemia is associated with high-risk disease and reflects antigen-driven, post-germinal center leukemogenic selection. *Blood* 111:5101–5108, 2008.

121. Baliakas P, Agathangelidis A, Hadzidimitriou A, et al: Not all IGHV3–21 chronic lymphocytic leukemias are equal: Prognostic considerations. *Blood* 125:856–859, 2015.

122. Gobessi S, Laurenti L, Longo PG, et al: ZAP-70 enhances B-cell-receptor signaling despite absent or inefficient tyrosine kinase activation in chronic lymphocytic leukemia and lymphoma B cells. *Blood* 109:2032–2039, 2007.

123. Crespo M, Bosch F, Villamor N, et al: ZAP-70 expression as a surrogate for immunoglobulin-variable-region mutations in chronic lymphocytic leukemia. *N Engl J Med* 348:1764–1775, 2003.

124. Corcoran M, Parker A, Orchard J, et al: ZAP-70 methylation status is associated with ZAP-70 expression status in chronic lymphocytic leukemia. *Haematologica* 90:1078–1088, 2005.

125. Cramer P, Hallek M: Prognostic factors in chronic lymphocytic leukemia—what do we need to know? *Nat Rev Clin Oncol* 8:38–47, 2011.

126. Claus R, Lucas DM, Ruppert AS, et al: Validation of ZAP-70 methylation and its relative significance in predicting outcome in chronic lymphocytic leukemia. *Blood* 124:42–48, 2014.

127. Letestu R, Levy V, Eclache V, et al: Prognosis of Binet stage A chronic lymphocytic leukemia patients: The strength of routine parameters. *Blood* 116:4588–4590, 2010.

128. Krober A, Seiler T, Benner A, et al: V(H) mutation status, CD38 expression level, genomic aberrations, and survival in chronic lymphocytic leukemia. *Blood* 100:1410–1416, 2002.

129. Deaglio S, Vaisitti T, Zucchetto A, et al: CD38 as a molecular compass guiding topographical decisions of chronic lymphocytic leukemia cells. *Semin Cancer Biol* 20:416–423, 2010.

130. Damle RN, Temburni S, Calissano C, et al: CD38 expression labels an activated subset within chronic lymphocytic leukemia clones enriched in proliferating B cells. *Blood* 110:3352–3359, 2007.

131. Thunberg U, Johnson A, Roos G, et al: CD38 expression is a poor predictor for VH gene mutational status and prognosis in chronic lymphocytic leukemia. *Blood* 97:1892–1894, 2001.

132. Zucchetto A, Benedetti D, Tripodo C, et al: CD38/CD31, the CCL3 and CCL4 chemokines, and CD49d/vascular cell adhesion molecule-1 are interchained by sequential events sustaining chronic lymphocytic leukemia cell survival. *Cancer Res* 69:4001–4009, 2009.

133. Zucchetto A, Bomben R, Dal Bo M, et al: CD49d in B-cell chronic lymphocytic leukemia: Correlated expression with CD38 and prognostic relevance. *Leukemia* 20:523–525; author reply 528–529, 2006.

134. Bulian P, Shanafelt TD, Fegan C, et al: CD49d is the strongest flow cytometry-based predictor of overall survival in chronic lymphocytic leukemia. *J Clin Oncol* 32:897–904, 2014.

135. Wierda WG, O'Brien S, Wang X, et al: Characteristics associated with important clinical end points in patients with chronic lymphocytic leukemia at initial treatment. *J Clin Oncol* 27:1637–1643, 2009.

136. Wierda WG, O'Brien S, Wang X, et al: Prognostic nomogram and index for overall survival in previously untreated patients with chronic lymphocytic leukemia. *Blood* 109:4679–4685, 2007.

137. Gentile M, Mauro FR, Rossi D, et al: Italian external and multicentric validation of the MD Anderson Cancer Center nomogram and prognostic index for chronic lymphocytic leukemia patients: Analysis of 1502 cases. *Br J Haematol* 167:224–232, 2014.

138. Montserrat E, Sanchez-Bisono J, Vinolas N, et al: Lymphocyte doubling time in chronic lymphocytic leukaemia: Analysis of its prognostic significance. *Br J Haematol* 62:567–575, 1986.

139. Matthews C, Catherwood MA, Morris TC, et al: Serum TK levels in CLL identify Binet stage A patients within biologically defined prognostic subgroups most likely to undergo disease progression. *Eur J Haematol* 77:309–317, 2006.

140. Magnac C, Porcher R, Davi F, et al: Predictive value of serum thymidine kinase level for Ig-V mutational status in B-CLL. *Leukemia* 17:133–137, 2003.

141. Hallek M, Langenmayer I, Nerl C, et al: Elevated serum thymidine kinase levels identify a subgroup at high risk of disease progression in early, nonsmoldering chronic lymphocytic leukemia. *Blood* 93:1732–1737, 1999.

142. Saka B, Aktan M, Sami U, et al: Prognostic importance of soluble CD23 in B-cell chronic lymphocytic leukemia. *Clin Lab Haematol* 28:30–35, 2006.

143. Molica S, Vitelli G, Levato D, et al: Elevated serum levels of soluble CD44 can identify a subgroup of patients with early B-cell chronic lymphocytic leukemia who are at high risk of disease progression. *Cancer* 92:713–719, 2001.

144. Christiansen I, Sundstrom C, Totterman TH: Elevated serum levels of soluble vascular cell adhesion molecule-1 (sVCAM-1) closely reflect tumour burden in chronic B-lymphocytic leukaemia. *Br J Haematol* 103:1129–1137, 1998.

145. Molica S, Vitelli G, Levato D, et al: Increased serum levels of matrix metalloproteinase-9 predict clinical outcome of patients with early B-cell chronic lymphocytic leukemia. *Eur J Haematol* 70:373–378, 2003.

146. Lai R, O'Brien S, Maushouri T, et al: Prognostic value of plasma interleukin-6 levels in patients with chronic lymphocytic leukemia. *Cancer* 95:1071–1075, 2002.

147. Wierda WG, Johnson MM, Do KA, et al: Plasma interleukin 8 level predicts for survival in chronic lymphocytic leukaemia. *Br J Haematol* 120:452–456, 2003.

148. Cimmino A, Calin GA, Fabbri M, et al: MiR-15 and miR-16 induce apoptosis by targeting BCL2. *Proc Natl Acad Sci U S A* 102:13944–13949, 2005.

149. Fabbri M, Bottoni A, Shimizu M, et al: Association of a microRNA/TP53 feedback circuitry with pathogenesis and outcome of B-cell chronic lymphocytic leukemia. *JAMA* 305:59–67, 2011.

150. Moussay E, Palissot V, Vallar L, et al: Determination of genes and microRNAs involved in the resistance to fludarabine in vivo in chronic lymphocytic leukemia. *Mol Cancer* 9:115, 2010.

151. Visone R, Rassenti LZ, Veronese A, et al: Karyotype-specific microRNA signature in chronic lymphocytic leukemia. *Blood* 114:3872–3879, 2009.

152. Rai KR, Sawitsky A, Cronkite EP, et al: Clinical staging of chronic lymphocytic leukemia. *Blood* 46:219–234, 1975.

153. Binet JL, Auquier A, Dighiero G, et al: A new prognostic classification of chronic lymphocytic leukemia derived from a multivariate survival analysis. *Cancer* 48:198–206, 1981.

154. Vasconcelos Y, Davi F, Levy V, et al: Binet's staging system and VH genes are independent but complementary prognostic indicators in chronic lymphocytic leukemia. *J Clin Oncol* 21:3928–3932, 2003.

155. Montserrat E, Marques-Pereira JP, Gallart MT, et al: Bone marrow histopathologic patterns and immunologic findings in B-chronic lymphocytic leukemia. *Cancer* 54:447–451, 1984.

156. Bruzzi JF, Macapinlac H, Tsimberidou AM, et al: Detection of Richter's transformation of chronic lymphocytic leukemia by PET/CT. *J Nucl Med* 47:1267–1273, 2006.

157. Falchi L, Keating MJ, Marom EM, et al: Correlation between FDG/PET, histology, characteristics, and survival in 332 patients with chronic lymphoid leukemia. *Blood* 123:2783–2790, 2014.

158. Pflug N, Bahlo J, Shanafelt TD, et al: Development of a comprehensive prognostic index for patients with chronic lymphocytic leukemia. *Blood* 124:49–62, 2014.

159. Chemotherapeutic options in chronic lymphocytic leukemia: A meta-analysis of the randomized trials. CLL Trialists' Collaborative Group. *J Natl Cancer Inst* 91:861–868, 1999.

160. Dighiero G, Maloum K, Desablens B, et al: Chlorambucil in indolent chronic lymphocytic leukemia. French Cooperative Group on Chronic Lymphocytic Leukemia. *N Engl J Med* 338:1506–1514, 1998.

161. Burgman MA, Busch R, Eichhorst B, et al: Overall survival in early stage chronic lymphocytic leukemia patients with treatment indication due to disease progression: Follow-Up Data of the CLL1 Trial of the German CLL Study Group (GCLLSG). *Blood* 122 (21), 2013.

162. Eichhorst B, Goede V, Hallek M: Treatment of elderly patients with chronic lymphocytic leukemia. *Leuk Lymphoma* 50:171–178, 2009.

163. Rai KR, Peterson BL, Appelbaum FR, et al: Fludarabine compared with chlorambucil as primary therapy for chronic lymphocytic leukemia. *N Engl J Med* 343:1750–1757, 2000.

164. Knospe WH, Loeb V Jr, Huguley CM Jr: Proceedings: Bi-weekly chlorambucil treatment of chronic lymphocytic leukemia. *Cancer* 33:555–562, 1974.

165. Sawitsky A, Rai KR, Glidewell O, et al: Comparison of daily versus intermittent chlorambucil and prednisone therapy in the treatment of patients with chronic lymphocytic leukemia. *Blood* 50:1049–1059, 1977.

166. Huguley CM Jr: Treatment of chronic lymphocytic leukemia. *Cancer Treat Rev* 4:261–273, 1977.

167. Shaklai S, Bairey O, Blickstein D, et al: Severe myelotoxicity of oral etoposide in heavily pretreated patients with non-Hodgkin's lymphoma or chronic lymphatic leukemia. *Cancer* 77:2313–2317, 1996.

168. Robak T, Szmigielska-Kaplon A, Blonski JZ, et al: Activity of cladribine combined with etoposide in heavily pretreated patients with indolent lymphoid malignancies. *Chemotherapy* 51:247–251, 2005.

169. Knauf WU, Lissichkov T, Aldaoud A, et al: Phase III randomized study of bendamustine compared with chlorambucil in previously untreated patients with chronic lymphocytic leukemia. *J Clin Oncol* 27:4378–4384, 2009.

170. Leoni LM, Bailey B, Reifert J, et al: Bendamustine (Treanda) displays a distinct pattern of cytotoxicity and unique mechanistic features compared with other alkylating agents. *Clin Cancer Res* 14:309–317, 2008.

171. Traynor K: Treanda approved for chronic lymphocytic leukemia. *Am J Health Syst Pharm* 65:793, 2008.

172. O'Brien S, Kantarjian H, Beran M, et al: Results of fludarabine and prednisone therapy in 264 patients with chronic lymphocytic leukemia with multivariate analysis-derived prognostic model for response to treatment. *Blood* 82:1695–1700, 1993.

173. Johnson S, Smith AG, Loffler H, et al: Multicentre prospective randomised trial of fludarabine versus cyclophosphamide, doxorubicin, and prednisone (CAP) for treatment of advanced-stage chronic lymphocytic leukaemia. The French Cooperative Group on CLL. *Lancet* 347:1432–1438, 1996.

174. Eichhorst BF, Busch R, Stilgenbauer S, et al: First-line therapy with fludarabine compared with chlorambucil does not result in a major benefit for elderly patients with advanced chronic lymphocytic leukemia. *Blood* 114:3382–3391, 2009.

175. Wijermans PW, Gerrits WB, Haak HL: Severe immunodeficiency in patients treated with fludarabine monophosphate. *Eur J Haematol* 50:292–296, 1993.

176. Bergmann L, Fenchel K, Jahn B, et al: Immunosuppressive effects and clinical response of fludarabine in refractory chronic lymphocytic leukemia. *Ann Oncol* 4:371–375, 1993.

177. Cohen RB, Abdallah JM, Gray JR, et al: Reversible neurologic toxicity in patients treated with standard-dose fludarabine phosphate for mycosis fungoides and chronic lymphocytic leukemia. *Ann Intern Med* 118:114–116, 1993.

178. Tosti S, Caruso R, D'Adamo F, et al: Severe autoimmune hemolytic anemia in a patient with chronic lymphocytic leukemia responsive to fludarabine-based treatment. *Ann Hematol* 65:238–239, 1992.

179. Bastion Y, Coiffier B, Dumontet C, et al: Severe autoimmune hemolytic anemia in two patients treated with fludarabine for chronic lymphocytic leukemia. *Ann Oncol* 3:171–172, 1992.

180. Vick DJ, Byrd JC, Beal CL, et al: Mixed-type autoimmune hemolytic anemia following fludarabine treatment in a patient with chronic lymphocytic leukemia/small cell lymphoma. *Vox Sang* 74:122–126, 1998.

181. Kielstein JT, Stadler M, Czock D, et al: Dialysate concentration and pharmacokinetics of 2F-Ara-A in a patient with acute renal failure. *Eur J Haematol* 74:533–534, 2005.

182. Byrd JC, Peterson B, Piro L, et al: A phase II study of cladribine treatment for fludarabine refractory B cell chronic lymphocytic leukemia: Results from CALGB Study 9211. *Leukemia* 17:323–327, 2003.

183. Sauter C, Lamanna N, Weiss MA: Pentostatin in chronic lymphocytic leukemia. *Expert Opin Drug Metab Toxicol* 4:1217–1222, 2008.

184. Ho AD, Thaler J, Stryckmans P, et al: Pentostatin in refractory chronic lymphocytic leukemia: A phase II trial of the European Organization for Research and Treatment of Cancer. *J Natl Cancer Inst* 82:1416–1420, 1990.

185. Dillman RO, Mick R, McIntyre OR: Pentostatin in chronic lymphocytic leukemia: A phase II trial of Cancer and Leukemia group B. *J Clin Oncol* 7:433–438, 1989.

186. Mulligan SP, Karlsson K, Stromberg M, et al: Cladribine prolongs progression-free survival and time to second treatment compared to fludarabine and high-dose chlorambucil in chronic lymphocytic leukemia. *Leuk Lymphoma* 55:2769–2777, 2014.

187. Tsimberidou AM, Wierda WG, Plunkett W, et al: Phase I-II study of oxaliplatin, fludarabine, cytarabine, and rituximab combination therapy in patients with Richter's syndrome or fludarabine-refractory chronic lymphocytic leukemia. *J Clin Oncol* 26:196–203, 2008.

188. Robertson LE, Hall R, Keating MJ, et al: High-dose cytosine arabinoside in chronic lymphocytic leukemia: A clinical and pharmacologic analysis. *Leuk Lymphoma* 10:43–48, 1993.

189. Raphael B, Andersen JW, Silber R, et al: Comparison of chlorambucil and prednisone versus cyclophosphamide, vincristine, and prednisone as initial treatment for chronic lymphocytic leukemia: Long-term follow-up of an Eastern Cooperative Oncology Group randomized clinical trial. *J Clin Oncol* 9:770–776, 1991.

190. Montserrat E, Alcala A, Alonso C, et al: A randomized trial comparing chlorambucil plus prednisone vs cyclophosphamide, melphalan, and prednisone in the treatment of chronic lymphocytic leukemia stages B and C. *Nouv Rev Fr Hematol* 30:429–432, 1988.

191. Prognostic and therapeutic advances in CLL management: The experience of the French Cooperative Group. French Cooperative Group on Chronic Lymphocytic Leukemia. *Semin Hematol* 24:275–290, 1987.

192. Friedenberg WR, Anderson J, Wolf BC, et al: Modified vincristine, doxorubicin, and dexamethasone regimen in the treatment of resistant or relapsed chronic lymphocytic leukemia. An Eastern Cooperative Oncology Group study. *Cancer* 71:2983–2989, 1993.

193. Keating MJ, O'Brien S, Lerner S, et al: Long-term follow-up of patients with chronic lymphocytic leukemia (CLL) receiving fludarabine regimens as initial therapy. *Blood* 92:1165–1171, 1998.

194. Elias L, Stock-Novack D, Head DR, et al: A phase I trial of combination fludarabine monophosphate and chlorambucil in chronic lymphocytic leukemia: A Southwest Oncology Group study. *Leukemia* 7:361–365, 1993.

195. O'Brien SM, Kantarjian HM, Cortes J, et al: Results of the fludarabine and cyclophosphamide combination regimen in chronic lymphocytic leukemia. *J Clin Oncol* 19:1414–1420, 2001.

196. Eichhorst BF, Busch R, Hopfinger G, et al: Fludarabine plus cyclophosphamide versus fludarabine alone in first-line therapy of younger patients with chronic lymphocytic leukemia. *Blood* 107:885–891, 2006.

197. Catovsky D, Richards S, Matutes E, et al: Assessment of fludarabine plus cyclophosphamide for patients with chronic lymphocytic leukaemia (the LRF CLL4 Trial): A randomised controlled trial. *Lancet* 370:230–239, 2007.

198. Robak T, Blonski JZ, Kasznicki M, et al: Cladribine with prednisone versus chlorambucil with prednisone as first-line therapy in chronic lymphocytic leukemia: Report of a prospective, randomized, multicenter trial. *Blood* 96:2723–2729, 2000.

199. Robak T, Blonski JZ, Kasznicki M, et al: Comparison of cladribine plus prednisone with chlorambucil plus prednisone in patients with chronic lymphocytic leukemia. Final report of the Polish Adult Leukemia Group (PALG CLL1). *Med Sci Monit* 11:PI71–9, 2005.

200. Laurencet F, Ballabeni P, Rufener B, et al: The multicenter trial SAKK 37/95 of cladribine, cyclophosphamide and prednisone in the treatment of chronic lymphocytic leukemias and low-grade non-Hodgkin's lymphomas. *Acta Haematol* 117:40–47, 2007.

201. Tefferi A, Li CY, Reeder CB, et al: A phase II study of sequential combination chemotherapy with cyclophosphamide, prednisone, and 2-chlorodeoxyadenosine in previously untreated patients with chronic lymphocytic leukemia. *Leukemia* 15:1171–1175, 2001.

202. Robak T, Blonski JZ, Wawrzyniak E, et al: Activity of cladribine combined with cyclophosphamide in frontline therapy for chronic lymphocytic leukemia with 17p13.1/TP53 deletion: Report from the Polish Adult Leukemia Group. *Cancer* 115:94–100, 2009.

203. Weiss MA, Maslak PG, Jurcic JG, et al: Pentostatin and cyclophosphamide: An effective new regimen in previously treated patients with chronic lymphocytic leukemia. *J Clin Oncol* 21:1278–1284, 2003.

204. Oken MM, Lee S, Kay NE, et al: Pentostatin, chlorambucil and prednisone therapy for B-chronic lymphocytic leukemia: A phase I/II study by the Eastern Cooperative Oncology Group study E1488. *Leuk Lymphoma* 45:79–84, 2004.

205. Robak T, Blonski JZ, Gora-Tybor J, et al: Cladribine alone and in combination with cyclophosphamide or cyclophosphamide plus mitoxantrone in the treatment of progressive chronic lymphocytic leukemia: Report of a prospective, multicenter, randomized trial of the Polish Adult Leukemia Group (PALG CLL2). *Blood* 108:473–479, 2006.

206. Bosch F, Ferrer A, Lopez-Guillermo A, et al: Fludarabine, cyclophosphamide and mitoxantrone in the treatment of resistant or relapsed chronic lymphocytic leukaemia. *Br J Haematol* 119:976–984, 2002.

207. Bosch F, Ferrer A, Villamor N, et al: Fludarabine, cyclophosphamide, and mitoxantrone as initial therapy of chronic lymphocytic leukemia: High response rate and disease eradication. *Clin Cancer Res* 14:155–161, 2008.

208. Osterborg A, Dyer MJ, Bunjes D, et al: Phase II multicenter study of human CD52 antibody in previously treated chronic lymphocytic leukemia. European Study Group of CAMPATH-1H Treatment in Chronic Lymphocytic Leukemia. *J Clin Oncol* 15:1567–1574, 1997.

209. Rai KR, Freter CE, Mercier RJ, et al: Alemtuzumab in previously treated chronic lymphocytic leukemia patients who also had received fludarabine. *J Clin Oncol* 20:3891–3897, 2002.

210. Keating MJ, Flinn I, Jain V, et al: Therapeutic role of alemtuzumab (Campath-1H) in patients who have failed fludarabine: Results of a large international study. *Blood* 99:3554–3561, 2002.

211. Kennedy B, Rawstron A, Carter C, et al: Campath-1H and fludarabine in combination are highly active in refractory chronic lymphocytic leukemia. *Blood* 99:2245–2247, 2002.

212. Lundin J, Porwit-MacDonald A, Rossmann ED, et al: Cellular immune reconstitution after subcutaneous alemtuzumab (anti-CD52 monoclonal antibody, CAMPATH-1H) treatment as first-line therapy for B-cell chronic lymphocytic leukaemia. *Leukemia* 18:484–490, 2004.

213. Hillmen P, Skotnicki AB, Robak T, et al: Alemtuzumab compared with chlorambucil as first-line therapy for chronic lymphocytic leukemia. *J Clin Oncol* 25:5616–5623, 2007.

214. Lundin J, Kimby E, Bjorkholm M, et al: Phase II trial of subcutaneous anti-CD52 monoclonal antibody alemtuzumab (Campath-1H) as first-line treatment for patients with B-cell chronic lymphocytic leukemia (B-CLL). *Blood* 100:768–773, 2002.

215. Karlsson C, Lundin J, Kimby E, et al: Phase II study of subcutaneous alemtuzumab without dose escalation in patients with advanced-stage, relapsed chronic lymphocytic leukemia. *Br J Haematol* 144:78–85, 2009.

216. Wendtner CM, Ritgen M, Schweighofer CD, et al: Consolidation with alemtuzumab in patients with chronic lymphocytic leukemia (CLL) in first remission—Experience on safety and efficacy within a randomized multicenter phase III trial of the German CLL Study Group (GCLLSG). *Leukemia* 18:1093–1101, 2004.

217. Hainsworth JD, Vazquez ER, Spigel DR, et al: Combination therapy with fludarabine and rituximab followed by alemtuzumab in the first-line treatment of patients with chronic lymphocytic leukemia or small lymphocytic lymphoma: A phase 2 trial of the Minnie Pearl Cancer Research Network. *Cancer* 112:1288–1295, 2008.

218. Schweighofer CD, Ritgen M, Eichhorst BF, et al: Consolidation with alemtuzumab improves progression-free survival in patients with chronic lymphocytic leukemia (CLL) in first remission: Long-term follow-up of a randomized phase III trial of the German CLL Study Group (GCLLSG). *Br J Haematol* 144:95–98, 2009.

219. Lin TS, Donohue KA, Byrd JC, et al: Consolidation therapy with subcutaneous alemtuzumab after fludarabine and rituximab induction therapy for previously untreated chronic lymphocytic leukemia: Final analysis of CALGB 10101. *J Clin Oncol* 28:4500–4506, 2010.

220. Awan FT, Lapalombella R, Trotta R, et al: CD19 targeting of chronic lymphocytic leukemia with a novel Fc-domain-engineered monoclonal antibody. *Blood* 115:1204–1213, 2010.

221. Weitzman J, Betancur M, Boissel L, et al: Variable contribution of monoclonal antibodies to ADCC in patients with chronic lymphocytic leukemia. *Leuk Lymphoma* 50:1361–1368, 2009.

222. Byrd JC, Kitada S, Flinn IW, et al: The mechanism of tumor cell clearance by rituximab in vivo in patients with B-cell chronic lymphocytic leukemia: Evidence of caspase activation and apoptosis induction. *Blood* 99:1038–1043, 2002.

223. Itala M, Geisler CH, Kimby E, et al: Standard-dose anti-CD20 antibody rituximab has efficacy in chronic lymphocytic leukaemia: Results from a Nordic multicentre study. *Eur J Haematol* 69:129–134, 2002.

224. Hainsworth JD, Litchy S, Barton JH, et al: Single-agent rituximab as first-line and maintenance treatment for patients with chronic lymphocytic leukemia or small lymphocytic lymphoma: A phase II trial of the Minnie Pearl Cancer Research Network. *J Clin Oncol* 21:1746–1751, 2003.

225. Byrd JC, Murphy T, Howard RS, et al: Rituximab using a thrice weekly dosing schedule in B-cell chronic lymphocytic leukemia and small lymphocytic lymphoma demonstrates clinical activity and acceptable toxicity. *J Clin Oncol* 19:2153–2164, 2001.

226. O'Brien SM, Kantarjian H, Thomas DA, et al: Rituximab dose-escalation trial in chronic lymphocytic leukemia. *J Clin Oncol* 19:2165–2170, 2001.

227. Carson KR, Focosi D, Major EO, et al: Monoclonal antibody-associated progressive multifocal leucoencephalopathy in patients treated with rituximab, natalizumab,

and efalizumab: A Review from the Research on Adverse Drug Events and Reports (RADAR) Project. *Lancet Oncol* 10:816–824, 2009.

228. Carson KR, Evens AM, Richey EA, et al: Progressive multifocal leukoencephalopathy after rituximab therapy in HIV-negative patients: A report of 57 cases from the Research on Adverse Drug Events and Reports project. *Blood* 113:4834–4840, 2009.

229. Coiffier B, Lepretre S, Pedersen LM, et al: Safety and efficacy of ofatumumab, a fully human monoclonal anti-CD20 antibody, in patients with relapsed or refractory B-cell chronic lymphocytic leukemia: A phase 1–2 study. *Blood* 111:1094–1100, 2008.

230. Rafiq S, Butchar JP, Cheney C, et al: Comparative assessment of clinically utilized CD20-directed antibodies in chronic lymphocytic leukemia cells reveals divergent NK cell, monocyte, and macrophage properties. *J Immunol* 190:2702–2711, 2013.

231. Teeling JL, French RR, Cragg MS, et al: Characterization of new human CD20 monoclonal antibodies with potent cytolytic activity against non-Hodgkin lymphomas. *Blood* 104:1793–1800, 2004.

232. Coiffier B, Losic N, Ronn BB, et al: Pharmacokinetics and pharmacokinetic/pharmacodynamic associations of ofatumumab, a human monoclonal CD20 antibody, in patients with relapsed or refractory chronic lymphocytic leukemia: A phase 1–2 study. *Br J Haematol* 150:58–71, 2010.

233. Wierda WG, Kipps TJ, Mayer J, et al: Ofatumumab as single-agent CD20 immunotherapy in fludarabine-refractory chronic lymphocytic leukemia. *J Clin Oncol* 28:1749–1755, 2010.

234. Hillmen P, Robak T, Janssens A, et al: Chlorambucil plus ofatumumab versus chlorambucil alone in previously untreated patients with chronic lymphocytic leukaemia (COMPLEMENT 1): A randomised, multicentre, open-label phase 3 trial. *Lancet* 9;385(9980):1873-83, 2015.

235. Wierda WG, Kipps TJ, Durig J, et al: Chemoimmunotherapy with O-FC in previously untreated patients with chronic lymphocytic leukemia. *Blood* 117:6450–6458, 2011.

236. Shanafelt T, Lanasa MC, Call TG, et al: Ofatumumab-based chemoimmunotherapy is effective and well tolerated in patients with previously untreated chronic lymphocytic leukemia (CLL). *Cancer* 119:3788–3796, 2013.

237. Kay NE, Geyer SM, Call TG, et al: Combination chemoimmunotherapy with pentostatin, cyclophosphamide, and rituximab shows significant clinical activity with low accompanying toxicity in previously untreated B chronic lymphocytic leukemia. *Blood* 109:405–411, 2007.

238. Mossner E, Brunker P, Moser S, et al: Increasing the efficacy of CD20 antibody therapy through the engineering of a new type II anti-CD20 antibody with enhanced direct and immune effector cell-mediated B-cell cytotoxicity. *Blood* 115:4393–4402, 2010.

239. Patz M, Isaeva P, Forcob N, et al: Comparison of the in vitro effects of the anti-CD20 antibodies rituximab and GA101 on chronic lymphocytic leukaemia cells. *Br J Haematol* 152:295–306, 2011.

240. Herter S, Herting F, Mundigl O, et al: Preclinical activity of the type II CD20 antibody GA101 (obinutuzumab) compared with rituximab and ofatumumab in vitro and in xenograft models. *Mol Cancer Ther* 12:2031–2042, 2013.

241. Bologna L, Gotti E, Manganini M, et al: Mechanism of action of type II, glycoengineered, anti-CD20 monoclonal antibody GA101 in B-chronic lymphocytic leukemia whole blood assays in comparison with rituximab and alemtuzumab. *J Immunol* 186:3762–3769, 2011.

242. Dalle S, Reslan L, Besseyre de Horts T, et al: Preclinical studies on the mechanism of action and the anti-lymphoma activity of the novel anti-CD20 antibody GA101. *Mol Cancer Ther* 10:178–185, 2011.

243. Alduaij W, Ivanov A, Honeychurch J, et al: Novel type II anti-CD20 monoclonal antibody (GA101) evokes homotypic adhesion and actin-dependent, lysosome-mediated cell death in B-cell malignancies. *Blood* 117:4519–4529, 2011.

244. Goede V, Fischer K, Busch R, et al: Obinutuzumab plus chlorambucil in patients with CLL and coexisting conditions. *N Engl J Med* 370:1101–1110, 2014.

245. Byrd JC, Pagel JM, Awan FT, et al: A phase 1 study evaluating the safety and tolerability of otlertuzumab, an anti-CD37 mono-specific ADAPTIR therapeutic protein in chronic lymphocytic leukemia. *Blood* 123:1302–1308, 2014.

246. Woyach JA, Awan F, Flinn IW, et al: A phase I trial of the Fc engineered CD19 antibody XmAb(R)5574 (MOR00208) demonstrates safety and preliminary efficacy in relapsed chronic lymphocytic leukemia. *Blood* 124:3553–3560, 2014.

247. Beckwith KA, Frissora FW, Stefanovski MR, et al: The CD37-targeted antibody-drug conjugate IMGN529 is highly active against human CLL and in a novel CD37 transgenic murine leukemia model. *Leukemia* 28:1501–1510, 2014.

248. Bargou R, Leo E, Zugmaier G, et al: Tumor regression in cancer patients by very low doses of a T cell-engaging antibody. *Science* 321:974–977, 2008.

249. Thornton PD, Matutes E, Bosanquet AG, et al: High dose methylprednisolone can induce remissions in CLL patients with p53 abnormalities. *Ann Hematol* 82:759–765, 2003.

250. Castro JE, Sandoval-Sus JD, Bole J, et al: Rituximab in combination with high-dose methylprednisolone for the treatment of fludarabine refractory high-risk chronic lymphocytic leukemia. *Leukemia* 22:2048–2053, 2008.

251. Castro JE, James DF, Sandoval-Sus JD, et al: Rituximab in combination with high-dose methylprednisolone for the treatment of chronic lymphocytic leukemia. *Leukemia* 23:1779–1789, 2009.

252. Smolej L, Doubek M, Panovska A, et al: Rituximab in combination with high-dose dexamethasone for the treatment of relapsed/refractory chronic lymphocytic leukemia. *Leuk Res* 36:1278–1282, 2012.

253. Byrd JC, Peterson BL, Morrison VA, et al: Randomized phase 2 study of fludarabine with concurrent versus sequential treatment with rituximab in symptomatic, untreated patients with B-cell chronic lymphocytic leukemia: Results from Cancer and Leukemia Group B 9712 (CALGB 9712). *Blood* 101:6–14, 2003.

254. Byrd JC, Rai K, Peterson BL, et al: Addition of rituximab to fludarabine may prolong progression-free survival and overall survival in patients with previously untreated chronic lymphocytic leukemia: An updated retrospective comparative analysis of CALGB 9712 and CALGB 9011. *Blood* 105:49–53, 2005.

255. Woyach JA, Ruppert AS, Heerema NA, et al: Chemoimmunotherapy with fludarabine and rituximab produces extended overall survival and progression-free survival in chronic lymphocytic leukemia: Long-term follow-up of CALGB study 9712. *J Clin Oncol* 29:1349–1355, 2011.

256. Robak T, Dmoszynska A, Solal-Celigny P, et al: Rituximab plus fludarabine and cyclophosphamide prolongs progression-free survival compared with fludarabine and cyclophosphamide alone in previously treated chronic lymphocytic leukemia. *J Clin Oncol* 28:1756–1765, 2010.

257. Wierda W, O'Brien S, Wen S, et al: Chemoimmunotherapy with fludarabine, cyclophosphamide, and rituximab for relapsed and refractory chronic lymphocytic leukemia. *J Clin Oncol* 23:4070–4078, 2005.

258. Keating MJ, O'Brien S, Albitar M, et al: Early results of a chemoimmunotherapy regimen of fludarabine, cyclophosphamide, and rituximab as initial therapy for chronic lymphocytic leukemia. *J Clin Oncol* 23:4079–4088, 2005.

259. Tam CS, O'Brien S, Wierda W, et al: Long-term results of the fludarabine, cyclophosphamide, and rituximab regimen as initial therapy of chronic lymphocytic leukemia. *Blood* 112:975–980, 2008.

260. Strati P, Wierda W, Burger J, et al: Myelosuppression after frontline fludarabine, cyclophosphamide, and rituximab in patients with chronic lymphocytic leukemia: Analysis of persistent and new-onset cytopenia. *Cancer* 119:3805–3811, 2013.

261. Benjamini O, Jain P, Trinh L, et al: Second cancers in patients with chronic lymphocytic leukemia who received frontline fludarabine, cyclophosphamide and rituximab therapy: Distribution and clinical outcomes. *Leuk Lymphoma* 1–8, 2014.

262. Hallek M, Fischer K, Fingerle-Rowson G, et al: Addition of rituximab to fludarabine and cyclophosphamide in patients with chronic lymphocytic leukaemia: A randomised, open-label, phase 3 trial. *Lancet* 376:1164–1174, 2010.

263. Stilgenbauer S, Schnaiter A, Paschka P, et al: Gene mutations and treatment outcome in chronic lymphocytic leukemia: Results from the CLL8 trial. *Blood* 123:3247–3254, 2014.

264. Tam CS, O'Brien S, Plunkett W, et al: Long-term results of first salvage treatment in CLL patients treated initially with FCR (fludarabine, cyclophosphamide, rituximab). *Blood* 124:3059–3064, 2014.

265. Foon KA, Boyiadzis M, Land SR, et al: Chemoimmunotherapy with low-dose fludarabine and cyclophosphamide and high dose rituximab in previously untreated patients with chronic lymphocytic leukemia. *J Clin Oncol* 27:498–503, 2009.

266. Lamanna N, Jurcic JG, Noy A, et al: Sequential therapy with fludarabine, high-dose cyclophosphamide, and rituximab in previously untreated patients with chronic lymphocytic leukemia produces high-quality responses: Molecular remissions predict for durable complete responses. *J Clin Oncol* 27:491–497, 2009.

267. Fischer K, Cramer P, Busch R, et al: Bendamustine combined with rituximab in patients with relapsed and/or refractory chronic lymphocytic leukemia: A multicenter phase II trial of the German Chronic Lymphocytic Leukemia Study Group. *J Clin Oncol* 29:3559–3566, 2011.

268. Fischer K, Cramer P, Busch R, et al: Bendamustine in combination with rituximab for previously untreated patients with chronic lymphocytic leukemia: A multicenter phase II trial of the German Chronic Lymphocytic Leukemia Study Group. *J Clin Oncol* 30:3209–3216, 2012.

269. Eichhorst B, Fink A, Busch R, et al: Frontline chemoimmunotherapy with fludarabine (F), cyclophosphamide (C), and rituximab (R) (FCR) shows superior efficacy in comparison to bendamustine (B) and rituximab (BR) in previously untreated and physically fit patients (pts) with advanced chronic lymphocytic leukemia (CLL): Final analysis of an international, randomized study of the German CLL Study Group (GCLLSG) (CLL10 Study). *ASH Abstracts* 2014 19, 2014.

270. Kay NE, Wu W, Kabat B, et al: Pentostatin and rituximab therapy for previously untreated patients with B-cell chronic lymphocytic leukemia. *Cancer* 116:2180–2187, 2010.

271. Bertazzoni P, Rabascio C, Gigli F, et al: Rituximab and subcutaneous cladribine in chronic lymphocytic leukemia for newly diagnosed and relapsed patients. *Leuk Lymphoma* 51:1485–1493, 2010.

272. Robak T, Smolewski P, Cebula B, et al: Rituximab plus cladribine with or without cyclophosphamide in patients with relapsed or refractory chronic lymphocytic leukemia. *Eur J Haematol* 79:107–113, 2007.

273. Robak T, Smolewski P, Cebula B, et al: Rituximab combined with cladribine or with cladribine and cyclophosphamide in heavily pretreated patients with indolent lymphoproliferative disorders and mantle cell lymphoma. *Cancer* 107:1542–1550, 2006.

274. Honigberg LA, Smith AM, Sirisawad M, et al: The Bruton tyrosine kinase inhibitor PCI-32765 blocks B-cell activation and is efficacious in models of autoimmune disease and B-cell malignancy. *Proc Natl Acad Sci U S A* 107:13075–13080, 2010.

275. Woyach JA, Smucker K, Smith LL, et al: Prolonged lymphocytosis during ibrutinib therapy is associated with distinct molecular characteristics and does not indicate a suboptimal response to therapy. *Blood* 123:1810–1817, 2014.

276. O'Brien S, Furman R, Coutre S, et al: Independent evaluation of ibrutinib efficacy 3 years post-initiation of monotherapy in patients with chronic lymphocytic leukemia/small lymphocytic leukemia including deletion 17p disease. *J Clin Oncol* 32:5s, 2014.

277. O'Brien S, Furman RR, Coutre SE, et al: Ibrutinib as initial therapy for elderly patients with chronic lymphocytic leukaemia or small lymphocytic lymphoma: An open-label, multicentre, phase 1b/2 trial. *Lancet Oncol* 15:48–58, 2014.

278. Byrd JC, Brown JR, O'Brien S, et al: Ibrutinib versus ofatumumab in previously treated chronic lymphoid leukemia. *N Engl J Med* 371:213–223, 2014.

279. Kamel S, Horton L, Ysebaert L, et al: Ibrutinib inhibits collagen-mediated but not ADP-mediated platelet aggregation. *Leukemia* 29:783–787, 2015.

280. Godiwala N, Maddocks K, Westbrook T, et al: Covariation of psychological and inflammatory variables in patients with chronic lymphocytic leukemia receiving ibrutinib. *J Clin Oncol* 32:5s, (suppl; abstr 7057), 2014.

281. Woyach JA, Furman RR, Liu TM, et al: Resistance mechanisms for the Bruton's tyrosine kinase inhibitor ibrutinib. *N Engl J Med* 370:2286–2294, 2014.

282. Burger JA, Keating MJ, Wierda WG, et al: Safety and activity of ibrutinib plus rituximab for patients with high-risk chronic lymphocytic leukaemia: A single-arm, phase 2 study. *Lancet Oncol* 15:1090–1099, 2014.

283. Herman SE, Gordon AL, Wagner AJ, et al: Phosphatidylinositol 3-kinase-delta inhibitor CAL-101 shows promising preclinical activity in chronic lymphocytic leukemia by antagonizing intrinsic and extrinsic cellular survival signals. *Blood* 116:2078–2088, 2010.

284. So L, Fruman DA: PI3K signalling in B- and T-lymphocytes: New developments and therapeutic advances. *Biochem J* 442:465–481, 2012.

285. Bunney TD, Katan M: Phosphoinositide signalling in cancer: Beyond PI3K and PTEN. *Nat Rev Cancer* 10:342–352, 2010.

286. Chantry D, Vojtek A, Kashishian A, et al: P110delta, a novel phosphatidylinositol 3-kinase catalytic subunit that associates with p85 and is expressed predominantly in leukocytes. *J Biol Chem* 272:19236–19241, 1997.

287. Furman RR, Sharman JP, Coutre SE, et al: Idelalisib and rituximab in relapsed chronic lymphocytic leukemia. *N Engl J Med* 370:997–1007, 2014.

288. Kharfan-Dabaja MA, Wierda WG, Cooper LJ: Immunotherapy for chronic lymphocytic leukemia in the era of BTK inhibitors. *Leukemia* 28:507–517, 2014.

289. Chanan-Khan A, Miller KC, Musial L, et al: Clinical efficacy of lenalidomide in patients with relapsed or refractory chronic lymphocytic leukemia: Results of a phase II study. *J Clin Oncol* 24:5343–5349, 2006.

290. Maddocks K, Ruppert AS, Browning R, et al: A dose escalation feasibility study of lenalidomide for treatment of symptomatic, relapsed chronic lymphocytic leukemia. *Leuk Res* 38:1025–1029, 2014.

291. Wendtner CM, Hillmen P, Mahadevan D, et al: Final results of a multicenter phase 1 study of lenalidomide in patients with relapsed or refractory chronic lymphocytic leukemia. *Leuk Lymphoma* 53:417–423, 2012.

292. Badoux XC, Keating MJ, Wen S, et al: Lenalidomide as initial therapy of elderly patients with chronic lymphocytic leukemia. *Blood* 118:3489–3498, 2011.

293. Chen CI, Bergsagel PL, Paul H, et al: Single-agent lenalidomide in the treatment of previously untreated chronic lymphocytic leukemia. *J Clin Oncol* 29:1175–1181, 2011.

294. Awan FT, Johnson AJ, Lapalombella R, et al: Thalidomide and lenalidomide as new therapeutics for the treatment of chronic lymphocytic leukemia. *Leuk Lymphoma* 51:27–38, 2010.

295. James DF, Werner L, Brown JR, et al: Lenalidomide and rituximab for the initial treatment of patients with chronic lymphocytic leukemia: A multicenter clinical-translational study from the chronic lymphocytic leukemia research consortium. *J Clin Oncol* 32:2067–2073, 2014.

296. Badoux XC, Keating MJ, Wen S, et al: Phase II study of lenalidomide and rituximab as salvage therapy for patients with relapsed or refractory chronic lymphocytic leukemia. *J Clin Oncol* 31:584–591, 2013.

297. Costa LJ, Fanning SR, Stephenson J Jr., et al: Sequential ofatumumab and lenalidomide for the treatment of relapsed and refractory chronic lymphocytic leukemia and small lymphocytic lymphoma. *Leuk Lymphoma* 1–15, 2014.

298. Shanafelt TD, Ramsay AG, Zent CS, et al: Long-term repair of T-cell synapse activity in a phase II trial of chemoimmunotherapy followed by lenalidomide consolidation in previously untreated chronic lymphocytic leukemia (CLL). *Blood* 121:4137–4141, 2013.

299. Lee BN, Gao H, Cohen EN, et al: Treatment with lenalidomide modulates T-cell immunophenotype and cytokine production in patients with chronic lymphocytic leukemia. *Cancer* 117:3999–4008, 2011.

300. Arumainathan A, Kalakonda N, Pettitt AR: Lenalidomide can be highly effective in chronic lymphocytic leukaemia despite T-cell depletion and deletion of chromosome 17p. *Eur J Haematol* 87:372–375, 2011.

301. Lapalombella R, Andritsos L, Liu Q, et al: Lenalidomide treatment promotes CD154 expression on CLL cells and enhances production of antibodies by normal B cells through a PI3-kinase-dependent pathway. *Blood* 115:2619–2629, 2010.

302. Porter DL, Levine BL, Kalos M, et al: Chimeric antigen receptor-modified T cells in chronic lymphoid leukemia. *N Engl J Med* 365:725–733, 2011.

303. Gill S, June CH: Going viral: Chimeric antigen receptor T-cell therapy for hematological malignancies. *Immunol Rev* 263:68–89, 2015.

304. Kalos M, Levine BL, Porter DL, et al: T cells with chimeric antigen receptors have potent antitumor effects and can establish memory in patients with advanced leukemia. *Sci Transl Med* 3:95ra73, 2011.

305. ABT-199 shows effectiveness in CLL. *Cancer Discov* 4:OF7, 2014.

306. Souers AJ, Leverson JD, Boghaert ER, et al: ABT-199, a potent and selective BCL-2 inhibitor, achieves antitumor activity while sparing platelets. *Nat Med* 19:202–208, 2013.

307. Topp MS, Kufer P, Gokbuget N, et al: Targeted therapy with the T-cell-engaging antibody blinatumomab of chemotherapy-refractory minimal residual disease in B-lineage acute lymphoblastic leukemia patients results in high response rate and prolonged leukemia-free survival. *J Clin Oncol* 29:2493–2498, 2011.

308. Stephens DM, Ruppert AS, Maddocks K, et al: Cyclophosphamide, alvocidib (flavopiridol), and rituximab, a novel feasible chemoimmunotherapy regimen for patients with high-risk chronic lymphocytic leukemia. *Leuk Res* 37:1195–1199, 2013.

309. Lin TS, Ruppert AS, Johnson AJ, et al: Phase II study of flavopiridol in relapsed chronic lymphocytic leukemia demonstrating high response rates in genetically high-risk disease. *J Clin Oncol* 27:6012–6018, 2009.

310. Fabre C, Gobbi M, Ezzili C, et al: Clinical study of the novel cyclin-dependent kinase inhibitor dinaciclib in combination with rituximab in relapsed/refractory chronic lymphocytic leukemia patients. *Cancer Chemother Pharmacol* 74:1057–1064, 2014.

311. Blachly JS, Byrd JC: Emerging drug profile: Cyclin-dependent kinase inhibitors. *Leuk Lymphoma* 54:2133–2143, 2013.

312. Magni M, Di Nicola M, Patti C, et al: Results of a randomized trial comparing high-dose chemotherapy plus Auto-SCT and R-FC in CLL at diagnosis. *Bone Marrow Transplant* 49:485–491, 2014.

313. Sutton L, Chevret S, Tournilhac O, et al: Autologous stem cell transplantation as a first-line treatment strategy for chronic lymphocytic leukemia: A multicenter, randomized, controlled trial from the SFGM-TC and GFLLC. *Blood* 117:6109–6119, 2011.

314. Tam CS, Khouri I: The role of stem cell transplantation in the management of chronic lymphocytic leukaemia. *Hematol Oncol* 27:53–60, 2009.

315. Peres E, Braun T, Krijanovski O, et al: Reduced intensity versus full myeloablative stem cell transplant for advanced CLL. *Bone Marrow Transplant* 44:579–583, 2009.

316. Doney KC, Chauncey T, Appelbaum FR, et al: Allogeneic related donor hematopoietic stem cell transplantation for treatment of chronic lymphocytic leukemia. *Bone Marrow Transplant* 29:817–823, 2002.

317. Dreger P, Schetelig J, Andersen N, et al: Managing high-risk CLL during transition to a new treatment era: Stem cell transplantation or novel agents? *Blood* 124:3841–3849, 2014.

318. Sorror ML, Storer BE, Sandmaier BM, et al: Five-year follow-up of patients with advanced chronic lymphocytic leukemia treated with allogeneic hematopoietic cell transplantation after nonmyeloablative conditioning. *J Clin Oncol* 26:4912–4920, 2008.

319. Dreger P, Dohner H, Ritgen M, et al: Allogeneic stem cell transplantation provides durable disease control in poor-risk chronic lymphocytic leukemia: Long-term clinical and MRD results of the German CLL Study Group CLL3X trial. *Blood* 116:2438–2447, 2010.

320. Khouri IF, Bassett R, Poindexter N, et al: Nonmyeloablative allogeneic stem cell transplantation in relapsed/refractory chronic lymphocytic leukemia: Long-term follow-up, prognostic factors, and effect of human leukocyte histocompatibility antigen subtype on outcome. *Cancer* 117:4679–4688, 2011.

321. Brown JR, Kim HT, Armand P, et al: Long-term follow-up of reduced-intensity allogeneic stem cell transplantation for chronic lymphocytic leukemia: Prognostic model to predict outcome. *Leukemia* 27:362–369, 2013.

322. Dreger P, Montserrat E; European Society for Blood and Marrow Transplantation (EBMT); European Research Initiative on CLL (ERIC): Where does allogeneic stem cell transplantation fit in the treatment of chronic lymphocytic leukemia? *Curr Hematol Malig Rep* 10:59–64, 2015.

323. Dreger P, Brand R, Milligan D, et al: Reduced-intensity conditioning lowers treatment-related mortality of allogeneic stem cell transplantation for chronic lymphocytic leukemia: A population-matched analysis. *Leukemia* 19:1029–1033, 2005.

324. Jaglowski SM, Ruppert AS, Heerema NA, et al: Complex karyotype predicts for inferior outcomes following reduced-intensity conditioning allogeneic transplant for chronic lymphocytic leukaemia. *Br J Haematol* 159:82–87, 2012.

325. Gratwohl A, Brand R, Niederwieser D, et al: Introduction of a quality management system and outcome after hematopoietic stem-cell transplantation. *J Clin Oncol* 29:1980–1986, 2011.

326. Giebel S, Labopin M, Mohty M, et al: The impact of center experience on results of reduced intensity: Allogeneic hematopoietic SCT for AML. An analysis from the Acute Leukemia Working Party of the EBMT. *Bone Marrow Transplant* 48:238–242, 2013.

327. Shanafelt TD, Kay NE, Rabe KG, et al: Hematologist/oncologist disease-specific expertise and survival: Lessons from chronic lymphocytic leukemia (CLL)/small lymphocytic lymphoma (SLL). *Cancer* 118:1827–1837, 2012.

328. Hodgson K, Ferrer G, Pereira A, et al: Autoimmune cytopenia in chronic lymphocytic leukaemia: Diagnosis and treatment. *Br J Haematol* 154:14–22, 2011.

329. Coad JE, Matutes E, Catovsky D: Splenectomy in lymphoproliferative disorders: A report on 70 cases and review of the literature. *Leuk Lymphoma* 10:245–264, 1993.

330. Seymour JF, Cusack JD, Lerner SA, et al: Case/control study of the role of splenectomy in chronic lymphocytic leukemia. *J Clin Oncol* 15:52–60, 1997.

331. Dearden C: Disease-specific complications of chronic lymphocytic leukemia. *Hematology Am Soc Hematol Educ Program* 450–456, 2008.

332. Byhardt RW, Brace KC, Wiernik PH: The role of splenic irradiation in chronic lymphocytic leukemia. *Cancer* 35:1621–1625, 1975.

333. Aabo K, Walbom-Jorgensen S: Spleen irradiation in chronic lymphocytic leukemia (CLL): Palliation in patients unfit for splenectomy. *Am J Hematol* 19:177–180, 1985.

334. van Mook WN, Fickers MM, Verschueren TA: Clinical and immunological evaluation of primary splenic irradiation in chronic lymphocytic leukemia: A study of 24 cases. *Ann Hematol* 80:216–223, 2001.

335. Chanana AD, Cronkite EP, Rai KR: The role of extracorporeal irradiation of blood in treatment of leukemia. *Int J Radiat Oncol Biol Phys* 1:539–548, 1976.

336. Wieselthier JS, Rothstein TL, Yu TL, et al: Inefficacy of extracorporeal photochemotherapy in the treatment of B-cell chronic lymphocytic leukemia: Preliminary results. *Am J Hematol* 41:123–127, 1992.

337. Chiappa S, Bonadonna G, Uslenghi C, et al: The role of endolymphatic radiotherapy in the treatment of chronic lymphatic leukaemia. *Br J Cancer* 20:480–484, 1966.

338. Cooper IA, Ding JC, Adams PB, et al: Intensive leukapheresis in the management of cytopenias in patients with chronic lymphocytic leukaemia (CLL) and lymphocytic lymphoma. *Am J Hematol* 6:387–398, 1979.

339. Cukierman T, Gatt ME, Libster D, et al: Chronic lymphocytic leukemia presenting with extreme hyperleukocytosis and thrombosis of the common femoral vein. *Leuk Lymphoma* 43:1865–1868, 2002.

340. Ali R, Ozkalemkas F, Ozkocaman V, et al: Successful labor in the course of chronic lymphocytic leukemia (CLL) and management of CLL during pregnancy with leukapheresis. *Ann Hematol* 83:61–63, 2004.

341. Cheson BD, Byrd JC, Rai KR, et al: Novel targeted agents and the need to refine clinical end points in chronic lymphocytic leukemia. *J Clin Oncol* 30:2820–2822, 2012.

342. Rawstron AC, Villamor N, Ritgen M, et al: International standardized approach for flow cytometric residual disease monitoring in chronic lymphocytic leukaemia. *Leukemia* 21:956–964, 2007.

343. Raponi S, Della Starza I, De Propris MS, et al: Minimal residual disease monitoring in chronic lymphocytic leukaemia patients. A comparative analysis of flow cytometry and ASO IgH RQ-PCR. *Br J Haematol* 166:360–368, 2014.

344. Bottcher S, Ritgen M, Pott C, et al: Comparative analysis of minimal residual disease detection using four-color flow cytometry, consensus IgH-PCR, and quantitative IgH PCR in CLL after allogeneic and autologous stem cell transplantation. *Leukemia* 18:1637–1645, 2004.

345. Rawstron AC, Bottcher S, Letestu R, et al: Improving efficiency and sensitivity: European Research Initiative in CLL (ERIC) update on the international harmonised approach for flow cytometric residual disease monitoring in CLL. *Leukemia* 27:142–149, 2013.

346. Provan D, Bartlett-Pandite L, Zwicky C, et al: Eradication of polymerase chain reaction-detectable chronic lymphocytic leukemia cells is associated with improved outcome after bone marrow transplantation. *Blood* 88:2228–2235, 1996.

347. Moreton P, Kennedy B, Lucas G, et al: Eradication of minimal residual disease in B-cell chronic lymphocytic leukemia after alemtuzumab therapy is associated with prolonged survival. *J Clin Oncol* 23:2971–2979, 2005.

348. Royle JA, Baade PD, Joske D, et al: Second cancer incidence and cancer mortality among chronic lymphocytic leukaemia patients: A population-based study. *Br J Cancer* 105:1076–1081, 2011.

349. Benjamini O, Jain P, Trinh L, et al: Second cancers in patients with Chronic Lymphocytic Leukemia who received frontline FCR therapy—Distribution and clinical outcomes. *Leuk Lymphoma* 1–28, 2014.

350. Travis LB, Curtis RE, Hankey BF, et al: Second cancers in patients with chronic lymphocytic leukemia. *J Natl Cancer Inst* 84:1422–1427, 1992.

351. Davis JW, Weiss NS, Armstrong BK: Second cancers in patients with chronic lymphocytic leukemia. *J Natl Cancer Inst* 78:91–94, 1987.

352. Brewer JD, Shanafelt TD, Otley CC, et al: Chronic lymphocytic leukemia is associated with decreased survival of patients with malignant melanoma and Merkel cell carcinoma in a SEER population-based study. *J Clin Oncol* 30:843–849, 2012.

353. Solomon BM, Rabe KG, Slager SL, et al: Overall and cancer-specific survival of patients with breast, colon, kidney, and lung cancers with and without chronic lymphocytic leukemia: A SEER population-based study. *J Clin Oncol* 31:930–937, 2013.

354. Quaglino D, Paterlini P, De Pasquale A, et al: Association of chronic lymphocytic leukaemia and multiple myeloma: Report of a case and review of the literature. *Haematologica* 67:576–588, 1982.

355. Pedersen-Bjergaard J, Petersen HD, Thomsen M, et al: Chronic lymphocytic leukaemia with subsequent development of multiple myeloma. Evidence of two B-lymphocyte clones and of myeloma-induced suppression of secretion of an M-component and of normal immunoglobulins. *Scand J Haematol* 21:256–264, 1978.

356. Jeha MT, Hamblin TJ, Smith JL: Coincident chronic lymphocytic leukemia and osteosclerotic multiple myeloma. *Blood* 57:617–619, 1981.

357. Maeshima AM, Taniguchi H, Nomoto J, et al: Secondary CD5+ diffuse large B-cell lymphoma not associated with transformation of chronic lymphocytic leukemia/small lymphocytic lymphoma (Richter syndrome). *Am J Clin Pathol* 131:339–346, 2009.

358. Tsiodras S, Samonis G, Keating MJ, et al: Infection and immunity in chronic lymphocytic leukemia. *Mayo Clin Proc* 75:1039–1054, 2000.

359. Hensel M, Kornacker M, Yammeni S, et al: Disease activity and pretreatment, rather than hypogammaglobulinaemia, are major risk factors for infectious complications in patients with chronic lymphocytic leukaemia. *Br J Haematol* 122:600–606, 2003.

360. Morrison VA: Infectious complications of chronic lymphocytic leukaemia: Pathogenesis, spectrum of infection, preventive approaches. *Best Pract Res Clin Haematol* 23:145–153, 2010.

361. Morra E, Nosari A, Montillo M: Infectious complications in chronic lymphocytic leukaemia. *Hematol Cell Ther* 41:145–151, 1999.

362. Wierda WG: Immunologic monitoring in chronic lymphocytic leukemia. *Curr Oncol Rep* 5:419–425, 2003.

363. Raanani P, Gafter-Gvili A, Paul M, et al: Immunoglobulin prophylaxis in chronic lymphocytic leukemia and multiple myeloma: Systematic review and meta-analysis. *Leuk Lymphoma* 50:764–772, 2009.

364. Boughton BJ, Jackson N, Lim S, et al: Randomized trial of intravenous immunoglobulin prophylaxis for patients with chronic lymphocytic leukaemia and secondary hypogammaglobulinaemia. *Clin Lab Haematol* 17:75–80, 1995.

365. Gamm H, Huber C, Chapel H, et al: Intravenous immune globulin in chronic lymphocytic leukaemia. *Clin Exp Immunol* 97 Suppl 1:17–20, 1994.

366. Sinisalo M, Aittoniemi J, Kayhty H, et al: Vaccination against infections in chronic lymphocytic leukemia. *Leuk Lymphoma* 44:649–652, 2003.

367. Sinisalo M, Aittoniemi J, Oivanen P, et al: Response to vaccination against different types of antigens in patients with chronic lymphocytic leukaemia. *Br J Haematol* 114:107–110, 2001.

368. Sinisalo M, Vilpo J, Itala M, et al: Antibody response to 7-valent conjugated pneumococcal vaccine in patients with chronic lymphocytic leukaemia. *Vaccine* 26:82–87, 2007.

369. Jurlander J, de Nully Brown P, Skov PS, et al: Improved vaccination response during ranitidine treatment, and increased plasma histamine concentrations, in patients with B cell chronic lymphocytic leukemia. *Leukemia* 9:1902–1909, 1995.

370. Tomczyk S, Bennett NM, Stoecker C, et al: Use of 13-valent pneumococcal conjugate vaccine and 23-valent pneumococcal polysaccharide vaccine among adults aged ≥65 years: Recommendations of the Advisory Committee on Immunization Practices (ACIP). *MMWR Morb Mortal Wkly Rep* 63:822–825, 2014.

371. Grohskopf LA, Olsen SJ, Sokolow LZ, et al: Prevention and control of seasonal influenza with vaccines: Recommendations of the Advisory Committee on Immunization Practices (ACIP)—United States, 2014–15 influenza season. *MMWR Morb Mortal Wkly Rep* 63:691–697, 2014.

372. Bridges CB, Coyne-Beasley T, Advisory Committee on Immunization Practices (ACIP); et al: Advisory Committee on Immunization Practices recommended immunization schedule for adults aged 19 years or older—United States, 2014. *MMWR Morb Mortal Wkly Rep* 63:110–112, 2014.

373. Ruzickova S, Pruss A, Odendahl M, et al: Chronic lymphocytic leukemia preceded by cold agglutinin disease: Intraclonal immunoglobulin light-chain diversity in V(H)4–34 expressing single leukemic B cells. *Blood* 100:3419–3422, 2002.

374. Kipps TJ, Carson DA: Autoantibodies in chronic lymphocytic leukemia and related systemic autoimmune diseases. *Blood* 81:2475–2487, 1993.

375. Zent CS, Ding W, Reinalda MS, et al: Autoimmune cytopenia in chronic lymphocytic leukemia/small lymphocytic lymphoma: Changes in clinical presentation and prognosis. *Leuk Lymphoma* 50:1261–1268, 2009.

376. Quinquenel A, Al Nawakil C, Baran-Marszak F, et al: Old DAT and new data: Positive direct antiglobulin test identifies a subgroup with poor outcome among chronic lymphocytic leukemia stage A patients. *Am J Hematol* 90:E5–E8, 2015.

377. Shvidel L, Tadmor T, Braester A, et al: Pathogenesis, prevalence, and prognostic significance of cytopenias in chronic lymphocytic leukemia (CLL): A retrospective comparative study of 213 patients from a national CLL database of 1,518 cases. *Ann Hematol* 92:661–667, 2013.

378. Ferrer G, Navarro A, Hodgson K, et al: MicroRNA expression in chronic lymphocytic leukemia developing autoimmune hemolytic anemia. *Leuk Lymphoma* 54:2016–2022, 2013.

379. Mauro FR, Gentile M, Foa R: Erythropoietin and chronic lymphocytic leukemia. *Rev Clin Exp Hematol* Suppl 1:21–31, 2002.

380. Bennett CL, Silver SM, Djulbegovic B, et al: Venous thromboembolism and mortality associated with recombinant erythropoietin and darbepoetin administration for the treatment of cancer-associated anemia. *JAMA* 299:914–924, 2008.

381. Jolliffe E, Romeril K: Eltrombopag for resistant immune thrombocytopenia secondary to chronic lymphocytic leukaemia. *Intern Med J* 44:697–699, 2014.

382. Cobcroft R: Pure red cell aplasia associated with small lymphocytic lymphoma. *Br J Haematol* 113:260, 2001.

383. Itala M, Kotilainen P, Nikkari S, et al: Pure red cell aplasia caused by B19 parvovirus infection after autologous blood stem cell transplantation in a patient with chronic lymphocytic leukemia. *Leukemia* 11:171, 1997.

384. Chikkappa G, Pasquale D, Zarrabi MH, et al: Cyclosporine and prednisone therapy for pure red cell aplasia in patients with chronic lymphocytic leukemia. *Am J Hematol* 41:5–12, 1992.

385. Ding W, Zent CS: Diagnosis and management of autoimmune complications of chronic lymphocytic leukemia/small lymphocytic lymphoma. *Clin Adv Hematol Oncol* 5:257–262, 2007.

386. Visco C, Barcellini W, Maura F, et al: Autoimmune cytopenias in chronic lymphocytic leukemia. *Am J Hematol* 89:1055–1062, 2014.

387. Visco C, Cortelezzi A, Moretta F, et al: Autoimmune cytopenias in chronic lymphocytic leukemia at disease presentation in the modern treatment era: Is stage C always stage C? *Leuk Lymphoma* 55:1261–1265, 2014.

388. Michallet AS, Rossignol J, Cazin B, et al: Rituximab-cyclophosphamide-dexamethasone combination in management of autoimmune cytopenias associated with chronic lymphocytic leukemia. *Leuk Lymphoma* 52:1401–1403, 2011.

389. Rossi D, Spina V, Deambrogi C, et al: The genetics of Richter syndrome reveals disease heterogeneity and predicts survival after transformation. *Blood* 117:3391–3401, 2011.

390. Parikh SA, Rabe KG, Call TG, et al: Diffuse large B-cell lymphoma (Richter syndrome) in patients with chronic lymphocytic leukaemia (CLL): A cohort study of newly diagnosed patients. *Br J Haematol* 162:774–782, 2013.

391. Rossi D, Gaidano G: Richter syndrome: Molecular insights and clinical perspectives. *Hematol Oncol* 27:1–10, 2009.

392. Mao Z, Quintanila-Martinez L, Raffeld M, et al: IgVH mutational status and clonality analysis of Richter's transformation: Diffuse large B-cell lymphoma and Hodgkin lymphoma in association with B-cell chronic lymphocytic leukemia (B-CLL) represent 2 different pathways of disease evolution. *Am J Surg Pathol* 31:1605–1614, 2007.

393. Rossi D, Cerri M, Capello D, et al: Biological and clinical risk factors of chronic lymphocytic leukaemia transformation to Richter syndrome. *Br J Haematol* 142:202–215, 2008.

394. Fangazio M, De Paoli L, Rossi D, et al: Predictive markers and driving factors behind Richter syndrome development. *Expert Rev Anticancer Ther* 11:433–442, 2011.

395. Rossi D, Spina V, Cerri M, et al: Stereotyped B-cell receptor is an independent risk factor of chronic lymphocytic leukemia transformation to Richter syndrome. *Clin Cancer Res* 15:4415–4422, 2009.

396. Rossi D, Rasi S, Spina V, et al: Different impact of NOTCH1 and SF3B1 mutations on the risk of chronic lymphocytic leukemia transformation to Richter syndrome. *Br J Haematol* 158:426–429, 2012.

397. Lee JN, Giles F, Huh YO, et al: Molecular differences between small and large cells in patients with chronic lymphocytic leukemia. *Eur J Haematol* 71:235–242, 2003.

398. Papajik T, Myslivecek M, Urbanova R, et al: 2-[18F]fluoro-2-deoxy-D-glucose positron emission tomography/computed tomography examination in patients with chronic lymphocytic leukemia may reveal Richter transformation. *Leuk Lymphoma* 55:314–319, 2014.

399. Noy A, Schoder H, Gonen M, et al: The majority of transformed lymphomas have high standardized uptake values (SUVs) on positron emission tomography (PET) scanning similar to diffuse large B-cell lymphoma (DLBCL). *Ann Oncol* 20:508–512, 2009.

400. Tsimberidou AM, Wierda WG, Wen S, et al: Phase I-II clinical trial of oxaliplatin, fludarabine, cytarabine, and rituximab therapy in aggressive relapsed/refractory chronic lymphocytic leukemia or Richter syndrome. *Clin Lymphoma Myeloma Leuk* 13:568–574, 2013.

401. Dabaja BS, O'Brien SM, Kantarjian HM, et al: Fractionated cyclophosphamide, vincristine, liposomal daunorubicin (DaunoXome), and dexamethasone (hyperCVXD) regimen in Richter's syndrome. *Leuk Lymphoma* 42:329–337, 2001.

402. Ohno T, Smir BN, Weisenburger DD, et al: Origin of the Hodgkin/Reed-Sternberg cells in chronic lymphocytic leukemia with "Hodgkin's transformation." *Blood* 91:1757–1761, 1998.

403. Ghani AM, Krause JR, Brody JP: Prolymphocytic transformation of chronic lymphocytic leukemia. A report of three cases and review of the literature. *Cancer* 57:75–80, 1986.

404. Kjeldsberg CR, Marty J: Prolymphocytic transformation of chronic lymphocytic leukemia. *Cancer* 48:2447–2457, 1981.

405. Parikh SA, Habermann TM, Chaffee KG, et al: Hodgkin transformation of chronic lymphocytic leukemia: Incidence, outcomes, and comparison to de novo Hodgkin lymphoma. *Am J Hematol* 90:334–338, 2015.

406. Bacher U, Kern W, Schoch C, et al: Discrimination of chronic lymphocytic leukemia (CLL) and CLL/PL by cytomorphology can clearly be correlated to specific genetic markers as investigated by interphase fluorescence in situ hybridization (FISH). *Ann Hematol* 83:349–355, 2004.

407. Lens D, Coignet LJ, Brito-Babapulle V, et al: B cell prolymphocytic leukaemia (B-PLL) with complex karyotype and concurrent abnormalities of the p53 and c-MYC gene. *Leukemia* 13:873–876, 1999.

408. Katayama I, Aiba M, Pechet L, et al: B-lineage prolymphocytic leukemia as a distinct clinicopathological entity. *Am J Pathol* 99:399–412, 1980.

409. van der Velden VH, Hoogeveen PG, de Ridder D, et al: B-cell prolymphocytic leukemia: A specific subgroup of mantle cell lymphoma. *Blood* 124:412–419, 2014.

410. Tatarczuch M, Blombery P, Seymour JF: De novo B-cell prolymphocytic leukemia with central nervous system involvement. *Leuk Lymphoma* 55:1665–1667, 2014.

411. Pamuk GE, Puyan FO, Unlu E, et al: The first case of de novo B-cell prolymphocytic leukemia with central nervous system involvement: Description of an unreported complication. *Leuk Res* 33:864–867, 2009.

412. Matutes E, Brito-Babapulle V, Swansbury J, et al: Clinical and laboratory features of 78 cases of T-prolymphocytic leukemia. *Blood* 78:3269–3274, 1991.

413. Mourad YA, Taher A, Chehal A, et al: Successful treatment of B-cell prolymphocytic leukemia with monoclonal anti-CD20 antibody. *Ann Hematol* 83:319–321, 2004.

414. Solh M, Rai KR, Peterson BL, et al: The impact of initial fludarabine therapy on transformation to Richter syndrome or prolymphocytic leukemia in patients with chronic lymphocytic leukemia: Analysis of an intergroup trial (CALGB 9011). *Leuk Lymphoma* 54:252–254, 2013.

415. Catovsky D, Wechsler A, Matutes E, et al: The membrane phenotype of T-prolymphocytic leukaemia. *Scand J Haematol* 29:398–404, 1982.

416. Matutes E, Catovsky D: Similarities between T-cell chronic lymphocytic leukemia and the small-cell variant of T-prolymphocytic leukaemia. *Blood* 87:3520–3521, 1996.

417. Matutes E, Catovsky D: CLL should be used only for the disease with B-cell phenotype. *Leukemia* 7:917–918, 1993.

418. Bennett JM, Catovsky D, Daniel MT, et al: Proposals for the classification of chronic (mature) B and T lymphoid leukaemias. French-American-British (FAB) Cooperative Group. *J Clin Pathol* 42:567–584, 1989.

419. Pileri SA, Milani M, Fraternali-Orcioni G, et al: From the R.E.A.L. classification to the upcoming WHO scheme: A step toward universal categorization of lymphoma entities? *Ann Oncol* 9:607–612, 1998.

420. Rawstron AC, Green MJ, Kuzmicki A, et al: Monoclonal B lymphocytes with the characteristics of "indolent" chronic lymphocytic leukemia are present in 3.5% of adults with normal blood counts. *Blood* 100:635–639, 2002.

421. Goldin LR, Lanasa MC, Slager SL, et al: Common occurrence of monoclonal B-cell lymphocytosis among members of high-risk CLL families. *Br J Haematol* 151:152–158, 2010.

422. Lanasa MC, Weinberg JB: Immunologic aspects of monoclonal B-cell lymphocytosis. *Immunol Res* 49:269–280, 2011.

423. Landgren O, Albitar M, Ma W, et al: B-cell clones as early markers for chronic lymphocytic leukemia. *N Engl J Med* 360:659–667, 2009.

424. Pangalis GA, Angelopoulou MK, Vassilakopoulos TP, et al: B-chronic lymphocytic leukemia, small lymphocytic lymphoma, and lymphoplasmacytic lymphoma, including Waldenström's macroglobulinemia: A clinical, morphologic, and biologic spectrum of similar disorders. *Semin Hematol* 36:104–114, 1999.

425. Sheibani K, Nathwani BN, Winberg CD, et al: Small lymphocytic lymphoma. Morphologic and immunologic progression. *Am J Clin Pathol* 84:237–243, 1985.

426. Elnenaei MO, Jadayel DM, Matutes E, et al: Cyclin D1 by flow cytometry as a useful tool in the diagnosis of B-cell malignancies. *Leuk Res* 25:115–123, 2001.

427. Matutes E, Carrara P, Coignet L, et al: FISH analysis for BCL-1 rearrangements and trisomy 12 helps the diagnosis of atypical B cell leukaemias. *Leukemia* 13:1721–1726, 1999.

428. Njue A, Colosia A, Trask PC, et al: Clinical efficacy and safety in relapsed/refractory mantle cell lymphoma: A systematic literature review. *Clin Lymphoma Myeloma Leuk* 15:1–12e7, 2015.

429. Campo E, Rule S: Mantle cell lymphoma: Evolving management strategies. *Blood* 125:48–55, 2015.

430. Chung SS, Kim E, Park JH, et al: Hematopoietic stem cell origin of BRAFV600E mutations in hairy cell leukemia. *Sci Transl Med* 6:238ra71, 2014.

431. Tiacci E, Trifonov V, Schiavoni G, et al: BRAF mutations in hairy-cell leukemia. *N Engl J Med* 364:2305–2315, 2011.

432. Summers TA, Jaffe ES: Hairy cell leukemia diagnostic criteria and differential diagnosis. *Leuk Lymphoma* 52 Suppl 2:6–10, 2011.

433. Maevis V, Mey U, Schmidt-Wolf G, et al: Hairy cell leukemia: Short review, today's recommendations and outlook. *Blood Cancer J* 4:e184, 2014.

434. Kansal R, Ross CW, Singleton TP, et al: Histopathologic features of splenic small B-cell lymphomas. A study of 42 cases with a definitive diagnosis by the World Health Organization classification. *Am J Clin Pathol* 120:335–347, 2003.

435. Reid R, Friedberg JW: Management of marginal zone lymphoma. *Oncology (Williston Park)* 27:840, 842, 844, 2013.

436. Sahin I, Leblebjian H, Treon SP, et al: Waldenstrom macroglobulinemia: From biology to treatment. *Expert Rev Hematol* 7:157–168, 2014.

437. Frenkel EP, Ligler FS, Graham MS, et al: Acute lymphocytic leukemic transformation of chronic lymphocytic leukemia: Substantiation by flow cytometry. *Am J Hematol* 10:391–398, 1981.

438. Douer D: Will novel agents for ALL finally change the natural history? *Best Pract Res Clin Haematol* 27:247–258, 2014.

439. Mathisen MS, Kantarjian H, Thomas D, et al: Acute lymphoblastic leukemia in adults: Encouraging developments on the way to higher cure rates. *Leuk Lymphoma* 54:2592–2600, 2013.

CHAPTER 93
HAIRY CELL LEUKEMIA

Michael R. Grever and Gerard Lozanski

SUMMARY

Hairy cell leukemia (HCL) is an uncommon form of adult chronic B-cell leukemia. Whereas the cell of origin is uncertain, at diagnosis the characteristic leukemic cells are found in the marrow, the blood, and the spleen. Patients present with fatigue, infections, and many have splenomegaly. They are often pancytopenic, or may have isolated cytopenias, and usually have monocytopenia. The leukemic cell in classic hairy cell leukemia (HCL-c) has a characteristic immunophenotypic profile (CD11c+, CD19+, CD20+[bright], CD22+, CD25+, CD103+, and CD123+ and CD27−). A variant of hairy cell leukemia (HCL-v), which occurs less frequently, has been identified as a separate entity. A genetic mutation, *BRAF V600E*, has been identified in the majority of patients with the classic form of this disease, but is not present in the variant. This mutation is also present in the hematopoietic stem cells of patients with HCL-c.

HCL is characterized by impaired marrow function and immunity leading to a high incidence of infectious complications. Both pentostatin and cladribine are effective in achieving durable complete remissions. Long-term studies demonstrate prolonged survival of patients, but the disease-free survival curves do not plateau suggesting that the disease is not cured but subject to relapse. Survival has markedly improved with the introduction of purine nucleoside analogues and is estimated to be 90 percent at 5-year followup. When patients relapse, high-quality remissions can be achieved with salvage therapy.

DEFINITION AND HISTORY

Cases of malignant diseases involving marrow that probably represented examples of hairy cell leukemia (HCL) were reported through the first half of the 20th century and designated by such terms as "lymphoid fibrosis." They had features characteristic of HCL including marrow replacement by mononuclear cells, marrow fibrosis, splenomegaly and anemia and thrombocytopenia. In 1958, Bouruncle, Wiseman, and Doan described this constellation of findings in a group of patients.[1] At that time there was no means to characterize the immunophenotype of malignant lymphoid cells and they called the disease "leukemic reticuloendotheliosis." In 1966, Schrek and Donnelly, described the distinctive feature of cytoplasmic projections that were evident on the blood cells in two cases of this disorder. They called these "hairy" cells.[1A] The

designation HCL has become universally accepted as the name of this lymphocytic neoplasm, characterized by infiltration of the marrow by malignant B-lymphocytes of a specific immunophenotype (see "Laboratory Features" below), often accompanied by reticular fibrosis, splenomegaly, anemia, thrombocytopenia, neutropenia, monocytopenia, and usually pancytopenia. Occasionally, there is an elevated total white cell count because of the abundance of malignant B-lymphocytes in the blood. Splenectomy was the sole therapeutic approach until the early observations of responses secondary to α-interferon and the purine analogues.[2,3] Whereas splenectomy improved the blood counts, the impact of this intervention was temporary, resulting in improvement of symptoms related to splenic sequestration. Most standard chemotherapy was ineffective and poorly tolerated. In 1984, Quesada described the benefits of daily α-interferon in achieving responses in seven patients with progressive HCL.[2] Three patients achieved a complete response, with the remaining four having partial responses. Extensive description of the effects of α-interferon on marrow showed improvement in granulopoiesis associated with increases in the number of both circulating granulocytes and platelets. While this approach was heralded as a major achievement in treating this disease, other opportunities emerged in the same time frame.

Grever and colleagues demonstrated that low-dose pentostatin was effective in achieving responses in patients with far-advanced low-grade B-cell malignancy.[4,5] Spiers reported the initial response of HCL to pentostatin in a limited number of patients,[3] which was followed by a larger study with a complete remission rate of 59 percent.[6] Kraut and colleagues subsequently showed that low-dose, less-intense, intermittent pentostatin produced a higher complete remission rate (approximately 89 percent) in patients with HCL.[7] Others confirmed these findings,[8] and a large prospective randomized trial of pentostatin versus α-interferon solidified that frontline therapy should be based upon a purine analogue.[9] Piro and colleagues reported that cladribine produced complete responses in 11 of 12 patients with this disease.[10] Numerous trials with cladribine confirmed that a single course of therapy was equally capable of inducing a high percentage of long-term complete responses.[11,12] However, the initial trials with cladribine excluded patients with an active infection.[10,11] Several studies using cladribine aimed at optimizing the remission rate and attempting to reduce myelosuppression showed that either 5 to 7 days of intravenous administration or subcutaneous injection produced responses, but these alternate approaches did not consistently reduce the risks for febrile neutropenia.[13–15] In contrast, the reported frequency of febrile neutropenia was less in a study using intermittent administration of pentostatin[9] compared to those reported with cladribine.[10] Consequently, either purine nucleoside analogue is now used to induce remission.

In patients with an active infection, it is advisable to control the infection before initiating immunosuppressive chemotherapy. However, if this is not possible then administration of either pentostatin alone or following α-interferon may be effective in controlling the underlying disease.[9,16] If α-interferon is initially used to improve the neutrophil count and control the leukemia, the subsequent use of pentostatin to achieve a complete remission is not compromised. Therefore, some investigators have initially treated patients with HCL complicated by infection with α-interferon, which was followed by pentostatin in an effort to reduce infectious complications.[16] While the use of filgrastim does reduce the degree and the duration of neutropenia, it does not reduce the number of febrile episodes in patients being treated with cladribine, in comparison to historical controls.[17] However, it may be helpful in treating serious infections in neutropenic patients with HCL who are in a precarious medical condition. The optimal management of actively infected patients with HCL requiring treatment is still challenging.

The remarkable advances in diagnosis and therapeutics with purine analogues over the past 25 years have clearly changed the natural history of this disease.[18] Patients may now lead a near-normal life, despite the likelihood of intermittent relapses requiring retreatment.[19,20] Although the risk for serious bacterial infection is greatest during initial therapy, there are some delayed risks associated with impaired recovery of T-lymphocyte cell numbers and function following administration of purine analogues.[19,21]

In patients who achieve a complete morphologic remission, the presence of minimal residual disease (MRD) has been repeatedly shown by immunohistochemical staining of the marrow.[19] Some patients in hematologic remission with MRD may live normal lives, and do not require retreatment unless there is deterioration in their blood counts.[22,23] Consequently, further research to define the optimal therapeutic approach and timing for evaluation of response is needed.

The excellent results achieved with purine nucleoside induction associated with high percentages of complete remission have contributed to the improvement in overall survival for patients with this disease.[20] Using Surveillance, Epidemiology, and End Results Program (SEER) data after 1984, extensive analysis over the past 3 decades shows a progressive improvement in patient survival with HCL. Despite these truly remarkable results, at least 40 percent of patients will relapse.[19] Many of these patients will be successfully retreated, but the failure of the disease-free survival curve to flatten attests to the fact that this disease has been controlled but not cured. Strategies to predict who will be prone to relapse will enable new treatments to be risk-stratified. Furthermore, new agents are being developed to successfully treat patients who have developed resistant disease.[19,24,25]

EPIDEMIOLOGY

HCL is a rare chronic B-cell lymphoid malignancy accounting for approximately 2 percent of adult leukemias. The estimated annual incidence in the United States is approximately 3.3 persons per million person-years in the United States.[24] The mean age at diagnosis is 55 years, but there is a wide range in age of onset.[20] Patients may present in their 20s and 30s, and a report on 88 patients who were diagnosed at age 40 or younger showed that these patients do well long-term.[26] Younger patients respond better to therapy, but may relapse and require retreatment in order to experience long-term survival benefits.[9,19] There is an unexplained male predominance with this disease with a ratio of 4:1 males to females. There is also an unexplained racial difference with more than 90 percent of patients being white.[20]

There is a bimodal presentation in age raising the possibility of different etiologies in the younger and older patient groups.[27] The search for causative relationships in the older subset of patients has included extensive investigation of environmental and occupational exposures.[28] There is a suggestion of increased cases associated with farming and in jobs with extensive exposure to insecticides. Extensive investigation of the risk for secondary malignancies identified an increased overall risk (standardized incidence ratio [SIR] 1.24) in a large population-based study according to SEER data from 1973 through 2000.[29] In this study of more than 3000 patients with HCL, three separate malignancies were identified as being of particular concern (SIR 6.61 Hodgkin lymphoma; SIR 5.03 non-Hodgkin lymphoma; and SIR 3.56 thyroid cancer). Whether or not these second malignancies are related to an immune deficit from the leukemia or a result of the therapy for the leukemia is unknown.

ETIOLOGY AND PATHOGENESIS

HCL represents a clonal population of leukemic cells predominantly infiltrating the marrow, the spleen, and the liver. These cells are characterized as mature activated memory B cells based upon their immunophenotypic profile.[30] The neoplastic cells in classic HCL (HCL-c)

have hypermutated immunoglobulin genes in approximately 90 percent of the cases.[31] In those patients who have unmutated immunoglobulin genes, the disease appears to be more aggressive, as is the case in chronic lymphocytic leukemia. Leukemic cells use a variety of VH gene families. In those patients showing a VH4–34 gene, the clinical course has also been noted to be less favorable.[32,33] Molecular parameters may have prognostic value. For example, patients with a mutation in p53 have been less responsive to purine analogue therapy. Therefore, characterization of the molecular and genetic profile of the leukemic cells may elucidate the cell of origin and have prognostic value with respect to clinical outcome and responsiveness to standard therapy.

The identification of a mutation in *BRAF V600E* in almost 100 percent of patients with HCL-c has had a major impact on classification of the previously defined subsets of this disease.[34] The leukemic cells from patients with the variant of HCL (HCL-v) express BRAF wild-type. This genetic difference confirms that these two entities are clearly unrelated with a completely separate clinical course and therapeutic responsiveness. It is interesting that the small subset of patients with an immunophenotype consistent with HCL-c, yet using VH4–34 rearrangement, appear to be BRAF wild-type, further suggesting that there are multiple unique clonal patterns with distinct clinical courses.[35] Despite immunophenotypic features consistent with HCL-c, the lack of expression of *BRAF V600E* identifies a clinical course unlike the highly responsive form of the leukemia.

The presence of *BRAF V600E* mutation appears to activate the MEK-ERK signaling pathway responsible for leukemic cell survival and proliferation. Downstream activation of pERK correlates with presence of this mutational pathway.[36] Hematopoietic stem cells expressing this mutation have been identified in the marrow of murine models of the disease,[37] as well as in the marrow of patients with HCL.[37] *BRAF V600E* in marrow stem cells may explain the impairment in normal hematopoiesis that occurs in HCL-c. Furthermore, cytokines secreted by the leukemic cells may be responsible for the areas of hypocellularity observed in some patients with HCL-c.[38,39] Alternatively, impaired hematopoiesis may result from inadequate growth factor production.[40] Pancytopenia may also result either from extensive marrow infiltration with leukemia or fibrosis induced by the overproduction of transforming growth factor (TGF)-β by leukemic cells.[41]

CLINICAL FEATURES

The most common presenting symptoms are weakness and fatigue, which occur in 50 percent of patients with HCL.[42] Although many patients also have an enlarged spleen, the gradual onset of symptoms is described as fullness in left abdomen, early satiety, and discomfort. Initially, Bouroncle reported that splenomegaly was found in 96 percent of patients.[1] However, more recently the percentage with a markedly enlarged spleen may be less at diagnosis because of earlier detection of the disease. Patients may present with a history of increased infections, and approximately 17 percent have an active infection at the time of diagnosis.[1] Bleeding manifestations are also noted in patients with severe thrombocytopenia. Patients may present with few symptoms, but an abnormal laboratory report suggesting a hematologic disorder may emerge during a routine health examination.

Infection has been the leading cause of death in patients with HCL, and accounted for 55 percent of the fatalities in a large longitudinal review of 725 patients in an Italian series.[43] In general, the infections occur as a result of granulocytopenia, monocytopenia, and impaired function of immune effector cells. Approximately 30 percent of patients are found to have a documented source of infection, but an equal number of suspected infections cannot be documented microbiologically.[44] Fever in this patient population should prompt a search for infection. It has been estimated that 48 percent of infections are caused by pyogenic organisms including *Staphylococcus aureus, Pseudomonas aeruginosa, Streptococcus pneumoniae, Escherichia coli, Klebsiella* pneumonia, and *Legionella* pneumophilia.[21] Multiple other organisms have been identified as a source of infection including *Aspergillus, Candida, Blastomyces, Histoplasma, Cryptococcus, Toxoplasmosis, Pneumocystis jiroveci,* and atypical mycobacteria.

While the majority of infections occur before effective treatment has been initiated, the additional risk of infection as a complication of treatment exists both immediately following therapy and for many months thereafter.[21] The purine nucleoside analogues that are used as a backbone of induction therapy can produce profound and prolonged myelosuppression. Because of the extensive marrow involvement with leukemia, the myeloid reserve is severely compromised at the initiation of therapy. Following effective therapy, the granulocytes gradually recover, but the purine nucleoside analogues usually induce a prolonged period of reduction in lymphoid cells, thus opportunistic infections resulting from compromised lymphocyte function may also emerge in the posttreatment period.[45] Once the patient has achieved a complete remission, the risks for infection become progressively less as the hematologic parameters improve. Full recovery of lymphocyte function following purine analogue therapy, however, may require several years.[46,47]

Unusual symptoms related to HCL may include bone pain and autoimmune complications.[48,49] Bone pain may be the result of lytic disease that can involve the spine, the femur, and other skeletal sites. Lytic bone disease can occur at any time during the course of the disease. Both magnetic resonance imaging (MRI) and computed tomography (CT) scans have been helpful in identifying these lesions even when plain films of involved areas are normal. Biopsies of bone lesions have confirmed the presence of hairy cells, and these manifestations may respond to effective treatment of the leukemia. Many of the patients with bone lesions respond to systemic treatment of the disease, but others require additional localized irradiation.

Diverse autoimmune findings in patients represent other unusual complications.[49,50] Patients may complain of migratory inflammatory episodes involving the joints and tenosynovial tissues. These painful inflammatory episodes are usually self-limited and resolve spontaneously but may be recurrent. Vasculitic skin lesions and erythema nodosum have been reported.[51] Autoimmune hemolytic anemia and thrombocytopenia have also been observed.[52–54] The autoimmune phenomena are not related to tumor burden, and may be present at initial diagnosis or occur anytime throughout the course of the disease. Finally, patients have also presented with paraneoplastic neurological syndromes.[55]

● LABORATORY FEATURES

Patients with HCL reviewed in a large Italian series had pancytopenia (77 percent) reflecting impaired hematopoiesis due to marrow infiltration and splenic sequestration.[21,43] Approximately 28.4 percent of patients had a hemoglobin less than 8.5 g/dL with 14.9 percent requiring a blood transfusion, 39 percent of patients had an absolute neutropenia (neutrophils <500/μL), and 72.6 percent had a platelet count less than 100,000. Jansen earlier developed prognostic criteria for HCL relating the degree of anemia and splenomegaly to survival.[56] The Jansen staging system was developed before the age of effective therapy. Nevertheless, a later study also showed that the degree of anemia in younger patients correlated with overall survival following therapy with pentostatin.[9] Most patients have monocytopenia. Many patients have morphologic evidence of "hairy cells" on blood films characterized by pale blue or gray cytoplasm with a serrated/ruffled border (Fig. 93–1). The nucleus is oval and often reniform in shape with spongy chromatin and indistinct nucleoli. In the past, cytochemical staining with tartrate-resistant

acid phosphatase (TRAP) was routinely performed since hairy cells are positive for this enzyme. However, this stain is technically difficult and was therefore replaced by immunohistochemical stains (IHC) for this enzyme. Moreover, a more definitive diagnosis can be made by flow cytometry identifying the characteristic immunophenotypic profile. HCL cells are strongly positive for CD20, and are positive for CD11c+, CD25+, CD103+, and CD123+. The leukemic cells are usually negative for CD5–, CD10–, CD27–, and CD43–. Consequently, it is essential to secure a comprehensive immunophenotypic profile of the leukemic cells, as even small monoclonal populations can be identified by multichannel flow cytometry in the blood (see Fig. 93–1).

MARROW BIOPSY

In establishing the diagnosis, a marrow biopsy should be obtained to evaluate the degree of marrow cellularity and the percentage of leukemic cell infiltration (Fig. 93–2).[57] In addition, marrow fibrosis is characteristic of this disease. The marrow cellularity can be quite variable. Some patients with this diagnosis have a severely hypocellular marrow, and this pattern could be misread as hypocellular or aplastic anemia.[57] More often, there is either infiltrative disease or diffuse marrow replacement with the characteristic mononuclear cells with nonoverlapping cellular borders. These cells have resembled a "fried egg–like" appearance. Immunohistochemical stains can be used to definitively identify the leukemic cells within the biopsy. Immunohistochemical staining of the marrow with anti-CD20 is most useful, followed by staining with annexin and DBA.44 monoclonal antibody to further narrow the differential diagnosis. The demonstration that the mutation *BRAF V600E* is found in the overwhelming majority of cells from patients with HCL-c has provided yet another confirmatory stain for this disease.[58]

Additional baseline laboratory tests to obtain before treatment include an assessment of renal function as both of the commonly used purine nucleoside analogues are excreted by a renal route. It is important to screen for evidence of previous hepatitis B as serious complications including acute liver injury have resulted from the use of immunosuppressive agents (e.g., rituximab).[59]

LABORATORY VALUES USEFUL IN PATIENT MONITORING

Serial complete blood count monitoring with attention to the absolute neutrophil count, the platelet count, and the hemoglobin is the most useful approach to follow the progress of HCL patients. As the expression of soluble interleukin-2 (IL-2) receptor correlates with tumor burden a baseline determination of the soluble IL-2 receptor may be important for following the course of the disease and its response to treatment.[60] Soluble CD22 also can be followed in a similar manner as a correlate of leukemic cell burden.[61,62]

● DIFFERENTIAL DIAGNOSIS

Several B-cell clinical entities can be considered when establishing a diagnosis of HCL-c. The World Health Organization (WHO) defined an HCL-v that is completely separate from the classic form of this disease.[19,39,58,64] The frequency of HCL-v is approximately 10 percent of HCL-c.[64] This rare chronic B-cell lymphoproliferative disorder is characterized by leukocytosis, lack of monocytopenia and neoplastic B cells with nucleoli and convoluted nuclei. The cytoplasm may have a shaggy edge, but the ruffled border is usually not circumferential as in HCL-c. The immunophenotype is characterized as CD25– and CD123– negative, annexin-1 negative, and negative for TRAP, both by cytochemical and by immunohistochemical methods. The *BRAF V600E* mutation is not present in this entity.[34] The clinical course of the disease is initially

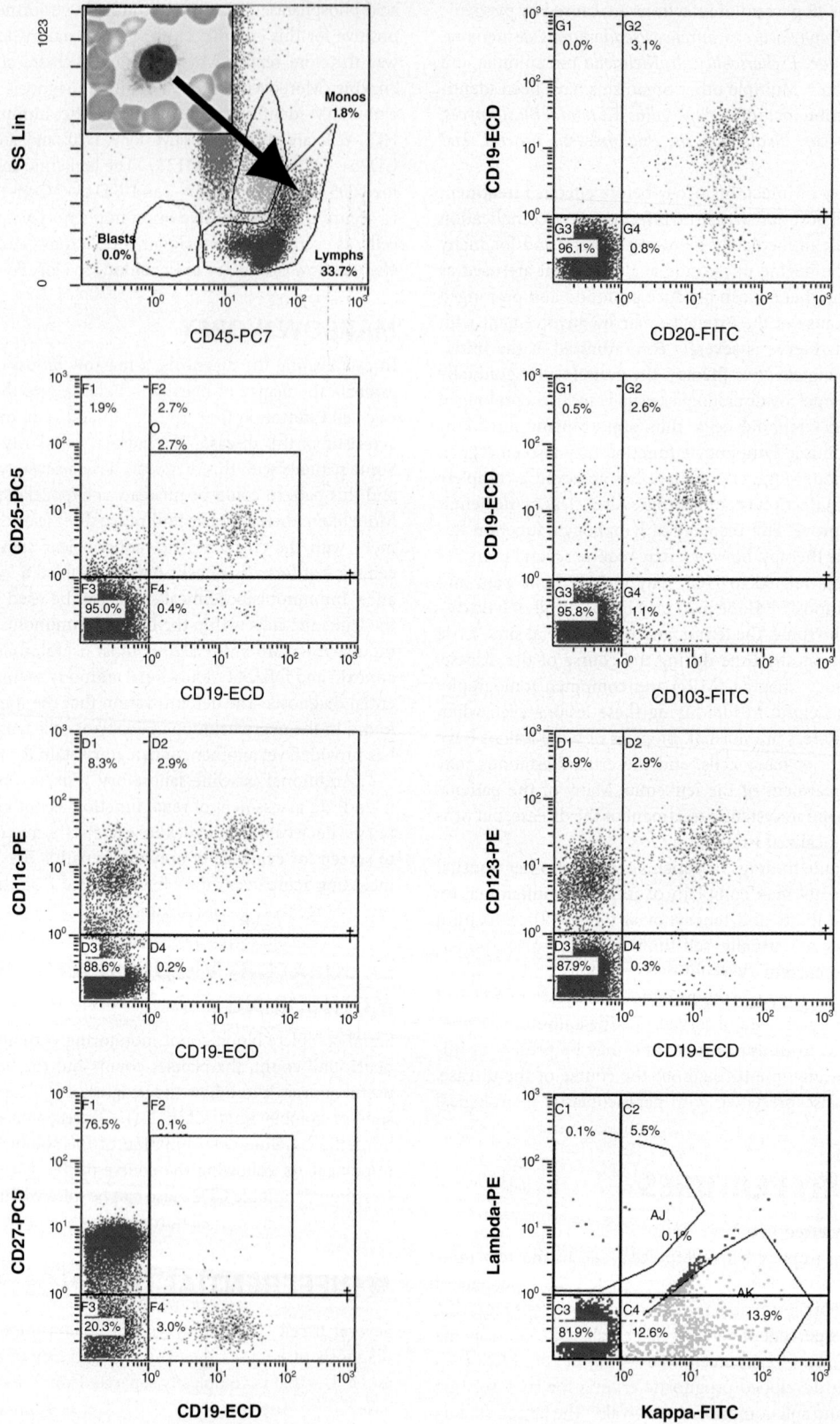

Figure 93–1. Hairy cell leukemia (HCL) immunophenotypic profiling should be performed using multiparametric flow cytometry analysis. Both blood and hemodilute marrow aspirates should be analyzed regardless of the number of leukemic cells seen on morphologic review of slides. Because of a very characteristic immunophenotype, definitive diagnosis of HCL can be rendered based on flow cytometric data even with a very low number of leukemic cells. As a result of their complex surface projections, hairy cells demonstrate moderate to high side scatter **(SC)** characteristics resulting in their shift on flow plots into the region typically occupied by monocytes. Hairy cells are positive for CD11c+, CD19+, CD20+, CD25+, CD103+, CD123+ and show κ light-chain restriction in this example. Hairy cells are negative for CD27–. Very rare cases of HCL may show positive staining for CD5 or CD10 antigens. It is important to note that while atypical, the expression of these antigens does not preclude a definitive diagnosis of HCL in cases with otherwise typical HCL immunophenotype.

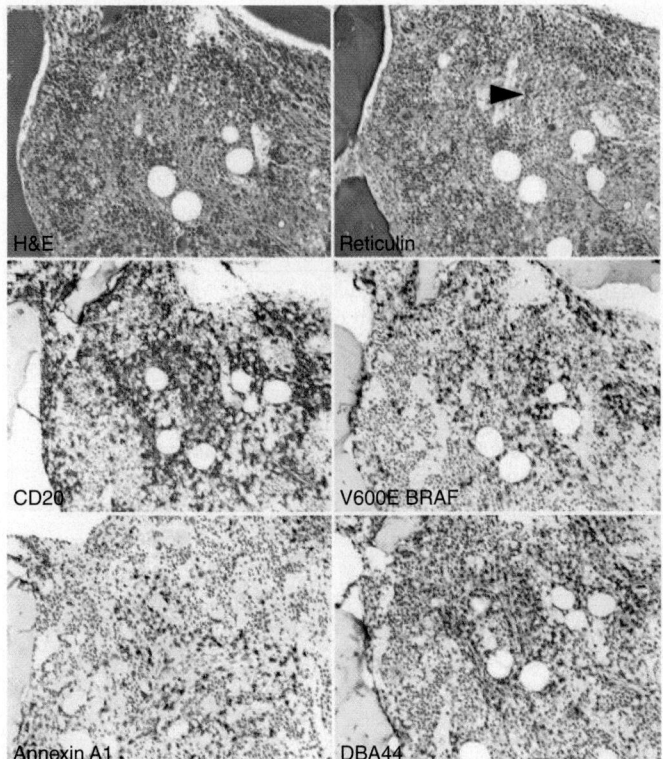

Figure 93–2. Marrow core biopsy is important in diagnosis of hairy cell leukemia (HCL) because marrow aspirates are frequently dry taps in HCL. This figure shows a marrow trephine biopsy involved by HCL. Hematoxylin-and-eosin (H&E) stained sections show a characteristic interstitial pattern of marrow infiltration by HCL. Leukemic cells are medium size with ample clear cytoplasm and centrally placed nuclei without nucleoli with "fried egg" morphology. Leukemic cells do not form discrete aggregates but are admixed with hematopoietic elements that often render their distinction from background erythroid precursors difficult. *Reticulin* stain shows reticulin fibrosis that is characteristically present in marrow involved by HCL and renders marrow difficult to aspirate resulting in frequent dry tap aspirates. *CD20* immunohistochemical stain highlights the extent of leukemic infiltrate. *V600E BRAF* immunohistochemical stain highlights leukemic cells that typically are positive for V600E BRAF mutation. *Annexin A1* immunohistochemical stain is positive in leukemic cells and is negative in background residual erythroid cells. *DBA44* immunohistochemical stain, while not absolutely specific, is always positive in HCL.

indolent, but eventually progresses with spleen and liver involvement. Some patients respond to splenectomy with temporary stabilization of the disease. Patients do not achieve durable responses with purine analogues as monotherapy, but may respond to immunotoxin conjugates (e.g., HA-22) or combined therapies with a purine analogue and a monoclonal antibody.[65,66]

Another entity that must be distinguished from HCL is splenic marginal zone lymphoma/splenic marginal zone lymphoma with villous lymphocytes.[64] This entity is a chronic B-cell neoplasm that involves the spleen, splenic hilar nodes, marrow and the blood. Patients may present with splenomegaly, anemia, and thrombocytopenia. The malignant cells in the blood are characterized by cytoplasmic villi/projections that are typically polar in distribution. The immunophenotypic profile is distinctly different than HCL-c. While the cells are positive for CD20, they are negative for CD25, annexin 1, and usually negative for CD103.

Splenic diffuse red pulp small B-cell lymphoma is an uncommon lymphoma that infiltrates the splenic red pulp in a diffuse pattern.[64] It can also involve the marrow and the blood. The malignant cells resemble those seen in splenic marginal lymphoma with villous lymphocytes. Patients usually have very large spleens, leukopenia, and thrombocytopenia. The immunophenotypic profile shows strong expression of CD20 and negative staining for CD25, CD11c, CD123, and annexin. This indolent lymphoma has been reported to respond to splenectomy.

There are patients with classic appearing HCL who have molecular features suggesting that there may be more than one molecular "variant" of this disease. For example, patients with a classic immunophenotype who are *BRAF V600E* mutation-negative and use the immunoglobulin VH4–34 have a worse prognosis than those with HCL-c, despite having identical immunophenotypic markers.[19,35] Patients with unmutated immunoglobulin gene rearrangement and those harboring a p53 mutation also have a worse prognosis, indicating that these molecular features potentially define yet another form of this disease.[31] Further study of the molecular prognostic features will hopefully identify information that will enable improvement in selection of appropriate therapy.[19] Establishing an accurate diagnosis of HCL or one of the clinical entities that mimic this disease by including a complete set of immunophenotypic and molecular markers is essential in selecting the best therapeutic option for each patient (Table 93–1).

●THERAPY

CRITERIA FOR INITIATION OF TREATMENT

Patients with HCL should be treated for symptoms related to the disease or for deterioration in blood counts. Patients may have symptoms associated with a markedly enlarged spleen. Excessive fatigue related either to the underlying disease or to the degree of anemia also warrant treatment. If the absolute neutrophil count is documented to be less than $1,000/\mu L$ or if the platelet count is confirmed to be less than $100,000/\mu L$, then consideration for treatment should be given rather than waiting until the patient's blood counts have deteriorated to very low levels. Many patients will have achieved these low hematologic parameters by the time of diagnosis, therefore meriting prompt therapy. Approximately 10 percent of patients with HCL-c may not meet these criteria, and can be followed for an extended period of time without therapy, albeit with close followup.[60,62,63]

If patients have had recurrent infections requiring antibiotics, it may be prudent to delay treatment for the HCL until after the infection has been controlled. After the infection is controlled, subsequent treatment with a purine analogue can be administered to secure a consolidated remission of the leukemia. These challenges highlight the importance of starting effective anti-leukemic therapy before the absolute neutrophil count deteriorates to a dangerous level.

STANDARD APPROACH

Patients may either be treated with cladribine or pentostatin (Table 93–2).[62,67,68] Cladribine has been approved for initial therapy, and pentostatin has been approved for second-line therapy. Cladribine has been administered by several routes on differing schedules. This agent is usually administered over 5 to 7 days, and the patient's blood counts need to be carefully monitored after this initial course. Initial studies administered cladribine as a continuous intravenous infusion for 7 days as a single course.[10] Subsequently, other investigators administered this agent as a daily intravenous infusion over 2 hours each day for 5 days.[68] Approximately 4 to 6 months after blood count recovery following cladribine, a marrow biopsy should be obtained to determine the quality of the response. The overall complete remission rate with this agent is reported to vary from 75 percent to 91 percent.[67,69,70]

Alternatively, if pentostatin is to be used for induction therapy, it is administered once every 2 weeks as a short intravenous injection

TABLE 93-1. Differential Diagnosis for Hairy Cell Leukemia

Characteristics	HCL	HCL-v	SMZL	SDRPSBL
Number of circulating malignant cells	Low	Moderate	Variable	Low
Monocytopenia	Present	Absent	Absent	Absent
Chromatin	Open	Condensed	Condensed	Condensed
Nucleolus	Absent	Prominent	Absent	Variable
Cytoplasm	Abundant with prominent circumferential hairy projections	Moderate to abundant with variably prominent circumferential hairy projections	Moderate to scant with variably prominent polar hairy projections	Moderate with variably prominent villous projections
Spleen involvement	Red pulp	Red pulp	White pulp	Red pulp
Marrow involvement	Interstitial, diffuse pattern, (fried egg morphology) Marrow reticulin fibrosis	Sinusoidal may be interstitial	Nodular may be intrasinusoidal	Intrasinusoidal, may be interstitial or nodular
Marrow reticulin fibrosis	Frequent and marked	Absent	Absent	Absent
Immunophenotype by flow cytometric analysis	CD11c+, CD19+, CD20+ bright, CD22+, CD25+, CD103+,CD123+, FMC7+, kappa or lambda (strong)	CD11c+, CD19+, CD20+, CD22+, CD27+, CD79b+, CD103+, FMC7+, kappa or lambda strong Negative for CD25–, CD123–	CD11c+, CD19+, CD20+, CD22+, CD27+, CD79b+, FMC7+, kappa or lambda strong Negative for CD25–, CD123–	CD11c+/–, CD103+/–, CD19+. CD20+, kappa or lambda+ Negative for CD25–, CD123–
Immunophenotype by immunohistochemistry	DBA44+ AnnexinA1+ Immuno-TRAP+ Cyclin D1+ Faint t-Bet+ V600E BRAF+	DBA44+ Annexin A1– Immuno-TRAP– Cyclin D_1– t-Bet– V600E BRAF–	DBA44+/– Annexin A1– Immuno-TRAP– Cyclin D_1– t-Bet– V600E BRAF–	DBA44+ Annexin A1– Immuno-TRAP– Cyclin D_1– t-Bet– V600E BRAF–
Recurrent mutation	V600E BRAF	None	None	None
Somatic hypermutation of immunoglobulin	>85% of cases	Mostly	>50% of cases	Variable

HCL, hairy cell leukemia; HCL-v, variant of hairy cell leukemia; SDRPSBL, splenic diffuse red pulp small B-cell lymphoma; SMZL, splenic marginal zone lymphoma; t-Bet, T-box transcription factor.

followed by administration of approximately a liter of fluid.[9,62] Weekly blood counts are monitored, and the second and subsequent doses are administered if the absolute granulocyte count has not decreased to dangerously low levels. Titrating these doses to be given every 2 to 3 weeks may lessen the degree of myelosuppression related to the agent.[62] After several reduced or delayed doses, the dose and schedule are returned to the standard dose of 4 mg/m² intravenous every 2 weeks in an effort to achieve complete remission. The complete remission rate to pentostatin with this approach approximated 75 percent in a multi-institutional study.[9] Patients may require 6 months or more of therapy with this agent. When the blood counts and the spleen have returned to normal, then a marrow biopsy should be performed to see if complete remission has been achieved by morphologic evaluation. This biopsy will serve as a baseline for evaluation of MRD. If there are no visible areas of HCL by morphologic criteria, then two additional doses are administered as consolidation.

MINIMAL RESIDUAL DISEASE

Although a complete remission is based upon recovery of blood counts, there must be no morphologic evidence of leukemic cells either in the

blood or the marrow.[19] MRD is defined as evidence of leukemic cells on the marrow biopsy that can be detected using IHC when there is no residual morphologic evidence of disease. IHC directed at markers on the leukemic cells may identify residual disease that is either diffusely infiltrating the marrow or localized. Antibodies directed at CD20, annexin, *BRAF V600E* (e.g., VE1), or DBA.44 will detect disease that is not identified morphologically.[19] In addition, detailed flow cytometric immunophenotypic analysis of either the blood or the marrow aspirate may be capable of identifying residual leukemia cells (e.g., positive for CD20+, CD11c+, CD103+, CD25+, CD123+ and negative for CD27–). Flow cytometry of the marrow may be negatively impacted by the difficulty in securing an aspirate that is not contaminated by blood. Consequently, identification of the extent of MRD using IHC on a marrow biopsy may be less adversely impacted by sampling error. Eradication of MRD may be achieved by adding additional therapy (e.g., administration of rituximab), but the necessity for this additional therapy must be considered.[71]

FOLLOWUP CARE

The advantages of achieving a complete remission have been stressed.[72] However, the therapy for this disease is immunosuppressive. Extensive

TABLE 93–2. Management of Hairy Cell Leukemia

Determine accurate diagnosis
- Marrow biopsy with immunohistochemical analysis
- Blood immunophenotypic characterization

Decision on initiation of therapy
- Approximately 10 percent can be carefully followed on "watch and wait" approach but majority of patients require treatment
- Determinants or symptoms prompting treatment: symptomatic splenomegaly or laboratory studies showing: absolute neutrophil count <1000/μL; hemoglobin <10 g/dL; or platelet count <100,000/μL

Important assessments before therapy for leukemia
- Presence or suspicion for infection
- Adequate renal function
- Previous exposure to hepatitis

Decision on frontline therapy
- Cladribine 0.1 mg/kg/day for 7 days continuous intravenous infusion[12,69,75]
- Cladribine 0.12 mg/kg/day for 5 days as 2-hour intravenous infusion vs. weekly infusion for 6 weeks[14]
- Pentostatin 4 mg/m² intravenous dose every 2 weeks until maximal response or failure[9,72,76]

Assessment of response
- Following induction therapy, a marrow biopsy to document quality of response and quantitate minimal residual disease (MRD)
- Methods for quantification of MRD with immunohistochemical stains and the optimal timing for MRD assessment are under investigation
- In general, response assessment after cladribine is recommended after 3 to 5 months. In contrast, response assessment following pentostatin is made at time of best clinical response

Clinical investigations for resistant hairy cell leukemia
- Alternate purine analogues alone or combined chemoimmunotherapy (e.g., bendamustine and rituximab)[77]
- Immunotoxin conjugates (e.g., moxetumomab pasudotox [HA22][73])
- BRAF V600E inhibitors (e.g., vemurafenib)[25,78]

Overall management strategies can be found in Refs. 62, 67, 71, and 79.

treatment to eradicate MRD may involve continued therapy with its attendant consequences of increased risk for infection or possibly a secondary malignancy. Consequently, clinical judgment must be exercised to achieve the optimal outcome for patients with this disease. An accurate assessment of response to therapy may best be made several months following completion of initial induction therapy.[71] In those who have achieved a complete response, careful followup is indicated. In those who had less than a complete remission, a determination will need to be made regarding salvage therapy versus close observation based upon blood count recovery.

THERAPY AT RELAPSE

The duration of response following initial therapy for HCL is variable. The criteria for retreatment can be based upon recurrence of clinical symptoms and on the status of the blood count.[62] A decision to restart therapy before progressive severe pancytopenia has returned is

important. Considering both the risks and benefits of additional therapy requires clinical judgment.

There are several therapeutic options for treating patients with either resistant disease or disease that had an early relapse following initial response. In general, if the patient achieved an initial response and subsequently relapses within 1 to 2 years, an alternate agent might be selected for retreatment.[62] Otherwise, retreatment with the initial therapy can be considered if the first remission was durable. Most patients will initially be treated with a purine nucleoside analogue. If there is an early relapse, the alternate purine analogue may be selected for reinduction. If patients initially received cladribine, pentostatin might be chosen for reinduction. In patients who demonstrate resistant disease, the identification of the *BRAF V600E* target has provided a therapeutic strategy involving an inhibitor (e.g., vemurafenib) as investigational therapy. Although patients have been reported to respond, this agent is not yet FDA-approved for this indication.[24,25] Furthermore, immunotoxin conjugates (e.g., HA22) have also been reported to produce remissions in patients with resistant disease.[73] The purine nucleoside analogues (cladribine and pentostatin) have also been effective in producing long-term salvage remissions in patients with HCL in relapse. In patients who have either resistant or relapsed disease, a combination of a purine analogue and a monoclonal antibody have also been used.[62,71]

● COURSE AND PROGNOSIS

The outlook for patients with HCL has markedly improved since its original description in 1958.[68] Patients can now anticipate a near normal life expectancy with the caveat that the disease will likely require close observation and retreatment for those who relapse. Survival at the end of 1 year is estimated to be approximately 88 percent with 5-year survival at 77 percent in one longitudinal population-based report.[21] Other long-term followup studies in the era of purine nucleoside therapy have identified similar results with 5-year survival being 90 percent and estimated 10-year survival at 81 percent.[72]

Whereas overall survival has improved, there is an increased risk of serious infection during the first year following diagnosis. The overall relative risk of a serious infection compared to a normal population is 2.59. This adjusted relative risk during the first year from diagnosis and treatment is 8.04.[21] The risk of serious infection is highest during the first year, and then declines toward normal in subsequent years. This indicates that patients should be followed very closely during the initial years following treatment. Full recovery of lymphocyte numbers and function after therapy may require several years. Consequently, physicians should follow their patients closely and document the recovery of these immune effectors cells. Patients should receive vaccinations utilizing dead or attenuated viral vaccines, and avoid "live" viral vaccines while in remission. Prompt attention to early signs of infection is important for health maintenance.

The results of clinical investigations have markedly improved the outcome for this patient population. Clinical relapse will likely occur because the current therapy controls the disease, but does not cure it.[74] Despite the enormous progress made in managing these patients, continued clinical investigation is warranted in an effort to achieve the best outcome with durable complete remissions and minimal risk of infection.

REFERENCES

1. Bouroncle B, Wiseman AG, Doan CA: Leukemic reticuloendotheliosis. *Blood* 13:609–630, 1958.
1A. Schrek R, Donnelly WJ: "Hairy" cells in blood in lymphoreticular neoplastic disease and "flagellated" cells of normal lymph nodes. *Blood* 27:199–211, 1966.
2. Quesada JR, Reuben J, Manning JT, et al: Alpha interferon for induction of remission in hairy-cell leukemia. *N Engl J Med* 310:15–18, 1984.

3. Spiers AS, Parekh SJ, Bishop MB: Hairy-cell leukemia: Induction of complete remission with pentostatin (2'-deoxycoformycin). *J Clin Oncol* 2:1336–1342, 1984.

4. Grever MR, Siaw MF, Jacob WF, et al: The biochemical and clinical consequences of 2'-deoxycoformycin in refractory lymphoproliferative malignancy. *Blood* 57:406–417, 1981.

5. Grever MR, Leiby JM, Kraut EH, et al: Low-dose deoxycoformycin in lymphoid malignancy. *J Clin Oncol* 3:1196–1201, 1985.

6. Spiers AS, Moore D, Cassileth PA, et al: Remissions in hairy-cell leukemia with pentostatin (2'-deoxycoformycin). *N Engl J Med* 316:825–830, 1987.

7. Kraut EH, Bouroncle BA, Grever MR: Pentostatin in the treatment of advanced hairy cell leukemia. *J Clin Oncol* 7:168–172, 1989.

8. Johnston JB, Eisenhauer E, Corbett WE, et al: Efficacy of 2'-deoxycoformycin in hairy-cell leukemia: A study of the National Cancer Institute of Canada Clinical Trials Group. *J Natl Cancer Inst* 80:765–769, 1988.

9. Grever M, Kopecky K, Foucar MK, et al: Randomized comparison of pentostatin versus interferon alfa-2a in previously untreated patients with hairy cell leukemia: An intergroup study. *J Clin Oncol* 13:974–982, 1995.

10. Piro LD, Carrera CJ, Carson DA, et al: Lasting remissions in hairy-cell leukemia induced by a single infusion of 2-chlorodeoxyadenosine. *N Engl J Med* 322:1117–1121, 1990.

11. Tallman MS, Hakimian D, Variakojis D, et al: A single cycle of 2-chlorodeoxyadenosine results in complete remission in the majority of patients with hairy cell leukemia. *Blood* 80:2203–2209, 1992.

12. Goodman GR, Burian C, Koziol JA, et al: Extended follow-up of patients with hairy cell leukemia after treatment with cladribine. *J Clin Oncol* 21:891–896, 2003.

13. Zenhausern R, Schmitz SF, Solenthaler M, et al: Randomized trial of daily versus weekly administration of 2-chlorodeoxyadenosine in patients with hairy cell leukemia: A multicenter phase III trial (SAKK 32/98). *Leuk Lymphoma* 50:1501–1511, 2009.

14. Robak T, Jamroziak K, Gora-Tybor J, et al: Cladribine in a weekly versus daily schedule for untreated active hairy cell leukemia: Final report from the Polish Adult Leukemia Group (PALG) of a prospective, randomized, multicenter trial. *Blood* 109:3672–3675, 2007.

15. Lauria F, Cencini E, Forconi F: Alternative methods of cladribine administration. *Leuk Lymphoma* 52 (Suppl 2):34–37, 2011.

16. Habermann TM, Andersen JW, Cassileth PA, et al: Sequential administration of recombinant interferon alpha and deoxycoformycin in the treatment of hairy cell leukaemia. *Br J Haematol* 80:466–471, 1992.

17. Saven A, Burian C, Adusumalli J, et al: Filgrastim for cladribine-induced neutropenic fever in patients with hairy cell leukemia. *Blood* 93:2471–2477, 1999.

18. Golomb HM: Hairy cell leukemia: Treatment successes in the past 25 years. *J Clin Oncol* 26:2607–2609, 2008.

19. Grever MR, Blachly JS, Andritsos LA: Hairy cell leukemia: Update on molecular profiling and therapeutic advances. *Blood Rev* 28:197–203, 2014.

20. Chandran R, Gardiner SK, Smith SD, et al: Improved survival in hairy cell leukaemia over three decades: A SEER database analysis of prognostic factors. *Br J Haematol* 163:407–409, 2013.

21. Teodorescu M, Engebjerg MC, Johansen P, et al: Incidence, risk of infection and survival of hairy cell leukaemia in Denmark. *Dan Med Bull* 57:A4216, 2010.

22. Sigal DS, Sharpe R, Burian C, et al: Very long-term eradication of minimal residual disease in patients with hairy cell leukemia after a single course of cladribine. *Blood* 115:1893–1896, 2010.

23. Tallman MS: Implications of minimal residual disease in hairy cell leukemia after cladribine using immunohistochemistry and immunophenotyping. *Leuk Lymphoma* 52 (Suppl 2):65–68, 2011.

24. Hall RD, Kudchadkar RR: BRAF mutations: Signaling, epidemiology, and clinical experience in multiple malignancies. *Cancer Control* 21:221–230, 2014.

25. Dietrich S, Glimm H, Andrulis M, et al: BRAF inhibition in refractory hairy-cell leukemia. *N Engl J Med* 366:2038–2040, 2012.

26. Rosenberg JD, Burian C, Waalen J, et al: Clinical characteristics and long-term outcome of young hairy cell leukemia patients treated with cladribine: A single-institution series. *Blood* 123:177–183, 2014.

27. Dores GM, Matsuno RK, Weisenburger DD, et al: Hairy cell leukaemia: A heterogeneous disease? *Br J Haematol* 142:45–51, 2008.

28. Orsi L, Delabre L, Monnereau A, et al: Occupational exposure to pesticides and lymphoid neoplasms among men: Results of a French case-control study. *Occup Environ Med* 66:291–298, 2009.

29. Hisada M, Chen BE, Jaffe ES, et al: Second cancer incidence and cause-specific mortality among 3104 patients with hairy cell leukemia: A population-based study. *J Natl Cancer Inst* 99:215–222, 2007.

30. Matutes E: Immunophenotyping and differential diagnosis of hairy cell leukemia. *Hematol Oncol Clin North Am* 20:1051–1063, 2006.

31. Forconi F, Sozzi E, Cencini E, et al: Hairy cell leukemias with unmutated IGHV genes define the minor subset refractory to single-agent cladribine and with more aggressive behavior. *Blood* 114:4696–4702, 2009.

32. Forconi F: Hairy cell leukaemia: Biological and clinical overview from immunogenetic insights. *Hematol Oncol* 29:55–66, 2011.

33. Arons E, Kreitman RJ: Molecular variant of hairy cell leukemia with poor prognosis. *Leuk Lymphoma* 52 (Suppl 2):99–102, 2011.

34. Tiacci E, Trifonov V, Schiavoni G, et al: BRAF mutations in hairy-cell leukemia. *N Engl J Med* 364:2305–2315, 2011.

35. Xi L, Arons E, Navarro W, et al: Both variant and IGHV4–34–expressing hairy cell leukemia lack the BRAF V600E mutation. *Blood* 119:3330–3332, 2012.

36. Tiacci E, Schiavoni G, Martelli MP, et al: Constant activation of the RAF-MEK-ERK pathway as a diagnostic and therapeutic target in hairy cell leukemia. *Haematologica* 98:635–639, 2013.

37. Chung SS, Kim E, Park JH, et al: Hematopoietic stem cell origin of BRAFV600E mutations in hairy cell leukemia. *Sci Transl Med* 6:238ra71, 2014.

38. Cawley JC: The pathophysiology of the hairy cell. *Hematol Oncol Clin North Am* 20:1011–1021, 2006.

39. Foucar K, Falini B, Catovsky D, Stein H: Hairy cell leukaemia, in *WHO Classification of Tumours of Haematopoietic and Lymphoid Tissues*, 4 ed, edited by Swerdlow SH, Campo E, Harris NL, et al, pp 188–190. IARC, Lyon, France, 2008.

40. Schwarzmeier JD, Hilgarth M, Nguyen ST, et al: Inadequate production of hematopoietic growth factors in hairy cell leukemia: Up-regulation of interleukin 6 by recombinant IFN-alpha *in vitro*. *Cancer Res* 56:4679–4685, 1996.

41. Shehata M, Schwarzmeier JD, Hilgarth M, et al: TGF-beta1 induces bone marrow reticulin fibrosis in hairy cell leukemia. *J Clin Invest* 113:676–685, 2004.

42. Hoffman MA: Clinical presentations and complications of hairy cell leukemia. *Hematol Oncol Clin North Am* 20:1065–1073, 2006.

43. Frassoldati A, Lamparelli T, Federico M, et al: Hairy cell leukemia: A clinical review based on 725 cases of the Italian Cooperative Group (ICGHCL). Italian Cooperative Group for Hairy Cell Leukemia. *Leuk Lymphoma* 13:307–316, 1994.

44. Lembersky BC, Golomb HM: Hairy cell leukemia: Clinical features and therapeutic advances. *Cancer Metastasis Rev* 6:283–300, 1987.

45. Morrison V: Infections in patients with leukemia and lymphoma. *Cancer Treat Res* 161:319–349, 2014.

46. Seymour JF, Kurzrock R, Freireich EJ, et al: 2-chlorodeoxyadenosine induces durable remissions and prolonged suppression of CD4+ lymphocyte counts in patients with hairy cell leukemia. *Blood* 83:2906–2911, 1994.

47. Tadmor T: Purine analog toxicity in patients with hairy cell leukemia. *Leuk Lymphoma* 52 (Suppl 2):38–42, 2011.

48. Herold CJ, Wittich GR, Schwarzinger I, et al: Skeletal involvement in hairy cell leukemia. *Skeletal Radiol* 17:171–175, 1988.

49. Westbrook CA, Golde DW: Autoimmune disease in hairy-cell leukaemia: Clinical syndromes and treatment. *Br J Haematol* 61:349–356, 1985.

50. Tadmor T, Polliack A: Unusual clinical manifestations, rare sites of involvement, and the association of other disorders with hairy cell leukemia. *Leuk Lymphoma* 52 (Suppl 2):57–61, 2011.

51. Anderson LA, Engels EA: Autoimmune conditions and hairy cell leukemia: An exploratory case-control study. *J Hematol Oncol* 3:35, 2010.

52. Hauswirth AW, Skrabs C, Schutzinger C, et al: Autoimmune hemolytic anemias, Evans' syndromes, and pure red cell aplasia in non-Hodgkin lymphomas. *Leuk Lymphoma* 48:1139–1149, 2007.

53. Mainwaring CJ, Walewska R, Snowden J, et al: Fatal cold anti-i autoimmune haemolytic anaemia complicating hairy cell leukaemia. *Br J Haematol* 109:641–643, 2000.

54. Moullet I, Salles G, Dumontet C, et al: Sever immune thrombocytopenic purpura and haemolytic anaemia in a hairy-cell leukaemia patient. *Eur J Haematol* 54:127–129, 1995.

55. Ozkan A, Taskapilioglu O, Bican A, et al: Hairy cell leukemia presenting with Guillain-Barre syndrome. *Leuk Lymphoma* 48:1048–1049, 2007.

56. Jansen J, Hermans J: Splenectomy in hairy cell leukemia: A retrospective multicenter analysis. *Cancer* 47:2066–2076, 1981.

57. Sharpe RW, Bethel KJ: Hairy cell leukemia: Diagnostic pathology. *Hematol Oncol Clin North Am* 20:1023–1049, 2006.

58. Wang XJ, Kim A, Li S: Immunohistochemical analysis using a BRAF V600E mutation specific antibody is highly sensitive and specific for the diagnosis of hairy cell leukemia. *Int J Clin Exp Pathol* 7:4323–4328, 2014.

59. Seetharam A, Perrillo R, Gish R: Immunosuppression in patients with chronic hepatitis B. *Curr Hepatol Rep* 13:235–244, 2014.

60. Golomb HM: Hairy cell leukemia: Lessons learned in twenty-five years. *J Clin Oncol* 1:652–656, 1983.

61. Matsushita K, Margulies I, Onda M, et al: Soluble CD22 as a tumor marker for hairy cell leukemia. *Blood* 112:2272–2277, 2008.

62. Grever MR: How I treat hairy cell leukemia. *Blood* 115:21–28, 2010.

63. Habermann TM: Splenectomy, interferon, and treatments of historical interest in hairy cell leukemia. *Hematol Oncol Clin North Am* 20:1075–1086, 2006.

64. Piris MA, Foucar K, Mollejo M, et al: Splenic B-cell lymphoma/leukaemia, unclassifiable, in *WHO Classification of Tumours of Haematopoietic and Lymphoid Tissues*, ed 4, edited by Swerdlow SH, Campo E, Harris NL, Jaffe ES, Pileri SA, Stein H, Thiele J, Vardiman JW, pp 191–193. IARC, Lyon, France, 2008.

65. Kreitman RJ, Wilson W, Calvo KR, et al: Cladribine with immediate rituximab for the treatment of patients with variant hairy cell leukemia. *Clin Cancer Res* 19:6873–6881, 2013.

66. Robak T: Hairy-cell leukemia variant: Recent view on diagnosis, biology and treatment. *Cancer Treat Rev* 37:3–10, 2011.

67. Naik RR, Saven A: My treatment approach to hairy cell leukemia. *Mayo Clin Proc* 87:67–76, 2012.

68. Golomb HM: Fifty years of hairy cell leukemia treatments. *Leuk Lymphoma* 52 (Suppl 2):3–5, 2011.

69. Chadha P, Rademaker AW, Mendiratta P, et al: Treatment of hairy cell leukemia with 2-chlorodeoxyadenosine (2-CdA): Long-term follow-up of the Northwestern University experience. *Blood* 106:241–246, 2005.

70. Gidron A, Tallman MS: 2-CdA in the treatment of hairy cell leukemia: A review of long-term follow-up. *Leuk Lymphoma* 47:2301–2307, 2006.

71. Jones G, Parry-Jones N, Wilkins B, et al: Revised guidelines for the diagnosis and management of hairy cell leukaemia and hairy cell leukaemia variant. *Br J Haematol* 156:186–195, 2012.

72. Flinn IW, Kopecky KJ, Foucar MK, et al: Long-term follow-up of remission duration, mortality, and second malignancies in hairy cell leukemia patients treated with pentostatin. *Blood* 96:2981–2986, 2000.

73. Kreitman RJ, Tallman MS, Robak T, et al: Phase I trial of anti-CD22 recombinant immunotoxin moxetumomab pasudotox (CAT-8015 or HA22) in patients with hairy cell leukemia. *J Clin Oncol* 30:1822–1828, 2012.

74. Grever MR: Hairy cell: Young living longer but not cured. *Blood* 123:150–151, 2014.

75. Saven A, Burian C, Koziol JA, et al: Long-term follow-up of patients with hairy cell leukemia after cladribine treatment. *Blood* 92:1918–1926, 1998.

76. Maloisel F, Benboubker L, Gardembas M, et al: Long-term outcome with pentostatin treatment in hairy cell leukemia patients. A French retrospective study of 238 patients. *Leukemia* 17:45–51, 2003.

77. Burotto M, Stetler-Stevenson M, Arons E, et al: Bendamustine and rituximab in relapsed and refractory hairy cell leukemia. *Clin Cancer Res* 19:6313–6321, 2013.

78. Maurer H, Haas P, Wengenmayer T, et al: Successful vemurafenib salvage treatment in a patient with primary refractory hairy cell leukemia and pulmonary aspergillosis. *Ann Hematol* 93:1439–1440, 2014.

79. Cornet E, Delmer A, Feugier P, et al: Recommendations of the SFH (French Society of Haematology) for the diagnosis, treatment and follow-up of hairy cell leukaemia. *Ann Hematol* 93:1977–1983, 2014.

CHAPTER 94
LARGE GRANULAR LYMPHOCYTIC LEUKEMIA

Pierluigi Porcu and Aharon G. Freud

SUMMARY

Indolent clonal proliferations of large granular lymphocytes (LGLs) can arise from either T cells or natural killer (NK) cells. These diseases show overlapping clinical, morphologic, immunophenotypic, and genetic features. T-cell large granular lymphocytic leukemia (T-LGLL) and the related provisional 2008 World Health Organization entity, chronic lymphoproliferative disorders of NK cells (CLPD-NK), are similarly defined as persistent (>6 months) and clonal expansions in blood LGLs, often without a clearly identifiable cause. These patients are typically older, present with single lineage or multilineage cytopenias, and often have clinical and laboratory features of autoimmunity or immune dysfunction. Autoimmune neutropenia, thrombocytopenia, hemolytic anemia, and occasionally pure red cell aplasia may occur. Patients with T-LGLL frequently have elevated rheumatoid factor and clinical hallmarks of rheumatoid arthritis. The diagnosis of LGL leukemia requires a high degree of suspicion and careful examination of the blood film, because a significant fraction of patients do not have an absolute lymphocytosis, although the proportion of LGLs is usually increased. Most patients with T-LGLL and fewer with CLPD-NK have chronic neutropenia, and approximately half of T-LGLL patients have neutrophil counts less than 0.5×10^9/L. Anemia is observed in approximately half of patients with T-LGLL. Morbidity and mortality usually result from recurrent infections secondary to chronic neutropenia, transfusion-related iron overload, and less frequently from disease acceleration and transformation into a more aggressive T/NK leukemia or lymphoma. The treatment approach generally consists of immune modulatory or immune suppressive drugs, such as weekly oral methotrexate, cyclophosphamide, cyclosporine, prednisone, and alemtuzumab.

Acronyms and Abbreviations: AICD, activation-induced cell death; ANKL, aggressive NK cell leukemia; CD, cluster of differentiation; CDR3, complementarity determining region 3; CLPD-NK, chronic lymphoproliferative disorders of NK cells; CMV, cytomegalovirus; CTL, cytotoxic T lymphocyte; EBV, Epstein-Barr virus; FS, Felty syndrome; HLA, human leukocyte antigen; HSTCL, hepatosplenic T-cell lymphoma; HTLV, human T-cell leukemia virus; IL, interleukin; KIR, killer immunoglobulin-like receptor; LGL, large granular lymphocyte; LGLL, large granular lymphocytic leukemia; NK, natural killer cell; NK-LGL, natural killer cell–large granular lymphocyte; PDGF, platelet-derived growth factor; PI3K, phosphatidylinositol 3′-kinase; RF, rheumatoid factor; STAT, signal transducer and activator of transcription; TCR, T-cell receptor; T-LGLL, T-cell large granular lymphocytic leukemia; WHO, World Health Organization.

DEFINITION AND HISTORY

Large granular lymphocytic leukemia (LGLL) was initially described in the 1970s,[1,2] and further characterized in 1985,[3] as a clonal disorder of cytotoxic cluster of differentiation (CD)8+ T-cells involving blood, marrow, liver, and spleen, and clinically manifesting as an indolent proliferation of large granular lymphocytes (LGLs). Normally LGLs comprise 10 to 15 percent of blood mononuclear cells and may be either surface CD3+ (T-cell) or surface CD3– (natural killer [NK] cell). The absolute number of LGLs in the blood of normal subjects is 0.2 to 0.4×10^9/L. According to the 2008 World Health Organization (WHO) Classification of Tumors of the Hematopoietic and Lymphoid Tissues, T-cell large granular lymphocytic leukemia (T-LGLL) is defined as a persistent (>6 months) and usually clonal expansion of surface CD3 (sCD3+) LGL without a clearly identifiable cause.[4] The corresponding NK cell type of LGLL (sCD3–, CD16+), referred to as chronic lymphoproliferative disorders of NK cells (CLPD-NK), was included as a provisional diagnosis in the 2008 WHO classification and is similarly defined.[5] LGLL represent 2 to 3 percent of mature lymphocytic leukemias.[4] CLPD-NK should be distinguished from the acute and often fulminant aggressive NK cell leukemia (ANKL),[6] which is associated with Epstein-Barr virus (EBV) infection of the neoplastic NK cells. In contrast to ANKL, both T-LGLL and CLPD-NK are clinically indolent and have a low risk of transformation into an aggressive malignancy. The main impact of LGLL on patients' lives, and the most common indication for therapy, derives from the occurrence and severity of single lineage or multilineage cytopenias and by the resultant infections and transfusion requirement.

ETIOLOGY AND PATHOGENESIS

The etiologies of T-LGLL and CLPD-NK are not definitively established. It has been postulated, based on the analysis of T-cell receptor (TCR) complementarity determining region 3 (CDR3) patterns and Vβ family usage, that chronic antigenic stimulation results in the proliferation and/or increased survival of LGLs. Moreover, leukemic T-LGL show characteristics of antigen-activated cytotoxic T lymphocytes (CTLs), suggesting that an initial step in T-LGLL could be an antigen-driven clonal expansion.[7-9] Clonal drift in the T-cell repertoire with a change in the dominant clone occurs in approximately one-third of cases during the course of the disease,[10] implying that a dynamic process of clonal expansion exists that may affect more than one T-cell family in the same patient. Early studies suggested a possible association with human T-cell leukemia viruses (HTLVs); however, most patients are not infected with this agent.[11] Some evidence implicates cytomegalovirus (CMV) as the inciting antigen in the rare CD4+ subset of LGLL, but its role in patients with the more typical CD8+ subtype of T-LGLL is not clear.[12]

In the absence of an exogenous antigenic drive, chronic immune dysregulation and aberrant cytokine production may lead to enhanced LGL survival and expansion and, therefore, contribute to the pathogenesis of LGLL. Patients with T-LGLL frequently have humoral immune abnormalities, including positive tests for rheumatoid factor (RF)—with or without clinical arthrosynovitis–antinuclear antibodies, antineutrophil cytoplasmic antibodies, polyclonal hypergammaglobulinemia, hypogammaglobulinemia, and circulating immune complexes (Table 94–1) .[13] The high incidence of autoimmunity in patients with LGLL and the fact that the autoimmune manifestations often precede the occurrence of LGL expansions suggest that sustained immune activation may contribute to the pathogenesis of LGLL. However, because the detection of asymptomatic expansions of LGL in the blood requires examination of a blood film or flow cytometry, this temporal association should be interpreted with caution.

TABLE 94–1. Clinical Features of T-Cell Large Granular Lymphocytic Leukemia

	Pandolfi[68] (1990)	Loughran[69] (1993)	Dhodapkar[70] (1994)	Semenzato[71] (1997)	Neben[72] (2003)	Bareau[48] (2010)
Number of patients	151	129	68	162	44	201
Median age	55	57	61	59	63	59
M/F	1.3	0.8	1	0.8	1.0	0.8
Symptomatic	72%	–	69%	–	73%	82%
Splenomegaly	50%	50%	19%	50%	35%	24%
Hepatomegaly	34%	23%	1%	32%	–	10%
Adenopathy	13%	1%	3%	13%	5%	6%
B symptoms	–	–	12%	–	–	7%
Infections	38%	39%	15%	56%	–	23%
Rheumatoid arthritis	12%	28%	26%	36%	20%	17%
Rheumatoid factor	–	57%	61%	43%	48%	41%
Antinuclear antibodies	–	38%	44%	38%	48%	48%
Autoimmune cytopenias	–	–	7%	9%	5%	7%
Lymphocytosis			29%			
LGL >4 × 10⁹/L	52%	52%	–	–	–	14%
LGL 1–4 × 10⁹/L	38%	40%	–	–	–	50%
LGL <1 × 10⁹/L	10%	8%	–	7%	–	36%
Neutropenia						
Moderate (<1.5 × 10⁹/L)	64%	84%	74%	–	52%	61%
Severe (0.5 × 10⁹/L)	7%	48%	40%	37%	41%	26%
Anemia						
Any severity	25%	49%	51%	26%	89%	24%
Severe (Hgb <8 g/dL)	37%	–	19%	–	36%	7%
Thrombocytopenia	9%	19%	20%	29%	36%	19%
LGL marrow infiltration	67%	88%	–	76%	83%	72%
Hypergammaglobulinemia	–	45%	5%	43%	–	35%
Monoclonal gammopathy	–	45%	8%	–	–	10%
Need for treatment	30%	73%	69%	33%	80%	44%
LGLL related death	14%	36%	8%	27%	–	7%

Hgb, hemoglobin; LGL, large granular lymphocyte; LGLL, large granular lymphocytic leukemia.

Modified with permission from Bareau B, Rey J, Hamidou M, et al: Analysis of a french cohort of patients with large granular lymphocyte leukemia: A report on 229 cases. *Haematologica* 95(9):1534–41, 2010.

Normal CTL homeostasis is maintained, in part, through activation-induced cell death (AICD). Leukemic T-LGL constitutively express high levels of Fas (CD95) and Fas ligand (CD178), yet are resistant to Fas-mediated death.[14] Some disease manifestations, such as neutropenia, are associated, at least in part, with circulating CD178 in these patients.[15] High levels of proinflammatory or prosurvival cytokines associated with sustained immune activation could account for at least part of the mechanism driving LGL leukemias.[16–19] Likewise, constitutive activation of survival signaling pathways could represent a central pathogenetic mechanism in LGLL. Evidence for the importance of signal transducer and activator of transcription (STAT)-3/Mcl-1, phosphatidylinositol 3′-kinase (PI3K)/AKT, and sphingolipid signaling leading to apoptotic resistance have all been demonstrated.[20–22]

Mutations in STAT3 were identified in approximately 40 percent of T-LGLL and in CLPD-NK, and STAT5b mutations have also been detected in T-LGLL.[23–26] Using a network modeling approach, it was also found that interleukin (IL)-15 and platelet-derived growth factor (PDGF) are the two key mediators controlling interactions amongst these survival pathways.[27] In a transgenic mouse model resulting in constitutive murine IL-15 production, there is clonal expansion of LGLs that show overlapping features with human LGLL diseases.[28,29]

Targeting of normal tissue by leukemic LGL may also play a role in disease pathogenesis. Lysis of endothelial cells resulting from activation of NK receptors via signaling partners DAP10 and DAP12 could explain development of pulmonary hypertension observed in some patients with LGL leukemia.[30]

HISTOLOGIC AND IMMUNOPHENOTYPIC FEATURES

The marrow biopsy in T-LGLL may be hypo-, normo-, or hypercellular, with often preserved trilineage hematopoiesis. There may be occasional nodules of reactive CD4+ and B lymphocytes as well as scattered LGL, which are better seen in the aspirate. The presence of interstitial and/or intrasinusoidal clusters of at least eight CD8+ and/or TIA-1+ LGLs or at least six granzyme B+ LGLs has been correlated with marrow involvement by LGLL.[31] Various superimposed findings may reflect secondary immune diseases such as granulocyte maturation arrest and absence of red cell precursors (red cell aplasia). T-LGL leukemia invariably affects the spleen, where the major findings are leukemic cell infiltration of the red pulp cords and sinuses, plasma cell hyperplasia, and prominent germinal centers (Fig. 94–1).[3,32] Hepatic sinusoids and portal areas are infiltrated by LGL. Lymph nodes usually are not involved but can have expanded paracortical areas containing plasma cells and LGLs.

T-LGLL and CLPD-NK share overlapping immunophenotypic features in that both often express the NK-associated markers CD16 and CD57. Aberrant expression of NKp46 (CD335), which is normally selectively expressed by NK cells, occurs in T-LGLL.[33] CD56, which is constitutively expressed by circulating NK cells in healthy individuals, may be downregulated in CLPD-NK, and its expression in T-LGLL may be associated with a less-favorable clinical course.[34] T-leukemic LGLs usually are CD3+, CD4–, CD8+, CD16+, CD56–, CD57+, and often human leukocyte antigen (HLA)-DR+. Less commonly, leukemic LGLs express CD4 with variable CD8 expression.[35] Leukemic T-LGL usually express the TCR αβ+ heterodimer, although cases with similar clinical features have been described that express the γδ TCR heterodimer.[36] In contrast to normal LGL of T-cell origin, leukemic LGL express significantly lower levels of CD5 and show abnormal killer immunoglobulin-like receptor (KIR) expression.[37] The neoplastic NK cells often demonstrate abnormal KIR expression with either complete absence of surface KIR or restricted KIR expression indicating outgrowth of a clonal population.[38]

CLINICAL AND LABORATORY FEATURES AT PRESENTATION

Table 94–1 summarizes the clinical features of T-LGLL, as reported in six large published series. Men and women are equally affected and median age at diagnosis is approximately 60 years. Only a minority of patients are less than 50 years old. Approximately one-third of patients with LGLL are asymptomatic at presentation and the diagnosis is made on an examination of the blood. The remainder of the patients typically present with symptoms related to neutropenia (80 percent), anemia (45 percent), or both. B symptoms are present only in 15 percent of patients. Physical examination reveals mild to moderate splenomegaly in 35 percent and hepatomegaly in up to 20 percent. Lymphadenopathy and skin involvement are rare. Pulmonary hypertension develops in occasional cases.[30] Rheumatoid arthritis is often a prominent feature of LGLL, sometimes resulting in a clinical picture that is difficult to distinguish from that of Felty syndrome (FS) (chronic arthritis, splenomegaly, and granulocytopenia in the background of longstanding seropositive rheumatoid arthritis) (Chaps. 56 and 65).[39] Clonal proliferations of LGL have been observed in patients with FS,[39] and it is likely that a significant subset of patients diagnosed with FS may in fact have T-LGLL. The distinction between FS and T-LGLL in patients with rheumatoid arthritis has generally been based on whether the LGL proliferation was monoclonal (LGLL) or polyclonal (FS). However, this distinction cannot always be made, and recent cases of FS with somatic STAT3 mutations

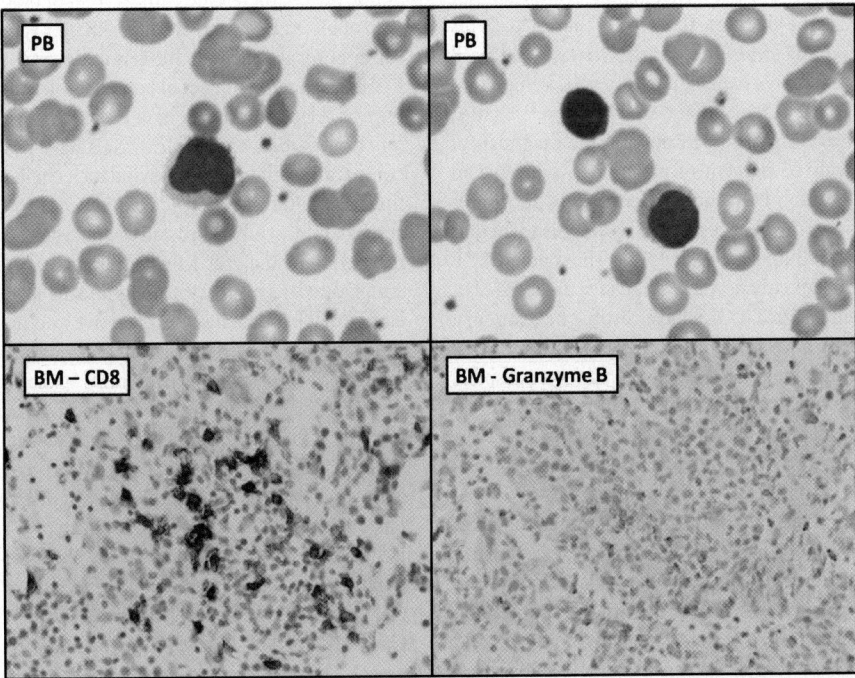

Figure 94–1. Morphology and immunohistochemical analysis of T-LGLL in peripheral blood and bone marrow. Upper panels show high powered images of circulating LGLs from a patient with T-LGLL (original magnification = 500X). Note for comparison the small lymphocyte next to the LGL in the right panel. LGLs are slightly larger than other lymphocytes, and they have more nuclear membrane irregularity, moderate amounts of pale blue cytoplasm, and fine cytoplasmic granules. The lower panels show foci of atypical clusters of CD8+ (left) and granzyme B+ (right) lymphocytes in the BM of a patient with T-LGLL (original magnification = 500X). The identification of atypical clusters of at least eight CD8+ and/or at least six granzyme B+ lymphocytes supports the diagnosis of LGLL in the appropriate clinical setting.[31] PB, peripheral blood; BM, bone marrow.

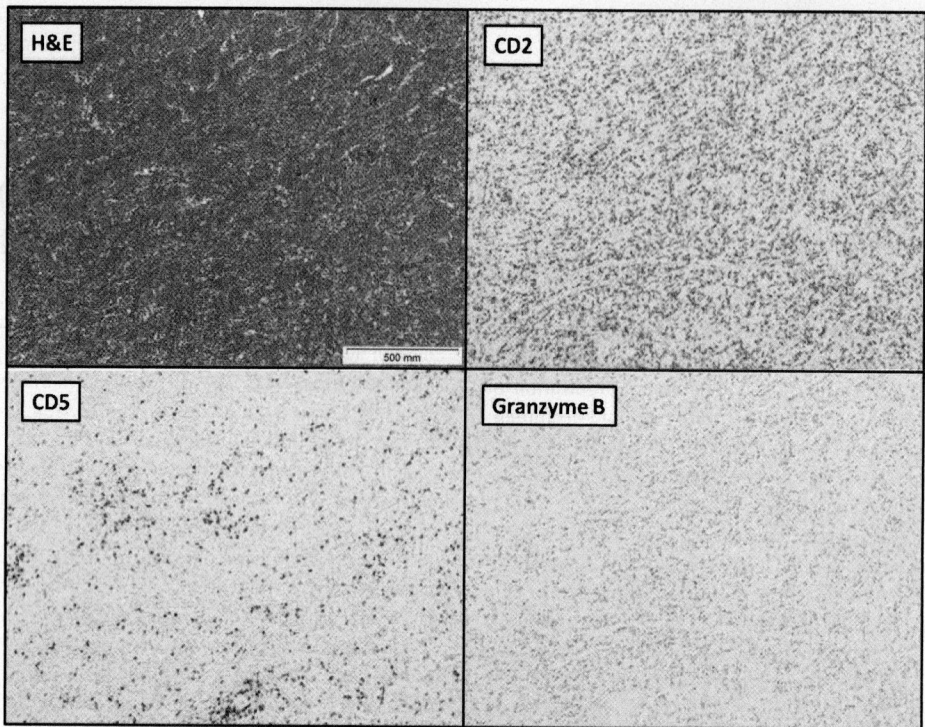

Figure 94–2. Morphology and immunohistochemical analysis of T-LGLL in the spleen. Panels demonstrate red pulp involvement in the spleen of a patient with T-LGLL (original magnification = 100X). In this example, lymphocytes are increased in the red pulp, which is expanded. Furthermore, by immunohistochemical analysis the lymphocytes show an aberrant immunophenotype with expression of CD2 and granzyme B but downregulation of the pan-T cell marker, CD5.

have been reported, suggesting that the two entities overlap also at the molecular level.[40]

The clinical presentation of CLPD-NK leukemia is very similar to that of T-LGLL[41] and must be distinguished from that of patients with aggressive NK-cell leukemia, who are younger, have systemic B symptoms, and typically have massive hepatosplenomegaly. Lymphadenopathy and gastrointestinal tract involvement are common.[42] Examination of the blood film is very important in making the diagnosis of T-LGLL because approximately 25 percent of patients do not have an increased total lymphocyte count.[13] LGL can be identified by morphology, although immunophenotyping is necessary to distinguish whether the LGLs are of T-cell or NK-cell lineage (Fig. 94–2). The median LGL count of patients with T-LGL leukemia is 4.2×10^9/L (see Table 94–1).

Most patients (70 percent) with T-LGLL have chronic neutropenia, and approximately 35 percent have neutrophil counts less than 0.5×10^9/L.[13] Recurrent bacterial infections of the upper and lower respiratory tract are observed in 30 percent of patients. Opportunistic infections, however, are uncommon. Anemia is observed in approximately 50 percent of cases of T-LGLL. Transfusion-dependent anemia occurs in approximately 20 percent of patients. More than one mechanism of anemia has been described, including autoimmune hemolytic anemia (Chap. 54), pure red cell aplasia (Chap. 36), and, rarely, aplastic anemia (Chap. 35).[3,43] LGLL is the most commonly associated disease in patients with pure red cell aplasia.[44] The role of LGL in the suppression of erythropoiesis in a patient with LGLL was established in vitro[45] and the role of T-cells is supported by response to antithymocyte globulin.[46] Thrombocytopenia, usually moderate, is seen in approximately 20 percent of patients. It may be immune-mediated (presence of antiplatelet antibodies) (Chap. 117), a result of splenic sequestration, and rarely secondary to amegakaryocytosis. Rare cases of amegakaryocytic thrombocytopenia or red cell aplasia have occurred and have responded to immunosuppressive.[3,47]

DIAGNOSTIC CRITERIA

While the characteristic clinical triad of blood cytopenias, clonal expansion of blood LGL, and elevated RF titer is now well recognized and useful in clinical practice, the definition of specific diagnostic criteria for LGLL has been a subject of considerable controversy. As a consequence, patient selection criteria have been inconsistent and inclusion rules for outcome studies and clinical trials have not been harmonized, making comparative interpretations of data a challenge. This fact likely explains the large differences in the frequency of specific clinical manifestations across LGLL studies and raises concerns about the validity of comparing outcome analyses from different centers. In the absence of molecular hallmarks, and with a significant level of overlap in clinical and laboratory features between reactive and neoplastic LGL proliferations, the diagnosis of LGLL hinges in part on the selection of the cut-off value for blood LGL levels. Historically, a diagnosis of LGLL required the detection of 2×10^9/L or greater blood LGL. However, there are patients with less than 2×10^9/L blood LGL that clearly have monoclonal CD8+ T-cell lymphoproliferations and display clinical and laboratory features, as well as outcomes, indistinguishable from LGLL. This finding has led to the adoption of less-restrictive criteria for the diagnosis of LGLL. Currently, the most commonly accepted blood LGL cutoff for a diagnosis of LGLL is greater than 0.5×10^9/L, with a TCR$\alpha\beta$+/CD3+/CD8+/CD57+ immunophenotype, lasting more than 6 months.[48] For CLPD-NK (CD3–/CD8+/CD16+ and/or CD16+/CD56+) the cutoff is greater than 0.75×10^9/L.

DIFFERENTIAL DIAGNOSIS

The diagnosis of LGLL should be considered in patients with chronic or cyclic neutropenia[49] and in patients with pure red cell aplasia or rheumatoid arthritis who have increased concentrations of LGL. HIV infection can lead to a mildly increased concentration of LGL cells; however, in these patients the LGLs are not monoclonal.[50] Reactive expansions in LGLs may also be seen in the settings of other viral infections such as CMV, postallogeneic stem cell transplantation, hyposplenism, and pharmacologic tyrosine kinase inhibition.[13,51,52] Molecular studies to identify a clonal *TCR* gene rearrangement may be helpful in distinguishing reactive from neoplastic LGL proliferations; however, reactive clonal T-cell LGL expansions can occur.[53,54] X-chromosome inactivation studies may be used to establish NK cell clonality in female patients.[55] The immunophenotypic features described above may be useful to screen for an aberrant LGL population; however, reactive TCRγδ+ T cells can show a similar pattern of surface expression including absence of CD4 with or without dim partial CD8 and expression of NK-associated markers such as CD56 expression.[56] The differential diagnosis also includes blood, marrow, and/or spleen involvement by other T-cell neoplasms. Often, the morphologic features in other T-cell neoplasms are more suggestive of malignancy compared to LGLL; however, this is not always the case. The clinical history is also important to consider. For example, both T-LGLL and hepatosplenic T-cell lymphoma (HSTCL) (Chap. 104) show a similar tissue distribution and with overlap in morphologic features. However, HSTCL is more common in young men, whereas T-LGLL typically affects older individuals without a predilection for gender. Moreover, whereas T-LGLL cells express TIA-1, perforin, and granzyme B cytolytic granules, HSTCL characteristically expresses TIA-1 but lacks perforin and granzyme B expression.[31,57,58] Consequently, close attention to these subtle details is important in evaluating a potential T-cell lymphoproliferative disorder.

● CLINICAL COURSE, THERAPY, AND PROGNOSIS

LGLL is typically a chronic, indolent, lymphoproliferative disorder with a 5-year survival close to 90 percent. Clinical symptoms and hematologic abnormalities are often only modestly to moderately severe, and many patients can remain infection-free and transfusion-independent for a long time. Therefore, treatment at diagnosis is not always indicated and, in the absence of curative strategies, the main goal of therapy for most patients is amelioration of the secondary clinical manifestations of the disease, rather than cytoreduction of leukemic LGL in the blood and marrow. For asymptomatic patients with modest neutropenia and anemia risk-versus-benefit analysis may not favor starting immediate treatment, and with no data supporting improved survival with early initiation of therapy, observation may be a better option. As in other chronic lymphoid neoplasms, therefore, it is important to define acceptable indications for therapy. These criteria typically include: (1) severe neutropenia (<0.5 × 10⁹/L) or moderate neutropenia (0.5 to 1.0 × 10⁹/L) with recurrent infections; (2) symptomatic or transfusion-dependent anemia; (3) moderately severe thrombocytopenia (<50 × 10⁹/L); and (4) associated autoimmune conditions requiring therapy.[59]

For patients who are symptomatic and exhibit one or more of the indications for treatment, the most commonly adopted approach is chronic immunosuppression with low-dose oral methotrexate (10 to 20 mg/week), cyclophosphamide (50 to 100 mg/day), or cyclosporine (variable daily doses, with or without monitoring of serum cyclosporine levels).[59,60] Response rates with each of these drugs are in the approximately 50 percent range, with time to response being from 2 to 12 weeks, and with acceptable and comparable safety profiles.[59] The optimal agent for initial therapy of LGLL is not currently known because these approaches have never been directly compared in a prospective fashion, and efficacy data come primarily from small, retrospective case series, often using different response criteria.[61–63] Prednisone (1 mg/kg)

may be briefly effective as a single agent or accelerate the initial response to one of the first-line immunosuppressive agent. Glucocorticoids, however, do not have long-term efficacy in LGLL and neutropenia generally recurs as soon as the medication is tapered. Because significant morbidity and mortality can result from chronic severe neutropenia[13] and transient responses to granulocyte- and granulocyte-monocyte colony-stimulating factors[64–66] have been reported, the judicious use of myeloid growth factors may be advantageous in patients before surgical procedures or during sepsis.

Methotrexate, cyclophosphamide, or cyclosporine, with or without prednisone, are usually effective in correcting the autoimmune cytopenias and the pure red cell aplasia associated with T-LGLL.[13] In cases of treatment failure with the three front-line therapies, the monoclonal antibody alemtuzumab (Campath-1H), which targets CD52 expressed on the surface of T-cell LGLL, has been effective in case reports and small case series, including patients with refractory red cell aplasia.[67]

Splenectomy has been reported to produce responses in up to 50 percent of patients with T-LGLL.[59] However, splenectomy should be considered only for patients with resistant disease who have persistent evidence of severe cytopenia or symptomatic splenomegaly.

Patients with chronic NK lymphocytosis usually do not require treatment.

REFERENCES

1. Brouet JC, Sasportes M, Flandrin G, et al: Chronic lymphocytic leukaemia of T-cell origin. Immunological and clinical evaluation in eleven patients. *Lancet* 2:890–893, 1975.
2. McKenna RW, Parkin J, Kersey JH, et al: Chronic lymphoproliferative disorder with unusual clinical, morphological, ultrastructural and membrane surface marker characteristics. *Am J Med* 62:588–596, 1977.
3. Loughran TP Jr, Kadin ME, Starkebaum G, et al: Leukemia of large granular lymphocytes: Association with clonal chromosomal abnormalities and autoimmune neutropenia, thrombocytopenia, and hemolytic anemia. *Ann Intern Med* 102:169–175, 1985.
4. Chan WC, Foucar K, Morice WG, Catovsky D: T-cell large granular lymphocytic leukaemia. in *WHO Classification of Tumours of Haematopoietic and Lymphoid Tissues, ed 4*, edited by SH Swerdlow, E Campo, NL Harris, ES Jaffe, SA Pileri, H Stein, J Thiele, JW Vardiman, pp 272–273. International Agency for Research on Cancer (IARC), Lyon, France, 2008.
5. Villamor NM, Morice WG., Chan WC, Foucar K: Chronic lymphoproliferative disorders of NK cells, in *WHO Classification of Tumours of Haematopoietic and Lymphoid Tissues, ed 4*, edited by SH Swerdlow, E Campo, NL Harris, ES Jaffe, SA Pileri, H Stein, J Thiele, JW Vardiman, pp 274–275. International Agency for Research on Cancer (IARC), Lyon, France, 2008.
6. JKC Chan, ES Jaffe, E Ralfkiaer, Y-H Ko: Aggressive NK-cell leukaemia, in *WHO Classification of Tumours of Haematopoietic and Lymphoid Tissues, ed 4*, edited by SH Swerdlow, E Campo, NL Harris, ES Jaffe, SA Pileri, H Stein, J Thiele, JW Vardiman, pp 276–277. International Agency for Research on Cancer (IARC), Lyon, France, 2008.
7. Wlodarski MW, Nearman Z, Jankowska A, et al: Phenotypic differences between healthy effector CTL and leukemic LGL cells support the notion of antigen-triggered clonal transformation in T-LGL leukemia. *J Leukoc Biol* 83:589–601, 2008.
8. Wlodarski MW, O'Keefe C, Howe EC, et al: Pathologic clonal cytotoxic T-cell responses: Nonrandom nature of the T-cell-receptor restriction in large granular lymphocyte leukemia. *Blood* 106:2769–2780, 2005.
9. Yang J, Epling-Burnette PK, Painter JS, et al: Antigen activation and impaired Fas-induced death-inducing signaling complex formation in T-large-granular lymphocyte leukemia. *Blood* 111:1610–1616, 2008.
10. Clemente MJ, Wlodarski MW, Makishima H, et al: Clonal drift demonstrates unexpected dynamics of the T-cell repertoire in T-large granular lymphocyte leukemia. *Blood* 118:4384–4393, 2011.
11. Duong YT, Jia H, Lust JA, et al: Short communication: Absence of evidence of HTLV-3 and HTLV-4 in patients with large granular lymphocyte (LGL) leukemia. *AIDS Res Hum Retroviruses* 24:1503–1505, 2008.
12. Rodriguez-Caballero A, Garcia-Montero AC, Barcena P, et al: Expanded cells in monoclonal TCR-alphabeta+/CD4+/NKa+/CD8-/+dim T-LGL lymphocytosis recognize hCMV antigens. *Blood* 112:4609–4616, 2008.
13. Lamy T, Loughran TP Jr: Clinical features of large granular lymphocyte leukemia. *Semin Hematol* 40:185–195, 2003.
14. Lamy T, Liu JH, Landowski TH, et al: Dysregulation of CD95/CD95 ligand-apoptotic pathway in CD3(+) large granular lymphocyte leukemia. *Blood* 92:4771–4777, 1998.
15. Liu JH, Wei S, Lamy T, et al: Chronic neutropenia mediated by Fas ligand. *Blood* 95:3219–3222, 2000.
16. Chen J, Petrus M, Bamford R, et al: Increased serum soluble IL-15ralpha levels in T-cell large granular lymphocyte leukemia. *Blood* 119:137–143, 2012.

17. Nearman ZP, Wlodarski M, Jankowska AM,: Immunogenetic factors determining the evolution of T-cell large granular lymphocyte leukaemia and associated cytopenias. *Br J Haematol* 136:237–248, 2007.

18. Zambello R, Facco M, Trentin L, et al: Interleukin-15 triggers the proliferation and cytotoxicity of granular lymphocytes in patients with lymphoproliferative disease of granular lymphocytes. *Blood* 89:201–211, 1997.

19. Zambello R, Trentin L, Cassatella MA, et al: IL-12 is involved in the activation of CD3+ granular lymphocytes in patients with lymphoproliferative disease of granular lymphocytes. *Br J Haematol* 92:308–314, 1996.

20. Epling-Burnette PK, Liu JH, Catlett-Falcone R, et al: Inhibition of STAT3 signaling leads to apoptosis of leukemic large granular lymphocytes and decreased MCL-1 expression. *J Clin Invest* 107:351–362, 2001.

21. Schade AE, Powers JJ, Wlodarski MW, Maciejewski JP: Phosphatidylinositol-3-phosphate kinase pathway activation protects leukemic large granular lymphocytes from undergoing homeostatic apoptosis. *Blood* 107:4834–4840, 2006.

22. Shah MV, Zhang R, Irby R, et al: Molecular profiling of LGL leukemia reveals role of sphingolipid signaling in survival of cytotoxic lymphocytes. *Blood* 112:770–781, 2008.

23. Jerez A, Clemente MJ, Makishima H, et al: Stat3 mutations unify the pathogenesis of chronic lymphoproliferative disorders of NK cells and T-cell large granular lymphocyte leukemia. *Blood* 120:3048–3057, 2012.

24. Koskela HL, Eldfors S, Ellonen P, et al: Somatic STAT3 mutations in large granular lymphocytic leukemia. *N Engl J Med* 366:1905–1913, 2012.

25. Rajala HL, Eldfors S, Kuusanmaki H, et al: Discovery of somatic STAT5b mutations in large granular lymphocytic leukemia. *Blood* 121:4541–4550, 2013.

26. Teramo A, Gattazzo C, Passeri F, et al: Intrinsic and extrinsic mechanisms contribute to maintain the JAK/STAT pathway aberrantly activated in T-type large granular lymphocyte leukemia. *Blood* 2013;121:3843–3854, S3841.

27. Zhang R, Shah MV, Yang J, et al: Network model of survival signaling in large granular lymphocyte leukemia. *Proc Natl Acad Sci U S A* 105:16308–16313, 2008.

28. Fehniger TA, Suzuki K, Ponnappan A, et al: Fatal leukemia in interleukin 15 transgenic mice follows early expansions in natural killer and memory phenotype CD8+ t cells. *J Exp Med* 193:219–231, 2001.

29. Mishra A, Liu S, Sams GH, et al: Aberrant overexpression of IL-15 initiates large granular lymphocyte leukemia through chromosomal instability and DNA hypermethylation. *Cancer Cell* 22:645–655, 2012.

30. Chen X, Bai F, Sokol L, et al: A critical role for DAP10 and DAP12 in CD8+ T cell-mediated tissue damage in large granular lymphocyte leukemia. *Blood* 113:3226–3234, 2009.

31. Morice WG, Kurtin PJ, Tefferi A, Hanson CA: Distinct bone marrow findings in T-cell granular lymphocytic leukemia revealed by paraffin section immunoperoxidase stains for CD8, TIA-1, and granzyme B. *Blood* 99:268–274, 2002.

32. Agnarsson BA, Loughran TP Jr, Starkebaum G, Kadin ME: The pathology of large granular lymphocyte leukemia. *Hum Pathol* 20:643–651, 1989.

33. Freud AG, Zhao S, Wei S, et al: Expression of the activating receptor, NKp46 (CD335), in human natural killer and T-cell neoplasia. *Am J Clin Pathol* 140:853–866, 2013.

34. Gentile TC, Uner AH, Hutchison RE, et al: CD3+, CD56+ aggressive variant of large granular lymphocyte leukemia. *Blood* 84:2315–2321, 1994.

35. Lima M, Almeida J, Dos Anjos Teixeira M, et al: TCRalphabeta+/CD4+ large granular lymphocytosis: A new clonal T-cell lymphoproliferative disorder. *Am J Pathol* 163:763–771, 2003.

36. Bourgault-Rouxel AS, Loughran TP Jr, Zambello R, et al: Clinical spectrum of gamma-delta+ T cell LGL leukemia: Analysis of 20 cases. *Leuk Res* 32:45–48, 2008.

37. Lundell R, Hartung L, Hill S, et al: T-cell large granular lymphocyte leukemias have multiple phenotypic abnormalities involving pan-T-cell antigens and receptors for MHC molecules. *Am J Clin Pathol* 124:937–946, 2005.

38. Morice WG, Kurtin PJ, Leibson PJ, et al: Demonstration of aberrant T-cell and natural killer-cell antigen expression in all cases of granular lymphocytic leukaemia. *Br J Haematol* 120:1026–1036, 2003.

39. Loughran TP Jr, Starkebaum G, Kidd P, Neiman P: Clonal proliferation of large granular lymphocytes in rheumatoid arthritis. *Arthritis Rheum* 31:31–36, 1988.

40. Schrenk KG, Krokowski M, Feller AC, et al: Clonal T-LGL population mimicking leukemia in Felty's syndrome—Part of a continuous spectrum of T-LGL proliferations? *Ann Hematol* 92:985–987, 2013.

41. Poullot E, Zambello R, Leblanc F, et al: Chronic natural killer lymphoproliferative disorders: Characteristics of an international cohort of 70 patients. *Ann Oncol* 25:2030–2035, 2014.

42. Cheung MM, Chan JK, Wong KF: Natural killer cell neoplasms: A distinctive group of highly aggressive lymphomas/leukemias. *Semin Hematol* 40:221–232, 2003.

43. Sokol L, Loughran TP Jr: Large granular lymphocyte leukemia. *Oncologist* 11:263–273, 2006.

44. Lacy MQ, Kurtin PJ, Tefferi A: Pure red cell aplasia: Association with large granular lymphocyte leukemia and the prognostic value of cytogenetic abnormalities. *Blood* 87:3000–3006, 1996.

45. Abkowitz JL, Kadin ME, Powell JS, Adamson JW: Pure red cell aplasia: Lymphocyte inhibition of erythropoiesis. *Br J Haematol* 63:59–67, 1986.

46. Abkowitz JL, Powell JS, Nakamura JM, et al: Pure red cell aplasia: Response to therapy with anti-thymocyte globulin. *Am J Hematol* 23:363–371, 1986.

47. Lai DW, Loughran TP Jr, Maciejewski JP, et al: Acquired amegakaryocytic thrombocytopenia and pure red cell aplasia associated with an occult large granular lymphocyte leukemia. *Leuk Res* 32:823–827, 2008.

48. Bareau B, Rey J, Hamidou M, et al: Analysis of a French cohort of patients with large granular lymphocyte leukemia: A report on 229 cases. *Haematologica* 95:1534–1541, 2010.

49. Loughran TP Jr, Hammond WP: Adult-onset cyclic neutropenia is a benign neoplasm associated with clonal proliferation of large granular lymphocytes. *J Exp Med* 164:2089–2094, 1986.

50. Zambello R, Trentin L, Agostini C, et al: Persistent polyclonal lymphocytosis in human immunodeficiency virus-1-infected patients. *Blood* 81:3015–3021, 1993.

51. Khan S, Myers K: Persistence of natural killer (NK) cell lymphocytosis with hyposplenism without development of leukaemia. *BMC Clin Pathol* 5:8, 2005.

52. Qiu ZY, Xu W, Li JY: Large granular lymphocytosis during dasatinib therapy. *Cancer Biol Ther* 15:247–255, 2014.

53. Rossi D, Franceschetti S, Capello D, et al: Transient monoclonal expansion of CD8+/CD57+ T-cell large granular lymphocytes after primary cytomegalovirus infection. *Am J Hematol* 82:1103–1105, 2007.

54. Wolniak KL, Goolsby CL, Chen YH, et al: Expansion of a clonal CD8+CD57+ large granular lymphocyte population after autologous stem cell transplant in multiple myeloma. *Am J Clin Pathol* 139:231–241, 2013.

55. Boudewijns M, van Dongen JJ, Langerak AW: The human androgen receptor X-chromosome inactivation assay for clonality diagnostics of natural killer cell proliferations. *J Mol Diagn* 9:337–344, 2007.

56. Inghirami G, Zhu BY, Chess L, Knowles DM: Flow cytometric and immunohistochemical characterization of the gamma/delta T-lymphocyte population in normal human lymphoid tissue and peripheral blood. *Am J Pathol* 136:357–367, 1990.

57. Belhadj K, Reyes F, Farcet JP, et al: Hepatosplenic gammadelta T-cell lymphoma is a rare clinicopathologic entity with poor outcome: Report on a series of 21 patients. *Blood* 102:4261–4269, 2003.

58. Lu CL, Tang Y, Yang QP, et al: Hepatosplenic T-cell lymphoma: Clinicopathologic, immunophenotypic, and molecular characterization of 17 Chinese cases. *Hum Pathol* 42:1965–1978, 2011.

59. Lamy T, Loughran TP Jr: How I treat LGL leukemia. *Blood* 117:2764–2774, 2011.

60. Dearden CE, Johnson R, Pettengell R, Devcreux S, et al: British Committee for Standards in Haematology: Guidelines for the management of mature T-cell and NK-cell neoplasms (excluding cutaneous T-cell lymphoma). *Br J Haematol* 153:451–485, 2011.

61. Loughran TP Jr, Kidd PG, Starkebaum G: Treatment of large granular lymphocyte leukemia with oral low-dose methotrexate. *Blood* 84:2164–2170, 1994.

62. Osuji N, Matutes E, Tjonnfjord G, et al: T-cell large granular lymphocyte leukemia: A report on the treatment of 29 patients and a review of the literature. *Cancer* 107:570–578, 2006.

63. Sood R, Stewart CC, Aplan PD, et al: Neutropenia associated with T-cell large granular lymphocyte leukemia: Long-term response to cyclosporine therapy despite persistence of abnormal cells. *Blood* 91:3372–3378, 1998.

64. Lamy T, LePrise PY, Amiot L, et al: Response to granulocyte-macrophage colony-stimulating factor (GM-CSF) but not to g-csf in a case of agranulocytosis associated with large granular lymphocyte (LGL) leukemia. *Blood* 85:3352–3353, 1995.

65. Kaneko Y, Ogawa Y, Hirata Y, et al: Agranulocytosis associated with granular lymphocyte leukaemia: Improvement of peripheral blood granulocyte count with human recombinant granulocyte colony-stimulating factor (G-CSF). *Br J Haematol* 74:121–122, 1990.

66. Thomssen C, Nissen C, Gratwohl A, et al: Agranulocytosis associated with t-gamma-lymphocytosis: No improvement of peripheral blood granulocyte count with human-recombinant granulocyte-macrophage colony-stimulating factor (GM-CSF). *Br J Haematol* 71:157–158, 1989.

67. Ru X, Liebman HA: Successful treatment of refractory pure red cell aplasia associated with lymphoproliferative disorders with the anti-CD52 monoclonal antibody alemtuzumab (Campath-1H). *Br J Haematol* 123:278–281, 2003.

68. Pandolfi F, Loughran TP Jr, Starkebaum G, et al: Clinical course and prognosis of the lymphoproliferative disease of granular lymphocytes. A multicenter study. *Cancer* 65:341–348, 1990.

69. Loughran TP Jr: Clonal diseases of large granular lymphocytes. *Blood* 82:1–14, 1993.

70. Dhodapkar MV, Li CY, Lust JA, et al: Clinical spectrum of clonal proliferations of T-large granular lymphocytes: A T-cell clonopathy of undetermined significance? *Blood* 84:1620–1627, 1994.

71. Semenzato G, Zambello R, Starkebaum G, et al: The lymphoproliferative disease of granular lymphocytes: updated criteria for diagnosis. *Blood* 89:256–260, 1997.

72. Neben MA, Morice WG, Tefferi A: Clinical features in T-cell vs. natural killer-cell variants of large granular lymphocyte leukemia. *Eur J Haematol* 71:263–265, 2003.

CHAPTER 95

GENERAL CONSIDERATIONS FOR LYMPHOMAS: EPIDEMIOLOGY, ETIOLOGY, HETEROGENEITY, AND PRIMARY EXTRANODAL DISEASE

Oliver W. Press and Marshall A. Lichtman*

SUMMARY

Lymphomas are a heterogeneous group of malignancies that originate from neoplastic transformation of lymphocytes that have undergone mutations that confer growth and survival advantages compared to their normal cellular counterparts. These neoplasms usually originate in lymph nodes or lymphatic tissue in other sites (extranodal lymphoma), and can be localized or widespread at the time of diagnosis. Men are affected more frequently than women and the risk of acquisition of most lymphomas increases logarithmically with age. Classification systems have considered the likely lymphoid progenitor that corresponds to the phenotype (immunotype) and genotype of the malignant cells in the transformed clone. The specific pathologic diagnosis is usually established by the appearance of the histopathology in tissue sections, the immunophenotypic profile of CD antigens expressed on affected lymphocytes, specific cytogenetic findings, especially

Acronyms and Abbreviations: ALCL, anaplastic large cell lymphoma; *ALK,* ALCL tyrosine kinase gene; ATLL, adult T-cell leukemia/lymphoma; CBC, complete blood count; CRu, complete remission unconfirmed; CT, computed tomography; DLBCL, diffuse large B-cell lymphoma; EBV, Epstein-Barr virus; FDG,2-fluorodeoxyglucose; HHV-8, human herpesvirus-8; HL, Hodgkin lymphoma; HTLV-1, human T-cell leukemia/lymphoma virus-1; iFISH, interphase fluorescence *in situ* hybridization; Ig, immunoglobulin; IWG, International Working Group; MALT, mucosa-associated lymphatic tissue; NCCN, National Cancer Center Network; NHL, non-Hodgkin lymphoma; NK, natural killer; PET, positron emission tomography; R-CHOP, rituximab-cyclophosphamide, hydroxydoxorubicin, vincristine (Oncovin), and prednisone; REAL, revised European-American classification of lymphoid neoplasm; RNA-seq, ribonucleic acid sequencing; SEER, Surveillance, Epidemiology, and End Results; TCE, trichloroethylene; *TCR,* T-cell receptor; WHO, World Health Organization.

*Kenneth A. Foon was a coauthor of this chapter for the 8th edition of *Williams Hematology* and significant portions of that chapter have been retained.

translocations (e.g., t[11;14]), immunocytochemical markers (e.g., cyclin D_1), and the specific tissue location (e.g., mucosa-associated lymphatic tissue). Although most lymphomas arise without an evident cause, *human T-cell leukemia/lymphoma virus I* (HTLV-1), *Epstein-Barr virus, hepatitis C virus, and human herpes virus-8* infections, as well as infections with the bacteria *Helicobacter pylori* and, perhaps, *Chlamydophila psittaci,* either are established as causal (e.g., HTLV-1) or have very strong associations with lymphoma incidence *(hepatitis C virus),* suggesting their role in causation. *HIV* is permissive by inducing severe immunodeficiency and setting the stage for an *Epstein-Barr virus*–induced or *human herpes virus-8*–induced lymphoma. These relationships may vary by geographic area. Several occupational and industrial exposures are suspected of being related to lymphoma incidence, for example, organochlorines, phenoxyacid herbicides, and others, but these associations have not been established with scientific certainty. At present, the estimated attributable risk of lymphoma from all suspected exogenous factors together is relatively small in proportion to the number of annual cases, leaving most cases without an apparent cause. There are wide discrepancies in the incidence of specific lymphoma subtypes in different geographic regions (e.g., follicular lymphoma is very common in the United States and very uncommon in East Asia). Primary extranodal lymphoma may involve virtually any tissue or organ. Depending on the site, important functional abnormalities may ensue (e.g., bilateral adrenal gland replacement and hypoadrenocorticism, hypothalamic–pituitary involvement and diabetes insipidus). Multidrug chemotherapy combinations in conjunction with lymphocyte-specific monoclonal antibody therapy form the foundation of current treatment paradigms for most lymphomas, though radiotherapy and surgical excision continue to play limited roles in selected circumstances, depending on the site and histopathology.

● DEFINITION AND HISTORY

Lymphomas are a heterogeneous group of malignancies of B cells, T cells, and, rarely, natural killer (NK) cells that usually originate in the lymph nodes, but may affect any organ of the body. Lymphoma previously was referred to as *lymphosarcoma* and its two major subtypes designated *reticulum cell sarcoma* and *giant follicular lymphoma* (Brill-Symmers disease).[1-3] In 1966, Rappaport[4] published a classification system based on the patterns of lymphoma cell growth, size, and shape that attempted to correlate morphology with clinical outcome. The classification proved to have some inaccuracies, such as the term *histiocytic lymphoma* to describe lymphoid tumors of large transformed lymphocytes that were not derived from the monocyte-macrophage lineage. Nonetheless, the Rappaport classification was an important milestone and became the most widely used classification in the United States. In 1974, Lukes and Collins proposed another classification system, which incorporated morphology with immunologic subtype, that was endorsed by the Committee on Nomenclature.[4] Another scheme, the Kiel classification, introduced by Karl Lennert and colleagues, had been more popular in Europe.[5] By the 1970s at least six classifications of lymphoma had been published, and the major ones included two in the United States, one in continental Europe, and one in the United Kingdom. There was no success in reaching a consensus classification that could be used worldwide. A National Cancer Institute study showed that there was poor reproducibility among different pathologists looking at the same slides and trying to classify the case of lymphoma using any existing scheme. In 1982, a Working Formulation sponsored by the National

Cancer Institute attempted to reconcile the large number of competing classifications then in use.[6] The Working Formulation was clinically useful and gained wide popularity. It divided the specific subtypes among high-grade, intermediate-grade, and low-grade lymphomas, focusing in part on the expected rate of progression, and not just on the phenotype of the case in question. With advances in our understanding of the immune system and lymphocyte progenitor developmental sequences, and the availability of monoclonal antibodies for subtyping lymphoid cells and lymphocyte gene profiling, a new classification schema became possible based on cell type, tissue of origin, immunophenotype, and genotype.

In 1994, a revised European-American classification of lymphoid neoplasms (the REAL classification) was proposed by the International Lymphoma Study Group (Chaps. 90 and 96).[7] This group distinguished three major categories of lymphoid malignancies, which included B-cell, T-cell, and Hodgkin lymphoma. Lymphomas were defined by morphologic, immunologic, and genetic techniques. Many of the lymphomas were associated with distinct clinical presentations, and cases that did not fit into defined entities were left unclassified. Further subclassification[8] divided each of the B-cell and T-cell lineages into (1) indolent lymphomas (low risk of rapid progression), (2) aggressive lymphomas (intermediate risk of progression), and (3) very aggressive lymphomas (high risk of progression). In 1995, a collaborative project of the European Association for Haematopathology and the Society for Hematopathology began to revise the REAL classification. In 2001, they published the World Health Organization (WHO) *Classification of Tumors of the Haematopoietic and Lymphoid Tissues* that is used in this chapter and represents the current worldwide consensus classification of malignancies that arise in a lymphocyte. In 2008, the WHO updated this classification (Chaps. 90 and 96).[9,10]

Emerging concepts in the staging, therapy, and response evaluation of lymphomas evolved in parallel with the changing nomenclature. Initial efforts to define the extent of disease involvement were undertaken primarily for Hodgkin lymphoma (HL) and ultimately led to the Ann Arbor classification,[11] which subdivided patients into four stages, each subclassified into A and B groups based on the presence of fevers greater than 38.3°C, weight loss, and drenching night sweats. The Ann Arbor system proved useful for decades and was subsequently applied also to non-Hodgkin lymphomas (NHLs). The Cotswold modification of the Ann Arbor Classification[12] first formally incorporated computed tomography (CT) into clinical staging paradigms and introduced the terms "X" for bulky disease and "complete remission unconfirmed" (CRu) to describe patients with a residual mass after treatment that most likely represented fibrous scar tissue. The sensitivity and accuracy of CT imaging of the abdomen rendered the "staging laparotomy" for assessment of the abdomen obsolete. The first universally accepted

response criteria for NHL were initially published in 1999 by the National Cancer Institute Working Group[13] and later revised in 2007 to incorporate positron emission tomography (PET), marrow immunohistochemistry and flow cytometry for response assessment.[14] PET/CT imaging rendered the CRu designation obsolete in 2007, because residual radiographic abnormalities could be accurately determined to be either residual active lymphoma or posttreatment fibrosis, based on the metabolic activity of the lesions. These criteria were critically reviewed and analyzed by working groups at the 11th and 12th International Conferences on Malignant Lymphoma in Lugano, Switzerland, in 2011 and 2013 and at the 4th International Workshops on Positron Emission Tomography in Lymphoma in Menton, France in 2012.[15,16] These international workshops were attended by leading hematologists, oncologists, radiation oncologists, pathologists, radiologists, and nuclear medicine physicians, representing all major lymphoma clinical trials groups and cancer centers in North America, Europe, Japan, and Australasia. Their deliberations culminated in the publication in 2014 of improved criteria for the initial evaluation, staging and response assessment for both HL and NHL[17] that are relevant for community physicians, investigator-led trials, cooperative groups, and registration trials. These new rules, known as the "Lugano Classification," depart substantially from older staging and evaluation systems as detailed later in this chapter.

● EPIDEMIOLOGY

Approximately 79,990 new cases of lymphoma were projected to be diagnosed and approximately 20,170 persons in the United States were expected to die of this disease in 2014.[18] These numbers represent 4.8 percent of the annual incidence of all cancers and 3.4 percent of annual cancer-related deaths. The most recent age-adjusted incidence rates per 100,000 population provided by Surveillance, Epidemiology, and End Results (SEER) Program of the United States National Cancer Institute are: 24.9 for white males, 17.4 for black males, 17.2 for white females, and 11.9 for black females.[19] The increased risk for men is similar to that found in other countries, although the incidence of NHL in the United States is approximately threefold that of several underdeveloped countries and twofold that of several comparable industrialized countries.[20] The risk of developing lymphoma is less in the United States among persons of African descent in comparison to those of European descent. An exponential increase in incidence in NHL among men and women occurs with increasing age (Fig.95–1). There are some notable exceptions to this overall trend, however, with lymphoblastic lymphoma occurring most commonly in children, Burkitt lymphoma in the 20- to 64-year-old age group, and primary mediastinal B-cell lymphoma developing at a median age of 35 years.[20]

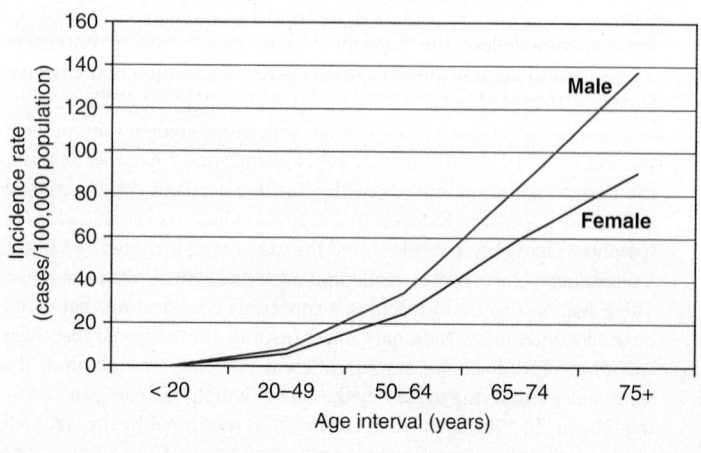

Figure 95–1. The graph depicts the rate of increase with age in non-Hodgkin lymphoma incidence among American males and females. This pattern is true for Americans of European or of African descent. *(Data from the Surveillance, Epidemiology, and End Results (SEER) Program (www.seer.cancer.gov) Research Data (1973-2011), National Cancer Institute, DCCPS, Surveillance Research Program, Surveillance Systems Branch, released April 2014, based on the November 2013 submission.; 2014.)*

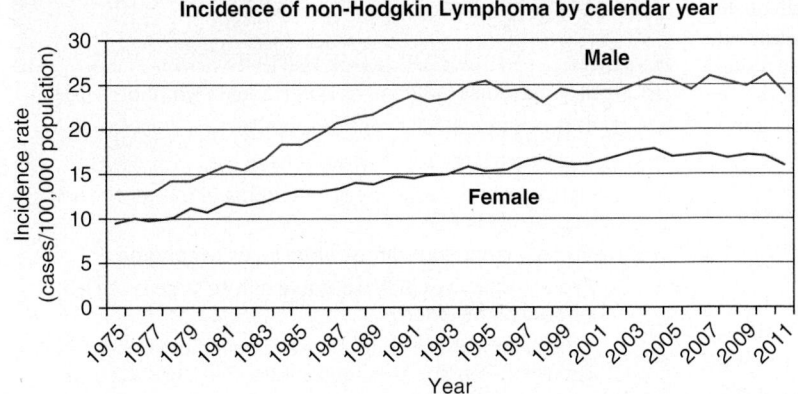

Incidence of non-Hodgkin Lymphoma by calendar year

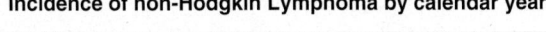

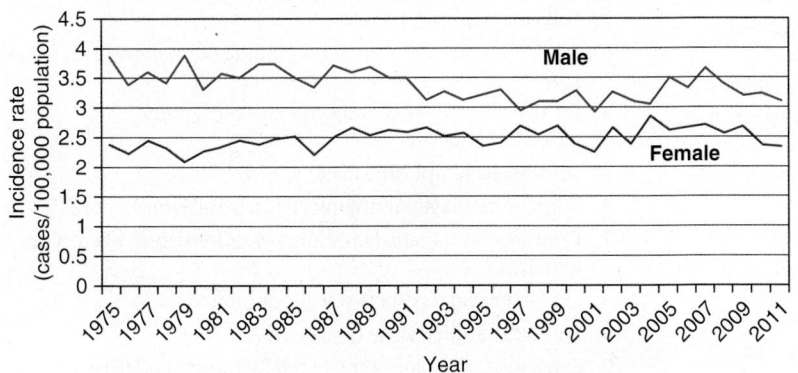

Incidence of non-Hodgkin Lymphoma by calendar year

Figure 95–2. Incidence of non-Hodgkin and Hodgkin lymphoma by calendar year. The incidence of non-Hodgkin lymphoma approximately doubled from the early 1970s to the mid-1990s in the United States and in other industrialized countries that tracked incidence of specific cancers. No satisfactory explanation has been uncovered for this change. The "epidemic" of lymphoma ended in the mid-1990s and the incidence curves have been "flat" since 1996. The increase in incidence was present in Americans of European and African descent and among men and women. In stark contrast and serving as an internal control, the incidence of Hodgkin lymphoma is essentially unchanged over that period of time. *(Data from the Surveillance, Epidemiology, and End Results (SEER) Program (www.seer.cancer.gov) Research Data (1973-2011), National Cancer Institute, DCCPS, Surveillance Research Program, Surveillance Systems Branch, released April 2014, based on the November 2013 submission.; 2014.)*

Follicular lymphoma represents approximately 25 percent of NHL cases in the United States, but is very uncommon in many developing countries and in Asia, especially in Japan and China.[21,22] The United States has a higher incidence of all lymphomas than does Japan, whereas the incidence of extranodal lymphoma is higher in Japan.[21,22] Burkitt lymphoma occurs most frequently in sub-Saharan Africa, whereas T-cell leukemia/lymphoma is most common in southwest Japan, the southeastern United States, northeastern South America, and the Caribbean basin.

The incidence of NHL increased dramatically in the last half of the 20th century in Europe, Asia, and in the United States.[20–22] From 1973 to 1990, inclusive, the increase in the United States was slightly more than 80 percent, or approximately 4 to 5 percent per year (Fig. 95–2). The increase in incidence started after World War II, but the best data in the United States were acquired after 1972. The increase affected men and women, all age groups except children, and most histologic types examined, though the greatest increase was in diffuse large B-cell lymphoma (DLBCL). The increased incidence per year reached a plateau in the early 1990s, except among women and older men where the incidence continued to rise.[21] Hardell has hypothesized that new chemicals synthesized during and after World War II accounted for increased incidence trends, with subsequent improvements in safety gear and regulatory restrictions resulting in stabilization in the last decade.[23] HIV was not prevalent in the human population when the increase first became apparent, although in later years HIV-related lymphoma may have played a part in increasing incidence rates. Orbital adnexal lymphoma and mantle cell lymphoma are exceptions to the recent plateau, with each still increasing at approximately 6 percent a year.[24,25]

Several occupations and industries and several potentially hazardous exposures, such as pesticides, herbicides, dyes, engine exhausts, and solvents, have been found in one study or another to be more frequent in lymphoma patients than "matched" healthy comparison groups.[21,26,27] The results often have been inconsistent from study to study. Expert opinion indicates that no workplace exposure has been conclusively linked to lymphoma,[28] although farming or living in a community in which farming is prevalent has been a frequent association with higher lymphoma incidence.[21,26,27]

Many publications have reported a slightly increased familial predisposition to the development of NHL, with an odds ratio of 1.5 in first-degree relatives of patients with NHL in a pooled analysis of 17 case control studies.[20,29–31] Nonsyndromic familial lymphoma refers to apparently healthy family members, unlike syndromic familial lymphoma in which immunodeficiency syndromes are the predisposing phenotype (e.g., Wiskott-Aldrich syndrome; see "Immunosuppression" below). The familial cases occur in different generations and among enough family members to strongly suggest that a predisposing unidentified gene results in an incidence above that in the population at large. Li-Fraumeni syndrome is such an example, involving germline mutations in *p53*. Alternatively, it is possible that family members inherit a susceptibility to an unidentified environmental lymphomagen.

●ETIOLOGY AND PATHOGENESIS

HISTOPATHOLOGIC HETEROGENEITY

Unlike other cancers, the malignancy referred to as "lymphoma" consists of nearly 80 phenotypes.[9] Because each subtype of lymphoma exhibits unique nuances in its natural history, therapeutic considerations, and prognosis, unequivocal establishment of the precise subtype of lymphoma is of paramount importance in a newly diagnosed patient.

The single most important test in a lymphoma patient is an adequate biopsy of affected tissue. In most cases, this should be an excisional lymph node biopsy, or generous incisional biopsy of an extranodal site. When the only sites of disease involvement are deep in the thorax or pelvis, rendering excisional node biopsy difficult, a core needle biopsy obtained with the assistance of ultrasound or CT guidance may be adequate. Fine-needle aspiration alone should never be used as the sole method of establishing the initial diagnosis of lymphoma,[17,32,33] because the precise subtyping of lymphomas requires examination of tissue architecture, not merely cytologic examination of isolated cells. Biopsies should be subjected to microscopic examination, flow cytometry of fresh cells, immunohistochemical examination of fixed tissue sections, and cytogenetic/interphase fluorescence *in situ* hybridization (iFISH) analysis.[33] In the near future, it is likely that genomic analyses using ribonucleic acid sequencing (RNA-seq) technology will also become important to define specific mutations permitting personalized selection of targeted agents capable of inhibiting deranged intracellular pathways.[34]

Table 95-1 lists the most prevalent phenotypes distinguishable by pathologists according to the current WHO classification system.[9,10] Approximately 88 percent of lymphomas originate in a cell that exhibits features most consistent with B lymphocyte derivation (B-cell CD surface antigens or immunoglobulin gene rearrangement). The remaining cases are lymphomas in which the phenotype and genotype are most closely related to T cells or NK cells (T-cell receptor [TCR] chain rearrangements or specific immunophenotypes). This heterogeneity is problematic for histopathologic diagnosis, classifying patients in clinical trials, and selecting therapy. It also makes studies of epidemiology and etiology more difficult. To understand acquired (environmental) or genetic causes of the type of lymphoma in question, the latter studies, to be insightful, must stratify the study group by specific histopathologic diagnosis. This requirement can be difficult if one is studying uncommon phenotypes.

The histopathologic diversity of lymphoma is the result of the complexity of the immune system; its wide distribution through many organs with highly specialized sites, such as mucosa-associated lymphatic tissue (MALT); its differentiation into T-lymphocyte, B-lymphocyte, and NK-lymphocytic lineages; its complex maturation through many progenitor cell levels; the concomitant sequential alterations in expression of immune complex genes and the myriad opportunities for transforming mutations; and the transforming effects of mutations in the many genes encoding immunoglobulin chains or the TCR. Thus, studies in prevalent subtypes of lymphoma such as follicular and DLBCL are more common than in uncommon or rare subtypes. In addition, epidemiologic or etiologic findings relevant to one subtype may not be relevant to another subtype or to lymphoma in general.

ENVIRONMENTAL FACTORS

An increased incidence of lymphoma has been observed, especially among farmers and gardeners but also in printers, woodworkers, dry cleaners, barbers and hairdressers, possibly from organic solvent exposure, especially to trichloroethylene (TCE), a solvent used in many industries.[20–22,26–28] The increased incidence in agricultural workers may be attributed to exposure to a variety of agents, including organochlorines, organophosphates, and phenoxyacid herbicides.[21,22] Despite many studies, an association with lymphoma incidence with herbicide or pesticide exposure has not reached the level of scientific certainty.[21] Indeed, evidence indicates that modest exposure to herbicides by adults who use such products in and around their homes is not likely to increase lymphoma risk,[35] although heavy occupational exposures remain under study. Large studies of two pesticides, chlorpyrifos[36] and glyphosate[37] showed no association with lymphoma incidence. In the former case,

TABLE 95–1. Histologic Subtypes and Relative Frequency of the Non-Hodgkin Lymphomas*

A. B-cell lymphomas (~88% of all non-Hodgkin lymphoma [NHL])
   1. Diffuse large B-cell lymphomas (30%)
      T-cell–rich large B-cell lymphoma
      Primary diffuse large B-cell lymphoma of the central nervous system
      Primary cutaneous diffuse large B-cell lymphoma
      Epstein-Barr virus (EBV)–positive diffuse large B-cell lymphoma of the elderly
      Diffuse large B-cell lymphoma arising in human herpesvirus (HHV)-8–associated multicentric Castleman disease
      Diffuse large B-cell lymphomas with features simulating Hodgkin lymphoma
   2. Follicular lymphoma (25%)
   3. Extranodal marginal zone lymphoma of mucosa-associated lymphatic tissue (MALT lymphoma) (7%)
   4. Small lymphocytic lymphoma-chronic lymphocytic leukemia (7%)
   5. Mantle cell lymphoma (5%)
   6. Primary mediastinal (thymic) large B-cell lymphoma (3%)
   7. Lymphoplasmacytic lymphoma–Waldenström macroglobulinemia (<2%)
   8. Nodal marginal zone B-cell lymphoma (<1.5%)
   9. Splenic marginal zone lymphoma (<1%)
   10. Extranodal marginal zone B-cell lymphoma (<1%)
   11. Intravascular large B-cell lymphoma (<1%)
   12. Primary effusion lymphoma (<1%)
   13. Primary cutaneous follicle center lymphoma (1%)
   14. Burkitt lymphoma–Burkitt leukemia (1.5%)
   15. Plasmablastic lymphoma (<1%)
   16. Lymphomatoid granulomatosis (<1%)

B. T- and natural killer (NK)–cell lymphomas (~12% of all NHL)
   1. Extranodal T- or NK-cell lymphoma
   2. Enteropathy-associated T-cell lymphoma
   3. Hepatosplenic T-cell lymphoma
   4. Subcutaneous panniculitis-like T-cell lymphoma
   5. Cutaneous T-cell lymphoma (Sézary syndrome and mycosis fungoides)
   6. Primary cutaneous γδT-cell lymphoma
   7. Anaplastic large cell lymphoma
   8. Angioimmunoblastic T-cell lymphoma
   9. Primary T-cell lymphoma unspecified

C. Immunodeficiency-associated lymphoproliferative disorders (see Table 95–2 for inherited diseases associated with immunodeficiencies and lymphoma)
   1. HIV-associated lymphoma
   2. Posttransplantation lymphoproliferative disorder
   3. Lymphoma associated with a primary immune disorder

*The parenthetical percentages are approximate but give some sense of the relative distribution of subtypes. The frequency of lymphoma varies depending on the geographic area under consideration. The frequencies cited here are approximate and related to those observed in the United States, the United Kingdom, or Western Europe. Rare subtypes are not listed.

Data from Swerdlow SH, Campo E, Harris NL, et al: *WHO classification of tumours of haematopoietic and lymphoid tissues,* 4th ed. Lyon: International Agency for Research on Cancer; 2008.

the relative risk of death from all causes, from any cancer, or from lymphoma was significantly less in the 22,000 applicators exposed to chlorpyrifos than in the 33,000 applicators not so exposed. It is possible that subsets of individuals may be susceptible to different exposures based on genetic differences (see "Interaction of Environment and Genotype" below) Indeed, preliminary studies using single nucleotide polymorphism–based analysis have linked lymphomagenesis with normal variations (polymorphisms) in genes involved in apoptosis, cell cycle regulation, lymphocyte development, and inflammation.[38–40] In some cases, polymorphic genes have been associated with specific morphologic subsets of lymphoma.[41] Dark hair dyes have also been associated with a moderately increased risk of follicular lymphoma in women.[42] A meta-analysis has demonstrated a dose–response relationship of NHL with cigarette smoking, with increasing NHL risk in heavy or long-duration smokers, possibly from a suppressive effect of smoking on the immune system.[20] Increased body mass index is associated with an increased risk of many cancers,[43,44] including lymphoma.[44–47] Indexes above 30 to 35 kg/m^2 (normal = 8.5 to 25 kg/m^2) are associated with an increased risk of lymphoma and a worse outcome after treatment. The risk factors discussed in this section have not been found uniformly in all studies of their association with lymphoma and should be considered provisional associations. In addition, as larger populations of patients with lymphoma, stratified by histologic type, are studied, it may become possible to dissect out etiologic relationships of exogenous exposures with specific subtypes of lymphoma but not others.

Small but significant increases in lymphoma are associated with radiation exposure. An increased incidence of lymphoma was reported in survivors of the atomic bombings in Hiroshima and Nagasaki who were near the hypocenter of the detonation.[48–51] An increased incidence of lymphomas also has been reported for individuals at the Chernobyl accident site who received radiation equivalent to that of the atomic bomb exposures in Japan.[52] Individuals treated a half century ago with radiation for ankylosing spondylitis also had a small increase in lymphoma incidence.[53] The relative risk of lymphoma with high-dose radiation is low and some still question the causal relationship.[54] Several studies have found an inverse relationship between an individual's exposure to ultraviolet light and lymphoma incidence (especially DLBCL).[55]

INTERACTION OF ENVIRONMENT AND GENOTYPE

Polymorphic immune gene variations have been identified as significant factors in the association of organochloride exposure with increased incidence of lymphoma in a large population of patients and matched controls.[56] Associations between all exposures and NHL risk were limited to the same genotypes for interferon-γ, *IFNG* (C-1615T) TT, and interleukin-4, *IL4* (5′-UTR, Ex1–168C→T) CC. Associations between PCB180 in plasma and dust and NHL risk were limited to the same genotypes for interleukin-16, *IL16* (3′-UTR, Ex22+871A→G) AA, interleukin-8, *IL8* (T-251A) TT, and interleukin-10, *IL10* (A-1082G) AG/GG. This result indicates that the relation between organochlorine exposure and NHL risk may be modified by particular variants in immune genes, supporting the concept of a gene-environment interaction for induction of NHL.

INFECTIOUS AGENTS

Human T-Cell Leukemia/Lymphoma Virus I

Adult T-cell leukemia/lymphoma (ATLL) provides the most compelling evidence for a viral etiology of lymphoma.[57] Human T-cell leukemia/lymphoma virus-1 (HTLV-1) is a C-type RNA tumor virus, isolated

from patients with ATLL.[58] HTLV-1 is an acquired retrovirus that is not related to other known animal retroviruses. HTLV-1 can immortalize lymphoid cells in culture and induce malignancy in an infected human host. The incidence of infection with HTLV-1 in endemic areas is very high, yet few of these infected patients develop ATLL. HTLV-1 also leads to a neurologic disorder called *tropical spastic paraparesis*.[59] Host determinants affect transformation of lymphocytes by HTLV-1, and these may be genetic factors.[58] Development of ATLL is associated with infection by the virus.[60] Serum specimens from Japanese patients with ATLL are positive for HTLV-1, as are serum samples from ATLL patients in the Caribbean, where ATLL is endemic.[61] The highest prevalence of ATLL in Japan is in the southern island of Kyushi, where 10 to 15 percent of the population has antibody to HTLV-1.[62] On the Japanese islands where ATLL is rare, the rate is less than 1 percent. These and additional data from the Caribbean, the southeastern United States, South America, and Africa indicate that ATLL clusters in regions where HTLV-1 is prevalent.[60,61] How these regions are linked is not known. One hypothesis is that HTLV-1 was brought to the Americas from Africa by the slave trade and then to the southern islands of Japan by trade between Japan and Africa.[61,63]

Host susceptibility, a shared environmental exposure, or both contribute to HTLV-1 infection. The prevalence of HTLV-1 antibodies in close family members is three to four times higher than in the corresponding normal population.[63,64] In some instances, cell cultures of antibody-positive, clinically normal patients yield HTLV-1 isolates.[64] Blood donors are routinely screened for antibodies to HTLV-1 to prevent transmission by this route.

Epstein-Barr Virus

Some B-cell lymphomas, including Burkitt lymphoma, posttransplantation lymphoma, and HIV-associated lymphomas (immunodeficiency-related Burkitt lymphoma, primary central nervous system lymphoma, primary effusion lymphoma, the immunoblastic-plasmacytoid type of DLBCL, and oral cavity plasmablastic lymphoma) may be caused by Epstein-Barr virus (EBV; Chaps. 98 and 102).[65] EBV is a DNA virus in the herpesvirus family that first was described in cultured lymphoblasts from patients with African Burkitt lymphoma.[66] EBV binds to the CD21 antigen (also the receptor for the C3d component of complement) on B lymphocytes.[67] It is capable of transforming B lymphocytes into lymphoblastoid cells that may proliferate perpetually in cell culture.[68] EBV is present in greater than 95 percent of cases of endemic Burkitt lymphoma and in approximately 20 percent of cases of nonendemic Burkitt lymphoma.[69,70] Malaria is holoendemic in regions where endemic Burkitt lymphoma exists.[71] A three-step process in the development of this lymphoma has been proposed[72,73]: (1) EBV initiates a polyclonal proliferation of B cells; (2) malaria or other infections further stimulate the proliferating B cells; and (3) the transforming B cells incur specific reciprocal translocations of chromosome 8 with chromosome 2, 14, or 22, resulting in a clonal expansion of B lymphocytes.

Extranodal NK/T-cell lymphoma, nasal type is mostly endemic to East Asia and is usually associated with EBV infection (Chap. 104). The EBV genome is typically detected in the lymphoma cells.[74,75] Geographic localization of extranodal NK/T-cell lymphoma matches the endemic distribution of EBV, suggesting the role of EBV in lymphomagenesis.

Human Herpesvirus-8

Human herpesvirus-8 (HHV-8) is associated with Kaposi sarcoma, Castleman disease, and primary effusion lymphoma, found most commonly in immunodeficient individuals infected with HIV.[65,76–79] HHV-8 is not a ubiquitous virus. It is mainly endemic in areas where classical or Kaposi sarcoma is of high prevalence, including the Mediterranean basin and East and Central Africa. In the latter areas, the HHV-8 seroprevalence can reach 80 percent in the adult population.[79] In the homosexual population (mainly in the United States and Europe), HHV-8 is principally transmitted during repeated sexual contacts, whereas in Africa it is mainly transmitted from mother to child and among siblings. Saliva seems to play a major role in HHV-8 transmission.[79] Posttransplantation primary effusion lymphoma is associated with HHV-8.[76]

Hepatitis Viruses B and C

Hepatitis B and C have been implicated in the pathogenesis of lymphoproliferative diseases.[80] In one study, 334 newly diagnosed lymphoma patients and 1014 controls had a serologic evaluation for the presence of prior hepatitis virus B or C infection.[81] The results suggested that hepatitis B seropositivity was significantly higher in patients with DLBCL and follicular lymphoma, and seropositivity for hepatitis C was significantly higher in DLBCL patients. A similar result was found in another study in Taiwan, an area with a high frequency of hepatitis B virus infection.[82] In two other studies, seropositivity for hepatitis C was significantly higher in patients with B-cell lymphomas.[83,84] Hepatitis C virus has a predilection for B cells. Hepatitis C virus RNA levels are significantly higher in B cells than CD4+ or CD8+ T cells or other cells in infected patients, and the virus is associated with immunopathologic reactions, such as cryoglobulinemia, and, not infrequently, clonality of infected B lymphocytes.[85] Hepatitis C virus infection may be associated with the onset of DLBCL, marginal zone lymphoma, and lymphoplasmacytic lymphoma, but not follicular lymphoma.[83]

Helicobacter pylori

Helicobacter pylori can cause marginal zone B-cell MALT lymphomas of the stomach and probably causes some of the higher-grade lymphomas, either from transformation of a MALT or *de novo* large cell lymphoma.[86–88] This spiral Gram-negative bacillus is the first bacterium demonstrated to cause a human neoplasm. It had been thought that the stomach was sterile because of the acid environment, but *H. pylori* had evolved to tolerate the environment, perhaps in part, because it secretes urease, an enzyme that converts urea to ammonia, making the microenvironment around the organism less acidic. Although the stomach has no endogenous lymphoid tissue, the latter develops in response to the organism, and ultimately the chronic inflammatory reaction can result in the transformation and selection of a mutant lymphocyte with a growth and survival advantage leading to a lymphoma (Chap. 101). Eradication of *H. pylori* with antibiotics early in the course of gastric MALT lymphoma can lead to regression of the lymphoma and permanent cure of the majority of afflicted patients.[89]

Chlamydophila psittaci

Ocular adnexal lymphomas are the most common tumor of the eye.[90,91] The majority of ocular adnexal lymphomas are extranodal, mucosa-associated lymphoid tissue lymphomas and have been linked to *Chlamydophila psittaci* infection in several reports. In one study, this organism was detected in lymphoma tissue in 75 percent of cases.[92] DNA was detected in conjunctival swabs and/or blood mononuclear cells from 50 percent of patients. Mononuclear phagocytes were the carriers of *C. psittaci* in this population of patients.[93] Confirmatory reports of the association of *C. psittaci* with adnexal ocular lymphoma have been published,[94,95] but other studies report no association.[96–98] These discrepant reports may be explained by the association of different organisms with ocular lymphoma in different geographic regions of the world.[99,100]

Other Bacteria

Other bacterial infestations have been found in association with lymphomas of MALT. *Campylobacter jejuni* and *Borrelia burgdorferi* have been connected to the onset of immunoproliferative disease of the small intestine and B-cell lymphoma of the skin.[101]

IMMUNOSUPPRESSION

Inherited

A number of the rare immunodeficiency syndromes tabulated in Table 95–2[82,102–123] result from gene mutations leading to deficiencies in cellular or humoral immunity or both. These syndromes have a paradoxically high frequency of autoantibodies but, more relevant to this discussion, an increased probability of developing a lymphoma. Because these syndromes are so uncommon, reliable assessment of the increased risk of lymphoma often has to be inferred. The increased risk of approximately 0.5 to 10 percent of patients, depending on the immunodeficiency disease in question, is several orders of magnitude above the risk in the general population (age-adjusted incidence rate in the United States younger than 65 years of age: males = 0.011 percent and females = 0.008 percent). With the exception of common variable immunodeficiency, the syndromes present in childhood and because several are X-chromosome-linked, males are affected more commonly than females. The lymphomas induced may result from a susceptibility to EBV and the lymphoproliferation may initially be polyclonal before evolving to a monoclonal tumor. Extranodal involvement appears to be more common than in persons with lymphoma who are immunocompetent. The initial manifestations of the immunodeficiency are usually infections or autoimmune abnormalities, such as immune cytopenias, and lymphoma is a later complication. We have included Li-Fraumeni syndrome in this cluster for convenience of presentation. This germline predisposition syndrome does not have an immunodeficiency phenotype as do all the other entries in Table 95–2. Rather, it is a nonsyndromic familial cancer syndrome transmitting susceptibility to mutations in *p53*. The cancers that occur in these families include lymphoma.

Acquired

A variety of types of immunosuppressed individuals develop lymphoma. Chapter 81 discusses AIDS-related lymphoma.[124] Posttransplantation lymphoproliferative diseases generally display B-cell lineage derivation, involvement of extranodal sites, aggressive histology and clinical behavior, and frequent association with EBV infection. The occurrence of immunoglobulin (Ig) V mutations in the overwhelming majority of posttransplantation lymphoproliferative disease indicates that malignant transformation targets germinal center B cells and their descendants, both in EBV-positive and EBV-negative cases.[125–127] Posttransplantation T-cell lymphomas may occur and often arise in extranodal sites, such as skin or central nervous system.[128,129]

The incidence and severity of lymphomas have increased with the introduction of immunosuppressive agents such as cyclosporine, infliximab, and etanercept for treatment of autoimmune diseases.

AUTOIMMUNITY

Several autoimmune disorders are risk factors for lymphoma, probably as a result of chronic immune stimulation leading to excessive B-cell proliferation as well as depressed regulatory T-cell function. The strongest associations are for primary Sjögren syndrome, systemic lupus erythematosus, and rheumatoid arthritis with relative risks of 18.8, 7.4, and 3.9, respectively.[20] Patients with Sjögren syndrome are especially susceptible to development of parotid gland marginal zone

TABLE 95–2. Inherited Syndromes Predisposing to Lymphoma

Syndrome	Inheritance	Description	Mechanism	Leukemia Type	References
	Altered Genes				
DNA REPAIR DEFECTS					
Ataxia telangiectasia	R	*ATM* homozygotes Dominant-negative missense mutations	Genomic instability Increased translocations in T cells formed at the time of V(D)J recombination	T-cell lymphoma, T-cell ALL, T-cell PLL, B-cell lymphoma	112, 115
Bloom	R	*BLM*	Genomic instability	ALL, lymphoma	107, 108
Nijmegen breakage	R	*NBS1*	Genomic instability Altered telomere maintenance	Lymphoid tumors, especially B-cell lymphoma	103, 109
TUMOR-SUPPRESSOR GENE DEFECT					
Li-Fraumeni*	D	*p53*	Defect in tumor suppressor	CLL, ALL, Hodgkin and Burkitt lymphoma	111, 120
IMMUNODEFICIENCY STATES					
Common variable immunodeficiency	R and D	Defect in CD40 signaling	Failure of B-cell maturation	Burkitt, MALT, other B-cell lymphomas, Hodgkin lymphoma	102, 240
Severe combined immunodeficiency disease (SCID)	R	*ADA*	Defective T-cell + B-cell function	B-cell lymphoma	113
Wiskott-Aldrich	X	*WASP*	Signaling and apoptosis	Hodgkin and non-Hodgkin lymphoma	117, 119
X-linked immunodeficiency with normal or increased immunoglobulin (Ig) M	X	*CD40L*	CD40 ligand defect on T cell	Hodgkin and non-Hodgkin lymphoma	116, 123
X-linked lymphoproliferative syndrome (XLP)	X	*SAP*	Defect in immune signaling	EBV-related B-cell lymphoma	110
APOPTOTIC DEFECT					
Autoimmune lymphoproliferative syndrome (ALPS)	D	*APT (FAS)*	Germline heterozygous *FAS* mutations; defective apoptosis	Lymphoma	106, 241
UNKNOWN DEFECT					
Dubowitz	R	Unknown	Unknown	ALL, lymphoma	105
Poland	D	May not be inherited	Unknown	ALL, lymphoma	104, 114, 118
Wilms tumor (WT)	D	Unknown	Unknown	ALL, Castleman disease	122

ALL, acute lymphocytic leukemia; CLL, chronic lymphocytic leukemia; D, dominant; EBV, Epstein-Barr virus; MALT, mucosa-associated lymphatic tissue lymphoma; R, recessive; T-PLL, T prolymphocytic leukemia; V(D)J, variable diversity joining; X, X-linked.

*Li-Fraumeni or Li-Fraumeni–like syndrome has been described in which a gene other than *p53* is mutated. *hCHK2* in particular has been described as etiologic.[242,243] We have not included these variants in the table because we are uncertain if lymphoma is one of the cancers for which susceptibility is increased.

Data from Segel GB, Lichtman MA: Familial (inherited) leukemia, lymphoma, and myeloma: an overview. *Blood Cells Mol Dis* 32:246-61, 2004.

lymphoma (1000-fold increased risk), DLBCL and follicular lymphomas (Fig. 95–3). Similarly, marginal zone lymphoma and DLBCL are the subtypes most likely to develop in patients with lupus.[130] DLBCL has also been reported in association with autoimmune hemolytic anemia. The risk of developing a T-cell lymphoma is increased for patients with celiac disease and psoriasis. Hashimoto thyroiditis is associated with an increased risk of thyroid marginal zone lymphoma, but may also have a higher risk of marginal zone lymphoma in other locations.[131] Sarcoidosis is an inflammatory (granulomatous) disorder that may predispose to lymphoma.[132]

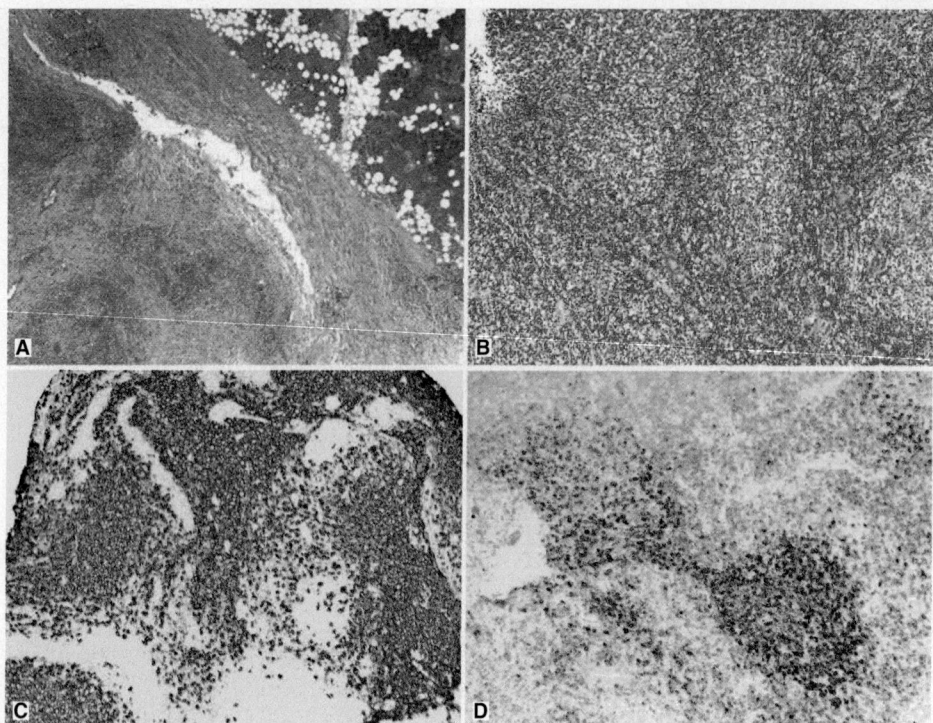

Figure 95–3. Primary extranodal follicular lymphoma in a parotid gland of a 67-year-old woman. **A.** Upper right corner shows normal salivary gland tissue adjacent to a lymphomatous follicular infiltrate with intense fibrosis. **B.** Lymphoma infiltrate with a vaguely nodular appearance. **C.** Nodular appearance better appreciated after immunohistochemical staining for the B-cell marker CD20. **D.** Lymphomatous follicles display over-expression for BCL2, which would not be seen in reactive germinal centers. Flow cytometric evaluation showed a monotypic CD10+ B-cell population with λ light-chain restriction and BCL2 expression on cytoplasmic staining (not shown). *(Used with permission from Raymond Felgar, University of Pittsburgh Medical Center.)*

CHROMOSOMAL TRANSLOCATIONS ASSOCIATED WITH HISTOPATHOLOGIC SUBTYPE

Chromosomal abnormalities involving all chromosomes may occur in lymphomas (Chap. 11). Lymphoid malignancies have a high frequency of translocation-inducing fusion genes. Usually they are of two types: one involving oncogenes that are activated by juxtaposition with *IgH* or *TCR* genes, or by formation of chimeric genes that constitutively activate mutant kinases or mutant transcription factors. The molecular alterations leading to translocations involving nonimmune genes are not known, whereas there is strong evidence that mistakes in V(D) J (variable diversity joining) recombinase activity are responsible for those translocations involving *IgH* or the *TCR* genes.[133]

As in translocations associated with childhood acute lymphocytic leukemia and adult chronic myelogenous leukemia (CML) and acute myelogenous leukemia, translocations involving t(14;18)(*IgH;BCL-2*) are found in healthy persons. Presumably, additional genetic events are required for transformation of a lymphocyte to occur. Alternatively, cells containing these translocations may be entering an apoptotic process, destined to be eliminated.[133]

FOLLICULAR LYMPHOMA

Approximately 85 percent of follicular lymphomas carry the chromosomal translocation t(14;18)(q32;q21) in which the *BCL-2* oncogene on chromosome 18q21 is brought in continuity with the immunoglobulin heavy-chain loci on 14q32,[134] resulting in overexpression of

the BCL-2 protein.[135] The accumulation of the BCL-2 protein permits accumulation of long-lived centrocytes, because the BCL-2 protein inhibits programmed cell death (apoptosis), leading to a longer cell life (Chap. 99).[136] The *BCL-2* rearrangement can be detected by the polymerase chain reaction or by iFISH testing (Chap. 99).

BURKITT LYMPHOMA

In Burkitt lymphoma, the common genetic abnormality is the translocation of the *MYC* oncogene from chromosome 8 to either the immunoglobulin heavy-chain region on chromosome 14, t(8;14)(q24;q32), or, less commonly, the κ region on chromosome 2, t(2;8)(p13;q24), or the λ region on chromosome 22, t(8;22)(q24;q11). In the African endemic cases, the breakpoint on chromosome 14 includes the heavy-chain joining region, suggesting translocation occurs before complete immunoglobulin gene rearrangement in an early B cell (Chap. 102). In nonendemic cases, the translocation involves the immunoglobulin heavy-chain switch region, suggesting translocation occurs at a later stage of B-cell development.[137] EBV genomes are demonstrated in the tumor cells in most of the African cases, in approximately one-third of the cases associated with AIDS,[138,139] but less frequently in non-African, nonimmune-deficient cases (Chap. 102).

ANAPLASTIC LARGE CELL LYMPHOMA

The translocation t(2;5)(p23;q35) of anaplastic large cell lymphoma (ALCL) involves the nucleophosmin (*NPM*) gene at 5p35 and the ALCL tyrosine kinase (*ALK*) gene at 2p23,[140] leading to expression of the novel fusion protein p80 that can be identified by immunohistochemical studies.[141]

This translocation has been identified in approximately 50 percent of systemic cases in adults and in a majority of pediatric cases of ALCL.[142,143] The t(2;5) translocation is rare in primary cutaneous ALCL, which is generally considered to be a different disease than systemic ALCL (Chap2. 103 and 104.)[144]

MARGINAL ZONE LYMPHOMA OF MUCOSA-ASSOCIATED LYMPHATIC TISSUE

t(11;18)(*API2-MALT1*), t(1;14)(*IGH-BCL10*), t(14;18)(*IGH-MALT1*), and t(3;14)(*IGH-FOXP1*) occur in marginal zone B-cell lymphoma of MALT of different sites. The first three chromosome translocations are specifically associated with the marginal zone lymphoma of MALT lymphomas and the oncogenic products of these translocations target the nuclear factor-κB pathway (Chap. 101).[101]

MANTLE CELL LYMPHOMA

t(11;14)(q13;q32) is present in the cells of most cases of mantle cell lymphoma and results in cyclin D1 upregulation. iFISH is the most useful test to identify the juxtaposition of the *CCND1* and *IGH* genes in mantle cell lymphoma (Chap. 100).[145]

● CLINICAL FEATURES

HISTORY AND PHYSICAL EXAMINATION

A complete history and physical examination are required in all patients with lymphoma to ascertain the distribution of lymphadenopathy, extranodal disease, and functional disturbances of affected organ systems. It is also important to document whether the patient has fever (i.e., temperature >38°C for 3 consecutive days), drenching night sweats, or metabolic wasting resulting in loss of more than 10 percent of body weight within the preceding 6 months. The presence of such "B" symptoms has unfavorable prognostic significance in HL, but recent analyses have shown that these "B symptoms" do not have independent prognostic significance for NHL, and current staging criteria no longer recommend assigning "A" or "B" designations when staging patients with NHL.[17] Fatigue, rash, pruritus, and alcohol-induced pain in patients with HL should also be noted, as their recurrence after treatment may herald disease relapse. During the physical examination, all enlarged lymph nodes (>1.5 cm) should be recorded. Involved nodes typically are nontender, firm, and rubbery. The throat should be examined for involvement of the oropharyngeal lymphoid tissue (Waldeyer ring). Aggressive lymphomas more likely involve extranodal sites, such as the skin and CNS (see "Primary Extranodal Lymphoma" below). Liver and spleen size should be assessed as well as palpation of the abdomen for evidence of enlargement of deep nodes (e.g., paraaortic, iliac).

STAGING

Optimal management of a patient with lymphoma relies not only on knowledge of the precise histopathologic subtype of lymphoma, but also on an appreciation of the degree of disease dissemination, determined by a sequence of diagnostic tests known as "staging." The 2014 recommendations from an international working group for the evaluation, staging and response assessment of lymphomas emphasize the emerging dominance of 2-fluorodeoxyglucose (FDG)-PET/CT for initial staging and "end of treatment" response assessment of all FDG-avid lymphomas (including HL, DLBCL, follicular lymphoma, mantle cell lymphoma, Burkitt lymphoma, ALCL, and most subtypes of peripheral T-cell lymphoma) (Fig. 95–4).[16,17] Contrast-enhanced CT imaging remains the standard for lymphoma subtypes that are not reliably

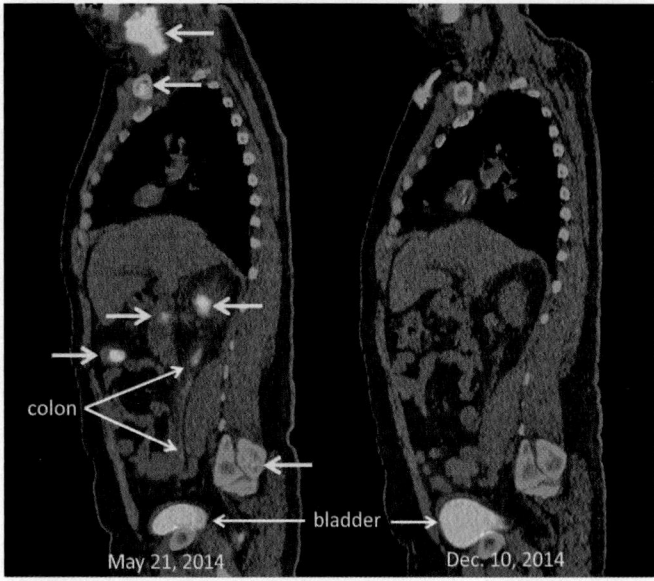

Figure 95–4. [18]Fluorine-deoxyglucose positron emission tomography/computed tomography (FDG-PET/CT) imaging of Burkitt lymphoma before and after successful therapy. At the time of initial diagnosis (May 21, 2014), hypermetabolic areas of avid FDG uptake were detected in a right cervical mass, clavicle, abdominal lymph nodes, stomach, and pelvic bones *(yellow arrows)* in this patient with stage IV lymphoma. Physiologic FDG activity is also seen in the colon and bladder *(white arrows)*. After completion of multiagent chemotherapy (December 10, 2014), there is no abnormal hypermetabolic activity in any of the original sites of disease, although physiologic FDG activity in the bowel and urinary system are still evident.

FDG-avid (e.g., most marginal zone lymphomas, chronic lymphocytic leukemia/small lymphocytic lymphoma, lymphoplasmacytic lymphoma/Waldenström macroglobulinemia, angioimmunoblastic T-cell lymphoma, mycosis fungoides, and cutaneous B-cell lymphomas). For FDG-avid lymphomas, PET/CT imaging has been shown to improve the accuracy of staging for both nodal and extranodal sites compared with CT imaging, leading to a change in stage in 10 to 30 percent of patients, usually as a result of upstaging. Alterations in the therapeutic plan occur in fewer patients and no impact on overall survival as a result of PET/CT imaging has been demonstrated; however, improved staging assures that fewer patients are undertreated or overtreated.[17] PET/CT is particularly important before consideration of radiation therapy for apparently localized disease, because identification of disease sites outside the radiation field by PET/CT entirely alters the treatment plan. The CT portion of a PET/CT scan may be performed with contrast enhancement at a full radiation dose to obtain a high-quality CT examination or without contrast using a lower radiation dose, which merely allows correction for the attenuation of radioactivity within the patient and to localize abnormalities seen on PET.

Full-dose, contrast-enhanced CT scans may identify additional findings, improve detection of abdominal or pelvic disease, permit radiation therapy planning in the treatment position, and are required for accurate nodal measurements on clinical trials. However, full-dose, contrast-enhanced CT scans entail additional radiation exposure and expense, and uncommonly change the overall management plan. Several international consensus groups have recommended that PET/CT with full-dose, contrast-enhanced CT scans be done at the time of initial diagnosis, but that if contrast-enhanced CT scans do not divulge additional sites of disease, that only low-dose, noncontrast PET/CT imaging be done at the end of treatment.[16]

Although marrow aspiration and biopsy have been standard in lymphoma staging in the past, the high sensitivity of PET/CT for marrow involvement has rendered this procedure unnecessary for patients with HL and DLBCL who have negative PET/CT imaging of the bones and marrow. Data for other histologies are currently insufficient and a single 2.5-cm core biopsy with flow cytometry and cytogenetics are still recommended for full staging of other subtypes.[16,17] Standard blood testing should also be performed, including a complete blood count (CBC) and chemistries. Lactate dehydrogenase and β_2-microglobulin are important serum prognostic markers that should be assessed at baseline for most lymphomas.[33,146] Table 95–3 lists the staging procedures that are currently recommended and the criteria used to assign a patient's stage (Table 95–4).[17]

At the completion of therapy, all diagnostic studies performed at baseline detecting evidence of disease are repeated for response evaluation. Current recommendations suggest that PET/CT imaging be interpreted using visual inspection according to a 5-point "Deauville scale" (Table 95–5).[15] Deauville scores of 1 to 2 on FDG-PET scans indicate metabolic activity in tumor sites less than in the mediastinal blood pool, signifying complete metabolic response and complete remission. In contrast, Deauville scores of 4 or 5 at the end of treatment,

---

TABLE 95–3. Staging Procedures for Lymphoma

Initial studies

  History and physical examination

  CBC

  Metabolic panel including renal and hepatic function

  Uric acid

  Lactate dehydrogenase and/or β_2-microglobulin

  Hepatitis B and C serologies (if rituximab therapy planned)

  HIV serology

  Tumor biopsy specimen with histopathology

  Flow cytometry of tumor specimen

  Immunohistochemistry of tumor specimen

  Cytogenetic analysis (including iFISH for lymphoma-associated translocations)

  PET/CT scans of neck, chest, abdomen, and pelvis (for FDG-avid lymphomas)

  Contrast-enhanced CT scans of neck, chest, abdomen, and pelvis (particularly for lymphomas that are not FDG-avid)

Additional studies (useful in selected cases)

  Marrow aspiration and biopsy

  Pregnancy testing in women of childbearing potential

  Immunoglobulin and *TCR* gene rearrangement studies

  Cardiac ejection fraction measurement (if anthracycline therapy planned)

  Magnetic resonance imaging of brain if neurologic signs or symptoms

  Cerebrospinal fluid analysis (including flow cytometry) for high-risk aggressive lymphomas or if neurologic signs or symptoms are present

  Gastrointestinal studies (imaging and endoscopy) if Waldeyer ring involvement, mantle cell lymphoma, or enteropathy associated lymphoma

CBC, complete blood count; CT, computed tomography; FDG, 2-fluorodeoxyglucose; iFISH, interphase fluorescence *in situ* hybridization; PET, positron emission tomography; TCR, T-cell receptor.

TABLE 95–4. The Lugano Staging System for Lymphomas[17]

Stage*	Involvement†	Extranodal (E) Status
LIMITED		
I	One nodal group involved	Single extranodal lesions without nodal involvement
II	Two or more nodal groups involved, on the same side of the diaphragm	Stage I or II nodal involvement with limited, contiguous extranodal extension
II bulky‡	As in II above, but with "bulky" disease	Not applicable
ADVANCED		
III	Involvement of nodal groups on both sides of the diaphragm§	Not applicable
IV	Diffuse involvement of a visceral organ not contiguous with an involved nodal site	Not applicable

CT, computed tomography; DLBCL, diffuse large B-cell lymphoma; FDG, 2-fluorodeoxyglucose; HL, Hodgkin lymphoma; NHL, non-Hodgkin lymphoma; PET, positron emission tomography.

*Stages are refined further for patients with HL by designating whether or not "B symptoms" are present, namely, fevers greater than 38.3°C, drenching night sweats, or unexplained weight loss of more than 10% of body mass over 6 months. Current recommendations discourage applying A and B designations to staging for patients with NHL because these features do not confer independent prognostic information.[17]

†Extent of disease is assessed by PET/CT imaging for FDG-avid lymphomas and by CT imaging for nonavid histologies.

‡A nodal mass of ≥10 cm, or greater than one-third of the transthoracic diameter at any level of thoracic vertebrae as determined by CT imaging is considered bulky disease for HL. There is no consensus on the size of "bulk" for NHL with a suggestion that 6 cm may be optimal for follicular lymphoma. Sizes between 6 cm and 10 cm have been advocated to define bulk for DLBCL.[17] Current recommendations are to record the longest measurement by CT scan and not employ the "X" notation to designate bulky disease. Stage II bulky disease may be considered to be either limited or advanced disease depending on histology and associated prognostic factors.

§Tonsils, Waldeyer ring, and spleen are considered nodal tissue in this staging system.

---

indicate residual abnormal metabolic activity, representing treatment failure (Table 95–6). A Deauville score of 3, indicating metabolic activity greater than the mediastinum but less than the liver, is indeterminant. Most patients with HL or DLBCL who have a Deauville score of 3 at the end of treatment have good outcomes, but careful followup of such patients is important.

The International Working Group (IWG) and the National Cancer Center Network (NCCN) have published recommendations for followup of patients in remission that vary by histology, whether a patient

TABLE 95–5. The Deauville 5-Point Scale for Assessment of Positron Emission Tomography/Computed Tomography Imaging in Lymphoma Patients[16]

Deauville Score	FDG Uptake*
1	No significant FDG uptake in tumor site(s) above background.
2	FDG uptake in tumor site(s) less than that in the mediastinal blood pool
3	FDG uptake in tumor site(s) greater than the mediastinum but less than the liver
4	FDG uptake in tumor site(s) moderately† higher than in the liver
5	FDG uptake in tumor site(s) markedly† higher than that in the liver and/or new FDG-avid lesions likely to be lymphoma
X	New areas of uptake unlikely to be related to lymphoma

FDG, 2-fluorodeoxyglucose.

*The Deauville 5-point scale scores the most intense uptake in a site of initial disease.

†It has been recommended that the Deauville score of 4 be applied to uptake in tumor site(s) that is less than twice as high as the maximum standard uptake value (SUV) in a large region of normal liver whereas the score of 5 be used if the tumor uptake is more than twice the maximum SUV in the liver.

is on a clinical trial or not, and by the clinical setting (e.g., initial vs. relapsed/refractory disease; complete response *or not*). For curable histologies such as HL and DLBCL, the likelihood of relapse decreases over time and visits are reduced from every 3 months during the first 2 years, to every 6 months for the next 3 years, and then annually thereafter. Incurable histologies are observed every 3 to 6 months, determined by pretreatment risk factors, whether the patient is being managed conservatively, and whether treatment has achieved a complete remission or not. At each visit, a history, physical examination, CBC, metabolic panel, and serum lactate dehydrogenase are performed. The role, if any, of surveillance radiographic imaging for patients in remission is controversial. All groups strongly discourage surveillance monitoring with PET/CT imaging for patients in remission because of the high rate of false-positive findings in this setting, which lead to unnecessary anxiety, expense, and biopsy procedures.[15–17,33] The Lugano IWG guidelines also discourage surveillance CT imaging for patients with HL and DLBCL in complete remission at the end of therapy. In contrast, NCCN guidelines recommend that contrast-enhanced CT imaging be performed no more frequently than every 6 months for 2 years after the end of therapy for DLBCL and HL, and then be discontinued.

● PRIMARY EXTRANODAL LYMPHOMA

Lymphomas involving extranodal sites most commonly occur simultaneously with nodal involvement, either at the time of diagnosis or during the course of the disease. Extranodal involvement that occurs as the only initial evidence of lymphoma after staging procedures is referred to as *primary extranodal lymphoma*. The presence of a tumor or mass outside of the lymph nodes is usually not considered lymphoma until a biopsy is done and the histopathology establishes the diagnosis. On the other hand, solitary extranodal lymphomas can occur in virtually any organ or tissue and should be considered in the differential diagnosis of

a solitary mass lesion anywhere. The histopathology of primary extranodal lymphoma is usually either marginal zone lymphoma of MALT or DLBCL. Follicular lymphoma and several other histologic subtypes of lymphoma may also occur. Therapy usually involves a combination of multidrug chemotherapy and a lymphocyte-directed monoclonal antibody, such as rituximab-cyclophosphamide, hydroxydoxorubicin, vincristine (Oncovin), and prednisone (R-CHOP). Selection of the best regimen depends on the histopathologic subtype of lymphoma and the location of the disease. Radiotherapy is used less commonly in the management of lymphoma than in the past because of concerns about induction of secondary malignancies and delayed cardiopulmonary toxicities, although it still has a role in treatment of localized, stages I to II lymphomas, and for consolidation of bulky adenopathy (>10 cm) in selected settings.

An unanswered pathogenetic question concerning primary extranodal lymphoma is the propensity for both sites of paired organs (e.g., ovaries, testicles, breasts, ocular adnexa, adrenal glands, kidneys, and ureters) to be affected simultaneously. It is also curious that several of these sites (e.g., kidney) are normally devoid of significant accumulations of lymphatic tissue. If the transformed lymphocyte arises outside these tissues, it must have a tropism for both paired organs, perhaps because of expression of site-specific adhesion molecules or addressins.[147]

CENTRAL NERVOUS SYSTEM

Primary lymphomas originating in and confined to the leptomeninges,[148] brain,[149–151] or spinal cord[152] are uncommon. They almost always are of an aggressive histologic subtype, usually DLBCL.[151,153] Spinal cord compression typically presents with back pain, followed by extremity weakness, paresis, and paralysis. Leptomeningeal spread may present with cranial nerve palsies and signs of meningeal irritation, for example, headache and stiff neck. Intracerebral mass lesions may present with headaches, lethargy, papilledema, focal neurologic signs, or seizures. Intracerebral lymphoma increased dramatically after the onset of the human immunodeficiency virus epidemic as a result of the association with AIDS-related aggressive lymphomas (Chap. 81). The incidence of intracerebral lymphoma has slowed in AIDS patients because of more successful antiviral therapy. Primary pituitary (or hypothalamic) extranodal lymphoma may result in hypopituitarism. Diabetes insipidus or anterior pituitary failure may occur. The lesion may invade the sella turcica or other neighboring bone and nervous tissue.[154–156]

EYE

Ophthalmic lymphoma, the most common orbital malignancy, includes lymphoma localized to the eyelid, conjunctiva, lacrimal sac, lacrimal gland, orbit, or intraocular space.[157–159] This location accounts for approximately 7 percent of all extranodal lymphomas.[160] The most frequent subtype is extranodal marginal zone lymphoma of MALT. Bilateral involvement occurs in 10 percent of cases. The most common site of ocular lesions is the periorbital soft tissues, particularly the conjunctival mucosal surfaces and the area surrounding the lacrimal gland. These lesions typically have a low-risk of progression and commonly have the histology of a marginal zone lymphoma of MALT or follicular center cell lymphoma and may be associated with *C. psittaci* (see "Infectious Agents" above). In a Danish study, approximately 50 percent of orbital and ocular adnexal lymphomas were of the marginal zone lymphoma of MALT subtype; DLBCL was the most common intraocularly.[91,160] Lymphoma arising in the lacrimal sac was usually DLBCL. There has been a striking increase in incidence rates for lymphoma of the eye over the past 30 years.[24,157–159,161] Patients with marginal zone lymphoma of MALT of the ocular orbit may relapse or have progression of disease after

TABLE 95–6. Revised Criteria for Lymphoma Response Assessment[17]

Response (By Site)	PET/CT-Based Response	CT-Based Response
Complete Remission	Complete metabolic response	Complete radiologic response
Lymph nodes and extranodal (E) sites	Deauville score of 1, 2, or 3 with or without a residual, imaged mass	Target nodes regress to ≤1.5 cm in longest diameter No extranodal sites
Nonmeasured lesion	Not applicable	Absent
Organ enlargement	Not applicable	Regress to normal
New lesions	None	None
Marrow	FDG-negative	Normal morphology
Partial Remission	Partial metabolic response	Partial radiologic response
Lymph nodes and extranodal (E) Sites	Deauville score of 4 or 5 with reduced uptake compared to baseline	≥50% decrease in the sums of the biperpendicular diameters (SPD) of up to 6 target measurable lesions
Nonmeasured lesion	Not applicable	Absent, normal, or regressed without increase
Organ enlargement	Not applicable	Spleen has regressed by ≥50% in length beyond normal
New lesions	None	None
Marrow	Reduced FDG uptake compared to baseline, but higher than in normal marrow	Not applicable
No Response or Stable Disease	No metabolic response	Stable disease
Lymph nodes and extranodal (E) sites	Score 4 or 5 without significant change in FDG uptake compared to baseline	<50% decrease in the sums of the biperpendicular diameters (SPD) of up to 6 target measurable lesions
Nonmeasured lesion	Not applicable	No increase consistent with progression
Organ enlargement	Not applicable	No increase consistent with progression
New lesions	None	None
Marrow	No change from baseline	Not applicable
Progressive Disease	Progressive metabolic disease	Progressive disease
Lymph nodes and extranodal (E) sites	Score 4 or 5 with significant increase in FDG uptake compared to baseline and/or new FDG-avid foci consistent with new lymphoma sites	Target lesions with an increase of >50% from nadir with a longest diameter of at least 1.5 cm. Increases must be by at least 0.5 cm for lesions <2.0 cm and by at least 1.0 cm for lesions >2.0 cm. New or recurrent splenomegaly
Nonmeasured lesion	None	New or clear progression of preexisting nonmeasured lesions
New lesions	New FDG-avid foci consistent with lymphoma and not suggestive of other etiologies (infection, inflammation)	A new lesion >1.0 cm (or if <1.0, must be demonstrated to be due to lymphoma by biopsy or other unequivocal method)
Marrow	New or recurrent FDG-avid foci	New or recurrent involvement

FDG, 2-fluorodeoxyglucose.

initial therapy and relapses can be found at extraocular sites.[91] Overall survival, however, was not significantly worse for patients with relapse. The frequency of translocations involving the *MALT1* and *IGH* gene loci is low in orbital marginal zone lymphoma of MALT (approximately 5 percent), but may predict increased risk of relapse.[160] The therapy for orbital marginal zone lymphoma is usually radiotherapy, which is curative in the majority of patients.[157] Anecdotal reports of responses to rituximab or rituximab postradiation suggest that rituximab may have a therapeutic role in low-grade lymphomas involving the eye. In the rare situation where DLBCL involves the periorbital soft tissue, treatment is determined by the distribution of the disease, but R-CHOP chemotherapy either alone or combined with local radiotherapy is standard.

Intraocular lymphomas are a rare presentation of lymphoma of the eye. Most cases are DLBCL. The diagnosis is established by a vitrectomy. There is an approximately 50 percent chance that the disease will be bilateral and the disease is frequently associated with brain or leptomeningeal involvement. The mainstay of therapy in the past has been local radiotherapy or intraocular injections of methotrexate or rituximab, but most patients treated in this manner relapse within the eye or brain. Standard chemotherapeutic agents administered intravenously (e.g., R-CHOP) typically do not penetrate the eye or brain, rendering these regimens ineffective. In recent years, many neuro-oncologists have advised treating intraocular lymphomas similarly to primary DLBCL of the brain with high-dose methotrexate based-chemotherapy with or without intrathecal treatment and/or whole-brain and eye radiotherapy. A large study conducted at 17 European centers has not confirmed the expected efficacy of this aggressive approach for vitreoretinal lymphoma, however.[158]

PARANASAL SINUSES

Localized NHL involving the nasal cavity and/or paranasal sinuses may be DLBCL, T-cell lymphoma, or NK/T-cell lymphoma.[74,162–168] The nasal cavity is the predominant site of involvement in T-cell and NK/T-cell lymphoma, whereas sinus involvement without nasal disease is common in B-cell lymphoma. Systemic B symptoms are more frequently observed in NK/T-cell lymphoma. Based on *in situ* hybridization studies, there is a strong association of EBV with NK/T-cell lymphoma. These lymphomas may involve the frontal, maxillary, ethmoid, and sphenoid sinuses and typically involve bone. They present with local pain, upper airway obstruction, rhinorrhea, facial swelling, or epistaxis. They may extend into the periorbital area causing proptosis, visual loss, or diplopia. These lymphomas typically are DLBCL in the United States and Western Europe and more often T- and NK-cell lymphomas in Asia. Nasal NK/T lymphomas are typically treated with combination chemotherapy including L-asparaginase plus radiotherapy.[162,169] In contrast, patients with primary sinus lymphoma usually have DLBCL. A series of 80 patients with primary sinonasal DLBCL treated with R-CHOP chemotherapy demonstrated a long-term progression-free survival rate of 50 to 60 percent, with only a single patient experiencing CNS relapse.[170]

SKIN

The three main types of cutaneous B-cell lymphomas are primary cutaneous marginal zone B-cell lymphoma, primary cutaneous follicular center lymphoma, and primary cutaneous large B-cell lymphoma (leg type) as defined by the WHO–European Organization for Research and Treatment of Cancer.[171] Primary cutaneous marginal zone B-cell and primary cutaneous follicle center lymphoma are indolent types with an excellent prognosis that should be treated primarily with nonaggressive therapies, including simple excision, glucocorticoid injections or local radiotherapy. Primary cutaneous large B-cell lymphoma (leg type) is a diffuse dermal infiltrate of neoplastic B cells with extension to both the papillary dermis and the subcutaneous fat.[172,173] It typically presents as a solitary soft-tissue mass and mimics a soft-tissue sarcoma until biopsy clarifies the diagnosis. It is an aggressive lymphoma that should be treated primarily with aggressive chemotherapy (Chap. 98). Chap. 103 discusses classical T-cell cutaneous lymphomas, particularly mycosis fungoides.

CHEST AND LUNG

Primary pulmonary lymphoma may present as a pulmonary nodule or mass and may be associated with hilar lymph node enlargement. The histopathology is usually marginal zone B-cell lymphoma of the mucosa-associated lymphoid tissue or DLBCL, though lymphomatoid granulomatosis may also present in this fashion.[174,175] Lung biopsy is usually required to make a definitive diagnosis. Pleural effusions may occur as a result of either central lymphatic obstruction or pleural seeding.

Primary chest wall lymphoma may present as local pain or may be accompanied by fever, sweating, and dyspnea. These masses usually require excisional or incisional biopsy. They may be associated with pleural effusions and involvement of neighboring ribs.[176]

Primary endobronchial lymphoma is a rare occurrence and may follow lung transplantation. It can lead to airway obstruction as an early sign.

HEART

Primary cardiac lymphoma may involve the heart or pericardium or both. Patients may present with dyspnea, edema, arrhythmia, or pericardial effusion. The effusion may result in cardiac tamponade. Lymphomatous masses may be found in the right atrium (most common), pericardium, right ventricle, left atrium, or left ventricle. Most cases are a B-cell lymphoma; less than 5 percent are of T-cell lineage.[177–179]

GASTROINTESTINAL TRACT

Gastrointestinal lymphoma is the most common form of extranodal lymphoma, accounting for one-third of cases.[180] The most commonly involved site is the stomach, followed by the small bowel, ileum, cecum, colon, and rectum. Lymphoma of the stomach typically causes dyspeptic symptoms and sometimes anorexia or early satiety. Hemorrhage is unusual but if present suggests a high-grade lymphoma. Diagnosis typically is made by endoscopic biopsy.[180,181] *H. pylori* infection has been implicated in the pathogenesis of MALT gastric lymphoma.[88] At endoscopy, mild to severe gastritis is common. Multiple biopsies are important to obtaining adequate material to determine the presence of *H. pylori*. MALT lymphoma is common, but DLBCL also may arise *de novo* or may be found in the background of a MALT lymphoma.[181] If both subtypes of lymphoma are present, the treatment should be directed at the large B-cell lymphoma.

In the bowel, the small intestine, rectum, and colon may be involved, in that order of frequency.[88,182] The intestinal location most often involved is the ileocecal region followed by small bowel, large bowel, and multiple intestinal sites.[182] Primary esophageal lymphoma is rare.[183] Primary colonic lymphoma is associated with symptoms of diarrhea, lower gastrointestinal bleeding, and nausea and vomiting secondary to low-grade obstruction. The most common disease location is the cecum, followed by the right colon, and the sigmoid colon.[184]

Rare cases of lymphoma may be confined to the liver. Right upper quadrant pain is the most common symptom. In about half of cases there is a history of previous inflammatory liver disease, such as hepatitis C.[185–188]

Primary extranodal lymphoma of the pancreas may present with abdominal pain, nausea, vomiting, obstructive jaundice, and weight loss, and very rarely signs of pancreatitis.[189–191]

The gallbladder may be the site of primary extranodal lymphoma and may present with right upper quadrant pain or other symptoms and signs consistent with cholecystitis.[192,193] It may extend into the bile ducts with jaundice and other signs of bile duct obstruction.[194]

GENITOURINARY

Testicular

Primary lymphoma of the testes typically presents as a painless enlargement of the testis in an older man (Fig. 95–5). A hydrocele may also be present.[195–198] The histologic type usually is a DLBCL. At presentation, two-thirds of cases are localized to the testicle or to the testicle and pelvic or abdominal lymph nodes. After orchiectomy has established the diagnosis, patients are staged with a special focus on the remaining testicle. If sonography of the remaining testicle demonstrates a solid mass, it should be assumed to be lymphoma. Patients presenting with

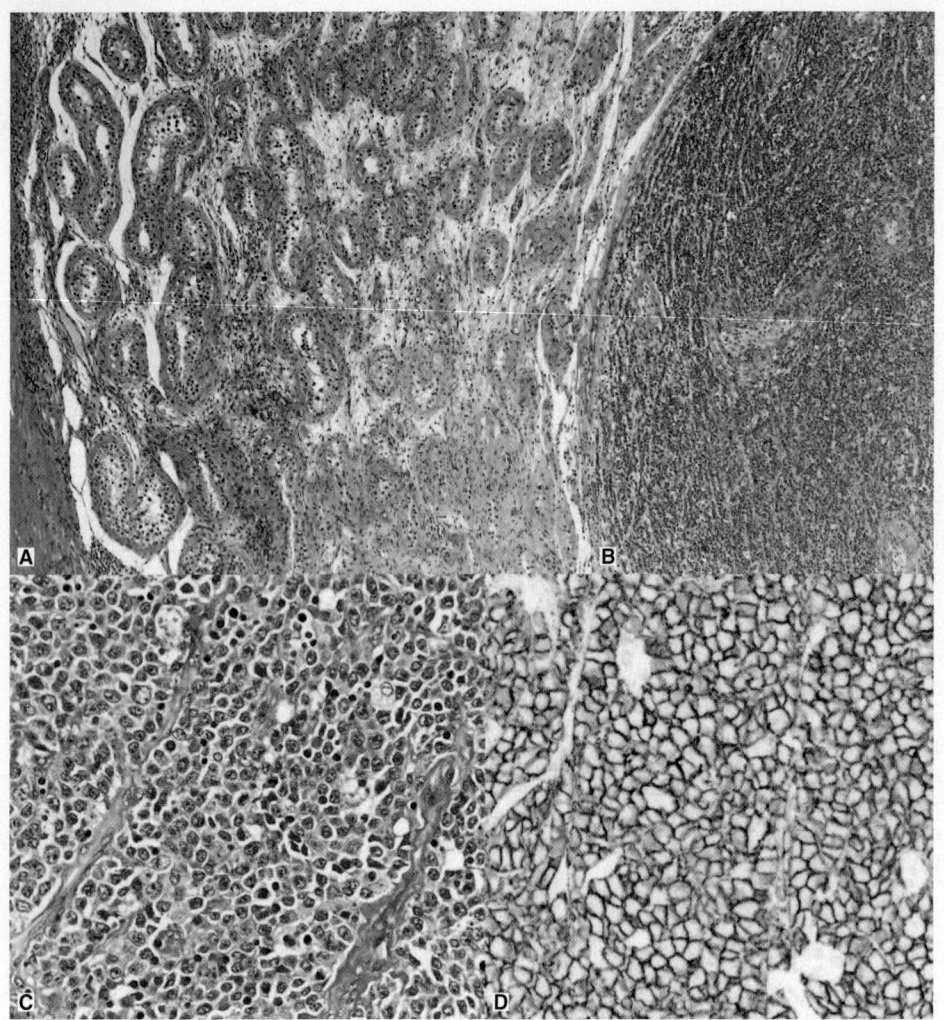

Figure 95–5. Primary extranodal diffuse large B-cell lymphoma in a testicular mass. **A.** Uninvolved area of testes. **B.** Area of testes replaced by an abnormal lymphocyte population. **C.** High-power view of the lymphoma cells. **D.** Positive immunohistochemistry staining for CD20. *(Used with permission from Raymond Felgar, University of Pittsburgh Medical Center.)*

testicular lymphoma have historically experienced a poorer prognosis compared to patients with other presentations of DLBCL, with relapses commonly occurring in either the CNS or contralateral testicle.[199] The current international standard of care consists of orchiectomy, R-CHOP chemotherapy given every 21 days for six cycles, intrathecal methotrexate, and locoregional radiotherapy to the contralateral testicle.[195,196] This combined modality approach has been shown to render an excellent 5-year progression-free survival rate of 74 percent.[196]

Ovary

Primary lymphoma of the ovary is often bilateral and presents as an abdominal mass with abdominal pain or palpation of a mass on physical examination.[200–205]

Uterus, Cervix, Genitalia

Cases of lymphoma limited to the uterus,[206–208] uterine cervix,[209,210] vagina, or vulva[211] can occur. Uterine and cervical lymphoma usually presents with an abdominal mass or vaginal bleeding. Lymphoma can develop within a uterine leiomyoma.[208]

Kidney

Lymphomatous involvement of both kidneys usually presents with renal insufficiency, which can be reversed with multidrug chemotherapy, or radiotherapy. Bilateral enlargement of the kidneys without

obstruction and other organ or nodal involvement and absence of other causes of renal failure are characteristic of primary renal lymphoma.[212–216] The origins of the lymphoma are perplexing as the kidney is thought to be devoid of lymphoid tissue. Both careful staging and postmortem examination have verified the absence of lymphoma in other sites. An increased association of renal cell carcinoma and primary renal lymphoma may exist.[215] Rarely, the lymphomatous involvement, although still solely extranodal, involves only the perirenal space.[217]

Ureter, Bladder, Prostate

Bilateral ureteral involvement with obstructive renal failure may occur.[218] Primary lymphoma of the bladder may rarely extend to the kidney. Usually it is localized and responds well to treatment.[219–221] Primary extranodal lymphoma may involve the prostate.[222,223]

SPLEEN

Primary splenic lymphoma is rare.[224,225] Concomitant marrow involvement is present in most cases. When primary to the spleen, the lymphoma may be principally confined to the red pulp and is usually consistent histopathologically with DLBCL or marginal zone lymphoma.[224] In the absence of lymph node involvement or splenic white pulp involvement at the time of diagnosis or during the course of the disease, it can be considered an "extranodal" splenic lymphoma.[225]

BONE

Primary bone lymphoma may involve any bone but usually affects the long bones.[226-229] The presentation is usually bone pain and the lesions are usually lytic when imaged.[226,228] When the skull is involved the lymphoma may invade the central nervous system.[227] Most patients exhibiting skeletal involvement are due to aggressive lymphomas, particularly DLBCL. Management generally involves R-CHOP chemotherapy with consolidative radiotherapy.[226]

BREAST

The clinical presentation of primary lymphoma of the female breast often mimics carcinoma of the breast. A small proportion of cases may be bilateral. The pathologic diagnosis is DLBCL in approximately 85 percent of cases.[230] BCL-2 expression is frequently present in the tumor cells. Small lymphocytic lymphoma, follicular lymphoma, and marginal zone lymphoma of mucosa-associated lymphoid tissue may also be the histopathologic diagnosis.[231,232] Staging may uncover either nodal involvement, marrow involvement or other extranodal sites with lymphoma in as many as half of cases. Approximately 10 percent of cases of primary breast lymphoma relapse in the central nervous system.[230,232]

ENDOCRINE GLANDS

Primary adrenal lymphoma usually present bilaterally and thus may lead to adrenal insufficiency. In the latter case, the presenting symptoms may be fatigue, asthenia, and other signs of hypoadrenocorticism.[233-236] Primary thyroid lymphoma often occurs in a gland afflicted by Hashimoto thyroiditis. Thus, it occurs more frequently in women than men. The patient may present with an enlarged thyroid (goiter) or have symptoms as a result of tracheal compression.[237-239] The histopathology may be DLBCL or marginal zone B-cell MALT lymphoma. Primary pituitary lymphoma is discussed under "Central Nervous System" above.

REFERENCES

1. Brill NE, Baehr G, Rosenthal N: Generalized giant lymph follicle hyperplasia of lymph nodes and spleen: A hitherto undescribed type. *JAMA* 84:668–671, 1925.
2. Ewing J: Endothelioma of lymph nodes. *J Med Res* 28:1–40.7, 1913.
3. Symmers D: Follicular lymphadenopathy with splenomegaly: A newly recognized disease of the lymphatic system. *Arch Pathol Lab Med* 3:816, 1927.
4. Lukes RJ, Craver LF, Hall TC, et al: Report of the nomenclature committee. *Cancer Res* 26:1311, 1966.
5. Lennert K, Mohri N, Stein H, et al: The histopathology of malignant lymphoma. *Br J Haematol* 31:193, 1975.
6. National Cancer Institute sponsored study of classifications of non-Hodgkin's lymphomas: Summary and description of a working formulation for clinical usage. The Non-Hodgkin's Lymphoma Pathologic Classification Project. *Cancer* 49:2112–2135, 1982.
7. Harris NL, Jaffe ES, Diebold J, et al: World Health Organization classification of neoplastic diseases of the hematopoietic and lymphoid tissues: Report of the Clinical Advisory Committee meeting-Airlie House, Virginia, November 1997. *J Clin Oncol* 17:3835–3849, 1999.
8. Hiddemann W, Longo DL, Coiffier B, et al: Lymphoma classification—The gap between biology and clinical management is closing. *Blood* 88:4085–4089, 1996.
9. Swerdlow SH, Campo E, Harris NL, et al: *WHO Classification of Tumours of Haematopoietic and Lymphoid Tissues*, ed 4. International Agency for Research on Cancer, Lyon, 2008.
10. Vardiman JW, Thiele J, Arber DA, et al: The 2008 revision of the World Health Organization (WHO) classification of myeloid neoplasms and acute leukemia: Rationale and important changes. *Blood* 114:937–951, 2009.
11. Carbone PP, Kaplan HS, Musshoff K, et al: Report of the Committee on Hodgkin's Disease Staging Classification. *Cancer Res* 31:1860–1861, 1971.
12. Lister TA, Crowther D, Sutcliffe SB, et al: Report of a committee convened to discuss the evaluation and staging of patients with Hodgkin's disease: Cotswolds meeting. *J Clin Oncol* 7:1630–1636, 1989.
13. Cheson BD, Horning SJ, Coiffier B, et al: Report of an international workshop to standardize response criteria for non-Hodgkin's lymphomas. NCI Sponsored International Working Group. *J Clin Oncol* 17:2454–2460., 1999.
14. Cheson BD, Pfistner B, Juweid ME, et al: Revised response criteria for malignant lymphoma. *J Clin Oncol* 25:579–586, 2007.
15. Kostakoglu L, Cheson BD: Current role of FDG PET/CT in lymphoma. *Eur J Nucl Med Mol Imaging* 41:1004–1027, 2014.
16. Barrington SF, Mikhaeel NG, Kostakoglu L, et al: Role of imaging in the staging and response assessment of lymphoma: Consensus of the International Conference on Malignant Lymphomas Imaging Working Group. *J Clin Oncol* 32:3048–3058, 2014.
17. Cheson BD, Fisher RI, Barrington SF, et al: Recommendations for initial evaluation, staging, and response assessment of Hodgkin and Non-Hodgkin lymphoma: The Lugano classification. *J Clin Oncol* 32:3059–3068, 2014.
18. Siegel R, Ma J, Zou Z, et al: Cancer statistics, 2014. *CA Cancer J Clin* 64:9–29, 2014.
19. Surveillance, Epidemiology, and End Results (SEER) Program (www.seer.cancer.gov) Research Data (1973–2011), National Cancer Institute, DCCPS, Surveillance Research Program, Surveillance Systems Branch, released April 2014, based on the November 2013 submission; 2014.
20. Skrabek P, Turner D, Seftel M: Epidemiology of non-Hodgkin lymphoma. *Transfus Apher Sci* 49:133–138, 2013.
21. Alexander DD, Mink PJ, Adami HO, et al: The non-Hodgkin lymphomas: A review of the epidemiologic literature. *Int J Cancer* 120 Suppl 12:1–39, 2007.
22. Chiu BC, Weisenburger DD: An update of the epidemiology of non-Hodgkin's lymphoma. *Clin Lymphoma* 4:161–168, 2003.
23. Hardell L, Eriksson M: Is the decline of the increasing incidence of non-Hodgkin lymphoma in Sweden and other countries a result of cancer preventive measures? *Environ Health Perspect* 111:1704–1706, 2003.
24. Moslehi R, Devesa SS, Schairer C, et al: Rapidly increasing incidence of ocular non-Hodgkin lymphoma. *J Natl Cancer Inst* 98:936–939, 2006.
25. Zhou Y, Wang H, Fang W, et al: Incidence trends of mantle cell lymphoma in the United States between 1992 and 2004. *Cancer* 113:791–798, 2008.
26. Karunanayake CP, McDuffie HH, Dosman JA, et al: Occupational exposures and non-Hodgkin's lymphoma: Canadian case-control study. *Environ Health* 7:44, 2008.
27. Schenk M, Purdue MP, Colt JS, et al: Occupation/industry and risk of non-Hodgkin's lymphoma in the United States. *Occup Environ Med* 66:23–31, 2009.
28. Blair A: Occupational exposures and non-Hodgkin lymphoma: Where do we stand? *Occup Environ Med* 63:1–3, 2006.
29. Lu Y, Sullivan-Halley J, Cozen W, et al: Family history of haematopoietic malignancies and non-Hodgkin's lymphoma risk in the California Teachers Study. *Br J Cancer* 100:524–526, 2009.
30. McDuffie HH, Pahwa P, Karunanayake CP, et al: Clustering of cancer among families of cases with Hodgkin lymphoma (HL), multiple myeloma (MM), non-Hodgkin's lymphoma (NHL), soft tissue sarcoma (STS) and control subjects. *BMC Cancer* 9:70, 2009.
31. Segel GB, Lichtman MA: Familial (inherited) leukemia, lymphoma, and myeloma: An overview. *Blood Cells Mol Dis* 32:246–261, 2004.
32. Hehn ST, Grogan TM, Miller TP: Utility of fine-needle aspiration as a diagnostic technique in lymphoma. *J Clin Oncol* 22:3046–3052, 2004.
33. Zelenetz AD, Gordon LI, Wierda WG, et al: Non-Hodgkin's lymphomas, version 4.2014. *J Natl Compr Canc Netw* 12:1282–1303, 2014.
34. Abrams J, Conley B, Mooney M, et al: National Cancer Institute's Precision Medicine Initiatives for the new National Clinical Trials Network. *Am Soc Clin Oncol Educ Book* 71–76, 2014.
35. Hartge P, Colt JS, Severson RK, et al: Residential herbicide use and risk of non-Hodgkin lymphoma. *Cancer Epidemiol Biomarkers Prev* 14:934–937, 2005.
36. Lee WJ, Alavanja MC, Hoppin JA, et al: Mortality among pesticide applicators exposed to chlorpyrifos in the Agricultural Health Study. *Environ Health Perspect* 115:528–534, 2007.
37. De Roos AJ, Blair A, Rusiecki JA, et al: Cancer incidence among glyphosate-exposed pesticide applicators in the Agricultural Health Study. *Environ Health Perspect* 113: 49–54, 2005.
38. Lan Q, Morton LM, Armstrong B, et al: Genetic variation in caspase genes and risk of non-Hodgkin lymphoma: A pooled analysis of 3 population-based case-control studies. *Blood* 114:264–267, 2009.
39. Morton LM, Purdue MP, Zheng T, et al: Risk of non-Hodgkin lymphoma associated with germline variation in genes that regulate the cell cycle, apoptosis, and lymphocyte development. *Cancer Epidemiol Biomarkers Prev* 18:1259–1270, 2009.
40. Wang SS, Purdue MP, Cerhan JR, et al: Common gene variants in the tumor necrosis factor (TNF) and TNF receptor superfamilies and NF-kB transcription factors and non-Hodgkin lymphoma risk. *PLoS One* 4:e5360, 2009.
41. Purdue MP, Lan Q, Wang SS, et al: A pooled investigation of Toll-like receptor gene variants and risk of non-Hodgkin lymphoma. *Carcinogenesis* 30:275–281, 2009.
42. Zhang Y, Sanjose SD, Bracci PM, et al: Personal use of hair dye and the risk of certain subtypes of non-Hodgkin lymphoma. *Am J Epidemiol* 167:1321–1331, 2008.
43. Becker S, Dossus L, Kaaks R: Obesity related hyperinsulinaemia and hyperglycaemia and cancer development. *Arch Physiol Biochem* 115:86–96, 2009.
44. Renehan AG, Tyson M, Egger M, et al: Body-mass index and incidence of cancer: A systematic review and meta-analysis of prospective observational studies. *Lancet* 371: 569–578, 2008.
45. Chiu BC, Soni L, Gapstur SM, et al: Obesity and risk of non-Hodgkin lymphoma (United States). *Cancer Causes Control* 18:677–685, 2007.
46. Maskarinec G, Erber E, Gill J, et al: Overweight and obesity at different times in life as risk factors for non-Hodgkin's lymphoma: The multiethnic cohort. *Cancer Epidemiol Biomarkers Prev* 17:196–203, 2008.
47. Willett EV, Morton LM, Hartge P, et al: Non-Hodgkin lymphoma and obesity: A pooled analysis from the InterLymph Consortium. *Int J Cancer* 122:2062–2070, 2008.

48. Anderson RE, Nishiyama H, Ii Y, et al: Pathogenesis of radiation-related leukaemia and lymphoma. Speculations based primarily on experience of Hiroshima and Nagasaki. *Lancet* 1:1060–1062, 1972.

49. Beebe GW, Kato H, Land CE: Studies of the mortality of A-bomb survivors: 6. Mortality and radiation dose, 1950–1974. *Radiat Res* 75:138–201, 1978.

50. Richardson DB, Sugiyama H, Wing S, et al: Positive associations between ionizing radiation and lymphoma mortality among men. *Am J Epidemiol* 169:969–976, 2009.

51. Shimizu Y, Kato H, Schull WJ: Risk of cancer among atomic bomb survivors. *J Radiat Res* 32 Suppl 2:54–63, 1991.

52. Kesminiene A, Evrard AS, Ivanov VK, et al: Risk of hematological malignancies among Chernobyl liquidators. *Radiat Res* 170:721–735, 2008.

53. Court-Brown WM, Doll R: Leukaemia and aplastic anaemia in patients irradiated for ankylosing spondylitis. *Spec Rep Ser Med Res Counc (G B)* 1–135, 1957.

54. Ron E: Ionizing radiation and cancer risk: Evidence from epidemiology. *Radiat Res* 150:S30–S41, 1998.

55. Boffetta P, van der Hel O, Kricker A, et al: Exposure to ultraviolet radiation and risk of malignant lymphoma and multiple myeloma—A multicentre European case-control study. *Int J Epidemiol* 37:1080–1094, 2008.

56. Colt JS, Rothman N, Severson RK, et al: Organochlorine exposure, immune gene variation, and risk of non-Hodgkin lymphoma. *Blood* 113:1899–1905, 2009.

57. Murata K, Yamada Y: The state of the art in the pathogenesis of ATL and new potential targets associated with HTLV-1 and ATL. *Int Rev Immunol* 26:249–268, 2007.

58. Poiesz BJ, Ruscetti FW, Gazdar AF, et al: Detection and isolation of type C retrovirus particles from fresh and cultured lymphocytes of a patient with cutaneous T-cell lymphoma. *Proc Natl Acad Sci U S A* 77:7415–7419, 1980.

59. Jacobson S, Raine CS, Mingioli ES, et al: Isolation of an HTLV-1-like retrovirus from patients with tropical spastic paraparesis. *Nature* 331:540–543, 1988.

60. Snoda S: Relationship of HTLV-I-related adult T-cell leukemia and HTLV-I-associated myelopathy to distinct HLA haplotypes. *Jikken Igaku* 5:769, 1987.

61. Wong-Staal F, Gallo RC: The family of human T-lymphotropic leukemia viruses: HTLV-I as the cause of adult T cell leukemia and HTLV-III as the cause of acquired immunodeficiency syndrome. *Blood* 65:253–263, 1985.

62. Blattner WA, Kalyanaraman VS, Robert-Guroff M, et al: The human type-C retrovirus, HTLV, in blacks from the Caribbean region, and relationship to adult T-cell leukemia/lymphoma. *Int J Cancer* 30:257–264, 1982.

63. Robert-Guroff M, Kalyanaraman VS, Blattner WA, et al: Evidence for human T cell lymphoma-leukemia virus infection of family members of human T cell lymphoma-leukemia virus positive T cell leukemia-lymphoma patients. *J Exp Med* 157:248–258, 1983.

64. Sarin PS, Aoki T, Shibata A, et al: High incidence of human type-C retrovirus (HTLV) in family members of a HTLV-positive Japanese T-cell leukemia patient. *Proc Natl Acad Sci U S A* 80:2370–2374, 1983.

65. Carbone A, Cesarman E, Spina M, et al: HIV-associated lymphomas and gamma-herpesviruses. *Blood* 113:1213–1224, 2009.

66. Epstein MA, Achong BG, Barr YM: Virus particles in cultured lymphoblasts from Burkitt's lymphoma. *Lancet* 1:702–703, 1964.

67. Nemerow GR, Wolfert R, McNaughton ME, et al: Identification and characterization of the Epstein-Barr virus receptor on human B lymphocytes and its relationship to the C3d complement receptor (CR2). *J Virol* 55:347–351, 1985.

68. Henle W, Diehl V, Kohn G, et al: Herpes-type virus and chromosome marker in normal leukocytes after growth with irradiated Burkitt cells. *Science* 157:1064–1065, 1967.

69. Andersson M, Klein G, Zeigler JL, et al: Association of Epstein-Barr viral genomes with American Burkitt lymphoma. *Nature* 260:357–359, 1976.

70. Potter M, Mushinski JF: Oncogenes in B-cell neoplasia. *Cancer Invest* 2:285–300, 1984.

71. Morrow RH Jr: Epidemiological evidence for the role of falciparum malaria in the pathogenesis of Burkitt's lymphoma. *IARC Sci Publ* 177–186, 1985.

72. Klein G: Lymphoma development in mice and humans: Diversity of initiation is followed by convergent cytogenetic evolution. *Proc Natl Acad Sci U S A* 76:2442–2446, 1979.

73. Klein G: Specific chromosomal translocations and the genesis of B-cell-derived tumors in mice and men. *Cell* 32:311–315, 1983.

74. Aozasa K, Takakuwa T, Hongyo T, et al: Nasal NK/T-cell lymphoma: Epidemiology and pathogenesis. *Int J Hematol* 87:110–117, 2008.

75. Suzuki R, Takeuchi K, Ohshima K, et al: Extranodal NK/T-cell lymphoma: Diagnosis and treatment cues. *Hematol Oncol* 26:66–72, 2008.

76. Dotti G, Fiocchi R, Motta T, et al: Primary effusion lymphoma after heart transplantation: A new entity associated with human herpesvirus-8. *Leukemia* 13:664–670, 1999.

77. Gessain A: [Human herpesvirus 8 (HHV-8): Clinical and epidemiological aspects and clonality of associated tumors] [in French]. *Bull Acad Natl Med* 192:1189–204; discussion 204–6, 2008.

78. Laurent C, Meggetto F, Brousset P: Human herpesvirus 8 infections in patients with immunodeficiencies. *Hum Pathol* 39:983–993, 2008.

79. Sullivan RJ, Pantanowitz L, Casper C, et al: HIV/AIDS: Epidemiology, pathophysiology, and treatment of Kaposi sarcoma-associated herpesvirus disease: Kaposi sarcoma, primary effusion lymphoma, and multicentric Castleman disease. *Clin Infect Dis* 47:1209–1215, 2008.

80. Hartridge-Lambert SK, Stein EM, Markowitz AJ, et al: Hepatitis C and non-Hodgkin lymphoma: The clinical perspective. *Hepatology* 55:634–641, 2012.

81. Okan V, Yilmaz M, Bayram A, et al: Prevalence of hepatitis B and C viruses in patients with lymphoproliferative disorders. *Int J Hematol* 88:403–408, 2008.

82. Chen MH, Hsiao LT, Chiou TJ, et al: High prevalence of occult hepatitis B virus infection in patients with B cell non-Hodgkin's lymphoma. *Ann Hematol* 87:475–480, 2008.

83. de Sanjose S, Benavente Y, Vajdic CM, et al: Hepatitis C and non-Hodgkin lymphoma among 4784 cases and 6269 controls from the International Lymphoma Epidemiology Consortium. *Clin Gastroenterol Hepatol* 6:451–458, 2008.

84. Schollkopf C, Smedby KE, Hjalgrim H, et al: Hepatitis C infection and risk of malignant lymphoma. *Int J Cancer* 122:1885–1890, 2008.

85. Inokuchi M, Ito T, Uchikoshi M, et al: Infection of B cells with hepatitis C virus for the development of lymphoproliferative disorders in patients with chronic hepatitis C. *J Med Virol* 81:619–627, 2009.

86. Isaacson PG: Update on MALT lymphomas. *Best Pract Res Clin Haematol* 18:57–68, 2005.

87. Isaacson PG, Spencer J: Gastric lymphoma and *Helicobacter pylori*. *Important Adv Oncol* 111–121, 1996.

88. Mbulaiteye SM, Hisada M, El-Omar EM: *Helicobacter pylori* associated global gastric cancer burden. *Front Biosci (Landmark Ed)* 14:1490–1504, 2009.

89. Stathis A, Chini C, Bertoni F, et al: Long-term outcome following *Helicobacter pylori* eradication in a retrospective study of 105 patients with localized gastric marginal zone B-cell lymphoma of MALT type. *Ann Oncol* 20:1086–1093, 2009.

90. Stefanovic A, Lossos IS: Extranodal marginal zone lymphoma of the ocular adnexa. *Blood* 114:501–510, 2009.

91. Sjo LD, Heegaard S, Prause JU, et al: Extranodal marginal zone lymphoma in the ocular region: Clinical, immunophenotypical, and cytogenetical characteristics. *Invest Ophthalmol Vis Sci* 50:516–522, 2009.

92. Ferreri AJ, Dolcetti R, Dognini GP, et al: *Chlamydophila psittaci* is viable and infectious in the conjunctiva and peripheral blood of patients with ocular adnexal lymphoma: Results of a single-center prospective case-control study. *Int J Cancer* 123:1089–1093, 2008.

93. Yoo C, Ryu MH, Huh J, et al: *Chlamydia psittaci* infection and clinicopathologic analysis of ocular adnexal lymphomas in Korea. *Am J Hematol* 82:821–823, 2007.

94. Chan CC, Shen D, Mochizuki M, et al: Detection of *Helicobacter pylori* and *Chlamydia pneumoniae* genes in primary orbital lymphoma. *Trans Am Ophthalmol Soc* 104:62–70, 2006.

95. Ponzoni M, Ferreri AJ, Guidoboni M, et al: Chlamydia infection and lymphomas: Association beyond ocular adnexal lymphomas highlighted by multiple detection methods. *Clin Cancer Res* 14:5794–5800, 2008.

96. Vargas RL, Fallone E, Felgar RE, et al: Is there an association between ocular adnexal lymphoma and infection with *Chlamydia psittaci*? The University of Rochester experience. *Leuk Res* 30:547–551, 2006.

97. Yakushijin Y, Kodama T, Takaoka I, et al: Absence of chlamydial infection in Japanese patients with ocular adnexal lymphoma of mucosa-associated lymphoid tissue. *Int J Hematol* 85:223–230, 2007.

98. Zhang GS, Winter JN, Variakojis D, et al: Lack of an association between *Chlamydia psittaci* and ocular adnexal lymphoma. *Leuk Lymphoma* 48:577–583, 2007.

99. Chanudet E, Zhou Y, Bacon CM, et al: *Chlamydia psittaci* is variably associated with ocular adnexal MALT lymphoma in different geographical regions. *J Pathol* 209:344–351, 2006.

100. Verma V, Shen D, Sieving PC, et al: The role of infectious agents in the etiology of ocular adnexal neoplasia. *Surv Ophthalmol* 53:312–331, 2008.

101. Du MQ: MALT lymphoma: Recent advances in aetiology and molecular genetics. *J Clin Exp Hematop* 47:31–42, 2007.

102. Cunningham-Rundles C, Bodian C: Common variable immunodeficiency: Clinical and immunological features of 248 patients. *Clin Immunol* 92:34–48, 1999.

103. Dembowska-Baginska B, Perek D, Brozyna A, et al: Non-Hodgkin lymphoma (NHL) in children with Nijmegen Breakage syndrome (NBS). *Pediatr Blood Cancer* 52:186–190, 2009.

104. Fokin AA, Robicsek F: Poland's syndrome revisited. *Ann Thorac Surg* 74:2218–2225, 2002.

105. Grobe H: [Dubowitz syndrome and acute lymphatic leukemia] [in German]. *Monatsschr Kinderheilkd* 131:467–468, 1983.

106. Holzelova E, Vonarbourg C, Stolzenberg MC, et al: Autoimmune lymphoproliferative syndrome with somatic Fas mutations. *N Engl J Med* 351:1409–1418, 2004.

107. Kaneko H, Inoue R, Fukao T, et al: Two Japanese siblings with Bloom syndrome gene mutation and B-cell lymphoma. *Leuk Lymphoma* 27:539–542, 1997.

108. Kaneko H, Kondo N: Clinical features of Bloom syndrome and function of the causative gene, BLM helicase. *Expert Rev Mol Diagn* 4:393–401, 2004.

109. Kruger L, Demuth I, Neitzel H, et al: Cancer incidence in Nijmegen breakage syndrome is modulated by the amount of a variant NBS protein. *Carcinogenesis* 28:107–111, 2007.

110. MacGinnitie AJ, Geha R: X-linked lymphoproliferative disease: Genetic lesions and clinical consequences. *Curr Allergy Asthma Rep* 2:361–367, 2002.

111. Malkin D, Li FP, Strong LC, et al: Germ line p53 mutations in a familial syndrome of breast cancer, sarcomas, and other neoplasms. *Science* 250:1233–1238, 1990.

112. Meyn MS: Ataxia-telangiectasia, cancer and the pathobiology of the ATM gene. *Clin Genet* 55:289–304, 1999.

113. Mustillo P, Bajwa RP, Termuhlen AM, et al: Tumor immune surveillance defect of X-linked severe combined immunodeficiency is not Epstein-Barr virus specific. *Pediatr Blood Cancer* 51:706–709, 2008.

114. Parikh PM, Karandikar SM, Koppikar S, et al: Poland's syndrome with acute lymphoblastic leukemia in an adult. *Med Pediatr Oncol* 16:290–292, 1988.

115. Perlman S, Becker-Catania S, Gatti RA: Ataxia-telangiectasia: Diagnosis and treatment. *Semin Pediatr Neurol* 10:173–182, 2003.
116. Rangel-Santos A, Wakim VL, Jacob CM, et al: Molecular characterization of patients with X-linked Hyper-IgM syndrome: Description of two novel CD40L mutations. *Scand J Immunol* 69:169–173, 2009.
117. Rengan R, Ochs HD: Molecular biology of the Wiskott-Aldrich syndrome. *Rev Immunogenet* 2:243–255, 2000.
118. Sackey K, Odone V, George SL, et al: Poland's syndrome associated with childhood non-Hodgkin's lymphoma. *Am J Dis Child* 138:600–601, 1984.
119. Shcherbina A, Candotti F, Rosen FS, et al: High incidence of lymphomas in a subgroup of Wiskott-Aldrich syndrome patients. *Br J Haematol* 121:529–530, 2003.
120. Srivastava S, Zou ZQ, Pirollo K, et al: Germ-line transmission of a mutated p53 gene in a cancer-prone family with Li-Fraumeni syndrome. *Nature* 348:747–749, 1990.
121. Cohen BJ, Moskowitz C, Straus D, et al: Cyclophosphamide/fludarabine (CF) is active in the treatment of mantle cell lymphoma. *Leuk Lymphoma* 42:1015–1022, 2001.
122. Vergin C, Cetingul N, Kavakli K, et al: A patient with WT syndrome and Castleman disease. *Acta Paediatr Jpn* 37:108–112, 1995.
123. Winkelstein JA, Marino MC, Ochs H, et al: The X-linked hyper-IgM syndrome: Clinical and immunologic features of 79 patients. *Medicine (Baltimore)* 82:373–384, 2003.
124. Dunleavy K, Wilson WH: How I treat HIV-associated lymphoma. *Blood* 119:3245–3255, 2012.
125. Capello D, Rossi D, Gaidano G: Post-transplant lymphoproliferative disorders: Molecular basis of disease histogenesis and pathogenesis. *Hematol Oncol* 23:61–67, 2005.
126. Dolcetti R: B lymphocytes and Epstein-Barr virus: The lesson of post-transplant lymphoproliferative disorders. *Autoimmun Rev* 7:96–101, 2007.
127. Taylor AL, Marcus R, Bradley JA: Post-transplant lymphoproliferative disorders (PTLD) after solid organ transplantation. *Crit Rev Oncol Hematol* 56:155–167, 2005.
128. Jamali FR, Otrock ZK, Soweid AM, et al: An overview of the pathogenesis and natural history of post-transplant T-cell lymphoma (corrected and republished article originally printed in Leukemia & Lymphoma, June 2007; 48(6): 1237–1241). *Leuk Lymphoma* 48:1780–1784, 2007.
129. Lok C, Viseux V, Denoeux JP, et al: Post-transplant cutaneous T-cell lymphomas. *Crit Rev Oncol Hematol* 56:137–145, 2005.
130. Ekstrom Smedby K, Vajdic CM, Falster M, et al: Autoimmune disorders and risk of non-Hodgkin lymphoma subtypes: A pooled analysis within the InterLymph Consortium. *Blood* 111:4029–4038, 2008.
131. Troch M, Woehrer S, Streubel B, et al: Chronic autoimmune thyroiditis (Hashimoto's thyroiditis) in patients with MALT lymphoma. *Ann Oncol* 19:1336–1339, 2008.
132. Ji J, Shu X, Li X, et al: Cancer risk in hospitalized sarcoidosis patients: A follow-up study in Sweden. *Ann Oncol* 20:1121–1126, 2009.
133. Brassesco MS: Leukemia/lymphoma-associated gene fusions in normal individuals. *Genet Mol Res* 7:782–790, 2008.
134. Ong ST, Le Beau MM: Chromosomal abnormalities and molecular genetics of non-Hodgkin's lymphoma. *Semin Oncol* 25:447–460, 1998.
135. Korsmeyer SJ: Bcl-2 initiates a new category of oncogenes: Regulators of cell death. *Blood* 80:879–886, 1992.
136. Hockenbery DM, Zutter M, Hickey W, et al: BCL2 protein is topographically restricted in tissues characterized by apoptotic cell death. *Proc Natl Acad Sci U S A* 88:6961–6965, 1991.
137. Neri A, Barriga F, Knowles DM, et al: Different regions of the immunoglobulin heavy-chain locus are involved in chromosomal translocations in distinct pathogenetic forms of Burkitt lymphoma. *Proc Natl Acad Sci U S A* 85:2748–2752, 1988.
138. Ballerini P, Gaidano G, Gong JZ, et al: Multiple genetic lesions in acquired immunodeficiency syndrome-related non-Hodgkin's lymphoma. *Blood* 81:166–176, 1993.
139. Hamilton-Dutoit SJ, Pallesen G, Franzmann MB, et al: AIDS-related lymphoma. Histopathology, immunophenotype, and association with Epstein-Barr virus as demonstrated by in situ nucleic acid hybridization. *Am J Pathol* 138:149–163, 1991.
140. Filippa DA, Ladanyi M, Wollner N, et al: CD30 (Ki-1)-positive malignant lymphomas: Clinical, immunophenotypic, histologic, and genetic characteristics and differences with Hodgkin's disease. *Blood* 87:2905–2917, 1996.
141. Morris SW, Kirstein MN, Valentine MB, et al: Fusion of a kinase gene, ALK, to a nucleolar protein gene, NPM, in non-Hodgkin's lymphoma. *Science* 263:1281–1284, 1994.
142. Downing JR, Shurtleff SA, Zielenska M, et al: Molecular detection of the (2;5) translocation of non-Hodgkin's lymphoma by reverse transcriptase-polymerase chain reaction. *Blood* 85:3416–3422, 1995.
143. Lopategui JR, Sun LH, Chan JK, et al: Low frequency association of the t(2;5) (p23;q35) chromosomal translocation with CD30+ lymphomas from American and Asian patients. A reverse transcriptase-polymerase chain reaction study. *Am J Pathol* 146:323–328, 1995.
144. DeCoteau JF, Butmarc JR, Kinney MC, et al: The t(2;5) chromosomal translocation is not a common feature of primary cutaneous CD30+ lymphoproliferative disorders: Comparison with anaplastic large-cell lymphoma of nodal origin. *Blood* 87:3437–3441, 1996.
145. Campbell LJ: Cytogenetics of lymphomas. *Pathology* 37:493–507, 2005.
146. Press OW, Unger JM, Rimsza LM, et al: A comparative analysis of prognostic factor models for follicular lymphoma based on a phase III trial of CHOP-rituximab versus CHOP + 131iodine-tositumomab. *Clin Cancer Res* 19:6624–6632, 2013.
147. Campbell JJ, Clark RA, Watanabe R, et al: Sézary syndrome and mycosis fungoides arise from distinct T-cell subsets: A biologic rationale for their distinct clinical behaviors. *Blood* 116:767–771, 2010.
148. Merlin E, Chabrier S, Verkarre V, et al: Primary leptomeningeal ALK+ lymphoma in a 13-year-old child. *J Pediatr Hematol Oncol* 30:963–967, 2008.
149. Nayak L, Batchelor TT: Recent advances in treatment of primary central nervous system lymphoma. *Curr Treat Options Oncol* 14:539–552, 2013.
150. Korfel A, Schlegel U: Diagnosis and treatment of primary CNS lymphoma. *Nat Rev Neurol* 9:317–327, 2013.
151. Ferreri AJ: How I treat primary CNS lymphoma. *Blood* 118:510–522, 2011.
152. Epelbaum R, Haim N, Ben-Shahar M, et al: Non-Hodgkin's lymphoma presenting with spinal epidural involvement. *Cancer* 58:2120–2124, 1986.
153. Paul T, Challa S, Tandon A, et al: Primary central nervous system lymphomas: Indian experience, and review of literature. *Indian J Cancer* 45:112–118, 2008.
154. Kozakova D, Machalekova K, Brtko P, et al: Primary B-cell pituitary lymphoma of the Burkitt type: Case report of the rare clinic entity with typical clinical presentation. *Cas Lek Cesk* 147:569–573, 2008.
155. Layden BT, Dubner S, Toft DJ, et al: Primary CNS lymphoma with bilateral symmetric hypothalamic lesions presenting with panhypopituitarism and diabetes insipidus. *Pituitary* 14:194–197, 2011.
156. Moshkin O, Muller P, Scheithauer BW, et al: Primary pituitary lymphoma: A histological, immunohistochemical, and ultrastructural study with literature review. *Endocr Pathol* 20:46–49, 2009.
157. Woolf DK, Ahmed M, Plowman PN: Primary lymphoma of the ocular adnexa (orbital lymphoma) and primary intraocular lymphoma. *Clin Oncol (R Coll Radiol)* 24:339–344, 2012.
158. Riemens A, Bromberg J, Touitou V, et al: Treatment strategies in primary vitreoretinal lymphoma: A 17-center European collaborative study. *JAMA Ophthalmol* 133:191–197, 2014.
159. Munch-Petersen HD, Rasmussen PK, Coupland SE, et al: Ocular adnexal diffuse large B-cell lymphoma: A multicenter international study. *JAMA Ophthalmol* 133:165–173, 2015.
160. Sjo LD: Ophthalmic lymphoma: Epidemiology and pathogenesis. *Acta Ophthalmol* 87 Thesis 1:1–20, 2009.
161. Sjo LD, Ralfkiaer E, Prause JU, et al: Increasing incidence of ophthalmic lymphoma in Denmark from 1980 to 2005. *Invest Ophthalmol Vis Sci* 49:3283–3288, 2008.
162. Corradini P, Marchetti M, Barosi G, et al: SIE-SIES-GITMO Guidelines for the management of adult peripheral T- and NK-cell lymphomas, excluding mature T-cell leukaemias. *Ann Oncol* 25:2339–2350, 2014.
163. Au WY, Weisenburger DD, Intragumtornchai T, et al: Clinical differences between nasal and extranasal natural killer/T-cell lymphoma: A study of 136 cases from the International Peripheral T-Cell Lymphoma Project. *Blood* 113:3931–3937, 2009.
164. Schmitz N, Trumper L, Ziepert M, et al: Treatment and prognosis of mature T-cell and NK-cell lymphoma: An analysis of patients with T-cell lymphoma treated in studies of the German High-Grade Non-Hodgkin Lymphoma Study Group. *Blood* 116:3418–3425, 2010.
165. Kim GE, Koom WS, Yang WI, et al: Clinical relevance of three subtypes of primary sinonasal lymphoma characterized by immunophenotypic analysis. *Head Neck* 26:584–593, 2004.
166. Oprea C, Cainap C, Azoulay R, et al: Primary diffuse large B-cell non-Hodgkin lymphoma of the paranasal sinuses: A report of 14 cases. *Br J Haematol* 131:468–471, 2005.
167. Mathews Griner LA, Guha R, Shinn P, et al: High-throughput combinatorial screening identifies drugs that cooperate with ibrutinib to kill activated B-cell-like diffuse large B-cell lymphoma cells. *Proc Natl Acad Sci U S A* 111:2349–2354, 2014.
168. Shohat I, Berkowicz M, Dori S, et al: Primary non-Hodgkin's lymphoma of the sinonasal tract. *Oral Surg Oral Med Oral Pathol Oral Radiol Endod* 97:328–331, 2004.
169. Yamaguchi M, Suzuki R, Kwong YL, et al: Phase I study of dexamethasone, methotrexate, ifosfamide, L-asparaginase, and etoposide (SMILE) chemotherapy for advanced-stage, relapsed or refractory extranodal natural killer (NK)/T-cell lymphoma and leukemia. *Cancer Sci* 99:1016–1020, 2008.
170. Lee GW, Go SI, Kim SH, et al: Clinical outcome and prognosis of patients with primary sinonasal tract diffuse large B-cell lymphoma treated with rituximab-cyclophosphamide, doxorubicin, vincristine and prednisone chemotherapy: A study by the Consortium for Improving Survival of Lymphoma. *Leuk Lymphoma* 1–7, 2014. [Epub ahead of print]
171. Willemze R, Dreyling M: Primary cutaneous lymphoma: ESMO clinical recommendations for diagnosis, treatment and follow-up. *Ann Oncol* 4 Suppl 4:115–118, 2009.
172. Levy A, Randall MB, Henson T: Primary cutaneous B-cell lymphoma, leg type restricted to the subcutaneous fat arising in a patient with dermatomyositis. *Am J Dermatopathol* 30:578–581, 2008.
173. Zhao J, Han B, Shen T, et al: Primary cutaneous diffuse large B-cell lymphoma (leg type) after renal allograft: Case report and review of the literature. *Int J Hematol* 89:113–117, 2009.
174. Hu YH, Hsiao LT, Yang CF, et al: Prognostic factors of Chinese patients with primary pulmonary non-Hodgkin's lymphoma: The single-institute experience in Taiwan. *Ann Hematol* 88:839–846, 2009.
175. Kennedy JL, Nathwani BN, Burke JS, et al: Pulmonary lymphomas and other pulmonary lymphoid lesions. A clinicopathologic and immunologic study of 64 patients. *Cancer* 56:539–552, 1985.
176. Tabatabai A, Hashemi M, Ahmadinejad M, et al: Primary chest wall lymphoma with no history of tuberculous pyothorax: Diagnosis and treatment. *J Thorac Cardiovasc Surg* 136:1472–1475, 2008.

177. Antoniades L, Eftychiou C, Petrou PM, et al: Primary cardiac lymphoma: Case report and brief review of the literature. *Echocardiography* 26:214–219, 2009.

178. Ikeda H, Nakamura S, Nishimaki H, et al: Primary lymphoma of the heart: Case report and literature review. *Pathol Int* 54:187–195, 2004.

179. Legault S, Couture C, Bourgault C, et al: Primary cardiac Burkitt-like lymphoma of the right atrium. *Can J Cardiol* 25:163–165, 2009.

180. Nakamura S, Matsumoto T: Gastrointestinal lymphoma: Recent advances in diagnosis and treatment. *Digestion* 87:182–188, 2013.

181. Psyrri A, Papageorgiou S, Economopoulos T: Primary extranodal lymphomas of stomach: Clinical presentation, diagnostic pitfalls and management. *Ann Oncol* 19:1992–1999, 2008.

182. Lee J, Kim WS, Kim K, et al: Intestinal lymphoma: Exploration of the prognostic factors and the optimal treatment. *Leuk Lymphoma* 45:339–344, 2004.

183. Zhu Q, Xu B, Xu K, et al: Primary non-Hodgkin's lymphoma in the esophagus. *J Dig Dis* 9:241–244, 2008.

184. Gonzalez QH, Heslin MJ, Davila-Cervantes A, et al: Primary colonic lymphoma. *Am Surg* 74:214–216, 2008.

185. Asagi A, Miyake Y, Ando M, et al: [Case of primary malignant lymphoma of the liver treated by R-CHOP therapy] [in Japanese]. *Nihon Shokakibyo Gakkai Zasshi* 106:389–396, 2009.

186. Chan WK, Tse EW, Fan YS, et al: Positron emission tomography/computed tomography in the diagnosis of multifocal primary hepatic lymphoma. *J Clin Oncol* 26:5479–5480, 2008.

187. Doi H, Horiike N, Hiraoka A, et al: Primary hepatic marginal zone B cell lymphoma of mucosa-associated lymphoid tissue type: Case report and review of the literature. *Int J Hematol* 88:418–423, 2008.

188. Kaneko F, Yokomori H, Sato A, et al: A case of primary hepatic non-Hodgkin's lymphoma with chronic hepatitis C. *Med Mol Morphol* 41:171–174, 2008.

189. Liakakos T, Misiakos EP, Tsapralis D, et al: A role for surgery in primary pancreatic B-cell lymphoma: A case report. *J Med Case Rep* 2:167, 2008.

190. Pagel JM, Lin Y, Hedin N, et al: Comparison of a tetravalent single-chain antibody-streptavidin fusion protein and an antibody-streptavidin chemical conjugate for pretargeted anti-CD20 radioimmunotherapy of B-cell lymphomas. *Blood* 108:328–336, 2006.

191. Sata N, Kurogochi A, Endo K, et al: Follicular lymphoma of the pancreas: A case report and proposed new strategies for diagnosis and surgery of benign or low-grade malignant lesions of the head of the pancreas. *JOP* 8:44–49, 2007.

192. Jelic TM, Barreta TM, Yu M, et al: Primary, extranodal, follicular non-Hodgkin lymphoma of the gallbladder: Case report and a review of the literature. *Leuk Lymphoma* 45:381–387, 2004.

193. Mitropoulos FA, Angelopoulou MK, Siakantaris MP, et al: Primary non-Hodgkin's lymphoma of the gall bladder. *Leuk Lymphoma* 40:123–131, 2000.

194. Ferluga D, Luzar B, Gadzijev EM: Follicular lymphoma of the gallbladder and extrahepatic bile ducts. *Virchows Arch* 442:136–140, 2003.

195. Cheah CY, Wirth A, Seymour JF: Primary testicular lymphoma. *Blood* 123:486–493, 2014.

196. Vitolo U, Chiappella A, Ferreri AJ, et al: First-line treatment for primary testicular diffuse large B-cell lymphoma with rituximab-CHOP, CNS prophylaxis, and contralateral testis irradiation: Final results of an international phase II trial. *J Clin Oncol* 29:2766–2772, 2011.

197. Fonseca R, Habermann TM, Colgan JP, et al: Testicular lymphoma is associated with a high incidence of extranodal recurrence. *Cancer* 88:154–161, 2000.

198. Vural F, Cagirgan S, Saydam G, et al: Primary testicular lymphoma. *J Natl Med Assoc* 99:1277–1282, 2007.

199. Zucca E, Conconi A, Mughal TI, et al: Patterns of outcome and prognostic factors in primary large-cell lymphoma of the testis in a survey by the International Extranodal Lymphoma Study Group. *J Clin Oncol* 21:20–27, 2003.

200. Yadav BS, George P, Sharma SC, et al: Primary non-Hodgkin lymphoma of the ovary. *Semin Oncol* 41:e19–e30, 2014.

201. Crawshaw J, Sohaib SA, Wotherspoon A, et al: Primary non-Hodgkin's lymphoma of the ovaries: Imaging findings. *Br J Radiol* 80:e155–e158, 2007.

202. Elharroudi T, Ismaili N, Errihani H, et al: Primary lymphoma of the ovary. *J Cancer Res Ther* 4:195–196, 2008.

203. Munoz Martin AJ, Perez Fernandez R, Vinuela Beneitez MC, et al: Primary ovarian Burkitt lymphoma. *Clin Transl Oncol* 10:673–675, 2008.

204. Pectasides D, Iacovidou I, Psyrri A, et al: Primary ovarian lymphoma: Report of two cases and review of the literature. *J Chemother* 20:513–517, 2008.

205. Ray S, Mallick MG, Pal PB, et al: Extranodal non-Hodgkin's lymphoma presenting as an ovarian mass. *Indian J Pathol Microbiol* 51:528–530, 2008.

206. Hamadani M, Kharfan-Dabaja M, Kamble R, et al: Marginal zone B-cell lymphoma of the uterus: A case report and review of the literature. *J Okla State Med Assoc* 99:154–156, 2006.

207. Latteri MA, Cipolla C, Gebbia V, et al: Primary extranodal non-Hodgkin lymphomas of the uterus and the breast: Report of three cases. *Eur J Surg Oncol* 21:432–434, 1995.

208. Merz H, Lange K, Koch BU, et al: Primary extranodal CD8 positive epitheliotropic T-cell lymphoma arising in a leiomyoma of the uterus. *BJOG* 110:527–529, 2003.

209. Gabriele A, Gaudiano L: Primary malignant lymphoma of the cervix. A case report. *J Reprod Med* 48:899–901, 2003.

210. Hanprasertpong J, Hanprasertpong T, Thammavichit T, et al: Primary non-Hodgkin's lymphoma of the uterine cervix. *Asian Pac J Cancer Prev* 9:363–366, 2008.

211. Sungurtekin U, Lacin S, Ayhan S: Primary genital non-Hodgkin lymphoma. *Aust N Z J Obstet Gynaecol* 38:346–349, 1998.

212. Brancato T, Alvaro R, Paulis G, et al: Primary lymphoma of the kidney: Case report and review of literature. *Clin Genitourin Cancer* 10:60–62, 2012.

213. Diskin CJ, Stokes TJ, Dansby LM, et al: Acute renal failure due to a primary renal B-cell lymphoma. *Am J Kidney Dis* 50:885–889, 2007.

214. James TC, Shaikh H, Escuadro L, et al: Bilateral primary renal lymphoma. *Br J Haematol* 143:1, 2008.

215. Kunthur A, Wiernik PH, Dutcher JP: Renal parenchymal tumors and lymphoma in the same patient: Case series and review of the literature. *Am J Hematol* 81:271–280, 2006.

216. Kuo CC, Li WY, Huang CC, et al: Primary renal lymphoma. *Br J Haematol* 144:628, 2009.

217. Mai KT, Burns BB, Isotalo P, et al: Primary extranodal perirenal malignant lymphoma. *Can J Urol* 5:599–602, 1998.

218. Kubota Y, Kawai A, Tsuchiya T, et al: Bilateral primary malignant lymphoma of the ureter. *Int J Clin Oncol* 12:482–484, 2007.

219. Horasanli K, Kadihasanoglu M, Aksakal OT, et al: A case of primary lymphoma of the bladder managed with multimodal therapy. *Nat Clin Pract Urol* 5:167–170, 2008.

220. Hughes M, Morrison A, Jackson R: Primary bladder lymphoma: Management and outcome of 12 patients with a review of the literature. *Leuk Lymphoma* 46:873–877, 2005.

221. Terzic T, Radojevic S, Cemerikic-Martinovic V, et al: Primary non-Hodgkin lymphoma of urinary bladder with nine years later renal involvement and absence of systemic lymphoma: A case report. *Med Oncol* 25:248–250, 2008.

222. Bostwick DG, Iczkowski KA, Amin MB, et al: Malignant lymphoma involving the prostate: Report of 62 cases. *Cancer* 83:732–738, 1998.

223. Jhavar S, Agarwal JP, Naresh KN, et al: Primary extranodal mucosa associated lymphoid tissue (MALT) lymphoma of the prostate. *Leuk Lymphoma* 41:445–449, 2001.

224. Kashimura M, Noro M, Akikusa B, et al: Primary splenic diffuse large B-cell lymphoma manifesting in red pulp. *Virchows Arch* 453:501–509, 2008.

225. Kehoe J, Straus DJ: Primary lymphoma of the spleen. Clinical features and outcome after splenectomy. *Cancer* 62:1433–1438, 1988.

226. Held G, Zeynalova S, Murawski N, et al: Impact of rituximab and radiotherapy on outcome of patients with aggressive B-cell lymphoma and skeletal involvement. *J Clin Oncol* 31:4115–4122, 2013.

227. Agrawal A, Sinha A: Lymphoma of frontotemporal region with massive bone destruction and intracranial and intraorbital extension. *J Cancer Res Ther* 4:203–205, 2008.

228. Bakhshi S, Singh P, Thulkar S: Bone involvement in pediatric non-Hodgkin's lymphomas. *Hematology* 13:348–351, 2008.

229. Catlett JP, Williams SA, O'Connor SC, et al: Primary lymphoma of bone: An institutional experience. *Leuk Lymphoma* 49:2125–2132, 2008.

230. Hosein PJ, Maragulia JC, Salzberg MP, et al: A multicentre study of primary breast diffuse large B-cell lymphoma in the rituximab era. *Br J Haematol* 165:358–363, 2014.

231. Giardini R, Piccolo C, Rilke F: Primary non-Hodgkin's lymphomas of the female breast. *Cancer* 69:725–735, 1992.

232. Validire P, Capovilla M, Asselain B, et al: Primary breast non-Hodgkin's lymphoma: A large single center study of initial characteristics, natural history, and prognostic factors. *Am J Hematol* 84:133–139, 2009.

233. Gu B, Ding Q, Xia G, et al: Primary bilateral adrenal non-Hodgkin's lymphoma associated with normal adrenal function. *Urology* 73:752–753, 2009.

234. Hernandez Marin B, Diaz Munoz de la Espada VM, Alvarez Alvarez R, et al: Adrenal failure caused by primary adrenal non-Hodgkin lymphoma: A case report and review of the literature] [in Spanish]. *An Med Interna* 25:131–133, 2008.

235. Nishiuchi T, Imachi H, Fujiwara M, et al: A case of non-Hodgkin's lymphoma primary arising in both adrenal glands associated with adrenal failure. *Endocrine* 35:34–37, 2009.

236. Zhou J, Ye D, Wu M, et al: Bilateral adrenal tumor: Causes and clinical features in eighteen cases. *Int Urol Nephrol* 41:547–551, 2009.

237. Derringer GA, Thompson LD, Frommelt RA, et al: Malignant lymphoma of the thyroid gland: A clinicopathologic study of 108 cases. *Am J Surg Pathol* 24:623–639, 2000.

238. Hwang YC, Kim TY, Kim WB, et al: Clinical characteristics of primary thyroid lymphoma in Koreans. *Endocr J* 56:399–405, 2009.

239. Skacel M, Ross CW, Hsi ED: A reassessment of primary thyroid lymphoma: High-grade MALT-type lymphoma as a distinct subtype of diffuse large B-cell lymphoma. *Histopathology* 37:10–18, 2000.

240. Chua I, Quinti I, Grimbacher B: Lymphoma in common variable immunodeficiency: Interplay between immune dysregulation, infection and genetics. *Curr Opin Hematol* 15:368–374, 2008.

241. Straus SE, Jaffe ES, Puck JM, et al: The development of lymphomas in families with autoimmune lymphoproliferative syndrome with germline Fas mutations and defective lymphocyte apoptosis. *Blood* 98:194–200, 2001.

242. Bell DW, Varley JM, Szydlo TE, et al: Heterozygous germ line hCHK2 mutations in Li-Fraumeni syndrome. *Science* 286:2528–2531, 1999.

243. Varley J: TP53, hChk2, and the Li-Fraumeni syndrome. *Methods Mol Biol* 222:117–129, 2003.

CHAPTER 96
PATHOLOGY OF LYMPHOMAS

Randy D. Gascoyne and Brian F. Skinnider

SUMMARY

The classification of malignant lymphomas has been a contentious issue during the past 50 years, undergoing numerous changes during its evolution. The recent World Health Organization (WHO) classification of lymphoid neoplasms has gained worldwide acceptance by both pathologists and oncologists. It provides a list of distinct diseases that are defined by a combination of morphologic, phenotypic, genetic, and clinical features, and attempts to correlate each disease with a cell of origin. Because the classification of lymphomas requires the integration of such diverse information, the diagnosis has become more complex compared to other solid malignancies. As a result, several ancillary studies have become useful in the diagnosis of lymphomas, which require special handling of biopsy material when a diagnosis of lymphoma is suspected. The WHO classification identifies three major categories of lymphoid malignancies: B-cell neoplasms, T and natural killer (NK) cell neoplasms, and Hodgkin lymphoma. Two major categories are identified within the B-cell and T/NK-cell neoplasms: precursor neoplasms and peripheral or mature neoplasms. Unlike previous lymphoma classifications, the WHO classification does not group different lymphomas by clinical outcome or histologic grade. It recognizes that each disease has distinctive clinical features and response to treatment and may have a spectrum of clinical aggressiveness that may correlate with histologic grade or gene expression patterns. The WHO classification recognizes that several of the diseases it describes are heterogenous and likely include two or more distinct diseases that cannot be identified based on current data, and remains open to incorporate new data as they become available. One such source of new data for classifying lymphoma is the study of gene expression profiling by complementary DNA microarray technology, which is providing new insights into the classification of diseases such as diffuse large B-cell lymphoma and chronic lymphocytic leukemia. Proteomic approaches will add further texture to the molecular taxonomy of lymphoma classification.

Acronyms and Abbreviations: ABC, activated B cell; ALCL, anaplastic large cell lymphoma; ALK, anaplastic lymphoma kinase; DLBCL, diffuse large B-cell lymphoma; EBV, Epstein-Barr virus; FISH, fluorescence *in situ* hybridization; GCB, germinal center B cell; IGH, immunoglobulin heavy chain; LP, lymphocyte predominant; MALT, mucosa-associated lymphoid tissue; NF-κB, nuclear factor-κB; NK, natural killer; PCR, polymerase chain reaction; PTCL, peripheral T-cell lymphoma; REAL, Revised European-American Lymphoma; WHO, World Health Organization; ZAP-70, zeta-associated protein of 70 kDa.

● HISTORICAL ASPECTS OF LYMPHOMA CLASSIFICATION

The classification of malignant lymphoma has been fraught with controversy during much of the 20th century, with much needed consensus reached during the past two decades. A detailed discussion of the history of lymphoma classification is beyond the scope of this chapter and can be found elsewhere.[1]

From Thomas Hodgkin's description in 1832 of what became known as Hodgkin's disease[2] to the first half of the 20th century, several types of lymphomas with distinctive morphologic and clinical features were described using a variety of terms, including lymphoma, lymphosarcoma, reticulum cell sarcoma, and giant follicular lymphoma.[1] However, many of the terms were not used uniformly, resulting in significant misunderstanding, particularly between pathologists and clinicians. Starting in the 1930s, several attempts were made to classify lymphomas and provide some uniformity of diagnosis, culminating in the Rappaport classification, initially published in 1956, which divided lymphomas based on growth pattern, cell type, and stage of differentiation.[3,4] Most importantly, this classification demonstrated clinical relevance, showing that lymphomas with a nodular pattern had a better prognosis than diffuse lymphomas.

In the 1960s and 1970s, an explosion of studies on the immune system had a profound effect on our understanding of lymphocyte biology and had a consequent effect on our understanding of malignant lymphomas. Normal lymphocytes could now be classified into distinct lineages (B, T, and natural killer [NK]), which could be determined by expression of lineage-specific surface antigens and eventually by genetic analysis of B- and T-cell receptors.[5,6] Several new lymphoma classification schemes were developed to incorporate the new immunologic data, the most important being the Kiel classification[7] (used primarily in Europe) and the Lukes and Collins classification[8] (used primarily in North America). By the 1970s, at least five classification schemes were widely used in different parts of the world. At the same time, clinical studies were beginning to show that some patients with aggressive lymphomas could be cured with combination chemotherapy.[9] Oncologists needed to interpret results of clinical trials performed in different institutions, a situation made difficult by the use of different classification schemes that were not easily translated among themselves.

The problem was addressed by the United States National Cancer Institute, which convened a large group of investigators to determine which classification scheme was best at predicting clinical outcome of lymphoma. None of the classification schemes was identified as predicting clinical outcome better than the other schemes. Therefore, pathologists were advised to continue using one of the six classification schemes studied, and a "Working Formulation" was developed so that oncologists could translate clinical data derived in different institutions using different classification schemes.[10] Lymphomas were divided into 10 categories based solely on morphologic features. To help clinicians deal with a large number of lymphoma subtypes, the lymphomas were further grouped into three clinical prognostic groups (clinical grades). Although the Working Formulation was not intended to be a standalone classification scheme, it was used as such by many institutions, particularly in North America.

However, increasing phenotypic and genotypic data were further defining several distinctive lymphoma subtypes. The Working Formulation lumped different lymphomas into broad categories that were obscuring the distinctive features of the newly described entities. The Working Formulation categories were based solely on morphologic features and were not able to incorporate new immunologic and molecular genetic data that were recognizing new types of lymphomas.

In the 1980s and 1990s, several new lymphoma entities were identified based on new immunologic and molecular genetic data. Although attempts were made to incorporate these new entities into the existing classification schemes,[11] problems with uniformity between different institutions persisted. A desire to eliminate the continued confusion ultimately led to a new approach to lymphoma classification proposed by the International Lymphoma Study Group that used all available information, including morphology, immunophenotype, genetic and clinical features, to define a list of distinctive entities that could be uniformly diagnosed by hematopathologists. The proposal was published in 1994 and was known as the Revised European-American Lymphoma (REAL) classification.[12] Importantly, this classification identified entities that had distinctive clinical features and could be reproducibly diagnosed by expert hematopathologists.[13]

● WORLD HEALTH ORGANIZATION CLASSIFICATION

In the late 1990s, a new World Health Organization (WHO) classification for lymphoproliferative disorders was being developed, based on the REAL classification. First published in 2001 (and revised in 2008), the WHO classification represented a consensus between an international group of more than 50 experienced hematopathologists, including contributions from a clinical advisory committee of hematologists and oncologists experienced in treating lymphomas.[14] The WHO classification (Table 96–1) identified several major categories, including

---

TABLE 96–1. The WHO Classification of Lymphoid Neoplasms

PRECURSOR LYMPHOID NEOPLASMS
- B lymphoblastic leukemia/lymphoma, NOS
- B lymphoblastic leukemia/lymphoma with recurrent genetic abnormalities
  - B lymphoblastic leukemia/lymphoma with t(9;22)(q34;q11.2); *BCR-ABL1*
  - B lymphoblastic leukemia/lymphoma with t(v;11q23); *MLL* rearranged
  - B lymphoblastic leukemia/lymphoma with t(12;21)(p13;q22); *TEL-AML1*
  - B lymphoblastic leukemia/lymphoma with hyperdiploidy
  - B lymphoblastic leukemia/lymphoma with hypodiploidy
  - B lymphoblastic leukemia/lymphoma with t(5;14)(q31;q32); *IL3-IGH*
  - B lymphoblastic leukemia/lymphoma with t(1;19)(q23;p13.3); *E2A-PBX1*
- T-lymphoblastic leukemia/lymphoma

MATURE B-CELL NEOPLASMS
- Chronic lymphocytic leukemia/small lymphocytic lymphoma
- B-cell prolymphocytic leukemia
- Splenic B-cell marginal zone lymphoma
- Hairy cell leukemia
- Splenic B-cell lymphoma/leukemia, unclassifiable
- Lymphoplasmacytic lymphoma
- Heavy-chain diseases
- Plasma cell neoplasms
- Extranodal marginal zone lymphoma of mucosa-associated lymphoid tissue (MALT lymphoma)
- Nodal marginal zone lymphoma
- Follicular lymphoma
- Primary cutaneous follicle center lymphoma
- Mantle cell lymphoma
- Diffuse large B-cell lymphoma (DLBCL), NOS
  - T-cell/histiocyte rich large B-cell lymphoma
  - Primary DLBCL of the CNS
  - Primary cutaneous DLBCL, leg type
  - EBV-positive DLBCL of the elderly
- DLBCL associated with chronic inflammation
- Lymphomatoid granulomatosis
- Primary mediastinal (thymic) large B-cell lymphoma

- Intravascular large B-cell lymphoma
- ALK-positive large B-cell lymphoma
- Plasmablastic lymphoma
- Large B-cell lymphoma arising in HHV-8–associated multicentric Castleman disease
- Primary effusion lymphoma
- Burkitt lymphoma
- B-cell lymphoma, unclassifiable, with features intermediate between DLBCL and Burkitt lymphoma
- B-cell lymphoma, unclassifiable, with features intermediate between DLBCL and classical Hodgkin lymphoma

MATURE T- AND NK-CELL NEOPLASMS
- T-cell prolymphocytic leukemia
- T-cell large granular lymphocytic leukemia
- Chronic lymphoproliferative disorder of NK cells
- Aggressive NK-cell leukemia
- EBV-positive T-cell lymphoproliferative diseases of childhood
- Adult T-cell leukemia/lymphoma
- Extranodal NK/T-cell lymphoma, nasal type
- Enteropathy-associated T-cell lymphoma
- Hepatosplenic T-cell lymphoma
- Subcutaneous panniculitis-like T-cell lymphoma
- Mycosis fungoides
- Sézary syndrome
- Primary cutaneous CD30-positive T-cell lymphoproliferative disorders
- Primary cutaneous peripheral T-cell lymphoma, rare subtypes
- Peripheral T-cell lymphoma, NOS
- Angioimmunoblastic T-cell lymphoma
- Anaplastic large cell lymphoma, ALK-positive
- Anaplastic large cell lymphoma, ALK-negative

HODGKIN LYMPHOMA
- Nodular lymphocyte predominant Hodgkin lymphoma
- Classical Hodgkin lymphoma
  - Nodular sclerosis classical Hodgkin lymphoma
  - Mixed cellularity classical Hodgkin lymphoma
  - Lymphocyte-rich classical Hodgkin lymphoma
  - Lymphocyte-depleted classical Hodgkin lymphoma

precursor lymphoid neoplasms, mature B-cell neoplasms, mature T- and NK-cell neoplasms, and Hodgkin lymphoma.

Distinctive lymphoma entities were identified based upon a combination of morphologic, immunophenotypic, genetic, and clinical features. The 2008 WHO classification includes several provisional entities and categories of unclassifiable neoplasms with features intermediate between two distinct entities. This allows the classification to retain flexibility so that new data that further identify distinct diseases within these entities can be incorporated. In distinction from the Working Formulation, lymphomas were not classified based on clinical outcome. The WHO classification agreed that each type of lymphoma that was identified by pathologic and clinical features could have a spectrum of clinical aggressiveness, and that lumping distinct entities into groups based on clinical outcome would inhibit the development of targeted therapeutic approaches. Therefore, the WHO classification represents a complete change from the Working Formulation, with the emphasis on pathologic classification rather than classification based on survival characteristics.

Genome-wide expression studies have been instrumental in further delineating distinctive subtypes of lymphomas of clinical relevance. Using complementary DNA microarray technology, the expression of thousands of genes at the mRNA level can be studied simultaneously and compared to other tumor samples.[15] Such studies have (1) defined more than one distinct entity in what was previously characterized as a morphologically homogeneous category, (2) identified distinct gene expression patterns that each encompasses a disease that may demonstrate morphologic heterogeneity, and (3) identified new surface molecules and signaling pathways that could provide targets for new therapeutic approaches. The impact of the new gene expression profiles is detailed in the sections on separate lymphomas below.

The WHO classification attempts to correlate each lymphoma to normal lymphocyte biology by postulating a cell of origin for each neoplasm. This correlation is particularly well-suited for B-cell lymphomas in which several distinct stages of normal B-cell development can be identified (Fig. 96–1) but is not as satisfying for T and NK neoplasms.

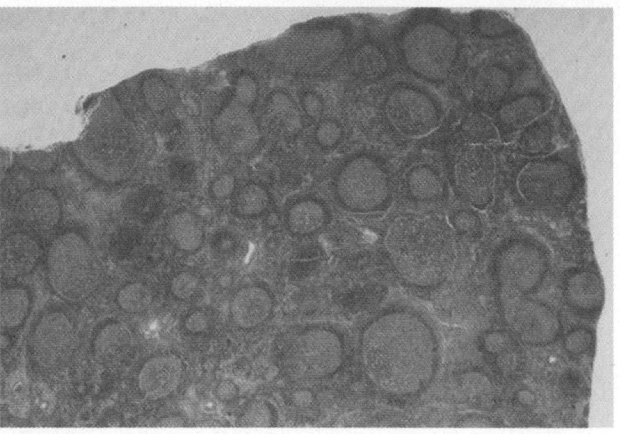

Figure 96–2. Reactive lymph node with follicular hyperplasia, characterized by numerous secondary lymphoid follicles with intact mantle zones.

Briefly, B-cell development begins in the marrow with precursor B lymphoblasts that differentiate into naïve B cells that circulate in the blood. The lymph node is the primary site where B cells encounter antigen, where naïve B cells colonize primary follicles and in mantle zones of secondary follicles (Figs. 96–2 to 96–4). Upon antigen stimulation, these cells undergo blast transformation and enter the germinal center reaction in the late primary immune response and the secondary immune response. In the germinal center, cells downregulate BCL2 (Fig. 96–5) and initially transform into intermediate-size cells (follicular B blasts), then into large centroblasts, and finally into small centrocytes (Figs. 96–6 and 96–7).[16] Cells that survive the germinal center upregulate BCL2 and either differentiate into short-lived plasma cells through an immunoblast stage or differentiate into memory cells that populate follicular marginal zones or recirculate in the blood. Several

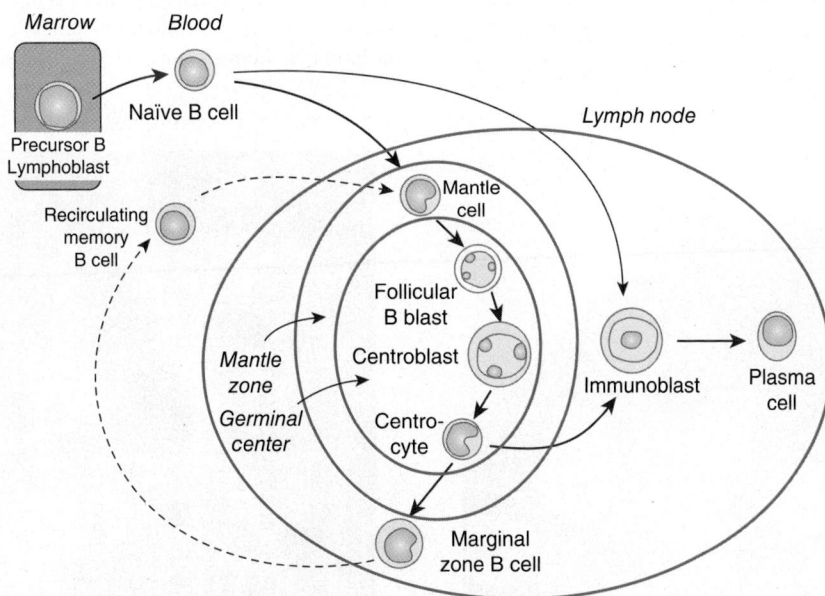

Figure 96–1. Stages of B-cell development. Precursor B lymphoblasts in the marrow differentiate into mature B cells that circulate in blood and colonize mantle zones of lymphoid follicles. Upon antigen stimulation, the cells can differentiate directly into immunoblasts (early primary immune response) or enter the germinal center reaction (late primary and secondary immune responses). In the germinal center, cells undergo blast transformation and progress to form large centroblasts, followed by small centrocytes. These cells differentiate into either antibody-secreting plasma cells through an immunoblast stage or memory B cells that can recirculate or localize to the marginal zones of lymphoid follicles.

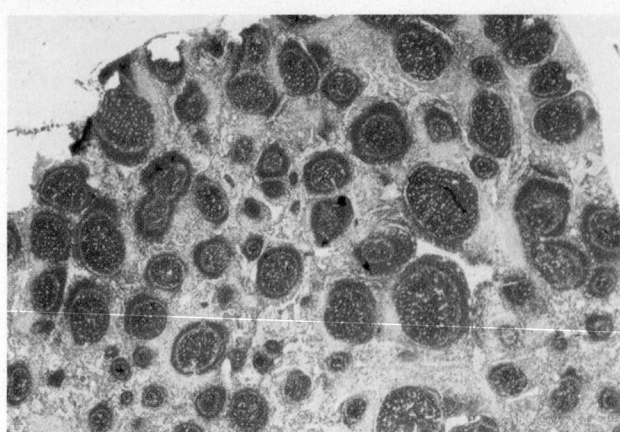

Figure 96–3. Same reactive lymph node as in Fig. 96–2 but stained with an antibody to CD20 (B-cell marker), showing B cells predominantly localized to the follicles.

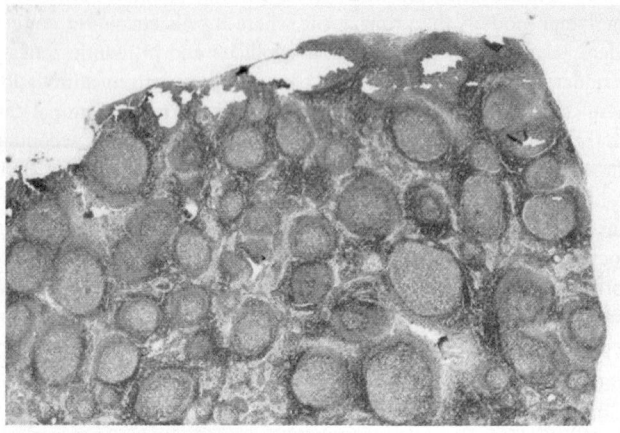

Figure 96–4. Same reactive lymph node as in Fig. 96–2 but stained with an antibody to CD3 (T-cell marker), showing T cells predominantly localized to the interfollicular areas.

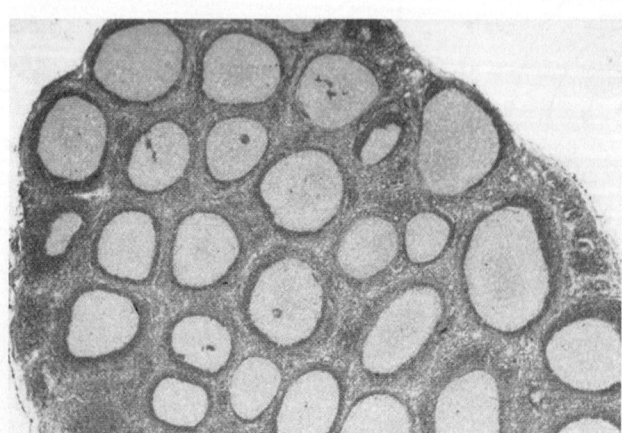

Figure 96–5. Same reactive lymph node as in Fig. 96–2 but stained with an antibody to the antiapoptotic protein BCL2. Note the negative staining of the germinal centers where most of the cells will die during the maturation process.

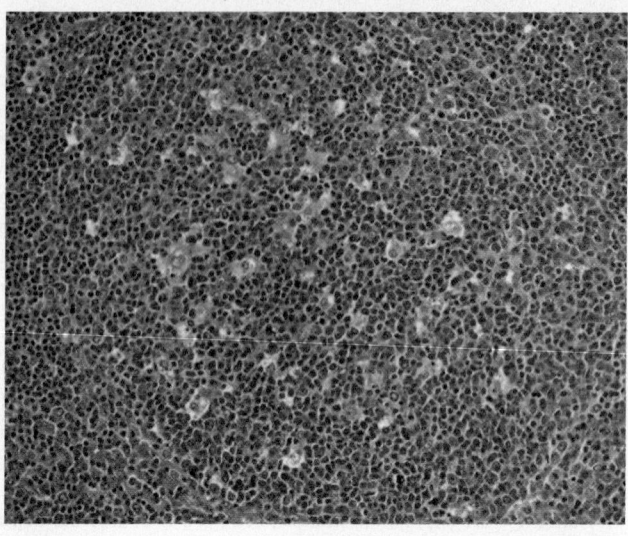

Figure 96–6. Reactive germinal center in a normal lymph node.

B-cell lymphomas can be correlated with these stages of development (Fig. 96–8) and are mentioned in the sections on separate lymphomas below.

● PRACTICAL CONSIDERATIONS IN THE DIAGNOSIS OF LYMPHOMA

Determining a benign from malignant lymphoid infiltrate often can be difficult because malignant lymphocytes in many lymphomas closely resemble their benign counterparts. Therefore, diagnosis commonly rests on demonstrating a combination of an abnormal architectural pattern, an abnormal immunophenotype, and evidence of lymphoid monoclonality. As a result, several ancillary special studies have become instrumental in the diagnosis and classification of lymphoma, requiring special handling of the biopsy material (Table 96–2). Whenever a diagnosis of lymphoma is considered clinically, the surgeon should perform

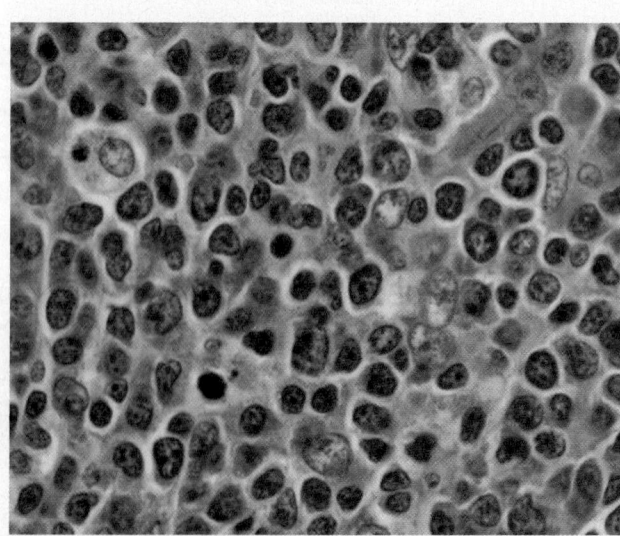

Figure 96–7. Spectrum of cells within the germinal center in a normal lymph node, ranging from small lymphocytes to larger cells with nucleoli.

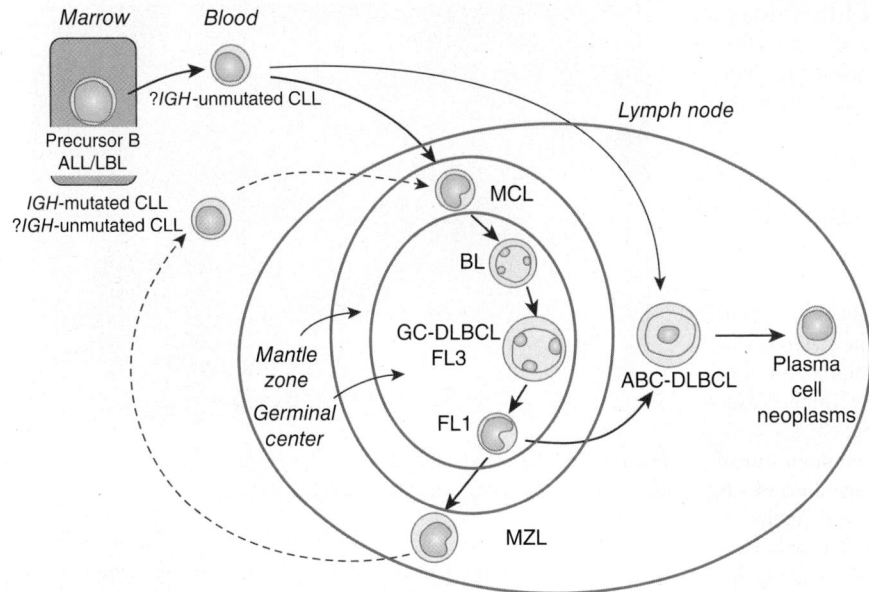

Figure 96–8. B-cell neoplasms correlate with different stages of development. ABC-DLBCL, activated B-cell type diffuse large B-cell lymphoma; ALL/LBL, acute lymphoblastic leukemia/lymphoblastic lymphoma; BL, Burkitt lymphoma; CLL, chronic lymphocytic leukemia; FL1, follicular lymphoma, grade 1; FL3, follicular lymphoma, grade 3; GC-DLBCL, germinal center type diffuse large B-cell lymphoma; MCL, mantle cell lymphoma; MZL, marginal zone lymphoma.

TABLE 96–2. Routine and Ancillary Studies for Lymphoma Diagnosis

Method	Applications	Type of Tissue Needed
Routine histology	Examination of routine sections will allow diagnosis of lymphoma in certain situations. In the remaining cases, the diagnosis will require the use of ancillary studies	Formalin-fixed
Immunohistochemistry	Immunophenotyping for lymphoma classification; can demonstrate B-cell clonality (light-chain restriction) and unique antigen expression in some cases	Formalin-fixed
Automated flow cytometry	Demonstration of B-cell clonality by surface immunoglobulin (Ig) light-chain restriction; immunophenotyping for lymphoma classification	Fresh tissue (single cell suspensions)
Polymerase chain reaction analysis	Demonstration of B- and T-cell clonality by Ig and T-cell receptor analyses; demonstration of lymphoma specific translocations (example: *BCL2* gene rearrangements)	Frozen tissue Can be performed on paraffin tissue, but may not yield amplifiable DNA in some cases
Cytogenetics	Demonstration of clonality; Demonstration of lymphoma-specific translocations	Sterile fresh tissue
Fluorescent *in situ* hybridization	Demonstration of lymphoma-specific translocations	Fresh tissue Can be performed on paraffin tissue, but yield is variable

an open biopsy of the largest involved lymph node. The lymph node should be removed intact whenever possible, because assessment of architecture is extremely important in the diagnosis and classification of lymphomas. The lymph node should be sent immediately to the pathology laboratory in the fresh state, at which time the pathologist allocates the tissue for fixation for routine histology and for special studies.

Automated flow cytometry on single-cell suspensions prepared from tissue samples is extremely helpful in demonstrating B-cell clonality by surface immunoglobulin light chain restriction. It also determines the expression pattern of surface markers helpful in subclassifying lymphomas, particularly lymphomas of small B cells.[17] A wide variety of antibodies that can be used on formalin-fixed tissue now are available, allowing accurate diagnosis and subclassification of lymphoma in most cases.

Molecular genetic techniques to determine B- or T-cell monoclonality or lymphoma-specific chromosomal translocations include polymerase chain reaction (PCR), Southern blot, fluorescence *in situ* hybridization (FISH), and cytogenetic analysis.[18] PCR and FISH can be performed on formalin-fixed tissue. Results from molecular genetic testing should be interpreted in conjunction with the morphologic and immunophenotypic data, as some benign reactive lymphoid proliferations show evidence of lymphoid monoclonality.[19]

The diagnosis of lymphoma has become more complex than the diagnosis of other malignancies because diagnosis of lymphoma rests on correlation of morphologic features with immunophenotype and genetic data in many cases. Because of the complexity of diagnosis and the relative infrequency of lymphoma in general pathology practice, a second review by a hematopathologist with expertise in lymphoma pathology is recommended. The second review can have a significant impact on the clinical management of patients.[20]

Whereas open biopsy of an involved lymph node is the most useful diagnostic procedure, core-needle biopsies and fine-needle aspiration can play a role in limited situations. Core-needle biopsy might be helpful in the diagnosis of deep-seated disease in the abdomen, allowing the patient to avoid a laparotomy. However, a definitive diagnosis by core biopsy is not always possible, necessitating an open biopsy. Fine-needle aspiration is not helpful in primary diagnosis of lymphoma,[21] but it may be helpful in detecting recurrence of a previously diagnosed lymphoma or in ruling out a nonhematolymphoid lesion causing lymphadenopathy. Although automated flow cytometry can be used in conjunction with cytologic examination to provide additional information for lymphoma diagnosis and classification, tissue biopsy generally is required before commencement of therapy.

● PRECURSOR B- AND T-CELL LYMPHOMAS/LEUKEMIAS

Lymphoblastic leukemia/lymphoma represents a malignancy of lymphoblasts, either of B or T lineage. They can present in the marrow (leukemia) or with predominant tissue involvement (lymphoma), but they are considered single-disease entities. Most cases of acute lymphoblastic leukemia are of B lineage, whereas most cases of lymphoblastic lymphoma are of T lineage, with the mediastinum being a common site of involvement. The morphologic features are the same regardless of site or lineage, consisting of small- to intermediate-size cells with finely dispersed nuclear chromatin, inconspicuous nucleoli, and scant cytoplasm (Fig. 96–9). Assessment of lineage and distinction from minimally differentiated acute myeloid leukemia require immunophenotypic data and may require molecular genetic analysis of B- and T-cell receptors. Lymphoblastic neoplasms are distinguished from other lymphomas by the expression of terminal deoxynucleotide transferase, which is specifically expressed at the lymphoblast stage of development.

The 2008 WHO classification includes several categories of B-lymphoblastic leukemia/lymphoma characterized by recurrent genetic abnormalities.[14] Many of these are associated with distinct clinical or pathologic features, have prognostic implications, or are considered biologically distinct entities.

● MATURE B-CELL NON-HODGKIN LYMPHOMAS

CHRONIC LYMPHOCYTIC LEUKEMIA/SMALL LYMPHOCYTIC LYMPHOMA

Chronic lymphocytic leukemia is a neoplasm of mature B lymphocytes characterized by blood and marrow involvement and commonly associated with lymph node involvement (Chap. 92). Small lymphocytic

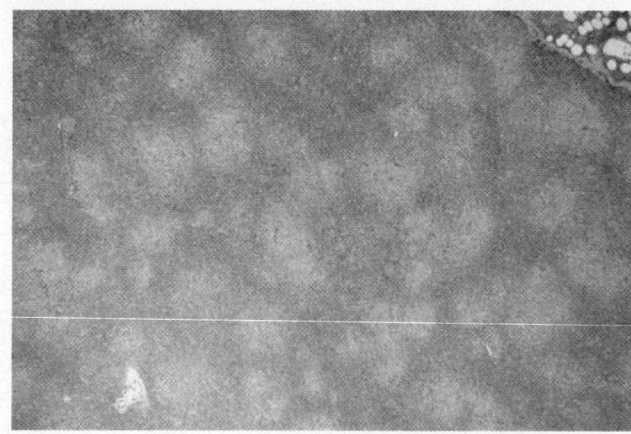

Figure 96–10. Small lymphocytic lymphoma with vague nodular appearance imparted by proliferation centers.

lymphoma is the nonleukemic form of the disease. Lymph nodes involved by chronic lymphocytic leukemia show a diffuse infiltrate of small mature lymphocytes admixed with prolymphocytes and paraimmunoblasts, which characteristically form ill-defined nodules known as *proliferation* or *growth centers* (Figs. 96–10 and 96–11). The B cells have a characteristic immunophenotype, demonstrating CD5 and CD23 expression and dim expression of CD20 and clonal immunoglobulin light chain. Studies have divided chronic lymphocytic leukemia into two distinct subtypes with distinct clinical behavior (Chap. 92). The type with the more favorable prognosis expresses mutated variable regions of the immunoglobulin heavy-chain (*IGH*) genes, whereas the other subtype expresses unmutated *IGH* genes. The *IGH* gene mutation status is reflected in differences in gene expression.[22,23] The gene encoding the zeta-associated protein of 70 kDa (ZAP-70) is one of these genes, which generally is expressed by leukemia cells that express unmutated *IGH* genes and hence can be used to discriminate between the two subtypes.[24] Certain cytogenetic abnormalities also correlate with clinical aggressiveness.[25]

Some cases of chronic lymphocytic leukemia/small lymphocytic lymphoma demonstrate plasmacytic features but are distinct from an entity known as *lymphoplasmacytic lymphoma*, which is characterized by a prominent component of plasmacytic lymphocytes and plasma

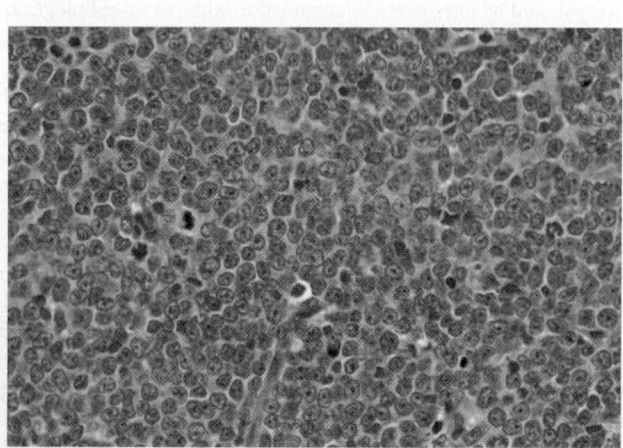

Figure 96–9. Lymphoblastic lymphoma of T-cell type, characterized by a diffuse proliferation of medium-size cells with finely distributed chromatin and high mitotic activity.

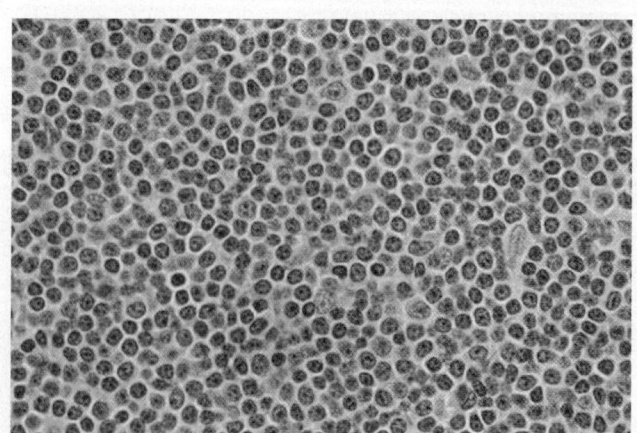

Figure 96–11. Small lymphocytic lymphoma, characterized by small lymphocytes with mature chromatin pattern. Note that individual lymphocytes in small lymphocytic lymphoma are morphologically indistinguishable from benign lymphocytes.

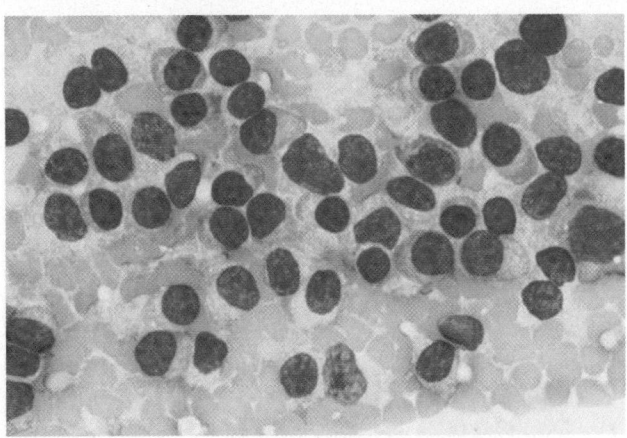

Figure 96–12. Imprint preparation of lymphoplasmacytic lymphoma demonstrating small lymphocytes and cells with plasmacytoid features (eccentric nuclei and bluish cytoplasm).

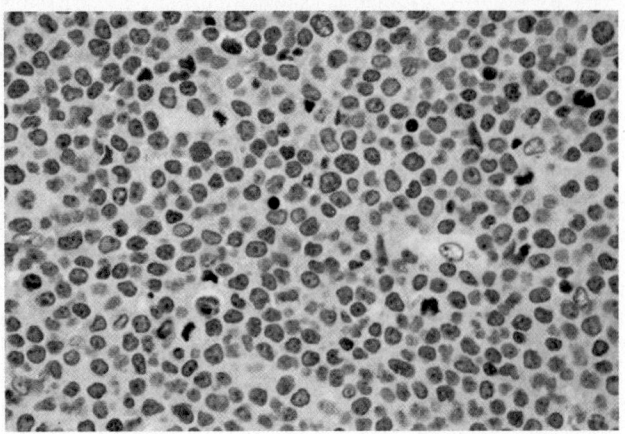

Figure 96–14. Mantle cell lymphoma with a diffuse pattern, characterized by a monomorphous infiltrate of small irregular lymphocytes with numerous mitotic figures.

cells (Fig. 96–12). These cases typically do not express CD5, less often involve blood, and often are associated with a monoclonal immunoglobulin M serum protein that can cause hyperviscosity or cryoglobulinemia (Waldenström macroglobulinemia). Somatic mutations in *MYD88* are a commonly recurring and highly specific feature of Waldenström macroglobulinemia.[26]

MANTLE CELL LYMPHOMA

Mantle cell lymphoma most commonly involves lymph nodes, but it can involve extranodal sites, including the gastrointestinal tract, as a clinical variant known as *lymphomatous polyposis* (Fig. 96–13). It typically is composed of a uniform population of small lymphocytes with cleaved nuclei and a virtual absence of large transformed cells (Fig. 96–14).[27,28] It most commonly has a diffuse growth pattern, but it can show a nodular or, more rarely, a mantle zone pattern (Fig. 96–15). The postulated cell of origin is the B cell of the inner mantle zone. The lymphoma cells coexpress CD5, as does chronic lymphocytic leukemia, but mantle cell lymphoma can be distinguished by lack of CD23 expression and expression of cyclin D1 (Fig. 96–16). Cyclin D1 expression results from the chromosomal translocation t(11;14)(q13;q32) characteristic of mantle cell lymphoma. Gene expression data have demonstrated a subset of mantle cell lymphomas that are cyclin D1–negative.[29] Some of these

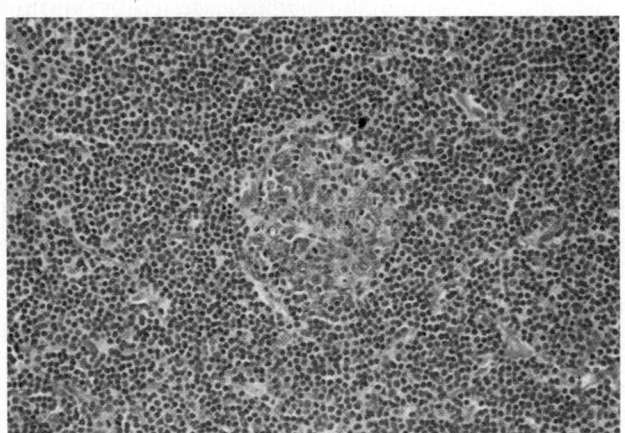

Figure 96–15. Mantle cell lymphoma with a mantle-zone pattern, characterized by monomorphous small lymphocytes surrounding a benign germinal center.

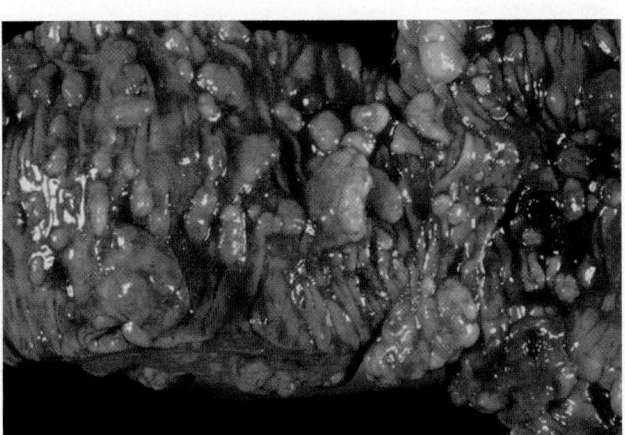

Figure 96–13. Large bowel involved with mantle cell lymphoma (multiple lymphomatous polyposis).

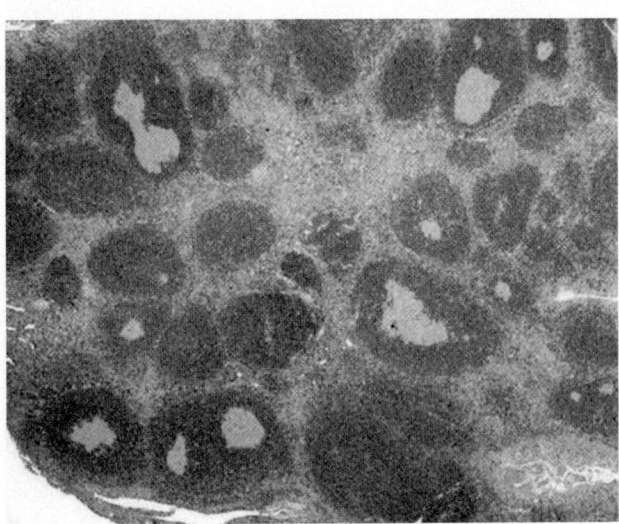

Figure 96–16. Mantle cell lymphoma with mantle-zone pattern stained with antibody to cyclin D1.

cyclin D1–negative cases have chromosomal translocations involving the cyclin D2 gene.[30] SOX11 expression is a highly specific immuno-histochemical marker for mantle cell lymphoma, and can identify cases that are negative for cyclin D1.[31] Overall, patients with mantle cell lymphoma have a median survival of approximately 3 years, but gene expression data that determine tumor cell proliferation are able to identify patient subsets that differ in median survival by more than 5 years[29] (Chap. 100).

Cyclin D1–positive lymphocytes in mantle zones can be an incidental finding in reactive lymphoid follicles, a condition referred to as *in situ* mantle cell lymphoma. These appear to have an indolent behavior and do not require treatment.[32]

FOLLICULAR LYMPHOMA

Follicular lymphoma is a proliferation of cells that correspond to normal germinal center cells,[33] retaining expression of germinal center markers (BCL6, CD10), and demonstrates a follicular architecture (Fig. 96–17) imparted by nodular aggregates of CD21-positive follicular dendritic cells. Follicular lymphomas are composed of a variable mixture of centrocytes (small cleaved cells) and centroblasts (large non-cleaved cells). They can be divided into three grades (grades 1 to 3) based on the number of centroblasts present. The most common is grade 1 (0–5 centroblasts per high-power microscopic field), previously known as *follicular small-cleaved-cell lymphoma* (Fig. 96–18). Both grade 1 and grade 2 tumors are indolent, and distinguishing between them is not required. Grade 3 follicular lymphoma (>15 centroblasts per high-power microscopic field) can be further divided into grade 3A (mixture of centroblasts and centrocytes) (Fig. 96–19) and grade 3B (solid sheets of centroblasts). Data have shown some molecular genetic differences between 3A and 3B cases, but further study is required because no significant clinical impact has been demonstrated.[34,35] Follicular lymphoma can have an accompanying diffuse component, and identification of a diffuse area of large cells (diffuse large B-cell lymphoma) indicates transformation to a more aggressive disease. Approximately 90 percent of follicular lymphoma demonstrate the t(14;18)(q32;q21) involving rearrangement of the *BCL2* gene, leading to the constitutive expression of the antiapoptotic BCL2 protein. Although BCL2 protein expression does not help distinguish follicular lymphoma from other lymphomas, it is a helpful feature in distinguishing it from reactive follicles that are BCL2-negative (Fig. 96–20).

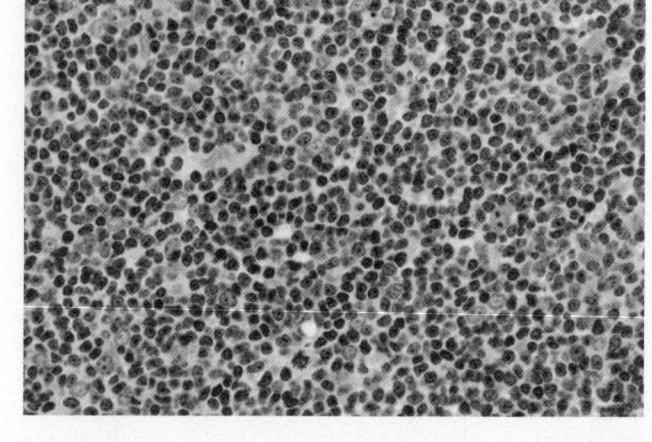

Figure 96–18. Center of a neoplastic follicle in grade 1 follicular lymphoma with almost exclusively small centrocytes.

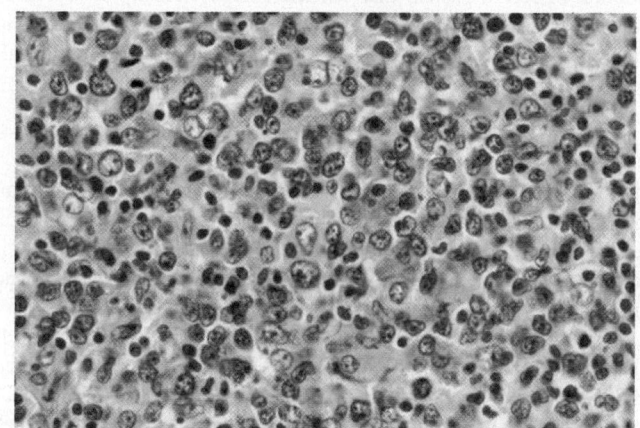

Figure 96–19. Grade 3A follicular lymphoma with >15 centroblasts per high-power field.

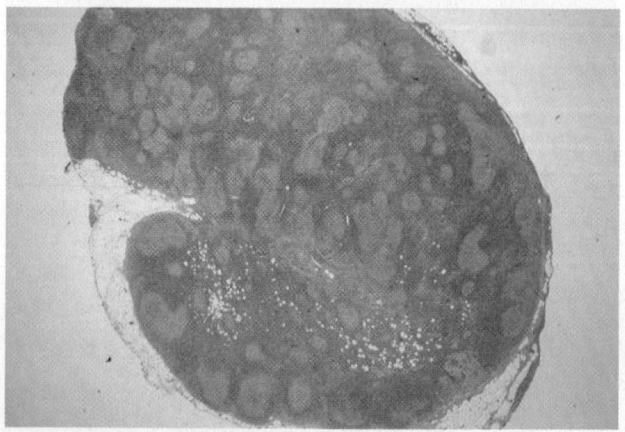

Figure 96–17. Grade 2 follicular lymphoma (low-power magnification), characterized by crowded follicles throughout the entire lymph node.

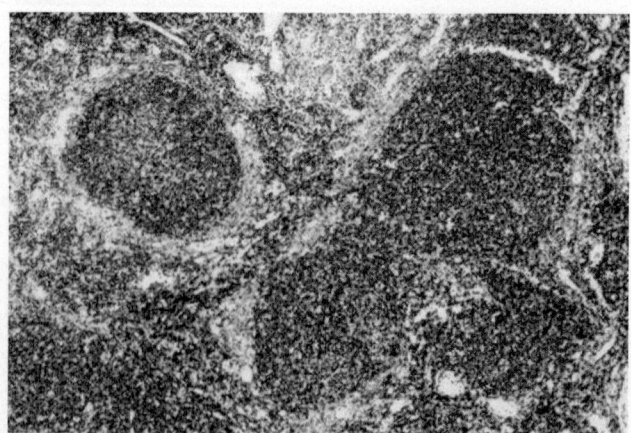

Figure 96–20. Positive BCL2 immunostain of a follicular lymphoma (contrast with Fig. 96–5).

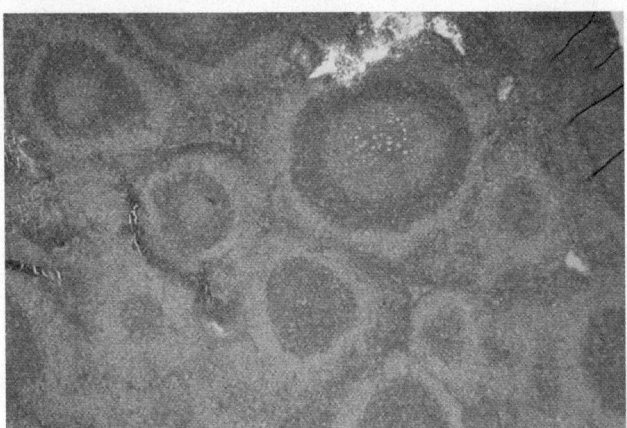

Figure 96–21. Lymph node involved by marginal zone B-cell lymphoma, in which the benign germinal centers and mantle zones are surrounded by expanded pale marginal zones.

Follicular lymphoma *in situ* is an entity where BCL2-positive germinal centers are present in an otherwise reactive lymph node. When it is distinguished from partial involvement by follicular lymphoma, follicular lymphoma *in situ* has a very low rate of progression to overt follicular lymphoma.[36]

MARGINAL ZONE B-CELL LYMPHOMAS

Marginal zone lymphomas are characterized by a proliferation of small lymphocytes, commonly with abundant pale cytoplasm (called *monocytoid B cells*) and plasmacytic features. The postulated cell of origin of these lymphomas is the postgerminal center B cell of the marginal zone at various anatomic sites. Marginal zone lymphomas can be divided into three distinct types based on site of presentation: (1) extranodal marginal zone lymphomas of mucosa-associated lymphoid tissue (MALT), (2) splenic marginal zone lymphomas,[37] and (3) nodal marginal zone lymphomas (Fig. 96–21).[38] This classification is supported by distinctive cytogenetic abnormalities in each entity. Extranodal lymphomas of the MALT type are the most common and arise in mucosal sites subject to longstanding chronic inflammation (Fig. 96–22), including chronic infection, the prototypical example being chronic *Helicobacter pylori*

infection of the stomach.[39] At early stages of development, many of these lymphomas respond to treatment with antibiotics to eradicate *H. pylori*, whereas later changes, including cases with chromosomal translocations activating genes involved in nuclear factor-κB (NF-κB) signaling,[40] lead to antigen-independent growth (Chap. 101).

DIFFUSE LARGE B-CELL LYMPHOMA

Diffuse large B-cell lymphoma (DLBCL) is characterized by a diffuse infiltrate of large B cells that can resemble centroblasts or immunoblasts (Figs. 96–23 and 96–24). The 2008 WHO classification identifies several types of large B-cell lymphoma, the most common type being DLBCL not otherwise specified, which constitutes 25 to 30 percent of all non-Hodgkin lymphomas.

Gene-expression data show that DLBCL is a heterogeneous disease consisting of at least three entities having distinct gene-expression profiles based on cell of origin: (1) cases with an expression profile similar to germinal center B cells (GCBs), (2) cases expressing genes typical of activated B cells (ABCs), and (3) cases with a different pattern referred to as "unclassifiable" that are neither GCB-type nor ABC-type (Fig. 96–25).[41] Importantly, clinical differences were apparent, with GCB-type cases having a significantly better prognosis compared to the other two types, even when clinical prognostic markers are considered (Chap. 98). Further studies confirmed these differences in the current era of therapy (including anti-CD20 antibody therapy), and identified

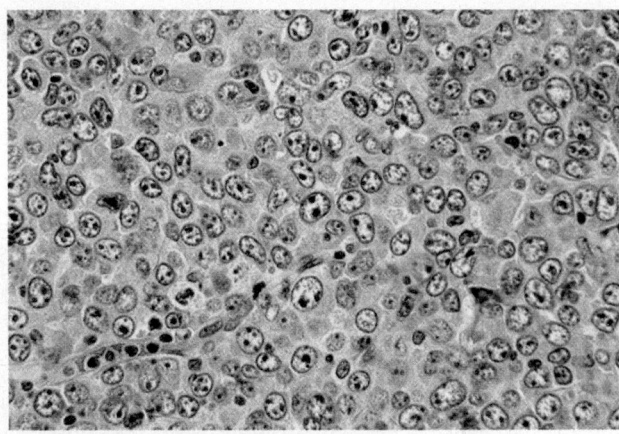

Figure 96–23. Diffuse large B-cell lymphoma.

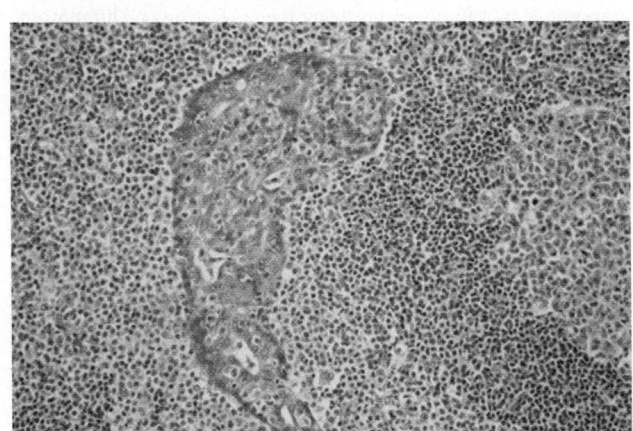

Figure 96–22. Salivary gland involved by mucosa-associated lymphoid tissue (MALT) lymphoma, showing a diffuse infiltrate of small lymphocytes with pale cytoplasm, infiltrating an enlarged salivary gland duct (lymphoepithelial lesion).

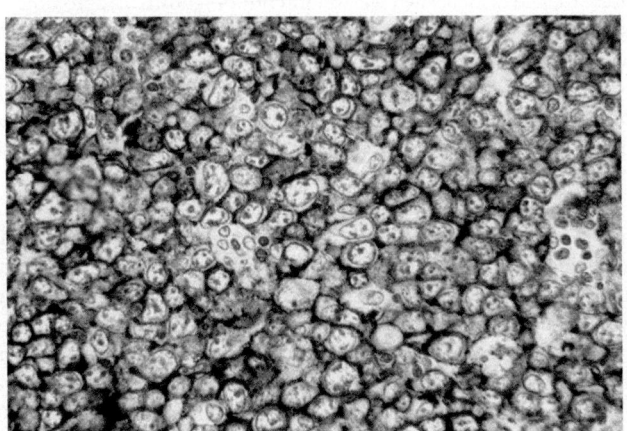

Figure 96–24. Diffuse large B-cell stained with antibody to CD20 (B-cell marker).

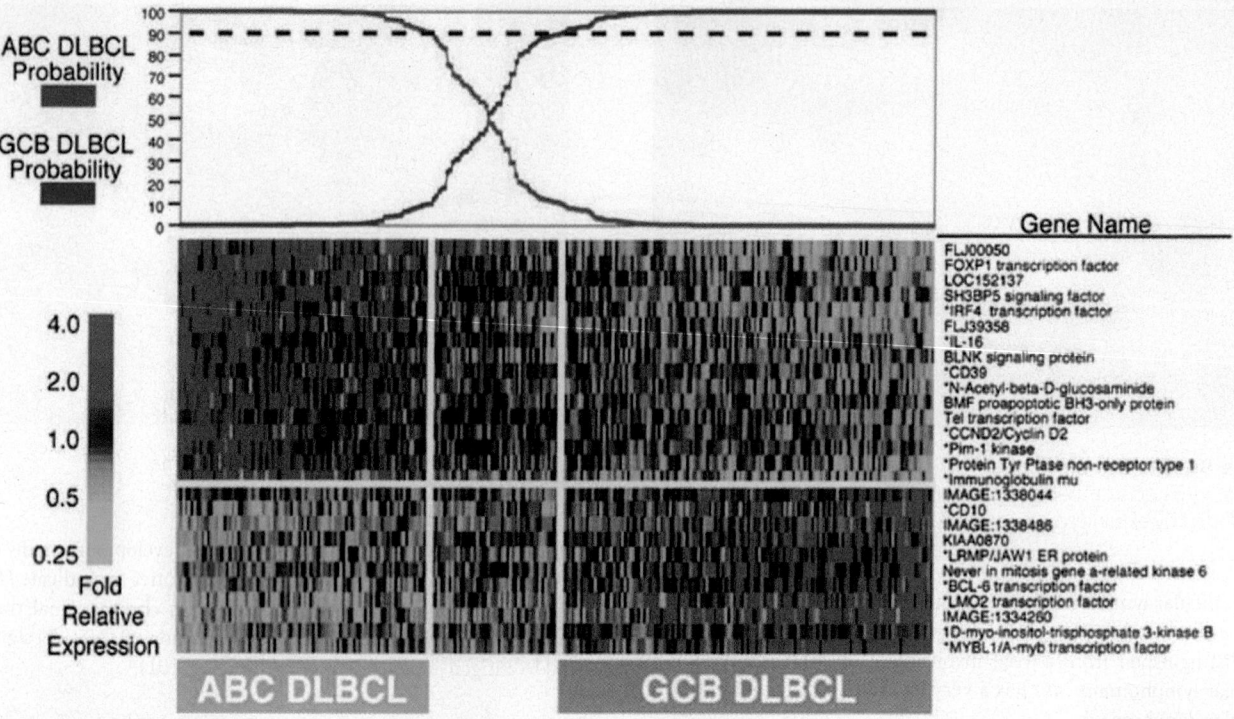

Figure 96–25. Gene-expression profiling diffuse large B-cell lymphoma (DLBCL), showing the subgroup discriminator used divide cases into germinal center B-cell–like (GCB) and activated B-cell–like (ABC). Each vertical column represents an individual patient and each horizontal row a unique gene. Red is relative overexpression of a gene and green relative underexpression. Using a probability of subgroup assignment of 90%, approximately 15% of cases are left unclassified (cases between the vertical yellow bars that are neither GCB or ABC). This approach allows one to analyze thousands of genes from a single patient in one experiment, and forms the basis of the new molecular classification of lymphoma. (*Reproduced with permission from Wright G, Tan B, Rosenwald A, et al: A gene expression-based method to diagnose clinically distinct subgroups of diffuse large B cell lymphoma,* Proc Natl Acad Sci U S A. *2003 Aug 19;100(17):9991–9996.*)

nonneoplastic cells in the microenvironment as important contributors to patient survival.[42] New therapies with selective activity in these subtypes of DLBCL are under development.[43] It has been suggested that division of DLBCL into clinically distinct groups may be determined by the expression profile of a limited number of genes using routine immunohistochemistry.[44] However, such an approach to classification is limited by problems of reproducibility of immunohistochemical staining and interpretation.[45] The study of gene expression patterns of a small number of genes using formalin-fixed paraffin-embedded material may provide a rapid and accurate method to classify DLBCL.[46]

Rearrangement of the *MYC* gene is present in 5 to 10 percent of DLBCLs, and is associated with an inferior prognosis.[47] Approximately half of these cases will also have a rearrangement involving the *BCL2* gene, referred to as a "double-hit" lymphoma. Such double-hit lymphomas have a very poor prognosis.[48] MYC protein expression is present in approximately 30 percent of DLBCLs, which may be independent of gene rearrangement. Concurrent expression of MYC and BCL2 in DLBCL is associated with an inferior prognosis.[49]

Mediastinal large B-cell lymphoma is a distinct subtype of DLBCL that has been separately identified in the WHO classification.[50] Patients with mediastinal lymphomas typically are younger than those with conventional DLBCL. The histology shows large cells with abundant cytoplasm associated with diffuse fibrosis (Fig. 96–26). Gene expression studies have demonstrated an expression profile that is distinct from conventional diffuse large B-cell lymphoma and shares some features with classic Hodgkin lymphoma (Fig. 96–27).[51,52] Indeed, the 2008 WHO classification recognizes that some cases of mediastinal lymphomas can have features that are intermediate between DLBCL and classical Hodgkin lymphoma.[14]

BURKITT LYMPHOMA

Burkitt lymphoma is a highly aggressive lymphoma characterized histologically by a diffuse infiltrate of intermediate-size cells with a high mitotic rate. The lymphomas commonly have significant spontaneous cell death (apoptosis), which results in a "starry sky" appearance caused by numerous macrophages that have engulfed the apoptotic debris (known as *tingible body macrophages*) (Figs. 96–28 and 96–29). The postulated cell of origin is the early follicular B blast cell of the germinal center. Virtually all cases of Burkitt lymphoma are characterized by chromosomal translocations involving the *MYC* gene on chromosome 8.

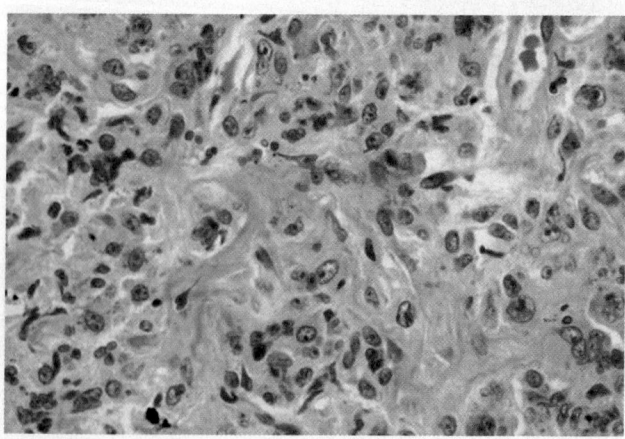

Figure 96–26. Primary mediastinal large B-cell lymphoma with sclerosis.

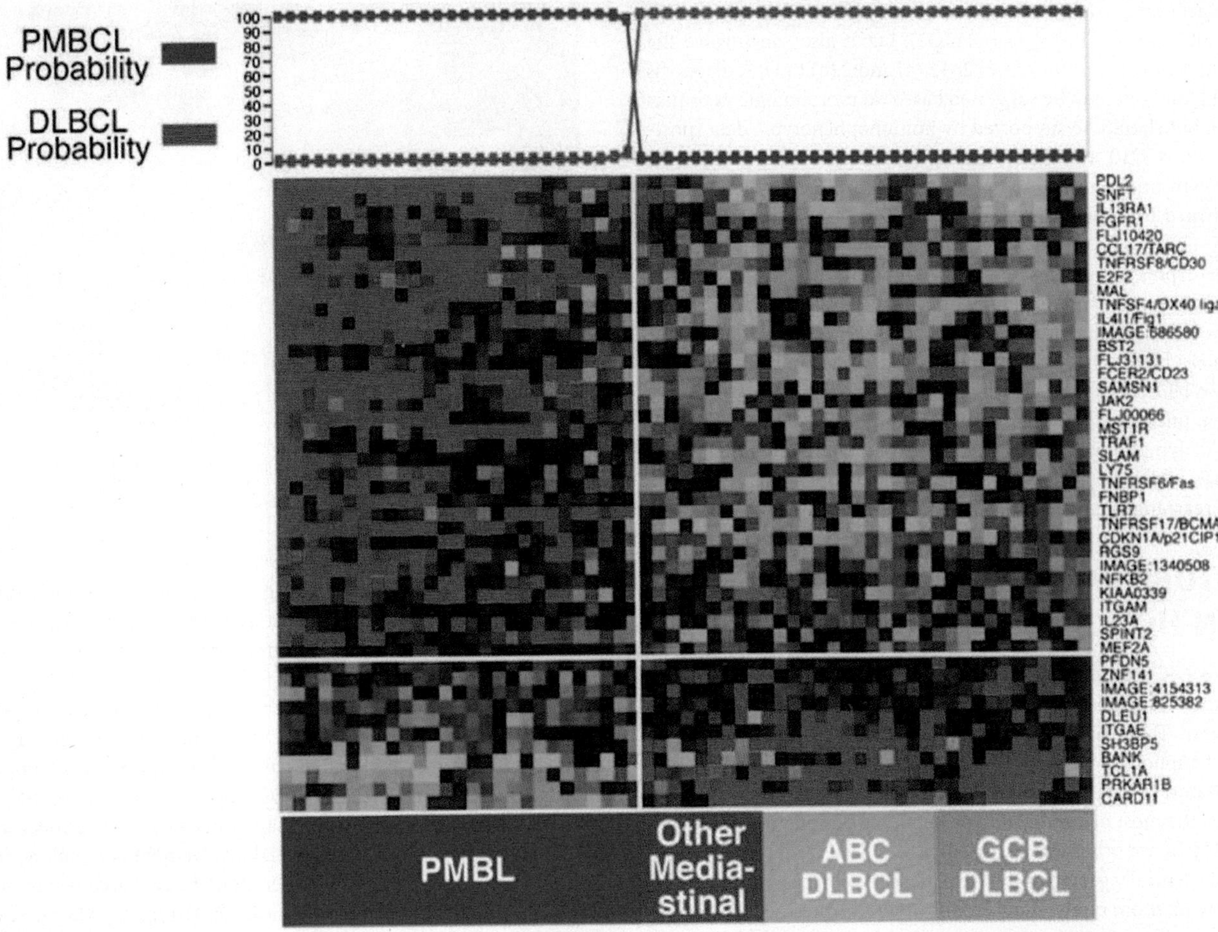

PMBCL Probability ▬

DLBCL Probability ▬

Figure 96–27. Gene-expression profiling of primary mediastinal large B-cell lymphoma (PMBCL), contrasting the expression profile with nodal diffuse large B-cell lymphomas (DLBCL). This figure shows numerous genes that are overexpressed in PMBCL *(red)*. Many of these genes are shared with classical Hodgkin lymphoma, suggesting a biologic overlap between these two diseases. Cases listed as "Other Mediastinal" refer to those cases of DLBCL with mediastinal involvement, but not felt to be typical of PMBCL. This is borne out by the gene-expression data, showing that these cases are more closely related to DLBCL rather than PMBCL. ABC, activated B cell; GCB, germinal center B cell. *(Reproduced with permission from Rosenwald A, Wright G, Leroy K, Yu X, et al: Molecular siagnosis of primary mediastinal B cell lymphoma identifies a clinically favorable subgroup of diffuse large B cell lymphoma related to Hodgkin Lymphoma. J Exp Med 15;198(6):851–862, 2003.)*

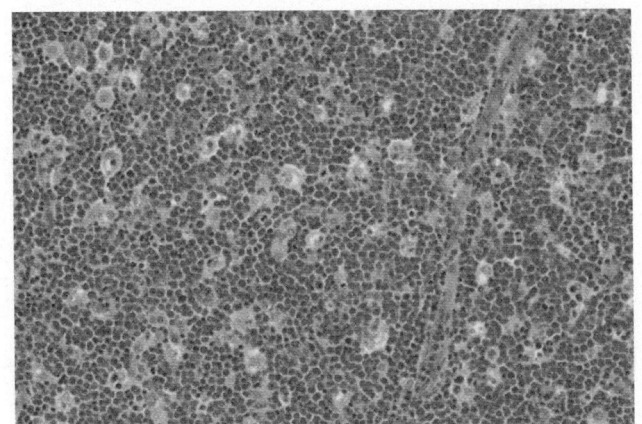

Figure 96–28. Burkitt lymphoma with starry-sky appearance, imparted by macrophages that have engulfed apoptotic debris of dying tumor cells.

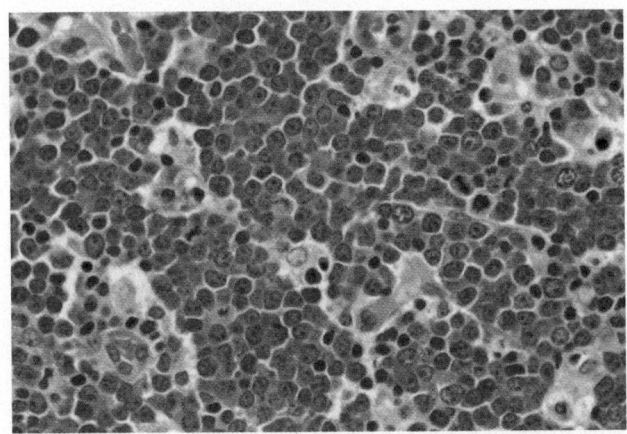

Figure 96–29. Burkitt lymphoma, characterized by a diffuse infiltrate of medium-size cells with small nucleoli and a high mitotic activity.

The *MYC* gene most commonly is translocated to the *IGH* gene on chromosome 14, resulting in t(8;14)(q24;q32), but it also can involve the light-chain genes on chromosomes 2p12 *(κ)* and 22q11 *(λ).* A diagnosis of Burkitt lymphoma can be suggested based on morphologic examination alone but should be supported by immunophenotypic data (positive for CD20, CD10, and BCL6; negative or focally weakly positive for BCL2; growth fraction near 100 percent as determined by Ki67 stain) and confirmed by molecular testing for *MYC* translocations whenever possible.

Gene-expression studies have shown that Burkitt lymphoma has a consistent gene-expression signature, but that there is not always correlation between the diagnosis based on gene-expression profiling and the diagnosis based on standard diagnostic testing.[53,54] To reflect this, the 2008 WHO classification recognizes a provisional entity of B-cell lymphoma, unclassifiable, with features intermediate between DLBCL and Burkitt lymphoma.[14] Many of these cases represent "double-hit" lymphomas, which carry a *MYC* gene rearrangement and another chromosomal rearrangement, often involving the *BCL2* gene.[48]

⬤ MATURE T-CELL AND NK CELL NON-HODGKIN LYMPHOMAS

T cells and NK cells share several immunophenotypic and functional features; therefore, these neoplasms are grouped together in the WHO classification. These lymphomas make up 10 to 15 percent of non-Hodgkin lymphomas in Western countries, with a higher incidence in Asia. Mature T-cell lymphomas comprise a heterogeneous group of neoplasms, the most common subtype being the peripheral T-cell lymphoma (PTCL) not otherwise specified.

PTCLs typically grow in a diffuse pattern that effaces normal nodal architecture or, more rarely, show expansion of the interfollicular areas. They show a diverse cytologic spectrum, with most cases showing a mixture of large- to intermediate-size cells and occasional cases showing predominantly small cells (Figs. 96–30 and 96–31). Cell type has no prognostic relevance. A reactive background consisting of eosinophils, plasma cells, and macrophages may be present, in which case the diagnosis of Hodgkin lymphoma may be entertained. Immunophenotypic data cannot prove clonality as in B-cell lymphomas, but evidence of an aberrant T-cell phenotype supports a diagnosis of T-cell lymphoma. Molecular techniques to demonstrate clonal rearrangement of T-cell receptor genes can be helpful in confirming the diagnosis. Gene-expression profiling has helped to delineate biologic and prognostic groups within

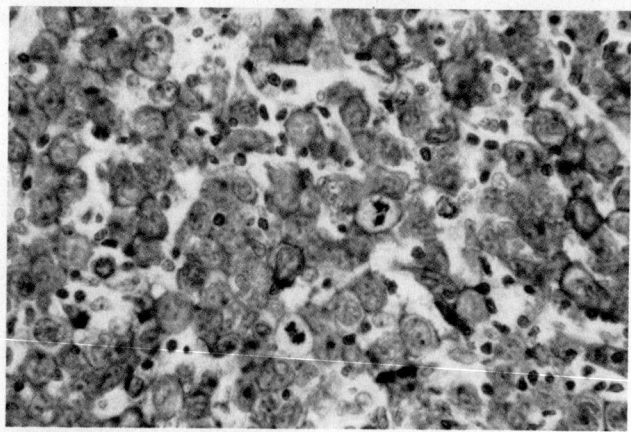

Figure 96–31. Peripheral T-cell lymphoma stained with antibody to CD3 (T-cell marker).

PTCL, not otherwise specified.[55] Angioimmunoblastic T-cell lymphoma is a mature T-cell lymphoma that typically presents with systemic symptoms and polyclonal hypergammaglobulinemia, and arises from a distinct subset of helper T cells, the follicular helper T cell.[56]

Anaplastic large cell lymphoma (ALCL) represents a unique subtype of T-cell lymphoma, particularly common in children. ALCL can show significant morphologic variability but typically is composed of large pleomorphic cells characterized by the presence of "hallmark" cells with horseshoe- or kidney-shaped nuclei and a perinuclear eosinophilic region (Fig. 96–32).[57] Partial involvement of lymph nodes can be limited to the sinuses, with obliteration of nodal architecture in later stages. ALCL is characterized by uniform, strong expression of CD30 (Fig. 96–33). The majority of cases express one or more T-cell antigens and demonstrate clonal T-cell receptor gene rearrangement.[57] ALCL is divided into two entities based on the expression of anaplastic lymphoma kinase (ALK) (Fig. 96–34). ALK-positive ALCL is most often seen in the first 3 decades of life and has a favorable prognosis compared to ALK-negative ALCL.[58,59] Expression of ALK is the result of chromosomal translocations involving the *ALK* gene on chromosome 2p23, the most common translocation being the t(2;5)(p23;q35) involving the nucleophosmin gene on chromosome 5.[60] ALK-negative ALCL is recognized as a provisional entity that is distinct from ALK-positive ALCL and PTCL, not otherwise specified.[61] Recently, additional genetic

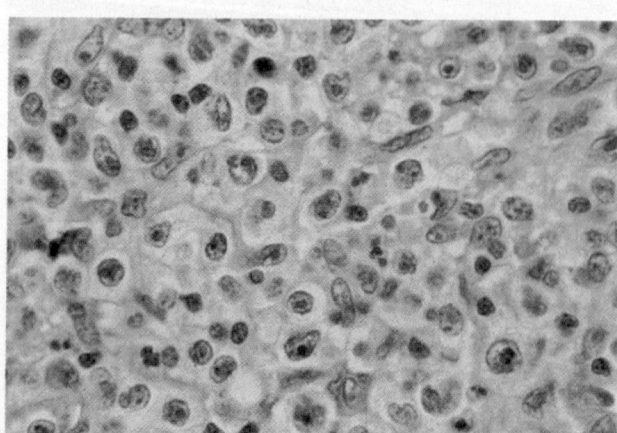

Figure 96–30. Peripheral T-cell lymphoma, unspecified, composed predominantly of large cells.

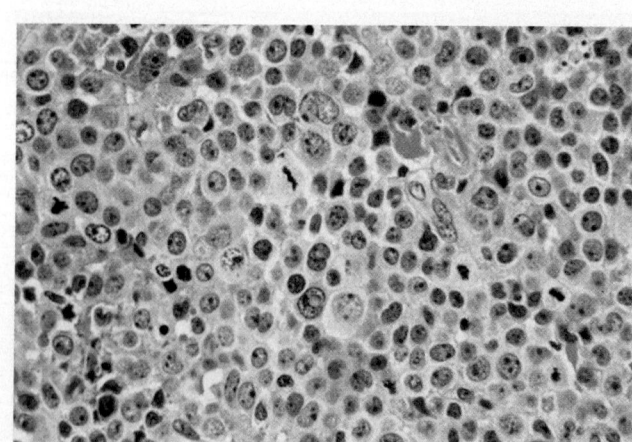

Figure 96–32. Anaplastic large cell lymphoma, T-cell type, containing a population of large cells with wreath-shaped nuclei and an eosinophilic perinuclear accentuation.

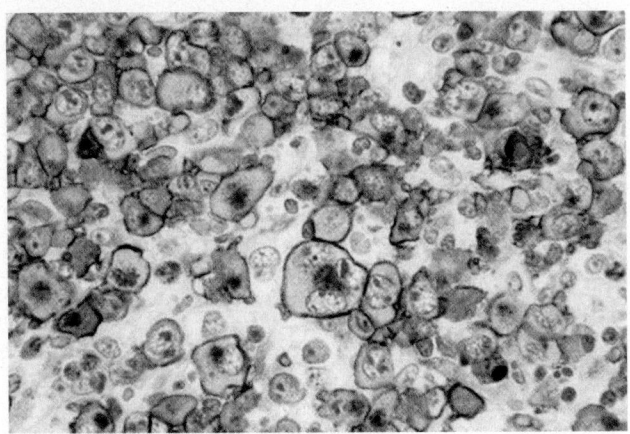

Figure 96–33. Anaplastic large cell lymphoma stained with antibody to CD30.

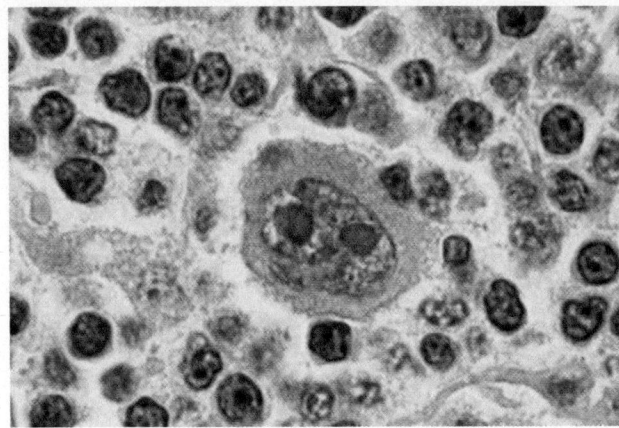

Figure 96–35. Diagnostic Reed-Sternberg cell in Hodgkin lymphoma.

abnormalities have been identified in ALK-negative ALCL, involving *DUSP22* and *TP63* genes.[62,63]

Other types of mature T/NK cell lymphomas are uncommon and include enteropathy-associated T-cell lymphoma (an aggressive T-cell lymphoma typically arising in the small bowel from a background of celiac disease) and extranodal NK/T-cell lymphoma, nasal type (an aggressive Epstein-Barr virus [EBV]-associated neoplasm commonly involving the nasal cavity). A detailed description of these specific lymphoma subtypes is beyond the scope of this chapter and can be found in the WHO classification.[14]

● HODGKIN LYMPHOMA

Hodgkin lymphoma consists of two distinct clinicopathologic entities: *classical Hodgkin lymphoma* (including four subtypes) and *nodular lymphocyte predominant Hodgkin lymphoma* (Chap. 97).

CLASSICAL HODGKIN LYMPHOMA

The neoplastic cell of classical Hodgkin lymphoma is the Reed-Sternberg cell, first described more than 100 years ago.[64,65] It is a large cell with two or more nuclei or nuclear lobes, each of which contains a large eosinophilic nucleolus (Fig. 96–35). The presence of Reed-Sternberg

cells alone is insufficient for a diagnosis of Hodgkin lymphoma, because cells with similar morphology can be seen in a variety of non-Hodgkin lymphomas and benign reactive conditions.[66] For a diagnosis of Hodgkin lymphoma, diagnostic Reed-Sternberg cells must be found in an appropriate background consisting of a variable polymorphous reactive infiltrate of inflammatory and accessory cells.[67]

Reed-Sternberg cells are derived from B cells in the vast majority of cases of classical Hodgkin lymphoma, as determined by clonal rearrangement of *IGH* genes.[68] However, Reed-Sternberg cells have lost most of their B-lineage antigens, including expression of immunoglobulin. Reed-Sternberg cells express CD30 in almost all cases of classical Hodgkin lymphoma and express CD15 in the majority (Figs. 96–36 and 96–37).[67] They typically are negative for CD45 (leukocyte common antigen) and positive for B-cell marker CD20 in 20 to 40 percent of cases, usually of variable intensity in a minority of cells. Classical Hodgkin lymphoma is associated with EBV in 20 to 40 percent of cases and is thought to play a role in the pathogenesis of these cases.[69] Reed-Sternberg cells express many cytokines and several members of the tumor necrosis factor receptor family (e.g., CD40, CD30).[70] The cytokines are thought to play a role in the recruitment of reactive infiltrate and to contribute to Reed-Sternberg cell proliferation and survival. The tumor necrosis factor receptor family members can be activated by ligands expressed by the surrounding reactive infiltrate, leading to proliferation and survival.

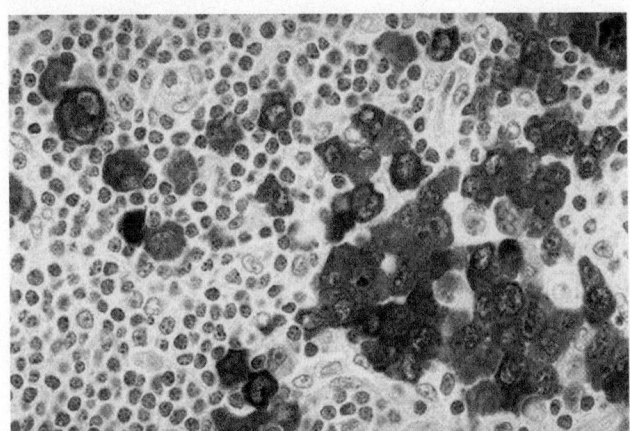

Figure 96–34. Anaplastic large cell lymphoma stained with antibody to ALK (anaplastic lymphoma kinase).

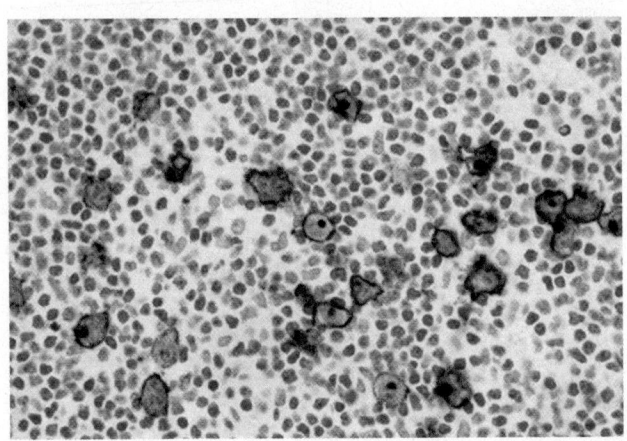

Figure 96–36. Classical Hodgkin lymphoma stained with antibody to CD30.

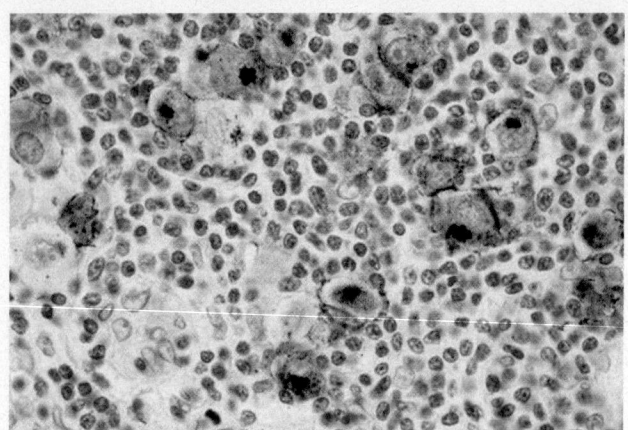

Figure 96–37. Classical Hodgkin lymphoma with Reed-Sternberg cells clearly identified with antibody to CD15.

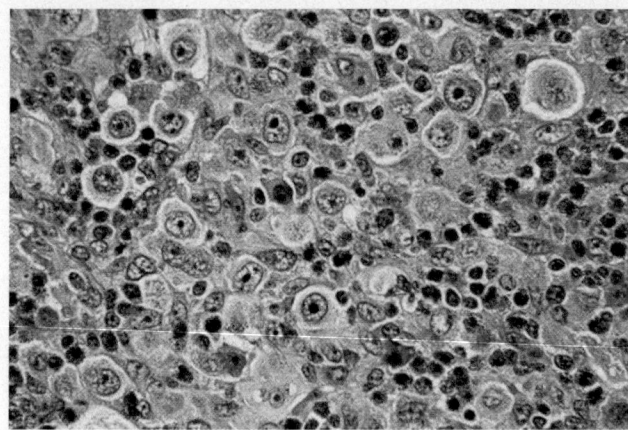

Figure 96–39. Mixed cellularity Hodgkin lymphoma.

The most common subtype of classical Hodgkin lymphoma is the nodular sclerosis variant. The variant is characterized by the presence of broad collagen bands dividing the tumor into nodules and by the presence of "lacunar" cells, mononuclear Reed-Sternberg variants that typically show retraction artifact so that the cells appear to be in lacunae (Fig. 96–38). These cells are found within a reactive infiltrate that typically includes prominent eosinophils and lymphocytes.

The second most common subtype is the mixed cellularity variant, which is characterized by Reed-Sternberg cells in a mixed inflammatory background without the broad collagen bands seen in nodular sclerosis (Fig. 96–39). Mixed cellularity cases are more commonly associated with EBV compared to the nodular sclerosis variant.

The lymphocyte-rich and lymphocyte-depleted subtypes of classical Hodgkin lymphoma are the least common, each representing approximately 5 percent of all cases. The lymphocyte-rich variant has a small number of Reed-Sternberg cells in a background of small lymphocytes with absent or rare eosinophils and neutrophils, typically in a nodular pattern. It is easily confused with nodular lymphocyte predominant Hodgkin lymphoma, so immunohistochemical stains to determine the immunophenotype of the Reed-Sternberg cells is required to make the distinction.[71,72] It can rarely have a diffuse growth pattern.

In the past, the lymphocyte-depleted variant had been divided into reticular and diffuse fibrosis types. The diffuse fibrosis variant is

characterized by a hypocellular infiltrate with prominent diffuse non-birefringent sclerosis accompanied by rare Reed-Sternberg cells and a minor reactive inflammatory component. The reticular variant showed an increased number of large atypical cells, commonly with bizarre multinucleated cells, with a minor reactive component. It now is recognized that the vast majority of these cases are cases of ALCL or DLBCL, and as such the diagnosis of the reticular variant of lymphocyte-depleted Hodgkin lymphoma is rare and should be made only in the presence of definitive supportive immunophenotypic data.

NODULAR LYMPHOCYTE PREDOMINANT HODGKIN LYMPHOMA

Nodular lymphocyte predominant Hodgkin lymphoma has several pathologic and clinical features that are distinct from classical Hodgkin lymphoma.[73] The malignant cells are known as lymphocyte predominant (LP) cells, large cells with a single nucleus that contains multilobated or folded features. They often are referred to as "popcorn" cells because they resemble popped kernels of corn (Fig. 96–40). Nucleoli typically are smaller than the nucleoli seen in classical Reed-Sternberg cells. They differ from Reed-Sternberg cells in classical Hodgkin lymphoma in that they retain expression of CD45 and B-lineage markers (CD20, immunoglobulin) and are negative for CD15 and CD30 (Fig. 96–41).[74] As the name implies, the cells have a complete or partial

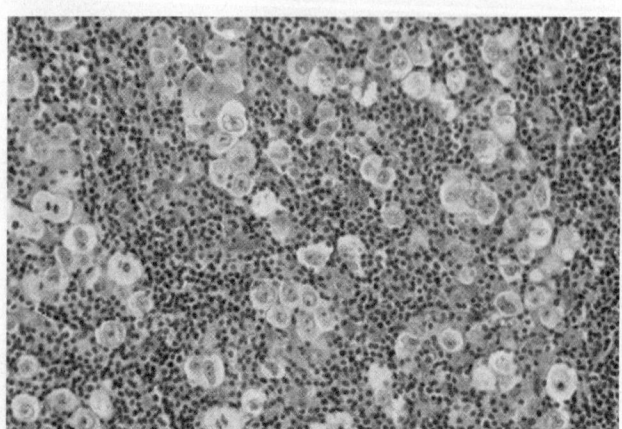

Figure 96–38. Classical Hodgkin lymphoma, nodular sclerosis type with characteristic lacunar cells.

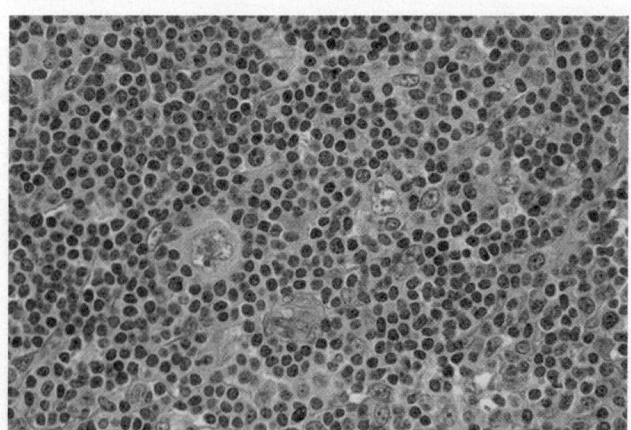

Figure 96–40. Nodular lymphocyte predominance Hodgkin lymphoma showing characteristic lymphocyte predominant (LP) cells (popcorn cells) in a background of small benign lymphocytes.

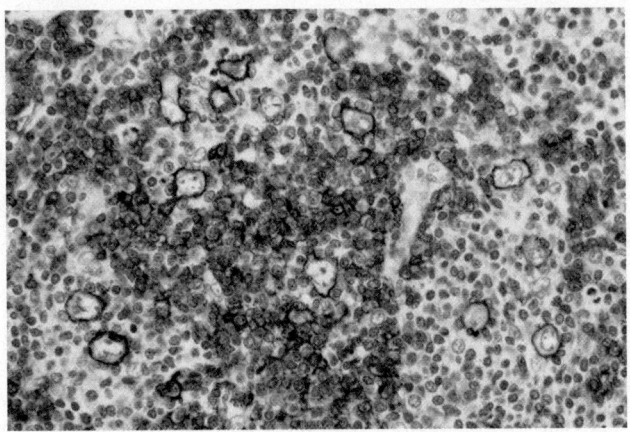

Figure 96–41. Nodular lymphocyte predominance Hodgkin lymphoma stained with antibody CD20. Note the positive staining of the lymphocyte predominant (LP) cells (popcorn cells).

nodular architectural pattern with a background consisting primarily of lymphocytes. Histiocytes are also a common feature, but neutrophils and eosinophils are absent or rare.

REFERENCES

1. Magrath IT: Historical perspective: The evolution of modern concepts of biology and management, in *The Non-Hodgkin's Lymphomas*, 2nd ed, edited by Magrath IT, p 47. Arnold, London, 1997.
2. Hodgkin T: On some morbid appearances of the absorbent glands and spleen. *Trans Med Soc Lond* 17:68, 1832.
3. Rappaport H, Winter W, Hicks E: Follicular lymphoma: A re-evaluation of its position in the scheme of malignant lymphoma, based on a survey of 253 cases. *Cancer* 9:792, 1956.
4. Rappaport H: *Tumors of the Hematopoietic System, Fasc 8.* Armed Forces Institute of Pathology, Washington, 1966.
5. Arnold A, Cossman J, Bakhshi A, et al: Immunoglobulin-gene rearrangements as unique clonal markers in human lymphoid neoplasms. *N Engl J Med* 309:1593, 1983.
6. Aisenberg AC, Krontiris TG, Mak TW, Wilkes BM: Rearrangement of the gene for the beta chain of the T-cell receptor in T-cell chronic lymphocytic leukemia and related disorders. *N Engl J Med* 313:529, 1985.
7. Gerard-Marchant R, Hamlin I, Lennert K, et al: Classification of non-Hodgkin's lymphoma. *Lancet* ii:406, 1974.
8. Lukes RJ, Collins RD: Immunologic characterization of human malignant lymphomas. *Cancer* 34(Suppl 4):1488, 1974.
9. Schein PS, Chabner BA, Canellos GP, et al: Potential for prolonged disease-free survival following combination chemotherapy of non-Hodgkin's lymphoma. *Blood* 43:181, 1974.
10. National Cancer Institute sponsored study of classifications of non-Hodgkin's lymphomas: Summary and description of a working formulation for clinical usage. The Non-Hodgkin's Lymphoma Pathologic Classification Project. *Cancer* 49:2112, 1982.
11. Stansfeld AG, Diebold J, Noel H, et al: Updated Kiel classification for lymphomas. *Lancet* 1:292, 1988.
12. Harris NL, Jaffe ES, Stein H, et al: A revised European-American classification of lymphoid neoplasms: A proposal from the International Lymphoma Study Group. *Blood* 84:1361, 1994.
13. A clinical evaluation of the International Lymphoma Study Group classification of non-Hodgkin's lymphoma. The Non-Hodgkin's Lymphoma Classification Project. *Blood* 89:3909, 1997.
14. Swerdlow SH, Campo E, Harris NL, et al: *WHO Classification of Tumours of Haematopoietic and Lymphoid Tissues*, 4th ed. IARC Press, Lyon, 2008.
15. Liang P, Pardee AB: Analyzing differential gene expression in cancer. *Nat Rev Cancer* 3:869, 2003.
16. MacLennan IC: Germinal centers. *Annu Rev Immunol* 12:117, 1994.
17. Jennings CD, Foon KA: Recent advances in flow cytometry: Application to the diagnosis of hematologic malignancy. *Blood* 90:2863, 1997.
18. Mauvieux L, Macintyre EA: Practical role of molecular diagnostics in non-Hodgkin's lymphomas. *Baillieres Clin Haematol* 9:653, 1996.
19. Collins RD: Is clonality equivalent to malignancy: Specifically, is immunoglobulin gene rearrangement diagnostic of malignant lymphoma? *Hum Pathol* 28:757, 1997.
20. Lester JF, Dojcinov SD, Attanoos RL, et al: The clinical impact of expert pathological review on lymphoma management: A regional experience. *Br J Haematol* 123:463, 2003.
21. Hajdu SI, Melamed MR: Limitations of aspiration cytology in the diagnosis of primary neoplasms. *Acta Cytol* 28:337, 1984.
22. Klein U, Tu Y, Stolovitzky GA, et al: Gene expression profiling of B cell chronic lymphocytic leukemia reveals a homogeneous phenotype related to memory B cells. *J Exp Med* 194:1625, 2001.
23. Rosenwald A, Alizadeh AA, Widhopf G, et al: Relation of gene expression phenotype to immunoglobulin mutation genotype in B cell chronic lymphocytic leukemia. *J Exp Med* 194:1639, 2001.
24. Wiestner A, Rosenwald A, Barry TS, et al: ZAP-70 expression identifies a chronic lymphocytic leukemia subtype with unmutated immunoglobulin genes, inferior clinical outcome, and distinct gene expression profile. *Blood* 101:4944, 2003.
25. Dohner H, Stilgenbauer S, Benner A, et al: Genomic aberrations and survival in chronic lymphocytic leukemia. *N Engl J Med* 343:1910, 2000.
26. Treon SP, Lian X, Yang G, et al: MYD88 L265P somatic mutation in Waldenström's macroglobulinemia. *N Engl J Med* 367:826, 2012.
27. Weisenburger DD, Armitage JO: Mantle cell lymphoma: An entity comes of age. *Blood* 87:4483, 1996.
28. Argatoff LH, Connors JM, Klasa RJ, et al: Mantle cell lymphoma: A clinicopathologic study of 80 cases. *Blood* 89:2067, 1997.
29. Rosenwald A, Wright G, Wiestner A, et al: The proliferation gene expression signature is a quantitative integrator of oncogenic events that predicts survival in mantle cell lymphoma. *Cancer Cell* 3:185, 2003.
30. Gesk S, Klapper W, Martin-Subero JI, et al: A chromosomal translocation in cyclin D1-negative/cyclin D2-positive mantle cell lymphoma fuses the CCND2 gene to the IGK locus. *Blood* 108:1109, 2006.
31. Mozos A, Royo C, Hartmann E, et al: SOX11 expression is highly specific for mantle cell lymphoma and identifies the cyclin D1-negative subtype. *Haematologica* 94:1555, 2009.
32. Carvajal-Cuenca A, Sua LF, Silva NM, et al: *In situ* mantle cell lymphoma: clinical implications of an incidental finding with indolent clinical behavior. *Haematologica* 97:270, 2012.
33. Jaffe ES, Shevach EM, Frank MM, et al: Nodular lymphoma: Evidence for origin from follicular B lymphocytes. *N Engl J Med* 290:813, 1974.
34. Bosga-Bouwer AG, van Imhoff GW, Boonstra R, et al: Follicular lymphoma grade 3B includes 3 cytogenetically defined subgroups with primary t(14;18) 3q27, or other translocations: t(14;18) and 3q27 are mutually exclusive. *Blood* 101:1149, 2003.
35. Ott G, Katzenberger T, Lohr A, et al: Cytomorphologic, immunohistochemical, and cytogenetic profiles of follicular lymphoma: 2 types of follicular lymphoma grade 3. *Blood* 99:3806, 2002.
36. Jegalian AG, Eberle FC, Pack SD, et al: Follicular lymphoma *in situ*: Clinical implications and comparisons with partial involvement by follicular lymphoma. *Blood* 118; 2976, 2011.
37. Thieblemont C, Felman P, Callet-Bauchu E, et al: Splenic marginal zone lymphoma: A distinct clinical and pathological entity. *Lancet Oncol* 4:95, 2003.
38. Nathwani BN, Drachenberg MR, Hernandez AM, et al: Nodal monocytoid B-cell lymphoma (nodal marginal-zone B-cell lymphoma). *Semin Hematol* 36:128, 1999.
39. Zucca E, Bertoni F, Roggero E, Cavalli F: The gastric marginal zone B cell lymphoma of MALT type. *Blood* 96:410, 2000.
40. Bertoni F, Cotter FE, Zucca E: Molecular genetics of extranodal marginal zone (MALT-type) B-cell lymphoma. *Leuk Lymphoma* 35:57, 1999.
41. Rosenwald A, Wright G, Chan WC, et al: The use of molecular profiling to predict survival after chemotherapy for diffuse large-B-cell lymphoma. *N Engl J Med* 346:1937, 2002.
42. Lenz G, Wright G, Dave SS, et al: Stromal gene signatures in large-B-cell lymphomas. *N Engl J Med* 359:2313, 2008.
43. Barton S, Hawkes EA, Wotherspoon A, Cunningham D: Are we ready to stratify treatment for diffuse large B-cell lymphoma using molecular hallmarks? *Oncologist* 17:1562, 2012.
44. Choi WWL, Weisenburger DD, Greiner TC, et al: A new immunostain algorithm classifies diffuse large B-cell lymphoma into molecular subtypes with high accuracy. *Clin Cancer Res* 15:5494, 2009.
45. De Jong D, Rosenwald A, Chhanabhai M, et al: Immunohistochemical prognostic markers in diffuse large B-cell lymphoma: Validation of tissue microarray as a prerequisite for broad clinical applications—A study from the Lunenburg Lymphoma Biomarker Consortium. *J Clin Oncol* 25:805, 2007.
46. Scott DW, Wright GW, Williams PM, et al: Determining cell-of-origin subtypes of diffuse large B-cell lymphoma using gene expression in formalin-fixed paraffin-embedded tissue. *Blood* 123:1214, 2014.
47. Savage KJ, Johnson NA, Ben-Neriah S, et al: *MYC* gene rearrangements are associated with a poor prognosis in diffuse large B cell lymphoma patients treated with R-CHOP chemotherapy. *Blood* 114:3533, 2009.
48. Aukema SM, Siebert R, Schuuring E, et al: Double-hit B-cell lymphomas. *Blood* 117:2319, 2011.
49. Johnson NA, Slack GW, Savage KS, et al: Concurrent expression of MYC and BCL2 in diffuse large B-cell lymphoma treated with rituximab plus cyclophosphamide, doxorubicin, vincristine, and prednisone. *J Clin Oncol* 30: 3452, 2012.
50. van Besien K, Kelta M, Bahaguna P: Primary mediastinal B-cell lymphoma: A review of pathology and management. *J Clin Oncol* 19:1855, 2001.
51. Rosenwald A, Wright G, Leroy K, et al: Molecular diagnosis of primary mediastinal B cell lymphoma identifies a clinically favorable subgroup of diffuse large B cell lymphoma related to Hodgkin lymphoma. *J Exp Med* 198:851, 2003.

52. Savage KJ, Monti S, Kutok JL, et al: The molecular signature of mediastinal large B-cell lymphoma differs from that of other diffuse large B-cell lymphomas and shares features with classical Hodgkin lymphoma. *Blood* 102:3871, 2003.

53. Dave SS, Fu K, Wright GW, et al: Molecular diagnosis of Burkitt's lymphoma. *N Engl J Med* 354:2431, 2006.

54. Hummel M, Bentink S, Berger H, et al: A biologic definition of Burkitt's lymphoma from transcriptional and genomic profiling. *N Engl J Med* 354:2419, 2006.

55. Iqbal J, Wright G, Wang C, et al: Gene expression signatures delineate biological and prognostic subgroups in peripheral T-cell lymphoma. *Blood* 123:2915, 2014.

56. Gaulard P, de Leval L. Follicular helper T cells: implications in neoplastic hematopathology. *Semin Diagn Pathol* 28:202, 2011.

57. Stein H, Foss HD, Durkop H, et al: CD30(+) anaplastic large cell lymphoma: A review of its histopathologic, genetic, and clinical features. *Blood* 96:3681, 2000.

58. Gascoyne RD, Aoun P, Wu D, et al: Prognostic significance of anaplastic lymphoma kinase (ALK) protein expression in adults with anaplastic large cell lymphoma. *Blood* 93:3913, 1999.

59. Benharroch D, Meguerian-Bedoyan Z, Lamant L, et al: ALK-positive lymphoma: A single disease with a broad spectrum of morphology. *Blood* 91:2076, 1998.

60. Duyster J, Bai RY, Morris SW: Translocations involving anaplastic lymphoma kinase (ALK). *Oncogene* 20:5623, 2001.

61. Savage KJ, Harris NL, Vose JM, et al: ALK-negative anaplastic large cell lymphoma (ALCL) is clinically and immunophenotypically different from both ALK-positive ALCL and peripheral T cell lymphoma, not otherwise specified: Report from the International Peripheral T-cell Lymphoma Project. *Blood* 111:5496, 2008.

62. Feldman AL, Dogan A, Smith DI, et al: Discovery of recurrent t(6;7)(p25.3;q32.3) translocations in ALK-negative anaplastic large cell lymphomas by massively parallel genomic sequencing. *Blood* 117:915, 2011.

63. Vasmatzis G, Johnson SH, Knudson RA, et al: Genome-wide analysis reveals recurrent structural abnormalities of *TP63* and other p53-related genes in peripheral T-cell lymphomas. *Blood* 120:2280, 2012.

64. Sternberg C: Uber eine Eigenartige unter dem Bilde der Pseudoleukamie verlaufende Tuberculose des lymphatischen Apparates. *Z Heilk* 19:21, 1898.

65. Reed DM: On the pathologic changes in Hodgkin's disease, with especial reference to its relation to tuberculosis. *Johns Hopkins Hosp Rep* 10:133, 1902.

66. Strum SB, Park JK, Rappaport H: Observation of cells resembling Sternberg-Reed cells in conditions other than Hodgkin's disease. *Cancer* 26:176, 1970.

67. Harris NL: Hodgkin's disease: Classification and differential diagnosis. *Mod Pathol* 12:159, 1999.

68. Kuppers R, Rajewsky K: The origin of Hodgkin and Reed/Sternberg cells in Hodgkin's disease. *Annu Rev Immunol* 16:471, 1998.

69. Jarrett RF, MacKenzie J: Epstein-Barr virus and other candidate viruses in the pathogenesis of Hodgkin's disease. *Semin Hematol* 36:260, 1999.

70. Skinnider BF, Mak TW: The role of cytokines in classical Hodgkin lymphoma. *Blood* 99:4283, 2002.

71. von Wasielewski R, Werner M, Fischer R, et al: Lymphocyte-predominant Hodgkin's disease. An immunohistochemical analysis of 208 reviewed Hodgkin's disease cases from the German Hodgkin Study Group. *Am J Pathol* 150:793, 1997.

72. Anagnostopoulos I, Hansmann ML, Franssila K, et al: European Task Force on Lymphoma project on lymphocyte predominance Hodgkin disease: Histologic and immunohistologic analysis of submitted cases reveals 2 types of Hodgkin disease with a nodular growth pattern and abundant lymphocytes. *Blood* 96:1889, 2000.

73. Mason DY, Banks PM, Chan J, et al: Nodular lymphocyte predominance Hodgkin's disease. A distinct clinicopathological entity. *Am J Surg Pathol* 18:526, 1994.

74. Chan WC: Cellular origin of nodular lymphocyte-predominant Hodgkin's lymphoma: Immunophenotypic and molecular studies. *Semin Hematol* 36:242, 1999.

CHAPTER 97
HODGKIN LYMPHOMA

Oliver W. Press*

SUMMARY

Classical Hodgkin lymphoma is derived by malignant transformation of a mature B cell at the germinal center stage of differentiation and is characterized pathologically by multinucleated Hodgkin and Reed-Sternberg cells embedded in a mixed infiltrate of nonneoplastic cells. Hodgkin and Reed-Sternberg cells contain monoclonal immunoglobulin gene rearrangements, but have lost most of the B-cell–specific expression program. Multiple signaling pathways and transcription factors are deregulated in Hodgkin lymphoma and genetic lesions involving the JAK-STAT and nuclear factor-κB pathways are commonly identified. Epstein-Barr virus is an important environmental factor in the pathogenesis of Hodgkin lymphoma, and also leads to activation of the nuclear factor-κB pathway. The inflammatory microenvironment promotes survival and allows escape of Hodgkin and Reed-Sternberg cells from immune attack. Morphologic and immunophenotypic features distinguish the four subtypes of classical Hodgkin lymphoma (accounting for 95 percent of cases) from nodular lymphocyte predominance Hodgkin lymphoma (accounting for 5 percent of cases). Hodgkin lymphoma spreads in a predictable, contiguous manner and is classified into four stages, I to IV. Hodgkin lymphoma is treated with the intent to cure the disease in all stages, and long-term survival exceeds 85 percent. Doxorubicin-containing chemotherapy plays a major role in treatment of all stages of the disease whereas radiotherapy is used selectively because of concerns for late toxicities. 18-Fluorodeoxyglucose positron emission tomography is a valuable diagnostic test for assessment of disease extent and response to treatment. High-dose therapy and autologous transplantation are effective in patients who have relapsed, and several promising new biologic agents are available, including brentuximab vedotin (an anti-CD30 antibody–drug conjugate) and nivolumab (an anti-PD1 blocking antibody). Concerns regarding late treatment effects guide therapy and followup decisions in Hodgkin lymphoma, which disproportionately affects adolescents and young adults. Major treatment challenges include the maintenance of high cure rates with fewer short-term and long-term complications, biomarker identification of the small refractory subgroup, and integration of biologic therapies into treatment paradigms.

DEFINITION AND HISTORY

Classical Hodgkin lymphoma (cHL) is a neoplasm of lymphoid tissue, in most cases derived from a germinal center B cell, defined by the presence of the malignant Hodgkin and Reed-Sternberg cells with a characteristic immunophenotype and appropriate cellular background. cHL accounts for 95 percent of cases and contains four histologic subtypes distinguished on the basis of microscopic appearance and relative proportions of Hodgkin and Reed-Sternberg cells, lymphocytes, and fibrosis (nodular sclerosis, mixed cellularity, lymphocyte-rich and lymphocyte-depleted; Table 97–1). Nodular lymphocyte-predominant Hodgkin lymphoma (NLPHL) represents the other major category, which is distinguished by Hodgkin and Reed-Sternberg variants termed *lymphocytic and histiocytic cells* that, unlike cHL, express typical B-lineage markers.

HISTORICAL ASPECTS

In his historic 1832 paper entitled *On Some Morbid Appearances of the Absorbent Glands and Spleen*, Thomas Hodgkin described the clinical histories and gross postmortem findings of seven cases of the disease that was later to bear his name.[1] In 1856, Samuel Wilks independently described 10 cases of "a peculiar enlargement of the lymphatic glands frequently associated with disease of the spleen," including four of Hodgkin's original cases.[2] Upon discovering Hodgkin's original report, he used the appellation "Hodgkin's Disease" in a subsequent series of 15 cases published in 1865.[2] Thirteen years after Hodgkin's original paper, the first cases of leukemia were described. Cases in which the neoplastic cells remained confined to the lymphatic system were described by Dreschfield (1892)[3] and Kundrat (1893)[4]; Kundrat gave the name *lymphosarcoma* to these cases. The description of additional members of the lymphoma–leukemia complex continued up to the present time.

Carl Sternberg (1898)[5] and Dorothy Reed (1902)[6] are credited with the first definitive and thorough descriptions of the pathology of cHL, although a number of investigators from England, Germany, and France had previously recognized the characteristic multinucleated giant cells. In 1926, Fox examined microscopic sections from the gross specimens preserved in the Gordon Museum of Guy's Hospital in London of three of Hodgkin's original cases.[7] It is remarkable that the preserved microanatomy allowed him to confirm the histopathologic diagnosis in two of these cases. Jackson and Parker made the first serious effort at the histopathologic classification of cHL, correlating their

*Sandra J. Horning, MD, was the author of this chapter for the 8th edition of *Williams Hematology* and significant portions of that chapter have been retained.

TABLE 97-1. Classification of Hodgkin Lymphoma

Histologic Subtype	Immunophenotype
Nodular lymphocyte-predominant	CD20+ CD30– CD15– Ig+
Classical	CD20–* CD30+ CD15+ Ig–
Nodular sclerosis	
Mixed cellularity	
Lymphocyte-rich	
Lymphocyte-depleted	

Ig, immunoglobulin.
*Infrequently positive.

findings with prognosis.[8] A second advance was made in 1966 when Lukes, Butler, and Hicks proposed a classification that related well to clinical presentation and course.[9] Their proposal was slightly modified into the Rye classification, in which four histopathologic subtypes were described: lymphocyte-predominant, nodular sclerosis, mixed cellularity, and lymphocyte-depleted. In the *World Health Organization Classification of Lymphoid Neoplasms*, the NLPHL subtype is clearly distinguished from cHL.[10] The "lymphocyte-rich" subtype of cHL was introduced in 1999.

Peters described a clinical staging system in 1950, emphasizing the diagnostic evaluation of the anatomic extent of disease.[11] In 1952, Kinmouth introduced lower-extremity lymphangiography that allowed roentgenologic visualization of the pelvic and retroperitoneal lymph nodes and was found to be far more sensitive than palpation or other radiographic methods.[12] The frequency of unsuspected splenic involvement was revealed in a group of 65 patients subjected to laparotomy and splenectomy with biopsy of splenic hilar, paraaortic and mesenteric nodes, and liver at Stanford University.[13] These diagnostic procedures led to improved understanding of the mode of dissemination of the disease and correlated well with prognosis, culminating in the modern concepts of staging codified at the Rye, New York, conference in 1965,[14] and further refined at the Workshop on the Staging of Hodgkin's Disease in Ann Arbor, Michigan, in 1971.[15]

Pusey (1902)[16] and Senn (1903)[17] were the first to report dramatic regressions of lymphadenopathy with exposure to X-rays, discovered by Roentgen in 1896. Based upon the nearly inevitable recurrence in untreated areas, Gilbert proposed the systematic treatment of both involved and uninvolved areas in 1939.[18] Peters (1950) is credited for the first demonstration of the curative potential of radiotherapy in her classic paper.[11] The development of megavoltage radiotherapy (doses >4000 cGy), as reported by Kaplan in 1962,[19] permitted the delivery of tumoricidal doses to virtually all lymphoid regions in the body within acceptable limits of normal tissue tolerance.

The chemotherapy of cHL originated as a byproduct of the wartime work on the mustard gases.[20,21] Following the initial work with the nitrogen mustards, antimetabolites were synthesized and a number of alkaloids and antibiotics extracted from various plant, fungus, and microbial sources became available for clinical use. DeVita and colleagues introduced the first highly effective combination chemotherapy, MOPP (mechlorethamine [nitrogen mustard], vincristine [Oncovin], procarbazine, and prednisone), based on experimental studies indicating the desirability of combining agents with non-overlapping toxicities.[22] Combination chemotherapy extended the curative potential for cHL to advanced disease. The ABVD (doxorubicin [Adriamycin], bleomycin, vinblastine, dacarbazine) regimen introduced by Bonadonna and colleagues represented another major advance.[23] Based on a more favorable safety profile and greater efficacy, ABVD replaced MOPP.

EPIDEMIOLOGY

The estimated incidence of Hodgkin lymphoma in the United States was 9190 cases in 2014, with equal incidences in Americans of European and African descent (2.9/100,000).[24] The disease has a median age of onset of 38 years with bimodal incidence peaks at ages 15 to 34 and older than age 60 years (Fig. 97–1).[25] The second incidence peak is smaller in Americans of European descent whereas it is more prominent in Americans of Hispanic descent.[24] Except for Americans of Asian descent, for whom the incidence has increased by 5.2 percent per year, the incidence of Hodgkin lymphoma has been stable in the United States from 1975 to 2011 (Fig. 97–2). The nodular sclerosis subtype predominates in young adults, whereas the mixed cellularity subtype is more common in the pediatric population and at older ages. There is a male predominance at all ages (~1.4:1).

Early studies associated an increased risk of Hodgkin lymphoma in the young adult population with high socioeconomic status.[26] Living in a rental home, sharing a bedroom, and attending daycare or nursery school and early parity in women have been associated with reduced risk. The relationship of incidence to neighborhood socioeconomic status was demonstrated in California for younger but not for older patients.[25] Although associations with occupational exposure to pesticides and lifestyle factors such as cigarette smoking have been reported, the aggregate data do not indicate consistent causal relationships with exogenous chemicals or toxins. A personal or family history of an autoimmune disorder, particularly sarcoidosis, has been associated with an increased risk of Hodgkin lymphoma.[27] Shared etiologic factors with multiple sclerosis have been suggested but these are thought to be of minor importance.

Geographic patterns vary for the three major age groups: the incidence of Hodgkin lymphoma is greater in childhood in less-developed countries, whereas the incidence peaks in young adulthood and is associated with more favorable histologic subtypes in developed countries.[28] Presence of the Epstein-Barr virus (EBV) in Hodgkin and Reed-Sternberg cells is more common in less-developed countries and in pediatric and older adult cases. The worldwide incidence of the disease is much lower in the Asian population, whether residing in the Far East or in the United States, although the reported rate in Vancouver, Canada, among

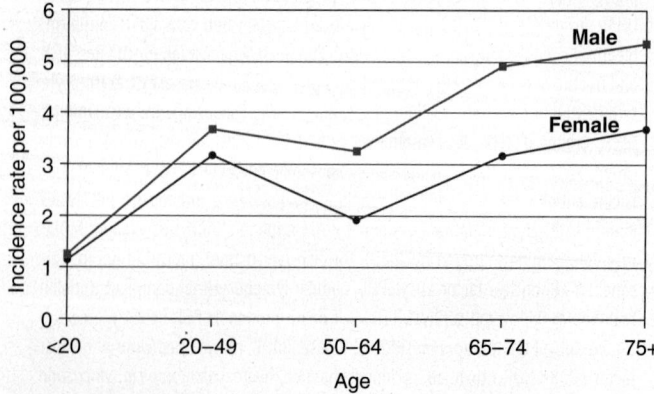

Figure 97-1. The graph depicts the incidence of Hodgkin lymphoma as a function of age among American males and females, 2000 to 2011. *(Data from the Surveillance, Epidemiology, and End Results (SEER) Program (www.seer.cancer.gov) Research Data (1973-2011), National Cancer Institute, DCCPS, Surveillance Research Program, Surveillance Systems Branch, released April 2014, based on the November 2013 submission; 2014.)*

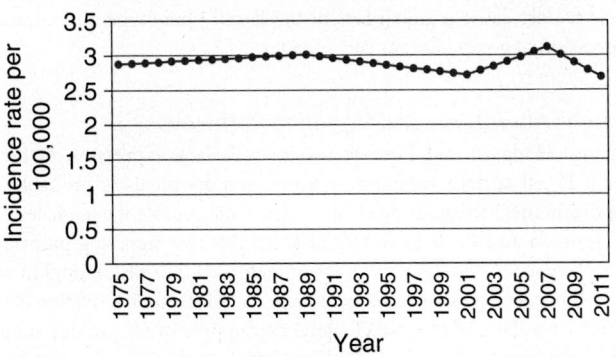

Figure 97–2. Incidence of Hodgkin lymphoma by calendar year. *(Data from the Surveillance, Epidemiology, and End Results (SEER) Program (www.seer.cancer.gov) Research Data (1973-2011), National Cancer Institute, DCCPS, Surveillance Research Program, Surveillance Systems Branch, released April 2014, based on the November 2013 submission; 2014.)*

immigrants of Chinese descent was higher than among Chinese residing in Hong Kong.[29,30] Together these data suggest a complex interaction among possible socioeconomic, environmental, immunologic, genetic, and infectious factors in the incidence of Hodgkin lymphoma.

POSSIBLE INFECTIOUS ETIOLOGY

Demographic features have long supported a "hygiene hypothesis" postulating that one or more subtypes of cHL represent delayed exposure to an infectious agent. In 1966, MacMahon proposed that the first age peak in young adults was infectious in nature, whereas the second peak resulted from causes similar to other lymphomas.[26] As noted above, socioeconomic status correlates with the first, but not the second, peak.[25] Several reports of clustering of cHL at the time of diagnosis suggested the possibility of infectious transmission.[31] The weaknesses of the retrospective methodology in these studies have been critically assessed, and further statistical analyses indicate that these likely occurred by chance alone.

A threefold increased risk of cHL in young adults is conferred by a prior history of serologically confirmed infectious mononucleosis. In addition, elevations in titers of EBV, the etiologic agent of infectious mononucleosis, have been reported in patients with cHL.[32,33] A large population study showed that people who developed the disease had abnormally high titers of EBV viral capsid antigen and early antigen in prediagnostic sera.[34] In two subsequent reports, a significantly increased risk of cHL after serologically verified infectious mononucleosis and limited to EBV-positive cases was reported in young adults.[35,36] The median incubation time was approximately 4.1 years.

EBV genomes have been detected in 30 to 50 percent of cHL tissues in developed countries, and EBV-associated cases are more common in cases with mixed cellularity histology, Hispanic ethnicity, and patients older than the age of 60 years.[37–39] Several studies report a high incidence of EBV association, 85 to 100 percent, in pediatric cHL in which geographic, ethnic, and racial factors have been implicated in the association.[37–39] The incidence of cHL is 10 to 20 times higher in patients with HIV infection than in the general population, and such cases typically have detectable EBV within Hodgkin and Reed-Sternberg cells.[40] In contrast to non-Hodgkin lymphoma, the incidence of cHL in the HIV-infected population has increased despite less-severe immunosuppression in the era of highly active antiretroviral therapy.[41,42]

GENETIC BASIS

Genetic susceptibility and familial aggregation appear to play a role in the incidence of cHL. The increased risk of the disease among identical,

but not fraternal, twins provides the strongest evidence for a genetic association.[43] cHL-prone families, with or without other forms of cancer, have been described in the literature and it is estimated that 4.5 percent of cases are familial.[44–46] The standard incidence ratio for age-specific familial risk from the Swedish Cancer Registry was higher for Hodgkin lymphoma (4.8) than any other neoplasm.[47] The relative risk for familial disease is stronger in individuals older than 40 years of age, males, and siblings, and a shared risk with chronic lymphocytic leukemia and non-Hodgkin lymphoma has been described.[46] An increased incidence in same sex siblings (eight- to 12-fold) versus opposite-sex siblings (1.3- to 1.4-fold) detected in the Swedish registry is consistent with older data and has been interpreted to be supportive of an environmental influence or a pseudoautosomal susceptibility gene located on a sex chromosome.[48–50]

Immunoregulatory genes within or near the major histocompatibility complex that may govern susceptibility to viral infections have been postulated to influence susceptibility to cHL, an hypothesis that is supported by the demonstration of lifelong, depressed cellular immunity in cHL patients and their healthy relatives.[51] Several groups described specific human leukocyte antigen (HLA) susceptibility or resistance regions, but these data have been relatively weak and sometimes inconsistent.[52]

ETIOLOGY AND PATHOGENESIS

ORIGIN OF THE REED-STERNBERG CELL

The histologic diagnosis of cHL is based on the recognition of the Reed-Sternberg cell in an appropriate cellular background. The classic Reed-Sternberg cell has a bilobed nucleus with prominent eosinophilic nucleoli separated by a clear space from the thickened nuclear membrane (Fig. 97–3; see also Chap. 96, Fig. 96–35). Mononuclear variants (Hodgkin cells) have similar nuclear characteristics and may represent Reed-Sternberg cells cut in a plane that shows only one lobe of the nucleus. Reed-Sternberg cells are not pathognomonic for cHL; they may be seen in reactive and other neoplastic conditions. Study of the Reed-Sternberg cell has been complicated by the fact that the neoplastic cells are sparsely interspersed among a reactive, mixed, nonclonal population of lymphocytes, eosinophils, histiocytes, plasma cells, and neutrophils. Difficulty characterizing the neoplastic cells, which account

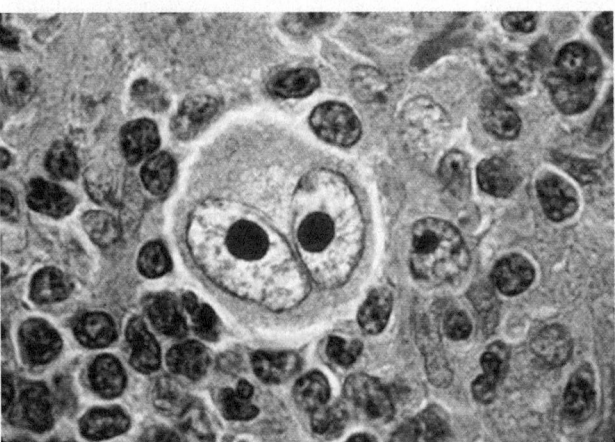

Figure 97–3. High magnification of lymph node section in a patient with Hodgkin lymphoma. A Reed-Sternberg cell is in the center of the field with the classical findings of giant size compared to background lymphocytes, binucleation, and prominent eosinophilic nucleoli.

for only 1 to 2 percent of the cellular composition, led to controversy regarding the etiology and pathogenesis of cHL for more than 150 years. Molecular analyses of single cells obtained by microdissection led to the discovery that cHL and NLPHL are both clonal disorders derived from germinal center B cells, in most cases.[53] The need to survive negative selection in the germinal center, the determination of genetic alterations and constitutive activity of key signaling pathways, and the involvement of EBV in a subset of cases have led to hypotheses concerning the malignant transformation events leading to the formation of Hodgkin/Reed-Sternberg cells. Application of additional genomic technology promises to clarify the molecular changes underlying malignant transformation and cellular proliferation.

Antigen Receptor Rearrangements

Reed-Sternberg cells and their mononuclear variants demonstrate inconsistent lineage-specific antigen expression that is unlike any other cell of the hematopoietic system. The origin of these cells was eventually determined through isolation of single cells by micromanipulation of histologic sections and analysis for immunoglobulin variable gene rearrangements.[53,54] Nearly all Hodgkin and Reed-Sternberg cells have rearranged and somatically mutated immunoglobulin VH genes, indicating a germinal center or postgerminal center origin of classic Hodgkin and Reed-Sternberg cells.[55-57] Extrapolating from the fact that a subset of these cells carries crippling mutations, it is possible that Hodgkin and Reed-Sternberg cells originate from a preapoptotic germinal center B cell with unfavorable mutations that has escaped negative selection. Rare cases of cHL with a clonal T-cell receptor gene rearrangement have been observed.[58] In contrast, single-cell analyses of NLPHL demonstrated clonal immunoglobulin gene rearrangements with ongoing mutations, an intraclonal diversity consistent with a germinal center origin of lymphocyte and histiocytic cells.[59-61]

Reprogramming of Hodgkin and Reed-Sternberg Cells

Hodgkin and Reed-Sternberg cells show a global loss of their B-cell phenotype, retaining only B-cell features associated with their interaction with T cells and their antigen-presenting function.[62] Furthermore, Hodgkin and Reed-Sternberg cells express markers of other lineages, including T cells, dendritic cells, cytotoxic cells, and myeloid cells. The lack of expression of numerous B-cell genes is the result of loss of transcription factor expression (OCT2, BOB1, PU.1) and epigenetic silencing.[63-65] The main B-cell lineage commitment factor, PAX5, is typically expressed, but its target genes are downregulated.[66,67] Reduced expression of target genes likely reflects the fact that B-cell genes are regulated by coordinated action of multiple transcription factors.

The heterogeneity of expression of myeloid, T-cell, dendritic cell, and other genes by Hodgkin and Reed-Sternberg cells is the result of many factors. Early B-cell factor 1 levels are low, de-repressing the expression of T-cell and myeloid genes and lowering transcription of B-cell–specific genes.[68] Notch 1, which plays a key role in promoting T-cell differentiation and inhibiting B-cell development, is expressed in Hodgkin and Reed-Sternberg cells.[69] Notch 1 also contributes to the expression of GATA2, a transcription factor required for proliferation and survival of hematopoietic stem cells.[70] The hematopoietic stem cell regulator polycomb G proteins are also expressed by Hodgkin and Reed-Sternberg cells and are thought to contribute to the expression of markers of different hematopoietic lineages.[71] The signal transducer and activation of transcription factors (STAT) 5A and STAT5B are implicated in Hodgkin and Reed-Sternberg reprogramming as they upregulate CD30 and downregulate B-cell–receptor expression.[72] Together,

these factors cause a global loss of the B-cell phenotype and aberrant expression of genes of other cell lineages.

Genetic Alterations and Signaling Pathways

Because Hodgkin and Reed-Sternberg cells lack expression of functional B-cell surface receptors, rescue from apoptosis is probably an important mechanism of survival.[53,73] The most prevalent genetic lesions in Hodgkin and Reed-Sternberg cells involve two signaling pathways: Janus kinase (JAK)-STAT and nuclear factor-κB (NF-κB). Hodgkin and Reed-Sternberg cells have frequent gains in JAK2 and inactivation of the negative regulator of JAK-STAT signaling, suppressor of cytokine signaling 1, resulting in enhanced cytokine signaling.[74,75] Genetic alterations in NF-κB include gains and amplifications of the NF-κB transcription factor REL in about half the cases of cHL.[76] Somatic mutations of the gene encoding the inhibitor of NF-κB (IκBα) occur in approximately 20 percent of cases.[77,78] Inactivating mutations and deletions of the gene encoding A20, a negative regulator of NF-κB, have been found in approximately 40 percent of cases, nearly all of which were EBV-negative.[79]

Autocrine and paracrine signaling events also contribute to constitutive activation of the JAK-STAT pathway and NF-κB transcription.[72] STAT factors are activated by autocrine means through expression of interleukins (ILs) 13 and 21 and their receptors by Hodgkin and Reed-Sternberg cells and augmented by NF-κB activity.[80-82] Receptor tyrosine kinases expressed in these cells may also contribute to STAT activation. The tumor necrosis factor receptor family, which includes CD30, CD40, transmembrane activator, calcium modulator, and cyclophilin ligand interactor (TACI), B-cell maturation antigen (BCMA), and receptor activator of NF-κB (RANK), is involved in NF-κB signaling through interactions with the cHL microenvironment or in an autocrine fashion.[83,84]

Multiple receptor tyrosine kinases are aberrantly expressed in Hodgkin and Reed-Sternberg cells, including platelet-derived growth factor receptor-α. In addition, deregulated and constitutive activation of the phosphoinositide 3′-kinase (PI3K)-AKT and extracellular signal-regulated kinase (ERK) pathways are implicated in Hodgkin and Reed-Sternberg cells. The activator protein 1 (AP1) transcription factors also appear to play a role, inducing target genes such as galectin 1 and CD30 in Hodgkin and Reed-Sternberg cells.

Several factors point to the pathogenetic role of EBV in approximately 40 percent of classical cHL. The viral proteins latent membrane protein 1 (LMP1) and latent membrane protein 2 (LMP2), in particular, appear to have hijacked signaling pathways to promote the survival of EBV-infected Hodgkin and Reed-Sternberg cells. LMP1 induces constitutive NF-κB signaling by mimicking the CD40 receptor and can activate JAK-STAT, PI3K, and AP1 signaling. LMP2 functions as a surrogate for the B-cell receptor. The role of EBV in the pathogenesis of cHL also is supported by the findings that (1) there is an inverse relationship between expression of multiple receptor tyrosine kinases and EBV expression, (2) there is an ability of EBV to rescue crippled germinal center B cells in the laboratory, (3) mutations preventing any B-cell receptor expression are in EBV-positive Hodgkin and Reed-Sternberg cells, and (4) there is an inverse relationship between mutations reducing the expression of the NF-κB regulator A20 and EBV-positive Hodgkin and Reed-Sternberg cells.

Overall, genetic alterations involving the JAK-STAT and NF-κB signaling pathways and further activation via autocrine or paracrine mechanisms interact to support the growth and survival of cHL cells. In the EBV-positive subset of patients, viral genes can provide the pathogenetic function of genetic lesions found in EBV-negative cases.

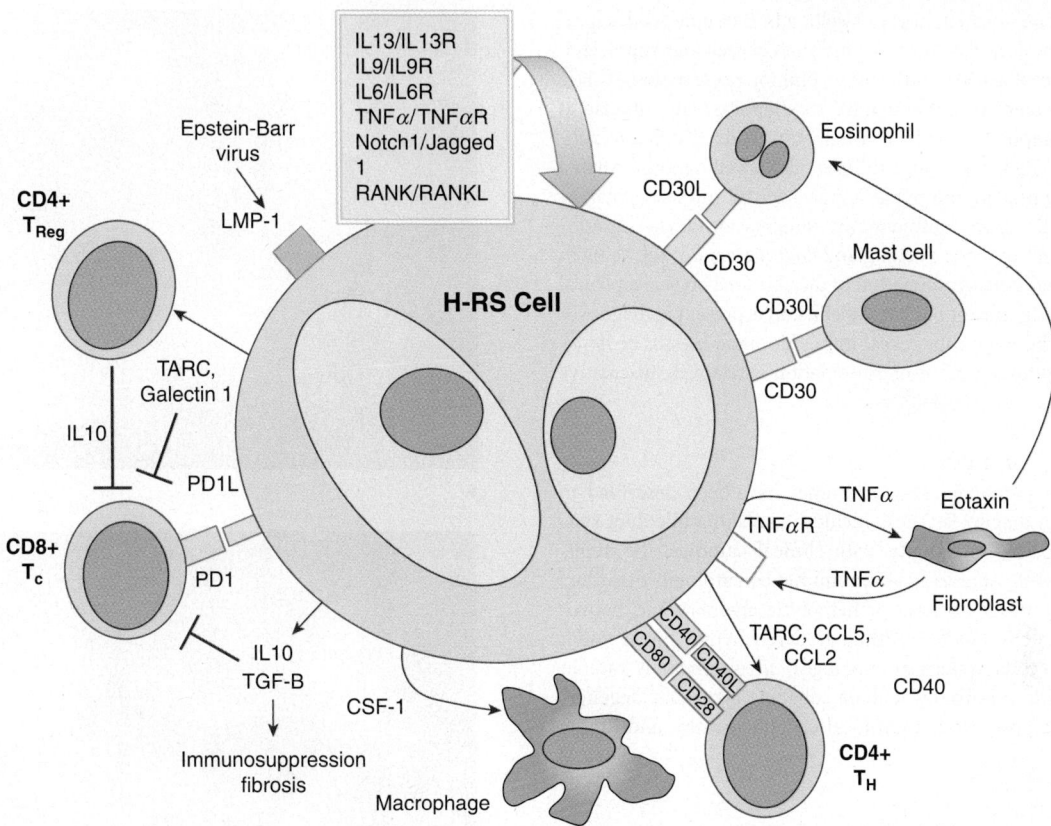

Figure 97–4. The Reed-Sternberg cell and its environment. In a network of highly complex interactions, Reed-Sternberg cells elaborate chemokines that attract a variety of cells, which cascade their influence on the microenvironment. Reed-Sternberg cells express ligands that play a role in autocrine and paracrine interactions and also produce a number of immunosuppressive factors (e.g., galectin 1) that directly contribute to a protumor, humoral T-helper 2 environment (see "Role of the Microenvironment" for further details).

ROLE OF THE MICROENVIRONMENT

The survival of Hodgkin and Reed-Sternberg cells appear to be dependent on their microenvironment, which represents 95 to 99 percent of the cellular composition of the tumor. Hodgkin and Reed-Sternberg cells attract T cells, B cells, neutrophils, plasma cells, eosinophils and mast cells by secreting chemokines (Fig. 97–4). For instance, CCL5, CCL17, and CCL22 attract T-helper 2 and T-regulatory cells. Other chemokines attract eosinophils and mast cells, and IL-8 attracts neutrophils. These chemokines may also have direct effects on Hodgkin and Reed-Sternberg cells. T cells represent the largest and probably most important population. CD4+ T cells trigger CD40 signaling and CD4+ T-regulatory cells have potent immunosuppressive activity against infiltrating cytotoxic T cells. Other interactions include activation of TACI and BCMA through their ligand production by neutrophils and activation of CD30 through CD30 ligand-expressing mast cells and eosinophils. Connective tissue cells and their products can be involved in complex interactions, such as the stimulation of fibroblasts via factors expressed by Hodgkin and Reed-Sternberg cells and the consequent secretion by these fibroblasts of eotaxin and CCL5, which attract eosinophils and T-regulatory cells to the cHL microenvironment.

The differentiation of CD4+ T cells to T-regulatory cells and the immunosuppressive features of the cHL microenvironment have received much attention. A hallmark of these changes is the shift from an antitumor, cytotoxic T-helper 1 response to a protumor, humoral T-helper 2 response. Hodgkin and Reed-Sternberg cells produce a number of immunosuppressive factors such as IL-10, transforming growth factor-β, galectin 1, and prostaglandin E$_2$. Hodgkin and Reed-Sternberg cells express programmed cell death protein 1 (PD1) ligand that binds and inhibits T-cell cytotoxic function.

⬤ CLINICAL FEATURES

PRESENTING MANIFESTATIONS

History and Physical Examination

Constitutional symptoms accompany the diagnosis of cHL in approximately 30 percent of cases. Fever in excess of 38°C, drenching night sweats, and weight loss exceeding 10 percent of baseline body weight during the 6 months preceding diagnosis are designated as symptomatic "B" disease. Fevers are usually of low grade and irregular. Rarely, a cyclic pattern of high fevers for 1 to 2 weeks alternating with afebrile periods of similar duration, known as Pel-Ebstein fever, is present at diagnosis and is virtually diagnostic of the disease.[85,86] Generalized pruritus, often accompanied by marked excoriation, may be present at diagnosis; but does not confer prognostic significance. Pain in involved lymph nodes immediately after the ingestion of alcohol is a curious complaint that occurs in fewer than 10 percent of patients but is nearly specific to cHL.[87] The etiology of these symptoms has been the subject of speculation, but remains largely unexplained. Patients with extensive intrathoracic disease may present with cough, chest pain, dyspnea, and, rarely, hemoptysis. Infrequently, patients present with bone pain, including the constellation of back pain accompanied by signs and symptoms of spinal cord compression.

Detection of an unusual mass or swelling in the superficial, supradiaphragmatic lymph nodes (60 to 70 percent cervical and supraclavicular, 15 to 20 percent axillary) is the most common presentation of cHL. Only 15 to 20 percent of patients have subdiaphragmatic disease at presentation.[88] Lymphadenopathy is usually nontender and has a "rubbery" consistency. By inspection, a diffuse, puffy swelling rather than a discrete mass may be apparent in the supraclavicular, infraclavicular, or anterior chest wall regions. Infrequently, compression of the superior vena cava will result in facial swelling and engorgement of the veins in the neck and upper chest. Auscultation of the chest may reveal a pleural effusion. Rarely, a significant pericardial effusion is present at diagnosis. Palpation of the abdomen may reveal intraabdominal masses or hepatosplenomegaly, although physical examination is relatively insensitive for detection of these abnormalities.

Paraneoplastic Findings

A number of rare paraneoplastic syndromes have been described in cHL at the time of diagnosis. These include "vanishing bile duct syndrome" and idiopathic cholangitis with clinical jaundice, the nephrotic syndrome with anasarca, autoimmune hematologic disorders (e.g., immune thrombocytopenia or hemolytic anemia), and neurologic signs and symptoms.[89–91] Although parenchymal involvement of the central nervous system or meningeal involvement is rare in cHL, paraneoplastic syndromes include subacute cerebellar degeneration, myelopathy, progressive multifocal encephalopathy, and limbic encephalitis.[91,92]

RADIOGRAPHIC FEATURES

Intrathoracic disease is present at diagnosis in two-thirds of patients. Mediastinal adenopathy is common in cHL, particularly in young women with the nodular sclerosis subtype.[93] Hilar adenopathy, pulmonary parenchymal involvement, pleural effusions, pericardial effusions, and chest wall masses may be appreciated by chest computed tomography (CT); these are more common in the presence of extensive mediastinal disease. CT of the abdomen and pelvis is routinely employed in the diagnostic evaluation of cHL. Although technologic advances have greatly increased the resolution of this technique and the subsequent detection of celiac, portal, splenic hilar, and mesenteric lymph nodes, the correlation with histologic involvement of the spleen, historically determined by laparotomy staging, has been disappointing.

Whole-body ^{18}F-fluorodeoxyglucose positron emission tomography (FDG-PET) has become standard in the staging of cHL (Fig. 97–5).[94,95] FDG-PET correlates well with CT evaluation and may demonstrate additional areas of disease, although this information uncommonly results in changes in stage or choice of initial therapy.[95,96] FDG-PET, however, is more sensitive to bone and hepatic disease and a diffuse increase in signal can be seen at diagnosis in patients with neutrophilia. FDG-PET imaging is superior to CT scanning in distinguishing active residual disease (increased glucose metabolism) from inactive residual tissue, a major problem in assessing remission status after treatment, and has been incorporated in formal revised response guidelines.[94,95] False-positive FDG-PET scans can be seen in the marrow during or at the end of treatment as a consequence of the chemotherapy effect or use of hematopoietic colony-stimulating factors. In followup, false-positive studies may be caused by thymic hyperplasia, granulomatous disease, or infectious disorders. In addition to evaluation of residual masses, FDG-PET has been incorporated in early response monitoring for risk stratification and, in clinical trials, to alter therapy.[96–102] The predictive accuracy of FDG-PET is dependent on expertise of the imaging staff and clinical correlation. In most situations, but particularly in FDG-PET, avid anatomic sites that were previously uninvolved or

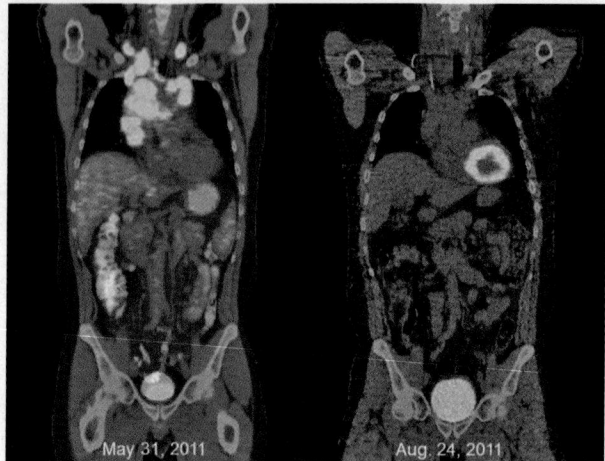

A

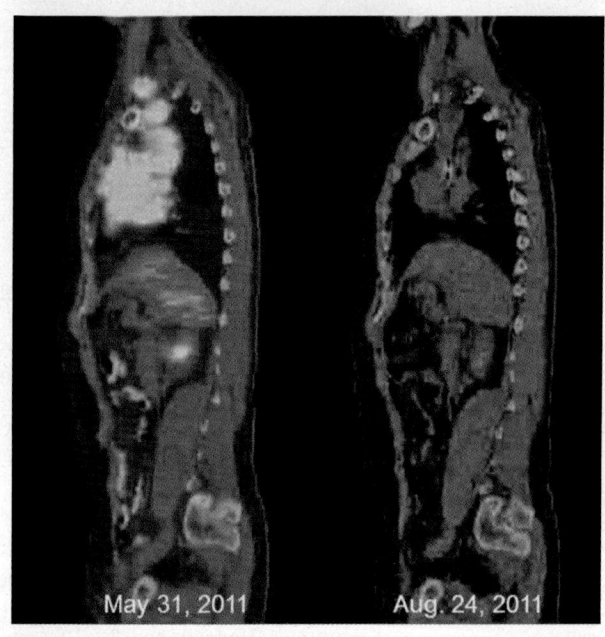

B

Figure 97–5. [18]Fluorodeoxyglucose positron emission tomography/computed tomography (FDG-PET/CT) imaging of classical Hodgkin lymphoma. **A.** Coronal views of whole-body FDG-PET/CT imaging performed before (May 31, 2011) and after (August 24, 2011) therapy for stage IIB classical Hodgkin lymphoma with Adriamycin, bleomycin, vinblastine, and dacarbazine (ABVD) chemotherapy and involved field radiotherapy. At the time of diagnosis, hypermetabolic areas of avid-FDG uptake were evident in bilateral cervical, supraclavicular, mediastinal, and hilar lymph nodes. Physiologic FDG uptake was visible in the colon and bladder. After completion of therapy, there was no abnormal hypermetabolic activity in any of the original sites of disease, although physiologic FDG activity was seen in the cardiac blood cardiac blood pool. **B.** Sagittal views of the same patient before (May 31, 2011) and after (August 24, 2011) therapy, showing resolution of hypermetabolism in all involved nodal sites. The patient has remained in complete remission since finishing therapy.

those without concomitant abnormality on CT scan, usually require tissue biopsy confirmation. Combined CT and FDG-PET technology is now standard for staging and posttreatment response evaluation and has resulted in improved anatomic definition of sites with increased signal.[94–96]

● CLINICAL AND PATHOLOGIC CORRELATION

NODULAR LYMPHOCYTE PREDOMINANCE SUBTYPE

There is a strong correlation between age at onset, the anatomic extent of disease and histologic subtype of Hodgkin lymphoma. Approximately 5 to 10 percent of patients present with NLPHL, which is considered to be a distinct subtype, discrete from cHL.[103,104] Progressive transformation of germinal centers may precede or follow NLPHL in other sites. The cellular composition is predominantly benign B lymphocytes with or without histiocytes. The characteristic multilobated, CD20+ lymphocyte and histiocytic cells are relatively abundant (see Chap. 96, Fig. 96–40). Patients most commonly present with stage I disease (70 percent) in peripheral lymph node sites, particularly in the axillae, and there is a 3 to 4:1 male predominance.[103,104] NLPHL may be associated with diffuse large B-cell non-Hodgkin lymphoma as a composite tumor or a large cell lymphoma may develop at a later date.[105,106] The large cell variant, T-cell–rich B-cell lymphoma, may be difficult to distinguish from NLPHL and may occur concurrently or subsequently (Chap. 98).[107]

NODULAR SCLEROSIS SUBTYPE

cHL is characterized by Hodgkin and Reed-Sternberg cells that express CD30 and CD15+ but usually not typical B-cell surface markers such as CD20 or CD79B. The nodular sclerosis subtype constitutes 40 to 70 percent of cHL and is distinguished by its distinctive clinical and histologic features. This subtype typically involves lower cervical, supraclavicular, and mediastinal lymph nodes in adolescents and young adults, particularly females. Approximately 70 percent of patients with the nodular sclerosis subtype present with limited stage disease. A characteristic histologic feature is the lacunar cell, a Reed-Sternberg variant that results from retraction of the cytoplasm of Hodgkin and Reed-Sternberg cells during formalin fixation (see Chap. 96, Fig. 96–38). Another typical feature is the thickened capsule and fibrous bands that divide the lymphoid tissue into cellular nodules.

MIXED CELLULARITY SUBTYPE

Mixed cellularity cHL involves both pediatric and older age groups and is more commonly associated with advanced stage disease, constitutional symptoms, and immunodeficiency. Approximately 30 to 50 percent of patients present with this histology. Classic Hodgkin and Reed-Sternberg cells are easily found amid a cellular background composed of lymphocytes, eosinophils, plasma cells, and histiocytes (see Chap. 96, Fig. 96–39). A worse prognosis has been reported for this subtype.[108]

LYMPHOCYTE-DEPLETED SUBTYPE

Lymphocyte-depleted cHL has two morphologic variants: reticular and diffuse fibrosis. The reticular variant contains abundant pleomorphic neoplastic cells whereas the diffuse fibrosis variant has a prominent fibroblastic proliferation with few normal lymphocytes. Hodgkin and Reed-Sternberg cells are sparse. The lymphocyte-depleted subtype presents in older patients with symptomatic, extensive disease, and may be associated with fever of unknown origin, jaundice, hepatosplenomegaly, or pancytopenia. Peripheral and mediastinal adenopathy is much less common than in other subtypes. Cases of cHL developing in the setting of HIV typically exhibit the lymphocyte-depleted morphology.

LYMPHOCYTE-RICH SUBTYPE

The lymphocyte-rich subtype of cHL was introduced by the World Health Organization classification in 1999 (see Table 97–1) following an expert pathology review of cases of NLPHL.[109] The two subtypes differ subtly on morphologic grounds, but the major difference is that the Hodgkin and Reed-Sternberg cells in lymphocyte-rich cHL exhibit the classic CD30+ CD20– immunophenotype. The presenting features are very similar although patients with the lymphocyte-rich subtype tend to be older compared with NLPHL patients.[109] A higher rate of multiple relapses and a more favorable prognosis upon relapse is characteristic of NLPHL.

● ANATOMIC DISTRIBUTION OF DISEASE

In approximately 70 percent of patients, cHL presents in the cervical nodes; in 12 percent, in the axillary nodes; and in 9 percent, in the inguinal nodes.[110] A small minority of patients presents exclusively with subdiaphragmatic disease. In an historical series of 285 consecutive, unselected, and untreated patients evaluated at Stanford University, involvement of abdominal lymph nodes and the spleen was documented in 272 upon laparotomy, a surgical diagnostic procedure in which the intraabdominal and pelvic lymph nodes are biopsied, the spleen is removed and examined pathologically in thin slices, the liver is biopsied by needle and wedge technique, and the marrow is biopsied. The frequency of splenic involvement at laparotomy in untreated patients averaged 37 percent in 17 published series.[110] Involvement of the spleen was strongly dependent on histologic subtype: it was involved in 60 percent of mixed cellularity and lymphocyte-depleted cases compared with 34 percent of nodular lymphocyte-predominant and nodular sclerosis cases. Hepatic and marrow disease were invariably associated with splenic involvement.

Two different theories, the "contiguity" theory of Kaplan and Rosenberg[111] and the "susceptibility" theory of Smithers,[112] have been proposed for the mode of spread of cHL. In support of the former, most cases of cHL appear to spread via lymphatic channels to contiguous lymphatic structures in a predictable, nonrandom pattern. Controversy has surrounded the mode of spread to the spleen, which lacks afferent lymphatics. When four or more lymph node regions are involved, spread by hematogenous distribution appears likely. Disseminated disease is more common in mixed cellularity and lymphocyte-depleted cases, consistent with the presence of reported vascular invasion.[113] Whereas vascular invasion is controversial, it is more common in the spleen than in lymph nodes and connotes a poor prognosis.[114]

● STAGING

Optimal management of Hodgkin lymphoma relies on knowledge of the extent of disease dissemination, which is determined by performing a careful physical examination, supplemented by laboratory tests and radiographic imaging studies (Chap. 95). This process, known as "staging," has been refined by a series of international working groups. The current 2014 Lugano staging system[94] is a refinement of the historical Ann Arbor classification[15] and assigns patients to one of four stages as indicated in Table 97–2. The classification for Hodgkin lymphoma is further refined by designating the presence or absence of constitutional "B" symptoms (fever >38°C, weight loss >10 percent of body weight, or drenching night sweats). Extranodal disease, representing extracapsular extension of lymph node disease that could be incorporated in a standard radiotherapy field, is distinguished from disseminated, stage IV disease. The correlation of this staging classification system with prognosis was extensively verified when radiotherapy served as the

TABLE 97–2. Staging System for Hodgkin Lymphoma

Stage

I. Involvement of a single lymph node region (I) or a single extra-lymphatic organ or site (I_E)

II. Involvement of two or more lymph node regions on the same side of the diaphragm alone (II) or with involvement of limited, contiguous extralymphatic organ or tissue (II_E)

III. Involvement of lymph node regions on both sides of the diaphragm (III), which may include the spleen (III_S) or limited, contiguous extralymphatic organ or site (III_E) or both (III_{ES})

IV. Multiple or disseminated foci of involvement of one or more extralymphatic organs or tissues, with or without associated lymph node involvement

Modifying Features

A. Asymptomatic

B. Drenching night sweats; fever >38°C; loss of more than 10% body weight in 6 months

C. Involvement of a single, contiguous or proximal extranodal site

Bulky disease is defined as a mass >10 cm or a mediastinal mass ration >0.33. The mediastinal mass ratio is the ratio of the maximal width of a mediastinal mass relative to the maximal width of the mediastinum, as measured by CT imaging.

principal treatment for all but stage IV disease. Recommended staging procedures for untreated patients have evolved with changes in therapy. Exploratory laparotomy and splenectomy, which historically advanced about one-third of clinical stages I and II patients to pathologic stages III and IV, is no longer performed. CT of the chest, abdomen, and pelvis and FDG-PET imaging provide sensitive delineation of involved sites, and the use of chemotherapy in all stages of disease has reduced the critical nature of detecting subclinical disease. Marrow involvement occurs in approximately 12 percent of new patients and is more common in patients of older age, advanced stage, less-favorable histology, or those with constitutional symptoms or immunodeficiency. Because the marrow is almost never involved in young, asymptomatic patients with favorable clinical stage I or II presentations, marrow biopsy may be omitted in staging such patients.

● LABORATORY FEATURES

There are no diagnostic laboratory features of cHL. A complete blood count may reveal granulocytosis, eosinophilia, lymphocytopenia, thrombocytosis, or anemia. Anemia is usually the result of "chronic disease," but rarely may be caused by hemolysis associated with a positive direct antiglobulin (Coombs) test. Thrombocytopenia may occur as a result of marrow involvement, hypersplenism or an immune mechanism. Immune neutropenia can occur in cHL. Cytopenias are particularly common in advanced-stage disease and the lymphocyte-depleted subtype. Elevation of the erythrocyte sedimentation rate (ESR) is most common in advanced disease and correlates with constitutional symptoms.[115,116] The degree of sedimentation rate elevation correlates with prognosis, particularly in limited-stage disease.[117] Although nonspecific, it may be a useful harbinger of recurrent disease if serially monitored. Serum lactate dehydrogenase levels are elevated in 35 percent of patients at diagnosis.[118,119] The alkaline phosphatase may be elevated in cHL, nonspecifically in limited disease, or in association with involvement of liver, bone, or marrow in advanced disease. Hypercalcemia is unusual in cHL and when present may be secondary to synthesis of

increased levels of 1,25-dihydroxyvitamin D by Hodgkin lymphoma cells.[120] A variety of other abnormalities have been reported, including hypoglycemia[121,122] resulting from autoantibodies to insulin receptors and hyponatremia resulting from inappropriate secretion of antidiuretic hormone.[123]

Anemia, granulocytosis, lymphopenia, and low serum albumin constitute four of seven adverse prognostic factors identified in advanced Hodgkin lymphoma by an international consortium.[124] Similar to the non-Hodgkin lymphomas, serum β_2-microglobulin levels correlate with tumor burden and prognosis in Hodgkin lymphoma.[125] Serum levels of cytokines including soluble CD30, IL-6, IL-10, and the IL-2 receptor, have been reported to correlate with constitutional symptoms and advanced disease.[126–129] Examination of pleural fluid in Hodgkin lymphoma may reveal transudative, exudative or chylous characteristics. Because cytology rarely yields diagnostic Hodgkin and Reed-Sternberg cells, the etiology is most often considered to be one of central lymphatic obstruction. Laboratory abnormalities, including abnormal liver function tests associated with marked enlargement of porta hepatis nodes and biliary obstruction or intrahepatic cholestasis, may be prominent in rare presentations of Hodgkin lymphoma.[130] Similarly, the nephrotic syndrome, characterized by edema, azotemia, hypoalbuminemia, and hyperlipidemia, may rarely be present at the time of diagnosis of Hodgkin lymphoma.[131]

● DIFFERENTIAL DIAGNOSIS

Clinically enlarged lymph nodes may be associated with a variety of infectious, inflammatory, autoimmune, and neoplastic disorders. Biopsy of unexplained, persistent, or recurrent adenopathy should be reviewed by an experienced hematopathologist. Distinction of cHL[132] from primary mediastinal B-cell lymphoma may be difficult based on both clinical and histologic features. Gene expression profiling studies suggest that these disorders are closely related pathogenetically.[132–135] Mixed cellularity Hodgkin lymphoma may demonstrate varied cellular and stromal compositions and must be distinguished from peripheral T-cell lymphoma and T-cell–rich, B-cell lymphoma, which can also be difficult to distinguish from NLPHL.[136] Immune markers of Hodgkin and Reed-Sternberg cells, such as CD30, CD20, and CD15, are invaluable for differential diagnosis (see Chap. 96, Figs. 96–36 and 96–41). Nonneoplastic conditions that simulate Hodgkin lymphoma include viral infections, particularly infectious mononucleosis. Depleted nodes of any histology, including the depleted phase of lymph nodes from HIV-infected patients, may resemble the diffuse fibrosis variant of lymphocyte-depleted Hodgkin lymphoma. Histologic assessment of extranodal sites depends upon the organ involved and whether there is a known diagnosis of cHL. Identification of typical Hodgkin and Reed-Sternberg cells in needle biopsies of liver and marrow biopsies are not required because the specimens for evaluation are typically very small.

● THERAPY

HISTORICAL PERSPECTIVE

Hodgkin lymphoma first became a curable neoplasm through the systematic study of the spread of the disease and the use of higher dose, extended field radiotherapy delivered with supervoltage techniques.[137] When used alone, radiotherapy doses to involved fields usually ranged from 3500 to 4400 cGy with prophylactic doses of 3000 to 3500 cGy to uninvolved tissues. The mantle, paraaortic region, and pelvis constitute the classic radiotherapy regions. With increased recognition of late effects, radiation therapy has been modified to reduce field size to areas of known or bulky disease and doses have been lowered, coincident with addition of systemic chemotherapy. Furthermore, initial disease reduction with chemotherapy results in less radiation exposure to the neck, female breast, heart, and lungs, all of which are anticipated to result in fewer late complications. Advances in radiotherapy techniques deliver more precise dose distributions, sparing normal tissues. The first modern combination chemotherapy program was the MOPP regimen devised by Devita and colleagues.[22] The national mortality figures for cHL decreased by more than 60 percent in the decade that followed the introduction of MOPP.[138] Bonadonna and colleagues developed an important alternative regimen for the treatment of cHL. ABVD, which was effective in the treatment of patients who had failed MOPP[139,140] and offered a more favorable toxicity profile. ABVD subsequently became the preferred primary chemotherapy regimen, alone or in combination with radiotherapy.[141,142] Of the multiple alternative chemotherapy regimens introduced for the treatment of advanced cHL, only the bleomycin, etoposide, doxorubicin, cyclophosphamide, vincristine, prednisone, procarbazine (BEACOPP) combination developed by Diehl and colleagues has demonstrated superior cure rates in multiple phase III studies.[143,144] Table 97-3 describes the drugs, doses, and schedules of combination chemotherapy programs effective in the management of Hodgkin lymphoma.

FAVORABLE, LIMITED-STAGE DISEASE

Favorable, limited-stage Hodgkin lymphoma is typically defined in North America as asymptomatic stage I or II supradiaphragmatic disease with no bulky sites. A more restrictive definition is used in Europe based on the number of Ann Arbor sites, ESR, age and extranodal sites, as well as bulky disease (Table 97-4).[143] Approximately 35 percent of stages I and II patients meet this more limited definition of favorable disease. For many years, extended-field (subtotal lymphoid) radiotherapy administered after staging laparotomy, was the treatment of choice for early stage, favorable Hodgkin lymphoma. A change in that standard was compelled by the observation that the overall mortality rate from other causes, particularly second cancers, exceeded deaths resulting from Hodgkin lymphoma at 15 to 20 years.[145] Early studies from Stanford University demonstrated that involved-field radiotherapy plus chemotherapy produced results equivalent or superior to wide-field radiotherapy.[146] Subsequently, several randomized trials demonstrated the superiority of involved-field radiotherapy plus anthracycline-containing chemotherapy compared to extended-field radiotherapy in early stage favorable Hodgkin lymphoma.[147,148]

The next series of clinical trials were designed to test the optimal number of cycles of chemotherapy and the volume and dose of radiotherapy when both modalities are used in limited Hodgkin lymphoma. The Milan Tumor Institute documented disease control in more than 95 percent of early stage cHL patients treated with four cycles of ABVD and radiotherapy, with no advantage seen for extended-field radiotherapy compared to involved-field radiotherapy.[149] Similarly, no advantage to more extensive radiation in combination with chemotherapy was observed in a German Hodgkin Study Group (GHSG) study.[150] A comparison of two versus four cycles of ABVD chemotherapy paired with 20 Gy or 30 Gy radiotherapy was made in a four-arm trial conducted by the GHSG, evaluating patients with "favorable" early stage cHL, defined as patients with two or fewer sites of disease, no masses larger than 10 cm, a normal ESR, and no extranodal sites of disease. This trial produced equivalent outstanding outcomes for all four arms, with 91 to 93 percent freedom from treatment failure after 5 years, and established two cycles of ABVD followed by 20 Gy of involved field radiotherapy as a new standard of care for early stage, favorable cHL. In a subsequent study, the GHSG evaluated eliminating drugs from the ABVD regimen,

randomizing patients between four cycles of ABVD, AV, ABV, or AVD plus 30 Gy involved-field radiotherapy. The AV and ABV arms were closed early because of clearly inferior outcomes, and subsequent analysis suggests that the AVD arm is also worse than the full four-drug combination.[151]

The high cure rate with current limited chemotherapy and low-dose radiotherapy creates a high standard for comparison with alternative treatment approaches. Nevertheless, considerable interest exists in devising management strategies omitting radiotherapy altogether, largely motivated by desires to avoid secondary malignancies and late cardiopulmonary complications.[145] This approach is particularly favored for women younger than age 30 years, who have a very high risk of developing breast cancer if treated with mediastinal radiotherapy.[145,152] Canellos and colleagues treated 71 patients with early stage, favorable cHL with six cycles of ABVD without radiotherapy and achieved a 5-year failure-free survival of 92 percent.[153] A single institution study of ABVD versus ABVD plus radiotherapy demonstrated no significant progression-free survival difference between the treatment arms, but this trial accrued relatively small numbers of patients.[154] A phase III North American study assigned 405 patients with previously untreated stage IA or IIA nonbulky Hodgkin lymphoma to treatment with ABVD alone for four to six cycles or subtotal nodal radiation therapy, with or without ABVD. Among those assigned to subtotal nodal radiation therapy, patients who had a favorable risk profile received subtotal nodal radiation therapy alone and patients with an unfavorable risk profile received two cycles of ABVD plus subtotal nodal radiation therapy. After a median followup of 11.3 years, the overall survival (OS) was 94 percent among those receiving ABVD alone, compared to 87 percent for those receiving subtotal nodal radiation therapy (p = 0.04). The rates of freedom from disease progression were 87 percent and 92 percent in the two groups, respectively (p = 0.05). The investigators concluded that treatment with ABVD therapy alone was superior because of a lower rate of death from secondary malignancies and other causes,[155] although critics have emphasized that the large fields and high doses of radiotherapy used in this trial are obsolete and that modern radiotherapy techniques would be anticipated to have much more favorable outcomes. In a European trial, the epirubicin, bleomycin, vinblastine, prednisone (EBVP) regimen was tested against the same chemotherapy plus 20- or 30-Gy involved-field radiotherapy.[156] Inferiority of the EBVP combination without radiotherapy resulted in the trial's early closure. A Cochrane meta-analysis of randomized controlled trials comparing chemotherapy alone with combined modality therapy concluded that adding radiotherapy to chemotherapy improves tumor control and OS in patients with early stage Hodgkin lymphoma.[157]

Current studies are focused on assessing the potential role of interim FDG-PET scanning as a means of identifying patients (PET-negative) for whom radiotherapy can be omitted. The European Organization for Research and Treatment of Cancer (EORTC), the Lymphoma Study Association (LySA), and Fondazione Italiana Linfomi (FIL) H10 trial randomized 1137 patients with untreated supradiaphragmatic clinical stage I/II cHL to either standard therapy or an experimental, PET-response-adapted approach. Patients on the trial were stratified into favorable and unfavorable cohorts based on the presence or absence of adverse risk factors (age ≥50 years, more than four involved nodal areas, presence of mediastinal bulk [mediastinum-to-thorax ratio ≥0.35], or ESR ≥50 mm without B symptoms or ESR ≥30 mm with B symptoms).[101] The favorable group was randomized to either standard therapy with three cycles of ABVD chemotherapy followed by involved nodal radiotherapy (30 Gy + 6 Gy boost), or "experimental therapy" in which patients whose interim PET scans after two cycles of ABVD were negative received two more cycles of ABVD (total of four cycles) but no radiotherapy. Patients in the experimental

TABLE 97–3. Combination Chemotherapy for Hodgkin Lymphoma

Drug	Dose (mg/m²)	Route	Schedule (Days Administered)	Cycle Length (Days)
ABVD				28
Doxorubicin	25	IV	1, 15	
Bleomycin	10	IV	1, 15	
Vinblastine	6	IV	1, 15	
Dacarbazine	375	IV	1, 15	
COPP				28
Cyclophosphamide	650	IV	1, 8	
Vincristine	1.4*	IV	1, 8	
Procarbazine	100	PO	1–14	
Prednisone	40	PO	1–14	
COPP/ABVD				28
Alternate cycles of COPP with ABVD				
BEACOPP (Standard)				21
Bleomycin	10	IV	8	
Etoposide	100	IV	1–3	
Doxorubicin	25	IV	1	
Cyclophosphamide	650	IV	1	
Vincristine	1.4*	IV	8	
Procarbazine	100	PO	1–7	
Prednisone	40	PO	1–14	
BEACOPP (Escalated)				21
Bleomycin	10	IV	8	
Etoposide	200	IV	1–3	
Doxorubicin	35	IV	1	
Cyclophosphamide	1250	IV	1	
Vincristine	1.4*	IV	8	
Procarbazine	100	PO	1–7	
Prednisone	40	PO	1–14	
G-CSF	(+)	SQ	8+	
BEACOPP (14-day)				14
Standard BEACOPP given every 14 days with growth factor support.				
STANFORD V				12 weeks
Nitrogen mustard	6	IV	day 1 on wk 1, 5, 9	
Doxorubicin	25	IV	day 1 on wk 1, 3, 5, 7, 9, 11	
Vinblastine	6	IV	day 1 on wk 1, 3, 5, 7, 9, 11	
Vincristine	1.4*	IV	day 1 on wk 2, 4, 6, 8, 10, 12	
Bleomycin	5	IV	day 1 on wk 2, 4, 6, 8, 10, 12	
Etoposide	60 × 2	IV	day 1 & 2 on wk 3, 7, 11	
Prednisone	40	PO	day 1 on wk 1–10, taper	
G-CSF for dose reduction, delay				

G-CSF, granulocyte colony-stimulating factor; SQ, subcutaneously.

*Capped at 2 mg.

TABLE 97–4. Prognostic Factors for Hodgkin Lymphoma

Limited Stage		Advanced Stage
EORTC	GHSG	International Collaborative Study
Adverse Prognostic Factors		Adverse Prognostic Factors
MMR ≥0.35	MMR ≥0.35	Age ≥45 years
ESR >30 if symptomatic	ESR >30 if symptomatic	Stage IV
ESR >50 if asymptomatic	ESR >50 if asymptomatic	Male sex
>3 Ann Arbor sites	>2 Ann Arbor sites	White blood count ≥15 × 10^9/L
Age ≥50	Extranodal disease	Lymphocyte count <0.6 × 10^9/L or <8%
	Massive splenic disease	Albumin <4 g/dL
Presence of any factor is considered unfavorable		Hemoglobin <10.5 g/dL
Two-thirds of limited stage patients have one or more adverse factors		Factors summed to yield the international prognostic score 75% of patients have a score of 1–3

EORTC, European Organization for the Research and Treatment of Cancer; ESR, erythrocyte sedimentation rate; GHSG, German Hodgkin Study Group; MMR, mediastinal mass ratio, which is the ratio of the maximal width of a mediastinal mass relative to the maximal width of the mediastinum, as measured by computed tomographic imaging.

arm who had FDG-avid foci of disease after two cycles of ABVD were switched to the BEACOPP-escalated regimen for 2 cycles followed by involved nodal radiotherapy. An independent data monitoring committee stopped the study after a median followup of 1.1 years because of inferior results in the experimental group, with a 1-year progression-free survival of only 94 percent compared to 100 percent in patients treated on the standard arm (p = 0.017). The independent data monitoring committee mandated that all patients on the experimental arm be crossed over to receive involved nodal radiotherapy.[101] Interestingly, the opposite conclusion was reached by investigators in England conducting a similarly designed trial, dubbed the "RAPID" trial.[102] In this study, patients with early stage cHL were given three cycles of ABVD followed by a PET scan. Patients who were PET-negative after three cycles of ABVD were randomized to either receive 30 Gy of involved field radiotherapy or no further treatment. Patients who were PET-positive after three cycles received a fourth cycle of ABVD followed by involved field radiotherapy. An intent-to-treat analysis of the randomized PET-negative population revealed a 3-year progression-free survival of 94.5 percent in the combined modality group compared to 90.8 percent in those receiving only three cycles of ABVD (p = 0.23). An analysis of the data according to the treatment actually received revealed a 3-year progression-free survival of 97 percent in the combined modality group compared to 90.7 percent in the ABVD-alone group (p = 0.03). There were no statistically significant differences in OS between the groups (97.1 vs. 99.5 percent, respectively; p = 0.07). The investigators conducting this trial concluded that the inferior progression-free survival in the group receiving ABVD alone was acceptable in order to avoid late complications associated with radiotherapy. In view of the conflicting conclusions derived from these two large phase III trials, the role of interim

FDG-PET/CT imaging in early stage cHL remains controversial. Nevertheless, the National Comprehensive Cancer Network has incorporated interim PET-imaging into their guidelines, suggesting that early stage cHL patients who are PET-negative after two cycles of ABVD may be treated with chemotherapy alone, without radiotherapy.[158]

UNFAVORABLE LIMITED-STAGE HODGKIN LYMPHOMA

Patients with "unfavorable" prognostic factors (large tumor bulk defined as a mass 10 cm or larger in diameter or more than one-third of the transthoracic diameter, an ESR of 50 or greater, three or more sites of tumor involvement, the presence of B symptoms, or the presence of extranodal sites [see Table 97–4]) require more intensive treatment than do patients not exhibiting any of these features.[158] The EORTC and the Groupe d'Etude des Lymphomes de l'Adulte (GELA) reported results from a randomized study (H9U) in which such "unfavorable" early stage patients were randomized to treatment with either four or six cycles of ABVD or six cycles of BEACOPP, each followed by 30-Gy involved-field radiotherapy.[156] No significant differences were observed among these three treatment arms, establishing four cycles of ABVD and 30 Gy of involved field radiotherapy as a standard of care for these patients. The GHSG subsequently randomized 1395 patients with unfavorable early stage Hodgkin lymphoma to four cycles of either ABVD or BEACOPP$_{baseline}$ followed by either 20 Gy or 30 Gy of involved field radiotherapy. In this study, four cycles of ABVD followed by 30 Gy of radiotherapy was the best approach, affording an 85 percent rate of "freedom from treatment failure" and an OS rate of approximately 95 percent after 5 years, while maintaining a favorable toxicity profile.[159] The administration of only 20 Gy of radiotherapy following ABVD was found to be clearly inferior to the other three treatment arms which all administered 30 Gy to this unfavorable group of patients. The subsequent GHSG HD14 study reported an advantage in progression-free survival for two cycles of escalated BEACOPP and two cycles of ABVD plus radiation therapy compared to four cycles of ABVD–radiation therapy, in a specified interim analysis, though no OS benefit was seen.[160] After 3 years, 90 percent of ABVD–radiation therapy patients were disease-free compared to 96 percent treated with the BEACOPP–ABVD–radiation therapy regimen. The EORTC//LySA/FIL H10 trial randomized both favorable and unfavorable early stage patients to either standard therapy or experimental, PET-response adapted therapy.[101] Of the 519 "unfavorable" patients evaluated in the interim analysis, 251 were randomized to standard ABVD for four cycles followed by 30 Gy of involved nodal radiotherapy, and 268 were randomized to PET-response adapted therapy. Patients on the experimental arm received six cycles of ABVD without any radiotherapy if the PET scan was negative after the second cycle of ABVD, whereas PET-positive patients were switched to BEACOPP$_{escalated}$ for 2 cycles followed by radiotherapy. An independent data safety monitoring board stopped this trial after a median followup of only 1.1 years because of worse outcomes on the experimental, PET-response adapted arm, with 16 relapses in 268 cases compared to only nine relapses of 251 cases on the standard arm (hazard ratio of 2.4; 95 percent confidence intervals 1.4 to 4.4).[101]

ADVANCED DISEASE

ABVD became the standard therapy for advanced Hodgkin lymphoma by proving to be superior to the MOPP chemotherapy and equal to, but less toxic than, hybrid or alternating combinations with MOPP.[141,142,161-164] Specifically, the incidence of secondary myelodysplasia, leukemia, and sterility was less with ABVD. The GHSG developed the BEACOPP regimen (see Table 97–3) based upon mathematical modeling that indicated a moderate increase in chemotherapy dose intensity would result in a significant increase in the cure rate. In the original HD9 study, BEACOPP was given in "standard" and "escalated" versions, the latter facilitated by granulocyte colony-stimulating factor use, and was compared with the cyclophosphamide, vincristine (Oncovin), procarbazine, prednisone (COPP)–ABVD regimen.[143] Patients with initial tumors equal to or greater than 5 cm or residual radiographic disease received 36-Gy radiotherapy after chemotherapy. The 5- and 10-year results demonstrated a significant progression-free and OS advantage for escalated BEACOPP compared to COPP–ABVD.[143,144] The cure rates in excess of 80 percent for escalated BEACOPP are the best ever recorded for a large phase III trial in advanced Hodgkin lymphoma. The superiority of escalated BEACOPP was observed regardless of the clinical international prognostic score.[124] Despite these outcomes, BEACOPP has not been universally accepted as the new standard in advanced Hodgkin lymphoma because of concerns about the acute toxicity, which includes greater need for hospitalization and transfusion, and late toxicity, which includes male and female sterility and an increased risk of secondary leukemia.[165-168] In addition, approximately two-thirds of patients received radiotherapy in the HD9 study. Two randomized clinical trials from Italy subsequently confirmed the superiority of BEACOPP over ABVD for the end point of progression-free survival.[169,170] In the first trial, BEACOPP (four escalated dose cycles plus two standard cycles) was compared to ABVD; all patients were to receive consolidation radiotherapy for bulky or residual disease. BEACOPP yielded significantly superior progression-free survival compared to ABVD although no difference in OS was observed.[169] In the second study, patients were randomized to ABVD versus four cycles of standard and four cycles of escalated BEACOPP with preplanned retreatment and high-dose therapy and autologous transplantation for treatment failures.[170] This study also showed a significantly higher progression-free survival for the BEACOPP arm but no difference in OS (Table 97–5). The EORTC 20012 Trial randomized patients with "high-risk" advanced stage Hodgkin lymphoma with an international prognostic scale score of 3 to 7[124] to treatment with either BEACOPP (four escalated cycles + four standard cycles) or ABVD.[171] Progression-free survival was improved in the BEACOPP arm but there was no statistically significant improvement in event-free or OS compared to ABVD.[171] In each of the four cited trials, the hazard ratio for relapse with BEACOPP was approximately 0.5. Standards of care in advanced Hodgkin lymphoma continue to be debated in view of the lack of a survival benefit with the BEACOPP program, which benefits approximately 15 percent of patients while exposing 100 percent of patients to more toxicity.

Efforts to reduce the risk of treatment-related morbidity of escalated BEACOPP have included studying the combination of four cycles of escalated and four cycles of standard BEACOPP and eliminating radiation therapy. In the GHSG HD12 trial, four standard cycles of BEACOPP plus four escalated cycles performed similarly to eight cycles of escalated BEACOPP, with freedom from treatment failure rates of 85 percent and 86 percent, respectively, 5 years after treatment. In this study, there was a slight trend for worse failure-free survival in patients with residual radiographic masses on end-of-treatment CT imaging who did not received consolidative radiotherapy (90 percent after 5 years with radiotherapy and 87 percent without it, p = 0.08).[172] The subsequent HD15 trial randomized 2182 patients with newly diagnosed advanced stage cHL to receive either eight cycles of BEACOPP$_{escalated}$, six cycles of BEACOPP$_{escalated}$, or eight cycles of the BEACOPP-14 regimen. Patients with a persistent mass after chemotherapy measuring 2.5 cm or larger that was FDG-avid on an end-of-treatment FDG-PET imaging received consolidative radiotherapy (30 Gy). Freedom from treatment failure was similar for all three treatment arms but 5-year OS was significantly better for patients receiving six cycles of BEACOPP$_{escalated}$ than

for 8 cycles of BEACOPP$_{escalated}$ (91.9 percent vs. 95.3 percent) as a result of higher treatment-related mortality and secondary malignancies with the latter regimen.[173]

Numerous investigations are underway to determine if interim PET scans can direct more-intensive treatment with escalated BEACOPP to the subgroup that benefits.[95,97,100,174,175] Likewise, interim and end-of-treatment PET scans are being used to direct the use of consolidative radiotherapy.[95,174-177] Although there is great enthusiasm regarding this approach to direct subsequent treatment, it is notable that the majority of patients remaining PET-positive after four cycles of escalated BEACOPP appear to be cured by the planned therapy, in contrast to findings with ABVD.[177]

The Stanford group took an alternate approach to advanced Hodgkin lymphoma by abbreviating the duration of therapy and reducing cumulative drug doses in the Stanford V regimen.[178] This approach appeared highly successful in institutional and phase II cooperative group trials; however, three randomized controlled trials have failed to show improved progression-free survival compared to standard ABVD chemotherapy.[179-181] The impressive efficacy of brentuximab vedotin in relapsed and refractory cHL[182,183] has also led to investigations into its incorporation into front-line regimens. This drug consists of an anti-CD30 monoclonal antibody conjugated to a highly potent antitubulin cytotoxic drug, monomethyl auristatin E. Phase I studies revealed unacceptable pulmonary toxicity when brentuximab vedotin was incorporated into the full ABVD regimen,[184] presumably as a result of augmenting the pulmonary toxicity of bleomycin. Omission of bleomycin, however, allows safe and effective combination therapy with brentuximab vedotin concurrently with AVD, with 96 percent of patients achieving complete remission.[184] An international phase III randomized comparison of standard ABVD versus brentuximab vedotin + AVD is underway for patients with advanced cHL.

The use of radiotherapy as a consolidation to combination chemotherapy in advanced cHL is controversial. Encouraging data from single institutions in adults and children were not borne out in randomized trials, some of which were criticized as underpowered. Furthermore, chemotherapy regimens have evolved over the time span of these studies. The application of 30 Gy involved-field radiotherapy to patients in complete remission after MOPP–ABV was studied in an adequately powered phase III trial.[185] No significant difference in failure-free survival was observed. Of note, all patients in partial remission received 40 Gy on this study and their outcome was not different from complete remission patients. The GHSG HD12 study randomized patients to observation or consolidation radiotherapy, with the incorporation of a central review panel, following BEACOPP. The final analysis of this study reported a slight decrease in the freedom from treatment failure if radiotherapy was omitted in patients who had persistent radiographic abnormalities on CT imaging after chemotherapy (90.4 percent vs. 87 percent after 5 years), but no difference was seen in patients with bulk disease in complete response after chemotherapy. Unfortunately, FDG-PET imaging was not routinely used in this trial.[172] The two Italian studies comparing ABVD with BEACOPP mentioned above routinely incorporated consolidation radiation therapy for residual or bulky disease.[169,186] The HD15 study limited the use of radiotherapy to patients with positive PET scans after four cycles of chemotherapy. With this approach, only 12 percent of patients received radiotherapy and the progression-free survival rate among PET-negative patients, who did not receive radiotherapy, was 96 percent after 1 year.[173] In sum, the data do not support the routine use of radiotherapy following a full course of chemotherapy in advanced Hodgkin lymphoma. However, the role of this potent treatment in patients with an early incomplete response or following a brief course of chemotherapy is likely to be more significant.[177,178]

TABLE 97–5. Selected Randomized Clinical Therapeutic Trials in Hodgkin Lymphoma

Study (Number of Patients)	Treatment	Failure-Free Survival (%)	Overall Survival (%)	Followup (Years)
LIMITED STAGE, FAVORABLE AND UNFAVORABLE				
Milan (140)[149]	4 ABVD + IFRT	94	94	12
	4 ABVD + STLI	93	96	
		p = NS	p = NS	
NCIC-ECOG (405)[155]	STLI	92	87	12
	4–6 ABVD	87	94	
		p = 0.006	p = NS	
LIMITED STAGE, FAVORABLE				
EORTC/GELA H9F (783)[156]	6 EBVP + 20-IFRT	84	98	4
	6 EBVP + 36-IFRT	87	98	
	6 EBVP	70	98	
		p ≤ 0.001	p = NS	
GHSG HD10 (1370)[278]	2 ABVD + 30-IFRT	86	94	8
	2 ABVD + 20-IFRT	86	95	
	4 ABVD + 30-IFRT	87	94	
	4 ABVD + 20-IFRT	90	95	
		p = NS	p = NS	
LIMITED STAGE, UNFAVORABLE				
EORTC/GELA H9U (808)[156]	6 ABVD + 30-IFRT	91	95	4
	4 ABVD + 30-IFRT	87	94	
	4 BEACOPP + 30-IFRT	90	93	
		p = NS	p = NS	
GHSG HD11 (1422)[159]	4 ABVD + 30-IFRT	85	94	
	4 ABVD + 20-IFRT	81*	94	
	4 BEACOPP + 30-IFRT	87	95	
	4 BEACOPP+ 20-IFRT	87	95	
ADVANCED STAGE				
GHSG HD9 (1201)[143]	8 COPP/ABVD + RT	64	75	10
	8 BEACOPP + RT	70	80	
	8 BEACOPP$_{escalated}$ + RT	82	86	
		p <0.0001	p <0.005	
US Intergroup (854)[181]	6–8 ABVD	74	88	5
	Stanford V	71	88	
		p = NS	p = NS	
Italian Intergroup (331)[170]	6–8 ABVD	73	84	7
	BEACOPP (4 escalated + 4 standard cycles)	85	89	
		p = 0.004	p = 0.39	

ABVD, doxorubicin, bleomycin, vinblastine, dacarbazine; BEACOPP, bleomycin, etoposide, doxorubicin, cyclophosphamide, vincristine, procarbazine, prednisone; COPP, cyclophosphamide, vincristine, procarbazine, prednisone; EBVP, epirubicin, bleomycin, vinblastine, prednisone; ECOG, Eastern Cooperative Oncology Group; EORTC, European Organization for the Research and Treatment of Cancer; GELA, Groupe d'Etude des Lymphomes de l'Adulte; GHSG, German Hodgkin Study Group; IFRT, involved-field radiotherapy; NCIC, National Cancer Institute of Canada; RT, radiotherapy; STLI, subtotal lymphoid irradiation.
*p = 0.03

NODULAR LYMPHOCYTE PREDOMINANT HODGKIN LYMPHOMA

NLPHL presents as asymptomatic, limited-stage disease in most (~80 percent) patients.[103,104,109] Peripheral lymph nodes in the neck, axilla, or groin are commonly involved as stage IA disease. The European Task Force on lymphoma reported a 96 percent complete response rate and 99 percent and 94 percent 8-year disease-specific survival for stages I and II disease, respectively.[109] Because of the low likelihood of occult disease in nodular lymphocyte-predominant Hodgkin lymphoma and the tendency for the disease to remain localized for years, regional radiation therapy is considered the treatment of choice for early stage disease.[104] Analyses from the GHSG demonstrate that outcomes with limited radiation therapy are comparable to the use of more extensive radiation and combined modality regimens.[187] For the 20 percent of patients who present with stage III or IV disease, most authorities advise treatment with ABVD-based chemotherapy following the paradigms developed for cHL,[104] although some contend that alkylator-based regimens such as rituximab, cyclophosphamide, hydroxydaunorubicin, vincristine (Oncovin), prednisone (R-CHOP) may be equally effective and less toxic.[188] Because of the consistent high level expression of the CD20 antigen on the surface of NLPHL cells, the monoclonal antibody rituximab has been tested in this entity. Initial studies were conducted using single-agent rituximab in relapsed and refractory cases and demonstrated response rates of 94 to 100 percent with median durations of remission of 33 to 60 months, with longer remissions observed when maintenance rituximab was used.[189,190] Based on these findings,, and the low toxicity of rituximab, some authorities have extrapolated its use to the frontline setting,[188] adding it to radiotherapy for stage I or II patients and to ABVD for stage III or IV disease, although few data been published concerning the frontline use of this agent in NLPHL.

RECURRENT DISEASE

Historically, patients with cHL who relapsed after a full course of chemotherapy had a low chance for cure with second-line treatment, with the duration of initial remission a significant predictor of subsequent response and relapse-free survival. High-dose therapy and autologous blood stem cell transplantation improved the outlook for such patients and is routinely employed in first relapse for most patients younger than age 65 years, based on institutional and phase III trial experience.[191,192] Cure rates with transplantation range from 40 to 60 percent with transplant-related mortality less than 5 percent.[193,194] High-dose regimens include BEAM (carmustine, etoposide, cytarabine, melphalan), CBV (cyclophosphamide, carmustine, etoposide), and total-body irradiation with cyclophosphamide and etoposide. Consolidation radiotherapy is often employed to sites of pretransplantation bulk disease. The superiority of any single transplant conditioning regimen has not been definitively established; however, the use of high-dose sequential therapy coupled with tandem autologous transplantation is being tested in randomized trials.[195,196] In most cases, second-line chemotherapy with ICE (ifosfamide, carboplatin, etoposide), GVD (gemcitabine, vinorelbine, liposomal doxorubicin), DHAP (dexamethasone, cytarabine, cisplatin), or brentuximab vedotin is used to achieve a minimal disease state prior to stem cell mobilization and transplantation.[197-199] Treatment failures following autologous transplantation present a challenge, with longevity directly related to the time to relapse after transplantation. Allogeneic transplantation in multiply recurrent Hodgkin lymphoma has been limited by significant transplant-related mortality, although long-term disease control has been observed in a small subset together with anecdotal evidence of a graft-versus-Hodgkin antitumor effect. Nonmyeloablative transplantation conditioning regimens reduce transplant-related

mortality but disease recurrence continues to present a major challenge, with failure-free survivals in the 20 to 30 percent range.[199-201]

As mentioned above, the anti-CD20 antibody rituximab achieves high response rates in relapsed NLPHL and can be used as retreatment or as an extended-treatment regimen.[189,202] Monoclonal antibodies directed against the CD30 antigen are well tolerated in classical Hodgkin lymphoma but have limited therapeutic value.[203] However, the anti-CD30 antibody–drug conjugate, brentuximab vedotin has major activity with 96 of 102 patients with relapsed or refractory cHL experiencing tumor shrinkage in a phase II clinical trial, including 75 percent with objective remissions and 34 percent with complete remissions.[183] The agent has also shown major efficacy when used as a bridge to allogeneic transplantation[204] or in patients relapsing after allogeneic stem cell transplantation.[205] The major toxicity of this agent when used as a single agent is peripheral neuropathy, though mild to moderate cytopenias also occur. Nivolumab and pembrolizumab are PD-1 blocking antibodies that have recently been shown to have remarkable efficacy in patients with relapsed or refractory cHL, with objective remission rates of up to 87 percent observed in trials enrolling heavily pretreated patients.[205A]

● COURSE AND PROGNOSIS

The goal of treatment for Hodgkin lymphoma is to cure the greatest number of patients with the fewest complications. Improvements in management have resulted in cure for a large majority of patients younger than age 65 years. Survival expectations at 10 years for patients diagnosed from 2006 to 2010 exceed 90 percent for patients to age 44 years, 80 percent for patients to age 54 years, and 70 percent for patients to age 64 years.[206] These outstanding results have been achieved by refining the use of radiotherapy and chemotherapy in the frontline setting and the development of improved secondary treatments for patients with persistent or relapsed disease. However, the late effects of treatment for Hodgkin lymphoma remain a concern for cured patients, and a small subset of patients has refractory disease.

CLINICAL PROGNOSTIC FACTORS

A number of complex prognostic factor schemes have been developed for limited Hodgkin lymphoma treated with radiotherapy alone (see Table 97–4). Massive mediastinal disease and constitutional symptoms have been consistently identified as independent predictors of relapse, whereas only older age was predictive of inferior survival. European and Canadian investigators incorporated gender, age, ESR, number of Ann Arbor disease sites, stage, and histology into stratifications for favorable, very favorable, and unfavorable disease categories. The EORTC defines four or more nodal sites, ESR greater than 50 in asymptomatic patients or ESR greater than 40 in symptomatic patients, and histology as indicators of intermediate disease, whereas the GHSG designates any one of the following: massive mediastinal disease, extranodal disease, ESR greater than 50 if asymptomatic and greater than 30 if symptomatic, and three or more nodal sites as intermediate disease (see Table 97–4). It is important to be aware of the variable eligibility criteria when interpreting the literature in early stage Hodgkin lymphoma and to note that these clinical variables are currently used to group patients for clinical investigations. The international prognostic score, based on seven factors (see Table 97–4), is used in advanced disease.[124,207] Each factor reduced the freedom from progression by approximately 7 percent. Only 7 percent of patients were in the worst prognostic group (five to seven factors) and the freedom from progression in this subset was 42 percent at 5 years. Consensus with regard to prognostic factors promotes uniformity in clinical trial design and provides a rationale for alternate approaches in high-risk subsets. The superiority of escalated BEACOPP was seen across the spectrum of the international prognostic score, but approximately 30 percent of high-risk (four to seven factors) patients experience treatment failure.[144] Alternately, the improvement in progression-free survival with BEACOPP over ABVD in an Italian study was limited to higher-risk patients.[169] Age has been a consistent adverse prognostic marker regardless of tumor burden, but recent gains eliminate this adverse factor up to approximately age 55 years.[208,209] Although less-intensive treatment may explain inferior results in a subset of patients, results in older patients are worse, even when the intensity of therapy is controlled.[209] The BEACOPP regimen was associated with unacceptable toxicity and demonstrated no advance over ABVD for patients older than age 65 years.[210]

Normal results from FDG-PET imaging at the completion of treatment confers a high negative predictive value, ranging from 81 to 100 percent.[176] The positive predictive value at the end of chemotherapy is more variable and is related to disease extent and use of radiotherapy.[176,211,212] There is great interest in FDG-PET imaging after one to three cycles of chemotherapy, as several studies indicate that negative results predict treatment success whereas positive results predict a high likelihood of treatment failure.[95,96,98,99] Numerous ongoing phase III clinical trials are designed to alter treatment based on early PET results with a goal of achieving high cure rates and minimizing toxicity.[100] PET status prior to autologous transplantation has also emerged as a dominant prognostic factor.[213]

Adverse prognostic factors identified for patients with relapsed cHL undergoing autologous stem cell transplantation include (1) duration of first complete remission less than 1 year, (2) failure to achieve a second complete remission with salvage chemotherapy prior to transplantation, (3) presence of B symptoms or extranodal sites of disease involvement, and (4) persistence of FDG-avidity on PET imaging prior to transplant.[213–215]

Patients with primary progressive Hodgkin lymphoma have the least-favorable prognosis. Fortunately, newer treatment approaches have reduced the proportion of patients in this category.

Clinical prognostic factors are surrogates for the underlying cellular and molecular biology of Hodgkin lymphoma. Serum levels of cytokines, including soluble CD30, a probable marker of tumor burden, and IL-10, a measure of immunosuppression related to the microenvironment, are associated with adverse prognosis independent of clinical features.[216] The chemokine CCL17, secreted by Hodgkin and Reed-Sternberg cells, is elevated in patients' sera and is being studied as a marker of response.[217,218] Multiple, but not all, investigators found BCL-2 expression to be of prognostic significance.[219–222] CD20 expression by Hodgkin and Reed-Sternberg cells has been associated with less-favorable outcomes in some, but not all, series.[223,224] Lack of HLA class II expression, which may allow immune escape of Hodgkin and Reed-Sternberg cells, was found to be an independent prognostic factor.[225] The prognostic significance of EBV association varies with age, conferring an adverse outcome in older individuals.[226,227] Furthermore, single nucleotide polymorphisms in HLA-A2 have been associated with risk of EBV-positive Hodgkin lymphoma.[52] A number of studies have focused on the inflammatory microenvironment of Hodgkin lymphoma. Increased numbers of T-regulatory cells have correlated with favorable outcomes and decreased numbers of markers for cytotoxic T cells have correlated with adverse outcomes in several series.[228–230] Similarly, heavy infiltration of cHL with macrophages (detected by immunohistocytochemical staining for CD68), is associated with poor outcome, presumably because of secretion of immunosuppressive cytokines.[231] Finally, a 23-gene expression signature that can be assessed in formalin-fixed paraffin embedded tissue biopsies has been shown to have major prognostic power in patients with cHL.[232] Together, these findings suggest an important interplay between characteristics of Hodgkin and Reed-Sternberg cells and the inflammatory environment.

COMPLICATIONS OF TREATMENT

The treatment of Hodgkin lymphoma is associated with important acute and chronic side effects. Although the acute complications of chemotherapy and radiotherapy may be troublesome, they are relatively easily managed. Late-treatment effects in the form of sterility, second malignancy, and cardiopulmonary disease are more serious and are known to contribute to shortened longevity for cured patients.[145,152,233,234] Excess mortality from second malignancies and cardiac disease increase with time and are currently the leading causes of death for cHL patients. As treatment has evolved, the risks of radiation-related complications has lessened but long latency periods and uncertainty regarding associations with lower doses make it difficult to predict individual risks. Recognition and understanding of these problems helps to shape primary treatment choice and facilitate optimal followup for survivors.

Acute leukemia and myelodysplasia were the initial second malignancies to be observed after successful treatment for Hodgkin lymphoma with MOPP chemotherapy.[235] The risk following MOPP was proportional to the cumulative dose of alkylating agents and was associated with recurring abnormalities of chromosomes 5 and 7.[235–237] Actuarial risks of approximately 5 percent with relative risks in excess of 100 have been reported over a 7- to 10-year period with alkylating agent-based therapies. The risk of secondary leukemia is greater in patients older than age 35 years. Prognosis for secondary leukemia is poor with survivals of less than 1 year.[238] The risk of acute leukemia is significantly less after ABVD chemotherapy,[141] although it is not absent. A large international study observed a significant reduction in excess absolute risk after 1984, presumably as a consequence of change in primary therapy.[238] However, acute leukemia may complicate Hodgkin lymphoma treatment with higher doses of etoposide and doxorubicin, such as in the BEACOPP regimen.[143,165,168] This form of leukemia tends to occur earlier and be associated with balanced translocations of chromosome 11. Patients who have received second-line therapies and autologous transplantation are at highest risk for myelodysplasia and secondary leukemia.

There is an increased relative risk of non-Hodgkin lymphomas after treatment for Hodgkin lymphoma.[239,240] These are diffuse, aggressive B-cell lymphomas that may occur early or late after treatment. There is no clear relationship to the type of primary treatment. The incidence of secondary lymphoma in a series of 5406 patients treated on GHSG protocols was 0.9 percent; prognosis was worse if lymphoma developed within 3 months of primary therapy.[241] Although prognosis was relatively poor in this series, the data antedated the routine use of rituximab in treatment regimens. It is not clear how non-Hodgkin lymphomas relate to treatment-related immunodeficiency, predisposition to B-cell malignancy, or a shared common cell of origin. Marginal zone lymphomas with identical B-cell receptor genes also have been identified.[242] Diffuse large B-cell lymphoma and its variants are most frequent in nodular lymphocyte-predominant Hodgkin lymphoma, where they have been found to be genetically related.[243]

An increased risk of solid cancers after treatment for Hodgkin lymphoma has long been recognized, and with time, these have emerged to account for 75 to 80 percent of all cases of second malignancy.[145,152,239] The risk is related to radiotherapy exposure, with tumors occurring in or at the edges of the radiation field. The most common solid tumors are breast, lung, and gastrointestinal malignancies. The latency for developing second cancers is an important consideration, as these typically develop after at least 10 years and continue to pose excess risk for as long as 30 years after treatment. Breast cancer is increased in women treated before age 30 years and is markedly increased in children and adolescents.[152,244–246] Case-control studies have examined the relationship of radiation dose to the breast and the risk of cancer, finding a 3.2-fold increased risk with doses greater than 4 Gy and an eightfold risk for doses greater than 40 Gy.[247,248] Elimination of routine axillary radiation, which is now standard, results in a 2.7-fold reduction in risk and it is anticipated that risks may further decline with current low-dose or nodal radiotherapy. Cofactors are important for defining the risks of second breast cancer, which are highest for women younger than age 30 years when irradiated and for those who continue to have normal menses.[249,250]

Lung cancer risk is greatest among patients who are older than 45 years of age when treated. Tobacco exposure has a multiplying effect and alkylating agent exposure also contributes to risk. Among patients with chest irradiation, a tobacco history, and alkylating chemotherapy, the lung cancer risk was 49-fold higher than in patients who had none of these exposures.[248] Alkylating agent chemotherapy independently increases risk of lung cancer with dose–response associations reported in population-based studies.[247,248,251]

Estimates of relative risks of cardiac mortality in Hodgkin lymphoma survivors range from 2.2- to sevenfold.[233,234,252,253] Mediastinal radiotherapy is associated with an increased risk of cardiac disease. An increased risk of death from coronary artery disease and acute myocardial infarction has been identified in adults and children.[245,253,254] Other types of cardiac disease are often asymptomatic, including valvular disease, conduction defects, and cardiomyopathy.[255,256] The risks of radiation-related heart disease do not appear to be influenced significantly by the addition of chemotherapy. The onset of increased risk is within 5 to 10 years. As risk is associated with the dose and volume of radiotherapy and the latency is 5 to 10 or more years, the hazards associated with current lower dose and smaller fields remain to be assessed.[252] Established cardiac risk factors, including hypertension, hypercholesterolemia, and smoking, significantly contribute to the subsequent risk of cardiac disease after therapy, offering opportunities to reduce individual risks.[257] A British report indicated an elevated risk of cardiac mortality of 7.8-fold following ABVD alone, which rose to 12.1-fold when given with mediastinal irradiation.[258] These results provide a cautionary note, but more data are needed and these results do not address cumulative exposures that are lower with modern therapy.

Noncoronary vascular complications have been reported after neck irradiation, with associations to dose greater than 36 Gy and cofactors of hypertension, diabetes and hypercholesterolemia.[259,260] In a retrospective cohort study, the standardized incidence ratio for was 2.2 for stroke and 3.1 for transient ischemic attack.[259] However, it is important to note that modern approaches to Hodgkin lymphoma therapy use lower radiation doses, smaller fields, and planning techniques that limit dose inhomogeneity and hot spots commonly seen in the neck area with older techniques.

Approximately 90 percent of males are permanently sterilized by six cycles of MOPP chemotherapy.[261] The risk is related to the cumulative dose of alkylating agents such that two to three cycles of MOPP result in azoospermia in approximately 50 percent of patients.[262] Female fertility after alkylating agent-based treatment is related to age at treatment as well as cumulative alkylating agent dose.[263,264] The ABVD combination is associated with temporary amenorrhea and azoospermia with full recovery noted in 50 to 95 percent of patients.[265,266] A case-control study found no significant reduction in fertility among women treated with ABVD.[267] In contrast, no men had normospermia following treatment with BEACOPP and amenorrhea occurred in more than 50 percent of women.[166,167,268] Several authors have described pregnancy outcome following treatment for Hodgkin lymphoma. No increase in birth defects or complications of pregnancy has been seen.[264]

Thyroid dysfunction is common after neck irradiation, reaching a risk of 47 percent at 26 years in the Stanford series.[269] Thus, patients at risk should be monitored during followup observation. Rarely, hyperthyroidism, Graves ophthalmopathy or thyroid neoplasms occur after neck radiotherapy.[269] Lhermitte sign, a transient complaint of an "electric shock" sensation produced by head flexion, is a common sequela of mantle radiotherapy.[270] The incidence of radiation pneumonitis depends on the volume of lung irradiated and the total dose. Symptoms include cough, dyspnea, and fever. Although prospective assessment of pulmonary function demonstrates reduction of lung volumes following mantle radiotherapy, recovery is seen in 12 to 24 months and symptomatic radiation pneumonitis is unusual.[271,272]

Full-dose radiation therapy interferes with normal growth and development in children. Current therapy programs use low-dose or no radiotherapy for all stages of disease. Overwhelming sepsis is a rare event in patients who have been splenectomized and treated for Hodgkin lymphoma, particularly children.[273,274] Vaccination against encapsulated organisms 10 to 14 days prior to the onset of treatment is advised. However, it must be recognized that neither vaccines nor antibiotic prophylaxis may provide adequate protection. Fatigue is commonly reported in Hodgkin lymphoma survivors and has been related to pulmonary function and peak oxygen uptake.[255,275]

With the high rates of cure currently attained in the management of Hodgkin lymphoma, reduction in late effects and quality of life assume even greater importance. Patient education is essential to promote healthy behaviors to reduce modifiable risk factors. In addition, early detection and prevention strategies for second cancers and cardiac disease should be considered in high-risk patients. However, the choice and efficacy of diagnostic testing, and their optimal timing and frequency, require further study.[276] Most of the documented late effects relate to outdated chemotherapy and radiotherapy protocols, and that modeling, as well as recent data, indicate that lesser exposures significantly reduce second cancer risk.[249,277] Modern therapies will likely further reduce the risks of late complications. It continues to be important to follow long-term survivors, and the contribution of genetic and environmental factors is an important ongoing area of inquiry.

REFERENCES

1. Hodgkin T: On some morbid appearances of the absorbent glands and spleen. *Med Chir Trans* 17:68–114, 1832.
2. Wilks S: Cases of lardaceous disease and some allied affections, with remarks. *Guys Hosp Rep* 17:103–132, 1856.
3. Dreschfeld J: Clinical lecture on acute Hodgkin's disease. *Br Med J* 1:893–896, 1892.
4. Kundrat H: Uber Lympho-Sarkomatosis. *Wien Klin Wochenschr* 6:211–234, 1893.
5. Sternberg C: Über eine eigenartige unter dem Bilde der Pseudoleukämie verlaufende Tuberculose des lymphatischen Apparates. *Ztschr Heilk* 19:21–90, 1898.
6. Reed D: On the pathological changes in Hodgkin's disease, with special reference to its relation to tuberculosis. *Johns Hopkins' Hosp Rep* 10:133–196, 1902.
7. Fox H: Remarks on microscopical preparations made from some of the original tissue described by Thomas Hodgkin, 1832. *Ann Med Hist* 8:370–374, 1926.
8. Jackson H, Parker F: *Hodgkin's Disease and Allied Disorders.* Oxford University Press, New York, 1947.
9. Lukes RJ, Craver LF, Hall TC, et al: Report of the nomenclature committee. *Cancer Res* 26:1311, 1966.
10. Swerdlow SH, Campo E, Harris NL, et al: *WHO Classification of Tumours of Haematopoietic and Lymphoid Tissues,* 4th ed. International Agency for Research on Cancer, Lyon, 2008.
11. Peters M: A study in survivals in Hodgkin's disease treated radiologically. *AJR Am J Roentgenol* 63:299–311, 1950.
12. Kinmonth JB: Lymphangiography in man; a method of outlining lymphatic trunks at operation. *Clin Sci (Lond)* 11:13–20, 1952.
13. Glatstein E, Guernsey JM, Rosenberg SA, et al: The value of laparotomy and splenectomy in the staging of Hodgkin's disease. *Cancer* 24:709–718, 1969.
14. Rosenberg SA: Report of the committee on the staging of Hodgkin's disease. *Cancer Res* 26:1225–1231, 1966.
15. Carbone PP, Kaplan HS, Musshoff K, et al: Report of the Committee on Hodgkin's Disease Staging Classification. *Cancer Res* 31:1860–1861, 1971.
16. Pusey W: Cases of sarcoma and of Hodgkin's disease treated by exposures to X-rays: A preliminary report. *JAMA* 38:166–196, 1902.
17. Senn N: Therapeutical value of Roentgen ray in treatment of pseudoleukemia. *NY Med J* 77:665–668, 1903.

18. Gilbert R: Radiotherapy in Hodgkin's disease (malignant granulomatosis): Anatomic and clinical foundations, governing principles, results. *AJR Am J Roentgenol* 41:198–241, 1939.
19. Kaplan HS: The radical radiotherapy of regionally localized Hodgkin's disease. *Radiology* 78:553–561, 1962.
20. Goodman LS, Wintrobe MM, et al: Nitrogen mustard therapy; use of methyl-bis (beta-chloroethyl) amine hydrochloride and tris (beta-chloroethyl) amine hydrochloride for Hodgkin's disease, lymphosarcoma, leukemia and certain allied and miscellaneous disorders. *JAMA* 132:126–132, 1946.
21. Jacobson LO, Spurr CL, et al: Nitrogen mustard therapy; studies on the effect of methyl-bis (beta-chloroethyl) amine hydrochloride on neoplastic diseases and allied disorders of the hemopoietic system. *JAMA* 132:263–271, 1946.
22. Devita VT Jr, Serpick AA, Carbone PP: Combination chemotherapy in the treatment of advanced Hodgkin's disease. *Ann Intern Med* 73:881–895, 1970.
23. Bonadonna G, Zucali R, Monfardini S, et al: Combination chemotherapy of Hodgkin's disease with Adriamycin, bleomycin, vinblastine, and imidazole carboxamide versus MOPP. *Cancer* 36:252–259, 1975.
24. Surveillance, Epidemiology, and End Results (SEER) Program (www.seer.cancer.gov) Research Data (1973–2011), National Cancer Institute, DCCPS, Surveillance Research Program, Surveillance Systems Branch, released April 2014, based on the November 2013 submission; 2014.
25. Clarke CA, Glaser SL, Keegan TH, et al: Neighborhood socioeconomic status and Hodgkin's lymphoma incidence in California. *Cancer Epidemiol Biomarkers Prev* 14:1441–1447, 2005.
26. MacMahon B: Epidemiology of Hodgkin's disease. *Cancer Res* 26:1189–1201, 1966.
27. Landgren O, Engels EA, Pfeiffer RM, et al: Autoimmunity and susceptibility to Hodgkin lymphoma: A population-based case-control study in Scandinavia. *J Natl Cancer Inst* 98:1321–1330, 2006.
28. Grufferman S, Delzell E: Epidemiology of Hodgkin's disease. *Epidemiol Rev* 6:76–106, 1984.
29. Au WY, Gascoyne RD, Gallagher RE, et al: Hodgkin's lymphoma in Chinese migrants to British Columbia: A 25-year survey. *Ann Oncol* 15:626–630, 2004.
30. Katanoda K, Yako-Suketomo H: Comparison of time trends in Hodgkin and non-Hodgkin lymphoma incidence (1973–97) in East Asia, Europe and USA, from cancer incidence in five continents Vol. IV–VIII. *Jpn J Clin Oncol* 38:391–393, 2008.
31. Vianna NJ, Greenwald P, Davies JN: Extended epidemic of Hodgkin's disease in high-school students. *Lancet* 1:1209–1211, 1971.
32. Kvale G, Hoiby EA, Pedersen E: Hodgkin's disease in patients with previous infectious mononucleosis. *Int J Cancer* 23:593–597, 1979.
33. Rosdahl N, Larsen SO, Clemmesen J: Hodgkin's disease in patients with previous infectious mononucleosis: 30 years' experience. *Br Med J* 2:253–256, 1974.
34. Mueller N, Evans A, Harris NL, et al: Hodgkin's disease and Epstein-Barr virus. Altered antibody pattern before diagnosis. *N Engl J Med* 320:689–695, 1989.
35. Alexander FE, Lawrence DJ, Freeland J, et al: An epidemiologic study of index and family infectious mononucleosis and adult Hodgkin's disease (HD): Evidence for a specific association with EBV+ve HD in young adults. *Int J Cancer* 107:298–302, 2003.
36. Hjalgrim H, Askling J, Rostgaard K, et al: Characteristics of Hodgkin's lymphoma after infectious mononucleosis. *N Engl J Med* 349:1324–1332, 2003.
37. Ambinder RF, Browning PJ, Lorenzana I, et al: Epstein-Barr virus and childhood Hodgkin's disease in Honduras and the United States. *Blood* 81:462–467, 1993.
38. Armstrong AA, Alexander FE, Cartwright R, et al: Epstein-Barr virus and Hodgkin's disease: Further evidence for the three disease hypothesis. *Leukemia* 12:1272–1276, 1998.
39. Glaser SL, Lin RJ, Stewart SL, et al: Epstein-Barr virus-associated Hodgkin's disease: Epidemiologic characteristics in international data. *Int J Cancer* 70:375–382, 1997.
40. Herndier BG, Sanchez HC, Chang KL, et al: High prevalence of Epstein-Barr virus in the Reed-Sternberg cells of HIV-associated Hodgkin's disease. *Am J Pathol* 142:1073–1079, 1993.
41. Biggar RJ, Jaffe ES, Goedert JJ, et al: Hodgkin lymphoma and immunodeficiency in persons with HIV/AIDS. *Blood* 108:3786–3791, 2006.
42. Powles T, Robinson D, Stebbing J, et al: Highly active antiretroviral therapy and the incidence of non-AIDS-defining cancers in people with HIV infection. *J Clin Oncol* 27:884–890, 2009.
43. Mack TM, Cozen W, Shibata DK, et al: Concordance for Hodgkin's disease in identical twins suggesting genetic susceptibility to the young-adult form of the disease. *N Engl J Med* 332:413–418, 1995.
44. Chang ET, Smedby KE, Hjalgrim H, et al: Family history of hematopoietic malignancy and risk of lymphoma. *J Natl Cancer Inst* 97:1466–1474, 2005.
45. Ferraris AM, Racchi O, Rapezzi D, et al: Familial Hodgkin's disease: A disease of young adulthood? *Ann Hematol* 74:131–134, 1997.
46. Goldin LR, Pfeiffer RM, Gridley G, et al: Familial aggregation of Hodgkin lymphoma and related tumors. *Cancer* 100:1902–1908, 2004.
47. Hemminki K, Li X, Czene K: Familial risk of cancer: Data for clinical counseling and cancer genetics. *Int J Cancer* 108:109–114, 2004.
48. Altieri A, Hemminki K: The familial risk of Hodgkin's lymphoma ranks among the highest in the Swedish Family-Cancer Database. *Leukemia* 20:2062–2063, 2006.
49. Grufferman S, Cole P, Smith PG, et al: Hodgkin's disease in siblings. *N Engl J Med* 296:248–250, 1977.
50. Horwitz MS, Mealiffe ME: Further evidence for a pseudoautosomal gene for Hodgkin's lymphoma: Reply to "The familial risk of Hodgkin's lymphoma ranks among the highest in the Swedish Family-Cancer Database" by Altieri A and Hemminki K. *Leukemia* 21:351, 2007.
51. Cimino G, Lo Coco F, Cartoni C, et al: Immune-deficiency in Hodgkin's disease (HD): A study of patients and healthy relatives in families with multiple cases. *Eur J Cancer Clin Oncol* 24:1595–1601, 1988.
52. Niens M, Jarrett RF, Hepkema B, et al: HLA-A*02 is associated with a reduced risk and HLA-A*01 with an increased risk of developing EBV+ Hodgkin lymphoma. *Blood* 110:3310–3315, 2007.
53. Kuppers R, Rajewsky K, Zhao M, et al: Hodgkin disease: Hodgkin and Reed-Sternberg cells picked from histological sections show clonal immunoglobulin gene rearrangements and appear to be derived from B cells at various stages of development. *Proc Natl Acad Sci U S A* 91:10962–10966, 1994.
54. Kuppers R, Roers A, Kanzler H: Molecular single cell studies of normal and transformed lymphocytes. *Cancer Surv* 30:45–58, 1997.
55. Bargou RC, Emmerich F, Krappmann D, et al: Constitutive nuclear factor-kappaB-RelA activation is required for proliferation and survival of Hodgkin's disease tumor cells. *J Clin Invest* 100:2961–2969, 1997.
56. Jox A, Zander T, Kuppers R, et al: Somatic mutations within the untranslated regions of rearranged Ig genes in a case of classical Hodgkin's disease as a potential cause for the absence of Ig in the lymphoma cells. *Blood* 93:3964–3972, 1999.
57. Kanzler H, Kuppers R, Hansmann ML, et al: Hodgkin and Reed-Sternberg cells in Hodgkin's disease represent the outgrowth of a dominant tumor clone derived from (crippled) germinal center B cells. *J Exp Med* 184:1495–1505, 1996.
58. Muschen M, Rajewsky K, Brauninger A, et al: Rare occurrence of classical Hodgkin's disease as a T cell lymphoma. *J Exp Med* 191:387–394, 2000.
59. Braeuninger A, Kuppers R, Strickler JG, et al: Hodgkin and Reed-Sternberg cells in lymphocyte predominant Hodgkin disease represent clonal populations of germinal center-derived tumor B cells. *Proc Natl Acad Sci U S A* 94:9337–9342, 1997.
60. Marafioti T, Hummel M, Anagnostopoulos I, et al: Origin of nodular lymphocyte-predominant Hodgkin's disease from a clonal expansion of highly mutated germinal-center B cells. *N Engl J Med* 337:453–458, 1997.
61. Ohno T, Stribley JA, Wu G, et al: Clonality in nodular lymphocyte-predominant Hodgkin's disease. *N Engl J Med* 337:459–465, 1997.
62. Schwering I, Brauninger A, Klein U, et al: Loss of the B-lineage-specific gene expression program in Hodgkin and Reed-Sternberg cells of Hodgkin lymphoma. *Blood* 101:1505–1512, 2003.
63. Re D, Muschen M, Ahmadi T, et al: Oct-2 and Bob-1 deficiency in Hodgkin and Reed Sternberg cells. *Cancer Res* 61:2080–2084, 2001.
64. Stein H, Marafioti T, Foss HD, et al: Down-regulation of BOB.1/OBF.1 and Oct2 in classical Hodgkin disease but not in lymphocyte predominant Hodgkin disease correlates with immunoglobulin transcription. *Blood* 97:496–501, 2001.
65. Ushmorov A, Leithauser F, Sakk O, et al: Epigenetic processes play a major role in B-cell-specific gene silencing in classical Hodgkin lymphoma. *Blood* 107:2493–2500, 2006.
66. Cobaleda C, Schebesta A, Delogu A, et al: Pax5: The guardian of B cell identity and function. *Nat Immunol* 8:463–470, 2007.
67. Foss HD, Reusch R, Demel G, et al: Frequent expression of the B-cell-specific activator protein in Reed-Sternberg cells of classical Hodgkin's disease provides further evidence for its B-cell origin. *Blood* 94:3108–3113, 1999.
68. Mathas S, Janz M, Hummel F, et al: Intrinsic inhibition of transcription factor E2A by HLH proteins ABF-1 and Id2 mediates reprogramming of neoplastic B cells in Hodgkin lymphoma. *Nat Immunol* 7:207–215, 2006.
69. Jundt F, Acikgoz O, Kwon SH, et al: Aberrant expression of Notch1 interferes with the B-lymphoid phenotype of neoplastic B cells in classical Hodgkin lymphoma. *Leukemia* 22:1587–1594, 2008.
70. Kumano K, Chiba S, Shimizu K, et al: Notch1 inhibits differentiation of hematopoietic cells by sustaining GATA-2 expression. *Blood* 98:3283–3289, 2001.
71. Dukers DF, van Galen JC, Giroth C, et al: Unique polycomb gene expression pattern in Hodgkin's lymphoma and Hodgkin's lymphoma-derived cell lines. *Am J Pathol* 164:873–881, 2004.
72. Scheeren FA, Diehl SA, Smit LA, et al: IL-21 is expressed in Hodgkin lymphoma and activates STAT5: Evidence that activated STAT5 is required for Hodgkin lymphoma-genesis. *Blood* 111:4706–4715, 2008.
73. Marafioti T, Hummel M, Foss HD, et al: Hodgkin and Reed-Sternberg cells represent an expansion of a single clone originating from a germinal center B-cell with functional immunoglobulin gene rearrangements but defective immunoglobulin transcription. *Blood* 95:1443–1450, 2000.
74. Joos S, Kupper M, Ohl S, et al: Genomic imbalances including amplification of the tyrosine kinase gene JAK2 in CD30+ Hodgkin cells. *Cancer Res* 60:549–552, 2000.
75. Weniger MA, Melzner I, Menz CK, et al: Mutations of the tumor suppressor gene SOCS-1 in classical Hodgkin lymphoma are frequent and associated with nuclear phospho-STAT5 accumulation. *Oncogene* 25:2679–2684, 2006.
76. Barth TF, Martin-Subero JI, Joos S, et al: Gains of 2p involving the REL locus correlate with nuclear c-Rel protein accumulation in neoplastic cells of classical Hodgkin lymphoma. *Blood* 101:3681–3686, 2003.
77. Cabannes E, Khan G, Aillet F, et al: Mutations in the IkBa gene in Hodgkin's disease suggest a tumour suppressor role for IkappaBalpha. *Oncogene* 18:3063–3070, 1999.
78. Emmerich F, Theurich S, Hummel M, et al: Inactivating I kappa B epsilon mutations in Hodgkin/Reed-Sternberg cells. *J Pathol* 201:413–420, 2003.

79. Schmitz R, Hansmann ML, Bohle V, et al: TNFAIP3 (A20) is a tumor suppressor gene in Hodgkin lymphoma and primary mediastinal B cell lymphoma. *J Exp Med* 206: 981–989, 2009.

80. Baus D, Pfitzner E: Specific function of STAT3, SOCS1, and SOCS3 in the regulation of proliferation and survival of classical Hodgkin lymphoma cells. *Int J Cancer* 118: 1404–1413, 2006.

81. Kapp U, Yeh WC, Patterson B, et al: Interleukin 13 is secreted by and stimulates the growth of Hodgkin and Reed-Sternberg cells. *J Exp Med* 189:1939–1946, 1999.

82. Lamprecht B, Kreher S, Anagnostopoulos I, et al: Aberrant expression of the Th2 cytokine IL-21 in Hodgkin lymphoma cells regulates STAT3 signaling and attracts Treg cells via regulation of MIP-3alpha. *Blood* 112:3339–3347, 2008.

83. Chiu A, Xu W, He B, et al: Hodgkin lymphoma cells express TACI and BCMA receptors and generate survival and proliferation signals in response to BAFF and APRIL. *Blood* 109:729–739, 2007.

84. Fiumara P, Snell V, Li Y, et al: Functional expression of receptor activator of nuclear factor kappaB in Hodgkin disease cell lines. *Blood* 98:2784–2790, 2001.

85. Ebstein WV: Das chronische Ruckfallsfieber, eine neu infectionskrankheit. *Berl Klin Wochenschr* 24:565, 1887.

86. Pel PK: Zur symptomatolgie der sogennanten pseudoleukamie. II. Pseudokeukamie oder chronischen Ruckfallsfieber? *Berl Klin Wochenschr* 24:844, 1887.

87. Atkinson K, Austin DE, McElwain TJ, et al: Alcohol pain in Hodgkin's disease. *Cancer* 37:895–899, 1976.

88. Rueffer U, Sieber M, Josting A, et al: Prognostic factors for subdiaphragmatic involvement in clinical stage I-II supradiaphragmatic Hodgkin's disease: A retrospective analysis of the GHSG. *Ann Oncol* 10:1343–1348, 1999.

89. Audard V, Larousserie F, Grimbert P, et al: Minimal change nephrotic syndrome and classical Hodgkin's lymphoma: Report of 21 cases and review of the literature. *Kidney Int* 69:2251–2260, 2006.

90. Barta SK, Yahalom J, Shia J, et al: Idiopathic cholestasis as a paraneoplastic phenomenon in Hodgkin's lymphoma. *Clin Lymphoma Myeloma* 7:77–82, 2006.

91. Cavalli F: Rare syndromes in Hodgkin's disease. *Ann Oncol* 9 Suppl 5:S109–S113, 1998.

92. Gerstner ER, Abrey LE, Schiff D, et al: CNS Hodgkin lymphoma. *Blood* 112:1658–1661, 2008.

93. Filly R, Bland N, Castellino RA: Radiographic distribution of intrathoracic disease in previously untreated patients with Hodgkin's disease and non-Hodgkin's lymphoma. *Radiology* 120:277–281, 1976.

94. Cheson BD, Fisher RI, Barrington SF, et al: Recommendations for initial evaluation, staging, and response assessment of Hodgkin and non-Hodgkin lymphoma: The Lugano classification. *J Clin Oncol* 32:3059–3068, 2014.

95. Barrington SF, Mikhaeel NG, Kostakoglu L, et al: Role of imaging in the staging and response assessment of lymphoma: Consensus of the International Conference on Malignant Lymphomas Imaging Working Group. *J Clin Oncol* 32:3048–3058, 2014.

96. Kostakoglu L, Cheson BD: Current role of FDG PET/CT in lymphoma. *Eur J Nucl Med Mol Imaging* 41:1004–1027, 2014.

97. Dann EJ, Bar-Shalom R, Tamir A, et al: Risk-adapted BEACOPP regimen can reduce the cumulative dose of chemotherapy for standard and high-risk Hodgkin lymphoma with no impairment of outcome. *Blood* 109:905–909, 2007.

98. Gallamini A, Hutchings M, Rigacci L, et al: Early interim 2-[18F]fluoro-2-deoxy-D-glucose positron emission tomography is prognostically superior to international prognostic score in advanced-stage Hodgkin's lymphoma: A report from a joint Italian-Danish study. *J Clin Oncol* 25:3746–3752, 2007.

99. Hutchings M, Loft A, Hansen M, et al: FDG-PET after two cycles of chemotherapy predicts treatment failure and progression-free survival in Hodgkin lymphoma. *Blood* 107:52–59, 2006.

100. Press OW, LeBlanc M, Rimsza LM, et al: A phase II trial of response-adapted therapy of stages III-IV Hodgkin lymphoma using early interim FDG-PET imaging: US Intergroup S0816. *Hematol Oncol* 31 (Suppl1):137, 2013.

101. Raemaekers JM, Andre MP, Federico M, et al: Omitting radiotherapy in early positron emission tomography-negative stage I/II Hodgkin lymphoma is associated with an increased risk of early relapse: Clinical results of the preplanned interim analysis of the randomized EORTC/LYSA/FIL H10 trial. *J Clin Oncol* 32:1188–1194, 2014.

102. Radford J, Barrington S, Counsell N, et al: Involved field radiotherapy versus no further treatment in patients with clinical stages IA and IIA Hodgkin lymphoma and a "negative" PET scan after 3 cycles ABVD: Results of the UK NCRI RAPID trial. *Blood* 120 (ASH Annual Meeting Abstracts): 547, 2012.

103. Nogova L, Reineke T, Brillant C, et al: Lymphocyte-predominant and classical Hodgkin's lymphoma: A comprehensive analysis from the German Hodgkin Study Group. *J Clin Oncol* 26:434–439, 2008.

104. Advani RH, Hoppe RT: How I treat nodular lymphocyte predominant Hodgkin lymphoma. *Blood* 122:4182–4188, 2013.

105. Miettinen M, Franssila KO, Saxen E: Hodgkin's disease, lymphocytic predominance nodular. Increased risk for subsequent non-Hodgkin's lymphomas. *Cancer* 51:2293–2300, 1983.

106. Sundeen JT, Cossman J, Jaffe ES: Lymphocyte predominant Hodgkin's disease nodular subtype with coexistent "large cell lymphoma." Histological progression or composite malignancy? *Am J Surg Pathol* 12:599–606, 1988.

107. Rudiger T, Gascoyne RD, Jaffe ES, et al: Workshop on the relationship between nodular lymphocyte predominant Hodgkin's lymphoma and T cell/histiocyte-rich B cell lymphoma. *Ann Oncol* 13 Suppl 1:44–51, 2002.

108. Allemani C, Sant M, De Angelis R, et al: Hodgkin disease survival in Europe and the U.S.: Prognostic significance of morphologic groups. *Cancer* 107:352–360, 2006.

109. Diehl V, Sextro M, Franklin J, et al: Clinical presentation, course, and prognostic factors in lymphocyte-predominant Hodgkin's disease and lymphocyte-rich classical Hodgkin's disease: Report from the European Task Force on Lymphoma Project on Lymphocyte-Predominant Hodgkin's Disease. *J Clin Oncol* 17:776–783, 1999.

110. Kaplan HS. *Hodgkin's Disease*, ed 2. Harvard University Press, Cambridge, MA, 1980.

111. Rosenberg SA, Kaplan HS: Evidence for an orderly progression in the spread of Hodgkin's disease. *Cancer Res* 26:1225–1231, 1966.

112. Smithers DW: Spread of Hodgkin's disease. *Lancet* 1:1262–1267, 1970.

113. Rappaport H, Berard CW, Butler JJ, et al: Report of the Committee on Histopathological Criteria Contributing to Staging of Hodgkin's Disease. *Cancer Res* 31:1864–1865, 1971.

114. Kirschner RH, Abt AB, O'Connell MJ, et al: Vascular invasion and hematogenous dissemination of Hodgkin's disease. *Cancer* 34:1159–1162, 1974.

115. Haybittle JL, Hayhoe FG, Easterling MJ, et al: Review of British National Lymphoma Investigation studies of Hodgkin's disease and development of prognostic index. *Lancet* 1:967–972, 1985.

116. Le Bourgeois JP, Tubiana M: The erythrocyte sedimentation rate as a monitor for relapse in patients with previously treated Hodgkin's disease. *Int J Radiat Oncol Biol Phys* 2:241–247, 1977.

117. Tubiana M, Henry-Amar M, van der Werf-Messing B, et al: A multivariate analysis of prognostic factors in early stage Hodgkin's disease. *Int J Radiat Oncol Biol Phys* 11: 23–30, 1985.

118. Friedenberg WR, Gatlin PF, Mazza JJ, et al: Prognostic value of serum lactic dehydrogenase level in Hodgkin's disease. *J Lab Clin Med* 103:489–490, 1984.

119. Schilling RF, McKnight B, Crowley JJ: Prognostic value of serum lactic dehydrogenase level in Hodgkin's disease. *J Lab Clin Med* 99:382–387, 1982.

120. Mercier RJ, Thompson JM, Harman GS, et al: Recurrent hypercalcemia and elevated 1,25-dihydroxyvitamin D levels in Hodgkin's disease. *Am J Med* 84:165–168, 1988.

121. Braund WJ, Naylor BA, Williamson DH, et al: Autoimmunity to insulin receptor and hypoglycaemia in patient with Hodgkin's disease. *Lancet* 1:237–240, 1987.

122. Walters EG, Tavare JM, Denton RM, et al: Hypoglycaemia due to an insulin-receptor antibody in Hodgkin's disease. *Lancet* 1:241–243, 1987.

123. Eliakim R, Vertman E, Shinhar E: Syndrome of inappropriate secretion of antidiuretic hormone in Hodgkin's disease. *Am J Med Sci* 291:126–127, 1986.

124. Hasenclever D, Diehl V: A prognostic score for advanced Hodgkin's disease. International Prognostic Factors Project on Advanced Hodgkin's Disease. *N Engl J Med* 339:1506–1514, 1998.

125. Dimopoulos MA, Cabanillas F, Lee JJ, et al: Prognostic role of serum beta 2-microglobulin in Hodgkin's disease. *J Clin Oncol* 11:1108–1111, 1993.

126. Kurzrock R, Redman J, Cabanillas F, et al: Serum interleukin 6 levels are elevated in lymphoma patients and correlate with survival in advanced Hodgkin's disease and with B symptoms. *Cancer Res* 53:2118–2122, 1993.

127. Nadali G, Vinante F, Ambrosetti A, et al: Serum levels of soluble CD30 are elevated in the majority of untreated patients with Hodgkin's disease and correlate with clinical features and prognosis. *J Clin Oncol* 12:793–797, 1994.

128. Pizzolo G, Chilosi M, Vinante F, et al: Soluble interleukin-2 receptors in the serum of patients with Hodgkin's disease. *Br J Cancer* 55:427–428, 1987.

129. Sarris AH, Kliche KO, Pethambaram P, et al: Interleukin-10 levels are often elevated in serum of adults with Hodgkin's disease and are associated with inferior failure-free survival. *Ann Oncol* 10:433–440, 1999.

130. Lieberman DA: Intrahepatic cholestasis due to Hodgkin's disease. An elusive diagnosis. *J Clin Gastroenterol* 8:304–307, 1986.

131. Routledge RC, Hann IM, Jones PH: Hodgkin's disease complicated by the nephrotic syndrome. *Cancer* 38:1735–1740, 1976.

132. Savage KJ, Monti S, Kutok JL, et al: The molecular signature of mediastinal large B-cell lymphoma differs from that of other diffuse large B-cell lymphomas and shares features with classical Hodgkin lymphoma. *Blood* 102:3871–3879, 2003.

133. Rosenwald A, Wright G, Leroy K, et al: Molecular diagnosis of primary mediastinal B cell lymphoma identifies a clinically favorable subgroup of diffuse large B cell lymphoma related to Hodgkin lymphoma. *J Exp Med* 198:851–862, 2003.

134. Kondratiev S, Duraisamy S, Unitt CL, et al: Aberrant expression of the dendritic cell marker TNFAIP2 by the malignant cells of Hodgkin lymphoma and primary mediastinal large B-cell lymphoma distinguishes these tumor types from morphologically and phenotypically similar lymphomas. *Am J Surg Pathol* 35:1531–1539, 2011.

135. Green MR, Monti S, Rodig SJ, et al: Integrative analysis reveals selective 9p24.1 amplification, increased PD-1 ligand expression, and further induction via JAK2 in nodular sclerosing Hodgkin lymphoma and primary mediastinal large B-cell lymphoma. *Blood* 116:3268–3277, 2010.

136. Brassesco MS: Leukemia/lymphoma-associated gene fusions in normal individuals. *Genet Mol Res* 7:782–790, 2008.

137. Kaplan HS, Rosenberg SA: The treatment of Hodgkin's disease. *Med Clin North Am* 50:1591–1610, 1966.

138. Feuer EJ, Kessler LG, Baker SG, et al: The impact of breakthrough clinical trials on survival in population based tumor registries. *J Clin Epidemiol* 44:141–153, 1991.

139. Santoro A, Bonadonna G: Prolonged disease-free survival in MOPP-resistant Hodgkin's disease after treatment with Adriamycin, bleomycin, vinblastine and dacarbazine (ABVD). *Cancer Chemother Pharmacol* 2:101–105, 1979.

140. Santoro A, Bonfante V, Bonadonna G: Salvage chemotherapy with ABVD in MOPP-resistant Hodgkin's disease. *Ann Intern Med* 96:139–143, 1982.

141. Duggan DB, Petroni GR, Johnson JL, et al: Randomized comparison of ABVD and MOPP/ABV hybrid for the treatment of advanced Hodgkin's disease: Report of an intergroup trial. *J Clin Oncol* 21:607–614, 2003.

142. Canellos GP, Niedzwiecki D, Johnson JL: Long-term follow-up of survival in Hodgkin's lymphoma. *N Engl J Med* 361:2390–2391, 2009.

143. Diehl V, Franklin J, Pfreundschuh M, et al: Standard and increased-dose BEACOPP chemotherapy compared with COPP-ABVD for advanced Hodgkin's disease. *N Engl J Med* 348:2386–2395, 2003.

144. Engert A, Diehl V, Franklin J, et al: Escalated-dose BEACOPP in the treatment of patients with advanced-stage Hodgkin's lymphoma: 10 years of follow-up of the GHSG HD9 study. *J Clin Oncol* 27:4548–4554, 2009.

145. Armitage JO: Early-stage Hodgkin's lymphoma. *N Engl J Med* 363:653–662, 2010.

146. Horning SJ, Hoppe RT, Hancock SL, et al: Vinblastine, bleomycin, and methotrexate: An effective adjuvant in favorable Hodgkin's disease. *J Clin Oncol* 6:1822–1831, 1988.

147. Ferme C, Eghbali H, Meerwaldt JH, et al: Chemotherapy plus involved-field radiation in early-stage Hodgkin's disease. *N Engl J Med* 357:1916–1927, 2007.

148. Press OW, LeBlanc M, Lichter AS, et al: Phase III randomized intergroup trial of subtotal lymphoid irradiation versus doxorubicin, vinblastine, and subtotal lymphoid irradiation for stage IA to IIA Hodgkin's disease. *J Clin Oncol* 19:4238–4244, 2001.

149. Bonadonna G, Bonfante V, Viviani S, et al: ABVD plus subtotal nodal versus involved-field radiotherapy in early-stage Hodgkin's disease: Long-term results. *J Clin Oncol* 22:2835–2841, 2004.

150. Engert A, Schiller P, Josting A, et al: Involved-field radiotherapy is equally effective and less toxic compared with extended-field radiotherapy after four cycles of chemotherapy in patients with early-stage unfavorable Hodgkin's lymphoma: Results of the HD8 trial of the German Hodgkin's Lymphoma Study Group. *J Clin Oncol* 21:3601–3608, 2003.

151. Behringer K, Borchmann P, Diehl V, et al: Impact of bleomycin and dacarbazine within the ABVD regimen in the treatment of early stage favorable Hodgkin lymphoma: Final results of the GHSG HD13 trial (abstract T033). *Haematologica* 98(Suppl 2):11, 2013.

152. Moskowitz CS, Chou JF, Wolden SL, et al: Breast cancer after chest radiation therapy for childhood cancer. *J Clin Oncol* 32:2217–2223, 2014.

153. Canellos GP, Abramson JS, Fisher DC, et al: Treatment of favorable, limited-stage Hodgkin's lymphoma with chemotherapy without consolidation by radiation therapy. *J Clin Oncol* 28:1611–1615, 2010.

154. Straus DJ, Portlock CS, Qin J, et al: Results of a prospective randomized clinical trial of doxorubicin, bleomycin, vinblastine, and dacarbazine (ABVD) followed by radiation therapy (RT) versus ABVD alone for stages I, II, and IIIA nonbulky Hodgkin disease. *Blood* 104:3483–3489, 2004.

155. Meyer RM, Gospodarowicz MK, Connors JM, et al: ABVD alone versus radiation-based therapy in limited-stage Hodgkin's lymphoma. *N Engl J Med* 366:399–408, 2012.

156. Noordijk EM, Thomas J, Ferme C: First results of the EORTC-GELA H9 randomized trials: The H9-F trial and H9u trial in patients with favorable or unfavorable early stage Hodgkin's lymphoma. *Proc Am Soc Clin Oncol* 23:6505a, 2005.

157. Herbst C, Rehan FA, Skoetz N, et al: Chemotherapy alone versus chemotherapy plus radiotherapy for early stage Hodgkin lymphoma. *Cochrane Database Syst Rev* 2:CD007110, 2011.

158. Hoppe RT, Advani RH, Ai WZ, et al: NCCN Clinical Practice Guidelines in Oncology (NCCN Guidelines) Hodgkin lymphoma V.2.2014: National Comprehensive Cancer Network, 2014. Available at NCCN.org. http://www.nccn.org/professionals/physician_gls/pdf/hodgkins.pdf. Last Accessed on August 25, 2015.

159. Eich HT, Diehl V, Gorgen H, et al: Intensified chemotherapy and dose-reduced involved-field radiotherapy in patients with early unfavorable Hodgkin's lymphoma: Final analysis of the German Hodgkin Study Group HD11 trial. *J Clin Oncol* 28:4199–4206, 2010.

160. Borchmann P, Engert A, Pluetschow A: Dose-intensified combined modality treatment with 2 cycles of BEACOPP escalated followed by 2 cycles of ABVD and involved field radiotherapy (IF-RT) is superior to 4 cycles of ABVD and IFRT in patients with early unfavourable Hodgkin lymphoma (HL): An analysis of the German Hodgkin Study Group (GHSG) HD14 trial. *ASH Annu Meet Abstr* 112:367, 2008.

161. Canellos GP, Anderson JR, Propert KJ, et al: Chemotherapy of advanced Hodgkin's disease with MOPP, ABVD, or MOPP alternating with ABVD. *N Engl J Med* 327:1478–1484, 1992.

162. Canellos GP, Niedzwiecki D: Long-term follow-up of Hodgkin's disease trial. *N Engl J Med* 346:1417–1418, 2002.

163. Connors JM, Klimo P, Adams G, et al: Treatment of advanced Hodgkin's disease with chemotherapy—comparison of MOPP/ABV hybrid regimen with alternating courses of MOPP and ABVD: A report from the National Cancer Institute of Canada clinical trials group. *J Clin Oncol* 15:1638–1645, 1997.

164. Viviani S, Bonadonna G, Santoro A, et al: Alternating versus hybrid MOPP and ABVD combinations in advanced Hodgkin's disease: Ten-year results. *J Clin Oncol* 14:1421–1430, 1996.

165. Eichenauer DA, Thielen I, Haverkamp H, et al: Therapy-related acute myeloid leukemia and myelodysplastic syndromes in patients with Hodgkin lymphoma: A report from the German Hodgkin Study Group. *Blood* 123:1658–1664, 2014.

166. Behringer K, Mueller H, Goergen H, et al: Gonadal function and fertility in survivors after Hodgkin lymphoma treatment within the German Hodgkin Study Group HD13 to HD15 trials. *J Clin Oncol* 31:231–239, 2013.

167. Sieniawski M, Reineke T, Nogova L, et al: Fertility in male patients with advanced Hodgkin lymphoma treated with BEACOPP: A report of the German Hodgkin Study Group (GHSG). *Blood* 111:71–76, 2008.

168. Wongso D, Fuchs M, Plutschow A, et al: Treatment-related mortality in patients with advanced-stage Hodgkin lymphoma: An analysis of the German Hodgkin Study Group. *J Clin Oncol* 31:2819–2824, 2013.

169. Federico M, Luminari S, Iannitto E, et al: ABVD compared with BEACOPP compared with CEC for the initial treatment of patients with advanced Hodgkin's lymphoma: Results from the HD2000 Gruppo Italiano per lo Studio dei Linfomi Trial. *J Clin Oncol* 27:805–811, 2009.

170. Viviani S, Zinzani PL, Rambaldi A, et al: ABVD versus BEACOPP for Hodgkin's lymphoma when high-dose salvage is planned. *N Engl J Med* 365:203–212, 2011.

171. Carde P, Karrasch M, Fortpied C, et al: BEACOPP (escalated × 4 + baseline × 4 cycles) vs ABVD (×8 cycles) in stage III-IV, high risk Hodgkin lymphoma (IPS >3). Intergroup Study 20012 (Abstract 8002). *J Clin Oncol* 30:510s, 2012.

172. Borchmann P, Haverkamp H, Diehl V, et al: Eight cycles of escalated-dose BEACOPP compared with four cycles of escalated-dose BEACOPP followed by four cycles of baseline-dose BEACOPP with or without radiotherapy in patients with advanced-stage Hodgkin's lymphoma: Final analysis of the HD12 trial of the German Hodgkin Study Group. *J Clin Oncol* 29:4234–4242, 2011.

173. Engert A, Haverkamp H, Kobe C, et al: Reduced-intensity chemotherapy and PET-guided radiotherapy in patients with advanced stage Hodgkin's lymphoma (HD15 trial): A randomised, open-label, phase 3 non-inferiority trial. *Lancet* 379:1791–1799, 2012.

174. Gallamini A, Kostakoglu L: Interim FDG-PET in Hodgkin lymphoma: A compass for a safe navigation in clinical trials? *Blood* 120:4913–4920, 2012.

175. Kostakoglu L, Gallamini A: Interim 18F-FDG PET in Hodgkin lymphoma: Would PET-adapted clinical trials lead to a paradigm shift? *J Nucl Med* 54:1082–1093, 2013.

176. Kobe C, Dietlein M, Franklin J, et al: Positron emission tomography has a high negative predictive value for progression or early relapse for patients with residual disease after first-line chemotherapy in advanced-stage Hodgkin lymphoma. *Blood* 112:3989–3994, 2008.

177. Markova J, Kobe C, Skopalova M, et al: FDG-PET for assessment of early treatment response after four cycles of chemotherapy in patients with advanced-stage Hodgkin's lymphoma has a high negative predictive value. *Ann Oncol* 20:1270–1274, 2009.

178. Horning SJ, Hoppe RT, Breslin S, et al: Stanford V and radiotherapy for locally extensive and advanced Hodgkin's disease: Mature results of a prospective clinical trial. *J Clin Oncol* 20:630–637, 2002.

179. Chisesi T, Federico M, Levis A, et al: ABVD versus Stanford V versus MEC in unfavourable Hodgkin's lymphoma: Results of a randomised trial. *Ann Oncol* 13 Suppl 1:102–106, 2002.

180. Hoskin PJ, Lowry L, Horwich A, et al: Randomized comparison of the Stanford V regimen and ABVD in the treatment of advanced Hodgkin's Lymphoma: United Kingdom National Cancer Research Institute Lymphoma Group Study ISRCTN 64141244. *J Clin Oncol* 27:5390–5396, 2009.

181. Gordon LI, Hong F, Fisher RI, et al: Randomized phase III trial of ABVD versus Stanford V with or without radiation therapy in locally extensive and advanced-stage Hodgkin lymphoma: An intergroup study coordinated by the Eastern Cooperative Oncology Group (E2496). *J Clin Oncol* 31:684–691, 2013.

182. Younes A, Bartlett NL, Leonard JP, et al: Brentuximab vedotin (SGN-35) for relapsed CD30-positive lymphomas. *N Engl J Med* 363:1812–1821, 2010.

183. Younes A, Gopal AK, Smith SE, et al: Results of a pivotal phase II study of brentuximab vedotin for patients with relapsed or refractory Hodgkin's lymphoma. *J Clin Oncol* 30:2183–2189, 2012.

184. Younes A, Connors JM, Park SI, et al: Brentuximab vedotin combined with ABVD or AVD for patients with newly diagnosed Hodgkin's lymphoma: A phase 1, open-label, dose-escalation study. *Lancet Oncol* 14:1348–1356, 2013.

185. Aleman BM, Raemaekers JM, Tirelli U, et al: Involved-field radiotherapy for advanced Hodgkin's lymphoma. *N Engl J Med* 348:2396–2406, 2003.

186. Gianni AM, Rambaldi A, Zinzani P: Comparable 3-year outcome following ABVD or BEACOPP first-line chemotherapy, plus pre-planned high-dose salvage, in advanced Hodgkin lymphoma (HL): A randomized trial of the Michelangelo, GITIL and IIL cooperative groups. *J Clin Oncol* 26: Abstract 8506, 2008.

187. Nogova L, Reineke T, Eich HT, et al: Extended field radiotherapy, combined modality treatment or involved field radiotherapy for patients with stage IA lymphocyte-predominant Hodgkin's lymphoma: A retrospective analysis from the German Hodgkin Study Group (GHSG). *Ann Oncol* 16:1683–1687, 2005.

188. Fanale M: Lymphocyte-predominant Hodgkin lymphoma: What is the optimal treatment? *Hematology Am Soc Hematol Educ Program* 2013:406–413, 2013.

189. Schulz H, Rehwald U, Morschhauser F, et al: Rituximab in relapsed lymphocyte-predominant Hodgkin lymphoma: Long-term results of a phase 2 trial by the German Hodgkin Lymphoma Study Group (GHSG). *Blood* 111:109–111, 2008.

190. Advani RH, Horning SJ, Hoppe RT, et al: Mature results of a phase II study of rituximab therapy for nodular lymphocyte-predominant Hodgkin lymphoma. *J Clin Oncol* 32:912–918, 2014.

191. Linch DC, Winfield D, Goldstone AH, et al: Dose intensification with autologous bone-marrow transplantation in relapsed and resistant Hodgkin's disease: Results of a BNLI randomised trial. *Lancet* 341:1051–1054, 1993.

192. Schmitz N, Pfistner B, Sextro M, et al: Aggressive conventional chemotherapy compared with high-dose chemotherapy with autologous haemopoietic stem-cell transplantation for relapsed chemosensitive Hodgkin's disease: A randomised trial. *Lancet* 359:2065–2071, 2002.

193. Nademanee A, O'Donnell MR, Snyder DS, et al: High-dose chemotherapy with or without total body irradiation followed by autologous bone marrow and/or peripheral blood stem cell transplantation for patients with relapsed and refractory Hodgkin's disease: Results in 85 patients with analysis of prognostic factors. *Blood* 85:1381–1390, 1995.

194. Stiff PJ, Unger JM, Forman SJ, et al: The value of augmented preparative regimens combined with an autologous bone marrow transplant for the management of relapsed or refractory Hodgkin disease: A Southwest Oncology Group phase II trial. *Biol Blood Marrow Transplant* 9:529–539, 2003.

195. Fung HC, Stiff P, Schriber J, et al: Tandem autologous stem cell transplantation for patients with primary refractory or poor risk recurrent Hodgkin lymphoma. *Biol Blood Marrow Transplant* 13:594–600, 2007.

196. Smith EP, Li H, Friedberg J, et al: SWOG S0410/BMT CTN 0703: A phase II trial of tandem autologous stem cell transplantation for patients with primary progressive or recurrent Hodgkin lymphoma. *Blood* 124 (ASH Annual Meeting Abstracts): 676, 2014.

197. Moskowitz CH, Bertino JR, Glassman JR, et al: Ifosfamide, carboplatin, and etoposide: A highly effective cytoreduction and peripheral-blood progenitor-cell mobilization regimen for transplant-eligible patients with non-Hodgkin's lymphoma. *J Clin Oncol* 17:3776–3785, 1999.

198. Bartlett NL, Niedzwiecki D, Johnson JL, et al: Gemcitabine, vinorelbine, and pegylated liposomal doxorubicin (GVD), a salvage regimen in relapsed Hodgkin's lymphoma: CALGB 59804. *Ann Oncol* 18:1071–1079, 2007.

199. Kuruvilla J, Keating A, Crump M: How I treat relapsed and refractory Hodgkin lymphoma. *Blood* 117:4208–4217, 2011.

200. Burroughs LM, O'Donnell PV, Sandmaier BM, et al: Comparison of outcomes of HLA-matched related, unrelated, or HLA-haploidentical related hematopoietic cell transplantation following nonmyeloablative conditioning for relapsed or refractory Hodgkin lymphoma. *Biol Blood Marrow Transplant* 14:1279–1287, 2008.

201. Sureda A, Robinson S, Canals C, et al: Reduced-intensity conditioning compared with conventional allogeneic stem-cell transplantation in relapsed or refractory Hodgkin's lymphoma: An analysis from the Lymphoma Working Party of the European Group for Blood and Marrow Transplantation. *J Clin Oncol* 26:455–462, 2008.

202. Horning S, Bartlett NL, Breslin S: Results of a prospective phase II trial of limited and extended rituximab treatment in nodular lymphocyte predominant Hodgkin's disease (NLPHD). *ASH Annu Meet Abstr* 110:644, 2007.

203. Forero-Torres A, Leonard JP, Younes A, et al: A Phase II study of SGN-30 (anti-CD30 mAb) in Hodgkin lymphoma or systemic anaplastic large cell lymphoma. *Br J Haematol* 146:171–179, 2009.

204. Illidge T, Bouabdallah R, Chen R, et al: Allogeneic transplant following brentuximab vedotin in patients with relapsed or refractory Hodgkin lymphoma and systemic anaplastic large cell lymphoma. *Leuk Lymphoma* 56:703–710, 2015.

205. Gopal AK, Ramchandren R, O'Connor OA, et al: Safety and efficacy of brentuximab vedotin for Hodgkin lymphoma recurring after allogeneic stem cell transplantation. *Blood* 120:560–568, 2012.

205a. Ansell SM, Lesokhin AM, Borrello I, et al: PD-1 blockade with nivolumab in relapsed or refractory Hodgkin's lymphoma. *N Engl J Med* 372:311–319, 2015.

206. Brenner H, Gondos A, Pulte D: Survival expectations of patients diagnosed with Hodgkin's lymphoma in 2006–2010. *Oncologist* 14:806–813, 2009.

207. Moccia AA, Donaldson J, Chhanabhai M, et al: International Prognostic Score in advanced-stage Hodgkin's lymphoma: Altered utility in the modern era. *J Clin Oncol* 30:3383–3388, 2012.

208. Brenner H, Gondos A, Pulte D: Ongoing improvement in long-term survival of patients with Hodgkin disease at all ages and recent catch-up of older patients. *Blood* 111:2977–2983, 2008.

209. Evens AM, Sweetenham JW, Horning SJ: Hodgkin lymphoma in older patients: An uncommon disease in need of study. *Oncology (Williston Park)* 22:1369–1379, 2008.

210. Ballova V, Ruffer JU, Haverkamp H, et al: A prospectively randomized trial carried out by the German Hodgkin Study Group (GHSG) for elderly patients with advanced Hodgkin's disease comparing BEACOPP baseline and COPP-ABVD (study HD9elderly). *Ann Oncol* 16:124–131, 2005.

211. Advani R, Maeda L, Lavori P, et al: Impact of positive positron emission tomography on prediction of freedom from progression after Stanford V chemotherapy in Hodgkin's disease. *J Clin Oncol* 25:3902–3907, 2007.

212. Sher DJ, Mauch PM, Van Den Abbeele A, et al: Prognostic significance of mid- and post-ABVD PET imaging in Hodgkin's lymphoma: The importance of involved-field radiotherapy. *Ann Oncol* 20:1848–1853, 2009.

213. Moskowitz CH, Matasar MJ, Zelenetz AD, et al: Normalization of pre-ASCT, FDG-PET imaging with second-line, non-cross-resistant, chemotherapy programs improves event-free survival in patients with Hodgkin lymphoma. *Blood* 119:1665–1670, 2012.

214. Moskowitz CH, Nimer SD, Zelenetz AD, et al: A 2-step comprehensive high-dose chemoradiotherapy second-line program for relapsed and refractory Hodgkin disease: Analysis by intent to treat and development of a prognostic model. *Blood* 97:616–623, 2001.

215. Moskowitz C: Risk-adapted therapy for relapsed and refractory lymphoma using ICE chemotherapy. *Cancer Chemother Pharmacol* 49 Suppl 1:S9–S12, 2002.

216. Casasnovas RO, Mounier N, Brice P, et al: Plasma cytokine and soluble receptor signature predicts outcome of patients with classical Hodgkin's lymphoma: A study from the Groupe d'Etude des Lymphomes de l'Adulte. *J Clin Oncol* 25:1732–1740, 2007.

217. Niens M, Visser L, Nolte IM, et al: Serum chemokine levels in Hodgkin lymphoma patients: Highly increased levels of CCL17 and CCL22. *Br J Haematol* 140:527–536, 2008.

218. Weihrauch MR, Manzke O, Beyer M, et al: Elevated serum levels of CC thymus and activation-related chemokine (TARC) in primary Hodgkin's disease: Potential for a prognostic factor. *Cancer Res* 65:5516–5519, 2005.

219. Brink AA, Oudejans JJ, van den Brule AJ, et al: Low p53 and high bcl-2 expression in Reed-Sternberg cells predicts poor clinical outcome for Hodgkin's disease: Involvement of apoptosis resistance? *Mod Pathol* 11:376–383, 1998.

220. Montalban C, Garcia JF, Abraira V, et al: Influence of biologic markers on the outcome of Hodgkin's lymphoma: A study by the Spanish Hodgkin's Lymphoma Study Group. *J Clin Oncol* 22:1664–1673, 2004.

221. Rassidakis GZ, Medeiros LJ, Vassilakopoulos TP, et al: BCL-2 expression in Hodgkin and Reed-Sternberg cells of classical Hodgkin disease predicts a poorer prognosis in patients treated with ABVD or equivalent regimens. *Blood* 100:3935–3941, 2002.

222. Vassallo J, Metze K, Traina F, et al: The prognostic relevance of apoptosis-related proteins in classical Hodgkin's lymphomas. *Leuk Lymphoma* 44:483–488, 2003.

223. Portlock CS, Donnelly GB, Qin J, et al: Adverse prognostic significance of CD20 positive Reed-Sternberg cells in classical Hodgkin's disease. *Br J Haematol* 125:701–708, 2004.

224. Tzankov A, Krugmann J, Fend F, et al: Prognostic significance of CD20 expression in classical Hodgkin lymphoma: A clinicopathological study of 119 cases. *Clin Cancer Res* 9:1381–1386, 2003.

225. Diepstra A, van Imhoff GW, Karim-Kos HE, et al: HLA class II expression by Hodgkin Reed-Sternberg cells is an independent prognostic factor in classical Hodgkin's lymphoma. *J Clin Oncol* 25:3101–3108, 2007.

226. Diepstra A, van Imhoff GW, Schaapveld M, et al: Latent Epstein-Barr virus infection of tumor cells in classical Hodgkin's lymphoma predicts adverse outcome in older adult patients. *J Clin Oncol* 27:3815–3821, 2009.

227. Keegan TH, Glaser SL, Clarke CA, et al: Epstein-Barr virus as a marker of survival after Hodgkin's lymphoma: A population-based study. *J Clin Oncol* 23:7604–7613, 2005.

228. Alvaro T, Lejeune M, Salvado MT, et al: Outcome in Hodgkin's lymphoma can be predicted from the presence of accompanying cytotoxic and regulatory T cells. *Clin Cancer Res* 11:1467–1473, 2005.

229. Alvaro-Naranjo T, Lejeune M, Salvado-Usach MT, et al: Tumor-infiltrating cells as a prognostic factor in Hodgkin's lymphoma: A quantitative tissue microarray study in a large retrospective cohort of 267 patients. *Leuk Lymphoma* 46:1581–1591, 2005.

230. Kelley TW, Pohlman B, Elson P, et al: The ratio of FOXP3+ regulatory T cells to granzyme B+ cytotoxic T/NK cells predicts prognosis in classical Hodgkin lymphoma and is independent of bcl-2 and MAL expression. *Am J Clin Pathol* 128:958–965, 2007.

231. Steidl C, Lee T, Shah SP, et al: Tumor-associated macrophages and survival in classic Hodgkin's lymphoma. *N Engl J Med* 362:875–885, 2010.

232. Scott DW, Chan FC, Hong F, et al: Gene expression-based model using formalin-fixed paraffin-embedded biopsies predicts overall survival in advanced-stage classical Hodgkin lymphoma. *J Clin Oncol* 31:692–700, 2013.

233. Hoppe RT: Hodgkin's disease: Complications of therapy and excess mortality. *Ann Oncol* 8 Suppl 1:115–118, 1997.

234. Ng AK, Bernardo MP, Weller E, et al: Long-term survival and competing causes of death in patients with early-stage Hodgkin's disease treated at age 50 or younger. *J Clin Oncol* 20:2101–2108, 2002.

235. Arseneau JC, Sponzo RW, Levin DL, et al: Nonlymphomatous malignant tumors complicating Hodgkin's disease. Possible association with intensive therapy. *N Engl J Med* 287:1119–1122, 1972.

236. Kaldor JM, Day NE, Clarke EA, et al: Leukemia following Hodgkin's disease. *N Engl J Med* 322:7–13, 1990.

237. Koontz MZ, Horning SJ, Balise R, et al: Risk of therapy-related secondary leukemia in Hodgkin lymphoma: The Stanford University experience over three generations of clinical trials. *J Clin Oncol* 31:592–598, 2013.

238. Schonfeld SJ, Gilbert ES, Dores GM, et al: Acute myeloid leukemia following Hodgkin lymphoma: A population-based study of 35,511 patients. *J Natl Cancer Inst* 98:215–218, 2006.

239. Tucker MA, Coleman CN, Cox RS, et al: Risk of second cancers after treatment for Hodgkin's disease. *N Engl J Med* 318:76–81, 1988.

240. van Leeuwen FE, Somers R, Taal BG, et al: Increased risk of lung cancer, non-Hodgkin's lymphoma, and leukemia following Hodgkin's disease. *J Clin Oncol* 7:1046–1058, 1989.

241. Rueffer U, Josting A, Franklin J, et al: Non-Hodgkin's lymphoma after primary Hodgkin's disease in the German Hodgkin Study Group: Incidence, treatment, and prognosis. *J Clin Oncol* 19:2026–2032, 2001.

242. Schmitz R, Renne C, Rosenquist R, et al: Insights into the multistep transformation process of lymphomas: IgH-associated translocations and tumor suppressor gene mutations in clonally related composite Hodgkin's and non-Hodgkin's lymphomas. *Leukemia* 19:1452–1458, 2005.

243. Huang JZ, Weisenburger DD, Vose JM, et al: Diffuse large B-cell lymphoma arising in nodular lymphocyte predominant Hodgkin lymphoma: A report of 21 cases from the Nebraska Lymphoma Study Group. *Leuk Lymphoma* 45:1551–1557, 2004.

244. Bhatia S, Robison LL, Oberlin O, et al: Breast cancer and other second neoplasms after childhood Hodgkin's disease. *N Engl J Med* 334:745–751, 1996.

245. Hancock SL, Donaldson SS, Hoppe RT: Cardiac disease following treatment of Hodgkin's disease in children and adolescents. *J Clin Oncol* 11:1208–1215, 1993.

246. Shapiro CL, Mauch PM: Radiation-associated breast cancer after Hodgkin's disease: Risks and screening in perspective. *J Clin Oncol* 10:1662–1665, 1992.

247. Swerdlow AJ, Barber JA, Hudson GV, et al: Risk of second malignancy after Hodgkin's disease in a collaborative British cohort: The relation to age at treatment. *J Clin Oncol* 18:498–509, 2000.

248. Travis LB, Gospodarowicz M, Curtis RE, et al: Lung cancer following chemotherapy and radiotherapy for Hodgkin's disease. *J Natl Cancer Inst* 94:182–192, 2002.

249. De Bruin ML, Sparidans J, van't Veer MB, et al: Breast cancer risk in female survivors of Hodgkin's lymphoma: Lower risk after smaller radiation volumes. *J Clin Oncol* 27:4239–4246, 2009.

250. van Leeuwen FE, Klokman WJ, Stovall M, et al: Roles of radiation dose, chemotherapy, and hormonal factors in breast cancer following Hodgkin's disease. *J Natl Cancer Inst* 95:971–980, 2003.

251. Swerdlow AJ, Schoemaker MJ, Allerton R, et al: Lung cancer after Hodgkin's disease: A nested case-control study of the relation to treatment. *J Clin Oncol* 19:1610–1618, 2001.

252. Eriksson F, Gagliardi G, Liedberg A, et al: Long-term cardiac mortality following radiation therapy for Hodgkin's disease: Analysis with the relative seriality model. *Radiother Oncol* 55:153–162, 2000.

253. Hancock SL, Hoppe RT, Horning SJ, et al: Intercurrent death after Hodgkin disease therapy in radiotherapy and adjuvant MOPP trials. *Ann Intern Med* 109:183–189, 1988.

254. Boivin JF, Hutchison GB, Lubin JH, et al: Coronary artery disease mortality in patients treated for Hodgkin's disease. *Cancer* 69:1241–1247, 1992.

255. Adams MJ, Lipsitz SR, Colan SD, et al: Cardiovascular status in long-term survivors of Hodgkin's disease treated with chest radiotherapy. *J Clin Oncol* 22:3139–3148, 2004.

256. Heidenreich PA, Hancock SL, Lee BK, et al: Asymptomatic cardiac disease following mediastinal irradiation. *J Am Coll Cardiol* 42:743–749, 2003.

257. Aleman BM, van den Belt-Dusebout AW, De Bruin ML, et al: Late cardiotoxicity after treatment for Hodgkin lymphoma. *Blood* 109:1878–1886, 2007.

258. Swerdlow AJ, Higgins CD, Smith P, et al: Myocardial infarction mortality risk after treatment for Hodgkin disease: A collaborative British cohort study. *J Natl Cancer Inst* 99:206–214, 2007.

259. De Bruin ML, Dorresteijn LD, van't Veer MB, et al: Increased risk of stroke and transient ischemic attack in 5-year survivors of Hodgkin lymphoma. *J Natl Cancer Inst* 101:928–937, 2009.

260. Hull MC, Morris CG, Pepine CJ, et al: Valvular dysfunction and carotid, subclavian, and coronary artery disease in survivors of Hodgkin lymphoma treated with radiation therapy. *JAMA* 290:2831–2837, 2003.

261. Chapman RM, Sutcliffe SB, Rees LH, et al: Cyclical combination chemotherapy and gonadal function. Retrospective study in males. *Lancet* 1:285–289, 1979.

262. da Cunha MF, Meistrich ML, Fuller LM, et al: Recovery of spermatogenesis after treatment for Hodgkin's disease: Limiting dose of MOPP chemotherapy. *J Clin Oncol* 2:571–577, 1984.

263. Chapman RM, Sutcliffe SB, Malpas JS: Cytotoxic-induced ovarian failure in women with Hodgkin's disease. I. Hormone function. *JAMA* 242:1877–1881, 1979.

264. Horning SJ, Hoppe RT, Kaplan HS, et al: Female reproductive potential after treatment for Hodgkin's disease. *N Engl J Med* 304:1377–1382, 1981.

265. Anselmo AP, Cartoni C, Bellantuono P, et al: Risk of infertility in patients with Hodgkin's disease treated with ABVD vs MOPP vs ABVD/MOPP. *Haematologica* 75:155–158, 1990.

266. Viviani S, Santoro A, Ragni G, et al: Gonadal toxicity after combination chemotherapy for Hodgkin's disease. Comparative results of MOPP vs ABVD. *Eur J Cancer Clin Oncol* 21:601–605, 1985.

267. Hodgson DC, Pintilie M, Gitterman L, et al: Fertility among female Hodgkin lymphoma survivors attempting pregnancy following ABVD chemotherapy. *Hematol Oncol* 25:11–15, 2007.

268. Behringer K, Breuer K, Reineke T, et al: Secondary amenorrhea after Hodgkin's lymphoma is influenced by age at treatment, stage of disease, chemotherapy regimen, and the use of oral contraceptives during therapy: A report from the German Hodgkin's Lymphoma Study Group. *J Clin Oncol* 23:7555–7564, 2005.

269. Hancock SL, Cox RS, McDougall IR: Thyroid diseases after treatment of Hodgkin's disease. *N Engl J Med* 325:599–605, 1991.

270. Carmel RJ, Kaplan HS: Mantle irradiation in Hodgkin's disease. An analysis of technique, tumor eradication, and complications. *Cancer* 37:2813–2825, 1976.

271. Horning SJ, Adhikari A, Rizk N, et al: Effect of treatment for Hodgkin's disease on pulmonary function: Results of a prospective study. *J Clin Oncol* 12:297–305, 1994.

272. Smith LM, Mendenhall NP, Cicale MJ, et al: Results of a prospective study evaluating the effects of mantle irradiation on pulmonary function. *Int J Radiat Oncol Biol Phys* 16:79–84, 1989.

273. Donaldson SS, Kaplan HS: Complications of treatment of Hodgkin's disease in children. *Cancer Treat Rep* 66:977–989, 1982.

274. Rosner F, Zarrabi MH: Late infections following splenectomy in Hodgkin's disease. *Cancer Invest* 1:57–65, 1983.

275. Knobel H, Havard Loge J, Lund MB, et al: Late medical complications and fatigue in Hodgkin's disease survivors. *J Clin Oncol* 19:3226–3233, 2001.

276. Carver JR, Shapiro CL, Ng A, et al: American Society of Clinical Oncology clinical evidence review on the ongoing care of adult cancer survivors: Cardiac and pulmonary late effects. *J Clin Oncol* 25:3991–4008, 2007.

277. Hodgson DC, Koh ES, Tran TH, et al: Individualized estimates of second cancer risks after contemporary radiation therapy for Hodgkin lymphoma. *Cancer* 110:2576–2586, 2007.

278. Engert A, Plutschow A, Eich HT, et al: Reduced treatment intensity in patients with early-stage Hodgkin's lymphoma. *N Engl J Med* 363:640–652, 2010.

CHAPTER 98
DIFFUSE LARGE B-CELL LYMPHOMA AND RELATED DISEASES

Stephen D. Smith and Oliver W. Press*

SUMMARY

Diffuse large B-cell lymphomas (DLBCLs) comprise a heterogeneous group of aggressive malignancies of large, transformed B lymphocytes. DLBCL is the most common lymphoma in the world and accounts for approximately 25 to 30 percent of lymphoma cases in the United States. The incidence increases with age, with a median age at presentation in the sixth decade. The disease typically presents as a rapidly growing mass that may involve either lymph node or extranodal sites, and often is associated with systemic symptoms. Approximately 50 to 60 percent of patients will present with advanced stage, disseminated disease. DLBCL is curable with combination chemotherapy. For localized disease, either three cycles of rituximab, cyclophosphamide, doxorubicin, vincristine, and prednisone (R-CHOP) plus involved-field radiation therapy or six cycles of (R-CHOP) is recommended, whereas for advanced stage DLBCL, six cycles of R-CHOP is appropriate. A large phase III intergroup trial testing whether a novel infusional regimen consisting of dose-adjusted rituximab, etoposide, prednisone, vincristine, cyclophosphamide, and doxorubicin (DA-R-EPOCH) is superior to standard R-CHOP has been completed, but the results not yet reported as of this writing. High-dose chemotherapy with autologous stem cell transplantation may be curative for patients with DLBCL that relapses after treatment with frontline chemotherapy.

Acronyms and Abbreviations: ABC, activated B-cell–like; ACVBP, doxorubicin (Adriamycin), cyclophosphamide, vindesine, bleomycin, prednisone; allo-HSCT, allogeneic hematopoietic stem cell transplantation; ASCT, autologous stem cell transplantation; BEAM, high-dose carmustine, etoposide, cytarabine, and melphalan; CHOP, cyclophosphamide, doxorubicin, vincristine, prednisone; CR, complete remission; CytaBOM, cytarabine, bleomycin, vincristine, methotrexate (with leucovorin rescue); DFS, disease-free survival; DLBCL, diffuse large B-cell lymphoma; EBV, Epstein-Barr virus; EFS, event-free survival; EPOCH, etoposide, prednisone, vincristine, cyclophosphamide, doxorubicin; ESHAP, etoposide, methylprednisolone, cytarabine, cisplatin; FDG, 18-fluorodeoxyglucose; GCB, germinal center B-cell–like; GELA, Group d'Etude des Lymphomes de l'Adulte; GVHD, graft-versus-host disease; ICE, ifosfamide, carboplatin, etoposide; IFRT, involved-field radiation therapy; Ig, immunoglobulin; LDH, lactate dehydrogenase; MACOP-B, high-dose methotrexate, doxorubicin, cyclophosphamide, vincristine, prednisone, bleomycin; m-BACOD, moderate-dose methotrexate, bleomycin, doxorubicin, cyclophosphamide, vincristine, dexamethasone; MOPP, mechlorethamine, vincristine, procarbazine, prednisone; OS, overall survival; PFS, progression-free survival; ProMACE, prednisone, methotrexate, doxorubicin, cyclophosphamide, etoposide; PTLD, posttransplantation lymphoproliferative disorder; R-CHOP, rituximab plus CHOP; R-EPOCH, rituximab plus EPOCH; R-ICE, rituximab plus ICE; VACOP-B, vincristine, doxorubicin, cyclophosphamide, etoposide, prednisone, and bleomycin; WHO, World Health Organization.

*This chapter contains elements from the chapter in the 8th edition of *Williams Hematology* written by Michael Boyiadzis and Kenneth A. Foon.

DEFINITION AND HISTORY

Diffuse large B-cell lymphomas (DLBCLs) comprise a heterogeneous group of aggressive malignancies of large, transformed B cells which cause diffuse effacement of the normal lymph node structure. DLBCL has masqueraded under a variety of colorful but misleading monikers in early lymphoma classification systems, including "reticulum cell sarcoma," and "diffuse histiocytic lymphoma," as described in an excellent recent review of the history of the lymphomas.[1] Distinct disease entities are distinguished based on morphologic, biologic, and clinical features as established by an international panel of experts on behalf of the World Health Organization (WHO, Table 98–1).[2] The disease can arise *de novo* or may transform from an indolent lymphoma, such as small lymphocytic lymphoma or follicular lymphoma.

EPIDEMIOLOGY

DLBCL is the most common B-cell lymphoid neoplasm in the United States and Europe and accounts for approximately 28 percent of all mature B-cell lymphomas.[3,4] Incidence varies by ethnicity, with Americans of European descent being more likely to develop DLBCL than Americans of African descent. Like most other lymphomas, there is a male predominance. The disease most commonly presents in late middle-aged and older persons with a median age at diagnosis of approximately 65 years. Because lymphoma incidence rates increased dramatically from the 1940s to the 1990s, numerous exogenous factors have been examined to ascertain if one or more play a role in pathogenesis of the disease, including herbicides (e.g., phenoxyacids), pesticides (e.g., organochlorines), organic solvents (e.g., toluene, benzene), dark hair dyes, body mass index, tobacco use, alcohol use, and inflammatory states. At this time, no inhalant, exposure, or ingestant has been unequivocally proven to increase the relative risk of DLBCL.[5]

ETIOLOGY AND PATHOGENESIS

DLBCL is a molecularly heterogeneous disease with multiple complex chromosomal translocations and genetic abnormalities as identified by cytogenetics, gene expression profiling, and whole-genome sequencing. The disease is derived from B cells whose immunoglobulin (Ig) genes have undergone somatic mutation in the lymph node germinal center.[6] Approximately 40 percent of cases in immunocompetent hosts and approximately 20 percent of HIV-related cases display *BCL6* rearrangements.[7–9] Chromosomal translocations involving band 3q27 lead to a truncated *BCL6* gene within its 5′ flanking region. Such truncations commonly occur within the first exon or first intron, leading to complete removal or truncation of the promoter sequences; the coding sequence is left intact.[10] In a small number of cases, the breakpoint is not located in the immediate proximity of the *BCL6* gene. Increased expression of *BCL6* occurs from a process termed *promoter substitution* by which heterologous promoters are juxtaposed to the *BCL6* coding

TABLE 98–1. Diffuse Large B-Cell Lymphoma: Variants and Subtypes[2]

I. Diffuse large B-cell lymphoma, NOS
   A. Common morphologic variants
      1. Centroblastic
      2. Immunoblastic
      3. Anaplastic
   B. Rare morphologic variants
   C. Molecular subgroups
      1. Germinal center B-cell–like
      2. Activated B-cell–like
   D. Immunohistochemical subgroups
      1. CD5-positive DLBCL
      2. Germinal center B-cell–like
      3. Nongerminal center B-cell–like

II. Diffuse large B-cell lymphoma subtypes
   A. T-cell/histiocyte-rich large B-cell lymphoma
   B. DLBCL associated with chronic inflammation*
   C. EBV-positive DLBCL of the elderly*

III. Related mature B-cell neoplasms
   A. Primary mediastinal (thymic) large B-cell lymphoma[15]
   B. Intravascular large B-cell lymphoma
   C. Primary cutaneous DLBCL, leg type*
   D. Lymphomatoid granulomatosis
   E. ALK-positive DLBCL
   F. Plasmablastic lymphoma (Chap. 81)
   G. Large B-cell lymphoma arising in HHV-8–associated multicentric Castleman disease (Chap. 81)*
   H. Primary effusion lymphoma (Chap. 81)

IV. Borderline cases
   A. B-cell lymphoma, unclassifiable, with features intermediate between diffuse large B-cell lymphoma and Burkitt lymphoma*
   B. B-cell lymphoma, unclassifiable, with features intermediate between diffuse large B-cell lymphoma and classical Hodgkin lymphoma

ALK, anaplastic lymphoma kinase; DLBCL, diffuse large B-cell lymphoma; EBV, Epstein-Barr virus; HHV, human herpes virus; NOS, not otherwise specified.

*These represent provisional entities or provisional subtypes of other neoplasms.

domain. This process occurs through reciprocal translocations between 3q27 and chromosomal partner sites, including 14q32 (IgH), 2p11 (Igκ), and 22q11 (Igλ).[10,11] The BCL6 protein mediates the specific binding of several transcription factors to DNA. It also may be involved in induction of germinal-center-associated functions, as it is expressed in germinal center B cells but not in plasma cells. Therefore, downregulation of BCL6 may be necessary for terminal differentiation of B cells to memory B cells and plasma cells.[12]

Approximately 30 percent of DLBCLs possess a t(14;18) translocation involving the Ig heavy-chain gene and BCL2. Such BCL2 gene rearrangements occur in DLBCL in either of two circumstances: (1) in DLBCLs arising by histologic transformation of a previous follicular lymphoma or (2) in de novo DLBCLs with a germinal center gene-expression profile. The presence of a p53 mutation in combination with BCL2 denotes that the tumor is derived from a histologic transformation of a prior follicular lymphoma.[13]

Normally, mutations in the variable region of the Ig genes confer antibody diversity in germinal center B cells. However, aberrant somatic hypermutation occurs in more than 50 percent of cases of DLBCL. Such alterations target multiple loci, including the protooncogenes PIM1, MYC, RhoH/TTF (ARHH), and PAX5.[11] The c-MYC gene rearrangement occurs in 10 percent of patients with DLBCL.

Gene-expression profiling studies have distinguished three molecular subtypes of DLBCL known as (1) germinal center B-cell–like (GCB), (2) activated B-cell–like (ABC), and (3) primary mediastinal B-cell lymphoma (PMBCL).[14–17] GCB DLBCLs are believed to arise from normal germinal center B cells, whereas ABC DLBCLs appear to arise from postgerminal center B cells that are arrested during plasmacytic differentiation, and PMBCLs arise from thymic B cells. These DLBCL subtypes arise by distinct pathogenetic mechanisms, as judged by high-resolution, genome-wide copy-number analysis coupled with gene-expression profiling.[18] Furthermore, genomic studies employing massively parallel sequencing (genome/exome/RNAseq) have demonstrated common recurrent mutations in histone modification and chromatin remodeling genes in the GCB-DLBCL subtype of DLBCL, whereas mutations affecting the B-cell signaling pathway and nuclear factor (NF)-κB family are typical of the ABC subtype of lymphoma, as summarized in Table 98–2.[19–23] In addition, GCB DLBCLs often exhibit amplification of the oncogenic microRNA (miRNA)-17–92 cluster and deletion of the tumor-suppressor PTEN, whereas these events are rare in the ABC-type of DLBCL.

●CLINICAL FEATURES

SIGNS AND SYMPTOMS

Patients with DLBCL typically present with rapidly enlarging, symptomatic, lymphatic masses, typically in the neck or abdomen. B symptoms (drenching night sweats, fever, weight loss) are observed in approximately 30 percent of patients. Extranodal disease occurs in approximately 40 percent of patients, most commonly involving the gastrointestinal tract or marrow.[24,25] Other sites that may be affected include the testis, bone, thyroid, salivary glands, skin, liver, breast, nasal cavity, paranasal sinuses, and CNS. DLBCL may cause local compression of vessels (e.g., superior vena cava syndrome) or airways (e.g., tracheobronchial compression) requiring urgent treatment.

Unusual symptoms and presentations occur with some subtypes of DLBCL, such as intravascular large B-cell lymphoma, which may present with unexplained fever, or primary effusion lymphoma, which may present in immunocompromised hosts with human herpesvirus-8 infection. Approximately 60 percent of patients present with disseminated DLBCL (stage III or IV). Marrow involvement occurs in approximately 15 percent of patients. Discordant disease in which the lymph nodes are involved with DLBCL but the marrow contains an indolent lymphoma may occur. This combination is not associated with a poorer prognosis but increases the risk of late relapse. CNS dissemination occurs more frequently in patients with multiple extranodal sites of disease, particular testicular, paranasal sinus or marrow involvement[26] and in patients with marked elevations of serum lactic dehydrogenase (LDH). Patients at high risk for CNS involvement should undergo an examination of spinal fluid by flow cytometry for clonal B cells, which is the most sensitive method for detection of CNS disease. Patients with involvement of Waldeyer ring have an increased risk of gastrointestinal lymphoma.

TABLE 98–2. Diffuse Large B-Cell Lymphoma Subtypes Are Distinguished By Distinct Mutations in the Cells of Origin[19-23]

GCB DLBCL			ABC DLBCL		
Mutation	Frequency	Effect	Mutation	Frequency	Effect
BCL2 translocation	25%	Antiapoptotic	PRDM1	50%	Differentiation block
EZH2 mutations	22%	Histone modification	A20 loss	20%	NF-κB activation
MEF2B mutations	22%	Chromatin remodeling	CD79B mutations	21%	NF-κB/BCR signaling
MYC translocation	5%	Proliferation	CARD 11 mutations	11%	NF-κB activation
TNFRSF14 mutations	13%	Immune escape	MYD88 mutations	29%	NF-κB /JAK-STAT signaling
GNA 12 & 13 mutations	29%	GTPases; B-cell homing			

ABC, activated B-cell–like; BCR, breakpoint cluster region; DLBCL, diffuse large B-cell lymphoma; GCB, germinal center B-cell–like; GTPase, guanosine triphosphatase; KAK, Janus kinase; NF-κB, nuclear factor kappaB; STAT, signal transducer and activator of transcription.

LABORATORY FEATURES

BLOOD AND MARROW

Lymphomatous involvement of the marrow occurs in approximately 10 to 20 percent of cases of DLBCL, with blood involvement noted on morphologic examination of blood films in approximately 3 to 8 percent of cases. These percentages are undoubtedly underestimates, and data using more sensitive tests, such as flow cytometry, are needed. Marrow involvement may lead to anemia, and in severe cases to leucopenia and thrombocytopenia, which may worsen when cytotoxic therapy is administered.

CELL IMMUNOPHENOTYPE

The malignant cells of DLBCL express monoclonal surface immunoglobulin with κ or λ light-chain restriction. IgM is the most commonly expressed isotype of surface immunoglobulin, although occasionally cells may be negative for surface immunoglobulin.[27] The lymphoma cells generally express the pan–B-cell antigens, CD19, CD20, CD22, PAX5, and CD79a, as well as the pan-hematopoietic antigen, CD45 and, less commonly, CD10 or CD5.[27,28] CD5-expressing DLBCLs appear to be more aggressive and have a worse prognosis.[29] CD10+ DLBCL may be difficult to distinguish from Burkitt lymphoma or from grade 3 follicular lymphoma.[30] When a mature CD10+ B-cell phenotype is identified by flow cytometry, distinction between these possibilities should be further evaluated by morphology and genetic studies. Adhesion molecules such as LFA-1 (leukocyte function-associated antigen-1; CD16/CD18) and CD44 are expressed in 50 to 75 percent of cases of DLBCL. CD44 is expressed in highly aggressive subsets of DLBCL and is associated with disseminated disease and a poor prognosis.[31]

HISTOPATHOLOGY

Lymph nodes affected by DLBCL are usually effaced by a diffuse infiltrate of large lymphocytes. Three cytologic patterns are commonly recognized, namely, centroblastic, immunoblastic, and anaplastic, which are distinguished based on the size of the cells, the number of nucleoli, the basophilia of the cytoplasm, and the presence of bizarre and pleomorphic nuclei. Other rare morphologic variants occur, for example, with myxoid or fibrillary appearances. Although the diffuse growth pattern of DLBCL can be distinguished on histologic sections from the nodular growth pattern of follicular lymphoma, this distinction is usually not possible in fine-needle aspirates, body fluids, blood, or marrow specimens. Furthermore, genotypic characteristics overlap between

follicular lymphoma and DLBCL, with the t(14;18)(q32;q21) translocation identified in approximately 20 percent of DLBCL and approximately 85 percent of follicular lymphomas (Chap. 99). The cells in DLBCL undergo immunoglobulin variable-region gene rearrangement and are commonly somatically mutated. Furthermore, isotype switch variants may occur.[32]

DIFFERENTIAL DIAGNOSIS

The differential diagnosis of DLBCL includes nonmalignant conditions characterized by immunoblastic infiltrates (infectious mononucleosis), nonlymphoid malignancies (carcinoma), and other lymphoma subtypes, including Hodgkin lymphoma (Chap. 97), lymphoblastic lymphoma, and Burkitt lymphoma (Chap 102). Adequate tissue sampling is crucial at the time of initial diagnosis, and excisional biopsies are strongly preferred to small core needle biopsies. Fine-needle aspirates are inadequate for securing a definitive diagnosis of DLBCL and are strongly discouraged. The presence of a neoplastic clone should be confirmed with molecular or and immunophenotypic studies in most cases.

THERAPY

GENERAL CONSIDERATIONS

DLBCL is commonly curable with combination chemotherapy regimens containing an anthracycline. The best outcomes are obtained in patients who receive full doses of chemotherapy on schedule, without dose attenuations or treatment delays. Before therapy is instituted, several factors should be evaluated, including the patient's clinical stage, symptoms, and the international prognostic index (IPI). In addition, response to therapy should be evaluated according to defined criteria.[33] Other considerations, such as the patient's age and comorbid conditions, are important before a therapeutic intervention is selected. Future trials and therapies may be precisely tailored to subgroups of DLBCL based on biologic features of the tumor, but detailed staging, recognition of important variants, and IPI score calculation presently form the cornerstone of patient assessment.

LIMITED STAGE DIFFUSE LARGE B-CELL LYMPHOMA (STAGES I AND II)

Localized disease occurs in approximately 30 percent of patients, and historically was treated with radiation therapy alone.[34] However, the 5-year disease-free survival with radiation therapy in stage I disease was

TABLE 98–3. Treatment of Limited-Stage Aggressive Lymphoma

Patient Population	Number of Patients	Treatment	5-Year OS (p value) (%)	Ref.
Stages I and II, nonbulky	401	8 cycles CHOP	72	41, 42
		vs.		
		3 cycles CHOP + IFRT	82 (p = 0.05)	
Bulky stages I, IE, II, and IIE	399	8 cycles CHOP	73*	43
		vs.		
		8 cycles CHOP + IFRT	87 (p = 0.24)	
Age >60 years, IPI O	576	4 cycles CHOP	72	44
		vs.		
		4 cycles CHOP + IFRT	68 (p = 0.5)	
Age <61 years, localized stages I and II, IPI O	647	ACVBP	90	45
		vs.		
		3 cycles CHOP + IFRT	87 (p <0.001)	
Stages I and II with IPI >O	60	R-CHOP + IFRT	92	46

CHOP, cyclophosphamide, doxorubicin, vincristine, and prednisone; IFRT, involved-field radiation therapy; IPI, international prognostic index; OS, overall survival; R-CHOP, rituximab, cyclophosphamide, doxorubicin, vincristine, and prednisone.

*OS for 172 complete remission patients randomized to observation versus involved-field radiation therapy.

only 50 percent, and in stage II disease was approximately 20 percent. Combining chemotherapy with radiation therapy improved the control of local disease and resulted in a lower rate of delayed dissemination.[35–40] The role of chemotherapy alone, and cyclophosphamide, doxorubicin, vincristine, and prednisone (CHOP) in particular, has been studied in several randomized trials (Table 98–3).

A Southwest Oncology Group study randomly assigned 401 patients with stage I and nonbulky stage II disease to receive either eight cycles of CHOP chemotherapy or three cycles of CHOP plus involved-field radiotherapy (IFRT).[41] The 5-year overall and progression-free survival (PFS) rates of the patients treated with the short-course, combined modality approach were significantly better (82 percent and 72 percent, respectively, p = 0.02) than outcomes among patients treated with chemotherapy alone (77 percent and 64 percent, respectively, p = 0.03). Cardiac and hematologic toxicity was greater in patients treated with eight cycles of CHOP without radiation therapy. A subset analysis using modified IPI criteria showed that patients with poor risk factors had a worse overall survival. However, with longer followup, failure-free survival curves overlapped at 7 years and the overall survival

(OS) curves overlapped at 9 years. The early treatment advantage of CHOP plus IFRT disappeared as a result of lymphoma recurrence between 5 and 10 years after therapy.[42]

In an Eastern Cooperative Oncology Group (ECOG) trial involving 399 patients with bulky stage I (mediastinal or retroperitoneal mass, or a mass >10 cm), stage IE, stage II, or stage IIE disease, patients who achieved complete remission (CR) after CHOP chemotherapy were randomized to observation or 30 Gy involved-field radiation.[43] All patients with partial remission received 40 Gy to the involved field and radiation to the contiguous noninvolved regions. Among 172 CR patients, the 6-year disease-free survival (DFS) was 73 percent for low-dose involved-field radiation versus 56 percent for CHOP followed by observation only (p = 0.05) without a survival difference between the two arms. After 6 years failure-free survival was 63 percent in patients in partial remission (PR), and conversion to CR with radiation therapy did not influence outcome. For patients in CR after eight cycles of CHOP, low-dose involved-field radiation prolonged DFS and provided local control, but did not influence survival.

In a Group d'Etude des Lymphomes de l'Adulte (GELA) study, 576 patients older than age 60 years with stages I and II disease and an IPI score of 0 were randomized to four cycles of CHOP with or without involved-field radiation (40 Gy).[44] The 5-year event-free survival (EFS) was 61 percent for patients treated with CHOP compared to 64 percent for patients treated with CHOP plus involved-field radiation, and the OS was 72 and 68 percent, respectively. In another GELA study, 647 patients younger than age 61 years with low-risk localized aggressive lymphoma were randomized to three cycles of CHOP followed by 30 to 40 Gy of involved-field radiation or doxorubicin (Adriamycin), cyclophosphamide, vindesine, bleomycin, and prednisone (ACVBP) chemotherapy followed by consolidation chemotherapy with methotrexate, ifosfamide, etoposide, and cytarabine.[45] The EFS (82 percent vs. 74 percent, p = 0.001) and OS (90 percent vs. 87 percent, p <0.001) were significantly better for patients given intensive chemotherapy alone compared to patients given CHOP chemotherapy plus radiation therapy. The ACVBP regimen cannot be given in the United States, however, because vindesine is not available.

These studies were conducted before the incorporation of rituximab into frontline regimens for DLBCL. Subsequently, in a phase II study, 60 patients older than age 60 years with at least one adverse risk factor as defined by the IPI (but excluding bulky stage II disease) received rituximab and CHOP (R-CHOP), followed by 40 to 46 Gy involved-field radiation.[46] PFS was 95 percent at 2 years and 88 percent at 4 years, and OS was 95 percent at 2 years and 92 percent at 4 years. PFS and OS for historical controls not treated with rituximab were 78 percent and 88 percent at 4 years, respectively. Additional, retrospective analyses suggest a role for radiotherapy in unselected DLBCL patients (including limited stage disease) treated with R-CHOP,[47] and in subsets age 61 to 80 years with bulky disease (7.5 cm or greater).[48]

Although the data available are not clearcut, at this time either three cycles of R-CHOP followed by 40 to 46 Gy of involved-field radiation or six cycles of R-CHOP without radiotherapy represent standard therapeutic options.

ADVANCED STAGE DIFFUSE LARGE B-CELL LYMPHOMA

Combination chemotherapy (mechlorethamine, vincristine, procarbazine, prednisone [MOPP]) proved so successful for treatment of Hodgkin lymphoma that similar regimens were soon explored for treatment of DLBCL, including cyclophosphamide, vincristine, procarbazine, and prednisone (C-MOPP; synonym: COPP)[49] and cyclophosphamide

750 mg/m² IV, doxorubicin 50 mg/m² IV, vincristine 1.4 mg/m,² and prednisone 100 mg orally administered daily for days 1 through 5 of each cycle (CHOP). Between 1972 and 1975, reports of CRs with long-lasting PFS with these regimens heralded the advent of curative therapy for patients with DLBCL, with CHOP administered every 21 days for six to eight cycles emerging as the most popular regimen in the United States for treatment of DLBCL (Table 98–4).

In an effort to improve upon the efficacy of CHOP, a number of intensified, multidrug combinations were developed. Early single-institution, single-armed trials showed promising results, including CR rates up to 80 percent and prolonged DFS rates of 60 percent.[50,51] Phase II trials of m-BACOD (moderate-dose methotrexate, bleomycin, doxorubicin, cyclophosphamide, vincristine, dexamethasone), Pro-MACE (prednisone, methotrexate, doxorubicin, cyclophosphamide,

TABLE 98–4. Combination Chemotherapy for Intermediate- and High-Grade Lymphoma

Regimen	Dose	Route	Days of Treatment	Interval Between Treatment Cycles (Days)	Cycles
R-CHOP-21					
Rituximab	375 mg/m²	IV	1	21	6–8
Cyclophosphamide	750 mg/m²	IV	1		
Doxorubicin	50 mg/m²	IV	1		
Vincristine	1.4 mg/m²	IV	1		
Prednisone	100 mg/day	PO	1–5		
CHOP-14					
Cyclophosphamide	750 mg/m²	IV	1	14	6–8
Doxorubicin	50 mg/m²	IV	1		
Vincristine	1.4 mg/m²	IV	1		
Prednisone	100 mg/day	PO	1–5		
Dose-adjusted R-EPOCH*					
Rituximab	375 mg/m²	IV	1	21	6–8
Etoposide	50 mg/m²/day	CIV	1–4 (96 hours)		
Doxorubicin	10 mg/m²/day	CIV	1–4 (96 hours)		
Vincristine	0.4 mg/day	CIV	1–4 (96 hours)		
Cyclophosphamide	750 mg/m²/day	IV	5		
Prednisone	60 mg/m²/day	PO	1–5		
ESHAP (for relapsed lymphoma)					
Etoposide	40 mg/m²	IV	1–4	21	
Methylprednisone	500 mg/m²	IV	1–5		
Cytarabine	2 mg/m²	IV	5		
Cisplatin	25 mg/m²	CIV	1–4		
DHAP (for relapsed lymphoma)					
Dexamethasone	40 mg/m²	PO or IV	1–4	21	
Cisplatin	100 mg/m²	CIV	1		
Cytarabine	2 gm/m²	IVq12h × 2 doses	2		
R±ICE (for relapsed lymphoma)					
Rituximab	375 mg/m²	IV	1	14	
Mesna	5000 mg/m²	IV	I (day 2)		
Carboplatin	AUC = 5 (maximum 800 mg)	IV	1 (day 2)		
Etoposide	100 mg/m²	IV	1–3		
Neulasta	6 mg	SQ	1 (day 4)		

AUC, area under the curve; CIV, continuous intravenous infusion; I-CHOP, intensified-CHOP; SQ, subcutaneously.

*Doses of etoposide, doxorubicin, and cyclophosphamide are increased 20% over the dose in the previous cycle if the nadir of the absolute neutrophil count in the previous cycle was ≥0.5 × 10⁹/L.

The reader is advised to verify drugs, doses, and administration schedules of these regimens.

etoposide)/CytaBOM (cytarabine, bleomycin, vincristine, methotrexate), and MACOP-B (high-dose methotrexate, doxorubicin, cyclophosphamide, vincristine, prednisone, bleomycin) appeared to show superior response rates compared to previously published results achieved with CHOP.[52] However, the benefits demonstrated in single-institution studies could not be replicated in multiinstitutional studies, or with extended followup. A prospective randomized study that compared m-BACOD with CHOP showed no difference in the CR rates, DFS, or OS.[53] Because of these conflicting data, a four-arm phase III study was conducted and enrolled patients in a randomized prospective trial comparing CHOP, m-BACOD, MACOP-B, and ProMACE/CytaBOM.[54] This landmark trial enrolled 897 patients with intermediate- or high-grade lymphoma, of whom 85 percent had diffuse or follicular large cell lymphoma. In the trial, each of these regimens produced equivalent results. The DFS was 35 to 40 percent with a 4-year survival of 36 percent in the patients who received CHOP, 34 percent in the m-BACOD group, 45 percent in those treated with ProMACE/CytaBOM, and 39 percent in the MACOP-B group (p = 0.14). CHOP chemotherapy was the safest regimen, with only 1 percent treatment-related mortality compared to 6 percent mortality with MACOP-B. In this randomized phase III trial, the more intensive regimens offered no improvement in the remission rate, DFS, or OS compared to the simpler and safer CHOP regimen. In retrospect, the improved complete response rates observed in the initial, single-institution phase II clinical trials of the augmented regimens appear to have been a result of enrollment of a disproportionate patients with favorable IPI scores.

In 2002, a major randomized clinical trial conducted by GELA demonstrated not only increased efficacy, but minimal added toxicity, with the addition of the monoclonal antibody rituximab to CHOP in older adults with DLBCL.[55,56] In this study, 399 patients 60 to 80 years of age with newly diagnosed DLBCL were randomized to receive either eight cycles of CHOP given every 21 days (CHOP-21) or the same chemotherapy with eight infusions of rituximab. The combination of CHOP and rituximab significantly improved the CR rate from 63 to 76 percent, EFS from 38 to 57 percent, and OS from 57 to 70 percent compared to CHOP-21 without rituximab. There were no differences in toxicity other than a higher risk of minor cardiac events, many of which were attributed to rituximab infusion reactions. These results were confirmed by an ECOG group trial, in which 632 older patients were treated with six to eight cycles of CHOP-21 and randomized to the same chemotherapy plus five infusions of rituximab.[57] In this study, 2-year failure-free survival was 53 percent after a median followup of 3.5 years in patients receiving R-CHOP compared to 46 percent for patients receiving CHOP alone. A second randomization in this trial suggested that patients who received R-CHOP did not benefit from maintenance rituximab therapy. In the RICOVER-60 study, 1222 elderly patients were randomized to six or eight cycles of CHOP given every 14 days with leukocyte growth factor support (CHOP-14) or six to eight cycles of R-CHOP-14.[58] Six cycles of R-CHOP-14 significantly improved EFS, PFS, and OS compared to six cycles of CHOP-14. No benefit was conferred by administering eight cycles of R-CHOP-14 rather than six cycles of R-CHOP-14.

The benefit of adding rituximab to CHOP-like chemotherapy in younger patients was subsequently confirmed by The Monoclonal Antibody Therapeutic International Trial (MInT) Group.[59] A total of 824 patients with a good prognosis and an age-adjusted IPI of 0 or 1, and stage II to IV disease or stage I with bulky adenopathy, were randomized to receive six cycles of a CHOP-like regimens or the same regimen plus rituximab. Patients with bulky (>5 cm) disease received additional radiotherapy to those areas. After a median observation time of 34 months, the addition of rituximab increased the EFS from 59 percent to 79 percent, and the OS from 84 percent to 93 percent, both

statistically significant findings (p <0.05). These results suggest that six cycles of rituximab with a CHOP-like regimen is the best therapy for young patients with good-prognosis DLBCL. Subset analysis suggested that patients with an IPI of zero and no bulky disease represent a very favorable subgroup with a 3-year EFS of 89 percent whereas patients with an age-adjusted IPI of 1 and bulky disease represent a less-favorable subgroup with only a 74 percent 3-year EFS.

Investigators have attempted to improve the efficacy of R-CHOP by reducing the time between doses to every 14 days (R-CHOP-14), thereby increasing the "dose-density." Unfortunately, three randomized trials have shown no improvement in EFS, PFS, or OS with R-CHOP-14 compared to R-CHOP-21, and the dose-dense regimen was associated with increased hematologic toxicity.[60,61] On the other hand, an intensified combination chemotherapy regimen developed for younger patients by GELA, known as R-ACVBP (rituximab, doxorubicin, cyclophosphamide, vindesine, bleomycin, and prednisone as induction, followed by consolidation, including methotrexate, etoposide, and cytarabine) was shown to have superior EFS (81 percent vs. 67 percent) and OS (92 percent vs. 84 percent) compared to R-CHOP-21 in a randomized trial of 379 DLBCL patients younger than the age of 60 years with an age-adjusted IPI of 1.[62] However, patients experienced a substantially higher risk of hematologic toxicity and serious adverse events with R-ACVBP (42 percent vs. 15 percent with R-CHOP).

In a novel strategy to enhance chemotherapy efficacy, investigators at the United States National Cancer Institute developed an infusional chemotherapy regimen known as EPOCH (containing etoposide, prednisone, vincristine, cyclophosphamide, and doxorubicin). In this regimen, vincristine, etoposide, and doxorubicin are administered by continuous infusion over 96 hours, and cyclophosphamide is administered as a bolus. The regimen is based on in vitro data that showed that lymphoma cells exhibited less chemotherapy resistance when exposed to prolonged low concentrations of vincristine, doxorubicin, and etoposide than when exposed to brief, higher concentrations of the same drugs.[63] EPOCH was initially evaluated in 131 patients with relapsed or refractory lymphoma and demonstrated a 74 percent overall response rate and tolerable toxicity.[64] Pharmacokinetics demonstrated considerable interpatient variability and suggested the need for dose adjustments to optimize outcomes for individual patients.[65] This observation led to incorporation of a dose-adjustment strategy based on the observed hematopoietic nadir with each cycle of treatment.[66] Fifty patients with previously untreated DLBCL were treated with dose-adjusted EPOCH and demonstrated a complete response rate of 92 percent with PFS and OS rates of 70 and 73 percent, respectively. In a subsequent trial, 72 patients with untreated DLBCL were treated with dose-adjusted EPOCH and rituximab with 5-year PFS and OS of 79 percent and 80 percent, respectively.[67] A randomized study comparing rituximab plus EPOCH (R-EPOCH) to R-CHOP in untreated DLBCL has recently been completed but the results have not yet been reported (Cancer and Leukemia Group B study 50303).[68]

In summary, R-CHOP administered every 21 days has emerged as the modern standard of care for DLBCL, based on the demonstration of superior outcomes and acceptable toxicity compared to CHOP in randomized clinical trials. Neither intensifying therapy by adding chemotherapy agents, nor altering dose density, have substantially improved upon the therapeutic ratio of the standard R-CHOP regimen. As a novel approach, infusional chemotherapy with dose-adjusted R-EPOCH remains under investigation in a prospective randomized trial in the United States. An improved understanding of the heterogeneous biology of DLBCL, and identification of tumor-defined prognostic subgroups with therapy modified accordingly, may soon permit tailored treatment approaches to maximize cure rates for the ABC and GCB subtypes.

ROLE OF HIGH-DOSE CHEMOTHERAPY AND AUTOLOGOUS STEM CELL TRANSPLANTATION IN INITIAL THERAPY

High-dose chemotherapy with autologous stem cell transplantation (ASCT) has been established as the standard of care for patients with relapsed, chemotherapy-sensitive aggressive lymphomas. However, the role of ASCT as part of initial treatment remains very contentious.[69–76] A recent phase III U.S. cooperative group study evaluated this question by enrolling 397 patients with high-intermediate and high-risk aggressive non-Hodgkin lymphoma who were treated with CHOP or R-CHOP and then randomized responders (N = 253) to ASCT or further chemotherapy alone.[75] The ASCT group achieved superior PFS after 2 years (69 percent vs. 55 percent for further chemotherapy, p = 0.005) but no difference in OS was observed (74 percent vs. 71 percent, p = 0.3). In an unplanned subgroup analysis, patients with high-risk DLBCL based on the IPI achieved superior PFS and OS with ASCT.

A meta-analysis evaluated the role of high-dose chemotherapy with ASCT as part of initial treatment.[77] Fifteen randomized control trials including 3079 patients were eligible for this meta-analysis. Overall treatment-related mortality was 6 percent in the ASCT group, which was not significantly different than with conventional chemotherapy. Thirteen studies including 2018 patients showed significantly higher CR rates in the group receiving ASCT (p = 0.004). However, ASCT did not have an effect on OS, when compared to conventional chemotherapy. Subgroup analysis of prognostic groups according to IPI did not show any survival difference between ASCT and chemotherapy alone in 12 trials. EFS also showed no significant difference between ASCT and conventional chemotherapy.

High-dose chemotherapy and ASCT is not routinely recommended as part of frontline therapy of DLBCL. Some authorities believe that high-risk DLBCL patients who achieve at least a PR with firstline therapy may achieve superior outcomes if consolidated with ASCT, but available data supporting this approach are flawed, preventing uniform adoption. Because abbreviated courses of chemotherapy prior to transplantation impair outcomes, patients should receive a full course of standard chemotherapy even if subsequent ASCT is planned.

RECURRENT AND REFRACTORY DIFFUSE LARGE B-CELL LYMPHOMA

Chemotherapy

Despite major advances in initial treatment of advanced DLBCL a substantial proportion of patients is either refractory to initial induction chemotherapy or relapses after chemotherapy. Relapse usually occurs within the first 2 years after diagnosis, and the probability of long-term survival among immunochemotherapy-treated patients who survive 2 years from DLBCL diagnosis without an event (relapse, retreatment, or death) is similar to age-matched controls.[78] Several second-line regimens have been evaluated in refractory and relapsed DLBCL with response rates of 50 to 70 percent, but none of these regimens has distinguished itself as the preferred regimen. The use of single agents, such as etoposide,[79] cytarabine,[80] mitoxantrone,[81] lenalidomide,[82] and paclitaxel,[83] result in response rates from 20 to 40 percent; however, responses to monotherapy are generally not long-lasting.

A prospective phase II study of EPOCH was examined in 131 patients with relapsed or resistant lymphoma.[64] In 125 assessable patients, 29 (23 percent) achieved complete responses and 60 (48 percent) achieved partial responses. Among 42 patients with resistant disease, 57 percent responded, and in 28 patients with relapsed lymphomas, 89 percent responded with 54 percent complete responses.

With a median followup of 76 months, the overall and EFSs were 17.5 and 7 months, respectively. In 33 patients with chemotherapy-sensitive, aggressive disease who did not receive ASCT, EFS was 19 percent at 36 months.

The addition of rituximab to the ifosfamide-carboplatin-etoposide (ICE) chemotherapy regimen (R-ICE) increased the CR rate of patients with relapsed or primary refractory DLBCL under consideration for ASCT.[84] The CR rate was 53 percent, significantly better than the 27 percent CR rate (p = 0.01) achieved among 147 similar, consecutive historical control patients with DLBCL treated with ICE. PFS for patients who underwent transplantation after R-ICE was marginally better than those of 95 consecutive historical control patients who underwent transplantation after ICE (54 percent vs. 43 percent, P = 0.25).

A prospective study of 122 patients with relapsed and refractory DLBCL evaluated the role of etoposide, methylprednisolone, cytarabine, and cisplatin (ESHAP).[85] Forty-five patients (37 percent) attained a CR and 33 (27 percent) attained a PR, for a total response rate of 64 percent. The median duration of CR was 20 months, with 28 percent in CR at 3 years. The overall median survival duration was 14 months with an OS rate of 31 per cent after 3 years. Only 10 percent of all patients were alive and disease free after 40 months, however.

A randomized trial of second-line chemotherapy was published in 2010, comparing three cycles of either R-ICE or R-DHAP (rituximab, dexamethasone, high-dose cytarabine, and cisplatin) before planned ASCT.[86] This study of 396 patients demonstrated no difference in terms of efficacy (response rate 64 percent vs. 63 percent) or survival (3-year OS 47 percent vs. 51 percent) with R-ICE or DHAP, respectively. In the absence of high-level evidence supporting one salvage regimen over another, treatment for relapsed/refractory DLBCL requires individualized consideration of comorbidities and patient factors.

Autologous Stem Cell Transplantation

The role of ASCT in relapsed DLBCL was demonstrated in a randomized trial of 109 patients who responded to salvage chemotherapy with the DHAP chemotherapy regimen and were randomly assigned to receive four courses of chemotherapy plus radiotherapy (54 patients) or radiotherapy plus intensive chemotherapy and ASCT (55 patients).[87] After 5 years, the EFS was 46 percent in the transplantation group and 12 percent in the chemotherapy/radiotherapy group (p = 0.001), and the rate of OS was 53 and 32 percent, respectively (p = 0.038). Patients with relapsed or primary refractory DLBCL who achieved CR before ASCT, had better outcomes than those who achieved only PR. Disease sensitivity at the time of ASCT and time from initial diagnosis to relapse remain key prognostic variables for predicting treatment outcome after standard ASCT.[86,87] Patients who undergo ASCT when the disease is resistant to the initial induction therapy have less than a 20 percent probability of durable DFS.

Allogeneic Hematopoietic Stem Cell Transplantation

Allogeneic hematopoietic stem cell transplantation (allo-HSCT) has also been used in patients with DLBCL. The European Bone Marrow Transplant Group performed a case-controlled study by matching 101 allo-HSCT patients with 101 ASCT patients.[88] The PFS was similar in both types of transplants (49 percent for allo-HSCT vs. 46 percent for ASCT). The overall relapse and progression rate for the allo-HSCT patients was 23 percent compared with 38 percent for the ASCT patients. This difference was not statistically significant. Nine patients who had undergone ASCT died from early procedure-related toxicity and 17 patients who had undergone allo-HSCT died from early procedure-related toxicity. To reduce the treatment-related mortality associated with allo-HSCT, nonmyeloablative preparative regimens were developed to minimize the toxicity associated with standard high-dose chemotherapy, achieve sufficient engraftment to prevent graft rejection and exploit the graft-versus-tumor effect of allo-HSCT. In a prospective study, 31 patients with DLBCL and one patient with Burkitt lymphoma received allo-HSCT following 2 Gy total-body irradiation with or without fludarabine.[89] Twenty-four patients had undergone prior ASCT. With a median followup of 45 months, 3-year OS and PFS were 45 percent and 35 percent, respectively. Three-year cumulative incidences of relapse and nonrelapse mortality were 41 percent and 25 percent, respectively. Cumulative incidences of acute graft-versus-host disease (GVHD) grades II to IV, grades III and IV, and chronic GVHD were 53, 19, and 47 percent, respectively. In another study, 48 consecutive patients with relapsed or refractory DLBCL (30 patients with *de novo* disease and 18 patients with transformed follicular lymphoma) underwent transplantation with an alemtuzumab-containing regimen.[90] The PFS and OS rates after 4 years were 48 and 47 percent, respectively. Seventeen percent of patients developed grades II to IV acute GVHD, and 13 percent experienced extensive chronic GVHD. Four-year estimated nonrelapse mortality was 32 percent, and relapse risk was 33 percent. Although these results are promising, allo-HSCT cannot be recommended before ASCT except in the context of a clinical trial.

Radioimmunotherapy

Radioimmunotherapy as monotherapy is not recommended for DLBCL but its role as part of a conditioning regimen prior to ASCT has been encouraging. A phase II trial evaluated the safety and efficacy of combining ^{90}Y-ibritumomab tiuxetan with high-dose carmustine, cytarabine, etoposide, and melphalan (BEAM) and ASCT in patients with lymphoma who were considered ineligible for total-body irradiation because of older age or prior radiotherapy.[91] The addition of ^{90}Y-ibritumomab tiuxetan to BEAM with ASCT was feasible and the toxicity and tolerability profile similar to that observed with BEAM alone. Similarly, ^{131}I-tositumomab (up to 0.75 Gy) was combined with BEAM followed by ASCT for the treatment of chemotherapy-resistant relapsed or refractory lymphoma. Short-term and long-term toxicities were similar to that in patients previously treated with BEAM alone, with an OS rate of 55 percent and an EFS rate of 39 percent.[92]

Summary of Approach to Patients with Relapsed Disease

Patients with relapsed disease should receive multidrug chemotherapy, such as R-ICE or R-DHAP. If chemosensitivity is demonstrated and no contraindications are present, ASCT should be performed. If patients are elderly or have comorbid conditions the goal should be palliation. Radiotherapy can be used to alleviate symptoms at particular sites of involvement in patients with relapsed DLBCL and single-agent therapy can be used but with low expected response rates and duration of responses.

● COURSE AND PROGNOSIS

INTERNATIONAL PROGNOSTIC INDEX

In 1993, a model was proposed to assign a prognosis to patients with aggressive lymphoma undergoing treatment with doxorubicin-containing chemotherapeutic regimens termed the *international prognostic index* (IPI).[93,94] The model used clinical data, including (1) tumor stage, (2) serum LDH level, (3) number of extranodal disease sites involved, (4) performance status, and (5) patient age. This model resulted in the IPI, which is used to forecast the behavior of aggressive lymphoma (Table 98–5 and Fig. 98-1). For patients younger than age 60 years, an age-adjusted IPI has been proposed in which all the factors of the IPI are

TABLE 98–5. International Prognostic Factor Index for Non-Hodgkin Lymphoma[93]

Risk factors
Age older than 60 years
Serum lactic dehydrogenase greater than twice normal
Performance status ≥2
Stage III or IV
Extranodal involvement at more than 1 site

Each factor accounts for 1 point, for a total score that ranges from 0 to 3 for patients younger than 61 years of age. The latter age-adjusted index includes all variables except for age and extranodal sites. For patients 61 years of age and older, a total score ranges from 0 to 5 and includes each variable shown in this table.

used, except for age and presence of extranodal sites. The 5-year survival rates for patients age 60 years or younger with IPI scores of 0, 1, 2, and 3 were 83, 69, 46, and 32 percent, respectively (Table 98–6).[93] To better estimate prognosis among modern DLBCL patients, a revision of the IPI was recently developed by the National Comprehensive Cancer Network (the NCCN-IPI).[95] This model employs the same five risk factors but uses a different scoring algorithm, and improves discrimination of groups treated with rituximab-containing chemoimmunotherapy.

GENE-EXPRESSION PROFILING AND DETERMINATION OF DIFFUSE LARGE B-CELL LYMPHOMA SUBTYPES

Gene-expression profiling has also been used to delineate groups of patients with DLBCL who may differ in their response to therapy and prognosis (Fig. 98–2).[14–17,96,97] Six genes identified by gene-expression analysis and detected by quantitative real-time polymerase chain reaction can identify three prognostic groups in patients with DLBCL.[98] The six genes that were used in this model occur in the germinal center B-cell signature (*LMO2, BCL6*), activated B-cell signature (*BCL2, CCND2, SCYA3*), and lymph node signature (*FN1*). In this study, expression of *LMO2, BCL6*, and *FN1* correlated with prolonged survival, whereas expression of *BCL2, CCND2*, and *SCYA3* correlated with short survival. Protein immunohistochemistry (IHC) has also been used to delineate DLBCL subtypes, but shows imperfect concordance with gene expression results.[96] Even though various algorithms have been developed for subtyping DLBCL by IHC, further refinement is needed prior to relying on IHC for management decisions and prognostication.

SERUM LACTIC DEHYDROGENASE AND β_2-MICROGLOBULIN

Patients with an elevated β_2-microglobulin level and high serum LDH have a poor prognosis, with a 26 percent survival compared to 81 percent survival in patients without elevation of either of these markers.[93,99]

PRESENCE OF *MYC* GENE REARRANGEMENT OR ELEVATED PROTEIN EXPRESSION

Approximately 10 percent of DLBCL patients harbor a translocation involving the *MYC* gene. Patients with a *MYC* rearrangement detected

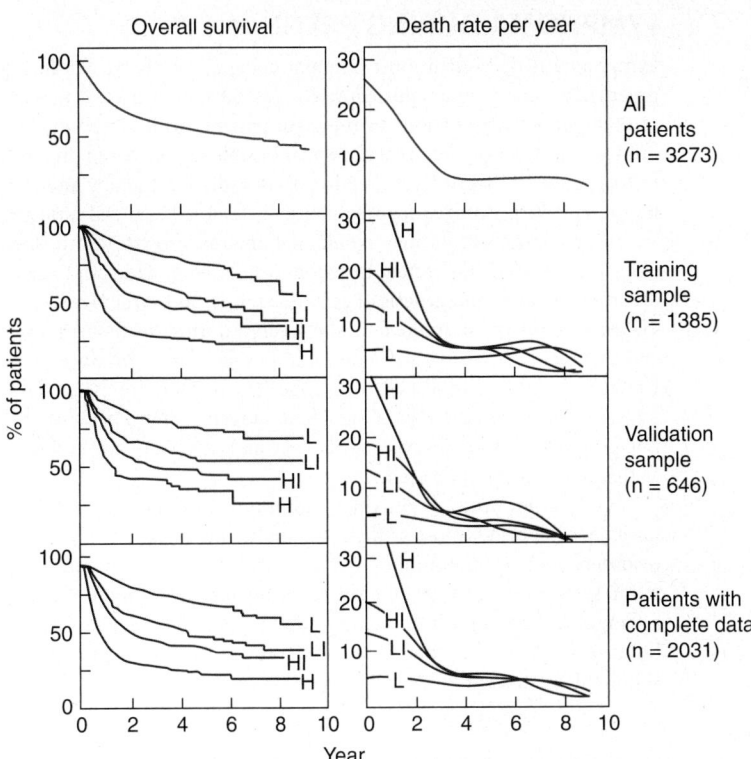

Figure 98–1. *(Left panels)* Kaplan-Meier survival curves for the four risk groups.[94] *(Right panels)* Death rates during the study period. Only 2031 of the 3273 patients had sufficient relevant information for classification according to the international index. H, high risk; HI, high-intermediate risk; L, low risk; LI, low-intermediate risk.

by fluorescence *in situ* hybridization (FISH) have been shown to have an inferior 5-year survival of 33 percent when treated with standard R-CHOP therapy, compared to 72 percent survival for those without *MYC* rearrangements.[100] Concurrent translocation of BCL2 or BCL6 is seen in a subset of cases. These "double-hit" lymphomas are often classified morphologically as "B-cell lymphoma, unclassifiable, with features intermediate between DLBCL and Burkitt lymphoma" using the 2008 WHO classification of lymphomas and have a very bad prognosis.[2] MYC protein overexpression by IHC is also associated with an inferior prognosis, particularly when accompanied by BCL2 protein overexpression.[101,102]

POSITRON EMISSION TOMOGRAPHY

Fluorine-18-fluorodeoxyglucose-positron emission tomography (FDG-PET) is used for initial staging and at the end of treatment (to assess remission status) in patients with DLBCL. FDG-PET is superior to computed tomography imaging in detecting nodal and extranodal sites of aggressive lymphoma, with the potential to alter stage, prognosis, and selection of therapy.[103] In addition, FDG-PET performed at the end of therapy is highly informative. A negative PET predicts a high probability of disease control, and is required to designate a CR by modern response criteria.[33,104] Other uses of PET in DLBCL are investigational or not routinely recommended.

TABLE 98–6. Outcome According to Risk Group Defined by the International Prognostic Index[93]

International Index	No. of Risk Factors	Complete Response Rate (%)	Relapse-Free Survival (%)		Survival (%)	
INTERNATIONAL PROGNOSTIC INDEX, ALL PATIENTS						
			2-Year	5-Year	2-Year	5-Year
Low	0 or 1	87	79	70	84	73
Low-intermediate	2	67	66	50	66	51
High-intermediate	3	55	59	49	54	43
High	4 or 5	44	58	40	34	26
AGE-ADJUSTED INTERNATIONAL INDEX, PATIENTS <61 YEARS OF AGE						
			2-Year	5-Year	2-Year	5-Year
Low	0	92	88	86	90	83
Low-intermediate	1	78	74	66	79	69
High-intermediate	2	57	62	53	59	46
High	3	46	61	58	37	32

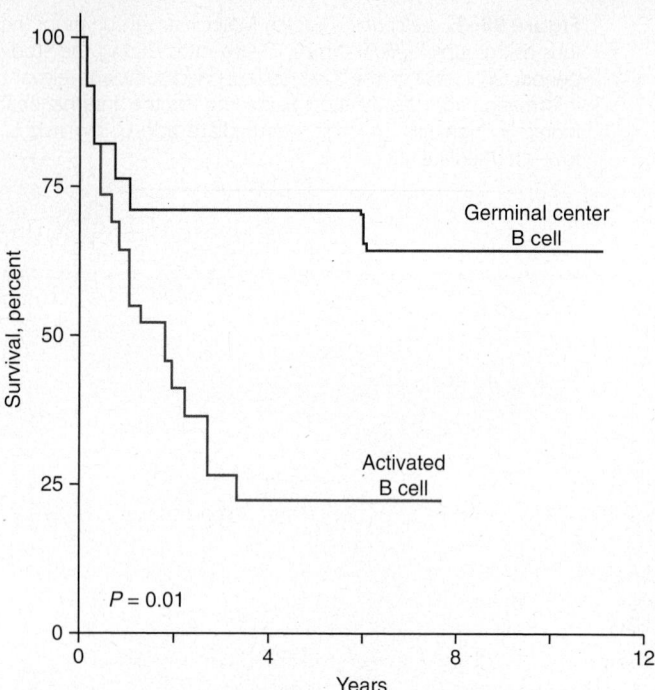

Figure 98–2. Overall survival in a group of patients with diffuse large B-cell lymphoma whose cell of origin was determined by gene-expression profiling.[14] Survival of patients with diffuse large B-cell lymphoma whose malignant cells were thought to arise from a germinal center B cell was significantly better than in patients whose cell of origin arose from activated B cells.

● PRESENTATION AND THERAPY FOR SPECIFIC DIFFUSE LARGE B-CELL LYMPHOMA SUBTYPES AND RELATED MATURE B-CELL NEOPLASMS

PRIMARY TESTICULAR LYMPHOMA

Primary testicular lymphoma represents 1 to 2 percent of all lymphomas, with an estimated incidence of 0.26 per 100,000 males per year.[105] Even though lymphomas account for only 1 to 7 percent of all testicular malignancies, they represent the most common testicular tumor in men older than 50 years of age. Histologically, 80 to 90 percent of primary testicular lymphomas are DLBCL, with a mean age at diagnosis of 68 years (range: 21 to 98 years).[106,107] Most patients present with stage I or II disease with isolated involvement of the right or left testis equal in frequency, whereas 6 percent of cases have bilateral involvement. Primary testicular lymphoma shows a tendency to disseminate to several extranodal sites, including the contralateral testis, CNS, skin, Waldeyer ring, lung, pleura, and soft tissues. Treatment using radiation therapy alone provides suboptimal disease control, even for patients with stage I disease. Chemotherapy without anthracyclines was shown to produce inferior results compared with regimens containing anthracyclines. Thus, R-CHOP is the regimen recommended by most lymphoma specialists following orchiectomy for testicular DLBCL, with a median OS of 4.4 years. Radiation therapy to the contralateral testis should also be administered.[105,108,109] CNS prophylaxis with intrathecal chemotherapy or high-dose methotrexate should be strongly considered because of the observed propensity for CNS relapses.

LYMPHOMA DURING PREGNANCY

Lymphoma is the fourth most frequent malignancy diagnosed during pregnancy, occurring in approximately 1 in 6000 deliveries.[110] Reports of therapeutic interventions in pregnant patients with lymphoma are limited, and management recommendations are largely based on small retrospective studies and case reports. Both radiation therapy and chemotherapy during pregnancy are potentially teratogenic. Fetal exposure to antineoplastic agents may result in impaired growth, diminished neurologic and/or intellectual function, decreased gonadal and reproductive function, mutagenesis of germline tissue, and carcinogenesis.[111] The risks of treatment to the fetus are greatest during the first trimester and therapeutic abortion is a consideration under these circumstances. CHOP during the second and third trimesters may be administered relatively safely with little risk of significant adverse fetal outcomes.[112,113] The prognosis of patients who receive optimal chemotherapy is similar to that of nonpregnant patients.[114]

Only a few cases of rituximab administration during pregnancy have been reported, most of them for the treatment of nonmalignant disorders such as autoimmune diseases. Patients with supradiaphragmatic stage I disease may be considered for localized radiotherapy as a temporary measure until the second trimester, when chemotherapy holds less risk for the fetus.[115] Patients in the second or third trimester should be treated with full-dose chemotherapy.

PRIMARY MEDIASTINAL LARGE B-CELL LYMPHOMA

Definition

Primary mediastinal large B-cell lymphoma arises in the mediastinal lymphatic structures, probably from a thymic B-cell precursor.

Epidemiology

This variant type of DLBCL accounts for approximately 3 percent of lymphomas, and is most commonly seen in young and middle-aged adults, with about two-thirds of cases occurring in females.

Clinical Features

The clinical presentation is typically with an anterior mediastinal mass that is locally invasive into neighboring tissues including the lungs and pericardium. Upper airway obstruction and superior vena cava syndrome occur in approximately 40 percent of patients.[116] Regional lymph nodes, especially the cervical chain, are often involved, but distant nodal involvement at presentation is uncommon with this entity. Relapses tend to be extranodal, including sites such as the liver, gastrointestinal tract, kidneys, ovaries, and CNS. Marrow involvement is very unusual.

Laboratory Features

PMBCL and Hodgkin lymphoma exhibit similar gene-expression profiles, raising questions about biologic relationships.[16,117] Sometimes bizarre multinucleated cells mimicking Reed-Sternberg cells are seen in PMBCL along with other morphologic features suggestive of Hodgkin lymphoma. Fibrotic bands may be prominent in biopsies, leading to the appellation "primary B-cell mediastinal lymphoma with sclerosis." IHC may be helpful in the differential diagnosis since primary mediastinal lymphoma expresses weak CD30, lacks CD15 antigen as seen in Hodgkin lymphoma, and expresses B-cell–associated antigens CD19, CD20, CD22, and CD79a.[118] Other useful markers include the melanocytic marker, HMB-45, keratin, and placental leukocyte alkaline phosphatase which can help distinguish PMBCL from sarcoma, melanoma, thymoma, and seminoma.

Therapy

Several regimens have been evaluated in PMBCL. A retrospective study compared the outcomes of 426 patients who had fibrotic tumor reactions (sclerosis) and previously untreated disease using CHOP-like regimens, third-generation (MACOP-B, VACOP-B [etoposide, doxorubicin, cyclophosphamide, vincristine, prednisone, and bleomycin], ProMACE CytaBOM) regimens, or high-dose chemotherapy with autologous hematopoietic stem cell transplantation.[119] With chemotherapy, the CR rates were 49, 51, and 53 percent with first-generation, third-generation, and high-dose chemotherapy treatments, respectively. All patients who achieved CR or PR had radiation therapy to the mediastinum. The final CR rates were 61 percent for CHOP-like regimens, 79 percent for MACOP-B and other regimens, and 75 percent for high-dose chemotherapy/autologous hematopoietic stem cell transplantation. Projected 10-year PFS rates were 35, 67, and 78 percent, respectively, and projected 10-year OS rates were 44, 71, and 77 percent, respectively.

In another retrospective study of 138 patients with PMBCL the effectiveness of two chemotherapy regimens (CHOP vs. MACOP-B/VACOP-B) and the role of mediastinal IFRT as consolidation were evaluated.[120] CR occurred in 51 percent of the CHOP group and 80 percent in MACOP-B/VACOP-B. EFS was 40 percent with CHOP and 76 percent in the MACOP-B/VACOP-B group. The addition of IFRT improved the outcome, regardless of the type of chemotherapy used. The incorporation of rituximab in the dose-adjusted EPOCH regimen, without radiotherapy consolidation, resulted in 97 percent OS and 93 percent EFS in a nonrandomized, phase II clinical trial.[121] Based on this study, which included 5-year followup data, many authorities believe that the dose-adjusted R-EPOCH regimen should be the preferred firstline regimen for this entity, without routine incorporation of radiotherapy.

LYMPHOMATOID GRANULOMATOSIS

Definition

Lymphomatoid granulomatosis is a rare lymphoproliferative disorder characterized by angiocentric and angiodestructive Epstein-Barr virus (EBV)–driven B-cell proliferation associated with extensive reactive T-cell infiltration.[2]

Epidemiology

Approximately two-thirds of cases occur in males. The median age of presentation is in the fifth decade of life, although pediatric cases occur.

Clinical Features

The lung is the most common site of involvement (90 percent), followed by the skin (25 to 50 percent), kidney (30 to 40 percent), liver (29 percent), and CNS (26 percent). The spleen and the lymph nodes are uncommonly involved.[122] Nearly all patients are symptomatic at presentation with cough, dyspnea, chest pain, fever, weight loss, and joint pain. Abdominal pain and diarrhea occur as a result of gastrointestinal involvement and various neurologic signs, including diplopia, ataxia, and mental status changes may occur as a result of CNS involvement. Skin manifestations are clinically diverse, and include ulcerations, plaques, and maculopapules, although subcutaneous nodules are most common.

Laboratory Features

Imaging Studies Pulmonary involvement typically involves bilateral, lower lobe nodules, which frequently cavitate. Nodules may also be found in the brain and kidney and other locations.

Histopathology The grading of lymphomatoid granulomatosis depends upon the proportion of EBV-positive B cells identified by *in situ* hybridization with an EBV-encoded RNA probe relative to the number of reactive lymphocytes in the background.[2] Grade 1 lesions contain a polymorphous lymphoid infiltrate without cytologic atypia. Large transformed lymphoid cells are absent or rare and EBV-positivity is detectable in only a few cells. Grade 2 lesions contain occasional large lymphoid cells or immunoblasts in a polymorphous background. *In situ* hybridization for EBV readily identifies EBV-positive cells, which are present at 5 to 20 per high-power field. Grade 3 lesions continue to show an inflammatory background, but contain frequent large atypical B cells that are CD20-positive. By *in situ* hybridization, EBV-positive cells are numerous (>50/high-power field).

Therapy and Prognosis

The clinical prognosis is variable in lymphomatoid granulomatosis with a median survival of 2 years.[123] Poor prognostic features include neurologic involvement and higher pathologic grade. The disease is uncommon and the optimal treatment regimen is unclear. In a prospective study, patients with grades I and II disease were treated with interferon-α, whereas those with grade III lesions received dose-adjusted R-EPOCH chemotherapy.[124] Among 27 patients with grade I or II disease treated with interferon-α, 56 percent were in continuous CR for a median of 52 months. Among grade III patients treated with dose-adjusted R-EPOCH, 40 percent achieved CR, with OS and PFS rates of 69 and 82 percent, respectively, after a median follow up of 46 months.

INTRAVASCULAR LARGE B-CELL LYMPHOMA

Definition

Intravascular large B-cell lymphoma is a rare type of extranodal large B-cell lymphoma characterized by selective growth of lymphoma cells within the lumina of vessels, sparing the large arteries and veins.[2]

Epidemiology

This tumor usually occurs in adults in the sixth and seventh decade. It occurs equally in men and women.

Clinical Features

The clinical manifestations of this lymphoma are extremely variable, with most symptoms related to the organs affected. Two major patterns of clinical presentation have been recognized: the first is in European countries with brain and skin involvement and the second in the Asian countries where patients typically present with multiorgan failure, hepatosplenomegaly, pancytopenia and hemophagocytic syndrome.[125–129] B symptoms (fever, drenching sweats, and weight loss) are common in both types. An isolated cutaneous variant almost unique to Western countries has been identified in females and is associated with a better prognosis.[125] In this variant, skin lesions range from single to striking clusters of nodules and tumors which may appear as violaceous plaques, erythematous nodules, or ulcerating tumors, which are often painful. These lesions commonly appear on the arms and legs, abdomen and breasts, but may occur anywhere.

Laboratory Features

There are no laboratory findings specific for intravascular B cell lymphoma. Increased LDH and β_2-microglobulin levels are observed in most patients. An elevated erythrocyte sedimentation rate and abnormalities in hepatic, renal, and thyroid function are also common.[130] Tumor cells express B-cell–associated antigens and occasionally express CD5.

Therapy

Anthracycline-based chemotherapy is the standard of care for this type of lymphoma and retrospective studies suggest that the addition of rituximab improves clinical outcomes.[131,132] One study analyzed 106 patients who received chemotherapy either with rituximab (R-chemotherapy, n = 49) or without rituximab (chemotherapy, n = 57).[132] The CR rate was 82 percent for patients in the R-chemotherapy group compared to 51 percent in the chemotherapy-alone group (p = 0.001). PFS and OS rates 2 years after diagnosis were 56 and 66 percent, respectively, in the R-chemotherapy group, compared with 27 and 46 percent for patients in the chemotherapy-alone group (p = 0.001 for PFS and p = 0.01 for OS). More intensive chemotherapy including high-dose methotrexate and/or high-dose cytarabine are recommended for patients with CNS involvement (e.g., R-CHOP with high-dose methotrexate). Many authorities believe that CNS prophylaxis is warranted even in cases of intravascular large cell lymphoma without demonstrable CNS disease at diagnosis, because of the high rate of CNS relapse.

POSTTRANSPLANT LYMPHOPROLIFERATIVE DISORDERS

Definition

Posttransplantation lymphoproliferative disorders (PTLD) result from lymphoid or plasmacytic proliferations that develop in the setting of solid-organ or marrow transplantation. Although PTLD represents an uncommon complication in transplant patients, it is a significant cause of morbidity and mortality.[133]

Epidemiology

The incidence of PTLD is approximately 1 to 2 percent in solid-organ transplant recipients, which is 30 to 50 times higher than the incidence of lymphoproliferative diseases in the immunocompetent general population.[134] There is a clear association between PTLD and the type of organ transplanted. Among the most commonly transplanted solid organs, heart, lung, and intestinal transplantation have the highest incidences of PTLD,[135] with the highest risk occurring in the first year after transplantation. The incidence of PTLD after blood or marrow transplantation is lower than after solid-organ transplantation and ranges from 0.5 to 1.0 percent in reported series.

Pathogenesis

The major risk factors that have been identified for the development of PTLD include EBV-positive serology pretransplantation, type of organ transplanted, and intensity of immunosuppressive regimen used.[136–138] The onset of posttransplantation lymphoma in most patients is related to B-cell proliferation induced by infection with EBV in the setting of chronic immunosuppression. The genome of the virus can be detected in the cells of the majority of cases.[139] However, in approximately 20 to 30 percent of cases the virus is undetectable in involved tissues.[140] Involvement of the lymph nodes, gastrointestinal tract, lungs, and liver are common with all types of allografts. The majority of PTLDs in solid-organ transplant recipients are of host origin. In contrast, the majority of PTLDs in hematopoietic stem cell allografts are of donor origin. Involvement of the grafted organ occurs in approximately 30 percent of patients and may lead to organ damage and fatal complications.[141]

Therapy

Management of PTLD is not uniform. A wide variety of approaches, including decreasing the dose of immunosuppressive drugs or administering antiviral therapy, interferon, intravenous immunoglobulin, adoptive therapy with EBV-specific cytotoxic T lymphocytes, chemotherapy, radiation, and rituximab therapy, have been reported. If feasible, reduction of immunosuppression is the first step in the management of such patients. Many cases of polyclonal PTLD resolve completely with a reduction in immunosuppressive therapy.[142] Patients with late PTLD

and more aggressive monoclonal PTLD are less likely to respond.[143] Rituximab has shown promising results in the treatment of CD20+ PTLD. In a multicenter prospective trial, 43 patients with previously untreated B-cell PTLD who failed to respond to tapering of immunosuppression, were treated with 4 weekly injections of rituximab at 375 mg/m^2.[144] The overall response rate was 44 percent, with an OS of 86 per cent after 80 days and 67 percent after 1 year. The only baseline factor predicting response at day 80 was a normal level of serum LDH. A retrospective study evaluated the efficacy and safety of chemotherapy salvage therapies in adult recipients of solid-organ transplants with a second progression of PTLD after initial therapy with rituximab.[145] CHOP therapy achieved a favorable overall response rate of 70 percent in this setting, indicating that PTLD generally remains chemotherapy-sensitive after progression following initial therapy with rituximab.

A prospective trial evaluated a stepwise treatment approach beginning with reduction of immunosuppression, then interferon-α, and finally chemotherapy with ProMACE-CytaBOM plus granulocyte-monocyte colony-stimulating factor.[146] Sixteen eligible patients began treatment with reduced immunosuppression. The response rate to reduced immunosuppression was zero of 16 CR and one of 16 PR (6 percent). Six of the 16 patients (38 percent) had documented rejection of the transplanted organ during the period of reduced immunosuppression. Eight of the 16 patients had documented progressive disease during the period of reduced immunosuppression. Thirteen patients underwent treatment with interferon, with two patients achieving CRs (15 percent) and two achieving PRs (15 percent). Seven eligible patients proceeded to ProMACE-CytaBOM chemotherapy with five (67 percent) attaining CR. Four of the five CRs experienced remission durations of more than 2 years. The median survival for the treatment cohort as a whole was 19 months, with a range of 5 days to 60+ months. Overall survival was 50 percent at 2 years, 44 percent at 4 years, and 24 percent at 8 years.

The following sequence is currently recommended for PTLD: The first intervention should be reduction in immunosuppression, followed by four weekly cycles of rituximab if reduction of the immunosuppression by itself is ineffective. If PTLD does not regress with these measures, then six cycles of R-CHOP are recommended.

T-CELL–HISTIOCYTE-RICH LARGE B-CELL LYMPHOMA

Definition

T-cell–histiocyte-rich large B-cell lymphoma is characterized by effacement of the architecture of the lymph node by a lymphohistiocytic infiltrate with a diffuse or vaguely nodular growth pattern.[2,147] There are a limited number of large atypical B cells occurring singly or in small clusters with a predominant background infiltrate composed of T cells and histiocytes, the latter usually of the nonepithelioid type.

Epidemiology

T-cell–histiocyte-rich large B-cell lymphoma accounts for less than 5 percent of all cases of DLBCL and occurs at a younger age on average. The median age of onset is in the fourth decade, compared to the sixth decade for DLBCL.[148–151] A male predominance is noted in most series, in contrast to DLBCL not otherwise specified, which occurs equally in men and women.

Clinical Features

This variant more often presents with advanced stage disease, B symptoms, an elevated LDH, splenic infiltration and multiple extranodal sites (especially the marrow and liver) compared to standard DLBCL.[148–150,152]

Therapy and Prognosis

When treated with CHOP-like regimens, most series suggest that the outcome for these patients is similar to patients with typical DLBCL,[149,151–154] with CR rates of approximately 60 percent, and 3-year and 5-year OS rates of 50 to 64 percent and 45 to 58 percent, respectively. Two case-control analyses have been performed comparing T-cell–histiocyte-rich large B-cell lymphoma and DLBCL with no differences in OS observed.[149,150] Based on these data, this subtype of large B-cell lymphoma should be treated in the same fashion as traditional DLBCL. Six cycles of R-CHOP for advanced disease is a reasonable initial approach to therapy.

PRIMARY CUTANEOUS DIFFUSE LARGE B-CELL LYMPHOMA, LEG TYPE

Definition

This lymphoma is a primary cutaneous lymphoma composed solely of large transformed B cells that exhibits a predilection for the skin of the leg.[2]

Epidemiology

Primary cutaneous DLBCLs of the leg type constitute approximately 4 percent of all primary cutaneous B-cell lymphomas.[2,155] The median age at the time of presentation is 60 to 70 years.

Clinical Features

These lymphomatous tumors affect the skin of the legs in most cases, but approximately 10 percent arise at other sites.[156–158] Multiple tumors, sometimes ulcerating, are associated with poorer prognosis. There are frequent relapses and extracutaneous dissemination may occur.

Laboratory Features

The malignant B cells in this entity usually express CD20, BCL2, and FOX-P1. FISH of the lymphoma cells often detects translocations involving *MYC, BCL6,* or *IGH* genes. Amplification of the *BCL2* gene is usually responsible for the high frequency of BCL2 overexpression. The t(14;18) translocation is generally not observed in this lymphoma variant. The gene-expression profile observed in this subtype suggests an activated B-cell origin.

Therapy

Anthracycline-containing chemotherapy with rituximab should be considered as initial therapy. The incorporation of rituximab improves the response rates and OS.[156–158] However, because of the advanced age of most patients with this variant at the time of diagnosis, aggressive combination chemoimmunotherapy may not be feasible due to patient frailty or comorbidities. In such circumstances, local radiation therapy or less-aggressive chemotherapy are reasonable.

ANAPLASTIC LYMPHOMA KINASE-POSITIVE LARGE B-CELL LYMPHOMA

Definition

Anaplastic lymphoma kinase (ALK)-positive large B-cell lymphoma is an uncommon neoplasm of large immunoblast-like B cells that stain for nuclear and/or cytoplasmic ALK protein.

Epidemiology

The average age at presentation is in the fourth decade with a male predilection. Most patients present with advanced stage disease.

Clinical Features

Patients with anaplastic DLBCL usually present with widespread disease, with cervical and mediastinal nodes being the most frequent sites of adenopathy, and the liver, spleen, bone and gastrointestinal tract being the most common sites of extranodal involvement.[159,160]

Laboratory Features

The immunoblastic cells of anaplastic DLBCL typically have a large central nucleolus and may exhibit maturation to plasmablastic cells. The lymphoma cells stain for the ALK protein by immunohistocytochemistry, usually with a granular cytoplasmic appearance though nuclear staining may also occur. These cells are usually negative for CD3, CD20, CD30, and CD79a. MUC1 mucin, a high-molecular-weight transmembrane glycoprotein, also known as epithelial membrane antigen and CD138 are usually strongly expressed by these cells. Monoclonal (light-chain restricted) IgA or IgG is generally present in the cytoplasm of the malignant cells. Occasional cases possess a t(2;17)(p23;q23) translocation that results in a clathrin-ALK fusion protein.

Therapy and Prognosis

The clinical course of ALK-positive large B-cell lymphoma is aggressive with a median survival time of 24 months. Because the tumors are usually negative for CD20, the utility of rituximab is dubious for this entity. Anthracycline-based chemotherapy is often inadequate and more intensive therapies should be considered.[159,160]

HUMAN IMMUNODEFICIENCY RELATED DIFFUSE LARGE B-CELL LYMPHOMA VARIANTS

Primary effusion lymphoma, plasmablastic lymphoma, and large B-cell lymphoma arising in human herpesvirus-8–associated multicentric Castleman disease usually develop in the setting of acquired immunodeficiency induced by HIV and are discussed in Chap. 81.

REFERENCES

1. Lichtman MA: Historical landmarks in the understanding of the lymphomas, in *Neoplastic Diseases of the Blood,* ed 5, edited by Wiernik PH, Goldman JM, Dutcher J, Kyle RA, p 789. Springer, New York, 2013.
2. Swerdlow SH, World Health Organization, International Agency for Research on Cancer, et al: *WHO Classification of Tumours of Haematopoietic and Lymphoid Tissues.* World Health Organization International Agency for Research on Cancer, Lyon, France 2008.
3. Fisher SG, Fisher RI: The epidemiology of non-Hodgkin's lymphoma. *Oncogene* 23:38, 2004.
4. Morton LM, Wang SS, Devesa SS, et al: Lymphoma incidence patterns by WHO subtype in the United States, 1992–2001. *Blood* 107:1, 2006.
5. Alexander DD, Mink PJ, Adami HO, et al: The non-Hodgkin lymphomas: A review of the epidemiologic literature. *Int J Cancer* 120:1, 2007.
6. Ye BH, Lista F, Lo Coco F, et al: Alterations of a zinc finger-encoding gene, BCL-6, in diffuse large-cell lymphoma. *Science* 262:5134, 1993.
7. Dalla-Favera R, Migliazza A, Chang CC, et al: Molecular pathogenesis of B cell malignancy: The role of BCL-6. *Curr Top Microbiol Immunol* 246:257, 1999.
8. Gaidano G, Lo Coco F, Ye BH, et al: Rearrangements of the BCL-6 gene in acquired immunodeficiency syndrome-associated non-Hodgkin's lymphoma: Association with diffuse large-cell subtype. *Blood* 84:2, 1994.
9. Lo Coco F, Ye BH, Lista F, et al: Rearrangements of the BCL6 gene in diffuse large cell non-Hodgkin's lymphoma. *Blood* 83:7, 1994.
10. Ye BH, Chaganti S, Chang CC, et al: Chromosomal translocations cause deregulated BCL6 expression by promoter substitution in B cell lymphoma. *EMBO J* 14:24, 1995.
11. Kaneita Y, Yoshida S, Ishiguro N, et al: Detection of reciprocal fusion 5′-BCL6/partner-3′ transcripts in lymphomas exhibiting reciprocal BCL6 translocations. *Br J Haematol* 113:3, 2001.
12. Chang CC, Ye BH, Chaganti RS, et al: BCL-6, a POZ/zinc-finger protein, is a sequence-specific transcriptional repressor. *Proc Natl Acad Sci U S A* 93:14, 1996.
13. Lo Coco F, Gaidano G, Louie DC, et al: p53 mutations are associated with histologic transformation of follicular lymphoma. *Blood* 82:3, 1993.
14. Alizadeh AA, Eisen MB, Davis RE, et al: Distinct types of diffuse large B-cell lymphoma identified by gene expression profiling. *Nature* 403:6769, 2000.
15. Rosenwald A, Wright G, Chan WC, et al: The use of molecular profiling to predict survival after chemotherapy for diffuse large-B-cell lymphoma. *N Engl J Med* 346:25, 2002.
16. Rosenwald A, Wright G, Leroy K, et al: Molecular diagnosis of primary mediastinal B cell lymphoma identifies a clinically favorable subgroup of diffuse large B cell lymphoma related to Hodgkin lymphoma. *J Exp Med* 198:6, 2003.

17. Wright G, Tan B, Rosenwald A, et al: A gene expression-based method to diagnose clinically distinct subgroups of diffuse large B cell lymphoma. *Proc Natl Acad Sci U S A* 100:17, 2003.

18. Lenz G, Wright GW, Emre NC, et al: Molecular subtypes of diffuse large B-cell lymphoma arise by distinct genetic pathways. *Proc Natl Acad Sci U S A* 105:36, 2008.

19. Morin RD, Johnson NA, Severson TM, et al: Somatic mutations altering EZH2 (Tyr641) in follicular and diffuse large B-cell lymphomas of germinal-center origin. *Nat Genet* 42:2, 2010.

20. Morin RD, Mendez-Lago M, Mungall AJ, et al: Frequent mutation of histone-modifying genes in non-Hodgkin lymphoma. *Nature* 476:7360, 2011.

21. Morin RD, Mungall K, Pleasance E, et al: Mutational and structural analysis of diffuse large B-cell lymphoma using whole-genome sequencing. *Blood* 122:7, 2013.

22. Davis RE, Ngo VN, Lenz G, et al: Chronic active B-cell-receptor signalling in diffuse large B-cell lymphoma. *Nature* 463:7277, 2010.

23. Ngo VN, Young RM, Schmitz R, et al: Oncogenically active MYD88 mutations in human lymphoma. *Nature* 470:7332, 2011.

24. Aviles A, Neri N, Huerta-Guzman J: Large bowel lymphoma: An analysis of prognostic factors and therapy in 53 patients. *J Surg Oncol* 80:2, 2002.

25. Paryani S, Hoppe RT, Burke JS, et al: Extralymphatic involvement in diffuse non-Hodgkin's lymphoma. *J Clin Oncol* 1:11, 1983.

26. van Besien K, Ha CS, Murphy S, et al: Risk factors, treatment, and outcome of central nervous system recurrence in adults with intermediate-grade and immunoblastic lymphoma. *Blood* 91:4, 1998.

27. Doggett RS, Wood GS, Horning S, et al: The immunologic characterization of 95 nodal and extranodal diffuse large cell lymphomas in 89 patients. *Am J Pathol* 115:2, 1984.

28. Stein H, Lennert K, Feller AC, Mason DY: Immunohistological analysis of human lymphoma: Correlation of histological and immunological categories. *Adv Cancer Res* 42:67, 1984.

29. Yamaguchi M, Seto M, Okamoto M, et al: *De novo* CD5+ diffuse large B-cell lymphoma: A clinicopathologic study of 109 patients. *Blood* 99:3, 2002.

30. Craig FE, Foon KA: Flow cytometric immunophenotyping for hematologic neoplasms. *Blood* 111:8, 2008.

31. Stauder R, Eisterer W, Thaler J, Gunthert U: CD44 variant isoforms in non-Hodgkin's lymphoma: A new independent prognostic factor. *Blood* 85:10, 1995.

32. Ottensmeier CH, Stevenson FK: Isotype switch variants reveal clonally related subpopulations in diffuse large B-cell lymphoma. *Blood* 96:7, 2000.

33. Cheson B, Pfistner B, Gascoyne R: Revised response criteria for malignant lymphoma. *J Clin Oncol* 25:5, 2007.

34. Chen MG, Prosnitz LR, Gonzalez-Serva A, Fischer DB: Results of radiotherapy in control of stage I and II non-Hodgkin's lymphoma. *Cancer* 43:4, 1979.

35. Jones SE, Miller TP, Connors JM: Long-term follow-up and analysis for prognostic factors for patients with limited-stage diffuse large-cell lymphoma treated with initial chemotherapy with or without adjuvant radiotherapy. *J Clin Oncol* 7:9, 1989.

36. Longo DL, Glatstein E, Duffey PL, et al: Treatment of localized aggressive lymphomas with combination chemotherapy followed by involved-field radiation therapy. *J Clin Oncol* 7:9, 1989.

37. Monfardini S, Banfi A, Bonadonna G, et al: Improved five year survival after combined radiotherapy-chemotherapy for stage I-II non-Hodgkin's lymphoma. *Int J Radiat Oncol Biol Phys* 6:2, 1980.

38. Nissen NI, Ersboll J, Hansen HS, et al: A randomized study of radiotherapy versus radiotherapy plus chemotherapy in stage I-II non-Hodgkin's lymphomas. *Cancer* 52:1, 1983.

39. Tondini C, Zanini M, Lombardi F, et al: Combined modality treatment with primary CHOP chemotherapy followed by locoregional irradiation in stage I or II histologically aggressive non-Hodgkin's lymphomas. *J Clin Oncol* 11:4, 1993.

40. Vokes EE, Ultmann JE, Golomb HM, et al: Long-term survival of patients with localized diffuse histiocytic lymphoma. *J Clin Oncol* 3:10, 1985.

41. Miller TP, Dahlberg S, Cassady JR, et al: Chemotherapy alone compared with chemotherapy plus radiotherapy for localized intermediate- and high-grade non-Hodgkin's lymphoma. *N Engl J Med* 339:1, 1998.

42. Miller TP, Leblanc M, Spier C, et al: CHOP alone compared to CHOP plus radiotherapy for early stage aggressive non-Hodgkin's lymphomas: Update of the Southwest Oncology Group (SWOG) randomized trial. *Blood* 98:11, 2001.

43. Horning SJ, Weller E, Kim K, et al: Chemotherapy with or without radiotherapy in limited-stage diffuse aggressive non-Hodgkin's lymphoma: Eastern Cooperative Oncology Group study 1484. *J Clin Oncol* 22:15, 2004.

44. Bonnet C, Fillet G, Mounier N, et al: CHOP alone compared with CHOP plus radiotherapy for localized aggressive lymphoma in elderly patients: A study by the Groupe d'Etude des Lymphomes de l'Adulte. *J Clin Oncol* 25:7, 2007.

45. Reyes F, Lepage E, Ganem G, et al: ACVBP versus CHOP plus radiotherapy for localized aggressive lymphoma. *N Engl J Med* 352:12, 2005.

46. Persky DO, Unger JM, Spier CM, et al: Phase II study of rituximab plus three cycles of CHOP and involved-field radiotherapy for patients with limited-stage aggressive B-cell lymphoma: Southwest Oncology Group study 0014. *J Clin Oncol* 26:14, 2008.

47. Phan J, Mazloom A, Medeiros L, et al: Benefit of consolidative radiation therapy in patients with diffuse large B-cell lymphoma treated with R-CHOP chemotherapy. *J Clin Oncol* 28:27, 2010.

48. Held G, Murawski N, Ziepert M, et al: Role of radiotherapy to bulky disease in elderly patients with aggressive B-cell lymphoma. *J Clin Oncol* 31:15, 2014.

49. DeVita VT Jr, Canellos GP, Chabner B, et al: Advanced diffuse histiocytic lymphoma, a potentially curable disease. *Lancet* 1:7901, 1975.

50. Gaynor ER, Ultmann JE, Golomb HM, Sweet DL: Treatment of diffuse histiocytic lymphoma (DHL) with COMLA (cyclophosphamide, Oncovin, methotrexate, leucovorin, cytosine arabinoside): A 10-year experience in a single institution. *J Clin Oncol* 3:12, 1985.

51. Schein PS, DeVita VT Jr, Hubbard S, et al: Bleomycin, Adriamycin, cyclophosphamide, vincristine, and prednisone (BACOP) combination chemotherapy in the treatment of advanced diffuse histiocytic lymphoma. *Ann Intern Med* 85:4, 1976.

52. Fisher RI, DeVita VT Jr, Hubbard SM, et al: Diffuse aggressive lymphomas: Increased survival after alternating flexible sequences of proMACE and MOPP chemotherapy. *Ann Intern Med* 98:3, 1983.

53. Gordon LI, Harrington D, Andersen J, et al: Comparison of a second-generation combination chemotherapeutic regimen (m-BACOD) with a standard regimen (CHOP) for advanced diffuse non-Hodgkin's lymphoma. *N Engl J Med* 327:19, 1992.

54. Fisher RI, Gaynor ER, Dahlberg S, et al: Comparison of a standard regimen (CHOP) with three intensive chemotherapy regimens for advanced non-Hodgkin's lymphoma. *N Engl J Med* 328:14, 1993.

55. Coiffier B, Lepage E, Briere J, et al: CHOP chemotherapy plus rituximab compared with CHOP alone in elderly patients with diffuse large-B-cell lymphoma. *N Engl J Med* 346:4, 2002.

56. Feugier P, Van Hoof A, Sebban C, et al: Long-term results of the R-CHOP study in the treatment of elderly patients with diffuse large B-cell lymphoma: A study by the Groupe d'Etude des Lymphomes de l'Adulte. *J Clin Oncol* 23:18, 2005.

57. Habermann TM, Weller EA, Morrison VA, et al: Rituximab-CHOP versus CHOP alone or with maintenance rituximab in older patients with diffuse large B-cell lymphoma. *J Clin Oncol* 24:19, 2006.

58. Pfreundschuh M, Schubert J, Ziepert M, et al: Six versus eight cycles of bi-weekly CHOP-14 with or without rituximab in elderly patients with aggressive CD20+ B-cell lymphomas: A randomised controlled trial (RICOVER-60). *Lancet Oncol* 9:2, 2008.

59. Pfreundschuh M, Trumper L, Osterborg A, et al: CHOP-like chemotherapy plus rituximab versus CHOP-like chemotherapy alone in young patients with good-prognosis diffuse large-B-cell lymphoma: A randomised controlled trial by the MabThera International Trial (MInT) Group. *Lancet Oncol* 7:5, 2006.

60. Cunningham D, Hawkes E, Jack A, et al: Rituximab plus cyclophosphamide, doxorubicin, vincristine, and prednisolone in patients with newly diagnosed diffuse large B-cell non-Hodgkin lymphoma: A phase 3 comparison of dose intensification with 14-day versus 21-day cycles. *Lancet* 381:9880, 2013.

61. Delarue R, Tilly H, Mounier N, et al: Dose-dense rituximab-CHOP compared with standard rituximab-CHOP in elderly patients with diffuse large B-cell lymphoma (the LNH03-6B study): a randomised phase 3 trial. *Lancet Oncol* 14:6, 2013.

62. Recher C, Coiffier B, Haioun C, et al: Intensified chemotherapy with ACVBP plus rituximab versus standard CHOP plus rituximab for the treatment of diffuse large B-cell lymphoma (LNH03-2B): An open-label randomised phase 3 trial. *Lancet* 378:9806, 2011.

63. Lai GM, Chen YN, Mickley LA, et al: P-glycoprotein expression and schedule dependence of Adriamycin cytotoxicity in human colon carcinoma cell lines. *Int J Cancer* 49:5, 1991.

64. Gutierrez M, Chabner BA, Pearson D, et al: Role of a doxorubicin-containing regimen in relapsed and resistant lymphomas: An 8-year follow-up study of EPOCH. *J Clin Oncol* 18:21, 2000.

65. Wilson WH, Bates SE, Fojo A, et al: Controlled trial of dexverapamil, a modulator of multidrug resistance, in lymphomas refractory to EPOCH chemotherapy. *J Clin Oncol* 13:8, 1995.

66. Wilson WH, Grossbard ML, Pittaluga S, et al: Dose-adjusted EPOCH chemotherapy for untreated large B-cell lymphomas: A pharmacodynamic approach with high efficacy. *Blood* 99:8, 2002.

67. Wilson WH, Dunleavy K, Pittaluga S, et al: Phase II study of dose-adjusted EPOCH and rituximab in untreated diffuse large B-cell lymphoma with analysis of germinal center and post-germinal center biomarkers. *J Clin Oncol* 26:16, 2008.

68. U.S. National Library of Medicine. ClinicalTrials.gov [online] 2014. Available from: http://clinicaltrials.gov/show/NCT00118209.

69. Haioun C, Lepage E, Gisselbrecht C, et al: Benefit of autologous bone marrow transplantation over sequential chemotherapy in poor-risk aggressive non-Hodgkin's lymphoma: Updated results of the prospective study LNH87–2. Groupe d'Etude des Lymphomes de l'Adulte. *J Clin Oncol* 15:3, 1997.

70. Kluin-Nelemans HC, Zagonel V, Anastasopoulou A, et al: Standard chemotherapy with or without high-dose chemotherapy for aggressive non-Hodgkin's lymphoma: Randomized phase III EORTC study. *J Natl Cancer Inst* 93:1, 2001.

71. Santini G, Salvagno L, Leoni P, et al: VACOP-B versus VACOP-B plus autologous bone marrow transplantation for advanced diffuse non-Hodgkin's lymphoma: Results of a prospective randomized trial by the non-Hodgkin's Lymphoma Cooperative Study Group. *J Clin Oncol* 16:8, 1998.

72. Verdonck LF, van Putten WL, Hagenbeek A, et al: Comparison of CHOP chemotherapy with autologous bone marrow transplantation for slowly responding patients with aggressive non-Hodgkin's lymphoma. *N Engl J Med* 332:16, 1995.

73. Gisselbrecht C, Lepage E, Molina T, et al: Shortened first-line high-dose chemotherapy for patients with poor-prognosis aggressive lymphoma. *J Clin Oncol* 20:10, 2002.

74. Haioun C, Lepage E, Gisselbrecht C, et al: Survival benefit of high-dose therapy in poor-risk aggressive non-Hodgkin's lymphoma: Final analysis of the prospective LNH87–2 protocol—A Groupe d'Etude des lymphomes de l'Adulte study. *J Clin Oncol* 18:16, 2000.

75. Kaiser U, Uebelacker I, Abel U, et al: Randomized study to evaluate the use of high-dose therapy as part of primary treatment for "aggressive" lymphoma. *J Clin Oncol* 20:22, 2002.

76. Stiff P, Unger J, Cook J, et al: Autologous transplantation as consolidation for aggressive non-Hodgkin's lymphoma. *N Engl J Med* 369:18, 2013.

77. Greb A, Bohlius J, Schiefer D, et al: High-dose chemotherapy with autologous stem cell transplantation in the first line treatment of aggressive non-Hodgkin lymphoma (NHL) in adults. *Cochrane Database Syst Rev* 1:CD004024, 2008.

78. Maurer M, Ghesquieres H, Jais J: Event-free survival at 24 months is a robust end point for disease-related outcome in diffuse large B-cell lymphoma treated with immunochemotherapy. *J Clin Oncol* 32:10, 2014.

79. Schmoll H: Review of etoposide single-agent activity. *Cancer Treat Rev* 9 Suppl:21, 1982.

80. Shipp MA, Takvorian RC, Canellos GP: High-dose cytosine arabinoside. Active agent in treatment of non-Hodgkin's lymphoma. *Am J Med* 77:5, 1984.

81. Bajetta E, Buzzoni R, Valagussa P, Bonadonna G: Mitoxantrone: An active agent in refractory non-Hodgkin's lymphomas. *Am J Clin Oncol* 11:2, 1988.

82. Wiernik PH, Lossos IS, Tuscano JM, et al: Lenalidomide monotherapy in relapsed or refractory aggressive non-Hodgkin's lymphoma. *J Clin Oncol* 26:30, 2008.

83. Rizzieri DA, Sand GJ, McGaughey D, et al: Low-dose weekly paclitaxel for recurrent or refractory aggressive non-Hodgkin lymphoma. *Cancer* 100:11, 2004.

84. Kewalramani T, Zelenetz AD, Nimer SD, et al: Rituximab and ICE as second-line therapy before autologous stem cell transplantation for relapsed or primary refractory diffuse large B-cell lymphoma. *Blood* 103:10, 2004.

85. Velasquez WS, McLaughlin P, Tucker S, et al: ESHAP—An effective chemotherapy regimen in refractory and relapsing lymphoma: A 4-year follow-up study. *J Clin Oncol* 12:6, 1994.

86. Gisselbrecht C, Glass B, Mounier N, et al: Salvage regimens with autologous transplantation for relapsed large B-cell lymphoma in the rituximab era. *J Clin Oncol* 28:27, 2010.

87. Philip T, Guglielmi C, Hagenbeek A, et al: Autologous bone marrow transplantation as compared with salvage chemotherapy in relapses of chemotherapy-sensitive non-Hodgkin's lymphoma. *N Engl J Med* 333:23, 1995.

88. Chopra R, Goldstone AH, Pearce R, et al: Autologous versus allogeneic bone marrow transplantation for non-Hodgkin's lymphoma: A case-controlled analysis of the European Bone Marrow Transplant Group Registry data. *J Clin Oncol* 10:11, 1992.

89. Rezvani AR, Norasetthada L, Gooley T, et al: Non-myeloablative allogeneic haematopoietic cell transplantation for relapsed diffuse large B-cell lymphoma: A multicentre experience. *Br J Haematol* 143:3, 2008.

90. Thomson KJ, Morris EC, Bloor A, et al: Favorable long-term survival after reduced-intensity allogeneic transplantation for multiple-relapse aggressive non-Hodgkin's lymphoma. *J Clin Oncol* 27:3, 2009.

91. Krishnan A, Nademanee A, Fung HC, et al: Phase II trial of a transplantation regimen of yttrium-90 ibritumomab tiuxetan and high-dose chemotherapy in patients with non-Hodgkin's lymphoma. *J Clin Oncol* 26:1, 2008.

92. Vose JM, Bierman PJ, Enke C, et al: Phase I trial of iodine-131 tositumomab with high-dose chemotherapy and autologous stem-cell transplantation for relapsed non-Hodgkin's lymphoma. *J Clin Oncol* 23:3, 2005.

93. A predictive model for aggressive non-Hodgkin's lymphoma. The International Non-Hodgkin's Lymphoma Prognostic Factors Project. *N Engl J Med* 329:14, 1993.

94. A clinical evaluation of the International Lymphoma Study Group classification of non-Hodgkin's lymphoma. The Non-Hodgkin's Lymphoma Classification Project. *Blood* 89:11, 1997.

95. Zhou Z, Sehn L, Rademaker A, et al: An enhanced international prognostic index (NCCN-IPI) for patients with diffuse large B-cell lymphoma treated in the rituximab era. *Blood* 123:6, 2014.

96. Hans CP, Weisenburger DD, Greiner TC, et al: Confirmation of the molecular classification of diffuse large B-cell lymphoma by immunohistochemistry using a tissue microarray. *Blood* 103:1, 2004.

97. Shipp MA, Ross KN, Tamayo P, et al: Diffuse large B-cell lymphoma outcome prediction by gene-expression profiling and supervised machine learning. *Nat Med* 8:1, 2002.

98. Lossos IS, Czerwinski DK, Alizadeh AA, et al: Prediction of survival in diffuse large-B-cell lymphoma based on the expression of six genes. *N Engl J Med* 350:18, 2004.

99. Swan F Jr, Velasquez WS, Tucker S, et al: A new serologic staging system for large-cell lymphomas based on initial beta 2-microglobulin and lactate dehydrogenase levels. *J Clin Oncol* 7:10, 1989.

100. Savage K, Johnson N, Ben-Neriah S, et al: MYC gene rearrangements are associated with a poor prognosis in diffuse large B-cell lymphoma patients treated with R-CHOP chemotherapy. *Blood* 114:17, 2009.

101. Kluk M, Chapuy B, Sinha P, et al: Immunohistochemical detection of MYC-driven diffuse large B-cell lymphomas. *PloS One* 7:4, 2012.

102. Johnson N, Slack G, Savage K, et al: Concurrent expression of MYC and BCL2 in diffuse large B-cell lymphoma treated with rituximab plus cyclophosphamide, doxorubicin, vincristine, and prednisone. *J Clin Oncol* 30:28, 2013.

103. Buchmann I, Reinhardt M, Elsner K, et al: 2-(fluorine-18)fluoro-2-deoxy-D-glucose positron emission tomography in the detection and staging of malignant lymphoma. A bicenter trial. *Cancer* 91:5, 2001.

104. Spaepen K, Stroobants S, Dupont P, et al: Prognostic value of positron emission tomography (PET) with fluorine-18 fluorodeoxyglucose ([18F]FDG) after first-line chemotherapy in non-Hodgkin's lymphoma: Is [18F]FDG-PET a valid alternative to conventional diagnostic methods? *J Clin Oncol* 19:2, 2001.

105. Zucca E, Conconi A, Mughal TI, et al: Patterns of outcome and prognostic factors in primary large-cell lymphoma of the testis in a survey by the International Extranodal Lymphoma Study Group. *J Clin Oncol* 21:1, 2003.

106. Gundrum JD, Mathiason MA, Derek BM, et al: Primary testicular diffuse large B-cell lymphoma: A population-based study on the incidence, natural history, and survival comparison with primary nodal counterpart before and after the introduction of rituximab. *J Clin Oncol* 27:5227, 2009.

107. Pingali S, Go RS, Gundrum JD, et al: Adult testicular lymphoma in the United States (1985–2004): Analysis of 3,669 cases from the National Cancer Data Base (NCDB). *J Clin Oncol* 26(15S):19503, 2008.

108. Fonseca R, Habermann TM, Colgan JP, et al: Testicular lymphoma is associated with a high incidence of extranodal recurrence. *Cancer* 88:1, 2000.

109. Visco C, Medeiros LJ, Mesina OM, et al: Non-Hodgkin's lymphoma affecting the testis: Is it curable with doxorubicin-based therapy? *Clin Lymphoma* 2:1, 2001.

110. Pentheroudakis G, Pavlidis N: Cancer and pregnancy: Poena magna, not anymore. *Eur J Cancer* 42:2, 2006.

111. Pereg D, Koren G, Lishner M: Cancer in pregnancy: Gaps, challenges and solutions. *Cancer Treat Rev* 34:4, 2008.

112. Pereg D, Koren G, Lishner M: The treatment of Hodgkin's and non-Hodgkin's lymphoma in pregnancy. *Haematologica* 92:9, 2007.

113. Aviles A, Diaz-Maqueo JC, Torras V, et al: Non-Hodgkin's lymphomas and pregnancy: Presentation of 16 cases. *Gynecol Oncol* 37:3, 1990.

114. Evens AM, Advani R, Press OW, et al: Lymphoma occurring during pregnancy: Antenatal therapy, complications, and maternal survival in a multicenter analysis. *J Clin Oncol* 31:32, 2013.

115. Resnik R: Cancer during pregnancy. *N Engl J Med* 341:2, 1999.

116. van Besien K, Kelta M, Bahaguna P: Primary mediastinal B-cell lymphoma: A review of pathology and management. *J Clin Oncol* 19:6, 2001.

117. Savage KJ, Monti S, Kutok JL, et al: The molecular signature of mediastinal large B-cell lymphoma differs from that of other diffuse large B-cell lymphomas and shares features with classical Hodgkin lymphoma. *Blood* 102:12, 2003.

118. Perrone T, Frizzera G, Rosai J: Mediastinal diffuse large-cell lymphoma with sclerosis. A clinicopathologic study of 60 cases. *Am J Surg Pathol* 10:3, 1986.

119. Zinzani PL, Martelli M, Bertini M, et al: Induction chemotherapy strategies for primary mediastinal large B-cell lymphoma with sclerosis: A retrospective multinational study on 426 previously untreated patients. *Haematologica* 87:12, 2002.

120. Todeschini G, Secchi S, Morra E, et al: Primary mediastinal large B-cell lymphoma (PMLBCL): Long-term results from a retrospective multicentre Italian experience in 138 patients treated with CHOP or MACOP-B/VACOP-B: *Br J Cancer* 90:2, 2004.

121. Dunleavy K, Pittaluga S, Maeda L, et al: Dose-adjusted EPOCH-rituximab therapy in primary mediastinal B-cell lymphoma. *N Engl J Med* 368:15, 2013.

122. Katzenstein AL, Carrington CB, Liebow AA: Lymphomatoid granulomatosis: A clinicopathologic study of 152 cases. *Cancer* 43:1, 1979.

123. Gitelson E, Al-Saleem T, Smith MR: Review: Lymphomatoid granulomatosis: Challenges in diagnosis and treatment. *Clin Adv Hematol Oncol* 7:1, 2009.

124. Dunleavy K, Janik J, Cohen J, et al: 16. Clinical-pathological correlations: 079 Study of the treatment and biology of lymphomatoid granulomatosis (LYG); a rare EBV lymphoproliferative disorder. *Ann Oncol* 16:v59, 2005.

125. Ferreri AJ, Campo E, Seymour JF, et al: Intravascular lymphoma: Clinical presentation, natural history, management and prognostic factors in a series of 38 cases, with special emphasis on the "cutaneous variant." *Br J Haematol* 127:2, 2004.

126. Ferreri AJ, Dognini GP, Campo E, et al: Variations in clinical presentation, frequency of hemophagocytosis and clinical behavior of intravascular lymphoma diagnosed in different geographical regions. *Haematologica* 92:4, 2007.

127. Murase T, Nakamura S: An Asian variant of intravascular lymphomatosis: An updated review of malignant histiocytosis-like B-cell lymphoma. *Leuk Lymphoma* 33:5, 1999.

128. Murase T, Nakamura S, Kawauchi K, et al: An Asian variant of intravascular large B-cell lymphoma: Clinical, pathological and cytogenetic approaches to diffuse large B-cell lymphoma associated with haemophagocytic syndrome. *Br J Haematol* 111:3, 2000.

129. Shimazaki C, Inaba T, Nakagawa M: B-cell lymphoma-associated hemophagocytic syndrome. *Leuk Lymphoma* 38:1, 2000.

130. Ponzoni M, Ferreri AJ, Campo E, et al: Definition, diagnosis, and management of intravascular large B-cell lymphoma: Proposals and perspectives from an international consensus meeting. *J Clin Oncol* 25:21, 2007.

131. Ferreri AJ, Dognini GP, Govi S, et al: Can rituximab change the usually dismal prognosis of patients with intravascular large B-cell lymphoma? *J Clin Oncol* 26:31, 2008.

132. Shimada K, Matsue K, Yamamoto K, et al: Retrospective analysis of intravascular large B-cell lymphoma treated with rituximab-containing chemotherapy as reported by the IVL study group in Japan. *J Clin Oncol* 26:19, 2008.

133. Oton AB, Wang H, Leleu X, et al: Clinical and pathological prognostic markers for survival in adult patients with post-transplant lymphoproliferative disorders in solid transplant. *Leuk Lymphoma* 49:9, 2008.

134. Adami J, Gabel H, Lindelof B, et al: Cancer risk following organ transplantation: A nationwide cohort study in Sweden. *Br J Cancer* 89:7, 2003.

135. Tsao L, Hsi ED: The clinicopathologic spectrum of posttransplantation lymphoproliferative disorders. *Arch Pathol Lab Med* 131:8, 2007.

136. Cockfield SM, Preiksaitis JK, Jewell LD, Parfrey NA: Post-transplant lymphoproliferative disorder in renal allograft recipients. Clinical experience and risk factor analysis in a single center. *Transplantation* 56:1, 1993.

137. Swinnen LJ, Costanzo-Nordin MR, Fisher SG, et al: Increased incidence of lymphoproliferative disorder after immunosuppression with the monoclonal antibody OKT3 in cardiac-transplant recipients. *N Engl J Med* 323:25, 1990.

138. Walker RC, Paya CV, Marshall WF, et al: Pretransplantation seronegative Epstein-Barr virus status is the primary risk factor for posttransplantation lymphoproliferative disorder in adult heart, lung, and other solid organ transplantations. *J Heart Lung Transplant* 14:2, 1995.

139. Hanto DW: Classification of Epstein-Barr virus-associated posttransplant lymphoproliferative diseases: Implications for understanding their pathogenesis and developing rational treatment strategies. *Annu Rev Med* 46:381, 1995.

140. Leblond V, Davi F, Charlotte F, et al: Posttransplant lymphoproliferative disorders not associated with Epstein-Barr virus: A distinct entity? *J Clin Oncol* 16:6, 1998.

141. Kew CE 2nd, Lopez-Ben R, Smith JK, et al: Posttransplant lymphoproliferative disorder localized near the allograft in renal transplantation. *Transplantation* 69:5, 2000.

142. Rees L, Thomas A, Amlot PL: Disappearance of an Epstein-Barr virus-positive posttransplant plasmacytoma with reduction of immunosuppression. *Lancet* 352:9130, 1998.

143. Tsai DE, Hardy CL, Tomaszewski JE, et al: Reduction in immunosuppression as initial therapy for posttransplant lymphoproliferative disorder: Analysis of prognostic variables and long-term follow-up of 42 adult patients. *Transplantation* 71:8, 2001.

144. Choquet S, Leblond V, Herbrecht R, et al: Efficacy and safety of rituximab in B-cell post-transplantation lymphoproliferative disorders: Results of a prospective multicenter phase 2 study. *Blood* 107:8, 2006.

145. Trappe R, Riess H, Babel N, et al: Salvage chemotherapy for refractory and relapsed posttransplant lymphoproliferative disorders (PTLD) after treatment with single-agent rituximab. *Transplantation* 83:7, 2007.

146. Swinnen LJ, LeBlanc M, Grogan TM, et al: Prospective study of sequential reduction in immunosuppression, interferon alpha-2B, and chemotherapy for posttransplantation lymphoproliferative disorder. *Transplantation* 86:2, 2008.

147. Achten R, Verhoef G, Vanuytsel L, De Wolf-Peeters C: T-cell/histiocyte-rich large B-cell lymphoma: A distinct clinicopathologic entity. *J Clin Oncol* 20:5, 2002.

148. Abramson JS: T-cell/histiocyte-rich B-cell lymphoma: Biology, diagnosis, and management. *Oncologist* 11:4, 2006.

149. Aki H, Tuzuner N, Ongoren S, et al: T-cell-rich B-cell lymphoma: A clinicopathologic study of 21 cases and comparison with 43 cases of diffuse large B-cell lymphoma. *Leuk Res* 28:3, 2004.

150. Bouabdallah R, Mounier N, Guettier C, et al: T-cell/histiocyte-rich large B-cell lymphomas and classical diffuse large B-cell lymphomas have similar outcome after chemotherapy: A matched-control analysis. *J Clin Oncol* 21:7, 2003.

151. Boudova L, Torlakovic E, Delabie J, et al: Nodular lymphocyte-predominant Hodgkin lymphoma with nodules resembling T-cell/histiocyte-rich B-cell lymphoma: Differential diagnosis between nodular lymphocyte-predominant Hodgkin lymphoma and T-cell/histiocyte-rich B-cell lymphoma. *Blood* 102:10, 2003.

152. Greer JP, Macon WR, Lamar RE, et al: T-cell-rich B-cell lymphomas: Diagnosis and response to therapy of 44 patients. *J Clin Oncol* 13:7, 1995.

153. McBride JA, Rodriguez J, Luthra R, et al: T-cell-rich B large-cell lymphoma simulating lymphocyte-rich Hodgkin's disease. *Am J Surg Pathol* 20:2, 1996.

154. Rodriguez J, Pugh WC, Cabanillas F: T-cell-rich B-cell lymphoma. *Blood* 82:5, 1993.

155. Willemze R, Jaffe ES, Burg G, et al: WHO-EORTC classification for cutaneous lymphomas. *Blood* 105:10, 2005.

156. Grange F, Beylot-Barry M, Courville P, et al: Primary cutaneous diffuse large B-cell lymphoma, leg type: Clinicopathologic features and prognostic analysis in 60 cases. *Arch Dermatol* 143:9, 2007.

157. Grange F, Maubec E, Bagot M, et al: Treatment of cutaneous B-cell lymphoma, leg type, with age-adapted combinations of chemotherapies and rituximab. *Arch Dermatol* 145:3, 2009.

158. Kodama K, Massone C, Chott A, et al: Primary cutaneous large B-cell lymphomas: Clinicopathologic features, classification, and prognostic factors in a large series of patients. *Blood* 106:7, 2005.

159. Beltran B, Castillo J, Salas R, et al: ALK-positive diffuse large B-cell lymphoma: Report of four cases and review of the literature. *J Hematol Oncol* 2:11, 2009.

160. Reichard KK, McKenna RW, Kroft SH: ALK-positive diffuse large B-cell lymphoma: Report of four cases and review of the literature. *Mod Pathol* 20:3, 2007.

CHAPTER 99
FOLLICULAR LYMPHOMA

Oliver W. Press

SUMMARY

Follicular Lymphoma (FL) is an indolent, neoplastic disorder of germinal center-derived B lymphocytes that afflicts approximately 14,000 people in the United States each year. It typically presents as a disseminated disorder with painless, diffuse lymphadenopathy and marrow infiltration, and may be associated with hepatosplenomegaly and circulating lymphoma cells in the blood. A characteristic translocation, t(14;18), is found in the cells of 85 percent of patients, which deregulates BCL2 protein expression and inhibits apoptosis of affected B cells. The cells typically express monoclonal surface immunoglobulin, CD10, CD19, CD20, CD22, CD45, and CD79a on their cell surface, but not CD5 or CD23. Patients are often asymptomatic at the time of presentation, and may live for many years in good health without therapy. On the other hand, most patients eventually develop progressive lymphadenopathy, causing symptoms mandating intervention. Many treatment regimens are effective at inducing remissions, including single-agent rituximab or chlorambucil; or several multidrug programs, including bendamustine plus rituximab (BR), rituximab, cyclophosphamide, vincristine, and prednisone (R-CVP); rituximab, cyclophosphamide, doxorubicin, vincristine, and prednisone (R-CHOP). None of these therapies, however, is considered curative and most patients eventually relapse with recurrent disease. Autologous and allogeneic hematopoietic cell transplantation (HCT) can induce prolonged remissions in many patients with relapsed FL, but the role of HCT in this disease is controversial. Histologic transformation to aggressive lymphoma occurs in 30 to 40 percent of patients, usually leading to death within a few years of transformation.

DEFINITION AND HISTORY

Follicular lymphoma (FL) is an indolent lymphoid neoplasm that is derived from mutated germinal center B cells and exhibits a nodular or follicular histologic pattern. It is typically composed of a mixture of small, cleaved follicle center cells (centrocytes) and large noncleaved follicle center cells (centroblasts). The disease has masqueraded under multiple monikers, including "nodular lymphoma" in the Rappaport classification, and "follicle center cell lymphoma" in the Working Formulation.[1] The current World Health Organization (WHO) classification proposes the terms *follicular lymphoma, grades 1, 2, and 3*, to differentiate cases based on the numbers of centroblasts per high-power microscopic field (see "Lymph Node Morphology and Lymphocyte Immunophenotype" below).[2]

EPIDEMIOLOGY

FL accounts for approximately 20 to 25 percent of adult non-Hodgkin lymphomas (NHLs) in the United States, with an annual incidence of approximately 14,000 new cases per year.[3,4] FL is most common in North America and Western Europe, and much less frequent in Eastern Europe, Asia, Africa, and in Americans of African descent.[2] The median age at diagnosis is 59 years, and the male-to-female ratio is 1:1.7. The disease is rare in persons younger than age 20 years, and pediatric cases appear to represent a separate disease entity that is typically localized, lacks the t(14;18) translocation and BCL2 expression, and has a very good prognosis.[5,6]

CLINICAL FEATURES

SYMPTOMS AND SIGNS

Patients with FL usually present with painless diffuse lymphadenopathy. Less frequently, patients may have vague abdominal complaints, including pain, early satiety, and increasing girth, which may be caused by a large abdominal mass or hepatosplenomegaly. Approximately 10 percent of patients present with B symptoms (fever, drenching night sweats, or loss of 10 percent of body weight). The disease usually is widespread at presentation, with involvement of multiple lymph node–bearing sites, liver, and spleen. The marrow is involved in 40 to 70 percent of patients at diagnosis. FL may occasionally present with primary involvement of extranodal sites, such as the skin, gastrointestinal tract, ocular adnexa, and breast, but CNS disease is rare, unless histologic transformation to diffuse large B-cell lymphoma has occurred.[2]

LABORATORY FEATURES

LYMPH NODE MORPHOLOGY AND LYMPHOCYTE IMMUNOPHENOTYPE

FL exhibits a predominantly nodular lymph node pattern, however, the neoplastic follicles are distorted and as the disease progresses, the malignant follicles efface the nodal architecture (see Chap. 96, Fig. 96–18), commonly resulting in the development of areas of diffuse involvement, which may predominate histologically. The WHO has developed a three-grade system for classifying FL according to the proportion of centroblasts detected microscopically: grade 1 lymphomas have 0 to 5 centroblasts, grade 2 lymphomas have 6 to 15 centroblasts, and grade 3 lymphomas have more than 15 centroblasts per high-power microscopic field (Fig. 99–1).[2] Grade 3 FL is further subdivided into grade 3A, in which some small centrocytes are present despite the predominance of centroblasts, and grade 3B, in which solid sheets of centroblasts are exclusively present and centrocytes are entirely absent.[2] Some, but not all, studies suggest that grades 1 and 2 lymphomas follow a more indolent course than grade 3 FL, and many authorities suggest that these lower grades should be treated more conservatively than grade 3 FL.[7] Other studies indicate a similar natural history for grades 1, 2, and 3A.[8]

Acronyms and Abbreviations: ADCC, antibody-dependent cellular cytotoxicity; BR, bendamustine and rituximab; CDC, complement-dependent cytotoxicity; CHOP, cyclophosphamide, doxorubicin, vincristine, prednisone; CR, complete response; CVP, cyclophosphamide, vincristine, prednisone; FCM, fludarabine, cyclophosphamide, mitoxantrone; FDG, fluoro-2-deoxyglucose; FL, follicular lymphoma; FND, fludarabine, mitoxantrone (Novantrone), dexamethasone; GELF, Groupe d'Etudes des Lymphomes Folliculaires; Gy, gray; HLA, histocompatibility locus antigen; IFN, interferon; IPI, international prognostic index; KLH, keyhole limpet hemocyanin; LDH, lactate dehydrogenase; NHL, non-Hodgkin lymphoma; ORR, overall response rate; OS, overall survival; PCR, polymerase chain reaction; PET, positron emission tomography; PFS, progression-free survival; PR, partial remission; ProMACE/MOPP, prednisone, methotrexate, doxorubicin, cyclophosphamide, etoposide, mechlorethamine, vincristine, procarbazine, prednisone; R-CHOP, rituximab plus CHOP; R-CVP, rituximab plus CVP; RIT, radioimmunotherapy; WHO, World Health Organization.

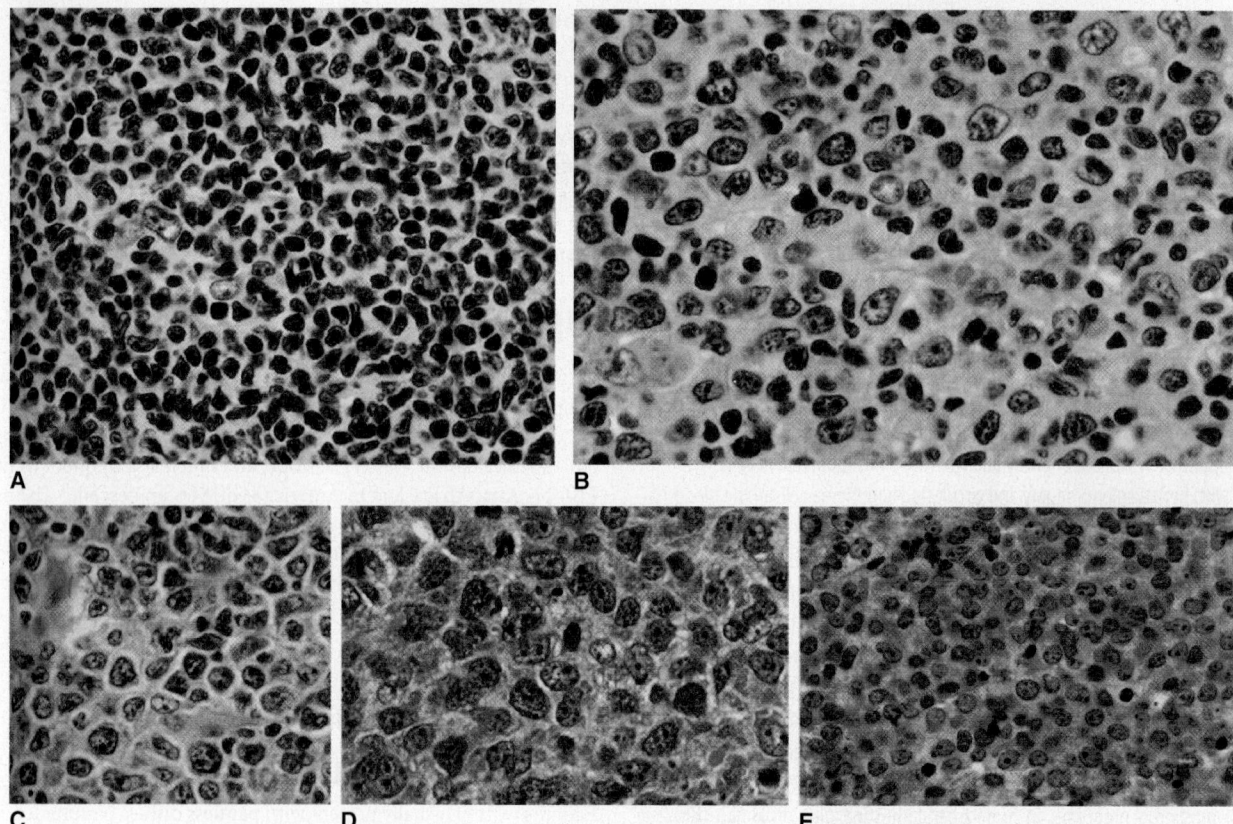

Figure 99–1. Follicular lymphoma grading is based on the relative proportions of small cells (centrocytes) and centroblasts (centroblasts). **A.** Grade 1 (0–5 centroblasts/high-powered field). **B.** Grade 2 (6–15 centroblasts/high-powered field). **C.** Grade 3A (>15 centroblasts/high-powered field). **D** and **E.** Grade 3B. See text for further definitions of grades 1, 2, 3A, and 3B. (*Reproduced with permission from Harris NL, Swerdlow SH, Jaffe ES, et al: Follicular Lymphoma, in WHO Classification of Tumours of Haematopoietic and Lymphoid Tissues, edited by Swerdlow SH, Campo E, Harris NL, et al: p 220–226. International Agency for Research on Cancer, Lyon, 2008.*)

Nearly all authorities now agree, however, that grade 3B FL behaves aggressively and should be treated with anthracycline-containing regimens (e.g., rituximab, cyclophosphamide, doxorubicin, vincristine, prednisone [R-CHOP]) similar to diffuse large B-cell lymphoma.[2] FL cells of all grades typically express monoclonal surface immunoglobulin, are positive for *BCL*-2, *BCL6*, and CD10, and express the pan–B-cell surface antigens CD19, CD20, CD22, and CD79a, but do not express CD5, CD23, CD11c, or CD43.

CYTOGENETICS

The classic cytogenetic finding detected in FL is the t(14;18)(q32;q21) translocation that juxtaposes the *BCL*-2 gene on band q21 of chromosome 18 with the immunoglobulin heavy-chain gene on band 32 of chromosome 14 (Fig. 99–2).[9] The immunoglobulin enhancer element results in amplified expression of the translocated gene product and, thus, overexpression of BCL-2 protein leading to inhibition of apoptosis of affected B cells. Quantitative real-time polymerase chain reaction (PCR) assays on blood and marrow can determine the number of t(14;18)-expressing cells and may be useful in predicting the outcome of therapy. The t(14;18) translocation is found in approximately 85 percent of patients in the United States, but the translocation is present in a significantly lower percentage of Asian patients afflicted with FL. Detection of the t(14;18) translocation in lymphoid cells is neither necessary nor sufficient for the diagnosis of FL. Small numbers of B cells harboring the t(14;18) translocation can be detected in the blood of 25 to 75 percent of healthy individuals, as well as in reactive lymph nodes and tonsils if

a very sensitive nested or reverse-transcription PCR assay is employed.[2] Additional cytogenetic abnormalities are found in the cells of 90 percent of patients with FL. The finding of multiple cytogenetic abnormalities is commonly associated with higher histologic grade and with the probability of transformation to aggressive lymphoma. A recent large, high-resolution, genome-wide copy-number analysis demonstrated that common recurrent chromosomal abnormalities include gains of chromosomes 2, 5, 6p, 7, 8, 12, 17q, 18, 21, and X and losses on 6q and 17p.[10] Frequent small abnormalities are also commonly observed, including

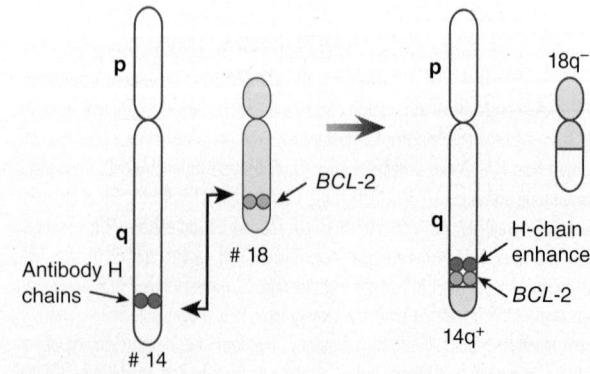

Figure 99–2. The t(14;18)(q32;q21) translocation juxtaposes the *BCL*-2 gene on band q21 of chromosome 18 with the immunoglobulin heavy-chain gene on band 32 of chromosome 14.

losses of 1p36.33–p36.31,6q23.3–q24.1, and 10q23.1–q25.1 and gains of 2p16.1–p15,8q24.13–q24.3, and 12q12–q13.13. Copy-number abnormalities more commonly observed in transformed FL include gains of 3q27.3–q28 and chromosome 11 and losses of 9p21.3 and 15q.[10] Important candidate genes whose expression is affected by these copy-number abnormalities includeTNFRSF14, PRDM16, TP73, and ARIDIA on chromosome 1p36; BCL10 on chromosome 1p; REL and BCL11A on 2p16; BCL6 on chromosome 3q27; histocompatibility locus antigen (HLA)-B, HLA-C, CCND3, and PRDM1 on chromosome 6p21; TNFAIP3 or PERP on chromosome 6q23; CARD11 on chromosome 7p22; MYC on chromosome 8q24; CDKN2A or CDKN2B on chromosome 9p21; STAT6 on 12q13.3; and MDM2 on 12q15.[10]

STAGING THE DISEASE

Evaluation of FL involves performance of a medical history, physical examination (with attention to the lymph nodes in Waldeyer ring and size and involvement of liver and spleen), laboratory testing (including a complete blood count, examination of the blood film and a differential white cell count, lactic dehydrogenase [LDH], β_2-microglobulin, comprehensive metabolic panel, serum uric acid level); lymph node biopsy; marrow aspiration and biopsy; flow cytometric analysis of blood, marrow, and lymph node cells; and computed tomography (CT) of the chest, abdomen, and pelvis.[7] Excisional lymph node biopsies are strongly preferred for the initial histologic diagnosis of FL, although in cases in which nodal masses are inaccessible, generous needle-core biopsies may suffice. The diagnosis should not be established merely on the basis of flow cytometry of the blood or marrow, or on cytologic examination of aspiration needle biopsies of lymph node or other tissue.[11] Hepatitis B serology should be assessed if rituximab therapy is contemplated, as hepatitis reactivation with rituximab may occasionally be life-threatening. In selected circumstances, additional CT scans of the neck, measurement of the cardiac ejection fraction, serum protein electrophoresis, quantitative immunoglobulins, and hepatitis C testing may be useful. Patients for whom chemotherapy is contemplated should receive counseling regarding contraception, fertility issues, and sperm or egg banking. The role of fluoro-2-deoxyglucose (FDG)-positron emission tomography (PET)/CT imaging in FL is rapidly evolving. Although PET/CT imaging was previously considered optional in FL, recent studies suggest that PET-negativity at the completion of induction chemotherapy is one of the most powerful predictors of both progression-free survival (PFS) and overall survival (OS) in this disease.[12]

● PROGNOSTIC FACTORS

CLINICAL AND LABORATORY VARIABLES

An international working group developed an international prognostic index (IPI) based on five independent variables (age, stage, LDH level, performance status, and number of extranodal sites) that affected OS of aggressive lymphoma patients treated with anthracycline-based combination chemotherapy.[13] The IPI was subsequently applied retrospectively to FL and found to be predictive of both OS and PFS for FL (as well as diffuse large B-cell lymphoma). Nevertheless, the IPI was considered to be suboptimal for segregating indolent lymphoma patients into prognostic categories because only 10 to 15 percent of patients with FL fall into the poor risk category using this index. To redress this deficiency, a French cooperative group conducted a detailed prognostic factor analysis of 4167 patients with FL diagnosed between 1985 and 1992 for whom prolonged followup was available to assess OS.[14] Five adverse prognostic factors were detected: age (>60 years vs. ≤60 years), Ann Arbor stage (III to IV vs. I to II), hemoglobin level (<120 g/L vs.

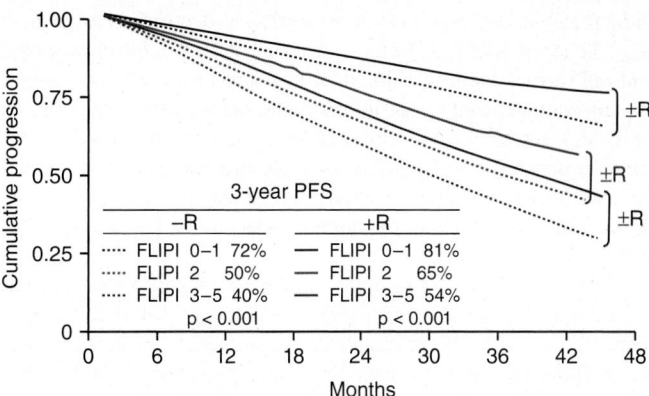

Figure 99–3. Progression-free survival (PFS) of 827 patients with FL stratified by the Follicular Lymphoma International Prognostic Index (FLIPI) into low risk (0 to 1 risk factors, 40% of patients, *black lines*), intermediate risk (2 risk factors, 33% of patients, *blue lines*), or high risk (3 to 5 risk factors, 27% of patients, *red lines*). Of the 827 patients, 267 were treated with chemotherapy regimens without rituximab *(dotted lines)* and 560 were treated with rituximab-containing regimens *(solid lines)*. *(Data from Federico M, Bellei M, Pro B: Revalidation of FLIPI in patients with follicular lymphoma registered in the F2 study and treated upfront with immunochemotherapy.* Proc Am Soc Clin Oncol 25:443s, 2007.)

≥120 g/L), number of nodal areas (>4 vs. ≤4), and serum LDH level (high vs. normal). Three risk groups were defined: low risk (zero to one adverse factors, 36% of patients), intermediate risk (two adverse factors, 37% of patients, hazard ratio [HR] = 2.3), and poor risk (three or more adverse factors, 27% of patients, HR = 4.3). The Follicular Lymphoma International Prognostic Index (FLIPI) discriminated outcomes for FL better than the IPI, both in the original cohort and in later studies evaluating patients treated with modern combined rituximab-chemotherapy regimens (Fig. 99–3).[15] A revised version of the FLIPI index (FLIPI2) was subsequently proposed to address perceived deficiencies in the original model.[16] The FLIPI2 model is also based on assessment of five adverse risk factors, namely the presence or absence of an elevated β_2-microglobulin level, the longest diameter of the largest involved lymph node (>6 cm), presence of marrow involvement, hemoglobin level less than 12 g/dL, and age older than 60 years. Although several studies have demonstrated the superiority of the FLIPI2 model compared to the original FLIPI model, it has not been widely adopted in North America. A simpler prognostic model was developed based solely on the baseline serum LDH and β_2-microglobulin level that has been shown to be superior to the original FLIPI model and equivalent to the FLIPI2 model in prognostic power for predicting outcomes for FL patients.[17, 18]

GENOMICS OF FOLLICULAR LYMPHOMA

New molecular approaches are revolutionizing our understanding of the pathogenesis of FL and providing insights into the pathways that might be targeted in the future by rationally designed therapies. Early gene-expression profiling studies of biopsy specimens from patients with untreated FL identified two gene-expression signatures that allowed construction of a survival predictor enabling segregation of patients into four quartiles with disparate median lengths of survival (13.6, 11.1, 10.8, and 3.9 years), independent of clinical prognostic variables.[19] One signature ("immune response 1") was associated with a good prognosis and included genes encoding T-cell markers (e.g., CD7, CD8B1, ITK, LEF1, and STAT4) as well as genes that are highly expressed in macrophages (e.g., ACTN1 and TNFSF13B). The "immune response 2" signature was associated with a poor prognosis and included genes known to be preferentially expressed in macrophages, dendritic cells, or both (e.g., *TLR5, FCGR1A, SEPT10, LGMN,* and *C3AR1*). Flow cytometry and cell sorting confirmed that these signatures reflected gene expression by nonmalignant tumor-infiltrating immune cells (CD19-negative cells) and not by the FL cells themselves (CD19-positive cells). The length of survival correlated with the molecular features of the nonmalignant immune cells present in the tumor at diagnosis and presumably reflected the robustness of the immune response mounted against the tumor.

"Next-generation sequencing" studies employing whole-genome or whole-exome sequencing and targeted mutational analyses have demonstrated that somatic mutations in epigenetic regulators are present in almost all cases of FL, including MLL2 (also known as KMT2D), a histone methyltransferase that is mutated in 89 percent of FL; CREBBP and EP300, two highly related histone and nonhistone acetyltransferases that act as transcriptional coactivators in multiple signaling pathways that are mutated in 30 percent and 11 percent of FL, respectively; EZH2, the catalytic subunit of PRC2 that catalyzes trimethylation of lysine 27 on histone H3, a repressive chromatin mark that is mutated in 27 percent of FL; and MEF2B, a calcium-regulated gene that cooperates with CREBBP and EP300 in acetylating histones that is mutated in 15 percent of FL.[20–24] Other mutational targets include genes involved in immune modulation (β_2-microglobulin, CD58, and TNFRSF14), Janus kinase (JAK)-signal transducer and activator of transcription (STAT) signaling (SOCS1 and STAT6) and B-cell receptor–nuclear factor (NF)-κB signaling (BCL10, CARD11 and CD79B).[22] Mutations in CREBBP and EP300 lesions are usually heterozygous, suggesting a haploinsufficient role in tumor suppression, apparently by impairing acetylation-mediated inactivation of the BCL6 oncoprotein and activation of the p53 tumor suppressor.[21] A unifying model of the genetic evolution of FL postulates that the t(14;18) translocation serves as a "founder mutation" that is succeeded by development of additional "driver mutations" (e.g., CREBBP), irrelevant "passenger" mutations, and accelerator mutations (TNFRSF14).[22,23] Disagreement exists over whether MLL2/KMT2D mutations are "driver" or "accelerator" mutations.[22,23] Mutations in EBF1 and in regulators of NF-κB signaling (e.g., MYD88, TNFAIP3) appear to be acquired at the time of histologic transformation to diffuse large B-cell lymphoma.[22]

●THERAPY

LIMITED STAGE I OR II FOLLICULAR LYMPHOMA

Radiotherapy

Patients with stage I or II FL represent only 10 to 30 percent of cases in most series.[2,4] Standard management for stage I or limited contiguous stage II FL involves the administration of involved field radiotherapy (35 to 40 Gray [Gy]).[7] Adjuvant chemotherapy does not appear to improve survival in this setting, although some studies suggest that combined chemoradiotherapy may improve PFS. A retrospective review of 177 patients with stage I or II and grade 1 or 2 FL reported a median survival of 14 years following radiation therapy as a single modality.[27] Approximately 50 percent of the patients were relapse-free after 5 to 10 years.

Observation

Excellent survival has also been observed in highly selected patients with early stage FL who received no initial therapy.[25] In a group of 43 patients, 56 percent were free from the requirement for treatment for at least 10 years and 86 percent were alive 10 years after diagnosis. Based on this study, many authorities have concluded that "watchful waiting" is an acceptable alternative to radiotherapy for stage I or II FL.

A watchful waiting approach may be particularly appropriate for certain variants of FL, such as FL presenting in the small intestine, which pursues a remarkably indolent course, rarely exhibits progressive growth, very rarely disseminates (two of 63 patients) and does not transform to high-grade disease.[26]

Chemoimmunotherapy

A large observational study, the National LymphoCare Study, assessed the outcomes of 471 patients with stage I FL according to treatment administered, including rituximab plus chemotherapy (28 percent of patients), radiotherapy alone (27 percent), observation (17 percent), systemic therapy + radiotherapy (13 percent), rituximab monotherapy (12 percent), and other treatments (3 percent).[28] This large, prospectively enrolled group of patients showed that national guidelines endorsing radiotherapy alone for stage I FL were not followed by practicing clinicians in the majority of cases. All treatment approaches resulted in excellent outcomes, though PFS was significantly better after a median followup of 57 months in patients treated with either rituximab plus chemotherapy (84 percent) or systemic therapy plus radiotherapy (96 percent) than in patients receiving radiotherapy alone (68 percent).[28] This study challenges the paradigm that radiotherapy alone should be the standard of care for patients with early stage indolent lymphoma, although the observational nature of this study, without randomization to treatment arm and the absence of differences in OS, attenuates the impact of the study.

ADVANCED STAGE FOLLICULAR LYMPHOMA

Observation Alone

Many patients with FL, particularly grades 1 or 2, will exhibit an indolent, asymptomatic course despite the absence of therapy. Because there is no conclusive evidence that survival of FL patients is improved by immediate institution of therapy, or that conventional management (other than allogeneic stem cell transplantation) can cure the disease, a "watch-and-wait" approach is often recommended for patients with extensive stage II or stage III or IV FL. In one study, survival was 82 percent at 5 years and 73 percent at 10 years after an initial strategy of observation alone, and the median time until therapy was required was 3 years.[29] Spontaneous regressions occurred in 23 percent of untreated patients. No differences in survival were observed in a trial of 309 patients randomized to initial watchful waiting or to chlorambucil.[30] In another trial, patients were randomized to either watchful waiting or to immediate aggressive combination chemotherapy with prednisone, methotrexate, doxorubicin, cyclophosphamide, etoposide, mechlorethamine, vincristine, procarbazine, prednisone (ProMACE/MOPP) chemotherapy followed by total nodal irradiation.[31] The OS rates for the two groups were similar, although the disease-free survival rate was naturally higher in the patients treated with combined modality therapy. Criteria established by the Groupe d'Etudes des Lymphomes Folliculaires (GELF) are useful to identify patients who may benefit from intervention rather than "watchful waiting." These criteria suggest that treatment is likely to be required for patients with a maximum diameter of any site of disease greater than 7 cm, more than three nodal sites greater than 3 cm in diameter, systemic B symptoms, a spleen size greater than 16 cm, pleural effusions, local compressive symptoms, circulating lymphoma cells, or cytopenias as a result of the lymphoma.[32]

Single-Agent Chemotherapy

FL patients can be palliated effectively with a variety of single chemotherapy agents (Table 99–1). Responses to single-agent therapy, such as chlorambucil, a nucleoside analogue, or bendamustine, range from 70 to 90 percent and may last for several years.[30,33]

TABLE 99–1. Therapeutic Regimens for Follicular Lymphoma

Agent(s)	Dose	Route	Days(s) of Treatment	Repeat Cycle at Day
SINGLE AGENTS				
Chlorambucil	0.08–0.12 mg/kg	PO	Daily	
	or 0.4–1.0 mg/kg	PO	1	28
Cyclophosphamide	50–100 mg/m²	PO	Daily	
	or 300 mg/m²	PO	1–5	28
Fludarabine	25 mg/m²/day	IV	1–5	28
Cladribine	0.1 mg/kg/day	IV (continuous)	1–7	28
	or 0.14 mg/kg/day	IV (2 h)	1–5	28
Bendamustine	70–120 mg/m²/day	IV	1, 2	21 or 28
Rituximab	375 mg/m²/day	IV	1, 8, 15, 22	
COMBINATION THERAPY				
Stanford CVP				
Cyclophosphamide	400 mg/m²	PO	1–5	21
Vincristine	1.4 mg/m² (maximum 2 mg)	IV	1	21
Prednisone	100 mg/m²	PO	1–5	21
R-CVP				
Rituximab	375 mg/m²	IV	1	21
Cyclophosphamide	750–1000 mg/m²	IV	1	21
Vincristine	1.4 mg/m² (maximum 2 mg)	IV	1	21
Prednisone	100 mg	PO	1–5	21
R-CHOP				
Rituximab	375 mg/m²	IV	1	21
Cyclophosphamide	750 mg/m²	IV	1	21
Doxorubicin	50 mg/m²	IV	1	
Vincristine	1.4 mg/m²	IV	1	
Prednisone	100 mg	PO	1–5	
FND				
Fludarabine	25 mg/m²	IV	1–3	28
Mitoxantrone	10 mg/m²	IV	1	
Dexamethasone	20 mg	IV or PO	1–5	

Monoclonal Antibody Therapy

Rituximab is a human–mouse chimeric monoclonal antibody that binds to the CD20 antigen that is expressed on nearly all normal and malignant B cells but not on other human tissues. After binding to B cells, rituximab induces cell death via antibody-dependent cellular cytotoxicity (ADCC), complement-fixation (complement-dependent cytotoxicity [CDC]), induction of apoptosis, and by facilitating cross-presentation of lymphoma-associated antigens by dendritic cells. Rituximab was approved by the FDA for therapy of indolent lymphomas based on the results of a pivotal trial that evaluated treatment of 166 patients with relapsed or refractory indolent lymphoma with four weekly infusions of 375 mg/m². The response rate was 48 percent, including a 6 percent complete response rate and a median time to progression of approximately 1 year.[34] The response rate to first-line therapy with rituximab in newly diagnosed FL is approximately 70 to 75 percent with a complete remission rate of 18 to 27 percent.[35,36] A second response to rituximab may be achieved in 40 percent of patients who relapse after an initial remission to rituximab.[37] Extended courses of rituximab or "rituximab maintenance" therapy have become popular. Various schedules are employed, including administration of one dose of 375 mg/m² every 2 months for 2 years (usually as part of frontline therapy), one dose every 3 months for 2 years (for relapsed patients), four doses every 6 months for 2 years, or one dose every 2 months for four doses.[38–42] No comparative studies of these disparate "maintenance" rituximab regimens have been performed. Several newer, humanized or fully human anti-CD20 monoclonal antibodies (ofatumumab, veltuzumab, obinutuzumab) have been engineered to exhibit superior ADCC, CDC, or improved induction of cell death. All are undergoing clinical trials to determine if they are superior to rituximab and one of them, obinutuzumab, has recently been approved for therapy of chronic lymphocytic leukemia

TABLE 99–2. Selected Randomized Studies of Chemotherapy Alone Versus Rituximab Plus Chemotherapy for First-Line Therapy of Follicular Lymphoma

Study	Treatment, No. of Patients	Median Followup (Months)	ORR (%)	CR (%)	Median TTP/TTF/EFS (Months)	OS (%)
Marcus[45]	CVP, 159	53	57	10	15	77
	R-CVP, 162		81	41	34	83
					p <0.0001	p = 0.0290
Hiddemann[46]	CHOP, 205	18	90	17	29	74
	R-CHOP, 223		96	20	NR	87
					p <0.001	p = 0.016
Herold[47]	MCP, 96	47	75	25	26	74
	R-MCP, 105		92	50	NR	87
					p <0.0001	p = 0.0096
Bachy[43]	CHVP-IFN, 183	100	73	63	34	69
	R-CHVP-IFN, 175		84	79	66	78 at 8 years
					p = 0.0004	p = 0.076
Hochster[44]	CVP, 158	36	82	22	16	92
	CVP + rituximab maintenance, 153		86	37	59	86 at 3 years
					P = 4.4×10^{-10}	p = 0.05 one sided

CR, complete response; CHOP, cyclophosphamide, doxorubicin, vincristine, prednisone; CHVP, cyclophosphamide, doxorubicin, teniposide, prednisone; CVP, cyclophosphamide, vincristine, prednisone; EFS, event-free survival; IFN, interferon; MCP, mitoxantrone, chlorambucil, prednisone; ORR, overall response rate; OS, overall survival; R, rituximab; TTF, time to treatment failure; TTP, time to progression.

(CLL) (but not FL). "Biosimilar" CD20 antibodies will also soon be available as an alternative to rituximab.

Rituximab Plus Chemotherapy

The introduction of rituximab into treatment protocols for FL has revolutionized the management of this disease. Multiple randomized, controlled clinical trials have documented the superiority of combining rituximab with chemotherapy compared to the use of chemotherapy alone in terms of overall response rates (ORRs), complete response (CR) rates, event-free survival (EFS), PFS, and OS (Table 99–2).[43–47] In one study, induction therapy consisting of eight cycles of rituximab,

cyclophosphamide, vincristine, and prednisone (R-CVP) was compared to eight cycles of CVP without rituximab in 321 patients with newly diagnosed FL (Fig. 99–4).[48] R-CVP was superior to CVP alone in terms of ORR (81 percent vs. 57 percent), CR rate (41 percent vs. 10 percent), time to progression (34 months vs. 15 months), time to treatment failure (27 months vs. 7 months), and OS (83 percent vs. 77 percent at 4 years, p = 0.029).[45] Similarly, R-CHOP was compared to CHOP for first-line treatment of 428 patients with advanced stage FL. R-CHOP exhibited a superior ORR (96 percent vs. 90 percent), time to treatment failure (p <0.001), duration of response (p = 0.001), and OS (p = 0.016) compared to CHOP alone.[46] Similar benefits have also

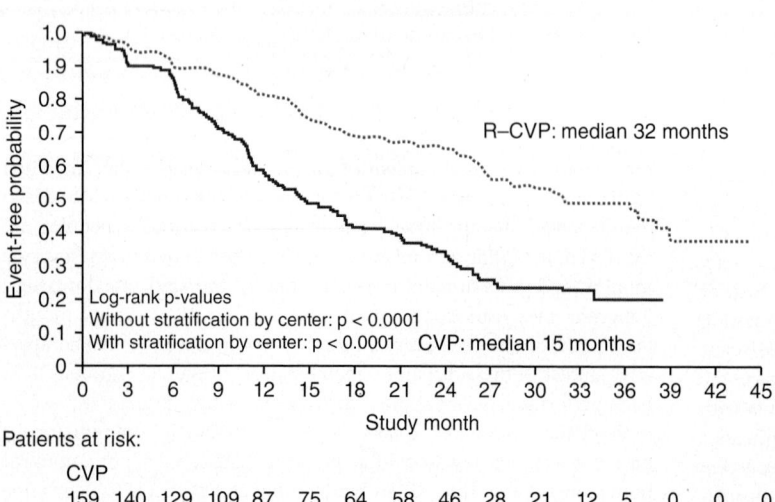

Figure 99–4. Time to disease progression, relapse, or death after a median followup of 30 months among 321 patients with grade 1 or 2 follicular lymphoma assigned to chemotherapy with CVP (cyclophosphamide, vincristine, prednisone) or with R-CVP (rituximab plus cyclophosphamide, vincristine, prednisone). *Solid line* represents CVP; *dotted line*, R-CVP. *(Reproduced with permission from Marcus R, Imrie K, Belch A, et al: CVP chemotherapy plus rituximab compared with CVP as first-line treatment for advanced follicular lymphoma.* Blood *105(4):1417–1423, 2005.)*

been reported for the addition of rituximab to other regimens for both frontline therapy and relapsed FL.[41,47,49,50] The selection of the "optimal" chemotherapy regimen to combine with rituximab remains hotly contentious.[51] Two recent large international phase III randomized studies compared the efficacy and toxicity of R-CVP, R-CHOP, and rituximab-fludarabine–based therapy, which until recently were the three most commonly employed regimens for frontline therapy of FL. Both trials demonstrated superior PFS for patients treated with R-CHOP or rituximab-fludarabine regimens than with R-CVP, although OS did not differ. Both studies also concluded that regimens with fludarabine and rituximab had significantly more hematologic toxicity and a higher risk of secondary malignancies than either R-CVP or R-CHOP, making fludarabine-based regimens less desirable. The investigators conducting these trials concluded that R-CHOP was the preferred regimen for FL, although some oncologists are hesitant to routinely employ R-CHOP in patients with indolent lymphomas because of its greater toxicity, including a 1 to 2 percent risk of cardiomyopathy, and the absence of a demonstrated OS advantage. These risks may be particularly justifiable, however, for patients with grade 3 FL, as many authorities believe anthracycline-based regimens may be curable for high-grade FL, which National Comprehensive Cancer Network (NCCN) guidelines advise treated identically to diffuse large B-cell lymphoma.[7] To further amplify the controversy, two recent randomized trials comparing bendamustine plus rituximab (BR) with R-CHOP show similar efficacy for the two regimens, and less toxicity for BR.[52,53] Although these studies have been criticized for methodologic flaws, they have been highly influential and have catapulted BR to prominence as the most popular frontline induction regimen for FL, with approximately 65 to 70 percent of FL patients in the United States and Europe currently receiving this regimen for frontline therapy.

Maintenance Rituximab

Despite the ability to induce long-lasting remissions in the majority of FL patients treated with chemoimmunotherapy regimens as outlined above, most patients will eventually relapse. Several strategies have emerged to prolong the remission durations and to delay lymphoma recurrence. The most popular approach is to administer extended courses of rituximab, also known as rituximab "maintenance" to forestall reappearance of FL. The PRIMA trial randomized 1217 patients with FL to either maintenance rituximab (375 mg/m^2 every 2 months for 2 years) or no maintenance therapy, following frontline induction therapy with R-CVP, R-CHOP, or rituximab, fludarabine, cyclophosphamide, and mitoxantrone (R-FCM).[42] This study convincingly demonstrated the superiority of 2 years of maintenance rituximab (PFS 74.9 percent) compared to observation alone after induction (PFS, 57.6 percent, p <0.0001), regardless of which induction chemotherapy regimen is used. Despite the marked improvement in PFS afforded by maintenance rituximab in PRIMA, however, there was no significant difference in OS between the rituximab maintenance and observation arms. Similar improvements in PFS but not OS have also been demonstrated for maintenance rituximab given for 2 years following rituximab monotherapy in the frontline setting[30] and following CHOP or R-CHOP induction in the relapsed setting.[54]

Radioimmunotherapy

Radiolabeled monoclonal antibodies targeting lymphoma-associated cell surface antigens, including idiotypic immunoglobulin, CD20, CD22, and HLA-DR, have emerged as effective and safe therapeutic agents for patients with FL.[55,56] Two radioimmunoconjugates targeting the CD20 antigen, [131]iodine-tositumomab (Bexxar) and [90]yttrium-ibritumomab tiuxetan (Zevalin), have been extensively tested in indolent lymphomas.[57–59] Radioimmunotherapy (RIT) is an attractive therapeutic option for

lymphomas because (1) many high-quality antibodies are available targeting pan–B-cell antigens expressed at high levels on lymphoma cells, (2) lymphomas are exquisitely sensitive to radiotherapy, and (3) cross-fire radiotherapy from β particles emitted by decaying radionuclides on targeted lymphoma cells can kill neighboring antigen-negative tumor cells (or inaccessible cells deep in tumor clumps), which would escape killing by nonradioactive antibodies. Several trials have demonstrated ORRs of 50 to 80 percent and CR rates of 15 to 40 percent in patients with relapsed or refractory indolent lymphoma treated with either [131]iodine-tositumomab or [90]yttrium-ibritumomab tiuxetan.[57,59,60] In a randomized study comparing treatment of patients with relapsed FL with either[90] Y-ibritumomab tiuxetan or rituximab, the ORR (86 percent vs. 55 percent) and the CR rate (30 percent vs. 15 percent) were both statistically superior in the group treated with the radioimmunoconjugate.[59] Similarly,[131] I-tositumomab was compared with unlabeled tositumomab in a randomized trial of relapsed indolent lymphoma and both the ORR (55 percent vs. 19 percent) and the CR rate (33 percent vs. 8 percent) were higher in patients receiving the radiolabeled antibody.[61]

Six phase II studies have studied frontline RIT for patients with newly diagnosed FL, either as a single agent or in combination with various chemotherapy regimens, including CVP, CHOP, and fludarabine. In all six studies, outstanding ORR rates (90 to 100 percent) and CR rates (50 to 96 percent) were observed with first-line RIT, with median PFSs in excess of 5 years in several of the studies.[62–64] A phase III randomized study evaluated the utility of consolidation therapy with[90] Y-ibritumomab tiuxetan for patients with FL in remission after frontline chemotherapy.[65] In this trial, 414 patients in either partial or complete remission after a variety of chemotherapy induction regimens (chlorambucil, CVP, CHOP, fludarabine or rituximab combinations) were randomized to either consolidation with RIT or to no consolidation. RIT dramatically improved the median PFS in the total patient population (36.5 months vs. 13.3 months, p <0.0001), and this advantage was observed regardless of whether patients were in partial remission (PR; 29.3 months vs. 6.2 months, p <0.0001) or CR (53.9 months vs. 29.5 months, p = 0.015) at the time of consolidation. Furthermore, RIT consolidation converted 77 percent of patients who were in PR after induction chemotherapy to CR following RIT. However, a recent study comparing six cycles of R-CHOP with six cycles of CHOP (without rituximab) followed by a single dose of[131] I-tositumomab (CHOP-RIT) demonstrated similar outcomes in both treatment arms.[17]

The major toxicity of RIT is myelosuppression, with cytopenic nadirs occurring 4 to 7 weeks after treatment and requiring 2 to 4 weeks for recovery. Growth factor administration and transfusions are required in approximately 20 percent of patients. Human antimouse antibodies (HAMA) may develop in the serum of approximately 1 percent of patients treated with[90] Y-labeled ibritumomab and in 10 percent of patients treated with[131] I-labeled tositumomab. A potential long-term concern with both radiolabeled antibody formulations is the potential development of myelodysplasia and acute leukemia as late complications. Hypothyroidism may also occur as a delayed toxicity of ^{131}I-labeled tositumomab in approximately 10 percent of patients.

Interferon-α$_2$

Interferon (IFN)-α$_2$ has been studied in 10 large phase III studies evaluating its utility in both the induction phase of treatment and for maintenance therapy. A meta-analysis of 1922 newly diagnosed patients with FL treated in these trials concluded that the addition of IFN-α$_2$ to induction chemotherapy did not significantly influence response rates, but did show a significant difference in favor of IFN-α$_2$ with regard to survival.[66] Results differed greatly from trial to trial and further analyses were carried out to define the circumstances in which IFN-α$_2$ prolonged OS. The survival advantage was seen when IFN-α$_2$ was given (1) in conjunction with relatively intensive initial chemotherapy (p = 0.00005), (2) at a dose of 5 million units or greater (p = 0.000002), (3) at a cumulative dose of 36 million units or greater per month (p = 0.000008), and (4) when given with induction chemotherapy rather than as maintenance therapy (p = 0.004).[66] With regard to remission duration, there was also a significant difference in favor of IFN-α_2, irrespective of the intensity of chemotherapy used, IFN dose, or whether IFN was given as a maintenance strategy or with chemotherapy. Despite these salutary findings, IFN is rarely employed to treat FL in the United States because of its unfavorable toxicity profile (asthenia, fatigue, flu-like symptoms, cytopenias) and because of the perception that rituximab confers similar or superior advantages with much less toxicity.

Idiotype Vaccines

The idiotypic immunoglobulin protein expressed on the surface of B lymphoma cells represents a true tumor-specific antigen and is an ideal target for immunotherapeutic strategies. Several groups have reported favorable phase II trials using idiotypic vaccines produced either by rescue hybridoma fusions or recombinant DNA approaches. The idiotypic immunoglobulin in most of the vaccines is coupled to keyhole limpet hemocyanin (KLH) and administered with sargramostim (granulocyte-macrophage colony-stimulating factor) to enhance immunogenicity. Specific immune responses are generated in approximately 50 percent of immunized FL patients who are in complete remission at the time of vaccination. Patients exhibiting immune responses to the vaccine experience longer remission durations and superior survival compared to patients failing to mount immune responses to the vaccine. Three phase III randomized trials have been conducted using idiotypic vaccination following induction therapy. Two of these studies found no statistical differences in PFS between an idiotypic KLH vaccine and a control vaccine.[67,68] The third study reported an improved disease-free survival for specifically vaccinated patients,[69] although the study has been criticized for a variety of methodologic imperfections.[68]

Hematopoietic Stem Cell Transplantation

The role of high-dose chemoradiotherapy and hematopoietic stem cell transplantation in the management of patients with FL remains highly controversial. Proponents of autologous stem cell transplantation for indolent NHL note the favorable outcome of a collaborative study of 121 adult patients conducted by St. Bartholomew's Hospital and the Dana-Farber Cancer Institute, where an apparent plateau in the remission duration curve was observed in 48 percent of patients with a median followup of 13.5 years.[70] Survival was longer in patients transplanted in second remission compared to those transplanted later in their disease course. The value of autologous stem cell transplantation was also tested in a randomized trial of 89 patients with relapsed FL (Fig. 99–5). Transplanted patients experienced a marked advantage in PFS and a marginal OS advantage compared to patients randomized to continued conventional salvage chemotherapy without transplantation.[71] When used as part of initial therapy for high-risk patients, randomized studies demonstrate a prolongation of PFS, but no improvement in OS.[72,73] Adverse outcomes associated with autologous stem cell transplantation include treatment-related mortality (3 to 5 percent) and a substantial increase in the incidence of secondary myelodysplasia and acute myelogenous leukemia, occurring in 7 to 19 percent of patients, particularly if total-body irradiation is employed in the conditioning regimen.

Allogeneic transplantation affords long-term PFS for approximately 40 to 50 percent of patients with relapsed FL, but widespread adoption of this approach has been hampered by transplant-related mortality ranging from 20 to 40 percent. Consequently, careful patient selection and informed consent are essential. When allogeneic and autologous stem cell transplantation are compared for patients with relapsed FL, the long-term survival rates are comparable.[74,75] Autologous stem cell transplantation is associated with a greater likelihood of dying from recurrent disease, and allogeneic stem cell transplantation results in a higher frequency of death from graft-versus-host disease, infection, and venoocclusive disease. Nonmyeloablative and reduced-intensity allogeneic transplantation conditioning regimens have been developed to exploit the benefit of a graft-versus-lymphoma effect while minimizing transplant-related morbidity and mortality. Preliminary results of this approach are encouraging, with 52 to 85 percent OS and 43 to 83 percent PFS after 3 to 11 years with 8 to 43 percent nonrelapse mortality.[76,77]

TRANSFORMED FOLLICULAR LYMPHOMA

Approximately 30 to 40 percent of patients with FL undergo documented transformation to a more aggressive histology, usually diffuse large B-cell lymphoma, with an annual rate of transformation of

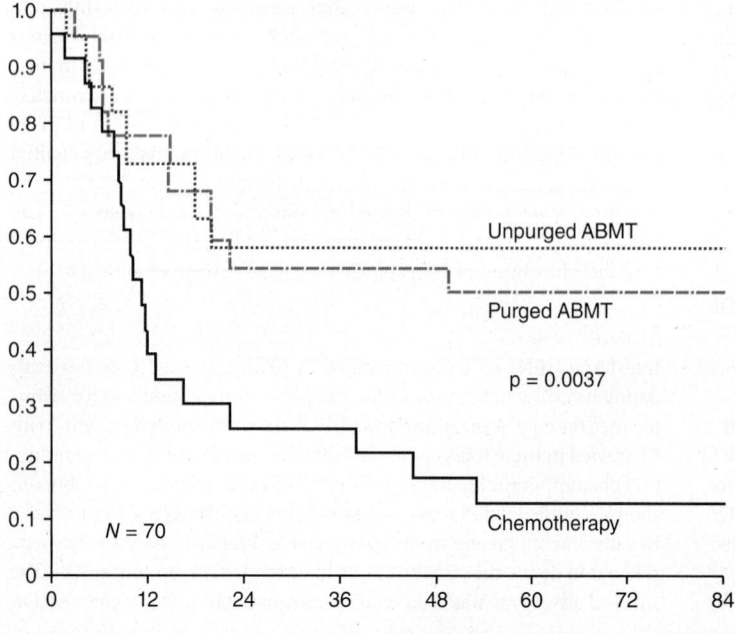

Figure 99–5. Progression-free survival of 70 patients with relapsed follicular lymphoma randomized to either conventional chemotherapy *(solid line)*, or to high-dose chemoradiotherapy with autologous marrow transplantation using either marrow purged to remove tumor cells *(long dashes)* or unpurged marrow *(short dashes)*. ABMT, autologous bone marrow transplantation. *(Reproduced with permission from Schouten HC, Qian W, Kvaloy S, et al: High-dose therapy improves progression-free survival and survival in relapsed follicular non-Hodgkin's lymphoma: results from the randomized European CUP trial. J Clin Oncol 21(21):3918–3927, 2003.)*

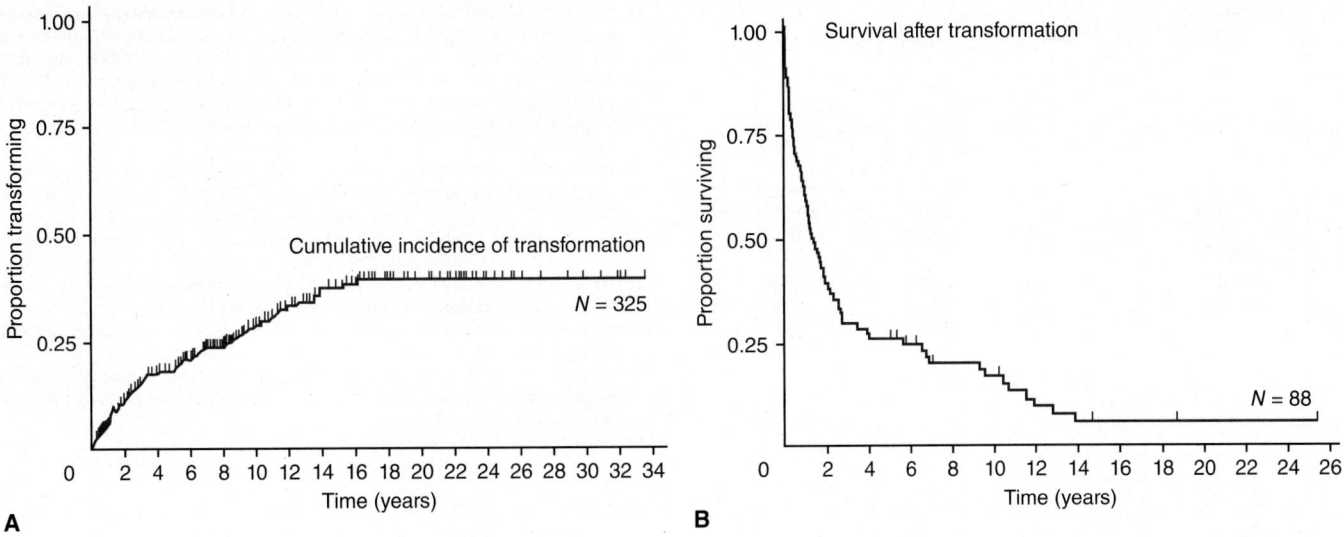

Figure 99–6. **A.** Transformation of follicular lymphoma (FL) to an histologic pattern compatible with rapid progression of disease. The line depicts the cumulative incidence of histologic transformation to a histologic pattern compatible with more rapid progression (e.g., diffuse large B-cell lymphoma) in 325 patients followed from the date of diagnosis of FL. **B.** The proportion of patients with FL surviving after transformation to a less-favorable histologic pattern. The graph shows the survival of the 88 patients from the date of their transformation to aggressive lymphoma. *(Reproduced with permission from Montoto S, Davies AJ, Matthews J, et al.: Risk and clinical implications of transformation of follicular lymphoma to diffuse large B-cell lymphoma. J Clin Oncol 25(17):2426–2433, 2007.)*

approximately 3 percent (Fig. 99–6A). Clinically, histologic transformation is characterized by the sudden explosive growth of a single lymph node site (or extranodal mass). Anthracycline-based chemotherapy (e.g., R-CHOP) is the most appropriate therapy for patients experiencing transformation, however, most studies indicate that the prognosis is poor despite aggressive management. Whereas 50 to 65 percent of patients presenting with *de novo* diffuse large B-cell lymphoma are cured with R-CHOP chemotherapy, less than 10 percent of patients with diffuse large B-cell lymphoma arising by transformation from FL will be cured by this regimen (Fig. 99–6B). Most series report median survivals of 6 to 20 months for patients undergoing transformation,[29,78–80] although one recent study reports a 50-month median survival, with particularly good survival in patients experiencing transformation more than 18 months after initial diagnosis of FL.[81] Because of the historically poor outcome of chemotherapy alone, some authorities advise either autologous or allogeneic stem cell transplantation following induction of remission with R-CHOP. A recent multicenter cohort study of 172 patients with transformed FL concluded that patients undergoing autologous stem cell transplantation had better outcomes than those treated with rituximab-containing chemotherapy alone. However, allogeneic transplantation did not improve outcomes compared with rituximab-containing chemotherapy because of high rates of transplant-related mortality.[82]

A PRAGMATIC APPROACH TO THERAPY OF FOLLICULAR LYMPHOMA

There is currently little consensus among lymphoma experts with regard to the optimal management of patients with either frontline or relapsed FL.[51] Therefore, at this time all patients with FL should be considered for entry into clinical trials to define the best regimens and to allow evaluation of the multitude of promising new drugs and antibodies that are now available. Patients who are ineligible for trials or who decline enrollment should receive individualized treatment. Patients with localized stage I or II disease may be offered local radiotherapy, observation or chemoimmunotherapy. Elderly patients with asymptomatic, stage III

or IV disease are best monitored with observation alone, particularly if their disease is of low volume and if they have multiple coexistent medical illnesses. Patients who are symptomatic, have cytopenias, massive splenomegaly, effusions, or bulky adenopathy should be treated with rituximab plus chemotherapy. Several regimens are acceptable including BR, R-CVP, and R-CHOP, with the latter regimen being most appropriate for young patients with aggressive presentations and rapidly growing bulky adenopathy, B symptoms or for patients with grade 3 FL. The roles of maintenance rituximab and consolidative RIT following initial induction chemoimmunotherapy of newly diagnosed patients are contentious. It appears that either rituximab maintenance for 2 years or a single dose of consolidative RIT with ^{90}Y-ibritumomab tiuxetan can prolong initial remission duration and PFS, but neither improves OS. Management of FL following relapse depends on the patient's initial treatment and the resultant remission duration. If the first remission lasts many years, the initial treatment regimen may again be used (except for anthracycline-containing regimens). If the initial remission is short, an alternative second-line regimen should be selected from among the many available options, including BR, R-CVP, R-CHOP, R-FND (rituximab, fludarabine, mitoxantrone [Novantrone], and dexamethasone), and RIT. In the near future, many additional attractive options will be available, including ibrutinib,[83,84] idelalisib,[85,86] ABT-199,[87,88] antibody–drug conjugates,[89] and adoptive immunotherapy with chimeric antigen receptor modified T lymphocytes.[90,91] Patients with a good performance status, who experience very short response durations, should be considered for autologous or allogeneic stem cell transplantation. Patients who undergo histologic transformation should receive R-CHOP and be offered the option of stem cell transplantation.

● COURSE AND PROGNOSIS

FL has been considered an indolent but incurable disease for which the median survival of approximately 10 years is minimally affected by medical interventions. This attitude is no longer valid, and survival of FL patients has been progressively increasing over the past 20 years (Fig. 99–7).[92–94] Much of the improvement in survival appears

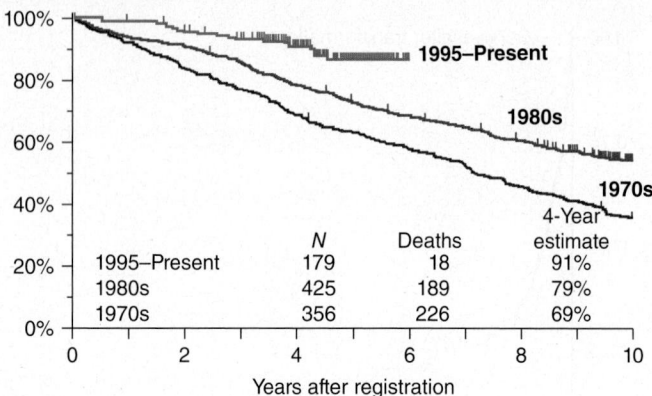

Figure 99–7. Improved survival of patients with follicular lymphoma treated by the Southwest Oncology Group. *(Reproduced with permission from Fisher RI, LeBlanc M, Press OW, et al: New treatment options have changed the survival of patients with follicular lymphoma.* J Clin Oncol *23(33):8447–8452, 2005.)*

attributable to the introduction of rituximab, better salvage therapies (bendamustine, RIT), improved supportive care measures, and the wider implementation of stem cell transplantation. Controversy persists over whether any of the grades of FL are curable with standard chemoimmunotherapy regimens, although it is clear that OS has improved significantly in the last decade. Further clinical research will settle these disputes and permit formulation of a consensus standard of care for the management of both newly diagnosed and relapsed FL.

REFERENCES

1. Siegel R, Ma J, Zou Z, et al: Cancer statistics, 2014. *CA Cancer J Clin* 64:9–29, 2014.
2. Harris NL, Swerdlow SH, Jaffe ES, et al: Follicular lymphoma, in *WHO Classification of Tumours of Haematopoietic and Lymphoid Tissues*, 4th edition, edited by SH Swerdlow, E Campo, NL Harris, ES Jaffe, SA Pileri, H Stein, J Thiele, JW Vardiman, pp 220–226. International Agency for Research on Cancer, Lyon, 2008.
3. Friedberg JW, Taylor MD, Cerhan JR, et al: Follicular lymphoma in the United States: First report of the national LymphoCare study. *J Clin Oncol* 27:1202–1208, 2009.
4. Groves FD, Linet MS, Travis LB, et al: Cancer surveillance series: Non-Hodgkin's lymphoma incidence by histologic subtype in the United States from 1978 through 1995. *J Natl Cancer Inst* 92:1240–1251, 2000.
5. Louissaint A Jr, Ackerman AM, Dias-Santagata D, et al: Pediatric-type nodal follicular lymphoma: An indolent clonal proliferation in children and adults with high proliferation index and no BCL2 rearrangement. *Blood* 120:2395–2404, 2012.
6. Liu Q, Salaverria I, Pittaluga S, et al: Follicular lymphomas in children and young adults: A comparison of the pediatric variant with usual follicular lymphoma. *Am J Surg Pathol* 37:333–343, 2013.
7. Zelenetz AD, Gordon LI, Wierda WG, et al: Non-Hodgkin's lymphomas, version 4.2014. *J Natl Compr Canc Netw* 12:1282–1303, 2014.
8. Miller TP, LeBlanc M, Grogan TM, et al: Follicular lymphomas: Do histologic subtypes predict outcome? *Hematol Oncol Clin North Am* 11:893–900, 1997.
9. Reed JC: Bcl-2-family proteins and hematologic malignancies: History and future prospects. *Blood* 111:3322–3330, 2008.
10. Bouska A, McKeithan TW, Deffenbacher KE, et al: Genome-wide copy-number analyses reveal genomic abnormalities involved in transformation of follicular lymphoma. *Blood* 123:1681–1690, 2014.
11. Hehn ST, Grogan TM, Miller TP: Utility of fine-needle aspiration as a diagnostic technique in lymphoma. *J Clin Oncol* 22:3046–3052, 2004.
12. Trotman J, Fournier M, Lamy T, et al: Positron emission tomography-computed tomography (PET-CT) after induction therapy is highly predictive of patient outcome in follicular lymphoma: Analysis of PET-CT in a subset of PRIMA trial participants. *J Clin Oncol* 29:3194–3200, 2011.
13. Shipp MA: A predictive model for aggressive non-Hodgkin's lymphoma. The International Non-Hodgkin's Lymphoma Prognostic Factors Project. *N Engl J Med* 329:987–994, 1993.
14. Solal-Celigny P, Roy P, Colombat P, et al: Follicular lymphoma international prognostic index. *Blood* 104:1258–1265, 2004.
15. Federico M, Bellei M, Pro B: Revalidation of FLIPI in patients with follicular lymphoma registered in the F2 study and treated upfront with immunochemotherapy. *Proc Am Soc Clin Oncol* 25:443s, 2007.

16. Federico M, Bellei M, Marcheselli L, et al: Follicular lymphoma international prognostic index 2: A new prognostic index for follicular lymphoma developed by the international follicular lymphoma prognostic factor project. *J Clin Oncol* 27:4555–4562, 2009.
17. Press OW, Unger JM, Rimsza LM, et al: Phase III randomized intergroup trial of CHOP plus rituximab compared with CHOP chemotherapy plus (131)iodine-tositumomab for previously untreated follicular non-Hodgkin lymphoma: SWOG S0016. *J Clin Oncol* 31:314–320, 2013.
18. Press OW, Unger JM, Rimsza LM, et al: A comparative analysis of prognostic factor models for follicular lymphoma based on a phase III trial of CHOP-rituximab versus CHOP + 131iodine-tositumomab. *Clin Cancer Res* 19:6624–6632, 2013.
19. Dave SS, Wright G, Tan B, et al: Prediction of survival in follicular lymphoma based on molecular features of tumor-infiltrating immune cells. *N Engl J Med* 351:2159–2169, 2004.
20. Morin RD, Mendez-Lago M, Mungall AJ, et al: Frequent mutation of histone-modifying genes in non-Hodgkin lymphoma. *Nature* 476:298–303, 2011.
21. Pasqualucci L, Dominguez-Sola D, Chiarenza A, et al: Inactivating mutations of acetyl-transferase genes in B-cell lymphoma. *Nature* 471:189–195, 2011.
22. Okosun J, Bodor C, Wang J, et al: Integrated genomic analysis identifies recurrent mutations and evolution patterns driving the initiation and progression of follicular lymphoma. *Nat Genet* 46:176–181, 2014.
23. Green MR, Gentles AJ, Nair RV, et al: Hierarchy in somatic mutations arising during genomic evolution and progression of follicular lymphoma. *Blood* 121:1604–1611, 2013.
24. Bodor C, Grossmann V, Popov N, et al: EZH2 mutations are frequent and represent an early event in follicular lymphoma. *Blood* 122:3165–3168, 2013.
25. Advani R, Rosenberg SA, Horning SJ: Stage I and II follicular non-Hodgkin's lymphoma: Long-term follow-up of no initial therapy. *J Clin Oncol* 22:1454–1459, 2004.
26. Schmatz AI, Streubel B, Kretschmer-Chott E, et al: Primary follicular lymphoma of the duodenum is a distinct mucosal/submucosal variant of follicular lymphoma: A retrospective study of 63 cases. *J Clin Oncol* 29:1445–1451, 2011.
27. Mac Manus MP, Hoppe RT: Is radiotherapy curative for stage I and II low-grade follicular lymphoma? Results of a long-term follow-up study of patients treated at Stanford University. *J Clin Oncol* 14:1282–1290, 1996.
28. Friedberg JW, Byrtek M, Link BK, et al: Effectiveness of first-line management strategies for stage I follicular lymphoma: Analysis of the National LymphoCare Study. *J Clin Oncol* 30:3368–3375, 2012.
29. Horning SJ, Rosenberg SA: The natural history of initially untreated low-grade non-Hodgkin's lymphomas. *N Engl J Med* 311:1471–1475, 1984.
30. Ardeshna KM, Smith P, Norton A, et al: Long-term effect of a watch and wait policy versus immediate systemic treatment for asymptomatic advanced-stage non-Hodgkin lymphoma: A randomised controlled trial. *Lancet* 362:516–522, 2003.
31. Young RC, Longo DL, Glatstein E, et al: The treatment of indolent lymphomas: Watchful waiting v aggressive combined modality treatment. *Semin Hematol* 25:11–16, 1988.
32. Brice P, Bastion Y, Lepage E, et al: Comparison in low-tumor-burden follicular lymphomas between an initial no-treatment policy, prednimustine, or interferon alfa: A randomized study from the Groupe d'Etude des Lymphomes Folliculaires. Groupe d'Etude des Lymphomes de l'Adulte. *J Clin Oncol* 15:1110–1117, 1997.
33. Friedberg JW, Cohen P, Chen L, et al: Bendamustine in patients with rituximab-refractory indolent and transformed non-Hodgkin's lymphoma: Results from a phase II multicenter, single-agent study. *J Clin Oncol* 26:204–210, 2008.
34. McLaughlin P, Grillo-Lopez AJ, Link BK, et al: Rituximab chimeric anti-CD20 monoclonal antibody therapy for relapsed indolent lymphoma: Half of patients respond to a four-dose treatment program. *J Clin Oncol* 16:2825–2833, 1998.
35. Colombat P, Salles G, Brousse N, et al: Rituximab (anti-CD20 monoclonal antibody) as single first-line therapy for patients with follicular lymphoma with a low tumor burden: Clinical and molecular evaluation. *Blood* 97:101–106, 2001.
36. Hainsworth JD: Rituximab as first-line systemic therapy for patients with low-grade lymphoma. *Semin Oncol* 27:25–29, 2000.
37. Davis TA, Grillo-Lopez AJ, White CA, et al: Rituximab anti-CD20 monoclonal antibody therapy in non-Hodgkin's lymphoma: Safety and efficacy of re-treatment. *J Clin Oncol* 18:3135–3143, 2000.
38. Ghielmini M, Schmitz SF, Cogliatti S, et al: Effect of single-agent rituximab given at the standard schedule or as prolonged treatment in patients with mantle cell lymphoma: A study of the Swiss Group for Clinical Cancer Research (SAKK). *J Clin Oncol* 23:705–711, 2005.
39. Hainsworth JD: Rituximab as first-line and maintenance therapy for patients with indolent non-Hodgkin's lymphoma: Interim follow-up of a multicenter phase II trial. *Semin Oncol* 29:25–29, 2002.
40. Hainsworth JD: First-line and maintenance treatment with rituximab for patients with indolent non-Hodgkin's lymphoma. *Semin Oncol* 30:9–15, 2003.
41. van Oers MH, Klasa R, Marcus RE, et al: Rituximab maintenance improves clinical outcome of relapsed/resistant follicular non-Hodgkin lymphoma in patients both with and without rituximab during induction: Results of a prospective randomized phase 3 intergroup trial. *Blood* 108:3295–3301, 2006.
42. Salles G, Seymour JF, Offner F, et al: Rituximab maintenance for 2 years in patients with high tumour burden follicular lymphoma responding to rituximab plus chemotherapy (PRIMA): A phase 3, randomised controlled trial. *Lancet* 377:42–51, 2011.
43. Bachy E, Houot R, Morschhauser F, et al: Long-term follow up of the FL2000 study comparing CHVP-interferon to CHVP-interferon plus rituximab in follicular lymphoma. *Haematologica* 98:1107–1114, 2013.
44. Hochster H, Weller E, Gascoyne RD, et al: Maintenance rituximab after cyclophosphamide, vincristine, and prednisone prolongs progression-free survival in advanced

indolent lymphoma: Results of the randomized phase III ECOG1496 Study. *J Clin Oncol* 27:1607–1614, 2009.

45. Marcus R, Imrie K, Solal-Celigny P, et al: Phase III study of R-CVP compared with cyclophosphamide, vincristine, and prednisone alone in patients with previously untreated advanced follicular lymphoma. *J Clin Oncol* 26:4579–4586, 2008.

46. Hiddemann W, Kneba M, Dreyling M, et al: Frontline therapy with rituximab added to the combination of cyclophosphamide, doxorubicin, vincristine, and prednisone (CHOP) significantly improves the outcome for patients with advanced-stage follicular lymphoma compared with therapy with CHOP alone: Results of a prospective randomized study of the German Low-Grade Lymphoma Study Group. *Blood* 106:3725–3732, 2005.

47. Herold M, Haas A, Srock S, et al: Rituximab added to first-line mitoxantrone, chlorambucil, and prednisolone chemotherapy followed by interferon maintenance prolongs survival in patients with advanced follicular lymphoma: An East German Study Group Hematology and Oncology Study. *J Clin Oncol* 25:1986–1992, 2007.

48. Marcus R, Imrie K, Belch A, et al: CVP chemotherapy plus rituximab compared with CVP as first-line treatment for advanced follicular lymphoma. *Blood* 105:1417–1423, 2005.

49. Forstpointner R, Dreyling M, Repp R, et al: The addition of rituximab to a combination of fludarabine, cyclophosphamide, mitoxantrone (FCM) significantly increases the response rate and prolongs survival as compared with FCM alone in patients with relapsed and refractory follicular and mantle cell lymphomas: Results of a prospective randomized study of the German Low-Grade Lymphoma Study Group. *Blood* 104:3064–3071, 2004.

50. Salles G, Mounier N, de Guibert S, et al: Rituximab combined with chemotherapy and interferon in follicular lymphoma patients: Results of the GELA-GOELAMS FL2000 study. *Blood* 112:4824–4831, 2008.

51. Press OW, Palanca-Wessels MC: Selection of first-line therapy for advanced follicular lymphoma. *J Clin Oncol* 31:1496–1498, 2013.

52. Rummel MJ, Niederle N, Maschmeyer G, et al: Bendamustine plus rituximab versus CHOP plus rituximab as first-line treatment for patients with indolent and mantle-cell lymphomas: An open-label, multicentre, randomised, phase 3 non-inferiority trial. *Lancet* 381:1203–1210, 2013.

53. Flinn IW, Van der Jagt RH, Kahl BS, et al: An open-label, randomized study of bendamustine and rituximab (BR) compared with rituximab, cyclophosphamide, vincristine, and prednisone (R-CVP) or rituximab, cyclophosphamide, doxorubicin, vincristine, and prednisone (R-CHOP) in first-line treatment of patients with advanced indolent non-Hodgkin's lymphoma (NHL) or mantle cell lymphoma (MCL): The Bright Study. *Blood* 123(19):2944–2952, 2014.

54. van Oers MH, Van Glabbeke M, Giurgea L, et al: Rituximab maintenance treatment of relapsed/resistant follicular non-Hodgkin's lymphoma: Long-term outcome of the EORTC 20981 phase III randomized intergroup study. *J Clin Oncol* 28:2853–2858, 2010.

55. Goldenberg DM, Sharkey RM: Advances in cancer therapy with radiolabeled monoclonal antibodies. *Q J Nucl Med Mol Imaging* 50:248–264, 2006.

56. Press OW: Evidence mounts for the efficacy of radioimmunotherapy for B-cell lymphomas. *J Clin Oncol* 26:5147–5150, 2008.

57. Kaminski MS, Estes J, Zasadny KR, et al: Radioimmunotherapy with iodine (131) I tositumomab for relapsed or refractory B-cell non-Hodgkin lymphoma: Updated results and long-term follow-up of the University of Michigan experience. *Blood* 96:1259–1266, 2000.

58. Witzig TE, Flinn IW, Gordon LI, et al: Treatment with ibritumomab tiuxetan radioimmunotherapy in patients with rituximab-refractory follicular non-Hodgkin's lymphoma. *J Clin Oncol* 20:3262–3269, 2002.

59. Witzig TE, Gordon LI, Cabanillas F, et al: Randomized controlled trial of yttrium-90-labeled ibritumomab tiuxetan radioimmunotherapy versus rituximab immunotherapy for patients with relapsed or refractory low-grade, follicular, or transformed B-cell non-Hodgkin's lymphoma. *J Clin Oncol* 20:2453–2463, 2002.

60. Witzig TE: The use of ibritumomab tiuxetan radioimmunotherapy for patients with relapsed B-cell non-Hodgkin's lymphoma. *Semin Oncol* 27:74–78, 2000.

61. Davis TA, Kaminski MS, Leonard JP, et al: The radioisotope contributes significantly to the activity of radioimmunotherapy. *Clin Cancer Res* 10:7792–7798, 2004.

62. Kaminski MS, Tuck M, Estes J, et al: 131I-tositumomab therapy as initial treatment for follicular lymphoma. *N Engl J Med* 352:441–449, 2005.

63. Leonard JP, Coleman M, Kostakoglu L, et al: Abbreviated chemotherapy with fludarabine followed by tositumomab and iodine I 131 tositumomab for untreated follicular lymphoma. *J Clin Oncol* 23:5696–5704, 2005.

64. Press OW, Unger JM, Braziel RM, et al: Phase II trial of CHOP chemotherapy followed by tositumomab/iodine I-131 tositumomab for previously untreated follicular non-Hodgkin's lymphoma: Five-year follow-up of Southwest Oncology Group Protocol S9911. *J Clin Oncol* 24:4143–4149, 2006.

65. Morschhauser F, Radford J, Van Hoof A, et al: 90Yttrium-ibritumomab tiuxetan consolidation of first remission in advanced-stage follicular non-Hodgkin lymphoma: Updated results after a median follow-up of 7.3 years from the international, randomized, phase III first-line indolent trial. *J Clin Oncol* 31:1977–1983, 2013.

66. Rohatiner AZ, Gregory WM, Peterson B, et al: Meta-analysis to evaluate the role of interferon in follicular lymphoma. *J Clin Oncol* 23:2215–2223, 2005.

67. Freedman A, Neelapu SS, Nichols C, et al: Placebo-controlled phase III trial of patient-specific immunotherapy with mitumprotimut-T and granulocyte-macrophage colony-stimulating factor after rituximab in patients with follicular lymphoma. *J Clin Oncol* 27:3036–3043, 2009.

68. Brody J, Kohrt H, Marabelle A, et al: Active and passive immunotherapy for lymphoma: Proving principles and improving results. *J Clin Oncol* 29:1864–1875, 2011.

69. Schuster SJ, Neelapu SS, Gause BL, et al: Vaccination with patient-specific tumor-derived antigen in first remission improves disease-free survival in follicular lymphoma. *J Clin Oncol* 29:2787–2794, 2011.

70. Rohatiner AZ, Nadler L, Davies AJ, et al: Myeloablative therapy with autologous bone marrow transplantation for follicular lymphoma at the time of second or subsequent remission: Long-term follow-up. *J Clin Oncol* 25:2554–2559, 2007.

71. Schouten HC, Qian W, Kvaloy S, et al: High-dose therapy improves progression-free survival and survival in relapsed follicular non-Hodgkin's lymphoma: Results from the randomized European CUP trial. *J Clin Oncol* 21:3918–3927, 2003.

72. Deconinck E, Foussard C, Milpied N, et al: High-dose therapy followed by autologous purged stem-cell transplantation and doxorubicin-based chemotherapy in patients with advanced follicular lymphoma: A randomized multicenter study by GOELAMS. *Blood* 105:3817–3823, 2005.

73. Lenz G, Dreyling M, Schiegnitz E, et al: Myeloablative radiochemotherapy followed by autologous stem cell transplantation in first remission prolongs progression-free survival in follicular lymphoma: Results of a prospective, randomized trial of the German Low-Grade Lymphoma Study Group. *Blood* 104:2667–2674, 2004.

74. Bierman PJ, Sweetenham JW, Loberiza FR, Jr., et al: Syngeneic hematopoietic stem-cell transplantation for non-Hodgkin's lymphoma: A comparison with allogeneic and autologous transplantation—The Lymphoma Working Committee of the International Bone Marrow Transplant Registry and the European Group for Blood and Marrow Transplantation. *J Clin Oncol* 21:3744–3753, 2003.

75. van Besien K, Loberiza FR, Jr., Bajorunaite R, et al: Comparison of autologous and allogeneic hematopoietic stem cell transplantation for follicular lymphoma. *Blood* 102:3521–3529, 2003.

76. Rezvani AR, Storer B, Maris M, et al: Nonmyeloablative allogeneic hematopoietic cell transplantation in relapsed, refractory, and transformed indolent non-Hodgkin's lymphoma. *J Clin Oncol* 26:211–217, 2008.

77. Khouri IF, Saliba RM, Erwin WD, et al: Nonmyeloablative allogeneic transplantation with or without 90yttrium ibritumomab tiuxetan is potentially curative for relapsed follicular lymphoma: 12-year results. *Blood* 119:6373–6378, 2012.

78. Al-Tourah AJ, Gill KK, Chhanabhai M, et al: Population-based analysis of incidence and outcome of transformed non-Hodgkin's lymphoma. *J Clin Oncol* 26:5165–5169, 2008.

79. Montoto S, Davies AJ, Matthews J, et al: Risk and clinical implications of transformation of follicular lymphoma to diffuse large B-cell lymphoma. *J Clin Oncol* 25:2426–2433, 2007.

80. Oviatt DL, Cousar JB, Collins RD, et al: Malignant lymphomas of follicular center cell origin in humans. V. Incidence, clinical features, and prognostic implications of transformation of small cleaved cell nodular lymphoma. *Cancer* 53:1109–1114, 1984.

81. Link BK, Maurer MJ, Nowakowski GS, et al: Rates and outcomes of follicular lymphoma transformation in the immunochemotherapy era: A report from the University of Iowa/Mayo Clinic Specialized Program of Research Excellence Molecular Epidemiology Resource. *J Clin Oncol* 31:3272–3278, 2013.

82. Villa D, Crump M, Panzarella T, et al: Autologous and allogeneic stem-cell transplantation for transformed follicular lymphoma: A report of the Canadian blood and marrow transplant group. *J Clin Oncol* 31:1164–1171, 2013.

83. Advani RH, Buggy JJ, Sharman JP, et al: Bruton tyrosine kinase inhibitor ibrutinib (PCI-32765) has significant activity in patients with relapsed/refractory B-cell malignancies. *J Clin Oncol* 31:88–94, 2013.

84. Wang ML, Rule S, Martin P, et al: Targeting BTK with ibrutinib in relapsed or refractory mantle-cell lymphoma. *N Engl J Med* 369:507–516, 2013.

85. Flinn IW, Kahl BS, Leonard JP, et al: Idelalisib, a selective inhibitor of phosphatidylinositol 3-kinase-delta, as therapy for previously treated indolent non-Hodgkin lymphoma. *Blood* 123:3406–3413, 2014.

86. Gopal AK, Kahl BS, de Vos S, et al: PI3Kdelta inhibition by idelalisib in patients with relapsed indolent lymphoma. *N Engl J Med* 370:1008–1018, 2014.

87. Davids MS, Letai A: ABT-199: Taking dead aim at BCL-2. *Cancer Cell* 23:139–141, 2013.

88. Souers AJ, Leverson JD, Boghaert ER, et al: ABT-199, a potent and selective BCL-2 inhibitor, achieves antitumor activity while sparing platelets. *Nat Med* 19:202–208, 2013.

89. Palanca-Wessels MC, Press OW: Advances in the treatment of hematologic malignancies using immunoconjugates. *Blood* 123:2293–2301, 2014.

90. Kochenderfer JN, Rosenberg SA: Treating B-cell cancer with T cells expressing anti-CD19 chimeric antigen receptors. *Nat Rev Clin Oncol* 10:267–276, 2013.

91. Budde LE, Berger C, Lin Y, et al: Combining a CD20 chimeric antigen receptor and an inducible caspase 9 suicide switch to improve the efficacy and safety of T cell adoptive immunotherapy for lymphoma. *PLoS One* 8:e82742, 2013.

92. Fisher RI, LeBlanc M, Press OW, et al: New treatment options have changed the survival of patients with follicular lymphoma. *J Clin Oncol* 23:8447–8452, 2005.

93. Liu Q, Fayad L, Cabanillas F, et al: Improvement of overall and failure-free survival in stage IV follicular lymphoma: 25 years of treatment experience at The University of Texas M.D. Anderson Cancer Center. *J Clin Oncol* 24:1582–1589, 2006.

94. Swenson WT, Wooldridge JE, Lynch CF, et al: Improved survival of follicular lymphoma patients in the United States. *J Clin Oncol* 23:5019–5026, 2005.

CHAPTER 100
MANTLE CELL LYMPHOMA

Martin Dreyling

SUMMARY

Mantle cell lymphoma is a distinct subtype of non-Hodgkin lymphoma with a pathognomonic chromosomal translocation t(11;14), leading to constitutive cyclin D1 overexpression. The clinical presentation usually is characterized by widespread disease, occurring more often in male patients older than age 60 years. Despite high initial response rates, early relapses occur frequently after conventional chemotherapy resulting in a median survival of only 3 to 5 years. However, 10 to 15 percent of patients present with a more indolent, chronic course. Dose-intensified treatment regimens containing cytarabine, rituximab, and autologous stem cell transplantation can achieve long-term remissions in patients fit enough to tolerate such aggressive therapy. For the majority of elderly patients, rituximab maintenance therapy can result in prolonged survival. Targeted approaches, including proteasome inhibitors, immunomodulatory drugs, and inhibitors of the B-cell receptor pathway, have proven highly efficacious in patients with relapsed disease and should be implemented in a multimodal treatment plan.

● DEFINITION AND HISTOLOGY

Mantle cell lymphoma (MCL) was originally named centrocytic lymphoma or subsumed under the term intermediate lymphocytic lymphoma. In 1992, the term *mantle cell lymphoma* was adopted for this entity because of morphologic and immunophenotypic similarities of the malignant cells to lymphocytes of the mantle zone of germinal centers.[1] In 1994, the term *mantle cell lymphoma* was incorporated into the revised European-American classification of the International Lymphoma Study Group, and remains a distinctive lymphoma subtype in the World Health Organization classification of malignant lymphoid disorders.[2,3]

Acronyms and Abbreviations: ASCT, autologous stem cell transplantation; ATM, ataxia-telangiectasia mutant; BR, bendamustine and rituximab; BTK, Bruton tyrosine kinase; CHOP, cyclophosphamide, doxorubicin, vincristine, and prednisone; CLL, chronic lymphocytic leukemia; DHAP, dexamethasone, high-dose cytarabine, and cisplatinum; E2F, elongation factor 2; LDH, lactate dehydrogenase; MCL, mantle cell lymphoma; MIPI, Mantle Cell Lymphoma International Prognostic Index; mTOR, mammalian target of rapamycin; MTX, methotrexate; NF-κB, nuclear factor-κB; PI3K, phosphoinositol 3′-kinase; PFS, progression-free survival; R-CHOP, rituximab, cyclophosphamide, doxorubicin, vincristine, and prednisone; R-CVP, rituximab, cyclophosphamide, vincristine, and prednisone; R-hyperCVAD, rituximab, hyperfractionated cyclophosphamide, vincristine, doxorubicin, and dexamethasone; sIg, secretory immunoglobulin; TBI, total-body irradiation.

Based on cytology, the classical form is characterized by small to intermediate-size cells with irregular, cleaved nuclei, dense chromatin, and indistinct nucleoli. A *small cell* variant, resembling chronic lymphocytic leukemia (CLL), may be associated with a more indolent course.[4] In contrast, the blastoid cell variant, including a blastic and a pleomorphic phenotype, displays a more aggressive clinical course.[3]

Histologically, MCL most frequently displays a diffuse infiltration of the lymph nodes, less commonly a nodular pattern, and, rarely, a mantle zone pattern, the latter of which may represent an earlier phase of the disease.[5] The immunophenotype of the cells resembles the lymphocytes in the mantle zone of normal germinal follicles, and is characterized by coexpression of B-cell antigens (CD19+, CD20+, CD22+, CD43+, CD79+, secretory immunoglobulin [sIg] M+, sIgD+) and the T-cell associated marker CD5+. Based on their predominantly pregerminal center origin, MCL cells stain strongly for the antiapoptotic protein BCL-2, but are negative for germinal center markers like CD10 and BCL-6.[3]

Because of the morphologic heterogeneity of MCL, detection of the MCL genetic hallmark, either by immunohistochemistry (cyclin D1 overexpression) or fluorescence *in situ* hybridization (chromosomal translocation t[11;14][q13;q32]) is crucial to confirm the diagnosis. In rare cases that are negative for cyclin D1, staining for SOX11, a transcription factor specifically expressed in more than 90 percent of MCL cases, may help to establish the diagnosis.[6]

● EPIDEMIOLOGY

MCL represents approximately 6 percent of all non-Hodgkin lymphomas, although a lower incidence has also been reported.[7,8] Between 1992 and 2004, the age-adjusted annual incidence more than doubled from about 0.3 to 0.7 cases per 100,000. The incidence is more than twice as high in males and increases with age. Median age at presentation is approximately 65 years. No specific etiologic agent has been associated with MCL.

● ETIOLOGY AND PATHOGENESIS

The chromosomal translocation t(11;14) results in overexpression of cyclin D1, a cell-cycle protein not normally expressed in lymphoid cells. The very rare cyclin D1–negative cases usually overexpress cyclin D2 or D3.[6] The cytogenetic abnormality t(11;14) is the primary event in the pathogenesis of MCL, facilitating the deregulation of the cell cycle at the G_1–S phase transition.[9] However, additional genetic events are required for the clinical manifestation of MCL. Thus, a low copy-number of the t(11;14) translocation has been found in the blood cells of 1 to 2 percent of healthy individuals without evidence of clinical disease.[10] Cytogenetic studies have identified frequent secondary genetic alterations that are involved in cell-cycle dysregulation and DNA repair, which may explain why MCL has one of the highest levels of genomic instability among the malignant lymphoid neoplasms. These genetic abnormalities include losses in chromosomes 1p13–p31, 2q13, 6q23–27, 8p21, 9p21, 10p14–15, 11q22–23, 13q11–13, 13q14–34, 17p13, and 22q12; gains in chromosomes 3q25, 4p12–13, 7p21–22, 8q21, 9q22, 10p11–12, 12q13, and 18q11q23; and high copy-number amplifications of certain chromosomal regions.[11]

Figure 100–1 depicts a proposed scheme relating genetic derangements with specific MCL subtypes. Cell-cycle dysregulation is a hallmark of MCL. The overexpressed cyclin D1 complexes with CDK4, which results in phosphorylation of the retinoblastoma gene *RB1* and release of elongation factor 2 (E2F) transcription factors and progression

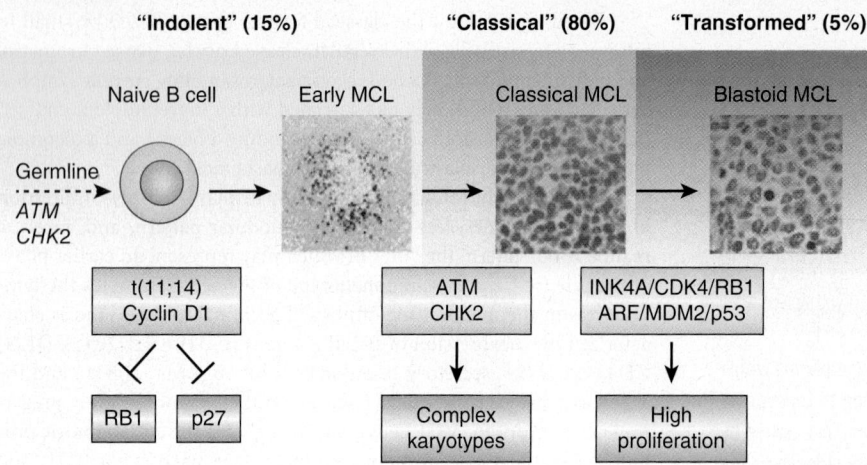

"Indolent" (15%)   "Classical" (80%)   "Transformed" (5%)

Figure 100–1. Proposed model of molecular pathogenesis of mantle cell lymphoma (MCL). The t(11;14) translocation leads to the constitutive deregulation of cyclin D1. Acquired inactivation of DNA damage response pathways may facilitate additional genetic alterations and the development of classical MCL. Further genetic alterations may target genes of the cell cycle and senescence regulatory pathways, leading to more proliferative and aggressive variants of MCL. (*Modified with permission from Jares P, Colomer D, Campo E: Genetic and molecular pathogenesis of mantle cell lymphoma: Perspectives for new targeted therapeutics. Nat Rev Cancer 7(10):750–762, 2007.*)

of the lymphoma cells into S-phase. In addition, mutation of the ataxia-telangiectasia mutant *(ATM)* gene facilitates genomic instability in lymphoma cells through impaired response to DNA damage. Phosphoinositol 3′-kinase (PI3K) and mammalian target of rapamycin (mTOR) are important downstream targets of this signaling pathway. Finally, specific gene alterations, namely *p53* or *p16/CDKN2*, are associated with the blastoid variant and poor clinical outcome.[12,13]

According to the characteristic cyclin D1 overexpression, molecular profiling has identified a *cell proliferation* gene signature that distinguishes patient subsets that differ by more than 5 years in median survival.[14] A five-gene model to predict survival in MCL based on formalin-fixed, paraffin-embedded tissue has been devised.[15] In the clinical setting, only Ki-67 expression, a cell-cycle–related protein, as determined by immunohistochemistry, has been prospectively confirmed as a reliable prognostic marker, which allows the identification of high-risk patients (Ki-67 >30 percent) who may qualify for more-aggressive therapeutic approaches.[5,16] This marker is independent of clinical features including the Mantle Cell Lymphoma International Prognostic Index (MIPI) score (see Clinical Features and Risk Factors[20,21] below).

CLINICAL FEATURES AND RISK FACTORS

MCL typically presents in an older male patient with lymphadenopathy in several sites (e.g., cervical, axillary, inguinal). The patient may be asymptomatic but some experience fever, night sweats, or weight loss (Table 100–1).[5,17] The spleen is enlarged in 40 percent of patients. Marrow is involved with MCL in the vast majority of patients, and 50 percent of patients present with blood involvement, sometimes with an overt leukemic phase.

In 25 percent of cases, there is symptomatic gastrointestinal involvement, typically presenting as *polyposis coli*.[18] Gastrointestinal symptoms may include abdominal pain and diarrhea, signs of small-bowel obstruction, or hematochezia. The intestinal polyps usually appear in the ileocecal region, and histopathologic analysis and immunocytochemistry are required to confirm the diagnosis of MCL involvement. Asymptomatic gastrointestinal involvement may be detected in up to 90 percent of cases; thus, endoscopy and histologic analysis of random biopsies are recommended, especially in the few cases with localized stage.

The frequency of CNS disease is low at first diagnosis but increases with subsequent relapses and correlates with elevated

TABLE 100–1. Patient Characteristics at Presentation (304 Cases)

Characteristic	Number
Age (years)	
<60	123
>60	178
Sex	
Male	230
Female	71
Stage	
I–II	23
III–IV	267
Status (World Health Organization)	
0–1	233
≥2	43
Lactate dehydrogenase	
Elevated	56
Normal	140
International Prognostic Index	
0–1	15
≥2	75
Marrow involvement	
Yes	207
No	81
B symptoms	
Yes	107
No	155
Extranodal involvement	
Yes	161
No	16

Data from Tiemann M, Schrader C, Klapper W, et al: European MCL Network: Histopathology, cell proliferation indices and clinical outcome in 304 patients with mantle cell lymphoma (MCL): A clinicopathological study from the European MCL Network. *Br J Haematol* 131(1):29–38, 2005.

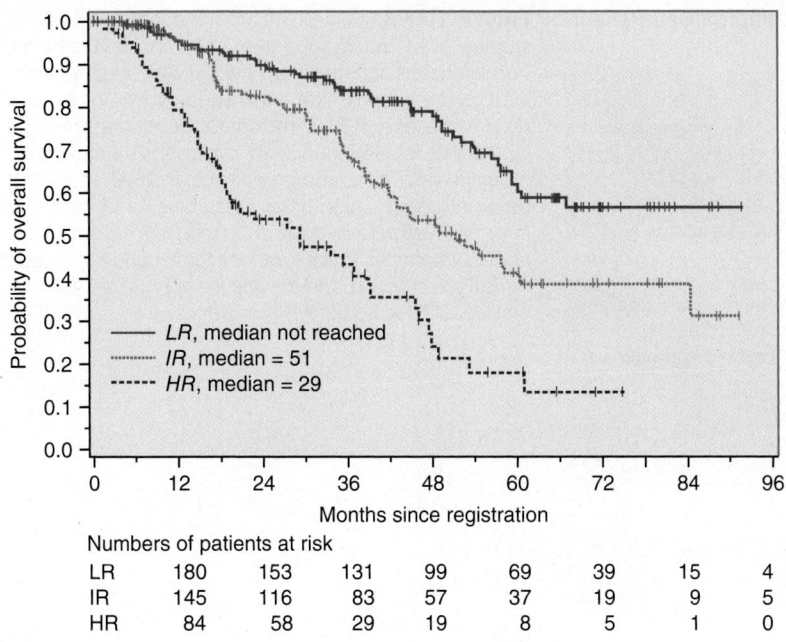

Figure 100–2. Overall survival according to Mantle Cell Lymphoma International Prognostic Index (MIPI). LR, low risk; IR, intermediate risk; HR, high risk. *(Reproduced with permission from Hoster E, Dreyling M, Klapper W, et al: German Low Grade Lymphoma Study Group (GLSG); European Mantle Cell Lymphoma Network: A new prognostic index (MIPI) for patients with advanced-stage mantle cell lymphoma. Blood 111(2):558–565, 2008.)*

lactate dehydrogenase (LDH), blastoid cytology, and cell proliferation (Ki-67).[19] There is no consensus on the need for CNS prophylaxis.

Prognostic parameters include the serum level of β_2-microglobulin and LDH, blastoid cytology, age, Ann Arbor stage, extranodal presentation, and constitutional symptoms, among others.[5] Most of these prognostic variables were determined retrospectively and are based on doxorubicin-containing regimens only. Thus, a prognostic model, the MIPI, was established, which implements four independent prognostic factors: age, performance status, LDH, and leukocyte count (Fig. 100–2).[20] This score has been confirmed in numerous series, including in a prospective study that corroborated the reliability of this score for various chemotherapy-based regimens.[21]

Based on frequent marrow involvement, detection of minimal residual disease with patient-specific primers allows the detection of one malignant cell in 10^5 to 10^6 background cells. A number of reports have confirmed a correlation between molecular residual disease and clinical recurrence.[22,23] This fact has been used in trials evaluating the value of preemptive treatment with rituximab prior to emergence of clinical evidence of recurrence.

● DIFFERENTIAL DIAGNOSIS

The clinical presentation of MCL may resemble CLL or other indolent nodal lymphomas. The immunophenotype of CLL is similar with coexpression of immunoglobulin (Ig) M and IgD, the B-cell–associated antigens CD19 and CD20, and aberrant expression of the T-cell antigen CD5. In contrast to MCL cells, however, CD23 is typically highly expressed in CLL. Like follicular lymphoma, MCL is positive for CD20 and BCL-2, but in contrast to follicular lymphoma, MCL is negative for CD10 and BCL-6. However, because these expression patterns vary, analysis of cyclin D1 overexpression or t(11;14) remains crucial to confirm or exclude the diagnosis of MCL.

● THERAPY

In general, MCL is still considered incurable and most patients follow an aggressive clinical course. However, 10 to 15 percent of patients may exhibit a more indolent evolution and may not require therapy for several years. These cases are commonly characterized by a nonnodal leukemic presentation with only marrow involvement and splenomegaly.[4] Sox-11 negativity may also identify some of these more indolent cases, although its role is controversial, as additional *p53* mutations may cause an aggressive clinical evolution (see Fig. 100–1).[25] Thus, the reliable diagnosis of indolent cases is difficult, and a short, watchful, waiting period under close observation seems to be appropriate in cases with low tumor burden.[26]

LOCALIZED STAGE

Localized disease with low tumor burden is rare. A small retrospective review has suggested long-term remissions after involved-field radiotherapy (30 to 36 Gray).[27] In contrast, in a randomized trial all patients relapsed within a year.[28] Thus, a shortened chemotherapy induction followed by radiation consolidation seems to be most appropriate.

ADVANCED STAGE

Conventional Chemotherapy

Because of the typical aggressive clinical presentation, anthracycline-containing chemotherapy has usually been applied to MCL in the past, although a small randomized trial did not confirm a major clinical benefit.[29] Complete remission rates are only 30 to 40 percent with cyclophosphamide, doxorubicin, vincristine, and prednisone (CHOP), typically with a short duration of response of 10 to 12 months.[30,31]

Combined Immunochemotherapy

Rituximab monotherapy achieves low response rates of approximately 25 percent, and should be used only in medically unfit patients who are not able to tolerate cytotoxic therapy (Fig. 100–3).[32] On the other hand, addition of rituximab to chemotherapy has been shown to significantly improve complete response rates, overall response rates, and overall survival in a systematic meta-analysis, making immunochemotherapy the standard of care, both in first-line and relapsed settings for patients with advanced stage MCL (Table 100–2).[33–43] In patients with an overt

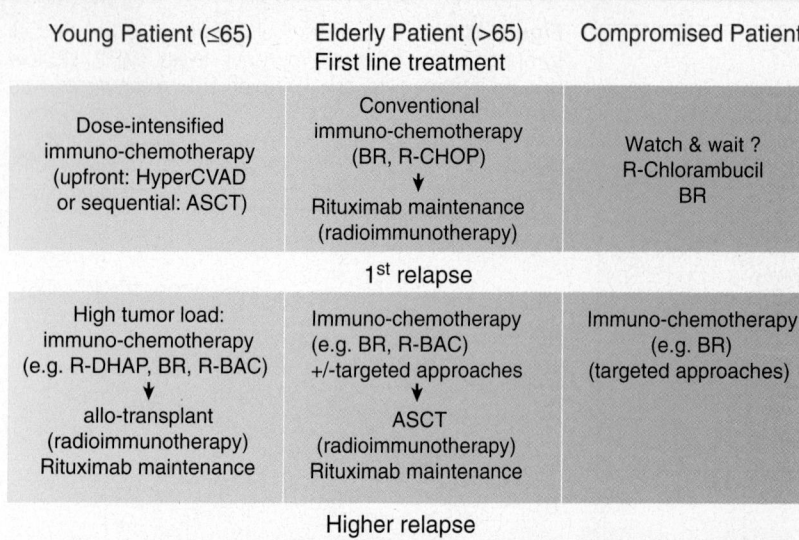

Young Patient (≤65) | Elderly Patient (>65) First line treatment | Compromised Patient

Dose-intensified immuno-chemotherapy (upfront: HyperCVAD or sequential: ASCT)

Conventional immuno-chemotherapy (BR, R-CHOP)
↓
Rituximab maintenance (radioimmunotherapy)

Watch & wait ? R-Chlorambucil BR

1st relapse

High tumor load: immuno-chemotherapy (e.g. R-DHAP, BR, R-BAC)
↓
allo-transplant (radioimmunotherapy) Rituximab maintenance

Immuno-chemotherapy (e.g. BR, R-BAC) +/-targeted approaches
↓
ASCT (radioimmunotherapy) Rituximab maintenance

Immuno-chemotherapy (e.g. BR) (targeted approaches)

Higher relapse

-Targeted approaches: Temsirolimus, Bortezomib, Ibrutinib, Lenalidomide (preferably in combination)
-Repeat previous therapy (long prior remissions)

Figure 100–3. Clinical recommendations outside of studies. ASCT, autologous stem cell transplantation; BR, bendamustine and rituximab; hyperCVAD, hyperfractionated cyclophosphamide, vincristine, doxorubicin, and dexamethasone; R-BAC, rituximab, bendamustine, and cytarabine; R-CHOP, rituximab, cyclophosphamide, doxorubicin, vincristine, and prednisone; R-DHAP, rituximab, dexamethasone, high-dose cytarabine, and cisplatin. *(Modified with permission from Dreyling M, European Mantle Cell Lymphoma Network: Mantle cell lymphoma: Biology, clinical presentation, and therapeutic approaches.* Am Soc Clin Oncol Educ Book *191–198, 2014.)*

leukemic phase and high lymphocyte counts of greater than $50 \times 10^9/L$, the first dose of rituximab should be delivered with caution because of the risk of tumor lysis syndrome or cytokine-release syndrome.

In a randomized trial, rituximab with CHOP considerably improved response rates (94 percent vs. 75 percent), and time to treatment failure in comparison to CHOP chemotherapy alone.[34] In contrast, rituximab with cyclophosphamide, vincristine, and prednisone (R-CVP) resulted in significantly inferior response rates and progression-free survival (PFS), and cannot be recommended in patients with MCL.[44] Similarly, fludarabine combinations result in prolonged cytopenias, and resulted in overall survival rates significantly inferior (46 percent vs. 62 percent at 4 years) to those achieved with rituximab, cyclophosphamide, doxorubicin, vincristine, and prednisone (R-CHOP) in a large prospective European trial.[39] In contrast, a bendamustine-based combination resulted in similar response rates (93 percent vs. 91 percent) and PFS in two randomized trials, but a more favorable toxicity profile, particularly with regard to alopecia and peripheral neuropathy, making the bendamustine and rituximab (BR) regimen the most commonly administered regimen currently, especially in elderly patients.[41,44] Finally, an intensified approach combining bendamustine with cytarabine resulted in impressive response rates (100 percent), but significant thrombocytopenia, suggesting that this regimen should be used only in young, fit patients.[42]

In conclusion, BR and R-CHOP represent the current standard approaches in older patients who represent the majority of MCL patients (see Fig. 100–3). Based on clinical presentation, BR may be preferable, especially in patients with CLL-like presentation, whereas CHOP seems to be appropriate in the more-aggressive cases with elevated LDH. Especially in blastoid variants, one might consider cytarabine-containing regimens based on the improved results in younger patients.[45] However, such an individualized approach has never been tested in a prospective fashion.

Maintenance/Consolidation

The concept of regular rituximab maintenance, previously established in follicular lymphoma, has also been investigated in MCL.[39]

After conventional R-CHOP induction, continuous antibody maintenance results in an impressive prolongation of both PFS (58 percent vs. 29 percent at 4 years) and overall survival (79 percent vs. 67 percent at 4 years) so that rituximab maintenance is now generally recommended.

Alternatively, radioimmunotherapy consolidation has been tested after a shortened R-CHOP induction. Again, survival rates seem to be prolonged with a median time to treatment failure of 31 months, but results seem to be inferior to ongoing rituximab maintenance, possibly because of the single-application scheme used with radioimmunotherapy.[40]

Intensive Chemotherapy with and without Stem Cell Transplantation

In several studies, either intensified upfront therapy or the addition of high-dose consolidation followed by autologous stem cell transplantation (ASCT) resulted in impressive survival rates (Table 100–3).[45–56] A randomized trial has proven that ASCT prolongs PFS in comparison to CHOP-like induction therapy alone (3.3 vs. 1.4 years).[46] In a subsequent meta-analysis, overall survival was also significantly prolonged by ASCT, independent of the addition of rituximab.[57] "*In vivo* purging" with a rituximab-containing induction regimen was shown to further improve long-term survival. Various studies have investigated the potential benefit of cytarabine-containing induction regimens (Table 100–3). Most importantly, a randomized trial demonstrated that the median PFS was almost doubled by the administration of the R-CHOP/DHAP (dexamethasone, high-dose cytarabine, and cisplatinum) regimen (7.6 vs. 3.8 years) compared to administration of R-CHOP alone prior to ASCT.[45] In contrast, a phase II study suggested that high-dose methotrexate (MTX) adds significant organ toxicity, but similar long term remissions could be also achieved with considerably reduced doses.[47]

A study-to-study comparison suggests a benefit of a total-body irradiation (TBI)–containing high-dose consolidation in patients with only partial remission after induction, whereas such benefit was not observed for the addition of conventionally dosed radioimmunotherapy.[58,59]

TABLE 100–2. Conventional Immuno-Chemotherapy for Mantle Cell Lymphoma

Author (Year)	Phase	Number of Patients	Regimen	ORR% (CR%)	Median PFS (Months)	2-Year OS (%)
Howard (2002)[33]	II	40	R-CHOP	96 (48)	17	95 (3 years)
Lenz (2005)[34]	III	112	CHOP	75 (7)	14 (TTF)	77
			R-CHOP	94 (34)	21 (TTF)	77
Herold (2008)[35]	III	90	MCP	63 (15)	18	52 (4 years)
			R-MCP	71 (32)	20	55 (4 years)
Gressin (2010)[37]	II	113	R-VAD-C	73 (48)	18 (no ASCT) 58 (ASCT)	62 (3 years)
Sachenes (2011)[38]	II	20	R-chlorambucil	95 (90)	89% (3 years)	95 (3 years)
Kenkra (2011)[36]	II	22	R-hyperCVAD R maintenance	77 (64)	38	62 (4 years)
Kluin-Nelemans (2012)[39]	III	485	R-CHOP	86 (34)	28 (TTF)	62 (4 years)
			R-FC	78 (40)	26 (TTF)	47 (4 years)
		274	I maintenance	NA	29% (4 year DR)	67 (4 years)
			R maintenance		58% (4 year DR)	79 (4 years)
Smith (2012)[40]	II	50	R-CHOP 90Y-Ibritumumab	64 (46)	31 (TTF)	73 (5 years)
Rummel (2013)[41]	III	94	R-CHOP	91 (30)	21	No difference
			BR	93 (40)	35	
Visco (2013)[42]	II	20	R-BAC	100 (95)	95% (2 years)	93
Ruan (2011)[93]	II	35	R-CHOP + bortezomib	91 (72)	44% (2 years)	86
Houot (2012)[99]	II	29	R-doxorubicin/ dexamethasone/ chlorambucil + bortezomib	79 (59)	26	69
Chang (2014)[59A]	II	75	R-hyperCVAD + bortezomib R maintenance	95 (68)	67% (3 years)	91 (3 years)
Robak (2015)[98]	III	487	R-CHOP	89 (53)	14	54 (4 years)
			R-CHP + bortezomib	92 (42)	25	64 (4 years)
Inwards (2014)[101]	I	17	R-cladribine + temsirolimus	94 (53)	19	65

ASCT, autologous stem cell transplantation; BR, bendamustine and rituximab; CR, complete response; MCP, mitoxantrone, chlorambucil, and prednisolone; ORR, overall response rate; OS, overall survival; PFS, progression-free survival; R-BAC, rituximab, bendamustine, and cytarabine; R-CHOP, rituximab, cyclophosphamide, doxorubicin, vincristine, and prednisone; R-CHP, rituximab, cyclophosphamide, doxorubicin, and prednisone; R-FC, rituximab, fludarabine, and cyclophosphamide; R-hyperCVAD, rituximab, hyperfractionated cyclophosphamide, vincristine, doxorubicin, and dexamethasone; R-MCP, rituximab, mitoxantrone, chlorambucil, and prednisone; TTF, time to treatment failure; 90Y, yttrium-90.

The upper panel includes six studies using immunochemotherapy; the lower panel includes five studies that combine rituximab with other drugs.

An interim analysis has suggested a benefit from subsequent rituximab maintenance, but further followup is necessary to confirm the superiority of this approach.[53]

Alternatively, upfront dose intensification may be applied. The rituximab plus hyperfractionated cyclophosphamide, vincristine, doxorubicin, and dexamethasone (R-hyperCVAD) regimen has achieved high complete response rates and long-term remissions in various trials.[54–56] However, this regimen is hampered by significant therapy-associated toxicity, including secondary malignancies, and should only be considered in young, fit patients.

RECURRENT AND REFRACTORY DISEASE

Salvage Chemotherapy

The inherent resistance of MCL to conventional doses of chemotherapy becomes especially apparent in relapsed disease. Conventional immunochemotherapy options, some of them highly effective in first line treatment, achieve only short term remissions in relapsed disease. (Table 100–4).[42,60–64] Thus, consolidation with ASCT deserves consideration if not already employed in the frontline setting. Unfortunately, long-term results of this approach in recurrent/refractory MCL are rather sobering.

TABLE 100–3. Dose-Intensified Immunochemotherapy of Mantle Cell Lymphoma

Author (Year)	Phase	Number of Patients	Regimen	ORR% (CR%)	Median PFS (Years)	OS (%)
Dreyling (2005)[46]	III	122	R-CHOP + ASCT	98 (81)	3.3	83 (3 years)
			R-CHOP + IFN	99 (37)	1.4	77 (3 years)
De Guibert (2006)[51]	II	17	R-DHAP + ASCT	100 (94)	76% (3 years)	75% (3 years)
		7	R-DHAP	86 (86)	NA	NA
Damon (2009)[47]	II	77	R-CHOP/MTX/Ara-C/etoposide + ASCT	88 (69)	56% (5 years)	64 (5 years)
van 't Veer (2009)[48]	II	87	R-CHOP/Ara-C + ASCT	70 (64)	36% (4 years)	56 (4 years)
Magni (2009)[52]	II	28	Sequential R-chemo + ASCT	100 (100)	57% (low risk)	76 (low risk)
					34% (high risk)	68 (high risk)
Geisler (2012)[49]	II	160	R-maxiCHOP/Ara-C + ASCT	96 (54)	7.4	58 (10 years)
Hermine (2012)[45]	III	455	R-CHOP + ASCT	97 (61)	3.8	67 (5 years)
			R-CHOP/DHAP + ASCT	98 (63)	7.3	74 (5 years)
Delarue (2013)[50]	II	60	R-CHOP/DHAP + ASCT	100 (96)	6.9	75 (5 years)
Le Gouill (2014)[53]	III	299	R-DHAP + ASCT	NA	83% (2 years)	93% (2 years)
			R-DHAP + ASCT + R maintenance	NA	93% (2 years)	95% (2 years)
Romaguera (2010)[54]	II	97	R-hyperCVAD	97 (87)	4.5	64 (10 years)
Merli (2012)[55]	II	60	R-hyperCVAD	83 (72)	61% (5 years)	73 (5 years)
Bernstein (2013)[56]	II	2013	R-hyperCVAD	86 (55)	4.8	63 (5 years)

Ara-C, cytarabine; ASCT, autologous stem cell transplantation; CR, complete response; DHAP, dexamethasone, high-dose cytarabine, and cisplatinum; IFN, interferon; MTX, methotrexate; ORR, overall response rate; OS, overall survival; PFS, progression-free survival; R, rituximab; R-CHOP, rituximab, cyclophosphamide, doxorubicin, vincristine, and prednisone; R-DHAP, rituximab, dexamethasone, high-dose cytarabine, and cisplatinum; R-hyperCVAD, rituximab, hyperfractionated cyclophosphamide, vincristine, doxorubicin, and dexamethasone; R-maxiCHOP, cyclophosphamide, hydroxydaunorubicin, vincristine, and prednisone.

The upper panel includes nine studies using sequential intensification with autologous stem cell transplantation (ASCT); the lower panel includes three studies that use upfront intensification.

In younger patients responding to salvage therapy, it is recommended to discuss the option of potentially curative allogeneic transplantation, based on the observed graft-versus-lymphoma activity in MCL. Reduced intensity conditioning may be applicable also in patients older than age 60 years, but is hampered by delayed toxicities, including chronic graft-versus-host disease and 20 to 25 percent treatment-related mortality.[65–68]

In elderly patients, one might consider rituximab maintenance if not administered previously. Alternatively, radioimmunotherapy consolidation has achieved long-term remissions in some patients, although efficacy as a single approach is limited with a median time to progression of only 5 months.[69,70]

Targeted Approaches

Chemotherapy alone has only short-term activity in relapsed disease, and therefore a number of targeted approaches have been investigated, especially in relapsed MCL, both as single agents and in combination with chemotherapy (see Tables 100–4 and 100–5).[71–97]

Proteasome Inhibitors Bortezomib, a first-generation proteosome inhibitor, is thought to exert its effect in part through alterations in the nuclear factor-κB (NF-κB). In relapsed disease, this single agent has shown response rates of 30 to 40 percent with a median PFS of approximately 6 months, which led to the first Federal Drug Administration approval of a targeted drug in relapsed MCL.[71–73] In subsequent trials, bortezomib was evaluated in combination with different chemotherapy regimens to further improve remission rates and avoid cumulative side effects (see Table 100–4).[88–93] Based on the encouraging data, a first-line trial has been completed. Substituting bortezomib for vincristine (within R-CHOP) led to an almost doubling of PFS.[98] In such a combined approach, bortezomib should be administered on only days 1 and 4 of each cycle to avoid cumulative thrombocytopenia.

Immunomodulatory Drugs Based on its oral formulation and its favorable tolerability, lenalidomide represents an attractive option, especially in the context of continuous treatment. After long-term efficacy was observed in multiple myeloma, various studies confirmed its benefit in relapsed MCL as well, with a response rate of 35 to 50 percent.[75–78] In a randomized phase II trial, this approach was superior to monochemotherapy (response rate 40 percent vs. 11 percent).[78] Other studies have investigated combining lenalidomide with chemotherapy.[94]

Mammalian Target of Rapamycin Inhibitors Temsirolimus has been registered by the European Union based on a randomized phase III trial proving its superiority compared to monochemotherapy in a highly refractory patient population (response rate, 22 percent vs. 2 percent).[81] Combining temsirolimus with chemotherapy resulted in objective responses in all evaluable patients in a phase I trial.[96]

TABLE 100-4. Conventional Immunochemotherapy of Relapsed Mantle Cell Lymphoma

Author (Year)	Phase	Number of Patients	Regimen	ORR% (CR%)	Median PFS (Months)	Median OS (Months)
Forstpointner (2004)[60]	III	24	FCM	46 (0)	4	11
		24	R-FCM	58 (29)	8	65% (2 years)
Rummel (2005)[61]	II	16	BR	75 (50)	18	NA
Robinson (2008)[62]	II	12	BR	92 (42)	19	NA
Weide (2007)[63]	II	18	BMR	78 (33)	21	60% (2 years)
Gironella (2012)[64]	II	28	R-GemOx	79 (75)	18	30
Visco (2013)[42]	II	20	R-BAC	80 (70)	87% (2 years)	93% (2 years)
Weigert (2009)[90]	Retrospective	8	R-Ara-C + bortezomib	50 (25)	5	16
Ruan (2010)[95]	II	22	R-PEP-C + bortezomib	73 (32)	10	45% (2 years)
Kouroukis (2011)[89]	II	25	Gemcitabine + bortezomib	60 (11)	11	NA
Friedberg (2011)[91]	II	7	BR + bortezomib	71 (NA)	NA	NA
Gerecitano (2011)[92]	II	10	R-CP + bortezomib	60 (50)	NA	NA
Furtado (2015)[88]	II	46				
			CHOP	48 (22)	8	12
			CHOP + bortezomib	83 (35)	17	36
Ruan (2010)[95]	II	22	R-PEP-C + thalidomide	73 (32)	10	45% (2 years)
Zaja[94]	II	42	BR + lenalidomide	79 (55)	68% (1year)	82% (1 year)
Hess (2015)[96]	I	11	BR + temsirolimus	91 (45)	22	92% (19 months)

BR, bendamustine and rituximab; BMR, bendamustine, mitoxantrone, rituximab; CHOP, cyclophosphamide, doxorubicin, vincristine, and prednisone; CR, complete response; FCM, fludarabine, cyclophosphamide, and mitoxantrone; ORR, overall response rate; OS, overall survival; PFS, progression-free survival; R-Ara-C, rituximab and cytarabine; R-BAC, rituximab, bendamustine, and cytarabine; R-CP, rituximab, cyclophosphamide, and prednisone; R-FCM, rituximab, fludarabine, cyclophosphamide, and mitoxantrone; R-GemOx, rituximab, gemcitabine, and oxaliplatin; R-PEP-C, rituximab, prednisone, etoposide, procarbazine, and cyclophosphamide.

The upper panel includes six studies using immunochemotherapy; the middle panel includes six studies that combine agents with bortezomib; the lower panel includes three studies combining rituximab with other therapies.

B-Cell Receptor Pathway Small molecules targeting the B-cell receptor have achieved remarkable response rates in relapsed MCL. The Bruton tyrosine kinase (BTK)-inhibitor, ibrutinib, exhibited a response rate of 68 percent in relapsed disease.[84] Combination with rituximab led to a response in all cases with low Ki-67, whereas in highly proliferating disease, this approach was only effective in half of the patients.[85] The compound is very well tolerated with only slight immunosuppression, bleeding, and atrial fibrillation being the predominant side effects. However, early relapses with a highly aggressive course have been observed. Combinations of ibrutinib with chemotherapy are being tested in the frontline setting.

Idelalisib achieves similar high response rates of 62 percent in MCL, although many of the remissions are short-lived.[86]

COURSE AND PROGNOSIS

The prospects for patients with MCL have significantly improved over the last few years based on advances in therapy, including the addition of rituximab and optimization of chemotherapy regimens, both according to tolerability (bendamustine) as well as efficacy (cytarabine, autologous transplantation; see Fig. 100–3). Accordingly, overall survival has been observed to improve from a median of 2.7 years in the 1980s to 5.8 years in the 1990s.[100]

Improved diagnostic tools, which allow the detection of pathognomonic cyclin D1 overexpression, show that MCL represents a spectrum of disease (see Fig. 100–1). Accordingly, a few patients may be followed with watchful waiting, whereas others present with a highly proliferative disease insensitive to conventionally dosed chemotherapy. In the majority of cases, initial responses are followed by a continuous relapse pattern, although remission durations have significantly improved as a result of improved frontline therapeutic approaches. The implementation of targeted therapies with proven efficacy in relapsed disease represents the current challenge in treatment of MCL (see Fig. 100–3). With the possible exception of ibrutinib, combined approaches are required to achieve high response rates and prolonged remission durations. In addition, predictive markers for distinct targeted therapies are urgently needed for more individualized treatment strategies which will allow patients to achieve optimal outcomes.

TABLE 100–5. Therapy for Relapsed Mantle Cell Lymphoma

Author (Year)	Phase	Number of Patients	Regimen	ORR% (CR%)	Median PFS (Months)	Median OS (Months)
Goy (2009)[71]	II	141	Bortezomib	33 (8)	7	24 months
Baiocchi (2011)[72]	II	13	R-bortezomib	29 (29)	2	NA
Lamm (2011)[73]	II	16	R-bortezomib/ dexamethasone	81 (44)	12	39
Kaufmann (2004)[74]	II	16	R-thalidomide	81 (31)	20	75% (3 years)
Zinzani (2013)[75]	II	57	Lenalidomide	35 (12)	4	19
Goy (2013)[76]	II	134	Lenalidomide	28 88)	4	19
Trneny (2014)[78]	II	170	Lenalidomide	40 (5)	9	28
		84	monochemotherapy	11 (0)	5	21
Wang (2012)[77]	II	44	R-lenalidomide	57 (36)	11	24
Witzig (2005)[79]	II	34	Temsirolimus 250 mg	38 (3)	7 (TTP)	12
Ansell (2008)[80]	II	27	Temsirolimus 25 mg	41 (4)	6 (TTP)	14
Hess (2009)[81]	III	162	Temsirolimus 175/75 mg	22 (2)	5	13
				6 (0)	3	10
			Temsirolimus 175/25 mg	2 (2)	2	10
			chemotherapy			
Ansell (2011)[82]	II	69	R-temsirolimus	59 (19)	10	30
Renner (2012)[83]	II	35	Everolimus	20 (6)	6	NA
Wang (2013)[84]	II	111	Ibrutinib	68 (21)	14	NA
Wang (2014)[85]	II		R-ibrutinib			
				100 (low Ki-67)	90% (1 year)	90% (1 year)
				50 (high Ki-67)	13.6	13.6
Kahl (2014)[86]	I	16	Idelalisib	62 (NA)	3 (RD)	NA
Davids (2013)[87]	I	8 MCL	Abt-199 (Venetoclax)	100	NA	NA

CR, complete response; NA, not available; ORR, overall response rate; OS, overall survival; PFS progression-free survival; R, rituximab; TTP, time to progression.

REFERENCES

1. Banks PM, Chan J, Cleary ML, et al: Mantle cell lymphoma. A proposal for unification of morphologic, immunologic, and molecular data. *Am J Surg Pathol* 16:637, 1992.
2. Harris NL, Jaffe ES, Stein H, et al: A revised European-American classification of lymphoid neoplasms: A proposal from the International Lymphoma Study Group. *Blood* 84:1361, 1994.
3. Swerdlow SH, Campo E, Harris NL, et al: *WHO Classification of Tumours of Haematopoietic and Lymphoid Tissues*, ed 4. International Agency for Research on Cancer, Lyon, France, 2008.
4. Fernández V, Salamero O, Espinet B, et al: Genomic and gene expression profiling defines indolent forms of mantle cell lymphoma. *Cancer Res* 70:1408, 2010.
5. Tiemann M, Schrader C, Klapper W, et al: European MCL Network: Histopathology, cell proliferation indices and clinical outcome in 304 patients with mantle cell lymphoma (MCL): A clinicopathological study from the European MCL Network. *Br J Haematol* 131:29, 2005.
6. Fu K, Weisenburger DD, Greiner TC, et al: Cyclin D1-negative mantle cell lymphoma: A clinicopathologic study based on gene expression profiling. *Blood* 106:4315, 2005.
7. A clinical evaluation of the International Lymphoma Study Group classification of non-Hodgkin's lymphoma. The Non-Hodgkin's Lymphoma Classification Project. *Blood* 89:3909, 1997.
8. Zhou Y, Wang H, Fang W, et al: Incidence trends of mantle cell lymphoma in the United States between 1992 and 2004. *Cancer* 113:791, 2008.
9. Jares P, Colomer D, Campo E: Genetic and molecular pathogenesis of mantle cell lymphoma: Perspectives for new targeted therapeutics. *Nat Rev Cancer* 7:750, 2007.
10. Hirt C, Schuler F, Dölken L, et al: G. Low prevalence of circulating t(11;14) (q13;q32)-positive cells in the peripheral blood of healthy individuals as detected by real-time quantitative PCR. *Blood* 104:904, 2004.
11. Cuneo A, Bigoni R, Rigolin GM, et al: Cytogenetic profile of lymphoma of follicle mantle lineage: Correlation with clinicobiologic features. *Blood* 93:1372, 1999.
12. Greiner TC, Moynihan MJ, Chan WC, et al: p53 mutations in mantle cell lymphoma are associated with variant cytology and predict a poor prognosis. *Blood* 87:4302, 1996.
13. Dreyling MH, Bullinger L, Ott G, et al: Alterations of the cyclin D1/p16-pRB pathway in mantle cell lymphoma. *Cancer Res* 57:4608, 1997.
14. Rosenwald A, Wright G, Wiestner A, et al: The proliferation gene expression signature is a quantitative integrator of oncogenic events that predicts survival in mantle cell lymphoma. *Cancer Cell* 3:185, 2003.
15. Hartmann E, Fernàndez V, Moreno V, et al: Five-gene model to predict survival in mantle-cell lymphoma using frozen or formalin-fixed, paraffin-embedded tissue. *J Clin Oncol* 26:4966, 2008.
16. Determann O, Hoster E, Ott G, et al: European Mantle Cell Lymphoma Network and the German Low Grade Lymphoma Study Group: Ki-67 predicts outcome in advanced-stage mantle cell lymphoma patients treated with anti-CD20 immunochemotherapy: Results from randomized trials of the European MCL Network and the German Low Grade Lymphoma Study Group. *Blood* 111:2385, 2008.
17. Dreyling M; European Mantle Cell Lymphoma Network: Mantle cell lymphoma: Biology, clinical presentation, and therapeutic approaches. *Am Soc Clin Oncol Educ Book* 191, 2014.
18. Romaguera JE, Medeiros LJ, Hagemeister FB, et al: Frequency of gastrointestinal involvement and its clinical significance in mantle cell lymphoma. *Cancer* 97:586, 2003. Erratum in: *Cancer* 97:3131, 2003.
19. Cheah CY, George A, Giné E, et al: European Mantle Cell Lymphoma Network: Central nervous system involvement in mantle cell lymphoma: Clinical features, prognostic factors and outcomes from the European Mantle Cell Lymphoma Network. *Ann Oncol* 24:2119, 2013.

20. Hoster E, Dreyling M, Klapper W, et al: German Low Grade Lymphoma Study Group (GLSG); European Mantle Cell Lymphoma Network: A new prognostic index (MIPI) for patients with advanced-stage mantle cell lymphoma. *Blood* 111:558, 2008.

21. Hoster E, Klapper W, Hermine O, et al: Confirmation of the mantle-cell lymphoma International Prognostic Index in randomized trials of the European Mantle-Cell Lymphoma Network. *J Clin Oncol* 32:1338, 2014.

22. Pott C, Schrader C, Gesk S, et al: Quantitative assessment of molecular remission after high-dose therapy with autologous stem cell transplantation predicts long-term remission in mantle cell lymphoma. *Blood* 107:2271, 2006.

23. Pott C, Hoster E, Delfau-Larue MH, et al: Molecular remission is an independent predictor of clinical outcome in patients with mantle cell lymphoma after combined immunochemotherapy: A European MCL intergroup study. *Blood* 115:3215, 2010.

24. Nygren L, Baumgartner Wennerholm S, Klimkowska M, et al: Prognostic role of SOX11 in a population-based cohort of mantle cell lymphoma. *Blood* 119:4215, 2012.

25. Martin P, Chadburn A, Christos P, et al: Outcome of deferred initial therapy in mantle-cell lymphoma. *J Clin Oncol* 27:1209, 2009.

26. Leitch HA, Gascoyne RD, Chhanabhai M, et al: Limited-stage mantle-cell lymphoma. *Ann Oncol* 10:1555, 2003.

27. Engelhard M, Unterhalt M, Hansmann M, et al: Follicular lymphoma, immunocytoma, and mantle cell lymphoma: Randomized evaluation of curative radiotherapy in limited stage nodal disease. *Ann Oncol* 19(Suppl 4):418, 2008.

28. Meusers P, Engelhard M, Bartels H, et al: Multicentre randomized therapeutic trial for advanced centrocytic lymphoma: Anthracycline does not improve the prognosis. *Hematol Oncol* 7:365, 1989.

29. Fisher RI, Dahlberg S, Nathwani BN, et al: A clinical analysis of two indolent lymphoma entities: Mantle cell lymphoma and marginal zone lymphoma (including mucosa-associated lymphoid tissue and monocytoid B-cell categories): A Southwest Oncology Group study. *Blood* 85:1075, 1995.

30. Hiddemann W, Unterhalt M, Herrmann R, et al: Mantle-cell lymphomas have more widespread disease and a slower response to chemotherapy compared with follicle-center lymphomas: Results of a prospective comparative analysis of the German Low-Grade Lymphoma Study Group. *J Clin Oncol* 16:1922, 1998.

31. Ghielmini M, Schmitz SF, Cogliatti S, et al: Effect of single-agent rituximab given at the standard schedule or as prolonged treatment in patients with mantle cell lymphoma: A study of the Swiss Group for Clinical Cancer Research (SAKK). *J Clin Oncol* 23:705, 2005.

32. Howard OM, Gribben JG, Neuberg DS, et al: Rituximab and CHOP induction therapy for newly diagnosed mantle-cell lymphoma: Molecular complete responses are not predictive of progression-free survival. *J Clin Oncol* 20:1288, 2002.

33. Lenz G, Dreyling M, Hoster E, et al: Immunochemotherapy with rituximab and cyclophosphamide, doxorubicin, vincristine, and prednisone significantly improves response and time to treatment failure, but not long-term outcome in patients with previously untreated mantle cell lymphoma: Results of a prospective randomized trial of the German Low Grade Lymphoma Study Group (GLSG) *J Clin Oncol* 23:1984, 2005.

34. Herold M, Haas A, Doerken B, et al: Immunochemotherapy (R-MCP) in advanced mantle cell lymphoma is not superior to chemotherapy (MCP) alone—50 months update of the OSHO phase III study (OSHO#39). *Ann Oncol* 19:abstr 12, 2008.

35. Kenkre VP1, Long WL, Eickhoff JC, et al: Maintenance rituximab following induction chemo-immunotherapy for mantle cell lymphoma: Long-term follow-up of a pilot study from the Wisconsin Oncology Network. *Leuk Lymphoma* 52:1675, 2011.

36. Gressin R, Caulet-Maugendre S, Deconinck E, et al: Evaluation of the (R)VAD+C regimen for the treatment of newly diagnosed mantle cell lymphoma. Combined results of two prospective phase II trials from the French GOELAMS group. *Haematologica* 95:1350, 2010.

37. Sachanas S, Pangalis GA, Vassilakopoulos TP, et al: Combination of rituximab with chlorambucil as first line treatment in patients with mantle cell lymphoma: A highly effective regimen. *Leuk Lymphoma* 52:387, 2011.

38. Kluin-Nelemans HC, Hoster E, Hermine O, et al: Treatment of older patients with mantle-cell lymphoma. *N Engl J Med* 367:520, 2012.

39. Smith MR, Li H, Gordon L, et al: Phase II study of rituximab plus cyclophosphamide, doxorubicin, vincristine, and prednisone immunochemotherapy followed by yttrium-90-ibritumomab tiuxetan in untreated mantle-cell lymphoma: Eastern Cooperative Oncology Group Study E1499. *J Clin Oncol* 30:3119, 2012.

40. Rummel MJ, Niederle N, Maschmeyer G, et al: Bendamustine plus rituximab versus CHOP plus rituximab as first-line treatment for patients with indolent and mantle-cell lymphomas: An open-label, multicentre, randomised, phase 3 non-inferiority trial. *Lancet* 381:1203, 2013.

41. Visco C, Finotto S, Zambello R, et al: Combination of rituximab, bendamustine, and cytarabine for patients with mantle-cell non-Hodgkin lymphoma ineligible for intensive regimens or autologous transplantation. *J Clin Oncol* 31:1442, 2013.

42. Schulz H, Bohlius JF, Trelle S, et al: Immunochemotherapy with rituximab and overall survival in patients with indolent and mantle cell lymphoma: A systematic review and meta-analysis. *J Natl Cancer Inst* 99:706, 2004.

43. Flinn IW, van der Jagt R, Kahl BS, et al: Randomized trial of bendamustine-rituximab or R-CHOP/R-CVP in first-line treatment of indolent NHL or MCL: The BRIGHT study. *Blood* 123:2944, 2014.

44. Hermine O, Hoster E, Walewski J, et al: Alternating courses of 3x CHOP and 3x DHAP plus rituximab followed by a high dose ARA-C containing myeloablative regimen and autologous stem cell transplantation (ASCT) increases overall survival when compared to 6 courses of CHOP plus rituximab followed by myeloablative radiochemotherapy

and ASCT in mantle cell lymphoma: Final analysis of the MCL Younger Trial of the European Mantle Cell Lymphoma Network (MCL net). (ASH Annual Meeting Abstracts) *Blood* 120:151, 2012.

45. Dreyling M, Lenz G, Hoster E, et al: Early consolidation by myeloablative radiochemotherapy followed by autologous stem cell transplantation in first remission significantly prolongs progression-free survival in mantle cell lymphoma: Results of a prospective randomized trial of the European MCL Network. *Blood* 105:2677, 2005.

46. Damon LE, Johnson JL, Niedzwiecki D, et al: Immunochemotherapy and autologous stem-cell transplantation for untreated patients with mantle-cell lymphoma: CALGB 59909. *J Clin Oncol* 27:6101, 2009.

47. van 't Veer MB, de Jong D, MacKenzie M, et al: High-dose Ara-C and beam with autograft rescue in R-CHOP responsive mantle cell lymphoma patients. *Br J Haematol* 144:524, 2009.

48. Geisler CH, Kolstad A, Laurell A, et al: Nordic Lymphoma Group: Nordic MCL2 trial update: Six-year follow-up after intensive immunochemotherapy for untreated mantle cell lymphoma followed by BEAM or BEAC + autologous stem-cell support: Still very long survival but late relapses do occur. *Br J Haematol* 158:355, 2012.

49. Delarue R, Haioun C, Ribrag V, et al: CHOP and DHAP plus rituximab followed by autologous stem cell transplantation in mantle cell lymphoma: A phase 2 study from the Groupe d'Etude des Lymphomes de l'Adulte. *Blood* 121:48, 2013.

50. de Guibert S, Jaccard A, Bernard M, et al: Rituximab and DHAP followed by intensive therapy with autologous stem-cell transplantation as first-line therapy for mantle cell lymphoma. *Haematologica* 91:425, 2006.

51. Magni M, Di Nicola M, Carlo-Stella C, et al: High-dose sequential chemotherapy and in vivo rituximab-purged stem cell autografting in mantle cell lymphoma: A 10-year update of the R-HDS regimen. *Bone Marrow Transplant* 43:509, 2009.

52. Le Gouill S, Thieblemont C, Oberic L, et al: Rituximab maintenance versus wait and watch after four courses of R-DHAP followed by autologous stem cell transplantation in previously untreated young patients with mantle cell lymphoma: First interim analysis of the phase III prospective Lyma Trial, a Lysa Study. (ASH Annual Meeting Abstracts) *Blood* 124:146, 2014.

53. Romaguera JE, Fayad LE, McLaughlin P, et al: Phase I trial of bortezomib in combination with rituximab-HyperCVAD alternating with rituximab, methotrexate and cytarabine for untreated aggressive mantle cell lymphoma. *Br J Haematol* 151:47, 2013, 2010.

54. Merli F, Luminari S, Ilariucci F, et al: Rituximab plus HyperCVAD alternating with high dose cytarabine and methotrexate for the initial treatment of patients with mantle cell lymphoma, a multicentre trial from Gruppo Italiano Studio Linfomi. *Br J Haematol* 156:346, 2012.

55. Bernstein SH, Epner E, Unger JM, et al: A phase II multicenter trial of hyperCVAD MTX/Ara-C and rituximab in patients with previously untreated mantle cell lymphoma; SWOG 0213. *Ann Oncol* 24:1587, 2013.

56. Hoster E, Metzner B, Forstpointner R, et al: Autologous stem cell transplantation and addition of rituximab independently prolong response duration in advanced stage mantle cell lymphoma. (ASH Annual Meeting Abstracts) *Blood* 114:880, 2009.

57. Hoster E, Geisler GH, Doorduijn JK, et al: Role of high-dose cytarabine and total body irradiation conditioning before autologous stem cell transplantation in mantle cell lymphoma—A comparison of Nordic MCL2, HOVON 45, and European MCL Younger Trials. (ASH Annual Meeting Abstracts) *Blood* 122:3367, 2013.

58. Kolstad A, Laurell A, Jerkeman M, et al: Nordic MCL3 study: 90Y-ibritumomab-tiuxetan added to BEAM/C in non-CR patients before transplant in mantle cell lymphoma. *Blood* 123(19):2953, 2014.

58A. Chang JE, Li H, Smith MR, et al: Phase 2 study of VcR-CVAD with maintenance rituximab for untreated mantle cell lymphoma: An Eastern Cooperative Oncology Group study (E1405). *Blood* 123(11):1665–1673, 2014.

59. Forstpointner R, Dreyling M, Repp R, et al: German Low-Grade Lymphoma Study Group: The addition of rituximab to a combination of fludarabine, cyclophosphamide, mitoxantrone (FCM) significantly increases the response rate and prolongs survival as compared with FCM alone in patients with relapsed and refractory follicular and mantle cell lymphomas: Results of a prospective randomized study of the German Low-Grade Lymphoma Study Group. *Blood* 104:3064, 2004.

60. Rummel MJ, Al-Batran SE, Kim SZ, et al: Bendamustine plus rituximab is effective and has a favorable toxicity profile in the treatment of mantle cell and low-grade non-Hodgkin's lymphoma. *J Clin Oncol* 23:3383, 2005.

61. Robinson KS, Williams ME, van der Jagt RH, et al: Phase II multicenter study of bendamustine plus rituximab in patients with relapsed indolent B-cell and mantle cell non-Hodgkin's lymphoma. *J Clin Oncol* 26:4473, 2008.

62. Weide R, Hess G, Köppler H, et al: High anti-lymphoma activity of bendamustine/mitoxantrone/rituximab in rituximab pretreated relapsed or refractory indolent lymphomas and mantle cell lymphomas. A multicenter phase II study of the German Low Grade Lymphoma Study Group (GLSG). *Leuk Lymphoma* 48:1299, 2007.

63. Gironella M, Lopez A, Merchan B, et al: Rituximab plus gemcitabine and oxaliplatin as salvage therapy in patients with relapsed/refractory mantle-cell lymphoma. (ASH Annual Meeting Abstracts) *Blood* 120:1627, 2012.

64. Tam CS, Bassett R, Ledesma C, et al: Mature results of the M. D. Anderson Cancer Center risk-adapted transplantation strategy in mantle cell lymphoma. *Blood* 113:4144, 2009.

65. Le Gouill S, Kröger N, Dhedin N, et al: Reduced-intensity conditioning allogeneic stem cell transplantation for relapsed/refractory mantle cell lymphoma: A multicenter experience. *Ann Oncol* 23:2695, 2012.

66. Hamadani M, Saber W, Ahn KW, et al: Allogeneic hematopoietic cell transplantation for chemotherapy-unresponsive mantle cell lymphoma: A cohort analysis from the center

for international blood and marrow transplant research. *Biol Blood Marrow Transplant* 19:625, 2013.

67. Zoellner A, Fritsch S, Prevalsek D, et al: Sequential therapy combining clofarabine and HLA-haploidentical hematopoietic stem cell transplantation in the treatment of refractory and advanced lymphoma: Feasibility, toxicity and early outcome. (ASH Annual Meeting Abstracts) *Blood* 122:4544, 2013.

68. Wang M, Oki Y, Pro B, et al: Phase II study of yttrium-90-ibritumomab tiuxetan in patients with relapsed or refractory mantle cell lymphoma. *J Clin Oncol* 27:5213, 2009.

69. Ferrero S, Pastore A, Forstpointner R, et al: Radioimmunotherapy in relapsed/refractory mantle cell lymphoma patients: Final results of a European MCL Network phase II trial. (ASH Annual Meeting Abstracts) *Blood* 122:4384, 2013.

70. Goy A, Bernstein SH, Kahl BS, et al: Bortezomib in patients with relapsed or refractory mantle cell lymphoma: Updated time-to-event analyses of the multicenter phase 2 PINNACLE study. *Ann Oncol* 20:520, 2009.

71. Baiocchi RA, Alinari L, Lustberg ME, et al: Phase 2 trial of rituximab and bortezomib in patients with relapsed or refractory mantle cell and follicular lymphoma. *Cancer* 117:2442, 2011.

72. Lamm W, Kaufmann H, Raderer M, et al: Bortezomib combined with rituximab and dexamethasone is an active regimen for patients with relapsed and chemotherapy-refractory mantle cell lymphoma. *Haematologica* 96:1008, 2011.

73. Kaufmann H, Raderer M, Wöhrer S, et al: Antitumor activity of rituximab plus thalidomide in patients with relapsed/refractory mantle cell lymphoma. *Blood* 104:2269, 2004.

74. Zinzani PL, Vose JM, Czuczman MS, et al: Long-term follow-up of lenalidomide in relapsed/refractory mantle cell lymphoma: subset analysis of the NHL-003 study. *Ann Oncol* 24:2892, 2013.

75. Goy A, Sinha R, Williams ME, et al: Single-agent lenalidomide in patients with mantle-cell lymphoma who relapsed or progressed after or were refractory to bortezomib: Phase II MCL-001 (EMERGE) study. *J Clin Oncol* 31:3688, 2013.

76. Wang M, Fayad L, Wagner-Bartak N, Zhang L, et al: Lenalidomide in combination with rituximab for patients with relapsed or refractory mantle-cell lymphoma: A phase 1/2 clinical trial. *Lancet Oncol* 13:716, 2012.

77. Trneny M, Lamy T, Walewski J, et al: Phase II randomized, multicenter study of lenalidomide vs best investigator's choice in relapsed/refractory mantle cell lymphoma: Results of the MCL-002 (SPRINT) Study. (ASH Annual Meeting Abstracts) *Blood* 124:626.

78. Witzig TE, Geyer SM, Ghobrial I, et al: Phase II trial of single-agent temsirolimus (CCI-779) for relapsed mantle cell lymphoma. *J Clin Oncol* 23:5347, 2005.

79. Ansell SM, Inwards DJ, Rowland KM Jr, et al: Low-dose, single-agent temsirolimus for relapsed mantle cell lymphoma: A phase 2 trial in the North Central Cancer Treatment Group. *Cancer* 113:508, 2008.

80. Hess G, Herbrecht R, Romaguera R, et al: Phase III study to evaluate temsirolimus compared with investigator's choice therapy for the treatment of relapsed or refractory mantle cell lymphoma. *J Clin Oncol* 27(23):3822–3829, 2009.

81. Ansell SM, Tang H, Kurtin PJ, et al: Temsirolimus and rituximab in patients with relapsed or refractory mantle cell lymphoma: A phase 2 study. *Lancet Oncol* 12:361, 2011.

82. Renner C, Zinzani PL, Gressin R, et al: A multicenter phase II trial (SAKK 36/06) of single-agent everolimus (RAD001) in patients with relapsed or refractory mantle cell lymphoma. *Haematologica* 97:1085, 2012.

83. Wang ML, Rule S, Martin P, et al: Targeting BTK with ibrutinib in relapsed or refractory mantle-cell lymphoma. *N Engl J Med* 369:507, 2013.

84. Wang ML, Hagemeister F, Westin JR, et al: Ibrutinib and rituximab are an efficacious and safe combination in relapsed mantle cell lymphoma: Preliminary results from a phase II. (ASH Annual Meeting Abstracts) *Blood* 124:627, 2014.

85. Kahl BS, Spurgeon SE, Furman RR, et al: A phase 1 study of the PI3Kδ inhibitor idelalisib in patients with relapsed/refractory mantle cell lymphoma (MCL). *Blood* 123:3398, 2014.

86. Davids MS, Seymour JF, Gerecitano JF, et al: The single-agent Bcl-2 inhibitor ABT-199 (GDC-0199) in patients with relapsed/refractory (R/R) non-Hodgkin lymphoma (NHL): Responses observed in all mantle cell lymphoma (MCL) patients. (ASH Annual Meeting Abstracts) *Blood* 122:1789, 2013.

87. Furtado M, Johnson R, Kruger A, et al: Addition of bortezomib to standard dose chop chemotherapy improves response and survival in relapsed mantle cell lymphoma. *Br J Haematol* 168:55, 2015.

88. Kouroukis CT, Fernandez LA, Crump M, et al: A phase II study of bortezomib and gemcitabine in relapsed mantle cell lymphoma from the National Cancer Institute of Canada Clinical Trials Group (IND 172). *Leuk Lymphoma* 52:394, 2011.

89. Weigert O, Weidmann E, Mueck R, et al A novel regimen combining high dose cytarabine and bortezomib has activity in multiply relapsed and refractory mantle cell lymphoma-long-term results of a multicenter observation study. *Leuk Lymphoma* 50:716, 2009.

90. Friedberg JW, Vose JM, Kelly JL, et al: The combination of bendamustine, bortezomib, and rituximab for patients with relapsed/refractory indolent and mantle cell non-Hodgkin lymphoma. *Blood* 117:2807, 2011.

91. Gerecitano J, Portlock C, Hamlin P, et al: Phase I trial of weekly and twice-weekly bortezomib with rituximab, cyclophosphamide, and prednisone in relapsed or refractory non-Hodgkin lymphoma. *Clin Cancer Res* 17:2493, 2011.

92. Ruan J, Martin P, Furman RR, et al: Bortezomib plus CHOP-rituximab for previously untreated diffuse large B-cell lymphoma and mantle cell lymphoma. *J Clin Oncol* 29:690, 2011.

93. Zaja F, Ferrero S, Stelitano C et al:. Rituximab, Lenalidomide, Bendamustine second line therapy in mantle cell lymphoma: a phase II study of the fondazione Italiana linfomi (FIL). *Hematol Oncol* 33(suppl 1):14, 2015.

94. Ruan J, Martin P, Coleman M, et al: Durable responses with the metronomic rituximab and thalidomide plus prednisone, etoposide, procarbazine, and cyclophosphamide regimen in elderly patients with recurrent mantle cell lymphoma. *Cancer* 116:2655, 2010.

95. Hess G, Keller U, Scholz CW, et al: Safety and efficacy of temsirolimus in combination with bendamustine and rituximab in relapsed mantle cell and follicular lymphoma. *Leukemia* 2015 Mar 13 [Epub ahead of print].

96. Lin TS, Blum KA, Fischer DB, et al: Flavopiridol, fludarabine, and rituximab in mantle cell lymphoma and indolent B-cell lymphoproliferative disorders. *J Clin Oncol* 28:418, 2010.

97. Robak T, Huang H, Jin J, et al: Bortezomib-based therapy for newly diagnosed mantle-cell lymphoma. *N Engl J Med* 372:944, 2015.

98. Houot R, Le Gouill S, Ojeda Uribe M, et al: Combination of rituximab, bortezomib, doxorubicin, dexamethasone and chlorambucil (RiPAD+C) as first-line therapy for elderly mantle cell lymphoma patients: results of a phase II trial from the GOELAMS. *Ann Oncol* 23:1555, 2012.

99. Herrmann A, Hoster E, Zwingers T, et al: Improvement of overall survival in advanced stage mantle cell lymphoma. *J Clin Oncol* 27:511, 2009.

100. Inwards DJ, Fishkin PA, LaPlant BR, et al: Phase I trial of rituximab, cladribine, and temsirolimus (RCT) for initial therapy of mantle cell lymphoma. *Ann Oncol* 25:2020, 2014.

CHAPTER 101
MARGINAL ZONE B-CELL LYMPHOMAS

Pier Luigi Zinzani and Alessandro Broccoli

SUMMARY

Indolent B-cell lymphomas deriving from the marginal zone include three specific entities: extranodal marginal zone (or mucosa-associated lymphoid tissue) lymphoma (EMZL), splenic marginal zone lymphoma (SMZL), and nodal marginal zone lymphoma (NMZL). The clinical and molecular characteristics are distinctive for each of these entities, although some phenotypic and genetic features are overlapping. EMZL is the most common entity, arising at virtually any extranodal site, commonly associated with chronic antigenic stimulation either as a result of an external infection (e.g., *Helicobacter pylori* in the stomach) or an autoimmune disease (as Sjögren syndrome or Hashimoto thyroiditis). SMZL accounts for approximately 20 percent of all marginal zone lymphomas, with patients typically presenting with an enlarged spleen and involvement of marrow and splenic hilar lymph nodes. NMZL is the least-common entity, representing approximately 10 percent of all marginal zone lymphomas and typically presenting with lymph node-based disease without splenic or extranodal site involvement.

● INTRODUCTION AND CLASSIFICATION

Marginal zone lymphomas (MZLs) represent a heterogeneous group of indolent lymphoproliferative disorders originating from memory B-lymphocytes, which are normally present in the marginal zone—that is, the outer part of the mantle zone—of the secondary lymphoid follicles. The spleen and the mucosa-associated lymphoid tissues (MALT) are the most frequently involved anatomic compartments; lymph nodes may also been involved, albeit rarely. The 2008 *World Health Organization (WHO) Classification of Tumours of Haematopoietic and Lymphoid Tissue* identifies three distinct subtypes of MZL based on the involved site, the clinical presentation and course of the disease, as well as the molecular profiles, namely, extranodal MZL of MALT type (also termed *extranodal marginal zone lymphoma* [EMZL]); splenic marginal zone lymphoma (SMZL); and nodal marginal zone lymphoma (NMZL).[1] In

addition, two provisional entities are recognized by the 2008 WHO classification: splenic diffuse red pulp lymphoma and hairy-cell leukemia variant, which represent two subtypes of splenic lymphomas with features overlapping with those of MZL.

In adults, MZLs account for 5 to 17 percent of all non-Hodgkin lymphomas (NHLs); MALT lymphoma is the most frequent overall, being the third most frequent NHL and representing 7 to 8 percent of all B-cell neoplasms. It mostly affects middle-aged adults, at a median age of 60 years, with a slight female preponderance and often in association with chronic antigenic stimulation, either as a consequence of a chronic infection or an autoimmune disease. Gastric MALT lymphoma is by far the most common clinical entity, displaying considerable geographic variability with a higher incidence in areas associated with a high incidence of *Helicobacter pylori* infection. SMZL and NMZL represent 20 percent and 10 percent of MZLs, respectively, accounting for less than 2 percent of all NHLs. The median age at disease onset is 65 years for SMZL, and between 50 and 60 years for NMZL.[2,3]

Each lymphoma subtype is presented and discussed separately in terms of epidemiology, etiology and pathogenesis, clinical presentation and treatment strategies.

● EXTRANODAL MARGINAL ZONE LYMPHOMA

DEFINITION

EMZL or MALT lymphoma is an extranodal lymphoma that arises both in organs with an anatomically well-defined MALT, such as the gut, the nasopharynx and the lung (in which MALT represents an acquired and specialized immunologic barrier associated with highly permeable mucosal sites in close contact with the external environment), and in sites which normally lack lymphoid tissue, but have accumulated B cells in response to a chronic infection or an autoimmune process, such as the salivary glands, the ocular adnexa (orbits, conjunctiva and lacrimal glands), the skin, the thyroid, the genitourinary tract (bladder, prostate, kidney, uterus), and the breasts.

EPIDEMIOLOGY

MALT lymphoma accounts for at least 50 percent of primary gastric lymphomas, typically presenting in middle-aged adults, with a female predominance. Gastric MALT lymphoma is particularly common in the north-eastern part of Italy, which is an area of high prevalence of *H. pylori* infection. In contrast, a specific subtype of small intestinal MALT lymphoma (termed *immunoproliferative small intestinal disease* [IPSID]) tends to be more frequent in the Middle East, on the Indian subcontinent, and in the Cape Region of South Africa.

ETIOLOGY AND PATHOGENESIS

Sustained antigenic stimulation, triggered either by a chronic infection or by an autoimmune process, induces an initially polyclonal B-cell proliferation, as well as the development of an inflammatory response, with the attraction of neutrophils, which release reactive oxygen species (ROS). ROS are genotoxic, and may induce a wide range of genetic abnormalities. Moreover, the prolonged proliferation of B-lymphocytes induced by a chronic lymphoproliferative stimulus may increase the risk of DNA damage (double-strand breaks and translocations), as a consequence of the genetic instability of B cells during somatic hypermutation and class-switch recombination. Genetic abnormalities tend to involve those genes related to the activation of nuclear factor-kappa B (NF-κB), a key transcription factor regulating the expression of several survival- and proliferation-related genes in B cells during immune responses. The constitutive activation of this signalling pathway results in uncontrolled B-cell proliferation and subsequent neoplastic transformation of the involved tissue.

The longstanding antigenic stimulation explains how lymphoid infiltrates—or an acquired MALT—may appear in extranodal sites normally lacking MALT. The MALT that organizes in proximity to an epithelium receives stimuli from the epithelium itself (as occurs in autoimmune disorders) or from antigens entering the lymphoid tissue through the epithelium or via the afferent lymphatics (as during exogenous infections).

Microbial species thought to be associated with MALT lymphoma include: *H. pylori* and *Helicobacter heilmannii*, hepatitis C virus (HCV), *Campylobacter jejuni*, *Borrelia burgdorferi*, and *Chlamydia psittaci*. These entities have been found to be related with the development of MALT lymphoma of the stomach, IPSID, cutaneous MALT lymphoma and orbital MALT lymphoma, respectively.[4-7] *H. pylori* has been documented as the etiologic agent in more than 90 percent of gastric MALT lymphoma, which arises from *H. pylori*–stimulated autoreactive B cells.[8] *H. pylori* can be demonstrated by histology, polymerase chain reaction, or urea breath test, and can be isolated and cultured. *H. pylori* appears to be a fundamental factor for the development of the disease, and its elimination often induces a remission of the lymphoma by itself without any other intervention, thus fulfilling all four of Koch's postulates and establishing the microorganism as the main etiologic factor. However, because only a minority of patients with an overt *H. pylori* infection develop the disease, it is obvious that the pathogenesis of gastric EMZL also depends on other, largely unknown factors, perhaps related to the host, the environment, or the virulence of the infecting *H. pylori* strain.

It has also been demonstrated that viable *C. psittaci* can be found not only in monocytes and macrophages infiltrating orbital MALT lymphoma, but also in patients' blood and conjunctiva, raising the possibility of microbial eradication and disease remission by antibiotic therapy with drugs such as doxycycline.[9]

Autoreactive B cells found in autoimmune diseases, such as those infiltrating the thyroid in Hashimoto thyroiditis, or the salivary glands in Sjögren syndrome, organize progressively into a well-developed MALT, mimicking lymphoproliferation and eventually evolving into an overt lymphoma. Patients with Sjögren syndrome have a 44-fold increased risk of developing lymphoma, and patients with Hashimoto thyroiditis have a 70-fold increased risk of thyroid lymphoma.[10,11]

GENETIC ABERRATIONS

Recurrent genomic lesions, including chromosomal translocations and unbalanced aberrations, can be detected in MALT lymphomas in up to 40 percent of the cases, depending on the specific aberration. The t(11;18)(q21;q21) translocation is the most common structural chromosomal abnormality in MALT lymphoma, being demonstrated in 15 to 40 percent of the cases, especially in gastric and lung MALT lymphoma.[12] Other chromosomal translocations include t(14;18)(q32;q21), t(1;14)(p22;q32) and t(3;14)(p13;q32), all involving the immunoglobulin heavy chain variable region *(IGHV)* gene on chromosome 14, and displaying a specific anatomic distribution (Table 101–1).[13] The presence of any of these chromosomal alterations correlates with a lack of any further genetic instability or chromosomal imbalances.

Current knowledge of the genetic lesions seen in MALT lymphoma suggest a model of multistage development and progression from a preneoplastic lesion to overt lymphoma. The accumulation of genetic abnormalities is associated with a loss of dependency from antigenic stimulation (with subsequent antibiotic resistance) and with possible histologic transformation.

CLINICAL FEATURES

EMZL mostly presents as Ann Arbor stage IE disease, which implies the sole involvement of the extranodal site of origin, with possible extension of the disease to tributary lymph nodes in close proximity to the affected organ. Marrow and peripheral lymph node infiltration is uncommon, observed in less than 20 percent of the cases at presentation. The stomach is the most commonly involved organ, accounting for approximately one-third of cases. Other typical presentations include the salivary glands, the orbits and the ocular adnexa, the thyroid, the lungs, the skin, the breasts, the liver, and other gastrointestinal sites, apart from the stomach. Disseminated disease can be documented in up to 25 percent of patients with gastric MALT lymphoma, although those with nongastrointestinal extranodal disease exhibit disseminated lymphoma in nearly half of the cases.[14] Gastric MALT lymphoma is often multifocal, which may explain the high rate of relapse in the gastric stump after surgical excision. Synchronous involvement of gastrointestinal and extraintestinal sites is detected in approximately 10 percent of cases.

Systemic lymphoma-related symptoms are generally uncommon, and the clinical aspects and presenting symptoms generally correlate with the primary location of the disease.

TABLE 101–1. Common Genetic Lesions in Mucosa-Associated Lymphoid Tissue Lymphoma

	Lesion	Genes	Frequency	Sites
Translocations	t(11;18)(q21;q21)	BIRC3-MALT1	15–40%	Stomach, lung
	t(14;18)(q32;q21)	IGHV-MALT1	20%	Lung, skin, ocular adnexa, salivary gland
	t(1;14)(p22;q32)	IGHV-BCL10	<5%	Stomach, lung
	t(3;14)(p13;q32)	IGHV-FOXP1	<5%	Unclear
Gains	+3; +3q		20–40%	No differences in sites
	+18; +18q		20–40%	No differences in sites
Losses	−6q23	TNFAIP3	15–30%	No differences in sites

BCL-10, B-cell CLL/lymphoma 10 gene; *BIRC3*, baculoviral IAP repeat-containing 3 gene; *FOXP1*, forkhead box P1 gene; *IGHV*, immunoglobulin heavy-chain variable region gene; *MALT1*, mucosa-associated lymphoid tissue translocation gene 1; *TNFAIP3*, tumor necrosis factor-α–induced protein 3 gene.

Gastric MALT lymphoma presents with nonspecific dyspepsia, epigastric pain, and nausea. Chronic bleeding may become evident with progressively worsening iron-deficiency anemia. The *antrum* is the most frequently involved portion of the organ, although any part of the stomach can be affected: intragastric nodularities, enlarged rugal folds, thickened gastric walls, irregularly shaped superficial erosions or shallow ulcers all represent macroscopic features of this lymphoma.

MALT lymphomas of the ocular adnexa most often arise in the orbit (40 percent of cases), with masses that cause progressive proptosis, periorbital edema and abnormalities in ocular motility and vision. The conjunctiva is the site of origin in approximately 35 to 40 percent of the cases, with bilateral involvement observed in nearly 15 percent of patients. More rarely, the lymphoma originates from the lacrimal gland (10 percent of the cases) or the eyelid.

Cutaneous MALT lymphoma generally presents with papules, plaques or nodules mainly involving the trunk and the upper limbs; the occurrence of multiple lesions affecting noncontiguous regions is, however, not infrequent. Lesions may show spontaneous remissions, but cutaneous relapses are the rule.

Immunoproliferative small intestinal disease, which is considered a special variant of intestinal MALT lymphoma, usually manifests with a severe and unremitting malabsorption. The lymphoma usually remains confined to the upper intestine and the regional lymph nodes, spreading beyond the abdomen only in advanced stages of the disease and upon transformation into high-grade lymphoma.

MORPHOLOGY

The neoplastic lymphocytes tend to infiltrate the marginal zone around reactive B-cell follicles, external to an intact follicular mantle. Their cytoplasm is pale, and they display small to medium-sized and irregularly shaped nuclei, with dispersed chromatin and inconspicuous nucleoli, either resembling germinal center centrocytes or monocytoid elements. Scattered, centroblast-like large cells may be present, although never predominant, as well as mature plasma cells in up to a third of cases. Lymphoepithelial lesions are characterized by invasion or necrotic destruction of the glandular epithelium by infiltrating lymphoma cells: they are highly characteristic of MALT lymphoma, particularly gastric MALT lymphoma (Fig. 101–1), although they are not pathognomonic. Germinal centers may also be colonized by MZL cells, thus conferring a vaguely nodular or follicular pattern; lymphoma cells may also undergo

a blastic or plasma cell differentiation. Upon immunohistochemistry, cells are CD20+, CD79a+, CD21+, and CD35+, lacking CD5, CD23, and CD10, typically expressing immunoglobulin (Ig) M (less often IgA or IgG), with an immunoglobulin light-chain restriction.

DIFFERENTIAL DIAGNOSIS

A distinction between reactive (i.e., acquired) and neoplastic MALT is sometimes difficult, especially for MALT lymphoma at early stages of evolution. The demonstration of clonality by virtue of light-chain restriction (on immunohistochemistry or flow cytometry) is of great diagnostic value. Other entities to be considered are other indolent B-cell lymphomas involving extranodal sites, such as mantle cell lymphoma, small lymphocytic lymphoma and follicular lymphoma. An extended immunohistochemical panel, including CD5, CD23, CD10, and cyclin D1, along with cytogenetic and molecular analysis is required to rule out other diagnoses.

STAGING PROCEDURES

A complete and detailed patient's history and a full physical exam, along with blood studies evaluating renal and liver function, lactate dehydrogenase (LDH), serum protein electrophoresis and immunofixation, and complete serology for HIV, HCV, and hepatitis B virus are considered mandatory.[15] Cryoglobulins should be measured in HCV-positive individuals. Computed tomography of the neck, chest, abdomen, and pelvis, as well as marrow aspiration and biopsy, are required. *H. pylori* status should always be evaluated on the gastric biopsy or through a urea breath test, and repeated after therapy if positive at baseline. Endoscopic ultrasound to evaluate the regional lymph nodes and gastric wall infiltration is also recommended in gastric MALT lymphoma. Fluorescence *in situ* hybridization for t(11;18) is optional, but useful to guide therapy. Involvement with *C. jejuni*, *C. psittaci*, or *B. burgdorferi* may be detected in tumor biopsies from intestine, ocular adnexa or skin, respectively, by polymerase chain reaction, immunohistochemistry or of *in situ* hybridization.

THERAPY

H. pylori eradication therapy should be administered to all patients with *H. pylori*–positive MALT lymphomas, independent of stage at presentation or histologic grade. The outcome of *H. pylori* eradication must be confirmed by urea breath test at least 6 weeks after eradication therapy, and at least 2 weeks after proton pump inhibitors withdrawal.

Antibiotic therapy is based on the epidemiology of the infection in the patient's country of residence, and should take into account locally expected antibiotic resistance patterns. The most common approach is based on three drugs: a proton pump inhibitor, in association with either amoxicillin or metronidazole, and clarithromycin, for 10 to 14 days.[16]

The role of surgery has been questioned, as gastric MALT lymphoma is generally multifocal, thus requiring an extensive (total or subtotal) gastrectomy, usually severely impairing the quality of life. Nevertheless, gastrectomy can be considered in cases with major hemorrhage, massive infiltration of the gastric walls (with an enhanced risk of perforation during chemotherapy), or pyloric stenosis.[17]

Patients with nongastric MALT lymphoma and gastric MALT lymphoma patients who fail to respond to *H. pylori* eradication or who have no evidence of *H. pylori* infection should be considered for alternative treatments. However, there is no evidence-based consensus delineating optimal alternative treatment strategies. Involved field radiation therapy (25 to 35 Gy) is a reasonable option for localized disease.[18,19] Chemotherapy or rituximab immunotherapy, or a combination of both, are

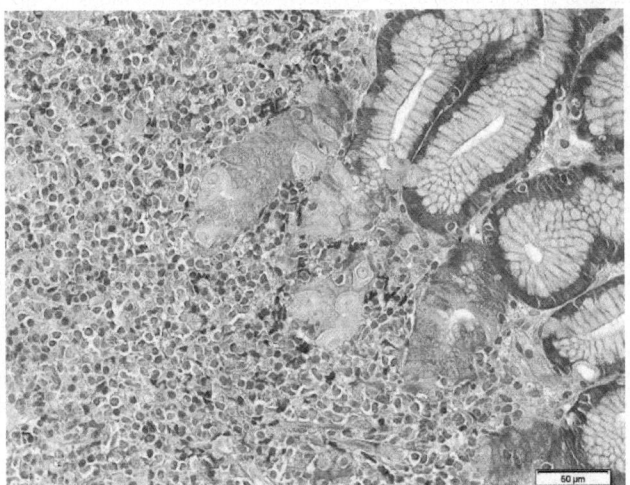

Figure 101–1. Gastric mucosa-associated lymphoid tissue lymphoma (Giemsa stain, magnification ×200). *(Used with permission of Dr. Claudio Agostinelli.)*

TABLE 101–2. Chemotherapy/Immunotherapy Experiences in Gastric Mucosa-Associated Lymphoid Tissue Lymphoma

Study	Patients	Early Stage	Treatment	Outcomes
Hammel[20]	24	71%	Cyclophosphamide or Chlorambucil	75% CR
Avilés[21]	83	100%	CHOP × 3 + CVP × 4	100% CR
Jäger[22]	19	100%	Cladribine	100% CR
Martinelli[23]	27	86%	Rituximab	46% CR; 31% PR
Raderer[24]	7	57%	R-CHOP/R-CNOP	100% CR
Conconi[25]	13	100%	Bortezomib	46% CR; 15% PR
Salar[26]	21	64%	Bendamustine + rituximab	94% CR; 6% PR

CHOP, cyclophosphamide, doxorubicin, vincristine, prednisone; CNOP, cyclophosphamide, mitoxantrone, vincristine, prednisone; CR, complete response; CVP, cyclophosphamide, vincristine, prednisolone; PR, partial response; R, rituximab.

effective in the treatment of all stages of disease (Table 101–2).[20–26] It is important to note that patients with the t(11;18) translocation are usually unresponsive to alkylating drugs if administered as single agents. Fludarabine has important antitumor activity,[27] especially when combined with rituximab,[28] as has the combination of chlorambucil plus rituximab.[29] Radioimmunotherapy with ^{90}Y-ibritumomab tiuxetan is also effective for patients with MALT lymphoma.[30]

COURSE AND PROGNOSIS

MALT lymphoma usually has a favorable outcome, with a 5-year overall survival greater than 85 percent in most series. The reported median time-to-progression seems to be more favorable for gastrointestinal MALT lymphomas than nongastrointestinal lymphomas; however, no significant differences in overall survival have been demonstrated between the two disease subgroups. Approximately 30 to 50 percent of patients with a *H. pylori*–positive gastric MALT lymphoma show persistent or progressive disease after *H. pylori* eradication with antibiotic therapy. Among complete responders, almost 15 percent relapse within 3 years, suggesting that additional therapies are required in a significant percentage of patients. Histologic transformation to diffuse large B-cell lymphoma has been reported in approximately 10 percent of the cases, usually as a late event that occurs independently from dissemination.

●SPLENIC MARGINAL ZONE LYMPHOMA

DEFINITION AND EPIDEMIOLOGY

SMZL is a mature B-cell neoplasm arising from postgerminal center lymphocytes and involving the white pulp follicles of the spleen, the splenic hilar lymph nodes, the marrow and often the blood, showing characteristic neoplastic lymphoid elements referred to as "villous lymphocytes." It accounts for 1 to 2 percent of all lymphomas, with a median age at diagnosis of nearly 65 years (range: 30 to 90 years) and a slight male predominance.

ETIOLOGY AND PATHOGENESIS

The precise pathogenesis of SMZL is unknown: the cell of origin is a marginal zone B cell, which is believed to be of postgerminal center origin, as demonstrated by the presence of somatic hypermutations in *IGHV* genes[31,32]; however, up to one-third of cases are nonmutated. Conversely, SMZL exhibits a low frequency of somatic mutations involving oncogenes such as *BCL-6*, *PAX5*, and *PIM1*, which suggests a pathway of differentiation that may not involve a transit through the germinal center.[33]

In cases of SMZL associated with chronic HCV infection, longstanding antigenic stimulation of B-lymphocytes as a result of the interaction of the viral E2 glycoprotein with CD81 on B cells is responsible for lymphocytes activation through the B-cell receptor (BCR), which ultimately leads to an increased rate of proliferation of B cells. Antiviral treatments can induce remissions of SMZL, thus proving the causative role of the infection in the pathogenetic process of HCV-related SMZL.[34] SMZL associated with chronic HCV infection is often associated with mixed cryoglobulinemia and the development of cryoglobulinemic vasculitis.

GENETIC ABERRATIONS AND MOLECULAR PATHOGENESIS

Cytogenetic abnormalities can be found in up to 80 percent of SMZL patients, most frequently consisting of complete or partial 3q trisomy (30 to 80 percent of cases) and gains of 12q (15 to 20 percent of patients). However, the most significant karyotype aberrations, considered typical of SMZL, are deletions or translocations involving 7q32, which are reported in nearly 40 percent of the cases. Other alterations involving chromosomes 8, 9p34, 12q23–24, 17p, and 18q, although not typical, are helpful for the diagnosis of SMZL.[35]

SMZL displays a characteristic transcriptional profile with a molecular signature consisting of over-expression of genes involved in the *AKT1*, *BCR*, and *NF-κB* signalling pathways. Mutations in signalling pathways involved in marginal zone B-cell development are also observed in nearly 60 percent of SMZL, with mutations of *NOTCH2* being the most frequent, accounting for 20 percent of the cases.[36] As these mutations are restricted to SMZL, they represent a potential diagnostic marker (and presumably a therapeutic target) for this lymphoma subtype.

CLINICAL FEATURES

Isolated and generally asymptomatic splenomegaly and cytopenias are the most significant clinical characteristics of this lymphoma. The majority of patients seek medical attention because of the presence of anemia and/or thrombocytopenia, mostly related to hypersplenism rather than marrow insufficiency as a consequence of disease infiltration. Lymphocytosis is always present, and basophilic villous cells in blood may also be found. Splenomegaly is detectable upon physical examination; dyspepsia and abdominal discomfort, due to the enlarged (or sometimes markedly enlarged) spleen, are often reported. Massive splenomegaly, frequently associated with small splenic hilar lymph nodes, is the typical feature of advanced cases.

Autoimmune phenomena can be associated with this lymphoma, a result of the production of autoantibodies sustained by the neoplastic clone. Hemolytic autoimmune anemia or immune thrombocytopenia are present in 10 to 15 percent of patients. In up to 40 percent, a serum monoclonal paraprotein can be detected.

MORPHOLOGY

A micronodular lymphoid infiltrate of small lymphocytes typically surrounds and replaces the splenic white pulp germinal centers in SMZL, with involvement of the red pulp also consistently observed. The malignant cells resemble those of marginal zone MALT lymphoma; although some are larger and resemble centroblasts or immunoblasts. Plasmacytic differentiation is usually appreciated within germinal centers. Neoplastic lymphocytes are typically CD20+, CD23–, CD38–, CD5–, CD10–, cyclin D1–, IgD+. Intertrabecular lymphoid nodules in the marrow mimic the morphology of tumor nodules in the spleen, with occasional reactive germinal centers surrounded by neoplastic cells. Neoplastic lymphocytes can usually be recognized in the blood,[37] with the classic villous morphology, characterized by the presence of polar small cytoplasmic projections (seen in only a subset of cells).

DIFFERENTIAL DIAGNOSIS

SMZL can be distinguished from other indolent lymphomas associated with splenomegaly by the integration of clinical, morphologic, immunohistochemical and genetic data. Both follicular lymphoma and mantle cell lymphoma may show a micronodular pattern of splenic involvement: however, the expression of both CD5 and cyclin D1 by mantle cell lymphoma and of CD10 by follicular lymphoma represent clear diagnostic clues differentiating these subtypes. A more challenging distinction is with lymphoplasmacytic lymphoma because plasmacytic differentiation is seen in 28 percent of cases of SMZL. The presence of a very large IgM paraprotein spike (>10 g/L) favors the diagnosis of lymphoplasmacytic lymphoma (LPL) rather than SMZL, though small IgM paraprotein spikes may also been seen in SMZL (<10 g/L usually).

THERAPY

Treatment is required only in symptomatic SMZL patients with massive splenomegaly causing pain, early satiety or cytopenias, defined as hemoglobin less than 100 g/L, platelets less than 80,000/μL, or neutrophils less than 1000/μL. Asymptomatic patients may be followed clinically without intervention for many years, since treatment does not influence survival.[15]

When treatment is indicated because of the occurrence of clinical symptoms, the recommended frontline therapy is splenectomy, which allows a rapid correction of anemia, thrombocytopenia and neutropenia—if present—and the removal of the dominant focus of the disease, even though such management does not influence marrow infiltration or blood lymphocytosis. Postsplenectomy partial remissions are generally stably maintained for years, and patients can remain asymptomatic, with a median time to next treatment of 8 years.[38]

Systemic therapy is required when major contraindications to surgery exist, in elderly patients, in those who relapse or progress after splenectomy and in case of advanced disseminated nodal disease or high-grade transformation. Rituximab, used both as a single agent or combined with chemotherapy, is highly effective in this subgroup of patients[41,42] and is preferred to splenectomy by some authorities. Chemotherapy regimens are based on alkylating agents (such as chlorambucil or cyclophosphamide), fludarabine or bendamustine.[39,40]

COURSE AND PROGNOSIS

The median overall survival for patients with SMZL is 5 to 10 years, although a median survival time of less than 4 years has been documented in a subset of patients presenting with advanced or aggressive disease (25 to 30 percent of cases). In 10 to 20 percent of cases, histologic transformation into a diffuse large B-cell lymphoma occurs.

A prognostic model has been recently developed and validated in a cohort of more than 300 patients[43] based on three variables: hemoglobin concentration (<120 g/L), LDH (if elevated at diagnosis), and albumin levels (<35 g/L). This model, although lacking therapeutic implications, allows stratification of patients into three risk-groups, including a low-risk group (no risk factors) with an 88 percent 5-year cause-specific survival rate, an intermediate-risk group (one risk factor) with a 73 percent 5-year cause-specific survival rate, and a high risk group (at least two risk factors) with a 50 percent cause-specific survival rate.

⬤ NODAL MARGINAL ZONE LYMPHOMA

DEFINITION AND EPIDEMIOLOGY

Nodal MZL is a mature, postgerminal center B-cell lymphoma, sharing many morphologic and immunohistochemical characteristics with EMZL and SMZL, although it is considered a distinct clinicopathologic subtype by the current WHO classification. It is a rare disease, accounting for less than 2 percent of all lymphomas, with a median age at onset of between 50 and 60 years. The association with autoimmune phenomena is weak for this lymphoma, in contrast to other MZLs.

GENETIC ABERRATIONS AND MOLECULAR PATHOGENESIS

No typical cytogenetic aberrations have been demonstrated for NMZL: among the reported abnormalities are gains of chromosomes 3, 7, 12, and 18, and structural rearrangements of chromosome 1, with breakpoints in 1q21 or 1p34.[44] Gain of several regions of chromosome 3 constitute a common marker of NMZL, occurring in 20 to 25 percent of patients, and are shared with patients presenting with EMZL. More than three-quarters of patients harbor somatic *IGHV* gene mutations, and show a biased use of *IGHV* segments 3 and 4. These mutations are equally seen in both HCV-positive and HCV-negative patients; however, *IGHV* gene segment 1–69 seems to be preferentially used in HCV-related cases, suggesting differential antigenic stimulation driving lymphoma B-cell precursor selection, and the possible pathogenic role of HCV itself.[45]

CLINICAL FEATURES

The majority of patients affected by NMZL present with disseminated peripheral and abdominal nodal involvement. Marrow infiltration is seen in less than half of the patients, and blood involvement is rare. Extranodal disease is absent, by definition and the presence of splenomegaly should suggest a diagnosis of SMZL. Performance status is generally good with lymphoma-related symptoms reported in 10 to 40 percent of the cases. A serum monoclonal component is detected in only 10 percent of patients.

MORPHOLOGY

Neoplastic elements within lymph nodes have a marginal zone pattern of infiltration, with residual follicles being well-preserved or expanded in some cases ("MALT-type" NMZL), diminished in other cases ("splenic-type" NMZL), or sometimes colonized by the lymphoma cells,

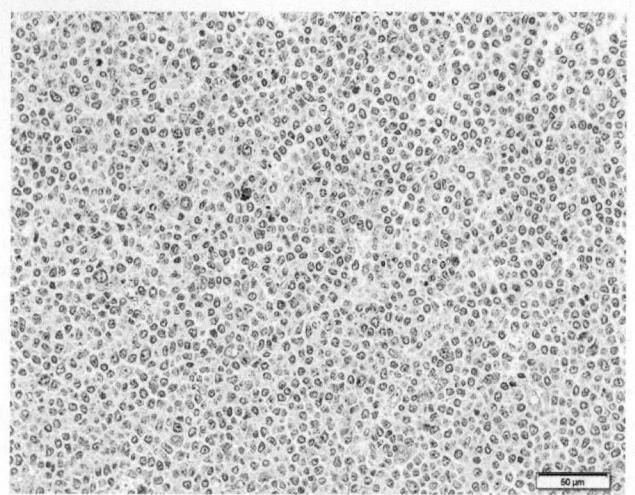

Figure 101–2. Nodal marginal zone lymphoma (Giemsa stain, magnification ×200). *(Used with permission of Dr. Claudio Agostinelli.)*

in which case marked plasmacytoid differentiation and a nodular or follicular growth pattern mimicking follicular lymphoma is often seen (Fig. 101–2).

DIFFERENTIAL DIAGNOSIS

Pediatric NMZL is a different clinical entity that arises in adolescent patients, with a striking predominance in males. Atypical cells within lymph nodes show a marked pleomorphism and an interfollicular distribution with marginal zones considerably expanded.[1] Patients generally present with localized stage I disease, which can be managed conservatively (surgical excision and observation), with low rates of disease recurrence.

The pathologic distinction between NMZL, LPL and follicular lymphoma with marginal zone differentiation can be difficult. Immunohistochemistry may be a useful diagnostic tool by demonstrating *BCL6* and CD10 expression in follicular lymphoma, whereas the demonstration of a large IgM paraprotein spike in the serum suggests LPL rather than NMZL.

THERAPY

No specific treatment consensus guidelines have been developed for NMZL, and patients are generally well managed according to treatment paradigms developed for follicular lymphoma and other indolent NHLs. In limited stage disease, surgery and radiotherapy are often appropriate, whereas immunochemotherapy is the most suitable option for patients presenting with symptomatic advanced stage disease.[15,46] Patients with concomitant HCV infection and no urgency for lymphoma treatment should receive antiviral treatment with interferon and ribavirin.[47] High-dose therapy and autologous stem cell transplantation can be considered for patients with aggressive presentations and short remission durations following standard immunochemotherapy regimens.[46]

COURSE AND PROGNOSIS

The average 5-year survival of NMZL is approximately 60 to 70 percent, with an estimated 5-year event-free survival of nearly 30 percent, thus indicating a high tendency of disease to relapse over time, albeit with rare involvement of extranodal sites.

REFERENCES

1. Swerdlow SH, Campo E, Harris NL, et al. (eds): *World Health Organization Classification of Tumours of Haematopoietic and Lymphoid Tissues.* IARC Press, Lyon, 2008.
2. Berger F, Felman P, Thieblemont C, et al: Non-MALT marginal zone B-cell lymphomas: A description of clinical presentation and outcome in 124 patients. *Blood* 95: 1950–1956, 2000.
3. Arcaini L, Lucioni M, Boveri E, Paulli M: Nodal marginal zone lymphoma: Current knowledge and future directions of an heterogeneous disease. *Eur J Haematol* 83: 165–174, 2009.
4. Ferreri AJ, Dolcetti R, Magnino S, et al: Chlamydial infection: The link with ocular adnexal lymphomas. *Nat Rev Clin Oncol* 6:658–669, 2009.
5. Lecuit M, Abachin E, Martin A, et al: Immunoproliferative small intestinal disease associated with *Campylobacter jejuni. N Engl J Med* 350:239–248, 2004.
6. Zucca E, Roggero E, Maggi-Solcà N, et al: Prevalence of *Helicobacter pylori* and hepatitis C virus infection among non-Hodgkin's lymphoma patients in southern Switzerland. *Haematologica* 85:147–153, 2000.
7. Roggero E, Zucca E, Mainetti C, et al: Eradication of *Borrelia burgdorferi* infection in primary marginal zone B-cell lymphoma of the skin. *Hum Pathol* 31:263–268, 2000.
8. O'Rourke JL: Gene expression profiling in Helicobacter-induced MALT lymphoma with reference to antigen drive and protective immunization. *J Gastroenterol Hepatol* 23(Suppl):S151–S156, 2008.
9. Ponzoni M, Ferreri AJ, Guidoboni M, et al: Chlamydia infection and lymphomas: Association beyond ocular adnexal lymphomas highlighted by multiple detection methods. *Clin Cancer Res* 14:5794–5800, 2008.
10. Derringer GA, Thompson LD, Frommelt RA, et al: Malignant lymphoma of the thyroid gland: A clinicopathologic study of 108 cases. *Am J Surg Pathol* 24:623–639, 2000.
11. Manganelli P, Fietta P, Quaini F: Hematologic manifestations of primary Sjögren's syndrome. *Clin Exp Rheumatol* 24:438–448, 2006.
12. Dierlamm J, Baens M, Wlodarska I, et al: The apoptosis inhibitor gene API2 and a novel 18q gene, MLT, are recurrently rearranged in the t(11;18)(q21;q21) associated with mucosa-associated lymphoid tissue lymphoma. *Blood* 93:3601–3609, 1999.
13. Kwee I, Rancoita PM, Rinaldi A, et al: Genomic profiles of MALT lymphomas: Variability across anatomical sites. *Haematologica* 96:1064–1066, 2011.
14. Troch M, Kiesewetter B, Raderer M: Recent developments in nongastric mucosa-associated lymphoid tissue lymphoma. *Curr Hematol Malig Rep* 6:216–221, 2011.
15. Dreyling M, Thieblemont C, Gallamini A, et al: ESMO consensus conferences: Guidelines on malignant lymphoma. Part 2: Marginal zone lymphoma, mantle cell lymphoma, peripheral T-cell lymphoma. *Ann Oncol* 24:857–877, 2013.
16. Chey WD, Wong BC: American College of Gastroenterology guideline on the management of *Helicobacter pylori* infection. *Am J Gastroenterol* 102:1808–1825, 2007.
17. Zinzani PL, Tani M, Barbieri E, et al: Utility of surgical resection with or without radiation therapy in patients with low-grade mucosa-associated lymphoid tissue lymphoma. *Haematologica* 88:830–831, 2003.
18. Yahalom J: MALT lymphomas: A radiation oncology view-point. *Ann Hematol* 80(Suppl 3):B100–B105, 2001.
19. Koch P, Probst A, Berdel WE, et al: Treatment results in localized primary gastric lymphoma: Data of patients registered within the German multicenter study (GIT NHL 02/96). *J Clin Oncol* 23:7050–7059, 2005.
20. Hammel P, Haioun C, Chaumette MT, et al: Efficacy of single-agent chemotherapy in low-grade B-cell mucosa-associated lymphoid tissue lymphoma with prominent gastric expression. *J Clin Oncol* 13:2524–2529, 1995.
21. Avilés A, Nambo MJ, Neri N, et al: Mucosa-associated lymphoid tissue (MALT) lymphoma of the stomach: Results of a controlled clinical trial. *Med Oncol* 22:57–62, 2005.
22. Jäger U, Neumeister P, Quehenberger F, et al: Prolonged clinical remission in patients with extranodal marginal zone B-cell lymphoma of the mucosa-associated lymphoid tissue type treated with cladribine: 6 year follow-up of a phase II trial. *Ann Oncol* 17:1722–1723, 2006.
23. Martinelli G, Laszlo D, Ferreri A, et al: Clinical activity of rituximab in gastric marginal zone non-Hodgkin's lymphoma resistant to or not eligible for anti-*Helicobacter pylori* therapy. *J Clin Oncol* 23:1979–1983, 2005.
24. Raderer M, Chott A, Drach J, et al: Chemotherapy for management of localised high grade gastric B-cell lymphoma: How much is necessary? *Ann Oncol* 13:1094–1098, 2002.
25. Conconi A, Martinelli G, Lopez-Guillermo A, et al: Clinical activity of bortezomib in relapsed/refractory MALT lymphomas: Results of a phase II study of the International Extranodal Lymphoma Study Group (IELSG). *Ann Oncol* 22:689–695, 2011.
26. Salar A, Domingo E, Canales M, et al: Bendamustine and rituximab as first line treatment for patients with MALT lymphoma. An interim report of a phase 2 trial in Spain (GELTAMO MALT-2008-01). *Ann Oncol* 22(Suppl 4):IV184, 2011.
27. Zinzani PL, Stefoni V, Musuraca G, et al: Fludarabine-containing chemotherapy as frontline treatment of nongastrointestinal mucosa-associated lymphoid tissue lymphoma. *Cancer* 100:2190–2194, 2004.
28. Zinzani PL, Pellegrini C, Broccoli A, et al: Fludarabine-mitoxantrone-rituximab regimen in untreated indolent non-follicular non-Hodgkin's lymphoma: Experience on 143 patients. *Hematol Oncol* 2014, in press. DOI: 10.1002/hon.2151. [Epub ahead of print]
29. Zucca E, Conconi A, Laszlo D, et al: Addition of rituximab to chlorambucil produces superior event-free survival in the treatment of patients with extranodal marginal-zone B-cell lymphoma: 5-year analysis of the IELSG-19 randomized study. *J Clin Oncol* 31:565–572, 2013.

30. Vanazzi A, Grana C, Crosta C, et al: Efficacy of ⁹⁰Yttrium-ibritumomab tiuxetan in relapsed/refractory extranodal marginal-zone lymphoma. *Hematol Oncol* 32:10–15, 2014.
31. Boveri E, Arcaini L, Merli M, et al: Bone marrow histology in marginal zone B-cell lymphomas: Correlation with clinical parameters and flow cytometry in 120 patients. *Ann Oncol* 20:129–136, 2009.
32. Zibellini S, Capello D, Forconi F, et al: Stereotyped patterns of B-cell receptor in splenic marginal zone lymphoma. *Haematologica* 95:1792–1796, 2010.
33. Traverse-Glehen A, Verney A, Baseggio L, et al: Analysis of BCL-6, CD95, PIM1, RHO/TTF and PAX5 mutations in splenic and nodal marginal zone B-cell lymphomas suggests a particular B-cell origin. *Leukemia* 21:1821–1824, 2007.
34. Hermine O, Lefrère F, Bronowicki JP, et al: Regression of splenic lymphoma with villous lymphocytes after treatment of hepatitis C virus infection. *N Engl J Med* 347:89–94, 2002.
35. Salido M, Baro C, Oscier D, et al: Cytogenetic aberrations and their prognostic value in a series of 330 splenic marginal zone B-cell lymphomas: A multicenter study of the Splenic B-Cell Lymphoma Group. *Blood* 116:1479–1488, 2010.
36. Rossi D, Trifonov V, Fangazio M, et al: The coding genome of splenic marginal zone lymphoma: Activation of NOTCH2 and other pathways regulating marginal zone development. *J Exp Med* 209:1537–1551, 2012.
37. Melo JV, Hegde U, Parreira A, et al: Splenic B cell lymphoma with circulating villous lymphocytes: Differential diagnosis of B cell leukaemias with large spleens. *J Clin Pathol* 40:642–651, 1987.
38. Thieblemont C, Felman P, Berger F, et al: Treatment of splenic marginal zone B-cell lymphoma: An analysis of 81 patients. *Clin Lymphoma* 3:41–47, 2002.
39. Tsimberidou AM, Catovsky D, Schlette E, et al: Outcomes in patients with splenic marginal zone lymphoma and marginal zone lymphoma treated with rituximab with or without chemotherapy or chemotherapy alone. *Cancer* 107:125–135, 2006.
40. Bennett M, Sharma K, Yegena S, et al: Rituximab monotherapy for splenic marginal zone lymphoma. *Haematologica* 90:856–858, 2005.
41. Lefrère F, Hermine O, Belanger C, et al: Fludarabine: An effective treatment in patients with splenic lymphoma with villous lymphocytes. *Leukemia* 14:573–575, 2000.
42. Cheson BD, Friedberg JW, Kahl BS, et al: Bendamustine produces durable responses with an acceptable safety profile in patients with rituximab refractory indolent non-Hodgkin lymphoma. *Clin Lymphoma Myeloma Leuk* 10:452–457, 2010.
43. Arcaini L, Lazzarino M, Colombo N, et al: Splenic marginal zone lymphoma: A prognostic model for clinical use. *Blood* 107:4643–4649, 2006.
44. Brynes RK, Almaguer PD, Leathery KE, et al: Numerical cytogenetic abnormalities of chromosomes 3, 7, and 12 in marginal zone B-cell lymphomas. *Mod Pathol* 9:995–1000, 1996.
45. Marasca R, Vaccai P, Luppi M, et al: Immunoglobulin gene mutations and frequent use of VH1-69 and VH4-34 segments in hepatitis C virus-positive and hepatitis C virus-negative nodal marginal zone B-cell lymphoma. *Am J Pathol* 159:253–261, 2001.
46. Thieblemont C, Coiffier B: Management of marginal zone lymphomas. *Curr Treat Options Oncol* 7:213–222, 2006.
47. Vallisa D, Bernuzzi P, Arcaini L, et al: Role of anti-hepatitis C virus (HCV) treatment in HCV-related, low-grade, B-cell, non-Hodgkin's lymphoma: A multicenter Italian experience. *J Clin Oncol* 23:468–473, 2005.

CHAPTER 102
BURKITT LYMPHOMA

Andrew G. Evans and Jonathan W. Friedberg

SUMMARY

Burkitt lymphoma is one of the highly aggressive B-cell lymphomas. It was the first tumor to be etiologically associated with (1) a virus, specifically Epstein-Barr virus, (2) a specific translocation involving the *MYC* oncogene, and (3) one of the first cancers shown to be curable by chemotherapy alone. It presents in three clinically distinct forms: endemic, sporadic, and immunodeficiency-associated. Burkitt lymphoma is an uncommon form of lymphoma in adults, with an incidence of approximately 1200 patients per year in the United States. Over the last decade, the definition of Burkitt lymphoma has been refined, largely as a consequence of improvements in immunohistochemical, cytogenetic, and molecular diagnostic techniques. Transcriptional profiling has more clearly defined Burkitt lymphoma at the molecular level, while whole-genome sequencing has expanded our understanding of the mutational landscape that underlies this disease. Despite these refinements in diagnostic criteria, the differential diagnosis includes several high-grade lymphomas, including a group of patients with a diagnosis defined by the World Health Organization as intermediate between Burkitt lymphoma and diffuse large B-cell lymphoma. Burkitt lymphoma is a highly curable malignancy in the modern therapeutic era. The majority of younger patients are cured with intensive chemotherapeutic regimens, and increasing efficacy has been demonstrated in older patients with reduced intensity treatments. Remaining challenges include the optimal management of older patients, the development of therapy for patients with relapsed or refractory disease, and the translation of gains made in treatment to the management of endemic disease.

DEFINITION AND HISTORY

Burkitt lymphoma (BL) may present in three distinct forms: endemic (African), sporadic, and immunodeficiency-associated.[1] The endemic form (eBL) is the most common pediatric tumor in sub-Saharan Africa

and other regions of the world where malaria is endemic. It typically presents in the jaw or maxilla, and is associated with Epstein-Barr virus (EBV) infection at an early age. Although there are reports dating to as early as 1910, it was Denis Burkitt who is credited with describing this malignancy in 1958 as a common tumor in children of Uganda.[2,3] Originally thought by Burkitt to be a sarcoma of the jaw, it was a pathologist named George O'Connor who, in 1960, concluded it was a lymphoma.[4] In 1964, while studying BL samples by electron microscopy, Sir Michael Anthony Epstein, Yvonne Barr, and Bert Achong discovered EBV when they recognized viral particles were present in tumor cells,[5] thus helping to launch the nascent field of tumor virology. Further studies of BL over many years led to epidemiologic associations with both EBV and malaria in Africa.[6,7] Tumors of a similar histologic appearance were subsequently identified in the United States, Middle East, and elsewhere (i.e., nonendemic regions) and termed *sporadic BL*. Sporadic cases were found to occur in older individuals, typically presented in the abdomen rather than the orofacial region, and were infrequently associated with EBV.[8] In 1985, a third class of BL was identified in immunosuppressed patients, most commonly as a result of infection with HIV.[9] BL was referred to as "small noncleaved cell lymphoma" according to the Kiel classification system proposed by Karl Lennert in 1977, but this designation is no longer used. In the mid-1970s, recurrent chromosomal translocations involving chromosomes 8 and 14 were described in BL,[10,11] paving the way for the identification of *MYC* as an important human oncogene when it was shown to be the translocation partner involved with immunoglobulin (Ig) heavy-chain and light-chain translocations.[12,13] Evolution in the diagnosis and treatment of BL has occurred over the past few decades. High cure rates are now achieved among pediatric and young adult populations in healthcare settings capable of delivering intensive combined chemotherapy regimens, both with and without B-cell–directed monoclonal antibody therapy (i.e., rituximab). In 2006, a "molecular signature" for BL was developed from gene-expression profiling (GEP) data,[14] and in 2012 the first whole-genome sequences were published.[15] Despite these scientific and technologic advances in our understanding of this historically important disease, translation of this information into specific targeted therapeutics for BL (i.e., inhibitors of known dysregulated pathways or mutated gene products) has yet to be realized.

EPIDEMIOLOGY

The endemic form of BL is found in equatorial Africa (as well as Brazil, Papua New Guinea, and other malaria-endemic regions), with a peak age incidence at 4 to 7 years, and is nearly twice as frequent in boys as in girls. In Africa it accounts for 20 percent of cancers in newborns to 14-year-olds, and for the majority of non-Hodgkin lymphomas (NHLs) in all age groups.[16] Infection by EBV is found in nearly 100 percent of patients with eBL, and higher titers are linked to increase risk of eBL.[7] Although not as close, there is an epidemiologic association with malaria,[17] in addition to other environmental factors.[16] Sporadic BL, defined as cases outside of endemic African regions, accounts for 1 to 2 percent of NHL, is higher in males than in females, and has a median age of 30 years. In the United States, BL exhibits a primarily a bimodal age distribution, with at least two incidence peaks of approximately 10 and 75 years of age (median age of approximately 30 years), as compared to other NHLs, which generally increase from childhood through adulthood.[18] Immunodeficiency-related BL increased in incidence during the AIDS epidemic; however, with improved antiretroviral therapy, the incidence has decreased in the United States and countries with access to effective therapy for HIV.

ETIOLOGY AND PATHOGENESIS

MOLECULAR GENETICS

Myc Overexpression and Gene-Expression Profiling

The unifying feature of all three types of BL is activation of the *MYC* gene via an Ig translocation leading to high levels of MYC protein, which activates transcription of a variety of genes involved in cell growth. Translocations are thought to occur via double-stranded DNA breaks that occur during normal class-switch reaction and somatic hypermutation in mature B-cell development, which, in turn, depends on activation-induced cytidine deaminase.[19] In addition, somatic point mutation of growth-regulatory genes (such as *MYC*) which are also caused by activation-induced cytidine deaminase may also play an important role.[20] The dominant role of *MYC* activation in BL pathogenesis is emphasized by the results of multiple independent gene-expression studies. GEP analysis is capable of distinguishing BL from diffuse large B-cell lymphoma (DLBCL), and this finding is predicated on identifying cases with highly expressed target genes of MYC, as well as markers of germinal center B cells, and lower expression of target genes of the nuclear factor (NF)-κB pathway.[21] In a separate study, a core group of eight cases of pediatric BL (fulfilling World Health Organization [WHO] criteria) were used to generate a molecular signature, and tumors that matched this expression pattern were termed "molecular BL" (mBL).[22] Additional characteristics of this group included lower cytogenetic complexity (including near total absence of translocations involving *BCL6* and/or *IGH-BCL2*) and the presence of *MYC* translocations involving Ig genes, rather than non-Ig partners, features which, again, distinguish BL from DLBCLs and other high-grade NHLs.

Next Generation Sequencing and ID3/TCF3 Mutations

Advanced sequencing analysis at the level of the whole genome, exome, and transcriptome has provided a more complete view of the spectrum of somatic mutations that occur in Burkitt lymphomagenesis and identified several recurring and previously unappreciated determinants of molecular pathogenesis. In addition to mutations in *MYC*, as many as 70 additional genes were found to be recurrently mutated in BL.[23] Mutations in *ID3*, *TCF3*, and *CCND3* are among the most common seen in multiple independent studies.[23–25] ID3 is a member of the inhibitor of DNA binding (ID) protein family, and it is a negative regulator of transcription factor TCF3. The presence of biallelic inactivating mutations and/or deletions of *ID3* suggests it serves as a tumor suppressor. TCF3, conversely, was shown to be essential for BL cell viability, and the presence of monoallelic mutations that result in substitutions among highly conserved amino acid residues suggests gain of function mutations in TCF3 may result. Overall, the mutational landscape for BL differs significantly from DLBCL. For example, relatively few *ID3* mutations were found among other B-cell lymphomas, even in those with *Ig-MYC* translocations.[24] *ID3* and/or *TCF3* mutations were also common among all three epidemiologic subtypes of BL. *CCND3* mutations were rare in eBL, but abundant in the other two subtypes.[25]

ALTERED IMMUNE STATUS AND INFECTION

HIV-Associated and Endemic Disease

Underlying immune alteration likely plays a role in at least two epidemiologic subtypes of BL (endemic and immunodeficiency-associated), although teasing apart the precise role of immune function in BL pathogenesis has proven challenging. Immunodeficiency-associated BL occurs predominantly in HIV-positive patients. Its occurrence does not directly correlate with CD4+ T cell status, and BL only rarely occurs with other forms of immunosuppression. BL is different from other EBV-associated lymphoproliferative disorders that occur with advanced HIV, yet is otherwise comparable to EBV-positive posttransplantation lymphoproliferative disorders (PTLDs) that arise in severely immunosuppressed solid-organ allograft recipients.[26] Rather, the clinical course and pathogenesis of immunodeficiency-associated BL more closely parallels that of sporadic BL in the immunologically intact patient. In eBL, the underlying immune alteration is probably multifactorial, may be influenced by chronic malnutrition, and may stem from chronic immune activation to various stimuli including holoendemic malaria, EBV, and possibly other environmental agents.[27,28]

Epstein-Barr Virus and Malaria

The clear epidemiologic and immunologic link to malaria and EBV-infection has led several investigators to characterize eBL as a "polymicrobial" disease.[29] Numerous biological mechanisms have been proposed to explain the etiologic link between eBL and each infection. For example, EBV may play a role prior to the MYC translocation event, simultaneously inducing proliferation (via Epstein-Barr nuclear antigen [EBNA]-2) and inhibiting apoptosis (via EBNA3A- and EBNA3C-induced epigenetic silencing of proapoptotic protein Bim [Bcl-2-interacting mediator of cell death], a key defender of MYC-induced tumorigenesis).[30] Alternatively, inhibition of apoptosis may be sustained in BL tumor cells as a result of EBNA-1 expression (the only latency-associated viral protein consistently expressed in BL), noncoding viral RNAs (including Epstein-Barr virus-encoded RNA [EBER] and microRNAs), or possibly as a result of epigenetic reprogramming.[31] Precise mechanisms for the role of malaria in eBL are less clear, but it has been shown that *Plasmodium* species can stimulate B cells in a polyclonal fashion,[32,33] the effects of which may modulate EBV transcriptional programs within infected B cells.[34] Malaria infection also modulates virus-specific T-cell responses to EBV.[35] By simultaneously expanding EBV-infected B cells, which may dysregulate the activation induced cytidine deaminase function and thereby increase the chance of acquiring a MYC translocation, while at the same time perturbing the host's antiviral immune response, malaria infection may serve as a critical facilitator that brings together these otherwise disparate pathologic events in a manner that predisposes specific populations to developing eBL.[36] Overall, these findings suggest that BL emerges in the setting of chronically altered but fundamentally intact immune system.

CLINICAL FEATURES

The endemic (African) form often presents as a jaw or facial bone tumor. It may spread to extranodal sites, especially to the marrow and meninges. Almost all cases are EBV-positive. The nonendemic or American form presents as an abdominal mass in approximately 65 percent of cases, often with ascites. Extranodal sites, such as the kidneys, gonads, breast, marrow, and CNS, may be involved. Involvement of the marrow and CNS is much more common in the nonendemic form. Patients with more than 25 percent marrow involvement with malignant cells often are referred to as having Burkitt cell leukemia (see Blood and Marrow below). In addition, in contrast to the endemic form, only 15 percent of the nonendemic cases are EBV-positive.

Immunodeficiency-related cases often involve the lymph nodes and are associated with EBV in 30 percent of the cases. Staging using the system modified for childhood BL (Murphy staging system, Table 102–1) may be used rather than the Ann Arbor system, given that BL is largely an extranodal lymphoma.

TABLE 102–1. Murphy Staging System for Burkitt Lymphoma

Stage I: Single nodal or extranodal site excluding mediastinum or abdomen

Stage II: Single extranodal tumor with regional nodal involvement

    Two extranodal tumors on one side of diaphragm

    Primary gastrointestinal tumor with or without associated mesenteric nodes

    Two or more nodal areas on one side of diaphragm

Stage IIR: Completely resected intraabdominal disease

Stage III: Two single extranodal tumors on opposite sides of diaphragm

    All primary intrathoracic tumors

    All paraspinal or epidural tumors

    All extensive primary intraabdominal disease

    Two or more nodal areas on opposite sides of diaphragm

Stage IIIA: Localized, nonresectable abdominal disease

Stage IIIB: Widespread multiorgan abdominal disease

Stage IV: Initial CNS or marrow involvement (<25%)

Adapted with permisison from Perkins AS, Friedberg JW: Burkitt lymphoma in adults. *Hematology Am Soc Hematol Educ Program* 341–348, 2008.

LABORATORY FEATURES

BLOOD AND MARROW

Patients with bulky disease may have Burkitt cells in marrow and blood with accompanying suppression of normal blood counts. Characteristic pathologic features of BL on smear preparation are intermediate-size cells with round nuclei, multiple nucleoli, strongly basophilic cytoplasm (a consequence of the abundant polyribosomes), and the presence of lipid-filled cytoplasmic vesicles, some of which overlie the nucleus (Fig. 102–1). Rare cases, more commonly in males, may present principally with marrow and blood involvement, so-called Burkitt cell leukemia variant (previously classified as acute lymphocytic leukemia–L3, according to the former French-American-British [FAB] classification).

The serum lactic dehydrogenase (LDH) is often elevated as a reflection of the high cell turnover, especially in patients with bulky disease.

HISTOPATHOLOGY AND CYTOLOGY

BL is characterized by monomorphic medium-size cells with round nuclei, multiple nucleoli, and basophilic cytoplasm.[37] Burkitt cells have a very high proliferative rate (≥95 percent as determined by Ki-67 staining) and frequent mitotic figures are usually present. BL has a diffuse pattern of growth comprised of intermediate-size B cells (12 μM

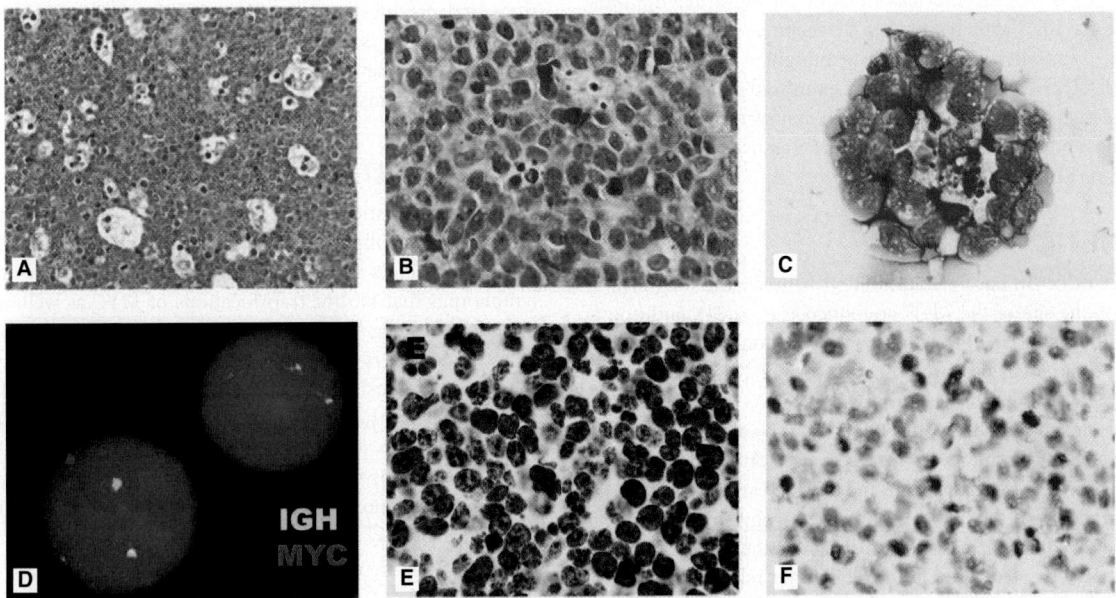

Figure 102–1. A. Lymph node biopsy section. A monomorphic population of Burkitt lymphoma (BL) cells interspersed with macrophages engorged with cellular debris as a result of the high cell turnover rate (high rate of apoptosis and cell proliferation). These "tingible body macrophages," a term derived from a description of phagocytized nuclear debris of small lymphocytes by macrophages in germinal centers of normal lymph nodes used more than 100 years ago, are embedded in the solid monomorphic infiltrate of Burkitt cells give rise to the "starry sky appearance," a descriptor commonly used in lymph node and marrow sections in BL. **B.** Tumor biopsy. High-powered image showing histologic detail of a monomorphic population of medium-size BL cells with rounded nuclei, relatively fine chromatin, multiple prominent nucleoli, and interspersed macrophages. **C.** Cytologic smear preparation demonstrating cluster of BL tumor cells, with characteristic vacuolated, deep-blue, basophilic cytoplasm, rounded nuclei, and multiple nucleoli. Note the associated tingible body macrophage at center. Similar cytologic features of tumor cells are seen on blood and marrow aspirate smear preparations. **D.** Fluorescence *in situ* hybridization (FISH) image demonstrating the presence of *IGH-MYC* translocation *(lower left hand cell)*. Colocalization of the IGH locus probe *(labeled green)* and MYC probe *(labeled red)* results in a fused yellow signal consistent with t(8:14) chromosomal translocation. The *upper right hand cell* shows a normal pattern of two red and two green nontranslocated alleles. **E.** Ki-67 immunoperoxidase stain of BL showing the very high prevalence of cells in the mitotic cycle (virtually all nuclei show the reddish-brown reaction product of the stain). The Ki-67 monoclonal antibody identifies a nuclear protein expressed throughout the cell cycle and is a marker of cell proliferative activity. **F.** MYC immunoperoxidase stain, demonstrating upregulated nuclear expression of MYC in virtually 100 percent of cells. *(A, reproduced with permission from* Lichtman's Atlas of Hematology, *www.accessmedicine.com. D, used with permission of Dr. A. Iqbal, University of Rochester.)*

diameter on a blood or marrow film) with a high nuclear-to-cytoplasmic ratio. Nuclear contours are round to oval without cleaves or folds, a key feature in the distinction from DLBCL. Nucleoli are typically multiple, small-to-intermediate in size, and the nuclear chromatin is relatively immature, being finely granular. Along with a high proliferation rate these cells are characterized by a high rate of spontaneous apoptosis leading to the characteristic "starry sky" pattern in marrow and lymph nodes—a monomorphic diffuse background of lymphoma cells that is interspersed with reactive macrophages engulfing cellular debris (so-called tingible-body macrophages) (see Fig. 102–1).

IMMUNOPHENOTYPE

BL cells are mature B cells, positive for CD19, CD20, CD22, and CD79a, and have monotypic surface IgM; they lack CD5 and CD23. BL cells also show immunologic similarity to germinal center cells of B-cell follicles rather than activated B cells, being positive for BCL6, CD10, Tcl1, and CD38, negative for Mum-1, CD44, CD138, TdT (terminal deoxynucleotidyl transferase), and importantly little to no expression of BCL2. However, germinal center cells markers are not specific for BL, since a significant proportion of DLBCL also has this germinal center cell signature.

EPSTEIN-BARR VIRUS STUDIES

Although EBV is associated with 98 percent of eBL, it is also seen in 20 percent of sporadic cases, and in 30 to 40 percent of HIV-associated cases.[38] It can be detected using *in situ* hybridization for EBER. Although EBV likely plays a key role in B-cell stimulation during a prelymphoma stage, the role for EBV after lymphoma development is unclear, as is whether EBV positivity is clinically meaningful. In EBV-positive endemic cases, CD21 (the EBV receptor) is expressed and is negative in most EBV-negative nonendemic BL cases. In contrast to primary effusion lymphomas and DLBCL, EBV-positive, HIV-associated BL does not express LMP1 or EBNA2.

CYTOGENETICS

Virtually all cases of BL have a translocation between the long arm of chromosome 8, the site of the *MYC* protooncogene (8q24), and one of three translocation partners: the Ig heavy-chain region on chromosome 14; the κ light-chain locus on chromosome 2; or the λ light-chain locus on chromosome 22. The translocations involving MYC can be detected by fluorescence *in situ* hybridization (FISH) using so-called MYC "break apart" probes: a set of two fluorescently tagged DNA probes of two different colors that hybridize to the upstream and downstream side of the gene. In an unperturbed gene, they hybridize together within interphase cells giving a composite color, whereas with translocation, the two fluorescently labeled probes are separated. A key feature of BL is the relative simplicity of their karyotype; in the majority of cases, the MYC translocation is the sole abnormality. This relatively limited degree of chromosomal change has been confirmed by microarray studies which can detect submicroscopic chromosomal alterations.[39,40] Among the few changes repeatedly seen by microarray, MYC amplification is found in mBL cases that lack Ig-MYC translocation. In general, this noncomplex cytogenetic profile for BL distinguishes it from DLBCL, which is among one of the primary considerations in the differential diagnosis with BL, as discussed below.

● DIFFERENTIAL DIAGNOSIS

DIFFUSE LARGE B-CELL LYMPHOMA

The primary pathologic diagnosis in the differential diagnosis of BL is DLBCL.[41] Since the publication of the 2008 WHO guidelines,[1] the diagnosis of BL has been refined and diagnostic criteria have been tightened. Although the majority of BL cases, even in the adult, possess all of the criteria for the diagnosis: high mitotic rate in an appropriate morphologic and immunophenotypic setting, together with an Ig-positive MYC translocation, significant overlap exists with DLBCL and a minority of cases do not fit neatly into the diagnosis of either. Typically, this arises because of the absence of key morphologic features in a lesion that otherwise resembles BL: a nonmonomorphic nuclear morphology; fewer tingible-body macrophages than is typical; or an abnormal immunophenotype. Terms that were once frequently used to describe such cases, such as "atypical" BL or "Burkitt-like lymphoma," have fallen out of favor for diagnostic purposes, and these cases may be best classified as an intermediate or unclassifiable B-cell lymphoma (see "B-Cell Lymphoma, Unclassifiable" below). Consequently the term "Burkitt lymphoma" is now reserved for a more pathologically uniform tumor type, and thus BL now arguably comprises one of the most homogeneous subtypes of aggressive B-cell NHL.

B-CELL LYMPHOMA, UNCLASSIFIABLE

To address the spectrum of overlapping clinicopathologic features exhibited by some cases that fall outside BL, the WHO developed a mixed classifier, termed "B-cell lymphoma, unclassifiable, (BCL-U) with features intermediate between diffuse large B-cell lymphoma and Burkitt lymphoma."[42] Although some propose that this category represents a distinct clinicopathologic entity, this designation is primarily reserved for cases with morphologic and/or immunophenotypic features that preclude more specific classification into either group. The BCL-U category is not intended simply to include otherwise conventional DLBCL that harbor a *MYC* translocation, or conversely BL for which a *MYC* translocation cannot be demonstrated.

DOUBLE-HIT LYMPHOMA

Another diagnostic term that has recently gained widespread use is "double-hit lymphoma" (DHL).[43] Although not a formal diagnostic category, DHL refers to a subset of aggressive mature B-cell (non-Burkitt) lymphomas that harbor translocations of *MYC* as well as at least one other protooncogene (most commonly *BCL2* or *BCL6*). Distinction of such a subset is warranted given that DHL, empirically, has among the worst prognosis of any NHL and patients may benefit from more intensive chemotherapy. The prognostic implication for DLBCLs that overexpress both MYC and BCL2 (i.e., "double-hit" patterns of protein expression as determined by immunohistochemistry) is similar.[44] Whereas DHL most frequently exhibits histomorphologic features of DLBCL or BCL-U, and the importance of BCL2 activity clearly distinguishes it from BL, the clinical aggressiveness of these tumors and critical importance of *MYC* dysregulation have prompted comparisons to BL.

B-CELL LYMPHOBLASTIC LYMPHOMA

Despite the fact that B-cell lymphoblastic lymphoma (B-LBL; a.k.a. B-cell acute lymphoblastic leukemia [B-ALL]) is a malignant neoplasm of immature B-cell precursors, numerous features warrant its consideration in the differential diagnosis with BL, including: anatomic distribution (marrow, soft tissues, and nodes), high proliferation index, overlapping histomorphology (medium-size round-cell morphology, finely dispersed nuclear chromatin, high nuclear-to-cytoplasmic ratio, and occasional "starry sky" pattern), immunophenotype (CD10-positive/CD20-variable), and propensity to occur in young patients. Distinctive features include the expression of TdT, absence of mature B-cell markers (e.g., surface immunoglobulin expression and BCL6), and the distinctive cytologic and flow cytometric features of immature blasts.

●THERAPY

GENERAL CONSIDERATIONS

BL is a highly aggressive tumor; however, therapy with multiagent chemotherapeutic programs results in excellent long-term remission rates and long-term survival of up to 85 percent of children. Applying the same chemotherapy regimens to adults has shown dramatically improved response rates.[45–47] Risk stratification allows patients with limited disease to be treated with less-intensive therapy than more advanced cases and still achieve very high responses, although the vast majority of patients present with advanced disease. Patients with extensive disease can achieve 80 percent long-term survival. The regimens employ multiple non–cross-resistant drugs used over a short period. These drugs include high-dose cyclophosphamide, methotrexate, vincristine, prednisone, high-dose methotrexate, high-dose cytarabine, etoposide, and sometimes ifosfamide. CNS prophylaxis therapy, either intrathecal or systemic, is given in almost all patients with BL. Radiation therapy does not play a role in the treatment of BL, and use of radiation therapy for limited-stage diseases is of no additional benefit.[48,49]

TUMOR LYSIS SYNDROME

The tumor lysis syndrome is a serious metabolic complication of rapidly growing tumors, of which BL is a classic example. The syndrome is the result of the rapid destruction of tumor cells, highly sensitive to chemotherapy, and can result in hyperuricemia, hyperkalemia, hyperphosphatemia, secondary hypocalcemia, metabolic acidosis, and renal failure. In tumors such as BL the cell death rate (and proliferative rate) may be so substantial in patients with bulky disease that the tumor lysis syndrome may occur before therapy, so-called spontaneous tumor lysis.[50] Spontaneous tumor lysis is a highly morbid phenomenon with a poor prognosis for a salutary outcome from therapy and a complication with a high death rate. It occurs in patients with a high body burden of tumor, usually with abdominal disease, a common situation in BL. Its principal manifestation is the combination of hyperuricemia and azotemia. In BL a critical part of therapy is recognizing incipient or overt spontaneous tumor lysis rapidly or preventing chemotherapy-induced tumor lysis. LDH has been used as a surrogate marker for risk of tumor lysis with a serum level twice the upper limit of normal for the laboratory in question being the threshold for urgent concern. The usual prophylactic therapy for this situation is carefully monitored hydration of at least 3 L of saline per day and either allopurinol or rasburicase to decrease serum uric acid concentration and thereby hyperuricosuria.

Rasburicase acts more quickly than allopurinol and should be used if risk is considered high or if evidence of spontaneous tumor lysis is present initially.[51,52] Continuous venovenous hemofiltration has also been very useful in allowing concomitant full-dose chemotherapy and preventing tumor lysis and renal failure.[53,54]

SPECIFIC REGIMENS

The specific regimens that have been developed to treat BL have historically been adapted from pediatric experience; Table 102–2 depicts representative trial results, including adult patients. There are no studies directly comparing these regimens, and comparison among the single-arm studies is difficult because of lack of uniform diagnostic criteria, staging, and the heterogeneous patient populations studied. In general, shorter durations of chemotherapy (i.e., 6 months) are as good as longer (18 months) periods of treatment. Other studies have shown a dramatically improved response with use of four cycles of chemotherapy as opposed to 15 cycles. BL has a high proliferative rate, so subsequent chemotherapy cycles should be started as soon as hematologic recovery occurs. Waiting for a fixed period between cycles may lead to regrowth of resistant tumor cells between cycles.

Cyclophosphamide, doxorubicin, vincristine, methotrexate, ifosfamide, etoposide, and high-dose cytarabine, with intrathecal cytarabine and methotrexate (CODOX-M/IVAC) is among the most commonly used regimens in the United States for adults with BL, based upon an initial favorable publication from the National Cancer Institute (NCI) indicating extremely high response rates.[45] Two subsequent, small, phase II trials have used this regimen with minor modifications, and have successfully enrolled greater numbers of older patients, demonstrating cure rates of approximately 64 percent.[55,56] These cure rates are substantially less than the initial report,[49] but still better than historical data with standard-dose regimens. A modification of this regimen in patients with aggressive lymphomas and high proliferative rate as measured by Ki-67 fraction has been proposed.[57] BL was strictly defined as the following: germinal center phenotype, BCL2-negative, MYC-rearrangement–positive, and absence of the t(14;18) or abnormalities at chromosome 3q27. Overall survival of the subgroup defined as BL was 67 percent in this group of older patients. Treatment-related mortality was 8 percent. Outcomes were similar among all age groups with the exception of patients older than age 65 years who clearly had an inferior prognosis. These results likely reflect the true outcome of this regimen in practice. Several groups have further modified this regimen with the addition of rituximab, demonstrating superior outcomes

TABLE 102–2. Outcome of Burkitt Lymphoma in Larger Studies			
Citation	**Regimen**	**No. of Patients**	**2-Year Outcome**
Hoelzer[71]	Short duration/dose intensive; pediatric NHL based	35	51% (estimated survival)
Magrath[45]	CODOX-M/IVAC	54	89% (actual survival)
Mead[57]	CODOX-M/IVAC	58	64% (progression-free survival)
Rizzieri[65]	Short duration/dose intensive with rituximab	105	74% (3-year event-free survival)
Thomas[64]	Hyper-CVAD with rituximab	31	89% (estimated survival)
Dunleavy[61]	Dose adjusted R-EPOCH	29	95% (event-free survival)
Evens[60]	R-CODOX-M/IVAC	25	80% (progression-free survival)

CODOX-M/IVAC, cyclophosphamide, doxorubicin, vincristine, methotrexate, ifosfamide, etoposide and high-dose cytarabine, with intrathecal cytarabine and methotrexate; hyper-CVAD, fractionated cyclophosphamide, vincristine, doxorubicin, dexamethasone; NHL, non-Hodgkin lymphoma; R-CODOX-M/IVAC, rituximab with CODOX-M/IVAC; R-EPOCH, etoposide, vincristine and doxorubicin, with bolus rituximab, cyclophosphamide and steroids.

compared with historical controls.[58–60] Based upon these findings and extrapolating from studies in other histologies of lymphoma, rituximab should be routinely incorporated in the treatment algorithms of BL.

The NCI has published an experience using a lower-intensity chemotherapy program consisting of infusional etoposide, vincristine and doxorubicin, with bolus rituximab, cyclophosphamide and steroids (dose-adjusted R-EPOCH). Nineteen patients with a median age of 25 years with generally favorable features (only 37 percent had elevated LDH, and only one patient had CNS disease) achieved a 95 percent rate of freedom from disease progression.[61] Intrathecal methotrexate was administered to all patients for CNS prophylaxis.

Other regimens used for the therapy of BL include fractionated cyclophosphamide, vincristine, doxorubicin, and dexamethasone (hyper-CVAD) alternating with high-dose methotrexate and cytarabine.[62] The outcome of patients at a single institution (M.D. Anderson Cancer Center) with BL treated with this regimen in combination with rituximab resulted in an overall survival of 89 percent with only one death.[63,64] The Cancer and Leukemia Group B has developed an intensive short duration regimen consisting of cyclophosphamide, ifosfamide, methotrexate, vincristine, cytarabine, etoposide and glucocorticoids. This regimen was combined with rituximab in a trial enrolling high risk patients with a median age of 43 years, with 74 percent event-free survival at 3 years.[65]

No advantage of autologous stem cell transplantation in patients with BL has been observed, although incorporating planned autologous transplantation into the initial therapeutic algorithm has been used with reasonable results.[66]

Historically, patients with HIV have been managed with less-intensive chemotherapy because of the concern of immunosuppression-related morbidity. In the highly active antiretroviral therapy (HAART) era, HIV-positive patients with BL should be treated similarly to nonimmunocompromised patients, and the dose-adjusted R-EPOCH regimen may be an excellent option for these patients. The rate of treatment failure in HIV-positive patients with BL was significantly lower with a highly aggressive protocol when compared with patients who were treated with less-aggressive chemotherapy. In addition, patients tolerated the aggressive protocol reasonably well, particularly when HAART therapy was incorporated into the regimen.[67]

● COURSE AND PROGNOSIS

To better define optimal therapy and outcome of adults with BL, an international effort focused on with a group of adult patients with BL.[68] Authors of 12 large treatment series (10 prospective; two retrospective) provided outcome information of patients enrolled on their clinical trials who were older than age 40 years. In this pooled analysis, patients older than age 40 years were underrepresented in the published literature, and had significantly inferior outcomes in 10 of the 12 series. Despite this, the majority of adult patients were cured using these regimens.

According to data from the NCI's Surveillance, Epidemiology, and End Results (SEER) program, up to 30 percent of BL diagnosis in the United States includes an "older" group of patients, age 60 years or older. Treatment options may be limited for this group of patients, as many older patients may not tolerate high-dose methotrexate and are not candidates for autologous transplantation. Although the number of older patients on the dose adjusted R-EPOCH trial was limited, this regimen has demonstrated safety in elderly patients with DLBCL. A confirmatory trial conducted in several centers is ongoing and enrolling older patients.

For patients with relapsed or refractory disease, autologous transplantation is best reserved for patients inadequately treated initially, as a consolidation procedure. Patients who relapse after appropriate therapy for BL tend to have highly treatment-resistant disease, with almost uniformly unfavorable outcome. These patients can be retreated with

chemotherapy and considered for allogeneic stem cell transplantation because autologous transplantation is often not beneficial in these patients.[69]

REFERENCES

1. Leoncini L, Raphael M, Stein H, et al: Burkitt lymphoma, in *WHO Classification of Tumours of the Haematopoietic and Lymphoid Tissues*, 4th ed, edited by SK Swerdlow, E Campo, NL Harris, ES Jaffe, SA Pileri, H Stein, J Thiele, and JW Vardiman, p 262–64. International Agency for Research on Cancer, Lyon, 2008.
2. Burkitt D: A sarcoma involving the jaws in African children. *Br J Surg* 46:218–223, 1958.
3. Magrath I: Denis Burkitt and the African lymphoma. *Ecancermedicalscience* 3:159, 2009.
4. O'Conor GT, Davies JN: Malignant tumors in African children. With special reference to malignant lymphoma. *J Pediatr* 56:526–535, 1960.
5. Epstein MA, Achong BG, Barr YM: Virus particles in cultured lymphoblasts from Burkitt's lymphoma. *Lancet* 1:702–703, 1964.
6. Wright DH: Burkitt's lymphoma: A review of the pathology, immunology, and possible etiologic factors. *Pathol Annu* 6:337–363, 1971.
7. de-Thé G, Geser A, Day NE, et al: Epidemiological evidence for causal relationship between Epstein-Barr virus and Burkitt's lymphoma from Ugandan prospective study. *Nature* 274:756–761, 1978.
8. Magrath I: The pathogenesis of Burkitt's lymphoma. *Adv Cancer Res* 55:133–270, 1990.
9. Kalter SP, Riggs SA, Cabanillas F, et al: Aggressive non-Hodgkin's lymphomas in immunocompromised homosexual males. *Blood* 66:655–659, 1985.
10. Manolov G, Manolova Y: Marker band in one chromosome 14 from Burkitt lymphomas. *Nature* 237:33–34, 1972.
11. Zech L, Haglund U, Nilsson K, Klein G: Characteristic chromosomal abnormalities in biopsies and lymphoid-cell lines from patients with Burkitt and non-Burkitt lymphomas. *Int J Cancer* 17:47–56, 1976.
12. Dalla-Favera R, Bregni M, Erikson J, et al: Human c-myc onc gene is located on the region of chromosome 8 that is translocated in Burkitt lymphoma cells. *Proc Natl Acad Sci U S A* 79:7824–7827, 1982.
13. Taub R, Kirsch I, Morton C, et al: Translocation of the c-myc gene into the immunoglobulin heavy chain locus in human Burkitt lymphoma and murine plasmacytoma cells. *Proc Natl Acad Sci U S A* 79:7837–7841, 1982.
14. Harris NL, Horning SJ: Burkitt's lymphoma—The message from microarrays. *N Engl J Med* 354:2495–2498, 2006.
15. Campo E: New pathogenic mechanisms in Burkitt lymphoma. *Nat Genet* 44:1288–1289, 2012.
16. Orem J, Mbidde EK, Lambert B, et al: Burkitt's lymphoma in Africa, a review of the epidemiology and etiology. *Afr Health Sci* 7:166–175, 2007.
17. Geser A, Brubaker G, Draper CC: Effect of a malaria suppression program on the incidence of African Burkitt's lymphoma. *Am J Epidemiol* 129:740–752, 1989.
18. Mbulaiteye SM, Anderson WF, Bhatia K, et al: Trimodal age-specific incidence patterns for Burkitt lymphoma in the United States, 1973–2005. *Int J Cancer* 126:1732–1739, 2010.
19. Dorsett Y, Robbiani DF, Jankovic M, et al: A role for AID in chromosome translocations between c-myc and the IgH variable region. *J Exp Med* 204:2225–2232, 2007.
20. Bhatia K, Huppi K, Spangler G, et al: Point mutations in the c-Myc transactivation domain are common in Burkitt's lymphoma and mouse plasmacytomas. *Nat Genet* 5:56–61, 1993.
21. Dave SS, Fu K, Wright GW, et al: Lymphoma/Leukemia Molecular Profiling Project: Molecular diagnosis of Burkitt's lymphoma. *N Engl J Med* 354:2431–2442, 2006.
22. Hummel M, Bentink S, Berger H, et al; Molecular Mechanisms in Malignant Lymphomas Network Project of the Deutsche Krebshilfe: A biologic definition of Burkitt's lymphoma from transcriptional and genomic profiling. *N Engl J Med* 354:2419–2430, 2006.
23. Love C, Sun Z, Jima D, et al: The genetic landscape of mutations in Burkitt lymphoma. *Nat Genet* 44:1321–1325, 2012.
24. Richter J, Schlesner M, Hoffmann S, et al: ICGC MMML-Seq Project: Recurrent mutation of the ID3 gene in Burkitt lymphoma identified by integrated genome, exome and transcriptome sequencing. *Nat Genet* 44:1316–1320, 2012.
25. Schmitz R, Young RM, Ceribelli M, et al: Burkitt lymphoma pathogenesis and therapeutic targets from structural and functional genomics. *Nature* 490:116–120, 2012.
26. Biggar RJ, Chaturvedi AK, Goedert JJ, Engels EA: HIV/AIDS Cancer Match Study: AIDS-related cancer and severity of immunosuppression in persons with AIDS. *J Natl Cancer Inst* 99:962–972, 2007.
27. Aka P, Vila MC, Jariwala A, et al: Endemic Burkitt lymphoma is associated with strength and diversity of Plasmodium falciparum malaria stage-specific antigen antibody response. *Blood* 122:629–635, 2013.
28. Mannucci S, Luzzi A, Carugi A, et al: EBV reactivation and chromosomal polysomies: Euphorbia tirucalli as a possible cofactor in endemic Burkitt lymphoma. *Adv Hematol* 2012:149780, 2012.
29. Rochford R, Cannon MJ, Moormann AM: Endemic Burkitt's lymphoma: A polymicrobial disease? *Nat Rev Microbiol* 3:182–187, 2005.
30. Thorley-Lawson DA, Allday MJ: The curious case of the tumour virus: 50 years of Burkitt's lymphoma. *Nat Rev Microbiol* 6:913–924, 2008.
31. Molyneux EM, Rochford R, Griffin B, et al: Burkitt's lymphoma. *Lancet* 379:1234–1244, 2012.

32. Donati D, Zhang LP, Chêne A, et al: Identification of a polyclonal B-cell activator in *Plasmodium falciparum. Infect Immun* 72:5412–5418, 2004.

33. Chêne A, Donati D, Guerreiro-Cacais AO, et al: A molecular link between malaria and Epstein-Barr virus reactivation. *PLoS Pathog* 3:e80, 2007.

34. Zauner L, Melroe GT, Sigrist JA, et al: TLR9 triggering in Burkitt's lymphoma cell lines suppresses the EBV BZLF1 transcription via histone modification. *Oncogene* 29:4588–4598, 2010.

35. Chattopadhyay PK, Chelimo K, Embury PB, et al: Holoendemic malaria exposure is associated with altered Epstein-Barr virus-specific CD8(+) T-cell differentiation. *J Virol* 87:1779–1788, 2013.

36. Torgbor C, Awuah P, Deitsch K, et al: A multifactorial role for *P. falciparum* malaria in endemic Burkitt's lymphoma pathogenesis. *PLoS Pathog* 10:e1004170, 2014.

37. Yano T, van Krieken JH, Magrath IT, et al: Histogenetic correlations between subcategories of small noncleaved cell lymphomas. *Blood* 79:1282–1290, 1992.

38. Brady G, MacArthur GJ, Farrell PJ: Epstein-Barr virus and Burkitt lymphoma. *J Clin Pathol* 60:1397–1402, 2007.

39. Lundin C, Hjorth L, Behrendtz M, et al: Submicroscopic genomic imbalances in Burkitt lymphomas/leukemias: Association with age and further evidence that 8q24/MYC translocations are not sufficient for leukemogenesis. *Genes Chromosomes Cancer* 52:370–377, 2013.

40. Scholtysik R, Kreuz M, Klapper W, et al: Detection of genomic aberrations in molecularly defined Burkitt's lymphoma by array-based, high resolution, single nucleotide polymorphism analysis. *Haematologica* 95:2047–2055, 2010.

41. Bellan C, Stefano L, Giulia de F, et al: Burkitt lymphoma versus diffuse large B-cell lymphoma: A practical approach. *Hematol Oncol* 28:53–56, 2010.

42. Jaffe ES, Pittaluga S: Aggressive B-cell lymphomas: A review of new and old entities in the WHO classification. *Hematology Am Soc Hematol Educ Program* 2011:506–514, 2011.

43. Lindsley RC, LaCasce AS: Biology of double-hit B-cell lymphomas. *Curr Opin Hematol* 19:299–304, 2012.

44. Green TM, Young KH, Visco C, et al: Immunohistochemical double-hit score is a strong predictor of outcome in patients with diffuse large B-cell lymphoma treated with rituximab plus cyclophosphamide, doxorubicin, vincristine, and prednisone. *J Clin Oncol* 30:3460–3467, 2012.

45. Magrath I, Adde M, Shad A, et al: Adults and children with small non-cleaved-cell lymphoma have a similar excellent outcome when treated with the same chemotherapy regimen. *J Clin Oncol* 14:925–934, 1996.

46. Rizzieri DA, Johnson JL, Niedzwiecki D, et al: Intensive chemotherapy with and without cranial radiation for Burkitt leukemia and lymphoma: Final results of Cancer and Leukemia Group B Study 9251. *Cancer* 100:1438–1448, 2004.

47. Soussain C, Patte C, Ostronoff M, et al: Small noncleaved cell lymphoma and leukemia in adults. A retrospective study of 65 adults treated with the LMB pediatric protocols. *Blood* 85:664–674, 1995.

48. Link MP, Donaldson SS, Berard CW, et al: Results of treatment of childhood localized non-Hodgkin's lymphoma with combination chemotherapy with or without radiotherapy. *N Engl J Med* 322:1169–1174, 1990.

49. Magrath IT, Haddy TB, Adde MA: Treatment of patients with high grade non-Hodgkin's lymphomas and central nervous system involvement: Is radiation an essential component of therapy? *Leuk Lymphoma* 21:99–105, 1996.

50. Hsu HH, Chan YL, Huang CC: Acute spontaneous tumor lysis presenting with hyperuricemic acute renal failure: Clinical features and therapeutic approach. *J Nephrol* 17:50–56, 2004.

51. Goldman SC, Holcenberg JS, Finklestein JZ, et al: A randomized comparison between rasburicase and allopurinol in children with lymphoma or leukemia at high risk for tumor lysis. *Blood* 97:2998–3003, 2001.

52. Hummel M, Reiter S, Adam K, et al: Effective treatment and prophylaxis of hyperuricemia and impaired renal function in tumor lysis syndrome with low doses of rasburicase. *Eur J Haematol* 80:331–336, 2008.

53. Choi KA, Lee JE, Kim YG, et al: Efficacy of continuous venovenous hemofiltration with chemotherapy in patients with Burkitt lymphoma and leukemia at high risk of tumor lysis syndrome. *Ann Hematol* 88:639–645, 2009.

54. Saccente SL, Kohaut EC, Berkow RL: Prevention of tumor lysis syndrome using continuous veno-venous hemofiltration. *Pediatr Nephrol* 9:569–573, 1995.

55. Lacasce A, Howard O, Lib S, et al: Modified magrath regimens for adults with Burkitt and Burkitt-like lymphomas: Preserved efficacy with decreased toxicity. *Leuk Lymphoma* 45:761–767, 2004.

56. Mead GM, Sydes MR, Walewski J, et al: An international evaluation of CODOX-M and CODOX-M alternating with IVAC in adult Burkitt's lymphoma: Results of United Kingdom Lymphoma Group LY06 study. *Ann Oncol* 13:1264–1274, 2002.

57. Mead GM, Barrans SL, Qian W, et al: A prospective clinicopathologic study of dose-modified CODOX-M/IVAC in patients with sporadic Burkitt lymphoma defined using cytogenetic and immunophenotypic criteria (MRC/NCRI LY10 trial). *Blood* 112:2248–2260, 2008.

58. Barnes JA, Lacasce AS, Feng Y, et al: Evaluation of the addition of rituximab to CODOX-M/IVAC for Burkitt's lymphoma: A retrospective analysis. *Ann Oncol* 22:1859–1864, 2011.

59. Corazzelli G, Frigeri F, Russo F, et al: RD-CODOX-M/IVAC with rituximab and intrathecal liposomal cytarabine in adult Burkitt lymphoma and "unclassifiable" highly aggressive B-cell lymphoma. *Br J Haematol* 156:234–244, 2012.

60. Evens AM, Carson KR, Kolesar J, et al: A multicenter phase II study incorporating high-dose rituximab and liposomal doxorubicin into the CODOX-M/IVAC regimen for untreated Burkitt's lymphoma. *Ann Oncol* 24:3076–3081, 2013.

61. Dunleavy K, Pittaluga S, Shovlin M, et al: Low-intensity therapy in adults with Burkitt's lymphoma. *N Engl J Med* 369:1915–1925, 2013.

62. Thomas DA, Cortes J, O'Brien S, et al: Hyper-CVAD program in Burkitt's-type adult acute lymphoblastic leukemia. *J Clin Oncol* 17:2461–2470, 1999.

63. Fayad L, Thomas D, Romaguera J: Update of the M. D. Anderson Cancer Center experience with hyper-CVAD and rituximab for the treatment of mantle cell and Burkitt-type lymphomas. *Clin Lymphoma Myeloma* 8 (Suppl 2):S57–S62, 2007.

64. Thomas DA, Faderl S, O'Brien S, et al: Chemoimmunotherapy with hyper-CVAD plus rituximab for the treatment of adult Burkitt and Burkitt-type lymphoma or acute lymphoblastic leukemia. *Cancer* 106:1569–1580, 2006.

65. Rizzieri DA, Johnson JL, Byrd JC, et al: Alliance for Clinical Trials In Oncology (ACTION): Improved efficacy using rituximab and brief duration, high intensity chemotherapy with filgrastim support for Burkitt or aggressive lymphomas: Cancer and Leukemia Group B study 10 002. *Br J Haematol* 165:102–111, 2014.

66. Song KW, Barnett MJ, Gascoyne RD, et al: Haematopoietic stem cell transplantation as primary therapy of sporadic adult Burkitt lymphoma. *Br J Haematol* 133:634–637, 2006.

67. Hoffmann C, Wolf E, Wyen C, et al: AIDS-associated Burkitt or Burkitt-like lymphoma: Short intensive polychemotherapy is feasible and effective. *Leuk Lymphoma* 47:1872–1880, 2006.

68. Kelly JL, Toothaker SR, Ciminello L, et al: Outcomes of patients with Burkitt lymphoma older than age 40 treated with intensive chemotherapeutic regimens. *Clin Lymphoma Myeloma* 9:307–310, 2009.

69. Grigg AP, Seymour JF: Graft versus Burkitt's lymphoma effect after allogeneic marrow transplantation. *Leuk Lymphoma* 43:889–892, 2002.

70. Perkins AS, Friedberg JW: Burkitt lymphoma in adults. *Hematology Am Soc Hematol Educ Program* 341–348, 2008.

71. Hoelzer D, Ludwig WD, Thiel E, et al: Improved outcome in adult B-cell acute lymphoblastic leukemia. *Blood* 87:495–508, 1996.

CHAPTER 103
CUTANEOUS T-CELL LYMPHOMA (MYCOSIS FUNGOIDES AND SÉZARY SYNDROME)

Larisa J. Geskin

SUMMARY

Cutaneous T-cell lymphoma (CTCL) is a heterogeneous group of malignant lymphomas that share the propensity for malignant T lymphocytes expressing cutaneous lymphocyte antigen to infiltrate the skin. Mycosis fungoides (MF) is the most common variant of CTCL, representing approximately 50 percent of all cases. Sézary syndrome (SS) is a leukemic variant of MF, affecting approximately 5 percent of patients with MF.[1] MF and SS are the most common malignant proliferations of mature memory T lymphocytes of the helper phenotype (CD4+CD45RO+),[2] which renders patients immunocompromised even at the earliest stages of the disease. Advanced stages are associated with severe immune suppression. Diagnosis is established by skin biopsy, followed by staging work up which includes radiologic imaging and pathologic evaluation of the lymph nodes, internal organs, blood, and marrow, as appropriate, according to presenting manifestations of the disease.

MF is divided into early and advanced stages for therapeutic and prognostic reasons. In early stages, the disease follows an indolent course and has a favorable prognosis. In advanced stages, the prognosis is poor. There are numerous therapeutic options. No treatment has been definitively proven to improve survival, but newer studies suggest that survival is longer than historically documented.[3,4] Multiagent chemotherapy is not a useful option because it is inferior to immune modulating and biologic therapies.[5]

Considering the overall protracted course of the disease, its indolent character, immunocompromised status of the patients, and absence of definitive therapy, aggressive multiagent chemotherapy contributing to immunosuppression should be reserved for end-stage palliation or as a bridge to stem cell transplantation with the goal of definitive cure.[6–8] There are several FDA-approved single agents for therapy of MF, which are safe and effective against the disease and may be used in the therapeutic ladder prior to multi-agent regimens.[9–11] Several single agents and combinations of new and older agents are in clinical trials now to test for efficacy in MF and SS. Because no single therapy is considered to be the standard of care for MF and SS, clinical trials remain a viable option for most patients. The goal of therapy is to induce long-term remissions without compromising patients' immunity and improvement of the quality of life.

DEFINITION AND HISTORY

In 1806, Baron Jean-Louis Alibert described a patient who presented with skin patches that grew into plaques and mushroom-like tumors and first coined the term *mycosis fungoides* (MF).[12] In 1938, Sézary and Bouvrain described a syndrome of pruritus, generalized exfoliative erythroderma, and abnormal hyperconvoluted lymphoid cells in the blood.[13] Today this condition is referred to as *Sézary syndrome* (SS), a condition seen in a subset of patients with MF.

Prior to the 1970s, cutaneous lymphomas were believed to be cutaneous counterparts of the systemic lymphomas. In 1975, Lutzner and associates[14] suggested the term *cutaneous T-cell lymphoma* (CTCL), recognizing that despite the significant similarities of malignant cell morphology and phenotype to systemic T-cell lymphomas, the cutaneous lymphomas represented distinct entities. Although this definition has helped to distinguish cutaneous lymphomas from systemic disease, it has also led to inappropriately using the umbrella term *CTCL* interchangeably with MF. Common World Health Organization (WHO)–European Organisation for Research and Treatment of Cancer (EORTC) classification was first developed in 2005[15] to resolve differences between various classifications (Table 103–1) and is currently accepted as the standard for CTCL staging and classification.[16]

EPIDEMIOLOGY

MF is twice as common in males as in females. The median age at diagnosis is 55 years. Americans of African descent have a higher incidence of MF and a poorer prognosis than Americans of European descent. MF occurs least often in Asians and Hispanics. Evidence for a genetic predisposition (germline transmission of susceptibility) in patients with CTCL is inconclusive. An approximately 6 percent increase in incidence of CTCL per decade was documented from the early 1970s to 1998, but the incidence subsequently leveled off and stabilized, with a current incidence of approximately one per 100,000.[17] Incidence is highly age-dependent, with the highest incidence of 3.6 per 100,000 of adults after the age of 70 years. Approximately 3000 new cases of MF are reported annually, comprising approximately 3 percent of all lymphomas. The mortality rate varies widely according to the stage of disease. Stage I mortality does not differ from the mortality of age-matched controls. However, stage IV patients have a 27 percent 5-year survival and 10 percent 15-year survival. Median survival of patients with SS is 1.5 years. The mortality rate of MF in the United States has been declining, possibly because of earlier diagnosis of the disease.[1,18]

TABLE 103–1. World Health Organization–European Organization for Research and Treatment of Cancer Classification of Primary Cutaneous T-Cell and Natural Killer Cell Lymphomas

I. Mycosis Fungoides (MF)

   A. MF variants and subtypes

      1. Folliculotropic MF

      2. Pagetoid reticulosis

      3. Granulomatous slack skin

II. Sézary Syndrome

III. Adult T-Cell Leukemia/Lymphoma

IV. Primary Cutaneous CD30+ Lymphoproliferative Disorders

   A. Primary cutaneous anaplastic large cell lymphoma

   B. Lymphomatoid papulosis

V. Subcutaneous Panniculitis-Like T-Cell Lymphoma

VI. Extranodal Natural Killer/T-Cell Lymphoma, Nasal Type

VII. Primary Cutaneous Peripheral T-Cell Lymphoma, Unspecified

   A. Primary cutaneous aggressive epidermotropic CD8+ T-cell lymphoma (provisional)

   B. Cutaneous γδ T-cell lymphoma (provisional)

   C. Primary cutaneous CD4+ small-/medium-size pleomorphic T-cell lymphoma (provisional)

VIII. Precursor Hematologic Neoplasm

   A. CD4+/CD56+ hematodermic neoplasm (blastic NK-cell lymphoma)

ETIOLOGY AND PATHOGENESIS

The etiologies of MF and SS are unknown, although epidemiologic features are suggestive of an infectious origin, including a predilection for elderly individuals and a higher-than-expected incidence in immune-suppressed patients.[19] However, studies to date have failed to reveal consistent associations between any particular infectious agent and CTCL, including novel infectious agents.[20] A "persistent antigen stimulation" hypothesis was proposed as an initial event after MF was observed to be a disease of mature CD4+ memory T cells, but the stimulating antigen is not known.[21,22] MF also may be viewed as a disease of immune dysregulation. Tumor progression is associated with decreased antigen-specific T-cell responses and impaired cell-mediated cytotoxicity. On the other hand, improved survival is associated with intact cell-mediated immunity. Progression of MF is associated with progressive T-helper type 2 (Th2) skewing and increased production of Th2 cytokines. This alteration accounts for many of the immune abnormalities associated with advanced MF, such as hypereosinophilia, increased serum immunoglobulin (Ig) A and IgE levels, impaired natural killer (NK) cell function, and impaired cellular immunity.[23,24] Late-stage MF and SS are associated with declining immunocompetence,[25] resulting in severe life-threatening infections, and a high incidence of secondary malignancies. The latter increase is not attributable to prior treatment with carcinogenic agents alone.[26] Fifty percent of deaths among patients with MF result from infections.

Environmental factors have been suggested in the etiology of CTCL in Europe,[27,28] but have not been confirmed by epidemiologic studies in the United States.

CLINICAL FEATURES

The clinical presentation of MF is highly variable. Cutaneous manifestations of the disease result from skin infiltration by malignant cutaneous lymphocyte antigen (CLA)-positive lymphocytes and depend on the extent of skin involvement. Patients initially may present with "chronic dermatitis" that is resistant to therapy, which is often misdiagnosed as spongiotic dermatitis (so-called eczema), "psoriasis-like dermatitis," or other chronic, nonspecific dermatoses, usually associated with pruritus. Histologically, diagnosis may be difficult, especially in the early stages of the disease and in its erythrodermic form, as the abnormal atypical infiltrate can be minimal and can be masked by normal inflammatory infiltrates in the skin, or it can be misinterpreted as a normal inflammatory infiltrate because of its mature CD4+ phenotype.

MF may progress through distinct stages of skin involvement, ranging from patch (Fig. 103–1A) to plaque (Fig. 103–1B) to tumor (Fig. 103–1C), but any type of lesion may progress or lesions may arise de novo. For descriptive purposes, the skin manifestations of MF are divided into patch stage (patch-only disease), plaque stage (both patches and plaques), and tumor stage (more than one tumor present, usually in the context of patches and plaques) (Fig. 103–1C). A *patch* is defined as a flat lesion with various degrees of erythema and fine scaling; it may be atrophic or poikilodermatous (Fig. 103–1D). A *plaque* is a well-demarcated erythematous, brownish, or violaceous lesion of at least 1 mm elevation with a variable amount of scale. Tumors are elevated at least 10 mm above the skin surface and may resemble a plaque or be dome shaped without significant scaling.

Distribution of the lesions depends on the clinical stage at presentation. In earlier stages, the lesions have a predilection for folds and non–sun-exposed body areas ("bathing trunk" distribution). In later stages, the lesions can affect the face, including development of ectropion, and other areas, such as palms and soles (keratoderma; see Fig. 103–1E). Tumors may be generalized, and ulceration is common. Progression through the stages is variable but commonly occurs over several years.[29] Lesions usually are associated with pruritus, which may range from mild to excruciatingly severe, leading to insomnia, weight loss, depression, and suicidal ideation. Pruritus is one of the most important quality-of-life issues for these patients.[30]

Erythrodermic skin involvement occurs in 5 percent of patients with MF. Manifestations range from very faint to severe, with significant scaling, keratoderma, painful fissures of the hands and feet, nail dystrophy, and nail loss leading to the patient's inability to walk and maintain daily activities. Severely inflamed skin serves as a breeding ground for bacteria and other pathogens, with resulting fevers, chills, and septicemia.[19,31] Peripheral edema of the extremities may be significant in the later stages and lead to cardiovascular compromise.

Depending on the stage of presentation, patients may present with nodal and/or blood involvement and/or visceral metastases. The earliest stages of MF (e.g., Stage IA and B), may pursue a waxing and waning course, with minimal symptoms and may not have any negative prognostic implications for a patient. The more advanced stages usually, but not inevitably, present with symptoms of the disease. The symptomatology usually reflects the site and severity of involvement and ranges from completely asymptomatic to severe pain, organ malfunction, or at the end stage disease, multi-organ failure.

LABORATORY FINDINGS

There is no definitive marker for MF or SS. The diagnosis of CTCL usually is established by correlating clinical and pathologic findings. Early lesions may show polymorphic infiltration (containing mixed

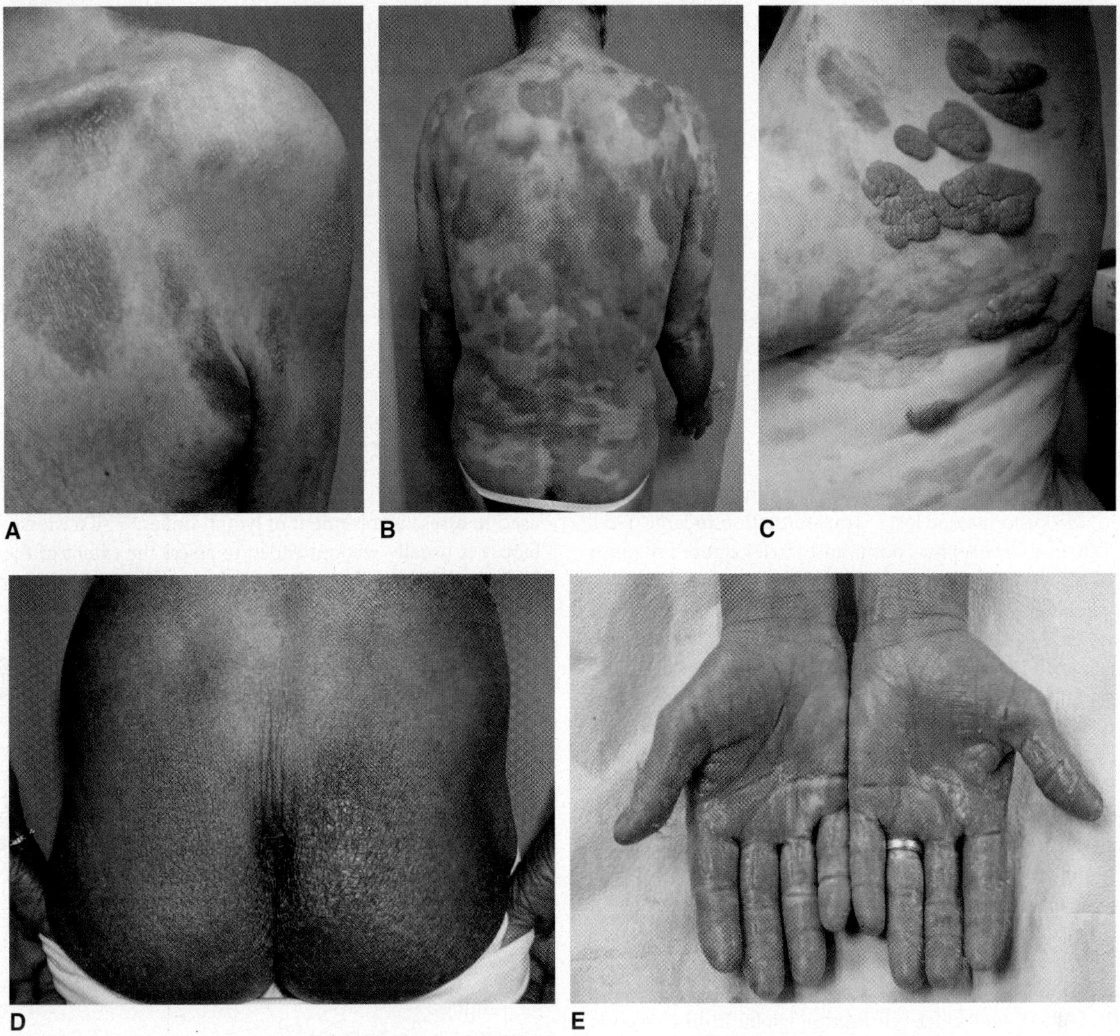

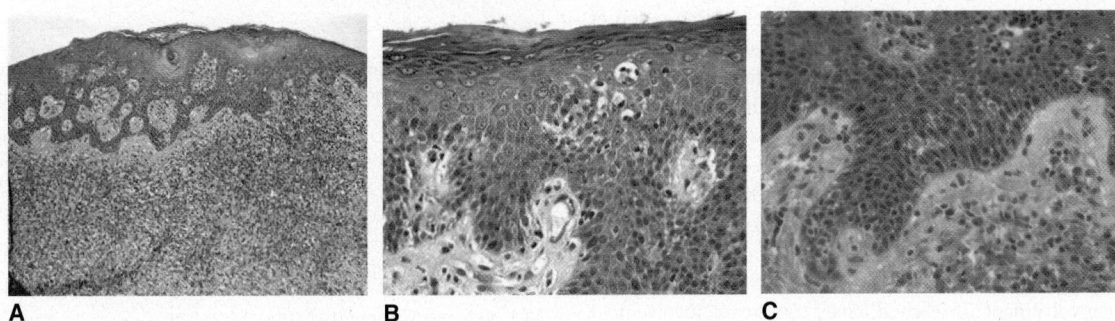

Figure 103–1. Mycosis fungoides. **A.** Erythematous atrophic patches with fine scale. **B.** Extensive patches and thicker plaques. **C.** Tumors on the background of preexisting patches and plaques. **D.** Poikiloderma. **E.** Keratoderma.

inflammatory cells) compatible with several benign dermatoses. Classically, MF lesions show superficial band-like (lichenoid) lymphocytic infiltrate (Fig. 103–2A). The lymphocytes may range from small to large, with characteristic convoluted (cerebriform) nuclei. The hallmark of the malignant infiltrate in MF is epidermotropism (presence of lymphocytes in the epidermis without spongiosis) with formation of

the epidermal clusters of lymphocytes around Langerhans cells termed *Pautrier microabscesses* (Fig. 103–2B). Atypical lymphocytes line up along the dermoepidermal junction and are surrounded by a halo artifact (Fig. 103–2C), which is an important feature of early disease.[32] Superficial dermal collagen may be thickened, so called ropey collagen. In more advanced stages, the infiltrate is less polymorphic,

Figure 103–2. Mycosis fungoides. Skin biopsies stained with hematoxylin and eosin. **A.** Lichenoid (band-like) lymphocytic infiltrate in the superficial dermis. **B.** Epidermotropic atypical lymphocytes lining the dermoepidermal junction in the absence of spongiosis-forming Pautrier microabscesses. Note, halo artifact around lymphocytes at the dermoepidermal junction. **C.** Atypical lymphocytes in the epidermis.

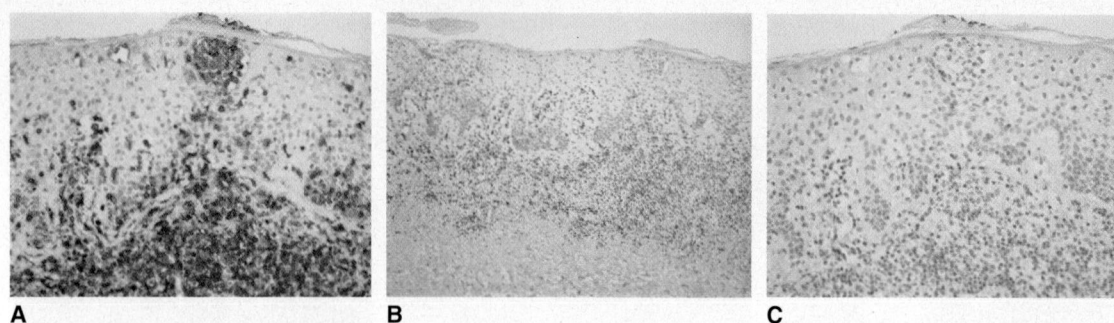

Figure 103–3. Mycoses fungoides. Immunohistochemistry. **A.** CD4+ lichenoid infiltrate in the superficial dermis. Note Pautrier microabscess in the epidermis. **B.** Few CD8+ cells are present. **C.** Loss of maturation marker CD7.

with a predominance of larger atypical cells extending deeper into the dermis; epidermotropism may be lost.[33] Transformation to large T-cell lymphoma (CD30+ or CD30–) may occur and carries a poor prognosis in the setting of MF.[34]

Immunophenotyping plays an important role in diagnosis. The cells usually are CD3+CD4+CD45RO+CD8–, a phenotype associated with mature helper-inducer T lymphocytes. Loss of maturation markers, such as CD7 and CD26 expression on CD4+ are important markers for malignant T lymphocytes.[35,36] The cells may express T-cell activation markers, such as HLA-DR or CD25 (interleukin [IL]-2 receptor). Clonal rearrangement of the T-cell receptor (TCR) Vβ gene can be identified in approximately 90 percent of advanced cases of MF, but in only 50 percent of early stage cases.[37] In rare instances, the classic clinical presentation of MF may be associated with an aberrant CD4 phenotype or may have CD4–dyCD8+ T-cell phenotype[38,39] (Fig. 103–3A to C). Recent molecular studies have identified several new markers, which may prove useful as positive markers of the disease, including thymocyte selection-associated high mobility group box factor (TOX), plastin (PLS3), and killer cell immunoglobulin-like receptor KIR3DL2.[40–43] Cytogenetic abnormalities are not consistently identified, but loss of heterozygosity on 10q and microsatellite instability may be seen in advanced-stage disease.[44] A possible association exists with homozygous deletion of PTEN and CDKN2A and tumor-suppressor genes on 10p and 9p chromosomes, respectively. These may be silenced with progression of disease.[45,46]

STAGING

MF is classified according to the widely accepted modified *tumor, node, metastasis, blood (TNMB) classification*, originally adopted in 1975 by the Mycosis Fungoides Cooperative Study Group[47,48] and revised to match modern developments in the field.[16] Accurate determination of the stage in MF and SS is of utmost importance because of its prognostic significance and critical role in selecting therapy. Cutaneous lesions are classified using the *T staging system* (Table 103–2). The area of the skin and type of the lesions were found to correlate with patient survival and are important prognostic predictors and need to be calculated at every visit to assess disease status.[49] Prognosis varies according to tumor burden. The presence of tumors (T3) may indicate a worse prognosis than erythroderma (T4).[18]

The extent of extracutaneous disease usually correlates with the extent of skin involvement. In early disease, significant involvement of lymph nodes and blood is unlikely. However, lymphadenopathy is present in more than half of patients as disease advances and increases with progressive cutaneous involvement. Lymph nodes are assigned *N category* in the TNMB staging of MF[16] (see Table 103–2). Computed

tomography (CT) and positron emission tomography (PET) scans are used to assess involvement of lymph nodes.[50,51] Excisional lymph node biopsy is usually recommended to assess the extent of the disease and nodal architecture, but other techniques, including fine-needle aspiration, are selectively used as well.[52]

TABLE 103–2. TNMB Classification of Mycosis Fungoides

T: Skin

T1: Limited patches, papules, or plaques covering <10% of the skin surface (T1a = patch only; T1b = plaques ± patches)

T2: Generalized patches, papules, or plaques covering 10% of the skin surface (T2a = patch only; T2b = plaques ± patches)

T3: At least one tumor (≥1 cm in diameter)

T4: Generalized erythroderma over at least 80% body surface area

N: Lymph nodes

N0: No clinically abnormal peripheral lymph nodes; biopsy not required

N1: Clinically abnormal peripheral lymph nodes; histopathology Dutch grade 1 or NCI LN0 to 2

N2: Clinically abnormal peripheral lymph nodes; histopathology Dutch grade 2 or NCI LN3

N3: Clinically abnormal peripheral lymph nodes; histopathology Dutch grades 3 to 4 or NCI LN4

NX: Clinically abnormal peripheral lymph nodes; no histologic confirmation

M: Visceral organs

M0: No visceral organ involvement

M1: Visceral organ involvement; requires histologic confirmation and specify organ

B: Blood

B0: Atypical circulating cells not present (<5%); specify "a" if flow cytometry is negative for clonal T lymphocytes or "b" if positive for clonal T lymphocytes

B1: Atypical circulating cells present (>5%, minimal blood involvement); specify "a" if flow cytometry is negative for clonal T lymphocytes or "b" if positive for clonal T lymphocytes

B2: Leukemia (≥1000 cells/μL, CD4 to CD8 ratio of 10 or higher, evidence of a T-cell clone in the blood)

NCI, National Cancer Institute.

T indicates the size of the tumor and whether it has invaded nearby tissue. N indicates the regional lymph nodes that are involved. M indicates distant metastasis. B indicates whether there are tumor cells in the blood.

TABLE 103-3. Revised Staging of Mycosis Fungoides and Sézary Syndrome[16]

	T	N	M	B
IA	1	0	0	0, 1
IB	2	0	0	0, 1
IIA	1, 2	1, 2	0	0, 1
IIB	3	0–2	0	0, 1
III	4	0–2	0	0, 1
IIIA	4	0–2	0	0
IIIB	4	0–2	0	1
IVA1	1–4	0–2	0	2
IVA2	1–4	3	0	0–2
IVB	1–4	0–3	1	0–2

See Table 103-2 for definitions of T1 to T4, N0 to N3, and M0 to M1.

Histopathologic examination of affected lymph nodes may show partial or complete effacement of normal architecture, with a monomorphic infiltrate of MF cells. However, in most cases, the nodal architecture is not effaced, and dermatopathic changes are present with varying numbers of atypical lymphocytes in the T-cell paracortical areas of the node. Even the presence of dermatopathic changes alone in the lymph nodes carries prognostic significance (see Tables 103–2 and 103–3).[53,54] Abnormal lymph nodes should be biopsied regardless of the T stage.

Metastatic disease (including patients with positive nodes) is the most significant prognostic predictor (see Tables 103–2 and 103–3). Patients with visceral involvement that includes liver, spleen, pleura, and lung have a median survival of less than 1 year.[55] Blood involvement may be an important predictor of progression and survival (Figs. 103–4 and 103–5).[56] The number of circulating Sézary cells increases with advancing disease, and the cells are particularly prominent in patients with generalized erythroderma. However, even in early stage disease, a high frequency of clonal T cells in the blood may be detected using a highly sensitive polymerase chain reaction (PCR) technique, suggesting that early systemic disease is common.[57] Blood involvement is rated as *B category* in the TNMB staging (see Table 103–2). For staging purposes, the B2 blood rating is equivalent to nodal involvement.[58,59] The B2 rating is defined as (1) a Sézary cell count of 1000 cells/mm³ or more; (2) a CD4-to-CD8 ratio of 10 or higher caused by an increase in circulating T cells and/or an aberrant loss or expression of pan–T-cell markers by flow cytometry; (3) increased lymphocyte counts with evidence of a T-cell clone in the blood determined by the Southern blot or PCR technique; or (4) a chromosomally abnormal T-cell clone. Malignant cells also can be detected using sensitive techniques such as cytogenetics or TCR gene rearrangement studies.[60-64] Patients with blood involvement have a higher likelihood of lymphadenopathy and visceral involvement. Marrow infiltration is infrequently detected by biopsy despite circulating malignant cells; it is identified at autopsy in 30 to 40 percent of cases. The cytologic appearance of the malignant cells in visceral organs is similar to that of the malignant cells in the skin.[65]

In the erythrodermic subset of MF, three T4 subsets can be identified (Table 103–4). In general, in SS, a triad of exfoliative erythroderma, generalized lymphadenopathy, and leukemia, has the worst prognosis among the forms of MF.

● DIFFERENTIAL DIAGNOSIS

Diagnosis of MF is based on a constellation of findings, which include clinical presentation, skin and lymph node biopsies (if indicated), and blood evaluation. A number of benign dermatoses can mimic MF or SS, and may even have TCR gene rearrangements.[66-69] Such benign conditions include psoriasis and psoriasiform dermatoses (such as pityriasis rubra pilaris, seborrheic dermatitis, contact dermatitis, and eczema), intertrigo, tinea, drug eruptions, and other conditions.

Cutaneous and systemic lymphomas other than MF should be considered in the differential diagnosis. Smoldering adult T-cell leukemia/lymphoma has a number of clinical features similar to MF, but it usually can be distinguished by the presence of antibodies to human T-lymphotropic virus type 1 (HTLV-1) and by other associated findings unusual in MF. However, this distinction may be difficult.[70,71]

Pagetoid reticulosis *(Woringer-Kolopp disease)* is a rare skin disorder that consists of solitary or localized cutaneous plaques. It affects young males almost exclusively. It has a benign course, and the prognosis is excellent.[72-74] It is an epidermal process, with the majority of atypical lymphocytes found within hyperplastic epidermis.[75] Although

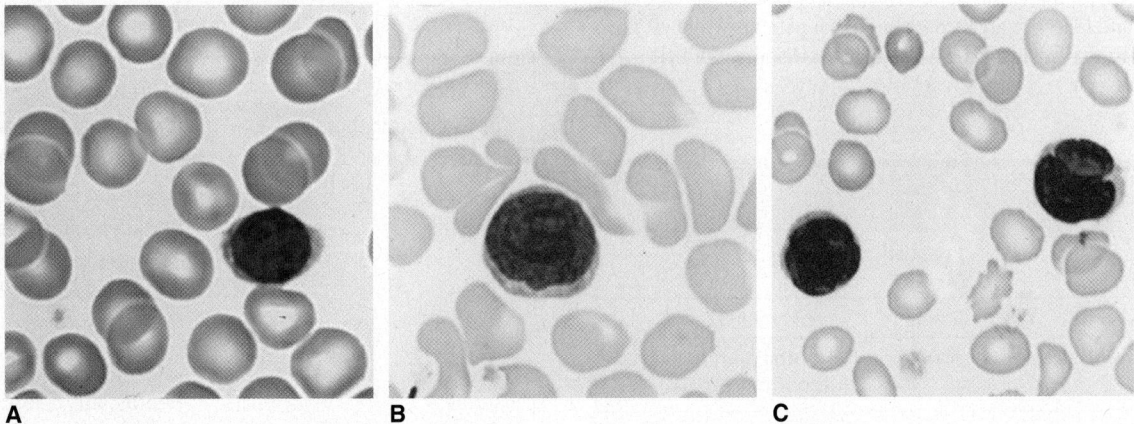

Figure 103–4. Blood lymphocytes. **A.** Normal small lymphocyte. **B.** Sézary cell. Note the nuclear swirls and the light microscopic appearance of the Sézary cell nucleus. Without careful inspection in cases of lymphocytosis, Sézary cells can be mistaken for small lymphocytes as seen in chronic lymphocytic leukemia. **C.** Blood lymphocytes from a patient with mycosis fungoides and disseminated disease involving marrow and blood. Note clefted appearance of the nucleus. *(Reproduced with permission from Lichtman's Atlas of Hematology, www.accessmedicine.com.)*

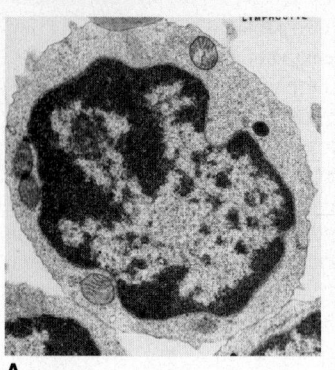
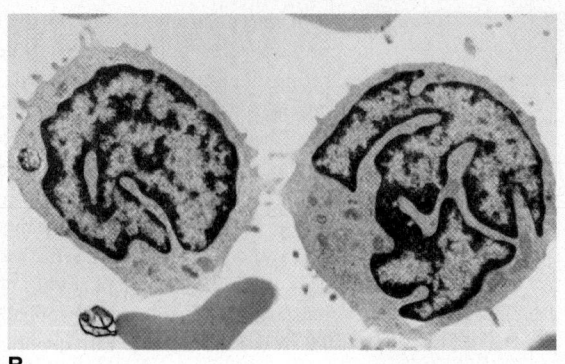

Figure 103–5. Transmission electron micrographs of lymphocytes. **A.** Normal lymphocyte. **B.** Two lymphocytes from a patient with Sézary cells in the blood. The latter have the striking cerebriform nuclear abnormalities characteristic of Sézary cells. (*Reproduced with permission from* Lichtman's Atlas of Hematology, *www.accessmedicine.com.*)

the disease usually is indolent and localized, some patients present with a disseminated form referred to as the *Ketron-Goodman variant*.[76] The histologic findings are similar to those found in Woringer-Kolopp disease, with predominantly epidermal involvement by malignant cells and a poor prognosis.[76] This variant is a disease of an activated T lymphocyte that only occasionally expresses the helper T-cell CD4 antigen.[77,78] Like MF, the neoplastic cells have TCR gene rearrangements.

Other mimics of CTCL, such as alopecia mucinosa, contact dermatitis, lichen planus, parapsoriasis, pediatric atopic dermatitis, pemphigus foliaceus, plaque psoriasis, pustular psoriasis, and tinea corporis, should be considered in the differential diagnosis. The diagnosis is made by appropriate investigation (e.g., potassium hydroxide skin prep) and skin biopsy. CD30+ (Ki-1) and CD30– lymphomas can mimic tumors of MF; they present as erythematous or violaceous nodules that ulcerate. The critical issue is to differentiate primary cutaneous CD30+ lymphoproliferative disorder from CD30+ large cell transformation of MF and from secondary cutaneous involvement caused by CD30+ nodal lymphoma. The course of CD30+ lymphomas of the skin is indolent, they carry a favorable prognosis and tend to regress spontaneously, whereas transformed MF and nodal lymphoma have poor prognoses. In rare instances, these lymphomas progress to systemic involvement and have the same prognosis as nodal CD30+ lymphomas.[79,80] Lymphomatoid papulosis (LyP) is a benign counterpart of CD30+ lymphoproliferative disorders of the skin with excellent prognosis. It usually presents as crops of recurrent pruritic or painful erythematous papules or nodules, which ulcerate and heal spontaneously. LyP usually runs a chronic course.[81] LyP may be associated with other malignancies, particularly MF and other lymphomas, in up to 10 percent of cases. Therefore close observation and followup are recommended for patients with LyP. Low-dose oral methotrexate is the drug of choice for treatment of LyP.

TABLE 103–4. Classification of Erythrodermic Cutaneous T-Cell Lymphoma

Erythrodermic Subset (T4)	Preexisting MF	Blood
Sézary syndrome	Rarely	Leukemia: B2
Erythrodermic mycosis Fungoides	Always	Normal or minimally abnormal: B0–B1
Erythrodermic cutaneous T-cell lymphoma, not otherwise specified	Absent	Normal or minimally abnormal: B0–B1

MF, mycosis fungoides.

●THERAPY

A variety of therapeutic modalities produce remissions in most patients with MF. In general, MF therapy is divided into (1) skin-directed therapy (SDT) and (2) systemic therapy (Table 103–5). SDT is the mainstream therapy in early disease but also is used as an adjunct in systemic disease. Therapeutic decisions may be difficult and heavily depend on the stage at presentation. Revised practice guidelines are available on National Comprehensive Cancer Network (NCCN) website (www.nccn.org). See Fig. 103–6 for an overview of the treatment algorithm for MF/SS. In view of the protracted course of the disease and lack of curative therapies, therapeutic decisions should generally be focused

TABLE 103–5. Therapeutic Option for Mycosis Fungoides and Sézary Syndrome

Skin-Directed Therapy	Systemic Therapy
Topical therapy	Immunomodulators
Topical glucocorticoids	Interferon-α
Nitrogen mustard (mechlorethamine)	Extracorporeal photophoresis (ECP)
Carmustine (BCNU, nitrosourea)	Antibodies/fusion proteins
Retinoids (bexarotene, tretinoin)	Denileukin diftitox (ONTAK, DAB$_{389}$–IL-2)
Topical tacrolimus (Protopic)	Alemtuzumab (Campath)
Imiquimod (Aldara)	Retinoids
Light therapy	Oral bexarotene (Targretin)
UVB and PUVA	Acitretin (Soriatane)
Photodynamic therapy	Isotretinoin (Accutane)
Electron beam	Histone deacetylase inhibitors
Localized	Vorinostat (Zolinza)
Total-skin	Romidepsin (Istodax)
	Chemotherapy (alone or in combinations)
	Oral prednisone, methotrexate, doxorubicin, cyclophosphamide; chlorambucil; pentostatin, cladribine, fludarabine, pralatrexate, several others

PUVA, psoralen and ultraviolet radiation of the A spectrum; UVB, ultraviolet radiation of the B spectrum.

Therapies for Cutaneous T-Cell Lymphomas

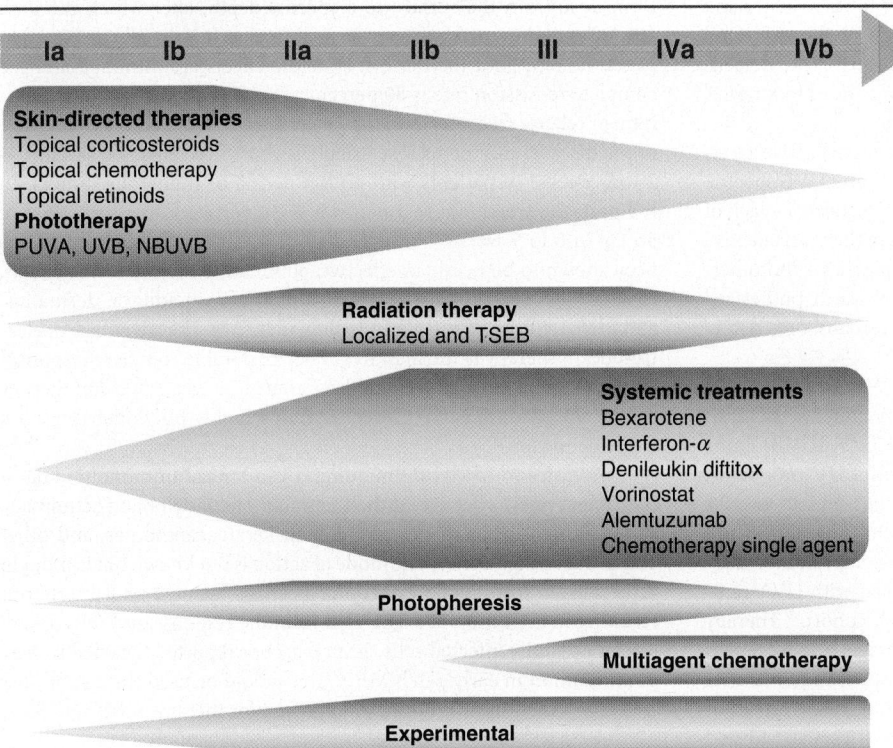

Figure 103–6. Cutaneous T-cell lymphoma treatment algorithm. NBUVB, narrowband ultraviolet B; PUVA, psoralen ultraviolet A; TSEB, total-skin electron beam; UVB, ultraviolet B.

on induction of long-term remissions with the least toxic agents and regimens. A number of highly effective monotherapies were recently shown to be safe and effective in patients with MF and SS in prospective clinical trials, leading to their approval by the FDA in the United States and abroad. Several novel agents are in clinical trials to test for their efficacy as monotherapy for MF. In addition, there are number of promising combination regimens being tested in clinical trials examining systemic multiagent therapies in advanced MF or SS to guide therapeutic decisions.

SKIN-DIRECTED THERAPIES

Topical Glucocorticoids

These agents are effective during early stages of MF. They are limited to temporary short-term use because of suppression of collagen synthesis (skin atrophy), striae formation, skin fragility, and secondary infections. The class of topical preparation depends on the area and the site of involvement. Ultrapotent topical glucocorticoids should not be used on the face, neck, and intertriginous areas. Topical steroids are rarely used as monotherapy, but may be effective as an additional modality for symptomatic relieve of pruritus.

Topical Tacrolimus (Protopic) Topical tacrolimus has been approved for use in atopic dermatitis. It is as effective as mid- to low-potency glucocorticoids for use on facial skin and intertriginous areas in patients with MF. A major advantage of tacrolimus compared with steroids is that it does not suppress collagen synthesis and therefore does not cause skin atrophy.[82] However, because the use of calcineurin inhibitors in CTCL is controversial,[83] tacrolimus use should be limited to short-term use on small areas.

Topical Nitrogen Mustard (Mechlorethamine Hydrochloride) Topical nitrogen mustard is a topical alkylating agent used predominantly in patients with early stages of the disease (stages IA and IB), but can be used as a part of combination therapy with systemic agents in advanced stages. Prior to FDA-approval of mechlorethamine hydrochloride 0.02 percent gel in 2013,[84] it was only available through certified compounding pharmacies in forms of solution, cream or ointment of various concentrations (0.01 to 0.04 percent). The major advantage of this topical therapy is its relatively low toxicity. Disadvantages include the inconvenience of daily application to large areas of skin, allergic reactions in up to half of cases,[85] the potential for development of skin cancer,[86] and the inability to cure the disease. Therapy is usually continued for up to 12 months in responders. Frequency then is reduced to every other day for an additional 1 to 2 years. Therapy is discontinued after 3 years or when cutaneous lesions disappear completely. Mechlorethamine should not be used together with ultraviolet A (UVA) or ultraviolet B (UVB) therapy because of cumulative carcinogenic effects on the skin and significant increase in risk for skin cancer and melanoma.

Topical Carmustine (*Bis*-Chloroethylnitrosourea [BCNU]) BCNU is not currently widely used for treatment of MF because of its severe irritant reactions and its absorption from the skin that results in systemic toxicity. The preparation ranges from 20 to 40 mg/dL in petrolatum ointment. It is applied at night and washed off in the morning. Monitoring includes biweekly complete blood counts to identify marrow suppression. Carmustine causes irreversible skin thinning, telangiectasias, and hyperpigmentation.[87]

Topical Retinoids Bexarotene (Targretin) 1 percent gel, is a topical retinoid (rexinoid) FDA-approved for treatment of MF patients who are refractory to at least one other topical therapy. It is a small lipophilic molecule related to vitamin A. It readily crosses the cytoplasmic membrane and binds to nuclear receptors (retinoid X receptors [RXRs]), resulting in changes in gene expression mediated through specific intracellular receptors, leading to maturating and apoptosis of malignant cells.[88] Complete responses of 20 percent and overall responses of 60 percent are reported.[89,90] It is applied in a thin layer to the patches and plaques twice daily. The major toxicity is irritation at the site. Oral administration of bexarotene is associated with severe birth defects. Considering potential absorption of the drug from the skin surface, bexarotene should not be given to pregnant women.

Phototherapy Phototherapy is a well-established effective treatment for MF, utilizing ultraviolet radiation of the UVA and UVB spectra. It is not FDA-approved for treatment of MF and SS because of a lack of prospective clinical trials, but is considered to be one of the most effective therapies for early disease (mainly patches and thin plaques). Phototherapy may result in complete clearing of the lesions. It was hypothesized that the mechanism of action of this therapy is Langerhans' cells depletion from the epidermis.[91]

The peak of therapeutic effectiveness of UVB is within 295 to 313 nm. Conventional broad band UVB lamps emit wavelengths ranging from 280 to 330 nm, but narrow band UVB (NBUVB) emits only wavelengths 311 to 312 nm, eliminating harmful UV rays below 300 nm, which can cause erythema or severe burning and increase the risk of skin cancer.[92–94] Similarly, excimer lasers emitting at 308 nm can be successfully used for hard to reach areas resistant to other therapy.[95] NBUVB may be a viable alternative to psoralen with UVA radiation (PUVA) with similar response rates in a small cohort.[96] Therapy should be instituted three times per week. On average, 6 to 12 weeks are required to achieve response. Maintenance therapy is required after a response occurs for at least 2 more months, but thereafter the maintenance regimen for various light sources is not well established and depends on the personal experience of the treating physician.

The UVA spectrum ranges from 320 to 400 nm, therefore UVA light penetrates deeper than UVB, into the dermis. Phototherapy involving UVA radiation is used with psoralen and is referred to as PUVA. Psoralen is a phototoxic furocoumarin activated by UVA light. In its active form, psoralen bonds covalently and irreversibly to DNA. Therefore, psoralen activated by UVA light affects cells primarily in the epidermis and papillary dermis. A 60 percent complete remission rate and long-term remissions (>10 years) have been reported with PUVA; patients with generalized erythroderma and tumors have lower response rates than patients with plaques.[97–99] Psoralen usually is given at a dose of 0.6 mg/kg orally, 2 hours before the UVA light therapy. Treatments initially are given three times per week. Maintenance therapy may be given every 2 to 4 weeks for an indefinite period. Adverse effects of PUVA therapy include mild nausea, pruritus, and sunburn-like changes, with atrophy and dry skin. PUVA is not cross-resistant with other treatment modalities. Disadvantages of PUVA therapy are its necessity to visit doctor's office frequently (from three times a week to once a month) and its expense. Long-term side effects include an increased incidence of skin cancers and melanoma.[100]

Photodynamic Therapy Photodynamic therapy is a photochemotherapy that utilizes two properties of porphyrins: their selective accumulation in tumor sites (e.g., 5-aminolevulinic acid) and their ability to generate cytotoxic oxygen species at the tumor site after red-light irradiation. 5-Aminolevulinic acid is a natural porphyrin precursor and upon irradiation is converted in the tumor to the highly photoactive endogenous protoporphyrin IX. Red-light irradiation is safe and penetrates deep in the tissue, allowing for treatment of thick tumors. Photodynamic therapy is especially useful in patients with limited skin area involved by few tumors. The main problem with the treatment is that the pain induced during irradiation limits its use for larger areas.[101,102] It is used for therapy of MF off-label.

Electron Beam Therapy Electron beam therapy is a highly effective form of treatment of MF and can be used as a localized therapy (LEBT) to specific sites or lesions, or as radiation of the entire skin surface (total skin electron beam therapy [TSEBT]). It delivers a uniform dose from the surface to a specific depth, after which the dose falls off rapidly, sparing deeper normal tissues. It is usually delivered to penetrate only into the dermis, systemic effects are minimal, and the complete remission rate is 80 percent.[3,103,104] Twenty percent of patients remain relapse free after 3 years. The relapse rate depends on the stage of the disease, and the relapse usually is short lived (may be as short as 2 to 3 weeks) in patients with erythroderma or numerous tumors. In the past, the treatment regimen was 4 Gy per week to a total dose of 36 Gy in 8 to 9 weeks. However, low-dose electron beam therapy has been shown to be nearly as effective, eliminating the usual side effects, such as alopecia, skin atrophy, destruction of skin adnexa, dermatitis, and increased risk of cutaneous malignancy.[105–108] The advantage of electron beam therapy is the high frequency of durable complete responses without systemic toxicity. Up to three courses of electron beam therapy can be safely administered when used in a highly fractionated fashion (1 Gy per dose).

Imiquimod (Aldara) Imiquimod is a topical immunomodulator that is extremely effective in the treatment of condylomata acuminata, actinic keratoses, basal cell carcinomas, keratoacanthomas, and other cutaneous malignancies. The mode of action is not known but is thought to be related to induction of tumor necrosis factor-α and interferons resulting in activation of a Th1-type immune response and rejection of cancer or virally infected cells. Several groups reported the effectiveness of imiquimod in early patch MF.[109,110] It should be used three times per week for 3 months. It is not FDA-approved for therapy of MF and SS.

SYSTEMIC THERAPY

Oral Retinoids

Bexarotene (Targretin) is an FDA-approved RXR-selective retinoid, or "rexinoid," for therapy of the MF. It is a first-line systemic agent for patients without contraindications to retinoids. At the currently FDA-approved dose of 300 mg/m²/day the overall response rate to bexarotene monotherapy ranges from 45 to 57 percent with at least 2 percent complete responses.[111,112] Higher doses are associated with higher response rates and shorter time to response, but also with a higher incidence of adverse events. All patients on bexarotene rapidly develop central hypothyroidism and hyperlipidemia (most significantly hypertriglyceridemia), requiring coadministration of thyroid supplements and lipid-lowering agents. Other rare adverse events include headaches, possibly a result of pseudotumor cerebri, leucopenia, and pruritus. The majority of side effects are laboratory findings and dose-dependent; bexarotene is usually well tolerated by the patients. Its use is recommended beginning with refractory or persistent stage IA disease as well as in more advanced stages (NCCN guidelines). Standard procedures for management of patients on bexarotene therapy are reviewed.[113] Bexarotene is safe to use long-term for maintenance therapy. Bexarotene and other retinoids are labeled pregnancy Category X, and must not be given to a pregnant woman or a woman who intends to become pregnant.

Other retinoids have been used for treatment of MF and SS, including isotretinoin, acitretin, etretinate (not available in United States), and all-*trans* retinoic acid (ATRA). Activity of these compounds in MF/SS has been demonstrated in case series or small open-label pilot studies, but there are no prospective studies formally evaluating these drugs.[114]

Histone Deacetylase Inhibitors Vorinostat is an oral histone deacetylase inhibitor (HDACi), which was FDA-approved for treatment of cutaneous manifestations of recurrent, refractory or persistent MF and SS in 2008 at the dose of 400 mg by mouth daily.[115] Vorinostat was evaluated in an open-label phase IIb clinical trial and was shown to have an overall response rate of 30 percent. No complete responses were observed on the clinical trial. Median time to relapse in patients with advanced disease was 56 days. Median time to progression was 4.9 months overall, and 9.8 months for stage IIB or higher responders. Overall, 32 percent of patients had pruritus relief. The most common drug-related adverse events were diarrhea (49 percent), fatigue (46 percent), nausea (43 percent), and anorexia (26 percent); most were grade 2 or lower but those grade 3 or higher included fatigue (5 percent), pulmonary embolism (5 percent), thrombocytopenia (5 percent), and nausea (4 percent).

Romidepsin is a selective HDACi given as an intravenous infusion. Romidepsin was FDA-approved for therapy of CTCL based on a phase IIB clinical trial documenting an overall response rate of 34 percent, with 6 percent complete responses.[116] The median duration of response was 13.7 months. Toxicities included nausea, vomiting, fatigue, and transient thrombocytopenia and granulocytopenia. Romidepsin was shown to have single-agent clinical activity with significant and durable responses in patients with CTCL.[116] HDACi may be excellent combinational agents, potentiating effects of other therapies, possessing a radio- and photosensitizing effects. Several clinical trials are on the way examining potential combinations, including electron beam.[106]

Interferon-α Interferon-α can be used as a single agent or combined with other systemic therapies. The response rate when interferon-α is used as a monotherapy is 50 to 70 percent at doses beginning at 3 to 5×10^6 units/day or three times per week, either subcutaneously or intralesionally.[117] Toxicity includes acute flu-like symptoms and fatigue. It is commonly used in combination with other immunotherapies (such as extracorporeal photopheresis [ECP] and phototherapy), but this practice is based on small case series and small prospective studies. It is not clear if combinations truly result in improved clinical outcomes.[10,118,119]

Extracorporeal Photopheresis PUVA can be delivered by an extracorporeal technique.[120,121] White cells are collected by leukapheresis, exposed to a photoactivating drug, and irradiated with UVA. The cells then are reinfused into the patient. The effect may be both a direct cytotoxic effect on the tumor cells and an immunologic effect by activating lymphocytes against the tumor cells. Photopheresis typically is administered every 2 to 4 weeks until clearance of disease. Side effects are minimal and may be related to fluid shifts during the procedure.[100] A recent retrospective review suggested a survival advantage for patients treated with ECP[122] and beneficial responses in patients with early stage MF.[123]

Monoclonal Antibodies Alemtuzumab (Campath-1H) is a humanized IgG1 monoclonal antibody that targets the CD52 antigen. A response rate of 50 percent has been reported in a small cohort of patients.[124,125] Low-dose alemtuzumab was shown to be safe and effective in very elderly SS patients.[126] Alemtuzumab effectively depletes leukemic cells from blood of these patients. Very low doses on an as needed basis were reported to be effective long-term in SS patients.[127] Numerous monoclonal antibodies are in clinical trials now as single agents and in combinations, including anti–PD-1 antibodies and anti-CCR4 antibody.

Monoclonal Antibody Conjugates Brentuximab vedotin (SGN-35) is an anti-CD30 antibody conjugated via a protease-cleavable linker to the potent antimicrotubule agent monomethyl auristatin E (MMAE). Following binding to CD30, brentuximab vedotin is rapidly internalized and transported to lysosomes where MMAE is released and binds to tubulin, leading to cell-cycle arrest and apoptosis. Brentuximab was recently FDA-approved for CD30+ cutaneous T-cell lymphomas, showing durable antitumor activity with a manageable safety profile in patients with relapsed/refractory primary cutaneous CD30-positive lymphoproliferative disorders.[128] The overall response rate was 73 percent, with 54 percent for MF and 100 percent for all other tumor types (LyP

and primary cutaneous anaplastic large cell lymphoma [PCALCL]). Response was not correlated with level of CD30 expression at baseline in MF. Peripheral sensory neuropathy is a significant adverse event associated with brentuximab vedotin administration. Neuropathy symptoms are cumulative and dose related. Multiple ongoing trials are currently evaluating brentuximab vedotin alone or in combination with other agents in relapsed/refractory patients, as well as patients with newly diagnosed disease.

Recombinant Fusion Proteins Denileukin diftitox (DD) is an IL-2 diphtheria toxin fusion protein, which had full FDA approval in October 2008 following a phase III randomized, double-blind, placebo-controlled trial.[129] The overall response rate was 37 percent at a dose of 9 μg/kg/day and 46 percent with 18 μg/kg/day, which was statistically significant (p = 0.002) compared to placebo. Patients receiving 18 μg/kg/day had a progression-free survival of 971+ days and duration of response of 220 days. Time to response was 92 days; time to treatment failure was 169 days. Importantly, 45 percent of best responses occurred during cycle 4 and beyond, suggesting that an appropriate trial of the drug is necessary to achieve optimal responses. All complete responses occurred after four or more cycles.[129] Side effects were numerous, including a capillary leak syndrome, infection, hepatitis, increased fluid retention, rash, shortness of breath, and flu-like symptoms such as chills, fever, weakness, bone and muscle pain, headache, nausea, and vomiting. Cardiac arrhythmias and thrombotic emergencies have been reported occasionally. Usually, adverse events are most severe during the first two cycles, diminishing as the treatments continue. DD manufacturing was discontinued and a new formulation of the same product is in clinical trials at this time.

Chemotherapy Several agents have been FDA-approved for therapy of various subsets of MF and SS.

Pralatrexate is a novel antifolate with high affinity for reduced folate carrier-1, which was recently FDA-approved for therapy of transformed MF (tMF). The recommended regimen was identified as 15 mg/m² a week for 3 of 4 weeks; the response rate was 45 percent.[130] The most common grade 3 adverse event (AE) was mucositis (17 percent); the only grade 4 AE was leukopenia (3 percent). MF patients were not able to tolerate the "lymphoma" dosage of pralatrexate (30 mg/m² a week for 6 of 7 weeks) because of intolerable toxicities, including severe mucositis. It was hypothesized that the higher incidence of mucositis was a result of distribution of malignant cells from the skin and mucosal surfaces beyond visible lesions resulting in "localized" tumor necrosis in the skin with collateral damage to surrounding tissues. Administration of a single 10 to 15 mg dose of leucovorin 24 hours following pralatrexate infusion, completely abrogated these side effects and allowed therapy with 30 mg/m² without sacrificing efficacy.[131]

Alkylating agents used to treat MF and SS include nitrogen mustard topically or systemic cyclophosphamide, or chlorambucil. Response rates of 60 percent, with 15 percent complete remissions, have been reported.[132,133] Similar results are obtained with methotrexate 2.5 to 10 mg/day orally[134]; bleomycin 7.5 to 15 mg intramuscularly given twice weekly; and doxorubicin 60 mg/m² intravenously given once per month.[135,136] Pegylated doxorubicin used in advanced MF has resulted in an overall response of 88 percent.[137] Purine analogues including fludarabine and pentostatin have response rates as high as 50 percent.[138–140] Gemcitabine has a similar response rate.[141] Neither single-agent or multiagent therapy cures MF. Chemotherapy with a single agent and polychemotherapy result in a higher incidence of transformation to large cell lymphoma, which carries a worse prognosis than the original diagnosis.[142,143] Because responses to therapy are generally higher after combination therapy, single-agent chemotherapy is used rarely. However, use of multiagent chemotherapy results in increased immunosuppression and an increased risk of serious infections, leading to death in the majority of patients who develop this complication.[144] Combination therapy produces objective responses in greater than 80 percent of patients and complete responses in approximately one fourth of cases.[99,145] The duration of remission varies, with a median of approximately 1 year. No long-term disease-free survival has been reported.

Combined Modality Therapy Several multidrug regimens reportedly improve clinical response in patients with MF, including combination of extracorporeal photophoresis with low-dose interferon-α and oral bexarotene; prednisone and fludarabine; and PUVA and oral bexarotene.[3,146]

Because in general MF is an indolent malignancy of T cells with excellent prognosis in early stages, the treatment should be conservative, with skin-directed therapies (nitrogen mustard, topical glucocorticoids, topical bexarotene) combined with light therapy, low-dose interferon, low-dose methotrexate, or other single-agent chemotherapy. The survival of patients treated with aggressive chemotherapy is not different from the survival of patients treated conservatively, but aggressive chemotherapy results in greater toxicity. Because no curative therapy exists, the goal of therapy is to prevent progression to more advanced stages and to preserve the patient's quality of life for as long as possible.

PROGNOSIS

Prognosis largely depends on the stage at presentation. Fifty percent of deaths among patients with MF result from infections. Septicemia and bacterial pneumonia are common; they usually are caused by *Staphylococcus* or *Pseudomonas* and develop from cutaneous lesions.[54] Herpes virus infections occur in up to 10 percent of patients with advanced MF. Progressive MF with widespread visceral involvement late in the course of the disease is the next most common cause of death.

PRIMARY CUTANEOUS ANAPLASTIC LARGE CELL LYMPHOMA

CLINICAL FINDINGS

CD30+ cutaneous lymphoproliferative disorders are the second most common CTCLs after MF and represent approximately 25 percent of CTCL cases.[81] PCALCL represents a spectrum of CD30+ lymphoproliferative disorders, including LyP and PCALCL as its malignant counterpart. It is defined by the presence of skin involvement without evidence of extracutaneous disease for at least 6 months after presentation.[13] Secondary involvement of lymph nodes may not necessarily be associated

with a worse prognosis.[14] In some cases, distinction between LyP and PCALCL cannot be made because of discrepancies between clinical features and histologic appearance. These cases are referred to as *borderline lesions*, and their classification should take into consideration their clinical behavior and appearance (Fig. 103–7A).

Other CD30+ cutaneous lymphoproliferative disorders include large cell transformation of MF, systemic anaplastic large cell lymphoma (ALCL), cutaneous NK/T-cell lymphoma, and Hodgkin lymphoma. Making the distinctions between these diagnoses is critical because management and prognosis are significantly different (see "Treatment" below). The descriptive term *anaplastic* could be omitted from the name of this lymphoma because these lymphomas may have an anaplastic, immunoblastic, or pleomorphic cell morphology. Regardless of pathologic type, these CD30+ large cell lymphomas have a similar clinical course, treatment, and prognosis.[81,147–149]

CD30+ PCALCL can occur at any age, with the peak incidence in patients in their 60s, with a slight male predominance.[79,150] PCALCL can occur anywhere on the body. The lesions are brownish to violaceous nodules or tumors, ranging in number from solitary (most commonly) to numerous with generalized involvement. They may regress spontaneously. Histopathologically, at least 75 percent of the large cells should express CD30. Most cases are CD4+, with loss of pan–T-cell markers CD2, CD3, and CD5. In rare cases, the cells are CD8+CD30+. In contrast to systemic ALCL, primary cutaneous large cell lymphoma is negative for CD15 and epithelial membrane antigen.[151] In addition, primary cutaneous large cell lymphoma usually does not express anaplastic lymphoma kinase-1 (ALK-1) or the t(2;5) chromosomal translocation.[152,153] Presence of ALK-1 in cutaneous lesions without systemic involvement does not carry a worse prognosis.

LYMPHOMATOID PAPULOSIS

LyP is the benign counterpart of primary cutaneous ALCL. It is characterized by crops of erythematous, dome-shaped papules or nodules that may ulcerate spontaneously. It regresses over a few months with minor sequelae such as scarring or atrophy (see Fig. 103–7B). The three main histologic types of LyP are A, B, and C. The infiltrate usually is wedge shaped with ulcer formation. The large atypical cells of type A resemble immunoblasts of Reed-Sternberg cells. These cells are surrounded by neutrophils and eosinophils. Type B cells resemble MF, with lichenoid lymphocytic infiltration of cells with cerebriform nuclei and some epidermotropism. Type C cells resemble ALCL, with sheets of large CD30+ cells in the infiltrate. The histologic distinction between LyP and the corresponding condition may be difficult, and clinical correlation is

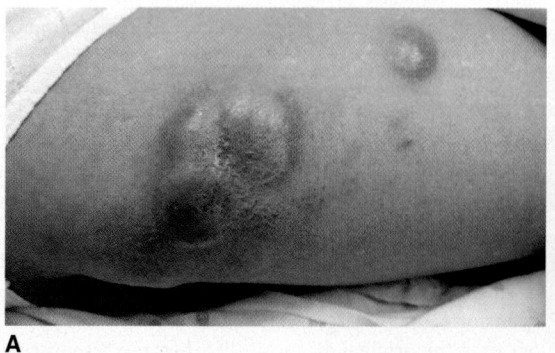

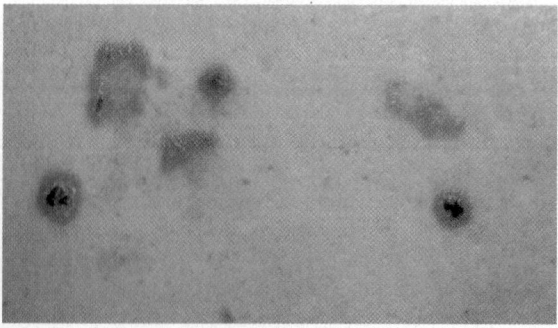

A
B

Figure 103–7. CD30+ lymphoproliferative disorders. **A.** Primary cutaneous anaplastic large cells lymphoma. Large cutaneous tumors on the anterior thigh. **B.** Lymphomatoid papulosis. Numerous small erythematous papules and small nodules. Some with necrotic centers in crops. Some lesions show spontaneous regression.

required.[154] In rare cases, LyP evolves into more aggressive primary cutaneous large cell lymphoma. In addition, a higher incidence of lymphoid and nonlymphoid malignancies is observed in patients with LyP.[155]

TREATMENT

LyP is extremely responsive to low-dose methotrexate therapy, requiring 10 to 15 mg orally weekly, with noticeable clinical response within a month. Brentuximab vedotin was shown to be highly effective in patients with PCALCL and LyP (see section Monoclonal Antibody Conjugates above). Other treatment options include oral PUVA therapy, retinoids, topical and systemic glucocorticoids, and intralesional and systemic interferon-α.[81,147,154] Treatment of primary cutaneous large cell lymphoma depends on the extent of skin involvement. In cases of solitary lesions, radiotherapy is often the best initial treatment modality. A combination of PUVA and interferon-α may be considered for more disseminated disease. Combination chemotherapy should be reserved for resistant cases.[81,147,156]

REFERENCES

1. Criscione VD, Weinstock MA: Incidence of cutaneous T-cell lymphoma in the United States, 1973–2002. *Arch Dermatol* 143:854–859, 2007.
2. Lorincz AL: Cutaneous T-cell lymphoma (mycosis fungoides). *Lancet* 347:871–876, 1996.
3. Duvic M, Apisarnthanarax N, Cohen DS, et al: Analysis of long-term outcomes of combined modality therapy for cutaneous T-cell lymphoma. *J Am Acad Dermatol* 49:35–49, 2003.
4. Ai WZ, Keegan TH, Press DJ, et al: Outcomes after diagnosis of mycosis fungoides and Sezary syndrome before 30 years of age: A population-based study. *JAMA Dermatol* 150:709–715, 2014.
5. Hughes CF, Khot A, McCormack C, et al: Lack of durable disease control with chemotherapy for mycosis fungoides and Sézary syndrome: A comparative study of systemic therapy. *Blood* 125:71–81, 2014.
6. Duarte RF, Canals C, Onida F, et al: Allogeneic hematopoietic cell transplantation for patients with mycosis fungoides and Sézary syndrome: A retrospective analysis of the Lymphoma Working Party of the European Group for Blood and Marrow Transplantation. *J Clin Oncol* 28:4492–4499, 2010.
7. Duvic M, Donato M, Dabaja B, et al: Total skin electron beam and non-myeloablative allogeneic hematopoietic stem-cell transplantation in advanced mycosis fungoides and Sézary syndrome. *J Clin Oncol* 28:2365–2372, 2010.
8. Shiratori S, Fujimoto K, Nishimura M, et al: Allogeneic hematopoietic stem cell transplantation following reduced-intensity conditioning for mycosis fungoides and Sézary syndrome. *Hematol Oncol* 2014. [Epub ahead of print]
9. Wilcox RA: Cutaneous T-cell lymphoma: 2014 update on diagnosis, risk-stratification, and management. *Am J Hematol* 89:837–851, 2014.
10. Humme D, Nast A, Erdmann R, et al: Systematic review of combination therapies for mycosis fungoides. *Cancer Treat Rev* 40:927–933, 2014.
11. Guenova E, Hoetzenecker W, Rozati S, et al: Novel therapies for cutaneous T-cell lymphoma: What does the future hold? *Expert Opin Investig Drugs* 23:457–467, 2014.
12. Alibert J: *Description des maladies de la peau observées à l'Hôpital Saint-Louis et exposition des meilleures méthodes suivies pour leur traitement.* Barrois l'aîné et fils, 1806.
13. Sezary A, Bouvrain Y: Erythrodermie avec présence de cellules monstrueses dans le derme et dans lang circulant. *Bull Soc Fr Dermatol Syphilig* 45, 1938.
14. Lutzner M, Edelson R, Schein P, et al: Cutaneous T-cell lymphomas: The Sézary syndrome, mycosis fungoides, and related disorders. *Ann Intern Med* 83:534–552, 1975.
15. Willemze R, Jaffe ES, Burg G, et al: WHO-EORTC classification for cutaneous lymphomas. *Blood* 105:3768–3785, 2005.
16. Olsen E, Vonderheid E, Pimpinelli N, et al: Revisions to the staging and classification of mycosis fungoides and Sézary syndrome: A proposal of the International Society for Cutaneous Lymphomas (ISCL) and the cutaneous lymphoma task force of the European Organization of Research and Treatment of Cancer (EORTC). *Blood* 110:1713–1722, 2007.
17. Korgavkar K, Xiong M, Weinstock M: Changing incidence trends of cutaneous T-cell lymphoma. *JAMA Dermatol* 149:1295–1299, 2013.
18. Kim YH, Liu HL, Mraz-Gernhard S, et al: Long-term outcome of 525 patients with mycosis fungoides and Sézary syndrome: Clinical prognostic factors and risk for disease progression. *Arch Dermatol* 139:857–866, 2003.
19. Mirvish JJ, Pomerantz RG, Falo LD Jr, et al: Role of infectious agents in cutaneous T-cell lymphoma: Facts and controversies. *Clin Dermatol* 31:423–431, 2013.
20. Dulmage BO, Feng H, Mirvish E, et al: Black cat in a dark room: Absence of a directly oncogenic virus does not eliminate the role of an infectious agent in CTCL pathogenesis. *Br J Dermatol* 172(5):1449–1451, 2015.
21. Burg G, Dummer R, Haeffner A, et al: From inflammation to neoplasia: Mycosis fungoides evolves from reactive inflammatory conditions (lymphoid infiltrates) transforming into neoplastic plaques and tumors. *Arch Dermatol* 137:949–952, 2001.
22. Tan RS, Butterworth CM, McLaughlin H, et al: Mycosis fungoides—A disease of antigen persistence. *Br J Dermatol* 91:607–616, 1974.
23. Kim EJ, Hess S, Richardson SK, et al: Immunopathogenesis and therapy of cutaneous T cell lymphoma. *J Clin Invest* 115:798–812, 2005.
24. Wong HK, Mishra A, Hake T, et al: Evolving insights in the pathogenesis and therapy of cutaneous T-cell lymphoma (mycosis fungoides and Sézary syndrome). *Br J Haematol* 155:150–166, 2011.
25. Yawalkar N, Ferenczi K, Jones DA, et al: Profound loss of T-cell receptor repertoire complexity in cutaneous T-cell lymphoma. *Blood* 102:4059–4066, 2003.
26. Smoller BR: Risk of secondary cutaneous malignancies in patients with long-standing mycosis fungoides. *J Am Acad Dermatol* 31:295, 1994.
27. Morales-Suarez-Varela MM, Olsen J, Johansen P, et al: Occupational risk factors for mycosis fungoides: A European multicenter case-control study. *J Occup Environ Med* 46:205–211, 2004.
28. Moreau JF, Buchanich JM, Geskin JZ, et al: Non-random geographic distribution of patients with cutaneous T-cell lymphoma in the Greater Pittsburgh Area. *Dermatol Online J* 20, 2014.
29. Talpur R, Singh L, Daulat S, et al: Long-term outcomes of 1,263 patients with mycosis fungoides and Sézary syndrome from 1982 to 2009. *Clin Cancer Res* 18:5051–5060, 2012.
30. Vij A, Duvic M: Prevalence and severity of pruritus in cutaneous T cell lymphoma. *Int J Dermatol* 51:930–934, 2012.
31. Nguyen V, Huggins RH, Lertsburapa T, et al: Cutaneous T-cell lymphoma and *Staphylococcus aureus* colonization. *J Am Acad Dermatol* 59:949–952, 2008.
32. Pimpinelli N, Olsen EA, Santucci M, et al: Defining early mycosis fungoides. *J Am Acad Dermatol* 53:1053–1063, 2005.
33. Naraghi ZS, Seirafi H, Valikhani M, et al: Assessment of histologic criteria in the diagnosis of mycosis fungoides. *Int J Dermatol* 42:45–52, 2003.
34. Benner MF, Jansen PM, Vermeer MH, et al: Prognostic factors in transformed mycosis fungoides: A retrospective analysis of 100 cases. *Blood* 119:1643–1649, 2012.
35. Jones D, Dang NH, Duvic M, et al: Absence of CD26 expression is a useful marker for diagnosis of T-cell lymphoma in peripheral blood. *Am J Clin Pathol* 115:885–892, 2001.
36. Bernengo MG, Novelli M, Quaglino P, et al: The relevance of the CD4+ CD26– subset in the identification of circulating Sézary cells. *Br J Dermatol* 144:125–135, 2001.
37. Delfau-Larue MH, Petrella T, Lahet C, et al: Value of clonality studies of cutaneous T lymphocytes in the diagnosis and follow-up of patients with mycosis fungoides. *J Pathol* 184:185–190, 1998.
38. Lu D, Patel KA, Duvic M, et al: Clinical and pathological spectrum of CD8-positive cutaneous T-cell lymphomas. *J Cutan Pathol* 29:465–472, 2002.
39. Santucci M, Pimpinelli N, Massi D, et al: Cytotoxic/natural killer cell cutaneous lymphomas. Report of EORTC Cutaneous Lymphoma Task Force Workshop. *Cancer* 97:610–627, 2003.
40. Morimura S, Sugaya M, Suga H, et al: TOX expression in different subtypes of cutaneous lymphoma. *Arch Dermatol Res* 306:843–849, 2014.
41. Dulmage BO, Geskin LJ: Lessons learned from gene expression profiling of cutaneous T-cell lymphoma. *Br J Dermatol* 169:1188–1197, 2013.
42. Zhang Y, Wang Y, Yu R, et al: Molecular markers of early-stage mycosis fungoides. *J Invest Dermatol* 132:1698–1706, 2012.
43. Moins-Teisserenc H, Daubord M, Clave E, et al: CD158k is a reliable marker for diagnosis of Sézary syndrome and reveals an unprecedented heterogeneity of circulating malignant cells. *J Invest Dermatol* 135:247–257, 2014.
44. Scarisbrick JJ, Woolford AJ, Russell-Jones R, et al: Loss of heterozygosity on 10q and microsatellite instability in advanced stages of primary cutaneous T-cell lymphoma and possible association with homozygous deletion of PTEN. *Blood* 95:2937–2942, 2000.
45. Navas IC, Algara P, Mateo M, et al: P16(INK4a) is selectively silenced in the tumoral progression of mycosis fungoides. *Lab Invest* 82:123–132, 2002.
46. Navas IC, Ortiz-Romero PL, Villuendas R, et al: P16(INK4a) gene alterations are frequent in lesions of mycosis fungoides. *Am J Pathol* 156:1565–1572, 2000.
47. Bunn PA Jr, Lamberg SI: Report of the Committee on Staging and Classification of Cutaneous T-Cell Lymphomas. *Cancer Treat Rep* 63:725–728, 1979.
48. Lamberg SI, Bunn PA Jr: Cutaneous T-cell lymphomas. Summary of the Mycosis Fungoides Cooperative Group-National Cancer Institute Workshop. *Arch Dermatol* 115:1103–1105, 1979.
49. Stevens SR, Ke MS, Parry EJ, et al: Quantifying skin disease burden in mycosis fungoides-type cutaneous T-cell lymphomas: The severity-weighted assessment tool (SWAT). *Arch Dermatol* 138:42–48, 2002.
50. Kumar R, Xiu Y, Zhuang HM, et al: 18F-fluorodeoxyglucose-positron emission tomography in evaluation of primary cutaneous lymphoma. *Br J Dermatol* 155:357–363, 2006.
51. Rosen ST, Gore R, Brennan J, et al: Evaluation of computed tomography and radionuclide scanning in the staging of cutaneous T-cell lymphoma. *Arch Dermatol* 122:884–886, 1986.
52. Vigliar E, Cozzolino I, Picardi M, et al: Lymph node fine needle cytology in the staging and follow-up of cutaneous lymphomas. *BMC Cancer* 14:8, 2014.
53. Bunn PA Jr, Huberman MS, Whang-Peng J, et al: Prospective staging evaluation of patients with cutaneous T-cell lymphomas. Demonstration of a high frequency of extracutaneous dissemination. *Ann Intern Med* 93:223–230, 1980.

54. Epstein EH Jr, Levin DL, Croft JD Jr, et al: Mycosis fungoides. Survival, prognostic features, response to therapy, and autopsy findings. *Medicine (Baltimore)* 51: 61–72, 1972.

55. Zackheim HS, Amin S, Kashani-Sabet M, et al: Prognosis in cutaneous T-cell lymphoma by skin stage: Long-term survival in 489 patients. *J Am Acad Dermatol* 40: 418–425, 1999.

56. Scarisbrick JJ, Whittaker S, Evans AV, et al: Prognostic significance of tumor burden in the blood of patients with erythrodermic primary cutaneous T-cell lymphoma. *Blood* 97:624–630, 2001.

57. Muche JM, Lukowsky A, Asadullah K, et al: Demonstration of frequent occurrence of clonal T cells in the peripheral blood of patients with primary cutaneous T-cell lymphoma. *Blood* 90:1636–1642, 1997.

58. Vonderheid EC, Pena J, Nowell P: Sézary cell counts in erythrodermic cutaneous T-cell lymphoma: Implications for prognosis and staging. *Leuk Lymphoma* 47:1841–1856, 2006.

59. Vonderheid EC, Bernengo MG, Burg G, et al: Update on erythrodermic cutaneous T-cell lymphoma: Report of the International Society for Cutaneous Lymphomas. *J Am Acad Dermatol* 46:95–106, 2002.

60. Bergman R: How useful are T-cell receptor gene rearrangement studies as an adjunct to the histopathologic diagnosis of mycosis fungoides? *Am J Dermatopathol* 21:498–502, 1999.

61. Cherny S, Mraz S, Su L, et al: Heteroduplex analysis of T-cell receptor gamma gene rearrangement as an adjuvant diagnostic tool in skin biopsies for erythroderma. *J Cutan Pathol* 28:351–355, 2001.

62. Delfau-Larue MH, Dalac S, Lepage E, et al: Prognostic significance of a polymerase chain reaction-detectable dominant T-lymphocyte clone in cutaneous lesions of patients with mycosis fungoides. *Blood* 92:3376–3380, 1998.

63. Poszepczynska-Guigne E, Bagot M, Wechsler J, et al: Minimal residual disease in mycosis fungoides follow-up can be assessed by polymerase chain reaction. *Br J Dermatol* 148:265–271, 2003.

64. Wood GS, Tung RM, Haeffner AC, et al: Detection of clonal T-cell receptor gamma gene rearrangements in early mycosis fungoides/Sézary syndrome by polymerase chain reaction and denaturing gradient gel electrophoresis (PCR/DGGE). *J Invest Dermatol* 103:34–41, 1994.

65. Long JC, Mihm MC: Mycosis fungoides with extracutaneous dissemination: A distinct clinicopathologic entity. *Cancer* 34:1745–1755, 1974.

66. Smith DI, Vnencak-Jones CL, Boyd AS: T-lymphocyte clonality in benign lichenoid keratoses. *J Cutan Pathol* 29:623–624, 2002.

67. Nihal M, Mikkola D, Horvath N, et al: Cutaneous lymphoid hyperplasia: A lymphoproliferative continuum with lymphomatous potential. *Hum Pathol* 34:617–622, 2003.

68. Holm N, Flaig MJ, Yazdi AS, et al: The value of molecular analysis by PCR in the diagnosis of cutaneous lymphocytic infiltrates. *J Cutan Pathol* 29:447–452, 2002.

69. Shieh S, Mikkola DL, Wood GS: Differentiation and clonality of lesional lymphocytes in pityriasis lichenoides chronica. *Arch Dermatol* 137:305–308, 2001.

70. Zucker-Franklin D: The role of human T cell lymphotropic virus type I tax in the development of cutaneous T cell lymphoma. *Ann N Y Acad Sci* 941:86–96, 2001.

71. Kikuchi A, Ohata Y, Matsumoto H, et al: Anti-HTLV-1 antibody positive cutaneous T-cell lymphoma. *Cancer* 79:269–274, 1997.

72. Palmer RA, Keefe M, Slater D, et al: Case 4: Pagetoid reticulosis (Woringer-Kolopp type) or unilesional mycosis fungoides (MF). *Clin Exp Dermatol* 27:345–346, 2002.

73. Wood GS, Weiss LM, Hu CH, et al: T-cell antigen deficiencies and clonal rearrangements of T-cell receptor genes in pagetoid reticulosis (Woringer-Kolopp disease). *N Engl J Med* 318:164–167, 1988.

74. Cohen EL: Woringer-Kolopp disease (pagetoid reticulosis). *Clin Exp Dermatol* 3: 447–450, 1978.

75. Scarabello A, Fantini F, Giannetti A, et al: Localized pagetoid reticulosis (Woringer-Kolopp disease). *Br J Dermatol* 147:806, 2002.

76. Nakada T, Sueki H, Iijima M: Disseminated pagetoid reticulosis (Ketron-Goodman disease): Six-year follow-up. *J Am Acad Dermatol* 47:S183–S186, 2002.

77. Fierro MT, Novelli M, Savoia P, et al: CD45RA+ immunophenotype in mycosis fungoides: Clinical, histological and immunophenotypical features in 22 patients. *J Cutan Pathol* 28:356–362, 2001.

78. Haghighi B, Smoller BR, LeBoit PE, et al: Pagetoid reticulosis (Woringer-Kolopp disease): An immunophenotypic, molecular, and clinicopathologic study. *Mod Pathol* 13:502–510, 2000.

79. Bekkenk MW, Geelen FA, van Voorst Vader PC, et al: Primary and secondary cutaneous CD30(+) lymphoproliferative disorders: A report from the Dutch Cutaneous Lymphoma Group on the long-term follow-up data of 219 patients and guidelines for diagnosis and treatment. *Blood* 95:3653–3661, 2000.

80. Bekkenk MW, Vermeer MH, Jansen PM, et al: Peripheral T-cell lymphomas unspecified presenting in the skin: Analysis of prognostic factors in a group of 82 patients. *Blood* 102:2213–2219, 2003.

81. Willemze R, Meijer CJ: Primary cutaneous CD30-positive lymphoproliferative disorders. *Hematol Oncol Clin North Am* 17:1319–1332, vii–viii, 2003.

82. Reitamo S, Rissanen J, Remitz A, et al: Tacrolimus ointment does not affect collagen synthesis: Results of a single-center randomized trial. *J Invest Dermatol* 111:396–398, 1998.

83. Pomerantz RG, Campbell LS, Jukic DM, et al: Posttransplant cutaneous T-cell lymphoma: Case reports and review of the association of calcineurin inhibitor use with posttransplant lymphoproliferative disease risk. *Arch Dermatol* 146:513–516, 2010.

84. Lessin SR, Duvic M, Guitart J, et al: Topical chemotherapy in cutaneous T-cell lymphoma: Positive results of a randomized, controlled, multicenter trial testing the efficacy and safety of a novel mechlorethamine, 0.02%, gel in mycosis fungoides. *JAMA Dermatol* 149:25–32, 2013.

85. Vonderheid EC, Van Scott EJ, Johnson WC, et al: Topical chemotherapy and immunotherapy of mycosis fungoides: Intermediate-term results. *Arch Dermatol* 113:454–462, 1977.

86. Du Vivier A, Vonderheid EC, Van Scott EJ, et al: Mycosis fungoides, nitrogen mustard and skin cancer. *Br J Dermatol* 99:61–63, 1978.

87. Zackheim HS, Epstein EH Jr, Grekin DA: Treatment of mycosis fungoides with topical BCNU. *Cancer Treat Rep* 63:623, 1979.

88. Pileri A, Delfino C, Grandi V, et al: Role of bexarotene in the treatment of cutaneous T-cell lymphoma: The clinical and immunological sides. *Immunotherapy* 5:427–433, 2013.

89. Kempf W, Kettelhack N, Duvic M, et al: Topical and systemic retinoid therapy for cutaneous T-cell lymphoma. *Hematol Oncol Clin North Am* 17:1405–1419, 2003.

90. Martin AG: Bexarotene gel: A new skin-directed treatment option for cutaneous T-cell lymphomas. *J Drugs Dermatol* 2:155–167, 2003.

91. Morison WL: *In vivo* effects of psoralens plus longwave ultraviolet radiation on immunity. *Natl Cancer Inst Monogr* 66:243–246, 1984.

92. Baron ED, Stevens SR: Phototherapy for cutaneous T-cell lymphoma. *Dermatol Ther* 16:303–310, 2003.

93. Ramsay DL, Lish KM, Yalowitz CB, et al: Ultraviolet-B phototherapy for early-stage cutaneous T-cell lymphoma. *Arch Dermatol* 128:931–933, 1992.

94. Samson Yashar S, Gielczyk R, Scherschun L, et al: Narrow-band ultraviolet B treatment for vitiligo, pruritus, and inflammatory dermatoses. *Photodermatol Photoimmunol Photomed* 19:164–168, 2003.

95. Deaver D, Cauthen A, Cohen G, et al: Excimer laser in the treatment of mycosis fungoides. *J Am Acad Dermatol* 70:1058–1060, 2014.

96. Drucker AM, Baibergenova A, Rosen CF, et al: Narrowband UVB as an effective substitute for psoralen plus UVA: Lessons from a psoralen shortage. *Photodermatol Photoimmunol Photomed* 28:267–268, 2012.

97. Gilchrest BA: Methoxsalen photochemotherapy for mycosis fungoides. *Cancer Treat Rep* 63:663–667, 1979.

98. Herrmann JJ, Roenigk HH Jr, Hurria A, et al: Treatment of mycosis fungoides with photochemotherapy (PUVA): Long-term follow-up. *J Am Acad Dermatol* 33:234–242, 1995.

99. Roenigk HH Jr, Kuzel TM, Skoutelis AP, et al: Photochemotherapy alone or combined with interferon alpha-2a in the treatment of cutaneous T-cell lymphoma. *J Invest Dermatol* 95:198S–205S, 1990.

100. Geskin L: ECP versus PUVA for the treatment of cutaneous T-cell lymphoma. *Skin Therapy Lett* 12:1–4, 2007.

101. Orenstein A, Haik J, Tamir J, et al: Photodynamic therapy of cutaneous lymphoma using 5-aminolevulinic acid topical application. *Dermatol Surg* 26:765–769; discussion 769–770, 2000.

102. Edstrom DW, Porwit A, Ros AM: Photodynamic therapy with topical 5-aminolevulinic acid for mycosis fungoides: Clinical and histological response. *Acta Derm Venereol* 81:184–188, 2001.

103. Jones GW, Kacinski BM, Wilson LD, et al: Total skin electron radiation in the management of mycosis fungoides: Consensus of the European Organization for Research and Treatment of Cancer (EORTC) Cutaneous Lymphoma Project Group. *J Am Acad Dermatol* 47:364–370, 2002.

104. Hoppe R: Total skin electron beam therapy in the management of mycosis fungoides, in *The Role of High Energy Electrons in the Treatment of Cancer*, edited by Vaeth M, p 80. S Karger, Basel, Switzerland, 1991.

105. Kazmierska J: Clinical results of the total skin electron irradiation of the mycosis fungoides in adults. Conventional fractionation and low dose schemes. *Rep Pract Oncol Radiother* 19:99–103, 2014.

106. Akilov OE, Grant C, Frye R, et al: Low-dose electron beam radiation and romidepsin therapy for symptomatic cutaneous T-cell lymphoma lesions. *Br J Dermatol* 167: 194–197, 2012.

107. Harrison C, Young J, Navi D, et al: Revisiting low-dose total skin electron beam therapy in mycosis fungoides. *Int J Radiat Oncol Biol Phys* 81:e651–7, 2011.

108. Kamstrup MR, Specht L, Skovgaard GL, et al: A prospective, open-label study of low-dose total skin electron beam therapy in mycosis fungoides. *Int J Radiat Oncol Biol Phys* 71:1204–1207, 2008.

109. Do JH, McLaughlin SS, Gaspari AA: Topical imiquimod therapy for cutaneous T-cell lymphoma. *Skinmed* 2:316–318, 2003.

110. Dummer R, Urosevic M, Kempf W, et al: Imiquimod induces complete clearance of a PUVA-resistant plaque in mycosis fungoides. *Dermatology* 207:116–118, 2003.

111. Duvic M, Hymes K, Heald P, et al: Bexarotene is effective and safe for treatment of refractory advanced-stage cutaneous T-cell lymphoma: Multinational phase II-III trial results. *J Clin Oncol* 19:2456–2471, 2001.

112. Duvic M, Martin AG, Kim Y, et al: Phase 2 and 3 clinical trial of oral bexarotene (Targretin capsules) for the treatment of refractory or persistent early-stage cutaneous T-cell lymphoma. *Arch Dermatol* 137:581–593, 2001.

113. Assaf C, Bagot M, Dummer R, et al: Minimizing adverse side-effects of oral bexarotene in cutaneous T-cell lymphoma: An expert opinion. *Br J Dermatol* 155:261–266, 2006.

114. Zhang C, Duvic M: Treatment of cutaneous T-cell lymphoma with retinoids. *Dermatol Ther* 19:264–271, 2006.

115. Olsen EA, Kim YH, Kuzel TM, et al: Phase IIb multicenter trial of vorinostat in patients with persistent, progressive, or treatment refractory cutaneous T-cell lymphoma. *J Clin Oncol* 25:3109–3115, 2007.

116. Piekarz RL, Frye R, Turner M, et al: Phase II multi-institutional trial of the histone deacetylase inhibitor romidepsin as monotherapy for patients with cutaneous T-cell lymphoma. *J Clin Oncol* 27:5410–5417, 2009.

117. Olsen EA: Interferon in the treatment of cutaneous T-cell lymphoma. *Dermatol Ther* 16:311–321, 2003.

118. Wozniak MB, Tracey L, Ortiz-Romero PL, et al: Psoralen plus ultraviolet A +/- interferon-alpha treatment resistance in mycosis fungoides: The role of tumour microenvironment, nuclear transcription factor-kappaB and T-cell receptor pathways. *Br J Dermatol* 160: 92–102, 2009.

119. Rupoli S, Goteri G, Pulini S, et al: Long-term experience with low-dose interferon-alpha and PUVA in the management of early mycosis fungoides. *Eur J Haematol* 75:136–145, 2005.

120. Edelson R, Berger C, Gasparro F, et al: Treatment of cutaneous T-cell lymphoma by extracorporeal photochemotherapy. Preliminary results. *N Engl J Med* 316:297–303, 1987.

121. Knobler R, Girardi M: Extracorporeal photochemoimmunotherapy in cutaneous T cell lymphomas. *Ann N Y Acad Sci* 941:123–138, 2001.

122. Knobler R, Duvic M, Querfeld C, et al: Long-term follow-up and survival of cutaneous T-cell lymphoma patients treated with extracorporeal photopheresis. *Photodermatol Photoimmunol Photomed* 28:250–257, 2012.

123. Talpur R, Demierre MF, Geskin L, et al: Multicenter photopheresis intervention trial in early-stage mycosis fungoides. *Clin Lymphoma Myeloma Leuk* 11:219–227, 2011.

124. Kennedy GA, Seymour JF, Wolf M, et al: Treatment of patients with advanced mycosis fungoides and Sézary syndrome with alemtuzumab. *Eur J Haematol* 71:250–256, 2003.

125. Lundin J, Hagberg H, Repp R, et al: Phase 2 study of alemtuzumab (anti-CD52 monoclonal antibody) in patients with advanced mycosis fungoides/Sézary syndrome. *Blood* 101:4267–4272, 2003.

126. Alinari L, Geskin L, Grady T, et al: Subcutaneous alemtuzumab for Sézary syndrome in the very elderly. *Leuk Res* 32:1299–1303, 2008.

127. Bernengo MG, Quaglino P, Comessatti A, et al: Low-dose intermittent alemtuzumab in the treatment of Sézary syndrome: Clinical and immunologic findings in 14 patients. *Haematologica* 92:784–794, 2007.

128. Mehra T, Ikenberg K, Moos RM, et al: Brentuximab as a treatment for CD30+ mycosis fungoides and Sézary syndrome. *JAMA Dermatol* 151:73–77, 2014.

129. Negro-Vilar A, Dziewanowska Z, Groves ES, et al: Efficacy and safety of denileukin diftitox (Dd) in a phase III, double-blind, placebo-controlled study of CD25+ patients with cutaneous T-cell lymphoma (CTCL). *J Clin Oncol* 25:8026, 2007.

130. Horwitz SM, Kim YH, Foss F, et al: Identification of an active, well-tolerated dose of pralatrexate in patients with relapsed or refractory cutaneous T-cell lymphoma. *Blood* 119:4115–4122, 2012.

131. Koch E, Story SK, Geskin LJ: Preemptive leucovorin administration minimizes pralatrexate toxicity without sacrificing efficacy. *Leuk Lymphoma* 54:2448–2451, 2013.

132. Van Scott EJ, Grekin DA, Kalmanson JD, et al: Frequent low doses of intravenous mechlorethamine for late-stage mycosis fungoides lymphoma. *Cancer* 36:1613–1618, 1975.

133. Van Scott EJ, Auerbach R, Clendenning WE: Treatment of mycosis fungoides with cyclophosphamide. *Arch Dermatol* 85:499–501, 1962.

134. Zackheim HS, Kashani-Sabet M, Hwang ST: Low-dose methotrexate to treat erythrodermic cutaneous T-cell lymphoma: Results in twenty-nine patients. *J Am Acad Dermatol* 34:626–631, 1996.

135. Spigel SC, Coltman CA, Jr: Therapy of mycosis fungoides with bleomycin. *Cancer* 32:767–770, 1973.

136. Levi JA, Diggs CH, Wiernik PH: Adriamycin therapy in advanced mycosis fungoides. *Cancer* 39:1967–1970, 1977.

137. Wollina U, Dummer R, Brockmeyer NH, et al: Multicenter study of pegylated liposomal doxorubicin in patients with cutaneous T-cell lymphoma. *Cancer* 98:993–1001, 2003.

138. Foss FM: Activity of pentostatin (Nipent) in cutaneous T-cell lymphoma: Single-agent and combination studies. *Semin Oncol* 27:58–63, 2000.

139. Kurzrock R: Therapy of T cell lymphomas with pentostatin. *Ann N Y Acad Sci* 941:200–205, 2001.

140. Quaglino P, Fierro MT, Rossotto GL, et al: Treatment of advanced mycosis fungoides/Sézary syndrome with fludarabine and potential adjunctive benefit to subsequent extracorporeal photochemotherapy. *Br J Dermatol* 150:327–336, 2004.

141. Zinzani PL, Baliva G, Magagnoli M, et al: Gemcitabine treatment in pretreated cutaneous T-cell lymphoma: Experience in 44 patients. *J Clin Oncol* 18:2603–2606, 2000.

142. Vonderheid EC: Treatment of cutaneous T cell lymphoma: 2001. *Recent Results Cancer Res* 160:309–320, 2002.

143. Abd-el-Baki J, Demierre MF, Li N, et al: Transformation in mycosis fungoides: The role of methotrexate. *J Cutan Med Surg* 6:109–116, 2002.

144. Kaye FJ, Bunn PA Jr, Steinberg SM, et al: A randomized trial comparing combination electron-beam radiation and chemotherapy with topical therapy in the initial treatment of mycosis fungoides. *N Engl J Med* 321:1784–1790, 1989.

145. Rosen ST, Foss FM: Chemotherapy for mycosis fungoides and the Sezary syndrome. *Hematol Oncol Clin North Am* 9:1109–1116, 1995.

146. Vonderheid EC: Treatment planning in cutaneous T-cell lymphoma. *Dermatol Ther* 16:276–282, 2003.

147. Kadin ME, Carpenter C: Systemic and primary cutaneous anaplastic large cell lymphomas. *Semin Hematol* 40:244–256, 2003.

148. Willemze R, Beljaards RC: Spectrum of primary cutaneous CD30 (Ki-1)-positive lymphoproliferative disorders. A proposal for classification and guidelines for management and treatment. *J Am Acad Dermatol* 28:973–980, 1993.

149. Bergman R, Marcus-Farber BS, Manov L, et al: Clinicopathologic reassessment of non-mycosis fungoides primary cutaneous lymphomas during 17 years. *Int J Dermatol* 41:735–743, 2002.

150. Tomaszewski MM, Moad JC, Lupton GP: Primary cutaneous Ki-1(CD30) positive anaplastic large cell lymphoma in childhood. *J Am Acad Dermatol* 40:857–861, 1999.

151. Gorczyca W, Tsang P, Liu Z, et al: CD30-positive T-cell lymphomas co-expressing CD15: An immunohistochemical analysis. *Int J Oncol* 22:319–324, 2003.

152. Jaffe ES: Anaplastic large cell lymphoma: The shifting sands of diagnostic hematopathology. *Mod Pathol* 14:219–228, 2001.

153. DeCoteau JF, Butmarc JR, Kinney MC, et al: The t(2;5) chromosomal translocation is not a common feature of primary cutaneous CD30+ lymphoproliferative disorders: Comparison with anaplastic large-cell lymphoma of nodal origin. *Blood* 87:3437–3441, 1996.

154. El Shabrawi-Caelen L, Kerl H, Cerroni L: Lymphomatoid papulosis: Reappraisal of clinicopathologic presentation and classification into subtypes A, B, and C. *Arch Dermatol* 140:441–447, 2004.

155. Wang HH, Myers T, Lach LJ, et al: Increased risk of lymphoid and nonlymphoid malignancies in patients with lymphomatoid papulosis. *Cancer* 86:1240–1245, 1999.

156. Liu HL, Hoppe RT, Kohler S, et al: CD30+ cutaneous lymphoproliferative disorders: The Stanford experience in lymphomatoid papulosis and primary cutaneous anaplastic large cell lymphoma. *J Am Acad Dermatol* 49:1049–1058, 2003.

CHAPTER 104
MATURE T-CELL AND NATURAL KILLER CELL LYMPHOMAS

Neha Mehta, Alison Moskowitz, and Steven Horwitz

SUMMARY

The mature T-cell and natural killer (NK)-cell lymphomas represent 10 to 15 percent of the non-Hodgkin lymphomas by incidence and comprise 23 clinicopathologic entities in the most recent classification. They include cutaneous T-cell lymphomas, discussed in Chap. 103, and systemic T-cells lymphomas, which are discussed here. The systemic T-cell lymphomas have highly variable courses and are typically aggressive and frequently less responsive to conventional chemotherapy than their B-cell counterparts. The most common systemic T-cell and NK-cell lymphomas worldwide include peripheral T-cell lymphoma, not otherwise specified (PTCL-NOS) and angioimmunoblastic T-cell lymphoma (AITL), representing 26 percent and 19 percent of systemic T-cell and NK-cell lymphomas, respectively. There is considerable geographic variation in the incidence of certain entities, such as adult T-cell leukemia/lymphoma (ATL) and extranodal NK/T-cell lymphoma (ENKTL). In view of the rarity of systemic T-cell and NK-cell disorders, large randomized trials are lacking to guide therapies. Treatment strategies are generally based upon the best data available, which includes prospective phase II studies and retrospective analyses. The most frequently used regimens for the more common entities, PTCL-NOS, AITL, and anaplastic large cell lymphoma (ALCL) are cyclophosphamide, doxorubicin, vincristine, prednisone (CHOP)-based, although long-term outcomes are often unsatisfactory. Therefore, ongoing clinical trials are aimed at improving upon CHOP by adding novel agents or using alternate regimens. Although controversial, patients are often considered for consolidation with autologous stem cell transplant in first remission to improve remission durations. Recently, targeted agents specific for particular T-cell and NK-cell lymphomas, such as brentuximab vedotin for ALCL and crizotinib for anaplastic lymphoma kinase (ALK)-positive ALCL, are now allowing the investigation of more individualized therapy for these entities. Furthermore, for a considerable number of the T-cell and NK-cell lymphoma entities, including ENKTL and ATL, CHOP-based therapy is ineffective, and treatment strategies are disease-specific. There is still much to learn about the biology and potential drug targets for these diseases and ongoing studies using gene expression profiling and genomics may help answer some of these questions. In addition, ongoing clinical trials evaluating disease-specific treatment approaches and employing novel and often targeted agents will hopefully lead to improved outcomes for patients with these diseases.

Acronyms and Abbreviations: AITL, angioimmunoblastic T-cell lymphoma; ALCL, anaplastic large cell lymphoma; ALK, anaplastic lymphoma kinase; ASCT, autologous stem cell transplantation; ATL, adult T-cell leukemia/lymphoma; BCCA, British Columbia Cancer Agency; CHOEP, cyclophosphamide, doxorubicin, vincristine, etoposide, prednisone; CHOP, cyclophosphamide, hydroxydaunorubicin (doxorubicin), vincristine (Oncovin), prednisone; CR, complete response; CT, computed tomography; DHAP, dexamethasone, cytarabine, cisplatinum; DSHNHL, German High-Grade Non-Hodgkin Lymphoma Study Group; EBV, Epstein-Barr virus; EFS, event-free survival; ENKTL, extranodal NK/T-cell lymphoma; FFS, failure-free survival; HTLV, human T-lymphotrophic virus; hyper-CVAD, cyclophosphamide, vincristine, doxorubicin, methotrexate, cytarabine; ICE, ifosfamide, carboplatin, etoposide; IVAC, ifosfamide, etoposide, cytarabine; IPI, International Prognostic Index; IPTCLP, International Peripheral T-Cell Lymphoma Project; LDH, lactate dehydrogenase; MACOP-B, high-dose methotrexate, doxorubicin, cyclophosphamide, vincristine, prednisone, bleomycin; NK, natural killer; ORR, overall response rate; OS, overall survival; PCR, polymerase chain reaction; PET, positron emission tomography; PFS, progression-free survival; PIT, prognostic Index for T-cell lymphoma; PR, partial response; PTCL, peripheral T-cell lymphoma; PTCL-NOS, peripheral T-cell lymphoma, not otherwise specified; SMILE, dexamethasone, methotrexate, ifosfamide, L-asparaginase, and etoposide; TCR, T-cell receptor.

● OVERVIEW OF MATURE T-CELL LYMPHOMAS

The peripheral T-cell lymphomas (PTCLs) represent approximately 10 to 15 percent of non-Hodgkin lymphomas and are made up of 23 heterogeneous diseases (Table 104–1).[1] The most common entities, peripheral T-cell lymphoma, not otherwise specified (PTCL-NOS), angioimmunoblastic T-cell lymphoma (AITL), anaplastic lymphoma kinase (ALK)-positive anaplastic large cell lymphoma (ALCL), and ALK-negative ALCL, account for approximately 60 percent of cases. This overview primarily pertains to these most common subtypes of PTCL and more detailed discussion of other subsets of PTCL follows this discussion.

As a result of the rarity of these disorders, there are no randomized controlled clinical trials to drive treatment decisions in PTCL. Our most comprehensive knowledge of the expected outcomes for patients with PTCL is mainly based upon three large retrospective series: the International Peripheral T-Cell Lymphoma Project (IPTCLP), the British Columbia Cancer Agency (BCCA) series, and a Swedish series which reported outcomes on 1314 cases, 199 cases, and 755 cases, respectively.[2-4] The prospective Comprehensive Oncology Measures for Peripheral T-Cell Lymphoma Treatment (COMPLETE) study is an ongoing registry of patients from the United States that has reported data on 253 subjects to date.[5] These registries underscore the geographical variations in the incidence of these disorders (Table 104–2).

DIAGNOSIS OF PERIPHERAL T-CELL LYMPHOMA

The diagnosis of PTCL is based on histologic features, immunophenotype, molecular studies, and clinical presentation. While B-cell lymphomas are often characterized by a specific immunophenotypic profile, T-cell lymphomas are often characterized by antigen aberrancy that may vary within a subtype or even during the course of the disease.[6,7] In the IPTCLP, a consensus diagnosis (three of four expert pathologists arriving at the same diagnosis) was reached only 74 to 81 percent of the time for ALK-negative ALCL, PTCL-NOS, and AITL. Diagnoses were significantly refined in 154 out of 1314 cases when clinical information was available.[3] In establishing the diagnosis of T-cell non-Hodgkin lymphoma, it is important to exclude a reactive process, particularly when the clinical picture is not congruent with the pathologic features, when the diagnostic biopsy is small, or when a clonal T-cell receptor (TCR) rearrangement is the primary or only reason for the diagnosis because reactive nonmalignant conditions often mimic PTCL.[8-10]

TABLE 104–1. 2008 WHO Classification of Mature T-Cell and Natural Killer–Cell Neoplasms (Excluding Primary Cutaneous Lymphomas)

Peripheral T-cell lymphoma, NOS
Angioimmunoblastic T-cell lymphoma
Anaplastic large cell lymphoma, ALK-positive
Anaplastic large cell lymphoma, ALK-negative
Enteropathy-associated T-cell lymphoma
Adult T-cell leukemia/lymphoma
Hydroa vacciniforme–like lymphoma
T-cell prolymphocytic leukemia
T-cell large granular lymphocytic leukemia
Hepatosplenic T-cell lymphoma
Extranodal NK/T-cell lymphoma, nasal type
Aggressive NK cell leukemia
Systemic EBV+ T-cell lymphoproliferative disease of childhood (associated with chronic active EBV infection)
Chronic lymphoproliferative disorder of NK cells*

ALK, anaplastic lymphoma kinase; EBV, Epstein-Barr virus; NK, natural killer; NOS, not otherwise specified.

*Provisional entities.

INITIAL WORKUP

In addition to routine physical examination, initial evaluation should include systemic imaging (computed tomography [CT] of the chest, abdomen, and pelvis with contrast or positron emission tomography [PET]-CT), marrow aspirate/biopsy, and laboratory evaluation (including complete blood count, lactate dehydrogenase or lactate dehydrogenase [LDH], comprehensive metabolic panel). Serologic testing for human T-cell lymphotrophic virus (HTLV)-1 is particularly important in establishing a new diagnosis of PTCL in a person from an endemic area as adult T-cell leukemia/lymphoma (ATL) represents approximately 9 percent of PTCL, is associated with a different prognosis, and usually requires alternative therapy.[3]

Evaluating Prognosis in Peripheral T-Cell Lymphoma

The International Prognostic Index (IPI) established for evaluating aggressive lymphomas has been effective in risk stratifying patients with PTCL, although the utility in AITL is less clear (Table 104–3).[11] The "prognostic index for T-cell lymphoma (PIT)," is an improved index developed specifically for PTCL that includes age, performance status, LDH level, and marrow involvement.[7,12] Other prognostic indices, such as the IPTCLP score, have been suggested for PTCL. Each has some value, although none provides a significant improvement over IPI in terms of impacting clinical management.[13] It is important to note that even patients identified as low risk by these indices often experience disappointing outcomes. For example, in the IPTCLP, the 5-year failure-free survival (FFS) for patients with 0 or 1 IPI risk factors were only 33 percent for PTCL-NOS and 34 percent for AITL. For this reason, the approach to management of PTCL patients usually does not differ significantly based on IPI alone. Nevertheless, in patients with ALK-positive ALCL, which tends to be more responsive to chemotherapy, the progression-free survivals for patients with zero/one, two, three, and four/five IPI risk factors are 80 percent, 60 percent, 40 percent and 25 percent, respectively.[14] Consequently, patients with higher risk ALK-positive ALCL may be treated similarly to those with the less-favorable PTCL histologies.

APPROACH TO INITIAL THERAPY

CHOP (cyclophosphamide, doxorubicin, vincristine, prednisone) chemotherapy remains the most commonly employed backbone for upfront therapy of PTCL, based on extrapolation from studies done in aggressive B-cell lymphomas. In the IPTCLP, more than 85 percent of patients received CHOP-based therapy, and in contrast to ALK-positive ALCL where the 5-year FFS was 60 percent, the 5-year FFS for PTCL-NOS, AITL, and ALK-negative ALCL, were only 20 percent, 18 percent, and 36 percent, respectively (see Table 104–3). Similar outcomes were observed in the BCCA series with 5-year progression-free survival (PFS) of 29 percent, 13 percent, and 28 percent for PTCL-NOS, AITL, and ALCL, respectively.[2] In the Swedish Registry study where 84 percent of patients were treated with CHOP-like therapy, 5-year PFSs were 21 percent, 20 percent, and 31 percent for PTCL-NOS, AITL, and ALK-negative ALCL, respectively, compared to 63 percent for ALK-positive ALCL.[4]

Several prospective clinical trials in PTCL are available to inform us on the expected response rate to CHOP. In a phase II study evaluating CHOP induction therapy followed by autologous stem cell

TABLE 104–2. Incidence of Lymphoma Subtypes By Geographic Region

Subtype	Registry	PTCL-NOS	AITL	ALCL, ALK+	ALCL, ALK–	NK/T	ATL	EATL
North America	IPTCL	34%	16%	16%	8%	5%	2%	6%
	BCCA	59%	5%	6%	9%	9%	NA*	5%
	COMPLETE	34%	15%	11%	8%	6%	2%	3%
Europe	IPTCL	34%	29%	6%	9%	4%	1%	9%
	Swedish	34%	14%	9%	15%	4%	NA*	9%
Asia	IPTCL	22%	18%	3%	3%	22%	25%	2%

AITL, angioimmunoblastic T-cell lymphoma; ALCL ALK–, anaplastic large cell lymphoma anaplastic lymphoma kinase negative; ALCL ALK+, anaplastic large cell lymphoma anaplastic lymphoma kinase positive; ATLL, adult T-cell leukemia/lymphoma; BCCA, British Columbia Cancer Agency; COMPLETE, Comprehensive Oncology Measures for Peripheral T-Cell Lymphoma Treatment; EATL, enteropathy-associated T-cell lymphoma; IPI, International Prognostic Index; IPTCL, International Peripheral T-Cell Lymphoma Project; NA, not available; NK/T, natural killer–cell/T-cell lymphoma; NOS, not otherwise specified; PTCL, peripheral T-cell lymphoma. *ATLL patients were excluded in both the BCCA and Swedish Registry Studies.

TABLE 104–3. Characteristics and Outcomes in Common Peripheral T-Cell Lymphoma Subtypes

PTCL Subtype	Number	Median Age	% IPI			5 Year OS*	5-Year PFS*	5-Year OS by IPI	
			0–1	2–3	4–5			0–1	4–5
PTCL-NOS									
IPTCL	229	60	28	57	15	32%	20%	50%	11%
BCCA	117	64	30	47	22	35%	29%	64%	22%
Swedish	256	69	17[†]	59[†]	24[†]	28%	21%	NA	NA
AITL									
IPTCL	213	65	14	59	28	32%	18%	56%	25%
BCCA	10	66	0	30	70	36%	13%	NA	NA
Swedish	104	70	4[†]	69[†]	27[†]	31%	20%	NA	NR
ALCL ALK−									
IPTCL	72	58	41	44	15	49%	36%	74%	13%
BCCA	18	55	44	22	33	34%	28%[‡‡]	66%[‡]	25%[‡]
Swedish	115	67	34	42	24	38%	31%	NA	NA
ALCL ALK+									
IPTCL	76	34	49	37	14	70%	60%	90%	33%
BCCA	12	32	67	25	8	58%	28%[‡]	66%[‡]	25%[‡]
Swedish	68	41	55[†]	39[†]	6[†]	79%	63%	NA	NA
EATL									
IPTCL	62	61	25	63	13	20%	4%	29%	15%
BCCA	9	61	0	30	70	22%	22%	NA	NA
Swedish	68	68	42	44	14	20%	18%	NA	NA
NK/T									
IPTCL	35	44	26	57	17	9%	6%	17%	20%
Extranasal	92	52	51	47	2	42%	29%	57%	0%
Nasal	17	47	47	24	29	24%	15%	38%	20%
BCCA	33	62	33	63	4	21%	14%	NA	NA
Swedish									

AITL, angioimmunoblastic T-cell lymphoma; ALCL ALK−, anaplastic large cell lymphoma anaplastic lymphoma kinase negative; ALCL ALK+, anaplastic large cell lymphoma anaplastic lymphoma kinase positive; BCCA, British Columbia Cancer Agency; EATL, enteropathy associated T-cell lymphoma; IPI, International Prognostic Index; IPTCL, International Peripheral T-Cell Lymphoma Project; NA, not available; NK/T, natural killer cell/T-cell lymphoma; NOS, not otherwise specified; OS, overall survival; PFS, progression-free survival; PTCL, peripheral T-cell lymphoma.

*Data from International T-cell lymphoma project in which >85% of patients received an anthracycline-based regimen without upfront transplant.

†Distribution of patients with the given IPI scores is based on the number of patients for whom the score could be completely calculated.

‡BCCA ALCL reported as both ALK + and −.

transplantation (ASCT) for untreated PTCL, the overall response rate (ORR) to CHOP was 79 percent with a complete response (CR) rate of 39 percent.[15] Similarly, a small phase III study of CHOP versus VIP-rABVD (etoposide, ifosfamide, cisplatin alternating with Adriamycin, bleomycin, vinblastine and dacarbazine) showed no significant difference in outcomes with an ORR of 70 percent and a CR rate of 35 percent.[16]

Although the majority of patients receive CHOP, there is currently no standard frontline treatment approach for PTCL, as there are no randomized data guiding a preferred approach. Many have sought to augment the efficacy of CHOP by adding agents to the CHOP backbone. Several phase II studies adding the anti-CD52 antibody, alemtuzumab, to CHOP demonstrated impressive CR rates of 65 to 71 percent. However, the addition of alemtuzumab conferred significant toxicity including Jacob-Creutzfeldt virus encephalitis, invasive aspergillosis, *Pneumocystis carinii* pneumonia, sepsis, Epstein-Barr virus (EBV)-related lymphoma and cytomegalovirus reactivation.[17–19]

Similarly, in a phase II study of denileukin diftitox plus CHOP, the ORR and CR rates were 65 percent and 55 percent, respectively; however three deaths occurred following one cycle of therapy and four other patients were taken off study because of toxicity.[20]

The German High-Grade non-Hodgkin Lymphoma Study Group (DSHNHL) evaluated the addition of etoposide to the CHOP regimen. They analyzed patients with PTCL treated on seven different prospective phase II or phase III protocols with either CHOP or CHOEP (cyclophosphamide, doxorubicin, vincristine, etoposide, prednisone).[21] Younger patients (<60 years old) with a normal LDH exhibited better outcomes if treated with CHOEP than with CHOP, with 3-year event-free survival (EFS) of 75.4 and 51 percent, respectively, although no difference in overall survival (OS) was observed. The benefits were greatest in the more favorable ALK-positive ALCL subtype but there was a trend toward improved EFS in favor of CHOEP in other subsets as well (p = 0.057). However, the addition of etoposide led to excessive toxicity in elderly patients. The Nordic group adopted CHOEP induction for subjects younger than age 60 years in a prospective study evaluating upfront stem cell transplantation for PTCL.[22] In this phase II study, patients received biweekly CHOEP followed by ASCT for the responders. The ORR to CHOEP was 82 percent with a CR rate of 51 percent. Although one must be cautious when comparing results from different study populations, these results appear superior to those reported by Reimer and colleagues for patients treated with CHOP followed by ASCT, who achieved CR in only 39 percent of cases.[15]

There are no randomized trials assessing the controversial approach of performing ASCT in first remission for PTCL, although several prospective studies suggest the benefit of this strategy. The aforementioned Nordic study enrolled 160 patients with PTCL, including 39 percent with PTCL-NOS, 19 percent with ALK-negative ALCL, and 19 percent with AITL, while excluding ALK-positive ALCL.[22] Patients were treated with CHOEP for six cycles (etoposide was omitted for patients >60 years of age) and those in CR or partial response (PR) proceeded to high-dose therapy with carmustine, etoposide, cytarabine, and melphalan (or cyclophosphamide) and ASCT. By intent-to-treat analysis, 71 percent of patients underwent ASCT and the 5-year OS and PFS were 51 percent and 44 percent. Reimer and colleagues conducted the second largest prospective study evaluating ASCT in first remission following CHOP, enrolling 83 patients.[15] A 3-year OS rate of 48 percent was observed by intent-to-treat analysis. For those who were transplanted (66 percent of patients enrolled) outcomes were considerably more favorable with a 3-year OS of 71 percent. In a retrospective analysis performed at Memorial Sloan Kettering Cancer Center to evaluate patients treated with the intent to transplant in first remission, interim PET imaging was found to be the most powerful predictor of outcome. Of the 53 percent of patients who had a negative interim PET scan after four cycles, 59 percent were progression free after 5 years, including 53 percent of those with IPI of 3 or greater.[23]

APPROACH TO RELAPSED OR REFRACTORY THERAPY

There are no randomized data or standard of care to guide treatment of patients with relapsed or refractory PTCL.[24] In the largest series of patients with PTCL-NOS, AITL, and ALCL treated from 1976 to 2010, those with relapsed or refractory disease who did not proceed to hematopoietic stem cell transplant demonstrated a median OS of 5.5 months.[26] However, the outlook for this patient population may improve as several new agents have been approved for this setting, including romidepsin, belinostat, and pralatrexate.[28,29] In addition, brentuximab vedotin is listed in the National Comprehensive Cancer Network (NCCN) compendium of appropriate therapeutic agents for CD30-positive T-cell lymphomas (Table 104–4).[30-33]

For patients who are transplantation-eligible, allogeneic transplantation should be considered in the relapsed/refractory setting. Once a donor is identified, intensive salvage chemotherapy options should be considered, including ICE (ifosfamide, carboplatin, etoposide) or DHAP (dexamethasone, cytarabine, cisplatinum), as they have a high potential to induce major remissions that will optimize outcomes after transplantation.[30] However, these regimens are generally only tolerated for three to four cycles and should be followed promptly by consolidation with transplantation. Both myeloablative and reduced intensity allogeneic stem cell transplantation have demonstrated up to 60 percent 3-year PFS.[37-39] The role of ASCT in relapsed/refractory PTCL is controversial. Several series suggest that ASCT rarely results in long-term disease control of PTCL, with the exception of patients with ALCL.[34,35] Other series, however, including registry data from the Center for International Blood and Marrow Transplant Research, report more salutary results for ASCT after relapse.[36]

For patients who are not transplantation-eligible, the goals of treatment are palliative, and therapy should be geared toward maintaining quantity and quality of life. Options for treatment include romidepsin, belinostat, pralatrexate, gemcitabine, bendamustine, and alemtuzumab.[26-29,40-42] In addition, brentuximab vedotin should be considered as the first choice for relapsed CD30-expressing ALCL patients, who have not previously received this agent.[21-33]

In view of the heterogeneity of PTCL, there is an increasing interest in individualizing therapy based on histology and other factors. For example, brentuximab vedotin, a CD30 antibody–drug conjugate, induced responses in patient with relapsed or refractory ALCL as well as those with CD30-positive AITL and PTCL-NOS.[32,33] Similarly, crizotinib, an ALK inhibitor, demonstrated significant activity in a small number of patients with relapsed ALK-positive ALCL and is being further investigated.[43-45] The histone deacetylase (HDAC) inhibitors, such as belinostat and romidepsin, appear to have preferential activity and duration of response in patients with AITL (see Table 104–4).[27,29]

Gene-expression profiling has identified molecular classifiers that improve classification and prognostication in ALK-negative ALCL, AITL, and PTCL-NOS.[46-49] Furthermore, additional translocations and recurrent mutations have been identified that may help better classify PTCLs and identify potential treatment targets. Next-generation sequencing has identified a novel translocation within ALK-negative ALCL, t(6;7),[50] which potentially identifies a unique entity within ALK-negative ALCL associated with a better prognosis.[51] This mutation typically leads to reduced expression of the *DUSP22* gene, which likely functions as a tumor suppressor. A translocation producing an *ITK-SYK* fusion gene, t(5;9), was initially found in a subset of PTCL-NOS cases.[52] SYK expression was subsequently evaluated in 141 PTCL cases by immunohistochemistry and found to be overexpressed in

TABLE 104–4. Overall Response Rate to Agents FDA Approved for Relapsed/Refractory Peripheral T-Cell Lymphoma

Subtype	Pralatrexate*	Romidepsin†	Belinostat‡	Brentuximab Vedotin§¶
PTCL-NOS	31%	29%	23%	33%
AITL	8%	30%	46%	50%
ALCL	29%	24%	15%	86%

AITL, angioimmunoblastic T-cell lymphoma; ALCL, anaplastic large cell lymphoma; PTCL, peripheral T-cell lymphoma; PTCL-NOS, peripheral T-cell lymphoma, not otherwise specified.

*Data extrapolated from OA O'Connor, B Pro, L Pinter-Brown, et al.[26]
†Data extrapolated from B Coiffier, B Pro, HM Prince, et al.[27]
‡Data extrapolated from S Horwitz, W Jurczak, A Van Hoof, et al.[29] and OA O'Connor, T Masszi, KJ Savage, et al.[28]
§Data extrapolated from B Pro, R Advani, P Brice, et al.[32] and SM Horwitz, RH Advani, NL Bartlett, et al.[32]
¶Brentuximab vedotin is National Comprehensive Cancer Network (NCCN) Compendium listed for relapsed/refractory CD30+ PTCL.

94 percent, although the translocation was only detected in 39 percent.[53] These findings suggest a potential role for SYK inhibitors in these cases.[54] Mutations involving the *TET2* gene appear to be common in AITL as well as PTCL-NOS expressing T-follicular helper (T_{FH}) cell markers; they are less frequent among the other PTCL-NOS cases (24 percent) and absent in ALCL.[55] *TET2* is involved in epigenetic control of transcription through DNA methylation and inactivating mutations of this gene were first identified in myeloid malignancies. These mutations signify a biologic connection between AITL and PTCL-NOS with AITL features (T_{FH}-like PTCL-NOS) and suggest a role for hypomethylating agents.

● PERIPHERAL T-CELL LYMPHOMA, NOT OTHERWISE SPECIFIED

DEFINITION

PTCLs that do not fit into any of the currently recognized histopathologic categories are designated PTCL, not otherwise specified (PTCL-NOS; Chap. 96.)

EPIDEMIOLOGY

PTCL-NOS is the most common of the mature T-cell neoplasms, representing approximately 25 to 30 percent of the total cases of T-cell lymphoma in Western countries.[56–58] In the United States, there are approximately 0.4 cases per 100,000 adults.[62] In Asia, PTCL-NOS accounts for 20 to 25 percent of cases mature T-cell neoplasms (see Table 104–2).[3,57] The median age of diagnosis is 60 years with a male predominance (2:1).[3,7]

CLINICAL FINDINGS

In general, patients with PTCL-NOS have aggressive, rapidly growing disease. Diffuse lymphadenopathy, constitutional symptoms, extranodal involvement, an elevated LDH level, and advanced stage disease are common.[56,57] Hepatomegaly and splenomegaly occur in 17 percent and 24 percent of patients, respectively. Stages I, II, III, and IV disease are observed in approximately 14 percent, 17 percent, 26 percent, and 43 percent of cases, respectively. The marrow is involved in approximately 20 percent of cases.[2,4] Pruritus, peripheral eosinophilia, hypercalcemia, and hemophagocytic syndrome may accompany PTCL.[60,61]

LABORATORY FINDINGS

Histopathology

The majority of cases arise in lymph nodes, which exhibit mixtures of small and large atypical lymphoid cells, typically admixed with an inflammatory background (Chap. 96).[62] The immunophenotype is typically that of a mature T-cell expressing either a CD4 or CD8 phenotype, most commonly CD4, although CD4/CD8 double-positive and double-negative cases have been reported.[6,63] Malignant cells are often characterized by antigen aberrancy that may vary from one patient to another or even vary during the course of the disease within a single patient.[6,7] Deletion of one or more pan–T-cell antigens is frequently observed,[64] along with rearrangements of the TCR.

TREATMENT AND PROGNOSIS

As discussed previously, patients with PTCL-NOS are most commonly treated with CHOP-based regimens, although there is no uniform standard of care for first-line treatment. Little prospective data exists for CHOP alone in PTCL, but based on clinical trials employing CHOP as a component of therapy, it appears that CHOP produces an ORR as high as 79 percent and a CR rate as high as 39 percent.[15] However, with CHOP alone long-term remissions are uncommon, with PFS rates of

20 to 30 percent seen in the larger retrospective series.[2–4] Efforts to improve the efficacy of first-line therapy by adding new agents to CHOP, such as alemtuzumab, bortezomib, or denileukin diftitox, have not clearly resulted in significant benefit.[20,12,19] The addition of etoposide to CHOP appears to provide some benefit over CHOP in more favorable young patients, according to a retrospective analysis of seven prospective studies conducted by the DSHNHL.[21] Moreover, in a prospective study of CHOEP followed by ASCT, the ORR to CHOEP was 82 percent, with 51 percent achieving a CR.[22] Newer agents approved in the relapsed setting, such as romidepsin and brentuximab vedotin, are currently being combined with CHOP-based regimens and compared to standard CHOP in ongoing phase III clinical trials.

Another strategy for improving frontline therapy for PTCL-NOS has been through consolidation with ASCT in first remission, as discussed in "Approach to Initial Therapy" above. Even though there are no randomized trials of ASCT in first remission, three prospective phase II trials support this approach.[15,22,23] The largest of these studies demonstrated 5-year OS and PFS of 47 percent and 38 percent, respectively in patients with PTCL-NOS.[22]

Allogeneic transplantation provides long-term disease control for a select group of patients with relapsed PTCL-NOS. Although transplant-related mortality is significant, retrospective studies have demonstrated up to 61 percent OS at 2 years in some trials. Consequently, allogeneic transplantation is often considered for fit patients who fail frontline therapy.[23,39,66]

Several promising new agents, including belinostat, bendamustine, gemcitabine, and alemtuzumab, have become available for the treatment of PTCL-NOS in the relapsed setting.[28,40–42] Pralatrexate, romidepsin, and belinostat are approved broadly for PTCL, with an approximately 20 to 30 percent ORR in large phase II studies (see Table 104–4).[27,71,72]

Overall, the 5-year FFS for PTCL-NOS is 20 percent with a 5-year OS of 32 percent in patients treated with CHOP-based therapy.[60] The IPI and PIT have been used to risk stratify patients with PTCL-NOS and estimate prognosis. For patients with PIT scores of 0, 1, 2, or 3 or greater, the 5-year FFSs are 34 percent, 22 percent, 13 percent, and 8 percent, respectively. For patients with IPI scores of 1 or less, 2, 3, or 4 or greater, 5-year FFSs are 36 percent, 18 percent, 15 percent, and 9 percent, respectively.[7] PIT scores have not been used to direct treatment decisions, however (see Table 104–3).[13,12]

● ANGIOIMMUNOBLASTIC T-CELL LYMPHOMA

DEFINITION

AITL was initially described as angioimmunoblastic lymphadenopathy with dysproteinemia in 1974. It is now known that these entities are identical.[1,68]

EPIDEMIOLOGY

AITL represents approximately 1 percent of all cases of lymphoma and approximately 20 percent of all T-cell lymphomas.[57] International series show that AITL represents a higher portion of T-cell lymphomas in Europe than North America or Asia.[3] The male-to-female ratio is approximately 1:1 and the median age at diagnosis is approximately 65 to 70 years.[3,4,7]

CLINICAL FINDINGS

Common features at presentation include B symptoms (fever, drenching sweats, and weight loss), generalized lymphadenopathy, rash, polyclonal hypergammaglobulinemia, blood eosinophilia, and autoimmune hemolytic anemia (direct Coombs positive). Some patients experience waxing and waning of symptoms over several years before a diagnosis is made. Patients with AITL can develop diffuse large B-cell lymphoma, which evolves from EBV-positive B cells, which usually are present in the lymphoid infiltrate. Emergence of diffuse large B-cell lymphoma can occur concomitantly with AITL at the time of diagnosis or may be the primary histology at relapse; therefore, repeat biopsies are strongly encouraged whenever relapse is suspected in order to guide therapy.[69,70]

LABORATORY FINDINGS

Histopathology

AITL is characterized histologically by effacement of the normal lymphoid architecture with a pleomorphic cellular infiltrate and proliferation of small arborizing blood vessels. Small lymphocytes, plasma cells, immunoblasts, histiocytes, and eosinophils infiltrate involved lymph nodes. As a result, the normal lymphoid architecture may be obliterated, with loss of germinal centers and extensive intranodal neovascularization and expansion of the follicular dendritic cell meshwork (CD21). Scattered EBV+ B cells are almost always present and reflect the accompanying immunodeficient state. The malignant cells are CD4+ $\alpha\beta$ T cells with TCR-β and -γ rearrangements[70-72] and express CD10, a marker typical for AITL, approximately 90 percent of the time.[73] Abnormal karyotypes involving the X chromosome and chromosomes 1, 3, and 5 are frequently found in AITL. A complex karyotype is a negative prognostic factor for AITL.[77] The normal counterpart of AITL is suspected to be the follicular T-helper cell based on genomic profiling, which reveals overexpression of specific markers, including CXCL13 and PD1.[74,75] A subset of PTCL-NOS exhibits a similar gene-expression profile, suggesting it may behave similarly.[76]

TREATMENT AND PROGNOSIS

Most patients with AITL are treated with CHOP-based regimens as discussed in the section Approach to Initial Therapy. The CR rate is similar to the rate observed with PTCL-NOS (approximately 50 to 60 percent). Nonrandomized data support upfront ASCT in patients who achieve a CR to first-line therapy.[22] Rare patients may be managed with glucocorticoid monotherapy, which can induce remissions, although responses are rarely sustained.[78] Responses to low-dose methotrexate and cyclosporine have also been reported.[79-81] Finally, response rates as high as 50 percent have been reported in CD30-positive relapsed/refractory AITL treated with brentuximab vedotin.[32]

Both the IPI and the PIT have been used to risk stratify patients but have not been used to direct therapy (see Table 104–3).[13,12,82] One group has reported that immunoglobulin A levels, age older than 60 years, more than one extranodal site of involvement, anemia, and thrombocytopenia may also be of prognostic value in this disease.[82]

● ANAPLASTIC LARGE CELL LYMPHOMA

DEFINITION

ALCL is defined as a CD30+ peripheral T-cell neoplasm. The disease has been provisionally subdivided into those that are ALK-positive (60 to 70 percent) or negative (30 to 40 percent).[1,83,84] In addition to the systemic form, there are primary cutaneous forms (Chap. 103), which generally behave in an indolent fashion, as well as a recently identified entity called breast implant–associated ALCL.[85,86]

EPIDEMIOLOGY

ALCL accounts for 6 to 24 percent of all T-cell lymphomas.[2-4] However, the prevalence of ALCL varies by geographic region (see Table 104–2).

ALK-positive ALCL accounts for 16 percent, 6 percent, and 3 percent of PTCL in North America, Europe, and Asia, respectively.[3] The median age of ALK-positive ALCL is 30 to 40 years old. Ninety percent of children with ALCL are ALK-positive.[83,87] In the United States and Asia, the ALK-positive phenotype is more common (ratio being 2:1 and 3:2, respectively), whereas in Europe the ALK-negative phenotype is more common (3:2).[3] Both diseases exhibit a slight male predominance. ALK-negative ALCL accounts for 8 percent, 9 percent, and 3 percent of PTCL in North America, Europe, and Asia, respectively.[3] The median age of presentation is 55 to 60 for ALK-negative ALCL.[3,14,67]

CLINICAL FEATURES

ALCL has an aggressive clinical course, frequently presenting with systemic symptoms, advanced disease, and extranodal localization. Patients with ALK-positive ALCL tend to be younger and have better performance statuses and lower serum LDH levels. Approximately 8 to 12 percent of patients with ALK-positive ALCL have morphologic evidence of marrow involvement.[2-4] The rate of detection of marrow involvement doubles when immunohistochemical staining techniques with anti-CD30 and anti-ALK antibodies are used.[88]

Patients with ALK-negative ALCL tend to be older, with higher LDH values, and worse performance status than ALK-positive cases. Extranodal presentations are more common in the ALK-negative population,[14] and include sites such as the marrow, liver, lung, and skin, but rarely the central nervous system. Marrow involvement occurs in 12 to 22 percent of cases of ALK-negative ALCL.[2-4]

A new clinical variant of ALK-negative ALCL associated with textured saline and silicone breast implants has been reported. Although the natural history and treatment course of this variant needs further elucidation, the clinical course seems to be less aggressive and patients with localized disease may be adequately treated merely by surgical removal of the implant and capsule.[85,89-91] In the largest series to date (60 patients), most presented with disease limited to the breast (83 percent), whereas 10 percent and 7 percent, respectively, presented with stage II and stage IV disease. Patients most commonly presented with an effusion within the breast and less frequently with a distinct breast mass.[85]

LABORATORY FEATURES

ALCL cells tend to grow cohesively and are found preferentially invading lymph node sinuses.[92] There are three morphologic variants based on the size of the neoplastic and admixed reactive cells[93]: the "common type," representing most cases, is characterized by large pleomorphic tumor cells; the "small cell variant," representing 5 to 10 percent of cases, has a dominant population of small- to medium-size tumor cells mixed with large anaplastic cells that stain for CD30 and ALK; and the "lymphohistiocytic variant," representing 5 to 10 percent of cases, that is closely related to the small cell variant and contains small neoplastic cells mixed with large anaplastic cells and a large number of histiocytes (Chap. 96).[94]

ALK-positive ALCL is characterized by a nonrandom t(2;5) (p23;q35) translocation resulting in fusion of the *NPM* and *ALK* genes.[95] The resultant *NPM-ALK* fusion gene encodes an 80-kDa chimeric protein NPM-ALK (p80) that functions as an oncogene in ALK-positive ALCL. Of note, other translocations resulting in ALK expression in ALK-positive ALCL have also been identified but are rarer.[50,96-102] Thus, ALK immunoreactivity is a highly specific marker for this disease.[83,84,96] Either T or null immunophenotypes may be observed in ALCL. The T-cell variant expresses pan-T antigens CD2, CD2, CD4, CD5, and CD7, whereas the null variant lacks both T-cell and B-cell antigens, but usually expresses cytotoxic molecules such as granzyme B and perforin, and has rearranged TCR genes, suggesting a T-cell origin.[102,103]

Genomic and proteomic cluster analyses strongly suggest that ALK-positive and ALK-negative ALCL are two distinct disease entities. CEBPB, PTPN12, SERPINA1, and BCL6 genes are typically overexpressed in ALK-positive ALCL, and CCR7, CNTFR, interleukin (IL)-21, and IL-22 are overexpressed in ALK-negative ALCL.[104] Based on comparative genomic hybridization and fluorescence *in situ* hybridization for TP53 and ATM loci, gains of 17p and 17q24, and losses of 4q13–q21 and 11q14 are more common in ALK-positive tumors, whereas gains of 1q and 6p21 are preferentially observed in ALK-negative tumors.[112] These differences are underscored by the different responses of these two entities to therapy.[87] Interestingly, cases of ALK-negative ALCL that express DUSP22 appear to have a similar prognosis to ALK-positive ALCL, while those with TP63 expression are associated with especially poor prognosis.[51]

TREATMENT AND PROGNOSIS

ALK-positive ALCL is the most chemosensitive of the T-cell lymphomas, with rates of survival and response similar to diffuse large B-cell lymphomas. ALCL is commonly seen in the pediatric age group, where intensive anthracycline-based chemotherapy regimens have been studied.[106,107] Approximately 90 percent of patients with ALK-positive ALCL treated with anthracycline-based chemotherapy achieve a tumor response, with 65 to 75 percent of pediatric patients remaining relapse-free after 5 years.[76,108] Among adults, treatment with CHOP-based therapy has remained the most commonly used approach as more intensive regimens, such as high-dose methotrexate, doxorubicin, cyclophosphamide, vincristine, prednisone, bleomycin (MACOP-B) and doxorubicin, cyclophosphamide, vindesine, bleomycin, and prednisone have not shown superiority to CHOP-based therapy.[67,109]

The IPI appears to be particularly helpful in risk-stratification of ALK-positive ALCL, with some authorities suggesting that patients with high risk ALK-positive ALCL should be treated similarly to those with other forms of PTCL (see Table 104–3).[2,3,110] The DSHNHL concluded in a retrospectively assessment of seven phase II and phase III trials that patients with ALK-positive ALCL who were 60 years of age or younger and had a normal LDH, had an improved EFS but not OS if treated with CHOP plus etoposide, rather than CHOP alone.[21] The Groupe d'Étude des Lymphomes de l'Adulte (GELA) group has suggested that the prognostic significance of ALK expression is limited to those older than age 40 years.[67] After relapse, it appears that patients can be cured with intensive salvage therapy (including ASCT) at a higher rate compared to other T-cell lymphomas.

Brentuximab vedotin, which combines an anti-CD30 antibody with monomethylauristatin E (MMAE) has demonstrated objective responses in more than 80 percent of patients with relapsed/refractory ALCL treated on a single-agent phase II trial.[32] The FDA approved brentuximab vedotin for the treatment of relapsed ALCL in 2011.[111] Brentuximab vedotin in combination with chemotherapy is being explored as a first-line therapy in ALCL. Crizotinib, an inhibitor of ALK tyrosine kinase that is FDA-approved for the treatment of ALK-positive non–small cell lung cancer, has demonstrated encouraging responses in small series of ALK-positive ALCL, leading to ongoing trials in relapsed/refractory ALCL.[44,45,112]

ALK-negative ALCL typically presents with unfavorable features, including stages III and IV disease, B-symptoms, high IPI scores, high LDH serum levels, and expression of TP63.[51,114,115] The disease typically pursues an aggressive clinical course and is less responsive to chemotherapy than ALK-positive ALCL. It has been common practice to treat patients with CHOP-like therapy, as with other forms of PTCL, as discussed in the previous section Approach to Initial Therapy. Similar to PTCL-NOS, consolidation with ASCT in first remission is often considered for ALK-negative ALCL based upon large prospective studies

suggesting improved remission durations.[22,15] The IPTCLP reported 5-year FFS and OS rates of 36 percent and 49 percent, respectively, for patients with ALK-negative ALCL (see Table 104–3).[3] CD56 expression has been shown to be an independent favorable prognostic factor for ALK-negative ALCL, as has expression of DUSP22.[51,113]

● ENTEROPATHY-ASSOCIATED T-CELL LYMPHOMA

DEFINITION

Enteropathy-associated intestinal T-cell lymphoma (EATL) is a mature T-cell lymphoma that presents within the gastrointestinal tract. The World Health Organization divided EATL into two variants—type I and type II—which are differentiated based on their histopathology.[116]

EPIDEMIOLOGY

EATL constitutes approximately 2 to 10 percent of all PTCL and incidence varies by geographic distribution.[2–4] The median patient age at diagnosis is 55 to 65 years with a slight male predisposition.[116,117] Type I EATL comprises 60 to 80 percent of cases,[116] is most common in patients who have underlying celiac disease, and is strongly associated with the human leukocyte antigen (HLA)-DQ2 haplotype. Among European patients with EATL, 80 percent have type I EATL.[116,118] Patients who have refractory celiac disease, which does not improve with a gluten-free diet, have a significantly higher risk of EATL. In particular, those with refractory celiac disease who demonstrate a clonal expansion of abnormal intraepithelial lymphocytes lacking CD3, CD8, and TCR markers, but expressing intracellular CD3, have a significantly higher risk of developing EATL.[117] In contrast, type II EATL, present in 20 to 40 percent of cases, is less frequently associated with celiac sprue and the HLA-DQ2 haplotype.[116,119]

CLINICAL FINDINGS

The majority of patients with EATL present with acute abdominal symptoms that often require urgent or emergent surgical procedures, resulting in diagnosis of the disease.[120] EATL typically presents with ulcerative lesions of the jejunum or ileum which may perforate, though other regions of the gastrointestinal tract may also be affected. As a result of the malabsorption that accompanies the disease, frequent presenting signs and symptoms include weight loss, diarrhea, nausea, and vomiting, accompanied by abdominal pain and bowel obstruction.[121] The course can be fulminant; death may occur during treatment secondary to the consequences of intestinal perforation. Extraintestinal presentation of EATL is rare, and there is little data on the manifestations of cutaneous, neuromeningeal, or pulmonary presentations. Systemic symptoms should be considered signs of clinical progression, although they occur in less than 30 percent of patients with EATL.[124,129]

LABORATORY FINDINGS

Histopathology

The two types of EATL are recognized on the basis of the specific immunophenotype: EATL type 1 is characterized by CD56 negativity and EATL type 2 exhibits CD56 expression.[119] The histology of EATL type I demonstrates mostly medium to large tumor cells with round or angulated vesicular nuclei, prominent nucleoli, and pale-staining cytoplasm. There is often a moderate to abundant infiltrate of eosinophils, histiocytes, and small lymphocytes.[123] EATL type 1 characteristically demonstrates the following immunophenotype: positive for CD3, CD7, CD103, and usually CD30, but negative for CD4, CD5, CD8, and CD56. The cells also exhibit a cytotoxic phenotype and are positive for perforin, granzyme B, and TIA-1.[124,125] EATL type 2 is characterized by a monomorphic infiltrate of small- to medium-size lymphocytes positive for CD3, CD8, CD56, and TCR-β, and negative for CD4. CD30 is often negative in EATL type 2.[119]

TREATMENT AND PROGNOSIS

CHOP chemotherapy has been used most widely for both type I and type II EATL, with a 5-year relapse FFS of 4 to 22 percent and a 5-year OS of approximately 20 percent.[2-4,116] The addition of etoposide to CHOP does not appear to confer additional benefit.[133] Even patients who initially respond to CHOP therapy usually relapse after a median interval of 6 months, with a median survival after relapse of approximately 6 months to 1 year.[116,121,126,12] In patients who are transplantation-eligible, high-dose chemotherapy followed by ASCT may improve outcomes.[15,127,128] The Scotland and Newcastle Group demonstrated that high-intensity therapy with CHOP alternating with IVE (ifosfamide, epirubicin, etoposide) and intermediate-dose methotrexate, followed by consolidation with ASCT resulted in a 5-year OS of 60 percent and PFS of 52 percent in the 50 percent of patients who were able to complete ASCT.[120] Many patients could not complete the course of chemotherapy, however, and there were a large number of complications, including gastrointestinal bleeding, small bowel perforation, and enterocolic fistulae. Twelve patients required either enteral or parental feeding.

Adverse prognostic factors include a history of celiac sprue, a large tumor mass (≥5 cm) at diagnosis, an elevated LDH, and a nonambulatory performance status.[116] The PIT score predicts both OS and FFS in EATL better than the IPI.[116]

● ADULT T-CELL LEUKEMIA/LYMPHOMA

DEFINITION

ATL is an uncommon lymphoproliferative neoplasm of mature CD4+CD25+ T-cells caused by infection with the retrovirus, HTLV-1, that was initially characterized in 1977.[130,131] These cells classically have a leukemic "flower-cell" appearance.[132] At least 5 percent of circulating abnormal T lymphocytes are required to diagnose ATL in patients without histologically proven tumor lesions.[133]

EPIDEMIOLOGY

The incidence of ATL in the United States is approximately 0.05 cases per 100,000 people.[134] The disease prevalence parallels the geographic distribution of the HTLV-1 virus, with the highest incidences occurring in southern Japan, the Caribbean, Central and South America, intertropical Africa, Romania, and northern Iran (see Table 104–2).[135-139] Among approximately 10 to 20 million HTLV-1 carriers, the lifetime risk of developing ATL is approximately 2.5 to 4 percent, with a mean latency of greater than 50 years.[134,137,139,140] HTLV-1 is transmitted through breastfeeding, blood products, and unprotected sexual intercourse. The overwhelming majority of ATL cases occur in patients infected during the early years of life,[141] In addition, the prolonged infection may increase chances of accruing subsequent mutations, and ultimately malignant transformation. The mean age of patients with adult T-cell leukemia/lymphoma is 62 years, without a gender predominance.[142,143]

CLINICAL FEATURES

Several clinical variants of ATL have been described: acute, lymphoma, chronic, and smoldering; these appear to have differing genomic alterations and different clinical courses.[133,143,144]

The acute variant of ATL represents 60 percent of cases and is characterized by patients who present with a leukemic presentation. An additional 20 percent of cases present with the lymphoma variant characterized by lymphadenopathy and less than 1 percent of leukemic cells in the blood. These subtypes exhibit an aggressive clinical course with a median survival of less than 1 year. The majority of patients present with hepatosplenomegaly (50 percent of cases), lymphadenopathy, elevated LDH, hypercalcemia (50 percent of cases), and visceral and cutaneous lesions. The marrow is involved in approximately 35 percent of cases.[143] Most patients have generalized lymphadenopathy, particularly in the retroperitoneal and hilar regions, though the nodes are often relatively small and mediastinal masses are rare. Extranodal sites of disease include the lung, liver, skin, gastrointestinal tract, and central nervous system, including cord myelopathy and spastic paraparesis.

In contrast to the acute and lymphoma forms, the smoldering form of adult T-cell leukemia/lymphoma typically presents with a predominance of skin lesions or lung infiltration without visceral or marrow disease, and minimal blood involvement (<5 percent of lymphocytes). Patients with chronic ATL present with leukocytosis with lymphadenopathy and organomegaly without an elevated LDH, or visceral involvement. Although smoldering and chronic ATL are characterized initially by indolent courses, the prognosis remains poor with a survival of 4.1 years and 49 percent progressing to acute ATL after a median of 18.8 months.[145]

Opportunistic infections are common in patients with adult T-cell leukemia/lymphoma, even indolent forms,[146] including *P. carinii*, strongyloides, and cryptococcal meningitis, as well as bacterial and other fungal infections.

LABORATORY FEATURES

Histopathology

The neoplastic cells are pleomorphic, have highly lobulated nuclei ("clover leaf" or "flower cell" appearances) with condensed nuclear chromatin, inconspicuous nucleoli, and a mature helper T-lymphocyte immunophenotype.[132] At least 5 percent of circulating abnormal T-lymphocytes are required to diagnose ATL in patients without histologically proven tumor lesions.[133] In approximately 20 percent of cases, nuclear lobulation is less pronounced, and the cells may be difficult to distinguish from Sézary cells. These cells express the surface T-cell lymphocytic markers CD2, CD4 and CD5, CD45RO, CD29, and TCR-αβ, and are usually negative for CD7, CD8, and CD26, and show reduced CD3 expression. The lymphocytic activation markers HLA-DP, -DQ, and -DR, and IL-2Rα (CD25) are always present, whereas terminal deoxynucleotidyl transferase is typically absent.[147] Rare immunophenotypic variants (CD4-negative, CD8-positive, double-positive or double-negative variants) have also been reported.[148-150] Although there are no specific chromosomal abnormalities diagnostic of ATL, the karyotype of ATL cells is usually complex in the aggressive variants of the disorder.[131] Clonal rearrangements of the TCR genes are typically present.[151-153]

Laboratory Analysis

Patients with aggressive forms of ATL commonly present with an elevated LDH and hypercalcemia.

TREATMENT AND PROGNOSIS

Overall, prognosis in ATL remains poor with a median survival of less than 1 year for patients with aggressive subtypes. A multivariate analysis of 126 patients with acute (13 percent) and lymphoma (87 percent) subtypes of ATL performed by the IPTCLP indicated that the IPI was the only independent predictor of OS.[142] Although smoldering and chronic ATL are characterized initially by indolent courses, the prognosis remains guarded with 5-year survivals of 40 percent and 50 percent, respectively; 49 percent of patients with the more indolent forms of ATL progress to acute ATL after a median time of 18.8 months.[145]

Despite its limited efficacy, cytotoxic chemotherapy remains the mainstay of therapy for this disease. A Japanese cooperative group developed a multidrug regimen called LSG15, which consists of seven cycles of VCAP (vincristine, cyclophosphamide, doxorubicin, and prednisone), AMP (doxorubicin, ranimustine, and prednisone), and VECP (vindesine, etoposide, carboplatin, and prednisone). LSG15 was evaluated in a phase II study that enrolled 96 patients with treatment-naïve acute type (n = 58), lymphoma type (n = 28) or unfavorable chronic type (n = 10) ATL. The ORR was 81 percent, with 35 percent CRs and 45 percent PRs.[154] In view of these results, a phase III trial of LSG15 versus biweekly CHOP was performed in a similar patient population and demonstrated a superior CR rate (40 percent vs. 25 percent) and 3-year OS (24 percent vs. 13 percent), favoring the intensive arm; however the median survival was only 13 months in the LSG15 arm.[155] These results highlight the inadequacy of CHOP in this disease, but the results seen with LSG15 leave significant room for improvement as well.

The role of antiviral therapy remains controversial. A recent meta-analysis of 254 patients with ATL demonstrated that there appears to be a benefit to first-line antiviral therapy, including interferon for patients with acute, chronic, and smoldering ATL, whereas patients with the lymphoma variant did not benefit. In patients with chronic and smoldering ATL treated with first-line antiviral therapy in combination with either chemotherapy or interferon, a 100 percent 5-year survival has been reported. In patients with leukemic ATL who were treated upfront with combined antiviral therapy and chemotherapy a 5-year OS of 28 percent was observed, compared to 10 percent in patients treated with first-line chemotherapy alone. Maintenance antiviral therapy also was reported to confer an improved OS in patients treated with first-line chemotherapy. These findings have not yet been prospectively validated, however.[156]

Additionally, mogamulizumab (anti-CCR4 monoclonal antibody) has been approved in Japan for the treatment of relapsed or refractory adult T-cell leukemia-lymphoma. In a multicenter phase II study of 28 patients with relapsed/refractory ATL, the ORR with mogamulizumab was 50 percent, with a median OS of 13.7 months.[157] A randomized phase II study of modified LSG15 with or without mogamulizumab confirmed that the combination was well tolerated and had a CR rate of 52 percent compared to 33 percent with LGS15 alone.[158]

A large nationwide Japanese retrospective report of 386 patients with ATL assessed the role of allogeneic hematopoietic stem cell transplantation in ATL and demonstrated a 3-year OS for entire cohort of 33 percent. Among patients who underwent related donor transplantation, donor HTLV-1 seropositivity adversely affected disease-associated mortality.[159] In patients who are transplantation-eligible, allogeneic transplantation is therefore an attractive option, but ASCT has been found to be ineffective in ATL.[160,161]

● HEPATOSPLENIC T-CELL LYMPHOMA

DEFINITION

Hepatosplenic T-cell lymphoma (HSTCL) is a rare lymphoma that infiltrates the spleen, liver, and marrow. In the majority of cases, cells consist of mature γ/δ T-cells, however, α/β HSTCL has also been reported.[1]

EPIDEMIOLOGY

HSTCL is a rare lymphoma representing 3 percent of all T-cell lymphomas.[162] This disease typically occurs in young males at a median age of 35 years.[7,163] Immunosuppression following solid-organ transplantation

or from use of anti–tumor necrosis factor-α or thiopurine agents (as are used for Crohn disease and other autoimmune diseases) has been implicated as a risk factor for this disease.[164,165]

CLINICAL FINDINGS

Patients commonly present with isolated hepatosplenomegaly without lymphadenopathy, frequently accompanied by cytopenias, B symptoms, and an elevated serum LDH.[57,163]

LABORATORY FINDINGS

Histopathology

Neoplastic cells localize to sinusoids in the spleen, liver, and marrow. The malignant lymphocytes typically express CD3, CD56, and TCR-δ, but are negative for CD4 and usually CD8.[166] Clonal rearrangement of the TCR-γ gene usually present, and in most cases the lymphoma cells have an isochromosome 7q [I⁷(q10)] along with trisomy 8, which also may be seen in the αβ variant of this disease.[167–169]

TREATMENT AND PROGNOSIS

HSTCL is characterized by an aggressive course, with a median survival of 16 months.[170] The optimal therapy for HSTCL is not known. Small patient series and anecdotal reports describe limited responsiveness and poor survival with CHOP and suggest better outcomes with other non–cross-resistant regimens such as ICE, hyper-CVAD (cyclophosphamide, vincristine, doxorubicin, methotrexate, cytarabine), or IVAC (ifosfamide, etoposide, cytarabine).[162,163,170–172] Successful treatment with pentostatin has been reported as well.[180] Consolidation with either allogeneic stem cell transplantation or ASCT is likely necessary to achieve long-term remission.[171]

● EXTRANODAL NATURAL KILLER/T-CELL LYMPHOMA

DEFINITION

Extranodal natural killer (NK)/T-cell lymphoma (ENKTL), nasal type previously known as lethal midline granuloma, malignant granuloma, or angiocentric lymphoma, is an uncommon subtype of T-cell lymphoma.

EPIDEMIOLOGY

ENKTL represents approximately 2 to 9 percent of T-cell lymphomas.[2–4,174–175] The disease typically afflicts middle-aged men, with a median age of 50 years at diagnosis, but may also affect children.[134,135] ENKTL occurs worldwide, with a strong geographic predilection for Asian populations from China, Japan, Korea, and Southeast Asia[177] and for Central and South American populations from Mexico,[178] Peru,[179] Argentina, and Brazil,[180] constituting 5 percent to 15 percent of lymphomas in these countries. Occasional case series have also been reported from Europe and North America (see Table 104–2).[181]

CLINICAL FEATURES

ENKTLs are almost exclusively extranodal.[177] Initial sites involved are often the nose and nasopharynx and occasionally the paranasal sinuses, tonsil, Waldeyer ring, and oropharynx. When nasal lymphomas destroy the floor of the nasal cavity, a characteristic hard-palate perforation is found.[182] Although they are usually localized, ENKTLs may disseminate to the skin, salivary glands, testis, and gastrointestinal tract. Interestingly, the lymphoma occasionally presents primarily in these sites without an apparent nasal primary. These "nonnasal" ENKTLs were thought to be more aggressive.[183] Modern imaging technology, such as PET/CT, shows that most, if not all, nonnasal lymphomas are associated with occult nasal primaries, and imply that they are disseminated nasal lymphomas.[184,185] With improved treatment strategies, primary sites of presentation are no longer an independent prognostic indicator.[186] Rarely, the lymphoma can evolve into NK-cell leukemia, which is characterized by widespread systemic dissemination and involvement of the marrow and blood.

LABORATORY FINDINGS

Histopathology

The histopathology shows angiocentric plesiomorphic small- or medium-size atypical lymphoid cells with vascular invasion and ischemic tissue necrosis. Marrow hemophagocytosis may be present. As NK and T cells share a common ontogeny, the malignant cells express CD2 and CD7 but are negative for surface CD3. They also express CD16, CD56, cytoplasmic CD3ε, and CD57, and often demonstrate clonal rearrangements in the TCR genes.[1,175,182] Neoplastic cells are invariably infected by EBV which is detected most reliably by in situ hybridization for EBV-encoded RNA (EBER), a diagnostic requisite.[177] Rare cases may not express CD56.[1]

Laboratory Assessments

EBV DNA polymerase chain reaction (PCR) measured in plasma has been found to correlate with tumor burden and serial EBV PCR monitoring is useful for assessing responses and disease recurrence.[187,188]

TREATMENT AND PROGNOSIS

Outcomes of localized NK/T-cell lymphoma are best with combined chemotherapy and radiation therapy. In studies of radiation therapy alone, 75 to 100 percent of patients respond; however, systemic relapse rates are as high as 25 to 40 percent.[189,190] Previously, patients were treated with CHOP-based therapy in combination with radiation with a CR rate of 59 percent and 3-year disease-free survival of 25 percent.[191–193] L-Asparaginase has a major single-agent activity in NK/T-cell lymphomas, and is incorporated into most modern regimens for this disease.[194] L-Asparaginase combined with gemcitabine, oxaliplatin, and radiation therapy exhibits an ORR of 96 percent and a local and systemic relapse rate of 10 to 15 percent in a phase I study.[195] Vincristine and prednisolone in combination with L-asparaginase produce an ORR of 89 percent when combined with radiation therapy. SMILE (dexamethasone, methotrexate, ifosfamide, L-asparaginase, and etoposide) in combination with radiation therapy demonstrates an 82 percent response rate with a CR rate of 78 percent.[186] L-Asparaginase has also been studied in combination with methotrexate and dexamethasone with an ORR of 78 percent.[197] In patients with localized ENKTL, it is standard to consolidate asparaginase-based chemotherapy with radiation therapy. In the setting of patients with advanced stage or relapsed/refractory disease, combination chemotherapy remains the standard treatment.[182] Studies of SMILE demonstrate an ORR of 25 to 80 percent in disseminated disease.[186,196] NK-cell leukemia is characterized by widespread systemic dissemination and involvement of the marrow and blood and is associated with an extremely poor survival measured only in weeks.

EBV DNA PCR measured in the plasma has been found to correlate with tumor burden and serial EBV PCR monitoring is useful for assessing responses and disease recurrence.[187,188] In view of the improved efficacy of L-asparaginase–based regimens, the role of ASCT remains unclear.

Even though the IPI has been found to be effective in risk stratification of ENKTL, Lee and colleagues have developed an NK/T-cell lymphoma-specific prognostic index that also predicts prognosis (see Table 104–3).[2,3,186] This model includes B-symptoms, elevated LDH, stage, and presence of regional lymph nodes. Those with no risk factors, one risk factor, two risk factors, and three or more risk factors had a 5-year OS of 81 percent, 64 percent, 34 percent, and 4 percent, respectively.[198]

SUBCUTANEOUS PANNICULITIS-LIKE T-CELL LYMPHOMA

Definition

Subcutaneous panniculitis-like T-cell lymphoma (SPTL) is a primary cutaneous T-cell lymphoma presenting with painful subcutaneous nodules.[199-202] The lesions consist of atypical lymphoid cells, and reactive histiocytes with admixed adipose tissue often associated with coagulation necrosis. Histologically, the cells express an α/β phenotype. The γ/δ phenotype of this disease is now classified as cutaneous γ/δ T-cell lymphoma.[1,202]

Epidemiology

As discussed in a worldwide retrospective analysis, SPTL is a rare disorder accounting for 0.9 percent all T-cell lymphomas.[7,203] SPTL is primarily a disorder of adults with an average age at diagnosis in the mid to late 30s, although cases have also been reported in children.[204] SPTL has a female predominance with a male to female ratio of 0.5.[204]

Clinical Features

Patients present with subcutaneous nodules that typically begin in the extremities and may spontaneously regress for a number of years, but eventually progress.[205] They may ulcerate, and patients may have systemic symptoms.

Laboratory Features

The lesions consist of atypical lymphoid cells, and reactive histiocytes with admixed adipose tissue often associated with coagulation necrosis. In most cases, the tumor is composed of mature CD8+ $\alpha\beta$ cytotoxic T cells that express TIA-1, granzymes, and perforin genes.[202,204,205]

Treatment and Prognosis

Responses to combination chemotherapy have been reported but are usually of short duration.[204–207] Responses to glucocorticoids, interferon-α, zidovudine, and cyclosporine also have been reported.[206,208,209] Therapy for this disease remains controversial. Although standard chemotherapy may be effective, CRs are rare. Single patient cases of successful allogeneic stem cell transplantation have been reported, but the rarity of this disease hampers further investigation of this modality.[210,211] The use of denileukin diftitox in two patients has been reported with evidence of activity, and bexarotene restored a clinical response in one of the patients after disease progression.[212] Single-agent bexarotene has also been shown to have significant clinical activity with an ORR of 82 percent.[213]

REFERENCES

1. Swerdlow SH, Harris NL, Jaffe ES, Pileri SA, Stein H, Thiele J, Vardiman JW, eds: WHO Classification of Tumours of Haematopoietic and Lymphoid Tissues, 4th ed. International Agency for Research on Cancer (IARC), Lyon, France, 2008.
2. Savage KJ, Chhanabhai M, Gascoyne RD, et al: Characterization of peripheral T-cell lymphomas in a single North American institution by the WHO classification. Ann Oncol 15:1467–1475, 2004.

3. Vose J, Armitage J, Weisenburger D, et al: International peripheral T-cell and natural killer/T-cell lymphoma study: Pathology findings and clinical outcomes. *J Clin Oncol* 26:4124–4130, 2008.

4. Ellin F, Landstrom J, Jerkeman M, et al: Real world data on prognostic factors and treatment in peripheral T-cell lymphomas: A study from the Swedish Lymphoma Registry. *Blood* 124:1570–1577, 2014.

5. Foss FM, Carson KR, Pinter-Brown L, et al: Comprehensive Oncology Measures for Peripheral T-Cell Lymphoma Treatment (COMPLETE): First detailed report of primary treatment. *Blood* 120, 2012.

6. Went P, Agostinelli C, Gallamini A, et al: Marker expression in peripheral T-cell lymphoma: A proposed clinical-pathologic prognostic score. *J Clin Oncol* 24:2472–2479, 2006.

7. Weisenburger DD, Savage KJ, Harris NL, et al: Peripheral T-cell lymphoma, not otherwise specified: A report of 340 cases from the International Peripheral T-cell Lymphoma Project. *Blood* 117:3402–3408, 2011.

8. Mansoor A, Pittaluga S, Beck PL, et al: NK-cell enteropathy: A benign NK-cell lymphoproliferative disease mimicking intestinal lymphoma: Clinicopathologic features and follow-up in a unique case series. *Blood* 117:1447–1452, 2011.

9. Weiss LM, Wood GS, Trela M, et al: Clonal T-cell populations in lymphomatoid papulosis. Evidence of a lymphoproliferative origin for a clinically benign disease. *N Engl J Med* 315:475–479, 1986.

10. Perry AM, Warnke RA, Hu Q, et al: Indolent T-cell lymphoproliferative disease of the gastrointestinal tract. *Blood* 122:3599–3606, 2013.

11. Federico M, Rudiger T, Bellei M, et al: Clinicopathologic characteristics of angioimmunoblastic T-cell lymphoma: Analysis of the international peripheral T-cell lymphoma project. *J Clin Oncol* 31:240–246, 2013.

12. Gallamini A, Stelitano C, Calvi R, et al: Peripheral T-cell lymphoma unspecified (PTCL-U): A new prognostic model from a retrospective multicentric clinical study. *Blood* 103:2474–2479, 2004.

13. Gutierrez-Garcia G, Garcia-Herrera A, Cardesa T, et al: Comparison of four prognostic scores in peripheral T-cell lymphoma. *Ann Oncol* 22:397–404, 2011.

14. Savage KJ, Harris NL, Vose JM, et al: ALK– anaplastic large-cell lymphoma is clinically and immunophenotypically different from both ALK+ ALCL and peripheral T-cell lymphoma, not otherwise specified: Report from the International Peripheral T-Cell Lymphoma Project. *Blood* 111:5496–5504, 2008.

15. Reimer P, Rudiger T, Geissinger E, et al: Autologous stem-cell transplantation as first-line therapy in peripheral T-cell lymphomas: Results of a prospective multicenter study. *J Clin Oncol* 27:106–113, 2009.

16. Simon A, Peoch M, Casassus P, et al: Upfront VIP-reinforced-ABVD (VIP-rABVD) is not superior to CHOP/21 in newly diagnosed peripheral T cell lymphoma. Results of the randomized phase III trial GOELAMS-LTP95. *Br J Haematol* 151:159–166, 2010.

17. Kluin-Nelemans HC, van Marwijk Kooy M, Lugtenburg PJ, et al: Intensified alemtuzumab-CHOP therapy for peripheral T-cell lymphoma. *Ann Oncol* 22:1595–1600, 2011.

18. Kim JG, Sohn SK, Chae YS, et al: Alemtuzumab plus CHOP as front-line chemotherapy for patients with peripheral T-cell lymphomas: A phase II study. *Cancer Chemother Pharmacol* 60:129–134, 2007.

19. Gallamini A, Zaja F, Patti C, et al: Alemtuzumab (Campath-1H) and CHOP chemotherapy as first-line treatment of peripheral T-cell lymphoma: Results of a GITIL (Gruppo Italiano Terapie Innovative nei Linfomi) prospective multicenter trial. *Blood* 110:2316–2323, 2007.

20. Foss FM, Sjak-Shie N, Goy A, et al: A multicenter phase II trial to determine the safety and efficacy of combination therapy with denileukin diftitox and cyclophosphamide, doxorubicin, vincristine and prednisone in untreated peripheral T-cell lymphoma: The CONCEPT study. *Leuk Lymphoma* 54:1373–1379, 2013.

21. Schmitz N, Trumper L, Ziepert M, et al: Treatment and prognosis of mature T-cell and NK-cell lymphoma: An analysis of patients with T-cell lymphoma treated in studies of the German High-Grade Non-Hodgkin Lymphoma Study Group. *Blood* 116:3418–3425, 2010.

22. d'Amore F, Relander T, Lauritzsen GF, et al: Up-front autologous stem-cell transplantation in peripheral T-cell lymphoma: NLG-T-01. *J Clin Oncol* 30:3093–3099, 2012.

23. Mehta N, Maragulia JC, Moskowitz A, et al: A retrospective analysis of peripheral T-cell lymphoma treated with the intention to transplant in the first remission. *Clin Lymphoma Myeloma Leuk* 13:664–670, 2013.

24. Lunning MA, Moskowitz AJ, Horwitz S: Strategies for relapsed peripheral T-cell lymphoma: The tail that wags the curve. *J Clin Oncol* 31:1922–1927, 2013.

25. Mak V, Hamm J, Chhanabhai M, et al: Survival of patients with peripheral T-cell lymphoma after first relapse or progression: Spectrum of disease and rare long-term survivors. *J Clin Oncol* 31:1970–1976, 2013.

26. O'Connor OA, Pro B, Pinter-Brown L, et al: Pralatrexate in patients with relapsed or refractory peripheral T-cell lymphoma: Results from the pivotal PROPEL study. *J Clin Oncol* 29:1182–1189, 2011.

27. Coiffier B, Pro B, Prince HM, et al: Results from a pivotal, open-label, phase II study of romidepsin in relapsed or refractory peripheral T-cell lymphoma after prior systemic therapy. *J Clin Oncol* 30:631–636, 2012.

28. O'Connor OA, Masszi T, Savage KJ, et al: Belinostat, a novel pan-histone deacetylase inhibitor (HDACi), in relapsed or refractory peripheral T-cell lymphoma (R/R PTCL): Results from the BELIEF trial [abstract]. *J Clin Oncol* 31:8507, 2013.

29. Horwitz S, Jurczak W, Van Hoof A, et al: Belinostat in relapsed or refractory peripheral T-cell lymphoma subtype angioimmunoblastic T-cell lymphoma: Results from the pivotal BELIEF trial. *Hematol Oncol* 31(Suppl 1):147, 2013.

30. Zelenetz A GL, Wierda WG, et al. NCCN Clinical Practice Guidelines in Oncology: Non-Hodgkin's Lymphomas. http://www.nccn.org/professionals/physician_gls/pdf/nhl.pdf: National Comprehensive Cancer Network; 2014:451.

31. Horwitz SM, Advani RH, Bartlett NL, et al: Objective responses in relapsed T-cell lymphomas with single-agent brentuximab vedotin. *Blood* 123:3095–3100, 2014.

32. Pro B, Advani R, Brice P, et al: Brentuximab vedotin (SGN-35) in patients with relapsed or refractory systemic anaplastic large-cell lymphoma: Results of a phase II study. *J Clin Oncol* 30:2190–2196, 2012.

33. Oki SH, Bartlett NL, Jacobsen E, et al: Safety and efficacy of brentuximab vedotin for treatment of relapsed or refractory mature T/NK-cell lymphomas. *Hematol Oncol* 31(Suppl 1):147, 2013.

34. Smith SD, Bolwell BJ, Rybicki LA, et al: Autologous hematopoietic stem cell transplantation in peripheral T-cell lymphoma using a uniform high-dose regimen. *Bone Marrow Transplant* 40:239–243, 2007.

35. Horwitz SM, Kewalramani T, Hamlin P, et al: Second-line therapy with ICE followed by high dose therapy and autologous stem cell transplantation for relapsed/refractory peripheral T-cell lymphoma: Minimal benefit when analyzed by intent to treat. *Blood (ASH Annual Meeting Abstracts)* 2005; 106: Abstract 2679.

36. Smith SM, Burns LJ, van Besien K, et al: Hematopoietic cell transplantation for systemic mature T-cell non-Hodgkin lymphoma. *J Clin Oncol* 31:3100–3109, 2013.

37. Le Gouill S, Milpied N, Buzyn A, et al: Graft-versus-lymphoma effect for aggressive T-cell lymphomas in adults: A study from the Societe Francaise de Greffe de Moelle et de Therapie Cellulaire. *J Clin Oncol* 26:2264–2271, 2008.

38. Jacobsen ED, Kim HT, Ho VT, et al: A large single-center experience with allogeneic stem-cell transplantation for peripheral T-cell non-Hodgkin lymphoma and advanced mycosis fungoides/Sézary syndrome. *Ann Oncol* 22:1608–1613, 2011.

39. Goldberg JD, Chou JF, Horwitz S, et al: Long-term survival in patients with peripheral T-cell non-Hodgkin lymphoma after allogeneic hematopoietic stem cell transplant. *Leuk Lymphoma* 53:1124–1129, 2012.

40. Zinzani PL, Venturini F, Stefoni V, et al: Gemcitabine as single agent in pretreated T-cell lymphoma patients: Evaluation of the long-term outcome. *Ann Oncol* 21:860–863, 2010.

41. Damaj G, Gressin R, Bouabdallah K, et al: Results from a prospective, open-label, phase II trial of bendamustine in refractory or relapsed T-cell lymphomas: The BENTLY trial. *J Clin Oncol* 31:104–110, 2013.

42. Enblad G, Hagberg H, Erlanson M, et al: A pilot study of alemtuzumab (anti-CD52 monoclonal antibody) therapy for patients with relapsed or chemotherapy-refractory peripheral T-cell lymphomas. *Blood* 103:2920–2924, 2004.

43. Farina F, Stasia A, Ceccon M, et al: High response rates to crizotinib in advanced, chemoresistant ALK+ lymphoma patients. *Blood* 122:368, 2013.

44. Gambacorti Passerini C, Farina F, Stasia A, et al: Crizotinib in advanced, chemoresistant anaplastic lymphoma kinase-positive lymphoma patients. *J Natl Cancer Inst* 106:djt378, 2014.

45. Mosse YP, Lim MS, Voss SD, et al: Safety and activity of crizotinib for paediatric patients with refractory solid tumours or anaplastic large-cell lymphoma: A Children's Oncology Group phase 1 consortium study. *Lancet Oncol* 14:472–480, 2013.

46. Odejide O, Weigert O, Lane AA, et al: A targeted mutational landscape of angioimmunoblastic T-cell lymphoma. *Blood* 123:1293–1296, 2014.

47. Iqbal J, Weisenburger DD, Greiner TC, et al: Molecular signatures to improve diagnosis in peripheral T-cell lymphoma and prognostication in angioimmunoblastic T-cell lymphoma. *Blood* 115:1026–1036, 2010.

48. Piccaluga PP, Fuligni F, De Leo A, et al: Molecular profiling improves classification and prognostication of nodal peripheral T-cell lymphomas: Results of a phase III diagnostic accuracy study. *J Clin Oncol* 31:3019–3025, 2013.

49. Criscione VD, Weinstock MA: Incidence of cutaneous T-cell lymphoma in the United States, 1973–2002. *Arch Dermatol* 143:854–859, 2007.

50. Feldman AL, Dogan A, Smith DI, et al: Discovery of recurrent t(6;7)(p25.3;q32.3) translocations in ALK-negative anaplastic large cell lymphomas by massively parallel genomic sequencing. *Blood* 117:915–919, 2011.

51. Parrilla Castellar ER, Jaffe ES, Said JW, et al: ALK-negative anaplastic large cell lymphoma is a genetically heterogeneous disease with widely disparate clinical outcomes. *Blood* 124:1473–1480, 2014.

52. Streubel B, Vinatzer U, Willheim M, et al: Novel t(5;9)(q33;q22) fuses ITK to SYK in unspecified peripheral T-cell lymphoma. *Leukemia* 20:313–318, 2006.

53. Feldman AL, Sun DX, Law ME, et al: Overexpression of Syk tyrosine kinase in peripheral T-cell lymphomas. *Leukemia* 22:1139–1143, 2008.

54. Attygalle AD, Feldman AL, Dogan A: ITK/SYK translocation in angioimmunoblastic T-cell lymphoma. *Am J Surg Pathol* 37:1456–1457, 2013.

55. Lemonnier F, Couronne L, Parrens M, et al: Recurrent TET2 mutations in peripheral T-cell lymphomas correlate with TFH-like features and adverse clinical parameters. *Blood* 120:1466–1469, 2012.

56. Rudiger T, Weisenburger DD, Anderson JR, et al: Peripheral T-cell lymphoma (excluding anaplastic large-cell lymphoma): Results from the Non-Hodgkin's Lymphoma Classification Project. *Ann Oncol* 13:140–149, 2002.

57. Vose JM: Peripheral T-cell non-Hodgkin's lymphoma. *Hematol Oncol Clin North Am* 22:997–1005, x, 2008.

58. Armitage JO, Weisenburger DD: New approach to classifying non-Hodgkin's lymphomas: Clinical features of the major histologic subtypes. Non-Hodgkin's Lymphoma Classification Project. *J Clin Oncol* 16:2780–2795, 1998.

59. Abouyabis AN, Shenoy PJ, Lechowicz MJ, et al: Incidence and outcomes of the peripheral T-cell lymphoma subtypes in the United States. *Leuk Lymphoma* 49:2099–2107, 2008.

60. Greer JP, York JC, Cousar JB, et al: Peripheral T-cell lymphoma: A clinicopathologic study of 42 cases. *J Clin Oncol* 2:788–798, 1984.

61. Alomari A, Hui P, Xu M: Composite peripheral T-cell lymphoma not otherwise specified, and B-cell small lymphocytic lymphoma presenting with hemophagocytic lymphohistiocytosis. *Int J Surg Pathol* 21:303–308, 2013.

62. Kim H, Jacobs C, Warnke RA, et al: Malignant lymphoma with a high content of epithelioid histiocytes: A distinct clinicopathologic entity and a form of so-called "Lennert's lymphoma." *Cancer* 41:620–635, 1978.

63. Gaulard P, Bourquelot P, Kanavaros P, et al: Expression of the alpha/beta and gamma/delta T-cell receptors in 57 cases of peripheral T-cell lymphomas. Identification of a subset of gamma/delta T-cell lymphomas. *Am J Pathol* 137:617–628, 1990.

64. Knowles DM: Immunophenotypic and antigen receptor gene rearrangement analysis in T cell neoplasia. *Am J Pathol* 134:761–785, 1989.

65. Kim SJ, Yoon DH, Kang HJ, et al: Bortezomib in combination with CHOP as first-line treatment for patients with stage III/IV peripheral T-cell lymphomas: A multicentre, single-arm, phase 2 trial. *Eur J Cancer* 48:3223–3231, 2012.

66. Kahl C, Leithauser M, Wolff D, et al: Treatment of peripheral T-cell lymphomas (PTCL) with high-dose chemotherapy and autologous or allogeneic hematopoietic transplantation. *Ann Hematol* 81:646–650, 2002.

67. Sibon D, Fournier M, Briere J, et al: Long-term outcome of adults with systemic anaplastic large-cell lymphoma treated within the Groupe d'Etude des Lymphomes de l'Adulte trials. *J Clin Oncol* 30:3939–3946, 2012.

68. Frizzera G, Moran EM, Rappaport H: Angio-immunoblastic lymphadenopathy with dysproteinaemia. *Lancet* 1:1070–1073, 1974.

69. Smith JL, Hodges E, Quin CT, et al: Frequent T and B cell oligoclones in histologically and immunophenotypically characterized angioimmunoblastic lymphadenopathy. *Am J Pathol* 156:661–669, 2000.

70. Willenbrock K, Roers A, Seidl C, et al: Analysis of T-cell subpopulations in T-cell non-Hodgkin's lymphoma of angioimmunoblastic lymphadenopathy with dysproteinemia type by single target gene amplification of T cell receptor-beta gene rearrangements. *Am J Pathol* 158:1851–1857, 2001.

71. Weiss LM, Strickler JG, Dorfman RF, et al: Clonal T-cell populations in angioimmunoblastic lymphadenopathy and angioimmunoblastic lymphadenopathy-like lymphoma. *Am J Pathol* 122:392–397, 1986.

72. Feller AC, Griesser H, Schilling CV, et al: Clonal gene rearrangement patterns correlate with immunophenotype and clinical parameters in patients with angioimmunoblastic lymphadenopathy. *Am J Pathol* 133:549–556, 1988.

73. Attygalle A, Al-Jehani R, Diss TC, et al: Neoplastic T cells in angioimmunoblastic T-cell lymphoma express CD10. *Blood* 99:627–633, 2002.

74. Yu H, Shahsafaei A, Dorfman DM: Germinal-center T-helper-cell markers PD-1 and CXCL13 are both expressed by neoplastic cells in angioimmunoblastic T-cell lymphoma. *Am J Clin Pathol* 131:33–41, 2009.

75. Dorfman DM, Brown JA, Shahsafaei A, et al: Programmed death-1 (PD-1) is a marker of germinal center-associated T cells and angioimmunoblastic T-cell lymphoma. *Am J Surg Pathol* 30:802–810, 2006.

76. de Leval L, Rickman DS, Thielen C, et al: The gene expression profile of nodal peripheral T-cell lymphoma demonstrates a molecular link between angioimmunoblastic T-cell lymphoma (AITL) and follicular helper T (TFH) cells. *Blood* 109:4952–4963, 2007.

77. Schlegelberger B, Zwingers T, Hohenadel K, et al: Significance of cytogenetic findings for the clinical outcome in patients with T-cell lymphoma of angioimmunoblastic lymphadenopathy type. *J Clin Oncol* 14:593–599, 1996.

78. Siegert W, Agthe A, Griesser H, et al: Treatment of angioimmunoblastic lymphadenopathy (AILD)-type T-cell lymphoma using prednisone with or without the COPBLAM/IMVP-16 regimen. A multicenter study. Kiel Lymphoma Study Group. *Ann Intern Med* 117:364–370, 1992.

79. Takemori N, Kodaira J, Toyoshima N, et al: Successful treatment of immunoblastic lymphadenopathy-like T-cell lymphoma with cyclosporin A. *Leuk Lymphoma* 35:389–395, 1999.

80. Gerlando Q, Barbera V, Ammatuna E, et al: Successful treatment of angioimmunoblastic lymphadenopathy with dysproteinemia-type T-cell lymphoma by combined methotrexate and prednisone. *Haematologica* 85:880–881, 2000.

81. Quintini G, Iannitto E, Barbera V, et al: Response to low-dose oral methotrexate and prednisone in two patients with angio-immunoblastic lymphadenopathy-type T-cell lymphoma. *Hematol J* 2:393–395, 2001.

82. Tokunaga T, Shimada K, Yamamoto K, et al: Retrospective analysis of prognostic factors for angioimmunoblastic T-cell lymphoma: A multicenter cooperative study in Japan. *Blood* 119:2837–2843, 2012.

83. Falini B, Bigerna B, Fizzotti M, et al: ALK expression defines a distinct group of T/null lymphomas ("ALK lymphomas") with a wide morphological spectrum. *Am J Pathol* 153:875–886, 1998.

84. Pulford K, Lamant L, Morris SW, et al: Detection of anaplastic lymphoma kinase (ALK) and nucleolar protein nucleophosmin (NPM)-ALK proteins in normal and neoplastic cells with the monoclonal antibody ALK1. *Blood* 89:1394–1404, 1997.

85. Miranda RN, Aladily TN, Prince HM, et al: Breast implant-associated anaplastic large-cell lymphoma: Long-term follow-up of 60 patients. *J Clin Oncol* 32:114–120, 2014.

86. Xu J, Wei S: Breast implant-associated anaplastic large cell lymphoma: Review of a distinct clinicopathologic entity. *Arch Pathol Lab Med* 138:842–846, 2014.

87. Gascoyne RD, Aoun P, Wu D, et al: Prognostic significance of anaplastic lymphoma kinase (ALK) protein expression in adults with anaplastic large cell lymphoma. *Blood* 93:3913–3921, 1999.

88. Fraga M, Brousset P, Schlaifer D, et al: Bone marrow involvement in anaplastic large cell lymphoma. Immunohistochemical detection of minimal disease and its prognostic significance. *Am J Clin Pathol* 103:82–89, 1995.

89. Lazzeri D, Agostini T, Bocci G, et al: ALK-1-negative anaplastic large cell lymphoma associated with breast implants: A new clinical entity. *Clin Breast Cancer* 11:283–296, 2011.

90. Lechner MG, Megiel C, Church CH, et al: Survival signals and targets for therapy in breast implant-associated ALK—Anaplastic large cell lymphoma. *Clin Cancer Res* 18:4549–4559, 2012.

91. Said SM, Reynolds C, Jimenez RE, et al: Amyloidosis of the breast: Predominantly AL type and over half have concurrent breast hematologic disorders. *Mod Pathol* 26:232–238, 2013.

92. Morris SW, Kirstein MN, Valentine MB, et al: Fusion of a kinase gene, ALK, to a nucleolar protein gene, NPM, in non-Hodgkin's lymphoma. *Science* 263:1281–1284, 1994.

93. Kadin ME: Anaplastic large cell lymphoma and its morphological variants. *Cancer Surv* 30:77–86, 1997.

94. Falini B: Anaplastic large cell lymphoma: Pathological, molecular and clinical features. *Br J Haematol* 114:741–760, 2001.

95. Rimokh R, Magaud JP, Berger F, et al: A translocation involving a specific breakpoint (q35) on chromosome 5 is characteristic of anaplastic large cell lymphoma ("Ki-1 lymphoma"). *Br J Haematol* 71:31–36, 1989.

96. Shin S, Kim J, Yoon SO, et al: ALK-positive anaplastic large cell lymphoma with TPM3-ALK translocation. *Leuk Res* 36:e143–e145, 2012.

97. Ma Z, Cools J, Marynen P, et al: Inv(2)(p23q35) in anaplastic large-cell lymphoma induces constitutive anaplastic lymphoma kinase (ALK) tyrosine kinase activation by fusion to ATIC, an enzyme involved in purine nucleotide biosynthesis. *Blood* 95:2144–2149, 2000.

98. Hernandez L, Pinyol M, Hernandez S, et al: TRK-fused gene (TFG) is a new partner of ALK in anaplastic large cell lymphoma producing two structurally different TFG-ALK translocations. *Blood* 94:3265–3268, 1999.

99. Lamant L, Dastugue N, Pulford K, et al: A new fusion gene TPM3-ALK in anaplastic large cell lymphoma created by a (1;2)(q25;p23) translocation. *Blood* 93:3088–3095, 1999.

100. Cools J, Wlodarska I, Somers R, et al: Identification of novel fusion partners of ALK, the anaplastic lymphoma kinase, in anaplastic large-cell lymphoma and inflammatory myofibroblastic tumor. *Genes Chromosomes Cancer* 34:354–362, 2002.

101. Touriol C, Greenland C, Lamant L, et al: Further demonstration of the diversity of chromosomal changes involving 2p23 in ALK-positive lymphoma: 2 cases expressing ALK kinase fused to CLTCL (clathrin chain polypeptide-like). *Blood* 95:3204–3207, 2000.

102. Krenacs L, Wellmann A, Sorbara L, et al: Cytotoxic cell antigen expression in anaplastic large cell lymphomas of T- and null-cell type and Hodgkin's disease: Evidence for distinct cellular origin. *Blood* 89:980–989, 1997.

103. Foss HD, Anagnostopoulos I, Araujo I, et al: Anaplastic large-cell lymphomas of T-cell and null-cell phenotype express cytotoxic molecules. *Blood* 88:4005–4011, 1996.

104. Lamant L, de Reynies A, Duplantier MM, et al: Gene-expression profiling of systemic anaplastic large-cell lymphoma reveals differences based on ALK status and two distinct morphologic ALK+ subtypes. *Blood* 109:2156–2164, 2007.

105. Salaverria I, Bea S, Lopez-Guillermo A, et al: Genomic profiling reveals different genetic aberrations in systemic ALK-positive and ALK-negative anaplastic large cell lymphomas. *Br J Haematol* 140:516–526, 2008.

106. Massimino M, Gasparini M, Giardini R: Ki-1 (CD30) anaplastic large-cell lymphoma in children. *Ann Oncol* 6:915–920, 1995.

107. Brugieres L, Deley MC, Pacquement H, et al: CD30(+) anaplastic large-cell lymphoma in children: Analysis of 82 patients enrolled in two consecutive studies of the French Society of Pediatric Oncology. *Blood* 92:3591–3598, 1998.

108. Laver JH, Kraveka JM, Hutchison RE, et al: Advanced-stage large-cell lymphoma in children and adolescents: Results of a randomized trial incorporating intermediate-dose methotrexate and high-dose cytarabine in the maintenance phase of the APO regimen: A Pediatric Oncology Group phase III trial. *J Clin Oncol* 23:541–547, 2005.

109. Zinzani PL, Martelli M, Magagnoli M, et al: Anaplastic large cell lymphoma Hodgkin's-like: A randomized trial of ABVD versus MACOP-B with and without radiation therapy. *Blood* 92:790–794, 1998.

110. Moskowitz AJ, Lunning MA, Horwitz SM: How I treat the peripheral T-cell lymphomas. *Blood* 123:2636–2644, 2014.

111. Foyil KV, Bartlett NL: Brentuximab vedotin and crizotinib in anaplastic large-cell lymphoma. *Cancer J* 18:450–456, 2012.

112. Gambacorti-Passerini C, Messa C, Pogliani EM: Crizotinib in anaplastic large-cell lymphoma. *N Engl J Med* 364:775–776, 2011.

113. Suzuki R, Kagami Y, Takeuchi K, et al: Prognostic significance of CD56 expression for ALK-positive and ALK-negative anaplastic large-cell lymphoma of T/null cell phenotype. *Blood* 96:2993–3000, 2000.

114. Ferreri AJ, Govi S, Pileri SA, et al: Anaplastic large cell lymphoma, ALK-negative. *Crit Rev Oncol Hematol* 85:206–215, 2013.

115. Rassidakis GZ, Sarris AH, Herling M, et al: Differential expression of BCL-2 family proteins in ALK-positive and ALK-negative anaplastic large cell lymphoma of T/null-cell lineage. *Am J Pathol* 159:527–535, 2001.

116. Delabie J, Holte H, Vose JM, et al: Enteropathy-associated T-cell lymphoma: Clinical and histological findings from the international peripheral T-cell lymphoma project. *Blood* 118:148–155, 2011.

117. Di Sabatino A, Biagi F, Gobbi PG, et al: How I treat enteropathy-associated T-cell lymphoma. *Blood* 119:2458–2468, 2012.
118. Catassi C, Bearzi I, Holmes GK: Association of celiac disease and intestinal lymphomas and other cancers. *Gastroenterology* 128:S79–S86, 2005.
119. Deleeuw RJ, Zettl A, Klinker E, et al: Whole-genome analysis and HLA genotyping of enteropathy-type T-cell lymphoma reveals 2 distinct lymphoma subtypes. *Gastroenterology* 132:1902–1911, 2007.
120. Sieniawski M, Angamuthu N, Boyd K, et al: Evaluation of enteropathy-associated T-cell lymphoma comparing standard therapies with a novel regimen including autologous stem cell transplantation. *Blood* 115:3664–3670, 2010.
121. Gale J, Simmonds PD, Mead GM, et al: Enteropathy-type intestinal T-cell lymphoma: Clinical features and treatment of 31 patients in a single center. *J Clin Oncol* 18:795–803, 2000.
122. Rohatiner A, d'Amore F, Coiffier B, et al: Report on a workshop convened to discuss the pathological and staging classifications of gastrointestinal tract lymphoma. *Ann Oncol* 5:397–400, 1994.
123. Domizio P, Owen RA, Shepherd NA, et al: Primary lymphoma of the small intestine. A clinicopathologic study of 119 cases. *Am J Surg Pathol* 17:429–442, 1993.
124. Bagdi E, Diss TC, Munson P, et al: Mucosal intra-epithelial lymphocytes in enteropathy-associated T-cell lymphoma, ulcerative jejunitis, and refractory celiac disease constitute a neoplastic population. *Blood* 94:260–264, 1999.
125. de Bruin PC, Connolly CE, Oudejans JJ, et al: Enteropathy-associated T-cell lymphomas have a cytotoxic T-cell phenotype. *Histopathology* 31:313–317, 1997.
126. Wohrer S, Chott A, Drach J, et al: Chemotherapy with cyclophosphamide, doxorubicin, etoposide, vincristine and prednisone (CHOEP) is not effective in patients with enteropathy-type intestinal T-cell lymphoma. *Ann Oncol* 15:1680–1683, 2004.
127. Bishton MJ, Haynes AP: Combination chemotherapy followed by autologous stem cell transplant for enteropathy-associated T cell lymphoma. *Br J Haematol* 136:111–113, 2007.
128. Jantunen E, Juvonen E, Wiklund T, et al: High-dose therapy supported by autologous stem cell transplantation in patients with enteropathy-associated T-cell lymphoma. *Leuk Lymphoma* 44:2163–2164, 2003.
129. Daum S, Ullrich R, Heise W, et al: Intestinal non-Hodgkin's lymphoma: A multicenter prospective clinical study from the German Study Group on Intestinal non-Hodgkin's Lymphoma. *J Clin Oncol* 21:2740–2746, 2003.
130. Uchiyama T, Yodoi J, Sagawa K, et al: Adult T-cell leukemia: Clinical and hematologic features of 16 cases. *Blood* 50:481–492, 1977.
131. Bunn PA Jr, Schechter GP, Jaffe E, et al: Clinical course of retrovirus-associated adult T-cell lymphoma in the United States. *N Engl J Med* 309:257–264, 1983.
132. Waldmann TA, Greene WC, Sarin PS, et al: Functional and phenotypic comparison of human T cell leukemia/lymphoma virus positive adult T cell leukemia with human T cell leukemia/lymphoma virus negative Sézary leukemia, and their distinction using anti-Tac. Monoclonal antibody identifying the human receptor for T cell growth factor. *J Clin Invest* 73:1711–1718, 1984.
133. Shimoyama M: Diagnostic criteria and classification of clinical subtypes of adult T-cell leukaemia-lymphoma. A report from the Lymphoma Study Group (1984–87). *Br J Haematol* 79:428–437, 1991.
134. Yamamoto JF, Goodman MT: Patterns of leukemia incidence in the United States by subtype and demographic characteristics, 1997–2002. *Cancer Causes Control* 19:379–390, 2008.
135. Abbaszadegan MR, Gholamin M, Tabatabaee A, et al: Prevalence of human T-lymphotropic virus type 1 among blood donors from Mashhad, Iran. *J Clin Microbiol* 41:2593–2595, 2003.
136. Paun L, Ispas O, Del Mistro A, et al: HTLV-I in Romania. *Eur J Haematol* 52:117–118, 1994.
137. Gessain A, Cassar O: Epidemiological aspects and world distribution of HTLV-1 infection. *Front Microbiol* 3:388, 2012.
138. Mahieux R, Gessain A: Adult T-cell leukemia/lymphoma and HTLV-1. *Curr Hematol Malig Rep* 2:257–264, 2007.
139. Kaplan J, Khabbaz R: The epidemiology of human T-lymphotropic virus types I and II. *Rev Med Virol* 3:137–148, 1993.
140. Franchini G, Nicot C, Johnson JM: Seizing of T cells by human T-cell leukemia/lymphoma virus type 1. *Adv Cancer Res* 89:69–132, 2003.
141. Cleghorn FR, Manns A, Falk R, et al: Effect of human T-lymphotropic virus type I infection on non-Hodgkin's lymphoma incidence. *J Natl Cancer Inst* 87:1009–1014, 1995.
142. Suzumiya J, Ohshima K, Tamura K, et al: The International Prognostic Index predicts outcome in aggressive adult T-cell leukemia/lymphoma: Analysis of 126 patients from the International Peripheral T-Cell Lymphoma Project. *Ann Oncol* 20:715–721, 2009.
143. Bazarbachi A, Suarez F, Fields P, et al: How I treat adult T-cell leukemia/lymphoma. *Blood* 118:1736–1745, 2011.
144. Oshiro A, Tagawa H, Ohshima K, et al: Identification of subtype-specific genomic alterations in aggressive adult T-cell leukemia/lymphoma. *Blood* 107:4500–4507, 2006.
145. Takasaki Y, Iwanaga M, Imaizumi Y, et al: Long-term study of indolent adult T-cell leukemia-lymphoma. *Blood* 115:4337–4343, 2010.
146. Moriyama K, Muranishi H, Nishimura J, et al: Immunodeficiency in preclinical smoldering adult T-cell leukemia. *Jpn J Clin Oncol* 18:363–369, 1988.
147. Takatsuki F YK, Hattori T.. Adult T-cell leukemia/lymphoma. In:, (ed. *Retrovirus Biology and Human Disease*, edited by Robert C Gallo and Flossie Wong-Staal, pp 147–159. Marcel Dekker, New York, 1990:.
148. Amagasaki T, Tomonaga Y, Yamada Y, et al: Adult T-cell leukemia with an unusual phenotype, Leu-2a positive and Leu-3a negative. *Blut* 50:209–211, 1985.
149. Takemoto S, Matsuoka M, Yamaguchi K, et al: A novel diagnostic method of adult T-cell leukemia: Monoclonal integration of human T-cell lymphotropic virus type I provirus DNA detected by inverse polymerase chain reaction. *Blood* 84:3080–3085, 1994.
150. Lorand-Metze I, Pombo-de-Oliveira MS: Adult T-cell leukemia (ATL) with an unusual immunophenotype and a high cellular proliferation rate. *Leuk Lymphoma* 22:523–526, 1996.
151. Flug F, Pelicci PG, Bonetti F, et al: T-cell receptor gene rearrangements as markers of lineage and clonality in T cell neoplasms. *Proc Natl Acad Sci U S A* 82:3460–3464, 1985.
152. Bertness V, Kirsch I, Hollis G, et al: T-cell receptor gene rearrangements as clinical markers of human T-cell lymphomas. *N Engl J Med* 313:534–538, 1985.
153. Waldmann TA, Davis MM, Bongiovanni KF, et al: Rearrangements of genes for the antigen receptor on T cells as markers of lineage and clonality in human lymphoid neoplasms. *N Engl J Med* 313:776–783, 1985.
154. Yamada Y, Tomonaga M, Fukuda H, et al: A new G-CSF-supported combination chemotherapy, LSG15, for adult T-cell leukaemia-lymphoma: Japan Clinical Oncology Group Study 9303. *Br J Haematol* 113:375–382, 2001.
155. Tsukasaki K, Utsunomiya A, Fukuda H, et al: VCAP-AMP-VECP compared with biweekly CHOP for adult T-cell leukemia-lymphoma: Japan Clinical Oncology Group Study JCOG9801. *J Clin Oncol* 25:5458–5464, 2007.
156. Bazarbachi A, Plumelle Y, Carlos Ramos J, et al: Meta-analysis on the use of zidovudine and interferon-alfa in adult T-cell leukemia/lymphoma showing improved survival in the leukemic subtypes. *J Clin Oncol* 28:4177–4183, 2010.
157. Ishida T, Joh T, Uike N, et al: Defucosylated anti-CCR4 monoclonal antibody (KW-0761) for relapsed adult T-cell leukemia-lymphoma: A multicenter phase II study. *J Clin Oncol* 30:837–842, 2012.
158. Jo T, Ishida T, Takemoto S, et al: Randomized phase II study of mogamulizumab (KW-0761) plus VCAP-AMP-VECP (mLSG15) versus mLSG15 alone for newly diagnosed aggressive adult T-cell leukemia-lymphoma (ATL). *J Clin Oncol* 31, 2013.
159. Hishizawa M, Kanda J, Utsunomiya A, et al: Transplantation of allogeneic hematopoietic stem cells for adult T-cell leukemia: A nationwide retrospective study. *Blood* 116:1369–1376, 2010.
160. Phillips AA, Willim RD, Savage DG, et al: A multi-institutional experience of autologous stem cell transplantation in North American patients with human T-cell lymphotropic virus type-1 adult T-cell lymphoma/leukemia suggests ineffective salvage of relapsed patients. *Leuk Lymphoma* 50:1039–1042, 2009.
161. Tsukasaki K, Maeda T, Arimura K, et al: Poor outcome of autologous stem cell transplantation for adult T cell leukemia/lymphoma: A case report and review of the literature. *Bone Marrow Transplant* 23:87–89, 1999.
162. Falchook GS, Vega F, Dang NH, et al: Hepatosplenic gamma-delta T-cell lymphoma: Clinicopathological features and treatment. *Ann Oncol* 20:1080–1085, 2009.
163. Weidmann E: Hepatosplenic T cell lymphoma. A review on 45 cases since the first report describing the disease as a distinct lymphoma entity in 1990. *Leukemia* 14:991–997, 2000.
164. Clarke CA, Morton LM, Lynch C, et al: Risk of lymphoma subtypes after solid organ transplantation in the United States. *Br J Cancer* 109:280–288, 2013.
165. Mason M, Siegel CA: Do inflammatory bowel disease therapies cause cancer? *Inflamm Bowel Dis* 19:1306–1321, 2013.
166. Farcet JP, Gaulard P, Marolleau JP, et al: Hepatosplenic T-cell lymphoma: Sinusal/sinusoidal localization of malignant cells expressing the T-cell receptor gamma delta. *Blood* 75:2213–2219, 1990.
167. Jonveaux P, Daniel MT, Martel V, et al: Isochromosome 7q and trisomy 8 are consistent primary, non-random chromosomal abnormalities associated with hepatosplenic T gamma/delta lymphoma. *Leukemia* 10:1453–1455, 1996.
168. Wang CC, Tien HF, Lin MT, et al: Consistent presence of isochromosome 7q in hepatosplenic T gamma/delta lymphoma: A new cytogenetic-clinicopathologic entity. *Genes Chromosomes Cancer* 12:161–164, 1995.
169. Kanavaros P, Farcet JP, Gaulard P, et al: Recombinative events of the T cell antigen receptor delta gene in peripheral T cell lymphomas. *J Clin Invest* 87:666–672, 1991.
170. Belhadj K, Reyes F, Farcet JP, et al: Hepatosplenic gammadelta T-cell lymphoma is a rare clinicopathologic entity with poor outcome: Report on a series of 21 patients. *Blood* 102:4261–4269, 2003.
171. Voss MH, Lunning MA, Maragulia JC, et al: Intensive induction chemotherapy followed by early high-dose therapy and hematopoietic stem cell transplantation results in improved outcome for patients with hepatosplenic T-cell lymphoma: A single institution experience. *Clin Lymphoma Myeloma Leuk* 13:8–14, 2013.
172. Tey SK, Marlton PV, Hawley CM, et al: Post-transplant hepatosplenic T-cell lymphoma successfully treated with HyperCVAD regimen. *Am J Hematol* 83:330–333, 2008.
173. Corazzelli G, Capobianco G, Russo F, et al: Pentostatin (2'-deoxycoformycin) for the treatment of hepatosplenic gammadelta T-cell lymphomas. *Haematologica* 90:ECR14, 2005.
174. Cheung MM, Chan JK, Wong KF: Natural killer cell neoplasms: A distinctive group of highly aggressive lymphomas/leukemias. *Semin Hematol* 40:221–232, 2003.
175. Chan JK: Natural killer cell neoplasms. *Anat Pathol* 3:77–145, 1998.
176. Liang X, Graham DK: Natural killer cell neoplasms. *Cancer* 112:1425–1436, 2008.
177. Kwong YL: Natural killer-cell malignancies: Diagnosis and treatment. *Leukemia* 19:2186–2194, 2005.
178. Aviles A, Diaz NR, Neri N, et al: Angiocentric nasal T/natural killer cell lymphoma: A single centre study of prognostic factors in 108 patients. *Clin Lab Haematol* 22:215–220, 2000.
179. Barrionuevo C, Zaharia M, Martinez MT, et al: Extranodal NK/T-cell lymphoma, nasal type: Study of clinicopathologic and prognosis factors in a series of 78 cases from Peru. *Appl Immunohistochem Mol Morphol* 15:38–44, 2007.

180. Laurini JA, Perry AM, Boilesen E, et al: Classification of non-Hodgkin lymphoma in Central and South America: A review of 1028 cases. *Blood* 120:4795–4801, 2012.

181. Li S, Feng X, Li T, et al: Extranodal NK/T-cell lymphoma, nasal type: A report of 73 cases at MD Anderson Cancer Center. *Am J Surg Pathol* 37:14–23, 2013.

182. Tse E, Kwong YL: How I treat NK/T-cell lymphomas. *Blood* 121:4997–5005, 2013.

183. Au WY, Weisenburger DD, Intragumtornchai T, et al: Clinical differences between nasal and extranasal natural killer/T-cell lymphoma: A study of 136 cases from the International Peripheral T-Cell Lymphoma Project. *Blood* 113:3931–3937, 2009.

184. Chan WK, Au WY, Wong CY, et al: Metabolic activity measured by F-18 FDG PET in natural killer-cell lymphoma compared to aggressive B- and T-cell lymphomas. *Clin Nucl Med* 35:571–575, 2010.

185. Khong PL, Pang CB, Liang R, et al: Fluorine-18 fluorodeoxyglucose positron emission tomography in mature T-cell and natural killer cell malignancies. *Ann Hematol* 87:613–621, 2008.

186. Kwong YL, Kim WS, Lim ST, et al: SMILE for natural killer/T-cell lymphoma: Analysis of safety and efficacy from the Asia Lymphoma Study Group. *Blood* 120:2973–2980, 2012.

187. Kwong YL, Anderson BO, Advani R, et al: Management of T-cell and natural-killer-cell neoplasms in Asia: Consensus statement from the Asian Oncology Summit 2009. *Lancet Oncol* 10:1093–1101, 2009.

188. Au WY, Pang A, Choy C, et al: Quantification of circulating Epstein-Barr virus (EBV) DNA in the diagnosis and monitoring of natural killer cell and EBV-positive lymphomas in immunocompetent patients. *Blood* 104:243–249, 2004.

189. Kim SJ, Kim WS: Treatment of localized extranodal NK/T cell lymphoma, nasal type. *Int J Hematol* 92:690–696, 2010.

190. Wang ZY, Li YX, Wang WH, et al: Primary radiotherapy showed favorable outcome in treating extranodal nasal-type NK/T-cell lymphoma in children and adolescents. *Blood* 114:4771–4776, 2009.

191. Cheung MM, Chan JK, Lau WH, et al: Primary non-Hodgkin's lymphoma of the nose and nasopharynx: Clinical features, tumor immunophenotype, and treatment outcome in 113 patients. *J Clin Oncol* 16:70–77, 1998.

192. Kim SJ, Kim K, Kim BS, et al: Phase II trial of concurrent radiation and weekly cisplatin followed by VIPD chemotherapy in newly diagnosed, stage IE to IIE, nasal, extranodal NK/T-cell lymphoma: Consortium for Improving Survival of Lymphoma study. *J Clin Oncol* 27:6027–6032, 2009.

193. Kim WS, Song SY, Ahn YC, et al: CHOP followed by involved field radiation: Is it optimal for localized nasal natural killer/T-cell lymphoma? *Ann Oncol* 12:349–352, 2001.

194. Yong W, Zheng W, Zhang Y, et al: L-Asparaginase-based regimen in the treatment of refractory midline nasal/nasal-type T/NK-cell lymphoma. *Int J Hematol* 78:163–167, 2003.

195. Wang L, Wang ZH, Chen XQ, et al: First-line combination of gemcitabine, oxaliplatin, and L-asparaginase (GELOX) followed by involved-field radiation therapy for patients with stage IE/IIE extranodal natural killer/T-cell lymphoma. *Cancer* 119:348–355, 2013.

196. Yamaguchi M, Kwong YL, Kim WS, et al: Phase II study of SMILE chemotherapy for newly diagnosed stage IV, relapsed, or refractory extranodal natural killer (NK)/T-cell lymphoma, nasal type: The NK-Cell Tumor Study Group study. *J Clin Oncol* 29:4410–4416, 2011.

197. Jaccard A, Gachard N, Marin B, et al: Efficacy of L-asparaginase with methotrexate and dexamethasone (AspaMetDex regimen) in patients with refractory or relapsing extranodal NK/T-cell lymphoma, a phase 2 study. *Blood* 117:1834–1839, 2011.

198. Lee J, Suh C, Park YH, et al: Extranodal natural killer T-cell lymphoma, nasal-type: A prognostic model from a retrospective multicenter study. *J Clin Oncol* 24:612–618, 2006.

199. Gonzalez CL, Medeiros LJ, Braziel RM, et al: T-cell lymphoma involving subcutaneous tissue. A clinicopathologic entity commonly associated with hemophagocytic syndrome. *Am J Surg Pathol* 15:17–27, 1991.

200. Takeshita M, Okamura S, Oshiro Y, et al: Clinicopathologic differences between 22 cases of CD56-negative and CD56-positive subcutaneous panniculitis-like lymphoma in Japan. *Hum Pathol* 35:231–239, 2004.

201. Paulli M, Berti E: Cutaneous T-cell lymphomas (including rare subtypes). Current concepts. II. *Haematologica* 89:1372–1388, 2004.

202. Willemze R, Hodak E, Zinzani PL, et al: Primary cutaneous lymphomas: ESMO Clinical Practice Guidelines for diagnosis, treatment and follow-up. *Ann Oncol* 24 Suppl 6:vi149–vi154, 2013.

203. Gallardo F, Pujol RM: Subcutaneous panniculitic-like T-cell lymphoma and other primary cutaneous lymphomas with prominent subcutaneous tissue involvement. *Dermatol Clin* 26:529–540, viii, 2008.

204. Willemze R, Jansen PM, Cerroni L, et al: Subcutaneous panniculitis-like T-cell lymphoma: Definition, classification, and prognostic factors: An EORTC Cutaneous Lymphoma Group Study of 83 cases. *Blood* 111:838–845, 2008.

205. Go RS, Wester SM: Immunophenotypic and molecular features, clinical outcomes, treatments, and prognostic factors associated with subcutaneous panniculitis-like T-cell lymphoma: A systematic analysis of 156 patients reported in the literature. *Cancer* 101:1404–1413, 2004.

206. Wang CY, Su WP, Kurtin PJ: Subcutaneous panniculitic T-cell lymphoma. *Int J Dermatol* 35:1–8, 1996.

207. Matsue K, Itoh M, Tsukuda K, et al: Successful treatment of cytophagic histiocytic panniculitis with modified CHOP-E. Cyclophosphamide, Adriamycin, vincristine, prednisone, and etoposide. *Am J Clin Oncol* 17:470–474, 1994.

208. Papenfuss JS, Aoun P, Bierman PJ, et al: Subcutaneous panniculitis-like T-cell lymphoma: Presentation of 2 cases and observations. *Clin Lymphoma* 3:175–180, 2002.

209. Springinsfeld G, Guillaume JC, Boeckler P, et al: [Two cases of subcutaneous panniculitis-like T-cell lymphoma (CD4- CD8+ CD56-)] [in French]. *Ann Dermatol Venereol* 136:264–268, 2009.

210. Perez-Persona E, Mateos-Mazon JJ, Lopez-Villar O, et al: Complete remission of subcutaneous panniculitic T-cell lymphoma after allogeneic transplantation. *Bone Marrow Transplant* 38:821–822, 2006.

211. Ichii M, Hatanaka K, Imakita M, et al: Successful treatment of refractory subcutaneous panniculitis-like T-cell lymphoma with allogeneic peripheral blood stem cell transplantation from HLA-mismatched sibling donor. *Leuk Lymphoma* 47:2250–2252, 2006.

212. Hathaway T, Subtil A, Kuo P, et al: Efficacy of denileukin diftitox in subcutaneous panniculitis-like T-cell lymphoma. *Clin Lymphoma Myeloma* 7:541–545, 2007.

213. Mehta N, Wayne AS, Kim YH, et al: Bexarotene is active against subcutaneous panniculitis-like T-cell lymphoma in adult and pediatric populations. *Clin Lymphoma Myeloma Leuk* 12:20–25, 2012.

CHAPTER 105
PLASMA CELL NEOPLASMS: GENERAL CONSIDERATIONS

Guido Tricot, Siegfried Janz, Kalyan Nadiminti, Erik Wendlandt, and Fenghuang Zhan

SUMMARY

Plasma cell neoplasms are tumors derived from an expansion of mutated mature B-cells and their precursors. These neoplasms include essential monoclonal gammopathy (synonym: monoclonal gammopathy of unknown significance; Chap. 106), smoldering myeloma (Chap. 107), myeloma (Chap. 107), solitary and extramedullary plasmacytomas (Chap. 107), light-chain amyloidosis (Chap. 108), and Waldenström macroglobulinemia (Chap. 109). The prototype of a malignant plasma cell neoplasm is myeloma, which is characterized by complex genetic alterations, best assessed by metaphase cytogenetics, fluorescence *in situ* hybridization analysis, and gene-expression profiling. The genetic changes are more akin to solid tumors than to hematologic malignancies. Interactions between myeloma cells and the marrow microenvironment affect the survival, proliferation, and drug resistance of myeloma cells, and the development of osteoporosis or osteolysis, which is a hallmark of myeloma. As in most malignancies, a cancer stem cell (e.g., myeloma stem cell) has been identified and is the most likely site of drug resistance, which almost invariably develops during treatment; such cells are not affected by the typical drugs one uses in patients with myeloma. The best prognostic markers in myeloma in order of importance are the presence of (1) specific cytogenetic abnormalities, (2) extent of the disease by appropriate imaging techniques, such as magnetic resonance imaging and/or combined positron emission and computed tomographic imaging, (3) the serum free light-chain level and kappa-to-lambda ratio, and (4) the use of the International Staging System. The development of several classes of drugs over the past decade in combination with transplantation, has improved therapeutic outcomes significantly in patients achieving an unequivocal complete remission. Thus, optimal techniques to assess minimal residual disease have also become important.

Acronyms and Abbreviations: AL, light-chain amyloidosis; BAFF, B-cell activating factor; BCR, B-cell receptor; BMSC, bone mesenchymal stem cell; BTK, Bruton tyrosine kinase; CDR, complementarity determining regions of the heavy chain; CR, complete remission; CSC, cancer stem cell; D, diversity immunoglobulin gene segment; FISH, fluorescence *in situ* hybridization; FLC, free light chain; GFR, glomerular filtration rate; ICAM-1, intercellular adhesion molecule 1; Ig, immunoglobulin; IGH, immunoglobulin heavy chain; IGF-1, insulin-like growth factor 1; IL, interleukin; IRAK, interleukin-1 receptor-associated kinase; JAK2/STAT3, Janus kinase 2/signal transducers and activators of transcription; J_H, joining region immunoglobulin gene segment; M, monoclonal; MBD, myeloma bone disease; MPC, multiparameter flow cytometry; MRD, minimal residual disease; MRI, magnetic resonance imaging; mSMART, Mayo stratification of myeloma and risk-adapted therapy; MYD, myeloid differentiation primary response gene; nCR, near complete remission; NEK2, a serine/threonine kinase; NF-κB, nuclear factor κB; OB, osteoblast; OC, osteoclast; OL, osteolytic lesion; OPG, osteoprotegerin; PCN, plasma cell neoplasm; PDGF, platelet-derived growth factor; PET/CT, ^{18}F-fluorodeoxyglucose positron emission tomography–computed tomography; pP-7, a hyperphosphorylated protein; RAG, recombinase-activating genes; RANK, receptor activator of NF-κB; RARα, retinoic receptor α; RB, retinoblastoma gene sCR, stringent complete remission; sIFE, serum immunofixation electrophoresis; SMM, smoldering myeloma; SP, side population; SPEP, serum protein electrophoresis; TGF-β, transforming growth factor β; TLR, toll-like receptor; TME, tumor microenvironment; TNF-α, tumor necrosis factor α; TRAF3, the adaptor molecule for toll receptor; uIFE, urine immunofixation electrophoresis; UPEP, urine protein electrophoresis; VCAM-1, vascular cell adhesion molecule 1; VEGF, vascular endothelial growth factor; V_H, the variable immunoglobulin gene segment.

● DEFINITION AND HISTORY

Plasma cell neoplasms (PCNs) are clonal B-cell tumors that range from stable disease without functional abnormalities (monoclonal gammopathy, synonym monoclonal gammopathy of unknown significance) to one of slowly proliferating plasma cells (smoldering myeloma [SMM]), to one resulting in end-organ compromise (myeloma). PCNs are accompanied by the synthesis and release into the plasma of a monoclonal (M) protein, and, in the case of myeloma, either diffuse osteoporosis or osteolytic lesions. Myeloma accounts for approximately 1 percent of all malignant diseases and 10 percent of hematologic malignancies.

Approximately two-thirds of patients presenting with an M protein have (1) monoclonal gammopathy (Chap. 106), whereas approximately 15 percent have (2) myeloma (Chap. 107). Other diseases associated with M-protein productions are (3) immunoglobulin light-chain amyloidosis (AL) (10 percent; Chap. 108) resulting from the deposition of immunoglobulin (Ig) fragments in visceral organs a consequence of extensive misfolding of these Ig fragments, (4) SMM (3 percent; Chap. 107), (5) Waldenström macroglobulinemia (3 percent; Chap. 109), (6) lymphoproliferative disorders (2 percent; Chap. 90), (7) solitary or extramedullary plasmacytomas (1 percent; Chap. 107) and (8) miscellaneous other diseases (2 percent).[3]

● NORMAL B-CELL DEVELOPMENT

B-cell development is discussed in detail in Chaps. 74 and 75. In brief, B-cell lymphopoiesis occurs initially in the marrow and in lymphoid tissues. In the marrow, the pro–B-cell, undergoes rearrangement of immunoglobulin heavy chain (IGH) genes and, then, is designated a pre–B-cell, which is characterized by the presence of cytoplasmic μ chains. Subsequent rearrangement of the light chain enables the cell to express surface IgM, the immature B lymphocyte phase of development. These cells leave the marrow and upon entering the blood express surface IgD, which then defines them as virgin B cells, also characterized by G_0 cell-cycle arrest. Virgin B cells enter the lymphoid tissue, where they are exposed to antigen-presenting cells, become activated when in contact with the corresponding antigen and differentiate into short-lived, low-affinity plasma cells or memory B-cells. These memory B-cells travel from the extra-follicular area of the lymph node to the primary follicles, where if confronted with an antigen, presented by follicular dendritic cells, a secondary response is induced. At this stage, primary follicles change into secondary follicles containing germinal centers. Through activation by an antigen, the memory B cells differentiate into centroblasts, resulting in Ig isotype switching and somatic mutations in the variable region of the immunoglobulin gene with the generation of high-affinity antibodies. Centroblasts progress to the centrocyte stage and reexpress surface Ig. The centrocytes with high-affinity antibodies differentiate into either memory B cells or plasmablasts, which then move to the marrow and terminally differentiate to plasma cells. Marrow plasma cells produce most of the plasma immunoglobulins and have a life span of approximately 3 weeks.

Three distinct gene segments, the variable (V_H), diversity (D), and joining region (J_H) genes, encode the variable region of the heavy chain, whereas two segments, variable ($V\kappa$ or $V\lambda$) and joining ($J\kappa$ or $J\lambda$) region genes, encode the variable fraction of the light chain. The IGH locus on chromosome 14q32 contains an estimated 100 to 150 V_H genes, 30 D, and six J_H gene segments. Because some of the V_H genes are nearly identical, it is likely that 60 to 70 V_H genes are available for rearrangement. These 60 to 70 genes belong to seven families (V_H 1 to 7) whose members have more than 80 percent sequence homology. Of the 75 known $V\kappa$ sequences, only 36 are potentially functional and of the 36 known $V\lambda$ sequences, only 24 are functional. Rearrangement of the V gene segments is dependent on the protein products of the recombinase-activating genes RAG-1 and RAG-2. Recombination of V genes starts in lymphoid progenitors within the IGH locus of either the maternal or paternal chromosome 14. If the initial V_H-D-J_H rearrangement yields a sequence that cannot be translated, then rearrangement of the IGH locus proceeds on the other allele. The presence on the B-cell surface of a fully assembled μ heavy chain rearrangement begins when one of the $V\kappa$ genes rearranges to one of the $J\kappa$ genes. If κ light-chain rearrangement is unsuccessful on both alleles, by default λ light chains will subsequently rearrange. The Ig heavy and light chains each contain three hypervariable complementarity determining regions segments, which are the areas of the immunoglobulin in direct contact with the antigen. In a process of trial and error, immunoglobulins increase their affinity for an antigen by a series of somatic mutations. The complementarity determining regions of the IGH (CDR) 3 is the most variable portion of the Ig molecule, because it not only contains somatic mutations as is the case for CDR 1 and CDR 2, but it also encompasses the 3' end of V_H, all of D, and the 5' end of J_H. It is, therefore, an ideal marker to detect a very small population of the malignant myeloma clone within a larger population of normal cells.

● ETIOLOGY AND PATHOGENESIS

ETIOLOGY OF PLASMA CELL NEOPLASM

Monoclonal Gammopathy

Although monoclonal gammopathy (Chap. 106) shares the same constellation of risk factors and cytogenetic abnormalities with myeloma, it is an antecedent neoplasm that may undergo clonal evolution to any one of the PCNs or to a B-cell lymphoma.[1] Two studies have reported that monoclonal gammopathy is a precursor to myeloma in virtually all cases.[23]

Retrospective population-based cohort studies have established that nearly 80 percent of cases of myeloma develop from IGH monoclonal gammopathy. The remaining 20 percent have serum free light chain (FLC) monoclonal gammopathy. The prevalence of FLC monoclonal gammopathy is 0.8 percent in the general population. It progresses to myeloma in a minority of patients at the rate of 0.3 percent per year,[3] much lower than the conventional monoclonal gammopathy progression rate of approximately 1 percent.

Factors such as chronic antigen stimulation and chemical exposure have been suspected in the development of monoclonal gammopathy and other PCNs. Some studies have found a positive association,[45] but the results have not been consistent and given our current understanding of the genetic precedents of myeloma, one would have to show a direct effect of such agents on the causal mutations involved.

A familial history of monoclonal gammopathy and myeloma has been reported to be a risk factor for developing the disease in first-degree relatives, including a population-based study from the Mayo Clinic. A twofold increased relative risk was noted for the development of monoclonal gammopathy among the first-degree relatives of myeloma and monoclonal gammopathy patients. In a large Swedish population study, among first-degree relatives of patients with monoclonal gammopathy, a threefold increased risk for both monoclonal gammopathy and myeloma, a fourfold risk of developing Waldenström macroglobulinemia, and a twofold risk of developing B-cell chronic lymphocytic leukemia was observed.[6] These observations support the role of both germline susceptibility genes and possibly immune-related phenomena in the causation.[7] Because of the extremely low lifetime-risk of developing myeloma in the general population (0.2 percent), it would be inefficient to screen the first-degree relatives of persons with myeloma or monoclonal gammopathy.

Hyperphosphorylated paratarg-7, a frequent autoantigenic target of human paraproteins, is linked to both familial and nonfamilial forms of monoclonal gammopathy and myeloma.[7] Paratarg-7 is the target of 15 percent of the monoclonal proteins of the IgA and IgG type, and 11 percent of IgM-monoclonal gammopathy or macroglobulinemia patients. All patients with paratarg-7–specific paraproteins were carriers of a hyperphosphorylated protein (pP-7); this hyperphosphorylation is inherited in a dominant fashion. Hyperphosphorylation is a result of inactivation of phosphatase 2A.[8] Hyperphosphorylated paratarg-7 carriers are most prevalent among Americans of African wdefined single risk factor for monoclonal gammopathy or myeloma in all ethnic groups[9] and is associated with a sixfold increased risk of IgM monoclonal gammopathy or macroglobulinemia.[10]

Nearly 50 percent of patients with monoclonal gammopathy have plasma cells with translocations involving the IGH locus on chromosome 14q32 and one of the five partner chromosomes: 11q13 (cyclin D1 gene), 4q16,3 (FGFR-2 and MMSET), 6q21 (CCND3), 16q23 (c-maf), and 20q11 (maf-B).[11–14]

Unfortunately, none of the molecular or chromosomal abnormalities associated with myeloma predict the evolution of monoclonal gammopathy to myeloma. Two clinical risk stratification models propose high-risk features that can predict progression from monoclonal gammopathy and SMM to myeloma.[15,16] While one model uses the type of immunoglobulin, quantity of M-protein, and the serum FLC ratio to determine the risk of progression, the other model is based on flow cytometry findings of aberrant plasma cells, marrow plasma cell percentage, DNA aneuploidy, and immune paresis (a decrease in noninvolved immunoglobulins).

Smoldering Myeloma

SMM is discussed in Chap. 107. In addition to the marrow plasma cell burden and quantitative M-protein (>3 g/dL), presence of light-chain proteinuria and IgA M-heavy chain were identified as separate risk factors predicting progression to active myeloma.[17–20] The median time of progression to myeloma has been reported to range between 3 and 8 years in low-risk groups, and between 1 and 2 years in high-risk groups.[17–22] Some studies have also investigated the use of magnetic resonance imaging (MRI) in detecting skeletal abnormalities not seen on a skeletal survey; time to progression to myeloma was much shorter in patients with focal lesions on the MRI[23] and these patients should be treated.

A number of models estimating the risk of progression to myeloma have been proposed. The presence of serum M-protein of greater than 3 g/dL, an FLC ratio outside the reference range of 0.125 to 8, and greater than 10 percent plasma cells in the marrow represents SMM with a high-risk of progression. Patients with these three risk factors had a cumulative risk of 76 percent of progression to myeloma within

5 years.[15,24] The risk of progression decreased to 51 percent in patients with two of the risk factors and to 25 percent in patients with a single risk factor.[24,25] Another clinical risk stratification model uses flow-cytometry of marrow aspirates. Using as risk factors (1) greater than 95 percent of all plasma cells being aberrant at diagnosis, (2) DNA aneuploidy, and (3) immune paresis, the presence of one, two, or three risk factors translated to 4, 46, and 72 percent risk of progression to myeloma with 5 years of observation, respectively.[16] Other researchers have found that in addition to the intrinsic, molecular, and cytogenetic abnormalities of the plasma cells, an angiogenic switch and immunologic factors play a key role in the transformation of SMM to established myeloma.[26]

Myeloma

The development of myeloma is a complex multistep process involving karyotypic instability, Ig translocations, cell-cycle abnormalities (cyclin Ds), and multiple other mutations[27] (Chap. 107). No molecular or chromosomal abnormalities can distinguish among monoclonal gammopathy, SMM, or myeloma at the time of diagnosis. Certain mutations occur in much higher frequencies in myeloma, such as p53 deletions, especially in refractory and extramedullary presentations,[12,28] N-RAS and K-RAS mutations, chromosome 1p deletion and gain of 1q21, and translocations involving MYC (8q24).[29-33] In whole-exome sequencing studies, intraclonal heterogeneity has been shown to be present at all stages of development—from monoclonal gammopathy to SMM to progressive myeloma.[39] Genetic complexity increases as the disease progresses to myeloma.

Effect of Endogenous Factors There is an increased relative risk of monoclonal gammopathy and myeloma in overweight and obese patients based on their body mass index (BMI). With the exception of elite athletes, a BMI of 25.0 to 29.9 kg/m^2 and 30 kg/m^2 or greater define overweight and obese individuals, respectively.[35-41] Fat tissue is a dynamic endocrine organ, secreting adipokines, hormones that play an important role in energy homeostasis and inflammation. Several adipokines, such as leptin and adiponectin, have been implicated in the development of cancer.[40] Adiponectin levels are inversely correlated with obesity. Adiponectin serum concentrations were lower in monoclonal gammopathy patients who subsequently developed myeloma. In the KaLwRij strain of C57 black mice, which is permissive to the growth of 5T myeloma, compared to the parental strain of C57B16, which is not, adiponectin gene expression is significantly lower than in the parental strain. An increased myeloma burden was found in adiponectin-deficient mice, while pharmacologic enhancement of circulating adiponectin resulted in apoptosis of myeloma cells and also prevented bone disease. Fat tissue is a principal source of interleukin (IL)-6, one of the principal growth and antiapoptotic cytokines acting on myeloma cells. Obese individuals have been shown to have shorter telomeres than nonobese individuals. Because telomeres protect chromosomes from injury, including undesirable translocations, this effect may also contribute the relationship of body mass with PCN.

Effect of Exogenous Factors Aspirin has been shown not only to reduce cancer incidence, but to also dramatically decrease cancer mortality, especially in colorectal cancer, esophageal, gastric cancer, breast cancer, prostate cancer, and lung cancer. Aspirin inhibits several pathways that are important in myeloma, including nuclear factor κB (NF-κB), AKT activation, and the BCL-2 family of proteins. Aspirin is used frequently as thromboprophylaxis in myeloma patients receiving immunomodulatory therapy. In a prospective study designed to examine whether regular aspirin use influences the risk of myeloma, participants taking 5 or more tablets of 325 mg per week had a 39 percent lower myeloma incidence than nonusers. The association appeared stronger in men than in women.[43] Aspirin inhibits proliferation and induces apoptosis of myeloma cell lines in vitro through regulation of

BCL-2 and BAX and suppression of vascular endothelial growth factor (VEGF). In addition, in vivo studies in mice showed that aspirin administration resulted in retardation of tumor growth and in increased survival.[44] A number of case-control and cohort studies have established that smoking has no association with the incidence of myeloma. Convincing evidence has not been found linking alcohol consumption to myeloma development.[45]

Occupation Many studies evaluated the potential role of exposure to certain occupations and/or toxin and the subsequent risk of myeloma development. Agricultural workers and farmers were studied in the United States and Europe. The majority of studies report an increase frequency of myeloma in agricultural workers, whereas other reports fail to find such a correlation.[46] Exposure to toxins such as organic solvents (e.g., toluene, benzene), pesticides, paints, and others products with trace benzene content have been investigated for an association with the incidence of myeloma, but the findings are inconsistent.[47]

Radiation Studies on the survivors of the atomic bombing in Japan have failed to establish a cause-and-effect relationship between high-dose radiation exposure and an increased incidence of myeloma.[48] Studies from the United Kingdom have reported no increased frequency of myeloma in workers exposed to ionizing radiation, nuclear plants, and/or plutonium.[45] In a large study in China of x-ray technicians, there were no reported cases of myeloma or plasma cells disorders.[49] Thus, radiation exposure is not linked to the risk of myeloma.

Chronic immune stimulation has not been shown to play a causative role in the etiology of myeloma. No link between infections, allergic conditions, or immunizations and the development of myeloma has been established. Patients with autoimmune disorders, in general, have not been found to have an excess risk of myeloma. Some studies report an increased risk of myeloma in HIV[50,51] and hepatitis C patients,[52] although more convincing data are needed to establish a cause-and-effect relationship.

Waldenström Macroglobulinemia

Etiology In a small study of 65 patients and 213 controls, a preceding autoimmune condition did not predict the development of Waldenström macroglobulinemia.[53] In contrast, many other studies have found such a link. In a large population-based study, that included 146,394 hepatitis C patients and 572,293 controls, a threefold increased risk of macroglobulinemia was observed along with a 20 to 30 percent increased risk of lymphoma.[54] In a study of 361 U.S. veterans with Waldenström macroglobulinemia after a 27-year followup, a two- to threefold increased risk of developing the disease was found in patients with autoimmune-related conditions, hepatitis, HIV infection, and rickettsiosis.[55] In two Swedish population-based studies, a personal history of autoimmune conditions and infections was associated with an increased risk of macroglobulinemia.[56]

Case-control studies and a large population-based study in Sweden have established the role of familial clustering of macroglobulinemia, thereby raising the concept of common susceptibility genes that could predispose to the disease.[53,57-61] In study of macroglobulinemia, 19 percent of patients had at least one identified first-degree relative with macroglobulinemia or a B-cell disorder.[60] In genome-wide linkage analyses of high-risk families with macroglobulinemia and IgM monoclonal gammopathy, the strongest linkage was found to be chromosomes 1q, 3q, 4q, and 6q.[58,60,62-64] In a gene-sequencing study performed on marrow cells of macroglobulinemia patients, a recurrent somatic mutation of the gene MYD88L265P on chromosome 3 that encodes signal transduction and innate immunity was found to be in approximately 91 percent of the patients tested.[60]

In a novel study using expression cloning, several common self-antigens designated Paratarg-7 were discovered.[10] When carriers of the phosphorylated forms of Paratarg-7 were studied, they were found to have a 6.5-fold higher risk of developing IgM monoclonal gammopathy or macroglobulinemia. The antigen causes continuous autostimulation of cognate T-helper cells, which, in turn, specifically activate B cells with high affinity to Paratarg-7.

●GENETIC ABNORMALITIES IN PLASMA CELL NEOPLASM

MYELOMA

Plasma cell differentiation begins in lymph nodes and in the spleen where cells undergo changes in gene expression and cell-surface molecules followed by migration to the marrow or mucosal lamina propria.[65] The development of plasma cells alters the cellular receptor landscape of the cell with the deletion of important B-cell receptors and the addition of receptors necessary for plasma cell function and antibody production. Changes to cellular receptors include downregulation of major histocompatibility complex (MHC) class II, CD19, CD21, and CD22.[66] Perhaps, the most important alterations during myeloma development are decreases of the B-cell receptor (BCR), CXCR5, and CCR7. In contrast, plasma cells upregulate CXCR4, CD138, and CD38 (Fig. 105–1).[66–68] Plasma cells also undergo changes to transcription factors highlighted by a decrease in PAX5, CIITA, and EBF.[66–70] Furthermore, plasma cells express genes that are present in B cells at low levels or not at all and are highlighted by increased expression of Blimp-1, IRF4, and XBP1, the only transcription factor exclusively required for plasma cell development.[71] For more information on plasma cell development (Chap. 74).

Early Genetic Events in Myeloma Genesis

Early genetic events in myeloma genesis include the accumulation of sequential genetic changes; however, the full mechanism remains elusive.[72] Protein kinases provide selective growth advantages to cells and, therefore, act as driver mutations, or inducers of early neoplastic events.[73] The dysregulation of the cyclin D genes exposes cells to additional proliferative stimuli and commonly occurs as a result of a translocation of the cyclin D gene to the Ig loci.[74] Activation-induced deaminase contributes to genetic instability through its involvement in induction of somatic mutations in the immunoglobulin genes and immunoglobulin translocations.[75] Although important, gene alterations

are not the only driving force in the development of PCN. Although ethnicity and genealogy affect the prevalence of monoclonal gammopathy,[76] they do not impact the rate of progression from monoclonal gammopathy to myeloma. Furthermore, there is a higher incidence in monoclonal gammopathy in relatives of myeloma patients than seen in the general public.[77,78] These results demonstrate that not only are there somatic mutations important to the development of PCNs, but genetic background also contributes to the likelihood of the development of plasma cell diseases.

Late Events in Myeloma Progression

Much focus has been placed on risk factors and early genetic events that can be used as diagnostic and prognostic markers. However, we are learning more about the genetic alterations that occur throughout disease progression. One of the more prominent discoveries focuses on the activation of NF-κB. Approximately 50 percent of myeloma patients exhibit canonical NF-κB activation.[79,80] NF-κB functions, in part, by regulating growth and survival within the myeloma cells; overexpression of positive regulators, such as NIK, NFKB1, NFKB2, and CD40, and inactivation of negative regulators, such as CLYD, TRAF2, TRAF3, and cIAP1/cIAP2, contribute to the constitutive activation of NF-κB within these cells.[80]

RAS mutations are also important contributors to the development of myeloma from monoclonal gammopathy. Oncogenic activation of RAS occurs through mutation of one of three different codons with mutations resulting in constitutively activated RAS. Less than 5 percent of cases of monoclonal gammopathy display mutations of RAS, whereas in newly diagnosed myeloma patients mutated RAS is found in nearly 40 percent of patient samples, suggesting that RAS may be associated with the conversion of monoclonal gammopathy to myeloma.[81–83]

p53, which regulates the cell cycle and acts as a tumor suppressor represents the most commonly inactivated tumor-suppressor gene in cancer.[84,85] In newly diagnosed PCNs, p53 mutations occur in 5 percent of patients. The frequency of p53 mutations increases with disease progression; while infrequent in newly diagnosed myelomas, 30 percent of plasma cell leukemia patients present with p53 mutations.[86,87] Furthermore, p53 mutations are negatively correlated with survival.[88] Similar in function to p53, the retinoblastoma (RB) gene regulates the cell cycle. RB functions by inhibiting the effects of the cyclin D proteins with the help of the p18^{INK4} proteins. However, overexpression of cyclin D or decreased expression of RB can lead to cell-cycle progression and neoplastic growth. Decreased expression of the two RB pathway regulators

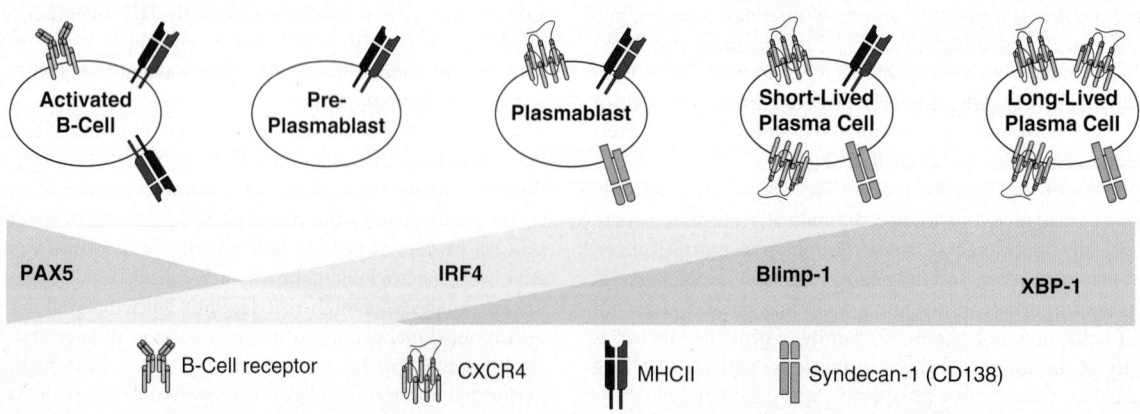

Figure 105–1. Overview of plasma cell differentiation. The differentiation of a plasma cell from a B-cell lineage occurs over a multistep process using plasmablast and short-lived plasma cell intermediates. Throughout the process, there is a profound change in gene expression and cell-surface markers, which allows for the identification of each stage based on the cell-surface marker expression and gene expression of transcription factors important to plasma cell differentiation. Depicted here are necessary changes to transcription factors and cell-surface markers that occur during each phase of plasma cell differentiation.

p18INK4a and p18INK4c can inhibit the regulatory effects of RB and result in cell-cycle release. Decreased expression of the two proteins is considered to be a late disease progression event.[76]

Genetic Expression Changes in Myeloma

Myeloma is genetically heterogeneous and more closely resembles solid tumors than other hematologic malignancies. Because of its high degree of tumor heterogeneity, myeloma gene-expression microarrays have proven invaluable to our understanding and treatment of myeloma. Four stratification models exist designed to classify myeloma based on the risk profile as determined by gene-expression profiles.[89] Of the four, one model has proven most reliable, as it retains its prognostic relevance with newer therapeutic regimens. This model compares the expression of 70 different genes to devise a scoring system that ranks a sample as high risk (13 percent of patients) or low risk.[90] Abnormalities of expression that map to chromosome 1 are disproportionately represented within the model, with an impressive number of upregulated genes mapping to 1q and a high percentage of downregulated genes mapping to 1p. The 70-gene model offers a reliable method for the detection of high-risk myeloma. However, it does not take into account all important genes related to myeloma. One important gene not found in this model is *MYC*, which is a transcription factor that influences the expression of many genes through the binding of consensus sequences within the noncoding region of genes. It is thought to regulate the expression of 15 percent of all genes.[91] *MYC* expression within myeloma and monoclonal gammopathy varies depending on the state of the disease. In high-risk monoclonal gammopathy and early stages of myeloma, the increase in *MYC* expression is primarily a result of a decrease in transcriptional regulation, whereas in late disease states, the 8q region encoding MYC translocates to the immunoglobulin loci, resulting in dysregulation of expression because of the influence of neighboring regulatory elements.[32]

Drug Resistance

Refractory myeloma has several causes, with dysregulation of gene expression contributing significantly to the overall development of drug resistance. The serine/threonine kinase NEK2 induces drug resistance in myeloma through the activation of efflux drug pumps.[92] Overexpression of *NEK2* results in the activation of the AKT pathway and subsequently of NF-κB, which results in the upregulation of ABC drug efflux transporters. Overexpression of the antiapoptotic molecule MCL-1 induces drug resistance through the inhibition of apoptosis.[93] More specifically, MCL-1 overexpression results in the inhibition of the proapoptotic BCL-2 family members, which results in blocking apoptosis.

Next-Generation Sequencing

Next-generation sequencing or deep sequencing relies on the ability to sequence large amounts of small DNA fragments quickly and assemble the output into a complete coherent data set. This technique is providing new insights into our understanding of existing neoplastic mechanisms and identifying novel mechanisms and genes that had evaded detection thus far. One of the first reports to use next-generation sequencing was from a study that compared 38 whole-tumor genomes from patients with myeloma to matched normal DNA.[94] Novel genes involved in histone methylation, protein translation and blood coagulation were identified. Mutations to the toll-like receptor (TLR) 4, the adaptor molecule TRAF3, and to the kinases CYLD, RIPK4, and BTRC also were discovered. A greater-than-anticipated change in NF-κB was observed, including identifying 11 mutated genes involved in the NF-κB pathway. Furthermore, the prognostic value of next-generation sequencing was tested by using the sequencing technology to detect minimal residual disease (MRD) in myeloma patient samples.[95]

Cytogenetic Microarrays

Fluorescence *in situ* hybridization (FISH) has become the gold standard for the detection and classification of myeloma. However, FISH cannot provide information about chromosomal abnormalities without the use of large scale panels of probes. Comparative genomic hybridization (CGH) arrays overcome some of the short falls of FISH technology by providing a genome-wide view of chromosomal changes, but do so at a reduced resolution of 10 to 20 megabases. To combat the low resolution of CGH arrays, small nucleotide polymorphism (SNP)-based technology has been employed. SNP arrays can detect copy number changes and have improved the resolution of CGH arrays to a submegabase level. An early report validated the use of SNP arrays by comparing its results to those obtained by FISH analysis using identical samples. Furthermore, uniparental disomy (UPD) was identified as prevalent in myeloma samples and may occur through several mechanisms, including mitotic nondisjunction and mitotic recombination.[96] A technical advance was the introduction of the Affymetrix Cyto Scan HD arrays. The Cyto Scan arrays incorporate the most up-to-date SNP library to generate a 2.6-million probe library across the human genome, allowing for resolution up to 50 kb. The technology has not been published in a myeloma study yet, but the resolution matches that of FISH and can provide a wealth of knowledge related to changes in copy number, mosaic chromosomes and loss of heterozygosity. Using these technologies numerous cytogenetic changes were identified that may be important for the development and progression of monoclonal gammopathy to myeloma.

● TECHNIQUES TO ASSESS CYTOGENETIC INFORMATION

FLUORESCENCE *IN SITU* HYBRIDIZATION

In PCNs, FISH has emerged as one of the most useful and reliable methods for the detection of chromosomal abnormalities and performing risk assessment on newly diagnosed patients. G-banding cytogenetic analysis requires actively dividing cells for identification of chromosomal changes, not commonly seen in plasma cells, whereas FISH analysis can overcome this limitation to an extent and detect structural abnormalities in non-dividing plasma cells.[97] A panel of FISH probes is used to query for commonly identified cytogenetic changes, including t(4;14), t(11;14), t(14;16), t(14;20), t(6;14), del(13q14), and del(17p13), and probes for hyperdiploidy (5, 7, 9, 11, 15, and 17). Cytogenetic abnormalities, using FISH, are observed in more than 90 percent of myeloma patients. Panels like the one described here provide essential information and paired with gene-expression profiles provides clinicians with essential data for diagnosis and the development of treatment regimens.

METAPHASE CYTOGENETICS

Approximately 30 percent of patients with newly diagnosed myeloma present with chromosomal abnormalities by metaphase cytogenetics, and this percentage increases to 50 percent in patients with relapsed myeloma. Cytogenetic changes broadly divide patients into one of two categories: patients with hyperdiploid chromosomal profile and non-hyperdiploid, encompassing hypodiploid and hypotetraploid cases. Hyperdiploid cytogenetic profiles are characterized by trisomies of many odd-numbered chromosomes, namely 3, 5, 7, 9, 15, 19, and 21 and are associated with a favorable outcome.[98] Nonhyperdiploid profiles are highly enriched with translocations at the IGH loci (14q32) with partner chromosomes, most importantly resulting in t(4;14), t(6;14), t(11;14), t(14;16), and t(14;20).[97] However, many of the translocations result in the activation of cell-cycle regulators and oncogenes like cyclin

D, MMSET and c-MAF, MAFB. In addition, amplification of chromosome 1q and deletions to chromosomes 13q and 17p are commonly seen within myeloma patients.[86] With regards to deletion of chromosome 17p, the number of patients presenting with this abnormality increases as the disease progresses.[85,96] To accommodate the variability in cytogenetic markers, researchers have developed diagnostic criteria to aid in the management of patients with a variety of cytogenetic abnormalities with prognostic value and will be discussed below.

CYTOGENETIC ABNORMALITIES AS PROGNOSTIC MARKERS IN PLASMA CELL NEOPLASM

One model has become the standard for myeloma prognostic risk assessment: The Mayo stratification of myeloma and risk-adapted therapy (mSMART).[99,100] Historically, risk assessment was categorized into two groups, standard or high-risk. The mSMART guidelines add an intermediate-risk subgroup to better assess the appropriate treatment regimen. The standard-risk group consists of patients presenting with either the t(6;14) or t(11;14) translocation as well as the hyperdiploid group, whereas the intermediate-risk group comprises patients presenting with the t(4;14) translocation and deletions of chromosome 13 or hypodiploidy; the high-risk group is made up of patients presenting with the t(14;16), the t(14;20), or deletion 17p13. Patients with deletion of chromosome 13 by metaphase cytogenetics (not by FISH) are also considered high risk. The mSMART guidelines do not take into account all cytogenetic abnormalities seen in myeloma samples. There has been considerable research performed to identify prognostic markers within patients, including mRNAs and cell-surface receptors such as CD20+ samples as a prognostic marker.[101] Chromosome 1 changes are important markers in myeloma; patients harboring the 1p deletion have a poor outcome.[102] The amplification of chromosome 1q has also been identified as an important locus in myeloma. Amplification of 1q21 is a poor prognosis marker in PCN and the frequency of 1q21 amplifications increases as the disease progresses.[30] Furthermore, studies have identified the chromosome 1q genes, NEK2 and CKS1B, as markers of aggressive disease and poor prognosis.[92,103] Presently, alterations to chromosome 1 are the only chromosomal markers not incorporated into the commonly accepted prognostic models.

GENETIC ABNORMALITIES IN IMMUNOGLOBULIN LIGHT-CHAIN AMYLOIDOSIS

The clonal plasma cell burden in AL is usually small and similar to that seen in patients with monoclonal gammopathy. Because the proliferation rate of plasma cells is very low, chromosomal aberrations need to be assessed by FISH analysis and not by conventional metaphase cytogenetics. Approximately 70 percent of patients with AL have FISH abnormalities, the most common being IgH translocations (48 percent), including t(11;14) and t(14;16). Other chromosomal abnormalities seen in AL include deletion 13/13q– and hyperdiploidy.[104] The t(11;14) occurs more frequently in AL (39 percent) than in monoclonal gammopathy or myeloma.[105] Although cases with t(4;14) abnormality have been reported, those are exceptional and deletion 17p13 is not seen in this form of amyloidosis. FISH analysis is important in this disease, because t(11;14) is associated with an inferior prognosis in amyloidosis in contrast to myeloma, where it is associated with a good prognosis. In another large study assessing the prognostic significance of cytogenetic abnormalities, t(11;14) was not associated with an inferior outcome, but gain of chromosome 1q21 clearly was.[106]

GENETIC ABNORMALITIES IN WALDENSTRÖM MACROGLOBULINEMIA

Alterations in one of myeloid differentiation primary response gene MYD88 have been identified in 90 percent of patients with macroglobulinemia.[107] MYD88 is an adaptor protein important in TLR and IL-1 receptor (IL-1R) signaling pathways. MYD88 is recruited to the activated receptor complex as a homodimer that complexes with the IL-1R–associated kinase (IRAK) 4 to activate IRAK 1. It leads to NF-κB activation via IκB α phosphorylation. Cell survival is enhanced by MYD88 overexpression, which leads to Bruton tyrosine kinase (BTK) phosphorylation. Combined use of IRAK and BTK inhibitors results in synergistic killing of MYD88-expressing macroglobulinemia cells. High rates of response have been observed in a clinical trial with a BTK inhibitor in relapsed and refractory patients.[108]

● THE MARROW MICROENVIRONMENT

The marrow microenvironment, discussed in detail in Chap. 5, provides a highly supportive tumor microenvironment (TME) for the development, growth, and survival of neoplastic cells in patients with myeloma. In the great majority of cases, the clonal expansion of these cells in the marrow is associated with increased blood vessel formation (neoangiogenesis) and, more importantly, myeloma bone disease (MBD).

Nonmalignant stromal cells in the marrow secrete cytokines and chemokines that promote myeloma cell growth and survival upon binding to specific receptors on the myeloma cell surface. Tumor promoters include IL-6, insulin-like growth factor 1 (IGF-1), VEGF, B-cell activating factor (BAFF), fibroblast growth factors (FGFs), stroma cell-derived factor 1α (SDF-1α, a.k.a. C-X-C motif chemokine 12 or CXCL12), and tumor necrosis factor α (TNF-α). Direct physical interaction of myeloma and marrow stromal cells by virtue of cell-to-cell adhesion may further enhance the cellular signaling pathways that are activated by cytokines and chemokines, thereby facilitating migration of myeloma cells to distant marrow and/or extramedullary sites (tumor dissemination). Myeloma-to-bone mesenchymal stem cell adhesion is also involved in the acquisition of drug resistance by tumor cells, underlying tumor relapse and/or refractory disease in patients with myeloma.[109]

HOMING AND ADHESION OF MYELOMA CELLS

Homing and adhesion of myeloma cells to the marrow microenvironment involves the CXCL12/CXCR4 pathway and a number of homo- or heterotypic adhesion factors, including CD44 (an anionic, nonsulfated glycosaminoglycan called hyaluronan), very-late antigen 4 (VLA-4, composed of integrins α_4 [CD49d] and β_1 [CD29]) and its receptor, vascular cell adhesion molecule 1 (VCAM-1, CD106), leukocyte function–associated antigen 1 (LFA-1, CD11a), neuronal cell–adhesion molecule (NCAM, CD56), intercellular adhesion molecule 1 (ICAM-1, CD54), and, importantly, syndecan 1 (CD138). Syndecan 1 is a transmembrane heparan sulfate–containing proteoglycan that is usually expressed at high levels on the myeloma cell surface. Syndecan 1-mediated adhesion of myeloma cells promotes adhesion-dependent drug resistance and bone resorption via expression of matrix metalloproteinases, among other mechanisms.

Adhesion of myeloma cells to mesenchymal cells activates pleiotropic cellular signal transduction pathways that mediate the proliferative and survival-enhancing response of myeloma cells upon interaction with the marrow microenvironment. Resistance of myeloma cells to cytotoxic drugs is also promoted. These pathways include NF-κB (nuclear factor kappa light-chain enhancer of activated B cells); PI3K/ AKT (phosphatidylinositol 3-kinase/protein kinase B/AKT oncogene),

RAS/RAF/MEK/ERK (rat sarcoma protein subfamily of small GTPase/ RAF protooncogene serine and threonine protein kinase/MAPK kinase/extracellular signal–regulated kinase) and JAK2/STAT3 (Janus kinase 2/signal transducers and activators of transcription 3). Engagement of these pathways results in upregulation of proteins that control cell cycle progression (e.g., D cyclins and Myc) and those that protect myeloma cells from programmed apoptotic cell death (e.g., BCL2, BCL-x$_L$, and MCL1).

The interplay of myeloma and mesenchymal cells is not the same in all subtypes of the disease. Instead, the genetic makeup of myeloma determines, in part, the interaction of tumor with the nonmalignant stromal cells in the marrow environment. For instance, myeloma cells harboring a MAF (v-MAF oncogene homologue)-activating chromosomal translocation, t(14;16), overexpress the adhesion factor, integrin β_7. This results in enhanced tumor cell adhesion to bone mesenchymal stem cells (BMSCs) relative to myeloma cells not containing a t(14;16).[110] Signaling pathways that govern interactions of myeloma and normal marrow cells also promote neoangiogenesis in the TME. The formation of new blood vessels, which is driven to a large extent by CXCL12/CXCR4 signaling and production of VEGF, B-FGFs, matrix metallopeptidases (MMPs), IGF-1, interleukins (e.g., IL-8, IL-1), angiopoietin 1, transforming growth factor β (TGF-β), platelet-derived growth factor (PDGF), and hepatocyte growth factor (HGF), is critical for myeloma progression and thus an important target of myeloma drug development.

MYELOMA BONE DISEASE

Increased bone resorption and suppressed bone formation leads to osteolytic lesions in patients with myeloma.[111,112] The main cytokines involved in that process are IL-6, receptor activator of NF-κB ligand (RANKL)/osteoprotegerin (OPG), BAFF, chemokine (C-C motif) ligand 3 (CCL3)/macrophage inflammatory protein (MIP)-1α, and VEGF. The main cell adhesion and integrin signaling pathways involved in that process are VLA-4/VCAM-1 and LFA-1/ICAM-1.[112,113] WNT/β-catenin signaling antagonists that inhibit osteoblast differentiation in myeloma also play an important role in the natural history of MBD. These include Dickkopf 1 (DKK1),[114] soluble-frizzled receptor-like proteins (sFRPs), and sclerostin. Inhibition of osteoblast differentiation drives the bone disease and, presumably, facilitates the expansion of myeloma cells[111] because upregulation of β-catenin–dependent osteoblast activity *in vivo* results in significant inhibition of myeloma cell growth,[116] relying on an ill-defined mechanism that appears to involve the small leucine-rich proteoglycan, decorin.[117]

RANK/RANKL/OPG PATHWAY

The receptor activator of NF-κB (RANK)/RANKL/OPG pathway is arguably one of the most important regulatory systems for homeostatic bone remodeling. RANK, a membrane-anchored signaling receptor of the TNF receptor family, is expressed on osteoclast (OC) precursors. Binding of its ligand, RANKL, expressed by osteoblasts (OBs) and BMSCs, induces osteoclastogenesis and activation of mature OCs. OPG, a soluble member of the TNF receptor family, is also produced by OBs and BMSCs. Because OPG acts as a soluble decoy receptor for RANKL, it blocks RANK-dependent OC maturation and activation. Thus, it is easy to understand that the ratio of RANKL and OPG significantly impacts the balance of bone resorption and bone deposition. Indeed, compared to normal individuals, marrow plasma of myeloma patients contains elevated levels of RANKL and reduced levels of OPG,[117] consistent with a proosteoclastogenic TME. Also, low serum levels of OPG correlate with advanced MBD in patients with myeloma.[118] In mouse models of MBD, treatment with OPG and OPG-like compounds prevented both bone destruction and myeloma growth *in vivo*.[119,120] Similarly, in patients with myeloma treated with thalidomide[121] or autologous stem cell transplantation[122] responding to therapy, the RANKL-to-OPG ratio normalized and bone resorption was inhibited. In aggregate, these findings indicate the RANK-RANKL-OPG axis is an important therapeutic target for MBD.

B-CELL ACTIVATION FACTOR

BAFF is a myeloma cell-promoting member of the TNF superfamily of proteins that is expressed by OCs and BMSCs. BAFF is significantly increased in the serum of patients with myeloma. In a preclinical study using a mouse model of myeloma, targeting BAFF by means of a neutralizing antibody led to reductions in tumor burden and osteolytic bone disease and increased survival.

DKK1 is an inhibitor of the WNT signaling pathway that plays a major role in MBD.[114] DKK1 inhibits OB differentiation and promotes OC maturation.[123] Patients responsive to myeloma drugs exhibit reduced serum levels of DKK1.

Activin A, a member of the TGF-β superfamily of proteins, activates a signaling pathway that results in phosphorylation of SMADs (homologues of *Drosophila*'s mothers against decapentaplegic [MAD] and *Caeno Rhabditis elegans*' small body size [SMA] proteins) followed by execution of a complex SMAD-dependent gene-expression program. Activin A is a stimulator of osteoclastogenesis and is overexpressed in myeloma.[124] IL-3, another stimulator of OCs, can induce the secretion of activin A by resident macrophages in the myeloma marrow microenvironment, providing a mechanism for the upregulation of activin A in patients with myeloma.[112] Levels of activin A in the marrow plasma of myeloma patients with osteolytic lesions (OLs) are increased.[125] RAP-011 is a soluble mouse activin A receptor that was shown to inhibit myeloma-like tumors and prevent OLs in laboratory mice.[124,126] Sotatercept (ACE-011), the human version of mouse RAP-011 is a soluble receptor of activin A and is undergoing clinical trials in patients with myeloma.

BRUTON TYROSINE KINASE

The metalloprotein, BTK, is a member of the Scr-related Tec family of protein kinases. BTK is a regulator of OC differentiation that is expressed in OCs (but not in OBs) and has been implicated in bone resorption. BTK is expressed in myeloma cells.[127,128] Genetic evidence indicates BTK may be crucial for neoplastic plasma cell development in laboratory mice.[129]

MYELOMA STEM CELL

Major progress has been made in the treatment of newly diagnosed myeloma patients with 80 percent achieving either a complete remission (CR) or near CR (nCR) and more than 50 percent surviving 10 years.[130] However, many patients ultimately relapse. Gene-expression profiles (GEPs) remain abnormal in myeloma patients with long-lasting remission (>10 years).[131] This finding suggests that the persistence of a myeloma cell population with low proliferative capacity and limited sensitivity to our most intensive therapies, points to the concept of a myeloma stem cell problem. There is no agreement on the specific phenotype of the myeloma stem cell, but side-population (SP) cells, which constitute a minor fraction of the myeloma cells, have the features of stem cells. Such cells have a greater clonogenic potential and drug resistance, whether isolated from myeloma cell lines or primary myeloma samples.[132,133] Many different groups have tried to identity the phenotype of myeloma stem cells. A drug-resistant subpopulation of memory B-cell–like cells with the CD138–/CD19+/CD27+ phenotype was identified and termed myeloma stem cells.[134,135] The CD138– cell population derived from myeloma cell lines contains significantly higher levels of ALDH, a marker for stem cells. In contrast to the CD138+ cells, the CD138– cells were not affected by the drugs we typically use in myeloma, such as lenalidomide, bortezomib, dexamethasone, and cyclophosphamide.[134] In an earlier study, human CD34+/CD45$_{low}$ clonotypic myeloma cells were shown to cause lytic bone lesions in a xenograft mouse model, and these CD34+ progenitors included approximately one-third of DNA aneuploid cells.[135,136] Mature CD138+ myeloma cell dedifferentiation to myeloma stem cells with a CD34+/CD138+/B7–/H1+ phenotype has been reported,[137] showing that myeloma cells have the plasticity to replenish the stem cell compartment if required, and that we should not think of stem cells as a static, but as a dynamic concept. CD38++/CD45– plasma cells proliferated successfully within an engrafted human fetal bone using the severe combined immune deficiency (SCID)-hu mouse model.[138,139] This could have been because of dedifferentiation of these more mature myeloma cells. It also has been demonstrated that the SP cells from different myeloma cell lines are able to generate more colonies than mature plasma cells. However, this SP cell population lacked correlation with CD138 expression.[132,133] To isolate multiple myeloma stem cells (MMSCs) from primary samples, we have relied on a functional characteristic of cancer stem cells, the ability to pump out the Hoechst dye, rather than on membrane markers, which are more likely to change with changing environmental conditions. To this functional marker, we have added a myeloma specific marker, either surface κ or λ light chain, based on the specific M-protein. Because drug-resistant myeloma cells are enriched in patients relapsing early after tandem autologous transplants, we compared GEPs at baseline and at relapse in 51 patients. The gene most differentially expressed at relapse was the retinoic receptor α (RARα). This receptor has two splice variants: α_1 and α_2. RARα_1 is present on all myeloma cells; RARα_2 expression is only present in one-third of newly diagnosed patients. The latter patients have a significantly inferior survival after tandem autotransplants.[140] In a subsequent study, we were able to show that increased RARα_2 expression conferred stem cell features to myeloma cells, such as increased drug resistance, increased clonogenic potential, activation of pathways typically found in a cancer stem cell (CSC) such as the Wnt and Hedgehog pathways, increased SP and ALDH levels, and increased expression of embryonic stem cell genes, such as Nanog, Oct4, and Sox2. These same characteristics were found in the SP+ and surface light-chain–restricted cells of primary myeloma samples. We also found that RARα_2 expressing CD138+ myeloma cells have a much higher expression of Oct4, Sox2, Nanog, TCF1, CCND1, and ABCC3. This indicates that RARα_2-positive myeloma cells show stem cell features and, therefore, have a worse outcome.[141]

● DIAGNOSIS OF PLASMA CELL NEOPLASM

TESTS OF SERUM

Because PCNs are B-cell malignancies derived from antibody-producing plasma cells in the marrow, which continue to secrete in the vast majority, an M-protein will be found in serum and/or urine in the majority of patients. The monoclonal protein is either an intact immunoglobulin or a component of the immunoglobulin. The most common types in myeloma are IgG and IgA; in Waldenström macroglobulinemia, it is IgM. The most common screening test to identify a serum M-protein is the serum protein electrophoresis (SPEP). While the quantity of M-protein is often considered a marker of tumor load, myeloma cells

are ineffective producers of immunoglobulins and produce 10 to 100 times less immunoglobulin per cell per day than a normal plasma cell. In addition, the more immature and more proliferative myeloma cells are, the less immunoglobulin per cell per day they secrete. In myeloma, there is an imbalance of heavy chains and light chains in favor of the light chains. In general, the more aggressive the myeloma, the more pronounced the imbalance in favor of excess light-chain secretion. The excess light chains cannot bind to heavy chains and can pass freely though the renal glomeruli. Monomeric FLC, characteristic κ, are cleared from the serum in 2 to 4 hours at 40 percent of the glomerular filtration rate (GFR), while dimeric FLC, typically λ, are cleared in 3 to 6 hours at 20 percent of GFR. Removal may take 2 to 3 days in patients with complete renal failure. This is in contrast to IgG, which has a plasma half-life of 21 days.

Although it has long been possible to measure the total amount (free plus bound to heavy chains) of light chains in the urine, our ability to measure serum FLCs became a reality early in the 21st century. This test is not only of high affinity and allows measurement of low concentrations of FLC, but it is also of high specificity and only measures unbound light chains. Serum FLC are several orders of magnitude lower than serum light chains bound to intact immunoglobulin and the test is based on an antibody that exclusively binds to an epitope of the FLC that is hidden if the light-chain molecule is bound to a heavy chain. Because the half-life of serum FLCs is much shorter than that of the intact immunoglobulin, serial serum FLCs allow assessment of success of therapy much earlier than serial M-protein levels. Patients with highest amount of light chains have the worst outcome.[142] The serum FLC ratio is an independent prognostic factor for progression of myeloma in monoclonal gammopathy and SMM.[143] Incorporation of serum FLCs into a staging system also improves risk stratification for patients with AL[144] and levels of serum FLCs correlate with tumor burden in macroglobulinemia..[145] The serum FLC assay is also an early indicator of relapse in myeloma. As explained above, both serum κ and λ concentrations increase with deteriorating renal function, but the ratio only changes slightly; with increasing renal failure the κ:λ ratio gradually increases. Diseases associated with generalized increased B-cell activation frequently have high concentrations of polyclonal immunoglobulins and high polyclonal FLC, but the κ:λ ratios will remain within normal range.

In addition to a SPEP and serum FLCs, it is important perform a serum immunofixation electrophoresis (sIFE) to identify the nature of the M-protein, and to measure the quantitative immunoglobulins. Many of the IgA and some of the IgG myelomas have their M-spike in the β-globulin region, where the M-protein level is less reliable because there is comigration of many other proteins. If an M-protein is identified on SPEP and sIFE does not identify the heavy chain, quantitative analysis of IgD and IgE should be performed. Most IgD myelomas are associated with lambda light chains.

TESTS OF URINE

A typical myeloma workup will have a 24-hour urine collection for total protein, urine protein electrophoresis (UPEP), urine M-protein, and urine immunofixation electrophoresis (uIFE). In contrast to the serum FLCs, the role of urine FLCs is much less clear and is generally not used. In the era of serum FLC assays, some experts believe that urine analysis can be eliminated. In a study by the Mayo Clinic of 428 patients, there were only two cases where a urinary monoclonal protein was missed by omitting urine analysis (0.5 percent). These two cases did not require any medical intervention.[146] When patients have a large amount of albuminuria in the presence of PCN with or without urine M-protein, the possibility of AL should be entertained, either primary AL or AL in the context of myeloma.

MARROW EXAMINATION

Marrow aspirate and biopsy are essential in the workup of PCN. It is best not to rely solely on a marrow aspirate. Myeloma cells have the tendency to form small or large clusters and myeloma is not evenly distributed throughout the marrow. The marrow may be falsely negative in the presence of overt myeloma. In a normal marrow with normal cellularity, there may be up to 2 percent plasma cells present. However, the percentage of plasma cells can be much higher in reactive marrows and hypoplastic or aplastic marrows in the absence of PCN. In a normal marrow, there can be some clustering of plasma cells around the blood vessels. However, the presence of larger clusters of plasma cells away from the blood vessels should alert one to the possibility of PCN, especially myeloma. In addition to the morphologic examination, the biopsy slides should be stained with a CD138 monoclonal antibody, which is a specific immune marker for plasma cells. If the diagnosis of PCN is not clear based on morphology and CD138 staining, *in situ* hybridization for cytoplasmic κ and λ should be used to evaluate whether the plasma cells are clonal (light-chain restricted).

It is customary to perform flow cytometry, metaphase cytogenetics, and FISH analysis on myeloma samples. Flow cytometry at diagnosis is mainly performed to identify aberrant surface markers on myeloma cells, which can be used subsequently to assess MRD. The identification of an accurate gating strategy is a critical component of a reproducible and sensitive immunophenotypic analysis. The best gating strategy uses a combination of CD38, CD138, CD45, and light scatter characteristics. The previously used gating method of CD38 and CD45 decreases the risk of contamination with other cells, but excludes the CD45+ cells, which can constitute the majority of the plasma cells. It is recommended that at least a four-color instrument be used, as at least two antigens (CD38 and CD138) are required after the initial analysis with CD138, CD38, CD45, and light scatter, to gate plasma cells accurately. When used for MRD, at least 100 neoplastic plasma cell events should be acquired. CD56 and CD19 should always be assessed. CD56 is negative on normal plasma cells but is positive on myeloma cells, while the opposite is true for CD19. It is also recommended to stain for CD117 and CD20, which are negative on normal plasma cells and can be aberrantly expressed on myeloma cells. CD28 and CD200 are negative or only weakly expressed on normal plasma cells, but can be strongly positive on myeloma cells, whereas CD27 and CD81 are strongly expressed on normal plasma cells, but weak or negative on myeloma cells. It is important to remember that there is no single marker that can systematically differentiate neoplastic cells from normal plasma cells. Also, the percentage of plasma cells detected by flow cytometry is typically lower than that found by morphology.[147] The importance of metaphase cytogenetics and FISH analysis was outlined above in the section Techniques to assess cytogenetic information. However, metaphase cytogenetic analysis remains important and is the best marker to differentiate between stroma-dependent (early) and stroma-independent (advanced) myeloma. The metaphases with normal cytogenetics obtained in most patients with myeloma are derived from the remaining normal hematopoietic elements and not from the myeloma cells. If myeloma cells are stroma-dependent, they will die soon after being removed from their supporting microenvironment, while stroma-independent myeloma cells are able to grow and divide in the absence of a supporting microenvironment.[148]

IMAGING STUDIES

Bone disease is present in 70 percent of patients with myeloma at diagnosis. A skeletal X-ray survey has long been considered the gold standard for assessing bone disease in myeloma. However, the sensitivity and specificity of a skeletal survey is low. At least 50 to 75 percent of trabecular bone must be lost to see a lytic lesion. The false-negative rate varies between 30 and 70 percent, which leads to significant underestimation in diagnosing and staging of patients with myeloma. The skeletal survey does not provide us with a direct image of the tumor cells, but rather with the consequence of tumor cells being present or having been present. Bone lesions in myeloma seldom heal and in most cases, there is no healing at all or at the most there is a sclerotic rim around the bone lesion. Therefore, a skeletal survey is not a good technique to assess response to treatment or to diagnose early recurrence of myeloma. Much better imaging techniques have become available in the form of ^{18}F-fluorodeoxyglucose positron emission tomography–computed tomography (PET/CT) and MRI. When used in combination, PET/CT scan and MRI were found to have specificity and a positive predictive value of virtually 100 percent, which is invaluable to clinicians assessing the efficacy of intensive and expensive treatment approaches with the goal to cure myeloma.[149]

Magnetic Resonance Imaging

Between CT and MRI the latter is the more specific test. A complete MRI examination should include a series of sequences to permit identification of focal and diffuse marrow involvement, including spin echo (T1 and T2 weighted), gradient echo (T2), and short T1 inversion recovery (STIR) sequences. MRI should include the axial bones with active hematopoiesis in adults (skull, spine, sternum, shoulders and upper humeri, pelvis, and upper femora). In a study from the University of Arkansas for Medical Sciences, using these parameters and including 611 myeloma patients treated uniformly with tandem transplants, 74 percent had focal myeloma lesions compared with 56 percent on skeletal survey and 52 percent of patients with negative skeletal surveys had focal lesions on the MRI. Resolution of the MRI focal lesions after treatment occurred slowly, but ultimately was seen in 60 percent of patients and conferred a superior overall survival.[150] MRI should be used routinely for the staging, prognosis and response assessment of patients treated with curative intent.

^{18}F-Fluorodeoxyglucose Positron Emission Tomography–Computed Tomography

One of the major advantages of the PET/CT scan is that it allows assessing the presence of extramedullary myeloma, which is present in 6 percent of the patients and associated with a significantly inferior overall survival based on two large studies. In a study of 239 patients receiving uniform therapy, the presence of more than three fluorodeoxyglucose (FDG)-avid focal lesions was associated with a significantly inferior overall and event-free survival. In contrast, complete FDG suppression prior to the first transplant conferred a significantly better outcome.[151] These data were confirmed in an Italian study including 192 patients.[152] A PET-CR occurs earlier than a clinical CR and a MRI-CR happens much later and less frequently.

OTHER IMPORTANT TESTS

β_2-Microglobulin

The serum β2-microglobulin (β2m) is one of the most important prognostic factors in myeloma; β2m is a small protein that associates with human leukocyte antigen class I and is almost exclusively catabolized in the kidneys. Its best-characterized function is to interact with and stabilize the tertiary structure of major histocompatibility complexn (MCH) class α chain. The main source of β2m in the serum is membrane turnover. It reflects tumor load and renal function; however, it predicts survival irrespective of renal function and Durie-Salmon stage.[153] The exact underlying biologic significance of β2m remains obscure, but interactions with drug resistance pathways may exist. β2m in high concentrations retards the generation of monocyte-derived dendritic cells.[154]

Serum $\beta 2m$ and albumin levels form the basis for the International Staging System, which has major prognostic significance.[99]

High-risk myeloma, defined by genetic abnormalities, is independent of the International Staging System and the latter had only significant prognostic value in patients with a low-risk gene expression profile and normal metaphase cytogenetics.[155]

Serum Lactic Dehydrogenase Levels

The significance of high serum lactate dehydrogenase (LDH) levels in the absence of any other cause, such as liver disease or hemolytic anemia, predicting poor prognosis has long been recognized in myeloma.[156] Although rarely observed in the early phase of the disease, marked elevations of LDH were detected in up to 20 percent of patients with disease progressing after vincristine, Adriamycin, and dexamethasone chemotherapy. High LDH levels were associated with hypercalcemia, elevated serum $\beta 2m$ levels, extramedullary manifestations, plasmablastic morphology, and short overall survival duration, despite marked (usually very transient) antitumor responses to high-dose therapy. The same poor prognosis was noted in patients with initially normal LDH levels in who marked LDH increments were induced by treatment, presumably resulting from tumor lysis syndrome as an indicator of rapidly proliferative myeloma.[156] Close correlations with plasma cell labeling index and plasmablastic morphology has been demonstrated.[157] Elevated serum LDH levels at diagnosis also emerged as a significant prognostic factor in an analysis of 155 newly diagnosed patients who received at least one course of high-dose therapy with autologous stem cell transplantation (ASCT), irrespective of the deletion of chromosome 13.[158]

MINIMAL RESIDUAL DISEASE

Methods to assess MRD include allele-specific oligonucleotide PCR (ASO-PCR), multiparameter flow cytometry (MPF), fluorescent-PCR (F-PCR) and high-throughput sequencing-based MRD assessment.

Allele-Specific Oligonucleotide Polymerase Chain Reaction

ASO-PCR can detect one clonal cell in 10^5 normal cells. It remains a costly and labor-intensive assay to perform because a specific probe needs to be generated for each patient and it is unsuccessful in approximately 30 percent of patients.[159] In a relatively small study of 40 patients who achieved either a CR or very good partial response after autologous transplantation and who received consolidation with bortezomib, thalidomide, and dexamethasone (VTD), eight patients achieved a molecular remission: two only in one sample and six had at least two consecutive negative samples. With a median followup of 26 months from study entry, no clinical relapses were seen in patients achieving a molecular remission, although one molecular relapse was seen, while eight clinical relapses occurred in patients not a achieving a molecular remission. Importantly, VTD consolidation decreased the tumor load further after transplantation.[161] In contrast to earlier held opinions that molecular remissions could only be obtained with allotransplantation, this study showed that molecular remission were also seen after autologous transplants followed by consolidation therapy with VTD.

Multiparameter Flow Cytometry

Multiparameter flow cytometry (MPC) has the advantage of being readily available and short turn-around time. It requires sophisticated analysis, but is automated. This technique can detect one clonal cell in 10^4 normal cells. In the MRC Myeloma 9 study, MRD was assessed by MPF in 397 patients who received an autotransplant and 245 patients who were treated with a nontransplantation approach. A six-color panel was applied. For pretreatment samples 100,000 events were acquired,

while for the posttreatment samples a minimum of 500,000 events were analyzed. In the transplantation group, absence of MRD at day 100 after transplantation, observed in 62 percent of patients, was highly predictive of a favorable outcome (progression-free survival [PFS]: p <0.001; overall survival [OS]: p = 0.018). This outcome advantage was seen irrespective of cytogenetic findings, but more clearly in patients with adverse cytogenetics (p <0.001 vs. p = 0.014). There was no complete agreement between immunofixation electrophoresis (IFE)-negative CR and absence of MRD by MPF. Approximately 15 percent of patients in CR still had measurable disease by MPF, while 25 percent of MRD-negative patients failed to achieve a CR by IFE. The effect of thalidomide maintenance therapy after transplantation was also assessed. The best outcomes were seen in patients who achieved MRD negativity and were maintained on thalidomide, while the outcome was worst in patients who failed to achieve MRD negativity and did not receive thalidomide maintenance. In the MRD-positive group at day 100, 28 percent of those receiving thalidomide became MRD-negative, while in those not receiving thalidomide maintenance only 3 percent became MRD-negative (p = 0.025). Finally, MRD assessment at the end of induction therapy in the nontransplantation group had no predictive value; only 15 percent of such patients became MRD-negative.[161] It should be noted that there is a large heterogeneity in assessing MRD by MPF in the United States in terms of events acquired and number of antibodies used.[162] If outcomes of therapies are based on MPF, it is critical that this technique becomes standardized and suitable quality controls are in place.

Fluorescent Polymerase Chain Reaction

F-PCR can detect one clonal cell in 10^3 normal cells and is thus less sensitive than ASO-PCR and MPF. However, F-PCR is rapid, affordable, and easy to perform. High-molecular-weight DNA is isolated from 500 μL of marrow. Three different multiplex PCRs are used: *IGH* D-J, *IGK* V-J, and KDE rearrangements. The clonal population is identified at diagnosis. Patient with a visible lack of a clonal peak identified at diagnosis were considered F-PCR–negative. MRD was assessed in 130 newly diagnosed myeloma patients. The test was informative in 91.5 percent of patients. MPC was used in parallel with F-PCR. After induction, 64 patients achieved a molecular response and 66 did not. Median PFS was 61 versus 36 months (p = 0.001). The corresponding PFS with MPC was 67 versus 42 months for MPC– and MPC+ patients (p = 0.005).[163]

High-Throughput Sequencing-Based Minimal Residual Disease Assessment

High-throughput sequencing-based MRD assessment relies on amplification and sequencing of immunoglobulin gene segments using consensus primers. It employs the IGH-VDJ$_H$, IGH-DJ$_H$, and IGK assays. The assay can detect one clonal cell in 10^6 normal cells and is 1 log more sensitive than ASO-PCR. The prognostic value of this test was assessed in 133 myeloma patients enrolled in the GEM myeloma trials and was compared to MPC and ASO-PCR. The test was informative in 91 percent of patients. Concordance between deep sequencing and MPC or ASO-PCR was 83 percent and 85 percent, respectively. Patients who were MRD– by deep sequencing had a significantly longer time to progression (80 vs. 31 months; p <0.0001). In CR patients, the time to progression remained significantly longer in MRD– patients (131 vs. 35 months; p = 0.0009).[95]

There is no doubt that assessment of MRD will receive more attention in the coming years to guide the clinicians in their treatment decisions and to individualize patient care. However, it should not be automatically concluded that MRD– obtained after continuation of aggressive therapy to ultimately reach MRD– status which was not achieved after a standard aggressive approach will have the same prognostic significance as MRD– obtained with standard intensive approaches. It will also be important to establish what degree of tumor reduction has the highest prognostic significance. Extremely sensitive techniques might not necessarily provide better prognostic information than somewhat less-sensitive techniques.

REFERENCES

1. Lindqvist EK, Goldin LR, Landgren O, et al: Personal and family history of immune-related conditions increase the risk of plasma cell disorders: A population based study. *Blood* 118:6284, 2011.
2. Landgren O, Kyle RA, Pfeiffer RM, et al: Monoclonal gammopathy of undetermined significance consistently precedes multiple myeloma: A prospective study. *Blood* 113:5412, 2009.
3. Weiss BM, Abadie J, Verma P, et al: A monoclonal gammopathy precedes multiple myeloma in most patients. *Blood* 113:5418, 2009.
4. Landgren O, Kyle RA, Hoppin JA, et al: Pesticide exposure and risk of monoclonal gammopathy of undetermined significance in the agricultural health study. *Blood* 113:6386, 2009.
5. Brown LM, Gridley G, Check D, Landgren O: Risk of multiple myeloma and monoclonal gammopathy of undetermined significance among white and black male United States veterans with prior autoimmune, infectious, inflammatory and allergic disorders. *Blood* 111:3388, 2008.
6. Landgren O, Kristinsson SY, Goldin LR, et al: Risk of plasma cell and lymphoproliferative disorders about 14621 first-degree relatives of 4458 patients with monoclonal gammopathy of undetermined significance in Sweden. *Blood* 114:791, 2009.
7. Vachon CM, Kyle RA, Therneau TM, et al: Increased risk of monoclonal gammopathy in first-degree relatives of patients with multiple myeloma or monoclonal gammopathy of undetermined significance. *Blood* 114:785, 2009.
8. Grass S, Pruess KD, Ahlgrimm M, et al: Association of dominantly inherited hyperphosphorylated paraprotein target with sporadic and familial multiple myeloma and monoclonal gammopathy of undetermined significance: A case control study. *Lancet Oncol* 10:950, 2009.
9. Preuss KD, Pfreundschuh M, Fadle N, et al: Hyperphosphorylation of autoantigenic targets of paraproteins is due to inactivations of PP2A. *Blood* 118:3340, 2011.
10. Zwick C, Held G, Augh M, et al: Over one-third of African American MGUS and multiple myeloma patients are carries of hyperphosphorylated paratarg-7, an autosomal dominantly inherited risk factor for MGUS/MM. *Int J Cancer* 135:934, 2014.
11. Fonseca R, Bailey RJ, Ahman, et al: Genomic abnormalities in monoclonal gammopathy of undetermined significance. *Blood* 100:1417, 2002.
12. Fonseca R, Barlogie B, Bataille R, et al: Genetics and cytogenetics of multiple myeloma: A workshop report. *Cancer Res* 64:1546, 2004.
13. Kuehl WM, Bergsagel PL: Multiple myeloma: Evolving genetic events and host interactions. *Nat Rev Cancer* 2:175, 2002.
14. Kuehl WM, Bergsagel PL: Chromosome translocations in multiple myeloma. *Oncogene* 20:5611, 2001.
15. Rajkumar SV, Kyle RA, Therneau TM, et al: Serum free light chain ratio is an independent risk factor for progression in monoclonal gammopathy of undetermined significance. *Blood* 106:812, 2005.
16. Perez-Persona E, Vidriales MB, Mateo G, et al: New criteria to identify risk of progression in monoclonal gammopathy of uncertain significance and smoldering multiple myeloma based on multiparameter flow cytometry analysis of bone marrow plasma cells. *Blood* 110:2586, 2007.
17. Cesana C, Klersy C, Barbarano L, et al: Prognostic factors for malignant transformation in monoclonal gammopathy of undetermined significance and smoldering multiply myeloma. *J Clin Oncol* 20:1625, 2002.
18. Facon T, Menard FJ, Chaux JL, et al: Prognostic factors in low tumor mass asymptomatic multiple myeloma: A report on 91 patients. *Am J Hematol* 48:71, 1995.
19. Wisloff F, Andersen P, Andersson TR, et al: Incidence and follow up of asymptomatic multiple myeloma. *Eur J Haematol* 47:338, 1991.
20. Weber DM, Dimopoulos MA, Moulopoulos LA, et al: Prognostic features of asymptomatic multiple myeloma. *Br J Haematol* 97:810, 1997.
21. Alexanian R, Barlogie B, Dixon D: Prognosis of asymptomatic multiple myeloma. *Arch Intern Med* 148:1963, 1988.
22. Dimopoulos MA, Moulopoulos A, Smith T, et al: Risk of disease progression in asymptomatic multiple myeloma. *Am J Med* 94:57, 1993.
23. Dimopoulos MA, Terpos E, Comenzo RL, et al: International myeloma working group consensus statement and guidelines regarding the current role of imaging techniques in the diagnosis and monitoring of multiple myeloma. *Leukemia* 23:1545, 2009.
24. Kyle RA, Remstein ED, Therneau TM, et al: Clinical course and prognosis of smoldering (asymptomatic) multiple myeloma. *N Engl J Med* 356:2582, 2007.
25. Dispenzieri A, Kyle RA, Katzmann JA, et al: Immunoglobulin free light chain ratio is an independent risk factor for progression of smoldering (asymptomatic) multiple myeloma. *Blood* 111:785, 2008.
26. Landgren O: Monoclonal gammopathy of undetermined significance of smoldering multiple myeloma: New insights into pathophysiology and epidemiology. *Hematology Am Soc Hematol Educ Program* 2010:295, 2010.
27. Hallek M, Bergsagel PL, Anderson KC: Multiple myeloma: Increasing evidence for a multistep transformation process. *Blood* 91:3, 1998.
28. Cheng WJ, Glebov O, Bergsagel PL, Kuehl WM: Genetic events in the pathogenesis of multiple myeloma. *Best Pract Res Clin Haematol* 20:571, 2007.
29. Chiecchio L, Dagrada GP, Protheroe RK, et al: Loss of 1p and rearrangement of MYC are associated with progression of smoldering myeloma to myeloma: Sequential analysis of a single case. *Haematologica* 94:1024, 2009.
30. Hanamura I, Stewart JP, Huang Y, et al: Frequent gain of chromosome band 1q21 in plasma cell dyscrasias detected by fluorescence *in situ* hybridization: Incidence increases from MGUS to relapse myeloma and is related to prognosis and disease progression following tandem stem-cell transplantation. *Blood* 108:1724, 2006.
31. Rosinol L, Carrio A, Blade J, et al: Comparative genomic hybridization identifies two variant of smoldering multiple myeloma. *Br J Haematol* 130:729, 2005.
32. Anguiano A, Tuchman SA, Acharya C, et al: Gene expression profiles of tumor biology provide a novel approach to prognosis and may guide the selection of therapeutic targets in multiple myeloma. *J Clin Oncol* 27:4197, 2009.
33. Avet-Loiseau H, Gerson F, Magrangeas F, et al: Rearrangements of the c-MYC oncogene are present in 15% of primary human multiple myeloma tumors. *Blood* 98:3082, 2001.
34. Walker BA, Wardell CP, Melchor L, et al: Intraclonal heterogeneity is a critical early event in the development of myeloma and precedes the development of clinical symptoms. *Leukemia* 28:384, 2014.
35. Landgren O, Rajkumar SV, Pfeiffer RM, Kyle RA, Katzmann JA, Dispenzieri A, et al: Obesity is associated with an increased risk of monoclonal gammopathy of undetermined significance (MGUS) among African-American and Caucasian women. *Blood* 116:1056, 2010.
36. Carson KR, Bates ML, Tomasson MH: The skinny on obesity and plasma cell myeloma: A review of the literature. *Bone Marrow Transplant* 49:1009, 2014.
37. Teras LR, Kitahara CM, Birmann BM, et al: Body size and multiple myeloma mortality: A pooled analysis of 20 prospective studies. *Br J Haematol* 166:667, 2014.
38. Murphy F, Kroll ME, Pirie K, et al: Body size in relation to incidence of subtypes of haematological malignancy in the prospective Million Women Study. *Br J Cancer* 108:2390, 2013.
39. Hofmann JN, Moore SC, Lim U, et al: Body mass index and physical activity at different ages and risk of multiple myeloma in the NIH-AARP diet and health study. *Am J Epidemiol* 177:776, 2013.
40. Wallin A, Larsson SC: Body mass index and risk of multiple myeloma: A meta-analysis of prospective studies. *Eur J Cancer* 47:1606, 2011.
41. Calle EE, Rodriguez C, Walker-Thurmond K, Thun MJ: Overweight, obesity, and mortality from cancer in a prospectively studied cohort of U.S. adults. *N Engl J Med* 348:1625, 2003.
42. Dhodapkar MV: Adipokines in MM: Time to trim the fat. *Blood* 118:5716, 2011.
43. Birmann BM, Giovannucci EL, Rosner BA, Colditz GA: Regular aspirin use and risk of multiple myeloma: A prospective analysis in the health professionals follow up study and nurses' health study. *Cancer Prev Res (Phila)* 7:33, 2014.
44. Ding J, Yuan L, Huang RB, Chen G: Aspirin inhibits proliferation and induces apoptosis of multiple myeloma cells through regulation of Bcl-2 and Bax and suppression of VEGF. *Eur J Haematol* 93:329, 2014.
45. Alexander DD, Mink PJ, Adami HO, et al: Multiple myeloma: A review of epidemiologic literature. *Int J Cancer* 120:40, 2007.
46. Mohamed-Ali V, Goodrick S, Rawesh A, et al: Subcutaneous adipose tissue releases IL-6 but not tumor necrosis factor-alpha, *in vivo*. *J Clin Endocrinol Metab* 82:4196, 1997.
47. Morgan GJ, Davies FE, Linet M: Myeloma aetiology and epidemiology. *Biomed Pharmacother* 56:223, 2002.
48. Hsu WL, Preston DL, Soda M, et al: The incidence of leukemia, lymphoma and multiple myeloma among atomic bomb survivors: 1950–2001. *Radiat Res* 179:361, 2013.
49. Wang JX, Boice JD, Li BX, et al: Cancer among medical diagnostic x-ray workers in China. *J Natl Cancer Inst* 80:344, 1988.
50. Goedert JJ, Cote TR, Virgo P, et al: Spectrum of AIDS-associated malignant disorders. *Lancet* 351:1833, 1988.
51. Grulich AE, Wan X, Law MG, et al: Risk of cancer in people with AIDS. *AIDS* 13:839, 1999.
52. Duberg A, Nordstrom M, Torner A, et al: Non-Hodgkin's lymphoma and other non-hepatic malignancies in Swedish patient with hepatitis C virus infection. *Hepatology* 41:652, 2005.
53. Linet MS, Humphrrey RL, Mehl ES, et al: A case control and family study of WM. *Leukemia* 7:1363, 1993.
54. Giordano TP, Henderson L, Landgren O, et al: Risk of non-Hodgkin lymphoma and lymphoproliferative precursor diseases in US veterans with hepatitis C virus. *JAMA* 297:2010, 2007.
55. Koshiol J, Gridley G, Engels EA, et al: Chronic immune stimulation and subsequent Waldenström macroglobulinemia. *Arch Intern Med* 168:1903, 2008.
56. Kristinsson SY, Koshiol J, Goldin LR, et al: Immune related and inflammatory conditions and risk of lymphoplasmacytic lymphoma or Waldenström macroglobulinemia. *J Natl Cancer Inst* 102:557, 2010.
57. Fine JM, Lambin P, Massari M, Leroux P: Malignant evolution of asymptomatic monoclonal IgM after seven and fifteen years in two siblings of a patient with Waldenström's macroglobulinemia. *Acta Med Scand* 211:237, 1982.
58. McMaster ML, Goldin LR, Bai Y, et al: Genome wide linkage screen for Waldenstrom macroglobulinemia susceptibility loci in high risk families. *Am J Hum Genet* 79:695, 2006.

59. Ogmundsdottir HM, Johannesson GM, Sceinsdottir S, et al: Familial macroglobuline-mia: Hyperactive B-cells but normal natural killer function. *Scand J Immunol* 40:195, 1994.
60. Treon SP, Hunter ZR, Aggarwal A, et al: Characterization of familial Waldenstrom's macroglobulinemia. *Ann Oncol* 17:488, 2006.
61. Kristinsson SY, Goldin LR, McMaster ML, et al: Risk of lymphoproliferative disorders among first-degree relatives of lymphoplasmacytic lymphoma/Waldenstrom macro-globulinemia patients: A population-based study in Sweden. *Blood* 112:3052, 2008.
62. McMaster ML: Familial Waldenstrom's macroglobulinemia. *Semin Oncol* 30:146, 2003.
63. Treon SP, Tripsas C, Hanzis C, et al: Familial disease predisposition impacts treatment outcome in patients with Waldenström macroglobulinemia. *Clin Lymphoma Myeloma Leuk* 12:433, 2012.
64. Royer RH, Koshoil J, Vasquez LG, et al: Differential characteristics of Waldenström macroglobulinemia according to patterns of familial aggregation. *Blood* 115:4464, 2010.
65. Zhan F, Tian E, Bumm K, et al: Gene expression profiling of human plasma cell differ-entiation and classification of multiple myeloma based on similarities to distinct stages of late-stage B-cell development. *Blood* 101:1128, 2003.
66. Silacci P, Mottet A, Steimle V, et al: Developmental extinction of major histocompati-bility complex class II gene expression in plasmocytes is mediated by silencing of the transactivator gene CIITA. *J Exp Med* 180:1329, 1994.
67. Calame KL: Plasma cells: Finding new light at the end of B cell development. *Nat Immunol* 2:1103, 2001.
68. Hargreaves DC, Hyman PL, Lu TT, et al: A coordinated change in chemokine respon-siveness guides plasma cell movements. *J Exp Med* 194:45, 2001.
69. Barberis A, Widenhorn K, Vitelli L, Busslinger M: A novel B-cell lineage-specific tran-scription factor present at early but not late stages of differentiation. *Genes Dev* 4:849, 1990.
70. Nutt SL, Eberhard D, Horcher M, et al: Pax5 determines the identity of B cells from the beginning to the end of B-lymphopoiesis. *Int Rev Immunol* 20:65, 2001.
71. Reimold AM, Iwakoshi NN, Manis J, et al: Plasma cell differentiation requires the tran-scription factor XBP-1. *Nature* 412:300, 2001.
72. Bergsagel PL, Kuehl WM: Molecular pathogenesis and a consequent classification of multiple myeloma. *J Clin Oncol* 23:6333, 2005.
73. Greenman C, Stephens P, Smith R, et al: Patterns of somatic mutation in human cancer genomes. *Nature* 446:153, 2007.
74. Bergsagel PL, Kuehl WM, Zhan F, Sawyer J, et al: Cyclin D dysregulation: An early and unifying pathogenic event in multiple myeloma. *Blood* 106:296, 2005.
75. Kotani A, Kakazu N, Tsuruyama T, et al: Activation-induced cytidine deaminase (AID) promotes B cell lymphomagenesis in Emu-cMyc transgenic mice. *Proc Natl Acad Sci U S A* 104:1616, 2007.
76. Landgren O, Kyle RA, Pfeiffer RM, et al: Monoclonal gammopathy of undetermined significance (MGUS) consistently precedes multiple myeloma: A prospective study. *Blood* 113:5412, 2009.
77. Kalff MW, Hijmans W: Immunoglobulin analysis in families of macroglobulinemia patients. *Clin Exp Immunol* 5:361, 1969.
78. Landgren O, Kristinsson SY, Goldin LR, et al: Risk of plasma cell and lymphoprolifer-ative disorders among 14621 first-degree relatives of 4458 patients with monoclonal gammopathy of undetermined significance in Sweden. *Blood* 114:791, 2009.
79. Annunziata CM, Davis RE, Demchenko Y, et al: Frequent engagement of the classical and alternative NF-kappaB pathways by diverse genetic abnormalities in multiple mye-loma. *Cancer Cell* 12:115, 2007.
80. Keats JJ, Fonseca R, Chesi M, et al: Promiscuous mutations activate the noncanonical NF-kappaB pathway in multiple myeloma. *Cancer Cell* 12:131, 2007.
81. Bezieau S, Devilder MC, Avet-Loiseau H, et al: High incidence of N and K-Ras acti-vating mutations in multiple myeloma and primary plasma cell leukemia at diagnosis. *Hum Mutat* 18:212, 2001.
82. Liu P, Leong T, Quam L, et al: Activating mutations of N- and K-ras in multiple mye-loma show different clinical associations: Analysis of the Eastern Cooperative Oncol-ogy Group Phase III Trial. *Blood* 88:2699, 1996.
83. Rasmussen T, Kuehl M, Lodahl M, et al: Possible roles for activating RAS mutations in the MGUS to MM transition and in the intramedullary to extramedullary transition in some plasma cell tumors. *Blood* 105:317, 2005.
84. Levine AJ: P53, the cellular gatekeeper for growth and division. *Cell* 88:323, 1997.
85. Matlashewski G, Lamb P, Pim D, et al: Isolation and characterization of a human p53 cDNA clone: Expression of the human p53 gene. *EMBO J* 3:3257, 1984.
86. Chng WJ, Price-Troska T, Gonzalez-Paz N, et al: Clinical significance of TP53 mutation in myeloma. *Leukemia* 21:582, 2007.
87. Neri A, Baldini L, Trecca D, et al: P53 gene mutations in multiple myeloma are associ-ated with advanced forms of malignancy. *Blood* 81:128, 1993.
88. Fonseca R, Harrington D, Oken MM, et al: Biological and prognostic significance of interphase fluorescence in situ hybridization detection of chromosome 13 abnormali-ties (delta13) in multiple myeloma: An eastern cooperative oncology group study. *Cancer Res* 62:715, 2002.
89. Klein B, Seckinger A, Moehler T, Hose D: Molecular pathogenesis of multiple mye-loma: Chromosomal aberrations, changes in gene expression, cytokine networks, and the bone marrow microenvironment. *Recent Results Cancer Res* 183:39, 2011.
90. Shaughnessy JD Jr, Zhan F, Burington BE, et al: A validated gene expression model of high-risk multiple myeloma is defined by deregulated expression of genes mapping to chromosome 1. *Blood* 109:2276, 2007.
91. Gearhart J, Pashos EE, Prasad MK: Pluripotency redux—Advances in stem-cell research. *N Engl J Med* 157:1469, 2007.
92. Zhou W, Yang Y, Xia J, et al: NEK2 induces drug resistance mainly through activation of efflux drug pumps and is associated with poor prognosis in myeloma and other cancers. *Cancer Cell* 23:48, 2013.
93. Pei XY, Dai Y, Felthousen J, et al: Circumvention of Mcl-1-dependent drug resistance by simultaneous Chk1 and MEK1/2 inhibition in human multiple myeloma cells. *PLoS One* 9:e89064, 2014.
94. Chapman MA, Lawrence MS, Keats JJ, et al: Initial genome sequencing and analysis of multiple myeloma. *Nature* 471:467, 2011.
95. Martinez-Lopez J, Lahuerta JJ, Pepin F, et al: Prognostic value of deep sequencing method for minimal residual disease detection in multiple myeloma. *Blood* 123:3073, 2014.
96. Walker BA, Leone PE, Jenner MW, et al: Integration of global SNP-based mapping and expression arrays reveals key regions, mechanisms, and genes important in the patho-genesis of multiple myeloma. *Blood* 108:1733, 2006.
97. Avet-Loiseau H, Attal M, Moreau P, et al: Genetic abnormalities and survival in multiple myeloma: The experience of the Intergroupe Francophone du Myelome. *Blood* 109:3489, 2007.
98. Van Wier S, Braggio E, Baker A, et al: Hypodiploid multiple myeloma is characterized by more aggressive molecular markers than non-hyperdiploid multiple myeloma. *Hae-matologica* 98:1586, 2013.
99. Greipp PR, San Miguel J, Durie BG, et al: International staging system for multiple myeloma. *J Clin Oncol* 23:3412, 2005.
100. Mikhael JR, Dingli D, Roy V, et al: Management of newly diagnosed symptomatic mul-tiple myeloma: Updated Mayo Stratification of Myeloma and Risk-Adapted Therapy (mSMART) consensus guidelines 2013. *Mayo Clin Proc* 88:360, 13.
101. Liu J, Gu Z, Yang Y, et al: A subset of CD20 MM patients without the t(11;14) are asso-ciated with poor prognosis and a link to aberrant expression of Wnt signaling. *Hematol Oncol* 32:215, 2014.
102. Ouyang J, Gou X, Ma Y, et al: Prognostic value of 1p deletion for multiple myeloma: A meta-analysis. *Int J Lab Hematol* 36:555, 2014.
103. Zhan F, Colla S, Wu X, et al: CKS1B, overexpressed in aggressive disease, regulates multiple myeloma growth and survival through SKP2- and p27Kip1-dependent and -independent mechanisms. *Blood* 109:4995, 2007.
104. Bryce AH, Ketterling RP, Gertz MA, et al: Translocation t(11;14) and survival of patients with light chain (AL) amyloidosis. *Haematologica* 94:380, 2009.
105. Fonseca R, Ahmann GJ, Jalal SM, et al: Chromosomal abnormalities in systemic amy-loidosis. *Br J Haematol* 103:704, 2002.
106. Bochtler T, Hegenbart U, Kunz C, et al: Gain of chromosome 1q21 is an independent adverse prognostic factor in light chain amyloidosis patients treated with melphalan/dexamethasone. *Amyloid* 21:9, 2014.
107. Poulain S, Roumier C, Decambron A, et al: MYD88 L265P mutation in Waldenstrom macroglobulinemia. *Blood* 121:4504, 2013.
108. Treon SP, Hunter ZR: A new era for Waldenstrom macroglobulinemia: MYD88 L265P. *Blood* 121:4434, 2013.
109. Anderson KC, Carrasco RD: Pathogenesis of myeloma. *Annu Rev Pathol* 6:249, 2011.
110. Hurt EM, Wiestner A, Rosenwald A, et al: Overexpression of c-maf is a frequent onco-genic event in multiple myeloma that promotes proliferation and pathological interac-tions with bone marrow stroma. *Cancer Cell* 5:191, 2004.
111. Hideshima T, Mitsiades C, Tonon G, et al: Understanding multiple myeloma pathogen-esis in the bone marrow to identify new therapeutic targets. *Nat Rev Cancer* 7:585, 2007.
112. Galson DL, Silbermann R, Roodman GD: Mechanisms of multiple myeloma bone disease. *Bonekey Rep* 1:135, 2012.
113. Damiano JS, Cress AE, Hazlehurst LA, et al: Cell adhesion mediated drug resistance (CAM-DR): Role of integrins and resistance to apoptosis in human myeloma cell lines. *Blood* 93:1658, 1999.
114. Tian E, Zhan F, Walker R, et al: The role of the Wnt-signaling antagonist DKK1 in the development of osteolytic lesions in multiple myeloma. *N Engl J Med* 349:2483, 2003.
115. Yaccoby S, Wezeman MJ, Zangari M, et al: Inhibitory effects of osteoblasts and increased bone formation on myeloma in novel culture systems and a myelomatous mouse model. *Haematologica* 91:192, 2006.
116. Webb SL, Edwards CM: Novel therapeutic targets in myeloma bone disease. *Br J Pharmacol* 171:3765, 2014.
117. Li X, Pennisi A, Yaccoby S: Role of decorin in the antimyeloma effects of osteoblasts. *Blood* 112:159, 2008.
118. Seidel C, Hjertner O, Abildgaard N, et al: Serum osteoprotegerin levels are reduced in patients with multiple myeloma with lytic bone disease. *Blood* 98:2269, 2001.
119. Croucher PI, Shipman CM, Lippitt J, et al: Osteoprotegerin inhibits the development of osteolytic bone disease in multiple myeloma. *Blood* 98:3534, 2001.
120. Pearse RN, Sordillo EM, Yaccoby S, et al: Multiple myeloma disrupts the TRANCE/osteoprotegerin cytokine axis to trigger bone destruction and promote tumor progres-sion. *Proc Natl Acad Sci U S A* 98:11581, 2001.
121. Terpos E, Mihou D, Szydlo R, et al: The combination of intermediate doses of thalido-mide with dexamethasone is an effective treatment for patients with refractory/relapsed multiple myeloma and normalizes abnormal bone remodeling, through the reduction of sRANKL/osteoprotegerin ratio. *Leukemia* 19:1969, 2005.
122. Terpos E, Politou M, Szydlo R, et al: Autologous stem cell transplantation normalizes abnormal bone remodeling and sRANKL/osteoprotegerin ratio in patients with multi-ple myeloma. *Leukemia* 18:1420, 2004.
123. Gunn WG, Conley A, Deininger L, et al: A crosstalk between myeloma cells and mar-row stromal cells stimulates production of DKK1 and interleukin-6: A potential role in the development of lytic bone disease and tumor progression in multiple myeloma. *Stem Cells* 24:986, 2006.

124. Vallet S, Mukherjee S, Vaghela N, et al: Activin A promotes multiple myeloma-induced osteolysis and is a promising target for myeloma bone disease. *Proc Natl Acad Sci U S A* 107:5124, 2010.

125. Terpos E, Kastritis E, Christoulas D, et al: Circulating activin-A is elevated in patients with advanced multiple myeloma and correlates with extensive bone involvement and inferior survival; no alterations post-lenalidomide and dexamethasone therapy. *Ann Oncol* 23:2681, 2012.

126. Chantry AD, Heath D, Mulivor AW, et al: Inhibiting activin-A signaling stimulates bone formation and prevents cancer-induced bone destruction *in vivo*. *J Bone Miner Res* 25:2633, 2010.

127. Tai YT, Chang BY, Kong SY, et al: Bruton tyrosine kinase inhibition is a novel therapeutic strategy targeting tumor in the bone marrow microenvironment in multiple myeloma. *Blood* 120:1877, 2012.

128. Rushworth SA, Bowles KM, Barrera LN, et al: BTK inhibitor ibrutinib is cytotoxic to myeloma and potently enhances bortezomib and lenalidomide activities through NF-kappaB. *Cell Signal* 25:106, 2013.

129. Potter M, Wax JS, Hansen CT, Kenny JJ: BALB/c.CBA/N mice carrying the defective Btk(xid) gene are resistant to pristane-induced plasmacytomagenesis. *Int Immunol* 11:1059, 1999.

130. Barlougie B, Attal M, Crowley J, et al: Long term follow up of autotransplantation trials for multiple myeloma: Update of protocols conducted by the intergroupe francophone du myeloma, southwest oncology group, and university of Arkansas for medical sciences. *J Clin Oncol* 28:1209, 2010.

131. Zhan F, Hardin J, Kordsmeier B, et al: Global gene expression profiling of multiple myeloma, monoclonal gammopathy of undetermined significance, and normal bone marrow plasma cells. *Blood* 99:1745, 2002.

132. Jakubikova J, Adamia S, Kost-Alimova M, et al: Lenalidomide targets clonogenic side population in multiple myeloma: Pathophysiologic and clinical implications. *Blood* 117:4409, 2011.

133. Nara M, Teshima K, Watanabe A, et al: Bortezomib reduces the tumorigenicity of multiple myeloma via down regulation of up regulated targets in clonogenic side population cells. *PLoS One* 8:e56954, 2013.

134. Matsui W, Wang Q, Barber JP, et al: Clonogenic multiple myeloma progenitors, stem cell properties, and drug resistance. *Cancer Res* 68:190, 2008.

135. Matsui W, Hugg CA, Wang Q, et al: Characterization of clonogenic multiple myeloma cells. *Blood* 103:2332, 2004.

136. Pilarski LM, Belch AR: Clonotypic myeloma cells able to xenograft myeloma to non-obese diabetic sever combined immunodeficient mice copurify with CD34 (+) hematopoietic progenitors. *Clin Cancer Res* 8:3198, 2002.

137. Kuranda K, Berthon C, Dupont C, et al: A subpopulation of malignant CD34+CD138+B7-H1+ plasma cells is present in multiple myeloma patients. *Exp Hematol* 28:124, 2010.

138. Yaccoby S, Barlogie B, Epstein J: Primary myeloma cells growing in SCID-hu mice: A model for studying the biology and treatment of myeloma and its manifestations. *Blood* 92:2908, 1998.

139. Yaccoby S, Epstein J: The proliferative potential of myeloma plasma cells manifest in the SCID-hu host. *Blood* 94:3576, 1999.

140. Wang S, Tricot G, Shi L, et al: RARalpha2 expression is associated with disease progression and plays a crucial role in efficacy of ATRA treatment in myeloma. *Blood* 114:600, 2009.

141. Yang Y, Shi J, Tolomelli G, et al: RARα2 expression confers myeloma stem cell features. *Blood* 122:1437, 2013.

142. Van Rhee F, Bolejack V, Hollmig K, et al: High serum-free light chain levels and their rapid reduction in response to therapy define an aggressive multiple myeloma subtype with poor prognosis. *Blood* 110:827, 2007.

143. Rajkumar SV, Kyle RA, Therneau TM, et al: Serum free light chain ratio is an independent risk factor for progression in monoclonal gammopathy of undetermined significance. *Blood* 106:812, 2005.

144. Kumar S, Dispenzieri A, Lac MQ, et al: Revised prognostic staging system for light chain amyloidosis incorporating cardiac biomarkers and serum free light chain measurements. *J Clin Oncol* 30:989, 2012.

145. Leleu Z, Moreau AS, Weller E, et al: Serum immunoglobulin free light chain correlates with tumor burden markers in Waldenstrom macroglobulinemia. *Leuk Lymphoma* 49:1104, 2008.

146. Katzmann JA, Dispenzieri A, Kyle RA, et al: Elimination of the need for urine studies in the screening algorithm for monoclonal gammopathies by using serum immunofixation and free light chain assays. *Mayo Clin Proc* 81:1575, 2006.

147. Rawstron AC, Orfao A, Beksac M, et al: Report of the European myeloma network on multiparametric flow cytometry in multiple myeloma and related disorders. *Haematologica* 93:431, 2008.

148. Zhan F, Sawyer J, Tricot G: The role of cytogenetics in myeloma. *Leukemia* 20:1484, 2006.

149. Shortt CP, Gleeson TG, Breen KA, et al: Whole-body MRI versus PET in assessment of multiple myeloma disease activity. *AJR Am J Roentgenol* 192:980, 2009.

150. Walker R, Barlogie B, Haessler J, et al: Magnetic resonance imaging in multiple myeloma: Diagnostic and clinical implications. *J Clin Oncol* 25:1121, 2007.

151. Bartel TB, Haessler J, Brown TLY, et al: F18-fluorodeoxyglucose positron emission tomography in the context of other imaging techniques and prognostic factors in multiple myeloma. *Blood* 114:2068, 2009.

152. Zamagni E, Patriarca F, Nanni C, et al: Prognostic relevance of 18-FDG PET/CT in newly diagnosed multiple myeloma patients treated with upfront autologous transplantation. *Blood* 118:5989, 2011.

153. Durie GM, Stock-Novak D, Salmon S, et al: Prognostic value of treatment serum B2 microglobulin in mycelia: A Southwest Oncology group study. *Blood* 4:823, 1990.

154. Xie J, Wang Y, Freeman ME, et al: β_2-microglobulin as a negative regulator of the immune system: High concentrations of the protein inhibit in vitro generation of functional dendritic cells. *Blood* 101:4005, 2003.

155. Waheed S, Shaughnessy JD, van Rhee F, et al: International staging system and metaphase cytogenetic abnormalities in the era of gene expression profiling data in multiple myeloma treated with total therapy 2 and 3 protocols. *Cancer* 117:1001, 2011.

156. Barlogie B, Smallwood L, Smith T, et al: High serum levels of lactic dehydrogenase identify a high-grade lymphoma-like myeloma. *Ann Intern Med* 110:521, 1989.

157. Fassas AB, Muwalla F, Berryman T, et al: Myeloma of the central nervous system: Association with high risk chromosomal abnormalities, plasmablastic morphology and extramedullary manifestations. *Br J Haematol* 117:103, 2002.

158. Fassas AB, van Rhee F, Tricot G: Predicting long term survival in multiple myeloma patients follow autotransplants. *Leuk Lymphoma* 44:211, 2003.

159. Tricot G: What is the significance of molecule remission in multiple myeloma? *Clin Adv Hematol Oncol* 5:91, 2007.

160. Ladetto M, Pagliano G, Ferrero S, et al: 3683 Major shrinking of residual tumor cell burden and achievement of molecule remission in myeloma patients undergoing post-transplant consolidation with bortezomib, thalidomide and dexamethasone: A qualitative and quantitative PCR study. *ASH.* 2008.

161. Rawstron AC, Child JA, de Tute RM, et al: Minimal residual disease assessed by multiparameter flow cytometry in multiple myeloma: Impact on outcome in the medical research council myeloma IX study. *J Clin Oncol* 31:2504, 2013.

162. Flanders A, Stetler-Stevenson, Landgren O: Minimal residual disease testing in multiple myeloma by flow cytometry: Major heterogeneity. *Blood* 122:1088, 2013.

163. Martinez-Lopez J, Fernandez-Redondo E, Garcia-Sanz, R, et al: Clinical applicability and prognostic significance of molecular response assess by fluorescent-PCR of immunoglobulin genes in multiple myeloma. Results from a GEM/PETHEMA study. *Br J Haematol* 163:581, 2013.

CHAPTER 106
ESSENTIAL MONOCLONAL GAMMOPATHY

Marshall A. Lichtman

SUMMARY

Essential monoclonal gammopathy is defined by two key features: (1) the presence of a monoclonal immunoglobulin or a monoclonal immunoglobulin light chain in the serum and (2) the absence of evidence for an overt malignancy of B lymphocytes or plasma cells (e.g., lymphoma, myeloma, or amyloidosis). The prevalence of essential monoclonal gammopathy depends on the demographic features in the population under study. In Americans of European descent, the prevalence increases from approximately 2 percent in individuals 50 years of age to approximately 7 percent in octogenarians. It is two to three times as prevalent in persons of African descent. The condition has been reported in association with a large variety of disorders, especially non-lymphocytic cancers. These coincidences are thought, in most cases, to be the chance concurrence of conditions that have a high prevalence in older persons. Some cases of essential monoclonal gammopathy are symptomatic because in those cases the immunoglobulin can interact with plasma proteins, blood cells, kidney, ocular structures, or neural tissue and cause serious dysfunction, for example, an acquired bleeding disorder, renal insufficiency, or an incapacitating neuropathy. In such cases, disability may be so great that attempts to remove the immunoglobulin by plasmapheresis and to suppress its production using immune or cytotoxic therapy can be warranted. Because myeloma or lymphoma may emerge at the time the monoclonal immunoglobulin is first detected, periodic evaluation of the patient is required to ascertain if essential monoclonal gammopathy is the appropriate diagnosis. Long-term followup at appropriate intervals is prudent to detect conversion from a stable, asymptomatic condition to a progressive lymphoma or myeloma, which occurs in approximately 0.5 to 1.0 percent of cases per year. In the absence of a symptomatic gammopathy or evolution to a progressive clonal gammopathy, periodic followup is all that is required.

DEFINITION AND HISTORY

The syndrome of essential monoclonal gammopathy has two important characteristics. The first feature is a plasma immunoglobulin (Ig) or Ig light chain that has the molecular features of the product of a single clone of B lymphocytes or plasma cells: homogeneous electrophoretic migration and a single light-chain type. The second feature is the absence of evidence of an overt neoplastic disorder of B lymphocytes or plasma cells, such as lymphoma, myeloma, macroglobulinemia, or amyloidosis.

Acronyms and Abbreviations: CD, cluster of differentiation; HLA, human leukocyte antigen; Ig, immunoglobulin; IL, interleukin.

The observations that Bence Jones proteinuria could precede the clinical signs of multiple myeloma by many years[1] and that hyperglobulinemia without evidence of multiple myeloma could occur in some patients[2] antedated the concept of monoclonal gammopathy as a syndrome. With the more frequent clinical application of zonal electrophoresis of plasma proteins during the 1950s and 1960s, patients were discovered who had a monoclonal Ig, either without an associated disease or with diseases such as nonlymphoid cancers, infections, and inflammatory disorders, which typically are not associated with a monoclonal proliferation of B lymphocytes.[3-10] The presence of a monoclonal Ig or monoclonal free light chain in serum, if it is not associated with an overt neoplastic disease of lymphocytes, is referred to as *essential monoclonal gammopathy*. Several synonyms for the syndrome have been used, particularly *monoclonal gammopathy* and *benign monoclonal gammopathy*.[6] *Monoclonal gammopathy of unknown significance* (MGUS) has become fashionable as a designation preferable to *benign monoclonal gammopathy* because approximately one quarter of patients eventually progress to myeloma, macroglobulinemia, amyloidosis, or a B-cell lymphoma over decades of observation.[10-12] The suffix "of unknown significance" was justified, it was argued, because one did not know in whom or when the progression might occur. Now the term "monoclonal gammopathy of renal significance" has been coined, arguing that in this case the monoclonal gammopathy is of significance. However, other organs (e.g., nerves, eyes, bones), plasma proteins, and blood cells, as well as kidneys, may be injured or inactivated by a monoclonal protein (see "Functional Impairment from a Monoclonal Protein" below) and we will have to have (an unnecessary) proliferation of such designations. The term *essential monoclonal gammopathy* seems best, because it neither highlights a benign process nor indicates that the risks of subsequent lymphoma or myeloma are unknown; that risk is universally appreciated. It is unnecessary to assign the postscript "of unknown significance" to the numerous well-defined benign neoplasms at risk of clonal evolution and progression, such as colonic adenomatous polyps, other adenomas, uterine leiomyomas, monoclonal B-cell lymphocytosis, and clonal sideroblastic anemia. Biologically, essential monoclonal gammopathy is one of many such well-defined examples of a stable ("benign") neoplasm with the potential to evolve through the acquisition of additional somatic mutations to a progressive neoplasm. More is known about its significance and pathobiology than perhaps any other benign neoplasm with a risk of clonal evolution to a malignant state.[12] As in all diseases, the physician should understand its pathobiology and act accordingly.

Table 106–1 presents an immunologic classification of essential monoclonal gammopathy.

EPIDEMIOLOGY

Monoclonal gammopathy can occur at any age, but it is unusual before puberty, and its frequency increases with age.[14,15] The frequency of a serum paraprotein using zonal electrophoresis is approximately 1 percent in persons older than age 25 years,[4] approximately 3 percent in those older than age 70 years,[4,9] and approximately 10 percent in those older than age 80 years.[3] A much higher prevalence of monoclonal gammopathy has been reported using more sensitive screening methods, such as isoelectric focusing or immunoblotting.[16,17] Prevalence rates differ in different geographic areas and have been somewhat lower in the United States (Minnesota),[15] Iceland,[18] and the Netherlands.[19] The frequency of monoclonal gammopathy is less in Japanese[20,21] and Chinese.[22] The prevalence rate among Africans[23] and Americans of African descent[15,24-27] is significantly greater than the rate among those of European descent in each comparative age group. Males are more frequently affected than females. Familial occurrence also has been described.[28-31]

TABLE 106–1. Types of Monoclonal Immunoglobulin Synthesized By B-Cell Clone in Essential Monoclonal Gammopathy

Serum IgG, IgA, IgM,[6–12] IgE,[63] IgD[64–66]
Serum IgG + IgA, IgG + IgM, IgG + IgA + IgM[67–70]
Serum Monoclonal κ or λ light chain*[71,97]

*Urinary monoclonal immunoglobulin light chain excretion (Bence Jones proteinuria) may accompany serum monoclonal light chain.

An increased incidence of monoclonal gammopathy may be associated with several occupational groups, including farmers and industrial workers, but such associations are not firmly established.[32] There is a higher frequency of monoclonal gammopathy among inhabitants of Nagasaki, Japan who were younger than age 20 years when exposed to high doses of radiation from the atomic bomb detonation in 1945 than among inhabitants with lower or no exposure or older than 20 years at time of exposure.[21]

There is a positive association of being overweight or obese with the incidence of a monoclonal gammopathy[33] and a similar positive association exists with the incidence of or mortality from myeloma.[34–36]

● ETIOLOGY AND PATHOGENESIS

Monoclonal gammopathy can be compared with any benign tumor, such as a colonic adenomatous polyp, which can remain the same size indefinitely or undergo malignant transformation at an unpredictable future time.

Monoclonal gammopathy is caused by the proliferation of a single B lymphocyte, a plasma cell progenitor, leading to a clonal population that reaches a steady-state at approximately 1 to 5×10^{10} cells. At this cell-population density, marrow lymphocyte or plasma cell prevalence is indistinguishable from that of normal marrow. IgG and IgA monoclonal gammopathy arise from somatically mutated postswitch preplasma cells and may have translocations involving the Ig heavy-chain region on chromosome 14. IgM monoclonal gammopathy arises from a mutated postgerminal center lymphocyte that does not have evidence of isotype switching.[37] Not surprisingly, these origins determine the phenotype of the clonal B-lymphocytic diseases that may evolve. For example, IgG or IgA monoclonal gammopathy tend to evolve into myeloma or plasmacytoma (plasma cell phenotypes) and IgM monoclonal gammopathies tend to evolve into lymphomas and Waldenström macroglobulinemia (lymphocytic phenotypes).

The expanded clone secretes monoclonal Ig at a rate per cell sufficient for detection by standard tests. The clonal expansion, however, does not cause osteolysis, hypercalcemia, inhibit hematopoietic proliferation and maturation, or impair differentiation of polyclonal B lymphocytes to plasma cells. Polyclonal Ig synthesis usually is normal, and patients do not incur an increased risk of infection. The cells in the stable (benign) clone do not accumulate further and do not elaborate significant amounts of osteoclast-activating factors that are responsible for bone destruction.

Despite these significant differences from myeloma in the behavior of the neoplastic B cells, cytogenetic abnormalities akin to those seen in myeloma may be present in plasma cells derived from patients with essential monoclonal gammopathy.[37–47] G-banding cytogenetic evaluation usually is normal in patients with monoclonal gammopathy, presumably related to the unavailability of cells in the cell cycle (metaphase). However, clones containing numerical abnormalities (e.g., trisomy or monosomy) and translocations have been identified with fluorescence *in situ* hybridization of interphase cells (see "Cytogenetic Analysis" below). The presence of clonal cytogenetic changes does not necessarily predict clonal evolution and progression. It was initially thought that 25 to 30 percent of patients with myeloma had an identified antecedent period of essential monoclonal gammopathy which underwent clonal evolution to myeloma[43,46]; whereas more recent studies suggest that an antecedent period of monoclonal gammopathy may precede all patients who develop myeloma.[48,49] The presence of clonal cytogenetic abnormalities does not correlate with such evolution, however.[37,38,45] Gene-expression studies of plasma cells isolated from normal marrow and marrow from patients with essential monoclonal gammopathy have identified several hundred genes that are differentially expressed.[50,51] The predominate finding was a gradient of overexpression of 41 of 52 genes studied in plasma cells from normal subjects, from patients with monoclonal gammopathy, and from patients with myeloma, respectively.[51] In addition, myeloma patients could be stratified into those with gene-expression profiles that were more or less similar to that of essential monoclonal gammopathy. The group more similar to monoclonal gammopathy constituted approximately 30 percent of myeloma patients.

Americans of African descent have a much higher frequency of an autosomal dominant inherited risk factor for monoclonal gammopathy and myeloma. Hyperphosphorylated paratarg-7 (pP-7) results from an inability to inactivate protein phosphatase 2A, which leads to the inability to dephosphorylate p-7 at serine 17. The pP-7 carrier state is associated with an increased risk of monoclonal gammopathy and myeloma. The carrier state is more than twice as prevalent in Americans of African descent as those of European descent and is much less prevalent in Americans of Asian descent than those of European descent, a gradient similar to the incidence of monoclonal gammopathy in those populations.[52]

Common single nucleotide polymorphisms at 2p23.3(rs6746082), 3p22.1(rs1052501), 3q26.2(rs10936599), 6p21.33(rs2285803), 7p15.3 (rs4487645), 17p11.2(rs4273077), and 22q13.1(rs877529) are associated with increased risk of myeloma. Similarly these polymorphisms independently increased the risk of monoclonal gammopathy. Polymorphism associations were independent; risk increased with a larger number of risk alleles carried, supporting a polygenic model of disease susceptibility to monoclonal gammopathy and, therefore, to myeloma.[53]

MYD88 L265 is a somatic mutation found in approximately 50 percent of individuals with IgM monoclonal gammopathy and in more than 90 percent of patients with Waldenström macroglobulinemia. It is thought to represent an early oncogenic event in monoclonal gammopathy contributing to evolution to macroglobulinemia.[54,55]

The C57BL mouse provides a model of essential monoclonal gammopathy. The frequency of monoclonal gammopathy increases with age in these mice.[56] The gammopathy can be transferred to either irradiated or nonirradiated mice by marrow or spleen cells.[57] The transfer can be accomplished only during the first four consecutive transplantations, and no effect is seen on the survival of the recipient compared with that of appropriate control animals. In contrast, if mouse B-cell lymphoma or myeloma cells are transplanted into normal mice, the engraftment frequency is higher than that of B cells from mice with essential monoclonal gammopathy. Passage from the original recipient to a new recipient is unlimited. Progressive disease develops, and survival of the recipient animals is impaired. Thus, an intrinsic difference exists in the growth potential (degree of malignancy) of these B-cell clones.[43] The frequency of monoclonal gammopathy increases with age, but progression to myeloma in the C57BL mouse is a rare event.[58] Studies in transgenic mice and their litter mates replicate the increased incidence of B-cell clones and gammopathy with aging.[59]

Occasionally, monoclonal gammopathy is the result of exaggerated production of natural antibody by a B-lymphocyte clone.[60] For example, patients with cold agglutinins may have monoclonal IgM for years. A few monoclonal IgM antibodies act as rheumatoid factors and may form cryoglobulins through complex formation with IgG molecules.

CLINICAL FEATURES

BLOOD CELLS AND MARROW

Blood counts and the marrow examination are normal. Notably anemia is not present and the proportion of plasma cells in marrow is less than 10 percent. Although an increased percent of plasma cells is the most constant morphologic feature of myeloma, the presence of cytologic atypia as judged by frequent binucleate plasma cells and large plasma cell nucleoli are findings more specific for myeloma.[61] Quantitative microscopy of the number of marrow microvessels per high-power field, using immunohistochemistry, indicates microvessel density on average is threefold greater than in normal persons, but far less than in patients with myeloma, although some overlap with myeloma occurs.[62]

CYTOGENETIC ANALYSIS

Hyperdiploidy, assessed by DNA content, is present in about half the cases and hypodiploidy is present in approximately 10 percent of cases of monoclonal gammopathy.[42] Use of interphase fluorescence *in situ* hybridization has uncovered numerical chromosome abnormalities in the plasma cells of more than 50 percent of subjects. Clones containing trisomy or monosomy involving chromosomes 3, 6, 7, 9, 11, 13, 17, and 18 have been identified.[38-41,44,45] Deletions of 13q14 are present in about one-quarter of patients and abnormalities involving 14q32, the site of the Ig heavy-chain genes, are present in approximately 60 percent of subjects.[38-41] Chromosomal changes do not appear to be correlated with progression.

MONOCLONAL PROTEIN

Characteristically, individuals are detected by the unexpected identification of a monoclonal IgG or light chain in the serum in the absence of symptoms or signs (e.g., anemia, marrow plasmacytosis, lymph node enlargement, plasmacytoma, bone lesions, or amyloid deposits) caused by diseases associated with monoclonal proteins.[6-10,60,63-71] Although classically a serum Ig or urine monoclonal light chain was the standard for diagnosis, the ability to measure serum free light chains with high specificity and sensitivity has replaced the necessity to measure urine light chain excretion for diagnosis as the latter is less sensitive than the former.[72]

Monoclonal IgG gammopathy occurs in approximately 70 percent of persons and IgM and IgA in approximately 20 percent and 10 percent, respectively. A few percent of persons may have biclonal or triclonal gammopathy (see Table 106–1).[6-10,12,60,63-71]

Most patients with essential monoclonal gammopathy have a monoclonal protein concentration of less than 30 g/L, but exceptions occur. The diagnosis reflects the sum of (1) the monoclonal protein level, (2) the marrow plasma cell concentration (<10 percent), (3) the absence of other features of progressive plasma cell neoplasm (e.g., hypercalcemia, osteolysis, otherwise unexplained anemia, otherwise unexplained renal disease), and (4) the absence of progression on periodic long-term followup.

A developing consensus favors measurement of serum protein gel electrophoresis and serum free light chain levels (and the $\kappa:\lambda$ ratio), and serum protein immunofixation electrophoresis without urinary Ig measurements to detect monoclonal gammopathies.[73-75]

Some pathologists are still reluctant to give up urinary measurements because of the uncommon occurrence of urinary monoclonal light chains in the absence of evidence of an abnormality of serum monoclonal light chains.[76] Followup of these cases has not shown any clinical consequence of these uncommon false-negative serum light-chain measurements. Serum protein gel electrophoresis has a limit of detection of approximately 0.03 g/dL, if the monoclonal protein migrates in the γ-globulin fraction. Small monoclonal proteins that migrate in the α- or β-globulin fraction are more difficult to identify on electrophoresis. Immunofixation electrophoresis is used to confirm a monoclonal protein found on gel electrophoresis. Immunofixation electrophoresis may also detect a monoclonal protein not evident on serum protein gel electrophoresis, usually because the protein is in too low a concentration or is embedded in the normal polyclonal α- or β-globulin peak. Monoclonal proteins identified by immunofixation electrophoresis may be transient (approximately 15 to 20 percent) and have a greater likelihood to progress to a disease if they are of an IgA or IgM isotype.[77] In the future, mass spectroscopy may be a more sensitive and specific method to identify monoclonal proteins.[78]

In individuals with a serum monoclonal IgG of less than 1.5 g/dL, especially if of an older age and with no overt end-organ abnormality, marrow examination and radiographic examination of the bones have a very low diagnostic yield and can be omitted. A presumptive diagnosis of essential monoclonal gammopathy can be made with reexamination at approximately 6 months and at appropriate intervals, thereafter.[79,80]

FUNCTIONAL IMPAIRMENT FROM A MONOCLONAL PROTEIN

Interaction with Plasma Protein or Blood Cells

Some patients have monoclonal proteins with antibody specificity directed against plasma or cell proteins, resulting in symptomatic pathophysiologic effects, such as immune hemolytic anemia,[81] acquired von Willebrand disease,[82-84] immune neutropenia,[85,86] and other functional manifestations[87-92] (Table 106–2).

Renal Injury

Occasional patients may have severe renal disease associated with monoclonal gammopathy.[93-100] The renal disease my take the form of a tubular disorder, mimicking Fanconi syndrome (glycosuria, hypouricemia, proteinuria, asymptomatic renal insufficiency)[93,96] or a glomerular deposition disorder resulting from the deleterious interaction of the monoclonal Ig or a light chain and the renal parenchyma resulting

TABLE 106–2. Functional Abnormalities Associated with Essential Monoclonal Gammopathy

Plasma protein and blood cell disturbances

Antierythrocyte antibodies,[81] acquired von Willebrand disease,[82-84] immune neutropenia,[85,86] cryoglobulinemia,[10] cryofibrinogenemia,[10] acquired C1 esterase inhibitor deficiency (angioedema),[10] acquired antithrombin,[87] insulin antibodies,[88,89] antiacetylcholine receptor antibodies,[90] "antiphospholipid" antibodies,[91] dysfibrinogenemia[92]

Renal disease[93-100]

Oculopathies[102-106]

Neuropathies[107-111]

Deep venous thrombosis[136,137]

in renal insufficiency.[94,95,97,100] The term "dangerous small B-cell clone" has been applied to a monoclonal gammopathy that can produce disease, often quite serious, without lymphoproliferation and progression of the neoplastic cell population. The principal approach to therapy is to attempt to suppress the small B-cell clone and, thereby, its monoclonal protein secretion with chemotherapy. Cyclophosphamide, thalidomide, bortezomib, or bendamustine are favored because they have much less renal toxicity than congeners such as melphalan or lenalidomide. A glucocorticoid and rituximab can, also, be useful.[100,101] One should also consider the possibility that the monoclonal protein may be secreted by a solitary plasmacytoma, which would be amenable to local radiation therapy. Thus, in the face of significant renal impairment a careful evaluation, including positron emission tomography, should be considered to exclude a solitary lesion. In exceptional cases, ablative therapy with an autologous hematopoietic stem cell transplant may be considered.[101]

Ophthalmic Injury

Corneal deposits of crystalline Ig[102,103] and a monoclonal copper binding Ig resulting in copper deposits in the eye,[104,105] each associated with classical monoclonal gammopathy, have led to loss of visual acuity. Remarkably, despite very high serum copper levels in the latter cases, no other organ damage ensued. Iritis, vitritus, and maculopathy with loss of visual acuity have also been described in association with a monoclonal gammopathy.[106]

NEUROPATHIES

Frequency of Occurrence

A significant association exists between the incidence of neuropathies and essential monoclonal gammopathy.[107-114] Approximately 10 percent of patients with idiopathic neuropathy have a monoclonal Ig, a frequency about eight times that of age-adjusted healthy comparison groups.[107-111] The frequency of neuropathy among patients with monoclonal gammopathy varies depending on the distribution of Ig classes, but is in the range of 3 to 5 percent. IgM monoclonal gammopathy has a significantly higher frequency of neuropathy than does IgG or IgA monoclonal gammopathy.[107,108]

Mechanisms of Nerve Damage

Monoclonal antibodies, especially IgM, can react with peripheral nerve myelin, specifically with myelin-associated glycoprotein, glycolipids, or sulfatides.[112-117] Although various antinerve antibodies are present in approximately 40 percent of patients with neuropathy and IgG monoclonal gammopathy, a similar frequency has been found in such patients without neuropathy.[118] Neuropathy in the absence of reactivity of the monoclonal protein with nerve antigens implies other mechanisms also operate to cause nerve damage.[107,109,116] Deposition of monoclonal protein in the epineurium has been proposed as an alternative mechanism of nerve injury.[119] Also, in one report, four of 16 patients with IgG monoclonal gammopathy and neuropathy had polyclonal, not monoclonal, antibodies against neurofilament protein.[116] In addition, a proportion of patients develop a detectable monoclonal protein after the onset of the neuropathy, sometimes years later.[118]

Signs and Symptoms

Patients with essential IgM monoclonal gammopathy and neuropathy can have dysesthesia of the hands and feet, loss of vibration and position sense, atrophy of distal muscles, ataxia, and intention tremor.[114,115,117] The monoclonal antibodies reactive with nerve antigens usually are of the IgM type. Serum often contains antibodies to myelin-associated glycoprotein.[107,108] In contrast, patients with IgG or IgA monoclonal gammopathy usually have chronic inflammatory demyelinating polyneuropathy;

a minority have sensory axonal or mixed neuropathy.[108,118,120-122] The neuropathy may be (1) mild with minor motor and/or sensory signs with or without mild functional impairment, (2) moderately disabling but with full range of activities, or (3) severely disabling, interfering with walking, dressing, and eating.[118] The course may be relapsing and remitting or progressive. IgA gammopathy is associated with dysautonomia.[123] The presence or absence of antibody to myelin-associated glycoprotein may have an effect on the specific nature of the neuropathic manifestations.[108,109,114-117]

Diagnostic Findings

Demyelinization is reflected in decreased nerve conduction velocity. Axonal loss is reflected in decreased sensory potentials.[109,113,114,120-124] Electromyography may show denervation of muscles.[109,113] Immunofluorescence studies of sural nerve or of skin biopsies may uncover Ig binding to nerve.[109,114] Morphologic studies of nerve biopsies may show decreased or absent myelinated fibers or axonal degeneration. A rare case of crystal formation in the epineurium has been described.[125]

Management

At least seven treatment approaches have been used to ameliorate the neuropathies: (1) intravenous Ig administration; (2) glucocorticoids alone; (3) immunoadsorption of perfused blood with staphylococcal protein A; (4) plasma exchange or plasmapheresis; (5) immunosuppressive cytotoxic chemotherapy, such as cyclophosphamide, chlorambucil, or fludarabine with or without added glucocorticoids; (6) rituximab (anti–cluster of differentiation [CD]20 antibody) to deplete B cells; and (7) high-dose cytotoxic therapy with autologous hematopoietic stem cell rescue.[107-109,117,118,124,126-135] In some cases, use of plasmapheresis has been followed by cytotoxic therapy in an effort to produce a sustained effect. Plasma exchange has shown benefit in a small clinical trial. The other modalities of treatment await such studies.[107] Response rates to each form of therapy are low and duration of response is variable,[109,118,126-131] but some patients obtain coincidental significant improvement for prolonged periods. A recommendation has been made to start therapy with intravenous Ig, especially in essential monoclonal IgM-associated neuropathy, because of the relative safety of this approach.[107] Mild symptoms and signs may not be an indication for treatment because of the low response rate and the potential noxious effects of therapy.[107]

COINCIDING DISORDERS

Monoclonal gammopathy unrelated to a clinically evident proliferation of B lymphocytes or plasma cells has been observed in association with a wide variety of conditions (Table 106–3).[136-201] Although they are grouped under the designation *monoclonal gammopathy with a coincidental disease*, few such reports have examined whether the coincidence is greater than expected in a control group matched for age and ethnicity, the two variables having the greatest impact on the incidence of monoclonal gammopathy. Non–B-cell malignancies, including solid tumors,[3,5,6,18,178-181] myeloproliferative disorders,[182-189] and Hodgkin and T-cell lymphomas,[190-193] are associated with monoclonal Ig. These relationships could result from various factors: (1) patients with a monoclonal Ig have an increased risk of developing cancer; (2) the monoclonal Ig is an antibody against some antigen associated with the cancer; (3) the monoclonal Ig is the product of cancer cells; or (4) coincidence. The last possibility is favored by two epidemiologic studies that found the same frequency of monoclonal gammopathy in a matched control group as in cancer patients.[9,18] Furthermore, when the monoclonal Ig is associated with a cancer, it usually persists after successful resection of the tumor. A convincing case for an association of acute myelogenous leukemia and myelodysplasia with monoclonal gammopathy was made

TABLE 106–3. Disorders Reported in Coincidence with Monoclonal Gammopathy

Axial bone fracture[138,139]

Connective tissue diseases and autoimmune diseases: Crohn disease, cryoglobulinemia, Hashimoto thyroiditis, lupus erythematosus, myasthenia gravis, pernicious anemia, polymyalgia rheumatica, psoriatic arthritis, rheumatoid arthritis, scleroderma, Sjögren disease[140-149]

Corneal and other ocular diseases: pseudo–Kayser-Fleischer ring,[243] corneal gammopathy[102-106,244]

Cutaneous diseases: Schnitzler syndrome, urticaria, hyperkeratotic spicules, pyoderma gangrenosum (neutrophilic dermatoses), psoriasis, scleromyxedema[150-156]

Diffuse idiopathic skeletal hyperostosis[157]

Endocrine diseases: hyperparathyroidism[158,159]

Gaucher disease, type I[160-162]

Hepatic disease: cirrhosis,[148] hepatitis,[163,164]

Hereditary spherocytosis[165]

Infectious diseases: bacterial endocarditis, *Corynebacterium* species, cytomegalovirus, Epstein-Barr virus, human immunodeficiency virus, *Mycobacterium tuberculosis*, purpura fulminans[19,148,166-169,212,215]

Metabolic disease: hyperlipidemia[170]

Neutropenia, chronic[85,86,171]

Osteoporosis[172,174,175]

Pituitary macroadenoma[173]

Pregnancy[174]

Systemic capillary leak syndrome[177]

Carcinomas: colon, lung, prostate, other[3,5,6,178-181]

Myeloproliferative diseases: acute and chronic myelogenous leukemia,[182-184] chronic neutrophilic leukemia, polycythemia vera[185-189]

T-cell lymphomas, Hodgkin lymphoma[190-193]

After chemotherapy, radiotherapy, or marrow, kidney, or liver transplantation[194-198,213-215]

Miscellaneous diseases[200-202]

Transient, monoclonal, or oligoclonal gammopathies[204-206]

Factitious hyperferremia[207]

Factitious increase in C-reactive protein[208]

Vitamin B_{12} deficiency[140,209]

by one group of scientists[183-184] but a large longitudinal study did not find this association.[12] Some observers propose that in clonal myeloid diseases the monoclonal protein reflects B-cell lineage involvement.

Chemotherapy, radiotherapy, organ or marrow transplantation,[194-199] and other miscellaneous disorders[5,7,10,24-26,147,148,200-202] are associated with a transient or persistent monoclonal Ig (see Table 106–3). The high prevalence of monoclonal proteins and associated diseases, especially after age 50 years, indicates some of these associations are coincidental. Thus, although surgical correction of hyperparathyroidism is associated with disappearance of the plasma monoclonal protein,[158] statistical studies of this disorder suggest a coincidental

relationship in most patients.[159] Gaucher disease type I has a higher-than-expected frequency of polyclonal (approximately 40 percent) and monoclonal (approximately 20 percent) gammopathy, and, probably, of myeloma.[160-162] Elaboration of proinflammatory cytokines, growth factors, and chemokines, several involved in B-cell function, is disturbed in type I Gaucher disease. An increase of interleukin (IL)-10 and pulmonary and activation-regulated chemokine is notable. A high frequency of B-cell clonality and IgH gene rearrangements have also been described.[162] The administration of recombinant glucocerebrosidase therapy may decrease the occurrence and progression of gammopathies.[161]

In inflammatory, autoimmune, and infectious diseases, the association is viewed as an unusual expansion of a restricted population of B lymphocytes. Following marrow transplantation, the presence of oligoclonal blood B-lymphocyte populations often reflects the process of reconstitution of the B-cell population.

● LABORATORY FEATURES

PLASMA AND URINARY MONOCLONAL IMMUNOGLOBULINS

The monoclonal protein usually is an IgG; however, IgM, IgA, IgD, and IgE, urinary light chains, double gammopathy involving IgA and IgG or IgM and IgA, and triple gammopathy can occur. Rare cases may have the isotype IgD or IgE (see Table 106–1).[12,63-66,178,203] By definition, no findings other than a serum monoclonal Ig or monoclonal light chain is present with no other features of a B-lymphocyte or plasma cell malignancy.

In monoclonal gammopathy of the IgG type, the concentration of monoclonal Ig usually is less than 3 g/dL. In the IgA or IgM type, the concentration usually is less than 2.5 g/dL.[10,12,203] However, dramatic exceptions to this rule exist. Occasional patients with essential monoclonal gammopathy have concentrations as high as 6 g/dL. Some patients have urinary monoclonal light chain excretion (Bence Jones proteinuria) as the sole manifestation of monoclonal gammopathy.[1,10] The amount of urinary light chains excreted occasionally is so large (>1.0 g/day) that renal dysfunction may develop.[93,96,97]

Most patients with myeloma or macroglobulinemia have significantly depressed nonmonoclonal Ig levels. For example, patients with IgG myeloma usually have very low IgA and IgM concentrations and a reduced polyclonal IgG level. Patients with monoclonal gammopathy usually have normal polyclonal Ig levels; and, if a decrease of their polyclonal Ig levels is present, it is usually not as severe as in myeloma.[10,12,203,210]

Depression of normal polyclonal immunoglobulin concentrations is considered one of several factors that may portend the likelihood of progression to a B-cell malignancy.

OLIGOCLONAL IMMUNOGLOBULINS

Oligoclonal or monoclonal serum Ig levels have been detected with high-resolution agarose gel electrophoresis in hospitalized patients with acute-phase reactions or polyclonal hyperglobulinemia.[206] Oligoclonal Ig bands are frequently seen in the cerebrospinal fluid and serum of patients with a variety of neurologic conditions, especially multiple sclerosis, when the fluids are analyzed by isoelectric focusing.[211] Patients with AIDS have B-cell activation and aberrancies of B-cell regulation. High-resolution electrophoresis indicates most AIDS patients with advanced disease have monoclonal or oligoclonal serum Ig bands. Persons with AIDS, lymphadenopathy syndrome, or antibody to the human immunodeficiency virus also have oligoclonal or monoclonal

Ig bands by standard zonal electrophoresis.[167,168] These monoclonal proteins are typically IgG. In about half the patients with AIDS who receive antiviral therapy the monoclonal protein disappears by 5 years of treatment.[212] Oligoclonal or monoclonal serum Ig has also been associated with Epstein-Barr virus infection and in patients after liver,[213] heart,[214] and marrow transplantation.[215]

LYMPHOCYTE AND PLASMA CELL PHENOTYPES

The concentration of plasma cells in the marrow is less than 10 percent, and the incorporation of tritiated thymidine into marrow plasma cells is negligible (<1 percent) in essential monoclonal gammopathy. Marrow plasma cells in monoclonal gammopathy do not express neural cell adhesion molecule (CD56), whereas myeloma cells strongly express this surface protein.[216] Blood T-lymphocyte subset levels are normal in monoclonal gammopathy, whereas CD4+ T-cell levels are lower and CD8+ T-cell levels higher in myeloma and macroglobulinemia.[217-220] Blood B-cell concentration is normal in monoclonal gammopathy, but often is decreased in myeloma patients. Clonally restricted, idiotype-positive blood B cells are characteristic of myeloma but not of monoclonal gammopathy.[221]

β_2-Microglobulin is the light chain of cell surface human leukocyte antigen (HLA) molecules and is present in low concentrations in normal serum. Its concentration in serum frequently is elevated in myeloma, and the magnitude of the elevation is positively correlated with tumor mass. β_2-Microglobulin concentration is not elevated in essential monoclonal gammopathy.[222,223]

The distinction between stable essential monoclonal gammopathy and emerging (so-called "larval") myeloma or low-infiltrate myeloma (so-called "smoldering" myeloma) with a very low tumor burden is not easily discerned except by following the patient's clinical status. This finding has not kept investigators from looking for a distinguishing test. More than 40 variables have been studied as an index for discriminating a stable (benign) from progressive (malignant) clone (Table 106–4). No single test is sufficiently sensitive and specific to be useful in an individual patient. Periodic examination of the patient is the best method for detecting the emergence of myeloma or lymphoma or a related disease. Measurement of the concentration of the serum monoclonal protein, serum polyclonal proteins, serum free Ig light chains, serum β_2-microglobulin, and hemoglobin concentration at appropriate intervals is required. The marrow should be reexamined if the monoclonal protein level increases or hemoglobin concentration decreases significantly. Practical and sensitive methods for measuring bone density would be an additional useful measure of stability or progression.

● COURSE, PROGNOSIS, AND THERAPY

Longitudinal studies have reported three major patterns of outcome for patients with essential monoclonal gammopathy.[10,224–226] Approximately 25 percent of patients do not progress to a lymphocytic neoplasm over 25 to 30 years of observation. In this group, occasional patients experience increases in monoclonal protein concentration of up to 50 percent of their initial diagnostic value. However, these patients restabilize and do not develop signs of myeloma, macroglobulinemia, amyloidosis, or lymphoma. About half of patients die of an unrelated cause over the 25- to 30-year period of observation. The remaining 25 percent of patients develop a plasmacytoma, myeloma, amyloidosis, macroglobulinemia, lymphoma, or chronic lymphocytic leukemia over several decades of observation. The occurrence of a lymphoma or myeloma in the latter group of patients continues to increase slowly without reaching a plateau. Evolution to a progressive clonal B-cell disorder has been observed

TABLE 106–4. Variables Used in an Attempt to Distinguish Essential Monoclonal Gammopathy from Myeloma or Lymphoma

LYMPHOCYTES AND IMMUNOGLOBULINS

Igκ light-chain expression[245]

Ig light chains in urine[245]

Polyclonal Ig serum concentration[245]

β_2-Microglobulin or C-reactive protein serum concentration[246]

Ig-secreting cells in blood[247]

Idiotype-reactive blood T lymphocytes[248,249]

CD4-to-CD8 lymphocyte ratio in blood or marrow[217,250,251]

Clonally restricted B lymphocytes[221,252–254]

Immunofluorescence of lymphocytes[218]

Natural killer cell frequency[255]

PLASMA CELLS

Frequency[6,7,9,10,15,203]

Morphology[219,256–258]

MB2 antibody reactivity[259]

Proliferative index[219,220,250,256,260]

Asynchronous replication[261]

DNA content or interphase fluorescent *in situ* hybridization[38,39,43,219,256]

Gene-expression profile[51,237]

Ratio of monoclonal CD19–/CD38+/CD56++ to polyclonal CD19+/CD38++/CD56– cells[262]

Blood or marrow concentration[10,219–221,253]

J chains[263]

Acid phosphatase[264]

Multidrug resistance expression[265]

CD19 expression[266]

CD56/neural cell adhesion molecule expression[216]

Proportion of CD19+/CD56– plasma cells in marrow[267]

5′ Nucleotidase[268]

BONE INTEGRITY

Magnetic resonance imaging[269,270]

Dual-energy x-ray absorptiometry[271]

Histomorphometry[272]

Urinary pyridinium-collagen complexes[273]

MISCELLANEOUS

Marrow microvessel density[62]

Neural cell adhesion molecules[274]

Serum IL-1β[275]

Serum IL-6, IL-10, soluble CD16, soluble IL-6 receptor, IL-1β[276–281]

Serum transforming growth factor-β[282]

Urinary deoxypyridinoline excretion rate[282]

Hemoglobin concentration[8,148,178]

Mononuclear cell E-cadherin gene methylation[283]

more than 25 years after the diagnosis of monoclonal gammopathy. The actuarial risk of progressing to a clonal B-cell malignancy for all classes of monoclonal protein is approximately 0.5 to 1.0 percent per year depending on the population studied.[12,224–226] IgM gammopathy usually progresses to lymphoma, macroglobulinemia, amyloidosis, or chronic lymphocytic leukemia.[227] Although one large study found that IgM monoclonal gammopathy evolved to a progressive clonal lymphoid disorder at a rate of approximately 1.5 percent per year,[228] two other large studies found no significant difference in the rate of progression when patients with IgG or IgM were compared.[229,230] IgG or IgA monoclonal gammopathy evolves principally into myeloma, plasmacytoma, or amyloidosis.[231,232] Several studies have found a somewhat higher progression rate in persons with IgA monoclonal gammopathy.[18,233]

Patients with a higher percentage of plasma cells in the marrow, higher monoclonal Ig levels at the time of diagnosis, lower levels of polyclonal Ig, an elevated erythrocyte sedimentation rate, a more disturbed serum light chain ratio, a lower relative proportion of CD19+ plasma cells, and more than one focal lesion in marrow as determined by whole-body magnetic resonance imaging evolve to a progressive clonal B-lymphocyte disease more frequently.[12,229–236] None of these variables have the specificity and sensitivity to be highly accurate in predicting the behavior of an individual patient. Neither the plasma cell gene-expression profile nor the cell population cytogenetic findings are sufficiently specific to predict progression from a stable to an unstable clone based on current studies.[41,237] These findings indicate, not surprisingly, that the qualitative leap is between normal, polyclonal plasma cells (B lymphocytes) and the emergence of a monoclonal population (either stable or progressively growing) and that the distinctions between the latter two states are subtle, complex, and as yet unidentified. In rare patients, the monoclonal protein appears transiently in relation to a disease (e.g., infection)[202,204,205] or disappears spontaneously even when not associated with a disease (clonal exhaustion).[3]

Generally, the diagnosis of essential monoclonal gammopathy cannot be made with certainty at the time of the initial evaluation. Periodic reexamination is required to document a stable clinical course. One of the most subtle interfaces is between essential monoclonal gammopathy and smoldering myeloma (Chap. 107). In the latter, the marrow plasma cell concentration is between 10 and 20 percent or the monoclonal protein concentration is greater than 3 g/dL or both. There is no anemia, increase in serum calcium, or evident bone or kidney disease.[238] Careful observation of patients with presumed essential monoclonal gammopathy should permit identification of those who are better categorized as smoldering myeloma. Although at this time treatment is not recommended for smoldering myeloma until progression, calls for clinical trials to assess whether early treatment may improve outcome have been made.[239] Therapy is not required for essential monoclonal gammopathy without a confirmed diagnosis of myeloma, macroglobulinemia, amyloidosis, or lymphoma with evidence of progressive disease. Therapy may be indicated, however, if the monoclonal protein interferes with the vital function of a normal plasma or tissue constituent, induces kidney disease, or is associated with a disabling neuropathy.

A better understanding and an ability to identify the somatic mutations that underlie the evolution of monoclonal gammopathy to a progressive and potentially fatal B-cell neoplasm may permit the application of therapy at an earlier time when curability or sustained remissions would be more frequent.[240–242]

REFERENCES

1. Prentiss RG Jr: Multiple myeloma with diffuse skeletal involvement: Case report. *Mil Surg* 80:294, 1937.
2. Waldenstrom JG: Incipient myelomatosis or essential hyperglobulinemia with fibrinogenopenia: A new syndrome? *Acta Med Scand* 117:216, 1944.
3. Hallen J: Frequency of "abnormal serum globulins" (M-components) in the aged. *Acta Med Scand* 173:737, 1963.
4. Axelsson U, Bachmann R, Hallen J: Frequency of pathological proteins (M-components) in 6995 sera from an adult population. *Acta Med Scand* 179:235, 1966.
5. Migliore PJ, Alexanian R: Monoclonal gammopathy in human neoplasia. *Cancer* 21:1127, 1968.
6. Ritzmann SE, Loukes D, Sakai H, et al: Idiopathic (asymptomatic) monoclonal gammopathies. *Arch Intern Med* 135:95, 1975.
7. Amies A, Ko HS, Pruzanski W: M-components: A review of 1242 cases. *Can Med Assoc J* 114:889, 1976.
8. Lindstrom FD, Dahlstrom V: Multiple myeloma or benign monoclonal gammopathy? A study of differential diagnostic criteria in 44 cases. *Clin Immunol Immunopathol* 10:168, 1978.
9. Salerin JP, Vicariot M, Deroff P, et al: Monoclonal gammopathies in the adult population of Finistère, France. *J Clin Pathol* 35:63, 1982.
10. Kyle RA: Monoclonal gammopathy of undetermined significance and solitary myeloma. *Hematol Oncol Clin North Am* 11:71, 1997.
11. Owen RG, Parapia LA, Higginson J, et al: Clinicopathological correlates of IgM paraproteinemias. *Clin Lymphoma* 1:39, 2000.
12. Turesson I, Kovalchik SA, Pfeiffer RM, et al: Monoclonal gammopathy of undetermined significance and risk of lymphoid and myeloid malignancies: 728 cases followed up to 30 years in Sweden. *Blood* 123:338, 2014.
13. Lichtman MA. Monoclonal gammopathy: Do we know its significance? *Blood Cells Mol Dis* 45:267, 2010.
14. Ligthart GL, Radl J, Corberand JX, et al: Monoclonal gammopathies in human aging: Increased occurrence with age and correlation with health status. *Mech Ageing Dev* 52:235, 1990.
15. Kyle RA, Rajkumar SV: Epidemiology of the plasma-cell disorders. *Best Pract Res Clin Haematol* 20:637, 2007.
16. Sinclair D, Sheehan T, Parrott DMV, Stott DI: The incidence of monoclonal gammopathy in a population over 45 years old determined by isoelectric focusing. *Br J Haematol* 67:745, 1986.
17. Radl J, Wels J, Hoogeven CM: Immunoblotting with (sub)class specific antibodies reveals a high frequency of monoclonal antibodies in persons thought to be immunodeficient. *Clin Chem* 34:1839, 1988.
18. Ögmundsdóttir HM, Haraldsdóttir V, M Jóhannesson G, et al: Monoclonal gammopathy in Iceland: A population-based registry and follow-up. *Br J Haematol* 118:166, 2002.
19. Ong F, Hermans J, Noordik EM, et al: A population-based registry on paraproteinaemia in the Netherlands. *Br J Haematol* 99:914, 1997.
20. Iwanaga M, Tagawa M, Tsukasaki K, et al: Prevalence of monoclonal gammopathy of undetermined significance: Study of 52,802 persons in Nagasaki City, Japan. *Mayo Clin Proc* 82:1474, 2007.
21. Iwanaga M, Tomonaga M. Prevalence of monoclonal gammopathy of undetermined significance in Asia: A viewpoint from Nagasaki atomic bomb survivors. *Clin Lymphoma Myeloma Leuk* 14:18, 2014.
22. Wu SP, Minter A, Costello R, et al: MGUS prevalence in an ethnically Chinese population in Hong Kong. *Blood* 121:2363, 2013.
23. Landgren O, Katzmann JA, Hsing AW, et al: Prevalence of monoclonal gammopathy of undetermined significance among men in Ghana. *Mayo Clin Proc* 82:1468, 2007.
24. Schecter GP, Shoff N, Chan C, et al: The frequency of monoclonal gammopathy in black and white veterans in a hospital population, in *Epidemiology and Biology of Multiple Myeloma*, edited by Obrams GI, Potter M, p 93. Springer-Verlag, New York, 1991.
25. Singh J, Dudley AW, Kulig KA: Increased incidence of monoclonal gammopathy of undetermined significance in blacks and its age-related differences with whites on the basis of a study of 397 men and one woman in a hospital setting. *J Lab Clin Med* 116:785, 1990.
26. Landgren O, Gridley G, Turesson I, et al: Risk of monoclonal gammopathy of undetermined significance (MGUS) and subsequent multiple myeloma among African American and white veterans in the United States. *Blood* 107:904, 2006.
27. Landgren O, Graubard BI, Katzmann JA, et al: Racial disparities in the prevalence of monoclonal gammopathies: A population-based study of 12 482 persons from the National Health and Nutritional Examination Survey. *Leukemia* 28:1537, 2014.
28. Bizzaro N, Pasini P: Familial occurrence of multiple myeloma and monoclonal gammopathy of undetermined significance in siblings. *Haematologica* 75:58, 1990.
29. Lynch HT, Sanger WG, Pirruccello S, et al: Familial multiple myeloma: A family study and review of the literature. *J Natl Cancer Inst* 94:1479, 2001.
30. Ögmundsdóttir HM, Haraldsdóttirm V, Jóhannesson GM, et al: Familiality of benign and malignant paraproteinemias. A population-based cancer-registry study of multiple myeloma families. *Haematologica* 90:66, 2005.
31. Ögmundsdóttir HM, Valgeirsdóttir S, Schiffhauer HR, et al: Familial predisposition to monoclonal gammopathies: Deviations in B-cell biology. *Clin Lymphoma Myeloma Leuk* 13:191, 2013.
32. Pasqualetti P, Collacciani A, Casole R: Risk of monoclonal gammopathy of undetermined significance. *Am J Hematol* 52:217, 1996.
33. Landgren O, Rajkumar SV, Pfeiffer RM, et al: Obesity is associated with an increased risk of monoclonal gammopathy of undetermined significance among black and white women. *Blood* 116:1056, 2010.
34. Lichtman MA: Obesity and the risk for a hematological malignancy: Leukemia, lymphoma, or myeloma. *Oncologist* 15:1083, 2006.

35. Wallin A, Larsson SC: Body mass index and risk of multiple myeloma: A meta-analysis of prospective studies. *Eur J Cancer* 47:1606, 2011.

36. Hofmann JN, Moore SC, Lim U, et al: Body mass index and physical activity at different ages and risk of multiple myeloma in the NIH-AARP diet and health study. *Am J Epidemiol* 177:776, 2013.

37. Fonesca R, Bailey RJ, Ahmann GJ, et al: Genomic abnormalities in monoclonal gammopathy of undetermined significance. *Blood* 100:1417, 2002.

38. Zandecki M, Lai JL, Genevieve F, et al: Several cytogenetic subclones may be identified within plasma cells from patients with monoclonal gammopathy of undetermined significance both at diagnosis and during the indolent course of the disease. *Blood* 90:3682, 1997.

39. Avet-Loiseau H, Facon T, Daviet A, et al: 14q32 translocations and monosomy 13 observed in monoclonal gammopathy of undetermined significance delineate a multistep process for the oncogenesis of multiple myeloma. *Cancer Res* 59:4546, 1999.

40. Königsberg R, Ackermann J, Kaufmann H, et al: Deletions of chromosome 13q in monoclonal gammopathy of undetermined significance. *Leukemia* 14:1975, 2000.

41. Schilling G, Dierlamm J, Hossfeld DK: Prognostic impact of cytogenetic aberrations in patients with multiple myeloma or monoclonal gammopathy of unknown significance. *Hematol Oncol* 23:102, 2005.

42. Brousseau M, Leleu X, Gerard J, et al: Hyperdiploidy is a common finding in monoclonal gammopathy of undetermined significance and monosomy 13 is restricted to these hyperdiploid patients. *Clin Cancer Res* 13:6026, 2007.

43. Avet-Loiseau H, Li J-Y, Morineau N: Monosomy 13 is associated with the transition of monoclonal gammopathy of undetermined significance to multiple myeloma. *Blood* 94:2583, 1999.

44. Bernasconi P, Cavigliano PM, Boni M, et al: Long-term follow up with conventional cytogenetics and band 13q14 interphase/metaphase *in situ* hybridization monitoring in monoclonal gammopathies of undetermined significance. *Br J Haematol* 118:545, 2002.

45. Rasillo A, Tabernero MD, Sanchez ML, et al: Fluorescence *in situ* hybridization analysis of aneuploidization patterns in monoclonal gammopathy of undetermined significance versus multiple myeloma and plasma cell leukemia. *Cancer* 97:601, 2003.

46. Zojer N, Ludwig H, Fiegi M, et al: Patterns of somatic mutations in VH genes reveal pathways of clonal transformations from MGUS to multiple myeloma. *Blood* 101:4137, 2003.

47. Lloveras E, Sole F, Florensa L, et al: Contribution of cytogenetics and *in situ* hybridization to the study of monoclonal gammopathy of undetermined significance. *Cancer Genet Cytogenet* 132:25, 2002.

48. Landgren O, Kyle RA, Pfeiffer RM, et al: Monoclonal gammopathy of undetermined significance (MGUS) consistently precedes multiple myeloma: A prospective study. *Blood* 113:5412, 2009.

49. Weiss BM, Abadie J, Verma P, et al: A monoclonal gammopathy precedes multiple myeloma in most patients. *Blood* 113:5418, 2009.

50. Davies FE, Dring AM, Li C, et al: Insights into the multistep transformation of MGUS to myeloma using microarray expression analysis. *Blood* 102:4504, 2003.

51. Zhan F, Hardin J, Kordesmeier B, et al: Global gene expression profiling of multiple myeloma, monoclonal gammopathy of undetermined significance, and normal bone marrow plasma cells. *Blood* 99:1745, 2002.

52. Zwick C, Held G, Auth M, et al: Over one-third of African-American MGUS and multiple myeloma patients are carriers of hyperphosphorylated paratarg-7, an autosomal dominantly inherited risk factor for MGUS/MM. *Int J Cancer* 135:934, 2014.

53. Weinhold N, Johnson DC, Rawstron AC, et al: Inherited genetic susceptibility to monoclonal gammopathy of unknown significance. *Blood* 123:2513, 2014.

54. Xu L, Hunter ZR, Yang G, et al: MYD88 L265P in Waldenström macroglobulinemia, immunoglobulin M monoclonal gammopathy, and other B-cell lymphoproliferative disorders using conventional and quantitative allele-specific polymerase chain reaction. *Blood* 121:2051, 2013.

55. Xu L, Hunter ZR, Yang G, et al: Detection of MYD88 L265P in peripheral blood of patients with Waldenström's macroglobulinemia and IgM monoclonal gammopathy of undetermined significance. *Leukemia* 28:1698, 2014.

56. Radl J, Hollander CF: Homogeneous immunoglobulins in sera of mice during aging. *J Immunol* 112:2271, 1974.

57. Radl J, De Glopper E, Schuit HR, Zurcher C: Idiopathic paraproteinemia: II. Transplantation of the paraprotein-producing clone from old to young 57B1/KaLwRij mice. *J Immunol* 122:609, 1979.

58. Radl J: Age-related monoclonal gammopathies: Clinical lessons from the aging C57BL mouse. *Immunol Today* 11:234, 1990.

59. van Arkel C, Hopstaken CM, Zurcher C, et al: Monoclonal gammopathies in aging mu, kappa-transgenic mice: Involvement of the B-1 cell lineage. *Eur J Immunol* 27:2436, 1997.

60. George G, Gilburd B, Schoenfeld Y: The emerging concept of pathogenic natural antibodies. *Hum Antibodies* 8:70, 1997.

61. Milla F, Oriol A, Aguilar J, et al: Usefulness and reproducibility of cytomorphic evaluations to differentiate myeloma from monoclonal gammopathies of unknown significance. *Am J Clin Pathol* 115:127, 2001.

62. Rajkumar SV, Mesa RA, Fonesca R, et al: Bone marrow angiogenesis in 400 patients with monoclonal gammopathy of undetermined significance, multiple myeloma, and primary amyloidosis. *Clin Cancer Res* 8:2210, 2002.

63. Ludwig H, Vormittag W: "Benign" monoclonal IgE gammopathy. *Br Med J* 281:539, 1980.

64. O'Connor ML, Rice DT, Buss DH, Muss HB: Immunoglobulin D benign monoclonal gammopathy. *Cancer* 68:611, 1991.

65. Kinoshita K, Nagai H, Murate T, et al: IgD monoclonal gammopathy of undetermined significance. *Int J Hematol* 65:169, 1997.

66. Galeazzi M, Frezzotti A, Paladini C, et al: A case of monoclonal gammopathy of undetermined significance (MGUS): Type IgD-lambda. *Clin Chem Lab Med* 51:e123, 2013.

67. Imhof JW, Balliux RE, Mul NA, Poen H: Monoclonal and diclonal gamma-pathies. *Acta Med Scand* 179(Suppl 455):102, 1966.

68. Jensen K, Jensen B, Olesen H: Three M-components in serum from an apparently healthy person. *Scand J Haematol* 4:485, 1967.

69. Kyle RA, Robinson RA, Katzmann JA: The clinical aspects of biclonal gammopathies: Review of 57 cases. *Am J Med* 71:999, 1981.

70. Riddell S, Traczyk Z, Paraskevas F, Israels LG: The double gammopathies: Clinical and immunological studies. *Medicine (Baltimore)* 65:135, 1986.

71. Kyle RA, Greipp PR: "Idiopathic" Bence Jones proteinuria. *N Engl J Med* 306:564, 1982.

72. Jenner E: Serum free light chains in clinical laboratory diagnostics. *Clin Chim Acta* 427:15, 2014.

73. Hill PG, Forsyth JM, Rai B, Mayne S: Serum free light chains: An alternative to the urine Bence Jones proteins screening test for monoclonal gammopathies. *Clin Chem* 52:1743, 2006.

74. Katzmann JA, Dispenzieri A, Kyle RA, et al: Elimination of the need for urine studies in the screening algorithm for monoclonal gammopathies by using serum immunofixation and free light chain assays. *Mayo Clin Proc* 81:1575, 2006.

75. Jagannath S: Value of serum free light chain testing for the diagnosis and monitoring of monoclonal gammopathies in hematology. *Clin Lymphoma Myeloma* 7:518, 2007.

76. Beetham R, Wassell J, Wallage MJ, et al: Can serum free light chains replace urine electrophoresis in the detection of monoclonal gammopathies? *Ann Clin Biochem* 44:516, 2007.

77. Murray DL, Seningen JL, Dispenzieri A, et al: Laboratory persistence and clinical progression of small monoclonal abnormalities. *Am J Clin Pathol* 138:609, 2012.

78. Barnidge DR, Dasari S, Botz CM, et al: Using mass spectrometry to monitor monoclonal immunoglobulins in patients with a monoclonal gammopathy. *J Proteome Res* 13:1419, 2014.

79. Mangiacavalli S, Cocito F, Pochintesta L, et al: Monoclonal gammopathy of undetermined significance: A new proposal of workup. *Eur J Haematol* 91:356, 2013.

80. Rajan AM, Rajkumar SV. Diagnostic evaluation of monoclonal gammopathy of undetermined significance. *Eur J Haematol* 91:561, 2013.

81. Kay NE, Gordon LI, Douglas SD: Autoimmune hemolytic anemia in association with monoclonal IgM(kappa) with anti-i activity. *Am J Med* 64:845, 1978.

82. Lamboley V, Zabraniecki L, Sie P, et al: Myeloma and monoclonal gammopathy of uncertain significance associated with acquired von Willebrand's syndrome. Seven new cases with a literature review. *Joint Bone Spine* 69:62, 2002.

83. Agarwal N, Klix MM, Burns CP: Successful management with intravenous immunoglobulins of acquired von Willebrand disease associated with monoclonal gammopathy of undetermined significance. *Ann Intern Med* 6:141:83, 2004.

84. Yujiri T, Nakamura Y, Oota I, et al: Acquired von Willebrand syndrome associated with monoclonal gammopathy of undetermined significance. *Ann Hematol* 93:1427, 2014.

85. Nocente R, Cammarota G, Gentiloni Silveri N, et al: A case of Sweet's syndrome associated with monoclonal immunoglobulin of IgG-lambda type and p-ANCA positivity. *Panminerva Med* 44:149, 2002.

86. Carrington PA, Walsh SE, Houghton JB: Benign paraproteinemia and immune neutropenia. *Clin Lab Haematol* 2:407, 1989.

87. Gabriel DA, Carr ME, Cook L, Roberts HR: Spontaneous antithrombin in a patient with benign paraprotein. *Am J Hematol* 25:85, 1987.

88. Sluiter WJ, Marrink J, Houwen B: Monoclonal gammopathy with an insulin binding IgG(K) M-component, associated with severe hypoglycaemia. *Br J Haematol* 62:679, 1986.

89. Wasada T, Eguei Y, Takayama S, et al: Insulin autoimmune syndrome associated with benign monoclonal gammopathy. *Diabetes Care* 12:147, 1989.

90. Ahlberg RE, Lefvert AK: Monoclonal gammopathy and antibody activity against the acetylcholine receptor. *Am J Hematol* 29:49, 1988.

91. Disdier P, Swiader L, Aillaud M-F, et al: Ig M monoclonal gammopathy, lymphoid proliferations and lupus anticoagulant. *Am J Med* 102:319, 1997.

92. Dear A, Brennan SO, Sheat MJ, et al: Acquired dysfibrinogenemia caused by monoclonal production of immunoglobulin lambda light chain. *Haematologica* 92:e111, 2007.

93. Maldonado JE, Velosa JA, Kyle RA, et al: Fanconi syndrome in adults: A manifestation of a latent form of myeloma. *Am J Med* 58:354, 1975.

94. Gavarotti P, Fortina F, Costa D, et al: Benign monoclonal gammopathy presenting with severe renal failure. *Scand J Haematol* 36:115, 1986.

95. Maes B, Vanwalleghem J, Kuypers D, et al: IgA antiglomerular basement membrane disease associated with bronchial carcinoma and monoclonal gammopathy. *Am J Kidney Dis* 33:E3, 1999.

96. Hashimoto T, Arakawa K, Ohta Y, et al: Acquired Fanconi syndrome with osteomalacia secondary to monoclonal gammopathy of undetermined significance. *Intern Med* 46:241, 2007.

97. Pozzi C, D'Amico M, Fogazzi GB, et al: Light chain deposition disease with renal involvement: Clinical characteristics and prognostic factors. *Am J Kidney Dis* 42:1154, 2003.

98. Merlini G, Stone MJ: Dangerous small B-cell clones. *Blood* 108:2520, 2006.

99. Leung N, Bridoux F, Hutchison CA, et al: Monoclonal gammopathy of renal significance: When MGUS is no longer undetermined or insignificant. *Blood* 120:4292, 2012.

100. Sethi S, Rajkumar SV: Monoclonal gammopathy-associated proliferative glomerulonephritis. *Mayo Clin Proc* 88:1284, 2013.

101. Fermand JP, Bridoux F, Kyle RA, et al: How I treat monoclonal gammopathy of renal significance (MGRS). *Blood* 122:3583, 2013.

102. Paladini I, Pieretti G, Giuntoli M, et al: Crystalline corneal deposits in monoclonal gammopathy: In-vivo confocal microscopy. *Semin Ophthalmol* 28:37, 2013.

103. Secundo W, Seifert P: Monoclonal corneal gammopathy: Topographic considerations. *Ger J Ophthalmol* 5:262, 1996.

104. Shah S, Espana EM, Margo CE: Ocular manifestations of monoclonal copper-binding immunoglobulin. *Surv Ophthalmol* 59:11, 2014.

105. Probst LE, Hoffman E, Cherian MG, et al: Ocular copper deposition associated with benign monoclonal gammopathy and hypercupremia. *Cornea* 15:94, 1996.

106. Saffra N, Rakhamimov A, Solomon WB, Scheers-Masters J: Monoclonal gammopathy of undetermined significance maculopathy. *Can J Ophthalmol* 48:e168, 2013.

107. Drappatz J, Batchelor T: Neurologic complications of plasma cell disorders. *Clin Lymphoma* 5:163, 2004.

108. Lozeron P, Adams D: Monoclonal gammopathy and neuropathy. *Curr Opin Neurol* 20:536, 2007.

109. Ropper AH, Gorsin KC: Neuropathies associated with paraproteinemia. *N Engl J Med* 338:1601, 1998.

110. Kissel JT, Mendell JR: Neuropathies associated with monoclonal gammopathies. *Neuromuscul Disord* 6:3, 1996.

111. Vallatt JM, Jauberteau MO, Bordessoule D, et al: Link between peripheral neuropathy and monoclonal dysglobulinemia: A study of 66 cases. *J Neurol Sci* 137:124, 1996.

112. Lee KW, Inghirami G, Spatz L, et al: The B-cells that express anti-MAG antibodies in neuropathy and non-malignant IgM monoclonal gammopathy belong to the CD5 subpopulation. *J Neuroimmunol* 31:83, 1991.

113. Cocito D, Durelli L, Isoardo G: Different clinical, electrophysiological and immunological features of CDIP associated with paraproteinemia. *Acta Neurol Scand* 108:274, 2003.

114. Chassande B, Léger J-M, Younes-Chennoufi AB, et al: Peripheral neuropathy associated with IgM monoclonal gammopathy: Correlation between M-protein antibody activity and clinical/electrophysiological features in 40 cases. *Muscle Nerve* 21:55, 1998.

115. Pestronk A, Li F, Bieser BS, et al: Anti-MAG antibodies. *Neurology* 44:1131, 1994.

116. Stubbs EB Jr, Lawlor MW, Richards MP, et al: Anti-neurofilament antibodies in neuropathy with monoclonal gammopathy of undetermined significance produce experimental motor nerve conduction block. *Acta Neuropathol* 105:109, 2003.

117. Ellie E, Vital A, Steck A, et al: Neuropathy associated with "benign" anti-myelin-associated glycoprotein IgM gammopathy: Clinical, immunological, neurophysiological pathological findings and response to treatment in 33 cases. *J Neurol* 243:34, 1996.

118. Di Troia A, Carpo M, Meucci N, et al: Clinical features and anti-neural reactivity in neuropathy associated with IgG monoclonal gammopathy of undetermined significance. *J Neurol Sci* 164:64, 1999.

119. Vallat JM, Magy L, Richard L, Piaser M, et al: Intranervous immunoglobulin deposits: An underestimated mechanism of neuropathy. *Muscle Nerve* 38:904, 2008.

120. Gorsin KC, Ropper AH: Axonal neuropathy associated with monoclonal gammopathy of undetermined significance. *J Neurol Neurosurg Psychiatry* 63:163, 1997.

121. Wilson JR, Stittsworth JD Jr, Fisher MA: Electrodiagnostic patterns in MGUS neuropathy. *Electromyogr Clin Neurophysiol* 41:409, 2001.

122. Nicholas G, Maisonobe T, Le Forestier N, et al: Proposed revised electrophysiological criteria for chronic inflammatory demyelinating polyradiculopathy. *Muscle Nerve* 25:26, 2002.

123. Jonsson V, Schroder HD, Trojaborg W, et al: Autoimmune reactions in patients with M-component and peripheral neuropathy. *J Intern Med* 232:185, 1992.

124. Gorsin KC, Allan G, Ropper AH: Chronic inflammatory demyelinating polyneuropathy: Clinical features and response to treatment in 67 consecutive patients with and without a monoclonal gammopathy. *Neurology* 48:321, 1997.

125. Vital A, Nedelec-Ciceri C, Vital C: Presence of crystalline inclusions in the peripheral nerve of a patient with IgA lambda monoclonal gammopathy of undetermined significance. *Neuropathology* 28:526, 2008.

126. Latov N: Pathogenesis and therapy of neuropathies associated with monoclonal gammopathies. *Ann Neurol* 37(Suppl 1):532, 1995.

127. Sghirlanzoni A, Solari A, Ciano C: Chronic inflammatory demyelinating polyradiculopathy: Long-term course and treatment of 60 patients. *Neurol Sci* 21:31, 2000.

128. Kiprov DD, Miller RG: Paraproteinemia associated with demyelinating polyneuropathy or myositis: Treatment with plasmapheresis and immunosuppressive drugs. *Artif Organs* 9:47, 1985.

129. Gorson KC: Clinical features, evaluation, and treatment of patients with polyneuropathy associated with monoclonal gammopathy of undetermined significance (MGUS). *J Clin Apher* 14:149, 1999.

130. Blume G, Pestronk A, Goodnough LT: Anti-MAG antibody-associated polyneuropathies: Improvement following immunotherapy with monthly plasma exchange and IV cyclophosphamide. *Neurology* 45:1577, 1995.

131. Oksenhendler E, Chevret S, Léger JM, et al: Plasma exchange and chlorambucil in polyneuropathy associated with monoclonal IgM gammopathy. *J Neurol Neurosurg Psychiatry* 59:243, 1995.

132. Lee YC, Came N, Schwarer A, Day B: Autologous peripheral blood stem cell transplantation for peripheral neuropathy secondary to monoclonal gammopathy of unknown significance. *Bone Marrow Transplant* 30:53, 2002.

133. Niermeijer JM, Eurelings M, Lokhorst H, et al: Neurologic and hematologic response to fludarabine treatment in IgM MGUS polyneuropathy. *Neurology* 67:2076, 2006.

134. Finsterer J: Treatment of immune-mediated, dysimmune neuropathies. *Acta Neurol Scand* 112:115, 2005.

135. Renaud S, Fuhr P, Gregor M, et al: High-dose rituximab and anti-MAG-associated polyneuropathy. *Neurology* 66:742, 2006.

136. Kristinsson SY, Fears TR, Gridley G, et al: Deep vein thrombosis following monoclonal gammopathy of undetermined significance (MGUS) and multiple myeloma. *Blood* 112:3582, 2008.

137. Auwerda JJ, Sonneveld P, de Maat MP, Leebeek FW: Prothrombotic coagulation abnormalities in patients with paraprotein-producing B-cell disorders. *Clin Lymphoma Myeloma* 7:462, 2007.

138. Melton LJ 3rd, Rajkumar SV, Khosla S, et al: Fracture risk in monoclonal gammopathy of undetermined significance. *J Bone Miner Res* 19:25, 2004.

139. Farr JN, Zhang W, Kumar SK, et al: Altered cortical microarchitecture in patients with monoclonal gammopathy of undetermined significance. *Blood* 123:647, 2014.

140. Burner E, Swahlen A, Cruchaud A: Nonmalignant monoclonal immunoglobulinemia, pernicious anemia, and gastric carcinoma: A model of immunologic dysfunction. *Am J Med* 60:1019, 1976.

141. Rowland LP, Osserman EF, Scharfman WB, et al: Myasthenia gravis with a myeloma-type gamma-G (IgG) immunoglobulin abnormality. *Am J Med* 46:599, 1969.

142. Ilfeld D, Barzilay J, Vana D, et al: IgG monoclonal gammopathy in four patients with polymyalgia rheumatica [letter]. *Ann Rheum Dis* 44:501, 1985.

143. Nanji AA: Monoclonal gammopathy associated with Crohn's disease during treatment with total parenteral nutrition. *JPEN J Parenter Enteral Nutr* 9:621, 1985.

144. Wallach D, Carado Y, Foldes C, Cottenot F: Dermatomyositis and monoclonal gammopathy. *Ann Dermatol Venereol* 112:783, 1985.

145. McFadden N, Ree K, Syland E, Larse TE: Scleredema adultorum associated with a monoclonal gammopathy and generalized hyperpigmentation. *Arch Dermatol* 123:629, 1987.

146. Oikarinen A, Ala-Kokko L, Palatsi R, et al: Scleroderma and paraproteinemia. *Arch Dermatol* 123:226, 1987.

147. Johnsson V, Svendsen B, Vostrup S, et al: Multiple autoimmune manifestations in monoclonal gammopathy of undetermined significance and chronic lymphocytic leukemia. *Leukemia* 10:327, 1996.

148. Kyle RA: Monoclonal gammopathy of unknown significance (MGUS). *Baillieres Clin Haematol* 8:761, 1995.

149. Kagaya M, Takahashi H: A case of type I cryoglobulinemia associated with a monoclonal gammopathy of undetermined significance (MGUS). *J Dermatol* 32:128, 2005.

150. de Koning HD, Bodar EJ, van der Meer JW, et al: Schnitzler syndrome: Beyond the case reports: Review and follow-up of 94 patients with an emphasis on prognosis and treatment. *Semin Arthritis Rheum* 37:137, 2007.

151. Ryan JG, de Koning HD, Beck LA, et al: IL-1 blockade in Schnitzler syndrome: *Ex vivo* findings correlate with clinical remission. *J Allergy Clin Immunol* 121:260, 2008.

152. Wayte JA, Rogers S, Powell FC: Pyoderma gangrenosum, erythema elevatum diutinum and Ig A monoclonal gammopathy. *Australas J Dermatol* 36:21, 1995.

153. Doutre MS, Beylot C, Bioulac P, Bezian JH: Monoclonal IgM and chronic urticaria: Two cases. *Ann Allergy* 58:413, 1987.

154. Samochocki Z, Szudzinski A: Gangrenous pyoderma in monoclonal IgA gammopathy and functional disorders of T lymphocytes. *Przegl Dermatol* 73:409, 1986.

155. Abraham Z, Feuerman EJ: IgA benign monoclonal gammopathy with recurrent self-healing skin tumors. *J Am Acad Dermatol* 21:1303, 1989.

156. Paul C, Fermaud J-P, Flageul B, et al: Hyperkeratotic spicules and monoclonal gammopathy. *J Am Acad Dermatol* 33:346, 1995.

157. Scutellari PN, Antinolfi G: Association between monoclonal gammopathy of undetermined significance (MGUS) and diffuse idiopathic skeletal hyperostosis (DISH). *Radiol Med (Torino)* 108:172, 2004.

158. Schnur MJ, Appel GB, Bilezikian JP: Primary hyperparathyroidism and benign monoclonal gammopathy. *Arch Intern Med* 137:1201, 1977.

159. Rao DS, Antonelli R, Kane KR, et al: Primary hyperparathyroidism and monoclonal gammopathy. *Henry Ford Hosp Med J* 39:41, 1991.

160. Schoenfeld Y, Berliner S, Pinkhas J, Beutler E: The association of Gaucher's disease and dysproteinemias. *Acta Haematol* 64:241, 1980.

161. de Fost M, Out TA, de Wilde FA, et al: Immunoglobulin and free light chain abnormalities in Gaucher disease type I: Data from an adult cohort of 63 patients and review of the literature. *Ann Hematol* 87:439, 2008.

162. Rodic P, Pavlovic S, Kostic T et al: Gammopathy and B lymphocyte clonality in patients with Gaucher type I disease. *Blood Cells Mol Dis* 50:222, 2013.

163. Andreone P, Zignego AL, Cursaro C, et al: Prevalence of monoclonal gammopathies in patients with hepatitis C virus infection. *Ann Intern Med* 129:294, 1998.

164. Hamazaaki K, Baba M, Hasegawa H, et al: Chronic hepatitis associated with monoclonal gammopathy of undetermined significance. *Gastroenterol Hepatol* 18:459, 2003.

165. Schafer AL, Miller JB, Lester EP, et al: Monoclonal gammopathy in hereditary spherocytosis: A possible pathogenetic relation. *Ann Intern Med* 88:45, 1978.

166. Danon F, Bussel A, Perol Y: Immunoglobulines monoclonales infections a cytomegalovirus et hémopathies malignes. *Ann Immunol (Paris)* 128A:83, 1977.

167. Papadopoulos NM, Lane HC, Costello R, et al: Oligoclonal immunoglobulins in patients with the acquired immunodeficiency syndrome. *Clin Immunol Immunopathol* 35:43, 1985.

168. Heriot K, Hallquist AE, Tomar RH: Paraproteinemia in patients with acquired immunodeficiency syndrome (AIDS) or lymphadenopathy syndrome (LAS). *Clin Chem* 31:1224, 1985.

169. Kouns DM, Marty AM, Sharpe RW: Oligoclonal bands in serum protein electrophoretograms of individuals with human immunodeficiency virus antibodies. *JAMA* 256:2343, 1986.

170. Johnston JD, Lumb PJ, Wierzbicki AS: Hyperlipidaemia in association with benign paraproteinemia. *Ann Clin Biochem* 34:697, 1997.

171. Papadaki HA, Eliopoulos DG, Ponticoglou C, Eliopoulos GD: Increased frequency of monoclonal gammopathy of undetermined significance in patients with nonimmune chronic idiopathic neutropenia syndrome. *Int J Hematol* 73:339, 2001.

172. Dizdar O, Erman M, Cankurtaran M, et al: Lower bone mineral density in geriatric patients with monoclonal gammopathy of undetermined significance. *Ann Hematol* 87:57, 2008.

173. Tucci A, Bonadonna S, Cattaneo C, et al: Transformation of MGUS to overt multiple myeloma: The possible role of pituitary microadenoma secreting high levels of insulin-like growth factor 1 (IGF-1). *Leuk Lymphoma* 44:543, 2003.

174. Chryssikkopoulos A, Dalamaga AL, Hassiakos D: Monoclonal gammopathy of unknown significance in pregnancy. *Clin Exp Obstet Gynecol* 24:31, 1997.

175. Buonocore E, Solmon A, Kerley HE: Pseudomyeloma. *Radiology* 95:41, 1970.

176. Maldonado JE, Riggs L, Bayrd ED: Pseudomyeloma. *Arch Intern Med* 135:267, 1975.

177. Xie Z, Ghosh CC, Patel R, et al: Vascular endothelial hyperpermeability induces the clinical symptoms of Clarkson disease (the systemic capillary leak syndrome). *Blood* 119:4321, 2012.

178. Kyle RA: Monoclonal gammopathy of unknown significance. *Curr Top Microbiol Immunol* 210:375, 1996.

179. Solomon A: Homogeneous (monoclonal) immunoglobulins in cancer. *Am J Med* 63:169, 1977.

180. Colls BM, Lorier MA: Immunocytoma, cancer, and other associations of monoclonal gammopathy: A review of 224 cases. *N Z Med J* 82:221, 1975.

181. Abdul M, Hassein NM: Gammopathy associated with advanced prostate cancer. *Urol Res* 23:185, 1995.

182. Landgren O, Mailankody S: Update on second primary malignancies in multiple myeloma: A focused review. *Leukemia* 28:1423, 2014.

183. Wu SP, Costello R, Hofmann JN, et al: MGUS prevalence in a cohort of AML patients. *Blood* 122:294, 2013.

184. Mailankody S, Pfeiffer RM, Kristinsson SY, et al: Risk of acute myeloid leukemia and myelodysplastic syndromes after multiple myeloma and its precursor disease (MGUS). *Blood* 118:4086, 2011.

185. Shoenfeld Y, Berliner S, Ayalone A, et al: Monoclonal gammopathy in patients with chronic and acute myeloid leukemia. *Cancer* 54:280, 1984.

186. Berner Y, Berrebi A: Myeloproliferative disorders and nonmyelomatous paraprotein. *Isr J Med Sci* 22:109, 1986.

187. Tosato F, Fossaluzza V, Rossi P, et al: Monoclonal gammopathy of undetermined significance in a case of primary thrombocythemia. *Haematologica* 71:417, 1986.

188. Economopoulos T, Economidou J, Papageorgiou E, et al: Monoclonal gammopathy in chronic myeloproliferative disorders. *Blut* 58:7, 1989.

189. Ito T, Kojima H, Otani K, et al: Chronic neutrophilic leukemia associated with monoclonal gammopathy of unknown significance. *Acta Haematol* 95:140, 1996.

190. Offit K, Macris NT, Hellman G, Rotterdam, HZ: Consecutive lymphoma with monoclonal gammopathy in a married couple. *Cancer* 57:277, 1986.

191. Venencie PY, Winkelmann RK, Puissant A, Kyle RA: Monoclonal gammopathy in Sézary syndrome: Report of three cases and review of the literature. *Arch Dermatol* 120:605, 1984.

192. Kamihira S, Taguchi H, Kinoshita K, Ichimaru M: Monoclonal gammopathy in adult T-cell leukemia/lymphoma: A report of three cases. *Jpn J Clin Oncol* 14:699, 1984.

193. Chisesi I, Capnist G, Barbui T: Two serum IgG M-components of differing light chain types in a case of Hodgkin's disease. *Acta Haematol* 55:250, 1976.

194. Hammarstrom L, Smith CIE: Frequent occurrence of monoclonal gammopathies with an imbalanced light-chain ratio following bone marrow transplantation. *Transplantation* 43:447, 1987.

195. Mitus AJ, Stein R, Rappeport JM, et al: Monoclonal and oligoclonal gammopathy after bone marrow transplantation. *Blood* 74:2764, 1989.

196. Passweg J, Thiel G, Bock HA: Monoclonal gammopathy after intense induction immunosuppression in renal transplant patients. *Nephrol Dial Transplant* 11:2461, 1996.

197. Badley AD, Portela DF, Patel R, et al: Development of monoclonal gammopathy precedes the development of Epstein-Barr virus-induced posttransplant lymphoproliferative disorder. *Liver Transpl Surg* 2:375, 1996.

198. Touchard G, Pasdeloup T, Parpeix J, et al: High prevalence and usual persistence of serum monoclonal immunoglobulins evidenced by sensitive methods in renal transplant recipients. *Nephrol Dial Transplant* 12:1199, 1997.

199. Ho JL, Polde PA, McEniry D, et al: Acquired immunodeficiency syndrome with progressive multifocal leukoencephalopathy and monoclonal B-cell proliferation. *Ann Intern Med* 100:693, 1984.

200. Nagler A, Ben-Arieh Y, Brenner B, et al: Eosinophilic fibrohistiocytic lesion of bone marrow associated with monoclonal gammopathy and osteolytic lesions. *Am J Hematol* 23:277, 1986.

201. Hineman VL, Phyliky RL, Banks PM: Angiofollicular lymph node hyperplasia and peripheral neuropathy: Association with monoclonal gammopathy. *Mayo Clin Proc* 57:379, 1982.

202. Radl J, VandenBerg A: Transitory appearance of homogeneous immunoglobulins—paraproteins—in children with severe combined immunodeficiency before and after transplantation, in *Protides of Biological Fluids*, vol 20, edited by Peeters H, p 203. Pergamon, Oxford, 1973.

203. Malacrida V, De-Francesco D, Banfi G, et al: Laboratory investigation of monoclonal gammopathy during 10 years of screening in a general hospital. *J Clin Pathol* 40:793, 1987.

204. DelCarpio J, Espinoza LR, Lauater S, Osterland CK: Transient monoclonal proteins in drug hypersensitivity reactions. *Am J Med* 66:1051, 1979.

205. Keshgegian AA: Prevalence of small monoclonal proteins in the serum of hospitalized patients. *Am J Clin Pathol* 77:436, 1982.

206. VanCamp B, Reynaerts PH, Naets JP, Radl J: Transient IgA$_1$-λ para-proteinemia during treatment of acute myeloblastic leukemia. *Blood* 55:21, 1980.

207. Bakker AJ, Kothman-Tijkotte MJ: Artifactually high concentration of iron determined in serum from a patient with a monoclonal immunoglobulin. *Clin Chem* 36:1517, 1990.

208. Yu A, Pira U: False increase in serum C-reactive protein caused by monoclonal IgM-lambda: A case report. *Clin Chem Lab Med* 39:983, 2001.

209. Baz R, Alemany C, Green R, Hussein MA: Prevalence of vitamin B$_{12}$ deficiency in patients with plasma cell dyscrasias: A retrospective review. *Cancer* 101:790, 2004.

210. Moller-Petersen J, Schmidt EB: Diagnostic value of the concentration of M-component in initial classification of monoclonal gammopathy. *Scand J Haematol* 26:295, 1986.

211. Link H, Kostulas V: Utility of isoelectric focusing of cerebrospinal fluid and serum of agarose evaluated for neurological patients. *Clin Chem* 29:810, 1983.

212. Ouedraogo DE, Makinson A, Vendrell JP, et al: Pivotal role of HIV and EBV replication in the long-term persistence of monoclonal gammopathy in patients on antiretroviral therapy. *Blood* 122:3030, 2013.

213. Pham H, Lemoine A, Sol O et al: Monoclonal and oligoclonal gammopathies in liver transplant recipients. *Transplantation* 58:253, 1994.

214. Myara I, Quenum G, Storogenko M, et al: Monoclonal and oligoclonal gammopathies in heart-transplant recipients. *Clin Chem* 37:1334, 1991.

215. Chiusolo P, Metafuni E, Cattani P, et al: Prospective evaluation of Epstein-Barr virus reactivation after stem cell transplantation: Association with monoclonal gammopathy. *J Clin Immunol* 30:894, 2010.

216. Ely SA, Knowles DM: Expression of CD56/neural adhesion molecule correlates with the presence of lytic bone lesions in multiple myeloma and distinguishes myeloma from monoclonal gammopathy of undetermined significance and lymphomas with plasmacytoid differentiation. *Am J Pathol* 160:1293, 2002.

217. San Miguel JF, Caballero MD, Gonzalez M: T-cell subpopulations in patients with monoclonal gammopathies: Essential monoclonal gammopathy, multiple myeloma and Waldenstrom macroglobulinemia. *Am J Hematol* 20:267, 1985.

218. Lindstrom FD, Hardy WR, Eberle BJ, Williams RC Jr: Multiple myeloma and benign monoclonal gammopathy: Differentiation by immunofluorescence of lymphocytes. *Ann Intern Med* 78:837, 1973.

219. Greipp PR, Kyle RA: Clinical, morphological and cell kinetic differences among multiple myeloma, monoclonal gammopathy of undetermined significance and smoldering myeloma. *Blood* 62:166, 1983.

220. Boccadoro M, Gavarotti P, Fossati G: Low plasma cell 3(H)-thymidine incorporation in MGUS, smoldering myeloma and remission phase myeloma: Reliable identification of patients not requiring therapy. *Br J Haematol* 58:689, 1984.

221. Billadeau D, Greipp P, Ahmann G, et al: Detection of B-cells clonally related to the tumor population in multiple myeloma and MGUS. *Curr Top Microbiol Immunol* 194:9, 1995.

222. Morrell A, Riesen W: Serum β_2-macroglobulin, serum creatinine and bone marrow plasma cells in benign and malignant monoclonal gammopathy. *Acta Haematol* 64:87, 1980.

223. Fine JM, Lambin P, Desjobert H: Serum neopterin and β_2-microglobulin concentrations in monoclonal gammopathies. *Acta Haematol Scand* 224:179, 1988.

224. Pasqualetti P, Festucci V, Collacciani A, Casale R: The natural history of monoclonal gammopathy of undetermined significance. *Acta Haematol* 97:174, 1997.

225. Gregersen H, Ibsen JS, Mellemkjaer L, et al: Mortality and causes of death in patients with monoclonal gammopathy of undetermined significance. *Br J Haematol* 112:353, 2001.

226. Kyle RA: A long-term study of the prognosis in monoclonal gammopathy of undetermined significance. *N Engl J Med* 346:564, 2002.

227. Morra E, Cesana C, Klersy C, et al: Clinical characteristics and factors predicting evolution of asymptomatic IgM monoclonal gammopathies and IgM-related disorders. *Leukemia* 18:1512, 2004.

228. Kyle RA, Therneau TM, Rajkumar SV, et al: Long-term follow-up of IgM monoclonal gammopathy of undetermined significance. *Blood* 102:3759, 2003.

229. Gregersen H, Mellemkjaer L, Ibsen JS, et al: The impact of M-component type and immunoglobulin concentration on risk of malignant transformation in patients with monoclonal gammopathy of undetermined significance. *Haematologica* 86:1172, 2001.

230. Montoto S, Rozman K, Rosinol L, et al: Malignant transformation in IgM monoclonal gammopathy of undetermined significance. *Semin Oncol* 30:178, 2003.

231. Van De Donk N, De Weerdt O, Eureling M, et al: Malignant transformation of monoclonal gammopathy of undetermined significance: Cumulative incidence and prognostic factors. *Leuk Lymphoma* 42:609, 2001.

232. Cesana C, Klersy C, Barbarano L, et al: Prognostic factors for malignant transformation in monoclonal gammopathy of undetermined significance and smoldering multiple myeloma. *J Clin Oncol* 15:1625, 2002.

233. Sackmann F, Pavlovsky MA, Corrado C, et al: Prognostic factors in monoclonal gammopathy of undetermined significance. *Haematologica* 93:153, 2008.

234. Rosiñol L, Cibeira MT, Montoto S, et al: Monoclonal gammopathy of undetermined significance: Predictors of malignant transformation and recognition of an evolving type characterized by a progressive increase in M protein size. *Mayo Clin Proc* 82:428, 2007.

235. Olteanu H, Wang HY, Chen W, et al: Immunophenotypic studies of monoclonal gammopathy of undetermined significance. *BMC Clin Pathol* 8:13, 2008.

236. Hillengass J, Weber MA, Kilk K, et al: Prognostic significance of whole-body MRI in patients with monoclonal gammopathy of undetermined significance. *Leukemia* 28:174, 2014.

237. Zhan F, Barlogie B, Arzoumanian V, et al: Gene-expression signature of benign monoclonal gammopathy evident in multiple myeloma is linked to good prognosis. *Blood* 109:1692, 2007.

238. Kyle RA, Rajkumar SV: Monoclonal gammopathy of undetermined significance and smoldering multiple myeloma. *Hematol Oncol Clin North Am* 21:1093, 2007.

239. Barlogie B, van Rhee F, Shaughnessy JD Jr, et al: Seven year median time to progression with thalidomide for smoldering myeloma: Partial response identifies subset requiring earlier salvage therapy for symptomatic disease. *Blood* 112:3122, 2008.

240. Cherry BM, Costello R, Zingone A, et al: Immunoparesis and monoclonal gammopathy of undetermined significance are disassociated in advanced age. *Am J Hematol* 88:89, 2013.

241. Bacher U, Haferlach T, Kern W, et al: Correlation of cytomorphology, immunophenotyping, and interphase fluorescence in situ hybridization in 381 patients with monoclonal gammopathy of undetermined significance and 301 patients with plasma cell myeloma. *Cancer Genet Cytogenet* 203:169, 2010.

242. Agarwal A, Ghobrial IM: Monoclonal gammopathy of undetermined significance and smoldering multiple myeloma: A review of the current understanding of epidemiology, biology, risk stratification, and management of myeloma precursor disease. *Clin Cancer Res* 19:985, 2013.

243. Probst LE, Hoffman E, Cherian MG, et al: Ocular copper deposition associated with benign monoclonal gammopathy and hypercupremia. *Cornea* 15:94, 1996.

244. Secundo W, Seifert P: Monoclonal corneal gammopathy: Topographic considerations. *Ger J Ophthalmol* 5:262, 1996.

245. Baldini L, Guffanti A, Cesana BM, et al: Role of different hematologic variables in defining the risk of malignant transformation in monoclonal gammopathy. *Blood* 87:92, 1996.

246. Bataille R: New insights in the clinical biology of multiple myeloma. *Semin Hematol* 34:23, 1997.

247. Witzig TE, Gonchoroff NJ, Katzmann JA, et al: Peripheral blood B cell labeling indices are a measure of disease activity in patients with monoclonal gammopathies. *J Clin Oncol* 6:1041, 1988.

248. Yi Q, Eriksson I, He W, et al: Idiotype-specific T lymphocytes in monoclonal gammopathies: Evidence for the presence of CD4+ and CD8+ subsets. *Br J Haematol* 96:338, 1997.

249. Yi Q, Osterborg A, Bergenbrant S, et al: Idiotype-reactive T-cell subsets and tumor load in monoclonal gammopathies. *Blood* 86:3043, 1995.

250. Halapi E, Werner A, Wahlstrom J, et al: T cell repertoire in patients with multiple myeloma and monoclonal gammopathy of undetermined significance: Clonal CD8+ T cell expansions are found preferentially in patients with a low tumor burden. *Eur J Immunol* 27:2245, 1997.

251. Corso A, Castelli G, Pagnucco G, et al: Bone marrow T-cell subsets in patients with monoclonal gammopathies: Correlation with clinical stage and disease. *Haematologica* 82:43, 1997.

252. Miguel-Garcia A, Matutes E, Tarin F, et al: Circulating Ki-67 positive lymphocytes in multiple myeloma and benign monoclonal gammopathy. *J Clin Pathol* 48:835, 1995.

253. Billadeau D, Van Ness B, Kimlinger T, et al: Clonal circulation cells are common in plasma cell proliferative disorders: A comparison of monoclonal gammopathy, smoldering myeloma, and active myeloma. *Blood* 88:289, 1996.

254. Isaksson E, Bjockholm M, Holm G, et al: Blood clonal B-cell excess in patients with monoclonal gammopathy of undetermined significance (MGUS): Association with malignant transformation. *Br J Haematol* 92:71, 1996.

255. Sawanoborj M, Suzuki K, Nakagawa Y, et al: Natural killer cell frequency and serum cytokine levels in monoclonal gammopathies: Correlation of bone marrow granular lymphocytes to prognosis. *Acta Haematol* 98:150, 1997.

256. Leo E, Kropff M, Lindemann A, et al: DNA aneuploidy, increased proliferation and nuclear area of plasma cells in monoclonal gammopathy of undetermined significance and multiple myeloma. *Anal Quant Cytol Histol* 17:113, 1995.

257. Pérez-Persona E, Vidriales MB, Mateo G, et al: New criteria to identify risk of progression in monoclonal gammopathy of uncertain significance and smoldering multiple myeloma based on multiparameter flow cytometry analysis of bone marrow plasma cells. *Blood* 110:2586, 2007.

258. Turesson I: Nucleolar size in benign and malignant plasma cell proliferation. *Acta Med Scand* 197:7, 1975.

259. Dehou MF, Schots R, Lacor P, Arras N, et al: Diagnostic and prognostic value of the MB2 monoclonal antibody in paraffin-embedded bone marrow sections of patients with multiple myeloma and monoclonal gammopathy of undetermined significance. *J Clin Pathol* 94:287, 1990.

260. French M, Fench P, Remy F, et al: Plasma cell proliferation in monoclonal gammopathy: Relations with other biologic variables—Diagnostic and prognostic significance. *Am J Med* 98:60, 1995.

261. Amiel A, Kirgner I, Gaber E, et al: Replication pattern in cancer: Asynchronous replication in multiple myeloma and in monoclonal gammopathy. *Cancer Genet Cytogenet* 108:32, 1999.

262. Almeida J, Orfao A, Mateo G, et al: Immunophenotype and DNA content characteristics of plasma cells in multiple myeloma and monoclonal gammopathy of undetermined significance. *Pathol Biol* 47:119, 1999.

263. Yasuda N, Kanoh T, Uchino H: J chain synthesis in human myeloma cells: Light and electron microscopic studies. *Clin Exp Immunol* 40:573, 1980.

264. Cassuto JP, Hammore JC, Pastorelli F, et al: Plasma cell acid phosphatase, a discriminative test for benign and malignant monoclonal gammopathies. *Biomedicine* 27:97, 1977.

265. Sonneveld P, Durie BGM, Lokhorst HM, et al: Analysis of multidrug-resistance (MDR-1) glycoprotein and CD56 expression to separate monoclonal gammopathy from multiple myeloma. *Br J Haematol* 83:63, 1993.

266. Zandecki N, Facon T, Bernard F, et al: CD19 and immunophenotype of bone marrow plasma cells in monoclonal gammopathy of undetermined significance. *J Clin Pathol* 48:548, 1995.

267. Sezer O, Heider U, Zavrski I, Possinger K: Differentiation of monoclonal gammopathy of undetermined significance and multiple myeloma using flow cytometric characteristics of plasma cells. *Haematologica* 86:837, 2001.

268. Majumdar G, Heard SE, Singh AK: Use of cytoplasmic 5′nucleotidase for differentiating malignant from benign monoclonal gammopathies. *J Clin Pathol* 43:891, 1990.

269. Van de Berg BC, Michaux L, Lecouvet FE, et al: Nonmyelomatous monoclonal gammopathy: Correlation of bone marrow MR images with laboratory findings and spontaneous clinical outcome. *Radiology* 202:249, 1997.

270. Bellaiche L, Laredo J-D, Lioté F, et al: Magnetic resonance appearance of monoclonal gammopathies of unknown significance and multiple myeloma. *Spine (Phila Pa 1976)* 22:2551, 1997.

271. Laroche M, Attal M, Pouilles JM, et al: Dual-energy x-ray absorption in patients with multiple myeloma and benign gammopathies. *Clin Exp Rheumatol* 14:108, 1996.

272. Bataille R, Chappard D, Basle M: Quantifiable excess of bone resorption in monoclonal gammopathy is an early symptom of malignancy: A prospective study of 87 bone biopsies. *Blood* 87:4762, 1996.

273. Pecherstorfer M, Seibel MJ, Woitge HW, et al: Bone resorption in multiple myeloma and in monoclonal gammopathy of undetermined significance: Quantification by urinary pyridinium cross-links of collagen. *Blood* 90:3743, 1997.

274. Ong F, Kaiser U, Seelen PJ, et al: Serum neural cell adhesion molecule differentiates multiple myeloma from paraproteinemias due to other causes. *Blood* 87:712, 1996.

275. Lacy MQ, Donovan KA, Heimbach JK, et al: Comparison of interleukin-1 beta expression by in situ hybridization in monoclonal gammopathy of undetermined significance and multiple myeloma. *Blood* 93:300, 1999.

276. Greco C, Ameglio F, Alvino S, et al: Selection of patients with monoclonal gammopathy of undetermined significance is mandatory for a reliable use of interleukin-6 and other nonspecific multiple myeloma serum markers. *Acta Haematol* 92:1, 1994.

277. Mathiot C, Mary JY, Tartour E, et al: Soluble CD16 (sCD16), a marker of malignancy in individuals with monoclonal gammopathy of undetermined significance (MGUS). *Br J Haematol* 95:660, 1996.

278. Gaillard JP, Bataille R, Brailly H, et al: Increased and highly stable levels of functional soluble interleukin-6 receptor levels in sera of patients with monoclonal gammopathy. *Eur J Immunol* 23:820, 1993.

279. DuVillard L, Guiguet M, Casasnovas R-O, et al: Diagnostic value of serum IL-6 level in monoclonal gammopathies. *Br J Haematol* 89:243, 1995.

280. Cozzolino F, Torcia M, Aldinucci D, et al: Production of interleukin-1 by bone marrow myeloma cells. *Blood* 74:380, 1989.

281. Donovan KA, Lacy MQ, Kline MP, et al: Contrast in cytokine expression between patients with monoclonal gammopathy of undetermined significance or multiple myeloma. *Leukemia* 12:593, 1998.

282. Diamond T, Levy S, Smith A, et al: Non-invasive markers of bone turnover and plasma cytokines differ in osteoporotic patients with multiple myeloma and monoclonal gammopathies of undetermined significance. *Intern Med* 31:272, 2001.

283. Seidl S, Ackerman J, Kaufmann H, et al: DNA methylation analysis identifies the E-cadherin gene as a potential marker of disease progression in patients with monoclonal gammopathy. *Cancer* 100:2598, 2004.

CHAPTER 107
MYELOMA

Elizabeth O'Donnell, Francesca Cottini, Noopur Raje, and Kenneth Anderson

SUMMARY

Myeloma derives from the proliferation of a clone of malignant plasma cells that secretes a complete and/or partial monoclonal immunoglobulin protein. It originates in most, perhaps all, cases from an antecedent monoclonal gammopathy (essential monoclonal gammopathy) that progresses by clonal evolution (acquisition of additional mutations) to a malignant B-cell malignancy, often myeloma, at a rate of 1 percent per year. Myeloma cells accumulate in the marrow microenvironment where contact with extracellular matrix and interaction with marrow accessory cells, such as osteoblasts, osteoclasts, and stromal cells, evokes cell growth and cell-survival signals, and contributes to resistance to therapy. Myeloma cells show a complex genomic phenotype, with chromosomal translocations and small copy number variations that affect patient prognosis. Patients with myeloma have signs resulting from marrow infiltration (anemia), bone destruction (bone pain, pathologic fractures), excessive immunoglobulin production and deposition (renal failure and amyloidosis-related symptoms), and immunosuppression (e.g., infection). Clinical manifestations of myeloma vary as a result of the heterogeneous biology, spanning the entire spectrum from indolent to highly aggressive disease with extramedullary features. Diagnostic workup of myeloma should include serum protein electrophoresis together with immunoglobulin immunofixation, serum-free light-chain assay, a 24-hour urine collection to quantitate urinary protein, basic blood metabolic panel including blood counts and renal function, and marrow aspirate or biopsy with fluorescence *in situ* hybridization and cytogenetic studies. Radiographic bone survey is used to detect osteopenia and bone lesions or impending fractures. Magnetic resonance imaging (MRI) is more sensitive than the bone survey, can identify early bone disease and extramedullary disease, and can distinguish myeloma from normal marrow, helping in quantifying the extent of the disease. Positron emission tomography coupled with computed tomography (PET-CT) detects metabolically active intramedullary or extramedullary myeloma foci and lytic bone lesions. The most common staging system for myeloma is the International Staging System, based on two parameters, serum β_2-microglobulin (β_2M) and albumin; three stages are defined and correlate with patient outcome. Serum levels of β_2M, C-reactive protein, number of circulating plasma cells and their labeling-index are related to patient prognosis. Other prognostic factors include the presence of specific chromosomal abnormalities (deletion of chromosome 17p and loss of chromosome 1p/gain of chromosome 1q), altered gene expression profiling, as well as MRI and PET-CT abnormalities. The introduction of the immunomodulatory drugs (IMiDs) thalidomide and lenalidomide and the proteasome inhibitor bortezomib have increased the 5-year relative survival rate to 45 percent, with some patients achieving long-term survival of more than 10 years. Melphalan-based autologous hematopoietic stem cell transplantation in combination with novel agents can achieve remarkable results in patients with good risk myeloma; patients who are not eligible for autologous transplant have traditionally been treated with melphalan and prednisone; novel agents such as bortezomib and lenalidomide are also active and well-tolerated also in this population. Consolidation and maintenance regimens based on lenalidomide as single agent or in combination with bortezomib have been evaluated to extend the duration of complete remission following autologous stem cell transplant. Finally, several novel agents can be used in the setting of relapsed/refractory disease including new proteasome inhibitors (carfilzomib, ixazomib, and marizomib), IMiDs (pomalidomide), histone deacetylase inhibitors (vorinostat, panabinostat, and ricolinostat), and monoclonal antibodies (daratumumab and elotuzumab).

Acronyms and Abbreviations: auto-HSCT, autologous hematopoietic stem cell transplantation; BMSCs, bone marrow stromal cells; β_2M, β_2-microglobulin; CALGB, Cancer and Leukemia Group B; CR, complete response; CRD, carfilzomib, lenalidomide, and dexamethasone; CT, computed tomography; CyBorD, cyclophosphamide, bortezomib, and dexamethasone; del, deletion; DLI, donor lymphocyte infusion; EBMT, European Bone Marrow Transplant Group; ECM, extracellular matrix; ECOG, Eastern Cooperative Oncology Group; EFS, event-free survival; EMP, extramedullary plasmacytoma; FISH, fluorescence *in situ* hybridization; GVHD, graft-versus-host disease; GVM, graft-versus-myeloma effect; IGF-1, insulin-like growth factor; ISS, International Staging System; LCDD, light-chain deposition disease; MG, essential monoclonal gammopathy; MGUS, monoclonal gammopathy of undetermined significance; MIP, macrophage inflammatory protein; MP, melphalan-prednisone; MRD, minimal residual disease; MRI, magnetic resonance imaging; MTD, maximum tolerated dose; ONJ, osteonecrosis of the jaw; ORR, overall response rate; OS, overall survival; PET, positron emission tomography; RVD, lenalidomide, bortezomib, and dexamethasone; SCID, severe combined immunodeficiency; sCR, stringent complete response; SMM, smoldering multiple myeloma; SOP, solitary osseous plasmacytoma; TGF-β, transforming growth factor-β; TTP, thrombotic thrombocytopenic purpura; VGPR, very good partial response; VTE, venous thromboembolism.

DEFINITION AND HISTORY

Myeloma is a disease characterized by clonal expansion of malignant plasma cells that accumulate in the marrow, leading to anemia and associated cytopenias, hypogammaglobulinemia, osteolytic bone disease, hypercalcemia, and renal dysfunction.[1] Symptoms are a result of tumor mass effects, cytokine release by myeloma cells, marrow stroma or bone cells, or deposition of myeloma proteins into target organs (amyloid light-chain [AL] amyloidosis and light-chain deposition disease [LCDD]). Myeloma is part of a spectrum of diseases called plasma cell dyscrasias that include the following conditions: essential monoclonal gammopathy (MG; also known as monoclonal gammopathy of undetermined significance [MGUS]), smoldering myeloma (Chap. 106); solitary plasmacytoma, located in the bone as isolated lytic lesion or in the soft tissues; macroglobulinemia (Chap. 109); AL amyloidosis and LCDD (Chap. 108); and very rare disorders, such as osteosclerotic myeloma (POEMS [polyneuropathy, organomegaly, endocrinopathy, M protein, and skin changes] syndrome), Castleman disease, and heavy chain diseases (α-heavy-chain disease, μ-heavy-chain disease, and γ-heavy chain disease) (Chap. 110). Myeloma derives from cells with plasma cell morphologic features, capable of producing immunoglobulin molecules (Chap. 75), which can be detected in the serum and/or urine by electrophoresis and immunofixation. By definition, plasma cell dyscrasias result from the expansion of monoclonal cells, with resultant monoclonal protein secretion; however, oligoclonal and polyclonal protein abnormalities accompany some conditions, such as Castleman disease.

EPIDEMIOLOGY

INCIDENCE AND PREVALENCE

Myeloma represents the second most common hematologic cancer, accounting for 1.4 percent of all cancers and 10 percent of hematologic malignancies, with a prevalence of 83,367 people in 2011.[2] The American Cancer Society has estimated that 24,050 new myeloma cases were diagnosed in the United States in 2014, of which approximately 11,090 will die. Most of the patients are diagnosed among people ages 65 to 74 years, with a median age at onset of 69 years; only 4 percent of cases occur before age 45 years. Men are affected more frequently than women (1.6:1 ratio) and individuals of African descent have twice the prevalence of myeloma as those of European descent. Conversely, individuals of Japanese and Spanish (Latino) descent have very low prevalence rates.[3-5] Myeloma is always preceded by a condition called MG, as has been demonstrated by long-term followup studies of a cohort of more than 70,000 banked serum samples from healthy subjects and from an independent military cohort.[6,7] MGUS is present in 3.2 to 4.0 percent of the general population,[8] developing years before the diagnosis of myeloma, at a rate of approximately 1 percent per year (Chap. 106).[9]

GENETIC PREDISPOSITION

The etiology and the mechanisms of myeloma progression are still largely unknown.[1] Several epidemiologic reports have demonstrated an increased risk of myeloma or MG (up to fourfold) in first-degree relatives of individuals affected by plasma cell dyscrasias.[10] Moreover, myeloma is associated with an increased risk of prostate cancer, melanoma, non-Hodgkin lymphoma, and chronic lymphocytic leukemia.[11] More than 100 myeloma families have been described from different geographic areas[12-14]; in one family, a germline mutation of the *CDKN2A* (*p16*) gene together with loss of heterozygosity of the other allele was identified as a rare low-penetrance genetic risk.[13] Genome-wide association studies have identified six single nucleotide polymorphisms (SNPs) at chromosomes 2p23.3, 3p22.1, 3q26.2, 6p21.33, 7p15.3, 17p11.2, and 22q13.1 that are associated with risk of myeloma. The identified genes (*DNMT3A, ULK4, TERC, PSORS1C1, CDCA7L/DNAH1, TNFRSF13B,* and *CBX7*) have never been validated as myeloma-driver genes.[15,16] These same SNPs have also been independently associated with development of MG, with the risk increasing with the number of alleles carried.[17] Moreover, the presence of hyperphosphorylated paratarg-7 (pP-7) carrier status has been reported as an autosomal dominantly inherited risk factor for MG and myeloma in a European population and in MG/myeloma cases in African Americans.[18,19]

LIFE STYLE AND OCCUPATIONAL FACTORS

Some epidemiologic studies, including a cohort study of Swedish and Finnish twins and a meta-analysis,[20,21] have shown an association between high body mass index and risk of myeloma.[22,23] Specifically, obese individuals have higher levels of cytokines, such as interleukin (IL)-6 and insulin-like growth factor (IGF-1), which also are produced by adipocytes and are potent growth factor for myeloma cells.[24] No consistent associations have been observed with any particular diet, alcohol consumption, or smoking.[25] Occupational exposure to pesticides, organic solvents (benzene, petroleum derivatives, styrene) or chronic radiation have been alleged to be associated with myeloma in some studies,[25,26] but refuted by others. Furthermore, the use of thorium dioxide (thorotrast), a contrast medium used in the 1950s for angiography, increases the risk of plasmacytomas up to fourfold.[27] Exposure to acute radiation, as in atomic bomb survivors increases the overall rate of MG

or myeloma after 15 to 20 years,[28] and accelerates MG transformation to myeloma.[29] People exposed to fresh wood, wood dust, or working in saw mill factories had an increased risk of myeloma in some studies.[30,31] Finally, associations between myeloma risk and autoimmune diseases (especially rheumatoid arthritis[32,33] or pernicious anemia[34]) or infections (HIV and hepatitis C[35,36]) have been proposed, based on a retrospective study among American male military veterans,[37,38] suggesting an immune-mediated mechanism for malignant transformation. Human herpes virus 8 DNA sequences responsible for Kaposi sarcoma and Castleman disease pathogenesis[39] have been reported by some investigators in marrow dendritic cells of myeloma patients, although other studies suggest that this is an epiphenomenon.[40,41]

ETIOLOGY AND PATHOGENESIS

CELL OF ORIGIN

Myeloma cells derive from postgerminal–center marrow plasmablasts/plasma cells (Fig. 107–1). Myeloma cell immunoglobulin heavy chain (IGH) variable genes present somatic mutations in the absence of intraclonal variation or ongoing somatic hypermutation, indicating antigen-contact selection in the germinal center.[42,43] The existence of a myeloma stem cell, that is a precursor with self-renewal capacity, has been proposed for a long time, given myeloma's low proliferative index and clonogenic efficiency. However, this remains a matter of debate.[44] Myeloma is a multistep process, always preceded by a MG phase.[6,7] MG cells share several similarities with myeloma, including a similar prevalence of hyperdiploidy and of the three primary IGH rearrangements

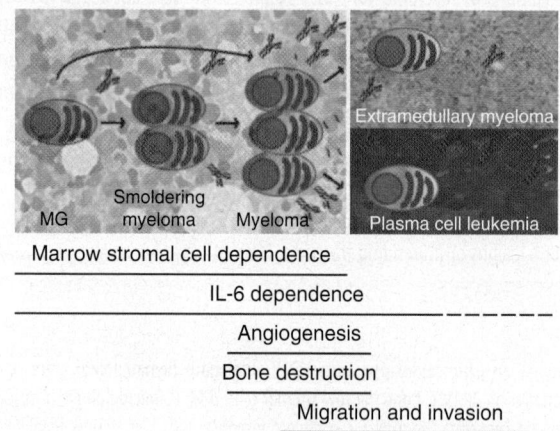

Figure 107–1. Myeloma stages, from essential monoclonal gammopathy (MG) to plasma cell leukemia. Myeloma evolves from a benign condition called essential monoclonal gammopathy (or monoclonal gammopathy of undetermined significance), with an annual rate of progression of 1 percent. In some patients, a stage called smoldering myeloma is sometimes evident, where there is a higher number of monoclonal plasma cells in the marrow, but still absence of symptoms. At early stages during the so-called intramedullary phase, myeloma cells are totally dependent on marrow microenvironment to survive and on interleukin (IL)-6 and other cytokines. During progression, myeloma cells can acquire the capability of growing without microenvironmental support and localize to other tissues (extramedullary disease) or circulate in the blood (secondary plasma cell leukemia). Active myeloma is characterized by onset of angiogenesis and bone lytic lesions in contrast to MG or smoldering myeloma; during late stages there is an increase in migration and invasion capabilities, as well as high proliferative rates.

[t(6;14), t(11;14), and t(14;16)]. However, chromosome 13 deletions, *RAS* mutations and non–immunoglobulin (Ig)-locus associated *MYC* translocations are more frequent in myeloma.[43] Indeed, the development of myeloma seems to necessitate an immortalizing event, such as a primary IGH translocation, an oncogene activation, or deregulation of a tumor suppressor, to occur in the germinal center during the switch recombination or somatic hypermutation, resulting in uncontrolled expansion of a long-lived plasmablast/plasma cell.[42] In early stages, myeloma cells are dependent on the growth support provided by bone marrow stromal cells (BMSCs) (intramedullary phase), but can become independent of their medullary environment at late stages (plasma cell leukemia). However, 15 to 70 percent of newly diagnosed myeloma patients, using conventional morphology techniques[45–51] or multiparametric flow cytometry[52] have circulating clonotypic myeloma cells (circulating tumor cells [CTCs]) in their blood, suggesting the presence of a "metastatic"/dissemination process that disseminates the disease hematogenously.[53] Moreover, the presence of CTCs in MG is a risk factor for myeloma progression,[54,55] as well as a poor prognostic factor in newly diagnosed or relapsed/refractory myeloma patients.[56,57] Myeloma CTCs share a similar phenotype to marrow myeloma cells, but are more quiescent, have better *in vitro* clonogenic capacity and have lower expression of integrin and adhesion molecules (including CD138) making them less dependent on marrow niches.[58]

GENOMIC ALTERATION

Abnormal Karyotype and Common Translocations

Myeloma is a heterogeneous disease with a complex genetic landscape, characterized by several numerical and structural aberrations, including abnormal karyotypes, chromosomal translocations and copy-number changes (Fig. 107–2 and Table 107–1).

Traditionally, myeloma patients have been divided into two subgroups: hyperdiploid cases with more than 46 but less than 76 chromosomes (34 to 60 percent of myeloma); and nonhyperdiploid cases, which include individuals with a hypodiploid (up to 44 to 45 chromosomes), pseudodiploid (44/45 or 46/47 chromosomes with gains or losses), and near-tetraploid karyotype.[59–61] Hyperdiploid patients, normally IgG kappa-type with bone involvement, show gains of odd-numbered chromosomes, including trisomies of chromosomes 15, 9, 5, 19, 3, 11, 7, and 21 (ordered by decreasing frequency), and have a favorable prognosis that can however be affected by the concomitant presence of additional abnormalities such as chr11 or chr1q gains or chr13 loss.[62,63] Fluorescence *in situ* hybridization (FISH) analysis is employed to detect five major primary IGH translocations in myeloma,[64] which occur more frequently in nonhyperdiploid patients (85 percent vs. <30 percent).[65] Primary translocations are caused by errors during normal DNA recombination in isotype class switching of terminally differentiated B cells. Conversely, IGH translocations involving chromosome 8p24 and 11q13 (called secondary translocations) result from errors in somatic hypermutation processes.[42] All of the translocations induce increased constitutive expression of specific oncogenes by their juxtaposition to immunoglobulin enhancer elements. The most frequent translocation (20 percent of cases) is t(11;14)(q13;q32),[66–68] leading to upregulation of cyclin D1, a crucial promoter of G_1-to-S transition via cyclin-dependent kinase (CDK)-4 or CDK6.[69,70] Rarely, cyclin D2 and cyclin D3 can be rearranged via t(12;14) (<1 percent) or t(6;14) translocations (2 percent of myeloma patients), respectively.[71] Even in the absence of translocations, cyclins D1, D2, and D3 are often upregulated, creating specific patient subgroups with different prognoses.[72] Specifically, the CD-1 subgroup (cyclin D1-high) responds well to treatment and has an increased frequency of early relapse but also has an excellent long-term survival, while the CD-2 subgroup (cyclin D3-high) exhibits a

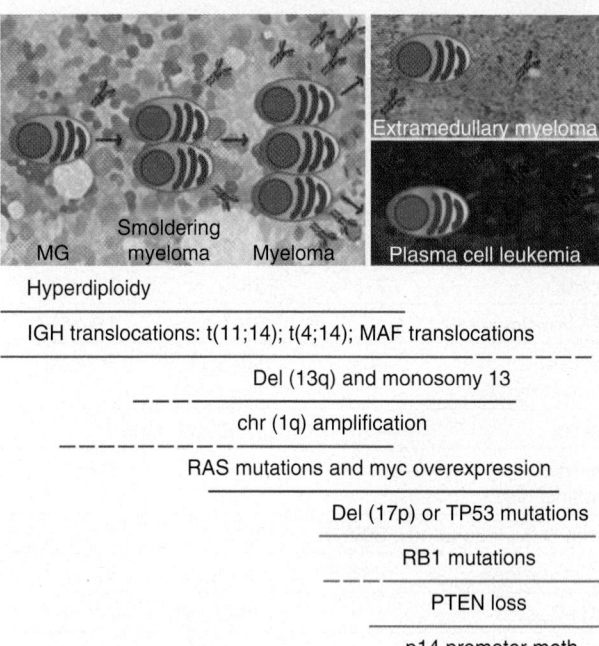

Hyperdiploidy

IGH translocations: t(11;14); t(4;14); MAF translocations

Del (13q) and monosomy 13

chr (1q) amplification

RAS mutations and myc overexpression

Del (17p) or TP53 mutations

RB1 mutations

PTEN loss

p14 promoter meth

Figure 107–2. Genomic aberrations, including karyotype abnormalities, chromosomal translocations, and copy number variations in essential monoclonal gammopathy (MG), myeloma, and plasma cell leukemia. Myeloma cells are characterized by several genomic aberrations, which combine differently in distinct patients. Hyperdiploidy and immunoglobin heavy-chain (IGH) translocations [t(11;14), t(4;14) and *MAF* translocations] are already present in the MG phase, a benign condition that can evolve to active myeloma with a rate of 1 percent per year. These abnormalities are not considered driver events in myeloma. Conversely, several groups have proposed other aberrancies, such as *MYC* translocations and increased *MYC* mRNA levels or *RAS* mutations as transforming events, because they are rare in MG and smoldering myeloma but common in myeloma. Also chromosome gains and losses, including deletion of chromosome 13q or monosomy 13, deletion of chromosome 1p, and amplification of chromosome 1q21 are seen more frequently in active myeloma, even though their role in myeloma progression is still not totally elucidated. Deletion of chromosome 17p or *TP53* mutations are rare at diagnosis, but present in advanced/relapsed settings, being associated with reduced response to treatment and unfavorable patient outcomes. The acquisition of independence from support by the marrow microenvironment is a feature of advanced myeloma, possibly leading to plasma cell accumulation in various organs (extramedullary disease) or in the blood (plasma cell leukemia). PTEN losses, methylations of p14 promoter, and RB1 inactivations are reported more frequently in plasma cell leukemia, suggesting a role in the development of extramedullary growth.

lymphoplasmacytoid morphology. Translocation t(4;14), a poor prognostic factor, pairs *MMSET/WHSC1*, a nuclear SET DOMAIN protein with *FGFR3* (fibroblast growth factor receptor), an oncogenic tyrosine kinase receptor in 15 percent of patients, often in association with chromosome 13 abnormalities.[73–76] MMSET is an H3K4-, H3K27-, H3K36-, and H4K20-specific histone methyltransferase, that causes global changes in chromatin status, favoring myeloma cellular and clonogenic growth, adhesion, and tumorigenicity,[75] while FGFR3 promotes myeloma cell proliferation via RAS-MAPK (mitogen-activated protein kinase) and STAT (signal transducer and activator of transcription) pathways.[77] Additionally, activating *FGFR3* mutations, mutually exclusive with RAS mutations, have also been reported in a small fraction of

TABLE 107–1. Common Genomic Aberrations in Essential Monoclonal Gammopathy, Myeloma, and Plasma Cell Leukemia*

Genetic Lesion	MG	Myeloma	Plasma Cell Leukemia
Hyperdiploidy	50%	60%	20%
t(11;14)	5–10%	20%	25–60%
t(4;14)	2–3%	15%	15–25%
MAF translocations		5%	15–35%
Del(13q)/ Monosomy 13	20%	50–60%	60–80%
Del(1p)	4%	7–40%	
Chr 1q21 amplification		40%	70%
Cyclin D dysregulation	60%	80%	
RAS mutations	<5%	30–50%	30%
FAM46C, DIS3		10–21%	
NF-κB activating mutations and CNVs		15–20%	
IGH *MYC* rearrangements	1–2%	15%	30–50%
UTX deletions and mutations		30%	
TP53 inactivations (mutations + del(17p))	5%	10–20%	20–80%
p18 and/or Rb inactivation		<5%	25–30%
p14 promoter methylation		<5%	25–30%
PTEN loss	0%	<2%	8–33%

CNV, copy number variant; IGH, immunoglobin heavy chain; MG, essential monoclonal gammopathy; NF-κB, nuclear factor-kappaB; Rb, retinoblastoma tumor-suppressor protein.

*Myeloma is a multistep process, progressing from an indolent MG stage, to overt myeloma to plasma cell leukemia. Hyperdiploidy and IGH translocations [t(11;14), t(4;14) and MAF translocations] are present at similar rates in MG and myeloma. Conversely, *MYC* secondary rearrangements, deletion 13p, chromosome 1 abnormalities, and *RAS* mutations are more common in active myeloma and they have been postulated as driver myeloma events. Plasma cell leukemia shows distinct abnormalities, including p14 promoter methylation and *PTEN* losses. Frequencies of common genomic aberrancies in plasma cell dyscrasias are reported. Blank spaces are left in case of unknown data.

patients.[78,79] *MAF* translocations, which include t(14;16) overexpressing c-*MAF*, t(14;20) which deregulates *MAFB*, and t(8;16) involving *MAFA* are relatively rare (5 percent, 2 percent, <1 percent of cases, respectively) but associated with poor prognosis.[80] c-MAF, MAFA, and MAFB are all transcription factors involved in proliferation, responsiveness to IL-6 and BMSC-MM (multiple myeloma) adhesion,[81] promoting cell-adhesion-mediated drug resistance (CAM-DR), via integrin α₇/E-cadherin interactions.[82] The prevalences of these three primary IGH rearrangements [t(6;14), t(11;14), and t(14;16)] are similar in MG, indicating the need of additional transforming events to precipitate active myeloma.[83–85]

Copy Number Alterations in Myeloma

Array comparative genomic hybridization (aCGH) analysis demonstrates numerous copy number alterations (CNAs) in myeloma cells. Deletion of chromosome 13, deletion of chromosome 17p13, and amplification of chromosome 1q21 are genomic aberrations associated with poor prognosis in myeloma patients.[86,87] Deletion of chromosome 13 affects 50 to 60 percent of newly diagnosed myeloma, is more frequent in the nonhyperdiploid group (>70 percent) in comparison to the hyperdiploid group and often cooccurs with t(4;14) or t(14;16) translocations.[88] Among other genes, *RB1* and the miRNA-15a/16–1 cluster are deregulated in this context and may play a role in myeloma pathogenesis. Despite being traditionally associated with a poor prognosis, the adverse impact of isolated chromosome 13 deletion is now controversial,[89] in view of the good response of such patients to bortezomib-based regimens and the close association of del13 with the t(4;14)(p16;q32) and hypodiploid karyotype.

Deletions of chromosome 17p involving the *TP53* locus are rare in newly diagnosed myeloma (5 to 10 percent), more common in relapsed and refractory cases (20 to 40 percent), and inevitably associated with negative prognosis, causing early relapse in patients treated with or without autologous stem cell transplantation. Mutations in *TP53* are also often present on the second allele.[90,91] Despite having an unfavorable prognosis, regimens containing bortezomib can increase the median progression-free survival (PFS) and 3 years of patients with TP53 mutations (17 percent to 69 percent [P = 0.028]) in comparison to non–bortezomib-containing regimens, as shown by the HOVON-65/GMMG-HD4 trial.[92] 1q21 amplification is detected by FISH in approximately 40 percent of newly diagnosed myeloma and in 70 percent of relapsed myeloma, and negatively affects overall survival (OS), with a cumulative effect based on the number of 1q21 locus copies.[93] Possible target genes of this lesion are *CKS1B*, a protein that regulates cyclin-dependent protein kinases, *PSMD4*, a proteasome subunit modulating response to bortezomib treatment, *MCL1* or *BCL9*.[93–95] Interestingly, a reported jumping translocation of 1q12 (JT1q12) can have a receptor chromosome *TP53* genomic locus, causing simultaneous gain of 1q21 and deletion of 17p.[96] Additionally, deletions of 1p, present in 7 to 40 percent of patients, are linked to reduced PFS and OS despite autologous stem cell transplantation.[97–99] *TP73, LAPTM5, CDKN2C*, a CDK inhibitor which interacts with CDK4 or CDK6 to regulate G_1/S phase, *MTF2, TMED5*, and *FAM46C* are candidate genes of the deletion. *FAM46C* loss or *FAM46C* mutations (evident in 15 percent of patients) are especially associated with shortened survival (median OS 25.7 months vs. 51.3 months, P = 0.004).[97,100] The biologic function of FAM46C is uncertain, although some data suggest it is related to mRNA stabilization. Other mutations include *MYC* rearrangements involving unbalanced translocations and insertions, small duplications, amplifications, and inversions on chromosome 8p24[101–104]; homozygous deletions of 11q22 locus resulting in loss of *YAP1, BIRC3*, and *BIRC2* genomic region[105–107]; chromosomes 4, 14, and 16 aberrations that disrupt *FGFR3, WWOX*, and *CYLD*; deletions or amplifications of chromosome 6; and homozygous deletions of Xp11.2 locus,[62,63] involving *UTX*, an histone H3 lysine 27 (H3K27) demethylase, which is also mutated in 10 percent myeloma,[100] are also common. The "purpose" of these multiple plasmin inhibitors is to guard against premature plasmin activation and subsequent degradation of fibrinogen, until intravascular fibrin begins to appear.

Somatic Mutations and Interclonal Diversity Myeloma evolves in a stepwise process, transforming from MG to smoldering myeloma to overt myeloma, where mutations accumulate, conferring either a growth advantage (driver mutations) or are functionally irrelevant (passenger mutations). So far, more than 300 myeloma patient DNA samples have been sequenced using whole-genome sequencing or whole-exome sequencing approaches.[100,108–113] Specifically, 11 genes are commonly mutated in myeloma reaching a standard significant threshold.[112] Five of them (*KRAS*, *NRAS*, *FAM46C*, *DIS3*, and *TP53*) are relatively frequent.[100,108] Approximately 30 to 50 percent of newly diagnosed patients have *RAS* mutations at codons 12 or 13,[82,114–117] often in association with t(11;14), but mutually exclusive with t(4;14) that constitutively activates the MAPK pathway via FGFR3 upregulation.[115,118,119] Because RAS mutations are rare in MG, they are considered a possible driver to progression.[120] Conversely, *TP53* mutations are a late event in myeloma,[91,121,122] an independent poor prognostic factor,[123] and are associated in one-third of patients with concomitant hemizygous deletion of chromosome 17.[90,124] Mutations in *FAM46C* and *DIS3*, genes possibly involved in RNA processing, are present in 10 to 21 percent of patients, often coupled with loss-of-heterozygosity in the remaining allele. Other significant genes are *BRAF* (4 percent of patients), *TRAF3*, *CYLD*, *RB1*, *PRDM1*, and *ACTG1*. *TRAF3* and *CYLD* mutations, together with homozygous deletions in BIRC2/BIRC3, NIK overexpression and mutations in other genes (*CARD11* and *MYD88*) contribute to constitutively activation of the NF-κB pathway.[100,105,107,112] Genes involved in protein homeostasis, the unfolded protein response, or lymphoid/plasma cell development, such as *PRDM1* involved in plasmacytic differentiation, and *XBP1*, *IRF4*, *LRRK2*, *SP140*, and *LTB* form a cluster of genes mutated in myeloma. Other recurrent mutated genes are *ROBO1*, a transmembrane receptor involved in β-catenin and MET signaling; *EGR1* transcription factor; *FAT3*, a transmembrane protein belonging to cadherin superfamily; and histone-modifying genes (*MLL*, *MLL2*, *MLL3*, *WHSC1/MMSET*, *WHSC1L1*, and *UTX*, among others).[100,108,112] Plasma cell leukemia patients possess different aberrancies, including p14^ARF promoter methylation, *PTEN* loss, *RB1* mutations and higher rates of *TP53* mutations and deletions.[125] Finally, a novel intriguing concept is the idea of intratumor heterogeneity in myeloma, where different subclones can emerge and become predominant following different mechanisms of evolution, including linear, branching, parallel or convergent evolution.[108,126] Clonal diversity is indeed a fundamental process akin to Darwinian selection, favoring cancer progression and adaptation to therapy. Next-generation sequencing analyses show that most patients have a subclonal structure at diagnosis, with one predominant clone and several others which can reappear at different stages or following treatment.[108,110,111] Gene-expression profiling of myeloma cells helps categorize patients into distinct subgroups[127,128] and can predict therapeutic responsiveness to specific drugs, although the role of specific genetic signatures in risk stratification is still under debate.[129]

ROLE OF MARROW MICROENVIRONMENT IN MYELOMA

The marrow microenvironment is composed of extracellular matrix (ECM) proteins, such as fibronectin, collagen, laminin and osteopontin; and cells, including hematopoietic stem cells, BMSCs, and endothelial cells, as well as osteoclasts and osteoblasts (Fig. 107–3) (Chap. 5).[130–133] Myeloma cells physically interact with ECM proteins and accessory cells to gain growth, survival, and drug resistance advantages. Among others, CD44, very-late antigen 4 (VLA4), neuronal adhesion molecule (NCAM), intercellular adhesion molecule (ICAM)-1, and syndecan 1 (CD138) mediate the adhesion of myeloma cells to the marrow and ECM, activating signaling pathways, such as nuclear factor-κB (NF-κB), to obtain CAM-DR to conventional chemotherapy.[134,135] In particular, CD138 (syndecan-1) is a transmembrane heparan sulphate bearing proteoglycan, expressed during the plasma cell stage of B-cell maturation, that can bind to type I collagen inducing expression of metalloproteinases, and promoting bone resorption and invasion.[136] Moreover, CD138 can be shed in the ECM, trapping growth-promoting and proangiogenic cytokines.[137,138] Increased soluble CD138 levels correlate with

tumor burden and poor outcomes.[139] The SDF-1/CXCR4 axis regulates specific homing of myeloma cells to the marrow, but also mobilization or marrow egress, being possibly accountable for the multifocal marrow localization and blood circulation of myeloma cells.[140,141] Moreover, other chemokine receptors, such as CXCR3, CCR1, CCR2, and CCR5 can be expressed by myeloma conferring different migration capabilities to medullary and extramedullary cells.[142] Accessory cells (BMSCs, endothelial cells, osteoclasts, and osteoblasts) secrete factors including IL-6,[143–146] IGF-1,[147–149] vascular endothelial growth factor (VEGF),[150,151] tumor necrosis factor-α (TNF-α),[152] fibroblast growth factor (FGF),[153] stromal cell-derived factor 1α (SDF-1α),[141] and B-cell activating factor (BAFF)[154]; all capable of promoting expression of survival factors such as NF-κB.[155] IL-6 and other survival signals also induce phosphatidylinositol 3′-kinase (PI3K)/AKT,[156,157] STAT3 and MAPK signaling (Fig. 107–3).[133] BMSCs, myeloma cells and osteoclasts also secrete growth factors and cytokines such as VEGF, basic fibroblast growth factor (bFGF), and IL-8, to promote marrow angiogenesis, which increases delivery of oxygen and nutrients to myeloma cells. Moreover, the same endothelial cells produce growth factors (IL-6 and IGF-1), to favor plasma cell survival[150,151,158,159] and express deregulated genes important for ECM and bone remodeling, cell adhesion, migration and resistance to apoptosis.[160] The degree of marrow angiogenesis, as assessed by microvessel density (MVD) is higher in active myeloma compared with MG[161] and is also related to myeloma proliferation and infiltration, negatively affecting patient prognosis.[162] Also lymphoid and myeloid cells are part of marrow microenvironment and can modulate myeloma survival. Myeloid cells, such as macrophages, mast cells and neutrophils control both pro- and antiinflammatory responses and regulate antigen presentation.[163] For instance, a specific group of myeloid cells, named myeloid-derived suppressor cells (MDSCs),[164] are highly represented in the marrow of myeloma individuals in comparison to healthy persons, and increase with disease progression, facilitating tumor development, growth, and immune escape, by blocking T-cell (CD8+ T and natural killer [NK] T) antitumor immune responses.[165]

BONE METABOLISM

The presence of osteolytic bone lesions, bone pain, increased risk of pathologic fractures and generalized bone loss (or osteoporosis) is a well-defined feature of myeloma.[166] Indeed, as myeloma burden increases, an imbalance between osteoblast and osteoclast activities ensues, with suppression of bone formation by osteoblasts and uncoupled activation of osteoclasts (Fig. 107–4).[167–169] The ligand for receptor activator of NF-κB (RANKL) binds to RANK receptor to stimulate osteoclast differentiation, formation and survival[170]; myeloma cells produce RANKL and upregulate RANKL expression in BMSCs and osteoblasts via direct contact interaction, signaling induction[171–173] or production of IL-7. Moreover, they promote suppression of osteoprotegerin (OPG),[174–176] a decoy receptor that normally prevents RANK–RANKL interaction[177,178] via soluble factors, integrin $α_4β_1$-vascular cell adhesion molecule (VCAM)-1 interaction,[179] production of Dickkopf-1(DKK1),[180] or inactivation by syndecan-mediated internalization into myeloma cells.[181] Interestingly, OPG levels are decreased in the serum of myeloma patients and correlate with lytic bone lesion development[182]; a high RANKL-to-OPG ratio is associated with worse prognosis.[183] Recombinant OPG constructs, soluble RANK, OPG peptidomimetics[175,178,184,185] and an anti-RANKL antibody, denosumab,[186–189] have been developed to modulate the RANKL/OPG axis and reduce osteoclast activity in myeloma. Macrophage inflammatory protein (MIP)-1α, or chemokine C-C motif ligand, is also produced by myeloma cells and promotes maturation of precursor cells into osteoclasts[190–192]; MIP-1α signals via CCR1 and CCR5 on osteoclasts and can further upregulate

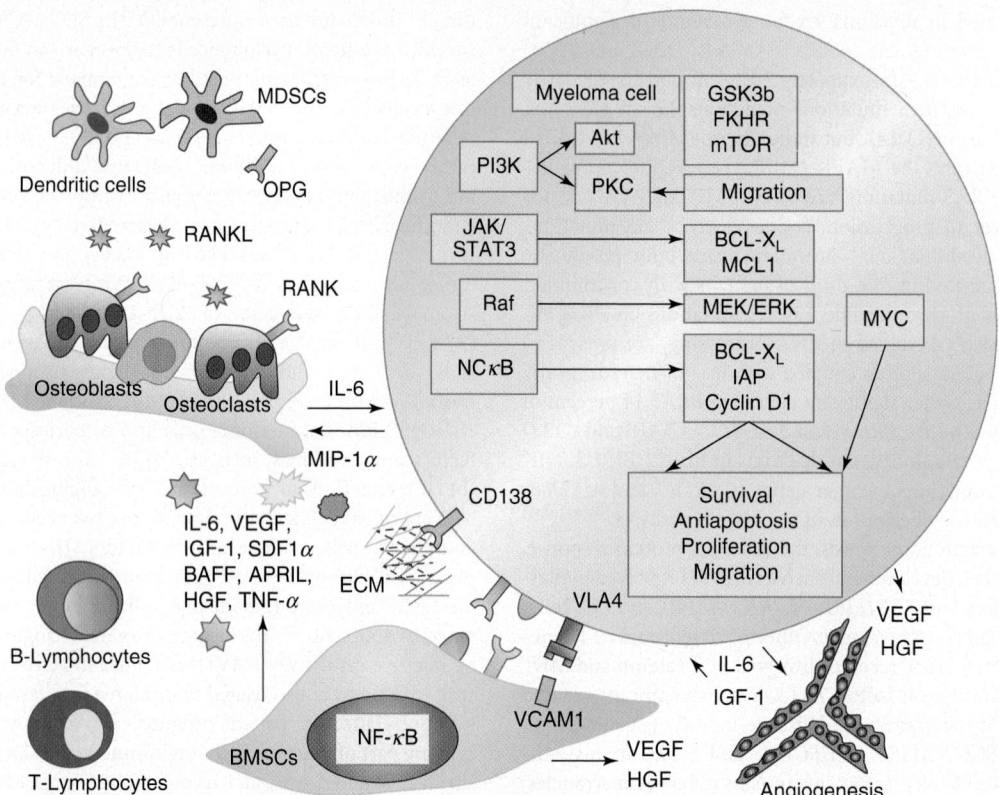

Figure 107–3. Myeloma cell interaction with extracellular matrix (ECM) and accessory cells in the marrow. Myeloma cells require support from bone marrow stromal cells (BMSCs) during early stage disease. Adhesion between myeloma cells and BMSCs favors myeloma cell survival, growth, and migration via release of cytokines (IL-6, VEGF, IGF-1, SDF1α, BAFF, APRIL, HGF, TNF-α) from both myeloma cells and BMSCs. Among others, extra-cellular signal-regulated kinase (ERK); Janus kinase 2 (JAK2)–signal transducer and activator of transcription 3 (STAT3); phosphatidylinositol 3′-kinase (PI3K)–Akt; nuclear factor-κB (NF-κB) and MYC are constitutively active in myeloma, promoting transcription or activation of important targets, including cytokines (IL-6, IGF-1, VEGF), antiapoptotic proteins (BCL-XL, IAP, MCL1), cell-cycle modulators (cyclin D1) and proteins involved in migration, invasion, and autophagy. NF-κB activation in both myeloma and BMSCs upregulates adhesion molecules (VCAM1, VLA4) to promote reciprocal binding. Proangiogenic factors, including VEGF and HGF are released from myeloma cells, BMSCs and marrow endothelial cells, to promote neoan-giogenesis and increase delivery of oxygen and nutrients to tumor cells. Cells from the innate and adaptive immune response, including B lympho-cytes, T lymphocytes, dendritic cells, and myeloid-derived suppressor cells, are also modulated by myeloma cells, creating an immunosuppressive microenvironment that promotes tumor survival and reduces antigen presenting capabilities. Receptor activator of NF-κB ligand (RANKL) and MIP-1α are produced by BMSCs and myeloma cells and trigger osteoclast activation via RANK receptor. Osteoprotegerin (OPG), a decoy receptor for RANKL secreted by osteoblasts and BMSCs to block RANKL–RANK ligand interaction and inhibit osteoclastogenesis, is reduced in myeloma patients. APRIL, a proliferation-inducing ligand; BAFF, B-cell activating factor; HGF, human growth factor; IGF-1, insulin-like growth factor; IL, interleukin; MIP, macro-phage inflammatory protein; SDF1α, stromal cell derived factor 1α; TNF, tumor necrosis factor; VCAM, vascular cell adhesion molecule; VEGF, vascular endothelial growth factor; VLA, very-late antigen.

RANKL in stromal cells.[190] MIP-1α levels are elevated in myeloma patients,[193,194] whereas MIP-1α silencing or blockade of CCR1 reduces bone disease in in vitro or animal models. IL-6,[195] parathyroid hor-mone-related peptide (PTHrP),[196,197] annexin II,[198] and the ephrinB2/EphB4 axis[199] also promote bone reabsorption. Osteoblast suppres-sion is another major player in myeloma bone disease: WNT signal-ing antagonists, including DKK1, frizzled related protein-2 (FRP-2),[200] and sclerostin (SOST),[201,202] interfere with osteoblast maturation. DKK1 is expressed by myeloma cells and can upregulate RANKL levels in osteoblasts, increasing osteoclast activity.[203–205] DKK1 levels are increased in the serum of myeloma patients,[206] and anti-DKK1 antibodies have been tested in animal studies[207–210] and are currently employed in clin-ical trials. Finally, high levels of Activin A, a member of transforming growth factor-beta (TGF-β) superfamily, IL-3 and IL-7 (via RUNX2/CBFA1 blockade) can inhibit bone formation and promote bone reab-sorption.[211–213] Furthermore, the bone niche itself supports myeloma cell survival and prevents TNF-α–mediated apoptosis by producing various

molecules.[167] Indeed, bisphosphonates not only block osteoclasts and modulate osteoblasts, but have an effect on tumor burden.[214] A similar effect is reported with OPG peptidomimetics and RANKL constructs in in vivo xenograft models.[215] Hence, bisphosphonates, especially zoledronic acid, are currently used in the clinic to reduce bone disease,[216,217] but are also associated with an increase in OS when compared to placebo based on a meta-analysis.[218] Markers of bone resorption and formation cor-relate with the extent of osteolytic disease.[219] Specifically, urine levels of pyridinoline (PYD) and deoxypyridinoline (DPD) crosslinks and serum levels of tartrate-resistant acid phosphatase isoform 5b (TRACP-5b), a resorption marker only produced by activated osteoclasts and of col-lagen degradation products, including the N-terminal crosslinking telopeptide of type I collagen (NTX), are elevated in myeloma patients compared with healthy controls and can predict early progression of bone disease in myeloma. Conversely, bone formation markers, such as bone alkaline phosphatase (bALP) and osteocalcin (OC), are reduced.[219]

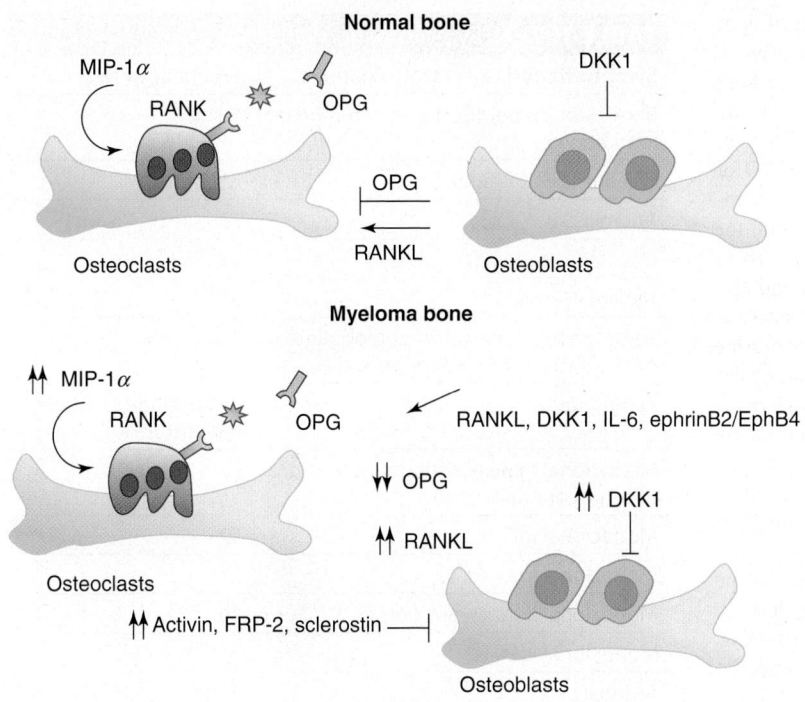

Figure 107–4. Mechanism of bone remodeling in normal conditions and in the presence of myeloma cells. The major factors affecting osteoclast and osteoblast activation, and thus the balance between bone formation and bone reabsorption, are illustrated in the upper panel. Receptor activator of nuclear factor-κB (RANK) receptor/receptor activator of nuclear factor-κB ligand (RANKL) and macrophage inflammatory protein (MIP)-1α stimulate osteoclastogenesis and osteoclast activity, while osteoprotegerin (OPG) acts a decoy receptor for RANKL, reducing its action. DKK1 (Dickkopf-1) is an inhibitor of osteoblast activity. In the presence of myeloma cells in the bone, the normal balance between osteoblasts and osteoclasts is totally inverted. Specifically, myeloma cells secrete factors to promote osteoclast activation, a result of upregulation of RANKL and MIP-1α, and to inhibit osteoblasts. Increased levels of DKK1, activin, FRP-2 (frizzled related protein-2), and sclerostin are evident in myeloma patients. In red are marked cytokines or receptors used as targets to treat myeloma bone disease. IL, interleukin.

PRECLINICAL MODELS OF MYELOMA

Novel therapies need to be tested in preclinical *in vitro/vivo* models capable of mimicking the role of human marrow microenvironment. In *in vitro* settings, myeloma cells are cocultured in liquid or semisolid systems together with different cytokines (IL-6, IGF-1, TNF-α) or with autologous BMSCs from patients. However, these systems do not truly recapitulate the marrow microenvironment[220–222] and *in vivo* models are necessary. Two main types of myeloma animal models have been exploited to study human myeloma biology and response to treatment: xenogeneic models in immunodeficient and humanized mice or syngeneic tumor models (Fig. 107–5).[223] The xenogeneic models require subcutaneous injection of tumor myeloma cells in severe combined immune deficiency (SCID) or nonobese diabetic (NOD)/SCID mice, which are immunocompromised. These models lack the complex marrow–myeloma interaction, but can still be used to explore myeloma homing and novel drugs. Conversely, the SCID-hu or the SCID-rab mice models recreate a look-alike microenvironment, able to sustain myeloma cell growth.[224] Specifically, primary myeloma cells or myeloma cell lines are grown in human fetal bone (the SCID-hu model) or rabbit bone (SCID-rab model), later implanted in SCID mice. Myeloma cells grow inside the implanted bones, or disseminate to the outer surface of the implanted bone, if they derive from patients with extramedullary disease. Moreover, these mice have circulating

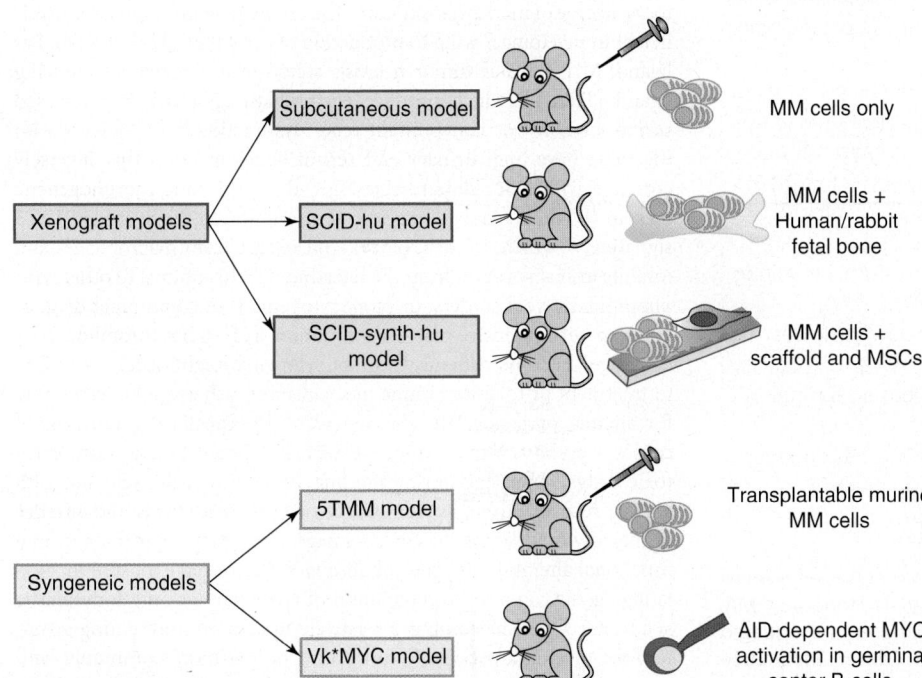

Figure 107–5. Preclinical models of myeloma. Xenogeneic and syngeneic models have been developed to study myeloma biology and test novel therapies. In xenogeneic models, human myeloma (MM) cells are injected subcutaneously, inside human/rabbit fetal bone or into synthetic scaffolds, previously coated with mesenchymal stromal cells (MSCs). In the last two types of models, a look-alike microenvironment, able to sustain myeloma cell growth, is present. Two types of syngeneic models have been established: the first one consists in the transplant of murine myeloma cells into other mice (5TMM), while the second one (Vκ*MYC mouse) is a genetically engineered mouse where MYC is activated in germinal center B-cells via an activation-induced cytidine deaminase (AID)-dependent mechanism. SCID, severe combined immune deficiency.

monoclonal immunoglobulins, osteolytic lesions, suppression of bone formation near myeloma foci and angiogenesis.[224,225] Studies propose novel xenogeneic models, where three-dimensional bone-like scaffolds are used instead of human fetal bone or rabbit bone.[226,227] Specifically, these scaffolds are internally coated with murine/human BMSCs or human mesenchymal stromal cells and then implanted in SCID or RAG2−/−γc−/− mice, to recapitulate the autologous marrow microenvironment *in vivo*. Myeloma cells are then loaded directly inside the scaffold or injected intracardiac to mimic myeloma homing. These models are more suitable for studying the microenvironment and also for drug testing, affording the opportunity to evaluate different stages or type of disease. Syngeneic tumor models include transplantable murine models like 5T33,[228,229] which are mostly representative of aggressive late-stage disease, as well as genetically engineered mouse models, such as the Vk*MYC mouse,[230] generated from the C57BL/6 mouse strain, which has a high incidence of spontaneous monoclonal gammopathy with aging, after activation-induced cytidine deaminase–dependent MYC activation in germinal center B-cells. This model exhibits high penetrance, clonal malignant plasma cells, which produce isotype class-switched immunoglobulins, a similar histology and immunophenotype to human myeloma, and delayed onset of renal failure, bone lesions, and anemia. The Vk*MYC mouse model has been used for drug testing, strongly paralleling the drug activity observed in myeloma patients.[230]

●CLINICAL AND LABORATORY FEATURES

Table 107–1 summarizes the signs and symptoms associated with myeloma. The International Myeloma Working Group has issued simplified criteria for the classification of myeloma and related disorders.[231,232] Symptomatic myeloma is diagnosed by evidence of organ or tissue impairment (end-organ damage) manifested by anemia, hypercalcemia, lytic bone lesions, renal insufficiency, hyperviscosity, amyloidosis, or recurrent infections, (commonly referred to as the "CRAB" criteria; namely, hyper*c*alcemia, *r*enal failure, *a*nemia, and *b*one lesions) (Tables 107–2 and 107–3; Fig. 107–6). Presence of these features necessitate immediate treatment for myeloma.

TABLE 107–2. Criteria for Diagnosis of Myeloma
1. Clonal bone marrow plasma cells ≥10% of biopsy-proven bony or extramedullary plasmacytoma
2. Any one or more of the following myeloma-defining events:
• Evidence of end-organ damage that can be attributed to the underlying plasma cell proliferative disorder, specifically:
• Hypercalcemia: serum calcium >0.25 mmol/L (>1 mg/dL) higher than the upper limit of normal or >2.75 mmol/L (>11 mg/dL)
• Renal insufficiency: creatinine clearance <40 mL per min or serum creatinine >177 μmol/L (>2 mg/dL)
• Anemia: hemoglobin value of >20 g/L below the lower limit of normal, or a hemoglobin value <100 g/L
• Bone lesions: one or more osteolytic lesions on skeletal radiography, CT, or PET-CTᐃ
• Any one or more of the following biomarkers of malignancy:
• Clonal bone marrow plasma cell percentage* ≥60%
• Involved: uninvolved serum free light chain ratio ≥100
• >1 focal lesions on MRI studies

Modified with permission from Rajkumar SV, Dimopoulos MA, Palumbo A, et al: International Myeloma Working Group updated criteria for the diagnosis of multiple myeloma. *Lancet Oncol* 2014 Nov;15(12):e538–e54.

TABLE 107–3. Symptomatic Myeloma[247]	
Symptoms and Laboratory Features	**Frequency (%)**
Bone pain (spine, chest, less common in long bones)	58
Weakness and fatigue	32
Anemia	73
Elevated creatinine	48
Hypercalcemia	28
Serum monoclonal immunoglobulin (Ig) peak on standard electrophoresis	82
Weight loss	24 (one-half of whom had lost ≥9 kg)
Monoclonal Ig peak on immunofixation of serum or urine	97
Monoclonal IgG	52
Monoclonal IgA	21
Monoclonal light chains only	16
Monoclonal IgD	2
Biclonal	2
Monoclonal IgM	0.5
Negative	6.5
Urinary monoclonal light chains	75
Marrow plasmacytosis >10%	90

Data from Kyle RA, Gertz MA, Witzig TE, et al: Review of 1027 patients with newly diagnosed multiple myeloma. Mayo Clin Proc 78:21–33, 2003.

HEMATOLOGIC ABNORMALITIES

Myelomatous involvement of the marrow typically causes anemia, which is present in more than two-thirds of patients with myeloma and relates to the degree of marrow infiltration. The erythropoietin response is insufficient in myeloma, owing to production of cytokines, (IL-1, TNF-β, Fas ligand, MIP-1α, and tumor necrosis factor–related apoptosis-inducing ligand [TRAIL], which produce erythroblast apoptosis),[233] increased serum viscosity, or concomitant renal dysfunction.[234–236] Patients with myeloma have high urinary and serum hepcidin levels that inversely correlate with hemoglobin values.[237,238] IL-6 and bone morphogenetic protein (BMP)-2 mediate hepcidin transcription in the liver via STAT3 signaling,[239] which, in turn, blocks iron release from macrophages and inhibits iron absorption from the intestine.[240,241] In contrast to other lymphoproliferative disorders, thrombocytopenia is uncommon at diagnosis, even with extensive marrow infiltration, as IL-6 has thrombopoietic activity.[242] In some patients, thrombocytopenia might occur secondary to treatment or to autoimmune mechanisms (such as those accounting for anemia or factor VIII deficiency[46,243–245]). Specifically, bortezomib causes a cyclic thrombocytopenia, with a different kinetic from cytotoxic drugs, appearing during the first 10 days of each cycle, but with a short recovery time, no cumulative or persistent effects and absence of marrow megakaryocyte toxic damage, as it primarily results from a functional alteration in platelet budding.[246] Prolonged exposure to alkylating agents can also promote onset of a concomitant myelodysplastic syndrome. Overt bleeding is a relatively uncommon presenting symptom for myeloma patients[247]; however it occurs more commonly with IgA paraproteins, in the presence of very high concentrations of serum

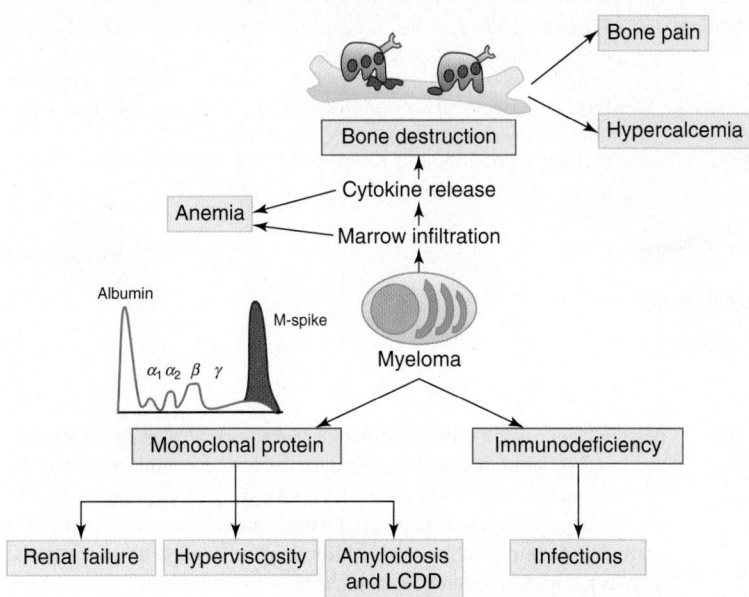

Figure 107–6. Summary of clinical manifestations of myeloma. Bone destruction, immunodeficiency, and presence of a monoclonal protein account for the main factors capable of inducing symptoms in myeloma patients. Anemia, hypercalcemia, bone pain, and renal failure represent the classical symptoms of myeloma presentation, together with increased risk of infections. Hyperviscosity and amyloid light-chain amyloidosis or light-chain deposition disease (LCDD) are less common presenting situations.

immunoglobins, high serum viscosity, and a prolonged bleeding time, with normal platelet counts, prothrombin time (PT), activated partial thromboplastin time (aPTT), and thrombin time.[248,249] Acquired von Willebrand factor (VWF) deficiency can develop[250] as a result of plasma VWF-neutralizing antibodies, antibodies binding to the VWF glycoprotein 1b binding domain, or interfering with VWF binding to collagen,[251,252] or immunoglobulins that nonspecifically coat platelets or bind to fibrin, preventing aggregation. An asymptomatic prolonged thrombin time can also be present,[253] as a result of interference with fibrin clot formation by the monoclonal protein[254]; in few cases, paraproteins recognizing thrombin and factor VIII have been reported.[253,255] Bleeding may also result from progression of disease, renal insufficiency, infections, therapy-related toxicity, invasive procedures, and anoxia/thrombosis in the capillary circulation. Bleeding is more common in systemic AL amyloidosis (15 to 41 percent of patients at diagnosis),[256–258] because of the deposition of free immunoglobin light chains forming insoluble fibrils in the small vessels or, more rarely, as a result of acquired factor X deficiency, related to absorption of factor X onto AL fibrils in the liver and spleen.[259,260] Amyloid splenic infiltration can cause hyposplenism and thrombocytosis.[260] An increased risk of venous thromboembolic events is typical of MG and myeloma patients.[261,262] Hypercoagulable states may result from the pro-inflammatory activity of IL-6, abnormal interactions between myeloma cells, BMSCs and endothelial cells,[263] paraprotein effects on fibrin polymerization and resistance to fibrinolysis, or rarely neutralizing antibodies against protein C, S,[264,265] or lupus anticoagulant[266] and acquired protein C resistance.[267] IMiDs, such as thalidomide and lenalidomide, have anti-angiogenic properties and are associated with an increased risk of venous thromboembolism (VTE), ranging from 5 percent[268] to 18 percent of treated patients,[269] especially when combined with high-dose dexamethasone, doxorubicin, or erythropoietic agents.[270–274] Warfarin and low-molecular-weight heparin play a role in primary and secondary VTE prevention,[275] but aspirin is normally used in patients treated with IMiDs and steroids, in view of the presence of increased aggregation between platelet and VWF antigens.[276–279]

IMMUNOGLOBULIN ABNORMALITIES

The majority of myeloma patients produce and secrete a monoclonal immunoglobulin (M-protein or M-spike) that can be detected by protein electrophoresis of the serum (SPEP) and/or of urine (UPEP) after

a 24-hour urine collection. The M-protein presents as a single narrow peak, migrating in the γ, or rarely β, region of the densitometer tracing. Myeloma cells can secrete immunoglobulin heavy chains plus light chains, light chains alone, or neither (nonsecretory myeloma). In this last case, cytoplasmic immunoglobulins are detected. Immunofixation analysis identifies the unique and specific immunoglobulin idiotypes.[47] Monoclonal IgG (usually >3.5 g/dL) is present in approximately 60 percent of myeloma patients, monoclonal IgA (typically >2 g/dL) in 20 percent of patients, monoclonal immunoglobulin light chains alone are detected in 20 percent of patients, while IgD, IgM, and biclonal myeloma are rare (5 percent of cases). A low M-spike concentration is particularly suggestive of IgD myeloma isotype. Light-chain myeloma patients should be followed by UPEP and urine immunofixation and present more often with renal failure or increased creatinine levels. Light-chain proteinuria is frequent especially in IgD myeloma (see Table 107–3). Traditionally, IgA and especially IgD isotypes have been considered prognostically unfavorable.[280,281] Their prognostic value has been confirmed in patients enrolled on Total Therapy 1, 2, and 3 protocols; IgD was of borderline significance, mainly because of its rarity, but was strongly associated with elevated β_2-microglobulin (β_2M) and lactic dehydrogenase (LDH) serum levels, reflecting high tumor burden.[282] Suppression of normal, polyclonal serum immunoglobulins resulting in total hypoglobulinemia and an increased risk of infection is present in 70 to 90 percent of patients. The κ light-chain isotype is twice as common as the λ isotype, except in IgD myeloma. The free light chain (FLC) assay (FREELITE assay) is a novel technique used to detect monoclonal FLCs, and provides a FLC κ:λ ratio (Fig. 107–7).[283] The κ:λ ratio is considered abnormal if less than 0.26 (λ-restricted Ig) or more than 1.65 (κ-restricted Ig).[284] Because the half-life of FLCs is only 2 to 4 hours, in contrast to the half-life of the entire immunoglobulin, which is 17 to 21 days, the FLC assay can be used to detect early treatment responses and should be evaluated routinely in patients with AL amyloidosis and oligosecretory myeloma.[285] A normal FLC ratio is also included in the criteria for stringent complete response (sCR).[8] The FLC ratio is considered a predictor of the risk of progression from MG or smoldering myeloma to active myeloma[286,287] and it has prognostic value, being related to tumor burden.[285] Indeed, high baseline FLC correlates with shorter survival in newly diagnosed myeloma patients despite achievement of complete response.[288,289] A rapid reduction in FLCs after therapy is

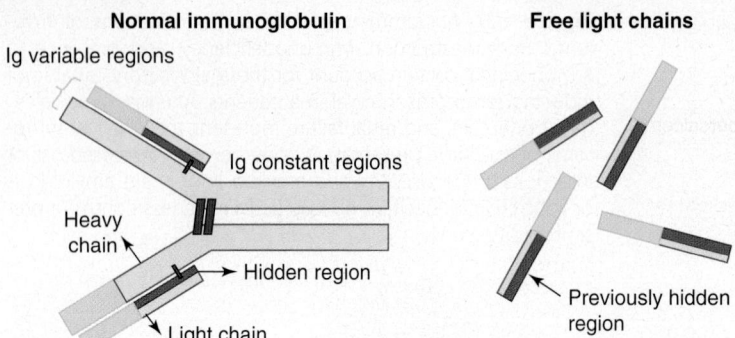

Normal immunoglobulin

Ig variable regions

Ig constant regions

Heavy chain

Hidden region

Light chain

Free light chains

Previously hidden region

Figure 107–7. Free light-chain assay description. Normal immunoglobulins are composed of two heavy chains and two light chains, which together form a constant region and a variable region, capable of recognizing specific antigens. The free light-chain assay is used to quantify the amount of free light chains in myeloma patients and to specifically recognize a "hidden" antigenic region (in *red*) that is normally not detectable from intact immunoglobulins.

also linked to inferior overall and event-free survival, suggesting the presence of highly proliferative myeloma cells, particularly sensitive to combination chemotherapy.[290]

MARROW FINDINGS

A marrow aspirate or biopsy showing plasmacytosis is a key component for the diagnosis of myeloma. The marrow can be evenly infiltrated (diffuse involvement) but more commonly displays considerable site-to-site variability (focal involvement).[291] The percentage of plasma cells can range from 10 percent to a virtual complete replacement of marrow. Occasionally, the biopsy specimen may contain a normal proportion of plasma cells as a result of the patchy marrow involvement. Myeloma diagnosis is also considered in the presence of less than 10 percent of chain restricted plasma cells if symptoms are reported or after histopathologic confirmation of an intraosseous or extraosseous plasmacytoma. By light microscopy, the morphologic appearance of myeloma

plasma cells can be indistinguishable from normal plasma cells, characterized by abundant basophilic cytoplasm and round, eccentrically located nuclei, with "clock-face" or "spoke-wheel" chromatin without nucleoli, or by bizarre plasma cells with giant cellular size, open chromatin, and punched nucleoli (indicating increased transcriptional activity), a high frequency of binucleate or multinucleate cells, and the presence of inclusion globules of condensed or crystallized cytoplasmic immunoglobulin, including Russell bodies (cherry-red refractive round bodies), multiple pale bluish-white, grape-like accumulations (Mott cells or Morula cells), crystalline rods, glycogen-rich IgA (flame cells), or other inclusions. These abnormal cells are characteristic of plasmablastic myeloma,[292,293] a poor prognostic type of myeloma with a high number of mitotic figures (Figs. 107–8 to 107–10).[294] Myeloma cells are clonal by definition and produce either κ or λ light chains, which are present in the cytoplasm but not on the membrane surface. A κ:λ ratio greater than 4:1 (normal 2:1[295]) or less than 1:2 is considered an index of κ or λ monoclonality, distinguishing this condition from reactive

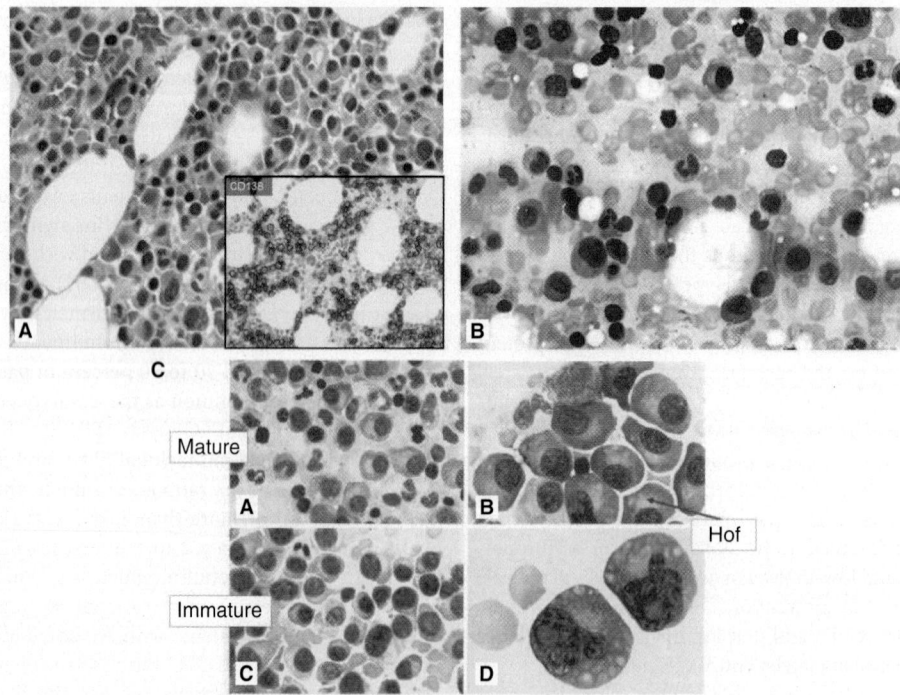

A

B

C

CD138

Mature

A

B

Immature

C

D

Hof

Figure 107–8. Marrow findings in myeloma. **A.** Marrow film. Infiltrate of neoplastic plasma cells (myeloma cells). These cells resemble normal plasma cells in their appearance with characteristic nuclear: cytoplasmic area ratio, blocky nuclear chromatin pattern, intense cytoplasmic basophilia, and a prominent "hof" or clear area (Golgi zone). CD138 immunohistochemistry staining is shown in the small box. **B.** Marrow film. Infiltrate of malignant plasma (myeloma) cells. **C(A).** Marrow section. Mature malignant plasma cells. **C(B).** Marrow film. Malignant plasma cells showing prominent perinuclear Golgi apparatus *(Hof)*. **C(C)** and **C(D).** Immature plasma cells with abnormal nuclei and size and aberrant morphology.

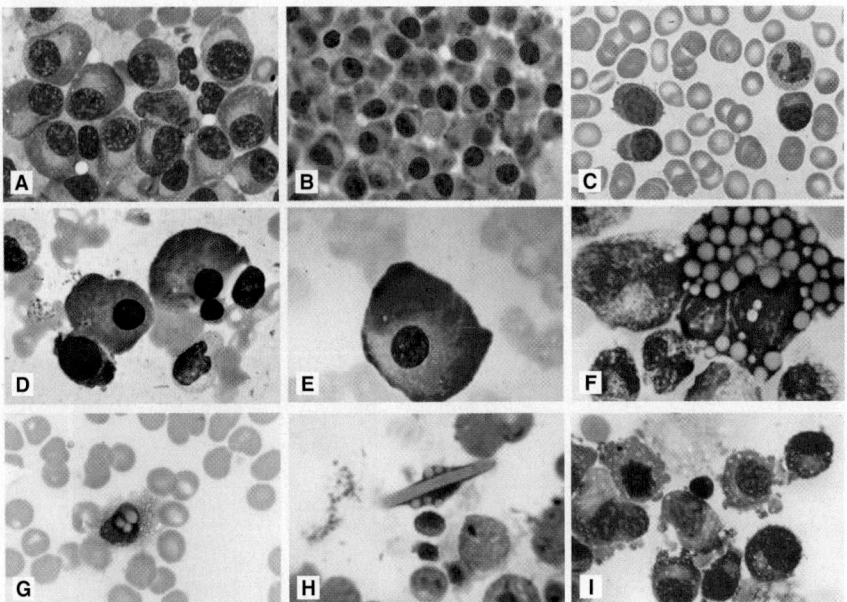

Figure 107–9. Myeloma: morphologic appearances. **A.** Marrow film showing replacement by malignant plasma (myeloma) cells. Note classical oval cell shape, eccentric nucleus, striking paranuclear clear area, deeply blue cytoplasm. **B.** Marrow biopsy section showing replacement by myeloma cells. **C.** Blood film in a patient with plasma cell leukemia. Three myeloma cells in the blood film field. **D** and **E.** Marrow films. Flaming-type giant myeloma cells. Reddish peripheral cytoplasmic coloration reflecting very high concentration of carbohydrate, characteristic of IgA myeloma. The peripheral cytoplasm contains numerous dilated cisterns of the endoplasmic reticulum distended with immunoglobulin. Flaming plasma cells may occasionally be found in IgG myeloma and in reactive plasmacytosis. **F.** Morula or Mott cell. Myeloma cell engorged with globules presumably containing immunoglobulin. These globules individually are referred to as Russell bodies and plasma cells may be found containing one, several, or many such bodies. **G.** Plasma cell with immunoglobulins containing globules overlying the nucleus but presumably cytoplasmic in location along with smaller cytoplasmic globular inclusions. **H.** Immunoglobulin crystal with several globules of immunoglobulin on either side. Note remarkable distortion of the cell to accommodate the crystal. **I.** Marrow film. Myeloma cells exhibiting cytoplasmic shedding. *(Reproduced with permission from* Lichtman's Atlas of *Hematology, www.accesmedicine.com.)*

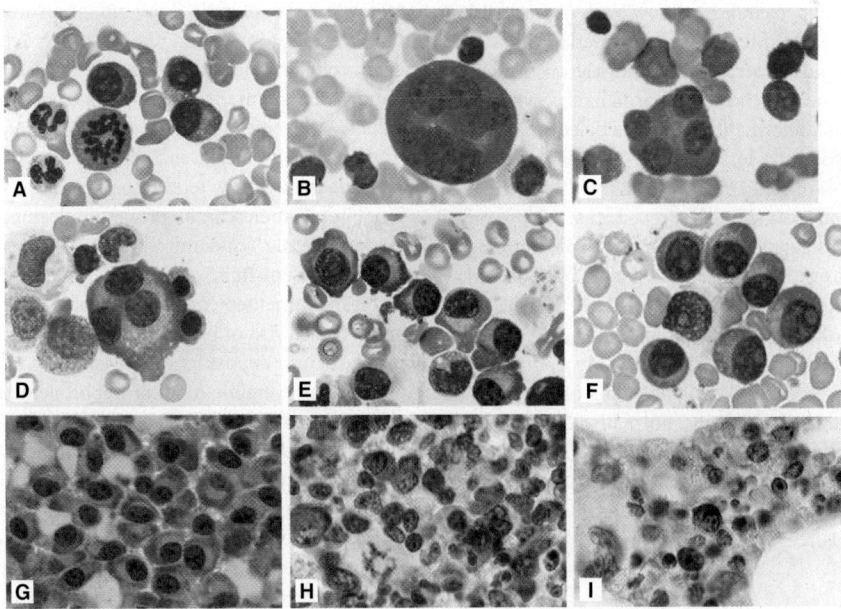

Figure 107–10. Myeloma: Additional morphologic appearances. **A.** Marrow film. Three characteristic malignant plasma (myeloma) cells and one in mitosis. **B.** Marrow film. Giant multinucleated myeloma cell. **C.** Marrow film. Tetranucleated myeloma cell. **D.** Marrow film. Trinucleated myeloma cell. **E.** Marrow film. Infiltrate of classical well-differentiated myeloma cells (plasma cell phenocopies). Eccentric nuclei, paranuclear clear zone, deeply blue (basophilic) peripheral cytoplasm. **F.** Infiltrate of immature myeloma cells with more circular than ovoid shapes, very large, prominent large nucleoli, less-intense basophilic cytoplasm, less-discrete paranuclear clear zone (plasmablasts). **G** to **I.** Marrow biopsy sections showing striking infiltrate of myeloma cells. **G.** Hematoxylin-and-eosin stain. **H.** Immunostained for κ light chains, showing frequently positive cells evident by deep rust color in cytoplasm. **I.** Immunostained for λ light chains showing negative reaction with rare positive cell. Approximately 20:1 κ:λ ratio. *(Reproduced with permission from* Lichtman's Atlas of Hematology, *www.accesmedicine.com.)*

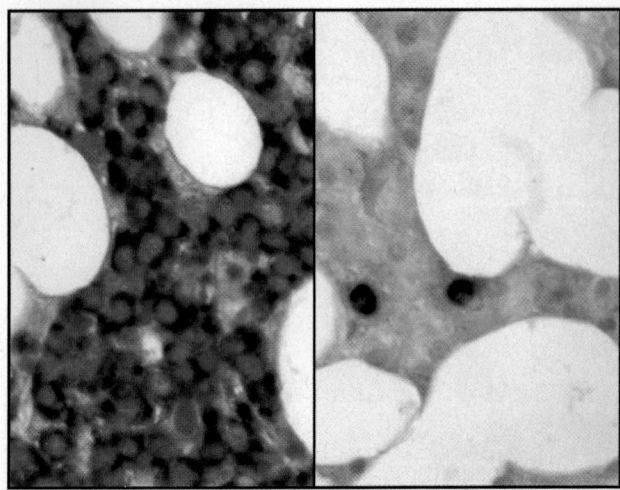

Figure 107–11. Kappa-lambda staining.

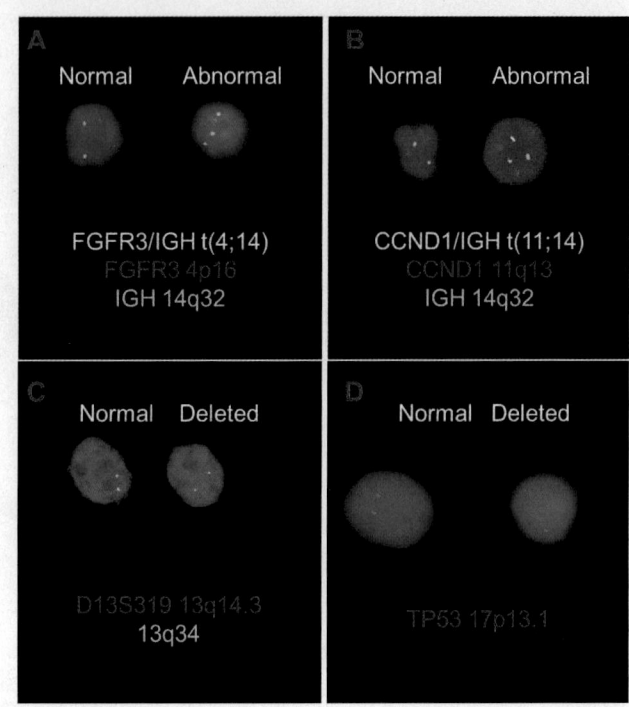

Figure 107–12. Common fluorescence *in situ* hybridization (FISH) abnormalities in myeloma. **A.** t(4;14). **B.** t(11;14). **C.** Deletion 13. **D.** Deletion 17p.

plasmacytosis.[296] Two-parameter flow cytometry staining for nuclear DNA content by propidium iodide and anti-κ and anti-λ light-chains can also be used to quantitate marrow involvement (Fig. 107–11).[297] Myeloma cells are normally CD138+, CD45–, CD38+, and CD19–[298], and are CD56+ in 70 percent of patients.[299-301] A few cases are CD20+[302] or CD117+ (KIT),[303] but responses to treatment with rituximab or imatinib mesylate are uncommon. If amyloid deposition is suspected, Congo red staining can be performed on the marrow biopsy, showing diffuse involvement or focal perivascular niche localization of amyloid protein. Microvessel density can be assessed by staining for endothelial markers such as CD131 and CD34 in specialized laboratories or during clinical trials.[304] Secondary myelodysplastic changes can rarely develop after prolonged treatment in myeloma patients, presenting with pancytopenia in the context of a hypercellular marrow, with characteristic FISH abnormalities (Chap. 87).[305,306] Metaphase cytogenetic studies and interphase FISH analysis should be performed routinely on myeloma cells at diagnosis to evaluate the presence of abnormal karyotypes and poor prognostic chromosomal abnormalities, such as deletion of chromosome 17, gain of chromosome 1q, loss of chromosome 1p, deletion of chromosome 13, and t(4;14) or t(14;16) translocations (Figs. 107–12 and 107–13).[63,307-310] Genetic analysis should be repeated at relapse only in patients initially classified as genetic standard-risk to rule out emergence of a more aggressive clone.[311] The plasma cell labeling index corresponds to the percentage of plasma cells in the S-phase of the cell cycle and is measured by immunofluorescence staining using an antibody against 5-bromo-2′-deoxyuridine, which is actively incorporated by DNA on marrow plasma cells. Actively cycling myeloma cells represent a small proportion of the total malignant cells, normally 0.5 percent on average,[312-317] with few patients with a labeling index of more than 5 percent.[318,319] This value has been proposed as a myeloma prognostic marker, as patients with a labeling index of more than 0.5 percent at diagnosis have a shorter event-free survival (EFS) and OS.[318]

RENAL DISEASE

Increased creatinine levels (>1.5 to 2.0 mg/dL) occur in 30 to 50 percent of myeloma patients at diagnosis, while overt renal failure requiring hemodialysis affects up to 10 percent of patients.[247] Renal insufficiency is related to two major causes: myeloma cast nephropathy (also called light-chain cast nephropathy or myeloma kidney) and hypercalcemia.[320] In myeloma cast nephropathy, the tubular absorptive capacity for light chains is overwhelmed, leading to the formation in the distal convoluted tubule (DCT) of the nephron of tubular casts. These tubular casts derive from the binding of precipitated light chains to Tamm-Horsfall mucoprotein (uromodulin) and can obstruct the DCT and parts of the ascending loop of Henle, initiating a giant cell reaction which leads to interstitial inflammation and fibrosis (interstitial nephritis).[321] The cast formation rate is strongly related to the urinary free-light chain concentration, which can be estimated by the amount of total proteinuria, based on the 24-hour urine collection or the serum light chain values. Conversely, the urine dipstick may be negative for protein as immunoglobulin light chains are often not detected by this technique. Lambda light chains tend to be more nephrotoxic than the κ type and renal impairment can be present with minimal λ light-chain secretion. Hypercalcemia (calcium >11 mg/dL), the second cause of nephropathy, is present in 15 percent of patients at diagnosis. Hypercalcemia creates volume depletion, natriuresis, and renal vasoconstriction, with an increased risk of prerenal azotemia; moreover, it can lead to intratubular calcium deposition, increasing the toxicity of filtered light chains or cause a reversible form of nephrogenic diabetes insipidus.[322] Light-chain glomerulopathy is caused by the deposition of immunoglobulins either in the form of amyloid or nonamyloid. In AL amyloidosis, light-chain immunoglobulin proteinuria is associated with glomerular damage, resulting into an overt nephrotic syndrome (Chap. 108).[323] Light chains are converted into insoluble fibrils or granular deposits inside the mesangial cells causing Congo red-positive amyloid accumulation, localized predominantly in the glomeruli. Vascular and tubular amyloid deposits are less common, but can cause narrowing of the vascular lumens or tubular dysfunction such as type 1 (distal) renal tubular acidosis or nephrogenic diabetes insipidus.[324] AL amyloidosis with renal dysfunction is more common in patients with λ light-chains, especially those with λ VI light-chain subgroup.[325] Kappa chains or heavy-chain fragments can form Congo red-negative nonfibrillar deposits with linear involvement of the basement membrane, in a condition called LCDD or, more generally, monoclonal immunoglobulin deposition disease

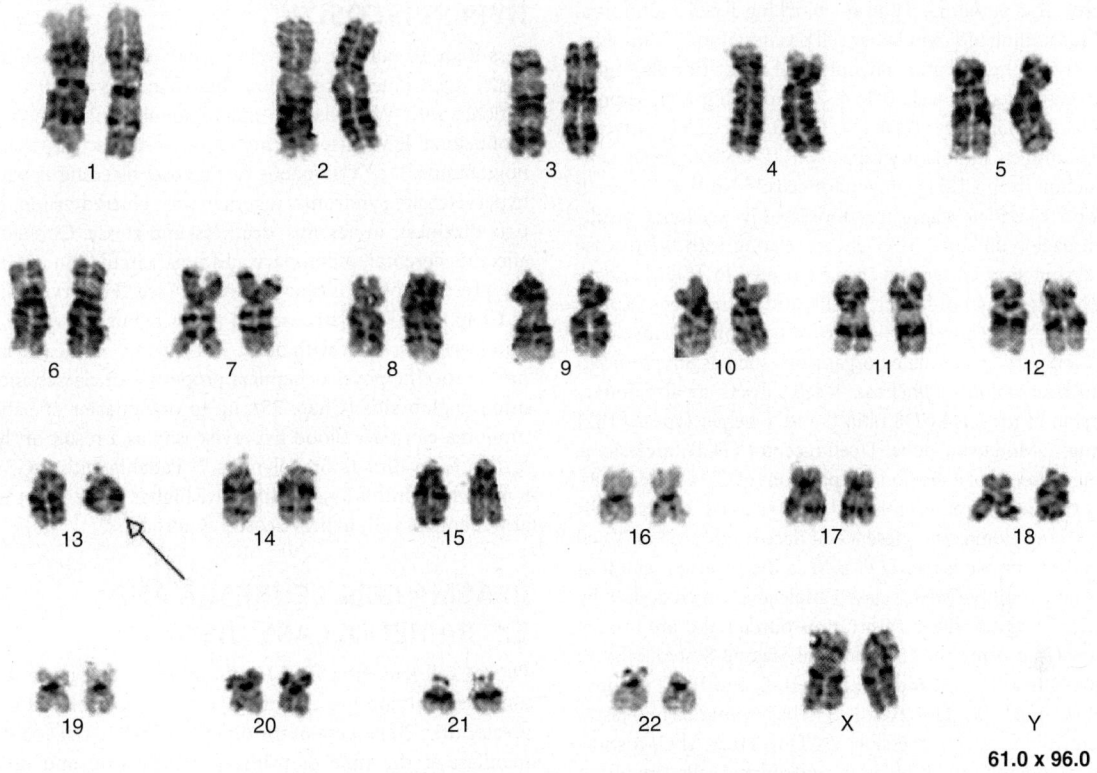

61.0 x 96.0

Figure 107–13. Abnormal karyotype in myeloma. Deletion of del(13)(q14q31).

(MIDD). The clinical presentation of LCDD is heralded by development of the nephrotic syndrome followed by renal failure or acquired Fanconi syndrome (more often associated with κ light-chain deposition). In these deposition diseases, the urine dipstick for protein is positive, as a result of the glomerular leakage of albumin.[256,324] Renal enlargement can be caused by AL amyloidosis (Chap. 108) or, less commonly, by renal plasmacytomas.[326] Renal vein thrombosis, hyperviscosity, dehydration, use of nephrotoxic drugs (antibiotics, nonsteroidal antiinflammatory drugs, imaging contrast agents—especially when rapidly infused),[327] hyperuricemia, or type I cryoglobulinemia can all induce or aggravate renal impairment in myeloma patients. Bisphosphonates, in particular, should be infused slowly, at adjusted doses, based on creatinine values. Renal biopsy is usually unnecessary, unless nephrotic syndrome is present. However, if systemic amyloidosis or, less likely, LCDD, is suspected, a subcutaneous fat aspirate or rectal biopsy should be performed first and tested for amyloid deposits.[320] Renal biopsy specimens should be processed fresh-frozen to allow for immunofixation studies, including electron microscopy and Congo red staining for amyloidosis. Supportive care associated with prompt initiation of antimyeloma treatment is the cornerstone of the management of renal impairment in myeloma. To correct hypercalcemia, aggressive hydration, use of calcitonin and a slow infusion of one single dose of a bisphosphonate is applied. Cytoreductive chemotherapy should be started as soon as possible. Rapid removal of light chains by plasma exchange is a controversial technique; the introduction of high cut-off hemodialysis, which employs novel dialysis filters capable of clearing away free-light chains, is showing promising results and improved patient outcomes.[328-330]

In general, myeloma renal impairment is reversible in approximately 50 percent of patients. Conversely, amyloid- and LCDD-related renal impairment tends to be stable or progressive. Patients presenting in acute renal failure have a high early mortality, with up to 30 percent dying within the first months. Improvements in renal function rarely occur after 6 months from diagnosis. Renal dysfunction is a negative prognostic factor, results in use of suboptimal therapies, longer hospitalization, and an increased risk of infection. Hence, patients who recover normal kidney function have a better outcome compared to those who do not.[331-333]

PAIN

Back or chest bone pain as result of vertebral or rib fractures at sites of osteopenia or from lytic bone lesions is present at the time of diagnosis in approximately 60 percent of patients.[247] The pain is usually worse with movement and at night. Pathologic fractures of long bones can ensue as well. Kyphosis or reduction of patient's height is another common feature. Localized pain can also derive from focal plasmacytomas, presenting as expanding masses compressing the spinal cord or nerve roots. Amyloid deposits can provoked painful mass effects, when localizing into nerve sheaths, as in amyloid-associated carpal tunnel syndrome.[334]

INFECTIONS

Myeloma patients are at an increased risk for infections that represent a leading cause of morbidity and mortality. Several aspects contribute to infection risk, including immune dysfunction in the innate and adaptive immune systems,[335] extrinsic factors, like type and duration of therapy (e.g., cytotoxic agents, glucocorticoids, lenalidomide, autologous/allogeneic hematopoietic stem cell transplantation), and physical factors, such as age, coexisting comorbidities, hypoventilation secondary to pathologic fractures, indwelling vascular catheters and impaired mucosal integrity. A broad immune dysfunction involving B lymphocytes, T lymphocytes, NK cells, and dendritic cells is noted in myeloma patients.[335-337] Specifically, myeloma cells or BMSCs can produce a series of immunologically molecules, such as TGF-β, IL-10, and IL-6. TGF-β and IL-10 suppress IL-2 autocrine pathways, blocking T-cell antitumoral responses[338-340] and stimulate T-regulatory cell proliferation.[341] Moreover, these cytokines sustain the immature phenotype of dendritic cells, highly specialized antigen-presenting cells (Chap. 21), reducing their expression of costimulatory molecules (HLA-DR, CD40, and CD80 antigens) and thereby their antigen stimulatory capacity.[342] IL-6 also inhibits dendritic cell production from CD34+ progenitor cells.[342] Normal CD19+ B lymphocytes at early and late stages are suppressed in myeloma, resulting in hypogammaglobulinemia, inversely correlating with the disease stage.[343] B-cell dysfunction in myeloma can be related to TGF-β effects, lack of stimulatory signals from helper T cells, and altered gene expression. Hypogammaglobulinemia is particularly responsible for a myeloma patients' susceptibility to encapsulated organisms, such as *Streptococcus pneumoniae* and *Haemophilus influenzae*. T-cell subsets are also abnormal, with inversion of the CD4:CD8 ratio[344] and T-helper type 2 (Th2) cell–type skewing.[345] Moreover, global T-cell receptor (TCR) diversity is reduced, with the presence of oligoclonal expansions of CD4+ and CD8+ T cells and TCR signaling is compromised[344,346,347]; $\chi\delta$T cells and NK cells are also aberrant in myeloma. The presence of decreased B cell or T cell counts can negatively impact survival.[348] β_2M is the invariant chain of the major histocompatibility (MHC) class 1 molecule, which is shed by myeloma cells. Its levels correlates with tumor burden and are important for patient staging using the International Staging System (ISS)[232] (see section Staging below). β_2M induces IL-6, IL-8, and IL-10 production and activation of STAT3. However, it also has immunosuppressive functions, by reducing surface expression of CD83, HLA-ABC, costimulatory molecules, and adhesion molecules on dendritic cells, impairing stimulatory dendritic-allospecific T-cell responses by inactivation of Raf/MEK/ERK cascade and NF-κB in dendritic cells.[349] Vaccines, prophylactic antibiotics or antivirals, and intravenous immunoglobulin are preventative measures apt to decrease infections among myeloma patients. Yearly influenza vaccines and a single pneumococcal vaccine at diagnosis is recommended, as myeloma patients can still mount a suboptimal immunologic response. Antiviral prophylaxis (e.g., acyclovir 400 mg twice daily or valacyclovir 500 mg once daily) is mandatory in patients treated with bortezomib combined with glucocorticoid regimens to prevent herpes zoster. Antibiotic prophylaxis is controversial. A study where patients were randomized on a 1:1:1 basis to receive either a daily quinolone, trimethoprim-sulfamethoxazole, or placebo for the first 2 months of treatment did not show a decreased incidence of serious infection (more severe than grade 3 and/or requiring hospitalization) nor of any infection within the first 2 months of treatment or any improvement in response rate or OS.[350] However, antibiotic prophylaxis with ciprofloxacin or trimethoprim-sulfamethoxazole might be still beneficial in selected patients, such as those patients with a history of repeated infections, those receiving more intense regimens or those with persistently low CD4+ counts to prevent *Pneumocystis carinii* pneumonia or other infections. Intravenous immunoglobulin (IVIG) infusion may be considered in patients with recurrent, serious infections despite antibiotic prophylaxis.

NEUROPATHY

Local myeloma growth can cause polyneuropathy by spinal cord or peripheral nerve compression, even though polyneuropathy is not a common presenting symptom, unless in the context of perineuronal or perivascular *(vasa nervorum)* amyloid deposition.[256] POEMS syndrome, or osteosclerotic myeloma, is an exception, where complete polyneuropathy is practically always present along with organomegaly, endocrinopathy, monoclonal gammopathy, and skin changes.[351,352] The pathogenesis of POEMS syndrome is largely unknown, but chronic overproduction of proinflammatory cytokines, such as VEGF, plays a major role.

HYPERVISCOSITY

Less than 10 percent of myeloma patients develop signs of hyperviscosity syndrome, a condition that manifests in 10 to 30 percent of patients with Waldenström macroglobulinemia (Chap. 109), because monoclonal IgMs display a higher intrinsic viscosity than other immunoglobulins.[353-355] Cutaneous or mucosal bleeding is very common in hyperviscosity syndrome, together with blurred vision, headache, vertigo, dizziness, nystagmus, deafness, and ataxia. Circulatory problems, affecting cerebral, pulmonary and renal circulation can rarely ensue in the presence of high blood viscosity (see "Hyperviscosity Syndrome" in Chap. 109).[356] Relative serum viscosity but not serum immunoglobulin levels correlates with onset and extent of clinical symptoms. Based on the specific physicochemical properties of classes and subclasses of immunoglobulins (Chap. 75), up to one-quarter of patients with IgA myeloma can have blood hyperviscosity as a result of the tendency of IgA to form dimers or polymers.[357] Patients with IgG$_3$ subclass myeloma, whose immunoglobulins have higher propensity to aggregate, can also manifest with hyperviscosity syndrome.[358]

PLASMA CELL LEUKEMIA AND EXTRAMEDULLARY DISEASE

Plasma cell leukemia (PCL) is diagnosed when more than 2000 myeloma cells/μL are present in the blood or plasmacytosis accounts for greater than 20 percent of the differential white cell count. PCL is rarely manifest at the time of primary presentation and more commonly arises from preexisting myeloma as end-stage disease. In this case, tumor cells have become microenvironment-independent and accumulate in the marrow, but also recirculate in the blood (extramedullary disease).[359-362] However, low levels of circulating plasma cells can be detected in the majority of myeloma patients. By definition, extramedullary disease (EMD) is the presence of a clonal plasmacytic infiltrate outside the marrow. Specifically, it is now considered EMD only if the infiltrate is present at anatomic sites distant from the bone or adjacent soft tissue, hence excluding cases where soft-tissue masses arise in contiguity with the marrow.[363] Indeed, in true EMD, plasma cells have an immature, plasmablastic morphology and have a high proliferative index. According to different clinical trials, 6.0 to 7.5 percent of patients screened with magnetic resonance imaging (MRI) or positron emission tomography–computed tomography (PET-CT) have EMD at the time of diagnosis.[364,365] Extramedullary masses can localize to several organs, including liver, lymph nodes, spleen, kidneys, breasts, pleura, meninges, and cutaneous sites, and are inevitably associated with elevated levels of LDH[366] and a poor response to treatment.[367-369] Leptomeningeal myelomatosis with abnormal cerebrospinal fluid findings is rare but can manifest at advanced stage.[370,371] EMD cells are often CD56– or [low], and present t(4;14) and del(17p) more commonly,[372,373] together with *TP53* mutations, TP53 nuclear localization,[110,374] or high expression levels of focal adhesion kinase (FAK1).[375] Additionally, it has been speculated that high-dose melphalan and modern salvage therapies can artificially increase the incidence of EMD as a result of longer duration of treatment, emergence of dormant cells, and poor penetration of the drugs to sanctuary sites like the central nervous system.[376]

SPINAL CORD COMPRESSION

Spinal cord compression can result from an extramedullary plasmacytoma or vertebral fracture and present acutely with severe back pain alongside with weakness or paresthesias of the lower extremities, or bladder/bowel incontinence. It should be considered a medical emergency, evaluated with MRI, and promptly treated with a combination of local radiotherapy, decompressive laminectomy, and systemic chemotherapy to avoid permanent deficits. Specifically, local radiotherapy using less than 30 Gy is potentially curative, in the presence of a solitary plasmacytoma; in patients with systemic disease, the DT-PACE regimen, which combines high-dose dexamethasone pulsing, as part of the combination with oral dexamethasone, daily thalidomide, and 4 days of continuous-infusion cisplatin, doxorubicin, cyclophosphamide, and etoposide, can provide effective treatment and should be followed by local radiation in the absence of symptom relief and lack of tumor shrinkage. If a singular vertebral collapse is evident without plasmacytoma, decompressive laminectomy is the treatment of choice.

INITIAL EVALUATION OF THE PATIENT WITH MYELOMA

Minimal evaluation requirements include a complete blood count with differential white cell count; examination of a blood film for the presence of rouleaux and circulating myeloma cells; a comprehensive serum metabolic panel for the detection of hypercalcemia, renal failure, serum $\beta_2 M$, C-reactive protein, and elevation of LDH (Table 107–4). Myeloma protein studies should include serum protein electrophoresis to quantitate the serum protein electrophoretic pattern in combination with nephelometric quantitation of immunoglobulin levels, serum-free light-chain assay, and a 24-hour urine collection to quantitate 24-hour total urinary protein and determine specific urinary proteins, such as light chains or Bence Jones protein, using urine electrophoresis.

Immunofixation of serum and urine is needed for the immunoglobulin heavy- and light-chain isotype determination. Serum-free light-chain assay is of particular use in the monitoring of patients with a plasma monoclonal immunoglobulin, the diagnosis and monitoring of patients who would otherwise be considered to have nonsecretory myeloma, and patients who only have light-chain proteinuria. Marrow aspiration and biopsy should include genetic studies (FISH and cytogenetics) and flow cytometry. Newer modalities such as mutational profiling and gene expression studies are being undertaken but are not yet standard of care tests. Radiographic examination usually comprises a metastatic bone survey to detect vertebral compression fractures, osteopenia, and impending fractures of long bones and pelvis. MRI and PET-CT are more sensitive than the bone survey, and better capture early bone disease, the extent of bone disease, and EMD. Both MRI and PET-CT findings have important prognostic implications.[209,364] These tests are now being used more frequently specifically in smoldering multiple myeloma (SMM) patients. Assessment of the heart by echocardiogram and electrocardiogram is useful in the right clinical context to detect cardiac amyloidosis and/or LCDD, and, in selected cases, cardiac MRI may be helpful to demonstrate myocardial infiltration. Measurement of brain natriuretic peptide and N-terminal prohormone B-type natriuretic peptide are useful screening tests to detect cardiac dysfunction caused by amyloidosis or LCDD.

STAGING

Multiple attempts have been made to define clinical and laboratory parameters that have prognostic significance in myeloma.[231,377,378] Of the many staging systems, the Salmon-Durie staging system was historically the most commonly used, however, it has been replaced by newer staging systems, which reflect better myeloma biology.[379] The Salmon-Durie system relates myeloma cell mass to the extent of bony disease, hemoglobin, and calcium levels, and the monoclonal immunoglobulin levels in serum and urine (Table 107–5). However, measurement of

---

TABLE 107–4. Assessment of Myeloma

Complete blood count and differential count; examination of blood film
Chemistry screen, including calcium, creatinine, lactate dehydrogenase, BNP, proBNP
β_2-Microglobulin, C-reactive protein
Serum protein electrophoresis, immunofixation, quantification of immunoglobulins, serum-free light chains
24-Hour urine collection for protein electrophoresis, immunofixation, quantification of immunoglobulins, including light chains
Marrow aspirate and trephine biopsy with metaphase cytogenetics, FISH, immunophenotyping; gene array, and plasma cell labeling index (if available)
Bone survey and MRI; PET-CT (if available)
Echocardiogram with assessment of diastolic function and measurement of interventricular septal thickness; EKG (if amyloidosis suspected)

BNP, brain natriuretic peptide; CT, computed tomography; EKG, electrocardiogram; FISH, fluorescence *in situ* hybridization; MRI, magnetic resonance imaging; PET, positron emission tomography; proBNP, prohormone B-type natriuretic peptide.

TABLE 107–5. Assessment of Myeloma Tumor Mass (Salmon-Durie)

I. High tumor mass (stage III) (>1.2×10^{12} myeloma cells/m^2)*
   One of the following abnormalities must be present:
   A. Hemoglobin <8.5 g/dL, hematocrit <25%
   B. Serum calcium >12 mg/dL
   C. Very high serum or urine myeloma protein production rates:
      1. IgG peak >7 g/dL
      2. IgA peak >5 g/dL
      3. Urine light chains >12 g/24 h
   D. >3 lytic bone lesions on bone survey (bone scan not acceptable)

II. Low tumor mass (stage I) (<0.6×10^{12} myeloma cells/m^2)*
   All of the following must be present:
   A. Hemoglobin >10.5 g/dL or hematocrit >32%
   B. Serum calcium normal
   C. Low serum myeloma protein production rates:
      1. IgG peak <5 g/dL
      2. IgA peak <3 g/dL
      3. Urine light chains <4 g/24 h
   D. No bone lesions or osteoporosis

III. Intermediate tumor mass (stage II) (0.6 to 1.2×10^{12} myeloma cells/m^2)*
   All patients who do not qualify for high or low tumor mass categories are considered to have intermediate tumor mass
   A. No renal failure (creatinine ≤2 mg/dL)
   B. Renal failure (creatinine >2 mg/dL)

*Estimated number of neoplastic plasma cells.

Reproduced with permission from Durie BG, Salmon SE: A clinical staging system for multiple myeloma. Correlation of measured myeloma cell mass with presenting clinical features, response to treatment, and survival. *Cancer* 1975 Sep;36(3):842–854.

TABLE 107-6. International Staging System

Stage I:	β_2M <3.5
	ALB ≥3.5
Stage II:	β_2M <3.5
	ALB <3.5
	or
	β_2M 3.5 to 5.5
Stage III:	β_2M >5.5

ALB, serum albumin in g/dL; β_2M, serum β_2-microglobulin in mg/L.[231]

Data from Greipp PR, San Miguel J, Durie BG, et al: International staging system for multiple myeloma. *J Clin Oncol* 2005 May 20;23(15):3412–3420.

bone disease by skeletal survey in myeloma is observer-dependent and potentially subjective.

The ISS is based on two widely available parameters—serum β_2M and albumin—and recognizes three stages (Table 107–6). Stage I is defined by β_2M less than 3.5 mg/L and albumin 3.5 g or greater/100 mL; stage III is characterized by a β_2M of 5.5 mg or greater/L.[231] The intermediate stage II has features of neither stage I nor III. β_2M correlates with tumor mass and impairment in renal function, whereas a low albumin reflects the effect of IL-6 produced by the microenvironment of myeloma cells on the liver.[380–382] The different ISS stages were predictive of outcome in an analysis of more than 11,000 patients receiving either standard therapies or melphalan-based high-dose therapy followed by autologous hematopoietic stem cell transplantation (auto-HSCT; Table 107–7). Although predictive of outcome, several shortcomings of the ISS include lack of accounting for cytogenetics and bone disease in patients.

IMAGING STUDIES

Imaging studies are an essential part of the diagnosis and management of myeloma. The standard of care in the initial staging of newly diagnosed myeloma is a complete skeletal survey, which includes a posteroanterior view of the chest; anteroposterior and lateral views of the cervical spine, thoracic spine, lumbar spine, humeri, femora, and skull; as well as, an anteroposterior view of the pelvis. Approximately

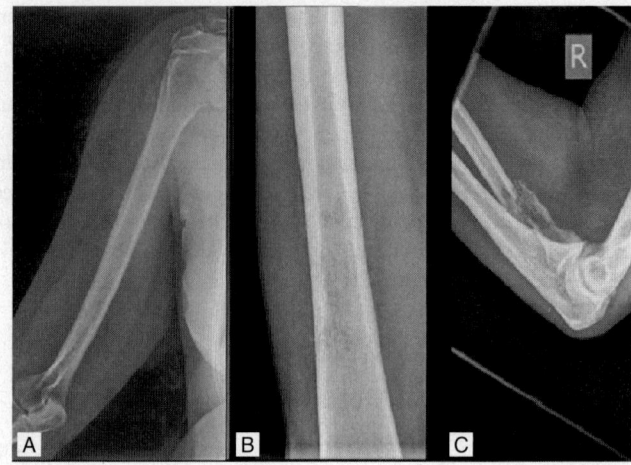

Figure 107–14. Plain x-rays of osteolytic lesions. Osteolytic lesions captured on plain x-rays or skeletal survey. **A.** Right humerus. **B.** Right femur. **C.** Right radius.

80 percent of patients with myeloma will have radiologic evidence of bone involvement on skeletal survey. Although widely employed, this modality has limitations. Roentgenographically detectable osteolytic lesions require at least 50 to 70 percent loss of bone mass,[383] and hence represent advanced bone destruction. Conventional x-rays have limited sensitivity and, consequently, may miss between 10 and 20 percent of early lytic lesions.[384] In addition, reproducibility of skeletal survey results is low and dependent on the expertise of the reveiwer.[385] Another limitation of plain x-rays is that they cannot be used to assess response to therapy as lytic lesions seldom show evidence of healing.[386] Although skeletal survey remains the gold standard for the initial evaluation of myeloma, there are limitations to this modality that necessitate the use of additional imaging modalities (Fig. 107–14).[387]

MRI is widely used in both newly diagnosed and relapsed myeloma and in the event of suspected cord compression. Whole-body MRI can give complementary information to skeletal survey and is recommended in patients with normal plain radiography, particularly when symptoms are present. Numerous studies demonstrate superior sensitivity of MRI when compared to both skeletal survey[388,389] and whole-body multidetector computed tomography (MDCT).[390] MRI also has

TABLE 107–7. Novel Agent Induction for Newly Diagnosed Transplant-Eligible Patients

Study	Regimen	No. of Patients	Cr/nCR (%)	ORR (%)	Outcome
Rajkumar et al.[414]	RD	223	18	79	OS 96% on Rd vs. 87% on RD at 1-year
	Rd	222	14	68	
Harousseau et al.[638]	VAD	121	6.4	62.8	PFS 36 mo Bd vs. 30 mo VAD at 32 mo
	Bd	121	14.8	78.5	
Reeder et al.[639]	CyBorD	33	39	88	N/A
Richardson et al.[418]	RVD	66	39	100	OS 97% at 18 mo
Jakubowiak et al.[421]	CRD	53	62	98	PFS 92% at 24 mo

Bd, bortezomib, low-dose dexamethasone; CRD, carfilzomib, lenalidomide, dexamethasone; CyBorD, cyclophosphamide, bortezomib, dexamethasone; N/A not available; OS-overall survival; PFS-progression free survival; RD, lenalidomide, high-dose dexamethasone; Rd, lenalidomide, low-dose dexamethasone; RVD, lenalidomide, Velcade, dexamethasone; VAD, vincristine, Adriamycin, dexamethasone.

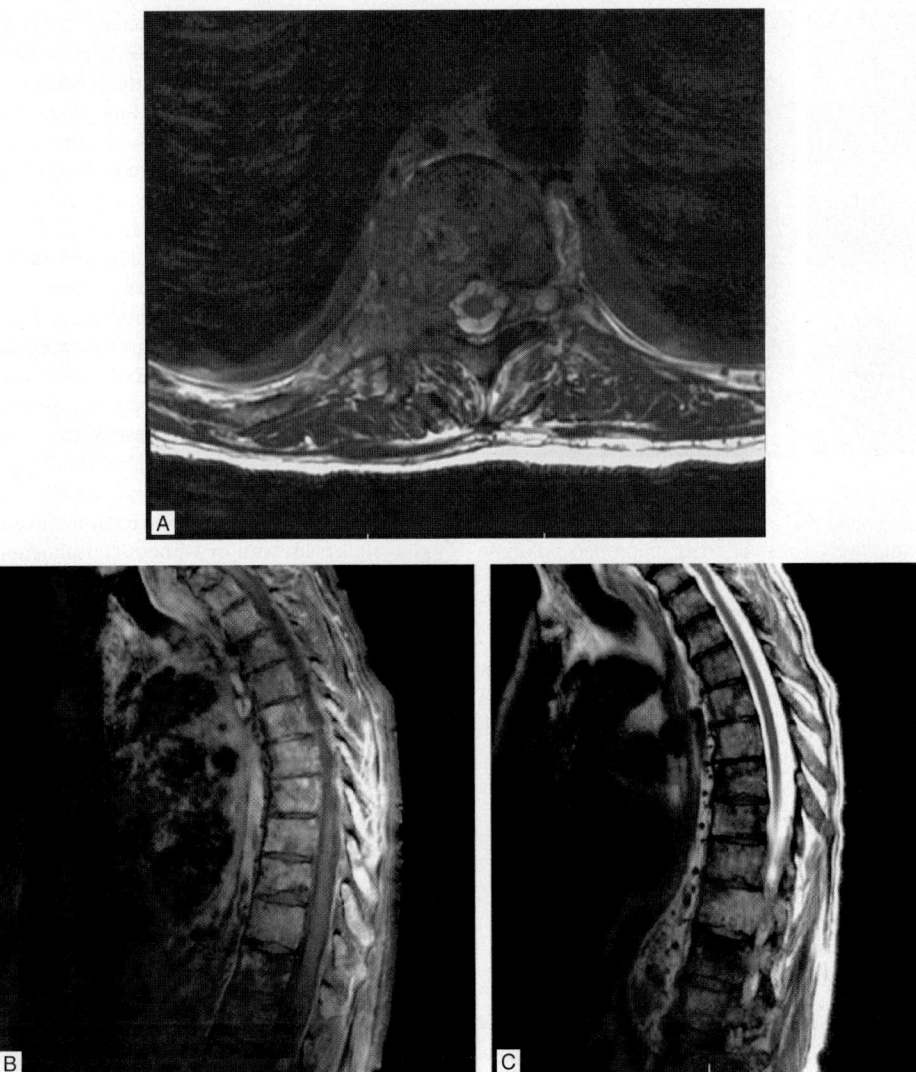

Figure 107–15 A. T2-weighted axial imaging of thoracic spine. Myelomatous lesion involves T11 vertebral body and extends into left posterior elements. **B.** T1-weighted sequencing. Sagittal view of thoracic spine demonstrating diffuse marrow replacement. **C.** T2-weighted sequencing. Sagittal view of thoracic spine. At T10, there is extraosseous extension of soft tissue within the paravertebral space on the right as well as the ventral epidural space and right lateral epidural space. Soft tissue extends laterally to partly efface the right T10–11 neural foramen.

the ability to discriminate myeloma from normal marrow. Specifically, MRI allows visualization of the medullary cavity and thus direct assessment of the extent of myeloma cell infiltration of the bone.[391] In the event of suspected spinal cord compression, MRI is the imaging modality of choice for its ability to provide an assessment of the level and extent of cord compression, the size of the tumor mass, and the extent to which it is compressing the epidural space (Fig. 107–15).[392] In the event that MRI is unavailable or contraindicated, urgent CT may be used for the evaluation of a potential cord compression.

PET, particularly in combination with CT, can be used for the detection of active myeloma. Multiple studies demonstrate that PET-CT is able to detect lesions at least 1 cm in diameter using a standard uptake value (SUV) cutoff of 2.5 to indicate the presence of disease.[393] The limitation of this technology is that subcentimeter lesions may not be detected.[394] In a prospective study comparing PET-CT, MRI, and whole-body x-rays in newly diagnosed myeloma patients, PET-CT was superior to plain films in 46 percent of patients, including 19 percent with negative x-rays. However, PET-CT scans of the spine and pelvis

failed to show abnormalities in 30 percent of patients in whom MRI had demonstrated an abnormal pattern of marrow involvement. On the other hand, PET-CT identified myelomatous lesions in areas that were out of the field of view of MRI in 35 percent of patients. The combination of these two modalities proved the most powerful with a detection rate of as high as 92 percent.[395] In a multivariate analysis, the same group also showed that persistent PET-CT positivity before and after primary therapy and subsequent high-dose therapy, is a predictor of prognosis in patients with symptomatic myeloma (Fig. 107–16).[396] CT, PET-CT, and MRI can be used for the diagnosis and assessment of soft-tissue masses.

DIFFERENTIAL DIAGNOSIS

If the initial laboratory evaluation indicates the presence of a monoclonal immunoglobulin in serum and/or urine, the finding requires further studies to distinguish among (1) MG; (2) solitary plasmacytoma of bone or soft tissue; (3) indolent myeloma; (4) immunoglobulin deposition

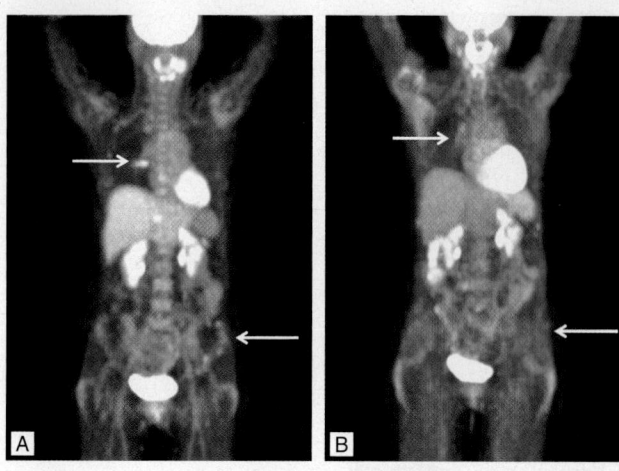

Figure 107–16. Positron emission tomography–computed tomography (PET-CT) imaging before **(A)** and after **(B)** initial therapy for newly diagnosed myeloma with interval resolution of fluorodeoxyglucose uptake.

diseases, such as primary amyloidosis or LCDD; and (5) symptomatic or progressive myeloma.[397] Table 107–5 lists the important studies that can be done to distinguish among these possibilities. Tables 107–1 through 107–4 indicate the findings of symptomatic myeloma. The International Myeloma Working Group has developed new standardized diagnostic criteria that have been widely adopted.[398]

●THERAPY

MANAGEMENT OF NEWLY DIAGNOSED MYELOMA

Myeloma therapy is in a period of dynamic change. The years since 1996 have seen dramatic advances in the treatment of myeloma, beginning with the publication of a randomized trial investigating the use of high-dose melphalan and autologous stem cell transplant in 1996,[399] followed by the introduction of IMiDs thalidomide,[400] lenalidomide,[401] and pomalidomide,[402] and the proteasome inhibitors bortezomib[403] and carfilzomib.[404,405] With these new treatments, the 5-year relative survival rate has increased in the Surveillance Epidemiology and End Results (SEER) database from 28.8 percent from the period of 1990 to 1992 to 34.7 percent in years 2002 to 2004 to 40.3 percent in years 2003 to 2007.[406,407] Previously, most of the survival benefit observed was in younger patients, but one analysis showed that patients older than the age of 70 years were deriving benefit as well.[406,407] Table 107–7 lists novel agents and combinations currently used for induction in transplant-eligible patients with newly diagnosed myeloma.

High-Dose Therapy

Every newly diagnosed myeloma patient should be assessed for fitness to undergo auto-HSCT. Although some centers use an age cutoff (usually age 65 years or younger), it is reasonable to take performance status, organ function, and comorbidities into account, rather than age, when deciding whether a patient is eligible. The rationale for the administration of high doses of alkylating agents (melphalan) followed by transplantation of syngeneic, allogeneic, and autologous marrow or blood progenitor cells (PBPCs), is based on the fact that myeloma is uniformly fatal and myeloma cells have demonstrated a dose–response curve to chemotherapy with a high proportion of patients achieving complete responses when higher doses of therapy are given.

High-dose chemoradiotherapy followed by transplantation of either autologous marrow or PBPCs has achieved high (40 percent) complete response (CR) rates, but the median duration of these responses has been only 2 to 3 years. The Intergroupe Francais du Myeloma (IFM 90), a national French study, first demonstrated the efficacy of auto-HSCT over conventional chemotherapy in 200 myeloma patients.[399] Several randomized trials and case-controlled studies have been performed and the results have been variable. For example, the Medical Research Council (MRC) randomized study confirmed a 12-month survival benefit for the transplanted arm.[408] In contrast, the U.S. Intergroup randomized trial was unable to confirm the benefits of transplantation.[409] Despite the use of aggressive approaches like transplantation, few, if any, patients are cured. To improve upon the results of high-dose chemotherapy, the French group has compared single versus double autografts and their data suggest that two sequential transplants may benefit a subset of patients with myeloma who did not achieve a complete remission after the first transplant.[410] This question is also being addressed by the ongoing phase III, multicenter trial of single autologous transplant with or without consolidation therapy versus tandem autologous transplant with lenalidomide maintenance (BMT CTN 0702).

Novel Agents

Beginning in the 1980s, the combination of vincristine, doxorubicin (Adriamycin), and dexamethasone (VAD) was used as the standard induction chemotherapy, but has been replaced by the advent of novel drugs.[271] Highly active regimens using IMiDs and proteasome inhibitors have replaced VAD. Two studies combined thalidomide with dexamethasone as initial therapy for myeloma and achieved rapid responses in two-thirds of patients, allowing for successful harvesting of blood stem cells for transplantation.[411,412] Thalidomide/dexamethasone has been compared with VAD and with dexamethasone, as initial therapy for patients prior to collection of autologous stem cells and transplantation. In a case-control analysis, Cavo and colleagues showed that thalidomide/dexamethasone achieved higher overall response rates[413] whereas a randomized phase III (Eastern Cooperative Oncology Group [ECOG]) trial showed statistically significantly higher response rates for thalidomide/dexamethasone than dexamethasone-treated patient cohorts.[271] This study provided the rationale for FDA approval of this regimen for initial treatment of myeloma. Moreover, early studies show 91 percent responses, including 6 percent complete and 32 percent near complete/very good partial responses to lenalidomide combined with dexamethasone.

Based on these promising results, a phase III trial in the United States headed by ECOG investigated the role of lenalidomide and dexamethasone in newly diagnosed myeloma. The study design allowed all patients to stay on-study for the first four cycles only for response assessment, after which patients could go off-study to proceed with stem cell transplantation. Published safety data from this trial found that combining lenalidomide with the low-dose dexamethasone regimen was preferable to the combination with high-dose dexamethasone, with a reduction in grade 3 or higher nonhematologic adverse events at (48 percent vs. 65 percent), including thromboembolism (12 percent vs. 26 percent), and infections (9 percent vs. 16 percent) in the two treatment arms of the trial.[414] The low-dose dexamethasone-containing regimen did lead to an increased occurrence of grade 3 or greater neutropenia (20 percent vs. 12 percent). Importantly, the combination with low-dose dexamethasone had a survival benefit over combination with high-dose dexamethasone, with a 1-year OS of 96 percent and 87 percent, respectively.[414,415] Prophylaxis against clotting with aspirin, Coumadin, or subcutaneous heparin, is needed when patients are treated with lenalidomide therapy.[269,270]

One study examined single-agent bortezomib[416] and a second tested bortezomib combined with dexamethasone as initial therapy[417]; in both studies, high frequency and extent of response were noted. In the phase I/II trials, the safety and efficacy of the combination of lenalidomide, bortezomib, and dexamethasone (RVD) were demonstrated.[418] The benefits of combination therapy with RVD as first-line therapy were documented in two phase II trials—the IFM 2008 trial and the EVOLUTION trial.[419,420] The overall response rate (ORR) after induction in the IFM trial was 97 percent (13 percent sCR, 16 percent CR, and 54 percent very good partial response [VGPR] or better). The EVOLUTION trial was designed to compare RVD with cyclophosphamide, bortezomib, and dexamethasone (CyBorD) in a randomized, multicenter setting. The ORR for the RVD arm after primary treatment followed by maintenance with bortezomib for four 6-week cycles was 85 percent (24 percent CR, 51 percent VGPR or better).

Carfilzomib is a second-generation proteosome inhibitor that binds to the proteasome in a highly selective and irreversible fashion. Although the drug was initially approved only for relapsed or refractory myeloma, carfilzomib is now being studied in the upfront setting.[404] In a dose-escalation study, the combination of carfilzomib, lenalidomide, and dexamethasone (CRD) has been evaluated at carfilzomib doses of 20, 27, and 36 mg/m^2 given on days 1, 2, 8, 9, 15, and 16 for eight cycles followed by days 1, 2, 15, and 16 with subsequent cycles. Lenalidomide was given at a dose of 25 mg on days 1 to 21 and dexamethasone at 40 mg weekly for cycles one to four, then 20 mg weekly for cycles five to eight, with cycles of 28 days.[421] After eight cycles, patients received the regimen every other week for eight cycles. After 24 cycles, maintenance with lenalidomide was recommended off-study. After a median of 12 cycles, 62 percent achieved at least a near CR and 42 percent a sCR. The 24-month PFS was estimated to be 92 percent. The toxicity profile was acceptable and notable for limited peripheral neuropathy.

Doublet, and especially triplet, regimens of novel drugs in combination with dexamethasone can induce complete remission rates comparable to transplantation regimens.[413,422] Examples of modern regimens include doublet combinations of lenalidomide and dexamethasone and bortezomib and dexamethasone, as well as, the triple combination of RVD, CyBorD, and CRD.

Combinations that include alkylating agents should be avoided as damage to normal hematopoietic stem cells can be incurred, which may render it impossible to collect stem cells for auto-HSCT.[423] Lenalidomide may also hamper the collection of stem cells, although stem cell mobilization with growth factors and chemotherapy may overcome the myelosuppressive effects of lenalidomide.[424–427] The number of cycles of treatment, especially with lenalidomide-containing regimens is limited to roughly four cycles before stem cell collection, as additional cycles may compromise stem cell harvesting.[424,428]

Combination therapy with novel drugs achieves complete remission rates comparable to those obtained with auto-HSCT. This has led to the design of ongoing studies that compare novel agents followed by auto-HSCT with novel agents followed by delayed auto-HSCT following disease relapse. Novel agents seem to be able to overcome some of the cytogenetic adverse prognostic factors such as del 13, t(4;14), and del 17p. However, it is premature to abandon auto-HSCT as the followup of clinical trials with new agents is too short to determine whether increased complete remission rates will translate into durable remissions and EFS and OS. Complete remission rates as a surrogate marker for eventual outcome may prove to be inadequate. NCT01208662 is a phase III, multicenter randomized trial of RVD versus high-dose treatment with stem cell transplantation (SCT) for myeloma patients up to age 65 years, which was designed to address this question of the role of autologous transplantation in the context of novel drugs. It is likely that autologous transplantation will add to the benefits noted with new drugs.

THERAPY FOR THE TRANSPLANTATION-INELIGIBLE PATIENT

The traditional age limit for auto-HSCT has been 65 years, although older patients should be considered for transplantation provided good organ function is present. Physiologic rather than chronologic age is more suitable for determining transplantation eligibility (Chap. 14).

Oral administration of melphalan and prednisone (MP) has been the standard of care for more than 5 decades in elderly myeloma patients. This form of therapy produces objective response in 50 to 60 percent of patients. The shortcomings of MP have stimulated investigators to use many combinations of chemotherapeutic agents. Several different combinations have been tested and two large overviews of more than 10,000 patients have demonstrated that MP had equivalent efficacy and survival to combination chemotherapy.[429,430] Consequently, MP remains a very reasonable treatment strategy for elderly myeloma patients. A number of new approaches promise to be improvements over MP, however. Palumbo and colleagues have incorporated the use of thalidomide in combination with MP in newly diagnosed patients with myeloma who are older than age 65 years.[431] The addition of thalidomide resulted in a 76 percent complete or partial response rate compared to 47 percent in the MP arm. This translated into a doubling of the 2-year EFS to 54 percent from 27 percent. Based on these data, melphalan, prednisone, and thalidomide (MPT) emerged as the standard of care for transplantation-ineligible patients. However, all studies showed an increase in adverse events in the MPT arm, including infections, neuropathy, and thromboembolism, suggesting that thromboprophylaxis and antimicrobial prophylaxis is required.[432] Melphalan, prednisone, and lenalidomide (MPR) is another effective regimen in this population. The GIMEMA–Italian Multiple Myeloma Network evaluated 54 patients with this combination. The maximum tolerated dose (MTD) was 0.18 mg/kg melphalan, 2 mg/kg prednisone, and 10 mg lenalidomide. In this study, 81 percent of patients achieved at least a partial response, 47.6 percent a VGPR, and 23.8 percent a CR. One-year OS was 100 percent.[433] A subsequent study evaluated the efficacy and safety of induction therapy with MPR followed by lenalidomide maintenance therapy (MPR-R), as compared with MPR or MP without maintenance therapy, in patients with newly diagnosed myeloma who were ineligible for transplantation. At a median followup of 30 months, the median PFS was 31 months for MPR-R versus 14 months for MPR and 13 months for MP. This benefit was observed in patients 65 to 75 years of age, but not in patients older than 75 years. Response rates were superior for the lenalidomide-containing regimen: 77 percent for MPR-R and 68 percent for MPR versus 5 percent with MP.[434]

Randomized trials of other novel agents, like bortezomib with MP, have proven benefits as well. For example, the VISTA trial compared the regimen of bortezomib, melphalan, and prednisone (VMP) to MP in patients who were not candidates for autologous SCT.[435] Overall survival was significantly improved in the VMP group versus MP group, with 3-year OS of 68.5 percent versus 54 percent, respectively.[436]

The FIRST trial, a randomized, phase III trial, compared continuous lenalidomide with low-dose dexamethasone (Rd) against lenalidomide with low-dose dexamethasone for 18 cycles (Rd18) and MPT for 12 cycles.[437] Median PFS for continuous Rd was 25.5 months versus 20.7 for Rd18 and 21.2 for MPT. The OS at 4 years was 59.4 percent for Rd versus 55.7 percent for Rd18 and 51.4 percent for MPT. In the continuous Rd arm, the ORR was 75.1 percent (15.1 percent CR, 28.4 percent VGPR) versus 73.4 in Rd18 (Cr 14.2 percent, VGPR 28.5 percent) and 32.3 percent MPT (CR 9.3 percent, VGPR 18.8 percent). The safety profile with continuous Rd was manageable as hematologic and nonhematologic adverse events were as expected for Rd and MPT. Notably, the incidence of hematologic second primary malignancies was lower with continuous

TABLE 107-8. Novel Agent Induction for Newly Diagnosed Transplantation-Ineligible Patients

Study	Regimen	No. of Patients	Median Followup (months)	Median OS (months)	Median PFS (months)
IFM 99-06[538]	MP	196	51.5	33.2	17.8
	MPT	125		51.6	27.5
	MEL100	126		38.3	19.4
IFM 01/01[640]	MPT	113	47.5	44	24.1
	MP	116		29.1	18.5
MM-015[434]	MPR-R	152	30	45.2	31
	MPR	153		NR	14
	MP	154		NR	13
VISTA[641]	VMP	344	60	56.4	N/A
	MP	338		43.1	N/A
FIRST[437]	Rd	536	37	59.4	25.5
	Rd18	541		55.7	20.7
	MPT	547		51.4	21.2

MEL 100, melphalan 100 mg/m²; MP, melphalan and prednisone; MPR, melphalan, prednisone, and lenalidomide; MPR-R, melphalan, prednisone, and lenalidomide induction followed by lenalidomide maintenance; MPT, melphalan, prednisone, and thalidomide; NR, not reached; OS, overall survival; PFS, progression-free survival; Rd, lenalidomide and low-dose dexamethasone continuously; Rd18, lenalidomide and low-dose dexamethasone for 18 cycles; VMP, bortezomib, melphalan, and prednisone.

Rd than MPT. In newly diagnosed transplantation-ineligible patients, the FIRST trial established continuous Rd as the new standard of care. There are ongoing trials evaluating three-drug combinations, including bortezomib, lenalidomide, and dexamethasone, at reduced doses and attenuated schedules in this population as well. Table 107-8 provides a summary of clinical trial results for novel agent induction regimen for newly diagnosed transplantation-ineligible patients.

MAINTENANCE THERAPY

Maintenance regimens have been proposed to extend the duration of complete remission following autologous SCT. The increased tolerability and efficacy of newer antimyeloma agents has increased the attractiveness and the applicability of this approach; previous attempts at maintenance therapy with older conventional chemotherapy agents such as melphalan or interferon were not beneficial.[438]

A meta-analysis of six randomized, controlled trials with 2786 patients, comparing thalidomide maintenance with other regimens after induction chemotherapy, demonstrated that patients receiving thalidomide maintenance had marginally better OS (hazard ratio [HR] 0.83, p = 0.07). The difference was most prominent in groups who received both thalidomide and glucocorticoids (HR 0.70, p = 0.02). Thalidomide improved PFS (HR 0.65, p <0.01) but was associated with a higher thrombotic risk (risk difference 0.024, p <0.05) and increased peripheral neuropathy (risk difference 0.072, p <0.01).[439]

Three randomized trials explored the use of lenalidomide as maintenance therapy, with two of the trials following autologous SCT[440,441] and one trial after 9 months of melphalan-based therapy in patients ineligible for high-dose treatment.[434] In all three trials, there was a near doubling in PFS with lenalidomide maintenance; for example, from 27 to 46 months in the Cancer and Leukemia Group B (CALGB) 100104 study.[441] Furthermore, the CALGB study showed an OS benefit with lenalidomide: 15 percent of the lenalidomide group had died compared to 23 percent in the placebo group (p <0.03) and at 3 years, the OS was

88 percent in the lenalidomide group compared to 80 percent in the placebo group.

A significant concern with maintenance therapy with lenalidomide is the risk of secondary malignancy. The risk of second primary cancers was roughly double in the maintenance group, (7.0 to 7.7 percent) compared to the placebo group (2.6 to 3.0 percent). The secondary cancers observed included both hematologic malignancies, such as acute myelogenous leukemia, and solid tumors. The risk of a secondary hematologic malignancy appears to be greatest when lenalidomide is given in combination with oral melphalan (HR 4.86, p <0.0001).[442] This increased risk of secondary malignancies and the risk-to-benefit ratio of maintenance therapy should be considered and discussed with the patient when initiating maintenance therapy.

Bortezomib has also been studied as maintenance therapy. In the HOVON-65/GMMG-HD4 study, bortezomib was given every 2 weeks and was associated with increasing the near CR and CR rate from 31 percent to 49 percent.[443] Table 107-9 summarizes maintenance trials.

CONSOLIDATION THERAPY

The use of a short course of consolidation therapy after autologous SCT increases the CR rate and relapse-free survival. Posttransplantation consolidation using the combination of bortezomib, thalidomide, and dexamethasone made it possible to convert 22 percent of VGPR into full, lasting molecular responses [Polymerase chain reaction, negavtive (PCR–)].[444] Enhanced rates of CR, ranging between 10 and 30 percent, have been reported with post–autologous SCT use of bortezomib and lenalidomide as single agents.[445,446] In the IFM 2008 pilot study (enrollment completed in December 2009), the usefulness and safety of posttransplantation consolidation with two cycles of the RVD regimen is being tested. Mature results from these trials will help to better define the role of consolidation in therapy for improving clinical outcomes after transplantation.

TABLE 107-9. Maintenance Therapies

Study	Regimen	No. of Patients	Outcome
IFM 2005-02[440]	Lenalidomide vs. placebo as maintenance following first or second ASCT	614	PFS 41 vs. 23 months
CALGB 100104[441]	Lenalidomide vs. placebo as maintenance therapy after ASCT	460	TTP 46 vs. 27 months
HOVON-65/GMMG-HD4[443]	VAD vs. PAD followed by ASCT, then thalidomide or bortezomib as maintenance	827	PFS 28 vs. 35 months

ASCT, autologous stem cell transplantation; CR, complete response; PAD, bortezomib, doxorubicin, and dexamethasone; PFS, progression-free survival; TTP, time to progression; VAD, vincristine, doxorubicin, and dexamethasone.

CONTINUOUS THERAPY

Data in the upfront setting, both in transplantation-eligible and transplantation-ineligible patients, suggest that continuous therapy may result in improved disease control.[447,448] Several clinical trials have demonstrated superiority of maintenance strategies using thalidomide, lenalidomide, and bortezomib in transplantation-eligible patients.

Thus far, the results from lenalidomide trials are perhaps the most convincing. The IFM 2005–02 and CALGB 100104 studies have both demonstrated a doubling of PFS,[440,441] although only the CALGB trial has suggested an OS advantage. Lenalidomide certainly fits the requirements of a maintenance drug for continued use in myeloma, as it is administered orally and is generally well tolerated. The FIRST trial, comparing continuous Rd with Rd for 18 cycles and MPT, demonstrated that continuous treatment with lenalidomide is superior to a finite therapy. Thrombotic thrombocytopenic purpura (TTP) for the Rd arm was 32.5 months versus 21.9 months for Rd18 and 23.9 months for MPT.[437] However, the risk of second primary malignancies, although low, does need to be discussed and balanced in the decision-making process when considering maintenance therapy with this agent.

As far as studies of patients with relapsed/refractory myeloma are concerned, treatment generally continues until disease progression.[449] However, the development of toxicities is the biggest challenge of continued therapy in this setting. Ultimately, duration of therapy must be balanced with the adverse events encountered by the patient.

As yet, the optimal duration of therapy is myeloma has not been defined. Data suggest that patients should receive continuous antimyeloma therapy as long as patients are benefitting and tolerating therapy without excessive toxicity.

APPROACH TO RELAPSED OR REFRACTORY PATIENTS

A number of options are available for the therapy of relapsing patients. If the relapse occurs more than 6 months after the discontinuation of the initial therapy, patients may be treated with the same primary therapy. Table 107–10 summarizes trials of novel treatment regimens for relapsed or refractory disease.

Proteasome Inhibitors

Two phase II studies, SUMMIT and CREST, demonstrated activity of bortezomib in relapsed or refractory myeloma patients.[403,450] An update of the 202 patients enrolled in the SUMMIT study showed median times to progression and duration of response of 7 and 13 months, respectively.[451] A similar analysis of the CREST study demonstrated 5-year survivals of 32 and 45 percent in patients treated with 1.0 mg/m²

and 1.3 mg/m² of bortezomib, respectively.[452] The randomized phase III APEX study comparing bortezomib with dexamethasone alone, found a median OS of 30 months in the bortezomib group versus 24 months in the dexamethasone group.[453,454] The addition of dexamethasone to bortezomib monotherapy improved response in 18 to 34 percent of patients.[455]

A next-generation proteasome inhibitor, carfilzomib, was granted accelerated FDA approval as a single agent for the treatment of patients who have received at least two prior lines of therapy based on the results of the phase II of single-agent carfilzomib twice weekly that showed an ORR of 23.7 percent in patients who had had a median of five prior lines of therapy. Median duration of response was 7.8 months and median OS was 15.6 months. The drug was well tolerated. The most common side effects were fatigue, anemia, nausea, and thrombocytopenia, with 12.4 percent reporting treatment-related peripheral neuropathy and cardiac.[404]

Oral proteasome inhibitors, ixazomib and oprozomib, are in clinical trials now and will likely gain approval. Ixazomib, has already demonstrated safety and efficacy in phase I trials in the relapsed, refractory population. Of 60 patients who had received a median of six prior regimens including bortezomib (83 percent), there were 41 evaluable patients. Responses included one VGPR, five partial response (PR), one minimal response (MR), and 15 with stable disease. Only 10 percent of patients had drug-related peripheral neuropathy and none were grade 3 or higher.[456] In a phase I/II trial, weekly ixazomib was evaluated in combination with standard dose lenalidomide and dexamethasone in patients with newly diagnosed myeloma. Preliminary results from 58 response-evaluable patients demonstrated a 93 percent ORR, with 67 percent of subjects achieving a very good response rate or better, including a CR rate of 24 percent.[457] Based on these results, ixazomib is being evaluated in combination with lenalidomide and dexamethasone in two large, international phase III trials—TOURMALINE MM1 for relapsed, refractory myeloma patients, and TOURMALINE MM2 for newly diagnosed patients. Oprozomib, another oral proteasome inhibitor, is also under investigation for the treatment of myeloma. These drugs could significantly impact the treatment of myeloma, allowing for completely oral treatment regimens and, consequently, completely outpatient care for patients. This could have a measurable quality-of-life benefit for patients, particularly in the elderly population, and may provide a convenient way of incorporating proteasome inhibitor-based maintenance strategies.

Immunomodulatory Drugs

Three IMiDs, thalidomide, lenalidomide, and pomalidomide, are FDA approved for the treatment of relapsed or refractory myeloma. Long-term followup of the first thalidomide trial showed that 10 years after

TABLE 107–10. Novel Therapies for Relapsed or Refractory Myeloma

Trial	Phase	Agent	No. of Patients	ORR (%)	OS (months)	Outcome (months)
Richardson et al.[454]	III	Bortezomib	669	43	29.8	TTP 6.2 vs. 3.5
		Dexamethasone		18	23.7	
Orlowski et al.[479]	III	Bort/PLD	646	44	76%*	TTP 9.3 vs. 6.5
		Bortezomib		41	65%*	
Weber et al.[462]	III	Lenalidomide	353	61	29.6	TTP 11.1 vs. 4.7
		Dexamethasone		20	20.2	
Dimopoulos et al.[401]	III	Lenalidomide	351	60	NR	TTP 11.3 vs. 4.7
		Dexamethasone		24	20.6	
Richardson et al.[642]	II	RVD	64	64	26	Median TTP 9.5
Siegel et al.[404]	II	Carfilzomib	266	24	15.6	Median PFS 3.7
San Miguel et al.[643]	III	Pom/LoDex	302	31	12.7	Median PFS 4.0 vs. 1.9
		Pom/HiDex		10	8.1	
Dimopoulos et al.[466]	III	Vor/Bort	637	56	NR	Median PFS 7.6 vs. 6.8
		Bort		41	28.1	
Richardson et al.[467]	III	Pan/Bort/Dex	768	61	NR	Duration of response 12 vs. 8.1
		Bort/Dex		55		
Lokhorst et al.[470]	I/II	Daratumumab	32	42†	NR	Median PFS NR
Lonial et al.[473]	II	Elo/Len/Dex	73	92‡	NR	Median PFS NR‡
Lentzsch et al.[476]	II	Benda/Len/Dex	29	52	NR	Median PFS 6.1

Benda, bendamustine; Bort, bortezomib; Dex, dexamethasone; Elo, elotuzumab; Hi, high dose; Lo, low dose; NR, not reported/reached; Pan, panobinostat; PLD, pegylated liposomal doxorubicin; Pom, pomalidomide; RVD, lenalidomide, bortezomib, and dexamethasone; Vor, vorinostat.

*At 15 months.

†Of those receiving a dose of ≥4 mg/kg.

‡Of those receiving dose of 10 mg/kg at 20.8 months.

initiation of therapy 17 of the original cohort of 169 patients were alive and 10 had an uninterrupted remission.[458] The combination of thalidomide and dexamethasone was superior to dexamethasone alone in several studies.[459–461] Patients who have had prior thalidomide exposure should probably be treated with one of the other novel agents. Furthermore, cytogenetic abnormalities predict for a poor long-term response to thalidomide.[268,458]

Lenalidomide is more potent than its predecessor, thalidomide, and is not associated with sedation, peripheral neuropathy, and severe constipation. In two large, randomized phase III trials, lenalidomide with high-dose dexamethasone produced a superior response and delayed time to progression compared to dexamethasone and placebo.[401,462] The combination of lenalidomide and dexamethasone had activity in both bortezomib-naïve and previously treated patients, in thalidomide-resistant patients, and after prior auto-HSCT. An analysis of the expanded access lenalidomide program, enrolling 1438 patients, showed that the combination of lenalidomide and dexamethasone had an acceptable safety profile, with less than 10 percent of patients experiencing pneumonia or deep vein thrombosis.[463]

Pomalidomide has also demonstrated potent antimyeloma effects. Several studies have evaluated pomalidomide in combination with low-dose dexamethasone in the relapsed population, culminating in the approval of pomalidomide 4 mg orally on days 1 to 21 of 28-day cycles until progression. The phase II, randomized, open-label study compared pomalidomide and low-dose dexamethasone with single-agent pomalidomide in patients with relapsed or refractory myeloma. Median PFS for the combination arm was 4.2 months compared to 2.7 months for monotherapy (HR 0.68, P = 0.003). The ORR was 33 percent with combination therapy versus 18 percent for pomalidomide alone. Median OS was 16.5 months versus 13.6 months, respectively. Refractoriness to lenalidomide and bortezomib did not affect outcomes with pomalidomide and dexamethasone.[464] In the phase III European study comparing pomalidomide and low-dose dexamethasone with high-dose dexamethasone alone, PFS at the interim analysis was 3.6 months in the combination arm compared to 1.8 months for dexamethasone alone (HR 0.45; P <0.001). The most common side effects seen were myelosuppression and infections.[465]

Histone Deacetylase Inhibitors

Histone deacetylase (HDAC) inhibitors are another class of drugs that have demonstrated activity in relapsed or refractory myeloma when used in combination with bortezomib. The phase III, randomized trial, called Vantage 088, showed the combination of vorinostat and bortezomib was active and well-tolerated. When this combination was compared with bortezomib alone, the ORR for vorinostat and bortezomib was 56.2 percent versus 40.6 percent for bortezomib alone (p <0.0001); similarly, PFS was 7.63 months compared to 6.83 months, respectively (p = 0.01).[466] Panobinostat has been combined with bortezomib and dexamethasone in a phase II study and compared with bortezomib and dexamethasone alone in the relapsed/refractory population. PFS was

12 months versus 8.1 months (p <0.0001) for patients treated with the triple therapy. ORR was 61 percent versus 55 percent and duration of response of 13.1 months versus 10.9 months. OS data is not yet mature. Common side effects included myelosuppression and diarrhea.[467] ACY-1215, a selective HDAC 6 inhibitor, is another well-tolerated HDAC inhibitor that is being studied in combination with both lenalidomide and bortezomib plus dexamethasone. The ORR in combination with lenalidomide and dexamethasone was 69 percent even though 13 of 16 patients had received prior lenalidomide and three of six were refractory to lenalidomide.[468] In combination with bortezomib and dexamethasone, the ORR was 60 percent.[469]

Monoclonal Antibodies

Several monoclonal antibodies have demonstrated activity in myeloma, including novel drugs targeting CD38, CS1, and BAFF. Daratumumab, a monoclonal anti-CD38 antibody, was granted Fast Track Designation and Breakthrough Therapy Designation by the FDA based on results of a phase I/II trial that demonstrated single-agent activity in relapsed, refractory myeloma. In the 4 mg or more/kg groups (n = 12), five PRs and three MRs were observed. Median PFS had not been reached by a data cutoff of 3.8 months.[470] Daratumumab is now being studied in combination with lenalidomide and dexamethasone in relapsed or refractory disease. SAR650984, another anti-CD38 antibody, had an ORR of 30.8 percent as a single agent in the dose-escalation study in relapsed or refractory (RR) patients at the MTD.[471]

Elotuzumab, a humanized monoclonal IgG$_1$ antibody directed against human CS1 (also known as CD2 subset-1, SLAMF7, CRACC, and CD319), a cell-surface antigen glycoprotein that is highly expressed on myeloma cells and normal plasma cells, has also been granted Breakthrough Therapy Designation by the FDA. In a phase I study, no objective responses were seen, although 26.5 percent had stable disease by European Bone Marrow Transplant Group (EBMT) myeloma response criteria.[472] In combination with lenalidomide and dexamethasone, objective responses were obtained in 82 percent (23 of 28) of treated patients. After a median followup of 16.4 months, the median time to progression was not reached for patients in the 20 mg/kg cohort who were treated until disease progression. An ORR of 92 percent and a median PFS of 33 months was observed after a median followup of 20.8 months at the 10 mg/kg dose which was the dose chosen for the phase III trial.[473] Phase I results of elotuzumab in combination with bortezomib and dexamethasone are also favorable. Phase I results demonstrate a PR or better in 48 percent of 27 evaluable patients with relapsed or refractory disease.[474]

Tabalumab, is a fully human monoclonal antibody designed to have neutralizing activity against both membrane-bound and soluble BAFF, has been combined with bortezomib and dexamethasone. In the phase I/II study, the ORR was 45.8 percent.[475] A phase II trials of this combination has been completed but results have not yet been reported.

Other Treatments

Bendamustine as a single-agent or in combination with lenalidomide and dexamethasone is another option for patients with relapsed or refractory myeloma. The combination of bendamustine, lenalidomide, and dexamethasone was evaluated in a phase I/II trial. The median PFS was 6.1 months, PR rate 52 percent, and VGPR rate 24 percent.[476] The MTD of bendamustine was 75 mg/m^2 as compared with prior studies using 100 mg/m^2. Toxicity was mainly hematologic arguing in favor of the lower dose, particularly in light of the fact that this population is heavily pretreated.[477]

Other regimens that have been explored include bortezomib and pegylated doxorubicin with or without thalidomide, bortezomib combined with thalidomide and dexamethasone, bendamustine with prednisone and thalidomide, and lenalidomide with doxorubicin and dexamethasone.[478–482] There are currently many new drugs in development that target novel pathways. For example, filanesib, a kinesin spindle protein inhibitor, has demonstrated activity in combination with lenalidomide and bortezomib.[483,484] Several other classes of novel drugs are currently under investigation including the bromodomain inhibitors, CDK inhibitors, and inhibitors of the ubiquitin pathway. Data generated from these early studies will provide a better understanding of how these new drugs will be incorporated into the continuum of myeloma care.[485–487]

Another area of interest and therapy development is the blockade of interactions between the tumor cells and immune cells. PD-1 and PD-L1 are two targets of interest. PD-1 is a molecule present on T cells that interacts with PD-L1 expressed on tumor cells. There are ongoing clinical trials exploring PD-1 blockade in combination with a dendritic cell/myeloma fusion vaccine in myeloma.[488]

The choice of therapy for relapsed or refractory patients depends on a number of factors, including time since last therapy, prior exposure to novel agents, alone or in combination, and drug-induced comorbidities, for example, neuropathy, renal malfunction, and loss of patient physiologic reserve. In the past decade, there has been a dramatic increase in the number of therapies available to patients with relapsed or refractory myeloma. This is a very dynamic area within oncology and will continue to evolve as more new therapies enter trials and gain approval.

ALLOGENEIC HEMATOPOIETIC STEM CELL TRANSPLANTATION

Allogeneic transplantation was seen as an attractive option to treat myeloma because it has the potential to be curative, provides a donor graft that is not contaminated with myeloma stem cells, and may establish a graft-versus-myeloma (GVM) effect that could eradicate any surviving myeloma cells.[489,490] Furthermore, molecular remissions have been observed, which predict for longer survival.[491,492] However, the early experience with myeloablative allogeneic transplantation has not been encouraging as a result of a high mortality, varying from 30 to 50 percent, despite improvements in patient selection and supportive care.[493–500]

Studies from Seattle[494,501] and the EBMT[502] have reported that some patients remain progression-free at long intervals after hematopoietic stem cell transplantation (HSCT). The EBMT has reported that actuarial OS was 32 percent at 4 years, and 28 percent at 7 years for the 72 (44 percent) patients who achieved CR after allografting.[496,497,503] However, overall PFS was 34 percent at 6 years, and few patients remain in continuing CR for more than 4 years post allograft. Favorable pre–marrow transplantation prognostic factors for both response and survival after marrow transplantation were female sex, IgA isotype, low serum β_2M, stage I disease at diagnosis, one line of previous treatment, and being in CR prior to marrow transplantation. Of major concern is the early 40 percent transplant-related mortality (50 percent in males) in the EBMT report,[495] which has subsequently been reduced to 20 to 30 percent as a consequence of better patient selection, early transplantation, and less pretransplantation treatment.[503] The actuarial probabilities of survival and progression-free survival were 0.50 +/– 0.21 and 0.43 +/– 0.17 at 4.5 years. Adverse prognostic factors included: transplantation more than 1 year after diagnosis; serum β_2M higher than 2.5 mg/dL at time of transplantation; female patients transplanted from male donors; having received more than eight cycles of chemotherapy; and Salmon-Durie stage III disease at presentation (see Table 107–5). Toxicity was substantial, with 35 (44 percent) patients dying of transplant-related causes within 100 days of marrow transplantation.[494,501]

Reduced-intensity conditioning regimens were introduced to reduce transplantation-related mortality and extend the age limit for allografting.[504–509] Autografting has been performed prior to nonmyeloablative transplantation by several investigators, demonstrating the feasibility of this approach to cytoreduce tumor and then enhance antimyeloma immunity.[510,511] Bruno and colleagues published a prospective trial of initial autologous SCT followed by mini-allogeneic transplantation versus double autologous transplantation.[512,513] The median OS was 80 months for allografting versus 54 months for double autografting. The CR rate after allografting was 55 percent versus 26 percent after double autograft. In contrast, a randomized trial in high-risk myeloma showed that the combination of autologous SCT followed by dose-reduced allogeneic transplantation (IFM 99–03) was not superior to tandem autotransplant (IFM 99–04).[514] BMT CTN 0102, also evaluated autologous SCT followed by second autologous versus nonmyeloablative allogeneic SCT. In both standard- and high-risk patients, nonmyeloablative allogeneic HSCT after auto-HSCT was not more effective than tandem auto-HSCT.[515,516] Bjorkstand and colleagues conducted a prospective study of single or tandem autologous SCT versus reduced-intensity allogeneic SCT based on availability of an human leukocyte antigen (HLA)-identical sibling. Long-term followup of 357 patients who received either autologous SCT (single or double) or autologous–allogeneic with HLA-identical sibling matched donor demonstrated that PFS was superior (35 percent versus 18 percent; p = 0.001) at 60 months for those receiving an autologous–allogeneic tandem transplantation. Nonrelapse mortality was 12 percent after autologous–allogeneic versus 3 percent in the autologous group (p <0.001) and the incidence of limited to extensive graft-versus-host disease (GVHD) was 31 percent and 23 percent.[517]

The use of allogeneic transplantation as salvage therapy, while feasible, is unlikely to be of significant benefit in a heavily pretreated population. The EBMT reported on the outcomes of 229 patients who received reduced-intensity conditioning allogeneic SCT. Transplant-related mortality at 1 year was 22 percent and 3-year OS and PFS were 41 percent and 21 percent, respectively, with 25 percent of patients developing extensive chronic GVHD.[518] The best outcomes were seen in patients who received a transplant in remission and early in the course of the disease. Adverse OS was associated with chemoresistant disease, transplantation more than 1 year after diagnosis, and in male patients transplanted with female donors.

In patients whose disease does not respond to or relapses after allogeneic SCT, donor lymphocyte infusion (DLI) can be considered. Molecular remissions are more common after allografting than after autografting,[492,519–521] and DLI can treat relapsed myeloma post allografting,[490,522,523] indicating a clinically significant GVM effect. In an effort to reduce toxicity and exploit GVM, CD4+ DLI have been used at 6 months post–CD6-depleted marrow allografting so as to enhance GVM and thereby improve outcome.[524] Although prophylactic DLI induces significant GVM responses after allogeneic marrow transplantation, only 58 percent of patients were able to receive DLI despite T-cell-depleted marrow transplantation.

Allografting should only be undertaken in the context of clinical trials, which aim to reduce chronic GVHD, separate GVM from GVHD, and amplify the GVM effect to improve outcome by ameliorating toxicity and maximizing the antimyeloma effect of immunologic effector cells.[525]

ADJUNCTIVE THERAPIES

Bone Disease

Bone involvement is one of the defining characteristics of myeloma, either as lytic lesions or diffuse osteopenia. Bisphosphonates, such as pamidronate and zoledronic acid, inhibit osteoclast activity and can palliate pain and prevent bone-related complications.[219,526,527] Hypercalcemia is associated with increased bone resorption in myeloma, and bisphosphonates also play a key role in the treatment of hypercalcemia. Zoledronic acid, which is more potent than pamidronate, is superior to pamidronate for the treatment of hypercalcemia.[528]

The International Myeloma Working Group (IMWG) and the National Comprehensive Cancer Network (NCCN) panels advocate the use of either pamidronate or zoledronic acid monthly for patients with myeloma and lytic bone disease. Both pamidronate and zoledronic acid are considered equally effective in reducing skeletal complications.[529,530] These guidelines recommend the use of pamidronate at 90 mg delivered intravenously for at least 4 hours or zoledronic acid at 4 mg intravenously for 15 minutes every 3 to 4 weeks for patients with myeloma and lytic bone disease.

In addition to playing an important supportive role, bisphosphonates may have a direct antitumor effect. The MRC Myeloma IX trial compared zoledronic acid to oral clodronic acid and found that zoledronic acid reduced mortality by 16 percent and increased median OS from 44.5 months to 50 months.[531] The benefit of zoledronic acid on skeletal morbidity was also seen in patients without bone lesions at baseline.[532]

A key concern with bisphosphonates, especially zoledronic acid, is the risk of osteonecrosis of the jaw (ONJ).[533] In the MRC Myeloma IX trial, the rate of ONJ was 4 percent.[531] Attention to dental hygiene and minimizing invasive procedures may reduce the risk of ONJ.[534]

Denosumab is a monoclonal antibody to RANK ligand that also inhibits osteoclasts; it showed promising activity in myeloma in a phase II trial.[188] Although denosumab was superior to zoledronic acid in patients with solid tumors and bone metastases, denosumab was inferior in a subset analysis of myeloma patients in a phase III trial.[187] However, interpretation is limited based on the small numbers in the trial. A larger phase III study (NCT01345019) focusing on patients with myeloma is ongoing.

Vertebroplasty (injection of methyl methacrylate or bone cement) and kyphoplasty (use of an inflatable balloon followed by instillation of bone cement) are percutaneous procedures for treating compression fractures, and have also been used in the setting of myeloma.[535,536]

Palliative Radiation Therapy

Radiation also plays a key role for palliation of painful bony lesions in myeloma. An estimated 38 percent of patients are expected to receive radiation over the course of their illness.[537] The primary indication for the use of radiation therapy is palliation of bone pain. Other indications include impending fracture, cord compression, or relief of symptoms associated with a mass (i.e., cranial nerve palsies, cosmesis or organ or joint dysfunction). Doses of 20 to 35 Gy can be used, but it is essential to consider ability to retreat when designing treatment fields, particularly of the spine. Doses of 20 Gy, delivered in either 5 or 10 fractions, typically provide adequate symptom relief.

EMERGENT COMPLICATIONS OF NEW MYELOMA THERAPY

Venous Thromboembolism

Patients with myeloma are at an increased risk for deep vein thrombosis and pulmonary embolism, particularly when known risk factors are present (history of VTE, immobilization, dehydration, other factors).[432] Genetic predispositions include high levels of homocysteine and deficiencies of antithrombin, protein C, and protein S, as well as mutations that predispose to thrombosis, such as the factor V Leiden allele and/or the prothrombin gene G20210A allele. Genetic abnormalities should be suspected with repeated episodes of VTE. The incidence of VTE is highest during the first 3 to 4 months following diagnosis and occurs in approximately 3 to 4 percent of patients receiving either dexamethasone alone or MP, but is much higher when newer agents are combined with dexamethasone and melphalan.[271,538,539] A number of procoagulant abnormalities have been described in myeloma, including endothelial damage, paraprotein interference with fibrin structure, elevated von Willebrand multimers, elevated factor VIII, decreased protein S, and acquired activated protein C resistance.[540,541] A SNP analysis discovered 18 polymorphisms associated with thalidomide-induced VTE. These polymorphisms were involved in pathways important for drug transport or metabolism, DNA repair, and cytokine pathways.[542] The precise mechanisms causing VTE in myeloma patients absent a known genetic predisposition remain elusive, but the type of therapy plays an important role.

The incidence of VTE with single-agent thalidomide is approximately 2 to 4 percent in newly diagnosed and in relapsed patients, comparable to that observed with dexamethasone alone or MP, implying that thalidomide alone does not increase the risk of VTE. However, the risk for VTE increases significantly when thalidomide is combined with dexamethasone, melphalan, doxorubicin, or cyclophosphamide, or with multiagent chemotherapy.[274,432] The MPT combination causes VTE in 12 to 20 percent of patients who do not receive anticoagulant prophylaxis, whereas the incidence of VTE with thalidomide and dexamethasone in newly diagnosed patients is 14 to 26 percent.[271,411,431,538] Most VTEs occur within the first 60 days of therapy, coinciding with maximum cytoreduction. In the Total Therapy 2 study, 22 percent of patients developed a VTE, 95 percent of which occurred in the first 12 months of therapy.[543] Oral regimens principally promote deep vein thrombosis or pulmonary embolism, whereas infusional regimens can give rise to central line–related thrombosis in approximately 50 percent of patients.[542]

Single-agent lenalidomide does not appear to increase VTE, at least not in the setting of myeloma relapse, but is associated with a marked increase in VTE risk when lenalidomide is combined with dexamethasone.[482] Three risk factors for lenalidomide-associated VTE are higher dexamethasone doses, administration of erythropoietin, and concomitant administration of other agents. When combined with cyclophosphamide, the incidence of lenalidomide-induced VTE was 14 percent.[544] Bortezomib did not seem to increase the risk of VTE, at least not in patients with relapsed or refractory disease.[272]

Prevention of VTE is based on the assessment for known risk factors for VTE: (1) myeloma-related (hyperviscosity, newly diagnosed status); (2) therapy-related (high-dose dexamethasone [≥480 mg/month], doxorubicin, multiagent chemotherapy); (3) individual factors (age, history of VTE, inherited thrombophilia, obesity, immobilization, central venous line, infections, surgery, administration of erythropoietin); and (4) factors related to comorbidities (acute infection, diabetes mellitus, cardiac or renal dysfunction). Therapy-related risk factors weigh highest in the risk equation for VTE. The following thromboprophylaxis is recommended: (1) acetylsalicylic acid (aspirin) in either a standard dose of 325 mg/day or in a low dose of 81 mg/day for patients with one or no risk factors or (2) low-molecular-weight heparin (LMWH) once a day, or full-dose warfarin for patients if two or more risk factors or therapy-related risks are present. The recommended duration of prophylaxis in general is 6 to 12 months.[432]

Therapy for VTE should begin with standard therapeutic doses of LMWH. Oral anticoagulation may be considered as a followup. If oral anticoagulation is deemed inappropriate in a given patient, LMWH should be continued as long as the patient is receiving antineoplastic therapy. The optimal duration of therapy is unknown but one study reported a recurrence of VTE of 10 percent in patients who had discontinued anticoagulant therapy,[545] suggesting that long-term prophylaxis

may be indicated in some patients. A survival benefit for patients who were anticoagulated for a VTE may suggest an additional effect of anticoagulants on the myelomatous process.[543]

Peripheral Neuropathy

Bortezomib-[546,547] and thalidomide-induced[548,549] peripheral neuropathy should be distinguished from other causes such as paraneoplastic neuropathies, antecedent chemotherapy with neurotoxic agents (vincristine or cisplatin), diabetes mellitus, and AL amyloidosis. Patients with AL amyloidosis of the peripheral nerves are especially sensitive to neurotoxic agents. Clinical findings include bilateral tingling, and numbness in the toes and/or fingers and/or pain ascending in the extremities when neurotoxic drug therapy is continued. Symptoms are typically in a glove-and-stocking distribution. Neurologic examination should evaluate sensory loss, deep tendon reflexes, and distal weakness, especially in the lower extremities. If significant weakness or asymmetry of signs is present, a neurologic consultation must be obtained along with electromyography and nerve conduction studies.

Bortezomib inhibits NF-κB activation, blocking the transcription of nerve growth factor–mediated neuron survival. Other proposed mechanisms for bortezomib-induced neuropathy include mitochondria and endoplasmic reticulum damage because of activation of the mitochondrial-based apoptotic pathway.[546,550,551] Second-generation, more selective proteasome inhibitors such as carfilzomib have a reduced neurotoxicity.[552] Grade 3 or 4 bortezomib-induced neurotoxicity occurs in approximately 20 percent of newly diagnosed patients and in 30 percent of patients with relapsing disease.[417,553,554] A 50 percent dose reduction should be made for bortezomib-induced grade 2 neuropathy while grade 3 or 4 neuropathy requires drug discontinuation. Improvement or resolution of symptoms has been reported in 3 months, whereas in other patients maximum improvement may take 2 years.[403,553,555,556] Subcutaneous dosing of bortezomib appears to be similarly effective to intravenous administration and has a significantly improved safety profile. When compared head-to-head, 38 percent of patients receiving bortezomib subcutaneously reported any grade of neuropathy compared to 53 percent when given IV (p = 0.044). By grade, 24 percent versus 41 percent (p = 0.012) had grade 2 or worse, and 6 percent versus 16 percent (p = 0.026) had grade 3 or worse when comparing subcutaneous with intravenous administration, respectively.[557] Subcutaneous administration is now the preferred route of administration based on these findings.

Daily thalidomide dose, dose intensity, cumulative dose 400 mg or greater, and duration of therapy are all implicated in the pathogenesis of thalidomide-induced neuropathy, which occurs in up to 75 percent of patients.[548,549,558–563] Dose reduction or cessation of therapy with the option of switching to lenalidomide will usually improve neuropathy, although resolution or improvement of neuropathy can take considerable time as thalidomide appears to induce an axonal-length-dependent neuropathy.[564] Symptomatic treatment for thalidomide- and bortezomib-induced neuropathy usually comprises gabapentin, pregabalin, or tricyclic antidepressants.

Osteonecrosis of the Jaw

ONJ is a severe "bone" disease, associated with bisphosphonate therapy that affects the jaws and typically presents as infection with necrotic bone in the mandible or maxilla. ONJ is characterized by the presence of exposed bone in the maxillofacial region that does not heal within 8 weeks. Although asymptomatic at times, ONJ usually presents as pain and/or numbness in the affected area, soft-tissue swelling, drainage, and tooth mobility. The exact cause of ONJ is not known and is likely to be multifactorial. The risk of developing ONJ increases with duration of bisphosphonate exposure and is 5 to 15 percent at 4 years.[565–567] A further predisposing factor for ONJ is invasive dental procedures such as extractions.[568,569] Approximately 50 percent of affected patients had dental work prior to developing ONJ.[569] A genome-wide SNP analysis has shown that a polymorphism in the cytochrome P450–2C polypeptide is associated with an increased risk of developing ONJ on bisphosphonate therapy, although the mechanism underlying this genetic predisposition to ONJ has as yet not been elucidated.[570,571] To prevent ONJ, patients should be referred for dental evaluation prior to commencing intravenous bisphosphonates and should be advised to maintain excellent oral hygiene and avoid dental procedures while receiving these agents.[534] Antibiotic prophylaxis before dental procedures may reduce the incidence of ONJ in patients receiving bisphosphonate therapy.[572] Management is usually conservative (discontinuation of bisphosphonates, limited debridement, antibiotic therapy, and topical mouth rinses).[573] Surgical resection of necrotic bone should be reserved for refractory cases. In a series of 97 patients, healing of ONJ was observed in 75 percent of patients. Patients who develop spontaneous ONJ have a significantly higher risk of nonhealing ONJ or recurrence.[568]

COURSE AND PROGNOSIS

MONITORING DISEASE MARKERS FOR DOCUMENTATION OF RESPONSE AND RELAPSE

The previously widely used criteria for assessing response developed by the EBMT Registry, also referred to as the EBMT criteria, have been supplanted by the International Uniform Response Criteria proposed by the IMWG (Table 107–11).[8,574] The IMWG response criteria incorporate the serum-free light-chain assay to allow for assessment of patients previously thought to have hyposecretory or nonsecretory disease. Stricter definitions of complete remission resulted in the inclusion of a category of stringent complete remission in which monoclonal plasma cells are not detectable in the marrow by immunohistochemistry or immunofluorescence and the free light-chain ratio is normal. The previously used near complete remission (only positivity by serum monoclonal immunoglobulin immunofixation) is now included in the new category of "very good partial response" and the previously used minor response category is eliminated.

Survival end points include PFS, EFS, and disease-free survival. PFS is the time from start of therapy to myeloma progression or death and includes all patients. It is being used as a surrogate for OS. In the case of EFS, precise definition of what constitutes an event is required (e.g., significant drug toxicity, death, etc.). Stable disease is no longer used as a measure of treatment efficacy, but rather time to progression, which is measured from the start of therapy and, importantly, includes all patients entered into clinical studies. Duration of a response is calculated from the onset of response and only counts the subgroup of responding patients. Long-term followup is recommended to fully evaluate the impact of novel treatment. Other limitations of the new criteria are that response is determined only by monoclonal immunoglobulin and marrow evaluation. Dynamic changes in skeletal events readily identified by modern imaging techniques such as MRI and PET-CT are excluded from response assessments.

Sequencing-based platforms, quantitative polymerase chain reaction, and multiparametric flow cytometry are now being employed to detect minimal residual disease (MRD) in patients attaining at least a VGPR after primary therapy which may be of significant prognostic value. Martinez-Lopez and colleagues reported the results of sequencing-based marrow evaluations on 133 patients in VGPR or better

TABLE 107–11. Uniform Response Criteria from the International Myeloma Working Group

Response Subcategory*	Response Criteria
CR	Negative immunofixation of the serum and urine and disappearance of any soft-tissue plasmacytomas and <5% plasma cells in marrow.[†]
sCR	CR as defined above plus
	Normal FLC ratio and
	Absence of clonal cells in marrow[†] by immunohistochemistry or immunofluorescence.[‡]
VGPR	Serum and urine M-protein detectable by immunofixation but not on electrophoresis or 90 or greater reduction in serum M-protein plus urine M-protein <100 mg per 24 h.
PR	>50% reduction of serum M-protein and reduction in 24-h urinary M-protein by >90% or to <200 mg per 24 h.
	If the serum and urine M-protein are unmeasurable, >50% decrease in the difference between involved and uninvolved FLC levels is required in place of the M-protein criteria.
	If serum and urine M-protein are unmeasurable, and serum-free light assay is also unmeasurable, >50% reduction in plasma cells is required in place of M-protein, provided baseline marrow plasma cell percentage was >30%.
	In addition to the above listed criteria, if present at baseline, a >50% reduction in the size of soft-tissue plasmacytomas is also required.
SD	Not meeting criteria for CR, VGPR, PR, or progressive disease.

CR, complete response; FLC, free light chain; M-protein, monoclonal protein; PR, partial response; sCR, stringent complete response; VGPR, very good partial response.

*All response categories require two consecutive assessments made at any time before the institution of any new therapy; CR, PR, and stable disease categories also require no known evidence of progressive or new bone lesions if radiographic studies were performed. Radiographic studies are not required to satisfy these response requirements.

[†]Confirmation with repeat marrow biopsy not needed.

[‡]Presence/absence of clonal cells is based upon the κ:λ ratio of >4:1 or <1:2. An abnormal κ:λ ratio by immunohistochemistry and/or immunofluorescence requires a minimum of 100 plasma cells for analysis.

NOTE: SD is not recommended for use as an indicator of response; stability of disease is best described by providing the time-to-progression estimates.

following primary therapy. In patients achieving a CR, the TTP was 131 months for MRD-negative patients compared to 35 months for MRD-positive patients. When stratified by level of MRD, the respective TTP medians were 27 months for MRD 10^{-3} or greater, 48 months for MRD 10^{-3} to 10^{-5}, and 80 months for MRD less than 10^{-5} (p = 0.003 to 0.0001).[575] Although not currently a standard of care, MRD assessment may play an important role in evaluating disease response in the future.

Disease features can change over the course of the disease. Not infrequently, clonal evolution occurs with successive relapses, resulting in the loss of previously secreted intact immunoglobulin and a switch to secretion of light-chains only ("Bence Jones escape") or entire loss of immunoglobulin-secretory capacity, often associated with extramedullary spread, best signified by increased LDH levels and lesions found on PET-CT examination. Occasionally, unexplained anemia or pancytopenia accompanies the disappearance of myeloma protein markers, necessitating prompt marrow examination to detect fulminant relapse.

Many induction regimens currently affect tumor cytoreduction rapidly, so that monoclonal immunoglobulin reduction of 50 percent or more is apparent within a few months of therapy. Thus, at least monthly myeloma protein evaluations should be performed during induction. After two to four induction cycles and prior to high-dose melphalan-based auto-HSCT, the disease is restaged, to include marrow examination with cytogenetics and MRI and/or PET-CT of indicator lesions in order to assess whether intramedullary or EMD has been reduced. Disease monitoring should be performed at least every month for the first year and at a minimum every other month thereafter. Marrow biopsy, including cytogenetic examinations, should be performed at the time of progression or change in therapy. Imaging should be performed annually or in the presence of new symptoms.

PROGNOSIS

The prognosis of myeloma is determined by three factors: (1) the host, (2) tumor biology and disease burden, and (3) the type of therapy applied. Host parameters, such as comorbidities, advanced age, frailty, and poor performance status, negatively impact overall outcome and increase treatment-related morbidity and mortality. With the advent of new drugs, used in combination or incorporated into high-dose melphalan-based auto-HSCT approaches, some poor prognostic factors can be overcome (see "Management of Newly Diagnosed Myeloma" above).

Advances in cytogenetics, gene-expression profiling, and imaging (MRI and PET-CT) have greatly increased our understanding of tumor biology and burden. Furthermore, such variables are more powerful prognostic indicators than standard prognostic variables.

Numerous individual parameters have been examined for their value as prognostic features. Higher labeling indices, serum IL-6 receptor levels, increased *RAS* mutations, more aggressive disease, and shortened survival has been reported in patients with plasmablastic morphology.[292] Serum β_2M represents the light chain of the MHC complex of the cell membrane. Increased serum β_2M results from secretion by tumors with a high growth fraction and rapid cell turnover rates. In patients with myeloma and normal renal function, rising serum β_2M predicts for progression.[301] The labeling index (LI), a measure of DNA synthesis by myeloma cells, predicts for survival. It is usually low (<1 percent) at diagnosis, higher at relapse, and lower in MG and indolent myeloma.[576]

Serum IL-6 levels appear to correlate both with stage of disease and survival.[577,578] IL-6 stimulates hepatocytes to produce acute phase proteins, such as C-reactive protein (CRP); CRP, therefore, may reflect the IL-6 level and proliferative status of marrow plasma cells. Indeed, CRP levels are significantly lower in patients with MG than in those with MM, and survival can be correlated with serum CRP level.[579] High serum levels of soluble IL-6 receptor (sIL-6R), hepatocyte growth factor,[580] and syndecan-1,[581] as well as low serum levels of hyaluronate,[582] are independent prognostic factors predicting poor outcome.

The percentage of circulating plasma cells in the blood and their labeling indices are independent prognostic factors for survival in myeloma after both conventional and high-dose therapy.[294,583] Circulating endothelial cells also correlate with disease course and response to

thalidomide.[584] Finally, circulating proteasome levels are an independent prognostic factor for survival.[585]

Many of these factors are interrelated and, therefore, of limited independent value. Using multivariate analysis, several groups have found that the best combination of variables to predict outcome was serum β_2M, reflecting both the tumor burden and the renal function; and the proliferative activity of plasma cells, evaluated by the LI or number of tumor cells in S-phase. Age and performance status also improves the prognostic assessment.[586,587]

Cytogenetic findings associated with poor outcome include hypodiploidy and deletion 17p13, the locus of the tumor-suppressor gene *TP53*.[308,309,372,588] Gains of chromosome 1q arm and loss of 1p occur in tandem duplications and jumping translocations of chromosome 1, and signify more aggressive and more advanced myeloma.[59,589-591] Combining hypodiploidy and high β_2M has also been used to identify patient populations with a poor outcome.[588,592] In contrast, hyperdiploidy, which accounts for almost half of the patients with abnormal cytogenetics and involves nonrandom gains of chromosomes 3, 5, 7, 9, 11, 15, 19, and 21, is associated with chemosensitive disease and better OS. Translocation t(11;14) also confers a better outcome.[101] Chromosome 13 deletions are present in more than 50 percent of patients with myeloma and are associated with poor prognosis; however, these deletions are also associated with MG,[83,89,307] and their role in transformation to myeloma is undefined at present. Chromosome 13 deletion is not prognostic for response to bortezomib, highlighting the importance of prognostic factors for particular therapies.[593]

Interphase FISH does not depend on cycling cells and increases the detection of abnormal cells to 80 to 90 percent.[594] Interphase FISH can also detect cytogenetically silent translocations, for example, t(4;14), t(14;16), and t(14;20), and can be performed on stored material. The above data suggest that analysis of metaphase cytogenetic abnormalities and FISH can identify patients who do not do well with auto-HSCT or standard therapies. Individual prognostication remains highly variable despite the application of these more sophisticated cytogenetic techniques. The Total Therapy 2 patient data set revealed that standard prognostic variables and metaphase cytogenetic had limited ability to account for outcome variability with hazard ratios not exceeding 2.0.[64,595,596]

Gene-expression profiling on newly diagnosed patients has allowed for the interpretation of outcome in the context of whole human genomic data. Gene-expression profiling not only has the ability to define disease pathogenesis, but also to identify both novel prognostic factors and potential therapeutic targets.[597,598] Using tumor cells from 532 newly diagnosed patients, Shaughnessy and colleagues defined a 70-gene model and a 17-gene subset that have the ability to identify high-risk disease.[599] In a study by the IFM, gene-expression profiles were generated for 250 newly diagnosed patients. The 15 most stable genes were used to construct a survival model. The 15-gene model demonstrated an improved ability to predict survival in newly diagnosed patients with myeloma treated with high-dose therapy. Specifically, this work demonstrated that high-risk patients have a 6.8-fold hazard ratio (95 percent confidence interval, 3.92 to 11.73; P <0.001) of death compared with low-risk patients. IFM 15-gene and University of Arkansas for Medical Sciences (UAMS) 17-gene models, when applied to their respective data sets, are powerful prognostic tools that can enhance the ISS for the identification of high-risk disease. The HOVON group developed a 92 gene signature which predicts for differential outcome.[600] These gene signatures are, however, not yet generalizable, as they have not been studied prospectively. Moreover, an analysis of signatures defined in Arkansas, IFM, Millennium, and HOVON studies shows that these signatures are not broadly useful in myeloma.[129]

These gene-expression profiling studies also identify mechanisms of sensitivity versus resistance to conventional and novel myeloma therapies.[601,602] For example, gene-expression profiling of patient tumor samples showed genes upregulated in patients responding to bortezomib compared to patients who did not respond. Hsp27 upregulation correlated with intrinsic or acquired bortezomib resistance (Chap. 109). Preclinical studies showed that p38[MAPK] inhibition downregulated Hsp27 expression and restored Velcade sensitivity in resistant myeloma cell lines and patient samples,[603] providing the basis for a trial combining these two agents.

Gene-expression profiling data should have an important impact on the interpretation of future clinical trials. Validated prognostic models from gene microarray data are now used for improved prognostication and will ultimately be used to assist in selecting therapy for individual patients.

Myeloma is a very complex disease at the genomic level. Parallel sequencing of paired and normal samples from 203 myeloma patients were performed and mutations were most frequently observed in *KRAS, NRAS, BRAF, FAM46C, TP53,* and *DIS3.*[112] The tumors demonstrated significant heterogeneity. Mutations were often present in subclonal populations and multiple mutations within the same pathway were observed within the same patient. Results of whole-exome sequencing, copy-number profiling, and cytogenetics of myeloma samples, including serial samples in 15 patients, demonstrated complex clonal evolution over time.[108] Moreover, clonal and subclonal heterogeneity within the same patient without the predominant clone did not necessarily translate into mRNA. These and other studies demonstrate the complexity of the myeloma genome underscoring a need for rapid identification of possible druggable oncogenic mutations to customize therapy for myeloma patients. Genomic analysis technology that can facilitate this understanding may prove valuable in the further development of effective targeted therapies. Future strategies of treatment may include the combination of targeted therapies with existing proteosome inhibitors and IMiDs. In addition, identification of mutations may provide important prognostic information. For example, *SP140* mutations were associated with increased risk of relapse suggesting that this gene may have prognostic features in myeloma.

● SPECIAL DISEASE MANIFESTATIONS

IGM MYELOMA

A rare diagnostic dilemma concerns the existence of an IgM myeloma entity that is distinct from Waldenström macroglobulinemia (histopathologic diagnosis, immunocytoma).[604,605] Upon examination, plasma cells, rather than the lymphoplasmacytic infiltrate, are seen to dominate the marrow of myeloma, whereas mastocytosis is a hallmark of immunocytoma. DNA aneuploidy and the presence of lytic bone lesions support a diagnosis of myeloma. Myeloma, also of the IgM isotype, is resistant to purine analogues, which are effective in Waldenström macroglobulinemia.[606,607]

SOLITARY PLASMACYTOMA

Plasmacytomas are collections of monoclonal plasma cells originating either in bone (solitary osseous plasmacytoma [SOP]) or in soft tissue (extramedullary plasmacytoma [EMP]). They comprise less than 10 percent of plasma cell dyscrasias. Indications of systemic disease such as marrow plasmacytosis, anemia, renal insufficiency, or multiple lytic or soft-tissue lesions must be excluded before the diagnosis of either SOP or EMP can be made. MRI can be useful to show additional marrow abnormalities consistent with myeloma.[608] The median age of diagnosis of either SOP or EMP is approximately 50 years, nearly 10 years younger than that for myeloma.[609–611] Although patients with SOP and EMP can both progress to myeloma, persons with SOP progress in the

majority of cases, in contrast to EMP, where only 50 percent eventually develop myeloma. The median survival of 86.4 months and 100.8 months for patients with SOP and EMP, respectively, is similar; however, PFS is markedly different, 16 percent for SOP patients versus 71 percent for EMP patients. The persistence of stable monoclonal Ig in the serum and/or urine after primary treatment of plasmacytoma does not necessitate additional therapy, as it does not influence survival or disease-free survival.[609] In contrast, rising monoclonal Ig levels in a patient with a history of either SOP or EMP should trigger a workup for either recurrent plasmacytoma or myeloma. It has been suggested, as is true for myeloma, that serum β_2M has prognostic value in patients with SOP. For example, 17 of 19 patients with elevated serum β_2M had transformation to myeloma and shorter survival (31 months) as compared with those with normal serum β_2M levels.[612]

Local therapy, primarily radiotherapy, with surgery as needed for structural anatomic support is the standard treatment for SOP and EMP.[609–611] Patients with soft-tissue solitary plasmacytomas can often be cured with appropriate local radiation (dose of at least 4.5 Gy). By contrast, this local treatment approach fails in the majority of patients with solitary plasmacytomas of bone.[613] The development of myeloma in such patients probably reflects multifocal systemic disease present at the outset and hitherto not detectable by standard radiographic imaging but readily by applying MRI[614] and PET-CT.[615]

The benefit of chemotherapy, either alone or in combination with radiotherapy and surgery, as primary therapy for SOP or EMP has not been proven. Moreover, the benefit of adjuvant chemotherapy, given to prevent recurrent disease and/or progression to myeloma, is also undefined. Disappearance of protein after involved-field radiotherapy predicts for long-term disease-free survival and possible cure.[613]

AMYLOID LIGHT-CHAIN AMYLOIDOSIS

When clinical features of congestive heart failure, nephrotic syndrome, malabsorption, coagulopathy, skin rash (oral mucosal rash, "raccoon's eyes") or neuropathy are present, a careful search for primary amyloidosis should be carried out (Chap. 108). LCDD may also have a similar clinical presentation. The primary difference between AL amyloidosis and LCDD is the difference in structure of the deposited protein; in AL amyloidosis it is fibrillar versus granular in LCDD. LCDD is usually associated with the κ light-chain subtype, whereas AL amyloidosis is associated with the λ light-chain subtype of myeloma.

Primary AL amyloidosis and immunoglobulin deposition diseases are best characterized functionally as MG with clinical manifestations because of normal tissue infiltration by these processes, although they can also accompany overt myeloma. Further workup following suspicion on clinical presentation depends on the organ of concern. Cardiac amyloidosis may be associated with low voltage on an electrocardiogram, arrhythmias, increased interventricular septal thickness greater than 12 mm, diastolic dysfunction or speckling on echocardiogram, and elevation of markers, such as B-type natriuretic peptide, N-terminal pro–B-type natriuretic protein, and cardiac troponin T.[616,617] Involvement of the gastrointestinal tract may present with decreased albumin and prealbumin. Renal involvement may present as nonspecific proteinuria with high total protein on 24-hour collection and low monoclonal immunoglobulin. Carpal tunnel syndrome and peripheral neuropathy may be a manifestation of amyloid, and nerve conduction studies may help in this diagnosis. Orthostatic hypotension also should alert to the possibility of systemic amyloidosis as a result of amyloid deposition in *vasa nervorum* of the autonomic nervous system or in adrenal glands resulting in hypoadrenalism. Occasionally, primary amyloidosis presents as tumors either mostly consisting of amyloid or mixed with plasmacytoma. Typically, MRI signals can distinguish plasmacytomas, which show hypointensity on T1-weighted images and hyperintensity on short tau inversion recovery (STIR)–weighted images, whereas amyloidoma-type lesions remain hypointense.

Appropriate biopsy techniques should be applied to clarify the presence and extent of accompanying amyloidosis or, similarly, LCDD in these patients. The diagnosis of AL amyloid (Chap. 108) often can be made by fine-needle aspiration of subcutaneous fat or by biopsy of the rectal mucosa,[618] although biopsy of accessible clinically involved tissue is preferable. AL amyloid also may be detectable on marrow biopsy.[252] Staining the tissue with Congo red may reveal perivascular amyloid with its classical apple-green birefringence when viewed under polarized light.[619] Thioflavin T is also a useful stain, producing intense yellow green fluorescence in AL amyloidosis. LCDD require immunofluorescence analysis of unfixed tissue; formalin fixation should be avoided whenever it is suspected.

Even though the tumor load is very low, patients with AL amyloidosis and immunoglobulin deposition disease suffer from the consequences of myeloma secretory products, even at relatively modest amounts, resulting in damage to kidneys, heart, gastrointestinal tract, liver, spleen, and peripheral and autonomic nerves. All current treatment targets the monoclonal plasma cell population and advances have paralleled the advances in treatment of myeloma. Whereas standard melphalan-prednisone has been only marginally effective, high-dose dexamethasone pulsing plus interferon, effecting more rapid and profound responses in myeloma, has also shown encouraging results in AL amyloidosis.[620] Similarly, positive results have been obtained with dexamethasone plus melphalan.[621] The Boston University group has pioneered the use of high-dose melphalan with auto-HSCT (see Fig. 107–16),[622] which is an effective regimen in carefully selected patients. In a study of 312 patients, high-dose melphalan (100 to 200 mg/m²) with auto-HSCT resulted in a median survival of 4.6 years with a treatment-related mortality of 13 percent.[623] There was also significant improvement in organ function. The role of allogeneic transplantation in AL amyloidosis is unclear.

Incorporation of the newer agents, such as the IMiDs and proteasome inhibitors, has shown promising results in the treatment of patients with AL amyloidosis in combination with other agents such as melphalan, dexamethasone, and cyclophosphamide. In phase II trials of lenalidomide in combination with dexamethasone 29 percent achieved a CR and 38 percent achieved a PR with an OR RF of 67 percent. Lenalidomide was given at a dose reduction of 15 mg/day because of poor tolerability at standard dose of 25 mg/day.[624] The safety and efficacy of the combination of pomalidomide and dexamethasone was also evaluated in a phase II clinical trial. Of 33 patients, the ORR was 48 percent. The time to response was 1.9 months and the median overall and PFS rates were 28 and 14 months, respectively. The most common side effects were fatigue and neutropenia.[625]

Bortezomib has also demonstrated efficacy and tolerability in the treatment of AL amyloidosis. In a phase II trial of 40 patients not achieving a CR after autologous SCT, 21 patients were treated with bortezomib and dexamethasone. Of the 12 evaluable patients at 1-year post–autologous SCT, ORR was 92 percent—67 percent achieved a CR and 50 percent had organ responses.[626] When used in combination with cyclophosphamide (CyBorD), high response rates are reported. Venner and colleagues evaluated the combination in 43 treatment-naïve patients. The overall hematologic response rate was 81.4 percent with CRs in 39.5 percent; 30 percent of patients reported peripheral neuropathy. This is likely attributable to the fact that dosing on this regimen was biweekly and the route of bortezomib administration was intravenous.[627]

Cardiac amyloid remains the most challenging clinical condition and is currently addressed with repeated cycles of dose-reduced melphalan (70 to 100 mg/m²) and stem cell support to avoid cardiac

catastrophes possibly linked to arrhythmias, caused by fluid overload or cytokines.[628] There is a prevailing misconception that high-dose dexamethasone pulsing, alone or with added thalidomide, even at low doses, is safer and better tolerated than appropriately dosed melphalan with stem cell support. Owing to its hematopoietic stem cell–compromising properties, melphalan, even at 50 to 70 mg/m², is still best administered in the context of autologous stem cell support.

SMOLDERING MYELOMA

Patients with smoldering myeloma have historically been followed without therapy.[629–631] At this time, there is no role for treating smoldering myeloma patients. Patients should be followed at close intervals of every 3 to 6 months and clinical trials should be offered where available.

At a median followup of 40 months in a small, randomized, prospective study of 125 patients with high-risk smoldering myeloma, treated with either lenalidomide and dexamethasone or observation,[632] TTP was not reached by the intervention arm compared to 21 months in the observation arm (p <0.001), and the 3-year OS was 94 percent versus 30 percent (p = 0.03). Despite these favorable finding, the high-risk criteria employed by this study are not those commonly used in practice. High-risk in this study was defined as having at least 10 percent marrow infiltration with plasma cells, a M-protein of 3 g/dL or greater, or a urinary Bence Jones protein level of more than 1 g/24 hours. Based on these criteria, some patients with active myeloma were classified as having high-risk smoldering myeloma, which may have contributed to the differences in the outcomes between the two arms of the trial. The IMWG has advised that those smoldering myeloma patients who have greater than 60 percent marrow plasma cells,[633] κ:λ FLC ratios greater than 100,[634] and two lesions on MRI or PET-CT imaging may benefit from therapy.[635–637] Further investigation of treatment in high-risk myeloma is warranted before changing the treatment paradigm in this population.

REFERENCES

1. Palumbo A, Anderson K: Multiple myeloma. *N Engl J Med* 364:1046–1060, 2011.
2. Borrow P, Lewicki H, Hahn BH, et al: Virus-specific CD8+ cytotoxic T-lymphocyte activity associated with control of viremia in primary human immunodeficiency virus type 1 infection. *J Virol* 68:6103–6110, 1994.
3. Cohen HJ, Crawford J, Rao MK, et al: Racial differences in the prevalence of monoclonal gammopathy in a community-based sample of the elderly. *Am J Med* 104:439–444, 1998.
4. Iwanaga M, Tagawa M, Tsukasaki K, et al: Prevalence of monoclonal gammopathy of undetermined significance: Study of 52,802 persons in Nagasaki City, Japan. *Mayo Clin Proc* 82:1474–1479, 2007.
5. Landgren O, Gridley G, Turesson I, et al: Risk of monoclonal gammopathy of undetermined significance (MGUS) and subsequent multiple myeloma among African American and white veterans in the United States. *Blood* 107:904–906, 2006.
6. Landgren O, Kyle RA, Pfeiffer RM, et al: Monoclonal gammopathy of undetermined significance (MGUS) consistently precedes multiple myeloma: A prospective study. *Blood* 113:5412–5417, 2009.
7. Weiss BM, Abadie J, Verma P, et al: A monoclonal gammopathy precedes multiple myeloma in most patients. *Blood* 113:5418–5422, 2009.
8. Durie BG, Harousseau JL, Miguel JS, et al: International uniform response criteria for multiple myeloma. *Leukemia* 20:1467–1473, 2006.
9. Kyle RA, Therneau TM, Rajkumar SV, et al: A long-term study of prognosis in monoclonal gammopathy of undetermined significance. *N Engl J Med* 346:564–569, 2002.
10. Vachon CM, Kyle RA, Therneau TM, et al: Increased risk of monoclonal gammopathy in first-degree relatives of patients with multiple myeloma or monoclonal gammopathy of undetermined significance. *Blood* 114:785–790, 2009.
11. Bourguet CC, Grufferman S, Delzell E, et al: Multiple myeloma and family history of cancer. A case-control study. *Cancer* 56:2133–2139, 1985.
12. Grosbois B, Jego P, Attal M, et al: Familial multiple myeloma: Report of fifteen families. *Br J Haematol* 105:768–770, 1999.
13. Lynch HT, Ferrara K, Barlogie B, et al: Familial myeloma. *N Engl J Med* 359:152–157, 2008.
14. Lynch HT, Sanger WG, Pirruccello S, et al: Familial multiple myeloma: A family study and review of the literature. *J Natl Cancer Inst* 93:1479–1483, 2001.

15. Chubb D, Weinhold N, Broderick P, et al: Common variation at 3q26.2, 6p21.33, 17p11.2 and 22q13.1 influences multiple myeloma risk. *Nat Genet* 45:1221–1225, 2013.

16. Morgan GJ, Johnson DC, Weinhold N, et al: Inherited genetic susceptibility to multiple myeloma. *Leukemia* 28:518–524, 2014.

17. Weinhold N, Johnson DC, Rawstron AC, et al: Inherited genetic susceptibility to monoclonal gammopathy of unknown significance. *Blood* 123:2513–2517; quiz 2593, 2014.

18. Grass S, Preuss KD, Ahlgrimm M, et al: Association of a dominantly inherited hyperphosphorylated paraprotein target with sporadic and familial multiple myeloma and monoclonal gammopathy of undetermined significance: A case-control study. *Lancet Oncol* 10:950–956, 2009.

19. Zwick C, Held G, Auth M, et al: Over one-third of African-American MGUS and multiple myeloma patients are carriers of hyperphosphorylated paratarg-7, an autosomal dominantly inherited risk factor for MGUS/MM. *Int J Cancer* 135:934–938, 2014.

20. Soderberg KC, Kaprio J, Verkasalo PK, et al: Overweight, obesity and risk of haematological malignancies: A cohort study of Swedish and Finnish twins. *Eur J Cancer* 45:1232–1238, 2009.

21. Wallin A, Larsson SC: Body mass index and risk of multiple myeloma: A meta-analysis of prospective studies. *Eur J Cancer* 47:1606–1615, 2011.

22. Calle EE, Rodriguez C, Walker-Thurmond K, et al: Overweight, obesity, and mortality from cancer in a prospectively studied cohort of U.S. adults. *N Engl J Med* 348:1625–1638, 2003.

23. Friedman GD, Herrinton LJ: Obesity and multiple myeloma. *Cancer Causes Control* 5:479–483, 1994.

24. Carson KR, Bates ML, Tomasson MH: The skinny on obesity and plasma cell myeloma: A review of the literature. *Bone Marrow Transplant* 49:1009–1015, 2014.

25. Alexander DD, Mink PJ, Adami HO, et al: Multiple myeloma: A review of the epidemiologic literature. *Int J Cancer* 120 Suppl 12:40–61, 2007.

26. Riedel DA, Pottern LM: The epidemiology of multiple myeloma. *Hematol Oncol Clin North Am* 6:225–247, 1992.

27. van Kaick G, Dalheimer A, Hornik S, et al: The German thorotrast study: Recent results and assessment of risks. *Radiat Res* 152:S64–S71, 1999.

28. Ichimaru M, Ishimaru T, Mikami M, et al: Multiple myeloma among atomic bomb survivors in Hiroshima and Nagasaki, 1950–1976: Relationship to radiation dose absorbed by marrow. *J Natl Cancer Inst* 69:323–328, 1982.

29. Neriishi K, Nakashima E, Suzuki G: Monoclonal gammopathy of undetermined significance in atomic bomb survivors: Incidence and transformation to multiple myeloma. *Br J Haematol* 121:405–410, 2003.

30. Eriksson M, Karlsson M: Occupational and other environmental factors and multiple myeloma: A population based case-control study. *Br J Ind Med* 49:95–103, 1992.

31. Kristensen P, Andersen A, Irgens LM, et al: Incidence and risk factors of cancer among men and women in Norwegian agriculture. *Scand J Work Environ Health* 22:14–26, 1996.

32. Isomaki HA, Hakulinen T, Joutsenlahti U: Excess risk of lymphomas, leukemia and myeloma in patients with rheumatoid arthritis. *J Chronic Dis* 31:691–696, 1978.

33. Raposo A, Peixoto D, Bogas M: Monoclonal gammopathy and rheumatic diseases. *Acta Reumatol Port* 39:12–18, 2014.

34. McShane CM, Murray LJ, Landgren O, et al: Prior autoimmune disease and risk of monoclonal gammopathy of undetermined significance and multiple myeloma: A systematic review. *Cancer Epidemiol Biomarkers Prev* 23:332–342, 2014.

35. Duberg AS, Nordstrom M, Torner A, et al: Non-Hodgkin's lymphoma and other nonhepatic malignancies in Swedish patients with hepatitis C virus infection. *Hepatology* 41:652–659, 2005.

36. Goedert JJ, Cote TR, Virgo P, et al: Spectrum of AIDS-associated malignant disorders. *Lancet* 351:1833–1839, 1998.

37. Brown LM, Gridley G, Check D, et al: Risk of multiple myeloma and monoclonal gammopathy of undetermined significance among white and black male United States veterans with prior autoimmune, infectious, inflammatory, and allergic disorders. *Blood* 111:3388–3394, 2008.

38. Gramenzi A, Buttino I, D'Avanzo B, et al: Medical history and the risk of multiple myeloma. *Br J Cancer* 63:769–772, 1991.

39. Soulier J, Grollet L, Oksenhendler E, et al: Kaposi's sarcoma-associated herpesvirus-like DNA sequences in multicentric Castleman's disease. *Blood* 86:1276–1280, 1995.

40. Chauhan D, Bharti A, Raje N, et al: Detection of Kaposi's sarcoma herpesvirus DNA sequences in multiple myeloma bone marrow stromal cells. *Blood* 93:1482–1486, 1999.

41. Rettig MB, Ma HJ, Vescio RA, et al: Kaposi's sarcoma-associated herpesvirus infection of bone marrow dendritic cells from multiple myeloma patients. *Science* 276:1851–1854, 1997.

42. Kuehl WM, Bergsagel PL: Multiple myeloma: Evolving genetic events and host interactions. *Nat Rev Cancer* 2:175–187, 2002.

43. Kuehl WM, Bergsagel PL: Molecular pathogenesis of multiple myeloma and its premalignant precursor. *J Clin Invest* 122:3456–3463, 2012.

44. Hajek R, Okubote SA, Svachova H: Myeloma stem cell concepts, heterogeneity and plasticity of multiple myeloma. *Br J Haematol* 163:551–564, 2013.

45. Bast EJ, van Camp B, Reynaert P, et al: Idiotypic peripheral blood lymphocytes in monoclonal gammopathy. *Clin Exp Immunol* 47:677–682, 1982.

46. Berenson J, Wong R, Kim K, et al: Evidence for peripheral blood B lymphocyte but not T lymphocyte involvement in multiple myeloma. *Blood* 70:1550–1553, 1987.

47. Mellstedt H, Holm G, Pettersson D, et al: Idiotype-bearing lymphoid cells in plasma cell neoplasia. *Clin Haematol* 11:65–86, 1982.

48. Pilarski LM, Jensen GS: Monoclonal circulating B cells in multiple myeloma. A continuously differentiating, possibly invasive, population as defined by expression of CD45 isoforms and adhesion molecules. *Hematol Oncol Clin North Am* 6:297–322, 1992.

49. Pilarski LM, Mant MJ, Ruether BA: Pre-B cells in peripheral blood of multiple myeloma patients. *Blood* 66:416–422, 1985.

50. Ruiz-Arguelles GJ, Katzmann JA, Greipp PR, et al: Multiple myeloma: Circulating lymphocytes that express plasma cell antigens. *Blood* 64:352–356, 1984.

51. Chen BJ, Epstein J: Circulating clonal lymphocytes in myeloma constitute a minor subpopulation of B cells. *Blood* 87:1972–1976, 1996.

52. Paiva B, Perez-Andres M, Vidriales MB, et al: Competition between clonal plasma cells and normal cells for potentially overlapping bone marrow niches is associated with a progressively altered cellular distribution in MGUS vs myeloma. *Leukemia* 25:697–706, 2011.

53. Ghobrial IM: Myeloma as a model for the process of metastasis: Implications for therapy. *Blood* 120:20–30, 2012.

54. Kumar S, Rajkumar SV, Kyle RA, et al: Prognostic value of circulating plasma cells in monoclonal gammopathy of undetermined significance. *J Clin Oncol* 23:5668–5674, 2005.

55. Bianchi G, Kyle RA, Larson DR, et al: High levels of peripheral blood circulating plasma cells as a specific risk factor for progression of smoldering multiple myeloma. *Leukemia* 27:680–685, 2013.

56. Nowakowski GS, Witzig TE, Dingli D, et al: Circulating plasma cells detected by flow cytometry as a predictor of survival in 302 patients with newly diagnosed multiple myeloma. *Blood* 106:2276–2279, 2005.

57. Peceliunas V, Janiulioniene A, Matuzeviciene R, et al: Circulating plasma cells predict the outcome of relapsed or refractory multiple myeloma. *Leuk Lymphoma* 53:641–647, 2012.

58. Paiva B, Paino T, Sayagues JM, et al: Detailed characterization of multiple myeloma circulating tumor cells shows unique phenotypic, cytogenetic, functional, and circadian distribution profile. *Blood* 122:3591–3598, 2013.

59. Cremer FW, Bila J, Buck I, et al: Delineation of distinct subgroups of multiple myeloma and a model for clonal evolution based on interphase cytogenetics. *Genes Chromosomes Cancer* 44:194–203, 2005.

60. Smadja NV, Fruchart C, Isnard F, et al: Chromosomal analysis in multiple myeloma: Cytogenetic evidence of two different diseases. *Leukemia* 12:960–969, 1998.

61. Zandecki M, Lai JL, Facon T: Multiple myeloma: Almost all patients are cytogenetically abnormal. *Br J Haematol* 94:217–227, 1996.

62. Carrasco DR, Tonon G, Huang Y, et al: High-resolution genomic profiles define distinct clinico-pathogenetic subgroups of multiple myeloma patients. *Cancer Cell* 9:313–325, 2006.

63. Walker BA, Leone PE, Chiecchio L, et al: A compendium of myeloma-associated chromosomal copy number abnormalities and their prognostic value. *Blood* 116:e56–e65, 2010.

64. Tabernero D, San Miguel JF, Garcia-Sanz M, et al: Incidence of chromosome numerical changes in multiple myeloma: Fluorescence in situ hybridization analysis using 15 chromosome-specific probes. *Am J Pathol* 149:153–161, 1996.

65. Fonseca R, Debes-Marun CS, Picken EB, et al: The recurrent IgH translocations are highly associated with nonhyperdiploid variant multiple myeloma. *Blood* 102:2562–2567, 2003.

66. Meeus P, Stul MS, Mecucci C, et al: Molecular breakpoints of t(11;14)(q13;q32) in multiple myeloma. *Cancer Genet Cytogenet* 83:25–27, 1995.

67. Raynaud SD, Bekri S, Leroux D, et al: Expanded range of 11q13 breakpoints with differing patterns of cyclin D1 expression in B-cell malignancies. *Genes Chromosomes Cancer* 8:80–87, 1993.

68. Ronchetti D, Finelli P, Richelda R, et al: Molecular analysis of 11q13 breakpoints in multiple myeloma. *Blood* 93:1330–1337, 1999.

69. Hoyer JD, Hanson CA, Fonseca R, et al: The (11;14)(q13;q32) translocation in multiple myeloma. A morphologic and immunohistochemical study. *Am J Clin Pathol* 113:831–837, 2000.

70. Soverini S, Cavo M, Cellini C, et al: Cyclin D1 overexpression is a favorable prognostic variable for newly diagnosed multiple myeloma patients treated with high-dose chemotherapy and single or double autologous transplantation. *Blood* 102:1588–1594, 2003.

71. Shaughnessy J Jr, Gabrea A, Qi Y, et al: Cyclin D3 at 6p21 is dysregulated by recurrent chromosomal translocations to immunoglobulin loci in multiple myeloma. *Blood* 98:217–223, 2001.

72. Bergsagel PL, Kuehl WM, Zhan F, et al: Cyclin D dysregulation: An early and unifying pathogenic event in multiple myeloma. *Blood* 106:296–303, 2005.

73. Gertz MA, Lacy MQ, Dispenzieri A, et al: Clinical implications of t(11;14)(q13;q32), t(4;14)(p16.3;q32), and −17p13 in myeloma patients treated with high-dose therapy. *Blood* 106:2837–2840, 2005.

74. Keats JJ, Reiman T, Maxwell CA, et al: In multiple myeloma, t(4;14)(p16;q32) is an adverse prognostic factor irrespective of FGFR3 expression. *Blood* 101:1520–1529, 2003.

75. Martinez-Garcia E, Popovic R, Min DJ, et al: The MMSET histone methyl transferase switches global histone methylation and alters gene expression in t(4;14) multiple myeloma cells. *Blood* 117:211–220, 2011.

76. Richelda R, Ronchetti D, Baldini L, et al: A novel chromosomal translocation t(4; 14) (p16.3; q32) in multiple myeloma involves the fibroblast growth-factor receptor 3 gene. *Blood* 90:4062–4070, 1997.

77. Chesi M, Brents LA, Ely SA, et al: Activated fibroblast growth factor receptor 3 is an oncogene that contributes to tumor progression in multiple myeloma. *Blood* 97:729–736, 2001.

78. Intini D, Baldini L, Fabris S, et al: Analysis of FGFR3 gene mutations in multiple myeloma patients with t(4;14). *Br J Haematol* 114:362–364, 2001.

79. Ronchetti D, Greco A, Compasso S, et al: Deregulated FGFR3 mutants in multiple myeloma cell lines with t(4;14): Comparative analysis of Y373C, K650E and the novel G384D mutations. *Oncogene* 20:3553–3562, 2001.

80. Chesi M, Bergsagel PL, Shonukan OO, et al: Frequent dysregulation of the c-maf proto-oncogene at 16q23 by translocation to an Ig locus in multiple myeloma. *Blood* 91:4457–4463, 1998.

81. Hurt EM, Wiestner A, Rosenwald A, et al: Overexpression of c-maf is a frequent oncogenic event in multiple myeloma that promotes proliferation and pathological interactions with bone marrow stroma. *Cancer Cell* 5:191–199, 2004.

82. Neri P, Ren L, Azab AK, et al: Integrin beta7-mediated regulation of multiple myeloma cell adhesion, migration, and invasion. *Blood* 117:6202–6213, 2011.

83. Avet-Loiseau H, Facon T, Daviet A, et al: 14q32 translocations and monosomy 13 observed in monoclonal gammopathy of undetermined significance delineate a multistep process for the oncogenesis of multiple myeloma. Intergroupe Francophone du Myelome. *Cancer Res* 59:4546–4550, 1999.

84. Drach J, Schuster J, Nowotny H, et al: Multiple myeloma: High incidence of chromosomal aneuploidy as detected by interphase fluorescence in situ hybridization. *Cancer Res* 55:3854–3859, 1995.

85. Zandecki M, Obein V, Bernardi F, et al: Monoclonal gammopathy of undetermined significance: Chromosome changes are a common finding within bone marrow plasma cells. *Br J Haematol* 90:693–696, 1995.

86. Avet-Loiseau H, Li C, Magrangeas F, et al: Prognostic significance of copy-number alterations in multiple myeloma. *J Clin Oncol* 27:4585–4590, 2009.

87. Sawyer JR: The prognostic significance of cytogenetics and molecular profiling in multiple myeloma. *Cancer Genet* 204:3–12, 2011.

88. Avet-Louseau H, Daviet A, Sauner S, et al: Chromosome 13 abnormalities in multiple myeloma are mostly monosomy 13. *Br J Haematol* 111:1116–1117, 2000.

89. Fonseca R, Harrington D, Oken MM, et al: Biological and prognostic significance of interphase fluorescence in situ hybridization detection of chromosome 13 abnormalities (delta13) in multiple myeloma: An Eastern Cooperative Oncology Group study. *Cancer Res* 62:715–720, 2002.

90. Lode L, Eveillard M, Trichet V, et al: Mutations in TP53 are exclusively associated with del(17p) in multiple myeloma. *Haematologica* 95:1973–1976, 2010.

91. Neri A, Baldini L, Trecca D, et al: P53 gene mutations in multiple myeloma are associated with advanced forms of malignancy. *Blood* 81:128–135, 1993.

92. Neben K, Lokhorst HM, Jauch A, et al: Administration of bortezomib before and after autologous stem cell transplantation improves outcome in multiple myeloma patients with deletion 17p. *Blood* 119:940–948, 2012.

93. Shaughnessy J: Amplification and overexpression of CKS1B at chromosome band 1q21 is associated with reduced levels of p27Kip1 and an aggressive clinical course in multiple myeloma. *Hematology* 10 Suppl 1:117–126, 2005.

94. Hanamura I, Stewart JP, Huang Y, et al: Frequent gain of chromosome band 1q21 in plasma-cell dyscrasias detected by fluorescence in situ hybridization: Incidence increases from MGUS to relapsed myeloma and is related to prognosis and disease progression following tandem stem-cell transplantation. *Blood* 108:1724–1732, 2006.

95. Wu KL, Beverloo B, Lokhorst HM, et al: Abnormalities of chromosome 1p/q are highly associated with chromosome 13/13q deletions and are an adverse prognostic factor for the outcome of high-dose chemotherapy in patients with multiple myeloma. *Br J Haematol* 136:615–623, 2007.

96. Sawyer JR, Tian E, Heuck CJ, et al: Jumping translocations of 1q12 in multiple myeloma: A novel mechanism for deletion of 17p in cytogenetically defined high-risk disease. *Blood* 123:2504–2512, 2014.

97. Boyd KD, Ross FM, Walker BA, et al: Mapping of chromosome 1p deletions in myeloma identifies FAM46C at 1p12 and CDKN2C at 1p32.3 as being genes in regions associated with adverse survival. *Clin Cancer Res* 17:7776–7784, 2011.

98. Leone PE, Walker BA, Jenner MW, et al: Deletions of CDKN2C in multiple myeloma: Biological and clinical implications. *Clin Cancer Res* 14:6033–6041, 2008.

99. Qazilbash MH, Saliba RM, Ahmed B, et al: Deletion of the short arm of chromosome 1 (del 1p) is a strong predictor of poor outcome in myeloma patients undergoing an autotransplant. *Biol Blood Marrow Transplant* 13:1066–1072, 2007.

100. Chapman MA, Lawrence MS, Keats JJ, et al: Initial genome sequencing and analysis of multiple myeloma. *Nature* 471:467–472, 2011.

101. Avet-Loiseau H, Gerson F, Magrangeas F, et al: Rearrangements of the c-myc oncogene are present in 15% of primary human multiple myeloma tumors. *Blood* 98:3082–3086, 2001.

102. Dib A, Gabrea A, Glebov OK, et al: Characterization of MYC translocations in multiple myeloma cell lines. *J Natl Cancer Inst Monogr* 39:25–31, 2008.

103. Gabrea A, Martelli ML, Qi Y, et al: Secondary genomic rearrangements involving immunoglobulin or MYC loci show similar prevalences in hyperdiploid and nonhyperdiploid myeloma tumors. *Genes Chromosomes Cancer* 47:573–590, 2008.

104. Shou Y, Martelli ML, Gabrea A, et al: Diverse karyotypic abnormalities of the c-myc locus associated with c-myc dysregulation and tumor progression in multiple myeloma. *Proc Natl Acad Sci U S A* 97:228–233, 2000.

105. Annunziata CM, Davis RE, Demchenko Y, et al: Frequent engagement of the classical and alternative NF-kappaB pathways by diverse genetic abnormalities in multiple myeloma. *Cancer Cell* 12:115–130, 2007.

106. Cottini F, Hideshima T, Xu C, et al: Rescue of Hippo coactivator YAP1 triggers DNA damage-induced apoptosis in hematological cancers. *Nat Med* 20:599–606, 2014.

107. Keats JJ, Fonseca R, Chesi M, et al: Promiscuous mutations activate the noncanonical NF-kappaB pathway in multiple myeloma. *Cancer Cell* 12:131–144, 2007.

108. Bolli N, Avet-Loiseau H, Wedge DC, et al: Heterogeneity of genomic evolution and mutational profiles in multiple myeloma. *Nat Commun* 5:2997, 2014.

109. Egan JB, Kortuem KM, Kurdoglu A, et al: Extramedullary myeloma whole genome sequencing reveals novel mutations in Cereblon, proteasome subunit G2 and the glucocorticoid receptor in multidrug resistant disease. *Br J Haematol* 161:748–751, 2013.

110. Egan JB, Shi CX, Tembe W, et al: Whole-genome sequencing of multiple myeloma from diagnosis to plasma cell leukemia reveals genomic initiating events, evolution, and clonal tides. *Blood* 120:1060–1066, 2012.

111. Keats JJ, Chesi M, Egan JB, et al: Clonal competition with alternating dominance in multiple myeloma. *Blood* 120:1067–1076, 2012.

112. Lohr JG, Stojanov P, Carter SL, et al: Widespread genetic heterogeneity in multiple myeloma: Implications for targeted therapy. *Cancer Cell* 25:91–101, 2014.

113. Schmidt J, Braggio E, Kortuem KM, et al: Genome-wide studies in multiple myeloma identify XPO1/CRM1 as a critical target validated using the selective nuclear export inhibitor KPT-276. *Leukemia* 27:2357–2365, 2013.

114. Corradini P, Ladetto M, Voena C, et al: Mutational activation of N- and K-ras oncogenes in plasma cell dyscrasias. *Blood* 81:2708–2713, 1993.

115. Liu P, Leong T, Quam L, et al: Activating mutations of N- and K-ras in multiple myeloma show different clinical associations: Analysis of the Eastern Cooperative Oncology Group Phase III Trial. *Blood* 88:2699–2706, 1996.

116. Matozaki S, Nakagawa T, Nakao Y, et al: RAS gene mutations in multiple myeloma and related monoclonal gammopathies. *Kobe J Med Sci* 37:35–45, 1991.

117. Paquette RL, Berenson J, Lichtenstein A, et al: Oncogenes in multiple myeloma: Point mutation of N-ras. *Oncogene* 5:1659–1663, 1990.

118. Bezieau S, Devilder MC, Avet-Loiseau H, et al: High incidence of N and K-Ras activating mutations in multiple myeloma and primary plasma cell leukemia at diagnosis. *Hum Mutat* 18:212–224, 2001.

119. Chng WJ, Gonzalez-Paz N, Price-Troska T, et al: Clinical and biological significance of RAS mutations in multiple myeloma. *Leukemia* 22:2280–2284, 2008.

120. Rasmussen T, Kuehl M, Lodahl M, et al: Possible roles for activating RAS mutations in the MGUS to MM transition and in the intramedullary to extramedullary transition in some plasma cell tumors. *Blood* 105:317–323, 2005.

121. Preudhomme C, Facon T, Zandecki M, et al: Rare occurrence of P53 gene mutations in multiple myeloma. *Br J Haematol* 81:440–443, 1992.

122. Ackermann J, Meidlinger P, Zojer N, et al: Absence of p53 deletions in bone marrow plasma cells of patients with monoclonal gammopathy of undetermined significance. *Br J Haematol* 103:1161–1163, 1998.

123. Drach J, Ackermann J, Fritz E, et al: Presence of a p53 gene deletion in patients with multiple myeloma predicts for short survival after conventional-dose chemotherapy. *Blood* 92:802–809, 1998.

124. Chng WJ, Price-Troska T, Gonzalez-Paz N, et al: Clinical significance of TP53 mutation in myeloma. *Leukemia* 21:582–584, 2007.

125. Tiedemann RE, Gonzalez-Paz N, Kyle RA, et al: Genetic aberrations and survival in plasma cell leukemia. *Leukemia* 22:1044–1052, 2008.

126. Melchor L, Brioli A, Wardell CP, et al: Single-cell genetic analysis reveals the composition of initiating clones and phylogenetic patterns of branching and parallel evolution in myeloma. *Leukemia* 28:1705–1715, 2014.

127. Zhan F, Barlogie B, Mulligan G, et al: High-risk myeloma: A gene expression based risk-stratification model for newly diagnosed multiple myeloma treated with high-dose therapy is predictive of outcome in relapsed disease treated with single-agent bortezomib or high-dose dexamethasone. *Blood* 111:968–969, 2008.

128. Mulligan G, Mitsiades C, Bryant B, et al: Gene expression profiling and correlation with outcome in clinical trials of the proteasome inhibitor bortezomib. *Blood* 109:3177–3188, 2007.

129. Amin SB, Yip WK, Minvielle S, et al: Gene expression profile alone is inadequate in predicting complete response in multiple myeloma. *Leukemia* 28:2229–2234, 2014.

130. Caligaris-Cappio F, Bergui L, Gregoretti MG, et al: Role of bone marrow stromal cells in the growth of human multiple myeloma. *Blood* 77:2688–2693, 1991.

131. Grigorieva I, Thomas X, Epstein J: The bone marrow stromal environment is a major factor in myeloma cell resistance to dexamethasone. *Exp Hematol* 26:597–603, 1998.

132. Hallek M, Bergsagel PL, Anderson KC: Multiple myeloma: Increasing evidence for a multistep transformation process. *Blood* 91:3–21, 1998.

133. Hideshima T, Mitsiades C, Tonon G, et al: Understanding multiple myeloma pathogenesis in the bone marrow to identify new therapeutic targets. *Nat Rev Cancer* 7:585–598, 2007.

134. Damiano JS, Cress AE, Hazlehurst LA, et al: Cell adhesion mediated drug resistance (CAM-DR): Role of integrins and resistance to apoptosis in human myeloma cell lines. *Blood* 93:1658–1667, 1999.

135. Damiano JS, Dalton WS: Integrin-mediated drug resistance in multiple myeloma. *Leuk Lymphoma* 38:71–81, 2000.

136. Ridley RC, Xiao H, Hata H, et al: Expression of syndecan regulates human myeloma plasma cell adhesion to type I collagen. *Blood* 81:767–774, 1993.

137. Borset M, Hjertner O, Yaccoby S, et al: Syndecan-1 is targeted to the uropods of polarized myeloma cells where it promotes adhesion and sequesters heparin-binding proteins. *Blood* 96:2528–2536, 2000.

138. Dhodapkar MV, Abe E, Theus A, et al: Syndecan-1 is a multifunctional regulator of myeloma pathobiology: Control of tumor cell survival, growth, and bone cell differentiation. *Blood* 91:2679–2688, 1998.

139. Dhodapkar MV, Kelly T, Theus A, et al: Elevated levels of shed syndecan-1 correlate with tumour mass and decreased matrix metalloproteinase-9 activity in the serum of patients with multiple myeloma. *Br J Haematol* 99:368–371, 1997.

140. Alsayed Y, Ngo H, Runnels J, et al: Mechanisms of regulation of CXCR4/SDF-1 (CXCL12)-dependent migration and homing in multiple myeloma. *Blood* 109:2708–2717, 2007.

141. Hideshima T, Chauhan D, Hayashi T, et al: The biological sequelae of stromal cell-derived factor-1alpha in multiple myeloma. *Mol Cancer Ther* 1:539–544, 2002.

142. Trentin L, Miorin M, Facco M, et al: Multiple myeloma plasma cells show different chemokine receptor profiles at sites of disease activity. *Br J Haematol* 138:594–602, 2007.

143. Hata H, Xiao H, Petrucci MT, et al: Interleukin-6 gene expression in multiple myeloma: A characteristic of immature tumor cells. *Blood* 81:3357–3364, 1993.

144. Kawano M, Hirano T, Matsuda T, et al: Autocrine generation and requirement of BSF-2/IL-6 for human multiple myelomas. *Nature* 332:83–85, 1988.

145. Klein B, Zhang XG, Jourdan M, et al: Paracrine rather than autocrine regulation of myeloma-cell growth and differentiation by interleukin-6. *Blood* 73:517–526, 1989.

146. Thomas X, Xiao HQ, Chang R, et al: Circulating B lymphocytes in multiple myeloma patients contain an autocrine IL-6 driven pre-myeloma cell population. *Curr Top Microbiol Immunol* 182:201–207, 1992.

147. Freund GG, Kulas DT, Mooney RA: Insulin and IGF-1 increase mitogenesis and glucose metabolism in the multiple myeloma cell line, RPMI 8226. *J Immunol* 151:1811–1820, 1993.

148. Vanderkerken K, Asosingh K, Braet F, et al: Insulin-like growth factor-1 acts as a chemoattractant factor for 5T2 multiple myeloma cells. *Blood* 93:235–241, 1999.

149. Mitsiades CS, Mitsiades NS, McMullan CJ, et al: Inhibition of the insulin-like growth factor receptor-1 tyrosine kinase activity as a therapeutic strategy for multiple myeloma, other hematologic malignancies, and solid tumors. *Cancer Cell* 5:221–230, 2004.

150. Podar K, Tai YT, Davies FE, et al: Vascular endothelial growth factor triggers signaling cascades mediating multiple myeloma cell growth and migration. *Blood* 98:428–435, 2001.

151. Podar K, Tai YT, Lin BK, et al: Vascular endothelial growth factor-induced migration of multiple myeloma cells is associated with beta 1 integrin- and phosphatidylinositol 3-kinase-dependent PKC alpha activation. *J Biol Chem* 277:7875–7881, 2002.

152. Hideshima T, Chauhan D, Schlossman R, et al: The role of tumor necrosis factor alpha in the pathophysiology of human multiple myeloma: Therapeutic applications. *Oncogene* 20:4519–4527, 2001.

153. Otsuki T, Yamada O, Yata K, et al: Expression of fibroblast growth factor and FGF-receptor family genes in human myeloma cells, including lines possessing t(4;14) (q16.3;q32. 3) and FGFR3 translocation. *Int J Oncol* 15:1205–1212, 1999.

154. Moreaux J, Legouffe E, Jourdan E, et al: BAFF and APRIL protect myeloma cells from apoptosis induced by interleukin 6 deprivation and dexamethasone. *Blood* 103:3148–3157, 2004.

155. Chauhan D, Uchiyama H, Akbarali Y, et al: Multiple myeloma cell adhesion-induced interleukin-6 expression in bone marrow stromal cells involves activation of NF-kappa B. *Blood* 87:1104–1112, 1996.

156. Hideshima T, Nakamura N, Chauhan D, et al: Biologic sequelae of interleukin-6 induced PI3-K/Akt signaling in multiple myeloma. *Oncogene* 20:5991–6000, 2001.

157. Pene F, Claessens YE, Muller O, et al: Role of the phosphatidylinositol 3-kinase/Akt and mTOR/P70S6-kinase pathways in the proliferation and apoptosis in multiple myeloma. *Oncogene* 21:6587–6597, 2002.

158. Gupta D, Treon SP, Shima Y, et al: Adherence of multiple myeloma cells to bone marrow stromal cells upregulates vascular endothelial growth factor secretion: Therapeutic applications. *Leukemia* 15:1950–1961, 2001.

159. Vacca A, Ribatti D, Presta M, et al: Bone marrow neovascularization, plasma cell angiogenic potential, and matrix metalloproteinase-2 secretion parallel progression of human multiple myeloma. *Blood* 93:3064–3073, 1999.

160. Ria R, Todoerti K, Berardi S, et al: Gene expression profiling of bone marrow endothelial cells in patients with multiple myeloma. *Clin Cancer Res* 15:5369–5378, 2009.

161. Rajkumar SV, Mesa RA, Fonseca R, et al: Bone marrow angiogenesis in 400 patients with monoclonal gammopathy of undetermined significance, multiple myeloma, and primary amyloidosis. *Clin Cancer Res* 8:2210–2216, 2002.

162. Kumar S, Gertz MA, Dispenzieri A, et al: Prognostic value of bone marrow angiogenesis in patients with multiple myeloma undergoing high-dose therapy. *Bone Marrow Transplant* 34:235–239, 2004.

163. Biswas SK, Mantovani A: Macrophage plasticity and interaction with lymphocyte subsets: Cancer as a paradigm. *Nat Immunol* 11:889–896, 2010.

164. Gabrilovich DI, Nagaraj S: Myeloid-derived suppressor cells as regulators of the immune system. *Nat Rev Immunol* 9:162–174, 2009.

165. Gorgun GT, Whitehill G, Anderson JL, et al: Tumor-promoting immune-suppressive myeloid-derived suppressor cells in the multiple myeloma microenvironment in humans. *Blood* 121:2975–2987, 2013.

166. Melton LJ 3rd, Kyle RA, Achenbach SJ, et al: Fracture risk with multiple myeloma: A population-based study. *J Bone Miner Res* 20:487–493, 2005.

167. Bataille R, Chappard D, Marcelli C, et al: Recruitment of new osteoblasts and osteoclasts is the earliest critical event in the pathogenesis of human multiple myeloma. *J Clin Invest* 88:62–66, 1991.

168. Taube T, Beneton MN, McCloskey EV, et al: Abnormal bone remodelling in patients with myelomatosis and normal biochemical indices of bone resorption. *Eur J Haematol* 49:192–198, 1992.

169. Raje N, Roodman GD: Advances in the biology and treatment of bone disease in multiple myeloma. *Clin Cancer Res* 17:1278–1286, 2011.

170. Li J, Sarosi I, Yan XQ, et al: RANK is the intrinsic hematopoietic cell surface receptor that controls osteoclastogenesis and regulation of bone mass and calcium metabolism. *Proc Natl Acad Sci U S A* 97:1566–1571, 2000.

171. Farrugia AN, Atkins GJ, To LB, et al: Receptor activator of nuclear factor-kappaB ligand expression by human myeloma cells mediates osteoclast formation *in vitro* and correlates with bone destruction *in vivo*. *Cancer Res* 63:5438–5445, 2003.

172. Lai FP, Cole-Sinclair M, Cheng WJ, et al: Myeloma cells can directly contribute to the pool of RANKL in bone bypassing the classic stromal and osteoblast pathway of osteoclast stimulation. *Br J Haematol* 126:192–201, 2004.

173. Sezer O, Heider U, Jakob C, et al: Human bone marrow myeloma cells express RANKL. *J Clin Oncol* 20:353–354, 2002.

174. Giuliani N, Bataille R, Mancini C, et al: Myeloma cells induce imbalance in the osteoprotegerin/osteoprotegerin ligand system in the human bone marrow environment. *Blood* 98:3527–3533, 2001.

175. Pearse RN, Sordillo EM, Yaccoby S, et al: Multiple myeloma disrupts the TRANCE/osteoprotegerin cytokine axis to trigger bone destruction and promote tumor progression. *Proc Natl Acad Sci U S A* 98:11581–11586, 2001.

176. Shipman CM, Croucher PI: Osteoprotegerin is a soluble decoy receptor for tumor necrosis factor-related apoptosis-inducing ligand/Apo2 ligand and can function as a paracrine survival factor for human myeloma cells. *Cancer Res* 63:912–916, 2003.

177. Simonet WS, Lacey DL, Dunstan CR, et al: Osteoprotegerin: A novel secreted protein involved in the regulation of bone density. *Cell* 89:309–319, 1997.

178. Croucher PI, Shipman CM, Lippitt J, et al: Osteoprotegerin inhibits the development of osteolytic bone disease in multiple myeloma. *Blood* 98:3534–3540, 2001.

179. Mori Y, Shimizu N, Dallas M, et al: Anti-alpha4 integrin antibody suppresses the development of multiple myeloma and associated osteoclastic osteolysis. *Blood* 104:2149–2154, 2004.

180. Qiang YW, Chen Y, Stephens O, et al: Myeloma-derived Dickkopf-1 disrupts Wnt-regulated osteoprotegerin and RANKL production by osteoblasts: A potential mechanism underlying osteolytic bone lesions in multiple myeloma. *Blood* 112:196–207, 2008.

181. Standal T, Seidel C, Hjertner O, et al: Osteoprotegerin is bound, internalized, and degraded by multiple myeloma cells. *Blood* 100:3002–3007, 2002.

182. Seidel C, Hjertner O, Abildgaard N, et al: Serum osteoprotegerin levels are reduced in patients with multiple myeloma with lytic bone disease. *Blood* 98:2269–2271, 2001.

183. Terpos E, Szydlo R, Apperley JF, et al: Soluble receptor activator of nuclear factor kappaB ligand-osteoprotegerin ratio predicts survival in multiple myeloma: Proposal for a novel prognostic index. *Blood* 102:1064–1069, 2003.

184. Heath DJ, Vanderkerken K, Cheng X, et al: An osteoprotegerin-like peptidomimetic inhibits osteoclastic bone resorption and osteolytic bone disease in myeloma. *Cancer Res* 67:202–208, 2007.

185. Body JJ, Greipp P, Coleman RE, et al: A phase I study of AMGN-0007, a recombinant osteoprotegerin construct, in patients with multiple myeloma or breast carcinoma related bone metastases. *Cancer* 97:887–892, 2003.

186. Ferguson C, Body R: Towards evidence-based emergency medicine: Best BETs from the Manchester Royal Infirmary. Use of aspirin in acute stroke. *Emerg Med J* 23:804–805, 2006.

187. Henry DH, Costa L, Goldwasser F, et al: Randomized, double-blind study of denosumab versus zoledronic acid in the treatment of bone metastases in patients with advanced cancer (excluding breast and prostate cancer) or multiple myeloma. *J Clin Oncol* 29:1125–1132, 2011.

188. Vij R, Horvath N, Spencer A, et al: An open-label, phase 2 trial of denosumab in the treatment of relapsed or plateau-phase multiple myeloma. *Am J Hematol* 84:650–656, 2009.

189. Yee AJ, Raje NS: Denosumab, a RANK ligand inhibitor, for the management of bone loss in cancer patients. *Clin Interv Aging* 7:331–338, 2012.

190. Abe M, Hiura K, Wilde J, et al: Role for macrophage inflammatory protein (MIP)-1alpha and MIP-1beta in the development of osteolytic lesions in multiple myeloma. *Blood* 100:2195–2202, 2002.

191. Choi SJ, Cruz JC, Craig F, et al: Macrophage inflammatory protein 1-alpha is a potential osteoclast stimulatory factor in multiple myeloma. *Blood* 96:671–675, 2000.

192. Han JH, Choi SJ, Kurihara N, et al: Macrophage inflammatory protein-1alpha is an osteoclastogenic factor in myeloma that is independent of receptor activator of nuclear factor kappaB ligand. *Blood* 97:3349–3353, 2001.

193. Hashimoto T, Abe M, Oshima T, et al: Ability of myeloma cells to secrete macrophage inflammatory protein (MIP)-1alpha and MIP-1beta correlates with lytic bone lesions in patients with multiple myeloma. *Br J Haematol* 125:38–41, 2004.

194. Terpos E, Politou M, Szydlo R, et al: Serum levels of macrophage inflammatory protein-1 alpha (MIP-1alpha) correlate with the extent of bone disease and survival in patients with multiple myeloma. *Br J Haematol* 123:106–109, 2003.

195. Adebanjo OA, Moonga BS, Yamate T, et al: Mode of action of interleukin-6 on mature osteoclasts. Novel interactions with extracellular Ca2+ sensing in the regulation of osteoclastic bone resorption. *J Cell Biol* 142:1347–1356, 1998.

196. Cafforio P, Savonarola A, Stucci S, et al: PTHrP produced by myeloma plasma cells regulates their survival and pro-osteoclast activity for bone disease progression. *J Bone Miner Res* 29:55–66, 2014.

197. Otsuki T, Yamada O, Kurebayashi J, et al: Expression and in vitro modification of parathyroid hormone-related protein (PTHrP) and PTH/PTHrP-receptor in human myeloma cells. *Leuk Lymphoma* 41:397–409, 2001.

198. D'Souza S, Kurihara N, Shiozawa Y, et al: Annexin II interactions with the annexin II receptor enhance multiple myeloma cell adhesion and growth in the bone marrow microenvironment. *Blood* 119:1888–1896, 2012.

199. Pennisi A, Ling W, Li X, et al: The ephrinB2/EphB4 axis is dysregulated in osteoprogenitors from myeloma patients and its activation affects myeloma bone disease and tumor growth. *Blood* 114:1803–1812, 2009.

200. Oshima T, Abe M, Asano J, et al: Myeloma cells suppress bone formation by secreting a soluble Wnt inhibitor, sFRP-2. *Blood* 106:3160–3165, 2005.

201. Brunetti G, Oranger A, Mori G, et al: Sclerostin is overexpressed by plasma cells from multiple myeloma patients. *Ann N Y Acad Sci* 1237:19–23, 2011.

202. Colucci S, Brunetti G, Oranger A, et al: Myeloma cells suppress osteoblasts through sclerostin secretion. *Blood Cancer J* 1:e27, 2011.

203. Giuliani N, Morandi F, Tagliaferri S, et al: Production of Wnt inhibitors by myeloma cells: Potential effects on canonical Wnt pathway in the bone microenvironment. *Cancer Res* 67:7665–7674, 2007.

204. Giuliani N, Rizzoli V: Myeloma cells and bone marrow osteoblast interactions: Role in the development of osteolytic lesions in multiple myeloma. *Leuk Lymphoma* 48:2323–2329, 2007.

205. Tian E, Zhan F, Walker R, et al: The role of the Wnt-signaling antagonist DKK1 in the development of osteolytic lesions in multiple myeloma. *N Engl J Med* 349:2483–2494, 2003.

206. Politou MC, Heath DJ, Rahemtulla A, et al: Serum concentrations of Dickkopf-1 protein are increased in patients with multiple myeloma and reduced after autologous stem cell transplantation. *Int J Cancer* 119:1728–1731, 2006.

207. Fulciniti M, Tassone P, Hideshima T, et al: Anti-DKK1 mAb (BHQ880) as a potential therapeutic agent for multiple myeloma. *Blood* 114:371–379, 2009.

208. Heath DJ, Chantry AD, Buckle CH, et al: Inhibiting Dickkopf-1 (Dkk1) removes suppression of bone formation and prevents the development of osteolytic bone disease in multiple myeloma. *J Bone Miner Res* 24:425–436, 2009.

209. Yaccoby S, Ling W, Zhan F, et al: Antibody-based inhibition of DKK1 suppresses tumor-induced bone resorption and multiple myeloma growth *in vivo*. *Blood* 109:2106–2111, 2007.

210. Pozzi S, Fulciniti M, Yan H, et al: *In vivo* and *in vitro* effects of a novel anti-Dkk1 neutralizing antibody in multiple myeloma. *Bone* 53:487–496, 2013.

211. Ehrlich LA, Chung HY, Ghobrial I, et al: IL-3 is a potential inhibitor of osteoblast differentiation in multiple myeloma. *Blood* 106:1407–1414, 2005.

212. Giuliani N, Colla S, Morandi F, et al: Myeloma cells block RUNX2/CBFA1 activity in human bone marrow osteoblast progenitors and inhibit osteoblast formation and differentiation. *Blood* 106:2472–2483, 2005.

213. Vallet S, Mukherjee S, Vaghela N, et al: Activin A promotes multiple myeloma-induced osteolysis and is a promising target for myeloma bone disease. *Proc Natl Acad Sci U S A* 107:5124–5129, 2010.

214. Pozzi S, Vallet S, Mukherjee S, et al: High-dose zoledronic acid impacts bone remodeling with effects on osteoblastic lineage and bone mechanical properties. *Clin Cancer Res* 15:5829–5839, 2009.

215. Vanderkerken K, De Leenheer E, Shipman C, et al: Recombinant osteoprotegerin decreases tumor burden and increases survival in a murine model of multiple myeloma. *Cancer Res* 63:287–289, 2003.

216. Mahindra A, Pozzi S, Raje N: Clinical trials of bisphosphonates in multiple myeloma. *Clin Adv Hematol Oncol* 10:582–587, 2012.

217. Terpos E, Berenson J, Raje N: Management of bone disease in multiple myeloma. *Expert Rev Hematol* 7:113–125, 2014.

218. Mhaskar R, Redzepovic J, Wheatley K, et al: Bisphosphonates in multiple myeloma: A network meta-analysis. *Cochrane Database Syst Rev* 5:CD003188, 2012.

219. Terpos E, Dimopoulos MA, Sezer O, et al: The use of biochemical markers of bone remodeling in multiple myeloma: A report of the International Myeloma Working Group. *Leukemia* 24:1700–1712, 2010.

220. Ferrarini M, Steinberg N, Ponzoni M, et al: *Ex-vivo* dynamic 3-D culture of human tissues in the RCCS bioreactor allows the study of multiple myeloma biology and response to therapy. *PLoS One* 8:e71613, 2013.

221. Kirshner J, Thulien KJ, Martin LD, et al: A unique three-dimensional model for evaluating the impact of therapy on multiple myeloma. *Blood* 112:2935–2945, 2008.

222. Zdzisinska B, Rolinski J, Piersiak T, et al: A comparison of cytokine production in 2-dimensional and 3-dimensional cultures of bone marrow stromal cells of multiple myeloma patients in response to RPMI8226 myeloma cells. *Folia Histochem Cytobiol* 47:69–74, 2009.

223. Mitsiades CS, Anderson KC, Carrasco DR: Mouse models of human myeloma. *Hematol Oncol Clin North Am* 21:1051–1069, viii, 2007.

224. Yaccoby S, Barlogie B, Epstein J: Primary myeloma cells growing in SCID-hu mice: A model for studying the biology and treatment of myeloma and its manifestations. *Blood* 92:2908–2913, 1998.

225. Pennisi A, Li X, Ling W, et al: The proteasome inhibitor, bortezomib suppresses primary myeloma and stimulates bone formation in myelomatous and nonmyelomatous bones *in vivo*. *Am J Hematol* 84:6–14, 2009.

226. Calimeri T, Battista E, Conforti F, et al: A unique three-dimensional SCID-polymeric scaffold (SCID-synth-hu) model for *in vivo* expansion of human primary multiple myeloma cells. *Leukemia* 25:707–711, 2011.

227. Groen RW, Noort WA, Raymakers RA, et al: Reconstructing the human hematopoietic niche in immunodeficient mice: Opportunities for studying primary multiple myeloma. *Blood* 120:e9–e16, 2012.

228. Manning LS, Berger JD, O'Donoghue HL, et al: A model of multiple myeloma: Culture of 5T33 myeloma cells and evaluation of tumorigenicity in the C57BL/KaLwRij mouse. *Br J Cancer* 66:1088–1093, 1992.

229. Vanderkerken K, Asosingh K, Croucher P, et al: Multiple myeloma biology: Lessons from the 5TMM models. *Immunol Rev* 194:196–206, 2003.

230. Chesi M, Robbiani DF, Sebag M, et al: AID-dependent activation of a MYC transgene induces multiple myeloma in a conditional mouse model of post-germinal center malignancies. *Cancer Cell* 13:167–180, 2008.

231. Greipp PR, San Miguel J, Durie BG, et al: International staging system for multiple myeloma. *J Clin Oncol* 23:3412–3420, 2005.

232. Kyle RA, Rajkumar SV: Criteria for diagnosis, staging, risk stratification and response assessment of multiple myeloma. *Leukemia* 23:3–9, 2009.

233. Silvestris F, Cafforio P, Tucci M, et al: Negative regulation of erythroblast maturation by Fas-L(+)/TRAIL(+) highly malignant plasma cells: A major pathogenetic mechanism of anemia in multiple myeloma. *Blood* 99:1305–1313, 2002.

234. Faquin WC, Schneider TJ, Goldberg MA: Effect of inflammatory cytokines on hypoxia-induced erythropoietin production. *Blood* 79:1987–1994, 1992.

235. Ludwig H, Pecherstorfer M, Leitgeb C, et al: Recombinant human erythropoietin for the treatment of chronic anemia in multiple myeloma and squamous cell carcinoma. *Stem Cells* 11:348–355, 1993.

236. Singh A, Eckardt KU, Zimmermann A, et al: Increased plasma viscosity as a reason for inappropriate erythropoietin formation. *J Clin Invest* 91:251–256, 1993.

237. Ganz T, Olbina G, Girelli D, et al: Immunoassay for human serum hepcidin. *Blood* 112:4292–4297, 2008.

238. Sharma S, Nemeth E, Chen YH, et al: Involvement of hepcidin in the anemia of multiple myeloma. *Clin Cancer Res* 14:3262–3267, 2008.

239. Maes K, Nemeth E, Roodman GD, et al: In anemia of multiple myeloma, hepcidin is induced by increased bone morphogenetic protein 2. *Blood* 116:3635–3644, 2010.

240. Verga Falzacappa MV, Vujic Spasic M, Kessler R, et al: STAT3 mediates hepatic hepcidin expression and its inflammatory stimulation. *Blood* 109:353–358, 2007.

241. Wrighting DM, Andrews NC: Interleukin-6 induces hepcidin expression through STAT3. *Blood* 108:3204–3209, 2006.

242. Kerr R, Stirling D, Ludlam CA: Interleukin 6 and haemostasis. *Br J Haematol* 115:3–12, 2001.

243. Glueck HI, Hong R: A circulating anticoagulant in gamma-1A-multiple myeloma: Its modification by penicillin. *J Clin Invest* 44:1866–1881, 1965.

244. Kelsey PR, Leyland MJ: Acquired inhibitor to human factor VIII associated with paraproteinaemia and subsequent development of chronic lymphatic leukaemia. *Br Med J* 285:174–175, 1982.

245. Wenz B, Friedman G: Acquired factor VIII inhibitor in a patient with malignant lymphoma. *Am J Med Sci* 268:295–299, 1974.

246. Lonial S, Waller EK, Richardson PG, et al: Risk factors and kinetics of thrombocytopenia associated with bortezomib for relapsed, refractory multiple myeloma. *Blood* 106:3777–3784, 2005.

247. Kyle RA, Gertz MA, Witzig TE, et al: Review of 1027 patients with newly diagnosed multiple myeloma. *Mayo Clin Proc* 78:21–33, 2003.

248. Lackner H: Hemostatic abnormalities associated with dysproteinemias. *Semin Hematol* 10:125–133, 1973.

249. Perkins HA, MacKenzie MR, Fudenberg HH: Hemostatic defects in dysproteinemias. *Blood* 35:695–707, 1970.

250. Federici AB, Mannucci PM: Diagnosis and management of acquired von Willebrand syndrome. *Clin Adv Hematol Oncol* 1:169–175, 2003.

251. Shinagawa A, Kojima H, Berndt MC, et al: Characterization of a myeloma patient with a life-threatening hemorrhagic diathesis: Presence of a lambda dimer protein inhibiting shear-induced platelet aggregation by binding to the A1 domain of von Willebrand factor. *Thromb Haemost* 93:889–896, 2005.

252. van Genderen PJ, Vink T, Michiels JJ: Acquired von Willebrand disease caused by an autoantibody selectively inhibiting the binding of von Willebrand factor to collagen. *Blood* 84:3378–3384, 1994.

253. Glaspy JA: Hemostatic abnormalities in multiple myeloma and related disorders. *Hematol Oncol Clin North Am* 6:1301–1314, 1992.

254. Coleman M, Vigliano EM, Weksler ME, et al: Inhibition of fibrin monomer polymerization by lambda myeloma globulins. *Blood* 39:210–223, 1972.

255. Nijziel MR, van Oerle R, Christella M, et al: Acquired resistance to activated protein C in breast cancer patients. *Br J Haematol* 120:117–122, 2003.

256. Kyle RA, Gertz MA: Primary systemic amyloidosis: Clinical and laboratory features in 474 cases. *Semin Hematol* 32:45–59, 1995.

257. Mumford AD, O'Donnell J, Gillmore JD, et al: Bleeding symptoms and coagulation abnormalities in 337 patients with AL-amyloidosis. *Br J Haematol* 110:454–460, 2000.

258. Yood RA, Skinner M, Rubinow A, et al: Bleeding manifestations in 100 patients with amyloidosis. *JAMA* 249:1322–1324, 1983.

259. Choufani EB, Sanchorawala V, Ernst T, et al: Acquired factor X deficiency in patients with amyloid light-chain amyloidosis: Incidence, bleeding manifestations, and response to high-dose chemotherapy. *Blood* 97:1885–1887, 2001.

260. Furie B, Greene E, Furie BC: Syndrome of acquired factor X deficiency and systemic amyloidosis in vivo studies of the metabolic fate of factor X. *N Engl J Med* 297:81–85, 1977.

261. Baron JA, Gridley G, Weiderpass E, et al: Venous thromboembolism and cancer. *Lancet* 351:1077–1080, 1998.

262. Srkalovic G, Cameron MG, Rybicki L, et al: Monoclonal gammopathy of undetermined significance and multiple myeloma are associated with an increased incidence of venothromboembolic disease. *Cancer* 101:558–566, 2004.

263. Zangari M, Elice F, Fink L, et al: Hemostatic dysfunction in paraproteinemias and amyloidosis. *Semin Thromb Hemost* 33:339–349, 2007.

264. Deitcher SR, Erban JK, Limentani SA: Acquired free protein S deficiency associated with multiple myeloma: A case report. *Am J Hematol* 51:319–323, 1996.

265. Gruber A, Blasko G, Sas G: Functional deficiency of protein C and skin necrosis in multiple myeloma. *Thromb Res* 42:579–581, 1986.

266. Yasin Z, Quick D, Thiagarajan P, et al: Light-chain paraproteins with lupus anticoagulant activity. *Am J Hematol* 62:99–102, 1999.

267. Zangari M, Saghafifar F, Anaissie E, et al: Activated protein C resistance in the absence of factor V Leiden mutation is a common finding in multiple myeloma and is associated with an increased risk of thrombotic complications. *Blood Coagul Fibrinolysis* 13:187–192, 2002.

268. Barlogie B, Desikan R, Eddlemon P, et al: Extended survival in advanced and refractory multiple myeloma after single-agent thalidomide: Identification of prognostic factors in a phase 2 study of 169 patients. *Blood* 98:492–494, 2001.

269. Knight R, DeLap RJ, Zeldis JB: Lenalidomide and venous thrombosis in multiple myeloma. *N Engl J Med* 354:2079–2080, 2006.

270. Rajkumar SV, Blood E: Lenalidomide and venous thrombosis in multiple myeloma. *N Engl J Med* 354:2079–2080, 2006.

271. Rajkumar SV, Blood E, Vesole D, et al: Phase III clinical trial of thalidomide plus dexamethasone compared with dexamethasone alone in newly diagnosed multiple myeloma: A clinical trial coordinated by the Eastern Cooperative Oncology Group. *J Clin Oncol* 24:431–436, 2006.

272. Richardson PG, Blood E, Mitsiades CS, et al: A randomized phase 2 study of lenalidomide therapy for patients with relapsed or relapsed and refractory multiple myeloma. *Blood* 108:3458–3464, 2006.

273. Zangari M, Anaissie E, Barlogie B, et al: Increased risk of deep-vein thrombosis in patients with multiple myeloma receiving thalidomide and chemotherapy. *Blood* 98:1614–1615, 2001.

274. Zangari M, Siegel E, Barlogie B, et al: Thrombogenic activity of doxorubicin in myeloma patients receiving thalidomide: Implications for therapy. *Blood* 100:1168–1171, 2002.

275. Minnema MC, Breitkreutz I, Auwerda JJ, et al: Prevention of venous thromboembolism with low molecular-weight heparin in patients with multiple myeloma treated with thalidomide and chemotherapy. *Leukemia* 18:2044–2046, 2004.

276. Baz R, Li L, Kottke-Marchant K, et al: The role of aspirin in the prevention of thrombotic complications of thalidomide and anthracycline-based chemotherapy for multiple myeloma. *Mayo Clin Proc* 80:1568–1574, 2005.

277. Hirsh J: Risk of thrombosis with lenalidomide and its prevention with aspirin. *Chest* 131:275–277, 2007.

278. Larocca A, Cavallo F, Bringhen S, et al: Aspirin or enoxaparin thromboprophylaxis for patients with newly diagnosed multiple myeloma treated with lenalidomide. *Blood* 119:933–939; quiz 1093, 2012.

279. Palumbo A, Cavo M, Bringhen S, et al: Aspirin, warfarin, or enoxaparin thromboprophylaxis in patients with multiple myeloma treated with thalidomide: A phase III, open-label, randomized trial. *J Clin Oncol* 29:986–993, 2011.

280. Blade J, Lust JA, Kyle RA: Immunoglobulin D multiple myeloma: Presenting features, response to therapy, and survival in a series of 53 cases. *J Clin Oncol* 12:2398–2404, 1994.

281. Krejci M, Buchler T, Hajek R, et al: Prognostic factors for survival after autologous transplantation: A single centre experience in 133 multiple myeloma patients. *Bone Marrow Transplant* 35:159–164, 2005.

282. Nair B, Waheed S, Szymonifka J, et al: Immunoglobulin isotypes in multiple myeloma: Laboratory correlates and prognostic implications in total therapy protocols. *Br J Haematol* 145:134–137, 2009.

283. Drayson M, Tang LX, Drew R, et al: Serum free light-chain measurements for identifying and monitoring patients with nonsecretory multiple myeloma. *Blood* 97:2900–2902, 2001.

284. Katzmann JA, Clark RJ, Abraham RS, et al: Serum reference intervals and diagnostic ranges for free kappa and free lambda immunoglobulin light chains: Relative sensitivity for detection of monoclonal light chains. *Clin Chem* 48:1437–1444, 2002.

285. Dispenzieri A, Kyle R, Merlini G, et al: International Myeloma Working Group guidelines for serum-free light chain analysis in multiple myeloma and related disorders. *Leukemia* 23:215–224, 2009.

286. Dispenzieri A, Kyle RA, Katzmann JA, et al: Immunoglobulin free light chain ratio is an independent risk factor for progression of smoldering (asymptomatic) multiple myeloma. *Blood* 111:785–789, 2008.

287. Rajkumar SV, Kyle RA, Therneau TM, et al: Serum free light chain ratio is an independent risk factor for progression in monoclonal gammopathy of undetermined significance. *Blood* 106:812–817, 2005.

288. Kyrtsonis MC, Vassilakopoulos TP, Kafasi N, et al: Prognostic value of serum free light chain ratio at diagnosis in multiple myeloma. *Br J Haematol* 137:240–243, 2007.

289. Snozek CL, Katzmann JA, Kyle RA, et al: Prognostic value of the serum free light chain ratio in newly diagnosed myeloma: Proposed incorporation into the international staging system. *Leukemia* 22:1933–1937, 2008.

290. van Rhee F, Bolejack V, Hollmig K, et al: High serum-free light chain levels and their rapid reduction in response to therapy define an aggressive multiple myeloma subtype with poor prognosis. *Blood* 110:827–832, 2007.

291. Bartl R, Frisch B, Fateh-Moghadam A, et al: Histologic classification and staging of multiple myeloma. A retrospective and prospective study of 674 cases. *Am J Clin Pathol* 87:342–355, 1987.

292. Greipp PR, Leong T, Bennett JM, et al: Plasmablastic morphology—An independent prognostic factor with clinical and laboratory correlates: Eastern Cooperative Oncology Group (ECOG) myeloma trial E9486 report by the ECOG Myeloma Laboratory Group. *Blood* 91:2501–2507, 1998.

293. Greipp PR, Raymond NM, Kyle RA, et al: Multiple myeloma: Significance of plasmablastic subtype in morphological classification. *Blood* 65:305–310, 1985.

294. Rajkumar SV, Fonseca R, Lacy MQ, et al: Plasmablastic morphology is an independent predictor of poor survival after autologous stem-cell transplantation for multiple myeloma. *J Clin Oncol* 17:1551–1557, 1999.

295. Hsu SM, Cossman J, Jaffe ES: Lymphocyte subsets in normal human lymphoid tissues. *Am J Clin Pathol* 80:21–30, 1983.

296. San Miguel JF, Gutierrez NC, Mateo G, et al: Conventional diagnostics in multiple myeloma. *Eur J Cancer* 42:1510–1519, 2006.

297. Barlogie B, Alexanian R, Dixon D, et al: Prognostic implications of tumor cell DNA and RNA content in multiple myeloma. *Blood* 66:338–341, 1985.

298. Bataille R, Robillard N, Pellat-Deceunynck C, et al: A cellular model for myeloma cell growth and maturation based on an intraclonal CD45 hierarchy. *Immunol Rev* 194:105–111, 2003.

299. Harada H, Kawano MM, Huang N, et al: Phenotypic difference of normal plasma cells from mature myeloma cells. *Blood* 81:2658–2663, 1993.

300. Rawstron AC, Orfao A, Beksac M, et al: Report of the European Myeloma Network on multiparametric flow cytometry in multiple myeloma and related disorders. *Haematologica* 93:431–438, 2008.

301. Van Camp B, Durie BG, Spier C, et al: Plasma cells in multiple myeloma express a natural killer cell-associated antigen: CD56 (NKH-1; Leu-19). *Blood* 76:377–382, 1990.

302. Robillard N, Avet-Loiseau H, Garand R, et al: CD20 is associated with a small mature plasma cell morphology and t(11;14) in multiple myeloma. *Blood* 102:1070–1071, 2003.

303. Ocqueteau M, Orfao A, Garcia-Sanz R, et al: Expression of the CD117 antigen (c-Kit) on normal and myelomatous plasma cells. *Br J Haematol* 95:489–493, 1996.

304. Kumar S, Fonseca R, Dispenzieri A, et al: Bone marrow angiogenesis in multiple myeloma: Effect of therapy. *Br J Haematol* 119:665–671, 2002.

305. Barlogie B, Tricot G, Haessler J, et al: Cytogenetically defined myelodysplasia after melphalan-based autotransplantation for multiple myeloma linked to poor hematopoietic stem-cell mobilization: The Arkansas experience in more than 3,000 patients treated since 1989. *Blood* 111:94–100, 2008.

306. Govindarajan R, Jagannath S, Flick JT, et al: Preceding standard therapy is the likely cause of MDS after autotransplants for multiple myeloma. *Br J Haematol* 95:349–353, 1996.

307. Konigsberg R, Zojer N, Ackermann J, et al: Predictive value of interphase cytogenetics for survival of patients with multiple myeloma. *J Clin Oncol* 18:804–812, 2000.

308. Seong C, Delasalle K, Hayes K, et al: Prognostic value of cytogenetics in multiple myeloma. *Br J Haematol* 101:189–194, 1998.

309. Tricot G, Sawyer JR, Jagannath S, et al: Unique role of cytogenetics in the prognosis of patients with myeloma receiving high-dose therapy and autotransplants. *J Clin Oncol* 15:2659–2666, 1997.

310. Zojer N, Konigsberg R, Ackermann J, et al: Deletion of 13q14 remains an independent adverse prognostic variable in multiple myeloma despite its frequent detection by interphase fluorescence in situ hybridization. *Blood* 95:1925–1930, 2000.

311. Ross FM, Avet-Loiseau H, Ameye G, et al: Report from the European Myeloma Network on interphase FISH in multiple myeloma and related disorders. *Haematologica* 97:1272–1277, 2012.

312. Boccadoro M, Massaia M, Dianzani U, et al: Multiple myeloma: Biological and clinical significance of bone marrow plasma cell labelling index. *Haematologica* 72:171–175, 1987.

313. Drewinko B, Alexanian R, Boyer H, et al: The growth fraction of human myeloma cells. *Blood* 57:333–338, 1981.

314. Durie BG, Salmon SE, Moon TE: Pretreatment tumor mass, cell kinetics, and prognosis in multiple myeloma. *Blood* 55:364–372, 1980.

315. Greipp PR, Witzig TE, Gonchoroff NJ, et al: Immunofluorescence labeling indices in myeloma and related monoclonal gammopathies. *Mayo Clin Proc* 62:969–977, 1987.

316. Latreille J, Barlogie B, Dosik G, et al: Cellular DNA content as a marker of human multiple myeloma. *Blood* 55:403–408, 1980.

317. Latreille J, Barlogie B, Johnston D, et al: Ploidy and proliferative characteristics in monoclonal gammopathies. *Blood* 59:43–51, 1982.

318. Greipp PR, Lust JA, O'Fallon WM, et al: Plasma cell labeling index and beta 2-microglobulin predict survival independent of thymidine kinase and C-reactive protein in multiple myeloma. *Blood* 81:3382–3387, 1993.

319. Witzig TE, Gonchoroff NJ, Katzmann JA, et al: Peripheral blood B cell labeling indices are a measure of disease activity in patients with monoclonal gammopathies. *J Clin Oncol* 6:1041–1046, 1988.

320. Dimopoulos MA, Kastritis E, Rosinol L, et al: Pathogenesis and treatment of renal failure in multiple myeloma. *Leukemia* 22:1485–1493, 2008.

321. Solomon A, Weiss DT, Kattine AA: Nephrotoxic potential of Bence Jones proteins. *N Engl J Med* 324:1845–1851, 1991.

322. Alexanian R, Barlogie B, Dixon D: Renal failure in multiple myeloma. Pathogenesis and prognostic implications. *Arch Intern Med* 150:1693–1695, 1990.

323. Kyle RA, Greipp PR: Amyloidosis (AL). Clinical and laboratory features in 229 cases. *Mayo Clin Proc* 58:665–683, 1983.

324. Buxbaum J: Mechanisms of disease: Monoclonal immunoglobulin deposition. Amyloidosis, light chain deposition disease, and light and heavy chain deposition disease. *Hematol Oncol Clin North Am* 6:323–346, 1992.

325. Solomon A, Frangione B, Franklin EC: Bence Jones proteins and light chains of immunoglobulins. Preferential association of the V lambda VI subgroup of human light chains with amyloidosis AL (lambda). *J Clin Invest* 70:453–460, 1982.

326. Zhang SQ, Dong P, Zhang ZL, et al: Renal plasmacytoma: Report of a rare case and review of the literature. *Oncol Lett* 5:1839–1843, 2013.

327. Reeves WB, Foley RJ, Weinman EJ: Nephrotoxicity from nonsteroidal anti-inflammatory drugs. *South Med J* 78:318–322, 1985.

328. Grima DT, Airia P, Attard C, et al: Modelled cost-effectiveness of high cut-off haemodialysis compared to standard haemodialysis in the management of myeloma kidney. *Curr Med Res Opin* 27:383–391, 2011.

329. Hutchison C, Sanders PW: Evolving strategies in the diagnosis, treatment, and monitoring of myeloma kidney. *Adv Chronic Kidney Dis* 19:279–281, 2012.

330. Hutchison CA, Cockwell P, Reid S, et al: Efficient removal of immunoglobulin free light chains by hemodialysis for multiple myeloma: *In vitro* and *in vivo* studies. *J Am Soc Nephrol* 18:886–895, 2007.

331. Blade J, Fernandez-Llama P, Bosch F, et al: Renal failure in multiple myeloma: Presenting features and predictors of outcome in 94 patients from a single institution. *Arch Intern Med* 158:1889–1893, 1998.

332. Kastritis E, Anagnostopoulos A, Roussou M, et al: Reversibility of renal failure in newly diagnosed multiple myeloma patients treated with high dose dexamethasone-containing regimens and the impact of novel agents. *Haematologica* 92:546–549, 2007.

333. Knudsen LM, Hjorth M, Hippe E: Renal failure in multiple myeloma: Reversibility and impact on the prognosis. Nordic Myeloma Study Group. *Eur J Haematol* 65:175–181, 2000.

334. Bjerrum OW, Rygaard-Olsen C, Dahlerup B, et al: The carpal tunnel syndrome and amyloidosis. A clinical and histological study. *Clin Neurol Neurosurg* 86:29–32, 1984.

335. Pratt G, Goodyear O, Moss P: Immunodeficiency and immunotherapy in multiple myeloma. *Br J Haematol* 138:563–579, 2007.

336. Jacobson DR, Zolla-Pazner S: Immunosuppression and infection in multiple myeloma. *Semin Oncol* 13:282–290, 1986.

337. Ullrich S, Zolla-Pazner S: Immunoregulatory circuits in myeloma. *Clin Haematol* 11:87–111, 1982.

338. Campbell JD, Cook G, Robertson SE, et al: Suppression of IL-2-induced T cell proliferation and phosphorylation of STAT3 and STAT5 by tumor-derived TGF beta is reversed by IL-15. *J Immunol* 167:553–561, 2001.

339. Cook G, Campbell JD: Immune regulation in multiple myeloma: The host-tumour conflict. *Blood Rev* 13:151–162, 1999.

340. Cook G, Campbell JD, Carr CE, et al: Transforming growth factor beta from multiple myeloma cells inhibits proliferation and IL-2 responsiveness in T lymphocytes. *J Leukoc Biol* 66:981–988, 1999.

341. Gorelik L, Flavell RA: Transforming growth factor-beta in T-cell biology. *Nat Rev Immunol* 2:46–53, 2002.

342. Ratta M, Fagnoni F, Curti A, et al: Dendritic cells are functionally defective in multiple myeloma: The role of interleukin-6. *Blood* 100:230–237, 2002.

343. Rawstron AC, Davies FE, Owen RG, et al: B-lymphocyte suppression in multiple myeloma is a reversible phenomenon specific to normal B-cell progenitors and plasma cell precursors. *Br J Haematol* 100:176–183, 1998.

344. Mills KH, Cawley JC: Abnormal monoclonal antibody-defined helper/suppressor T-cell subpopulations in multiple myeloma: Relationship to treatment and clinical stage. *Br J Haematol* 53:271–275, 1983.

345. Ogawara H, Handa H, Yamazaki T, et al: High Th1/Th2 ratio in patients with multiple myeloma. *Leuk Res* 29:135–140, 2005.

346. Mariani S, Coscia M, Even J, et al: Severe and long-lasting disruption of T-cell receptor diversity in human myeloma after high-dose chemotherapy and autologous peripheral blood progenitor cell infusion. *Br J Haematol* 113:1051–1059, 2001.

347. Mozaffari F, Hansson L, Kiaii S, et al: Signalling molecules and cytokine production in T cells of multiple myeloma-increased abnormalities with advancing stage. *Br J Haematol* 124:315–324, 2004.

348. Kay NE, Leong TL, Bone N, et al: Blood levels of immune cells predict survival in myeloma patients: Results of an Eastern Cooperative Oncology Group phase 3 trial for newly diagnosed multiple myeloma patients. *Blood* 98:23–28, 2001.

349. Xie J, Wang Y, Freeman ME 3rd, et al: Beta 2-microglobulin as a negative regulator of the immune system: High concentrations of the protein inhibit *in vitro* generation of functional dendritic cells. *Blood* 101:4005–4012, 2003.

350. Vesole DH, Oken MM, Heckler C, et al: Oral antibiotic prophylaxis of early infection in multiple myeloma: A URCC/ECOG randomized phase III study. *Leukemia* 26:2517–2520, 2012.

351. Miralles GD, O'Fallon JR, Talley NJ: Plasma-cell dyscrasia with polyneuropathy. The spectrum of POEMS syndrome. *N Engl J Med* 327:1919–1923, 1992.

352. Waldenstrom JG, Adner A, Gydell K, et al: Osteosclerotic "plasmocytoma" with polyneuropathy, hypertrichosis and diabetes. *Acta Med Scand* 203:297–303, 1978.

353. Preston FE, Cooke KB, Foster ME, et al: Myelomatosis and the hyperviscosity syndrome. *Br J Haematol* 38:517–530, 1978.

354. Pruzanski W, Watt JG: Serum viscosity and hyperviscosity syndrome in IgG multiple myeloma. Report on 10 patients and a review of the literature. *Ann Intern Med* 77:853–860, 1972.

355. Somer T: Rheological basis of the hyperviscosity syndrome of plasma cell dyscrasias: A review. *Bibl Anat* 13:105–106, 1975.

356. Stone MJ, Bogen SA: Evidence-based focused review of management of hyperviscosity syndrome. *Blood* 119:2205–2208, 2012.

357. Chandy KG, Stockley RA, Leonard RC, et al: Relationship between serum viscosity and intravascular IgA polymer concentration in IgA myeloma. *Clin Exp Immunol* 46:653–661, 1981.

358. Capra JD, Kunkel HG: Aggregation of gamma-G3 proteins: Relevance to the hyperviscosity syndrome. *J Clin Invest* 49:610–621, 1970.

359. Bichel J, Effersoe P, Gormsen H, et al: Leukemic myelomatosis (plasma cell leukemia); a review with report of four cases. *Acta Radiol* 37:196–207, 1952.

360. Garcia-Sanz R, Orfao A, Gonzalez M, et al: Primary plasma cell leukemia: Clinical, immunophenotypic, DNA ploidy, and cytogenetic characteristics. *Blood* 93:1032–1037, 1999.

361. Noel P, Kyle RA: Plasma cell leukemia: An evaluation of response to therapy. *Am J Med* 83:1062–1068, 1987.

362. van de Donk NW, Lokhorst HM, Anderson KC, et al: How I treat plasma cell leukemia. *Blood* 120:2376–2389, 2012.

363. Weinstock M, Ghobrial IM: Extramedullary multiple myeloma. *Leuk Lymphoma* 54:1135–1141, 2013.

364. Bartel TB, Haessler J, Brown TL, et al: F18-fluorodeoxyglucose positron emission tomography in the context of other imaging techniques and prognostic factors in multiple myeloma. *Blood* 114:2068–2076, 2009.

365. Short KD, Rajkumar SV, Larson D, et al: Incidence of extramedullary disease in patients with multiple myeloma in the era of novel therapy, and the activity of pomalidomide on extramedullary myeloma. *Leukemia* 25:906–908, 2011.

366. Barlogie B, Smallwood L, Smith T, et al: High serum levels of lactic dehydrogenase identify a high-grade lymphoma-like myeloma. *Ann Intern Med* 110:521–525, 1989.

367. Usmani SZ, Heuck C, Mitchell A, et al: Extramedullary disease portends poor prognosis in multiple myeloma and is over-represented in high-risk disease even in the era of novel agents. *Haematologica* 97:1761–1767, 2012.

368. Varettoni M, Corso A, Pica G, et al: Incidence, presenting features and outcome of extramedullary disease in multiple myeloma: A longitudinal study on 1003 consecutive patients. *Ann Oncol* 21:325–330, 2010.

369. Cherng NC, Asal NR, Kuebler JP, et al: Prognostic factors in multiple myeloma. *Cancer* 67:3150–3156, 1991.

370. Chamberlain MC, Glantz M: Myelomatous meningitis. *Cancer* 112:1562–1567, 2008.

371. Chang H, Sloan S, Li D, et al: Multiple myeloma involving central nervous system: High frequency of chromosome 17p13.1 (p53) deletions. *Br J Haematol* 127:280–284, 2004.

372. Fassas AB, Spencer T, Sawyer J, et al: Both hypodiploidy and deletion of chromosome 13 independently confer poor prognosis in multiple myeloma. *Br J Haematol* 118:1041–1047, 2002.

373. Rasche L, Bernard C, Topp MS, et al: Features of extramedullary myeloma relapse: High proliferation, minimal marrow involvement, adverse cytogenetics: A retrospective single-center study of 24 cases. *Ann Hematol* 91:1031–1037, 2012.

374. Sheth N, Yeung J, Chang H: P53 nuclear accumulation is associated with extramedullary progression of multiple myeloma. *Leuk Res* 33:1357–1360, 2009.

375. Wang SY, Hao HL, Deng K, et al: Expression levels of phosphatase and tensin homolog deleted on chromosome 10 (PTEN) and focal adhesion kinase in patients with multiple myeloma and their relationship to clinical stage and extramedullary infiltration. *Leuk Lymphoma* 53:1162–1168, 2012.

376. Raanani P, Shpilberg O, Ben-Bassat I: Extramedullary disease and targeted therapies for hematological malignancies—Is the association real? *Ann Oncol* 18:7–12, 2007.

377. Bataille R, Durie BG, Grenier J, et al: Prognostic factors and staging in multiple myeloma: A reappraisal. *J Clin Oncol* 4:80–87, 1986.

378. Gassmann W, Pralle H, Haferlach T, et al: Staging systems for multiple myeloma: A comparison. *Br J Haematol* 59:703–711, 1985.

379. Durie BG, Salmon SE: A clinical staging system for multiple myeloma. Correlation of measured myeloma cell mass with presenting clinical features, response to treatment, and survival. *Cancer* 36:842–854, 1975.

380. Bataille R, Grenier J, Sany J: Beta-2-microglobulin in myeloma: Optimal use for staging, prognosis, and treatment—a prospective study of 160 patients. *Blood* 63:468–476, 1984.

381. Garewal H, Durie BG, Kyle RA, et al: Serum beta 2-microglobulin in the initial staging and subsequent monitoring of monoclonal plasma cell disorders. *J Clin Oncol* 2:51–57, 1984.

382. Child JA, Norfolk DR, Cooper EH: Serum beta 2-microglobulin in myelomatosis. *Br J Haematol* 63:406–407, 1986.

383. Resnick D KM: Plasma cell dyscrasias, in *Bone and Joint Imaging*. Elsevier: Canada, 2004.

384. Collins CD: Multiple myeloma. *Cancer Imaging* 4:S47–S53, 2004.

385. Singh J, Fairbairn KJ, Williams C, et al: Expert radiological review of skeletal surveys identifies additional abnormalities in 23% of cases: Further evidence for the value of myeloma multi-disciplinary teams in the accurate staging and treatment of myeloma patients. *Br J Haematol* 137:172–173, 2007.

386. Wahlin A, Holm J, Osterman G, et al: Evaluation of serial bone X-ray examination in multiple myeloma. *Acta Med Scand* 212:385–387, 1982.

387. Collins CD: Problems monitoring response in multiple myeloma. *Cancer Imaging* 5:S119–S126, 2005.

388. Ludwig H, Fruhwald F, Tscholakoff D, et al: Magnetic resonance imaging of the spine in multiple myeloma. *Lancet* 2:364–366, 1987.

389. Ghanem N, Lohrmann C, Engelhardt M, et al: Whole-body MRI in the detection of bone marrow infiltration in patients with plasma cell neoplasms in comparison to the radiological skeletal survey. *Eur Radiol* 16:1005–1014, 2006.

390. Baur-Melnyk A, Buhmann S, Becker C, et al: Whole-body MRI versus whole-body MDCT for staging of multiple myeloma. *AJR Am J Roentgenol* 190:1097–1104, 2008.

391. Baur-Melnyk A, Buhmann S, Durr HR, et al: Role of MRI for the diagnosis and prognosis of multiple myeloma. *Eur J Radiol* 55:56–63, 2005.

392. Joffe J, Williams MP, Cherryman GR, et al: Magnetic resonance imaging in myeloma. *Lancet* 1:1162–1163, 1988.

393. Nosas-Garcia S, Moehler T, Wasser K, et al: Dynamic contrast-enhanced MRI for assessing the disease activity of multiple myeloma: A comparative study with histology and clinical markers. *J Magn Reson Imaging* 22:154–162, 2005.

394. Bredella MA, Steinbach L, Caputo G, et al: Value of FDG PET in the assessment of patients with multiple myeloma. *AJR Am J Roentgenol* 184:1199–1204, 2005.

395. Zamagni E, Nanni C, Patriarca F, et al: A prospective comparison of 18F-fluorodeoxyglucose positron emission tomography-computed tomography, magnetic resonance imaging and whole-body planar radiographs in the assessment of bone disease in newly diagnosed multiple myeloma. *Haematologica* 92:50–55, 2007.

396. Zamagni E, Patriarca F, Nanni C, et al: Prognostic relevance of 18-F FDG PET/CT in newly diagnosed multiple myeloma patients treated with up-front autologous transplantation. *Blood* 118:5989–5995, 2011.

397. International Myeloma Working G: Criteria for the classification of monoclonal gammopathies, multiple myeloma and related disorders: A report of the International Myeloma Working Group.. *Br J Haematol* 121:749, 2003.

398. Avet-Loiseau H, Durie BG, Cavo M, et al: Combining fluorescent *in situ* hybridization data with ISS staging improves risk assessment in myeloma: An International Myeloma Working Group collaborative project. *Leukemia* 27:711–717, 2013.

399. Attal M, Harousseau JL, Stoppa AM, et al: A prospective, randomized trial of autologous Bone Marrow Transplant and chemotherapy in multiple myeloma. Intergroupe Francais du Myelome. *N Engl J Med* 335:91–97, 1996.

400. Singhal S, Mehta J, Desikan R, et al: Antitumor activity of thalidomide in refractory multiple myeloma. *N Engl J Med* 341:1565–1571, 1999.

401. Dimopoulos M, Spencer A, Attal M, et al: Lenalidomide plus dexamethasone for relapsed or refractory multiple myeloma. *N Engl J Med* 357:2123–2132, 2007.

402. Richardson PG, Siegel D, Baz R, et al: Phase 1 study of pomalidomide MTD, safety, and efficacy in patients with refractory multiple myeloma who have received lenalidomide and bortezomib. *Blood* 121:1961–1967, 2013.

403. Richardson PG, Barlogie B, Berenson J, et al: A phase 2 study of bortezomib in relapsed, refractory myeloma. *N Engl J Med* 348:2609–2617, 2003.

404. Siegel DS, Martin T, Wang M, et al: A phase 2 study of single-agent carfilzomib (PX-171-003-A1) in patients with relapsed and refractory multiple myeloma. *Blood* 120:2817–2825, 2012.

405. Vij R, Siegel DS, Jagannath S, et al: An open-label, single-arm, phase 2 study of single-agent carfilzomib in patients with relapsed and/or refractory multiple myeloma who have been previously treated with bortezomib. *Br J Haematol* 158:739–748, 2012.

406. Brenner H, Gondos A, Pulte D: Recent major improvement in long-term survival of younger patients with multiple myeloma. *Blood* 111:2521–2526, 2008.

407. Pulte D, Gondos A, Brenner H: Improvement in survival of older adults with multiple myeloma: Results of an updated period analysis of SEER data. *Oncologist* 16:1600–1603, 2011.

408. Child JA, Morgan GJ, Davies FE, et al: High-dose chemotherapy with hematopoietic stem-cell rescue for multiple myeloma. *N Engl J Med* 348:1875–1883, 2003.

409. Barlogie B, Kyle RA, Anderson KC, et al: Standard chemotherapy compared with high-dose chemoradiotherapy for multiple myeloma: Final results of phase III US Intergroup Trial S9321. *J Clin Oncol* 24:929–936, 2006.

410. Attal M, Harousseau JL, Facon T, et al: Single versus double autologous stem-cell transplantation for multiple myeloma. *N Engl J Med* 349:2495–2502, 2003.

411. Rajkumar SV, Hayman S, Gertz MA, et al: Combination therapy with thalidomide plus dexamethasone for newly diagnosed myeloma. *J Clin Oncol* 20:4319–4323, 2002.

412. Weber D, Rankin K, Gavino M, et al: Thalidomide alone or with dexamethasone for previously untreated multiple myeloma. *J Clin Oncol* 21:16–19, 2003.

413. Cavo M, Zamagni E, Tosi P, et al: Superiority of thalidomide and dexamethasone over vincristine-doxorubicindexamethasone (VAD) as primary therapy in preparation for autologous transplantation for multiple myeloma. *Blood* 106:35–39, 2005.

414. Rajkumar SV, Jacobus S, Callander NS, et al: Lenalidomide plus high-dose dexamethasone versus lenalidomide plus low-dose dexamethasone as initial therapy for newly diagnosed multiple myeloma: An open-label randomised controlled trial. *Lancet Oncol* 11:29–37, 2010.

415. Lacy MQ, Gertz MA, Dispenzieri A, et al: Long-term results of response to therapy, time to progression, and survival with lenalidomide plus dexamethasone in newly diagnosed myeloma. *Mayo Clin Proc* 82:1179–1184, 2007.

416. Richardson PG, Schlossman R, Mitsiades C, et al: Emerging trends in the clinical use of bortezomib in multiple myeloma. *Clin Lymphoma Myeloma.* 6:84–88, 2005.

417. Jagannath S, Barlogie B, Berenson JR, et al: Bortezomib in recurrent and/or refractory multiple myeloma. Initial clinical experience in patients with impaired renal function. *Cancer* 103:1195–1200, 2005.

418. Richardson PG, Weller E, Lonial S, et al: Lenalidomide, bortezomib, and dexamethasone combination therapy in patients with newly diagnosed multiple myeloma. *Blood* 116:679–686, 2010.

419. Kumar S, Flinn I, Richardson PG, et al: Randomized, multicenter, phase 2 study (EVOLUTION) of combinations of bortezomib, dexamethasone, cyclophosphamide, and lenalidomide in previously untreated multiple myeloma. *Blood* 119:4375–4382, 2012.

420. Roussel M, Facon T, Moreau P, et al: Firstline treatment and maintenance in newly diagnosed multiple myeloma patients. *Recent Results Cancer Res* 183:189–206, 2011.

421. Jakubowiak AJ, Dytfeld D, Griffith KA, et al: A phase 1/2 study of carfilzomib in combination with lenalidomide and low-dose dexamethasone as a frontline treatment for multiple myeloma. *Blood* 120:1801–1809, 2012.

422. Lokhorst HM, Schmidt-Wolf I, Sonneveld P, et al: Thalidomide in induction treatment increases the very good partial response rate before and after high-dose therapy in previously untreated multiple myeloma. *Haematologica* 93:124–127, 2008.

423. de la Rubia J, Blade J, Lahuerta JJ, et al: Effect of chemotherapy with alkylating agents on the yield of CD34+ cells in patients with multiple myeloma. Results of the Spanish Myeloma Group (GEM) Study. *Haematologica* 91:621–627, 2006.

424. Kumar S, Dispenzieri A, Lacy MQ, et al: Impact of lenalidomide therapy on stem cell mobilization and engraftment post-peripheral blood stem cell transplantation in patients with newly diagnosed myeloma. *Leukemia* 21:2035–2042, 2007.

425. Mark T, Stern J, Furst JR, et al: Stem cell mobilization with cyclophosphamide overcomes the suppressive effect of lenalidomide therapy on stem cell collection in multiple myeloma. *Biol Blood Marrow Transplant* 14:795–798, 2008.

426. Mazumder A, Kaufman J, Niesvizky R, et al: Effect of lenalidomide therapy on mobilization of peripheral blood stem cells in previously untreated multiple myeloma patients. *Leukemia* 22:1280–1281; author reply 1281–1282, 2008.

427. Popat U, Saliba R, Thandi R, et al: Impairment of filgrastim-induced stem cell mobilization after prior lenalidomide in patients with multiple myeloma. *Biol Blood Marrow Transplant* 15:718–723, 2009.

428. Paripati H, Stewart AK, Cabou S, et al: Compromised stem cell mobilization following induction therapy with lenalidomide in myeloma. *Leukemia* 22:1282–1284, 2008.

429. Combination chemotherapy versus melphalan plus prednisone as treatment for multiple myeloma: An overview of 6,633 patients from 27 randomized trials. Myeloma Trialists' Collaborative Group. *J Clin Oncol* 16:3832–3842, 1998.

430. Gregory WM, Richards MA, Malpas JS: Combination chemotherapy versus melphalan and prednisolone in the treatment of multiple myeloma: An overview of published trials. *J Clin Oncol* 10:334–342, 1992.

431. Palumbo A, Bringhen S, Caravita T, et al: Oral melphalan and prednisone chemotherapy plus thalidomide compared with melphalan and prednisone alone in elderly patients with multiple myeloma: Randomised controlled trial. *Lancet* 367:825–831, 2006.

432. Palumbo A, Rajkumar SV, Dimopoulos MA, et al: Prevention of thalidomide- and lenalidomide-associated thrombosis in myeloma. *Leukemia* 22:414–423, 2008.

433. Palumbo A, Falco P, Corradini P, et al: Melphalan, prednisone, and lenalidomide treatment for newly diagnosed myeloma: A report from the GIMEMA—Italian Multiple Myeloma Network. *J Clin Oncol* 25:4459–4465, 2007.

434. Palumbo A, Hajek R, Delforge M, et al: Continuous lenalidomide treatment for newly diagnosed multiple myeloma. *N Engl J Med* 366:1759–1769, 2012.

435. San Miguel JF, Schlag R, Khuageva NK, et al: Bortezomib plus melphalan and prednisone for initial treatment of multiple myeloma. *N Engl J Med* 359:906–917, 2008.

436. Mateos MV, Richardson PG, Schlag R, et al: Bortezomib plus melphalan and prednisone compared with melphalan and prednisone in previously untreated multiple myeloma: Updated follow-up and impact of subsequent therapy in the phase III VISTA trial. *J Clin Oncol* 28:2259–2266, 2010.

437. Facon TD, Dispenzieri M, Catalano A, et al: Initial phase 3 results of the FIRST (Frontline Investigation of Lenalidomide + Dexamethasone versus Standard Thalidomide) Trial (MM-020/IFM 0701) in newly diagnosed multiple myeloma (NDMM) patients ineligible for stem cell transplantation. ASH 2013 Annual Meeting Abstract 2, 2013.

438. Ludwig H, Durie BG, McCarthy P, et al: IMWG consensus on maintenance therapy in multiple myeloma. *Blood* 119:3003–3015, 2012.

439. Kagoya Y, Nannya Y, Kurokawa M: Thalidomide maintenance therapy for patients with multiple myeloma: Meta-analysis. *Leuk Res* 36:1016–1021, 2012.

440. Attal M, Lauwers-Cances V, Marit G, et al: Lenalidomide maintenance after stem-cell transplantation for multiple myeloma. *N Engl J Med* 366:1782–1791, 2012.

441. McCarthy PL, Owzar K, Hofmeister CC, et al: Lenalidomide after stem-cell transplantation for multiple myeloma. *N Engl J Med* 366:1770–1781, 2012.

442. Palumbo A, Bringhen S, Kumar SK, et al: Second primary malignancies with lenalidomide therapy for newly diagnosed myeloma: A meta-analysis of individual patient data. *Lancet Oncol* 15:333–342, 2014.

443. Sonneveld P, Schmidt-Wolf IG, van der Holt B, et al: Bortezomib induction and maintenance treatment in patients with newly diagnosed multiple myeloma: Results of the randomized phase III HOVON-65/GMMG-HD4 trial. *J Clin Oncol* 30:2946–2955, 2012.

444. Ladetto M, PaglianoG, Avonto I, et al: Consolidation with bortezomib, thalidomide and dexamethasone induces molecular remissions in autografted multiple myeloma patients. *Blood* 110:163a, 2007.

445. Mellqvist UH, Gimsing P, Hjertner O, et al: Bortezomib consolidation after autologous stem cell transplantation in multiple myeloma: A Nordic Myeloma Study Group randomized phase 3 trial. *Blood* 121:4647–4654, 2013.

446. Attal M, Lauwers-Cances V, Marit G, et al: Lenalidomide maintenance after stem-cell transplantation for multiple myeloma. *N Engl J Med* 366:1782–1791, 2012.

447. Attal M, Roussel M: Maintenance therapy for myeloma: How much, how long, and at what cost? *Am Soc Clin Oncol Educ Book* 32:515–522, 2012.

448. Palumbo A, Attal M, Roussel M: Shifts in the therapeutic paradigm for patients newly diagnosed with multiple myeloma: Maintenance therapy and overall survival. *Clin Cancer Res* 17:1253–1263, 2011.

449. Ludwig H, Sonneveld P: Disease control in patients with relapsed and/or refractory multiple myeloma: What is the optimal duration of therapy? *Leuk Res* 36 Suppl 1:S27–S34, 2012.

450. Jagannath S, Barlogie B, Berenson J, et al: A phase 2 study of two doses of bortezomib in relapsed or refractory myeloma. *Br J Haematol* 127:165–172, 2004.

451. Richardson PG, Barlogie B, Berenson J, et al: Extended follow-up of a phase II trial in relapsed, refractory multiple myeloma: Final time-to-event results from the SUMMIT trial. *Cancer* 106:1316–1319, 2006.

452. Jagannath S, Barlogie B, Berenson JR, et al: Updated survival analyses after prolonged follow-up of the phase 2, multicenter CREST study of bortezomib in relapsed or refractory multiple myeloma. *Br J Haematol* 143:537–540, 2008.

453. Richardson PG, Sonneveld P, Schuster MW, et al: Bortezomib or high-dose dexamethasone for relapsed multiple myeloma. *N Engl J Med* 352:2487–2498, 2005.

454. Richardson PG, Sonneveld P, Schuster M, et al: Extended follow-up of a phase 3 trial in relapsed multiple myeloma: Final time-to-event results of the APEX trial. *Blood* 110:3557–3560, 2007.

455. Mikhael JR, Belch AR, Prince HM, et al: High response rate to bortezomib with or without dexamethasone in patients with relapsed or refractory multiple myeloma: Results of a global phase 3b expanded access program. *Br J Haematol* 144:169–175, 2009.

456. Kumar SK, Bensinger WI, Zimmerman TM, et al: Weekly MLN9708, an investigational oral proteasome inhibitor (PI), in relapsed/refractory multiple myeloma (MM): Results from a phase I study after full enrollment. *J Clin Oncol* 31, 2013.

457. Richardson PG, Hofmeister CC, Rosenbaum CA, et al: Twice-weekly oral MLN9708 (Ixazomib Citrate), an investigational proteasome inhibitor, in combination with lenalidomide (len) and dexamethasone (Dex) in patients (Pts) with newly diagnosed multiple myeloma (MM): Final phase 1 results and phase 2 data. *Blood* Abstract 535, 2013.

458. van Rhee F, Dhodapkar M, Shaughnessy JD Jr, et al: First thalidomide clinical trial in multiple myeloma: A decade. *Blood* 112:1035–1038, 2008.

459. Palumbo A, Giaccone L, Bertola A, et al: Low-dose thalidomide plus dexamethasone is an effective salvage therapy for advanced myeloma. *Haematologica* 86:399–403, 2001.

460. Dimopoulos MA, Zervas K, Kouvatseas G, et al: Thalidomide and dexamethasone combination for refractory multiple myeloma. *Ann Oncol* 12:991–995, 2001.

461. Anagnostopoulos A, Weber D, Rankin K, et al: Thalidomide and dexamethasone for resistant multiple myeloma. *Br J Haematol* 121:768–771, 2003.

462. Weber DM, Chen C, Niesvizky R, et al: Lenalidomide plus dexamethasone for relapsed multiple myeloma in North America. *N Engl J Med* 357:2133–2142, 2007.

463. Chen C, Reece DE, Siegel D, et al: Expanded safety experience with lenalidomide plus dexamethasone in relapsed or refractory multiple myeloma. *Br J Haematol* 146:164–170, 2009.

464. Richardson PG, Siegel DS, Vij R, et al: Pomalidomide alone or in combination with low-dose dexamethasone in relapsed and refractory multiple myeloma; a randomized phase 2 study. *Blood* 123:1826–1832, 2014.

465. Dimopoulos ML, Moreau M, P et al: Pomalidomide in combination with low-dose dexamethasone; demonstrates significant progression free survival and overall survival advantage, in relapsed/refractory MM: A phase 3, multicenter, randomized, open-label study. *Blood* 120, 2012.

466. Dimopoulos M, Siegel DS, Lonial S, et al: Vorinostat or placebo in combination with bortezomib in patients with multiple myeloma (VANTAGE 088): A multicentre, randomised, double-blind study. *Lancet Oncol* 14:1129–1140, 2013.

467. Richardson PG, Yoon V, S et al: Panorama 1: A randomized double-blind, phase 3 study of panobinostat or placebo plus bortezomib and dexamethasone in relapsed or refractory multiple myeloma. *J Clin Oncol* 32:suppl: Abstract 8510, 2014.

468. Yee AV, P, Bensinger, W et al: ACY-1215, a selective histone deacetylase (HDAC) 6 inhibitor, in combination with lenalidomide and dexamethasone, is well tolerated with dose-limiting toxicity in patients with multiple myeloma (MM) at doses demonstrating biologic activity: Interim results of a phase Ib trial. *Blood* 2013.

469. Raje NV, Hari D, p et al: ACY-1215, a selective histone deacetylase (HDAC) 6 inhibitor: Interim results of combination therapy with multiple myeloma. *Blood* 2013.

470. Lokhorst HP, Gimsing T, P et al: Phase I/II dose-escalation study of daratumumab in patients with relapsed or refractory multiple myeloma. *J Clin Oncol* 31:suppl: Abstract 8512, 2013.

471. Martin TG, Strickland SA, Glenn M, et al: SAR650984, a CD38 monoclonal antibody in patients with selected CD38+ hematological malignancies—Data from a dose-escalation phase I study. *Blood* 2013.

472. Zonder JA, Mohrbacher AF, Singhal S, et al: A phase 1, multicenter, open-label, dose escalation study of elotuzumab in patients with advanced multiple myeloma. *Blood* 120:552–559, 2012.

473. Lonial S, Vij R, Harousseau JL, et al: Elotuzumab in combination with lenalidomide and low-dose dexamethasone in relapsed or refractory multiple myeloma. *J Clin Oncol* 30:1953–1959, 2012.

474. Jakubowiak AJ, Benson DM, Bensinger W, et al: Phase I trial of anti-CS1 monoclonal antibody elotuzumab in combination with bortezomib in the treatment of relapsed/refractory multiple myeloma. *J Clin Oncol* 30:1960–1965, 2012.

475. Raje NF, Faber E, Richardson P, et al: Phase 1 study of tabalumab, a human anti-BAFF antibody and bortezomib in patients with previously-treated multiple myeloma. *Blood* 2012.

476. Lentzsch S, O'Sullivan A, Kennedy RC, et al: Combination of bendamustine, lenalidomide, and dexamethasone (BLD) in patients with relapsed or refractory multiple myeloma is feasible and highly effective: Results of phase 1/2 open-label, dose escalation study. *Blood* 119:4608–4613, 2012.

477. Knop S, Straka C, Haen M, et al: The efficacy and toxicity of bendamustine in recurrent multiple myeloma after high-dose chemotherapy. *Haematologica* 90:1287–1288, 2005.

478. Chanan-Khan AA, Niesvizky R, Hohl RJ, et al: Phase III randomised study of dexamethasone with or without oblimersen sodium for patients with advanced multiple myeloma. *Leuk Lymphoma* 50:559–565, 2009.

479. Orlowski RZ, Nagler A, Sonneveld P, et al: Randomized phase III study of pegylated liposomal doxorubicin plus bortezomib compared with bortezomib alone in relapsed or refractory multiple myeloma: Combination therapy improves time to progression. *J Clin Oncol* 25:3892–3901, 2007.

480. Pineda-Roman M, Zangari M, van Rhee F, et al: VTD combination therapy with bortezomib-thalidomide-dexamethasone is highly effective in advanced and refractory multiple myeloma. *Leukemia* 22:1419–1427, 2008.

481. Ponisch W, Rozanski M, Goldschmidt H, et al: Combined bendamustine, prednisolone and thalidomide for refractory or relapsed multiple myeloma after autologous stem-cell transplantation or conventional chemotherapy: Results of a phase I clinical trial. *Br J Haematol* 143:191–200, 2008.

482. Palumbo A, Dimopoulos M, San Miguel J, et al: Lenalidomide in combination with dexamethasone for the treatment of relapsed or refractory multiple myeloma. *Blood Rev* 23:87–93, 2009.

483. Lonial SS, Shah J, Zonder JA, et al: Prolonged survival and improved response rates with ARRY-520 (Filanesib) in relapsed/refractory multiple myeloma (RRMM) patients with low α-1 acid glycoprotein (AAG) levels: Results from a phase 2 study. *Blood* Abstract 653, 2013.

484. Chari AH, Htut M, Zonder JA, et al: A phase 1 study of ARRY-520 (Filanesib) with bortezomib (BTZ) and dexamethasone (DEX) in relapsed or refractory multiple myeloma (RRMM). *Blood* 2013.

485. Santo L, Vallet S, Hideshima T, et al: AT7519, a novel small molecule multi-cyclin-dependent kinase inhibitor, induces apoptosis in multiple myeloma via GSK-3beta activation and RNA polymerase II inhibition. *Oncogene* 29:2325–2336, 2010.

486. Chaidos A, Caputo V, Gouvedenou K, et al: Potent antimyeloma activity of the novel bromodomain inhibitors I-BET151 and I-BET762. *Blood* 123:697–705, 2014.

487. Chauhan D, Tian Z, Nicholson B, et al: A small molecule inhibitor of ubiquitin-specific protease-7 induces apoptosis in multiple myeloma cells and overcomes bortezomib resistance. *Cancer Cell* 22:345–358, 2012.

488. Rosenblatt JA, Avivi I, Vasir D, et al: Blockade of PD-1 in combination with dendritic cell/myeloma fusion cell vaccination following autologous stem cell transplantation. *Blood* 2013.

489. Lokhorst HM, Schattenberg A, Cornelissen JJ, et al: Donor leukocyte infusions are effective in relapsed multiple myeloma after allogeneic bone marrow transplant. *Blood* 90:4206–4211, 1997.

490. Tricot G, Vesole DH, Jagannath S, et al: Graft-versus-myeloma effect: Proof of principle. *Blood* 87:1196–1198, 1996.

491. Bird JM, Russell NH, Samson D: Minimal residual disease after bone marrow transplant for multiple myeloma: Evidence for cure in long-term survivors. *Bone Marrow Transplant* 12:651–654, 1993.

492. Corradini P, Voena C, Tarella C, et al: Molecular and clinical remissions in multiple myeloma: Role of autologous and allogeneic transplantation of hematopoietic cells. *J Clin Oncol* 17:208–215, 1999.

493. Alyea E, Weller E, Schlossman R, et al: Outcome after autologous and allogeneic stem cell transplantation for patients with multiple myeloma: Impact of graft-versus-myeloma effect. *Bone Marrow Transplant* 32:1145–1151, 2003.

494. Bensinger WI, Buckner CD, Anasetti C, et al: Allogeneic marrow transplantation for multiple myeloma: An analysis of risk factors on outcome. *Blood* 88:2787–2793, 1996.

495. Bjorkstrand BB, Ljungman P, Svensson H, et al: Allogeneic bone marrow transplant versus autologous stem cell transplantation in multiple myeloma: A retrospective case-matched study from the European Group for Blood and Marrow Transplantation. *Blood* 88:4711–4718, 1996.

496. Gahrton G, Tura S, Ljungman P, et al: Allogeneic bone marrow transplant in multiple myeloma. European Group for Bone Marrow Transplant. *N Engl J Med* 325:1267–1273, 1991.

497. Gahrton G, Tura S, Ljungman P, et al: Prognostic factors in allogeneic bone marrow transplant for multiple myeloma. *J Clin Oncol* 13:1312–1322, 1995.

498. Hunter HM, Peggs K, Powles R, et al: Analysis of outcome following allogeneic haemopoietic stem cell transplantation for myeloma using myeloablative conditioning—evidence for a superior outcome using melphalan combined with total body irradiation. *Br J Haematol* 128:496–502, 2005.

499. Reece DE, Shepherd JD, Klingemann HG, et al: Treatment of myeloma using intensive therapy and allogeneic bone marrow transplant. *Bone Marrow Transplant* 15:117–123, 1995.

500. Varterasian M, Janakiraman N, Karanes C, et al: Transplantation in patients with multiple myeloma: A multicenter comparative analysis of peripheral blood stem cell and allogeneic transplant. *Am J Clin Oncol* 20:462–466, 1997.

501. Bensinger WI, Demirer T, Buckner CD, et al: Syngeneic marrow transplantation in patients with multiple myeloma. *Bone Marrow Transplant* 18:527–531, 1996.

502. Gahrton G, Svensson H, Bjorkstrand B, et al: Syngeneic transplantation in multiple myeloma-a case-matched comparison with autologous and allogeneic transplantation. European Group for Blood and Marrow Transplantation. *Bone Marrow Transplant* 24:741–745, 1999.

503. Gahrton G, Svensson H, Cavo M, et al: Progress in allogenic bone marrow and peripheral blood stem cell transplantation for multiple myeloma: A comparison between transplants performed 1983–93 and 1994–8 at European Group for Blood and Marrow Transplantation centres. *Br J Haematol* 113:209–216, 2001.

504. Giralt S, Estey E, Albitar M, et al: Engraftment of allogeneic hematopoietic progenitor cells with purine analog-containing chemotherapy: Harnessing graft-versus-leukemia without myeloablative therapy. *Blood* 89:4531–4536, 1997.

505. Slavin S, Nagler A, Naparstek E, et al: Nonmyeloablative stem cell transplantation and cell therapy as an alternative to conventional bone marrow transplant with lethal

cytoreduction for the treatment of malignant and nonmalignant hematologic diseases. *Blood* 91:756–763, 1998.

506. Garban F, Attal M, Rossi JF, et al: Immunotherapy by non-myeloablative allogeneic stem cell transplantation in multiple myeloma: Results of a pilot study as salvage therapy after autologous transplantation. *Leukemia* 15:642–646, 2001.

507. McSweeney PA, Niederwieser D, Shizuru JA, et al: Hematopoietic cell transplantation in older patients with hematologic malignancies: Replacing high-dose cytotoxic therapy with graft-versus-tumor effects. *Blood* 97:3390–3400, 2001.

508. Michallet M, Bilger K, Garban F, et al: Allogeneic hematopoietic stem-cell transplantation after nonmyeloablative preparative regimens: Impact of pretransplantation and posttransplantation factors on outcome. *J Clin Oncol* 19:3340–3349, 2001.

509. Mohty M, Fegueux N, Exbrayat C, et al: Reduced intensity conditioning: Enhanced graft-versus-tumor effect following dose-reduced conditioning and allogeneic transplantation for refractory lymphoid malignancies after high-dose therapy. *Bone Marrow Transplant* 28:335–339, 2001.

510. Bensinger WI, Maloney D, Storb R: Allogeneic hematopoietic cell transplantation for multiple myeloma. *Semin Hematol* 38:243–249, 2001.

511. Kroger N, Schwerdtfeger R, Kiehl M, et al: Autologous stem cell transplantation followed by a dose-reduced allograft induces high complete remission rate in multiple myeloma. *Blood* 100:755–760, 2002.

512. Bruno B, Rotta M, Patriarca F, et al: A comparison of allografting with autografting for newly diagnosed myeloma. *N Engl J Med* 356:1110–1120, 2007.

513. Bruno B, Rotta M, Patriarca F, et al: Nonmyeloablative allografting for newly diagnosed multiple myeloma: The experience of the Gruppo Italiano Trapianti di Midollo. *Blood* 113:3375–3382, 2009.

514. Garban F, Attal M, Michallet M, et al: Prospective comparison of autologous stem cell transplantation followed by dose-reduced allograft (IFM99–03 trial) with tandem autologous stem cell transplantation (IFM99–04 trial) in high-risk de novo multiple myeloma. *Blood* 107:3474–3480, 2006.

515. Krishnan A, Pasquini MC, Logan B, et al: Tandem autologous stem cell transplants (auto-auto) with or without maintenance therapy versus single autologous transplant followed by HLA-matched sibling non-myeloablative allogeneic stem cell transplant (auto-allo) for patients (pts) with high risk (HR) multiple myeloma (MM): Results from the Blood and Marrow Transplant Clinical Trials Network (BMT-CTN) 0102 Trial. *Blood* (ASH Annual Meeting Abstracts) 116:Abstract 526, 2010.

516. Krishnan A, Pasquini MC, Logan B, et al: Autologous haemopoietic stem-cell transplantation followed by allogeneic or autologous haemopoietic stem-cell transplantation in patients with multiple myeloma (BMT CTN 0102): A phase 3 biological assignment trial. *Lancet Oncol* 12:1195–1203, 2011.

517. Bjorkstrand B, Iacobelli S, Hegenbart U, et al: Tandem autologous/reduced-intensity conditioning allogeneic stem-cell transplantation versus autologous transplantation in myeloma: Long-term follow-up. *J Clin Oncol* 29:3016–3022, 2011.

518. Crawley C, Lalancette M, Szydlo R, et al: Outcomes for reduced-intensity allogeneic transplantation for multiple myeloma: An analysis of prognostic factors from the Chronic Leukaemia Working Party of the EBMT. *Blood* 105:4532–4539, 2005.

519. Cavo M, Terragna C, Martinelli G, et al: Molecular monitoring of minimal residual disease in patients in long-term complete remission after allogeneic stem cell transplantation for multiple myeloma. *Blood* 96:355–357, 2000.

520. Martinelli G, Terragna C, Zamagni E, et al: Molecular remission after allogeneic or autologous transplantation of hematopoietic stem cells for multiple myeloma. *J Clin Oncol* 18:2273–2281, 2000.

521. Willems P, Verhagen O, Segeren C, et al: Consensus strategy to quantitate malignant cells in myeloma patients is validated in a multicenter study. Belgium-Dutch Hematology-Oncology Group. *Blood* 96:63–70, 2000.

522. Alyea EP, Soiffer RJ, Canning C, et al: Toxicity and efficacy of defined doses of CD4(+) donor lymphocytes for treatment of relapse after allogeneic bone marrow transplant. *Blood* 91:3671–3680, 1998.

523. Verdonck LF, Lokhorst HM, Dekker AW, et al: Graft-versus-myeloma effect in two cases. *Lancet* 347:800–801, 1996.

524. Alyea E, Weller E, Schlossman R, et al: T-cell–depleted allogeneic bone marrow transplant followed by donor lymphocyte infusion in patients with multiple myeloma: Induction of graft-versus-myeloma effect. *Blood* 98:934–939, 2001.

525. van Rhee F: Con: Allogeneic transplantation in multiple myeloma. *Clin Adv Hematol Oncol* 4:391–394, 2006.

526. Berenson J: Pamidronate in the treatment of osteolytic bone lesions in multiple myeloma patients—The American experience. *Br J Clin Pract Suppl* 87:5–7; discussion 13–14, 1996.

527. Rosen LS, Gordon D, Kaminski M, et al: Zoledronic acid versus pamidronate in the treatment of skeletal metastases in patients with breast cancer or osteolytic lesions of multiple myeloma: A phase III, double-blind, comparative trial. *Cancer J* 7:377–387, 2001.

528. Major P, Lortholary A, Hon J, et al: Zoledronic acid is superior to pamidronate in the treatment of hypercalcemia of malignancy: A pooled analysis of two randomized, controlled clinical trials. *J Clin Oncol* 19:558–567, 2001.

529. Terpos E, Morgan G, Dimopoulos MA, et al: International Myeloma Working Group recommendations for the treatment of multiple myeloma-related bone disease. *J Clin Oncol* 31:2347–2357, 2013.

530. National Comprehensive Cancer Network: *NCCN Clinical Practice Guidelines in Oncology Multiple Myeloma.* Version 2.2010, 2014. http://www.nccn.org/professionals/physician_gls/pdf/myeloma.pdf. Last accesse August 2015.

531. Morgan GJ, Davies FE, Gregory WM, et al: First-line treatment with zoledronic acid as compared with clodronic acid in multiple myeloma (MRC Myeloma IX): A randomised controlled trial. *Lancet* 376:1989–1999, 2010.

532. Morgan GJ, Child JA, Gregory WM, et al: Effects of zoledronic acid versus clodronic acid on skeletal morbidity in patients with newly diagnosed multiple myeloma (MRC Myeloma IX): Secondary outcomes from a randomised controlled trial. *Lancet Oncol* 12:743–752, 2011.

533. Woo SB, Hellstein JW, Kalmar JR: Narrative [corrected] review: Bisphosphonates and osteonecrosis of the jaws. *Ann Intern Med* 144:753–761, 2006.

534. Dimopoulos MA, Kastritis E, Bamia C, et al: Reduction of osteonecrosis of the jaw (ONJ) after implementation of preventive measures in patients with multiple myeloma treated with zoledronic acid. *Ann Oncol* 20:117–120, 2009.

535. Dudeney S, Lieberman IH, Reinhardt MK, et al: Kyphoplasty in the treatment of osteolytic vertebral compression fractures as a result of multiple myeloma. *J Clin Oncol* 20:2382–2387, 2002.

536. Fourney DR, Schomer DF, Nader R, et al: Percutaneous vertebroplasty and kyphoplasty for painful vertebral body fractures in cancer patients. *J Neurosurg* 98:21–30, 2003.

537. Featherstone C, Delaney G, Jacob S, et al: Estimating the optimal utilization rates of radiotherapy for hematologic malignancies from a review of the evidence: Part II-leukemia and myeloma. *Cancer* 103:393–401, 2005.

538. Facon T, Mary JY, Hulin C, et al: Melphalan and prednisone plus thalidomide versus melphalan and prednisone alone or reduced-intensity autologous stem cell transplantation in elderly patients with multiple myeloma (IFM 99–06): A randomised trial. *Lancet* 370:1209–1218, 2007.

539. Palumbo A, Ambrosini MT, Benevolo G, et al: Bortezomib, melphalan, prednisone, and thalidomide for relapsed multiple myeloma. *Blood* 109:2767–2772, 2007.

540. Zangari M, Saghafifar F, Mehta P, et al: The blood coagulation mechanism in multiple myeloma. *Semin Thromb Hemost* 29:275–282, 2003.

541. Auwerda JJ, Sonneveld P, de Maat MP, et al: Prothrombotic coagulation abnormalities in patients with newly diagnosed multiple myeloma. *Haematologica* 92:279–280, 2007.

542. Johnson DC, Corthals S, Ramos C, et al: Genetic associations with thalidomide mediated venous thrombotic events in myeloma identified using targeted genotyping. *Blood* 112:4924–4934, 2008.

543. Zangari M, Barlogie B, Cavallo F, et al: Effect on survival of treatment-associated venous thromboembolism in newly diagnosed multiple myeloma patients. *Blood Coagul Fibrinolysis* 18:595–598, 2007.

544. Morgan GJ, Schey SA, Wu P, et al: Lenalidomide (Revlimid), in combination with cyclophosphamide and dexamethasone (RCD), is an effective and tolerated regimen for myeloma patients. *Br J Haematol* 137:268–269, 2007.

545. Baglin T, Luddington R, Brown K, et al: Incidence of recurrent venous thromboembolism in relation to clinical and thrombophilic risk factors: Prospective cohort study. *Lancet* 362:523–526, 2003.

546. Argyriou AA, Iconomou G, Kalofonos HP: Bortezomib-induced peripheral neuropathy in multiple myeloma: A comprehensive review of the literature. *Blood* 112:1593–1599, 2008.

547. Richardson PG, Sonneveld P, Schuster MW, et al: Reversibility of symptomatic peripheral neuropathy with bortezomib in the phase III APEX trial in relapsed multiple myeloma: Impact of a dose-modification guideline. *Br J Haematol* 144:895–903, 2009.

548. Mileshkin L, Stark R, Day B, et al: Development of neuropathy in patients with myeloma treated with thalidomide: Patterns of occurrence and the role of electrophysiologic monitoring. *J Clin Oncol* 24:4507–4514, 2006.

549. Plasmati R, Pastorelli F, Cavo M, et al: Neuropathy in multiple myeloma treated with thalidomide: A prospective study. *Neurology* 69:573–581, 2007.

550. Pei XY, Dai Y, Grant S: Synergistic induction of oxidative injury and apoptosis in human multiple myeloma cells by the proteasome inhibitor bortezomib and histone deacetylase inhibitors. *Clin Cancer Res* 10:3839–3852, 2004.

551. Landowski TH, Megli CJ, Nullmeyer KD, et al: Mitochondrial-mediated disregulation of Ca2+ is a critical determinant of Velcade (PS-341/bortezomib) cytotoxicity in myeloma cell lines. *Cancer Res* 65:3828–3836, 2005.

552. Dikic I, Crosetto N, Calatroni S, et al: Targeting ubiquitin in cancers. *Eur J Cancer* 42:3095–3102, 2006.

553. Badros A, Goloubeva O, Dalal JS, et al: Neurotoxicity of bortezomib therapy in multiple myeloma: A single-center experience and review of the literature. *Cancer* 110:1042–1049, 2007.

554. Caravita TP, Spagnoli M, A, et al: Neuropathy in multiple myeloma patients treated with bortezomib: A multicenter experience. *Blood* Abstract 4823, 2007.

555. Richardson PG, Briemberg H, Jagannath S, et al: Frequency, characteristics, and reversibility of peripheral neuropathy during treatment of advanced multiple myeloma with bortezomib. *J Clin Oncol* 24:3113–3120, 2006.

556. Chen CI, Kouroukis CT, White D, et al: Bortezomib is active in patients with untreated or relapsed Waldenström's macroglobulinemia: A phase II study of the National Cancer Institute of Canada Clinical Trials Group. *J Clin Oncol* 25:1570–1575, 2007.

557. Moreau P, Pylypenko H, Grosicki S, et al: Subcutaneous versus intravenous administration of bortezomib in patients with relapsed multiple myeloma: A randomised, phase 3, non-inferiority study. *Lancet Oncol* 12:431–440, 2011.

558. Richardson P, Schlossman R, Jagannath S, et al: Thalidomide for patients with relapsed multiple myeloma after high-dose chemotherapy and stem cell transplantation: Results of an open-label multicenter phase 2 study of efficacy, toxicity, and biological activity. *Mayo Clin Proc* 79:875–882, 2004.

559. Ghobrial IM, Rajkumar SV: Management of thalidomide toxicity. *J Support Oncol* 1:194–205, 2003.

560. Bastuji-Garin S, Ochonisky S, Bouche P, et al: Incidence and risk factors for thalidomide neuropathy: A prospective study of 135 dermatologic patients. *J Invest Dermatol* 119:1020–1026, 2002.

561. Briani C, Zara G, Rondinone R, et al: Thalidomide neurotoxicity: Prospective study in patients with lupus erythematosus. *Neurology* 62:2288–2290, 2004.

562. Offidani M, Corvatta L, Marconi M, et al: Common and rare side-effects of low-dose thalidomide in multiple myeloma: Focus on the dose-minimizing peripheral neuropathy. *Eur J Haematol* 72:403–409, 2004.

563. Tosi P, Zamagni E, Cellini C, et al: Neurological toxicity of long-term (>1 yr) thalidomide therapy in patients with multiple myeloma. *Eur J Haematol* 74:212–216, 2005.

564. Apfel SC, Zochodne DW: Thalidomide neuropathy: Too much or too long? *Neurology* 62:2158–2159, 2004.

565. Dimopoulos MA, Kastritis E, Anagnostopoulos A, et al: Osteonecrosis of the jaw in patients with multiple myeloma treated with bisphosphonates: Evidence of increased risk after treatment with zoledronic acid. *Haematologica* 91:968–971, 2006.

566. Zervas K, Verrou E, Teleioudis Z, et al: Incidence, risk factors and management of osteonecrosis of the jaw in patients with multiple myeloma: A single-centre experience in 303 patients. *Br J Haematol* 134:620–623, 2006.

567. Badros A, Weikel D, Salama A, et al: Osteonecrosis of the jaw in multiple myeloma patients: Clinical features and risk factors. *J Clin Oncol* 24:945–952, 2006.

568. Badros A, Terpos E, Katodritou E, et al: Natural history of osteonecrosis of the jaw in patients with multiple myeloma. *J Clin Oncol* 26:5904–5909, 2008.

569. Clarke BM, Boyette J, Vural E, et al: Bisphosphonates and jaw osteonecrosis: The UAMS experience. *Otolaryngol Head Neck Surg* 136:396–400, 2007.

570. Sarasquete ME, Garcia-Sanz R, Marin L, et al: Bisphosphonate-related osteonecrosis of the jaw is associated with polymorphisms of the cytochrome P450 CYP2C8 in multiple myeloma: A genome-wide single nucleotide polymorphism analysis. *Blood* 112:2709–2712, 2008.

571. Terpos E, Dimopoulos MA: Genetic predisposition for the development of ONJ. *Blood* 112:2596–2597, 2008.

572. Montefusco V, Gay F, Spina F, et al: Antibiotic prophylaxis before dental procedures may reduce the incidence of osteonecrosis of the jaw in patients with multiple myeloma treated with bisphosphonates. *Leuk Lymphoma* 49:2156–2162, 2008.

573. Khan AA, Sandor GK, Dore E, et al: Canadian consensus practice guidelines for bisphosphonate associated osteonecrosis of the jaw. *J Rheumatol* 35:1391–1397, 2008.

574. Blade J, Samson D, Reece D, et al: Criteria for evaluating disease response and progression in patients with multiple myeloma treated by high-dose therapy and haemopoietic stem cell transplantation. Myeloma Subcommittee of the EBMT. European Group for Blood and Marrow Transplant. *Br J Haematol* 102:1115–1123, 1998.

575. Martinez-Lopez J, Lahuerta JJ, Pepin F, et al: Prognostic value of deep sequencing method for minimal residual disease detection in multiple myeloma. *Blood* 123:3073–3079, 2014.

576. Greipp PR: Prognosis in myeloma. *Mayo Clin Proc* 69:895–902, 1994.

577. Bataille R, Jourdan M, Zhang XG, et al: Serum levels of interleukin 6, a potent myeloma cell growth factor, as a reflect of disease severity in plasma cell dyscrasias. *J Clin Invest* 84:2008–2011, 1989.

578. Ludwig H, Nachbaur DM, Fritz E, et al: Interleukin-6 is a prognostic factor in multiple myeloma. *Blood* 77:2794–2795, 1991.

579. Bataille R, Boccadoro M, Klein B, et al: C-reactive protein and beta-2 microglobulin produce a simple and powerful myeloma staging system. *Blood* 80:733–737, 1992.

580. Seidel C, Borset M, Turesson I, et al: Elevated serum concentrations of hepatocyte growth factor in patients with multiple myeloma. The Nordic Myeloma Study Group. *Blood* 91:806–812, 1998.

581. Seidel C, Sundan A, Hjorth M, et al: Serum syndecan-1: A new independent prognostic marker in multiple myeloma. *Blood* 95:388–392, 2000.

582. Dahl IM, Turesson I, Holmberg E, et al: Serum hyaluronan in patients with multiple myeloma: Correlation with survival and Ig concentration. *Blood* 93:4144–4148, 1999.

583. Witzig TE, Gertz MA, Lust JA, et al: Peripheral blood monoclonal plasma cells as a predictor of survival in patients with multiple myeloma. *Blood* 88:1780–1787, 1996.

584. Zhang H, Vakil V, Braunstein M, et al: Circulating endothelial progenitor cells in multiple myeloma: Implications and significance. *Blood* 105:3286–3294, 2005.

585. Jakob C, Egerer K, Liebisch P, et al: Circulating proteasome levels are an independent prognostic factor for survival in multiple myeloma. *Blood* 109:2100–2105, 2007.

586. Blade J, Kyle RA, Greipp PR: Presenting features and prognosis in 72 patients with multiple myeloma who were younger than 40 years. *Br J Haematol* 93:345–351, 1996.

587. San Miguel JF, Garcia-Sanz R, Gonzalez M, et al: A new staging system for multiple myeloma based on the number of S-phase plasma cells. *Blood* 85:448–455, 1995.

588. Smadja NV, Bastard C, Brigaudeau C, et al: Hypodiploidy is a major prognostic factor in multiple myeloma. *Blood* 98:2229–2238, 2001.

589. Le Baccon P, Leroux D, Dascalescu C, et al: Novel evidence of a role for chromosome 1 pericentric heterochromatin in the pathogenesis of B-cell lymphoma and multiple myeloma. *Genes Chromosomes Cancer* 32:250–264, 2001.

590. Sawyer JR, Tricot G, Mattox S, et al: Jumping translocations of chromosome 1q in multiple myeloma: Evidence for a mechanism involving decondensation of pericentromeric heterochromatin. *Blood* 91:1732–1741, 1998.

591. Sawyer JR, Tricot G, Lukacs JL, et al: Genomic instability in multiple myeloma: Evidence for jumping segmental duplications of chromosome arm 1q. *Genes Chromosomes Cancer* 42:95–106, 2005.

592. Facon T, Avet-Loiseau H, Guillerm G, et al: Chromosome 13 abnormalities identified by FISH analysis and serum beta2-microglobulin produce a powerful myeloma staging system for patients receiving high-dose therapy. *Blood* 97:1566–1571, 2001.

593. Berenson JR, Jagannath S, Barlogie B, et al: Safety of prolonged therapy with bortezomib in relapsed or refractory multiple myeloma. *Cancer* 104:2141–2148, 2005.

594. Fonseca R, Barlogie B, Bataille R, et al: Genetics and cytogenetics of multiple myeloma: A workshop report. *Cancer Res* 64:1546–1558, 2004.

595. Haessler J, Shaughnessy JD, Jr., Zhan F, et al: Benefit of complete response in multiple myeloma limited to high-risk subgroup identified by gene expression profiling. *Clin Cancer Res* 13:7073–7079, 2007.

596. Shaughnessy J, Tian E, Sawyer J, et al: High incidence of chromosome 13 deletion in multiple myeloma detected by multiprobe interphase FISH. *Blood* 96:1505–1511, 2000.

597. Plowright EE, Li Z, Bergsagel PL, et al: Ectopic expression of fibroblast growth factor receptor 3 promotes myeloma cell proliferation and prevents apoptosis. *Blood* 95:992–998, 2000.

598. Zhan F, Hardin J, Kordsmeier B, et al: Global gene expression profiling of multiple myeloma, monoclonal gammopathy of undetermined significance, and normal bone marrow plasma cells. *Blood* 99:1745–1757, 2002.

599. Shaughnessy JD Jr, Zhan F, Burington BE, et al: A validated gene expression model of high-risk multiple myeloma is defined by deregulated expression of genes mapping to chromosome 1. *Blood* 109:2276–2284, 2007.

600. Kuiper R, Broyl A, de Knegt Y, et al: A gene expression signature for high-risk multiple myeloma. *Leukemia* 26:2406–2413, 2012.

601. Chauhan D, Auclair D, Robinson EK, et al: Identification of genes regulated by dexamethasone in multiple myeloma cells using oligonucleotide arrays. *Oncogene* 21:1346–1358, 2002.

602. Mitsiades N, Mitsiades CS, Poulaki V, et al: Molecular sequelae of proteasome inhibition in human multiple myeloma cells. *Proc Natl Acad Sci U S A* 99:14374–14379, 2002.

603. Hideshima T, Podar K, Chauhan D, et al: P38 MAPK inhibition enhances PS-341 (bortezomib)-induced cytotoxicity against multiple myeloma cells. *Oncogene* 23:8766–8776, 2004.

604. Kyle RA, Garton JP: The spectrum of IgM monoclonal gammopathy in 430 cases. *Mayo Clin Proc* 62:719–731, 1987.

605. Avet-Loiseau H, Garand R, Lode L, et al: Translocation t(11;14)(q13;q32) is the hallmark of IgM, IgE, and nonsecretory multiple myeloma variants. *Blood* 101:1570–1571, 2003.

606. Dimopoulos MA, Panayiotidis P, Moulopoulos LA, et al: Waldenström's macroglobulinemia: Clinical features, complications, and management. *J Clin Oncol* 18:214–226, 2000.

607. Dhodapkar MV, Jacobson JL, Gertz MA, et al: Prognostic factors and response to fludarabine therapy in patients with Waldenström macroglobulinemia: Results of United States intergroup trial (Southwest Oncology Group S9003). *Blood* 98:41–48, 2001.

608. Moulopoulos LA, Dimopoulos MA, Weber D, et al: Magnetic resonance imaging in the staging of solitary plasmacytoma of bone. *J Clin Oncol* 11:1311–1315, 1993.

609. Frassica DA, Frassica FJ, Schray MF, et al: Solitary plasmacytoma of bone: Mayo Clinic experience. *Int J Radiat Oncol Biol Phys* 16:43–48, 1989.

610. Knowling MA, Harwood AR, Bergsagel DE: Comparison of extramedullary plasmacytomas with solitary and multiple plasma cell tumors of bone. *J Clin Oncol* 1:255–262, 1983.

611. Wiltshaw E: The natural history of extramedullary plasmacytoma and its relation to solitary myeloma of bone and myelomatosis. *Medicine (Baltimore)* 55:217–238, 1976.

612. Aviles A, Huerta J, Zepeda G, et al: Serum beta 2 microglobulin in solitary plasmocytomata. *Blood* 76:1663, 1990.

613. Dimopoulos MA, Moulopoulos LA, Maniatis A, et al: Solitary plasmacytoma of bone and asymptomatic multiple myeloma. *Blood* 96:2037–2044, 2000.

614. Moulopoulos LA, Maris TG, Papanikolaou N, et al: Detection of malignant bone marrow involvement with dynamic contrast-enhanced magnetic resonance imaging. *Ann Oncol* 14:152–158, 2003.

615. Durie BG, Waxman AD, D'Agnolo A, et al: Whole-body (18)F-FDG PET identifies high-risk myeloma. *J Nucl Med* 43:1457–1463, 2002.

616. Hind CR, Gibson DG, Lavender JP, et al: Non-invasive demonstration of cardiac involvement in acquired forms of systemic amyloidosis. *Lancet* 1:1417, 1984.

617. Palladini G, Campana C, Klersy C, et al: Serum N-terminal pro-brain natriuretic peptide is a sensitive marker of myocardial dysfunction in AL amyloidosis. *Circulation* 107:2440–2445, 2003.

618. Libbey CA, Skinner M, Cohen AS: Use of abdominal fat tissue aspirate in the diagnosis of systemic amyloidosis. *Arch Intern Med* 143:1549–1552, 1983.

619. Cooper JT, Bacon CP: A histochemical construct of the amyloid fibril in *Amyloidosis* edited by EARS, p 31. John Wright and Sons, Bristol, UK, 1983.

620. Dhodapkar MV, Jagannath S, Vesole D, et al: Treatment of AL-amyloidosis with dexamethasone plus alpha interferon. *Leuk Lymphoma* 27:351–356, 1997.

621. Palladini G, Perfetti V, Obici L, et al: Association of melphalan and high-dose dexamethasone is effective and well tolerated in patients with AL (primary) amyloidosis who are ineligible for stem cell transplantation. *Blood* 103:2936–2938, 2004.

622. Dispenzieri A, Kyle RA, Lacy MQ, et al: Superior survival in primary systemic amyloidosis patients undergoing peripheral blood stem cell transplantation: A case-control study. *Blood* 103:3960–3963, 2004.

623. Skinner M, Sanchorawala V, Seldin DC, et al: High-dose melphalan and autologous stem-cell transplantation in patients with AL amyloidosis: An 8-year study. *Ann Intern Med* 140:85–93, 2004.

624. Sanchorawala V, Wright DG, Rosenzweig M, et al: Lenalidomide and dexamethasone in the treatment of AL amyloidosis: Results of a phase 2 trial. *Blood* 109:492–496, 2007.

625. Dispenzieri A, Buadi F, Laumann K, et al: Activity of pomalidomide in patients with immunoglobulin light-chain amyloidosis. *Blood* 119:5397–5404, 2012.

626. Landau HH, Hassoun H, Cohen AD, et al: Adjuvant bortezomib and dexamethasone following high-risk melphalan and stem cell transplant in systemic AL amyloidosis [abstract]. *J Clin Oncol* 27:Abstract 8540, 2009.

627. Venner CP, Lane T, Foard D, et al: Cyclophosphamide, bortezomib, and dexamethasone therapy in AL amyloidosis is associated with high clonal response rates and prolonged progression-free survival. *Blood* 119:4387–4390, 2012.

628. Comenzo RL, Gertz MA: Autologous stem cell transplantation for primary systemic amyloidosis. *Blood* 99:4276–4282, 2002.

629. Alexanian R: Localized and indolent myeloma. *Blood* 56:521–525, 1980.

630. Kyle RA, Greipp PR: Smoldering multiple myeloma. *N Engl J Med* 302:1347–1349, 1980.

631. Dimopoulos MA, Moulopoulos A, Smith T, et al: Risk of disease progression in asymptomatic multiple myeloma. *Am J Med* 94:57–61, 1993.

632. Mateos MV, Hernandez MT, Giraldo P, et al: Lenalidomide plus dexamethasone for high-risk smoldering multiple myeloma. *N Engl J Med* 369:438–447, 2013.

633. Rajkumar SV, Larson D, Kyle RA: Diagnosis of smoldering multiple myeloma. *N Engl J Med* 365:474–475, 2011.

634. Larsen JT, Kumar SK, Dispenzieri A, et al: Serum free light chain ratio as a biomarker for high-risk smoldering multiple myeloma. *Leukemia* 27:941–946, 2013.

635. Hillengass J, Fechtner K, Weber MA, et al: Prognostic significance of focal lesions in whole-body magnetic resonance imaging in patients with asymptomatic multiple myeloma. *J Clin Oncol* 28:1606–1610, 2010.

636. Hillengass J, Landgren O: Challenges and opportunities of novel imaging techniques in monoclonal plasma cell disorders: Imaging "early myeloma." *Leuk Lymphoma* 54:1355–1363, 2013.

637. Landgren O: Monoclonal gammopathy of undetermined significance and smoldering multiple myeloma: Biological insights and early treatment strategies. *Hematology Am Soc Hematol Educ Program* 2013:478–487, 2013.

638. Harousseau JL, Attal M, Avet-Loiseau H, et al: Bortezomib plus dexamethasone is superior to vincristine plus doxorubicin plus dexamethasone as induction treatment prior to autologous stem-cell transplantation in newly diagnosed multiple myeloma: Results of the IFM 2005–01 phase III trial. *J Clin Oncol* 28:4621–4629, 2010.

639. Reeder CB, Reece DE, Kukreti V, et al: Cyclophosphamide, bortezomib and dexamethasone induction for newly diagnosed multiple myeloma: High response rates in a phase II clinical trial. *Leukemia* 23:1337–1341, 2009.

640. Hulin C, Facon T, Rodon P, et al: Efficacy of melphalan and prednisone plus thalidomide in patients older than 75 years with newly diagnosed multiple myeloma: IFM 01/01 trial. *J Clin Oncol* 27:3664–3670, 2009.

641. San Miguel JF, Schlag R, Khuageva NK, et al: Persistent overall survival benefit and no increased risk of second malignancies with bortezomib-melphalan-prednisone versus melphalan-prednisone in patients with previously untreated multiple myeloma. *J Clin Oncol* 31:448–455, 2013.

642. Richardson PG, Xie W, Jagannath S, et al: Phase II trial of lenalidomide, bortezomib, and dexamethasone in patients (pts) with relapsed and relapsed/refractory multiple myeloma (MM): Updated efficacy and safety data after >2 years of follow-up. *Blood* (ASH Annual Meeting Abstracts) 116:Abstract 3049, 2010.

643. San Miguel J, Weisel K, Moreau P, et al: Pomalidomide plus low-dose dexamethasone versus high-dose dexamethasone alone for patients with relapsed and refractory multiple myeloma (MM-003): A randomised, open-label, phase 3 trial. *Lancet Oncol* 14:1055–1066, 2013.

CHAPTER 108
IMMUNOGLOBULIN LIGHT-CHAIN AMYLOIDOSIS

Morie A. Gertz, Taimur Sher, Angela Dispenzieri, and Francis K. Buadi

SUMMARY

Amyloidosis should be considered in any patient presenting with nephrotic range proteinuria; infiltrative cardiomyopathy or heart failure with preserved ejection fraction; hepatomegaly without specific imaging findings; or peripheral neuropathy, particularly if a monoclonal protein is present; as well as any patient with atypical multiple myeloma.

When a patient is seen with a relevant syndrome, the patient should have immunofixation of serum and urine proteins and measurement of κ and λ immunoglobulin free light chains. If all of these tests are normal, it is unlikely that the patient has immunoglobulin light-chain (AL) amyloidosis.

If any of the above tests are positive, further investigation for amyloidosis should be undertaken. The diagnostic test of choice is subcutaneous fat aspiration; marrow biopsy is the second best procedure. With these two tests, 83 percent of patients will have a positive result when stained with Congo red under green birefringence.

All patients with biopsy proven amyloidosis should have the deposits analyzed by laser capture microdissection mass spectroscopy to definitively classify the exact protein subunit composing the amyloid. This technique does not distinguish between systemic and localized amyloidosis, however.

The prognosis in AL amyloidosis is determined by three tests: (1) the N-terminal probrain natriuretic peptide, (2) serum troponin, and (3) the difference between the involved and uninvolved immunoglobulin free light chains. These three tests can be combined to stage the patient from stage 1 through stage 4.

Treatment of AL amyloidosis involves either standard systemic chemotherapy or high-dose chemotherapy with autologous stem cell transplantation. Fit patients who are expected to have low morbidity with transplantation should undergo this approach. The majority of patients, however, will not be candidates for transplantation and should be treated with traditional systemic chemotherapy; with the cyclophosphamide, bortezomib, and dexamethasone regimen currently favored by many investigators.

DEFINITION AND HISTORY

Amyloidosis is a heterogeneous group of diseases characterized by tissue infiltration with misfolded protein precursors as amyloid material. For nearly 100 years, amyloid has been defined by its staining properties. Divry and Florkin first used Congo red to detect amyloid in the

Acronyms and Abbreviations: CRAB, calcemia, renal insufficiency, anemia, or bone disease; CyBorD, cyclophosphamide, bortezomib, and dexamethasone; MRI, magnetic resonance imaging; NT-ProBNP, N-terminal probrain natriuretic peptide; TTR, transthyretin.

brain of patients with Alzheimer disease.[1] Amyloid deposits are always extracellular and, under the light microscope, appear amorphous and pink when seen after standard hematoxylin-and-eosin staining. All amyloid deposits bind Congo red dye and demonstrate green birefringence under polarized light,[2] and this test remains the standard diagnostic procedure required to confirm a diagnosis of amyloidosis. Under the electron microscope, amyloid consists of rigid, linear, nonbranching fibrils of 9.5 nm diameter.[3] Historically, amyloid was defined based on whether there was a family history (inherited), whether it was the result of a chronic inflammatory condition (secondary), or whether it was idiopathic (primary). Today, amyloidosis is classified based on the protein subunit composition of the deposits. The term "primary amyloid" is archaic and should not be used. Instead, such cases should be called "immunoglobulin light-chain (AL) amyloidosis," reflecting the fact that they represent a systemic plasma cell dyscrasia. The subunit classification is important because AA amyloidosis (secondary) can be the consequence of sustained inflammation but can also be inherited, as in familial Mediterranean fever. Inherited forms of amyloidosis are generally composed of mutant transthyretin (TTR) but can also be a consequence of mutations in apolipoprotein, fibrinogen, and gelsolin.[4] Senile systemic amyloidosis, primarily a cardiac disorder, is being increasingly recognized, and is caused by deposition of wild-type TTR as amyloid material in patients older than age 60 years.[5] Table 108–1 lists the nomenclature of the various forms of amyloidosis. Practicing hematologists and oncologists are not likely to see patients with forms of amyloidosis other than immunoglobulin light-chain (AL) amyloidosis. This is the only form that is responsive to chemotherapy and is the focus of this chapter; additionally, the term *amyloidosis*, unless specified otherwise, refers to *AL amyloidosis*.

EPIDEMIOLOGY

Amyloidosis is rare, with an incidence of eight per million persons per year with a median age at diagnosis of 67 years.[11] This makes it one-sixth as common as myeloma and twice as common as Waldenström macroglobulinemia. Conversely, a practicing oncologist should see approximately one light-chain amyloid patient for every six patients with myeloma in the oncologist's practice. If this is not the case, there is a significant likelihood that the disease is going unrecognized.

ETIOLOGY AND PATHOGENESIS

The fibrils of immunoglobulin light chain amyloid are composed, in most patients, of fragments of immunoglobulin light chains. A normal immunoglobulin light chain has a molecular weight of approximately 25 kDa, but the immunoglobulin light chains found in amyloid deposits usually range from 8 kDa to 15 kDa. The fragment size is important because it usually reflects the deletion of the constant region of the immunoglobulin light chain, making immunohistochemistry a poor technique to identify the fibril type in paraffin-embedded tissues.[6] A fraction of patients have immunoglobulin heavy chain amyloid deposits where fragments of immunoglobulin G, A, or M heavy chains comprise the basic subunit. Whereas AL amyloidosis represents approximately 62 percent of all amyloid patients, immunoglobulin heavy-chain amyloidosis represents less than 1 percent of all patients.[7]

There is clearly something "amyloidogenic" about the immunoglobulin light chains in patients with AL amyloidosis. Unlike monoclonal gammopathy and myeloma where the κ:λ ratio is 2:1, in AL amyloidosis, the κ:λ ratio is 1:3, suggesting an intrinsic propensity of λ light chains to form amyloid. Moreover, the subgroup λ_{VI} is exclusively found in patients with AL amyloidosis.[8] When the light chains

TABLE 108–1. Nomenclature of Amyloidosis

Amyloid Type	Subunit Protein	Clinical Organ Involvement
AL (κ or λ) or AH	Immunoglobulin light or heavy chain May be localized or systemic	Heart Kidney Liver Nerve
AA	Secondary serum amyloid A	Kidney Gastrointestinal Thyroid
ATTR (age related)	Senile systemic transthyretin	Heart Carpal tunnel
ATTR (mutant)	Familial transthyretin	Heart Nerve
A Lect-2	Leukocyte chemotactic factor No mutation found	Kidney
A Ins	Insulin localized to injection sites	Skin
A Fib	Fibrinogen A-2 mutation	Kidney
A β_2M	β_2-Microglobulin Chronic dialysis	Soft tissue Joints spine

are extracted from the urine of patients with myeloma and injected into mice, amyloid deposits are not seen. However, when the light chains from patients with amyloidosis are extracted from the urine and injected into mice, they will develop amyloidosis.[8] The exact structural characteristics that lead to the misfolding of the α helical protein into the amyloid β-pleated sheet configuration are unknown. Patients with amyloidosis are classified into those with myeloma and those without myeloma. The percentage of plasma cells present in the marrow at the time of diagnosis is prognostic and predicts outcome in patients with amyloidosis.[9] As a result, the percentage of plasma cells in the marrow may dictate alternate therapeutic considerations at diagnosis (see "Therapy" below). Overt myeloma with CRAB criteria (hypercalcemia, renal insufficiency, anemia, or bone disease) is uncommon in AL amyloidosis. However, an elevation in the percentage of plasma cells in the marrow of patients without CRAB criteria confers the same adverse prognosis as observed in patients who have overt symptomatic myeloma, and these groups can be considered as a single cohort of myeloma-associated amyloidosis. Patients who do not have myeloma at presentation have almost no chance of developing myeloma later in the course of their disease.[10] The plasma cells in the marrow of patients with amyloidosis tend to be nonproliferative and frequently lack the karyotypic abnormalities typically seen in myeloma, such as –17p, t(4;14), and –13. A translocation 11;14 is commonly seen in amyloidosis and appears to confer an inferior outcome. Circulating plasma cells detectable by flow cytometry are uncommonly seen relative to their frequency in myeloma[12]

●CLINICAL FEATURES

Unfortunately, the symptoms of amyloidosis are vague and often non-specific. Physical findings, when present, can be highly specific but are only present in a minority of patients. For a disease this rare, it

is important for clinicians to have an operational approach to avoid inappropriate resource utilization. Only 1 percent of patients with AL amyloidosis are younger than age 40 years. Consequently, it would be unlikely for younger patients to have AL amyloidosis, although this age group regularly can be seen with secondary systemic amyloidosis. The majority of patients with AL amyloidosis are males (66 percent), unlike myeloma, where the male-to-female is 52:48.[15]

The most common symptoms reported by patients with amyloidosis are fatigue, weight loss, and lower-extremity edema. Unfortunately, these symptoms are too nonspecific to be used as a trigger to screen patients, as the yield for these vague symptoms would be very low. The mechanism underlying fatigue in this disorder is usually amyloid heart disease, which can be an extremely subtle diagnosis and is discussed further under the specific amyloid syndromes. Weight loss accompanying amyloidosis can be impressive, and may exceed 20 kg. This usually results in an investigation for occult malignancy; but even if blind biopsies are performed, the diagnosis may be overlooked if a specific request for amyloid stains is not made to the pathologist. Lower-extremity edema may be attributable to nephrotic range proteinuria, hypoalbuminemia, and transudation of serum into the extracellular space. Edema may also be seen from high filling pressures caused by the restrictive cardiomyopathy, which, again, can easily be overlooked because of the subtle diagnostic testing required. These patients are often treated empirically with diuretics until cardiac dysfunction becomes more evident.

The physical findings of amyloidosis are present in only one patient in six. Periorbital purpura is frequently cited as a diagnostic finding and, when present, is useful but is only seen in 15 percent of patients (Fig. 108–1). Sometimes the purpura is subtle and can only be seen with the patient's eyes closed. Even when purpura is present, it may lead to an evaluation of a coagulopathy or platelet dysfunction, which would invariably be negative in this setting. Purpura not only is seen on the eyelids but also on the face, neck, and anterior chest above the nipple line. Enlargement of the tongue is seen in approximately one person in eight (Fig. 108–2). Dental indentations on the underside of the tongue are characteristic. Often the patient will have sudden-onset of sleep apnea syndrome as a result of occlusion of the airway by the enlarged tongue when the patient is supine.[16] Even when diagnostic findings are present, their significance is often missed, leading in many cases to tongue biopsy with a preoperative suspicion of tongue cancer. Most patients with enlargement of the tongue will also have palpable submandibular lymphadenopathy, usually caused by displacement of the nodes by the enlarged base of the tongue; although amyloid infiltration of the submandibular gland may also result in a firm palpable mass in the submandibular region. Hepatomegaly is seen in approximately 20 percent

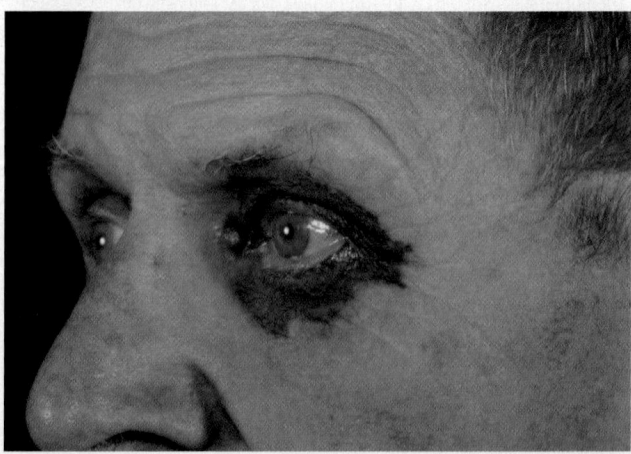

Figure 108–1. Amyloid purpura.

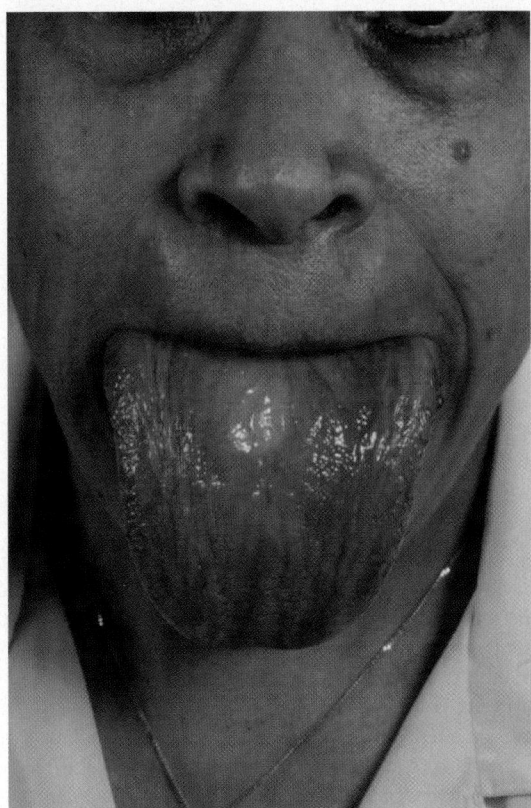

Figure 108–2. Macroglossia as a result of amyloid infiltration.

TABLE 108–2. Amyloid Syndromes Seen at the Mayo Clinic

	% Present
Kidney	67
Heart	47
Peripheral nerve	12
Liver	12
Autonomic nerve	4
Carpal tunnel	12
Tongue	9

Table 108–2 gives the frequency of amyloid syndromes seen in patients at the Mayo Clinic. If an oncologist sees a patient with one of these five syndromes, or an internist is faced with an undiagnosed patient, laboratory evaluation is indicated, as outlined below.

LABORATORY FEATURES

The best screening tests for initial evaluation of patients with suspected amyloidosis are immunoelectrophoresis and immunofixation of both serum and urine and a serum immunoglobulin free light-chain assay (both κ and λ). Systemic immunoglobulin AL amyloidosis is a plasma cell dyscrasia, and 99 percent of patients will have a detectable abnormality of one of these three tests, reflecting synthesis by a clonal population of plasma cells in the marrow. If an immunoglobulin protein is detected, further investigation for amyloidosis as described in the next section ("Differential Diagnosis") should proceed. If a systemic plasma cell dyscrasia and an immunoglobulin light chain cannot be confirmed, three possibilities exist: (1) the patient does not have amyloidosis, (2) the patient does not have systemic amyloidosis, or (3) the amyloidosis is not immunoglobulin light chain in type and reflects a different protein subunit.

The serum free light-chain assay is a critically important test. It not only heightens the suspicion of the presence of immunoglobulin AL amyloidosis, it also is prognostic and vital to staging the patient. The serum immunoglobulin free light chain is part of the response evaluation for this disease. A screening serum protein electrophoresis is insufficient as a screening technique because a visible M-spike is seen in less than half of patients because of the high prevalence of primary light-chain proteinemia.

Finding a monoclonal protein in the serum or in the urine of a patient with heavy albuminuria often obviates the need for a renal biopsy. A patient with free light chains in the serum or urine and proteinuria can have only one of three disorders: (1) myeloma cast nephropathy, (2) AL amyloidosis, or (3) Randall-type immunoglobulin deposition disease (κ).

Screening for a light-chain immunoglobulin is the best noninvasive approach when confronted with a patient with any of the five syndromes listed in Table 108–2. If amyloid is present but the light chains are normal, strong consideration of referral to a specialty center to further clarify the underlying form of amyloidosis should be considered.

DIFFERENTIAL DIAGNOSIS

Once a clinician has begun an evaluation of a patient with a compatible clinical syndrome and an immunoglobulin abnormality has been detected, a biopsy is required to confirm the diagnosis before therapy should commence. Although imaging of amyloid deposits with various

of patients and may be due to direct infiltration of the liver, which will cause a firm markedly enlarged liver.[17] In some patients, however, the liver enlargement is a reflection of high venous filling pressures in the right-sided cardiac chambers and represents chronic passive congestion. Patients rarely have periarticular infiltration of the shoulders producing the so-called shoulder pad sign, a baseball-shaped enlargement of the anterior soft tissues of the shoulder. A rare patient will develop temporal artery infiltration and develop classic jaw claudication, as well as limb, buttock, and calf claudication.[18] On questioning, many patients will have xerostomia from infiltration of the minor salivary glands; and at some centers, biopsy of the minor salivary glands is a preferred technique for the diagnosis of amyloidosis.[19]

● AMYLOID SYNDROMES

Because the symptoms of amyloidosis are highly nonspecific and the physical findings are specific but not very sensitive, an operational approach is required to ascertain which patients need investigation for amyloidosis. We recommend screening for AL amyloidosis when a patient is seen with any of the following clinical syndromes:

- Nephrotic range proteinuria with any serum creatinine level
- Infiltrative cardiomyopathy or heart failure with preserved ejection fraction. A normal ejection fraction does not exclude AL amyloidosis
- Hepatomegaly or alkaline phosphatase elevation without specific imaging abnormalities
- A mixed axonal demyelinating peripheral sensory, motor or autonomic neuropathy, particularly when associated with a monoclonal gammopathy
- A patient with myeloma with symptoms that are not typical of the disease, particularly profound, unexplained fatigue

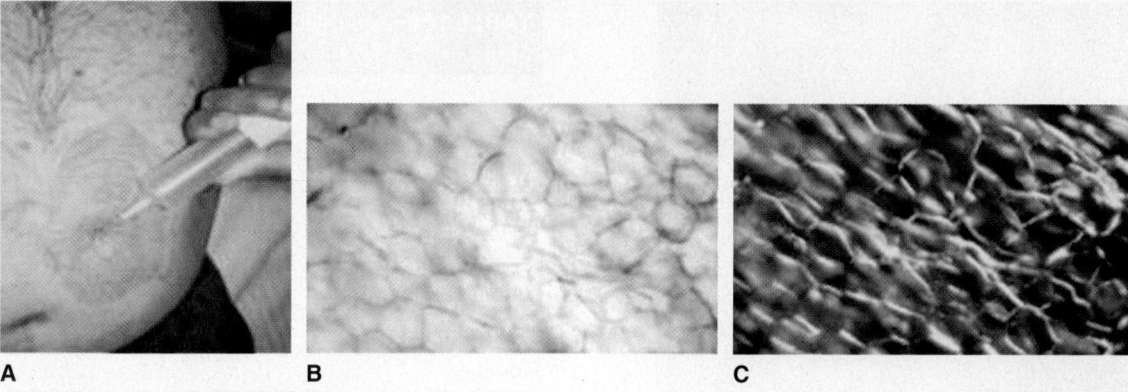

Figure 108–3. Technique and results of subcutaneous fat aspiration. **A.** Procedural technique. **B.** Fat stained with Congo red, note the preserved interstices of the fat cells. **C.** Viewed under polarized light to demonstrate green birefringence.

radionuclides, most notably anti–serum amyloid P component, continue to be explored and used in practice, they are not a substitute for histologic confirmation of the presence of amyloidosis.[20–22] In a patient with renal, cardiac, hepatic, or peripheral nerve amyloidosis, it is straight forward to establish the diagnosis by kidney, heart, liver, or nerve biopsy, but this is unnecessary in the majority of patients. Subcutaneous fat aspiration is a bedside office procedure done with local anesthesia and does not require an incision (Fig. 108–3). An excellent YouTube video has been produced by the Boston Medical Center on the technique (https://www.youtube.com/watch?v=tctYTmxd9gQ). Typically, fat aspirations are reviewed at a specialty center unless the pathology department regularly processes fatty tissue. The fat is not paraffin-embedded and, therefore, it is subject to overfixation, trapping of Congo red dye, and the possibility of inadequate controls.[23] Fat aspiration is positive in three-quarters of patients with amyloidosis.

A second tissue easily stained for amyloid is the marrow. Because AL amyloidosis patients will have a plasma cell dyscrasia, a marrow examination is clinically indicated to quantify the number of plasma cells in the marrow. Congo red staining of marrow blood vessels can detect amyloid deposits in half of patients with AL amyloidosis. Combining the two techniques (marrow and fat pad aspiration), establishes a diagnosis in 85 percent of afflicted patients. Minor salivary gland biopsy, endoscopic gastric biopsy, rectal biopsy, and skin biopsy can also be used to establish the diagnosis. If the clinical suspicion of AL amyloidosis is strong and these biopsies are negative, it is appropriate to biopsy the affected organ.

Once tissue containing Congo red has been identified, it becomes imperative that the protein subunit be determined. Historically, immunohistochemistry has been used to identify the type of amyloid, but immunohistochemistry can be challenging because only those protein subunits for which antisera exist can be detected.[24,25] Second, particularly in AL amyloidosis, the reactive epitope may have been deleted during the process of amyloid fibril formation and, frequently, the background staining is high, particularly in kidney tissues. Third, because the protein in amyloid misfolds, even if the epitopes are present, they may be hidden deep within the deposits and may be inaccessible to commercial antisera. Not only can immunohistochemistry be unreliable, it can be misleading. It is therefore recommended that laser capture of the amyloid deposit be performed routinely followed by mass spectroscopic analysis.[26–28] The subunit protein can be identified by this approach in the majority of cases. Even in patients who have a false-positive Congo red stain, this technique is useful because it will not identify amyloid-related peptides upon analysis. With this technique, one is able to confirm the presence of AL amyloidosis, which represents slightly less than two-thirds of patients seen with amyloidosis. A full quarter of patients with amyloid deposits are composed of amyloidogenic transthyretin (ATTR) (inherited) or wild-type amyloid (senile systemic). Less than 4 percent are amyloid A (AA) and approximately 4 percent represent ALect2 amyloidosis, which deposits in the kidney and causes proteinuria. Other forms of amyloid, which are often localized, are seen in less than 1 percent of patients. A particularly important form of localized amyloid occurs at the sites of subcutaneous insulin injections in diabetics. Crystalline insulin can form amyloid, which can cause discolored firm deposits which, when biopsied, will be Congo red–positive, but by mass spectroscopic analysis, can be confirmed to be insulin. Other forms of systemic amyloidosis for which systemic chemotherapy is contraindicated include fibrinogen A-α amyloidosis, and amyloid caused by apolipoprotein-A1, and gelsolin.

One additional advantage, particularly for those patients who have TTR amyloidosis is that mass spectroscopy not only identifies the protein, in most instances, it can confirm whether the protein is wild-type or a mutant. We still recommend that patients who have mutant TTR seen on mass spectroscopy have this confirmed by DNA sequencing of a blood sample, which is a readily available commercial test, to confirm the findings on mass spectroscopy. We have investigated a small number of patients in whom an amyloid syndrome was strongly suspected, a subcutaneous fat aspirate was not definitively positive, yet mass spectroscopic analysis demonstrated peptides in the tissue that are associated with amyloid including apolipoprotein-E and serum amyloid P component. When a pathologist makes a diagnosis of amyloid in tissue sections, the clinicians are required to ask what type of amyloidosis it represents. Although not widely available, mass spectroscopic analysis is the most sensitive and specific technique for identifying the amyloid subunit protein.

DIAGNOSIS AND CLINICAL CHARACTERIZATION OF ORGAN-SPECIFIC SYNDROMES

Kidney

Kidney involvement is seen in 45 percent of patients with immunoglobulin AL amyloidosis. It is conspicuously absent in the majority of patients with TTR amyloidosis until late in the disease. Renal involvement is virtually universal in systemic AA amyloidosis as well as ALect2 amyloidosis and A-fib α amyloidosis. Amyloid is seen in 2.5 percent of all renal biopsies. When limited to nondiabetics older than age 50 years, amyloid deposits will be found in 10 percent of renal biopsies.[29]

These patients present with the typical four features of the nephrotic syndrome: (1) nephrotic range proteinuria, (2) hypoalbuminemia, (3) hyperlipidemia, and (4) edema. Nearly a third of patients with renal amyloidosis have at least a 1-year history of dramatic elevations of cholesterol and triglycerides. These are often managed with statin-type medication and dietary modification without consideration that a dramatic (>100 mg/dL) rise in cholesterol and triglycerides may be caused by heavy proteinuria. In the majority of patients, the glomerular filtration rate (GFR) is preserved until sustained proteinuria has been present for years. Only a small percentage of patients, usually with interstitial but not glomerular amyloid, present with renal insufficiency in the absence of heavy proteinuria.[30]

The management of the lower-extremity edema is primarily diuretic therapy. However, excessive diuretic use, particularly in patients with cardiac amyloidosis, can aggravate already reduced intravascular volume. Diuretics can also compromise renal blood flow, increase orthostatic hypotension, and reduce cardiac filling pressures necessary for adequate cardiac output in patients that have "stiff heart syndrome." The threat of continuous proteinuria in amyloidosis is damage to the tubular system. One-third of patients with renal amyloidosis will ultimately require dialysis or renal transplantation.[31] The serum creatinine level at the time of presentation is the best predictor of which patients are most likely to require dialysis. Clearly, the best method for prevention of the need for dialysis is effective therapy of the underlying plasma cell dyscrasia. There are no reported differences between outcomes for those patients receiving hemodialysis and those receiving peritoneal dialysis.

In rare instances, patients have profound depression of the serum albumin below 1 g/dL. These patients often will be disabled by anasarca. In situations where intractable edema and anasarca makes management next to impossible, renal ablation has been performed to stop the urinary protein leak, normalize the serum oncotic pressure, and resolve the edema. Multiple techniques have been reported, including nephrectomy, ligation of the renal artery, and bilateral ureteral clips. In some patients, the early initiation of dialysis, even with a normal estimated GFR, can result in anuria and restoration of normal serum albumin levels.[32]

The correlation between the amount of amyloid detected and the degree of renal dysfunction is poor. The urinary sediment is nonspecific, shows fat and fatty casts, but generally does not contain red cell casts. The most common cause of death in patients with renal amyloidosis is progressive cardiac dysfunction from infiltrative amyloid cardiomyopathy.

Heart

Unlike most cardiac disorders, which are caused by a loss of systolic function, the restrictive cardiomyopathy caused by amyloid infiltration results in poor relaxation (so-called stiff heart syndrome) and poor filling during diastole so that the ventricular chamber has a low end-diastolic volume, which results in reduced stroke volume and a reduced cardiac output. This constitutes a classic example of heart failure with preserved systolic function. In fact, the majority of patients with amyloidosis have an echocardiographically normal ejection fraction until late in the disease.[5] Cardiac amyloid is found in 40 to 50 percent of patients at diagnosis and is responsible for nearly 90 percent of deaths. It is the most challenging syndrome to diagnose because of the lack of specificity of its symptoms. Fatigue and dyspnea on exertion are often not associated with cardiac disease in the presence of amyloid (1) because of the lack of radiographic changes of cardiomegaly, pleural effusions, and pulmonary vascular redistribution; (2) because echocardiography will demonstrate preserved ejection fraction; and (3) because coronary angiography is invariably normal.[33] This triad often leads to a diagnosis

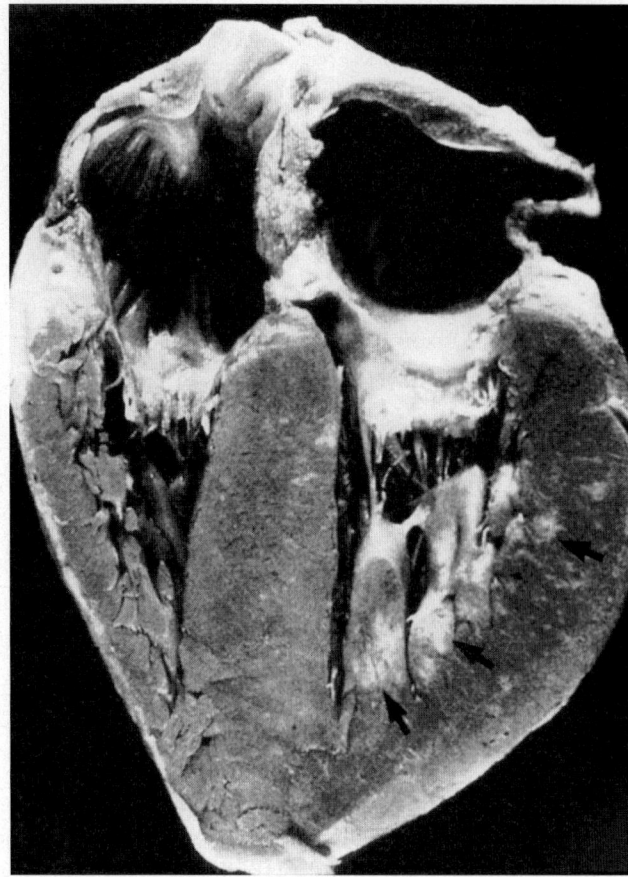

Figure 108–4. Amyloid heart disease. Note thickening of heart walls from infiltration. White patches were responsible for the designation "lardaceous change."

of noncardiac dyspnea. Even when amyloid infiltrates the myocardial wall and causes it to be thickened, it is often misattributed to hypertensive heart disease (hypertrophy) rather than infiltration (Fig. 108–4). Electrocardiographic abnormalities, including pseudoinfarction and low voltage, are quite common but are frequently overlooked, whereas a pseudoinfarction pattern is misattributed to ischemic heart disease.

The supportive care of patients with cardiac amyloidosis can be strikingly different from that of ischemic or valvular heart disease. There is no evidence that afterload reduction with angiotensin-converting enzyme inhibitors or angiotensin II receptor blockers benefits patients with relaxation abnormalities, and dyspnea and reduced exercise tolerance frequently increase in patients treated with these medications. Fatigue and dyspnea on exertion can also be exacerbated when β blockers are used for rate or rhythm control.

In addition to standard echocardiography, accurate diagnosis of cardiac amyloid requires Doppler flow studies to demonstrate the rapid decline in velocity of blood inflow into the ventricular chambers and optimally conducted cardiac strain studies that demonstrate a decline in the rate of fractional shortening of the ventricular chamber. Patients with unexplained fatigue and/or dyspnea on exertion should have immunofixation of the serum and urine and free light-chain testing to assess for possible light-chain amyloid. However, even if light chain-testing is negative, age related amyloidosis may still be present because of the deposition of wild-type TTR in the heart.[34] This typically occurs in patients older than age 60 years, predominantly men, half of whom will also have carpal tunnel syndrome.[35,36] Wild-type TTR amyloidosis will not be detected by screening for serum and urine light chains, and

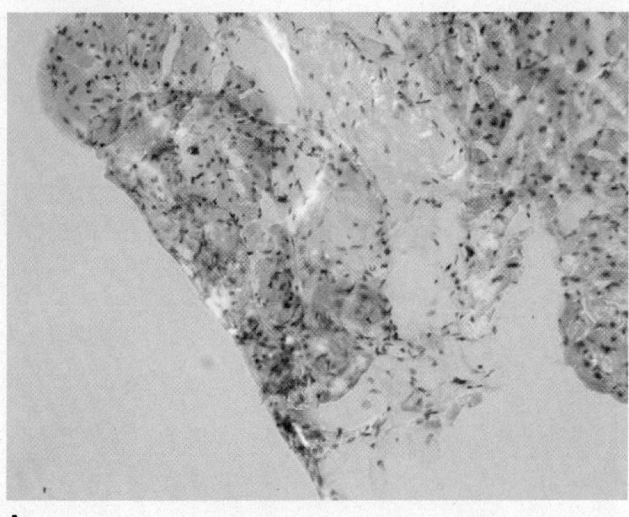

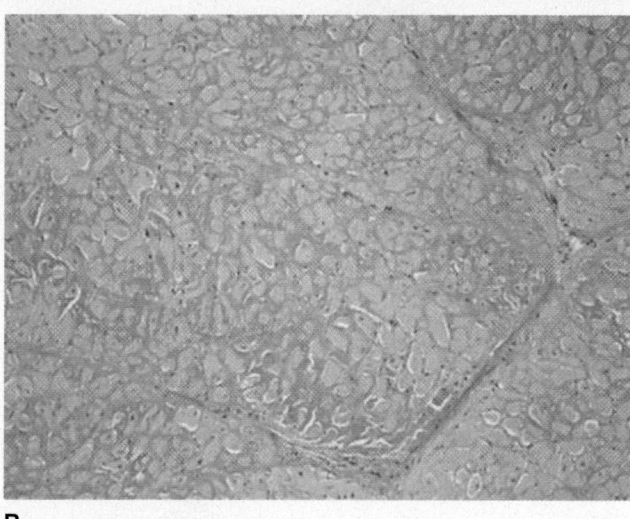

Figure 108–5. A. Polarized micrograph of Congo red–stained endomyocardial biopsy demonstrates birefringence in the involved area. **B.** Light micrograph of hematoxylin-and-eosin–stained slide of the same specimen demonstrating amyloid as extracellular eosinophilic amorphous material.

subcutaneous fat aspiration has a lower sensitivity than in AL amyloidosis. These patients require recognition by echocardiography, magnetic resonance imaging (MRI), or endomyocardial biopsy to establish a diagnosis (Fig. 108-5).

Early diagnosis of cardiac amyloid is imperative because it is this group that is responsible for the majority of the early deaths with this disorder. In our experience, 40 percent of newly diagnosed patients with AL amyloidosis will succumb to the disease within the first year; and this percentage has not changed over a quarter century.

Echocardiography remains the most useful test for the imaging and diagnosis of amyloid; however, it is not particularly useful for serial monitoring of patients for response or progression after treatment. The technique still suffers from interobserver variability, and the calculations of the septal thickness can vary substantially on serial measurements. Conversely, a septal thickness greater than 15 mm would be rare with hypertensive cardiomyopathy and would be limited to either amyloidosis or hypertrophic cardiomyopathy. Interestingly, the degree of cardiac infiltration in senile systemic and familial amyloid cardiomyopathy is substantially greater than that seen in AL amyloidosis. A patient with AL amyloidosis with a septal thickness greater than 18 mm will generally have significant disability related to cardiac failure. Patients with TTR amyloidosis, both mutant and wild-type, will frequently have septal thicknesses in the range of 25 mm with minimal symptomatology. The old echocardiographic finding of granular sparkling appearance is little used today. Other echocardiographic clues include thickening of the right ventricle and reduction in left ventricular chamber size.[37] Late consequences of cardiac involvement include valvular thickening and valvular regurgitation. Repair of the valve will not result in meaningful improvement in the patient's aerobic exercise capacity. The restriction to flow seen in restrictive cardiomyopathy can be confused with restrictive pericardial disease; and occasionally, patients have undergone pericardiectomies without benefit.[38] Endomyocardial biopsy is highly sensitive in the diagnosis of cardiac amyloidosis; and if five specimens are taken, recognition of the diagnosis is virtually certain. Patients with cardiac amyloidosis have poor atrial function and a high incidence of atrial standstill. Atrial and atrial appendage thrombi are well recognized and are potential sources of cardiac embolism.[39] Rare patients can develop amyloid deposition in the coronary microcirculation resulting in true

ischemic symptomatology and angina with normal epicardial coronary artery anatomy.[40]

Sudden death remains a problem in patients with amyloidosis.[41] The placement of an implantable defibrillator may not reduce the risk of sudden death.[42] Electromechanical dissociation is a common occurrence and the ability of a fibrillating amyloid heart to be appropriately shocked internally and establish hemodynamic stability has not been established.[43]

Diuretic therapy remains the mainstay of management for cardiac amyloidosis; but in these patients with noncompliant ventricular chambers, higher than normal filling pressures are often required to open the ventricle and fill it with blood. Aggressive diuretic therapy will often reduce preload, and this can result in drops in systolic blood pressure, reduced renal blood flow, and syncope.[44]

Familial amyloid cardiomyopathy is rare, but one special TTR mutant known as TTRVal122Ile requires awareness. In a prospective study of cord blood samples, this mutation was found in 3 percent of newborns of American parents of African descent. This compared with a prevalence of 0.44 percent in Americans of European descent and 0 percent of Americans of Hispanic descent. The degree of penetrance of this mutation at the clinical level has not been determined; however, in view of the high incidence and prevalence of this genetic abnormality, the diagnosis of cardiac amyloidosis in Americans of African descent warrants early analysis of the DNA for this mutation.[45,46]

Cardiac biomarkers play an important role in the prognosis of amyloid as well as in its functional assessment.[47] Both the B-natriuretic peptide and troponin levels predict outcomes in patients with amyloidosis and are important parts of the staging system for this disease.[48] Staging involves assigning a point for any of the following characteristics: difference between the involved and uninvolved free light chain of greater than 180 mg/L; for a cardiac troponin T level greater than 0.025 ng/mL; and for the N-terminal of the prohormone brain natriuretic peptide (NT-proBNP) level greater than 1800 pg/mL. This creates four stages with median survivals ranging from 6 months (stage 4) to 60 months (stage 1). Serialized measurements of the NT-proBNP also have been used to define response and progression and, in fact, have supplanted the use of serial echocardiography to assess changes over time, both in following the natural history as well as assessing response

TABLE 108–3. Suggested Testing of a Known Amyloid Patient

If mass spectroscopy identifies light-chain amyloid:

   Consider localized amyloidosis (bladder, larynx, skin, bronchi)

If systemic (visceral involvement) perform the following tests:

- Alkaline phosphatase
- Aspartate aminotransferase
- β_2-Microglobulin
- Bilirubin
- Calcium
- Creatinine
- Glucose
- Complete blood count
- Immunoglobulin free light chains
- Immunofixation and electrophoresis
- Serum and 24-hour urine
- Quantitative immunoglobulins
- N-terminal probrain natriuretic peptide
- Troponin T
- Factor X level
- Chest x-ray
- Electrocardiogram
- Echocardiogram
- Doppler and strain imaging
- Creatinine clearance

If mass spectroscopy identifies transthyretin (TTR) amyloid, perform these tests:

- Echocardiogram
- Doppler and strain imaging
- Familial amyloidosis genetic testing (mass spectroscopy of serum TTR; if abnormal, TTR gene sequencing)

to therapeutic interventions.[49–51] All patients who present with amyloidosis, whether or not cardiac disease is suspected, should have cardiac biomarkers performed. Table 108–3 lists the suggested diagnostic tests to perform when a patient with amyloidosis is seen.

Contrast-enhanced cardiac MRI is increasingly being used in the assessment of cardiac amyloid. Cardiac MRI (Fig. 108–6) can measure the thickness of the myocardium accurately and, after gadolinium injection, can demonstrate delayed subendocardial enhancement that can be quite specific for cardiac amyloidosis.[52,53] Phase-contrast MRI provides information on flow dynamics, diastolic filling parameters, and mitral peak in-flow velocity.[54] By providing a functional assessment, this technique can help establish an early diagnosis and has the potential to assess response to therapy. MRI cannot be used in the presence of a pacemaker or defibrillator or if there is renal insufficiency, because gadolinium is contraindicated. Radionuclide scanning is being explored for amyloidosis. Technetium pyrophosphate is a sensitive marker for the presence of ATTR amyloidosis, both wild-type and mutant, whereas uptake is not seen in AL amyloidosis.[55] A recent small study assessing ^{11}C-labeled Pittsburgh Compound-B (^{11}C-PiB)–based positron emission tomography (PET) imaging identified cardiac amyloid deposits in all patients with light chain amyloidosis and ATTR and was negative in controls.[56] Therefore, nuclear imaging in the future may not only help

confirm cardiac involvement by amyloidosis, but also help differentiate one type versus another.

Liver

Liver infiltration from amyloid can be seen in up to one-quarter of patients with AL amyloidosis.[17] These patients will present with hepatomegaly, elevation of the serum alkaline phosphatase with normal or near-normal transaminases and bilirubin. Half of the patients with hepatic amyloidosis have renal amyloidosis, which dominates the clinical syndrome. When a patient presents with hepatomegaly and imaging shows no filling defects, the presence of proteinuria, a monoclonal protein, or the presence of Howell–Jolly bodies in a blood film indicative of hyposplenism are highly suggestive of amyloidosis. Most patients have symptoms consistent with chronic liver disease, early satiety, anorexia, and unexplained weight loss. It is common to find spider telangiectasias on the upper chest. Portal hypertension and ascites are uncommon, however.[57] Rare instances of both hepatic and splenic rupture have been reported.[58] The diagnosis can usually be established with fat aspiration and marrow biopsy, but a liver biopsy is safe and does not have a higher risk of bleeding complications than in other patients with liver disease.

Nervous System

Amyloid, by virtue of its deposition in the vasa nervorum, causes a mixed axonal and demyelinating peripheral neuropathy. The neuropathy is symmetric, tends to ascend beginning in the toes, and eventually involves the upper extremities. It causes paresthesias, often painful dysesthesias, and eventually causes motor loss. Approximately half of the patients have an associated carpal tunnel syndrome, and approximately one-quarter have associated autonomic features including orthostatic hypotension, autonomic dysmotility of the gastrointestinal tract, including vomiting because of pseudoobstruction and alternating constipation with diarrhea, often intractable, and bladder abnormalities, including overflow incontinence and incomplete emptying.[59,60] The progression of amyloid neuropathy is slow, and it is common to have delays of 2 to 3 years before a diagnosis is established. Electromyography is not particularly useful in the early diagnosis because amyloid preferentially affects the small unmyelinated fibers of the extremities, which are not well assessed with standard electrodiagnostic studies. Patients with an unexplained peripheral neuropathy who are not diabetic should have immunofixation of serum and urine and a free light-chain assay performed. A positive finding requires the consideration of amyloidosis in the differential; although, for patients who have an immunoglobulin (Ig) M monoclonal protein, the possibility that the IgM is directly responsible for neuropathy in the absence of amyloid is significant. Sural nerve biopsies can usually detect the amyloid deposits, but there are reports in the literature of sural nerve biopsies having missed proven amyloidosis.[61] Mass spectroscopic analysis of the amyloid deposits is particularly important because of the high prevalence of neuropathy in patients with non-AL amyloidosis.

THERAPY

Treatment of amyloidosis has improved significantly with the introduction of novel agents and refinements in autologous stem cell transplantation. For years, the regimen of melphalan and prednisone was the standard of therapy, but the response rate never exceeded 25 percent, and the impact on survival was unimpressive. Melphalan and prednisone therapy has now been supplanted by the use of melphalan and dexamethasone, which has a very low therapy-related mortality and can be administered to patients with cardiac and renal failure as well as frail patients. The 5-year actuarial survival in patients treated with

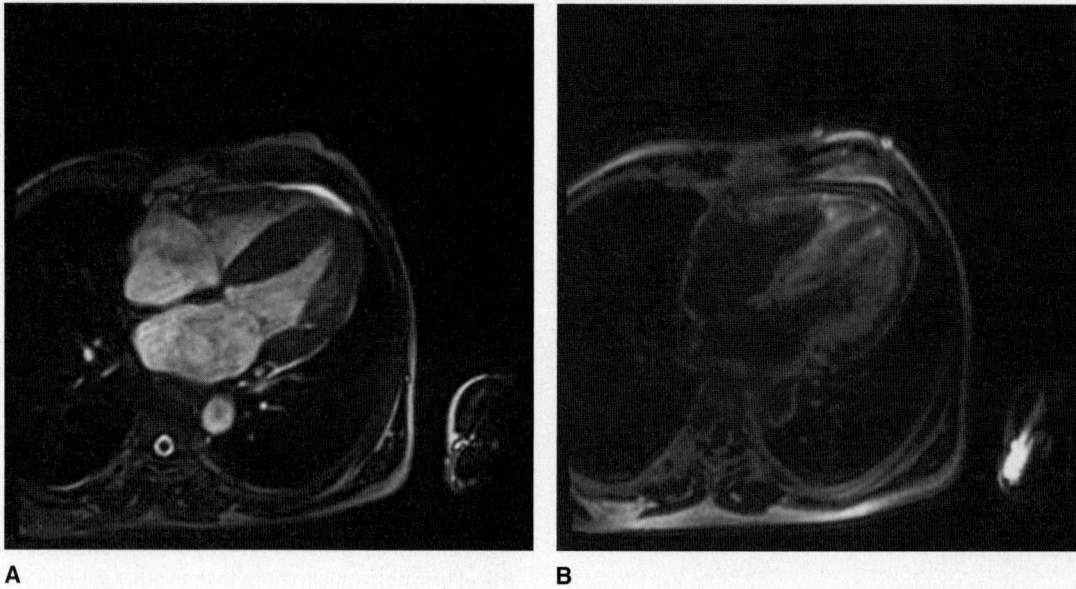

Figure 108–6. **A.** Magnetic resonance imaging demonstrating thickened interventricular septum from amyloid infiltration. **B.** Delayed gadolinium enhancement on subendocardial tissue is characteristic of amyloid cardiomyopathy.

melphalan and dexamethasone is 50 percent but is highly dependent on the enrolled population. Median responses as short as 10.5 and 17.5 months have been reported and are a function of the proportion of patients with advanced cardiac amyloid enrolled. Retreatment with melphalan and dexamethasone after an initial response also can be successful. It is often difficult to interpret results in phase 2 trials because of patient heterogeneity. Stratification of patients, based on the staging mentioned above, is important in reporting outcomes. Melphalan and dexamethasone should be considered the standard of care in patients that are not eligible for stem cell transplantation.[66]

AUTOLOGOUS STEM CELL TRANSPLANT

Most experts believe that autologous stem cell transplantation is the treatment of choice for patients with amyloidosis who do not have severe end-organ dysfunction, even though this approach has not been proven superior to conventional chemotherapy in prospective randomized trials or meta-analyses. However, it must be recognized that no more than 20 percent of patients with amyloidosis are eligible for stem cell transplantation. Currently, the therapy-related mortality at the Mayo Clinic is 2.5 percent (three out of 120), and the 10-year overall survival is 43 percent. Significant improvements in organ function and quality of life are commonly observed following stem cell transplantation and are strongly correlated with attainment of a very good partial response or better.[67-69] To reduce treatment-related mortality, current patient selection for transplantation includes age younger than 70 years, serum creatinine less than 1.8 mg/dL, serum troponin T less than 0.06, and an NT-proBNP less than 5000 pg/mL. The median age at the time of transplantation at the Mayo Clinic is 57 years. The median percent plasma cells in the marrow of transplanted patients is 7 percent, and the median urinary protein loss is just under 4 g/day. Seventy percent of patients who receive autologous stem cell transplantation have predominant renal involvement, 12 percent have peripheral neuropathy, and 14 percent have liver involvement. Patients with advanced cardiac involvement are generally excluded from transplantation, although half of transplanted patients have mild to moderate cardiac involvement as assessed by biomarkers and echocardiogram.

Blood stem cells are generally mobilized using leukocyte growth factors alone without cytotoxic chemotherapy to avoid hemodynamic deterioration during the mobilization process. A median of two aphereses are required to collect adequate stem cells for transplantation. The standard conditioning regimen is melphalan 200 mg/m^2, although the dose may be reduced for multiorgan involvement, age, and frailty. Induction chemotherapy is not generally administered prior to autologous stem cell transplantation, although this approach is considered in patients with significant marrow plasmacytosis, because of data suggesting an inferior outcome in such patients. In 2013, 40 percent of patients were transplanted at the Mayo Clinic without requiring hospitalization, and of the 60 percent of patients who were hospitalized, the median hospital stay was 6 days. Leukocyte growth factors are not routinely used after transplantation because they increase fluid retention. A partial response or better is seen in 75 percent of patients. Complete hematologic responses are documented in 40 percent of patients. Organ responses are seen in 50 percent of patients transplanted at the Mayo Clinic. Median survival for complete responders has not been reached, whereas patients with partial response or better have a median survival of 107 months. Predictors of outcome following autologous stem cell transplantation include cardiac biomarkers, NT-proBNP, and troponin.[70]

IMMUNOMODULATORY DRUGS

The combination of melphalan, dexamethasone, and lenalidomide has been reported for the treatment of AL amyloidosis. The maximum tolerated dose of lenalidomide was found to be 15 mg. Melphalan doses lower than those recommended for myeloma patients are used (0.18 mg/kg/day for 4 days every 28 days), with a complete response rate of 42 percent, an overall response rate of 58 percent, and a 2-year overall survival of 81 percent. Prophylaxis against deep venous thrombosis is required when lenalidomide is used. A combination of cyclophosphamide, thalidomide, and dexamethasone is safe and effective. In a risk-adapted all-oral therapy, 75 patients (with PS was 0-1) were treated, with a hematologic response in 74 percent, of which 21 percent were complete. The 3-year estimated overall survival was 82 percent, and grade 2 toxicity was seen in 52 percent. Lenalidomide and dexamethasone have been used in amyloidosis in a fashion identical to that used for multiple myeloma. It is important to remember that lenalidomide can increase the level of NT-proBNP and may actually aggravate heart failure.[71] Additionally, the typical dose of lenalidomide used to treat multiple myeloma is not well tolerated by AL patients and treatment should be initiated at a dose of no more than 15 mg daily. There is a high discontinuation rate of lenalidomide within the first three cycles. Myelosuppression, skin rash, and fatigue are common. In a study of lenalidomide and dexamethasone in patients who had failed melphalan and bortezomib, two patients died prior to first-response evaluation and 50 percent experienced grade 3 or greater toxicity. The hematologic response rate was 41 percent. The median overall survival was 14 months. Cyclophosphamide, lenalidomide, and dexamethasone have been used in the treatment of amyloidosis with lenalidomide at 15 mg per day and cyclophosphamide 100 mg per day. A partial response or greater was observed in 55 percent of patients, with complete responses in 8 percent, organ responses in 40 percent, and a 2-year overall survival of 41 percent. Cyclophosphamide, lenalidomide, and dexamethasone hematologic response rates ranged from 40 to 77 percent in three different studies. Complete responses did not exceed 10 percent. Lenalidomide toxicity was substantial and included fatigue and fluid retention.

Pomalidomide has been used with dexamethasone in relapsed amyloidosis. In a population of 33 evaluable patients, the response rate was 48 percent with a median time to response of 2 months. Organ improvement was found in 15 percent. The progression-free survival was 14 months; overall survival was 28 months.[72]

Bortezomib is highly active in the treatment of amyloidosis.[73] The combination with dexamethasone in untreated patients produces a 47 percent complete response rate, with higher responses seen in patients treated with twice-weekly bortezomib. The cardiac response rate is 29 percent. Hematologic responses are associated with cardiac response as measured by a reduction in NT-proBNP. Bortezomib also has been used with melphalan and dexamethasone, as well as cyclophosphamide with dexamethasone.[74] The CyBorD (cyclophosphamide, bortezomib, and dexamethasone) regimen was reported by the Mayo Clinic as a retrospective review of 17 patients with responses seen in 94 percent (71 percent complete, 24 percent partial) and a median time to response of 2 months.[75] In many published trials, patients with severe cardiac involvement were excluded; as a consequence, it is difficult to determine the efficacy of bortezomib in this difficult subgroup.[76] In one study of 38 patients with advanced cardiac disease using reduced doses of twice-weekly bortezomib and dexamethasone, 18 of 38 patients died during therapy; 21 patients achieved a hematologic response after a median of three cycles. In a series of 35 patients treated with bortezomib-dexamethasone with subsequent addition of cyclophosphamide, 86 percent achieved a rapid response. A second trial of cyclophosphamide-bortezomib-dexamethasone resulted in hematologic responses in 68 percent and a 1-year overall survival of 65 percent. Because bortezomib has been reported to increase the severity of heart failure in myeloma, it is clearly a concern that requires monitoring in patients. The oral proteasome inhibitor MLN9708, ixazomib, is currently under investigation.

Bortezomib and dexamethasone have been used as consolidation therapy following stem cell transplantation.[77] Forty patients were transplanted with risk-adapted melphalan; patients with less than a complete response received consolidation with bortezomib-dexamethasone. Survivals at 12 and 24 months post treatment were 88 and 82 percent, respectively. Of the original 40 patients, 23 received consolidation, and their response was enhanced in 20 (86 percent). Organ response occurred in 70 percent at 24 months. The use of bortezomib-dexamethasone consolidation following stem cell transplantation can help deepen the response in patients that do not achieve a complete response.

● COURSE AND PROGNOSIS

In spite of the introduction of new agents, late diagnosis, particularly of cardiac amyloid, remains a major barrier to improvement in the overall survival of patients; and despite recent improvements in survival, 40 percent of patients succumb to the disease within the first year after diagnosis, and this early mortality has not changed in 30 years. Patients can have a hematologic response and still die of end-organ damage because it is impossible to repair the tissue damage that has occurred prior to diagnosis.[64,65] The prognosis in amyloidosis is determined by two primary factors. The first is the extent of cardiac involvement, and the second is the plasma cell burden seen in these patients. The former, historically measured by echocardiography, is more reproducibly measured by the use of cardiac biomarkers. The percentage of plasma cells in the marrow has an important impact on prognosis.[9,62] The best surrogate and the most reproducible way to measure the plasma cell burden is to look at the difference between the involved and uninvolved light chains in the serum (dFLC). A four-stage prognostic model has been developed using measurements of NT-proBNP, troponin, and serum free light chains. One point each is assigned for a troponin T level of 0.025 ng/mL or greater, an NT-proBNP greater than 1800 pg/mL, and a free light chain difference of greater than 180 mg/L. This provides almost four equal-size groups (if you have none of the 3 its stage 1; if you have 1 its stage 2; if you have 2 its stage 3 and if you have all 3 its stage 4) with median overall survivals of 94, 40, 14, and 6 months, respectively. These serum tests are currently the standard for assessing prognosis in amyloidosis. Assessing response in amyloidosis is a twofold process. First, the hematologic response is assessed by determining the reduction of the plasma cell burden and of the production of precursor amyloid light chains achieved by systemic therapy. There are four classes of response: (1) complete remission defined by negative immunofixation of serum and urine and a normal immunoglobulin free light-chain ratio; (2) a very good partial response that requires the difference between involved and uninvolved serum free light chain be less than 40 mg/L; (3) a partial response is defined as a 50 percent decrease from baseline in the dFLC; and (4) failure to respond includes all other patients. Light-chain assessment is not only the ideal method for measuring response because of the rapid decline in levels if therapy is effective, but it is better than the intact immunoglobulin as a measure of response when both are present.[63] Although hematologic response is the first goal, the purpose of therapy is preservation of organ function. Therefore, to have a meaningful impact, an organ response should be seen. Current data indicate that organ response rates are directly linked to hematologic response rates; and the deeper the hematologic response, the more likely there will be an organ response. A renal response is defined as a 50 percent decrease in 24-hour urine protein. The decrease must be no less than 0.5 g/day without a change in serum creatinine. A 50 percent increase in urinary protein loss to at least 1 g/day or a 25 percent worsening of creatinine clearance is indicative of progression. Cardiac response is defined primarily by changes in the NT-proBNP. A 30 percent reduction in the NT-proBNP, a minimum of 300 ng/L in patients whose baseline NT-proBNP is greater than 650 ng/L, constitutes a response. However, we have seen patients in whom fluctuations of the NT-proBNP of as much as 30 percent can occur as a result of changes in diuretics or the development of superimposed pulmonary infections that are unrelated to true changes in cardiac function; consequently, some caution is warranted in interpreting the results. An improvement in New York Heart Association class by two stages from 4 to 2 or 3 to 1 also is considered a response. Historically, echocardiography has been used to assess response, but interobserver variability has rendered it less useful and echocardiography is not currently part of response criteria. Cardiac progression constitutes a 30 percent increase in NT-proBNP, a minimum increase of 300 ng/dL. Finally, liver response is defined as a 50 percent reduction in the abnormal alkaline phosphatase value, with progression defined as a 50 percent increase of alkaline phosphatase above the lowest recorded value. Currently, consensus criteria to define response in soft tissues, the gastrointestinal tract, the tongue, the lung, or the peripheral nerve do not exist for AL amyloidosis.

REFERENCES

1. Bobon J: [Professor Paul Divry 1889–1967] [in French]. *Acta Neurol Psychiatr Belg* 67(2):143–148, 1967.
2. Steensma DP: "Congo" red: Out of Africa? *Arch Pathol Lab Med* 125(2):250–252, 2001.
3. Cohen AS, Calkins E: Electron microscopic observations on a fibrous component in amyloid of diverse origins. *Nature* 183(4669):1202–1203, 1959.
4. Murakami T, Uchino M, Ando M: Genetic abnormalities and pathogenesis of familial amyloidotic polyneuropathy. *Pathol Int* 45(1):1–9, 1995.
5. Esplin BL, Gertz MA: Current trends in diagnosis and management of cardiac amyloidosis. *Curr Probl Cardiol* 38(2):53–96, 2013.
6. Fernandez-Flores A: A review of amyloid staining: Methods and artifacts. *Biotech Histochem* 86(5):293–301, 2011.
7. Picken MM: Non-light-chain immunoglobulin amyloidosis: Time to expand or refine the spectrum to include light+heavy chain amyloidosis? *Kidney Int* 83(3):353–356, 2013.
8. del Pozo Yauner L, Ortiz E, Sanchez R, et al: Influence of the germline sequence on the thermodynamic stability and fibrillogenicity of human lambda 6 light chains. *Proteins* 72(2):684–692, 2008.
9. Kourelis TV, Kumar SK, Gertz MA, et al: Coexistent multiple myeloma or increased bone marrow plasma cells define equally high-risk populations in patients with immunoglobulin light chain amyloidosis. *J Clin Oncol* 31(34):4319–4324, 2013.
10. Madan S, Dispenzieri A, Lacy MQ, et al: Clinical features and treatment response of light chain (AL) amyloidosis diagnosed in patients with previous diagnosis of multiple myeloma. *Mayo Clin Proc* 85(3):232–238, 2010.
11. Kyle RA, Linos A, Beard CM, et al: Incidence and natural history of primary systemic amyloidosis in Olmsted County, Minnesota, 1950 through 1989. *Blood* 79(7):1817–1822, 1992.
12. Pardanani A, Witzig TE, Schroeder G, et al: Circulating peripheral blood plasma cells as a prognostic indicator in patients with primary systemic amyloidosis. *Blood* 101(3):827–830, 2003.
13. Fonseca R, Ahmann GJ, Jalal SM, et al: Chromosomal abnormalities in systemic amyloidosis. *Br J Haematol* 103(3):704–710, 1998.
14. Bryce AH, Ketterling RP, Gertz MA, et al: Translocation t(11;14) and survival of patients with light chain (AL) amyloidosis. *Haematologica* 94(3):380–386, 2009.
15. Kyle RA, Gertz MA: Primary systemic amyloidosis: Clinical and laboratory features in 474 cases. *Semin Hematol* 32(1):45–59, 1995.
16. Lesser BA, Leeper KV Jr, Conway W. Obstructive sleep apnea in amyloidosis treated with nasal continuous positive airway pressure. *Arch Intern Med* 148(10):2285–2287, 1988.
17. Park MA, Mueller PS, Kyle RA, et al: Primary (AL) hepatic amyloidosis: Clinical features and natural history in 98 patients. *Medicine (Baltimore)* 82(5):291–298, 2003.
18. Neri A, Rubino P, Macaluso C, Gandolfi SA: Light-chain amyloidosis mimicking giant cell arteritis in a bilateral anterior ischemic optic neuropathy case. *BMC Ophthalmol* 13:82, 2013.
19. Foli A, Palladini G, Caporali R, et al: The role of minor salivary gland biopsy in the diagnosis of systemic amyloidosis: Results of a prospective study in 62 patients. *Amyloid* 18 (Suppl 1):80–82, 2011.
20. Aljaroudi WA, Desai MY, Tang WH, et al: Role of imaging in the diagnosis and management of patients with cardiac amyloidosis: State of the art review and focus on emerging nuclear techniques. *J Nucl Cardiol* 21(2):271–283, 2014.
21. Glaudemans AW, Slart RH, Noordzij W, et al: Utility of 18F-FDG PET(/CT) in patients with systemic and localized amyloidosis. *Eur J Nucl Med Mol Imaging* 40(7):1095–1101, 2013.
22. Hazenberg BP, van Rijswijk MH, Lub-de Hooge MN, et al: Diagnostic performance and prognostic value of extravascular retention of 123I-labeled serum amyloid P component in systemic amyloidosis. *J Nucl Med* 48(6):865–872, 2007.
23. Shidham VB, Hunt B, Jardeh SS, et al: Performing and processing FNA of anterior fat pad for amyloid. *J Vis Exp* (44), 2010.
24. Linke RP: On typing amyloidosis using immunohistochemistry. Detailed illustrations, review and a note on mass spectrometry. *Prog Histochem Cytochem* 47(2):61–132, 2012.
25. Schonland SO, Hegenbart U, Bochtler T, et al: Immunohistochemistry in the classification of systemic forms of amyloidosis: A systematic investigation of 117 patients. *Blood* 119(2):488–493, 2012.
26. Sethi S, Vrana JA, Theis JD, et al: Laser microdissection and mass spectrometry-based proteomics aids the diagnosis and typing of renal amyloidosis. *Kidney Int* 82(2):226–234, 2012.
27. Brambilla F, Lavatelli F, Di Silvestre D, et al: Reliable typing of systemic amyloidoses through proteomic analysis of subcutaneous adipose tissue. *Blood* 119(8):1844–1847, 2012.
28. Vrana JA, Gamez JD, Madden BJ, et al: Classification of amyloidosis by laser microdissection and mass spectrometry-based proteomic analysis in clinical biopsy specimens. *Blood* 114(24):4957–4959, 2009.
29. von Hutten H, Mihatsch M, Lobeck H, et al: Prevalence and origin of amyloid in kidney biopsies. *Am J Surg Pathol* 33(8):1198–1205, 2009.
30. Said SM, Sethi S, Valeri AM, et al: Renal amyloidosis: Origin and clinicopathologic correlations of 474 recent cases. *Clin J Am Soc Nephrol* 8(9):1515–1523, 2013.
31. Gertz MA, Leung N, Lacy MQ, et al: Clinical outcome of immunoglobulin light chain amyloidosis affecting the kidney. *Nephrol Dial Transplant* 24(10):3132–3137, 2009.
32. Duda SH, Raible RT, Risler T, et al: [Therapeutic bilateral renal artery embolization in the nephrotic syndrome] [in German]. *Dtsch Med Wochenschr* 119(3):58–62, 1994.
33. Sher T, Gertz MA: Recent advances in the diagnosis and management of cardiac amyloidosis. *Future Cardiol* 10(1):131–146, 2014.
34. Guan J, Mishra S, Falk RH, Liao R: Current perspectives on cardiac amyloidosis. *Am J Physiol Heart Circ Physiol* 302(3):H544–H552, 2012.
35. Suresh R, Grogan M, Maleszewski JJ, et al: Advanced cardiac amyloidosis associated with normal interventricular septal thickness: An uncommon presentation of infiltrative cardiomyopathy. *J Am Soc Echocardiogr* 27(4):440–447, 2014.
36. Falk RH: Senile systemic amyloidosis: Are regional differences real or do they reflect different diagnostic suspicion and use of techniques? *Amyloid* 19 Suppl 1:68–70, 2012.
37. Leone O, Longhi S, Quarta CC, et al: New pathological insights into cardiac amyloidosis: Implications for non-invasive diagnosis. *Amyloid* 19(2):99–105, 2012.
38. Singh V, Fishman JE, Alfonso CE: Primary systemic amyloidosis presenting as constrictive pericarditis. *Cardiology* 118(4):251–255, 2011.
39. Dubrey S, Pollak A, Skinner M, Falk RH: Atrial thrombi occurring during sinus rhythm in cardiac amyloidosis: Evidence for atrial electromechanical dissociation. *Br Heart J* 74(5):541–544, 1995.
40. Morin J, Schreiber WE, Lee C: Sudden death due to undiagnosed primary amyloidosis. *J Forensic Sci* 58(Suppl 1):S250–S252, 2013.
41. Dubrey SW, Rosser G, Dahdal MT, Gillmore JD: Diagnostic dilemma and sudden death outcome: A case of amyloid cardiomyopathy. *Clin Med* 12(6):596–597, 2012.
42. Dhoble A, Khasnis A, Olomu A, Thakur R: Cardiac amyloidosis treated with an implantable cardioverter defibrillator and subcutaneous array lead system: Report of a case and literature review. *Clin Cardiol* 32(8):E63–E65, 2009.
43. Lin G, Dispenzieri A, Kyle R, et al: Implantable cardioverter defibrillators in patients with cardiac amyloidosis. *J Cardiovasc Electrophysiol* 24(7):793–798, 2013.
44. Mohty D, Damy T, Cosnay P, et al: Cardiac amyloidosis: Updates in diagnosis and management. *Arch Cardiovasc Dis* 106(10):528–540, 2013.
45. Yamashita T, Hamidi Asl K, Yazaki M, Benson MD: A prospective evaluation of the transthyretin Ile122 allele frequency in an African-American population. *Amyloid* 12(2):127–130, 2005.
46. Afolabi I, Hamidi Asl K, Nakamura M, et al: Transthyretin isoleucine-122 mutation in African and American blacks. *Amyloid* 7(2):121–125, 2000.
47. Dispenzieri A, Gertz MA, Kumar SK, et al: High sensitivity cardiac troponin T in patients with immunoglobulin light chain amyloidosis. *Heart* 100(5):383–388, 2014.
48. Kumar S, Dispenzieri A, Lacy MQ, et al: Revised prognostic staging system for light chain amyloidosis incorporating cardiac biomarkers and serum free light chain measurements. *J Clin Oncol* 30(9):989–995, 2012.
49. Girnius S, Seldin DC, Cibeira MT, Sanchorawala V: New hematologic response criteria predict survival in patients with immunoglobulin light chain amyloidosis treated with high-dose melphalan and autologous stem-cell transplantation. *J Clin Oncol* 31(21):2749–2750, 2013.
50. Leung N, Glavey SV, Kumar S, et al: A detailed evaluation of the current renal response criteria in AL amyloidosis: Is it time for a revision? *Haematologica* 98(6):988–992, 2013.
51. Palladini G, Dispenzieri A, Gertz MA, et al: New criteria for response to treatment in immunoglobulin light chain amyloidosis based on free light chain measurement and cardiac biomarkers: Impact on survival outcomes. *J Clin Oncol* 30(36):4541–4549, 2012.
52. White JA, Kim HW, Shah D, et al: CMR imaging with rapid visual T1 assessment predicts mortality in patients suspected of cardiac amyloidosis. *JACC Cardiovasc Imaging* 7(2):143–156, 2014.
53. Mesquita D, Nobre C, Thomas B, et al: Cardiac amyloidosis: Diagnosis using delayed enhancement cardiac magnetic resonance imaging sequences. *Rev Port Cardiol* 32(11):941–945, 2013.
54. Gerbaud E, Lederlin M, Laurent F: Value of phase-sensitive inversion recovery sequence to perform and analyse late gadolinium enhancement in cardiac amyloidosis. *Arch Cardiovasc Dis* 102(12):859–860, 2009.
55. Glaudemans AW, van Rheenen RW, van den Berg MP, et al: Bone scintigraphy with technetium-hydroxymethylene diphosphonate allows early diagnosis of cardiac involvement in patients with transthyretin-derived systemic amyloidosis. *Amyloid* 21(1):35–44, 2014.
56. Antoni G, Lubberink M, Estrada S, et al: In vivo visualization of amyloid deposits in the heart with 11C-PIB and PET. *J Nucl Med* 54(2):213–220, 2013.
57. Norero B, Perez-Ayuso RM, Duarte I, et al: Portal hypertension and acute liver failure as uncommon manifestations of primary amyloidosis. *Ann Hepatol* 13(1):142–149, 2013.
58. Mousa AY, Abu-Halimah S, Alhalbouni S, et al: Amyloidosis and spontaneous hepatic bleeding, transcatheter therapy for hepatic parenchymal bleeding with massive intraperitoneal hemorrhage: A case report and review of the literature. *Vascular* 22(5):356–360, 2014.
59. Shin SC, Robinson-Papp J. Amyloid neuropathies. *Mt Sinai J Med* 79(6):733–748, 2012.
60. Adams D, Lozeron P, Lacroix C: Amyloid neuropathies. *Curr Opin Neurol* 25(5):564–572, 2012.
61. Rajani B, Rajani V, Prayson RA: Peripheral nerve amyloidosis in sural nerve biopsies: A clinicopathologic analysis of 13 cases. *Arch Pathol Lab Med* 124(1):114–118, 2000.

62. Dinner S, Witteles W, Witteles R, et al: The prognostic value of diagnosing concurrent multiple myeloma in immunoglobulin light chain amyloidosis. *Br J Haematol* 161(3):367–372, 2013.

63. Kumar SK, Dispenzieri A, Lacy MQ, et al: Changes in serum-free light chain rather than intact monoclonal immunoglobulin levels predicts outcome following therapy in primary amyloidosis. *Am J Hematol* 86(3):251–255, 2011.

64. Gatt ME, Palladini G: Light chain amyloidosis 2012: A new era. *Br J Haematol* 160(5):582–598, 2013.

65. Chari A, Barley K, Jagannath S, Osman K: Safety and efficacy of triplet regimens in newly diagnosed light chain amyloidosis. *Clin Lymphoma Myeloma Leuk* 13(1):55–61, 2013.

66. Palladini G, Milani P, Foli A, et al: Oral melphalan and dexamethasone grants extended survival with minimal toxicity in AL amyloidosis: Long-term results of a risk-adapted approach. *Haematologica* 99(4):743–750, 2014.

67. Dispenzieri A, Seenithamby K, Lacy MQ, et al: Patients with immunoglobulin light chain amyloidosis undergoing autologous stem cell transplantation have superior outcomes compared with patients with multiple myeloma: A retrospective review from a tertiary referral center. *Bone Marrow Transplant* 48(10):1302–1307, 2013.

68. Gertz MA, Dispenzieri A: Immunoglobulin light-chain amyloidosis: Growing recognition, new approaches to therapy, active clinical trials. *Oncology (Williston Park)* 26(2):152–161, 2012.

69. Schonland SO, Dreger P, de Witte T, Hegenbart U: Current status of hematopoietic cell transplantation in the treatment of systemic amyloid light-chain amyloidosis. *Bone Marrow Transplant* 47(7):895–905, 2012.

70. Gertz MA, Lacy MQ, Dispenzieri A, et al: Autologous stem cell transplant for immunoglobulin light chain amyloidosis: A status report. *Leuk Lymphoma* 51(12):2181–2187, 2010.

71. Dispenzieri A, Dingli D, Kumar SK, et al: Discordance between serum cardiac biomarker and immunoglobulin-free light-chain response in patients with immunoglobulin light-chain amyloidosis treated with immune modulatory drugs. *Am J Hematol* 85(10):757–759, 2010.

72. Dispenzieri A, Buadi F, Laumann K, et al: Activity of pomalidomide in patients with immunoglobulin light-chain amyloidosis. *Blood* 119(23):5397–5404, 2012.

73. Dubrey SW, Reece DE, Sanchorawala V, et al: Bortezomib in a phase 1 trial for patients with relapsed AL amyloidosis: Cardiac responses and overall effects. *QJM* 104(11):957–970, 2011.

74. Sher T, Hayman SR, Gertz MA: Treatment of primary systemic amyloidosis (AL): Role of intensive and standard therapy. *Clin Adv Hematol Oncol* 10(10):644–651, 2012.

75. Mikhael JR, Schuster SR, Jimenez-Zepeda VH, et al: Cyclophosphamide-bortezomib-dexamethasone (CyBorD) produces rapid and complete hematologic response in patients with AL amyloidosis. *Blood* 119(19):4391–4394, 2012.

76. Yamasaki S, Muta T, Higo T, et al: Ventricular fibrillation after bortezomib therapy in a patient with systemic amyloidosis. *Hematol Rep* 5(3):e12, 2013.

77. Landau H, Hassoun H, Rosenzweig MA, et al: Bortezomib and dexamethasone consolidation following risk-adapted melphalan and stem cell transplantation for patients with newly diagnosed light-chain amyloidosis. *Leukemia* 27(4):823–828, 2013.

CHAPTER 109
MACROGLOBULINEMIA

Steven P. Treon, Jorge J. Castillo, Zachary R. Hunter, and Giampaolo Merlini

SUMMARY

Waldenström macroglobulinemia (WM) is an indolent B-cell neoplasm manifested by the accumulation of clonal immunoglobulin (Ig) M secreting lymphoplasmacytic cells. MYD88[L265P] and CXCR4 WHIM (warts, hypogammaglobulinemia, infections, myelokathexis)-like somatic mutations are present in more than 90 percent, and 30 to 35 percent of WM patients, respectively, and impact disease presentation, treatment outcome, and/or overall survival. Familial predisposition is common in WM. Asymptomatic patients should be observed. Patients with disease-related hemoglobin of less than 10g/dL, platelets less than 100×10^9/L, bulky adenopathy and/or organomegaly, symptomatic hyperviscosity, peripheral neuropathy, amyloidosis, cryoglobulinemia, cold-agglutinin disease, or transformed disease should be considered for therapy. Plasmapheresis should be used for patients with symptomatic hyperviscosity, and prerituximab for those with high serum IgM levels to preempt a symptomatic IgM flare. The treatment choice should take into account specific goals of therapy, necessity for rapid disease control, risk of treatment-related neuropathy, immunosuppression and secondary malignancies, and planning for future autologous stem cell transplantation. Frontline treatments include rituximab alone or combined with alkylating agents (bendamustine, cyclophosphamide), proteasome inhibitors (bortezomib, carfilzomib), or nucleoside analogues (fludarabine, cladribine). In case of relapsed or treatment-resistant patients, an alternative frontline regimen or autologous stem cell transplantation can be considered. Novel targeted agents for the treatment of WM include everolimus and ibrutinib.

DEFINITION AND HISTORY

Waldenström macroglobulinemia (WM) is a lymphoid neoplasm resulting from the accumulation, predominantly in the marrow, of a clonal population of lymphocytes, lymphoplasmacytic cells, and plasma cells, which secrete a monoclonal immunoglobulin (Ig) M.[1] WM corresponds to lymphoplasmacytic lymphoma (LPL) as defined in the Revised European-American Lymphoma (REAL) and World Health Organization (WHO) classification systems.[2,3] Most cases of LPL are WM; less than 5 percent of cases are IgA-secreting, IgG-secreting, or nonsecreting LPL.

In 1944, Jan Waldenström, a Swedish physician-scientist, reported in *Acta Medica Scandinavica* three cases of a disease, he presciently thought was related to myeloma but for the absence of bone involvement and the scarcity of plasma cells in the infiltrate of small lymphocytes. He noted the increase in plasma protein concentration, marked increased serum viscosity, exaggerated bleeding and retinal hemorrhages, and virtually every other feature of the disorder in his case descriptions. In collaboration with a colleague, he showed, using ultracentrifugation and electrophoresis, that the abundant abnormal protein had a molecular weight of approximately 1 million and was not an aggregate of smaller proteins. The disease, which he described with such thoroughness, was later named in his honor.

EPIDEMIOLOGY

The age-adjusted incidence rate of WM is 3.4 per 1 million among males and 1.7 per 1 million among females in the United States. It increases in incidence geometrically with age.[4,5] The incidence rate is higher among Americans of European descent. Americans of African descent represent approximately 5 percent of all patients.

Genetic factors play a role in the pathogenesis of WM. Approximately 20 percent of WM patients are of Ashkenazi-Jewish ethnic background.[6] Familial disease has been reported commonly, including multigenerational clustering of WM and other B-cell lymphoproliferative diseases.[7–10] Approximately 20 percent of 257 sequential patients with WM presenting to a tertiary referral center had a first-degree relative with either WM or another B-cell disorder.[9] Familial clustering of WM with other immunologic disorders, including hypogammaglobulinemia and hypergammaglobulinemia (particularly polyclonal IgM), autoantibody production (particularly to the thyroid), and manifestation of hyperactive B cells has also been reported in relatives without WM.[9,10] Increased expression of the *BCL-2* gene with enhanced survival has been observed in B cells from familial patients and their family members.[10]

The role of environmental factors is uncertain, but chronic antigenic stimulation from infections and certain drug or chemical exposures have been considered but have not reached a level of scientific certainty. Hepatitis C virus (HCV) infection was implicated in WM causality in some series, but in a study of 100 consecutive WM patients in whom serologic and molecular diagnostic studies for HCV infection were performed, no association was found.[11–13]

PATHOGENESIS

NATURE OF THE WALDENSTRÖM MACROGLOBULINEMIA CLONE

Examination of the B-cell clone(s) found in the marrow of WM patients reveals a range of differentiation from small lymphocytes with large focal deposits of surface immunoglobulins, to lymphoplasmacytic cells, to mature plasma cells that contain intracytoplasmic IgM (Fig. 109–1).[14] Circulating clonal B cells are often detectable in patients with WM, although lymphocytosis is uncommon.[15,16] WM cells express the monoclonal IgM, and some clonal cells also express surface IgD.[17] The characteristic immunophenotypic profile of WM lymphoplasmacytic cells includes the expression of the pan–B-cell markers CD19, CD20 (including FMC7), CD22, and CD79.[17,18] Expression of CD5, CD10, and CD23 can be present in 10 to 20 percent of cases, and their presence does not exclude the diagnosis of WM.[19] Multiparameter flow cytometric analysis has also identified CD25 and CD27 as being characteristic of the WM clone, and found that a CD22[dim]/CD25[+]/CD27[+]/IgM[+] population may be present among clonal B lymphocytes in patients with

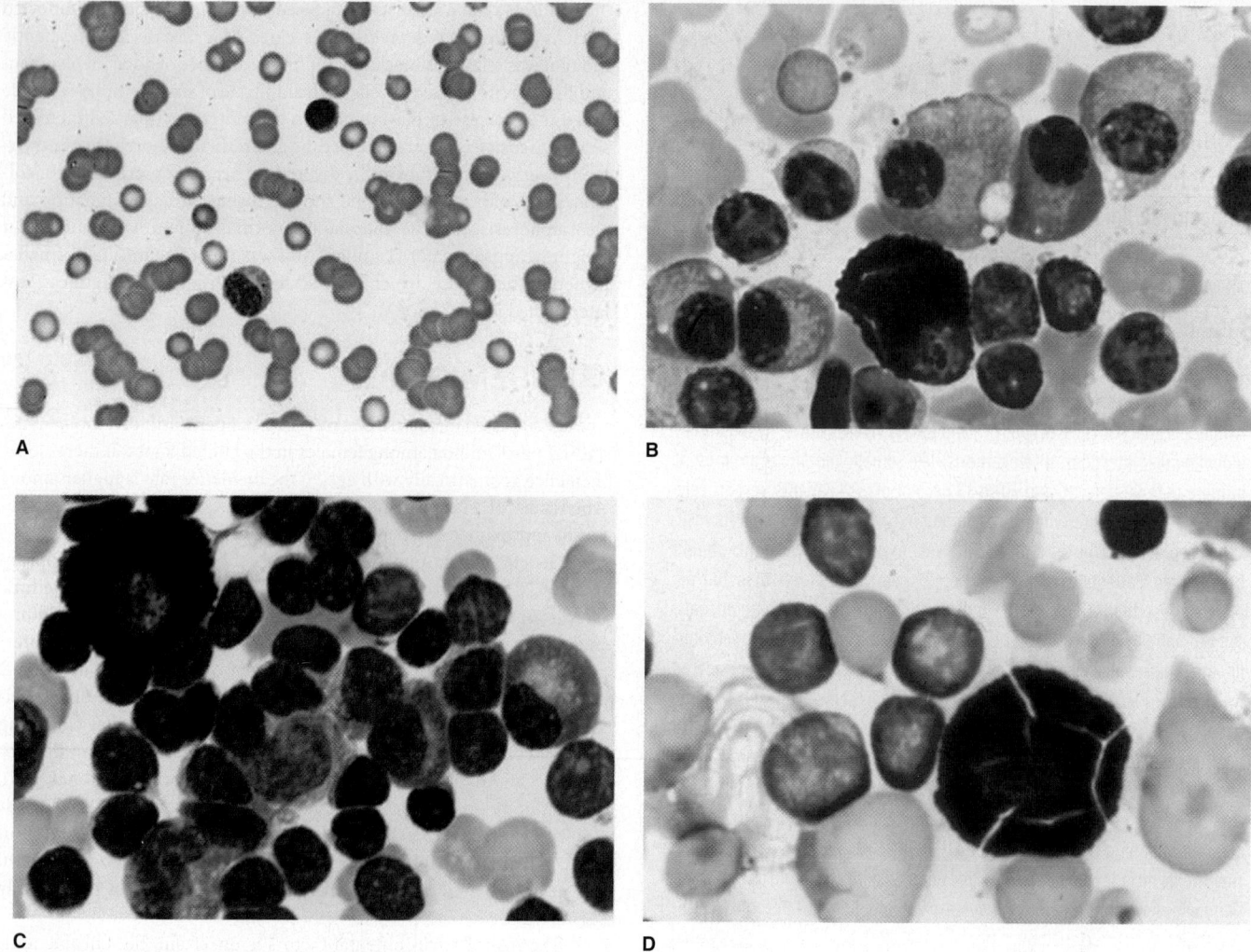

Figure 109–1. Waldenström macroglobulinemia. **A.** Blood film displaying the characteristic pathologic rouleaux seen as a result of the red cell aggregating properties of immunoglobulin M. **B.** Marrow film showing characteristic infiltrate of lymphocytes, lymphoplasmacytic cells, and plasma cells. A mast cell is evident lower center. Although not specific for this disease, mast cells are commonly present in the marrow. **C.** Marrow film showing infiltrate of lymphocytes with occasional plasma cells and a mast cell. **D.** Marrow film showing lymphocytic infiltrate with a "cracked" mast cell sometimes seen in this disease. The fraction of plasma cells varies as shown by the somewhat higher proportion in **(B)** as compared to **(C)** and **(D)**. Lymphocytes and lymphoplasmacytic cells predominate. *(Reproduced with permission from Lichtman's Atlas of Hematology, www.accessmedicine.com.)*

essential monoclonal gammopathy (synonym: monoclonal gammopathy of unknown significance [MGUS]) of the IgM type who ultimately progressed to WM.[20]

Somatic mutations in immunoglobulin genes are present with an increased frequency of nonsynonymous as compared to silent mutations in complement determining regions, along with somatic hypermutation, thereby supporting a postgerminal center derivation for the WM B-cell clone in most patients.[21,22] A strong preferential usage of *VH3/JH4* gene families without intraclonal variation, and without evidence for any isotype-switched transcripts is present.[23,24] These data support an IgM+ and/or IgM+IgD+ memory B-cell origin for most cases of WM.

In contrast to myeloma plasma cells, no recurrent translocations have been described in WM, which can help to distinguish WM from IgM myeloma cases, as IgM myeloma cases often exhibit t11;14 translocations.[25,26] Despite the absence of IgH translocations, recurrent chromosomal abnormalities are present in WM cells. These include deletions in chromosome 6q21–23 in 40 to 60 percent of WM patients, with concordant gains in 6p in 41 percent of 6q-deleted patients.[27–30] In a series of 174 untreated WM patients, 6q deletions, followed by trisomy 18, 13q

deletions, 17p deletions, trisomy 4, and 11q deletions, were observed.[30] Deletion of 6q and trisomy 4 were associated with adverse prognostic markers in this series. As 6q deletions represent the most recurrent cytogenetic finding in WM cases, there has been interest in identifying the region of minimal deletion and possible target genes within this region. Two putative gene candidates within this region are *TNFAIP3*, a negative regulator of nuclear factor kappa B signaling (NFκB), and *PRDM1*, a master regulator of B-cell differentiation.[29,31] The removal of a NFκB-negative regulator is of particular interest as the phosphorylation and translocation of NFκB into the nucleus is a crucial event for WM cell survival.[32] The success of proteasome inhibitor therapy in WM may occur because the degradation of negative regulators of NFκB, such as the inhibitor of kappa B (IκB), is blocked[33,34].

MUTATION IN MYD88

A highly recurrent somatic mutation (MYD88[L265P]) was first identified in WM patients by whole-genome sequencing (WGS), and confirmed by multiple studies through Sanger sequencing and/or allele-specific polymerase chain reaction (PCR) assays.[35–40] MYD88[L265P] is expressed in 90 to 95 percent of WM cases when more sensitive allele-specific PCR has been employed, using both CD19-sorted and unsorted marrow cells.[36–40] By comparison, MYD88[L265P] was absent in myeloma samples, including IgM myeloma, and was expressed in a small subset (6 to 10 percent) of marginal zone lymphoma patients, who surprisingly have WM-related features.[36–38,41] By PCR assays, 50 to 80 percent of IgM MGUS patients, also express MYD88[L265P], and expression of this mutation was associated with increased risk for malignant progression.[36–38,42] The presence of MYD88[L265P] in IgM MGUS patient suggests a role for this mutation as an early oncogenic driver, and other mutations and/or copy number alterations leading to abnormal gene expression are likely to promote disease progression.[29]

The impact of MYD88[L265P] to growth and survival signaling in WM cells has been addressed in several studies (Fig. 109–2). Knockdown of MYD88 decreased survival of MYD88[L265P]-expressing WM cells, whereas survival was enhanced by knock-in of MYD88[L265P] versus wild-type MYD88.[43] The discovery of a mutation in MYD88 is significant given its role as an adaptor molecule in toll-like receptor (TLR) and interleukin-1 receptor (IL-1R) signaling.[44] All TLRs except for TLR3 use MYD88 to facilitate their signaling. Following TLR or IL-1R stimulation, MYD88 is recruited to the activated receptor complex as a homodimer which then complexes with IRAK4 and activates IRAK1 and IRAK2.[45–47] Tumor necrosis factor receptor–associated factor 6 is then activated by IRAK1 leading to NFκB activation via IκBα phosphorylation.[48] Use of inhibitors of MYD88 pathway led to decreased IRAK1 and IκBα phosphorylation, as well as survival of MYD88[L265P] expressing WM cells. These observations are of particular relevance to WM since NFκB signaling is important for WM growth and survival.[49] Bruton tyrosine kinase (BTK) is also activated by MYD88[L265P].[43] Activated BTK coimmunoprecipitates with MYD88 that could be abrogated by use of a BTK kinase inhibitor, and overexpression of MYD88[L265P], but not wild-type(WT) MYD88, triggers BTK activation. Knockdown of MYD88 by lentiviral transfection or use of a MYD88 homodimerization inhibitor also abrogated BTK activation in MYD88[L265P]-mutated WM cells.

CXCR4[WHIM] Mutations

The second most common somatic mutation after MYD88[L265P] revealed by WGS was found in the C-terminus of the CXCR4 receptor. These mutations are present in 30 to 35 percent of WM patients, and impact serine phosphorylation sites that regulate CXCR4 signaling by its only known ligand, stromal cell-derived factor (SDF)-1a (CXCL12).[29,50–52] The location of somatic mutations found in the C-terminus of CXCR4 in WM are similar to those observed in the germline of patients with WHIM (warts, hypogammaglobulinemia, infections, and myelokathexis) syndrome, a congenital immunodeficiency disorder characterized by chronic noncyclic neutropenia.[53] Patients with WHIM syndrome exhibit impaired CXCR4 receptor internalization following SDF-1a stimulation, which results in persistent CXCR4 activation and myelokathexis.[54]

In WM patients, two classes of CXCR4 mutations occur in the C-terminus. These include nonsense (CXCR4[WHIM/NS]) mutations, which truncate the distal 15- to 20-amino-acid region, and frameshift (CXCR4[WHIM/FS]) mutations, which compromise a region of up to 40 amino acids in the C-terminal domain.[29,50] Nonsense and frameshift mutations are almost equally divided among WM patients with CXCR4 somatic mutations, and more than 30 different types of CXCR4[WHIM] mutations have been identified in WM patients.[29,50] Preclinical studies with WM cells engineered to express nonsense and frameshift CXCR4[WHIM]-mutated receptors have shown enhanced and sustained AKT and extracellular signal-regulated kinase (ERK) signaling following SDF-1a relative to CXCR4[WT] (see Fig. 109–2), as well increased cell migration, adhesion, growth and survival, and drug resistance of WM cells.[51,55,56]

Other Somatic Events

Many copy number alterations have been revealed in WM patients that impact growth and survival pathways. Frequent loss of *HIVEP2* (80 percent) and *TNFAIP3* (50 percent) genes that are negative regulators of NFκB expression (Fig. 109–2), as well as LYN (70 percent) and IBTK (40 percent) that modulate B-cell receptor (BCR) signaling have been

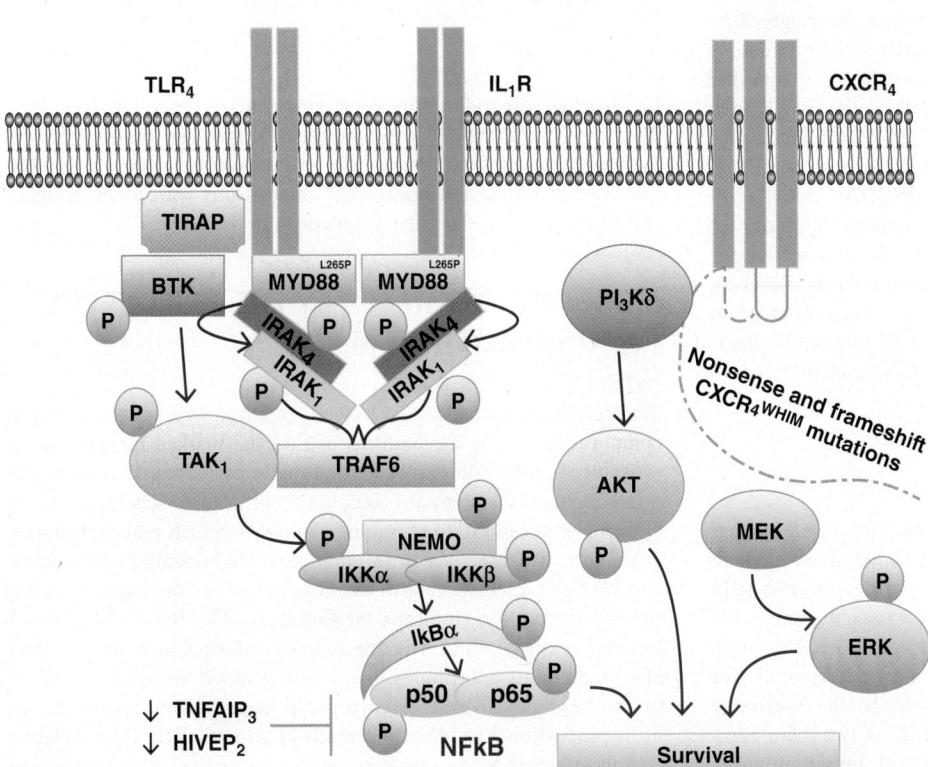

Figure 109–2. MYD88[L265P] and CXCR4[WHIM] mutations are highly prevalent in patients with Waldenström macroglobulinemia, and trigger transcriptional factors that include nuclear factor κB (NFκB), AKT, and extracellular signal-regulated kinase (ERK) that support the growth and survival of lymphoplasmacytic cells.

revealed by WGS.[29] WGS has also revealed common defects in chromatin remodeling with somatic mutations in ARID1A present in 17 percent, and loss of ARID1B in 70 percent of WM patients. Both ARID1A and ARID1B are members of the SWI/SNF family of proteins, and are thought to exert their effects via p53 and CDKN1A regulation. TP53 is mutated in 7 percent of sequenced WM genomes, while PRDM2 and TOP1 that participate in TP53-related signaling are deleted in 80 percent and 60 percent of WM patients, respectively.[29] Taken together, somatic events that contribute to impaired DNA damage response are also common in WM.

Impact of Waldenström Macroglobulinemia Genomics on Clinical Presentation

MYD88 and CXCR4 mutations are important determinants of the clinical presentation of WM patients. Significantly higher marrow disease involvement, serum IgM levels, and symptomatic disease requiring therapy, including hyperviscosity syndrome was observed in those patients with $MYD88^{L265P}CXCR4^{WHIM/NS}$ mutations.[50] Patients with $MYD88^{L265P}CXCR4^{WHIM/FS}$ or $MYD88^{L265P}CXCR4^{WT}$ had intermediate marrow and serum IgM levels; those with $MYD88^{WT}CXCR4^{WT}$ showed the lowest marrow disease burden. Fewer patients with $MYD88^{L265P}$ and $CXCR4^{WHIM/FS}$ or $CXCR4^{WHIM/NS}$, compared to $MYD88^{L265P}CXCR4^{WT}$ presented with adenopathy, further delineating differences in disease tropism based on CXCR4 status. Despite the more-aggressive presentation associated with $CXCR4^{WHIM/NS}$ genotype, risk of death was not impacted by CXCR4 mutation status. Risk of death was found to be 10-fold higher in patients with $MYD88^{WT}$ versus $MYD88^{L265P}$ genotype.[50]

MARROW MICROENVIRONMENT

Increased numbers of mast cells are found in the marrow of WM patients, wherein they are usually admixed with tumor cell aggregates (see Fig. 109–1).[14,18,57] The role of mast cells in WM was investigated in one study wherein coculture of primary autologous or mast cell lines with WM cells resulted in dose-dependent WM cell proliferation and/or tumor colony formation, through CD40 ligand (CD40L) signaling.[57] WM cells release soluble CD27 (sCD27), which may be triggered by cleavage of membrane-bound CD27 by matrix metalloproteinase 8 (MMP8).[58] sCD27 levels are elevated in the serum of WM patients, and follow disease burden in mice engrafted with WM cells, as well as in WM patients.[60] sCD27 triggers the upregulation of CD40L and a proliferation-inducing ligand (APRIL) on mast cells derived from WM patients, and mast cell lines through its receptor CD70. Modeling in mice engrafted with a CD70-blocking antibody shows inhibition of tumor cell growth, suggesting that WM cells require a microenvironmental support system for their growth and survival.[59] High levels of CXCR4 and very late antigen-4 (VLA-4) have also been observed in WM cells.[60] In blocking experiments studies, CXCR4 supported migration of WM cells, while VLA-4 contributed to adhesion of WM cells to marrow stromal cells.[60]

●CLINICAL FEATURES

Table 109–1 presents the clinical and laboratory findings at time of diagnosis of WM in one large institutional study.[16] Unlike most indolent lymphomas, splenomegaly and lymphadenopathy are uncommon (≤15 percent). Purpura is frequently associated with cryoglobulinemia and in rare circumstances with light-chain (AL) amyloidosis (Chap. 108). Hemorrhagic and neuropathic manifestations are multifactorial (see "Immunoglobulin M–Related Neuropathy" below). The morbidity associated with WM is caused by the concurrence of two main components: tissue infiltration by neoplastic cells and, importantly, the

TABLE 109–1. Clinical and Laboratory Findings for 356 Consecutive Newly Diagnosed Patients with Waldenström Macroglobulinemia

	Median	Range	Normal Reference Range
Age (years)	58	32–91	NA
Gender (male/female)	215/141		NA
Marrow involvement (% of area on slide)	30	5–95	NA
Adenopathy (% of patients)	15		NA
Splenomegaly (% of patients)	10		NA
IgM (mg/dL)	2620	270–12,400	40–230
IgG (mg/dL)	674	80–2770	700–1600
IgA (mg/dL)	58	6–438	70–400
Serum viscosity (cp)	2.0	1.1–7.2	1.4–1.9
Hematocrit (%)	35	17–45	35–44
Platelet count (× 10⁹/L)	275	42–675	155–410
White cell count (× 10⁹/L)	6.4	1.7–22	3.8–9.2
β_2M (mg/dL)	2.5	0.9–13.7	0–2.7
LDH (U/mL)	313	61–1701	313–618

β_2M, β_2-microglobulin; cp, centipoise; LDH, lactic dehydrogenase; NA, not applicable.

Data from patients seen at the Dana Farber Cancer Institute, Boston, MA.

physicochemical and immunologic properties of the monoclonal IgM. As shown in Table 109–2, the monoclonal IgM can produce clinical manifestations through several different mechanisms related to its physicochemical properties, nonspecific interactions with other proteins, antibody activity, and tendency to deposit in tissues.[61–63]

MORBIDITY MEDIATED BY THE EFFECTS OF IMMUNOGLOBULIN M

Hyperviscosity Syndrome

The increased plasma IgM levels leads to blood hyperviscosity and its complications.[64] The mechanisms behind the marked increase in the resistance to blood flow and the resulting impaired transit through the microcirculatory system are complex.[64–67] The main determinants are (1) a high concentration of monoclonal IgMs, which may form aggregates and may bind water through their carbohydrate component; and (2) their interaction with blood cells. Monoclonal IgM increases red cell aggregation (rouleaux formation; see Fig. 109–1) and red cell internal viscosity while reducing red cell deformability. The presence of cryoglobulins contributes to increasing blood viscosity, as well as to the tendency to induce erythrocyte aggregation. Serum viscosity is proportional to IgM concentration up to 30 g/L, then increases sharply at higher levels. Increased plasma viscosity may also contribute

TABLE 109–2. Physicochemical and Immunological Properties of the Monoclonal Immunoglobulin M Protein in Waldenström's Macroglobulinemia

Properties of IgM Monoclonal Protein	Diagnostic Condition	Clinical Manifestations
Pentameric structure	Hyperviscosity	Headaches, blurred vision, epistaxis, retinal hemorrhages, leg cramps, impaired mentation, intracranial hemorrhage
Precipitation on cooling	Cryoglobulinemia (type I)	Raynaud phenomenon, acrocyanosis, ulcers, purpura, cold urticaria
Autoantibody activity to myelin-associated glycoprotein, ganglioside M₁, sulfatide moieties on peripheral nerve sheaths	Peripheral neuropathies	Sensorimotor neuropathies, painful neuropathies, ataxic gait, bilateral foot drop
Autoantibody activity to IgG	Cryoglobulinemia (type II)	Purpura, arthralgia, renal failure, sensorimotor neuropathies
Autoantibody activity to red blood cell antigens	Cold agglutinins	Hemolytic anemia, Raynaud phenomenon, acrocyanosis, livedo reticularis
Tissue deposition as amorphous aggregates	Organ dysfunction	Skin: bullous skin disease, papules, Schnitzler syndrome
		Gastrointestinal: diarrhea, malabsorption, bleeding
		Kidney: proteinuria, renal failure (light-chain component)
Tissue deposition as amyloid fibrils (light-chain component most commonly)	Organ dysfunction	Fatigue, weight loss, edema, hepatomegaly, macroglossia, organ dysfunction of involved organs (heart, kidney, liver, peripheral sensory and autonomic nerves)

Ig, immunoglobulin.

to inappropriately low erythropoietin production, which is the major reason for anemia in these patients.[67] Renal synthesis of erythropoietin is inversely correlated with plasma viscosity. Clinical manifestations are related to circulatory disturbances that can be best appreciated by ophthalmoscopy, which shows distended and tortuous retinal veins, hemorrhages, and papilledema (Fig. 109–3).[68] Symptoms usually occur when the monoclonal IgM concentration exceeds 50 g/L or when serum viscosity is greater than 4.0 centipoises (cp), but there is individual variability, with some patients showing no evidence of hyperviscosity even at 10 cp.[64] The most common symptoms are oronasal mucosal bleeding, visual disturbances because of retinal bleeding, and dizziness that rarely may lead to stupor or coma. Heart failure can be aggravated, particularly in the elderly, owing to increased blood viscosity, expanded plasma volume, and anemia. Inappropriate red cell transfusion can exacerbate hyperviscosity and may precipitate cardiac failure.

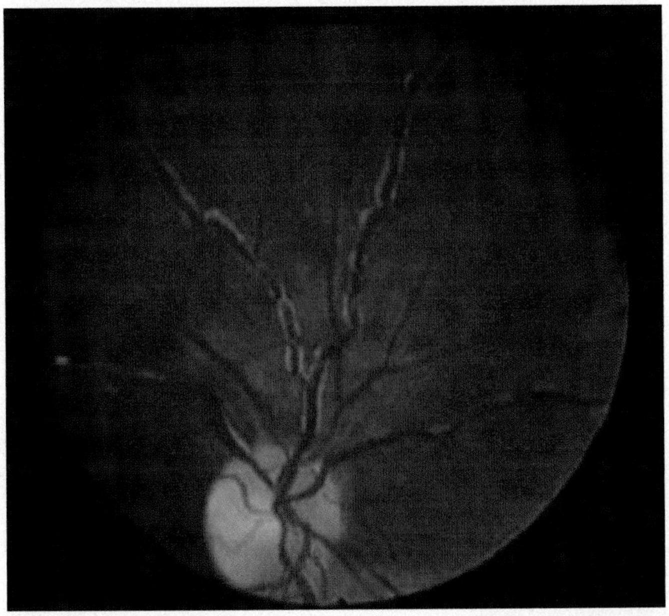

Cryoglobulinemia

The monoclonal IgM can behave as a cryoglobulin in up to 20 percent of patients, and is usually type I and asymptomatic in most cases.[16,64,70] Cryoprecipitation is mainly dependent on the concentration of monoclonal IgM; for this reason plasmapheresis or plasma exchange are commonly effective in this condition. Symptoms result from impaired blood flow in small vessels and include Raynaud phenomenon, acrocyanosis, and necrosis of the regions most exposed to cold, such as the tip of the nose, ears, fingers, and toes (Fig. 109–4), malleolar ulcers, purpura, and cold urticaria. Renal manifestations are infrequent. Mixed cryoglobulins (type II) consisting of IgM–IgG complexes may be associated with hepatitis C infections.[70]

Autoantibody Activity

Monoclonal IgM may exert its pathogenic effects through specific recognition of autologous antigens, the most notable being nerve constituents, immunoglobulin determinants, and red blood cell antigens.

Immunoglobulin M–Related Neuropathy

IgM-related peripheral neuropathy is common in WM patients, with estimated prevalence rates of 5 to 40 percent.[71-73] Approximately 8 percent of idiopathic neuropathies are associated with a monoclonal gammopathy, with a preponderance of IgM (60 percent) followed by IgG (30 percent) and IgA (10 percent) (Chap. 106).[74,75] The nerve damage is mediated by diverse pathogenetic mechanisms: (1) IgM antibody activity toward nerve constituents causing demyelinating polyneuropathies;

Figure 109–3. Funduscopic examination of a patient with Waldenström macroglobulinemia with hyperviscosity-related changes, including dilated retinal vessels, hemorrhages, and "venous sausaging." The white material at the edge of the veins may be cryoglobulin. *(Used with permission of Marvin J. Stone, MD.)*

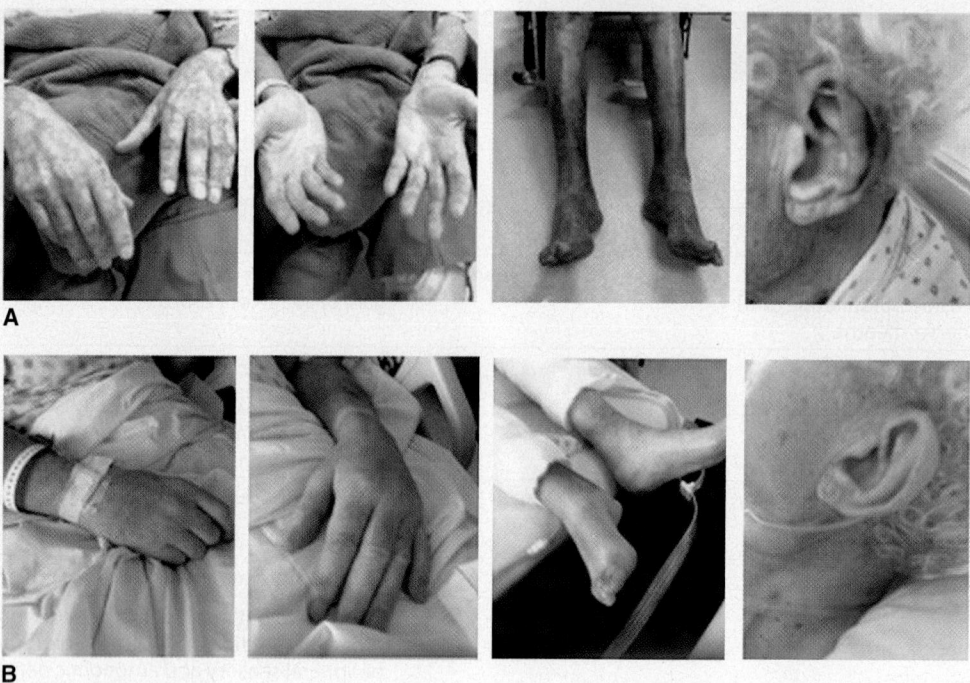

Figure 109–4. Cryoglobulinemia manifesting with severe acrocyanosis in a patient with Waldenström macroglobulinemia before **(A)** and following warming and plasmapheresis **(B)**.

(2) endoneurial granulofibrillar deposits of IgM without antibody activity, associated with axonal polyneuropathy; (3) occasionally by tubular deposits in the endoneurium associated with IgM cryoglobulin; and, rarely, (4) by amyloid deposits or by neoplastic cell infiltration of nerve structures.[73,76] Half of the patients with IgM neuropathy have a distinctive clinical syndrome that is associated with antibodies against a minor 100-kDa glycoprotein component of nerve known as the myelin-associated glycoprotein (MAG). Anti-MAG antibodies are generally monoclonal IgMκ, and usually also exhibit reactivity with other glycoproteins or glycolipids that share antigenic determinants with MAG.[77–79] The anti–MAG-related neuropathy is typically distal and symmetrical, affecting both motor and sensory functions; it is slowly progressive with a long period of stability.[72,80] Most patients present with sensory complaints (paresthesias, aching discomfort, dysesthesias, or lancinating pains), imbalance and gait ataxia, owing to lack proprioception; leg muscles atrophy in advanced stage. Patients with predominantly demyelinating sensory neuropathy in association with monoclonal IgM to gangliosides with disialosyl moieties, such as GD1b, GD3, GD2, GT1b, and GQ1b, have also been reported.[81,82] Anti-GD1b and anti-GQ1b antibodies were associated with sensory ataxic neuropathy. These antiganglioside monoclonal IgMs present core clinical features of chronic ataxic neuropathy sometimes with present ophthalmoplegia and/or red blood cell cold agglutinating activity. The disialosyl epitope is also present on red blood cell glycophorins, thereby accounting for the red cell cold agglutinin activity of anti-Pr2 specificity.[83,84] Monoclonal IgM proteins that bind to gangliosides with a terminal trisaccharide moiety, including ganglioside M_2 (GM_2) and GalNac-GD1A, are associated with chronic demyelinating neuropathy and severe sensory ataxia, unresponsive to glucocorticoids.[85] Antiganglioside IgM proteins may also cross-react with lipopolysaccharides of *Campylobacter jejuni*, whose infection is known to precipitate the Miller-Fisher syndrome, a variant of the Guillain-Barré syndrome.[86] Thus, molecular mimicry may play a role in this condition. Antisulfatide monoclonal IgM proteins, associated with sensory-sensorimotor neuropathy, have been detected in 5 percent of

patients with IgM monoclonal gammopathy and neuropathy.[87] Motor neuron disease has been reported in patients with WM and monoclonal IgM with anti-GM_1 and sulfoglucuronyl paragloboside activity.[88] Polyneuropathy, organomegaly, endocrinopathy, M protein, and skin changes (the POEMS syndrome) are rare in patients with WM.[89]

Cold Agglutinin Hemolytic Anemia

Monoclonal IgM may have cold agglutinin activity, that is, it can recognize specific red cell antigens at temperatures below 37°C, producing chronic hemolytic anemia. This disorder occurs in less than 10 percent of WM patients and is associated with cold agglutinin titers greater than 1:1000 in most cases.[90] The monoclonal component is usually an IgMκ and reacts most commonly with red cell I/i antigens, resulting in complement fixation and activation.[91,92] Mild to moderate chronic hemolytic anemia can be exacerbated after cold exposure. Hemoglobin usually remains above 70 g/L. The hemolysis is usually extravascular, mediated by removal of C3b opsonized red cells by the mononuclear phagocyte system, primarily in the liver. Intravascular hemolysis from complement destruction of red blood cell membrane is infrequent. The agglutination of red cells in the skin circulation also causes Raynaud syndrome, acrocyanosis, and livedo reticularis. Macroglobulins with the properties of both cryoglobulins and cold agglutinins with anti-Pr specificity can occur. These properties may have as a common basis the binding of the sialic acid-containing carbohydrate present on red blood cell glycophorins and on Ig molecules. Several other macroglobulins with antibody activity toward autologous antigens (e.g., phospholipids, tissue and plasma proteins) and foreign ligands have also been described.

Immunoglobulin M Tissue Deposition

The monoclonal protein can deposit in several tissues as amorphous aggregates. Linear deposition of monoclonal IgM along the skin basement membrane is associated with bullous skin disease.[93] Amorphous IgM deposits in the dermis result in IgM storage papules on the extensor surface of the extremities, referred to as macroglobulinemia cutis.[94] Deposition of monoclonal IgM in the lamina propria and/or submucosa of the intestine may be associated with diarrhea, malabsorption, and gastrointestinal bleeding.[95,96] Kidney involvement is less common and less severe in WM than in myeloma, probably because the amount of light chain excreted in the urine is generally lower in WM than in myeloma and because of the absence of contributing factors, such as hypercalcemia. Urinary cast nephropathy, however, has occurred in WM.[97] On the other hand, the IgM macromolecule is more susceptible to being trapped in the glomerular loops where ultrafiltration presumably contributes to its precipitation, forming subendothelial deposits of aggregated IgM proteins that occlude the glomerular capillaries.[98] Mild and reversible proteinuria may result and most patients are asymptomatic. The deposition of monoclonal light chain as fibrillar amyloid deposits (AL amyloidosis) is uncommon in patients with WM.[99] Clinical expression and prognosis are similar to those of other AL amyloidosis patients with involvement of heart (44 percent), kidneys (32 percent), liver (14 percent), lungs (10 percent), peripheral or autonomic nerves (38 percent), and soft tissues (18 percent). The incidence of cardiac and pulmonary involvement is higher in patients with monoclonal IgM than with other immunoglobulin isotypes. The association of WM with reactive amyloidosis has been documented rarely.[100,101] Simultaneous occurrence of fibrillary glomerulopathy, characterized by glomerular deposits of wide noncongophilic fibrils and amyloid deposits, has been described.[102]

MANIFESTATIONS RELATED TO TISSUE INFILTRATION BY NEOPLASTIC CELLS

Tissue infiltration by neoplastic cells is uncommon but can involve various organs and tissues, including the liver, spleen, lymph nodes, lungs, gastrointestinal tract, kidneys, skin, eyes, and central nervous system.

Lung

Pulmonary involvement in the form of masses, nodules, diffuse infiltrate, or pleural effusions is uncommon; the overall incidence of pulmonary and pleural findings is approximately 4 percent.[103-105] Cough is the most common presenting symptom, followed by dyspnea and chest pain. Chest radiographic findings include parenchymal infiltrates, confluent masses, and effusions.

Gastrointestinal Tract

Malabsorption, diarrhea, bleeding, or obstruction may indicate involvement of the gastrointestinal tract at the level of the stomach, duodenum, or small intestine.[106-109]

Renal System

In contrast to myeloma, infiltration of the kidney interstitium with lymphoplasmacytoid cell can occur in WM, and renal or perirenal masses are not uncommon.[110,111]

Skin

The skin can be the site of dense lymphoplasmacytic infiltrates, similar to that seen in the liver, spleen, and lymph nodes, forming cutaneous plaques and, rarely, nodules.[112] Chronic urticaria and IgM gammopathy are the two cardinal features of the Schnitzler syndrome, which is not usually associated initially with clinical features of WM, although evolution to WM is not uncommon.[113] Thus, close followup of these patients is important.

Joints

Invasion of articular and periarticular structures by WM malignant cells is rarely reported.[114]

Eye

The neoplastic cells can infiltrate the periorbital structures, lacrimal gland, and retroorbital lymphoid tissues, resulting in ocular nerve palsies.[115,116]

Central Nervous System

Direct infiltration of the central nervous system by monoclonal lymphoplasmacytic cells as infiltrates or as tumors constitutes the rarely observed Bing-Neel syndrome, characterized clinically by confusion, memory loss, disorientation, and motor dysfunction (reviewed in Ref. 117).

● LABORATORY FINDINGS

BLOOD ABNORMALITIES

Anemia is the most common finding in patients with symptomatic WM and is caused by a combination of factors: decrease in red cell survival, impaired erythropoiesis, moderate plasma volume expansion, hepcidin production leading to iron reutilization defect, and blood loss from the gastrointestinal tract.[16,118,119] Blood films are usually normocytic and normochromic, and rouleaux formation is often pronounced (see Fig. 109-1). Mean red cell volume may be elevated spuriously owing to erythrocyte aggregation. In addition, the hemoglobin estimate can be inaccurate, that is, falsely high, because of interaction between the monoclonal protein and the diluent used in some automated analyzers.[120] Leukocyte and platelet counts are usually within the reference range at presentation, although patients may occasionally present with severe thrombocytopenia. Monoclonal B-lymphocytes expressing surface IgM and late-differentiation B-cell markers are uncommonly detected in blood by flow cytometry. A raised erythrocyte sedimentation rate is almost always present and may be the first clue to the presence of the macroglobulinemia. The clotting abnormality detected most frequently is prolongation of thrombin time. AL amyloidosis should be suspected in all patients with nephrotic syndrome, cardiomyopathy, hepatomegaly, or peripheral neuropathy. Diagnosis requires the demonstration of green birefringence under polarized light of amyloid deposits stained with Congo red.

MARROW FINDINGS

Central to the diagnosis of WM is the demonstration, by trephine biopsy, of marrow infiltration by a lymphoplasmacytic cell population characterized by small lymphocytes with evidence of plasmacytoid and plasma cell maturation (see Fig. 109-1).[1,14] The pattern of marrow infiltration may be diffuse, interstitial, or nodular, usually with an intertrabecular pattern of infiltration. A solely paratrabecular pattern of infiltration is unusual and should raise the possibility of follicular lymphoma.[1] The marrow cell immunophenotype should be confirmed by flow cytometry and/or immunohistochemistry. The cell immunoprofile: sIgM+CD19+CD20+CD22+CD79+ is characteristic of WM.[14,120,121] Up to 20 percent of cases may express either CD5, CD10, or CD23.[19] In these cases, chronic lymphocytic leukemia and mantle cell lymphoma should be excluded. "Intranuclear" periodic acid-Schiff–positive inclusions (Dutcher-Fahey bodies)[122] consisting of IgM deposits in the perinuclear space, and sometimes in intranuclear vacuoles, may be seen occasionally in lymphoid cells. An increased number of mast cells, usually in association with the lymphoid aggregates is commonly found, and their presence may help in differentiating WM from other B-cell lymphomas (Fig. 109-5).[14] MYD88[L265P] testing of marrow samples has been incorporated into many clinical laboratories, and may help in clarifying the diagnosis of WM from other IgM-secreting entities.[35-39] The use of blood B cells may also permit determination of MYD88[L265P] status by allele-specific PCR assays, particularly in untreated WM patients.

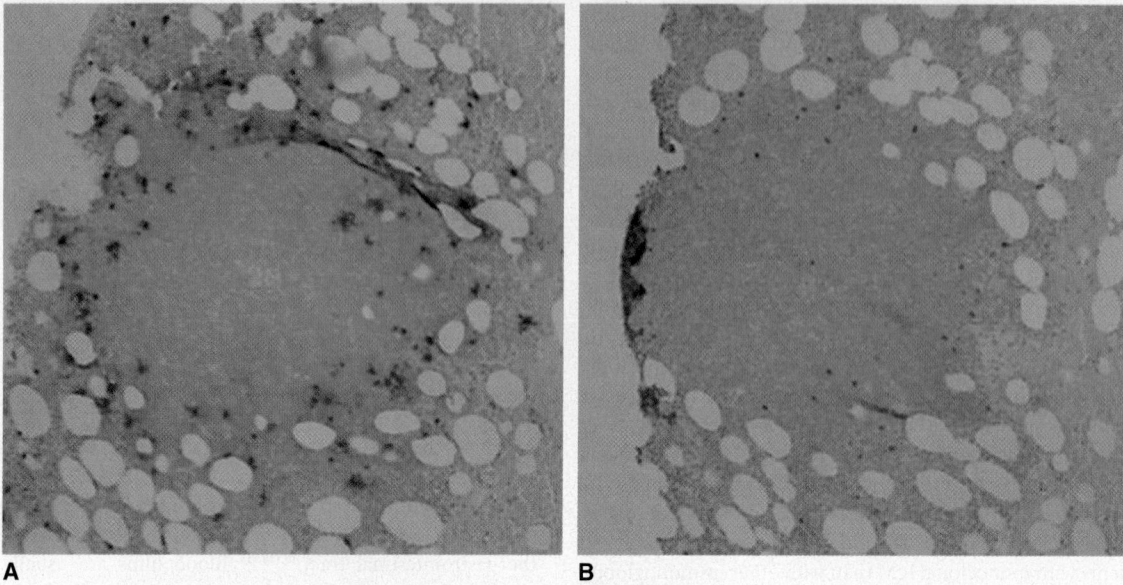

Figure 109–5. Marrow clot section. **A.** Tryptase-staining mast cells surrounding a nodule of lymphoplasmacytic cells in a patient with Waldenström macroglobulinemia. **B.** Mast cells in the same section exhibit strong CD40 ligand signaling, which has been shown to support (at least in part) the growth and survival of lymphoplasmacytic cells.

IMMUNOLOGIC ABNORMALITIES

High-resolution electrophoresis combined with immunofixation of serum and urine is recommended for identification and characterization of the IgM monoclonal protein. The light chain of the monoclonal IgM is κ in 75 to 80 percent of patients. More than one M component may be present. The concentration of the serum monoclonal protein is very variable but in most cases lies within the range of 15 to 45 g/L. Densitometry should be adopted to determine IgM levels for serial evaluations because nephelometry is unreliable and shows large laboratory variation. The presence of cold agglutinins or cryoglobulins may affect determination of IgM levels and, therefore, testing for cold agglutinins and cryoglobulins should be performed at diagnosis. If present, subsequent serum samples should be analyzed at 37°C for determination of serum monoclonal IgM level. Although Bence Jones proteinuria is frequently present, it exceeds 1 g/24 h in only 3 percent of cases. Whereas IgM levels are elevated in WM patients, IgA and IgG levels are most often depressed and do not recover after successful treatment.[123]

SERUM VISCOSITY

Because of its large size (almost 1,000,000 daltons), most IgM molecules are retained within the intravascular compartment and can exert an undue effect on serum viscosity.[64] Serum viscosity can be measured if the patient has signs or symptoms of hyperviscosity syndrome, although serum viscosity levels are erratic because of a lack of standardization in most clinical laboratories.[16] As such, inferences derived from serum IgM levels may be more reliable. Patients typically become symptomatic at serum viscosity levels of 4 cp and above, which relates to serum IgM levels above 6000 mg/dL.[124,125] Patients may be symptomatic at lower serum viscosity and IgM levels, and in these patients cryoglobulins may be present. Recurring nosebleeds, headaches, and visual disturbances are common symptoms in patients with symptomatic hyperviscosity.[16] Funduscopy is an important indicator of clinically relevant hyperviscosity. Among the first clinical signs of hyperviscosity are the appearance of peripheral and midperipheral dot and blot-like hemorrhages in the retina, which are best appreciated with indirect ophthalmoscopy and

scleral depression.[68] In more severe cases of hyperviscosity, dot, blot, and flame-shaped hemorrhages can appear in the macular area along with markedly dilated and tortuous veins with focal constrictions resulting in "venous sausaging," as well as papilledema. The effects of hyperviscosity are mediated by the blood viscosity as a result of IgM-red cell interactions but measurement of serum viscosity is much simpler than is blood viscosity and is not shear rate dependent so easier to related to clinical manifestations.

IMAGING

Magnetic resonance imaging (MRI) of the spine in conjunction with computed tomography (CT) of the abdomen and pelvis are useful in evaluating the disease status.[126] Marrow involvement can be documented by MRI studies of the spine in more than 90 percent of patients; CT of the abdomen and pelvis demonstrates enlarged nodes in approximately 40 percent of WM patients.[126]

LYMPH NODE BIOPSY

Lymph node biopsy may show preserved architecture or replacement by infiltration of neoplastic cells with lymphoplasmacytoid, lymphoplasmacytic, or polymorphous cytologic patterns.

POLYMERASE CHAIN REACTION

The residual disease after high-dose chemotherapy with allogeneic or autologous stem-cell rescue can be monitored by PCR-based methods using primers specific for the monoclonal Ig variable regions.

●TREATMENT

DECIDING ON INITIATING TREATMENT

As part of the Second International Workshop on Waldenström Macroglobulinemia, a consensus panel was organized to recommend criteria for the initiation of therapy in patients with WM.[127] The panel recommended that initiation of therapy should not be based on the IgM level per se, as this may not correlate with the clinical manifestations of WM.

The consensus panel did, however, agree that initiation of therapy is appropriate for patients with constitutional symptoms, such as recurrent fever, night sweats, fatigue as a consequence of anemia, or weight loss. Progressive symptomatic lymphadenopathy and/or splenomegaly provide additional reasons to begin therapy. Anemia with a hemoglobin value of 10 g/dL or less or a platelet count of 100×10^9/L or less owing to marrow infiltration, also justifies treatment. Certain complications, such as hyperviscosity syndrome, symptomatic sensorimotor peripheral neuropathy, systemic amyloidosis, renal insufficiency, or symptomatic cryoglobulinemia, may also be indications for therapy.[16,127]

INITIAL THERAPY

The International Workshops on Waldenström Macroglobulinemia have also formulated consensus recommendations for both initial therapy and therapy for refractory disease based on the best available evidence. The most recent recommendations emerged from the Seventh International Workshop on Waldenström Macroglobulinemia.[128] Individual patient considerations, including the presence of cytopenias, need for more rapid disease control, age, and candidacy for autologous transplant therapy, should be taken into account in making the choice of the drugs to use. For patients who are candidates for autologous stem cell transplantation, which typically is reserved for those patients younger than 70 years of age, the panel recommended that exposure to alkylating agents or nucleoside analogues should be limited. The use of nucleoside analogues should be approached cautiously in patients with WM as there appears to be an increased risk for the development of disease transformation, as well as myelodysplasia and acute myelogenous leukemia.

Oral Alkylating Agents

Oral alkylating drugs, alone and in combination therapy with glucocorticoids, have been extensively evaluated in the treatment of WM. Chlorambucil has been administered on both a continuous (i.e., daily dose schedule) and an intermittent schedule. Patients receiving chlorambucil on a continuous schedule typically receive 0.1 mg/kg per day, whereas on the intermittent schedule patients typically receive 0.3 mg/kg for 7 days, every 6 weeks. In a prospective randomized study, no significant difference in the overall response rate between these schedules was observed,[129] although the median response duration was greater for patients receiving intermittent-dose versus continuous-dose chlorambucil (46 vs. 26 months). Despite the favorable median response duration in this study for use of the intermittent schedule, no difference in the median overall survival was observed. Moreover, an increased incidence for development of myelodysplasia and acute myelogenous leukemia with the intermittent (three of 22 patients) versus the continuous (zero of 24 patients) chlorambucil schedule prompted the preference for use of continuous chlorambucil dosing. The use of glucocorticoids in combination with alkylating agent therapy has also been explored. Chlorambucil (8 mg/m²) plus prednisone (40 mg/m²) given orally for 10 days, every 6 weeks, resulted in a major response (i.e., reduction of IgM by more than 50 percent) in 72 percent of patients.[130] Alkylating agent regimens employing melphalan and cyclophosphamide in combination with glucocorticoids also have been examined.[131,132] This approach produced slightly higher overall response rates and response durations, although the benefit of these more complex regimens over chlorambucil remains to be demonstrated. Pretreatment factors associated with shorter survival in the entire population of patients receiving single-agent chlorambucil were age older than age 60 years, male sex, hemoglobin less than 10 g/dL, leukocytes less than 4×10^9/L, and platelets less than 150×10^9/L. Organomegaly, signs of hyperviscosity, renal failure, monoclonal IgM level, blood lymphocytosis, and percentage of marrow lymphoid cells were not significantly correlated with survival.[133] Additional factors to be taken into account in considering alkylating

agent therapy for patients with WM include necessity for more rapid disease control given the slow response, as well as consideration for preserving stem cells in patients who are candidates for autologous stem cell transplantation therapy. A large randomized study showed an inferior response rate and time to progression in WM patients receiving chlorambucil versus fludarabine, as well as a higher incidence of secondary malignancies in the former. Neutropenia was, however, more pronounced in those patients on fludarabine.[134]

Nucleoside Analogue Therapy

Cladribine administered as a single agent by continuous intravenous infusion, by 2-hour daily infusion, or by subcutaneous bolus injections for 5 to 7 days has resulted in major responses in 40 to 90 percent of patients who received primary therapy, whereas in the previously treated patients, responses have ranged from 38 to 54 percent.[135-141] Median time to achievement of response in responding patients following cladribine ranged from 1.2 to 5 months. The overall response rate with daily infusion of fludarabine, administered mainly on 5-day schedules, in previously untreated and treated patients, ranged from 38 to 100 percent and 30 to 40 percent, respectively,[142-147] similar to the responses to cladribine. Median time to achievement of response for fludarabine (3 to 6 months) was also similar to cladribine. In general, response rates and durations of responses have been greater for patients receiving nucleoside analogues as initial therapy, although in several studies in which both untreated and previously treated patients were enrolled, no difference in the overall response rate was reported.

Myelosuppression commonly occurs following prolonged exposure to either of the nucleoside analogues. A sustained decrease in both CD4+ and CD8+ T lymphocytes, measured 1 year following initiation of therapy, is notable.[135-137] Treatment-related mortality as a consequence of myelosuppression and/or opportunistic infections attributable to immunosuppression occurred in up to 5 percent of all treated patients in some series with nucleoside analogues.

Factors predicting for a better response to nucleoside analogues include younger age at start of treatment (<70 years), higher pretreatment hemoglobin (>95 g/L), higher platelet count (>75 × 10⁹/L), disease relapsing off therapy, and a long interval between first-line therapy and initiation of a nucleoside analogue in relapsing patients.[135,140,146] There are limited data on the use of an alternate nucleoside analogue in previously treated patients among whom disease relapsed or who had resistance when not on cladribine or fludarabine therapy.[148,149] Three of four (75 percent) patients responded to cladribine after progression following an unmaintained remission to fludarabine, whereas only one of 10 (10 percent) with disease resistant to fludarabine responded to cladribine.[148] A response in two of six patients (33 percent) and disease stabilization in the remaining patients to fludarabine, in spite of an inadequate response or progressive disease, following cladribine therapy has been reported.[149]

Harvesting autologous blood stem cells succeeded on the first attempt in 14 of 15 patients who did not receive nucleoside analogue therapy as compared to two of six patients who received a nucleoside analogue.[150] A sevenfold increase in transformation to an aggressive lymphoma and a threefold increase in the development of myelodysplasia or acute myelogenous leukemia were observed among patients who received a nucleoside analogue versus other therapies for their WM.[151] A meta-analysis of several trials in which patients were treated with nucleoside analogues in WM patients, included patients who had previously received an alkylating agent, and showed a crude incidence of approximately 8 percent for development of disease transformation and of approximately 5 percent for development of myelodysplasia or acute myelogenous leukemia.[152] None of the risk factors—that is, gender, age, family history of WM, or B-cell malignancies, typical markers of tumor burden and prognosis, type of nucleoside analogue therapy (cladribine vs. fludarabine), time from diagnosis to nucleoside analogue use, nucleoside analogue treatment as primary or salvage therapy, or treatment with an oral alkylator (i.e., chlorambucil)—predicted for the occurrence of transformation or development of myelodysplasia or acute myelogenous leukemia in patients treated with a nucleoside analogue.[152]

CD20-Directed Antibody Therapy

Rituximab is a chimeric monoclonal antibody that targets CD20, a widely expressed antigen on lymphoplasmacytic cells in WM.[153] Several retrospective and prospective studies indicated that rituximab, when used at standard doses (i.e., 4 weekly intravenous infusions of 375 mg/m²) induced major responses in approximately 30 percent of previously treated and untreated patients.[154,155] Even patients who achieved minor responses benefited from rituximab by improved hemoglobin and platelet counts, and reduction of lymphadenopathy and/or splenomegaly.[154] The median time to treatment failure in these studies was found to range from 8 to 27+ months. Patients on an extended rituximab schedule consisting of four weekly courses at 375 mg/m² per week, repeated 3 months later by another 4-week course have demonstrated major response rates of approximately 45 percent, with time to progression estimates of 16+ to 29+ months.[156,157]

In many WM patients, a transient increase or flare of the serum IgM may occur immediately following initiation of rituximab treatment.[156,158,159] Such an increase does not herald treatment failure and most patients will return to their baseline serum IgM level by 12 weeks. Some patients continue to show a prolonged increase in IgM despite an apparent reduction in their marrow tumor cells. However, patients with baseline serum IgM levels of greater than 50 g/dL or serum viscosity of greater than 3.5 cp may be particularly at risk for a hyperviscosity-related event and plasmapheresis should be considered in these patients in advance of rituximab therapy.[158] Because of the decreased likelihood of response in patients with higher IgM levels, as well as the possibility that serum IgM and blood viscosity levels may abruptly rise, rituximab monotherapy should not be used as sole therapy for the treatment of patients at risk for hyperviscosity signs and symptoms.[128,156,157]

Time to response after rituximab is slow and exceeds 3 months on the average. The time to best response in one study was 18 months.[157] Patients with baseline serum IgM levels of less than 60 g/dL are more likely to respond, regardless of the underlying marrow involvement by tumor cells.[156,157] An analysis of 52 patients who were treated with single-agent rituximab found the objective response rate was significantly lower in patients who had either low serum albumin (<35 g/L) or a serum monoclonal protein greater than 40 g/L.[160] The presence of both adverse prognostic factors was associated with a short time to progression (3.6 months). Patients who had normal serum albumin and relatively low serum monoclonal protein levels derived a substantial benefit from rituximab with a time to progression exceeding 40 months.

A correlation between polymorphisms at position 158 in the FcγRIIIa receptor (CD16), an activating Fc receptor on important effector cells that mediate antibody-dependent cell-mediated cytotoxicity, and rituximab response was observed in WM patients.[161] Individuals may encode either the amino acid valine or phenylalanine at position 158 in the FcγRIIIa receptor. WM patients who carried the valine amino acid (either in a homozygous or heterozygous pattern) had a fourfold higher major response rate (i.e., 50 percent decline in serum IgM levels) to rituximab versus those patients who expressed phenylalanine in a homozygous pattern.

Proteasome Inhibitors

Both bortezomib and carfilzomib have been evaluated in prospective studies in patients with WM, although the latter only in combination therapy (discussed below). In a retrospective study, 10 patients with refractory or relapsed WM were treated with bortezomib administered intravenously at a dose of 1.3 mg/m² on days 1, 4, 8, and 11 in a 21-day cycle for a total of four cycles. Most patients had been exposed to all active agents for WM and eight patients had received three or more regimens. Six of these patients achieved a partial response which occurred at a median of 1 month. The median time to progression in the responding patients is expected to exceed 11 months. Peripheral neuropathy occurred in three patients and one patient developed severe paralytic ileus in this series.[162] In a prospective study among 27 relapsed or refractory patients who received up to eight cycles of bortezomib at 1.3 mg/m² on days 1, 4, 8, and 11, median serum IgM levels declined significantly from 4.7 g/dL to 2.1 g/dL.[33] The overall response rate was 85 percent, with 10 and 13 patients achieving a minor (≥25 percent) and major (≥50 percent) decrease in IgM level. Responses occurred at a median of 1.4 months. The median time to progression for all responding patients in this study was 7.9 (range: 3.0 to 21.4+) months, and the most common grades III/IV toxicities were sensory neuropathies (22.2 percent), leukopenia (18.5 percent), neutropenia (14.8 percent), dizziness (11.1 percent), and thrombocytopenia (7.4 percent). Sensory neuropathies resolved or improved in nearly all patients following cessation of therapy. Twenty-seven patients with both untreated (44 percent) and previously treated (56 percent) disease received bortezomib, using the standard schedule until they either demonstrated progressive disease or two cycles beyond a complete response or stable disease.[163] The overall response rate was 78 percent, with major responses observed in 44 percent of patients. Sensory neuropathy occurred in 20 patients following two to four cycles of therapy. Among the 20 patients developing a neuropathy, 14 showed resolution or improvement 2 to 13 months after therapy.

Combination Therapies

Because rituximab is not myelosuppressive, its combination with chemotherapy has been explored. A regimen of rituximab, cladribine, and cyclophosphamide used in 17 previously untreated patients resulted in a partial response in 94 percent of WM patients, including a complete response in 18 percent.[164] No patient had relapsed with a median followup of 21 months. The combination of rituximab and fludarabine used in 43 patients of whom 32 (75 percent) were previously untreated, led to an overall response rate of 95.3 percent, with 83 percent of patients achieving a major response (i.e., 50 percent reduction in disease burden).[165] The median time to progression was 51.2 months in this series, and was longer for those patients who were previously untreated and for those achieving a very good partial remission (i.e., 90 percent reduction in disease) or better. Hematologic toxicity was common: grade 3 neutropenia and thrombocytopenia observed in 27 and four patients, respectively. Two deaths occurred in this study from pneumonia. Secondary malignancies including transformation to aggressive lymphoma and development of myelodysplasia or acute myelogenous leukemia were observed in six patients in this series. The addition of rituximab to fludarabine and cyclophosphamide has also been explored in previously treated patients, of whom four of five patients had a response.[166] In another combination study, rituximab along with pentostatin and cyclophosphamide given to 13 patients with untreated and previously treated WM or LPL resulted in a major response in 77 percent of patients.[167] The combination of rituximab, dexamethasone, and cyclophosphamide was used as primary therapy to treat 72 patients with WM in whom a major response was observed in 74 percent of patients in this study, and the 2-year progression-free survival was 67 percent.[168] Therapy was well tolerated, although one patient died of interstitial pneumonia.

Two studies examined cyclophosphamide, doxorubicin, vincristine, and prednisone (CHOP) in combination with rituximab (R-CHOP). In a randomized trial involving 69 patients, most of whom had WM, the addition of rituximab to CHOP resulted in a higher overall response rate (94 percent vs. 67 percent) and median time to progression (63 vs. 22 months) in comparison to patients treated with

CHOP alone.[169] R-CHOP was also used in 13 WM patients, 10 of whom had relapsed or refractory disease.[170] Among 13 evaluable patients, 10 patients achieved a major response (77 percent), including three complete and seven partial remissions. Two other patients achieved a minor response. In a retrospective study of symptomatic WM patients who received either R-CHOP; rituximab, cyclophosphamide, vincristine, and prednisone (R-CVP); or cyclophosphamide, prednisone, and rituximab (R-CP) and were similar in most pretreatment variables, the overall response rates to therapy were comparable among all three treatment groups—R-CHOP (96 percent), R-CVP (88 percent), and R-CP (95 percent)—although there was a trend for more complete remissions among patients treated with R-CVP and R-CHOP.[171] Adverse events attributed to therapy showed a higher incidence for neutropenic fever and treatment related neuropathy for R-CHOP and R-CVP versus R-CP. The results of this study suggest that in WM, the use of R-CP may provide analogous treatment responses to more intense cyclophosphamide-based regimens while minimizing treatment-related complications. The extended alkylator bendamustine has also been evaluated in combination with rituximab in both untreated, as well as previously treated WM patients. A randomized study by the German STiL Group examined bendamustine plus rituximab (BR) versus R-CHOP in patients with untreated, indolent B-cell lymphomas including WM.[172] Patients with WM in this study showed similar overall responses (96 percent vs. 94 percent), although progression-free survival was significantly longer (69 vs. 29 months) in patients who received BR versus R-CHOP. Treatment was also better tolerated in patients receiving BR. In the relapsed or refractory setting, an overall response rate of 83 percent was observed with bendamustine in combination with a CD20 monoclonal antibody.[173] The median time to progression was 13 months in this study. Prolonged myelosuppression was more common in patients who received prior nucleoside analogues.

The use of two cycles of oral cyclophosphamide along with subcutaneous cladribine to 37 patients with previously untreated WM led to a partial response in 84 percent of patients and the median duration of response was 36 months.[164] Fludarabine in combination with intravenous cyclophosphamide resulted in partial responses in six of 11 (55 percent) WM patients with either primary refractory disease or who had relapsed on treatment.[174] The combination of fludarabine plus cyclophosphamide was also evaluated in 49 patients, 35 of whom were previously treated. Seventy-eight percent of the patients achieved a response, and the median time to treatment failure was 27 months.[175] Hematologic toxicity was frequent, and three patients died of treatment-related toxicities. Two important findings in this study were the development of acute leukemia in two patients, histologic transformation to diffuse large B-cell lymphoma in one patient, and two cases of solid malignancies (prostate and melanoma), as well as failure to mobilize stem cells in 4 of 6 patients.

The combination of bortezomib, dexamethasone, and rituximab (BDR) as primary therapy in patients with WM resulted in an overall response rate of 96 percent, and a major response rate of 83 percent.[176] The incidence of grade 3 neuropathy was approximately 30 percent, but was reversible in most patients following discontinuation of therapy. An increased incidence of herpes zoster was also observed prompting the prophylactic use of antiviral therapy. Alternative schedules for administration of bortezomib (i.e., once weekly at higher doses) in combination with rituximab in patients with WM have achieved overall response rates of 80 to 90 percent.[177,178] The European Myeloma Network (EMN) recently showed that transitioning bortezomib from twice weekly intravenous dosing during the first cycle to weekly administration thereafter reduced grade 3 neuropathy to less than 10 percent in patients treated with BDR.[179] There have been no studies addressing the safety and efficacy of subcutaneous bortezomib use in WM.

Carfilzomib which is associated with a low risk of treatment-related peripheral neuropathy has been evaluated in combination with rituximab and dexamethasone (CaRD) in WM patients.[34] Carfilzomib was administered intravenously at 20 mg/m² (cycle one), then 36 mg/m² (cycles two to six), together with dexamethasone (20 mg) on days 1, 2, 8, and 9 as part of a 21-day cycle. As part of this regimen, rituximab 375 mg/m² was given on days 2 and 9 every 21 days. Maintenance therapy was given 8 weeks following induction therapy with intravenous carfilzomib (36 mg/m²) and dexamethasone (20 mg) administered on days 1 and 2 and rituximab 375 mg/m² on day 2 every 8 weeks for up to eight cycles. Overall response rate with this regimen was 87.1 percent (one complete response, 10 very good partial responses, 10 partial responses, and six minimal responses) and was not impacted by MYD88[L265P] or CXCR4[WHIM] mutation status. With a median followup of 15.4 months, 20 patients remained progression free. Grade 2 or higher toxicities included asymptomatic hyperlipasemia (41.9 percent), reversible neutropenia (12.9 percent), and cardiomyopathy in one patient (3.2 percent) with multiple risk factors. Treatment-related neuropathy, which was grade 2, occurred in one patient (3.2 percent). Declines in serum IgA and IgG were common, and some patients required intravenous gammaglobulin therapy for recurring sinus and bronchial infections.

Novel Therapeutics

The use of Ibrutinib was recently approved by the FDA for the treatment of symptomatic patients with WM. Ibrutinib targets BTK, a target of ibrutinib that is activated by MYD88[L265P].[43] In a multicenter study that examined the role of ibrutinib in previously treated (median: two prior therapies, 40 percent refractory) WM patients, the overall response rate was 91 percent.[180] Patients on this study received 420 mg/day of ibrutinib by mouth. Posttherapy, median serum IgM levels declined from 3610 to 915 mg/dL; hemoglobin rose from 10.5 to 13.5 g/dL; and marrow involvement declined from 60 percent to 25 percent. Decreased or resolved adenopathy was observed in 60 percent of patients with extramedullary disease, and five of nine patients with IgM-related peripheral neuropathy had symptomatic improvement. The 24-month estimate for progression-free and overall survival was 70 percent and 95 percent, respectively. Although major response rates were lower in patients with MYD88[WT] and CXCR4[WHIM] mutations, it is not recommended that genotyping be used to select which patients should go on ibrutinib until further data is available. Grade 2 or higher treatment-related toxicities included neutropenia (25 percent) and thrombocytopenia (14 percent), which were more common in heavily pretreated patients; atrial fibrillation associated with a prior history of arrhythmia (5 percent); and bleeding associated with procedures and marine oil supplements (3 percent). Serum IgA and IgG levels were unchanged following treatment with ibrutinib, and treatment-related infections were infrequent.

Everolimus is an oral inhibitor of the mammalian target of rapamycin (mTOR) pathway that is active in WM. A multicenter study examined everolimus in 60 previously treated patients that showed an overall response rate (ORR) of 73 percent, with 50 percent of patients attaining a major response.[181] The median progression-free survival in this study was 21 months. Grade 3 or higher related toxicities were observed in 67 percent of patients, with cytopenias constituting the most common toxicity. Pulmonary toxicity occurred in 5 percent of patients, and dose reductions as a result of toxicity occurred in 52 percent of patients. A clinical trial examining the activity of everolimus in 33 previously untreated patients with WM has also been reported that included serial marrow biopsies in response assessment.[182] The ORR in this study was 72 percent, including partial or better responses in 60 percent of patients. However, discordance between serum IgM levels upon which consensus criteria for response are based, and marrow disease response were common and complicated response assessment. In a few patients, discontinuation of everolimus led to rapid increases in serum IgM levels, and symptomatic hyperviscosity. Grade 2 or higher hematologic and nonhematologic toxicities in this study that were related to everolimus were predominately hematologic, including anemia (40 percent), thrombocytopenia (12 percent), and neutropenia (18 percent). Nonhematologic toxicities included oral ulcerations (27 percent), which improved with oral dexamethasone swish and spit solution, and pneumonitis (15 percent), which led to treatment discontinuation.

Maintenance Therapy

A large retrospective study examined the categorical responses outcome of rituximab-naïve patients who were either observed or received maintenance rituximabwere .[183] Categorical responses improved after induction therapy in 42 percent of patients who received maintenance rituximab versus 10 percent in patients on observation. Additionally, both progression-free survival (56.3 vs. 28.6 months) and overall survival (>120 vs. 116 months) were longer in patients who received maintenance rituximab. Improved progression-free survival was evident despite previous treatment status or induction with rituximab, either alone or in combination therapy. Best serum IgM response was also lower and hematocrit higher in those patients who received maintenance rituximab. Among patients who received maintenance rituximab therapy, an increased number of infectious events, predominantly grade 1 or 2 sinusitis and bronchitis were observed, along with lower serum IgA and IgG levels. A prospective study examining the role of maintenance rituximab was also initiated by the German STiL group.[184] In this study, patients received up to six cycles of bendamustine and rituximab, and responders randomized to either observation or maintenance rituximab every 2 months for 2 years. Enrollment for this study is complete and response outcome for maintenance rituximab therapy is awaited.

HIGH-DOSE THERAPY AND STEM CELL TRANSPLANTATION

The European Bone Marrow Transplant Registry reported the largest experience for both autologous as well as allogeneic stem cell transplantation (SCT) in WM.[185,186] Among 158 WM patients receiving an autologous SCT, which included primarily relapsed or refractory patients, the 5-year progression-free and overall survival rate was 39.7 percent and 68.5 percent, respectively.[185] Nonrelapse mortality at 1 year was 3.8 percent. Chemorefractory disease, and the number of prior lines of therapy at time of the autologous SCT were the most important prognostic factor for progression-free and overall survival. In the allogeneic SCT experience from the European Bone Marrow Transplant, the long-term outcome of 86 WM patients was reported.[186] A total of 86 patients received allograft by either myeloablative or reduced-intensity conditioning. The median age of patients in this series was 49 years, and 47 patients had three or more previous lines of therapy. Eight patients failed prior autologous SCT. Fifty-nine patients (68.6 percent) had chemotherapy-sensitive disease at the time of allogeneic SCT. Nonrelapse mortality at 3 years was 33 percent for patients receiving a myeloablative transplant, and 23 percent for those who received reduced-intensity conditioning. The overall response rate was 75.6 percent. The relapse rates at 3 years were 11 percent for myeloablative, and 25 percent for reduced-intensity conditioning recipients. Five-year progression-free and overall survival for WM patients who received a myeloablative allogeneic SCT were 56 percent and 62 percent, respectively, and for patients who received reduced intensity conditioning were 49 percent and 64 percent, respectively. The occurrence of chronic graft-versus-host disease was associated with improved progression-free survival, and suggested the existence of a clinically relevant graft-versus-WM effect in this study.

● RESPONSE CRITERIA IN WALDENSTRÖM MACROGLOBULINEMIA

Table 109–3 summarizes the response categories and criteria for progressive disease in WM based on the most recent consensus recommendations.[187] The term *overall response* is used to characterize all responses, including minor responses. Major responses only include partial, very good partial, and complete responses. The attainment of very good partial or complete responses is associated with improved progression-free survival.[155,165,176,179,188] Response assessments in WM rely primarily on serum IgM or IgM paraprotein levels, although complete responses require disappearance of the IgM monoclonal protein, and resolution of marrow and/or extramedullary WM disease.[187] An important concern with the use of IgM as a surrogate marker of disease is that it can fluctuate, independent

TABLE 109–3. Summary of Consensus Response Criteria for Waldenstrom's Macroglobulinemia[187]

Complete Response	CR	Absence of serum monoclonal IgM protein by immunofixation.
		Normal serum IgM level.
		Complete resolution of extramedullary disease, i.e., lymphadenopathy/splenomegaly if present at baseline.
		Morphologically normal marrow aspirate and trephine biopsy.
Very Good Partial Response	VGPR	Monoclonal IgM protein is detectable.
		90% reduction in serum IgM level from baseline, or normalization of serum IgM level.
		Complete resolution of extramedullary disease, i.e., lymphadenopathy/splenomegaly if present at baseline.
		No new signs or symptoms of active disease.
Partial Response	PR	Monoclonal IgM protein is detectable.
		≥50% but <90% reduction in serum IgM level from baseline.
		Reduction in extramedullary disease, i.e., lymphadenopathy/splenomegaly if present at baseline.
		No new signs or symptoms of active disease.
Minor Response	MR	Monoclonal IgM protein is detectable.
		≥25% but <50% reduction in serum IgM level from baseline.
		No new signs or symptoms of active disease.
Stable Disease	SD	Monoclonal IgM protein is detectable.
		<25% reduction and <25% increase in serum IgM level from baseline.
		No progression in extramedullary disease, i.e., lymphadenopathy/splenomegaly.
		No new signs or symptoms of active disease.
Progressive Disease	PD	>25% increase in serum IgM level from lowest nadir (requires confirmation) and/or progression in clinical features attributable the disease.

Reproduced with permission from Owen RG, Kyle RA, Stone MJ, et al: Response Assessment in Waldenström macroglobulinemia. *Br J Haematol* 160(2):171–176, 2013.

of tumor-cell killing with some agents. By way of example, rituximab can induce a flare in serum IgM levels, whereas everolimus, bortezomib, and ibrutinib can suppress IgM levels independent of tumor-cell killing in some patients, a finding referred to as IgM discordance.[158,159,162,181,183,189] Moreover, with selective B-cell–depleting agents such as rituximab and alemtuzumab, residual IgM-producing plasma cells are spared and continue to persist, thus potentially skewing the relative response and assessment to treatment.[190] sCD27 levels have been investigated as an alternative surrogate marker in WM given their correlation with WM disease burden, and may remain a faithful marker of disease in patients experiencing a rituximab-related IgM flare, as well as after plasmapheresis.[59,191] The use of quantitative allele-specific PCR assays to assess serial MYD88[L265P] burden in WM patients is also under investigation.[36,38]

● COURSE AND PROGNOSIS

WM typically presents as an indolent disease. The presence of 6q deletions may have prognostic significance, although this is disputed.[20,21] Age is an important prognostic factor (>65 years),[192–194] but is influenced by comorbidities. Anemia that reflects both marrow involvement and the serum level of the IgM monoclonal protein (because of the impact of IgM on intravascular fluid retention) has emerged as a strong adverse prognostic factor with hemoglobin levels of less than 9 to 12 g/dL associated with decreased survival in several series.[192–194]

Other cytopenias also may be significant predictors of survival.[193] The precise level of cytopenias with prognostic significance has not been determined. Some series have identified a platelet count of less than 100 to 150 × 10^9/L and a granulocyte count of less than 1.5 × 10^9/L as independent prognostic factors.[193,194] The number of cytopenias in a given patient has been proposed as a prognostic factor.[193] Serum albumin levels also correlate with survival in WM patients in some studies, using multivariate analyses.[193,195] Elevated serum β_2-microglobulin levels (>3.0 to 3.5 g/dL) have also shown strong prognostic correlation in WM.[193–196] Several scoring systems have been proposed based on these analyses (Table 109–4), including the WM International Prognostic Scoring System (WM IPSS) which incorporates five adverse covariates: advanced age (>65 years), hemoglobin less than or equal to 11.5 g/dL, platelet count less than or equal to 100 × 10^9/L, β_2-microglobulin greater than 3 mg/L, and serum monoclonal protein concentration greater than 7 g/dL.[197] Among 537 WM patients evaluated in the development of WM IPSS, low-risk patients (27 percent) presented with none or one of the adverse characteristics and advanced age, intermediate-risk patients (38 percent) with two adverse characteristics or only advanced age, and high-risk patients (35 percent) with more than two adverse characteristics. Five-year survival rates for these patients were 87 percent, 68 percent, and 36 percent, respectively. Importantly, the WM IPSS retained its prognostic significance in subgroups defined by age, treatment with alkylating agent and nucleoside analogues. Recent data from the

TABLE 109–4. Prognostic Scoring Systems in Waldenström Macroglobulinemia

Study	Adverse Prognostic Factors	Number of Groups	Survival
Gobbi and colleagues[185]	Hgb <9 g/dL	0–1 prognostic factors	Median: 48 months
	Age >70 years	2–4 prognostic factors	Median: 80 months
	Weight loss		
	Cryoglobulinemia		
Morel and colleagues[186]	Age ≥65 years	0–1 prognostic factors	5 year: 87% of patients
	Albumin <4 g/dL	2 prognostic factors	5 year: 62%
	Number of cytopenias:	3–4 prognostic factors	5 year: 25%
	Hgb <12 g/dL		
	Platelets <150 × 10^9/L		
	WBC <4 × 10^9/L		
Dhodapkar and colleagues[187]	β_2M ≥3 g/dL	β_2M <3 mg/dL + Hgb ≥12 g/dL	5 year: 87% of patients
	Hgb <12 g/dL	β_2M <3 mg/dL + Hgb <12 g/dL	5 year: 63%
	IgM <4 g/dL	β_2M ≥3 mg/dL + IgM ≥4 g/dL	5 year: 53%
		β_2M ≥3 mg/dL + IgM <4 g/dL	5 year: 21%
Application of International Staging System Criteria for Myeloma to WM Dimopoulos and colleagues[188]	Albumin ≤3.5 g/dL	Albumin ≥3.5 g/dL + β_2M <3.5 mg/dL	Median: NR
	β_2M ≥3.5 mg/L	Albumin ≤3.5 g/dL + β_2M <3.5 or	Median: 116 months
		β_2M 3.5–5.5 mg/dL	Median: 54 months
		β_2M >5.5 mg/dL	
International Prognostic Scoring System for WM Morel and colleagues[190]	Age >65 year	0–1 prognostic factors (excluding age)	5 year: 87% of patients
	Hgb <11.5 g/dL	2 prognostic factors (or age >65 years)	5 year: 68%
	Platelets <100 × 10^9/L	3–5 prognostic factors	5 year: 36%
	β_2M >3 mg/L		
	IgM >7 g/dL		

β_2M, β_2-microbloulin; Hgb, hemoglobulin; NR, not reported; WBC, white blood cell count.

Surveillance, Epidemiology, and End Results (SEER) database involving 7744 WM patients showed that the relative survival of WM patients has improved over time. Patients diagnosed during the years 2001 to 2010 had higher 5-year (78 percent vs. 67 percent) and 10-year (66 percent vs. 49 percent) relative survival rates versus patients diagnosed during the years 1980 to 2000.[198] A Greek study that included 345 patients with WM failed to show any overall or cause-specific survival improvement in recent years, although the study might have been too underpowered to detect any expected benefit.[199] A Swedish study of 1555 patients diagnosed with WM between 1980 and 2005 showed that the 5-year relative survival rate improved from 57 percent in 1980 to 1985 to 78 percent in 2001 to 2005.[200]

REFERENCES

1. Owen RG, Treon SP, Al-Katib A, et al: Clinicopathological definition of Waldenström's macroglobulinemia: Consensus Panel Recommendations from the Second International Workshop on Waldenström's macroglobulinemia. *Semin Oncol* 30:110, 2003.
2. Harris NL, Jaffe ES, Stein H, et al: A revised European-American classification of lymphoid neoplasms: A proposal from the International Lymphoma Study Group. *Blood* 84:1361, 1994.
3. Harris NL, Jaffe ES, Diebold J, et al: The World Health Organization classification of neoplastic diseases of the hematopoietic and lymphoid tissues. Report of the Clinical Advisory Committee meeting, Airlie House, Virginia, November, 1997. *Ann Oncol* 10:1419, 1999.
4. Groves FD, Travis LB, Devesa SS, et al: Waldenström's macroglobulinemia: Incidence patterns in the United States, 1988–1994. *Cancer* 82:1078, 1998.
5. Herrinton LJ, Weiss NS: Incidence of Waldenström's macroglobulinemia. *Blood* 82:3148, 1993.
6. Hanzis C, Ojha RP, Hunter Z, et al: Associated malignancies in patients with Waldenström's macroglobulinemia and their kin. *Clin Lymphoma Myeloma Leuk* 11:88, 2011.
7. Bjornsson OG, Arnason A, Gudmunosson S, et al: Macroglobulinaemia in an Icelandic family. *Acta Med Scand* 203:283, 1978.
8. Renier G, Ifrah N, Chevailler A, et al: Four brothers with Waldenström's macroglobulinemia. *Cancer* 64:1554, 1989.
9. Treon SP, Hunter ZR, Aggarwal A, et al: Characterization of familial Waldenström's macroglobulinemia. *Ann Oncol* 17:488, 2006.
10. Ogmundsdottir HM, Sveinsdottir S, Sigfusson A, et al: Enhanced B cell survival in familial macroglobulinaemia is associated with increased expression of Bcl-2. *Clin Exp Immunol* 117:252, 1999.
11. Santini GF, Crovatto M, Modolo ML, et al: Waldenström macroglobulinemia: A role of HCV infection? *Blood* 82:2932, 1993.
12. Silvestri F, Barillari G, Fanin R, et al: Risk of hepatitis C virus infection, Waldenström's macroglobulinemia, and monoclonal gammopathies. *Blood* 88:1125, 1996.
13. Leleu X, O'Connor K, Ho A, et al: Hepatitis C viral infection is not associated with Waldenström's macroglobulinemia. *Am J Hematol* 82:83, 2007.
14. Swerdlow SH, Campo E, Harris NL, et al., eds: *WHO Classification of Tumours of Haematopoietic and Lymphoid Tissues*, 4th ed. IARC, Lyon, 2008.
15. Smith BR, Robert NJ, Ault KA. In Waldenström's macroglobulinemia the quantity of detectable circulating monoclonal B lymphocytes correlates with clinical course. *Blood* 61:911, 1983.
16. Treon SP. How I treat Waldenström's macroglobulinemia. *Blood* 114:2375, 2009.
17. Preud'homme JL, Seligmann M. Immunoglobulins on the surface of lymphoid cells in Waldenström's macroglobulinemia. *J Clin Invest* 51:701, 1972.
18. San Miguel JF, Vidriales MB, Ocio E, et al: Immunophenotypic analysis of Waldenström's macroglobulinemia. *Semin Oncol* 30:187, 2003.
19. Hunter ZR, Branagan AR, Manning R, et al: CD5, CD10, and CD23 expression in Waldenström's macroglobulinemia. *Clin Lymphoma* 5:246, 2005.
20. Paiva B, Montes MC, García-Sanz R, et al: Multiparameter flow cytometry for the identification of the Waldenström's clone in IgM MGUS and Waldenström's Macroglobulinemia: New criteria for differential diagnosis and risk stratification. *Leukemia* 28:166, 2013.
21. Wagner SD, Martinelli V, Luzzatto L: Similar patterns of V kappa gene usage but different degrees of somatic mutation in hairy cell leukemia, prolymphocytic leukemia, Waldenström's macroglobulinemia, and myeloma. *Blood* 83:3647, 1994.
22. Aoki H, Takishita M, Kosaka M, Saito S. Frequent somatic mutations in D and/or JH segments of Ig gene in Waldenström's macroglobulinemia and chronic lymphocytic leukemia (CLL) with Richter's syndrome but not in common CLL. *Blood* 85:1913, 1995.
23. Shiokawa S, Suehiro Y, Uike N, Muta K, Nishimura J: Sequence and expression analyses of mu and delta transcripts in patients with Waldenström's macroglobulinemia. *Am J Hematol* 68:139, 2001.
24. Sahota SS, Forconi F, Ottensmeier CH, et al: Typical Waldenström macroglobulinemia is derived from a B-cell arrested after cessation of somatic mutation but prior to isotype switch events. *Blood* 100:1505, 2002.
25. Ackroyd S, O'Connor SJM, Owen RG: Rarity of IgH translocations in Waldenström macroglobulinemia. *Cancer Genet Cytogenet* 163:77, 2005.
26. Avet-Loiseau H, Garand R, Lode L, et al: 14q32 translocations discriminate IgM multiple myeloma from Waldenström's macroglobulinemia. *Semin Oncol* 30:153, 2003.
27. Braggio E, Keats JJ, Leleu X, et al: High-resolution genomic analysis in Waldenström's macroglobulinemia identifies disease-specific and common abnormalities with marginal zone lymphomas. *Clin Lymphoma Myeloma* 9:39, 2009.
28. Schop RF, Kuehl WM, Van Wier SA, et al: Waldenström macroglobulinemia neoplastic cells lack immunoglobulin heavy chain locus translocations but have frequent 6q deletions. *Blood* 100:2996, 2002.
29. Hunter ZR, Xu L, Yang G, et al: The genomic landscape of Waldenström's macroglobulinemia is characterized by highly recurring MYD88 and WHIM-like CXCR4 mutations, and small somatic deletions associated with B-cell lymphomagenesis. *Blood* 123:1637, 2014.
30. Nguyen-Khac F, Lambert J, Chapiro E, et al: Chromosomal aberrations and their prognostic value in a series of 174 untreated patients with Waldenström's macroglobulinemia. *Haematologica* 98:649, 2013.
31. Braggio E, Keats JJ, Leleu X, et al: Identification of copy number abnormalities and inactivating mutations in two negative regulators of nuclear factor-kappaB signaling pathways in Waldenström's macroglobulinemia. *Cancer Res* 69:3579, 2009.
32. Leleu X, Eeckhoute J, Jia X, et al: Targeting NF-kappaB in Waldenström macroglobulinemia. *Blood* 111:5068, 2008.
33. Treon SP, Hunter ZR, Matous J, et al: Multicenter clinical trial of bortezomib in relapsed/refractory Waldenström's macroglobulinemia: results of WMCTG Trial 03-248. *Clin Cancer Res* 13:3320, 2007.
34. Treon SP, Tripsas CK, Meid K, et al: Carfilzomib, rituximab and dexamethasone (CaRD) is active and offers a neuropathy-sparing approach for proteasome-inhibitor based therapy in Waldenström's macroglobulinemia. *Blood* 124:503, 2014.
35. Treon SP, Xu L, Yang G, et al: MYD88 L265P somatic mutation in Waldenström's macroglobulinemia. *N Engl J Med* 367:826, 2012.
36. Xu L, Hunter Z, Yang G, et al: MYD88 L265P in Waldenström macroglobulinemia, immunoglobulin M monoclonal gammopathy, and other B-cell lymphoproliferative disorders using conventional and quantitative allele-specific polymerase chain reaction. *Blood* 121:2051, 2013.
37. Varettoni M, Arcaini L, Zibellini S, et al: Prevalence and clinical significance of the MYD88 L265P somatic mutation in Waldenström macroglobulinemia, and related lymphoid neoplasms. *Blood* 121: 2522, 2013.
38. Jiménez C, Sebastián E, Del Carmen Chillón M, et al: MYD88 L265P is a marker highly characteristic of, but not restricted to, Waldenström's macroglobulinemia. *Leukemia* 27:1722, 2013.
39. Poulain S, Roumier C, Decambron A, et al: MYD88 L265P mutation in Waldenström macroglobulinemia. *Blood* 121: 4504, 2013.
40. Ansell SM, Hodge LS, Secreto FJ, et al: Activation of TAK1 by MYD88 L265P drives malignant B-cell growth in Non-Hodgkin lymphoma. *Blood Cancer J* 4:e183, 2014.
41. Ngo VN, Young RM, Schmitz R, et al: Oncogenically active MYD88 mutations in human lymphoma. *Nature* 470:115, 2011.
42. Landgren O, Staudt L: MYD88 L265P somatic mutation in IgM MGUS. *N Engl J Med* 367:2255, 2012.
43. Yang G, Zhou Y, Liu X, et al: A mutation in MYD88 (L265P) supports the survival of lymphoplasmacytic cells by activation of Bruton tyrosine kinase in Waldenström macroglobulinemia. *Blood* 122:1222, 2013.
44. Watters T, Kenny EF, O'Neill LAJ: Structure, function and regulation of the Toll/IL-1 receptor adaptor proteins. *Immunol Cell Biol* 85: 411, 2007.
45. Cohen L, Henzel WJ, Baeuerie PA. IKAP is a scaffold protein of the IkappaB kinase complex. *Nature* 395:292, 1998.
46. Loiarro M, Gallo G, Fanto N, et al: Identification of critical residues of the MYD88 death domain involved in the recruitment of downstream kinases. *J Biol Chem* 284: 28093, 2009.
47. Lin SC, Lo YC, Wu H: Helical assembly in the MYD88-IRAK4-IRAK2 complex in TLR/IL-1R signaling. *Nature* 465:885, 2010.
48. Kawagoe T, Sato S, Matsushita K, et al: Sequential control of Toll-like receptor dependent responses by IRAK1 and IRAK2. *Nat Immunol* 9:684, 2008.
49. Leleu X, Eeckhoute J, Jia X, et al: Targeting NF-kappaB in Waldenström macroglobulinemia. *Blood* 111: 5068, 2008.
50. Treon SP, Cao Y, Xu L, et al: Somatic mutations in MYD88 and CXCR4 are determinants of clinical presentation and overall survival in Waldenström macroglobulinemia. *Blood* 123:2791, 2014.
51. Roccaro A, Sacco A, Jiminez C, et al: C1013G/CXCR4 acts as a driver mutation of tumor progression and modulator of drug resistance in lymphoplasmacytic lymphoma. *Blood* 123:4120, 2014.
52. Poulain S, Roumier C, Doye E, et al: Genomic landscape of CXCR4 mutations in Waldenström's macroglobulinemia. *Blood* (ASH Annual Meeting Abstracts) 122(21) Abstract 1610, 2014.
53. Busillo JM, Amando S, Sengupta R, et al: Site-specific phosphorylation of CXCR4 is dynamically regulated by multiple kinases and results in differential modulation of CXCR4 signaling. *J Biol Chem* 285:7805, 2010.
54. Dotta L, Tassone L, Badolato R. Clinical and genetic features of warts, hypogammaglobulinemia, infections and myelokathexis (WHIM) syndrome. *Curr Mol Med* 11:317, 2011.
55. Cao Y, Hunter ZR, Liu X, et al: The WHIM-like CXCR4(S338X) somatic mutation activates AKT and ERK, and promotes resistance to ibrutinib and other agents used in the treatment of Waldenström's macroglobulinemia. *Leukemia* 29:169, 2015.

56. Cao Y, Hunter ZR, Liu X, et al: CXCR4 WHIM-like frameshift and nonsense mutations promote ibrutinib resistance but do not supplant MYD88 L265P directed signaling in Waldenström macroglobulinaemia cells. *Br J Haematol* 168:701, 2015.
57. Tournilhac O, Santos DD, Xu L, et al: Mast cells in Waldenström's macroglobulinemia support lymphoplasmacytic cell growth through CD154/CD40 signaling. *Ann Oncol* 17:1275, 2006.
58. Zhou Y, Liu X, Xu L, et al: Matrix metalloproteinase-8 is overexpressed in Waldenström's macroglobulinemia cells, and specific inhibition of this metalloproteinase blocks release of soluble CD27. *Clin Lymphoma Myeloma Leuk* 11:172, 2011.
59. Ho AW, Hatjiharissi E, Ciccarelli BT, et al: CD27–CD70 interactions in the pathogenesis of Waldenström macroglobulinemia. *Blood* 112:4683, 2008.
60. Ngo HT, Leleu X, Lee J, et al: SDF-1/CXCR4 and VLA-4 interaction regulates homing in Waldenström macroglobulinemia. *Blood* 112:150, 2008.
61. Merlini G, Farhangi M, Osserman EF: Monoclonal immunoglobulins with antibody activity in myeloma, macroglobulinemia and related plasma cell dyscrasias. *Semin Oncol* 13:350, 1986.
62. Farhangi M, Merlini G: The clinical implications of monoclonal immunoglobulins. *Semin Oncol* 13:366, 1986.
63. Marmont AM, Merlini G: Monoclonal autoimmunity in hematology. *Haematologica* 76:449, 1991.
64. Mackenzie MR, Babcock J: Studies of the hyperviscosity syndrome. II: Macroglobulinemia. *J Lab Clin Med* 85:227, 1975.
65. Gertz MA, Kyle RA: Hyperviscosity syndrome. *J Intensive Care Med* 10:128, 1995.
66. Kwaan HC, Bongu A: The hyperviscosity syndromes. *Semin Thromb Hemost* 25:199, 1999.
67. Singh A, Eckardt KU, Zimmermann A, et al: Increased plasma viscosity as a reason for inappropriate erythropoietin formation. *J Clin Invest* 91:251, 1993.
68. Menke MN, Feke GT, McMeel JW, et al: Hyperviscosity-related retinopathy in Waldenström's macroglobulinemia. *Arch Ophthalmol* 124:1601, 2006.
69. Merlini G, Baldini L, Broglia C, et al: Prognostic factors in symptomatic Waldenström's macroglobulinemia. *Semin Oncol* 30:211, 2003.
70. Stone MJ: Waldenström's macroglobulinemia: hyperviscosity syndrome and cryoglobulinemia. *Clin Lymphoma Myeloma* 9:97, 2009.
71. Dellagi K, Dupouey P, Brouet JC, et al: Waldenström's macroglobulinemia and peripheral neuropathy: A clinical and immunologic study of 25 patients. *Blood* 62:280, 1983.
72. Nobile-Orazio E, Marmiroli P, Baldini L, et al: Peripheral neuropathy in macroglobulinemia: Incidence and antigen-specificity of M proteins. *Neurology* 37:1506, 1987.
73. Treon SP, Hanzis C, Ioakimidis L, et al: Clinical characteristics and treatment outcome of disease-related peripheral neuropathy in Waldenström's macroglobulinemia (WM). *J Clin Oncol* 28:15s (Abstract 8114), 2010.
74. Nemni R, Gerosa E, Piccolo G, Merlini G: Neuropathies associated with monoclonal gammopathies. *Haematologica* 79:557, 1994.
75. Ropper AH, Gorson KC: Neuropathies associated with paraproteinemia. *N Engl J Med* 338:1601, 1998.
76. Vital A: Paraproteinemic neuropathies. *Brain Pathol* 11:399, 2001.
77. Latov N, Braun PE, Gross RB, et al: Plasma cell dyscrasia and peripheral neuropathy: Identification of the myelin antigens that react with human paraproteins. *Proc Natl Acad Sci U S A* 78:7139, 1981.
78. Chassande B, Leger JM, Younes-Chennoufi AB, et al: Peripheral neuropathy associated with IgM monoclonal gammopathy: Correlations between M-protein antibody activity and clinical/electrophysiological features in 40 cases. *Muscle Nerve* 21:55, 1998.
79. Weiss MD, Dalakas MC, Lauter CJ, et al: Variability in the binding of anti-MAG and anti-SGPG antibodies to target antigens in demyelinating neuropathy and IgM paraproteinemia. *J Neuroimmunol* 95:174, 1999.
80. Latov N, Hays AP, Sherman WH: Peripheral neuropathy and anti-MAG antibodies. *Crit Rev Neurobiol* 3:301, 1988.
81. Dalakas MC, Quarles RH: Autoimmune ataxic neuropathies (sensory ganglionopathies): Are glycolipids the responsible autoantigens? *Ann Neurol* 39:419, 1996.
82. Eurelings M, Ang CW, Notermans NC, et al: Antiganglioside antibodies in polyneuropathy associated with monoclonal gammopathy. *Neurology* 57:1909, 2001.
83. Ilyas AA, Quarles RH, Dalakas MC, et al: Monoclonal IgM in a patient with paraproteinemic polyneuropathy binds to gangliosides containing disialosyl groups. *Ann Neurol* 18:655, 1985.
84. Willison HJ, O'Leary CP, Veitch J, et al: The clinical and laboratory features of chronic sensory ataxic neuropathy with anti-disialosyl IgM antibodies. *Brain* 124:1968, 2001.
85. Lopate G, Choksi R, Pestronk A: Severe sensory ataxia and demyelinating polyneuropathy with IgM anti-GM$_2$ and GalNAc-GD1A antibodies. *Muscle Nerve* 25:828, 2002.
86. Jacobs BC, O'Hanlon GM, Breedland EG, et al: Human IgM paraproteins demonstrate shared reactivity between *Campylobacter jejuni* lipopolysaccharides and human peripheral nerve disialylated gangliosides. *J Neuroimmunol* 80:23, 1997.
87. Nobile-Orazio E, Manfredini E, Carpo M, et al: Frequency and clinical correlates of antineural IgM antibodies in neuropathy associated with IgM monoclonal gammopathy. *Ann Neurol* 36:416, 1994.
88. Gordon PH, Rowland LP, Younger DS, et al: Lymphoproliferative disorders and motor neuron disease: An update. *Neurology* 48:1671, 1997.
89. Pavord SR, Murphy PT, Mitchell VE: POEMS syndrome and Waldenström's macroglobulinaemia. *J Clin Pathol* 49:181, 1996.
90. Crisp D, Pruzanski W: B-cell neoplasms with homogeneous cold-reacting antibodies (cold agglutinins). *Am J Med* 72:915, 1982.
91. Pruzanski W, Shumak KH: Biologic activity of cold-reacting autoantibodies (first of two parts). *N Engl J Med* 297:538, 1977.
92. Pruzanski W, Shumak KH: Biologic activity of cold-reacting autoantibodies (second of two parts). *N Engl J Med* 297:583, 1977.
93. Whittaker SJ, Bhogal BS, Black MM: Acquired immunobullous disease: A cutaneous manifestation of IgM macroglobulinaemia. *Br J Dermatol* 135:283, 1996.
94. Daoud MS, Lust JA, Kyle RA, Pittelkow MR: Monoclonal gammopathies and associated skin disorders. *J Am Acad Dermatol* 40:507, 1999.
95. Gad A, Willen R, Carlen B, et al: Duodenal involvement in Waldenström's macroglobulinemia. *J Clin Gastroenterol* 20:174, 1995.
96. Case records of the Massachusetts General Hospital. Weekly clinicopathological exercises. Case 3–1990. A 66-year-old woman with Waldenström's macroglobulinemia, diarrhea, anemia, and persistent gastrointestinal bleeding. *N Engl J Med* 322:183, 1990.
97. Isaac J, Herrera GA: Cast nephropathy in a case of Waldenström's macroglobulinemia. *Nephron* 91:512, 2002.
98. Morel-Maroger L, Basch A, Danon F, et al: Pathology of the kidney in Waldenström's macroglobulinemia. Study of sixteen cases. *N Engl J Med* 283:123, 1970.
99. Gertz MA, Kyle RA, Noel P: Primary systemic amyloidosis: A rare complication of immunoglobulin M monoclonal gammopathies and Waldenström's macroglobulinemia. *J Clin Oncol* 11:914, 1993.
100. Moyner K, Sletten K, Husby G, Natvig JB: An unusually large (83 amino acid residues) amyloid fibril protein AA from a patient with Waldenström's macroglobulinaemia and amyloidosis. *Scand J Immunol* 11:549, 1980.
101. Gardyn J, Schwartz A, Gal R, et al: Waldenström's macroglobulinemia associated with AA amyloidosis. *Int J Hematol* 74:76, 2001.
102. Dussol B, Kaplanski G, Daniel L, et al: Simultaneous occurrence of fibrillary glomerulopathy and AL amyloid. *Nephrol Dial Transplant* 13:2630, 1998.
103. Rausch PG, Herion JC: Pulmonary manifestations of Waldenström macroglobulinemia. *Am J Hematol* 9:201, 1980.
104. Fadil A, Taylor DE: The lung and Waldenström's macroglobulinemia. *South Med J* 91:681, 1998.
105. Kyrtsonis MC, Angelopoulou MK, Kontopidou FN, et al: Primary lung involvement in Waldenström's macroglobulinaemia: Report of two cases and review of the literature. *Acta Haematol* 105:92, 2001.
106. Kaila VL, el Newihi HM, Dreiling BJ, et al: Waldenström's macroglobulinemia of the stomach presenting with upper gastrointestinal hemorrhage. *Gastrointest Endosc* 44:73, 1996.
107. Yasui O, Tukamoto F, Sasaki N, et al: Malignant lymphoma of the transverse colon associated with macroglobulinemia. *Am J Gastroenterol* 92:2299, 1997.
108. Rosenthal JA, Curran WJ Jr, Schuster SJ: Waldenström's macroglobulinemia resulting from localized gastric lymphoplasmacytoid lymphoma. *Am J Hematol* 58:244, 1998.
109. Recine MA, Perez MT, Cabello-Inchausti B, et al: Extranodal lymphoplasmacytoid lymphoma (immunocytoma) presenting as small intestinal obstruction. *Arch Pathol Lab Med* 125:677, 2001.
110. Veltman GA, van Veen S, Kluin-Nelemans JC, et al: Renal disease in Waldenström's macroglobulinaemia. *Nephrol Dial Transplant* 12:1256, 1997.
111. Moore DF Jr, Moulopoulos LA, Dimopoulos MA: Waldenström macroglobulinemia presenting as a renal or perirenal mass: Clinical and radiographic features. *Leuk Lymphoma* 17:331, 1995.
112. Mascaro JM, Montserrat E, Estrach T, et al: Specific cutaneous manifestations of Waldenström's macroglobulinaemia. A report of two cases. *Br J Dermatol* 106:17, 1982.
113. Schnitzler L, Schubert B, Boasson M, et al: Urticaire chronique, lésions osseuses, macroglobulinémie IgM: Maladie de Waldenström? *Bull Soc Fr Dermatol Syphiligr* 81:363, 1974.
114. Roux S, Fermand JP, Brechignac S, et al: Tumoral joint involvement in multiple myeloma and Waldenström's macroglobulinemia—Report of 4 cases. *J Rheumatol* 23:2175, 1996.
115. Orellana J, Friedman AH: Ocular manifestations of multiple myeloma, Waldenström's macroglobulinemia and benign monoclonal gammopathy. *Surv Ophthalmol* 26:157, 1981.
116. Ettl AR, Birbamer GG, Philipp W: Orbital involvement in Waldenström's macroglobulinemia: Ultrasound, computed tomography and magnetic resonance findings. *Ophthalmologica* 205:40, 1992.
117. Civit T, Coulbois S, Baylac F, et al: [Waldenström's macroglobulinemia and cerebral lymphoplasmacytic proliferation: Bing and Neel syndrome. Apropos of a new case.] [in French] *Neurochirurgie* 43:245, 1997.
118. Ciccarelli BT, Patterson CJ, Hunter ZR, et al: Hepcidin is produced by lymphoplasmacytic cells and is associated with anemia in Waldenström's macroglobulinemia. *Clin Lymphoma Myeloma Leuk* 11:160, 2011.
119. Treon SP, Tripsas C, Ciccarelli BT, et al: Patients with Waldenström macroglobulinemia commonly present with iron deficiency and those with severely depressed transferrin saturation levels show response to parenteral iron administration. *Clin Lymphoma Myeloma Leuk* 13:241, 2013.
120. Owen RG, Barrans SL, Richards SJ, et al: Waldenström macroglobulinemia. Development of diagnostic criteria and identification of prognostic factors. *Am J Clin Pathol* 116:420, 2001.
121. Feiner HD, Rizk CC, Finfer MD, et al: IgM monoclonal gammopathy/Waldenström's macroglobulinemia: A morphological and immunophenotypic study of the bone marrow. *Mod Pathol* 3:348, 1990.
122. Dutcher TF, Fahey JL: The histopathology of macroglobulinemia of Waldenström. *J Natl Cancer Inst* 22:887, 1959.

123. Hunter ZR, Manning RJ, Hanzis C, et al: IgA and IgG hypogammaglobulinemia in Waldenström's macroglobulinemia. *Haematologica* 95:470, 2010.

124. Stone MJ, Bogen SA: Evidence-based focused review of management of hyperviscosity syndrome. *Blood* 119:2205, 2012.

125. Menke MN, Treon SP: Hyperviscosity syndrome, in *Clinical Malignant Hematology*, edited by M Sekeres, M Kalaycio, B Bolwell, p 937. McGraw Hill, New York, 2007.

126. Mouloupoulos LA, Dimopoulos MA, Varma DG, et al: Waldenström macroglobulinemia: MR imaging of the spine and CT of the abdomen and pelvis. *Radiology* 188:669, 1993.

127. Kyle RA, Treon SP, Alexanian R, et al: Prognostic markers and criteria to initiate therapy in Waldenström's macroglobulinemia: Consensus Panel Recommendations from the Second International Workshop on Waldenström's macroglobulinemia. *Semin Oncol* 30:116, 2003.

128. Dimopoulos MA, Kastritis E, Owen RG et al: Treatment recommendations for patients with Waldenström macroglobulinemia (WM) and related disorders: IWWM-7 consensus. *Blood* 124:1404, 2014.

129. Kyle RA, Greipp PR, Gertz MA, et al: Waldenström's macroglobulinaemia: A prospective study comparing daily with intermittent oral chlorambucil. *Br J Haematol* 108:737, 2000.

130. Dimopoulos MA, Alexanian R: Waldenström's macroglobulinemia. *Blood* 83:1452, 1994.

131. Petrucci MT, Avvisati G, Tribalto M, et al: Waldenström's macroglobulinaemia: Results of a combined oral treatment in 34 newly diagnosed patients. *J Intern Med* 226:443, 1989.

132. Case DC Jr, Ervin TJ, Boyd MA, Redfield DL: Waldenström's macroglobulinemia: Long-term results with the M-2 protocol. *Cancer Invest* 9:1, 1991.

133. Facon T, Brouillard M, Duhamel A, et al: Prognostic factors in Waldenström's macroglobulinemia: A report of 167 cases. *J Clin Oncol* 11:1553, 1993.

134. Leblond V, Johnson S, Chevret S, et al: Results of a randomized trial of chlorambucil versus fludarabine for patients with Waldenström macroglobulinemia, marginal zone lymphoma, or lymphoplasmacytic lymphoma. *J Clin Oncol* 31:301, 2013.

135. Dimopoulos MA, Kantarjian H, Weber D, et al: Primary therapy of Waldenström's macroglobulinemia with 2-chlorodeoxyadenosine. *J Clin Oncol* 12:2694, 1994.

136. Delannoy A, Ferrant A, Martiat P, et al: 2-Chlorodeoxyadenosine therapy in Waldenström's macroglobulinaemia. *Nouv Rev Fr Hematol* 36:317, 1994.

137. Fridrik MA, Jager G, Baldinger C, et al: First-line treatment of Waldenström's disease with cladribine. Arbeitsgemeinschaft Medikamentose Tumortherapie. *Ann Hematol* 74:7, 1997.

138. Liu ES, Burian C, Miller WE, Saven A: Bolus administration of cladribine in the treatment of Waldenström macroglobulinaemia. *Br J Haematol* 103:690, 1998.

139. Hellmann A, Lewandowski K, Zaucha JM, et al: Effect of a 2-hour infusion of 2-chlorodeoxyadenosine in the treatment of refractory or previously untreated Waldenström's macroglobulinemia. *Eur J Haematol* 63:35, 1999.

140. Betticher DC, Hsu Schmitz SF, Ratschiller D, et al: Cladribine (2-CDA) given as subcutaneous bolus injections is active in pretreated Waldenström's macroglobulinaemia. Swiss Group for Clinical Cancer Research (SAKK). *Br J Haematol* 99:358, 1997.

141. Dimopoulos MA, Weber D, Delasalle KB, et al: Treatment of Waldenström's macroglobulinemia resistant to standard therapy with 2-chlorodeoxyadenosine: Identification of prognostic factors. *Ann Oncol* 6:49, 1995.

142. Dimopoulos MA, O'Brien S, Kantarjian H, et al: Fludarabine therapy in Waldenström's macroglobulinemia. *Am J Med* 95:49, 1993.

143. Foran JM, Rohatiner AZ, Coiffier B, et al: Multicenter phase II study of fludarabine phosphate for patients with newly diagnosed lymphoplasmacytoid lymphoma, Waldenström's macroglobulinemia, and mantle-cell lymphoma. *J Clin Oncol* 17:546, 1999.

144. Thalhammer-Scherrer R, Geissler K, Schwarzinger I, et al: Fludarabine therapy in Waldenström's macroglobulinemia. *Ann Hematol* 79:556, 2000.

145. Dhodapkar MV, Jacobson JL, Gertz MA, et al: Prognostic factors and response to fludarabine therapy in patients with Waldenström macroglobulinemia: Results of United States intergroup trial (Southwest Oncology Group S9003). *Blood* 98:41, 2001.

146. Zinzani PL, Gherlinzoni F, Bendandi M, et al: Fludarabine treatment in resistant Waldenström's macroglobulinemia. *Eur J Haematol* 54:120, 1995.

147. Leblond V, Ben Othman T, Deconinck E, et al: Activity of fludarabine in previously treated Waldenström's macroglobulinemia: A report of 71 cases. Groupe Cooperatif Macroglobulinemie. *J Clin Oncol* 16:2060, 1998.

148. Dimopoulos MA, Weber DM, Kantarjian H, et al: 2-Chlorodeoxyadenosine therapy of patients with Waldenström macroglobulinemia previously treated with fludarabine. *Ann Oncol* 5:288, 1994.

149. Lewandowski K, Halaburda K, Hellmann A: Fludarabine therapy in Waldenström's macroglobulinemia patients treated previously with 2-chlorodeoxyadenosine. *Leuk Lymphoma* 43:361, 2002.

150. Popat U, Saliba R, Thandi R, et al: Impairment of filgrastim-induced stem cell mobilization after prior lenalidomide in patients with multiple myeloma. *Biol Blood Marrow Transplant* 15:718, 2009.

151. Leleu XP, Manning R, Soumerai JD, et al: Increased incidence of transformation and myelodysplasia/acute leukemia in patients with Waldenström macroglobulinemia treated with nucleoside analogs. *J Clin Oncol* 27:250, 2009.

152. Leleu X, Tamburini J, Roccaro A, et al: Balancing risk versus benefit in the treatment of Waldenström's macroglobulinemia patients with nucleoside analogue based therapy. *Clin Lymphoma Myeloma* 9:71, 2009.

153. Treon SP, Kelliher A, Keele B, et al: Expression of serotherapy target antigens in Waldenström's macroglobulinemia: Therapeutic applications and considerations. *Semin Oncol* 30:248, 2003.

154. Treon SP, Agus DB, Link B, et al: CD20-Directed antibody-mediated immunotherapy induces responses and facilitates hematologic recovery in patients with Waldenström's macroglobulinemia. *J Immunother* 24:272, 2001.

155. Gertz MA, Rue M, Blood E, et al: Multicenter phase 2 trial of rituximab for Waldenström macroglobulinemia (WM): An Eastern Cooperative Oncology Group Study (E3A98). *Leuk Lymphoma* 45:2047, 2004.

156. Dimopoulos MA, Zervas C, Zomas A, et al: Treatment of Waldenström's macroglobulinemia with rituximab. *J Clin Oncol* 20:2327, 2002.

157. Treon SP, Emmanouilides C, Kimby E, et al: Extended rituximab therapy in Waldenström's Macroglobulinemia. *Ann Oncol* 16:132, 2005.

158. Treon SP, Branagan AR, Hunter Z, et al: Paradoxical increases in serum IgM and viscosity levels following rituximab in Waldenström's macroglobulinemia. *Ann Oncol* 15:1481, 2004.

159. Ghobrial IM, Fonseca R, Greipp PR, et al: Initial immunoglobulin M "flare" after rituximab therapy in patients with Waldenström macroglobulinemia: An Eastern Cooperative Oncology Group Study. *Cancer* 101:2593, 2004.

160. Dimopoulos MA, Anagnostopoulos A, Zervas C, et al: Predictive factors for response to rituximab in Waldenström's macroglobulinemia. *Clin Lymphoma* 5:270, 2005.

161. Treon SP, Hansen M, Branagan AR, et al: Polymorphisms in FcγRIIIA (CD16) receptor expression are associated with clinical responses to rituximab in Waldenström's macroglobulinemia. *J Clin Oncol* 23:474, 2005.

162. Dimopoulos MA, Anagnostopoulos A, Kyrtsonis MC, et al: Treatment of relapsed or refractory Waldenström's macroglobulinemia with bortezomib. *Haematologica* 90:1655, 2005.

163. Chen CI, Kouroukis CT, White D, et al: Bortezomib is active in patients with untreated or relapsed Waldenström's macroglobulinemia: A phase II study of the National Cancer Institute of Canada Clinical Trials Group. *J Clin Oncol* 25:1570, 2007.

164. Weber DM, Dimopoulos MA, Delasalle K, et al: 2-chlorodeoxyadenosine alone and in combination for previously untreated Waldenström's macroglobulinemia. *Semin Oncol* 30:243, 2003.

165. Treon SP, Branagan AR, Ioakimidis L, et al: Long-term outcomes to fludarabine and rituximab in Waldenström's macroglobulinemia. *Blood* 113:3673, 2009.

166. Tam CS, Wolf MM, Westerman D, et al: Fludarabine combination therapy is highly effective in first-line and salvage treatment of patients with Waldenström's macroglobulinemia. *Clin Lymphoma Myeloma* 6:136, 2005.

167. Hensel M, Villalobos M, Kornacker M, et al: Pentostatin/cyclophosphamide with or without rituximab: An effective regimen for patients with Waldenström's macroglobulinemia/lymphoplasmacytic lymphoma. *Clin Lymphoma Myeloma* 6:131, 2005.

168. Dimopoulos MA, Anagnostopoulos A, Kyrtsonis MC, et al: Primary treatment of Waldenström's macroglobulinemia with dexamethasone, rituximab and cyclophosphamide. *J Clin Oncol* 25:3344, 2007.

169. Buske C, Hoster E, Dreyling MH, et al: The addition of rituximab to front-line therapy with CHOP (R-CHOP) results in a higher response rate and longer time to treatment failure in patients with lymphoplasmacytic lymphoma: Results of a randomized trial of the German Low-Grade Lymphoma Study Group (GLSG). *Leukemia* 23:153, 2009.

170. Treon SP, Hunter Z, Branagan A: CHOP plus rituximab therapy in Waldenström's macroglobulinemia. *Clin Lymphoma Myeloma* 5:273, 2005.

171. Ioakimidis L, Patterson CJ, Hunter ZR, et al: Comparative outcomes following CP-R, CVP-R and CHOP-R in Waldenström's macroglobulinemia. *Clin Lymphoma Myeloma* 9:62, 2009.

172. Rummel M, Niederle N, Maschmeyer G, et al: Bendamustine plus rituximab versus CHOP plus rituximab as first-line treatment for patients with indolent and mantle-cell lymphomas: an open-label, multicentre, randomised, phase 3 non-inferiority trial. *Lancet* 381:1203, 2013.

173. Treon SP, Hanzis C, Tripsas C, et al: Bendamustine therapy in patients with relapsed or refractory Waldenström's macroglobulinemia. *Clin Lymphoma Myeloma Leuk* 211:133, 2011.

174. Dimopoulos MA, Hamilos G, Efstathiou E, et al: Treatment of Waldenström's macroglobulinemia with the combination of fludarabine and cyclophosphamide. *Leuk Lymphoma* 44:993, 2003.

175. Tamburini J, Levy V, Chateilex C, et al: Fludarabine plus cyclophosphamide in Waldenström's macroglobulinemia: Results in 49 patients. *Leukemia* 19:1831, 2005.

176. Treon SP, Ioakimidis L, Soumerai JD, et al: Primary therapy of Waldenström's macroglobulinemia with bortezomib, dexamethasone and rituximab. *J Clin Oncol* 27:3830, 2009.

177. Ghobrial IM, Matous J, Padmanabhan S, et al: Phase II trial of combination of bortezomib and rituximab in relapsed and/or refractory Waldenström's macroglobulinemia. *Blood* 112:832, 2008.

178. Agathocleous A, Rohatiner A, Rule S, et al: Weekly versus twice weekly bortezomib given in conjunction with rituximab in patients with recurrent follicular lymphoma, mantle cell lymphoma, and Waldenström's macroglobulinemia. *Br J Haematol* 151:346, 2010.

179. Dimopoulos MA, García-Sanz R, Gavriatopoulou M, et al: Primary therapy of Waldenström macroglobulinemia (WM) with weekly bortezomib, low-dose dexamethasone, and rituximab (BDR): Long-term results of a phase 2 study of the European Myeloma Network (EMN). *Blood* 122:3276, 2013.

180. Treon SP, Tripsas CK, Meid K, et al: Ibrutinib in previously treated Waldenstrom's Macroglobulinemia. *N Engl J Med* 372(15):1430, 2015.

181. Ghobrial IM, Witzig TE, Gertz M, et al: Long-term results of the phase II trial of the oral mTOR inhibitor everolimus (RAD001) in relapsed or refractory Waldenström macroglobulinemia. *Am J Hematol*; 89:237, 2014.

182. Treon SP, Tripsas CK, Meid K, et al: Prospective, multicenter study of the mTOR inhibitor everolimus (RAD001) as primary therapy in Waldenström's macroglobulinemia. *Blood* 2013; 122:1822.

183. Treon SP, Hanzis, C, Manning, RJ, et al: Maintenance rituximab is associated with improved clinical outcome in rituximab naïve patients with Waldenström's macroglobulinemia who respond to a rituximab containing regimen. *Br J Haematol* 2011; 154:357–62.

184. Rummel MJ, Lerchenmüller C, Greil R, et al: Bendamustine-rituximab induction followed by observation or rituximab maintenance for newly diagnosed patients with Waldenström's macroglobulinemia: results from a prospective, randomized, multicenter study (StiL NHL 7–2008). *Blood* 2012; 120: 2739.

185. Kyriakou C, Canals C, Sibon D, et al: High-dose therapy and autologous stem-cell transplantation in Waldenström macroglobulinemia: The Lymphoma Working Party of the European Group for Blood and Marrow Transplantation. *J Clin Oncol* 28:2227, 2010.

186. Kyriakou C, Canals C, Cornelissen JJ, et al: Allogeneic stem-cell transplantation in patients with Waldenström macroglobulinemia: report from the Lymphoma Working Party of the European Group for Blood and Marrow Transplantation. *J Clin Oncol* 28:4926, 2010.

187. Owen RG, Kyle RA, Stone MJ, et al: Response Assessment in Waldenström macroglobulinemia. *Br J Haematol* 160:171, 2013.

188. Treon SP, Yang G, Hanzis C, et al: Attainment of complete/very good partial response following rituximab based therapy is an important determinant to progression-free survival and is impacted by polymorphisms in FCGR3A in Waldenström macroglobulinaemia. *Br J Haematol* 154:223, 2011.

189. Strauss SJ, Maharaj L, Hoare S, et al: Bortezomib therapy in patients with relapsed or refractory lymphoma: Potential correlation of *in vitro* sensitivity and tumor necrosis factor alpha response with clinical activity. *J Clin Oncol* 24:2105, 2006.

190. Varghese AM, Rawstron AC, Ashcroft J, et al: Assessment of bone marrow response in Waldenström's macroglobulinemia. *Clin Lymphoma Myeloma* 9:53, 2009.

191. Ciccarelli BT, Yang G, Hatjiharissi E, et al: Soluble CD27 is a faithful marker of disease burden and is unaffected by the rituximab induced IgM flare, as well as plasmapheresis in patients with Waldenström's macroglobulinemia. *Clin Lymphoma Myeloma* 9:56, 2009.

192. Gobbi PG, Bettini R, Montecucco C, et al: Study of prognosis in Waldenström's macroglobulinemia: A proposal for a simple binary classification with clinical and investigational utility. *Blood* 83:2939, 1994.

193. Morel P, Monconduit M, Jacomy D, et al: Prognostic factors in Waldenström macroglobulinemia: A report on 232 patients with the description of a new scoring system and its validation on 253 other patients. *Blood* 96:852, 2000.

194. Dhodapkar MV, Jacobson JL, Gertz MA, et al: Prognostic factors and response to fludarabine therapy in patients with Waldenström macroglobulinemia: Results of United States intergroup trial (Southwest Oncology Group S9003). *Blood* 98:41, 2001.

195. Dimopoulos M, Gika D, Zervas K, et al: The international staging system for multiple myeloma is applicable in symptomatic Waldenström's macroglobulinemia. *Leuk Lymphoma* 45:1809, 2004.

196. Anagnostopoulos A, Zervas K, Kyrtsonis M, et al: Prognostic value of serum beta 2-microglobulin in patients with Waldenström's macroglobulinemia requiring therapy. *Clin Lymphoma Myeloma* 7:205, 2006.

197. Morel P, Duhamel A, Gobbi P, et al: International prognostic scoring system for Waldenström macroglobulinemia. *Blood* 113:4163, 2009.

198. Castillo JJ, Olszewski A, Cronin AM, et al: Survival trends in Waldenström macroglobulinemia: An analysis of the Surveillance, Epidemiology and End Results database. *Blood* 123:3999, 2014.

199. Kastritis S, Kyrtsonis MC, Hatjiharissi E, et al: No significant improvement in the outcome of patients with Waldenström macroglobulinemia treated over the last 25 years. *Am J Hematol* 86:479, 2011.

200. Kristinsson SY, Eloranta S, Dickman PW, et al: Patterns of survival in lymphoplasmacytic lymphoma/Waldenström macroglobulinemia: a population based study of 1,555 patients diagnosed in Sweden from 1980 to 2005. *Am J Hematol* 88:60, 2013.

CHAPTER 110
HEAVY-CHAIN DISEASE

Dietlind L. Wahner-Roedler and Robert A. Kyle

SUMMARY

The heavy-chain diseases (HCDs) are B-cell lymphoplasmacytic proliferative disorders in which neoplastic cells produce monoclonal immunoglobulins (Ig) consisting of truncated heavy chains (HCs) without attached light chains. The complex abnormalities of HCD proteins and the usual lack of normal light chains are a result of several distinct gene alterations, including somatic mutations, deletions, and insertions. HCDs involving the three main immunoglobulin classes have been described: a-HCD is the most common and has the most uniform presentation; γ- and μ-HCDs have variable clinical presentations and histopathologic features. The diagnosis is established from immunofixation of serum, urine, or secretory fluids in the case of a-HCD or by immunohistologic analysis of the proliferating lymphoplasmacytic cells in nonsecretory disease. Treatment of a-HCD consists of antibiotics. If there is no response to antibiotics or if aggressive lymphoma is diagnosed, chemotherapy is indicated. Treatment of γ- and μ-HCDs depends on the underlying clinicopathologic features rather than on the presence of the abnormal protein. Table 110–1 summarizes the features of the HCDs.

γ-HEAVY-CHAIN DISEASE DEFINITION AND HISTORY

γ-Heavy-chain disease (HCD) is not a specific cytopathologic process; rather, it is a biochemical expression of a mutant B-cell clone. The disease should be considered a serologically determined entity with a variety of clinical and histopathologic features. It is defined by the recognition of monoclonal deleted gamma (γ) chains devoid of light chains.[1]

The first case of γ-HCD was described in 1964 by Franklin and colleagues,[2] who observed a homogeneous band between γ- and β-globulin in an African American patient with generalized lymphadenopathy. Comparison of the proteins in the urine to those in the serum showed that they were the same, a suggestion of the presence of a low-molecular-weight serum γ-globulin, which then was shown to be a fragment of a γ-heavy chain (HC). Since this first description, more than 130 patients with γ-HCD have been described in the literature.[3–5]

EPIDEMIOLOGY

γ-HCD has been described throughout the world. Although initially γ-HCD was reported to occur equally in men and women,[4] there was a clear predominance of women in a more recent series of 23 patients.[5] The median age at diagnosis in that series was 68 years (range: 42 to 87 years).

Acronyms and Abbreviations: $C_H 1$ (2, 3, 4), constant region 1 (2, 3, 4); D, diversity; HC, heavy chain; HCD, heavy-chain disease; Ig, immunoglobulin; IPSID, immunoproliferative small intestinal disease; J, joining; V, variable.

ETIOLOGY AND PATHOGENESIS

The etiology of γ-HCD is unknown.

CLINICAL FEATURES

Originally, γ-HCD was considered to be a lymphomatous illness. However, γ-HCD has various clinical and pathologic features that can be divided into three broad categories, as described below.

DISSEMINATED LYMPHOPROLIFERATIVE DISEASE

Disseminated lymphoproliferative disease is present in most patients at the time of diagnosis, and various series have reported it in 57 percent to 66 percent of patients.[4–6] In two different series,[4,5] lymphadenopathy was present in 56 percent and 62 percent of patients, splenomegaly in 38 percent and 52 percent, and hepatomegaly in 8 percent and 37 percent at the time of diagnosis.

LOCALIZED PROLIFERATIVE DISEASE

In approximately 25 percent of patients, the lymphoproliferative process is localized, which may be extramedullary or may involve only the marrow.[4,5] Cutaneous involvement is the most frequently reported extramedullary presentation.[4,5] Patients may present with extramedullary plasmacytoma of the thyroid or parotid gland or an oropharyngeal mass[5] and hypertrophic spinal pachymeningitis.[7]

NO APPARENT PROLIFERATIVE DISEASE

A proliferative lymphoplasmacytic disease is not apparent in 9 percent to 17 percent of patients. In most of these patients, an underlying autoimmune disorder has been reported. Autoimmune disorders with or without underlying lymphoid proliferation include rheumatoid arthritis, autoimmune cytopenias, systemic lupus erythematosus, Sjögren syndrome, myasthenia gravis, thyroiditis, and vasculitis.[5]

LABORATORY FEATURES

MOLECULAR BIOLOGY AND GENETICS

Most γ-HCD proteins are dimers of truncated HCs devoid of light chains. The molecular weight of the monomeric unit varies from 27,000 to 49,000. The length of the truncated γ chain varies, but usually it is one-half to three-fourths the length of the normal γ chain. Structural analysis of the defective monoclonal γ-HC of 23 patients with γ-HCD showed several characteristic features (Fig. 110–1). The proteins usually begin with a normal variable region. In most cases, this sequence is short and interrupted by a large deletion encompassing the remainder of the variable region, although four of the HCs shown in Fig. 110–1 appear to have retained most or all of their variable (V), diversity (D), and joining (J) sequences. In all γ-HCD proteins, the entire constant region 1 ($C_H 1$) domain is also deleted, with normal sequence beginning at the hinge or occasionally at the $C_H 2$ domain. $C_H 1$ is responsible for light-chain binding. In the absence of an associated light chain, the $C_H 1$ domain binds to heat shock protein 78 (HC binding protein), and the HC undergoes proteasomal degradation rather than secretion.

In two cases of γ-HCD (OMM and RIV), genomic sequence data are available (Fig. 110–2). The presence of large deletions in the switch/$C_H 1$ regions of these two γ-HCD genes explains why the corresponding HCD proteins lack $C_H 1$. Because the normal $C_H 1$ acceptor splice site is deleted, the donor splice of the leader, or the J region, is spliced directly

TABLE 110–1. Summary of Features of the Heavy-Chain Diseases

Features	Types of Heavy-Chain Diseases		
	α	γ	μ
Year described	1968	1964	1969
Incidence	Rare	Very rare	Very rare
Age at diagnosis	Young adult (<30 years)	Older adult (60–70 years)	Older adult (50–60 years)
Demographics	Mediterranean region	Worldwide	Worldwide
Structurally abnormal monoclonal protein	IgA	IgG	IgM
MGUS phase	No	Rarely	Rarely
Urine monoclonal light chain	No	No	Yes
Urine abnormal heavy chain	Small amounts	Often present	Infrequent
Sites involved	Small intestine, mesenteric lymph nodes	Lymph nodes, marrow, spleen	Lymph nodes, marrow, liver, spleen
Pathology	Extranodal marginal zone lymphoma (MALT or IPSID)	Lymphoplasmacytoid lymphoma	Small lymphocytic lymphoma, CLL
Associated diseases	Infection, malabsorption	Autoimmune diseases	None
Therapy	Antibiotics, chemotherapy	Chemotherapy	Chemotherapy

CLL, chronic lymphocytic leukemia; Ig, immunoglobulin; IPSID, immunoproliferative small intestinal disease; MALT, mucosa-associated lymphoid tissue; MGUS, monoclonal gammopathy of undetermined significance.

Adapted with permission from Witzig TE, Wahner-Roedler DL: Heavy chain disease. *Curr Treat Options Oncol* 3(3):247–254, 2002.

to the next available functional acceptor splice site at the beginning of the hinge or C_H2 domain.

SERUM AND URINE PROTEIN FINDINGS

The serum protein electrophoretic pattern is extremely variable. A monoclonal peak is detected in 60 percent to 86 percent of patients.[4,5] When present, it is most commonly in the β_1 or β_2 region. The median value of the monoclonal spike at diagnosis in 19 patients was 1.59 g/dL (range: 0.40 to 3.91 g/dL).[5] The diagnosis is established by immunofixation of the serum and a concentrated urine specimen. A modified immunoselection technique for the diagnosis of HCD has been described.[8] In one case of γ-HCD, low concentrations of free HCs in serum were detected by capillary zone electrophoresis coupled with immunosubtraction.[9] A heavy/light chain assay to identify truncated immunoglobulin (Ig) HCs was used on serum samples from 15 patients with known γ-HCD. By this method, 20 percent of these patients were shown to also have small amounts of monoclonal free light chains.[10] The amount of HCD protein in the urine usually is small (<1 g/24 h) but may reach 20 g/24 h. An occasional patient with Bence Jones proteinuria has been described.[5]

No standard has been established to identify the subclass of the HC fragment. In reported cases in which the HC fragment subclass has been studied, different methods have been used, ranging from Ouchterlony in the earlier cases to indirect immunofluorescence staining, immunoblotting, amino acid sequence, immunoselection, and enzyme-linked immunosorbent assay.[11] IgG subclass distribution shows a lower-than-expected incidence of IgG_2. The most common subclass is IgG_1, which occurs in 65 percent of cases. IgG_3 has been identified in 27 percent of patients, IgG_4 in 5 percent, and IgG_2 in 3 percent.[4] Although biclonal gammopathy has been reported in 1 percent to 8 percent of all patients with serum monoclonal components, the association between

γ-HCD and another monoclonal protein is much higher. In a series of 23 patients with γ-HCD, 7 percent had an IgM-λ intact monoclonal Ig.[5] No association between γ-HCD and monoclonal IgA has been described, although the IgG-IgA association was the most frequent in several series of biclonal gammopathies. One patient described in the literature was unique in that the serum contained two deleted γ chains of different subclasses (IgG_1 and IgG_2).[12]

HEMATOLOGIC ABNORMALITIES

Anemia is frequent. It is usually normochromic, normocytic, and moderate. Coombs-positive autoimmune hemolytic anemia has been reported in several cases and may be associated with thrombocytopenia (Evans syndrome). The total and differential leukocyte counts are usually normal. Lymphocytosis may occur, and an occasional patient presents with chronic lymphocytic leukemia. In some cases, rare plasmacytoid lymphocytes or plasma cells have been noted in the blood. Plasma cell leukemia has been reported in two patients.[13,14]

Marrow aspirates and biopsy specimens often show an increase of plasma cells, lymphocytes, or plasmacytoid lymphocytes, similar to the marrow findings in Waldenström macroglobulinemia. The typical marrow features of myeloma or chronic lymphocytic leukemia are rare. An unusual concurrence of T-cell large granular lymphocytic leukemia with γ-HCD has been reported.[15] Marrow changes consistent with a myeloproliferative neoplasm have been noted in a few patients.[5]

OTHER FEATURES

Bone lesions are rare in γ-HCD. Cytogenetic studies have seldom been reported. No unique abnormalities or characteristics of lymphoma have been found.

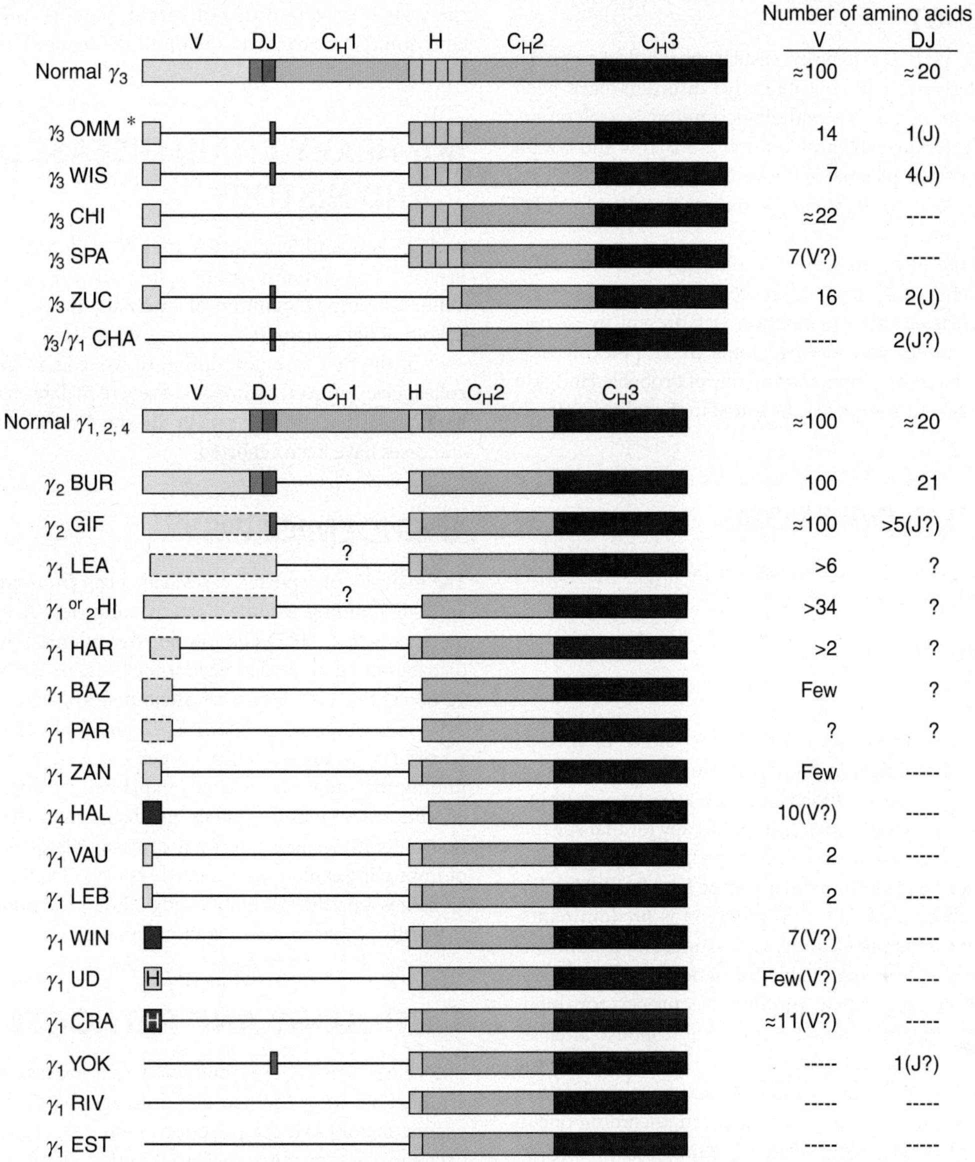

Number of amino acids
V DJ
V DJ CH1 H CH2 CH3
Normal γ3 ≈100 ≈20
γ3 OMM * 14 1(J)
γ3 WIS 7 4(J)
γ3 CHI ≈22 -----
γ3 SPA 7(V?) -----
γ3 ZUC 16 2(J)
γ3/γ1 CHA ----- 2(J?)
V DJ CH1 H CH2 CH3
Normal γ1, 2, 4 ≈100 ≈20
γ2 BUR 100 21
γ2 GIF ≈100 >5(J?)
γ1 LEA ? >6 ?
γ1 or 2HI ? >34 ?
γ1 HAR >2 ?
γ1 BAZ Few ?
γ1 PAR ? ?
γ1 ZAN Few -----
γ4 HAL 10(V?) -----
γ1 VAU 2 -----
γ1 LEB 2 -----
γ1 WIN 7(V?) -----
γ1 UD H Few(V?) -----
γ1 CRA H ≈11(V?) -----
γ1 YOK ----- 1(J?)
γ1 RIV ----- -----
γ1 EST ----- -----

Figure 110–1. Structure of various deleted γ-heavy-chain disease (HCD) proteins compared with that of normal chains. *Structure shown is a primary synthetic product synthesized by the HCD cells. Serum protein was modified after synthesis and did not contain any amino acids before the hinge. H, indicates heterogeneous amino acid sequences; H, unusual and heterogeneous amino acid sequences; ■, unusual amino acid sequences; boxes, coding regions; lines, deletions; dashed lines, likely structures for which sequence data are missing; ?, probable missing domain based on molecular weight and partial protein structure analysis; V, variable region; D, diversity segment; J, joining region; H, hinge region; C_H1, C_H2, C_H3, constant regions of heavy chains. OMM,[66] WIS,[67] CHI,[68] SPA,[69] ZUC,[70] CHA,[71] BUR,[72] GIF,[73] LEA,[74] HI,[75] HAR,[74] BAZ,[76] PAR,[77] ZAN,[78] HAL,[79] VAU,[80] LEB,[80] WIN,[81] UD,[82] CRA,[83] YOK,[84] RIV,[85] EST.[86]

L V DJ S CH1 H CH2 CH3
Normal γ3 gene
LVJ S CH1 H CH2 CH3
OMM γ3 gene
LVJ H CH2 CH3
OMM primary synthetic protein
OMM serum protein
L V DJ S CH1 H CH2 CH3
Normal γ1 gene
L I V I J Del S CH1 H CH2 CH3
RIV γ1 gene
LH CH2 CH3
RIV primary synthetic protein
RIV serum protein

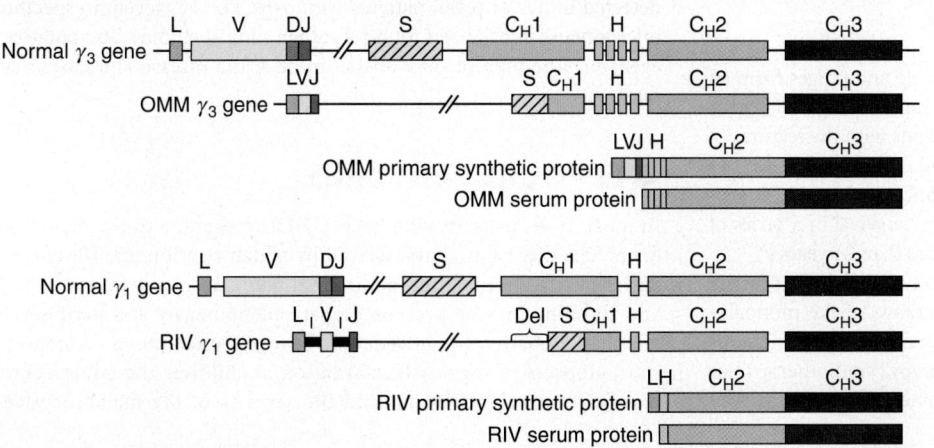

Figure 110–2. Structure of two genes coding for γ-heavy-chain-disease proteins compared with that of normal γ_3 and γ_1 genes. Boxes indicate coding regions; ▨, switch region; ▬, inserted noncoding sequence; lines, intervening (noncoding) sequences; L, leader region; V, variable region; D, diversity segment; J, joining region; S, switch region; H, hinge region; C_H1, C_H2, C_H3, constant regions of heavy chains; I, inserted sequence; Del, deleted sequence. OMM,[66] RIV.[85]

HISTOPATHOLOGY

In contrast to α-HCD, γ-HCD has no consistent morphologic pattern and a variety of underlying lymphoproliferative disorders have been described.[16] The most frequent histopathologic finding is a pleomorphic malignant lymphoplasmacytic proliferation in marrow and lymph nodes. These lymphocytoid plasma cells express pan–B-cell markers and cytoplasmic γ-HC without light chains and are negative for CD5 and CD10.[17]

Lymphoma without any consistent morphologic type was diagnosed in 18 (38 percent) of 47 patients in whom lymph nodes were examined. A lymphoplasmacytic proliferation was present in 36 percent and hyperplastic nodes and plasmacytoma in 11 percent each; there was one case of Hodgkin lymphoma and one of probable Hodgkin lymphoma.[6] Plasmacytic infiltration may be found in the salivary glands or thyroid.[4,5,18]

DIFFERENTIAL DIAGNOSIS

All patients presenting with a lymphoplasmacytic proliferative disorder should be evaluated for γ-HCD.

THERAPY

Because γ-HCD is a heterogeneous condition, the choice of therapy depends on the clinical findings. In an asymptomatic patient with a monoclonal γ-HC, no therapy is indicated. Any associated autoimmune disease should be managed with standard therapy for that specific disease type. In symptomatic patients with a low-grade lymphoplasmacytic malignancy, a trial of chlorambucil may be beneficial. Melphalan and prednisone can be used, if the proliferation is predominantly plasmacytic. A trial of cyclophosphamide, vincristine, and prednisone with or without doxorubicin is reasonable for patients with evidence of a progressive lymphoplasmacytic proliferative process or high-grade lymphoma. One patient achieved a complete response after six courses of fludarabine.[19] Successful treatment of γ-HCD with low-dose etoposide has been reported.[20] CD20 expression has been analyzed in only seven cases and was detected in six of the seven, including one in which CD20 expression appeared transient.[5,21-23] Rituximab monotherapy was given in two cases, resulting in clinical responses in both.[5,21] In two other cases, a combination of rituximab with chemotherapy had an antitumor effect in lymphoplasmacytic-type γ-HCD.[22,24] In localized extramedullary plasmacytomas treated with radiation[4] or surgical removal (or both), complete clinical and serologic remission has been achieved.

COURSE AND PROGNOSIS

The clinical course of γ-HCD is extremely variable and ranges from an asymptomatic, benign, or transient process to a rapidly progressive neoplasm leading to death within a few weeks. Patients with the features of only a monoclonal gammopathy have remained clinically well for 2 to 7 years of followup.[5,25] Spontaneous disappearance of the γ-HCD protein has been reported.[4] The median duration of survival in a series of 23 patients was 7.4 years (range: 1 month to more than 21 years).[5]

The amount of serum γ-HCD protein usually parallels the severity of the associated malignant process. Disappearance of the monoclonal component from serum and urine associated with apparent complete response has been induced by chemotherapy,[19] radiotherapy,[4] or surgical removal of a localized process. In some instances, however, the γ-HCD protein does not vary in parallel with the associated process, and relapse can occur without the reappearance of the pathologic protein.[4]

α-HEAVY-CHAIN DISEASE DEFINITION AND HISTORY

α-HCD is a proliferative disorder of B-lymphoid cells involving the IgA secretory immune system, especially the gastrointestinal tract. It is defined by the recognition of internally deleted monoclonal α chains devoid of light chains.

In the first case description of α-HCD, in 1968 by Seligman and colleagues,[26] an Arab woman had severe malabsorption resulting from a lymphoplasmacytic infiltrate in the small bowel. Since then, more than 400 cases have been reported.

EPIDEMIOLOGY

The majority of reported cases have been from northern Africa, Israel, and surrounding Middle Eastern countries. A common variable for patients with α-HCD is a low socioeconomic status. In a study of the distribution of monoclonal gammopathies in Tunisia published in 1990, 17 percent of 198 cases were attributed to α-HCD.[27] In a later study of 270 cases observed between 1992 and 2000 at the university hospital of Sfax in Tunisia, only 2.2 percent were attributed to α-HCD,[28] a finding that might be partially explained by improved socioeconomic conditions. Similarly, a persistent decrease in the incidence of immunoproliferative small intestinal disease (IPSID) since 1986 as a result of improving sanitation has been reported from Iran[29] and Greece.[30] α-HCD has a predilection for young adults. The prevalence of the disease is slightly higher in males than in females.

ETIOLOGY AND PATHOGENESIS

The cause of α-HCD is unknown. The disease might be considered a model showing the complex interactions of the environment with genetic factors and the infection–immunity–cancer interrelationships originating from the same proliferating clone. Although the mechanisms leading to the development of a clonal population synthesizing the structurally abnormal IgA are still speculative, the lymphoplasmacytic infiltration of the intestinal mucosa is likely a response of the alimentary tract immune system to protracted luminal antigenic stimulation. A causal relationship between infection and pathogenesis is supported by the observation that α-HCD can respond to broad-spectrum antibiotics. Using molecular strategies, *Campylobacter jejuni* was detected in five of seven patients with α-HCD.[31] However, no specific microorganism has been found in other clinical studies. The putative agent may be present only at the onset of the disease and absent at diagnosis.

CLINICAL FEATURES

In most cases, patients who have α-HCD present with the digestive form. The disease is characterized by malabsorption manifested by diarrhea, weight loss, and abdominal pain. Ascites, tetany, edema, and clubbing may be present. Hepatosplenomegaly and peripheral lymphadenopathy are infrequent. Fever is uncommon. Amenorrhea, alopecia, and growth retardation in children and adolescents correlate with the duration and the severity of the malabsorptive

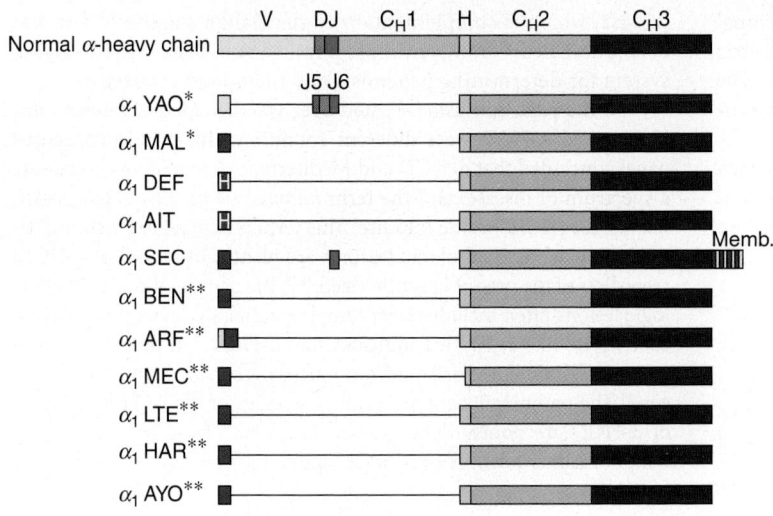

Figure 110–3. Structure of various α-heavy-chain disease (HCD) proteins compared with that of normal chain. *Structures shown are primary synthetic products synthesized by the HCD cells. Serum proteins were modified after synthesis and did not contain any amino acids before the hinge. **Structures shown are deduced amino acid sequences determined by complementary DNA sequencing. ▯, indicates unusual and heterogeneous amino acid sequences; ▮, unusual amino acid sequences; boxes, coding regions; lines, deletion; V, variable region; D, diversity segment; J, joining region; H, hinge region; C_H1, C_H2, C_H3, constant regions of heavy chains; Memb., membrane exon. YAO,[87] MAL,[88] DEF,[89] AIT,[90] SEC,[91] BEN,[92] ARF,[92] MEC,[92] LTE,[92] HAR,[92] AYO.[92]

process. α-HCD may be confined to the respiratory tract, but this is extremely rare, as is a lymphomatous form characterized by generalized lymphadenopathy. α-HCD has been reported in a patient with a goiter from a plasmacytoma of the thyroid[32] and in a patient with polyneuropathy, organomegaly, endocrinopathy, monoclonal protein, and skin lesions (POEMS).[33]

●LABORATORY FEATURES

MOLECULAR BIOLOGY AND GENETICS

Most α-HCD proteins consist of multiple polymers. The molecular weight of the basic monomeric unit varies from 29,000 to 34,000. The length of the basic polypeptide subunit differs from patient to patient and in most instances is between one-half and three-fourths that of a normal α chain. Sequence data are available for several α-HCD proteins (Fig. 110–3). In all cases of α-HCD studied, the α-HCD protein belonged to the α_1 subclass. Common features of the defective α chain include deleted V regions, missing C_H1 domains, and the absence of light chains. Most of the proteins have short, non–Ig-related sequences of unknown origin at the amino terminus. The complete sequences of the genes encoding 3 α-HCD proteins are shown in Fig. 110–4. These

three genes show striking similarity in their position and extent of the two main deletions, which encompass sequences in the V/J and the switch/C_H1 region.

SERUM, URINE, AND INTESTINAL FLUID PROTEIN FINDINGS

In contrast to other monoclonal gammopathies, the characteristic sharp spike of a monoclonal gammopathy is not found on serum protein electrophoresis in α-HCD. In about half of cases, an abnormal broad band is found in the α_2- or β-globulin region, which is probably related to polymerization of the α chains. In the other half of cases, serum protein electrophoresis shows no evidence of an abnormal protein. Identification of the α-HCD protein depends on immunoselection or immunofixation. The pathologic protein may easily escape detection by immunoelectrophoresis when its serum concentration is low. In most patients, the α-HCD protein can be found in the serum. During the course of the disease, the progressive diminution of mature plasma cells and their replacement by immature immunoblasts likely is followed by a progressive decrease in the serum concentration of α-HCD protein. α-HCD protein hyposecretion also may be found during the early stage of the disease.

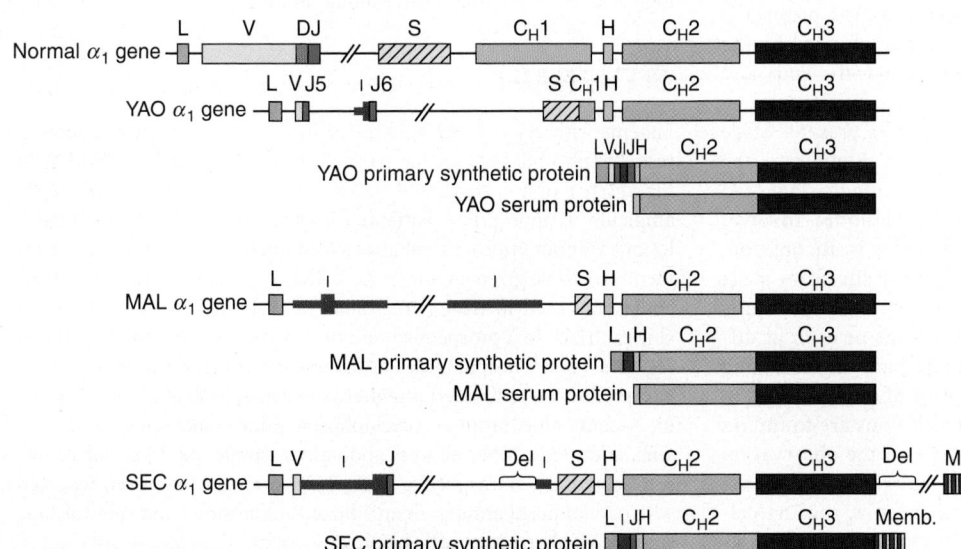

Figure 110–4. Structure of three genes coding for different α_1-heavy-chain disease proteins compared with that of normal α_1 gene. Boxes indicate coding regions; ▨, switch region; ▮, inserted coding sequence; ▬, inserted noncoding sequence; lines, intervening (noncoding) sequences; L, leader region; V, variable region; D, diversity segment; J, joining region; S, switch region; H, hinge region; C_H1, C_H2, C_H3, constant regions of heavy chains; I, inserted sequence; Del, deleted sequence; Memb., membrane exon. YAO,[87] MAL,[88] SEC.[91]

In most cases, the α-HCD protein also is found in the jejunal secretions.[34] α-HCD protein has been found in the intestinal or gastric fluid in a few cases when it was undetectable in serum and urine. The concentration of α-HCD protein in the urine is low. Bence Jones proteinuria has never been documented.

Synthesis of the α-HCD protein by the proliferating cells has been demonstrated by immunohistochemical or immunocytochemical methods and by biosynthesis studies *in vitro*.[35] These techniques are helpful in the recognition of nonsecreting forms of α-HCD.

HEMATOLOGIC AND METABOLIC ABNORMALITIES

Mild to moderate anemia is often found. Hypokalemia, hypocalcemia, hypomagnesemia, and hypoalbuminemia are common. The intestinal isoenzyme fraction of the alkaline phosphatase level may be increased. Results of tests to indicate malabsorption are usually positive.

IMAGING PROCEDURES

Abnormal radiographic findings of the small intestine include hypertrophic and pseudopolypoid mucosal folds, occasionally associated with strictures and filling defects. The extent of the disease should be evaluated with computed tomography.

ENDOSCOPY

α-HCD intestinal lesions nearly always affect the duodenum and jejunum, making endoscopy with biopsy a useful tool in the evaluation of patients in whom α-HCD is suspected. Several endoscopic patterns have been defined. The infiltrated pattern is the most specific, followed by the nodular pattern. Other primary lesions (ulcerations, mosaic pattern, and mucosal fold thickening alone) are nonspecific.

HISTOPATHOLOGY

In the digestive form of α-HCD, the proliferation involves at least the proximal half of the small intestine and adjacent mesenteric lymph nodes. The whole length of the small bowel, the gastric, and the colorectal mucosae that belong to the IgA secretory system may be involved.

The disease progresses in three histopathologic stages according to Galian and colleagues.[36] In stage A, a mature plasmacytic or lymphoplasmacytic infiltration of the mucosal lamina propria is noted. Villous atrophy is variable. Stage B is characterized by the presence of atypical plasmacytic or lymphoplasmacytic cells and more or less atypical immunoblast-like cells extending at least to the submucosa. Subtotal or total villous atrophy is present. Stage C corresponds to an immunoblastic lymphoma. Similar to the changes described in the small intestine, three histologic stages (A, B, C) have been described in the mesenteric lymph nodes. Involvement of liver, spleen, and peripheral lymph nodes is uncommon. The histologic lesions may progress at any given site from stage A to stage B or from stage B to stage C. However, different stages can be found at the same time in different organs or even at different sites in the same organ. Thus, accurate pathologic staging of α-HCD requires a laparotomy with sampling of multiple sites in all patients with α-HCD in whom no stage C lesions are found on peroral biopsy. This recommendation is based on the observation that mesenteric lymph nodes may harbor malignant lymphoma when the intestinal mucosa reveals only a benign-appearing cellular infiltrate that one might be tempted to treat with antibiotics alone.[37] A staging system based on anatomical spread of the

disease, which is complementary to the Galian staging system has been published;[38] however, most physicians use the Galian staging system for determining prognosis and therapeutic strategies.

In the past, confusion existed over whether Mediterranean lymphoma and α-HCD were different conditions. In 1976, a consensus panel concluded that α-HCD and Mediterranean lymphoma constitute a spectrum of disease, and the term *immunoproliferative small intestinal disease* (IPSID) came into use. This term is applied to small intestinal lesions whose pathologic features are identical to those of α-HCD, regardless of the type of Ig synthesized.[34,39] The pattern of α-HCD pathologic lesions often includes clear lymphoepithelial lesions composed of centrocytic-like cells. This indicates that α-HCD can be considered a subtype of lymphoma arising from mucosa-associated lymph node tissue.[40] The pathologic changes in the few cases of the respiratory form of α-HCD are poorly documented. In a case of the lymph node or lymphomatous form, lymph node biopsy showed diffuse plasmacytic lymphoma.

CYTOGENETICS

Cytogenetic abnormalities have been found in the lymphoid cells of patients with α-HCD. The clonal proliferation in this disease appears to be associated with frequent alterations of chromosome 14 at band q32 resulting from translocations that differ from those observed in the vast majority of other lymphomas. Abnormal karyotypes were reported in three of four patients.[41] Two patients had a rearrangement of 14q32 resulting from a t(9;14)(p11;q32) and a t(2;14)(p12;q32). Cloning and sequencing of the der(14) breakpoint of a chromosome translocation involving the 14q32 Ig locus in 1 of these patients suggested that the translocation originated from a local pairing of the two chromosomes, 9 and 14.[42] One case showed complex rearrangements, including t(5;9). No abnormalities were found in the intestinal tumor of the fourth case with immunoblastic lymphoma.

● DIFFERENTIAL DIAGNOSIS

The digestive form of α-HCD must be differentiated from lymphoma, although this is an uncommon diagnosis in the age range typical of α-HCD. Other causes of malabsorption need to be considered, especially celiac disease. Enteric presentation of γ-HCD, variable immunodeficiency, and acquired immunodeficiency syndrome with clinicopathologic features simulating IPSID should be excluded.

● THERAPY

Patients with stage A lesions limited to the bowel and to the mesenteric lymph nodes should be treated initially with oral antibiotics. In the absence of a documented parasite, tetracycline, metronidazole, or ampicillin is appropriate. Patients with stage B or C lesions or stage A lesions without improvement after a 6-month course of antibiotic treatment should be given chemotherapy. The treatment regimens are those commonly used to treat lymphoma. There have been few controlled clinical trials. In a prospective randomized study, a doxorubicin-based regimen (cyclophosphamide, doxorubicin hydrochloride, vincristine, and prednisone) provided a higher response rate than a non–doxorubicin-containing protocol (cyclophosphamide, vincristine, procarbazine, and prednisone) or total abdominal irradiation.[43] Similar results were noted in a retrospective study.[44] Good results have been reported with cyclophosphamide, doxorubicin, teniposide, and prednisone, sometimes alternating with bleomycin, vinblastine, and doxorubicin[45] and with cyclophosphamide, epidoxorubicin, vincristine, prednisolone, ifosfamide, methotrexate, etoposide (VP-16), and dexamethasone.[46] Surgical resection should be considered for focal or bulky transmural lymphomatous tumors and extramedullary plasmacytoma. Autologous hematopoietic stem cell transplantation has been recommended for patients with advanced or refractory disease,[34] but to our knowledge there are no reports in the literature demonstrating the usefulness of this approach. Previous trials have not incorporated immunotherapy with rituximab, an anti-CD20 monoclonal antibody, in the management of IPSID. As expected, the centrocyte-like cells are CD20-positive, but the plasma cells are not. In light of the extreme plasma cell differentiation and the plasmacytic nature of large-cell IPSID lymphoma, there is interest in investigating the value of treating patients with IPSID with the novel agents (thalidomide, lenalidomide, bortezomib, pomalidomide, or carfilzomib).

COURSE AND PROGNOSIS

The course of α-HCD is variable but generally progressive in the absence of therapy. Followup should include a periodic search for α-HCD protein in serum and urine and, if negative, in the intestinal secretions. Bowel radiography, ultrasonography, and esophagogastroduodenojejunal endoscopy should be performed. A second-look laparotomy may be necessary.[34] Relapses may occur after treatment at any stage of the disease. The long-term prognosis for patients with α-HCD remains imprecise because of the lack of large series with prolonged followup. In a small prospective Tunisian study,[45] including eight patients with stage A disease and 15 with stages B and C, the survival of the total group was 90 percent at 2 years. A series from Turkey[47] reported 5-year treatment results of 23 patients with IPSID, including five with secretion of α chains. In patients with stage A disease, tetracycline yielded a 71 percent complete response. The 5-year overall survival rate for the entire group was 70 percent. However, the median overall survival for 3 patients with immunoblastic lymphoma was only 7 months.

Thirteen patients were studied who had IPSID associated with α-HCD.[48] Six patients, two with high-grade lymphoma and four with low-grade disease, received chemotherapy or radiotherapy or both. One patient died at 76 months, and five were alive at an average of 92 months. Five patients with low-grade disease received conservative therapy (antibiotics and in some cases prednisone). All five patients were alive at an average of 40 months after presentation. Three of these five patients achieved remission at 5, 6, and 27 months. Two of the five patients had persistent disease at 20 and 25 months. Two patients did not receive treatment and died of high-grade lymphoma.

Another study[49] described six patients who had α-HCD with lymphoma. All patients responded poorly to chemotherapy; the median duration of survival was 10.5 months.

A subsequent study[50] described 12 patients with secretory and nonsecretory IPSID. Six patients presented with stage A disease. Four patients responded to antibiotic or glucocorticoid therapy. In two patients, stage A disease evolved into stage C. Three patients presented with stage B disease. Two of these patients responded completely to chemotherapy, and the third refused treatment and died after 16 months. Three patients with stage C disease at diagnosis received aggressive combination chemotherapy and remained in complete remission with a median followup of 2.2 years.

Preliminary results suggest that flow cytometric analysis of S-phase fraction[51] and certain immunomarkers, such as syndecan, Bcl6, and p53,[52] may be useful prognostic indicators in the clinical management of patients with IPSID. Patients with a poor prognosis have a higher fraction of cells in S phase, lower syndecan-1 expression, and higher Bcl6 expression than those with a good prognosis.

μ-HEAVY-CHAIN DISEASE DEFINITION AND HISTORY

μ-HCD is a proliferative disorder of B lymphocytes defined by the recognition of monoclonal deleted μ-HCs. In the first reported case, in 1969 by Forte and colleagues,[53] the patient had chronic lymphocytic leukemia. Since then, approximately 34 additional cases have been reported.[54-57]

EPIDEMIOLOGY

μ-HCD is extremely rare. In a series of 27 patients, the majority were white (76 percent) and male (55 percent). The median age at diagnosis in 27 patients was 57.5 years (range: 15 to 80 years).[54]

ETIOLOGY AND PATHOGENESIS

The cause of μ-HCD is unknown.

CLINICAL FEATURES

The most common presenting symptoms of patients with μ-HCD are those of a lymphoproliferative malignancy. An associated lymphoplasmacytic proliferative disorder was noted in 22 of 27 patients at some time during the disease and designated as chronic lymphocytic leukemia, lymphoma, Waldenström macroglobulinemia, or myeloma.[54] μ-HCD protein has been described in one patient each with systemic lupus erythematosus, hepatic cirrhosis, hepatosplenomegaly with ascites, pulmonary infection, splenomegaly with pancytopenia,[54] and myelodysplasia.[55] Three cases of μ-HCD associated with amyloidosis have been reported.[58]

Splenomegaly and hepatomegaly are common in μ-HCD and were noted in 21 of 22 and 15 of 21 patients, respectively.[54] Peripheral lymphadenopathy was described in 10 of 25 patients.[54]

LABORATORY FEATURES

MOLECULAR BIOLOGY AND GENETICS

The molecular weight of the μ-HCD protein determined in eight patients ranged from 26,500 to 158,000. The higher molecular weights are thought to be the result of polymerization of the μ-chain fragments. The μ-HCD fragments from 6 patients were subjected to detailed chemical analysis. Figure 110-5 depicts the structure of these six μ-HCD proteins compared with that of normal μ-HC. The V_H domain is absent in all cases. The normal sequence began with C_H1 in three cases, C_H2 in two cases, and C_H3 in one case. There are sequence data for only 1 gene coding for a μ-HCD protein (Fig. 110-6).

SERUM AND URINE PROTEIN FINDINGS

A monoclonal spike was found on serum protein electrophoresis in less than half of a series of patients with μ-HCD (eight of 19).[54] The diagnosis of μ-HCD is made by documentation of the abnormal HC. Immunofixation of both serum and urine should be done. When these procedures yield ambiguous results, two-dimensional gel electrophoresis is a useful additional tool. The combination of capillary immunotyping electrophoresis and high-resolution two-dimensional electrophoresis has been used successfully for the detection of μ-HCD in one patient,[59]

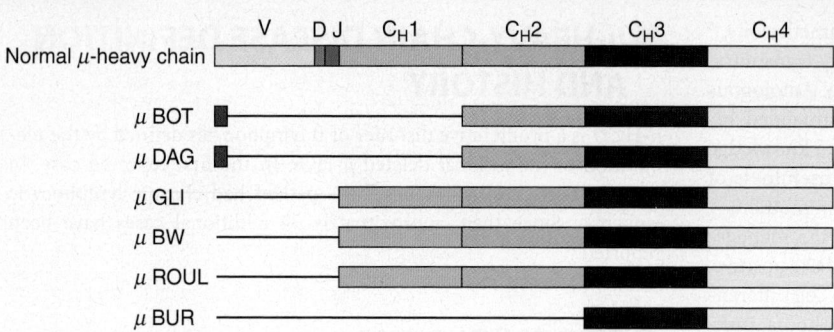

Figure 110–5. Structure of various deleted μ-heavy-chain disease proteins compared with that of normal chain. ■, indicates unusual amino acid sequences; boxes, coding regions; lines, deletions; V, variable region; D, diversity segment; J, joining region; C$_H$1, C$_H$2, C$_H$3, C$_H$4, constant regions of heavy chains. BOT,[93] DAG,[94] GLI,[95] BW,[96] ROUL,[97] BUR.[98]

whereas in another capillary zone electrophoresis failed to detect the μ-HCD protein.[60] Three of 33 reported patients with μ-HCD had a biclonal gammopathy. Hypogammaglobulinemia was noted in 10 of 22 patients.[54] Hypergammaglobulinemia with a polyclonal pattern in the γ-globulin fraction was described in one case.[55] In contrast to γ- and α-HCD in which there usually is no detectable monoclonal light chain in the serum and urine, Bence Jones proteinuria was found in more than half the cases of μ-HCD (14 of 22 patients).[54] μ-HCD protein was found in the urine of only two patients.[54] Three cases of nonsecretory μ-HCD have been reported.[61–63] μ-HCs were documented by immunofluorescence on the cell surface of proliferating lymphocytes in 1 case and in marrow plasma cells of two others.

HEMATOLOGIC ABNORMALITIES

Anemia is frequent, but lymphocytosis and thrombocytopenia are uncommon. One patient had a positive direct antiglobulin test.[55] Examination of the marrow usually shows an increase in lymphocytes, plasma cells, or plasmacytoid lymphocytes. Plasmacytosis was noted in 18 of 20 cases; in 13 of these, vacuolated plasma cells were found.[54] The presence of vacuolated plasma cells in the marrow of a patient with a lymphoplasmacytic proliferative disorder should always suggest the possibility of μ-HCD.

OTHER FEATURES

Lytic bone lesions were described in three of 15 patients[54] and osteoporosis was mentioned in three others. No cytogenetic studies have been reported.

HISTOPATHOLOGY

In a literature review that included 27 documented cases of μ-HCD, 22 patients (81 percent) had an associated lymphoplasmacytic proliferative disorder designated as chronic lymphocytic leukemia, lymphoma, Waldenström macroglobulinemia, or myeloma.[54]

● DIFFERENTIAL DIAGNOSIS

The differential diagnosis of μ-HCD includes all lymphoplasmacytic proliferative disorders. Without a suspicion for the disease, μ-HCD is difficult to diagnose. The finding of Bence Jones proteinuria in a patient with a lymphoproliferative disorder and vacuolated plasma cells in the marrow deserves further investigation for possible μ-HCD.

● THERAPY

There is no specific therapy for μ-HCD. The finding of a μ-HCD protein in the serum of an apparently normal patient should be considered to represent monoclonal gammopathy of undetermined significance, and the patient should be followed closely for the development of a symptomatic lymphoplasmacytic proliferative disorder. Once this develops, chemotherapy is indicated. Various agents have been used. Initially, a combination of cyclophosphamide, vincristine, and prednisone with or without doxorubicin is a reasonable choice. The use of fludarabine has been reported in two patients with μ-HCD; one had an "apparent hematologic response,"[64] and the other had a partial response.[56] Vincristine, cyclophosphamide, prednisolone, and doxorubicin in combination with rituximab led to complete resolution of tumoral lesions in one patient with μ-HCD.[65]

● COURSE AND PROGNOSIS

The course of μ-HCD is variable. Because of the rarity of the disease, no large series of patients treated systematically in a single center has been reported. The median duration of survival from the time of diagnosis is 24 months (range: <1 month to 11 years).[54] Because several of the reported patients had findings consistent with μ-HCD before recognition of the μ-HCD protein, the course is probably longer than reported in most patients. In one patient, the hematologic abnormalities became normal and the μ-HC disappeared after 2 years without specific treatment.

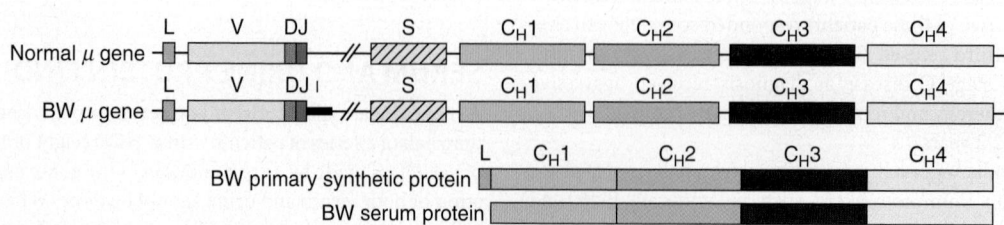

Figure 110–6. Structure of a gene coding for a μ-heavy-chain disease protein compared with that of normal μ gene. Boxes indicate coding regions; ▨, switch region; ■, inserted noncoding sequence; L, leader region; V, variable region; D, diversity segment; J, joining region; S, switch region; C$_H$1, C$_H$2, C$_H$3, C$_H$4, constant regions of heavy chains; I, inserted sequence. BW.[96]

REFERENCES

1. Corcos D, Osborn MJ, Matheson LS: B-cell receptors and heavy chain diseases: Guilty by association? *Blood* 117:6991, 2011.

2. Franklin EC, Lowenstein J, Bigelow B, Meltzer M: Heavy chain disease: A new disorder of serum gamma-globulins: Report of the first case. *Am J Med* 37:332, 1964.

3. Fermand JP, Brouet JC: Heavy-chain diseases. *Hematol Oncol Clin North Am* 13:1281, 1999.

4. Fermand JP, Brouet JC, Danon F, Seligmann M: Gamma heavy chain "disease": Heterogeneity of the clinicopathologic features: Report of 16 cases and review of the literature. *Medicine (Baltimore)* 68:321, 1989.

5. Wahner-Roedler DL, Witzig TE, Loehrer LL, Kyle RA: Gamma-heavy-chain disease: Review of 23 cases. *Medicine (Baltimore)* 82:236, 2003.

6. Wester SM, Banks PM, Li CY: The histopathology of gamma heavy-chain disease. *Am J Clin Pathol* 78:427, 1982.

7. Yunokawa K, Hagiyama Y, Mochizuki Y, et al: Hypertrophic spinal pachymeningitis associated with heavy-chain disease: Case report. *J Neurosurg Spine* 7:459, 2007.

8. Sun T, Peng S, Narurkar L: Modified immunoselection technique for definitive diagnosis of heavy-chain disease. *Clin Chem* 40:664, 1994.

9. Luraschi P, Infusino I, Zorzoli I, et al: Heavy chain disease can be detected by capillary zone electrophoresis. *Clin Chem* 51:247, 2005.

10. Kaleta E, Kyle R, Clark R, Katzmann J: Analysis of patients with γ-heavy chain disease by the heavy/light chain and free light chain assays. *Clin Chem Lab Med* 52:665, 2014.

11. Lee MT, Parwani A, Humphrey R, et al: Gamma heavy chain disease in a patient with diabetes and chronic renal insufficiency: Diagnostic assessment of the heavy chain fragment. *J Clin Lab Anal* 22:146, 2008.

12. Lebreton JP, Fontaine M, Rousseaux J, et al: Deleted IgG1 and IgG2 H chains in a patient with an IgG subclass imbalance. *Clin Exp Immunol* 47:206, 1982.

13. Keller H, Spengler GA, Skvaril F, et al: [Heavy chain disease: A case of IgG-heavy-chain-fragment and IgM-type K-paraproteinemia with plasma cell leukemia] [in German]. *Schweiz Med Wochenschr* 100:1012, 1970.

14. Woods R, Blumenschein GR, Terry WD: A new type of human gamma heavy chain disease protein: Immunochemical and physical characteristics. *Immunochemistry* 7:373, 1970.

15. Zhang L, Sotomayor EM, Papenhausen PR, et al: Unusual concurrence of T-cell large granular lymphocytic leukemia with Franklin disease (gamma heavy chain disease) manifested with massive splenomegaly. *Leuk Lymphoma* 54:205, 2013.

16. Bieliauskas S, Tubbs RR, Bacon CM, et al: Gamma heavy-chain disease: Defining the spectrum of associated lymphoproliferative disorders through analysis of 13 cases. *Am J Surg Pathol* 36:534, 2012.

17. Grogan TM, Muller-Hermelink HK, Van Camp B, et al: Plasma cell neoplasms, in *World Health Organization Classification of Tumours: Pathology and Genetics of Tumours of Haematopoietic and Lymphoid Tissues*, edited by Jaffe ES, Harris NL, Stein H, Vardiman JW, p 154. IARC Press, Lyon, France, 2001.

18. Tan JN, Kroll MH, O'Hara CJ, et al: Gamma heavy chain disease in a patient with underlying lymphoplasmacytic lymphoma of the thyroid: Report of a case and comparison with other reported cases with thyroid involvement. *Clin Chim Acta* 413:1696, 2012.

19. Agrawal S, Abboudi Z, Matutes E, Catovsky D: First report of fludarabine in gamma-heavy chain disease. *Br J Haematol* 88:653, 1994.

20. Ishikawa K, Hirai M, Tsutsumi H, et al: [Successful treatment of heavy-chain disease with etoposide] [in Japanese]. *Nippon Ronen Igakkai Zasshi* 34:221, 1997.

21. Munshi NC, Digumarthy S, Rahemtullah A: Case records of the Massachusetts General Hospital: Case 13–2008: A 46-year-old man with rheumatoid arthritis and lymphadenopathy. *N Engl J Med* 358:1838, 2008.

22. Takano H, Nagata K, Mikoshiba M, et al: Combination of rituximab and chemotherapy showing anti-tumor effect in gamma heavy chain disease expressing CD20. *Am J Hematol* 83:938, 2008.

23. Jacobson E, Sharp G, Rimmer J, MacPherson B: A 59-year-old woman with immunotactoid glomerulopathy, heavy-chain disease, and non-Hodgkin lymphoma. *Arch Pathol Lab Med* 128:689, 2004.

24. Inoue D, Matsushita A, Kiuchi M, et al: Successful treatment of -heavy-chain disease with rituximab and fludarabine. *Acta Haematol* 128:139, 2012.

25. Galanti LM, Doyen C, Vander Maelen C, et al: Biological diagnosis of a gamma-1-heavy chain disease in an asymptomatic patient. *Eur J Haematol* 54:202, 1995.

26. Seligmann M, Danon F, Hurez D, et al: Alpha-chain disease: A new immunoglobulin abnormality. *Science* 162:1396, 1968.

27. Makni S, Zouari R, Barbouch MR, et al: [Monoclonal gammopathies in Tunisia] [in French]. *Rev Fr Transfus Hemobiol* 33:31, 1990.

28. Mseddi-Hdiji S, Haddouk S, Ben Ayed M, et al: [Monoclonal gammopathies in Tunisia: Epidemiological, immunochemical and etiological analysis of 288 cases] [in French]. *Pathol Biol (Paris)* 53:19, 2005.

29. Lankarani KB, Masoompour SM, Masoompour MB, et al: Changing epidemiology of IPSID in southern Iran. *Gut* 54:311, 2005.

30. Economidou I, Manousos ON, Triantafillidis JK, et al: Immunoproliferative small intestinal disease in Greece: Presentation of 13 cases including two from Albania. *Eur J Gastroenterol Hepatol* 18:1029, 2006.

31. Lecuit M, Abachin E, Martin A, et al: Immunoproliferative small intestinal disease associated with *Campylobacter jejuni*. *N Engl J Med* 350:239, 2004.

32. Tracy RP, Kyle RA, Leitch JM: Alpha heavy-chain disease presenting as goiter. *Am J Clin Pathol* 82:336, 1984.

33. Kim SK, Park IK, Park BH, et al: A case report: Isolated α heavy chain monoclonal gammopathy in a patient with polyneuropathy, organomegaly, endocrinopathy, monoclonal gammopathy and skin change syndrome. *Int J Clin Pract Suppl* 147:26, 2005.

34. Rambaud JC, Halphen M, Galian A, Tsapis A: Immunoproliferative small intestinal disease (IPSID): Relationships with alpha-chain disease and "Mediterranean" lymphomas. *Springer Semin Immunopathol* 12:239, 1990.

35. Tashiro T, Sato H, Takahashi T, et al: Non-secretory alpha chain disease involving stomach, small intestine and colon. *Intern Med* 34:255, 1995.

36. Galian A, Lecestre MJ, Scotto J, et al: Pathological study of alpha-chain disease, with special emphasis on evolution. *Cancer* 39:2081, 1977.

37. Al-Saleem T, Al-Mondhiry H: Immunoproliferative small intestinal disease (IPSID): A model for mature B-cell neoplasms. *Blood* 105:2274, 2005.

38. Salem PA, Estephan FF: Immunoproliferative small intestinal disease: Current concepts. *Cancer J* 11:374, 2005.

39. Martin IG, Aldoori MI: Immunoproliferative small intestinal disease: Mediterranean lymphoma and alpha heavy chain disease. *Br J Surg* 81:20, 1994.

40. Isaacson PG: Gastrointestinal lymphoma. *Hum Pathol* 25:1020, 1994.

41. Berger R, Bernheim A, Tsapis A, et al: Cytogenetic studies in four cases of alpha chain disease. *Cancer Genet Cytogenet* 22:219, 1986.

42. Pellet P, Tsapis A, Brouet JC: Alpha heavy chain disease of patient MAL: Structure of the non-functional rearranged alpha gene translocated on chromosome 9. *Eur J Immunol* 20:2731, 1990.

43. Khojasteh A, Saalabian MJ, Haghshenass M: Randomized comparison of abdominal irradiation (AI) vs CHOP vs C-MOPP for the treatment of immunoproliferative small intestinal disease (IPSID) associated lymphoma (AL) [abstract]. *Proc Annu Meeting Am Soc Clin Oncol.* 2:207, 1983.

44. Salimi M, Spinelli JJ: Chemotherapy of Mediterranean abdominal lymphoma: Retrospective comparison of chemotherapy protocols in Iranian patients. *Am J Clin Oncol* 19:18, 1996.

45. Ben-Ayed F, Halphen M, Najjar T, et al: Treatment of alpha chain disease: Results of a prospective study in 21 Tunisian patients by the Tunisian-French Intestinal Lymphoma Study Group. *Cancer* 63:1251, 1989.

46. Hubmann R, Kaiser W, Radaszkiewicz T, et al: Malabsorption associated with a high-grade-malignant non-Hodgkin's lymphoma, alpha-heavy-chain disease and immunoproliferative small intestinal disease. *Z Gastroenterol* 33:209, 1995.

47. Akbulut H, Soykan I, Yakaryilmaz F, et al: Five-year results of the treatment of 23 patients with immunoproliferative small intestinal disease: A Turkish experience. *Cancer* 80:8, 1997.

48. Price SK: Immunoproliferative small intestinal disease: A study of 13 cases with alpha heavy-chain disease. *Histopathology* 17:7, 1990.

49. Shih LY, Liaw SJ, Dunn P, Kuo TT: Primary small-intestinal lymphomas in Taiwan: Immunoproliferative small-intestinal disease and nonimmunoproliferative small-intestinal disease. *J Clin Oncol* 12:1375, 1994.

50. Malik IA, Shamsi Z, Shafquat A, et al: Clinicopathological features and management of immunoproliferative small intestinal disease and primary small intestinal lymphoma in Pakistan. *Med Pediatr Oncol* 25:400, 1995.

51. Demirer T, Uzunalimoglu O, Anderson T, et al: Flow cytometric measurement of proliferation-associated nuclear antigen P105 and DNA content in immuno-proliferative small intestinal disease (IPSID). *J Surg Oncol* 58:25, 1995.

52. Vaiphei K, Kumari N, Sinha SK, et al: Roles of syndecan-1, bcl6 and p53 in diagnosis and prognostication of immunoproliferative small intestinal disease. *World J Gastroenterol* 12:3602, 2006.

53. Forte FA, Prelli F, Yount W, et al: Heavy chain disease of the µ type: Report of the first case. *Blood* 1970 Aug;36(2):137–44.

54. Wahner-Roedler DL, Kyle RA: Mu-heavy chain disease: Presentation as a benign monoclonal gammopathy. *Am J Hematol* 40:56, 1992.

55. Witzens M, Egerer G, Stahl D, et al: A case of mu heavy-chain disease associated with hyperglobulinemia, anemia, and a positive Coombs test. *Ann Hematol* 77:231, 1998.

56. Yanai M, Maeda A, Watanabe N, et al: Successful treatment of mu-heavy chain disease with fludarabine monophosphate: A case report. *Int J Hematol* 79:174, 2004.

57. Cogne M, Aucouturier P, Brizard A, et al: Complete variable region deletion in a mu heavy chain disease protein (ROUL): Correlation with light chain secretion. *Leuk Res* 17:527, 1993.

58. Kinoshita K, Yamagata T, Nozaki Y, et al: Mu-heavy chain disease associated with systemic amyloidosis. *Hematology* 9:135, 2004.

59. Maisnar V, Tichy M, Stulik J, et al: Capillary immunotyping electrophoresis and high resolution two-dimensional electrophoresis for the detection of mu-heavy chain disease. *Clin Chim Acta* 389:171, 2008.

60. Marien G, Verhoef G, Bossuyt X: Detection of heavy chain disease by capillary zone electrophoresis. *Clin Chem* 51:1302, 2005.

61. Gordon J, Hamblin TJ, Smith JL, et al. A human B-cell lymphoma synthesizing and expressing surface mu-chain in the absence of detectable light chain. *Blood* 58:552, 1981.

62. Guglielmo P, Granata P, Di Raimondo F, et al: "Mu" heavy chain type "non-excretory" myeloma. *Scand J Haematol* 29:36, 1982.

63. Leglise MC, Briere J, Abgrall JF, Hurez D: [Non-secretory myeloma of heavy mu-chain type] [in French]. *Nouv Rev Fr Hematol* 25:103, 1983.

64. Preud'homme JL, Bauwens M, Dumont G, et al: Cast nephropathy in mu heavy chain disease. *Clin Nephrol* 48:118, 1997.

65. Maeda A, Mori M, Torii S, et al: Multiple extranodal tumors in mu-heavy chain disease. *Int J Hematol* 84:286, 2006.

66. Alexander A, Anicito I, Buxbaum J: Gamma heavy chain disease in man: Genomic sequence reveals two noncontiguous deletions in a single gene. *J Clin Invest* 82:1244, 1988.

67. Frangione B, Rosenwasser E, Prelli F, Franklin EC: Primary structure of human gamma 3 immunoglobulin deletion mutant: Gamma 3 heavy-chain disease protein Wis. *Biochemistry* 19:4304, 1980.

68. Frangione B: A new immunoglobulin variant: Gamma3 heavy chain disease protein CHI. *Proc Natl Acad Sci U S A* 73:1552, 1976.

69. Frangione B, Franklin EC: Correlation between fragmented immunoglobulin genes and heavy chain deletion mutants. *Nature* 281:600, 1979.

70. Wolfenstein-Todel C, Frangione B, Prelli F, Franklin EC: The amino acid sequence of "heavy chain disease" protein ZUC: Structure of the Fc fragment of immunoglobulin G3. *Biochem Biophys Res Commun* 71:907, 1976.

71. Arnaud P, Wang AC, Gianazza E, et al: Gamma heavy chain disease protein CHA: Immunological and structural studies. *Mol Immunol* 18:379, 1981.

72. Prelli F, Frangione B: Franklin's disease: Ig gamma 2 H chain mutant BUR. *J Immunol* 148:949, 1992.

73. Cooper SM, Franklin EC, Frangione B: Molecular defect in a gamma-2 heavy chain. *Science* 176:187, 1972.

74. Frangione B, Franklin EC, Smithies O: Unusual genes at the aminoterminus of human immunoglobulin variants. *Nature* 273:400, 1978.

75. Terry WD, Ohms J: Implications of heavy chain disease protein sequences for multiple gene theories of immunoglobulin synthesis. *Proc Natl Acad Sci U S A* 66:558, 1970.

76. Smith LL, Barton BP, Garver FA, et al: Physicochemical and immunochemical properties of gamma l heavy chain disease protein BAZ. *Immunochemistry* 15:323, 1978.

77. Rabin BS, Moon J: Clinical findings in a case of newly defined gamma heavy chain disease protein. *Clin Exp Immunol* 14:563, 1973.

78. Franklin EC, Prelli F, Frangione B: Human heavy chain disease protein WIS: Implications for the organization of immunoglobulin genes. *Proc Natl Acad Sci U S A* 76:452, 1979.

79. Frangione B, Lee L, Haber E, Bloch KJ: Protein Hal: Partial deletion of a "γ" immunoglobulin gene(s) and apparent reinitiation at an internal AUG codon. *Proc Natl Acad Sci U S A* 70:1073, 1973.

80. Franklin EC, Kyle R, Seligmann M, Frangione B: Correlation of protein structure and immunoglobulin gene organization in the light of two new deleted heavy chain disease proteins. *Mol Immunol* 16:919, 1979.

81. Hauke G, Schiltz E, Bross KJ, et al: Unusual sequence of immunoglobulin L-chain rearrangements in a gamma heavy chain disease patient. *Scand J Immunol* 36:463, 1992.

82. Sala P, Tonutti E, Pizzolitto S, et al: Immunochemical and structural characterization of an IgG1 heavy chain disease. *Ric Clin Lab* 19:59, 1989.

83. Franklin EC, Frangione B: The molecular defect in a protein (CRA) found in gamma-1 heavy chain disease, and its genetic implications. *Proc Natl Acad Sci U S A* 68:187, 1971.

84. Nabeshima Y, Ikenaka T: N- and C-terminal amino acid sequences of a gamma-heavy chain disease protein YOK. *Immunochemistry* 13:245, 1976.

85. Guglielmi P, Bakhshi A, Cogne M, et al: Multiple genomic defects result in an alternative RNA splice creating a human gamma H chain disease protein. *J Immunol* 141:1762, 1988.

86. Biewenga J, Frangione B, Franklin EC, van Loghem E: A gamma l heavy-chain disease protein (EST) lacking the entire VH and CH1 domains. *Scand J Immunol* 11:601, 1980.

87. Bentaboulet M, Mihaesco E, Gendron MC, et al: Genomic alterations in a case of alpha heavy chain disease leading to the generation of composite exons from the JH region. *Eur J Immunol* 19:2093, 1989.

88. Tsapis A, Bentaboulet M, Pellet P, et al: The productive gene for alpha-H chain disease protein MAL is highly modified by insertion-deletion processes. *J Immunol* 143:3821, 1989.

89. Wolfenstein-Todel C, Mihaesco E, Frangione B: "Alpha chain disease" protein def: Internal deletion of a human immunoglobulin A1 heavy chain. *Proc Natl Acad Sci U S A* 71:974, 1974.

90. Wolfenstein-Todel C, Mihaesco E, Frangione B: Variant of a human immunoglobulin: "alpha chain disease" protein AIT. *Biochem Biophys Res Commun* 65:47, 1975.

91. Cogne M, Preud'homme JL: Gene deletions force nonsecretory alpha-chain disease plasma cells to produce membrane-form alpha-chain only. *J Immunol* 145:2455, 1990.

92. Fakhfakh F, Dellagi K, Ayadi H, et al: Alpha heavy chain disease alpha mRNA contain nucleotide sequences of unknown origins. *Eur J Immunol* 22:3037, 1992.

93. Barnikol-Watanabe S, Mihaesco E, Mihaesco C, et al: The primary structure of mu-chain-disease protein BOT: Peculiar amino-acid sequence of the N-terminal 42 positions. *Hoppe Seylers Z Physiol Chem* 365:105, 1984.

94. Mihaesco C, Ferrara P, Guillemot JC, et al: A new extra sequence at the amino terminal of a mu heavy chain disease protein (DAG). *Mol Immunol* 27:771, 1990.

95. Franklin EC, Frangione B, Prelli F: The defect in mu heavy chain disease protein GLI. *J Immunol* 116:1194, 1976.

96. Bakhshi A, Guglielmi P, Siebenlist U, et al: A DNA insertion/deletion necessitates an aberrant RNA splice accounting for a mu heavy chain disease protein. *Proc Natl Acad Sci U S A* 83:2689, 1986.

97. Cogne M, Aucouturier P, Brizard A, et al: Complete variable region deletion in a mu heavy chain disease protein (ROUL): Correlation with light chain secretion. *Leuk Res* 17:527, 1993.

98. Lebreton JP, Ropartz C, Rousseaus J, et al: Immunochemical and biochemical study of a human Fcmu-like fragment (mu-chain disease). *Eur J Immunol* 5:179, 1975.

Part XII Hemostasis and Thrombosis

111. Megakaryopoiesis and Thrombopoiesis 1815

112. Platelet Morphology, Biochemistry, and Function 1829

113. Molecular Biology and Biochemistry of the Coagulation Factors and Pathways of Hemostasis.............. 1915

114. Control of Coagulation Reactions.....1949

115. Vascular Function in Hemostasis......1967

116. Classification, Clinical Manifestations, and Evaluation of Disorders of Hemostasis 1985

117. Thrombocytopenia...................1993

118. Heparin-Induced Thrombocytopenia.. 2025

119. Reactive Thrombocytosis.............2035

120. Hereditary Qualitative Platelet Disorders 2039

121. Acquired Qualitative Platelet Disorders 2073

122. The Vascular Purpuras 2097

123. Hemophilia A and Hemophilia B......2113

124. Inherited Deficiencies of Coagulation Factors II, V, V+VIII, VII, X, XI, and XIII.... 2133

125. Hereditary Fibrinogen Abnormalities .. 2151

126. von Willebrand Disease 2163

127. Antibody-Mediated Coagulation Factor Deficiencies 2183

128. Hemostatic Alterations in Liver Disease and Liver Transplantation 2191

129. Disseminated Intravascular Coagulation 2199

130. Hereditary Thrombophilia...........2221

131. The Antiphospholipid Syndrome 2233

132. Thrombotic Microangiopathies.......2253

133. Venous Thrombosis 2267

134. Atherothrombosis: Disease Initiation, Progression, and Treatment 2281

135. Fibrinolysis and Thrombolysis 2303

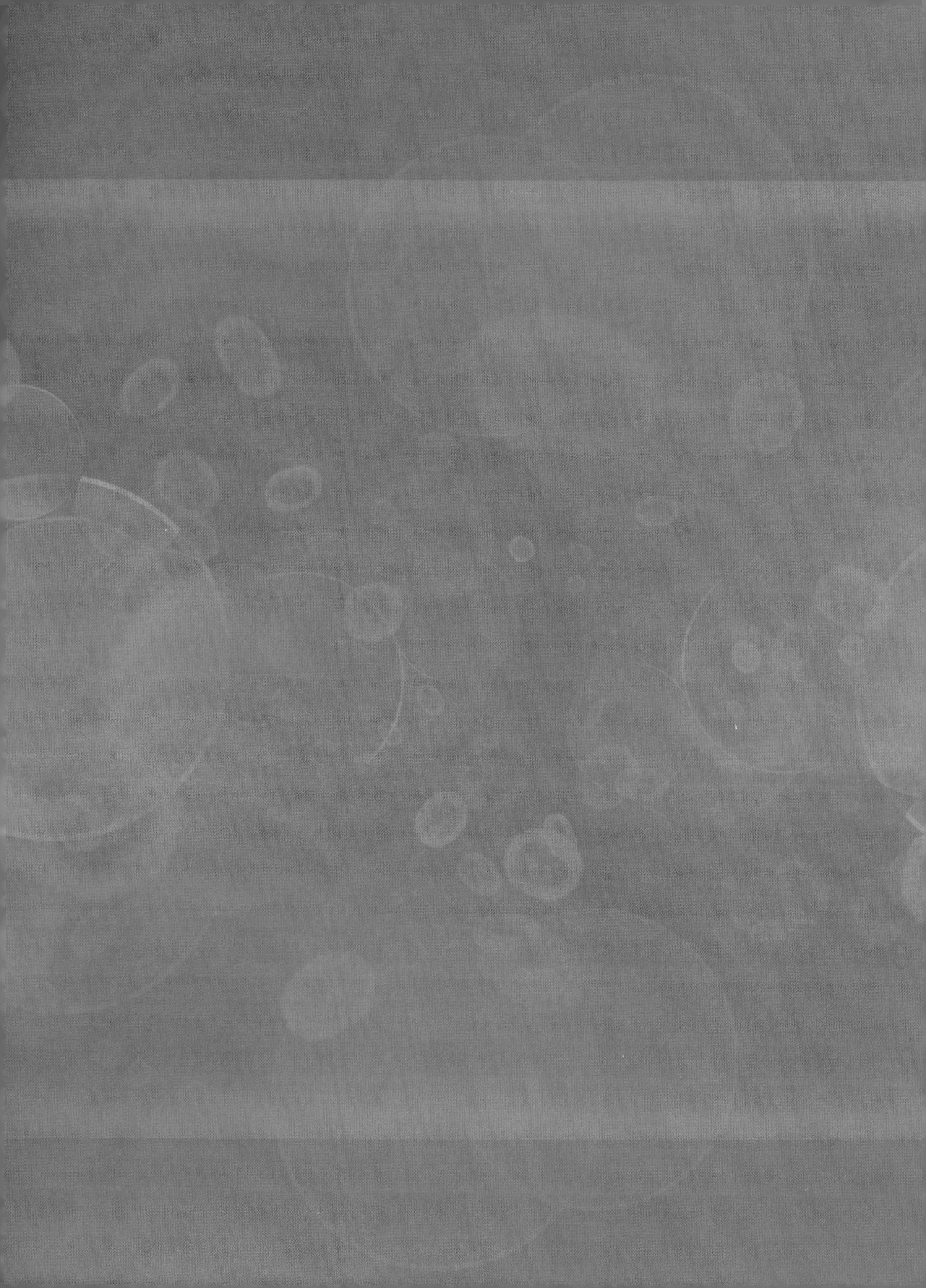

CHAPTER 111
MEGAKARYOPOIESIS AND THROMBOPOIESIS

Kenneth Kaushansky

SUMMARY

Each day the adult human produces approximately 1×10^{11} platelets, a level of production that can increase 10- to 20-fold in times of increased demand and an additional five- to 10-fold under the stimulation of exogenous thrombopoietin mimetic drugs. Production of platelets depends on the proliferation and differentiation of hematopoietic stem and progenitor cells to cells committed to the megakaryocyte lineage, their maturation to large, polyploid megakaryocytes, and their final fragmentation into platelets. The external influences that impact megakaryopoiesis and thrombopoiesis are a supportive marrow stroma consisting of endothelial and other cells, matrix glycosaminoglycans, and a family of protein hormones and cytokines, including thrombopoietin, stem cell factor, and stromal cell-derived factor-1. The role of the cytokines essential for these processes has been defined, the transcription factors critical for megakaryocyte development identified, the molecular mechanisms that underlie the two most unusual aspects of thrombopoiesis—endomitosis and proplatelet formation—have been studied, and reagents to specifically modify platelet production have been generated. This chapter focuses on the development of megakaryocytes, their precursors and their progeny, and the hematopoietic growth factors and transcriptionally active molecules that control the survival, proliferation, and differentiation of these cells.

KINETICS OF THROMBOPOIESIS

The circulatory life span of a platelet is approximately 10 days in humans with normal platelet counts, but somewhat shorter in patients with moderate (7 days) to severe (5 days) thrombocytopenia, as a higher proportion of the total-body platelet mass is consumed in the day-to-day function of maintaining vascular integrity.[1] Based on a "normal" level of 200,000 platelets/μL, a blood volume of 5 L, and a half-life of 10 days, 1×10^{11} platelets per day are produced. If 1 megakaryocyte produces approximately 1000 platelets, approximately 1×10^8 megakaryocytes are generated in the marrow each day.

Several independent lines of evidence indicate the transit time from megakaryocyte progenitor cell to release of platelets into the circulation ranges from 4 to 7 days. For example, following platelet apheresis, the platelet count falls, recovers substantially by day 4, and completely

recovers by day 7.[2] In most physiologic and pathologic states, the platelet count is inversely related to plasma thrombopoietin levels. For example, liver failure is associated with moderate thrombocytopenia as a result of splenomegaly and thrombopoietin deficiency. Within the first week following orthotopic liver transplantation, the platelet count rises substantially, with kinetics matching those of thrombopoietin infusion.[3,4] These findings indicate expansion of the megakaryocyte mass takes from 3 to 4 days following a thrombopoietin stimulus in humans and, coupled with the approximate 12 hours required for platelet release,[5] results in a relatively brisk response to thrombocytopenia.

CELLULAR PHYSIOLOGY OF THROMBOPOIESIS

Platelets form by fragmentation of megakaryocyte membrane extensions termed *proplatelets*, in a process that consumes nearly the entire cytoplasmic complement of membranes, organelles, granules, and soluble macromolecules. Although at first controversial, as the process was initially observed only *in vitro*, *in situ* microscopic studies have identified proplatelet formation and fragmentation in living animals.[6] Each megakaryocyte is estimated to give rise to 1000 to 3000 platelets[7] before the residual nuclear material is engulfed and eliminated by marrow macrophages. This process has been extensively reviewed.[8] The continuum of megakaryocyte development is arbitrarily divided into four stages. The major criteria differentiating these stages are the quality of the cytoplasm and the size, lobulation, and chromatin pattern of the nucleus (Table 111–1).

MEGAKARYOBLAST

Stage I megakaryocytes, also termed *megakaryoblasts*, account for approximately 20 percent of all cells destined to form platelets. These cells in human marrow are 8 to 24 μm in spherical diameter (i.e., the actual size *in vivo*, as opposed to the apparent size of a cell on a flattened marrow smear), contain a relatively large, minimally indented nucleus with loosely organized chromatin and multiple nucleoli, and scant basophilic cytoplasm containing a small Golgi complex, a few mitochondria and α granules, and abundant free ribosomes (Fig. 111–1).

Surface Adhesion Molecule Expression

Although elegant experiments clearly demonstrated that the gene for integrin α_{IIb} is expressed as early as the erythroid-megakaryocytic progenitor stage[9] and possibly in the common myeloid progenitor, the cell-surface protein becomes demonstrable and functionally important only at the early stages of megakaryocyte development. Integrin $\alpha_{IIb}\beta_3$ is an integral transmembrane protein of two subunits, but only the α subunit is megakaryocyte-lineage specific. Absence of integrin $\alpha_{IIb}\beta_3$ leads to Glanzmann thrombasthenia resulting from failure of the defective platelets to engage fibrinogen and other adhesive ligands during hemostasis (Chap. 120). Megakaryocytes and platelets contain in their cytoplasmic membranes approximately twice the amount of integrin $\alpha_{IIb}\beta_3$ as is present on the cell surface. The granule compartment serves as a mobilizable pool that is exteriorized upon platelet activation. During the early and midstages of megakaryocyte development, the granule content of integrin rises. Moreover, as developing megakaryocytes do not synthesize but contain fibrinogen in their α-granules and cells from patients with Glanzmann thrombasthenia do not, integrin $\alpha_{IIb}\beta_3$ clearly begins to function, at least at the level of fibrinogen binding and uptake, long before platelet formation.

The glycoprotein (GP) Ib-IX complex is expressed only slightly after the appearance of integrin $\alpha_{IIb}\beta_3$.[10] Although endothelial cells reportedly express GPIb,[11] its levels are very low; otherwise, GPIb is the

TABLE 111–1. Maturation Stages of Megakaryocytes

Term	Size (μM)	Morphology
Megakaryoblast (stage I)	>10	Lobed nucleus, basophilic cytoplasm
Basophilic megakaryocyte (stage II)	>20	Horseshoe-shaped nucleus, basophilic cytoplasm, azurophilic granules around centrosome
Granular megakary-ocyte (stage III)	>25–50	Large multilobed nucleus, acidophilic cytoplasm, numerous azurophilic granules
Mature megakaryo-cyte (stage IV)	>25–50	Pyknotic nucleus, groups of 10–12 azurophilic granules

second most abundant megakaryocyte-specific protein. Glycoprotein V also is expressed in complex with GPIb and GPIX, in a ratio of 1:2:2.[12] However, the genetic elimination of GPV has little effect on platelet adhesion,[13] and unlike GPIb and GPIX, no mutations of GPV are associated with Bernard-Soulier disease (Chap. 120).[14] Therefore, GPV does

not appear to be required for the GPIb-V-IX complex to function as a von Willebrand factor receptor. Rather, GPV is a target of thrombin, potentially playing a role in platelet activation.[15]

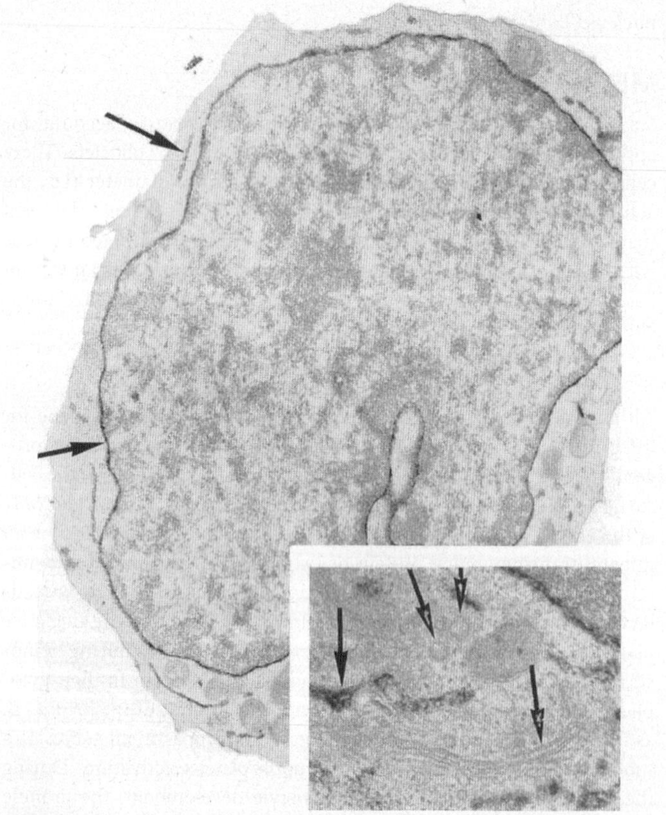

Demarcation Membranes

Another feature of the megakaryoblast is the initial development of demarcation membranes, which begin as invaginations of the plasma membrane and ultimately develop into a highly branched interconnected system of channels that course through the cytoplasm. The demarcation membrane system is in open communication with the extracellular space, based on studies using electron dense tracers.[16] Biochemical analysis indicates the composition of these membranes is very similar to the plasma membrane at each stage of megakaryocyte development. Over the 72 hours required for stage III/IV cells to develop from megakaryoblasts, the demarcation membrane system grows substantially. The demarcation membrane system provides the material necessary for development of proplatelet processes, structures that form in stage IV megakaryocytes and give rise upon fragmentation to mature platelets.[8,17]

Endomitosis

One of the most characteristic features of megakaryocyte development is endomitosis, a unique form of mitosis in which the DNA is repeatedly replicated in the absence of nuclear or cytoplasmic division. The resultant cells are highly polyploid. Endomitosis begins in megakaryoblasts (Fig. 111–2) following the many standard cell divisions required

Figure 111–1. Electron micrograph of a normal human megakaryoblast stained for platelet peroxidase. The small cell (<9 μm) exhibits dense platelet peroxidase in the perinuclear space and endoplasmic reticulum *(arrows)* (magnification ×12,150). *(Inset)* Enlargement of the Golgi zone. The Golgi saccules and vesicles are devoid of platelet peroxidase *(open arrows)*, whereas the endoplasmic reticulum contains platelet peroxidase activity *(closed arrow)* (magnification ×25,000). *(Used with permission of Dr. J. Breton-Gorius.)*

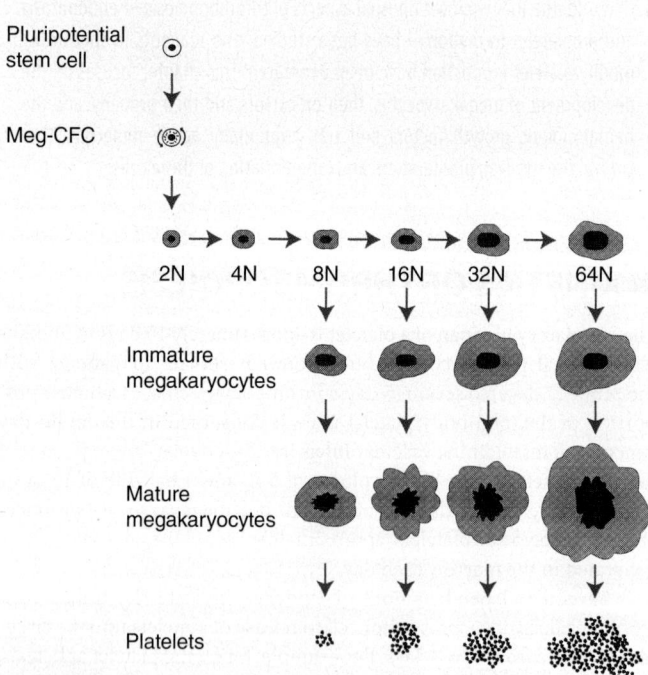

Figure 111–2. Origin and development of megakaryocytes. The pluripotential stem cell produces a progenitor committed to megakaryocyte differentiation (colony-forming unit–megakaryocyte [CFU-MK]), which can undergo mitosis. Eventually the CFU-MK stops mitosis and enters endomitosis. During endomitosis, neither cytoplasm nor nucleus divides, but DNA replication proceeds and gives rise to immature polyploid progenitors, which then enlarge and mature into morphologically identifiable, mature megakaryocytes that shed platelets. This figure does not necessarily imply that endomitosis and platelet formation are sequential but they can occur simultaneously. Meg-CFC, megakaryocyte colony-forming cells.

to expand the number of megakaryocytic precursor cells and is completed by the end of stage II megakaryocyte development.[18] During the endomitotic phase, each cycle of DNA synthesis produces an exact doubling of all the chromosomes, resulting in cells containing DNA content from eight to 128 times the normal chromosomal complement in a single, highly lobated nucleus. Although poorly understood for many years, the ability to produce large numbers of normal megakaryocytes in culture has started to shed light on this enigmatic process. Endomitosis is not simply the absence of mitosis but rather consists of recurrent cycles of aborted mitoses.[19] Cell-cycle kinetics in endomitotic cells also are unusual, characterized by a short G_1 phase, a relatively normal DNA synthesis phase, a short G_2 phase, and a very short endomitosis phase.[20] During the endomitosis phase, megakaryocytic chromosomes condense, the nuclear membrane breaks down, and multiple (at advanced stages) mitotic spindles form upon which the replicated chromosomes assemble. However, following initial chromosomal separation, individual chromosomes fail to complete their normal migration to opposite poles of the cell, the spindle dissociates, the nuclear membrane reforms around the entire chromosomal complement, and the cell again enters G_1 phase.

Regulation of Gene Expression

The promoters for integrin α_{IIb}, GPIb, GPVI, GPIX, and platelet factor-4 genes have been the focus of several studies and are active at the megakaryoblast stage of development. Consensus sequences for both GATA-1 and members of the Ets family of transcription factors (e.g., Fli-1) are present in the 5′ flanking regions of these genes, deletion of which reduces or eliminates reporter gene expression,[21–24] at least in mature hematopoietic cells. MafB also enhances GATA-1 and Ets activity during megakaryoblast differentiation,[25] induced by activation of ERK1/2, one of the primary downstream events of thrombopoietin stimulation.[26]

Another target of GATA-1 in megakaryocytes is polyphosphate-4-phosphatase (P4P), which was first identified by subtraction cloning between normal and GATA-1 knockdown megakaryocytes.[27] One of the unexplained features of megakaryocytes in GATA-1 knockdown mice is that, rather than massive cell death as seen in GATA-1–deficient erythroid progenitors,[28] the aberrantly developing megakaryoblasts in GATA-1 knockdown marrow are highly abundant and proliferate *in vitro* far more than control cells.[29] P4P catalyzes hydrolysis of the D-4 position phosphate of $PI_{3,4}P$ and $PI_{3,4,5}P$. These membrane phospholipids are products of phosphoinositol 3′-kinase (PI3K) action on membrane phospholipids, and they play an important role in the proliferative and survival response to megakaryocyte growth factors. When reintroduced into the knockdown mice, P4P diminishes the exuberant growth characteristic of the knockdown cells.[27] These findings are similar to the phenotype of cells from PTEN or SHIP knockout mice, enzymes that hydrolyze the D-3 and D-5 positions of $PI_{3,4,5}P$.

Another transcription factor vital for megakaryoblast differentiation is RUNX1 (also termed CBFA2 and AML1), the gene responsible for thrombocytopenia seen in familial platelet disorder/predisposition to acute myelogenous leukemia (Chap. 119).[30] In this disorder, haploinsufficiency of RUNX1 is associated with thrombocytopenia. As its genetic elimination in mice leads to significant maturation defects in the megakaryocyte lineage,[31] the human disorder almost certainly results from this genetic alteration. During normal megakaryoblast differentiation, RUNX1 levels rise and, conversely, fall during erythroid differentiation. In response to phosphorylation by ERK1/2, RUNX1, in complex with CBFβ and together with GATA-1, induces integrin α_{IIb} and integrin α_2 expression in megakaryoblast-like cells,[32] providing the beginnings of a molecular explanation for megakaryocyte development.

Cytokine Dependency

The cytokines, hormones, and chemokines that affect the survival and proliferation of megakaryoblasts include thrombopoietin, interleukin (IL)-3, stem cell factor (also termed mast cell growth factor, steel factor, and *c-kit* ligand), and the chemokine CXCL12 (previously termed stromal cell-derived factor [SDF]-1). Thrombopoietin is the most critical (for additional details, see the more extensive discussion in "Hormones and Cytokines" below), as genetic elimination of the *TPO* gene in mice leads to circulating platelet levels approximately 10 percent of normal. Homozygous or complex heterozygous mutation of the gene encoding the thrombopoietin receptor cMPL leads to congenital amegakaryocytic thrombocytopenia, in which platelet levels are approximately 10 percent of normal because of a near absence of megakaryocytic progenitors and megakaryoblasts (Chap. 117). The importance of stem cell factor to megakaryoblast development is revealed by experimental findings both *in vitro* and *in vivo*. Genetic reduction in expression of stem cell factor or its receptor *c-kit* leads to a 50 percent reduction in circulating platelet levels.[33] The cytokine acts in synergy with thrombopoietin to enhance megakaryocyte production in semisolid and suspension culture systems.[34] Evidence that IL-3 contributes to normal or accelerated megakaryopoiesis *in vivo* is weak. Genetic elimination of the IL-3 gene fails to affect platelet counts, even when combined with thrombopoietin receptor deficiency,[35] but the cytokine can induce growth of marrow progenitors into colonies containing immature megakaryocytes *in vitro* in the absence of thrombopoietin.[36] The chemokine CXCL12 appears to play a role in megakaryocyte proliferation. *In vitro*, the chemokine acts in synergy with thrombopoietin to support the survival and proliferation of megakaryocyte progenitors.[37] The combination of fibroblast growth factor (FGF)-4 and CXCL12 restores megakaryopoiesis in *TPO* and *c-mpl* null mice.[38]

Signal Transduction

The survival and proliferation of megakaryoblasts depends on at least two thrombopoietin-induced signaling pathways: PI3K and mitogen-activated protein kinase (MAPK; Chap. 17). In the presence of chemical inhibitors of PI3K, the favorable effects of thrombopoietin on megakaryocyte progenitor survival and proliferation are eliminated,[39] although constitutively activating this pathway is not sufficient for thrombopoietin-induced growth. MAPK is another important signaling pathway stimulated by thrombopoietin. Using purified marrow megakaryocytic progenitors and model cell lines, several groups showed that inhibition of MAPK blocks megakaryoblast maturation[26,40–42] because of its effect of activating Ets transcription factors.

STAGE II MEGAKARYOCYTES

Stage II megakaryocytes contain a lobulated nucleus and more abundant, but less intensely basophilic, cytoplasm. Ultrastructurally, the cytoplasm contains more abundant α granules and organelles. The demarcation membrane system begins to expand at this stage of development. Stage II megakaryocytes measure up to 30 μm in diameter, constitute approximately 25 percent of marrow megakaryocytes, and are the stage of development during which endomitosis is most prominent, generating cells displaying ploidy values of 8N to 64N.

Endomitosis

Whereas megakaryoblasts are generally thought to be able to expand by cell division, at an early stage of their maturation, the cells begin to undergo endomitosis, in which cells diverge from the normal cell cycle during mid- to late anaphase. Like normally mitotic cells, endomitotic megakaryocytes condense their chromatin into chromosomes, form a spindle, dissolve the nuclear membrane, and assemble the chromosomes on a metaphase plate, then the chromosomes begin to separate during early anaphase. However, rather than the dividing chromosomes migrating to opposite poles of the cell to allow the formation of a cleavage furrow, the chromosomes quickly decondense, the nuclear membrane reforms around the entire chromosomal complement, and the endomitotic cells reenter G_1 phase followed by S phase. A number of attempts to understand this process at the biochemical level have involved leukemic cell lines. Alterations in cyclin B, cdc2, cell-cycle kinase inhibitors, and aurora kinases have been claimed to be responsible for endomitosis.[43,44] Unfortunately, although these hypotheses possibly explain the polyploidy in various leukemic cell lines, the hypotheses have not been substantiated in studies of normal endomitotic megakaryocytes.[19,45] Endomitosis departs from a normal mitotic cell cycle at the late anaphase stage, when furrow invagination aborts short of cell abscission.[46] Additional studies indicate that disordered localization of the small G-protein RhoA may be responsible for this property.[46] Confirmation that a decrease in proper RhoA function is critical for endomitosis comes from the, genetic elimination of RhoA from the megakaryocytic lineage; *RhoA* null megakaryocytes display enhanced polyploidy, although the released platelets are characterized by abnormal membrane rheology, resulting in their rapid clearance from the circulation.[47] Proper RhoA localization is controlled by its activation by the RhoA guanosine triphosphate (GTP) exchange factor (GEF) ECT2; ECT2 is down-modulated during the switch from mitosis to endomitosis in megakaryocytes, providing a mechanistic explanation for the onset of endomitosis.[48]

Cytoplasmic Development

Early in megakaryocyte development, the cytoplasm acquires a rich network of microfilaments and microtubules. Toward stages III and IV, the proteins accumulate in the cell periphery, creating an organelle poor peripheral zone. Biochemically, the megakaryocyte cytoskeleton is composed of actin, α-actinin, filamin, nonmuscle myosin (including the product of the *MYH9* gene), mutated in several giant platelet thrombocytopenic syndromes[49] (Chap. 117), β_1-tubulin, talin, and several other actin-binding proteins. Like platelets, megakaryocytes can respond to external stimuli by changing shape, transporting organelles around the cytoplasm, and secreting granules. These functions are dependent on the microfilament and microtubule systems of the cell. In addition, microtubules play a vital role during the later stages of platelet formation.[50]

Regulation of Gene Expression

As discussed earlier, GATA-1 is vital for committing primitive multipotent progenitors to the erythroid–megakaryocyte pathway. However, the transcription factor also is critical later in megakaryopoiesis, for cytoplasmic development. The first convincing evidence that GATA proteins affect megakaryocyte development came from overexpression studies of *GATA-1* in a leukemic cell line, in which the transcription factor led to partial megakaryocytic differentiation.[51] Reduction in *GATA-1* expression also impairs cytoplasmic development in murine megakaryocytes, reducing demarcation membranes and platelet-specific granules.[29] Additional transcription factors expressed during stage II megakaryocyte development include RUNX-1, Tal1, and Fli1, but these transcription factors appear to play far greater a role in megakaryocyte maturation and platelet formation, and are discussed in "Stage III/IV Megakaryocytes" below.

Platelet Granule Formation

Although more prominent in later stages of differentiation (Fig. 111–3), platelet-specific α granules first begin to form adjacent to the Golgi apparatus as 300- to 500-nm round or oval organelles in stage II megakaryocytes. Three distinct compartments are recognized in α granules:

(1) a central, electron-dense nucleoid, containing fibrinogen, platelet factor-4, β-thromboglobulin, transforming growth factor (TGF)-β_1, vitronectin, and tissue plasminogen activator–like plasminogen activator; (2) a peripheral zone, containing tubules and von Willebrand factor (arranged much like that seen in endothelial cell Weibel-Palade bodies); and (3) the granule membrane, containing many of the critical platelet receptors for cell rolling (P-selectin), firm adhesion (GPIb-V-IX), and aggregation (integrin $\alpha_{IIb}\beta_3$). Proteins present in α granules arise from *de novo* megakaryocyte synthesis (e.g., GPIb-V-IX, GPIV, integrin $\alpha_{IIb}\beta_3$, von Willebrand factor, P-selectin, β-thromboglobulin, platelet-derived growth factor), nonspecific pinocytosis of environmental proteins (albumin and immunoglobulin G), or cell surface membrane receptor-mediated uptake from the environment (e.g., fibrinogen, fibronectin, factor V). Insights into platelet granule formation have come from a molecular understanding of Hermansky-Pudlak syndrome (HPS). In this disorder, characterized by oculocutaneous albinism and a qualitative platelet bleeding disorder, a complex of at least eight proteins form in various granule-associated complexes such as the biogenesis of lysosome-related organelles complexes, which affect δ granule formation.[52] These complexes are thought to be involved in cargo transport of a number of subcellular granules, such as lysosomes, melanosomes, and platelet δ granules.

STAGE III/IV MEGAKARYOCYTES

Continued cytoplasmic maturation characterizes stage III/IV megakaryocyte development (Fig. 111–4). Cells are extremely large (40 to 60 μm in diameter) and display a low nuclear-to-cytoplasmic ratio. Cytoplasmic basophilia disappears as cells progress from stage III to stage IV. The demarcation membrane system gradually replaces the endoplasmic reticulum and Golgi apparatus during the final stages of maturation. The nucleus usually is eccentrically placed. Although the nucleus sometimes appears as several distinct nuclei in biopsy sections, it remains highly lobulated but single at all stages of megakaryocyte development. In occasional marrow sections (Fig. 111–4C), neutrophils or other marrow cells are seen transiting through the cytoplasm of the mature megakaryocyte, a process termed *emperipolesis*, and is of no pathologic significance.

Proplatelet Formation

Careful microscopic studies have localized marrow megakaryocytes to the abluminal surface of sinusoidal endothelial cells. In specially prepared specimens, the megakaryocytes can be seen issuing long, slender cytoplasmic processes between endothelial cells and into the sinusoidal lumen, structures termed *proplatelet processes* (Fig. 111–5).[53] The processes have been reproduced *in vitro* and *in vivo*.[6] The processes consist of a β-tubulin cytoskeleton and highway, transporting organelles and platelet constituents from the megakaryocyte to the terminal projection, the nascent platelet.[17]

Membrane Composition

Most of the specific characteristics of platelet membranes are present at stages III and IV of megakaryocyte development. Megakaryocyte membrane lipid composition progressively changes through development, achieving approximately four times the content of phospholipids and cholesterol as found in immature cells. Megakaryocytes contain approximately the same amounts of membrane neutral and phospholipid as platelets, but contain relatively more phosphatidylinositol and less phosphatidylserine and arachidonic acid.

Regulation of Gene Expression

One transcription factor that plays an important role in the final stages of megakaryocyte maturation is nuclear factor-E2. Initially described as

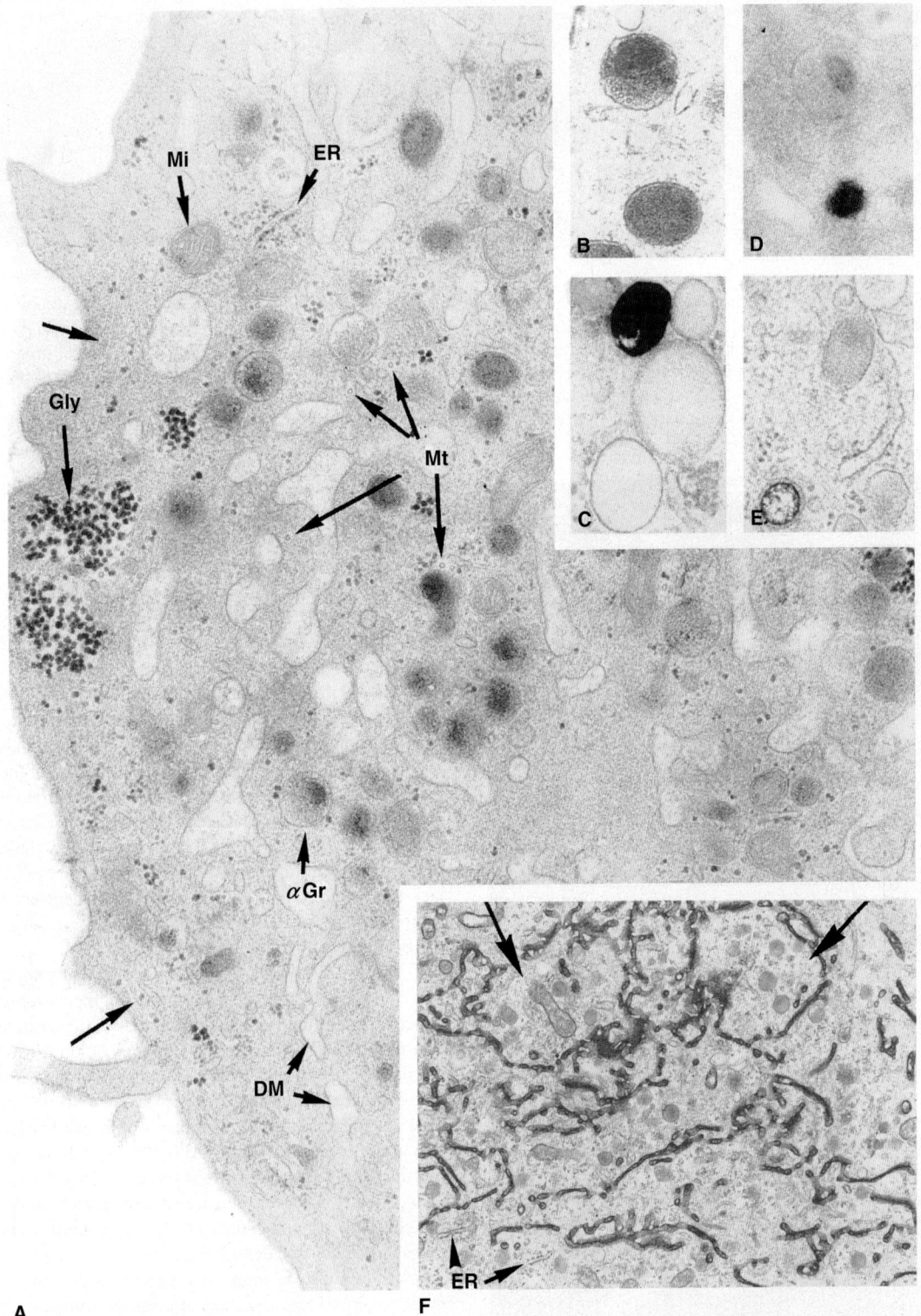

Figure 111–3. A. Ultrastructure of the cytoplasm of a mature megakaryocyte. The majority of the granules are *a* granules (*a*Gr) exhibiting dense nucleoid. Demarcation membranes (DM) are slightly dilated. Transverse sections of microtubules (Mt) are dispersed. At the periphery, a longitudinal microtubule runs under the cell membrane *(arrows)*. Dense aggregates of glycogen (Gly), small cisternae of endoplasmic reticulum (ER), and free ribosomes are seen (magnification ×30,320). **B.** Morphology of an *a* granule. Dense nucleoid is located at the *top*. In a clear zone at the opposite pole, four transverse sections of tubular structures are adjacent to the granule membrane (magnification ×37,200). **C.** Dense body can be distinguished from *a* granule by the black deposit when calcium is added to the fixative (magnification ×37,200). **D.** Cytochemical detection of acid phosphatase using β-glycophosphate as substrate and cerium as a trapping agent. Dense cerium–phosphate precipitates are present in lysosomal granules, whereas *a* granules are unreactive (magnification ×37,200). **E.** Microperoxisome visualized using alkaline thiaminobenzidine. Note the small size of a reactive granule compared to the *a* granule. **F.** Distribution of a dense tracer filling the lumen of the demarcation membrane system in a maturing megakaryocyte *(arrows)*. In contrast to the demarcation membrane system, which is open to the extracellular space, the endoplasmic reticulum (ER) is not labeled (magnification ×9700). *(Used with permission of Dr. J. Breton-Gorius.)*

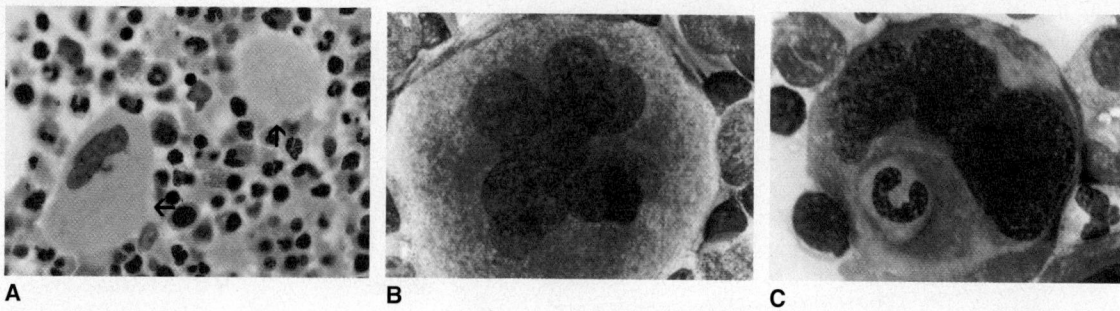

Figure 111–4. Megakaryocyte morphology. **A.** Normal human marrow biopsy. Two megakaryocytes are evident. In one case the section is through the cell at the level of the nuclei *(horizontal arrow)*, and in the other it is through the cytoplasm above or below the nucleus *(vertical arrow)*. **B.** Normal human marrow aspirate. Mature (stage III) megakaryocyte with a multilobated nucleus and abundant cytoplasm. **C.** Normal human marrow aspirate. Mature megakaryocyte with a neutrophil embedded in the cytoplasm. Many ultrastructural studies have confirmed that this appearance represents marrow cells entering the canalicular system of megakaryocyte cytoplasm through its opening to the exterior of the cell (emperipolesis). *(Reproduced with permission from Lichtman's Atlas of Hematology, www.accessmedicine.com.)*

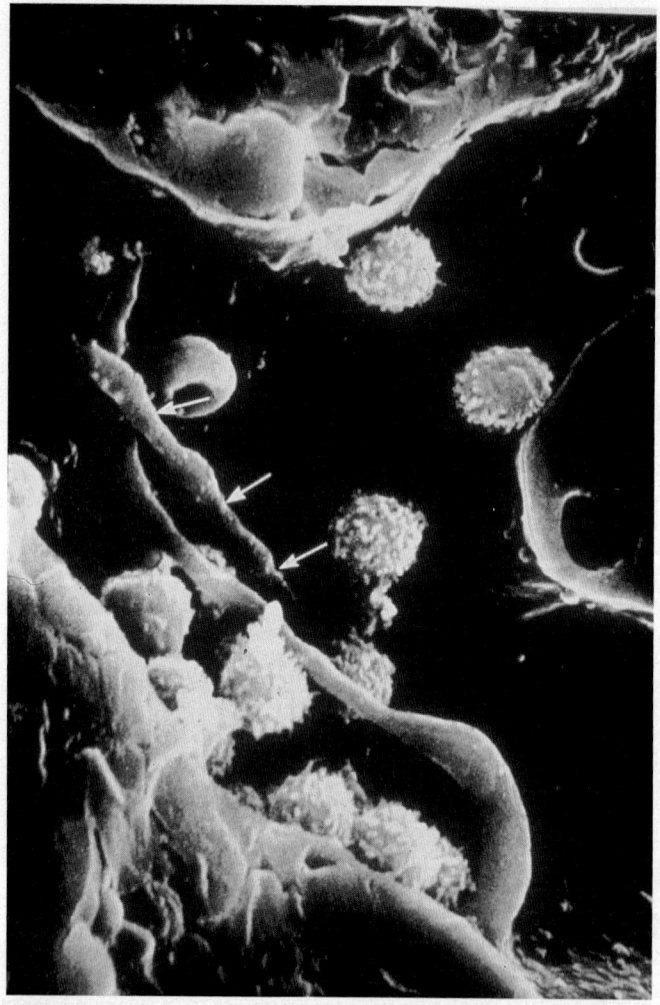

Figure 111–5. Megakaryocyte proplatelet processes in the marrow sinusoid. Scanning electron micrograph showing the luminal view of the confluence of two marrow sinusoids with two proplatelet processes protruding through the lining endothelial cells. One of the processes has intermittent constrictions *(arrows)*, indicating potential sites for platelet formation. Other cells depicted include lymphocytes and erythrocytes (magnification ×3000). *(Reproduced with permission from Becker RP, De Bruyn P: The transmural passage of blood cells into myeloid sinusoids and the entry of platelets into sinusoidal circulation; a scanning electron microscope investigation, Am J Anat 1976 Feb;145(2):183-205.)*

an erythroid-specific, heterodimeric protein belonging to the basic leucine zipper family of transcription factors, NF-E2 is composed of a ubiquitously expressed p18 subunit, and a 45-kDa protein (p45) expressed only in erythroid cells and megakaryocytes.[54] NF-E2 binds to tandem AP-1–like motifs, such as those seen in the second deoxyribonuclease (DNAse) hypersensitive site of the β-globin locus control region, and is required for β-globin expression.[55] However, genetic elimination of p45 failed to significantly affect erythropoiesis. Rather, p45-deficient mice display prominent alterations in megakaryocyte development and severe thrombocytopenia,[56] leading to death from widespread hemorrhage soon after birth. Examination of the animals reveals modest expansion of marrow megakaryocytes but failure of the cells to produce platelets because of defects in cytoplasmic maturation, including substantial reductions in platelet granules and demarcation membranes. Thus, the loss of either GATA-1 or NF-E2 results in failure of late aspects of cellular maturation. As p45 NF-E2 is induced by GATA-1/FOG,[57] the lack of cytoplasmic development in GATA-deficient mice likely is an indirect effect. The role of transcription factors in late megakaryopoiesis has been reviewed.[58]

Nearly all studies of megakaryopoiesis have focused on the marrow. The final stages of megakaryocyte fragmentation also are proposed to occur in the lung, at least for some cells, a theory based on the finding that platelet levels in pulmonary venous blood exceed those found in the pulmonary artery.[59] Whether this process represents the migration and fragmentation of intact megakaryocytes in the lung or merely the final size reduction of large fragments of megakaryocyte cytoplasm that also are released into the blood is not clear. Some data exist supporting the notion that lung megakaryocytes contribute to blood platelet production.[60] However, in mice administered high doses of thrombopoietin, with platelet counts as high as 4 million/μm^3, neither intact megakaryocytes nor denuded nuclei were found in the lungs of these animals.[61] One study found that canine lungs contain 2.5 megakaryocytes per cm^2.[62] Extrapolation of these data suggest human lungs contain approximately 6000 megakaryocytes, only enough to account for a small proportion (<0.1 percent) of daily platelet production.

PLATELET FORMATION

Numerous studies have indicated thrombopoietin is the primary regulator of megakaryocyte maturation.[36,63] However, despite the importance of the hormone for generation of fully mature megakaryocytes from which platelets arise, elimination of the cytokine during the final stages of platelet formation is not detrimental.[64] Although proplatelet formation is possible under serum-free conditions,[65] most investigators have reported the presence of plasma and/or an integrin ligand-containing substratum (e.g., fibronectin or vitronectin) stimulates the process substantially.[64,66] These findings suggest external signals probably are required for normal platelet formation. One report suggests the thrombin–antithrombin complex with or without high-density lipoprotein particles mediates the favorable effect of plasma on proplatelet formation,[67] although other data suggest prothrombin and its conversion to thrombin by megakaryocytes inhibit the process.[68] Although the cytokine(s) required for this process is not known, activation of protein kinase Cα clearly is necessary for the process to occur.[66]

Platelet formation involves massive reorganization of megakaryocyte cytoskeletal components, including actin and tubulin, during a highly active, motile process in which the termini of the process branch and issue platelets.[5] The size of the individual platelets formed is of interest. Unfortunately, little is known about this aspect of platelet formation except that tubulin is proposed to act as a measuring device for the proper site to pinch off platelets from proplatelet processes. The mechanism of platelet formation clearly must be affected in some way by the transcription factor GATA-1, the GPIb-IX complex, the Wiskott-Aldrich syndrome protein, and platelet myosin, as defects in each of these genes leads to unusually large or small platelets (Chap. 117).[69,70] Finally, localized cytoplasmic membrane proteolysis, a sublethal form of apoptosis, likely plays a role in initiating the final stages of platelet formation.[71]

● EXTRINSIC REGULATION OF MEGAKARYOCYTE PRODUCTION

HORMONES AND CYTOKINES

Several cytokines, first identified using alternate hematopoietic activity assays, affect megakaryocyte development. IL-3, granulocyte-macrophage colony-stimulating factor, and stem cell factor support the proliferation of megakaryocytic progenitors in plasma-containing cultures.[72–74] In 1994, several groups reported the purification and/or cloning of thrombopoietin.[75] This cytokine clearly is the primary regulator of megakaryopoiesis but cannot explain thrombopoiesis in its entirety.

Interleukin-3

IL-3 is a 25- to 30-kDa protein produced almost exclusively by T lymphocytes.[76] The mature human protein contains 133 amino acids, but N-linked carbohydrate modification accounts for the larger than expected Mr of the cytokine. Granulocyte-macrophage colony-stimulating factor is an 18- to 30-kDa protein also produced by T lymphocytes. However, endothelial cells, monocytes, and fibroblasts also produce the protein and, like IL-3, granulocyte-macrophage colony-stimulating factor is highly modified with both N-linked and O-linked carbohydrate.[77] Although the two proteins display essentially no primary sequence homology, their tertiary structures are highly related,[78] and the receptors for the two cytokines share a common subunit.[79] However, the physiologic relevance of IL-3 and granulocyte-macrophage colony-stimulating factor for steady-state thrombopoiesis is uncertain. Administration of the cytokines to mice or humans has only minimal effects on thrombopoiesis, and genetic elimination of either has no impact on megakaryopoiesis, even when combined with elimination of other thrombopoietic cytokines.[80,81]

Interleukin-6 and Related Cytokines

IL-6, cloned by several groups using multiple assays (hepatocyte growth, myeloma cell growth, immunoglobulin secretion, antiviral activity), enhances megakaryocyte maturation. IL-6 is a 26-kDa polypeptide produced by T lymphocytes, fibroblasts, macrophages, and stromal cells in response to inflammatory stimuli.[82] The mature protein is composed of 184 amino acids, contains two disulfide bonds, and displays both N-linked and O-linked carbohydrate modification. Although IL-6 alone fails to affect in vitro megakaryopoiesis, it augments the number of megakaryocyte colonies obtained in the presence of IL-3 or stem cell factor[83] and exerts primarily a differentiating effect.[84,85] Administration of IL-6 to mice or nonhuman primates or patients results in a modest thrombocytosis.[86–88] These findings suggest IL-6 contributes to megakaryopoiesis in vivo, a conclusion supported by its production by tumor cells in selected cases of paraneoplastic thrombocytosis.[89] However, genetic elimination of the cytokine fails to significantly affect basal platelet production.[90] Evidence suggests the cytokine affects platelet production indirectly[91] by stimulating thrombopoietin production.

IL-6 acts through a heterodimeric receptor, composed of a signaling subunit, termed GP130, and an affinity-converting subunit, termed IL-6Rα. GP130 also acts as the signaling subunit for several other cytokines, including IL-11 and leukemia inhibitory factor. Therefore, the finding that these cytokines also stimulate megakaryopoiesis in a manner similar to that of IL-6 is not surprising. IL-11 and leukemia inhibitory factor act in synergy with IL-3 or stem cell factor to augment megakaryocyte formation. IL-11 is a 23-kDa polypeptide, initially cloned from a gibbon marrow stromal cell line, whose activity can support the proliferation of an IL-6–responsive myeloma cell line.[92,93] Leukemia inhibitory factor displays a wide range of activities,[94] including (1) inducing the acute phase hepatic response, (2) inducing an adrenergic-to-cholinergic switch in neurons, (3) inhibiting lipoprotein lipase in adipocytes, and (4) maintaining pluripotentiality in embryonic cells.

Like IL-6, IL-11 and leukemia inhibitory factor enhance megakaryocytic maturation in vitro[95,96] and augment the effects of IL-3 and stem cell factor on primitive hematopoietic cells. Consistent with the in vitro findings, administration of either recombinant IL-11 or leukemia inhibitory factor to rodents, nonhuman primates, or humans produces modest thrombocytosis.[97–100] Despite the in vitro and in vivo findings, genetic elimination of either leukemia inhibitory factor or the IL-11 receptor has no effect on thrombopoiesis,[101] even when combined with elimination of the thrombopoietin receptor.[102]

Stem Cell Factor

In contrast to the hematopoietic cytokine family, stem cell factor is more closely related to other hematopoietic proteins that utilize protein tyrosine kinase receptors, such as macrophage colony-stimulating factor and the flt-3 ligand.[103] Nevertheless, stem cell factor stimulates megakaryocyte colony growth when used in combination with other cytokines.[104] Moreover, genetic elimination of its receptor c-kit reduces megakaryocyte production[105] and the rebound thrombocytosis that occurs following immunosuppressive therapy.[106,107]

Stem cell factor was first identified using several different biologic assays (in addition to this term, the cytokine has been dubbed c-kit ligand, mast cell growth factor, and steel factor).[108] Later studies indicate the cytokine acts primarily on primitive cells of the hematopoietic, melanogenic, and germ cell lineages. Stem cell factor is a dimeric protein composed of two identical noncovalently linked polypeptides. The soluble form monomer contains 165 residues,[109] derived by proteolytic cleavage of a membrane-bound splice form of the molecule.[110] The membrane bound form is more active than the soluble cytokine, as intracellular signaling in response to membrane-bound stem cell factor is prolonged in receptor-bearing cells.[111] Moreover, a naturally occurring mutant allele of the gene (Sl^d), which allows production of the soluble but not the membrane-bound form of the cytokine, results in a phenotype nearly identical to deletion of the entire locus,[112] again pointing to the importance of the membrane-bound form present on marrow stromal cells.

Flt-3 Ligand

The flt-3 ligand initially was identified as a ligand for a novel member of the protein tyrosine kinase family of receptors.[103] This growth factor also affects megakaryocyte formation. Like stem cell factor, to which it is most closely related, flt-3 ligand is found in both soluble and membrane-bound forms, is a noncovalently linked dimer, and affects primarily primitive hematopoietic cells.[113] Although several studies have shown that flt-3 ligand used alone does not support megakaryocyte colony formation, some studies suggest it works in synergy with other megakaryocyte stimulatory agents to augment the proliferation of megakaryocytic progenitor cells in culture.[114,115] Administration of flt-3 ligand to mice expands the number of marrow and splenic progenitor cells that can give rise to megakaryocytes *in vitro*.[116] However, genetic elimination of either flt-3 ligand or its receptor does not produce a platelet phenotype.

Thrombopoietin

The term *thrombopoietin* was first coined in 1958 to describe the primary regulator of platelet production.[117] A major impetus to the discovery of thrombopoietin in 1986 was the identification of the myeloproliferative leukemia virus (MPLV), which induces a vast expansion of hematopoietic cells.[118] The responsible viral oncogene was characterized in 1990,[119] and its cellular homologue c-*Mpl* was cloned in 1992.[120] Based on the presence of two copies of the hematopoietic cytokine receptor motif[121] and the ability of a fusion of c-Mpl and the IL-4 receptor to signal in factor dependent cells,[122] c-*Mpl* clearly encoded a growth factor receptor, but its ligand was not known. Using three distinct strategies, four separate groups were able to clone complementary DNA for the corresponding hormone and report their results in 1994 (reviewed in Ref. 75). The gene for thrombopoietin encodes a 36-kDa polypeptide,[123] which also is predicted to be extensively posttranslationally modified, resulting in an approximately 50- to 70-kDa protein.

Thrombopoietin bears striking homology to erythropoietin, the primary regulator of erythropoiesis, within the aminoterminal half of the predicted polypeptide. The two proteins are more closely related than any other two cytokines within the hematopoietic cytokine family, sharing 20 percent identical amino acids, an additional 25 percent conservative substitutions, and identical positions of three of the four cysteine residues. Unlike any of the other cytokines in the family, thrombopoietin contains a 181-residue carboxyl-terminal extension, which bears homology to no known proteins. Two functions have been assigned to this region: it prolongs the circulatory half-life of the hormone,[3] and it aids in its secretion from the cells that normally synthesize the hormone.[124]

The biologic activities of thrombopoietin have been demonstrated *in vitro* and *in vivo*, in mice, rats, dogs, nonhuman primates, and man. Incubation of marrow cells with thrombopoietin stimulates megakaryocyte survival and proliferation, alone and in combination with other cytokines.[34] *In vivo*, thrombopoietin stimulates platelet production in a log-linear manner to levels 10-fold higher than baseline[3,61,125] without affecting the blood red or white cell counts. In addition, because of its effect on hematopoietic stem cells (Chap. 16), the number of erythroid and myeloid progenitors and mixed myeloid progenitors in marrow and spleen also are increased,[126,127] an effect that is particularly impressive when the hormone is administered following myelosuppressive therapy.[126,128,129] This effect likely results from the synergy between thrombopoietin and the other hematopoietic cytokines circulating at high levels in this condition.

Based on genetic studies, thrombopoietin clearly is the primary regulator of thrombopoiesis. Elimination of either the c-*Mpl* or *Tpo* gene leads to profound thrombocytopenia in mice as a result of a greatly reduced number of megakaryocyte progenitors, mature megakaryocytes,

and the reduced polyploidy of the remaining megakaryocytes.[130] A similar result occurs in humans. Patients with congenital amegakaryocytic thrombocytopenia (CAMT) display numerous homozygous or compound heterozygous nonsense or severe missense mutations of the thrombopoietin receptor c-*Mpl* (Chap. 117).[131,132] The effect of thrombopoietin on hematopoietic stem cells is particularly revealed by consideration of children with CAMT. Within 5 years of birth, nearly every patient with CAMT develops aplastic anemia as a result of stem cell exhaustion.

The thrombopoietin gene displays an unusual 5′ flanking structure. Unlike the majority of genes that initiate translation of the encoded polypeptide with the first ATG codon present in the mRNA, thrombopoietin translation initiates at the eighth ATG codon located within the third exon of a full-length transcript.[133] However, because the eighth ATG of thrombopoietin mRNA is embedded in the short, open reading frame of the seventh ATG, its translation is particularly inefficient because of the mechanism of ribosomal initiation.[134] As such, little thrombopoietin protein is produced for any given amount of mRNA. Although this molecular arrangement has no known physiologic consequences, it forms the basis for an unusual form of disease, a disorder of translation efficiency. Four cases of autosomal dominant familial thrombocytosis have been linked to mutations in the region surrounding the initiation codon. In two families, a single mutation in different nucleotides of the intron 3 splice donor sequence results in alternate splicing of the primary thrombopoietin transcript, eliminating the seventh and eighth ATG codons, creating a new aminoterminus by fusing of the fifth open reading frame with the thrombopoietin coding sequence. This novel thrombopoietin mRNA is efficiently translated, resulting in supraphysiologic levels of hormone production and nonclonal expansion of thrombopoiesis.[135,136] In another mutant thrombopoietin allele, deletion of a single nucleotide within the seventh open reading frame leads to its fusion with the thrombopoietin coding sequence and now enhanced translation of thrombopoietin from the seventh ATG codon.[137] A fourth mutation has been described within the seventh open reading frame, leading to premature termination of that short peptide, preventing its interference with translation initiation from the usual eighth initiation codon,[138] again enhancing thrombopoietin production (reviewed in Ref. 139). Of note, while reactive thrombocytosis is not thought to lead to hypercoagulability (Chap. 119), several patients in these pedigrees developed thromboses, raising the physiologic question of why should chronic stimulation of platelets with enhanced levels of thrombopoietin lead to hypercoagulability.

The physiologic regulation of thrombopoietin production has received much attention. Experimental induction of immune-mediated thrombocytopenia results in relatively rapid restoration of platelet levels, followed by a brief period of rebound thrombocytosis.[140] In these experimental cases and in most naturally occurring cases of thrombocytopenia, plasma hormone concentrations vary inversely with platelet counts, rising to maximal levels within 24 hours of onset of profound thrombocytopenia.[141] Two non–mutually exclusive models have been advanced to explain these findings. In the first model, thrombopoietin production is constitutive, but its consumption, and hence the level remaining in the blood to affect megakaryopoiesis, is determined by the mass of c-Mpl receptors present on platelets and megakaryocytes accessible to the plasma.[142] In this way, states of thrombocytosis result in increased thrombopoietin consumption (by the expanded platelet mass of c-Mpl receptors), reducing megakaryopoiesis. Conversely, thrombocytopenia reduces blood thrombopoietin destruction, resulting in elevated blood levels of the hormone that drive megakaryopoiesis and platelet recovery. This model is based on one of the mechanisms regulating macrophage colony-stimulating factor levels.[143] The invariable levels of thrombopoietin-specific mRNA present in the liver and kidney of experimental animals and patients with thrombocytopenia or thrombocytosis support this model.[144,145] Moreover, thrombopoietin knockout mice display a gene dosage effect.[146] Platelet levels in heterozygous mice are intermediate between that seen in wild-type and nullizygous animals, suggesting active regulation of the remaining thrombopoietin allele cannot compensate for the mild (60 percent of normal) thrombocytopenia induced by the loss of one allele.

A second model suggests thrombopoietin expression is a regulated event. Very-low platelet levels can induce thrombopoietin-specific mRNA production. Several studies show that thrombopoietin mRNA levels are modulated in response to moderate to severe thrombocytopenia, at least in the marrow.[145,147] The signal(s) responsible for this form of thrombopoietin regulation is being uncovered, but is, at least in part, mediated by transcriptional enhancement.[148] CD40 ligand, platelet-derived growth factor, FGF, TGF-β, platelet factor-4, and thrombospondin modulate thrombopoietin production from marrow stromal cells.[149,150]

The human thrombopoietin gene 5′ flanking region lacks a TATA box or CAAT motif and directs transcription initiation at multiple sites over a 50-nucleotide region.[151] Reporter gene analysis in a hepatocyte cell line identified an Ets2 transcription factor-binding motif responsible for high-level expression of the gene. The 5′ flanking region also includes SP-1, AP-2, and nuclear factor-κB binding sites,[152] although the contribution of these transcription factors to thrombopoietin gene expression, either under steady-state or inflammatory conditions, has not been studied.

CXCL12 (Stromal Cell-Derived Factor-1)

Chemokines are members of a rapidly growing class of molecules that play multiple roles in blood cell physiology.[153] Initially defined as substances that induce leukocyte chemotaxis, four classes of the 8- to 12-kDa polypeptides have been recognized, based on the spacing of cysteine residues close to the aminoterminus of the proteins. An equally rapidly growing family of chemokine receptors also has been discovered, classified by the subfamily of chemokines they serve. All chemokine receptors are members of the seven-transmembrane family of receptors that signal through heterotrimeric G proteins.

Most work has been conducted with the CC and CXC subfamilies of chemokines, molecules that display modest inhibitory effects on cell proliferation when used alone and potent effects when used in combination on hematopoietic progenitors at all levels of development.[154] On many levels, the CXC chemokine CXCL12 (previously termed SDF-1) and its receptor CXCR4 are notable exceptions to the many features shared by most members of the chemokine and chemokine receptor families. For example, although all the other genes for the known CXC chemokines reside on the long arm of human chromosome 14, CXCL12 localizes to the long arm of chromosome 10.[155] Moreover, most chemokine receptors can be activated by multiple ligands. For example, the chemokine CCL3 (macrophage inflammatory protein [MIP]-1α) can bind and activate CCR1 and CCR5, and IL-8 can bind both CXCR1 and CXCR2.[156] In contrast, as the phenotype of genetic elimination of both CXCR4 and CXCL12 are almost identical,[157,158] CXCR4 appears to be the only receptor for CXCL12, and CXCL12 is the only ligand for CXCR4.

The marrow stroma is the primary source of CXCL12, and most of the cell types known to express CXCR4 are hematopoietic in origin. One of the major phenotypes in CXCL12- or CXCR4-deficient neonatal mice is marrow aplasia, thought to be secondary to failure of perinatal hematopoietic stem cell homing (Chap. 16).[159] In addition, megakaryocytes display CXCR4[160] and migrate in response to an CXCL12 concentration gradient.[161] Several groups have shown that CXCL12 augments thrombopoietin-induced megakaryocyte growth in suspension culture.[37,160] Later studies have shown the synergy between

CXCL12 and other stimuli on megakaryocyte growth extends to cell surface adhesion.[38]

Transforming Growth Factor-β

In addition to the many positive regulators of megakaryopoiesis, several substances down-modulate their development. Five isoforms of TGF-β have been identified, all disulfide-linked homodimers each containing 112 residues.[162] TGF-β_1 is the predominant type of TGF found in hematopoietic tissues. Platelet α granules are a particularly rich source of the cytokine. In general, transforming growth factors are inhibitors of hematopoiesis,[163,164] particularly of megakaryocyte development.[165,166] The best understood TGF-β growth inhibitory effects are exerted on cell-cycle progression. After binding to one of five receptors, two pathways that block cell-cycle progression are activated. pRb is hypophosphorylated,[167] antagonizing the effects of G_1-phase cyclin-dependent kinases, and cell-cycle inhibitors, including p27 and p15^{INK}, are upregulated, affecting cell-cycle progression.[168,169] In contrast to these negative effects of TGF-β on cell proliferation, the cytokine enhances megakaryocyte differentiation.

Interferon-α

A second class of cytokines that negatively impact thrombopoiesis are the interferons (IFNs), proteins first defined by their ability to induce an antiviral state in mammalian cells.[170] Biochemical fractionation has revealed three classes of IFNs: IFN-α, a family of 17 distinct but highly homologous molecules; IFN-β, a single molecule more distantly related to the various isoforms of IFN-α; and IFN-γ, a unique molecule that shares functional properties but not structure with the others. IFNs exert profound inhibitory effects on hematopoiesis.[171]

The genes for the IFN-α/β subfamily cluster on the short arm of chromosome 9 and encode 165- to 172-residue polypeptides, of which 35 percent are invariant across the family of IFN-α molecules. IFNs of the α/β type are produced by transcriptional upregulation in fibroblasts and leukocytes in response to viruses and other infectious agents and to inflammatory cytokines. Once bound to the IFN receptors, a cascade of kinases and intracellular mediators are triggered, initiated by JAKs (Janus family kinases), STAT (signal transducer and activator of transcription) factors, and p38 MAPK (Chap. 17), resulting in changes in gene transcription.

IFN-α inhibits megakaryopoiesis, the clinical use of which is responsible for modest to severe thrombocytopenia in a significant number of patients undergoing therapy for chronic viral hepatitis.[172,173] The mechanisms responsible for the inhibitory effect of IFN-α are multifactorial. Some studies suggest a direct inhibitory effect of IFN-α on growth factor-induced proliferation pathways. For example, the cytokine augments double-stranded RNA-activated protein kinase activity, inhibiting translation initiation factor-2, implicating reduction of the growth factor-induced protein synthesis necessary for growth factor response.[174] IFN-β induces expression of the cell-cycle inhibitor p27^{Kip1}, arresting cells in G_0/G_1.[175] Other studies have demonstrated IFN-α induces a SOCS (suppressor of cytokine signaling)-1–based feedback mechanism that cross-reacts and depresses thrombopoietin signaling.[176] Thus, in addition to the multiple positive mediators of megakaryopoiesis, several cytokines block the process and can lead to thrombocytopenia.

MEGAKARYOCYTE MICROENVIRONMENT

Chapter 5 details the role of the marrow microenvironment in hematopoiesis. This chapter discusses only aspects particularly vital for megakaryocyte growth. The cellular concentration within the marrow is estimated to be 10^9/mL. Consequently, cell–cell and cell–matrix interactions will occur.[177] A particularly important interaction for thrombopoiesis is between the marrow sinusoidal endothelial cell and the mature megakaryocyte. Studies using *in situ* videomicroscopy indicate that proplatelet processes extend through the sinusoids into the vascular lumen, where the shear stress of flowing blood liberates single platelets.[6] Marrow stromal cells influence hematopoiesis in a number of other ways, perhaps the most prominent through production of several cytokines that positively or negatively affect megakaryocyte growth.[145,178–180] Stromal cells are the origin of a number of extracellular matrix proteins and glycomucins that either directly affect hematopoietic cells or indirectly affect hematopoietic cells by binding growth factors and presenting them in a functional context.[181,182] Stromal cells also bear ligands for Notch proteins, cell-surface receptors that are critical mediators of cell fate decisions.[183] Notch and its ligands Delta and Jagged play important roles as regulators of hematopoietic progenitor cell proliferation[184] and play a potential role in influencing the lineage fate choice between erythropoiesis and megakaryopoiesis.[185] Cell–cell interactions mediated by integrins present on hematopoietic cells and counterreceptors on stromal cells are very important for megakaryopoiesis,[186] both by bringing hematopoietic cells into close proximity to stromal cells producing soluble or cell-bound cytokines and more directly by triggering or augmenting intracellular signaling, promoting entry into the cell cycle, and preventing programmed cell death.

● THERAPEUTIC MANIPULATION OF THROMBOPOIESIS BY NATURALLY OCCURRING CYTOKINES

Thrombocytopenia is a major clinical problem with multiple origins (Chap. 117). Primary marrow diseases, certain infections, and solid tumors with a high propensity for marrow metastases directly affect platelet production. Nearly all leukemias, advanced lymphomas, and myelomas ultimately cause thrombocytopenia by this mechanism. Hypersplenism and thrombopoietin deficiency contribute to platelet sequestration and reduced platelet production in patients with hepatic failure. Consumptive coagulopathies, initiated by infection, tumors, or severe injury, can be responsible for severe thrombocytopenia. In other patients, autoimmune thrombocytopenia arises during the course of disease or is a primary disease. However, the most common cause of significant thrombocytopenia is iatrogenic: the use of potentially curative or palliative chemotherapy or radiation therapy in patients with malignancy. An estimated 300,000+ persons yearly worldwide undergo courses of chemotherapy adequate to produce clinically significant thrombocytopenia. Recovery from the marrow suppressive effects of most chemotherapeutic agents occurs within 1 to 3 weeks following discontinuation of therapy. However, some agents, including mitomycin C or nitrosoureas, can produce prolonged periods of marrow suppression. Moreover, the widespread use of IFN-α for chronic hepatitis C infection adds large numbers of patients who experience thrombocytopenia as a dose-limiting toxicity. Tumor- or treatment-related thrombocytopenia often delays much needed additional therapy, may necessitate potentially complicated platelet transfusions (Chap. 139), and causes significant morbidity and occasional mortality. Given the increased understanding of the humoral basis for megakaryopoiesis and thrombopoiesis, numerous attempts have been made to manipulate these processes for therapeutic benefit.

INTERLEUKIN-11

IL-11 augments the growth of megakaryocytic progenitors in the presence of IL-3[187,188] and acts to promote megakaryocyte maturation rather than proliferation.[189,190] The preclinical effects of IL-11 were evaluated in mice, rats, and subhuman primates and revealed moderate activity in normal animals and following cytoreductive therapy.[98,191,192]

The first clinical trials of IL-11 were reported in abstract form in 1993 and 1994.[193,194] Randomized clinical trials were reported a few years later.[195–197] Most studies reported IL-11 ameliorated drug-induced thrombocytopenia. For example, IL-11 administered to patients with advanced stages of breast cancer undergoing multiple courses of anthracycline-based chemotherapy significantly reduced the need for platelet transfusions by 27 percent. However, use of the drug in patients undergoing autologous stem cell transplantation did not enhance platelet recovery or other indices of hematopoiesis. Although chemical evidence of an acute-phase response was noted in many of the patients treated in these studies, the drug was generally well tolerated, even though fluid retention has been a significant side effect, often necessitating concomitant use of diuretics. IL-11 (oprelvekin, Neumega) was approved by the Food and Drug Administration in 1998 for use in patients undergoing chemotherapy who have evidence of previous drug-induced thrombocytopenia (Chap. 119).

INTERFERON-α

As noted in "Hormones and Cytokines" above, IFN suppresses hematopoiesis and thrombopoiesis by multiple mechanisms. As a consequence, IFN-α has been used to reduce platelet counts in patients with many forms of myeloproliferative disease. The first reported clinical trial was performed in patients with a mixture of these disorders. The trial found the mean platelet count decreased significantly from 1050×10^9/L to 340×10^9/L.[198] Long-term therapy with IFN also was shown to be effective and safe.[199] From these and other studies, IFN (2 to 5 million units 3 times per week) clearly effectively reduces the platelet count toward normal in most patients with myeloproliferative disease. More aggressive regimens (2 to 6 million units daily) result in complete hematologic remissions but with no evidence that the clonal disorder responsible has been affected.[200] Not surprisingly, reduced energy level, weight loss, myalgia, and depression have been consistently reported, forcing discontinuation of the drug in approximately one-third of patients taking low to moderate doses of various forms of IFN-α.[201] Of some concern and possibly related to its effects on the immune system, a significant number of patients treated with IFN for thrombocytosis have developed antibodies to the administered drug, with subsequent reduced efficacy.[202]

THROMBOPOIETIN

Clinically, the most important activity of thrombopoietin likely is its effects on megakaryopoiesis, potentially ameliorating the thrombocytopenia that occurs in natural and iatrogenic states of marrow failure. In this regard, a number of promising results in preclinical trials of the cytokine were reported.[126,128,129,203] In general, in rodent, dog, and nonhuman primates, almost every model of myelosuppression or immune-mediated platelet destruction has responded favorably to parenteral administration of thrombopoietin. In addition to the favorable effects on platelet recovery, many of these studies also reported enhanced recovery or hematopoietic progenitors of all lineages, accelerated recovery of erythrocytes or leukocytes, or both. The only exception to these generally favorable results has been reported in animal models of stem cell transplantation, where negligible to minimal acceleration of blood cell recovery was found, unless the stem cell donor was treated with the hormone.[204,205]

A number of clinical trials in patients with cancer undergoing cytotoxic therapy have been conducted. Results were varied, with the hormone helpful in many patients,[206–208] but not in all clinical situations.[209,210] In general, the hormone has been useful in patients who were administered moderately aggressive chemotherapeutic regimens that produce clinically important thrombocytopenia. However, the hormone has not been helpful in the setting of high-dose, prolonged cytotoxic therapy, as in the treatment of acute myelogenous leukemia, or in stem cell transplantation, unless, as in the animal studies, it is administered to the stem cell donor.[211] Thrombopoietin also reportedly increases platelet levels in patients with immune-mediated thrombocytopenia.[212] The timing of drug administration can significantly impact both the total amount of drug required and its efficacy.[213] For example, administration of one dose of drug before and once following myelo-suppressive therapy was as effective as any other multidose regimen. This regimen resulted in significant reductions in nadir platelet counts and the need for platelet transfusion during chemotherapy cycles supplemented with thrombopoietin. Nevertheless, use of a modified form of recombinant thrombopoietin is associated with antibody formation to the drug, which cross-reacts with and neutralizes the native hormone, resulting in thrombocytopenia.[214] Although this effect has not been reported with a nonmodified recombinant thrombopoietin, most efforts using thrombopoietin in patients with thrombocytopenia are focusing on small peptide or organic mimics that bind to and activate the thrombopoietin receptor (reviewed in Ref. 218).[215-217] Both types of thrombopoietin mimetic agents have been tested in clinical trials (Chap. 117). Two lead indications have been tested; primary immune thrombocytopenia (ITP) and IFN-induced thrombocytopenia in patients being treated for chronic hepatitis C infection. The results of these trials have been very promising. For example, in a randomized control phase III clinical trial of a peptibody bearing four copies of a c-Mpl receptor-stimulating peptide on an immunoglobulin scaffold, 84 percent of heavily pretreated patients with ITP responded to treatment, with rates being slightly lower or higher depending on whether they had previously undergone splenectomy.[219] Likewise, the administration of a small, orally available organic thrombopoietin mimetic to patients with ITP resulted in 81 percent of patients achieving a platelet count above 50×10^9/L.[220] These studies have led to FDA approval of the two thrombopoietin agonists for use in patients with ITP. The same molecule was administered to patients with modest hepatic insufficiency undergoing IFN/ribavirin therapy for hepatitis C; 75 percent of such patients were able to complete 3 months of therapy without IFN dose reduction, compared to 6 percent of patients given placebo.[221]

Thrombopoietin mimics have also been tested in combination with other agents for the treatment of chronic ITP. For example, the combination of recombinant human thrombopoietin plus rituximab results in higher response rates and longer duration of response than rituximab alone.[222]

A number of studies have suggested that thrombopoietin mimics could lead to marrow fibrosis, particularly if used for long periods of time. For example, in a series of patients treated with several different thrombopoietin mimics over 60 patients were shown to develop modest degrees of marrow fibrosis, that progressed with time.[223] Careful study of these patients will be required to assess the true incidence and predictors of such complications of therapy.

REFERENCES

1. Hanson SR, Slichter SJ: Platelet kinetics in patients with bone marrow hypoplasia: Evidence for a fixed platelet requirement. *Blood* 66:1105, 1985.
2. Dettke M, Hlousek M, Kurz M, et al: Increase in endogenous thrombopoietin in healthy donors after automated plateletpheresis. *Transfusion* 38:449, 1998.
3. Harker LA, Marzec UM, Hunt P, et al: Dose-response effects of pegylated human megakaryocyte growth and development factor on platelet production and function in nonhuman primates. *Blood* 88:511, 1996.
4. O'Malley CJ, Rasko JE, Basser RL, et al: Administration of pegylated recombinant human megakaryocyte growth and development factor to humans stimulates the production of functional platelets that show no evidence of *in vivo* activation. *Blood* 88:3288, 1996.
5. Machlus KR, Italiano JE Jr: The incredible journey: From megakaryocyte development to platelet formation. *J Cell Biol* 201:785, 2013.
6. Junt T, Schulze H, Chen Z, et al: Dynamic visualization of thrombopoiesis within bone marrow. *Science* 317:1767, 2007.
7. Harker LA, Finch CA: Thrombokinetics in man. *J Clin Invest* 48:963, 1969.
8. Machlus KR, Italiano JE Jr: The incredible journey: From megakaryocyte development to platelet formation. *J Cell Biol* 201:785, 2013.
9. Tronik-Le Roux D, Roullot V, Schweitzer A, et al: Suppression of erythro-megakaryocytopoiesis and the induction of reversible thrombocytopenia in mice transgenic for the thymidine kinase gene targeted by the platelet glycoprotein alpha IIb promoter. *J Exp Med* 181:2141, 1995.
10. Debili N, Robin C, Schiavon V, et al: Different expression of CD41 on human lymphoid and myeloid progenitors from adults and neonates. *Blood* 97:2023, 2001.
11. Wu G, Essex DW, Meloni FJ, et al: Human endothelial cells in culture and *in vivo* express on their surface all four components of the glycoprotein Ib/IX/V complex. *Blood* 90:2660, 1997.
12. Hickey MJ, Hagen FS, Yagi M, Roth GJ: Human platelet glycoprotein V: Characterization of the polypeptide and the related Ib-V-IX receptor system of adhesive, leucine-rich glycoproteins. *Proc Natl Acad Sci U S A* 90:8327, 1993.
13. Kahn ML, Diacovo TG, Bainton DF, et al: Glycoprotein V-deficient platelets have undiminished thrombin responsiveness and do not exhibit a Bernard-Soulier phenotype. *Blood* 94:4112, 1999.
14. Lopez JA, Andrews RK, Afshar-Kharghan V, Berndt MC: Bernard-Soulier syndrome. *Blood* 91:4397, 1998.
15. Ramakrishnan V, DeGuzman F, Bao M, et al: A thrombin receptor function for platelet glycoprotein Ib-IX unmasked by cleavage of glycoprotein V. *Proc Natl Acad Sci U S A* 98:1823, 2001.
16. Breton-Gorius J, Reyes F: Ultrastructure of human bone marrow cell maturation. *Int Rev Cytol* 46:251, 1976.
17. Italiano JE Jr, Shivdasani RA: Megakaryocytes and beyond: The birth of platelets. *J Thromb Haemost* 1:1174, 2003.
18. Ebbe S, Stohlman F Jr: Megakaryocytopoiesis in the rat. *Blood* 26:20, 1965.
19. Vitrat N, Cohen-Solal K, Pique C, et al: Endomitosis of human megakaryocytes are due to abortive mitosis. *Blood* 91:3711, 1998.
20. Odell TT Jr, Reiter RS: Generation cycle of rat megakaryocytes. *Exp Cell Res* 53:321, 1968.
21. Tijssen MR, Ghevaert C. Transcription factors in late megakaryopoiesis and related platelet disorders. *J Thromb Haemost* 11:593, 2013.
22. Bastian LS, Kwiatkowski BA, Breininger J, et al: Regulation of the megakaryocytic glycoprotein IX promoter by the oncogenic Ets transcription factor Fli-1. *Blood* 93:2637, 1999.
23. Ramachandran B, Surrey S, Schwartz E: Megakaryocyte-specific positive regulatory sequence 5′ to the human PF4 gene. *Exp Hematol* 23:49, 1995.
24. Furihata K, Kunicki TJ: Characterization of human glycoprotein VI gene 5′ regulatory and promoter regions. *Arterioscler Thromb Vasc Biol* 22:1733, 2002.
25. Sevinsky JR, Whalen AM, Ahn NG: Extracellular signal-regulated kinase induces the megakaryocyte GPIIb/CD41 gene through MafB/Kreisler. *Mol Cell Biol* 24:4534, 2004.
26. Rojnuckarin P, Drachman JG, Kaushansky K: Thrombopoietin-induced activation of the mitogen-activated protein kinase (MAPK) pathway in normal megakaryocytes: Role in endomitosis. *Blood* 94:1273, 1999.
27. Vyas P, Norris FA, Joseph R, et al: Inositol polyphosphate 4-phosphatase type I regulates cell growth downstream of transcription factor GATA-1. *Proc Natl Acad Sci U S A* 97:13696, 2000.
28. Pevny L, Simon MC, Robertson E, et al: Erythroid differentiation in chimaeric mice blocked by a targeted mutation in the gene for transcription factor GATA-1. *Nature* 349:257, 1991.
29. Shivdasani RA, Fujiwara Y, McDevitt MA, Orkin SH: A lineage-selective knockout establishes the critical role of transcription factor GATA-1 in megakaryocyte growth and platelet development. *EMBO J* 16:3965, 1997.
30. Song WJ, Sullivan MG, Legare RD, et al: Haploinsufficiency of CBFA2 causes familial thrombocytopenia with propensity to develop acute myelogenous leukaemia. *Nat Genet* 23:166, 1999.
31. Ichikawa M, Asai T, Saito T, et al: AML-1 is required for megakaryocytic maturation and lymphocytic differentiation, but not for maintenance of hematopoietic stem cells in adult hematopoiesis. *Nat Med* 10:299, 2004.
32. Elagib KE, Racke FK, Mogass M, et al: RUNX1 and GATA-1 coexpression and cooperation in megakaryocytic differentiation. *Blood* 101:4333, 2003.
33. Ebbe S, Phalen E, Stohlman F Jr: Abnormalities of megakaryocytes in W-WV mice. *Blood* 42:857, 1973.
34. Broudy VC, Lin NL, Kaushansky K: Thrombopoietin (c-mpl ligand) acts synergistically with erythropoietin, stem cell factor, and interleukin-11 to enhance murine megakaryocyte colony growth and increases megakaryocyte ploidy in vitro. *Blood* 85:1719, 1995.
35. Gainsford T, Roberts AW, Kimura S, et al: Cytokine production and function in cmpl–deficient mice: No physiologic role for interleukin-3 in residual megakaryocyte and platelet production. *Blood* 92:2745, 1998.
36. Kaushansky K, Broudy VC, Lin N, et al: Thrombopoietin, the Mp1 ligand, is essential for full megakaryocyte development. *Proc Natl Acad Sci U S A* 92:3234, 1995.

37. Hodohara K, Fujii N, Yamamoto N, Kaushansky K: Stromal cell-derived factor-1 (SDF-1) acts together with thrombopoietin to enhance the development of megakaryocytic progenitor cells (CFU-MK). *Blood* 95:769, 2000.
38. Avecilla ST, Hattori K, Heissig B, et al: Chemokine-mediated interaction of hematopoietic progenitors with the bone marrow vascular niche is required for thrombopoiesis. *Nat Med* 10:64, 2004.
39. Geddis AE, Fox NE, Kaushansky K: Phosphatidylinositol 3-kinase is necessary but not sufficient for thrombopoietin-induced proliferation in engineered Mp1-bearing cell lines as well as in primary megakaryocytic progenitors. *J Biol Chem* 276:34473, 2001.
40. Miyazaki R, Ogata H, Kobayashi Y: Requirement of thrombopoietin-induced activation of ERK for megakaryocyte differentiation and of p38 for erythroid differentiation. *Ann Hematol* 80:284, 2001.
41. Pettiford SM, Herbst R: The protein tyrosine phosphatase HePTP regulates nuclear translocation of ERK2 and can modulate megakaryocytic differentiation of K562 cells. *Leukemia* 17:366, 2003.
42. Dorsey JF, Cunnick JM, Mane SM, Wu J: Regulation of the Erk2-Elk1 signaling pathway and megakaryocytic differentiation of Bcr-Abl(+) K562 leukemic cells by Gab2. *Blood* 99:1388, 2002.
43. Zhang Y, Nagata Y, Yu G, et al: Aberrant quantity and localization of Aurora-B/AIM-1 and survivin during megakaryocyte polyploidization and the consequences of Aurora-B/AIM-1-deregulated expression. *Blood* 103:3717, 2004.
44. Carow CE, Fox NE, Kaushansky K: Kinetics of endomitosis in primary murine megakaryocytes. *J Cell Physiol* 188:291, 2001.
45. Geddis AE, Kaushansky K: Megakaryocytes express functional aurora kinase B in endomitosis. *Blood* 104:1017, 2004.
46. Geddis AE, Fox NE, Tkachenko E, Kaushansky K: Endomitotic megakaryocytes that form a bipolar spindle exhibit cleavage furrow ingression followed by furrow regression. *Cell Cycle* 6:455, 2007.
47. Suzuki A, Shin JW, Wang Y, et al: RhoA is essential for maintaining normal megakaryocyte ploidy and platelet generation. *PLoS One* 8:e69315, 2013.
48. Gao Y, Smith E, Ker E, et al: Role of RhoA-specific guanine exchange factors in regulation of endomitosis in megakaryocytes. *Dev Cell* 22:573, 2012.
49. Seri M, Cusano R, Gangarossa S, et al: Mutations in MYH9 result in the May-Hegglin anomaly, and Fechtner and Sebastian syndromes. The May-Hegglin/Fechtner Syndrome Consortium. *Nat Genet* 26:103, 2000.
50. Hartwig J, Italiano J Jr: The birth of the platelet. *J Thromb Haemost* 1:1580, 2003.
51. Visvader JE, Elefanty AG, Strasser A, Adams JM: GATA-1 but not SCL induces megakaryocytic differentiation in an early myeloid line. *EMBO J* 11:4557, 1992.
52. Huizing M, Parkes JM, Helip-Wooley A, White JG, Gahl WA: Platelet alpha granules in BLOC-2 and BLOC-3 subtypes of Hermansky-Pudlak syndrome. *Platelets* 18:150, 2007.
53. Tavassoli M, Aoki M: Localization of megakaryocytes in the bone marrow. *Blood Cells* 15:3, 1989.
54. Andrews NC, Erdjument-Bromage H, Davidson MB, et al: Erythroid transcription factor NF-E2 is a haematopoietic-specific basic-leucine zipper protein. *Nature* 362:722, 1993.
55. Bean TL, Ney PA: Multiple regions of p45 NF-E2 are required for beta-globin gene expression in erythroid cells. *Nucleic Acids Res* 25:2509, 1997.
56. Shivdasani RA, Rosenblatt MF, Zucker-Franklin D, et al: Transcription factor NF-E2 is required for platelet formation independent of the actions of thrombopoietin/MGDF in megakaryocyte development. *Cell* 81:695, 1995.
57. Querfurth E, Schuster M, Kulessa H, et al: Antagonism between C/EBPbeta and FOG in eosinophil lineage commitment of multipotent hematopoietic progenitors. *Genes Dev* 14:2515, 2000.
58. Tijssen MR, Ghevaert C. Transcription factors in late megakaryopoiesis and related platelet disorders. *J Thromb Haemost* 11:593, 2013.
59. Howell WH DD: The production of blood platelets in the lungs. *J Exp Med* 65:177, 1939.
60. Slater DN, Trowbridge EA, Martin JF: The megakaryocyte in thrombocytopenia: A microscopic study which supports the theory that platelets are produced in the pulmonary circulation. *Thromb Res* 31:163, 1983.
61. Kaushansky K, Lok S, Holly RD, et al: Promotion of megakaryocyte progenitor expansion and differentiation by the c-Mpl ligand thrombopoietin. *Nature* 369:568, 1994.
62. Kaufman RM, Airo R, Pollack S, et al: Origin of pulmonary megakaryocytes. *Blood* 25:767, 1965.
63. Harker LA, Marzec UM, Kelly AB: Effects of Mpl ligands on platelet production and function in nonhuman primates. *Stem Cells* 16(Suppl 2):107, 1998.
64. Choi ES, Nichol JL, Hokom MM, et al: Platelets generated in vitro from proplatelet-displaying human megakaryocytes are functional. *Blood* 85:402, 1995.
65. Norol F, Vitrat N, Cramer E, et al: Effects of cytokines on platelet production from blood and marrow CD34+ cells. *Blood* 91:830, 1998.
66. Rojnuckarin P, Kaushansky K: Actin reorganization and proplatelet formation in murine megakaryocytes: The role of protein kinase C alpha. *Blood* 97:154, 2001.
67. Ishida Y, Yano K, Ito T, et al: Purification of proplatelet formation (PPF) stimulating factor: Thrombin/antithrombin III complex stimulates PPF of megakaryocytes in vitro and platelet production in vivo. *Thromb Haemost* 85:349, 2001.
68. Hunt P, Hokom MM, Wiemann B, et al: Megakaryocyte proplatelet-like process formation in vitro is inhibited by serum prothrombin, a process which is blocked by matrix-bound glycosaminoglycans. *Exp Hematol* 21:372, 1993.
69. Geddis AE, Kaushansky K: Inherited thrombocytopenias: Toward a molecular understanding of disorders of platelet production. *Curr Opin Pediatr* 16:15, 2004.
70. Eckly A, Strassel C, Freund M, et al: Abnormal megakaryocyte morphology and proplatelet formation in mice with megakaryocyte-restricted MYH9 inactivation. *Blood* 113(14):3182, 2009.
71. De Botton S, Sabri S, Daugas E, et al: Platelet formation is the consequence of caspase activation within megakaryocytes. *Blood* 100:1310, 2002.
72. Quesenberry PJ, Ihle JN, McGrath E: The effect of interleukin 3 and GM-CSA-2 on megakaryocyte and myeloid clonal colony formation. *Blood* 65:214, 1985.
73. Kaushansky K, O'Hara PJ, Berkner K, et al: Genomic cloning, characterization, and multilineage growth-promoting activity of human granulocyte-macrophage colony-stimulating factor. *Proc Natl Acad Sci U S A* 83:3101, 1986.
74. Briddell RA, Bruno E, Cooper RJ, et al: Effect of c-kit ligand on in vitro human megakaryocytopoiesis. *Blood* 78:2854, 1991.
75. Kaushansky K: Thrombopoietin: The primary regulator of platelet production. *Blood* 86:419, 1995.
76. Yang YC, Ciarletta AB, Temple PA, et al: Human IL-3 (multi-CSF): Identification by expression cloning of a novel hematopoietic growth factor related to murine IL-3. *Cell* 47:3, 1986.
77. Wong GG, Witek JS, Temple PA, et al: Human GM-CSF: Molecular cloning of the complementary DNA and purification of the natural and recombinant proteins. *Science* 228:810, 1985.
78. Feng Y, Klein BK, Vu L, et al: 1H 13C, and 15N NMR resonance assignments, secondary structure, and backbone topology of a variant of human interleukin-3. *Biochemistry* 34:6540, 1995.
79. Lopez AF, Eglinton JM, Gillis D, et al: Reciprocal inhibition of binding between interleukin 3 and granulocyte-macrophage colony-stimulating factor to human eosinophils. *Proc Natl Acad Sci U S A* 86:7022, 1989.
80. Scott CL, Robb L, Mansfield R, et al: Granulocyte-macrophage colony-stimulating factor is not responsible for residual thrombopoiesis in Mpl null mice. *Exp Hematol* 28:1001, 2000.
81. Chen Q, Solar G, Eaton DL, de Sauvage FJ: IL-3 does not contribute to platelet production in c-Mpl–deficient mice. *Stem Cells* 16(Suppl 2):31, 1998.
82. Kishimoto T: The biology of interleukin-6. *Blood* 74:1, 1989.
83. Quesenberry PJ, McGrath HE, Williams ME, et al: Multifactor stimulation of megakaryocytopoiesis: Effects of interleukin 6. *Exp Hematol* 19:35, 1991.
84. Williams N, De Giorgio T, Banu N, et al: Recombinant interleukin 6 stimulates immature murine megakaryocytes. *Exp Hematol* 18:69, 1990.
85. Mei RL, Burstein SA: Megakaryocytic maturation in murine long-term bone marrow culture: Role of interleukin-6. *Blood* 78:1438, 1991.
86. Ishibashi T, Kimura H, Shikama Y, et al: Interleukin-6 is a potent thrombopoietic factor in vivo in mice. *Blood* 74:1241, 1989.
87. Asano S, Okano A, Ozawa K, et al: In vivo effects of recombinant human interleukin-6 in primates: Stimulated production of platelets. *Blood* 75:1602, 1990.
88. van Gameren MM, Willemse PH, Mulder NH, et al: Effects of recombinant human interleukin-6 in cancer patients: A phase I–II study. *Blood* 84:1434, 1994.
89. Blay JY, Favrot M, Rossi JF, Wijdenes J: Role of interleukin-6 in paraneoplastic thrombocytosis. *Blood* 82:2261, 1993.
90. Bernad A, Kopf M, Kulbacki R, et al: Interleukin-6 is required in vivo for the regulation of stem cells and committed progenitors of the hematopoietic system. *Immunity* 1:725, 1994.
91. Kaser A, Brandacher G, Steurer W, et al: Interleukin-6 stimulates thrombopoiesis through thrombopoietin: Role in inflammatory thrombocytosis. *Blood* 98:2720, 2001.
92. Du X, Williams DA: Interleukin-11: Review of molecular, cell biology, and clinical use. *Blood* 89:3897, 1997.
93. Gough NM: Molecular genetics of leukemia inhibitory factor (LIF) and its receptor. *Growth Factors* 7:175, 1992.
94. Hilton DJ: LIF: Lots of interesting functions. *Trends Biochem Sci* 17:72, 1992.
95. Debili N, Masse JM, Katz A, et al: Effects of the recombinant hematopoietic growth factors interleukin-3, interleukin-6, stem cell factor, and leukemia inhibitory factor on the megakaryocytic differentiation of CD34+ cells. *Blood* 82:84, 1993.
96. Teramura M, Kobayashi S, Hoshino S, et al: Interleukin-11 enhances human megakaryocytopoiesis in vitro. *Blood* 79:327, 1992.
97. Metcalf D, Nicola NA, Gearing DP: Effects of injected leukemia inhibitory factor on hematopoietic and other tissues in mice. *Blood* 76:50, 1990.
98. Neben TY, Loebelenz J, Hayes L, et al: Recombinant human interleukin-11 stimulates megakaryocytopoiesis and increases peripheral platelets in normal and splenectomized mice. *Blood* 81:901, 1993.
99. Farese AM, Myers LA, MacVittie TJ: Therapeutic efficacy of recombinant human leukemia inhibitory factor in a primate model of radiation-induced marrow aplasia. *Blood* 84:3675, 1994.
100. Gordon MS, McCaskill-Stevens WJ, Battiato LA, et al: A phase I trial of recombinant human interleukin-11 (Neumega rhIL-11 growth factor) in women with breast cancer receiving chemotherapy. *Blood* 87:3615, 1996.
101. Nandurkar HH, Robb L, Tarlinton D, et al: Adult mice with targeted mutation of the interleukin-11 receptor (IL11Ra) display normal hematopoiesis. *Blood* 90:2148, 1997.
102. Gainsford T, Nandurkar H, Metcalf D, et al: The residual megakaryocyte and platelet production in c-Mpl–deficient mice is not dependent on the actions of interleukin-6, interleukin-11, or leukemia inhibitory factor. *Blood* 95:528, 2000.
103. Lyman SD, James L, Vanden Bos T, et al: Molecular cloning of a ligand for the flt3/flk-2 tyrosine kinase receptor: A proliferative factor for primitive hematopoietic cells. *Cell* 75:1157, 1993.

104. Avraham H, Vannier E, Cowley S, et al: Effects of the stem cell factor, c-kit ligand, on human megakaryocytic cells. *Blood* 79:365, 1992.

105. Ebbe S, Phalen E, Stohlman F Jr: Abnormalities of megakaryocytes in S1-S1d mice. *Blood* 42:865, 1973.

106. Arnold J, Ellis S, Radley JM, Williams N: Compensatory mechanisms in platelet production: The response of Sl/Sld mice to 5-fluorouracil. *Exp Hematol* 19:24, 1991.

107. Hunt P, Zsebo KM, Hokom MM, et al: Evidence that stem cell factor is involved in the rebound thrombocytosis that follows 5-fluorouracil treatment. *Blood* 80:904, 1992.

108. Broudy VC: Stem cell factor and hematopoiesis. *Blood* 90:1345, 1997.

109. Langley KE, Bennett LG, Wypych J, et al: Soluble stem cell factor in human serum. *Blood* 81:656, 1993.

110. Cheng HJ, Flanagan JG: Transmembrane kit ligand cleavage does not require a signal in the cytoplasmic domain and occurs at a site dependent on spacing from the membrane. *Mol Biol Cell* 5:943, 1994.

111. Miyazawa K, Williams DA, Gotoh A, et al: Membrane-bound Steel factor induces more persistent tyrosine kinase activation and longer life span of c-kit gene-encoded protein than its soluble form. *Blood* 85:641, 1995.

112. Flanagan JG, Chan DC, Leder P: Transmembrane form of the kit ligand growth factor is determined by alternative splicing and is missing in the Sld mutant. *Cell* 64:1025, 1991.

113. Lyman SD, Jacobsen SE: C-kit ligand and Flt3 ligand: Stem/progenitor cell factors with overlapping yet distinct activities. *Blood* 91:1101, 1998.

114. Ramsfjell V, Borge OJ, Veiby OP, et al: Thrombopoietin, but not erythropoietin, directly stimulates multilineage growth of primitive murine bone marrow progenitor cells in synergy with early acting cytokines: Distinct interactions with the ligands for c-kit and FLT3. *Blood* 88:4481, 1996.

115. Piacibello W, Garetto L, Sanavio F, et al: The effects of human FLT3 ligand on *in vitro* human megakaryocytopoiesis. *Exp Hematol* 24:340, 1996.

116. Brasel K, McKenna HJ, Morrissey PJ, et al: Hematologic effects of flt3 ligand *in vivo* in mice. *Blood* 88:2004, 1996.

117. Kelemen E CI, Tanos B: Demonstration and some properties of human thrombopoietin in thrombocythemic sera. *Acta Haematol* 20:350, 1958.

118. Wendling F, Varlet P, Charon M, Tambourin P: MPLV: A retrovirus complex inducing an acute myeloproliferative leukemic disorder in adult mice. *Virology* 149:242, 1986.

119. Souyri M, Vigon I, Penciolelli JF, et al: A putative truncated cytokine receptor gene transduced by the myeloproliferative leukemia virus immortalizes hematopoietic progenitors. *Cell* 63:1137, 1990.

120. Vigon I, Mornon JP, Cocault L, et al: Molecular cloning and characterization of MPL, the human homolog of the v-Mpl oncogene: Identification of a member of the hematopoietic growth factor receptor super-family. *Proc Natl Acad Sci U S A* 89:5640, 1992.

121. Cosman D: The hematopoietin receptor superfamily. *Cytokine* 5:95, 1993.

122. Skoda RC, Seldin DC, Chiang MK, et al: Murine c-Mpl: A member of the hematopoietic growth factor receptor superfamily that transduces a proliferative signal. *EMBO J* 12:2645, 1993.

123. Lok S, Kaushansky K, Holly RD, et al: Cloning and expression of murine thrombopoietin cDNA and stimulation of platelet production *in vivo*. *Nature* 369:565, 1994.

124. Linden HM, Kaushansky K: The glycan domain of thrombopoietin enhances its secretion. *Biochemistry* 39:3044, 2000.

125. Basser RL, Rasko JE, Clarke K, et al: Thrombopoietic effects of pegylated recombinant human megakaryocyte growth and development factor (PEG-rHuMGDF) in patients with advanced cancer. *Lancet* 348:1279, 1996.

126. Kaushansky K, Broudy VC, Grossmann A, et al: Thrombopoietin expands erythroid progenitors, increases red cell production, and enhances erythroid recovery after myelosuppressive therapy. *J Clin Invest* 96:1683, 1995.

127. Farese AM, Hunt P, Boone T, MacVittie TJ: Recombinant human megakaryocyte growth and development factor stimulates thrombocytopoiesis in normal nonhuman primates. *Blood* 86:54, 1995.

128. Akahori H, Shibuya K, Obuchi M, et al: Effect of recombinant human thrombopoietin in nonhuman primates with chemotherapy-induced thrombocytopenia. *Br J Haematol* 94:722, 1996.

129. Neelis KJ, Hartong SC, Egeland T, et al: The efficacy of single-dose administration of thrombopoietin with coadministration of either granulocyte/macrophage or granulocyte colony-stimulating factor in myelosuppressed rhesus monkeys. *Blood* 90:2565, 1997.

130. Gurney AL, Carver-Moore K, de Sauvage FJ, Moore MW: Thrombocytopenia in c-Mpl–deficient mice. *Science* 265:1445, 1994.

131. van den Oudenrijn S, Bruin M, Folman CC, et al: Mutations in the thrombopoietin receptor, Mpl, in children with congenital amegakaryocytic thrombocytopenia. *Br J Haematol* 110:441, 2000.

132. Ballmaier M, Germeshausen M, Schulze H, et al: C-mpl mutations are the cause of congenital amegakaryocytic thrombocytopenia. *Blood* 97:139, 2001.

133. Sohma Y, Akahori H, Seki N, et al: Molecular cloning and chromosomal localization of the human thrombopoietin gene. *FEBS Lett* 353:57, 1994.

134. Morris D: *Cis*-Acting mRNA structures in gene-specific translational control, in *Post-Transcriptional Gene Regulation*, edited by Harford JB, Morris DR, p 165. Wiley-Liss, New York, 1997.

135. Wiestner A, Schlemper RJ, Van der Maas AP, Skoda RC: An activating splice donor mutation in the thrombopoietin gene causes hereditary thrombocythaemia. *Nat Genet* 18:49, 1998.

136. Jorgensen MJ, Raskind WH, Wolff JF, et al: Familial thrombocytosis associated with overproduction of thrombopoietin due to a novel splice donor site mutation. *Blood* 92:205a, 1998.

137. Kondo T, Okabe M, Sanada M, et al: Familial essential thrombocythemia associated with one-base deletion in the 5′-untranslated region of the thrombopoietin gene. *Blood* 92:1091, 1998.

138. Ghilardi N, Wiestner A, Kikuchi M, et al: Hereditary thrombocythaemia in a Japanese family is caused by a novel point mutation in the thrombopoietin gene. *Br J Haematol* 107:310, 1999.

139. Cazzola M, Skoda RC: Translational pathophysiology: A novel molecular mechanism of human disease. *Blood* 95:3280, 2000.

140. Odell TT Jr, McDonald TP, Detwiler TC: Stimulation of platelet production by serum of platelet-depleted rats. *Proc Soc Exp Biol Med* 108:428, 1961.

141. Nichol JL, Hokom MM, Hornkohl A, et al: Megakaryocyte growth and development factor. Analyses of in vitro effects on human megakaryopoiesis and endogenous serum levels during chemotherapy-induced thrombocytopenia. *J Clin Invest* 95:2973, 1995.

142. Kuter DJ, Rosenberg RD: The reciprocal relationship of thrombopoietin (c-Mpl ligand) to changes in the platelet mass during busulfan-induced thrombocytopenia in the rabbit. *Blood* 85:2720, 1995.

143. Bartocci A, Mastrogiannis DS, Migliorati G, et al: Macrophages specifically regulate the concentration of their own growth factor in the circulation. *Proc Natl Acad Sci U S A* 84:6179, 1987.

144. Emmons RV, Reid DM, Cohen RL, et al: Human thrombopoietin levels are high when thrombocytopenia is due to megakaryocyte deficiency and low when due to increased platelet destruction. *Blood* 87:4068, 1996.

145. McCarty JM, Sprugel KH, Fox NE, et al: Murine thrombopoietin mRNA levels are modulated by platelet count. *Blood* 86:3668, 1995.

146. de Sauvage FJ, Carver-Moore K, Luoh SM, et al: Physiological regulation of early and late stages of megakaryocytopoiesis by thrombopoietin. *J Exp Med* 183:651, 1996.

147. Sungaran R, Markovic B, Chong BH: Localization and regulation of thrombopoietin mRNA expression in human kidney, liver, bone marrow, and spleen using in situ hybridization. *Blood* 89:101, 1997.

148. McIntosh B, Kaushansky K: Marrow stromal production of thrombopoietin is regulated by transcriptional mechanisms in response to platelet products. *Exp Hematol* 36:799, 2008.

149. Solanilla A, Dechanet J, El Andaloussi A, et al: CD40-ligand stimulates myelopoiesis by regulating flt3-ligand and thrombopoietin production in bone marrow stromal cells. *Blood* 95:3758, 2000.

150. Sungaran R, Chisholm OT, Markovic B, et al: The role of platelet alpha-granular proteins in the regulation of thrombopoietin messenger RNA expression in human bone marrow stromal cells. *Blood* 95:3094, 2000.

151. Kamura T, Handa H, Hamasaki N, Kitajima S: Characterization of the human thrombopoietin gene promoter. A possible role of an Ets transcription factor, E4TF1/GABP. *J Biol Chem* 272:11361, 1997.

152. Chang MS, McNinch J, Basu R, et al: Cloning and characterization of the human megakaryocyte growth and development factor (MGDF) gene. *J Biol Chem* 270:511, 1995.

153. Rollins BJ: Chemokines. *Blood* 90:909, 1997.

154. Broxmeyer HE, Mantel CR, Aronica SM: Biology and mechanisms of action of synergistically stimulated myeloid progenitor cell proliferation and suppression by chemokines. *Stem Cells* 15(Suppl 1):69, discussion 15(Suppl 1):78, 1997.

155. Shirozu M, Nakano T, Inazawa J, et al: Structure and chromosomal localization of the human stromal cell-derived factor 1 (SDF1) gene. *Genomics* 28:495, 1995.

156. Luster AD: Chemokines—Chemotactic cytokines that mediate inflammation. *N Engl J Med* 338:436, 1998.

157. Nagasawa T, Hirota S, Tachibana K, et al: Defects of B-cell lymphopoiesis and bone-marrow myelopoiesis in mice lacking the CXC chemokine PBSF/SDF-1. *Nature* 382:635, 1996.

158. Ma Q, Jones D, Borghesani PR, et al: Impaired B-lymphopoiesis, myelopoiesis, and derailed cerebellar neuron migration in CXCR4- and SDF-1-deficient mice. *Proc Natl Acad Sci U S A* 95:9448, 1998.

159. Aiuti A, Webb IJ, Bleul C, et al: The chemokine SDF-1 is a chemoattractant for human CD34+ hematopoietic progenitor cells and provides a new mechanism to explain the mobilization of CD34+ progenitors to peripheral blood. *J Exp Med* 185:111, 1997.

160. Wang JF, Liu ZY, Groopman JE: The alpha-chemokine receptor CXCR4 is expressed on the megakaryocytic lineage from progenitor to platelets and modulates migration and adhesion. *Blood* 92:756, 1998.

161. Hamada T, Mohle R, Hesselgesser J, et al: Transendothelial migration of megakaryocytes in response to stromal cell-derived factor 1 (SDF-1) enhances platelet formation. *J Exp Med* 188:539, 1998.

162. Daopin S, Piez KA, Ogawa Y, Davies DR: Crystal structure of transforming growth factor-beta 2: An unusual fold for the superfamily. *Science* 257:369, 1992.

163. Keller JR, Mantel C, Sing GK, et al: Transforming growth factor beta 1 selectively regulates early murine hematopoietic progenitors and inhibits the growth of IL-3-dependent myeloid leukemia cell lines. *J Exp Med* 168:737, 1988.

164. Dybedal I, Jacobsen SE: Transforming growth factor beta (TGF-beta), a potent inhibitor of erythropoiesis: Neutralizing TGF-beta antibodies show erythropoietin as a potent stimulator of murine burst-forming unit erythroid colony formation in the absence of a burst-promoting activity. *Blood* 86:949, 1995.

165. Ishibashi T, Miller SL, Burstein SA: Type beta transforming growth factor is a potent inhibitor of murine megakaryocytopoiesis *in vitro*. *Blood* 69:1737, 1987.

166. Kuter DJ, Gminski DM, Rosenberg RD: Transforming growth factor beta inhibits megakaryocyte growth and endomitosis. *Blood* 79:619, 1992.

167. Laiho M, DeCaprio JA, Ludlow JW, et al: Growth inhibition by TGF-beta linked to suppression of retinoblastoma protein phosphorylation. *Cell* 62:175, 1990.

168. Polyak K, Kato JY, Solomon MJ, et al: P27Kip1, a cyclin-Cdk inhibitor, links transforming growth factor-beta and contact inhibition to cell cycle arrest. *Genes Dev* 8:9, 1994.

169. Teofili L, Martini M, Di Mario A, et al: Expression of p15(ink4b) gene during megakaryocytic differentiation of normal and myelodysplastic hematopoietic progenitors. *Blood* 98:495, 2001.

170. Theofilopoulos AN, Baccala R, Beutler B, Kono DH: Type I interferons (alpha/beta) in immunity and autoimmunity. *Annu Rev Immunol* 23:307, 2005.

171. Broxmeyer HE, Cooper S, Rubin BY, Taylor MW: The synergistic influence of human interferon-gamma and interferon-alpha on suppression of hematopoietic progenitor cells is additive with the enhanced sensitivity of these cells to inhibition by interferons at low oxygen tension *in vitro. J Immunol* 135:2502, 1985.

172. Fattovich G, Giustina G, Favarato S, Ruol A: A survey of adverse events in 11,241 patients with chronic viral hepatitis treated with alfa interferon. *J Hepatol* 24:38, 1996.

173. Dusheiko G: Side effects of alpha interferon in chronic hepatitis C. *Hepatology* 26(Suppl 1):112S, 1997.

174. Jaster R, Tschirch E, Bittorf T, Brock J: Interferon-alpha inhibits proliferation of Ba/F3 cells by interfering with interleukin-3 action. *Cell Signal* 11:769, 1999.

175. Kuniyasu H, Yasui W, Kitahara K, et al: Growth inhibitory effect of interferon-beta is associated with the induction of cyclin-dependent kinase inhibitor p27Kip1 in a human gastric carcinoma cell line. *Cell Growth Differ* 8:47, 1997.

176. Wang Q, Miyakawa Y, Fox N, Kaushansky K: Interferon-alpha directly represses megakaryopoiesis by inhibiting thrombopoietin-induced signaling through induction of SOCS-1. *Blood* 96:2093, 2000.

177. Long MW: Blood cell cytoadhesion molecules. *Exp Hematol* 20:288, 1992.

178. Toksoz D, Zsebo KM, Smith KA, et al: Support of human hematopoiesis in long-term bone marrow cultures by murine stromal cells selectively expressing the membrane-bound and secreted forms of the human homolog of the steel gene product, stem cell factor. *Proc Natl Acad Sci U S A* 89:7350, 1992.

179. Yang L, Yang YC: Regulation of interleukin (IL)-11 gene expression in IL-1 induced primate bone marrow stromal cells. *J Biol Chem* 269:32732, 1994.

180. Linenberger ML, Jacobson FW, Bennett LG, et al: Stem cell factor production by human marrow stromal fibroblasts. *Exp Hematol* 23:1104, 1995.

181. Gordon MY, Riley GP, Watt SM, Greaves MF: Compartmentalization of a haematopoietic growth factor (GM-CSF) by glycosaminoglycans in the bone marrow microenvironment. *Nature* 326:403, 1987.

182. Roberts R, Gallagher J, Spooncer E, et al: Heparan sulphate bound growth factors: A mechanism for stromal cell mediated haemopoiesis. *Nature* 332:376, 1988.

183. Artavanis-Tsakonas S, Matsuno K, Fortini ME: Notch signaling. *Science* 268:225, 1995.

184. Karanu FN, Murdoch B, Miyabayashi T, et al: Human homologues of Delta-1 and Delta-4 function as mitogenic regulators of primitive human hematopoietic cells. *Blood* 97:1960, 2001.

185. Lam LT, Ronchini C, Norton J, et al: Suppression of erythroid but not megakaryocytic differentiation of human K562 erythroleukemic cells by notch-1. *J Biol Chem* 275:19676, 2000.

186. Fox NE, Kaushansky K: Engagement of integrin a4b1 enhances thrombopoietin-induced megakaryopoiesis. *Exp Hematol* 33:94, 2005.

187. Bruno E, Briddell RA, Cooper RJ, Hoffman R: Effects of recombinant interleukin 11 on human megakaryocyte progenitor cells. *Exp Hematol* 19:378, 1991.

188. Neben S, Turner K: The biology of interleukin 11. *Stem Cells* 11(Suppl 2):156, 1993.

189. Burstein SA, Mei RL, Henthorn J, et al: Leukemia inhibitory factor and interleukin-11 promote maturation of murine and human megakaryocytes *in vitro. J Cell Physiol* 153:305, 1992.

190. Yonemura Y, Kawakita M, Masuda T, et al: Synergistic effects of interleukin 3 and interleukin 11 on murine megakaryopoiesis in serum-free culture. *Exp Hematol* 20:1011, 1992.

191. Yonemura Y, Kawakita M, Masuda T, et al: Effect of recombinant human interleukin-11 on rat megakaryopoiesis and thrombopoiesis *in vivo*: Comparative study with interleukin-6. *Br J Haematol* 84:16, 1993.

192. Schlerman FJ, Bree AG, Kaviani MD, et al: Thrombopoietic activity of recombinant human interleukin 11 (rHuIL-11) in normal and myelosuppressed nonhuman primates. *Stem Cells* 14:517, 1996.

193. Gordon MS SG, Battiato L, et al: The *in vivo* effects of subcutaneously (SC) administered recombinant human interleukin-11 (Neumega rhIL-11 growth factor; rhIL-11) in women with breast cancer (BC). *Blood* 82(Suppl 1):498a, 1993.

194. Champlin RE MR, Kaye JA, et al: Recombinant human interleukin eleven (rhIL-11) following autologous BMT for breast cancer. *Blood* 84(suppl 1):395a, 1994.

195. Tepler I, Elias L, Smith JW 2nd, et al: A randomized placebo-controlled trial of recombinant human interleukin-11 in cancer patients with severe thrombocytopenia due to chemotherapy. *Blood* 87:3607, 1996.

196. Isaacs C, Robert NJ, Bailey FA, et al: Randomized placebo-controlled study of recombinant human interleukin-11 to prevent chemotherapy-induced thrombocytopenia in patients with breast cancer receiving dose-intensive cyclophosphamide and doxorubicin. *J Clin Oncol* 15:3368, 1997.

197. Vredenburgh JJ, Hussein A, Fisher D, et al: A randomized trial of recombinant human interleukin-11 following autologous bone marrow transplantation with peripheral blood progenitor cell support in patients with breast cancer. *Biol Blood Marrow Transplant* 4:134, 1998.

198. Tichelli A, Gratwohl A, Berger C, et al: Treatment of thrombocytosis in myeloproliferative disorders with interferon alpha-2a. *Blut* 58:15, 1989.

199. Gisslinger H, Ludwig H, Linkesch W, et al: Long-term interferon therapy for thrombocytosis in myeloproliferative diseases. *Lancet* 1:634, 1989.

200. Sacchi S, Gugliotta L, Papineschi F, et al: Alfa-interferon in the treatment of essential thrombocythemia: Clinical results and evaluation of its biological effects on the hematopoietic neoplastic clone. Italian Cooperative Group on ET. *Leukemia* 12:289, 1998.

201. Taylor PC, Dolan G, Ng JP, et al: Efficacy of recombinant interferon-alpha (rIFN-alpha) in polycythaemia vera: A study of 17 patients and an analysis of published data. *Br J Haematol* 92:55, 1996.

202. Tornebohm-Roche E, Merup M, Lockner D, Paul C: Alpha-2a interferon therapy and antibody formation in patients with essential thrombocythemia and polycythemia vera with thrombocytosis. *Am J Hematol* 48:163, 1995.

203. Hokom MM, Lacey D, Kinstler OB, et al: Pegylated megakaryocyte growth and development factor abrogates the lethal thrombocytopenia associated with carboplatin and irradiation in mice. *Blood* 86:4486, 1995.

204. Fibbe WE, Heemskerk DP, Laterveer L, et al: Accelerated reconstitution of platelets and erythrocytes after syngeneic transplantation of bone marrow cells derived from thrombopoietin pretreated donor mice. *Blood* 86:3308, 1995.

205. Molineux G, Hartley C, McElroy P, et al: Megakaryocyte growth and development factor accelerates platelet recovery in peripheral blood progenitor cell transplant recipients. *Blood* 88:366, 1996.

206. Fanucchi M, Glaspy J, Crawford J, et al: Effects of polyethylene glycol conjugated recombinant human megakaryocyte growth and development factor on platelet counts after chemotherapy for lung cancer. *N Engl J Med* 336:404, 1997.

207. Vadhan-Raj S, Murray LJ, Bueso-Ramos C, et al: Stimulation of megakaryocyte and platelet production by a single dose of recombinant human thrombopoietin in patients with cancer. *Ann Intern Med* 126:673, 1997.

208. Basser RL, Underhill C, Davis I, et al: Enhancement of platelet recovery after myelosuppressive chemotherapy by recombinant human megakaryocyte growth and development factor in patients with advanced cancer. *J Clin Oncol* 18:2852, 2000.

209. Archimbaud E, Ottmann OG, Yin JA, et al: A randomized, double-blind, placebo-controlled study with pegylated recombinant human megakaryocyte growth and development factor (PEG-rHuMGDF) as an adjunct to chemotherapy for adults with *de novo* acute myeloid leukemia. *Blood* 94:3694, 1999.

210. Bolwell B, Vredenburgh J, Overmoyer B, et al: Phase 1 study of pegylated recombinant human megakaryocyte growth and development factor (PEG-rHuMGDF) in breast cancer patients after autologous peripheral blood progenitor cell (PBPC) transplantation. *Bone Marrow Transplant* 26:141, 2000.

211. Somlo G, Sniecinski I, Ter Veer A, et al: Recombinant human thrombopoietin in combination with granulocyte colony-stimulating factor enhances mobilization of peripheral blood progenitor cells, increases peripheral blood platelet concentration, and accelerates hematopoietic recovery following high-dose chemotherapy. *Blood* 93:2798, 1999.

212. Nomura S, Dan K, Hotta T, et al: Effects of pegylated recombinant human megakaryocyte growth and development factor in patients with idiopathic thrombocytopenic purpura. *Blood* 100:728, 2002.

213. Vadhan-Raj S, Patel S, Bueso-Ramos C, et al: Importance of predosing of recombinant human thrombopoietin to reduce chemotherapy-induced early thrombocytopenia. *J Clin Oncol* 21:3158, 2003.

214. Li J, Yang C, Xia Y, et al: Thrombocytopenia caused by the development of antibodies to thrombopoietin. *Blood* 98:3241, 2001.

215. Kimura T, Kaburaki H, Tsujino T, et al: A non-peptide compound which can mimic the effect of thrombopoietin via c-Mpl. *FEBS Lett* 428:250, 1998.

216. de Serres M, Yeager RL, Dillberger JE, et al: Pharmacokinetics and hematological effects of the PEGylated thrombopoietin peptide mimetic GW395058 in rats and monkeys after intravenous or subcutaneous administration. *Stem Cells* 17:316, 1999.

217. Broudy VC, Lin NL: AMG531 stimulates megakaryopoiesis *in vitro* by binding to Mpl. *Cytokine* 25:52, 2004.

218. Kaushansky K: Hematopoietic growth factor mimetics. *Ann N Y Acad Sci* 938:131, 2001.

219. Kuter DJ, Bussel JB, Lyons RM, et al: Efficacy of romiplostim in patients with chronic immune thrombocytopenic purpura: A double-blind randomised controlled trial. *Lancet* 371:395, 2008.

220. Bussel JB, Cheng G, Saleh MN, et al: Eltrombopag for the treatment of chronic idiopathic thrombocytopenic purpura. *N Engl J Med* 357:2237, 2007.

221. McHutchison JG, Dusheiko G, Shiffman ML, et al: Eltrombopag for thrombocytopenia in patients with cirrhosis associated with hepatitis C. *N Engl J Med* 357:2227, 2007.

222. Qin P, Dong X, Li J, et al: Recombinant human thrombopoietin and rituximab vs. rituximab monotherapy in corticosteroid resistant primary immune thrombocytopenia: A multicenter randomized controlled study. *American Society of Hematology annual meeting*, abstract 329, 2013.

223. Ghanima W, Geyer JT, Lee CS, et al: Bone marrow fibrosis in 66 immune thrombocytopenia patients treated with thrombopoietin receptor agonists: A single center long-term follow-up. *Haematologica* 99:937, 2014.

CHAPTER 112
PLATELET MORPHOLOGY, BIOCHEMISTRY, AND FUNCTION

Susan S. Smyth, Sidney Whiteheart, Joseph E. Italiano Jr., Paul Bray, and Barry S. Coller

SUMMARY

The approximately 1 trillion platelets that circulate in an adult human are small anucleate cell fragments adapted to adhere to damaged blood vessels, to aggregate with one another, and to facilitate the generation of thrombin. These actions contribute to hemostasis by producing a platelet plug and then reinforcing plug strength by the action of thrombin converting fibrinogen to fibrin strands. To accomplish these tasks, platelets have surface receptors that can bind adhesive glycoproteins; these include the GPIb/IX/V complex, which supports platelet adhesion by binding von Willebrand factor, especially under conditions of high shear, and the $a_{IIb}\beta_3$ (GPIIb/IIIa) receptor, which is platelet-specific and mediates platelet aggregation by binding fibrinogen and/or von Willebrand factor. Other receptors for adhesive glycoproteins (integrin $a_2\beta_1$ [GPIa/IIa], GPVI, and perhaps others for collagen; integrin $a_5\beta_1$ [GPIc*/IIa] for fibronectin; integrin $a_6\beta_1$ [GPIc/IIa] for laminin; and CLEC-2 for podoplanin) also contribute to platelet adhesion, but their precise contributions are less-well defined. Activated platelets express both surface P-selectin, which mediates interactions with leukocytes, and CD40 ligand, which activates a number of proinflammatory cells, and release chemokines and a soluble form of CD40 ligand, thus initiating an inflammatory reaction. Platelet coagulant activity results from the exposure of negatively charged phospholipids on the surface of platelets and the generation of platelet microparticles, along with release and activation of platelet factor V and perhaps exposure of specific receptors for activated coagulation factor. Platelets change shape with activation as a result of a complex reorganization of the platelet membrane skeleton and cytoskeleton. With activation, platelets undergo release of a granules, dense bodies, and lysosomes, the contents of which work to restore vascular integrity. The activation process involves a number of receptors for agonists such as adenosine diphosphate, epinephrine, thrombin, collagen, thromboxane (TX) A_2, vasopressin, serotonin, platelet activating factor, lysophosphatidic acid, sphingosine-1-phosphate, and thrombospondin, as well as several signal transduction pathways, including phosphoinositide metabolism, arachidonic acid release and conversion into TXA_2, and phosphorylation of a number of different target proteins. Increases in intracellular calcium result from, and further contribute to, platelet activation. Platelet activation results in a change in the conformation of the integrin $a_{IIb}\beta_3$ receptor, leading to high affinity ligand binding and platelet aggregation.

Platelets also act as storehouses for a variety of molecules that affect platelet function, inflammation, innate immunity, cell proliferation, vascular tone, fibrinolysis, and wound healing; these agents are actively released upon platelet activation. Other vasoactive and platelet activating substances are newly synthesized when platelets are activated. Through cooperative biochemical interactions, platelets can communicate with, and are affected by, other blood cells and endothelial cells.

Quantitative and qualitative disorders of platelets produce hemorrhagic diatheses (Chaps. 119 to 122). In pathologic states, uncontrolled platelet thrombus formation can lead to vasoocclusion and ischemic tissue necrosis, as, for example, in myocardial infarction and stroke (Chap. 135). Platelets may also facilitate tumor cell growth and metastasis.

Acronyms and Abbreviations: AA, arachidonic acid; ADAM, a disintegrin and metalloprotease; ADMIDAS, adjacent to metal ion-dependent adhesion site; AngII, angiotensin II; APP, amyloid precursor protein; AP3, activator protein 3; BTK, Bruton tyrosine kinase; CIB, calcium and integrin binding protein; CLEC, C-type lectin-like receptor; COX, cyclooxygenase; DAG, diacylglycerol; DTS, dense tubular system; EDTA, ethylenediaminetetraacetic acid; EGF, epidermal growth factor; EMMPRIN, matrix metalloproteinase inducer; ERK, extracellular signal-regulated kinase; FAK, focal adhesion kinase; FOG, friend of GATA; FERM, four point one, ezrin, radixin, and moesin; Gas, growth arrest-specific gene; GP, glycoprotein; GPCR, G-protein–coupled receptor; GPI, glycosylphosphatidylinositol; GSK, glycogen synthase kinase; HDL, high-density lipoprotein; HPETE, hydroxyeicosatetraenoic acid; hTRPC, human canonical transient receptor potential; ICAM, intercellular adhesion molecule; IL, interleukin; IP₃, inositol-1,4,5-trisphosphate; ITAM, immunoreceptor tyrosine-based activation motif; ITIM, immunoreceptor tyrosine-based inhibitory motif; ITSM, immunoreceptor tyrosine-based switch motif; JAM, junctional adhesion molecule; LAMP, lysosome-associated membrane protein; LDL, low-density lipoprotein; LIBS, ligand-induced binding site; LIMBS, ligand-associated metal binding site; LOX, lipoxygenase; LPA, lysophosphatidic acid; LPC, lysophosphatidyl choline; LPS, lipopolysaccharide; LT, leukotriene; LX, lipoxin; MAPK, mitogen-activated protein kinase; MIDAS, metal ion-dependent adhesion site; miRNA, microRNA; MLC, myosin light chain; MMP, matrix metalloproteinase; MRP, myeloid-related protein; MVB, multivesicular body; NAP, neutrophil-activating peptide; NET, neutrophil extracellular trap; NMR, nuclear magnetic resonance; NO, nitric oxide; PAF, platelet-activating factor; PAR, protease-activated receptor; PDGF, platelet-derived growth factor; PDI, protein disulfide isomerase; PDZ, postsynaptic density protein (PSD95), *Drosophila* disk large tumor suppressor (Dlg1), and zonula occludens-1 protein (zo-1); PECAM, platelet-endothelial cell adhesion molecule; PG, prostaglandin; PH, pleckstrin homology; PI, phosphoinositol; PIPK, phosphoinositol phosphate kinase; PIP₂, phosphoinositol 4,5-bisphosphate; PKC, protein kinase C; PL, phospholipase; PNH, paroxysmal nocturnal hemoglobinuria; PPAR, peroxisome proliferator-activated receptors; PSGL, P-selectin glycoprotein ligand; PTB, phosphotyrosine binding; RIAM, Rap1GTP-interacting adapter molecule; SERT, serotonin transporter; SNP, single nucleotide polymorphism; S1P, sphingosine-1-phosphate; SR, scavenger receptor; STIM, stromal interaction molecule; SyMBS, synergy metal binding site; TFPI, tissue factor pathway inhibitor; TGF, transforming growth factor; TLR, toll-like receptor; TLT, TREM-like transcript; TNF, tumor necrosis factor; TP, thromboxane prostanoid receptor; TRAIL, TNF-related apoptosis-inducing ligand; TREM, triggering receptors expressed on myeloid cells; TSP, thrombospondin; TX, thromboxane; VASP, vasodilator-stimulated protein; VEGF, vascular endothelial growth factor; VWF, von Willebrand factor; WASP, Wiskott-Aldrich syndrome protein.

OVERVIEW OF PLATELET ADHESION, AGGREGATION, AND PLATELET THROMBUS FORMATION

The hemostatic system is under elaborate control mechanisms lest the response be either inadequate to meet the hemorrhagic challenge or result in inappropriate thrombosis in response to trivial provocation. Evolutionary pressures have probably favored a more active hemostatic system as individuals with more active hemostatic systems were more likely to avoid death from hemorrhage prior to attaining sexual maturity or in association with childbirth. Our active hemostatic system may be less-well adapted to our modern age, which is characterized by long life spans and progressive vascular disease, given that the deposition of a platelet-fibrin thrombus on a damaged atherosclerotic plaque is the cause of most myocardial infarctions and many strokes.

The platelet's major function is to seal openings in the vascular tree. It is appropriate, therefore, that the initiating signal for platelet deposition and activation is exposure of underlying portions of the blood vessel wall that are normally concealed from circulating platelets by an intact endothelial lining (Fig.112–1).[1] Additional parameters that probably control the platelet response are: (1) the depth of injury, with deeper damage exposing more platelet-reactive materials and tissue factor (Chap. 115); (2) the vascular bed, with the blood vessels serving mucocutaneous tissues especially dependent on platelets for hemostasis, in contrast to the vascular beds in muscles and joints, which rely more on the coagulation mechanism; (3) the age of the individual, because the composition of the blood vessel wall probably changes with age; (4) the hematocrit, because increased numbers of erythrocytes enhance platelet interactions with the blood vessel wall by forcing platelets to the periphery of the bloodstream (as the erythrocytes disproportionately occupy the axial region), by imparting radially directed energy to platelets as the erythrocytes engage in flip-flop motions, and perhaps by releasing the platelet activator adenosine diphosphate (ADP) at sites of vascular injury[2–4]; and (5) the speed of blood flow and the size of the blood vessel, which will determine the number of platelets passing by a single point in a given time interval, the amount of time a platelet has to interact with the blood vessel wall or other platelets, the rate of dilution of platelet activating agents, and the forces tending to pull a platelet from the vessel wall or another platelet (shear rate).[2,4–6] The vasospastic response that accompanies vascular injury, to which platelets contribute by release of thromboxane (TX) A_2 and serotonin, probably plays a key role in decreasing hemorrhage and facilitating platelet and fibrin deposition via its effect on blood flow.

The initial adhesion of platelets occurs to the adhesive proteins within the subendothelial layer immediately subjacent to the endothelium[1,5] or to activated endothelium. The platelet expresses many receptors that participate in adhesive interactions (Table 112–1). Intravital microscopy and *ex vivo* flow chamber studies indicate that discoid platelets that show minimal or no evidence of activation can form the initial layers of platelet aggregates when laminar flow is disrupted by a stenotic lesion, but that stable thrombus development requires the generation and/or release of soluble activators.[6] Membrane tethers, which can undergo restructuring and stabilization, are important in achieving interactions with matrix proteins and other platelets.

The shear rate differentially affects platelet adhesion to surfaces.[3,4,7–12] Shear rates, which reflect the differences in flow velocity

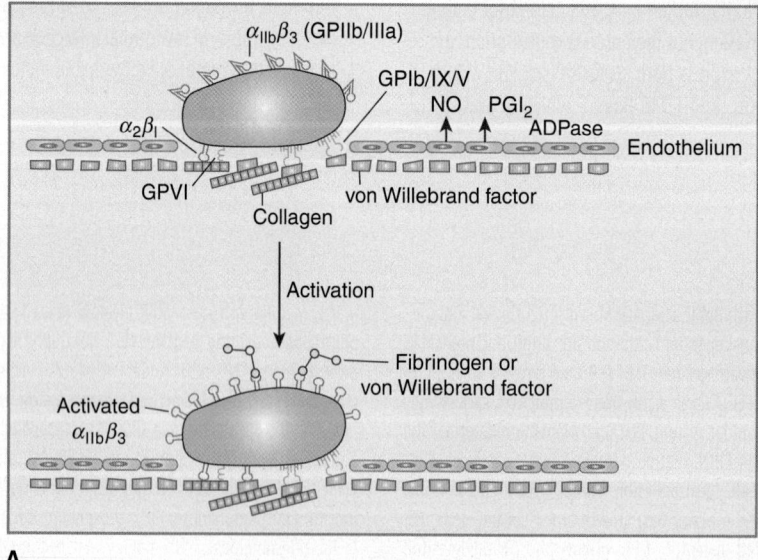

A

Figure 112–1. Platelet adhesion, activation, aggregation, and platelet-leukocyte interactions. **A.** Endothelial cells limit platelet deposition because they separate platelets from the adhesive proteins in the subendothelial area, produce two inhibitors of platelet function (nitric oxide [NO] and prostacyclin [PGI₂]), and contain a potent enzyme (CD39) that can digest adenosine diphosphate (ADP) released from platelets. Platelet adhesion is initiated by loss of endothelial cells (or, in the case of an atherosclerotic lesion, rupture or erosion of the plaque), which exposes adhesive glycoproteins such as collagen and von Willebrand factor (VWF) in the subendothelium. In addition, VWF and perhaps other adhesive glycoproteins in plasma deposit in the damaged area, in part by binding to collagen. Platelets adhere to the subendothelium via receptors that bind to the adhesive glycoproteins. Glycoprotein (GP) Ib binding to VWF plays a prominent role, but integrin $\alpha_2\beta_1$ (GPIa/IIa) and GPVI binding to collagen and other platelet receptors (see Table 112–4) probably helso play a role. After platelets adhere, they undergo an activation process that leads to a conformational change in integrin $\alpha_{IIb}\beta_3$ receptors involving headpiece extension and leg separation (see Fig.112–5), resulting in their ability to bind with high-affinity select multivalent adhesive proteins, most prominently fibrinogen and VWF, including the VWF that binds to collagen in the subendothelial area.

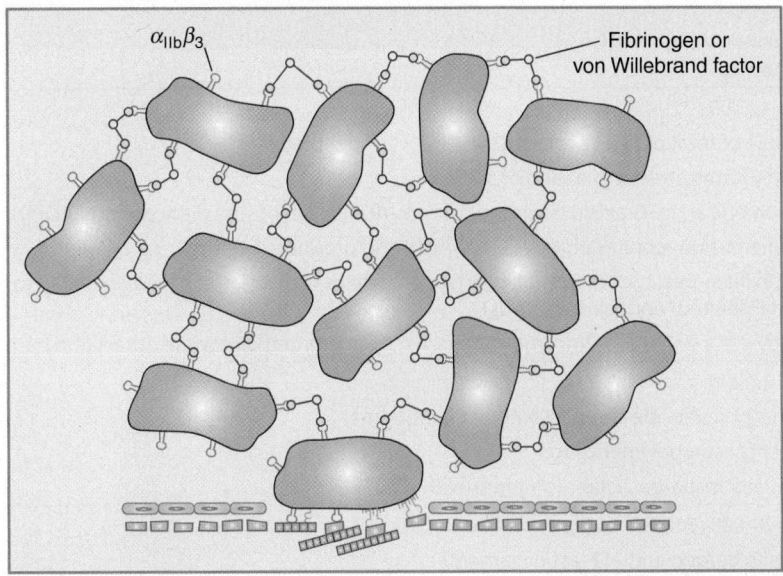

B

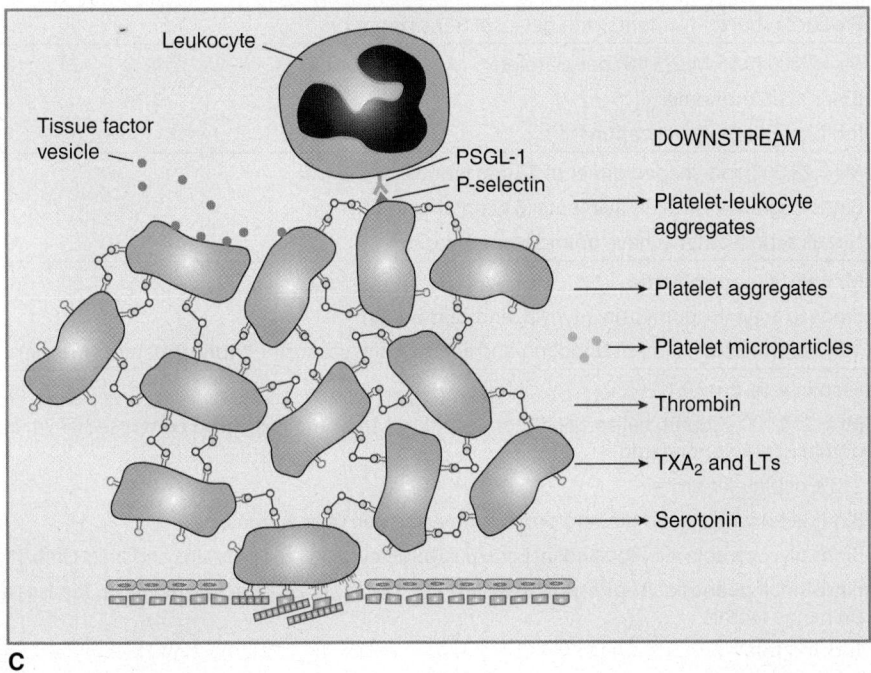

C

Figure 112–1. B. Platelet aggregation occurs when the multivalent adhesive glycoproteins bind simultaneously to integrin $\alpha_{IIb}\beta_3$ receptors on two different platelets, resulting in receptor crosslinking. Clustering of the receptors probably also contributes to the stability of the aggregates (not shown). **C.** After platelets adhere and aggregate, they help to initiate coagulation by binding tissue factor-containing vesicles circulating in the plasma, exposing negatively charged phospholipids on their surface (not shown), releasing platelet factor V (not shown), and releasing procoagulant microparticles. Activated platelets also express P-selectin on their surface, which leads to recruitment of leukocytes via interactions between platelet P-selectin and P-selectin glycoprotein ligand-1 (PSGL-1) expressed on the surface of leukocytes. Other interactions between platelets and leukocytes are detailed in Fig. 112–9. Thrombus formation is a dynamic cyclical process, with platelets repeatedly adhering, aggregating, and then breaking off and embolizing downstream. Platelet–leukocyte aggregates, platelet aggregates, platelet microparticles, thrombin, thromboxane A_2 (TXA$_2$), leukotrienes (LTs), and serotonin probably all go downstream and affect the microvasculature. Ultimately, the vessel either becomes fully occluded or loses its thrombogenic reactivity; that is, it becomes passivated.

as a function of distance from the blood vessel wall, vary considerably throughout the vasculature, being highest in small arterioles and lowest in large arteries and veins; very high rates are observed at the tips of severely stenotic atherosclerotic arteries.[6,11,12] Very high shear rates can cause platelets to aggregate via a mechanism that involves von Willebrand factor (VWF) binding to glycoprotein (GP) Ib/IX followed by intracellular signaling, leading to activation of integrin $\alpha_{IIb}\beta_3$.[13–16] Platelets contribute more significantly to arterial thrombi than to venous thrombi, perhaps as a result of differences in the shear rates in the different beds.[5]

TABLE 112–1. Platelet Cytoskeletal Proteins*

Protein	Properties
Actin[1811]	$Mr = 42,000$
	20–30% of total platelet protein (0.55 M; 2×10^6 per platelet)
	β and γ forms present at a ratio of 5:1
	Monomeric actin (G-actin) bound to calcium-ATP (or adenosine diphosphate [ADP])
	Polymerization requires energy (ATP→ADP) and produces F-actin
	F-actin filaments: two strands of intertwined helices with polarity based on ability to interact with myosin fragment ("pointed" and "barbed" ends)
	Steady-state polymerization: monomers lost from pointed end while others join barbed end ("treadmilling")
Profilin[1812]	$Mr = 15,200$
	Forms 1:1 reversible complex with actin monomer
	Prevents actin polymerization
	May help "recharge" actin monomers with ATP
Gelsolin[1813]	$Mr = 81,000$ (5 μM; 2×10^4 per platelet)
	Binds to barbed end of F-actin filaments
	Severs actin filaments
	Facilitates nucleation
	Produces shorter filaments with gel→sol transformation
Thymosin β_4[267,268]	$Mr = 5000$ (0.55 M; 2×10^6 per platelet)
	Binds actin monomer
	Inhibits actin polymerization
Tropomyosin[1814]	$Mr = 28,000$; rod-shaped dimer of 35-nm length
	Binds to groove on actin filaments (6 actins:1 tropomyosin)
	Not all actin filaments have bound tropomyosin
Caldesmon[1815]	$Mr = 80,000$; asymmetric
	Binds to actin, tropomyosin, myosin, and calmodulin
	May control actin filament bundling and actomyosin adenosine triphosphatase (ATPase)
Filamin A (X) and B (3) (actin-binding protein)[133,154,216,249,1816,1817]	Filamin A-to-B = 10:1
	$Mr = 260,000$ subunit; tail-to-tail dimer; elongated 162-nm flexible rod composed of 24 immunoglobulin-like domains; phosphorylated
	2–3% of platelet protein
	Binds actin with 1 actin binding protein molecule per 14 actin molecules
	Binds glycoprotein (GP) Ibα and integrin β subunit cytoplasmic domains and links GPIb/IX to actin
	Binds small guanosine triphosphatases (GTPases) ralA, ras, rho, Cdc-42, as well as kinases and phosphatases, and exchange factors
	Trio and Toll
	Crosslinks actin filaments to form a gel
	Dephosphorylation leads to loss of activity
Migfilin[142,1818]	$Mr = 50,000$; binds kindling-2 and vasodilator-stimulated protein (VASP)
	Can displace filamin from β_3 cytoplasmic domain, facilitating binding of talin
Talin[142,245,1818–1820]	$Mr = 235,000$
	3% of platelet protein
	Binds to β_3 integrin cytoplasmic tail to activate $\alpha_{IIb}\beta_3$; also binds vinculin and α-actinin; cleaved and activated by calpain
α-Actinin[1812]	$Mr = 100,000$ and 102,000; dimer
	Binds actin at 1:10 stoichiometry; binds Ca^{2+}
	Forms gel with F-actin; cooperates with actin-binding protein; promotes actin polymerization
Vinculin[269,1821,1822]	$Mr = 130,000$
	Binds to talin; may link actin to membrane proteins at adhesion sites

(Continued)

TABLE 112–1. Platelet Cytoskeletal Proteins* (Continued)

Protein	Properties
Myosin II[1823,1824]	$M_r = 480,000$ ($2 \times 200,000$; $2 \times 20,000$; $2 \times 16,000$)
	2–5% of platelet protein; 325×111-nm filaments
	Myosin light chain ($M_r = 20,000$); phosphorylated; required for ATPase activity
Myosin light-chain kinase[1825]	$M_r = 105,000$
	Phosphorylates myosin light chain and activates actomyosin ATPase leading to contraction
Calmodulin[1826]	$M_r = 17,000$
	Binds four calciums and activates myosin light-chain kinase
CapZ[154,216]	$M_r = 36,000$ and $32,000$ ($5\,\mu M$; 2×10^4 per platelet)
	Heterodimer
	Binds barbed ends of actin filaments
Cofilin[154,216]	$M_r = 20,000$
	Accelerates depolymerization of actin filaments
Fimbrin (L-plastin)	$M_r = 68,000$
	Bundles actin filaments
	Found in microvilli
VASP[154,216]	$M_r = 50,000$
	Tetrameric
	Binds profilin, vinculin, zyxin
GTPases[154,229,249]	Cdc42–filopodia
	Rho–stress fibers
	Rac–lamellipods and ruffles
	Rap1b–$\alpha_{IIb}\beta_3$ control
Tyrosine kinases	pp60[src]
	pp125[Fak]–$\alpha_{IIb}\beta_3$ signaling
	pp72[syk]–GPVI signaling
Adaptor proteins	14–3–3ζ–binds to GPIbα
	Pleckstrin–phosphorylated on activation
PI kinases	PI-3 kinase
	PI$_4$P-5 kinase
Spectrin	α,β heterodimers form head to head tetramers
	Bind to actin filaments
α,γ Adducins	Cap barbed ends of actin filaments and bind to spectrin
	Phosphorylated with platelet activation and cleaved by calpain

*See Refs. 216, 249, 261, 266, and 1827.

Platelets also interact directly with exposed collagen, including types I, III, and VI, via GPVI and integrin $\alpha_2\beta_1$ (GPIa/IIa), or perhaps one or more of the many other receptors implicated in platelet-collagen interactions (e.g., CD36 [GPIV], p65).[17–29] The interaction of platelets with collagen is most evident at relatively low shear rates. Depending on the vascular bed, available adhesive glycoproteins, and shear conditions, it is likely that various combinations of platelet receptors, including GPIbα, integrin $\alpha_2\beta_1$ (GPIa/IIa), GPVI, and integrin $\alpha_{IIb}\beta_3$ act in concert to transform the tethering and slow translocation of platelets initiated by GPIbα interacting with VWF into stable platelet adhesion.[1,3,4,8,10,16,25,28]

For platelet plug formation to occur, platelets must undergo activation as well as adhesion. Adhesion of platelets to subendothelial structures, in particular VWF at high shear, may itself lead to platelet activation, including the generation of TXA_2, release of ADP and serotonin, and activation of the integrin $\alpha_{IIb}\beta_3$ receptors on the luminal side of the platelet so that they adopt their high-affinity ligand-binding conformation(s).[10] These positive feedback mechanisms insure an adequate hemostatic response. Depending on the nature of the surface to which they adhere, platelets also undergo variable spreading reactions and become anchored by a process that at least partially involves integrin $\alpha_{IIb}\beta_3$ ligation and clustering, leading to "outside-in" signaling, cytoskeletal reorganization, and tyrosine phosphorylation; these reactions also contribute to initiating the release reaction.[30–36] In addition, platelet activators, such as ADP, are released or synthesized at the site of vascular injury, resulting in a local response. Cooperative biochemical interactions between erythrocytes and platelets may enhance platelet activation.[37]

Activated luminal integrin $\alpha_{IIb}\beta_3$ receptors on adherent platelets bind VWF, fibrinogen, and other adhesive glycoproteins, and await the interaction with another platelet, which itself may have undergone activation of its integrin $\alpha_{IIb}\beta_3$ receptors as a result of exposure to released

ADP and TXA_2. Alternatively, a platelet may become activated and bind VWF or fibrinogen while still circulating, in which case the platelet-ligand complex may bind directly to an activated integrin $\alpha_{IIb}\beta_3$ receptor on the luminal surface. The binding of adhesive ligands to platelet receptors then repeats itself, resulting in the recruitment of additional layers of platelets, and ultimately the formation of a hemostatic plug. Intravital videomicroscopy of the mesenteric and cremasteric circulations of mice after endothelial cell damage demonstrates that, at least in these vascular beds, platelet thrombus formation is initially a very dynamic process, with many platelets depositing but then embolizing.[38] The thrombus grows relatively slowly compared to what its growth would be if all of the platelets that deposited remained attached to the surface.[39–41]

The integrin $\alpha_{IIb}\beta_3$ receptor occupies a central role in determining the extent of platelet aggregation, in part because it is present at an extraordinarily high density on the platelet surface (approximately 50,000 receptors per platelet, such that receptors are probably less than 20 nm apart).[30,42–45] This permits it to rapidly initiate platelet aggregation. On the other hand, the receptor is not in its high-affinity ligand-binding state on resting platelets but rather needs to be activated by agonists, including ADP, serotonin, thrombin, collagen, and TXA_2, that are localized to sites of vascular injury.[34,44,46] As a result, platelets can circulate in plasma containing high concentrations of the integrin $\alpha_{IIb}\beta_3$ ligands fibrinogen and VWF without ongoing platelet thrombus formation. The agonists that activate the integrin $\alpha_{IIb}\beta_3$ receptor are likely to work in combination in vivo. In fact, the mixture of agonists present is likely to change as the process unfolds, with collagen perhaps more important at the beginning, thrombin more important later on, and the other agonists in varying mixtures throughout. The platelet activation effects of multiple agonists may be additive or synergistic, depending on the mechanism(s) involved.[47,48]

A number of mechanisms stabilize platelet aggregates. These include absence of fibrinogen (presumably limiting fibrin formation),[41] leptin,[49–51] CD40 ligand,[52] growth arrest-specific gene 6 product (Gas6) and its receptors (Axl, Sky, and Mer),[53–57] Eph kinases and ephrins,[58] factor XII,[59] plasminogen activator inhibitor-1 and vitronectin,[50] or inhibition of select regions of fibrinogen.[60]

Activated platelets can facilitate thrombin generation by one or more different mechanisms, including recruitment of bloodborne tissue factor, synthesis or activation of tissue factor, formation of procoagulant microvesicles, exposure of activated factor V, exposure of negatively charged phospholipids, and perhaps activation of the contact system. The thrombin thus generated further activates platelets, leading to more extensive degranulation; it also further activates coagulation and initiates the deposition of fibrin strands that reinforce the platelet thrombus and serve as sites for additional VWF deposition.[61] Thrombin also helps to consolidate the plug by initiating platelet-mediated clot retraction (see section "Platelet Shape Change, Spreading, Contraction and Clot Retraction" below). Finally, thrombin affects the surface membrane receptors, down-regulating GPIb/IX and upregulating integrin $\alpha_{IIb}\beta_3$, perhaps facilitating the transition from platelet adhesion to platelet aggregation.[62–65]

Release of vasoactive and mitogenic agents, as well as chemokines, from platelets contributes to the inflammatory response, as does the appearance of P-selectin on the surface of activated platelets and endothelial cells, because P-selectin and other platelet receptors recruit leukocytes to the damaged region.[66–68] Finally, after contributing to hemostasis and initiating an inflammatory response, platelet-fibrin thrombi eventually resolve, most likely by a combination of embolization, fibrinolysis, and macrophage removal of debris.

Several inhibitory factors serve to balance platelet activation and thus prevent excessive platelet deposition. The dilutional effects of flowing blood are probably most important; thus, alterations in the surface of the blood vessel that produce local areas of stasis in which platelets

and coagulation factors may concentrate are prothrombogenic.[2,5] Endothelial cells can synthesize two potent inhibitors of platelet activation, prostacyclin and nitric oxide (Chap. 115).[69–72] Generation of prostacyclin at sites of vascular injury or inflammation may provide a mechanism to limit platelet accumulation. Nitric oxide, which is synthesized by endothelial cells, is a potent inhibitor of ex vivo platelet adhesion and aggregation. Endothelial cells and lymphocytes also have CD39, an ecto-ATP diphosphohydrolase (ecto-ADPase) that can digest ATP and ADP to adenosine monophosphate (AMP), and thus limit the effects of released ADP.[73,74] They also have CD73, which can convert AMP into the platelet inhibitor adenosine.

● PLATELET MORPHOLOGY AND BIOCHEMISTRY

MICROSCOPIC APPEARANCE

On films made from blood anticoagulated with the strong calcium chelating agent ethylenediaminetetraacetic acid (EDTA) and treated with Wright stain, platelets appear as small bluish-gray, oval-to-round shaped cell fragments with several purple-red granules. The mean diameter of platelets varies in different individuals, ranging from approximately 1.5 to 3.0 μm, approximately one-third to one-fourth that of erythrocytes. There is also considerable variability in the size of platelets in a single individual, with occasional platelets in normal blood samples having diameters greater than half the diameter of erythrocytes. Overall, platelet size appears to follow a log normal distribution with an average volume of approximately 7 fL.[75] When unanticoagulated blood is used to prepare blood films, platelets undergo variable activation and spreading, and thus platelet aggregates are commonly seen; platelets from such specimens may demonstrate three or four very long finger-like processes extending out from the body of the platelet (filopodia), and some platelets may be devoid of granules.

Electron microscopy reveals a fuzzy coat (glycocalix) extending 14 to 20 nm from the platelet surface, which is thought to be composed of membrane GPs, glycolipids, mucopolysaccharides, and adsorbed plasma proteins (Fig. 112–2).[76] Platelets move in an electric field as if they have a net negative surface charge; sialic acid residues attached to proteins and lipids are major contributors to this negative charge.[77] The electrostatic repulsion created by the negative surface charge may help prevent resting platelets from attaching to each other or to negatively charged endothelial cells.

Indentations on the platelet surface are thought to be the openings of the open canalicular system, which is an elaborate channel system composed of invaginations of the plasma membrane that extend throughout the platelet (see Fig. 112–2 and "Membrane Systems" below). The contents of platelet granules can gain access to the outside when the granules fuse with either the plasma membrane or any region of the open canalicular system. Similarly, glycoproteins contained within granule membranes can join the plasma membrane after granule fusion with either the plasma membrane or the open canalicular system.

MEMBRANE SYSTEMS

The Plasma Membrane

The plasma membrane is a trilaminar unit composed of a bilayer of phospholipids embedded with cholesterol, glycolipids, and glycoproteins.[76,78] Platelets prepared by the freeze–fracture technique demonstrate more intramembranous particles embedded in the outer platelet membrane leaflet than in the inner leaflet, which is the reverse of findings in erythrocytes; this observation presumably reflects the many external receptors that mediate platelet interactions. The plasma membrane is

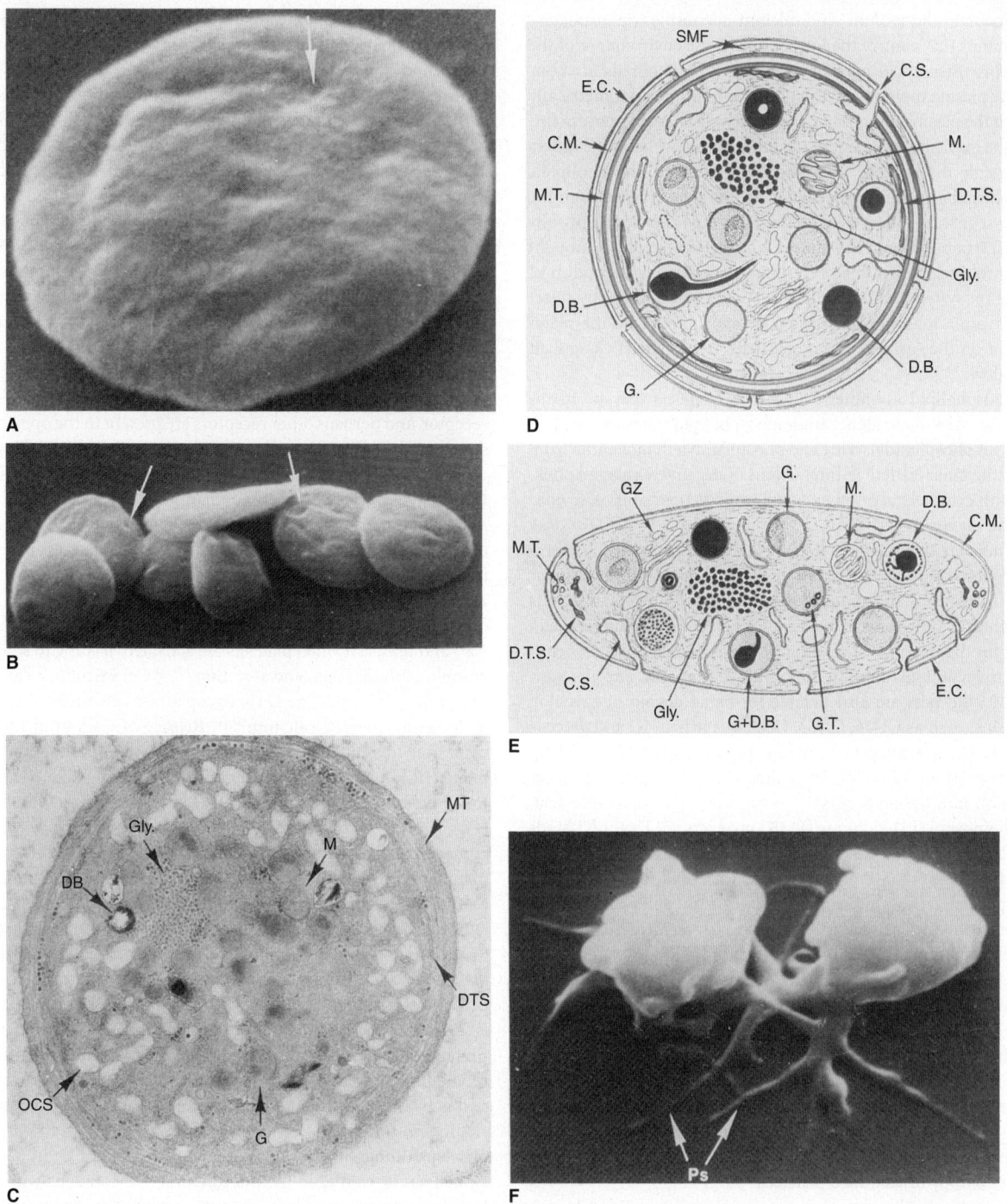

Figure 112–2. A and **B.** Discoid platelets. The lentiform shape of blood platelets is well preserved in samples fixed in glutaraldehyde and critical point dried for study in the scanning electron microscope. The indentations apparent on the otherwise smooth surfaces of the platelets *(arrows)* indicate sites where channels of the open canalicular system (OCS) communicate with the cell exterior. (Magnification: **A,** ×13,200; **B,** ×35,000.) **C, D,** and **E.** Ultrastructural features observed in thin sections of discoid platelets cut in the equatorial plane (**C** and **D**) or cross-section (**E**). Components include the exterior coat *(E.C.)*, trilaminar unit membrane *(CM)*, and submembrane area containing the specialized filaments of the membrane skeleton *(SMF)*. The plasma membrane indentations form the walls of the channels of the surface-connected open canalicular system *(C.S.* and *OCS)*. The circumferential band of microtubules *(M.T.)* is seen as a continuous band beneath the plasma membrane on the equatorial section and as small open cylinders at the ends of the platelet on the cross-section. Glycogen granules *(Gly)* are prominent punctate structures in the cytoplasm, and residual Golgi zones *(GZ)* can also be identified. Organelles include mitochondria *(M.)*, dense bodies *(D.B.)*, and *a* granules *(G.)*, many of which have regions of electron density (nucleoids). The dense tubular system *(D.T.S.)*, the platelet equivalent of the sarcoplasmic reticulum sequesters calcium. (Magnification: **C,** ×30,000.) **F.** Platelet shape change. Platelets exposed to adenosine diphosphate and then fixed and examined by scanning electron microscopy. The platelets lose their discoid shape and become spiny spheres with long extensions, variably referred to as *filopodia* or *pseudopodia*. (Magnification: ×17,000.) *(Reproduced with permission from Bloom AL, et al:* Hemostasis and Thrombosis, *Edinburgh: Churchill Livingstone; 1994.)*

thought to contain the sodium- and calcium-adenosine triphosphatase (ATPase) pumps that control the intracellular ionic environment of the platelet. Approximately 60 percent of platelet phospholipids are contained in the plasma membrane. The phospholipids are asymmetrically organized in the plasma membrane; the negatively charged phospholipids are almost exclusively present in the inner leaflet, whereas the others are more evenly distributed.[79] The negatively charged phospholipids, especially phosphatidylserine, are able to accelerate several steps in the coagulation sequence and so their presence in the inner leaflet of resting platelets, separated from the plasma coagulation factors, is thought to be a control mechanism for preventing inappropriate activation of the coagulation system.[80,81] During platelet activation induced by select agonists, the aminophospholipids may become exposed on the platelet surface or on the surface of microparticles (see "Platelet Coagulant Activity" below).[80-83]

The phospholipid asymmetry in resting platelets may be maintained by an ATP-dependent aminophospholipid translocase that actively moves phosphatidylserine and phosphatidylethanolamine from the outer to the inner leaflet.[80,84] Interactions of negatively charged phospholipids with cytoskeletal or other cytoplasmic elements may also contribute to the asymmetry.[80,81,85,86]

Lipid rafts are dynamic, cholesterol- and sphingolipid-rich membrane microdomains that are important in signaling and intracellular trafficking. In platelets the cholesterol-to-phospholipid molar ratio is twofold higher in rafts than in bulk membranes, with sphingomyelin accounting for the majority of total raft lipids.[87] Platelet lipid rafts contain the marker proteins flotillin 1, flotillin 2, stomatin, and the ganglioside GM_1; the rafts are also notable for being devoid of caveolin. Other proteins, such as CD36, CD63, CD9, integrin $\alpha_{IIb}\beta_3$, and glucose transporter (GLUT)-3, are present in rafts prepared from resting platelets.[87] Upon activation of GPVI, Fc gamma chain, FcγRIIa, and GPIb/IX/V partition into the lipid rafts,[88,89] as do c-Src,[90] phosphatidic acid, and phosphoinositol (PI) 3′-kinase (PI3K) products.[87,91] Factor XI binds to extracellularly-oriented lipid rafts and undergoes activation.[92] The calcium entry channel hTRPc1 is associated with lipid rafts in platelets and, upon platelet activation, contributes to calcium entry that is regulated by the state of intracellular calcium stores (store-mediated calcium entry).[93] The functionally detrimental effects of chilling platelets are thought to be mediated, at least in part, by the temperature-dependent coalescence of platelet lipid rafts.[94]

Open Canalicular System The surface-connected open canalicular system is an elaborate series of conduits that begin as indentations of the plasma membrane and tunnel throughout the interior of the platelet.[76,95,96] Tracer studies demonstrate that the open canalicular system is contiguous with the exterior of the platelet, even though elements of the open canalicular system may appear as closed vesicles or vacuoles by electron microscopy of sectioned platelets.[76,95-97]

The open canalicular system may serve several functions. It provides a mechanism for entry of external elements into the interior of the platelet. It also provides a potential route for the release of granule contents to the outside, eliminating the need for granule fusion with the plasma membrane itself.[97,98] This latter function is especially important because, under most circumstances, platelet granules appear to move to the center of the platelet upon platelet activation rather than to the periphery.[76,95,99] Controversy remains, however, regarding the relative frequency with which secretion occurs via the open canalicular system versus direct fusion with the plasma membrane.[76,95,100]

The open canalicular system also represents an extensive internal store of membrane. Both filopodia formation and platelet spreading after adhesion require a dramatic increase in surface plasma membrane compared to the plasma membrane of resting platelets, and it is not possible for new membrane to be synthesized during the short time-course

of these phenomena. Thus, the membrane of the open canalicular system most likely contributes to the increase in plasma membrane under these conditions; the membranes of α granules, dense bodies, and, to a lesser extent, lysosomes may also contribute, but only if the stimulus is sufficient to induce the fusion of these organelles with the plasma membrane (release reaction). Finally, the membrane of the open canalicular system may serve as a storage site for plasma membrane glycoproteins. For example, under certain conditions, platelet activation by thrombin leads to a consistent, selective loss of GPIb/IX from the platelet surface and data from electron microscopy indicate that the GPIb/IX becomes sequestered in the open canalicular system.[63,64,101] Plasmin may produce a similar phenomenon.[101,102] Platelet activation leads to an increase in surface integrin $\alpha_{IIb}\beta_3$, and although much of this receptor is thought to derive from α-granule membranes, at least some may come from integrin $\alpha_{IIb}\beta_3$ in the membranes of dense bodies and the open canalicular system.[101,103] Similarly, GPVI, the $P2Y_1$ ADP receptor, and the TXA_2 receptor, and perhaps other receptors are present in the open canalicular system and can be recruited to the platelet surface with activation.[104,105]

Dense Tubular System/Sarcoplasmic Reticulum The dense tubular system (DTS) is a closed-channel network of residual endoplasmic reticulum characterized histocytochemically by the presence of peroxidase activity.[76,106-108] The channels of the DTS are less extensive than those of the open canalicular system and tend to cluster in regions in close approximation to the open canalicular system.[76] The DTS is analogous to the sarcoplasmic reticulum of muscle because it can sequester Ca^{2+} and release it when platelets are activated, leading to shape change, granule centralization, and secretion.[109,110] Calreticulin, a calcium binding protein found in the DTS/sarcoplasmic reticulum, probably helps to sequester ionized calcium.[111,112] Release of Ca^{2+} from the DTS/sarcoplasmic reticulum involves the binding of inositol-1,4,5-trisphosphate (IP_3), a messenger molecule formed during signal transduction, to IP_3 type II receptors on the DTS/sarcoplasmic reticulum membrane (Fig. 112–3).[113,114] Cyclic AMP inhibits Ca^{2+} release from the DTS/sarcoplasmic reticulum, either by enhancing the calcium pumping mechanism[115] or by inhibiting release induced by IP_3.[116] NO inhibits Ca^{2+} uptake by the DTS/sarcoplasmic reticulum at high concentrations and stimulates uptake at low concentrations by effects on the calcium ATPase(s) SERCA26 and SERCA3.[117,118] Depletion of intracellular calcium stores activates store-operated calcium entry (SOCE) into platelets (reviewed in Ref. 119). The depletion of Ca^{2+} from the DTS/sarcoplasmic reticulum is sensed by stromal interaction molecule 1 (STIM1), a transmembrane protein with a Ca^{2+} binding motif (EF hand) in the DTS/sarcoplasmic reticulum.[120-122] Loss of Ca^{2+} binding to STIM1 results in translocation and activation of Orai1, a calcium release activated calcium (CRAC) channel in the plasma membrane,[123,124] that allows Ca^{2+} entry into the platelet. Although mice with defects in STIM1 and OraiI have demonstrated abnormalities in platelet function,[120-122] humans with mutations in these proteins have had immune dysfunction, but no overt hemostatic or thrombotic abnormalities.[125-127] The human canonical transient receptor potential 1 (hTRPC1) has also been implicated in regulating platelet SOCE, but mice deficient in this protein do not have a defect in platelet Ca^{2+} entry.[128-130]

The DTS membrane is also probably a major site of prostaglandin and TX synthesis[109,131]; in fact, the peroxidase activity used to identify the DTS is an enzymatic component of prostaglandin synthesis.[131,132]

Cytoskeletal Elements

The discoid shape of the resting platelet is maintained by a well-defined and highly specialized cytoskeleton. This system of molecular struts and girders preserves the shape and integrity of the platelet as it encounters high shear forces in the circulation. The platelet cytoskeleton is operationally defined as proteins that are insoluble in the presence of the

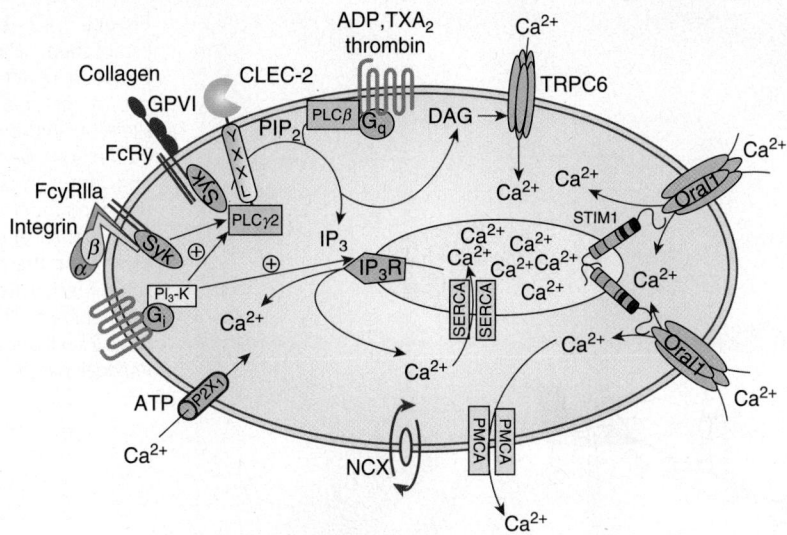

Figure 112–3. Platelet calcium homeostasis. Upon receptor activation different phospholipase (PL) C isoforms hydrolyze phosphatidylinositol-4,5-bisphosphate (PIP$_2$) to inositol-1,4,5-trisphosphate (IP$_3$) and diacylglycerol (DAG). IP$_3$ releases Ca^{2+} from the intracellular stores in the dense tubular system (DTS)/sarcoplasmic reticulum. The transmembrane protein stromal interaction molecule 1 (STIM1) senses the reduction in Ca^{2+} through a decrease in Ca^{2+} occupancy of its EF hand domain, and then opens Orai1 Ca^{2+} channels in the plasma membrane, a process called store-operated calcium entry, whereas DAG mediates calcium entry through canonical transient receptor potential channel 6 (TRPC6). Additionally, a direct receptor-operated calcium (ROC) channel, P2X$_1$, and a Na$^+$/Ca^{2+} exchanger (NCX) contribute to the elevation in Ca^{2+} in the platelet cytoplasm. The counteracting mechanisms to replenish DTS/sarcoplasmic reticulum Ca^{2+} stores involve Ca^{2+} adenosine triphosphatases (ATPases) (SERCAs). Plasma membrane Ca^{2+} ATPases (PMCAs) pump Ca^{2+} through the plasma membrane out of the cell. ADP, adenosine diphosphate; CLEC-2, C-type lectin-like receptor 2; FcRγ, Fc receptor γ chain; FcγRIIa, Fc γ receptor IIa; GPVI, glycoprotein VI; IP$_3$R, IP$_3$-receptor; PI$_3$-K, phosphatidylinositol 3-kinase; Syk, spleen tyrosine kinase. Because of controversies about the localization and role of TRPC1 in the literature, this protein is not depicted in the figure. (*Adapted with permission from Varga-Szabo D, Braun A, Nieswandt B: Calcium signaling in platelets.* J Thromb Haemost 7(7):1057–1066, 2009.)

nonionic detergent Triton X-100 under defined ionic conditions. The three major cytoskeletal elements are the spectrin membrane skeleton, the marginal microtubule coil, and the actin cytoskeleton.

Membrane Skeleton The plasma membrane and open canalicular system of the resting platelet are supported by a highly structured cytoskeletal system (see Figs. 112–2 and 112–4). This two-dimensional network, located just beneath the plasma membrane, has remarkable structural resemblance to its red blood cell counterpart. Thus, both involve the self-assembly of elongated spectrin strands that interconnect through their binding to actin filaments, generating triangular pores. Platelets contain approximately 2000 molecules of spectrin.[133–136] The spectrin network coats the cytoplasmic surfaces of both the plasma membrane and the open canalicular system. In contrast to the erythrocyte membrane skeleton, however, in which spectrin molecules connect on short actin filaments, in platelets, spectrin joins into a network by binding to the ends of actin filaments in close apposition to the plasma membrane. As a result, the spectrin lattice is assembled into a continuous network by its association with actin filaments. Moreover, tropomodulins, which are abundant in erythrocytes, are not expressed at significant levels in platelets and thus are unlikely to play a role in capping the pointed ends of actin filaments. Instead, these ends appear to be free in resting platelets. Finally, the protein adducin is abundantly expressed in platelets and appears to cap the majority of the barbed ends of the filaments making up the resting platelet cytoskeleton.[137] This serves to target them to the spectrin-based membrane skeleton, as the affinity of spectrin for adducin-actin complexes is greater than for either adducin or actin alone.[138–140]

The platelet spectrin-actin filament network is fortified by interactions with filamin A (actin binding protein), a noncovalent dimer of two identical Mr 280,000 protein subunits that fastens GPIb/IX/V complexes to the sides of actin filaments. By interacting with both the transmembrane glycoprotein GPIbα and the actin immediately below the membrane, filamin A connects these components to the spectrin network and the resulting membrane cytoskeleton, probably contributing to the platelet's discoid shape. In addition, the association of GPIbα with the membrane skeleton restricts the expansion of the spectrin network and probably helps to organize receptors into linear arrays on the platelet surface, thus enhancing receptor cooperation (see Fig.112–4).[133] Filamin also binds to the cytoplasmic domains of the β$_3$ subunits of integrin receptors and this keeps the receptor in a low affinity state.[141–143] Other proteins that have been found in the membrane skeleton include talin, vinculin, dystrophin-related protein, molecules implicated in signal transduction, and several isoenzymes of protein kinase C.[133]

Talin has been implicated in controlling integrin α$_{IIb}$β$_3$ activation, by binding to the cytoplasmic domain of integrin β$_3$ when phosphorylated and/or cleaved by calpain (see "Integrin α$_{IIb}$β$_3$" below and Fig. 112–4).[144–148] Migfilin (filamin-binding LIM protein-1) is a 373-amino-acid protein of Mr 50,000 that can displace filamin from the integrin β$_3$ cytoplasmic domain, thus facilitating talin binding and activation. Moreover, joining integrin α$_{IIb}$β$_3$ to the membrane skeleton via an integrin β$_3$ linkage creates the possibility for an actin–myosin contraction process to supply sufficient force to integrin α$_{IIb}$β$_3$ to induce conformational changes in the receptor that result in high affinity ligand binding.[149] The protein vimentin (Mr 58,000), which is an important component of intermediate filaments, is present in platelets and contributes to the membrane cytoskeleton. When platelets are activated, vitronectin–plasminogen activator inhibitor-1 (PAI-1) complexes bind to surface vimentin where they are strategically located to inhibit fibrinolysis.[150] With platelet activation, integrins α$_{IIb}$β$_3$ and α$_2$β$_1$ join the cytoskeleton. Thus, the cytoskeleton may affect whether receptors are free to move in the plane of the membrane; it may also have a role in moving certain receptors from the surface to the interior of platelets and

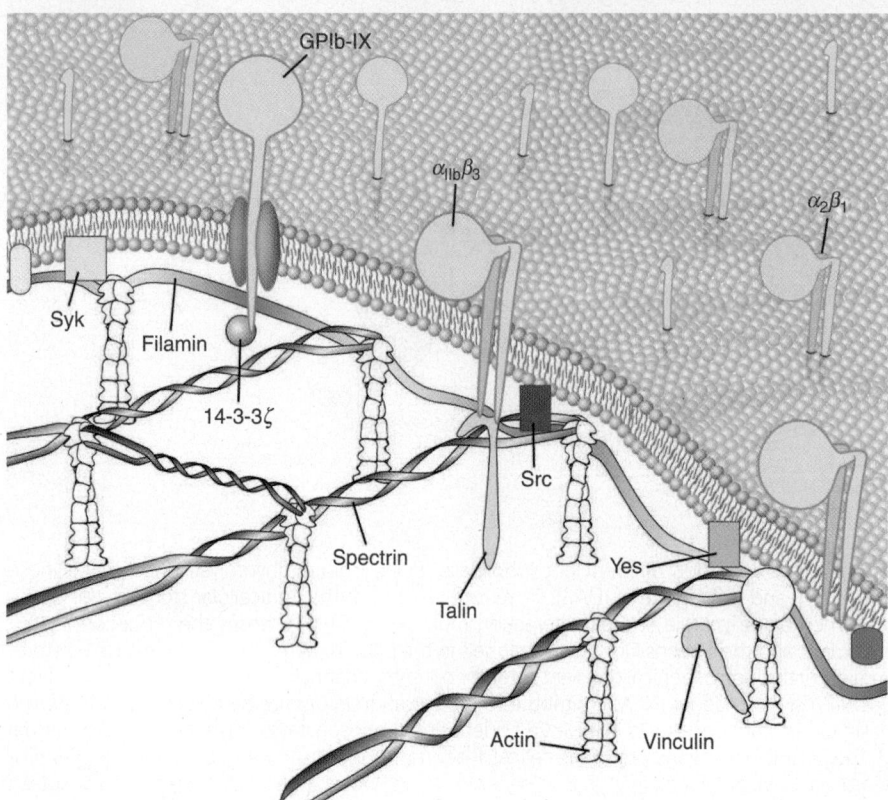

Figure 112–4. Diagrammatic depiction of established and hypothetical connections between select platelet transmembrane glycoproteins and the underlying membrane skeleton. Although evidence exists for direct interactions between IIb 3 with talin and Src and between GPIb with 14–3–3 and filamin, the remainder of the interactions are only hypothetical and are based on the recovery of proteins in the membrane skeleton fraction of solubilized platelets. *(Adapted with permission from Colman RW:* Hemostasis and Thrombosis: Basic Principles and Clinical Practice, *4th edition. Philadelphia, PA: Williams & Wilkins; 2001.)*

vice versa via the open canalicular system.[101,133] The membrane skeleton may also be important in platelet spreading after adhesion.

Microtubules One of the most distinguishing features of the resting platelet is its marginal microtubule coil (see Fig. 112–2). Located below the plasma membrane, it plays an important role in platelet formation from megakaryocytes and maintaining the platelet's discoid shape.[76,151–153] Microtubules are the largest cytoskeletal filaments (25 nm) and are comprised of hollow polarized polymers composed of 13 protofilaments made up of $\alpha\beta$ tubulin dimers (each of Mr 110,000) that associate with several high-molecular-weight proteins (microtubule-associated proteins).[153–155] Motor proteins of the dynein and kinesin families are also associated with microtubules.[156–158] In cells, $\alpha\beta$ tubulin subunits are in dynamic equilibrium with assembled microtubules such that reversible cycles of assembly and disassembly of microtubules are frequently observed.[159] The critical concentration for tubulin polymerization is 5 μM, which is well below the tubulin concentration in platelets (70 μM) and thus 60 percent of platelet tubulin is present as polymer.[154,160] On cross-section, approximately eight to 12 separate hollow structures are observed at the tapered ends of the platelet (see Fig. 112–2). Direct visualization of microtubule assembly in resting mouse platelets indicates that the circumferential coil in platelets is composed of at least 8 actively polymerizing microtubules.[159] Microtubule dynamics allows for necessary changes in platelet shape that occur during the platelet life span and with activation. Tubulin is acetylated in resting platelets and undergoes deacetylation by histone deacetylase (HDAC) 6 with activation in association with the dissolution of the marginal band.[161,162]

Platelets contain four different tubulin isoforms (β_1, β_2, β_4, β_5), but β_1 is dominant and is specific for megakaryocytes and platelets. Targeted gene deletion of β_1 tubulin in mice results in thrombocytopenia and abnormal platelet and microtubule morphology.[153] β_1-Tubulin–deficient platelets are spherical in shape, probably as a result of having defective

marginal bands with fewer (approximately two to three) than normal (approximately eight) microtubule coils.[163] A heterozygous polymorphism of human β_1-tubulin (Q43P) has been described in association with macrothrombocytopenia,[164] but it is probably not causal,[165] and individuals homozygous for the Q43P variant have low platelet counts, abnormal platelet ultrastructure, and decreased tubulin, but normal platelet length, width, and area.[166] A heterozygous β_1-tubulin mutation (R207H) in a strategically located region of the molecule has been reported in association with macrothrombocytopenia as has an F260S[167] mutation and an R318W mutation[165] (Chap. 120).[168]

Actin Filaments Actin is the most abundant of all platelet proteins, with 2 million molecules expressed per platelet (0.5 mM).[169] Like tubulin, actin is in dynamic monomer-polymer equilibrium, with 40 percent of the actin subunits polymerized to form 2000 to 5000 linear actin filaments in resting platelets (Fig. 112–5). The rest of the actin in the platelet cytoplasm is maintained in storage as a 1:1 complex with β_4-thymosin; this stored actin is converted to filaments during platelet activation to drive cell spreading.[170] Thus, actin filaments crisscross the interior of the cell, interconnected at various points into a rigid cytoplasmic network by abundantly expressed actin crosslinking proteins, including filamin and α-actinin.[171–173] Filamin exists in solution as homodimers of subunits that themselves are elongated strands composed primarily of 24 repeats, each approximately 100 amino acids in length, that are folded into immunoglobulin (Ig) G-like β barrels.[174,175] There are three filamin genes and they are located on the X chromosome, chromosome 3, and chromosome 7.[176,177] Filamin A and filamin B are expressed in platelets, with filamin A accounting for approximately 90 percent of total filamin.

Filamin is a prototypical scaffolding protein that attracts binding partners, including the small guanosine triphosphatase (GTPase), RalA, Rac, Rho, and Cdc42,[178] and positions them adjacent to the plasma membrane.[179] Approximately 90 percent of the filamin in resting

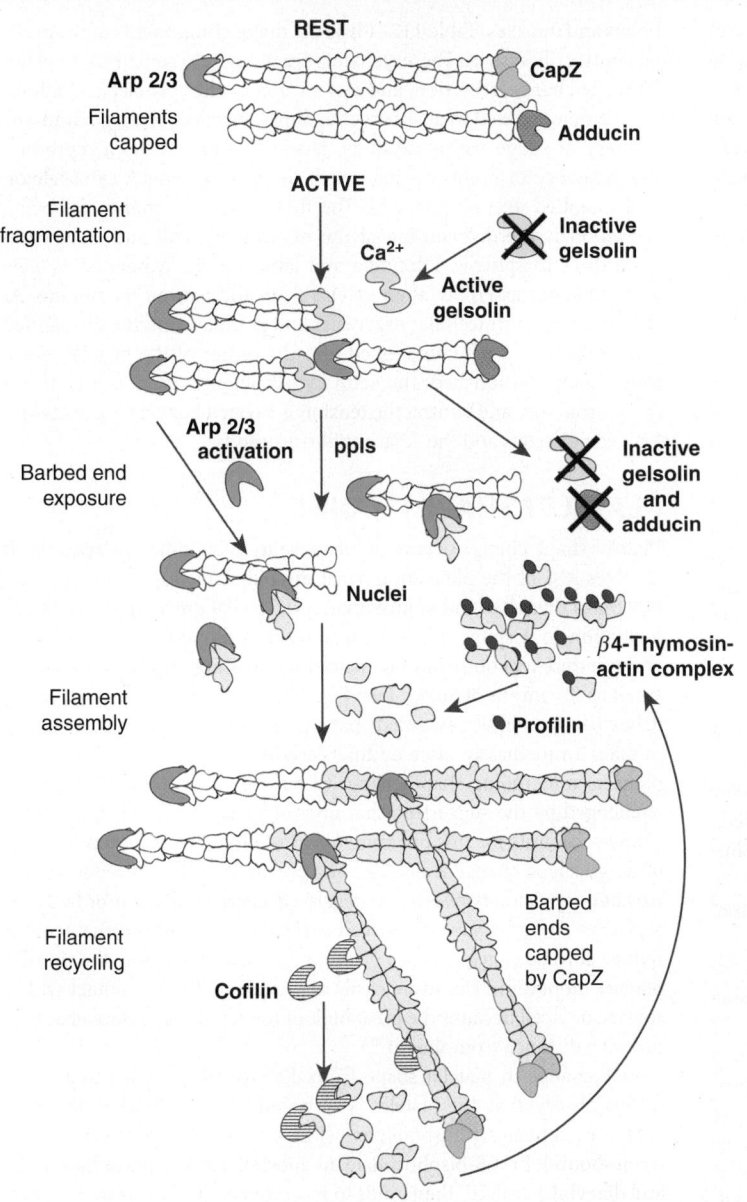

Figure 112–5. Control of platelet actin assembly. *(Rest)* Forty percent of the actin in the resting cell is filamentous. The rest of the actin is soluble (60 percent) and is in a 1:1 complex with β_4-thymosin. Filaments are stable because they are capped on their barbed ends by capZ. *(Active)* Shape change begins when calcium rises into the micromolar level and gelsolin becomes active. Gelsolin binds to actin filaments, interdigitates, and causes filaments to fragment. After fragmentation, gelsolin remains bound to the barbed filament end. Assembly of actin begins when capping proteins are dissociated from the barbed ends of the filament fragments formed in the rounding step by polyphosphoinositides (ppls) and when the actin-related protein (ARP2/3) complex in platelets is activated to nucleate de novo filaments. Actin monomers, stored in complex with β_4-thymosin, are the source of the actin for this polymerization event. Transfer of actin from β_4-thymosin to the barbed ends of actin filaments is facilitated by profilin. Once assembly is complete, capZ recaps the barbed filament ends. *(Adapted with permission from Michelson A: Platelets. 2nd edition. Boston, MA: Academic Press/Elsvevier; 2007.)*

platelets interacts with the cytoplasmic tail of the GPIbα subunit of the GPIb-IX-V complex via a binding site in filamin's second rod domain (repeats 17 to 20).[180,181] This interaction has three consequences. First, it positions filamin's self-association domain and associated partner proteins at the plasma membrane while presenting filamin's actin-binding sites into the cytoplasm. Second, because a large fraction of filamin is also bound to actin, it aligns the GPIb-IX-V complexes into rows on the plasma membrane surface of the platelet over the underlying actin filaments. Third, because the filamin linkages between actin filaments and the GPIb-IX-V complex pass through the pores of the spectrin lattice, it restrains the molecular movement of the spectrin strands in this lattice and holds the lattice in compression. The filamin–GPIbα connection is essential for the formation and release of discoid platelets by megakaryocytes, as platelets lacking this connection are produced in lower numbers and the ones that are produced are abnormally large and fragile. Platelets deficient in GPIb (Bernard-Soulier syndrome; Chap. 120) are very large, perhaps as a result of abnormalities in organizing the cytoskeleton.

PLATELET ENERGY METABOLISM

Platelets have sizable stores of glycogen that can often be seen on electron microscopy (see Fig. 112–2). Glycogen can be broken down into glucose 1-phosphate, and platelets can also take up glucose from their surrounding medium. Platelet glycolysis rates significantly exceed those of erythrocytes and skeletal muscle.[182] Oxidative metabolism probably contributes to energy production in resting platelets, but it has been estimated that less than 1 percent of the pyruvate produced by glycolysis actually enters the citric acid cycle. The remainder is either converted to lactate or remains as pyruvate; both leave the platelet.[183] Platelet mitochondria are capable of oxidation of fatty acids, but its importance to energy production is unclear.[184-187] Platelets can actively metabolize acetate, which has been exploited to improve platelet storage conditions.[185,188] Amino acids may also serve as energy sources and feed into the citric acid cycle, but their contributions are uncertain.

As in all cells, ATP consumption by platelets is partially devoted to maintaining ionic and osmotic homeostasis.[189,190] In addition, the continuous polymerization and depolymerization of actin involves conversion of ATP to ADP, and this may account for as much as 40 percent of the ATP consumption in resting platelets.[191] The continuous polymerization and depolymerization of tubulin that occurs in the coil of resting platelet involves conversion of guanosine triphosphate (GTP) to guanosine diphosphate (GDP), and thus consumes energy.[159] Continuing dephosphorylation and rephosphorylation of phosphatidylinositols, which are important in signal transduction, has been estimated to consume as much as 7 percent of the total ATP produced.[192] Protein phosphorylation also occurs as an ongoing process, but its fractional use of ATP is not clear in resting cells. Platelet stimulation leads to a marked increase in both glycolytic activity and oxidative ATP production, perhaps as a result of the abrupt decrease in ATP that occurs with platelet activation or the increase in cytoplasmic pH.[187] The increased ATP appears to be used, at least in part, for phosphatidylinositide and protein phosphorylation.

Platelet stimulation is accompanied by a marked increase in both glycolytic activity and oxidative ATP production, perhaps through a feedback mechanism in response to the abrupt decrease in ATP that occurs with platelet activation or as a result of the increase in cytoplasmic pH.[193] The increased ATP appears to be utilized, at least in part, in phosphoinositide phosphorylation and protein phosphorylation.

Organelles

Peroxisomes In platelets, some of the main metabolic functions of peroxisomes include fatty acid β-oxidation, plasmalogen (a phospholipid) synthesis, and synthesis of platelet-activating factor (PAF).[194] They contain acyl-CoA:dihydroxyacetone phosphate acyltransferase, which catalyzes the first step in the synthesis of ether-containing phospholipids. Deficiencies of this enzymatic activity have been identified in the cerebrorenal Zellweger syndrome, and the platelet activity can be used to diagnose the disorder.[195,196]

Mitochondria Platelets contain approximately four to seven mitochondria of relatively small size, often located near the plasma membrane; they are involved in oxidative energy metabolism.[197–199] Control of mitochondrial Bcl-2 family proteins, including Bcl-x1 and Bak, directly affects a platelet's life span and alterations in these proteins can produce thrombocytopenia (Chaps. 111 and 117).[200] Release of mitochondria upon platelet activation, either in microparticles or free in the circulation, may contribute to inflammation and nonhemolytic transfusion reactions.[199] Abnormalities of mitochondrial enzymes, including the reduced form of nicotinamide adenine dinucleotide (NADH) coenzyme Q reductase (complex I), have been implicated in the pathophysiology of aging and several neurodegenerative disorders, including Alzheimer disease, schizophrenia, and some forms of Parkinson disease. Assays of platelet mitochondrial enzyme levels have been used in these studies.[201–206] In addition, hyperglycemia-induced mitochondrial superoxide generation may contribute to the enhanced platelet aggregation observed in diabetes.[207] Loss of the mitochondrial inner leaflet potential has been associated with surface expression of platelet procoagulant activity and coated platelet formation (see "Platelet Coagulant Activity" below).[208–211]

● PLATELET SHAPE CHANGE, SPREADING, CONTRACTION, AND CLOT RETRACTION

OVERVIEW

The cytoskeleton establishes the platelets native structure and its ability to respond to stimuli through changes in shape and force generation; as such, the cytoskeleton can be considered analogous to an animal's

bones and muscles. Table 112–1 lists the major components of the platelet contractile system. These elements are thought to contribute to platelet shape change, secretion, and clot retraction after platelet activation.

When exposed to a variety of agonists, platelets undergo dramatic changes in shape within seconds. Shape change follows a reproducible sequence of events during which the resting platelet cytoskeleton is dismantled and reorganized. The first noticeable change following activation is the dismantling of the microtubule coil and conversion from discs to spheres. Filopodia and lamellipodia, generated by new actin filament assembly, then extend from the plasma membrane. At the same time, intracellular organelles and granules, and the dismantled microtubule coil, are compressed into the center of the platelet. Once shape change is finished, the actin cytoskeleton is used as a platform for contraction, and contractile tension is exerted between platelets and between platelets and the adjacent fibrin strands.

PLATELET SHAPE CHANGE

Platelet shape change occurs in response to many different agonists. It involves loss of the platelet's normal discoid shape (approximately 1.5 to 2.5 μm diameter and approximately 0.5 to 0.9 μm width) and transformation to a spiny sphere with long, thin filopodia extending several micrometers out from the platelet and ending in points that are as small as 0.1 μm in diameter (see Fig. 112–2).[95,212] In the aggregometer, it has been generally assumed that the initial decrease in light transmission immediately after adding certain agonists is a reflection of platelets undergoing shape change,[213] but this interpretation has been challenged by the suggestion that microaggregation rather than shape change accounts for this phenomenon.[214] Although the reason platelets undergo shape change is unclear, one possibility is that it reduces electrostatic repulsion between two negatively charged platelets or between a platelet and a negatively charged surface or cell without the need to reduce surface charge density. Thus, after changing shape, the tip of a platelet filopodium can more easily approach and make contact with a surface or a cell because the great bulk of the repulsive surface charge is now at a distance from the tip.[215]

A change in platelet shape from disk to sphere is the first event that is observed as the platelet is activated. Agonist binding to select receptors activates phospholipase (PL) Cβ, which hydrolyzes membrane-bound PI-4,5-bisphosphate to inositol-1,4,5-triphosphate (IP$_3$) and diacylglycerol. IP$_3$ then binds to receptors on the DTS/sarcoplasmic reticulum, generating a rise in cytosolic calcium concentrations to 5 to 10 μM. While calcium can influence the activity of many actin-binding proteins, one of the major proteins that is activated is gelsolin, which is present in platelets at a concentration of approximately 5 μM. Actin filaments in resting platelets are relatively stable because their barbed ends (the end from which they can grow by adding additional actin monomers), are capped with the protein CapZ and α,γ-adducins (see Fig. 112–5). Calcium-activated gelsolin both severs existing actin filaments and caps the newly created barbed ends. This increases the number of actin filaments by an estimated 10-fold, and substitutes gelsolin for CapZ and α,γ-adducins as the actin filament capping protein.[216] Severing of actin filaments that interact with the planar lattice composed of filamin A (actin binding protein), GPIb/IX, and spectrin in the membrane cytoskeleton releases the constraints on the spectrin network. This allows the membrane skeleton to swell (but not produce filopodia) (see Fig. 112–5) by incorporating into the plasma membrane the membranes from the open canalicular system, and later the membranes from the granules that release their contents.

The protrusive force for lamellipodia and filopodia formation comes from new actin polymerization, such that there is a doubling of actin filament content. This burst of actin filament assembly is powered by the generation of barbed-end nucleation sites after receptor activation. These nucleation sites are generated *de novo* by the activation of the Arp2/3 complex or by the exposure of the barbed ends of preexisting filaments.[217] Because barbed ends have a higher affinity for actin molecules than do the actin sequestering proteins, they have the capacity to initiate actin filament polymerization.

Platelets contain two proteins whose main function is to bind and sequester actin monomers. The first is profilin, which is present at a concentration of 50 μM. Profilin can sequester actin monomers from the pointed ends of actin filaments, but not the barbed ends. Profilin also functions as a major transfer factor in actin filament polymerization. The second and more abundant protein involved in sequestration of actin monomers and stimulation of the polymerization of actin is thymosin-β_4. With a platelet concentration of 55 mM, it is equimolar to actin. Thymosin-β_4 binds actin molecules with an affinity that is greater than that of the pointed end of the actin filament, allowing it to compete effectively for molecules from the pointed end. Thymosin-β_4 has a lower affinity for actin monomer than actin has for the barbed end of the filament, resulting in filament assembly when barbed ends are free. Thymosin-β_4 maintains a large pool of unpolymerized actin, and 60 percent of the total actin in the platelet is bound to thymosin-β_4. The affinity of thymosin-β_4 for actin monomer is regulated by the nucleotide that is bound to actin.[218]

The platelet actin assembly reaction that follows the addition of agonists starts when free barbed ends are formed (see Fig. 112–5). Barbed ends are generated by the uncapping of filament ends and the *de novo* assembly of filaments by the Arp 2/3 complex. Platelets contain high concentrations of barbed-end capping proteins that regulate the accessibility of these ends to regulate actin dynamics. Platelets contain 5 μM each of gelsolin[219] and capZ,[220] and 3 mM of adducin.[221] Uncapping of the actin filaments appears to be accomplished by the inactivation of capping proteins by phosphoinositides that are produced during platelet activation, including PI-3,4-bisphosphate ($PI_{3,4}P_2$), $PI_{4,5}P_2$, and $PI_{3,4,5}P_3$.[216] The uncapped actin filaments act as nuclei onto which actin monomers (which are maintained in an available pool by association with thymosin-β_4) can assemble on the barbed ends of the filaments. Profilin accelerates actin polymerization by facilitating the transfer of actin from the actin-thymosin-β_4 complex to the barbed ends of the actin filaments. In addition to exposing new filament ends as a source of nuclei, new nucleation sites are generated by activation by the Arp 2/3 complex. The Arp 2/3 complex mimics the pointed ends of actin filaments and stimulates barbed-end assembly of actin filaments. The Arp 2/3 complex is made up of seven polypeptides, two of which have actin-related sequences, Arp2 and Arp3.[222,223] Platelets contain high concentrations of the Arp2/3 complex (2 to 10 μM). Approximately 30 percent of the Arp2/3 complex is bound to the resting platelet cytoskeleton. Once platelets are activated, the Arp2/3 complex redistributes to the cytoskeleton, increasing three-fold and concentrating in the lamellipodial zone of actin filament assembly. Several signaling pathways regulate the activity of the Arp2/3 complex, including Wiskott-Aldrich syndrome protein (WASP) family members. Mutations in the *WASP* gene result in Wiskott-Aldrich syndrome, an inherited X-linked recessive disorder characterized by thrombocytopenia and T-cell immunodeficiency (see Chap.121).

Simultaneous with these changes, the peripheral microtubule coil becomes constricted and fragmented, and is ultimately compressed into the center of the cell. As the filopodia form, the platelet's granules and organelles move to the center, surrounded by the microtubule coil, resulting in an increase in electron density. Activation of myosin II via phosphorylation of myosin light chain kinase, contributes to the inward contractile force by its interaction with the actin fibers.

PLATELET SPREADING AND SURFACE-INDUCED ACTIVATION

After platelets adhere to surfaces, they undergo variable degrees of spreading and activation. The patterns of spreading and activation depend primarily on the protein surface on which they spread, with collagen consistently inducing the most activation.[224,225] In addition to the nature of the surface, the protein density, especially in the case of fibrinogen, can dramatically affect the signaling systems that are activated in the adherent platelets.[226] Activation can result in release of granule contents and exposure of activated integrin $\alpha_{IIb}\beta_3$ receptors on the luminal surface of the platelets, where they are strategically located to bind adhesive glycoprotein ligands that can recruit additional platelets.[227] If the surface density of platelets is sufficient, the platelets can also enter into lateral associations, which appear to depend on integrin $\alpha_{IIb}\beta_3$.[228] In general, platelet spreading results in the development of broad lamellipodia rather than spike-like filopodia (see Fig. 112–2).[216,229] The different morphologies of platelet spreading reflect differences in the organization of the network of actin filaments. Ultrastructural examination of lamellipodia reveals them to be replete with actin filaments that are organized into orthogonal networks. This organization is established by the actin filament crosslinking protein filamin A. In contrast, filopodia contain long actin filaments that are organized as tight bundles. These structural differences reflect the different signals initiated by the adhesion process, and both PIs and the small GTPase molecules Rac and Cdc42 appear to be particularly important in this process.[154] In platelets, Rac is activated by thrombin receptor ligation and it stimulates actin filament uncapping.[230] Proteins that have been implicated in organizing the tips of the filopodia where the actin bundles attach to the plasma membrane are the small GTPase Cdc42, the exchange protein WASP, vinculin, vasodilator-stimulated protein (VASP), zyxin, and profilin.[111] Pleckstrin, a platelet protein that is phosphorylated during platelet activation, appears to participate in this process by binding to PIs and affecting Rac via an exchange factor.[231,232] Platelets from mice deficient in pleckstrin have a defect in granule secretion, integrin $\alpha_{IIb}\beta_3$ activation, and aggregation mediated by protein kinase C. Thrombin can overcome this abnormality via a pathway involving PI3K.[233] Signaling after adhesion results from the assembly of protein complexes on the cytoplasmic surfaces of the receptor(s) involved in the adhesion process, including focal adhesion kinase (FAK), which is activated by integrin ligation and colocalizes with a number of cytoskeletal proteins. Deletion of FAK in megakaryocytes and platelets results in defects in platelet spreading.[234] These complexes then initiate local cytoskeletal rearrangements as well as the generation of signaling molecules that act throughout the platelet to produce a variety of effects, including the translation of new proteins.[235-238] The nature and extent of the signaling may determine whether the adherent platelets recruit additional platelets or white blood cells. In particular, the conversion of spread platelets to a microvesiculated procoagulant form has been associated with the recruitment of neutrophils.[239] Additionally, spread platelets can assemble fibronectin matrix on their surface, which may be important in stabilizing platelet-platelet interactions.[240]

Membrane glycoproteins are affected by cytoskeletal rearrangements associated with platelet shape change and spreading. Activation of platelets in suspension under certain conditions results in movement of GPIb/IX receptors from the surface of platelets to the open canalicular system.[241,242] With adherent platelets, the GPIb internalization is much slower.[111] The initial effect of activation on integrin $\alpha_{IIb}\beta_3$ is an approximate doubling of these receptors on the plasma membranes, as preassembled receptors in α granules, and perhaps dense bodies and the open canalicular system, join the plasma membrane. Inside-out activation of integrin $\alpha_{IIb}\beta_3$ has been associated with cytoskeletal changes, in particular, the binding of talin to the integrin β_3 cytoplasmic domain.[243-246] Tyrosine kinases, including FAK,[33,247] and Src,[247] may play a role in this process, along with cortactin, a protein of Mr 85 kDa that is phosphorylated on tyrosine, and small GTP binding proteins such as Rho, Rac, and Cdc42.[216,229,248,249] When the attachment of integrin $\alpha_{IIb}\beta_3$ to the cytoskeleton includes actin and myosin, the force produced by the cytoskeleton on the integrin may supply the energy to produce the conformational changes that lead to higher ligand binding affinity.[250] After activation, more integrin $\alpha_{IIb}\beta_3$ molecules become associated with the cytoskeleton, and this presumably reflects the interaction with talin and other cytoskeletal proteins and ligand-induced integrin clustering, resulting in the development of protein complexes, including cytoskeletal proteins, on the cytoplasmic surface of the receptor.[237,245,251] When ligand-coated beads are added to adherent platelets and bind to integrin $\alpha_{IIb}\beta_3$ receptors, the beads are transported to the center of the platelets, indicating that the cytoskeleton can move integrin receptors that have bound ligand.[252,253]

Platelets contain calpains, which are calcium-dependent, sulfhydryl-containing, neutral proteases composed of two subunits that preferentially cleave cytoskeletal proteins, in particular filamins and talin,[229,254] but have also been reported to cleave the cytoplasmic domain of integrin β_3, and a number of molecules involved in signaling, including kinases and phosphatases (see "Calcium-Dependent Proteases [Calpains]" below). μ-Calpain requires micromolar calcium and m-calpain requires millimolar calcium for activation. It has been proposed that calpains are involved in cytoskeletal reorganization upon platelet activation, specifically via cleavage of the integrin β_3 cytoplasmic tail and talin upon ligand engagement.[245,255-257] Calpain cleavage of the integrin β_3 cytoplasmic tail may switch the function of the integrin from promoting platelet spreading to mediating clot retraction.[258] Calpains have also been implicated in platelet spreading, microparticle formation, and the generation of platelet coagulant activity.[229,256,259] Mice lacking μ-calpain have reduced platelet aggregation and clot retraction, but normal bleeding time.[260]

PLATELET CONTRACTION AND CLOT RETRACTION

The contractile mechanism involving actin and myosin is thought to facilitate granule secretion, but the details remain obscure.[261,262] In fact, mice with nearly complete disruption of the platelet heavy-chain myosin gene, *Myh9*, have a defect in secretion, but only in response to low concentrations of select agonists.[263] The cytoskeleton of resting platelets consists of the membrane skeleton described above, which lies just beneath the membrane, and a lacy cytoplasmic actin filament network composed of 2000 to 5000 linear actin polymers, which also contains α-actin, filamins (actin binding proteins) A and B, tropomyosin, vinculin, and caldesmon.[176,177,248,249,264-268] The contractile response is also thought to be initiated by an increase in cytosolic calcium, which results in the formation of a calcium-calmodulin complex that then activates myosin light-chain kinase; phosphatases and cyclic adenosine monophosphate (cAMP) kinase can modulate this response. After the initial platelet shape change, actin becomes organized centrally into thick filamentous masses, where it probably associates with phosphorylated myosin filaments.[269,270] The centralization of organelles within a contractile ring correlates with secretion.[95] There is controversy, however, as to whether platelets secrete their granular contents by fusion with the open canalicular system in the center of the platelet or by direct fusion with the plasma membrane, or both.[95,100]

When blood initially clots *in vitro*, the fibrin mesh extends throughout, trapping virtually all of the serum in a gel-like state. If platelets are present, within minutes to hours, the clot retracts,

extruding a very large fraction of the serum.[271] This process is thought to mimic *in vivo* phenomena that result in consolidation of thrombi and perhaps enhancement of wound healing. Clot retraction has also been implicated in decreasing porosity and solute transport so as to concentrate intrathrombus thrombin,[272] as well as decreasing the efficiency of thrombolysis, which may partially account for the resistance of platelet-rich thrombi to fibrinolytic agents.[273] The platelet requirement for clot retraction is indisputable as is a requirement for integrin $\alpha_{IIb}\beta_3$ and a contractile mechanism involving actin and myosin.[274,275] In fact, nearly complete selective disruption of the myosin *Myh9* gene in murine megakaryocytes gives rise to a phenotype characterized by macrothrombocytopenia; absence of clot retraction; reduced secretion in response to low concentrations of agonists, but not high concentrations; prolonged bleeding time; and protection from thrombus formation.[263] The mice do not, however, spontaneously bleed.[263] Myosin activation involves phosphorylation of the myosin light chain, a process that is governed by calcium-regulated myosin light-chain kinase activity and Rho kinase–regulated myosin phosphatase activity. Calpain-cleavage of the cytoplasmic tail of integrin β_3 may promote RhoA activity and serve a molecular switch to convert platelet spreading to clot retraction.[258] Other signaling molecules appear to contribute to clot retraction, including the Eph kinase EphB2,[276] protein phosphatase 2B,[277] and PI3K.[278] Despite these data, no model describing the details of the clot retraction process has gained acceptance.[279] Proposed mechanisms include movement of platelet filopodia along fibrin strands, tugging of fibrin strands by filopodia, and internalization of fibrin by the action of the membrane skeleton.[274,275,279-282]

Platelet integrin $\alpha_{IIb}\beta_3$ is required for clot retraction, as demonstrated by studies of patients with Glanzmann thrombasthenia (Chap. 121) and studies of normal platelets in the presence of agents that block either the integrin $\alpha_{IIb}\beta_3$ receptor[280,283-288] or the fibrinogen γ-chain C-terminal sequence that mediates interactions with the integrin.[289] It also requires disulfide bond exchange[290] and the tyrosine residues on the integrin β_3 subunit that are phosphorylated upon platelet activation and contribute to outside-in signaling.[291] Clot retraction correlates temporally with an integrin $\alpha_{IIb}\beta_3$-dependent decrease in protein tyrosine phosphorylation, presumably via activation of one or more phosphatases,[292] and may require both integrin-mediated mitogen-activated protein kinase (MAPK) activation[293] and translation of proteins such as Bcl-3, with the latter facilitated by ligand binding to integrin $\alpha_{IIb}\beta_3$.[294] Results with integrin $\alpha_{IIb}\beta_3$ antagonists demonstrate, however, differences in their ability to inhibit clot retraction that do not correlate with their ability to block fibrinogen binding to platelets,[280,287] and patients with Glanzmann thrombasthenia differ in the extent of their defect in clot retraction. Some integrin $\alpha_{IIb}\beta_3$ mutations, such as integrin β_3 L262P, interfere with interactions with fibrinogen but do not prevent interactions with fibrin and clot retraction.[295] Of particular note, fibrinogen lacking the γ-chain C-terminal sequence (amino acids 400 to 411) that mediates binding to platelet integrin $\alpha_{IIb}\beta_3$, as well as the two Arg-Gly-Asp (RGD)-containing regions in fibrinogen, is still capable of supporting clot retraction.[296,297] It is well established that when fibrinogen converts to fibrin, new sites become exposed on the surface of the molecule. Therefore, one possible explanation for this paradox is that additional or alternative integrin binding sequences in the fibrinogen γ-chain (e.g., 316 to 322, 370 to 383, or other regions) may be able to mediate clot retraction.[298,299] Potential binding sites for the γ370 to 381 sequence, which is better expressed on fibrin than fibrinogen, on the integrin α_{IIb} β-propeller region, were identified and peptides from these regions inhibit clot retraction.[300] Factor XIII also plays an important role in clot retraction; it has been proposed to mediate the translocation of the fibrinogen/fibrin–integrin $\alpha_{IIb}\beta_3$ complex to sphingomyelin-rich lipid rafts in the platelet membrane as well as crosslink the complex to cytoskeletal and contractile elements.[301,302] It is also possible that GPIb/IX contributes to clot retraction by virtue of the binding of GPIbα to the thrombin and/or VWF bound to the fibrin.[303,304] Thus, while integrin $\alpha_{IIb}\beta_3$ is required for clot retraction, the process is not a simple reflection of fibrinogen binding to integrin $\alpha_{IIb}\beta_3$.

● PLATELET SECRETORY MACHINERY AND SECRETION

Platelets possess secretory granules and mechanisms for cargo release to amplify responses to stimuli and influence the surrounding environment. Platelet granule structures include α- and dense granules, lysosomes, and peroxisomes.

SECRETORY ORGANELLES

Lysosomes

Lysosomes are produced from the endosomal membrane system through a complex mechanism involving membrane and protein sorting and trafficking.[305] Platelets lysosomes contain acid hydrolases typical of these organelles (e.g., β-glucuronidase, cathepsins, aryl sulfatase, β-hexosaminidase, β-galactosidase, endoglucosidase [heparitinase], β-glycerophosphatase, elastase, and collagenase).[197] With activation, platelets secrete some of these enzymes; however, lysosomal contents are more slowly and less completely released than are those from α granules and dense bodies.[306–308] Thus, stronger agonists are required to induce lysosomal enzyme release than release from the other granules, and their appearance on the platelet plasma membrane serves as a marker of high-level platelet activation.[309,310] The elastase and collagenase activities released from platelet lysosomes may contribute to vascular damage at sites of platelet thrombus formation.[311] The heparitinase may be able to cleave heparin-like molecules from the surface of endothelial cells, and the resulting soluble molecules appear to inhibit growth of smooth muscle cells.[312]

Dense Bodies

Platelets contain approximately three to eight electron-dense organelles, 20 to 30 nm in diameter (see Fig. 112–2).[76,262] The intrinsic electron density of dense bodies when viewed as unstained whole mounts derives from their high content of calcium[76,197]; the granules are also dense when viewed by transmission electron microscopy because they are highly osmophilic.[262] Dense granules contain high concentrations of serotonin, which is taken up from plasma by a plasma membrane carrier and then trapped in the dense bodies.[262] Trapping of serotonin may occur as a result of the lower pH (approximately 6.1) maintained in dense granules as a result of the action of a proton pumping ATPase on the dense-body membrane.[262] ADP and ATP are also highly concentrated in dense bodies.[197] There is more ADP than ATP in the dense bodies (ATP to ADP ratio = 2:3), which is the reverse of their relative concentrations in the cytoplasm (ATP to ADP ratio = 8:1). As there is little connection between the pools of adenine nucleotides in the cytoplasm and the dense bodies, they have been respectively designated as the *metabolic* and *storage pools* of adenine nucleotides.[197] Storage of adenine nucleotides at such a high concentration in dense bodies appears to be achieved by stacking the ATP and ADP purine rings vertically in aggregates that are stabilized by the interactions of calcium ions with the polyphosphate groups.[313,314] The planar hydroxyindole rings of serotonin may also enter these stacks, providing a molecular basis for the trapping mechanism. Trapping of serotonin must differ from that of adenine nucleotides, however, because dense granule serotonin exchanges readily with external serotonin.[197] Transport and delivery of platelet-derived serotonin may play an important role in a variety of

biologic phenomena including vasospasm, platelet coagulant activity, and liver regeneration.[315]

The membrane of dense granules contains glycoproteins that are also found on the plasma membrane and the membranes of α granules and lysosomes, including CD36, LAMP-2, CD63, P-selectin, $\alpha_{IIb}\beta_3$, and GPIb/IX. Abnormalities of eight different genes have been implicated in the Hermansky Pudlak syndrome (HPS) (Chap. 121), an autosomal disorder characterized by a deficiency of dense bodies, and so these genes are presumed to participate in dense body formation. As with lysosomes, dense bodies are thought to derive from endosomes, via different types of multivesicular bodies (MVBs). The eight genes associated with HPS are thought to affect sorting and/or trafficking of membrane structures through participation in protein complexes that mediate these phenomena.[316,317] These complexes include three biogenesis of lysosome-related organelles complexes (BLOCs) and the activator protein 3 (AP3) complex.[305] Similarly, the product of the *LYST* gene, which is abnormal in some patients with Chediak-Higashi syndrome (who also have abnormal dense bodies), has been proposed to associate with the dense granule membrane (Chap. 121).[318] The *LYST* gene product may associate with the AP3 complex.[305]

The abnormalities of *in vitro* platelet function in patients with HPS suggest that released dense granule contents contribute to platelet activation through a positive feedback mechanism. Release of ADP, which is a potent platelet activator, and serotonin, a weaker agonist (see section "Signaling Pathways in Platelets" below), probably account for most of the positive feedback effects on platelet aggregation. ATP is a partial antagonist of ADP-induced activation, but as ATP is rapidly catabolized to ADP in plasma ($T_{1/2}$ = 1.5 min), and ADP is rapidly catabolized to AMP ($T_{1/2}$ = 4 min) and then to adenosine,[197] a platelet inhibitor,[319] it is difficult to predict the overall effect of ATP release. Adding to the complexity *in vivo* is the presence of an ecto-ADPase (CD39; ecto-ADPase) present on endothelial and lymphoid cells, which can metabolize ATP and ADP to AMP and thus probably limits the amount of ADP present.[74] ATP released from platelets may also serve as a high energy phosphate source for platelet ecto-protein kinases, which can phosphorylate several proteins, including CD36 (GPIV).[320–322]

α Granules

An important platelet function is storage and release of a variety of bioactive substances packaged in α granules. α Granules are the most abundant granule type of platelets, numbering approximately 50 to 80 per platelet.[323,324] They are approximately 200 nm in diameter on cross-section and demonstrate internal variation in electron density, often with an eccentric area of accentuated electron density, termed a *nucleoid*, in which β-thromboglobulin, platelet factor 4 (PF4), and proteoglycans are concentrated (see Fig. 112–2).[325] The more electron-lucent areas contain tubular elements in which VWF, multimerin, and factor V are preferentially localized.[76] Proteomic analysis of the releasate of activated human platelets has identified more than 300 proteins, most of which are stored within α granules.[326–328] The list of α-granule proteins includes adhesive proteins, coagulation factors, protease inhibitors, chemokines, and angiogenesis regulatory proteins. Some of the most important proteins present in α granules are described in detail below. Platelets contain distinct subpopulations of α granules that undergo differential release of α-granule cargo during activation. For example, some α granules contain proangiogenic proteins, such as vascular endothelial growth factor (VEGF), whereas others contain antiangiogenic factors, such as endostatin (Fig. 112–6).[329] These two subclasses of α granules can be differentially induced to undergo degranulation by exposure of human platelets to agonists specific for either protease-activated receptor (PAR)-1 or PAR-4. Fibrinogen and VWF are localized

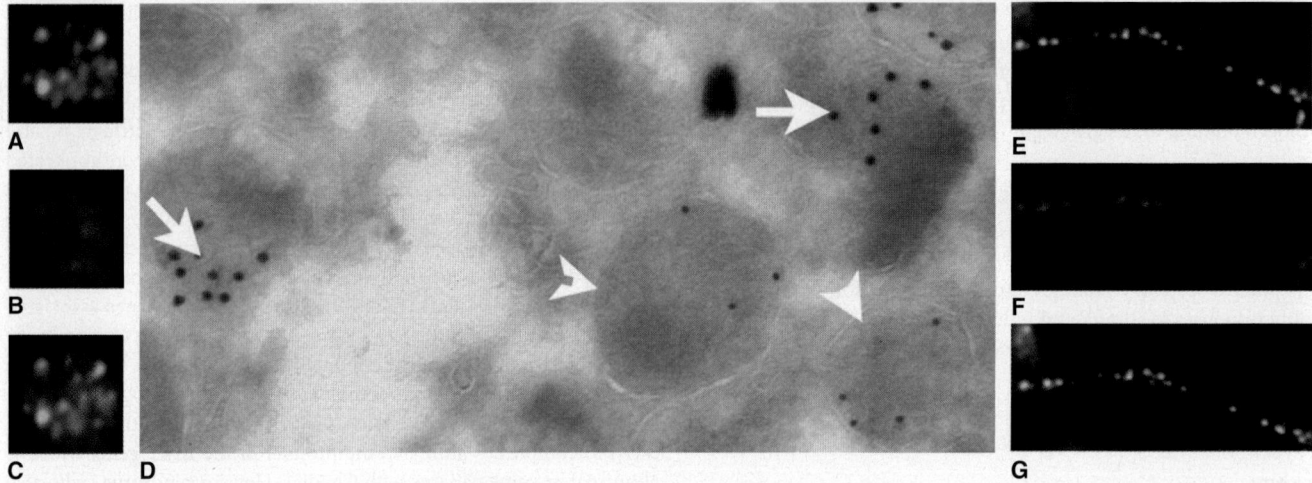

Figure 112–6. Platelets contain separate and distinct α-granule populations. **A, B,** and **C.** Specific pro- and antiangiogenic regulators organize into separate, distinct α granules in resting platelets. Double immunofluorescence microscopy of resting platelets using antibodies against vascular endothelial growth factor (VEGF) **(A)** and endostatin **(B)** and an overlay **(C)**. **D.** Localization of proteins in resting, human platelets using immunoelectron microscopy of ultrathin cryosections. Double immunogold labeling on platelet sections was performed with the use of anti-VEGF antibody and antiendostatin antibodies. Large gold particles representing anti-VEGF staining (15 nm, *arrows*) are evident on one population of α granules and small gold particles (5 nm) representing endostatin staining are abundantly present on a different population of α granules (*arrowheads*). **E, F,** and **G.** Pro- and antiangiogenic regulatory proteins are also segregated into separate, distinct α granules in megakaryocyte proplatelets. Megakaryocytes generate platelets by remodeling their cytoplasm into long proplatelet extensions, which serve as assembly lines for platelet production. Distinct α granules are visualized along proplatelets. Shown is a double immunofluorescence microscopy experiment of proplatelets using antibodies against VEGF **(E)** and endostatin **(F)**, and an overlay **(G)**. *(Reproduced with permission from Italiano, J.E., Jr., et al., Angiogenesis is regulated by a novel mechanism: pro- and antiangiogenic proteins are organized into separate platelet alpha granules and differentially released, Blood 1;111(3):1227–1233, 2008.)*

in separate α granules,[330] and glass activation of platelets results in the selective release of the fibrinogen-containing granules.

The α granule acquires its protein content by both biosynthesis (predominantly at the megakaryocyte level) and endocytosis (at both the megakaryocyte and circulating platelet levels). Small amounts of virtually all plasma proteins are nonspecifically taken up into α granules, and thus the plasma levels of these proteins determines their platelet levels.[331,332] For example, the α-granule pool of immunoglobulins contains most of the platelet immunoglobulin; therefore, total platelet immunoglobulin is more affected by changes in plasma immunoglobulin levels than by changes in surface immunoglobulin.[331,332]

The cell biologic pathways that regulate α-granule assembly are not fully understood, but several studies suggest MVBs play a crucial intermediary role in α-granule biogenesis.[316,333] These membranous sacs, containing numerous small vesicles, develop from budding vesicles in the Golgi complex within megakaryocytes and can interact with endocytic vesicles. They are abundant in immature megakaryocytes and decrease in number with cellular maturation, suggesting that they are the precursors of α granules and/or dense bodies. MVBs may also function as a sorting hub to rout proteins into distinct classes of α granules.

The platelet-specific proteins (PF4 and the β-thromboglobulin family) are present in α granules at concentrations that are approximately 20,000 times higher than their plasma concentrations (when each is expressed as a fraction of total protein in platelets or plasma, respectively).[334,335] These Mr 7000 to 11,000 proteins all bind to heparin, but with varying affinities. They also share amino acid sequence homology with each other and with other members of the "intercrine-cytokine" family of molecules, such as interleukin (IL)-8 (neutrophil-activating peptide 1 [NAP1]), which are active in inflammation, cell growth, and malignant transformation.[336–338]

PF4 is a CXC chemokine (CXCL4) that does not contain the Glu-Leu-Arg (ELR) conserved sequence.[339,340] It binds to heparin with high affinity and can neutralize heparin's anticoagulant activity.[335,341–343]

PF4 tetramers complex with a proteoglycan carrier.[344,345] Specific PF4 lysine residues (amino acids 61, 62, 65, and 66) are implicated in its binding to heparin, and X-ray crystallography indicates that these lysines are on the surface of the PF4 tetramer and interact with negatively charged heparin molecules that wind around this core.[346–348]

After PF4 is released from platelets, it binds to heparin-like molecules on the surface of endothelial cells.[346] Heparin administration can mobilize this endothelial-bound pool of PF4 into the circulation.[346] PF4-heparin complexes and PF4-heparin-like molecule complexes on endothelial cells have been implicated as the target antigens in heparin-induced thrombocytopenia with thrombosis.[349,350] PF4 also binds to hepatocytes, which take it up and catabolize it.[351] PF4 is a weak neutrophil and fibroblast attractant.[340,352] It inhibits angiogenesis, perhaps through inhibition of endothelial cell proliferation.[353] A large number of other activities have been ascribed to PF4, including histamine release from basophils[354]; inhibition of both tumor growth[353] and megakaryocyte maturation[355–357]; reversal of immunosuppression[352,358]; enhancement of fibroblast attachment to substrata[359]; potentiation of platelet aggregation[360]; inhibition of contact activation[361]; and enhancement of both polymorphonuclear leukocyte responsiveness to the activating peptide f-Met-Leu-Phe and monocyte responsiveness to lipopolysaccharide.[362,363]

The β-thromboglobulin family of proteins are CXC chemokines that contain the conserved Glu-Leu-Arg (ELR) sequence.[340] They include platelet basic protein, low-affinity PF4 (connective tissue-activating peptide III [CTAP-III]), β-thromboglobulin, and β-thromboglobulin-F (NAP2, CXCL7).[334,364–366] All of these proteins share the same carboxy terminus but differ in the length of their amino termini, presumably as a result of proteolytic digestion of the parent molecule, platelet basic protein. These proteins bind to heparin but with lower affinity than PF4, and thus neutralize heparin less well. Unlike PF4, they are cleared from the circulation by the kidney rather than the liver.[367] CTAP-III is a weak fibroblast mitogen, and β-thromboglobulin is a chemoattractant for fibroblasts.[340] β-thromboglobulin-F NAP2 (CXCL7) binds to CXCR2 and is chemotactic for granulocytes and activates them to undergo endocytosis.[339,340,366] Platelet α granules also contain additional chemokines that can variably activate leukocytes and platelets.[339]

The biochemistry of the adhesive glycoproteins contained in α granules and others variably present in plasma and extracellular matrix is described in Table 112–2 and in other chapters (e.g., Chaps. 113 and 125 for fibrinogen and Chap.126 for VWF). Their relative concentrations in α granules varies significantly. Their localization in platelet α granules allows them to achieve high local concentrations when released from platelets at the site of vascular injury.

Multimerin comprises a family of disulfide-linked homomultimers, ranging in molecular weight from 450,000 to many millions.[368] The Mr 450,000 multimer is thought to be a trimer of a single subunit of either Mr 167,000[369] or Mr 155,000[368] that is synthesized in megakaryocytes and endothelial cells and stored in the electron-lucent region of α granules in platelets and dense-core granules in endothelial cells.[370] It colocalizes with VWF in platelets, but not endothelial cells. Although multimerin's multimeric structure is similar to that of VWF, the deduced amino acid sequence of its subunit is not homologous to that of VWF.[368] The prepromultimerin subunit contains 1228 amino acids. It undergoes glycosylation and proteolysis during synthesis. It is composed of a number of domains, including an aminoterminal region that includes an RGD sequence, coiled coil sequences, epidermal growth factor (EGF)-like domains, and a carboxyterminal globular head similar to that found in the complement protein C1q. Multimerin binds both factor V and factor Va, and all of the biologically active factor V in platelets is bound to multimerin.[325] With thrombin activation of platelets, factor V separates from multimerin, and the higher molecular weight multimerin multimers bind to platelets. Multimerin does not circulate in plasma at an appreciable concentration, but it may act as an adhesive extracellular matrix protein.

Fibrinogen is concentrated in α granules as judged by the ratio of platelet-to-plasma fibrinogen. Megakaryocytes do not appear to synthesize fibrinogen; instead, it is taken up from plasma by a process that involves the $\alpha_{IIb}\beta_3$ receptor.[371] Because fibrinogen molecules that contain altered sequences in the γ chain are not stored in α granules, even when the molecules are heterodimeric (i.e., contain one normal and one abnormal γ chain), it is possible that uptake requires simultaneous binding of a single fibrinogen molecule to two different $\alpha_{IIb}\beta_3$ receptors via the γ-chain carboxyterminal sequence (see $\alpha_{IIb}\beta_3$ in the section "Platelet Membrane Glycoproteins" below and Chap. 121).[371,372]

The VWF stored in platelet α granules appears to contribute to hemostasis because in certain pathologic states it correlates better with bleeding symptoms than does plasma VWF concentration (Chap. 126). VWF is synthesized in megakaryocytes and endothelial cells. The multimeric structure of platelet VWF is thought to reflect endothelial VWF more nearly than plasma VWF, as higher Mr multimers are present.

Fibronectin is present in α granules, but no clear role in platelet function under normal conditions has been identified for this adhesive protein. Paradoxically, in murine models fibronectin has been reported to both support platelet thrombus formation and inhibit platelet aggregation and thrombus formation[41,373]; the former effect may be mediated by insoluble fibronectin fibrils whereas the latter may be mediated by soluble fibronectin.[374]

Vitronectin, which gets its name from its propensity to bind to glass, also binds to PAI-1, the urokinase receptor (uPAR), collagen, and heparin; it also forms ternary complexes with serine proteases and serpins in the coagulation and complement systems. It is present in platelets at levels that suggest it is concentrated,[375] but it does not appear to be synthesized in megakaryocytes. The binding of PAI-1 with vitronectin stabilizes PAI-1 in its active conformation, and it has been proposed that

only the approximately 5 percent of PAI-1 complexed with vitronectin in platelet α granules is active.[150] Mice deficient in vitronectin have been reported to be protected from, or have a predisposition to develop, thrombosis, depending on the method of inducing thrombosis.[376–378]

Thrombospondin-1 is unique among the adhesive glycoproteins in blood in that it is present almost exclusively inside the platelet.[379–381] It constitutes approximately 20 percent of the released platelet proteins. Thrombospondin-1 is synthesized by megakaryocytes, cultured endothelial cells, and other cultured cells.[382,383] Although integrin $\alpha_{IIb}\beta_3$, GPIb/IX, integrin $\alpha_V\beta_3$, proteoglycans, integrin-associated protein (CD47 or IAP), and CD36 (GPIV) have all been implicated as receptors for thrombospondin,[384–390] CD47 appears to be most important in initiating platelet activation by thrombospondin (see "Signaling Pathways in Platelet Activation and Aggregation" below).[386,387,391] The phosphorylation state of CD36 (GPIV) may affect its ability to bind thrombospondin.[385] Thrombospondin contains an RGD (RGD) sequence, which may contribute to its binding to platelets, but other regions are probably also involved.[381,392] The conformation of thrombospondin varies with the calcium concentration of the surrounding environment. Thrombospondin can interact with many other adhesive glycoproteins, including fibronectin and fibrinogen,[210,393,394] and it is a component of the extracellular matrix.[395] Thrombospondin appears to stabilize platelet aggregates that are formed[396]; it may also act as a negative regulator of angiogenesis, modulate fibrinolysis, and contribute to activation of latent transforming growth factor (TGF)-β_1 released from platelets (see below in this section).[397,398]

Platelets contribute approximately 20 percent of the factor V present in whole blood, with nearly all of it in α granules.[399–401] Human platelet factor V appears to be taken up from plasma rather than being synthesized in megakaryocytes, which is in stark contrast to the situation in mice. When stored in α granules, factor V associates with multimerin.[402,403] Platelet-derived factor V appears to undergo unique posttranslational modifications and proteolytic activation, resulting in resistance to protein C-catalyzed inactivation.[404–406] Evidence from patients with inhibitors and deficiencies of plasma and platelet factor V indicate that platelet-derived factor V has an important role in hemostasis.[399,407,408] Platelets undergo microvesiculation when activated, and the microvesicles, which are rich in factor V, are potent promoters of coagulation.[409]

Protein S (Chap. 114), plasminogen activator-1 (Chap. 135), and α_2-plasmin inhibitor (Chap. 135) are also contained in α granules and can be released from platelets. Similarly, tissue factor pathway inhibitor (TFPI; Chap. 114), α_1-protease inhibitor, and C-1 inhibitor (Chap. 114) have also been identified in α granules.

Gas6 is a 75-kDa vitamin K-dependent protein that contains γ-carboxyglutamic acids and is similar in structure to protein S.[410,411] Gas6 was originally isolated as a growth arrest-specific gene from quiescent fibroblasts, but subsequently was found to enhance platelet aggregation and secretion in response to several agonists.[412] Mice deficient in Gas6 have abnormalities in platelet aggregation and are protected from experimental thrombosis.[412] Gas6 is present in α granules and secreted with platelet activation. Platelets also express Mer, a tyrosine kinase receptor for Gas6, and mice deficient in Mer demonstrate both abnormalities in platelet aggregation and protection from thrombosis, but not to the same extent as mice deficient in Gas6.[413,414] Other Gas6 receptors in the same family as Mer also appear to contribute to platelet thrombus stability.[413–417]

Platelet-derived growth factor (PDGF) is a disulfide-linked dimeric molecule of approximately Mr 30,000 that is mitogenic for smooth muscle cells.[418] Platelet α granules contain a mixture of the homodimer PDGF-BB (30 percent) and the heterodimer PDGF-AB (70 percent); the different forms appear to have different functional activities.[419] PDGF may play a role in normal cell proliferation, as well

TABLE 112–2. Adhesive Glycoproteins

Protein	Subunit, κ Da	Unusual 1° Structural Features & Modifications	Domain Homologies & Binding Regions	Mature Protein Composition	Mature Protein M_r	Known Interactions
Collagens	95–180	Gly-Pro-X repeating sequence Hydroxylysine Hydroxyproline	RGD Right-handed triple helix	Tropocollagen = 3 chains		Variable Thrombospondin
Type I	$a_1(I)$ $a_2(I)$		DGEA† VWFC	$[a_1(I)]_2 a_2(I)$ (major component) $[a_1(I)]_3$		Fibronectin von Willebrand factor
Type III	$a_1(III)$		VWFC	$[a_1(III)]_3$		
Type VI	$a_1(VI)$ $a_2(VI)$ $a_3(VI)$		3 VWFA 3 VWFA 12 VWFA	$a_1(VI)a_2(VI)a_3(VI)$		
von Willebrand factor	220 (2050 amino acids)	Large propeptide (741 amino acids); A, B, C, D, E repeats	$a_{IIb}\beta_3$ – RGD 1789–1791 I Domains GPIb – 230–310	Dimer = protomer Multimers of protomers from 2–~40 via disulfide bonds	880,000– ~20,000,000	Collagen Heparin Factor VIII Fibrin
Fibrinogen	Aα = 63 (625 amino acids) Bβ = 56 (461 amino acids) γ = 47 (427 amino acids)	Alternately spliced γ chains Phosphorylation of Aα	2 RGDs in Aα (95–97 and 572–574) $a_v\beta_3$ – RGD 572–574 $a_{IIb}\beta_3$–C-terminal γ-chain dodecamer (400–411)	2 Aα, 2 Bβ, 2 γ via disulfide bonds	340,000	Thrombospondin ?Collagen Staphylococci Factor XIII Thrombin
Vitronectin	1 chain = 75 (458 amino acids) 2 chain = 65 + 10 via disulfide bonds	Met → Thr polymorphism	RGD Somatomedin B 2 Hemopexin	Same as subunits	75,000 and 65,000+10,000	Glass Plastic Heparin Serine protease: serpin complexes PAI-1 uPAR Factor XIII
Fibronectin	220 (2355 amino acids)	Types I, II, and III repeats Alternately spliced forms	RGD (1493–1495)	Heterodimer via disulfide bonds	440,000	Fibrin Heparin Collagen DNA Staphylococci
Thrombospondin 1	180 (1150 amino acids)		RGD (?functional) VTCG† $a_1(I)$ Collagen Epidermal growth factor Malaria antigen	Trimer via disulfide bonds	450,000	Calcium Plasminogen Collagen Fibrinogen Histidine-rich glycoprotein Fibronectin Laminin Heparin
Osteopontin	32 (298 amino acids)	Phosphorylation Sulfation	RGD			Hydroxyapatite Plaque components
Laminin	A = 400 B_1 = 215 (1765 amino acids) B_2 = 205 (1576 amino acids)		YIGSR† RGD (?functional) EGF	A, B_1, B_2, via disulfide bonds	850,000	Collagen type IV Nidogen/entactin Osteonectin Heparin sulfate C1q Plasminogen Plasmin
Multimerin	155 or 167 kDa	Large prepro-peptide (1228 amino acids)	RGD in N-terminal region EGF		450,000– ~5,000,000	Factor V

EGF, epidermal growth factor; PAI-1, plasminogen activator-1; RDG, arginine-glycine-aspartic acid sequence; uPAR, urine-type plasminogen activator receptor; VWFA, VWFC, von Willebrand factor A and C repeats.

Known Platelet Receptors	Electron Microscopy Structure	Plasma Concentration, mcg/mL	Platelet Concentration,* mcg/mL	Ratio Platelet/ Plasma	Sites of Synthesis
$\alpha_2\beta_1$ (GPIa/IIa; CD49b/ CD29; VLA-2) GPVI GPIV (CD36)?	Tropocollagen = rodlike coil, 15 × 3000; other forms have variable degrees of fibril formation	–	–	–	Fibroblasts
GPIb (CD42b, c) $\alpha_{IIb}\beta_3$ (GPIIb/IIIa; CD41/ CD61)	Elliptical, nodular coil, length 5000, but with some 11,000 Å	10	34	3.4	Endothelial cells Megakaryocytes
$\alpha_{IIb}\beta_3$ (GPIIb/IIIa; CD41/ CD61) $\alpha_V\beta_3$ (CD51/CD61)	Trinodular, asymmetrical; 475 Å diameter	3000	7300	2.4	Hepatocytes
$\alpha_{IIb}\beta_3$ (GPIIb/IIIa; CD41/ CD61) $\alpha_V\beta_3$ (CD51/CD61)		350	800	2.3	?Hepatocytes
$\alpha_5\beta_1$ (GPIc*/IIa (CD49e/ CD29; VLA-5) $\alpha_{IIb}\beta_3$ (GPIIb/IIIa; CD41/ CD61)	Extended antiparallel dimeric structure	300	315	1.1	Hepatocytes Fibroblasts ?Endothelial cells Megakaryocytes Monocytes, etc.
GPIV (CD36) $\alpha_{IIb}\beta_3$ (GPIIb/IIIa; CD41/ CD61)? Integrin associated protein (CD47)	3 Asymmetrical dumbbells, joined near smaller globular domains	0.16	4900	30,625	Megakaryocytes Many cultured cells
$\alpha_V\beta_3$		–	–	–	Bone ?Other cells
$\alpha_6\beta_1$ (GPIc/IIa; CD49/ CD29; VLA-6)	Cross-like structure	–	–	–	Fibroblasts Many other cell types
Unknown	Unknown	–	–	–	Megakaryocytes Endothelial cells

*Assumes 10^{11} platelets per mL of packed platelets.

†DGEA, VTCG, and YIGSR are other amino acid sequences involved in function.

as in the development of atherosclerosis, tumor growth, wound repair, and fibroproliferative responses.[420-422] After it was discovered in platelets and termed PDGF, other tissues were found to produce the same factor; thus, despite its name, PDGF is not exclusively derived from platelets. PDGF is structurally related to the transforming protein p28[sis] of simian sarcoma virus,[423,424] and its receptor is in the tyrosine kinase family.[425] Recombinant human PDGF-BB (becaplermin) is approved as adjunctive therapy to improve healing of foot ulcerations in diabetics.[426]

Platelets contain high concentrations of VEGF, an important stimulator of angiogenesis, and can release VEGF after stimulation *in vitro* and during the hemostatic response to a bleeding time wound.[427-429] Megakaryocytes express mRNA of the three VEGF isoforms (121, 165, and 189 amino acids),[430] and by immunoblot VEGF protein bands of apparent molecular weights 34,000 and 44,000 are identifiable in platelets.[431] Platelets and megakaryocytes also express the gene transcript for the VEGF receptor termed KDR.[432] Another endothelial growth factor structurally related to VEGF, VEGF-C, has also been identified in platelets.[433] Platelet levels of VEGF have been reported to be increased in malignancies, and so elevated levels of platelet VEGF may be a cancer biomarker.[434,435] Platelet VEGF has also been postulated to play in role in tumor growth[436] and proliferative retinopathy in sickle cell disease.[437,438]

EGF has also been identified in platelets, but the kinetics of its release upon thrombin or collagen stimulation differs from that of other granule proteins.[439]

Platelets contain the highest levels of all peripheral tissues of amyloid precursor protein (APP), which contains the sequence for the self-aggregating 40- to 43-amino-acid-residue peptide, Aβ, that has been strongly implicated in the pathogenesis of Alzheimer disease.[440,441] The isoforms containing the Kunitz protease inhibitor domain (APP 770 and APP 751) predominate in platelets. Although synthesized as a membrane protein, platelet APP is cleaved by α-, β-, and γ-secretase activities, producing all of the fragments produced by neurons, as well as the soluble sAPPα, sAPPβ, and Aβ peptides, and the corresponding remaining C-terminal membrane-associated fragments.[440,442,443] Calpain, which is present in platelets, can also cleave platelet APP.[444] Approximately 90 percent of platelet APP is soluble and stored in α granules, but full-length APP surface expression is increased threefold by thrombin stimulation.[445] Platelets are the major source of plasma sAPPs and Aβ.[443,446] APPs released by platelets are potent inhibitors of factor XIa[447] and IXa,[448,449] and also can inhibit platelet aggregation induced by ADP or epinephrine. In contrast, Aβ appears to enhance ADP-induced platelet aggregation and support platelet adhesion. It is possible, but not certain, that plasma Aβ contributes to brain Aβ in Alzheimer disease.[441] Patients with Alzheimer disease have been reported to display altered platelet APP metabolism.[450-455]

Factor XIII is present in the cytoplasm of platelets; it differs from plasma factor XIII in having only the "a" subunits (Chap. 113).[456-459] Platelet factor XIII accounts for approximately 50 percent of total blood factor XIII,[456,457] and platelet factor XIII may contribute to the plasma pool.[460] Upon platelet activation, factor XIII redistributes to the platelet periphery where it associates with the cytoskeleton and crosslinks filamin and vinculin.[461] It may also crosslink thymosin β_4 to fibrin after thrombin stimulation[462] and, in concert with calpain, decrease integrin $\alpha_{IIb}\beta_3$ adhesive function in thrombus formation on collagen.[463] Transglutaminase-mediated conjugation of serotonin to α-granule proteins after platelet stimulation with collagen and thrombin results in the generation of a subpopulation of platelets that are coated with fibrinogen, thrombospondin, factor V, VWF, and fibronectin, either directly through ligand-receptor interactions or through interactions between the serotonin conjugates and platelet surface fibrinogen or thrombospondin (COAT platelets).[464,465]

Platelet α granules contain a high concentration of TGF-β_1, an Mr 25,000 homodimeric protein that promotes the growth of certain cells and inhibits the growth of others.[466-469] For example, TGF-β can increase thrombopoietin production by marrow stromal cells. In turn, thrombopoietin induces both increased megakaryocyte production and megakaryocyte expression of TGF-β receptors. The interaction of TGF-β with these receptors then results in inhibition of megakaryocyte maturation.[470] TGF-β_1 also induces synthesis of extracellular matrix proteins, PAI-1, and metalloproteinases. It has been implicated in wound healing, malignancy, and tissue fibrosis.[471] In addition, TGF-β_1 has been reported to enhance platelet aggregation through a nontranscriptional effect.[472] Migration of endothelial cells is inhibited by TGF-β_1, but it acts as a chemoattractant for monocytes and fibroblasts. TGF-β exists in three isoforms (TGF-β_1, TGF-β_2, and TGF-β_3), but platelets contain only TGF-β_1. TGF-β_1 released from platelets can stimulate smooth muscle cells to express and release VEGF, thus perhaps supporting reendothelialization after vascular injury.[473]

TGF-β_1 released from platelets is inactive (latent) because it is complexed with the remaining portion of its precursor protein (latency-associated peptide [LAP]).[474] LAP, in turn, is covalently coupled to another protein, the latent TGF-β–binding protein-1 (LTBP-1), which localizes the complex to the extracellular matrix.[475] Activation of latent TGF-β_1 is a complex process that is thought to involve a conformational change in LAP that results in altering its ability to shield the active site in TGF-β_1.[475] Activation of latent TGF-β_1 can be achieved by several different mechanisms, including acidification; proteolysis by plasmin, a furin-like enzyme, or other enzymes; traction produced by LTBP-1 binding to extracellular matrix and LAP interaction with integrin $\alpha_V\beta_6$ or $\alpha_V\beta_8$; interaction with thrombospondin-1 or a small peptide derived from thrombospondin-1; or exposure to stirring or shear.[475-479] The interaction of LAP with integrin receptors via its RGD sequence probably plays a dominant role as mice with a mutation in this sequence have a phenotype like that of TGF-β_1 null mice.[480] The ability of thrombospondin-1 to activate TGF-β_1 is of special interest because both TGF-β_1 and thrombospondin-1 are present in α granules. However, data from mice suggest a minor role for platelet thrombospondin in either TGF-β_1 packaging or activation.[481-483] Only a very small percentage of the TGF-β_1 released from platelets with thrombin stimulation becomes activated, but this amount is sufficient to activate synthesis of PAI-1.[479,481,482,484] Based on animals models, TGF-β_1 released from platelets has been implicated in promoting tumor metastases and cardiac fibrosis in response to constriction of the aorta or aortic valve stenosis.[485-487] Active TGF-β can bind to three different cell surface proteins, a proteoglycan (β-glycan), and two serine/threonine kinases.[471,485-488]

Platelets may also release proteins that affect the uptake of oxidized low-density lipoproteins by macrophages, furnishing another potential link between platelet activation and atherosclerosis.[489]

Exosomes

In addition to the contents of α granules, activated platelets release both microparticles (see "Platelet Coagulant Activity" below), which are derived from the plasma membrane, and exosomes, which are internal membrane MVBs.[490] Exosomes are smaller than microparticles (40 to 100 nm vs. 100 to 1000 nm), enriched in CD63 and tetraspanins (see section "Platelet Membrane Glycoproteins" below), and relatively deficient in membrane proteins such as GPIb/IX and platelet-endothelial cell adhesion molecule (PECAM)-1. Unlike microparticles, exosomes are not highly procoagulant as judged by their inability to bind prothrombin or factor X, or to present negatively charged phospholipids on their surface. They may, however, contain NAD(P)H oxidase activity, which has the potential to generate reactive oxygen species that contribute to endothelial cell apoptosis in sepsis.[491]

PLATELET SECRETION

An intricate pathway of protein–protein interactions has been proposed for platelet secretion in which granules tether and dock to the inner leaflet of the plasma membrane, after which fusion of the two opposing lipid bilayers mediates cargo release.[492] Docking and tethering are thought to be, in part, mediated by small GTP-binding proteins of the Rab family. Platelets have been reported to contain at least 11 Rabs, although only a few have been shown to be functionally relevant. Rab27s a and b are important for both granule biogenesis and secretion,[493] while Rab 4 appears to have a role in secretion.[494] The α-granule–associated Rab6 was shown to be phosphorylated upon thrombin stimulation in a protein kinase C (PKC)-dependent manner and phosphorylation seems to increase its GTP-loading.[495]

Platelet granule–plasma membrane fusion is analogous to exocytosis in neurons, where detailed studies have shown the importance of a core set of integral membrane proteins called soluble *N*-ethylmaleimide-sensitive factor (NSF) attachment protein receptors (SNAREs).[496] It is generally accepted that vesicle/granule-target membrane fusion is governed by the binding of a SNARE from the cargo-containing granule or vesicle (v-SNARE), with a heteromeric protein complex in the target membrane (t-SNAREs). The resulting, *trans*-bilayer complex is minimally sufficient for membrane fusion.[497] In human platelets, the v-SNAREs are vesicle-associated membrane protein (VAMP)-2/synaptobrevin, VAMP-3/cellubrevin, VAMP-7/TI-VAMP, and VAMP-8/endobrevin, with the latter being most abundant.[498-502] There are two classes of t-SNAREs: the synaptosome-associated protein (SNAP)-23/25/29 type and the syntaxin type. Human platelets contain syntaxins 2, 4, 7, and 11[498-502] as well as SNAP-23, -25, and -29.[503,504] Functional studies using *in vitro* assays and genetically engineered mice, have established that VAMP-8 is the primary v-SNARE required for secretion from all three classes of platelet granules.[501,502] VAMP-2 or VAMP-3 can also play a role at higher levels of stimulation. As for t-SNAREs, SNAP-23 and syntaxin 2 are required for each secretion event. Syntaxin 4 appears to also play a role, but only in α granule and lysosome release.[505-508]

Although the SNARE proteins are sufficient to mediate membrane fusion, they do so inefficiently and thus require accessory proteins to control where and when they interact. Many of these regulators may be sensitive to second messengers such as diacylglycerol (DAG) and Ca^{2+}, while others are substrates for kinases, such as PKC. The Munc18 family (a, b, and c) control syntaxins and are critical for platelet secretion.[509-511] Studies show that Munc18a and c are phosphorylated by PKC upon platelet activation and that this affects Munc18/syntaxin binding affinity.[510,511] At least two members of the Munc13 family are present in platelets (Munc13–1 and Munc13–4) (Schraw TD, Ren Q, and Whiteheart SW, unpublished data).[512] Munc13–4 appears to be important for dense granule release and functions through its interactions with Rab27.[513,514] Munc13s have Ca^{2+} and DAG binding sites and thus may be regulated by the secondary messengers generated during platelet activation.

Munc13–4 has drawn particular attention based on its involvement in familial hemophagocytic lymphohistiocytosis (FHL) and Griscelli syndrome. Munc13–4 is mutated in type 3 FHL[515] and interacts with the protein mutated in type 2 Griscelli syndrome, namely Rab27a.[516] One feature common to both diseases is the inability of T-cells to properly organize the cytotoxic synapse required for toxin secretion and target cell killing.[515] For FHL patients, it is not clear whether they have bleeding-time defects as they generally receive marrow transplants very early in life.

PLATELET EXOCYTOSIS

Platelet granule–plasma membrane fusion is mechanistically analogous to exocytosis in neurons and other secretory cell types, where detailed studies have demonstrated the importance of a core set of integral membrane proteins called SNAREs.[517,518] It is generally accepted that vesicle/granule-target membrane fusion, and thus granule content release, require the binding of a SNARE from the cargo-containing granule or v-SNARE, with a heteromeric protein complex in the t-SNAREs. The resulting, *trans*-bilayer complex is minimally sufficient for membrane fusion.[519] In human platelets, the detectable v-SNAREs are VAMP-2/synaptobrevin, VAMP-3/cellubrevin, VAMP-4, VAMP-5, VAMP-7/TI-VAMP, and VAMP-8/endobrevin, with VAMP-8 being most abundant.[501,502,520-523] There are two classes of t-SNAREs: the SNAP-23/25/29 type and the syntaxin type. Human platelets contain syntaxins 2, 4, 6, 7, 8, 11, 12, 16, 17, and 18.[501,502,520-524] SNAP-23, -25, and -29 are all detectable, but SNAP-23 is the most abundant.[521,525,526] Functional studies, using *in vitro* assays and genetically altered mice, established that VAMP-8 is the primary v-SNARE required for secretion from all three classes of platelet granules; however, platelets lacking VAMP-8 do release their contents at attenuated rates, suggesting roles for other VAMPs.[502] Differential usage of the VAMPs may allow platelets to fine tune their release of cargo. For t-SNAREs, patients with FHL4, who are deficient in syntaxin 11, show robust platelet secretion defects from all three granule types.[527] Studies of mouse platelets suggest a minor role for syntaxin 8[524] but loss of syntaxin 2 and/or syntaxin 4 had no effect.[527] Syntaxins form a heterodimeric complex with SNAP-23/25–like t-SNAREs. In platelets, SNAP-23 is the critical family member, based on its abundance and results from *in vitro* assays.[505,506,528] SNAP-23 phosphorylation, by IκB kinase (IKK), is important for SNARE complex assembly, membrane fusion, and secretion. Platelet-specific loss of IKK or its pharmacological inhibition leads to bleeding.[529]

Although the SNARE proteins mediate membrane fusion, they do so inefficiently and thus require accessory proteins to control where, when, and how they interact. Many of these regulators are sensitive to second messengers (e.g., calcium). The Sec1/Munc18 (SM) proteins are syntaxin chaperones that control how the t-SNAREs interact with other SNAREs.[510,530-533] Although several isoforms are present, only Munc18b is important for platelet exocytosis.[530,532,534] It chaperones syntaxin 11 and is defective in FHL5 patients. Other SM proteins (e.g. Vps33a/b) are important for granule biogenesis.[535,536] Another syntaxin regulator, tomosyn1/syntaxin binding protein 5 (STXBP5), binds to syntaxin/SNAP-23 heterodimers and affects access to v-SNAREs.[537] Genome-wide association studies (GWAS) suggest that alterations in STXBP5 are linked to venous thrombosis risk resulting from increased plasma VWF.[537-539] Surprisingly, mice lacking STXBP5 have a severe arterial bleeding diathesis as a result of their defective platelet secretion.[537,539]

Munc13 family members contain binding sites for calcium, phosphatidylserine, DAG, and calmodulin.[540] Two major family members, Munc13–2 and Munc13–4, are detectable in platelets, although only Munc13–4 is functionally relevant.[521,541] Munc13s are generally thought to be docking factors that localize granules for membrane fusion. Both FHL3 patients and the Unc13d^{jinx} mouse strain lack Munc13–4 and have robust granule-release defects and bleeding diatheses.[541,542] Munc13–4 binds to a small GTP-binding protein called Rab27, which is also important for platelet exocytosis and is defective in Griscelli syndrome.[543] Another Rab27-binding protein, called synaptotagmin-like protein 4/granuphilin, is also reported to be important for platelet exocytosis.[544]

Three types of FHL are caused by defects in genes encoding proteins that are important in platelet secretion: Munc13–4/FHL3, syntaxin 11/FHL4, and Munc18b/FHL5. Rab27a is defective in a related disease, Griscelli syndrome. One feature common to both diseases is the inability of T cells to properly organize the cytotoxic synapse required for toxin secretion and target cell killing. This suggests that these T-cell populations and platelets share common secretory machinery elements. For FHL patients, it is unclear whether bleeding or defective platelet function can be used as diagnostic criteria, but they have been reported as symptoms.[545]

PLATELET GENOMICS, THE PLATELET TRANSCRIPTOME, AND PLATELET PROTEOMICS

PLATELET GENOMICS

The *Homo sapiens* genome is comprised of approximately 3.2 billion base pairs and has approximately 3.5 million single nucleotide polymorphisms (SNPs) that occur at frequencies of 1 percent or greater, but continued sequencing of more genomes indicates there are at least an additional 43 million rare or "private" SNPs. dbSNP (www.ncbi.nlm.nih.gov/projects/SNP) maintains information about sequence variation, allele frequencies, differences in frequencies between populations of different ethnicity and their functional consequences. New technologies, such as next-generation sequencing, and new analytic methodologies have driven and continue to drive expansion of genomics at a very rapid pace. Both epidemiologic and experimental approaches have been and are used to assess significance and functionality of platelet gene variants and gene expression, including genetic epidemiology, biochemistry, cell biology, physiology, and animal studies.

GENE VARIANTS ASSOCIATED WITH DISEASE

Candidate Genes

Because platelets play a central role in acute ischemic syndromes, antiplatelet therapy is a mainstay of therapy. Platelets may also contribute to the pathophysiology of the chronic process of atherosclerosis,[546] although the data are less consistent than with thrombosis. The earliest platelet genetic association studies considered associations between atherothrombotic disease outcomes and candidate platelet gene variants that altered amino acids in platelet membrane adhesion receptors. Numerous studies reported associations between myocardial infarction and stroke with SNPs in integrin β_3 *(ITGB3)*, integrin α_2 *(ITGA2)*, and GPIbα *(GP1BA)* and GPVI *(GP6)*.[547] In these relatively small studies, positive associations were more likely to be observed in patients with acute thrombosis and less likely in patients with stable atherosclerosis.

However, there were inconsistent and conflicting results in these candidate studies.

Genome-Wide Associations Studies

No unbiased GWAS has been performed using documented arterial thrombosis as the clinical phenotype, but many have been performed with coronary artery disease (CAD). Multiple studies have demonstrated that the Chr9p21.3 locus is associated with both myocardial infarction (MI) and CAD. A meta-analysis of all CAD GWAS studies that included 63,746 patients with acute and chronic CAD and 130,681 controls identified 46 loci meeting genome-wide significance.[548] These loci explain less than 11 percent of CAD heritability and although a substantial proportion of the identified genes regulate lipid metabolism and inflammation, most loci are not located in previously well-known or well-characterized platelet genes. Few of these loci have been tested for functional effects in platelets. There are numerous possible explanations for the non-association with well-studied platelet candidate genes, including small platelet gene effect sizes in under-powered heterogeneous clinical phenotypes.[549]

Whole-Exome Sequencing

Whole exome-sequencing is well-suited to identify variants in protein-coding genes and was used to identify *NBEAL2* as the causative gene in the gray platelet syndrome.[550,551]

Pharmacogenetics

The *CYP2C19*2* allele (681G>A; rs4244285) causes a loss of function of the CYP2C19 enzyme and reduced platelet inhibition by clopidogrel as a result of decreased conversion to the active metabolite.[552] It could account for approximately 12 percent of the variation in platelet inhibition in response to clopidogrel.[553] Several large meta-analyses have shown the loss-of-function *CYP2C19*2* allele is associated with both stent thrombosis and cardiovascular ischemic events or death in patients undergoing percutaneous coronary interventions.[554,555]

GENE VARIANTS ASSOCIATED WITH PLATELET TRAITS

Many cellular pathways in multiple tissues contribute to the pathogenic processes resulting in an atherothrombotic event (Fig. 112–7),

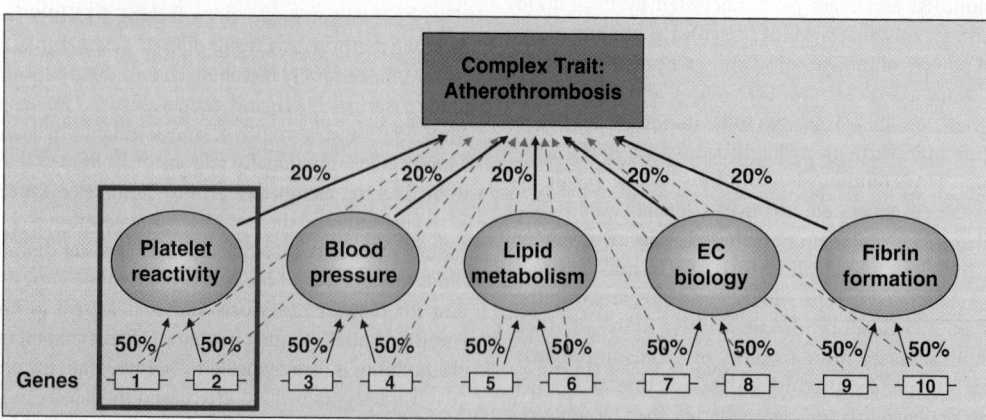

Figure 112–7. Intermediate phenotypes in association studies. Atherothrombosis is a complex phenotype that is regulated by many intermediate traits, of which platelet reactivity is only one. Because a large number of genes contribute to multiple traits, the effect of any one gene on atherothrombotic events, such as myocardial infarction, is small. This highly simplified diagram assumes five traits each contribute 20 percent to the complex trait *(heavy solid arrows)* and two different genes equally regulate each intermediate trait. Thus, each gene contributes 50 percent to the intermediate trait *(thin arrows)*, but only 10 percent to the clinical end point *(faint dashed arrows)*. Thus, for any given sample size, there is more power to detect genetic associations with intermediate phenotypes than with complex traits. *(Reproduced with permission from Bray PF: Platelet genomics beats the catch-22. Blood 13;114(7):1286–1287, 2009.)*

increasing the "noise" in genetic epidemiology studies testing for associations with complex phenotypes. The use of intermediate phenotypes as outcomes in genetic association studies has enhanced power to detect gene associations because the number of genes potentially responsible for the phenotype is reduced, thereby increasing the fraction of the variance explained by any single factor or gene. Despite large interindividual variability in platelet reactivity, light transmission aggregometry has been shown to be reproducible and heritable, with the reproducibility persisting for years.[556,557]

Candidate Functional Platelet Genes

The Leu33Pro variant of integrin β_3 (rs5918 of *ITGB3*) is responsible for human platelet alloantigen 1a/b (Pl[A1]/Pl[A2]).[558] Fibrinogen and prothrombin binding is enhanced to the Pro[33] isoform of purified integrin $\alpha_{IIb}\beta_3$.[559] Compared to cell lines expressing Leu33 variant of integrin, Pro33 cells have increased adhesion, spreading, actin cytoskeletal reorganization and migration under static[560,561] and shear conditions.[562] This prothrombotic phenotype of Pro33 is mediated by *enhanced outside-in platelet signaling* through integrin $\alpha_{IIb}\beta_3$.[563,564] Notably, this variant does *not* affect inside-out signaling, as assessed by standard platelet light transmission aggregometry of human platelets.[565] Additional support for the prothrombotic nature of the Pro33 variant of integrin β_3 comes from mice made homozygous for Pro33. These animals have reduced bleeding, increased *in vivo* thrombosis and enhanced outside-in integrin $\alpha_{IIb}\beta_3$ signaling, but normal inside-out signaling.[566]

Laboratory evidence for functional effects of genetic variants in the gene encoding GPIbβ has been inconsistent. Variants in the two platelet collagen receptors, GPVI and integrin α_2 subunit (of integrin $\alpha_2\beta_1$) alter receptor expression and adhesion to collagen using *in vitro* perfusion assays.[567–569] Functional variants in the genes encoding FcγRIIA (*FCGR2A*), P2Y$_{12}$ (*P2RY12*), GPIV (*CD36*), and PAR-1 (*F2R*) have also been reported.

Associations between SNPs in 97 hematopoietic cell genes were tested and 17 novel associations with platelet responses to crosslinked collagen-related peptide (CRP) and ADP were identified, including genes encoding cell surface receptors (*CD36, GP6, ITGA2, PEAR1,* and *P2Y12*), kinases (*JAK2, MAP2K2, MAP2K4,* and *MAPK14*), and other signaling molecules (*GNAZ, VAV3, ITPR1,* and *FCERG1*).[570] Variants at the Chr9p21.3 locus are associated with the platelet aggregation response to low (0.5 mcg/mL) but not higher concentrations of collagen in a large cohort with two replication studies.[571]

Genome-Wide Association Studies

The first GWAS reported for platelet reactivity tested association of 2.5 million SNPs with platelet aggregation responses to ADP, collagen, and epinephrine.[565] The primary cohorts were generally healthy, European-ancestry populations from the Framingham Heart Study (FHS) (n = 2753) and the GeneSTAR cohorts (n = 1238). SNPs at seven loci (*PEAR1, MRVI1, SHH, ADRA2A, PIK3CG, JMJD1C,* and *GP6*) met genome-wide statistical significance and were replicated in an African-ancestry cohort (n = 840). A second platelet function GWAS identified SNPs in *SVIL* (encodes supervillin) as associated with closure time in the *in vitro* platelet function analyzer PFA-100.[572] Human platelet gene expression studies and data with *Svil −/−* mice demonstrated an inhibitory role for supervillin in platelet adhesion and thrombus formation under high-shear but not low-shear conditions. A meta-analysis by the HaemGen consortium of 66,867 individuals identified 43 and 25 loci associated with platelet number and mean platelet volume (MPV), respectively.[573] These loci accounted for 4.8 percent of the phenotypic variance in platelet number and 9.9 percent in MPV and included well-known platelet regulators (*ITGA2B, GP1BA,* and *F2R*). These investigators identified

11 of the genes as novel regulators of blood cell formation using gene silencing in *Danio rerio* and *Drosophila melanogaster*.

● PLATELET GENE EXPRESSION

TRANSCRIPTOMICS

The *Homo sapiens* genome includes approximately 21,000 protein-coding genes (genome build GRCh38). To date, more than 10 times this number of protein-coding transcripts have been identified, primarily as a result of alternate exon splicing, and more are being continually discovered. Platelets from healthy subjects contain approximately 2.20 femtograms (fg) of total RNA per cell, which is approximately 1000-fold less than nucleated blood cells. Platelets can splice pre-mRNA into mature mRNA, which is translated into proteins.[574,575] Characterization of the transcriptome enables quantitative assessment of gene expression in the tissue of interest and identification of alternately spliced transcripts. Genome-wide transcriptome studies have enabled dissection of the molecular basis of inherited platelet disorders and a better understanding of the relationship between gene expression and megakaryocyte and platelet differentiation. In addition, platelet RNA profiles may have utility as biomarkers.[576]

Technologic advances have greatly facilitated understanding the platelet transcriptome. Early studies using serial analysis of gene expression and microarrays estimated approximately 6000 mRNAs in the human platelet.[577,578] Platelet RNA-sequencing (RNA-seq) has demonstrated an unexpected complexity to the transcriptome and substantive differences between the human and mouse platelet transcriptome.[579] The exquisite sensitivity of RNA-seq provided estimates of approximately 9,000 protein-coding genes in platelets (Fig. 112–8),[580,581] although only approximately 7800 are commonly expressed[582] in human platelets. Approximately half of the transcripts in platelets encode mitochondrial genes.[581] Platelet mitochondrial mRNAs are inversely correlated with subject age,[582] and mitochondrial function may regulate platelet apoptosis[583] and support optimal platelet function during storage,[584] but platelet mitochondria diseases have not been described. The S-shaped curves in Fig. 112–8 illustrate several features of the human platelet transcriptome: (1) estimates of expressed protein-coding genes are more similar amongst different subjects for high abundance genes (leftwards in Fig. 112–8) and (2) there is substantial interindividual variation in total transcript estimates when considering the less abundant genes (rightward in Fig. 112–9). Furthermore, it is not known what is the biologically relevant copy number of transcripts in any cell, and the arbitrary choice of "threshold" could dramatically affect the number of reported genes expressed in platelets. Transcriptomes of *primary* megakaryocytes have not been determined, but RNA profiling of megakaryocytes derived from cultured CD34+ hematopoietic stem cells has identified transcripts that are differentially expressed upon differentiation and between normal subjects and patients with essential thrombocytosis (ET).[585,586]

Platelet mRNAs Associated with Disease

Platelet mRNA profiling in patients with acute ST-segment-elevation MI and stable CAD demonstrated that *S100A9* (myeloid-related protein-14 [MRP-14]) was expressed at higher levels in patients than controls.[587] This discovery was validated in the Women's Health Study and PROVE IT-TIMI 22 trials.[587,588] Platelet mRNA expression profiling can distinguish essential thrombocythemia (ET) patients from healthy subjects[589] and levels of *HIST1H1A, SRP72, C20orf103,* and *CRYM* can predict JAK2 V617F–negative ET in 87 percent of patients.[590] mRNA expression profiling identified reduced *MYL9* transcripts in platelets of

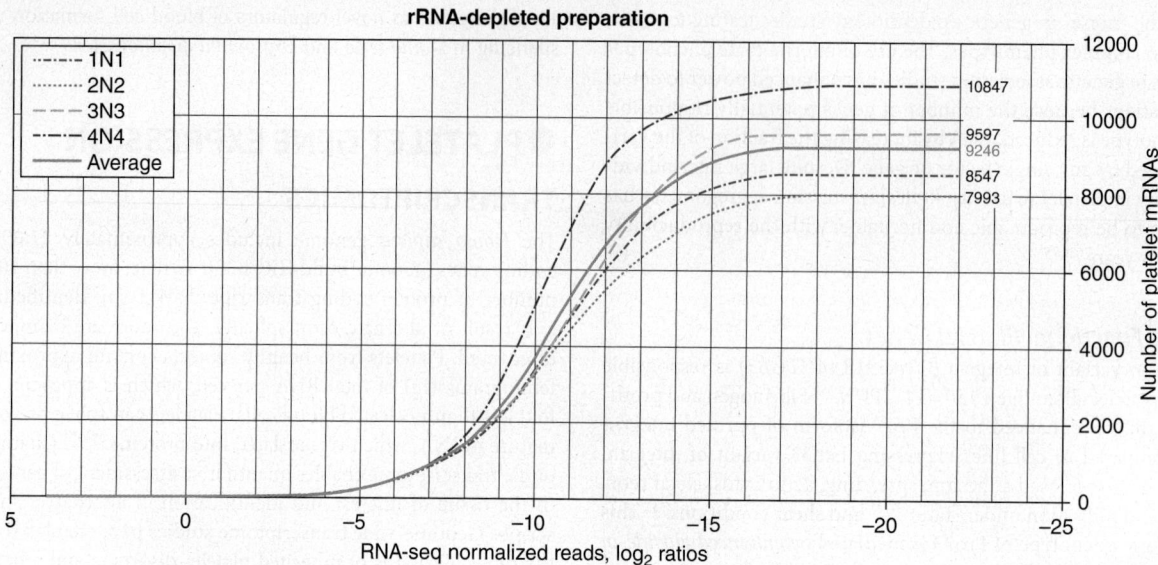

Figure 112–8. Estimates of platelet expressed mRNAs. Platelet total RNA was extracted from four normal donors, depleted of ribosomal RNA (rRNA) and subjected to RNA-seq. The number of platelet-expressed mRNAs *(y axis)* was plotted against RNA-seq read number in log2 ratios normalized to β-actin. *(Reproduced with permission from Bray, P.F., et al: The complex transcriptional landscape of the anucleate human platelet. BMC Genomics 16;14:1, 2013.)*

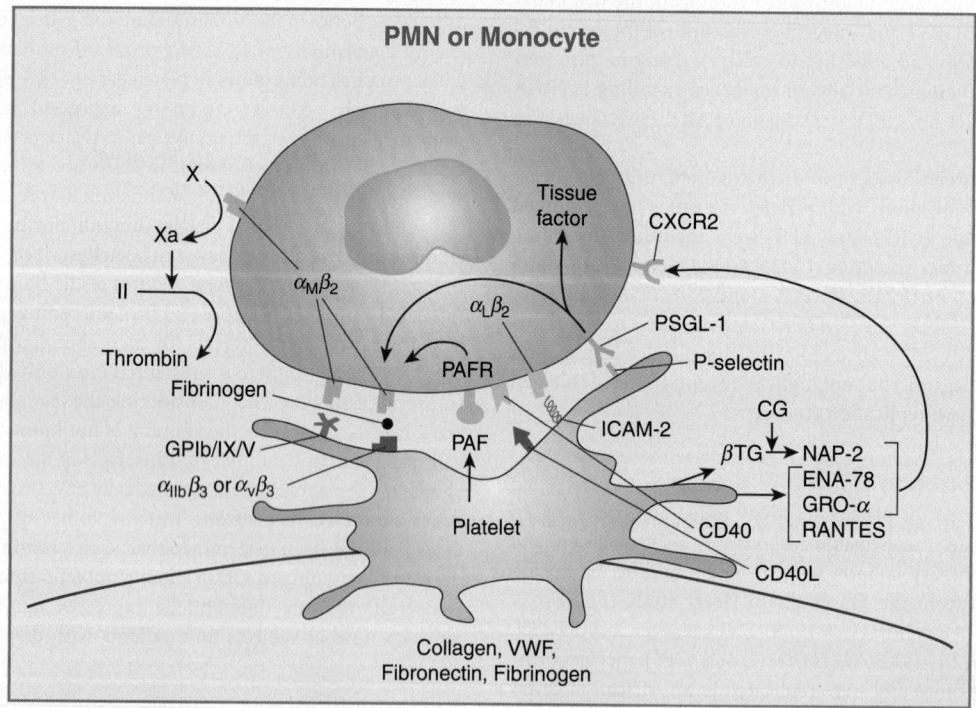

Figure 112–9. Platelet–leukocyte interactions. A number of interactions can occur between platelets and leukocytes, including neutrophils and monocytes. The interaction between platelet P-selectin and leukocyte P-selectin glycoprotein ligand-1 (PSGL-1) probably is the most important initial interaction (and can lead to tissue factor synthesis by monocytes), but fibrinogen binding simultaneously to activated $\alpha_M\beta_2$ on leukocytes and either $\alpha_{IIb}\beta_3$ or $\alpha_v\beta_3$ on platelets may play a role under certain circumstances. Platelets can release platelet-activating factor (PAF), which can interact with a PAF receptor (PAFR) on leukocytes, leading to $\alpha_M\beta_2$ activation and binding of fibrinogen and factor X. Leukocyte $\alpha_M\beta_2$ can also interact with platelet junctional adhesion molecule-3 (JAM-3) or GPIb. Platelets can release chemokines (e.g., ENA-78, GRO-α, and RANTES [regulated upon activation, normal T-cell expressed and secreted]), and β-thromboglobulin (βTG) released by platelets can be converted by leukocyte cathepsin G (CG) into the potent chemotactic CXC chemokine NAP-2. Some of the chemokines, in turn, activate leukocytes by binding to the chemokine receptor CXCR2. Platelets also contain the potent immune-stimulating molecule CD40 ligand (CD40L), and both express it on the platelet surface and release it into the circulation upon platelet activation. The interaction between thrombospondin and CD36 molecules on both platelets and some leukocytes and the presence of CD40 on platelets are not shown. VWF, von Willebrand factor.

a patient with an inherited platelet defect.[591] Platelet RNA-seq was also used to identify *NBEAL2* as causing the gray platelet syndrome.[592]

Platelet mRNAs Associated with Platelet Traits

An unbiased genome-wide platelet RNA expression study identified an association between expression of *PEAR1* with and platelet activation.[593] A similar approach identified 290 differentially expressed transcripts between hyperreactive *versus* hyporeactive platelets.[594] mRNA and protein levels of VAMP-8, a critical v-SNARE involved in platelet granule secretion, were significantly higher in hyperreactive platelets. Another study identified 63 genes differentially expressed according to platelet activation by ADP and/or CRP.[595] Two of these genes, *COMMD7* and *LRRFIP1*, were associated with early-onset MI.[595] The Platelet RNA and Expression-1 (PRAX1) study phenotyped platelet function and performed genome-wide platelet RNA expression profiling on 70 black and 84 white subjects.[596] PAR4-mediated platelet aggregation and calcium mobilization were greater in black subjects than white subjects. A novel platelet gene encoding phosphatidylcholine transfer protein (PC-TP) showed a strong correlation with race and with PAR-4 reactivity and a PC-TP–specific inhibitor blocked PAR-4– but not PAR-1–mediated platelet aggregation. This finding underscores the genetic basis for interindividual variation in platelet function and the potential need to consider race and genetic factors when treating patients with anti-platelet therapies.

Platelet Noncoding RNAs

The best studied of the noncoding RNAs are microRNAs (miRNAs), which regulate expression of more than 60 percent of protein coding genes.[597,598] Human platelets express approximately 200 annotated miRNAs, some of which are differentially expressed according to platelet reactivity and may predict platelet responsiveness to activation,[599] and some of which are differentially expressed by age, gender, and race.[582,596] Indirect evidence indicates strong correlations between megakaryocyte and platelet miRNA levels.[600] *miR-155* maintains megakaryocyte progenitors in an undifferentiated state,[601] whereas *miR-150* and *miR-125b-2* drive megakaryocyte differentiation.[602,603] Loss of expression of *miR-145* in the 5q– syndrome leads to an increase in the megakaryocyte Fli-1 transcription factor, thus enhancing megakaryocyte production.[604]

Platelet miRNA profiles are more stable than mRNA profiles and are useful as biomarkers.[576] Levels of *miR-26b* and *miR-28* are associated with myeloproliferative neoplasms,[605,606] whereas levels of *miR-10a*, *miR-148a*, and *miR-490–5p* discriminate ET from secondary thrombocytosis.[607] Specific sets of platelet miRNAs have associated with MI.[608,609] Antiplatelet therapies alter platelet miRNA levels.[610,611] Relationships between platelet miRNAs, mRNAs, and physiology in the same subjects permit prediction of miRNA function and discovery of novel platelet genes.[599] This approach identified *PRKAR2B* as associated with platelet reactivity, and a functional effect was confirmed in murine platelets lacking *Prkar2b*.[599] A similar approach was used to demonstrate platelet *miR-376c* levels were higher in white subjects compared to black subjects and these levels correlated with *PCTP* mRNA, PC-TP protein and platelet PAR-4 reactivity.[596] *miR-376c* directly targets the *PCTP* 3′UTR and represses its expression.[596]

PROTEOMICS

Disease pathophysiology is dictated by the effects of proteins, including their levels, structures and posttranslational modifications. Cataloging platelet proteomes in health and disease and under different activation states provides information not achievable from genomics or transcriptomics, including protein isoforms, localization, stoichiometry, and posttranslational modifications. Early proteome-wide studies of platelet

lysates utilized two-dimensional gel electrophoresis (2D-GE).[612] However, technologic advances using nongel approaches with proteolytic peptide analyses have largely replaced 2D-GE, and include surface-enhanced laser desorption/ionization (SELDI), isotope-coded affinity tags (iCAT), and isotope tags for relative and absolute quantification (iTRAQ).[613,614] These improved technologies have provided an estimate of approximately 20 million protein molecules per platelet and have updated estimates of the number of detectable different proteins in the platelet proteome to nearly 5000.[615] Pathway and gene ontology analyses reveal most highly expressed platelet proteins localize to the cytoplasm, with substantial percentages in the membrane or secretome,[616] and fall into expected functional categories of cytoskeletal rearrangement, membrane trafficking, and intracellular signal transduction.[615]

Platelet protein levels are regulated by mRNA translation in megakaryocytes and platelets, uptake of plasma proteins, and protein degradation,[574,617] although the relative contribution of each mechanism to the platelet proteome in health and disease is unknown. The dynamic nature of the platelet proteome is illustrated by alterations with disease, aging, gender, and other environmental factors,[616] as well as differential sorting of proteins between megakaryocytes and platelets.[618] Infectious agents, such as dengue virus, stimulate blood platelet mRNA translation into protein.[619] Posttranslational modifications of platelet proteins, such as phosphorylation, have critical effects on platelet activation. Platelets from healthy individuals exhibit marked interindividual variation in function,[556] and unbiased genome-wide approaches have identified variation in proteins regulating the corresponding function.[594] Components of protein ubiquitination and degradation have been identified in platelets, but their function is poorly understood.

Cataloging the Platelet Proteome

Most platelet proteomic analyses to date have studied platelets from small numbers of healthy donors. Analyses of resting whole platelets have provided global protein profiles.[612,620] Fractionation of platelet lysates has been used to assess the α granule,[621] dense granule,[622] and membrane proteomes.[623,624] Proteins with posttranslational modifications have been identified for phosphorylation,[625,626] palmitoylation,[627] and glycosylation.[628] After platelet activation, hundreds of proteins have been identified in releasates (secretomes)[629,630] and microparticles.[631,632]

Platelet Proteome Association Studies

Platelet proteome-wide analyses were used to identify *NBEAL2* as the gene responsible for the gray platelet syndrome[551] and to unravel the molecular basis of the Quebec platelet disorder.[633] Differentially expressed platelet proteins involved in integrin $\alpha_{IIb}\beta_3$ signaling were observed in the myelodysplastic syndrome.[634] Proteomic approaches have consistently identified platelet septin and actin as increasing over time in storage.[635–637] A small study suggested platelet protein posttranslational modifications may be associated with acute coronary syndromes.[638]

Relationship Between Platelet Proteome and Transcriptome

Transcriptomic approaches have identified about twice as many genes expressed in platelets as have proteomic approaches, primarily because the former has greater sensitivity. Correlations between 10 platelet RNA-seqs and the most quantitatively robust proteomic analyses to date has been reported.[639] Most (87.8 percent) proteins had a detectable corresponding mRNA and the relative abundances showed a significantly positive, albeit weak, correlation. Platelet proteins that lack a corresponding mRNA are likely to be taken up from plasma rather than being synthesized in megakaryocytes, and include fibrinogen, albumin, and immunoglobulins, all of which were suspected to fall into this category based on other studies.[640] Platelet mRNAs that lack a corresponding protein may be vestigial from the megakaryocyte. Some of these could be translated subsequently by the platelet under physiologic demands. Combining "multiomic" data with phenotyping can provide important insights as demonstrated by a study in which transcriptomic and proteomic analysis identified six platelet transcripts associated with aspirin resistance.[641] The expression of these genes was associated with death or MI. In addition, platelet phenotyping and genome-wide genotyping and platelet mRNA and miRNA profiling led to the identification of novel protein-coding and noncoding transcripts associated with platelet activation.[596]

PLATELET COAGULANT ACTIVITY

In resting platelets, negatively charged phospholipids, including phosphatidyl serine (PS) and phosphatidylethanolamine (PE), are almost exclusively present in the inner leaflet of the cell membrane and phosphatidylcholine predominates in the outer leaflet. This asymmetry is maintained by ATP-dependent "flippase" transporters, which restrict PS to the inner membrane surface and "floppases," which promote outward-directed lipid transport.[84,85,642,643] When platelets are activated by strong agonists, negatively charged phospholipids redistribute to the outer leaflet of the platelet plasma membrane. This involves a putative calcium-dependent "scramblase" that transports lipids bidirectionally and, when active, collapses membrane asymmetry and results in PS exposure on the outer leaflet. The eight transmembrane domain containing protein TMEM16F serves as a Ca^{2+}-activated, nonselective cation channel that is crucial for Ca^{2+}-dependent phospholipid scrambling and PS exposure on activated platelets.[644]

Platelet activation with strong agonists also results in the formation of microparticles, which are particularly rich in surface-exposed negatively charged phospholipids. Microparticles also are rich in factor Va and thus actively support thrombin generation.[82,645,646] Microparticle formation can be induced *in vitro* by activation of platelets with ionophore A23187, complement C5b-9, or the combination of thrombin and collagen; by adding tissue factor to recalcified platelet-rich plasma; or by high shear stress.[645,647–652] Elevations of cytosolic Ca^{2+}, calpain activation, cytoskeletal reorganization, protein phosphorylation, and phospholipid translocation have all been implicated in microparticle formation.

The biologic relevance of platelet microparticles is supported by the finding of increased circulating levels of platelet microparticles in patients with activated coagulation and fibrinolysis, diabetes mellitus, sickle cell anemia, human immunodeficiency virus infection, unstable angina, heparin-induced thrombocytopenia with thrombosis, and respiratory distress syndrome.[645,653] Microparticles can bind to fibrin thrombi via one or more of the receptors present on their surface, including integrin $\alpha_{IIb}\beta_3$, GPIb/IX, P-selectin, and possibly P-selectin glycoprotein ligand (PSGL)-1.[654]

Microparticles bind factors VIII, Va, and Xa, allowing them to form both the factor Xase and prothrombinase complexes on their surface.[645] They can also bind protein S and facilitate inactivation of factors Va and VIIIa which could serve an anticoagulant function.[655,656] In addition, microparticles can activate platelets by supplying arachidonic acid.

Evidence supporting the importance of platelet microparticle formation to platelet coagulant activity has been gathered from observations of patients who have significant bleeding diatheses in association with defects in platelet microparticle formation (Scott syndrome; Chap. 121).[657–659] Platelets from the most intensively studied patient had an impaired ability to accelerate the activation of both factor X and prothrombin. In addition, this patient's platelets exhibited both abnormal factor V binding and abnormal exposure of negatively charged phospholipids.

Activated platelets synthesize tissue factor by splicing pre-mRNA into mature mRNA and then translating the tissue factor protein.[660,661] Additionally, platelet thrombi can recruit tissue factor from blood by binding leukocyte-derived, tissue factor-containing microparticles or by binding an alternatively spliced, soluble form of tissue factor.[466,472,662–665] The interaction between PSGL-1 on the surface of leukocyte-derived microparticles and P-selectin on the surface of activated platelets appears to play an important role in the binding of microparticles to platelet thrombi.[664] Interactions between platelets and leukocytes, and perhaps leukocyte-derived microparticles, reportedly enhance ("de-encrypt" or decrypt) tissue factor activity, probably by supplying negatively charged phospholipids[666] and/or the oxidoreductase enzyme protein disulfide isomerase (PDI).[667]

Platelet dense granules contain polyphosphate, a linear polymer of inorganic phosphate synthesized by inositol hexakisphosphate 6 kinase. Polyphosphates are released during platelet activation and promote clot formation. Polyphosphates affect many steps in coagulation. Polyphosphates accelerate factor V and factor XII[668] and alter the structure of fibrin clots. In the presence of polyphosphates, fibrin clots have thicker fibers and are more resistant to fibrinolysis.[669] In contrast to bacterial polyphosphates, which are long-chain structures, platelet polyphosphates have shorter chain length and are more effective in increasing factor V and TFPI activity.

Incontrovertible evidence exists that platelets accelerate thrombin formation.[658,659,670–672] Platelets accelerate the activation of factor X by factors IXa and VIIIa and the activation of prothrombin by factors Xa and Va.[659,670] However, only a subpopulation of platelets develops a procoagulant phenotype with activation, as only a fraction of activated platelets display high levels of factors Va and Xa, termed "coat" platelets.[464,465,670,673] The assembly of the factor IXa/factor VIIIa/platelet complex increases the catalytic efficiency of factor X activation (k_{cat}/K_m [turnover number/Michaelis-Menten dissociation constant]) by a factor of 2.4×10^6.[670] Prothrombin binds to approximately 20,000 sites on activated platelets with a K_D equal to its plasma concentration (approximately 0.15 μM).[674] Integrin $\alpha_{IIb}\beta_3$ binds prothrombin through its RGD domain, and may contribute to the localization of prothrombin to the surface of unactivated and activated platelets.[675]

In addition to accelerating coagulation, the binding of activated coagulation factors to the surface of platelets appears to protect them from inactivation by inhibitors in plasma and platelets.[399] The bleeding diathesis in patients with Quebec platelet syndrome, who have proteolysis of their platelet α-granule factor V, supports the potential importance of platelet factor V in normal hemostasis (Chap. 121), as do the studies of another patient with abnormal platelet factor V.[659]

Other connections between platelets and the coagulation system include: (1) the presence of fibrinogen in platelet α granules and perhaps on the surface of platelets, where it is strategically located for interactions with locally generated thrombin[371,399]; (2) the presence of intracellular VWF and the binding of extracellular VWF to platelets (via GPIb/X and integrin $\alpha_{IIb}\beta_3$), with the potential colocalization of factor VIII attached to the VWF (Chap. 126); (3) activation of factor XI by thrombin on the platelet surface,[676,677] with the dimeric structure of factor XI allowing it to interact both with the platelet and factor IX simultaneously[678]; (4) a factor XI-like protein associated with platelet membranes, which may be an alternatively spliced form of factor XI lacking exon V; the level of this factor appears to correlate better with hemorrhagic symptoms than does the level of plasma factor XI[399,679]; (5) the presence of cytoplasmic factor XIII (Chap. 113); (6) the presence of inhibitors of coagulation (α_1-protease inhibitor, C-1 inhibitor, TFPI, the thrombin inhibitor protease nexin I, and the factors IXa and XIa inhibitor protease nexin II or β-APP)[399,448]; and (7) promotion of factor XII activation by ADP-treated platelets.[399]

● PLATELETS AND THROMBOLYSIS

The interactions between platelets and the fibrinolytic system are complex; Table 112–3 contains a partial listing of reported findings.[680–684] Both profibrinolytic[398,685–692] and antifibrinolytic[693–701] effects of platelets have been described, and so it is difficult to predict the net effect. Since platelet-rich thrombi are known to resist thrombolysis in animal models, the antifibrinolytic effects of platelets appear to predominate *in vivo*.[702]

TABLE 112–3. Platelets and Thrombolysis
Profibrinolytic effects of platelets
Tissue plasminogen activator (t-PA) and single-chain urokinase-type t-PA identified on or in platelets.
Unactivated platelets bind plasminogen, and binding is enhanced by thrombin.
Thrombospondin, a plasminogen-binding protein, is expressed on the surface of platelets after activation.
Activation of plasminogen by t-PA is enhanced by platelets.
Clot lysis is enhanced by platelets in some model systems.
Antifibrinolytic effects of platelets
Plasminogen activator inhibitor-1 and α_2-antiplasmin are present in platelet granules.
Platelets contain protease nexin-1, a serpin that inhibits plasminogen activators and plasmin.
Platelets contain factor XIII, which can crosslink fibrin, making it resist fibrinolysis, and can crosslink α_2-antiplasmin to fibrin, enhancing its antifibrinolytic effects.
Platelets contain tissue factor pathway inhibitor-2, which inhibits tissue plasminogen activator.
Platelet $\alpha_{IIb}\beta_3$ can bind plasma factor XIIIa directly or indirectly, localizing it to the site of thrombus formation.
Platelets facilitate clot retraction, which diminishes the efficiency of fibrinolysis.
Platelet-activating effects of thrombolytic agents
Streptokinase and t-PA activate platelets *in vivo* and *in vitro*.
Plasmin, at high doses, can aggregate platelets.
Thrombolytic agents may paradoxically generate the potent platelet agonist thrombin or release it from thrombi.
Thrombolytic agents may blunt the prostacyclin increase that accompanies acute thrombosis.
Platelet-inhibiting effects of thrombolytic agents
Plasmin, at low doses, can inhibit platelet activation and aggregation.
Platelets can be disaggregated by t-PA by selective lysis of platelet-bound fibrinogen.
Plasmin can cause redistribution and/or cleavage of platelet glycoprotein Ib.
Inhibition of platelet aggregation by the depletion of plasma fibrinogen, if severe, and generation of fibrin (ogen) degradation products.
Proteolysis of plasma von Willebrand factor.
Prolongation of the bleeding time.

Adapted with permission from Fozzard HA, et al: *The Heart and Cardiovascular System*. New York, NY: Raven Press; 1991.

The effects of fibrinolytic agents on platelets are similarly complex. For example, there is considerable evidence that fibrinolytic agents can activate platelets soon after administration,[703–709] via either a direct effect of plasmin,[710–713] perhaps acting on PAR-4[714] or an indirect effect through the paradoxical generation of thrombin.[683,715–718] Interpretation of the latter studies are complicated by the ability of tissue plasminogen activator to release fibrinopeptides from fibrinogen, one of the biomarkers used to assess thrombin activation.[719]

Stimulation of platelets by thrombolytic agents may prolong the time required for reperfusion of thrombosed blood vessels and may contribute to reocclusion after successful reperfusion.[680,720] In animal models and in humans, potent antiplatelet agents can, in fact, speed reperfusion, abolish reocclusion, and diminish the size of myocardial infarcts.[721–723] In human studies, the benefits of combining integrin $\alpha_{IIb}\beta_3$ antagonists with fibrinolytic agents in enhancing coronary thrombolysis have been counterbalanced by an increase in major hemorrhage.[724] Combining a potent integrin $\alpha_{IIb}\beta_3$ antagonist with a reduced dose of a fibrinolytic agent in acute ST-elevation MI when patients are rapidly treated with percutaneous coronary intervention has demonstrated evidence for more rapid reperfusion, but clinical benefit has been variable and bleeding has been increased.[725,726] In experimental models of stroke, paradoxically, early treatment with integrin $\alpha_{IIb}\beta_3$ antagonists reduces the hemorrhage associated with thrombolytic therapy, perhaps by preventing platelet aggregation in the microcirculation and the release of agents that can damage the vasculature and diminish its integrity.[727–729] In human studies, however, a potent integrin $\alpha_{IIb}\beta_3$ antagonist given alone did not improve clinical outcomes.[730,731]

With prolonged use of thrombolytic agents, inhibition of platelet function can occur via a variety of mechanisms.[102,707,708,732–744] These effects may contribute to some of the hemorrhagic phenomena observed with this therapy. One proposed mechanism is that the thrombolytic agents make platelets refractory to further stimulation by agonists.

● PLATELETS IN INFLAMMATION AND INFECTION

Leukocytes can bind to activated platelets and in model systems transmigrate through a platelet monolayer (reviewed in Ref. 745; see Fig. 112–9). Animal models and studies of human tissue demonstrate that within hours after vascular injury, leukocytes become enmeshed in platelet thrombi and/or transiently form a monolayer on top of adherent or aggregated platelets.[746,747] These interactions may be important at sites of vascular injury or inflammation where leukocytes have been shown to deposit on adherent and aggregated platelets. Platelet recruitment of leukocytes has been associated with a number of systemic and inflammatory processes in animal models, including the development of intimal hyperplasia after vascular injury,[748] ischemia–reperfusion injury, alloimmunity-mediated transplant rejection,[749] obesity,[750] and acute lung injury.[751] By depositing chemokines such as CCL5 (also termed RANTES [regulated upon activation, normal T-cell expressed and secreted]) on activated endothelium[752,753] or by direct interactions with leukocytes,[754] platelets may also enhance leukocyte recruitment to inflamed or atherosclerotic endothelium and thereby promote the development and progression of atherosclerosis.

Many mechanisms of platelet–leukocyte interactions have been defined, but the initial interaction appears to be mediated primarily by the interaction between P-selectin (CD62P) expressed on the surface of activated platelets and PSGL-1 on the surface of neutrophils and monocytes.[755–761] P-selectin–PSGL-1 interactions are characterized by rapid on-and-off rates that promote tethering and rolling of leukocytes along adherent platelets. In addition to PSGL-1, leukocyte CD24 may also bind P-selectin. The transient P-selectin–mediated interactions are stabilized by subsequent contacts mediated, in large part, by activation of leukocyte β_2 integrins. Platelet surface-immobilized and released chemokines promote firm leukocyte adhesion and arrest by acting through G-protein–coupled receptors to activate leukocyte β_2 integrins. Platelets can synthesize and release PAF, which can activate leukocyte $\alpha_M\beta_2$. CCL5 and the CXC chemokines ENA-78 and GRO-α, released by activated platelets, can also activate leukocytes. The chemokine neutrophil-activating peptide-2 (NAP-2) can be produced by the action of leukocyte cathepsin G on β-thromboglobulin secreted by platelets.[762,763] Activated $\alpha_M\beta_2$ on leukocytes can interact with platelet GPIbα[764] as well as with platelet-bound fibrinogen via a region(s) on the γ chain (amino acids 190 to 202,[765] and 377 to 395). Thrombospondin may serve as a bridging molecule between CD36 (GPIV) receptors, which are expressed on both platelets and mononuclear cells.[766] Platelets also have intercellular adhesion molecule (ICAM)-2 on their surface, which is a ligand for the leukocyte integrin receptor $\alpha_L\beta_2$; although this ligand-receptor interaction appears to have only a minor role in platelet–leukocyte adhesion, it may be more important in leukocyte tethering.[763] Platelet junctional adhesion molecule (JAM)3 has also been suggested as a counterreceptor for leukocyte $\alpha_M\beta_2$.[767] The immunoreceptor tyrosine-based activation motif (ITAM)-associated receptors GPVI and C-type lectin-like receptor-2 (CLEC-2) also promote platelet–leukocyte interactions during inflammation via their respective counterreceptors matrix metalloproteinase inducer (EMMPRIN) on neutrophils and macrophages and podoplanin on inflammatory macrophages.

Transcellular metabolism of eicosanoids can result in production of unique products (Fig. 112–10) and leukocytes can modify platelet activation.[768] In a complementary fashion, the intimate relationship between leukocytes and platelets allows the latter to contribute to the inflammatory response, including the release of chemokines that can activate leukocytes; PDGF can affect fibroblast and smooth muscle cells; TGF-β_1 both stimulates and inhibits cellular growth; and PF4 primes neutrophils and has antiangiogenic activity. Platelets synthesize the cytokine IL-1β, an important mediator of the inflammatory response.[769] Platelets contain FcγIIA receptors that can localize IgG and immune complexes, resulting in complement activation. Platelets express CD40L on their surface after activation, and this molecule can interact with CD40, a member of the tumor necrosis factor (TNF) receptor family, on leukocytes and endothelial cells, leading to their activation and their elaboration of a number of proinflammatory molecules[770–772] (see "CD40 Ligand (CD40L, CD154) and CD40"). Platelet CD40L also promotes procoagulant activity in endothelial cells.[773] Finally, platelet–leukocyte interactions can promote the generation of reactive oxygen species, but platelets can also generate signals to stop their production.[774]

Platelet–leukocyte interactions may be important in the initiation of coagulation and fibrin formation through a P-selectin–dependent pathway. In fact, platelet–leukocyte aggregates facilitate thrombin generation to a greater extent than either platelets or leukocytes alone.[775,776] Coincubation of platelets and leukocytes generates tissue factor activity, in part, through P-selectin–PSGL-1 interactions. The induction of tissue factor activity involves both *de novo* protein synthesis and exposure ("deencryption") of latent tissue factor. The latter may occur by P-selectin–mediated production of tissue factor containing microparticles from leukocytes. Real-time imaging of platelet thrombus formation *in vivo* indicates that tissue factor accumulates in growing thrombi before leukocytes become associated with the thrombus. The accumulation of tissue factor and fibrin formation in thrombi depend on both platelet P-selectin and PSGL-1. These observations, coupled with the finding of bloodborne tissue factor antigen in the circulation,[777] has led to a model in which platelet P-selectin recruits tissue factor-containing leukocyte microparticles to platelet-rich thrombi.[778] Neutrophil-derived microparticles express active integrin $\alpha_M\beta_2$, which can interact with platelets by binding to GPIbα. This, in turn, can initiate platelet P-selectin expression, which will enhance the interactions with neutrophil microparticles containing the counterreceptor PSGL-1.[779] In mice, increases in soluble P-selectin levels promote a procoagulant state associated with elevated levels of leukocyte-derived microparticles,[780] and a P-selectin–immunoglobulin chimeric molecule can increase levels of leukocyte-derived microparticles *in vitro* and normalize the bleeding time in hemophilia A mice.[781]

Several clinical observations support a potential role for platelet–leukocyte interactions in vascular disease, including the presence of circulating platelet–leukocyte aggregates in patients with unstable angina[782] and after coronary artery angioplasty[783]; in the latter situation, the presence of such aggregates appears to confer a worse prognosis for ischemic vascular complications.[783] Circulating platelet–leukocyte aggregates are perhaps the most sensitive indicator of systemic platelet activation, reflecting the expression of P-selectin on the surface of platelets.[784] Analysis of polymorphisms of PSGL-1 involving variable numbers of tandem repeats indicates that the longer PSGL-1 molecules are better able to form platelet–leukocyte aggregates; in some, but not all, studies, the longer molecules were associated with increased risk of some forms of thrombotic vascular disease.[785–790] The S100 calcium-modulated protein family member MRP-14 (also known as S100A9), which is abundant in neutrophils and released by activated platelets, promotes platelet thrombus, at least in part through CD36.[791]

Platelets can contribute to both innate and adaptive immunity in several ways. Bacterial endotoxin binding to toll-like receptors can activate platelets (see "Toll-Like Receptors[1,2,4,6,9]"), enhance platelet–neutrophil interactions, and promote bacterial trapping by stimulating the production of neutrophil extracellular traps (NETs) composed of DNA, histones, and enzymes that degrade pathogens.[792–794] The production of NETs confers resistance to a variety of pathogens, including Gram-positive (*Staphylococcus aureus*, *Streptococcus pneumoniae*, and Group A streptococci) and Gram-negative (*Salmonella typhimurium*, *Shigella flexneri*, and *Escherichia coli*) bacteria. A number of Gram-positive bacteria can activate and aggregate platelets and the platelet immune receptor RcγRIIA, integrin $\alpha_{IIb}\beta_3$, Src, and Syk, along with PF4, ADP, and TXA$_2$ all play a role in the process.[795] Platelets release mitochondria, which are related to bacteria in composition, when activated either in microparticles or free into plasma, where they associate with neutrophils and the platelet enzyme PLA2 IIA, which hydrolyzes mitochondrial and bacterial membranes, releasing a variety of proinflammatory molecules, including mitochondrial DNA, arachidonic acid, and lysophospholipids that are themselves capable of initiating NET formation.[796] Release of platelet mitochondria during storage for transfusion has been suggested as being a contributor to platelet-associated nonhemolytic transfusion reactions.[796]

Thrombocytopenia is often present in association with bloodborne bacterial infections (sepsis) and the severity of the thrombocytopenia mirrors the severity of the infection and prognosis. Platelet factor V contributes to resistance to Group A streptococcal infection[797] by promoting thrombin generation and fibrin deposition, which may help to wall off the bacteria.[797] Platelets also influence the function of lymphocytes.[798] They enhance cytolytic T-cell proliferation and antibody production by B cells. Platelets can inhibit the responses of helper T-cells, and via release of TGF-β_1, increase regulatory T (Treg) cells. Finally, platelets can bind to malarial-infected erythrocytes and both suppress the growth of the parasites and destroy the intraerythrocytic malarial parasites.[799]

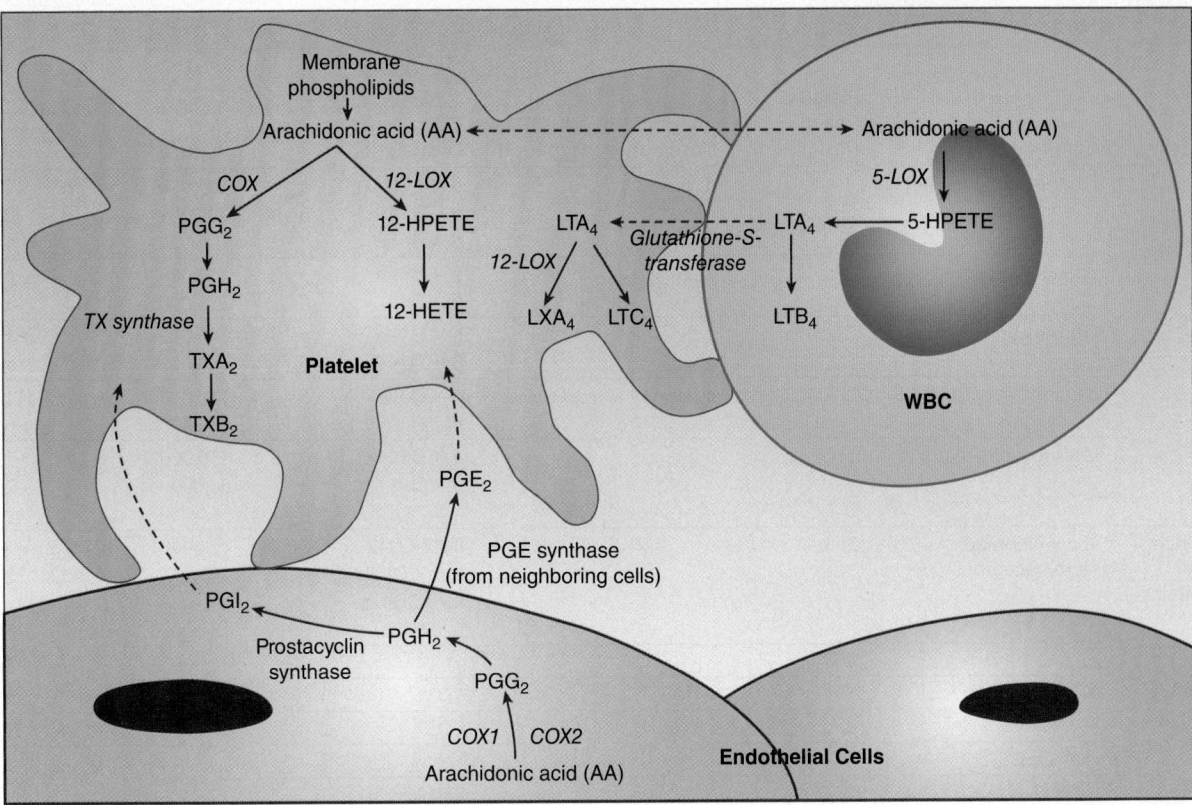

Figure 112–10. Select aspects of transcellular eicosanoid metabolism. At sites of platelet-white blood cell (WBC) interactions, free arachidonic acid (AA) can be generated by both activated platelets and leukocytes and exchanged between the cells. In the platelet, cyclooxygenase 1 (COX-1), the target for aspirin, generates the major AA-metabolite prostaglandin (PG) G$_2$, the precursor for PGH$_2$ that, in turn, is converted by thromboxane (TX) synthase to TXA$_2$. TXA$_2$ and PGH$_2$ promote platelet activation and inflammation through binding to thromboprostanoid (TP) receptors. TXA$_2$ is rapidly converted to TXB$_2$. Platelets also express platelet-type 12-lipoxygenase (LOX) that converts AA to the relatively unstable intermediate 12-hydroper-oxy-5,8,10,14-eicosatetraenoic acid (12-HPETE), which is subsequently converted to 12-hydroxyeicosatetraenoic acid (12-HETE). Platelets from most mammalian species do not possess 5-LOX and, therefore, cannot generate leukotriene A$_4$ (LTA$_4$) from AA. However, LTA$_4$ produced by leukocytes can be transferred to interacting platelets, where it can be metabolized by glutathione-S-transferase to LTC$_4$ or by platelet 12-LOX to the antiinflammatory mediator lipoxin (LXA$_4$). In endothelial cells, AA can also be released from membrane phospholipids, but unlike in the platelet, it is sequentially metabolized by COX-1 or COX-2 and prostacyclin synthase to PGI$_2$, which inhibits platelet activation by effects on the platelet inhibitory prostanoid (IP) receptor. Endothelial cells can also serve as a source of PGH$_2$ that is metabolized by PGE synthase to PGE$_2$. At high concentrations, PGE$_2$ inhibits platelet activation, and at lower concentrations (<10^{-6} M), it activates platelets through the EP3 receptor. *(Used with permission of Matt Hazard, Teaching and Academic Support Center, The University of Kentucky.)*

PLATELETS IN VESSEL INTEGRITY AND DEVELOPMENT

Platelets are essential to maintain the integrity of the vasculature, especially in inflammatory sites, although the mechanisms are not fully understood. Platelets store a number of barrier-stabilizing cytokines and growth factors that may be released constitutively or in a stimulus-dependent manner, including sphingosine-1-phosphate (S1P), which is essential for barrier function, ADP, serotonin, VEGF, and thrombospondin. While platelet G-protein–coupled signaling is essential for hemostasis and thrombosis after vascular injury, these pathways do not appear to be required for hemostasis during inflammation. And functional platelet ITAM motif receptors, CLEC-2 and GPVI, are required to maintain vascular integrity during inflammation, likely by triggering a unique response in the setting of inflammation.[800]

The partitioning between lymphatic and blood vessels during development requires normal platelet function. Platelets regulate lymphangiogenesis, at least in part, through interactions between platelet CLEC-2 and podoplanin on lymphatic endothelial cells. In addition, downstream ITAM signaling, mediated by Syk, SLP-76, and PLCγ$_2$, is also required.

Platelet activation along lymphatic endothelium may result in secretion of angiogenic factors. Importantly, platelet adhesion may result in intravascular hemostasis that promotes the lymphovenous junction, in that mouse embryos lacking CLEC-2, podoplanin, Syk, or SLP-76 display blood-filled lymphatic vessels. The requirement for platelets in maintaining blood–lymphatic separation extends beyond embryogenesis into adulthood. Importantly, the requirement for lymphovenous hemostasis are different from arterial and venous hemostasis, likely because of the low-flow, low-shear environment and intact lymphatic endothelium.

PLATELET MEMBRANE GLYCOPROTEINS

Platelet membrane glycoproteins mediate most of the interactions between platelets and their external environment. Receptors can receive signals from outside the platelet and transmit signals inside. In addition, glycoprotein receptors receive signals from inside the platelet that affect their external domain functions. Platelet glycoprotein receptors are grouped into several different receptor families (integrins, leucine-rich glycoproteins, immunoglobulin cell adhesion molecules, selectins, tetraspanins, and seven-transmembrane domain receptors; see Table 112–4).

TABLE 112-4. Important Platelet Surface Proteins

Gene Family	Common Name	Platelet Chain Designation	Integrin Designation	VLA[+] Designation	CD[+] Designation		M_r Non-Reduced		Reduced
Integrin	Fibrinogen/receptor		$\alpha_{IIb}\beta_3$		$\alpha_{IIb}\beta_3$-CD41a α_{IIb}-CD41b β_3-CD61	α_{IIb} β_3	145,000 90,000	$\alpha_{IIb}\alpha$ $\alpha_{IIb}\beta$	125,000 23,000 114,000
	Collagen receptor	GPIa/IIa	$\alpha_2\beta_1$	VLA-2	α_2-CD49b β_1-CD29	α_2 β_1	150,000 138,000		148,000
	Fibronectin receptor	CPIc*/IIa	$\alpha_5\beta_1$	VLA-5	α_5-CD49e β_1-CD29	α_5 β_1	140,000 138,000		148,000
	Laminin receptor	GPIc/IIa	$\alpha_6\beta_1$	VLA-6	α_6-CD49f β_1-CD29	α_6 β_1	140,000 138,000		148,000
	Vitronectin receptor	α_v/GPIIIa	$\alpha_v\beta_3$		α_v-CD51 β_3-CD61	α_v β_3	150,000 90,000	α_v α_v	125,000 25,000 114,000
Leucine-rich repeat glycoproteins	von Willebrand factor receptor	GPIb/Ix			Ib/Ix-CD42 Ib/a-CD42b Ib/β-CD42c Ix-CD42a	GPIb GPIX	170,000 17,000	GPIbα GPIbβ	145,000 22,000 17,000
	GPV					GPV	82,000		82,000
Immunoglobulin family cell adhesion modecules	PECAM-I				CD31		130,000		
	Fcγ-RII				CD32		40,000		
	HLA-Class 1								
	ICAM-2				CD102				59,000
	GPVI						62,000		65,000
	IAP				CD47		50,000		
Selectins	P-Selectin (GMP 140; PADGEM)				CD62P		140,000		
Tetraspanins	p24				CD9 CD63		24,000		
	PETA-3				CD151		27,000		
	Lamp 3 (granulophysin)				CD63		53,000		
Miscellaneous	GPIV				CD36		88,000		
	CLEC-2				CD94				
	TLR(1-6)								
	Lamp 1				CD107a		110,000		
	Lamp 2				CD107b		120,000		
	67 kDa Laminin receptor						67,000		
	ADP P2X1 receptor						70,000		
	Leukosialin, sialophorin				CD43		90,000		
Seven trans-membrane domain (G protein-linked)	PAR-1						70,000		
	PAR-4								
	Thromboxane A$_2$ receptor								55,000
	α_2-Adrenergic receptor								64,000
	Vasopressin receptor						125,000		
	ADP P2Y$_1$ receptor								
	ADP P2Y$_{12}$ receptor								
	Serotonin 5-HT2A						53,000		

Fib, fibrinogen; Fn, fibronectin; GP, glycoprotein; HLA, human leukocyte antigen; IAP, integrin-associated protein; ICAM, intercellular adhesion molecule; lamp, lysosome-associated membrane protein; PAR, protease-activated receptor; PECAM, platelet-endothelial cell adhesion molecule; PSGL-1, P-selectin glycoprotein ligand-1; TSP, thrombospondin; TX, thromboxane; Vn, vironectin; vwf, von Willebrand factor.

Amino Acids	Carbohydrate	Lipid	Phosphorylated	Chromosome	Ligands	Platelet Specific	Function	Molecules on Platelet Surface (S) or Internal (I)
α_{IIb}1039	+	−	−	17	Fib, VWF, Fn, Vn, ?TSP	+	Adhesion, aggregation, protein trafficking	(S)80,000
$\beta_3$762	+	−	+	17		+		(I)40,000
$\alpha_2$1152				5	Collagen	−	Adhesion	(S)1000
$\beta_1$778				10		−		
$\alpha_5$1008				12	Fn	−	Adhesion	(S)1000
$\beta_1$778				10				
$\alpha_6$1067				2	Laminin	−	Adhesion	(S)1,000
$\beta_1$778				10				
α_v1048				2	Vn, Fib, VWF, Fn, ?TSP, Osp	−	?Adhesion, ?Protein trafficking	(S)100
GPIIIa 762	+	−		17				
GPIbα610(8)*	+	−	−	1	VWF, Thrombin	+?	Adhesion (high shear), ?thrombin activation	(S)25,000
GPIbβ181(1)*	+	+	+	22		+?		(S)25,000
GPIX 160(1)*	+	+		3		+?		(S)25,000
GPV 544(15)*	+	+	+	3		+?		(S) 12,500
PECAM-1 738	+	?	+	17	Heparin	−	?Adhesion	(S) 8000
FcγRII 324	+		+	1	Immune complexes	−	Immune complex binding	(s) ~1000
HLA	+			6	−		Histocompatibility	(S)
ICAM-2 274				17	LFA-1	−	Platelet-leukocyte adhesion	(S) 2600
GPVI 316	+	−		?	Collagen	+	Activation	(S) ~2000
IAP 287	+			3	TSP	−	Activation	
P-Selectin 830	+	+	+	1	Sialyl-le^x PSGL-1		Platelet-leukocyte adhesion	(I) 20,000
CD9 228	+				?	−	Activation	(S) 40,000
CD151 253	+	−	−	11	?	−	Activation	(I) ~2000
Lamp 3 238	+							(I) 10,000
GPIV 471	+		+	7	Collagen, TSP	−	Adhesion	(S) 20,000
CLEC-2 229	+		+	12	Podoplanin	−	adhesion/activation	
TLR					Pathogen-associated molecular patterns	−	activation	
Lamp 1 389	+			13	?	−	?	(I) 1200
Lamp 2 381	+			X	?			
67 kDa ?295				X	Laminin	−	Adhesion	
P2X$_1$ 399	+			17	ATP, ADP	−	Activation	(S) 13–130
CD43 400	+		+	16	ICAM-1	−	Adhesion	
PAR-1 425				5	Thrombin	−	Activation	(S) ~1800
PAR-4 385	+		+	19	Thrombin	−	Activation	
TXA$_2$ 343				19	PGH$_2$/thromboxane A$_2$	−	Activation	~200
α_2-Adrenergin 450				10	Epinephrine	−	Activation	~250
Vasopressin 418				?x	Vasopressin	−	Activation	~75
P2Y$_1$ 373	+			3	ADP	−	Activation	
P2Y$_{12}$ 342				3	ADP	+	Activation	
5-HT2A	+		+	13	Serotonin	−	activation	

*Number of leucine-rich repeats.

†CD, cluster of differentiation (see Chap. 15); VLA, very-late antigen.

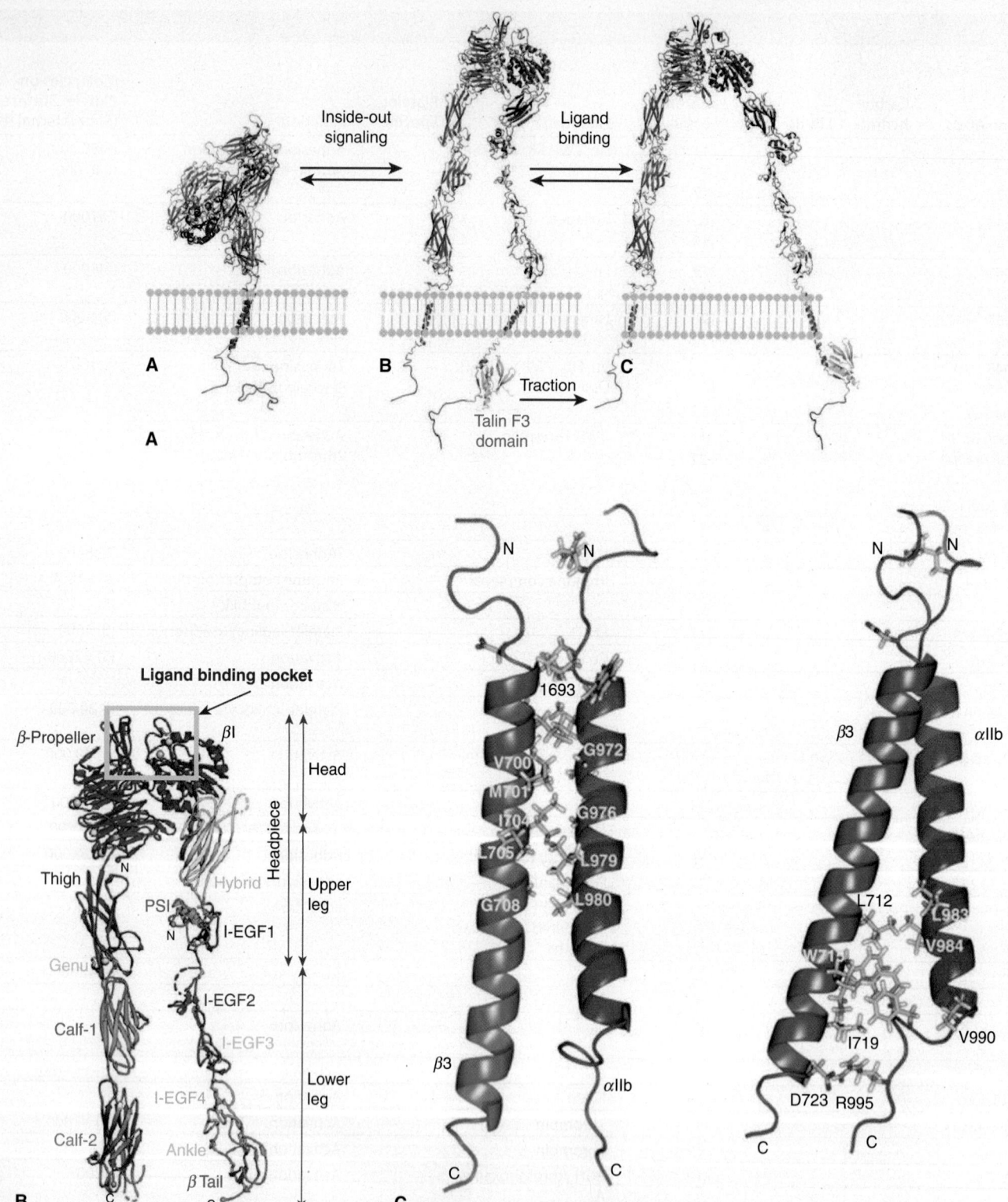

Figure 112–11. $a_{IIb}\beta_3$ Integrin structure and activation. **A.** Model for $a_{IIb}\beta_3$ integrin inside-out activation and outside-in signaling. The a subunit is in *blue* and the β subunit is in *red*. The bent, inactive receptor is depicted in (A). Under resting condition, the integrin β_3 cytoplasmic domain appears to interact with filamin. Cellular stimulation induces migfilin to displace filamin from the integrin β_3 cytoplasmic domain as well as a conformational change in talin that alters the interactions between the talin head and rod domains and exposes the talin head domain. The FERM F3 domain in the head then binds to the integrin β_3 cytoplasmic domain, which unclasps the inter-subunit cytoplasmic and transmembrane domains from their complex with the integrin β_3 cytoplasmic and transmembrane domains. Kindlin-3 binding to the integrin β_3 cytoplasmic domain may facilitate talin binding and appears to be required for the conversion to the high-affinity state. The binding of talin then leads to separation of the ectodomain subunit tails and may diminish the interaction of the integrin headpiece with the tails. Although small ligands can bind to the receptor without headpiece extension, the large glycoprotein ligands may require extension to facilitate access to the ligand binding site. Extension (B) may occur spontaneously after leg separation, or may result from traction force exerted on the integrin β_3 cytoplasmic domain via talin's association with the cytoskeleton

One member of the integrin family, integrin $\alpha_{IIb}\beta_3$, is virtually unique to platelets (and their precursors, megakaryocytes), whereas the leucine-rich glycoproteins GPIb/IX and GPV appear to have highly restricted but not uniquely platelet expression patterns, including cytokine-activated endothelial cells.[801,802] All of the other receptors are expressed more widely on other cell types.

INTEGRINS

Integrin receptors are heterodimeric complexes composed of an α subunit containing three or four divalent cation binding domains and a β subunit rich in disulfide bonds. Both subunits are transmembrane glycoproteins and are coded by different genes. There are at least 18 α subunits and eight β subunits.[43,803,804] Three major families of integrin receptors are recognized based on the β subunit: β_1, β_2, and β_3. Integrins are widely distributed on different cell types, and each integrin demonstrates unique ligand-binding properties. Integrin receptors mediate interactions between cells and proteins or proteins on cells; they are also involved in protein trafficking in cells. Integrin receptors can also transduce messages from outside the cell to inside the cell, and from inside the cell to outside the cell.

Integrin $\alpha_{IIb}\beta_3$ (Also Termed GPIIb/IIIa, Fibrinogen Receptor, and CD41/CD61)

The integrin $\alpha_{IIb}\beta_3$ complex, a member of the β_3 integrin receptor family, is the dominant platelet receptor, with 80,000 to 100,000 receptors present on the surface of a resting platelet (Fig. 112–11).[805–812] Another 20,000 to 40,000 receptors are present inside platelets, primarily in α-granule membranes, but also in dense bodies and membranes lining the open canalicular system; these receptors are able to join the plasma membrane when platelets are activated and undergo the release reaction.[813–815] On average, integrin $\alpha_{IIb}\beta_3$ receptors are less than 20 nm apart on the platelet surface and thus are among the most densely expressed adhesion/aggregation receptors present on any cell type.

On resting platelets, integrin $\alpha_{IIb}\beta_3$ has low affinity for fibrinogen in solution, but when platelets are activated with ADP, epinephrine, thrombin, or other agonists, integrin $\alpha_{IIb}\beta_3$ binds fibrinogen relatively strongly.[808,816] Activation induces changes in the integrin $\alpha_{IIb}\beta_3$ receptor itself that are responsible for the change in fibrinogen-binding affinity, but changes in the microenvironment surrounding integrin $\alpha_{IIb}\beta_3$ may also be involved. The integrin $\alpha_{IIb}\beta_3$ receptors in α granules appear to cycle to and from the plasma membrane.[817] This recycling helps to explain the ability of the integrin to take up fibrinogen from plasma and transport it to α granules, where it is concentrated.[375,818]

Data from other integrin receptors identified a cell recognition sequence composed of RGD in the ligand fibronectin,[819,820] and this same sequence is important in ligand binding to integrins $\alpha_v\beta_3$ and $\alpha_{IIb}\beta_3$. Fibrinogen contains one RGD sequence near the carboxy terminus of each of the two Aα chains (amino acids 572 to 574) and another at amino acids 95 to 97.[821] In addition, the carboxyterminal 12 amino acid region of each of the two γ chains (amino acids 400 to 411) contains a sequence that includes Lys-Gln-Ala-Gly-Asp-Val, which is the most important in the binding of fibrinogen to platelets.[822–826] VWF contains an RGD sequence in its carboxyterminal domain and that region mediates the binding to integrin $\alpha_{IIb}\beta_3$.[809,810,812] Small, synthetic peptides containing the RGD or γ-chain sequence inhibit the binding of fibrinogen to platelets, and these observations have been exploited to produce therapeutic agents (tirofiban and eptifibatide) to inhibit platelet thrombus formation[827] (Chap. 134). Similarly, monoclonal antibodies that inhibit binding of ligands to integrin $\alpha_{IIb}\beta_3$ have been developed and a mouse/human chimeric Fab fragment of one of them has been developed into a drug (abciximab) that is an effective antiplatelet agent.

The binding of fibrinogen to integrin $\alpha_{IIb}\beta_3$ appears to be a multistep process[808,828–833]: (1) the initial interaction is most likely via the γ-chain carboxyterminal region(s) and divalent cation-dependent[823–826]; (2) subsequent interactions enhance the binding and internalization of the fibrinogen[834] and render it irreversible, even when divalent cations are removed[835]; (3) binding of fibrinogen induces changes in the receptor that can be recognized by antibodies (ligand-induced binding sites [LIBSs])[442,826]; (4) binding of fibrinogen to integrin $\alpha_{IIb}\beta_3$ induces changes in fibrinogen (receptor-induced binding sites) that can be recognized by antibodies and may involve exposure of the Aα chain Arg-Gly-Asp-Phe sequence at amino acids 95 to 98[836,837]; and (5) fibrinogen binding induces receptor clustering.[251,838]

By electron microscopy, the receptors have a globular head of 8×12 nm and two 18-nm long tails representing the carboxyterminal regions of each subunit, including their hydrophobic transmembrane domains.[839,840] Crystallographic, electron microscopic, electron and neutron scattering, and biochemical data from integrin $\alpha_{IIb}\beta_3$ and the related integrin $\alpha_v\beta_3$ receptor indicate that the unactivated receptors are in a bent conformation and that activation involves both extension of the receptor head and a swing out motion in the β_3 subunit.[149,827,841–853] A three-dimensional reconstruction of integrin $\alpha_{IIb}\beta_3$ in a lipid bilayer nano disc from negative-stain electron microscopy images supports a compact conformation of the inactive receptor, but unlike the crystal structure of the ectodomain, the legs are not parallel and straight.[848]

Integrin $\alpha_{IIb}\beta_3$ shares the same basic structural features of all integrin receptors (Table 112–4).[30,848] The α subunit, α_{IIb}, is a transmembrane

---

and actin-myosin contractile force. Ligand binding to the integrin is associated with a swing out motion of the integrin β_3 hybrid domain from the $\beta A(I)$ domain (C), which results in both increased ligand affinity via alterations in the ADMIDAS (adjacent to metal ion-dependent adhesion site) and MIDAS (metal ion-dependent adhesion site) regions of integrin β_3 and greater leg separation. This conformational change may initiate outside-in signaling. The ligated integrins may then cluster (not shown). The structure in panel (A) is based on the crystal structure of the ectodomain (PDB 3FCS)[250] and the nuclear magnetic resonance (NMR) structure of the transmembrane and cytoplasmic domains (PDB 2K9J).[894] The structure in (B) is based on the same ectodomain crystal structure, but with extension at the genus of the subunits (PDB 3FCS),[250] the NMR structures of the separated transmembrane and cytoplasmic domains,[894] and the structure of the complex between the β_3 cytoplasmic domain and the talin F3 domain (PDB 2H7E).[896] The structure in (C) is based on crystal structure of the liganded receptor (PDB 2VDN) headpiece,[827] the extended structure of ectodomain (PDB3FCS),[250] and the monomeric transmembrane structures connected to unstructured cytosolic tails. **B.** Domain structure of structure of integrin $\alpha_{IIb}\beta_3$. The individual domains and the ligand binding pocket are identified in the model of the extended integrin. I-EGF, Integrin epidermal growth factor; PSI, plexins, semaphorins, integrins. **C.** The integrin transmembrane complex. Selected views of the NMR structure of the α_{IIb} (red) and β_3 (blue) transmembrane complex. The *left* panel depicts contacts involved in the outer membrane clasp and the *right* panel depicts the contacts involved in the inner membrane clasp. Note that after the integrin α_{IIb} helical region ends at V990, the next 5 residues (GFFKR) reenter the membrane; the two aromatic F residues make hydrophobic contacts with β_3 and α_{IIb} R995 makes a salt bridge with integrin β_3 D723. (A, reproduced with permission from Lau TL, Kim C, Ginsberg MH, et al: The structure of the integrin alphaIIbbeta3 transmembrane complex explains integrin transmembrane signalling. EMBO J 28(9):1351–1361, 2009. B, reproduced with permission from Zhu, J, et al: Structure of a complete integrin ectodomain in a physiologic resting state and activation and deactivation by applied forces. Mol Cell 32(6):849–861, 2008. C, reproduced with permission from Lau TL, Kim C, Ginsberg MH, et al: The structure of the integrin alphaIIbbeta3 transmembrane complex explains integrin transmembrane signalling. EMBO J 28(9):1351–1361, 2009.)

protein with four characteristic divalent cation-binding sites (see Fig. 112–11). The mature protein contains 1008 amino acids[43,854] with one transmembrane domain; during processing, it is cleaved into a heavy chain and a light chain connected by a disulfide bond. The β subunit, β_3, contains 762 amino acids and is rich in cysteine residues, with a characteristic cysteine-rich region near its transmembrane domain.[43,855] The integrin α_{IIb} and β_3 cytoplasmic tails consist of 20 and 47 amino acids, respectively. The genes coding for α_{IIb} and β_3 are very close to each other on chromosome 17 at q21.32, but are not so close as to share common regulatory domains.[856,857] Both proteins are synthesized in megakaryocytes and join to form a calcium-dependent, noncovalent complex in the rough endoplasmic reticulum.[858] Calnexin probably serves as a chaperone for integrin α_{IIb},[859] but it is unclear which chaperone(s) are involved in integrin β_3 folding and/or integrin $\alpha_{IIb}\beta_3$ complex formation. The integrin $\alpha_{IIb}\beta_3$ complex subsequently undergoes further processing in the Golgi apparatus, where the carbohydrate structures undergo maturation and the pro-GPIIb molecule is cleaved into its heavy and light chains by furin or a similar enzyme.[860,861] Approximately 15 percent of the mass of both integrins α_{IIb} and β_3 are composed of carbohydrate.[862] The mature integrin $\alpha_{IIb}\beta_3$ complex is then transported to the plasma membrane or the membranes of α granules or dense bodies. If integrins α_{IIb} and β_3 do not form a proper complex, either because of a structural abnormality in either subunit or the failure to synthesize one of the subunits, the subunit(s) that are synthesized are rapidly degraded and so are not expressed on the membrane surface (Chap. 121). Degradation of integrin α_{IIb} appears to involve retro-translocation from the endoplasmic reticulum into the cytoplasm, ubiquitination, and proteolysis by the megakaryocyte proteasome.[859]

Both integrins α_{IIb} and β_3 are composed of a series of domains (see Fig. 112–11). The aminoterminal region of integrin α_{IIb} contains a seven-blade β-propeller domain, and each blade is composed of four β strands connected by loops. The propeller interacts with the βA (I-like) domain of integrin β_3, forming the globular head region observed in electron micrographs. The four calcium ions bound by the propeller domain interact with β hairpin loops in blades four to seven that extend away from the interface with integrin β_3. In addition, there is a unique integrin α_{IIb} cap subdomain made up of four loops from blades one to three that are unique to α_{IIb} and contribute to its ligand binding specificity. The remainder of the extracellular components of integrin α_{IIb} are made up of a thigh, genu (knee-like), and two calf domains,[250] much like the structure of the related integrin α_v subunit.[841,844] The cytoplasmic domain of integrin α_{IIb} interacts with the cytoplasmic domain of integrin β_3 and the interaction is important in controlling activation of the holoreceptor.[863–866] The cytoplasmic domain of integrin α_{IIb} has a GFFKR sequence near the membrane that is thought to control inside-out activation of the integrin receptors because mutations or deletions in this region result in the receptor adopting a conformation with high affinity for fibrinogen.[867–871] A number of studies using mutagenesis and nuclear magnetic resonance (NMR) identified different structures for the transmembrane and cytoplasmic domains, and differences in the relative roles of heterodimeric and homodimeric associations.[864,872–875] Disrupting the conformation of this region also results in a constitutively high-affinity receptor,[876,877] which has led to the conclusion that inside-out activation of integrin $\alpha_{IIb}\beta_3$ requires separation of the transmembrane and cytoplasmic domains, but it remains possible that more subtle changes in the cytoplasmic and transmembrane domains may be sufficient.[848]

The integrin β_3 subunit domains are not linearly arranged because the first domain (PSI [plexins, semaphorins, and integrins]) was subjected to the insertion of a hybrid domain, which itself was subjected to the insertion of a βA (I-like) domain; the latter domain is homologous to the VWF A domain and integrin I domains, both of which bind ligands (see Fig. 112–11).[827,878] The double insertion in the PSI

domain explains why there is a "long range" disulfide bond extending from C13 to C435; thus, even though the βA domain makes contact with the integrin α_{IIb} propeller (via Arg261 and other residues that interact with two rings of hydrophobic residues in the integrin α_{IIb} "cage"), it is not the aminoterminus of the molecule. The PSI domain contains Leu33, which defines the Pl^{A1} (HPA-1a) specificity, as opposed to the alloantigen Pl^{A2} (HPA-1b), which is produced by a Pro33 polymorphism (Chap. 137). The integrin β_3 leg is composed of four integrin EGF domains that are rich in disulfide bonds. In the crystal structure, this region interacts with the integrin α_{IIb} stalk region and the globular head in the bent, unactivated receptor, but these interactions are less prominent in the three-dimensional reconstruction of the inactive receptor not in the activated receptor.[250,827,848] Mutations in the integrin EGF domains, including cysteine residues, can activate the receptor as can the binding of monoclonal antibodies.[879–882] The importance of the normal disulfide bond pairings in integrin β_3 is further supported by data demonstrating that certain reducing agents can cause activation of integrin $\alpha_{IIb}\beta_3$, fibrinogen binding, and platelet aggregation,[883,884] and an enzyme capable of catalyzing the exchange of thiol groups and disulfide in proteins (PDI) has been identified on the surface of platelets and in platelet releasates.[883,885–887] Thiol-disulfide exchange in integrins $\alpha_{IIb}\beta_3$ and $\alpha_v\beta_3$ is implicated as a contributor to clot retraction.[888] Moreover, regions in integrin β_3 itself have the same consensus sequence (CGXC) present in PDI that is thought to mediate the catalysis.[889] One model suggests that integrin $\alpha_{IIb}\beta_3$ can achieve a low level of activation without alterations in disulfide bonds, but that maximal activation requires PDI or similar activity along with a source of thiols such as plasma glutathione or a membrane NAD(P)H oxidoreductase system.[883] Inhibition of PDI and other enzymes that mediate thiol-disulfide exchange (ERp57, ERp5) reduces platelet thrombus formation.[890,891] It is still unclear, however, whether disulfide bond alterations contribute to activation *in vivo* under physiologic or pathologic conditions.

Transmembrane domain structures of integrin α_{IIb} and integrin β_3 have been proposed based on NMR and structural modeling studies.[871,873,874,892–896] Because the integrin α_{IIb} transmembrane helix is shorter than the integrin β_3 helix, they traverse the membrane at an angle of approximately 25 degrees. The association of the integrin α_{IIb} and integrin β_3 ectodomains near the site of entry into the membrane results in the transmembrane helices being directly juxtaposed in the region of the membrane closest to the ectodomain (outer membrane clasp). Near the cytoplasmic end of the membrane the helices are held together by an inner membrane clasp composed of the integrin α_{IIb} residues immediately after the end of the helix (GFFKR), with the membrane reimmersion of F992 and F993 filling the gap and interacting with integrin β_3 W715 and I719, with integrin α_{IIb} R995 creating a salt bridge with integrin β_3 723 and perhaps residue 726.[897,898] Of note, these regions are conserved in many other integrins receptors and so the basic mechanism may be common to many of the receptors.

Inside-out signaling is accomplished by the talin F3 domain binding to the integrin β_3 cytoplasmic domain, which is proposed to disrupt the inner membrane clasp.[34,244,245,863,865,866,869,870,872,876,892,899,900] This may be facilitated by migfilin displacing filamin from the integrin β_3 cytoplasmic domain as the latter interaction may prevent talin binding.[901] Talin binding results in dissociation of the transmembrane helices and reorganization of the cytoplasmic region of integrin β_3 into a more extended helix. Integrin $\alpha_{IIb}\beta_3$ ectodomain chain separation, headpiece extension, and integrin β_3 swing out then follow, either spontaneously or as a result of the traction force generated by the cytoskeleton on integrin β_3 through talin.[149] Outside-in signaling is presumed to be initiated by loss of ectodomain interactions between the membrane-proximal regions of integrins α_{IIb} and β_3, perhaps as a result of ligand binding producing even greater integrin β_3 swing out, resulting in disruption of the outer membrane clasp and subsequent dissociation of the transmembrane helices. This potentially may facilitate the interaction of the cytoplasmic domains with cytoskeletal elements and signaling molecules.

The integrin β_3 tail also contains two NXXY motifs and Y747 and Y759 within one of these motifs are phosphorylated upon platelet aggregation, thus producing docking sites for signaling molecules.[235] Studies in mice and in recombinant systems demonstrate a role for the sites in clot retraction and platelet aggregate stability.[291,902]

A number of proteins have been shown to bind to the cytoplasmic domains of integrin α_{IIb} and/or β_3, either directly or through interactions with other proteins, including signaling molecules (Src, Shc, FAK, paxillin, and ILK, all of which bind to integrin β_3), cytoskeletal proteins (kindlin-3, skelemin, α-actin, and myosin, which bind to integrin β_3, and filamin and talin, which bind to integrins α_{IIb} and/or β_3), and other proteins (β_3-endonexin and CD98, which bind to integrin β_3, and CIB and calreticulin, which bind to α_{IIb}) (Fig. 112–12).[244,866,903–919] These interactions are important in mediating inside-out signaling and outside-in signaling.[235] JAM-A is a negative regulator of outside-in activation by integrin $\alpha_{IIb}\beta_3$ that acts by regulating activation of Src.[920] Similarly, PECAM-1 serves as an inhibitor of integrin $\alpha_{IIb}\beta_3$ activation through a sequential phosphorylation mechanism.[921,922] Force on the integrin β_3 cytoplasmic domain by actin–myosin action may supply the energy for the conformational change in integrin $\alpha_{IIb}\beta_3$ from bent to extended.[250]

The junction between the integrin α_{IIb} propeller and the β_3 βA (I-like) domain is the site of ligand binding to integrin $\alpha_{IIb}\beta_3$ (see Fig. 112–11). This region of integrin β_3 contains three divalent cation binding sites: MIDAS (metal ion-dependent adhesion site), ADMIDAS (adjacent to MIDAS), and SyMBS (synergy metal binding site).[250] The latter was previously termed the ligand-associated metal binding site (LIMBS) based on the crystal structure of integrin $\alpha_V\beta_3$.[844,845]

The crystal structure of integrin $\alpha_V\beta_3$ demonstrated that an RGD peptide bound primarily via interactions between the Arg in the peptide and two Asp residues (D150 and D218) in integrin α_V and between the Asp in the peptide and the MIDAS cation.[845] The binding pocket in integrin $\alpha_{IIb}\beta_3$ is similar but differs in that only one Asp in integrin α_{IIb} (D224) is available to interact with an Arg (or Lys as in the fibrinogen γ-chain peptide), the distance between D224 in integrin α_{IIb} and the MIDAS cation is longer, and a cap subdomain of the integrin α_{IIb} propeller contributes Phe160 to a hydrophobic exosite in combination with Tyr190.[149,827] As a result, the pocket is able to accommodate the longer

fibrinogen γ-chain C-terminal peptide better, with the peptide's Asp and C-terminal Val carboxyls interacting with the MIDAS and ADMIDAS cations, respectively.[826] It also explains why integrin $\alpha_{IIb}\beta_3$ can bind peptides containing the longer Lys residue (KGD peptides).[923] Crystal structures are also available for the integrin $\alpha_{IIb}\beta_3$ receptor with the drugs eptifibatide and tirofiban, which are effective antithrombotic agents because of their ability to block ligand binding to integrin $\alpha_{IIb}\beta_3$, and demonstrate specificity for integrin $\alpha_{IIb}\beta_3$ compared to integrin $\alpha_V\beta_3$.[827] The basis of the specificity of these agents involves in part their interaction with the integrin α_{IIb}-specific exosite and the greater length between their positive and negative charges.[827] The third integrin $\alpha_{IIb}\beta_3$ antagonist drug, abciximab, is a chimeric murine monoclonal antibody Fab fragment. Its epitope has been localized to a region on integrin β_3 very close to the MIDAS, suggesting that it works by steric interference with ligand binding, disruption of the binding pocket, or both mechanisms.

Two major conformational changes in integrin $\alpha_{IIb}\beta_3$ have been described in association with activation: headpiece extension and integrin β_3 hybrid and PSI domain swing-out (see Fig. 112–11).[250,827,853] Headpiece extension can contribute to ligand binding by enhancing access to the binding site; it can also contribute to platelet aggregation by extending the receptor out further from the platelet surface,[924] thus facilitating the ability of fibrinogen to bridge between platelets.[846] The integrin β_3 hybrid and PSI domain swing-out motion appears to enhance ligand binding, but the precise mechanism is unclear.[826,847,850] Swing-out is associated with movement of the ADMIDAS metal ion and the α_1-β_1 loop toward the MIDAS with the latter movement stabilized by the interaction of two backbone nitrogens in the α_1-β_1 loop with the ligand carboxyl oxygen, thus reinforcing the binding to the MIDAS metal ion.[149,826] Mutations that produce swing-out of the hybrid and PSI domains result in constitutive ligand binding to integrin $\alpha_{IIb}\beta_3$.[925]

Binding of fibrinogen to platelet integrin $\alpha_{IIb}\beta_3$ leads to platelet aggregation, presumably via crosslinking of integrin molecules on two different platelets by fibrinogen.[840] The dimeric and relatively rigid structure of fibrinogen, and the location of the binding sites at the ends of the γ chains are all consistent with such a model as the two binding sites on a single fibrinogen molecule are probably more than 45 nm apart. Soon after fibrinogen binds, it can be dissociated from the platelet by chelating the divalent cations, but the binding becomes irreversible within an hour.[835] Fibrinogen binding alone is not sufficient for platelet aggregation, but the events necessary after fibrinogen binding, which

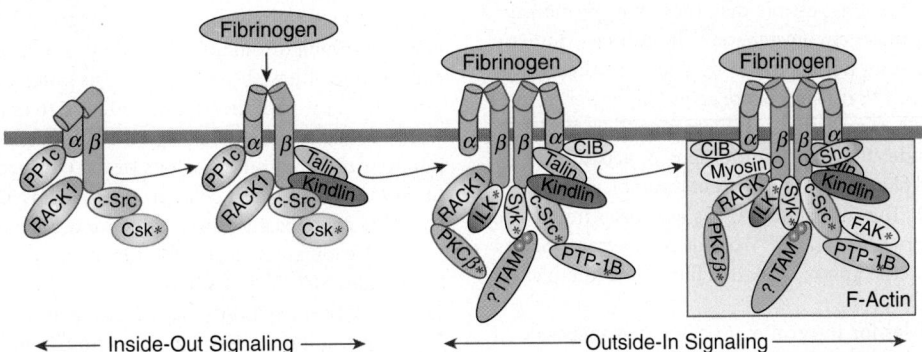

Figure 112–12. Protein interactions with the cytoplasmic domains of $\alpha_{IIb}\beta_3$ regulate inside-out and outside-in signaling. Shown are some, but not all, of the proteins reported to associate with the $\alpha_{IIb}\beta_3$ cytoplasmic domains, many in a dynamic fashion. Some are associated with resting platelets, while others are recruited to, or dissociate from, the integrin during inside-out or outside-in signaling, leading to F-actin assembly. In addition, several proteins with enzymatic function become activated *(asterisks)* after fibrinogen binding to $\alpha_{IIb}\beta_3$. Not shown are the many additional adapter molecules, enzymes, and substrates that may become recruited through more indirect interactions. CIB, calcium and integrin-binding 1; Csk, c-Src tyrosine kinase; ILK, integrin-linked kinase; ITAM, a yet-to-be identified protein with one or more immunoreceptor tyrosine activation motifs; PKCβ, protein kinase Cβ; PP1c, protein phosphatase 1c; RACK1, receptor for activated C kinase 1; Syk, spleen tyrosine kinase. *(Reproduced with permission from Coller, B.S. and S.J. Shattil, The GPIIb/IIIa (integrin alphaIIbbeta3) odyssey: A technology-driven saga of a receptor with twists, turns, and even a bend. Blood 112(8):3011–3025, 2008.)*

probably include ligand- and/or cytoskeletal-mediated receptor clustering, are not well understood.[95,835,926,927] After ligands bind to integrin $\alpha_{IIb}\beta_3$, "outside-in" signaling through the integrin can occur, resulting in a number of phosphorylation events, changes in the platelet cytoskeleton, platelet spreading, and even initiation of protein translation.[236,237,928]

In addition to fibrinogen, several other proteins can bind to integrin $\alpha_{IIb}\beta_3$ on activated platelets, including VWF, fibronectin, vitronectin, thrombospondin, and prothrombin[390,675,929]; each of these contains an RGD sequence in the region implicated in the initial interaction with platelets. There are subtle differences in the binding of each of these ligands, however, with regard to divalent cation preference and competent activating agents. The binding of all of these other ligands can also be inhibited by RGD-containing peptides, indicating a common requirement for the interaction between the RGD sequence in the protein and the RGD-binding site in integrin $\alpha_{IIb}\beta_3$.[930,931]

Platelet aggregation measured in the aggregometer *ex vivo* depends upon fibrinogen binding to integrin $\alpha_{IIb}\beta_3$. It is less clear whether fibrinogen is the most important ligand supporting platelet aggregation *in vivo* since studies performed in model systems under flowing conditions indicate that VWF is the major ligand at higher shear rates.[932] Even in the aggregometer, VWF can partially substitute for fibrinogen if the fibrinogen concentration is very low.[933] *In vivo*, mice deficient in both VWF and fibrinogen still make platelet thrombi in response to vascular injury.[934–936] Although fibronectin was initially implicated in supporting the development of such thrombi, mice deficient in fibrinogen, VWF, and fibronectin have paradoxically increased platelet aggregation and thrombus formation, suggesting that fibronectin may play an inhibiting role in thrombus formation under certain circumstances.[373]

Although resting platelets do not bind soluble fibrinogen (or other adhesive glycoproteins) to an appreciable extent, they can adhere to fibrinogen immobilized on a surface.[825,937] This activation-independent adhesion may be from alterations in the structure of fibrinogen when it is immobilized on a surface.[836,938] Alternatively, there may always be a few integrin $\alpha_{IIb}\beta_3$ receptors that are transiently in the proper conformation to bind fibrinogen, and immobilization may result in high local density of fibrinogen and favorable kinetics for adhesion. Finally, it is possible that even low-affinity fibrinogen interactions with integrin $\alpha_{IIb}\beta_3$ are sufficient to initiate integrin interactions with the cytoskeleton such that actin-myosin-induced contraction provides the energy required for the conformational changes needed to achieve higher affinity binding.[250]

Fibrinogen and/or fibrin have been identified on the surface of damaged blood vessels; thus it is possible that integrin $\alpha_{IIb}\beta_3$ mediates platelet adhesion under those circumstances.[939] In contrast, integrin $\alpha_{IIb}\beta_3$ on resting platelets does not appear to be able to mediate adhesion to VWF or fibronectin[940]; if platelets are activated, however, integrin $\alpha_{IIb}\beta_3$ can support adhesion to these glycoproteins.[930] In models of platelet accumulation under flowing conditions, $\alpha_{IIb}\beta_3$ acts in synergy with GPIb/IX, VWF, and fibrinogen at the apex of thrombi, where shear forces are greatest.[28,941,942] The integrin $\alpha_{IIb}\beta_3$ has also been implicated in platelet spreading after adhesion,[227,228,943] and it is necessary for clot retraction (see above) and the uptake of plasma fibrinogen into platelet α granules.[818,944]

Less-well-defined roles for integrin $\alpha_{IIb}\beta_3$ have been suggested in the binding of plasminogen,[688] calcium transport across the platelet membrane,[945–947] IgE binding to platelets leading to parasite cytotoxicity,[948] and interactions with the *Borrelia* species spirochetes that cause Lyme disease[949] and hantavirus.[950] Integrin $\alpha_{IIb}\beta_3$ also mediates factor XIIIa binding to platelets, but this is primarily as a result of factor XIII's association with fibrinogen.[456] Factor XIIIa and calpain have also been implicated in limiting platelet–platelet interactions after activation by adhesion to collagen.[951]

Integrin $\alpha_2\beta_1$ (Also Termed GPIa/IIa, Collagen Receptor, VLA-2 and CD49b/CD29)

Integrin $\alpha_2\beta_1$ (GPIa/IIa) is widely distributed on different cell types and can mediate adhesion to collagen.[19,20,952–957] The integrin α_2 subunit (GPIa) contains a region of 220 amino acids inserted in the aminoterminal β-propeller region (I domain) that is homologous to similar regions in other proteins that are known to interact with collagen, including VWF and cartilage matrix protein.[958] This region has a MIDAS and crystallographic data of the α_2 I domain in complex with a CRP containing the type I collagen sequence GFOGER (where O indicates hydroxyproline) demonstrated that the glutamic acid in the peptide coordinates Mg^{2+} binding in the MIDAS.[959–961] The integrin $\alpha_2\beta_1$ I domain can assume a variety of conformations, going from inactive (closed), through intermediate or low affinity, to active high affinity.[952,962]

Both integrin $\alpha_2\beta_1$ and GPVI appear to participate in platelet interactions with collagen.[963–965] Bleeding defects have been described in patients with decreased levels of integrin $\alpha_2\beta_1$ and GPVI, but the precise contributions of the decreases in these receptors is uncertain (Chap. 121). Although integrin $\alpha_2\beta_1$ is capable of supporting adhesion to collagen without exogenous activators, like integrin $\alpha_{IIb}\beta_3$, it appears to be able to increase its affinity for ligand in response to inside-out activation.[966,967] Potential initiators of integrin $\alpha_2\beta_1$ activation include signaling after GPVI interaction with collagen and GPIb-mediated adhesion to VWF, perhaps acting via actin polymerization.[959,968–970] Thus, one possible scenario is that following GPIb-mediated adhesion to VWF and collagen adhesion and activation mediated by GPVI, integrin $\alpha_2\beta_1$ may promote firm adhesion to collagen, stabilize thrombus growth on collagen, and promote procoagulant activity.[971,972] In addition, the affinity of integrin $\alpha_2\beta_1$ may also be modulated by alterations in disulfide bonds since inhibition of platelet PDI and sulfhydryl blocking agents inhibit integrin $\alpha_2\beta_1$-mediated platelet adhesion to type I collagen and to the related peptide GFOGER.[883,973] The state of the collagen may also influence whether integrin $\alpha_2\beta_1$ or GPVI mediates the interaction with collagen, because GPVI appears to mediate adhesion to fibrillar collagen whereas integrin $\alpha_2\beta_1$ preferentially adheres to collagen that has been treated with partial protease digestion.[28,974]

Ligand binding to integrin $\alpha_2\beta_1$ is enhanced in the presence of magnesium or manganese and is inhibited by calcium, and thus the conditions in human blood, where calcium concentrations are higher than those of magnesium, do not provide optimal cation concentrations for the receptor's function.[975] Integrin $\alpha_2\beta_1$ can, however, mediate platelet adhesion to collagen in heparinized blood[956,975] and inhibitors of integrin $\alpha_2\beta_1$ inhibit thrombus formation in animal models.[976–978] Regions of collagen type I have been implicated as potential binding sites for integrin $\alpha_2\beta_1$[979]; the peptide sequence 502 to 516 of collagen type I α_1 chain, which contains a Gly-Glu-Arg (GER) sequence, may be of particular importance,[980] but other regions of the collagen molecule may also be important.[981] In type III collagen, amino acids 522 to 528 of fragment α_1 (III) CB4 contains a binding region for $\alpha_2\beta_1$.[982]

Three different alleles for the integrin α_2 gene, which differ at nucleotides 807 (T or C) and 1648 (G or A), have been described.[983] The 807 substitution does not affect the amino acid sequence, but the 1648 substitution causes a change from Glu to Lys, resulting in the Br^b and Br^a alloantigens (HPA-5a and HPA-5b) (Chap. 137). Allele 1 (T-G) is present in 39 percent of individuals, allele 2 (C-G) in 53 percent, and allele 3 (C-A) in 7 percent.[984,985] Individuals with allele 1 have higher integrin $\alpha_2\beta_1$ platelet density than individuals with allele 2, and individuals with allele 3 have the lowest density; the density of integrin $\alpha_2\beta_1$ correlates with platelet deposition on collagen under flow. The association of these polymorphisms with cardiovascular disease morbidity and mortality, including the risk of developing MI[986,987] and stroke,[988] has been extensively study without firm conclusions, although there is some suggestion that they may be associated with cardiovascular risk.[983,989–992]

Integrin $\alpha_2\beta_1$ is probably linked to the membrane skeleton.[993] Its ligand specificity appears to be determined by the cell on which it is expressed, since on endothelial cells it functions as a laminin receptor as well as a collagen receptor.[994,995] Engagement of integrin $\alpha_2\beta_1$ is capable of initiating platelet protein synthesis.[236] Integrin $\alpha_2\beta_1$ has been implicated in megakaryocyte development and platelet formation. In particular, loss of activated integrin $\alpha_2\beta_1$ receptors on the surface of megakaryocytes, as a result of interacting with collagen, has been implicated in the transition from the marrow to the peripheral circulation,[967] and conditional targeting of megakaryocyte and platelet integrin $\alpha_2\beta_1$ in mice is associated with reduced MPV.[996]

Integrin $\alpha_5\beta_1$ (Also Termed GPIc*/IIa, Fibronectin Receptor, VLA-5 and CD49e/CD29)

Integrin $\alpha_5\beta_1$ is a receptor that is expressed on a wide variety of different cells and mediates adhesion to fibronectin.[804,819,820] It is important for interactions with extracellular matrix, and data from cells other than platelets indicate a role for this receptor in developmental biology and metastasis formation. The RGD sequence in fibronectin is crucial for cell adhesion, but other regions in fibronectin probably also contribute. RGD-containing peptides can inhibit cell adhesion mediated by integrin $\alpha_5\beta_1$. As with other integrin receptors, adhesion depends on the presence of divalent cations. Integrin $\alpha_5\beta_1$ is competent to mediate adhesion of resting platelets to fibronectin,[997,998] but its affinity may be modulated by activation.[999] The biologic role of this receptor on platelets is not clear. Although it may be involved in hemostasis and/or thrombosis, it is also possible that its function is primarily related to megakaryocyte binding to marrow matrix and proplatelet formation.[1000] Integrin $\alpha_5\beta_1$ is not the only fibronectin receptor on platelets, since with appropriate activation, integrin $\alpha_{IIb}\beta_3$ can also bind fibronectin.[804,1001]

Integrin $\alpha_6\beta_1$ (Also Termed GPIc/IIa, Laminin Receptor, VLA-6 and CD49f/CD29)

Platelet adhesion to select laminins, which are variably found in basement membranes and extracellular matrix, can be mediated by integrin $\alpha_6\beta_1$.[804,1002–1004] Because VWF can bind to some laminins, GPIb can also contribute to platelet adhesion to laminin.[1002] This adhesion is best demonstrated with magnesium and manganese; calcium does not support adhesion. This receptor is competent on resting platelets, but its role in platelet physiology is not clear. Mice deficient in integrin $\alpha_6\beta_1$ do not bleed pathologically but are protected against thrombosis.[1002] The integrin appears to be able to signal in platelets via PI3 kinase to induce morphologic changes.[1005] An approximate Mr 67,000 laminin receptor has also been identified on platelets; this receptor is present on other cells as well.[1006]

Integrin $\alpha_v\beta_3$ (Also Termed Vitronectin Receptor and CD51/CD61)

Integrin $\alpha_v\beta_3$ receptor shares the same β subunit as integrin $\alpha_{IIb}\beta3$ (GPIIb/IIIa) (see Fig. 112–11).[804,855,1007–1009] The integrin α_v and α_{IIb} subunits display 36 percent sequence identity.[1010] Integrin $\alpha_v\beta_3$ differs dramatically, however, from integrin $\alpha_{IIb}\beta_3$ in its platelet surface density, because there are only approximately 50 to 100 integrin $\alpha_v\beta_3$ receptors per platelet.[1011] The crystal structure of the external domains of integrin $\alpha_v\beta_3$ alone and in complex with a peptide containing the RGD cell recognition sequence found in a number of ligands have been solved at high resolution.[844,845] Such RGD peptides inhibit ligand binding to integrin $\alpha_v\beta_3$. The most important findings were: (1) the receptor adopts a bent conformation in which the globular headpiece composed of the

N-terminal β-propeller region of α_v and the βA (I-like) domain of integrin β_3, lies near the legs of the integrin α_v and β_3 subunits, and (2) the RGD peptide binds to the headpiece with the Arg (R) making contact with integrin α_v and the Asp (D) making contact with the MIDAS domain in β_3. Current evidence suggests that the bent conformation is the inactive one and that activation results in extension of the headpiece and pivoting between the integrin β_3, βA and hybrid domains in association with leg separation.[827,843,1007,1009] Integrin $\alpha_v\beta_3$ can mediate adhesion to vitronectin, but only in the presence of magnesium or manganese, not calcium.[1011] It can also mediate interactions with fibrinogen, VWF, prothrombin, and thrombospondin.[389,1012–1015] Platelet stimulation can activate integrin $\alpha_v\beta_3$, analogous to activation of integrins $\alpha_{IIb}\beta_3$ and $\alpha_2\beta_1$. Activated integrin $\alpha_v\beta_3$ may uniquely mediate adhesion to osteopontin, a protein found in high concentrations in atherosclerotic plaque.[1016] The receptor's role in platelet physiology is not defined, but it may contribute to the development of platelet coagulant activity.[1017]

The integrin $\alpha_v\beta_3$ receptor is also present on endothelial cells,[822,1013] osteoclasts,[1018] smooth muscle cells and other cells; it has been implicated in bone resorption,[1019–1021] endothelial–matrix interactions,[822,1013] lymphoid cell apoptosis,[1022] neovascularization,[1023] tumor angiogenesis,[1023–1025] intimal hyperplasia after vascular injury,[1026–1028] sickle cell disease,[1029–1031] focal segmental glomerulosclerosis[1032,1033] and scleroderma.[1034]

The presence or absence of integrin $\alpha_v\beta_3$ on the platelets of patients with Glanzmann thrombasthenia can help localize the abnormality to either integrin α_{IIb} (if integrin $\alpha_v\beta_3$ is present in normal or increased amounts) or integrin β_3 (if integrin $\alpha_v\beta_3$ is reduced or absent) (Chap. 121).

LEUCINE-RICH REPEAT GLYCOPROTEIN RECEPTORS

GPIb/GPIX/V (CD42)

GPIb is composed of GPIbα (CD42b) (610 amino acids) disulfide-bonded to two GPIbβ subunits (CD42c) (122 amino acids).[801,1035–1043] GPIb appears to exist on the surface of platelets in a 1:1 complex with GPIX (160 amino acids) and a 2:1 complex with GPV (Fig. 112–13). The GPIbα gene is on the short arm of chromosome 17 and the GPIbβ gene is on the long arm of chromosome 22. The GPIX gene is on the long arm of chromosome 3.[1044–1046] GPIX is required for efficient surface expression of GPIb,[1047] but beyond that, its function is unknown. GPIb/IX is expressed on megakaryocytes and platelets; there is controversy as to whether GPIb/IX is expressed on endothelial cells, either constitutively or after cytokine activation.[802] The promoters for GPIb/IX lack TATA or CAAT boxes, but contain binding sites for the GATA and ETS families of transcription factors, which, along with the expression of the cofactor FOG (friend of GATA-1), may account for the limited expression of GPIb/IX.[1048–1056]

A genetic polymorphism in GPIbα affects the number of repeating 13-amino-acid units (1, 2, 3, or 4) and produces changes in the molecular weight of GPIbα.[1057] The 2 repeat variant is most common, but there is considerable ethnic variation in the frequency of the different numbers of repeats. This molecular weight polymorphism has been linked to the Sib and Ko alloantigens, which have been localized to a T→M variation at amino acid 145 of GPIbα, with M associated with either 3 or 4 repeats and T associated with either 1 or 2 repeats.[984] Some, but not all reports suggest an association between the alleles with the larger number of repeats and vascular disease.[983,991,1058,1059] Two other GPIbα polymorphisms have been described: (1) C or T at position –5 from the ATG start codon (RS system), and (2) a nucleotide dimorphism at the third bases of the codon for Arg 358.[1038,1060,1061] A C at position –5 is

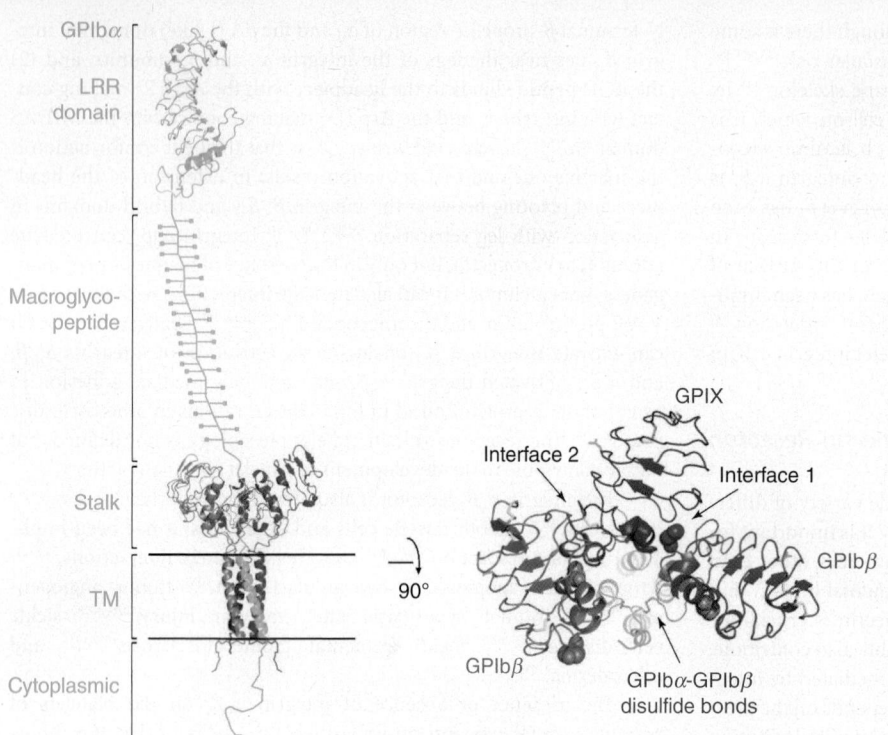

Figure 112–13. The organization of GPIb/IX complex. GPIbα *(green)*, GPIbβ *(blue)*, and GPIX *(purple)* subunits are colored differently. *Left:* A cartoon illustration of the GPIb/IX complex largely drawn in ribbon diagrams. Various parts of GPIbα are labeled on the left. *Right:* The top view of the membrane-proximal portion of GPIb/IX that contains the stalk region of GPIbα, the extracellular domains of GPIbβ and GPIX, and a portion of the transmembrane (TM) helical bundle. The disulfide bonds between GPIbα and GPIbβ are highlighted in *red*. Side chains of Tyr106 in GPIbβ are shown in *blue spheres*, one of which is located at the interface 1 between GPIbβ and GPIX. Residue Pro74 in GPIbβ are shown in *orange spheres*, one of which is located at or close to the interface 2. *(Reproduced with permission from Li R and Emsley J: The organizing principle of the platelet glycoprotein Ib-IX-V complex, J Thromb Haemost 2013 Apr;11(4):605-614.)*

present in only 8 to 17 percent of individuals, and more closely resembles the sequence surrounding the ATG start codon (Kozak sequence) considered optimal for translation. In fact, this polymorphism is associated with higher levels of platelet surface GPIb, and may be a risk factor for ischemic vascular disease.[1062-1070] GPIb has been implicated as a target antigen in autoimmune thrombocytopenia and in quinine and quinidine-induced thrombocytopenia (Chap. 117).

GPIbα has a large number of O-linked carbohydrate chains terminating in sialic acid residues,[1071] and the latter contribute significantly to the negative charge of the platelet membrane.[215] Electron micrographic analysis indicates that GPIb exists as a long flexible rod (approximately 60 nm) with two globular domains of approximately 9 and 16 nm.[1072] Thus, GPIb probably extends much further out from the platelet's surface than does integrin $\alpha_{IIb}\beta_3$, which may account for its primacy in platelet adhesion, as well as the increased risk of cardiovascular disease in individuals with longer GPIb molecules because of an increased number of 13-amino-acid repeats. The long extension may also make it susceptible to conformational changes induced by shear forces.[801] The extracellular region of GPIbα is readily cleaved by a variety of proteases, including platelet calpains,[1073] yielding a soluble fragment named *glycocalicin* that circulates in normal plasma at 1 to 3 mg/L.[1074] *In vivo*, platelet shedding of glycocalicin from GPIbα is mediated by a disintegrin and metalloprotease (ADAM)-17 (also termed TACE) cleaving a juxtamembrane sequence[1075,1076]; shedding is controlled by GPIbβ interactions with an unidentified protein, calpain, and reactive oxygen species.[1077-1079] Levels of plasma glycocalicin correlate with platelet production and thus can been used to differentiate thrombocytopenia based on decreased platelet production from thrombocytopenia as a result of increased platelet destruction.[1080-1085]

GPIbβ and GPIX have free sulfhydryl groups in their cytoplasmic domains that undergo palmitoylation, at least in part, further anchoring the protein to the membrane.[1086,1087] The penultimate serine residue at the C-terminus of GPIbα is phosphorylated, providing an attachment site for the signal-complex protein 14–3–3ζ.[1088] Similarly, GPIbβ can

undergo phosphorylation of Ser 166 in its cytoplasmic domain as a result of protein kinase A activation via cAMP, providing another binding site for 14–3–3ζ (see Fig. 112–13).[1089-1091] The cytoplasmic domain of GPIbα connects GPIb to filamin A (actin-binding protein), thus connecting GPIb to the platelet cytoskeleton.[993,1092,1093] Coordinated expression of GPIbα and filamin is required for efficient expression of both proteins and imbalances result in abnormalities in platelet size.[1094,1095] Alterations in the cytoskeleton can affect GPIb functional activity.[1096-1098] 14–3–3ζ can bind PI3 kinase and has been implicated in GPIb-mediated intracellular signaling that results in integrin $\alpha_{IIb}\beta_3$ activation; Lyn; Vav, Rac1, Alet, and Lim kinase-1 also have been implicated in GPIb/IX–mediated signaling.[9,1099-1101] GPIb also appears to be in close proximity to FcγRIIA and the Fc receptor γ-chain, two receptors that can initiate signaling via tyrosine phosphorylation of their cytoplasmic ITAM sequences by Src family kinases and recruitment of the tyrosine kinase syk.[1102-1105] Engagement of GPIb by VWF may lead to clustering of GPIb-IX–V complexes in glycolipid-enriched microdomains or lipid rafts, which may serve to concentrate signaling molecules; clustering also increases ligand avidity.[1106]

GPIbα has eight leucine-rich repeats in the aminoterminal region of its extracellular domain, whereas GPIbβ and GPIX have one each.[1039,1042,1045] These repeats are consensus sequences of 24 amino acids with seven regularly spaced leucines; well-defined disulfide loop sequences flank the repeats.[801] Similar leucine-rich repeats are present in a variety of other proteins.

Crystal structures of the N-terminus of GPIbα (amino acid residue 1–305) alone, and in complex with native and mutated A1 domains of VWF provide important information on the interactions between these proteins (Fig. 112–14).[1107,1108] This region of GPIbα adopts a curved shape made up of an N-terminal β-hairpin flanking sequence (finger) containing a C4-C17 disulfide loop (H1-D18), eight leucine-rich repeats (K19-W204), a β-switch region (V227-S241), and a C-terminal sulfated anionic region (D269-D287), with Y276, Y278, and Y279 undergoing posttranslation sulfation.[1108-1110] The VWF-A1 domain,

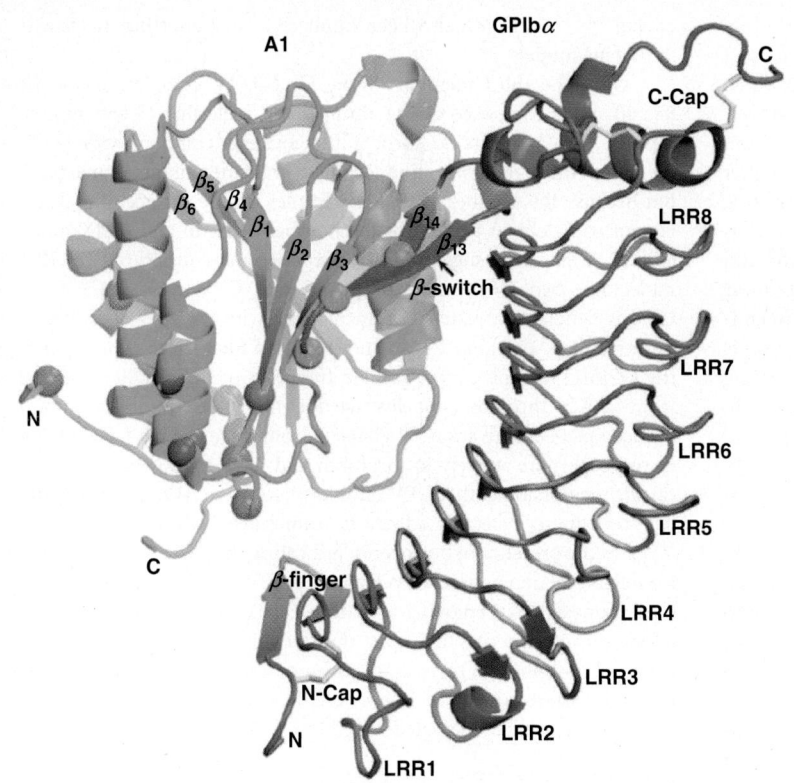

Figure 112–14. Structural, binding, and mutational features of the A1 domain (cyan) bound to GPIbα (magenta). Disulfides are in yellow stick. The A1-GPIbα complex forms a super β-sheet at the interface between the A1 β3 and GPIbα β14 strands. Platelet-type von Willebrand disease (VWD) mutations (green Cα atom spheres) stabilize the β-switch in its bound over its unbound conformation. VWD type 2B mutations (red Cα spheres) locate distal from the GPIbα interface, near to the A2 termini where elongational force is applied. VWD type 2B mutations are hypothesized to stabilize an alternative, high-affinity conformation. A region of GPIbα that is important for interaction with A1 in high shear [leucine-rich repeats (LRR) 3-5] and with ristocetin is shown in gray. *(Adapted with permission from Li R and Emsley J: The organizing principle of the platelet glycoprotein Ib-IX-V complex,* J Thromb Haemost *2013 Apr;11(4):605-614.)*

which has alternating β strands and α helices organized into a central β-sheet surround by amphiphatic α helices, interacts with the concave face of GPIbα with two areas of tight interactions, at the N-terminal β-hairpin + first leucine-rich repeat (with VWF A1 domain loops $α_1β_2$, $β_3α_2$, and $α_3β_4$), and a more extensive interaction at leucine-rich repeats 5 to 8 + the β switch region (with VWF A1 domain helix $α_3$, loop $α_3β_4$, and strand $β_3$). The structure of the VWF A1 domain when not bound to GPIbα differs from that of the bound VWF A1 in that the $α_1β_2$ loop protrudes in a way that would prevent interaction with GPIbα.[1108] This observation and others related to differences in the ability of different-sized fragments of VWF and GPIbα to interact indicate that other regions of both proteins probably contribute to both the binding and activation of the receptor. The crystal structure of GPIbα with the naturally occurring mutation M239V in the β-hairpin region that results in platelet-type (pseudo-) von Willebrand disease (Chap. 126) has also been obtained,[1109] and demonstrates a more stable β-hairpin conformation, which probably accounts for the approximately sixfold increase in binding affinity, primarily through an increase in the association rate. Leucine-rich repeats 3 to 5 do not demonstrate interaction with the normal VWF A domain in the crystal structure, but they are important in ristocetin-induced platelet agglutination, and platelet adhesion at high shear; they do participate to some extent in crystal structures with gain of function mutations in VWF A1.[1107,1111,1112] It has been proposed that hydrodynamic forces produced at high shear alter the A1 domain and expose regions that interact with these repeats in GPIb.[1113] Other natural and site-directed mutation causing the platelet-type von Willebrand disease pattern of enhanced VWF binding (G233V, V234G, D235V, K237V) also affect the β-hairpin region. A number of Bernard-Soulier syndrome mutations that cause loss of VWF binding to GPIbα localize to the concave face of leucine-rich repeats 5, 6, and 7 (L129P, A156V, and L179del) and to the sides of leucine-rich repeat 2 (C65R and L57P).[1110]

The GPIb ectodomain crystal structure has been determined, confirming the four predicted conserved disulfide bonds (C1-C7, C5-C14,

C68-C93, and C70-C116), along with the unpaired C122, which cross-links to GPIbα.[1114] The two former disulfides are in the N-capping region and the two latter are in the C-capping region flanking the single leucine-rich repeat.[1040] Using a chimeric GPIbβ/GPIX ectodomain protein, the likely contacts between GPIb and GPIX were identified. The structure proposed is a tetramer of one GPIbα, two GPIbβs, and one GPIX in which GPIX interacts with one of the GPIbβ molecules.[1037,1040,1043]

Plasma VWF will not bind to GPIb under static conditions unless the antibiotic ristocetin or the snake venom botrocetin is added. The mechanism by which ristocetin induces VWF binding to GPIb is unclear, but effects on VWF as well as on platelet surface charge have been described, and dimerization of ristocetin molecules and multimerization of VWF, as well as stabilization of an A1 domain conformation with high affinity for GPIb have also been implicated.[801,1113,1115–1118] Botrocetin binds to VWF, exposing the site that binds to GPIb.[1119] Peptide studies implicate the anionic, sulfated tyrosine region of GPIb as the binding site for botrocetin-treated VWF.[801]

Unlike integrin $α_{IIb}β_3$, which requires intact, activated platelets to bind to VWF, GPIb-mediated VWF binding does not require platelet activation or even platelet metabolic integrity, because fixed platelets are readily agglutinated in the presence of VWF and either ristocetin or botrocetin.[1116] This observation forms the basis of the assay of plasma VWF activity.

Platelets will adhere to VWF when the latter is immobilized on a surface, even in the absence of ristocetin or botrocetin.[1116,1120–1122] Under these circumstances, the VWF is believed to undergo a conformational change that allows for direct interactions. It may not, however, be necessary to propose a change in VWF conformation as the interaction between VWF and GPIb appears to have both high association and dissociation rates, permitting tethering and translocation on a surface coated with a high density of VWF, but minimal interaction in fluid phase.[809] Similarly, VWF associated with fibrin can interact with platelet GPIb without ristocetin or botrocetin.[61,1123] The C1C2 domains of VWF appears to contain a fibrin binding site.[304]

Shear stress is an important factor in GPIb-mediated adhesion of platelets to immobilized VWF and subendothelial surfaces.[1042,1113,1120–1122,1124,1125] Platelets deficient in GPIb or platelets in which GPIb has been blocked with monoclonal antibodies[1122,1124] adhere poorly to subendothelial surfaces at all shear rates, but the defect in blood from patients with von Willebrand disease is manifest primarily at higher shear rates.[10,11,1122] In what may be a related phenomenon, subjecting platelets to high shear stresses can induce platelet aggregation, which is mediated by VWF binding to GPIb, followed by platelet activation and integrin $\alpha_{IIb}\beta_3$-dependent platelet aggregation.[13,15,1126] Whether the shear rates generated *in vivo* in stenotic blood vessels are of sufficient magnitude and duration to produce a similar degree of platelet activation is unknown. It is also uncertain as to whether the effect of shear is acting on GPIb, on VWF, or on both,[15,801,809,1042] but shear-induced changes in the structure of VWF, leading to a more extended conformation and conformational changes in the A1 domain, have been defined.[1113,1127] GPIb forms catch bonds with VWF, meaning that increasing force first prolongs and then shortens bond lifetimes.[1113,1128]

GPIb also functions as a platelet binding site for thrombin.[801,1129,1130] The regions between amino acids 216 and 240 and amino acids 269 and 287 were proposed as thrombin binding sites based on biochemical data, with the latter region demonstrating similarity to hirudin, a thrombin-binding protein.[801,1131] Sulfation of the three tyrosine residues in the latter region is particularly important for thrombin binding.[1093]

Two somewhat different crystal structures of the interactions between thrombin and the negatively charged tail region of GPIb have been reported, but in both cases two molecules of thrombin bind to each GPIb molecule using different regions on thrombin (exosites I and II). This raises the possibility that free thrombin or thrombin adherent to fibrin can cluster GPIb/IX/V complexes.[1132]

Binding of thrombin to platelet GPIb appears to contribute to thrombin-induced activation of platelets, even when PAR-1 and PAR-4 are desensitized, and platelets lacking GPIb (Bernard-Soulier syndrome) do, in fact, have blunted responses to thrombin. GPIb has been proposed as the high-affinity binding site for thrombin,[1129,1133] but there are only approximately 50 high-affinity thrombin-binding sites and approximately 25,000 GPIb molecules per platelet,[1129,1130] raising the possibility that only the subpopulation of GPIb molecules in lipid rafts are able to function in activating platelets.[1134] Binding of thrombin to GPIb may also facilitate its effect on one or more of the other thrombin receptors, and there is experimental support for this hypothesis.[1135,1136]

GPIb has also been demonstrated to interact with P-selectin in a cation-independent manner.[764,1035,1093] Although GPIb shares a number of features with the P-selectin ligand, PSGL-1 (both are sialomucins and have analogous anionic/sulfated tyrosine sequences), the interaction between GPIb and P-selectin appears to be more like the interaction between P-selectin and heparin.[1035,1093] In inflamed mesenteric venules in animals, platelets are observed to roll on the activated endothelium[1137] and so it is possible that platelet GPIb interacts with endothelial P-selectin in this interaction.[1093] PSGL-1, a well-documented ligand for P-selectin on leukocytes, has also been identified on the surface of platelets,[1138] and so may also contribute to this interaction.

GPIbα also binds to high molecular weight kininogen and factor XII, and both of these interactions interfere with thrombin-induced platelet activation.[1139,1140] Factor XI also binds to GPIbα, where it undergoes activation by thrombin.[1141] Activated leukocyte integrin $\alpha_M\beta_2$, also can bind to GPIbα via the I-domain of the integrin,[1142] and this interaction has been proposed to play an important role in transmigration of leukocytes through platelet thrombi at sites of vascular injury. GPIb plays complex roles in inflammation and endotoxemia in murine models, demonstrating both proinflammatory and antiinflammatory

effects.[1143,1144] GPIb has also been implicated in supporting metastases in murine models.[1145]

GPV, the third member of the GPIb/IX/V complex, has a Mr 82,000 and is composed of 544 amino acids, including 15 leucine-rich repeats. GPV appears to form a noncovalent complex with GPIb, mediated through association of their transmembrane domains,[1146] but because the number of GPV molecules on the surface of platelets is approximately 50 percent of the number of GPIb and GPIX molecules,[1147] it has been suggested that the basic unit consists of two GPIb molecules, two GPIX molecules, and one GPV molecule.[801,1035,1038] GPV is deficient in platelets from patients with Bernard-Soulier syndrome (Chap. 121), but GPV is not required for surface expression of the GPIb/IX complex.[1148] A soluble fragment of Mr 69,000 is cleaved from GPV by thrombin, but cleavage does not correlate with thrombin-induced platelet activation.[1149] Platelets from mice lacking GPV appear to respond more actively to thrombin and ADP than wild-type mice, raising the possibility that GPV inhibits platelet activation.[1150] The platelets from these mice also adhere to immobilized VWF and can bind VWF in the presence of botrocetin, indicating that GPV is not required for the interaction between VWF and the GPIb/IX/V complex.[1150] It has been proposed that removing a portion of GPV by thrombin proteolysis allows thrombin access to GPIbα, thus facilitating its ability to activate platelets. In support of this model, thrombin's ability to activate platelets does not require proteolytic activity if GPV is absent, suggesting a direct nonproteolytic effect mediated via GPIbα.[1151]

IMMUNOGLOBULIN FAMILY OF CELL-SURFACE ADHESION RECEPTORS AND THEIR ASSOCIATED MEMBRANE PROTEINS

Platelet-Endothelial Cell Adhesion Molecule-1 (Also Termed CD31)

PECAM-1 is a transmembrane glycoprotein of the immunoglobulin gene family with six immunoglobulin-like domains of the C2 group and a Mr 130,000.[1152–1155] In addition to platelets and endothelial cells, PECAM-1 is expressed on monocytes, myeloid cells, and some lymphocyte subsets. There are approximately 8000 PECAM-1 molecules on the surface of platelets.[1156] PECAM promotes homophilic interactions via a homophilic binding domain in the immunoglobin-like repeats. The cytoplasmic tail of PECAM is 118 amino acids in length and contains a palmitoylation site (C595), an immunoreceptor tyrosine-based inhibitory motif (ITIM) including Y663, an immunoreceptor tyrosine-based switch motif (ITSM) including Y686, and a lipid-interacting α helix that contains Y686 and S702, which undergoes inducible phosphorylation.[1152,1157] Upon phosphorylation, the ITIMs recruit and activate phosphatases, such as SHP-2 and to a lesser extent SHP-1, SHIP, and PP2A,[1158] via their SH2 domains.[1152] PECAM-1 undergoes homotypic interactions that lead to signaling and crosslinking.[1159] PECAM-1 activation overall thus induces inhibitory activity as the phosphatases counteract the effects of stimulating kinases, but are complex and agonist specific. PECAM-1 activation decreases platelet responses to ADP and thrombin and PECAM-1 platelet expression correlates inversely with platelet sensitivity to these agonists.[1160] PECAM-1 also negatively regulates collagen-induced platelet activation mediated by the ITAM-bearing GPVI/FcRγ-chain complex, GPIb/IX/V signaling, and laminin-induced activation.[1159] Platelets from mice lacking PECAM-1 are hyperresponsive to subthreshold doses of collagen, and when compared to wild-type mice, form larger platelet thrombi on VWF and in experimental settings *in vivo*.

Crosslinking PECAM-1 molecules on the platelet surface with antibodies enhances platelet adhesion and aggregate formation, suggesting that under certain circumstances PECAM-1 might be a costimulatory agonist, working in concert with platelet integrin $\alpha_{IIb}\beta_3$.[1161] Moreover, mice lacking PECAM-1 can undergo normal inside-out activation of integrin $\alpha_{IIb}\beta_3$, but have a partial defect in integrin $\alpha_{IIb}\beta_3$-mediated outside-in signaling.[1162] PECAM-1 crosslinking may also lead to GPIb internalization, resulting in decreased platelet adhesion.[1163]

In endothelial cells, PECAM-1 is localized to the contact areas between endothelial cells, in the lateral border recycling compartment, where it is involved in controlling stimulus-specific transmigration of leukocytes.[1155,1164] It appears to be capable of both homotypic and heterotypic interactions, with the latter mediated by CD177 on neutrophils (and perhaps glycosaminoglycans, integrin $\alpha_V\beta_3$, or CD38) interacting with the fifth or sixth PECAM-1 immunoglobulin domain.[1155,1165] PECAM-1 engagement triggers signaling and leukocyte integrin receptor activation that facilitates transmigration, with activation of the laminin receptor, integrin $\alpha_6\beta_1$, of particular importance. Endothelial PECAM-1 is also important in maintaining vascular integrity and endothelial and leukocyte PECAM-1 mediate both proinflammatory and antiinflammatory phenomena in model systems.[1155]

Triggering Receptors Expressed on Myeloid Cells–Like Transcript-1

Triggering receptors expressed on myeloid cells (TREM)-like transcript-1 (TLT-1) is a receptor whose external domain is homologous to those in the family termed TREM. Like those receptors, it contains a single V-set immunoglobulin domain, but its cytoplasmic domain is much longer, is palmitoylated and carries a canonical ITIM capable of becoming phosphorylated and binding the Src homology-containing protein, tyrosine phosphate-1 (SHP-1).[627,1166] The phosphatase can then dephosphorylate signaling molecules, leading to inhibition of platelet activation. PECAM-1 has a similar ability to bind SHP-1. TLT appears to be restricted in expression to platelets and megakaryocytes. It is primarily in α-granule membranes in resting platelets and joins the plasma membrane when platelets are activated.

GPVI

GPVI is a Mr 62,000 transmembrane glycoprotein of 316 amino acids.[18,804,1167,1168] It belongs to the immunoglobulin superfamily, and is the major platelet signaling receptor for collagen. It may also mediate platelet interactions with monocytes by binding the ligand EMMPRIN.[1169] GPVI on the platelet surface exists in a complex with Fc receptor (FcR) γ-chain. Because the latter is a dimer, two GPVI molecules associate with one FcR γ-chain, forming a high-affinity complex.[1168] The GPVI extracellular region contains two immunoglobulin C2-like domains and its transmembrane domain contains an Arg residue that is essential for association with the FcRγ-chain. The 51-amino-acid cytoplasmic domain contains a proline-rich sequence that binds SH3 (Src homology 3) domains of Src family tyrosine kinases. GPVI signals through the FcRγ-chain, which contains an ITAM. An unpaired thiol in the cytoplasmic tail of GPVI can undergo oxidation, resulting in homodimer formation,[1170] required for high-affinity interactions with collagen peptides and GPVI-mediated signaling.[1171,1172] Resting platelets have approximately 29 percent of their GPVI molecules in dimers and interactions with CRPs or thrombin activation increase the percentage of GPVI in dimers.[1171] When GPVI binds collagen, the ITAM domain of the FcRγ-chain becomes phosphorylated by the Src kinases Fyn and/or Lyn, resulting in the formation of large complex of signal-transducing proteins (for a discussion of the role of GPVI as a receptor for collagen, see "Signaling Pathways in Platelets" below.).[1041,1104] GPVI is required for stable platelet thrombus formation on collagen surfaces *in vitro*. Mice lacking GPVI have a relatively mild phenotype and are protected from

thrombosis in some but not all experimental models. GPVI and FcRγ-chain appear to play important roles in ferric chloride-mediated arterial thrombosis in mice, but not in laser-induced thrombosis, perhaps because the former, but not the latter, injury elicits collagen exposure along the damaged vessel. Inherited and acquired defects in human platelet GPVI have been reported (Chap. 121) and the associated bleeding disorders have been variably described as mild to severe.[1172–1176] Two alternatively spliced forms and several polymorphisms have been identified for GPVI and variably linked to alterations in platelet function or risk of thrombotic disease.[1177,1178]

Fc Receptor γ-Chain

The FcRγ-chain[1179] exists as a homodimer of Mr 20,000 that physically and functionally associates with GPVI[1180] and GPIb/IX.[1102] In mouse platelets, the absence of FcRγ-chain results in lack of surface expression of GPVI. The FcRγ-chain, along with FcγRIIA, are the only known platelet proteins with ITAMs.[1104] Phosphorylation of the ITAM domain serves to recruit proteins with Src homology 2 (SH2) domains, which are essential for collagen-mediated signaling through the GPVI/FcRγ-chain pathway.[1041,1104,1181] The FcRγ-chain may also contribute to GPIb/IX-mediated intracellular signaling after VWF binding.[1035,1102,1105]

Fcγ Receptor IIA (FcγRIIA, Also Termed CD32)

The FcγRIIA is a low affinity immunoglobulin receptor of Mr 40,000 that is widely distributed on hematopoietic cells.[804] Three different mRNA transcripts (A, B, and C) make similar FcγRIIA molecules[1182] and these are preferentially expressed on different cells. FcγRIIA contains an ITAM domain and thus may be important for signaling by its associated proteins, including GPIb and select integrins, as well as through direct stimulation by immune complexes. Crosslinking of FcγRIIA initiates tyrosine phosphorylation, PI metabolism, activation of PLCγ_2, calcium signaling, and cytoskeletal rearrangements.[960,961] FcγRIIA appears to be in close proximity to the GPIb/IX/V complex in lipid rafts,[212] and signal transduction that accompanies VWF binding to GPIb may be mediated at least in part through FcγRIIA.[885,971] FcγRIIA is also be important in mediating integrin $\alpha_{IIb}\beta_3$ outside-in signaling, including effects on platelet spreading, clot retraction, and thrombus formation.[1183,1184] Platelet 12(S)-lipoxygenase (LOX) is required for platelet activation mediated by FcγRIIA.[1185]

The FcγRIIA on platelets may bind immune complexes generated in certain diseases, and by engaging these complexes the platelets may become sensitized to other stimuli.[1186–1188] It may also provide a second binding site for antibodies that bind to platelets via their antibody-binding site (see "CD9" below). This second interaction can potentially lead to bridging between platelets, with the antibody binding to an antigen on one platelet and an FcγRIIA receptor on another platelet.[1189] It is also possible that antibodies can bind to both an antigen and an FcγRIIA on a single platelet. These interactions can lead to platelet activation through engagement of FcγRIIA, followed by crosslinking of FcγRIIA receptors, which can lead to tyrosine phosphorylation, PI metabolism, activation of PLCγ_2, calcium signaling, and cytoskeletal rearrangements.[1190,1191] This type of interaction appears to play an important role in heparin-induced thrombocytopenia (Chap. 117). FcγRIIA undergoes proteolysis when platelets are activated and FcγRIIA proteolysis has been proposed as an assay for heparin-induced thrombocytopenia.[1192,1193] Cooperation between FcγRIIA and C1q receptor has been reported.[1194] A variety of viruses and bacteria can interact with, and activate platelets and this is variably mediated by FcγRIIA, with or without immunoglobulin.[795,1195,1196] FcγRIIA may also contribute to cancer cell activation in platelets.[1197]

FcγRIIA expression on platelets shows considerable variation among individuals (approximately 600 to 1500 molecules per platelet), and this variation correlates with FcγRIIA-mediated function.[1188] This variation in receptor density may explain individual differences in immune-mediated disorders such as heparin-induced thrombocytopenia with thrombosis.[1198] An H131R polymorphism within FcγRIIA affects the binding of different IgG subclasses.[1199,1200] The H131R polymorphism may also have clinical significance because the R131 allele is associated with increased binding of activation-dependent antibodies to platelets.[1201] A variety of associations have been identified between the H131ER polymorphism and different aspects of heparin-induced thrombocytopenia and immune thrombocytopenia, but the data differ from study to study and no consensus has yet emerged.[1202–1207]

Intercellular Adhesion Molecule-2 (CD102)

ICAM-2, a member of the immunoglobulin family of receptors, is an endothelial cell ligand for the β_2-integrin $\alpha_L\beta_2$ (LFA-1) on lymphocytes and myeloid cells.[1208] Approximately 2600 ICAM-2 molecules are present on platelets, distributed on the membrane surface and open canalicular system.[1208] Platelet ICAM-2 may contribute to platelet-leukocyte interactions (see "Platelet–Leukocyte Interactions" below).

FcεRI

Platelets express the high affinity IgE receptor FcεRI and appear to participate in both defense against parasitic diseases, including malaria, and allergic phenomena.[799,1209–1211]

Junctional Adhesion Molecule-A (A Also Termed F11)

JAM-A was identified on platelets by the ability of a monoclonal antibody directed against the receptor to initiate platelet activation via crosslinking to FcγRIIA.[1212–1216] It is phosphorylated during platelet activation and loss of JAM-A in a mouse model results in a prothrombotic phenotype.[1217] JAM-A appears to inhibit outside-in signaling via integrin $\alpha_{IIb}\beta_3$ by recruiting Csk, which, in turn, phosphorylates Src at Y529.[1217,1218] It is also able to interact with the integrin $\alpha_L\beta_1$ receptor on leukocytes, and in endothelial cells it participates in tight junction formation and leukocyte recruitment and transmigration.[920]

Junctional Adhesion Molecule-C

The JAM-C transmembrane protein has an Mr of 43,000 and 279 amino acids. It contains two C2-type immunoglobulin domains in its extracellular domain and three potential tyrosine phosphorylation sites in its cytoplasmic domain.[767,920] JAM-C is expressed on platelets but not granulocytes, monocytes, lymphocytes, or erythrocytes. It shares 32 percent homology with JAM-A. Based on monoclonal antibody binding studies, platelets contain approximately 1600 copies of JAM-C. Platelet JAM-C acts as a counterreceptor for leukocyte integrins $\alpha_M\beta_2$ and $\alpha_X\beta_2$ and contributes to platelet–leukocyte interactions under some conditions.[767] Its precise role in platelet physiology is uncertain, but it has been implicated in binding CD34 stem cells.[1219]

LECTIN-CONTAINING RECEPTORS

P-Selectin (Also Termed GMP140, PADGEM, and CD62P)

P-selectin, which has a Mr of 140,000, is a glycoprotein present in α-granule membranes in resting platelets that joins the plasma membrane when platelets are activated.[759,1220–1222] Approximately 13,000 P-selectin molecules are detected by antibodies on the surface of activated platelets. The expression of P-selectin on circulating platelets has, therefore, been used as an indicator of their *in vivo* activation.[1223,1224] It is also present in the Weibel-Palade body membranes of endothelial cells; as in platelets, it joins the plasma membrane when endothelial cells are activated.[759,1222]

P-selectin has a modular structure in which the aminoterminal region has a calcium-dependent lectin domain that binds carbohydrates. Adjacent to the lectin domain is an EGF domain, followed by nine repeats that are homologous to complement regulatory proteins ("sushi" domains), a transmembrane domain, and a cytoplasmic domain.[759,1220] The cytoplasmic domain contains Ser, Thr, Tyr, and His residues that can be phosphorylated. In addition, a Cys residue becomes acylated with stearic or palmitic acid. Alternatively spliced forms of P-selectin may be produced in which sushi domains are omitted. The selectin family also includes E-selectin (ELAM-1; CD62E), which is expressed on the surface of activated endothelial cells, and L-selectin (LAM-1; CD62L), which is expressed on the surface of myeloid and lymphoid cells.[1225]

Soluble P-selectin is present in plasma from humans and mice. Alternative splicing generates a soluble form of human P-selectin that lacks the transmembrane domain.[1226] In mice, at least a portion of soluble P-selectin is derived from proteolytic cleavage of surface P-selectin by an unidentified protease.[1227]

Recognition of ligand by P-selectin requires specific carbohydrate and protein structures. Fucose and sialic acid are important carbohydrate components, with sialyl-3-fucosyl-N-acetyllactosamine (SLe^x; CD15S) a preferred ligand structure.[756,1228–1230] Myeloid and tumor cell sulfatides may also act as ligands for P-selectin.[1231,1232] PSGL-1, a mucin-like transmembrane glycoprotein homodimer (Mr 220,000) expressed on neutrophils, monocytes, lymphocytes, and to a small extent on platelets, is an important ligand for P-selectin.[1138,1233–1235] Both sulfation of tyrosine residues contained in an anionic region and branched fucosylation of O-linked carbohydrates are required for optimal binding to P-selectin.

P-selectin can mediate the attachment of neutrophils and monocytes to platelets and endothelial cells. Thus, neutrophils and monocytes may be recruited to sites of vascular injury where platelets deposit and become activated (see "Platelet–Leukocyte Interactions" below). Platelet P-selectin can also recruit procoagulant monocyte-derived microparticles containing both PSGL-1 and tissue factor to growing thrombi *in vivo*.[1236] Binding of P-selectin to PSGL-1 on monocytes can trigger tissue factor synthesis[1237] and infusing a P-selectin chimeric molecule into mice results in the generation of procoagulant microparticles.[781] In a reciprocal fashion, P-selectin engagement of PSGL-1 may lead to platelet activation.[1238] Soluble P-selectin may also promote a prothrombotic state in humans by increasing tissue factor–expressing microparticles in plasma. Indeed, the risk of future cardiovascular events is elevated in apparently healthy women with the highest levels of soluble P-selectin.[1239]

In intact blood vessels, the rapid on and off rates of the interactions between PSGL-1 on neutrophils and P-selectin on endothelial cells allows leukocytes to roll on the endothelium, the first step in leukocyte transmigration (Chap. 66).[1240] The rapid upregulation of P-selectin after endothelial cell activation allows for a quick response. Platelets have been reported to roll on activated endothelium, and this appears to result from an interaction between endothelial P-selectin and perhaps either platelet GPIbα[1093,1137] or platelet PSGL-1.[1138,1241] Upon their corelease from endothelial Weibel-Palade bodies, P-selectin may tether ultralarge VWF to the surface of activated endothelium, and thereby promote platelet GPIbα-mediated platelet rolling.[1242]

Genetic and pharmacologic targeting of P-selectin or PSGL-1 in experimental animal models suggests that these receptors may modulate thrombolysis, sickle cell vasoocclusion, restenosis, deep venous thrombosis, cerebral ischemia and infarction, atherosclerosis, metastasis, and thrombotic glomerulonephritis (reviewed in Refs. 1243 to 1246).

C-Type Lectin-Like Receptor-2

Podoplanin is a sialoglycoprotein present on a variety of tumor cells, lymphatic endothelial cells, kidney podocytes, lung epithelial cells, lymph node stromal cells, and the choroid plexus epithelium that can aggregate platelets.[1247–1250] Its receptor on platelets is CLEC-2, a C-type lectin-like receptor selectively expressed on megakaryocytes and platelets (approximately 2,000 copies per platelet) that binds podoplanin and the snake venom platelet-activating protein rhodocytin.[1251–1253] The cytoplasmic tail of CLEC-2 contains an atypical ITAM (hemITAM) with a single YITL sequence that can be tyrosine phosphorylated by Src kinases when platelets are activated. Because CLEC-2 exists as a dimer, it can supply two ITAMS and lead to activation of Syk and, ultimately, PLCγ_2.[1254] This signaling system is similar to that of GPVI in combination with the FcRγ-chain. Activation of CLEC-2 leads to proteolytic cleavage of GPVI and FcγRIIa.[1255] In experimental tumor models, inhibiting the podoplanin/CLEC-2 system reduces metastases.[1256] CLEC-2 interaction with podoplanin on lymphatic endothelial cells, followed by platelet activation and CLEC-2-podoplanin clustering, is required for the separation of blood and lymph vessels during development.[1257–1259] CLEC-2 also plays a role in lymph node development and maintenance.[1260] HIV-1 can also bind to CLEC-2.

TETRASPANINS

Tetraspanins are a family of four-transmembrane-domain-containing proteins that have conserved Cys residues that form crucial disulfide bonds. The extracellular and intracellular loops in these proteins contain many motifs that mediate interactions with other proteins.[1261] While the specific function(s) of tetraspanins is not yet clear, these proteins are able to associate with several membrane proteins and have been reported to modulate integrin function, perhaps in part by organizing membrane and intercellular signaling molecules in cholesterol-associated microdomains distinct from lipid rafts.[1262] CD9, CD63, and CD151 have juxtamembrane Cys residues that can be palmitoylated and this modification may contribute to assembly of complexes with other proteins and localization to lipid microdomains.[1263] Studies in mice implicate CD151 and TSSC6 in outside-in signaling of integrin $\alpha_{IIb}\beta_3$.[1264] Oligomers of tetraspanins are known to facilitate the formation of larger complexes of membrane proteins that could serve as scaffolds for several platelet signaling events.[1265] CD9 is the most abundant platelet tetraspanin (approximately 40,000 molecules per platelet), followed by CD151, Tspan9, and CD63.[1266] The levels of TSSC6 are not known.

CD9 (5H9; BA2; P24; GIG2; MIC3; MRP-1; BTCC-1; DRAP-27; TSPAN29)

CD9 is a 228-amino-acid tetraspanin that is present on platelets, endothelial cells, smooth muscle cells, cultured fibroblasts, some lymphoblasts, eosinophils, basophils, and other cells.[1267–1269] It colocalizes with integrin $\alpha_{IIb}\beta_3$ on the inner surface of α granules in resting platelets and on pseudopods of activated platelets.[1270] Binding of monoclonal antibodies specific for CD9 to platelets results in platelet aggregation by triggering phosphatidylinositol metabolism via a mechanism that also requires binding to the platelet FcγRIIA receptor.[1271–1273] The platelet activation induced by the binding of such antibodies requires external calcium and results in an association between CD9 and integrin $\alpha_{IIb}\beta_3$.[1274] CD9 has been proposed to play a role in microparticle release from platelets.[1275] Studies in mice lacking CD9 suggest that CD9 is a negative regulator of integrin $\alpha_{IIb}\beta_3$ signaling, as the mice have enhanced platelet aggregation, fibrinogen binding, and thrombus formation.[1276]

CD63 (Also Termed Granulophysin and LAMP-3)

CD63 (Mr 53,000) appears to be present in both lysosomal and dense granule membranes in platelets.[310,1263,1277] CD63 is also present in Weibel-Palade bodies in endothelial cells, the lysosomal membranes of a variety of other cells, as well as the membranes of melanosomes.

It appears on the surface membrane when platelets are activated, making it a useful marker for platelet activation.[310,1224] CD63 colocalizes with integrin $\alpha_{IIb}\beta_3$ and CD9 on the surface of activated platelets in a process that appears to require CD63 palmitoylation.[1263] CD63 is markedly reduced or absent from the dense bodies of patients with Hermansky-Pudlak syndrome,[1277] who have oculocutaneous albinism and a defect in platelet dense bodies (Chap. 121). The amino acid sequence of CD63 has been deduced from complementary DNA (cDNA) cloning.[1278]

CD151 (Also Termed GP27, MER2, RAPH, SFA1, PETA-3, and TSPAN24)

CD151, a glycoprotein of Mr 27,000 is present on platelets, endothelial cells, and many other cells.[1279–1281] Antibodies to CD151, like those to CD9, can initiate platelet aggregation by binding to both CD151 and FcγRIIA.[1280] The role of CD151 in platelet physiology remains to be firmly established but it may participate with FcγRIIA as a signal transduction complex.[1280] CD151 appears to functionally associate with integrin $\alpha_{IIb}\beta_3$ and, in mice, loss of CD151 impairs platelet aggregation, clot retraction,[1282] and thrombus formation.[1283]

TSSC6 (PHMX, PHEMX FLJ17158, FLJ97586, MGC22455, TSPAN32)

TSSC6 is a 340-amino-acid tetraspanin that is expressed in marrow, spleen, thymus, and several hematopoietic cell types.[898] It is present in platelets and has been reported to interact with integrin $\alpha_{IIb}\beta_3$. Mice deficient in TSSC6 display a slightly prolonged bleeding time and a significantly increased rebleeding.[1265] Platelets lacking TSSC6 show impaired aggregation and clot retraction.

GLYCOSYLPHOSPHATIDYLINOSITOL-ANCHORED PROTEINS (CD55, CD59, CD109, PRION PROTEIN)

At least five separate platelet proteins are attached to the membrane through a GPI link. These include proteins involved in complement regulation (CD55, decay accelerating factor, and CD59, membrane inhibitor of reactive lysis)[1284]; CD109, a Mr 170,000 protein present on platelets, endothelial cells, hematopoietic cells, and fibroblasts that carries both ABO oligosaccharides and an alloantigen (HPA-15, Gov) involved in neonatal isoimmune thrombocytopenia[1285,1286]; and a Mr 500,000 protein of unknown identity. Patients with paroxysmal nocturnal hemoglobinuria (PNH) have abnormalities in the GPI anchor and thus variably lack all of the GPI-linked proteins. The diagnosis of PNH can be established by assessing platelet expression of these proteins.[897,1287,1288] Patients with PNH have been reported to have platelet function abnormalities,[1287] raising the possibility that one or more of these proteins has a role in platelet function, but no specific platelet function roles have yet been assigned to the proteins. Of particular interest is the presence of the normal prion protein, which is a Mr 27,000 to 30,000 GPI-linked protein that is both upregulated and shed from the platelet surface with platelet activation.[1289–1292] In fact, platelets contain the majority of the prion protein present in normal blood.

TYROSINE KINASE RECEPTORS

Eph Kinases and Ephrin Ligands

Eph kinase receptors comprise the largest family of cell surface-associated tyrosine kinases with 14 members identified in mammals. Eph kinases have a conserved structure consisting of an N-terminal extracellular ephrin-binding domain, two fibronectin type II repeats, and intracellular kinase, sterile α motif (SAM), and PDZ binding domains [defined by the first three proteins to display this protein–protein domain, post synaptic density protein (PSD95), *Drosophila* disk large tumor suppressor (Dlg1), and zonula occludens-1 protein (zo-1)]. A total of eight ephrins have been identified that serve as cell-surface ligands for the Eph kinases. In general, Eph A kinases recognize ephrins that contain a GPI anchor (ephrin A family), while Eph B kinases bind to ligands with a transmembrane domain (ephrin B family). The Eph receptors and the ephrins appear to signal bidirectionally at sites of cell-to-cell contact. Platelets contain Eph kinases EphA4 and EphB1, and their ligand ephrin B1, as well as EphB2.[276,1293] Messenger RNA for ephrinA3 has also been detected in platelets, but confirmation of the presence of ephrinA3 protein in platelets is lacking. Forced clustering of either Eph kinases or ephrins in platelets promotes cytoskeletal reorganization, adhesion, granule secretion, and Rap1b activation in concert with other platelet stimuli.[1293,1294] Eph kinase–ephrin interactions may stabilize platelet aggregates and thrombus formation after platelet–platelet contact has occurred.[276,1295]

Thrombopoietin Receptor (c-mpl, CD110)

The thrombopoietin receptor (c-mpl; Mr 80 to 85,000) is expressed at low levels on platelets (approximately 25 to 224 per platelet) and binds thrombopoietin with high affinity. (K_D approximately 0.50 nM).[1296-1299] Steady-state plasma levels of thrombopoietin are maintained, in part, by platelets and megakaryocytes, which bind thrombopoietin via the thrombopoietin receptor and then internalize and degrade the growth factor. Additional mechanisms for regulation of thrombopoietin levels have been described (Chap. 111). Although its major function is to stimulate megakaryocyte growth and maturation (Chap. 111), thrombopoietin also is able to sensitize platelets to activation by agonists.[1300-1305] Mutations of the receptor have been associated with inherited thrombocytopenia (Chap. 117) and myeloproliferative neoplasms (Chaps. 83 to 85).[1306,1307] It can also contribute to hematopoiesis through effects on hematopoietic stem cells and other progenitors.

SCAVENGER RECEPTORS

CD36 (GPIV)

CD36 (GPIV) is a Mr 88,000 glycoprotein that is highly, but variably, expressed on platelets (approximately 20,000 copies per platelet).[1308-1313] The nucleotide sequence of CD36 (GPIV) cDNA encodes a protein of 471 residues with a predicted Mr of 53,000 and 10 potential N-linked glycosylation sites,[1314] accounting for the difference between predicted and experimentally determined Mr. It is unusual in having two putative transmembrane domains and two short cytoplasmic tails. The cytoplasmic regions may associate with intracellular tyrosine kinases of the Src family and undergo phosphorylation.[1315] Antibodies to CD36 (GPIV) have been reported to produce neonatal alloimmune thrombocytopenia (Chap. 117).[1316] Biochemical data suggest that it may form dimers and multimers.[1317] Increased platelet surface expression of CD36 (GPIV) has been described in patients with myeloproliferative neoplasms.[1318] CD36 (GPIV) is also expressed on phagocytic cells (with the exception of neutrophils), fat and muscle cells, cardiac myocytes, and microvascular endothelial cells. The phosphorylation status of the extracellular region of the protein may control its ligand-binding properties,[1319] offering a potential explanation for some of the variable results obtained under different conditions.[1308,1319,1320]

CD36 (GPIV) plays an important role in long-chain fatty acid transport in the heart, fat, and muscle, and may contribute to atherosclerosis and insulin sensitivity.[1321,1322] Oxidized low-density lipoproteins (LDL), which can be produced by the effects of endothelial cell or platelet nitric oxide (NO) on LDL, bind to CD36 and, perhaps in concert with scavenger receptor (SR)-A, can increase platelet reactivity

to agonists via signal transduction mediated in part by Src kinases and a MAPK.[1323-1325] The variability in platelet CD36 expression may account for the variability in platelet hyperreactivity in response to elevated levels of oxidized LDL.[1326] CD36 can also mediate microparticle binding to platelets, which augments platelet-mediated thrombosis in model systems.[1327] Thus, CD36 has been reported to contribute to atherogenesis, diabetes, the metabolic syndrome, angiogenesis, and inflammation.[1328-1331] CD36 also interacts with the S100 calcium-modulated protein family member myeloid-related protein (MRP)-14 (also known as S100A9), which can be released from activated neutrophils and platelets. It has been proposed as a platelet receptor for thrombospondin[1332] and collagen,[1333,1334] but the functional significance of these interactions remains unclear because individuals who lack CD36 on an inherited basis (Nak^a-negative) do not have a bleeding disorder[1335] (Chap. 121). CD36 may play a role in the thrombospondin-mediated interaction reported between platelets and sickle erythrocytes,[1336] apoptosis, innate immunity, and in the binding of *Plasmodium falciparum*-infected erythrocytes to endothelial cells and monocytes.[1310,1314]

Scavenger Receptor-BI (SCARB1; CLA-I)

The class B SR-BI (CLA-I) is related to CD36 and is expressed on platelets, endothelial cells, and hepatocytes.[1313] It transports the cholesteryl esters from high-density lipoprotein (HDL) cholesterol and facilitates bidirectional flux of free cholesterol between cells and lipoproteins. Oxidized, but not unoxidized, HDL can inhibit platelet aggregation via binding to SR-BI.[1337] SR-BI has many other lipid ligands, however, and it is uncertain how these interact under physiologic conditions. A number of mutations are associated with elevated HDL levels.[1338] A heterozygous missense mutation has been associated with increased platelet unesterified cholesterol and both increased and decreased platelet function.[1338] Mouse studies indicate that disrupting the SR in nonhematopoietic tissues can affect platelet function via alterations in plasma lipids and alterations in the platelet SR can protect against hyperactivity induced by increased platelet cholesterol content.[1326]

MISCELLANEOUS

CD40 Ligand (CD40L, CD154) and CD40

CD40 ligand (CD40L, CD154) is a trimeric transmembrane protein (Mr 33,000) of the tumor-necrosis family that localizes to α granules in resting platelets and rapidly appears on the surface of platelets upon activation. Within minutes to hours of platelet activation, an Mr 18,000 fragment of CD40L is released from the platelet surface, perhaps mediated in part by matrix metalloproteinase (MMP-2) bound to integrin $\alpha_{IIb}\beta_3$.[1339] This soluble form of CD40L circulates as a trimer. The bulk of soluble CD40L in plasma is derived from activated platelets and, hence, can serve as a marker for platelet activation *in vivo*. Elevated levels of soluble CD40L are observed in acute coronary syndromes, following percutaneous coronary intervention, in the setting of coronary artery bypass surgery, and in peripheral vascular disease[1340] (reviewed in Refs. 1341 and 1342). Soluble CD40L activates neutrophil integrin $\alpha_M\beta_2$, enhances neutrophil adhesion, and induces the neutrophil oxidative burst.[1343] Moreover, elevated levels of soluble CD40L are associated with recurrent cardiovascular events in the setting of acute coronary syndromes[1340,1344] and restenosis following percutaneous coronary intervention.[1345] CD40L and, to a lesser extent, its counterreceptor CD40 have been implicated in the progression of atherosclerosis in animal models.[1346,1347]

The extracellular portion of CD40L binds to CD40, a Mr 48,000 transmembrane receptor. Approximately 600 to 1000 copies of CD40 are present on both resting and activated platelets,[1348] and while CD40L has been reported to initiate platelet activation via binding to CD40,[1349] the functional significance of CD40–CD40L interactions in platelet physiology remains to be determined. CD40L also contains a KGD sequence (RGD in mice) that has been implicated in binding to integrin $\alpha_{IIb}\beta_3$. In mice, CD40L–$\alpha_{IIb}\beta_3$ interactions appear to stabilize thrombus growth,[1348] perhaps by activating receptor mediated signaling.[1350] Additionally, integrin $\alpha_{IIb}\beta_3$ antagonists block the release of soluble CD40L from activated platelets. Both platelet-associated and soluble CD40L may stimulate leukocytes to release proinflammatory cytokines; CD40L may also inhibit endothelial cell migration after vascular injury.[1351] The inhibitory effects of CD40L on reendothelialization may partially explain why elevated levels of soluble CD40L are associated with higher rates of clinical restenosis.[1345] Finally, platelet CD40L may modulate adaptive immunity by serving as a costimulatory signal for antigen presenting cells.[1352,1353]

Fas Ligand, LIGHT and TRAIL

Fas ligand (FasL), LIGHT (also termed TNF superfamily member 14), and TNF-related apoptosis-inducing ligand (TRAIL), along with CD40L, belong to the TNF family of cytokines.[1354] With activation, platelets express FasL, LIGHT, and TRAIL on their surface and release soluble forms of these receptors,[1354–1356] analogous to activation-dependent CD40L platelet expression and release. The receptor Fas (Apo-1, CD95), is expressed on a wide variety of normal and malignant cells. Engagement of Fas by FasL initiates signaling that results in apoptosis, and this process is important in embryonic development, cellular hemostasis, and immune regulation.[1354] The surface-expressed FasL on platelets is biologically active and can initiate apoptosis. The soluble form of FasL may act as an inhibitor of apoptosis induced by surface-expressed FasL.[1354] Similarly, platelet-derived LIGHT is biologically active and can initiate inflammatory responses in monocytes and endothelial cells.[1356]

Lysosome-Associated Membrane Proteins 1 and 2 (CD107a, CD107b)

LAMP-1 and LAMP-2 are lysosome-associated membrane proteins that are approximately 30 percent homologous and constitute approximately 50 percent of lysosomal membrane proteins.[1357] They are integral membrane glycoproteins of Mr 110,000 and 120,000, respectively, that are contained within lysosomal membranes.[1358] When platelets undergo the release reaction, they join the plasma membrane. Each protein has two extracellular disulfide-bonded loops containing 36 to 38 amino acids. The loops are separated by a region rich in Pro and Ser that shares homology with the hinge region of IgA. There are multiple N-linked glycosylation sites on each glycoprotein and they contain more than 60 percent carbohydrate. Among the carbohydrate residues are polylactosaminoglycans that may possess sialylated Lewis^x structures, which are thought to interact with selectins. LAMP-1 and LAMP-2 play roles in control of lysosome fusion in autophagosomes and phagosomes.[1357]

C1q Receptors

Platelets have several receptors for C1q, a Mr 460,000 glycoprotein composed of six globular domains attached to a short collagen-like triple helix.[1359–1361] One is for the collagen-like domain (cC1qR, Mr 60,000 to 67,000 nonreduced and 72,000 to 75,000 reduced), and another is for the globular domain (gC1qR, Mr 28,000 to 33,000).[1362,1363] A third receptor of Mr 126,000 enhances phagocytosis.[1364] C1q circulates with C1r and C1s as a calcium-dependent complex, but interaction with immune complexes leads ultimately to dissociation of the complex and release of free C1q, with its collagen-like domain exposed. cC1qR has sequence homology to calreticulin and can modulate platelet-collagen interactions at low collagen concentrations. It may also localize

immune complexes, and when crosslinked by aggregated C1q, it can initiate platelet activation, aggregation, secretion, and expression of platelet coagulant activity.[1365,1366] Thus, the binding of C1q monomers to platelets inhibits collagen-induced platelet aggregation but has little effect on platelet adhesion to collagen.[1367] C1q multimers support platelet adhesion and can induce aggregation via activation of integrin $\alpha_{IIb}\beta_3$.[1368] C1q can also augment platelet aggregation induced by aggregated IgG.[1194] The gC1qR may self-associate to form a doughnut-shaped ternary complex.[1369] In addition to binding C1q, this receptor can bind *S. aureus* protein A on endothelial cells, where it functions as a receptor for high-molecular-weight kininogen.[1363] It may, therefore, participate in contact activation.

GMP-33 (Thrombospondin N-Terminal Fragment)

A Mr 33,000 α-granule membrane protein was initially identified as an activation-dependent protein that joins the plasma membrane when platelets undergo the release reaction. Approximately 4000 antibody molecules directed against GMP-33 bind to resting platelets, and 19,000 bind to activated platelets.[1370] Subsequent studies identified this antigen as a membrane-associated fragment from the N-terminal of thrombospondin.[1371]

Leukosialin, Sialophorin (CD43)

Leukosialin, a glycoprotein of Mr 90,000, may act as a ligand for ICAM-1.[1372] It is expressed on myeloid and some lymphoid cells. Abnormalities in leukosialin have been described in Wiskott-Aldrich syndrome (Chap. 121).

Toll-Like Receptors 1, 2, 4, 6, 9

Toll-like receptors (TLRs) are involved in innate immunity by virtue of their ability to sense products of protozoa, fungi, viruses, and bacteria, including endotoxin (lipopolysaccharide [LPS]), and then activate intracellular signaling pathways to initiate the inflammatory response.[1373] TLRs 1, 2, 4, 6, and 9 have been identified in platelets.[1373,1374] Activation of TLR-1 and TLR-2 can lead to platelet activation via a GPVI-like mechanism with TLR-4 through the nuclear factor (NF)-κB pathway.[1375] All of the components of the LPS signaling complex, including relatively high levels of TLR-4[1376] and CD14, MD2, and MyD88, have been identified in platelets. LPS binding to platelets stimulates secretion and potentiates agonist-activation by signaling thru the TLR-4 complex.[1377] LPS binding to platelet TLR-4 causes release of CD40L[1378] and modulates the release of cytokines by platelets.[1379,1380] In experimental animal models, TLR-4 may mediate LPS-induced microvascular thrombosis and thrombocytopenia.[1376,1381] TLR-4–null mice have prolonged times to vasoocclusion after vascular injury, but endothelial TLR-4 rather than platelet TLR-4 seems to be more important in supporting platelet thrombus formation.[1382] The interactions of LPS, produced by toxigenic *E. coli*, with platelet TLR-4 has been proposed to contribute to the pathophysiology of hemolytic uremic syndrome.[1378] Ligand binding to platelet TLR-4 also promotes platelet–neutrophil interactions, neutrophil activation, and along with TLR-2, the formation of NETs, which capture and sequester bacteria from the circulation.[792,1383] Activation of TLR-9 with protein adducts leads to Src-dependent platelet activation.[1374]

Peroxisome Proliferator-Activated Receptors

Peroxisome proliferator-activated receptors (PPARs) belong to a nuclear hormone receptor family of ligand-activated transcription factors.[1384] PPARγ is one of the three PPAR family members and is widely expressed in white adipose tissue, macrophages, B and T lymphocytes, smooth muscle cells, fibroblasts, and endothelial cells. It has been implicated in metabolism, insulin responsiveness, adipocyte differentiation, immune function, and inflammation. The thiazolidinedione class of insulin-sensitizing drugs used to treat type 2 diabetic patients act by binding PPARγ. Both PPARβ/δ and PPARγ are present in platelets. PPARγ agonists decrease thrombin-induced platelet aggregation and release of ATP, TX, and CD40L.[1384] Thus, PPARγ appears to downregulate platelet activation. Activated platelets release PPARγ complexed with the retinoid X receptor.[1385] Treatment with select thiazolidinediones has been associated with reductions in markers of platelet activation, including aggregation and P-selectin expression. PPARβ ligands synergize with NO to inhibit platelet function.[1386,1387] The antiplatelet effects of the calcium channel blocker nifedipine may be mediated through PPAR receptors.[348]

Matrix Metalloproteinases

Platelets contain a number of MMPs, as well as MMP activators and inhibitors.[1388,1389] MMP-1 can be activated by collagen and, in turn, cleave PAR-1 at a site two amino acids N-terminal to the site of thrombin cleavage.[1390] This cleavage, like thrombin's, activates PAR-1 by activating a tethered ligand. Thus, MMP-1 can augment collagen-induced platelet activation mediated by GPVI and integrin $\alpha_2\beta_1$. MMP-2 cleavage has been implicated in enhancing platelet aggregation via cleavage of talin and activation of integrin $\alpha_{IIb}\beta_3$.[1389] It exists in an inactive form in resting platelets and it is cleaved into its active form when platelets are activated, probably by platelet-type von Willebrand disease (MT1-MMP).[1391] It then moves to the surface via binding to integrin $\alpha_{IIb}\beta_3$ and may then go on to cleave CD40 ligand.[1339] MMP-2 is released into the coronary circulation of patients with acute coronary syndromes.[1392] ADAM-17 (TACE) is important in the cleavage of GPIb and the release glycocalicin.[1076] MMP-9, which is increased in plasma in models of sepsis, can also cleave platelet CD40L.[1393] Other related proteins in platelets include MMP-9 and -14, ADAM-10, and tissue inhibitor of metalloproteinase (TIMP)- 1, -2, and -3. Platelets also contain ADAMTS-13, which cleaves VWF, thus controlling hemostasis and thrombosis (Chap. 126).

● SIGNALING PATHWAYS IN PLATELETS

OVERVIEW

Platelets generally circulate in a quiescent state, but are poised to be activated in response to a variety of agonists that become available at sites of vascular injury or ruptured atherosclerotic plaques. Agonists differ in their intrinsic ability to produce these phenomena, and added complexity derives from differences in dose responses to each agonist and the synergistic effects of agonists used in combination. Agonists are diverse and include small and large soluble molecules, enzymes, and immobilized adhesive glycoproteins. They can be classified as either "strong" or "weak," depending on whether full activation, including the release reaction, can be initiated without the augmenting effect of platelet aggregation itself. Low doses of strong agonists behave like weak agonists. Most agonists are released, synthesized, or formed at the site of vascular injury, and this undoubtedly serves to localize the response.

Agonists bind to receptors of two general categories: seven-transmembrane G-protein–coupled receptors and receptors that can initiate phosphorylation of target proteins (Fig. 112–15). In both cases, a sequence of signaling events ultimately leads to platelet activation. Physiologic responses of platelets to agonists lead to the activation of the integrin $\alpha_{IIb}\beta_3$ receptor to a high-affinity ligand binding state and subsequent platelet aggregation. Moreover, binding of ligands to platelets and platelet aggregation itself further propagates signals that are required for stabilization of the platelet aggregates and clot retraction. In this section, the major agonists, receptors, and signaling pathways involved in early stages of platelet activation that lead to shape change, granule secretion, and platelet aggregation, as well as postaggregation signaling events are described.

AGONIST-INDUCED PLATELET ACTIVATION

Many platelet agonists initiate platelet activation by binding to seven-transmembrane heterotrimeric G-protein–coupled receptors (see Fig. 112–15).[1394] When such receptors are activated, the Gα subunit exchanges GDP for GTP and dissociates from the β/γ complex. The free Gα subunit, and in some cases, the β/γ complex can activate some relatively common downstream pathways and initiate positive feedback loops. Activation of these pathways is usually intertwined. One common pathway involves the activation of one or more isozymes of PLC, leading to phosphoinositide hydrolysis. Three classes of PLC (β, γ, and δ), have been described, and multiple isozymes exist within each class.[1395] The best-studied PLCs in platelets include PLCβ and PLCγ_2. PLCβ is often activated downstream of the seven-transmembrane, G-protein–coupled, receptor family, whereas PLCγ_2 can be activated by phosphorylation on tyrosine, which is a downstream signal from other types of agonist receptors. PLC of either type hydrolyzes phospholipids between the glycerol backbone and the phosphate moiety; the PLCβ class is relatively specific for phosphoinositides, whereas PLCγ can cleave other types of phospholipids as well. The hydrolysis of one particular phosphoinositide, PI 4,5-bisphosphate (PIP$_2$), by either class of PLC is critical in platelet function, since it results in the formation of two important products, IP$_3$ and DAG. IP$_3$ binds to specific receptors on the DTS/sarcoplasmic reticulum, causing a release of intracellular Ca^{2+}. Increases in intracellular Ca^{2+} are important for activation of a number of signaling enzymes and proteins involved in cytoskeletal reorganization. Increases in calcium are also important in granule fusion and the release reaction. DAG binds to PKC and participates in its conversion to an active enzyme. For many agonists, activation of one or more of the multiple isozymes of PKC is an obligatory step in the conversion of integrin $\alpha_{IIb}\beta_3$ to a high affinity fibrinogen receptor and subsequent platelet aggregation.[918,1396,1397] One consequence of PKC activation is to cause the release of ADP from dense granules. Released ADP acts at its own seven-transmembrane G-protein–coupled receptor(s) to potentiate the action of numerous agonists. The precise mechanism(s) by which PKC causes integrin $\alpha_{IIb}\beta_3$ activation, however, remains unclear.

Activation of a number of receptors also leads to the activation of PLA$_2$, which releases arachidonic acid from membrane lipid stores. Arachidonic acid is rapidly converted to prostaglandin (PG) products, PGH$_2$ and TXA$_2$, which are themselves potent activators of platelet aggregation.

Adenosine Diphosphate: P2Y$_1$, P2Y$_{12}$, P2X$_1$

Platelets express receptors for both ADP and ATP. Both nucleotides are present in platelet dense granules and are secreted when platelets are activated by adequate concentrations of most, if not all, agonists. Another source of these nucleotides is the red blood cell (RBC); damaged RBCs or those subjected to high shear stress, may release ADP and ATP, increasing their local concentrations. ADP is an especially important physiologic agonist, not only because it can induce platelet aggregation independent of other agonists, but because secreted ADP contributes significantly to the full aggregation response induced by many other agonists. This has been convincingly demonstrated in experimental systems in which secreted ADP is rapidly degraded or inhibited. Moreover, submaximal concentrations of ADP synergize with other agonists, and this has been best studied with epinephrine. ADP induces or contributes to a variety of responses in platelets: shape change, granule release, TXA$_2$ production, activation of integrin $\alpha_{IIb}\beta_3$, and platelet aggregation.[1398,1399] Recent pharmacologic and cloning and sequencing studies suggest that ADP exerts its full effect on platelets through at least two different receptors. These receptors, P2Y$_1$ and P2Y$_{12}$, are G-protein–coupled, and are responsible for most of the physiologic effects of ADP.[1400]

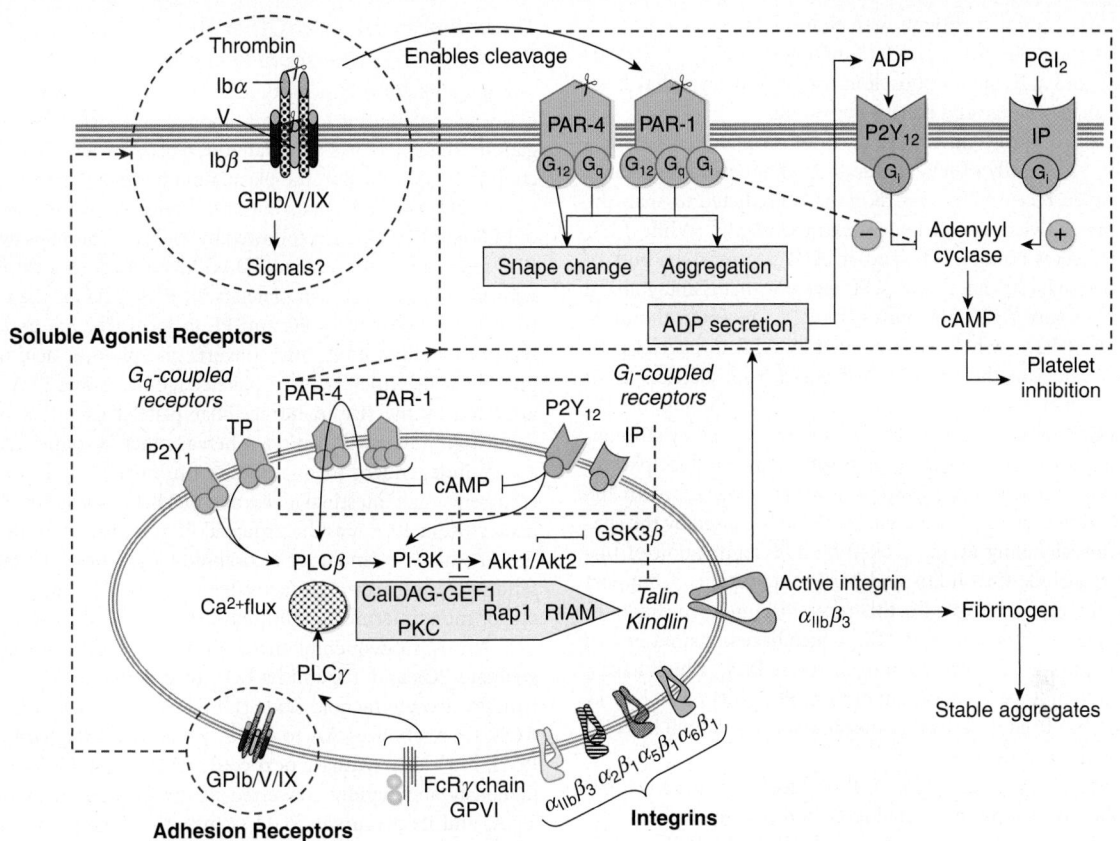

Figure 112–15. Role of G-protein–coupled receptors in platelet activation. Under basal conditions, prostacyclin produced by endothelial cells inhibits platelet activation by binding to its platelet receptor IP and increasing cyclic adenosine monophosphate (cAMP). When the endothelium is denuded, collagen interaction with GPVI can initiate signaling via the FcRγ-chain. In addition, the GPIb/V/IX complex can mediate adhesion of platelets to the newly exposed or deposited von Willebrand factor. This, in turn, can lead to platelet activation directly by a pathway not shown. GPIb/V/IX can also contribute to platelet activation by thrombin by facilitating the cleavage of protease-activated receptor (PAR)-1. Not shown is another pathway to PAR-1 cleavage and activation via collagen-induced release of matrix metalloproteinase (MMP)-1. In concert with PAR-4, cleaved PAR-1 initiates intracellular signaling pathways through molecular switches from the G_q, G_{12}, and G_i protein families. This results in adenosine diphosphate (ADP) secretion and subsequent activation of both $P2Y_{12}$, and $P2Y_1$. A number of signals can also initiate the synthesis of thromboxane (TX) A_2, which can exit from the platelet and activate the same or other platelets by binding to its own receptor, TP. Ultimately, activation of phospholipase C (PLC) β and γ, and released calcium (Ca^{2+}) initiate a series of steps that terminate in talin and kindlin binding to the cytoplasmic domain of β_3 and activation of the glycoprotein (GP) $\alpha_{IIb}\beta_3$ receptor to its high affinity ligand binding state. CalDAG-GEF1, calcium and diacylglycerol-regulated guanine-nucleotide exchange factor 1; PKC, protein kinase C; RIAM, Rap1-guanosine triphosphate (GTP)-interacting adapter molecule. *(Reproduced with permission from Smyth SS, Woulfe DS, Weitz JI, et al: G-protein-coupled receptors as signaling targets for antiplatelet therapy.* Arterioscler Thromb Vasc Biol *29(4):449–457, 2009.)*

The platelet $P2Y_{12}$ receptor, which is the target of the thienopyridine class of drugs (ticlopidine, clopidogrel, prasugrel, and ticagrelor) that are used in the treatment of acute coronary syndromes and peripheral vascular disease, as well as to prevent thrombosis following percutaneous vascular interventions, has been cloned and sequenced.[1401] It couples to Gαi[1402–1404] to inhibit adenylyl cyclases, a class of enzymes that produce cAMP, which, in turn, activates type A protein kinases that inhibit platelet activation by a variety of effects. VASP is phosphorylated in response to $P2Y_{12}$-mediated activation of protein kinase A and so the extent of VASP phosphorylation in response to a combination of ADP and an agent that stimulates cAMP formation can be used as a marker for receptor blockade (see "Nitric Oxide" below). Decreases in cAMP level alone are likely insufficient to activate platelets,[1405,1406] and ADP-activation of platelets requires synergistic effects between the signaling pathways of the $P2Y_1$ and $P2Y_{12}$ receptors (and perhaps the $P2X_1$ ATP receptor.) Regulation of $P2Y_{12}$ is complex and involves homologous desensitization, internalization, and recycling.[1407] Studies of $P2Y_{12}$ knockout mice demonstrate that $P2Y_{12}$ contributes to multiple steps during thrombosis, including platelet adhesion and activation, thrombus growth, and thrombus stability.[1408] Platelets obtained from $P2Y_{12}$-deficient mice respond only weakly to ADP and less vigorously than normal to other agonists such as collagen and thrombin.[1409] A minor $P2Y_{12}$ haplotype (H2) has been associated with enhanced ADP-induced platelet aggregation, as well as resistance to the antiplatelet effects of clopidogrel.[1410,1411]

The platelet $P2Y_1$ receptor, the other G-protein–coupled ADP receptor on platelets, has been cloned and sequenced and a high-resolution crystal structure demonstrating two disparate ligand binding sites is available.[1412] Data from experiments with inhibitors of $P2Y_1$ and mice lacking $P2Y_1$ suggest that stimulation of this receptor is necessary, but not sufficient, to induce platelet aggregation. Thus, platelets from $P2Y_1$-null mice are unable to change shape or aggregate in response to ADP; however, ADP activation does cause a decrease in cAMP via its effects on $P2Y_{12}$.[1413,1414] $P2Y_1$ couples to heterotrimeric G-proteins containing Gαq. The importance of Gαq can be inferred from the observation that platelets from mice that do not express Gαq do not aggregate in response to ADP and that patients with abnormalities in Gαq have a bleeding disorder and abnormal platelet function (Chap. 121).[1415] Activation of PLCβ and subsequent phosphoinositide hydrolysis has been linked to both shape change and platelet activation.

P2X$_1$, the third purine nucleotide receptor on platelets is P2X$_1$ a member of the P2X family of ligand-gated ion channels rather than a G-protein–coupled receptor.[1416] This receptor is predicted to span the plasma membrane twice and is largely extracellular.[1417] While P2X$_1$ has been described as both an ATP and an ADP receptor, the bulk of current evidence suggests that it is an ATP receptor that is antagonized by ADP.[1418,1419] Because ATP antagonizes the P2Y$_{12}$ receptor, the overall contribution of P2X$_1$, which is stimulated by ATP, to platelet activation, is not clear. Nonetheless, ATP is released from platelets upon stimulation with agonists such as collagen[1420] and ATP binding to P2X$_1$ causes a rapid Ca^{2+} influx.[1421] However, Ca^{2+} influx induced by stimulation of this receptor alone appears to be insufficient to induce platelet shape change or aggregation.[1405] It does, however, synergize with the P2Y platelet ADP receptors.[1421] This synergy is likely caused by the specific downstream signaling events evoked by ATP stimulation of this receptor, which include Ca^{2+} influx and MAPK activation.[1420] Support for a biologically important role for this receptor comes from data in both mice with targeted deletions of P2X$_1$, which have impaired *in vivo* thrombus formation,[1422] and mice that overexpress P2X$_1$, which have a prothrombotic phenotype.[1423] A variant of P2X$_1$ P(2X1del), which lacks 17 amino acids, has been described in megakaryocyte-like cell lines,[1424] but its functional role is uncertain.[1418,1419]

Several antiplatelet agents inhibit ADP-induced platelet activation. Thus, metabolites of ticlopidine, clopidogrel, and prasugrel inhibit the P2Y$_{12}$ receptor[1425] (Chap. 134), whereas soluble CD39 catabolizes ADP and ATP.[1426]

Epinephrine: α2A Adrenergic Receptors

When added to platelet-rich plasma, epinephrine uniquely-initiates a first phase of aggregation without first inducing shape-change; after a plateau period, a second wave of aggregation occurs. The ability of epinephrine to synergize with other agonists, such as ADP, is well documented, but there is controversy as to whether epinephrine, in the absence of released ADP or TXA$_2$, is sufficient to initiate platelet aggregation.[1427-1429] Epinephrine can cause an elevation in intracellular Ca^{2+}, even in aspirin-treated platelets,[1427] possibly by opening an external channel or causing release of calcium from membrane sources[1428,1429]; it does not appear to mobilize intracellular Ca^{2+} or generate measurable amounts of IP$_3$. Analysis of the purified epinephrine receptor and its nucleotide sequence identified it as a seven-transmembrane, G-protein–coupled, α2A adrenergic receptor of Mr 64,000.[1430,1431] It couples to Gαi family members, primarily Gαz, to inhibit adenylyl cyclase and thus prevent formation of cAMP.[1432] The reduction in cAMP caused by epinephrine is probably not sufficient, however, to initiate platelet aggregation, and it is likely that other effectors are required for platelet activation.[1433-1436] Platelets from a patient with a chronic bleeding disorder contained reduced amounts of Gαi1 and displayed impaired epinephrine-induced aggregation, suggesting that Gαi1 may also contribute to epinephrine-mediated responses.[1437] Polymorphisms of the α2A adrenergic receptor have been associated with enhanced platelet reactivity and signaling.[1438,1439]

The physiologic and pathologic significance of epinephrine-induced platelet activation remain unclear, but there is a possibility that sympathetic stimulation may contribute to enhanced platelet activation.[1440] In particular, in animal models, infusion of epinephrine can enhance platelet thrombus formation and can overcome the inhibition produced by aspirin.[1441,1442] Increased sympathetic tone may thus account for the resistance to antiplatelet agents during acute coronary syndromes.[1443]

Thromboxane A$_2$ and Other Arachidonic Acid Metabolites: Thromboxane Prostanoid Receptor

The metabolism of arachidonic acid (AA) to TXA$_2$ is a fundamental pathway contributing to agonist-induced platelet activation and aggregation. Many agonists stimulate the release of AA from phosphatidylcholine (PC) and PE in the plasma membrane.[1444] Most AA is released by the action of PLA$_2$, but some is also released by the concerted actions of PLC and DAG kinase, followed by PLA$_2$ and perhaps by the action of PLC followed by the action of DAG lipase. PLA$_2$ is a cytosolic enzyme, with multiple isoforms in platelets.[1445] PLA$_2$ acts on the C2 position of triacylglycerols such as PC and PE to form free AA and the resulting lysophospholipid. PLA$_2$ also converts phosphatidic acid into lysophosphatidic acid, which is also a platelet agonist. Some PLA$_2$ isozymes are activated by the rise in intracellular platelet Ca^{2+} that occurs during agonist-stimulated activation, whereas other isozymes are activated in a Ca^{2+}-independent manner. Studies in mice[1446] and in a patient with recurrent small intestinal ulcers and platelet dysfunction[1447] have identified cytosolic PLA$_2$α as the principal PL responsible for the liberation of the AA that is essential for eicosanoid biosynthesis in platelets. Ligand binding to integrin α$_{IIb}$β$_3$ activates cytosolic PLA$_2$α, perhaps through one or more intermediary proteins.[1448]

AA is subsequently metabolized by cyclooxygenase (COX) to generate PGs and TX and by LOX to generate leukotrienes (LTs) and hydroxyeicosatetraenoic acids (HPETEs). The main COX in platelets, COX-1, metabolizes AA to PGG$_2$, which is subsequently converted to PGH$_2$.[1449,1450] TX synthase next converts PGH$_2$ to TXA$_2$, which is spontaneously and rapidly converted to the inactive metabolite, TXB$_2$.[1451] TXA$_2$ and its precursor, PGH$_2$, can both stimulate platelet TX receptors to induce platelet aggregation.[1451-1453] An inducible COX (COX-2) is present in many cells involved in mediating the inflammatory response and megakaryocytes, but only trace amounts are present in normal platelets.[1454,1455] COX inhibitors such as aspirin inhibit platelet function by inhibiting COX-1 and decreasing TXA$_2$ production.[1451] It has been hypothesized that some patients whose platelets are resistant to aspirin inhibition may have increased amounts of COX-2, which is not as readily inhibited by aspirin as COX-1.[1452] Selective COX-2 inhibitor drugs are associated with increased risk of thrombosis and this is ascribed to their inhibition of endothelial cell prostacyclin production without the compensatory inhibition of TXA production via COX-1.[1456]

TXA$_2$ is a potent platelet agonist that exerts its effects via interaction with specific members of the thromboxane prostanoid receptor (TP) family of G-protein–coupled receptors. There are two TP isoforms in human platelets (TPα and TPβ), which arise from alternative splicing of exon 3 of the TP gene; TPβ, but not TPα, undergoes agonist-induced internalization.[1457] Although both TPα and TPβ mRNA can be detected in platelet lysates, it appears that TPα is the dominant form.[1458] The TXA$_2$ receptor has been localized to the platelet plasma membrane and on sodium dodecylsulfate (SDS)-polyacrylamide gel electrophoresis it migrates as a broad band of Mr 55,000 to 57,000,[1459,1460] the range a result of variability in glycosylation.[1458] Pharmacologic studies suggest the existence of two distinct TXA$_2$ receptor subtypes based on differing affinities for agonist ligands. The low-affinity binding sites may mediate platelet aggregation and granule secretion, whereas the high-affinity sites seem to be associated with platelet shape change.[1461] Studies of TP-deficient mice demonstrate that this gene locus is responsible for most, if not all, the biologic effects attributed to TXA$_2$.[1462] Bleeding times in these mice are prolonged, confirming the importance of this pathway in normal hemostasis. Platelet aggregation to collagen, but not ADP, is delayed, demonstrating the importance of TXA$_2$ production to the collagen response in platelets. TXA$_2$ pathways activate Gαq,[1415,1463] Gα12 and Gα13,[1464,1465] Gα11,[1466] and Gαi2.[1467,1468] Activation of Gαq is essential for aggregation and secretion whereas the Gα12/13-pathways contribute to shape change and aggregation.[1469-1471] It is unclear whether TP directly couples to GαI[1472] or activates this pathway indirectly via released ADP.[1467,1470] A significant portion of PGH$_2$/TXA$_2$-induced platelet aggregation is actually mediated by secreted ADP, because ADP scavenger systems inhibit aggregation induced by a stable PGH$_2$/TXA$_2$ analogue either partially (30 percent)[1473] or totally.[1472]

AA can also be converted to LTs and lipoxins by the sequential actions of LOX and other enzymes. Platelets from most animal species lack 5-LOX, but possess 12-LOX. Consequently, AA liberated by cytosolic PLA$_2$α can be oxygenated by 12-LOX to generate 12-HPETE, an unstable intermediate that is reduced by glutathione peroxidase or other mechanisms to generate HETE. The generation of 12-HPETE in platelets is slower and more sustained than the generation of TXA.[1474] Platelets from mice deficient in the platelet-type 12-LOX are hypersensitive to stimulation by ADP, suggesting an inhibitory role for this pathway in platelet activation by ADP.[1475] 12-LOX activity in platelets can be regulated by signaling through the GPVI collagen receptor.[1476] Because they lack 5-LOX, platelets do not generate LTB$_4$, nor do they appear to possess LTB$_4$ receptors.[1477] However, they participate in LT and lipoxin (LX) generation through transcellular metabolism involving leukocytes. Leukocyte metabolism of AA, some of which may be derived from platelets, by 5-LOX generates LTA$_4$, which is then released and can be transformed by glutathione-*S*-transferase in platelets to LTC$_4$.[1478] The generation of LTC$_4$ by platelets requires P-selectin–mediated adhesion to leukocytes.[1479] Leukocyte-derived LTA$_4$ can also be converted by platelets to the antiinflammatory metabolite LXA$_4$ by the actions of 12-LOX in platelets.[1480]

Thrombin

Thrombin is derived from the inactive zymogen, prothrombin, which circulates in plasma. When acted upon by the prothrombinase complex (FXa, FVa, Ca^{2+}) assembled on the membrane of activated platelets and other cells, prothrombin is cleaved into thrombin[1481] (Chap. 113), one of the most potent platelet agonists. The proteolytic activity of thrombin is required for its role as a platelet agonist.[1482] Thrombin activates PAR-1, a seven-transmembrane G-protein–coupled receptor on platelets and other cells,[514,1483,1484] by cleaving an extracellular 41-amino-acid peptide from the N-terminus of the receptor (Fig. 112–16). Removal of this peptide results in a new aminoterminus, which acts as a "tethered ligand," by binding to another region of PAR-1 to activate the receptor and initiate signal transduction. Short peptides modeled after the "tethered ligand" region (e.g., SFLLRN) also activate PAR-1 signaling. The 41-amino-acid cleavage product of PAR-1 can also induce platelet aggregation by a poorly defined mechanism.[1485] PAR-1 can also be cleaved to an active form by MMP-1 when platelets are stimulated with collagen, but the cleavage site is two amino acids N-terminal to the thrombin cleavage.[1390] A crystal structure of PAR-1 bound to vorapaxar, a small molecule antagonist recently approved for secondary prophylaxis of cardiovascular disease,[1486] has been solved and provides insights into PAR-1 activation by the SFLLRN-tethered ligand.[1487]

Cloning of PAR-1 and gene deletion experiments in mice led to the discovery of additional members of the PAR family[1483,1488,1489]: PAR-1 and PAR-4 are the main thrombin signaling receptors on human platelets; PAR-3 and PAR-4 mediate thrombin activation on mouse platelets; and PAR-2 is a receptor for trypsin and other proteases. Short endogenous peptide sequences that function as selective agonists have been identified for PAR-1 (SFLLR), PAR-2 (SLIGK), and PAR-4 (GYPGQV). On human platelets, a full response to thrombin requires both PAR-1 and PAR-4.[1489,1490] The receptors display distinct kinetics of activation and desensitization; PAR-1 mediates a substantial portion of thrombin signaling, but PAR-4 contributes at high doses of thrombin.[1490-1493] PAR-3 and PAR-4 serve as thrombin receptors on murine platelets,[1488] where PAR-4 is the primary signaling molecule[1494] and PAR-3 functions

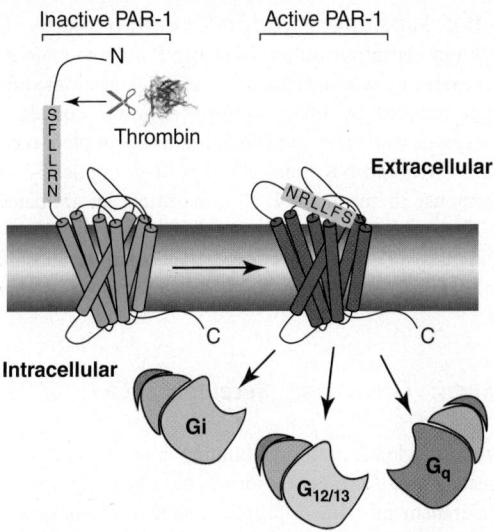

Figure 112–16. Protease-activated receptor (PAR)-1 activation by thrombin. Thrombin cleaves PAR-1 N-terminus and exposes a new N-terminal peptide SFLLRN, which can bind to and activate the transmembrane core of PAR-1. PAR-1 can activate several G proteins, including G$_i$, G$_{12/13}$, and G$_q$. *(Reproduced with permission from Zhang C, Srinivasan Y, Arlow DH, et al: High-resolution crystal structure of human protease-activated receptor 1.* Nature *492(7429):387–392, 2012.)*

as a cofactor for the cleavage and activation of PAR-4 by thrombin.[1495] Deficiency of either PAR-4 or PAR-3 results in a bleeding defect and protection from experimental thrombosis in mice.[1494,1496]

When platelets are exposed to a subaggregating concentration of thrombin, they become relatively insensitive to subsequent stimulation with an aggregating concentration of thrombin, a process termed homologous desensitization. This involves rapid receptor internalization and alterations in the thrombin receptor signaling systems.[1497] Trafficking of the thrombin receptor to lysosomes is dictated by the amino acid sequence in the cytoplasmic tail of PAR-1 and requires phosphorylation. In comparison with PAR-1, activation-dependent internalization of PAR-4 occurs to a lesser extent and termination of PAR-4 signaling occurs more slowly,[1493] resulting in distinct patterns of signaling through each receptor.

PAR-1 activation can be either proinflammatory or antiinflammatory, depending on the dose of thrombin. PAR-1 activation in nonhematopoietic cells contributes to the innate immune response to viral infection with influenza A and coxsackievirus B3 in animal models[1499] but in other models PAR-1 activation enhances influenza A pathogenicity in response to severe infection and PAR-1 deficiency offers protection.[1500] Thus, the relative roles of platelet PAR-1 and tissue-specific PAR-1 in viral infections are complex.[1501]

Thrombin can bind to GPIbα, and platelets from patients lacking the GPIb/IX complex (Bernard-Soulier syndrome) have decreased thrombin-induced platelet aggregation (Chap. 121). A region on GPIbα with three sulfated tyrosines and a large number of anionic amino acids, with homology to the high-affinity thrombin inhibitor hirudin, contains the thrombin binding site.[1132,1502] Tertiary structures of the extracellular, aminoterminal domain of GPIbα bound to thrombin indicate that two thrombin molecules interact with each GPIbα.[1503,1504] This bivalent interaction may allow thrombin to serve as a bridge linking GPIbα receptors on the same or adjacent platelets.[1132,1502] Binding of thrombin to GPIb may also enhance activation via PAR-1. Thrombin can activate platelets via interaction with GPIb even when both PAR-1 and PAR-4 have been desensitized, and there may be a still unidentified mechanism by which thrombin activates platelets independent of PAR-1, PAR-4, and GPIb.[1505]

Tachykinins: Substance P and Endokinins A and B

The tachykinin neurotransmitter substance P induces platelet aggregation and the release reaction at micromolar concentrations and enhances aggregation induced by other agonists at lower concentrations.[1506] Platelets express two seven-transmembrane G-coupled–receptors for substance P (NK_1 and NK_2) and NK_1 has been implicated in mediating the response to substance P.[1507] In addition, an amidated peptide from the C-terminus of the related tachykinins, endokinins A and B (GKASQFFGLM-NH_2), initiates platelet aggregation. Substance P has also been identified in platelets and platelets secrete substance P when activated.

Chemokines: Chemokine Receptors CCR1, CCR3, CCR4, CXCR1, CXCR4

Based on monoclonal antibody binding and/or mRNA expression studies, platelets and/or megakaryocytes have been reported to express the seven-transmembrane G-protein–coupled chemokine receptors CCR1, CCR3, CCR4, CXCR1, and CXCR4 (reviewed in Refs. 762 and 1508). These receptors may play a role in megakaryopoiesis and platelet production. In addition, a number of chemokines, in particular PF4 (CXCL4), CXCL12, CCL13, and CCL22, have been variably found to be able to either augment platelet activation and aggregation induced by other agonists, or to actually fully initiate platelet adhesion, activation, and aggregation. Because high concentrations of the chemokines relative to plasma concentrations are required to demonstrate these effects, it is unclear what role these receptors play in platelet physiology, but it is possible that local chemokine levels are higher in areas of inflammation.

Lipid Mediators (Platelet-Activating Factor, Lysophosphatidic Acid, and Sphingosphine-1-Phosphate)

PAF (a mixture of 1-O-hexadecyl-2-acetyl-sn-glycero-3-phosphocholine and 1-O-octadecyl-2-acetyl-sn-glycero-3-phosphocholine[1509]) is a phospholipid ether produced by platelets, leukocytes, and other cells. PAF is a potent platelet agonist and mediator of inflammation. Cellular responses to PAF are mediated by a specific seven-transmembrane G-protein–coupled receptor.[1510,1511] PAF induces G-protein–dependent inhibition of adenylyl cyclase and activation of PLC,[1512] which cause phosphoinositide turnover, leading to the activation of PKC and an increase in intracellular Ca^{2+}.[1511] PAF also indirectly activates PLA_2, which causes release of AA from the platelet membrane.[1513] All of these effects contribute to the overall platelet response to PAF. PAF is catabolized by PAF acetylhydrolase and this enzyme may play an important role in inflammation and atherosclerosis.[1514]

LDLs activate human platelets, and oxidized LDLs are more potent platelet activators. One active component in oxidized LDLs is oxidized phosphatidylcholine ($oxPC_{36}$), which increases with diet-induced hyperlipidemia. $oxPC_{36}$ signals through CD36[1325] via phosphorylation of the MAPKs p38 and c-Jun N-terminal kinase.[1323] Platelet activation by oxidized LDLs in the absence of hyperlipidemia may also require SR A.[1324] Increases in levels of $oxPC_{36}$ with hyperlipidemia may provide an explanation for observations that atherogenic mice have a prothrombotic phenotype as indicated in vivo by decreased tail-bleed time and propensity to thrombosis in response to either ferric chloride or photochemical injury, and in vitro by increased platelet aggregation.[1325,1515]

Activated platelets likely contribute to lysophosphatidic acid (LPA) generation in blood[1516] via lysophospholipase D (lysoPLD)-catalyzed hydrolysis of a lysophosphatidyl choline (LPC).[1517] Autotaxin, initially identified as a tumor-cell derived motility factor, appears to be responsible for the majority of lysoPLD activity in serum; it is also responsible for the formation of LPA from LPC[1518] and release of autotaxin from platelets may promote tumor cell metastasis through the generation of

LPA.[1519] Mild oxidation of LDL generates LPA, and the LPA component of oxidized LDL in the lipid-rich thrombogenic core of atherosclerotic lesions exposed during plaque rupture may be an important platelet activator.[1520]

In human platelets, LPA elicits shape change,[1521] platelet-monocyte aggregate formation,[1522] and fibronectin-matrix assembly[1523]; it also potentiates ADP-induced platelet aggregation. LPA signaling pathways couple by activation of the small G-protein Rho,[1521] Src kinase activity, and calcium entry,[1524] with little activation of Gq-dependent pathways.[1525] Some of the platelet responses to LPA in whole blood are attenuated by $P2Y_1$ and $P2Y_{12}$ receptor antagonists, suggesting that released ADP may play an important role in mediating aspects of the response to LPA.[1524] The platelet receptor(s) responsible for LPA signaling are not known.

S1P is a weaker activator of platelets than LPA and requires high concentrations (>10 μM) to induce platelet aggregation,[1526] raising the possibility that a contaminant or a S1P-derived metabolite may account for its biologic activity.[1527] S1P elicits platelet shape change,[1528] activates protein kinases, and stimulates fibronectin matrix assembly.[1523] Paradoxically, S1P has also been reported to inhibit thrombin- and epinephrine-induced platelet aggregation.[1529]

Serotonin

Platelets serve as the major serotonin (5-hydroxytryptophan [5HT]) storage site in the circulation because they have the capacity to take it up actively and store it in dense granules. The release of serotonin from dense granules during platelet activation may amplify platelet aggregation and granule release. Serotonergic receptors, which are seven-transmembrane G-protein–coupled receptors, exist in seven main subfamilies termed $5HT_1$ to $5HT_7$.[1530] The receptor that mediates serotonin's effects on platelet function is of the $5HT_{2A}$ subtype and is identical to the $5HT_{2A}$ receptor present in the brain frontal cortex.[1531-1534] The $5HT_2$ receptor-blocking compound ketanserin antagonizes serotonin's stimulatory effects on platelets and neurons.[1535] Two naturally occurring amino acid substitutions have been identified in the receptor.[1536] Platelets from patients heterozygous for the H452Y polymorphism have a blunted calcium response when stimulated with serotonin compared to platelets from patients homozygous for H452.[1536] Silent polymorphisms in the $5HT_{2A}$ gene (T102C in exon 1 and −1438A/G in the promoter region) have been correlated with nonfatal acute MIs and enhanced $5HT_{2A}$ receptor-mediated small platelet aggregate formation.[1537] Many studies have been performed correlating platelet serotonin transporter activity and $5HT_{2A}$ receptors with a number of neuropsychiatric disorders.[1538-1542] There is some concern, however, about the correlation between $5HT_{2A}$ receptors on platelets and those in the brain.[1543] Hyperresponsive $5HT_{2A}$ receptors have been implicated in the association between depression and increased risk of cardiovascular events.[1544]

Addition of serotonin in micromolar concentrations to platelets in vitro causes elevation of intracellular calcium, PLC activation, protein phosphorylation, and mild aggregation.[1545,1546] In whole blood, serotonin does not itself cause platelet aggregation, but it does enhance aggregation induced by ADP and thrombin.[1547] Serotonin released from platelets can cause vasoconstriction of blood vessels that have suffered endothelial damage,[1548] further promoting thrombus formation. Inhibition of serotonin's action has a favorable effect in animal models of thrombosis and vascular damage, but it is not clear whether the benefit derives from effects on platelet aggregation or vasoconstriction.[1549] Mice deficient in serotonin have prolonged bleeding times, suggesting a physiologic role for serotonin in hemostasis.[1550]

A role for serotonin in linking procoagulant proteins to activated platelets has been described. Serotonin can attach via a transglutaminase-dependent reaction to multiple substrates, including fibrinogen, VWF, thrombospondin, fibronectin, and α_2-antiplasmin. These serotonylated proteins then associate to a subpopulation of activated platelets termed "coated" platelets, perhaps via interactions with fibrinogen or thrombospondin.[1550,1551] Tissue transglutaminase in platelets can also catalyze the addition of serotonin to the small G-proteins Rab4 and RhoA in a reaction that renders them constitutively active and promotes α-granule secretion.[1552]

The serotonin transporter (SERT), which takes up and releases serotonin, contributes to platelet stores of serotonin. Expression of SERT is required for normal ADP- and thrombin-mediated aggregation of mouse platelets.[1553] Furthermore, SERT activity is enhanced by ligand binding to integrin $\alpha_{IIb}\beta_3$. Case reports have suggested an association between the use of a serotonin reuptake inhibitor and bleeding abnormalities.[1554] Reports conflict as to whether these antidepressants may protect from MI or reduce the complications of acute thrombosis. In mice, platelet release of serotonin is essential for liver regeneration following partial hepatectomy.[1555]

Vasopressin: V_1-Type Receptor

Vasopressin interacts with platelets to induce shape change, aggregation, and dense granule release.[1556] These events follow an induced rise in intracellular calcium and PLC activation.[1557] The platelet binding site is classified pharmacologically as a V_1-type receptor,[1558] and radiolabeled vasopressin binds with a K_D of 1 to 10 nM.[1559] Unlike the case with V_2 receptors that activate adenylate cyclase, the V_1 receptors appear to activate PLC,[1560] perhaps via coupling through Gαq11.[1561] There are fewer than 100 binding sites for vasopressin per platelet,[1562] and there is controversy as to whether physiologic concentrations of vasopressin are sufficiently high to activate platelets directly[1563,1564]; even if vasopressin does not directly activate platelets, it may be able to enhance platelet activation induced by other agonists. Vasopressin V_{1a} receptor antagonists inhibit vasopressin-induced platelet aggregation.[1565,1566]

Angiotensin II: AT1-Type Receptor

Platelets express angiotensin II (AngII) AT1-type receptors.[1567] AngII treatment of platelet-rich plasma results in shape change but not platelet aggregation.[1568,1569] Infusion of AngII into normal volunteers results in platelet activation as assessed by plasma β-thromboglobulin levels and platelet surface expression of P-selectin and fibrinogen binding sites.[1570] Certain AT1 receptor antagonists, such as losartan and irbesartan, competitively inhibit TXA$_2$ receptors on platelets.[1569,1571,1572] AT1 receptor antagonists stimulate NO release from isolated platelets.[1573] In hypertensive rats treated with losartan, platelet function appears to be attenuated,[1574] but data in humans on the effects of administering AT1 receptor antagonists are inconsistent.[1575-1578]

Thrombospondin: Integrin-Associated Protein (Cd47)

Thrombospondin (TSP), a large disulfide-bonded trimer (subunit Mr 160,000), is both a platelet α-granule protein and an extracellular matrix protein present in the subendothelium. TSP is rapidly released from platelets upon thrombin stimulation. In addition to its role as an adhesive protein, TSP also functions as an agonist to stimulate integrin $\alpha_{IIb}\beta_3$-mediated platelet aggregation.[386,1579] Multiple potential TSP receptors are present on platelets, including CD36, integrins $\alpha_{IIb}\beta_3$ and $\alpha_v\beta_3$, and integrin-associated protein (termed CD47). Of these receptors, CD47 is most strongly implicated as the major signaling receptor in response to TSP. CD47 was first discovered as a protein that copurifies with integrins, including integrins $\alpha_{IIb}\beta_3$,[386] $\alpha_v\beta_3$[1580] and $\alpha_2\beta_1$.[1581] The sequence of CD47 indicates that it has a single immunoglobulin-like extracellular domain, five membrane spanning regions, and a short cytoplasmic tail.[391,1579,1580] CD47 probably generates signals independent of integrins and affects integrin function via downstream effects. CD47 couples

physically and functionally to the large G-protein, GαI,[1582] which is of note because all known large G-proteins couple to receptors with seven rather than five transmembrane spanning regions. Further downstream signaling probably involves the activation of tyrosine kinases, including Syk, Lyn, and Fak, as well as PLCγ2.[1583] Studies of mice with targeted deletions of CD47 indicate that it may block the inhibitory effects of NO on platelets,[1584] which may contribute to its role in stimulating platelet adhesion to activated endothelium under low shear rates.[1585]

How other TSP binding sites on platelets contribute to the overall response induced by TSP is not clear. CD36 copurifies with several tyrosine kinases, including Fyn, Lyn, and Yes.[1315] However, whether TSP binding to CD36 activates these kinases and whether they then contribute to the observed platelet response is unknown.

TSP also functions as a reductase for VWF; in α granules it appears to reduce VWF multimer size.[1586,1587] In contrast, TSP also binds to the A3 domain of plasma VWF, where it competes for ADAMTS-13 binding, thus slowing the rate of VWF cleavage, thus favoring large multimers.[1587] TSP also makes a small, but significant, contribution to the conversion of latent TGF-β_1 released from platelets to active TGF-β_1.[478]

Collagen: GPVI and Integrin $\alpha_2\beta_1$

Upon vascular injury, collagens in the subendothelium become exposed to flowing blood and promote both platelet attachment and activation, thereby contributing to normal hemostasis. Collagen is also one of the most thrombogenic substances in atherosclerotic plaques, and upon plaque rupture it is believed to contribute to platelet aggregation and thrombus formation, leading to ischemic damage (Fig. 112–17).[1588] The types of collagen present in the subendothelium include: I, III, IV, V, VI, VIII, and XIII,[1589] the most abundant being types I and III (greater than 95 percent). Under conditions that mimic physiologic blood flow, platelets adhere tightly to collagen types I, III, and IV, weakly to types VI, VII, and VIII, and not at all to type V. However, under static conditions, platelets can adhere to types I to VIII.[1335] Collagens are normally acid insoluble fibers, but can form spiral microfibrils when subjected to proteolysis. Differences in the nature of the collagen surface influence its recognition by platelets.[1590]

Collagen-induced platelet activation probably involves multiple receptors, most notably GPVI and integrin $\alpha_2\beta_1$, with indirect activation of PAR-1 via activation of MMP-1.[1390] GPVI is a Mr 62,000 glycoprotein from the immunoglobulin superfamily[1591-1594] that functions in concert with the FcRγ-chain, with the latter initiating intracellular signaling.[804,1167,1168,1595-1598] Other collagen receptors on platelets include CD36[1309] and a Mr 65,000 protein termed GP65.[1599] The I (inserted) domain in the α_2 subunit of integrin $\alpha_2\beta_1$ is homologous to a number of collagen-binding domains in other proteins and mediates adhesion of the receptor to collagen. Integrin $\alpha_2\beta_1$ recognizes spiral microfibrils, but not the acid insoluble form of collagen in which the monomers assume a banded pattern.[1590] The potential interrelation of all of the collagen receptors is unknown, but GPVI appears to be responsible for platelet interactions with insoluble collagens and GPVI and $\alpha_2\beta_1$ work in concert to recognize collagen spiral microfibrils, perhaps by assembling intracellular proteins into complexes.[964,1600,1601]

GPVI exists as both monomer and dimer in a stable physical complex with the dimeric FcRγ-chain; FcRγ-chain is absent from GPVI-deficient platelets.[1168,1171,1180] The tertiary structure of GPVI revealed a dimeric structure with parallel orientation of the collagen binding domains, separated by a distance (5.5 nm) that matches the orientation of the collagen triple helix.[1596] Molecular docking studies suggested that collagen interacts with a shallow groove on the surface. The addition of either collagen or an antibody that can crosslink GPVI induces tyrosine phosphorylation of the FcRγ-chain.[1180] The kinases contributing to this event are probably Fyn and/or Lyn.[1041,1104,1602] Tyrosine phosphorylation

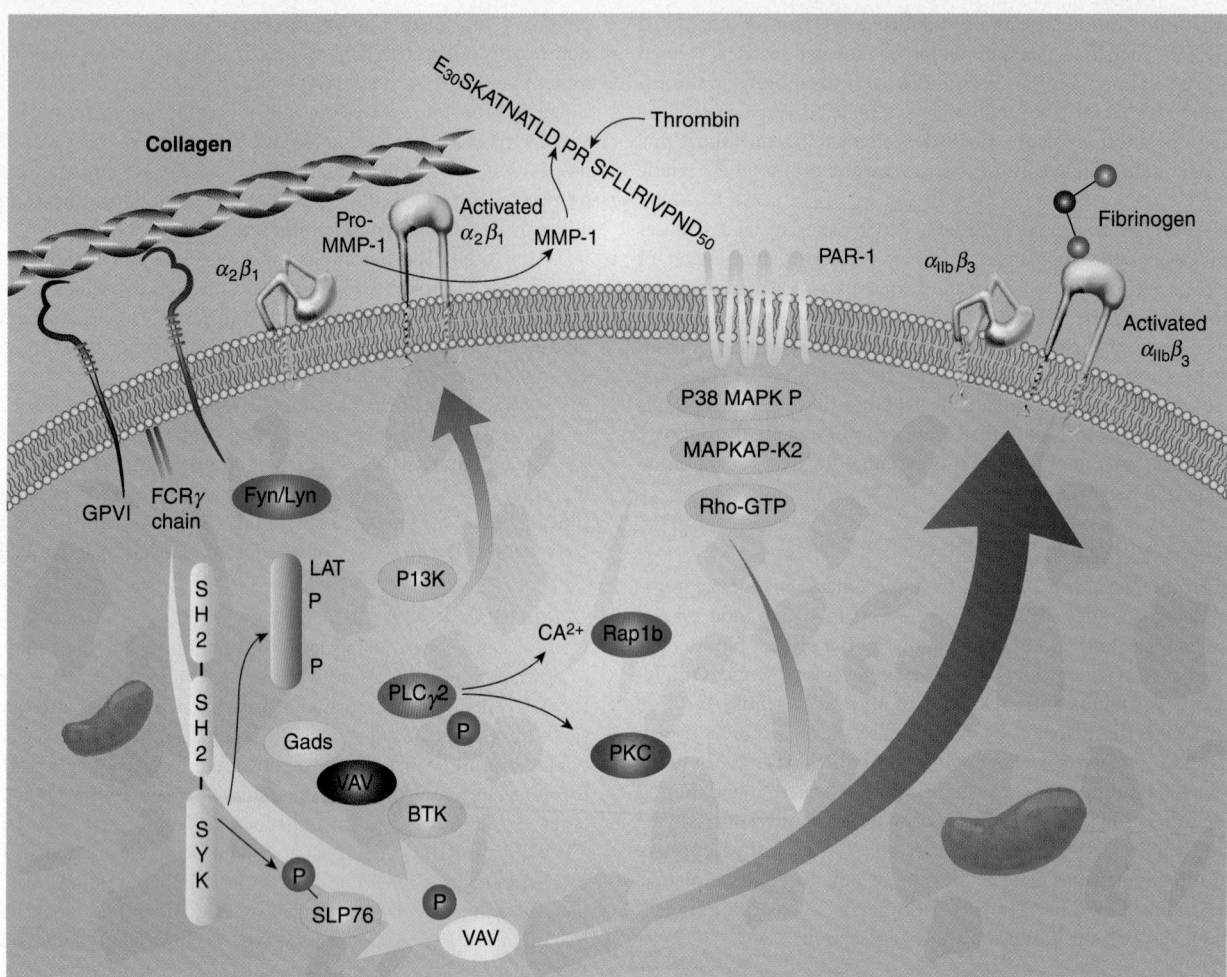

Figure 112–17. Collagen activation of platelets. The platelet collagen receptor GPVI is physically and functionally coupled to the immunoreceptor tyrosine-based activation motif (ITAM)-containing FcRγ-chain. Upon collagen binding to GPVI, GPVI dimerizes as a result of oxidation of intracytoplasmic thiol groups (not shown) and then tyrosine motifs within the FcRγ-chain are phosphorylated (P) by the Src family kinase Fyn. This action initiates a chain of events that includes recruitment of the tyrosine kinase Syk, which is phosphorylated and activated by Fyn and Lyn, and phosphorylation of adaptor proteins LAP and SLP76. A signaling cascade activates Bruton tyrosine kinase (BTK), phospholipase C (PLC)-2, protein kinase C (PKC), and phosphoinositol 3'-kinase (PI3K). Ultimately integrins $\alpha_2\beta_1$ and $\alpha_{IIb}\beta_3$ are converted to a high-affinity ("active") state. Activation of $\alpha_2\beta_1$ promotes firm adhesion to collagen and reinforces intracellular signaling pathways.

of the ITAM on the FcRγ-chain increases the motif's affinity for proteins containing SH2 domains, resulting in the recruitment of such proteins to the FcRγ-chain.[1041,1104] The nonreceptor tyrosine kinase Syk contains two adjacent SH2 domains and a tyrosine kinase domain. In platelets from normal mice, Syk physically associates with the FcRγ-chain and becomes phosphorylated and activated after collagen stimulation,[1180] whereas in platelets from mice lacking FcRγ-chain, collagen is unable to induce Syk phosphorylation and activation.[1597] Similarly, in platelets lacking GPVI or in platelets in which integrin $\alpha_2\beta_1$ is blocked, collagen-induced Syk phosphorylation is also inhibited, demonstrating that GPVI, integrin $\alpha_2\beta_1$, and Syk all participate in the platelet response to collagen. The β subunit of the integrin $\alpha_2\beta_1$ also displays Tyr residues spaced in a manner reminiscent of an ITAM motif, and thus it is possible that Syk might also associate with this collagen receptor. In addition to Syk,[1603] Src also becomes tyrosine phosphorylated in response to collagen. Although Src is an abundant kinase in platelets, its role in platelet signaling is unclear, as mice lacking Src do not suffer from any obvious bleeding disorder.[1605] Syk, on the other hand, appears to play a critical role in collagen activation of platelets as platelets from mice lacking Syk do not aggregate or undergo secretion in response to collagen.[1597]

Collagen stimulation of platelets also results in tyrosine phosphorylation and activation of PLCγ₂,[1606] and activation of this enzyme causes PI hydrolysis, leading to integrin $\alpha_{IIb}\beta_3$ activation. PLCγ₂ activation occurs downstream of Syk, as evidenced by the findings that collagen is unable to activate PLCγ₂ in platelets pretreated with a Syk-selective inhibitor[1607] or in platelets from Syk knockout mice.[1597] It is unknown whether Syk activates PLCγ₂ directly, but Bruton tyrosine kinase (BTK) might be positioned between Syk and PLCγ₂ because patients lacking BTK not only exhibit the B-cell deficiency X-linked agammaglobulinemia, but also show reduced platelet responsiveness to collagen and diminished phosphorylation of PLCγ₂.[1608] Signaling via GPVI also activates the other major collagen receptor integrin $\alpha_2\beta_1$,[1609,1610] perhaps via talin binding to the β₁ cytoplasmic domain,[245] elimination of an inhibitory influence of the α₂ cytoplasmic domain,[245] and/or extracellular disulfide exchange.[973]

Intermediate events of GPVI signaling involve the activation of a small G-protein, Rap-1, which has been implicated in integrin activation in platelets and megakaryocytes.[1611] Full GPVI-induced Rap-1 activation appears to involve both release of ADP (acting on the P2Y₁₂ ADP receptor) and ADP receptor-independent pathways.[1612] GPVI signaling also results in the activation of at least one negative regulator of platelet function, c-CBL, which is tyrosine phosphorylated and activated downstream of Src kinases. Platelets deficient in c-CBL show enhanced aggregation responses in response to GPVI engagement.[1613] While much of the GPVI-mediated signaling occurs via the associated FcRγ, the cytoplasmic domain of GPVI also contains a highly basic region that binds calmodulin and a Pro-rich region that binds Src kinases, which also appear to contribute to GPVI-mediated signaling.[1614] GPVI signaling also leads to the generation of reactive oxygen species.[1615]

Integrin $\alpha_2\beta_1$ can also signal in response to collagen, independent of GPVI and induce phosphorylation and activation of many of the same signaling components attributed to the GPVI-induced signaling cascade, such as Src, Syk, SLP-76, and PLC2. Other components include plasma membrane calcium ATPase and FAK.[1616] However, separate studies indicate that integrin $\alpha_2\beta_1$ must be in an active conformation in order to participate in this signaling.[967,1617] Thus it appears that collagen-induced signaling via GPVI activates integrin $\alpha_2\beta_1$, allowing both receptors to participate in the signaling necessary for a full response to collagen.[1617]

The inactive form of MMP-1 (proMMP-1) is associated with integrin $\alpha_2\beta_1$,[1390] as well as integrin $\alpha_{IIb}\beta_3$.[1618] With collagen activation, MMP-1 becomes activated and then can cleave the N-terminal region of PAR-1, resulting in the generation of a new N-terminal that can insert into the receptor and initiate downstream signaling through the p38 MAPK, Rho-GTP pathway. Of note, the cleavage of PAR-1 by MMP-1 is at a site two amino acids N-terminal to the cleavage site of thrombin. The combined activation of PAR-1, integrin $\alpha_2\beta_1$, and GPVI may account for the high thrombogenicity of collagen surfaces.

The levels of GPVI and integrin $\alpha_2\beta_1$ expressed on platelets vary among individuals, but it is unclear whether there is a correlation between the levels of expression of each of them.[983,1619-1621] The level of expression of these receptors correlates with the ability of platelets to be stimulated by collagen. GPVI is present on the membranes of the open canalicular system and α granules, but these pools are not detectable on the surface of resting platelets. These pools merge with the plasma membrane pool in stimulated platelets, increasing the apparent surface expression of GPVI by approximately 60 percent.[1622]

CD36 can also bind collagen and antibodies to CD36 partially inhibit platelet adhesion to collagen.[1623,1624] Platelets from patients lacking CD36 responded normally to collagen in one study,[1625] but showed a minor defect in adhesion to collagen under flow conditions in another.[1626]

Platelets stimulated with collagen exhibit several distinct responses. Although elevated cAMP levels normally inhibit platelet aggregation, collagen-stimulated platelets are relatively resistant to inhibition by cAMP.[1627] This may be related to the fact that collagen stimulates the PLCγ isotype, which is insensitive to cAMP-mediated inhibition, whereas other agonists such as thrombin stimulate PLCβ, which is inhibited by cAMP. In addition, phosphatase inhibition decreases collagen-, but not thrombin- or ADP-induced platelet aggregation,[1628] suggesting that one or more phosphatases are critical in collagen-induced platelet aggregation.

GPIb/IX/V

The GPIb/IX/V complex promotes the initial interactions of platelets with VWF, particularly under conditions of high shear, resulting in platelet tethering. GPIb/IX/V can also initiate signals that activated the integrin $\alpha_{IIb}\beta_3$ receptor, resulting in firm platelet adhesion and aggregation.[1035] Some of the first evidence that the GPIb/IX/V complex could serve as a signaling receptor came from studies in which antibodies to integrin $\alpha_{IIb}\beta_3$ partially inhibited ristocetin-induced

platelet aggregation.[284] Subsequently, ristocetin-mediated interaction of VWF with platelets was observed to cause PIP_2 metabolism, activation of PKC, and an increase in intracellular Ca^{2+}. Likewise, shear forces initiate signaling through the binding of VWF to GPIb/IX/V.[1629] In heterologous systems such as Chinese hamster ovary (CHO) cells expressing both GPIb/IX and integrin $\alpha_{IIb}\beta_3$, occupancy of GPIb/IX by VWF can lead to activation of $\alpha_{IIb}\beta_3$.[1630,1631] In platelets, the GPIb/IX/V complex associates with signaling proteins with ITAM motifs, such the FcγRIIA receptor[1632] and FcRγ-chain[1105]; however, engagement of GPIb/IX/V alone is sufficient to activate integrin $\alpha_{IIb}\beta_3$.[1633] The signaling pathway triggered by engagement of GPIb/IX/V is incompletely understood but appears to involve activation of Src[1523,1633,1634] and PI3K, and recruitment of the adaptor proteins SLP-76 and ADAP (SLAP-130).[1633] The result is activation of PLC_2,[1635] PKC, and integrin $\alpha_{IIb}\beta_3$. Signaling through the GPIb/IX/V complex also causes release of AA and generation of TXA_2. A cyclic guanosine monophosphate (cGMP) and MAPK-dependent pathway for GPIb/IX-mediated activation of integrin $\alpha_{IIb}\beta_3$ has also been reported.[1636] The GPIb/IX/V complex binds several intracellular proteins, including filamin (actin binding protein),[1092] calmodulin,[1637] and 14-3-3ζ.[1090,1638,1639] Activation of c-RAF by 14-3-3ζ may link GPIb/IX/V signaling to the MAPK signaling pathway; moreover, protein 14-3-3ζ exists as a dimer, which may allow it to bridge and dimerize GPIb molecules.[1639] In CHO cells, clustering of GPIb/IX promotes stable adhesion via integrin $\alpha_{IIb}\beta_3$.[1640]

The GPIb/IX/V complex also appears to be involved in transmitting at least one cAMP-dependent inhibitory signal. Thus, elevated cAMP, which activates protein kinase A (PKA), induces phosphorylation of GPIbβ on Ser 166.[1091] Elevated cAMP also normally inhibits agonist-induced platelet actin polymerization. However, in platelets from patients with Bernard-Soulier syndrome, which lack GPIb/IX/V, actin polymerization proceeds normally after collagen stimulation, even when cAMP is elevated, suggesting that cAMP-mediated phosphorylation of GPIbβ may be required for the cAMP-mediated inhibition.[1641]

GPV, a Mr 82,000 membrane-spanning protein that is a member of the leucine-rich repeat family and complexes with GPIb/IX, is a substrate for thrombin.[1642] GPV-null platelets display enhanced responses to thrombin[1150] and GPV-null mice have accelerated thrombus growth in response to vascular injury.[1643] Proteolytically inactive thrombin selectively activates mouse platelets lacking GPV and induces thrombosis in GPV-deficient but not wild-type mice.[1151] Together, these observations suggest that GPV may function as a negative regulator of thrombin signaling through GPIb/IX, and in its absence, thrombin may function as a ligand for GPIb/IX.

ADDITIONAL INTERMEDIATE SIGNALING MOLECULES

Calcium

Elevation of intracellular Ca^{2+} has a multitude of effects on platelet physiology.[1435,1644] The concentration of Ca^{2+} in resting platelets (100 to 500 nM) is very low compared to the plasma concentration of Ca^{2+} (approximately 2 mM). Exposure of platelets to most agonists is accompanied by a rapid, transient rise in the intracellular free Ca^{2+} concentration to micromolar levels, followed by a less-rapid return to normal resting levels. The cytoplasmic Ca^{2+} concentration at any given time is a result of the rates of passive Ca^{2+} influx, active Ca^{2+} extrusion across the plasma membrane, and both active release and/or uptake of Ca^{2+} by the DTS/sarcoplasmic reticulum (see "Dense Tubular System/Sarcoplasmic Reticulum" above), which is a Ca^{2+} storage depot in platelets analogous to the sarcoplasmic reticulum in muscle. Active Ca^{2+} extrusion and uptake of Ca^{2+} are mediated by several pumps (see Fig. 112-3). The cytosolic pool of Ca^{2+} turns over rapidly as a result of a plasma membrane

Na$^+$/Ca^{2+} antiporter, whereas the DTS/sarcoplasmic reticulum contains a more slowly exchanging pool of Ca^{2+} regulated by a Ca^{2+}/Mg^{2+} ATPase (sarco-/endoplasmic reticulum Ca^{2+}-ATPase 3 [SERCA3]), a pump that also appears to be located in the plasma membrane.[1645] During agonist stimulation, most Ca^{2+} enters the platelet cytosolic compartment through receptor-operated calcium channels (reviewed in Ref. 1646) in the plasma membrane. Collagen, for example, causes Na$^+$ entry into platelets, which reverses the Na$^+$/Ca^{2+} antiporter to promote Ca^{2+} entry, thus contributing to platelet aggregation.[1647] Release of intracellular Ca^{2+} from the DTS/sarcoplasmic reticulum also occurs rapidly in response to agonist stimulation, in large a result of the IP$_3$ generated as part of the phosphoinositide cycle.[1646,1648] The release of internal stores of Ca^{2+} results in translocation of STIM1 from the DTS/sarcoplasmic reticulum, followed by activation of the plasma membrane Ca^{2+} channel OraiI, leading to store-operated Ca^{2+} entry.[119] Calcium entry is also supported by TRPC6 mediating non–store-operated mechanisms, induced by DAG.[93,119,1646] The role of TRPC1 remains to be defined.[93,119,1646] Integrin $\alpha_{IIb}\beta_3$ may also participate in Ca^{2+} entry.[1649]

An intracellular rise of Ca^{2+} levels induces numerous downstream events, including activation of Ca^{2+}-sensitive forms of PLA$_2$[1650] and PKC[1651]; calmodulin-dependent enzymes such as myosin light-chain kinase, which phosphorylates myosin light chain[1652] and promotes cytoskeletal rearrangements required for platelet shape change; and gelsolin, which facilitates actin severing and rearrangement, secretion, and aggregation. In addition, Ca^{2+} probably plays a direct role in controlling the secretory machinery, which mediates the membrane fusion events that result in degranulation and the release reaction. Calcium-dependent proteases or calpains also become activated and play an important role in postaggregation events. The Ca^{2+} binding protein CIB (calcium and integrin binding protein)[1653] binds to the membrane proximal region of α_{IIb}[1654] and contributes to platelet spreading.[31]

Phosphoinositide 3'-Kinases

PI3Ks are a family of lipid kinases that phosphorylate the D-3 hydroxyl group of the myoinositol ring of phosphoinositides.[1655,1656] Class I PI3Ks are heterodimeric protein complexes containing both adaptor and catalytic subunits that use PI, PI(4)P, and PI(4,5)P$_2$ as substrates to form PI(3)P, PI(3,4)P$_2$, and PI(3,4,5)P$_3$, respectively. Class Ia (PI3Kα, PI3Kβ, and PI3Kδ) and class Ib (PI3Kγ) have distinct subunits and regulatory features. The catalytic subunit of class Ia PI3K is a Mr 110,000 to 120,000 protein; the adaptor subunit, p85 (PI3K p85α), has two SH2 domains, a breakpoint cluster region homology domain, a Pro-rich region, and a single SH3 domain. Members of this class of PI3K possess intrinsic serine-threonine protein kinase activity in addition to lipid kinase activity, and they appear to be regulated, at least in part, by binding of the p85 subunit to tyrosine-phosphorylated proteins. Although platelets possess PI3Kα and PI3Kδ, the main class Ia member that is thought to contribute to platelet function is PI3Kβ. PI3Kγ has been isolated from platelets and neutrophils and contains both regulatory (p101) and (p110γ) subunits; the latter is activated by the β/γ subunit of heterodimeric G proteins. Both isoforms of PI3K appear to associate with the platelet cytoskeleton after agonist activation.

In platelets, 3-phosphorylated phosphoinositides are produced in response to a variety of agonists, including thrombin, TXA$_2$, LPA, ADP, and collagen, and may mediate early signaling events that precede integrin $\alpha_{IIb}\beta_3$ activation, as well as late events involved in stabilizing fibrinogen binding and platelet aggregation.[1655–1657] Thrombin stimulates rapid accumulation of PI(3,4,5)P$_3$ and PI(3,4)P$_2$[1658] and late production of Ptdlns(3,4)P$_2$; the latter requires fibrinogen binding to $\alpha_{IIb}\beta_3$ and calpain activity.[1659] Collagen promotes the association of class Ia PI3K via the SH2 domains with tyrosine-phosphorylated forms of FcRγ-chain and the regulatory protein, linker-for-activator T cells, to modulate PI3K.[1660]

Platelets from mice lacking PI3K p85α aggregate normally to ADP, thrombin, U46619 and phorbol esters, but display impaired responses to collagen and CRP and diminished tyrosine phosphorylation of the PI3K effectors Btk, Tec, Akt, and PLCγ_2.[1661] FcγRIIA-induced platelet aggregation requires PI3K activity, which is upstream of PLCγ_2 in the pathway.[1662] Genetic deletion of PI3Kβ in mice results in embryonic lethality, but mice possessing a kinase dead form of the enzyme have been generated. Platelets from these mice have defects in G-protein–coupled receptor (GPCR)-, collagen-, and integrin-mediated signaling pathways.[1663] Platelets from mice lacking PI3Kγ isoform aggregate normally to thrombin and collagen but have impaired responses to ADP, and PI3Kγ-deficient mice are protected from ADP-induced thromboembolism.[1664] Platelets from mice expressing a kinase dead form of PI3Kγ have defective GPCR-induced activation of Rap1 and aggregation, but normal responses through GPVI-activated pathways.[1663] A working model to explain the observations is that PI3Kβ serves as a common intermediary of signals elicited by GPCR, collagen, and integrin ligation, whereas PI3Kγ primarily affects GPCR-initiated pathways. Many of the biologic actions of PI3K are mediated by their phospholipid products, which bind to specific sequences in proteins. The pleckstrin homology (PH) domains (approximately 100-amino-acids long) present in pleckstrin and other platelet proteins involved in signal transduction, recognize either PI(3,4)P$_2$ or PI(3,4,5)P$_3$. Binding of PI(3,4,5)P$_3$ to the aminoterminal PH domain in PLCγ enhances its activity.[1666] PI(3,4,5)P$_3$ binding to PH domains in BTK[1667] targets BTK to the plasma membrane, where it is further phosphorylated and activated.[1668] PI(3,4)P$_2$ or PI(3,4,5)P$_3$ binding to the PH domains in the serine/threonine kinase Akt (or protein kinase B) changes the conformation of Akt, permitting it to become activated by phosphorylation on Ser and Thr by Akt-kinase (PDK1).[1669,1670] Akt activation is biphasic, occurring before and after platelet aggregation.[1659] Two isoforms of Akt are present in human platelets (Akt1 and Akt2).[1671] The Akt isoforms have multiple substrates in platelets. One prominent substrate is glycogen synthase kinase (GSK)-3β, which is inactivated by Akt-mediated phosphorylation. GSK-3β suppresses platelet function and thrombosis in mice.[1672] Akt activation also stimulates NO production and resultant protein kinase G (PKG)-dependent degranulation.[1673] Finally, Akt has been implicated in activation of a cAMP-dependent phosphodiesterase (PDE3A), which plays a role in reducing platelet cAMP levels after thrombin stimulation.[1674] Each of these Akt-mediated events is expected to contribute to platelet activation. Deficiency of Akt2 in mice impairs platelet aggregation, secretion, and fibrinogen binding in response to low doses of thrombin and U46619, but has minimal effects on collagen signaling.[1675] Akt2 null mice have normal bleeding times, but are protected from experimental thrombosis, as are mice with a deficiency of Akt1.[1675,1676] Interestingly, in platelets containing either kinase dead PI3Kβ or PI3Kγ, activation of Akt by ADP was abolished, and yet under the same condition, aggregation was only modestly affected,[1663] which raises questions about the role of Akt in these events.

Small G Proteins

Overview The Ras superfamily of small GTPases are intracellular transducers that act as "on–off" switches to facilitate the response to extracellular stimuli. Platelets contain members of the Ras subfamily (Ras, Ral, and Rap), the Rho subfamily (Rho, Rac, and Cdc42), the Rab subfamily (Rab 1, 3, 4, 6, 8, 11, 27, 31, 32),[1677–1680] and the Arf subfamily (Arf1 or 3 and 6).[1681]

Rho family GTPases are regulators of cytoskeletal remodeling: Cdc42 for filopodia formation, Rac for lamellipodia and membrane ruffling, and Rho for focal adhesion and stress fiber formation.[1682,1683] Platelets have Cdc42,[1684] Rac1,[1685] and RhoA.[1679] Resting platelets have very low levels of the GTP-bound forms of these GTPases,[1686–1688] but all are converted to their GTP-bound states upon platelet activation.[1689,1690] Thus, receptor-mediated signaling activates Rho family GTPases. Cdc42 and Rac1 are activated at a very early phase of stimulation (approximately 10 sec) and reach maximal activation 30 seconds after stimulation with collagen, thrombin, or ADP.[1687,1688,1690,1691] This temporal response is consistent with an early role for these GTPases in filopodia and lamellipodia formation. Integrin-dependent secondary signaling is required for full activation of RhoA,[1686] but not Cdc42 or Rac1,[1687,1690] suggesting a role for RhoA in both early (adhesion/aggregation) and late (clot retraction) stages of platelet activation. More detailed descriptions of each subfamily follows.

Ras Platelets contain at least one Ras isoform (H-Ras).[1692] Despite its intensively studied functions in proliferation, differentiation, and cell survival in nucleated cells,[1693,1694] the exact role of Ras and its signaling in platelets is unclear. Platelets do contain most of the downstream Ras effectors: Raf-1, MEK (MAPK/ERK kinase), and ERK (extracellular signal-regulated kinase).[1695] Ras and ERK are both known to be activated upon platelet stimulation.[1696]

Rho Inactivation of RhoA with C3 exoenzyme treatment inhibits agonist induced shape change,[1697–1699] adhesion/aggregation,[1686,1698,1700,1701] and formation of focal adhesions.[1701] Platelets treated with the exoenzyme also show decreased stress fibers formation, a process mediated by Rho kinase-dependent phosphorylation of myosin light chain (MLC).[1686,1697,1700]

Rac In nucleated cells, Rac1 functions in actin remodeling *via* activation of three downstream effectors; phosphatidylinositol 4-phosphate 5-kinase type Iα, p21-Cdc42/Rac-activated kinase, and suppressor of cyclic AMP receptor/WASP-family verprolin-homologous protein.[1702] The roles of Rac1 in lamellipodia formation and aggregation have been examined using platelets from mice lacking Rac1. Rac1 deletion does not affect platelet production[1703–1705] or filopodia formation, but does affect lamellipodia formation upon stimulation with thrombin and collagen.[1704] Aggregation was diminished in Rac1−/− platelets when stimulated with low-dose of thrombin or collagen, or when subjected to shear stress under flow condition.[1704,1705]

Cdc42 The assessment of Cdc42 function in platelets is less clear. Wiskott-Aldrich syndrome is caused by a defect in WASP, which is a downstream effector of Cdc42. However, the platelets from affected individuals have normal shape change, including filopodia formation and Arp2/3 activation (Chap. 121).[1706] One study suggested that Cdc42 might function in GPVI-mediated integrin $\alpha_2\beta_1$ activation and subsequent platelet adhesion on collagen-coated surfaces.[969]

Rap Rap GTPases participate in cell adhesion, cell–cell junction formation, and the development of cell polarity in nucleated cells.[1707] In platelets, Rap1a, Rap1b, and Rap2 are all activated upon platelet stimulation.[1708,1709] Platelets from Rap1b−/− mice have a defect in platelet aggregation and decreased integrin $\alpha_{IIb}\beta_3$ activation upon platelet stimulation with ADP or PAR-4 peptide.[1710] With the discovery of the important role of CalDAG-GEF1, an exchange factor for Rap1 in platelet function, Rap1's role in integrin signaling has been a major focus of research.[1711] Platelets lacking CalDAG-GEF1 have decreased Rap1B activation and integrin $\alpha_{IIb}\beta_3$ activation.[1712] Integrin $\alpha_{IIb}\beta_3$ activation could be completely blocked by treating CalDAG-GEF1−/− platelets with a PKC inhibitor, suggesting that CalDAG-GEF1 and PKC function independently to activate integrin $\alpha_{IIb}\beta_3$.[1713] Studies using CHO cells reconstituted with integrin $\alpha_{IIb}\beta_3$, talin, and Rap1GTP-interacting adapter molecule (RIAM) showed that Rap1GTP-dependent talin recruitment to integrin β_3 by RIAM is required for integrin $\alpha_{IIb}\beta_3$ activation.[1714] The function of Rap2 remains to be determined; CalDAG-GEF1 does not interact with it.[1715]

Ral In nucleated cells, Ral GTPases (RalA and RalB) are thought to function in regulated exocytosis by recruiting a multisubunit complex termed "exocyst" for targeting secretory vesicles to specific plasma membrane domains.[1716] Both RalA and RalB in platelets are associated with platelet dense granules,[1717] and become rapidly activated in a Ca2+-dependent manner upon platelet activation.[1718] A recombinant Ral-interacting domain of Sec5, a downstream effector of RalA in exocyst complex, inhibits serotonin release from platelet dense bodies, suggesting a role for Ral exocyst in platelet granule release.[1719]

Rab Rab GTPases are the largest family of small GTPases; 63 members are detected in the human genome.[1720] They are highly compartmentalized to different organelle membranes and function by coordinating vesicle transport, including vesicle formation and tethering to their target compartments.[1720] Rab proteins have been shown to play roles in both granule biogenesis and secretion.

Arf Arf family GTPases, in nucleated cells, function in secretory and cytoskeletal processes. Platelets contain Arf1 or 3 and Arf6. Functional studies of Arf6 show that unlike other platelet GTPases, it is in the GTP-bound state in resting platelets and there is a conversion to the GDP-bound state upon platelet activation.[1681] Inhibitors of this transition disrupt aggregation, secretion, and clot retraction. Further analysis suggests that the Arf6-GTP to Arf6-GDP transition is required for activation of Rho family proteins in platelets.

Calcium-Dependent Proteases (Calpains)

After ligand binding, integrin clustering, and platelet aggregation, neutral, cysteine proteases termed *calpains* become activated by a rise in intracellular Ca2+.[229] The most important and best-studied calpains in platelets are: μ-calpain (calpain-1), which is activated by micromolar concentrations of Ca2+ and accounts for 80 percent of the Cys protease activity in platelets, and m-calpain (calpain-2), which requires millimolar levels of Ca2+ for activation.[1721] Each calpain consists of a common Mr 30,000 regulatory subunit paired with a unique catalytic subunit of Mr 80,000. Activated μ-calpain cleaves numerous proteins,[229] including cytoskeletal proteins (e.g., filamin [actin binding protein], talin, WASP, and cortactin), tyrosine kinases (e.g., BTK, Src, Syk, and FAK), tyrosine phosphatases (e.g., protein tyrosine phosphatase 1B [PTP1B also called PTPN1], SHP-1, and PTPMEG), as well as other important platelet proteins (e.g., integrin β_3, SNAP-23, Vav, PLC-β), and certain isoforms of PKC.[1721] Cleavage of talin by calpain *in vitro* enables talin to activate integrin $\alpha_{IIb}\beta_3$,[148] but the role of calpain in activation of integrin $\alpha_{IIb}\beta_3$ by talin in intact platelets is uncertain. Calpain also appears to be upstream of, and able to affect, the activation of the small G proteins Rac and RhoA. Calpain's role in platelet secretion has not been defined, although it is clear that the t-SNARE, SNAP-23 is inactivated by calpain-mediate cleavage.[1722] Thus calpains, through their effects on structural and signaling molecules, appear to affect multiple aspects of platelet function. Mice deficient in μ-calpain demonstrate abnormal platelet aggregation, decreased clot retraction, and reduced tyrosine phosphorylation of several platelet proteins, including the β subunit of integrin $\alpha_{IIb}\beta_3$. These abnormalities in platelet function can be reversed by inhibition of tyrosine phosphatases or by deletion of PTP1B, suggesting that μ-calpain's effects on platelet kinases and phosphatases may be central to its role in platelet function.[1723]

Inside-Out Activation of Integrin $\alpha_{IIb}\beta_3$ and Outside-in Signaling By Activated Integrin $\alpha_{IIb}\beta_3$

The active state of integrin $\alpha_{IIb}\beta_3$ is defined as the conformation that is competent to bind large, soluble, adhesive proteins, such as fibrinogen and VWF, with relatively high affinity. Precise regulation of the activation state of integrin $\alpha_{IIb}\beta_3$ is essential for maintenance of normal hemostasis, such that integrin $\alpha_{IIb}\beta_3$ activation only occurs upon vascular injury. Crystallographic and electron microscope studies suggest that the extracellular portion of both integrin $\alpha_{IIb}\beta_3$ and the related integrin $\alpha_V\beta_3$, are in a bent conformation when inactive and an extended conformation when activated.[149,843,844] The activation state of integrin $\alpha_{IIb}\beta_3$ is controlled by the cytoplasmic domains of this integrin in concert with specific intracellular binding proteins. Thus, under basal conditions, interactions between the cytoplasmic domains of integrins α_{IIb} and β_3 maintain the receptor in the resting state. Interrupting the interactions between the cytoplasmic domains results in long range conformational changes that convert the extracellular portion of the integrin to an active state.[1724] Interactions between regions of the integrins α_{IIb} and β_3 transmembrane and cytoplasmic domains near the membrane involve upper and lower membrane clasps and a salt bridge between acidic and basic amino acid residues of each subunit (see "Integrin $\alpha_{IIb}\beta_3$" above).[871,894,1725,1726] Mutations that disrupt these interactions result in integrin $\alpha_{IIb}\beta_3$ activation.[871,894,1726] Cytoskeletal restraints appear to further maintain integrin $\alpha_{IIb}\beta_3$ in an inactive conformation, because treatment of platelets with low doses of the actin depolymerizing agents activate the integrin.[243] Upon agonist activation, the binding of the cytoskeletal linking proteins talin and kindlin to integrin β_3 may play a key role in the conversion of integrin $\alpha_{IIb}\beta_3$, as well as several other integrins, to an active conformation.[245] One model suggests that filamin binding to the β subunit cytoplasmic tail maintains the receptor in an inactive state by presenting talin binding. The cytoskeletal adapter protein migfilin can displace filamin from the integrin β_3 subunit and facilitate the binding of talin.[901] Talin itself can exist in a conformation that is either less or more favorable for binding to integrin β_3 at multiple sites. The affinity of talin for β integrins increases in response to PI(4,5)P$_2$ binding to talin.[1727] PIP$_2$ may be generated locally from PI via the enzyme phosphatidylinositol phosphate kinase type 1γ, which can bind to talin.[1728,1729] Talin is composed of a Mr 47,000 head domain and a Mr 190,000 rod domain. The head contains a "FERM" domain named for the proteins four point one (4.1), ezrin, radixin, and moesin, that promotes specific interactions with cytoplasmic regions of multiple proteins. The F3 region of the FERM domain, which resembles a phosphotyrosine binding (PTB) domain,[1730] binds sequentially to membrane distal and proximal regions of integrin β_3 in addition to establishing electrostatic interactions with the lipid head groups, disrupting its interaction with the membrane and integrin α_{IIb}.[244,871,894,896,1730–1734] This binding site is not available when PI phosphate kinase (PIPK)I is bound to talin, so presumably any prebound PIPKI would be displaced from talin upon talin interaction with integrin β_3.[1735] After talin binding the reorganization of the transmembrane and intracytoplasmic domains disrupt the interaction of integrins α_{IIb} and β_3 and this is transmitted to the ectodomain.[871,894,1724] The β_3 cytoplasmic domain can also bind proteins that connect it to the cytoskeleton such as α-actinin, ICAP1, filamin, Src, and skelemin, and so it has been proposed that interactions of the integrin β_3 subunit with the actin–myosin contraction apparatus via the cytoskeleton may supply the energy needed to adopt the extended conformation of integrin $\alpha_{IIb}\beta_3$ with the swing out of the of integrin β_3 hybrid domain away from the of βA (I-like) domain.[250] The rod-like region of talin has also been reported to interact with integrin β_3,[1736] and an unknown region of talin has been reported to interact with integrin α_{IIb}.[1737] While these interactions may serve to stabilize or subsequently cluster the integrin, their exact roles are unknown.

Members of the kindlin family of focal adhesion proteins that contain PTB domains serve as integrin activators,[1738–1740] perhaps functioning to facilitate talin–integrin interactions. Kindlin-2 binds the C-terminus of integrin β_3 in a region containing the conserved TS(752) T sequence and NITY(759) motif and acts synergistically with talin to promote integrin $\alpha_{IIb}\beta_3$ activation in a recombinant expression system.[1738] Whereas kindlin-2 is widely distributed, kindlin-3 expression is limited to hematopoietic cells, including platelets. Genetic deletion of kindlin-3 in mice results in a severe bleeding phenotype and defective activation

of integrin $\alpha_{IIb}\beta_3$ on platelets.[1741] Mutations in kindlin-3 have been described in patients with leukocyte adhesion deficiency-III, which is characterized by abnormalities in leukocyte and platelet integrin activation and function (Chap. 121).[1742–1745] In fact, the bleeding symptoms are even more severe than those in Glanzmann thrombasthenia and the platelet aggregation defects are similar. Mutational analysis also identified the NXXY motif (Tyr795) and preceding threonine-region in kindlin binding to integrin β_1.[1746] Finally, based on model systems, it has been proposed that α_{IIb} transmembrane and cytoplasmic domains from adjacent integrin $\alpha_{IIb}\beta_3$ receptors may form homodimers and integrin β_3 transmembrane and cytoplasmic domains may form homotrimers, resulting in stabilization of the activated state and clustering of integrin $\alpha_{IIb}\beta_3$ receptors,[251,1747] but it is not clear that these interactions are favored under biologic conditions.[871,894]

Platelet aggregation is commonly described as progressing through two phases: an initial reversible aggregation phase, which is often the response observed with low concentrations of agonists, followed by a stronger, irreversible phase. The irreversible phase of aggregation correlates with TXA$_2$ production and platelet secretion of ADP. Fibrinogen binding to integrin $\alpha_{IIb}\beta_3$ and the platelet–platelet contacts that occur during the initial phase of aggregation initiate specific signal transduction events, resulting in positive feedback loops that promote irreversible aggregation, maintain secretion, and initiate later events like clot retraction.[291]

Fibrinogen or VWF binding to the extracellular region of integrin $\alpha_{IIb}\beta_3$ transmits long-range conformational changes to the integrin cytoplasmic domains, perhaps via a pivot action between the integrin β_3 βA (I-like) and hybrid domains[827] that induce signaling from outside the platelet to inside the platelet (outside-in signaling).[876,879] These conformational changes, along with integrin clustering,[838] are likely to be the basis for outside-in signal transduction through integrin $\alpha_{IIb}\beta_3$, perhaps by altering the association of the cytoplasmic domains with one another and initiating recruitment of proteins with enzymatic activity to the cytoplasmic tails, forming complexes capable of generating signaling molecules.

One important signaling molecule that is constitutively associated with the integrin β_3 cytoplasmic tail is the tyrosine kinase, Src.[1748–1750] Src binds to the C-terminus of the integrin in resting platelets via its SH3 domain independent of its catalytic activity.[1748] This pool of Src in unstimulated platelets appears to exist in a minimally active state with its activity suppressed in part by the Src regulator Csk, which phosphorylates Src at Tyr 529. Platelet adhesion to fibrinogen increases the Src activity associated with integrin $\alpha_{IIb}\beta_3$ in part because of the dissociation of Csk and subsequent dephosphorylation of Src 529.[1750] Full Src activation occurs upon integrin $\alpha_{IIb}\beta_3$ clustering and transphosphorylation of Src on Tyr 418. Src activation is required for several subsequent signaling events such as the activation of the tyrosine kinase Syk. Syk, along with Src, is required for platelet spreading on fibrinogen.[1748] Syk binds to unphosphorylated integrin β_3 via its N-terminus.[1751,1752] Some of these events have now been visualized in living platelets.[1753] Negative regulators of Src activation include PECAM-1, which can recruit the protein tyrosine phosphatases SHP-1 and SHP-2 via its ITIMs[1749,1754–1757]; carcinoembryonic antigen-related cell adhesion molecule-1, which also possess ITIMs[1758]; and perhaps G6b-B[1759–1761] and TLT-1.[1166]

When platelets are aggregated in response to one of multiple agonists, the integrin β_3 cytoplasmic domain becomes phosphorylated on Tyr.[902,910] Two sites of potential tyrosine phosphorylation exist on the β_3 cytoplasmic domain and both may be utilized. Several molecules have been identified that bind specifically to the tyrosine-phosphorylated cytoplasmic domain of integrin β_3. A synthetic integrin β_3 cytoplasmic domain peptide containing phosphate groups on the two candidate Tyr residues binds to the contractile protein myosin,[902] and this interaction may facilitate the transmission of cytoskeletal tension from inside the platelet to outside, and thus initiate clot retraction. Recombinant, mutated integrin β_3 that cannot be phosphorylated is unable to support extensive clot retraction when expressed in a cell line.[902] Other proteins that bind to the diphosphorylated integrin β_3 cytoplasmic domain include the SHC adapter proteins,[906] which also become tyrosine phosphorylated during platelet aggregation. Therefore, it is possible that the SHC adapter proteins may link diphosphorylated integrin β_3 to the MAPK pathway.[906,1762] Mice containing mutated integrin β_3 molecules that cannot be phosphorylated exhibit a mild bleeding disorder as evidenced by occasional rebleeding of tail cuts. Moreover platelets derived from these mice form abnormally loose thrombi when activated by shear forces.[1763] Other integrin β_3 cytoplasmic domain binding proteins have been described, including skelemin, a member of a family of proteins that regulate myosin,[914] and talin.

Some signaling events that occur downstream of integrin $\alpha_{IIb}\beta_3$ require only integrin clustering, whereas other events require clustering, ligand binding, and/or platelet aggregation. For example, the tyrosine kinase Syk becomes activated in response to integrin $\alpha_{IIb}\beta_3$ clustering, independent of cytoskeletal assembly, whereas activation of the tyrosine kinase FAK requires integrin clustering, ligand binding and cytoskeletal assembly.[1764] In studies conducted in cell lines, activation of Syk downstream of integrin $\alpha_{IIb}\beta_3$ leads to phosphorylation of Vav1, a guanine nucleotide exchange factor for Rac, and lamellipodia formation. Syk and Vav1 cooperate to activate Jun N-terminal kinase, ERK2, and Akt.[1764] These pathways are also likely to be involved in postaggregation events in the platelet.

Proteins other than the well-described integrin $\alpha_{IIb}\beta_3$ ligands fibrinogen and VWF also induce signaling events via binding to integrin $\alpha_{IIb}\beta_3$. One such protein is CD40L, a TNF family member that is expressed on a variety of cells including activated platelets. Platelets are also the major source of a soluble form of CD40L.[1765] In addition to binding to its classical receptor, CD40, CD40L also binds to integrin $\alpha_{IIb}\beta_3$ on platelets and induces signaling events[1350] that are required for normal arterial thrombus formation in mice.[1348] CD40L may also initiate platelet aggregation by binding to CD40 on platelets.[1349]

INHIBITORY PATHWAYS IN PLATELETS

Prostaglandins

Prostaglandins that inhibit platelet activation include PGE_2 (at high concentrations) and PGI_2 (at low concentrations) (also termed *prostacyclin*) (reviewed in Refs. 1766 and 1767). In the vasculature, the endothelium produces PGI_2 and PGE_2, which are important in maintaining vascular patency.[1768] Inhibition is initiated by the binding of these PGs to their own specific GPCR.[1769,1770] PG receptor occupancy converts the $G\alpha$ subunit to the GTP bound, active form, which then activates adenylyl cyclase. Adenylyl cyclase catalyzes the formation of cAMP. The exact amount of cAMP present in the cell is also determined by its rate of breakdown by phosphodiesterases (PDEs). Biochemical studies and studies from gene targeted mice support a primary role for PDE3A in platelets.[1771-1773] Therefore, agents that inhibit PDE, such as theophylline, caffeine, and the drug cilostazol, also elevate cAMP levels in platelets and other cells.[1774] cAMP then activates PKA, which phosphorylates specific target proteins. PKA inhibits platelet activation by several pathways. One mechanism involves PKA-dependent phosphorylation of VASP (discussed under "Nitric Oxide" below). A separate mechanism involves the phosphorylation and inhibition of $G\alpha13$, which couples to the TXA_2 receptor, thus impairing this activation pathway.[1775] Also, PKA phosphorylates $GPIb\beta$ on Ser 166, and negatively regulates the ability of GPIb to bind VWF.[1776] In addition, PKA may phosphorylate and inhibit the IP_3 receptor, which would repress agonist-induced intracellular

Ca^{2+}-mobilization.[1777] PI metabolism is also affected, as the activities of both PLC and PLA_2 are suppressed.[1778] Moreover, PKA also phosphorylates Raf kinase on three sites, which inhibits Raf kinase function in part by inhibiting its binding to the activating protein RasGTP.[1779,1780] Finally, the small G protein, Rap1b, which contributes to integrin $\alpha_{IIb}\beta_3$ activation,[1611] is phosphorylated by PKA,[1781] although it appears that this phosphorylation event does not inhibit platelet function[1782] and may, in fact, contribute to Rap1b activation.[1783]

Paradoxically, in contrast to the inhibitory effects of high levels of PGE_2, low levels of PGE_2 ($<10^{-6}$ M) potentiate agonist-induced platelet aggregation by acting via the EP3 receptor to decrease intraplatelet cAMP levels.[1784,1785] Mice lacking the EP3 receptor are protected from AA-induced thrombosis[1786]; thus it is possible that PGE_2 present in atherosclerotic lesions contributes to atherothrombosis.

Nitric Oxide

NO is synthesized from L-arginine by NO synthase in endothelial cells, platelets, and other cells. The formation of NO is enhanced at sites of shear stress and by platelet agonists (e.g., thrombin or ADP),[1787] and it readily diffuses into platelets.[1788,1789] Similar to PGI_2 or PGE_2, NO pretreatment of platelets inhibits platelet activation and can reverse platelet aggregation soon after initiation. However, NO works not by elevating cAMP, but instead by increasing cGMP.[1790] NO synthase activity in platelets increases during platelet activation, suggesting that NO production is a normal negative feedback mechanism that limits further platelet aggregation. NO and PGI_2 act together synergistically to inhibit platelet activation.[1791]

Elevation in intracellular cGMP levels activates cGMP-dependent PKG, whose downstream targets include ERK and the TXA_2 receptor.[1792] In mice, the absence of PKG results in enhanced platelet accumulation along damaged vessels after ischemic injury, supporting an important role for PKG in platelet deposition.[1793] VASP, a member of the Pro-rich, actin-regulatory Ena/VASP protein family, is phosphorylated in response to elevations in either cAMP or cGMP[1794] and both PKA and PKG phosphorylate VASP *in vitro*.[1795] A role for VASP in inhibition of platelet function was established in studies of VASP-deficient mice: platelets obtained from the mice display increased P-selectin expression and integrin $\alpha_{IIb}\beta_3$ activation in response to agonists,[1796] and platelet adhesion at sites of vascular injury or atherosclerosis is enhanced in VASP-deficient mice.[1797] The enhanced platelet adhesion in VASP-null mice is not corrected by NO, suggesting that VASP may be a key negative regulator of platelet function in the cGMP-mediated pathways.

Elevation in intracellular cGMP can also increase cAMP levels via inhibition of PDE activity.[1798] This crosstalk between cGMP and cAMP-dependent pathways may synergize to contribute to the inhibitory effects of NO on platelet function.

CD39 (ATP Diphosphohydrolase; Ecto-ADPase)

Vascular endothelium regulates platelet function by producing prostacyclin and NO, as well as by expressing CD39 NTPDase1, a plasma membrane-associated ectonucleotide (ATP diphosphohydrolase; ATPase; ecto-ADPase; EC 3.6.1.5) that converts extracellular ATP to ADP, and ADP to AMP.[1799-1801] CD39 limits the platelet-activating effects of ADP released by damaged tissues, RBCs, and activated platelets; furthermore, AMP generated by CD39 is degraded by an ecto-5′-nucleotidase (CD73; EC 3.1.3.5) to adenosine, an inhibitor of ADP-induced platelet activation, that increases cAMP binding to the A2a adenosine receptor on platelets.[1802] Adenosine deaminase (EC 3.5.4.4) degrades adenosine to inosine. CD39 is a Mr 95,000 cell-surface glycoprotein expressed on endothelial cells, subsets of activated natural killer (NK) cells, B cells, monocytes, and T cells. Small amounts may also be on platelets and erythrocytes. It is present in the lymphocytes in chronic lymphocytic leukemia, which may partially account for the thromboprotection noted in that disorder.[1803] CD39 is localized to lipid raft-like caveolae in the plasma membrane, and the cholesterol content may control enzymatic activity. It contains two putative transmembrane regions separated by an extracellular domain with six glycosylation sites and apyrase-like regions that confer the ecto-ADPase activity. A related molecule, ATP- and ATPase 2, which is found on the basolateral surface of endothelial cells, the adventitia of some blood vessels, and microvascular pericytes, is relatively selective for ATP, and thus it has the capacity to increase platelet aggregation by enhancing the production of ADP from ATP.[1799] The physiologic roles of the NTPDases are complex because of their production of variably prothrombotic and antithrombotic agents. It has been postulated that recruitment of microparticles enriched in mono-cyte CD39/NTPDase1 to thrombi could contribute to the limitation of the size of platelet thrombi. A role for CD39/NTPDase1 in ischemia reperfusion and allograft rejection has also been proposed. Mouse mod-els support the potential of modulating graft rejection and thrombosis by using gene therapy to increase CD39/NTPDase1. A soluble recombi-nant form of CD39 inhibits platelet aggregation and recruitment *in vitro* and may have potential as an anti-thrombotic agent *in vivo*.[1804]

REFERENCES

1. Ruggeri ZM: Platelets in atherothrombosis. *Nat Med* 8(11):1227–1234, 2002.
2. Goldsmith HL, Turitto VT: Rheological aspects of thrombosis and haemostasis: Basic principles and applications. ICTH-Report—Subcommittee on Rheology of the International Committee on Thrombosis and Haemostasis. *Thromb Haemost* 55(3): 415–435, 1986.
3. de Groot PG, JJ Sixma: Perfusion chambers, in *Platelets*, edited by AD Michelson:, pp 575–586. Academic Press, San Diego, 2007.
4. Savage, Ruggeri ZM: Platelet thrombus formation in flowing blood, in *Platelets*, edited by AD Michelson:, pp 359–376. Academic Press, San Diego, 2007.
5. Coller B: Platelets in cardiovascular thrombosis and thrombolysis, in *The Heart and Cardiovascular System*, edited by HA Fozzard, AM Katz, HE Morgan, E Haber: pp 219–273. Raven Press, New York, 1991.
6. Jackson SP, Nesbitt WS, Westein E: Dynamics of platelet thrombus formation. *J Thromb Haemost* 7 Suppl 1:17–20, 2009.
7. Roth GJ: Developing relationships: Arterial platelet adhesion, glycoprotein Ib, and leucine-rich glycoproteins. *Blood* 77(1):5–19, 1991.
8. Ruggeri ZM: Structure and function of von Willebrand factor. *Thromb Haemost* 82(2):576–584, 1999.
9. Andrews RK, et al: The glycoprotein Ib-IX-V complex in platelet adhesion and signal-ing. *Thromb Haemost* 82(2):357–364, 1999.
10. Ruggeri ZM: Von Willebrand factor, platelets and endothelial cell interactions. *J Thromb Haemost* 1(7):1335–1342, 2003.
11. Savage B, Ruggeri ZM: Platelet thrombus formation in flowing blood, in *Platelets*, edited by AD Michelson: p 215. Academic Press, San Diego, 2002.
12. Mailhac A, et al: Effect of an eccentric severe stenosis on fibrin(ogen) deposition on severely damaged vessel wall in arterial thrombosis. Relative contribution of fibrin(ogen) and platelets. *Circulation* 90(2):988–996, 1994.
13. Moake JL, et al: Involvement of large plasma von Willebrand factor (VWF) multimers and unusually large VWF forms derived from endothelial cells in shear stress-induced platelet aggregation. *J Clin Invest* 78(6):1456–1461, 1986.
14. Ikeda Y, et al: The role of von Willebrand factor and fibrinogen in platelet aggregation under varying shear stress. *J Clin Invest* 87(4):1234–1240, 1991.
15. Ruggeri ZM: Mechanisms of shear-induced platelet adhesion and aggregation. *Thromb Haemost* 70(1):119–123, 1993.
16. Andrews RK, Lopez JA, Berndt MC: The GPIb-IX-V complex, *Platelets*, edited by AD M, pp 145–164. Academic Press, San Diego, 2007.
17. Chiang TM, Rinaldy A, Kang AH: Cloning, characterization, and functional studies of a nonintegrin platelet receptor for type I collagen. *J Clin Invest* 100(3):514–521, 1997.
18. Clemetson JM, et al: The platelet collagen receptor glycoprotein VI is a member of the immunoglobulin superfamily closely related to FcalphaR and the natural killer receptors. *J Biol Chem* 274(41):29019–29024, 1999.
19. Clemetson KJ: Platelet collagen receptors: A new target for inhibition? *Haemostasis* 29(1):16–26, 1999.
20. Coller BS, et al: Collagen-platelet interactions: Evidence for a direct interaction of collagen with platelet GPIa/IIa and an indirect interaction with platelet GPIIb/IIIa mediated by adhesive proteins. *Blood* 74(1):182–192, 1989.
21. Gruner S, et al: Multiple integrin-ligand interactions synergize in shear-resistant platelet adhesion at sites of arterial injury in vivo. *Blood* 102(12):4021–4027, 2003.
22. Kato K, et al: The contribution of glycoprotein VI to stable platelet adhesion and throm-bus formation illustrated by targeted gene deletion. *Blood* 102(5):1701–1707, 2003.
23. Kuijpers MJ, et al: Complementary roles of glycoprotein VI and alpha2beta1 integrin in collagen-induced thrombus formation in flowing whole blood ex vivo. *FASEB J* 17(6):685–687, 2003.
24. Matsuno K, et al: Inhibition of platelet adhesion to collagen by monoclonal anti-CD36 antibodies. *Br J Haematol* 92(4):960–967, 1996.
25. Nakamura T, et al: Activation of the GP IIb-IIIa complex induced by platelet adhe-sion to collagen is mediated by both alpha2beta1 integrin and GP VI. *J Biol Chem* 274(17):11897–11903, 1999.
26. Nieswandt B, Watson SP: Platelet-collagen interaction: Is GPVI the central receptor? *Blood* 102(2):449–461, 2003.
27. Saelman EU, et al: Platelet adhesion to collagen types I through VIII under condi-tions of stasis and flow is mediated by GPIa/IIa (alpha 2 beta 1-integrin). *Blood* 83(5): 1244–1250, 1994.
28. Savage B, Almus-Jacobs F, Ruggeri ZM: Specific synergy of multiple substrate-receptor interactions in platelet thrombus formation under flow. *Cell* 94(5):657–666, 1998.
29. Watson SP: Collagen receptor signaling in platelets and megakaryocytes. *Thromb Hae-most* 82(2):365–376, 1999.
30. Coller BS, Shattil SJ: The GPIIb/IIIa (integrin alphaIIbbeta3) odyssey: A technology-driven saga of a receptor with twists, turns, and even a bend. *Blood* 112(8):3011–3025, 2008.
31. Naik UP, Naik MU: Association of CIB with GPIIb/IIIa during outside-in signaling is required for platelet spreading on fibrinogen. *Blood* 102(4):1355–1362, 2003.
32. Patel D, et al: Dynamics of GPIIb/IIIa-mediated platelet-platelet interactions in plate-let adhesion/thrombus formation on collagen in vitro as revealed by videomicroscopy. *Blood* 101(3):929–936, 2003.
33. Shattil SJ: Regulation of platelet anchorage and signaling by integrin alpha IIb beta 3. *Thromb Haemost* 70(1):224–228, 1993.
34. Shattil SJ: Signaling through platelet integrin alpha IIb beta 3: Inside-out, outside-in, and sideways. *Thromb Haemost* 82(2):318–325, 1999.
35. Shattil SJ, Newman PJ: Integrins: Dynamic scaffolds for adhesion and signaling in platelets. *Blood* 104(6):1606–1615, 2004.
36. Weiss HJ, Turitto VT, Baumgartner HR: Further evidence that glycoprotein IIb-IIIa mediates platelet spreading on subendothelium. *Thromb Haemost* 65(2):202–205, 1991.
37. Santos MT, et al: Enhancement of platelet reactivity and modulation of eicosanoid production by intact erythrocytes. A new approach to platelet activation and recruit-ment. *J Clin Invest* 87(2):571–580, 1991.
38. Dubois C, Atkinson B, Furie B, Furie B: Real-time imaging of platelets during thrombus formation, in *Platelets*, edited by AD M, pp 611–626. Academic Press, San Diego, 2007.
39. Celi A, et al: Thrombus formation: Direct real-time observation and digital analysis of thrombus assembly in a living mouse by confocal and widefield intravital microscopy. *J Thromb Haemost* 1(1):60–68, 2003.
40. Denis C, et al: A mouse model of severe von Willebrand disease: Defects in hemostasis and thrombosis. *Proc Natl Acad Sci U S A* 95(16):9524–9529, 1998.
41. Ni H, et al: Persistence of platelet thrombus formation in arterioles of mice lacking both von Willebrand factor and fibrinogen. *J Clin Invest* 106(3):385–392, 2000.
42. Peerschke EI: The platelet fibrinogen receptor. *Semin Hematol* 22(4):241–259, 1985.
43. Phillips DR, et al: The platelet membrane glycoprotein IIb-IIIa complex. *Blood* 71(4): 831–843, 1988.
44. Plow EF, Ginsberg MH: Cellular adhesion: GPIIb-IIIa as a prototypic adhesion recep-tor. *Prog Hemost Thromb* 9:117–156, 1989.
45. Plow EF, Pesho MM, Ma YQ: Integrin αIIbβ3, in *Platelets* edited by AD Michelson. San Diego, Academic Press: 165–178, 2007.
46. Peerschke EI: Ca+2 mobilization and fibrinogen binding of platelets refractory to ade-nosine diphosphate stimulation. *J Lab Clin Med* 106(2):111–122, 1985.
47. Steen VM, Holmsen H: Synergism between thrombin and epinephrine in human platelets: Different dose-response relationships for aggregation and dense granule secretion. *Thromb Haemost* 54(3):680–683, 1985.
48. Ware JA, Smith M, Salzman EW: Synergism of platelet-aggregating agents. Role of elevation of cytoplasmic calcium. *J Clin Invest* 80(1):267–271, 1987.
49. Giandomenico G, et al: The leptin receptor system of human platelets. *J Thromb Hae-most* 3(5):1042–1049, 2005.
50. Konstantinides S, et al: Leptin-dependent platelet aggregation and arterial throm-bosis suggests a mechanism for atherothrombotic disease in obesity. *J Clin Invest* 108(10):1533–1540, 2001.
51. Konstantinides S, et al: Inhibition of endogenous leptin protects mice from arterial and venous thrombosis. *Arterioscler Thromb Vasc Biol* 24(11):2196–2201, 2004.
52. Andre P, et al: CD40L stabilizes arterial thrombi by a beta3 integrin—Dependent mechanism. *Nat Med* 8(3):247–252, 2002.
53. Angelillo-Scherrer A, et al: Role of Gas6 receptors in platelet signaling during thrombus stabilization and implications for antithrombotic therapy. *J Clin Invest* 115(2):237–246, 2005.
54. Balogh I, et al: Analysis of Gas6 in human platelets and plasma. *Arterioscler Thromb Vasc Biol* 25(6):1280–1286, 2005.
55. Gould WR, et al: Gas6 receptors Axl, Sky and Mer enhance platelet activation and regulate thrombotic responses. *J Thromb Haemost* 3(4):733–741, 2005.
56. Maree AO, et al: Growth arrest specific gene (GAS) 6 modulates platelet thrombus for-mation and vascular wall homeostasis and represents an attractive drug target. *Curr Pharm Des* 13(26):2656–2661, 2007.
57. Saller F, et al: Role of the growth arrest-specific gene 6 (gas6) product in thrombus stabilization. *Blood Cells Mol Dis* 36(3):373–378, 2006.

58. Prevost N, et al: Eph kinases and ephrins support thrombus growth and stability by regulating integrin outside-in signaling in platelets. *Proc Natl Acad Sci U S A* 102(28):9820–9825, 2005.

59. Renne T, et al: Defective thrombus formation in mice lacking coagulation factor XII. *J Exp Med* 202(2):271–281, 2005.

60. Jirouskova M, et al: Antibody blockade or mutation of the fibrinogen gamma-chain C-terminus is more effective in inhibiting murine arterial thrombus formation than complete absence of fibrinogen. *Blood* 103(6):1995–2002, 2004.

61. Loscalzo J, Inbal A, Handin RI: Von Willebrand protein facilitates platelet incorporation in polymerizing fibrin. *J Clin Invest* 78(4):1112–1119, 1986.

62. Deckmyn H, et al: Inhibitors of the interactions between collagen and its receptors on platelets. *Handb Exp Pharmacol* 2012(210):311–337.

63. George JN, et al: Platelet surface glycoproteins. Studies on resting and activated platelets and platelet membrane microparticles in normal subjects, and observations in patients during adult respiratory distress syndrome and cardiac surgery. *J Clin Invest* 78(2):340–348, 1986.

64. Michelson AD: Thrombin-induced down-regulation of the platelet membrane glycoprotein Ib-IX complex. *Semin Thromb Hemost* 18(1):18–27, 1992.

65. Michelson AD, Barnard MR: Thrombin-induced changes in platelet membrane glycoproteins Ib, IX, and IIb-IIIa complex. *Blood* 70(5):1673–1678, 1987.

66. McEver RP: Properties of GMP-140, an inducible granule membrane protein of platelets and endothelium. *Blood Cells* 16(1):73–80; discussion 80–83, 1990.

67. McEver RP, et al: GMP-140, a platelet alpha-granule membrane protein, is also synthesized by vascular endothelial cells and is localized in Weibel-Palade bodies. *J Clin Invest* 84(1):92–99, 1989.

68. McEver R: P-selectin/PSGL-1 and other interactions between platelets, leukocytes, and endothelium, in *Platelets*, edited by AD M, p 231. Academic Press, San Diego, 2007.

69. Loscalzo J: Nitric oxide insufficiency, platelet activation, and arterial thrombosis. *Circ Res* 88(8):756–762, 2001.

70. Luscher TF: Platelet-vessel wall interaction: Role of nitric oxide, prostaglandins and endothelins. *Bailllieres Clin Haematol* 6(3):609–627, 1993.

71. Mitchell JA, et al: Role of nitric oxide and prostacyclin as vasoactive hormones released by the endothelium. *Exp Physiol* 93(1):141–147, 2008.

72. Rex S, Freedman JE: Inhibition of platelet function by the endothelium, in *Platelets*, edited by AD Michelson, pp 251–280. Academic Press, San Diego, 2007.

73. Marcus AJ, et al: The endothelial cell ecto-ADPase responsible for inhibition of platelet function is CD39. *J Clin Invest* 99(6):1351–1360, 1997.

74. Marcus AJ, et al: Inhibition of platelet function by an aspirin-insensitive endothelial cell ADPase. Thromboregulation by endothelial cells. *J Clin Invest* 88(5):1690–1696, 1991.

75. Holme S, et al: Light scatter and total protein signal distribution of platelets by flow cytometry as parameters of size. *J Lab Clin Med* 112(2):223–231, 1988.

76. White J: Anatomy and structural organization of the platelet, in *Hemostasis and Thrombosis: Basic Principles and Clinical Practice*, edited by RW Colman, VJ Marder, EW Salzman, p 397. JB Lippincott, Philadelphia, 1993.

77. Coller BS: Biochemical and electrostatic considerations in primary platelet aggregation. *Ann N Y Acad Sci* 416:693–708, 1983.

78. van Joost T, et al: Purpuric contact dermatitis to benzoyl peroxide. *J Am Acad Dermatol* 22(2 Pt 2):359–361, 1990.

79. Schick P: Megakaryocyte and platelet lipids, in *Hemostasis and Thrombosis: Basic Principles and Clinical Practice*, edited by RW Colman, VJ Marder, EW Salzman, p 574. JB Lippincott, Philadelphia, 1993.

80. Heemskerk JW, Bevers EM, Lindhout T: Platelet activation and blood coagulation. *Thromb Haemost* 88(2):186–193, 2002.

81. Solum NO: Procoagulant expression in platelets and defects leading to clinical disorders. *Arterioscler Thromb Vasc Biol* 19(12):2841–2846, 1999.

82. Sims PJ, et al: Complement proteins C5b-9 cause release of membrane vesicles from the platelet surface that are enriched in the membrane receptor for coagulation factor Va and express prothrombinase activity. *J Biol Chem* 263(34):18205–18212, 1988.

83. Sims PJ, et al: Assembly of the platelet prothrombinase complex is linked to vesiculation of the platelet plasma membrane. Studies in Scott syndrome: An isolated defect in platelet procoagulant activity. *J Biol Chem* 264(29):17049–17057, 1989.

84. Bevers EM, et al: Exposure of endogenous phosphatidylserine at the outer surface of stimulated platelets is reversed by restoration of aminophospholipid translocase activity. *Biochemistry* 28(6):2382–2387, 1989.

85. Comfurius P, Bevers EM, Zwaal RF: The involvement of cytoskeleton in the regulation of transbilayer movement of phospholipids in human blood platelets. *Biochim Biophys Acta* 815(1):143–148, 1985.

86. Tuszynski GP, et al: The platelet cytoskeleton contains elements of the prothrombinase complex. *J Biol Chem* 259(11):6947–6951, 1984.

87. Bodin S, Tronchere H, Payrastre B: Lipid rafts are critical membrane domains in blood platelet activation processes. *Biochim Biophys Acta* 1610(2):247–257, 2003.

88. Locke D, et al: Lipid rafts orchestrate signaling by the platelet receptor glycoprotein VI. *J Biol Chem* 277(21):18801–18809, 2002.

89. Shrimpton CN, et al: Localization of the adhesion receptor glycoprotein Ib-IX-V complex to lipid rafts is required for platelet adhesion and activation. *J Exp Med* 196(8):1057–1066, 2002.

90. Heijnen HF, et al: Concentration of rafts in platelet filopodia correlates with recruitment of c-Src and CD63 to these domains. *J Thromb Haemost* 1(6):1161–1173, 2003.

91. Bodin S, et al: Production of phosphatidylinositol 3,4,5-trisphosphate and phosphatidic acid in platelet rafts: Evidence for a critical role of cholesterol-enriched domains in human platelet activation. *Biochemistry* 40(50):15290–15299, 2001.

92. Baglia FA, et al: The glycoprotein Ib-IX-V complex mediates localization of factor XI to lipid rafts on the platelet membrane. *J Biol Chem* 278(24):21744–21750, 2003.

93. Brownlow SL, et al: A role for hTRPC1 and lipid raft domains in store-mediated calcium entry in human platelets. *Cell Calcium* 35(2):107–113, 2004.

94. Lopez JA, I. del Conde, Shrimpton CN: Receptors, rafts, and microvesicles in thrombosis and inflammation. *J Thromb Haemost* 3(8):1737–1744, 2005.

95. White JG: Anatomy and structural organization of the platelet, in *Hemostasis and Thrombosis: Basic Principles and Clinical Practice*, edited by RW Colman, VJ Marder, EW Salzman, pp 397–413. JB Lippincott, Philadelphia, 1993.

96. Behnke O: The morphology of blood platelet membrane systems. *Ser Haematol* 3(4):3–16, 1970.

97. White JG: Electron microscopic studies of platelet secretion. *Prog Hemost Thromb* 2:49, 1974.

98. Suzuki H, Yamazaki H, Tanoue K: Immunocytochemical studies on co-localization of alpha-granule membrane alphaIIbbeta3 integrin and intragranular fibrinogen of human platelets and their cell-surface expression during the thrombin-induced release reaction. *J Electron Microsc (Tokyo)* 52(2):183–195, 1970.

99. Stenberg PE, Shuman MA, Levine SP, Bainton DF: Redistribution of α granules and their contents in thrombin-stimulated platelets. *J Cell Biol* 98:748–760, 1984.

100. Ginsberg MH, Taylor L, Painter RG: The mechanism of thrombin-induced platelet factor 4 secretion. *Blood* 55:661, 1980.

101. Nurden P, Heilmann E, Paponneau A, Nurden A: Two-way trafficking of membrane glycoproteins on thrombin-activated human platelets. *Semin Hematol* 1994;31(3):240–250, 1980.

102. Michelson AD, Barnard MR: Plasmin-induced redistribution of platelet glycoprotein Ib. *Blood* 76(10):2005–2010, 1990.

103. Suzuki H, Nakamura S, Itoh Y, et al: Immunocytochemical evidence for the translocation of α-granule membrane glycoprotein IIb/IIIa (integrin αIIbβ3) of human platelets to the surface membrane during the release reaction. *Histochemistry* 97:381–388, 1992.

104. Suzuki H, Murasaki K, Kodama K, Takayama H: et al: Intracellular localization of glycoprotein VI in human platelets and its surface expression upon activation. *Br J Haematol* 121(6):904–912, 2003.

105. Nurden P, Poujol C, Winckler J, et al: Immunolocalization of P2Y1 and TPalpha receptors in platelets showed a major pool associated with the membranes of alpha-granules and the open canalicular system. *Blood* 101(4):1400–1408, 2003.

106. Breton-Gorius, J, Guichard J: Ultrastructural localization of peroxidase activity in human platelets and megakaryocytes. *Am J Pathol* 66:277, 1986.

107. Cramer EM: Platelets and megakaryocytes: Anatomy and structural organization, in *Hemostasis and Thrombosis: Basic Principles in Clinical Practice*, edited by RW Colman, J Hirsh, V J Marder, AW Clowes and J N George, et al, pp 411–428. Lippincott, Williams & Wilkins: Philadelphia, 2001.

108. White JG: Interaction of membrane systems in blood platelets. *Am J Pathol* 66(2):295–312, 1972.

109. Menashi S, Davis C, Crawford N: Calcium uptake associated with an intracellular membrane fraction prepared from human blood platelets by high-voltage, free-flow electrophoresis. *FEBS Lett* 140:298, 1982.

110. Robblee LS, Shepro D, Belamarich FA: Calcium uptake and associated adenosine triphosphate activity of isolated platelet membranes. *J Gen Physiol* 61:462, 1973.

111. Hartwig JH: Platelet morphology, in *Thrombosis and Hemorrhage*, edited by J Loscalzo, AI Schafer, pp 207–228. Williams & Wilkins, Baltimore, 1999.

112. Michalak M, Mariani P, Opas M: Calreticulin, a multifunctional Ca2+ binding chaperone of the endoplasmic reticulum. *Biochem Cell Biol* 76(5):779–785, 1998.

113. Brownlow SL, Sage SO: Rapid agonist-evoked coupling of type II Ins(1,4,5)P3 receptor with human transient receptor potential (hTRPC1) channels in human platelets. *Biochem J* 375(Pt 3):697–704, 2003.

114. van Gorp RM, et al: Irregular spiking in free calcium concentration in single, human platelets. Regulation by modulation of the inositol trisphosphate receptors. *Eur J Biochem* 269(5):1543–1552, 2002.

115. Käser-Glanzmann R, Jakábová M, George JN, Lüscher EF: Further characterization of calcium accumulating vesicles from human blood platelets. *Biochim Biophys Acta* 542:357, 1978.

116. Tertyshnikova S, Fein A: Inhibition of inositol 1,4,5-trisphosphate-induced Ca2+ release by cAMP- dependent protein kinase in a living cell. *Proc Natl Acad Sci U S A* 1998;95(4):1613–1617, 1978.

117. Pernollet MG, Lantoine F, Devynck MA: Nitric oxide inhibits ATP-dependent Ca^{2+} uptake into platelet membrane vesicles. *Biochem Biophys Res Commun* 222(3):780–785, 1996.

118. Teijeiro RG, et al: Calcium efflux from platelet vesicles of the dense tubular system. Analysis of the possible contribution of the Ca^{2+} pump. *Mol Cell Biochem* 199(1–2):7–14, 1999.

119. Bergmeier W, Stefanini L: Novel molecules in calcium signaling in platelets. *J Thromb Haemost* 7(Suppl 1):187–190, 2009.

120. Dziadek MA, Johnstone LS: Biochemical properties and cellular localisation of STIM proteins. *Cell Calcium* 42(2):123–132, 2007.

121. Grosse J, et al: An EF hand mutation in Stim1 causes premature platelet activation and bleeding in mice. *J Clin Invest* 117(11):3540–3550, 2007.

122. Varga-Szabo D, et al: The calcium sensor STIM1 is an essential mediator of arterial thrombosis and ischemic brain infarction. *J Exp Med* 205(7):1583–1591, 2008.

123. Bergmeier W, et al: R93W mutation in Orai1 causes impaired calcium influx in platelets. *Blood* 113(3):675–678, 2009.

124. Braun A, et al: Orai1 (CRACM1) is the platelet SOC channel and essential for pathological thrombus formation. *Blood* 113(9):2056–2063, 2009.

125. Feske S, et al: A mutation in Orai1 causes immune deficiency by abrogating CRAC channel function. *Nature* 441(7090):179–185, 2006.

126. Feske S, et al: Severe combined immunodeficiency due to defective binding of the nuclear factor of activated T cells in T lymphocytes of two male siblings. *Eur J Immunol* 26(9):2119–2126, 1996.

127. Picard C, et al: STIM1 mutation associated with a syndrome of immunodeficiency and autoimmunity. *N Engl J Med* 360(19):1971–1980, 2009.

128. Redondo PC, et al: Intracellular Ca2+ store depletion induces the formation of macromolecular complexes involving hTRPC1, hTRPC6, the type II IP3 receptor and SERCA3 in human platelets. *Biochim Biophys Acta* 1783(6):1163–1176, 2008.

129. Sage SO, Brownlow SL, Rosado JA: TRP channels and calcium entry in human platelets. *Blood* 100(12):4245–4246, 2002.

130. Varga-Szabo D, et al: Store-operated Ca(2+) entry in platelets occurs independently of transient receptor potential (TRP) C1. *Pflugers Arch* 457(2):377–387, 2008.

131. Gerrard JM, White JG, Rao GH, Townsend D: Localization of platelet prostaglandin production in the platelet dense tubular system. *Am J Pathol* 83(2):283–298, 1976.

132. Picot D, Loll PJ, Garavito RM: The X-ray crystal structure of the membrane protein prostaglandin H2 synthase-1. *Nature* 1994;367(6460):243–249, 1976.

133. Fox JE: The platelet cytoskeleton. *Thromb Haemost* 70(6):884–893, 1993.

134. Fox JE, et al: Identification of a membrane skeleton in platelets. *J Cell Biol* 106(5):1525–1538, 1988.

135. Fox JE, et al: Spectrin is associated with membrane-bound actin filaments in platelets and is hydrolyzed by the Ca2+-dependent protease during platelet activation. *Blood* 69(2):537–545, 1987.

136. Hartwig JH, DeSisto M: The cytoskeleton of the resting human blood platelet: Structure of the membrane skeleton and its attachment to actin filaments. *J Cell Biol* 112(3):407–425, 1991.

137. Barkalow KL, et al: Alpha-adducin dissociates from F-actin and spectrin during platelet activation. *J Cell Biol* 161(3):557–570, 2003.

138. Kaiser HW, O'Keefe E, Bennett V: Adducin: Ca++-dependent association with sites of cell-cell contact. *J Cell Biol* 109(2):557–569, 1989.

139. Kuhlman PA, et al: A new function for adducin. Calcium/calmodulin-regulated capping of the barbed ends of actin filaments. *J Biol Chem* 271(14):7986–7991, 1996.

140. Matsuoka Y, Li X, Bennett V: Adducin: Structure, function and regulation. *Cell Mol Life Sci* 57(6):884–895, 2000.

141. Calderwood DA, et al: Increased filamin binding to beta-integrin cytoplasmic domains inhibits cell migration. *Nat Cell Biol* 3(12):1060–1068, 2001.

142. Ithychanda SS, et al: Migfilin, a molecular switch in regulation of integrin activation. *J Biol Chem* 284(7):4713–4722, 2009.

143. Kiema T, et al: The molecular basis of filamin binding to integrins and competition with talin. *Mol Cell* 21(3):337–347, 2006.

144. Tadokoro S, et al: Talin binding to integrin beta tails: A final common step in integrin activation. *Science* 302(5642):103–106, 2003.

145. Tremuth L, et al: A fluorescence cell biology approach to map the second integrin-binding site of talin to a 130-amino acid sequence within the rod domain. *J Biol Chem* 279(21):22258–22266, 2004.

146. Ulmer TS, et al: NMR analysis of structure and dynamics of the cytosolic tails of integrin alpha IIb beta 3 in aqueous solution. *Biochemistry* 40(25):7498–7508, 2001.

147. Vinogradova O, et al: A structural mechanism of integrin alpha(IIb)beta(3) "inside-out" activation as regulated by its cytoplasmic face. *Cell* 110(5):587–597, 2002.

148. Yan B, et al: Calpain cleavage promotes talin binding to the beta 3 integrin cytoplasmic domain. *J Biol Chem* 276(30):28164–28170, 2001.

149. Zhu J, et al: Structure of a complete integrin ectodomain in a physiologic resting state and activation and deactivation by applied forces. *Mol Cell* 32(6):849–861, 2008.

150. Podor TJ, et al: Vimentin exposed on activated platelets and platelet microparticles localizes vitronectin and plasminogen activator inhibitor complexes on their surface. *J Biol Chem* 277(9):7529–7539, 2002.

151. Cramer EM, et al: Ultrastructure of platelet formation by human megakaryocytes cultured with the Mpl ligand. *Blood* 89(7):2336–2346, 1997.

152. Italiano JE Jr, et al: Blood platelets are assembled principally at the ends of proplatelet processes produced by differentiated megakaryocytes. *J Cell Biol* 147(6):1299–1312, 1999.

153. Italiano JE, JH Hartwig: Megakaryocyte development and platelet formation, in *Platelets*, edited by A Michelson, p 23. Academic Press, San Diego, 2007.

154. Hartwig J: Platelet structure, in *Platelets*, edited by A Michelson, p 75. Academic Press, San Diego, 2007.

155. Crawford N, Scrutton MC: Biochemistry of the blood platelet, in *Haemostasis and Thrombosis*, edited by AL Bloom, DP Thomas, EGD Tuddenham, p 89. Churchill Livingstone, London, England, 1994.

156. Miki H, Okada Y, Hirokawa N: Analysis of the kinesin superfamily: Insights into structure and function. *Trends Cell Biol* 15(9):467–476, 2005.

157. Pfister KK, et al: Genetic analysis of the cytoplasmic dynein subunit families. *PLoS Genet* 2(1):e1.

158. Sheetz MP: Microtubule motor complexes moving membranous organelles. *Cell Struct Funct* 1996;21(5):369–373, 2006.

159. Patel-Hett S, et al: Visualization of microtubule growth in living platelets reveals a dynamic marginal band with multiple microtubules. *Blood* 111(9):4605–4616, 2008.

160. Kenney DM, Linck RW: The cytoskeleton of unstimulated blood platelets: Structure and composition of the isolated marginal microtubular band. *J Cell Sci* 78:1–22, 1985.

161. Aslan JE, et al: Histone deacetylase 6-mediated deacetylation of alpha-tubulin coordinates cytoskeletal and signaling events during platelet activation. *Am J Physiol Cell Physiol* 305(12):C1230–9, 2013.

162. Sadoul K, et al: HDAC6 controls the kinetics of platelet activation. *Blood* 120(20):4215–4218, 2012.

163. Italiano JE Jr, et al: Mechanisms and implications of platelet discoid shape. *Blood* 101(12):4789–4796, 2003.

164. Freson K, et al: The TUBB1 Q43P functional polymorphism reduces the risk of cardiovascular disease in men by modulating platelet function and structure. *Blood* 106(7):2356–2362, 2005.

165. Kunishima S, et al: Mutation of the beta1-tubulin gene associated with congenital macrothrombocytopenia affecting microtubule assembly. *Blood* 113(2):458–461, 2009.

166. Navarro-Nunez L, et al: Rare homozygous status of P43 beta1-tubulin polymorphism causes alterations in platelet ultrastructure. *Thromb Haemost* 105(5):855–863, 2011.

167. Kunishima S, et al: TUBB1 mutation disrupting microtubule assembly impairs proplatelet formation and results in congenital macrothrombocytopenia. *Eur J Haematol* 92(4):276–282, 2014.

168. Kunishima S, et al: Mutation of the beta1-tubulin gene associated with congenital macrothrombocytopenia affecting microtubule assembly. *Blood* 113(2):458–461, 2009.

169. Nachmias VT, Yoshida K: The cytoskeleton of the blood platelet: A dynamic structure. *Adv Cell Biol* 2: 181–211, 1988.

170. Safer D, Nachmias VT: Beta thymosins as actin binding peptides. *Bioessays* 16(8):590, 1994.

171. Rosenberg S, Stracher A: Effect of actin-binding protein on the sedimentation properties of actin. *J Cell Biol* 1982;94(1):51–55, 1988.

172. Rosenberg S, Stracher A, Burridge K: Isolation and characterization of a calcium-sensitive alpha-actinin-like protein from human platelet cytoskeletons. *J Biol Chem* 256(24):12986–12991, 1981.

173. Rosenberg S, Stracher A, Lucas RC: Isolation and characterization of actin and actin-binding protein from human platelets. *J Cell Biol* 91(1):201–211, 1981.

174. Fucini P, et al: The repeating segments of the F-actin cross-linking gelation factor (ABP-120) have an immunoglobulin-like fold. *Nat Struct Biol* 4(3):223–230, 1997.

175. Gorlin JB, et al: Human endothelial actin-binding protein (ABP-280, nonmuscle filamin): A molecular leaf spring. *J Cell Biol* 111(3):1089–1105, 1990.

176. Gorlin JB, et al: Actin-binding protein (ABP-280) filamin gene (FLN) maps telomeric to the color vision locus (R/GCP) and centromeric to G6PD in Xq28. *Genomics* 17(2):496–498, 1993.

177. Takafuta T, et al: Human beta-filamin is a new protein that interacts with the cytoplasmic tail of glycoprotein Ibalpha. *J Biol Chem* 273(28):17531–17538, 1998.

178. Ohta Y, et al: The small GTPase RalA targets filamin to induce filopodia. *Proc Natl Acad Sci U S A* 96(5):2122–2128, 1999.

179. Stossel TP, et al: Filamins as integrators of cell mechanics and signalling. *Nat Rev Mol Cell Biol* 2(2):138–145, 2001.

180. Kovacsovics TJ, Hartwig JH: Thrombin-induced GPIb-IX centralization on the platelet surface requires actin assembly and myosin II activation. *Blood* 87(2):618–629, 1996.

181. Meyer SC, et al: Identification of the region in actin-binding protein that binds to the cytoplasmic domain of glycoprotein Ibalpha. *J Biol Chem* 272(5):2914–2919, 1997.

182. Karpatkin S, Langer RM: Biochemical energetics of simulated platelet plug formation. Effect of thrombin, adenosine diphosphate, and epinephrine on intra- and extracellular adenine nucleotide kinetics. *J Clin Invest* 47(9):2158–2168, 1968.

183. Akkerman JW, et al: A novel technique for rapid determination of energy consumption in platelets. Demonstration of different energy consumption associated with three secretory responses. *Biochem J* 210(1):145–155, 1983.

184. Akkerman JW, Holmsen H: Interrelationships among platelet responses: Studies on the burst in proton liberation, lactate production, and oxygen uptake during platelet aggregation and Ca2+ secretion. *Blood* 57(5):956–966, 1981.

185. Guppy M, et al: Fuel choices by human platelets in human plasma. *Eur J Biochem* 244(1):161–167, 1997.

186. Holmsen H, Farstad M: Energy metabolism, in *Platelet Responses and Metabolism*, edited by H Holmsen, p 245. CRC Press, Boca Raton, FL, 1987.

187. Akkerman JWN, Verhgoeven AJM: Energy metabolism and function, in *Platelet Responses and Metabolism*, edited by H Holmsen, p 69. CRC Press, Boca Raton, FL, 1987.

188. Shimizu T, Murphy S: Roles of acetate and phosphate in the successful storage of platelet concentrates prepared with an acetate-containing additive solution. *Transfusion* 33(4):304–310, 1993.

189. Dean WL: Structure, function and subcellular localization of a human platelet Ca2+-ATPase. *Cell Calcium* 10(5):289–297, 1989.

190. Simons ER, Greenberg-Sperssky SM: Transmembrane monovalent cation gradients, in *Platelet Responses and Metabolism*, edited by H Holmsen, p 31. CRC Press, Boca Raton, FL, 1987.

191. Daniel JL, et al: Nucleotide exchange between cytosolic ATP and F-actin-bound ADP may be a major energy-utilizing process in unstimulated platelets. *Eur J Biochem* 156(3):677–684, 1986.

192. Verhoeven AJ, et al: Turnover of the phosphomonoester groups of polyphosphoinositol lipids in unstimulated human platelets. *Eur J Biochem* 166(1):3–9, 1987.

193. Akkerman JW, Holmsen H, Driver HA: Platelet aggregation and Ca2+ secretion are independent of simultaneous ATP production. *FEBS Lett* 100(2):286–290, 1979.

194. van den Bosch H, de Vet EC, Zomer AW: The role of peroxisomes in ether lipid synthesis. Back to the roots of PAF. *Adv Exp Med Biol* 416:33–40, 1996.

195. van den Bosch H, et al: Ether lipid synthesis and its deficiency in peroxisomal disorders. *Biochimie* 75(3–4):183–189, 1993.

196. Wanders RJ, et al: Deficiency of acyl-CoA:dihydroxyacetone phosphate acyltransferase in thrombocytes of Zellweger patients: A simple postnatal diagnostic test. *Clin Chim Acta* 151(3):217–221, 1985.

197. Holmsen H: Platelet secretion and energy metabolism, in *Hemostasis and Thrombosis: Basic Principles and Clinical Practice*, edited by RW Colman, VJ Marder, EW Salzman, p 524. JB Lippincott, Philadelphia, 1993.

198. Shuster RC, Rubenstein AJ, Wallace DC: Mitochondrial DNA in anucleate human blood cells. *Biochem Biophys Res Commun* 155(3):1360–1365, 1988.

199. Boudreau LH, et al: Platelets release mitochondria serving as substrate for bactericidal group IIA-secreted phospholipase A2 to promote inflammation. *Blood* 124(14):2173–2183, 2014.

200. Mason KD, et al: Programmed anuclear cell death delimits platelet life span. *Cell* 128(6):1173–1186, 2007.

201. Cardoso SM, et al: Cytochrome c oxidase is decreased in Alzheimer's disease platelets. *Neurobiol Aging* 25(1):105–110, 2004.

202. Dror N, et al: State-dependent alterations in mitochondrial complex I activity in platelets: A potential peripheral marker for schizophrenia. *Mol Psychiatry* 7(9):995–1001, 2002.

203. Lenaz G, et al: Mitochondrial complex I defects in aging. *Mol Cell Biochem* 174(1–2):329–333, 1997.

204. Lenaz G, et al: Mitochondrial bioenergetics in aging. *Biochim Biophys Acta* 1459(2–3):397–404, 2000.

205. Mancuso M, et al: Decreased platelet cytochrome c oxidase activity is accompanied by increased blood lactate concentration during exercise in patients with Alzheimer disease. *Exp Neurol* 182(2):421–426, 2003.

206. Schapira AH: Mitochondrial dysfunction in neurodegenerative disorders. *Biochim Biophys Acta* 1366(1–2):225–233, 1998.

207. Yamagishi SI, et al: Hyperglycemia potentiates collagen-induced platelet activation through mitochondrial superoxide overproduction. *Diabetes* 50(6):1491–1494, 2001.

208. Dale GL, Friese P: Bax activators potentiate coated-platelet formation. *J Thromb Haemost* 4(12):2664–2669, 2006.

209. Jobe SM, et al: Critical role for the mitochondrial permeability transition pore and cyclophilin D in platelet activation and thrombosis. *Blood* 111(3):1257–1265, 2008.

210. Leung R, et al: Persistence of procoagulant surface expression on activated human platelets: Involvement of apoptosis and aminophospholipid translocase activity. *J Thromb Haemost* 5(3):560–570, 2007.

211. Remenyi G, et al: Role of mitochondrial permeability transition pore in coated-platelet formation. *Arterioscler Thromb Vasc Biol* 25(2):467–471, 2005.

212. Nachmias VT: Platelet and megakaryocyte shape change: Triggered alterations in the cytoskeleton. *Semin Hematol* 20(4):261–281, 1983.

213. Maurer-Spurej E, Devine DV: Platelet aggregation is not initiated by platelet shape change. *Lab Invest* 2001;81(11):1517–1525, 1983.

214. Born GV: Quantification of the morphological reaction of platelets to aggregating agents and of its reversal by aggregation inhibitors. *J Physiol* 280:193–212, 1978.

215. Coller BS: Biochemical and electrostatic considerations in primary platelet aggregation. *Ann N Y Acad Sci* 416:693.

216. Hartwig JH, et al: The elegant platelet: Signals controlling actin assembly. *Thromb Haemost* 82:392–398, 1984, 1999.

217. Falet H, et al: Importance of free actin filament barbed ends for Arp2/3 complex function in platelets and fibroblasts. *Proc Natl Acad Sci U S A* 99(26):16782–16787, 2002.

218. Carlier MF, et al: Tbeta 4 is not a simple G-actin sequestering protein and interacts with F-actin at high concentration. *J Biol Chem* 271(16):9231–9239, 1996.

219. Lind SE, Yin HL, Stossel TP: Human platelets contain gelsolin. A regulator of actin filament length. *J Clin Invest* 69(6):1384–1387, 1982.

220. Barkalow K, Hartwig JH: The role of actin filament barbed-end exposure in cytoskeletal dynamics and cell motility. *Biochem Soc Trans* 23(3):451–456, 1995.

221. Barkalow K, et al: A-Adducin dissociates from F-actin filaments and spectrin during platelet activation. *J Cell Biol* 161:557–570, 2003.

222. Machesky LM, Gould KL: The Arp2/3 complex: A multifunctional actin organizer. *Curr Opin Cell Biol* 11(1):117–121, 1999.

223. Mullins RD, Heuser JA, Pollard TD: The interaction of Arp2/3 complex with actin: Nucleation, high affinity pointed end capping, and formation of branching networks of filaments. *Proc Natl Acad Sci U S A* 95(11):6181–6186, 1998.

224. Heemskerk JW, et al: Collagen but not fibrinogen surfaces induce bleb formation, exposure of phosphatidylserine, and procoagulant activity of adherent platelets: Evidence for regulation by protein tyrosine kinase-dependent Ca2+ responses. *Blood* 90(7):2615–2625, 1997.

225. Watson SP: Collagen receptor signaling in platelets and megakaryocytes. *Thromb Haemost* 82(2):365–376, 1999.

226. Jirouskova M, Jaiswal JK, Coller BS: Ligand density dramatically affects integrin alpha IIb beta 3-mediated platelet signaling and spreading. *Blood* 109(5260):5269, 2007.

227. Coller BS, et al: Studies of activated GPIIb/IIIa receptors on the luminal surface of adherent platelets. Paradoxical loss of luminal receptors when platelets adhere to high density fibrinogen. *J Clin Invest* 92:2796–2806, 1999, 1993.

228. Patel D, et al: The dynamics of GPIIb/IIIa-mediated platelet-platelet interactions in platelet adhesion/thrombus formation on collagen in vitro as revealed by videomicroscopy. *Blood* 101:929–936, 2003.

229. Fox JE: On the role of calpain and Rho proteins in regulating integrin-induced signaling. *Thromb Haemost* 82(2):385–391, 1999.

230. Hartwig JH, et al: Thrombin receptor ligation and activated Rac uncap actin filament barbed ends through phosphoinositide synthesis in permeabilized human platelets. *Cell* 1995;82(4):643–653, 1999.

231. Lemmon MA, Ferguson KM, Abrams CS: Pleckstrin homology domains and the cytoskeleton. *FEBS Lett* 513(1):71–76, 2002.

232. Ma AD, Abrams CS: Pleckstrin homology domains and phospholipid-induced cytoskeletal reorganization. *Thromb Haemost* 82(2):399–406, 1999.

233. Lian L, Wang Y, Flick M, et al: Loss of pleckstrin defines a novel pathway for PKC-mediated exocytosis. *Blood* 113(15):3577–3584, 2009.

234. Hitchcock IS, et al: Roles of focal adhesion kinase (FAK) in megakaryopoiesis and platelet function: Studies using a megakaryocyte lineage specific FAK knockout. *Blood* 111(2):596–604, 2008.

235. Coller BS, Shattil SJ: The GPIIb/IIIa (integrin alphaIIbbeta3) odyssey: A technology-driven saga of a receptor with twists, turns, and even a bend. *Blood* 112(8):3011–3025, 2008.

236. Pabla R, et al: Integrin-dependent control of translation: Engagement of integrin alphaIIbbeta3 regulates synthesis of proteins in activated human platelets. *J Cell Biol* 144(1):175–184, 1999.

237. Shattil SJ: Signaling through platelet integrin αIIbβ3: Inside-out, outside-in and sideways. *Thromb Haemost* 82(2):318–325, 1999.

238. Shattil SJ, Newman PJ: Integrins: Dynamic scaffolds for adhesion and signaling in platelets. *Blood* 104(6):1606–1615, 2004.

239. Kulkarni S, et al: Conversion of platelets from a proaggregatory to a proinflammatory adhesive phenotype: Role of PAF in spatially regulating neutrophil adhesion and spreading. *Blood* 110(6):1879–1886, 2007.

240. Cho J, Mosher DF: Role of fibronectin assembly in platelet thrombus formation. *J Thromb Haemost* 4(7):1461–1469, 2006.

241. George JN, et al: Platelet surface glycoproteins. Studies on resting and activated platelets and platelet membrane microparticles in normal subjects, and observations in patients during adult respiratory distress syndrome and cardiac surgery. *J Clin Invest* 78:340–348, 1986.

242. Michelson AD: Thrombin-induced down-regulation of the platelet membrane glycoprotein Ib-IX complex. *Semin Thromb Hemost* 18:18–27, 1992.

243. Bennett JS, et al: The platelet cytoskeleton regulates the affinity of the integrin alpha(IIb)beta(3) for fibrinogen. *J Biol Chem* 274(36):25301–25307, 1999.

244. Patil S, et al: Identification of a talin-binding site in the integrin beta(3) subunit distinct from the NPLY regulatory motif of post-ligand binding functions. The talin n-terminal head domain interacts with the membrane-proximal region of the beta(3) cytoplasmic tail. *J Biol Chem* 274(40):28575–28583, 1999.

245. Tadokoro S, et al: Talin binding to integrin beta tails: A final common step in integrin activation. *Science* 302(5642):103–106, 2003.

246. Yan B, et al: Calpain cleavage promotes talin binding to the beta 3 integrin cytoplasmic domain. *J Biol Chem* 276(30):28164–28170, 2001.

247. Shattil SJ, Brugge JS: Protein tyrosine phosphorylation and the adhesive functions of platelets. *Curr Opin Cell Biol* 3:869–879, 1991.

248. Fox JE: The platelet cytoskeleton. *Thromb Haemost* 70(6):884–893, 1993.

249. Fox JE: Platelet cytoskeleton, in *Hemostasis and Thrombosis: Basic Principles and Clinical Practice*, edited by RW Colman, J Hirsh, VJ Marder, AW Clowes, JN George, pp 429–446. Lippincott, Williams & Wilkins, Philadelphia, 2001.

250. Zhu J, Luo BH, Xiao T, et al: Structure of a complete integrin ectodomain in a physiologic resting state and activation and deactivation by applied forces. *Mol Cell* 32(6):849–861, 2008.

251. Li R, et al: Activation of integrin alphaIIbbeta3 by modulation of transmembrane helix associations. *Science* 300(5620):795–798, 2003.

252. Olorundare OE, Simmons SR, Albrecht RM: Cytochalasin D and E: Effects on fibrinogen receptor movement and cytoskeletal reorganization in fully spread, surface-activated platelets: A correlative light and electron microscopic investigation. *Blood* 79(1):99–109, 1992.

253. White JG: Induction of patching and its reversal on surface-activated human platelets. *Br J Haematol* 76(1):108–115, 1990.

254. Fox JE, et al: Identification of two proteins (actin-binding protein and P235) that are hydrolyzed by endogenous Ca++-dependent protease during platelet aggregation. *J Biol Chem* 260:1060–1066, 1985.

255. Fox JE, Reynolds CC, Phillips DR: Calcium-dependent proteolysis occurs during platelet aggregation. *J Biol Chem* 258(16):9973–9981, 1983.

256. Fox JE, et al: Evidence that activation of platelet calpain is induced as a consequence of binding of adhesive ligand to the integrin, glycoprotein IIb-IIIa. *J Cell Biol* 120(6):1501–1507, 1993.

257. Xi X, et al: Critical roles for the COOH-terminal NITY and RGT sequences of the integrin beta3 cytoplasmic domain in inside-in and outside-in signaling. *J Cell Biol* 162(2):329–339, 2003.

258. Flevaris P, et al: A molecular switch that controls cell spreading and retraction. *J Cell Biol* 179(3):553–565, 2007.

259. Dachary-Prigent J, et al: Annexin V as a probe of aminophospholipid exposure and platelet membrane vesiculation: A flow cytometry study showing a role for free sulfhydryl groups. *Blood* 81:2554–2565, 1993.

260. Azam M, et al: Disruption of the mouse mu-calpain gene reveals an essential role in platelet function. *Mol Cell Biol* 21(6):2213–2220, 2001.

261. Furman MI, Gardner TM, Goldschmidt-Clermont PJ: Mechanisms of cytoskeletal reorganization during platelet activation. *Thromb Haemost* 70(1):229–232, 1993.

262. McNicol A, Israels SJ: Platelet dense granules: Structure, function and implications for haemostasis. *Thromb Res* 1999;95(1):1–18, 1993.

263. Leon C, et al: Megakaryocyte-restricted MYH9 inactivation dramatically affects hemostasis while preserving platelet aggregation and secretion. *Blood* 110(9): 3183–3191, 2007.

264. Escolar G, Krumwiede M, White JG: Organization of the actin cytoskeleton of resting and activated platelets in suspension. *Am J Pathol* 123:86–94, 1986.

265. Fox JE, et al: Actin filament content and organization in unstimulated platelets. *J Cell Biol* 98:1985.

266. Hartwig JH: Platelet structure, in *Platelets*, edited by AD Michelson, pp 75–97. Academic Press, San Diego, 2007, 1984.

267. Nachmias VT, Yoshida K: The cytoskeleton of the blood platelets: A dynamic structure. *Adv Cyclic Nucleotide Res* 2:181–211, 1999.

268. Weber A, et al: Interaction of thymosin-β-4 with muscle and platelet actin. Implications for actin sequestration in resting platelets. *Biochemistry* 31(27):6179–6185, 1992.

269. Gonnella PA, Nachmias VT: Platelet activation and microfilament bundling. *J Biol Chem* 89:146, 1981.

270. Nachmias VT: Cytoskeleton of human platelets at rest and after spreading. *J Cell Biol* 86:795, 1980.

271. Budtz-Olsen OE: *Clot Retraction*. Charles C Thomas, Springfield, 1951.

272. Stalker TJ, et al: A systems approach to hemostasis: 3. Thrombus consolidation regulates intrathrombus solute transport and local thrombin activity. *Blood* 124(11): 1824–1831, 2014.

273. Kunitada S, FitzGerald GA, Fitzgerald DJ: Inhibition of clot lysis and decreased binding of tissue-type plasminogen activator as a consequence of clot retraction. *Blood* 79(6):1420–1427, 1992.

274. Cohen I, Gerrard JM, White JG: Ultrastructure of clots during isometric contraction. *J Cell Biol* 91:775.

275. Pollard TD, et al: Contractile proteins in platelet activation and contraction. *Ann N Y Acad Sci* 283:218, 1977.

276. Vaiyapuri S, et al: EphB2 regulates contact-dependent and contact-independent signaling to control platelet function. *Blood* 2015;125(4):720–730, 1982.

277. Khatlani T, et al: The beta isoform of the catalytic subunit of protein phosphatase 2B restrains platelet function by suppressing outside-in alphaII b beta3 integrin signaling. *J Thromb Haemost* 12(12):2089–2101, 2014.

278. Yi W, Li Q, Shen J, et al: Modulation of platelet activation and thrombus formation using a pan-PI3K inhibitor S14161. *PLoS One* 9(8):e102394, 2014.

279. Cohen I: The mechanism of clot retraction, in *Platelet Membrane Glycoproteins*, edited by JN George, AT Nurden, DR Phillips, pp 299–323. Plenum Press, New York, 1985, 2014.

280. Carr ME Jr, et al: Glycoprotein IIb/IIIa blockade inhibits platelet-mediated force development and reduces gel elastic modulus. *Thromb Haemost* 73:499–505, 1995.

281. Leistikow EA: Platelet internalization in early thrombogenesis. *Semin Thromb Hemost* 22(3):289–294, 1996.

282. Morgenstern E, Daub M, Dierichs R: A new model for *in vitro* clot formation that considers the mode of the fibrin(ogen) contacts to platelets and the arrangement of the platelet cytoskeleton. *Ann N Y Acad Sci* 936:449–455, 2001.

283. Braaten JV, Jerome WG, Hantgan RR: Uncoupling fibrin from integrin receptors hastens fibrinolysis at the platelet-fibrin interface. *Blood* 83:982–993, 1994.

284. Coller BS, et al: A murine monoclonal antibody that completely blocks the binding of fibrinogen to platelets produces a thrombasthenic-like state in normal platelets and binds to glycoproteins IIb and/or IIIa. *J Clin Invest* 72:325–338, 1983.

285. Collet JP, et al: A structural and dynamic investigation of the facilitating effect of glycoprotein IIb/IIIa inhibitors in dissolving platelet-rich clots. *Circ Res* 90(4):428–434, 2002.

286. Huang TC, et al: Differential effects of c7E3 Fab on thrombus formation and rt-PA-mediated thrombolysis under flow conditions. *Thromb Res* 102(5):411–425, 2001.

287. Mousa SA, Khurana S, Forsythe MS: Comparative *in vitro* efficacy of different platelet glycoprotein IIb/IIIa antagonists on platelet-mediated clot strength induced by tissue factor with use of thromboelastography: Differentiation among glycoprotein IIb/IIIa antagonists. *Arterioscler Thromb Vasc Biol* 20(4):1162–1167, 2000.

288. Seiffert D, et al: Regulation of clot retraction by glycoprotein IIb/IIIa antagonists. *Thromb Res* 108(2–3):181–189, 2002.

289. Jirouskova M, et al: A hamster antibody to the mouse fibrinogen gamma chain inhibits platelet-fibrinogen interactions and FXIIIa-mediated fibrin cross-linking, and facilitates thrombolysis. *Thromb Haemost* 86(4):1047–1056, 2001.

290. Mor-Cohen R, et al: Disulfide bond exchanges in integrins alphaIIbbeta3 and alphavbeta3 are required for activation and post-ligation signaling during clot retraction. *Thromb Res* 133(5):826–836, 2014.

291. Law DA, et al: Integrin cytoplasmic tyrosine motif is required for outside-in alphaIIb-beta3 signalling and platelet function. *Nature* 401:808–811, 1999.

292. Osdoit S, Rosa JP: Fibrin clot retraction by human platelets correlates with alpha(IIb) beta(3) integrin-dependent protein tyrosine dephosphorylation. *J Biol Chem* 276(9):6703–6710, 2001.

293. Flevaris P, et al: Two distinct roles of mitogen-activated protein kinases in platelets and a novel Rac1-MAPK-dependent integrin outside-in retractile signaling pathway. *Blood* 113(4):893–901, 2009.

294. Weyrich AS, et al: MTOR-dependent synthesis of Bcl-3 controls the retraction of fibrin clots by activated human platelets. *Blood* 109(5):1975–1983, 2007.

295. Ward CM, Kestin AS, Newman PJ: A Leu262Pro mutation in the integrin beta(3) subunit results in an alpha(IIb)-beta(3) complex that binds fibrin but not fibrinogen. *Blood* 96(1):161–169, 2000.

296. Rooney MM, et al: The contribution of the three hypothesized integrin-binding sites in fibrinogen to platelet-mediated clot retraction. *Blood* 92(7):2374–2381, 1998.

297. Rooney MM, Parise LV, Lord ST: Dissecting clot retraction and platelet aggregation. Clot retraction does not require an intact fibrinogen gamma chain C terminus. *J Biol Chem* 271(15):8553–8555, 1996.

298. Podolnikova NP, et al: Identification of a novel binding site for platelet integrins alpha IIb beta 3 (GPIIbIIIa) and alpha 5 beta 1 in the gamma C-domain of fibrinogen. *J Biol Chem* 278(34):32251–32258, 2003.

299. Remijn JA, Ijsseldijk MJ, de Groot PG: Role of the fibrinogen gamma-chain sequence gamma316–322 in platelet-mediated clot retraction. *J Thromb Haemost* 1(10): 2245–2246, 2003.

300. Podolnikova NP, et al: The interaction of integrin alphaIIbbeta3 with fibrin occurs through multiple binding sites in the alphaIIb beta-propeller domain. *J Biol Chem* 289(4):2371–2383, 2014.

301. Kasahara K, et al: Clot retraction is mediated by factor XIII-dependent fibrin-alphaIIbbeta3-myosin axis in platelet sphingomyelin-rich membrane rafts. *Blood* 122(19):3340–3348, 2013.

302. Munday AD, Lopez JA: Factor XIII: Sticking it to platelets. *Blood* 122(19):3246–3247, 2013.

303. Dubois C, et al: Thrombin binding to GPIbalpha induces platelet aggregation and fibrin clot retraction supported by resting alphaIIbbeta3 interaction with polymerized fibrin. *Thromb Haemost* 89(5):853–865, 2003.

304. Keuren JF, et al: Von Willebrand factor C1C2 domain is involved in platelet adhesion to polymerized fibrin at high shear rate. *Blood* 103(5):1741–1746, 2004.

305. Huizing M, et al: Disorders of lysosome-related organelle biogenesis: Clinical and molecular genetics. *Annu Rev Genomics Hum Genet* 9:359–386, 2008.

306. Holmsen H, Kaplan KL, Dangelmaier CA: Differential energy requirements for platelet responses. A simultaneous study of aggregation, three secretory processes, arachidonate liberation, phosphatidylinositol breakdown and phosphatidate production. *Biochem J* 208(1):9–18, 1982.

307. Verhoeven AJ, Mommersteeg ME, Akkerman JW: Quantification of energy consumption in platelets during thrombin-induced aggregation and secretion. Tight coupling between platelet responses and the increment in energy consumption. *Biochem J* 221(3):777–787, 1984.

308. Ciferri S, et al: Platelets release their lysosomal content *in vivo* in humans upon activation. *Thromb Haemost* 83(1):157–164, 2000.

309. Abrams C, Shattil SJ: Immunological detection of activated platelets in clinical disorders. *Thromb Haemost* 65(5):467–473, 1991.

310. Nieuwenhuis HK, et al: Studies with a monoclonal antibody against activated platelets: Evidence that a secreted 53,000-molecular weight lysosome-like granule protein is exposed on the surface of activated platelets in the circulation. *Blood* 70(3):838–845, 1987.

311. Zhang ZG: Dynamic platelet accumulation at the site of the occluded middle cerebral artery and in downstream microvessels is associated with loss of microvascular integrity after embolic middle cerebral artery occlusion. *Brain Res* 912(2):181–194, 2001.

312. Castellot JJ Jr, et al: Inhibition of vascular smooth muscle cell growth by endothelial cell-derived heparin. Possible role of a platelet endoglycosidase. *J Biol Chem* 257(21):11256–11260, 1982.

313. Ugurbil K, Fukami MH, Holmsen H: 31P NMR studies of nucleotide storage in the dense granules of pig platelets. *Biochemistry* 23(3):409–416, 1984.

314. Ugurbil K, Holmsen H, Shulman RG: Adenine nucleotide storage and secretion in platelets as studied by 31P nuclear magnetic resonance. *Proc Natl Acad Sci U S A* 76(5):2227–2231, 1979.

315. Lesurtel M, et al: Platelet-derived serotonin mediates liver regeneration. *Science* 312(5770):104–107, 2006.

316. Gunay-Aygun M, Huizing M, Gahl WA: Molecular defects that affect platelet dense granules. *Semin Thromb Hemost* 30(5):537–547, 2004.

317. Youssefian T, Cramer EM: Megakaryocyte dense granule components are sorted in multivesicular bodies. *Blood* 95(12):4004–4007, 2000.

318. Nagle DL, et al: Identification and mutation analysis of the complete gene for Chediak-Higashi syndrome. *Nat Genet* 14(3):307–311, 1996.

319. FitzGerald GA, Dipyridamole. *N Engl J Med* 316(20):1247–1257, 1987.

320. Hatmi M, et al: Evidence for cAMP-dependent platelet ectoprotein kinase activity that phosphorylates platelet glycoprotein IV (CD36). *J Biol Chem* 271(40):24776–24780, 1996.

321. Kalafatis M, et al: Phosphorylation of factor Va and factor VIIIa by activated platelets. *Blood* 81(3):704–719, 1993.

322. Naik UP, Kornecki E, Ehrlich YH: Phosphorylation and dephosphorylation of human platelet surface proteins by an ecto-protein kinase/phosphatase system. *Biochim Biophys Acta* 1092(2):256–264, 1991.

323. Harrison P, Cramer EM: Platelet alpha-granules. *Blood Rev* 7(1):52–62, 1993.

324. Reed G: Platelet secretion, in *Platelets*, edited by A Michelson A, p 309. Academic Press, San Diego, 2007.

325. Hayward CP, et al: Factor V is complexed with multimerin in resting platelet lysates and colocalizes with multimerin in platelet alpha-granules. *J Biol Chem* 270(33):19217–19224, 1995.

326. Coppinger JA, et al: Characterization of the proteins released from activated platelets leads to localization of novel platelet proteins in human atherosclerotic lesions. *Blood* 103(6):2096–2104, 2004.

327. Maynard DM, et al: Proteomic analysis of platelet alpha-granules using mass spectrometry. *J Thromb Haemost* 5(9):1945–1955, 2007.

328. McRedmond JP, et al: Integration of proteomics and genomics in platelets: A profile of platelet proteins and platelet-specific genes. *Mol Cell Proteomics* 3(2):133–144, 2004.

329. Italiano JE Jr, Richardson JL, Patel-Hett S, et al: Angiogenesis is regulated by a novel mechanism: Pro- and antiangiogenic proteins are organized into separate platelet alpha granules and differentially released. *Blood* 111(3):1227–1233, 2008.

330. Sehgal S, Storrie B: Evidence that differential packaging of the major platelet granule proteins von Willebrand factor and fibrinogen can support their differential release. *J Thromb Haemost* 5(10):2009–2016, 2007.

331. George JN: Platelet immunoglobulin G: Its significance for the evaluation of thrombocytopenia and for understanding the origin of alpha-granule proteins. *Blood* 76(5):859–870, 1990.

332. George JN, Platelet IgG: Measurement, interpretation, and clinical significance. *Prog Hemost Thromb* 10:97–126, 1991.

333. Heijnen HF, et al: Multivesicular bodies are an intermediate stage in the formation of platelet alpha-granules. *Blood* 91(7):2313–2325, 1998.

334. Niewiarowski S: Secreted platelet proteins, in *Haemostasis and Thrombosis*, edited by AL Bloom, DP Thomas, EGD Tuddenham, p 167. Churchill Livingstone, London, England, 1994.

335. Niewiarowski S, Holt JC, Cook JJ: Biochemistry and physiology of secreted platelet proteins, in *Hemostasis and Thrombosis: Basic Principles and Clinical Practice*, edited by RW Colman, VJ Marder, EW Salzman, p 546. JB Lippincott, Philadelphia, 1993.

336. Brown KD, et al: A family of small inducible proteins secreted by leukocytes are members of a new superfamily that includes leukocyte and fibroblast-derived inflammatory agents, growth factors, and indicators of various activation processes. *J Immunol* 142(2):679–687, 1989.

337. Kawahara RS, Deuel TF: Platelet-derived growth factor-inducible gene JE is a member of a family of small inducible genes related to platelet factor 4. *J Biol Chem* 264(2):679–682, 1989.

338. Oppenheim JJ, et al: Properties of the novel proinflammatory supergene "intercrine" cytokine family. *Annu Rev Immunol* 9:617–648, 1991.

339. Gear AR, Camerini D: Platelet chemokines and chemokine receptors: Linking hemostasis, inflammation, and host defense. *Microcirculation* 10(3–4):335–350, 2003.

340. Rollins BJ: Chemokines. *Blood* 90(3):909–928, 1997.

341. Handin RI, Cohen HJ: Purification and binding properties of human platelet factor four. *J Biol Chem* 251(14):4273–4282, 1976.

342. Loscalzo J, Melnick B, Handin RI: The interaction of platelet factor four and glycosaminoglycans. *Arch Biochem Biophys* 240(1):446–455, 1985.

343. Rucinski B, et al: Human platelet factor 4 and its C-terminal peptides: Heparin binding and clearance from the circulation. *Thromb Haemost* 63(3):493–498, 1990.

344. Barber AJ, Käser-Glanzmann R, Jakábová M, Lüscher EF: Chromatography of chondroitin sulfate proteoglycan carrier for heparin neutralizing activity (platelet factor 4) released from human blood platelets. *Biochim Biophys Acta* 286.

345. Huang SS, Huang JS, Deuel TF: Proteoglycan carrier of human platelet factor 4. Isolation and characterization. *J Biol Chem* 1982;257(19):11546–11550, 1972.

346. Busch C, et al: Binding of platelet factor 4 to cultured human umbilical vein endothelial cells. *Thromb Res* 19(1–2):129–137, 1980.

347. Clore GM, Gronenborn AM: Three-dimensional structures of alpha and beta chemokines. *FASEB J* 9(1):57–62, 1995.

348. Cowan SW, et al: Binding of heparin to human platelet factor 4. *Biochem J* 234(2):485–488, 1986.

349. Visentin GP, et al: Antibodies from patients with heparin-induced thrombocytopenia/thrombosis are specific for platelet factor 4 complexed with heparin or bound to endothelial cells. *J Clin Invest* 93(1):81–88, 1994.

350. Warkentin TE, Heparin-induced thrombocytopenia. *Curr Hematol Rep* 1(1):63–72, 2002.

351. Rucinski B, et al: Uptake and processing of human platelet factor 4 by hepatocytes. *Proc Soc Exp Biol Med* 186(3):361–367, 1987.

352. Deuel TF, et al: Platelet factor 4 is chemotactic for neutrophils and monocytes. *Proc Natl Acad Sci U S A* 78(7):4584–4587, 1981.

353. Maione TE, et al: Inhibition of angiogenesis by recombinant human platelet factor-4 and related peptides. *Science* 247(4938):77–79, 1990.

354. Brindley LL, Sweet JM, Goetzl EJ: Stimulation of histamine release from human basophils by human platelet factor 4. *J Clin Invest* 72(4):1218–1223, 1983.

355. Gewirtz AM, et al: Inhibition of human megakaryocytopoiesis in vitro by platelet factor 4 (PF4) and a synthetic COOH-terminal PF4 peptide. *J Clin Invest* 83(5):1477–1486, 1989.

356. Han ZC, et al: Platelet factor 4 inhibits human megakaryocytopoiesis *in vitro*. *Blood* 75(6):1234–1239, 1990.

357. Lambert MP, et al: Platelet factor 4 is a negative autocrine *in vivo* regulator of megakaryopoiesis: Clinical and therapeutic implications. *Blood* 110(4):1153–1160, 2007.

358. Katz IR, et al: Protease-induced immunoregulatory activity of platelet factor 4. *Proc Natl Acad Sci U S A* 83(10):3491–3495, 1986.

359. Beyth RJ, Culp LA: Complementary adhesive responses of human skin fibroblasts to the cell-binding domain of fibronectin and the heparan sulfate-binding protein, platelet factor-4. *Exp Cell Res* 155(2):537–548, 1984.

360. Capitanio AM, et al: Interaction of platelet factor 4 with human platelets. *Biochim Biophys Acta* 839(2):161–173, 1985.

361. Dumenco LL, et al: Inhibition of the activation of Hageman factor (factor XII) by platelet factor 4. *J Lab Clin Med* 112(3):394–400, 1988.

362. Aziz KA, Cawley JC, Zuzel M: Platelets prime PMN via released PF4: Mechanism of priming and synergy with GM-CSF. *Br J Haematol* 91(4):846–853, 1995.

363. Engstad CS, et al: A novel biological effect of platelet factor 4 (PF4): Enhancement of LPS-induced tissue factor activity in monocytes. *J Leukoc Biol* 58(5):575–581, 1995.

364. Castor CW, Miller JW, Walz DA: Structural and biological characteristics of connective tissue activating peptide (CTAP-III), a major human platelet-derived growth factor. *Proc Natl Acad Sci U S A* 80(3):765–769, 1983.

365. Holt JC, et al: Characterization of human platelet basic protein, a precursor form of low-affinity platelet factor 4 and beta-thromboglobulin. *Biochemistry* 25(8):1988–1996, 1986.

366. Walz A, et al: Effects of the neutrophil-activating peptide NAP-2, platelet basic protein, connective tissue-activating peptide III and platelet factor 4 on human neutrophils. *J Exp Med* 170(5):1745–1750, 1989.

367. Bastl CP, et al: Role of kidney in the catabolic clearance of human platelet antiheparin proteins from rat circulation. *Blood* 57(2):233–238, 1981.

368. Hayward CP: Multimerin: A bench-to-bedside chronology of a unique platelet and endothelial cell protein—from discovery to function to abnormalities in disease. *Clin Invest Med* 20(3):176–187, 1997.

369. Polgar J, et al: Platelet glycoprotein Ia* is the processed form of multimerin—isolation and determination of N-terminal sequences of stored and released forms. *Thromb Haemost* 80(4):645–648, 1998.

370. Hayward CP, et al: Studies of multimerin in human endothelial cells. *Blood* 91(4):1304–1317, 1998.

371. Harrison P: Platelet alpha-granular fibrinogen. *Platelets* 3(1):1–10, 1992.

372. Harrison P, Wilbourn BR, Saundry RH, et al: Absence of the γ-Leu 427 (γ′) variant in the platelet alpha-granular fibrinogen pool supports the role of glycoprotein IIb/IIIa in mediating fibrinogen uptake into platelets/megakaryocytes. *Blood* 79(12):3394–3395, 1992.

373. Reheman A, et al: Plasma fibronectin depletion enhances platelet aggregation and thrombus formation in mice lacking fibrinogen and von Willebrand factor. *Blood* 2009;113(8):1809–1817, 1992.

374. Cho J, Mosher DF: Role of fibronectin assembly in platelet thrombus formation. *J Thromb Haemost* 4(7):1461–1469, 2006.

375. Coller BS, et al: Platelet fibrinogen and vitronectin in Glanzmann thrombasthenia: Evidence consistent with specific roles for glycoprotein IIb/IIIA and alpha v beta 3 integrins in platelet protein trafficking. *Blood* 78(10):2603–2610, 1991.

376. Eitzman DT, et al: Plasminogen activator inhibitor-1 and vitronectin promote vascular thrombosis in mice. *Blood* 95(2):577–580, 2000.

377. Fay WP, et al: Vitronectin inhibits the thrombotic response to arterial injury in mice. *Blood* 93(6):1825–1830, 1999.

378. Konstantinides S, et al: Plasminogen activator inhibitor-1 and its cofactor vitronectin stabilize arterial thrombi after vascular injury in mice. *Circulation* 103(4):576–583, 2001.

379. Adams JC, Lawler J, The thrombospondins. *Int J Biochem Cell Biol* 36(6):961–968, 2004.

380. Baenziger NL, Brodie GN, Majerus PW: A thrombin-sensitive protein of human platelet membranes. *Proc Natl Acad Sci U S A* 68(1):240–243, 1971.

381. Lawler J, Hynes RO: The structure of human thrombospondin, an adhesive glycoprotein with multiple calcium-binding sites and homologies with several different proteins. *J Cell Biol* 103(5):1635–1648, 1986.

382. Mosher DF, Doyle MJ, Jaffe EA: Synthesis and secretion of thrombospondin by cultured human endothelial cells. *J Cell Biol* 93(2):343–348, 1982.

383. Schwartz BS: Monocyte synthesis of thrombospondin. The role of platelets. *J Biol Chem* 264(13):7512–7517, 1989.

384. Aiken ML, et al: Effects of OKM5, a monoclonal antibody to glycoprotein IV, on platelet aggregation and thrombospondin surface expression. *Blood* 76(12):2501–2509, 1990.

385. Asch AS, et al: Analysis of CD36 binding domains: Ligand specificity controlled by dephosphorylation of an ectodomain. *Science* 262(5138):1436–1440, 1993.

386. Chung J, Gao AG, Frazier WA: Thrombospondin acts via integrin-associated protein to activate the platelet integrin alphaIIbbeta3. *J Biol Chem* 272(23):14740–14746, 1997.

387. Chung J, et al: Thrombospondin-1 acts via IAP/CD47 to synergize with collagen in alpha2beta1-mediated platelet activation. *Blood* 94(2):642–648, 1999.

388. Jurk K, et al: Thrombospondin-1 mediates platelet adhesion at high shear via glycoprotein Ib (GPIb): An alternative/backup mechanism to von Willebrand factor. *FASEB J* 17(11):1490–1492, 2003.

389. Lawler J, Hynes RO: An integrin receptor on normal and thrombasthenic platelets that binds thrombospondin. *Blood* 74(6):2022–2027, 1989.

390. Plow EF, et al: Related binding mechanisms for fibrinogen, fibronectin, von Willebrand factor, and thrombospondin on thrombin-stimulated human platelets. *Blood* 66(3):724–727, 1985.

391. Gao AG, et al: Integrin-associated protein is a receptor for the C-terminal domain of thrombospondin. *J Biol Chem* 271(1):21–24, 1996.

392. Lawler J, Hynes RO: The structure of human thrombospondin, an adhesive glycoprotein with multiple calcium binding sites and homologies with several different proteins. *J Cell Biol* 103:1635–1648, 1986.

393. Elzie CA, Murphy-Ullrich JE: The N-terminus of thrombospondin: The domain stands apart. *Int J Biochem Cell Biol* 36(6):1090–1101, 2004.

394. Tuszynski GP, et al: The interaction of human platelet thrombospondin with fibrinogen. Thrombospondin purification and specificity of interaction. *J Biol Chem* 260(22):12240–12245, 1985.

395. Dardik R, Lahav J: Functional changes in the conformation of thrombospondin-1 during complexation with fibronectin or heparin. *Exp Cell Res* 248(2):407–414, 1999.

396. Leung LL: Role of thrombospondin in platelet aggregation. *J Clin Invest* 74(5):1764–1772, 1984.

397. Schultz-Cherry S, Murphy-Ullrich JE: Thrombospondin causes activation of latent transforming growth factor-beta secreted by endothelial cells by a novel mechanism. *J Cell Biol* 122(4):923–932, 1993.

398. Silverstein RL, et al: Complex formation of platelet thrombospondin with plasminogen. Modulation of activation by tissue activator. *J Clin Invest* 74(5):1625–1633, 1984.

399. Bouchard BA, et al: Interactions between platelets and the coagulation system, in *Platelets*, edited by AD Michelson, p 229. Academic Press, San Diego, 2002.

400. Chesney CM, Pifer D, Colman RW: Subcellular localization and secretion of factor V from human platelets. *Proc Natl Acad Sci U S A* 78:5180–5184, 1981.

401. Tracy PB, Eide LL, Bowie EJ, et al: Radioimmunoassay of factor V in human plasma and platelets. *Blood* 60(1):59–63, 1982.

402. Camire RM, et al: Secretable human platelet-derived factor V originates from the plasma pool. *Blood* 1998;92(9):3035–3041, 1982.

403. Yang TL, et al: Biosynthetic origin and functional significance of murine platelet factor V. *Blood* 102(8):2851–2855, 2003.

404. Gould WR, Silveira JR, Tracy PB: Unique in vivo modifications of coagulation factor V produce a physically and functionally distinct platelet-derived cofactor: Characterization of purified platelet-derived factor V/Va. *J Biol Chem* 279(4):2383–2393, 2004.

405. Kane WH, Mruk JS, Majerus PW: Activation of coagulation factor V by a platelet protease. *J Clin Invest* 70:1092–1100, 1982.

406. Tracy PB, Nesheim ME, Mann KG: Proteolytic alterations of factor Va bound to platelets. *J Biol Chem* 662:669, 1983.

407. Nesheim ME, et al: Isolation and study of an acquired inhibitor of human coagulation factor V. *J Clin Invest* 405:415, 1986.

408. Tracy PB, et al: Factor V (Quebec): A bleeding diathesis associated with a qualitative platelet factor V deficiency. *J Clin Invest* 74:1221–1228, 1983, 1984.

409. Bode AP, et al: Association of factor V activity with membranous vesicles released from human platelets: Requirement for platelet stimulation. *Thromb Res* 39:49–61, 1985.

410. Manfioletti G, et al: The protein encoded by a growth arrest-specific gene (gas6) is a new member of the vitamin K-dependent proteins related to protein S, a negative coregulator in the blood coagulation cascade. *Mol Cell Biol* 13(8):4976–4985, 1993.

411. Melaragno MG, Fridell YW, Berk BC: The Gas6/Axl system: A novel regulator of vascular cell function. *Trends Cardiovasc Med* 9(8):250–253, 1999.

412. Angelillo-Scherrer A, et al: Deficiency or inhibition of Gas6 causes platelet dysfunction and protects mice against thrombosis. *Nat Med* 7(2):215–221, 2001.

413. Chen C, et al: Mer receptor tyrosine kinase signaling participates in platelet function. *Arterioscler Thromb Vasc Biol* 24(6):1118–1123, 2004.

414. Gould WR, et al: Gas6 receptors Axl, Sky and Mer enhance platelet activation and regulate thrombotic responses. *J Thromb Haemost* 3(4):733–741, 2005.

415. Angelillo-Scherrer A, et al: Role of Gas6 receptors in platelet signaling during thrombus stabilization and implications for antithrombotic therapy. *J Clin Invest* 115(2):237–246, 2005.

416. Maree AO, et al: Growth arrest specific gene (GAS) 6 modulates platelet thrombus formation and vascular wall homeostasis and represents an attractive drug target. *Curr Pharm Des* 13(26):2656–2661, 2007.

417. Saller F, et al: Role of the growth arrest-specific gene 6 (gas6) product in thrombus stabilization. *Blood Cells Mol Dis* 36(3):373–378, 2006.

418. Deuel TF, Huang SS, Huang JS: Platelet derived growth factor: Purification, characterization and role in normal and abnormal cell growth, in *Biochemistry of Platelets*, edited by DR Phillips, MA Shuman, pp 347–375. Academic, London, 1986.

419. Heldin CH, Westermark B: Platelet-derived growth factor: Three isoforms and two receptor types. *Trends Genet* 5(4):108–111, 1989.

420. Berk BC, Alexander RW: Vasoactive effects of growth factors. *Biochem Pharmacol* 38:219, 1989.

421. Madtes DK, Raines EW, Ross R: Modulation of local concentrations of platelet-derived growth factor. *Am Rev Respir Dis* 140:1118, 1989.

422. Ross R: Peptide regulatory factors. Platelet-derived growth factor. *Lancet* 1:1179, 1989.

423. Doolittle RF, et al: Simian sarcoma virus onc gene, v-sis, is derived from the gene (or genes) encoding a platelet-derived growth factor. *Science* 22:275, 1983.

424. Waterfield MD, et al: Platelet-derived growth factor is structurally related to the putative transforming protein p28-sis of simian sarcoma virus. *Nature* 304:35, 1983.

425. Williams LT: Signal transduction by the platelet-derived growth factor receptor. *Science* 89. 24:1564–1570, 1989.

426. Nagai MK, Embil JM: Becaplermin: Recombinant platelet derived growth factor, a new treatment for healing diabetic foot ulcers. *Expert Opin Biol Ther* 2(2):211–218, 2002.

427. Maloney JP, Silliman CC, Ambruso DR, et al: In vitro release of vascular endothelial growth factor during platelet aggregation. *Am J Physiol* 275(3 Pt 2):H1054–H1061, 1998.

428. Webb NJ, et al: Vascular endothelial growth factor (VEGF) is released from platelets during blood clotting: Implications for measurement of circulating VEGF levels in clinical disease. *Clin Sci (Lond)* 94(4):395–404, 1998.

429. Weltermann A, et al: Large amounts of vascular endothelial growth factor at the site of hemostatic plug formation in vivo. *Arterioscler Thromb Vasc Biol* 19(7):1757–1760, 1999.

430. Mohle R, et al: Constitutive production and thrombin-induced release of vascular endothelial growth factor by human megakaryocytes and platelets. *Proc Natl Acad Sci U S A* 94(2):663–668, 1997.

431. Amirkhosravi A, et al: Blockade of GPIIb/IIIa inhibits the release of vascular endothelial growth factor (VEGF) from tumor cell-activated platelets and experimental metastasis. *Platelets* 10:285–292, 1999.

432. Katoh O, et al: Expression of the vascular endothelial growth factor (VEGF) receptor gene, KDR, in hematopoietic cells and inhibitory effect of VEGF on apoptotic cell death caused by ionizing radiation. *Cancer Res* 55(23):5687–5692, 1995.

433. Wartiovaara U, et al: Peripheral blood platelets express VEGF-C and VEGF which are released during platelet activation. *Thromb Haemost* 80(1):171–175, 1998.

434. Italiano JE Jr, et al: Angiogenesis is regulated by a novel mechanism: Pro- and antiangiogenic proteins are organized into separate platelet alpha granules and differentially released. *Blood* 111(3):1227–1233, 2008.

435. Salven P, Orpana A, Joensuu H: Leukocytes and platelets of patients with cancer contain high levels of vascular endothelial growth factor. *Clin Cancer Res* 5(3):487–491, 1999.

436. Verheul HM, Pinedo HM: Tumor growth: A putative role for platelets? *Oncologist* 3(2):II, 1998.

437. Cao J, et al: Angiogenic factors in human proliferative sickle cell retinopathy. *Br J Ophthalmol* 83(7):838–846, 1999.

438. Solovey A, et al: Sickle cell anemia as a possible state of enhanced anti-apoptotic tone: Survival effect of vascular endothelial growth factor on circulating and unanchored endothelial cells. *Blood* 93(11):3824–3830, 1999.

439. Kiuru J, et al: Cytoskeleton-dependent release of human platelet epidermal growth factor. *Life Sci* 49(26):1997–2003, 1991.

440. Bush AI, Martins RN, Rumble B, et al: The amyloid precursor protein of Alzheimer's disease is released by human platelets. *J Biol Chem* 265(26):15977–15983, 1990.

441. Li Q, Beyreuther K, Masters CL: Alzheimer's disease, in *Platelets*, edited by AD Michelson, pp 779–789. Academic Press, San Diego, 2007.

442. Li Q, et al: Products of the Alzheimer's disease amyloid precursor protein generated by β-secretase are present in human platelets, and secreted upon degranulation. *Amer J Alzheimer's Dis*, 13:236–244, 1998.

443. Li QX, et al: Secretion of Alzheimer's disease Abeta amyloid peptide by activated human platelets. *Lab Invest* 78(4):461–469, 1998.

444. Li QX, et al: Proteolytic processing of Alzheimer's disease beta A4 amyloid precursor protein in human platelets. *J Biol Chem* 270(23):14140–14147, 1995.

445. Li QX, et al: Membrane-associated forms of the beta A4 amyloid protein precursor of Alzheimer's disease in human platelet and brain: Surface expression on the activated human platelet. *Blood* 84(1):133–142, 1994.

446. Van Nostrand WE, et al: Protease nexin-2/amyloid beta-protein precursor in blood is a platelet-specific protein. *Biochem Biophys Res Commun* 175(1):15–21, 1991.

447. Scandura JM, et al: Progress curve analysis of the kinetics with which blood coagulation factor XIa is inhibited by protease nexin-2. *Biochemistry* 36(2):412–420, 1997.

448. Schmaier AH, et al: Factor IXa inhibition by protease nexin-2/amyloid beta-protein precursor on phospholipid vesicles and cell membranes. *Biochemistry* 34(4):1171–1178, 1995.

449. Schmaier AH, et al: Protease nexin-2/amyloid β protein precursor. A tight-binding inhibitor of coagulation factor IXa. *J Clin Invest* 92(5):2540–2545, 1993.

450. Baskin F, et al: Platelet APP isoform ratios correlate with declining cognition in AD. *Neurology* 54(10):1907–1909, 2000.

451. Borroni B, et al: Microvascular damage and platelet abnormalities in early Alzheimer's disease. *J Neurol Sci* 203–204:189–193, 2002.

452. Davies TA, et al: Non-age related differences in thrombin responses by platelets from male patients with advanced Alzheimer's disease. *Biochem Biophys Res Commun* 194(1):537–543, 1993.

453. Davies TA, et al: Moderate and advanced Alzheimer's patients exhibit platelet activation differences. *Neurobiol Aging* 18(2):155–162, 1997.

454. Di Luca M, et al: Differential level of platelet amyloid beta precursor protein isoforms: An early marker for Alzheimer disease. *Arch Neurol* 55(9):1195–1200, 1998.

455. Rosenberg RN, et al: Altered amyloid protein processing in platelets of patients with Alzheimer disease. *Arch Neurol* 54(2):139–144, 1997.

456. Devine DV, Bishop PD: Platelet-associated factor XIII in platelet activation, adhesion, and clot stabilization. *Semin Thromb Hemost* 22(5):409–413, 1996.

457. McDonagh J, et al: Factor XIII in human plasma and platelets. *J Clin Invest* 48(5):940–946, 1969.

458. Adany R, Bardos H: Factor XIII subunit A as an intracellular transglutaminase. *Cell Mol Life Sci* 60(6):1049–1060, 2003.

459. Lorand L, Graham RM: Transglutaminases: Crosslinking enzymes with pleiotropic functions. *Nat Rev Mol Cell Biol* 4(2):140–156, 2003.

460. Inbal A, et al: Platelets but not monocytes contribute to the plasma levels of factor XIII subunit A in patients undergoing autologous peripheral blood stem cell transplantation. *Blood Coagul Fibrinolysis* 15(3):249–253, 2004.

461. Serrano K, Devine DV: Intracellular factor XIII crosslinks platelet cytoskeletal elements upon platelet activation. *Thromb Haemost* 88(2):315–320, 2002.

462. Huff T, et al: Thymosin beta4 is released from human blood platelets and attached by factor XIIIa (transglutaminase) to fibrin and collagen. *FASEB J* 16(7):691–696, 2002.

463. Kulkarni S, Jackson SP: Platelet factor XIII and calpain negatively regulate integrin alpha IIbbeta3 adhesive function and thrombus growth. *J Biol Chem* 279(29):30697–30706, 2004.

464. Szasz R, Dale GL: Thrombospondin and fibrinogen bind serotonin-derivatized proteins on COAT-platelets. *Blood* 100(8):2827–2831, 2002.

465. Szasz R, Dale GL: COAT platelets. *Curr Opin Hematol* 10(5):351–355, 2003.

466. Leask A: TGFbeta, cardiac fibroblasts, and the fibrotic response. *Cardiovasc Res* 74(2):207–212, 2007.

467. Massague J: TGFbeta in Cancer. *Cell* 134(2):215–230, 2008.

468. Rubtsov YP, Rudensky AY: TGFbeta signalling in control of T-cell-mediated self-reactivity. *Nat Rev Immunol* 7(6):443–453, 2007.

469. ten Dijke P, Arthur HM: Extracellular control of TGFbeta signalling in vascular development and disease. *Nat Rev Mol Cell Biol* 8(11):857–869, 2007.

470. Sakamaki S, et al: Transforming growth factor-beta1 (TGF-beta1) induces thrombopoietin from bone marrow stromal cells, which stimulates the expression of TGF- beta receptor on megakaryocytes and, in turn, renders them susceptible to suppression by TGF-beta itself with high specificity. *Blood* 94(6):1961–1970, 1999.

471. Shi Y, Massague J: Mechanisms of TGF-beta signaling from cell membrane to the nucleus. *Cell* 113(6):685–700, 2003.

472. Hoying JB, et al: Transforming growth factor beta1 enhances platelet aggregation through a non-transcriptional effect on the fibrinogen receptor. *J Biol Chem* 274(43):31008–31013, 1999.

473. Kronemann N, et al: Aggregating human platelets stimulate expression of vascular endothelial growth factor in cultured vascular smooth muscle cells through a synergistic effect of transforming growth factor-beta(1) and platelet-derived growth factor(AB). *Circulation* 100(8):855–860, 1999.

474. Koda Y, et al: Protein kinase C subtypes in tissues derived from neural crest. *Brain Res* 518(1–2):334–336, 1990.

475. Annes JP, Munger JS, Rifkin DB: Making sense of latent TGFbeta activation. *J Cell Sci* 116(Pt 2):217–224, 2003.

476. Lawler J, Hynes RO: The structure of human thrombospondin, an adhesive glycoprotein with multiple calcium-binding sites and homologies with several different proteins. *J Cell Biol* 103:1635.

477. Schultz-Cherry S, Murphy-Ullrich JE: Thrombospondin causes activation of latent transforming growth factor- beta secreted by endothelial cells by a novel mechanism. *J Cell Biol* 1993;122(4):923–932, 1986.

478. Ahamed J, Janczak CA, Wittkowski KM, Coller BS: *In vitro* and *in vivo* evidence that thrombospondin-1 (TSP-1) contributes to stirring- and shear-dependent activation of platelet-derived TGF-β1. *PLoS One* 4(8):e6608, 2009.

479. Blakytny R, Ludlow A, Martin GE, et al: Latent TGF-beta1 activation by platelets. *J Cell Physiol* 199(1):67–76, 2004.

480. Yang Z, et al: Absence of integrin-mediated TGFbeta1 activation *in vivo* recapitulates the phenotype of TGFbeta1-null mice. *J Cell Biol* 176(6):787–793, 2007.

481. Abdelouahed M, et al: Activation of platelet-transforming growth factor beta-1 in the absence of thrombospondin-1. *J Biol Chem* 275(24):17933–17936, 2000.

482. Ahamed J, et al: *In vitro* and *in vivo* evidence for shear-induced activation of latent transforming growth factor-beta1. *Blood* 112(9):3650–3660, 2008.

483. Crawford SE, et al: Thrombospondin-1 is a major activator of TGF-beta1 *in vivo*. *Cell* 93(7):1159–1170, 1998.

484. Slivka SR, Loskutoff DJ: Platelets stimulate endothelial cells to synthesize type 1 plasminogen activator inhibitor. Evaluation of the role of transforming growth factor beta. *Blood* 77(5):1013–1019, 1991.

485. Labelle M, Begum S, Hynes RO: Direct signaling between platelets and cancer cells induces an epithelial-mesenchymal-like transition and promotes metastasis. *Cancer Cell* 20(5):576–590, 2011.

486. Meyer A, et al: Platelet TGF-beta1 contributions to plasma TGF-beta1, cardiac fibrosis, and systolic dysfunction in a mouse model of pressure overload. *Blood* 119(4):1064–1074, 2012.

487. Wang W, et al: Association between shear stress and platelet-derived transforming growth factor-beta1 release and activation in animal models of aortic valve stenosis. *Arterioscler Thromb Vasc Biol* 34(9):1924–1932, 2014.

488. Lin HY, et al: Expression cloning of the TGF-beta type II receptor, a functional transmembrane serine/threonine kinase. *Cell* 68(4):775–785, 1992.

489. Fuhrman B, Brook GJ, Aviram M: Proteins derived from platelet alpha granules modulate the uptake of oxidized low density lipoprotein by macrophages. *Biochim Biophys Acta* 1127(1):15–21, 1992.

490. Heijnen HF, et al: Activated platelets release two types of membrane vesicles: Microvesicles by surface shedding and exosomes derived from exocytosis of multivesicular bodies and alpha-granules. *Blood* 94(11):3791–3799, 1999.

491. Janiszewski M, et al: Platelet-derived exosomes of septic individuals possess proapoptotic NAD(P)H oxidase activity: A novel vascular redox pathway. *Crit Care Med* 32(3):818–825, 2004.

492. Ren Q, Ye S, Whiteheart SW: The platelet release reaction: Just when you thought platelet secretion was simple. *Curr Opin Hematol* 15(5):537–541, 2008.

493. Tolmachova T, et al: Rab27b regulates number and secretion of platelet dense granules. *Proc Natl Acad Sci U S A* 104(14):5872–5877, 2007.

494. Shirakawa R, et al: Small GTPase Rab4 regulates Ca2+-induced alpha-granule secretion in platelets. *J Biol Chem* 275(43):33844–33849, 2000.

495. Fitzgerald ML, Reed GL: Rab6 is phosphorylated in thrombin-activated platelets by a protein kinase C-dependent mechanism: Effects on GTP/GDP binding and cellular distribution. *Biochem J* 342(Pt 2):353–360, 1999.

496. Sudhof TC, Rothman JE: Membrane fusion: Grappling with SNARE and SM proteins. *Science* 323(5913):474–477, 2009.

497. Weber T, et al: SNAREpins: Minimal machinery for membrane fusion. *Cell* 92(6):759–772, 1998.

498. Bernstein AM, Whiteheart SW: Identification of a cellubrevin/vesicle associated membrane protein 3 homologue in human platelets. *Blood* 93(2):571–579, 1999.

499. Graham GJ, Ren Q, Dilks JR, et al: Endobrevin/VAMP-8-dependent dense granule release mediates thrombus formation *in vivo*. *Blood* 114(5):1083–1090, 2009.

500. Lemons PP, et al: Regulated secretion in platelets: Identification of elements of the platelet exocytosis machinery. *Blood* 90(4):1490–1500, 1997.

501. Polgar J, Chung SH, Reed GL: Vesicle-associated membrane protein 3 (VAMP-3) and VAMP-8 are present in human platelets and are required for granule secretion. *Blood* 100(3):1081–1083, 2002.

502. Ren Q, et al: Endobrevin/VAMP-8 is the primary v-SNARE for the platelet release reaction. *Mol Biol Cell* 18(1):24–33, 2007.

503. Flaumenhaft R, et al: Proteins of the exocytotic core complex mediate platelet alpha-granule secretion. Roles of vesicle-associated membrane protein, SNAP-23, and syntaxin 4. *J Biol Chem* 274(4):2492–2501, 1999.

504. Polgar J, et al: Phosphorylation of SNAP-23 in activated human platelets. *J Biol Chem* 278(45):44369–44376, 2003.

505. Chen D, et al: Molecular mechanisms of platelet exocytosis: Role of SNAP-23 and syntaxin 2 in dense core granule release. *Blood* 95(3):921–929, 2000.

506. Chen D, et al: Molecular mechanisms of platelet exocytosis: Role of SNAP-23 and syntaxin 2 and 4 in lysosome release. *Blood* 96(5):1782–1788, 2000.

507. Flaumenhaft R, Furie B, Furie BC: Alpha-granule secretion from alpha-toxin permeabilized, MgATP-exposed platelets is induced independently by H+ and Ca2+. *J Cell Physiol* 179(1):1–10, 1999.

508. Lemons PP, Chen D, Whiteheart SW: Molecular mechanisms of platelet exocytosis: Requirements for alpha-granule release. *Biochem Biophys Res Commun* 267(3):875–880, 2000.

509. Houng A, Polgar J, Reed GL: Munc18-syntaxin complexes and exocytosis in human platelets. *J Biol Chem* 278(22):19627–19633, 2003.

510. Reed GL, Houng AK, Fitzgerald ML: Human platelets contain SNARE proteins and a Sec1p homologue that interacts with syntaxin 4 and is phosphorylated after thrombin activation: Implications for platelet secretion. *Blood* 93(8):2617–2626, 1999.

511. Schraw TD, et al: A role for Sec1/Munc18 proteins in platelet exocytosis. *Biochem J* 374(Pt 1):207–217, 2003.

512. Shirakawa R, et al: Munc13–4 is a GTP-Rab27-binding protein regulating dense core granule secretion in platelets. *J Biol Chem* 279(11):10730–10737, 2004.

513. Shirakawa R, et al: Purification and functional analysis of a Rab27 effector munc 13–4 using a semi-intact platelet dense-granule secretion assay. *Methods Enzymol* 403:778–788, 2005.

514. Vu TK, Hung DT, Wheaton VI, Coughlin SR: Molecular cloning of a functional thrombin receptor reveals a novel proteolytic mechanism of receptor activation. *Cell* 64:1057–1068, 1991.

515. Feldmann J, et al: Munc13–4 is essential for cytolytic granules fusion and is mutated in a form of familial hemophagocytic lymphohistiocytosis (FHL3). *Cell* 115(4):461–473, 2003.

516. Neeft M, et al: Munc13–4 is an effector of rab27a and controls secretion of lysosomes in hematopoietic cells. *Mol Biol Cell* 16(2):731–741, 2005.

517. Jahn R, Fasshauer D: Molecular machines governing exocytosis of synaptic vesicles. *Nature* 490(7419):201–207, 2012.

518. Rizo J, Sudhof TC: The membrane fusion enigma: SNAREs, Sec1/Munc18 proteins, and their accomplices—Guilty as charged? *Annu Rev Cell Dev Biol* 28:279–308, 2012.

519. Weber T, et al: SNAREpins: Minimal machinery for membrane fusion. *Cell* 92(6):759–772, 1998.

520. Bernstein AM, Whiteheart SW: Identification of a cellubrevin/vesicle associated membrane protein 3 homologue in human platelets. *Blood* 93(2):571–579, 1999.

521. Burkhart JM, et al: Systematic and quantitative comparison of digest efficiency and specificity reveals the impact of trypsin quality on MS-based proteomics. *J Proteomics* 75(4):1454–1462, 2012.

522. Graham GJ, et al: Endobrevin/VAMP-8-dependent dense granule release mediates thrombus formation in vivo. *Blood* 114(5):1083–1090, 2009.

523. Lemons PP, et al: Regulated secretion in platelets: Identification of elements of the platelet exocytosis machinery. *Blood* 90(4):1490–1500, 1997.

524. Golebiewska EM, et al: Syntaxin 8 regulates platelet dense granule secretion, aggregation, and thrombus stability. *J Biol Chem* 290(3):1536–1545, 2015.

525. Flaumenhaft R, et al: Proteins of the exocytotic core complex mediate platelet alpha-granule secretion. Roles of vesicle-associated membrane protein, SNAP-23, and syntaxin 4. *J Biol Chem* 274(4):2492–2501, 1999.

526. Polgar J, et al: Phosphorylation of SNAP-23 in activated human platelets. *J Biol Chem* 278(45):44369–44376, 2003.

527. Ye S, et al: Syntaxin-11, but not syntaxin-2 or syntaxin-4, is required for platelet secretion. *Blood* 120(12):2484–2492, 2012.

528. Lemons PP, Chen D, Whiteheart SW: Molecular mechanisms of platelet exocytosis: Requirements for alpha-granule release. *Biochem Biophys Res Commun* 267(3):875–880, 2000.

529. Karim ZA, et al: IkappaB kinase phosphorylation of SNAP-23 controls platelet secretion. *Blood* 121(22):4567–4574, 2013.

530. Al Hawas R, et al: Munc18b/STXBP2 is required for platelet secretion. *Blood* 120(12):2493–2500, 2012.

531. Houng A, Polgar J, Reed GL: Munc18-syntaxin complexes and exocytosis in human platelets. *J Biol Chem* 278(22):19627–19633, 2003.

532. Schraw TD, et al: Platelets from Munc18c heterozygous mice exhibit normal stimulus-induced release. *Thromb Haemost* 92(4):829–837, 2004.

533. Schraw TD, et al: A role for Sec1/Munc18 proteins in platelet exocytosis. *Biochem J* 374(Pt 1):207–217, 2003.

534. Sandrock K, et al: Platelet secretion defect in patients with familial hemophagocytic lymphohistiocytosis type 5 (FHL-5). *Blood* 116(26):6148–6150, 2010.

535. Suzuki T, et al: The mouse organellar biogenesis mutant buff results from a mutation in Vps33a, a homologue of yeast vps33 and *Drosophila* carnation. *Proc Natl Acad Sci U S A* 100(3):1146–1150, 2003.

536. Urban D, et al: The VPS33B-binding protein VPS16B is required in megakaryocyte and platelet alpha-granule biogenesis. *Blood* 120(25):5032–5040, 2012.

537. Ye S, et al: Platelet secretion and hemostasis require syntaxin-binding protein STXBP5. *J Clin Invest* 124(10):4517–4528, 2014.

538. Lillicrap D, Syntaxin-binding protein 5 exocytosis regulation: Differential role in endothelial cells and platelets. *J Clin Invest* 124(10):4231–4233, 2014.

539. Zhu Q, et al: STXBP5 regulates endothelial exocytosis, plasma VWF levels, and platelet endothelial interactions. *Clin Invest* 124(10):4503–4516, 2014.

540. James DJ, Martin TF: CAPS and Munc13: CATCHRs that SNARE Vesicles. *Front Endocrinol (Lausanne)* 4:187, 2013.

541. Ren Q, et al: Munc13–4 is a limiting factor in the pathway required for platelet granule release and hemostasis. *Blood* 2010;116(6):869–877, 2013.

542. Nakamura L, et al: First characterization of platelet secretion defect in patients with familial hemophagocytic lymphohistiocytosis type 3 (FHL-3). *Blood* 125(2):412–414, 2015.

543. Barral DC, et al: Functional redundancy of Rab27 proteins and the pathogenesis of Griscelli syndrome. *J Clin Invest* 110(2):247–257, 2002.

544. Hampson A, O'Connor A, Smolenski A: Synaptotagmin-like protein 4 and Rab8 interact and increase dense granule release in platelets. *J Thromb Haemost* 11(1):161–168, 2013.

545. Janka GE: Familial and acquired hemophagocytic lymphohistiocytosis. *Annu Rev Med* 63:233–246, 2012.

546. Lindemann S, et al: Platelets, inflammation and atherosclerosis. *J Thromb Haemost* 5 (Suppl 1):203–211, 2007.

547. Bray PF: Platelet glycoprotein polymorphisms as risk factors for thrombosis. *Curr Opin Hematol* 7(5):284–289, 2000.

548. Deloukas P, et al: Large-scale association analysis identifies new risk loci for coronary artery disease. *Nat Genet* 45(1):25–33, 2013.

549. Bray PF, Jones CI, Soranzo N, Ouwehand WH: Platelet genomics, in *Platelets*, edited by A Michelson, Editor. Academic Press, San Diego, 2012.

550. Albers CA, et al: Exome sequencing identifies NBEAL2 as the causative gene for gray platelet syndrome. *Nat Genet* 43(8):735–737, 2011.

551. Gunay-Aygun M, et al: NBEAL2 is mutated in gray platelet syndrome and is required for biogenesis of platelet alpha-granules. *Nat Genet* 43(8):732–734, 2011.

552. Hulot JS, et al: Cytochrome P450 2C19 loss-of-function polymorphism is a major determinant of clopidogrel responsiveness in healthy subjects. *Blood* 108(7):2244–2247, 2006.

553. Shuldiner AR, et al: Association of cytochrome P450 2C19 genotype with the antiplatelet effect and clinical efficacy of clopidogrel therapy. *JAMA* 302(8):849–857, 2009.

554. Mega JL, et al: Reduced-function CYP2C19 genotype and risk of adverse clinical outcomes among patients treated with clopidogrel predominantly for PCI: A meta-analysis. *JAMA* 304(16):1821–1830, 2010.

555. Holmes MV, et al: CYP2C19 genotype, clopidogrel metabolism, platelet function, and cardiovascular events: A systematic review and meta-analysis. *JAMA* 306(24):2704–2714, 2011.

556. Yee D, et al: Platelet hyperreactivity to submaximal epinephrine: Biologic and clinical correlates. 106(8):2723–2729, 2005.

557. Bray PF, et al: Heritability of platelet function in families with premature coronary artery disease. *J Thromb Haemost* 2007;5(8):1617–1623, 2005.

558. Newman PJ, Derbes RS, Aster RH: The human platelet alloantigens, PlA1 and PlA2, are associated with a leucine33/proline33 amino acid polymorphism in membrane glycoprotein IIIa, and are distinguishable by DNA typing. *J Clin Invest* 83(5):1778–1781, 1989.

559. Vijayan KV, et al: Fibrinogen and prothrombin binding is enhanced to the Pro33 isoform of purified integrin alphaIIbbeta3. *J Thromb Haemost* 4(4):905–906, 2006.

560. Vijayan KV, et al: The Pl(A2) polymorphism of integrin beta(3) enhances outside-in signaling and adhesive functions. *J Clin Invest* 105(6):793–802, 2000.

561. Sajid M, et al: PlA polymorphism of integrin beta 3 differentially modulates cellular migration on extracellular matrix proteins. *Arterioscler Thromb Vasc Biol* 22(12):1984–1989, 2002.

562. Vijayan KV, et al: Shear stress augments the enhanced adhesive phenotype of cells expressing the Pro33 isoform of integrin beta3. *FEBS Lett* 540(1–3):41–46, 2003.

563. Vijayan KV, et al: Enhanced activation of mitogen-activated protein kinase and myosin light chain kinase by the Pro33 polymorphism of integrin beta 3. *J Biol Chem* 278(6):3860–3867, 2003.

564. Vijayan KV, et al: The Pro33 isoform of integrin beta3 enhances outside-in signaling in human platelets by regulating the activation of serine/threonine phosphatases. *J Biol Chem* 280(23):21756–21762, 2005.

565. Johnson AD, et al: Genome-wide meta-analyses identifies seven loci associated with platelet aggregation in response to agonists. *Nat Genet* 42(7):608–613, 2010.

566. Oliver KH, et al: Pro32Pro33 mutations in the integrin beta3 PSI domain result in alphaIIbbeta3 priming and enhanced adhesion: Reversal of the hypercoagulability phenotype by the Src inhibitor SKI-606. *Mol Pharmacol* 85(6):921–931, 2014.

567. Kritzik M, et al: Nucleotide polymorphisms in the alpha2 gene define multiple alleles that are associated with differences in platelet alpha2 beta1 density. *Blood* 92(7):2382–2388, 1998.

568. Roest M, et al: Platelet adhesion to collagen in healthy volunteers is influenced by variation of both alpha(2)beta(1) density and von Willebrand factor. *Blood* 96(4):1433–1437, 2000.

569. Joutsi-Korhonen L, et al: The low-frequency allele of the platelet collagen signaling receptor glycoprotein VI is associated with reduced functional responses and expression. *Blood* 101(11):4372–4379, 2003.

570. Jones CI, et al: A functional genomics approach reveals novel quantitative trait loci associated with platelet signaling pathways. *Blood* 114(7):1405–1416, 2009.

571. Musunuru K, et al: Association of single nucleotide polymorphisms on chromosome 9p21.3 with platelet reactivity: A potential mechanism for increased vascular disease. Circulation. *Circ Cardiovasc Genet* 3(5):445–453, 2010.

572. Edelstein LC, et al: Human genome-wide association and mouse knockout approaches identify platelet supervillin as an inhibitor of thrombus formation under shear stress. *Circulation* 125(22):2762–2771, 2012.

573. Gieger C, et al: New gene functions in megakaryopoiesis and platelet formation. *Nature* 480(7376):201–208, 2011.

574. Weyrich AS, et al: Protein synthesis by platelets: Historical and new perspectives. *J Thromb Haemost* 7(2):241–246, 2009.

575. Denis MM, et al: Escaping the nuclear confines: Signal-dependent pre-mRNA splicing in anucleate platelets. *Cell* 122(3):379–391, 2005.

576. Edelstein LC, et al: MicroRNAs in platelet production and activation. *J Thromb Haemost* 11 Suppl 1:340–350, 2013.

577. Gnatenko DV, et al: Transcript profiling of human platelets using microarray and serial analysis of gene expression. *Blood* 101(6):2285–2293, 2003.

578. Bugert P, et al: Messenger RNA profiling of human platelets by microarray hybridization. *Thromb Haemost* 90(4):738–748, 2003.

579. Schubert S, Weyrich AS, Rowley JW: A tour through the transcriptional landscape of platelets. *Blood* 124(4):493–502, 2014.

580. Rowley JW, et al: Genome-wide RNA-seq analysis of human and mouse platelet transcriptomes. *Blood* 118(14):e101–e111, 2011.

581. Bray PF, McKenzie SE, Edelstein LC, et al: The complex transcriptional landscape of the anucleate human platelet. *BMC Genomics* 14(1):1, 2013.

582. Simon LM, Edelstein LC, Nagalla S, et al: Human platelet microRNA-mRNA networks associated with age and gender revealed by integrated plateletomics. *Blood* 123(16):e37–e45, 2014.

583. Wang Z, et al: The role of mitochondria-derived reactive oxygen species in hyperthermia-induced platelet apoptosis. *PLoS One* 8(9):e75044, 2013.

584. Hayashi T, Tanaka S, Hori Y, et al: Role of mitochondria in the maintenance of platelet function during in vitro storage. *Transfus Med* 21(3):166–174, 2011.

585. Shim MH, et al: Gene expression profile of primary human CD34+CD38lo cells differentiating along the megakaryocyte lineage. *Exp Hematol* 32(7):638–648, 2004.

586. Tenedini E, et al: Gene expression profiling of normal and malignant CD34-derived megakaryocytic cells. *Blood* 104(10):3126–3135, 2004.

587. Healy AM, et al: Platelet expression profiling and clinical validation of myeloid-related protein-14 as a novel determinant of cardiovascular events. *Circulation* 113(19):2278–2284, 2006.

588. Morrow DA, et al: Myeloid-related protein 8/14 and the risk of cardiovascular death or myocardial infarction after an acute coronary syndrome in the Pravastatin or Atorvastatin Evaluation and Infection Therapy: Thrombolysis in Myocardial Infarction (PROVE IT-TIMI 22) trial. *Am Heart J* 155(1):49–55, 2008.

589. Gnatenko DV, et al: Platelets express steroidogenic 17beta-hydroxysteroid dehydrogenases. Distinct profiles predict the essential thrombocythemic phenotype. *Thromb Haemost* 94(2):412–421, 2005.

590. Gnatenko DV, et al: Class prediction models of thrombocytosis using genetic biomarkers. *Blood* 115(1):7–14, 2010.

591. Sun L, et al: Decreased platelet expression of myosin regulatory light chain polypeptide (MYL9) and other genes with platelet dysfunction and CBFA2/RUNX1 mutation: Insights from platelet expression profiling. *J Thromb Haemost* 5(1):146–154, 2007.

592. Kahr WH, et al: Mutations in NBEAL2, encoding a BEACH protein, cause gray platelet syndrome. *Nat Genet* 43(8):738–740, 2011.

593. Nanda N, et al: Platelet endothelial aggregation receptor 1 (PEAR1), a novel epidermal growth factor repeat-containing transmembrane receptor, participates in platelet contact-induced activation. *J Biol Chem* 280(26):24680–24689, 2005.

594. Kondkar AA, et al: VAMP8/endobrevin is overexpressed in hyperreactive human platelets: Suggested role for platelet microRNA. *J Thromb Haemost* 8(2):369–378, 2010.

595. Goodall AH, et al: Transcription profiling in human platelets reveals LRRFIP1 as a novel protein regulating platelet function. *Blood* 116(22):4646–4656, 2010.

596. Edelstein LC, Simon LM, Montoya RT, et al: Racial differences in human platelet PAR4 reactivity reflect expression of PCTP and miR-376c. *Nat Med* 19(12):1609–1616, 2013.

597. Carninci P, et al: The transcriptional landscape of the mammalian genome. *Science* 309(5740):1559–1563, 2005.

598. Bartel DP: MicroRNAs: Target recognition and regulatory functions. *Cell* 136(2): 215–233, 2009.

599. Nagalla S, et al: Platelet microRNA-mRNA coexpression profiles correlate with platelet reactivity. *Blood* 117(19):5189–5197, 2011.

600. Edelstein LC, Bray PF: MicroRNAs in platelet production and activation. *Blood* 117(20):5289–5296, 2011.

601. Georgantas RW 3rd, et al: CD34+ hematopoietic stem-progenitor cell microRNA expression and function: A circuit diagram of differentiation control. *Proc Natl Acad Sci U S A* 104(8):2750–2755, 2007.

602. Lu J, et al: MicroRNA-mediated control of cell fate in megakaryocyte-erythrocyte progenitors. *Dev Cell* 14(6):843–853, 2008.

603. Klusmann JH, et al: MiR-125b-2 is a potential oncomiR on human chromosome 21 in megakaryoblastic leukemia. *Genes Dev* 24(5):478–490, 2010.

604. Kumar MS, et al: Coordinate loss of a microRNA and protein-coding gene cooperate in the pathogenesis of 5q- syndrome. *Blood* 118(17):4666–4673, 2011.

605. Bruchova H, Merkerova M, Prchal JT: Aberrant expression of microRNA in polycythemia vera. *Haematologica* 93(7):1009–1016, 2008.

606. Girardot M, et al: MiR-28 is a thrombopoietin receptor targeting microRNA detected in a fraction of myeloproliferative neoplasm patient platelets. *Blood* 116(3):437–445, 2010.

607. Xu X, et al: Systematic analysis of microRNA fingerprints in thrombocythemic platelets using integrated platforms. *Blood* 120(17):3575–3585, 2012.

608. Zampetaki A, et al: Prospective study on circulating MicroRNAs and risk of myocardial infarction. *J Am Coll Cardiol* 60(4):290–299, 2012.

609. Gidlof O, et al: Platelets activated during myocardial infarction release functional miRNA, which can be taken up by endothelial cells and regulate ICAM1 expression. *Blood* 121(19):3908–3917, S1–S26, 2013.

610. Willeit P, et al: Circulating MicroRNAs as novel biomarkers for platelet activation. *Circ Res* 2013.

611. de Boer HC, et al: Aspirin treatment hampers the use of plasma microRNA-126 as a biomarker for the progression of vascular disease. *Eur Heart J* 34(44):3451–3457, 2013.

612. Garcia A, et al: Extensive analysis of the human platelet proteome by two-dimensional gel electrophoresis and mass spectrometry. *Proteomics* 4(3):656–668, 2004.

613. Garcia A, Senis YA: *Platelet Proteomics: Principles, Analysis, and Applications*. John Wiley & Sons, Hoboken, NJ, 2011.

614. Thon JN, Devine DV: Translation of glycoprotein IIIa in stored blood platelets. *Transfusion* 47(12):2260–2270, 2007.

615. Burkhart JM, et al: The first comprehensive and quantitative analysis of human platelet protein composition allows the comparative analysis of structural and functional pathways. *Blood* 120(15):e73–e82, 2012.

616. Smith MC, Schwertz H, Zimmerman GA, Weyrich AS: The platelet proteome, in *Platelets*, edited by A Michelson. Academic Press, San Diego, 2012.

617. Booyse F, Rafelson ME Jr: *In vitro* incorporation of amino-acids into the contractile protein of human blood platelets. *Nature* 215(5098):283–284, 1967.

618. Cecchetti L, et al: Megakaryocytes differentially sort mRNAs for matrix metalloproteinases and their inhibitors into platelets: A mechanism for regulating synthetic events. *Blood* 118(7):1903–1911, 2011.

619. Hottz ED, Lopes JF, Freitas C, et al: Platelets mediate increased endothelium permeability in dengue through NLRP3-inflammasome activation. *Blood* 122(20): 3405–3414, 2013.

620. Martens L, et al: The human platelet proteome mapped by peptide-centric proteomics: A functional protein profile. *Proteomics* 5(12):3193–3204, 2005.

621. Zufferey A, et al: Characterization of the platelet granule proteome: Evidence of the presence of MHC1 in alpha-granules. *J Proteomics* 101:130–140, 2014.

622. Hernandez-Ruiz L, et al: Organellar proteomics of human platelet dense granules reveals that 14-3-3zeta is a granule protein related to atherosclerosis. *J Proteome Res* 6(11):4449–4457, 2007.

623. Senis YA, et al: A comprehensive proteomics and genomics analysis reveals novel transmembrane proteins in human platelets and mouse megakaryocytes including G6b-B, a novel immunoreceptor tyrosine-based inhibitory motif protein. *Mol Cell Proteomics* 6(3):548–564, 2007.

624. Lewandrowski U, et al: Platelet membrane proteomics: A novel repository for functional research. *Blood* 114(1):e10–e19, 2009.

625. Maguire PB, et al: Identification of the phosphotyrosine proteome from thrombin activated platelets. *Proteomics* 2(6):642–648, 2002.

626. Garcia A, et al: A global proteomics approach identifies novel phosphorylated signaling proteins in GPVI-activated platelets: Involvement of G6f, a novel platelet Grb2-binding membrane adapter. *Proteomics* 6(19):5332–5343, 2006.

627. Dowal L, et al: Proteomic analysis of palmitoylated platelet proteins. *Blood* 118(13):e62–e73, 2011.

628. Lewandrowski U, et al: Enhanced N-glycosylation site analysis of sialoglycopeptides by strong cation exchange prefractionation applied to platelet plasma membranes. *Mol Cell Proteomics* 6(11):1933–1941, 2007.

629. Coppinger JA, et al: Characterization of the proteins released from activated platelets leads to localization of novel platelet proteins in human atherosclerotic lesions. *Blood* 103(6):2096–2104, 2004.

630. Piersma SR, et al: Proteomics of the TRAP-induced platelet releasate. *J Proteomics* 72(1):91–109, 2009.

631. Garcia BA, et al: The platelet microparticle proteome. *J Proteome Res* 4(5):1516–1521, 2005.

632. Capriotti AL, et al: Proteomic characterization of human platelet-derived microparticles. *Anal Chim Acta* 776:57–63, 2013.

633. Maurer-Spurej E, et al: The value of proteomics for the diagnosis of a platelet-related bleeding disorder. *Platelets* 19(5):342–351, 2008.

634. Frobel J, et al: Platelet proteome analysis reveals integrin-dependent aggregation defects in patients with myelodysplastic syndromes. *Mol Cell Proteomics* 12(5): 1272–1280, 2013.

635. Snyder EL, et al: Protein changes occurring during storage of platelet concentrates. A two-dimensional gel electrophoretic analysis. *Transfusion* 27(4):335–341, 1987.

636. Thiele T, et al: Profiling of alterations in platelet proteins during storage of platelet concentrates. *Transfusion* 47(7):1221–1233, 2007.

637. Thon JN, et al: Comprehensive proteomic analysis of protein changes during platelet storage requires complementary proteomic approaches. *Transfusion* 48(3):425–435, 2008.

638. Parguina AF, Grigorian-Shamajian L, Agra RM, et al: Proteins involved in platelet signaling are differentially regulated in acute coronary syndrome: A proteomic study. *PLoS One* 5(10):e13404, 2010.

639. Londin ER, Hatzimichael E, Loher P, et al: The human platelet: Strong transcriptome correlations among individuals associate weakly with the platelet proteome. *Biol Direct* 9:3, 2014.

640. Handagama PJ, Shuman MA, Bainton DF: Incorporation of intravenously injected albumin, immunoglobulin G, and fibrinogen in guinea pig megakaryocyte granules. *J Clin Invest* 1989;84(1):73–82, 2010.

641. Voora D, et al: Aspirin exposure reveals novel genes associated with platelet function and cardiovascular events. *J Am Coll Cardiol* 62(14):1267–1276, 2013.

642. Bevers EM, et al: Lipid translocation across the plasma membrane of mammalian cells. *Biochim Biophys Acta* 1439(3):317–330, 1999.

643. Pomorski T, Menon AK: Lipid flippases and their biological functions. *Cell Mol Life Sci* 63(24):2908–2921, 2006.

644. Yang H, et al: TMEM16F Forms a Ca(2+)-activated cation channel required for lipid scrambling in platelets during blood coagulation. *Cell* 151(1):111–122, 2012.

645. Barry OP, FitzGerald GA: Mechanisms of cellular activation by platelet microparticles. *Thromb Haemost* 82:794–800, 1999.

646. Thiagarajan P, Tait JF: Collagen-induced exposure of anionic phospholipid in platelets and platelet-derived microparticles. *J Biol Chem* 266:24302–24307, 1991.

647. Bouchard BA, et al: Effector cell protease receptor-1, a platelet activation-dependent membrane protein, regulates prothrombinase-catalyzed thrombin generation. *J Biol Chem* 272(14):9244–9251, 1997.

648. Enjeti AK, Lincz LF, Seldon M: Microparticles in health and disease. *Semin Thromb Hemost* 34(7):683–691, 2008.

649. Hultin MB: Modulation of thrombin-mediated activation of factor VIII:C by calcium ions, phospholipid, and platelets. *Blood* 66(1):53–58, 1985.

650. Miyazaki Y, et al: High shear stress can initiate both platelet aggregation and shedding of procoagulant containing microparticles. *Blood* 88(9):3456–3464, 1996.

651. Nesheim ME, et al: On the existence of platelet receptors for factors V(a) and factor VIII (a). *Thromb Haemost* 70:80–85, 1993.

652. Piccin A, Murphy WG, Smith OP: Circulating microparticles: Pathophysiology and clinical implications. *Blood Rev* 21(3):157–171, 2007.

653. George JN, et al: Platelet surface glycoproteins. Studies on resting and activated platelets and platelet membrane microparticles in normal subjects, and observations in patients during adult respiratory distress syndrome and cardiac surgery. *J Clin Invest* 78(2):340–348, 1986.

654. Siljander P, Carpen O, Lassila R: Platelet-derived microparticles associate with fibrin during thrombosis. *Blood* 87(11):4651–4663, 1996.

655. Dahlback B, Wiedmer T, Sims PJ: Binding of anticoagulant vitamin K-dependent protein S to platelet-derived microparticles. *Biochemistry* 31(51):12769–12777, 1992.

656. Tans G, et al: Comparison of anticoagulant and procoagulant activities of stimulated platelets and platelet-derived microparticles. *Blood* 77(12):2641–2648, 1991.

657. Toti F, et al: Scott syndrome, characterized by impaired transmembrane migration of procoagulant phosphatidylserine and hemorrhagic complications, is an inherited disorder. *Blood* 87(4):1409–1415, 1996.

658. Weiss HJ, Scott syndrome-a disorder of platelet coagulant activity. *Semin Hematol* 31(4):312–319, 1994.

659. Weiss HJ, Lages B: Platelet prothrombinase activity and intracellular calcium responses in patients with storage pool deficiency, glycoprotein IIb-IIIa deficiency, or impaired platelet coagulant activity—a comparison with Scott syndrome. *Blood* 89(5):1599–1611, 1997.

660. Panes O, et al: Human platelets synthesize and express functional tissue factor. *Blood* 109(12):5242–5250, 2007.

661. Schwertz H, et al: Signal-dependent splicing of tissue factor pre-mRNA modulates the thrombogenicity of human platelets. *J Exp Med*J Exp Med 203(11):2433–2440, 2006.

662. Freedman JE, et al: Deficient platelet-derived nitric oxide and enhanced hemostasis in mice lacking the NOSIII gene. *Circ Res* 84(9):1416–1421, 1999.

663. Iafrati MD, Vitseva O, Tanriverdi K, et al: Compensatory mechanisms influence hemostasis in setting of eNOS deficiency. *Am J Physiol Heart Circ Physiol* 288(4):H1627–H1632, 2005.

664. Marjanovic JA, et al: Stimulatory roles of nitric-oxide synthase 3 and guanylyl cyclase in platelet activation. *J Biol Chem* 280(45):37430–37438, 2005.

665. Ozuyaman B, et al: Endothelial nitric oxide synthase plays a minor role in inhibition of arterial thrombus formation. *Thromb Haemost* 93(6):1161–1167, 2005.

666. Osterud B: The role of platelets in decrypting monocyte tissue factor. *Semin Hematol* 38(4 Suppl 12):2–5, 2001.

667. Reinhardt C, et al: Protein disulfide isomerase acts as an injury response signal that enhances fibrin generation via tissue factor activation. *J Clin Invest* 118(3):1110–1122, 2008.

668. Smith SA, et al: Polyphosphate modulates blood coagulation and fibrinolysis. *Proc Natl Acad Sci U S A* 103(4):903–908, 2006.

669. Smith SA, Morrissey JH: Polyphosphate enhances fibrin clot structure. *Blood* 112(7):2810–2816, 2008.

670. Bouchard BA, et al: Interactions between platelets and the coagulation system, in *Platelets*, edited by AD Michelson, pp 377–402. Academic Press, San Diego, 2007.

671. Swords NA, Tracy PB, Mann KG: Intact platelet membranes, not platelet-released microvesicles, support the procoagulant activity of adherent platelets. *Arterioscler Thromb* 13(11):1613–1622, 1993.

672. Zwaal RFA, Comfurius P, Bevers EM: Platelet procoagulant activity and microvesicle formation. Its putative role of hemostasis and thrombosis. *Biochim Biophys Acta* 1180:1–8, 1992.

673. Alberio L, et al: Surface expression and functional characterization of alpha-granule factor V in human platelets: Effects of ionophore A23187, thrombin, collagen, and convulxin. *Blood* 95(5):1694–1702, 2000.

674. Scandura JM, Ahmad SS, Walsh PN: A binding site expressed on the surface of activated human platelets is shared by factor X and prothrombin. *Biochemistry* 35(27):8890–8902, 1996.

675. Byzova TV, Plow EF: Networking in the hemostatic system. Integrin alphaiibbeta3 binds prothrombin and influences its activation. *J Biol Chem* 272(43):27183–27188, 1997.

676. Baglia FA, Walsh PN: Thrombin-mediated feedback activation of factor XI on the activated platelet surface is preferred over contact activation by factor XIIa or factor XIa. *J Biol Chem* 275(27):20514–20519, 2000.

677. Oliver JA, et al: Thrombin activates factor XI on activated platelets in the absence of factor XII. *Arterioscler Thromb Vasc Biol.*, 19(1):170–177, 1999.

678. Gailani D, et al: Model for a factor IX activation complex on blood platelets: Dimeric conformation of factor XIa is essential. *Blood* 97(10):3117–3122, 2001.

679. Walsh PN: Platelets and factor XI bypass the contact system of blood coagulation. *Thromb Haemost* 82:234–242, 1999.

680. Coller BS: Platelets and thrombolytic therapy. *N Engl J Med* 322:33–42, 1990.

681. Coller BS: Augmentation of thrombolysis with antiplatelet drugs. Overview. *Coron Artery Dis* 6:911–914, 1995.

682. Kolev K, Machovich R: Molecular and cellular modulation of fibrinolysis. *Thromb Haemost* 89(4):610–621, 2003.

683. Korbut R, Gryglewski RJ: Platelets in fibrinolytic system. *J Physiol Pharmacol* 46(4):409–418, 1995.

684. Maron BA, Loscalzo J: The role of platelets in fibrinolysis, in *Platelets*, edited by AD Michelson, pp 415–430. Academic Press, San Diego, 2007.

685. Carroll RC, et al: Plasminogen, plasminogen activator and platelets in the regulation of clot lysis. *J Lab Clin Med* 100:986–996, 1982.

686. de Haan J, van Oeveren W: Platelets and soluble fibrin promote plasminogen activation causing downregulation of platelet glycoprotein Ib/IX complexes: Protection by aprotinin. *Thromb Res* 92(4):171–179, 1998.

687. Jeanneau C, Sultan Y: Tissue plasminogen activator in human megakaryocytes and platelets: Immunocytochemical localization, immunoblotting and zymographic analysis. *Thromb Haemost* 19:529–534, 1988.

688. Miles LA, et al: Plasminogen interacts with human platelets through two distinct mechanisms. *J Clin Invest* 77:2001–2009, 1986.

689. Miles LA, Plow EF: Binding and activation of plasminogen on the platelet surface. *J Biol Chem* 260:4303–4311, 1985.

690. Park S, et al: Demonstration of single chain urokinase-type plasminogen activator on human platelet membrane. *Blood* 73:1421–1425, 1989.

691. Stricker RB, et al: Activation of plasminogen by tissue plasminogen activator on normal and thrombasthenic platelets: Effects on surface proteins and platelet aggregation. *Blood* 68:275–280, 1986.

692. Thorsen S, Brakman P, Astrup T: Influence of platelets on fibrinolysis: A critical review, in *Hematologic Reviews*, edited by JL Ambrole, pp 123–179. Marcel Dekker, New York, 1972.

693. Binder BR, et al: Plasminogen activator inhibitor 1: Physiological and pathophysiological roles. *News Physiol Sci* 17:56–61, 2002.

694. Cox AD, Devine DV: Factor XIIIa binding to activated platelets is mediated through activation of glycoprotein IIb-IIIa. *Blood* 83:1006–1016, 1994.

695. Erickson LA, Ginsberg MH, Loskutoff DJ: Detection and partial characterization of an inhibitor of plasminogen activator in human platelets. *J Clin Invest* 74:1465–1472, 1984.

696. Fay WP, et al: Platelets inhibit fibrinolysis in vitro by both plasminogen activator inhibitor-1 dependent and independent mechanisms. *Blood* 83:351–356, 1994.

697. Francis CW, Marder VJ: Rapid formation of large molecular weight alpha-polymers in cross-linked fibrin induced by high factor XIII concentrations: Role of platelet factor XIII. *J Clin Invest* 80:1459–1465, 1987.

698. Kawasaki T, et al: Vascular release of plasminogen activator inhibitor-1 impairs fibrinolysis during acute arterial thrombosis in mice. *Blood* 96(1):153–160, 2000.

699. Kruithof EKO, Tran-Thang C, Bachmann F: Studies on the release of plasminogen activator inhibitor from human platelets. *Thromb Haemost* 55:201–205, 1986.

700. Plow EF, Collen D: The presence and release of α2-antiplasmin from human platelets. *Blood* 58:1069–1074, 1981.

701. Smariga PE, Maynard JR: Purification of a platelet protein which stimulates fibrinolytic inhibition and tissue factor in human fibroblasts. *J Biol Chem* 257:11960–11965, 1982.

702. Jang IK, et al: Differential sensitivity of erythrocyte-rich and platelet-rich arterial thrombi to lysis with recombinant tissue-type plasminogen activator. A possible explanation for resistance to coronary thrombolysis. *Circulation* 79:920–928, 1989.

703. Fitzgerald DJ, et al: Marked platelet activation *in vivo* after intravenous streptokinase in patients with acute myocardial infarction. *Circulation* 77:142–150, 1988.

704. Fitzgerald DJ, Wright F, FitzGerald GA: Increased thromboxane biosynthesis during coronary thrombolysis: Evidence that platelet activation and thromboxane A2 modulate the response to tissue-type plasminogen activator *in vivo*. *Circ Res* 65:83–94, 1989.

705. Kerins DM, et al: Platelet and vascular function during coronary thrombolysis with tissue-type plasminogen activator. *Circulation* 80:1718–1725, 1990.

706. Ohlstein EH, et al: Tissue-type plasminogen activator and streptokinase induce platelet hyperaggregability in the rabbit. *Thromb Res* 46:575–585, 1987.

707. Penny WF, Ware JA: Platelet activation and subsequent inhibition by plasmin and recombinant tissue-type plasminogen activator. *Blood* 79(1):91–98, 1992.

708. Rudd MA, et al: Temporal effects of thrombolytic agents on platelet function in vivo and their modulation by prostaglandins. *Circ Res* 67(5):1175–1181, 1990.

709. Shebuski RJ: Principles underlying the use of conjunctive agents with plasminogen activators. *Ann N Y Acad Sci* 667:382–394, 1992.

710. Ervin AL, Peerschke EI: Platelet activation by sustained exposure to low-dose plasmin. *Blood Coagul Fibrinolysis* 12(6):415–425, 2001.

711. Ishii-Watabe A, et al: On the mechanism of plasmin-induced platelet aggregation. Implications of the dual role of granule ADP. *Biochem PharmacolAm Rev Respir Dis* 59(11):1345–1355, 2000.

712. Niewiarowski S, Senyi AF, Gillies P: Plasmin-induced platelet aggregation and platelet release reaction. *J Clin Invest* 52:1647–1659, 1973.

713. Schafer AI, et al: Platelet protein phosphorylation, elevation of cytosolic calcium, and inositol phospholipid breakdown in platelet activation induced by plasmin. *J Clin Invest* 78:73–79, 1986.

714. Quinton TM, et al: Plasmin-mediated activation of platelets occurs by cleavage of protease-activated receptor 4. *J Biol Chem* 279(18):18434–18439, 2004.

715. Eisenberg PR, Sherman LA, Jaffe AS: Paradoxic elevation of fibrinopeptide A after streptokinase: Evidence for continued thrombosis despite intense fibrinolysis. *J Am Coll Cardiol* 10:527–529, 1987.

716. Leopold JA, Loscalzo J: Platelet activation by fibrinolytic agents: A potential mechanism for resistance to thrombolysis and reocclusion after successful thrombolysis. *Coron Artery Dis* 6(12):923–929, 1995.

717. Owen J, et al: Thrombolytic therapy with tissue plasminogen activator or streptokinase induces transient thrombin activity. *Blood* 72:616–620, 1988.

718. Szczeklik A: Thrombin generation in myocardial infarction and hypercholesterolemia: Effects of aspirin. *Thromb Haemost* 74(1):77–80, 1995.

719. Weitz JI, et al: Human tissue-type plasminogen activator releases fibrinopeptides A and B from fibrinogen. *J Clin Invest* 82:1700–1707, 1988.

720. Coller BS: Platelets in cardiovascular thrombosis and thrombolysis, in *The Heart and Cardiovascular System*, edited by HA Fozzard, Jennings RB, Katz AM, Morgan HE, Haber E, pp 219–273. Raven Press, New York, 1991.

721. Coller BS: Inhibitors of the platelet glycoprotein IIb/IIIa receptor as conjunctive therapy for coronary artery thrombolysis. *Coron Artery Dis* 3:1016–1029, 1992.

722. Eccleston D, Topol EJ: Inhibitors of platelet glycoprotein IIb/IIIa as augmenters of thrombolysis. *Coron Artery Dis* 6(12):947–955, 1995.

723. O'Donnell CJ, Jonas MA, Hennekens CH: Aspirin augmentation of the efficacy of thrombolysis. *Coron Artery Dis* 6(12):936–939, 1995.

724. Topol EJ: Reperfusion therapy for acute myocardial infarction with fibrinolytic therapy or combination reduced fibrinolytic therapy and platelet glycoprotein IIb/IIIa inhibition: The GUSTO V randomised trial. *Lancet* 357(9272):1905–1914, 2001.

725. Di Mario C, Dudek D, Piscione F, et al: Immediate angioplasty versus standard therapy with rescue angioplasty after thrombolysis in the Combined Abciximab REteplase Stent Study in Acute Myocardial Infarction (CARESS-in-AMI): An open, prospective, randomised, multicentre trial. *Lancet* 371(9612):559–568, 2008.

726. Ellis SG, et al: Facilitated PCI in patients with ST-elevation myocardial infarction. *N Engl J Med* 358(21):2205–2217, 2008.

727. Lapchak PA, et al: The nonpeptide glycoprotein IIb/IIIa platelet receptor antagonist SM-20302 reduces tissue plasminogen activator-induced intracerebral hemorrhage after thromboembolic stroke. *Stroke* 33(1):147–152, 2002.

728. Zhang L, et al: Adjuvant treatment with a glycoprotein IIb/IIIa receptor inhibitor increases the therapeutic window for low-dose tissue plasminogen activator administration in a rat model of embolic stroke. *Circulation* 107(22):2837–2843, 2003.

729. Zhang ZG, et al: Dynamic platelet accumulation at the site of the occluded middle cerebral artery and in downstream microvessels is associated with loss of microvascular integrity after embolic middle cerebral artery occlusion. *Brain Res* 912(2):181–194, 2001.

730. Adams HP Jr, et al: Emergency administration of abciximab for treatment of patients with acute ischemic stroke: Results of an international phase III trial: Abciximab in Emergency Treatment of Stroke Trial (AbESTT-II). *Stroke* 39(1):87–99, 2008.

731. Mandava P, Thiagarajan P, Kent TA: Glycoprotein IIb/IIIa antagonists in acute ischaemic stroke: Current status and future directions. *Drugs* 68(8):1019–1028, 2008.

732. Adelman B, et al: Plasmin effect on platelet glycoprotein Ib-von Willebrand factor interactions. *Blood* 64:32–40, 1985.

733. Adnot S, et al: Plasmin: A possible physiological modulator of human platelet adenylate cyclase system. *Clin Sci* 72:467–473, 1987.

734. Federici AB, et al: Proteolysis of von Willebrand factor in patients undergoing thrombolytic therapy. *Circulation* 78(Suppl.II):II–120-(Abs).

735. Gimple LW, et al: Correlation between template bleeding times and spontaneous bleeding during treatment of acute myocardial infarction with recombinant tissue-type plasminogen activator. *Circulation* 80:581–588, 1988, 1989.

736. Johnstone MT, et al: Bleeding time prolongation with streptokinase and its reduction with 1- desamino-8-D-arginine vasopressin. *Circulation* 82(6):2142–2151, 1990.

737. Kamat SG, Schafer AI: Antiplatelet effects of fibrinolytic agents: A potential contributor to the hemostatic defect after thrombolysis. *Coron Artery Dis* 6(12):930–935, 1995.

738. Kowalski E, Kopec M, Wegrzynowicz Z: Influence of fibrinogen degradation products (FDP) on platelet aggregation, adhesiveness and viscous metamorphosis. *Thromb Diath Haemorrh* 10:406–423, 1963.

739. Loscalzo J, Vaughan DE: Tissue plasminogen activator promotes platelet disaggregation in plasma. *J Clin Invest* 79:1749–1754, 1987.

740. Michelson AD, et al: Effect of in vivo infusion of recombinant tissue-type plasminogen activator on platelet glycoprotein Ib. *Thromb Res* 60(5):421–424, 1990.

741. Schafer AL, Adelman B: Plasmin inhibition of platelet function and of arachidonic acid metabolism. *J Clin Invest* 75:456–461, 1985.

742. Schafer AL, et al: Synergistic inhibition of platelet activation by plasmin and prostaglandin I2. *Blood* 69:1504–1507, 1987.

743. Shin Y, et al: Binding of von Willebrand factor cleaving protease ADAMTS13 to Lys-plasmin(ogen). *J Biochem* 152(3):251–258, 2012.

744. Tersteeg C, et al: Plasmin cleavage of von Willebrand factor as an emergency bypass for ADAMTS13 deficiency in thrombotic microangiopathy. *Circulation* 129(12):1320–1331, 2014.

745. Coller BS: Binding of abciximab to $\alpha_v\beta_3$ and activated $\alpha_M\beta_2$ receptors: With a review of platelet-leukocyte interactions. *Thromb Haemost* 82(2):326–336, 1999.

746. Farb A, et al: Pathology of acute and chronic coronary stenting in humans. *Circulation* 99(1):44–52, 1999.

747. Merhi Y, et al: Selectin blockade reduces neutrophil interaction with platelets at the site of deep arterial injury by angioplasty in pigs. *Arterioscler Thromb Vasc Biol* 19(2):372–377, 1999.

748. Smyth SS, et al: β3-integrin-deficient mice, but not P-selectin-deficient mice, develop intimal hyperplasia after vascular injury: Correlation with leukocyte recruitment to adherent platelets 1 hour after injury. *Circulation* 103:2501–2507, 2001.

749. Wehner J, et al: Antibody and complement in transplant vasculopathy. *Circ Res* 100(2):191–203, 2007.

750. Nishimura S, et al: In vivo imaging in mice reveals local cell dynamics and inflammation in obese adipose tissue. *J Clin Invest* 118(2):710–721, 2008.

751. Bozza FA, et al: Amicus or adversary: Platelets in lung biology, acute injury, and inflammation. *Am J Respir Cell Mol Biol* 40(2):123–134, 2009.

752. Schober A, et al: Deposition of platelet RANTES triggering monocyte recruitment requires P-selectin and is involved in neointima formation after arterial injury. *Circulation* 106(12):1523–1529, 2002.

753. von Hundelshausen P, et al: RANTES deposition by platelets triggers monocyte arrest on inflamed and atherosclerotic endothelium. *Circulation* 103(13):1772–1777, 2001.

754. Huo Y, et al: Circulating activated platelets exacerbate atherosclerosis in mice deficient in apolipoprotein E. *Nat Med* 9(1):61–67, 2003.

755. Diacovo TG, et al: Neutrophil rolling, arrest, and transmigration across activated, surface-adherent platelets via sequential action of P-selectin and the beta 2-integrin CD11b/CD18. *Blood* 88(1):146–157, 1996.

756. Hamburger SA, McEver RP: GMP-140 mediates adhesion of stimulated platelets to neutrophils. *Blood* 75(3):550–554, 1990.

757. Kirchhofer D, Riederer MA, Baumgartner HR: Specific accumulation of circulating monocytes and polymorphonuclear leukocytes on platelet thrombi in a vascular injury model. *Blood* 89(4):1270–1278, 1997.

758. Konstantopoulos K, et al: Venous levels of shear support neutrophil-platelet adhesion and neutrophil aggregation in blood via P-selectin and beta2-integrin. *Circulation* 98(9):873–882, 1998.

759. Larsen E, et al: PADGEM protein: A receptor that mediates the interaction of activated platelets with neutrophils and monocytes. *Cell* 59(2):305–312, 1989.

760. Sheikh S, Nash GB: Continuous activation and deactivation of integrin CD11b/CD18 during de novo expression enables rolling neutrophils to immobilize on platelets. *Blood* 87(12):5040–5050, 1996.

761. Yeo EL, Sheppard JA, Feuerstein IA: Role of P-selectin and leukocyte activation in polymorphonuclear cell adhesion to surface adherent activated platelets under physiologic shear conditions (an injury vessel wall model). *Blood* 83(9):2498–2507, 1994.

762. Gear AR, Camerini D: Platelet chemokines and chemokine receptors: Linking hemostasis, inflammation, and host defense. *Microcirculation* 10(3–4):335–350, 2003.

763. Weber C, Springer TA: Neutrophil accumulation on activated, surface-adherent platelets in flow is mediated by interaction of Mac-1 with fibrinogen bound to alphaIIbbeta3 and stimulated by platelet-activating factor. *J Clin Invest* 100(8):2085–2093, 1997.

764. Romo GM, et al: The glycoprotein Ib-IX-V complex is a platelet counterreceptor for P-selectin. *J Exp Med* 190(6):803–814, 1999.

765. Altieri DC, Plescia J, Plow EF: The structural motif glycine 190-valine 202 of the fibrinogen gamma chain interacts with CD11b/CD18 integrin (alpha M beta 2, Mac-1) and promotes leukocyte adhesion. *J Biol Chem* 268(3):1847–1853, 1993.

766. Silverstein RL, Asch AS, Nachman RL: Glycoprotein IV mediates thrombospondin-dependent platelet-monocyte and platelet-U937 cell adhesion. *J Clin Invest* 84:546–552, 1989.

767. Santoso S, et al: The junctional adhesion molecule 3 (JAM-3) on human platelets is a counterreceptor for the leukocyte integrin Mac-1. *J Exp Med* 196(5):679–691, 2002.

768. Marcus AJ, Safier LB: Thromboregulation: Multicellular modulation of platelet reactivity in hemostasis and thrombosis. *FASEB J* 7(6):516–522, 1993.

769. Lindemann S, et al: Activated platelets mediate inflammatory signaling by regulated interleukin 1beta synthesis. *J Cell Biol* 154(3):485–490, 2001.

770. Alderson MR, et al: CD40 expression by human monocytes: Regulation by cytokines and activation of monocytes by the ligand for CD40. *J Exp Med* 178(2):669–674, 1993.

771. Henn V, et al: CD40 ligand on activated platelets triggers an inflammatory reaction of endothelial cells. *Nature* 391(6667):591–594, 1998.

772. Yellin MJ, et al: Functional interactions of T cells with endothelial cells: The role of CD40L-CD40-mediated signals. *J Exp Med* 182(6):1857–1864, 1995.

773. Slupsky JR, et al: Activated platelets induce tissue factor expression on human umbilical vein endothelial cells by ligation of CD40. *Thromb Haemost* 80(6):1008–1014, 1998.

774. Del PD, et al: The plasma membrane redox system in human platelet functions and platelet-leukocyte interactions. *Thromb Haemost* 101(2):284–289, 2009.

775. Goel MS, Diamond SL: Neutrophil enhancement of fibrin deposition under flow through platelet-dependent and -independent mechanisms. *Arterioscler Thromb Vasc Biol* 21(12):2093–2098, 2001.

776. Goel MS, Diamond SL: Neutrophil cathepsin G promotes prothrombinase and fibrin formation under flow conditions by activating fibrinogen-adherent platelets. *J Biol Chem* 278(11):9458–9463, 2003.

777. Giesen PL, et al: Blood-borne tissue factor: Another view of thrombosis. *Proc Natl Acad Sci U S A* 96(5):2311–2315, 1999.

778. Furie B, Furie BC: Role of platelet P-selectin and microparticle PSGL-1 in thrombus formation. *Trends Mol Med* 10(4):171–178, 2004.

779. Pluskota E, et al: Expression, activation, and function of integrin alphaMbeta2 (Mac-1) on neutrophil-derived microparticles. *Blood* 112(6):2327–2335, 2008.

780. Andre P, et al: Pro-coagulant state resulting from high levels of soluble P-selectin in blood. *Proc Natl Acad Sci U S A* 97(25):13835–13840, 2000.

781. Hrachovinova I, et al: Interaction of P-selectin and PSGL-1 generates microparticles that correct hemostasis in a mouse model of hemophilia A. *Nat Med* 9(8):1020–1025, 2003.

782. Ott I, et al: Increased neutrophil-platelet adhesion in patients with unstable angina. *Circulation* 94(6):1239–1246, 1996.

783. Mickelson JK, et al: Leukocyte activation with platelet adhesion after coronary angioplasty: A mechanism for recurrent disease? *J Am Coll Cardiol* 28(2):345–353, 1996.

784. Michelson AD, et al: Circulating monocyte-platelet aggregates are a more sensitive marker of in vivo platelet activation than platelet surface P-selectin: Studies in baboons, human coronary intervention, and human acute myocardial infarction. *Circulation* 104(13):1533–1537, 2001.

785. Bugert P, et al: The variable number of tandem repeat polymorphism in the P-selectin glycoprotein ligand-1 gene is not associated with coronary heart disease. *J Mol Med (Berl)* 81(8):495–501, 2003.

786. Diz-Kucukkaya R, et al: P-selectin glycoprotein ligand-1 VNTR polymorphisms and risk of thrombosis in the antiphospholipid syndrome. *Ann Rheum Dis* 66(10):1378–1380, 2007.

787. Lozano ML, et al: Polymorphisms of P-selectin glycoprotein ligand-1 are associated with neutrophil-platelet adhesion and with ischaemic cerebrovascular disease. *Br J Haematol* 115(4):969–976, 2001.

788. Ozben B, et al: The association of P-selectin glycoprotein ligand-1 VNTR polymorphisms with coronary stent restenosis. *J Thromb Thrombolysis* 23(3):181–187, 2007.

789. Roldan V, et al: Short alleles of P-selectin glycoprotein ligand-1 protect against premature myocardial infarction. *Am Heart J* 148(4):602–605, 2004.

790. Tauxe C, et al: P-selectin glycoprotein ligand-1 decameric repeats regulate selectin-dependent rolling under flow conditions. *J Biol Chem* 283(42):28536–28545, 2008.

791. Wang Y, et al: Platelet-derived S100 family member myeloid-related protein-14 regulates thrombosis. *J Clin Invest* 124(5):2160–2171, 2014.

792. Clark SR, et al: Platelet TLR4 activates neutrophil extracellular traps to ensnare bacteria in septic blood. *Nat Med* 13(4):463–469, 2007.

793. Geddings JE, Mackman N: New players in haemostasis and thrombosis. *Thromb Haemost* 111(4):570–574, 2014.

794. Martinod K, Wagner DD: Thrombosis: Tangled up in NETs. *Blood* 123(18):2768–2776, 2014.

795. Arman M, et al: Amplification of bacteria-induced platelet activation is triggered by FcgammaRIIA, integrin alphaIIbbeta3, and platelet factor 4. *Blood* 123(20):3166–3174, 2014.

796. Boudreau LH, et al: Platelets release mitochondria serving as substrate for bactericidal group IIA-secreted phospholipase A2 to promote inflammation. *Blood* 124(14):2173–2183, 2014.

797. Sun H, et al: Reduced thrombin generation increases host susceptibility to group A streptococcal infection. *Blood* 113(6):1358–1364, 2009.

798. Li N, Platelet-lymphocyte cross-talk. *J Leukoc Biol* 83(5):1069–1078, 2008.

799. McMorran BJ, et al: Platelets kill intraerythrocytic malarial parasites and mediate survival to infection. *Science* 323(5915):797–800, 2009.

800. Boulaftali Y, et al: Platelet immunoreceptor tyrosine-based activation motif (ITAM) signaling and vascular integrity. *Circ Res* 114(7):1174–1184, 2014.

801. Lopez JA: The platelet glycoprotein Ib-IX complex. *Blood Coagul Fibrinolysis* 5(1):97–119, 1994.

802. Wu G, et al: Human endothelial cells in culture and in vivo express on their surface all four components of the glycoprotein Ib/IX/V complex. *Blood* 90(7):2660–2669, 1997.

803. Hynes RO, Integrins: Bidirectional, allosteric signaling machines. *Cell* 110(6):673–687, 2002.

804. Kasirer-Friede A, Kahn ML, Shattil SJ: Platelet integrins and immunoreceptors. *Immunol Rev* 218:247–264, 2007.

805. Bennett JS, Berger BW, Billings PC: The structure and function of platelet integrins. *J Thromb Haemost* 7 Suppl 1:200–205, 2009.

806. Bledzka K, Smyth SS, Plow EF: Integrin alphaIIbbeta3: From discovery to efficacious therapeutic target. *Circ Res* 114(8):1189–1200, 2013.

807. Phillips DR, et al: The platelet membrane glycoprotein IIb-IIIa complex. *Blood* 71:831–843, 1988.

808. Plow EF, Ginsberg MH: Cellular adhesion: GPIIb-IIIa as a prototypic adhesion receptor. *Prog Hemost Thromb* 9:117–156, 1989.

809. Ruggeri ZM: Structure and function of von Willebrand factor. *Thromb Haemost* 82:576–584, 1999.

810. Savage B, Ruggeri ZM: Platelet thrombus formation in flowing blood, in *Platelets*, edited by AD Michelson, p 215. Academic Press, San Diego, 2002.

811. Wagner CL, et al: Analysis of GPIIb/IIIa receptor number by quantification of 7E3 binding to human platelets. *Blood* 88:907–914, 1996.

812. Zhou YF, et al: Sequence and structure relationships within von Willebrand factor. *Blood* 120(2):449–458, 2012.

813. Cramer ER, et al: α Granule pool of glycoprotein IIb-IIIa in normal and pathologic platelets and megakaryocytes. *Blood* 75:1220–1227, 1990.

814. Woods VL Jr, Wolff LE, Keller DM: Resting platelets contain a substantial centrally located pool of glycoprotein IIb-IIIa complexes which may be accessible to some but not other extracellular proteins. *J Biol Chem* 261:15242–15251, 1986.

815. Youssefian T, et al: Platelet and megakaryocyte dense granules contain glycoproteins Ib and IIb-IIIa. *Blood* 89(11):4047–4057, 1997.

816. Peerschke EI: The platelet fibrinogen receptor. *Semin Hematol* 22(4):241–259, 1985.

817. Wencel-Drake JD: Plasma membrane GPIIb/IIIa. Evidence for a cycling receptor pool. *Am J Clin Pathol* 136:61–70, 1990.

818. Harrison P: Platelet α-granular fibrinogen. *Platelets* 3:1–10, 1992.

819. Hynes RO: Integrins: A family of cell surface receptors. *Cell* 48:549–554, 1987.

820. Ruoslahti E: Fibronectin and its receptors. *Annu Rev Biochem* 57:375–413, 1988.

821. Doolittle RF, et al: The amino acid sequence of the alpha-chain of human fibrinogen. *Nature* 280:464, 1979.

822. Cheresh DA, et al: Recognition of distinct adhesive sites on fibrinogen by related integrins on platelets and endothelial cells. *Cell* 58:945–953, 1988, 1989.

823. Farrell DH, Thiagarajan P: Binding of recombinant fibrinogen mutants to platelets. *J Biol Chem* 269(1):226–231, 1994.

824. Farrell DH, et al: Role of fibrinogen α and γ chain sites in platelet aggregation. *Proc Natl Acad Sci U S A* 89(22):10729–10732, 1992.

825. Savage B, Ruggeri ZM: Selective recognition of adhesive sites in surface-bound fibrinogen by glycoprotein IIb-IIIa on nonactivated platelets. *J Biol Chem* 266(17):11227–11233, 1991.

826. Springer TA, Zhu J, Xiao T: Structural basis for distinctive recognition of fibrinogen gammaC peptide by the platelet integrin alphaIIbbeta3. *J Cell Biol* 182(4):791–800, 2008.

827. Xiao T, et al: Structural basis for allostery in integrins and binding to fibrinogen-mimetic therapeutics. *Nature* 432:59–67, 2004.

828. Goldsmith HL, et al: Time and force dependence of the rupture of glycoprotein IIb-IIIa-fibrinogen bonds between latex spheres. *Biophys J* 78(3):1195–1206, 2000.

829. Hsieh CF, et al: Stepped changes of monovalent ligand-binding force during ligand-induced clustering of integrin alphaIIB beta3. *J Biol Chem* 281(35):25466–25474, 2006.

830. Huber W, et al: Determination of kinetic constants for the interaction between the platelet glycoprotein IIb-IIIa and fibrinogen by means of surface plasmon resonance. *Eur J Biochem* 227(3):647–656, 1995.

831. Litvinov RI, et al: Multi-step fibrinogen binding to the integrin (alpha)IIb(beta)3 detected using force spectroscopy. *Biophys J* 89(4):2824–2834, 2005.

832. Muller B, et al: Two-step binding mechanism of fibrinogen to alpha IIb beta 3 integrin reconstituted into planar lipid bilayers. *J Biol Chem* 268(9):6800–6808, 1993.

833. Peerschke EI: Reversible and irreversible binding of fibrinogen to platelets. *Platelets* 8(5):311–317, 1997.

834. Wencel-Drake JD, et al: Internalization of bound fibrinogen modulates platelet aggregation. *Blood* 87(2):602–612, 1996.

835. Peerschke EIB: Events occurring after thrombin-induced fibrinogen binding to platelets. *Semin Thromb Hemost* 18:34–43, 1992.

836. Ugarova TP, et al: Conformational changes in fibrinogen elicited by its interaction with platelet membrane glycoprotein GPIIb-IIIa. *J Biol Chem* 268:21080–21087, 1993.

837. Zamarron C, Ginsberg MH, Plow EF: A receptor-induced binding site in fibrinogen elicited by its interaction with platelet membrane glycoprotein IIb-IIIa. *J Biol Chem* 266:17106–17111, 1991.

838. Hato T, Pampori N, Shattil SJ: Complementary roles for receptor clustering and conformational change in the adhesive and signaling functions of integrin alphaIIb beta3. *J Cell Biol* 141(7):1685–1695, 1998.

839. Carrell NA, et al: Structure of human platelet membrane glycoproteins IIb and IIIa as determined by electron microscopy. *J Biol Chem* 260:1743–1749, 1985.

840. Weisel JW, et al: Examination of the platelet membrane glycoprotein IIb-IIIa complex and its interaction with fibrinogen and other ligands by electron microscopy. *J Biol Chem* 267(23):16637–16643, 1992.

841. Arnaout M, Goodman S, Xiong J: Coming to grips with integrin binding to ligands. *Curr Opin Cell Biol* 14(5):641–651, 2002.

842. Arnaout MA: Integrin structure: New twists and turns in dynamic cell adhesion. *Immunol Rev* 2002;186(1):125–140, 2002.

843. Takagi J, et al: Global conformational rearrangements in integrin extracellular domains in outside-in and inside-out signaling. *Cell* 110:599–607, 2002.

844. Xiong JP, et al: Crystal structure of the extracellular segment of integrin alphaVbeta3. *Science* 294(5541):339–345, 2001.

845. Xiong JP, et al: Crystal structure of the extracellular segment of integrin alpha Vbeta3 in complex with an Arg-Gly-Asp ligand. *Science* 296(5565):151–155, 2002.

846. Blue R, et al: Effects of limiting extension at the alphaIIb genu on ligand binding to integrin alphaIIbbeta3. *J Biol Chem* 285(23):17604–17613, 2010.

847. Cheng M, Li J, Negri A, Coller BS: Swing-out of the beta3 hybrid domain is required for alphaIIbbeta3 priming and normal cytoskeletal reorganization, but not adhesion to immobilized fibrinogen. *PLoS One* 8(12):e81609, 2013.

848. Choi WS, et al: Three-dimensional reconstruction of intact human integrin alphaIIbbeta3: New implications for activation-dependent ligand binding. *Blood* 2013;122(26):4165–4171, 2013.

849. Eng ET, et al: Intact alphaIIbbeta3 integrin is extended after activation as measured by solution X-ray scattering and electron microscopy. *J Biol Chem* 286(40):35218–35226, 2011.

850. Kamata T, et al: Structural requirements for activation in alphaIIb beta3 integrin. *J Biol Chem* 285(49):38428–38437, 2010.

851. Nogales A, et al: Three-dimensional model of human platelet integrin alphaIIb beta3 in solution obtained by small angle neutron scattering. *J Biol Chem* 285(2):1023–1031, 2010.

852. Ye F, et al: Recreation of the terminal events in physiological integrin activation. *J Cell Biol* 188(1):157–173, 2010.

853. Zhu J, et al: Structure-guided design of a high affinity platelet integrin αIIbβ3 receptor antagonist that disrupts Mg2+ binding to the MIDAS. *Sci Transl Med* 4:1–12, 2012.

854. Poncz M, et al: Structure of the platelet membrane glycoprotein IIb. Homology to the alpha subunits of the vitronectin and fibronectin membrane receptors. *J Biol ChemJ Biol Chem* 262(18):8476–8482, 1987.

855. Fitzgerald LA, et al: Protein sequence of endothelial glycoprotein IIIa derived from a cDNA clone. Identity with platelet glycoprotein IIIa and similarity to "integrin." *J Biol Chem* 262(9):3936–3939, 1987.

856. Bray PF, et al: Physical linkage of the genes for platelet membrane glycoproteins IIb and IIIa. *Proc Natl Acad Sci U S A* 85(22):8683–8687, 1988.

857. Thornton MA, et al: The human platelet alphaIIb gene is not closely linked to its integrin partner beta3. *Blood* 94(6):2039–2047, 1999.

858. Steiner B, et al: Ca+2 dependent structural transitions of the platelet glycoprotein IIb-IIIa complex. Preparation of stable glycoprotein IIb and IIIa monomers. *J Biol Chem* 266:14986–14991, 1991.

859. Mitchell WB, et al: AlphaIIbbeta3 biogenesis is controlled by engagement of alphaIIb in the calnexin cycle via the N15-linked glycan. *Blood* 107(7):2713–2719, 2006.

860. Duperray A, et al: Biosynthesis and assembly of platelet GPIIb-IIIa in human megakaryocytes: Evidence that assembly between pro-GPIIb and GPIIIa is a prerequisite for expression of the complex on the cell surface. *Blood* 74:1603–1611, 1989.

861. O'Toole TE, et al: Efficient surface expression of platelet GPIIb-IIIa requires both subunits. *Blood* 74(1):14–18, 1989.

862. McEver RP, Baenziger JU, Majerus PW: Isolation and structural characterization of the polypeptide subunits of membrane glycoprotein IIb-IIIa from human platelets. *Blood* 59:80.

863. Haas TA, Plow EF: The cytoplasmic domain of alphaIIb beta3. A ternary complex of the integrin alpha and beta subunits and a divalent cation. *J Biol Chem* 1996;271(11):6017–6023, 1996.

864. Kim C, Lau TL, Ulmer TS, Ginsberg MH: Interactions of platelet integrin alphaIIb and beta3 transmembrane domains in mammalian cell membranes and their role in integrin activation. *Blood* 113(19):4747–4753, 2009.

865. Muir TW, et al: Design and chemical synthesis of a neoprotein structural model for the cytoplasmic domain of a multisubunit cell-surface receptor: Integrin alpha IIb beta 3 (platelet GPIIb-IIIa). *Biochemistry* 33(24):7701–7708, 1994.

866. Vallar L, et al: Divalent cations differentially regulate integrin alphaIIb cytoplasmic tail binding to beta3 and to calcium- and integrin-binding protein. *J Biol Chem* 274(24):17257–17266, 1999.

867. Hughes PE, et al: Breaking the integrin hinge. A defined structural constraint regulates integrin signaling. *J Biol Chem* 271(12):6571–6574, 1996.

868. Li A, et al: Integrin alphaII b tail distal of GFFKR participates in inside-out alphaII b beta3 activation. *J Thromb Haemost* 12(7):1145–1155, 2014.

869. O'Toole TE, et al: Integrin cytoplasmic domains mediate inside-out signal transduction. *J Cell Biol* 124(6):1047–1059, 1994.

870. O'Toole TE, et al: Modulation of the affinity of integrin αIIbβ3 (GPIIb-IIIa) by the cytoplasmic domain of alpha IIb. *Science* 254(5033):845–847, 1991.

871. Zhu J, et al: The structure of a receptor with two associating transmembrane domains on the cell surface: Integrin alphaIIbbeta3. *Mol Cell* 34(2):234–249, 2009.

872. Kim M, Carman CV, Springer TA: Bidirectional transmembrane signaling by cytoplasmic domain separation in integrins. *Science* 301(5640):1720–1725, 2003.

873. Li W, et al: A push-pull mechanism for regulating integrin function. *Proc Natl Acad Sci U S A* 102(5):1424–1429, 2005.

874. Luo BH, et al: Disrupting integrin transmembrane domain heterodimerization increases ligand binding affinity, not valency or clustering. *Proc Natl Acad Sci U S A* 102(10):3679–3684, 2005.

875. Partridge AW, et al: Transmembrane domain helix packing stabilizes integrin alphaIIbbeta3 in the low affinity state. *J Biol Chem* 280(8):7294–7300, 2005.

876. Leisner TM, et al: Bidirectional transmembrane modulation of integrin alphaIIbbeta3 conformations. *J Biol Chem* 274(18):12945–12949, 1999.

877. Vinogradova O, et al: A Structural mechanism of integrin alpha(IIb)beta(3) "inside-out" activation as regulated by its cytoplasmic face. *Cell* 110(5):587.

878. Xiong JP, Stehle T, Goodman SL, Arnaout MA: A novel adaptation of the integrin PSI domain revealed from its crystal structure. *J Biol Chem* 279(39):40252–40254, 2004.

879. Du X, et al: Long range propagation of conformational changes in integrin alpha IIb beta 3. *J Biol Chem* 268(31):23087–23092, 1993 [published erratum appears in *J Biol Chem* 269(15):11673, 1994].

880. Frelinger AL 3ed, Du XP, Plow EF, Ginsberg MH: Monoclonal antibodies to ligand-occupied conformers of integrin alpha IIb beta 3 (glycoprotein IIb-IIIa) alter receptor affinity, specificity, and function. *J Biol Chem* 266:17106–17111, 1991.

881. Kamata T, et al: Critical cysteine residues for regulation of integrin alphaIIbbeta3 are clustered in the epidermal growth factor domains of the beta3 subunit. *Biochem J* 378(Pt 3):1079–1082, 2004.

882. Kashiwagi H, et al: A mutation in the extracellular cysteine-rich repeat region of the beta3 subunit activates integrins alphaIIbbeta3 and alphaVbeta3. *Blood* 93(8):2559–2568, 1999.

883. Essex DW: The role of thiols and disulfides in platelet function. *Antioxid Redox Signal* 6(4):736–746, 2004.

884. Zucker MB, Masiello NC: Platelet aggregation caused by dithiothreitol. *Thromb Haemost* 51(1):119–124, 1984.

885. Chen K, Detwiler TC, Essex DW: Characterization of protein disulphide isomerase released from activated platelets. *Br J Haematol* 90(2):425–431, 1995.

886. Essex DW, Chen K, Swiatkowska M: Localization of protein disulfide isomerase to the external surface of the platelet plasma membrane. *Blood* 86(6):2168–2173, 1995.

887. Essex DW, Li M: Redox control of platelet aggregation. *Biochemistry* 42(1):129–136, 2003.

888. Mor-Cohen R, et al: Disulfide bond exchanges in integrins alphaIIbbeta3 and alphavbeta3 are required for activation and post-ligation signaling during clot retraction. *Thromb Res* 133(5):826–836, 2014.

889. O'Neill S, et al: The platelet integrin alpha IIbeta 3 has an endogenous thiol isomerase activity. *J Biol Chem* 275(47):36984–36990, 2000.

890. Furie B, Flaumenhaft R: Thiol isomerases in thrombus formation. *Circ Res* 114(7):1162–1173, 2014.

891. Wang L, et al: Platelet-derived ERp57 mediates platelet incorporation into a growing thrombus by regulation of the alphaIIbbeta3 integrin. *Blood* 122(22):3642–3650, 2013.

892. Provasi D, Negri A, Coller BS, Filizola M: Talin-driven inside-out activation mechanism of platelet αIIbβ3 integrin probed by multimicrosecond, all-atom molecular dynamics simulations. *Proteins* 82(12):3231–3240, 2014.

893. Gottschalk KE: A coiled-coil structure of the alphaIIbbeta3 integrin transmembrane and cytoplasmic domains in its resting state. *Structure* 13(5):703–712, 2005.

894. Lau TL, Kim C, Ginsberg MH, Ulmer TS: The structure of the integrin alphaIIb-beta3 transmembrane complex explains integrin transmembrane signalling. *EMBO J* 28(9):1351–1361, 2009.

895. Luo BH, Springer TA, Takagi J: A specific interface between integrin transmembrane helices and affinity for ligand. *PLoS Biol* 2(6):776–786, 2004.

896. Wegener KL, et al: Structural basis of integrin activation by talin. *Cell* 128(1):171–182, 2007.

897. Hernandez-Campo PM, et al: Comparative analysis of different flow cytometry-based immunophenotypic methods for the analysis of CD59 and CD55 expression on major peripheral blood cell subsets. *Cytometry* 50(3):191–201, 2002.

898. Robb L, et al: Molecular characterisation of mouse and human TSSC6: Evidence that TSSC6 is a genuine member of the tetraspanin superfamily and is expressed specifically in haematopoietic organs. *Biochim Biophys Acta* 1522(1):31–41, 2001.

899. Hughes PE, et al: Breaking the integrin hinge. A defined structural constraint regulates integrin signaling. *J Biol Chem* 271(12):6571–6574, 1996.

900. Anthis NJ, Wegener KL, Ye F, et al: The structure of an integrin/talin complex reveals the basis of inside-out signal transduction. *EMBO J* 28(22):3623–3632, 2009.

901. Ithychanda SS, Das M, Ma YQ, et al: Migfilin, a molecular switch in regulation of integrin activation. *J Biol Chem* 284(7):4713–4722, 2009.

902. Jenkins AL, et al: Tyrosine phosphorylation of the beta3 cytoplasmic domain mediates integrin-cytoskeletal interactions. *J Biol Chem* 273(22):13878–13885, 1998.

903. Jones CI, et al: Integrin-linked kinase regulates the rate of platelet activation and is essential for the formation of stable thrombi. *J Thromb Haemost* 12(8):1342–1352, 2014.

904. Calderwood DA, Shattil SJ, Ginsberg MH: Integrins and actin filaments: Reciprocal regulation of cell adhesion and signaling. *J Biol Chem* 275(30):22607–22610, 2000.

905. Calderwood DA, et al: The talin head domain binds to integrin beta subunit cytoplasmic tails and regulates integrin activation. *J Biol Chem* 274:28071–28074, 1999.

906. Cowan KJ, Law DA, Phillips DR: Identification of shc as the primary protein binding to the tyrosine-phosphorylated beta 3 subunit of alpha IIbbeta 3 during outside-in integrin platelet signaling. *J Biol Chem* 275(46):36423–36429, 2000.

907. Eigenthaler M, et al: A conserved sequence motif in the integrin beta3 cytoplasmic domain is required for its specific interaction with beta3-endonexin. *J Biol Chem* 272(12):7693–7698, 1997.

908. Hannigan GE, et al: Regulation of cell adhesion and anchorage-dependent growth by a new beta 1-integrin-linked protein kinase. *Nature* 379(6560):91–96, 1996.

909. Loh E, Qi W, Vilaire G, Bennett JS: Effect of cytoplasmic domain mutations on the agonist-stimulated ligand binding activity of the platelet integrin alphaIIbbeta3. *J Biol Chem* 271(47):30233–30241, 1966.

910. Law DA, Nannizzi-Alaimo L, Phillips DR: Outside-in integrin signal transduction. Alpha IIb beta 3-(GP IIb IIIa) tyrosine phosphorylation induced by platelet aggregation. *J Biol Chem* 271(18):10811–10815, 1996.

911. Leung-Hagesteijn CY, et al: Cell attachment to extracellular matrix substrates is inhibited upon downregulation of expression of calreticulin, an intracellular integrin alpha-subunit-binding protein. *J Cell Sci* 107(Pt 3):589–600, 1994.

912. Naik UP, Patel PM, Parise LV: Identification of a novel calcium-binding protein that interacts with the integrin alphaIIb cytoplasmic domain. *J Biol Chem* 272(8):4651–4654, 1997.

913. Otey CA, Pavalko FM, Burridge K: An interaction between alpha-actinin and the beta 1 integrin subunit *in vitro*. *J Cell Biol* 111(2):721–729, 1990.

914. Reddy KB, et al: Identification of an interaction between the m-band protein skelemin and beta3-integrin subunits. Colocalization of a skelemin-like protein with beta1- and beta3-integrins in non-muscle cells. *J Biol Chem* 273(52):35039–35047, 1998.

915. Rojiani MV, et al: *In vitro* interaction of a polypeptide homologous to human Ro/SS-A antigen (calreticulin) with a highly conserved amino acid sequence in the cytoplasmic domain of integrin alpha subunits. *Biochemistry* 30(41):9859–9866, 1991.

916. Schaller MD, et al: Focal adhesion kinase and paxillin bind to peptides mimicking beta integrin cytoplasmic domains. *J Cell Biol* 130(5):1181–1187, 1995.

917. Shattil SJ, et al: Beta 3-endonexin, a novel polypeptide that interacts specifically with the cytoplasmic tail of the integrin beta 3 subunit. *J Cell Biol* 131(3):807–816, 1995.

918. Shock DD, et al: Calcium-dependent properties of CIB binding to the integrin alphaIIb cytoplasmic domain and translocation to the platelet cytoskeleton. *Biochem J* 342(Pt 3):729–735, 1999.

919. Zent R, et al: Class- and splice variant-specific association of CD98 with integrin beta cytoplasmic domains. *J Biol Chem* 275(7):5059–5064, 2000.

920. Naik UP, Eckfeld K: Junctional adhesion molecule 1 (JAM-1). *J Biol Regul Homeost Agents* 17(4):341–347, 2003.

921. Ming Z, et al: Lyn and PECAM-1 function as interdependent inhibitors of platelet aggregation. *Blood* 117(14):3903–3906, 2011.

922. Tourdot BE, et al: Immunoreceptor tyrosine-based inhibitory motif (ITIM)-mediated inhibitory signaling is regulated by sequential phosphorylation mediated by distinct nonreceptor tyrosine kinases: A case study involving PECAM-1. *Biochemistry* 52(15):2597–2608, 2013.

923. Scarborough RM, et al: Design of potent and specific integrin antagonists. Peptide antagonists with high specificity for glycoprotein IIb-IIIa. *J Biol Chem* 268:1066–1073, 1993.

924. Beer JH, Springer KT, Coller BS: Immobilized Arg-Gly-Asp (RGD) peptides of varying lengths as structural probes of the platelet GPIIb/IIIa receptor. *Blood* 79:117–128, 1992.

925. Luo BH, Springer TA, Takagi J: Stabilizing the open conformation of the integrin headpiece with a glycan wedge increases affinity for ligand. *Proc Natl Acad Sci U S A* 100(5):2403–2408, 2003.

926. Heilmann E, et al: Thrombin-induced platelet aggregates have a dynamic structure: Time-dependent redistribution of GPIIb/IIIa complexes and secreted adhesive proteins. *Arterioscler Thromb* 11:704–718, 1991.

927. Isenberg WM, McEver RP, Phillips DR, et al: The platelet fibrinogen receptor: An immunogold-surface replica study of agonist-induced ligand binding and receptor clustering. *J Cell Biol* 104(6):1655–1663, 1987.

928. Prevost N, Shattil SJ: Outside-in signaling by integrin αIIbβ3, in *Platelets*, edited by AD Michelson, pp 347–350. Academic Press, San Diego, 2007.

929. Asch E, Podack E: Vitronectin binds to activated human platelets and plays a role in platelet aggregation. *J Clin Invest* 85(5);1372–1378, 1990.

930. Haverstick DM, et al: Inhibition of platelet adhesion to fibronectin, fibrinogen, and von Willebrand factor substrates by a synthetic tetrapeptide derived from the cell-binding domain of fibronectin. *Blood* 66:946–952, 1990, 1985.

931. Plow EF, D'Souza SE, Ginsberg MH: Ligand binding to GPIIb-IIIa: A status report. *Semin Thromb Hemost* 18(3):324–332, 1992.

932. Weiss HJ, et al: Fibrinogen-independent platelet adhesion and thrombus formation on subendothelium mediated by glycoprotein IIb-IIIa complex at high shear rate. *J Clin Invest* 83:288–297, 1989.

933. Schullek J, Jordan J, Montgomery RR: Interaction of von Willebrand factor with human platelets in the plasma milieu. *J Clin Invest* 73:421–428, 1984.

934. Ni H, et al: Persistence of platelet thrombus formation in arterioles of mice lacking both von Willebrand factor and fibrinogen. *J Clin Invest* 106(3):385–392, 2000.

935. Ni H, et al: Control of thrombus embolization and fibronectin internalization by integrin alpha IIb beta 3 engagement of the fibrinogen gamma chain. *Blood* 102(10):3609–3614, 2003.

936. Ni H, et al: Plasma fibronectin promotes thrombus growth and stability in injured arterioles. *Proc Natl Acad Sci U S A* 100(5):2415–2419, 2003.

937. Coller BS: Interaction of normal, thrombasthenic, and Bernard-Soulier platelets with immobilized fibrinogen: Defective platelet-fibrinogen interaction in thrombasthenia. *Blood* 55:169–178, 1980.

938. Moskowitz KA, Kudryk B, Coller BS: Fibrinogen coating density affects the conformation of immobilized fibrinogen: Implications for platelet adhesion and spreading. *Thromb Haemost* 79(4):824–831, 1998.

939. Hatton MW, Moar SL, Richardson M: Deendothelialization *in vivo* initiates a thrombogenic reaction at the rabbit aorta surface. Correlation of uptake of fibrinogen and antithrombin III with thrombin generation by the exposed subendothelium. *Am J Pathol* 135(3):499–508, 1989.

940. Savage B, Ruggeri ZM: Selective recognition of adhesive sites in surface-bound fibrinogen by glycoprotein IIb-IIIa on nonactivated platelets. *J Biol Chem* 266:11227–11233, 1991.

941. Goto S, et al: Distinct mechanisms of platelet aggregation as a consequence of different shearing flow conditions. *J Clin Invest* 101(2):479–486, 1998.

942. Ruggeri ZM, Dent JA, Saldivar E: Contribution of distinct adhesive interactions to platelet aggregation in flowing blood. *Blood* 94(1):172–178, 1999.

943. Weiss HJ, Turitto VT, Baumgartner HR: Further evidence that glycoprotein IIb-IIIa mediates platelet spreading on subendothelium. *Thromb Haemost* 65(2):202–205, 1991.

944. Coller BS, et al: Platelet fibrinogen and vitronectin in Glanzmann thrombasthenia: Evidence consistent with specific roles for glycoprotein IIb/IIIA and $\alpha V \beta 3$ integrins in platelet protein trafficking. *Blood* 78:2603–2610, 1991.

945. Peerschke EI, Grant RA, Zucker MB: Decreased association of 45-calcium with platelets unable to aggregate due to thrombasthenia or prolonged calcium deprivation. *Br J Haematol* 46:247–256, 1980.

946. Powling MJ, Hardisty RM: Glycoprotein IIb-IIIa complex and Ca++ influx into stimulated platelets. *Blood* 66(3):731–734, 1985.

947. Rybak ME, Renzulli LA: Effect of calcium channel blockers on platelet GPIIb-IIIa as a calcium channel in liposomes: Comparison with effects on the intact platelet. *Thromb Haemost* 67:131–136, 1985, 1991.

948. Ameisen JC, et al: A role for glycoprotein IIb-IIIa complexes in the binding of IgE to human platelets and platelet IgE-dependent cytolytic function. *Br J Haematol* 64:21–32, 1986.

949. Coburn J, Barthold SW, Leong JM: Diverse Lyme disease spirochetes bind integrin alpha IIb beta 3 on human platelets. *Infect Immun* 62(12):5559–5567, 1994.

950. Gavrilovskaya IN, et al: Cellular entry of hantaviruses which cause hemorrhagic fever with renal syndrome is mediated by beta3 integrins. *J Virol* 73(5):3951–3959, 1999.

951. Kulkarni S, Jackson SP: Platelet factor XIII and calpain negatively regulate integrin alphaIIbbeta3 adhesive function and thrombus growth. *J Biol Chem* 279(29):30697–30706, 2004.

952. Madamanchi A, Santoro SA, Zutter MM: Alpha2beta1 Integrin. *Adv Exp Med Biol* 819:41–60, 2014.

953. Barnes MJ, Knight CG, Farndale RW: The collagen-platelet interaction. *Curr Opin Hematol* 5(5):314–320, 1998.

954. Kunicki DJ, Nugent DJ, Staats SJ, et al: The human fibroblast II extracellular matrix receptor mediates platelet adhesion to collagen and is identical to the platelet glycoprotein Ia-IIa complex. *J Biol Chem* 263(10):4516–4519, 1988.

955. Pischel KD, et al: Use of the monoclonal antibody 12F1 to characterize the differentiation antigen VLA-2. *J Immunol* 138:226–233, 1988, 1987.

956. Saelman EU, et al: Platelet adhesion to collagen types I through VIII under conditions of stasis and flow is mediated by GPIa/IIa ($\alpha 2 \beta 1$-integrin). *Blood* 83(5):1244–1250, 1994.

957. Staatz WD, et al: The membrane glycoprotein Ia-IIa (VLA-2) complex mediates the Mg++-dependent adhesion of platelets to collagen. *J Cell Biol* 108:1917–1924, 1989.

958. Takada Y, Hemler ME: The primary structure of the VLA-2/collagen receptor $\alpha 2$ subunit (platelet GPIa): Homology to other integrins and the presence of a possible collagen-binding domain. *J Cell Biol* 109:397–407, 1987.

959. Clemetson KJ: Platelet receptors, in *Platelets*, edited by AD Michelson, pp 65–84. Academic Press, San Diego, 2002.

960. Emsley J, et al: Crystal structure of the I domain from integrin alpha2beta1. *J Biol Chem* 272(45):28512–28517, 1997.

961. Emsley J, et al: Structural basis of collagen recognition by integrin alpha2beta1. *Cell* 101(1):47–56, 2000.

962. Tulla M, et al: Effects of conformational activation of integrin alpha 1I and alpha 2I domains on selective recognition of laminin and collagen subtypes. *Exp Cell Res* 314(8):1734–1743, 2008.

963. Barnes MJ: The collagen platelet interaction, in *Collagen in Health and Disease*, edited by J Weiss J, MJV Jayson, pp. 179–197. Collagen in Health and Disease, Churchill Livingstone, Edinburgh, London, 1982.

964. Nieuwenhuis HK, et al: Human blood platelets showing no response to collagen fail to express surface glycoprotein Ia. *Nature* 318:470–472, 1985.

965. Sarratt KL, et al: GPVI and alpha2beta1 play independent critical roles during platelet adhesion and aggregate formation to collagen under flow. *Blood* 106(4):1268–1277, 2005.

966. Nissinen L, et al: Novel alpha2beta1 integrin inhibitors reveal that integrin binding to collagen under shear stress conditions does not require receptor preactivation. *J Biol Chem* 287(53):44694–44702, 2012.

967. Zou Z, Schmaier AA, Cheng L, et al: Negative regulation of activated alpha2 integrins during thrombopoiesis. *Blood* 113(25):6428–6439, 2009.

968. Cruz MA, et al: The platelet glycoprotein Ib-von Willebrand factor interaction activates the collagen receptor alpha2beta1 to bind collagen: Activation-dependent conformational change of the alpha2-I domain. *Blood* 105(5):1986–1991, 2005.

969. Pula G, Poole AW: Critical roles for the actin cytoskeleton and cdc42 in regulating platelet integrin alpha2beta1. *Platelets* 19(3):199–210, 2008.

970. Schoolmeester A, et al: Monoclonal antibody IAC-1 is specific for activated alpha-2beta1 and binds to amino acids 199 to 201 of the integrin alpha2 I-domain. *Blood* 104(2):390–396, 2004.

971. He L, et al: The contributions of the alpha 2 beta 1 integrin to vascular thrombosis *in vivo*. *Blood* 102(10):3652–3657, 2003.

972. Kuijpers MJ, et al: Complementary roles of glycoprotein VI and alpha2beta1 integrin in collagen-induced thrombus formation in flowing whole blood *ex vivo*. *FASEB J* 17(6):685–687, 2003.

973. Lahav J, et al: Enzymatically catalyzed disulfide exchange is required for platelet adhesion to collagen via integrin alpha2beta1. *Blood* 102(6):2085–2092, 2003.

974. Savage B, Ginsberg MH, Ruggeri ZM: Influence of fibrillar collagen structure on the mechanisms of platelet thrombus formation under flow. *Blood* 94(8):2704–2715, 1999.

975. Coller BS, et al: Collagen-platelet interactions: Evidence for a direct interaction of collagen with platelet GPIa/IIa and an indirect interaction with platelet GPIIb/IIa mediated by adhesive proteins. *Blood* 74:182–192, 1989.

976. Deckmyn H, De Meyer SF, Broos K, Vanhoorelbeke K: Inhibitors of the interactions between collagen and its receptors on platelets. *Handb Exp Pharmacol* (210):311–337, 2012.

977. Miller MW, et al: Small-molecule inhibitors of integrin alpha2beta1 that prevent pathological thrombus formation via an allosteric mechanism. *Proc Natl Acad Sci U S A* 106(3):719–724, 2009.

978. Nissinen L, et al: A small-molecule inhibitor of integrin alpha2 beta1 introduces a new strategy for antithrombotic therapy. *Thromb Haemost* 103(2):387–397, 2010.

979. Staatz WD, et al: The $\alpha 2 \beta 1$ integrin cell surface collagen receptor binds to the $\alpha 1$(I)-CB3 peptide of collagen. *J Biol Chem* 265:4778–4781, 1990.

980. Knight CG, et al: Identification in collagen type I of an integrin alpha2 beta1-binding site containing an essential GER sequence. *J Biol Chem* 273(50):33287–33294, 1998.

981. Santoro SA, et al: Distinct determinants on collagen support $\alpha 2 \beta 1$ integrin- mediated platelet adhesion and platelet activation. *Cell Regul* 2(11):905–913, 1991.

982. Verkleij MW, et al: Adhesive domains in the collagen III fragment alpha1(III)CB4 that support alpha2b. *Thromb Haemost* 82(3):1137–1144, 1999.

983. Yee DL, Bray PF: Clinical and functional consequences of platelet membrane glycoprotein polymorphisms. *Semin Thromb Hemost* 30(5):591–600, 2004.

984. Bray PF: Integrin polymorphisms as risk factors for thrombosis. *Thromb Haemost* 82:337–344, 1999.

985. Kritzik M, et al: Nucleotide polymorphisms in the alpha2 gene define multiple alleles that are associated with differences in platelet alpha2 beta1 density. *Blood* 92(7):2382–2388, 1998.

986. Moshfegh K, et al: Association of two silent polymorphisms of platelet glycoprotein Ia/IIa receptor with risk of myocardial infarction: A case-control study. *Lancet* 353(9150):351–354, 1999.

987. Santoso S, et al: Association of the platelet glycoprotein Ia C807T gene polymorphism with nonfatal myocardial infarction in younger patients. *Blood* 93(8):2449–2453, 1999.

988. Carlsson LE, et al: The alpha2 gene coding sequence T807/A873 of the platelet collagen receptor integrin alpha2beta1 might be a genetic risk factor for the development of stroke in younger patients. *Blood* 93(11):3583–3586, 1999.

989. Matsubara Y, et al: Association between diabetic retinopathy and genetic variations in alpha2beta1 integrin, a platelet receptor for collagen. *Blood* 95(5):1560–1564, 2000.

990. Roest M, et al: Homozygosity for 807 T polymorphism in alpha(2) subunit of platelet alpha(2)beta(1) is associated with increased risk of cardiovascular mortality in high-risk women. *Circulation* 102(14):1645–1650, 2000.

991. Vijayan KV, Bray PF: Molecular mechanisms of prothrombotic risk due to genetic variations in platelet genes: Enhanced outside-in signaling through the Pro33 variant of integrin beta3. *Exp Biol Med (Maywood)* 231(5):505–513, 2006.

992. von Beckerath N, et al: Glycoprotein Ia gene C807T polymorphism and risk for major adverse cardiac events within the first 30 days after coronary artery stenting. *Blood* 95(11):3297–3301, 2000.

993. Fox JE: Linkage of a membrane skeleton to integral membrane glycoproteins in human platelets. Identification of one of the glycoproteins as glycoprotein Ib. *J Clin Invest* 76:1673–1683, 1985.

994. Elices MJ, Hemler ME: The human integrin VLA-2 is a collagen receptor on some cells and a collagen/laminin receptor on others. *Proc Natl Acad Sci U S A* 86(24):9906–9910, 1989.

995. Kirchhofer D, Languino LR, Ruoslahti E, Pierschbacher MD: Alpha 2 beta 1 integrins from different cell types show different binding specificities. *J Biol Chem* 265(2):615–618, 1990.

996. Habart D, Cheli Y, Nugent DJ,: Conditional knockout of integrin alpha2beta1 in murine megakaryocytes leads to reduced mean platelet volume. *PLoS One* 8(1):e55094, 2013.

997. Piotrowicz RS, et al: Glycoprotein Ic-IIa functions as an activation-independent fibronectin receptor on human platelets. *J Cell Biol* 106:1359–1364, 1988.

998. Wayner EA, Carter WG, Piotrowicz RS, Kunicki TJ: The function of multiple extracellular matrix receptors in mediating cell adhesion to extracellular matrix: Preparation of monoclonal antibodies to the fibronectin receptor that specifically inhibit

cell adhesion of fibronectin and react with platelet glycoproteins Ic-IIa. *J Cell Biol* 107(5):1881–1891, 1988.

999. Garcia AJ, Huber F, Boettiger D: Force required to break alpha5beta1 integrin-fibronectin bonds in intact adherent cells is sensitive to integrin activation state. *J Biol Chem* 273(18):10988–10993, 1998.

1000. Matsunaga T, et al: Potentiated activation of VLA-4 and VLA-5 accelerates proplatelet-like formation. *Ann Hematol* 91(10):1633–1643, 2012.

1001. Plow EF, et al: Related binding mechanisms for fibrinogen, fibronectin, von Willebrand factor and thrombospondin on thrombin-stimulated human platelets. *Blood* 66:724–727, 1985.

1002. Schaff M, et al: Integrin alpha6beta1 is the main receptor for vascular laminins and plays a role in platelet adhesion, activation, and arterial thrombosis. *Circulation* 128(5):541–552, 2013.

1003. Hindriks G, et al: Platelet adhesion to laminin: Role of Ca2+ and Mg2+ ions, shear rate, and platelet membrane glycoproteins. *Blood* 79(4):928–935, 1992.

1004. Sonnenberg A, Modderman PW, Hogervorst F: Laminin receptor on platelets is the integrin VLA-6. *Nature* 336:487–489, 1988.

1005. Chang JC, et al: The integrin alpha6beta1 modulation of PI3K and Cdc42 activities induces dynamic filopodium formation in human platelets. *J Biomed Sci* 12(6):881–898, 2005.

1006. Tandon NN, et al: Interaction of human platelets with laminin and identification of the 67 kDa laminin receptor on platelets. *Biochem J Biochem* 274:535–542, 1991.

1007. Arnaout MA, Goodman SL, Xiong JP: Structure and mechanics of integrin-based cell adhesion. *Curr Opin Cell Biol* 19(5):495–507, 2007.

1008. Hynes RO: Integrins. Bidirectional, allosteric signaling machines. *Cell* 110(6):673–687, 2002.

1009. Luo BH, Carman CV, Springer TA: Structural basis of integrin regulation and signaling. *Annu Rev Immunol* 25:619–647, 2002, 2007.

1010. Fitzgerald LA, et al: Comparison of cDNA-derived protein sequences of the human fibronectin and vitronectin receptor α subunits and platelet glycoprotein IIb. *Biochemistry* 26:8158–8165, 1987.

1011. Coller BS, et al: Platelet vitronectin receptor expression differentiates Iraqi-Jewish from Arab Patients with Glanzmann thrombasthenia in Israel. *Blood* 77:75–83, 1991.

1012. Byzova TV, Plow EF: Activation of alphaVbeta3 on vascular cells controls recognition of prothrombin. *J Cell Biol* 143(7):2081–2092, 1998.

1013. Charo IF, Bekeart LS, Phillips DR: Platelet glycoprotein IIb-IIIa-like proteins mediate endothelial cell attachment to adhesive proteins and the extracellular matrix. *J Biol Chem* 262:9935–9938, 1987.

1014. Kieffer N, et al: Adhesive properties of the β3 integrins. Comparison of GPIIb-IIIa and the vitronectin receptor individually expressed in human melanoma cells. *J Cell Biol* 113:451–461, 1991.

1015. Lam SC, et al: Isolation and characterization of a platelet membrane protein related to the vitronectin receptor. *J Biol Chem* 264:3742–3749, 1989.

1016. Bennett JS, et al: Agonist-activated alphavbeta3 on platelets and lymphocytes binds to the matrix protein osteopontin. *J Biol Chem*, 272(13):8137–8140, 1997.

1017. Reverter JC, et al: Inhibition of platelet-mediated, tissue factor-induced thrombin generation by the mouse/human chimeric 7E3 antibody. Potential implications for the effect of c7E3 Fab treatment on acute thrombosis and "clinical restenosis." *J Clin Invest* 98(3):863–874, 1996.

1018. Beckstead JH, Stenberg PE, McEver RP, et al: Immunohistochemical localization of membrane and alpha-granule proteins in human megakaryocytes: Application to plastic-embedded bone marrow biopsy specimens. *Blood* 67(2):285–293, 1986.

1019. Davies J, et al: The osteoclast functional antigen, implicated in the regulation of bone resorption is biochemically related to the vitronectin receptor. *J Cell Biol* 109:1817, 1989.

1020. Feng X, et al: A Glanzmann's mutation in beta 3 integrin specifically impairs osteoclast function. *J Clin Invest* 2001;107(9):1137–1144, 1986.

1021. McHugh KP, et al: Mice lacking beta3 integrins are osteosclerotic because of dysfunctional osteoclasts. *J Clin Invest* 105(4):433–440, 2000.

1022. Savill J, et al: Vitronectin receptor-mediated phagocytosis of cells undergoing apoptosis. *Nature* 343(6254):170–173, 1990.

1023. Brooks PC, Clark RA, Cheresh DA: Requirement of vascular integrin αVβ3 for angiogenesis. *Science* 264(5158):569–571, 1994.

1024. Trikha M, et al: CNTO 95 a fully human monoclonal antibody that inhibits alphav integrins, has antitumor and antiangiogenic activity *in vivo. Int J Cancer* 110(3):326–335, 2004.

1025. Varner JA, Cheresh DA: Integrins and cancer. *Curr Opin Cell Biol* 8:724–730, 1996.

1026. Choi ET, et al: Inhibition of neointimal hyperplasia by blocking αVβ3 integrin with a small peptide antagonist GpenGRGDSPCA. *J Vasc Surg* 19:125–134, 1994.

1027. Sajid M, Stouffer GA: The role of alpha(v)beta3 integrins in vascular healing. *Thromb Haemost* 87(2):187–193, 2002.

1028. Stouffer GA, Smyth SS: Effects of thrombin on interactions between beta3-integrins and extracellular matrix in platelets and vascular cells. *Arterioscler Thromb Vasc Biol* 23(11):1971–1978, 2003.

1029. Kaul DK: Sickle red cell adhesion: Many issues and some answers. *Transfus Clin Biol* 15(1–2):51–55, 2008.

1030. Kaul DK, et al: Monoclonal antibodies to alphaVbeta3 (7E3 and LM609) inhibit sickle red blood cell-endothelium interactions induced by platelet-activating factor. *Blood* 95(2):368–374, 2000.

1031. Belcher JD, et al: Heme triggers TLR4 signaling leading to endothelial cell activation and vaso-occlusion in murine sickle cell disease. *Blood* 123(3):377–390, 2014.

1032. Amann K, et al: Beneficial effects of integrin alphavbeta3-blocking RGD peptides in early but not late phase of experimental glomerulonephritis. *Nephrol Dial Transplant* 27(5):1755–1768, 2012.

1033. Reiser J: Circulating permeability factor suPAR: From concept to discovery to clinic. *Trans Am Clin Climatol Assoc* 124:133–138, 2013.

1034. Gerber EE, et al: Integrin-modulating therapy prevents fibrosis and autoimmunity in mouse models of scleroderma. *Nature* 503(7474):126–130, 2013.

1035. Andrews RK, Lopez JA, Berndt MC: The GPIb-IX-V complex, in Platelets, edited by AD Michelson, pp 145–164. Academic Press, San Diego, 2007.

1036. Clemetson KJ, Clemetson JM: Platelet GPIb complex as a target for anti-thrombotic drug development. *Thromb Haemost* 99(3):473–479, 2008.

1037. Li R, Emsley J: The organizing principle of the platelet glycoprotein Ib-IX-V complex. *J Thromb Haemost* 11(4):605–614, 2013.

1038. Lopez JA, et al: Bernard-Soulier syndrome. *Blood* 91(12):4397–4418, 1998.

1039. Lopez JH, et al: The α and β chains of human platelet glycoprotein Ib are both transmembrane proteins containing a leucine-rich amino acid sequence. *Proc Natl Acad Sci U S A* 85:2135–2139, 1988.

1040. McEwan PA, et al: Quaternary organization of GPIb-IX complex and insights into Bernard-Soulier syndrome revealed by the structures of GPIbbeta and a GPIbbeta/GPIX chimera. *Blood* 118(19):5292–5301, 2011.

1041. Ozaki Y, et al: Platelet GPIb-IX-V-dependent signaling. *J Thromb Haemost* 3(8):1745–1751, 2005.

1042. Roth GJ: Developing relationships: Arterial platelet adhesion, glycoprotein Ib, and leucine-rich glycoproteins. *Blood* 77:5–19, 1991.

1043. Zhou L, Yang W, Li R: Analysis of inter-subunit contacts reveals the structural malleability of extracellular domains in platelet glycoprotein Ib-IX complex. *J Thromb Haemost* 12(1):82–89, 2014.

1044. Du X, Beutler L, Ruan C, et al: Glycoprotein Ib and glycoprotein IX are fully complexed in the intact platelet membrane. *Blood* 69(5):1524–1527, 1987.

1045. Hickey MJ, Deaven LL, Roth GJ: Human platelet glycoprotein IX. Characterization of cDNA and localization of the gene to chromosome 3. *FEBS Lett* 274:189–192, 1987, 1991.

1046. Hickey MJ, Williams SA, Roth GJ: Human platelet GPIX: An adhesive prototype of leucine-rich glycoproteins with flank-center-flank structures. *Proc Natl Acad Sci U S A* 86:6773–6777, 1989.

1047. Lopez JA, et al: Efficient plasma membrane expression of a functional platelet glycoprotein Ib-IX complex requires the presence of its three subunits. *J Biol Chem* 267:12851–12859, 1992.

1048. Bastian LS, et al: Analysis of the megakaryocyte glycoprotein IX promoter identifies positive and negative regulatory domains and functional GATA and Ets sites. *J Biol Chem* 271(31):18554–18560, 1996.

1049. Block KL, Poncz M: Platelet glycoprotein IIb gene expression as a model of megakaryocyte-specific expression. *Stem Cells*, 13(2):135–145, 1995.

1050. Hashimoto Y, Ware J: Identification of essential GATA and Ets binding motifs within the promoter of the platelet glycoprotein Ib alpha gene. *J Biol Chem* 270(41):24532–24539, 1995.

1051. Krause DS, Perkins AS: Gotta find GATA a friend. *Nat Med* 3(9):960–961, 1997.

1052. Lemarchandel V, et al: GATA and Ets cis-acting sequences mediate megakaryocyte-specific expression. *Mol Cell Biol* 13(1):668–676, 1993.

1053. Martin F, et al: The transcription factor GATA-1 regulates the promoter activity of the platelet glycoprotein IIb gene. *J Biol Chem* 268(29):21606–21612, 1993.

1054. Prandini MH, et al: Characterization of a specific erythromegakaryocytic enhancer within the glycoprotein IIb promoter. *J Biol Chem* 267(15):10370–10374, 1992.

1055. Tsang AP, et al: FOG, a multitype zinc finger protein, acts as a cofactor for transcription factor GATA-1 in erythroid and megakaryocytic differentiation. *Cell* 90(1):109–119, 1997.

1056. Uzan G, et al: Tissue-specific expression of the platelet GPIIb gene. *J Biol Chem* 266(14):8932–8939, 1991.

1057. Lopez JA, Ludwig EW, McCarthy BJ: Polymorphism of human glycoprotein Ibα results from a variable number of repeats of a 13-amino acid sequence in the mucin-like macroglycopeptide region. Structure function implications. *J Biol Chem* 267:10055–10061, 1992.

1058. Carlsson LE, et al: Polymorphisms of the human platelet antigens HPA-1, HPA-2, and HPA-5 on the platelet receptors for fibrinogen (GPIIb/IIIa), von Willebrand factor (GPIb/IX), and collagen (GPIa/IIa) are not correlated with an increased risk for stroke. *Stroke* 28(7):1392–1395, 1997.

1059. Shanker J, et al: Platelet function and antiplatelet therapy in cardiovascular disease: Implications of genetic polymorphisms. *Curr Vasc Pharmacol* 9(4):479–489, 2011.

1060. Kaski S, Kekomaki R, Partanen J: Systematic screening for genetic polymorphism in human platelet glycoprotein Ibalpha. *Immunogenetics* 44(3):170–176, 1996.

1061. Suzuki K, et al: StyI polymorphism at nucleotide 1610 in the human platelet glycoprotein Ib alpha gene. *Jpn J Hum Genet* 41(4):419–421, 1996.

1062. Afshar-Kharghan V, et al: Kozak sequence polymorphism of the glycoprotein (GP) Ibalpha gene is a major determinant of the plasma membrane levels of the platelet GP Ib- IX-V complex. *Blood* 94(1):186–191, 1999.

1063. Baker RI, et al: Platelet glycoprotein Ibalpha Kozak polymorphism is associated with an increased risk of ischemic stroke. *Blood* 98(1):36–40, 2001.

1064. Carlsson LE, et al: Platelet receptor and clotting factor polymorphisms as genetic risk factors for thromboembolic complications in heparin-induced thrombocytopenia. *Pharmacogenetics* 13(5):253–258, 2003.

1065. Douglas H, et al: Platelet membrane glycoprotein Ibalpha gene -5T/C Kozak sequence polymorphism as an independent risk factor for the occurrence of coronary thrombosis. *Heart* 87(1):70–74, 2002.

1066. Jilma-Stohlawetz P, et al: Glycoprotein Ib polymorphisms influence platelet plug formation under high shear rates. *Br J Haematol* 120(4):652–655, 2003.

1067. Kenny D, et al: Platelet glycoprotein Ib alpha receptor polymorphisms and recurrent ischaemic events in acute coronary syndrome patients. *J Thromb Thrombolysis* 13(1):13–19, 2002.

1068. Meisel C, et al: Role of Kozak sequence polymorphism of platelet glycoprotein Ibalpha as a risk factor for coronary artery disease and catheter interventions. *J Am Coll Cardiol* 38(4):1023–1027, 2001.

1069. Ozelo MC, et al: Platelet glycoprotein Ibα polymorphisms modulate the risk for myocardial infarction. *Thromb Haemost* 92(2):384–386, 2004.

1070. Rosenberg N, et al: Effects of platelet membrane glycoprotein polymorphisms on the risk of myocardial infarction in young males. *Isr Med Assoc J* 4(6):411–414, 2002.

1071. Tsuji T, et al: The carbohydrate moiety of human platelet glycocalicin. *J Biol Chem* 258(10):6335–6339, 1983.

1072. Fox JEB, Aggerbeck LP, Berndt MC: Structure of the glycoprotein Ib-IX complex from platelet membranes. *J Biol Chem* 263:4882–4890, 1988.

1073. Solum NO, et al: Platelet glycocalicin: Its membrane association in solvent and aqueous media. *Biochim Biophys Acta* 597:235–246, 1990.

1074. Coller BS, et al: Evidence that glycocalicin circulates in normal plasma. *J Clin Invest* 73:794–799, 1984.

1075. Liang X, et al: Specific inhibition of ectodomain shedding of glycoprotein Ibalpha by targeting its juxtamembrane shedding cleavage site. *J Thromb Haemost* 11(12):2155–2162, 2013.

1076. Bergmeier W, et al: Tumor necrosis factor-alpha-converting enzyme (ADAM17) mediates GPIbalpha shedding from platelets *in vitro* and *in vivo*. *Circ Res* 95(7):677–683, 2004.

1077. Mo X, et al: Transmembrane and trans-subunit regulation of ectodomain shedding of platelet glycoprotein Ibalpha. *J Biol Chem* 285(42):32096–32104, 2010.

1078. Wang Z, et al: The role of calpain in the regulation of ADAM17-dependent GPIbalpha ectodomain shedding. *Arch Biochem Biophys* 495(2):136–143, 2010.

1079. Zhang P, et al: The role of intraplatelet reactive oxygen species in the regulation of platelet glycoprotein Ibalpha ectodomain shedding. *Thromb Res* 132(6):696–701, 2013.

1080. Beer JH, Buchi L, Steiner B, Glycocalicin: A new assay—the normal plasma levels and its potential usefulness in selected diseases. *Blood* 83:691–702, 1994.

1081. Himmelfarb J, et al: Elevated plasma glycocalicin levels and decreased ristocetin-induced platelet agglutination in hemodialysis patients. *Am J Kidney Dis* 32(1):132–138, 1998.

1082. Kunishima S, et al: Rapid detection of plasma glycocalicin by a latex agglutination test. A useful adjunct in the differential diagnosis of thrombocytopenia. *Am J Clin Pathol* 100(5):579–584, 1993.

1083. Kurata Y, et al: Diagnostic value of tests for reticulated platelets, plasma glycocalicin, and thrombopoietin levels for discriminating between hyperdestructive and hypoplastic thrombocytopenia. *Am J Clin Pathol* 115(5):656–664, 2001.

1084. Steffan A, et al: Glycocalicin in the diagnosis and management of immune thrombocytopenia. *Eur J Haematol* 61(2):77–83, 1998.

1085. Steinberg MH, Kelton JG, Coller BS: Plasma glycocalicin. An aid in the classification of thrombocytopenic disorders. *N Engl J Med* 317(17):1037–1042, 1987.

1086. Kalomiris EL, Coller BS: Thiol-specific probes indicate that the alpha chain of platelet glycoprotein Ib is a transmembrane protein with a reactive endofacial sulfhydryl group. *Biochemistry* 24:5430–5436, 1985.

1087. Muszbek L, Laposata M: Glycoprotein Ib and glycoprotein IX in human platelets are acylated with palmitic acid through thioester linkages. *J Biol Chem* 264(17):9716–9719, 1989.

1088. Du X, Fox JE, Pei S: Identification of a binding sequence for the 14–3-3 protein within the cytoplasmic domain of the adhesion receptor, platelet glycoprotein Ib alpha. *J Biol Chem* 271(13):7362–7367, 1996.

1089. Andrews RK, et al: Binding of purified 14–3-3 zeta signaling protein to discrete amino acid sequences within the cytoplasmic domain of the platelet membrane glycoprotein Ib-IX-V complex. *Biochemistry* 37(2):638–647, 1998.

1090. Calverley DC, Kavanagh TJ, Roth GJ: Human signaling protein 14–3-3zeta interacts with platelet glycoprotein Ib subunits Ibalpha and Ibbeta. *Blood* 91(4):1295–1303, 1998.

1091. Wardell MR, et al: Platelet glycoprotein Ib beta is phosphorylated on serine 166 by cyclic AMP-dependent protein kinase. *J Biol Chem* 264(26):15656–15661, 1989.

1092. Andrews RK, Fox JE: Identification of a region in the cytoplasmic domain of the platelet membrane glycoprotein Ib-IX complex that binds to purified actin-binding protein. *J Biol Chem* 267(26):18605–18611, 1992.

1093. Andrews RK, et al: The glycoprotein Ib-IX-V complex in platelet adhesion and signaling. *Thromb Haemost* 82:357–364, 1999.

1094. Falet H: New insights into the versatile roles of platelet FlnA. *Platelets* 24(1):1–5, 2013.

1095. Kanaji T, et al: GPIbalpha regulates platelet size by controlling the subcellular localization of filamin. *Blood* 119(12):2906–2913, 2012.

1096. Coller BS: Inhibition of von Willebrand factor-dependent platelet function by increased platelet cyclic AMP and its prevention by cytoskeleton-disrupting agents. *Blood* 57:846–855, 1981.

1097. Coller BS: Effects of tertiary amine local anesthetics on von Willebrand factor-dependent platelet function: Alteration of membrane reactivity and degradation of GPIb by a calcium-dependent protease(s). *Blood* 248:1355–1357, 1982.

1098. Dong JF, et al: The cytoplasmic domain of glycoprotein (GP) Ibalpha constrains the lateral diffusion of the GP Ib-IX complex and modulates von Willebrand factor binding. *Biochemistry* 36(41):12421–12427, 1997.

1099. Delaney MK, et al: The role of Rac1 in glycoprotein Ib-IX-mediated signal transduction and integrin activation. *Arterioscler Thromb Vasc Biol* 32(11):2761–2768, 2012.

1100. Estevez B, et al: LIM kinase-1 selectively promotes glycoprotein Ib-IX-mediated TXA2 synthesis, platelet activation, and thrombosis. *Blood* 121(22):4586–4594, 2013.

1101. Munday AD, Berndt MC, Mitchell CA: Phosphoinositide 3-kinase forms a complex with platelet membrane glycoprotein Ib-IX-V complex and 14–3-3zeta. *Blood* 96(2):577–584, 2000.

1102. Falati S, Edmead CE, Poole AW: Glycoprotein Ib-V-IX, a receptor for von Willebrand factor, couples physically and functionally to the Fc receptor γ-chain, Fyn, and Lyn to activate human platelets. *Blood* 94(5):1648–1656, 1999.

1103. Sullam PM, et al: Physical proximity and functional interplay of the glycoprotein Ib-IX-V complex and the Fc receptor FcgammaRIIA on the platelet plasma membrane. *J Biol Chem* 273(9):5331–5336, 1998.

1104. Watson SP, et al: The role of ITAM- and ITIM-coupled receptors in platelet activation by collagen. *Thromb Haemost* 86(1):276–288, 2001.

1105. Wu Y, et al: Role of Fc receptor gamma-chain in platelet glycoprotein Ib-mediated signaling. *Blood* 97(12):3836–3845, 2001.

1106. Ozaki Y, Suzuki-Inoue K, Inoue O: Platelet receptors activated via mulitimerization: Glycoprotein VI, GPIb-IX-V, and CLEC-2. *J Thromb Haemost* 11 Suppl 1:330–339, 2013.

1107. Blenner MA, Dong X, Springer TA: Structural basis of regulation of von Willebrand factor binding to glycoprotein Ib. *J Biol Chem* 289(9):5565–5579, 2014.

1108. Dumas JJ, et al: Crystal structure of the wild-type von Willebrand factor A1-glycoprotein Ibalpha complex reveals conformation differences with a complex bearing von Willebrand disease mutations. *J Biol Chem* 279(22):23327–23334, 2004.

1109. Huizinga EG, et al: Structures of glycoprotein Ibalpha and its complex with von Willebrand factor A1 domain. *Science* 297(5584):1176–1179, 2002.

1110. Uff S, et al: Crystal structure of the platelet glycoprotein Ib(alpha) N-terminal domain reveals an unmasking mechanism for receptor activation. *J Biol Chem* 277(38):35657–35663, 2002.

1111. Shen Y, et al: Leucine-rich repeats 2–4 (Leu60-Glu128) of platelet glycoprotein Ibalpha regulate shear-dependent cell adhesion to von Willebrand factor. *J Biol Chem* 281(36):26419–26423, 2006.

1112. Shen Y, et al: Requirement of leucine-rich repeats of glycoprotein (GP) Ibalpha for shear-dependent and static binding of von Willebrand factor to the platelet membrane GP Ib-IX-V complex. *Blood* 95(3):903–910, 2000.

1113. Springer TA, von Willebrand factor, Jedi knight of the bloodstream. *Blood* 124(9):1412–1425, 2014.

1114. Tang J, et al: Mutation in the leucine-rich repeat C-flanking region of platelet glycoprotein Ibbeta impairs assembly of von Willebrand factor receptor. *Thromb Haemost* 92(1):75–88, 2004.

1115. Berndt MC, et al: Identification of aspartic acid 514 through glutamic acid 542 as a glycoprotein Ib-IX complex receptor recognition sequence in von Willebrand factor. Mechanism of modulation of von Willebrand factor by ristocetin and botrocetin. *Biochemistry* 31(45):11144–11151, 1992.

1116. Coller BS: Platelet von Willebrand factor interactions, in *Platelet Glycoproteins*, edited by J George, D Phillips, A Nurden, pp 215–244. Plenum, New York, 1985.

1117. Papi M, et al: Ristocetin-induced self-aggregation of von Willebrand factor. *Eur Biophys J* 39(12):1597–1603, 2010.

1118. Scott JP, Montgomery RR, Retzinger GS: Dimeric ristocetin flocculates proteins, binds to platelets, mediates von Willebrand factor-dependent agglutination of platelets. *J Biol Chem* 266(13):8149–8155, 1991.

1119. Andrews RK, et al: Purification of botrocetin from *Bothrops jararaca* venom. Analysis of the botrocetin-mediated interaction between von Willebrand factor and the human platelet membrane glycoprotein Ib-IX complex. *Biochemistry* 28(21):8317–8326, 1989.

1120. Olson JD, et al: Adhesion of platelets to purified solid-phase von Willebrand factor: Effect of wall shear rate, ADP, thrombin, and ristocetin. *J Lab Clin Med* 114:6–18, 1989.

1121. Ruggeri ZM, Von Willebrand factor, platelets and endothelial cell interactions. *J Thromb Haemost* 1(7):1335–1342, 2003.

1122. Sixma JJ: Interaction of blood platelets with the vessel wall, in *Haemostasis and Thrombosis*, edited by AL Bloom, CD Forbes, DP Thomas, EGD Tuddenham, pp 259–285. Churchill Livingstone, London, England, 1994.

1123. Parker RI, Gralnick HR: Fibrin monomer induces binding of endogenous VWF to the glycocalicin portion of platelet glycoprotein Ib. *Blood* 70:1589–1594, 1987.

1124. Sakariassen KS, et al: Role of platelet membrane glycoproteins and von Willebrand factor in adhesion of platelets to subendothelium and collagen. *Ann N Y Acad Sci* 516:52–65, 1987.

1125. Sakariassen KS, et al: The role of platelet membrane glycoproteins Ib and IIb-IIIa in platelet adherence to human artery subendothelium. *Br J Haematol* 63:681–691, 1986.

1126. Ikeda Y, et al: Importance of fibrinogen and platelet membrane glycoprotein IIb/IIIa in shear-induced platelet aggregation. *Thromb Res* 51:157–163, 1988.

1127. Siediecki CA, et al: Shear-dependent changes in the three-dimensional structure of human von Willebrand factor. *Blood* 88(8):2939–2950, 1996.

1128. Yago T, et al: Platelet glycoprotein Ibalpha forms catch bonds with human WT VWF but not with type 2B von Willebrand disease VWF. *J Clin Invest* 118(9):3195–3207, 2008.

1129. Jamieson GA: The activation of platelets by thrombin: A model for activation by high and moderate affinity receptor pathways. *Prog Clin Biol Res* 283:137–158, 1988.

1130. Ruggeri Z: The platelet glycoprotein Ib-IX complex. *Prog Hemost Thromb* 10:35–68, 1991.

1131. Katagiri Y, et al: Localization of von Willebrand factor and thrombin-interactive domains in human platelet glycoprotein Ib. *Thromb Haemost* 63:122–126, 1990.

1132. Zarpellon A, et al: Binding of alpha-thrombin to surface-anchored platelet glycoprotein Ib(alpha) sulfotyrosines through a two-site mechanism involving exosite I. *Proc Natl Acad Sci U S A* 108(21):8628–8633, 2011.

1133. Harmon JT, Jamieson GA: The glycocalicin portion of platelet glycoprotein Ib expresses both high and moderate affinity receptor sites of thrombin. A soluble radioreceptor assay for the injection of thrombin with platelets. *J Biol Chem* 261:13224–13229, 1986.

1134. Shrimpton CN, et al: Localization of the adhesion receptor glycoprotein Ib-IX-V complex to lipid rafts is required for platelet adhesion and activation. *J Exp Med Medicine (Baltimore)* 196(8):1057–1066, 2002.

1135. Adam F, et al: Thrombin-induced platelet PAR4 activation: Role of glycoprotein Ib and ADP. *J Thromb Haemost* 1(4):798–804, 2003.

1136. De Candia E, et al: Binding of thrombin to glycoprotein Ib accelerates the hydrolysis of Par-1 on intact platelets. *J Biol Chem* 276(7):4692–4698, 2001.

1137. Frenette PS, et al: Platelet-endothelial interactions in inflamed mesenteric venules. *Blood* 91(4):1318–1325, 1998.

1138. Frenette PS, et al: P-Selectin glycoprotein ligand 1 (PSGL-1) is expressed on platelets and can mediate platelet-endothelial interactions *in vivo*. *J Exp Med* 191(8):1413–1422, 2000.

1139. Bradford HN, et al: Human kininogens regulate thrombin binding to platelets through the glycoprotein Ib-IX-V complex. *Blood* 90(4):1508–1515, 1997.

1140. Bradford HN, Pixley RA, Colman RW: Human factor XII binding to the glycoprotein Ib-IX-V complex inhibits thrombin-induced platelet aggregation. *J Biol Chem* 275(30):22756–22763, 2000.

1141. Baglia FA, et al: Factor XI binding to the platelet glycoprotein Ib-IX-V complex promotes factor XI activation by thrombin. *J Biol Chem* 277(3):1662–1668, 2002.

1142. Simon DI, et al: Platelet glycoprotein Ibα is a counterreceptor for the leukocyte integrin Mac-1 (CD11b/CD18). *J Exp Med* 192(2):193–204, 2000.

1143. Corken A, et al: Platelet glycoprotein Ib-IX as a regulator of systemic inflammation. *Arterioscler Thromb Vasc Biol* 34(5):996–1001, 2014.

1144. Yin H, et al: Role for platelet glycoprotein Ib-IX and effects of its inhibition in endotoxemia-induced thrombosis, thrombocytopenia, and mortality. *Arterioscler Thromb Vasc Biol* 33(11):2529–2537, 2013.

1145. Jain S, et al: Platelet glycoprotein Ib alpha supports experimental lung metastasis. *Proc Natl Acad Sci U S A* 104(21):9024–9028, 2007.

1146. Mo X, et al: Transmembrane domains are critical to the interaction between platelet glycoprotein V and glycoprotein Ib-IX complex. *J Thromb Haemost* 10(9):1875–1886, 2012.

1147. Modderman PW, et al: Glycoproteins V and Ib-IX form a noncovalent complex in the platelet membrane. *J Biol Chem* 267:364–369, 1992.

1148. Dong JF, Gao S, Lopez JA: Synthesis, assembly, and intracellular transport of the platelet glycoprotein Ib-IX-V complex. *J Biol Chem* 273(47):31449–31454, 1998.

1149. McGowan EB, Ding A, Detwiler TC: Correlation of thrombin-induced glycoprotein V hydrolysis and platelet activation. *J Biol Chem* 258:11243.

1150. Ramakrishnan V, et al: Increased thrombin responsiveness in platelets from mice lacking glycoprotein V. *Proc Natl Acad Sci U S A* 1999;96(23):13336–13341, 1983.

1151. Ramakrishnan V, et al: A thrombin receptor function for platelet glycoprotein Ib-IX unmasked by cleavage of glycoprotein V. *Proc Natl Acad Sci U S A* 98(4):1823–1828, 2001.

1152. Jones CI, Moraes LA, Gibbins JM: Regulation of platelet biology by platelet endothelial cell adhesion molecule-1. *Platelets* 23(5):331–335, 2012.

1153. Newman PJ, et al: PECAM-1 (CD31) cloning and relation to adhesion molecules of the immunoglobulin gene superfamily. *Science* 247:1219–1222, 1990.

1154. Novinska MS, et al: PECAM-1, in *Platelets*, edited by AD Michelson, pp 221–230. Academic Press, San Diego, 2002.

1155. Privratsky JR, Newman DK, Newman PJ: PECAM-1: Conflicts of interest in inflammation. *Life Sci* 87(3–4):69–82, 2010.

1156. Metzelaar MJ, et al: Biochemical characterization of PECAM-1 (CD31 antigen) on human platelets. *Thromb Haemost* 66(6):700–707, 1991.

1157. Paddock C, et al: Residues within a lipid-associated segment of the PECAM-1 cytoplasmic domain are susceptible to inducible, sequential phosphorylation. *Blood* 117(22):6012–6023, 2011.

1158. Jackson DE, et al: The protein-tyrosine phosphatase SHP-2 binds platelet/endothelial cell adhesion molecule-1 (PECAM-1) and forms a distinct signaling complex during platelet aggregation. Evidence for a mechanistic link between PECAM-1- and integrin-mediated cellular signaling. *J Biol Chem* 272(11):6986–6993, 1997.

1159. Crockett J, Newman DK, Newman PJ: PECAM-1 functions as a negative regulator of laminin-induced platelet activation. *J Thromb Haemost* 8(7):1584–1593, 2010.

1160. Jones CI, et al: PECAM-1 expression and activity negatively regulate multiple platelet signaling pathways. *FEBS Lett* 583(22):3618–3624, 2009.

1161. Varon D, et al: Platelet/endothelial cell adhesion molecule-1 serves as a costimulatory agonist receptor that modulates integrin-dependent adhesion and aggregation of human platelets. *Blood* 91(2):500–507, 1998.

1162. Wee JL, Jackson DE: The Ig-ITIM superfamily member PECAM-1 regulates the "outside-in" signaling properties of integrin alpha(IIb)beta3 in platelets. *Blood* 106(12):3816–3823, 2005.

1163. Jones CI, et al: Platelet endothelial cell adhesion molecule-1 inhibits platelet response to thrombin and von Willebrand factor by regulating the internalization of glycoprotein Ib via AKT/glycogen synthase kinase-3/dynamin and integrin alphaIIbbeta3. *Arterioscler Thromb Vasc Biol* 34(9):1968–1976, 2014.

1164. Albelda SM, et al: Molecular and cellular properties of PECAM-1 (endoCAM/CD31): A novel vascular cell-cell adhesion molecule. *J Cell Biol* 114(5):1059–1068, 1991.

1165. DeLisser HM, et al: Platelet/endothelial cell adhesion molecule-1 (CD31)-mediated cellular aggregation involves cell surface glycosaminoglycans. *J Biol Chem* 268(21):16037–16046, 1993.

1166. Washington AV, et al: A TREM family member, TLT-1, is found exclusively in the alpha-granules of megakaryocytes and platelets. *Blood* 104(4):1042–1047, 2004.

1167. Kahn ML, Platelet-collagen responses: Molecular basis and therapeutic promise. *Semin Thromb Hemost* 30(4):419–425, 2004.

1168. Moroi M, Jung SM: Platelet glycoprotein VI: Its structure and function. *Thromb Res* 114(4):221–233, 2004.

1169. Schulz C, et al: EMMPRIN (CD147/basigin) mediates platelet-monocyte interactions in vivo and augments monocyte recruitment to the vascular wall. *J Thromb Haemost* 9(5):1007–1019, 2011.

1170. Arthur JF, et al: Platelet receptor redox regulation. *Platelets* 19(1):1–8, 2008.

1171. Jung SM, et al: Constitutive dimerization of glycoprotein VI (GPVI) in resting platelets is essential for binding to collagen and activation in flowing blood. *J Biol Chem* 287(35):30000–30013, 2012.

1172. Matus V, et al: An adenine insertion in exon 6 of human GP6 generates a truncated protein associated with a bleeding disorder in four Chilean families. *J Thromb Haemost* 11(9):1751–1759, 2013.

1173. Arthur JF, Dunkley S, Andrews RK: Platelet glycoprotein VI-related clinical defects. *Br J Haematol* 139(3):363–372, 2007.

1174. Dumont B, et al: Absence of collagen-induced platelet activation caused by compound heterozygous GPVI mutations. *Blood* 114(9):1900–1903, 2009.

1175. Hermans C, et al: A compound heterozygous mutation in glycoprotein VI in a patient with a bleeding disorder. *J Thromb Haemost* 7(8):1356–1363, 2009.

1176. Nurden P, et al: An acquired inhibitor to the GPVI platelet collagen receptor in a patient with lupus nephritis. *J Thromb Haemost* 7(9):1541–1549, 2009.

1177. Ezumi Y, Uchiyama T, Takayama H, Molecular cloning, genomic structure, chromosomal localization, and alternative splice forms of the platelet collagen receptor glycoprotein VI. *Biochem Biophys Res Commun* 277(1):27–36, 2000.

1178. Kotulicova D, et al: Variability of GP6 gene in patients with sticky platelet syndrome and deep venous thrombosis and/or pulmonary embolism. *Blood Coagul Fibrinolysis* 23(6):543–547, 2012.

1179. Gibbins J, et al: Tyrosine phosphorylation of the Fc receptor gamma-chain in collagen- stimulated platelets. *J Biol Chem* 271(30):18095–18099, 1996.

1180. Tsuji M, et al: A novel association of Fc receptor gamma-chain with glycoprotein VI and their co-expression as a collagen receptor in human platelets. *J Biol Chem* 272(38):23528–23531, 1997.

1181. Chacko GW, et al: Clustering of the platelet Fc gamma receptor induces noncovalent association with the tyrosine kinase p72syk. *J Biol Chem* 269(51):32435–32440, 1994.

1182. Qiu WQ, et al: Organization of the human and mouse low-affinity Fc gamma R genes: Duplication and recombination. *Science* 248(4956):732–735, 1990.

1183. Boylan B, et al: Identification of FcgammaRIIa as the ITAM-bearing receptor mediating alphaIIbbeta3 outside-in integrin signaling in human platelets. *Blood* 112(7):2780–2786, 2008.

1184. Zhi H, et al: Cooperative integrin/ITAM signaling in platelets enhances thrombus formation in vitro and in vivo. *Blood* 121(10):1858–1867, 2013.

1185. Yeung J, et al: Platelet 12-LOX is essential for FcgammaRIIa-mediated platelet activation. *Blood* 124(14):2271–2279, 2014.

1186. Berlacher MD, et al: FcgammaRIIa ligation induces platelet hypersensitivity to thrombotic stimuli. *Am J Pathol* 182(1):244–254, 2013.

1187. Rosenfeld SI, et al: Human platelet Fc receptor for immunoglobulin G. Identification as a 40,000-molecular-weight membrane protein shared by monocytes. *J Clin Invest* 76(6):2317–2322, 1985.

1188. Rosenfeld SI, et al: Human Fc gamma receptors: Stable inter-donor variation in quantitative expression on platelets correlates with functional responses. *J Immunol* 138(9):2869–2873, 1987.

1189. Anderson GP JG. van de Winkel, Anderson CL: Anti-GPIIb/IIIa (CD41) monoclonal antibody-induced platelet activation requires Fc receptor-dependent cell-cell interaction. *Br J Haematol* 79(1):75–83, 1991.

1190. Gratacap MP, et al: Phosphatidylinositol 3,4,5-trisphosphate-dependent stimulation of phospholipase C-gamma2 is an early key event in FcgammaRIIA-mediated activation of human platelets. *J Biol Chem* 273(38):24314–24321, 1998.

1191. Hildreth JE, Derr D, Azorsa DO: Characterization of a novel self-associating Mr 40,000 platelet glycoprotein. *Blood* 77(1):121–132, 1991.

1192. Nazi I, Arnold DM, Smith JW, et al: FcgammaRIIa proteolysis as a diagnostic biomarker for heparin-induced thrombocytopenia. *J Thromb Haemost* 11(6):1146–1153, 2013.

1193. Nazi I, et al: The association between platelet activation and FcgammaRIIa proteolysis. *J Thromb Haemost* 9(4):885–887, 2011.

1194. Peerschke EI, Ghebrehiwet B: C1q augments platelet activation in response to aggregated Ig. *J Immunol* 159(11):5594–5598, 1997.

1195. Boilard E, et al: Influenza virus H1N1 activates platelets through FcgammaRIIA signaling and thrombin generation. *Blood* 123(18):2854–2863, 2014.

1196. Tilley DO, et al: Glycoprotein Ibalpha and FcgammaRIIa play key roles in platelet activation by the colonizing bacterium, *Streptococcus oralis. J Thromb Haemost* 11(5): 941–950, 2013.

1197. Mitrugno A, et al: A novel and essential role for FcgammaRIIa in cancer cell-induced platelet activation. *Blood* 123(2):249–260, 2014.

1198. Chong BH, et al: Increased expression of platelet IgG Fc receptors in immune heparin-induced thrombocytopenia. *Blood* 81(4):988–993, 1993.

1199. Parren PW, et al: On the interaction of IgG subclasses with the low affinity Fc gamma RIIa (CD32) on human monocytes, neutrophils, and platelets. Analysis of a functional polymorphism to human IgG2. *J Clin Invest* 90(4):1537–1546, 1992.

1200. Warmerdam PA, et al: Polymorphism of the human Fc gamma receptor II (CD32): Molecular basis and functional aspects. *Immunobiology* 185(2–4):175–182, 1992.

1201. Chen J, et al: Platelet FcgammaRIIA His131Arg polymorphism and platelet function: Antibodies to platelet-bound fibrinogen induce platelet activation. *J Thromb Haemost* 1(2):355–362, 2003.

1202. Carlsson LE, et al: Heparin-induced thrombocytopenia: New insights into the impact of the FcgammaRIIa-R-H131 polymorphism. *Blood* 92(5):1526–1531, 1998.

1203. Denomme GA, et al: Activation of platelets by sera containing IgG1 heparin-dependent antibodies: An explanation for the predominance of the Fc gammaRIIa "low responder" (his131) gene in patients with heparin-induced thrombocytopenia. *J Lab Clin Med* 130(3):278–284, 1997.

1204. Gruel Y, et al: The homozygous FcgammaRIIIa-158V genotype is a risk factor for heparin-induced thrombocytopenia in patients with antibodies to heparin-platelet factor 4 complexes. *Blood* 104(9):2791–2793, 2004.

1205. Kannan M, et al: An update on the prevalence and characterization of H-PF4 antibodies in Asian-Indian patients. *Semin Thromb Hemost* 35(3):337–343, 2009.

1206. Trikalinos TA, Karassa FB, Ioannidis JP: Meta-analysis of the association between low-affinity Fcgamma receptor gene polymorphisms and hematologic and autoimmune disease. *Blood* 98(5):1634–1635, 2001.

1207. Williams Y, et al: Correlation of platelet Fc gammaRIIA polymorphism in refractory idiopathic (immune) thrombocytopenic purpura. *Br J Haematol* 101(4):779–782, 1998.

1208. Diacovo TG, et al: A functional integrin ligand on the surface of platelets: Intercellular adhesion molecule-2. *J Clin Invest* 94(3):1243–1251, 1994.

1209. Hasegawa S, et al: Functional expression of the high affinity receptor for IgE (FcepsilonRI) in human platelets and its' intracellular expression in human megakaryocytes. *Blood* 93(8):2543–2551, 1999.

1210. Joseph M, et al: Expression and functions of the high-affinity IgE receptor on human platelets and megakaryocyte precursors. *Eur J Immunol* 27(9):2212–2218, 1997.

1211. Kasperska-Zajac A, Rogala B: Platelet function in anaphylaxis. *J Investig Allergol Clin Immunol* 16(1):1–4, 2006.

1212. Gupta SK, Pillarisetti K, Ohlstein EH: Platelet agonist F11 receptor is a member of the immunoglobulin superfamily and identical with junctional adhesion molecule (JAM): Regulation of expression in human endothelial cells and macrophages. *IUBMB Life* 50(1):51–56, 2000.

1213. Kornecki E, et al: Activation of human platelets by a stimulatory monoclonal antibody. *J Biol Chem* 265(17):10042–10048, 1990.

1214. Naik UP, et al: Characterization and chromosomal localization of JAM-1, a platelet receptor for a stimulatory monoclonal antibody. *J Cell Sci* 114(Pt 3):539–547, 2001.

1215. Sobocka MB, et al: Cloning of the human platelet F11 receptor: A cell adhesion molecule member of the immunoglobulin superfamily involved in platelet aggregation. *Blood* 95(8):2600–2609, 2000.

1216. Sobocki T, et al: Genomic structure, organization and promoter analysis of the human F11R/F11 receptor/junctional adhesion molecule-1/JAM-A. *Gene* 366(1):128–144, 2006.

1217. Naik MU, et al: JAM-A protects from thrombosis by suppressing integrin alphaIIbbeta3-dependent outside-in signaling in platelets. *Blood* 119(14):3352–3360, 2012.

1218. Naik MU, Caplan JL, Naik UP: Junctional adhesion molecule-A suppresses platelet integrin alphaIIbbeta3 signaling by recruiting Csk to the integrin-c-Src complex. *Blood* 123(9):1393–1402, 2014.

1219. Stellos K, et al: Expression of junctional adhesion molecule-C on the surface of platelets supports adhesion, but not differentiation, of human CD34 cells *in vitro. Cell Physiol Biochem* 29(1–2):153–162, 2012.

1220. McEver RP: Properties of GMP-140, an inducible granule membrane protein of platelets and endothelium. *Blood Cells* 16:73–83, 1990.

1221. McEver RP, P-selectin/PSGL-1 and other interactions between platelets, leukocytes, and endothelium, in *Platelets*, edited by AD Michelson, p 231. Academic Press, San Diego, 2007.

1222. McEver RP, Beckstead JH, Moore KL, et al: GMP-140, a platelet -granule membrane protein, is also synthesized by vascular endothelial cells and is localized in Weibel-Palade bodies. *J Clin Invest* 84(1):92–99, 1989.

1223. Yong AS, et al: Intracoronary shear-related up-regulation of platelet P-selectin and platelet-monocyte aggregation despite the use of aspirin and clopidogrel. *Blood* 2011;117(1):11–20, 1989.

1224. Abrams C, Shattil SJ: Immunological detection of activated platelets in clinical disorders. *J Thromb Haemost* 65(5):467–473, 1991.

1225. Haskard DO: Adhesive proteins, in *Haemostasis and Thrombosis*, edited by AL Bloom, CD Forbes, DP Thomas, EGD Tuddenham, pp 233–257. Churchill Livingstone, England, 1994.

1226. Ishiwata N, et al: Alternatively spliced isoform of P-selectin is present *in vivo* as a soluble molecule. *J Biol Chem* 269(38):23708–23715, 1994.

1227. Hartwell DW, et al: Role of P-selectin cytoplasmic domain in granular targeting in vivo and in early inflammatory responses. *J Cell Biol* 143(4):1129–1141, 1998.

1228. Geng JG, et al: Rapid neutrophil adhesion to activated endothelium mediated by GMP-140. *Nature* 343:757–760, 1990.

1229. Handa K, et al: Selectin GMP-140 (CD62;PADGEM) binds to sialosyl-Le(a) and sialosyl-Le(x), and sulfated glycans modulate this binding. *Biochem Biophys Res Commun* 181:1223–1230, 1991.

1230. Polley MJ, et al: CD62 and endothelial cell-leukocyte adhesion molecule I (ELAM-1) recognize the same carbohydrate ligand, sialyl-Lewisx. *Proc Natl Acad Sci U S A* 88:6224–6228, 1991.

1231. Aruffo A, et al: CD62/P-selectin recognition of myeloid and tumor cell sulfatides. *Cell* 67:35–44, 1991.

1232. Stone JP, Wagner DD: P-selectin mediates adhesion of platelets to neuroblastoma and small cell lung cancer. *J Clin Invest* 92:804–813, 1993.

1233. McEver RP, Cummings RD: Perspectives series: Cell adhesion in vascular biology. Role of PSGL-1 binding to selectins in leukocyte recruitment. *J Clin Invest* 100(3):485–491, 1997.

1234. Sako D, et al: Expression cloning of a functional glycoprotein ligand for P-selectin. *Cell* 75(6):1179–1186, 1993.

1235. Yang J, Furie BC, Furie B: The biology of P-selectin glycoprotein ligand-1: Its role as a selectin counterreceptor in leukocyte-endothelial and leukocyte-platelet interaction. *Thromb Haemost* 81(1):1–7, 1999.

1236. Falati S, et al: Accumulation of tissue factor into developing thrombi in vivo is dependent upon microparticle P-selectin glycoprotein ligand 1 and platelet P-selectin. *J Exp Med* 197(11):1585–1598, 2003.

1237. Celi A, et al: P-selectin induces the expression of tissue factor on monocytes. *Proc Natl Acad Sci U S A* 91(19):8767–8771, 1994.

1238. Theoret JF, et al: P-selectin ligation induces platelet activation and enhances microaggregate and thrombus formation. *Thromb Res* 128(3):243–250, 2011.

1239. Ridker PM, Buring JE, Rifai N, Soluble P-selectin and the risk of future cardiovascular events. *Circulation* 103(4):491–495, 2001.

1240. Mayadas TN, et al: Leukocyte rolling and extravasation are severely compromised in P selectin-deficient mice. *Cell* 74(3):541–554, 1993.

1241. Frenette PS, et al: Platelets roll on stimulated endothelium *in vivo*: An interaction mediated by endothelial P-selectin. *Proc Natl Acad Sci U S A* 92(16):7450–7454, 1995.

1242. Padilla A, et al: P-selectin anchors newly released ultralarge von Willebrand factor multimers to the endothelial cell surface. *Blood* 103(6):2150–2156, 2004.

1243. Cambien B, Wagner DD: A new role in hemostasis for the adhesion receptor P-selectin. *Trends Mol Med* 10(4):179–186, 2004.

1244. Ludwig RJ, Schon MP, Boehncke WH: P-selectin: A common therapeutic target for cardiovascular disorders, inflammation and tumour metastasis. *Expert Opin Ther Targets* 11(8):1103–1117, 2007.

1245. Polanowska-Grabowska R, et al: P-selectin-mediated platelet-neutrophil aggregate formation activates neutrophils in mouse and human sickle cell disease. *Arterioscler Thromb Vasc Biol* 30(12):2392–2399, 2010.

1246. Polgar J, Matuskova J, Wagner DD: The P-selectin, tissue factor, coagulation triad. *J Thromb Haemost* 3(8):1590–1596, 2005.

1247. Navarro-Nunez L, et al: The physiological and pathophysiological roles of platelet CLEC-2. *Thromb Haemost* 109(6):991–998, 2013.

1248. Ozaki Y, Suzuki-Inoue K, Inoue O: Novel interactions in platelet biology: CLEC-2/podoplanin and laminin/GPVI. *J Thromb Haemost* 7(Suppl 1):191–194, 2009.

1249. Schacht V, et al: T1alpha/podoplanin deficiency disrupts normal lymphatic vasculature formation and causes lymphedema. *EMBO J* 22(14):3546–3556, 2003.

1250. Tsuruo T, Fujita N: Platelet aggregation in the formation of tumor metastasis. *Proc Jpn Acad Ser B Phys Biol Sci* 84(6):189–198, 2008.

1251. Christou CM, et al: Renal cells activate the platelet receptor CLEC-2 through podoplanin. *Biochem J* 411(1):133–140, 2008.

1252. Gitz E, et al: CLEC-2 expression is maintained on activated platelets and on platelet microparticles. *Blood* 124(14):2262–2270, 2014.

1253. Suzuki-Inoue K, et al: Involvement of the snake toxin receptor CLEC-2, in podoplanin-mediated platelet activation, by cancer cells. *J Biol Chem* 282(36):25993–26001, 2007.

1254. Watson AA, et al: The platelet receptor CLEC-2 is active as a dimer. *Biochemistry* 48(46):10988–10996, 2009.

1255. Gitz E, et al: CLEC-2 expression is maintained on activated platelets and on platelet microparticles. *Blood* 124(14):2262–2270, 2014.

1256. Lowe KL, Navarro-Nunez L, Watson SP: Platelet CLEC-2 and podoplanin in cancer metastasis. *Thromb Res* 129 Suppl 1:S30–S37, 2012.

1257. Bertozzi CC, et al: Platelets regulate lymphatic vascular development through CLEC-2-SLP-76 signaling. *Blood* 116(4):661–670, 2010.

1258. Pollitt AY, et al: Syk and Src family kinases regulate C-type lectin receptor 2 (CLEC-2)-mediated clustering of podoplanin and platelet adhesion to lymphatic endothelial cells. *J Biol Chem* 289(52):35695–35710, 2014.

1259. Suzuki-Inoue K, et al: Essential *in vivo* roles of the C-type lectin receptor CLEC-2: Embryonic/neonatal lethality of CLEC-2-deficient mice by blood/lymphatic misconnections and impaired thrombus formation of CLEC-2-deficient platelets. *J Biol Chem* 285(32):24494–24507, 2010.

1260. Benezech C, et al: CLEC-2 is required for development and maintenance of lymph nodes. *Blood* 123(20):3200–3207, 2014.

1261. Hemler ME: Tetraspanin functions and associated microdomains. *Nat Rev Mol Cell Biol* 6(10):801–811, 2005.

1262. Israels SJ, McMillan-Ward EM: Platelet tetraspanin complexes and their association with lipid rafts. *Thromb Haemost* 98(5):1081–1087, 2007.

1263. Israels SJ, McMillan-Ward EM: Palmitoylation supports the association of tetraspanin CD63 with CD9 and integrin alphaIIbbeta3 in activated platelets. *Thromb Res* 125(2):152–158, 2010.

1264. Goschnick MW, Jackson DE: Tetraspanins-structural and signalling scaffolds that regulate platelet function. *Mini Rev Med Chem* 7(12):1248–1254, 2007.

1265. Goschnick MW, et al: Impaired "outside-in" integrin alphaIIbbeta3 signaling and thrombus stability in TSSC6-deficient mice. *Blood* 108(6):1911–1918, 2006.

1266. Protty MB, et al: Identification of Tspan9 as a novel platelet tetraspanin and the collagen receptor GPVI as a component of tetraspanin microdomains. *Biochem J* 417(1):391–400, 2009.

1267. Boucheix C, et al: Molecular cloning of the CD9 antigen. A new family of cell surface proteins. *J Biol Chem* 266(1):117–122, 1991.

1268. Hato T, et al: Exposure of platelet fibrinogen receptors by a monoclonal antibody to CD9 antigen. *Blood* 72(1):224–229, 1988.

1269. Lanza F, et al: CDNA cloning and expression of platelet p24/CD9. Evidence for a new family of multiple membrane-spanning proteins. *J Biol Chem* 266(16):10638–10645, 1991.

1270. Brisson C, et al: Co-localization of CD9 and GPIIb-IIIa (alpha IIb beta 3 integrin) on activated platelet pseudopods and alpha-granule membranes. *Histochem J*, 29(2): 153–165, 1997.

1271. Hato T, et al: Induction of platelet Ca2+ influx and mobilization by a monoclonal antibody to CD9 antigen. *Blood* 75(5):1087–1091, 1990.

1272. Jennings LK, et al: The activation of human platelets mediated by anti-human platelet p24/CD9 monoclonal antibodies. *J Biol Chem* 265:3815–3822, 1990.

1273. Worthington RE, Carroll RC, Boucheix C: Platelet activation by CD9 monoclonal antibodies is mediated by the Fc gamma II receptor. *Br J Haematol* 74(2):216–222, 1990.

1274. Slupsky JR, et al: Evidence that monoclonal antibodies against CD9 antigen induce specific association between CD9 and the platelet glycoprotein IIb-IIIa complex. *J Biol Chem* 264(21):12289–12293, 1989.

1275. Dale GL, Remenyi G, Friese P: Tetraspanin CD9 is required for microparticle release from coated-platelets. *Platelets* 20(6):361–366, 2009.

1276. Mangin PH, et al: CD9 negatively regulates integrin alphaIIbbeta3 activation and could thus prevent excessive platelet recruitment at sites of vascular injury. *J Thromb Haemost* 7(5):900–902, 2009.

1277. Nishibori M, et al: The protein CD63 is in platelet dense granules, is deficient in a patient with Hermansky-Pudlak syndrome, and appears identical to granulophysin. *J Clin Invest* 91:1775–1782, 1993.

1278. Metzelaar MJ, et al: CD63 antigen. A novel lysosomal membrane glycoprotein, cloned by a screening procedure for intracellular antigens in eukaryotic cells. *J Biol Chem* 266(5):3239–3245, 1991.

1279. Fitter S, et al: Molecular cloning of cDNA encoding a novel platelet-endothelial cell tetra-span antigen, PETA-3. *Blood* 86(4):1348–1355, 1995.

1280. Roberts JJ, et al: Platelet activation induced by a murine monoclonal antibody directed against a novel tetra-span antigen. *Br J Haematol* 89(4):853–860, 1995.

1281. Sincock PM, Mayrhofer G, Ashman LK: Localization of the transmembrane 4 superfamily (TM4SF) member PETA-3 (CD151) in normal human tissues: Comparison with CD9, CD63, and alpha5beta1 integrin. *J Histochem Cytochem* 45(4):515–525, 1997.

1282. Lau LM, et al: The tetraspanin superfamily member, CD151 regulates outside-in integrin alphaIIbbeta3 signalling and platelet function. *Blood* 104(8):2368–2375, 2004.

1283. Orlowski E, et al: A platelet tetraspanin superfamily member, CD151, is required for regulation of thrombus growth and stability in vivo. *J Thromb Haemost* 7(12): 2074–2084, 2009.

1284. Polgar J, et al: Additional GPI-anchored glycoproteins on human platelets that are absent or deficient in paroxysmal nocturnal haemoglobinuria. *FEBS Lett* 327(1): 49–53, 1993.

1285. Hwang SM, Kim MJ, Chang HE, et al: Human platelet antigen genotyping and expression of CD109 (human platelet antigen 15) mRNA in various human cell types. *Biomed Res Int* 2013:946403, 2013.

1286. Kelton JG, et al: ABH antigens on human platelets: Expression on the glycosyl phosphatidylinositol-anchored protein CD109. *J Lab Clin Med* 1998;132(2):142–148, 2013.

1287. Grunewald M, et al: The platelet function defect of paroxysmal nocturnal haemoglobinuria. *Platelets* 15(3):145–154, 2004.

1288. Jin JY, et al: Glycosylphosphatidyl-inositol (GPI)-linked protein deficiency on the platelets of patients with aplastic anaemia and paroxysmal nocturnal haemoglobinuria: Two distinct patterns correlating with expression on neutrophils. *Br J Haematol* 96(3):493–496, 1997.

1289. Barclay GR, et al: Distribution of cell-associated prion protein in normal adult blood determined by flow cytometry. *Br J Haematol* 107(4):804–814, 1999.

1290. Holada K, et al: Increased expression of phosphatidylinositol-specific phospholipase C resistant prion proteins on the surface of activated platelets. *Br J Haematol* 103(1):276–282, 1998.

1291. MacGregor I, et al: Application of a time-resolved fluoroimmunoassay for the analysis of normal prion protein in human blood and its components. *Vox SangVox Sang* 77(2):88–96, 1999.

1292. Starke R, Cramer E, Harrison P: Expression of cell-associated prion protein on normal human platelets. *Br J Haematol* 110(3):748–750, 2000.

1293. Prevost N, et al: Interactions between Eph kinases and ephrins provide a mechanism to support platelet aggregation once cell-to-cell contact has occurred. *Proc Natl Acad Sci U S A* 99(14):9219–9224, 2002.

1294. Prevost N, et al: Signaling by ephrinB1 and Eph kinases in platelets promotes Rap1 activation, platelet adhesion, and aggregation via effector pathways that do not require phosphorylation of ephrinB1. *Blood* 103(4):1348–1355, 2004.

1295. Prevost N, et al: Eph kinases and ephrins support thrombus growth and stability by regulating integrin outside-in signaling in platelets. *Proc Natl Acad Sci U S A* 102(28):9820–9825, 2005.

1296. dem Borne AE, et al: Thrombopoietin and its receptor: Structure, function and role in the regulation of platelet production. *Baillieres Clin Haematol* 11(2):409–426, 1998.

1297. Fielder PJ, et al: Human platelets as a model for the binding and degradation of thrombopoietin. *Blood* 89(8):2782–2788, 1997.

1298. Kaushansky K, Thrombopoietin: A tool for understanding thrombopoiesis. *J Thromb Haemost* 1(7):1587–1592, 2003.

1299. Kaushansky K: Historical review: Megakaryopoiesis and thrombopoiesis. *Blood* 111(3):981–986, 2008.

1300. Chen J, et al: Regulation of platelet activation *in vitro* by the c-Mpl ligand, thrombopoietin. *Blood* 86(11):4054–4062, 1995.

1301. Ezumi Y, Takayama H, Okuma M: Thrombopoietin, c-Mpl ligand, induces tyrosine phosphorylation of Tyk2, JAK2, and STAT3, and enhances agonists-induced aggregation in platelets *in vitro*. *FEBS Lett* 374(1):48–52, 1995.

1302. Kojima H, et al: Modulation of platelet activation *in vitro* by thrombopoietin. *Thromb Haemost* 74(6):1541–1545, 1995.

1303. Kubota Y, et al: Thrombopoietin modulates platelet activation *in vitro* through protein-tyrosine phosphorylation. *Stem Cells*, 14(4):439–444, 1996.

1304. Oda A, et al: Thrombopoietin primes human platelet aggregation induced by shear stress and by multiple agonists. *Blood* 87(11):4664–4670, 1996.

1305. Rodriguez-Linares B, Watson SP: Thrombopoietin potentiates activation of human platelets in association with JAK2 and TYK2 phosphorylation. *Biochem J* 316 (Pt 1):93–98, 1996.

1306. Fox NE, et al: Compound heterozygous c-Mpl mutations in a child with congenital amegakaryocytic thrombocytopenia: Functional characterization and a review of the literature. *Exp Hematol* 37(4):495–503, 2009.

1307. Kilpivaara O, Levine RL: JAK2 and MPL mutations in myeloproliferative neoplasms: Discovery and science. *Leukemia* 22(10):1813–1817, 2008.

1308. Aiken ML, et al: Effects of OKM5, a monoclonal antibody to glycoprotein IV, on platelet aggregation and thrombospondin surface expression. *Blood* 76(12):2501–2509, 1990.

1309. Daviet L, McGregor JL: Vascular biology of CD36: Roles of this new adhesion molecule family in different disease states. *Thromb Haemost* 78(1):65–69, 1997.

1310. Febbraio M, Silverstein RL: CD36: Implications in cardiovascular disease. *Int J Biochem Cell Biol* 39(11):2012–2030, 2007.

1311. Legrand C, Pidard D, Beiso P, et al: Interaction of a monoclonal antibody to glycoprotein IV (CD36) with human platelets and its effect on platelet function. *Platelets* 2(2):99–105, 1991.

1312. Tandon NN, et al: Isolation and characterization of platelet glycoprotein IV (CD36). *J Biol Chem* 1989;264(13):7570–7575, 1991.

1313. Valiyaveettil M, Podrez EA: Platelet hyperreactivity, scavenger receptors and atherothrombosis. *J Thromb Haemost* 7(Suppl 1):218–221, 2009.

1314. Oquendo P, Hundt E, Lawler J, Seed B: CD36 directly mediates cytoadherence of *Plasmodium falciparum* infected erythrocytes. *Cell* 58(1):95–101, 1989.

1315. Huang MM, et al: Membrane glycoprotein IV (CD36) is physically associated with the Fyn, Lyn, and Yes protein-tyrosine kinases in human platelets. *Proc Natl Acad Sci U S A* 88(17):7844–7848, 1991.

1316. Taketani T, et al: Neonatal isoimmune thrombocytopenia caused by type I CD36 deficiency having novel splicing isoforms of the CD36 gene. *Eur J Haematol* 81(1):70–74, 2008.

1317. Thorne RF, et al: CD36 forms covalently associated dimers and multimers in platelets and transfected COS-7 cells. *Biochem Biophys Res Commun* 240(3):812–818, 1997.

1318. Thibert V, et al: Increased platelet CD36 constitutes a common marker in myeloproliferative disorders. *Br J Haematol* 91(3):618–624, 1995.

1319. Asch AS, et al: Analysis of CD36 binding domains: Ligand specificity controlled by dephosphorylation of an ectodomain. *Science* 262(5138):1436–1440, 1993.

1320. Aiken JW, Ginsberg MH, Plow EF: Mechanisms for expression of thrombospondin on the platelet surface. *Semin Thromb Hemost* 13:307–316, 1987.

1321. Collot-Teixeira S, et al: CD36 and macrophages in atherosclerosis. *Cardiovasc Res* 75(3):468–477, 2007.

1322. Yamashita S, et al: Physiological and pathological roles of a multi-ligand receptor CD36 in atherogenesis; insights from CD36-deficient patients. *Mol Cell Biochem* 299(1–2):19–22, 2007.

1323. Chen K, et al: A specific CD36-dependent signaling pathway is required for platelet activation by oxidized low-density lipoprotein. *Circ Res* 102(12):1512–1519, 2008.

1324. Korporaal SJ, et al: Platelet activation by oxidized low density lipoprotein is mediated by CD36 and scavenger receptor-A. *Arterioscler Thromb Vasc Biol* 27(11):2476–2483, 2007.

1325. Podrez EA, et al: Platelet CD36 links hyperlipidemia, oxidant stress and a prothrombotic phenotype. *Nat Med* 13(9):1086–1095, 2007.

1326. Ma Y, Ashraf MZ, Podrez EA: Scavenger receptor BI modulates platelet reactivity and thrombosis in dyslipidemia. *Blood* 116(11):1932–1941, 2010.

1327. Ghosh A, et al: Platelet CD36 mediates interactions with endothelial cell-derived microparticles and contributes to thrombosis in mice. *J Clin Invest* 118(5):1934–1943, 2008.

1328. Hajjar DP, Gotto AM: Targeting CD36: Modulating inflammation and atherogenesis. *Curr Atheroscler Rep* 5(3):155–156, 2003.

1329. Hirano K, et al: Pathophysiology of human genetic CD36 deficiency. *Trends Cardiovasc Med* 13(4):136–141, 2003.

1330. Pravenec M, Kurtz TW: Genetics of Cd36 and the hypertension metabolic syndrome. *Semin Nephrol* 22(2):148–153, 2002.

1331. Su X, Abumrad NA: Cellular fatty acid uptake: A pathway under construction. *Trends Endocrinol Metab* 20(2):72–77, 2009.

1332. Asch AS, et al: Isolation of the thrombospondin membrane receptor. *J Clin Invest* 79:1054–1061, 1987.

1333. Diaz-Ricart M, et al: Antibodies to CD36 (GPIV) inhibit platelet adhesion to subendothelial surfaces under flow conditions. *Arterioscler Thromb Vasc Biol* 16(7):883–888, 1996.

1334. Tandon NN, Kralisz U, Jamieson GA: Identification of glycoprotein IV (CD36) as a primary receptor for platelet-collagen adhesion. *J Biol Chem* 264:7576–7583, 1989.

1335. Saelman EU, et al: Platelet adhesion to collagen and endothelial cell matrix under flow conditions is not dependent on platelet glycoprotein IV. *Blood* 83(11):3240–3244, 1994.

1336. Wun T, et al: Platelet-erythrocyte adhesion in sickle cell disease. *J Investig Med* 47(3):121–127, 1999.

1337. Valiyaveettil M, et al: Oxidized high-density lipoprotein inhibits platelet activation and aggregation via scavenger receptor BI. *Blood* 111(4):1962–1971, 2008.

1338. Chadwick AC, Sahoo D: Functional genomics of the human high-density lipoprotein receptor scavenger receptor BI: An old dog with new tricks. *Curr Opin Endocrinol Diabetes Obes* 20(2):124–131, 2013.

1339. Choi WS, Jeon OH, Kim DS: CD40 ligand shedding is regulated by interaction between matrix metalloproteinase-2 and platelet integrin alpha(IIb)beta(3). *J Thromb Haemost* 8(6):1364–1371, 2010.

1340. Heeschen C, et al: Soluble CD40 ligand in acute coronary syndromes. *N Engl J Med* 348(12):1104–1111, 2003.

1341. Andre P, et al: Platelet-derived CD40L: The switch-hitting player of cardiovascular disease. *Circulation* 106(8):896–899, 2002.

1342. Aukrust P, Damas JK, Solum NO: Soluble CD40 ligand and platelets: Self-perpetuating pathogenic loop in thrombosis and inflammation? *J Am Coll Cardiol* 43(12):2326–2328, 2004.

1343. Jin R, Yu S, Song Z, et al: Soluble CD40 ligand stimulates CD40-dependent activation of the β2 integrin Mac-1 and protein kinase C zeda (PKCζ) in neutrophils: Implications for neutrophil-platelet interactions and neutrophil oxidative burst. *PLoS One* 8(6):e64631, 2013.

1344. Varo N, de Lemos JA, Libby P, et al: Soluble CD40L: Risk prediction after acute coronary syndromes. *Circulation* 108(9):1049–1052, 2003.

1345. Cipollone F, et al: Preprocedural level of soluble CD40L is predictive of enhanced inflammatory response and restenosis after coronary angioplasty. *Circulation* 108(22):2776–2782, 2003.

1346. Lievens D, et al: Platelet CD40L mediates thrombotic and inflammatory processes in atherosclerosis. *Blood* 116(20):4317–4327, 2010.

1347. Pamukcu B, et al: The CD40-CD40L system in cardiovascular disease. *Ann Med* 43(5):331–340, 2011.

1348. Andre P, et al: CD40L stabilizes arterial thrombi by a beta3 integrin-dependent mechanism. *Nat Med* 8(3):247–252, 2002.

1349. Inwald DP, et al: CD40 is constitutively expressed on platelets and provides a novel mechanism for platelet activation. *Circ Res* 92(9):1041–1048, 2003.

1350. Prasad KS, et al: Soluble CD40 ligand induces beta3 integrin tyrosine phosphorylation and triggers platelet activation by outside-in signaling. *Proc Natl Acad Sci U S A* 100(21):12367–12371, 2003.

1351. Urbich C, et al: CD40 ligand inhibits endothelial cell migration by increasing production of endothelial reactive oxygen species. *Circulation* 106(8):981–986, 2002.

1352. Czapiga M, Kirk AD, Lekstrom-Himes J: Platelets deliver costimulatory signals to antigen-presenting cells: A potential bridge between injury and immune activation. *Exp Hematol* 32(2):135–139, 2004.

1353. Elzey BD, et al: Platelet-mediated modulation of adaptive immunity. A communication link between innate and adaptive immune compartments. *Immunity* 19(1):9–19, 2003.

1354. Ahmad R, et al: Activated human platelets express Fas-L and induce apoptosis in Fas-positive tumor cells. *J Leukoc Biol* 69(1):123–128, 2001.

1355. Crist SA, et al: Expression of TNF-related apoptosis-inducing ligand (TRAIL) in megakaryocytes and platelets. *Exp Hematol* 32(11):1073–1081, 2004.

1356. Otterdal K, et al: Platelet-derived LIGHT induces inflammatory responses in endothelial cells and monocytes. *Blood* 108(3):928–935, 2006.

1357. Saftig P, Schroder B, Blanz J: Lysosomal membrane proteins: Life between acid and neutral conditions. *Biochem Soc Trans* 38(6):1420–1423, 2010.

1358. Silverstein RL, Febbraio M: Identification of lysosome-associated membrane protein-2 as an activation-dependent platelet surface glycoprotein. *Blood* 80(6):1470–1475, 1992.

1359. Ghebrehiwet B, et al: GC1q-R/p33, a member of a new class of multifunctional and multicompartment cellular proteins, is involved in inflammation and infection. *Immunol Rev* 180:65–77, 2001.

1360. Peerschke EI, Ghebrehiwet B: Platelet receptors for the complement component C1q: Implications for hemostasis and thrombosis. *Immunobiology* 199(2):239–249, 1998.

1361. Peerschke EIB, Ghebrehiwet B: Human blood platelets possess specific binding sites for C1q. *J Immunol* 138:1537–1541, 1987.

1362. Ghebrehiwet B, et al: Isolation, cDNA cloning, and overexpression of a 33-kD cell surface glycoprotein that binds to the globular "heads" of C1q. *J Exp Med* 179(6):1809–1821, 1994.

1363. Herwald H, et al: Isolation and characterization of the kininogen-binding protein p33 from endothelial cells. Identity with the gC1q receptor. *J Biol Chem* 271(22):13040–13047, 1996.

1364. Nepomuceno RR, Tenner AJ: C1qRP, the C1q receptor that enhances phagocytosis, is detected specifically in human cells of myeloid lineage, endothelial cells, and platelets. *J Immunol* 160(4):1929–1935, 1998.

1365. Peerschke EI, Reid KB, Ghebrehiwet B: Platelet activation by C1q results in the induction of alpha IIb/beta 3 integrins (GPIIb-IIIa) and the expression of P-selectin and procoagulant activity. *J Exp Med* 178(2):579–587, 1993.

1366. Skoglund C, et al: C1q induces a rapid up-regulation of P-selectin and modulates collagen- and collagen-related peptide-triggered activation in human platelets. *Immunobiology* 215(12):987–995, 2010.

1367. Peerschke EIB: Platelet membrane receptors for the complement component C1q. *Semin Hematol* 31:320–328, 1994.

1368. Peerschke EIB, et al: Platelet activation by C1q results in the induction of αIIbβ3 integrins (GPIIb-IIIa) and the expression of P-selectin and procoagulant activity. *J Exp Med* 178:579–587, 1993.

1369. Jiang J, et al: Crystal structure of human p32, a doughnut-shaped acidic mitochondrial matrix protein. *Proc Natl Acad Sci U S A* 96(7):3572–3577, 1999.

1370. Metzelaar MJ, et al: Identification of a 33-Kd protein associated with the alpha-granule membrane (GMP-33) that is expressed on the surface of activated platelets. *Blood* 79(2):372–379, 1992.

1371. Damas C, et al: The 33-kDa platelet alpha-granule membrane protein (GMP-33) is an N-terminal proteolytic fragment of thrombospondin. *Thromb Haemost* 86(3):887–893, 2001.

1372. Rosenstein Y, et al: CD43, a molecule defective in Wiskott-Aldrich syndrome, binds ICAM-1. *Nature* 354(6350):233–235, 1991.

1373. Koupenova M, Mick E, Mikhalev E, et al: Sex differences in platelet toll-like receptors and their association with cardiovascular risk factors. *Arterioscler Thromb Vasc Biol* 35(4):1030–1037, 2015.

1374. Panigrahi S, et al: Engagement of platelet toll-like receptor 9 by novel endogenous ligands promotes platelet hyperreactivity and thrombosis. *Circ Res* 112(1):103–112, 2013.

1375. Rivadeneyra L, et al: Regulation of platelet responses triggered by Toll-like receptor 2 and 4 ligands is another non-genomic role of nuclear factor-kappaB. *Thromb Res* 133(2):235–243, 2014.

1376. Semple JW, et al: Platelet-bound lipopolysaccharide enhances Fc receptor-mediated phagocytosis of IgG-opsonized platelets. *Blood* 109(11):4803–4805, 2007.

1377. Zhang G, et al: Lipopolysaccharide stimulates platelet secretion and potentiates platelet aggregation via TLR4/MyD88 and the cGMP-dependent protein kinase pathway. *J Immunol* 182(12):7997–8004, 2009.

1378. Stahl AL, et al: Lipopolysaccharide from enterohemorrhagic Escherichia coli binds to platelets through TLR4 and CD62 and is detected on circulating platelets in patients with hemolytic uremic syndrome. *Blood* 108(1):167–176, 2006.

1379. Cognasse F, et al: Toll-like receptor 4 ligand can differentially modulate the release of cytokines by human platelets. *Br J Haematol* 141(1):84–91, 2008.

1380. Scott T, Owens MD: Thrombocytes respond to lipopolysaccharide through Toll-like receptor-4, and MAP kinase and NF-kappaB pathways leading to expression of interleukin-6 and cyclooxygenase-2 with production of prostaglandin E2. *Mol Immunol* 45(4):1001–1008, 2008.

1381. Stark RJ, Aghakasiri N, Rumbaut RE: Platelet-derived Toll-like receptor 4 (Tlr-4) is sufficient to promote microvascular thrombosis in endotoxemia. *PLoS One* 7(7):e41254, 2012.

1382. Ren MP, et al: Endothelial cells but not platelets are the major source of Toll-like receptor 4 in the arterial thrombosis and tissue factor expression in mice. *Am J Physiol Regul Integr Comp Physiol* 307(7):R901–R907, 2014.

1383. Gould TJ, Vu TT, Swystun LL, et al: Neutrophil extracellular traps promote thrombin generation through platelet-dependent and platelet-independent mechanisms. *Arterioscler Thromb Vasc Biol* 34(9):1977–1984, 2014.

1384. Akbiyik F, et al: Human bone marrow megakaryocytes and platelets express PPARgamma, and PPARgamma agonists blunt platelet release of CD40 ligand and thromboxanes. *Blood* 104(5):1361–1368, 2004.

1385. Ray DM, et al: Peroxisome proliferator-activated receptor gamma and retinoid X receptor transcription factors are released from activated human platelets and shed in microparticles. *Thromb Haemost* 99(1):86–95, 2008.

1386. Ali FY, et al: Role of nuclear receptor signaling in platelets: Antithrombotic effects of PPARbeta. *FASEB J* 20(2):326–328, 2006.

1387. Borchert M, et al: Review of the pleiotropic effects of peroxisome proliferator-activated receptor gamma agonists on platelet function. *Diabetes Technol Ther* 9(5):410–420, 2007.

1388. Santos-Martinez MJ, et al: Matrix metalloproteinases in platelet function: Coming of age. *J Thromb Haemost* 6(3):514–516, 2008.

1389. Soslau G, et al: Intracellular matrix metalloproteinase-2 (MMP-2) regulates human platelet activation via hydrolysis of talin. *Thromb Haemost* 111(1):140–153, 2014.

1390. Trivedi V, et al: Platelet matrix metalloprotease-1 mediates thrombogenesis by activating PAR1 at a cryptic ligand site. *Cell* 137(2):332–343, 2009.

1391. Choi WS, et al: MMP-2 regulates human platelet activation by interacting with integrin alphaIIbbeta3. *J Thromb Haemost* 6(3):517–523, 2008.

1392. Gresele P, et al: Platelets release matrix metalloproteinase-2 in the coronary circulation of patients with acute coronary syndromes: Possible role in sustained platelet activation. *Eur Heart J* 32(3):316–325, 2011.

1393. Rahman M, et al: Platelet shedding of CD40L is regulated by matrix metalloproteinase-9 in abdominal sepsis. *J Thromb Haemost* 11(7):1385–1398, 2013.

1394. Stalker TJ, et al: Platelet signaling. *Handb Exp Pharmacol* (210):59–85, 2012.

1395. Pawelczyk T: Isozymes delta of phosphoinositide-specific phospholipase C. *Acta Biochim Pol* 46(1):91–98, 1999.

1396. Hirata T, et al: Two thromboxane A2 receptor isoforms in human platelets. Opposite coupling to adenylyl cyclase with different sensitivity to Arg60 to Leu mutation. *J Clin Invest* 97(4):949–956, 1996.

1397. Murphy CT, Westwick J: Selective inhibition of protein kinase C. Effect on platelet-activating-factor-induced platelet functional responses. *Biochem J* 283(Pt 1):159–164, 1992.

1398. Cattaneo M: The platelet P2 receptors, in *Platelets*, edited by AD Michelson, 201–220. Academic Press, San Diego, 2007.

1399. Kunapuli SP: Funcional characterization of platelet ADP. *Platelets* 9:343–351, 1998.

1400. Murugappa S, Kunapuli SP: The role of ADP receptors in platelet function. *Front Biosci* 11:1977–1986, 2006.

1401. Moheimani F, Jackson DE: P2Y12 receptor: Platelet thrombus formation and medical interventions. *Int J Hematol* 96(5):572–587, 2012.

1402. Conley PB, Delaney SM: Scientific and therapeutic insights into the role of the platelet P2Y12 receptor in thrombosis. *Curr Opin Hematol* 10(5):333–338, 2003.

1403. Dorsam RT, Kunapuli SP: Central role of the P2Y12 receptor in platelet activation. *J Clin Invest* 113(3):340–345, 2004.

1404. Hollopeter G, et al: Identification of the platelet ADP receptor targeted by antithrombotic drugs. *Nature* 409(6817):202–207, 2001.

1405. Jin J, Daniel JL, Kunapuli SP: Molecular basis for ADP-induced platelet activation. II. The P2Y1 receptor mediates ADP-induced intracellular calcium mobilization and shape change in platelets. *J Biol Chem* 273(4):2030–2034, 1998.

1406. Mills DC, et al: Clopidogrel inhibits the binding of ADP analogues to the receptor mediating inhibition of platelet adenylate cyclase. *Arterioscler Thromb* 12(4):430–436, 1992.

1407. Cunningham MR, Nisar SP, Mundell SJ: Molecular mechanisms of platelet P2Y(12) receptor regulation. *Biochem Soc Trans* 41(1):225–230, 2013.

1408. Andre P, et al: P2Y12 regulates platelet adhesion/activation, thrombus growth, and thrombus stability in injured arteries. *J Clin Invest* 112(3):398–406, 2003.

1409. Foster CJ, et al: Molecular identification and characterization of the platelet ADP receptor targeted by thienopyridine antithrombotic drugs. *J Clin Invest* 107(12):1591–1598, 2001.

1410. Fontana P, et al: Adenosine diphosphate-induced platelet aggregation is associated with P2Y12 gene sequence variations in healthy subjects. *Circulation* 108(8):989–995, 2003.

1411. Staritz P, et al: Platelet reactivity and clopidogrel resistance are associated with the H2 haplotype of the P2Y(12)-ADP receptor gene. *Int J Cardiol* 133(3):341–345, 2009.

1412. Zhang D, Gao ZG, Zhang K: et al: Two disparate ligand-binding sites in the human P2Y1 receptor. *Nature* 520(7547):317–321, 2015.

1413. Fabre JE, et al: Decreased platelet aggregation, increased bleeding time and resistance to thromboembolism in P2Y1-deficient mice. *Nat Med* 5(10):1199–1202, 1999.

1414. Leon C, et al: Defective platelet aggregation and increased resistance to thrombosis in purinergic P2Y(1) receptor-null mice. *J Clin Invest* 104(12):1731–1737, 1999.

1415. Offermanns S, et al: Defective platelet activation in G alpha(q)-deficient mice. *Nature* 389(6647):183–186, 1997.

1416. MacKenzie AB, Mahaut-Smith MP, Sage SO: Activation of receptor-operated cation channels via P2X1 not P2T purinoceptors in human platelets. *J Biol Chem* 271(6):2879–2881, 1996.

1417. Valera S, et al: A new class of ligand-gated ion channel defined by P2x receptor for extracellular ATP. *Nature* 371(6497):516–519, 1994.

1418. Oury C, et al: Does the P(2X1del) variant lacking 17 amino acids in its extracellular domain represent a relevant functional ion channel in platelets? *Blood* 99(6):2275–2277, 2002.

1419. Vial C, et al: Lack of evidence for functional ADP-activated human P2X1 receptors supports a role for ATP during hemostasis and thrombosis. *Blood* 102(10):3646–3651, 2003.

1420. Oury C, et al: P2X(1)-mediated activation of extracellular signal-regulated kinase 2 contributes to platelet secretion and aggregation induced by collagen. *Blood* 100(7):2499–2505, 2002.

1421. Vial C, et al: A study of P2X1 receptor function in murine megakaryocytes and human platelets reveals synergy with P2Y receptors. *Br J Pharmacol* 135(2):363–372, 2002.

1422. Hechler B, et al: A role of the fast ATP-gated P2X1 cation channel in thrombosis of small arteries in vivo. *J Exp Med* 198(4):661–667, 2003.

1423. Oury C, et al: Overexpression of the platelet P2X1 ion channel in transgenic mice generates a novel prothrombotic phenotype. *Blood* 101(10):3969–3976, 2003.

1424. Greco NJ, et al: Novel structurally altered P(2X1) receptor is preferentially activated by adenosine diphosphate in platelets and megakaryocytic cells. *Blood* 98(1):100–107, 2001.

1425. Raju NC, Eikelboom JW, Hirsh J, Platelet ADP-receptor antagonists for cardiovascular disease: Past, present and future. *Nat Clin Pract Cardiovasc Med* 5(12):766–780, 2008.

1426. Herbert JM, Savi P: P2Y12, a new platelet ADP receptor, target of clopidogrel. *Semin Vasc Med* 3(2):113–122, 2013.

1427. Banga HS, et al: Activation of phospholipases A and C in human platelets exposed to epinephrine: Role of glycoproteins IIb/IIIa and dual role of epinephrine. *Proc Natl Acad Sci U S A* 83(23):9197–9201, 1986.

1428. Lanza F, et al: Epinephrine potentiates human platelet activation but is not an aggregating agent. *Am J Physiol* 255(6 Pt 2):1276–1288, 1988.

1429. Shattil SJ, Budzynski A, Scrutton MC: Epinephrine induces platelet fibrinogen receptor expression, fibrinogen binding, and aggregation in whole blood in the absence of other excitatory agonists. *Blood* 73(1):150–158, 1989.

1430. Kobilka BK, et al: Cloning, sequencing, and expression of the gene coding for the human platelet alpha 2-adrenergic receptor. *Science* 238(4827):650–656, 1987.

1431. Regan JW, et al: Purification and characterization of the human platelet alpha 2-adrenergic receptor. *J Biol Chem* 261(8):3894–3900, 1986.

1432. Yang J, et al: Loss of signaling through the G protein, Gz, results in abnormal platelet activation and altered responses to psychoactive drugs. *Proc Natl Acad Sci U S A* 97(18):9984–9989, 2000.

1433. Haslam RJ, et al: Cyclic nucleotides in platelet function. *Thromb Haemost* 40(2):232–240, 1978.

1434. Homcy CJ, Graham RM: Molecular characterization of adrenergic receptors. *Circ Res* 56(5):635–650, 1985.

1435. Salzman EW, Ware JA: Ionized calcium as an intracellular messenger in blood platelets. *Prog Hemost Thromb* 9:177–202, 1989.

1436. Yang J, et al: Signaling through Gi family members in platelets. Redundancy and specificity in the regulation of adenylyl cyclase and other effectors. *J Biol Chem* 277(48):46035–46042, 2002.

1437. Patel YM, et al: Evidence for a role for Galphai1 in mediating weak agonist-induced platelet aggregation in human platelets: Reduced Galphai1 expression and defective Gi signaling in the platelets of a patient with a chronic bleeding disorder. *Blood* 101(12):4828–4835, 2003.

1438. Freeman K, et al: Genetic polymorphism of the alpha 2-adrenergic receptor is associated with increased platelet aggregation, baroreceptor sensitivity, and salt excretion in normotensive humans. *Am J Hypertens* 8(9):863–869, 1995.

1439. Small KM, et al: An asn to lys polymorphism in the third intracellular loop of the human alpha 2A-adrenergic receptor imparts enhanced agonist-promoted Gi coupling. *J Biol Chem* 275(49):38518–38523, 2000.

1440. von KR, Dimsdale JE: Effects of sympathetic activation by adrenergic infusions on hemostasis in vivo. *Eur J Haematol* 65(6):357–369, 2000.

1441. Bertha BG, Folts JD: Inhibition of epinephrine-exacerbated coronary thrombus formation by prostacyclin in the dog. *J Lab Clin Med* 103:204–214, 1984.

1442. Folts JD, Rowe GG: Epinephrine potentiation of in vivo stimuli reverses aspirin inhibition of platelet thrombus formation in stenosed canine coronary arteries. *Thromb Res* 50:507–516, 1988.

1443. Sibbing D, et al: Platelet function in clopidogrel-treated patients with acute coronary syndrome. *Blood Coagul Fibrinolysis* 18(4):335–339, 2007.

1444. Marcus A: Platelet eicosanoid metabolism, in *Hemostasis and Thrombosis: Basic Principles and Clinical Practice*, edited by RW Colman, Hirsch J, Marder VJ, Salzman EW, pp 676–688. JB Lippincott, Philadelphia, 1987.

1445. Puri RN: Phospholipase A2: Its role in ADP- and thrombin-induced platelet activation mechanisms. *Int J Biochem Cell Biol* 30(10):1107–1122, 1998.

1446. Wong DA, et al: Discrete role for cytosolic phospholipase A(2)alpha in platelets: Studies using single and double mutant mice of cytosolic and group IIA secretory phospholipase A(2). *J Exp Med* 196(3):349–357, 2002.

1447. Adler DH, Cogan JD, Phillips JA 3rd, et al: Inherited human cPLA(2alpha)deficiency is associated with impaired eicosanoid biosynthesis, small intestinal ulceration, and platelet dysfunction. *J Clin Invest* 118(6):2121–2131, 2008.

1448. Prevost N, et al: Group IVA cytosolic phospholipase A2 (cPLA2alpha) and integrin alphaIIbbeta3 reinforce each other's functions during alphaIIbbeta3 signaling in platelets. *Blood* 113(2):447–457, 2009.

1449. Crofford LJ: COX-1 and COX-2 tissue expression: Implications and predictions. *J Rheumatol* 24(Suppl 49):15–19, 1997.

1450. Warner TD, Mitchell JA: Cyclooxygenases: New forms, new inhibitors, and lessons from the clinic. *FASEB J* 18(7):790–804, 2004.

1451. Dubois RN, et al: Cyclooxygenase in biology and disease. *FASEB J* 12(12):1063–1073, 1998.

1452. Smith JB, Willis AL: Aspirin selectively inhibits prostaglandin production in human platelets. *Nat New Biol* 231(25):235–237, 1971.

1453. Svensson J, Hamberg M, Samuelsson B: On the formation and effects of thromboxane A2 in human platelets. *Acta Physiol Scand* 98(3):285–294, 1976.

1454. Rocca B, et al: Cyclooxygenase-2 expression is induced during human megakaryopoiesis and characterizes newly formed platelets. *Proc Natl Acad Sci U S A* 99(11):7634–7639, 2002.

1455. Weber AA, Zimmermann KC, Meyer-Kirchrath J, Schrör K: Cyclooxygenase-2 in human platelets as a possible factor in aspirin resistance. *Lancet* 353(9156):900, 1999.

1456. Funk CD, FitzGerald GA: COX-2 inhibitors and cardiovascular risk. *J Cardiovasc Pharmacol* 50(5):470–479, 2007.

1457. Parent JL, et al: Internalization of the TXA2 receptor alpha and beta isoforms. Role of the differentially spliced COOH terminus in agonist-promoted receptor internalization. *J Biol Chem* 274(13):8941–8948, 1999.

1458. Habib A, FitzGerald GA, Maclouf J: Phosphorylation of the thromboxane receptor alpha, the predominant isoform expressed in human platelets. *J Biol Chem* 274(5):2645–2651, 1999.

1459. Kim SO, et al: Purification of the human blood platelet thromboxane A2/prostaglandin H2 receptor protein. *Biochem Pharmacol* 43(2):313–322, 1992.

1460. Ushikubi F, et al: Purification of the thromboxane A2/prostaglandin H2 receptor from human blood platelets. *J Biol Chem* 264(28):16496–16501, 1989.

1461. Takahara K, et al: The response to thromboxane A2 analogues in human platelets. Discrimination of two binding sites linked to distinct effector systems. *J Biol Chem* 265(12):6836–6844, 1990.

1462. Thomas DW, et al: Coagulation defects and altered hemodynamic responses in mice lacking receptors for thromboxane A2. *J Clin Invest* 102(11):1994–2001, 1998.

1463. Gabbeta J, et al: Platelet signal transduction defect with Ga subunit dysfunction and diminished Gaq in a patient with abnormal platelet responses. *Proc Natl Acad Sci U S A* 94(16):8750–8755, 1997.

1464. Allan CJ, et al: Characterization of the cloned HEL cell thromboxane A2 receptor: Evidence that the affinity state can be altered by G alpha 13 and G alpha q. *J Pharmacol Exp Ther* 277(2):1132–1139, 1996.

1465. Djellas Y, et al: Identification of Galpha13 as one of the G-proteins that couple to human platelet thromboxane A2 receptors. *J Biol Chem* 274(20):14325–14330, 1999.

1466. Nakahata N, et al: Gq/11 communicates with thromboxane A2 receptors in human astrocytoma cells, rabbit astrocytes and human platelets. *Res Commun Mol Pathol Pharmacol* 87(3):243–251, 1995.

1467. Paul BZ, Jin J, Kunapuli SP: Molecular mechanism of thromboxane A(2)-induced platelet aggregation. Essential role for p2t(ac) and alpha(2a) receptors. *J Biol Chem* 274(41):29108–29114, 1999.

1468. Ushikubi F, Nakamura K, Narumiya S: Functional reconstitution of platelet thromboxane A2 receptors with Gq and Gi2 in phospholipid vesicles. *Mol Pharmacol* 46(5):808–816, 1994.

1469. Dorsam RT, et al: Coordinated signaling through both G12/13 and G(i) pathways is sufficient to activate GPIIb/IIIa in human platelets. *J Biol Chem* 277(49):47588–47595, 2002.

1470. Klages B, et al: Activation of G12/G13 results in shape change and Rho/Rho-kinase-mediated myosin light chain phosphorylation in mouse platelets. *J Cell Biol* 144(4):745–754, 1999.

1471. Nieswandt B, et al: Costimulation of Gi- and G12/G13-mediated signaling pathways induces integrin alpha IIbbeta 3 activation in platelets. *J Biol Chem* 277(42):39493–39498, 2002.

1472. Pulcinelli FM, et al: Protein kinase C activation is not a key step in ADP-mediated exposure of fibrinogen receptors on human platelets. *FEBS Lett* 364(1):87–90, 1995.

1473. Knezevic I, Dieter JP, Le Breton GC: Mechanism of inositol 1,4,5-trisphosphate-induced aggregation in saponin-permeabilized platelets. *J Pharmacol Exp Ther* 260(3):947–955, 1992.

1474. Nugteren DH: Arachidonate lipoxygenase in blood platelets. *Biochim Biophys Acta* 380(2):299–307, 1975.

1475. Johnson EN, Brass LF, Funk CD: Increased platelet sensitivity to ADP in mice lacking platelet-type 12-lipoxygenase. *Proc Natl Acad Sci U S A* 95(6):3100–3105, 1998.

1476. Coffey MJ, et al: Platelet 12-lipoxygenase activation via glycoprotein VI: Involvement of multiple signaling pathways in agonist control of H(P)ETE synthesis. *Circ Res* 94(12):1598–1605, 2004.

1477. Dasari VR, Jin J, Kunapuli SP: Distribution of leukotriene B4 receptors in human hematopoietic cells. *Immunopharmacology* 48(2):157–163, 2000.

1478. Maclouf JA, Murphy RC: Transcellular metabolism of neutrophil-derived leukotriene A4 by human platelets. A potential cellular source of leukotriene C4. *J Biol Chem* 263(1):174–181, 1988.

1479. Maugeri N, et al: Polymorphonuclear leukocyte-platelet interaction: Role of P-selectin in thromboxane B2 and leukotriene C4 cooperative synthesis. *Thromb Haemost* 72(3):450–456, 1994.

1480. Levy BD, et al: Agonist-induced lipoxin A4 generation: Detection by a novel lipoxin A4-ELISA. *Lipids* 28(12):1047–1053, 1993.

1481. Ofosu FA, Liu L, Freedman J: Control mechanisms in thrombin generation. *Semin Thromb Hemost* 22(4):303–308, 1996.

1482. Phillips DR: Thrombin interaction with human platelets. Potentiation of thrombin-induced aggregation and release by inactivated thrombin. *Thromb Diath Haemorrh* 32(1):207–215, 1974.

1483. Bahou W: Thrombin receptors, in *Platelets*, edited by AD Michelson, pp 179–200. Academic Press, San Diego, 2007.

1484. Hung DT, et al: Cloned platelet thrombin receptor is necessary for thrombin-induced platelet activation. *J Clin Invest* 89(4):1350–1353, 1992.

1485. Furman MI, et al: The cleaved peptide of the thrombin receptor is a strong platelet agonist. *Proc Natl Acad Sci U S A* 95(6):3082–3087, 1998.

1486. Cho JR, et al: Unmet needs in the management of acute myocardial infarction: Role of novel protease-activated receptor-1 antagonist vorapaxar. *Vasc Health Risk Manag* 10:177–188, 2014.

1487. Zhang C, et al: High-resolution crystal structure of human protease-activated receptor 1. *Nature* 492(7429):387–392, 2012.

1488. Ishihara H, et al: Antibodies to protease-activated receptor 3 inhibit activation of mouse platelets by thrombin. *Blood* 91(11):4152–4157, 1998.

1489. Kahn ML, et al: A dual thrombin receptor system for platelet activation. *Nature* 394(6694):690–694, 1998.

1490. Kahn ML, et al: Protease-activated receptors 1 and 4 mediate activation of human platelets by thrombin. *J Clin Invest* 103(6):879–887, 1999.

1491. Andrade-Gordon P, et al: Design, synthesis, and biological characterization of a peptide-mimetic antagonist for a tethered-ligand receptor. *Proc Natl Acad Sci U S A* 96(22):12257–12262, 1999.

1492. Covic L, Gresser AL, Kuliopulos A: Biphasic kinetics of activation and signaling for PAR1 and PAR4 thrombin receptors in platelets. *Biochemistry* 39(18):5458–5467, 2000.

1493. Shapiro MJ, et al: Protease-activated receptors 1 and 4 are shut off with distinct kinetics after activation by thrombin. *J Biol Chem* 275(33):25216–25221, 2000.

1494. Sambrano GR, et al: Role of thrombin signalling in platelets in haemostasis and thrombosis. *Nature* 413(6851):74–78, 2001.

1495. Nakanishi-Matsui M, et al: PAR3 is a cofactor for PAR4 activation by thrombin. *Nature* 404(6778):609–613, 2000.

1496. Weiss EJ, et al: Protection against thrombosis in mice lacking PAR3. *Blood* 100(9):3240–3244, 2002.

1497. Hoxie JA, et al: Internalization and recycling of activated thrombin receptors. *J Biol Chem* 268(18):13756–13763, 1993.

1498. Trejo J, Coughlin SR: The cytoplasmic tails of protease-activated receptor-1 and substance P receptor specify sorting to lysosomes versus recycling. *J Biol Chem* 274(4):2216–2224, 1999.

1499. Antoniak S, et al: PAR-1 contributes to the innate immune response during viral infection. *J Clin Invest* 123(3):1310–1322, 2013.

1500. Khoufache K, et al: PAR1 contributes to influenza A virus pathogenicity in mice. *J Clin Invest* 123(1):206–214, 2013.

1501. Berri F, et al: Switch from protective to adverse inflammation during influenza: Viral determinants and hemostasis are caught as culprits. *Cell Mol Life Sci* 71(5):885–898, 2014.

1502. Ruggeri ZM, et al: Unravelling the mechanism and significance of thrombin binding to platelet glycoprotein Ib. *Thromb Haemost* 104(5):894–902, 2010.

1503. Celikel R, et al: Modulation of alpha-thrombin function by distinct interactions with platelet glycoprotein Ibalpha. *Science* 301(5630):218–221, 2003.

1504. Dumas JJ, et al: Crystal structure of the GpIbalpha-thrombin complex essential for platelet aggregation. *Science* 301(5630):222–226, 2003.

1505. Lova P, et al: Thrombin induces platelet activation in the absence of functional protease activated receptors 1 and 4 and glycoprotein Ib-IX-V. *Cell Signal* 22(11):1681–1687, 2010.

1506. Gibbins JM: Tweaking the gain on platelet regulation: The tachykinin connection. *Atherosclerosis* 2008.

1507. Graham GJ, et al: Tachykinins regulate the function of platelets. *Blood* 104(4):1058–1065, 2004.

1508. Gleissner CA, von HP, Ley K: Platelet chemokines in vascular disease. *Arterioscler Thromb Vasc Biol* 28(11):1920–1927, 2008.

1509. McIntyre TM, Zimmerman GA, Prescott SM: Biologically active oxidized phospholipids. *J Biol Chem* 274(36):25189–25192, 1999.

1510. Honda Z, et al: Cloning by functional expression of platelet-activating factor receptor from guinea-pig lung. *Nature* 349(6307):342–346, 1991.

1511. Nakamura M, et al: Molecular cloning and expression of platelet-activating factor receptor from human leukocytes. *J Biol Chem* 266(30):20400–20405, 1991.

1512. Carlson SA, Chatterjee TK, Fisher RA: The third intracellular domain of the platelet-activating factor receptor is a critical determinant in receptor coupling to phosphoinositide phospholipase C-activating G proteins. Studies using intracellular domain minigenes and receptor chimeras. *J Biol Chem* 271(38):23146–23153, 1996.

1513. Chao W, et al: Protein tyrosine phosphorylation and regulation of the receptor for platelet-activating factor in rat Kupffer cells. Effect of sodium vanadate. *Biochem J* 288(Pt 3):777–784, 1992.

1514. Stafforini DM: Biology of platelet-activating factor acetylhydrolase (PAF-AH, lipoprotein associated phospholipase A2). *Cardiovasc Drugs Ther* 23(1):73–83, 2009.

1515. Eitzman DT, et al: Hyperlipidemia promotes thrombosis after injury to atherosclerotic vessels in apolipoprotein E-deficient mice. *Arterioscler Thromb Vasc Biol* 20(7):1831–1834, 2000.

1516. Sano T, et al: Multiple mechanisms linked to platelet activation result in lysophosphatidic acid and sphingosine 1-phosphate generation in blood. *J Biol Chem* 277(24):21197–21206, 2002.

1517. Smyth SS, et al: Roles of lysophosphatidic acid in cardiovascular physiology and disease. *Biochim Biophys Acta* 1781(9):563–570, 2008.

1518. Umezu-Goto M, et al: Autotaxin has lysophospholipase D activity leading to tumor cell growth and motility by lysophosphatidic acid production. *J Cell Biol* 158(2):227–233, 2002.

1519. Leblanc R, et al: Interaction of platelet-derived autotaxin with tumor integrin alphaVbeta3 controls metastasis of breast cancer cells to bone. *Blood* 124(20):3141–3150, 2014.

1520. Siess W, et al: Lysophosphatidic acid mediates the rapid activation of platelets and endothelial cells by mildly oxidized low density lipoprotein and accumulates in human atherosclerotic lesions. *Proc Natl Acad Sci U S A* 96(12):6931–6936, 1999.

1521. Retzer M, Essler M: Lysophosphatidic acid-induced platelet shape change proceeds via Rho/Rho kinase-mediated myosin light-chain and moesin phosphorylation. *Cell Signal* 12(9–10):645–648, 2000.

1522. Haseruck N, et al: The plaque lipid lysophosphatidic acid stimulates platelet activation and platelet-monocyte aggregate formation in whole blood: Involvement of P2Y1 and P2Y12 receptors. *Blood* 103(7):2585–2592, 2004.

1523. Olorundare OE, et al: Assembly of a fibronectin matrix by adherent platelets stimulated by lysophosphatidic acid and other agonists. *Blood* 98(1):117–124, 2001.

1524. Maschberger P, et al: Mildly oxidized low density lipoprotein rapidly stimulates via activation of the lysophosphatidic acid receptor Src family and Syk tyrosine kinases and Ca2+ influx in human platelets. *J Biol Chem* 275(25):19159–19166, 2000.

1525. Siess W: Athero- and thrombogenic actions of lysophosphatidic acid and sphingosine-1-phosphate. *Biochim Biophys Acta* 1582(1–3):204–215, 2002.

1526. Motohashi K, et al: Identification of lysophospholipid receptors in human platelets: The relation of two agonists, lysophosphatidic acid and sphingosine 1-phosphate. *FEBS Lett* 468(2–3):189–193, 2000.

1527. Siess W, Tigyi G: Thrombogenic and atherogenic activities of lysophosphatidic acid. *J Cell Biochem* 92(6):1086–1094, 2004.

1528. Yatomi Y, et al: Sphingosine-1-phosphate: A platelet-activating sphingolipid released from agonist-stimulated human platelets. *Blood* 86(1):193–202, 1995.

1529. Nugent D, Xu Y: Sphingosine-1-phosphate: Characterization of its inhibition of platelet aggregation. *Platelets* 11(4):226–232, 2000.

1530. Hoyer D, et al: International Union of Pharmacology classification of receptors for 5-hydroxytryptamine (Serotonin). *Pharmacol Rev* 46(2):157–203, 1994.

1531. Allen JA, Yadav PN, Roth BL: Insights into the regulation of 5-HT2A serotonin receptors by scaffolding proteins and kinases. *Neuropharmacology* 55(6):961–968, 2008.

1532. Cook EH Jr, et al: Primary structure of the human platelet serotonin 5-HT2A receptor: Identify with frontal cortex serotonin 5-HT2A receptor. *J Neurochem* 63(2):465–469, 1994.

1533. De Clerck F, et al: Evidence for functional 5-HT2 receptor sites on human blood platelets. *Biochem PharmacolAm Rev Respir Dis* 33(17):2807–2811, 1984.

1534. Roth BL, et al: 5-Hydroxytryptamine2-family receptors (5-hydroxytryptamine2A, 5-hydroxytryptamine2B, 5-hydroxytryptamine2C): Where structure meets function. *Pharmacol Ther* 79(3):231–257, 1998.

1535. Leysen JE, et al: Identification of nonserotonergic [3H]ketanserin binding sites associated with nerve terminals in rat brain and with platelets; relation with release of biogenic amine metabolites induced by ketans. *J Pharmacol Exp Ther* 244(1):310–321, 1988.

1536. Ozaki N, et al: A naturally occurring amino acid substitution of the human serotonin 5- HT2A receptor influences amplitude and timing of intracellular calcium mobilization. *J Neurochem* 68(5):2186–2193, 1997.

1537. Shimizu M, et al: Serotonin-2A receptor gene polymorphisms are associated with serotonin-induced platelet aggregation. *Thromb Res* 112(3):137–142, 2003.

1538. Arora RC, Meltzer HY: Serotonin2 receptor binding in blood platelets of schizophrenic patients. *Psychiatry Res* 47(2):111–119, 1993.

1539. Coccaro EF, et al: Impulsive aggression in personality disorder correlates with platelet 5- HT2A receptor binding. *Neuropsychopharmacology* 16(3):211–216, 1997.

1540. Pandey GN: Altered serotonin function in suicide. Evidence from platelet and neuroendocrine studies. *Ann N Y Acad Sci* 836:182–200, 1997.

1541. Tomiyoshi R, et al: Serotonin-induced platelet intracellular Ca2+ responses in untreated depressed patients and imipramine responders in remission. *Biol Psychiatry* 45(8):1042–1048, 1999.

1542. Wolfe BE, Metzger J, Jimerson DC: Research update on serotonin function in bulimia nervosa and anorexia nervosa. *Psychopharmacol Bull* 33(3):345–354, 1997.

1543. Cho R, et al: Relationship between central and peripheral serotonin 5-HT2A receptors: A positron emission tomography study in healthy individuals. *Neurosci Lett* 261(3):139–142, 1999.

1544. Schins A, et al: Increased coronary events in depressed cardiovascular patients: 5-HT2A receptor as missing link? *Psychosom Med* 65(5):729–737, 2003.

1545. de Chaffoy de Courcelles D, Leysen JE, De Clerck F, et al: Evidence that phospholipid turnover is the signal transducing system coupled to serotonin-S2 receptor sites. *J Biol Chem* 260(12):7603–7608, 1985.

1546. Erne P, Pletscher A: Rapid intracellular release of calcium in human platelets by stimulation of 5-HT2-receptors. *Br J Pharmacol* 84(2):545–549, 1985.

1547. Li N, et al: Effects of serotonin on platelet activation in whole blood. *Blood Coagul Fibrinolysis* 8(8):517–523, 1997.

1548. Houston DS, Shepherd JT, Vanhoutte PM: Aggregating human platelets cause direct contraction and endothelium- dependent relaxation of isolated canine coronary arteries. Role of serotonin, thromboxane A2, and adenine nucleotides. *J Clin Invest* 78(2):539–544, 1986.

1549. Golino P, et al: Mediation or reocclusion by thromboxane A2 and serotonin after thrombolysis with tissue-type plasminogen activator in a canine preparation of coronary thrombosis. *Circulation* 77:678–684, 1988.

1550. Alberio LJ, Clemetson KJ: All platelets are not equal: COAT platelets. *Curr Hematol Rep* 3(5):338–343, 2004.

1551. Dale GL, et al: Stimulated platelets use serotonin to enhance their retention of procoagulant proteins on the cell surface. *Nature* 415(6868):175–179, 2002.

1552. Walther DJ, et al: Serotonylation of small GTPases is a signal transduction pathway that triggers platelet alpha-granule release. *Cell* 115(7):851–862, 2003.

1553. Carneiro AM, et al: Interactions between integrin alphaIIbbeta3 and the serotonin transporter regulate serotonin transport and platelet aggregation in mice and humans. *J Clin Invest* 118(4):1544–1552, 2008.

1554. McCloskey DJ, et al: Selective serotonin reuptake inhibitors: Measurement of effect on platelet function. *Transl Res* 151(3):168–172, 2008.

1555. Lesurtel M, et al: Platelet-derived serotonin mediates liver regeneration. *Science* 312(5770):104–107, 2006.

1556. Haslam RJ, Rosson GM: Aggregation of human blood platelets by vasopressin. *Am J Physiol* 223(4):958–967, 1972.

1557. Pollock WK, MacIntyre DE: Desensitization and antagonism of vasopressin-induced phosphoinositide metabolism and elevation of cytosolic free calcium concentration in human platelets. *Biochem J* 234(1):67–73, 1986.

1558. Thomas ME, Osmani AH, Scrutton MC: Some properties of the human platelet vasopressin receptor. *Thromb Res* 32(6):557–566, 1983.

1559. Thibonnier M, Roberts JM: Characterization of human platelet vasopressin receptors. *J Clin Invest* 76(5):1857–1864, 1985.

1560. Siess W, et al: Activation of V1-receptors by vasopressin stimulates inositol phospholipid hydrolysis and arachidonate metabolism in human platelets. *Biochem J* 233(1):83–91, 1986.

1561. Thibonnier M, Goraya T, Berti-Mattera L: G protein coupling of human platelet V1 vascular vasopressin receptors. *Am J Physiol* 264(5 Pt 1):C1336–C1344, 1993.

1562. Berrettini WH, et al: Human platelet vasopressin receptors. *Life Sci* 1982;30(5):425–432, 1993.

1563. Siess W: Molecular mechanisms of platelet activation. *Physiol Rev* 69(1):58–178, 1989.

1564. Wun T, Paglieroni T, Lachant NA: Physiologic concentrations of arginine vasopressin activate human platelets *in vitro*. *Br J Haematol* 92(4):968–972, 1996.

1565. Gunnet JW, et al: Pharmacological characterization of RWJ-676070, a dual vasopressin V1(A)/V(2) receptor antagonist. *Eur J Pharmacol* 590(1–3):333–342, 2008.

1566. Serradeil-Le Gal C, et al: Nonpeptide vasopressin receptor antagonists: Development of selective and orally active V1a, V2 and V1b receptor ligands. *Prog Brain Res* 139:197–210, 2002.

1567. Crabos M, Bertschin S, Bühler FR, et al: Identification of AT1 receptors on human platelets and decreased angiotensin II binding in hypertension. *J Hypertens Suppl* 11 Suppl 5:S230–S231, 1993.

1568. Jagroop IA, Mikhailidis DP: Angiotensin II can induce and potentiate shape change in human platelets: Effect of losartan. *J Hum Hypertens* 2000;14(9):581–585, 1993.

1569. Lopez-Farre A, et al: Angiotensin II AT(1) receptor antagonists and platelet activation. *Nephrol Dial Transplant* 16 Suppl 1:45–49, 2001.

1570. Larsson PT, Schwieler JH, Wallen NH: Platelet activation during angiotensin II infusion in healthy volunteers. *Blood Coagul Fibrinolysis* 11(1):61–69, 2000.

1571. Li P, et al: Novel angiotensin II AT(1) receptor antagonist irbesartan prevents thromboxane A(2)-induced vasoconstriction in canine coronary arteries and human platelet aggregation. *J Pharmacol Exp Ther* 292(1):238–246, 2000.

1572. Monton M, et al: Comparative effects of angiotensin II AT-1-type receptor antagonists in vitro on human platelet activation. *J Cardiovasc Pharmacol* 35(6):906–913, 2000.

1573. Kalinowski L, et al: Angiotensin II AT1 receptor antagonists inhibit platelet adhesion and aggregation by nitric oxide release. *Hypertension* 40(4):521–527, 2002.

1574. Jimenez AM, et al: Inhibition of platelet activation in stroke-prone spontaneously hypertensive rats: Comparison of losartan, candesartan, and valsartan. *J Cardiovasc Pharmacol* 37(4):406–412, 2001.

1575. Owens P, et al: Comparison of antihypertensive and metabolic effects of losartan and losartan in combination with hydrochlorothiazide—A randomized controlled trial. *J Hypertens* 18(3):339–345, 2000.

1576. Schieffer B, et al: Comparative effects of AT1-antagonism and angiotensin-converting enzyme inhibition on markers of inflammation and platelet aggregation in patients with coronary artery disease. *J Am Coll Cardiol* 44(2):362–368, 2004.

1577. Serebruany VL, et al: Valsartan inhibits platelet activity at different doses in mild to moderate hypertensives: Valsartan Inhibits Platelets (VIP) trial. *Am Heart J* 151(1):92–99, 2006.

1578. Yamada K, Hirayama T, Hasegawa Y: Antiplatelet effect of losartan and telmisartan in patients with ischemic stroke. *J Stroke Cerebrovasc Dis* 16(5):225–231, 2007.

1579. Dorahy DJ, et al: Stimulation of platelet activation and aggregation by a carboxyl-terminal peptide from thrombospondin binding to the integrin-associated protein receptor. *J Biol Chem* 272(2):1323–1330, 1997.

1580. Lindberg FP, et al: Molecular cloning of integrin-associated protein: An immunoglobulin family member with multiple membrane-spanning domains implicated in alpha v beta 3-dependent ligand binding. *J Cell Biol* 123(2):485–496, 1993.

1581. Wang XQ, Frazier WA: The thrombospondin receptor CD47 (IAP) modulates and associates with alpha2 beta1 integrin in vascular smooth muscle cells. *Mol Biol Cell* 9(4):865–874, 1998.

1582. Frazier WA, et al: The thrombospondin receptor integrin-associated protein (CD47) functionally couples to heterotrimeric Gi. *J Biol Chem* 274(13):8554–8560, 1999.

1583. Chung J, Gao AG, Frazier WA: Thrombospondin acts via integrin-associated protein to activate the platelet integrin alphaIIbbeta3. *J Biol Chem* 272(23):14740–14746, 1997.

1584. Isenberg JS, et al: Thrombospondin-1 stimulates platelet aggregation by blocking the antithrombotic activity of nitric oxide/cGMP signaling. *Blood* 111(2):613–623, 2008.

1585. Lagadec P, et al: Involvement of a CD47-dependent pathway in platelet adhesion on inflamed vascular endothelium under flow. *Blood* 101(12):4836–4843, 2003.

1586. Pimanda JE, et al: The von Willebrand factor-reducing activity of thrombospondin-1 is located in the calcium-binding/C-terminal sequence and requires a free thiol at position 974. *Blood* 100(8):2832–2838, 2002.

1587. Pimanda JE, et al: Role of thrombospondin-1 in control of von Willebrand factor multimer size in mice. *J Biol Chem* 279(20):21439–21448, 2004.

1588. van Zanten GH, et al: Increased platelet deposition on atherosclerotic coronary arteries. *J Clin Invest* 93(2):615–632, 1994.

1589. van der Rest, M, Garrone R: Collagen family of proteins. *FASEB J* 5(13):2814–2823, 1991.

1590. Ruggeri ZM, Mendolicchio GL: Adhesion mechanisms in platelet function. *Circ Res* 100(12):1673–1685, 2007.

1591. Clemetson JM, et al: The platelet collagen receptor glycoprotein VI is a member of the immunoglobulin superfamily closely related to FcalphaR and the natural killer receptors. *J Biol Chem* 274(41):29019–29024, 1999.

1592. Ichinohe T, et al: Collagen-stimulated activation of Syk but not c-Src is severely compromised in human platelets lacking membrane glycoprotein VI. *J Biol Chem* 272(1):63–68, 1997.

1593. Ishibashi T, et al: Functional significance of platelet membrane glycoprotein p62 (GP VI), a putative collagen receptor. *Int J Hematol* 62(2):107–115, 1995.

1594. Kehrel B, et al: Glycoprotein VI is a major collagen receptor for platelet activation: It recognizes the platelet-activating quaternary structure of collagen, whereas CD36, glycoprotein IIb/IIIa, and von Willebrand factor do not. *Blood* 91(2):491–499, 1998.

1595. Clemetson KJ, Clemetson JM: Platelet receptors, in *Platelets*, edited by AD Michelson, pp 117–143. Academic Press, San Diego, 2007.

1596. Horii K, Kahn ML, Herr AB: Structural basis for platelet collagen responses by the immune-type receptor glycoprotein VI. *Blood* 108(3):936–942, 2006.

1597. Poole A, et al: The Fc receptor gamma-chain and the tyrosine kinase Syk are essential for activation of mouse platelets by collagen. *EMBO J* 16(9):2333–2341, 1997.

1598. Smethurst PA, et al: Identification of the primary collagen-binding surface on human glycoprotein VI by site-directed mutagenesis and by a blocking phage antibody. *Blood* 103(3):903–911, 2004.

1599. Chiang TM, Collagen-platelet interaction: Platelet non-integrin receptors. *Histol Histopathol* 14(2):579–585, 1999.

1600. Keely PJ, Parise LV: The alpha2beta1 integrin is a necessary co-receptor for collagen-induced activation of Syk and the subsequent phosphorylation of phospholipase Cgamma2 in platelets. *J Biol Chem* 271(43):26668–26676, 1996.

1601. Sugiyama T, et al: A novel platelet aggregating factor found in a patient with defective collagen-induced platelet aggregation and autoimmune thrombocytopenia. *Blood* 69:1712–1720, 1987.

1602. Briddon SJ, Watson SP: Evidence for the involvement of p59fyn and p53/56lyn in collagen receptor signalling in human platelets. *Biochem J* 338(Pt 1):203–209, 1999.

1603. Fujii C, et al: Involvement of protein-tyrosine kinase p72syk in collagen-induced signal transduction in platelets. *Eur J Biochem* 226(1):243–248, 1994.

1604. Shattil SJ, Ginsberg MH, Brugge JS: Adhesive signaling in platelets. *Curr Opin Cell Biol* 6(5):695–704, 1994.

1605. Soriano P, et al: Targeted disruption of the c-src proto-oncogene leads to osteopetrosis in mice. *Cell* 64(4):693–702, 1991.

1606. Daniel JL, Dangelmaier C, Smith JB: Evidence for a role for tyrosine phosphorylation of phospholipase Cg2 in collagen-induced platelet cytosolic calcium mobilization. *Biochem J* 302:617–622, 1994.

1607. Keely PJ, Parise LV: The alpha2beta1 integrin is a necessary co-receptor for collagen-induced activation of Syk and the subsequent phosphorylation of phospholipase Cgamma2 in platelets. *J Biol Chem* 271(43):26668–26676, 1996.

1608. Quek LS, Bolen J, Watson SP: A role for Bruton's tyrosine kinase (Btk) in platelet activation by collagen. *Curr Biol* 8(20):1137–1140, 1998.

1609. Jung SM, Moroi M: Platelet collagen receptor integrin alpha2beta1 activation involves differential participation of ADP-receptor subtypes P2Y1 and P2Y12 but not intracellular calcium change. *Eur J Biochem* 268(12):3513–3522, 2001.

1610. Wang Z, Leisner TM, Parise LV: Platelet alpha2beta1 integrin activation: Contribution of ligand internalization and the alpha2-cytoplasmic domain. *Blood* 102(4):1307–1315, 2003.

1611. Bertoni A, et al: Relationships between Rap1b, affinity modulation of integrin alpha IIbbeta 3, and the actin cytoskeleton. *J Biol Chem* 277(28):25715–25721, 2002.

1612. Larson MK, et al: Identification of P2Y12-dependent and -independent mechanisms of glycoprotein VI-mediated Rap1 activation in platelets. *Blood* 101(4):1409–1415, 2003.

1613. Auger JM, et al: C-Cbl negatively regulates platelet activation by glycoprotein VI. *J Thromb Haemost* 1(11):2419–2426, 2003.

1614. Locke D, et al: Fc Rgamma-independent signaling by the platelet collagen receptor glycoprotein VI. *J Biol Chem* 278(17):15441–15448, 2003.

1615. Qiao J, et al: An acquired defect associated with abnormal signaling of the platelet collagen receptor glycoprotein VI. *Acta Haematol* 128(4):233–241, 2012.

1616. Inoue O, et al: Integrin alpha2beta1 mediates outside-in regulation of platelet spreading on collagen through activation of Src kinases and PLCgamma2. *J Cell Biol* 160(5):769–780, 2003.

1617. Chen H, Kahn ML: Reciprocal signaling by integrin and nonintegrin receptors during collagen activation of platelets. *Mol Cell Biol* 23(14):4764–4777, 2003.

1618. Galt SW, et al: Outside-in signals delivered by matrix metalloproteinase-1 regulate platelet function. *Circ Res* 90(10):1093–1099, 2002.

1619. Best D, et al: GPVI levels in platelets: Relationship to platelet function at high shear. *Blood* 102(8):2811–2818, 2003.

1620. Chen H, et al: The platelet receptor GPVI mediates both adhesion and signaling responses to collagen in a receptor density-dependent fashion. *J Biol Chem* 277(4):3011–3019, 2002.

1621. Furihata K, et al: Variation in human platelet glycoprotein VI content modulates glycoprotein VI-specific prothrombinase activity. *Arterioscler Thromb Vasc Biol* 21(11):1857–1863, 2001.

1622. Suzuki H, et al: Intracellular localization of glycoprotein VI in human platelets and its surface expression upon activation. *Br J Haematol* 121(6):904–912, 2003.

1623. Matsuno K, et al: Inhibition of platelet adhesion to collagen by monoclonal anti-CD36 antibodies. *Br J Haematol* 92(4):960–967, 1996.

1624. Nakamura T, et al: Platelet adhesion to type I collagen fibrils: Role of GPVI in divalent cation-dependent and -independent adhesion and thromboxane A2 generation. *J Biol Chem* 273:4338–4344, 1998.

1625. Daniel JL, et al: Collagen induces normal signal transduction in platelets deficient in CD36 (platelet glycoprotein IV). *Thromb Haemost* 71:353–356, 1994.

1626. az-Ricart M, et al: Platelets lacking functional CD36 (glycoprotein IV) show reduced adhesion to collagen in flowing whole blood. *Blood* 82(2):491–496, 1993.

1627. Smith JB, et al: Cytosolic calcium as a second messenger for collagen-induced platelet responses. *Biochem J* 288(Pt 3):925–929, 1992.

1628. Greenwalt DE, Tandon NN: Platelet shape change and Ca2+ mobilization induced by collagen, but not thrombin or ADP, are inhibited by phenylarsine oxide. *Br J Haematol* 88(4):830–838, 1994.

1629. Chow TW, et al: Shear stress-induced von Willebrand factor binding to platelet glycoprotein Ib initiates calcium influx associated with aggregation. *Blood* 80(1):113–120, 1992.

1630. Gu M, et al: Analysis of the roles of 14–3–3 in the platelet glycoprotein Ib-IX-mediated activation of integrin alpha(IIb)beta(3) using a reconstituted mammalian cell expression model. *J Cell Biol* 147(5):1085–1096, 1999.

1631. Zaffran Y, et al: Signaling across the platelet adhesion receptor glycoprotein Ib-IX induces alpha IIbbeta 3 activation both in platelets and a transfected Chinese hamster ovary cell system. *J Biol Chem* 275(22):16779–16787, 2000.

1632. Sullam PM, et al: Physical proximity and functional interplay of the glycoprotein Ib-IX-V complex and the Fc receptor FcgammaRIIA on the platelet plasma membrane. *J Biol Chem* 273(9):5331–5336, 1998.

1633. Kasirer-Friede A, et al: Signaling through GP Ib-IX-V activates alphaIIbbeta3 independently of other receptors. *Blood* 103(9):3403–3411, 2004.

1634. Marshall SJ, et al: GPIb-dependent platelet activation is dependent on Src kinases but not MAP kinase or cGMP-dependent kinase. *Blood* 103(7):2601–2609, 2004.

1635. Mangin P, et al: Signaling role for phospholipase C gamma 2 in platelet glycoprotein Ib alpha calcium flux and cytoskeletal reorganization. Involvement of a pathway distinct from FcR gamma chain and Fc gamma RIIA. *J Biol Chem* 278(35):32880–32891, 2003.

1636. Li Z, et al: A stimulatory role for cGMP-dependent protein kinase in platelet activation. *Cell* 112(1):77–86, 2003.

1637. Andrews RK, et al: Interaction of calmodulin with the cytoplasmic domain of the platelet membrane glycoprotein Ib-IX-V complex. *Blood* 98(3):681–687, 2001.

1638. Du X, et al: Association of a phospholipase A2 (14–3–3 protein) with the platelet glycoprotein Ib-IX complex. *J Biol Chem* 269(28):18287–18290, 1994.

1639. Ohtsuka Y, et al: Chronic oral antigen exposure induces lymphocyte migration in anaphylactic mouse intestine. *Pediatr Res* 44(5):791–797, 1998.

1640. Kasirer-Friede A, et al: Lateral clustering of platelet GP Ib-IX complexes leads to up-regulation of the adhesive function of integrin alpha IIbbeta 3. *J Biol Chem* 277(14):11949–11956, 2002.

1641. Fox JE, Berndt MC: Cyclic AMP-dependent phosphorylation of glycoprotein Ib inhibits collagen-induced polymerization of actin in platelets. *J Biol Chem* 264(16):9520–9526, 1989.

1642. Phillips DR, Agin PP: Thrombin-induced alterations in the surface structure of the human platelet plasma membrane. *Ser Haematol* 6(3):292–310, 1973.

1643. Ni H, et al: Increased thrombogenesis and embolus formation in mice lacking glycoprotein V. *Blood* 98(2):368–373, 2001.

1644. Rink TJ: Cytosolic calcium in platelet activation. *Experientia* 44(2):97–100, 1988.

1645. Kovacs T, et al: All three splice variants of the human sarco/endoplasmic reticulum Ca2+-ATPase 3 gene are translated to proteins: A study of their co-expression in platelets and lymphoid cells. *Biochem J* 358(Pt 3):559–568, 2001.

1646. Hassock SR, et al: Expression and role of TRPC proteins in human platelets: Evidence that TRPC6 forms the store-independent calcium entry channel. *Blood* 100(8):2801–2811, 2002.

1647. Roberts DE, McNicol A, Bose R: Mechanism of collagen activation in human platelets. *J Biol Chem* 279:19421–19430, 2004.

1648. Jones GD, Gear AR: Subsecond calcium dynamics in ADP- and thrombin-stimulated platelets: A continuous-flow approach using indo-1. *Blood* 71(6):1539–1543, 1988.

1649. Rybak ME, Renzulli LA: Effect of calcium channel blockers on platelet GPIIb-IIIa as a calcium channel in liposomes: Comparison with effects on the intact platelet. *Thromb Haemost* 67(1):131–136, 1992.

1650. Dessen A, et al: Crystal structure of human cytosolic phospholipase A2 reveals a novel topology and catalytic mechanism. *Cell* 97(3):349–360, 1999.

1651. Khan WA, et al: Selective regulation of protein kinase C isoenzymes by oleic acid in human platelets. *J Biol Chem* 268(7):5063–5068, 1993.

1652. Scholey JM, Taylor KA, and J. Kendrick-Jones, Regulation of non-muscle myosin assembly by calmodulin-dependent light chain kinase. *Nature* 287(5779):233–235, 1980.

1653. Naik MU, Naik UP: Calcium-and integrin-binding protein regulates focal adhesion kinase activity during platelet spreading on immobilized fibrinogen. *Blood* 102(10):3629–3636, 2003.

1654. Barry WT, et al: Molecular basis of CIB binding to the integrin alpha IIb cytoplasmic domain. *J Biol Chem* 277(32):28877–28883, 2002.

1655. Zhang J, et al: Phosphoinositide 3-kinase gamma and p85/phosphoinositide 3-kinase in platelets. Relative activation by thrombin receptor or beta-phorbol myristate acetate and roles in promoting the ligand-binding function of alphaIIbbeta3 integrin. *J Biol Chem* 271(11):6265–6272, 1996.

1656. Rittenhouse SE, Phosphoinositide 3-kinase activation and platelet function. *Blood* 88(12):4401–4414, 1996.

1657. Hartwig JH, et al: D3 phosphoinositides and outside-in integrin signaling by glycoprotein IIb-IIIa mediate platelet actin assembly and filopodial extension induced by phorbol 12-myristate 13-acetate. *J Biol Chem* 271(51):32986–32993, 1996.

1658. Kucera GL, Rittenhouse SE: Human platelets form 3-phosphorylated phosphoinositides in response to α-thrombin, U46619, or GTPgammaS. *J Biol Chem* 265:5345–5348, 1990.

1659. Banfic H, Downes CP, Rittenhouse SE: Biphasic activation of PKBalpha/Akt in platelets. Evidence for stimulation both by phosphatidylinositol 3,4-bisphosphate, produced via a novel pathway, and by phosphatidylinositol 3,4,5-trisphosphate. *J Biol Chem* 273(19):11630–11637, 1998.

1660. Gibbins JM, et al: The p85 subunit of phosphatidylinositol 3-kinase associates with the Fc receptor gamma-chain and linker for activator of T cells (LAT) in platelets stimulated by collagen and convulxin. *J Biol Chem* 273(51):34437–34443, 1998.

1661. Watanabe N, et al: Functional phenotype of phosphoinositide 3-kinase p85alpha-null platelets characterized by an impaired response to GP VI stimulation. *Blood* 102(2):541–548, 2003.

1662. Gratacap MP, et al: Phosphatidylinositol 3,4,5-trisphosphate-dependent stimulation of phospholipase C-gamma2 is an early key event in FcgammaRIIA-mediated activation of human platelets. *J Biol Chem* 273(38):24314–24321, 1998.

1663. Canobbio I, Stefanini L, Cipolla L, et al: Genetic evidence for a predominant role of PI3Kbeta catalytic activity in platelets. *Blood* 114(10):2193–2196, 2009.

1664. Hirsch E, et al: Resistance to thromboembolism in PI3Kgamma-deficient mice. *FASEB J* 15(11):2019–2021, 2001.

1665. Leevers SJ, Vanhaesebroeck B, Waterfield MD: Signalling through phosphoinositide 3-kinases: The lipids take centre stage. *Curr Opin Cell Biol* 11(2):219–225, 1999.

1666. Bae YS, et al: Activation of phospholipase C-gamma by phosphatidylinositol 3,4,5-trisphosphate. *J Biol Chem* 273(8):4465–4469, 1998.

1667. Salim K, et al: Distinct specificity in the recognition of phosphoinositides by the pleckstrin homology domains of dynamin and Bruton's tyrosine kinase. *EMBO J* 15(22):6241–6250, 1996.

1668. Li Z, et al: Phosphatidylinositol 3-kinase-gamma activates Bruton's tyrosine kinase in concert with Src family kinases. *Proc Natl Acad Sci U S A* 94(25):13820–13825, 1997.

1669. Alessi DR, et al: Characterization of a 3-phosphoinositide-dependent protein kinase which phosphorylates and activates protein kinase Balpha. *Curr Biol* 7(4):261–269, 1997.

1670. Stokoe D, et al: Dual role of phosphatidylinositol-3,4,5-trisphosphate in the activation of protein kinase B. *Science* 277(5325):567–570, 1997.

1671. Kroner C, Eybrechts K, Akkerman JW: Dual regulation of platelet protein kinase B. *J Biol Chem* 275(36):27790–27798, 2000.

1672. Li D, August S, Woulfe DS: GSK3beta is a negative regulator of platelet function and thrombosis. *Blood* 111(7):3522–3530, 2008.

1673. Stojanovic A, et al: A phosphoinositide 3-kinase-AKT-nitric oxide-cGMP signaling pathway in stimulating platelet secretion and aggregation. *J Biol Chem* 281(24):16333–16339, 2006.

1674. Zhang W, Colman RW: Thrombin regulates intracellular cyclic AMP concentration in human platelets through phosphorylation/activation of phosphodiesterase 3A. *Blood* 110(5):1475–1482, 2007.

1675. Woulfe D, et al: Defects in secretion, aggregation, and thrombus formation in platelets from mice lacking Akt2. *J Clin Invest* 113(3):441–450, 2004.

1676. Chen J, De S, Damron DS, et al: Impaired platelet response to thrombin and collagen in AKT-1 deficient mice. *Blood* 104(6):1703–1710, 2004.

1677. Bao X, et al: Molecular cloning, bacterial expression and properties of Rab31 and Rab32. *Eur J Biochem* 269(1):259–271, 2002.

1678. Karniguian A, Zahraoui A, Tavitian A: Identification of small GTP-binding rab proteins in human platelets: Thrombin-induced phosphorylation of rab3B, rab6, and rab8 proteins. *Proc Natl Acad Sci U S A* 90(16):7647–7651, 1993.

1679. Richards-Smith B, et al: Analyses of proteins involved in vesicular trafficking in platelets of mouse models of Hermansky Pudlak syndrome. *Mol Genet Metab* 68(1):14–23, 1999.

1680. Wilson SM, et al: A mutation in Rab27a causes the vesicle transport defects observed in ashen mice. *Proc Natl Acad Sci U S A* 97(14):7933–7938, 2000.

1681. Choi W, Karim ZA, Whiteheart SW: Arf6 plays an early role in platelet activation by collagen and convulxin. *Blood* 107(8):3145–3152, 2006.

1682. Bishop AL, Hall A: Rho GTPases and their effector proteins. *Biochem J* 348 Pt 2:241–255, 2000.

1683. Hall A: Rho GTPases and the actin cytoskeleton. *Science* 279(5350):509–514, 1998.

1684. Polakis PG, Snyderman R, Evans T: Characterization of G25K, a GTP-binding protein containing a novel putative nucleotide binding domain. *Biochem Biophys Res Commun* 160(1):25–32, 1989.

1685. Polakis PG, et al: Identification of the ral and rac1 gene products, low molecular mass GTP-binding proteins from human platelets. *J Biol Chem* 264(28):16383–16389, 1989.

1686. Schoenwaelder SM, et al: RhoA sustains integrin alpha IIbbeta 3 adhesion contacts under high shear. *J Biol Chem* 277(17):14738–14746, 2002.

1687. Soulet C, et al: Characterisation of Rac activation in thrombin- and collagen-stimulated human blood platelets. *FEBS Lett* 507(3):253–258, 2001.

1688. Vidal C, et al: Cdc42/Rac1-dependent activation of the p21-activated kinase (PAK) regulates human platelet lamellipodia spreading: Implication of the cortical-actin binding protein cortactin. *Blood* 100(13):4462–4469, 2002.

1689. Moers A, Wettschureck N, Offermanns S: G13-mediated signaling as a potential target for antiplatelet drugs. *Drug News Perspect* 17(8):493–498, 2004.

1690. Soulet C, et al: A differential role of the platelet ADP receptors P2Y1 and P2Y12 in Rac activation. *J Thromb Haemost* 3(10):2296–2306, 2005.

1691. Azim AC, et al: Activation of the small GTPases, rac and cdc42, after ligation of the platelet PAR-1 receptor. *Blood* 95(3):959–964, 2000.

1692. Shock DD, et al: Ras activation in platelets after stimulation of the thrombin receptor, thromboxane A2 receptor or protein kinase C. *Biochem J* 321 (Pt 2):525–530, 1997.

1693. Omerovic J, et al: Ras isoform abundance and signalling in human cancer cell lines. *Oncogene* 27(19):2754–2762, 2008.

1694. Omerovic J, Laude AJ, Prior IA: Ras proteins: Paradigms for compartmentalised and isoform-specific signalling. *Cell Mol Life Sci* 64(19–20):2575–2589, 2007.

1695. Tulasne D, Bori T, Watson SP: Regulation of RAS in human platelets. Evidence that activation of RAS is not sufficient to lead to ERK1–2 phosphorylation. *Eur J Biochem* 269(5):1511–1517, 2002.

1696. Shock DD, et al: Ras activation in platelets after stimulation of the thrombin receptor, thromboxane A2 receptor or protein kinase C. *Biochem J* 321(Pt 2):525–530, 1997.

1697. Bauer M, et al: Dichotomous regulation of myosin phosphorylation and shape change by Rho-kinase and calcium in intact human platelets. *Blood* 94(5):1665–1672, 1999.

1698. Morii N, et al: A rho gene product in human blood platelets. II. Effects of the ADP-ribosylation by botulinum C3 ADP-ribosyltransferase on platelet aggregation. *J Biol Chem* 267(29):20921–20926, 1992.

1699. Nemoto Y, et al: A rho gene product in human blood platelets. I. Identification of the platelet substrate for botulinum C3 ADP-ribosyltransferase as rhoA protein. *J Biol Chem* 267(29):20916–20920, 1992.

1700. Klages B, et al: Activation of G12/G13 results in shape change and Rho/Rho-kinase- mediated myosin light chain phosphorylation in mouse platelets. *J Cell Biol* 144(4):745–754, 1999.

1701. Leng L, et al: RhoA and the function of platelet integrin alphaIIbbeta3. *Blood* 91(11):4206–4215, 1998.

1702. Schwartz M: Rho signalling at a glance. *J Cell Sci* 117(Pt 23):5457–5458, 2004.

1703. Akbar H, et al: Genetic and pharmacologic evidence that Rac1 GTPase is involved in regulation of platelet secretion and aggregation. *J Thromb Haemost* 5(8):1747–1755, 2007.

1704. McCarty OJ, et al: Rac1 is essential for platelet lamellipodia formation and aggregate stability under flow. *J Biol Chem* 280(47):39474–39484, 2005.

1705. Pleines I, et al: Rac1 is essential for phospholipase C-gamma2 activation in platelets. *Pflugers Arch* 457(5):1173–1185, 2009.

1706. Falet H, et al: Normal Arp2/3 complex activation in platelets lacking WASp. *Blood* 100(6):2113–2122, 2002.

1707. Kooistra MR, Dube N, Bos JL: Rap1: A key regulator in cell-cell junction formation. *J Cell Sci* 120(Pt 1):17–22, 2007.

1708. Franke B, Akkerman JW, Bos JL: Rapid Ca2+-mediated activation of Rap1 in human platelets. *EMBO J* 16(2):252–259, 1997.

1709. Greco F, et al: Activation of the small GTPase Rap2B in agonist-stimulated human platelets. *J Thromb Haemost* 2(12):2223–2230, 2004.

1710. Chrzanowska-Wodnicka M, et al: Rap1b is required for normal platelet function and hemostasis in mice. *J Clin Invest* 115(3):680–687, 2005.

1711. Eto K, et al: Megakaryocytes derived from embryonic stem cells implicate CalDAG-GEFI in integrin signaling. *Proc Natl Acad Sci U S A* 99(20):12819–12824, 2002.

1712. Crittenden JR, et al: CalDAG-GEFI integrates signaling for platelet aggregation and thrombus formation. *Nat Med* 10(9):982–986, 2004.

1713. Cifuni SM, Wagner DD, Bergmeier W: CalDAG-GEFI and protein kinase C represent alternative pathways leading to activation of integrin alphaIIbbeta3 in platelets. *Blood* 112(5):1696–1703, 2008.

1714. Watanabe N, et al: Mechanisms and consequences of agonist-induced talin recruitment to platelet integrin alphaIIbbeta3. *J Cell Biol* 181(6):1211–1222, 2008.

1715. Cullen PJ, Lockyer PJ: Integration of calcium and Ras signalling. *Nat Rev Mol Cell Biol* 3(5):339–348, 2002.

1716. Bodemann BO, White MA: Ral GTPases and cancer: Linchpin support of the tumorigenic platform. *Nat Rev Cancer* 8(2):133–140, 2008.

1717. Mark BL, Jilkina O, Bhullar RP: Association of Ral GTP-binding protein with human platelet dense granules. *Biochem Biophys Res Commun* 225(1):40–46, 1996.

1718. Wolthuis RM, et al: Activation of the small GTPase Ral in platelets. *Mol Cell Biol* 18(5):2486–2491, 1998.

1719. Kawato M, et al: Regulation of platelet dense granule secretion by the Ral GTPase-exocyst pathway. *J Biol Chem* 283(1):166–174, 2008.

1720. Zerial M, McBride H: Rab proteins as membrane organizers. *Nat Rev Mol Cell Biol* 2(2):107–117, 2001.

1721. Kuchay SM, Chishti AH: Calpain-mediated regulation of platelet signaling pathways. *Curr Opin Hematol* 14(3):249–254, 2007.

1722. Lai KC, Flaumenhaft R: SNARE protein degradation upon platelet activation: Calpain cleaves SNAP-23. *J Cell Physiol* 194(2):206–214, 2003.

1723. Kuchay SM, et al: Double knockouts reveal that protein tyrosine phosphatase 1B is a physiological target of calpain-1 in platelets. *Mol Cell Biol* 27(17):6038–6052, 2007.

1724. Vinogradova O, et al: Membrane-mediated structural transitions at the cytoplasmic face during integrin activation. *Proc Natl Acad Sci U S A* 101(12):4094–4099, 2004.

1725. Haas TA, Plow EF: The cytoplasmic domain of alphaIIb beta3. A ternary complex of the integrin alpha and beta subunits and a divalent cation. *J Biol Chem* 271(11):6017–6026, 1996.

1726. Hughes PE, et al: Breaking the integrin hinge. A defined structural constraint regulates integrin signaling. *J Biol Chem* 271(12):6571–6574, 1996.

1727. Martel V, et al: Conformation, localization, and integrin binding of talin depend on its interaction with phosphoinositides. *J Biol Chem* 276(24):21217–21227, 2001.

1728. Di Paolo G, et al: Recruitment and regulation of phosphatidylinositol phosphate kinase type 1 gamma by the FERM domain of talin. *Nature* 420(6911):85–89, 2002.

1729. Ling K, et al: Type I gamma phosphatidylinositol phosphate kinase targets and regulates focal adhesions. *Nature* 420(6911):89–93, 2002.

1730. Calderwood DA, et al: The phosphotyrosine binding-like domain of talin activates integrins. *J Biol Chem* 277(24):21749–21758, 2002.

1731. Akkerman JW, Holmsen H: Interrelationships among platelet responses: Studies on the burst in protein liberation, lactate production and oxygen uptake during platelet aggregation and Ca2+ secretion. *Blood* 57(5):956–966, 1981.

1732. Garcia-Alvarez B, et al: Structural determinants of integrin recognition by talin. Mol. *Cell* 2003;11(1):49–58, 1981.

1733. van Joost T, et al: Purpuric contact dermatitis to benzoyl peroxide. *J Am Acad Dermatol* 22(2 Pt 2):359–361, 1990.

1734. Wegener KL, Campbell ID: Transmembrane and cytoplasmic domains in integrin activation and protein-protein interactions (review). *Mol Membr Biol* 25(5):376–387, 2008.

1735. Ling K, et al: Tyrosine phosphorylation of type Igamma phosphatidylinositol phosphate kinase by Src regulates an integrin-talin switch. *J Cell Biol* 163(6):1339–1349, 2003.

1736. Xing B, Jedsadayanmata A, Lam SC: Localization of an integrin binding site to the C terminus of talin. *J Biol Chem* 276(48):44373–44378, 2001.

1737. Knezevic I, Leisner TM, Lam SC: Direct binding of the platelet integrin alphaIIbbeta3 (GPIIb-IIIa) to talin. Evidence that interaction is mediated through the cytoplasmic domains of both alphaIIb and beta3. *J Biol Chem* 271(27):16416–16421, 1996.

1738. Ma YQ, et al: Kindlin-2 (Mig-2): A co-activator of beta3 integrins. *J Cell Biol* 181(3):439–446, 2008.

1739. Montanez E, et al: Kindlin-2 controls bidirectional signaling of integrins. *Genes Dev* 22(10):1325–1330, 2008.

1740. Moser M, et al: Kindlin-3 is essential for integrin activation and platelet aggregation. *Nat Med* 14(3):325–330, 2008.

1741. Moser M, et al: Kindlin-3 is essential for integrin activation and platelet aggregation. *Nat Med* 14(3):325–330, 2008.

1742. Kuijpers TW, van de Vijver E, Weterman MA, et al: LAD-1/variant syndrome is caused by mutations in FERMT3. *Blood* 113(19):4740–4746, 2009.

1743. Malinin NL, et al: A point mutation in KINDLIN3 ablates activation of three integrin subfamilies in humans. *Nat Med* 15(3):313–318, 2009.

1744. Mory A, Feigelson SW, Yarali N, et al: Kindlin-3: A new gene involved in the pathogenesis of LAD-III. *Blood* 112(6):2591, 2008.

1745. Svensson L, et al: Leukocyte adhesion deficiency-III is caused by mutations in KINDLIN3 affecting integrin activation. *Nat Med* 15(3):306–312, 2009.

1746. Harburger DS, Bouaouina M, Calderwood DA: Kindlin-1 and -2 directly bind the C-terminal region of beta integrin cytoplasmic tails and exert integrin-specific activation effects. *J Biol Chem* 284(17):11485–11497, 2009.

1747. Li R, et al: Oligomerization of the integrin alphaIIbbeta3: Roles of the transmembrane and cytoplasmic domains. *Proc Natl Acad Sci U S A* 98(22):12462–12467, 2001.

1748. Arias-Salgado EG, et al: Src kinase activation by direct interaction with the integrin beta cytoplasmic domain. *Proc Natl Acad Sci U S A* 100(23):13298–13302, 2003.

1749. Newman DK: The Y's that bind: Negative regulators of Src family kinase activity in platelets. *J Thromb Haemost* 7(Suppl 1):195–199, 2009.

1750. Obergfell A, Eto K, Mocsai A, et al: Coordinate interactions of Csk, Src, and Syk kinases with [alpha]IIb[beta]3 initiate integrin signaling to the cytoskeleton. *J Cell Biol* 157(2):265–275, 2002.

1751. Woodside DG, et al: Activation of Syk protein tyrosine kinase through interaction with integrin beta cytoplasmic domains. *Curr Biol* 11(22):1799–1804, 2001.

1752. Woodside DG, et al: The N-terminal SH2 domains of Syk and ZAP-70 mediate phosphotyrosine-independent binding to integrin beta cytoplasmic domains. *J Biol Chem* 277(42):39401–39408, 2002.

1753. De Virgilio M, Kiosses WB, Shattil SJ: Proximal, selective, and dynamic interactions between integrin alphaIIbbeta3 and protein tyrosine kinases in living cells. *J Cell Biol* 2004.

1754. Falati S, et al: Platelet PECAM-1 inhibits thrombus formation *in vivo. Blood* 107(2):535–541, 2006.

1755. Newman EA: New roles for astrocytes: Regulation of synaptic transmission. *Trends Neurosci* 26(10):536–542, 2003.

1756. Newman PJ, Newman DK: Signal transduction pathways mediated by PECAM-1: New roles for an old molecule in platelet and vascular cell biology. *Arterioscler Thromb Vasc Biol* 23(6):953–964, 2003.

1757. Patil S, Newman DK, Newman PJ: Platelet endothelial cell adhesion molecule-1 serves as an inhibitory receptor that modulates platelet responses to collagen. *Blood* 97(6):1727–173, 20012.

1758. Wong C, et al: CEACAM1 negatively regulates platelet-collagen interactions and thrombus growth in vitro and in vivo. *Blood* 2009;113(8):1818–1828, 2009.

1759. Mori J, et al: G6b-B inhibits constitutive and agonist-induced signaling by glycoprotein VI and CLEC-2. *J Biol Chem* 283(51):35419–35427, 2008.

1760. Newland SA, et al: The novel inhibitory receptor G6B is expressed on the surface of platelets and attenuates platelet function *in vitro. Blood* 109(11):4806–4809, 2007.

1761. Senis YA, et al: A comprehensive proteomics and genomics analysis reveals novel transmembrane proteins in human platelets and mouse megakaryocytes including G6b-B, a novel immunoreceptor tyrosine-based inhibitory motif protein. *Mol Cell Proteomics* 6(3):548–564, 2007.

1762. Kumar G, et al: The membrane immunoglobulin receptor utilizes a Shc/Grb2/hSOS complex for activation of the mitogen-activated protein kinase cascade in a B-cell line. *Biochem J* 307(Pt 1):215–223, 1995.

1763. Law DA, et al: Integrin cytoplasmic tyrosine motif is required for outside-in alphaIIbbeta3 signalling and platelet function. *Nature* 401(6755):808–811, 1999.

1764. Miranti CK, et al: Identification of a novel integrin signaling pathway involving the kinase Syk and the guanine nucleotide exchange factor Vav1. *Curr Biol* 8(24):1289–1299, 1998.

1765. Prasad KS, et al: The platelet CD40L/GP IIb-IIIa axis in atherothrombotic disease. *Curr Opin Hematol* 10(5):356–361, 2003.

1766. Majerus PW: Arachidonate metabolism in vascular disorders. *J Clin Invest* 72(5):1521–1525, 1983.

1767. Moncada S, Whittle BJ: Biological actions of prostacyclin and its pharmacological use in platelet studies. *Adv Exp Med Biol* 192:337–358, 1985.

1768. Marcus AJ: The role of lipids in platelet function: With particular reference to the arachidonic acid pathway. *J Lipid Res* 19:793–826, 1978.

1769. Katsuyama M, et al: Cloning and expression of a cDNA for the human prostacyclin receptor. *FEBS Lett* 344(1):74–78, 1994.

1770. Kunapuli SP, et al: Cloning and expression of a prostaglandin E receptor EP3 subtype from human erythroleukaemia cells. *Biochem J* 298 (Pt 2):263–267, 1994.

1771. Feijge MA, et al: Control of platelet activation by cyclic AMP turnover and cyclic nucleotide phosphodiesterase type-3. *Biochem Pharmacol* 67(8):1559–1567, 2004.

1772. Hung SH, et al: New insights from the structure-function analysis of the catalytic region of human platelet phosphodiesterase 3A: A role for the unique 44-amino acid insert. *J Biol Chem* 281(39):29236–29244, 2006.

1773. Sun B, et al: Role of phosphodiesterase type 3A and 3B in regulating platelet and cardiac function using subtype-selective knockout mice. *Cell Signal* 19(8):1765–1771, 2007.

1774. Chapman TM, Goa KL: Cilostazol: A review of its use in intermittent claudication. *Am J Cardiovasc Drugs* 3(2):117–138, 2003.

1775. Manganello JM, et al: Protein kinase A-mediated phosphorylation of the Galpha13 switch I region alters the Galphabetagamma13-G protein-coupled receptor complex and inhibits Rho activation. *J Biol Chem* 278(1):124–130, 2003.

1776. Bodnar RJ, et al: Regulation of glycoprotein Ib-IX-von Willebrand factor interaction by cAMP-dependent protein kinase-mediated phosphorylation at Ser 166 of glycoprotein Ib(beta). *J Biol Chem* 277(49):47080–47087, 2002.

1777. Cavallini L, et al: Prostacyclin and sodium nitroprusside inhibit the activity of the platelet inositol 1,4,5-trisphosphate receptor and promote its phosphorylation. *J Biol Chem* 271:5545–5551, 1996.

1778. Nishimura T, et al: Antiplatelet functions of a stable prostacyclin analog, SM-10906 are exerted by its inhibitory effect on inositol 1,4,5-trisphosphate production and cytosolic Ca2++ increase in rat platelets stimulated by thrombin. *Thromb Res* 79:307–317, 1995.

1779. Cook SJ, McCormick F: Inhibition by cAMP of Ras-dependent activation of Raf. *Science* 262:1069–1072, 1993.

1780. Dumaz N, Marais R: Protein kinase A blocks Raf-1 activity by stimulating 14-3-3 binding and blocking Raf-1 interaction with Ras. *J Biol Chem* 278(32):29819–29823, 2003.

1781. Fischer TH, et al: The localization of the cAMP-dependent protein kinase phosphorylation site in the platelet rat protein, rap 1B. *FEBS Lett* 2832:173–176, 1991.

1782. Siess W, Grunberg B: Phosphorylation of rap1B by protein kinase A is not involved in platelet inhibition by cyclic AMP. *Cell Signal* 5(2):209–214, 1993.

1783. Lou L, et al: cAMP inhibition of Akt is mediated by activated and phosphorylated Rap1b. *J Biol Chem* 277(36):32799–32806, 2002.

1784. Fabre JE, et al: Activation of the murine EP3 receptor for PGE2 inhibits cAMP production and promotes platelet aggregation. *J Clin Invest* 107(5):603–610, 2001.

1785. Shio H, Ramwell P: Effect of prostaglandin E 2 and aspirin on the secondary aggregation of human platelets. *Nat New Biol* 236(63):45–46, 1972.

1786. Gross S, et al: Vascular wall-produced prostaglandin E2 exacerbates arterial thrombosis and atherothrombosis through platelet EP3 receptors. *J Exp Med* 204(2):311–320, 2007.

1787. Luscher TF, et al: Difference between endothelium-dependent relaxation in arterial and in venous coronary bypass grafts. *N Engl J Med* 319(8):462–467, 1988.

1788. Goretski J, Hollocher TC: Trapping of nitric oxide produced during denitrification by extracellular hemoglobin. *J Biol Chem* 263(5):2316–2323, 1988.

1789. Loscalzo J, Welch G: Nitric oxide and its role in the cardiovascular system. *Prog Cardiovasc Dis* 38(2):87–104, 1995.

1790. Mellion BT, et al: Evidence for the inhibitory role of guanosine 3′, 5′-monophosphate in ADP-induced human platelet aggregation in the presence of nitric oxide and related vasodilators. *Blood* 57(5):946–955, 1981.

1791. Radomski MW, Palmer RM, Moncada S: Modulation of platelet aggregation by an L-arginine-nitric oxide pathway. *Trends Pharmacol Sci* 12(3):87–88, 1991.

1792. Wang GR, et al: Mechanism of platelet inhibition by nitric oxide: In vivo phosphorylation of thromboxane receptor by cyclic GMP-dependent protein kinase. *Proc Natl Acad Sci U S A* 95(9):4888–4893, 1998.

1793. Massberg S, et al: Increased adhesion and aggregation of platelets lacking cyclic guanosine 3′,5′-monophosphate kinase I. *J Exp Med* 189(8):1255–1264, 1999.

1794. Aszodi A, et al: The vasodilator-stimulated phosphoprotein (VASP) is involved in cGMP- and cAMP-mediated inhibition of agonist-induced platelet aggregation, but is dispensable for smooth muscle function. *EMBO J* 18(1):37–48, 1999.

1795. Butt E, et al: CAMP- and cGMP-dependent protein kinase phosphorylation sites of the focal adhesion vasodilator-stimulated phosphoprotein (VASP) *in vitro* and in intact human platelets. *J Biol Chem* 269(20):14509–14517, 1994.

1796. Hauser W, et al: Megakaryocyte hyperplasia and enhanced agonist-induced platelet activation in vasodilator-stimulated phosphoprotein knockout mice. *Proc Natl Acad Sci U S A* 96(14):8120–8125, 1999.

1797. Massberg S, et al: Enhanced *in vivo* platelet adhesion in vasodilator-stimulated phosphoprotein (VASP)-deficient mice. *Blood* 103(1):136–142, 2004.

1798. Maurice DH, Haslam RJ: Molecular basis of the synergistic inhibition of platelet function by nitrovasodilators and activators of adenylate cyclase: Inhibition of cyclic AMP breakdown by cyclic GMP. *Mol Pharmacol* 37(5):671–681, 1990.

1799. Atkinson B, et al: Ecto-nucleotidases of the CD39/NTPDase family modulate platelet activation and thrombus formation: Potential as therapeutic targets. *Blood Cells Mol Dis* 36(2):217–222, 2006.

1800. Kaczmarek E, et al: Identification and characterization of CD39/vascular ATP diphosphohydrolase. *J Biol Chem* 271(51):33116–33122, 1996.

1801. Marcus AJ, et al: The endothelial cell ecto-ADPase responsible for inhibition of platelet function is CD39. *J Clin Invest* 99(6):1351–1360, 1997.

1802. Le F, et al: Characterization and chromosomal localization of the human A2a adenosine receptor gene: ADORA2A. *Biochem Biophys Res Commun* 223(2):461–467, 1996.

1803. Pulte D, Olson KE, Broekman MJ, et al: CD39 activity correlates with stage and inhibits platelet reactivity in chronic lymphocytic leukemia. *J Transl Med* 5:23, 2007.

1804. Gayle RB 3rd, Maliszewski CR, Gimpel SD, et al: Inhibition of platelet function by recombinant soluble ecto-ADPase/CD39. *J Clin Invest* 101(9):1851–1859, 1998.

1805. White JG: Platelet ultrastructure, in *Hemostasis and Thrombosis*, edited by AL Bloom, CD Forbes, P Duncan, EGD Tuddenham, pp 49–88. Churchill Livingstone, Edinburgh, 1994.

1806. Varga-Szabo D, Braun A, Nieswandt B: Calcium signaling in platelets. *J Thromb Haemost* 7(7):1057–1066, 2009.

1807. Bray PF: Platelet genomics beats the catch-22. *Blood* 114(7):1286–1287, 2009.

1808. Bray PF, McKenzie SE, Edelstein LC, et al: The complex transcriptional landscape of the anucleate human platelet. *BMC Genomics* 14:1, 2013.

1809. Smyth SS, Woulfe DS, Weitz JI, et al: G-protein-coupled receptors as signaling targets for antiplatelet therapy. *Arterioscler Thromb Vasc Biol* 29(4):449–457, 2009.

1810. Zhang C, Srinivasan Y, Arlow DH, et al: High-resolution crystal structure of human protease-activated receptor 1. *Nature* 492(7429):387–392, 2012.

1811. Pollard TD, Actin. *Curr Opin Cell Biol* 2:33–40, 1990.

1812. Vandekerckhove J: Actin-binding proteins. *Curr Opin Cell Biol* 2:41–50, 1990.

1813. Weeds AG, et al: Preparation and characterization of pig plasma and platelet gelsolins. *Eur J Biochem* 161:69–76, 1986.

1814. Smillie LB: Structure and function of tropomyosins from muscle and non-muscle. *Trends Biochem Sci* 4:151, 1979.

1815. Vandekerckhove J: Structural principles of actin-binding proteins. *Curr Opin Cell Biol* 1(1):15–22, 1989.

1816. Chen M, Stracher A: In situ phosphorylation of platelet actin-binding protein by cAMP-dependent protein kinase stabilizes it against proteolysis by calpain. *J Biol Chem* 264:14282–14289, 1989.

1817. Lind SE, Stossel TP: The microfilament network of the platelet. *Prog Hemost Thromb* 6:63–84, 1982.

1818. He P, Zhang H, Yun CC: IRBIT, inositol 1,4,5-triphosphate (IP3) receptor-binding protein released with IP3, binds Na+/H+ exchanger NHE3 and activates NHE3 activity in response to calcium. *J Biol Chem* 283(48):33544–33553, 2008.

1819. Beckerle MC, et al: Activation-dependent redistribution of the adhesion plaque protein, talin, in intact human platelets. *J Cell Biol* 109:3333–3346, 1989.

1820. O'Halloran T, Beckerle MC, Burridge K: Identification of talin as a major cytoplasmic protein implicated in platelet activation. *Nature* 317:449–451, 1985.

1821. Koteliansky VE, Gneushev GN, Glukhova MA, et al: Identification and isolation of vinculin from platelets. *FEBS Lett* 165(1):26–30, 1984.

1822. Langer B, Gonnella PA, Nachmias VT: Alpha-actinin and vinculin in normal and thrombasthenic platelets. *Blood* 63(3):606–614, 1984.

1823. Lucas RC, et al: The isolation and characterization of a cytoskeleton and a contractile apparatus from platelets., in *Protides of Biological Fluids*, edited by H Peeters, pp 465–470. Pergamon Press, New York, 1975.

1824. Wang LL, Bryan J: Isolation of calcium-dependent platelet proteins that interact with actin. *Cell* 25(3):637–649, 1981.

1825. Hathaway DR, Adelstein RS: Human platelet myosin light chain kinase requires the calcium binding protein calmodulin for activity. *Proc Natl Acad Sci U S A* 76:1653, 1979.

1826. Wolff DJ, Brostrom CO: Proterties and functions of the calcium-dependent regulator protein. *Adv Cyclic Nucleotide Res* 11:27, 1979.

1827. Daniel JL: Platelet contractile proteins, in *Hemostasis and Thrombosis: Basic Principles and Clinical Practice*, edited by RW Colman, J Hirsh, VJ Marder, EW Salzman, pp 557–573. JB Lippincott, Philadelphia, 1993.

CHAPTER 113

MOLECULAR BIOLOGY AND BIOCHEMISTRY OF THE COAGULATION FACTORS AND PATHWAYS OF HEMOSTASIS

Mettine H. A. Bos, Cornelis van 't Veer, and Pieter H. Reitsma

SUMMARY

The coagulation cascade consists of a complex network of reactions that are essential for the conversion of zymogens into enzymes and of inactive pro-cofactors into cofactors. Most of these reactions take place on a membrane surface, which restricts coagulation to the site of injury. Upon initiation, these reactions serve to produce the fibrin that is necessary for the formation of a stable hemostatic plug. In addition, these reactions provide feedback loops that limit and localize thrombus formation and regulate thrombus resolution. This chapter highlights key biochemical characteristics of the individual coagulation factors, essential aspects regarding their synthesis, and the clinical importance of acquired or inherited variations that affect their quantity or function. The coagulation factors are grouped as (1) the vitamin K-dependent zymogens (prothrombin, factor VII, factor IX, factor X, and protein C); (2) the procoagulant cofactors (factor V, factor VIII); (3) the soluble cofactors (protein S, von Willebrand factor); (4) factor XI and the contact system (factor XII, prekallikrein, and high-molecular weight kininogen); (5) the cell-associated cofactors (tissue factor, thrombomodulin, endothelial protein C receptor); (6) the fibrin network (fibrin[ogen], factor XIII, thrombin-activatable fibrinolysis inhibitor); and (7) inhibitors of coagulation (antithrombin, tissue factor pathway inhibitor, protein Z/protein Z-dependent protease inhibitor). Table 113–1 summarizes the major features of the coagulation factors addressed in this chapter. The final sections of this chapter present an overview of the coagulation cascade in which the pathways of hemostasis including the contribution of endothelial cells, blood platelets, and immune cells are described.

MOLECULAR BIOLOGY AND BIOCHEMISTRY OF THE COAGULATION FACTORS

THE VITAMIN K–DEPENDENT ZYMOGENS: PROTHROMBIN, FACTOR VII, FACTOR IX, FACTOR X, AND PROTEIN C

The vitamin K-dependent zymogens circulate in an inactive state and require proteolytic activation to function as a serine protease. All share a similar domain structure of a C-terminal serine protease domain and an N-terminal γ-carboxy glutamic acid (Gla) domain, which are connected by two epidermal growth factor (EGF)-like domains or kringle domains (Fig. 113–1). Each protein domain has a well-defined function and facilitates substrate recognition, interaction with protein cofactors, or binding to a negatively charged lipid surface, such as that of activated platelets or endothelial cells, thereby restricting coagulation to the site of injury. The latter is mediated via the Gla domain, a domain that is characteristic to the vitamin K–dependent proteins.

The high level of protein and gene homology suggests that the vitamin K–dependent zymogens originate from a common ancestral gene as a result of gene duplications.[1] Exon shuffling and tandem duplication may account for the generation of the ancestral gene, in which the functional domains that are encoded by a single exon each were combined and duplicated.[2] This process may also account for the presence of the kringle domains as opposed to EGF-like domains in prothrombin.

The Gla domain refers to the 42-residue region located in the N-terminus of the mature protein that comprises 9 to 12 glutamic acid residues that are posttranslationally γ-carboxylated into Gla residues by a specific γ-glutamyl carboxylase in the endoplasmatic reticulum of hepatocytes.[3] This γ-carboxylase requires oxygen, carbon dioxide, and the reduced form of vitamin K for its action, hence the name vitamin K–dependent proteins. For each Glu residue that is carboxylated, one molecule of reduced vitamin K is converted to the epoxide form (Fig. 113–2). Vitamin K epoxide reductase converts the epoxide form of vitamin K back to the reduced form.[4] Warfarin and related 4-hydroxy-coumarin–containing molecules inhibit the activity of vitamin K epoxide reductase, thereby preventing vitamin K recycling and inhibiting γ-carboxylation. This results in a heterogeneous population of circulating undercarboxylated forms of the vitamin K–dependent proteins with reduced activity. Because warfarin blocks the reductase and not the carboxylase, the inhibitory effect of warfarin can be (temporarily) reversed by administration of vitamin K. Recognition by and interaction with γ-carboxylase is facilitated by the propeptide sequence that is located C-terminal to the signal peptide. The propeptide is highly conserved among the vitamin K–dependent proteins, and amino acids at positions −18, −17, −16, −15, and −10 are critical to recognition by the γ-carboxylase.[5,6] Following γ-carboxylation, the propeptide is removed through limited proteolysis prior to secretion of the mature protein.

A correctly γ-carboxylated Gla domain is essential for interaction of the vitamin K–dependent proteins with phosphatidylserine, a negatively charged phospholipid. Under normal conditions, phosphatidylserine is not exposed on the outer membrane leaflet of cells. However, in activated endothelial cells or platelets, phosphatidylserine is part of the extracellular cell surface where it supports blood coagulation reactions. The Gla domain interacts with the anionic cell surface in a calcium-dependent manner. These calcium ions are coordinated by Gla residues and induce a conformational change in the Gla domain that is characterized by the appearance of a hydrophobic surface loop

TABLE 113-1. Characteristics of Coagulation Proteins

	Protein	Plasma Concentration		Mr	Plasma Half-Life
		(μg/mL)	(nmol/L)	(kDa)	(Hours)
ZYMOGENS					
+ Gla domain	Prothrombin (factor II)	100	1400	72	60
	Factor VII	0.5	10	50	3–6
	Factor IX	5	90	55	18–24
	Factor X	10	170	59	34–40
	Protein C	4	65	62	6–8
– Gla domain	Factor XI	5	30	160	60–80
	Factor XII	40	500	80	50–70
	Prekallikrein	40	490	85	35
	Factor XIIIA*†	-	–	83	–
	Factor XIIIB*	7	94	76.5	–
	Factor XIII	30	94	320	240
	TAFI	4–15	70–275	60	–
COFACTORS					
Soluble	Factor V†	5-10	20	330	12–36
	Factor VIII	0.2	0.7	300	8–12
	VWF	varies	10	500–20,000	8–12
	Protein S‡	25	350	75	42
	Protein Z§	2.5	40	62	60
	HK	80	670	120	150
Cellular	Tissue factor	–	–	47	–
	Thrombomodulin	-	–	78	–
	EPCR	–	–	49	–
STRUCTURAL PROTEIN	Fibrinogen	2500	7400	340	72–120
	Aα chain	–	–	66.5	–
	Bβ chain	–	-	52	–
	γ Chain	–	–	46.5	–
INHIBITORS	Antithrombin	150	2500	58	60–72
	TFPIα¶	0.01	0.25	40	0.03
	ZPI§	4	60	72	60

EPCR, endothelial protein C receptor; HK, high-molecular-weight kininogen; TAFI, thrombin-activatable fibrinolysis inhibitor; TFPI, full-length tissue factor pathway inhibitor; VWF, von Willebrand factor; ZPI, protein Z–dependent protease inhibitor.

*All of the factor XIIIA chain is in complex with factor XIIIB chain; only half of factor XIIIB is in complex with factor XIIIA, the rest is free in plasma.

†Platelets carry significant amounts of factor XIIIA and factor V (20% of circulating factor V).

‡Approximately 60% of protein S is in complex with C4b-binding protein; the remainder circulates as free protein S.

§ZPI circulates in complex with protein Z.

¶TFPI circulates in plasma at 2.5 nM in multiple forms; only 10% of circulating TFPI is the full-length TFPIα.

(Fig. 113–3). Membrane binding by the Gla domain occurs when this hydrophobic surface loop penetrates into the hydrophobic portion of the phospholipid bilayer, which is facilitated by the interaction of the Gla-bound calcium ions with the phosphate head groups of phosphatidylserine.[7,8] It has been shown that the phosphate head groups of exposed phosphatidylethanolamine are also capable of coordinating calcium ions, thereby contributing to the interaction of the Gla domains with the negatively charged membrane surface.[9]

The serine protease domains of the vitamin K–dependent proteins are highly homologous, as they bear a chymotrypsin-like fold and display trypsin-like activity.[10] Once activated, they cleave peptide bonds following a positively charged amino acid (Lys or Arg). Activation proceeds through proteolysis at one or more sites N-terminal to the serine protease domain (see Fig. 113–1). Subsequently, the newly formed N-terminus inserts into the serine protease domain to form a salt bridge with an Asp residue, which is associated with conformational

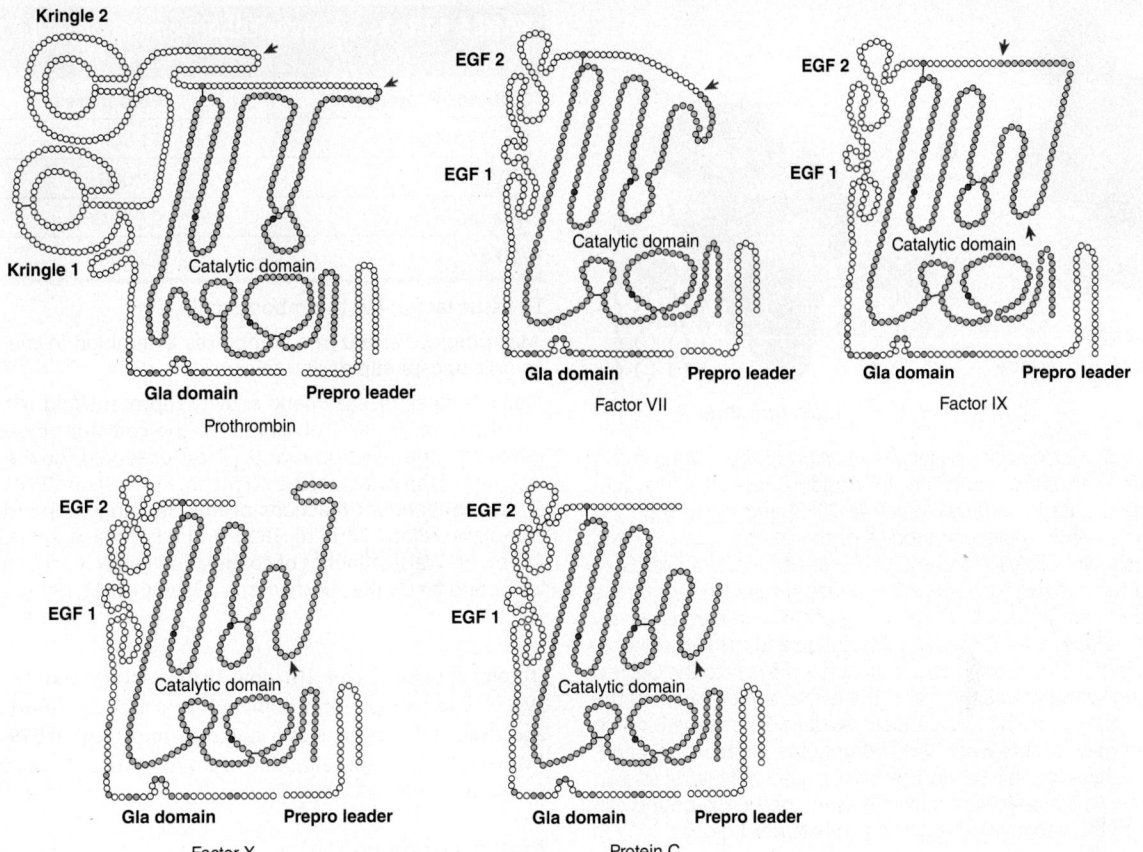

Figure 113–1. Vitamin K–dependent schematic of the vitamin K–dependent zymogens. Each circle represents an amino acid. The prepro leader sequence contains the signal peptide as well as the propeptide that directs γ-carboxylation of glutamic acid (Gla) residues. Cleavage of the prepro sequence from the mature protein is indicated by the separation between the two. The Gla domains are indicated with the Gla residues in *blue*. Prothrombin has a finger loop followed by two kringle domains. Factors VII, IX, X, and protein C have epidermal growth factor (EGF)-like domains. Prothrombin, factor VII, and factor IX circulate as single-chain molecules. Factor X and protein C circulate as two chains that are disulfide linked. All have homologous serine protease ("catalytic") domains (shown in *light red*), in which the active site His, Asp, and Ser residues are indicated in *dark red*. Cleavages that convert the zymogen to an active enzyme are indicated by the *red arrows*. In factor IX, factor X, and protein C, the released activation peptide is indicated in *yellow*. After proteolytic activation, all of the molecules are two-chain disulfide-linked molecules, with the cysteines forming a disulfide bridge *(black line)* indicated in *green*. All catalytic domains but that of prothrombin remain attached to the Gla domain following activation.

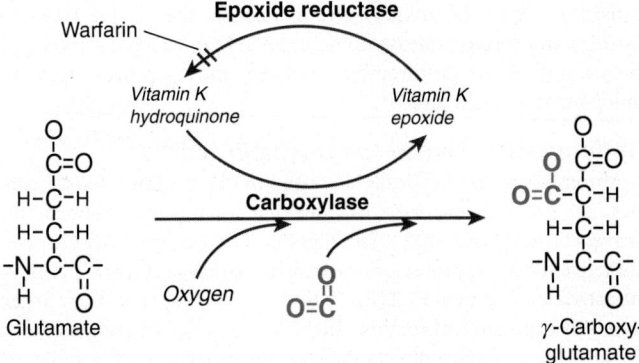

Figure 113–2. Vitamin K–dependent γ-carboxylation. Glutamic acid residues are converted to γ-carboxy glutamic acid (Gla) residues by a specific γ-carboxylase. This reaction requires oxygen, carbon dioxide (shown in *green*), and reduced vitamin K in the form of a hydroquinone. Carbon dioxide is incorporated onto the γ-carbon, providing a second carboxylate group on that residue. In the process of this reaction, reduced vitamin K is converted to an epoxide. Reduced vitamin K is recycled by a specific epoxide reductase, a reaction that can be blocked by warfarin and warfarin analogues.

changes in the serine protease domain. These lead to an optimal configuration of the active site through alignment of the active site residues His, Ser, and Asp, and to formation of the substrate-binding exosites, allowing for substrate conversion. The substrate-binding exosites are unique to each vitamin K–dependent protease and are responsible for their highly specific substrate recognition and associated function in coagulation.

Interaction of the vitamin K–dependent proteases with specific cofactors on a (anionic) membrane surface (Table 113–2) further enhances substrate recognition, as the cofactors interact with both the protease and the substrate, bridging the two together. This results in a dramatic enhancement of the catalytic activity (Table 113–3), thereby making the cofactor–protease complex the physiologic relevant enzyme. The increase in catalytic rate has also been attributed to a cofactor-induced conformational change in the protease.[11] However, whether this molecular mechanism holds true for all cofactor–protease complexes remains to be determined. Tissue factor is the cofactor for factor VIIa, factor VIIIa is the cofactor for factor IXa, and factor Va is the cofactor for factor Xa, while thrombin does not require a cofactor for its procoagulant activity. However, upon association with the cofactor thrombomodulin, thrombin's specificity is changed from procoagulant

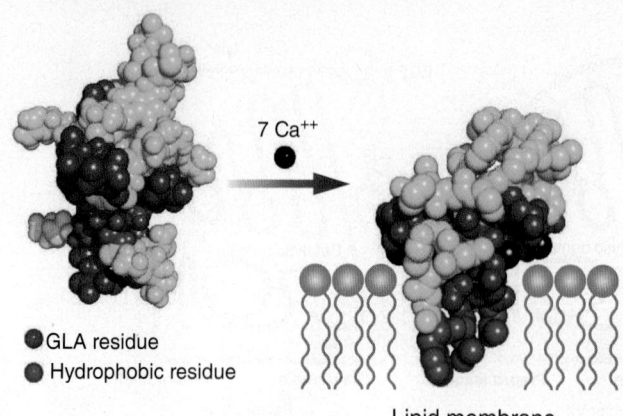

- GLA residue
- Hydrophobic residue

Lipid membrane

Figure 113–3. Calcium-dependent association of the glutamic acid (Gla) domain with the anionic phospholipid surface. Non–calcium bound [Protein Data Bank (PDB) structure 2PF2] and calcium bound (PDB structure 1WHE) molecular models of the Gla domain of prothrombin are shown. Circles represent amino acids, with the Gla (GLA) residues indicated in *red*. Hydrophobic residues involved in membrane insertion are shown in *blue*. In the absence of calcium, the negatively charged Gla residues are exposed to the solution and the hydrophobic residues are buried. Association of calcium ions (in *black*) to the Gla residues provides sufficient energy to alter the overall conformation of the Gla domain and expose the hydrophobic residues. Membrane binding by the Gla domain occurs when this hydrophobic surface loop penetrates into the hydrophobic portion of the phospholipid bilayer (drawn schematically), which is facilitated by interaction of the Gla-bound calcium ions with the negatively charged phosphate head groups.

to anticoagulant (cleaving and activating protein C). The complexes are also named for their physiologic substrate: the factor VIIIa–factor IXa complex is termed the "tenase" or "intrinsic tenase" complex; the tissue factor–factor VIIa complex is termed the "extrinsic tenase" complex; and the factor Va–factor Xa complex is termed the "prothrombinase" complex.

PROTHROMBIN (FACTOR II)

Prothrombin, or factor II, which was discovered by Pekelharing in 1894, is one of the four coagulation factors that were described by Paul Morawitz in 1905, in addition to fibrinogen (factor I), thromboplastin

TABLE 113–2. Protease–Cofactor Complexes

Protease	Cofactor	Substrate	Cellular Location
Factor VIIa	Tissue factor	Factor IX Factor X	Many cells*
Factor IXa	Factor VIIIa	Factor X	Platelets
Factor Xa	Factor Va	Prothrombin	Platelets
Thrombin	Thrombomodulin	Protein C	Endothelium
Activated protein C	Protein S	Factor Va Factor VIIIa	Endothelium

*Tissue factor is constitutively expressed on many extravascular cells (e.g., stromal cells, epithelial cells, astrocytes) and is induced by inflammatory mediators in many other cells (e.g., monocytes, endothelial cells).

TABLE 113–3. Cofactor Enhancement of Serine Protease Activity

Cofactor-Protease*	Fold Increase†
TM-Thrombin	11,000
TF-VIIa	31,000
VIIIa-IXa	9,000,000
Va-Xa	390,000

TF, tissue factor; TM, thrombomodulin.

*Macromolecular enzyme complexes assembled in the presence of anionic phospholipids and calcium.

†Relative rates of enzymatic activity represent fold increase of the reaction rate (k_{cat}/Km) observed for the cofactor-protease complex relative to the reaction rate (k_{cat}/Km) observed for the protease in absence of the cofactor (see KG Mann, ME Nesheim, WR Church, et al: Surface-dependent reactions of the vitamin K–dependent enzyme complexes. *Blood* 76:1–16, 1990; and R Rawala-Sheikh, SS Ahmad, B Ashby, PN Walsh: Kinetics of coagulation factor X activation by platelet-bound factor IXa. *Biochemistry* 29:2606–2611,1990).

(thrombokinase, factor III, now tissue factor), and calcium (factor IV).[12,13] The zymogen prothrombin is primarily synthesized in the liver and circulates in plasma as a single-chain protein of 579 amino acids (Mr ≈72,000) at a concentration of 1.4 µM with a plasma half-life of 60 hours (see Table 113–1).

Protein Structure

Prothrombin is composed of fragment 1 (F1), fragment 2 (F2), and the serine protease domain. F1 consists of the Gla domain, which comprises 10 Gla residues, and the kringle 1 domain; F2 contains the kringle 2 domain (see Fig. 113–1). The two kringle domains, which replace the EGF-like domains present in most vitamin K–dependent zymogens, are conserved secondary protein structures that fold into large loops that are stabilized by three disulfide bonds and schematically resemble a Danish pastry called a "kringle." Their primary function is to bind other proteins such as the cofactor Va and serine protease factor Xa that activate prothrombin.

Other than γ-carboxylation of Glu residues, prothrombin is post-translationally modified via *N*-glycosylation in the kringle 1 (Asn78, Asn143) and serine protease domains (Asn373), which contributes to the stability of the prothrombin precursor during processing in the endoplasmatic reticulum.[14,15]

Prothrombin Activation and Thrombin Activity

Prothrombin is proteolytically activated by the prothrombinase complex (i.e., factor Va, factor Xa, calcium, and anionic phospholipids) that cleaves at Arg271 and Arg320 (see Fig. 113–1). Cleavage at Arg320 opens the active site of the protease domain, while cleavage at Arg271 removes the activation fragment F1.2 (F1.2). Both cleavages are necessary to generate procoagulant α-thrombin (IIα) (Fig. 113–4). The composition of the membrane surface directs the cleavage order in prothrombin and the formation of either the zymogen prethrombin 2 (initial cleavage at Arg271) or the proteolytically active intermediate meizothrombin (initial cleavage at Arg320).[16,17] Meizothrombin has impaired procoagulant activity as compared to α-thrombin, but superior anticoagulant activity as it displays increased thrombomodulin-dependent protein C activation, which is likely facilitated by membrane binding of meizothrombin through its Gla domain.[18] The snake venom protease Ecarin is capable of generating meizothrombin specifically through proteolysis at Arg323 only. However, this meizothrombin is instable as a result of autocatalysis

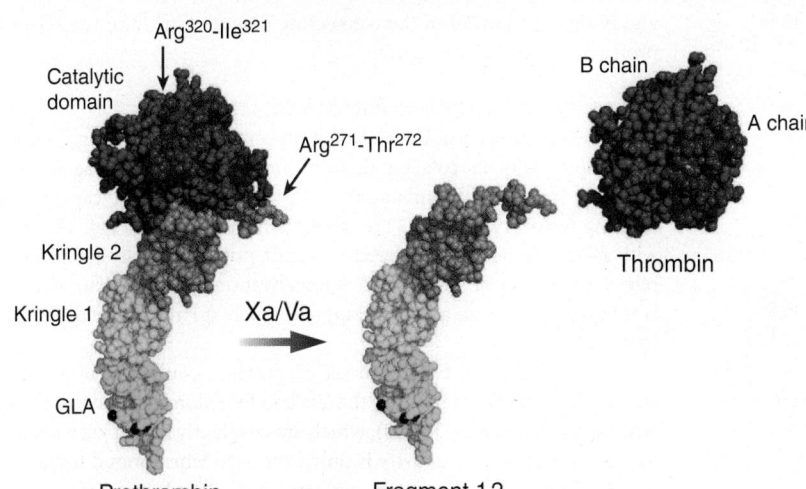

Figure 113–4. Prothrombin to thrombin conversion. A molecular model of prothrombin comprising the γ-carboxy glutamic acid (Gla; GLA) domain, both kringle domains, and the catalytic domain is shown (PDB structures 2PF2, 1HAG, 1A0H, 1HAI). Gla domain-bound calcium ions are indicated in *black*. Cleavage by the factor Va-Xa complex at Arg271 and Arg320 releases thrombin (with the A chain and catalytically active B chain) from the rest of the molecule (fragment 1.2).

at Arg155, thereby removing the Gla domain containing F1. The so formed meizo-des-F1 can be converted to thrombin by prothrombinase, but at a slower rate as it is incapable of membrane binding. Assessment of F1.2 levels reflects prothrombin activation and is commonly used as a marker for thrombin generation.

Thrombin (IIα) is a two-chain serine protease (Mr ≈37,000) comprising a light chain of 49 residues (A chain; Mr ≈6000) that is covalently linked to the catalytic heavy chain of 259 residues (B chain; Mr ≈31,000). Thrombin's main function is to induce the formation of a fibrin clot by removing fibrinopeptides A and B from fibrinogen to form fibrin monomers, which then spontaneously polymerize. In addition, thrombin is able to cleave a wide variety of substrates with high specificity, which is mediated via its negatively charged, deep active site cleft and via the anion binding exosites I and II that specifically interact with cofactors and/or substrates.[19] The dynamic structural conformation of thrombin allows for binding to diverse ligands, and the subsequent ligand-induced conformational stabilization, known as thrombin allostery, regulates and controls thrombin activity.[20,21]

Thrombin initiates important procoagulant pathways by proteolytic activation of the cofactors V and VIII and zymogen factor XI that collectively amplify thrombin and fibrin formation, and by activating factor XIII that crosslinks and stabilizes the fibrin polymers. Another procoagulant function of thrombin is to inhibit fibrinolysis by proteolytic activation of the thrombin-activatable fibrinolysis inhibitor (TAFI), a reaction enhanced by the endothelial-bound cofactor thrombomodulin. Thrombin also has an anticoagulant function and upon binding to the cofactor thrombomodulin, it is capable of proteolytically activating protein C, which inactivates the cofactors Va and VIIIa.

Thrombin activates the seven-transmembrane domain, G-protein–coupled protease-activated receptors (PARs) PAR1, PAR3, and PAR4 that are expressed on a wide range of cell types in the vasculature by proteolytic cleavage of their N-terminal extracellular domains.[22–25] Thrombin is one of the strongest platelet activators *in vivo* and activates platelet-expressed PAR1 and PAR4.[25] The platelet glycoprotein (GP) Ib (GPIb) serves as a cofactor for thrombin in PAR1 cleavage (Chap. 112). Thrombin-mediated activation of endothelial-PAR1 triggers release of von Willebrand factor (VWF) and P-selectin, which promote rolling and adhesion of platelets and leukocytes. In addition, this stimulates the endothelial production of platelet-activating factor, a potent platelet and leukocyte activator, as well as the production of chemokines, cyclooxygenase (COX)-2, and prostaglandins.[25] Thrombin-mediated PAR activation is not only critical for coagulation, but also plays an important role

in inflammatory and proliferative responses associated with vascular injury, such as in atherosclerosis and cancer.[26]

The physiologic inhibitors of thrombin are the serine protease inhibitors (serpins) antithrombin, heparin cofactor II, protein C inhibitor, and protease nexin 1, with antithrombin being the primary plasma inhibitor. For all four serpins, the rate of thrombin inhibition can be accelerated by glycosaminoglycans, such as heparin (Table 113–4), through mutual binding to the serpin and thrombin (see Fig. 113–2), which ensures rapid inhibition of thrombin at the intact endothelial cell surface where heparin-like glycosaminoglycans are found.

Heparin and heparin-derivatives are clinically used as anticoagulants to inhibit thrombin via antithrombin. Hirudin, which originates from the salivary glands of medicinal leeches, and its recombinant and synthetic derivatives are potent and highly specific inhibitors that directly target the active site and exosite I of thrombin.[27] The target-specific oral anticoagulant dabigatran also inhibits thrombin directly with high specificity and reversibly binds the active site of thrombin.[27,28]

TABLE 113–4. Antithrombin Inhibition of Coagulation Proteases

Second-Order Association Rate Constants (M⁻¹s⁻¹)			
Protease	– Heparin	+ H5	+ UFH
Thrombin	7.7×10^3	1.5×10^4	4.7×10^7
Factor Xa	2.6×10^3	7.6×10^5	6.6×10^6
Factor IXa	58	3.1×10^4	6.2×10^6
TF-Factor VIIa	33	4.9×10^3	1.5×10^4
Factor XIa	3.6×10^2	1.1×10^3	1.8×10^5
Factor XIIa	39	1.9×10^3	6.6×10^4
APC	0.08	1.9	2.1

APC, activated protein C; TF, tissue factor.

The association rate constants characterizing the antithrombin inhibition of coagulation proteases in the absence of heparin or accelerated by H5, the synthetic pentasaccharide fondaparinux, or UFH, unfractionated heparin, which comprises long heparin molecules. *In vivo*, natural glycosaminoglycan molecules on endothelium and other cells accelerate the rate of inhibition. (See ST Olson, R Swanson, E Raub-Segall, et al.[321])

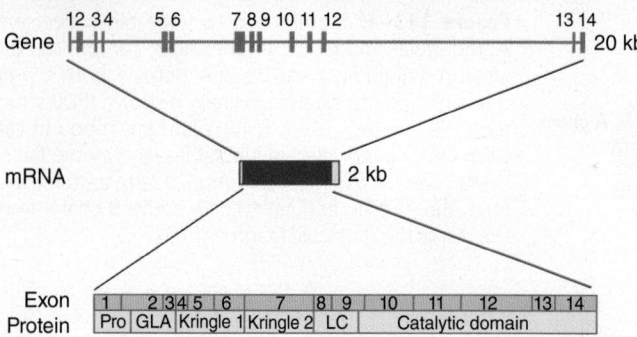

Figure 113–5. Relationship of gene structure to protein structure in prothrombin. The exons, introns, mRNA, and protein structure are as indicated. The mRNA is 2 kb with small 5′ and 3′ untranslated regions (shown in *light blue*). In the protein, Pro indicates the prepro leader sequence, GLA indicates the γ-carboxy glutamic acid (Gla) domain, Kringles 1 and 2 are indicated, LC indicates the light chain (also known as the A chain), and the serine protease (catalytic) domain is indicated.

Gene Structure and Variations

Prothrombin is encoded by a gene *(F2)* on chromosome 11p11.2 that is approximately 20 kb long.[29] The coding sequence is divided over 14 exons that range in size from 25 to 315 bp (Fig. 113–5). The reference sequence of prothrombin mRNA comprises 2018 bases. There are no common, well characterized, splicing variants with known biology.

Homozygosity or compound heterozygosity for loss of function mutations in the prothrombin gene leads to a bleeding tendency. This condition is quite rare with perhaps one case per 2,000,000 newborns.[30] Heterozygous carriers of loss-of-function mutations are without a bleeding phenotype. Mutations have been characterized in a relatively small number of cases with homozygous or compound heterozygous prothrombin deficiency (consult the human gene mutation database at http://www.hgmd.org for details). The majority of mutations underlying prothrombin deficiency are missense mutations, but several small deletions/insertions have also been reported.

Gain-of-function mutations in the prothrombin gene increase thrombotic risk. The best known variation is G20210A.[31] This variation of the last nucleotide preceding the poly(A)-tail of the mature mRNA has an effect on 3′-end mRNA processing and increases the level of prothrombin in plasma by approximately 10 to 20 percent in heterozygous individuals.[32] This relatively small increase in the level of prothrombin results in a two- to threefold enhanced risk for venous thrombosis. Homozygotes for the G20210A variation are quite rare, and the risk associated with homozygosity has not been measured with certainty. The G20210A variation is relatively common in whites, with a strong south-north gradient in that the variation is most common in southern Europe.[33]

FACTOR VII

Factor VII, which was discovered around 1950,[34] is synthesized in the liver and circulates in plasma as a single-chain zymogen of 406 amino acids (Mr ≈50,000) at a concentration of 10 nM with a short plasma half-life of 3 to 6 hours (see Table 113–1).

Protein Structure

Factor VII consists of a Gla domain with 10 Gla residues, two EGF-like domains, a connecting region, and the serine protease domain (see Fig. 113–1). Calcium coordination in EGF-1 is mediated by partial hydroxylation of Asn63 and O-linked fucosylation of Ser60.[35] Further posttranslational modifications of factor VII consist of O-linked (Ser52 in EGF-1)

and N-linked (Asn154 in the connecting region, Asn322 in the serine protease domain) glycosylation.

Factor VII Activation and Factor VIIa Activity

Factor VII is proteolytically activated once it has formed a high-affinity complex with its cofactor tissue factor. A number of coagulation proteases including thrombin and factors IXa and XIIa are capable of cleaving factor VII at Arg152 to generate factor VIIa (see Fig. 113–1), with factor Xa being considered the most potent and physiologically relevant activator of factor VII.[36] Autoactivation can also occur, which is initiated by minute amounts (approximately 0.1 nM) of preexisting factor VIIa.[37]

Factor VIIa is a two-chain serine protease composed of a light chain (Mr ≈20,000) comprising the Gla and EGF domains and the catalytic heavy chain (Mr ≈30,000), which are covalently linked via a disulfide bond. Factor VIIa activity is only expressed when bound to tissue factor, which induces an active conformation of the factor VIIa serine protease domain (Fig. 113–6).[11] Factor VIIa interacts with tissue factor via its Gla and EGF domains.

The tissue factor–factor VIIa complex activates both coagulation factors IX and X, which is considered to be the main initiating step of the extrinsic pathway of coagulation. In addition, the tissue factor–factor VIIa (–factor Xa) complex is not only critical to processes in coagulation, but also to wound healing, angiogenesis, tissue remodeling, and inflammation through proteolytic activation of PAR2.[38-40]

The ternary tissue factor–factor VIIa–factor Xa complex is inhibited by the tissue factor pathway inhibitor (TFPI). Tissue factor–factor VIIa is also inhibited by antithrombin, but only in the presence of heparin (see Table 113–4).

Gene Structure and Variations

The gene encoding factor VII *(F7)* is located on chromosome 13q34, is almost 15 kb in length, and comprises 9 exons (Fig. 113–7). The canonical mRNA encoding factor VII comprises 3000 bases.[41] Alternatively spliced transcript variants encoding multiple isoforms have been observed, but their biology is not well characterized.[42]

Inherited factor VII deficiency is a rare autosomal recessive disorder that affects approximately one in 500,000 newborns.[30] Factor VII deficiency is the most common of the inherited rare bleeding disorders,

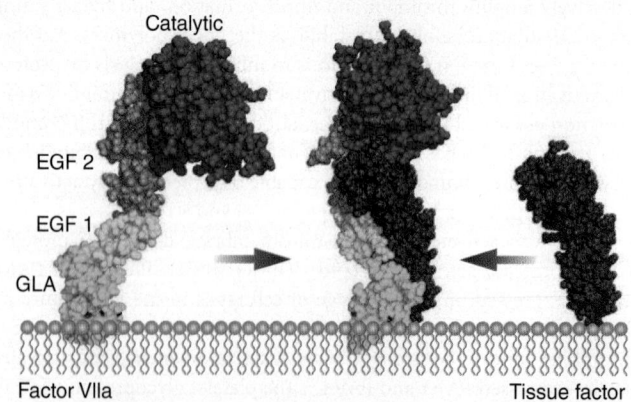

Figure 113–6. The tissue factor–factor VIIa complex. A molecular model of factor VIIa (PDB structures 1QHK, 1WHF, 1RFN, 1DAN) and the crystal structures of the tissue factor–factor VIIa complex (PDB structure 1DAN) and the extracellular domain of tissue factor (PDB structure 2HFT) are shown. The γ-carboxy glutamic acid (Gla; GLA) domain, epidermal growth factor (EGF)-like domains 1 and 2, and serine protease (catalytic) domain of factor VIIa are indicated. Binding to tissue factor alters the overall structure of factor VIIa.

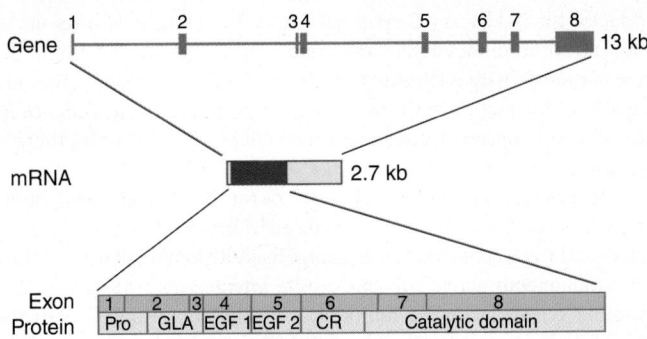

Figure 113–7. Relationship of gene structure to protein structure in factor VII. The exons, introns, mRNA, and protein structure are as indicated. The mRNA is 2.7 kb with a small 5′ untranslated region and a relatively large 3′ untranslated region *(light blue)*. In the protein, Pro indicates the prepro leader sequence, GLA indicates the γ-carboxy glutamic acid (Gla) domain, and epidermal growth factor (EGF)-1 and -2, as well as the serine protease (catalytic) domain, are indicated. CR indicates the connecting region that comprises the site of proteolytic activation.

although the reported prevalences vary between countries. Homozygotes and compound heterozygotes develop a hemorrhagic diathesis that may vary from mild to severe.

The human gene mutation database (http://www.hgmd.org) lists 258 mutations in the factor VII gene. The majority of these are missense mutations, but splicing and regulatory mutations also occur. Small deletions account for almost 10 percent of the documented mutations. Other gross gene abnormalities appear to be uncommon.

The factor VII gene harbors many common polymorphisms of which three are notable: Arg353Gln in the catalytic domain, a 10-bp insertion in the promotor region, and a variable number of 37 bp repeats in intron 7.[43] The minor alleles of these polymorphisms are associated with decreased levels of factor VII and explain up to 30 percent of the variation in activated factor VII levels. Furthermore, the minor alleles have been claimed to lower the risk of myocardial infarction. However, this finding has not led to routine genotyping in the management of this disorder. The relationship between factor VII levels, factor VII polymorphisms, and venous thrombosis has not been established with certainty.

FACTOR IX

Factor IX was originally reported in 1952 as "Christmas factor," named after one of the first identified hemophilia B patients.[34,44] Factor IX is synthesized in the liver and circulates in plasma as a single-chain zymogen of 415 amino acids (Mr ≈55,000) at a concentration of 90 nM with a half-life of 18 to 24 hours (see Table 113–1).

Protein Structure

Factor IX consists of a Gla domain, two EGF-like domains, a 35-residue activation peptide, and the serine protease domain (see Fig. 113–1). The Gla domain contains 12 Gla residues, of which the 11th and 12th Gla (Glu36 and Glu40) are not evolutionary conserved in other vitamin K–dependent proteins and are not essential for normal factor IX function.[45]

Factor IX comprises several posttranslational modifications that are not only important for its structure and function, but are also involved in the plasma clearance and distribution of factor IX.[35] Factor IX is sulfated at Tyr155 and phosphorylated at Ser158 in the activation peptide. Hydroxylation of Asp64 in EGF 1 mediates calcium binding, and while only approximately 40 percent of total plasma factor IX carries this modification, complete absence because of a point mutation

at this position dramatically reduces factor IX activity resulting in hemophilia B.[46,47] An O-linked fucose (Ser61) and glucose (Ser63) are found in the EGF 1 domain, in addition to several O-linked glycans in the activation peptide (Thr159, Thr169, Thr172, and Thr179). Further modification of the activation peptide includes N-linked glycosylation of Asn residues 157 and 167, which modulates the circulating levels of factor IX.[48-50]

Factor IX binds with high affinity to the extracellular matrix component collagen IV via residue Lys5 in the Gla domain.[51,52] Although factor IX variants incapable of collagen IV binding exhibit a greater recovery, collagen IV association generates an extravascular reservoir of factor IX that enables prolonged action of factor IX at a hemostatic relevant region.

Factor IX Activation and Factor IXa Activity

Limited proteolysis of factor IX at both Arg145 and Arg180 by either the tissue factor–factor VIIa complex or factor XIa results in the release of the activation peptide and generation of factor IXa (see Fig. 113–1). Cleavage at Arg180 generates factor IXaα, which displays catalytic activity toward synthetic substrates only, whereas fully active factor IXaβ is formed following cleavage at Arg145.[53,54]

Factor IXa is a two-chain serine protease (Mr ≈45,000) that is composed of a light chain of 145 residues (Mr ≈17,000) and the catalytic heavy chain of 235 residues (Mr ≈28,000), which are covalently linked via a disulfide bond.

Factor IXa has a low catalytic efficiency as a result of impaired access of substrates to the active site that results from steric and electrostatic repulsion.[55] Reversible interaction with the cofactor VIIIa on anionic membranes and subsequent factor X binding leads to rearrangement of the regions surrounding the active site and proteolytic factor X activation.

The primary plasma inhibitor of factor IXa is the serpin antithrombin, and this inhibition is enhanced by heparin (see Table 113–4), which induces a conformational change in antithrombin that is required for simultaneous active site and exosite interactions with factor IXa.[56]

Gene Structure and Variations

The gene encoding factor IX *(F9)* is located on chromosome Xq27.1 and covers nearly 25 kb.[57] It is divided into eight exons from which a mature mRNA molecule is transcribed with an ultimate length of 2802 bases (Fig. 113–8).

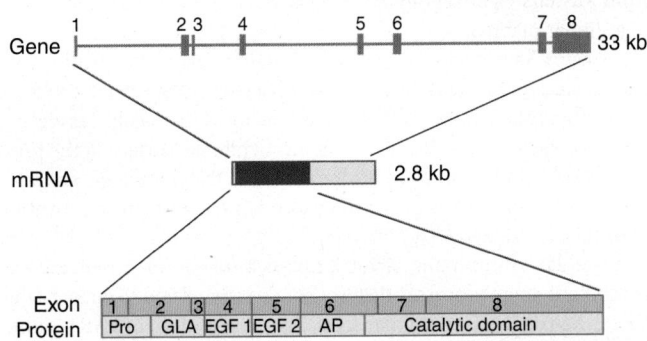

Figure 113–8. Relationship of gene structure to protein structure in factor IX. The exons, introns, mRNA, and protein structure are as indicated. The mRNA is 2.8 kb with a small 5′ untranslated region and a relatively large 3′ untranslated region *(light blue)*. In the protein, Pro indicates the prepro leader sequence, GLA indicates the γ-carboxy glutamic acid (Gla) domain, and epidermal growth factor (EGF)-1 and -2, as well as the serine protease (catalytic) domain are indicated. AP indicates the activation peptide that is released after cleavage of two bonds.

A defect or deficiency in factor IX leads to hemophilia B. Chapter 123 discusses the prevalence, clinical characteristics, and molecular genetics of hemophilia B in detail.

Conversely, increased levels of factor IX are a strong risk factor for venous thrombosis.[58] This is in agreement with a rare gain of function mutation (Arg335Leu; factor IX Padua), which renders the protein hyperfunctional and is associated with familial early-onset thrombophilia.[59]

FACTOR X

Factor X was originally reported in the late 1950s as the "Stuart-Prower factor," named after the first two identified factor X–deficient patients.[60-62] Factor X is primarily synthesized in the liver and circulates in plasma as a two-chain zymogen of 445 amino acids (Mr ≈59,000) at a concentration of 170 nM with a half-life of 34 to 40 hours (see Table 113–1).

Protein Structure

Factor X is synthesized as a single-chain precursor and during intracellular processing, the three-amino acid peptide Arg140-Lys141-Arg142 is excised. The resulting two-chain zymogen consists of a light chain (Mr ≈16,000), comprising the Gla domain with 11 Gla residues and the EGF domains, which is linked via a disulfide bond to the heavy chain (Mr ≈42,000) that consists of a 52-residue activation peptide and the serine protease domain (see Fig. 113–1).

Hydroxylation of Asp63 mediates calcium binding to the EGF 1 domain and orients the Gla domain, which is essential for factor X clotting activity.[35] N-linked glycosylation of the activation peptide residues Asn181 and Asn191 has been implicated in prolonging the factor X half-life.[63] Further posttranslational modification of factor X consists of O-linked glycosylation at Thr159 and Thr171 in the activation peptide and Thr443 in the serine protease domain. There is some evidence that glycosylation of the human factor X activation peptide may also contribute to substrate recognition by the intrinsic or extrinsic factor X-activating complex.[64,65]

Factor X Activation and Factor Xa Activity

Factor X is proteolytically activated by either the factor VIIIa–factor IXa ("intrinsic tenase") or the tissue factor–factor VIIa ("extrinsic tenase") enzyme complexes following cleavage at Arg194 in the heavy chain (see Fig. 113–1). This results in the release of the activation peptide and generation of factor Xa, also known as factor Xaα. A snake venom protease from Russell's viper venom (RVV-X) is capable of generating factor Xa in a similar manner.

Factor Xa consists of the Gla and EGF domains-comprising light chain (Mr ≈16,000) and the catalytic heavy chain (Mr ≈29,000) that are covalently linked via a disulfide bond. Factor Xa reversibly associates with its cofactor factor Va on an anionic membrane surface in the presence of calcium ions to form prothrombinase, the physiologic activator of prothrombin. Factor Xa is also involved in the proteolytic activation of factors V, VII, and VIII.[66-68]

Similar to thrombin, factor Xa plays a role in other biologic and pathophysiologic processes that are not directly related to coagulation. Factor Xa triggers intracellular signaling via activation of PAR1 and/or PAR2. Factor Xa cleaves PAR2 by itself as well as in complex with tissue factor–factor VIIa. These direct cellular effects of factor Xa contribute to wound healing, tissue remodeling, inflammation, angiogenesis, and atherosclerosis, among others.[26,69]

Further autocatalytic cleavage at Arg429 near the C-terminus of the factor Xa heavy chain leads to release of a 19-residue peptide, yielding the enzymatically active factor Xaβ.[70-72] Plasmin-mediated cleavage

of factor Xa at adjacent C-terminal Arg or Lys residues also results in the generation of factor Xaβ and factor Xaβ derivatives.[73,74] While the coagulation activity is eliminated in the factor Xaβ derivatives, they are capable of interacting with the zymogen plasminogen and enhance its tissue plasminogen activator-mediated conversion to plasmin, thereby promoting fibrinolysis.[75]

A primary plasma inhibitor of factor Xa is the serpin antithrombin, and this inhibition is enhanced by heparin (see Table 113–4), which induces a conformational change in antithrombin that is required for simultaneous active site and exosite interactions with factor Xa.[76] Another potent factor Xa inhibitor is TFPI, which inhibits both the ternary tissue factor–factor VIIa–factor Xa complex as well as free factor Xa, for which protein S functions as a cofactor.[77,78] Free factor Xa is also inhibited by the protein Z/protein Z–dependent protease inhibitor (ZPI) complex on membranes.[79]

Low-molecular-weight heparin and synthetic derivatives (e.g. fondaparinux) are clinically used as anticoagulants to enhance factor Xa inhibition by antithrombin specifically. The target-specific oral anticoagulants rivaroxaban, apixaban, edoxaban, and analogues directly inhibit both free factor Xa and prothrombinase complex-assembled factor Xa with high specificity through a high-affinity, reversible interaction with the factor Xa active site.[80-83]

Gene Structure and Variations

The gene encoding factor X *(F10)* is located on chromosome 13q34 and spans almost 27 kb.[84] The 8 exons in the factor X gene give rise to a mature mRNA of 1560 bases (Fig. 113–9). There are no common alternative splice variants with known biology.

Loss of function mutations in the factor X gene lead to a rare bleeding disorder with a recessive mode of inheritance. Factor X deficiency occurs in approximately one in every 1,000,000 newborns. Most cases of documented factor X deficiency experience serious bleeding problems. In fact, factor X deficiency may be the most severe of the rare congenital bleeding disorders.[30] Well over 100 mutations have been documented in cases with factor X deficiency (http://www.hgmd.org). The majority of these mutations are missense and nonsense mutations.

Gain-of-function mutations in factor X could potentially increase thrombotic risk, but such mutations have not been documented. There

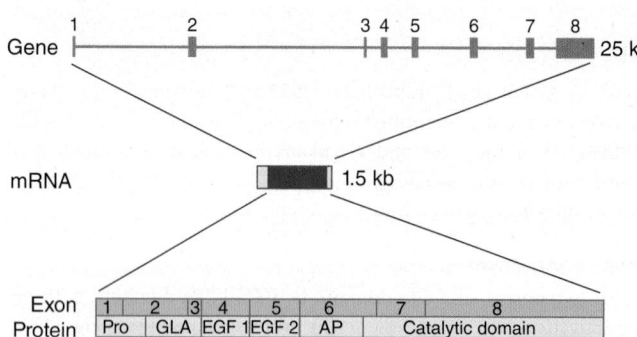

Figure 113–9. Relationship of gene structure to protein structure in factor X. The exons, introns, mRNA, and protein structure are as indicated. The mRNA is 1.5 kb with a relatively large 5′ untranslated region and a small 3′ untranslated region. In the protein, Pro indicates the pre-pro leader sequence, GLA indicates the γ-carboxy glutamic acid (Gla) domain, and epidermal growth factor (EGF)-1 and -2, as well as the serine protease (catalytic) domain, are indicated. AP indicates the activation peptide. Before secretion, cleavage in this domain processes factor X to the two-chain mature zymogen. A second cleavage releases the activation peptide and generates factor Xa activity.

is uncertainty about whether common gene variations influence the level of factor X in plasma.[85]

PROTEIN C

Protein C, which plays a central role in the anticoagulant pathway, was discovered in 1960, and being the third protein peak ("peak C") observed in a vitamin K–dependent plasma protein purification, it was named protein C.[86,87] Protein C is synthesized in the liver and circulates in plasma as a two-chain zymogen of 417 amino acids (Mr ≈62,000) at a concentration of 65 nM with a half-life of 6 to 8 hours (see Table 113–1).

Protein Structure

Protein C is synthesized as a single-chain precursor and during intracellular processing amino acids Lys146-Arg147 are excised. The resulting two-chain zymogen consists of a light chain (Mr ≈21,000) comprising the Gla domain with nine Gla residues and the EGF domains, which is linked via a disulfide bond to the heavy chain (Mr ≈41,000) that consists of the 12-residue activation peptide and the serine protease domain (see Fig. 113–1).

In addition to γ-carboxylation, protein C is hydroxylated at Asp71 in the EGF-1 domain, which coordinates calcium binding.[35] N-linked glycosylation of Asn97 in EGF-1 and Asn248, Asn313, and Asn329 in the serine protease domain are important for efficient protein secretion, proteolytic processing of Lys146-Arg147, and proteolytic activation.[88–90] Some of the total plasma protein C is not glycosylated at either Asn329 (β-protein C) or at both Asn329 and Asn248 (γ-protein C), of which the impact on protein function remains unclear.[91]

Protein C Activation and Activated Protein C Activity

Protein C is proteolytically activated by α-thrombin in complex with the endothelial cell surface protein thrombomodulin following cleavage at Arg169 (see Fig. 113–1). The activation peptide is released and the mature serine protease activated protein C (APC) is formed. Activation of protein C is enhanced by its localization on the endothelial surface through association with the endothelial cell protein C receptor (EPCR).[92] Several snake venom proteases (RVV-X and Protac) are also capable of activating protein C.

APC consists of the disulfide-linked light chain comprising the Gla and EGF domains (Mr ≈21,000) and the catalytic heavy chain (Mr ≈32,000). In complex with its cofactor protein S, APC proteolytically inactivates factors Va and VIIIa in a calcium- and membrane-dependent manner. Intact factor V has been reported to function as a cofactor for the inactivation of factor VIIIa in the presence of protein S.[93]

Downregulation of thrombin formation through inactivation of these cofactors seems to occur preferentially on the endothelial cell surface as opposed to that of platelets,[94] where it prevents coagulation and potential thrombosis. However, protein C activation is also accelerated by platelet factor 4 (PF4), which is secreted by activated platelets. Upon interaction with the Gla domain of protein C, PF4 modifies the conformation of protein C, thereby enhancing its affinity for the thrombomodulin-thrombin complex.[95] This ensures APC generation in close proximity of the injury site where platelets are activated, which serves to impede dissemination of coagulation.

APC also plays a major role in the cytoprotective pathway to prevent vascular damage and stress.[96] These activities include antiapoptotic activity, antiinflammatory activity, alterations of gene-expression profiles, and endothelial barrier stabilization. Most of these functions require binding to EPCR and PAR1 cleavage.

APC is primarily inhibited by the heparin-dependent serpin protein C inhibitor and by plasminogen activator inhibitor-1 (PAI-1). Because PAI-1 is the major inhibitor of tissue plasminogen

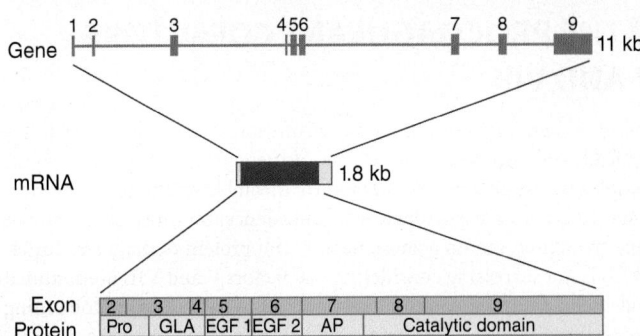

Figure 113–10. Relationship of gene structure to protein structure in protein C. The exons, introns, mRNA, and protein structure are as indicated. The mRNA is 1.8 kb with a small 5′ untranslated region coded for by exon 1 and a relatively small 3′ untranslated region *(light blue)*. In the protein, Pro indicates the prepro leader sequence, GLA indicates the γ-carboxy glutamic acid (Gla) domain, and epidermal growth factor (EGF)-1 and -2, as well as the serine protease (catalytic) domain, are indicated. AP indicates the activation peptide. Before secretion, cleavage in this domain processes protein C to the two-chain mature zymogen. A second cleavage releases the activation peptide and generates activated protein C.

activator, inhibition through complex formation with APC contributes to enhanced fibrinolysis. Chapter 114 discusses these and other factors that attenuate the anticoagulant activity of APC.

Gene Structure and Variations

The protein C gene *(PROC)* is located on chromosome 2q14.3 and spans almost 11 kb.[97] The gene is divided into nine exons and the mature mRNA has a length of 1790 bases (Fig. 113–10). There are no alternative mRNA species with known biology.

Loss-of-function mutations cause protein C deficiency. In homozygous or compound heterozygous form this leads to life-threatening purpura fulminans at birth which, if left untreated, is fatal.[98] In cases where there is still some protein C activity detectable, symptoms may be much milder.

Heterozygous protein C deficiency increases the risk of venous thrombosis. This is true for most deficiencies of natural anticoagulants and sets them apart from rare bleeding disorders where heterozygosity for loss of function mutations is mostly asymptomatic. The risk for venous thrombosis is increased approximately 10-fold in heterozygotes for protein C deficiency, albeit that the risk estimates vary considerably between studies.[99] Family studies in particular suggest a high risk, whereas case-control studies may show markedly lower estimates.[100]

Heterozygous protein C deficiency can be categorized as type I or type II. In type I deficiency, antigen levels are approximately 50 percent of normal, whereas in type II deficiency, antigen levels are (near) normal but activity levels are decreased by 50 percent.

The genetic basis of protein C deficiency, consistent with what is observed in general for congenital loss of function disorders, is heterogeneous. In line with this, more than 300 mutations have been documented and are tracked in the human gene mutation database (http://www.hgmd.org). Two-thirds of these documented mutations are missense or nonsense.

Several common polymorphisms, in particular in the promotor region of the protein C gene, are known to have a small but measurable effect on plasma protein C levels. Alleles of these polymorphisms that are associated with lower protein C levels are also associated with an increased thrombotic risk, albeit that the effect is small.[101] Therefore, it is not surprising that measurement of these polymorphisms have not found any clinical application.

●THE PROCOAGULANT COFACTORS V AND VIII

Factors V and VIII both function as cofactors in coagulation and dramatically enhance the catalytic rate of their macromolecular enzyme complexes, resulting in the generation of thrombin and factor Xa, respectively. Apart from their functional equivalence, they also share similar gene structures, amino acid sequences, and protein domain structures, which is not surprising considering that factors V and VIII are assumed to descend from the common ancestral A1-A2-A3 domain-containing copper-binding plasma protein ceruloplasmin through a gene duplication event.[102] After acquiring C-type domains as well as the central B domain, a second gene duplication ultimately separated the ancestral genes of factors V and VIII.

Factors V and VIII undergo similar mechanisms of intracellular processing in the endoplasmic reticulum (ER) and Golgi apparatus. Trafficking through this early secretory pathway involves interaction of factors V and VIII with a receptor complex that consists of the mannose-binding lectin-1 gene product LMAN1 (also called ER-Golgi intermediate compartment (ERGIC)-53) and multiple coagulation deficiency protein 2 (MCFD2).[103] Defects or deficiencies in one of the two subunits of the receptor complex can result in a combined deficiency of factors V and VIII (Chap. 124).

FACTOR V

In 1943, Norwegian physician Paul Owren discovered the fifth coagulation factor thus far known and named it factor V.[104–106] Factor V is synthesized in the liver and circulates in plasma as a large single-chain procofactor of 2196 amino acids (Mr ≈330,000) at a concentration of 20 nM with a half-life of 12 to 36 hours (see Table 113–1).

Approximately 20 percent of the total factor V in blood is stored in the α-granules of platelets. Although it was originally thought that megakaryocytes synthesize factor V, studies in humans indicate that platelet factor V originates from plasma through endocytic uptake.[107–109] Platelet factor V is modified intracellularly such that it is functionally unique compared to its plasma-derived counterpart. It is partially activated, more resistant to inactivation by APC, and has several different posttranslational modifications.[110]

Platelet factor V is associated with the large multimeric protein multimerin.[111] Multimerin has a massive repeating structure, with some of the multimers having molecular weights of several million daltons. Although the function of this platelet factor V-specific multimeric chaperon protein is similar to that of VWF, the multimeric chaperon protein of factor VIII in plasma, multimerin and VWF share no structural homology.

Following platelet activation, platelet factor V becomes available at the site of injury and can reach local concentrations that exceed the factor V plasma concentration by more than 100-fold.[112] Interestingly, the origin of factor V in mouse platelets differs from humans in that it is synthesized in megakaryocytes and stored into the α-granules before platelets are released from the marrow.[113,114]

Protein Structure

Factor V has an A1-A2-B-A3-C1-C2 domain structure (Fig. 113–11). The three A-type domains share significant homology with those of ancestral ceruloplasmin as well as with the factor VIII A domains (approximately 50 percent sequence identity). The two C-type domains belong to the family of discoidin domains, which are generally involved in cell adhesion, and share approximately 55 percent sequence identity with the factor VIII C domains. The C domains mediate binding to the anionic phospholipid surface, thereby localizing factor V to the site of injury and facilitating interaction with factor Xa and prothrombin.[115–118] In contrast, the large central B domain of factor V shows weak homology to the factor VIII B domain or to any other known protein domain. However, this domain comprises so-called basic and acidic regions that are highly conserved throughout evolution and serve to negatively regulate factor V function and prevent activity of the procofactor.[119,120]

Factor V undergoes extensive posttranslational modifications, including sulfation, phosphorylation, and N-linked glycosylation.[35,121] Sulfation at sites in the A2 and B domain are involved in the thrombin-mediated proteolytic activation of factor V.[122] Phosphorylation at Ser692 in the A2 domain enhances the APC-dependent inactivation of the cofactor Va.[123] N-linked glycosylation occurs throughout the whole protein; however, the majority of carbohydrates are linked to Asn residues within the B domain and play a role in the LMAN1-MCDF2 receptor complex-mediated trafficking of factor V from the ER to the Golgi in the early secretory pathway.[103] Partial glycosylation at Asn2181 in the C2 domain of factor V results in a lower binding affinity for negatively charged membranes of the glycosylated form, thereby reducing the factor V procoagulant activity, particularly at low phospholipid concentrations.[124,125] Furthermore, factor V comprises several disulfide bonds that are important for the three-dimensional structure of the A and C domains.[121]

Factor V Procofactor Activation and Factor Va Cofactor Function

Sequential proteolytic cleavage of the procofactor factor V at Arg709, Arg1018, and Arg1545 in the B domain results in release of the inhibitory constraints exerted by the B domain and in the generation of the heterodimeric cofactor Va (see Fig. 113–11).[126] Maximal cofactor activity correlates with cleavage at Arg1545, which is consistent with the observation that a snake venom protease from RVV-V, which cleaves only at Arg1545, results in full activation. Thrombin has generally been recognized to be the principal activator of factor V. However, recent findings suggest that in the initiation phase of coagulation factor V is primarily activated by factor Xa.[127] Factor Xa initially cleaves factor V at Arg1018, followed by proteolysis at Arg709 and Arg1545.[128]

Factor Va is composed of a heavy chain (Mr ≈105,000) comprising the A1-A2 domains and the A3-C1-C2 light chain (Mr ≈74,000), which are noncovalently associated via calcium ions. Factor Va is a nonenzymatic cofactor within the prothrombinase complex that greatly accelerates the ability of factor Xa to rapidly convert prothrombin to thrombin.[129] APC catalyzes the inactivation of factor Va by cleavage at the main sites Arg306 and Arg506, upon which the cleaved A2 fragment

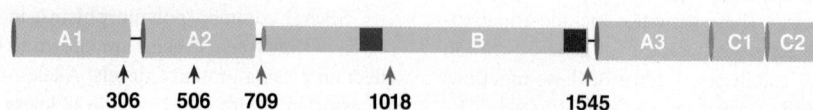

Figure 113–11. The domain structure of factor V. Schematic A1-A2-B-A3-C1-C2 domain representation of factor V. Thrombin cleavage sites (Arg709, Arg1018, Arg1545) are indicated by *green arrows*, and activated protein C (APC) cleavage sites (Arg306, Arg506) by *red arrows*. The *blue* and *red* boxes in the B domain represent the basic and acidic region, respectively, that are highly conserved throughout evolution and serve to negatively regulate factor V function and prevent activity of the procofactor V.

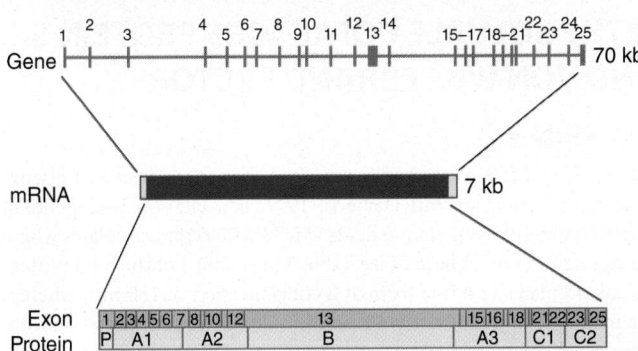

Figure 113–12. Relationship of gene structure to protein structure in factor V. The exons, introns, mRNA, and protein structure are as indicated. The mRNA is 7 kb with some 5′ and 3′ untranslated sequences *(light blue)*. In the protein, P indicates the propeptide leader sequence, and the A1-A2-B-A3-C1-C2 domains are indicated.

dissociates and factor Va can no longer associate with factor Xa.[130] A common Arg506Gln mutation in factor V leads to resistance to inactivation by APC (factor V Leiden) and is associated with an increased risk of venous thromboembolism (Chap. 133).[131]

Both factor V and an alternatively spliced isoform of factor V (factor V-short), which lacks the major part of the B domain (residues 756 to 1458) and normally circulates in low abundance, interact with full-length TFPI (TFPIα), most likely through the acidic B domain region.[132,133] The linkage of factor V and TFPIα is considered to attenuate the bleeding phenotype in factor V–deficient patients, as the low TFPIα levels in these patients allow the residual platelet factor V to be sufficient for coagulation.[132,134] Conversely, increased factor V–short expression caused by an A2440G mutation in the factor V gene leads to a dramatic increase in plasma TFPIα, resulting in a bleeding disorder.[133]

Gene Structure and Variations

The gene for factor V (*F5*) is located on chromosome 1q23. It is located very close to the genes for the selectin family of leukocyte adhesion molecules. The factor V gene spans approximately 70 kb and consists of 25 exons (Fig. 113–12). The gene structure is very similar to that of the factor VIII gene, with exon–intron boundaries occurring at exactly the same location in 21 out of 24 cases.[135]

Homozygosity or compound heterozygosity for loss-of-function mutations in the factor V gene lead to a bleeding disorder (termed *parahemophilia* or *Owren parahemophilia*).[136] At the time of writing, 152 mutations in the factor V gene have been collected in the human gene mutation database (www.hgmd.org).

Gain-of-function mutations in the factor V gene increase the risk of thrombosis. This is particularly the case for venous thrombosis and not so much for arterial thrombosis. In whites, the most common gain-of-function mutation in the factor V gene is factor V Leiden (Arg-506Gln), which leads to a plasma abnormality known as APC resistance (Chap. 133).[137,138]

FACTOR VIII

Factor VIII (antihemophilic factor) was first discovered in 1937, but it was not until 1979 that its purification by Tuddenham and coworkers led to the molecular identification of the protein.[139,140] Factor VIII is synthesized as a single-chain preprocofactor of 2351 amino acids and, subsequent to intracellular processing, is secreted as a series of metal ion-linked heterodimers due to proteolysis at the A3-B junction and differential processing in the central B domain (Fig. 113–13). The mature factor VIII procofactor comprises 2332 amino acids (Mr ≈300,000) and circulates in a high-affinity complex with its carrier protein VWF at a concentration of approximately 0.7 nM and a circulatory half-life of 8 to 12 hours (see Table 113–1). Complex formation with VWF protects factor VIII from proteolytic degradation, premature ligand binding, and rapid clearance from the circulation.

The primary source of factor VIII is the liver,[141,142] but extrahepatic synthesis of factor VIII also occurs.[143,144] While contradictory evidence exists on the cellular origin of both hepatic and extrahepatic factor VIII synthesis, recent studies in mice support that endothelial cells from many tissues and vascular beds synthesize factor VIII, with a large contribution from hepatic sinusoidal endothelial cells.[145–147] This is consistent with observations on factor VIII expression in human endothelial cells from the liver and lung.[148,149]

Factor VIII is less-efficiently secreted from the cell as compared to factor V, because it interacts with the ER-chaperon proteins calnexin and calreticulin, whereas factor V interacts with calreticulin only.[150] Both chaperons preferentially interact with GPs comprising monoglucosylated N-linked oligosaccharides and promote correct folding of proteins that enter the secretory pathway and target misfolded proteins for degradation. Factor VIII, but not factor V, also interacts with the ER-chaperon immunoglobulin-binding protein (BiP/GRP78), which appears to enhance the stability of factor VIII, but also retards its secretion.[151] Factor VIII trafficking from the ER to the Golgi is mediated via the LMAN1-MCDF2 receptor complex, similar to factor V.[103]

Several clearance receptors are responsible for actively removing factor VIII from the circulation, which include the low-density lipoprotein (LDL) receptor-related protein 1 (LRP1), the LDL receptor, and receptors that specifically interact with carbohydrate structures on factor VIII.[152–156]

Protein Structure

The A1-A2-B-A3-C1-C2 domain structure of factor VIII shares significant homology with factor V except in the B domain region (see Fig. 113–13). In contrast to factor V, the factor VIII B domain is dispensable for procoagulant activity. The mature factor VIII procofactor comprises a variably sized heavy chain (A1-A2-B; Mr ≈200,000 to 90,000 depending on the extent of proteolysis) and a light chain (A3-C1-C2; Mr ≈80,000). The C-terminal regions of the A1 and A2 domains and the N-terminal portion of the A3 domain contain short segments of 30 to 40 negatively charged residues known as the a1, a2, and a3 regions. Interaction with VWF is facilitated by the a3 region and C1 domain.[157,158] The C domains mediate binding to the anionic phospholipid surface, thereby localizing factor VIII to the site of injury and facilitating interaction with factor IXa and factor X.[159–161]

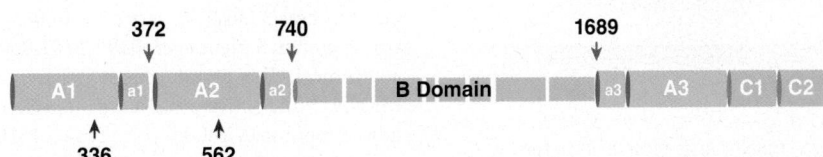

Figure 113–13. The domain structure of factor VIII. Schematic A1-a1-A2-a2-B-a3-A3-C1-C2 domain representation of factor VIII. The acidic regions denoted by a1, a2, and a3 are indicated, thrombin cleavage sites (Arg372, Arg740, Arg1689) are indicated by *green arrows*, and activated protein C (APC) cleavage sites (Arg336, Arg562) by *red arrows*. The variably sized B domain as a result of differential proteolytic processing is indicated.

Factor VIII is heavily glycosylated and the majority of the *N*-linked glycosylation sites are found in the B domain, which mediate interaction with the chaperons calnexin and calreticulin and, in part, with the LMAN1–MCDF2 receptor complex.[103,150,162] Sulfation of tyrosine residues is required for optimal activation by thrombin, maximal activity in complex with factor IXa, and maximal affinity of factor VIIIa for VWF.[35,163] Factor VIII comprises two phosphorylation sites that are located in the A1 (Thr351) and B (Ser1657) domains.

Factor VIII Procofactor Activation and Factor VIIIa Cofactor Function

Thrombin and factor Xa are the principal activators of the procofactor VIII and generate the cofactor VIIIa through sequential proteolysis at Arg740, Arg372, and Arg1689.[126,164–166] The heterotrimeric factor VIIIa is composed of the A1 (Mr ≈50,000), A2 (Mr ≈43,000), and the A3-C1-C2 light chain (Mr ≈73,000) subunits (see Fig. 113–13). The A1 and A3-C1-C2 subunits are noncovalently linked through calcium ions, whereas A2 is associated with weak affinity primarily by electrostatic interactions.[167,168] Once activated, factor VIIIa functions as a cofactor for factor IXa in the phospholipid-dependent conversion of factor X to factor Xa. The rapid and spontaneous loss of factor VIIIa cofactor activity is attributed to A2 domain dissociation from the heterotrimer.[167,168] Additional proteolysis by APC, factor Xa, or factor IXa also results in the downregulation of factor VIIIa cofactor activity.[169]

Gene Structure and Variations

The factor VIII encoding gene (*F8*) is situated at chromosome Xq28. The factor VIII gene contains 26 exons (Fig. 113–14), one more than factor V, because exon 5 of factor V corresponds to exons 5 and 6 of the factor VIII gene.[170] In addition, the gene for factor VIII is much larger than that of factor V, spanning approximately 190 kb. This is largely because six of the introns in the factor VIII gene are much larger than the corresponding *F5* introns. The mRNA for factor VIII is also much larger than the factor V mRNA because of a 1.8 kb 3′-untranslated region.

A defect or deficiency in factor VIII leads to hemophilia A. Chapter 123 discusses the prevalence, clinical characteristics, and molecular genetics of hemophilia A in detail.

High levels of factor VIII are a common and strong risk factor for venous thrombosis. It has been suspected that certain genetic variations in the factor VIII gene might play a role in determining the level of factor VIII; however, such variations have not been identified.[171] The ABO blood group does play a role in determining the level of factor VIII, but probably indirectly through an effect on the level of VWF.[172,173]

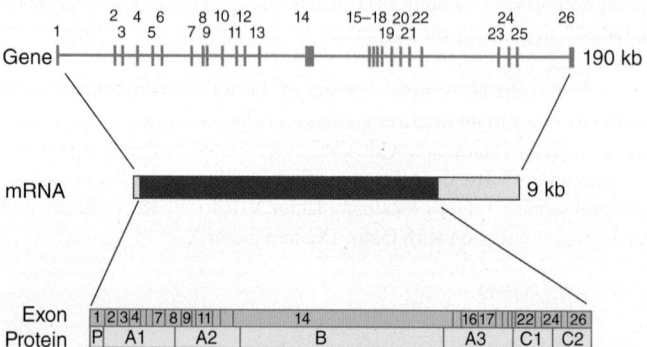

Figure 113–14. Relationship of gene structure to protein structure in factor VIII. The exons, introns, mRNA, and protein structure are as indicated. The mRNA is 9 kb with home 5′ untranslated sequence and a large 3′ untranslated region (*light blue*). In the protein, P indicates the propeptide leader sequence, and the A1-A2-B-A3-C1-C2 domains are indicated.

●THE SOLUBLE COFACTORS PROTEIN S AND VON WILLEBRAND FACTOR

PROTEIN S

Protein S, which is named after the city (Seattle) where it was discovered by the group of Earl Davie in 1977, is a vitamin K–dependent single-chain GP of 635 amino acids (Mr ≈75,000) that circulates with a plasma half-life of 42 hours (see Table 113–1). Part of the total protein S pool circulates in a free form at a concentration of 150 nM, whereas the majority (approximately 60 percent; 200 nM) circulates bound to the complement regulatory protein C4b–binding protein (C4BP). Protein S is primarily synthesized in the liver by hepatocytes, in addition to endothelial cells, megakaryocytes, testicular Leydig cells, and osteoblasts.[174–178]

Protein Structure

The protein structure of protein S differs from the other vitamin K–dependent proteins as it lacks a serine protease domain and, consequently, is not capable of catalytic activity. Protein S is composed of a Gla domain comprising 11 Gla residues, a thrombin-sensitive region (TSR), four EGF domains, and a C-terminal sex hormone–binding globulin (SHBG)-like region that consists of two laminin G-type domains (Fig. 113–15). The SHBG-like domain is involved in the interaction with the β-subunit of C4BP.

Apart from γ-carboxylation of Glu residues, protein S is posttranslationally modified via N-glycosylation in the second laminin G-type domain of the SHBG-like region (Asn458, Asn468, Asn489). β-Hydroxylation of Asp95 or Asn residues (Asn136, Asn178, Asn217) in each EGF domain allows for calcium binding that orients the four EGF domains relative to each other.[35]

Protein S Cofactor Function

Free protein S serves as a cofactor for APC in the proteolytic inactivation of factors Va and VIIIa.[179,180] Interaction of protein S with APC on a negatively charged membrane surface alters the location of the APC active site relative to factor Va,[181] which accounts for the selective protein S-dependent rate enhancement of APC cleavage at Arg306 in factor Va.[182] C4BP-bound protein S also exerts a similar stimulatory effect on Arg306 cleavage, albeit to lower extent, whereas it inhibits the initial APC-mediated factor Va cleavage at Arg506, resulting in an overall inhibition of factor Va inactivation.[183] Cleavage of the TSR by thrombin and/or factor Xa results in a loss of APC-cofactor activity.[184] Protein S also functions as a cofactor for TFPIα in the inhibition of factor Xa, which is mediated by the SHBG-like region in protein S.[77,185]

Protein S has been implied to play a role in phagocytosis of apoptotic cells, cell survival, activation of innate immunity, vessel integrity and angiogenesis, and local invasion and metastasis through interaction with a family of protein tyrosine kinase receptors referred to as Tyro-3, Axl and Mer (TAM) receptors.[186,187]

Gene Structure and Variations

The gene encoding protein S (*PROS1*) is located on the long arm of chromosome 3 (3q11.1), very close to the centromere. A highly homologous protein S pseudogene (*PROSP*) is located on the other side of the centromere. This pseudogene is inactive, as it is not transcribed into mRNA.[188] The active protein S gene encompasses 15 exons and covers a little more than 100 kb (Fig. 113–16). The mRNA sequence consists of 3560 bases. Several alternative transcripts have been identified, but none of these have known biology.

Loss-of-function mutations in *PROS1* lead to protein S deficiency. Several cases of homozygous and compound heterozygous protein S

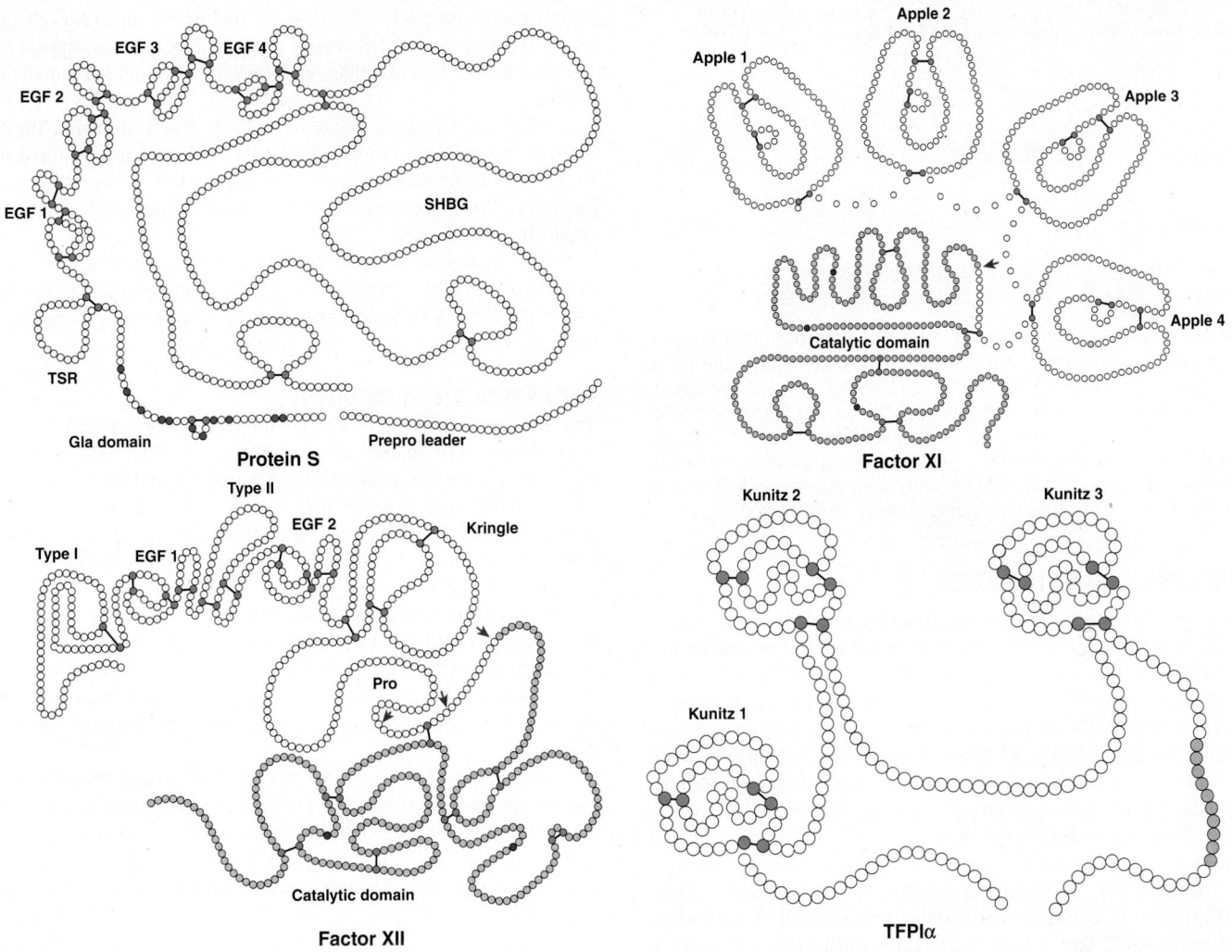

Figure 113–15. Protein S, factor XI, factor XII, and tissue factor pathway inhibitor (TFPI). Schematic of protein S, factor XI, factor XII, and TFPIα. Each *circle* represents an amino acid. For protein S: the prepro leader sequence comprising the signal peptide as well as the propeptide is indicated, the γ-carboxy glutamic acid (Gla) domain is indicated with the Gla residues in *blue*, TSR represents the thrombin-sensitive region, the four epidermal growth factor (EGF) domains are indicated, and SHBG represents the sex hormone–binding globulin-like region. For factor XI: the four apple domains are indicated, and the serine protease (catalytic) domain is shown. Cys321 in the apple 4 domain that forms a disulfide link with Cys321 in the other factor XI subunit, thereby mediating dimerization, is indicated in *yellow*. For factor XII: types I and II represent the fibronectin types I and II domains, the two EGF-like domains are indicated, the kringle domain is indicated, Pro indicates the proline-rich region, and the serine protease (catalytic) domain is indicated. For TFPIα: the three Kunitz domains are indicated and the C-terminal sequence of basic residues is indicated in *light blue*. Factors XI and XII have homologous serine protease ("catalytic") domains (shown in *light red*), in which the active site His, Asp, and Ser residues are indicated in *dark red*. Cleavages that convert the zymogens factor XI and factor XII to an active enzyme are indicated by the *red arrows*. Cysteine residues that form a disulfide bridge *(black line)* are indicated in *green*.

deficiency have been described with extremely low protein S levels. These very rare cases suffer from life-threatening purpura fulminans at birth.[189]

Much more common are heterozygous deficiencies of protein S, which can be categorized into three types of deficiency. Type I deficiency is characterized by antigen levels that are approximately 50 percent of normal. In type II deficiency, antigen levels are (near) normal while activity levels are decreased by 50 percent. Type III deficiency is defined by a low level of free protein S. In keeping with this classification, clinical chemistry laboratories may offer a protein S activity assay, free antigen assay, or total antigen assay (or a combination thereof). These assays are not without problems and the evaluation of protein S levels is fraught with complications that need careful attention before a final diagnosis can be made.[190]

The genetic basis of protein S deficiency is highly heterogeneous and there are more than 200 entries in the human gene mutation database (www.hgmd.org). Most of these are missense mutations. However, protein S deficiency is often characterized by gross gene deletions, that sometimes even involve neighboring genes.[191] The reason for this preponderance of gross gene abnormalities remains unknown.

It is commonly assumed that protein S deficiency increases venous thrombotic risk by 10-fold.[100] This assertion is mainly based on studies in thrombophilic families. In population-based case-control studies, however, the risk increase appears to be much more modest, if present at all.[192] The reason for this discrepancy between family and population-based studies remains enigmatic. The findings argue against including tests for protein S deficiency in a thrombophilia workup of venous thrombosis cases with a negative family history.

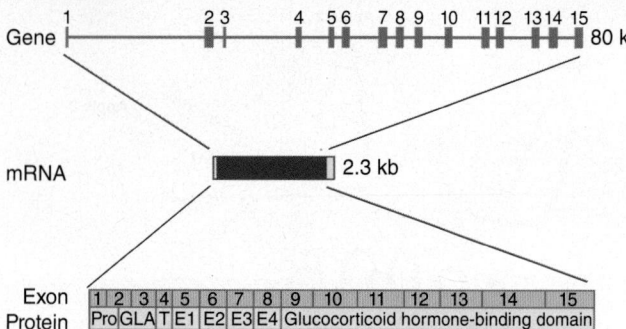

Figure 113–16. Relationship of gene structure to protein structure in protein S. The exons, introns, mRNA, and protein structure are as indicated. The mRNA is 2.3 kb with small 5′ and 3′ untranslated regions *(light blue)*. In the protein, Pro indicates the prepro leader sequence, GLA indicates the γ-carboxy glutamic acid (Gla) domain, T indicates the thrombin-sensitive region; E indicates the epidermal growth factor (EGF)-like domains, and the glucocorticoid hormone-binding domain represents the sex hormone–binding globulin (SHBG)-like domain.

VON WILLEBRAND FACTOR

Chapter 126 discusses the structure, function, and molecular biology of VWF in detail. VWF is a large multimeric GP that is required for normal platelet adhesion to components of the vessel wall and that serves as a carrier for factor VIII. It is exclusively synthesized in megakaryocytes and endothelial cells and stored in specialized organelles in platelets and endothelial cells. Release of VWF multimers from these organelles follows upon a stimulus or via unstimulated basal secretion from endothelial cells.[193] VWF multimers circulate at a concentration of 10 nM with a half-life of 8 to 12 hours (see Table 113–1). Clearance of VWF multimers is mainly mediated by macrophages from the liver and spleen.[194]

Large VWF multimers are cleaved by the plasma protease ADAMTS-13 (a disintegrin and metalloproteinase with thrombospondin motifs 13).[195] This cleavage produces the smaller size VWF multimers that circulate in plasma. Reduced ADAMTS-13 activity is linked to various microangiopathies with increased platelet activity.

Protein Structure

The precursor protein of VWF is composed of a 22-residue signal peptide and of a proVWF protein comprising 2791 amino acids that has 14 distinct domains in the order of D1-D2-D′-D3-A1-A2-A3-D4-B1-B2-B3-C1-C2-CK.[196] Upon translocation to the ER, the signal peptide is cleaved off, and the proVWF dimerizes in a tail-to-tail fashion through cysteines in its cysteine knot (CK) domain..During transit through the Golgi apparatus, proVWF dimers multimerize in a head-to-head fashion through the formation of disulfide bonds between cysteine residues in the D3 domain. At the same time, D1 and D2 domains are cleaved off as a single fragment to form the VWF propeptide (741 amino acids), while the remaining domains comprising 2050 amino acid residues and up to 22 carbohydrate chains form mature VWF. In the *trans*-Golgi network, the VWF propeptide promotes mature VWF to assemble into high-molecular-weight multimers (Mr ≈500,000 to 20,000,000). These multimers subsequently aggregate into tubular structures that are packaged into α-granules in megakaryocytes and into Weibel-Palade bodies in endothelial cells.

von Willebrand Factor Function

Upon exocytosis from Weibel-Palade bodies and at high shear rates, multimeric VWF unrolls from a globular to a filamental conformation (often called *VWF strings*), up to many microns long, which becomes a high-affinity surface for the platelet GPIb–V–IX complex. Large VWF multimers are more active than smaller multimers, which is explained by the fact that the former contain multiple domains that support the interactions between platelets, endothelial cells, and subendothelial collagen.

VWF binds to matrix collagens via its A1 and A3 domains. The A1 domain also mediates binding to platelet GPIb, which is required for the fast capture of platelets.[197] Platelet adhesion to VWF is further supported by VWF immobilization on a surface (collagen, other platelets) and by high shear stress.

VWF complexes with factor VIII through the first 272 residues in the N-terminal region of the mature VWF protein subunit,[198] thereby protecting factor VIII from proteolytic degradation, premature ligand binding, and rapid clearance from the circulation.

Gene Structure and Variations

The VWF gene *(VWF)* is located on chromosome 12p13.3, spans approximately 180 kb, and contains 52 exons.[199] The VWF mRNA is 8.7 kb long. There are no alternative transcripts with known biology. A partially inactive pseudogene that includes exons 23 to 34 is located on chromosome 22p11–13.[199] The VWF gene is very polymorphic, which makes it sometimes difficult to distinguish between disease causing mutations and neutral gene variations.

Qualitative or quantitative deficiencies in VWF cause von Willebrand disease (VWD), a mild to severe bleeding disorder. Quantitative deficiency of VWF leads to type 1 or type 3 VWD, whereas functional defects lead to type 2 VWD. Type 1 VWD is the most common form, but type 3 VWD is the most severe. Chapter 126 discusses VWD in detail.

High levels of VWF are a risk factor for venous and arterial thrombosis. Genome-wide association studies led to the identification of several genomic loci that influence the level of VWF, including the VWF gene itself, the ABO blood group, *STXB5*, and *SCARA5*.[200] Polymorphisms in several of these loci are also associated with thrombotic risk.[201]

⬤ FACTOR XI AND THE CONTACT SYSTEM

FACTOR XI

Factor XI, which was discovered in the early 1950s,[202,203] is synthesized in the liver and secreted as a single-chain zymogen of 607 amino acids (Mr ≈80,000). In the circulation, factor XI is found as a homodimer (Mr ≈160,000) at a concentration of 30 nM with a plasma half-life of 60 to 80 hours (see Table 113–1). All factor XI homodimers circulate in complex with high-molecular-weight kininogen (HK).[204] HK is thought to mediate binding of factor XI to negatively charged surfaces, thereby facilitating factor XI activation.[205] There is conflicting evidence suggesting that HK may be also involved in the interaction of factor XI with the activated platelet surface via GPIb.[206]

Protein Structure

Each factor XI subunit comprises four apple domains and a serine protease domain (see Fig. 113–15). The apple domains are structured by three disulfide bonds and form a disk-like platform on which the serine protease domain rests.[207] The dimerization of two factor XI subunits is mediated by interactions between the two apple 4 domains that involve a disulfide bond between the Cys321 residues, hydrophobic interactions, and a salt bridge, of which only the latter two are required for dimerization.[206] The domain structure of factor XI is highly similar to that of the monomer prekallikrein (PK), the zymogen of the protease kallikrein, which also circulates in complex with HK.[206]

Factor XI does not bear a Gla domain and thus does not require γ-carboxylation to exert its procoagulant activity. *N*-linked glycosylation occurs at three sites in the apple 1, 2, and 4 domains (Asn82, Asn114, Asn335) and at two sites in the serine protease domain (Asn432, Asn473).

Factor XI Activation and Activity

Activation of a factor XI subunit to factor XIa proceeds through proteolysis at Arg369 in the N-terminal region of the serine protease domain and yields two-chain activated factor XIa. There are several catalysts capable of factor XI activation, which include the contact factor XIIa, thrombin, or factor XIa itself in the presence of negatively charged surfaces.[208,209] However, their mechanisms differ as factor XI must be a dimer to be activated by factor XIIa, whereas thrombin and factor XIa lack this requirement.[210] An activated factor XI dimer may comprise either one (1/2-factor XIa) or two factor XIa subunits.[211]

Following activation of factor XI, binding sites for the substrate factor IX become available in the apple 3 domain and serine protease domain of factor XIa.[212,213] Factor XIa proteolytically activates factor IX to factor IXa in a calcium-dependent but phospholipid-independent manner. Both forms of the factor XIa dimer as well as monomeric factor XIa activate factor IX in a similar manner.[211]

Accumulating evidence supports the notion that factor XIa–dependent activation of factor XI is not essential to normal hemostasis, but is important in pathologic thrombus formation.[214–216] Thrombin-mediated activation of factor XI, on the other hand, seems most significant under conditions of low tissue factor and is assumed to enhance clot stability through thrombin-activation of TAFI.[217,218]

Factor XI has been reported to interact with platelet GPIb, which is mediated through a site within the apple 3 domain, and to platelet apolipoprotein E receptor 2 (ApoER2).[219,220] It has been proposed that the dimeric structure allows for simultaneous interaction with the platelet by one subunit, thereby localizing factor XI to the site of clot formation, while binding to factor IX with the other subunit.[221]

Factor XIa function is regulated by the serpins protease nexin 1, antithrombin, C1-inhibitor, α_1-protease inhibitor, protein Z–dependent protease inhibitor, and α_2-antiplasmin.[216,222] Platelets also contain a factor XIa inhibitor, the Kunitz-type inhibitor protease nexin 2.[223]

Gene Structure and Variations

The human factor XI gene *(F11)* is 23 kb in length and is localized to chromosome 4q35. It consists of 15 exons and 14 introns (Fig. 113–17). Each of the four apple domains is encoded by two exons. The serine protease domain is encoded by five exons, with an organization similar to the homologous protein PK.

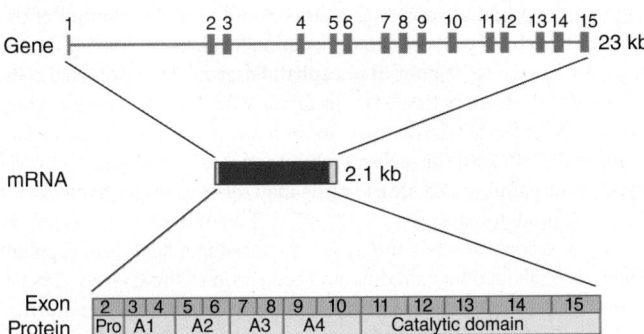

Figure 113–17. Relationship of gene structure to protein structure in factor XI. The exons, introns, mRNA, and protein structure are as indicated. The mRNA is 2.1 kb with small 5' and 3' untranslated regions *(light blue)*. In the protein, Pro indicates the prepro leader sequence, A1 to A4 indicate apple domains 1 to 4, and the serine protease (catalytic) domain is indicated.

Deficiencies of factor XI in humans can lead to a bleeding tendency, although not as severe as in hemophilia A or B.[224] Deficiency of factor XI is relatively common among Ashkenazi Jews in Israel.[225] The human gene mutation database lists 232 mutations in the factor XI gene (www.hgmd.org).

Increased levels of factor XI are a risk factor for venous thrombosis.[226] Genetic variations in the form of common single nucleotide polymorphisms (SNPs) seem to play a role in determining the level of factor XI and contribute to thrombotic risk.[227]

● THE CONTACT SYSTEM: FACTOR XII, PREKALLIKREIN, AND HIGH-MOLECULAR WEIGHT KININOGEN

Factor XII, HK, and PK are part of the contact system in blood coagulation, which is triggered following contact activation of factor XII mediated via a negatively charged surface. PK is synthesized in the liver, circulates as a zymogen, and is highly homologous to factor XI (see Table 113–1). Conversion into the serine protease proceeds through limited proteolysis by activated factor XII, and the generated kallikrein reciprocally activates more factor XII. HK, which is also synthesized in the liver, is a nonenzymatic cofactor that circulates in complex with factor XI or PK (see Table 113–1). HK is cleaved at two sites by kallikrein to release the bioactive nonapeptide bradykinin, a potent vasodilator.

The contact system is at the basis of the activated partial thromboplastin time (APTT) assay that is widely used in clinical practice. In this clinical laboratory test, the negatively charged surface is provided by reagents such as glass, kaolin, celite, or ellagic acid. Factor XIIa activates factor XI, which then activates factor IX. Despite HK and PK being required for a normal APTT, they appear to be dispensable for coagulation *in vivo*.[228] Individuals who are deficient in any of these factors do not have a bleeding tendency, even after significant trauma or surgery. However, factor XII, HK, and PK do participate in bacteremia or inflammatory responses in acute-phase reactions that do not involve the coagulation, but the classical complement system.[228]

FACTOR XII

Factor XII was originally reported in 1955 as the "Hageman factor," named after the first identified factor XII–deficient patient.[229] Factor XII is synthesized in the liver and circulates in plasma as a single-chain zymogen of 596 amino acids (Mr ≈80,000) at a concentration of 500 nM with a half-life of 50 to 70 hours (see Table 113–1).

Protein Structure

Factor XII, which is homologous to plasminogen activators, consists of an N-terminal fibronectin type I domain, an EGF-like domain, a fibronectin type II domain, a second EGF-like domain, a kringle domain, a proline-rich region, and a C-terminal serine protease domain (see Fig. 113–15). The proline-rich region is unique to factor XII, as it is not found in any of the other serine proteases.

Factor XII comprises an *O*-linked fucose in EGF 1 (Thr90), *N*-linked glycosylation sites in the kringle domain (Asn230) and the serine protease domain (Asn414), and several *O*-linked glycosylation sites in the kringle domain and proline-rich region.[230,231]

Factor XII Activation and Activity

Limited proteolysis by kallikrein at Arg353 in factor XII yields the activated two-chain α-factor XIIa, in which the heavy chain (the fibronectin types I and II domains, both EGF domains, the kringle domain, and proline-rich region; Mr ≈52,000) and light chain (serine protease domain; Mr ≈28,000) are linked via a Cys340–Cys467 disulfide bond (see Fig. 113–15). Once activated, α-factor XIIa activates factor XI to factor XIa. Furthermore, α-factor XIIa activates PK, thereby contributing to its own feedback activation.[232]

Factor XII is also known to acquire α-factor XIIa activity upon contact with a negatively charged surface, the latter inducing a conformational change in factor XII.[233] This conformational change induces a limited amount of proteolytic activity in factor XII, known as autoactivation.[234,235] Furthermore, the surface-induced active conformation of factor XII is suggested to enhance the proteolytic conversion to α-factor XIIa.[236] The fibronectin types I and II domains, EGF-2, the kringle domain, and the proline-rich region are reported to contribute to interaction with a negatively charged surface.[237–240] These naturally occurring surfaces include platelet polyphosphate (poly-P), microparticles derived from platelets and erythrocytes, RNA, and collagen.[241–244]

Further cleavage of α-factor XIIa by kallikrein at Arg334 and Arg343 in the light chain (proline-rich region) results in the generation of β-factor XIIa, which comprises a nine-residue heavy-chain fragment that is disulfide-linked to the light chain.[230] Given the absence of the heavy chain, β-factor XIIa does not interact with anionic surfaces. Even though β-factor XIIa is still capable of activating PK, it no longer activates factor XI.[245]

Despite its contribution to fibrin formation *in vitro*, factor XII has long been considered to be dispensable for coagulation *in vivo*, because factor XII deficiency is not associated with a bleeding.[229,246] However, newer *in vivo* studies indicate that factor XII contributes to surface-induced pathologic thrombosis via activation of factor XI.[215,242,247,248]

The serpin C1 inhibitor is the main plasma inhibitor of α-factor XIIa and β-factor XIIa. In addition, antithrombin (AT) and PAI-1 also inhibit factor XIIa activity. Conditions in which the factor XIIa activity is not properly controlled, such as in C1 inhibitor deficiency states or in case of a constitutively active form of factor XIIa, can result in the disorder hereditary angioedema.[249]

Gene Structure and Variations

The gene for factor XII is located on chromosome 5q35.3, spans approximately 12 kb, and contains 14 exons.[250] The intron–exon structure of the gene is similar to the plasminogen activator family of serine proteases. Portions of the gene are homologous to domains found in fibronectin and tissue-type plasminogen activator.

Loss-of-function mutations in the factor XII gene do not cause clinical symptoms in the form of a bleeding tendency in homozygous or compound heterozygous individuals, although they have a prolonged APTT.

Several common allelic variations in the factor XII gene have been examined to determine whether these variations influence plasma factor XII levels and whether these are associated with thrombotic risk. Best studied is a 46C>T transition four nucleotides upstream of the start codon. TT homozygotes have lower plasma factor XII levels than CC homozygotes, but there was no relationship with risk for venous thrombosis or myocardial infarction.[251]

●THE CELL-ASSOCIATED COFACTORS TISSUE FACTOR, THROMBOMODULIN, AND ENDOTHELIAL PROTEIN C RECEPTOR

TISSUE FACTOR

Tissue factor, also known as thromboplastin or CD142, is the cellular receptor and cofactor for factors VII and VIIa (see Fig. 113–6) and was first described in 1905.[12] Tissue factor is expressed in extravascular tissue, particularly fibroblasts and smooth muscle cells, where it serves as a hemostatic "envelope," poised to activate coagulation upon vascular damage. Generally, tissue factor is not exposed to the blood, but endothelial cells and adhered leukocytes may express tissue factor in response to injury or stimuli such as endotoxin or cytokines.

Protein Structure

Although many of the coagulation factors share some degree of homology, the structure of tissue factor is unique. It is the only procoagulant protein that is an integral membrane protein and shares structural homology with class II interferon receptors. Tissue factor consists of 263 amino acids (Mr ≈47,000) and comprises a 219-residue extracellular domain, a 23-residue hydrophobic transmembrane portion, and a short 21-residue intracellular tail.[252] The extracellular domain is made up of two fibronectin type III domains, which each comprise a disulfide bond (Cys49–Cys57, Cys186–Cys209). Elimination of the second disulfide link distorts the coagulant activity of tissue factor.

Tissue Factor Activation and Cofactor Function

The tissue factor–factor VIIa complex is generally acknowledged to be the major physiologic initiator of blood coagulation. The process of coagulation is initiated when an injury ruptures a vessel and allows blood to come into contact with extravascular tissue factor. Escape of blood from the vessel allows factor VII to bind to extravascular tissue factor and initiate coagulation. However, it is very likely that in the absence of injury, tissue factor located in close proximity of the vessels is already associated with factor VIIa.[253] An injury allows the extravascular tissue factor–factor VIIa complexes to come into contact with blood and initiate thrombin generation on activated platelet surfaces. Interaction of tissue factor with factor VII induces conformational changes in the serine protease domain of factor VIIa (see Fig. 113–6), thereby allowing the latter to proteolytically activate factors IX and X.[11]

Tissue factor does not require proteolytic activation to express its activity. However, it appears that tissue factor can occur in an inactive or "encrypted" state, and procoagulant activity follows after an appropriate stimulus. Even though the exact nature of the molecular mechanism remains to be identified, several models explaining tissue factor decryption have been put forward.

Originally, it was assumed that tissue factor encryption–decryption depends on the phospholipid environment, with decryption following upon expression of negatively charged phosphatidylserine on the membrane surface. Interaction of tissue factor with phosphatidylserine restricts the orientation of the tissue factor–factor VIIa complex, thereby ensuring correct alignment of the factor VIIa active site with the membrane-bound substrates factors X and IX.[254] Encryption of tissue factor has been proposed to occur upon localization into lipid rafts, which are known to be poor in phosphatidylserine. In endothelial cells, assembly of the ternary tissue factor–factor VIIa–factor X complex does result in tissue factor translocation to caveolae, which renders tissue factor inactive.[255] In addition, cell-membrane anchoring of tissue factor via acylation of palmitic and stearic acids may serve to target tissue factor to specific lipid domains.[256]

In a second model, the tissue factor–dependent procoagulant activity is explained by oxidation and reduction of the Cys186–Cys209 bond. This disulfide bond is less stable because of its strained conformation, and disruption of this link may cause conformational changes that alter the affinity of tissue factor for factor VIIa.[257,258] The breaking and formation of this disulfide link is suggested to be modulated by protein disulfide isomerases.[255]

A final model assumes that decryption relies on the dimerization of tissue factor. Like other members of the class II interferon receptors, tissue factor is capable of dimerization in a manner determined by the

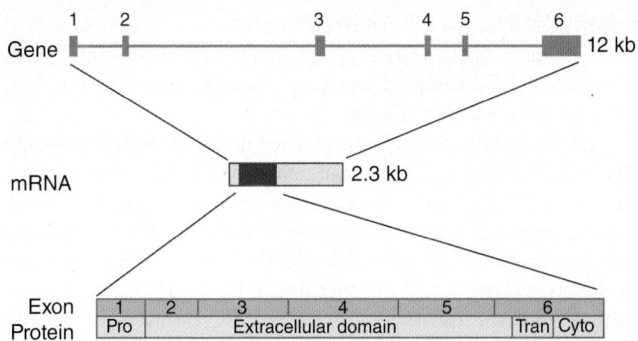

Figure 113–18. Relationship of gene structure to protein structure in tissue factor. The exons, introns, mRNA, and protein structure are as indicated. The mRNA is 2.3 kb with a 5′ untranslated region and a large 3′ untranslated region (*light blue*). Pro indicates the prepro leader sequence, the extracellular domain is indicated, Tran indicates the transmembrane region, and Cyto indicates the cytoplasmic domain.

redox (oxidation-reduction) environment and the exposure of phosphatidylserine. However, both monomeric and dimeric forms of tissue factor appear to possess procoagulant activity.[255]

Tissue factor is not only the primary initiator of the extrinsic pathway of coagulation, it also supports activation of PAR2 on endothelial cells and smooth muscle cells. Activation of PAR2 by the tissue factor–factor VIIa(–factor Xa) complex is not necessarily directly relevant for coagulation, but it is currently speculated that this event is important for wound healing, angiogenesis, tissue remodeling, and inflammation.[38–40]

Gene Structure and Variations

The human tissue factor gene is located on chromosome 1p21-p22. The DNA sequence of the tissue factor gene has been determined and consists of six exons and five introns that span approximately 12 kb (Fig. 113–18).

The primary transcript encoding full-length tissue factor contains six exons, but an alternatively spliced form of tissue factor (asTF) also exists in which exon 5 is spliced out. Because of a 3′ frameshift mutation, the full-length tissue factor transmembrane and cytoplasmic tail are replaced with a hydrophobic C-terminal domain, which renders the asTF soluble. asTF is expressed in lung, pancreas, placenta, heart, endothelium, and monocytes.[259–261] Although the level of asTF in human plasma may be substantial and amounts to 10 to 30 percent of total tissue factor,[262] it remains a matter of debate whether asTF contributes to coagulation.

In theory, variations in the tissue factor gene could influence thrombotic and bleeding risk. There are claims that polymorphisms in the tissue factor gene influence thrombotic risk but these claims have not been sufficiently confirmed.[263]

No relationship between loss-of-function mutations and bleeding has been described. This is perhaps not surprising in view of the fact that mice lacking tissue factor die early in gestation.

THROMBOMODULIN

Thrombomodulin, which was first identified by Esmon and colleagues in the early 1980s,[264,265] is a predominantly endothelial transmembrane protein and functions as an endothelial receptor for thrombin. In addition to endothelium, thrombomodulin has also been detected on a number of other cell types, including megakaryocytes, monocytes, and neuthrophils.[266]

Protein Structure

Mature single-chain thrombomodulin comprises 557 residues (Mr ≈78,000) and is composed of a lectin-like domain, a hydrophobic region, six EGF-like domains, a serine- and threonine-rich region, a transmembrane domain, and a 23-residue cytoplasmic tail. The highly charged lectin-like domains bear homology to the C-type lectins. Post-translational modifications include five *N*-linked glycosylation sites that are located in the lectin-like and EGF-4 and -5 domains. *O*-linked glycosylation in the serine- and threonine-rich region (Ser474) supports attachment of a glycosaminoglycan, a chondroitin sulfate moiety, which forms a low-affinity binding site for thrombin.

Thrombomodulin Cofactor Function

Thrombomodulin interacts with thrombin through its EGF-5 and -6 domains in a calcium-dependent manner.[267] As a result, thrombin's procoagulant exosite I is shielded, which causes thrombin's specificity to switch to the anticoagulant substrate protein C, requiring EGF domains 4 to 6 of thrombomodulin, and to TAFI, requiring EGF-3 to -6.[268] Thrombomodulin enhances the thrombin-dependent activation of protein C more than 1000-fold.

As a result of the relatively large endothelial surface area in capillary beds, the thrombomodulin-dependent activation of protein C proceeds efficiently in the microcirculation, which serves a major role in preventing thrombosis from occurring on intact endothelium.[269] In larger vessels where the endothelial surface area-blood volume ration is low, the presence of EPCR aids in the interaction with and presentation of protein C to the thrombomodulin-thrombin complex.[270]

Thrombomodulin also enhances the thrombin-mediated conversion of single-chain urokinase-type plasminogen activator to thrombin-cleaved two-chain urokinase-type plasminogen activator, which interferes with the generation of plasmin. Furthermore, thrombomodulin is a negative regulator of PAR signaling, as thrombomodulin-bound thrombin is incapable of PAR activation.[271] Based on this and because thrombomodulin is the cofactor responsible for APC generation, thrombomodulin plays an important role, albeit indirect, as an antiinflammatory protein. A direct contribution to suppress inflammation has been attributed to the lectin-like domains and hydrophobic region of thrombomodulin, independent of its anticoagulant activity.[272]

Protein C inhibitor is an effective inhibitor of the thrombomodulin-thrombin complex.[273]

Proteolysis of thrombomodulin by neutrophil-derived metalloproteinases and possibly rhomboids results in the generation of soluble thrombomodulin.[274] Normal plasma levels of soluble thrombomodulin are 3 to 50 ng/mL, but may increase as a result of vascular damage associated with infection, sepsis, or inflammation.[274]

Gene Structure and Variations

The human thrombomodulin gene (*THBD*) is located on chromosome 20p11.2, spans approximately 3.5 kb, and consists of a single exon (Fig. 113–19). Intronless genes are uncommon in eukaryotes and include rhodopsin, angiogenin, mitochondrial genes, interferons α- and β-adrenergic receptors. Intronless genes represent recent additions to the genome, created mostly by retroposition of processed mRNAs with retained functionality. Genetic variation in thrombomodulin has been studied in conjunction with venous thrombosis, bleeding and atypical hemolytic uremic syndrome (aHUS).

There are early reports that mutations in thrombomodulin are present in patients with venous thrombosis, but it was difficult to prove causality.[275] More recent work that made use of thrombomodulin sequencing in relatively large studies support the putative relationship between thrombomodulin function and venous thrombosis.[276] Such

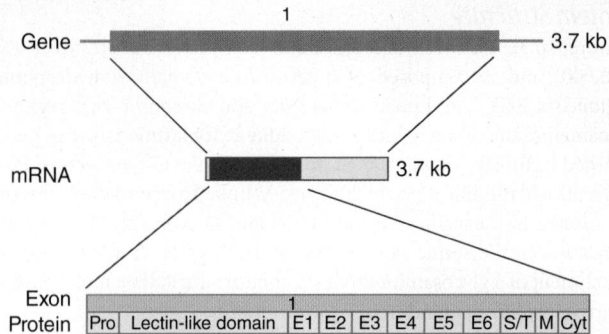

Figure 113–19. Relationship of gene structure to protein structure in thrombomodulin. The thrombomodulin gene has no introns. The exon, mRNA, and protein structure are as indicated. The mRNA is 3.7 kb, with a small 5′ untranslated region and a large 3′ untranslated region *(light blue)*. In the protein, Pro indicates the prepro leader sequence, the lectin-like domain is indicated, E indicates the epidermal growth factor (EGF)-like domains, S/T indicates the serine- and threonine-rich region, M indicates the transmembrane region, and Cyt indicates the cytoplasmic domain.

mutations, however, do not explain a large proportion of the heritability of venous thrombosis as they seem to be quite rare.

Recently a novel thrombomodulin mutation, p.Cys537Stop, was described in a family with a history of posttraumatic bleeding.[277] The endogenous thrombin potential was markedly reduced at low tissue factor concentrations in heterozygous carriers. Plasma thrombomodulin levels were elevated (433 to 845 ng/mL, normal range 2 to 8 ng/mL), and the addition of exogenous protein C further decreased thrombin generation. It was surmised that as a consequence of the premature stop codon, the truncated thrombomodulin is shed from the endothelial surface into the blood plasma, which would promote systemic protein C activation, thereby explaining the bleeding phenotype.

Missense mutations in thrombomodulin were also reported in patients with aHUS and this involvement in aHUS is probably related to the role of thrombomodulin in the complement system.[278] Thrombomodulin binds to C3b and factor H and negatively regulates complement by accelerating factor I-mediated inactivation of C3b. In addition, by promoting activation of TAFI, thrombomodulin also accelerates the inactivation of C3a and C5a. Thrombomodulin variants associated with aHUS had diminished capacity to inactivate C3b and to activate TAFI and were thus less protected from activated complement, thereby providing an explanation for their involvement in aHUS.

ENDOTHELIAL PROTEIN C RECEPTOR

The EPCR, a single-chain transmembrane receptor discovered in 1995 by Fukodome and Esmon,[279] binds both protein C and APC. EPCR increases the rate of activation of protein C[92] and alters the function of APC from anticoagulant to cytoprotective.[280] EPCR is mainly expressed by endothelial cells but also by leukocytes and other cell types.

Protein Structure

EPCR is homologous to CD1 and major histocompatibility class I proteins and folds with a β-sheet platform supporting two α-helical regions that form the potential binding pocket for protein C and APC. The mature protein (Mr ≈49,000) consists of 223 amino acids and is glycosylated through four N-linked glycosylation sites (Asn30, Asn47, Asn119, Asn155). EPCR contains a 25-residue long C-terminal transmembrane region with a short 3-residue cytoplasmic tail.

Endothelial Protein C Receptor Function

EPCR enhances the activation of membrane-bound protein C by the thrombomodulin–thrombin complex,[92] thereby enhancing the APC-mediated anticoagulant pathway.

APC bound to membrane-associated or soluble EPCR is disabled in its anticoagulant capacity. Instead, EPCR-bound APC activates PAR1 in an alternative manner by noncanonical cleavage at a Arg46,[281] resulting in an increased barrier function of endothelial cells mediated via the β-Arrestin/PI3K (phosphatidylinositide 3′-kinase)/AKT/Rac1 pathway. This is in contrast to the barrier-disruptive Arg41 cleavage of PAR1 by thrombin that activates the G-protein/ERK (extracellular regulated kinase) 1.2/RhoA pathway.[281]

EPCR is essential at the maternal–embryonic interface on trophoblast giant cells where it prevents fibrin formation. Consequently, complete EPCR deficiency leads to embryonic lethality. EPCR-deficient embryos rescued by the presence of EPCR in the trophoblast are viable and thrive, which seems to indicate that EPCR is not essential to blood circulation, at least in mice.[282] Additional ligands for EPCR have been discovered such as factor VIIa, *Plasmodium falciparum* erythrocyte membrane protein, and the V(γ)4V(δ)5 T-cell receptor.[283] These additional ligands indicate potential involvement of EPCR in the therapeutic effect of factor VIIa in hemophilia patients, and roles for EPCR in malaria, cytomegalovirus infection, and cancer.

Gene Structure and Variations

The chromosomal location of the EPCR gene *(PROCR)* is 20q11.2 and it contains four exons and spans 6 kb. Exon 1 encodes for the 5′-untranslated region and the signal peptide; exons 2 and 3 encode for almost the entire extracellular region; and exon 4 encodes for the transmembrane domain and cytoplasmic tail. One single mRNA encodes the centrosomal protein CCD41 and EPCR. Deletion of the signal sequence confers the centrosomal location of CCD41, while the unprocessed protein is incorporated into cell membranes as EPCR.

Variants of EPCR with reduced protein C affinity or increased cellular shedding are reported to be associated with unprovoked venous thromboembolism.[284]

⬤THE FIBRIN NETWORK: FIBRIN(OGEN), FACTOR XIII, AND THROMBIN-ACTIVATABLE FIBRINOLYSIS INHIBITOR

FIBRINOGEN

Fibrinogen, when converted to fibrin, forms the structural meshwork that consolidates an initial platelet plug into a solid hemostatic clot. Fibrinogen is synthesized in the liver and circulates in a concentration of approximately 7.4 μM. The plasma half-life of fibrinogen is 3 to 5 days, with only a small proportion of the catabolism caused by consumption.[285] Fibrinogen is also found in the α-granules of platelets. It was initially assumed that megakaryocytes synthesized fibrinogen. However, although some γ-chain transcripts are present in marrow precursors, it appears that most of the fibrinogen found within platelets is taken up from the plasma by endocytosis.[286,287]

Protein Structure

Chapter 135 provides a detailed description of the biochemistry of fibrinogen and of fibrin formation and degradation. Fibrinogen is a dimeric GP (Mr ≈340,000) and each of the two subunits contains three disulfide-linked polypeptide chains that are referred to as the Aα (Mr ≈66,500), Bβ (Mr ≈52,000), and γ (Mr ≈46,500) chains. A trinodular model of fibrinogen structure has been established from the crystal structure of fibrinogen (Fig. 113–20).[288]

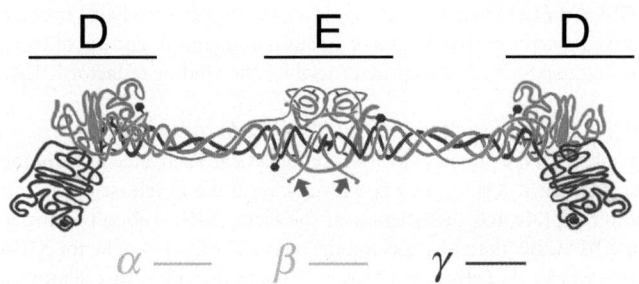

Figure 113–20. Structure of fibrinogen. Fibrinogen is a dimer. Each monomer consists of three chains: Aα shown in *light blue*, Bβ shown in *pink*, and γ shown in *dark blue*. The disulfides that link the two monomers are in the central E domain. The D domains consist primarily of the C-terminal regions of the Bβ and γ chains. The helical region connecting the two domains consists of all three chains intertwined. *(Reproduced with permission from Côté HC, Lord ST, Pratt KP: Gamma-Chain dysfibrinogenemias: Molecular structure-function relationships of naturally occurring mutations in the gamma chain of human fibrinogen. Blood 92(7):2195–2212, 1998.)*

Because human fibrinogen is subject to modification at a number of different sites both during and after biosynthesis, the fibrinogen present in the circulation is a heterogeneous mixture of molecules. These normal variants are caused by alternative splicing, modification of certain amino acids by sulfation, phosphorylation, and hydroxylation, different degrees of glycosylation, and proteolysis. It has been estimated that the number of nonidentical fibrinogen molecules that can be produced by these mechanisms is in excess of 1 million.[289] Some of these variations may have significant functional consequences. For example, the level of one variant of fibrinogen with an alternatively spliced γ chain (fibrinogen-γ') is associated with a risk of venous thrombosis.[290]

Fibrinogen Activation and Fibrin Function

Thrombin binds to the central domain of fibrinogen and proteolytically releases two fibrinopeptides A (Aα, residues 1 to 16) and two fibrinopeptides B (Bβ, residues 1 to 14) from each fibrinogen molecule.[291] Release of the fibrinopeptides exposes binding sites in the E domain that have complementary sites in the D domains of other fibrin monomers.[292,293] These complementary binding sites lead to the initial formation of two-stranded protofibrils with a half-staggered overlap configuration (Fig. 113–21). Protofibrils then aggregate into thick fibers that branch into a meshwork of interconnected thick fibers.[294] The half-staggered overlap of the fibrin monomers gives a characteristic cross-banded pattern on electron micrographs.[295]

During fibrin monomer polymerization, other plasma proteins also bind to the surface of the developing meshwork. These include elements of the fibrinolytic system and a variety of adhesive proteins, such as fibronectin, thrombospondin, and VWF. These surface proteins influence the generation, crosslinking, and lysis of fibrin. Fibrin(ogen) also has specific integrin-binding sites that are essential for platelet binding. The thrombin that initiates fibrin polymerization also activates factor XIII, which stabilizes the fibrin polymer by crosslinking. Factor XIIIa also crosslinks other bound proteins, for example, PAI-1, vitronectin, fibronectin, and α_2-antiplasmin, to the fibrin network.

Once formed, the fibrin mesh can be degraded by the fibrinolytic system. Plasmin cleaves fibrin and fibrinogen in an ordered sequence at arginyl and lysyl bonds, giving rise to a series of soluble degradation products.[296] In this process, the crosslink between two D fragments remains intact, resulting in the formation of a fragment consisting of two D domains and one E domain, called D-dimer. Circulating D-dimer concentrations are often measured as a surrogate marker of activated coagulation.

In addition to its obvious procoagulant role in stabilizing the initial platelet hemostatic plug, fibrin can also act as an important inhibitor of thrombin generation. Fibrin functions as "antithrombin I" by sequestering thrombin in the developing fibrin clot, and also by reducing the catalytic activity of fibrin-bound thrombin.[297]

Gene Structure and Variations

The genes for the three chains of fibrinogen are found within a 50-kb region on chromosome 4 at q23-q32 (Fig. 113–22). The genomic sequences show a high degree of homology, suggesting they were derived through duplication of a common ancestral gene. The homology extends to sites upstream of the gene, suggesting that common regulatory elements may reside in these areas, thus helping to coordinate synthesis of the three chains.

The physiologic importance of fibrinogen is underscored by the bleeding diathesis associated with afibrinogenemia and some dysfibrinogenemias (Chap. 125). Other dysfibrinogenemias are associated with thromboembolic disease. Although afibrinogenemia is associated with a bleeding tendency, it is usually not as severe as classical hemophilia.

FACTOR XIII

The GP factor XIII is a protransglutaminase that, upon activation, crosslinks and stabilizes fibrin clots.[298] Plasma factor XIII is a heterotetramer consisting of two factor XIIIA subunits (731 amino acids; Mr ≈83,000) bound to two factor XIIIB subunits (641 amino

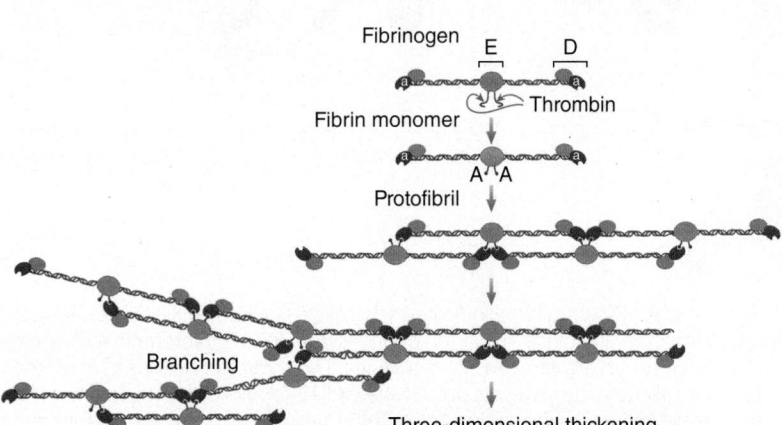

Figure 113–21. Cleavage of fibrinogen and polymerization of fibrin. The structure of fibrinogen is indicated schematically. Cleavage sites for fibrinopeptide A by thrombin are shown. Cleavage of the B peptide is not shown in this figure. Release of fibrinopeptide A exposes binding sites in the E domain that match complementary sites in the D domain. Fibrin monomers polymerize by half-staggered overlaps. Polymerization can also lead to branched structures. *(Reproduced with permission from Côté HC, Lord ST, Pratt KP: Gamma-Chain dysfibrinogenemias: Molecular structure-function relationships of naturally occurring mutations in the gamma chain of human fibrinogen. Blood 92(7):2195–2212, 1998.)*

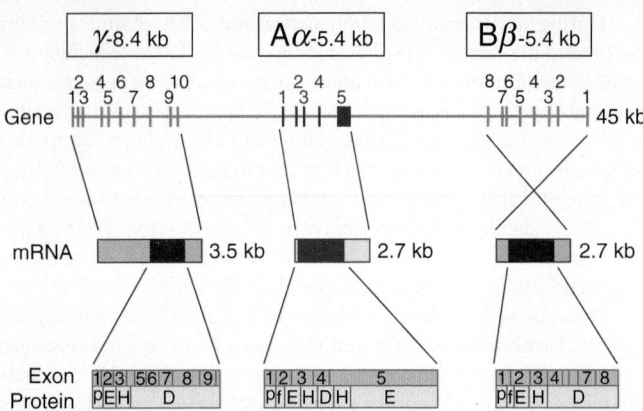

Figure 113–22. Relationship of gene structure to protein structure in fibrinogen. The exons, introns, mRNA, and protein structure for the three chains of fibrinogen are shown. The Bβ chain is translated in the opposite direction from the Aα and γ chains. Lighter colors in the mRNA indicate 5′ and 3′ untranslated regions. In the proteins, P designates the prepro leader sequence, f designates fibrinopeptide (A in Aα and B in Bβ), E designates residues in the E domain, H designates residues in the helical connecting region, and D designates residues in the D domain.

acids; Mr ≈76,500) that circulates in plasma as an A2B2 complex (Mr ≈320,000) at a concentration of 94 nM with a plasma half-life of 10 days (Fig. 113–23; see Table 113–1). Factor XIII circulates in plasma associated to fibrinogen via interaction of the factor XIIIB subunit with the fibrinogen γ′ chain.

The A and B subunits of factor XIII are synthesized and expressed separately and assemble in the circulation to the heterotetramer factor XIII-A2B2.[299] Factor XIIIA is synthesized in monocytes/macrophages, megakaryocytes, and hepatocytes, whereas factor XIIIB is synthesized exclusively in the liver and kidney.

Protein Structure

The factor XIIIA subunit consists of an activation peptide, a β-sandwich, a catalytic transglutaminase, and two β-barrel domains.[298] Factor

XIIIB acts as a carrier protein providing the long plasma half-life of factor XIII. Factor XIIIB consists of 10 Sushi domains in tandem, of which the first two Sushi domains are crucial for the binding to factor XIIIA.

Factor XIII Activation and Factor XIIIa Activity

Factor XIIIA is a proenzyme that is proteolytically activated by thrombin via cleavage at Arg37 (see Fig. 113–23), resulting in release of the activation peptide and dissociation of the factor XIIIB subunit from factor XIII-A2B2, thereby exposing the active site Cys314 of factor XIIIA. Cofactors for the activation of factor XIIIA by thrombin are calcium and fibrin(ogen). Platelets only contain the factor XIIIA (cfactor XIII-A2) dimer that is activated intracellularly in a proteolytic-independent manner through a rise in cytosolic calcium and subsequent conformational change before secretion by the stimulated platelet (see Fig. 113–23).[300]

Activation of factor XIII by thrombin is not a late event in blood coagulation, as it is activated with the same velocity by thrombin as the cleavage of the fibrinopeptides of fibrinogen.[301] Factor XIII can also be alternatively activated and inactivated by neutrophil elastase.[302]

Factor XIIIa consists of a factor XIII-A2 dimer comprising two activated factor XIIIA subunits that result from either thrombin-activation (factor XIIIa*) or conformational-activation (factor XIIIa°). The transglutaminase activity of factor XIIIa crosslinks a γ-carbon of glutamine in one protein chain to the ε-amino group of lysine in another protein chain in a reaction named transamidation. The specificity of factor XIIIa crosslinking of proteins stems mainly from the recognition by factor XIIIa of specific glutamines, while the crosslink to lysine appears to be random and limited to the ones that are in the vicinity.

When thrombin cleaves the fibrinopeptides A and B of fibrinogen molecules, the binding site on the central E domain for the D domain of other fibrin molecules is uncovered. This initiates lateral aggregation of protofibrils and fiber formation. Factor XIIIa stabilizes the forming of protofibrils by linking two γ chains in adjacent D domains in fibrin polymers. Binding of Arg158 in one subunit of the factor XIIIa dimer to the αC region residue AαGlu396 of fibrin facilitates crosslinking via αC chains to a next fibrin molecule by the other activated factor XIIIA subunit in factor XIIIa.[303]

The crosslinking of fibrin γ-chains or α-chains by factor XIIIa has independent and specific effects on clot formation and structure.

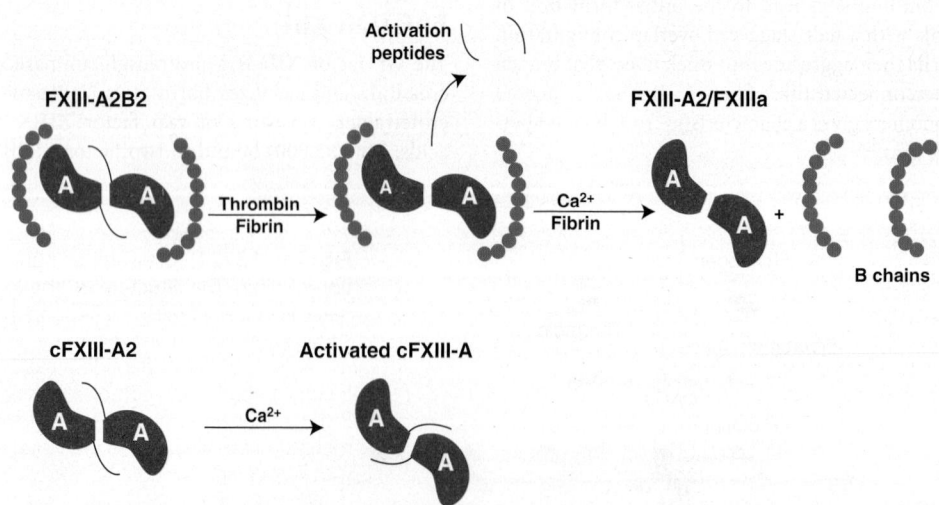

Figure 113–23. Factor XIII (FXIII) activation. The structure of the FXIIIA and FXIIIB subunits are indicated schematically. Plasma FXIII (FXIII-A2B2) consists of two FXIIIA (A, in red) subunits bound to two FXIIIB (in green) subunits. Cleavage of the activation peptides from FXIIIA by thrombin releases the FXIIIB subunits (B chains) and induces a conformational change in the FXIIIA subunits that opens the active site. This thrombin cleaved form of FXIIIA is known as FXIIIa or FXIIIa. Cellular FXIII (cFXIII-A2) found in platelets and macrophages consists only of the FXIIIA2 (cFXIII-A2) dimer. Before release by activated platelets, the cFXIII-A2 dimer becomes activated by an increase in intracellular calcium ions (Ca2+) that induces the active conformation without proteolysis of the activation peptide. This calcium activated form of cFXIIIA (cFXIII-A) is known as FXIIIa.

Crosslinks stabilize a clot by incorporation of the plasmin inhibitor α_2-antiplasmin which makes it resistant to fibrinolytic attack by plasmin.[304]

Several other processes during clotting are factor XIII-dependent, among which red blood cell incorporation in clots,[305] complement factor 3 (C3) crosslinking to fibrin,[306] and clot retraction by platelets.[307] Factor XIII also plays a role in the functioning of multiple adhesive and contractile proteins and in angiotensin type I receptor crosslinking.[308] Fetal specific crosslinking of Fas by factor XIII dampens apoptosis, suggesting that factor XIII may play a role in cell survival prenatally.[309] Related to its expression by monocytes/macrophages, factor XIII levels may drop after inhibition of IL-6 receptor signalling by tocilizumab.[310] Besides its crucial role in hemostasis, factor XIII has important functions during tissue regeneration and infection.[311] Factor XIII is necessary to prevent bleeding/stroke, maintain pregnancy, and aids in wound healing.[298]

Gene Structure and Function

The factor XIIIA chain gene *(F13A1)* has been localized to chromosome 6 p25.1.[312] It contains 15 exons, and is larger than 160 kb (Fig. 113–24). The fibrin-binding domain is encoded by exons 2 to 12. The active site, with its reactive thiol at Cys314, is present in exon 7. The gene encoding the factor XIIIB *(F13B)* chain has been localized to chromosome 1q31.3. It has 12 exons and is approximately 28 kb (Fig. 113–25).[313] Each Sushi domain is encoded by a single exon. The regulation of factor XIIIB expression is poorly understood. A total of 30 potential start sites are located upstream of the initial methionine.

Homozygosity or compound heterozygosity for loss-of-function mutations in the factor XIIIA or XIIIB genes leads to a severe bleeding disorder that is rare (1 in 2,000,000 of the population).[314] Factor XIII–deficient newborns often present with bleeding from the umbilical cord. The natural course is characterized by a life-long bleeding tendency and spontaneous miscarriages in affected women. Acquired factor XIII deficiency by development of an inhibitory antibody may lead to fatal bleeding if not treated.[315]

Mutations underlying factor XIII deficiency are more commonly found in the gene encoding factor XIIIA than the one encoding factor XIIIB. In accordance with this, the human gene mutation database lists 107 mutations in the factor XIIIA gene and 19 mutations in the factor XIIIB gene. Mutations in the gene encoding factor XIIIB often lead low levels of both factor XIII subunits. This is probably because free factor XIIIA has a short plasma half-life.

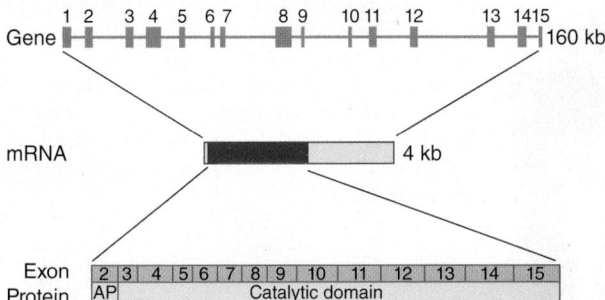

Figure 113–24. Relationship of gene structure to protein structure in the factor XIIIA chain. The exons, mRNA, and protein structure of the factor XIIIA chain are shown. The mRNA is 4 kb with some 5′ untranslated sequence coded in exon 1 and a large 3′ untranslated region *(light blue)*. In the protein, AP indicates the activation peptide, and the catalytic domain is indicated.

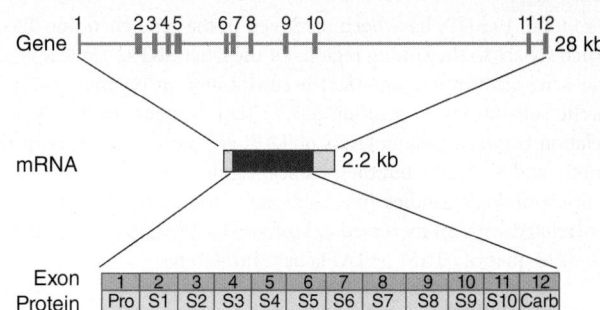

Figure 113–25. Relationship of gene structure to protein structure in the factor XIIIB chain. The exons, introns, mRNA, and protein structure are as indicated. The mRNA is 2.2 kb with small 3′ and 5′ untranslated noncoding regions *(light blue)*. In the protein, Pro indicates the propeptide, S1 to S10 indicates the Sushi 1 to 10 domains, and the C-terminal region is indicated by Carb.

A Val34Leu polymorphism associated with fatal atherothrombotic ischemic stroke results in a faster factor XIIIA activation rate by thrombin, which affects clot structure.[316]

THROMBIN-ACTIVATABLE FIBRINOLYSIS INHIBITOR

TAFI is the zymogen of a zinc-bound metalloprotease, and is also known as carboxypeptidase B, R, or U. TAFI is synthesized in the liver. Most TAFI present in the blood is in the plasma compartment, which circulates at 70 to 275 nM (see Table 113–1).

Protein Structure

TAFI is a 401-amino-acid proenzyme ($M_r \approx 60,000$) and consists of an N-terminal activation peptide (residues 1 to 76), a linker region (residues 77 to 92), and a catalytic domain (residues 93 to 401). Twenty percent of the protein mass of TAFI is accounted for by carbohydrate side chains that are attached to four sites within the activation peptide (Asn22, Asn51, Asn63) and linker region (Asn86). The active site residues (Glu271, Arg125) and zinc-binding residues (His67, Glu70, His196) in TAFI are conserved between other members of the carboxypeptidase A family.

Thrombin-Activatable Fibrinolysis Inhibitor Activation and Thrombin-Activatable Fibrinolysis Inhibitor-a Activity

TAFI is proteolytically activated by plasmin or thrombin, reactions that are accelerated 1000-fold when thrombin is bound to thrombomodulin. Both enzymes cleave TAFI at Arg92 to give rise to activated TAFI (TAFIa; $M_r \approx 37,000$) upon release of the activation peptide. TAFIa catalyzes removal of C-terminal lysine and arginine residues from fibrin and fibrin cleavage products. These residues are important for binding and activation of plasminogen, and removal of these residues by TAFIa reduces formation of plasmin on clots resulting in decreased clot lysis.

TAFIa may also have an antiinflammatory role as it can efficiently cleave C-terminal arginines of anaphylatoxins such as bradykinin and the complement activation peptides C3a and C5a.

Inhibitors of TAFIa have not been identified. Rather, the primary regulatory mechanism of TAFI activity involves its intrinsic thermal instability with a half-life of less than 15 minutes at 37°C.

Gene Structure and Variations

The gene for TAFI *(CPB2)* has been localized to 13q14.13. The gene contains 11 exons with 10 introns and spans 48 kb. Homozygosity or compound heterozygosity for mutations in the gene encoding TAFI have not been described.

In total, 19 SNPs have been identified in the gene encoding TAFI, of which six are in the coding region. Of the latter SNPs, two lead to an amino acid substitution: an Ala/Thr substitution at position 147 and a Thr/Ile substitution at position 325.[317] There appears to be a strong correlation between plasma levels of TAFI and polymorphisms in the promoter and 3′-region, but their clinical significance is unclear.

Epidemiologic studies have indicated that elevated TAFI levels are correlated with an increased risk of venous thrombosis, albeit that methods to quantify TAFI or TAFIa have limitations.[318]

● INHIBITORS OF COAGULATION: ANTITHROMBIN, TISSUE FACTOR PATHWAY INHIBITOR, AND PROTEIN Z/PROTEIN Z–DEPENDENT PROTEASE INHIBITOR

ANTITHROMBIN

AT was previously known as AT III as a result of a classification of several AT activities in plasma discovered in the 1950s.[319] AT is mainly synthesized in the liver and circulates in plasma as a single-chain GP of 432 amino acids (Mr ≈58,000) at a concentration of 2.5 μM with a half-life of 60 to 70 hours (see Table 113–1). AT is a member of the large serpin family and is known as SERPINC1 in the systematic nomenclature.

Protein Structure

AT consists of an N-terminal heparin-binding domain, a carbohydrate-rich domain, and a C-terminal serine protease-binding region that comprises the long, flexible, and surface-exposed reactive center loop. Structural stability is provided by three disulfide bonds, two of which are located in the N-terminal region and one in the serine protease-binding region. Posttranslational modifications comprise four

N-glycosylation sites, with three in the carbohydrate-rich domain (Asn96, Asn135, Asn155) and one in the serine protease-binding region (Asn192).

Antithrombin Function

The primary proteases targeted by AT are thrombin, factor Xa, and factor IXa. In addition, AT also inhibits factors XIa and XIIa, as well as tissue factor–factor VIIa; however, the latter is only inhibited in the presence of heparin.

Similar to other serpins, AT acts as a "suicide" substrate for its target proteases. These cleave at site Arg393 in the reactive center loop of AT, upon which AT is, unlike normal substrates, not released, but forms a 1:1 covalent complex with the protease, thereby blocking the active site. This complex is facilitated by a conformational change of the reactive center loop that folds into the N-terminal region of AT. By doing so, the covalently attached protease is dragged along, resulting in distortion of its serine protease domain and effectively converting the protease back into a zymogen-like state.[320]

Heparin and related molecules, such as endothelial-bound glycosaminoglycans, dramatically accelerate the rate of protease inhibition by AT (see Table 113–4) through two distinct mechanisms that characterize inhibition of either factors IXa and Xa or thrombin (Fig. 113–26). In case of the former, binding of a specific pentasaccharide sequence in heparin results in a conformational change in the reactive center loop of AT, which allows for enhanced access by the target protease and is known as allosteric activation of AT (Fig. 113–26, *middle panel*).[320] This results in a 500-fold acceleration of inhibition of factors IXa and Xa.[321] The pentasaccharide sequence is present in all forms of heparin including low-molecular-weight heparin and fondaparinux, a synthetic pentasaccharide. Heparin-accelerated thrombin inhibition involves bridging of AT to the protease, which serves to align the two molecules and enhances the rate of complex formation (Fig. 113–26, *right panel*).[322,323] This mechanism, also known as the template mechanism, requires longer heparin molecules found in unfractionated

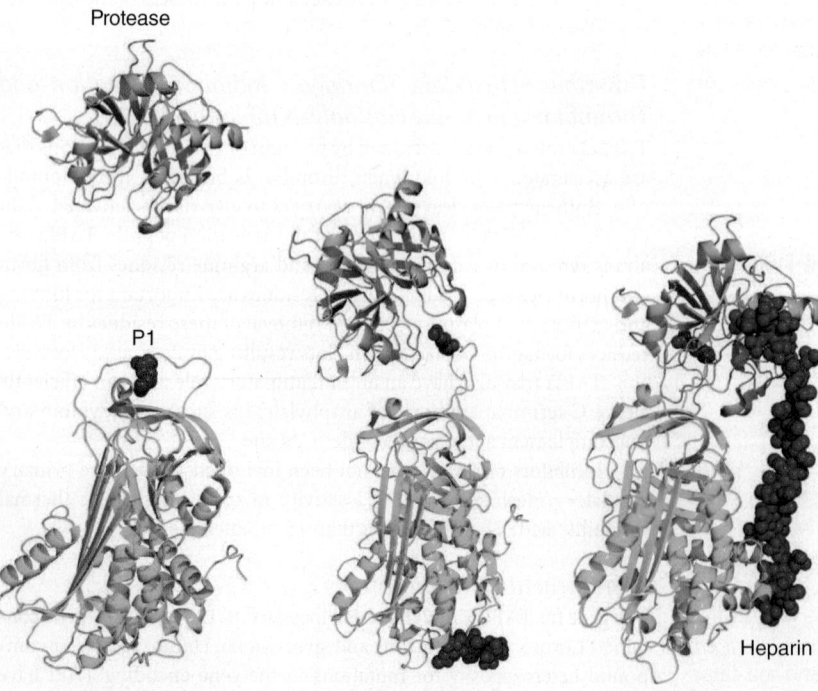

Figure 113–26. Effect of glycosaminoglycans on antithrombin inhibition. *Left panel:* Structures of thrombin (PDB structure 1TB6, *cyan*) and antithrombin (PDB structure 1T1F, *green*) with Arg393 (P1 residue, *red*) in the reactive center loop of antithrombin are shown. *Middle panel:* Binding of a specific pentasaccharide sequence (low-molecular-weight heparin [LMWH], *blue*) to antithrombin (PDB structure 2GD4) alters the conformation of the reactive center loop, thereby increasing exposure of the P1 residue and allowing for access of the target protease (allosteric activation). *Right panel:* A long heparin molecule *(blue)* interacts with both thrombin and antithrombin (PDB structure 1TB6), which aligns the two molecules and enhances the rate of complex formation (template mechanism).

Protease

P1

Antithrombin   LMWH   Heparin

heparin (UFH). Heparin-bridging of AT also contributes to some extent to the AT-mediated inhibition of factors IXa and Xa, but the majority of rate enhancement is provided by the allosteric activation of AT.

Protease–AT complexes are cleared from the circulation by lipoprotein receptor-related protein (LRP)-1–mediated endocytosis in the liver.[324,325]

Gene Structure and Variations

The 13.5-kb AT gene (SERPINC1) is localized on chromosome 1q25.1 and consists of seven exons. The cDNA is 1395 bp long, whereas the mRNA is approximately 1.4 kb.

Because of its essential role as an inhibitor of coagulation, individuals who are heterozygous for loss-of-function mutations are at increased risk for thrombosis. The prevalence of this condition in the general population is approximately one in 5000 individuals,[326] while it occurs in approximately 5 percent of patients with a history of thromboembolic disease.[327] AT deficiency can be categorized into type I and type II deficiencies.[328] Type I deficiency is characterized by reduced plasma levels of AT; however, homozygous type I deficiency is not compatible with life. Type II deficiency covers all functional AT defects.

The human gene mutation database (www.hgmd.org) lists 274 mutations. Mutations resulting in type I deficiency consist of large deletions, frameshift mutations, premature stop codons, splice-site mutations, and missense mutations. Mutations observed in type II deficiency impair heparin binding or affect the overall protein structure. Chapters 130 and 133 provide a more detailed description of the clinical significance of AT deficiency.

TISSUE FACTOR PATHWAY INHIBITOR

TFPI is a Kunitz-type protease inhibitor that inhibits factor Xa and tissue factor–factor VIIa activity and was discovered by Broze and Miletich in 1987.[329] TFPI circulates in plasma at 2.5 nM in multiple forms of which the majority is either truncated at the C-terminus or lipoprotein-associated. Only 10 percent of the circulating TFPI is the full-length TFPIα form of 276 amino acids (Mr ≈40,000; see Table 113–1).[330] The half-life of TFPIα in the circulation is only 2 minutes because it readily associates with the vessel wall endothelium.

Protein Structure

Full-length TFPIα consists of three tandem Kunitz domains and a C-terminus that contains a basic region (see Fig. 113–15).[331] However, TFPI is very heterogeneous as a result of proteolysis and alternative splicing. The latter gives rise to TFPIβ that lacks the third Kunitz domain and C-terminus, but instead includes a sequence that facilitates anchorage to the endothelial cell membrane via GPI linkage.[332]

Endothelial cells and platelets are the main producers of TFPI, with endothelial cells expressing both TFPIα and β, while platelets only produce TFPIα that is secreted upon platelet activation. Although a significant fraction of TFPIβ is GPI-linked to the endothelial cells, it is also found in plasma. In vivo, most of the full-length TFPIα appears to be bound to endothelial heparan sulphate proteoglycans through its positively charged C-terminus. This because total plasma TFPI levels rise by approximately threefold upon heparin treatment, which is completely attributable to an increase in TFPIα. In addition, TFPIα also circulates in complex with factor V.

Tissue Factor Pathway Inhibitor Function

The physiologic relevance of TFPI stems from its ability to regulate tissue factor–dependent coagulation as well as its direct inhibition of factor factor Xa. TFPI inhibits the tissue factor–factor VIIa complex in a two-step mechanism. TFPI will bind via its second Kunitz domain to the active site of factor Xa, thereby inhibiting the proteolytic capacity of

factor Xa.[331] This step is accelerated profoundly via protein S through interactions with the third Kunitz domain of TFPI.[333,334] The following step is the inhibition of the catalytic activity of tissue factor–factor VIIa complexes by formation of the quaternary tissue factor–factor VIIa–factor Xa–TFPI complex. This complex formation depends on the binding of Kunitz 1 to the factor VIIa active site. Overall, the effects of TFPI as regulator of tissue factor–initiated thrombin generation appear to depend on the fast protein S-dependent TFPI interaction with factor Xa.[333]

TFPI that is truncated at the C-terminus is effective in inhibiting tissue factor–factor VIIa activity; however, this seems to occur too slow to control thrombin generation at least in vitro. In contrast, inhibition of tissue factor–factor VIIa activity by GPI-anchored TFPIβ is effective and independent of protein S.[332] GPI-anchored TFPIβ also acts as an inhibitor of tissue factor–factor VIIa signaling by PARs, a function that TFPIα seems to lack.

TFPI may prevent prothrombinase formation by factor Xa in the presence of the procofactor factor V, factor V that is partially activated by factor Xa, or platelet factor V.[335] However, the factor Va–factor Xa prothrombinase complex is not inhibited by TFPI as a result of competition by prothrombin.

The heterogeneity and different activities of the multiple forms of TFPI have frustrated the measurement of TFPI for clinical purposes. However, tests that estimate the free full-length form in plasma indicate an association of low TFPIα levels with venous thrombosis.[336] Low levels of TFPIα are observed in protein S–deficient patients, which may be the result of a lack of association of TFPI with protein S in the circulation and faster clearance of free TFPIα.[337] High TFPIα levels have been observed in patients with increased expression of a splice variant of factor V, known as factor V-short. Factor V-short, which lacks the major part of the B domain, interacts with the basic C-terminus of TFPIα, most likely through the acidic B domain region in factor V.[132,133] Increased factor V-short levels lead to a dramatic increase in plasma TFPIα, resulting in a bleeding disorder.[133]

TFPI activity is downregulated by proteolysis at the C-terminus, upon which the basic C-terminal region or the third Kunitz domain are removed, thereby impairing inhibition of factor Xa and tissue factor–factor VIIa. Complete inactivation of TFPI is observed after proteolysis by the neutrophil derived proteases elastase and cathepsin G, which also cleave in between Kunitz 1 and 2. In this way, tissue factor–factor VIIa activity may be protected or reactivated during inflammatory processes.[338]

The in vivo relevance of TFPI was shown by the sensitization of rabbits to tissue factor–triggered disseminated intravascular coagulation after immunodepletion of TFPI.[339] Furthermore, mice lacking the first Kunitz domain of TFPI are not viable.[340]

Gene Structure and Variations

The human TFPI gene (TFPI) is located on chromosome 2q31-q32.1 and has nine exons that span 70 kb. TFPI is synthesized in two alternatively spliced forms, α and β.[332] TFPIβ is formed by an alternative splice event after exon 7 such that TFPIβ lacks the third Kunitz domain and instead has a unique C-terminus. Exon 2 appears to downregulate translation of the TFPIβ splice variant by a unique interaction with a sequence in the 3′-end of the TFPIβ mRNA.

Homozygosity or compound heterozygosity for loss of function mutations in the gene encoding TFPI has not been described. Several genetic polymorphisms have been identified and their relationship with venous thrombosis has been investigated. There is one report describing that a T33C polymorphism in intron 7 is highly associated with total TFPI antigen and protects against venous thrombosis,[341] but this relationship with thrombosis was not confirmed in a subsequent study.[342]

PROTEIN Z/PROTEIN Z–DEPENDENT PROTEASE INHIBITOR

ZPI is a serine protease inhibitor (Mr ≈72,000; SERPINA10 in the systematic nomenclature) that inhibits coagulation factors Xa and XIa. ZPI circulates in plasma at 60 nM with a half-life of 60 hours (see Table 113–1).[343] The ZPI-dependent inhibition of factor Xa is enhanced in the presence of protein Z.[79] Protein Z is a vitamin K–dependent plasma GP (Mr ≈62,000) that circulates at 40 nM (see Table 113–1). In normal plasma, which has a molar excess of ZPI over protein Z, all protein Z circulates in complex with ZPI.[344]

Protein Structure

ZPI displays 25 to 30 percent homology with other serpins such as AT. Based on this homology, Tyr387 was predicted and confirmed as P1 residue in the reactive center loop of ZPI and shown pivotal for inhibition of factor Xa.[345] Unlike other serpins, the N-terminal region of ZPI contains a very acidic domain.

Protein Z consists of a Gla domain, a hydrophobic region, and two EGF-like domains. Even though the C-terminal region of protein Z contains a domain that is homologous to the serine protease domains of the other Gla-containing proteins, it lacks the His and Ser active site residues characteristic for trypsin-like serine proteases.[346] Thus, protein Z has no protease activity.

Protein Z/Protein Z–Dependent Protease Inhibitor Function

The protein Z–ZPI complex associates with anionic phospholipid membranes in a calcium-dependent manner mediated by the Gla domain of protein Z, which facilitates formation of the ternary protein Z–ZPI–factor Xa complex. Furthermore, protein Z has also been suggested to induce conformational changes in ZPI, resulting in alignment of the reactive center loop and P1 site of ZPI with the factor Xa active site.[347] Together, these effects of protein Z enhance the inhibitory activity of ZPI to factor Xa by 1000-fold. In contrast, ZPI inactivation of factor XIa is protein Z–independent.[79] Similar to other serpins, ZPI acts as a "suicide" substrate. However, factors Xa and XIa eventually cleave ZPI at the P1 residue Tyr387, which results in release of a 4.2-kDa C-terminal ZPI peptide.[79]

The combination of protein Z and ZPI dramatically delays the initiation and reduces the ultimate rate of thrombin generation in mixtures containing prothrombin, factor V, phospholipids, and calcium. However, in similar mixtures containing factor Va, protein Z and ZPI do not inhibit thrombin generation.[79] Thus, the major effect of protein Z and ZPI is to dampen the coagulation response prior to the formation of the prothrombinase complex.

In mice, protein Z and ZPI deficiency is associated with a prothrombotic phenotype and both deficiencies dramatically increase mortality in animals with the factor V Leiden mutation. This indicates that protein Z and ZPI deficiency may be risk factors for thrombotic disease in humans.[348] Indeed, low protein Z levels appear weakly associated with thrombosis and ischemic stroke in subgroups of some small studies. However, these studies lack power to show a definite interaction with vascular disease.[349] Other studies demonstrate a possible association of protein Z and ZPI mutations with thrombosis and pregnancy complications.[350]

Gene Structure and Variations

The chromosomal location of the ZPI gene (SERPINA10) is 14q32.13. The gene encodes six exons and spans almost 10 kb. The gene for protein Z (PROZ) is on the long arm of chromosome 13 (q34) in close proximity to the genes for factor X and factor VII. The protein Z gene spans 14 kb and consists of nine exons. The intron/exon boundaries are identical to

the other Gla-containing coagulation proteins. There is an alternative exon that codes for a unique peptide of 22 amino acids in the prepro leader sequence. The gene is transcribed into a 1.6-kb mRNA.

Several mutations and polymorphisms have been described for the gene encoding ZPI,[351] but the association between such gene variations and risk of venous thrombosis has not been established with certainty.[352]

The human gene mutation database lists nine loss-of-function mutations in the protein Z gene. The relationship between these mutations and disease is uncertain at best, but a relationship with ischemic stroke and recurrent fetal loss cannot be excluded.[353–355]

PATHWAYS OF HEMOSTASIS

Early Coagulation Schemes

With the accumulated knowledge of the biochemistry of hemophilia it was recognized in the 1960s that blood coagulation was regulated by a sequential series of steps in which activation of one clotting factor led to the activation of another, finally leading to a burst of thrombin generation.[356,357] Each clotting factor was thought to exist as a proenzyme that could be converted to an active enzyme.

Since then the original waterfall reaction scheme of enzymes has been modified extensively. Factors V and VIII were identified as nonenzymatic procofactors for factors Xa and IXa, respectively, and the subsequent clotting events were divided into so-called extrinsic and intrinsic systems (Fig. 113–27). The extrinsic system was shown to consist of factor VIIa and tissue factor, the latter being viewed as extrinsic to the circulating blood. The tissue factor pathway could be activated in clotting tests by a brain tissue extract. The factor XII–dependent intrinsic system could even be activated by china clay (kaolin) and was viewed as being intravascular. Both pathways activate factor X, which, in complex with the activated cofactor Va, converts prothrombin to thrombin.

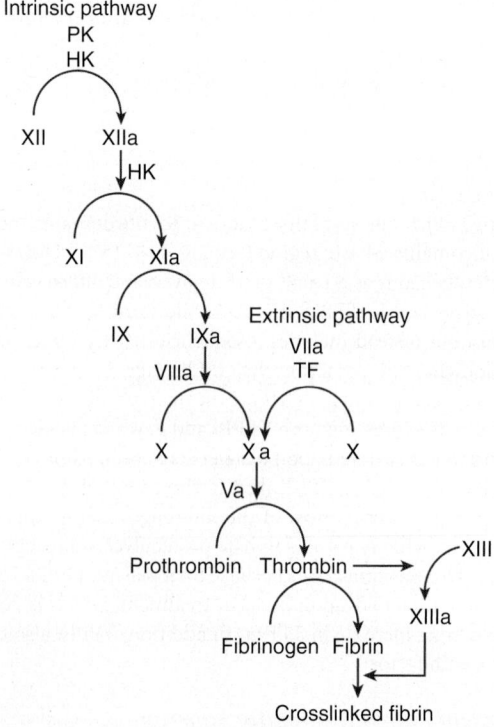

Figure 113–27. Cascade model of coagulation. This model shows successive activation of coagulation factors proceeding from the top of the schematic to thrombin generation and fibrin formation at the bottom of the schematic. The intrinsic and extrinsic pathways are indicated. HK, high-molecular-weight kininogen; PK, prekallikrein; TF, tissue factor.

Although these earlier concepts of coagulation were extremely valuable, investigators recognized that the intrinsic and extrinsic systems could not operate independently. The pivotal role of factor XII for the initiation of intrinsic thrombin generation and lack of bleeding tendency of factor XII deficient individuals was inconsistent with the extreme bleeding associated with a deficiency in factor VIII or IX, participants of the same intrinsic pathway, which urged investigators to search for additional links in the cascades.

Revision of the Coagulation Scheme

Key to the revision of the coagulation model was the purification and characterization of the transmembrane protein tissue factor.[358,359] A crucial observation was that the tissue factor–factor VIIa complex not only activates factor X, but also factor IX.[360] This showed that factor VIII or IX deficiencies, which result in hemophilia A or B, respectively, are in fact abnormalities of the tissue factor–factor VIIa pathway, even though factors VIII and IX are components of the intrinsic system. With the notion that traces of tissue factor–factor VIIa are rapidly inactivated by TFPI, it became clear that factor VIIIa–factor IXa activity is necessary to sustain hemostatic factor Xa and thrombin generation.[361–364] The embryonic lethality caused by both tissue factor as well as TFPI deficiency in mice underscores the importance of tissue factor–mediated thrombin generation and the control thereof.[340,365] Finally, it was observed that thrombin could directly activate factor XI,[366] thus providing an amplification loop once thrombin generation has been initiated: thrombin

→ factor XIa → factor IXa → FXa → thrombin. This model explains the mild bleeding tendency observed in factor XI–deficient patients and the absence of bleeding in factor XII–deficient individuals. A revised coagulation scheme is depicted in Fig. 113–28. This scheme builds on the conclusion that the major initiating event in hemostasis *in vivo* is the formation of the tissue factor–factor VIIa complex at the site of injury.[367]

It was also recognized that *in vivo* coagulation is regulated by control mechanisms, one of which is the localization of the coagulation reactions to cell surfaces. In addition, earlier and more recent observations emphasized the importance of plasma inhibitors targeting each step of the coagulation process. These include (1) TFPI, which controls tissue factor–factor VIIa and factor Xa activity in cooperation with protein S,[331,333] (2) thrombomodulin and APC, which inactivate thrombin and factors Va and VIIIa, the latter also in cooperation with protein S,[368] (3) AT, which inhibits thrombin and other coagulation proteases,[369] and (4) ZPI, which inhibits factor Xa on phospholipid surfaces in cooperation with protein Z prior to incorporation of factor Xa into the prothrombinase complex.[79] See also Fig. 113–28 for an overview of the inhibitory mechanisms of coagulation.

Most of the essential pathways of tissue factor–dependent thrombin generation and inhibitory control have been captured in a mathematical model based on the empirically derived rate constants of the individual reactions.[370] Completion and refinement of such models will aid our understanding of the biochemistry of the coagulation reactions on artificial membranes, given that the enzymatic events on

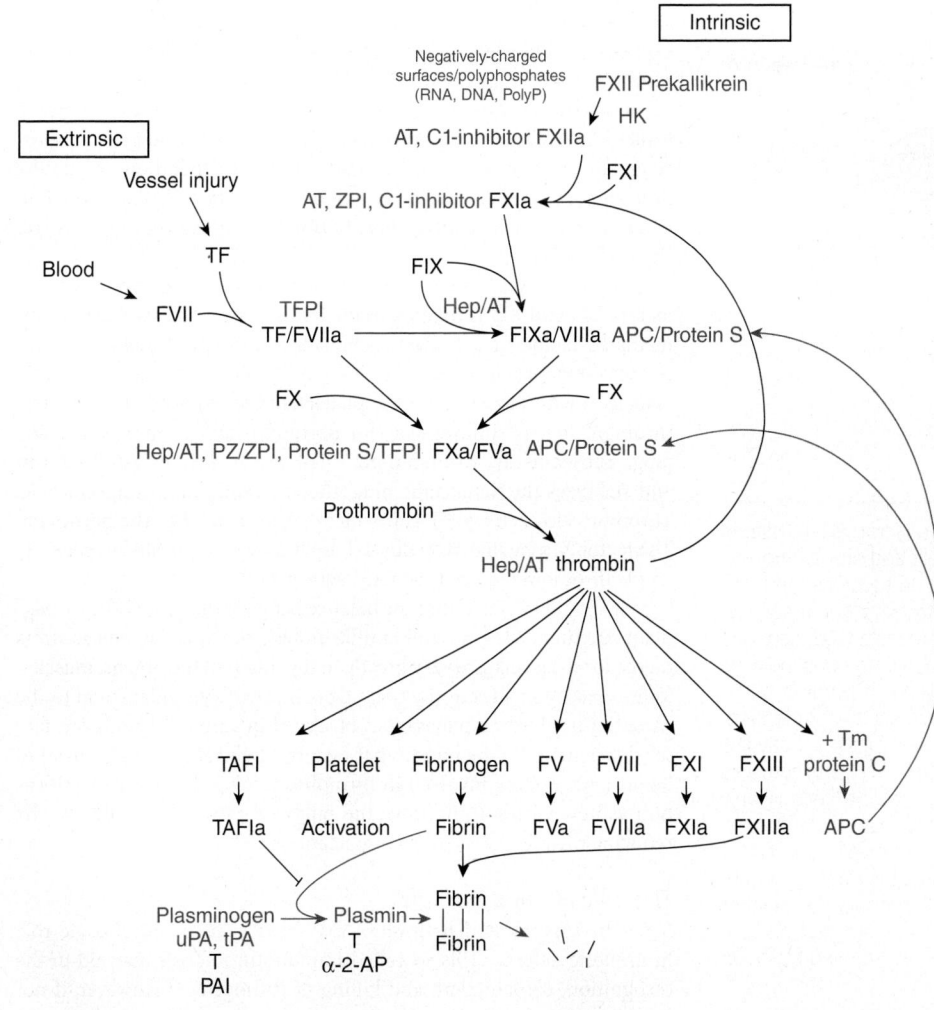

Figure 113–28. Revised model of coagulation. Schematic overview of the coagulation reactions in which several revisions have been made as compared to the classic cascade model of coagulation. The tissue factor–factor VIIa complex of the extrinsic pathway also activates factor IX, and thrombin activates factor XI, in a positive feedback loop. The factor IX–dependent amplification of factor Xa generation is necessary for hemostatic fibrin formation at low tissue factor concentrations, because tissue factor–factor VIIa–mediated factor X activation is inhibited by tissue factor pathway inhibitor (TFPI). Procoagulant extrinsic pathway components are indicated in *black*, the part of the intrinsic coagulation pathway that is not necessary for hemostasis is indicated in *gray*. Anticoagulant mediators are indicated in *red*. AP, antiplasmin; APC, activated protein C; AT, antithrombin; Hep, heparin; HK, high-molecular-weight kininogen; PAI, plasminogen activator inhibitor; PZ, protein Z; TAFI, thrombin-activatable fibrinolysis inhibitor; TF, tissue factor; Tm, thrombomodulin; tPA, tissue plasminogen activator; uPA, urokinase plasminogen activator; ZPI, protein Z–dependent protease inhibitor.

cellular membranes under (reduced) flow are still complicated, which hampers their incorporation into a mathematical model.[370]

A Cell-Based Scheme of Coagulation

The goal of coagulation is to produce a fibrin clot that seals the site of injury in the vessel wall. This process is initiated when tissue factor–bearing cells are exposed to blood at the damaged site. Tissue factor is anchored to cells via a transmembrane domain and acts as a receptor for plasma factor VII. Both trace amounts of factor VIIa as well as zymogen factor VII that is rapidly converted to factor VIIa by factor Xa and/or autoactivation bind to tissue factor. Tissue factor is expressed around vessels and in the epithelium, where it forms a "hemostatic envelope." The tissue factor surrounding the vessels may already be in complex with factor VIIa, even in the absence of an injury.[253]

The tissue factor–factor VIIa complex catalyzes two very important reactions: (1) activation of factor X to factor Xa and (2) activation of factor IX to IXa. The initial factors Xa and IXa formed on tissue factor–bearing cells may have distinct functions in initiating the process of blood coagulation.[371] When a vessel is damaged, the blood delivers platelets to the site of injury. These bind to extravascular matrix components to produce the primary hemostatic plug and become partially activated in the process. The platelets are consequently localized in close proximity to active tissue factor–factor VIIa complexes.

The factor Xa formed on the tissue factor–bearing cell interacts with factor Va to form prothrombinase complexes that generate small amounts of thrombin (Fig. 113–29). Although this amount of thrombin may not be sufficient to clot fibrinogen, it is sufficient to initiate events

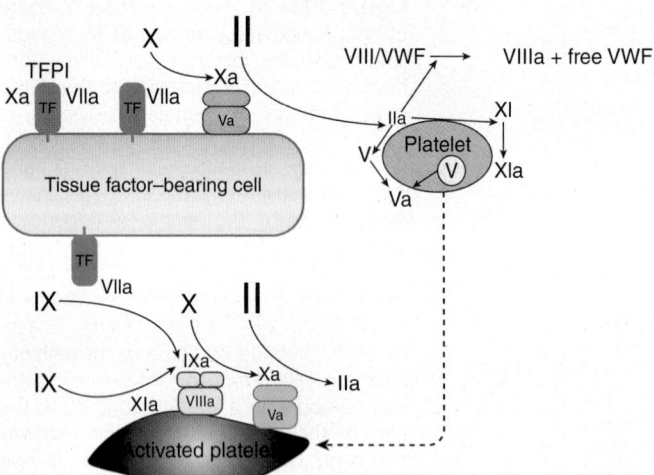

Figure 113–29. Cellular model of tissue factor–factor VIIa–mediated thrombin generation on tissue factor–bearing cells and propagation on platelets. After the initial generation of factor Xa on tissue factor–bearing cells, subsequent factor Xa generation is shutdown when tissue factor pathway inhibitor (TFPI) reacts with factor Xa to inactivate the tissue factor–factor VIIa complex. The small amount of thrombin generated on the tissue factor–bearing cell plays a critical role in priming platelets for subsequent coagulation steps. This thrombin activates platelets, releases factor V from platelet α-granules, activates factor V, activates factor VIII and releases it from von Willebrand factor (VWF), and activates factor XI. Factor IXa, generated on tissue factor–bearing cells, is only slowly inhibited by plasma inhibitors and can therefore make its way to the primed platelet surface where it binds to factor VIIIa. This factor VIIIa–IXa complex activates factor X on the platelet surface. The generated factor Xa complexes with factor Va and subsequently activates prothrombin, which leads to the burst of thrombin generation responsible for cleaving fibrinogen. Additional factor IXa is supplied by factor XIa on the platelet surface.

that "prime" the clotting system for a subsequent burst of thrombin generation. Experiments using tissue factor–activated whole blood and cell-based systems have shown that platelets can be activated by thrombin that is generated by direct tissue factor–factor VIIa activation of factor Xa.[371-373] The small amounts of factor Va required for prothrombinase assembly are likely provided by activated platelets, by factor Xa activation, or potentially by noncoagulation proteases secreted by the tissue factor–bearing cells.[335,374,375]

The small amounts of thrombin generated are capable of accomplishing the following: (1) activating platelets; (2) activating factor V; (3) activating factor VIII and dissociating factor VIII from VWF; and (4) activating factor XI (see Fig. 113–29).[366,372,373] The activity of the factor Xa formed by the tissue factor–factor VIIa complex will be mostly restricted to the tissue factor–bearing surface because free factor Xa that diffuses off the cell surface is rapidly inhibited by TFPI, AT, and/or the protein Z–ZPI complex. Factor IXa, on the other hand, will most likely act on activated platelets in close proximity to the tissue factor–bearing cell. This is because factor IXa can diffuse to adjacent cell surfaces as it is not inhibited by TFPI and ZPI, while the rate of factor IXa inhibition by AT is much lower than that of factor Xa (see Table 113–4).

The Role of Activated Platelets

Platelets also play a major role in localizing clotting reactions to the site of injury, as they adhere and aggregate at the same location where tissue factor is exposed to blood. Platelet localization and activation are mediated by VWF, thrombin, platelet receptors, and vessel wall components such as collagen (Chap. 112). Once platelets are activated, the cofactors Va and VIIIa are rapidly localized to the platelet membrane surface (see Fig. 113–29). Cofactor binding is mediated in part by the exposure of phosphatidylserine on the platelet membrane, a process resulting from a flip-flop mechanism whereby phosphatidylserine on the inner leaflet of the membrane bilayer flips to the outer membrane leaflet.[376] Endothelial cells, platelets, and leukocytes also generate procoagulant microvesicles that sustain thrombin generation. While the procoagulant characteristics of microvesicles have been studied in detail *in vitro*, their relative contribution to coagulation *in vivo* is still subject of debate.

Factor Xa generation is amplified on platelets by localization of factors IXa and XIa through specific binding sites,[377,378] and thrombin-mediated factor XI activation is enhanced by poly-P that is released by activated platelets (see Fig. 113–29).[379] Once formed, factor Xa associates with factor Va on the platelet surface to generate a burst of thrombin that is sufficient to clot fibrinogen and form a hemostatic plug. Subsequently, thrombin-activated factor XIII crosslinks fibrin and stabilizes the hemostatic plug, thereby rendering it impermeable. Thrombin also activates TAFI, which helps to stabilize the fibrin clot. The factor XIa-mediated feedback loop has been implicated to generate ample thrombin required for TAFI activation.[380]

It should be noted that the balance between the pro- and anticoagulant reactions, the pro- and antifibrinolytic potential, as well as stress on the local vasculature vary greatly in the different the organs, muscles, joints, and other sites in the body. This is probably fundamental to the variation in bleeding phenotypes observed in various coagulation factor deficiencies.[381] The notion that factors XI and XII are not crucial to hemostasis, but are involved in thrombosis, has led to their identification as new targets to improve the safety of anticoagulant therapy by reducing the risk of bleeding complications.[382,383]

The Role of Immune Cells

It has become clear that thrombi may have a major physiologic role in immune defense. This so-called immunothrombosis may aid in the recognition, containment, and killing of pathogens.[384] However, if not

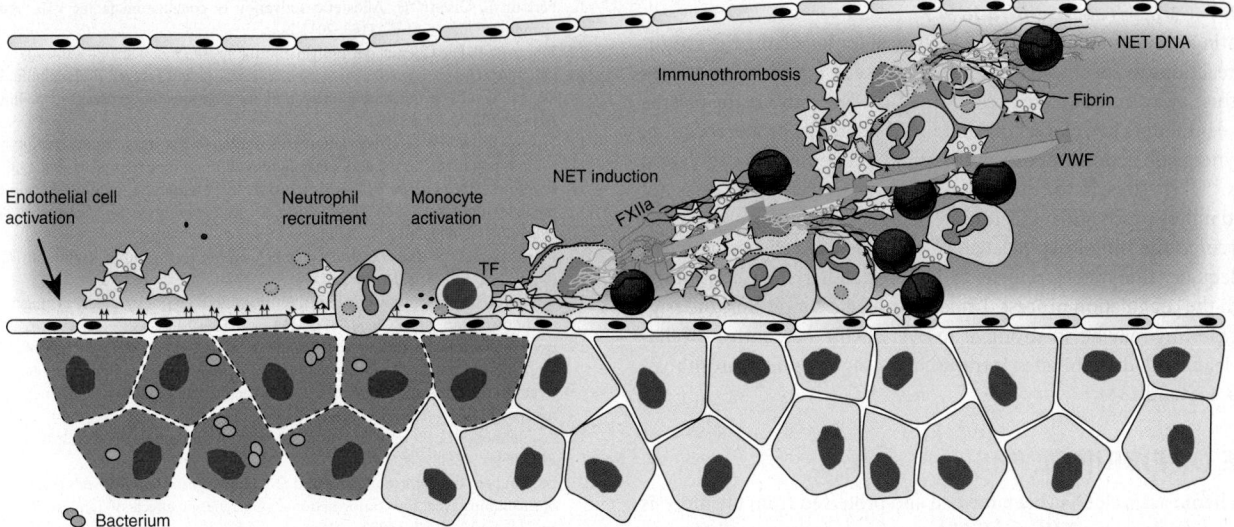

Figure 113–30. The role of immune cells: immunothrombosis. Endothelial cell activation by perturbation or infection causes neutrophil adhesion and monocyte activation. Induced tissue factor (TF) expression causes initial fibrin formation, while neutrophil activation by platelet interactions results in depolymerization of the DNA that bursts out the neutrophil as a mesh-generating neutrophil extracellular trap (NET). NETs may trap bacteria as innate immune defense, but also cause thrombosis by DNA-dependent factor XII activation and histone-dependent platelet activation. Furthermore, von Willebrand factor (VWF) may interact with DNA, which enhances platelet interaction with NETs.

controlled, it may contribute to thrombosis.[385] Figure 113–30 provides an overview of immunothrombosis.

The tight link between immune host defense and thrombosis is further demonstrated by the fact that immune cells play an active role in clot formation through several processes. First, monocytes express tissue factor upon activation by pathogens, which leads to thrombin generation by the extrinsic pathway.[386] Second, activated endothelium recruits neutrophils and, as a result of platelet-neutrophil interplay, neutrophil extracellular traps (NETs) can be formed,[387] which consist of decondensated chromatin fibers and DNA released by neutrophils.[388] NET-related proteins, such as histones and neutrophil elastase, activate platelets and inactivate TFPI, respectively, with both processes driving clot formation.[338,389] Moreover, NET DNA activates factor XII, resulting in enhanced thrombus formation mediated by the intrinsic pathway.[385] NETs also interact with VWF, which facilitates platelet binding to NETs.

The decondensation of chromatin that contributes to NET formation is caused by PAD4 relocalization to the neutrophil nucleus where it citrullinates histones. This results in unwinding of the DNA, which subsequently bursts out of the neutrophil.[388] The crucial role that PAD4-mediated NET formation may play in thrombosis has been shown in a physiologically relevant inferior vena cava thrombosis model in mice.[385,390] Consistent with this, NETs have been shown to be an integral component of human thrombi.[391] The notion that DNA is involved in pathologic thrombus formation opens doors to alternative ways of anticoagulation.

The Role of Endothelial Cells

Once a blood clot is formed to seal the injury, the clotting process must be terminated to avoid thrombotic occlusion in the adjacent, nonperturbed vascular bed. If the coagulation reactions are not controlled, clotting could occur throughout the entire vasculature, even after a modest procoagulant stimulus.

Endothelial cells play a major role in confining the coagulation reactions to the site of injury and preventing clot extension to areas where the endothelium is intact (Chap. 115). Endothelial cells have two major types of anticoagulant/antithrombotic activities, as illustrated in

Fig. 113–31. First, the protein C/protein S/thrombomodulin/EPCR system is activated in response to thrombin generation. This was demonstrated by Hanson and colleagues who showed that thrombin infusion *in vivo* is anticoagulant in a protein C–dependent manner.[392] This indicates that thrombin present at sites other than that of vascular damage is able to generate APC, which subsequently inactivates the cofactors Va and VIIIa, thereby terminating or preventing downstream thrombin generation.

Second, the protease inhibitors AT and TFPI are bound to heparan sulfates expressed on the endothelial surface, where they can inactivate proteases.[393] GPI-anchored TFPIβ may also play a role in controlling intravascular thrombin generation.[332] Furthermore, endothelial cells inhibit platelet activation by releasing the inhibitors prostacyclin (PGI₂) and nitric oxide (NO), as well as degrading adenosine diphosphate (ADP) by their membrane ecto-ADPase, CD39.[394]

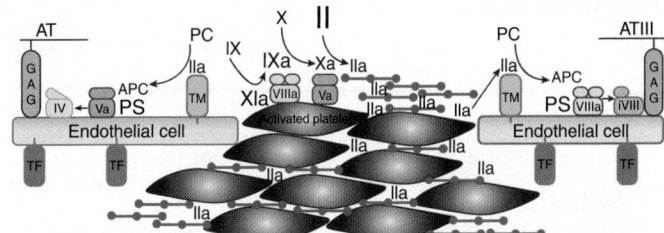

Figure 113–31. The role of endothelial cells. Activated coagulation proteins generated on platelets localized to the site of injury need to be confined to the site of injury. Activated coagulation factors that move to an endothelial cell surface are rapidly inhibited by antithrombin (AT), which is associated with glycosaminoglycans (GAG) on the endothelial surface. Furthermore, thrombin that reaches the endothelial cell surface binds to thrombomodulin (TM). Once bound, thrombin can no longer cleave fibrinogen. Instead, this thrombin activates protein C (APC), leading to the formation of APC–protein S (PS) complexes on the endothelial cell surface. APC-PS on the endothelial cell surface inactivates the procoagulant cofactors Va (to IV) and VIIIa (to iVIII). PC, protein C; TF, tissue factor.

Role of Plasma Protease Inhibitors

Circulating protease inhibitors are also critical for localizing the coagulation reactions to specific cell surfaces by directly inhibiting proteases that diffuse away from the site of clot formation. Not only are the plasma protease inhibitors key players in confining a clot to the proper location, their synergistic action imposes a threshold effect on the coagulation process.[363,395,396] Thus, in the presence of inhibitors, coagulation does not proceed unless procoagulant factors are generated in sufficient amounts to overcome the inhibitory mechanisms. In case the triggering event is inadequate, the system returns to baseline rather than continuing through the coagulation process. Under pathologic conditions, the trigger for clotting may be so strong as to overwhelm the control mechanisms, leading to disseminated intravascular coagulation or thrombosis (Chaps. 129 and 133).

ROLE OF FIBRINOLYSIS

Once a hemostatic clot has been formed and protected from fibrinolysis by the action of factor XIII and TAFI, some provision must be made for its eventual removal as wound healing takes place. Dissolution of clots is accomplished by the fibrinolytic system, as discussed in detail in Chap. 135.

The Concept of Basal Coagulation and Anticoagulation

The coagulation process only proceeds when enough thrombin is generated on or near the tissue factor–bearing cell to trigger activation of platelets and cofactors. One may wonder, however, if minute hemostatic plugs are not constantly formed throughout the body to maintain the integrity of the vasculature. Indeed, a low level of coagulation factor activation probably occurs at all times.[397] More than 30 years ago, it was shown that fibrinopeptides are continuously cleaved from fibrinogen at low levels in normal individuals.[398] Minute amounts of factor VIIa as well as the activation peptides of factors IX and X have also been demonstrated to circulate in the bloodstream of normal individuals.[399-401] This is known as basal coagulation or idling. Basal activation of coagulation factors likely results from minor injuries that occur during normal daily activities. The basal coagulation must be balanced by basal activity of the anticoagulation and fibrinolytic systems. This is evidenced by the presence of low levels of the protein C activation peptide and tissue plasminogen activator activity in normal individuals.[402]

REFERENCES

1. Davidson CJ, Hirt RP, Lal K, et al: Molecular evolution of the vertebrate blood coagulation network. *Thromb Haemost* 89:420–428, 2003.
2. Patthy L: Evolution of the proteases of blood coagulation and fibrinolysis by assembly from modules. *Cell* 41:657–663, 1985.
3. Wu SM, Cheung WF, Frazier D, Stafford DW: Cloning and expression of the cDNA for human gamma-glutamyl carboxylase. *Science* 254:1634–1636, 1991.
4. Li T, Chang C-Y, Jin D-Y, et al: Identification of the gene for vitamin K epoxide reductase. *Nature* 427:541–544, 2004.
5. Jorgensen MJ, Cantor AB, Furie BC, et al: Recognition site directing vitamin K-dependent gamma-carboxylation resides on the propeptide of factor IX. *Cell* 48:185–191, 1987.
6. Huber P, Schmitz T, Griffin J, et al: Identification of amino acids in the gamma-carboxylation recognition site on the propeptide of prothrombin. *J Biol Chem* 265:12467–12473, 1990.
7. Falls LA, Furie BC, Jacobs M, et al: The omega-loop region of the human prothrombin gamma-carboxyglutamic acid domain penetrates anionic phospholipid membranes. *J Biol Chem* 276:23895–23902, 2001.
8. Huang M, Rigby AC, Morelli X, et al: Structural basis of membrane binding by Gla domains of vitamin K-dependent proteins. *Nat Struct Biol* 10:751–756, 2003.
9. Tavoosi N, Davis-Harrison RL, Pogorelov TV, et al: Molecular determinants of phospholipid synergy in blood clotting. *J Biol Chem* 286:23247–23253, 2011.
10. Bode W, Mayr I, Baumann U, et al: The refined 1.9 A crystal structure of human alpha-thrombin: Interaction with D-Phe-Pro-Arg chloromethylketone and significance of the Tyr-Pro-Pro-Trp insertion segment. *EMBO J* 8:3467–3475, 1989.
11. Persson E, Olsen OH: Allosteric activation of coagulation factor VIIa. *Front Biosci (Landmark Ed)* 16:3156–3163, 2011.
12. Morawitz P: Die Chemie der Blutgerinnung. *Ergeb Physiol* 4:307–422, 1905.
13. Quick AJ: *Hemorrhagic Diseases,* pp 451–490. Lea and Febiger, Philadelphia, 1957.
14. Degen SJ: The prothrombin gene and its liver-specific expression. *Semin Thromb Hemost* 18:230–242, 1992.
15. Wu W, Suttie JW: N-glycosylation contributes to the intracellular stability of prothrombin precursors in the endoplasmic reticulum. *Thromb Res* 96:91–98, 1999.
16. Bradford HN, Orcutt SJ, Krishnaswamy S: Membrane binding by prothrombin mediates its constrained presentation to prothrombinase for cleavage. *J Biol Chem* 288:27789–27800, 2013.
17. Krishnaswamy S: The transition of prothrombin to thrombin. *J Thromb Haemost* 11 (Suppl 1):265–276, 2013.
18. Bradford HN, Krishnaswamy S: Meizothrombin is an unexpectedly zymogen-like variant of thrombin. *J Biol Chem* 287:30414–30425, 2012.
19. Bode W, Turk D, Karshikov A: The refined 1.9-A X-ray crystal structure of D-Phe-Pro-Arg chloromethylketone-inhibited human alpha-thrombin: Structure analysis, overall structure, electrostatic properties, detailed active-site geometry, and structure-function relationships. *Protein Sci* 1:426–471, 1992.
20. Lechtenberg BC, Freund SM, Huntington JA: An ensemble view of thrombin allostery. *Biol Chem* 393:889–898, 2012.
21. Lechtenberg BC, Johnson DJ, Freund SM, Huntington JA: NMR resonance assignments of thrombin reveal the conformational and dynamic effects of ligation. *Proc Natl Acad Sci U S A* 107:14087–14092, 2010.
22. Vu TK, Hung DT, Wheaton VI, Coughlin SR: Molecular cloning of a functional thrombin receptor reveals a novel proteolytic mechanism of receptor activation. *Cell* 64:1057–1068, 1991.
23. Ishihara H, Connolly AJ, Zeng D, et al: Protease-activated receptor 3 is a second thrombin receptor in humans. *Nature* 386:502–506, 1997.
24. Xu WF, Andersen H, Whitmore TE, et al: Cloning and characterization of human protease-activated receptor 4. *Proc Natl Acad Sci U S A* 95:6642–6646, 1998.
25. Coughlin SR: Protease-activated receptors in hemostasis, thrombosis and vascular biology. *J Thromb Haemost* 2005:1800–1814.
26. Spronk HM, de Jong AM, Crijns HJ, et al: Pleiotropic effects of factor Xa and thrombin: What to expect from novel anticoagulants. *Cardiovasc Res* 101:344–351, 2014.
27. Coppens M, Eikelboom JW, Gustafsson D, et al: Translational success stories: Development of direct thrombin inhibitors. *Circ Res* 111:920–929, 2012.
28. Hauel NH, Nar H, Priepke H, et al: Structure-based design of novel potent nonpeptide thrombin inhibitors. *J Med Chem* 45:1757–1766, 2002.
29. Royle NJ, Irwin DM, Koschinsky ML, et al: Human genes encoding prothrombin and ceruloplasmin map to 11p11-q12 and 3q21–24, respectively. *Somat Cell Mol Genet* 13:285–292, 1987.
30. Peyvandi F, Bolton-Maggs PH, Batorova A, De Moerloose P: Rare bleeding disorders. *Haemophilia* 18 (Suppl 4):148–153, 2012.
31. Poort SR, Rosendaal FR, Reitsma PH, Bertina RM: A common genetic variation in the 3′-untranslated region of the prothrombin gene is associated with elevated plasma prothrombin levels and an increase in venous thrombosis. *Blood* 88:3698–3703, 1996.
32. Gehring NH, Frede U, Neu-Yilik G, et al: Increased efficiency of mRNA 3′ end formation: A new genetic mechanism contributing to hereditary thrombophilia. *Nat Genet* 28:389–392, 2001.
33. Rosendaal FR, Doggen CJ, Zivelin A, et al: Geographic distribution of the 20210 G to A prothrombin variant. *Thromb Haemost* 79:706–708, 1998.
34. Giangrande PLF: Six characters in search of an author: The history of the nomenclature of coagulation factors. *Br J Haematol* 121:703–712, 2003.
35. Hansson K, Stenflo J: Post-translational modifications in proteins involved in blood coagulation. *J Thromb Haemost* 3:2633–2648, 2005.
36. Butenas S, Mann KG: Kinetics of human factor VII activation. *Biochemistry* 35:1904–1910, 1996.
37. Neuenschwander PF, Fiore MM, Morrissey JH: Factor VII autoactivation proceeds via interaction of distinct protease-cofactor and zymogen-cofactor complexes. Implications of a two-dimensional enzyme kinetic mechanism. *J Biol Chem* 268:21489–21492, 1993.
38. Camerer E, Huang W, Coughlin SR: Tissue factor- and factor X-dependent activation of protease-activated receptor 2 by factor VIIa. *Proc Natl Acad Sci U S A* 97:5255–5260, 2000.
39. Hoffman M, Monroe DM: The multiple roles of tissue factor in wound healing. *Front Biosci (Schol Ed)* 4:713–721, 2012.
40. Riewald M, Ruf W: Mechanistic coupling of protease signaling and initiation of coagulation by tissue factor. *Proc Natl Acad Sci U S A* 98:7742–7747, 2001.
41. O'Hara PJ, Grant FJ: The human factor VII gene is polymorphic due to variation in repeat copy number in a minisatellite. *Gene* 66:147–158, 1988.
42. Berkner K, Busby S, Davie E, et al: Isolation and expression of cDNAs encoding human factor VII. *Cold Spring Harb Symp Quant Biol* 51(Pt 1):531–541, 1986.
43. Girelli D, Russo C, Ferraresi P, et al: Polymorphisms in the factor VII gene and the risk of myocardial infarction in patients with coronary artery disease. *N Engl J Med* 343:774–780, 2000.
44. Biggs R, Douglas AS, MacFarlane RG, et al: Christmas disease: A condition previously mistaken for haemophilia. *Br Med J* 2:1378–1382, 1952.
45. Gillis S, Furie BC, Furie B, et al: gamma-Carboxyglutamic acids 36 and 40 do not contribute to human factor IX function. *Protein Sci* 6:185–196, 1997.

46. Winship PR, Dragon AC: Identification of haemophilia B patients with mutations in the two calcium binding domains of factor IX: Importance of a beta-OH Asp 64—Asn change. *Br J Haematol* 77:102–109, 1991.

47. Rallapalli PM, Kemball-Cook G, Tuddenham EG, et al: An interactive mutation database for human coagulation factor IX provides novel insights into the phenotypes and genetics of hemophilia B. *J Thromb Haemost* 11:1329–1340, 2013.

48. Begbie ME, Mamdani A, Gataiance S, et al: An important role for the activation peptide domain in controlling factor IX levels in the blood of haemophilia B mice. *Thromb Haemost* 94:1138–1147, 2005.

49. Bolt G, Bjelke JR, Hermit MB, et al: Hyperglycosylation prolongs the circulation of coagulation factor IX. *J Thromb Haemost* 10:2397–2398, 2012.

50. Brooks AR, Sim D, Gritzan U, et al: Glycoengineered factor IX variants with improved pharmacokinetics and subcutaneous efficacy. *J Thromb Haemost* 11:1699–1706, 2013.

51. Cheung WF, Hamaguchi N, Smith KJ, Stafford DW: The binding of human factor IX to endothelial cells is mediated by residues 3–11. *J Biol Chem* 267:20529–20531, 1992.

52. Cheung WF, van den Born J, Kühn K, et al: Identification of the endothelial cell binding site for factor IX. *Proc Natl Acad Sci U S A* 93:11068–11073, 1996.

53. Lenting PJ, ter Maat H, Clijsters PP, et al: Cleavage at arginine 145 in human blood coagulation factor IX converts the zymogen into a factor VIII binding enzyme. *J Biol Chem* 270:14884–14890, 1995.

54. Lindquist PA, Fujikawa K, Davie EW: Activation of bovine factor IX (Christmas factor) by factor XIa (activated plasma thromboplastin antecedent) and a protease from Russell's viper venom. *J Biol Chem* 253:1902–1909, 1978.

55. Zögg T, Brandstetter H: Activation mechanisms of coagulation factor IX. *Biol Chem* 390:391–400, 2009.

56. Johnson DJD, Langdown J, Huntington JA: Molecular basis of factor IXa recognition by heparin-activated antithrombin revealed by a 1.7-A structure of the ternary complex. *Proc Natl Acad Sci U S A* 107:645–650, 2010.

57. Camerino G, Grzeschik KH, Jaye M, et al: Regional localization on the human X chromosome and polymorphism of the coagulation factor IX gene (hemophilia B locus). *Proc Natl Acad Sci U S A* 81:498–502, 1984.

58. van Hylckama Vlieg A, van der Linden IK, Bertina RM, Rosendaal FR: High levels of factor IX increase the risk of venous thrombosis. *Blood* 95:3678–3682, 2000.

59. Simioni P, Tormene D, Tognin G, et al: X-linked thrombophilia with a mutant factor IX (factor IX Padua). *N Engl J Med* 361:1671–1675, 2009.

60. Denson K: Electrophoretic studies of the Prower factor: A blood coagulation factor which differs from factor VII. *Br J Haematol* 4:313–325, 1957.

61. Telfer TP, Denson KW, Wright DR: A new coagulation defect. *Br J Haematol* 2:308–316, 1956.

62. Hougie C, Barrow EM, Graham JB: Stuart clotting defect. I. Segregation of an hereditary hemorrhagic state from the heterogeneous group heretofore called stable factor (SPCA, proconvertin, factor VII) deficiency. *J Clin Invest* 36:485–496, 1957.

63. Gueguen P, Cherel G, Badirou I, et al: Two residues in the activation peptide domain contribute to the half-life of factor X *in vivo*. *J Thromb Haemost* 8:1651–1653, 2010.

64. Rudolph AE, Mullane MP, Porche-Sorbet R, et al: The role of the factor X activation peptide: A deletion mutagenesis approach. *Thromb Haemost* 88:756–762, 2002.

65. Yang L, Manithody C, Rezaie AR: Functional role of O-linked and N-linked glycosylation sites present on the activation peptide of factor X. *J Thromb Haemost* 7:1696–1702, 2009.

66. Rao LV, Rapaport SI: Activation of factor VII bound to tissue factor: A key early step in the tissue factor pathway of blood coagulation. *Proc Natl Acad Sci U S A* 85:6687–6691, 1988.

67. Monkovic DD, Tracy PB: Activation of human factor V by factor Xa and thrombin. *Biochemistry* 29:1118–1128, 1990.

68. Neuenschwander PF, Jesty J: Thrombin-activated and factor Xa-activated human factor VIII: Differences in cofactor activity and decay rate. *Arch Biochem Biophys* 296:426–434, 1992.

69. Borensztajn K, Peppelenbosch MP, Spek CA: Factor Xa: At the crossroads between coagulation and signaling in physiology and disease. *Trends Mol Med* 14:429–440, 2008.

70. Jesty J, Spencer AK, Nemerson Y: The mechanism of activation of factor X. Kinetic control of alternative pathways leading to the formation of activated factor X. *J Biol Chem* 249:5614–5622, 1974.

71. Fujikawa K, Titani K, Davie EW: Activation of bovine factor X (Stuart factor): Conversion of factor Xaalpha to factor Xabeta. *Proc Natl Acad Sci U S A* 72:3359–3363, 1975.

72. Pryzdial EL, Kessler GE: Kinetics of blood coagulation factor Xaalpha autoproteolytic conversion to factor Xabeta. Effect on inhibition by antithrombin, prothrombinase assembly, and enzyme activity. *J Biol Chem* 271:16621–16626, 1996.

73. Pryzdial EL, Kessler GE: Autoproteolysis or plasmin-mediated cleavage of factor Xaalpha exposes a plasminogen binding site and inhibits coagulation. *J Biol Chem* 271:16614–16620, 1996.

74. Grundy JE, Lavigne N, Hirama T, et al: Binding of plasminogen and tissue plasminogen activator to plasmin-modulated factor X and factor Xa. *Biochemistry* 40:6293–6302, 2001.

75. Talbot K, Meixner SC, Pryzdial ELG: Enhanced fibrinolysis by proteolysed coagulation factor Xa. *Biochim Biophys Acta* 1804:723–730, 2010.

76. Johnson DJD, Li W, Adams TE, Huntington Ja. Antithrombin-S195A factor Xa-heparin structure reveals the allosteric mechanism of antithrombin activation. *EMBO J* 25:2029–2037, 2006.

77. Hackeng TM, Seré KM, Tans G, Rosing J: Protein S stimulates inhibition of the tissue factor pathway by tissue factor pathway inhibitor. *Proc Natl Acad Sci U S A* 103:3106–3111, 2006.

78. Ndonwi M, Broze G: Protein S enhances the tissue factor pathway inhibitor inhibition of factor Xa but not its inhibition of factor VIIa-tissue factor. *J Thromb Haemost* 6:1044–1046, 2008.

79. Han X, Fiehler R, Broze GJ Jr: Characterization of the protein Z-dependent protease inhibitor. *Blood* 96:3049–3055, 2000.

80. Roehrig S, Straub A, Pohlmann J, et al: Discovery of the novel antithrombotic agent 5-chloro-N-({(5S)-2-oxo-3- [4-(3-oxomorpholin-4-yl)phenyl]-1,3-oxazolidin-5-yl}methyl)thiophene- 2-carboxamide (BAY 59-7939): An oral, direct factor Xa inhibitor. *J Med Chem* 48:5900–5908, 2005.

81. Pinto DJ, Orwat MJ, Koch S, et al: Discovery of 1-(4-methoxyphenyl)-7-oxo-6-(4-(2-oxopiperidin-1-yl)phenyl)-4,5,6,7-tetrahydro-1H-pyrazolo[3,4-c]pyridine-3-carboxamide (apixaban, BMS-562247), a highly potent, selective, efficacious, and orally bioavailable inhibitor of blood coagulation factor Xa. *J Med Chem* 50:5339–5356, 2007.

82. Furugohri T, Isobe K, Honda Y, et al: DU-176b, a potent and orally active factor Xa inhibitor: *In vitro* and *in vivo* pharmacological profiles. *J Thromb Haemost* 6:1542–1549, 2008.

83. Perzborn E, Roehrig S, Straub A, et al: The discovery and development of rivaroxaban, an oral, direct factor Xa inhibitor. *Nat Rev Drug Discov* 10:61–75, 2011.

84. Scambler PJ, Williamson R: The structural gene for human coagulation factor X is located on chromosome 13q34. *Cytogenet Cell Genet* 39:231–233, 1985.

85. de Visser MC, Poort SR, Vos HL, et al: Factor X levels, polymorphisms in the promoter region of factor X, and the risk of venous thrombosis. *Thromb Haemost* 85:1011–1017, 2001.

86. Mammen EF, Thomas WR, Seegers WH: Activation of purified prothrombin to autoprothrombin I or autoprothrombin II (platelet cofactor II or autoprothrombin II-A). *Thromb Diath Haemorrh* 5:218–249, 1960.

87. Stenflo J: A new vitamin K-dependent protein. *J Biol Chem* 251:355–363, 1976.

88. Foster DC, Yoshitake S, Davie EW: The nucleotide sequence of the gene for human protein C. *Proc Natl Acad Sci U S A* 82:4673–4677, 1985.

89. Grinnell BW, Walls JD, Gerlitz B: Glycosylation of human protein C affects its secretion, processing, functional activities, and activation by thrombin. *J Biol Chem* 266:9778–9785, 1991.

90. McClure DB, Walls JD, Grinnell BW: Post-translational processing events in the secretion pathway of human protein C, a complex vitamin K-dependent antithrombotic factor. *J Biol Chem* 267:19710–19717, 1992.

91. Preston R, Rawley O: Elucidating the role of carbohydrate determinants in regulating hemostasis: Insights and opportunities. *Blood* 121:3801–3810, 2013.

92. Stearns-Kurosawa DJ, Kurosawa S, Mollica JS, Ferrell GL, Esmon CT: The endothelial cell protein C receptor augments protein C activation by the thrombin-thrombomodulin complex. *Proc Natl Acad Sci U S A* 93:10212–10216, 1996.

93. Shen L, Dahlback B: Factor V and protein S as synergistic cofactors to activated protein C in degradation of factor VIIIa. *J Biol Chem* 269:18735–18738, 1994.

94. Oliver JA, Monroe DM, Church FC, et al: Activated protein C cleaves factor Va more efficiently on endothelium than on platelet surfaces. *Blood* 100:539–546, 2002.

95. Slungaard A, Fernandez JA, Griffin JH, et al: Platelet factor 4 enhances generation of activated protein C *in vitro* and *in vivo*. *Blood* 102:146–151, 2003.

96. Bouwens EA, Stavenuiter F, Mosnier LO: Mechanisms of anticoagulant and cytoprotective actions of the protein C pathway. *J Thromb Haemost* 11 Suppl 1:242–253, 2013.

97. Foster DC, Yoshitake S, Davie EW: The nucleotide sequence of the gene for human protein C. *Proc Natl Acad Sci U S A* 82:4673–4677, 1985.

98. Branson HE, Katz J, Marble R, Griffin JH: Inherited protein C deficiency and coumarin-responsive chronic relapsing purpura fulminans in a newborn infant. *Lancet* 2:1165–1168, 1983.

99. Reitsma PH: Protein C deficiency: From gene defects to disease. *Thromb Haemost* 78:344–350, 1997.

100. Lijfering WM, Christiansen SC, Rosendaal FR, Cannegieter SC: Contribution of high factor VIII, IX and XI to the risk of recurrent venous thrombosis in factor V Leiden carriers. *J Thromb Haemost* 7:1944–1946, 2009.

101. Spek CA, Koster T, Rosendaal FR, et al: Genotypic variation in the promoter region of the protein C gene is associated with plasma protein C levels and thrombotic risk. *Arterioscler Thromb Vasc Biol* 15:214–218, 1995.

102. Davidson CJ, Tuddenham EG, McVey JH: 450 Million years of hemostasis. *J Thromb Haemost* 1:1487–1494, 2003.

103. Zheng C, Zhang B: Combined deficiency of coagulation factors V and VIII: An update. *Semin Thromb Hemost* 39:613–620, 2013.

104. Owren PA: The coagulation of blood: Investigations on a new clotting factor. *Acta Med Scand* 128 (Suppl 194), 1947.

105. Owren PA: Parahaemophilia. Haemorrhagic diathesis due to absence of a previously unknown clotting factor. *Lancet* 1:446–448, 1947.

106. Stormorken H: The discovery of factor V: A tricky clotting factor. *J Thromb Haemost* 1:206–213, 2003.

107. Camire RM, Pollak ES, Kaushansky K, Tracy PB: Secretable human platelet-derived factor V originates from the plasma pool. *Blood* 92:3035–3041, 1998.

108. Thomassen MC, Castoldi E, Tans G, et al: Endogenous factor V synthesis in megakaryocytes contributes negligibly to the platelet factor V pool. *Haematologica* 88:1150–1156, 2003.

109. Bouchard BA, Williams JL, Meisler NT, et al: Endocytosis of plasma-derived factor V by megakaryocytes occurs via a clathrin-dependent, specific membrane binding event. *J Thromb Haemost* 3:541–551, 2005.

110. Gould WR, Silveira JR, Tracy PB: Unique *in vivo* modifications of coagulation factor V produce a physically and functionally distinct platelet-derived cofactor: Characterization of purified platelet-derived factor V/Va. *J Biol Chem* 279:2383–2393, 2004.

111. Hayward CP: Multimerin: A bench-to-bedside chronology of a unique platelet and endothelial cell protein—from discovery to function to abnormalities in disease. *Clin Invest Med* 20:176–187, 1997.

112. Nesheim ME, Nichols WL, Cole TL, et al: Isolation and study of an acquired inhibitor of human coagulation factor V. *J Clin Invest* 77:405–415, 1986.

113. Sun H, Yang TL, Yang A, et al: The murine platelet and plasma factor V pools are biosynthetically distinct and sufficient for minimal hemostasis. *Blood* 102:2856–2861, 2003.

114. Yang TL, Pipe SW, Yang A, Ginsburg D: Biosynthetic origin and functional significance of murine platelet factor V. *Blood* 102:2851–2855, 2003.

115. Ortel TL, Devore-Carter D, Quinn-Allen M, Kane WH: Deletion analysis of recombinant human factor V. Evidence for a phosphatidylserine binding site in the second C-type domain. *J Biol Chem* 267:4189–4198, 1992.

116. Adams TE, Hockin MF, Mann KG, Everse SJ: The crystal structure of activated protein C-inactivated bovine factor Va: Implications for cofactor function. *Proc Natl Acad Sci U S A* 101:8918–8923, 2004.

117. Peng W, Quinn-Allen Ma, Kane WH: Mutation of hydrophobic residues in the factor Va C1 and C2 domains blocks membrane-dependent prothrombin activation. *J Thromb Haemost* 3:351–354, 2005.

118. Stoilova-McPhie S, Parmenter CD, Segers K, et al: Defining the structure of membrane-bound human blood coagulation factor Va. *J Thromb Haemost* 6:76–82, 2008.

119. Bos MH, Camire RM: A bipartite autoinhibitory region within the B-domain suppresses function in factor V. *J Biol Chem* 287:26342–26351, 2012.

120. Bunce MW, Bos MH, Krishnaswamy S, Camire RM: Restoring the procofactor state of factor Va-like variants by complementation with B-domain peptides. *J Biol Chem* 288:30151–30160, 2013.

121. Mann KG, Kalafatis M: Factor V: A combination of Dr Jekyll and Mr Hyde. *Blood* 101:20–30, 2003.

122. Pittman DD, Tomkinson KN, Michnick D, et al: Posttranslational sulfation of factor V is required for efficient thrombin cleavage and activation and for full procoagulant activity. *Biochemistry* 33:6952–6959, 1994.

123. Kalafatis M: Identification and partial characterization of factor Va heavy chain kinase from human platelets. *J Biol Chem* 273:8459–8466, 1998.

124. Kim SW, Ortel TL, Quinn-Allen MA, et al: Partial glycosylation at asparagine-2181 of the second C-type domain of human factor V modulates assembly of the prothrombinase complex. *Biochemistry* 38:11448–11454, 1999.

125. Nicolaes GA, Villoutreix BO, Dahlbäck B: Partial glycosylation of Asn2181 in human factor V as a cause of molecular and functional heterogeneity. Modulation of glycosylation efficiency by mutagenesis of the consensus sequence for N-linked glycosylation. *Biochemistry* 38:13584–13591, 1999.

126. Camire RM, Bos MH: The molecular basis of factor V and VIII procofactor activation. *J Thromb Haemost* 7:1951–1961, 2009.

127. Schuijt TJ, Bakhtiari K, Daffre S, et al: Factor Xa activation of factor V is of paramount importance in initiating the coagulation system: Lessons from a tick salivary protein. *Circulation* 128:919–966, 2013.

128. Thorelli E, Kaufman RJ, Dahlback B: Cleavage requirements for activation of factor V by factor Xa. *Eur J Biochem* 247:12–20, 1997.

129. Mann KG, Nesheim ME, Church WR, et al: Surface-dependent reactions of the vitamin K-dependent enzyme complexes. *Blood* 76:1–16, 1990.

130. Mann KG, Hockin MF, Begin KJ, Kalafatis M: Activated protein C cleavage of factor Va leads to dissociation of the A2 domain. *J Biol Chem* 272:20678–20683, 1997.

131. Bertina RM, Koeleman BP, Koster T, et al: Mutation in blood coagulation factor V associated with resistance to activated protein C. *Nature* 369:64–67, 1994.

132. Duckers C, Simioni P, Spiezia L, et al: Low plasma levels of tissue factor pathway inhibitor in patients with congenital factor V deficiency. *Blood* 112:3615, 2008.

133. Vincent L, Tran S: Coagulation factor V A2440G causes east Texas bleeding disorder via TFPIα. *J Clin Invest* 123:3777–3787, 2013.

134. Duckers C, Simioni P, Spiezia L, et al: Residual platelet factor V ensures thrombin generation in patients with severe congenital factor V deficiency and mild bleeding symptoms. *Blood* 115:879–886, 2010.

135. Cripe LD, Moore KD, Kane WH: Structure of the gene for human coagulation factor V. *Biochemistry* 31:3777–3785, 1992.

136. Owren PA: Parahaemophilia; haemorrhagic diathesis due to absence of a previously unknown clotting factor. *Lancet* 1:446–448, 1947.

137. Dahlbäck B, Carlsson M, Svensson PJ: Familial thrombophilia due to a previously unrecognized mechanism characterized by poor anticoagulant response to activated protein C: Prediction of a cofactor to activated protein C. *Proc Natl Acad Sci U S A* 90:1004–1008, 1993.

138. Bertina RM, Koeleman BP, Koster T, et al: Mutation in blood coagulation factor V associated with resistance to activated protein C. *Nature* 369:64–67, 1994.

139. Patek AJ, Taylor FH: Hemophilia. II. Some properties of a substance obtained from normal human plasma effective in accelerating the coagulation of hemophilic blood. *J Clin Invest* 16:113–124, 1937.

140. Tuddenham EG, Trabold NC, Collins JA, Hoyer LW: The properties of factor VIII coagulant activity prepared by immunoadsorbent chromatography. *J Lab Clin Med* 93:40–53, 1979.

141. Shaw E, Giddings JC, Peake IR, Bloom AL: Synthesis of procoagulant factor VIII, factor VIII related antigen and other coagulation factors by the isolated perfused rat liver. *Br J Haematol* 41:585–596, 1979.

142. Bontempo FA, Lewis JH, Gorenc TJ, et al: Liver transplantation in hemophilia A. *Blood* 69:1721–1724, 1987.

143. Lamont PA, Ragni MV: Lack of desmopressin (DDAVP) response in men with hemophilia A following liver transplantation. *J Thromb Haemost* 3:2259–2263, 2005.

144. Madeira C, Layman R, de Vera M, et al: Extrahepatic factor VIII production in transplant recipient of hemophilia donor liver. *Blood* 113:5364–5366, 2009.

145. Kumaran V, Benten D, Follenzi A, et al: Transplantation of endothelial cells corrects the phenotype in hemophilia A mice. *J Thromb Haemost* 3:2022–2031, 2005.

146. Everett L, Cleuren A: Murine coagulation factor VIII is synthesized in endothelial cells. *Blood* 123:3697–3706, 2014.

147. Fahs SA, Hille MT, Shi Q, et al: A conditional knockout mouse model reveals endothelial cells as the principal and possibly exclusive source of plasma factor VIII. *Blood* 123:3706–3714, 2014.

148. Jacquemin M, Neyrinck A, Hermanns M, et al: FVIII production by human lung microvascular endothelial cells. *Blood* 108:515–518, 2006.

149. Shahani T, Covens K, Lavend'homme R, et al: Human liver sinusoidal endothelial cells but not hepatocytes contain factor VIII. *J Thromb Haemost* 12:36–42, 2014.

150. Pipe SW, Morris JA, Shah J, Kaufman RJ: Differential interaction of coagulation factor VIII and factor V with protein chaperones calnexin and calreticulin. *J Biol Chem* 273:8537–8544, 1998.

151. Swaroop M, Moussalli M, Pipe SW, Kaufman RJ: Mutagenesis of a potential immunoglobulin-binding protein-binding site enhances secretion of coagulation factor VIII. *J Biol Chem* 272:24121–24124, 1997.

152. Lenting PJ, Neels JG, van den Berg BM, et al: The light chain of factor VIII comprises a binding site for low density lipoprotein receptor-related protein. *J Biol Chem* 274:23734–23739, 1999.

153. Saenko EL, Yakhyaev AV, Mikhailenko I, et al: Role of the low density lipoprotein-related protein receptor in mediation of factor VIII catabolism. *J Biol Chem* 274:37685–37692, 1999.

154. Bovenschen N, Rijken DC, Havekes LM, et al: The B domain of coagulation factor VIII interacts with the asialoglycoprotein receptor. *J Thromb Haemost* 3:1257–1265, 2005.

155. Bovenschen N, Mertens K, Hu L, et al: LDL receptor cooperates with LDL receptor-related protein in regulating plasma levels of coagulation factor VIII in vivo. *Blood* 106:906–912, 2005.

156. Pegon JN, Kurdi M, Casari C, et al: Factor VIII and von Willebrand factor are ligands for the carbohydrate-receptor Siglec-5. *Haematologica* 97:1855–1863, 2012.

157. Leyte A, Verbeet MP, Brodniewicz-Proba T, et al: The interaction between human blood-coagulation factor VIII and von Willebrand factor. Characterization of a high-affinity binding site on factor VIII. *Biochem J* 257:679–683, 1989.

158. Saenko EL, Scandella D: The acidic region of the factor VIII light chain and the C2 domain together form the high affinity binding site for von Willebrand factor. *J Biol Chem* 272:18007–18014, 1997.

159. Gilbert GE, Kaufman RJ, Arena AA, et al: Four hydrophobic amino acids of the factor VIII C2 domain are constituents of both the membrane-binding and von Willebrand factor-binding motifs. *J Biol Chem* 277:6374–6381, 2002.

160. Meems H, Meijer A, Cullinan D, et al: Factor VIII C1 domain residues Lys 2092 and Phe 2093 contribute to membrane binding and cofactor activity. *Blood* 114:3938–3947, 2009.

161. Bloem E, van den Biggelaar M, Wroblewska A, et al: Factor VIII C1 domain spikes 2092–2093 and 2158–2159 comprise regions that modulate cofactor function and cellular uptake. *J Biol Chem* 288:29670–29679, 2013.

162. Cunningham MA, Pipe SW, Zhang B, et al: LMAN1 is a molecular chaperone for the secretion of coagulation factor VIII. *J Thromb Haemost* 1:2360–2367, 2003.

163. Michnick DA, Pittman DD, Wise RJ, Kaufman RJ: Identification of individual tyrosine sulfation sites within factor VIII required for optimal activity and efficient thrombin cleavage. *J Biol Chem* 269:20095–20102, 1994.

164. Vehar GA, Keyt B, Eaton D, et al: Structure of human factor VIII. *Nature* 312:337–342, 1983.

165. Eaton D, Rodriguez H, Vehar GA: Proteolytic processing of human factor VIII. Correlation of specific cleavages by thrombin, factor Xa, and activated protein C with activation and inactivation of factor VIII coagulant activity. *Biochemistry* 25:505–512, 1986.

166. Newell JL, Fay PJ: Proteolysis at Arg740 facilitates subsequent bond cleavages during thrombin-catalyzed activation of factor VIII. *J Biol Chem* 282:25367–25375, 2007.

167. Fay PJ, Haidaris PJ, Smudzin TM: Human factor VIIIa subunit structure. Reconstruction of factor VIIIa from the isolated A1/A3-C1-C2 dimer and A2 subunit. *J Biol Chem* 266:8957–8962, 1991.

168. Lollar P, Parker ET: Structural basis for the decreased procoagulant activity of human factor VIII compared to the porcine homolog. *J Biol Chem* 266:12481–12486, 1991.

169. Fay PJ: Activation of factor VIII and mechanisms of cofactor action. *Blood Rev* 18:1–15, 2004.

170. Gitschier J, Wood WI, Goralka TM, et al: Characterization of the human factor VIII gene. *Nature* 312:326–330, 1984.

171. Kamphuisen PW, Eikenboom JC, Rosendaal FR, et al: High factor VIII antigen levels increase the risk of venous thrombosis but are not associated with polymorphisms in the von Willebrand factor and factor VIII gene. *Br J Haematol* 115:156–158, 2001.

172. Preston AE, Barr A: The plasma concentration of factor VIII in the normal population. II. The effects of age, sex and blood group. *Br J Haematol* 10:238–245, 1964.

173. Morelli VM, De Visser MC, Vos HL, et al: ABO blood group genotypes and the risk of venous thrombosis: Effect of factor V Leiden. *J Thromb Haemost* 3:183–185, 2005.

174. Fair DS, Marlar RA: Biosynthesis and secretion of factor VII, protein C, protein S, and the protein C inhibitor from a human hepatoma cell line. *Blood* 67:64–70, 1986.

175. Fair DS, Marlar RA, Levin EG: Human endothelial cells synthesize protein S. *Blood* 67:1168–1171, 1986.

176. Ogura M, Tanabe N, Nishioka J, et al: Biosynthesis and secretion of functional protein S by a human megakaryoblastic cell line (MEG-01). *Blood* 70:301–306, 1987.

177. Dahlbäck B: Protein S and C4b-binding protein: Components involved in the regulation of the protein C anticoagulant system. *Thromb Haemost* 66:49–61, 1991.

178. Maillard C, Berruyer M, Serre CM, et al: Protein-S, a vitamin K-dependent protein, is a bone matrix component synthesized and secreted by osteoblasts. *Endocrinology* 130:1599–1604, 1992.

179. Walker FJ: Regulation of activated protein C by a new protein. A possible function for bovine protein S. *J Biol Chem* 255:5521–5524, 1980.

180. van de Poel RH, Meijers JC, Bouma BN: C4b-binding protein inhibits the factor V-dependent but not the factor V-independent cofactor activity of protein S in the activated protein C-mediated inactivation of factor VIIIa. *Thromb Haemost* 85:761–765, 2001.

181. Yegneswaran S, Wood GM, Esmon CT, Johnson AE: Protein S alters the active site location of activated protein C above the membrane surface. A fluorescence resonance energy transfer study of topography. *J Biol Chem* 272:25013–25021, 1997.

182. Rosing J, Hoekema L, Nicolaes GA, et al: Effects of protein S and factor Xa on peptide bond cleavages during inactivation of factor Va and factor VaR506Q by activated protein C. *J Biol Chem* 270:27852–27858, 1995.

183. Maurissen LF, Thomassen MC, Nicolaes GA, et al: Re-evaluation of the role of the protein S-C4b binding protein complex in activated protein C-catalyzed factor Va-inactivation. *Blood* 111:3034–3041, 2008.

184. Dahlback B: The tale of protein S and C4b-binding protein, a story of affection. *Thromb Haemost* 98:90–96, 2007.

185. Reglińska-Matveyev N, Andersson H, Rezende S, et al: TFPI cofactor function of protein S: Essential role of the protein S SHBG-like domain. *Blood* 123:3979–3988, 2014.

186. Suleiman L, Négrier C, Boukerche H: Protein S: A multifunctional anticoagulant vitamin K-dependent protein at the crossroads of coagulation, inflammation, angiogenesis, and cancer. *Crit Rev Oncol Hematol* 88:637–654, 2013.

187. van der Meer JH, van der Poll T, van 't Veer C: TAM receptors, Gas6, and protein S: Roles in inflammation and hemostasis. *Blood* 123:2460–2470, 2014.

188. Ploos van Amstel HK, Reitsma PH, van der Logt CP, Bertina RM: Intron-exon organization of the active human protein S gene PS alpha and its pseudogene PS beta: Duplication and silencing during primate evolution. *Biochemistry* 29:7853–7861, 1990.

189. Gómez E, Ledford MR, Pegelow CH, et al: Homozygous protein S deficiency due to a one base pair deletion that leads to a stop codon in exon III of the protein S gene. *Thromb Haemost* 71:723–726, 1994.

190. Marlar RA, Gausman JN: Protein S abnormalities: A diagnostic nightmare. *Am J Hematol* 86:418–421, 2011.

191. Pintao MC, Garcia AA, Borgel D, et al: Gross deletions/duplications in PROS1 are relatively common in point mutation-negative hereditary protein S deficiency. *Hum Genet* 126:449–456, 2009.

192. Pintao MC, Ribeiro DD, Bezemer ID, et al: Protein S levels and the risk of venous thrombosis: Results from the MEGA case-control study. *Blood* 122:3210–3219, 2013.

193. Giblin JP, Hewlett LJ, Hannah MJ: Basal secretion of von Willebrand factor from human endothelial cells. *Blood* 112:957–964, 2008.

194. van Schooten CJ, Shahbazi S, Groot E, et al: Macrophages contribute to the cellular uptake of von Willebrand factor and factor VIII *in vivo*. *Blood* 112:1704–1712, 2008.

195. Furlan M, Robles R, Lammle B: Partial purification and characterization of a protease from human plasma cleaving von Willebrand factor to fragments produced by *in vivo* proteolysis. *Blood* 87:4223–4234, 1996.

196. Bonthron DT, Handin RI, Kaufman RJ, et al: Structure of pre-pro-von Willebrand factor and its expression in heterologous cells. *Nature* 324:270–273, 1986.

197. Huizinga EG, Tsuji S, Romijn RA, et al: Structures of glycoprotein Ibalpha and its complex with von Willebrand factor A1 domain. *Science* 297:1176–1179, 2002.

198. Foster PA, Fulcher CA, Marti T, et al: A major factor VIII binding domain resides within the amino-terminal 272 amino acid residues of von Willebrand factor. *J Biol Chem* 262:8443–8446, 1987.

199. Mancuso DJ, Tuley EA, Westfield LA, et al: Human von Willebrand factor gene and pseudogene: Structural analysis and differentiation by polymerase chain reaction. *Biochemistry* 30:253–269, 1991.

200. Smith NL, Chen MH, Dehghan A, et al: Novel associations of multiple genetic loci with plasma levels of factor VII, factor VIII, and von Willebrand factor: The CHARGE (Cohorts for Heart and Aging Research in Genome Epidemiology) Consortium. *Circulation* 121:1382–1392, 2010.

201. Smith NL, Rice KM, Bovill EG, et al: Genetic variation associated with plasma von Willebrand factor levels and the risk of incident venous thrombosis. *Blood* 117:6007–6011, 2011.

202. Aggeler PM, White SG, Glendening MB, et al: Plasma thromboplastin component (PTC) deficiency; a new disease resembling hemophilia. *Proc Soc Exp Biol Med* 79:692–694, 1952.

203. Rosenthal RL, Dreskin OH, Rosenthal N: New hemophilia-like disease caused by deficiency of a third plasma thromboplastin factor. *Proc Soc Exp Biol Med* 82:171–174, 1953.

204. Thompson RE, Mandle R, Kaplan AP: Association of factor XI and high molecular weight kininogen in human plasma. *J Clin Invest* 60:1376–1380, 1977.

205. Kurachi K, Fujikawa K, Davie EW: Mechanism of activation of bovine factor XI by factor XII and factor XIIa. *Biochemistry* 19:1330–1338, 1980.

206. Emsley J, McEwan PA, Gailani D: Structure and function of factor XI. *Blood* 115:2569–2577, 2010.

207. Papagrigoriou E, McEwan PA, Walsh PN, Emsley J: Crystal structure of the factor XI zymogen reveals a pathway for transactivation. *Nat Struct Mol Biol* 13:557–558, 2006.

208. Bouma B, Griffin JH: Human blood coagulation factor XI. Purification, properties, and mechanism of activation by activated factor XII. *J Biol Chem* 252:6432, 1977.

209. Naito K, Fujikawa K: Activation of human blood coagulation factor XI independent of factor XII. Factor XI is activated by thrombin and factor XIa in the presence of negatively charged surfaces. *J Biol Chem* 266:7353–7358, 1991.

210. Geng Y, Verhamme I, Smith S: The dimeric structure of factor XI and zymogen activation. *Blood* 121:3962–3970, 2013.

211. Smith SB, Verhamme IM, Sun M-F, et al: Characterization of novel forms of coagulation factor XIa: Independence of factor XIa subunits in factor IX activation. *J Biol Chem* 283:6696–6705, 2008.

212. Sun Y, Gailani D: Identification of a factor IX binding site on the third apple domain of activated factor XI. *J Biol Chem* 271:29023–29028, 1996.

213. Sinha D, Marcinkiewicz M, Navaneetham D, Walsh PN: Macromolecular substrate-binding exosites on both the heavy and light chains of factor XIa mediate the formation of the Michaelis complex required for factor IX-activation. *Biochemistry* 46:9830–9839, 2007.

214. Kravtsov DV, Matafonov A, Tucker EI, et al: Factor XI contributes to thrombin generation in the absence of factor XII. *Blood* 114:452, 2009.

215. Cheng Q, Tucker E, Pine M, et al: A role for factor XIIa–mediated factor XI activation in thrombus formation in vivo. *Blood* 116:3981–3990, 2010.

216. He R, Chen D, He S: Factor XI: Hemostasis, thrombosis, and antithrombosis. *Thromb Res* 129:541–550, 2012.

217. von dem Borne PA, Cox LM, Bouma BN: Factor XI enhances fibrin generation and inhibits fibrinolysis in a coagulation model initiated by surface-coated tissue factor. *Blood Coagul Fibrinolysis* 17:251–257, 2006.

218. von dem Borne PA, Meijers JC, Bouma BN: Feedback activation of factor XI by thrombin in plasma results in additional formation of thrombin that protects fibrin clots from fibrinolysis. *Blood* 86:3035–3042, 1995.

219. Baglia FA, Gailani D, López JA, Walsh PN: Identification of a binding site for glycoprotein Ibalpha in the Apple 3 domain of factor XI. *J Biol Chem* 279:45470–45476, 2004.

220. White-Adams TC, Berny MA, Tucker EI, et al: Identification of coagulation factor XI as a ligand for platelet apolipoprotein E receptor 2 (ApoER2). *Arterioscler Thromb Vasc Biol* 29:1602–1607, 2009.

221. Gailani D, Ho D, Sun MF, et al: Model for a factor IX activation complex on blood platelets: Dimeric conformation of factor XIa is essential. *Blood* 97:3117–3122, 2001.

222. Knauer DJ, Majumdar D, Fong PC, Knauer MF: SERPIN regulation of factor XIa. The novel observation that protease nexin 1 in the presence of heparin is a more potent inhibitor of factor XIa than C1 inhibitor. *J Biol Chem* 275:37340–37346, 2000.

223. Cronlund AL, Walsh PN: A low molecular weight platelet inhibitor of factor XIa: Purification, characterization, and possible role in blood coagulation. *Biochemistry* 31:1685–1694, 1992.

224. Ragni MV, Sinha D, Seaman F, et al: Comparison of bleeding tendency, factor XI coagulant activity, and factor XI antigen in 25 factor XI-deficient kindreds. *Blood* 65:719–724, 1985.

225. Asakai R, Chung DW, Davie EW, Seligsohn U: Factor XI deficiency in Ashkenazi Jews in Israel. *N Engl J Med* 325:153–158, 1991.

226. Meijers JC, Tekelenburg WL, Bouma BN, et al: High levels of coagulation factor XI as a risk factor for venous thrombosis. *N Engl J Med* 342:696–701, 2000.

227. Bezemer ID, Bare LA, Doggen CJ, et al: Gene variants associated with deep vein thrombosis. *JAMA* 299:1306–1314, 2008.

228. Maas C, Oschatz C, Renne T: The plasma contact system 2.0. *Semin Thromb Hemost* 37:375–381, 2011.

229. Ratnoff O, Colopy J: A familial hemorrhagic trait associated with a deficiency of a clot-promoting fraction of plasma. *J Clin Invest* 34:602–613, 1955.

230. McMullen BA, Fujikawa K: Amino acid sequence of the heavy chain of human alpha-factor XIIa (activated Hageman factor). *J Biol Chem* 260:5328–5341, 1985.

231. Harris RJ, Ling VT, Spellman W: O-linked fucose is present in the first epidermal growth factor domain of factor XII but not protein C. *J Biol Chem* 15:5102–5107, 1992.

232. Cochrane CG, Revak SD, Wuepper KD: Activation of Hageman factor in solid and fluid phases. A critical role of kallikrein. *J Exp Med* 138:1564–1583, 1973.

233. Samuel M, Pixley RA, Villanueva MA, et al: Human factor XII (Hageman factor) autoactivation by dextran sulfate. Circular dichroism, fluorescence, and ultraviolet difference spectroscopic studies. *J Biol Chem* 267:19691–19697, 1992.

234. Engel R, Brain CM, Paget J, et al: Single-chain factor XII exhibits activity when complexed to polyphosphate. *J Thromb Haemost* 12:1513–1522, 2014.

235. Ratnoff OD, Saito H: Amidolytic properties of single-chain activated Hageman factor. *Proc Natl Acad Sci U S A* 76:1461–1463, 1979.

236. Griffin JH: Role of surface in surface-dependent activation of Hageman factor (blood coagulation factor XII). *Proc Natl Acad Sci U S A* 75:1998–2002, 1978.

237. Clarke BJ, Côté HC, Cool DE, et al: Mapping of a putative surface-binding site of human coagulation factor XII. *J Biol Chem* 264:11497–11502, 1989.

238. Citarella F, Ravon DM, Pascucci B, et al: Structure/function analysis of human factor XII using recombinant deletion mutants. Evidence for an additional region involved in the binding to negatively charged surfaces. *Eur J Biochem* 238:240–249, 1996.

239. Citarella F, te Velthuis H, Helmer-Citterich M, Hack CE: Identification of a putative binding site for negatively charged surfaces in the fibronectin type II domain of human factor XII—An immunochemical and homology modeling approach. *Thromb Haemost* 84:1057–1065, 2000.

240. Beringer DX, Kroon-Batenburg LMJ. The structure of the FnI-EGF-like tandem domain of coagulation factor XII solved using SIRAS. *Acta Crystallogr Sect F Struct Biol Cryst Commun* 69:94–102, 2013.

241. Kannemeier C, Shibamiya A, Nakazawa F, et al: Extracellular RNA constitutes a natural procoagulant cofactor in blood coagulation. *Proc Natl Acad Sci U S A* 104:6388–6393, 2007.

242. van der Meijden PE, Munnix IC, Auger JM, et al: Dual role of collagen in factor XII–dependent thrombus formation. *Blood* 114:881–891, 2014.

243. Muller F, Mutch NJ, Schenk WA, et al: Platelet polyphosphates are proinflammatory and procoagulant mediators in vivo. *Cell* 139:1143–1156, 2009.

244. van der Meijden PE, van Schilfgaarde M, van Oerle R, et al: Platelet- and erythrocyte-derived microparticles trigger thrombin generation via factor XIIa. *J Thromb Haemost* 10:1355–1362, 2012.

245. Revak SD, Cochrane CG, Bouma BN, Griffin JH: Surface and fluid phase activities of two forms of activated Hageman factor produced during contact activation of plasma. *J Exp Med* 147:719–729, 1978.

246. Lämmle B, Wuillemin WA, Huber I, et al: Thromboembolism and bleeding tendency in congenital factor XII deficiency—A study on 74 subjects from 14 Swiss families. *Thromb Haemost* 65:117–121, 1991.

247. Renne T, Pozgajova M, Gruner S, et al: Defective thrombus formation in mice lacking coagulation factor XII. *J Exp Med* 202:271–281, 2005.

248. Matafonov A, Leung PY, Gailani AE, et al: Factor XII inhibition reduces thrombus formation in a primate thrombosis model. *Blood* 123:1739–1747, 2014.

249. Cichon S, Martin L, Hennies HC, et al: Increased activity of coagulation factor XII (Hageman factor) causes hereditary angioedema type III. *Am J Hum Genet* 79:1098–1104, 2006.

250. Cool DE, MacGillivray RT: Characterization of the human blood coagulation factor XII gene. Intron/exon gene organization and analysis of the 5′-flanking region. *J Biol Chem* 262:13662–13673, 1987.

251. Johnson CY, Tuite A, Morange PE, et al: The factor XII -4C>T variant and risk of common thrombotic disorders: A HuGE review and meta-analysis of evidence from observational studies. *Am J Epidemiol* 173:136–144, 2011.

252. Morrissey JH, Gregory SA, Mackman N, Edgington TS: Tissue factor regulation and gene organization. *Oxf Surv Eukaryot Genes* 6:67–84, 1989.

253. Hoffman M, Colina CM, McDonald AG, et al: Tissue factor around dermal vessels has bound factor VII in the absence of injury. *J Thromb Haemost* 5:1403–1408, 2007.

254. Banner DW, D'Arcy A, Chene C, et al: The crystal structure of the complex of blood coagulation factor VIIa with soluble tissue factor. *Nature* 380:41–46, 1996.

255. Versteeg HH, Heemskerk JW, Levi M, Reitsma PH: New fundamentals in hemostasis. *Physiol Rev* 93:327–358, 2013.

256. Dorfleutner A, Ruf W: Regulation of tissue factor cytoplasmic domain phosphorylation by palmitoylation. *Blood* 102:3998–4005, 2003.

257. van den Hengel LG, Kocaturk B, Reitsma PH, et al: Complete abolishment of coagulant activity in monomeric disulfide-deficient tissue factor. *Blood* 118:3446–3448, 2011.

258. Rehemtulla A, Ruf W, Edgington TS: The integrity of the cysteine 186-cysteine 209 bond of the second disulfide loop of tissue factor is required for binding of factor VII. *J Biol Chem* 266:10294–10299, 1991.

259. Bogdanov VY, Balasubramanian V, Hathcock J, et al: Alternatively spliced human tissue factor: A circulating, soluble, thrombogenic protein. *Nat Med* 9:458–462, 2003.

260. Szotowski B, Antoniak S, Poller W, et al: Procoagulant soluble tissue factor is released from endothelial cells in response to inflammatory cytokines. *Circ Res* 96:1233–1239, 2005.

261. Szotowski B, Goldin-Lang P, Antoniak S, et al: Alterations in myocardial tissue factor expression and cellular localization in dilated cardiomyopathy. *J Am Coll Cardiol* 45:1081–1089, 2005.

262. Goldin-Lang P, Tran QV, Fichtner I, et al: Tissue factor expression pattern in human non-small cell lung cancer tissues indicate increased blood thrombogenicity and tumor metastasis. *Oncol Rep* 20:123–128, 2008.

263. Luyendyk JP, Tilley RE, Mackman N: Genetic susceptibility to thrombosis. *Curr Atheroscler Rep* 8:193–197, 2006.

264. Esmon NL, Owen WG, Esmon CT: Isolation of a membrane-bound cofactor for thrombin-catalyzed activation of protein C. *J Biol Chem* 257:859–864, 1982.

265. Esmon CT, Owen WG: The discovery of thrombomodulin. *J Thromb Haemost* 2:209–213, 2004.

266. Conway EM: Thrombomodulin and its role in inflammation. *Semin Immunopathol* 34:107–125, 2012.

267. Light DR, Glaser CB, Betts M, et al: The interaction of thrombomodulin with Ca2+. *Eur J Biochem* 262:522–533, 1999.

268. Adams TE, Huntington JA: Thrombin-cofactor interactions: Structural insights into regulatory mechanisms. *Arterioscler Thromb Vasc Biol* 26:1738–1745, 2006.

269. Cadroy Y, Diquelou A, Dupouy D, et al: The thrombomodulin/protein C/protein S anticoagulant pathway modulates the thrombogenic properties of the normal resting and stimulated endothelium. *Arterioscler Thromb Vasc Biol* 17:520–527, 1997.

270. Laszik Z, Mitro A, Taylor FB Jr, et al: Human protein C receptor is present primarily on endothelium of large blood vessels: Implications for the control of the protein C pathway. *Circulation* 96:3633–3640, 1997.

271. Lafay M, Laguna R, Le Bonniec BF, et al: Thrombomodulin modulates the mitogenic response to thrombin of human umbilical vein endothelial cells. *Thromb Haemost* 79:848–852, 1998.

272. Van de Wouwer M, Conway EM: Novel functions of thrombomodulin in inflammation. *Crit Care Med* 32(Suppl 5):S254–S261, 2004.

273. Rezaie AR, Cooper ST, Church FC, Esmon CT: Protein C inhibitor is a potent inhibitor of the thrombin-thrombomodulin complex. *J Biol Chem* 270:25336–25339, 1995.

274. Martin FA, Murphy RP, Cummins PM: Thrombomodulin and the vascular endothelium: Insights into functional, regulatory, and therapeutic aspects. *Am J Physiol Heart Circ Physiol* 304:H1585–H1597, 2013.

275. Ohlin AK, Norlund L, Marlar RA: Thrombomodulin gene variations and thromboembolic disease. *Thromb Haemost* 78:396–400, 1997.

276. Tang L, Wang HF, Lu X, et al: Common genetic risk factors for venous thrombosis in the Chinese population. *Am J Hum Genet* 92:177–187, 2013.

277. Langdown J, Luddington RJ, Huntington JA, Baglin TP: A hereditary bleeding disorder resulting from a premature stop codon in thrombomodulin (p.Cys537Stop). *Blood* 124:1951–1956, 2014.

278. Delvaeye M, Noris M, De Vriese A, et al: Thrombomodulin mutations in atypical hemolytic-uremic syndrome. *N Engl J Med* 361:345–357, 2009.

279. Fukudome K, Esmon CT: Molecular cloning and expression of murine and bovine endothelial cell protein C/activated protein C receptor (EPCR). The structural and functional conservation in human, bovine, and murine EPCR. *J Biol Chem* 270:5571–5577, 1995.

280. Mosnier LO, Zlokovic BV, Griffin JH: The cytoprotective protein C pathway. *Blood* 109:3161–3172, 2007.

281. Mosnier LO, Sinha RK, Burnier L, et al: Biased agonism of protease-activated receptor 1 by activated protein C caused by noncanonical cleavage at Arg46. *Blood* 120:5237–5246, 2012.

282. Li W, Zheng X, Gu JM, , et al: Extraembryonic expression of EPCR is essential for embryonic viability. *Blood* 106:2716–2722, 2005.

283. Mohan Rao LV, Esmon CT, Pendurthi UR: Endothelial cell protein C receptor: A multiliganded and multifunctional receptor. *Blood* 124:1553–1562, 2014.

284. Wu C, Dwivedi DJ, Pepler L, et al: Targeted gene sequencing identifies variants in the protein C and endothelial protein C receptor genes in patients with unprovoked venous thromboembolism. *Arterioscler Thromb Vasc Biol* 33:2674–2681, 2013.

285. Collen D, Tytgat GN, Claeys H, Piessens R: Metabolism and distribution of fibrinogen. I. Fibrinogen turnover in physiological conditions in humans. *Br J Haematol* 22:681–700, 1972.

286. Handagama PJ, Shuman MA, Bainton DF: In vivo defibrination results in markedly decreased amounts of fibrinogen in rat megakaryocytes and platelets. *Am J Pathol* 137:1393–1399, 1990.

287. Louache F, Debili N, Cramer E, et al: Fibrinogen is not synthesized by human megakaryocytes. *Blood* 77:311–316, 1991.

288. Côté HC, Lord ST, Pratt KP: gamma-Chain dysfibrinogenemias: Molecular structure-function relationships of naturally occurring mutations in the gamma chain of human fibrinogen. *Blood* 92:2195–2212, 1998.

289. Henschen AH: Human fibrinogen—Structural variants and functional sites. *Thromb Haemost* 70:42–47, 1993.

290. Uitte de Willige S, de Visser MC, Houwing-Duistermaat JJ, et al: Genetic variation in the fibrinogen gamma gene increases the risk for deep venous thrombosis by reducing plasma fibrinogen gamma' levels. *Blood* 106:4176–4183, 2005.

291. Blomback B: Studies on fibrinogen: Its purification and conversion into fibrin. *Acta Physiol Scand Suppl* 43:1–51, 1958.

292. Olexa SA, Budzynski AZ: Evidence for four different polymerization sites involved in human fibrin formation. *Proc Natl Acad Sci U S A* 77:1374–1378, 1980.

293. Kaczmarek E, McDonagh J: Thrombin binding to the A alpha-, B beta-, and gamma-chains of fibrinogen and to their remnants contained in fragment E. *J Biol Chem* 263:13896–13900, 1988.

294. Weisel JW, Phillips GN Jr, Cohen C: The structure of fibrinogen and fibrin: II. Architecture of the fibrin clot. *Ann N Y Acad Sci* 408:367–379, 1983.

295. Hantgan R, Fowler W, Erickson H, Hermans J: Fibrin assembly: A comparison of electron microscopic and light scattering results. *Thromb Haemost* 44:119–124, 1980.

296. Marder VJ, Budzynski AZ: The structure of the fibrinogen degradation products. *Prog Hemost Thromb* 2:141–174, 1974.

297. Mosesson MW: Update on antithrombin I (fibrin). *Thromb Haemost* 98:105–108, 2007.

298. Komaromi I, Bagoly Z, Muszbek L: Factor XIII: Novel structural and functional aspects. *J Thromb Haemost* 9:9–20, 2011.

299. Souri M, Koseki-Kuno S, Takeda N, et al: Administration of factor XIII B subunit increased plasma factor XIII A subunit levels in factor XIII B subunit knock-out mice. *Int J Hematol* 87:60–68, 2008.

300. Muszbek L, Haramura G, Polgar J: Transformation of cellular factor XIII into an active zymogen transglutaminase in thrombin-stimulated platelets. *Thromb Haemost* 73:702–705, 1995.

301. Brummel KE, Paradis SG, Butenas S, Mann KG: Thrombin functions during tissue factor-induced blood coagulation. *Blood* 100:148–152, 2002.

302. Bagoly Z, Fazakas F, Komaromi I, et al: Cleavage of factor XIII by human neutrophil elastase results in a novel active truncated form of factor XIII A subunit. *Thromb Haemost* 99:668–674, 2008.

303. Smith KA, Pease RJ, Avery CA, et al: The activation peptide cleft exposed by thrombin cleavage of FXIII-A(2) contains a recognition site for the fibrinogen alpha chain. *Blood* 121:2117–2126, 2013.

304. Fraser SR, Booth NA, Mutch NJ: The antifibrinolytic function of factor XIII is exclusively expressed through alpha(2)-antiplasmin cross-linking. *Blood* 117:6371–6374, 2011.

305. Aleman MM, Byrnes JR, Wang JG, et al: Factor XIII activity mediates red blood cell retention in venous thrombi. *J Clin Invest* 124:3590–3600, 2014.

306. Hoppe B: Fibrinogen and factor XIII at the intersection of coagulation, fibrinolysis and inflammation. *Thromb Haemost* 112:649–658, 2014.

307. Kasahara K, Souri M, Kaneda M, et al: Impaired clot retraction in factor XIII A subunit-deficient mice. *Blood* 115:1277–1279, 2010.

308. Richardson VR, Cordell P, Standeven KF, Carter AM: Substrates of factor XIII-a: Roles in thrombosis and wound healing. *Clin Sci (Lond)* 124:123–137, 2013.

309. Kikuchi H, Kuribayashi F, Imajoh-Ohmi S: Down-regulation of Fas-mediated apoptosis by plasma transglutaminase factor XIII that catalyzes fetal-specific cross-link of the Fas molecule. *Biochem Biophys Res Commun* 443:13–17, 2014.

310. Mokuda S, Murata Y, Sawada N, et al: Tocilizumab induced acquired factor XIII deficiency in patients with rheumatoid arthritis. *PLoS One* 8:e69944, 2013.

311. Soendergaard C, Kvist PH, Seidelin JB, Nielsen OH: Tissue-regenerating functions of coagulation factor XIII. *J Thromb Haemost* 11:806–816, 2013.

312. Weisberg LJ, Shiu DT, Greenberg CS, et al: Localization of the gene for coagulation factor XIII a-chain to chromosome 6 and identification of sites of synthesis. *J Clin Invest* 79:649–652, 1987.

313. Bottenus RE, Ichinose A, Davie EW: Nucleotide sequence of the gene for the b subunit of human factor XIII. *Biochemistry* 29:11195–11209, 1990.

314. Muszbek L, Bagoly Z, Cairo A, Peyvandi F: Novel aspects of factor XIII deficiency. *Curr Opin Hematol* 18:366–372, 2011.

315. Ichinose A: Factor XIII is a key molecule at the intersection of coagulation and fibrinolysis as well as inflammation and infection control. *Int J Hematol* 95:362–370, 2012.

316. Shemirani AH, Antalfi B, Pongracz E, et al: Factor XIII-A subunit Val34Leu polymorphism in fatal atherothrombotic ischemic stroke. *Blood Coagul Fibrinolysis* 25:364–368, 2014.

317. Foley JH, Kim PY, Mutch NJ, Gils A: Insights into thrombin activatable fibrinolysis inhibitor function and regulation. *J Thromb Haemost* 11 Suppl 1:306–315, 2013.

318. van Tilburg NH, Rosendaal FR, Bertina RM: Thrombin activatable fibrinolysis inhibitor and the risk for deep vein thrombosis. *Blood* 95:2855–2859, 2000.

319. Seegers WH, Johnson JF, Fell C: An antithrombin reaction to prothrombin activation. *Am J Physiol* 176:97–103, 1954.

320. Huntington JA: Serpin structure, function and dysfunction. *J Thromb Haemost* 9 Suppl 1:26–34, 2011.

321. Olson ST, Swanson R, Raub-Segall E, et al: Accelerating ability of synthetic oligosaccharides on antithrombin inhibition of proteinases of the clotting and fibrinolytic systems. Comparison with heparin and low-molecular-weight heparin. *Thromb Haemost* 92:929–939, 2004.

322. Olson ST, Bjork I: Predominant contribution of surface approximation to the mechanism of heparin acceleration of the antithrombin-thrombin reaction. Elucidation from salt concentration effects. *J Biol Chem* 266:6353–6364, 1991.

323. Li W, Johnson DJ, Esmon CT, Huntington JA: Structure of the antithrombin-thrombin-heparin ternary complex reveals the antithrombotic mechanism of heparin. *Nat Struct Mol Biol* 11:857–862, 2004.

324. Pizzo SV: Serpin receptor 1: A hepatic receptor that mediates the clearance of antithrombin III-proteinase complexes. *Am J Med* 87(3B):10S–14S, 1989.

325. Kounnas MZ, Church FC, Argraves WS, Strickland DK: Cellular internalization and degradation of antithrombin III-thrombin, heparin cofactor II-thrombin, and alpha 1-antitrypsin-trypsin complexes is mediated by the low density lipoprotein receptor-related protein. *J Biol Chem* 271:6523–6529, 1996.

326. Tait RC, Walker ID, Perry DJ, et al: Prevalence of antithrombin deficiency in the healthy population. *Br J Haematol* 87:106–112, 1994.

327. Harper PL, Luddington RJ, Daly M, et al: The incidence of dysfunctional antithrombin variants: Four cases in 210 patients with thromboembolic disease. *Br J Haematol* 77:360–364, 1991.

328. Lane DA, Bayston T, Olds RJ, et al: Antithrombin mutation database: 2nd (1997) update. For the Plasma Coagulation Inhibitors Subcommittee of the Scientific and Standardization Committee of the International Society on Thrombosis and Haemostasis. *Thromb Haemost* 77:197–211, 1997.

329. Broze GJ Jr, Miletich JP: Isolation of the tissue factor inhibitor produced by HepG2 hepatoma cells. *Proc Natl Acad Sci U S A* 84:1886–1890, 1987.

330. Novotny WF, Girard TJ, Miletich JP, Broze GJ Jr: Purification and characterization of the lipoprotein-associated coagulation inhibitor from human plasma. *J Biol Chem* 264:18832–18837, 1989.

331. Girard TJ, Warren LA, Novotny WF, et al: Functional significance of the Kunitz-type inhibitory domains of lipoprotein-associated coagulation inhibitor. *Nature* 338:518–520, 1989.

332. Wood JP, Ellery PE, Maroney SA, Mast AE: Biology of tissue factor pathway inhibitor. *Blood* 123:2934–2943, 2014.

333. Hackeng TM, Sere KM, Tans G, Rosing J: Protein S stimulates inhibition of the tissue factor pathway by tissue factor pathway inhibitor. *Proc Natl Acad Sci U S A* 103:3106–3111, 2006.

334. Ndonwi M, Tuley EA, Broze GJ Jr: The Kunitz-3 domain of TFPI-alpha is required for protein S-dependent enhancement of factor Xa inhibition. *Blood* 116:1344–1351, 2010.

335. Wood JP, Bunce MW, Maroney SA, et al: Tissue factor pathway inhibitor-alpha inhibits prothrombinase during the initiation of blood coagulation. *Proc Natl Acad Sci U S A* 110:17838–17843, 2013.

336. Dahm A, Van Hylckama Vlieg A, Bendz B, et al: Low levels of tissue factor pathway inhibitor (TFPI) increase the risk of venous thrombosis. *Blood* 101:4387–4392, 2003.

337. Castoldi E, Simioni P, Tormene D, et al: Hereditary and acquired protein S deficiencies are associated with low TFPI levels in plasma. *J Thromb Haemost* 8:294–300, 2010.

338. Massberg S, Grahl L, von Bruehl ML, et al: Reciprocal coupling of coagulation and innate immunity via neutrophil serine proteases. *Nat Med* 16:887–896, 2010.

339. Sandset PM, Warn-Cramer BJ, Rao LV, et al: Depletion of extrinsic pathway inhibitor (EPI) sensitizes rabbits to disseminated intravascular coagulation induced with tissue factor: Evidence supporting a physiologic role for EPI as a natural anticoagulant. *Proc Natl Acad Sci U S A* 88:708–712, 1991.

340. Huang ZF, Higuchi D, Lasky N, Broze GJ Jr: Tissue factor pathway inhibitor gene disruption produces intrauterine lethality in mice. *Blood* 90:944–951, 1997.

341. Ameziane N, Seguin C, Borgel D, et al: The -33T—>C polymorphism in intron 7 of the TFPI gene influences the risk of venous thromboembolism, independently of the factor V Leiden and prothrombin mutations. *Thromb Haemost* 88:195–199, 2002.

342. Opstad TB, Eilertsen AL, Hoibraaten E, et al: Tissue factor pathway inhibitor polymorphisms in women with and without a history of venous thrombosis and the effects of postmenopausal hormone therapy. *Blood Coagul Fibrinolysis* 21:516–521, 2010.

343. Han X, Fiehler R, Broze GJ Jr: Isolation of a protein Z-dependent plasma protease inhibitor. *Proc Natl Acad Sci U S A* 95:9250–9255, 1998.

344. Tabatabai A, Fiehler R, Broze GJ Jr: Protein Z circulates in plasma in a complex with protein Z-dependent protease inhibitor. *Thromb Haemost* 85:655–660, 2001.

345. Han X, Huang ZF, Fiehler R, Broze GJ Jr: The protein Z-dependent protease inhibitor is a serpin. *Biochemistry* 38:11073–11078, 1999.

346. Sejima H, Hayashi T, Deyashiki Y, et al: Primary structure of vitamin K-dependent human protein Z. *Biochem Biophys Res Commun* 171:661–668, 1990.

347. Huang X, Yan Y, Tu Y, et al: Structural basis for catalytic activation of protein Z-dependent protease inhibitor (ZPI) by protein Z. *Blood* 120:1726–1733, 2012.

348. Zhang J, Tu Y, Lu L, et al: Protein Z-dependent protease inhibitor deficiency produces a more severe murine phenotype than protein Z deficiency. *Blood* 111:4973–4978, 2008.

349. Al-Shanqeeti A, van Hylckama Vlieg A, Berntorp E, et al: Protein Z and protein Z-dependent protease inhibitor. Determinants of levels and risk of venous thrombosis. *Thromb Haemost* 93:411–413, 2005.

350. Almawi WY, Al-Shaikh FS, Melemedjian OK, Almawi AW: Protein Z, an anticoagulant protein with expanding role in reproductive biology. *Reproduction* 146:R73–R80, 2013.

351. Van de Water N, Tan T, Ashton F, et al: Mutations within the protein Z-dependent protease inhibitor gene are associated with venous thromboembolic disease: A new form of thrombophilia. *Br J Haematol* 127:190–194, 2004.

352. Young LK, Birch NP, Browett PJ, et al: Two missense mutations identified in venous thrombosis patients impair the inhibitory function of the protein Z dependent protease inhibitor. *Thromb Haemost* 107:854–863, 2012.

353. McQuillan AM, Eikelboom JW, Hankey GJ, et al: Protein Z in ischemic stroke and its etiologic subtypes. *Stroke* 34:2415–2419, 2003.

354. Dossenbach-Glaninger A, van Trotsenburg M, Helmer H, et al: Association of the protein Z intron F G79A gene polymorphism with recurrent pregnancy loss. *Fertil Steril* 90:1155–1160, 2008.

355. Grandone E, Colaizzo D, Cappucci F, et al: Protein Z levels and unexplained fetal losses. *Fertil Steril* 82:982–983, 2004.

356. Macfarlane RG: An enzyme cascade in the blood clotting mechanism, and its function as a biochemical amplifier. *Nature* 202:498–499, 1964.

357. Davie EW, Ratnoff OD: Waterfall sequence for intrinsic blood clotting. *Science* 145:1310–1312, 1964.

358. Pitlick FA, Nemerson Y: Purification and characterization of tissue factor apoprotein. *Methods Enzymol* 45:37–48, 1976.

359. Mackman N, Morrissey JH, Fowler B, Edgington TS: Complete sequence of the human tissue factor gene, a highly regulated cellular receptor that initiates the coagulation protease cascade. *Biochemistry* 28:1755–1762, 1989.

360. Osterud B, Rapaport SI: Activation of factor IX by the reaction product of tissue factor and factor VII: Additional pathway for initiating blood coagulation. *Proc Natl Acad Sci U S A* 74:5260–5264, 1977.

361. Repke D, Gemmell CH, Guha A, et al: Hemophilia as a defect of the tissue factor pathway of blood coagulation: Effect of factors VIII and IX on factor X activation in a continuous-flow reactor. *Proc Natl Acad Sci U S A* 87:7623–7627, 1990.

362. van 't Veer C, Hackeng TM, Delahaye C, et al: Activated factor X and thrombin formation triggered by tissue factor on endothelial cell matrix in a flow model: Effect of the tissue factor pathway inhibitor. *Blood* 84:1132–1142, 1994.

363. van 't Veer C, Mann KG: Regulation of tissue factor initiated thrombin generation by the stoichiometric inhibitors tissue factor pathway inhibitor, antithrombin-III, and heparin cofactor-II. *J Biol Chem* 272:4367–4377, 1997.

364. Hilden I, Lauritzen B, Sorensen BB, et al: Hemostatic effect of a monoclonal antibody mAb 2021 blocking the interaction between FXa and TFPI in a rabbit hemophilia model. *Blood* 119:5871–5878, 2012.

365. Carmeliet P, Mackman N, Moons L, et al: Role of tissue factor in embryonic blood vessel development. *Nature* 383:73–75, 1996.

366. Gailani D, Broze GJ Jr: Factor XI activation in a revised model of blood coagulation. *Science* 253:909–912, 1991.

367. Nemerson Y: The tissue factor pathway of blood coagulation. *Semin Hematol* 29:170–176, 1992.

368. Esmon CT: The protein C pathway. *Chest* 124(Suppl 3):26S–32S, 2003.

369. Holmer E, Kurachi K, Soderstrom G: The molecular-weight dependence of the rate-enhancing effect of heparin on the inhibition of thrombin, factor Xa, factor IXa, factor XIa, factor XIIa and kallikrein by antithrombin. *Biochem J* 193:395–400, 1981.

370. Brummel-Ziedins KE, Everse SJ, Mann KG, Orfeo T: Modeling thrombin generation: Plasma composition based approach. *J Thromb Thrombolysis* 37:32–44, 2014.

371. Monroe DM, Hoffman M, Roberts HR: Platelets and thrombin generation. *Arterioscler Thromb Vasc Biol* 22:1381–1389, 2002.

372. Cawthern KM, van 't Veer C, Lock JB, et al: Blood coagulation in hemophilia A and hemophilia C. *Blood* 91:4581–4592, 1998.

373. Monroe DM, Roberts HR, Hoffman M: Platelet procoagulant complex assembly in a tissue factor-initiated system. *Br J Haematol* 88:364–371, 1994.

374. Schuijt TJ, Bakhtiari K, Daffre S, et al: Factor Xa activation of factor V is of paramount importance in initiating the coagulation system: Lessons from a tick salivary protein. *Circulation* 128:254–266, 2013.

375. Allen DH, Tracy PB: Human coagulation factor V is activated to the functional cofactor by elastase and cathepsin G expressed at the monocyte surface. *J Biol Chem* 270:1408–1415, 1995.

376. Williamson P, Bevers EM, Smeets EF, et al: Continuous analysis of the mechanism of activated transbilayer lipid movement in platelets. *Biochemistry* 34:10448–10455, 1995.

377. Yang X, Walsh PN: An ordered sequential mechanism for factor IX and factor IXa binding to platelet receptors in the assembly of the Factor X-activating complex. *Biochem J* 390(Pt 1):157–167, 2005.

378. White-Adams TC, Berny MA, Tucker EI, et al: Identification of coagulation factor XI as a ligand for platelet apolipoprotein E receptor 2 (ApoER2). *Arterioscler Thromb Vasc Biol* 29:1602–1607, 2009.

379. Choi SH, Smith SA, Morrissey JH: Polyphosphate is a cofactor for the activation of factor XI by thrombin. *Blood* 118:6963–6970, 2011.

380. von dem Borne PA, Bajzar L, Meijers JC, et al: Thrombin-mediated activation of factor XI results in a thrombin-activatable fibrinolysis inhibitor-dependent inhibition of fibrinolysis. *J Clin Invest* 99:2323–2327, 1997.

381. Mackman N: Tissue-specific hemostasis in mice. *Arterioscler Thromb Vasc Biol* 25:2273–2281, 2005.

382. Kenne E, Renne T: Factor XII: A drug target for safe interference with thrombosis and inflammation. *Drug Discov Today* 19:1459–1464, 2014.

383. Buller HR, Bethune C, Bhanot S, et al: Factor XI antisense oligonucleotide for prevention of venous thrombosis. *N Engl J Med* 372:232–240, 2015.

384. Engelmann B, Massberg S: Thrombosis as an intravascular effector of innate immunity. *Nat Rev Immunol* 13:34–45, 2013.

385. von Bruhl ML, Stark K, Steinhart A, et al: Monocytes, neutrophils, and platelets cooperate to initiate and propagate venous thrombosis in mice *in vivo. J Exp Med* 209:819–835, 2012.

386. Broze GJ Jr: Binding of human factor VII and VIIa to monocytes. *J Clin Invest* 70:526–535, 1982.

387. Clark SR, Ma AC, Tavener SA, et al: Platelet TLR4 activates neutrophil extracellular traps to ensnare bacteria in septic blood. *Nat Med* 13:463–469, 2007.

388. Wang Y, Li M, Stadler S, et al: Histone hypercitrullination mediates chromatin decondensation and neutrophil extracellular trap formation. *J Cell Biol* 184:205–213, 2009.

389. Semeraro F, Ammollo CT, Morrissey JH, et al: Extracellular histones promote thrombin generation through platelet-dependent mechanisms: Involvement of platelet TLR2 and TLR4. *Blood* 118:1952–1961, 2011.

390. Martinod K, Demers M, Fuchs TA, et al: Neutrophil histone modification by peptidylarginine deiminase 4 is critical for deep vein thrombosis in mice. *Proc Natl Acad Sci U S A* 110:8674–8679, 2013.

391. Savchenko AS, Martinod K, Seidman MA, et al: Neutrophil extracellular traps form predominantly during the organizing stage of human venous thromboembolism development. *J Thromb Haemost* 12:860–870, 2014.

392. Hanson SR, Griffin JH, Harker LA, et al: Antithrombotic effects of thrombin-induced activation of endogenous protein C in primates. *J Clin Invest* 92:2003–2012, 1993.

393. de Agostini AI, Watkins SC, Slayter HS, et al: Localization of anticoagulantly active heparan sulfate proteoglycans in vascular endothelium: Antithrombin binding on cultured endothelial cells and perfused rat aorta. *J Cell Biol* 111:1293–1304, 1990.

394. Marcus AJ, Broekman MJ, Drosopoulos JH, et al: The endothelial cell ecto-ADPase responsible for inhibition of platelet function is CD39. *J Clin Invest* 99:1351–1360, 1997.

395. van 't Veer C, Golden NJ, Kalafatis M, Mann KG: Inhibitory mechanism of the protein C pathway on tissue factor-induced thrombin generation. Synergistic effect in combination with tissue factor pathway inhibitor. *J Biol Chem* 272:7983–7994, 1997.

396. Jesty J, Beltrami E: Positive feedbacks of coagulation: Their role in threshold regulation. *Arterioscler Thromb Vasc Biol* 25:2463–2469, 2005.

397. Brakman P, Albrechtsen OK, Astrup T: A comparative study of coagulation and fibrinolysis in blood from normal men and women. *Br J Haematol* 12:74–85, 1966.

398. Nossel HL, Yudelman I, Canfield RE, et al: Measurement of fibrinopeptide A in human blood. *J Clin Invest* 54:43–53, 1974.

399. Bauer KA, Kass BL, ten Cate H, et al: Detection of factor X activation in humans. *Blood* 74:2007–2015, 1989.

400. Bauer KA, Kass BL, ten Cate H, et al: Factor IX is activated in vivo by the tissue factor mechanism. *Blood* 76:731–736, 1990.

401. Morrissey JH: Tissue factor modulation of factor VIIa activity: Use in measuring trace levels of factor VIIa in plasma. *Thromb Haemost* 74:185–188, 1995.

402. Conard J, Bauer KA, Gruber A, et al: Normalization of markers of coagulation activation with a purified protein C concentrate in adults with homozygous protein C deficiency. *Blood* 82:1159–1164, 1993.

CHAPTER 114
CONTROL OF COAGULATION REACTIONS

Laurent O. Mosnier and John H. Griffin

SUMMARY

The blood coagulation system, like a powerful idling engine, is always active and generating thrombin at very low levels, poised for explosive thrombin generation. Positive feedback activation of factors V, VII, VIII, and XI imparts special threshold properties to blood coagulation, making the coagulant response nonlinearly responsive to stimuli. Overt blood coagulation represents a threshold system with apparent all-or-none responses to various levels of stimuli, and an ensemble of opposing reactions determines the ultimate upregulation and downregulation of thrombin generation both locally and systemically. Cellular and humoral anticoagulant mechanisms synergize with plasma coagulation inhibitors to prevent massive thrombin generation in the absence of a substantial procoagulant stimulus. This chapter highlights mechanisms that inhibit blood coagulation, with an emphasis on defects of plasma proteins that cause hereditary thrombophilias. Major thrombophilic defects involve the anticoagulant protein C pathway, comprising multiple cofactors or effectors that additionally include thrombomodulin, endothelial protein C receptor, protein S, high-density lipoprotein, and factor V. Activated protein C exerts multiple protective homeostatic actions, including proteolytic inactivation of factors Va and VIIIa, as well as direct cell-signaling activities involving protease activated receptors 1 and 3, endothelial cell protein C receptor, integrin CD11b/CD18, and apolipoprotein E receptor 2. The factor V Leiden variant causes hereditary activated protein C resistance by impairing the ability of the protein C pathway to inhibit coagulation because it cannot properly cleave factor Va Leiden. Plasma protease inhibitors are also key to block coagulation. Antithrombin inhibits thrombin and factors Xa, IXa, XIa, and XIIa, in reactions stimulated by physiologic heparan sulfate or pharmacologic heparins. Tissue factor pathway inhibitor neutralizes the extrinsic coagulation pathway factors VIIa and Xa. Other plasma protease inhibitors can also neutralize various coagulation proteases.

Control of coagulation reactions is essential for normal hemostasis. As part of the tangled web of host defense systems that respond to vascular injury, the blood coagulation factors (Chap. 113) act in concert with the endothelium and blood cells, especially platelets, to generate a protective fibrin-platelet clot, forming a hemostatic plug. Pathologic thrombosis occurs when the protective

clot is extended beyond its beneficial size, when a clot occurs inappropriately at sites of vascular disease, or when a clot embolizes to other sites in the circulatory bed. For normal hemostasis, both procoagulant and anticoagulant factors must interact with the vascular components and cell surfaces, including the vessel wall (Chap. 115) and platelets (Chap. 112). Moreover, the action of the fibrinolytic system must be integrated with coagulation reactions for timely formation and dissolution of blood clots (Chap. 135). This chapter on control of coagulation highlights the major physiologic mechanisms for downregulation of blood coagulation reactions and the plasma proteins that inhibit blood coagulation, with an emphasis on those mechanisms whose defects are clinically significant based on insights gleaned from consideration of the hereditary thrombophilias (Chap. 130). Chapter 113 provides a complete description of blood coagulation factors and hemostatic pathways.

● BLOOD COAGULATION PATHWAYS AND THE PROTEIN C PATHWAYS

Although decades have elapsed since the elaboration of the cascade model[1,2] for blood coagulation (see Chap. 113, Fig. 113–27), the basic outline of sequential conversions of protease zymogens to active serine proteases is still useful, albeit with important modifications (see Chap. 113, Fig. 113–28), to represent blood coagulation reactions. The major conceptual advances for procoagulant pathways in the past two decades emphasize both positive and negative feedback reactions affecting thrombin generation as depicted in Fig. 114–1.

In positive feedback reactions, procoagulant thrombin activates platelets and factors V, VIII, and XI (Chap. 113).[3–5] Small amounts of thrombin can be generated by trace amounts of tissue factor via the extrinsic pathway. Subsequently, thrombin can activate factors XI, VIII, and V, thereby stimulating each of the steps in the intrinsic pathway, thereby amplifying thrombin generation (see Fig. 114–1).

In negative feedback reactions, anticoagulant activated protein C (APC) that is generated on endothelial cell surfaces[6–8] (Fig. 114–2) downregulates coagulation (see Figs. 114–1 and 114–3). Furthermore, APC can exert direct cytoprotective effects on cells via reactions that involve certain receptors, including endothelial cell protein C receptor (EPCR) and protease-activated receptor-1 (PAR-1) (Fig. 114–4), PAR-3, integrin CD11b/CD18, and possibly apolipoprotein E receptor 2 (apoER2).[7,8] APC's cytoprotective effects include antiinflammatory and antiapoptotic activities, as well as alterations of gene-expression profiles and stabilization of endothelial barriers (see "Activated Protein C Activities" below). Because inflammation, apoptosis, and vascular barrier breakdown contribute significantly to reactions that promote thrombin generation, such direct cytoprotective effects of APC on cells indirectly downregulate thrombin generation.[7,8]

For APC generation by the protein C cellular pathway, binding of thrombin to thrombomodulin converts the bound thrombin from a procoagulant enzyme to an anticoagulant enzyme that converts the protein C zymogen to an anticoagulant serine protease, APC (see Figs. 114–1 and 114–2). This surface-dependent reaction is enhanced by the EPCR that binds protein C.[6,9,10] With the aid of its nonenzymatic cofactor, protein S, as well as other potential lipid and protein cofactors, APC inactivates factors Va and VIIIa by highly selective proteolysis, yielding inactive (i) cofactors, that is, factors V_i and VIII$_i$ (see Fig. 114–3 and Chap. 113, Figs. 113–11 and 113–13). Protein S also can directly inhibit factors VIIIa, Xa, and Va.[11–13] Thus, APC and protein S inhibit multiple steps in the intrinsic coagulation pathway.

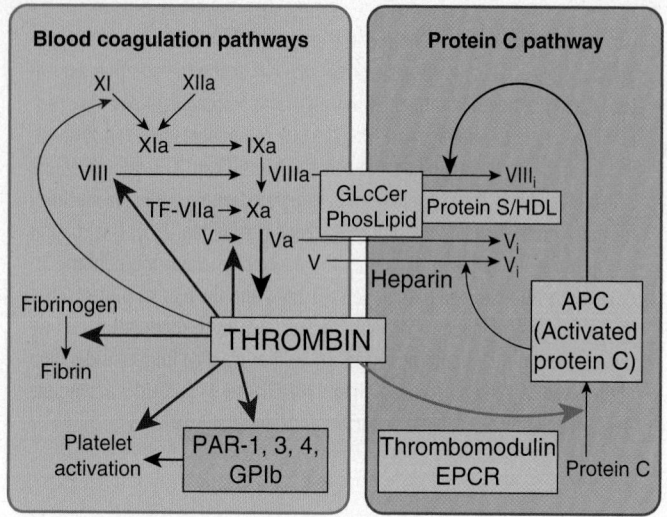

Figure 114–1. Blood coagulation pathways and protein C anticoagulant pathway. Thrombin can be either a procoagulant *(left)* or an anticoagulant *(right)*, depending on cofactors and surfaces. Coagulant thrombin clots fibrinogen and activates platelets and factors V, VIII, XI, and XIII. Conversion of zymogen protein C to the active protease, APC, by thrombomodulin-bound thrombin is enhanced by endothelial protein C receptor (EPCR). APC with its nonenzymatic cofactor, protein S, inactivates factors Va and VIIIa by highly selective proteolysis (e.g., at Arg506 and Arg306 in factor Va), yielding inactivated (i) factors V_i and VIII_i. This anticoagulant action may be enhanced by phospholipid (PhosLipid) surfaces on platelets, endothelial cells, or their microparticles. High-density lipoprotein (HDL) can also provide protein S–dependent anticoagulant APC-cofactor activity. Similarly, neutral glycosphingolipids such as glucosylceramide (GLcCer) can enhance APC anticoagulant activity. GPIb, glycoprotein Ib; PAR, protease-activated receptor. *(Adapted with permission from Griffin JH: Blood coagulation. The thrombin paradox.* Nature *378(6555):337–338, 1995.)*

At each step in the coagulation pathways, each clotting protease can be inhibited by one or more plasma protease inhibitors in reactions stimulated by negatively charged glycosaminoglycans such as heparan sulfate or heparin (see "Inhibition of Coagulation Proteases by Protease

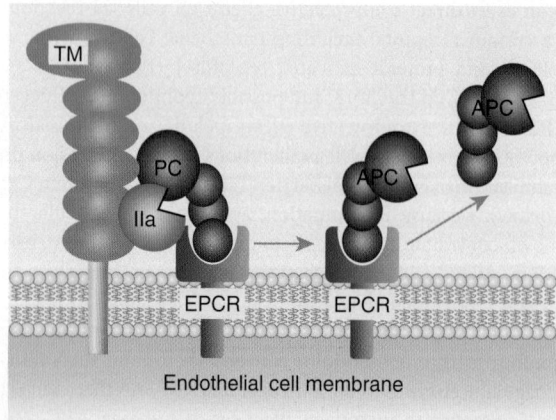

Figure 114–2. Protein C activation on endothelial cell surface. On an endothelial surface, activated protein C (APC) generation follows binding of protein C (PC) to endothelial protein C receptor (EPCR) where PC is activated by limited proteolysis by the thrombin (IIa)–thrombomodulin (TM) complex. This action of thrombin liberates a dodecapeptide (residues 158 to 169) from protein C to generate the multifunctional protease APC. *(Adapted with permission from Mosnier LO, Zlokovic BV, Griffin JH: The cytoprotective protein C pathway.* Blood *109(8):3161–3172, 2007.)*

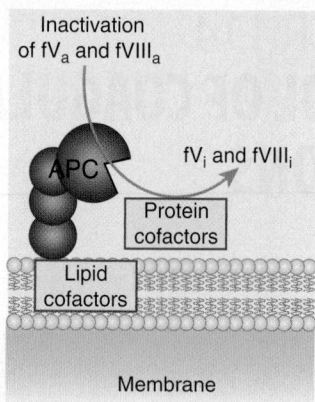

Figure 114–3. Activated protein C (APC) exerts its anticoagulant activity by proteolytic inactivation of factors Va and VIIIa on membrane surfaces containing phospholipids that are derived from cells, lipoproteins, or cellular microparticles. A variety of lipid and protein cofactors (see Fig. 114–1 legend and text) accelerate the inactivation of factors Va and VIIIa to yield the irreversibly inactivated factors Vi and VIIIi. *(Adapted with permission from Mosnier LO, Zlokovic BV, Griffin JH: The cytoprotective protein C pathway.* Blood *109(8):3161–3172, 2007.)*

Inhibitors" below). Given the highly nonlinear nature of the coagulation pathways with both positive and negative feedback reactions, synergy between the protein C pathway and plasma protease inhibitors is important for regulating thrombin generation.

There is continuous activation of coagulation factors at a basal physiologic low level. Plasma from all normal subjects contains circulating active enzymes, factor VIIa,[14] and APC,[15] as well as various polypeptide fragments generated by the action of clotting proteases, namely fibrinopeptides,[16,17] prothrombin fragment 1+2,[18] and activation peptides for factors IX and X.[19,20] The presence of multiple clotting factors that require positive feedback activation (e.g., factors V, VIII, XI, and VII)

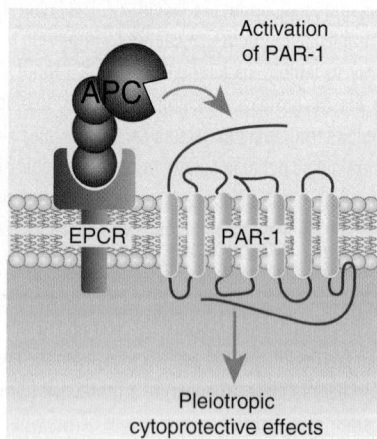

Figure 114–4. Paradigm for activated protein C (APC)'s initiation of cell signaling and multiple cytoprotective effects. Direct effects of APC on cells are initiated by activation of the G-protein–coupled receptor, protease-activated receptor-1 (PAR-1), by endothelial protein C receptor (EPCR)-bound APC. The γ-carboxyglutamic acid (GLA) domain of APC binds to EPCR to help position APC's protease domain for efficient cleavage of the extracellular N-terminal tail of PAR-1, which results in G-protein–coupled receptor activation and subsequent antiinflammatory and antiapoptotic effects, alterations of gene expression profiles, and stabilization of endothelial junctions. *(Adapted with permission from Mosnier LO, Zlokovic BV, Griffin JH: The cytoprotective protein C pathway.* Blood *109(8):3161–3172, 2007.)*

imparts special threshold properties to the blood coagulation pathways, making the coagulant response nonlinearly responsive to stimuli. Theoretical analysis of blood coagulation as a threshold system suggests there can be an all-or-none response to various levels of stimulation, depending on the ensemble of activating and inhibitory reactions that defines upregulation and downregulation of thrombin generation.[21,22] The coagulation system is active, but idling, and is poised for extensive and explosive generation of thrombin. Because of synergy among various cellular and humoral anticoagulant mechanisms that establish a threshold system, the presence of multiple coagulation inhibitors with complementary modes of action prevents massive thrombin generation in the absence of a substantial procoagulant stimulus.

● HEREDITARY DEFICIENCIES ASSOCIATED WITH THROMBOTIC DISEASE

Evidence for the physiologic importance of specific factors for controlling coagulation reactions comes from clinical observations and animal model studies. Major identified genetic risk factors for venous thrombosis involve protein structural defects in factor V, protein C, protein S, and antithrombin (Chap. 130). There are also gene regulatory defects associated with thrombotic disease, such as the G20210A polymorphism in the prothrombin gene that causes elevated levels of prothrombin, and defects in protein C gene regulatory elements that decrease the expression of protein C. Deficiencies of thrombomodulin might also be associated with increased risk of arterial thrombosis. Association of hereditary abnormalities of EPCR with increased risks of thrombosis has been suggested, but this remains somewhat controversial.

● PROTEIN C PATHWAY COMPONENTS

Figure 114–5 is a schematic of the structures of protein C, protein S, thrombomodulin, and EPCR. These proteins contain multiple domains, each of which may mediate different molecular functions. Values for the molecular weight, normal plasma concentration, chromosomal location, and gene structures of these factors are given in Table 114–1. Factors Va and VIIIa, as substrates of APC, are also participants in the reactions of the anticoagulant protein C pathway. Moreover, factor V, but not factor V Leiden, appears to act as an APC cofactor for the inactivation of factor VIIIa (see "Factor V as Activated Protein C Cofactor" below).[23]

PROTEIN C

In 1976, Stenflo designated a bovine plasma vitamin K–dependent protein that eluted in the third peak (peak C) from an anion exchange column as bovine "protein C."[24] Protein C, actually previously described as the anticoagulant factor autoprothrombin II-A,[25] is a plasma serine protease zymogen that can be converted to an active serine protease by the action of thrombin.

Protein C is synthesized in the liver as a polypeptide precursor of 461 residues, with a prepropeptide of 42 amino acids that contains the signal for carboxylation of Glu residues by a carboxylase that forms nine γ-carboxyglutamic acid (GLA) residues and secretion of the mature protein.[26–28] The mature glycoprotein of Mr 62,000 contains 419 residues (see Chap. 113, Fig. 113–1 and Fig. 114–5) and N-linked carbohydrate, and the majority of the secreted protein C molecules are cleaved by a furin-like endoprotease that releases Lys156-Arg157 and generates a two-chain zymogen that circulates in plasma at 65 nM (4 mcg/mL).[29] The heavy and light chains of plasma protein C are covalently linked by a disulfide bond that keeps the serine protease globular domain (residues 170 to 419) covalently tethered to the N-terminal string of three domains, the GLA domain and the epidermal growth factor (EGF)-like domains EGF1 and EGF2.[26–30]

The GLA domain of protein C (residues 1 to 42) and APC is important for a number of functions, including binding to phospholipid-containing membranes (see Chap. 113, Fig. 113–3), thrombomodulin, and EPCR; thus, incomplete carboxylation impairs the functional anticoagulant activity of APC.[31–33] The two EGF modules in the light chain may contribute to interactions of APC with protein S and of protein C with thrombomodulin.

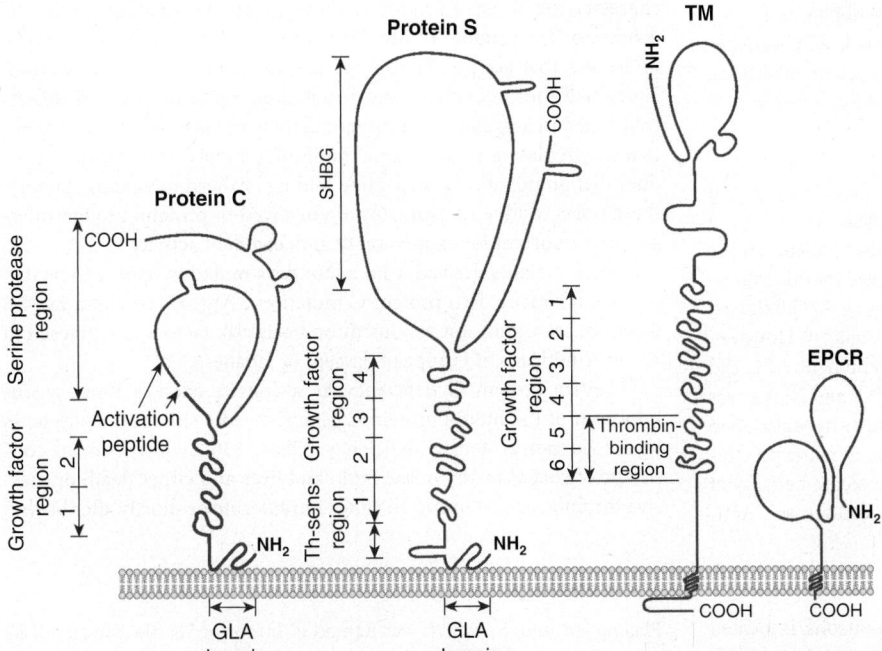

Figure 114–5. Membrane-bound protein C, protein S, thrombomodulin (TM) and endothelial cell protein C receptor (EPCR). Each protein is a multidomain protein that extends above the surface of cell membranes, and different domains mediate different functions of each protein. Protein C and protein S can bind reversibly to phospholipid membranes through their NH$_2$-terminal γ-carboxyglutamic acid (GLA) domains which contain nine or 11 GLA residues that bind four to six Ca^{2+} ions. TM and EPCR are integral membrane proteins that are embedded in cell membranes by a single hydrophobic transmembrane sequence. *(Adapted with permission from Esmon CT: The roles of protein C and thrombomodulin in the regulation of blood coagulation. J Biol Chem 264(9):4743–4746, 1989.)*

TABLE 114–1. Characteristics of Blood Coagulation Regulatory Molecules

	Molecular Weight (kDa)	Plasma Concentration (mcg/mL)	Half-Life (h)	Chromosome	Gene (kb)	Exon (N)	Function
Protein C	62	4	6	2q13–14	11	9	Anticoagulant protease
Protein S	75	26	42	3p11.1–11.2	80	15	Activated protein C (APC)-cofactor and coagulation inhibitor
Thrombomodulin	60–105	0.020	ND	20p11.2–cen	3.7	1	Receptor for thrombin/protein C
Endothelial protein C receptor (EPCR)	46	0.098	ND	20q11.2	6	4	Receptor for protein C/APC
Protease-activated receptor-1 (PAR-1)	68	NA	NA	5q13	27	2	G-protein–coupled receptor
Antithrombin	58	150	70	1q23–25	14	7	Protease inhibitor
Tissue factor pathway inhibitor (TFPI)	34	0.1	ND	2q31–32.1	85	9	Protease inhibitor
Heparin cofactor II	66	70	60	22q11	16	5	Protease inhibitor
Protein Z	70	1.7	60	13q34		9	Plasma protein
Protein Z–dependent protease inhibitor (ZPI)	72	1.5		14q32.13		5	Protease inhibitor

NA, not applicable; ND, not determined.

The serine protease domain of protein C is homologous to other trypsin-like proteases, and three-dimensional modeling[34] and X-ray crystallographic structures[30] reflect the structural similarity of APC to members of the serine protease family of which chymotrypsin is the prototype (see Mather and colleagues[30] for conversion of protein C to chymotrypsin numbering). APC's trypsin-like protease domain exerts its anticoagulant activity by highly specific interactions with factors Va and VIIIa followed by cleavage at only two Arg-containing peptide bonds in factors Va and VIIIa (see "Factors Va and VIIIa as Substrates for Activated Protein C" below). These stereo-specific interactions involve both the APC enzymatic active site region and a number of APC residues that are termed *exosites* because they are not located in the immediate vicinity of APC's enzymatic active site. Such APC exosites are essential for specific recognition of the macromolecular substrates, factors Va and VIIIa as well as recognition of cellular APC receptors.[35–44]

Protein C and Activated Protein C Therapy

Purified plasma protein C concentrate (Ceprotin) is FDA-approved for treating protein C–deficient patients.[45] Recombinant APC (Xigris) reduced all-cause 28-day mortality in severe sepsis adult patients in the PROWESS phase III trial in 2001 and was FDA-approved for this indication.[46] This successful therapy of adult severe sepsis using APC followed preclinical antithrombotic and sepsis studies in baboons.[47,48] However, a decade later, in the PROWESS-SHOCK trial, recombinant APC did not reduce mortality in adult severe sepsis patients,[49–51] and Xigris was withdrawn from the market. Animal injury model studies have also shed light on *in vivo* mechanisms for APC beneficial effects in many preclinical injury models and in many models the pharmacologic benefits of APC appear to be independent of APC's anticoagulant actions (see "Activated Protein C Direct Cellular Activities" below).[7,8]

Protein C Gene

The protein C gene, comprising nine exons and eight introns, is located on chromosome 2q14–21 and spans 11 kb (see Chap. 113, Fig. 113–10,

and Table 114–1).[52] The protein C gene is homologous to the genes for factors VII, IX, and X (Chap. 113).

Protein C Mutations

Hereditary protein C deficiency associated with thrombosis is caused by numerous mutations (see protein C mutation databases).[53,54] Based on three-dimensional structures of the protein C, the structural basis for hereditary protein C defects has been rationalized.[34,55,56] Most mutations that cause type I protein C deficiency, characterized by parallel reductions in activity and antigen, involve amino acid residues that form the hydrophobic cores of the two folded globulin-like domains that are characteristic of serine proteases. These mutations destabilize either the process or the product of protein folding, and they result in unstable molecules that are poorly secreted and/or exhibit a very short circulatory half-life. In contrast, most mutations that cause type II defects (reduced anticoagulant or enzymatic activity but normal antigen levels), that is, circulating dysfunctional molecules, involve polar surface residues that do not affect polypeptide folding or thermodynamic stability; these polar residues presumably are involved in protein–protein interactions important for expression of anticoagulant activity.

Rare variants derived from a founder's mutation appear to be distinctive for races. Two protein C mutations, Arg147Trp and a Lys150 deletion, are significant venous thrombosis risk factors in Chinese but not in Americans of European descent or Japanese.[57–59]

Severe protein C deficiency as a consequence of homozygous knockout of the mouse protein C gene showed a similar phenotype as severe human protein C deficiency (Chap. 130), with perinatal consumptive coagulopathy in the brain and liver and either death or massive thrombosis that occurred either intrauterine or shortly after birth.[60]

PROTEIN S

Plasma "protein S," which was named in honor of Seattle, the city of its discovery, is a vitamin K–dependent glycoprotein[61] that is synthesized by hepatocytes, neuroblastoma cells, kidney cells, testis, megakaryo-cytes, and endothelial cells, and is also found in platelet α-granules.[62]

Protein S is synthesized as a precursor protein of 676 amino acids, which gives rise to a mature secreted single-chain glycoprotein of 635 residues with three *N*-linked carbohydrate side chains (see Fig. 114–5).[63,64] Eleven GLA residues in the N-terminal region of mature protein S contribute to Ca^{2+}-mediated binding of the protein to phospholipid membranes. The thrombin-sensitive region, residues 47 to 72, follows the GLA-domain (see Fig. 114–5).

The C-terminal region of protein S, residues 270 to 635, the sex hormone–binding globulin-like (SHBG) region contains binding sites for C4b-binding protein (see "Activated Protein C–Independent Anticoagulant Activity of Protein S" below)[65] and for factor V, as well as factor Va.[66,67] Protein S, like the homologous gas6, also binds to receptor tyrosine kinases, for example, Axl, and initiates cell signaling, and the SHBG region binds the receptor.[68] Thus, for the expression of its multiple activities, different domains of protein S exhibit a number of different binding sites for different proteins.

Protein S Gene

The protein S gene, comprising 15 exons and 14 introns, is located on chromosome 3p11.1–11.2 and spans 80 kb (see Fig. 113–16 and Table 114–1).[69,70] The protein S gene has limited homology with other genes for vitamin K–dependent factors in the GLA and EGF domains and notable homology of the region coding for residues 240 to 635 with genes of the SHBG family. Humans contain a protein S pseudogene that contains several stop codons and is not translated and that is located very near the normal protein S gene on chromosome 3.

Protein S Mutations

The molecular basis for hereditary protein S deficiency associated with venous thrombosis (Chap. 130) is linked to more than 100 different mutations.[71] A protein S polymorphism that is strongly linked to risk for venous thrombosis in Japanese subjects is known as protein S Tokushima. It involves K155E, which ablates APC-cofactor activity.[57,72] But the K155E apparently is not present in Americans of European ancestry or Chinese populations, thus mirroring the presence of factor V Leiden and prothrombin G20210A that are risk factors in Americans of European decent but not in the Japanese, Chinese, or Americans of African descent populations.[73] Another single nucleotide polymorphism present in approximately 1 percent of Americans of European descent is S460P, which is designated protein S Heerlen; it results in absence of *N*-linked carbohydrate on Asn458 but has no accepted significant functional consequence.[74]

THROMBOMODULIN

Thrombomodulin was discovered as an endothelial cell surface receptor that binds protein C and thrombin, thereby accelerating protein C activation.[75–78] Binding of thrombin to thrombomodulin converts thrombin from a procoagulant enzyme to an anticoagulant enzyme because thrombomodulin-bound thrombin loses its normal ability to clot fibrinogen or activate platelets.[79,80] Thrombomodulin is a multidomain transmembrane protein comprising an N-terminal lectin-like domain, six EGF domains, a Ser/Thr-rich region, a single membrane-spanning sequence, and an intracellular C-terminal tail (see Fig. 114–5).[5–8,75–83] EGF domains 4, 5, and 6 are essential for activation of protein C, with the latter two domains binding thrombin and the first domain binding protein C. The mature protein has 557-amino-acid residues and variable amounts of *N*- and *O*-linked carbohydrate modifications that cause variability in molecular size. Glycosaminoglycans, notably chondroitin sulfate, covalently attached to the Ser/Thr-rich region, contribute to the functional properties of thrombomodulin by enhancing either

protein C activation by thrombin or by accelerating neutralization of thrombin by protease inhibitors. Modulation of the substrate specificity of thrombin by thrombomodulin involves conformational changes in thrombin caused by binding of thrombomodulin.

Low levels of soluble thrombomodulin circulate in plasma, presumably as a result of limited proteolysis of the protein near its transmembrane cell surface anchor. The functional significance of circulating thrombomodulin is unknown, although variations in its plasma level arise in different clinical conditions.

Recombinant soluble thrombomodulin has been developed for its potential therapeutic value for disseminated intravascular coagulation and has been approved for this indication in Japan.[77,84]

Thrombomodulin Gene

The thrombomodulin gene, which lacks introns, is located on chromosome 20p11.2 and spans 3.7 kb (see Chap. 113, Fig. 113–19, Fig. 114–5, and Table 114–1).[77,82] Deletion of the thrombomodulin gene in mice is embryonically lethal.[85] Downregulation of thrombomodulin gene expression is promoted by a variety of inflammatory agents, including endotoxin, interleukin-1, and tumor necrosis factor (TNF)-α, whereas its expression is upregulated by retinoic acid.[5–8,86,87] Generally, thrombomodulin is a key member among the counterbalancing factors that contribute to inflammation, thrombin generation, and coagulation in the endothelium.

Thrombomodulin Mutations

Thrombomodulin mutations are well documented in atypical hemolytic uremic syndrome patients,[78,88] and they may also be associated with an increased risk of arterial thrombosis and myocardial infarction. In contrast, there is less supportive data for association with risk for venous thrombosis (Chap. 130).[89–92] Atypical hemolytic uremic syndrome is strongly linked to excessive complement activation, and thrombomodulin's lectin-like domain inhibits complement activation.[77,93] Furthermore, besides promoting protein C activation by thrombin, thrombomodulin also supports activation of the carboxypeptidase, also known as thrombin-activatable fibrinolysis inhibitor (TAFI) that is a potent inactivator of bradykinin and of the activated complement components, C3a and C5a.[94–96]

ENDOTHELIAL PROTEIN C RECEPTOR

EPCR binds both protein C and APC with similar affinities through their GLA domains and mediates multiple activities of this zymogen or its activated protease, APC.[9,10,33,86,97–107] The mature EPCR glycoprotein contains 221-amino-acid residues and *N*-linked carbohydrate, giving an Mr of 46,000. EPCR is an integral membrane protein that is homologous to CD1/major histocompatibility complex class I molecules. The N-terminus is part of an extracellular domain, which is connected to a single transmembrane sequence that is followed by a short Arg-Arg-Cys-COOH cytoplasmic tail (see Fig. 114–5). The cytoplasmic tail can be palmitoylated, and this modification may help localize EPCR to certain lipid rafts or caveolae. The three-dimensional structure of EPCR determined by X-ray crystallography or inferred by molecular modeling established that the GLA domain of protein C and APC binds to EPCR.[107,108] EPCR on endothelial surfaces enhances by greater than fivefold the rate of activation of protein C by thrombin–thrombomodulin (see Fig. 114–2). EPCR is also required for the cytoprotective activities of APC by promoting the cleavage of PAR-1 by APC to induce cell-signaling pathways (see Fig. 114–4). Notably, the cytoprotective actions of APC are completely independent of its anticoagulant activity and are based on cell signaling actions (see "Activated Protein C Direct Cellular Activities" below).[7,8,109–111]

The presence of functional EPCR on the cell surface is regulated by two mechanisms, namely generation of EPCR and clearance of EPCR.

Inflammatory mediators induce EPCR ectodomain shedding from the endothelial cell surface by metalloproteinase TNF-α converting enzyme (known as "TACE").[112] The soluble EPCR ectodomain is found in normal human plasma at 100 ng/mL; however, carriers of the H3 EPCR haplotype that includes a Ser219Gly polymorphism (rs867186) have threefold higher soluble EPCR plasma levels.[113] Higher plasma levels of soluble EPCR are found in patients with disseminated intravascular coagulation or systemic lupus erythematosus, although plasma EPCR levels are not correlated with pathology-related alterations in circulating thrombomodulin levels.[114] Soluble EPCR binds the protein C and APC via their GLA domains with an affinity similar to the membrane-bound receptor. Because binding of the APC GLA domain to negatively charged phospholipid membranes is required for its anticoagulant activity, soluble EPCR at relatively high levels in purified reaction mixtures inhibits the anticoagulant action of APC against factor Va, although it does not block the reaction of APC with protease inhibitors.[10,86,99,115]

The EPCR crystal structure surprisingly revealed a single phospholipid molecule bound in a surface groove on the protein.[107] Secreted phospholipase A₂ group V can modify the lipid in EPCR and cause EPCR to lose its ability to bind protein C and APC.[116,117] The presence of functional EPCR on the cell surface has important implications for thrombotic and inflammatory vascular disease because EPCR inactivation *in vivo* increases susceptibility to thrombotic and inflammatory diseases.[10,86,97]

The physiologic requirement for EPCR in mice was established by the embryonic lethality observed for knockout of the murine EPCR gene.[118]

EPCR has functionally important interactions with multiple molecules beyond protein C and APC. It binds factor VII and factor VIIa.[10] Furthermore, EPCR was recently implicated to play a potentially important role in the pathogenesis of severe malaria.[119-122]

Endothelial Protein C Receptor Gene

The EPCR gene, comprising four exons and three introns, is located on human chromosome 20q11.2 and spans 6 kb (see Table 114–1).[123]

PROTEASE-ACTIVATED RECEPTOR-1

PAR-1, discovered as a high-affinity human platelet receptor for thrombin,[124] is the prototype of a four-member subfamily of G-protein–coupled receptors that share an unusual mechanism of activation, namely activation by proteases.[124-130] Each PAR contains seven transmembrane helical domains and an extracellular N-terminal tail that is cleaved by an activating protease such that the newly generated aminoterminus is a tethered ligand that triggers activation of the coupled G-protein. Human platelets employ PAR-1 and PAR-4 for activation by thrombin whereas, curiously, murine platelets that are devoid of PAR-1 require PAR-3 and PAR-4 for thrombin's normal effects.[125,131] PAR-1 is activated by various plasma proteases[132-135] and is generally required for APC's cytoprotective activities (see "Cellular Receptors for Physiologic Effects of Activated Protein C on Cells" below).[7,8,110,111]

Protease-Activated Receptor-1 Gene

The PAR-1 gene contains only two introns, is located on chromosome 5q13, and spans 25 kb (see Table 114–1).[125] Much is known about many factors that can either upregulate or downregulate the PAR-1 gene.[124-130]

● ACTIVATION OF PROTEIN C

Protein C is activated from zymogen to active protease as a result of cleavage by thrombin at the Arg169–Leu170 peptide bond in a reaction that is accelerated by thrombomodulin and EPCR (see Fig. 114–2 and "Thrombomodulin" above).[5,7,8,76,81,86] Thrombin infusions into animals

generate anticoagulant activity because of APC.[136,137] Interestingly, thrombin infusion into hyperlipidemic monkeys with atherosclerosis generates less APC and causes a poorer *ex vivo* response to APC compared with normolipidemic control monkeys,[138] showing that hyperlipidemia and vascular disease can affect protein C activation.

Ischemia causes protein C activation *in vivo*. A brief occlusion of the left anterior descending coronary artery in pigs results in APC generation.[139] During cerebral ischemia in humans undergoing routine endarterectomy, APC increases in the venous cerebral blood.[140] Protein C is significantly activated during cardiopulmonary bypass, mainly during the minutes immediately after aortic unclamping in the ischemic vascular beds.[141] Streptokinase therapy for acute myocardial infarction increases circulating APC.[142]

Circulating APC concentration in normal human subjects is highly correlated with circulating levels of protein C zymogen.[143] Based on protein C infusion studies in protein C-deficient subjects, the level of circulating APC is strongly determined by the concentration of protein C.[144] EPCR appears to be required for normal protein C activation in response to thrombin infusions in experimental animals.[145] EPCR and thrombomodulin must be in close proximity on cell surfaces (see Fig. 114–2), although this has yet to be experimentally demonstrated.

Thrombomodulin and EPCR appear to differ markedly in their relative distribution densities on blood vessels as the former is abundantly present in the small blood vessels but less so in large vessels, whereas the latter is more abundant in large vessels than in small vessels.[85,86,146,147] Low levels of thrombomodulin are expressed in brain,[148] and brain-specific activation of protein C in humans occurs during carotid occlusion.[140]

Proteolytic cleavage and activation of protein C can also be effected by meizothrombin, plasmin, or factor Xa.[149-153] On the surface of cultured endothelial cells, negatively charged sulfated polysaccharides in the presence of phospholipid vesicles containing phosphatidylethanolamine can enhance the rate of protein C activation by factor Xa to approach the protein C activation rate of thrombin:thrombomodulin.[152] No data yet indicate whether protein C activation by meizothrombin, plasmin, or factor Xa is physiologically relevant.

Protein C activation is stimulated by platelet factor 4. Both *in vitro* and *in vivo* data imply that platelet factor 4 may play a physiologic role in enhancing APC generation and influencing the activities of the protein C system.[154-157]

● ACTIVATED PROTEIN C ACTIVITIES

The clinical phenotype of severe protein C deficiency in neonatal purpura fulminans implies that APC exerts multiple physiologically essential activities, including potent anticoagulant and antiinflammatory actions (Chap. 130). Recent advances establish that APC's antiinflammatory actions are but one manifestation of its ability to interact directly with cell receptors to provide multiple cytoprotective activities.[7,8,110,111] These two distinct types of activities of APC—intravascular anticoagulant activity and initiation of cell signaling—are mediated by different sets of molecular interactions, and both types of activities are clinically relevant.

ACTIVATED PROTEIN C ANTICOAGULANT ACTIVITY

Mechanisms for APC's direct anticoagulant activity involve factors V and VIII, the two homologous coagulation cofactors that circulate as inactive molecules and that are converted to active cofactors by limited proteolysis (see Chap. 113, Figs. 113–11 and 113–13). APC circulates at 40 pM (picomolars) in normal humans, and there is an inverse correlation between fibrinopeptide A, the product that is cleaved from fibrinogen by thrombin, and APC levels in healthy nonsmoking adults, suggesting APC is a significant regulator of basal thrombin activity.[15,158]

Factors V and VIII are synthesized as large single-chain precursor coagulation cofactors of Mr 330,000, consisting of three homologous A domains (A1, A2, and A3) and two homologous C domains (C1 and C2) with a very large intervening, generally nonhomologous domain, designated the *B domain,* that connects the A2 and A3 domains (Chap. 113). Activation of the inactive precursor form of the two cofactors V and VIII involves limited proteolysis.[23,159–164] Factor V activation involves cleavages at Arg709, Arg1018, and Arg1545 by thrombin, factor Xa, or other proteases.[23,164–168] Cleavage at Arg1545 is the key step for generating factor Va activity because this proteolysis releases the B domain that blocks binding of factor Xa to factor Va.[164,169] The various forms of factor Va (see Chap. 113, Fig. 113–11) are composed of two polypeptide chains, one bearing the A1-A2 domains and the other bearing the A3-C1-C2 domains. Although generally similar to factor V activation, factor VIII activation (see Fig. 113–13) involves formation of a heterotrimer of polypeptide chains containing the A1 domain, the A2 domain, and the A3-C1-C2 domains, respectively. In contrast to heterodimeric factor Va, heterotrimeric factor VIIIa is intrinsically unstable as a consequence of spontaneous dissociation of the A2 domain.[170]

Factors Va and VIIIa as Substrates for Activated Protein C
Irreversible proteolytic inactivation of factors Va and VIIIa by APC can be accomplished by proteolysis at Arg506 and Arg306 in factor Va and Arg562 and Arg336 in factor VIIIa (see Chap. 113, Figs. 113–11 and 113–13).[23,171–173] Currently, the most common identifiable venous thrombosis risk factor involves a mutation of Arg506 to Gln in factor V that results in APC resistance (Chap. 130). The complexities of APC-dependent inactivation of factor Va and VIIIa are compounded by the number of different molecular forms of Va and VIIIa that can be generated by limited proteolysis by a variety of proteases and by their differing susceptibilities to APC and to the different APC cofactors.

Activated Protein C Resistance
APC resistance is defined as an abnormally reduced anticoagulant response of a plasma sample to APC (Chap. 130) and can be caused by many potential abnormalities in the protein C anticoagulant pathway. Such abnormalities could include defective APC cofactors, defective APC substrates, or other molecules that interfere with the normal functioning of the protein C anticoagulant pathway (e.g., autoantibodies against APC, APC cofactors, or APC substrates).

A report of familial venous thrombosis associated with APC resistance without any identifiable defect in four Swedish families[174] led to an intensive search for a genetic explanation that was soon found to involve replacement of G by A at nucleotide 1691 in exon 10 of the factor V gene which causes the amino acid replacement of Arg506 by Gln.[175–177] This factor V variant, like the prothrombin variant nt G20210A, arose in a single white founder some 18,000 to 29,000 years ago[178,179] and is known as *Gln506-factor V* or *factor V Leiden.* This mutation is currently a common, but not the only, cause of APC resistance (Chap. 130).

The molecular mechanism for APC resistance of Gln506-factor V is based on the fact that the variant molecule is inactivated 10 times slower than normal Arg506-factor Va.[23,177,180–182] The variant factor Va exhibits only a partial resistance to APC because cleavage at Arg306 in factor Va also occurs, causing complete loss of factor Va activity.

Plasma and recombinant factor V can exist in two biochemically distinct forms, designated *factor V1* and *factor V2* that differ in *N*-linked carbohydrate on Asn2181, near the phospholipid binding region of the C2 domain as factor V2 has none.[183,184] Because the *N*-linked carbohydrate appears to decrease the apparent affinity of factor V1 or Va1 for

phospholipid, it reduces the specific clotting activity and susceptibility to APC. Normal plasma contains a mixture of factors V1 and V2. Removal of the carbohydrate attached to factor V increases the rate of inactivation of factor Va by APC, although the clinical significance of this phenomenon is unknown.[185]

APC resistance with no identifiable genetic or acquired abnormalities is well described in patients with venous and arterial thrombosis and, at least for research purposes, should be therefore examined in patients with a suspected thrombophilia. Further studies are needed to identify the causes of APC resistance in such patients.[186–188] One major challenge involves defining the normal range for the clotting assays that are actually used to characterize APC resistance and the multiple plasma analytes or nonplasma assay components that are present in the assays. For example, activated partial thromboplastin time-based assays are not equivalently sensitive as are dilute tissue-factor-based assays to plasma high-density lipoprotein (HDL) levels or oral contraceptive use.[189–191] Plasma variables, such as elevated prothrombin levels,[192,193] may affect the response to APC by inhibiting APC anticoagulant actions. Endogenous thrombin potential assays involving dilute tissue factor as the procoagulant initiator provide additional tools for defining and characterizing APC resistance and extend the tools for shedding light on the gray area of APC resistance found in some thrombosis patients that is not linked to currently known factors.

ACTIVATED PROTEIN C ANTICOAGULANT COFACTORS
APC anticoagulant activity is enhanced by a number of factors that may be termed *APC anticoagulant cofactors*; these include Ca^{2+} ions; certain, but not all, phospholipids; protein S; factor V; certain glycosphingolipids; and HDL.

Phospholipids as Activated Protein C Cofactors
Certain phospholipids, such as phosphatidylserine, phosphatidylethanolamine, and cardiolipin, enhance the anticoagulant activity of APC. In addition, phosphatidylethanolamine and cardiolipin stimulate the APC anticoagulant pathway activities much more than they stimulate the procoagulant pathway activities.[194–197]

Protein S as Activated Protein C Cofactor
Protein S structure–activity relationships are informed by much biochemical work and the large number of mutations.[71,198] Protein S, as an anticoagulant APC cofactor, forms a 1:1 complex with APC and enhances by 10- to 20-fold the rate of APC's cleavage at Arg306 in factor Va but not the Arg506 cleavage.[181,182] Part of the mechanism for this activity of protein S may be related to its ability to bring the active site of APC closer to the plane of the phospholipid membrane on which the APC–protein S complex is located when the complex is formed.[199,200] Protein S also facilitates the action of APC against factor VIIIa.[201] Protein S enhances APC's action, in part at least, by ablating the ability of factor Xa to protect factor Va from APC.[202] The GLA domain, thrombin-sensitive region, and EGF1 and EGF2 domains of protein S are implicated in binding APC for expression of anticoagulant activity by the APC–protein S complex.[198,203–206] Cleavage of the thrombin-sensitive region by thrombin abolishes normal binding of protein S to phospholipid and its normal APC-cofactor anticoagulant activity.[205,207]

Factor V as Activated Protein C Cofactor
Factor V apparently can have anticoagulant as well as procoagulant properties because it enhances the anticoagulant action of APC against factors VIIIa and Va in a reaction in which protein S acts synergistically with factor V.[23,208–211] Cleavage at Arg1545, which optimizes factor

Va procoagulant activity, ablates the molecule's anticoagulant cofactor activity. However, when factor V is cleaved at Arg506 by APC, its APC cofactor activity is increased 10-fold. This suggests that Gln506-factor V has two potential prothrombotic defects, namely, resistance of the variant factor Va to APC inactivation and resistance of the variant factor V to activation of its APC cofactor function.[23,209–211]

High-Density Lipoprotein as Activated Protein C Cofactor

HDL can exert antithrombotic activity through multiple mechanisms.[212] HDL enhances the anticoagulant activity of APC both in plasma and in purified reaction mixtures, and this APC cofactor activity requires protein S and involves, at least in part, stimulation of APC's cleavage at Arg306 in factor Va.[189,190] HDL is heterogeneous in both protein and lipid composition, and the components responsible for this activity have not been identified, although large HDL, but not small HDL, possesses APC anticoagulant cofactor activity.[190] Venous thrombosis in males and in subjects experiencing venous thrombosis recurrence are associated with a pattern of dyslipoproteinemia and low HDL, consistent with the hypothesis that deficiency of large HDL is a risk factor for venous thrombosis.[213,214]

Glycosphingolipids as Activated Protein C Cofactors

Although both procoagulant and anticoagulant reactions are markedly enhanced by the presence of negatively charged phospholipid surfaces *in vitro*, certain lipoproteins, for example, HDL,[189] and certain lipids, for example, glycosphingolipids and sphingosine,[215–218] selectively enhance anticoagulant reactions in plasma. Plasma glucosylceramide deficiency is a biomarker and may be a potential risk factor for venous thrombosis.[215] Sphingosine and several of its common analogues are potent inhibitors of thrombin generation in plasma and on cell surfaces because they inhibit interactions between factors Va and Xa.[218] Further studies are needed to characterize the anticoagulant or procoagulant properties of minor abundance plasma and their significance for clinical thrombotic events.

ACTIVATED PROTEIN C DIRECT CELLULAR ACTIVITIES

As noted in Chap. 113, control of coagulation reactions does not occur in the absence of an integrated host defense system that involves a number of biologic processes involving multiple overlapping and integrated pathways. Reactions of the innate and acquired immune system including inflammatory processes, blood coagulation reactions, fibrinolysis, and thrombotic processes are intertwined *in vivo* via multiple molecular and cellular mechanisms.[5,7,8,81,86,87,212,219,220] In addition to its anticoagulant activity, APC acts directly on cells to cause multiple cytoprotective effects. Cytoprotective actions of APC include antiapoptotic and antiinflammatory activities, beneficial changes in gene-expression profiles, and endothelial barrier stabilization. These cytoprotective activities of APC generally require EPCR, involve APC's ability to activate PAR-1, and may also require additional receptors such as PAR-3, sphingosine-1-phosphate receptor 1, integrin CD11b/CD18, apoER2, EGF receptor, and/or Tie2.[7,8,86,110,221–227]

Pharmacologic APC infusions showed benefits in numerous animal injury model systems, with the most informative animal studies to date being in sepsis models and in neuroprotection experiments.[7,8,37,40,111,226,227] Protein engineering permitted the molecular dissection of APC's anticoagulant activity from its cytoprotective activities[7,8,37,40–44,228] and led to proof of principle that APC's cell signaling activities are both necessary and most likely sufficient for reducing lethality in murine septic shock models[42,229] and for providing neuroprotective effects in ischemic stroke models.[226,227,230–232] Notably, recombinant APC mutants that have little anticoagulant activity (<10 percent) but normal cell-signaling activity

are able to convey beneficial effects in multiple injury and disease models with diminished risks for bleeding that would be anticipated with wild-type APC therapy.[8,40–44]

Activated Protein C Neuroprotective Effects

Neuroprotective effects of APC have been convincingly demonstrated in rodent ischemic stroke models and N-methyl-D-aspartate (NMDA) excitotoxic injury models.[8,223,226,227,231,233–242] APC not only provides direct cytoprotection *in vitro* and *in vivo* for brain endothelium against ischemic injury but also directly protects neurons against NMDA-induced excitotoxic injury both *in vivo* and *in vitro*. APC mutants with reduced anticoagulant activity were as neuroprotective as wild-type APC, and certain cellular receptors were required for APC's neuroprotection, strongly implying that neuroprotection by APC involves its actions directly on the endothelium and on neurons. Remarkably, in the ischemic penumbra in a murine stroke model, APC caused neovascularization and neurogenesis.[223,240,243–245] The extensive preclinical studies on APC's neuroprotective effects paved the pathway for translation of the 3K3A-APC variant to potential neuroprotective therapy for acute ischemic stroke.[246,247] Because of the greatly reduced anticoagulant activity of 3K3A-APC (<10 percent of normal), high-dose bolus dosing in healthy volunteers can achieve circulating APC levels that are 100-fold higher than those used in the PROWESS or PROWESS-SHOCK sepsis trials without notable anticoagulant effects.[46,49,246]

Cellular Receptors for Physiologic Effects of Activated Protein C on Cells

The ability of exogenously administered APC to alter gene-expression profiles of cultured endothelial cells, to stabilize endothelial barriers, to reduce lethality caused by endotoxin in murine sepsis models, to prevent apoptosis of stressed endothelial cells, and to provide neuroprotection requires EPCR and PAR-1, strongly supporting the EPCR–PAR-1 cell-signaling pathway as key for APC's pharmacologic benefits (see Fig. 114–4).[7,8,40–43,221,225,229,233,234,236,237,244,248–251]

Although few details are known about intracellular mechanisms for APC's multiple cytoprotective actions, some mechanistic details for APC's cell signaling have become clear, as depicted in Fig. 114–6.[8] Multiple considerations help explain how PAR-1 can mediate thrombin's disruption of endothelial barrier leading to vascular leakage while, paradoxically, the same receptor mediates APC's endothelial barrier protection, preventing vascular leakage.[249,250] First, PAR-1–mediated APC signaling occurs in caveolae microdomains that contain EPCR whereas PAR-1–mediated thrombin signaling is not limited to caveolae (Fig. 114–6).[252,253] Second, different cleavages in the extracellular N-terminus of PAR-1, either at the canonical Arg41 thrombin-cleavage site (i.e., widely recognized as the essential thrombin cleavage site) or at the novel Arg46 APC-cleavage site, results in very different signaling initiated by different tethered N-terminal peptide sequences which begin at either residue 42 or residue 47.[124,254,255] Third, following thrombin cleavage at Arg41, PAR-1 initiates signaling involving G proteins, extracellular signal-regulated kinase (ERK)1/2 and RhoA, whereas, following APC cleavage at Arg46, PAR-1 initiates signaling involving β-arrestin-2, phosphatidylinositide 3′-kinase (PI3K)/Akt, and Rac1.[256] Fourth, peptides mimicking the N-terminus of cleaved PAR-1 are peptide agonists with pharmacologic effects resembling those of the respective proteases that cleave PAR-1 differentially. For example, "thrombin receptor activating peptides (TRAPs)" that begin with Ser 42 promote G-protein–mediated signaling similar to thrombin. In contrast, peptides that begins with Asn 47 (TR47) promote APC-like signaling.[254] TRAP but not TR47 promotes ERK1/2 phosphorylation on endothelial cells whereas TR47 but not TRAP promotes Akt phosphorylation.[254] The different and opposite induction of signaling pathways is also mirrored in different and

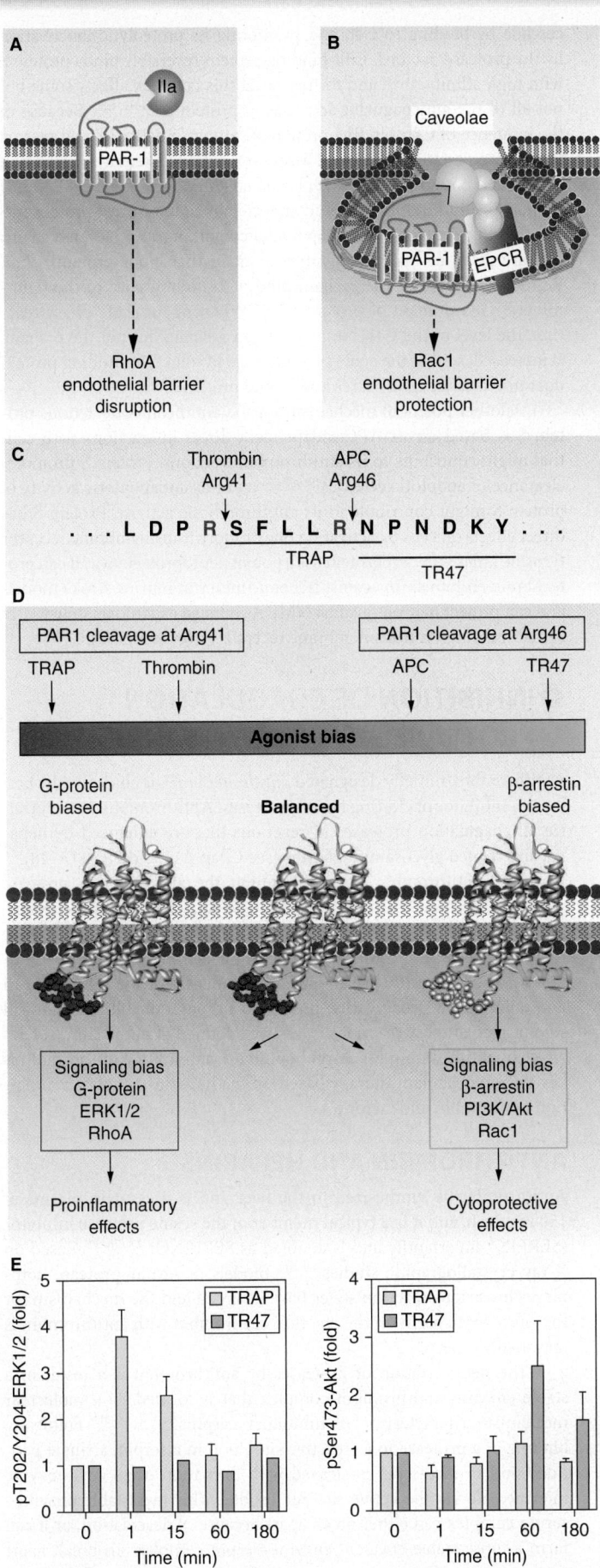

Figure 114–6. Biased protease-activated receptor (PAR)-1 signaling dependent on activation by thrombin or activated protein C (APC). Activation of PAR-1 by thrombin results in endothelial barrier-disruptive signaling (**A**) but activation of PAR-1 by APC in caveolae that also contain endothelial cell protein C receptor (EPCR) results in endothelial barrier-protective signaling (**B**).[252,253] The different PAR-1 signaling induced by thrombin and APC are caused by different proteolysis cleavage sites in PAR-1 for thrombin and APC.[254] Thrombin activates PAR-1 by cleavage at Arg41 (**C**). Synthetic agonist peptides with the N-terminal tethered-ligand sequence beginning with residue 42 are known as TRAP (thrombin receptor-activating peptide) and cause thrombin-like effects on cells. APC activates PAR-1 by cleavage at Arg46 (**C**). A synthetic agonist peptide with the N-terminal tethered-ligand sequence beginning with residue 47 (TR47) causes APC-like effects on cells. Activation of PAR-1 by thrombin or TRAP induces PAR-1 conformations such that the intracellular loops of PAR-1 preferentially interact with G proteins (termed "G-protein biased") resulting in G-protein–dependent signaling whereas activation of PAR-1 by APC or TR47 induces PAR-1 conformations that preferentially interact with β-arrestin-2 (termed "β-arrestin biased") resulting in β-arrestin-2–dependent signaling (**D**).[254,256] The implication of biased PAR-1 signaling are evident by the differences in phosphorylation of extracellular signal-regulated kinase (ERK)1/2 compared to Akt because TRAP, but not TR47, induces phosphorylation of ERK1/2, whereas TR47 but not TRAP induces phosphorylation of Akt (**E**).[254] (*Reproduced with permission of Griffin JH, Zlokovic BV, Mosnier LO: Activated protein C: Biased for translation.* Blood *125(19):2898–2907, 2015.*)

opposite functional effects, as thrombin peptide and TRAP cause endothelial barrier disruption and proinflammatory effects whereas APC and the TR47 peptide cause barrier-protective and antiinflammatory effects. Thus, PAR-1 displays biased signaling depending on the activation cleavage sites and the generated tethered-ligand with absolutely opposing outcomes for the cell, the tissue, and the host depending on which coagulation system protease, thrombin or APC, is cleaving PAR-1.

Other receptors are recognized that may also play key roles for APC's beneficial signaling effects, including PAR-3 and sphingosine-1-phosphate receptor-1.[249,250,257,258] ApoER2 can initiate Disabled-1-dependent pathway activation of the PI3K-Akt cell-survival pathway, which may ultimately help explain additional aspects of APC's cytoprotection.[259]

Although most studies demonstrating the cell-signaling activities of APC have focused on pharmacologic levels of APC, several reports of murine injury models demonstrate the physiologic importance of cell signaling by endogenous APC,[260-262] implying that defects in APC's endogenous cytoprotective actions might have pathophysiologic relevance. Future investigations on APC cellular receptors and on intracellular mechanisms involved in the protein C cellular pathway will likely provide novel clinical insights with diagnostic and therapeutic potential.

INHIBITION OF ACTIVATED PROTEIN C

Blood contains circulating APC in a well-defined normal concentration range that contributes to antithrombotic surveillance mechanisms and possibly to homeostatic cell signaling.[15,142,144] Circulating APC levels are determined by the balance between countervailing mechanisms for APC generation and for APC inhibition and clearance. APC generation is influenced by protein C zymogen levels, endogenous thrombin generation, and the availability of thrombomodulin and EPCR. Clearance of circulating APC is based on inhibition of APC by protease inhibitors and clearance of APC:inhibitor complexes.[263-269] The major plasma inhibitors of APC include α_1-antitrypsin, protein C inhibitor, and α_2-macroglobulin.

ACTIVATED PROTEIN C–INDEPENDENT ANTICOAGULANT ACTIVITY OF PROTEIN S

Because hereditary protein S deficiency[270,271] is strongly linked to increased venous thrombosis risk (Chap. 130), protein S is a significant physiologic anticoagulant factor.[71,198] In addition to its anticoagulant cofactor activity for APC, protein S can also inhibit coagulation reactions independently of APC. Several plausible mechanisms have been described for protein S's anticoagulant activity independent of APC. First, protein S can bind directly to procoagulant factors Xa and Va and thereby inhibit directly the activity of the prothrombinase complex.[11-13] The thrombin-sensitive region and the EGF3 domains of protein S (see Fig. 114–5) likely bind factor Xa, contributing to APC-independent anticoagulant activity.[206,272,273] Second, protein S can also bind factor VIIIa and inhibit activation of factor X by factor IXa–factor VIIIa complexes.[274-276] Third, protein S binds tissue factor pathway inhibitor (TFPI) and enhances its ability to inhibit factor Xa.[277-279] Zn^{2+} ions might play a key role for APC-independent protein S activity.[280] It is not easy to decipher the relative importance of each of these or other mechanisms for APC-independent anticoagulant activities of protein S or to establish their physiologic relevance, but infusions of protein S without APC are antithrombotic in baboon thrombosis models.[281]

The activities of protein S can be strongly influenced by C4b-binding protein, a plasma protein that enhances inactivation of the complement

cascade by binding to C4b and promoting its proteolytic inactivation by the protease, factor I. C4b-binding protein reversibly binds protein S with high affinity,[282-284] and formation of this complex affects some but not all of the anticoagulant activities of protein S.[71,198,271,285] Because of the influence of C4b-binding protein on protein S activities and plasma levels, interpretation of clinical assays for protein S requires evaluation of free and bound protein S as plasma contains approximately 240 nM protein S–C4b-binding protein complexes and 120 nM free protein S.[283] C4b-binding protein is a heteropolymer containing six or seven α chains that are disulfide-linked to a single β chain that binds protein S.[286,287] Residues 30 to 45 of the β chain bind with high affinity to the C-terminal SHBG domain of protein S.[65,288,289] During an acute phase reaction, the level of the C4b-binding protein α chain, but not the β chain, is increased, so that the acute phase change in total C4b-binding protein does not alter the level of free and bound protein S.[290]

Another potential mechanism for the antithrombotic actions protein S is based on its APC-independent direct interactions with cells that might contribute to its antithrombotic actions. Protein S promotes clearance of apoptotic cells,[68,71,198,291-294] and this antiapoptotic activity of protein S might contribute to its antithrombotic activity. Protein S has direct effects on cells by activating one or more transmembrane receptor tyrosine kinases.[68,198,292] Protein S is a potent neuroprotectant as it can protect brain endothelium against ischemic injury in murine stroke models and can protect neurons against NMDA-induced excitotoxic injury, presumably acting via transmembrane receptor tyrosine kinases.[295-299]

INHIBITION OF COAGULATION PROTEASES BY PROTEASE INHIBITORS

Antithrombin, initially designated *antithrombin III*, is clinically the best known inhibitor of clotting factor proteases. Antithrombin can neutralize all coagulation proteases in reactions that are enhanced by heparin and related glycosaminoglycans (see Chap. 113 and Fig. 113–28).[300] However, antithrombin does not inhibit the anticoagulant protease APC. TFPI can neutralize factors VIIa and Xa, proteases of the extrinsic coagulation pathway.[277,278,301-303] In addition, other plasma protease inhibitors such as α_1-antitrypsin, heparin cofactor II, protein C inhibitor, α_2-macroglobulin, or protein Z–dependent protease inhibitor, can neutralize various coagulation proteases, although the ultimate clinical significance of these reactions is less-well defined than the clinical relevance of antithrombin for thrombophilia (Chap. 130). Antithrombin is key for anticoagulant therapy based on the heparin-stimulated inhibition of thrombin and factor Xa.

ANTITHROMBIN AND HEPARINS

Antithrombin is synthesized in the liver and is present in plasma at 150 mcg/mL, and it is a typical member of the serine protease inhibitor (SERPIN) superfamily and is denoted as SERPINC1.[300,304-306] Based on X-ray crystallographic studies,[307-311] models of serpin–protease complexes in various reaction states have emerged and the mechanism for the effects of heparin on the reaction of thrombin with antithrombin is reasonably clear.

The neutralization of proteases by antithrombin is a result of a stable enzyme–antithrombin complex that is formed by a molecular mechanism characteristic of inhibitory serpins.[304-307,309-312] Following binding of a protease to a "reactive site" loop in a serpin, a single peptide bond in the serpin is cleaved with formation of an acyl-enzyme intermediate via the active site Ser residue. This metastable enzyme–serpin complex can either break apart because of deacylation, or it can form a more stable covalent enzyme–serpin complex. To break apart the enzyme–serpin covalent complex, deacylation liberates the cleaved product and regenerates the active site Ser residue of the protease. However, serpins have an ability to undergo major conformational changes following cleavage at the reactive site residue that can distort that protease's active site region and lock the enzyme into the protease–serpin complex in which both the serpin and the protease are essentially deformed.[304–307,309–312] The dominant structural feature of native serpins is a large five-stranded β-sheet that defines the structure of an ellipsoidal protein. Following cleavage at the reactive residue in the reactive center loop by a protease, this extended loop is able to partially or completely insert itself into the five-stranded β-sheet, forming a very stable six-stranded β-sheet. If this insertion reaction proceeds before deacylation occurs, then the protease remains covalently attached to the reactive center P1 residue through the protease's active site Ser residue, and a stable covalent protease–inhibitor complex with each protein in an altered conformation is formed.[307,308]

Heparin enhancement of the rate of reaction between antithrombin and thrombin or other clotting factors is caused by two distinct effects of heparin, one involving conformational effects on antithrombin and the other involving "approximation" effects on both antithrombin and thrombin.[300,307,308,311–315] For the first effect, a particular pentasaccharide sequence within heparin binds antithrombin and potently causes a conformational change that converts antithrombin from its native state of moderate reactivity to a conformation with relatively high reactivity. This pentasaccharide contains a specific sulfated sequence of glucosamine and iduronic acid residues,[300,307,308,311–315] and when it is present in a large heparin molecule, in low-molecular-weight heparin, or in a synthetic pentasaccharide, it alters antithrombin conformation and greatly accelerates the reaction of antithrombin, especially with factor Xa. Synthetic pentasaccharides, such as fondaparinux, which are analogues of the naturally occurring sequence, are often termed to be indirect factor Xa inhibitors and have significant clinical utility. For the second mechanistic effect, namely the approximation effect, unfractionated heparin or low-molecular-weight heparins simultaneously bind to antithrombin and the target protease to promote frequent and geometrically productive encounters between protease and inhibitor, thus increasing the reaction rate. Heparan sulfates to some extent can also act in this manner.

The mature antithrombin polypeptide chain contains 432-amino-acid residues after cleavage of a propeptide from a 464-amino-acid-residue precursor.[316] It has four sites for N-linked carbohydrate attachment, one of which (Asn135) is variably glycosylated, giving rise to a β-isoform that has higher affinity for heparin.[317,318] Heparin binding to antithrombin is mediated by a number of positively charged Arg and Lys residues in the N-terminal region of the molecule, including Lys11, Arg13, Arg47, Lys114, Lys125, and Arg129, whereas the reactive center loop containing the scissile peptide bond at Arg393-Ser394 is near the C-terminus.[311]

ANTITHROMBIN GENE

The antithrombin gene comprising seven exons and six introns spans 13.4 kb and is located on chromosome 1q23–25 (see Table 114–1).[319,320]

ANTITHROMBIN MUTATIONS

Hereditary deficiencies of antithrombin are risk factors for venous thrombosis (Chap. 130). More than 100 different antithrombin mutations are associated with thrombosis. An extensive database of mutations is published[321] and is available at http://www1.imperial.ac.uk/departmentofmedicine/divisions/experimentalmedicine/haematology/coag/antithrombin/.

Mutations that cause antithrombin deficiency are scattered throughout the gene. Molecular defects can be classified as type I, characterized by parallel decreases in antigen and activity, or type II, characterized by circulating dysfunctional molecules such that plasma has decreased functional activity but normal or near-normal antigen levels. Type II defects are further classified based on whether the dysfunction involves only reactive center defects that can be tested in the absence of heparin, only heparin-binding defects that can be tested only in the presence of heparin, or both of these defects (pleiotropic effects). Reactive center defects carry the largest risk of thrombosis, whereas heparin-binding defects are associated with less risk of venous thrombosis (Chap. 130).

● TISSUE FACTOR PATHWAY INHIBITOR

TFPI, also known as *lipoprotein-associated coagulation inhibitor* or *extrinsic pathway inhibitor*, has a predicted mature protein sequence of 276 residues and a Mr of 34,000. However, TFPI is a complex protein and has at least three isoforms in blood vessels.[277,301–303,322–327] There are two alternatively spliced forms of TFPI designated TFPIα and TFPIβ (Fig. 114–7).[323,324]

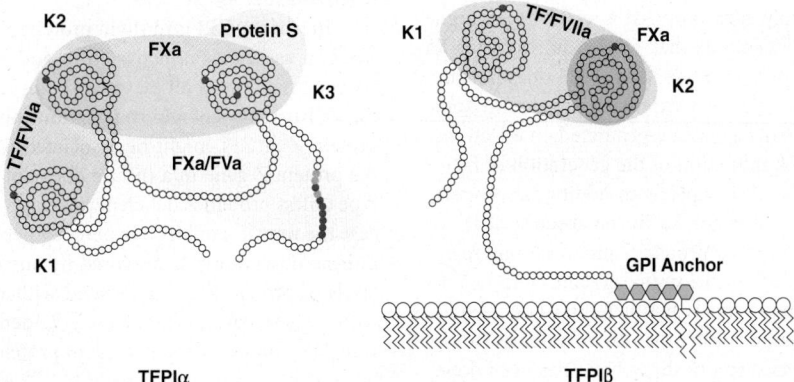

Figure 114–7. Tissue factor pathway inhibitor (TFPI) exists in multiple forms, TFPIα and TFPIβ, because of alternative splicing. Mature, full-length TFPIα is a multivalent protease inhibitor containing three Kunitz-type protease inhibitor domains (**K1**, **K2**, and **K3**) and a highly positively charged basic amino acid cluster near the C-terminus *(blue circles)*. TFPIβ contains K1 and K2 but lacks K3 and the basic amino acid cluster, but it can acquire a glycosylphosphatidylinositol (GPI) moiety that anchors it to cell membranes. As indicated by color overlays, K1 and K2 inhibit factor (**F**) VIIa and FXa, respectively. Both TFPIα and TFPIβ can form a quaternary complex with tissue factor (**TF**), FVIIa and FXa. However, TFPIα but not TFPIβ can interact with protein S or certain forms of FVa/FV via K3 or the positive amino acid cluster, respectively. Via such interactions, protein S or FVa/FV can promote inhibition of FXa with no involvement of FVIIa or tissue factor. TFPIα is the predominant form in plasma, whereas TFPIβ is the predominant form on the endothelium. *(Reproduced with permission from Wood JP, Ellery PE, Maroney SA, Mast AE: Biology of tissue factor pathway inhibitor. Blood 123(19):2934–2943, 2014.)*

TFPIα is the full-length mature protein that contains an acidic N-terminal sequence, three homologous but distinct Kunitz-type protease inhibitor domains (K1, K2, K3), and a C-terminal positively charged basic amino acid sequence (Fig. 114–7). TFPIβ contains K1 and K2 but an unrelated sequence replaces the K3 domain and the C-terminus. TFPIβ can be covalently modified by addition of glycosylphosphatidylinositol (GPI) that localizes TFPIβ to cell membranes (Fig. 114–7). Some TFPI in plasma is present as a disulfide-linked heterodimer of TFPI–apolipoprotein A-II,[327,328] but the functional significance of the apoA-II appendage is unknown. TFPI in its multiple forms is a significant inhibitor of the coagulation pathways that can function synergistically with the protein C pathway and antithrombin to suppress thrombin generation.

TFPI is synthesized by endothelial cells, megakaryocytes, and smooth muscle cells.[301-303] Free TFPI in plasma is TFPIα but it is a minor fraction of the amount of TFPI in blood vessels. More than half of TFPIα in plasma is associated with lipoproteins, especially HDL and low-density lipoprotein. TFPIα is also the main form within platelet and it is secreted by activated platelets. A substantial amount of TFPIα is released from the vessel wall when heparin is infused.[329] TFPIβ is membrane bound, especially to endothelium, because of its GPI anchor.

The interaction of TFPI with lipoproteins reduces its anticoagulant activity measured *in vitro* though the physiologic significance of TFPI's binding to various lipoproteins remains uncertain. In addition to binding lipoproteins, TFPIα but not TFPIβ binds to protein S and to certain forms of factor Va/factor V.[277-279,330-333] Different regions of TFPIα, namely the K3 domain or the basic amino acid cluster, respectively, are responsible for binding protein S or factors Va/V (see Fig. 114–7). Inhibition of factor Xa by TFPIα is accelerated by protein S and by certain but not all forms of factor Va (see below).

TFPI neutralizes factors Xa and VIIa by multiple complicated mechanisms.[277,301-303] In each mechanism, the K1 domain binds and inhibits factor VIIa while the K2 domain inhibits factor Xa (see Fig. 114–7). No protease has yet been identified as the target of the K3 protease inhibitor domain. In one mechanism, initially the K2 domain of TFPI reacts with and inhibits the enzyme activity of factor Xa. Subsequently, this binary complex reacts with factor VIIa in the tissue factor–factor VIIa complex to form a quaternary protein complex on a membrane with both proteases neutralized. In an alternative proposed scheme, TFPI first reacts with factor VIIa in a tissue factor–factor VIIa complex that has generated factor Xa, and thereafter it rapidly reacts with factor Xa before it can dissociate from the ternary tissue factor–factor VIIa–factor Xa complex. Possibly each proposal is valid. Some argue that because some kinetic studies showed that TFPI requires factor Xa for kinetically favorable reactions with factor VIIa, TFPI does not shut off the initiation of the extrinsic pathway by tissue factor until some significant though small amount of factor Xa is generated, in which case TFPI provides negative feedback inhibition of the generation of factor Xa by the factor VIIa–tissue factor complex. An additional property of TFPIα involves its inhibition of factor Xa in the absence of factor VIIa, and this reaction is accelerated by protein S and by certain forms of factor Va.[277-279,330-333] In contrast to the anticoagulant factors, antithrombin, protein C, and protein S, for which hereditary deficiencies are linked to significantly increased risk for venous thrombosis (Chap. 130), no clear pattern for increased risk of thrombosis has been definitively established for TFPI deficiency in humans. In mice, knockout of TFPI is embryonically lethal.[334] In a highly informative kindred that presented with a serious bleeding diathesis, highly elevated plasma TFPI levels were linked to increased bleeding risk, indicating that TFPI functions in man as a physiologically significant inhibitor of coagulation.[322,332] The genetic mutation causing elevated plasma TFPI levels was in the factor V gene, not the TFPI gene. The mutated factor V, named "factor V-short," has a higher affinity for TFPIα than wild-type factor

V, thereby binding more TFPIα and prolonging its half-life. Factor V-short may also enhance inhibition of factor Xa by TFPI with the effect of increasing bleeding risk. This genetic disorder, as well as previous studies showing that inhibition of TFPI reduced bleeding in preclinical hemophilia models, lends support for ongoing efforts to develop TFPI inhibitors for reducing bleeding in some hemophilia subjects, especially those with anti–factor VIII inhibitors.

TFPI GENE

The sequence of TFPI was established from cloning of its complementary DNA. The gene contains nine exons, spans 85 kb, and is located on chromosome 2q31–32.1 (see Table 114–1).[335,336]

● OTHER PROTEASE INHIBITORS

HEPARIN COFACTOR II

Heparin cofactor II, a serpin whose inhibitory activity is enhanced by dermatan sulfate, inhibits thrombin *in vivo* and *in vitro* by an approximation mechanism.[337-340] A few reports link heparin cofactor II deficiency to venous thrombosis, but no significant clinical relevance has been established.[341] Curiously, a severe heparin cofactor II deficiency was reported in an asymptomatic subject.[342] Some studies imply that heparin cofactor II may play significant roles in arterial vascular wall processes, but definitive mechanisms remain to be elucidated.

PROTEIN Z–DEPENDENT PROTEASE INHIBITOR

Protein Z–dependent protease inhibitor (ZPI) is a plasma serpin that inhibits factors Xa, XIa, and IXa, but not factor XIIa or thrombin.[343-350] Protein Z, which is a vitamin K–dependent protein that contains a GLA domain, two EGF-like domains, and a protease-like domain,[351] stimulates factor Xa inhibition by ZPI. Curiously, the protease-like domain of protein Z lacks any protease activity because it has mutations at two of the three active site triad residues. The major hypothesis for stimulation of inhibition of factor Xa by protein Z is based on a structural model in which three proteins assemble on a phospholipid membrane via the two GLA domains (see Fig. 114–7).[351] In this putative ternary complex, the protease-like domain and the second EGF-like domain of protein Z bind ZPI in an alignment that facilitates reaction of factor Xa with the reactive center loop of ZPI.

In plasma, ZPI is in slight protein molar excess over protein Z with which it associates noncovalently, and it has been speculated, but not proven, that almost all plasma protein Z is associated with ZPI.[352-357] If the ZPI is a physiologic coagulation inhibitor, the deficiency of either protein Z or ZPI might be associated with thrombosis. Knocking out the protein Z gene in a mouse does not produce a remarkable phenotype unless protein Z deficiency coexists with factor V Leiden, in which case the mouse exhibits a hypercoagulable, prothrombotic state.[353] This murine observation is mirrored by one clinical report that subnormal levels of protein Z are associated with venous thrombosis in subjects who are heterozygous for factor V Leiden.[354] Some associations between venous thrombosis and defects in protein Z or ZPI have been reported but not uniformly confirmed.[352,354-357] An association with peripheral arterial disease was reported.[358] However, to date no convincing pattern between thrombosis and defects in either protein Z or ZPI has been firmly established.

OTHER MINOR PROTEASE INHIBITORS

Thrombin in plasma can be inhibited not only by antithrombin but also by α_2-macroglobulin, an acute-phase reactant. No association between defects in bleeding or thrombosis has been confirmed for this inhibitor. In purified reaction mixtures, protein C inhibitor also efficiently neutralizes thrombin in the presence of thrombomodulin,[359] although no studies show that this is a physiologic reaction or that it is associated with thrombosis.

REFERENCES

1. MacFarlane RG: An enzyme cascade in the blood clotting mechanism and its function as a biochemical amplifier. *Nature* 202:498–499, 1964.
2. Davie EW, Ratnoff OD: Waterfall sequence for intrinsic blood clotting. *Science* 145(3638):1310–1312, 1964.
3. Furie B, Furie BC: Mechanisms of thrombus formation. *N Engl J Med* 359(9):938–949, 2008.
4. Lammle B, Griffin JH: Formation of the fibrin clot: The balance of procoagulant and inhibitory factors. *Clin Haematol* 14(2):281–342, 1985.
5. van de Wouwer M, Collen D, Conway EM: Thrombomodulin-protein C-EPCR system: Integrated to regulate coagulation and inflammation. *Arterioscler Thromb Vasc Biol* 24(8):1374–1383, 2004.
6. Griffin JH: The thrombin paradox. *Nature* 378(6555):337–338, 1995.
7. Mosnier LO, Zlokovic BV, Griffin JH: The cytoprotective protein C pathway. *Blood* 109(8):3161–3172, 2007.
8. Griffin JH, Zlokovic BV, Mosnier LO: Activated protein C: Biased for translation. *Blood* 125(19):2898–2907, 2015.
9. Fukudome K, Esmon CT: Identification, cloning, and regulation of a novel endothelial cell protein C/activated protein C receptor. *J Biol Chem* 269(42):26486–26491, 1994.
10. Rao LV, Esmon CT, Pendurthi UR: Endothelial cell protein C receptor: A multiliganded and multifunctional receptor. *Blood* 124(10):1553–1562, 2014.
11. Heeb MJ, Mesters RM, Tans G, et al: Binding of protein S to factor Va associated with inhibition of prothrombinase that is independent of activated protein C. *J Biol Chem* 268(4):2872–2877, 1993.
12. Heeb MJ, Rosing J, Bakker HM, et al: Protein S binds to and inhibits factor Xa. *Proc Natl Acad Sci U S A* 91(7):2728–2732, 1994.
13. Hackeng TM, van 't Veer C, Meijers JC, Bouma BN: Human protein S inhibits prothrombinase complex activity on endothelial cells and platelets via direct interactions with factors Va and Xa. *J Biol Chem* 269(33):21051–21058, 1994.
14. Morrissey JH, Macik BG, Neuenschwander PF, Comp PC: Quantitation of activated factor VII levels in plasma using a tissue factor mutant selectively deficient in promoting factor VII activation. *Blood* 81(3):734–744, 1993.
15. Gruber A, Griffin JH: Direct detection of activated protein C in blood from human subjects. *Blood* 79(9):2340–2348, 1992.
16. Nossel HL, Yudelman I, Canfield RE, et al: Measurement of fibrinopeptide A in human blood. *J Clin Invest* 54(1):43–53, 1974.
17. Nossel HL: Radioimmunoassay of fibrinopeptides in relation to intravascular coagulation and thrombosis. *N Engl J Med* 295(8):428–432, 1976.
18. Bauer KA, Rosenberg RD: The pathophysiology of the prethrombotic state in humans: Insight gained from studies using markers of hemostatic system activation. *Blood* 70(2):343–350, 1987.
19. Bauer KA, Kass BL, ten Cate H, et al: Detection of factor X activation in humans. *Blood* 74(6):2007–2015, 1989.
20. Bauer KA, Kass BL, ten Cate H, et al: Factor IX is activated *in vivo* by the tissue factor mechanism. *Blood* 76(4):731–736, 1990.
21. Jesty J, Beltrami E, Willems G: Mathematical analysis of a proteolytic positive-feedback loop: Dependence of lag time and enzyme yields on the initial conditions and kinetic parameters. *Biochemistry* 32(24):6266–6274, 1993.
22. Beltrami E, Jesty J: Mathematical analysis of activation thresholds in enzyme-catalyzed positive feedbacks: Application to the feedbacks of blood coagulation. *Proc Natl Acad Sci U S A* 92(19):8744–8748, 1995.
23. Nicolaes GAF, Dahlbäck B: Factor V and thrombotic disease: Description of a Janus-faced protein. *Arterioscler Thromb Vasc Biol* 22(4):530–538, 2002.
24. Stenflo J: A new vitamin K-dependent protein. Purification from bovine plasma and preliminary characterization. *J Biol Chem* 251(2):355–363, 1976.
25. Seegers WH, Novoa E, Henry RL, Hassouna HI: Relationship of "new" vitamin K-dependent protein C and "old" autoprothrombin II-a. *Thromb Res* 8(5):543–552, 1976.
26. Kisiel W: Human plasma protein C: Isolation, characterization, and mechanism of activation by alpha-thrombin. *J Clin Invest* 64(3):761–769, 1979.
27. Foster DC, Davie EW: Characterization of a cDNA coding for human protein C. *Proc Natl Acad Sci U S A* 81(15):4766–4770, 1984.
28. Beckmann RJ, Schmidt RJ, Santerre RF, et al: The structure and evolution of a 461 amino acid human protein C precursor and its messenger RNA, based upon the DNA sequence of cloned human liver cDNAs. *Nucleic Acids Res* 13(14):5233–5247, 1985.
29. Griffin JH, Evatt B, Zimmerman TS, et al: Deficiency of protein C in congenital thrombotic disease. *J Clin Invest* 68(5):1370–1373, 1981.
30. Mather T, Oganessyan V, Hof P, et al: The 2.8 Å crystal structure of Gla-domainless activated protein C. *EMBO J* 15(24):6822–6831, 1996.
31. Kurosawa S, Galvin JB, Esmon NL, Esmon CT: Proteolytic formation and properties of functional domains of thrombomodulin. *J Biol Chem* 262(5):2206–2212, 1987.
32. Jhingan A, Zhang L, Christiansen WT, Castellino FJ: The activities of recombinant gamma-carboxyglutamic-acid-deficient mutants of activated human protein C toward human coagulation factor Va and factor VIII in purified systems and in plasma. *Biochemistry* 33(7):1869–1875, 1994.
33. Regan LM, Mollica JS, Rezaie AR, Esmon CT: The interaction between the endothelial cell protein C receptor and protein C is dictated by the gamma-carboxyglutamic acid domain of protein C. *J Biol Chem* 272(42):26279–26284, 1997.
34. Greengard JS, Fisher CL, Villoutreix B, Griffin JH: Structural basis for type I and type II deficiencies of antithrombotic plasma protein C: Patterns revealed by three-dimensional molecular modelling of mutations of the protease domain. *Proteins* 18(4):367–380, 1994.
35. Gale AJ, Heeb MJ, Griffin JH: The autolysis loop of activated protein C interacts with factor Va and differentiates between the Arg506 and Arg306 cleavage sites. *Blood* 96(2):585–593, 2000.
36. Friedrich U, Nicolaes GAF, Villoutreix BO, Dahlbäck B: Secondary substrate-binding exosite in the serine protease domain of activated protein C important for cleavage at Arg-506 but not at Arg-306 in factor Va. *J Biol Chem* 276(25):23105–23108, 2001.
37. Rezaie AR: Exosite-dependent regulation of the protein C anticoagulant pathway. *Trends Cardiovasc Med* 13(1):8–15, 2003.
38. Gale AJ, Griffin JH: Characterization of a thrombomodulin binding site on protein C and its comparison to an activated protein C binding site for factor Va. *Proteins* 54(3):433–441, 2004.
39. Gale AJ, Tsavaler A, Griffin JH: Molecular characterization of an extended binding site for coagulation factor Va in the positive exosite of activated protein C. *J Biol Chem* 277(32):28836–28840, 2002.
40. Mosnier LO, Gale AJ, Yegneswaran S, Griffin JH: Activated protein C variants with normal cytoprotective but reduced anticoagulant activity. *Blood* 104(6):1740–1745, 2004.
41. Mosnier LO, Yang XV, Griffin JH: Activated protein C mutant with minimal anticoagulant activity, normal cytoprotective activity, and preservation of thrombin activable fibrinolysis inhibitor-dependent cytoprotective functions. *J Biol Chem* 282(45):33022–33033, 2007.
42. Mosnier LO, Zampolli A, Kerschen EJ, et al: Hyper-antithrombotic, non-cytoprotective Glu149Ala-activated protein C mutant. *Blood* 113(23):5970–5978, 2009.
43. Bae JS, Yang L, Manithody C, Rezaie AR: Engineering a disulfide bond to stabilize the calcium-binding loop of activated protein C eliminates its anticoagulant but not its protective signaling properties. *J Biol Chem* 282(12):9251–9259, 2007.
44. Yang L, Bae JS, Manithody C, Rezaie AR: Identification of a specific exosite on activated protein C for interaction with protease activated receptor 1. *J Biol Chem* 282(35):25493–25500, 2007.
45. Dreyfus M, Magny JF, Bridey F, et al: Treatment of homozygous protein C deficiency and neonatal purpura fulminans with a purified protein C concentrate. *N Engl J Med* 325(22):1565–1568, 1991.
46. Bernard GR, Vincent JL, Laterre PF, et al: Efficacy and safety of recombinant human activated protein C for severe sepsis. *N Engl J Med* 344(10):699–709, 2001.
47. Gruber A, Griffin JH, Harker LA, Hanson SR: Inhibition of platelet-dependent thrombus formation by human activated protein C in a primate model. *Blood* 73(3):639–642, 1989.
48. Taylor FB Jr, Chang AC, Esmon CT, et al: Protein C prevents the coagulopathic and lethal effects of Escherichia coli infusion in the baboon. *J Clin Invest* 79(3):918–925, 1987.
49. Ranieri VM, Thompson BT, Barie PS, et al: Drotrecogin Alfa (Activated) in Adults with Septic Shock. *N Engl J Med* 366(22):2055–2064, 2012.
50. Kalil AC, LaRosa SP: Effectiveness and safety of drotrecogin alfa (activated) for severe sepsis: A meta-analysis and metaregression. *Lancet Infect Dis* 12(9):678–686, 2012.
51. Christiaans SC, Wagener BM, Esmon CT, Pittet JF: Protein C and acute inflammation: A Clinical and biologic perspective. *Am J Physiol Lung Cell Mol Physiol* 305(7):L455–L466, 2013.
52. Foster DC, Yoshitake S, Davie EW: The nucleotide sequence of the gene for human protein C. *Proc Natl Acad Sci U S A* 82(14):4673–4677, 2013.
53. D'Ursi P, Marino F, Caprera A, et al: ProCMD: A database and 3D web resource for protein C mutants. *BMC Bioinformatics* 8(Suppl 1):S11, 2007.
54. Saunders RE, Perkins SJ: CoagMDB: A database analysis of missense mutations within four conserved domains in five vitamin K-dependent coagulation serine proteases using a text-mining tool. *Hum Mutat* 29(3):333–344, 2008.
55. Greengard JS, Griffin JH, Fisher CL: Possible structural implications of 20 mutations in the protein C protease domain. *Thromb Haemost* 72(6):869–873, 1994.
56. Rovida E, Merati G, D'Ursi P, et al: Identification and computationally-based structural interpretation of naturally occurring variants of human protein C. *Hum Mutat* 28(4):345–355, 2007.
57. Yin T, Miyata T: Dysfunction of protein C anticoagulant system, main genetic risk factor for venous thromboembolism in northeast Asians. *J Thromb Thrombolysis* 37(1):56–65, 2014.
58. Tang L, Lu X, Yu JM, et al: PROC c.574_576del polymorphism: A common genetic risk factor for venous thrombosis in the Chinese population. *J Thromb Haemost* 10(10):2019–2026, 2012.
59. Ding Q, Yang L, Hassanian SM, Rezaie AR: Expression and functional characterisation of natural R147W and K150del variants of protein C in the Chinese population. *Thromb Haemost* 109(4):614–624, 2013.
60. Jalbert LR, Rosen ED, Moons L, et al: Inactivation of the gene for anticoagulant protein C causes lethal perinatal consumptive coagulopathy in mice. *J Clin Invest* 102(8):1481–1488, 1998.
61. DiScipio RG, Davie EW: Characterization of protein S, a gamma-carboxyglutamic acid containing protein from bovine and human plasma. *Biochemistry* 18(5):899–904, 1979.

62. Schwarz HP, Heeb MJ, Wencel-Drake JD, Griffin JH: Identification and quantitation of protein S in human platelets. *Blood* 66(6):1452–1455, 1985.

63. Lundwall A, Dackowski W, Cohen E, et al: Isolation and sequence of the cDNA for human protein S, a regulator of blood coagulation. *Proc Natl Acad Sci U S A* 83(18):6716–6720, 1986.

64. Hoskins J, Norman DK, Beckmann RJ, Long GL: Cloning and characterization of human liver cDNA encoding a protein S precursor. *Proc Natl Acad Sci U S A* 84(2):349–353, 1987.

65. Fernández JA, Heeb MJ, Griffin JH: Identification of residues 413–433 of plasma protein S as essential for binding to C4b-binding protein. *J Biol Chem* 268(22):16788–16794, 1993.

66. Heeb MJ, Kojima Y, Rosing J, et al: C-terminal residues 621–635 of protein S are essential for binding to factor Va. *J Biol Chem* 274(51):36187–36192, 1999.

67. Nyberg P, Dahlback B, Garcia de FP: The SHBG-like region of protein S is crucial for factor V-dependent APC-cofactor function. *FEBS Lett* 433(1–2):28–32, 1998.

68. van der Meer JH, van der Poll T, van 't Veer C: TAM receptors, Gas6 and protein S: Roles in inflammation and hemostasis. *Blood* 123(16):2460–2469, 2014.

69. Ploos van Amstel JK, van der Zanden AL, Bakker E, et al: Two genes homologous with human protein S cDNA are located on chromosome 3. *Thromb Haemost* 58(4):982–987, 1987.

70. Schmidel DK, Tatro AV, Phelps LG, et al: Organization of the human protein S genes. *Biochemistry* 29(34):7845–7852, 1990.

71. Garcia de Frutos P, Fuentes-Prior P, Hurtado B, Sala N: Molecular basis of protein S deficiency. *Thromb Haemost* 98(3):543–556, 2007.

72. Kimura R, Honda S, Kawasaki T, et al: Protein S-K196E mutation as a genetic risk factor for deep vein thrombosis in Japanese patients. *Blood* 107(4):1737–1738, 2006.

73. Pecheniuk NM, Elias DJ, Xu X, Griffin JH: Failure to validate association of gene polymorphisms in EPCR, PAR-1, FSAP and protein S Tokushima with venous thromboembolism among Californians of European ancestry. *Thromb Haemost* 99(2):453–455, 2008.

74. Bertina RM, Ploos van Amstel HK, van Wijngaarden A, et al: Heerlen polymorphism of protein S, an immunologic polymorphism due to dimorphism of residue 460. *Blood* 76(3):538–548, 1990.

75. Esmon CT, Owen WG: Identification of an endothelial cell cofactor for thrombin catalyzed activation of protein C. *Proc Natl Acad Sci U S A* 78(4):2249–2252, 1981.

76. Esmon CT, Owen WG: The discovery of thrombomodulin. *J Thromb Haemost* 2(2):209–213, 2004.

77. Morser J: Thrombomodulin links coagulation to inflammation and immunity. *Curr Drug Targets* 13(3):421–431, 2012.

78. Conway EM: Thrombomodulin and its role in inflammation. *Semin Immunopathol* 34(1):107–125, 2012.

79. Esmon CT, Esmon NL, Harris KW: Complex formation between thrombin and thrombomodulin inhibits both thrombin-catalyzed fibrin formation and factor V activation. *J Biol Chem* 257(14):7944–7947, 1982.

80. Esmon NL, Carroll RC, Esmon CT: Thrombomodulin blocks the ability of thrombin to activate platelets. *J Biol Chem* 258(20):12238–12242, 1983.

81. Esmon CT: The roles of protein C and thrombomodulin in the regulation of blood coagulation. *J Biol Chem* 264(9):4743–4746, 1989.

82. Jackman RW, Beeler DL, Fritze L, et al: Human thrombomodulin gene is intron depleted: Nucleic acid sequences of the cDNA and gene predict protein structure and suggest sites of regulatory control. *Proc Natl Acad Sci U S A* 84(18):6425–6429, 1987.

83. Sadler JE, Lentz SR, Sheehan JP, et al: Structure-function relationships of the thrombin-thrombomodulin interaction. *Haemostasis* 23 Suppl 1:183–193, 1993.

84. Saito H, Maruyama I, Shimazaki S, et al: Efficacy and safety of recombinant human soluble thrombomodulin (ART-123) in disseminated intravascular coagulation: Results of a phase III, randomized, double-blind clinical trial. *J Thromb Haemost* 5(1):31–41, 2007.

85. Healy AM, Rayburn HB, Rosenberg RD, Weiler H: Absence of the blood-clotting regulator thrombomodulin causes embryonic lethality in mice before development of a functional cardiovascular system. *Proc Natl Acad Sci U S A* 92(3):850–854, 1995.

86. Esmon CT: Inflammation and the activated protein C anticoagulant pathway. *Semin Thromb Hemost* 32(Suppl 1):49–60, 2006.

87. Schouten M, Wiersinga WJ, Levi M, van der Poll T: Inflammation, endothelium, and coagulation in sepsis. *J Leukoc Biol* 83(3):536–545, 2008.

88. Delvaeye M, Noris M, de Vriese A, et al: Thrombomodulin mutations in atypical hemolytic-uremic syndrome. *N Engl J Med* 361(4):345–357, 2009.

89. Norlund L, Holm J, Zoller B, Ohlin AK: A common thrombomodulin amino acid dimorphism is associated with myocardial infarction. *Thromb Haemost* 77(2):248–251, 1997.

90. Ireland H, Kunz G, Kyriakoulis K, et al: Thrombomodulin gene mutations associated with myocardial infarction. *Circulation* 96(1):15–18, 1997.

91. Doggen CJ, Kunz G, Rosendaal FR, et al: A mutation in the thrombomodulin gene, 127G to A coding for Ala25Thr, and the risk of myocardial infarction in men. *Thromb Haemost* 80(5):743–748, 1998.

92. Wu KK: Soluble thrombomodulin and coronary heart disease. *Curr Opin Lipidol* 14(4):373–375, 2003.

93. van de Wouwer M, Plaisance S, de Vriese A, et al: The lectin-like domain of thrombomodulin interferes with complement activation and protects against arthritis. *J Thromb Haemost* 4(8):1813–1824, 2006.

94. Mosnier LO, Bouma BN: Regulation of fibrinolysis by thrombin activatable fibrinolysis inhibitor, an unstable carboxypeptidase B that unites the pathways of coagulation and fibrinolysis. *Arterioscler Thromb Vasc Biol* 26(11):2445–2453, 2006.

95. Foley JH, Kim PY, Mutch NJ, Gils A: Insights into thrombin activatable fibrinolysis inhibitor function and regulation. *J Thromb Haemost* 11 Suppl 1:306–315, 2013.

96. Myles T, Nishimura T, Yun TH, et al: Thrombin activatable fibrinolysis inhibitor, a potential regulator of vascular inflammation. *J Biol Chem* 278(51):51059–51067, 2003.

97. Bouwens EA, Stavenuiter F, Mosnier LO: Mechanisms of anticoagulant and cytoprotective actions of the protein C pathway. *J Thromb Haemost* 11(Suppl 1):242–253, 2013.

98. Fukudome K, Esmon CT: Molecular cloning and expression of murine and bovine endothelial cell protein C/activated protein C receptor (EPCR). The structural and functional conservation in human, bovine, and murine EPCR. *J Biol Chem* 270(10):5571–5577, 1995.

99. Regan LM, Stearns-Kurosawa DJ, Kurosawa S, et al: The endothelial cell protein C receptor. Inhibition of activated protein C anticoagulant function without modulation of reaction with proteinase inhibitors. *J Biol Chem* 271(29):17499–17503, 1996.

100. Fukudome K, Kurosawa S, Stearns-Kurosawa DJ, et al: The endothelial cell protein C receptor. Cell surface expression and direct ligand binding by the soluble receptor. *J Biol Chem* 271(29):17491–17498, 1996.

101. Stearns-Kurosawa DJ, Kurosawa S, Mollica JS, et al: The endothelial cell protein C receptor augments protein C activation by the thrombin-thrombomodulin complex. *Proc Natl Acad Sci U S A* 93(19):10212–10216, 1996.

102. Xu J, Esmon NL, Esmon CT: Reconstitution of the human endothelial cell protein C receptor with thrombomodulin in phosphatidylcholine vesicles enhances protein C activation. *J Biol Chem* 274(10):6704–6710, 1999.

103. Fukudome K, Ye X, Tsuneyoshi N, et al: Activation mechanism of anticoagulant protein C in large blood vessels involving the endothelial cell protein C receptor. *J Exp Med* 187(7):1029–1035, 1998.

104. Liang Z, Rosen ED, Castellino FJ: Nucleotide structure and characterization of the murine gene encoding the endothelial cell protein C receptor. *Thromb Haemost* 81(4):585–588, 1999.

105. Ye X, Fukudome K, Tsuneyoshi N, et al: The endothelial cell protein C receptor (EPCR) functions as a primary receptor for protein C activation on endothelial cells in arteries, veins, and capillaries. *Biochem Biophys Res Commun* 259(3):671–677, 1999.

106. Simmonds RE, Lane DA: Structural and functional implications of the intron/exon organization of the human endothelial cell protein C/activated protein C receptor (EPCR) gene: Comparison with the structure of CD1/major histocompatibility complex alpha1 and alpha2 domains. *Blood* 94(2):632–641, 1999.

107. Oganesyan V, Oganesyan N, Terzyan S, et al: The crystal structure of the endothelial protein C receptor and a bound phospholipid. *J Biol Chem* 277(28):24851–24854, 2002.

108. Villoutreix BO, Blom AM, Dahlbäck B: Structural prediction and analysis of endothelial cell protein C/activated protein C receptor. *Protein Eng* 12(10):833–840, 1999.

109. Rezaie AR: Protease-activated receptor signalling by coagulation proteases in endothelial cells. *Thromb Haemost* 112(5): 876–882, 2014.

110. McKelvey K, Jackson CJ, Xue M: Activated protein C: A regulator of human skin epidermal keratinocyte function. *World J Biol Chem* 5(2):169–179, 2014.

111. Danese S, Vetrano S, Zhang L, et al: The protein C pathway in tissue inflammation and injury: Pathogenic role and therapeutic implications. *Blood* 115(6):1121–1130, 2010.

112. Qu D, Wang Y, Esmon NL, Esmon CT: Regulated endothelial protein C receptor shedding is mediated by tumor necrosis factor-alpha converting enzyme/ADAM17. *J Thromb Haemost* 5(2):395–402, 2007.

113. Qu D, Wang Y, Song Y, et al: The Ser219—>Gly dimorphism of the endothelial protein C receptor contributes to the higher soluble protein levels observed in individuals with the A3 haplotype. *J Thromb Haemost* 4(1):229–235, 2006.

114. Kurosawa S, Stearns-Kurosawa DJ, Carson CW, et al: Plasma levels of endothelial cell protein C receptor are elevated in patients with sepsis and systemic lupus erythematosus: Lack of correlation with thrombomodulin suggests involvement of different pathological processes. *Blood* 91(2):725–727, 1998.

115. Kurosawa S, Stearns-Kurosawa DJ, Hidari N, Esmon CT: Identification of functional endothelial protein C receptor in human plasma. *J Clin Invest* 100(2):411–418, 1997.

116. Lopez-Sagaseta J, Puy C, Tamayo I, et al: SPLA2-V inhibits EPCR anticoagulant and antiapoptotic properties by accommodating lysophosphatidylcholine or PAF in the hydrophobic groove. *Blood* 119(12):2914–2921, 2012.

117. Tamayo I, Velasco SE, Puy C, et al: SPLA2-V impairs EPCR-dependent protein C activation and accelerates thrombosis *in vivo*. *J Thromb Haemost* 12(11):1921–1927, 2014.

118. Gu JM, Crawley JT, Ferrell G, et al: Disruption of the endothelial cell protein C receptor gene in mice causes placental thrombosis and early embryonic lethality. *J Biol Chem* 277(45):43335–43343, 2002.

119. Lau CK, Turner L, Jespersen JS, et al: Structural conservation despite huge sequence diversity allows EPCR binding by the pfemp1 family implicated in severe childhood malaria. *Cell Host Microbe* 17(1):118–129, 2015.

120. Turner L, Lavstsen T, Berger SS, et al: Severe malaria is associated with parasite binding to endothelial protein C receptor. *Nature* 498(7455):502–505, 2013.

121. Moxon CA, Wassmer SC, Milner DA Jr, et al: Loss of endothelial protein C receptors links coagulation and inflammation to parasite sequestration in cerebral malaria in African children. *Blood* 122(5):842–851, 2013.

122. Aird WC, Mosnier LO, Fairhurst RM: *Plasmodium falciparum* picks (on) EPCR. *Blood* 123(2):163–167, 2014.

123. Hayashi T, Nakamura H, Okada A, et al: Organization and chromosomal localization of the human endothelial protein C receptor gene. *Gene* 238(2):367–373, 1999.

124. Vu TK, Hung DT, Wheaton VI, Coughlin SR: Molecular cloning of a functional thrombin receptor reveals a novel proteolytic mechanism of receptor activation. *Cell* 64(6):1057–1068, 1991.

125. Kahn ML, Nakanishi-Matsui M, Shapiro MJ, et al: Protease-activated receptors 1 and 4 mediate activation of human platelets by thrombin. *J Clin Invest* 103(6):879–887, 1999.

126. Coughlin SR: Thrombin signaling and protease-activated receptors. *Nature* 407(6801): 258–264, 2000.

127. Macfarlane SR, Seatter MJ, Kanke T, et al: Proteinase-Activated Receptors. *Pharmacol Rev* 53(2):245–282, 2001.

128. Steinhoff M, Buddenkotte J, Shpacovitch V, et al: Proteinase-activated receptors: Transducers of proteinase-mediated signaling in inflammation and immune response. *Endocr Rev* 26(1):1–43, 2005.

129. Leger AJ, Covic L, Kuliopulos A: Protease-activated receptors in cardiovascular diseases. *Circulation* 114(10):1070–1077, 2006.

130. Traynelis SF, Trejo J: Protease-activated receptor signaling: New roles and regulatory mechanisms. *Curr Opin Hematol* 14(3):230–235, 2007.

131. Nakanishi-Matsui M, Zheng YW, Sulciner DJ, et al: PAR3 is a cofactor for PAR4 activation by thrombin. *Nature* 404(6778):609–613, 2000.

132. Sidhu TS, French SL, Hamilton JR: Differential signaling by protease-activated receptors: Implications for therapeutic targeting. *Int J Mol Sci* 15(4):6169–6183, 2014.

133. Hollenberg MD, Mihara K, Polley D, et al: Biased signalling and proteinase-activated receptors (PARs): Targeting inflammatory disease. *Br J Pharmacol* 171(5):1180–1194, 2014.

134. Bahou WF: Protease-activated receptors. *Curr Top Dev Biol* 54:343–369, 2003.

135. Austin KM, Covic L, Kuliopulos A: Matrix metalloproteases and PAR1 activation. *Blood* 121(3):431–439, 2013.

136. Comp PC, Jacocks RM, Ferrell GL, Esmon CT: Activation of protein C in vivo. *J Clin Invest* 70(1):127–134, 1982.

137. Hanson SR, Griffin JH, Harker LA, et al: Antithrombotic effects of thrombin-induced activation of endogenous protein C in primates. *J Clin Invest* 92(4):2003–2012, 1993.

138. Lentz SR, Fernandez JA, Griffin JH, et al: Impaired anticoagulant response to infusion of thrombin in atherosclerotic monkeys associated with acquired defects in the protein C system. *Arterioscler Thromb Vasc Biol* 19(7):1744–1750, 1999.

139. Snow TR, Deal MT, Dickey DT, Esmon CT: Protein C activation following coronary artery occlusion in the in situ porcine heart. *Circulation* 84(1):293–299, 1991.

140. Macko RF, Killewich LA, Fernández JA, et al: Brain-specific protein C activation during carotid artery occlusion in humans. *Stroke* 30(3):542–545, 1999.

141. Petaja J, Pesonen E, Fernandez JA, et al: Cardiopulmonary bypass and activation of antithrombotic plasma protein C. *J Thorac Cardiovasc Surg* 118(3):422–429, 1999.

142. Gruber A, Pal A, Kiss RG, et al: Generation of activated protein C during thrombolysis. *Lancet* 342(8882):1275–1276, 1993.

143. Macko RF, Ameriso SF, Gruber A, et al: Impairments of the protein C system and fibrinolysis in infection-associated stroke. *Stroke* 27(11):2005–2011, 1996.

144. Conard J, Bauer KA, Gruber A, et al: Normalization of markers of coagulation activation with a purified protein C concentrate in adults with homozygous protein C deficiency. *Blood* 82(4):1159–1164, 1993.

145. Taylor FB Jr, Peer GT, Lockhart MS, et al: Endothelial cell protein C receptor plays an important role in protein C activation in vivo. *Blood* 97(6):1685–1688, 2001.

146. Ishii H, Salem HH, Bell CE, et al: Thrombomodulin, an endothelial anticoagulant protein, is absent from the human brain. *Blood* 67(2):362–365, 1986.

147. Bajaj MS, Kuppuswamy MN, Manepalli AN, Bajaj SP: Transcriptional expression of tissue factor pathway inhibitor, thrombomodulin and von Willebrand factor in normal human tissues. *Thromb Haemost* 82:1047–1052, 1999.

148. Wong VL, Hofman FM, Ishii H, Fisher M: Regional distribution of thrombomodulin in human brain. *Brain Res* 556(1):1–5, 1991.

149. Hackeng TM, Tans G, Koppelman SJ, et al: Protein C activation on endothelial cells by prothrombin activation products generated in situ: Meizothrombin is a better protein C activator than alpha-thrombin. *Biochem J* 319(Pt 2):399–405, 1996.

150. Varadi K, Philapitsch A, Santa T, Schwarz HP: Activation and inactivation of human protein C by plasmin. *Thromb Haemost* 71(5):615–621, 1994.

151. Haley PE, Doyle MF, Mann KG: The activation of bovine protein C by factor Xa. *J Biol Chem* 264(27):16303–16310, 1989.

152. Rezaie AR: Rapid activation of protein C by factor Xa and thrombin in the presence of polyanionic compounds. *Blood* 91(12):4572–4580, 1998.

153. Shim K, Zhu H, Westfield LA, Sadler JE: A recombinant murine meizothrombin precursor, prothrombin R157A/R268A, inhibits thrombosis in a model of acute carotid artery injury. *Blood* 104(2):415–419, 2004.

154. Slungaard A, Fernández JA, Griffin JH, et al: Platelet factor 4 enhances generation of activated protein C in vitro and in vivo. *Blood* 102(1):146–151, 2003.

155. Slungaard A, Key NS: Platelet factor 4 stimulates thrombomodulin protein C-activating cofactor activity. A structure-function analysis. *J Biol Chem* 269(41):25549–25556, 1994.

156. Kowalska MA, Zhao G, Zhai L, et al: Modulation of protein C activation by histones, platelet factor 4, and heparinoids: New insights into activated protein C formation. *Arterioscler Thromb Vasc Biol* 34(1):120–126, 2014.

157. Kowalska MA, Rauova L, Poncz M: Role of the platelet chemokine platelet factor 4 (PF4) in hemostasis and thrombosis. *Thromb Res* 125(4):292–296, 2010.

158. Fernandez JA, Petaja J, Gruber A, Griffin JH: Activated protein C correlates inversely with thrombin levels in resting healthy individuals. *Am J Hematol* 56(1):29–31, 1997.

159. Pellequer JL, Gale AJ, Griffin JH, Getzoff ED: Homology models of the C domains of blood coagulation factors V and VIII: A proposed membrane binding mode for FV and FVIII C2 domains. *Blood Cells Mol Dis* 24(4):448–461, 1998.

160. Autin L, Steen M, Dahlbäck B, Villoutreix BO: Proposed structural models of the prothrombinase (FXa-FVa) complex. *Proteins* 63(3):440–450, 2006.

161. Adams TE, Hockin MF, Mann KG, Everse SJ: The crystal structure of activated protein C-inactivated bovine factor Va: Implications for cofactor function. *Proc Natl Acad Sci U S A* 101(24):8918–8923, 2004.

162. Lechtenberg BC, Murray-Rust TA, Johnson DJ, et al: Crystal structure of the prothrombinase complex from the venom of *Pseudonaja textilis*. *Blood* 122(16):2777–2783, 2013.

163. Lee CJ, Wu S, Pedersen LG: A proposed ternary complex model of prothrombinase with prothrombin: Protein-protein docking and molecular dynamics simulations. *J Thromb Haemost* 9(10):2123–2126, 2011.

164. Camire RM, Kalafatis M, Tracy PB: Proteolysis of factor V by cathepsin G and elastase indicates that cleavage at Arg1545 optimizes cofactor function by facilitating factor Xa binding. *Biochemistry* 37(34):11896–11906, 1998.

165. Steen M, Dahlbäck B: Thrombin-mediated proteolysis of factor V resulting in gradual B-domain release and exposure of the factor Xa-binding site. *J Biol Chem* 277(41):38424–38430, 2002.

166. Toso R, Camire RM: Removal of B-domain sequences from factor V rather than specific proteolysis underlies the mechanism by which cofactor function is realized. *J Biol Chem* 279(20):21643–21650, 2004.

167. Thorelli E, Kaufman RJ, Dahlbäck B: Cleavage requirements for activation of factor V by factor Xa. *Eur J Biochem* 247(1):12–20, 1997.

168. Camire RM: A new look at blood coagulation factor V. *Curr Opin Hematol* 18(5):338–342, 2011.

169. Bos MH, Camire RM: A bipartite autoinhibitory region within the B-domain suppresses function in factor V. *J Biol Chem* 287(31):26342–26351, 2012.

170. Fay PJ: Regulation of factor VIIIa in the intrinsic factor Xase. *Thromb Haemost* 82(2):193–200, 1999.

171. Marlar RA, Kleiss AJ, Griffin JH: Mechanism of action of human activated protein C, a thrombin dependent anticoagulant enzyme. *Blood* 59:1067–1072, 1982.

172. Fulcher CA, Gardiner JE, Griffin JH, Zimmerman TS: Proteolytic inactivation of human factor VIII procoagulant protein by activated human protein C and its analogy with factor V. *Blood* 63(2):486–489, 1984.

173. Kalafatis M, Rand MD, Mann KG: The mechanism of inactivation of human factor V and human factor Va by activated protein C. *J Biol Chem* 269(50):31869–31880, 1994.

174. Dahlbäck B, Carlsson M, Svensson PJ: Familial thrombophilia due to a previously unrecognized mechanism characterized by poor anticoagulant response to activated protein C: Prediction of a cofactor to activated protein C. *Proc Natl Acad Sci U S A* 90(3):1004–1008, 1993.

175. Bertina RM, Koelleman BPC, Koster T, et al: Mutations in blood coagulation factor V associated with resistance to activated protein C. *Nature* 369(6475):64–67, 1994.

176. Greengard JS, Sun X, Xu X, et al: Activated protein C resistance caused by Arg506Gln mutation in factor Va. *Lancet* 343(8909):1361–1362, 1994.

177. Sun X, Evatt B, Griffin JH: Blood coagulation factor Va abnormality associated with resistance to activated protein C in venous thrombophilia. *Blood* 83(11):3120–3125, 1994.

178. Zivelin A, Griffin JH, Xu X, et al: A single genetic origin for a common Caucasian risk factor for venous thrombosis. *Blood* 89(2):397–402, 1997.

179. Zivelin A, Mor-Cohen R, Kovalsky V, et al: Prothrombin 20210G>A is an ancestral prothrombotic mutation that occurred in whites approximately 24,000 years ago. *Blood* 107(12):4666–4668, 2006.

180. Heeb MJ, Kojima Y, Greengard JS, Griffin JH: Activated protein C resistance: Molecular mechanisms based on studies using purified Gln506-factor V. *Blood* 85(12):3405–3411, 1995.

181. Rosing J, Hoekema L, Nicolaes GAF, et al: Effects of protein S and factor Xa on peptide bond cleavages during inactivation of factor Va and factor Va R506Q by activated protein C. *J Biol Chem* 270(46):27852–27858, 1995.

182. Gale AJ, Xu X, Pellequer JL, et al: Interdomain engineered disulfide bond permitting elucidation of mechanisms of inactivation of coagulation factor Va by activated protein C. *Protein Sci* 11(9):2091–2101, 2002.

183. Rosing J, Bakker HM, Thomassen MC, et al: Characterization of two forms of human factor Va with different cofactor activities. *J Biol Chem* 268(28):21130–21136, 1993.

184. Nicolaes GAF, Villoutreix BO, Dahlbäck B: Partial glycosylation of Asn2181 in human factor V as a cause of molecular and functional heterogeneity. Modulation of glycosylation efficiency by mutagenesis of the consensus sequence for N-linked glycosylation. *Biochemistry* 38(41):13584–13591, 1999.

185. Fernández JA, Hackeng TM, Kojima K, Griffin JH: The carbohydrate moiety of factor V modulates inactivation by activated protein C. *Blood* 89(12):4348–4354, 1997.

186. Fisher M, Fernández JA, Ameriso SF, et al: Activated protein C resistance in ischemic stroke not due to factor V arginine506—>glutamine mutation. *Stroke* 27(7):1163–1166, 1996.

187. de Visser MCH, Rosendaal FR, Bertina RM: A reduced sensitivity for activated protein C in the absence of factor V Leiden increases the risk of venous thrombosis. *Blood* 93(4):1271–1276, 1999.

188. Rodeghiero F, Tosetto A: Activated protein C resistance and factor V Leiden mutation are independent risk factors for venous thromboembolism. *Ann Intern Med Intern Med* 130(8):643–650, 1999.

189. Griffin JH, Kojima K, Banka CL, et al: High-density lipoprotein enhancement of anticoagulant activities of plasma protein S and activated protein C. *J Clin Invest* 103(2):219–227, 1999.

190. Fernandez JA, Deguchi H, Banka CL, et al: Re-evaluation of the anticoagulant properties of high-density lipoprotein. *Arterioscler Thromb Vasc Biol* 35(3):570–572, 2015.

191. Curvers J, Thomassen MC, Nicolaes GAF, et al: Acquired APC resistance and oral contraceptives: Differences between two functional tests. *Br J Haematol* 105(1):88–94, 1999.

192. Smirnov MD, Safa O, Esmon NL, Esmon CT: Inhibition of activated protein C anticoagulant activity by prothrombin. *Blood* 94(11):3839–3846, 1999.

193. Brugge JM, Tans G, Rosing J, Castoldi E: Protein S levels modulate the activated protein C resistance phenotype induced by elevated prothrombin levels. *Thromb Haemost* 95(2):236–242, 2006.

194. Bakker HM, Tans G, Janssen-Claessen T, et al: The effect of phospholipids, calcium ions and protein S on rate constants of human factor Va inactivation by activated human protein C. *Eur J Biochem* 208(1):171–178, 1992.

195. Smirnov MD, Esmon CT: Phosphatidylethanolamine incorporation into vesicles selectively enhances factor Va inactivation by activated protein C. *J Biol Chem* 269(2):816–819, 1994.

196. Smirnov MD, Triplett DT, Comp PC, et al: On the role of phosphatidylethanolamine in the inhibition of activated protein C activity by antiphospholipid antibodies. *J Clin Invest* 95(1):309–316, 1995.

197. Fernández JA, Kojima K, Petäjä J, et al: Cardiolipin enhances protein C pathway anticoagulant activity. *Blood Cells Mol Dis* 26(2):115–123, 2000.

198. Rezende SM, Simmonds RE, Lane DA: Coagulation, inflammation, and apoptosis: Different roles for protein S and the protein S-C4b binding protein complex. *Blood* 103(4):1192–1201, 2004.

199. Yegneswaran S, Smirnov MD, Safa O, et al: Relocating the active site of activated protein C eliminates the need for its protein S cofactor. A fluorescence resonance energy transfer study. *J Biol Chem* 274(9):5462–5468, 1999.

200. Yegneswaran S, Wood GM, Esmon CT, Johnson AE: Protein S alters the active site location of activated protein C above the membrane surface. A fluorescence resonance energy transfer study of topography. *J Biol Chem* 272(40):25013–25021, 1997.

201. Koedam JA, Meijers JCM, Sixma JJ, Bouma BN: Inactivation of human factor VIII by activated protein C. Cofactor activity of protein S and protective effect of von Willebrand factor. *J Clin Invest* 82(4):1236–1243, 1988.

202. Solymoss S, Tucker MM, Tracy PB: Kinetics of inactivation of membrane-bound factor Va by activated protein C. Protein S modulates factor Xa protection. *J Biol Chem* 263(29):14884–14890, 1988.

203. Dahlbäck B, Hildebrand B, Malm J: Characterization of functionally important domains in human vitamin K-dependent protein S using monoclonal antibodies. *J Biol Chem* 265(14):8127–8135, 1990.

204. Saller F, Villoutreix BO, Amelot A, et al: The gamma-carboxyglutamic acid domain of anticoagulant protein S is involved in activated protein C cofactor activity, independently of phospholipid binding. *Blood* 105(1):122–130, 2005.

205. Saller F, Kaabache T, Aiach M, et al: The protein S thrombin-sensitive region modulates phospholipid binding and the gamma-carboxyglutamic acid-rich (Gla) domain conformation in a non-specific manner. *J Thromb Haemost* 4(3):704–706, 2006.

206. Heeb MJ, Mesters RM, Fernandez JA, et al: Plasma protein S residues 37–50 mediate its binding to factor Va and inhibition of blood coagulation. *Thromb Haemost* 110(2):275–282, 2013.

207. Walker FJ: Regulation of vitamin K-dependent protein S. Inactivation by thrombin. *J Biol Chem* 259:10335–10339, 1984.

208. Varadi K, Rosing J, Tans G, et al: Factor V enhances the cofactor function of protein S in the APC-mediated inactivation of factor VIII: Influence of the factor V^R506Q mutation. *Thromb Haemost* 76(2):208–214, 1996.

209. Thorelli E, Kaufman RJ, Dahlbäck B: Cleavage of factor V at Arg 506 by activated protein C and the expression of anticoagulant activity of factor V. *Blood* 93(8):2552–2558, 1999.

210. Cramer TJ, Gale AJ: The anticoagulant function of coagulation factor V. *Thromb Haemost* 107(1):15–21, 2012.

211. Cramer TJ, Griffin JH, Gale AJ: Factor V Is an anticoagulant cofactor for activated protein C during inactivation of factor Va. *Pathophysiol Haemost Thromb* 37(1):17–23, 2010.

212. Mineo C, Deguchi H, Griffin JH, Shaul PW: Endothelial and antithrombotic actions of HDL. *Circ Res* 98(11):1352–1364, 2006.

213. Deguchi H, Pecheniuk NM, Elias DJ, et al: High-density lipoprotein deficiency and dyslipoproteinemia associated with venous thrombosis in men. *Circulation* 112(6):893–899, 2005.

214. Eichinger S, Pecheniuk NM, Hron G, et al: High-density lipoprotein and the risk of recurrent venous thromboembolism. *Circulation* 115(12):1609–1614, 2007.

215. Deguchi H, Fernández JA, Pabinger I, et al: Plasma glucosylceramide deficiency as potential risk factor for venous thrombosis and modulator of anticoagulant protein C pathway. *Blood* 97(7):1907–1914, 2001.

216. Deguchi H, Fernández JA, Griffin JH: Neutral glycosphingolipid-dependent inactivation of coagulation factor Va by activated protein C and protein S. *J Biol Chem* 277(11):8861–8865, 2002.

217. Yegneswaran S, Deguchi H, Griffin JH: Glucosylceramide, a neutral glycosphingolipid anticoagulant cofactor, enhances the interaction of human- and bovine-activated protein C with negatively charged phospholipid vesicles. *J Biol Chem* 278(17):14614–14621, 2003.

218. Deguchi H, Yegneswaran S, Griffin JH: Sphingolipids as bioactive regulators of thrombin generation. *J Biol Chem* 279(13):12036–12042, 2004.

219. Esmon CT: Interactions between the innate immune and blood coagulation systems. *Trends Immunol* 25(10):536–542, 2004.

220. Levi M, van der Poll T, Buller HR: Bidirectional relation between inflammation and coagulation. *Circulation* 109(22):2698–2704, 2004.

221. Riewald M, Ruf W: Protease-activated receptor-1 signaling by activated protein C in cytokine perturbed endothelial cells is distinct from thrombin signaling. *J Biol Chem* 280(20):19808–19814, 2005.

222. Kerschen EJ, Hernandez I, Zogg M, et al: Activated protein C targets CD8+ dendritic cells to reduce the mortality of endotoxemia in mice. *J Clin Invest* 120(9):3167–3178, 2010.

223. Guo H, Zhao Z, Yang Q, et al: An activated protein C analog stimulates neuronal production by human neural progenitor cells via a PAR1-PAR3-S1PR1-Akt pathway. *J Neurosci* 33(14):6181–6190, 2013.

224. Xue M, Chow SO, Dervish S, et al: Activated protein C enhances human keratinocyte barrier integrity via sequential activation of epidermal growth factor receptor and tie2. *J Biol Chem* 286(8):6742–6750, 2011.

225. Riewald M, Petrovan RJ, Donner A, et al: Activation of endothelial cell protease activated receptor 1 by the protein C pathway. *Science* 296(5574):1880–1882, 2002.

226. Mosnier LO, Zlokovic BV, Griffin JH: Cytoprotective-selective activated protein C therapy for ischaemic stroke. *Thromb Haemost* 112(5):883–892, 2014.

227. Zlokovic BV, Griffin JH: Cytoprotective protein C pathways and implications for stroke and neurological disorders. *Trends Neurosci* 34(4):198–209, 2011.

228. Wildhagen KC, Lutgens E, Loubele ST, et al: The structure-function relationship of activated protein C. Lessons from natural and engineered mutations. *Thromb Haemost* 106(6):1034–1045, 2011.

229. Kerschen EJ, Fernandez JA, Cooley BC, et al: Endotoxemia and sepsis mortality reduction by non-anticoagulant activated protein C. *J Exp Med* 204(10):2439–2448, 2007.

230. Wang Y, Sinha RK, Mosnier LO, et al: Neurotoxicity of the anticoagulant-selective E149A-activated protein C variant after focal ischemic stroke in mice. *Blood Cells Mol Dis* 51(2):104–108, 2013.

231. Guo H, Singh I, Wang Y, et al: Neuroprotective activities of activated protein C mutant with reduced anticoagulant activity. *Eur J Neurosci* 29(6):1119–1130, 2009.

232. Wang Y, Thiyagarajan M, Chow N, et al: Differential neuroprotection and risk for bleeding from activated protein C with varying degrees of anticoagulant activity. *Stroke* 40(5):1864–1869, 2008.

233. Cheng T, Liu D, Griffin JH, et al: Activated protein C blocks p53-mediated apoptosis in ischemic human brain endothelium and is neuroprotective. *Nat Med* 9(3):338–342, 2003.

234. Cheng T, Petraglia AL, Li Z, et al: Activated protein C inhibits tissue plasminogen activator-induced brain hemorrhage. *Nat Med* 12(11):1278–1285, 2006.

235. Griffin JH, Fernández JA, Liu D, et al: Activated protein C and ischemic stroke. *Crit Care Med* 32(5 Suppl):S247–S253, 2004.

236. Guo H, Liu D, Gelbard H, et al: Activated protein C prevents neuronal apoptosis via protease activated receptors 1 and 3. *Neuron* 41(4):563–572, 2004.

237. Liu D, Cheng T, Guo H, et al: Tissue plasminogen activator neurovascular toxicity is controlled by activated protein C. *Nat Med* 10(12):1379–1383, 2004.

238. Shibata M, Kumar SR, Amar A, et al: Anti-inflammatory, antithrombotic, and neuroprotective effects of activated protein C in a murine model of focal ischemic stroke. *Circulation* 103(13):1799–1805, 2001.

239. Wang Y, Zhang Z, Chow N, et al: An activated protein C analog with reduced anticoagulant activity extends the therapeutic window of tissue plasminogen activator for ischemic stroke in rodents. *Stroke* 43(9):2444–2449, 2012.

240. Wang Y, Zhao Z, Chow N, et al: Activated protein C analog promotes neurogenesis and improves neurological outcome after focal ischemic stroke in mice via protease activated receptor 1. *Brain Res* 1507:97–104, 2013.

241. Wang Y, Zhao Z, Chow N, et al: Activated protein C analog protects from ischemic stroke and extends the therapeutic window of tissue-type plasminogen activator in aged female mice and hypertensive rats. *Stroke* 44(12):3529–3536, 2013.

242. Zlokovic BV: Neurodegeneration and the neurovascular unit. *Nat Med* 16(12):1370–1371, 2010.

243. Petraglia AL, Marky AH, Walker C, et al: Activated protein C is neuroprotective and mediates new blood vessel formation and neurogenesis after controlled cortical impact. *Neurosurgery* 66(1):165–171, 2010.

244. Thiyagarajan M, Fernandez JA, Lane SM, et al: Activated protein C promotes neovascularization and neurogenesis in postischemic brain via protease-activated receptor 1. *J Neurosci* 28(48):12788–12797, 2008.

245. Walker CT, Marky AH, Petraglia AL, et al: Activated protein C analog with reduced anti-coagulant activity improves functional recovery and reduces bleeding risk following controlled cortical impact. *Brain Res* 1347:125–131, 2010.

246. Lyden P, Levy H, Weymer S, et al: Phase 1 safety, tolerability and pharmacokinetics of 3K3A-APC in healthy adult volunteers. *Curr Pharm Des* 19(42):7479–7485, 2013.

247. Williams PD, Zlokovic BV, Griffin JH, et al: Preclinical safety and pharmacokinetic profile of 3K3A-APC, a novel, modified activated protein C for ischemic stroke. *Curr Pharm Des* 18(27):4215–4222, 2012.

248. Mosnier LO, Griffin JH: Inhibition of staurosporine-induced apoptosis of endothelial cells by activated protein C requires protease activated receptor-1 and endothelial cell protein C receptor. *Biochem J* 373(Pt 1):65–70, 2003.

249. Feistritzer C, Riewald M: Endothelial barrier protection by activated protein C through PAR1-dependent sphingosine 1-phosphate receptor-1 crossactivation. *Blood* 105(8):3178–3184, 2005.

250. Finigan JH, Dudek SM, Singleton PA, et al: Activated protein C mediates novel lung endothelial barrier enhancement: Role of sphingosine 1-phosphate receptor transactivation. *J Biol Chem* 280(17):17286–17293, 2005.

251. Schuepbach RA, Feistritzer C, Fernandez JA, et al: Protection of vascular barrier integrity by activated protein C in murine models depends on protease-activated receptor-1. *Thromb Haemost* 101(4):724–733, 2009.

252. Bae JS, Yang L, Rezaie AR: Receptors of the protein C activation and activated protein C signaling pathways are colocalized in lipid rafts of endothelial cells. *Proc Natl Acad Sci U S A* 104(8):2867–2872, 2007.

253. Russo A, Soh UJ, Paing MM, et al: Caveolae are required for protease-selective signaling by protease-activated receptor-1. *Proc Natl Acad Sci U S A* 106(15):6393–6397, 2009.

254. Mosnier LO, Sinha RK, Burnier L, et al: Biased agonism of protease-activated receptor 1 by activated protein C caused by non-canonical cleavage at Arg46. *Blood* 120(26):5237–5246, 2012.

255. Scarborough RM, Naughton MA, Teng W, et al: Tethered ligand agonist peptides. Structural requirements for thrombin receptor activation reveal mechanism of proteolytic unmasking of agonist function. *J Biol Chem* 267(19):13146–13149, 1992.

256. Soh UJ, Trejo J: Activated protein C promotes protease-activated receptor-1 cytoprotective signaling through beta-arrestin and dishevelled-2 scaffolds. *Proc Natl Acad Sci U S A* 108(50):E1372–E1380, 2011.

257. Burnier L, Mosnier LO: Novel mechanisms for activated protein C cytoprotective activities involving non-canonical activation of protease-activated receptor 3. *Blood* 122(5):807–816, 2013.

258. Stavenuiter F, Mosnier LO: Non-canonical PAR3 activation by factor Xa identifies a novel pathway for Tie2 activation and stabilization of vascular integrity. *Blood* 124(23):3480–3489, 2014.

259. Yang XV, Banerjee Y, Fernandez JA, et al: Activated protein C ligation of ApoER2 (LRP8) causes Dab1-dependent signaling in U937 cells. *Proc Natl Acad Sci U S A* 106(1):274–279, 2009.

260. Xu J, Ji Y, Zhang X, et al: Endogenous activated protein C signaling is critical to protection of mice from lipopolysaccharide induced septic shock. *J Thromb Haemost* 7(5):851–856, 2009.

261. Alabanza LM, Esmon NL, Esmon CT, Bynoe MS: Inhibition of endogenous activated protein C attenuates experimental autoimmune encephalomyelitis by inducing myeloid-derived suppressor cells. *J Immunol* 191(7):3764–3777, 2013.

262. Kager LM, Joost WW, Roelofs JJ, et al: Endogenous protein C has a protective role during Gram-negative pneumosepsis (melioidosis). *J Thromb Haemost* 11(2):282–292, 2013.

263. Heeb MJ, Gruber A, Griffin JH: Identification of divalent metal ion-dependent inhibition of activated protein C by alpha 2-macroglobulin and alpha 2-antiplasmin in blood and comparisons to inhibition of factor Xa, thrombin, and plasmin. *J Biol Chem* 266(26):17606–17612, 1991.

264. Heeb MJ, Griffin JH: Physiologic inhibition of human activated protein C by alpha 1-antitrypsin. *J Biol Chem* 263(24):11613–11616, 1988.

265. Heeb MJ, Espana F, Griffin JH: Inhibition and complexation of activated protein C by two major inhibitors in plasma. *Blood* 73(2):446–454, 1989.

266. Espana F, Vicente V, Tabernero D, et al: Determination of plasma protein C inhibitor and of two activated protein C-inhibitor complexes in normals and in patients with intravascular coagulation and thrombotic disease. *Thromb Res* 59(3):593–608, 1990.

267. Espana F, Gilabert J, Aznar J, et al: Complexes of activated protein C with alpha 1-antitrypsin in normal pregnancy and in severe preeclampsia. *Am J Obstet Gynecol* 164 (5 Pt 1):1310–1316, 1991.

268. Scully MF, Toh CH, Hoogendoorn H, et al: Activation of protein C and its distribution between its inhibitors, protein C inhibitor, alpha 1-antitrypsin and alpha 2-macroglobulin, in patients with disseminated intravascular coagulation. *Thromb Haemost* 69(5):448–453, 1993.

269. Bhiladvala P, Strandberg K, Stenflo J, Holm J: Early identification of acute myocardial infarction by activated protein C–protein C inhibitor complex. *Thromb Res* 118(2):213–219, 2006.

270. Schwarz HP, Fischer M, Hopmeier P, et al: Plasma protein S deficiency in familial thrombotic disease. *Blood* 64(6):1297–1300, 1984.

271. Comp PC, Nixon RR, Cooper MR, Esmon CT: Familial protein S deficiency is associated with recurrent thrombosis. *J Clin Invest* 74(6):2082–2088, 1984.

272. Stenberg Y, Muranyi A, Steen C, et al: EGF-like module pair 3–4 in vitamin K-dependent protein S: Modulation of calcium affinity of module 4 by module 3, and interaction with factor X. *J Mol Biol* 293(3):653–665, 1999.

273. Yegneswaran S, Hackeng TM, Dawson PE, Griffin JH: The thrombin-sensitive region of protein S mediates phospholipid-dependent interaction with factor Xa. *J Biol Chem* 283(48):33046–33052, 2008.

274. van 't Veer C, Hackeng TM, Biesbroeck D, et al: Increased prothrombin activation in protein S-deficient plasma under flow conditions on endothelial cell matrix: An independent anticoagulant function of protein S in plasma. *Blood* 85(7):1815–1821, 1995.

275. Koppelman SJ, Hackeng TM, Sixma JJ, Bouma BN: Inhibition of the intrinsic factor X activating complex by protein S: Evidence for a specific binding of protein S to factor VIII. *Blood* 86:1062–1071, 1995.

276. Koppelman SJ, van 't Veer C, Sixma JJ, Bouma BN: Synergistic inhibition of the intrinsic factor X activation by protein S and C4b-binding protein. *Blood* 86(7):2653–2660, 1995.

277. Peraramelli S, Rosing J, Hackeng TM: TFPI-dependent activities of protein S. *Thromb Res* 129 Suppl 2:S23–S26, 2012.

278. Ndonwi M, Tuley EA, Broze GJ Jr: The Kunitz-3 domain of TFPI-alpha is required for protein S-dependent enhancement of factor Xa inhibition. *Blood* 116(8):1344–1351, 2010.

279. Hackeng TM, Sere KM, Tans G, Rosing J: Protein S stimulates inhibition of the tissue factor pathway by tissue factor pathway inhibitor. *Proc Natl Acad Sci U S A* 103(9):3106–3111, 2006.

280. Heeb MJ, Prashun D, Griffin JH, Bouma BN: Plasma protein S contains zinc essential for efficient activated protein C-independent anticoagulant activity and binding to factor Xa, but not for efficient binding to tissue factor pathway inhibitor. *FASEB J* 23(7):2244–2253, 2009.

281. Heeb MJ, Marzec U, Gruber A, Hanson SR: Antithrombotic activity of protein S infused without activated protein C in a baboon thrombosis model. *Thromb Haemost* 107(4):690–698, 2012.

282. Dahlback B: Purification of human C4b-binding protein and formation of its complex with vitamin K-dependent protein S. *Biochem J* 209(3):847–856, 1983.

283. Griffin JH, Gruber A, Fernández JA: Reevaluation of total, free, and bound protein S and C4b-binding protein levels in plasma anticoagulated with citrate or hirudin. *Blood* 79(12):3203–3211, 1992.

284. Schwarz HP, Muntean W, Watzke H, et al: Low total protein S antigen but high protein S activity due to decreased C4b-binding protein in neonates. *Blood* 71(3):562–565, 1988.

285. Maurissen LF, Thomassen MC, Nicolaes GA, et al: Re-evaluation of the role of the protein S-C4b binding protein complex in activated protein C-catalyzed factor Va-inactivation. *Blood* 111(6):3034–3041, 2008.

286. Hillarp A, Dahlbäck B: Novel subunit in C4b-binding protein required for protein S binding. *J Biol Chem* 263(25):12759–12764, 1988.

287. Hillarp A, Hessing M, Dahlback B: Protein S binding in relation to the subunit composition of human C4b-binding protein. *FEBS Lett* 259(1):53–56, 1989.

288. Fernandez JA, Griffin JH: A protein S binding site on C4b-binding protein involves beta chain residues 31–45. *J Biol Chem* 269(4):2535–2540, 1994.

289. Fernández JA, Griffin JH, Chang GT, et al: Involvement of amino acid residues 423–429 of human protein S in binding to C4b-binding protein. *Blood Cells Mol Dis* 24(2):101–112, 1998.

290. Garcia de Frutos P, Alim RI, Hardig Y, et al: Differential regulation of alpha and beta chains of C4b-binding protein during acute-phase response resulting in stable plasma levels of free anticoagulant protein S. *Blood* 84(3):815–822, 1994.

291. Anderson HA, Maylock CA, Williams JA, et al: Serum-derived protein S binds to phosphatidylserine and stimulates the phagocytosis of apoptotic cells. *Nat Immunol* 4(1):87–91, 2003.

292. Prasad D, Rothlin CV, Burrola P, et al: TAM receptor function in the retinal pigment epithelium. *Mol Cell Neurosci* 33(1):96–108, 2006.

293. Uehara H, Shacter E: Auto-oxidation and oligomerization of protein S on the apoptotic cell surface is required for Mer tyrosine kinase-mediated phagocytosis of apoptotic cells. *J Immunol* 180(4):2522–2530, 2008.

294. McColl A, Bournazos S, Franz S, et al: Glucocorticoids induce protein S-dependent phagocytosis of apoptotic neutrophils by human macrophages. *J Immunol* 183(3):2167–2175, 2009.

295. Liu D, Guo H, Griffin JH, et al: Protein S confers neuronal protection during ischemic/hypoxic injury in mice. *Circulation* 107(13):1791–1796, 2003.

296. Fernandez JA, Heeb MJ, Xu X, et al: Species-specific anticoagulant and mitogenic activities of murine protein S. *Haematologica* 94(12):1721–1731, 2009.

297. Zhu D, Wang Y, Singh I, et al: Protein S controls hypoxic/ischemic blood-brain barrier disruption through the TAM receptor Tyro3 and sphingosine 1-phosphate receptor. *Blood* 115(23):4963–4972, 2010.

298. Zhong Z, Wang Y, Guo H, et al: Protein S protects neurons from excitotoxic injury by activating the TAM receptor Tyro3-phosphatidylinositol 3-kinase-Akt pathway through its sex hormone-binding globulin-like region. *J Neurosci* 30(46):15521–15534, 2010.

299. Guo H, Barrett TM, Zhong Z, et al: Protein S blocks the extrinsic apoptotic cascade in tissue plasminogen activator/N-methyl D-aspartate-treated neurons via Tyro3-Akt-F-KHRL1 signaling pathway. *Mol Neurodegener* 6(1):13, 2011.

300. Gray E, Hogwood J, Mulloy B: The anticoagulant and antithrombotic mechanisms of heparin. *Handb Exp Pharmacol* (207):43–61, 2012.

301. Broze GJ Jr, Girard TJ: Tissue factor pathway inhibitor: Structure-function. *Front Biosci (Landmark Ed)* 17:262–280, 2012.

302. Winckers K, ten Cate H, Hackeng TM: The role of tissue factor pathway inhibitor in atherosclerosis and arterial thrombosis. *Blood Rev* 27(3):119–132, 2013.

303. Wood JP, Ellery PE, Maroney SA, Mast AE: Biology of tissue factor pathway inhibitor. *Blood* 123(19):2934–2943, 2014.

304. Gettins PG: Serpin structure, mechanism, and function. *Chem Rev* 102(12):4751–4804, 2002.

305. Whisstock JC, Bottomley SP: Molecular gymnastics: Serpin structure, folding and misfolding. *Curr Opin Struct Biol* 16(6):761–768, 2006.

306. Rau JC, Beaulieu LM, Huntington JA, Church FC: Serpins in thrombosis, hemostasis and fibrinolysis. *J Thromb Haemost* 5 Suppl 1:102–115, 2007.

307. Huntington JA: Serpin structure, function and dysfunction. *J Thromb Haemost* 9 (Suppl 1):26–34, 2011.

308. Huntington JA: Thrombin inhibition by the serpins. *J Thromb Haemost* 11 (Suppl 1):254–264, 2013.

309. Schreuder HA, de Boer B, Dijkema R, et al: The intact and cleaved human antithrombin III complex as a model for serpin-proteinase interactions. *Nat Struct Biol* 1(1):48–54, 1994.

310. Skinner R, Abrahams JP, Whisstock JC, et al: The 2.6 A structure of antithrombin indicates a conformational change at the heparin binding site. *J Mol Biol* 266(3):601–609, 1997.

311. Li W, Johnson DJ, Esmon CT, Huntington JA: Structure of the antithrombin-thrombin-heparin ternary complex reveals the antithrombotic mechanism of heparin. *Nat Struct Mol Biol* 11(9):857–862, 2004.

312. Huber R, Carell RW: Implications of the three dimensional structure of α_1-antitrypsin for the structure and function of serpins. *Biochemistry* 28:8951–8966, 1989.

313. Choay J, Petitou M, Lormeau JC, et al: Structure-activity relationship in heparin: A synthetic pentasaccharide with high affinity for antithrombin III and eliciting high anti-factor Xa activity. *Biochem Biophys Res Commun* 116(2):492–499, 1983.

314. Bourin MC, Lindahl U: Glycosaminoglycans and the regulation of blood coagulation. *Biochem J* 289(Pt 2):313–330, 1993.

315. Hirsh J, O'Donnell M, Eikelboom JW: Beyond unfractionated heparin and warfarin: Current and future advances. *Circulation* 116(5):552–560, 2007.

316. Olds RJ, Lane DA, Chowdhury V, et al: Complete nucleotide sequence of the antithrombin gene: Evidence for homologous recombination causing thrombophilia. *Biochemistry* 32(16):4216–4224, 1993.

317. Picard V, Ersdal-Badju E, Bock SC: Partial glycosylation of antithrombin III asparagine-135 is caused by the serine in the third position of its N-glycosylation consensus sequence and is responsible for production of the beta-antithrombin III isoform with enhanced heparin affinity. *Biochemistry* 34(26):8433–8440, 1995.

318. Turko IV, Fan B, Gettins PG: Carbohydrate isoforms of antithrombin variant N135Q with different heparin affinities. *FEBS Lett* 335(1):9–12, 1993.

319. Chandra T, Stackhouse R, Kidd VJ, Woo SL: Isolation and sequence characterization of a cDNA clone of human antithrombin III. *Proc Natl Acad Sci U S A* 80(7):1845–1848, 1983.

320. Prochownik EV, Markham AF, Orkin SH: Isolation of a cDNA clone for human antithrombin III. *J Biol Chem* 258(13):8389–8394, 1983.

321. Lane DA, Bayston T, Olds RJ, et al: Antithrombin mutation database: 2nd (1997) update. For the Plasma Coagulation Inhibitors Subcommittee of the Scientific and Standardization Committee of the International Society on Thrombosis and Haemostasis. *Thromb Haemost* 77(1):197–211, 1997.

322. Broze GJ Jr, Girard TJ: Factor V, tissue factor pathway inhibitor, and east Texas bleeding disorder. *J Clin Invest* 123(9):3710–3712, 2013.

323. Chang JY, Monroe DM, Oliver JA, Roberts HR: TFPIbeta, a second product from the mouse tissue factor pathway inhibitor (TFPI) gene. *Thromb Haemost* 81(1):45–49, 1999.

324. Zhang J, Piro O, Lu L, Broze GJ Jr: Glycosyl phosphatidylinositol anchorage of tissue factor pathway inhibitor. *Circulation* 108(5):623–627, 2003.

325. Piro O, Broze GJ Jr: Comparison of cell-surface TFPIalpha and beta. *J Thromb Haemost* 3(12):2677–2683, 2005.

326. Girard TJ, Warren LA, Novotny WF, et al: Functional significance of the Kunitz-type inhibitory domains of lipoprotein-associated coagulation inhibitor. *Nature* 338(6215):518–520, 1989.

327. Lesnik P, Vonica A, Guerin M, et al: Anticoagulant activity of tissue factor pathway inhibitor in human plasma is preferentially associated with dense subspecies of LDL and with HDL and with Lp(a). *Arterioscler Thromb* 13(7):1066–1075, 1993.

328. Novotny WF, Girard TJ, Miletich JP, Broze GJ Jr: Purification and characterization of the lipoprotein-associated coagulation inhibitor from human plasma. *J Biol Chem* 264(31):18832–18837, 1989.

329. Sandset PM, Abildgaard U, Larsen ML: Heparin induces release of extrinsic coagulation pathway inhibitor (EPI). *Thromb Res* 50(6):803–813, 1988.

330. Ndonwi M, Girard TJ, Broze GJ Jr: The C-terminus of tissue factor pathway inhibitor alpha is required for its interaction with factors V and Va. *J Thromb Haemost* 10(9):1944–1946, 2012.

331. Castoldi E, Simioni P, Tormene D, et al: Hereditary and acquired protein S deficiencies are associated with low TFPI levels in plasma. *J Thromb Haemost* 8(2):294–300, 2010.

332. Vincent LM, Tran S, Livaja R, et al: Coagulation factor VA2440G causes east Texas bleeding disorder via TFPIalpha. *J Clin Invest* 123(9):3777–3787, 2013.

333. Duckers C, Simioni P, Spiezia L, et al: Low plasma levels of tissue factor pathway inhibitor in patients with congenital factor V deficiency. *Blood* 112(9):3615–3623, 2008.

334. Huang ZF, Broze G Jr: Consequences of tissue factor pathway inhibitor gene-disruption in mice. *Thromb Haemost* 78(1):699–704, 1997.

335. van der Logt CP, Reitsma PH, Bertina RM: Intron-exon organization of the human gene coding for the lipoprotein-associated coagulation inhibitor: The factor Xa dependent inhibitor of the extrinsic pathway of coagulation. *Biochemistry* 30(6):1571–1577, 1991.

336. Girard TJ, Eddy R, Wesselschmidt RL, et al: Structure of the human lipoprotein-associated coagulation inhibitor gene. Intro/exon gene organization and localization of the gene to chromosome 2. *J Biol Chem* 266(8):5036–5041, 1991.

337. Tollefsen DM, Majerus DW, Blank MK: Heparin cofactor II. Purification and properties of a heparin-dependent inhibitor of thrombin in human plasma. *J Biol Chem* 257(5):2162–2169, 1982.

338. Aihara K: Heparin cofactor II attenuates vascular remodeling in humans and mice. *Circ J* 74(8):1518–1523, 2010.

339. Tollefsen DM: Vascular dermatan sulfate and heparin cofactor II. *Prog Mol Biol Transl Sci* 93:351–372, 2010.

340. Rau JC, Mitchell JW, Fortenberry YM, Church FC: Heparin cofactor II: Discovery, properties, and role in controlling vascular homeostasis. *Semin Thromb Hemost* 37(4):339–348, 2011.

341. Bertina RM, van der Linden IK, Engesser L, et al: Hereditary heparin cofactor II deficiency and the risk of development of thrombosis. *Thromb Haemost* 57(2):196–200, 1987.

342. Corral J, Aznar J, Gonzalez-Conejero R, et al: Homozygous deficiency of heparin cofactor II: Relevance of P17 glutamate residue in serpins, relationship with conformational diseases, and role in thrombosis. *Circulation* 110(10):1303–1307, 2004.

343. Broze GJJ: Protein Z-dependent regulation of coagulation. *Thromb Haemost* 86(1):8–13, 2001.

344. Heeb MJ, Cabral KM, Ruan L: Down-regulation of factor IXa in the factor Xase complex by protein Z-dependent protease inhibitor. *J Biol Chem* 280(40):33819–33825, 2005.

345. Choi Q, Kim JE, Hyun J, et al: Contributions of procoagulants and anticoagulants to the international normalized ratio and thrombin generation assay in patients treated with warfarin: Potential role of protein Z as a powerful determinant of coagulation assays. *Thromb Res* 132(1):e70–e75, 2013.

346. Bolkun L, Galar M, Piszcz J, et al: Plasma concentration of protein Z and protein Z-dependent protease inhibitor in patients with haemophilia A. *Thromb Res* 131(3):e110–e113, 2013.

347. Huang X, Yan Y, Tu Y, et al: Structural basis for catalytic activation of protein Z-dependent protease inhibitor (ZPI) by protein Z. *Blood* 120(8):1726–1733, 2012.

348. Vasse M: The protein Z/protein Z-dependent protease inhibitor complex. Systemic or local control of coagulation? *Hamostaseologie* 31(3):155–158, 160–154, 2011.

349. Huang X, Rezaie AR, Broze GJ Jr, Olson ST: Heparin is a major activator of the anticoagulant serpin, protein Z-dependent protease inhibitor. *J Biol Chem* 286(11):8740–8751, 2011.

350. Sofi F, Cesari F, Abbate R, et al: A meta-analysis of potential risks of low levels of protein Z for diseases related to vascular thrombosis. *Thromb Haemost* 103(4):749–756, 2010.

351. Wei Z, Yan Y, Carrell RW, Zhou A: Crystal structure of protein Z-dependent inhibitor complex shows how protein Z functions as a cofactor in the membrane inhibition of factor X. *Blood* 114(17):3662–3667, 2009.

352. Corral J, Gonzalez-Conejero R, Hernandez-Espinosa D, Vicente V: Protein Z/Z-dependent protease inhibitor (PZ/ZPI) anticoagulant system and thrombosis. *Br J Haematol* 137(2):99–108, 2007.

353. Yin ZF, Huang ZF, Cui JS, et al: Prothrombotic phenotype of protein Z deficiency. *Proc Natl Acad Sci U S A* 97(12):6734–6738, 2000.

354. Kemkes-Matthes B, Nees M, Kuhnel G, et al: Protein Z influences the prothrombotic phenotype in Factor V Leiden patients. *Thromb Res* 106(4–5):183–185, 2002.

355. Van de Water N, Tan T, Ashton F, et al: Mutations within the protein Z-dependent protease inhibitor gene are associated with venous thromboembolic disease: A new form of thrombophilia. *Br J Haematol* 127(2):190–194, 2004.

356. Vasse M: Protein Z, a protein seeking a pathology. *Thromb Haemost* 100(4):548–556, 2008.

357. Dentali F, Gianni M, Lussana F, et al: Polymorphisms of the Z protein protease inhibitor and risk of venous thromboembolism: A meta-analysis. *Br J Haematol* 143(2):284–287, 2008.

358. Sofi F, Cesari F, Tu Y, et al: Protein Z-dependent protease inhibitor and protein Z in peripheral arterial disease patients. *J Thromb Haemost* 7(5):731–735, 2009.

359. Rezaie AR, Cooper ST, Church FC, Esmon CT: Protein C inhibitor is a potent inhibitor of the thrombin-thrombomodulin complex. *J Biol Chem* 270(43):25336–25339, 1995.

CHAPTER 115
VASCULAR FUNCTION IN HEMOSTASIS

Katherine A. Hajjar, Aaron J. Marcus*, and
William Muller

SUMMARY

Blood vessels, especially their endothelial lining, play a critical role in the maintenance of vascular fluidity, arrest of hemorrhage (hemostasis), prevention of occlusive vascular phenomena (thrombosis), and regulation of inflammatory cell processes. The endothelium extends to all recesses of the body and maintains an intimate association with flowing blood and blood cells. However, endothelial cell morphologies, gene-expression profiles, and functions vary among different vascular beds. For example, in straight arterial segments, but not at branch points or curvatures of the arteries or veins, endothelial cells align themselves in parallel to the direction of blood flow. Similarly, endothelial cells in post capillary venules are primarily responsible for mediating adhesion and transmigration of leukocytes, whereas arteriolar endothelium is important for regulation of vasomotor tone. Proteomic studies have revealed that endothelial cells have the unique capacity to express and elaborate thromboregulatory molecules, which can be classified according to their chronologic appearance following vascular injury. Early thromboregulators appear prior to thrombin formation and late thromboregulators arrive after thrombin has formed. This chapter reviews some of the mechanisms by which the vascular wall regulates hemostasis, and discuss their implications for vascular health and disease (Table 115–1).

Acronyms and Abbreviations: APC, activated protein C; Apo, apolipoprotein; APS, antiphospholipid syndrome; C5a, complement factor 5a; CAM, cell adhesion molecule; COX, cyclooxygenase; DAG, diacylglycerol; DDAVP, deamino D-arginine vasopressin; EPCR, endothelial protein C receptor; GMP, guanosine monophosphate; IL, interleukin; IP_3, inositol triphosphate; Lp(a), lipoprotein(a); NFκB, nuclear factor kappa B; NO, nitric oxide; NOS, nitric oxide synthase; PAF, platelet-activating factor; PDGF, platelet-derived growth factor; PECAM, platelet endothelial cell adhesion molecule; PGI_2, prostacyclin; PGIS, prostacyclin synthase; PSGL, P-selectin glycoprotein ligand; scu-PA, single-chain urokinase-type plasminogen activator; TAFI, thrombin-activatable fibrinolysis inhibitor; TF, tissue factor; TFPI, tissue factor pathway inhibitor; TM, thrombomodulin; TNF, tumor necrosis factor; t-PA, tissue-type plasminogen activator; VWF, von Willebrand factor.

*Dr. Aaron Marcus died on May 6, 2015

● VASCULAR FUNCTION IN HEMOSTASIS: INTRODUCTION

The endothelium represents a dynamic interface between flowing blood and the vessel wall, and produces a variety of factors that regulate blood fluidity (Fig. 115–1). Endothelial cells are subject to unique shear stress forces, to soluble factors in the blood, and to signals emanating from cells in the circulation, vascular wall, and tissues, all of which create region-specific phenotypes.[1-3] In addition to modulating vascular permeability and fragility, the endothelium regulates the fluid state of blood through its thromboresistant nature, profibrinolytic properties, and antiinflammatory potential. These activities maintain vascular patency.[4]

ENDOTHELIAL CELL HETEROGENEITY

The heterogeneity of endothelial cells is mediated by two mechanisms.[5,6] First, extracellular biochemical and biomechanical signals trigger posttranscriptional and/or posttranslational changes that vary across the vascular tree. Second, certain site-specific properties of the endothelium are genetically programmed, and therefore, independent of the extracellular milieu. This phenotypic variability serves at least two important purposes: (1) It allows endothelial cells to meet the specific metabolic needs of the surrounding tissue. For example, the tight junctions of the blood–brain barrier protect neurons from fluctuations in composition of the aqueous blood supply, whereas the fenestrated discontinuous endothelium of hepatic sinusoids allows ready access of nutrient-rich portal venous blood for the metabolic systems in hepatocytes; and (2) phenotypic variability provides endothelial cells with site-specific mechanisms for thriving within many different microenvironments. For example, endothelial cells in the inner medulla of the kidney must survive the relatively hypoxic and hyperosmolar local environment, whereas endothelial cells in the pulmonary capillary bed have adapted to an oxygen-rich environment.

A rapid endothelial cell response is required for sudden environmental perturbations. Translational control mechanisms, which are more immediate than transcriptional changes, provide regulatory responses for up to 10 percent of genes expressed in endothelial cells.[7] Because of their close association with both flowing blood and solid tissues, endothelial cells are subject to a broad spectrum of agonistic and inhibitory external signals that frequently require rapid functional and phenotypic responses. Clinically, such stimuli are associated with sepsis, inflammation, ischemia–reperfusion injury, and direct mechanical vascular trauma induced clinically by stents, balloon catheters, and graft procedures.

ENDOTHELIAL PRODUCTION OF THROMBOREGULATORY MOLECULES

Thromboregulatory compounds, such as eicosanoids, nitric oxide, and the ecto-ATP/Dase-1/CD39, control platelet and vascular reactivity during the early stages of thrombus formation (Table 115–2).[8] Eicosanoids are hydrocarbon compounds derived from essential fatty acids in the diet. The most important endothelial eicosanoid is prostacyclin (PGI_2), which blocks platelet reactivity, induces vascular relaxation, and stimulates cytokine production.[9] Nitric oxide (NO) is a naturally occurring gas released from vascular endothelial cells in response to binding of vasodilators to endothelial cell membrane receptors. Thus, it is a short-lived vasodilator and inhibitor of platelet reactivity. By

TABLE 115–1. Chronology of Endothelial Cell Thromboregulators

Early thromboregulators
  Nitric oxide (NO)
  Eicosanoids (prostacyclin and prostaglandin D_2)
  Endothelial cell CD39/ENTPDase1
  Endothelin
Late thromboregulators
  Endothelin
  Antithrombin
  Endothelial cell/heparin proteoglycans
  Tissue factor pathway inhibitor
  Thrombomodulin-protein C-protein S pathway
  Fibrinolytic system (plasminogen activators, inhibitors, and receptors)
  Inflammatory thromboregulators
  Thrombomodulin-protein C-protein S pathway
  Cellular adhesion molecules
  Selectins

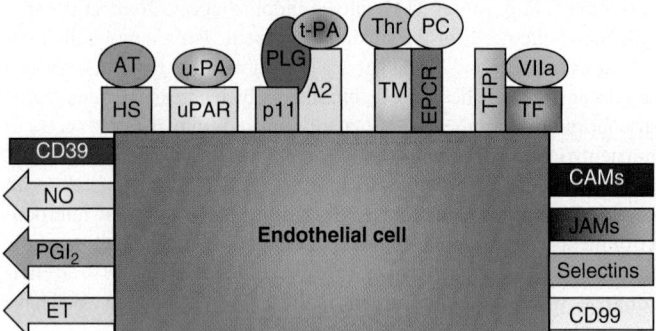

Figure 115–1. Schematic of endothelial cell thromboregulatory molecules. Products that are secreted and exert their effects in the fluid phase are represented by *arrows*. Cell-surface–associated molecules are shown as *rectangles*. Metabolites synthesized by endothelial cells are indicated. Thromboregulators that modulate platelet activation, recruitment, and blood vessel contractility are shown on the *left*. Agents that regulate components of the coagulation cascade and/or fibrinolytic system are located at the *top*. Inflammatory molecules whose expression or activity is directed by inflammatory mediators are shown at the *right*. A2, annexin 2; AT, antithrombin; CAMs, cellular adhesion molecules; CD39, endothelial cell ecto-ADPase/CD39; EPCR, endothelial cell protein C receptor; ET, endothelin; FVIIa, factor VIIa; HS, heparan sulfate; JAMs, junctional adhesion molecules; NO, nitric oxide; PC, protein C; PGI$_2$, prostacyclin; PLG, plasminogen; TF, tissue factor; TFPI, tissue factor pathway inhibitor; TM, thrombomodulin; t-PA, tissue plasminogen activator; u-PA, urokinase plasminogen activator; uPAR, urokinase plasminogen activator receptor. These components are discussed further in the text.

activating guanylate cyclase, the resulting increase in cyclic guanylate monophosphate (GMP) inhibits platelet function and induces vascular relaxation.[10,11] Endothelial cell ecto-ATP/Dase-1/CD39 is a membrane-associated apyrase that metabolizes adenosine diphosphate (ADP) in the primary platelet releasate, preventing further platelet activation and recruitment.[12,13]

Late thromboregulators produced by endothelial cells act either to prevent excessive thrombin generation or to promote lysis of intravascular thrombi (see Table 115–1). Antithrombin, a natural anticoagulant, acts as an inhibitor of thrombin and factor Xa in the circulation. Endothelial cell heparan proteoglycans act as cofactors for antithrombin. The tissue factor pathway inhibitor (TFPI) inhibits the complex between factor VIIa and tissue factor (TF). The thrombomodulin/endothelial cell protein C receptor (EPCR)/protein C system in the vascular wall regulates hemostasis through inactivation of procoagulant cofactors, and antiinflammatory activity.[14] The fibrinolytic system is intimately involved with the vascular endothelium because endothelial cells not only synthesize and secrete tissue plasminogen activator (t-PA), but also regulate formation of plasmin from its precursor, plasminogen, through the expression of receptors.[15] Impairment of fibrinolytic potential can play a central role in the etiology of occlusive vascular disease.[16] Finally, endothelial cell adhesion molecules, including the cell adhesion molecules (CAMs: mucosal addressin cell adhesion molecule [MAdCAM]-1, intercellular adhesion molecule [ICAM]-1, vascular cell adhesion molecule [VCAM]-1, and platelet endothelial cell adhesion molecule [PECAM]-1) and the selectins (P- and E-selectin), are glycoproteins that modulate multiple interactions between the endothelium and various classes of circulating leukocytes, thereby modulating vascular patency.[17] Together, these mechanisms define *thromboregulation*, the processes by which blood cells and cells of the vessel wall, through their close proximity, interact to facilitate or inhibit thrombus formation.[18]

The physiologic defense systems that render endothelial surfaces and blood cells antithrombotic can be overwhelmed by excessive shear stress, increased turbulence, injury, inflammation, and severe atherosclerosis.[19] These events transform the endothelial cells into a prothrombotic and antifibrinolytic phenotype,[20] which is accompanied by upregulation of leukocyte and endothelial CAMs, increased expression of TF, and accumulation of monocytes/macrophages in the vessel wall.[21] These events commonly occur at the site of fissured atherosclerotic plaques in the coronary and cerebrovascular circulation.[22] Because the eicosanoids such as PGI$_2$ (prostaglandin [PG]I$_2$), as well as NO, and the ecto-ATP/Dase-1/CD39 group reach peak activity very early in the hemostatic/thrombotic cascade (Figs. 115–2 to 115–4), they represent potential targets for therapeutic intervention in the sequence of events beginning with platelet activation, and leading to coagulation, thrombosis, and atherogenesis.[21,22] Finally, functional and physical contacts between platelets and endothelial cells are of critical importance for the maintenance of vascular integrity and cell permeability.[1,23]

TABLE 115–2. Early Pro- and Antithrombotic Thromboregulators Associated with Human Endothelial Cells

Class	Type	Site of Action	Aspirin Sensitivity	Mode of Action
Eicosanoids	PGI$_2$, PGD$_2$	Fluid phase autacoid	Sensitive	Elevation of platelet cAMP
Nitrovasodilators	EDRF/NO	Fluid phase autacoid	Insensitive	Elevation of platelet cGMP
Ectonucleotidases	CD39/ENTPD1	Endothelial cell surface	Insensitive	Enzymatic removal of secreted ADP
Thromboxane	TXA$_2$	Fluid phase vasoconstrictor	Sensitive	Lowers platelet cAMP and platelet agonist
Endothelins	ET-1, ET-2	Fluid phase vasoconstrictor	Insensitive	Direct vasoconstrictor peptide

ADP, adenosine diphosphate; cAMP, cyclic adenosine monophosphate; cGMP, cyclic guanosine monophosphate; EDRF, endothelium-derived relaxing factor; ET, endothelin; NO, nitric oxide; PGD$_2$, prostaglandin D$_2$; PGI$_2$, prostacyclin; TXA$_2$, thromboxane A$_2$.

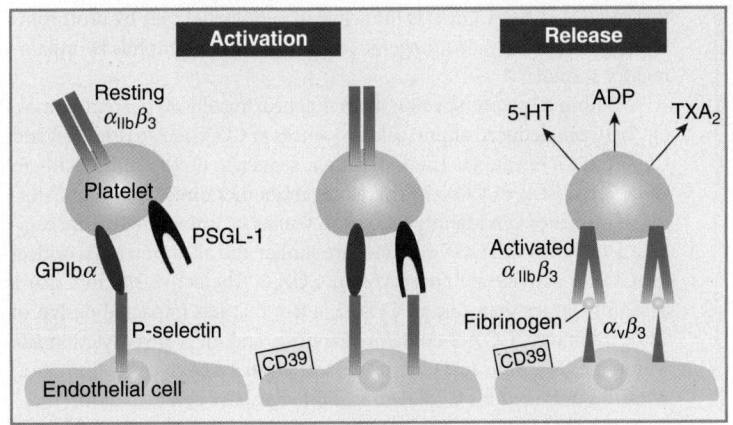

Figure 115–2. Following injury to the blood vessel wall, platelets adhere to the damaged surface of the endothelial cell. Concomitant with adhesion platelets and endothelial cells become activated. P-selectin is expressed on the endothelial cell surface. Platelet surface receptors glycosylphosphatidylinositol (GPI)bα and P-selectin glycoprotein ligand (PSGL)-1 interact with endothelial P-selectin, thereby mediating platelet rolling. Firm adhesion is mediated by the integrin $\alpha_{IIb}\beta_3$. In parallel with these intercellular events, platelet activation and release occur. The enzyme CD39 on the endothelial surface modulates the ambient concentration of adenosine diphosphate (ADP) by metabolizing it.[7,8] 5-HT, 5-hydroxytryptamine; TXA$_2$, thromboxane A$_2$. (*Adapted with permission from Gawaz M, Langer H, May AE: Platelets in inflammation and atherogenesis.* J Clin Invest 11(12):3378–3384, 2005.)

THE EICOSANOID PATHWAY IN BIOLOGY AND MEDICINE: CELL–CELL INTERACTIONS AND TRANSCELLULAR METABOLISM

Dietary fatty acids give rise to arachidonic acid, the starting point for synthesis of other eicosanoids. Originating from different cells, intermediates in the arachidonic acid pathway can interact with each other to produce new products with new biologic activities. Oxygenation and further enzymatic transformation of arachidonic acid gives rise to eicosanoids (formerly classified as PGs) and hydroxy acids, such as the leukotrienes. Eicosanoids are autocoids, an important group of transient, physiologically active endogenous substances, that act within the immediate environment of the cell, where they promote or inhibit a biologic function.[24] These autacoids have a very short life span and may act within a few seconds, a phenomenon that is clinically important but difficult to study experimentally.

In 1975, Hamberg and colleagues discovered that a new eicosanoid, PGI$_2$, was derived from arachidonic acid in endothelial cells.[25] Soon thereafter, Moncada realized that the effects of PGI$_2$ opposed those of

thromboxane, namely vasodilation and inhibition of platelet aggregation.[26,27] The biologic half-life of PGI$_2$ was found to be 10 to 20 seconds. In addition, it was determined that the first step in arachidonic acid oxidation and conversion, which is carried out by cyclooxygenase (COX)-1, is inhibited by aspirin (acetylsalicylic acid), which donates an acetyl group that inactivates COX-1 and inhibits platelet function.[28]

BIOSYNTHESIS OF PROSTACYCLIN IN ENDOTHELIAL CELLS

PGI$_2$ is the major and most important eicosanoid produced by endothelial cells. A broad range of stimuli, including hormones, biochemicals, or physical forces such as shear stress can elicit release of PGI$_2$. Kinetic studies revealed two distinct patterns of PGI$_2$ production: (1) rapid release, independent of new COX-1 mRNA or protein synthesis, and (2) slower production reflecting increased COX-2 expression.

In the case of rapid stimulation of PGI$_2$ production, as induced by thrombin, histamine, bradykinin, and ionophore, the response plateaus at 10 minutes.[29] These agonists activate phospholipase C which generates inositol trisphosphate (IP$_3$) and diacylglycerol (DAG). The released IP$_3$ induces an elevation of intracellular calcium, which translocates phospholipase A to the outer portion of the nuclear envelope and

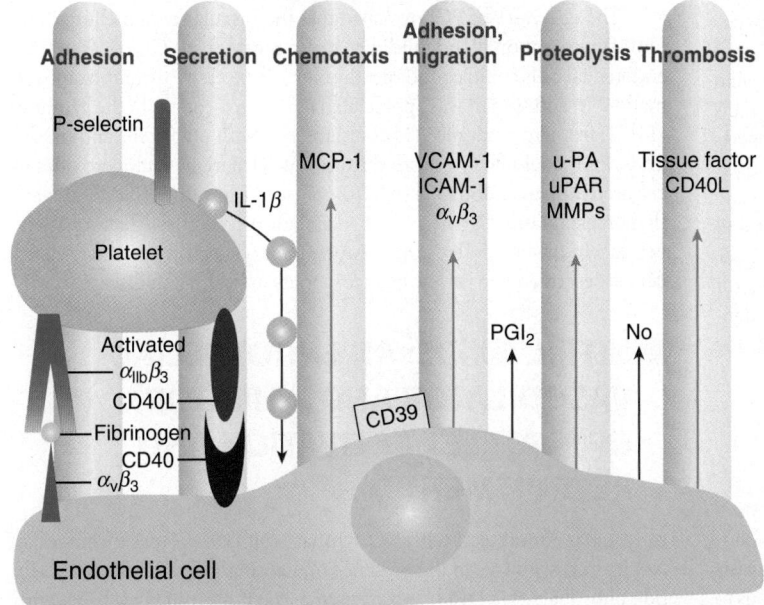

Figure 115–3. Adherent activated platelets induce an inflammatory response in endothelial cells. Platelet adhesion involving $\alpha_{IIb}\beta_3$ induces exposure of P-selectin (CD62P) and release of platelet CD40 ligand (CD40L) and interleukin (IL)-1β which then stimulate endothelial cells to respond with an inflammatory reaction that supports prothrombotic and proatherogenic alterations in the endothelium. IL-8 and MCP-1 (monocyte chemoattractant protein-1) are the principal chemoattractants for neutrophils and monocytes. ICAM, intercellular adhesion molecule; MMP, matrix metalloproteinase; u-PA, urokinase plasminogen activator; uPAR, urokinase plasminogen activator receptor; VCAM, vascular cell adhesion molecule. (*Adapted with permission from Gawaz M, Langer H, May AE: Platelets in inflammation and atherogenesis.* J Clin Invest 11(12): 3378–3384, 2005.)

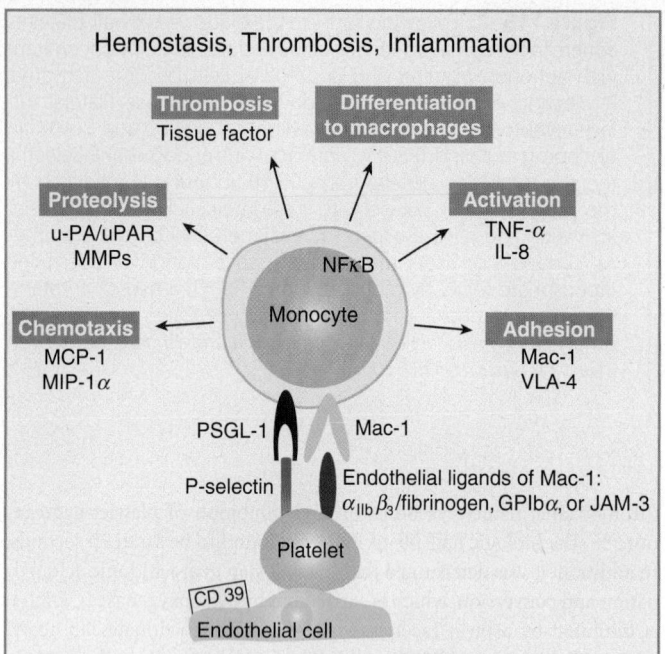

Figure 115–4. Adherent/activated platelets promote an inflammatory response in monocytes. The platelets mainly interact with monocyte P-selectin glycoprotein ligand (PSGL)-1 with monocytic PSGL-1 via P-selectin and with monocyte Mac-1 ($\alpha_M\beta_2$) via $\alpha_{IIb}\beta_3$ (and fibrinogen bridging) or glycosylphosphatidylinositol (GPI)ba. Through this mechanism platelets initiate monocyte secretion of chemokines, cytokines, and procoagulant tissue factor. These serve to upregulate and activate adhesion receptors and proteases. In parallel, they induce monocyte differentiation into macrophages. Therefore platelet-monocyte interactions provide a prothrombotic and atherogenic milieu at the vascular wall, which can eventually support plaque formation. IL, interleukin; JAM, junctional adhesion molecule; MCP, monocyte chemoattractant protein; MIP, macrophage inhibitory protein; MMP, matrix metalloproteinase; NFκB, nuclear factor kappa B; u-PA, urokinase plasminogen activator; uPAR, urokinase plasminogen activator receptor; TNF, tumor necrosis factor; VLA, very late antigen. *(Adapted with permission from Gawaz M, Langer H, May AE: Platelets in inflammation and atherogenesis. J Clin Invest 11(12):3378–3384, 2005.)*

endoplasmic reticulum. Phospholipase A then couples functionally to COX-1, which is located on the luminal membrane. Prostacyclin synthase (PGIS) colocalizes with COX-1 in endothelial cells. Activated phospholipase A2 (cPLA2) catalyzes the release of arachidonic acid from membrane phospholipids, and the free arachidonate interacts with COX-1 and is converted to the endoperoxide PGH_2. PGIS converts prostaglandin H_2 (PGH_2) to PGI_2. The half-life of COX-1 is approximately 10 minutes, whereupon it autoinactivates.

Stimulation of PGI_2 production by proinflammatory cytokines and growth factors, such as lipopolysaccharide (LPS), interleukin (IL)-1β, tumor necrosis factor (TNF)-α, and platelet-derived growth factor (PDGF), is a slower, more sustained process.[29] In response to these agonists, PGI_2 production occurs within 30 to 60 minutes, and parallels the time course of production induced by COX-2, but not COX-1.

THE TWO ISOFORMS OF PROSTACYCLIN G/H SYNTHASE

The recognition that there was a constitutive and an inducible cyclooxygenase (COX-1 and COX-2, respectively), was a major advance.[30] Cloning studies of an immediate to early response gene from 3T3 fibroblasts revealed that the COX-2 complementary DNA was highly homologous to

that of COX-1.[30–34] COX-2 is inducible in endothelial cells by prothrombotic, inflammatory, or mitogenic stimuli, and in neutrophils by inflammatory stimuli.[35,36]

Within a specific species, there is approximately 60 percent homology between deduced amino acid sequences of COX-1 (576 residues) and COX-2 (587 residues). The C-terminal sequence of 18 amino acids in COX-2 is absent in COX-1. Therefore, antibodies directed at this C-terminal sequence can identify COX-2 in tissues by immunoblot. The catalytic activity of both COX enzymes are similar and all amino acids critical for COX-1 activity are conserved in COX-2. The active site in COX-1 is slightly larger than that of COX-2, a fact that has impacted design of COX inhibitors. COX-2 contains mannose, and an *N*-glycosylation site within the 18-amino acid C-terminal sequence. An *N*-glycosylation site at Asn410 is required for COX-1 to fold into its active conformation.

The gene for COX-1 is located on chromosome 9 and spans 22 kb of genomic DNA, while the gene for COX-2 is located on chromosome 1 and spans 8 kb of DNA. Transcription of COX-2 proceeds via several signaling mechanisms initiated by cyclic adenosine monophosphate (cAMP)/protein kinase A, protein kinase C, tyrosine kinases, and pathways activated by growth factors, endotoxin, and cytokines.[33,37–39] The discoveries of COX-1 and COX-2 were of great importance and have led to new concepts concerning the structure and function of COX-induced autacoids.[40]

PROSTACYCLIN AS AN AUTACOID

PGI_2 is released from stimulated endothelial cells by a broad range of agonists, and plays a critical role in the maintenance of vascular integrity by promoting thromboresistance and inhibiting inflammatory responses in the vasculature. Production of PGI_2 is dynamically regulated to meet the challenges arising from frequent prothrombotic and proinflammatory events.[29] As an autacoid, PGI_2 has a half-life of 3 minutes, whereupon it undergoes chemical hydrolysis to 6-keto-$PGF_1\alpha$. It acts on the type I platelet PG receptor (IP) by increasing cAMP levels in a paracrine manner.[41] IP is a 7-transmembrane, G-protein– and adenylyl cyclase–coupled receptor. The latter binds to and activates protein kinase A (PKA), resulting in inhibition of platelet activation and recruitment.[42] Physical or chemical perturbation of endothelial cells results in enhanced PGI_2 production, which increases platelet cAMP resulting in abolition of platelet shape change, inhibition of platelet secretion and recruitment, and impaired binding of von Willebrand factor (VWF) and fibrinogen to the platelet surface. PGI_2 also inhibits platelet adhesion to subendothelium, especially at high shear rates.[43]

The discovery of PGI_2 revealed that the vascular endothelium had a protective effect on blood fluidity.[2,8] It also meant that PGI_2 released from endothelial cells could counteract the effect of excessive thromboxane formation. In addition, it was appreciated that intermediates in the synthesis of PGI_2 from arachidonic acid could interact with other cells and tissues. Thus, PGI_2 could be synthesized from platelet-derived endoperoxides by cultured human endothelial cells.[44] Because of a low threshold for toxicity (hypotension and diarrhea), PGI_2 does not display a satisfactory therapeutic window. An interesting compendium of eicosanoid-related disorders is described in a review on eicosanoids in health and disease.[45]

● NITRIC OXIDE: AN ENDOTHELIAL VASODILATOR AND INHIBITOR OF PLATELET ACTIVATION AND RECRUITMENT

In vascular endothelial cells, NO synthase (NOS) catalyzes formation of NO from L-arginine, in the presence of nicotinamide adenine dinucleotide phosphate (NADPH) and oxygen.[46] The L-arginine is subsequently converted to citrulline and NO. The endothelial cell isoform of NO synthase (eNOS or the NOS3 gene product) functions constitutively, and is further activated by receptor-agonists that elevate intracellular calcium. Major stimuli include ADP, thrombin, bradykinin, and shear stress.[43] Shear forces induce transcriptional activation of the eNOS gene because its promoter contains a shear response consensus sequence (GAGACC). The NO that forms activates guanylate cyclase, thereby generating cyclic GMP. NO becomes oxidized to nitrite and then to nitrate, which is measurable in blood samples. NO in the circulation is rapidly inactivated by erythrocytes.[11,47,48] NO has a vasodilatory effect on the pulmonary vasculature, and, in patients with congestive heart failure, its inhalation decreases pulmonary hypertension and increases pulmonary ventilation.[10,11,47–54] Acetylcholine released by activated nerve terminals in the vessel wall activate the endothelial cell to produce and release NO. This NO effect also explains the action of nitroglycerin, which has long been used to treat patients with angina resulting from coronary artery disease.[54]

Importantly, production of NO by endothelial cells is impaired in the presence of the thiol-containing amino acid, homocysteine. Cynomolgus monkeys with diet-induced hyperhomocysteinemia demonstrated reduced blood flow in the lower extremity and an impaired response to endothelial cell-dependent vasodilators.[51] Similarly, production of NO by endothelial cells *in vitro* is significantly inhibited in the presence of homocysteine, possibly by a mechanism involving impairment of the enzyme glutathione peroxidase.[52,53]

STRUCTURE AND BIOCHEMICAL PROPERTIES OF NITRIC OXIDE SYNTHASE

There are two isoforms of NOS, the constitutive form (eNOS), synthesized by the endothelial cell and regulated by Ca^{2+} and calmodulin, and the cytokine-inducible, posttranscriptionally regulated form (iNOS).[47] Both constitutive and inducible forms are mainly cytosolic, although a membrane-bound constitutive NOS isoform containing a myristoylation consensus sequence has been isolated from bovine aortic endothelial cells.[43] eNOS has a molecular mass of 144 kDa and shares 57 percent amino acid sequence identity with neuronal NOS. The cofactor (6R-tetrahydro-L-biopterin [H_4B]) participates in inducible and constitutive NOS isoform reactions. It is thought that H_4B stabilizes the enzyme in a manner allowing for maximum activity of the NOS subunit to which the pterin binds.[10,11,47,54]

BLOCKADE OF PLATELET AGGREGATION AND SECRETION BY NITRIC OXIDE

Platelet activation and recruitment in response to all agonists, such as ADP, collagen, epinephrine, and thrombin, is blocked by NO. Blockade also occurs *in vivo* via formation of NO from endothelium.[10] Importantly, the inhibitory action of NO is not affected by aspirin either *in vivo* or *ex vivo*. Therefore, NO production is not caused by participation of endothelial cell eicosanoids.

In addition to eNOS, the *NOS3* gene product, endothelial cells stimulated by agonists such as cytokines express the inducible form of NO synthase, iNOS, the *NOS2* gene product. Through this mechanism, NO can further inhibit platelet reactivity and reduce basal vessel tone by inducing relaxation of vascular smooth muscle. The biochemical basis for the reaction is that NO binds to the heme prosthetic group of guanylyl cyclase. The inhibitory effect of NO on platelet activation can be monitored by measuring surface expression of P-selectin. The ability of NO to inhibit mobilization of intracellular platelet calcium results in reduction of the conformational changes in platelet membrane glycoprotein (GP)IIb/IIIa, an absolute requirement for fibrinogen binding

and subsequent platelet aggregation. There is a broad spectrum of other effects of NO, including inhibition of leukocyte adhesion to endothelial cell surfaces, inhibition of smooth muscle migration, and reduction of smooth muscle cell proliferation. These phenomena suggest that secretion of NO into the microenvironment is a major component of the response to vascular injury[43]

● INHIBITION OF PLATELET ACTIVATION AND RECRUITMENT BY ECTO-ATP/DASE1-CD39

In addition to the platelet inhibition by PGI_2 and NO, endothelial cells inhibit platelet function via the action of endothelial cell ecto-ATP/Dase-1/CD39, an ecto-apyrase with ADPase and adenosine triphosphatase (ATPase) activities. The cluster designation symbol for this compound is CD39, the product of the *ENTPD1*, ectonucleotide triphosphate diphosphohydrolase gene.[55] CD39 is localized mainly in endothelial cells and leukocytes. In endothelial cells, CD39 is located on the cell surface with the major portion of the molecule facing the vessel lumen.[12,13,56] The enzyme has both N- and C-terminal transmembrane regions with small cytosolic portions anchoring the molecule.[57] In addition to CD39, CD73 (5'-nucleotidase) is present on vascular cells and converts the adenosine monophosphate (AMP) generated from CD39 metabolism to adenosine (Fig. 115–5). In contrast to all other known platelet inhibitors, acting in concert with CD73, CD39 can convert the local environment from a prothrombotic ADP/ATP-rich entity to an antithrombotic adenosine-rich environment.[58] This phenomenon was evident from observations that platelets became unresponsive to all agonists when in motion or in proximity to endothelial cells, even when eicosanoid and NO production were blocked.[2] Importantly, CD39 and CD73 do not exert their action on the platelet *per se* but act in series to metabolize ATP and ADP secreted from activated platelets to AMP and hence to adenosine.[13,59] ADP released from activated platelets is metabolized by CD39, thereby inhibiting ADP-induced platelet activation, release and aggregation (Fig. 115–5).

Most platelet agonists initiate secretion of dense granule contents within 15 to 20 seconds. The enhanced metabolism of ATP and ADP by therapeutically administered soluble CD39 would also reduce secondary autoamplification and recruitment, and, consequently, thrombus formation.[9,27,60] Because CD39 and CD73 are probably acting together, they will theoretically increase levels of endogenous adenosine and elevate the threshold for platelet activation in the local microenvironment. In a murine model, soluble CD39 administration ameliorates the extent of stroke and reverses excessive platelet reactivity without bleeding complications, even if administered 3 hours following stroke induction.[61] Therapeutic benefit of soluble CD39 has also been demonstrated in animal models of cardiac ischemia,[62] in the development of atherosclerosis,[63] regulation of leukocyte proinflammatory activity,[64] inhibition of metastasis,[65] and in transplantation medicine.[66] That the preclinical therapeutic use of soluble CD39 could abrogate thrombosis without inducing the hemorrhage seen with the use of existing antiplatelet therapies[67] could provide a therapeutic advantage over existing therapies for thrombotic disorders, including those who are resistant to existing therapeutic paradigms.[9] CD39 represents a major control system for blood fluidity.[68]

● THE PROTEIN C PATHWAY

The protein C pathway[69] plays a critical role in the prevention of thrombosis and is an integral part of the host inflammatory response. This pathway is initiated on the endothelial cell surface when thrombin

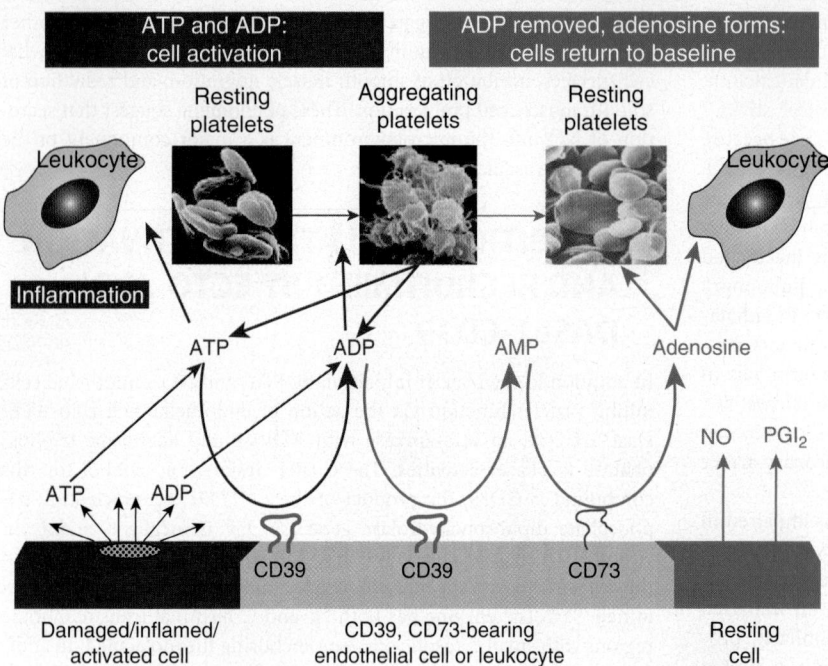

Figure 115–5. Released platelet adenosine diphosphate (ADP) is a major control system for hemostasis: ADP → adenosine monophosphate (AMP) → adenosine. Perturbation of endothelial cells, as a consequence of vascular injury, initiates the release of newly synthesized prostacyclin as well as nitric oxide, both of which inhibit platelet reactivity in the fluid phase. The apyrase CD39 is a cell-associated inhibitory thromboregulator. CD39 is substrate-activated and, in concert with CD39, CD73 brings the reaction to completion with the formation of adenosine.[309,310] The early metabolic deletion of ADP from the system may serve as a biologic safeguard to avoid excessive platelet accumulation, which would result in thrombosis.[21,22,309,310] NO, nitric oxide; PGI$_2$, prostacyclin.

combines with the endothelial receptor protein thrombomodulin (TM). Although thrombin is capable of slowly activating protein C, this reaction is markedly inhibited in the presence of physiologic concentrations of calcium ions. Upon binding of thrombin to TM, the rate of protein C activation is dramatically enhanced and becomes dependent on the presence of calcium. The detailed biochemistry of this activation reaction has been reviewed elsewhere.[70] Another protein found predominantly in large vessels, the EPCR, can bind protein C and further augment its activation by the thrombin–TM complex.[70] Activated protein C (APC) can dissociate from EPCR and interact with protein S on either the endothelial cell or other membrane surface to exert its anticoagulant function. The function of APC can be found in several reviews.[14,71-73]

By far, the best known function of TM is its role in protein C activation. When thrombin is bound to TM, it is no longer able to clot fibrinogen, activate platelets, activate factors V and VIII,[74] or interact with the protease-activated receptors.[75,76] Instead, thrombin-TM acts as a direct anticoagulant. TM also promotes the activation by thrombin of the plasma thrombin-activatable fibrinolysis inhibitor (TAFI).[77] TAFI inhibits plasmin-mediated fibrinolysis by removing carboxy-terminal lysine residues from fibrin, thereby reducing available binding sites for plasminogen and t-PA. In addition, TAFI is the major enzyme responsible for the removal of a C-terminal arginine from complement factor 5a (C5a),[78,79] leading to the inactivation of this potent anaphylotoxin generated during complement activation. Other vasoactive substances may also be inactivated by this enzyme. TM also accelerates the proteolytic inactivation of prourokinase (also called single-chain urokinase-type plasminogen activator [scu-PA]) by thrombin,[80,81] which may affect both fibrinolysis and tissue remodeling.[82] Despite these antifibrinolytic effects of TM, many *in vivo* experiments have demonstrated that soluble TM infusion results in a net antithrombotic and/or antiinflammatory effect.[83]

Independent of its effect on hemostasis, TM is essential to normal fetal development. When the TM gene is deleted by homologous recombination in mice, embryos die on day 8.5, prior to the development of a functional cardiovascular system,[84] implying that TM has functions in addition to its anticoagulant and antifibrinolytic properties. Both TM[85]

and EPCR[86] are highly expressed on the giant trophoblast cells of the placenta. If TM expression is maintained on these cells, the TM null embryos survive past this blockade point.[87,88]

The EPCR is a 220-amino-acid, type 1 transmembrane protein.[89-92] EPCR has two extracellular domains that show structural homology with the α and β domains of major histocompatibility complex (MHC) class 1 molecules, most notably the CD1d family. Because there are three Cys residues in the extracellular domain, the possibility of cross-linking with another protein exists. The cytoplasmic domain of human EPCR is only three amino acids long, Arg-Arg-Cys. The terminal Cys can be acylated with palmitate, which may have functional consequences.[93] Both protein C and APC bind to EPCR with similar affinity, approximately 30 nM.[89] Binding requires the presence of calcium and is enhanced in the presence of magnesium ions. In addition, a soluble form of EPCR found normally in plasma[94] is also capable of binding both protein C and APC with equivalent affinity.

EPCR augments protein C activation by the thrombin–TM complex *in vitro* and *in vivo*, primarily by decreasing the K$_m$ (Michaelis-Menten dissociation constant) for protein C.[70,95,96] Just as thrombin changes its function from procoagulant to anticoagulant when it binds to TM, it appears that APC bound to EPCR undergoes a similar switch from anticoagulant to antiinflammatory molecule.[97,98] Unfortunately, however, early studies that suggested a possible therapeutic role for APC in human sepsis have not been borne out in clinical trials.[99] Deletion of the EPCR gene by homologous recombination leads to early embryonic lethality around day 9.5,[100] at which time EPCR is highly expressed in the giant trophoblasts of the placenta, but not in the embryo itself.[86] In contrast to TM knockout animals,[101] the placentas of EPCR knockout embryos show significant fibrin deposition at the fetal maternal interface.

●VASCULAR FIBRINOLYSIS

Plasmin, the major clot-dissolving protease in humans, is formed upon the cleavage of a single peptide bond within the zymogen plasminogen (Chap. 135). This tightly regulated reaction is strongly influenced by cells of the blood vessel wall, including endothelial cells, smooth muscles cells, and macrophages, which express plasminogen activators, plasminogen activator inhibitors, and fibrinolytic receptors.

ENDOTHELIAL CELL PRODUCTION OF FIBRINOLYTIC PROTEINS

In 1958, Todd demonstrated that human blood vessels possess fibrinolytic activity that is dependent upon an intact endothelium.[102,103] We now know that the endothelium is the principal source of t-PA *in vivo* where it appears to be highly restricted to small blood vessels in specific anatomic locations, a pattern that likely reflects the heterogeneity of endothelial cells as they respond to a myriad of tissue-specific cues.[104,105] In the baboon, for example, sites of t-PA production include 7 to 30 μm precapillary arterioles and postcapillary venules, but not large arteries and veins.[106] In the mouse lung, similarly, bronchial, but not pulmonary, endothelial cells express t-PA.[107] Moreover, enhanced expression of t-PA at branch points of pulmonary blood vessels may reflect stimulation by laminar shear stress.[108] In addition, peripheral sympathetic neurons that invest the walls of small arteries may represent a significant source of circulating t-PA.[109]

Although *in vitro* studies suggest that t-PA expression in cultured endothelial cells is regulated by a wide array of factors, only a few of these pathways have been confirmed *in vivo*. Thrombin,[110] histamine,[111,112] oxygen radicals,[113] phorbol myristate acetate,[114] DDAVP (deamino D-arginine vasopressin),[115] and butyric acid liberated from dibutyryl cAMP[116] all increase t-PA mRNA in cultured endothelial cells. Both thrombin and histamine appear to act via receptor-mediated activation of the protein kinase C pathway.[105] Laminar shear stress stimulates both t-PA secretion[117] and steady-state mRNA levels.[118] Hyperosmotic stress and repetitive stretch also enhance t-PA expression.[119,120] In addition, differentiating agents, such as retinoids,[121,122] stimulate transcription of t-PA in endothelial cells *in vitro*.

In vivo, the circulating half-life of t-PA is approximately 5 minutes. Infusion of DDAVP, bradykinin, platelet-activating factor (PAF), endothelin, or thrombin is associated with an acute release of t-PA, and a burst of fibrinolytic activity can be detected within minutes.[123] In the mouse lung, exposure to hyperoxia leads to 4.5-fold upregulation of t-PA mRNA in small-vessel endothelial cells.[107] In humans, infusion of TNF into patients with malignancy is associated with an increase in plasma t-PA.[123] Deficient release of t-PA in response to venous occlusion in humans is associated with deep venous thrombosis,[124] as well as atrophie blanche and other cutaneous vasculitides.[125]

In vivo, urokinase plasminogen activator (u-PA) is not a product of resting endothelium,[126] but is produced primarily by renal tubular epithelium.[127] Expression of u-PA mRNA in endothelium, however, is strongly stimulated during wound repair and physiologic angiogenesis within ovarian follicles, corpus luteum, and maternal decidua.[128] Endothelial cells passaged in culture do synthesize u-PA,[129] and expression of its mRNA is stimulated by TNF-α by 5- to 30-fold.[130] Small increases in u-PA have also been observed *in vitro* in response to IL-1 and LPS.[131–133]

The association of u-PA with the blood vessel wall appears to reflect its association with the u-PA receptor (uPAR) which may fulfill a variety of nonproteolytic functions ranging from directed cell migration to cellular adhesion, differentiation, and proliferation (Fig. 115–6).[134] In the adult mouse, uPAR mRNA is not normally detected by *in situ* hybridization in the endothelium of either large or small blood vessels.[135] However, upon stimulation with endotoxin, expression is detected in endothelium lining aorta, as well as arteries, veins, and capillaries in heart, kidney, brain, and liver,[135] and in renal tubular epithelial cells.[127]

Plasminogen activator inhibitor (PAI)-1 is likely to function as a major regulator of plasmin generation in the vicinity of the endothelial cell. Thrombin, IL-1, transforming growth factor β, TNF, lipoprotein(a) (Lp[a]), and LPS all induce dramatic increases in steady state PAI-1 message levels.[110,131,132,136,137] Heparin-binding growth factor 1 reduces

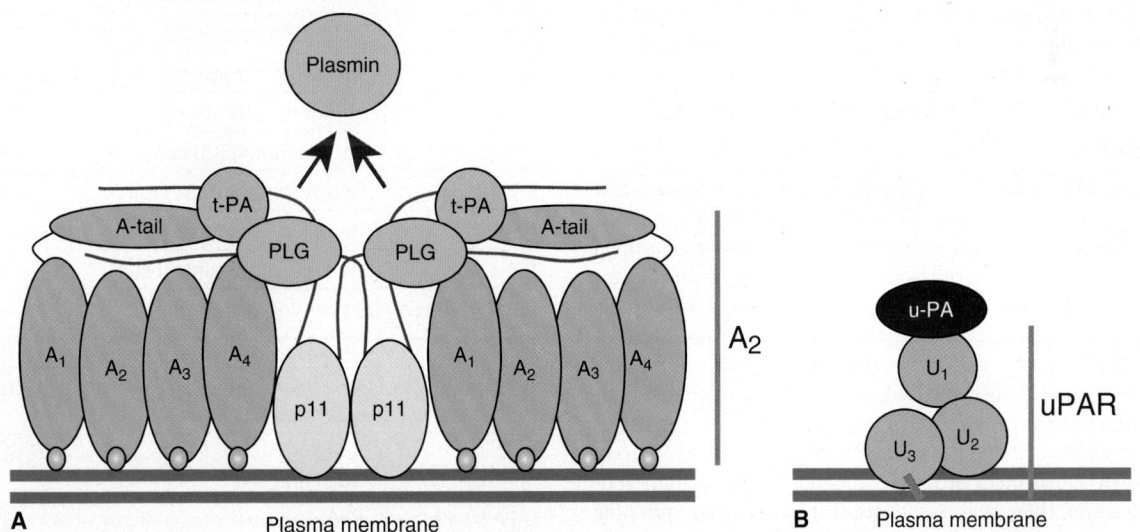

Figure 115–6. Schematic of principal endothelial cell fibrinolytic receptors. **A.** The annexin A2/S100A10 heterotetrameric complex. Annexin A2 consists of a hydrophilic aminoterminal tail domain (A-Tail, approximately 3 kDa), and a membrane-oriented carboxyl terminal core domain (approximately 33 kDa).[311,312] The tail domain contains residues required for tissue-type plasminogen activator (t-PA) binding. The core domain is composed of four homologous annexin repeats (A1, A2, A3, and A4), each consisting of five a-helical regions that contribute to calcium-dependent phospholipid binding sites. Repeat 2 appears to be most important for the interaction of annexin A2 with the endothelial cell surface. Plasminogen (PLG) binding requires lysine residue 307 within helix C of repeat 4. **B.** Urokinase plasminogen activator receptor (uPAR) is a 55- to 60-kDa, glycosylphosphatidylinositol-linked protein that consists of three disulfide-linked domains (U1, U2, U3).[314] Domain 1 contains sequences required for urokinase plasminogen activator (u-PA) binding, while domains 2 and 3 mediate the receptor's interaction with matrix proteins such as vitronectin. Domain 3 contains glycosylphosphatidylinositol-linked membrane anchor. (*A, adapted with permission from Gerke V, Creutz CE, Moss SE: Annexins: linking Ca2+ signalling to membrane dynamics. Nat Rev Mol Cell Biol 6(6):449–461.*)

PAI-1 mRNA production by cultured endothelial cells, but has no effect on t-PA.[138] Thus, synthesis and secretion of PAI-1 by the endothelial cell *in vitro* appears to be regulated independently of t-PA.

In vivo, elevated levels of circulating PAI-1 have been linked epidemiologically to risk for myocardial infarction.[124] Although the liver is the major source of plasma PAI-1, endothelial expression of PAI-1 is detected near neovascular sprouts during decidual neovascularization in the ovary.[128] In addition, inflammatory cytokines are powerful stimuli for induction of PAI-1 in a variety of tissues including liver, as injection of TNF in both rats and humans with active malignancy results in a striking increase plasma concentrations of PAI-1.[105,123]

The endothelial cell coreceptor for t-PA and plasminogen, the annexin A2/S100A10 complex (see Fig. 115–6), appears to be expressed constitutively *in vivo* by endothelial cells in a wide variety of tissues in the chicken,[139] mouse,[140] rat,[141] and human.[142] Annexin A2 is upregulated transcriptionally by hypoxia both *in vivo* and in endothelial cells *in vitro,*[143] and by nerve growth factor in neuronal-like PC12 cells.[144] In addition, the *in vitro* transition of human monocyte to macrophage is associated with a severalfold increase in both annexin A2 protein and steady state mRNA expression.[145]

The evidence that the annexin A2 system plays a role in maintaining vascular patency includes the findings that (1) overexpression of annexin A2 in blast cells in acute promyelocytic leukemia blast cells increases plasmin production and contributes to hyperfibrinolytic bleeding,[146–149] (2) systemic injection of annexin A2 diminishes thrombotic vascular occlusion resulting from vascular injury in experimental animals,[150] (3) annexin A2–deficient mice display fibrin deposition on microvessels and impaired clearance of arterial thrombi following vascular injury,[151] (4) high titer antibodies directed against annexin A2 are associated with thrombosis in antiphospholipid syndrome and in individuals with cerebral venous thrombosis,[152,153] and (5) that polymorphisms in the *ANXA2* gene are associated with cerebral vascular occlusion and osteonecrosis of bone in patients with sickle cell disease.[154–156] Whether defects in S100A10, which could serve either as a chaperone for annexin A2 or as a direct binding site for plasminogen,[157] might also be associated with these clinical entities remains to be determined.

NONFIBRINOLYTIC VASCULAR FUNCTIONS OF PLASMIN

Although not yet demonstrated *in vivo,* plasmin may inactivate factor Va *in vitro* by cleaving both the heavy and light chains of this 168-kDa protein, in a manner that is distinct from the action of activated protein C.[158,159] Plasmin can also inactivate factor VIIIa, a procoagulant cofactor that is structurally related to factor Va.[160] In addition, platelet GPIIb/IIIa and GPIb, the cell surface receptors for fibrinogen and VWF, respectively, are both plasmin substrates.[161,162] Thus, plasmin formation in the vicinity of a hemostatic plug could lead to impaired adhesion and poor aggregation in response to agonists. *In vivo,* prolonged bleeding times were found in patients 90 minutes after t-PA infusion for thrombolysis, suggesting early impairment of platelet function upon plasmin generation.[163] However, there is also evidence that platelets may promote thrombotic reocclusion following successful thrombolytic therapy.[164]

FIBRINOLYTIC FUNCTION IN VASCULAR INJURY

Transgenic mouse models of vascular disease have helped to elucidate the complex role of the fibrinolytic system in atherosclerosis (Table 115–3).[165,166] In mice, the general effects of plasminogen deficiency include runting, fibrin deposition in intra- and extravascular locations, and premature death.[167,168] In addition, the mice display

TABLE 115–3. The Fibrinolytic System in Cardiovascular Disease—Transgenic Mouse Models

Genotype	Result	Reference(s)
Atherogenesis:		
PLG$^{-/-}$ ApoE$^{-/-}$	Increased atherogenesis	178
t-PA$^{-/-}$ ApoE$^{-/-}$	Unchanged atherogenesis	179
u-PA$^{-/-}$ ApoE$^{-/-}$	Unchanged atherogenesis	179
PAI-1$^{-/-}$ ApoE$^{-/-}$	Decrease in early plaque size; increase in advanced plaque size	180–182
Transplant arteriosclerosis:		
PLG$^{-/-}$	Reduced leukocyte invasion in transplantation model; reduced extent of disease	185
Coronary ligation:		
u-PA$^{-/-}$	Protection from ventricular rupture; but poor revascularization and late death from heart failure	186
t-PA$^{-/-}$	No protection	186
uPAR$^{-/-}$	No protection	186
Aortic aneurysm:		
u-PA$^{-/-}$ ApoE$^{-/-}$	Protected	179
t-PA$^{-/-}$ ApoE$^{-/-}$	Not protected	179
Early oxidative injury:		
PAI-1$^{-/-}$	Attenuated thrombotic occlusion (Rose Bengal)	194
PAI-1$^{-/-}$	Attenuated thrombotic occlusion (FeCl$_3$)	195
u-PA$^{-/-}$	Increased thrombosis (FeCl$_3$)	196
t-PA$^{-/-}$	Increased thrombosis (FeCl$_3$)	196
A2$^{-/-}$	Increased thrombosis (FeCl$_3$)	155
Restenosis with prominent thrombosis:		
PAI-1$^{-/-}$	No neointima (Cu cuff)	199
PAI-1$^{-/-}$	Reduced neointima (ligation)	317
PAI-1$^{-/-}$	Reduced neointima (FeCl$_3$)	317
PAI-1$^{-/-}$ ApoE$^{-/-}$	Reduced neointima (FeCl$_3$)	198
Restenosis without prominent thrombosis:		
PLG$^{-/-}$	Reduced neointima (electrical)	187, 188
t-PA$^{-/-}$	No change (electrical or mechanical)	187, 189
u-PA$^{-/-}$	Reduced neointima (electrical or mechanical)	187, 189
u-PA$^{-/-}$ t-PA$^{-/-}$	Reduced neointima (electrical or mechanical)	187, 189
uPAR$^{-/-}$	No change (electrical)	190
PAI-1$^{-/-}$	Increased neointima (ligation)	318
PAI-1$^{-/-}$	Increased neointima (electrical or mechanical)	191

A2, annexin A2; ApoE, apolipoprotein E; PAI-1, plasminogen-activator inhibitor-1; PLG, plasminogen; t-PA, tissue-type plasminogen activator; u-PA, urokinase plasminogen activator; uPAR, u-PA receptor.

impaired healing of cutaneous wounds,[169] a response that appears to depend largely on the fibrinolytic action of plasmin as loss of fibrinogen eliminates these defects.[170] Mice doubly deficient in plasminogen and apolipoprotein E (ApoE) showed an increased predisposition to atherosclerosis compared to animals deficient in ApoE alone (Fig. 115–7A).[171] Mice with ApoE deficiency combined with deficiency of either u-PA or t-PA showed the same predilection for early fatty streaks and advanced plaques as was observed in mice with isolated ApoE deficiency, suggesting that complete elimination of plasmin generating activity is required to exacerbate the proatherogenic state.[172] Finally, mice doubly deficient in ApoE and PAI-1 exhibit no change in early plaque size at the aortic root,[173,174] decreased early plaque size at the carotid bifurcation,[173,174] but increased advanced plaque size with accelerated deposition of matrix.[175]

Once the atherosclerotic plaque is established, plasmin may affect its evolution by mediating invasion of leukocytes (see Table 115–3).[176] In the peritoneal cavity, recruitment of inflammatory cells is profoundly influenced by the presence or absence of plasminogen.[177] In transplant-associated arteriosclerosis, the extent of disease is significantly reduced in plasminogen-deficient mice, reflecting, at least in part, reduced influx of macrophages, with an associated reduction in medial necrosis, fragmentation of elastic laminae, and remodeling of the adventitia.[178] Thus, the role of plasmin in degrading fibrin and other matrix constituents in the early lesion limits atherosclerosis, whereas its ability to promote cellular invasion later on appears to promote atherogenesis.

During aortic aneurysm formation in mice, deficiency of u-PA, but not t-PA, was associated with reduced medial destruction and impaired activation of downstream plasmin-dependent matrix metalloproteinases (Fig. 115–7B and Table 115–3).[172] Similarly, u-PA–, but not t-PA–, deficient mice were protected from cardiac rupture secondary to ventricular aneurysm. In this study, temporary administration of PAI-1 or the general matrix metalloproteinase inhibitor, tissue inhibitor of metalloproteinase (TIMP)-1, completely protected wild-type mice from aortic rupture, reinforcing the concept that plasmin-based protease activity promotes aneurysm progression.[179]

Vascular remodeling may occur following acute arterial injury induced by interventions for vascular compromise, leading to vascular restenosis (Fig. 115–7C and Table 115–3). This process reflects leukocyte invasion, proliferation and migration of smooth muscle cells, deposition of extracellular matrix, and reendothelialization. Electrical or mechanical injury studies in gene-targeted mice indicate that neointima formation, an initial step in restenosis, requires intact expression of plasminogen and u-PA, but not t-PA.[180–182] Interestingly, loss of uPAR has no effect on neointima formation,[183] whereas loss of PAI-1 is associated with increased neointimal stenosis.[184,185] In these injury models, which do not induce severe thrombosis, it is thought that vascular occlusion, reflecting migration of smooth muscle cells and leukocytes, is impaired when fibrinolytic potential is attenuated.[186]

In the ferric chloride, Rose Bengal, and copper cuff models, on the other hand, thrombosis is observed within minutes of arterial injury (see Fig. 115–7 and Table 115–3). In these systems, deficiency of PAI-1 is associated with later and less-extensive thrombotic occlusion of the injured artery,[187,188] while loss of u-PA is associated with more rapid and more significant thrombotic occlusion.[189] At the same time, the absence of PAI-1 led to reduced vascular stenosis, regardless of whether ApoE was absent[190,191] or present.[192,193] In balloon-injured rat carotid arteries, finally, transduction of a PAI-1–expressing gene led to increased restenosis of the vessel, again suggesting that clearance of the initial thrombus may have longterm effects on vessel patency and neointima formation.[194] In these models, the predominant effect of the fibrinolytic system may be to clear the initial thrombus, which may provide a provisional scaffolding for later restenosis.

● FIBRINOLYTIC ASSEMBLY AND VASCULAR DISEASE

Endothelial cells use receptors, primarily uPAR and the annexin A2/S100A10 system, to assemble the fibrinolytic system on their surface (Chap. 135; Fig. 115–6). Recent evidence suggests that impairment of receptor-mediated fibrinolytic assembly may lead to vascular compromise.

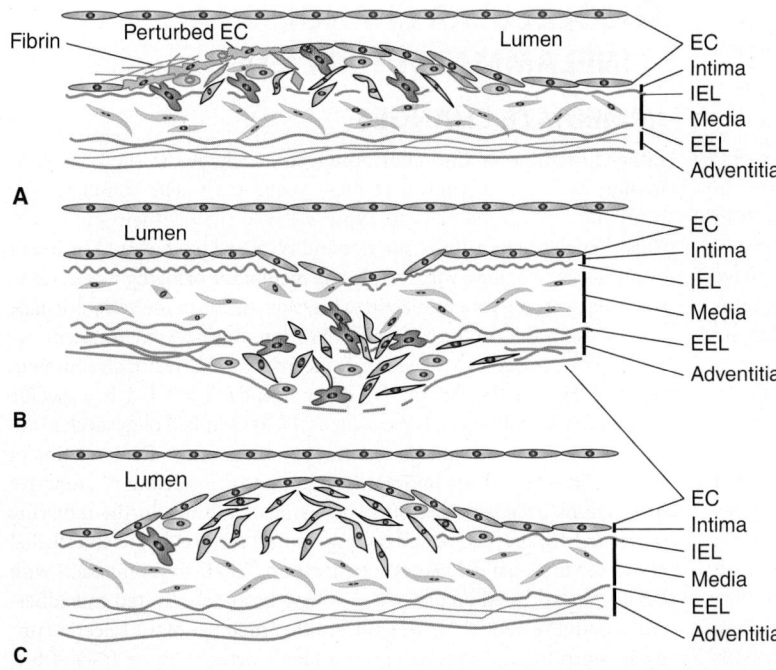

Figure 115–7. Working model for the actions of the fibrinolytic system in vascular disease. **A.** Plaque formation. Atheromatous plaque is thought to form in response to endothelial cell (EC) *(orange)* injury or perturbation. Following the initial injury, perturbed endothelial cells may fail to clear fibrin on the blood vessel surface, and may also promote adhesion and invasion of leukocytes *(blue)*. In addition, smooth muscle cells arising in the tunica media invade the developing plaque within the intima *(green)*. Endothelial cells may utilize cell-surface receptors for focal activation of plasmin to maintain a thromboresistant vascular surface. Leukocytes, macrophages, and smooth muscle cells may use plasmin to migrate into the evolving plaque (cells outlined in *red*). **B.** Aneurysm. Fragmentation and dissolution of the elastic laminae of the arterial wall may occur may occur upon matrix metalloproteinase activation via plasmin-dependent pathways, possibly mediated by smooth muscle cells. Cells migrating outward toward the adventitial surface of the vessel induce further matrix degradation, and the potential for rupture. **C.** Restenosis. In response to vascular injury, smooth muscle cells proliferate and, together with leukocytes, invade the subendothelial space establishing a thickened neointima that compromises vascular patency. In all three scenarios, cell migration is thought to require plasmin activity, possibly in association with cell surfaces. EEL, external elastic lamina; IEL, internal elastic lamina.

LIPOPROTEIN(A)

Lp(a) is a low-density lipoprotein (LDL)-like particle that is an independent risk factor for atherosclerosis.[195-197] In addition to the apolipoprotein B-100 found on LDL, Lp(a) contains a disulfide-linked moiety called apolipoprotein(a) [apo(a)]. Apo(a) shares a remarkable degree of homology with plasminogen, as it possesses multiple tandem repeats of a kringle IV-like domain, a single domain resembling kringle V, and a pseudoprotease domain.[198,199] Plasminogen and apo(a), furthermore, are closely linked on chromosome 6 and appear to have arisen from a common ancestral gene.[200]

Whereas Lp(a) levels are only transiently responsive to diet,[201,202] plasma levels appear to be subject to mendelian inheritance.[203-205] Plasma Lp(a) concentrations correlate inversely with the ratio of kringle IV to kringle V encoding domains within the apo(a) gene,[206,207] such that larger apo(a) gene products are associated with lower plasma concentrations of apo(a). In addition, Lp(a) is an acute phase reactant in the postsurgical and post–myocardial infarction setting,[204] and in patients with cancer,[205] suggesting a role for soluble inflammatory mediators in regulating its synthesis or assembly. Apo(a) possesses a high-affinity lysine binding site within kringle 4 that closely resembles that of kringle 1 of plasminogen,[208] and kringle 37 of the originally cloned apo(a) resembles the lysine-binding plasminogen kringle 4 of plasminogen.[209] *In vivo*, Lp(a) colocalizes histologically with fibrin in atheromatous tissue.[210]

When apo(a) is overexpressed in transgenic mice,[211] cell-associated plasmin activity is reduced such that the animals are resistant to t-PA thrombolysis.[212] Three potential explanations for the prothrombotic, proatherogenic effect of Lp(a) include (1) the observation that both Lp(a) and apo(a) inhibit Lys-plasminogen binding to endothelial cells (half-maximal inhibitory dose [ID_{50}] = 36-fold excess),[213] and to annexin A2,[214] with affinity similar to that for plasminogen[215-217]; (2) endothelial cell exposure to Lp(a) *in vitro* enhances expression of PAI-1[137]; and (3) Lp(a) may act as a competitive inhibitor of t-PA in the presence of fibrinogen,[218] or as an uncompetitive inhibitor of the fibrin-dependent enhancement of t-PA–induced plasmin generation.[219] Overexpression of Lp(a) in mice receiving a high-fat diet results in atherosclerosis-like lesions containing anti-apo(a) cross-reactive material.[220] Deposition of both lipid and apo(a) was reduced in mice expressing apo(a) in which lysine binding sites had been mutated.[221] Thus, lysine binding sites of apo(a) appear to allow it to compete with plasminogen for cell surface receptors, thereby increasing atherogenicity.

HOMOCYSTEINE

Homocysteine is a thiol-containing amino acid that accumulates in nutritional deficiencies of vitamin B_6, vitamin B_{12}, or folic acid, or in inherited abnormalities of cystathionine β-synthase, methylene tetrahydrofolate reductase, or methionine synthase.[222] Multiple studies have shown homocysteine to be an independent risk factor for atherosclerosis,[223] venous thromboembolism, and death.[224] Homocysteine lowering in patients with inborn errors of homocysteine metabolism leads to a striking reduction in cardiovascular morbidity, but supplementation with B vitamins in patients with established cardiovascular disease is of no benefit.[225] *In vitro*, homocysteine-treated endothelial cells bound approximately 50 percent less t-PA than untreated cells, and activated approximately 50 percent less plasminogen.[226] Mass spectrometry studies indicate that homocysteine directly disables the t-PA binding domain of annexin A2 by forming a covalent adduction product with cysteine 9 within the tail domain of purified annexin A2, thus inhibiting its ability to bind t-PA.[227] Mice on a high homocysteine-generating diet, moreover, displayed dysfunctional annexin A2, and loss of both fibrinolytic and angiogenic potential. This phenotype mimicked that of

annexin A2-deficient mice, and was overcome upon intravenous infusion of unmodified annexin A2.[228]

ANTIPHOSPHOLIPID SYNDROME

Antiphospholipid syndrome (APS) is an autoimmune disorder characterized by thrombosis, recurrent pregnancy loss, and persistently positive antiphospholipid antibodies.[229,230] Compared to patients with lupus erythematosus, nonimmune thrombosis, or healthy controls, a relatively high proportion of patients with APS and severe thrombosis (22 percent) has antibodies directed against annexin A2. Antiannexin A2 antibodies may block t-PA–dependent cell-surface plasmin generation, and also induce expression of procoagulant molecules, such as TF.[152] These events may require crosslinking of β_2-GPI bound to closely associated cell-surface A2,[231,232] and signaling via myeloid differentiation protein 88 (MyD88) and nuclear factor kappa B (NFκB)-dependent pathway.[233] Additional evidence shows that A2 is required for the pathogenic effects of antiphospholipid antibodies in mice.[234] High-titer antiannexin A2 antibodies are also associated with cerebral vein thrombosis in patients without the full diagnostic criteria for APS.[153]

● ROLE OF ADHESION MOLECULES

A proinflammatory environment is also prothrombotic. Endothelial cells express molecules that regulate binding of leukocytes to their surface during inflammation. These interactions have both direct and indirect roles in hemostasis and thrombosis, and, in some cases, interactions of leukocytes and platelets with inflamed endothelial cells feed forward to promote thrombosis.[235] Moreover, the inflammatory response itself results in the expression of adhesion molecules and mediators that secondarily promote hemostasis. In addition, membrane microparticles derived from platelets, leukocytes, and perhaps endothelium, provide circulating sources of TF, proinflammatory lipids, and other molecules that have the potential to regulate thrombosis and inflammation at a distance from the primary site.[236-240]

● MOLECULAR CHANGES IN AN INFLAMMATORY MILIEU

IMMEDIATE CHANGES

Either histamine or thrombin produced locally at the site of inflammation by degranulation of resident tissue mast cells stimulates the overlying endothelial cells to express P-selectin on their surfaces.[241] This change occurs within minutes and is caused by the rapid fusion of Weibel-Palade bodies, with the plasma membrane bringing P-selectin to the surface. Along with P-selectin expression, fusion of the Weibel-Palade bodies also results in the release of VWF into the local environment.

P-selectin serves as a leukocyte receptor for P-selectin glycoprotein ligand (PSGL)-1, L-selectin, and other ligands.[242] PSGL-1 is a specific sialomucin containing sialylated, fucosylated *O*-linked oligosaccharides as well as an unusual sulfated tyrosine residue motif.[243] Dimerization of PSGL-1 is required for optimal recognition of P-selectin.[244] Adhesive interactions between P-selectin and its ligands result in the tethering of passing leukocytes to, and rolling on, the surface of the endothelial cell as the first step in leukocyte emigration. PSGL-1 also interacts with P-selectin expressed on platelets that have become activated and adherent to endothelium.[45,245] L-selectin, another member of the selectin family, is constitutively expressed on most leukocytes. It binds to sialylated, fucosylated GP ligands expressed by endothelial cells in response to inflammation, as well as to CD34 constitutively expressed by cells of the high endothelial venules.

Adhesion of leukocytes to the endothelium at the site of inflammation results in their rolling along the luminal surface, which slows their movement and brings them into contact with a wide variety of chemical mediators that trigger the next stage of leukocyte emigration—tight adhesion to the endothelial surface. These mediators include surface-bound chemokines,[246] new adhesion molecules expressed by the endothelium in response to inflammatory cytokines,[247] PAF,[248] soluble chemokines,[249] and ligands that crosslink leukocyte CD31[250-252] and seem to work by stimulating the activation of leukocyte integrin adhesion molecules by so-called inside-out signaling. This process involves a conformational change and/or clustering of the two chains of these heterodimeric surface molecules such that the affinity or avidity, respectively, for their ligands on the surfaces of endothelial cells is increased.[253] The ligands identified are members of a third family of adhesion molecules, the immunoglobulin gene superfamily.[254]

Table 115–4 lists some of the more common leukocyte/endothelial CAM pairs participating in the inflammatory response. It is interesting to note that the mucosal addressin MAdCAM-1, a unique molecule expressed by endothelial cells of high endothelial venules of mesenteric

lymph nodes and Peyer patches, has structural features of both a mucin and an immunoglobulin superfamily molecule. It can bind both L-selectin and the leukocyte integrin $\alpha_4\beta_7$, expressed by a subset of memory T cells. It is believed to interact with L-selectin through its mucin (carbohydrate) domain and with $\alpha_4\beta_7$ through its immunoglobulin domains. Until recently, identified protein ligands for L-selectin (MAdCAM-1 and CD34) have been demonstrated to bind to L-selectin only in the context of lymphocyte homing, although recent evidence now suggests that they may play a role in rolling during inflammation.[255] Interestingly, intravital microscopy shows that leukocytes may roll on already adherent leukocytes and platelets through the interactions of L-selectin and PSGL-1 to amplify the inflammatory process.[256,257]

PAF is made and secreted acutely by leukocytes, mast cells, and endothelial cells at the site of inflammation. PAF (1-alkyl-2-acetyl-*sn*-glycero-3-phosphocholine) is produced enzymatically from phosphatidyl choline in the plasma membrane. Although its role as an activator of neutrophils in this environment has been established,[248] it appears to be a relatively weak agonist of platelet activation in this location.

Adherent leukocytes migrate to nearby interendothelial junctions by repeated cycles of adhesion in the front and disadhesion in the rear.[254,258] At the junction, additional distinct molecular interactions

TABLE 115–4. Common Leukocyte–Endothelial Cell Adhesion Molecule Pairs in Inflammation

Leukocyte Molecule	CD and Integrin Nomenclature	Leukocytes Expressing	Action	Endothelial Counter Ligand	CD Number
L-selectin	CD62L	PMN, Mo, T, B, NK	Tethering, rolling	MAdCAM-1*	Pending
				GP105–120	CD34
PSGL-1	CD162	PMN, Mo, T, B, NK	Tethering, rolling	P-selectin	CD62P
Sialyl LewisX ESL-1[†], CLA[†]	CD15s	PMN, Mo, T, B, NK	Tethering, rolling	E-selectin	CD62E
LFA-1	CD11a/CD18	PMN, Mo, T, B, NK	Tight adhesion	ICAM-1	CD54
	$(\alpha_L\beta_2)$			ICAM-2	CD102
				ICAM-3	CD50
			Adhesion, diapedesis	JAM-A	Pending
Mac-1	CD11b/CD18	PMN, Mo, NK	Tight adhesion	ICAM-1	CD54
VLA-4	CD49d/CD29	Mo, B, Eo[‡] > NK, T	Tight adhesion[§] Rolling	VCAM-1	CD106
PECAM-1	CD31	PMN, Mo, NK Subsets of T	Diapedesis	PECAM-1	CD31
CD99	CD99	All leukocytes to varying degrees	Diapedesis	CD99	CD99
JAM-C?	Pending	T	Diapedesis	JAM-C?	Pending

B, B lymphocytes; CLA, cutaneous lymphocyte antigen; Eo, eosinophils; ESL-1, E-selectin ligand; GP, glycoprotein; ICAM, intercellular adhesion molecule; JAM, junctional adhesion molecule; MAdCAM-1, mucosal addressin cell-adhesion molecule; Mo, monocytes; NK, natural killer cells; PECAM, platelet endothelial adhesion molecule; PMN, polymorphonuclear neutrophils; PSGL, P-selectin glycoprotein ligand; T, T lymphocytes; VCAM, vascular cell adhesion molecule; VLA, very-late antigen.

PMN, neutrophils;*MAdCAM-1 and CD34 have been shown to be important for homing of T cells to lymph nodes via high endothelial venules. The protein structures bearing the L-selectin ligands, including CD15s, at sites of inflammation have not been identified.

[†]ESL-1, a protein with homology to fibroblast growth factor receptor, has been identified in mice. CLA, a molecule on the surface of skin-homing T cells related to PSGL-1, directs them to skin via E-selectin expressed on dermal venules.

[‡]Expression of VLA-4 on granulocytes is limited to eosinophils and basophils. Adult human neutrophils do not express it under normal circumstances.

[§]Although VLA-4/VCAM-1 interactions are generally thought to be important for tight adhesion of leukocytes to endothelium, there are reports[319,320] that leukocytes can use VLA-4 to roll on endothelial VCAM-1, as well.

between leukocytes and endothelial cells regulate transendothelial migration for the vast majority of neutrophils, monocytes, and natural killer (NK) cells. Transendothelial migration and the nomenclature of the junctional adhesion molecule (JAM) family are reviewed elsewhere.[17,259,260] PECAM/CD31 on the leukocyte contacts the same molecule concentrated at the endothelial junctions in a homophilic manner.[261-263] Although the relevant signal(s) transduced by this interaction remain unclear, a transient rise in endothelial cell intracellular calcium is required for transmigration.[264] Blocking the function of either leukocyte PECAM or endothelial cell PECAM arrests the leukocyte poised over the junction,[263,265,266] a phenotype very similar to that seen when the rise in intracellular calcium is blocked by the chelator, bis(2-amino-5-methylphenoxy)ethane-N,N,N',N'-tetraacetic acid tetraacetoxymethyl ester (MAPTAM).[264]

Because anti-PECAM reagents never block diapedesis completely, PECAM-independent pathways of transendothelial migration must exist. The leukocyte integrins $\alpha_4\beta_1$ (very-late antigen [VLA]-4) and $\alpha_L\beta_2/\alpha_M\beta_2$ (lymphocyte function-associated antigen [LFA]-1/macrophage [Mac]-1) and their endothelial counter-receptors VCAM-1 and ICAM-1, have been implicated in transmigration.[254] Interaction of leukocyte LFA-1 with JAM-A on endothelial cells has also been implicated in leukocyte recruitment.[267] Antibodies directed against JAM-C also blocked migration of lymphocytes across endothelial cell monolayers, implicating its role in lymphocyte migration.[268] In addition, under certain specialized conditions, there appear to be pathways across the endothelial cell that bypass the intercellular junction.[269,270]

CD99 is a GP expressed on leukocytes, platelets, and erythrocytes, and concentrated at the endothelial cell borders. CD99 controls a step in diapedesis distal to the step controlled by PECAM both *in vitro* and in vivo,[271-273] by interfering with homophilic interaction between leukocyte CD99 and endothelial cell CD99-arrested monocytes. Their leading edges were below the endothelial cell monolayer, while their trailing uropods remained on the apical surface of the endothelial cell.

At the onset of most acute inflammatory responses, vascular permeability transiently increases as a result of histamine release. The endothelial junctions are soon re-established, and the junctions are closed to the leukocytes that arrive at the scene over the next hour. Studies performed both *in vivo* and *in vitro* indicate that, during subsequent diapedesis, leukocytes penetrate the vessel wall without further compromising the vascular permeability barrier.[264,274] Cortactin-deficient mice, for example, have constitutively leaky vascular junctions in the postcapillary venule circulation, and an exaggerated response to histamine, yet leukocyte recruitment is diminished because of inefficient clustering of ICAM-1,[275] which prevents exposure of subendothelial collagen and VWF deposits to circulating platelets. Although PECAM-1 has no known role in binding platelets to endothelial cells, it has been hypothesized to maintain the tight apposition of endothelial cells and leukocytes during diapedesis.[263]

ACUTE CHANGES

In addition to stimulating endothelial cell immediate responses, cytokines and inflammatory mediators released at the site of inflammation activate new endothelial cell genetic programs. Within several hours of exposure to mediator, *de novo* synthesis of mRNA and protein establishes an inflammatory endothelial cell phenotype that is both procoagulant and proadhesive.

Inflammatory cytokines such as TNF-α and IL-1 induce endothelial cell surface expression of several important CAMs. Expression of E-selectin peaks at 4 to 6 hours *in vitro*, but may be maintained by interferon (IFN)-γ for several days *in vivo*.[276,277] E-selectin mediates the slow rolling of leukocytes bearing sialylated, fucosylated carbohydrate

receptors similar to sialylated Lewis X antigen.[278] Endothelial cell P-selectin stimulated by thrombin or histamine is transient, but can be prolonged to hours or days by IL-3, IL-4, or oncostatin M stimulation of human endothelium, and by TNF-α stimulation of murine, but not human endothelium.[279-282]

In general, expression of the immunoglobulin superfamily members ICAM-1 and VCAM-1 is induced by the same stimuli that induce E-selectin. Some specializations exist, at least *in vitro*. For example, IL-4 induces VCAM-1 but not E-selectin or ICAM-1 in microvascular endothelial cells.[283,284] These molecules serve as counter-receptors for the leukocyte integrins in the tight adhesion step.

CHRONIC CHANGES

Stimulation of endothelial cells over several days with IFN-γ leads to surface expression of MHC class II molecules (human leukocyte antigen [HLA]-DR and -DQ). In human tissues such as skin and gut, class II is commonly seen even in the absence of overt inflammation, and is thought to be a result of chronic exposure of these sites to subclinical inflammation and antigenic stimulation. When costimulatory molecules such as CD40, ICAM-1, or LFA-3 are induced by inflammatory stimuli, the endothelial cell becomes capable (at least *in vitro*) of acting as an antigen presenting cell that can stimulate CD4+ memory T cells. This mechanism may stimulate graft rejection by the host when the endothelium belongs to an organ graft with foreign MHC class II.[285-287]

In contrast, the expression of the adhesion molecule ICAM-2 does not change in response to inflammatory mediators. PECAM-1 shows a unique expression pattern in response to IFN-γ *in vitro*[288] and *in vivo*,[289] as its distribution becomes diffuse over the surface of the cell, rather than being concentrated at intercellular borders. *In vitro* chronic exposure of human umbilical vein endothelial cells to a combination of IFN-γ and TNF-α at relatively high doses leads to a decrease in total PECAM-1 expression.[290] Such a response has not been described to date *in vivo*.

ADHESION MOLECULES IN A THROMBOTIC MILIEU

Activation of the hemostatic system exposes leukocytes to ligands that promote their adhesion and recruitment to the vessel wall. For example, *in vitro* thrombin induces E-selectin expression and IL-8 secretion by human umbilical vein endothelial cells.[291] These changes are classically induced by inflammatory cytokines such as IL-1 and TNF-α. Table 115–5 lists some mediators that could have dual roles in inflammation and hemostasis/thrombosis.

LEUKOCYTE–PLATELET AND ENDOTHELIAL CELL–PLATELET INTERACTIONS

Activated platelets bind to circulating lymphocytes in a P-selectin–dependent manner. This interaction can facilitate leukocyte rolling on the endothelium[292] and also allows homing of lymphocytes to peripheral lymph nodes in the absence of L-selectin, because P-selectin on the adherent platelets will interact with the peripheral lymph node addressin.[293] *In vitro*, neutrophils are capable of rolling on immobilized platelets via PSGL-1 on the leukocyte interacting with degranulated P-selectin on the platelet membranes.[294] Moreover, $\alpha_M\beta_2$ (CD11b/CD18)-dependent arrest and tight adhesion of neutrophils to bound platelets following P-selectin–dependent rolling has been described.[294,295] The endothelial ligand for this is not known. ICAM-2 has been found on the surface of activated platelets, but it is not a ligand for $\alpha_M\beta_2$. In

TABLE 115–5. Dual Roles of Inflammatory Mediators in Thrombosis and Hemostasis

Mediator	Role in Inflammation	Role in Thrombosis or Hemostasis
Histamine, thrombin	P-selectin expression induced on vascular endothelium	Degranulation of Weibel-Palade bodies; extrusion of VWF
Platelet-activating factor	Activation of leukocyte integrins	Activation of platelets
Expression of P-selectin glycoprotein ligand 1 (PSGL-1)	Adhesion of leukocytes to endothelial P-selectin	Adhesion of platelets to adherent leukocytes via P-selectin bidirectionally
Adherent platelets	Leukocyte rolling on platelet P-selectin; tight adhesion to platelet membrane component	Thrombosis
Fibrinogen	Adhesion of leukocytes to fibrinogen via CD11b/CD18	Bridging of platelets to VWF and matrix via α_{IIb}/β_{III}
Thrombin	Induction of E-selectin expression and IL-8 secretion by endothelial cells	Fibrinogen formation and platelet aggregation
Leukocyte Integrin CD11b/CD18	Adhesion of leukocytes to endothelium; phagocytosis CD11b/CD18	Binding and activation of factor X, adhesion of platelets via GPIbα; adhesion of platelets via JAM-C

GP, glycoprotein; IL, interleukin; JAM, junctional adhesion molecule; VWF, von Willebrand factor.

fact, antibodies against neither ICAM-2 nor its neutrophil receptor α_L (CD11) blocked this adhesion.[295,296] On the other hand, neutrophil $\alpha_M\beta_2$ reportedly binds to fibrinogen, which may be present on the surfaces of activated platelets bound to $\alpha_{IIb}\beta_3$ (GPIIb/IIIa). Two additional platelet surface molecules, GPIbα and JAM-C, have been demonstrated as ligands for leukocyte CD11b/CD18. GPIbα is part of the GP1b–IX–V complex,[297,298] and JAM-C was originally described as a component of epithelial and endothelial cell tight junctions.

Platelets can interact with activated endothelial cells. Platelets express PSGL-1 and can use this expression to interact with P-selectin on the surfaces of activated endothelial cells.[299] Activated platelets can also bind to endothelial cells via fibrinogen, fibrin, or VWF, forming a molecular bridge between platelet GPIIb/IIIa and endothelial cell integrin $\alpha_v\beta_3$ and ICAM-1.

Ultralarge VWF molecules are stored in Weibel-Palade bodies and released upon inflammatory endothelial cell activation. Ultralarge VWF molecules are normally cleaved by endothelial cell-surface proteases, notably the metalloprotease ADAMTS13 (a disintegrin and metalloprotease with thrombospondin repeats 13). Data in mice suggest that ADAMTS13 plays a homeostatic role in dampening inflammation.[300] In ADAMTS13-deficient mice, platelets bound to ultralarge VWF molecules on the endothelial surface and supported slower leukocyte rolling on venules at rest and greater leukocyte extravasation in models of inflammation.[300]

LEUKOCYTE–ENDOTHELIAL CELL MATRIX INTERACTIONS THAT PROMOTE COAGULATION

The same proinflammatory stimuli that stimulate *de novo* expression of E-selectin and VCAM-1, and augment expression of ICAM-1 for the recruitment of leukocytes, may stimulate synthesis and expression of TF by endothelial cells.[301] Furthermore, adhesion of monocytic cell lines to cytokine-activated endothelial cells in culture leads to rapidly increased TF-related procoagulant activity. This effect is partially blocked by a monoclonal antibody directed against E-selectin on endothelium and is mimicked by crosslinking Le^X on the monocyte cell lines.[302] A similar increase in TF gene expression can be induced by crosslinking α_4 or β_1 integrin chains, the components of VLA-4 on monocytic cell lines.[303]

During prolonged interaction of peripheral blood monocytes with human endothelial cells, monocytes that migrated across endothelial cell monolayers expressed functional cell surface TF.[304] Over the next several days, approximately half of these monocytes differentiated into immature dendritic cells bearing even higher levels of TF, and migrated back across the intact endothelial cell monolayer. This migration could be blocked by soluble fragments of TF. Therefore, in this system, TF was hypothesized to support both adhesion and a possible procoagulant role.[304]

Leukocytes that bind to P-selectin exposed on the surfaces of platelets on adherent thrombi promote the conversion of fibrinogen to fibrin.[305] The leukocyte integrin CD11b/CD18 has been shown to bind fibrinogen.[306] The same integrin has a conformational form that binds coagulation factor X.[307] Monocytic cells are capable of activating the bound factor X to factor Xa when activated,[308] defining a pathway for activation of factor X that is independent of TF.

REFERENCES

1. Nachman RL, Rafii S: Platelets, petechiae, and preservation of the vascular wall. *N Engl J Med* 359:1261–1270, 2008.
2. Marcus AJ, Broekman MJ, Drosopoulos JH, et al: Heterologous cell-cell interactions: Thromboregulation, cerebroprotection and cardioprotection by CD39 (NTPDase-1). *J Thromb Haemost* 1:2497–2509, 2003.
3. Furie B, Furie BC: Mechanisms of thrombus formation. *N Engl J Med* 359:938–949, 2008.
4. Kanthi YM, Sutton NR, Pinsky DJ: CD39: Interface between vascular thrombosis and inflammation. *Curr Atheroscler Rep* 16:425, 2014.
5. Aird WC: Phenotypic heterogeneity of the endothelium: I. Structure, function, and mechanisms. *Circ Res* 100:158–173, 2007.
6. Aird WC: Phenotypic heterogeneity of the endothelium: II. Representative vascular beds. *Circ Res* 100:174–190, 2007.
7. Brant-Zawadzki PB, Schmid DI, Jiang H, et al: Translational control in endothelial cells. *J Vasc Surg* 45 Suppl A:A8–A14, 2007.
8. Marcus AJ, Safier LB, Hajjar KA, et al: Inhibition of platelet function by an aspirin-insensitive endothelial cell ADPase. Thromboregulation by endothelial cells. *J Clin Invest* 88:1690–1696, 1991.
9. Marcus AJ, Broekman MJ, Drosopoulos JH, et al: Role of CD39 (NTPDase-1) in thromboregulation, cerebroprotection, and cardioprotection. *Semin Thromb Hemost* 31:234–246, 2005.
10. Broekman MJ, Eiroa AM, Marcus AJ: Inhibition of human platelet reactivity by endothelium-derived relaxing factor from human umbilical vein endothelial cells in suspension. Blockade of aggregation and secretion by an aspirin-insensitive mechanism. *Blood* 78:1033–1040, 1991.
11. Moncada S, Higgs EA: Molecular mechanisms and therapeutic strategies related to nitric oxide. *FASEB J* 9:1319–1330, 1995.
12. Kaczmarek E, Koziak K, Sevigny J, et al: Identification and characterization of CD39 vascular ATP diphosphohydrolase. *J Biol Chem* 271:33116–33122, 1996.
13. Marcus AJ, Broekman MJ, Drosopoulos JHF, et al: The endothelial cell ecto-ADPase responsible for inhibition of platelet function is CD39. *J Clin Invest* 99:1351–1360, 1997.
14. Esmon CT: Inflammation and the activated protein C anticoagulant pathway. *Semin Thromb Hemost* 32 Suppl 1:49–60, 2006.
15. Flood EC, Hajjar KA: The annexin A2 system and vascular homeostasis. *Vascul Pharmacol* 54:59–67, 2011.
16. Lisman T, De Groot PG, Meijers JC, Rosendaal FR: Reduced plasma fibrinolytic potential is a risk factor for venous thrombosis. *Blood* 105:1102–1105, 2005.

17. Muller WA: Mechanisms of leukocyte transendothelial migration. *Annu Rev Pathol* 6:323–344, 2011.
18. Marcus AJ, Safier LB: Thromboregulation: Multicellular modulation of platelet reactivity in hemostasis and thrombosis. *FASEB J* 7:516–522, 1993.
19. Ross R: Atherosclerosis: An inflammatory disease. *N Engl J Med* 340:115–126, 1999.
20. Garlanda C, Dejana E: Heterogeneity of endothelial cells: Specific markers. *Arterioscler Thromb Vasc Biol* 17:1193–1202, 1999.
21. Gawaz M, Langer H, May AE: Platelets in inflammation and atherogenesis. *J Clin Invest* 115:3378–3384, 2005.
22. May AE, Langer H, Seizer P, et al: Platelet-leukocyte interactions in inflammation and atherothrombosis. *Semin Thromb Hemost* 33:123–127, 2007.
23. Brass LF, Zhu L, Stalker TJ: Novel therapeutic targets at the platelet vascular interface. *Arterioscler Thromb Vasc Biol* 28(3):s43–s50, 2008.
24. Marcus AJ: Transcellular metabolism of eicosanoids. *Prog Hemost Thromb* 8:127–142, 1986.
25. Hamberg M, Svensson J, Samuelsson B: Thromboxanes: A new group of biologically active compounds derived from prostaglandin endoperoxides. *Proc Natl Acad Sci U S A* 72:2994–2998, 1975.
26. Moncada S, Gryglewski R, Bunting S, Vane JR: An enzyme isolated from arteries transforms prostaglandin endoperoxides to an unstable substance that inhibits platelet aggregation. *Nature* 263:663–665, 1976.
27. Woulfe D, Yang J, Brass L: ADP and platelets: The end of the beginning. *J Clin Invest* 107:1503–1505, 2001.
28. Al-Mondhiry H, Marcus AJ, Spaet TH: On the mechanism of platelet function inhibition by acetylsalicylic acid. *Proc Soc Exp Biol Med* 133:632–636, 1970.
29. Wu KK, Aird WC: Endothelial eicosanoids, in *Endothelial Biomedicine*, pp 1004–1014. Cambridge University Press, Cambridge, 2009.
30. McAdam BF, Catella-Lawson F, Mardini IA, et al: Systemic biosynthesis of prostacyclin by cyclooxygenase (COX)-2: The human pharmacology of a selective inhibitor of COX-2. *Proc Natl Acad Sci U S A* 96:272–277, 1999.
31. Herschman HR: Prostaglandin synthase 2. *Biochim Biophys Acta* 1299:125–140, 1996.
32. Maclouf J, Folco G, Patrono C: Eicosanoids and iso-eicosanoids: Constitutive, inducible and transcellular biosynthesis in vascular disease. *Thromb Haemost* 79:691–705, 1998.
33. Smith WL, DeWitt DL: Prostaglandin endoperoxide H synthases-1 and -2. *Adv Immunol* 62:167–215, 1996.
34. Xie WL, Chipman JG, Robertson DL, et al: Expression of a mitogen-responsive gene encoding prostaglandin synthase is regulated by mRNA splicing. *Proc Natl Acad Sci U S A* 88:2692–2696, 1991.
35. Kurumbail RG, Stevens Am, Gierse JK, et al: Structural basis for selective inhibition of cyclooxygenase-2 by anti-inflammatory agents. *Nature* 384:644–648, 1996 [published erratum appears in *Nature* 385(6616):555, 1997].
36. Pouliot M, Gilbert C, Borgeat P, et al: Expression and activity of prostaglandin endoperoxide synthase-2 in agonist-activated human neutrophils. *FASEB J* 12:1109–1123, 1998.
37. DeWitt DL, Smith WL: Cloning of sheep and mouse prostaglandin endoperoxide synthases. *Methods Enzymol* 187:469–479, 1990.
38. Dubois RN, Abramson SB, Crofford L, et al: Cyclooxygenase in biology and disease. *FASEB J* 12:1063–1073, 1998.
39. Lipsky LPE, Abramson SB, Crofford L, et al: The classification of cyclooxygenase inhibitors. *J Rheumatol* 25:2298–2303, 1998.
40. Marnett LJ: The COXIB experience: A look in the rear-view mirror. *Annu Rev Pharmacol Toxicol* 49:265–290, 2008.
41. Moncada S, Vane JR: Pharmacology and endogenous roles of prostaglandin endoperoxides, thromboxane A2, and prostacyclin. *Pharmacol Rev* 30:293–331, 1978.
42. Narumiya S, FitzGerald GA: Genetic and pharmacologic analysis prostanoid receptor function. *J Clin Invest* 108:25–30, 2001.
43. Cines DB, Pollak ES, Buck CA, et al: Endothelial cells in physiology and in the pathophysiology of vascular disorders. *Blood* 91:3527–3561, 1998.
44. Marcus AJ, Weksler BB, Jaffe EA, Broekman MJ: Synthesis of prostacyclin from platelet-derived endoperoxides by cultured human endothelial cells. *J Clin Invest* 66:979–986, 1980.
45. Smyth SS, McEver RP, Weyrich AS, et al: Platelet functions beyond hemostasis. *J Thromb Haemost* 7:1759–1766, 2009.
46. Pepine CJ: Impact of nitric oxide on cardiovascular medicine: Untapped potential utility. *Am J Med* 122:S10–S15, 2009.
47. Marletta MA: Nitric oxide synthase structure and mechanism. *J Biol Chem* 268:12231–12234, 1993.
48. Moncada S, Palmer RMJ, Higgs EA. Nitric oxide: Physiology, pathophysiology, and pharmacology. *Pharmacol Rev* 43:109–142, 1991.
49. Furchgott RF, Zawadzki JV: The obligatory role of endothelial cells in the relaxation of arterial smooth muscle by acetylcholine. *Nature* 288:373–376, 1980.
50. Matsumoto A, Momomura S, Sugiura S, et al: Effect of inhaled nitric oxide on gas exchange in patients with congestive heart failure. *Ann Intern Med* 130:40–44, 1999.
51. Lentz SR, Sobey CG, Piegers DJ, et al: Vascular dysfunction in monkeys with diet-induced hyperhomocyst(e)inemia. *J Clin Invest* 98:24–29, 1996.
52. Stamler JS, Osborne JA, Jaraki O, et al: Adverse vascular effects of homocysteine are modulated by endothelium-derived relaxing factor and related oxides of nitrogen. *J Clin Invest* 91:308–318, 1993.
53. Upchurch GR Jr, Welch GN, Fabian AJ, et al: Homocyst(e)ine decrease bioavailable nitric oxide by a mechanism involving glutathione peroxidase. *J Biol Chem* 272:17012–17017, 1997.
54. Voetsch B, Loscalzo J: Genetic determinants of arterial thrombosis. *Arterioscler Thromb Vasc Biol* 24:216–229, 2004.
55. Robson SC, Sevigny J, Zimmermann H: The E-NTPDase family of ectonucleotidases: Structure function relationships and pathophysiological significance. *Purinergic Signal* 2:409–430, 2006.
56. Gayle RB, Maliszewski CR, Gimpel SD, et al: Inhibition of platelet function by recombinant soluble ecto-ADPase/CD39. *J Clin Invest* 101:1851–1859, 1998.
57. Handa M, Guidotti G: Purification and cloning of a soluble ATP-diphosphohydrolase (apyrase) from potato tubers (Solanum tuberosum). *Biochem Biophys Res Commun* 218:916–923, 1996.
58. Hyman MC, Ptrovic-Djergovic D, Visovatti SH, et al: Self-regulation of inflammatory cell trafficking in mice by the leukocyte surface apyrase CD39. *J Clin Invest* 119:1136–1149, 2009.
59. Colgan S, Eltzschig H, Eckle T, Thompson L: Physiological roles for ecto-5′-nucleotidase (CD73). *Purinergic Signal* 2:351–360, 2006.
60. Atkinson BT, Jarvis GE, Watson SP: Activation of GPVI by collagen is regulated by alpha2beta1 and secondary mediators. *J Thromb Haemost* 1:1278–1287, 2003.
61. Pinsky DJ, Broekman MJ, Peschon JJ, et al: Elucidation of the thromboregulatory role of CD39/ectoapyrase in the ischemic brain. *J Clin Invest* 109:1031–1040, 2002.
62. Marcus AJ, Broekman MJ, Drosopoulos JHF, et al: Metabolic control of excessive extracellular nucleotide accumulation by CD39/ectonucleotidase-1: Implications for ischemic vascular diseases. *J Pharmacol Exp Ther* 305:9–16, 2003.
63. Koziak K, Bojakowska M, Robson SC, et al: Overexpression of CD39/nucleoside triphosphate diphosphohydrolase-1 decreases smooth muscle cell proliferation and prevents neointima formation after angioplasty. *J Thromb Haemost* 6:1191–1197, 2008.
64. Deaglio S, Dwyer KM, Gao W, et al: Adenosine generation catalyzed by CD39 and CD73 expressed on regulatory T cells mediates immune suppression. *J Exp Med* 204:1257–1265, 2007.
65. Uluckan O, Eagleton MC, Floyd DH, et al: APT102, a novel ADPase, cooperates with aspirin to disrupt bone metastasis in mice. *J Cell Biochem* 104:1311–1323, 2008.
66. Dwyer KM, Robson SC, Nandurkar HH, et al: Thromboregulatory manifestations in human CD39 transgenic mice and the implications for thrombotic disease and transplantation. *J Clin Invest* 113:1440–1446, 2004.
67. Serebruany VL, Malinin AI, Ferguson JJ, et al: Bleeding risks of combination vs. single antiplatelet therapy: A meta-analysis of 18 randomized trials comprising 129,314 patients. *Fundam Clin Pharmacol* 22:315–321, 2008.
68. Fung CY, Marcus AJ, Broekman MJ, Mahaut-Smith MP: P2X1 receptor inhibition and soluble CD39 administration as novel approaches to widen the cardiovascular therapeutic window. *Trends Cardiovasc Med* 19:1–5, 2009.
69. Esmon CT, Owen WG: Identification of an endothelial cell cofactor for thrombin-catalyzed activation of protein C. *Proc Natl Acad Sci U S A* 78:2249–2252, 1981.
70. Stearns-Kurosawa DJ, Kurosawa S, Mollica JS, et al: The endothelial cell protein C receptor augments protein C activation by the thrombin-thrombomodulin complex. *Proc Natl Acad Sci U S A* 93:10212–10216, 1996.
71. Esmon CT: Protein C pathway in sepsis. *Ann Med* 34:598–605, 2002.
72. Esmon CT: Inflammation and thrombosis. *J Thromb Haemost* 1:1343–1348, 2003.
73. Esmon CT: The protein C pathway. *Chest* 124(3 Suppl):26S–32S, 2003.
74. Esmon CT: The roles of protein C and thrombomodulin in the regulation of blood coagulation. *J Biol Chem* 264:4743–4746, 1989.
75. Grinnell BW, Berg DT: Surface thrombomodulin modulates thrombin receptor responses on vascular smooth muscle cells. *Am J Physiol* 270:H603–H609, 1996.
76. Lafay M, Laguna R, Le Bonniec BF, et al: Thrombomodulin modulates the mitogenic response to thrombin of human umbilical vein endothelial cells. *Thromb Haemost* 79:848–852, 1998.
77. Bajzar L, Manuel R, Nesheim M: Purification and characterization of TAFI, a thrombin activatable fibrinolysis inhibitor. *J Biol Chem* 270:14477–14484, 1995.
78. Campbell WD, Okada N, Okada H: Carboxypeptidase R is an inactivator of complement-derived inflammatory peptides and an inhibitor of fibrinolysis. *Immunol Rev* 180:162–167, 2001.
79. Ikeguchi H, Fujita Y, Kato T, et al: Effects of human soluble thrombomodulin on experimental glomerulonephritis. *Kidney Int* 61:490–501, 2002.
80. de Munk GA, Groeneveld E, Rijken DC: Acceleration of the thrombin inactivation of single chain urokinase-type plasminogen activator (pro-urokinase) by thrombomodulin. *J Clin Invest* 88:1680–1684, 1991.
81. Molinari A, Giogetti C, Lansen J, et al: Thrombomodulin is a cofactor for thrombin degradation of recombinant single-chain urokinase plasminogen activator *in vitro* and in a perfused rabbit heart model. *Thromb Haemost* 67:226–232, 1992.
82. Preissner KT, May AE, Wohn KD, et al: Molecular crosstalk between adhesion receptors and proteolytic cascades in vascular remodeling. *Thromb Haemost* 78:88–95, 1997.
83. Esmon CT, Scriver CR, Beaudet AL, et al: Anticoagulant protein C/thrombomodulin pathway, in *The Metabolic and Molecular Bases of Inherited Disease*, 8th ed, edited by Scriver CR, Beaudet AL, Valle D, Sly WS, Childs B, Kinzler KW, and Vogelstein B, pp 4327–4343. McGraw-Hill New York, 2001.
84. Healy AM, Hancock WW, Christie PD, et al: Intravascular coagulation activation in a murine model of thrombomodulin deficiency: Effects of lesion size, age, and hypoxia on fibrin deposition. *Blood* 263:15815–15822, 1988.
85. Weiler-Guettler H, Aird WC, Rayburn H, et al: Developmentally regulated gene expression of thrombomodulin in postimplantation mouse embryos. *Development* 122:2271–2281, 1996.
86. Crawley JT, Gu AM, Ferrell G, Esmon CT: Distribution of endothelial cell protein C/activated protein C receptor (EPCR) during mouse embryo development. *Thromb Haemost* 88:259–266, 2002.

87. Isermann B, Hendrickson SB, Hutley K, et al: Tissue-restricted expression of thrombomodulin in the placenta rescues thrombomodulin-deficient mice from early lethality and reveals a secondary developmental block. *Development* 128:827–838, 2001.

88. Isermann B, Hendrickson SB, Zogg M, et al: Endothelium-specific loss of murine thrombomodulin disrupts the protein C anticoagulant pathway and causes juvenile-onset thrombosis. *J Clin Invest* 108:537–546, 2001.

89. Fukodome K, Esmon CT: Identification, cloning, and regulation of a novel endothelial cell protein C/activated protein C receptor. *J Biol Chem* 269:26486–26491, 1994.

90. Esmon CT, Gu J, Xu J, et al: Regulation and functions of the protein C anticoagulant pathway. *Haematologica* 84:363–368, 1999.

91. Esmon CT, Xu J, Gu J, et al: Endothelial protein C receptor. *Thromb Haemost* 82:251–258, 1999.

92. Esmon CT: The endothelial cell protein C receptor. *Curr Opin Hematol* 13:382–385, 2006.

93. Xu J, Liaw PC, Esmon CT: A novel transmembrane domain of the endothelial cell protein C receptor (EPCR) dictates receptor localization of sphingolipid-cholesterol rich regions on plasma membrane while EPCR palmitoylation modulates intracellular trafficking patterns. *Thromb Haemost* 1999.

94. Kurosawa S, Stearns-Kurosawa DJ, Hidari N, Esmon CT: Identification of functional endothelial protein C receptor in human plasma. *J Clin Invest* 100:411–418, 1997.

95. Fukodome K, Ye X, Tsuneyoshi N, et al: Activation mechanism of anticoagulant protein C in large blood vessels involving the endothelial cell protein C receptor. *J Exp Med* 187:1029–1035, 1998.

96. Taylor FB Jr, Peer GT, Lockhart MS: Endothelial cell protein C receptor plays an important role in protein C activation *in vivo*. *Blood* 97:1685–1688, 2001.

97. Esmon CT, Taylor FB, Snow TR: Inflammation and coagulation: Linked processes potentially regulated through a common pathway mediated by protein C. *Thromb Haemost* 66:160–165, 1991.

98. Esmon CT, Schwarz HP: An update on clinical and basic aspects of the protein C anticoagulant pathway. *Trends Cardiovasc Med* 5:141–148, 1995.

99. Ranieri VM, Thompson BT, Barie PS, et al: Drotrecogin alfa (activated) in adults with septic shock. *N Engl J Med* 366:2055–2064, 2012.

100. Gu JM, Crawley JTB, Ferrell G, et al: Disruption of the endothelial cell protein C receptor gene in mice causes placental thrombosis and early embryonic lethality. *J Biol Chem* 277:43335–43343, 2002.

101. Weiler H, Isermann B: Thrombomodulin. *J Thromb Haemost* 1:1515–1524, 2003.

102. Todd AS: Fibrinolysis autographs. *Nature* 181:495–496, 1958.

103. Todd AS: Localization of fibrinolytic activity in tissues. *Br Med Bull* 20:210–212, 1964.

104. Augustin HG, Kozian DH, Johnson RC: Differentiation of endothelial cells: Analysis of the constitutive and activated endothelial cell phenotypes. *Bioessays* 16:901–906, 1994.

105. van Hinsbergh VW, Kooistra T, Emeis JJ, Koolwijk P: Regulation of plasminogen activator production by endothelial cells: Role in fibrinolysis and local proteolysis. *Int J Radiat Biol* 60:261–272, 1991.

106. Levin EG, del Zoppo GJ: Localization of tissue plasminogen activator in the endothelium of a limited number of vessels. *Am J Pathol* 144:855–861, 1994.

107. Levin EG, Santell L, Osborn KG: The expression of endothelial tissue plasminogen activator in vivo: A function defined by vessel size and anatomic location. *J Cell Sci* 110:139–148, 1997.

108. Levin EG, Osborn KG, Schleuning WD: Vessel-specific gene expression in the lung: Tissue plasmingen activator is limited to bronchial arteries and pulmonary vessels of discrete size. *Chest* 114:68S, 1998.

109. O'Rourke J, Jiang X, Hao Z, Cone RE, Hand AR: Distribution of sympathetic tissue plasminogen activator (tPA) to a distant microvasculature. *J Neurosci* 79:727–733, 2005.

110. Dichek D, Quertermous T: Thrombin regulation of mRNA levels of tissue plasminogen activator inhibitor-1 in cultured human umbilical vein endothelial cells. *Blood* 74:222–228, 1989.

111. Hanss M, Collen D: Secretion of tissue-type plasminogen activator and plasminogen activator inhibitor by cultured human endothelial cells: Modulation by thrombin, endotoxin, and histamine. *J Lab Clin Med* 109:97–104, 1987.

112. Levin EG, Santell L: Stimulation and desensitization of tissue plasminogen activator release from human endothelial cells. *J Biol Chem* 263:9360–9365, 1988.

113. Shatos MA, Doherty JM, Orfeo T, et al: Modulation of the fibrinolytic response of cultured human vascular endothelium by extracellularly generated oxygen radicals. *J Biol Chem* 267:597–601, 1992.

114. Levin EG, Marotti KR, Santell L: Protein kinase C and the stimulation of tissue plasminogen activator release from human endothelial cells. *J Biol Chem* 264:16030–16036, 1989.

115. Cugno M, Uziel L, Fabrizi I, et al: Fibrinolytic response in normal subjects to venous occlusion and DDAVP infusion. *Thromb Res* 56:625–634, 1989.

116. Kooistra T, van den Berg J, Tons A, et al: Butyrate stimulates tissue type plasminogen activator synthesis in cultured human endothelial cells. *Biochem J* 247:605–612, 1987.

117. Diamond SL, Eskin SG, McIntire LV: Fluid flow stimulates tissue plasminogen activator secretion by cultured human endothelial cells. *Science* 243:1483–1485, 1989.

118. Diamond SL, Sharefkin JB, Dieffenbach C, et al: Tissue plasminogen activator messenger RNA levels increase in cultured human endothelial cells exposed to laminar shear stress. *J Cell Physiol* 143:364–371, 1990.

119. Levin EG, Santell L, Saljooque F: Hyperosmotic stress stimulates tissue plasminoeg activator expression by a PKC-dependent pathway. *Am J Physiol* 265:C387–C396, 1993.

120. Iba T, Shin T, Sonoda T, et al: Stimulation of endothelial secretion of tissue-type plasminogen activator by repetitive stretch. *J Surg Res* 50:457–460, 1991.

121. Thompson EA, Nelles L, Collen D: Effect of retinoic acid on the synthesis of tissue-type plasminogen activator and plasminogen activator inhibitor 1 in human endothelial cells. *Eur J Biochem* 201:627–632, 1991.

122. Bulens F, Ibanez-Tallon I, Van Acker P, et al: Retinoic acid induction of human tissue-type plasminogen activator gene expression via a direct repeat element (DR5) located at −7 kilobases. *J Biol Chem* 270:7167–7175, 1995.

123. van Hinsbergh VW, Bauer KA, Kooistra T, et al: Progress of fibrinolysis during tumor necrosis factor infusions in humans. Concomitant increase in tissue-type plasminogen activator, plasminogen activator inhibitor type-1, and fibrin(ogen) degradation products. *Blood* 76:2284–2289, 1990.

124. Hamsten A, Wiman B, De Faire U, Blomback M: Increased plasma levels of a rapid inhibitor of tissue plasminogen activator in young survivors of myocardial infarction. *N Engl J Med* 313:1557–1563, 1985.

125. Pizzo SV, Murray JC, Gonias SL: Atrophie blanche: A disorder associated with defective release of tissue plasminogen activator. *Arch Pathol Lab Med* 110:517–519, 1986.

126. Kristensen P, Larson LI, Nielsen LS, et al: Human endothelial cells contain one type of plasminogen activator. *FEBS Lett* 168:33–37, 1984.

127. Yamamoto K, Loskutoff DJ: Fibrin deposition in tissues from endotoxin-treated mice correlates with decreases in the expression of urokinase-type but not tissue-type plasminogen activator. *J Clin Invest* 97:2440–2451, 1996.

128. Bacharach E, Itin A, Keshet E: *In vivo* patterns of expression of urokinase and its inhibitor PAI-1 suggest a concerted role in regulating phsyiological angiogenesis. *Proc Natl Acad Sci U S A* 89:10686–10690, 1992.

129. Booyse FM, Scheinbuks J, Radek J, et al: Immunological identification and comparision of plasminogen activator forms in cultured normal human endothelial cells and smooth muscle cells. *Thromb Res* 24:495–504, 1981.

130. van Hinsbergh VW, van den Berg EA, Fiers W, Dooijewaard G: Tumor necrosis factor induces the production of urokinase-type plasminogen activator by human endothelial cells. *Blood* 75:1991–1998, 1990.

131. Sawdey M, Podor TJ, Loskutoff DJ: Regulation of type-1 plasminogen activator inhibitor gene expression in cultured bovine aortic endothelial cells. *J Biol Chem* 264:10396–10401, 1989.

132. van den Berg EA, Sprengers ED, Jaye M, et al: Regulation of plasminogen activator inhibitor-1 mRNA in human endothelial cells. *Thromb Haemost* 60:63–67, 1988.

133. Ellis V, Scully MF, Kakkar VV: Plasminogen activation by single-chain urokinase in functional isolation. *J Biol Chem* 262:14998–15003, 1987.

134. Blasi F, Carmeliet P: uPAR: A versatile signalling orchestrator. *Nat Rev Mol Cell Biol* 3:932–943, 2002.

135. Almus-Jacobs F, Varki N, Sawdey MS, Loskutoff DJ: Endotoxin stimulates expression of the murine urokinase receptor gene in vivo. *Am J Pathol* 147:688–698, 1995.

136. Medina R, Socher SH, Han JH, Friedman PA: Interleukin-1, endotoxin, or tumor necrosis factor/cachectin enhance the level of plasminogen activator inhibitor messenger RNA in bovine aortic endothelial cells. *Thromb Res* 54:41–52, 1989.

137. Etingin OR, Hajjar DP, Hajjar KA, et al: Lipoprotein(a) regulates plasminogen activator inhibitor-1 expression in endothelial cells. *J Biol Chem* 266:2459–2465, 1990.

138. Konkle B, Ginsburg D: The addition of endothelial cell growth factor and heparin to human endothelial cell cultures decrease plasminogen activator. *J Clin Invest* 82:579, 1988.

139. Greenberg ME, Brackenbury R, Edelman GM: Changes in the distribution of the 34-kdalton tyrosine kinase substrate during differentiation and maturation of chicken tissues. *J Cell Biol* 98:473–486, 1984.

140. Hamre KM, Chepenik KP, Goldowitz D: The annexins: Specific markers of midline structures and sensory neurons in the developing murine central nervous system. *J Comp Neurol* 352:421–435, 1995.

141. Gould KL, Cooper JA, Hunter T: The 46,000-dalton tyrosine kinase substrate is widespread, whereas the 36,000-dalton substrate is only expressed at high levels in certain rodent tissues. *J Cell Biol* 98:487–497, 1984.

142. Dreier R, Schmid KW, Gerke V, Riehemann K: Differential expression of annexins I, II, and IV in human tissues: An immunohistochemical study. *Histochem Cell Biol* 110:137–148, 1998.

143. Huang B, Deora AB, He K, et al: Hypoxia-inducible factor-1 drives annexin A2 system-mediated perivascular fibrin clearance in oxygen-induced retinopathy in mice. *Blood* 118(10):2918–2929, 2011.

144. Jacovina AT, Zhong F, Khazanova E, et al: Neuritogenesis and the nerve growth factor-induced differentiation of PC-12 cells requires annexin II-mediated plasmin generation. *J Biol Chem* 276:49350–49358, 2001.

145. Brownstein C, Deora AB, Jacovina AT, et al: Annexin II mediates plasminogen-dependent matrix invasion by human monocytes: Enhanced expression by macrophages. *Blood* 103:317–324, 2004.

146. Menell JS, Cesarman GM, Jacovina AT, et al: Annexin II and bleeding in acute promyelocytic leukemia. *N Engl J Med* 340:994–1004, 1999.

147. Tallman MS, Abutalib SA, Altman JK: The double hazard of thrombophilia and bleeding in acute promyelocytic leukemia. *Semin Thromb Hemost* 33:330–338, 2007.

148. Stein E, McMahon B, Kwaan H, et al: The coagulopathy of acute promyelocytic leukaemia revisited. *Best Pract Res Clin Haematol* 22:152–163, 2009.

149. Liu Y, Wang Z, Jiang M, et al: The expression of annexin II and its role in the fibrinolytic activity in acute promyelocytic leukemia. *Leuk Res* 35:879–884, 2011.

150. Ishii H, Yoshida M, Hiraoka M, et al: Recombinant annexin II modulates impaired fibrinolytic activity *in vitro* and in rat carotid artery. *Circ Res* 89:1240–1245, 2001.

151. Ling Q, Jacovina AT, Deora AB, et al: Annexin II is a key regulator of fibrin homeostasis and neoangiogenesis. *J Clin Invest* 113:38–48, 2004.

152. Cesarman-Maus G, Rios-Luna NP, Deora AB, et al: Autoantibodies against the fibrinolytic receptor, annexin 2, in antiphospholipid syndrome. *Blood* 107:4375–4382, 2006.

153. Cesarman-Maus G, Cantu-Brito C, Barinagarrementeria F, et al: Autoantibodies against the fibrinolytic receptor, annexin A2, in cerebral venous thrombosis. *Stroke* 42:501–503, 2011.

154. Sebastiani P, Ramoni MF, Nolan V, et al: Genetic dissection and prognostic modeling of overt stroke in sickle cell anemia. *Nat Genet* 37:435–440, 2005.

155. Flanagan JM, Frohlich DM, Howard TA, et al: Genetic predictors for stroke in children with sickle cell anemia. *Blood* 117:6681–6684, 2011.

156. Baldwin CT, Nolan VG, Wyszynski DF, et al: Association of klotho, bone morphogenetic protein 6, and annexin A2 polymorphisms with sickle cell disease. *Blood* 106:372–375, 2005.

157. Surette AP, Madureira PA, Phipps KD, et al: Regulation of fibrinolysis by S100A10 *in vivo*. *Blood* 118:3172–3181, 2011.

158. Omar MN, Mann KG: Inactivation of factor Va by plasmin. *J Biol Chem* 262:9750–9755, 1987.

159. Esmon CT: The regulation of natural anticoagulant pathways. *Science* 235:1348–1352, 1987.

160. McKee PA, Anderson JC, Switzer ME: Molecular structural studies of human factor VIII. *Ann N Y Acad Sci* 240:8–33, 1975.

161. Stricker RB, Wong D, Shiu DT, et al: Activation of plasminogen by tissue plasminogen activator on normal and thrombasthenic platelets: Effects on surface proteins and platelet aggregation. *Blood* 68:275–280, 1986.

162. Adelman B, Michelson AD, Greenberg J, Handin RI: Proteolysis of platelet glycoprotein by plasmin is facilitated by plasmin lysine-binding regions. *Blood* 68:1280–1284, 1986.

163. Gimple LW, Gold HK, Leinbach RC, et al: Correlation between template bleeding times and spontaneous bleeding during treatment of acute myocardial infarction with recombinant tissue type plasminogen activator. *Blood* 80:581–588, 1989.

164. Coller BS: Platelets and thrombolytic therapy. *N Engl J Med* 322:33–42, 1990.

165. Fay WP, Garg N, Sunkar M: Vascular function of the plasminogen activation system. *Arterioscler Thromb Vasc Biol* 27:1231–1237, 2007.

166. Libby P, Aikawa M, Jain MK: Vascular endothelium and atherosclerosis. *Handb Exp Pharmacol* 176 Part 2:285–306, 2006.

167. Ploplis VA, Carmeliet P, Vazirzadeh S, et al: Effects of disruption of the plasminogen gene on thrombosis, growth, and health in mice. *Circulation* 92:2585–2593, 1995.

168. Bugge TH, Flick MJ, Daugherty CC, Degen JL: Plasminogen deficiency causes severe thrombosis but is compatible with development and reproduction. *Genes Dev* 9:794–807, 1995.

169. Romer J, Bugge TH, Pyke C, et al: Impaired wound healing in mice with a disrupted plasminogen gene. *Nat Med* 2:287–292, 1996.

170. Bugge TH, Kombrinck KW, Flick MJ, et al: Loss of fibrinogen rescues mice from the pleiotropic effects of plasminogen deficiency. *Cell* 87:709–719, 1996.

171. Xiao Q, Danton MJS, Witte DP, et al: Plasminogen deficiency accelerates vessel wall disease in mice predisposed to atherosclerosis. *Proc Natl Acad Sci U S A* 94:10335–10340, 1997.

172. Carmeliet P, Moons L, Lijnen R, et al: Urokinase-generated plasmin activates matrix metalloproteinases during aneurysm formation. *Nat Genet* 17:439–444, 1997.

173. Eitzman DT, Westrick RJ, Xu Z, et al: Plasminogen activator inhibitor-1 deficiency protects against atherosclerosis progression in the mouse carotid artery. *Blood* 96:4212–4215, 2000.

174. Sjoland H, Eitzman DT, Gordon D, et al: Atherosclerosis progression in LDL receptor-deficient and apolipoprotein E-deficient mice is independent of genetic alterations in plasminogen activator inhibitor-1. *Arterioscler Thromb Vasc Biol* 20:846–852, 1999.

175. Luttun A, Lupu F, Storkebaum E, et al: Lack of plasminogen activator inhibitor-1 promotes growth and abnormal remodeling of advanced atherosclerotic plaque in apolipoprotein E-deficient mice. *Arterioscler Thromb Vasc Biol* 22:499–505, 2002.

176. Plow EF, Ploplis VA, Busuttil S, et al: A role of plasminogen in atherosclerosis and restenosis models in mice. *Thromb Haemost* 82 Suppl:4–7, 1999.

177. Ploplis VA, French EL, Carmeliet P, et al: Plasminogen deficiency differentially affects recruitment of inflammatory cell populations in mice. *Blood* 91:2005–2009, 1998.

178. Moons L, Wi C, Ploplis V, et al: Reduced transplant arteriosclerosis in plasminogen-deficient mice. *J Clin Invest* 102:1788–1797, 1998.

179. Heymans S, Luttun A, Nuyens D, et al: Inhibition of plasminogen activators or matrix metalloproteinases prevents cardiac rupture but impairs therapeutic angiogenesis and causes cardiac failure. *Nat Med* 5:1135–1142, 1999.

180. Lijnen HR, Van Hoef B, Lupu F, et al: Function of the plasminogen/plasmin and matrix metalloproteinase systems after vascular injury in mice with targeted inactivation of fibrinolytic system genes. *Arterioscler Thromb Vasc Biol* 18:1035–1045, 1998.

181. Carmeliet P, Moons L, Ploplis VA, et al: Impaired arterial neointima formation in mice with disruption of the plasminogen gene. *J Clin Invest* 99:200–208, 1997.

182. Carmeliet P, Moons L, Herbert JM, et al: Urokinase but not tissue plasminogen activator mediates arterial neointima formation in mice. *Circ Res* 81:829–839, 1997.

183. Carmeliet P, Moons L, Dewerchin M, et al: Receptor-independent role of urokinase-type plasminogen activator in pericellular plasmin and matrix metalloproteinase proteolysis during vascular wound healing in mice. *J Cell Biol* 140:233–245, 1998.

184. Carmeliet P, Moons L, Lijnen R, et al: Inhibitory role of plasminogen activator inhibitor-1 in arterial wound healing amd neointima formation. *Circulation* 96:3180–3191, 1997.

185. de Waard V, Armitage RJ, Carmeliet P, et al: Plasminogen activator inhibitor-1 and vitronectin protect against stenosis in a murine carotid ligation model. *Arterioscler Thromb Vasc Biol* 22:1978–1983, 2002.

186. Konstantinides S, Schafer K, Loskutoff DJ: Do PAI-1 and vitronectin promote or inhbiit neointima formation? *Arterioscler Thromb Vasc Biol* 22:1943–1945, 2002.

187. Eitzman DT, Westrick RJ, Nabel EG, Ginsburg D: Plasminogen activator inhibitor-1 and vitronectin promote vascular thrombosis in mice. *Blood* 95:577–580, 2000.

188. Konstantinides S, Schafer K, Thinnes T, Loskutoff DJ: Plasminogen activator inhibitor-1 and its cofactor vitronectin stabilize arterial thrombi following vascular injury in mice. *Circulation* 103:576–583, 2001.

189. Schafer K, Konstantinides S, Riedel C, et al: Different mechanisms of increased luminal stenosis after arterial injury in mice deficient for urokinase- or tissue-type plasminogen activator. *Circulation* 106:1847–1852, 2002.

190. Schafer K, Muller K, Hecker A, et al: Enhanced thrombosis in atherosclerosis-prone mice is associated with increased arterial expression of plasmingen activator. *Arterioscler Thromb Vasc Biol* 23:2097–2103, 2003.

191. Zhu Y, Farrehi PM, Fay WP: Plasminogen activator inhibitor type 1 enhances neointima formation after oxidative vascular injury in atherosclerosis-prone mice. *Circulation* 103:3105–3110, 2001.

192. Ploplis VA, Cornelissen I, Sandoval-Cooper MJ, et al: Remodeling of the vessel wall after copper-induced injury is highly attenuated in mice with a total deficiency of plasminogen activator inhibitor-1. *Am J Pathol* 158:107–117, 2001.

193. Peng L, Bhatia N, Parker AC, et al: Endogenous vitronectin and plasminogen activator inhibitor-1 promote neointima formation in murine carotid arteries. *Arterioscler Thromb Vasc Biol* 22:934–939, 2002.

194. DeYoung MB, Tom C, Dichek DA: Plasminogen activator inhibitor type 1 increases neointima formation in balloon-injured rat carotid arteries. *Circulation* 104:1972–1981, 2001.

195. Scanu AM, Fless GM: Lipoprotein(a) heterogeneity and biologic relevance. *J Clin Invest* 85:1709–1715, 1990.

196. Utermann G: The mysteries of lipoprotein(a). *Science* 246:904–910, 1989.

197. Loscalzo J: Lipoprotein(a), a unique risk factor for atherothrombotic disease. *Arteriosclerosis* 10:672–679, 1990.

198. Hajjar KA, Nachman RL: The role of lipoprotein(a) in atherogenesis and thrombosis. *Annu Rev Med* 47:423–442, 1996.

199. McLean JW, Tomlinson JE, Kuang WJ, et al: CDNA sequence of human apolipoprotein(a) is homologous to plasminogen. *Nature* 330:132–137, 1987.

200. Weitkamp LR, Guttormsen SA, Schultz JS: Linkage between the loci for the Lp(a) lipoprotein (Lp) and plasminogen (PLG). *Hum Genet* 79:80–82, 1988.

201. Neven L, Khalil A, Pfaffinger D, et al: Rhesus monkey model of familial hypercholesterolemia: Relation between plasma Lp(a) levels, apo(a) isoforms and LDL-receptor function. *J Lipid Res* 31:633–643, 1990.

202. Pfaffinger D, Schuelke J, Kim C, et al: Relationship between apo(a) isoforms and Lp(a) density in subjects with different apo(a) phenotype: A study before and after a fatty meal. *J Lipid Res* 32:679–683, 1991.

203. Utermann G, Menzel HJ, Kraft HG, Duba HC, Kemmler HG, Seitz C: Lp(a) glycoprotein phenotypes. *J Clin Invest* 80:458–465, 1987.

204. Maeda S, Abe A, Seishima M, et al: Transient changes of serum lipoprotein(a) as an acute phase protein. *Atherosclerosis* 78:145–150, 1989.

205. Wright LC, Sullivan DR, Muller M, et al: Elevated apolipoprotein(a) levels in cancer patients. *Int J Cancer* 43:241–244, 1989.

206. Gavish D, Azrolan N, Breslow JL: Fish oil reduces plasma Lp(a) levels and affects post-prandial association of apo(a) with triglyceride rich lipoproteins. *J Clin Invest* 84:2021–2027, 1989.

207. Koschinsky ML, Beisiegel U, Henne-Bruns D, et al: Apolipoprotein(a) size heterogeneity is related to variable number of repeat sequences in its mRNA. *Biochemistry* 29:640–644, 1990.

208. Lerch PG, Rickli EE, Lergier W, Gillessen D: Localization of individual lysine-binding regions in human plasminogen and investiations on their complex-forming properties. *Eur J Biochem* 107:7–13, 1980.

209. Armstrong VW, Harrach B, Robenek H, et al: Heterogeneity of human lipoprotein Lp(a): Cytochemical and biochemical studies on the interaction of two Lp(a) species with the LDL receptor. *J Lipid Res* 31:429–441, 1990.

210. Wolf K, Rith M, Niendorf A, et al: Thrombosis: Cellular elements of the vasculature. *Circulation* 80:522, 1989.

211. Grainger DJ, Kemp PR, Liu AC, et al: Activation of transforming growth factor-beta is inhibited in transgenic apolipoprotein(a) mice. *Nature* 370:460–462, 1994.

212. Palabrica TM, Liu AC, Aronovitz MJ, et al: Antifibrinolytic activity of apolipoprotein(a) *in vivo*: Human apolipoprotein(a) transgenic mice are resistant to tissue plasminogen activator-mediated thrombolysis. *Nat Med* 1:256–259, 1995.

213. Petros AM, Ramesh V, Llinas M: NMR studies of aliphatic ligand binding to human plasminogen kringle 4. *Biochemistry* 28:1368–1376, 1989.

214. Hajjar KA: The endothelial cell tissue plasminogen activator receptor: Specific interaction with plasminogen. *J Biol Chem* 266:21962–21970, 1991.

215. Hajjar KA, Gavish D, Breslow J, Nachman RL: Lipoprotein(a) modulation of endothelial cell surface fibrinolysis and its potential role in atherosclerosis. *Nature* 339:303–305, 1989.

216. Gonzales-Gronow M, Edelberg JM, Pizzo SV: Further characterization of the cellular plasminogen binding site: Evidence that plasminogen 2 and lipoprotein a compete for the same site. *Biochemistry* 28:2374–2377, 1989.

217. Miles LA, Fless GM, Levin EG, et al: A potential basis for the thrombotic risks associated with lipoprotein(a). *Nature* 339:301–303, 1989.

218. Edelberg JM, Gonzalez-Gronow M, Pizzo SV: Lipoprotein(a) inhibition of plasminogen activation by tissue-type plasminogen activator. *Thromb Res* 57:155–162, 1990.

219. Loscalzo J, Weinfeld M, Fless G, Scanu AM: Lipoprotein(a), fibrin binding, and plasminogen activation. *Arteriosclerosis* 10:240–245, 1990.

220. Lawn RM, Wade DP, Hammer RE, et al: Atherogenesis in transgenic mice expressing human apolipoprotein(a). *Nature* 360:670–672, 1992.

221. Boonmark NW, Lou XJ, Schwartz K, et al: Modification of apolipoprotein(a) lysine binding site reduces atherosclerosis in transgenic mice. *J Clin Invest* 100:558–564, 1997.

222. Kraus JP: Molecular basis of phenotype expression in homocystinuria. *J Inherit Metab Dis* 17:383–390, 1994.

223. Boushey CJ, Beresford SAA, Omenn GS, Motulsky AG: A quantitative assessment of plasma homocysteine as a risk factor for vascular disease. *JAMA* 274:1049–1057, 1995.

224. Refsum H, Ueland PM, Nygard O, Vollset SE: Homocysteine and cardiovascular disease. *Annu Rev Med* 49:31–62, 1998.

225. Ueland PM, Loscalzo J: Homocysteine and cardiovascular risk: The perils of reductionism in a complex system. *Clin Chem* 58:1623–1625, 2012.

226. Hajjar KA: Homocysteine-induced modulation of tissue plasminogen activator binding to its endothelial cell membrane receptor. *J Clin Invest* 91:2873–2879, 1993.

227. Hajjar KA, Mauri L, Jacovina AT, et al: Tissue plasminogen activator binding to the annexin II tail domain: Direct modulation by homocysteine. *J Biol Chem* 273: 9987–9993, 1998.

228. Jacovina AT, Deora AB, Ling Q, et al: Homocysteine inhibits neoangiogenesis in mice through blockade of annexin A2-dependent fibrinolysis. *J Clin Invest* 119:3384–3394, 2009.

229. Miyakis S, Lockshin MD, Atsumi T, et al: International consensus statement on an update of the classification criteria for definite antiphospholipid syndrome (APS). *J Thromb Haemost* 4:295–306, 2006.

230. Cockrell E, Espinola RG, McCrae KR: Annexin A2: Biology and relevance to the antiphospholipid syndrome. *Lupus* 17:943–951, 2008.

231. Ma K, Simantov R, Zhang JC, et al: High affinity binding of beta 2-glycoprotein I to human enodthelial cells is mediated by annexin II. *J Biol Chem* 275:15541–15548, 2000.

232. Zhang J, McCrae KR: Annexin A2 mediates endothelial cell activation by antiphospholipid/anti-beta2 glycoprotein I antibodies. *Blood* 105:1964–1969, 2005.

233. Raschi E, Testoni C, Bosisio D, et al: Role of the My88 transduction signaling pathway in endothelial activation by antiphospholipid antibodies. *Blood* 101:3295–3500, 2003.

234. Romay-Penabad Z, Montiel-Manzano MG, Pappalardo E, et al: Pathogenic effects of antiphospholipid antibodies are ameliorated in annexin A2 deficient mice. *Blood* i114:3074–3083, 2009.

235. von Bruhl ML, Stark K, Steinhart A, et al: Monocytes, neutrophils, and platelets cooperate to initiate and propagate venous thrombosis in mice *in vivo*. *J Exp Med* 209:819–835, 2012.

236. Polgar J, Matuskova J, Wagner DD: The P-selectin, tissue factor, coagulation triad. *J Thromb Haemost* 3:1590–1596, 2005.

237. Ardoin SP, Shanahan JC, Pisetsky DS: The role of microparticles in inflammation and thrombosis. *Scand J Immunol* 66:159–165, 2007.

238. George FD: Microparticles in vascular diseases. *Thromb Res* 122:S55–S59, 2008.

239. Lechner D, Weltermann A: Circulating tissue factor-exposing microparticles. *Thromb Res* 122:S47–S54, 2008.

240. Peerschke EI, Yin W, Ghebrehiwet B: Platelet mediated complement activation. *Adv Exp Med Biol* 632:81–91, 2008.

241. Muller WA: Leukocyte-endothelial cell interactions in leukocyte transmigration and the inflammatory response. *Trends Immunol* 24:326–333, 2003.

242. Angiari S, Donnarumma T, Rossi B, et al: TIM-1 glycoprotein binds the adhesion receptor P-selectin and mediates T cell trafficking during inflammation and autoimmunity. *Immunity* 40:542–553, 2014.

243. Wilkins PP, Moore KL, McEver RP, Cummings RD: Tyrosine sulfation of P-selectin glycoprotein ligand-1 is required for high affinity binding to P-selectin. *J Biol Chem* 270:22677–22680, 1995.

244. Snapp KR, Craig R, Herron M, et al: Dimerization of P-selectin glycoprotein ligand-1 (PSGL-1) required for optimal recognition of P-selectin. *J Cell Biol* 142:263–270, 1998.

245. Lalor P, Nash GB: Adhesion of flowing leucocytes to immobilized platelets. *Br J Haematol* 89.

246. Tanaka Y, Adams DH, Hubscher S, et al: T-cell adhesion induced by proteoglycan-immobilized cytokine MIP-1 beta. *Nature* 361:79–82, 1995, 1993.

247. Lo SK, Lee S, Ramos RA, et al: Endothelial-leukocyte adhesion molecule 1 stimulates the adhesive activity of leukocyte integrin CD3 (CD11B/CD18, Mac-1, alpha m beta 2) on human neutrophils. *J Exp Med* 173:1493–1500, 1991.

248. Lorant DE, Patel KD, McIntyre TM, et al: Coexpression of GMP-140 and PAF by endothelium stimulated by histamine or thrombin: A juxtacrine system for adhesion and activation of neutrophils. *J Cell Biol* 115:223–234, 1991.

249. Huber AR, Kunkel SL, Todd RF, Weiss SL: Regulation of transendothelial neutrophil migration by endogenous interleukin-8. *Science* 254:99–102, 1991.

250. Tanaka Y, Albelda SM, Horgan KJ, et al: CD31 expressed on distinctive T cell subsets is a preferential amplifier of beta 1 integrin-mediated adhesion. *J Exp Med* 176:245–253, 1992.

251. Piali L, Albelda SM, Baldwin HS, et al: Murine platelet endothelial cell adhesion molecule (PECAM-1/CD31) modulates beta2 integrins on lymphokine-activated killer cells. *Eur J Immunol* 23:2464–2471, 1993.

252. Berman ME, Muller WA: Ligation of platelet/endothelial cell adhesion molecule 1 (PECAM-1/CD31) on monocytes and neutrophils increases binding capacity of leukocyte CR3 (CD11b/CD18). *J Immunol* 154:299–307, 1995.

253. Hynes RO: Integrins: Versatility, modulation, and signalling in cell adhesion. *Cell* 69:11–25, 1992.

254. Carlos TM, Harlan JM: Leukocyte-endothelial cell adhesion molecules. *Blood* 84:2068–2101, 1994.

255. Miles A, Liaskou E, Eksteen B, et al: CCL25 and CCL28 promote alpha4 beta7-integrin-dependent adhesion of lymphocytes to MAdCAM-1 under shear flow. *Am J Physiol Gastrointest Liver Physiol* 294:G1257–G1267, 2008.

256. Bargatze RF, Kurk S, Butcher EC, Jutila MA: Neutrophils roll on adherent neutrophils bound to cytokine-induced endothelial cells via L-selectin on the rolling cells. *J Exp Med* 180:1785–1792, 1994.

257. Walcheck B, Moore KL, McEver RP, Kishimoto TK: Neutrophil-neutrophil interactions under hydrodynamic shear stress involve L-selectin and PSGL-1. *J Clin Invest* 98:1081–1087, 1996.

258. Muller WA: Migration of leukocytes across the vascular intima. Molecules and mechanisms. *Trends Cardiovasc Med* 5:15–20, 1995.

259. Sullivan DP, Muller WA: Neutrophil and monocyte recruitment by PECAM, CD99, and other molecules via the LBRC. *Semin Immunopathol* 36:193–209, 2014.

260. Ley K, Laudanna C, Cybulsky MI, Nourshargh S: Getting to the site of inflammation: The leukocyte adhesion cascade updated. *Nat Rev Immunol* 7:678–689, 2007.

261. Muller WA, Ratti CM, McDonnell SL, Cohn ZA: A human endothelial cell-restricted, externally disposed plasmalemmal protein enriched in intercellular junctions. *J Exp Med* 170:399–414, 1989.

262. Newman PJ, Berndt MC, Gorski J, et al: PECAM-1 (CD31) cloning and relation to adhesion molecules of the immunoglobulin gene superfamily. *Science* 247:1219–1222, 1990.

263. Muller WA, Weigl SA, Deng X, Phillips DM: PECAM-1 is required for transendothelial migration of leukocytes. *J Exp Med* 178:449–460, 1993.

264. Huang AJ, Manning JE, Bandak TM, et al: Endothelial cell cytosolic free calcium regulates neutrophil migration across monolayers of endothelial cells. *J Cell Biol* 120:1371–1380, 1993.

265. Liao F, Ali J, Greene T, Muller WA: Soluble domain 1 of platelet-endothelial cell adhesion molecule (PECAM) is sufficient to block transendothelial migration in vitro and in vivo. *J Exp Med* 185:1349–1357, 1997.

266. Liao F, Huynh HK, Eiroa A, et al: Migration of monocytes across endothelium and passage through extracellular matrix involve separate molecular domains of PECAM-1. *J Exp Med* 182:1337–1343, 1995.

267. Ostermann G, Weber KSC, Zernecke A, et al: JAM-1 is a ligand for the b2 integrin LFA-1 involved in transendothelial migration of leuocytes. *Nat Immunol* 3:151–158, 2002.

268. Johnson-Leger C, Aurrand-Lions M, Beltraminelli N, et al: Junctional adhesion molecule-2 (JAM-2) promotes lymphocyte transendothelial migration. *Blood* 100:2479–2486, 2002.

269. Feng D, Nagy JA, Pyne K, et al: Neutrophils emigrate from venules by a transendothelial cell pathway in response to fMLP. *J Exp Med* 187:903–915, 1999.

270. Carman CV, Springer TA: Trans-cellular migration: Cell-cell contacts get intimate. *Curr Opin Cell Biol* 20:533–540, 2008.

271. Bixel MG, Petri B, Khandoga AG, et al: A CD99-related antigen on endothelial cells mediates neutrophil, but not lymphocyte extravasation *in vivo*. *Blood* 109:5327–5336, 2009.

272. Dufour EM, Deroche A, Bae Y, Muller WA: CD99 is essential for leukocyte diapedesis in vivo. *Cell Commun Adhes* 15:351–363, 2008.

273. Schenkel AR, Mamdouh Z, Chen X, et al: CD99 plays a major role in the migration of monocytes through endothelial junctions. *Nat Immunol* 3:2479–2486, 2002.

274. Marchesi VT, Florey HW: Electron micrographic observations on the emigration of leukocytes. *Q J Exp Physiol Cogn Med Sci* 45:343–347, 1960.

275. Schnoor M, Lai FP, Zarbock A, et al: Cortactin deficiency is associated with reduced neutrophil recruitment but increased vascular permeability *in vivo*. *J Exp Med* 208:1721–1735, 2011.

276. Leeuwenberg JFM, von Asmuth EJ, Jeunhomme TM, Buurman WA: IFN-gamma regulates the expression of the adhesion molecule ELAM-1 and IL-6 production by human endothelial cells in vitro. *J Immunol* 145:2110–2114, 1990.

277. Strindall J, Lundblad A, Pahlsson P: Interferon-gamma enhancement of E-selectin expression on endothelial cells is inhbiited by monensin. *Scand J Immunol* 46:338–343, 1997.

278. Ley K, Arbones ML, Bosse R, et al: Sequential contribution of L- and P-selectin to leukocyte rolling *in vivo*. *J Exp Med* 181:669–675, 1995.

279. Khew-Goodall Y, Butcher E, Litwin MS, et al: Chronic expression of P-selectin on endothelial cells stimulated by the T-cell cytokine, interleukin-3. *Blood* 87:1432–1438, 1999.

280. Yao L, Pan J, Setiadi H, et al: Interleukin-4 or oncostatin M induces a prolonged increase in P-selectin mRNA and protein in human endthelial cells. *J Exp Med* 184:81–92, 1996.

281. Jung U, Ley K: Regulation of E-selectin, P-selectin, and intercellular adhesion molecule-1 expression in mouse cremaster vasculature. *Microcirculation* 4:311–319, 1997.

282. Pan J, Xia L, Yao L, McEver RP: Tumor necrosis factor-alpha- or lipopolysaccharide-induced expression of the murine P-selectin gene in endothelial cells involves novel kappaB sites and a variant activating transcription factor/cAMP response element. *J Biol Chem* 273:10067–10077, 1998.

283. Masinovsky B, Urdal D, Gallatin WM: IL-4 acts synergistically with IL-1 beta to promote lymphocyte adhesion to microvascular endothelium by induction of vascular cell adhesion molecule-1. *J Immunol* 145:2886–2895, 1990.

284. Blease K, Seybold J, Adcock IM, et al: Interleukin-4 and lipopolysaccharide synergize to induce vascular adhesion molecule-1 expression in human lung microvascular endothelial cells. *Am J Respir Cell Mol Biol* 18:620–630, 1998.

285. Pober JS, Collins T, Gimbrone M, et al: Inducible expression of class II major histocompatibility complex antigens and the immunogenicity of vascular endothelium. *Transplantation* 41:141–146, 1986.

286. Savage CO, Hughes CC, McIntyre BW, et al: Human CD4+ cells proliferate to HLA-DR+ allogeneic vascular endothelium. Identification of accessory interactions. *Transplantation* 56:128–134, 1993.

287. Pober JS, Orosz CG, Rose ML, Savage CO: Can graft endothelial cells initiate a host anti-graft immune response? *Transplantation* 61:343–349, 1996.

288. Romer LH, McLean NV, Horng-Chin Y, et al: IFN-gamma and TNF-alpha induce redistribution of PECAM-1 (CD31) on human endothelial cells. *J Immunol* 154:6582–6592, 1995.

289. Tang Q, Hendricks RL: Interferon gamma regulates platelet endothelial cell adhesion molecule-1 expression and neutrophil infiltration into herpes simplex virus-infected mouse corneas. *J Exp Med* 184:1435–1447, 1996.

290. Rival Y, Del Maschio A, Rabiet MJ, et al: Inhibition of platelet endothelial cell adhesion molecule-1 synthesis and leukocyte transmigration in endothelial cells by the combined action of TNF-alpha and IFN-gamma. *J Immunol* 157:1233–1241, 1996.

291. Kaplanski G, Fabrigoule M, Boulay V, et al: Thrombin induces endothelial type II activation *in vitro*: IL-1 and TNF-alpha-independent IL-8 secretion and E-selectin expression. *J Immunol* 158:5435–5441, 1997.

292. Diacovo TG, Puri KD, Warnock RA, et al: Platelet-mediated lymphocyte delivery to high endothelial venules. *Science* 273:252–255, 1996.

293. Diacovo TG, Catalina MD, Siegelman MH, Von Adrian UH: Circulating activated platelets reconstitute lymphocyte homing and immunity in L-selectin-deficient mice. *J Exp Med* 187:197–204, 1998.

294. Buttrum SM, Hatton R, Nash GB: Selectin-mediated rolling of neutrophils on immobilized platelets. *Blood* 82:1165–1174, 1993.

295. Diacovo TG, Roth SJ, Buccola JM, et al: Neutrophil rolling, arrest, and transmigration across activated, surface-adherent platelets via sequential action of P-selectin and the beta 2-integrin CD11b/CD18. *Blood* 88:146–157, 1996.

296. Diacovo TG, de Fougerolles AR, Bainton DF, Springer TA: A functional integrin ligand on the surface of platelets: Intercellular adhesion molecule-2. *J Clin Invest* 94:1243–1251, 1994.

297. Simon DI, Chen Z, Xu H, et al: Platelet glycoprotein Iba is a counterreceptor for the leukocyte integrin Mac-1 (CD11b/CD18). *J Exp Med* 192:193–214, 2000.

298. Santoso S, Sachs UJ, Kroll H, et al: The junctional adhesion molecule 3 (JAM-3) on human platelets is a counterreceptor for the leukocyte integrin Mac-1. *J Exp Med* 196:679–691, 2002.

299. Frenette PS, Denis CV, Weiss L, et al: P-selectin glycoprotein ligand 1 (PSGL-1) is expressed on platelets and can mediate platelet-endothelial interactions *in vivo*. *J Exp Med* 191:1413–1422, 2000.

300. Chauhan AK, Kisucka J, Brill A, et al: ADAMTS13: A new link between thrombosis and inflammation. *J Exp Med* 205:2065–2074, 2008.

301. Altieri DC: Coagulation assembly on leukocytes in transmembrane sugnaling and cell adhesion. *Blood* 81:569–579, 1993.

302. Lo SK, Cheung A, Zheng Q, Silverstein RL: Induction of tissue factor in monocytes by adhesion to endothelial cells. *J Immunol* 154:4768–4777, 1995.

303. Fan ST, Mackman N, Cui MZ, Edgington TS: Integrin regulation of an inflammatory effector gene: Direct induction of the tissue factor promoter by engagement of beta1 or alpha4 integrin chains. *J Immunol* 154:3266–3274, 1995.

304. Randolph GJ, Luther T, Albrecht S, et al: Role of tissue factor adhesion of mononuclear phagocytes to and trafficking through endothelium. *Blood* 92:4167–4177, 1998.

305. Palabrica T, Lobb R, Furie BC, et al: Leukocyte accumulation promoting fibrin deposition is mediated in vivo by P-selectin on adherent platelets. *Nature* 359:848–851, 1992.

306. Wright SD, Weitz JI, Huang AJ, et al: Complement receptor type (CR3, CD11b/CD18) of human polymorphonuclear leukocytes recognizes fibrinogen. *Proc Natl Acad Sci U S A* 85:7734–7738, 1988.

307. Altieri DC, Morrisey JH, Edgington TS: Adhesive receptor Mac-1 coordinates the activation of factor X on stimulated cells of monocytic and myeloid differentiation: An alternative initiation of the coagulation protease cascade. *Proc Natl Acad Sci U S A* 85:7462–7466, 1988.

308. Altieri DC, Edgington TS: The saturable high affinity association of factor X to ADP-stimulated monocytes defines a novel function of the Mac-1 receptor. *J Biol Chem* 263:7007–7015, 1988.

309. Macfarlane RG: An enzyme cascade in the blood clotting mechanism, and its function as a biochemical amplifier. *Nature* 202:498–499, 1964.

310. Davie EW, Ratnoff OD: Waterfall sequence for intrinsic blood clotting. *Science* 145:1310–1312, 1964.

311. Huber R, Berendes R, Burger A, et al: Crystal and molecular structure of human annexin V after refinement: Implications for structure, membrane binding and ion channel formation of the annexin family of proteins. *J Mol Biol* 223:683–704, 1992.

312. Huang KS, Wallner BP, Mattaliano RJ, et al: Two human 35 kd inhibitors of phospholipase A2 are related to substrates of pp60 v-src and of the epidermal growth factor receptor/kinase. *Cell* 46:191–199, 1986.

313. Gerke V, Creutz CE, Moss SE: Annexins: Linking Ca++ signalling to membrane dynamics. *Nat Rev Mol Cell Biol* 6:449–461, 2005.

314. Blasi F, Conese M, Moller LB, et al: The urokinase receptor: Structure, regulation and inhibitor-mediated internalization. *Fibrinolysis* 8:182–188, 1994.

CHAPTER 116
CLASSIFICATION, CLINICAL MANIFESTATIONS, AND EVALUATION OF DISORDERS OF HEMOSTASIS

Marcel Levi, Uri Seligsohn, and Kenneth Kaushansky

SUMMARY

Evaluation of a hemostatic disorder is commonly initiated when (1) a patient or referring physician suspects a bleeding tendency, (2) a bleeding tendency is discovered in one or more family members, (3) an abnormal coagulation assay result is obtained from an individual as part of a routine examination, (4) an abnormal assay result is obtained from a patient during preparation for surgery, or (5) a patient has unexplained diffuse bleeding during or after surgery or following trauma. Evaluation of a possible hemostatic disorder in each of these scenarios is a stepwise process that requires knowledge of the various classes of hemostatic disorders commonly found under the particular circumstances. The patient's history, the results of physical examination, and an initial set of hemostatic tests usually enable a tentative diagnosis. However, more specific tests are commonly necessary to make a definitive diagnosis. This chapter reviews the necessary steps.

CLASSIFICATION OF HEMOSTATIC DISORDERS

Hemostatic disorders can conveniently be classified as either hereditary or acquired (Table 116–1). Alternatively, hemostatic disorders can be classified according to the mechanism of the defect. Of the acquired disorders, the thrombocytopenias are the most frequently encountered entities. Thrombocytopenias can result from reduced production of platelets, excessive destruction caused by antibodies or other consumptive processes, or pooling of platelets in the spleen, as in hypersplenism (Chap. 119); however, if hypersplenism is the sole cause of a hemostatic disorder, it is rarely severe enough to cause pathologic bleeding.

BLEEDING HISTORY

The bleeding history is a crucial element in the evaluation of a patient with a hemorrhagic disorder. The bleeding history helps define the subsequent diagnostic approach and the likelihood of future bleeding.

Acronyms and Abbreviations: aPTT, activated partial thromboplastin time; DIC, disseminated intravascular coagulation; ELISA, enzyme-linked immunosorbent assay; PT, prothrombin time; RCF, ristocetin cofactor.

Eliciting and interpreting all of the relevant information requires a systematic and methodical approach. The following points are worth considering:

1. Patients vary in their responses to hemorrhagic symptoms. Some patients ignore significant symptoms, whereas other patients are highly sensitive to even minor symptoms. When asked in standardized questionnaires, many normal, healthy people indicate they have excessive bleeding or bruising.[1,2] Therefore, some experts believe the question "Do you bruise easily?" is virtually worthless. Women are more likely to respond that they have excessive bleeding or bruising than are men.

2. Patients with severe hemorrhagic disorders invariably have very abnormal bleeding histories, for example, severe hemophilia A or hemophilia B, type 3 (homozygous) von Willebrand disease, and Glanzmann thrombasthenia. Importantly, these patients may experience spontaneous bleeding episodes.

3. The diagnostic value of any specific symptom varies in the different disorders. Therefore, recognizing typical patterns of bleeding is important (Table 116–2). Unprovoked hemarthroses and muscle hemorrhages suggest one of the hemophilias, whereas mucocutaneous bleeding (epistaxis, gingival bleeding, menorrhagia) are more characteristic of patients with qualitative platelet disorders, thrombocytopenia, or von Willebrand disease.

4. Assessing the extent of hemorrhage against the background of any trauma or provocation that may have elicited the hemorrhage is important. If a patient has never had a significant hemostatic challenge, such as tooth extraction, surgery, trauma, or childbirth, the lack of a significant bleeding history is much less valuable in excluding a mild hemorrhagic disorder. For example, a significant percentage of patients with mild von Willebrand disease or mild forms of hemophilia may have negative bleeding histories,[1] even though they may be at considerable risk for excessive bleeding after surgery or other interventions. Thus, these diagnoses must be considered even in elderly patients if their first severe hemostatic challenge occurs at that age.

5. Obtaining objective confirmation of the subjective information conveyed in the bleeding history is valuable. Objective data include (1) previous hospital or physician visits for bleeding symptoms, (2) results of previous laboratory evaluations, (3) previous transfusions of blood products for bleeding episodes, and (4) a history of anemia and/or previous treatment with iron.

6. Although self-administered questionnaires may provide useful background information, they cannot substitute for a dialogue between the physician and the patient. Thus, history taking in general, but especially in the often subtle histories related to hemostatic disorders, is an intellectually active process involving data collection, hypothesis development, new question formulation, additional data gathering, and new hypothesis development. However, this iterative procedure has its limitations even when it is carefully pursued.[3,4]

7. A medication history is a crucial component of the bleeding history, with particular attention to nonprescription drugs, such as aspirin and nonsteroidal antiinflammatory agents, which may affect bleeding symptoms. A medication history is especially important in patients with thrombocytopenia, because drug-induced thrombocytopenia is common (Chap. 120 and see Table 116–1). Medication also may affect hemostasis through deleterious effects on the liver or kidney functions. The increased use of herbal and alternative medicines poses particular problems, because patients may not readily share information about what they are taking, and the dose they are taking of any particular active ingredient may

TABLE 116-1. Classification of Disorders of Hemostasis

Major Types	Disorders	Examples
Acquired	Thrombocytopenias	Autoimmune and alloimmune, drug-induced, hypersplenism, hypoplastic (primary, myelosuppressive therapy, myelophthisic marrow infiltration), disseminated intravascular coagulation (DIC), thrombotic thrombocytopenic purpura, hemolytic-uremic syndrome (Chaps. 117, 129, and 132)
	Liver diseases	Cirrhosis, acute hepatic failure, liver transplantation (Chap. 128), thrombopoietin deficiency
	Renal failure	
	Vitamin K deficiency	Malabsorption syndrome, hemorrhagic disease of the newborn, prolonged antibiotic therapy, malnutrition, prolonged biliary obstruction
	Hematologic disorders	Acute leukemias (particularly promyelocytic), myelodysplasias, monoclonal gammopathies, essential thrombocythemia (Chaps. 85–87 and 106)
	Acquired antibodies against coagulation factors	Neutralizing antibodies against factors V, VIII, and XIII, accelerated clearance of antibody-factor complexes, e.g., acquired von Willebrand disease, hypoprothrombinemia associated with antiphospholipid antibodies (Chaps. 126, 127, and 131)
	DIC	Acute (sepsis, malignancies, trauma, obstetric complications) and chronic (malignancies, giant hemangiomas, retained products of conception) (Chap. 129)
	Drugs	Antiplatelet agents, anticoagulants, antithrombins, and thrombolytic, hepatotoxic, and nephrotoxic agents (Chaps. 25 and 133–135)
	Vascular	Nonpalpable purpura ("senile," solar, and factitious purpura), use of corticosteroids, vitamin C deficiency, child abuse, thromboembolic, purpura fulminans; palpable-purpura (Henoch-Schönlein, vasculitis, dysproteinemias; Chap. 122), amyloidosis
Inherited	Deficiencies of coagulation factors	Hemophilia A (factor VIII deficiency), hemophilia B (factor IX deficiency), deficiencies of fibrinogen factors II, V, VII, X, XI, and XIII and von Willebrand disease (Chaps. 123–126)
	Platelet disorders	Glanzmann thrombasthenia, Bernard-Soulier syndrome, platelet granule disorders (Chap. 120)
	Fibrinolytic disorders	α_2-Antiplasmin deficiency, plasminogen activator inhibitor-1 deficiency (Chap. 135)
	Vascular	Hemorrhagic telangiectasias (Chap. 122)
	Connective tissue disorders	Ehlers-Danlos syndrome (Chap. 122)

be difficult to determine. *Ginkgo biloba* and ginseng are the most commonly used herbals that can cause platelet dysfunction and induce bleeding.[5] Other dietary supplements can display similar effects.[5,6]

8. A nutrition history should be obtained to assess the likelihood of (1) vitamin K deficiency, especially if the patient also is taking broad-spectrum antibiotics, (2) vitamin C deficiency, especially if the patient has skin bleeding consistent with scurvy (perifollicular purpura), and (3) general malnutrition and/or malabsorption.

9. Several tissues have an increased local fibrinolytic activity. Such tissues include the urinary tract, endometrium, and mucous membranes of the nose and oral cavity. These sites are particularly likely to have prolonged oozing of blood after trauma in patients with hemostatic abnormalities. Excessive bleeding following tooth extraction is one of the most common manifestations. Bleeding resulting from defects in fibrin crosslinking (factor XIII deficiency) or fibrinolytic defects may often manifest as delayed bleeding after trauma.

10. Bleeding isolated to a single organ or system (e.g., hematuria, hematemesis, melena, hemoptysis, or recurrent nosebleeds) is less likely to result from a hemostatic abnormality than from a local cause such as neoplasm, ulcer, or angiodysplasia. Thus, careful anatomic evaluation of the involved organ or system should be performed.

11. Bleeding may result from blood vessel disorders such as hereditary hemorrhagic telangiectasias, Cushing disease, scurvy, or Ehlers-Danlos syndrome. Many primary dermatologic disorders also have a purpuric or hemorrhagic component and must also be considered in the differential diagnosis (Chap. 122).

12. A family history is particularly important when hereditary disorders are considered. Patients usually will not spontaneously offer a history of consanguinity, so specific inquiry should be made about this possibility. A diagram of the patient's genealogic tree, extending back at least two generations, should be included to document consideration of genetic disorders. A sex-linked pattern of inheritance is consistent with hemophilia A or B (Chap. 123). An autosomal dominant pattern is characteristic of most forms of von Willebrand disease (Chap. 126). An autosomal recessive pattern is typical for all other coagulation factor deficiencies (Chap. 124), inherited platelet disorders (Chap. 120), and the rare, severe (homozygous), type 3 von Willebrand disease. Population genetic information may be helpful; for example, the higher prevalence of factor XI deficiency in Ashkenazi Jews (Chap. 124).

13. The history should include information on diseases and organs that may affect hemostasis, such as cirrhosis, renal insufficiency, myeloproliferative neoplasms (e.g., essential thrombocythemia), acute leukemia, myelodysplasia, systemic lupus erythematosus, and Gaucher disease.

TABLE 116-2. Clinical Manifestations Typically Associated with Specific Hemostatic Disorders

Clinical Manifestations	Hemostatic Disorders
Mucocutaneous bleeding	Thrombocytopenias, platelet dysfunction, von Willebrand disease
Cephalhematomas in newborns, hemarthroses, hematuria, and intramuscular, intracerebral, and retroperitoneal hemorrhages	Severe hemophilias A and B, severe deficiencies of factor VII, X, or XIII, severe type 3 von Willebrand disease, afibrinogenemia
Injury-related bleeding and mild spontaneous bleeding	Mild and moderate hemophilias A and B, severe factor XI deficiency, moderate deficiencies of fibrinogen and factors II, V, VII, or X, combined factors V and VIII deficiency, α_2-antiplasmin deficiency
Bleeding from stump of umbilical cord and habitual abortions	Afibrinogenemia, hypofibrinogenemia, dysfibrinogenemia, factor XIII deficiency
Impaired wound healing	Factor XIII deficiency
Facial purpura in newborns	Glanzmann thrombasthenia, severe thrombocytopenia
Recurrent severe epistaxis and chronic iron deficiency anemia	Hereditary hemorrhagic telangiectasias

● CLINICAL MANIFESTATIONS

Individual hemorrhagic symptoms often require detailed analysis before the significance of the symptoms and the resulting diagnosis or therapy can be determined. Some of the more common symptoms are discussed below, and Table 116–2 summarizes clinical manifestations that are typical for specific hemostatic disorders.

1. Epistaxis is one of the most common signs of platelet disorders and von Willebrand disease. It also is the most common symptom of hereditary hemorrhagic telangiectasia. In the latter condition, epistaxis almost always becomes more severe with advancing age. Epistaxis is not uncommon in normal children, but it usually resolves before puberty. Dry air heating systems can provoke epistaxis even in otherwise normal individuals. Bleeding confined to a single nostril more likely results from a local vascular problem than a systemic coagulopathy.

2. Gingival hemorrhage is very common in patients with both qualitative and quantitative platelet abnormalities and von Willebrand disease. Occasional gum bleeding occurs in normal individuals, especially if they use a hard bristle tooth brush and dental hygiene procedures. Thus, establishing whether the bleeding is excessive may be difficult. Frequent gingival hemorrhage can occur in individuals with normal hemostasis if they have gingivitis.

3. Oral mucous membrane bleeding in the form of blood blisters is a common manifestation of severe thrombocytopenia. Such bleeding usually has a predilection for sites where teeth can traumatize the inner surface of the cheek.

4. Skin hemorrhage in the form of petechiae and ecchymoses are common manifestations of hemostatic disorders. However, skin hemorrhage also is common among individuals without hemostatic disorders. Excessive bruising is more common in women than men. Moreover, women frequently note that the severity of their bruising varies with the phase of their menstrual cycle, although the most severe phase of the cycle may differ in different women. Features that help establish the severity of skin hemorrhage include the size of the bruises, the frequency of bruising, whether the bruises occur spontaneously or only with trauma, and the appearance of bruises on regions of the body that usually are not traumatized, such as the trunk and back. The color of the bruise may yield information. Red bruises on the extensor surfaces of the arms and hands indicate loss of supporting tissues, as occurs in Cushing syndrome, glucocorticoid therapy, senile purpura, and damage from chronic sun exposure. Jet-black bruises may be caused by warfarin-induced skin necrosis and similar disorders. Easy bruising can also occur in patients with Ehlers-Danlos syndrome manifested by distensible skin or extraordinary ligament laxness, and in patients with hyperflexibility of the thumb.[8]

5. Tooth extractions are common hemostatic challenges and may be helpful in defining the risk of bleeding. Molar extractions are greater hemostatic challenges than extractions of other teeth. Objective data regarding excessive bleeding based on the need for blood products or the need to pack or suture the extraction site are valuable.

6. Excessive bleeding in response to razor nicks is common in patients with platelet disorders or von Willebrand disease.

7. Hemoptysis almost never is the presenting symptom of a bleeding disorder and is rare even in patients with serious bleeding disorders. However, blood-tinged sputum in association with upper respiratory tract infections may be more common in patients with hemostatic disorders.

8. Hematemesis, like hemoptysis, almost never is the presenting symptom of a hemostatic disorder. However, a hemostatic disorder may lead to hematemesis because of an anatomic abnormality in the upper gastrointestinal tract and bleeding may be more severe than expected. Some hemostatic disorders more likely result in hematemesis because of a combination of effects, such as liver disease with deficient synthesis of coagulation proteins and with esophageal varices and aspirin ingestion with gastritis.

9. Hematuria is rarely the presenting symptom of a hemostatic disorder except for the hemophilias. However, hemostatic disorders can exacerbate hematuria caused by other disorders, including simple urinary tract infections.

10. Rectal bleeding in individuals with normal hemostasis most often results from hemorrhoids. However, von Willebrand disease and platelet disorders may contribute to repeated episodes of rectal bleeding when associated with a number of different underlying causes, including diverticula, hemorrhoids, or angiodysplasia. Melena is also only rarely the presenting symptom of a hemorrhagic disorder. However, repeated episodes of melena may occur in patients with hemorrhagic disorders.

11. Menorrhagia is common in women with platelet disorders and von Willebrand disease. In general, menstrual bleeding is considered excessive if the patient indicates she has heavy flow for more than 3 days or total flow for more than 7 days. However, an objective distinction between menorrhagia (loss of more than 80 mL blood per period) and normal blood loss can only be made by a visual assessment technique using pictorial charts of towels or tampons.[7]

12. Postpartum hemorrhage. Childbirth poses a considerable hemostatic challenge. Consequently, patients with bleeding disorders commonly manifest excessive bleeding during or after labor necessitating blood transfusion. An exception may be mild and moderate von Willebrand disease due to the vast increase in von Willebrand factor during pregnancy.

13. Habitual spontaneous abortions raise the possibility that the patient has a quantitative or qualitative abnormality of fibrinogen (Chap. 125), factor XIII deficiency (Chap. 124), or the antiphospholipid syndrome (Chap. 131). There is also an association between infertility and spontaneous abortion in patients with inherited thrombophilia (Chap. 130).

14. Hemarthroses are the hallmark abnormality in the hemophiliac; they are rare in other disorders except in severe factor VII deficiency and type 3 von Willebrand disease (Chaps. 124 and 126). Because discoloration of the skin overlying the joint with hemarthroses does not occur, patients may not recognize that their symptoms (pain, swelling, and limitation of motion) are caused by bleeding into their joints.

15. Excessive hemorrhage associated with surgical procedures is common in patients with hemorrhagic disorders. Procedures involving tissues with increased local fibrinolytic activity like urinary tract, nose, tonsils and oral cavity are particularly prone to bleed.

16. Excessive bleeding following circumcision is common in males with severe hemostatic disorders such as hemophilia A, hemophilia B, or Glanzmann thromboasthenia, and often is the patient's first symptom.

17. Bleeding from the umbilical stump is characteristic of factor XIII deficiency (Chap. 124) and afibrinogenemia (Chap. 125).

PHYSICAL EXAMINATION

Physical examination is essential for identifying signs of bleeding or their sequelae and for signs of a possible underlying disorder that can cause the hemostatic derangement (see Table 116–1). Careful examination of the skin is essential for detecting petechiae and ecchymoses. These signs may be prominent on the legs, where the hydrostatic pressure is greatest, or around the hair follicles in vitamin C deficiency.

Telangiectasias may range from pinpoint erythematous dots that blanch with pressure to classic cherry angiomata ranging in size up to several centimeters. Many normal individuals develop increasing numbers of telangiectasias with aging. Patients with hereditary hemorrhagic telangiectasia have more florid lesions that characteristically affect the vermilion border of the lips and the tongue (including the underside of the tongue), but not all patients have these classic features. Thus, a systematic search of the integument is necessary. Spider telangiectasias found in patients with chronic liver disease have a more splotchy and serpiginous appearance than the telangiectasias associated with hereditary hemorrhagic telangiectasia. In addition, the telangiectasias tend to be concentrated on the shoulders, chest, and face.

Chapter 122 details the differential diagnosis of nonpalpable purpuras and palpable purpuras. Hematomas, ecchymoses, and protracted oozing should be sought at venipuncture sites, injection sites, and arterial and venous catheter insertion sites. Joint deformities and limited joint mobility are suggestive of severe hemophilia A or B, severe deficiency of factor VII, or type 3 von Willebrand disease (Chaps. 123, 124, and 126). Hyperelasticity of the skin and hyperextensibility of joints are typical of Ehlers-Danlos syndrome, and hyperextensibility of only the thumb probably is a variant.[8]

EVALUATION BASED ON BLEEDING HISTORY, PHYSICAL EXAMINATION, AND BASIC LABORATORY TESTS

The patient's history and results of physical examination provide important information on the likelihood of the patient having a hemostatic defect and the possible cause of the defect, if one is present.

However, performing an initial set of widely available and inexpensive tests, including prothrombin time (PT), activated partial thromboplastin time (aPTT), and platelet count, is important for the following reasons: (1) The patient's history sometimes is unreliable; (2) the patient may have a mild hemostatic abnormality that has not manifested itself for lack of hemostatic challenge; (3) the patient may have developed an acquired hemostatic defect that has remained asymptomatic; and (4) the tests may reveal more than one abnormality.[9]

Figure 116–1 shows a series of algorithms that integrate the patient's bleeding history and the results of the initial hemostatic tests. A prolonged aPTT as a sole abnormality can be caused by a deficiency of factor VIII, IX, XI, or XII; presence of heparin; or by an inhibitor, which can be either factor specific, such as an antibody against factor VIII, or factor nonspecific, such as the presence of heparin or a lupus anticoagulant (Fig. 116–1A). A prolonged PT as the sole finding can indicate a factor VII deficiency, a mild vitamin K deficiency, or the presence of an inhibitor (Fig. 116–1B). Abnormalities of both PT and aPTT may indicate a deficiency of fibrinogen, prothrombin, factor V or factor X, an inhibitor to one of these factors, or a combined deficiency of coagulation factors (Fig. 116–1C).

To distinguish between a deficiency state and the presence of an inhibitor, repeating the abnormal test, the PT and/or aPTT, using a 1:1 mixture of the patient's plasma and normal plasma is useful. If the mixture normalizes the prolonged PT or aPTT, a deficiency state is likely, as most coagulation tests are calibrated to produce a normal result if each of the relevant factor levels are 50 percent of normal or greater. If the mixture still yields a significantly prolonged PT or aPTT, an inhibitor probably is present. Some inhibitors, such as antibodies to factor VIII, require time to inhibit the factor VIII activity in the assay, whereas other inhibitors, such as lupus anticoagulant or heparin, do not. Consequently, incubating the mixture for 1 or 2 hours at 37°C before performing the coagulation assay is desirable.

When none of the initial test results (PT, aPTT, and platelet count) is abnormal and the patient exhibits bleeding manifestations, ristocetin cofactor (RCF) or von Willebrand factor activity and examination of the blood film can be helpful for distinguishing among various candidate hemostatic abnormalities. The bleeding time is not used anymore because the test is highly operator and situational (room temperature, skin circulation, etc.) dependent and is not sufficiently reliable to be useful in the diagnostic process. Instead, many laboratories have introduced the platelet function analyzer (PFA) to detect qualitative defects in primary hemostasis. Figure 116–2 shows an algorithm that includes these secondary tests. Patients with type 1 and type 2 von Willebrand disease often have normal findings on initial laboratory tests because factor VIII levels are sufficiently high (>30 U/dL) for a normal aPTT result (Chap. 126). Examination of the blood film is helpful for distinguishing between Bernard-Soulier syndrome and von Willebrand disease because giant platelets are characteristic of the former (Chap. 120). Distinguishing mild-type von Willebrand disease from normal is difficult because levels of von Willebrand factor in the normal population is highly variable, partly accounted for by differing von Willebrand factor levels in individuals with different ABO blood types. In fact, some investigators have questioned whether patients with von Willebrand factor levels as low as 35 percent should be labeled as having von Willebrand disease.[10] The likelihood of having von Willebrand disease is a function of bleeding history, the von Willebrand factor level, and the number of first-degree family members with reduced von Willebrand factor levels.[11]

The ristocetin-induced platelet aggregation test is useful for distinguishing type 2B and platelet-type von Willebrand disease from the other types of von Willebrand disease. In type 2B and platelet-type von Willebrand disease, an enhanced response to low concentrations

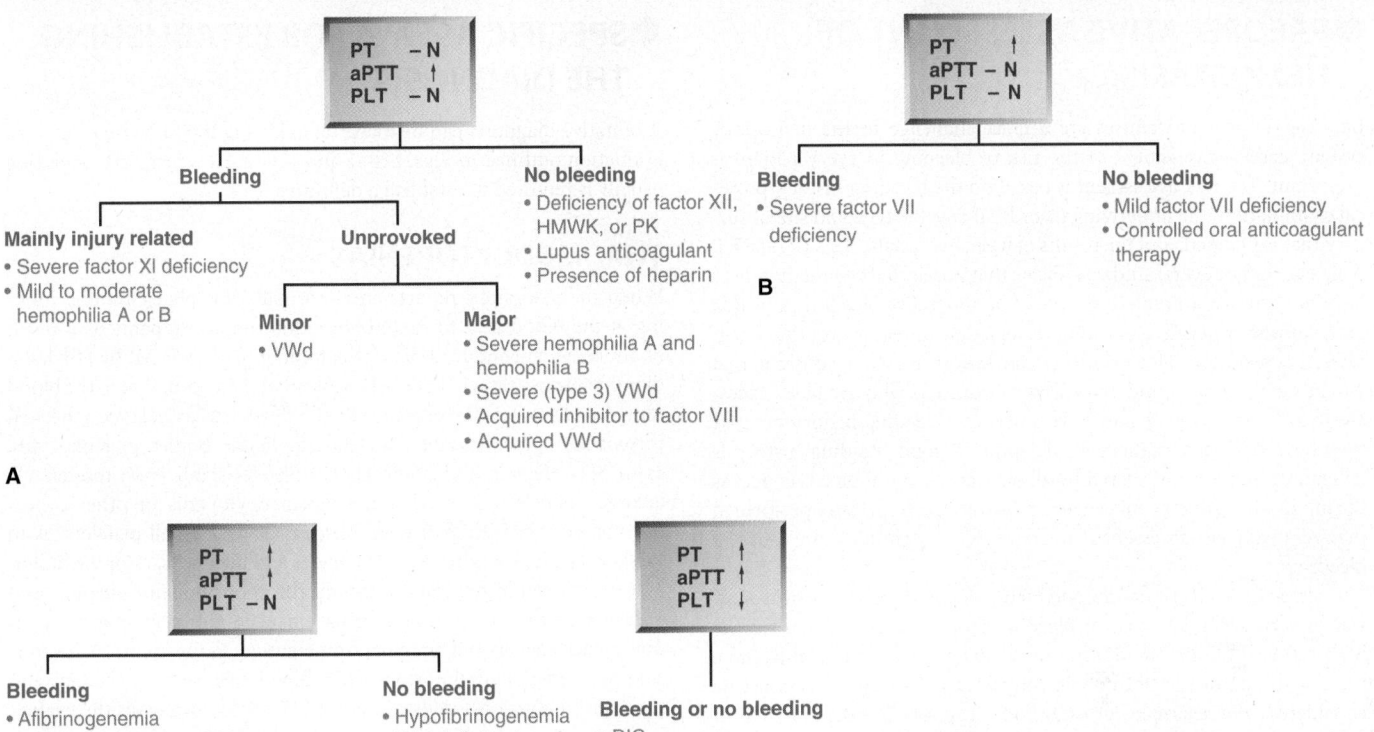

Figure 116–1. Measures for establishing a tentative diagnosis of a hemostatic disorder using basic tests of hemostasis and the patient's history of bleeding. ↓, Decrease; ↑, increase; aPTT, activated partial thromboplastin time; BT, bleeding time; DIC, disseminated intravascular coagulation; HMKK, high-molecular-weight kininogen; N, normal; PK, prekallikrein; PLT, platelets; PT, prothrombin time; VWD, von Willebrand disease.

of ristocetin is observed, whereas in the other types of von Willebrand disease, a decreased response is found. Total absence of platelet aggregates in a blood film prepared from non–anticoagulated blood and absent clot retraction are characteristic of Glanzmann thrombasthenia (Chap. 120).

Another simple test that may be useful for distinguishing among hemostatic disorders is the thrombin time (i.e., time for plasma to clot after adding thrombin). The thrombin time is prolonged in (1) afibrinogenemia, hypofibrinogenemia, and dysfibrinogenemias (Chap. 125), (2) the presence of heparin, (3) disseminated intravascular coagulation (DIC) causing increased levels of fibrin(ogen) degradation products, which inhibit fibrin monomer polymerization (see Fig. 116–1D and Chap. 129), and (4) patients with amyloidosis and an immunoglobulin inhibitor of thrombin.[12]

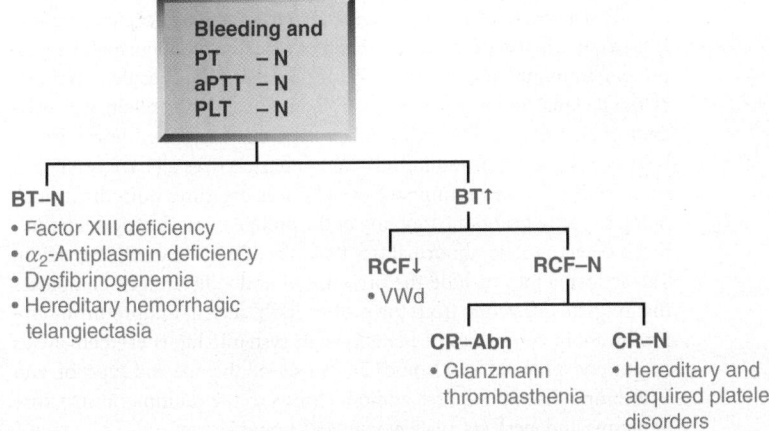

Figure 116–2. Tentative diagnoses in patients with bleeding manifestations and normal primary hemostatic tests using secondary tests. ↓, Decrease; ↑, increase; Abn, abnormal; aPTT, activated partial thromboplastin time; BT, bleeding time; CR, clot retraction; N, normal; PK, prekallikrein; PLT, platelets; PT, prothrombin time; RCF, ristocetin cofactor activity; VWD, von Willebrand disease.

PREOPERATIVE ASSESSMENT OF HEMOSTASIS

Because surgical procedures are a great challenge to the hemostatic system, careful assessment of the risk of bleeding in every patient is important. The risk assessment is based on the bleeding history, physical examination, the underlying disorder if any, the type and site of surgery that is planned, and the results of basic hemostatic tests (PT, aPTT, platelet count). Several studies indicate that unselected coagulation tests have no significant predictive value of perioperative bleeding, and that patients with a negative bleeding history do not require routine coagulation screening.[13] However, this conclusion does not consider that patients with mild to moderate bleeding disorders who can bleed excessively following surgery may have a negative bleeding history because they have not been challenged; obtaining a good bleeding history is an expertise that is not shared by all physicians; and if bleeding occurs during or after surgery for whatever reason, the basic tests performed preoperatively are an essential reference for determining the cause of bleeding.

Table 116–3 lists low-risk and high-risk conditions. A critical analysis of each potential cause of bleeding should be undertaken for the high-risk conditions. In addition to the extent of the surgical trauma, the magnitude of the fibrinolytic activity at the surgical site must be considered. For example, prostatectomy carries considerable risk of prolonged bleeding because of the presence of high fibrinolytic activity in the urine. Some surgical procedures can be anticipated to cause hemostatic abnormalities, such as operations in which extracorporeal circulation is used (because the extracorporeal circuits and/or the anticoagulation cause platelet dysfunction) and operations on patients with extensive malignancies or brain injury, which can give rise to DIC. Finally, the ability to institute local hemostatic measures should be considered. Thus, liver, lung, and kidney biopsies, although considered minor procedures, have a significant risk of bleeding because local measures, such as direct pressure, cannot be used to control bleeding.

TABLE 116-3. Evaluation of Bleeding Risk During Surgery

Assessed Factor	Risk of Bleeding	
	Low	High
Bleeding history	Negative	Positive[*]
Underlying conditions that compromise hemostasis (see Table 116–1)	Absent	Present
Initial hemostatic tests	Normal	Abnormal
Type of surgery	Minor	Major
	Not expected to induce a hemostatic defect at a site without local fibrinolysis	Expected to induce a hemostatic defect[†] at a site with local fibrinolysis[‡]
	Local hemostatic measures effective	Local hemostatic measures ineffective[§]

[*]Spontaneous bleeding episodes or injury-related hemorrhage.

[†]Open heart surgery or brain surgery.

[‡]Prostatectomy, tonsillectomy, oral or nasal surgery.

[§]Liver, lung, or kidney biopsy.

SPECIFIC ASSAYS FOR ESTABLISHING THE DIAGNOSIS

A tentative diagnosis can be made by following the stepwise process of evaluation outlined in Figs. 116–1 and 116–2. However, further testing usually is required to establish a definitive diagnosis.

THROMBOCYTOPENIAS

When the laboratory reports an abnormally low platelet count, looking at the blood film to exclude pseudothrombocytopenia as a result of anticoagulant-induced platelet clumping (e.g., induced by ethylenediaminetetraacetic acid [EDTA]) is essential.[14] Examination of the blood film also can reveal the presence of giant platelets, as in some inherited thrombocytopenias; giant platelets and Döhle bodies in leukocytes, as in May-Hegglin and other MYH9 platelet syndromes; moderately enlarged platelets, as in immune thrombocytopenia or other conditions associated with shortened platelet survival; small platelets, as in Wiskott-Aldrich syndrome; schistocytes and burr cells, as in the hemolytic uremic syndrome and thrombotic thrombocytopenic purpura, and occasionally in DIC; rouleaux formation, as in monoclonal gammopathies; macrocytosis and/or hypersegmentation, as in vitamin B_{12} or folic acid deficiency; and abnormal white blood cells, as in leukemias and myeloproliferative disorders. Chapter 117 further discusses the evaluation and differential diagnosis of the thrombocytopenias.

FACTOR DEFICIENCIES

Coagulation factors usually are assayed by measuring their clotting activity. The most common assays analyze the ability of dilutions of the patient's plasma to correct the clotting time of a plasma known to be deficient in the factor being measured (substrate plasma). The results are compared to the ability of dilutions of a normal reference plasma to correct the abnormality in the substrate plasma. The activities of factors II, V, VII, and X usually are determined in PT-based assays, whereas the activities of factors VIII, IX, XI, and XII, prekallikrein, and high-molecular-weight kininogen are measured in aPTT-based assays. The plasma level of fibrinogen most commonly is measured by assessing the time required for thrombin to clot the patient's diluted plasma (Clauss method).[15] Several assays of transglutaminase activity are available for measuring factor XIII activity,[16] but a simple qualitative test based on dissolving a fibrin clot in 5 M urea usually is sufficient (Chap. 124). The RCF function of von Willebrand factor can be measured by the ability of the patient's plasma to support the agglutination of a suspension of formaldehyde-fixed normal platelets by ristocetin.[17] This activity is defined as *RCF activity*. As with the coagulation factor assays, the results using patient plasma are compared to the results obtained with a normal reference plasma.

To determine whether a coagulation factor activity deficiency results from a quantitative decrease in protein or a qualitative abnormality in the protein, immunologic assays can be performed using specific polyclonal or monoclonal antibodies to assess the presence of the protein, independent of its function. Electroimmunoassays, enzyme-linked immunosorbent assays (ELISAs), and immunoradiometric assays all have been used successfully. Crossed immunoelectrophoresis measures both the immunologic reactivity and the mobility of the protein in an electric field; thus, it can detect protein abnormalities that affect electrophoretic migration. The abnormalities include the presence of antibody–antigen complexes that migrate differently from the protein itself, such as antiprothrombin–prothrombin complexes in patients with systemic lupus erythematosus or antiphospholipid syndrome. Diagnosis of the specific type of von Willebrand disease requires additional tests of the multimeric structure of plasma and, perhaps, platelet von Willebrand factor.

INHIBITORS TO COAGULATION FACTORS

If an inhibitor is suspected as a result of a prolonged PT or aPTT performed on a 1:1 mixture of the patient's plasma and normal plasma, further studies can help define the nature of the inhibitor and its titer. Among inhibitors that do not require incubation (i.e., immediate-type), perhaps the most common cause is the presence of heparin in the sample. This cause can be verified by finding a prolonged thrombin time on a test of the patient's plasma that is corrected with toluidine blue or other agents that neutralize heparin. The lupus anticoagulant also does not require incubation, and several methods for its detection are available (Chap. 131). However, with lupus anticoagulant, the PT usually is less prolonged than is the aPTT, and aPTT reagents have markedly different sensitivity to lupus-type anticoagulant depending on the amount of phosphatidyl serine present in each reagent.

Immunoglobulin inhibitors to specific coagulation factors may develop either after factor replacement therapy in patients with inherited deficiencies of coagulation factors (Chaps. 123 and 124) or spontaneously in patients without factor deficiencies (Chap. 127). Antibodies that neutralize factor activity frequently can be detected by incubating the patient's plasma with normal plasma, usually for 2 hours at 37°C, and then assaying the specific factor. The Bethesda assay originally was designed to quantify factor VIII inhibitors but can be modified to detect other inhibitors of coagulation factors (Chap. 123).[18] Some inhibitors do not directly neutralize clotting activity; instead they reduce factor levels by forming complexes with coagulation factors, which then are rapidly cleared from the circulation. Such plasmas do not produce prolonged clotting times when mixed 1:1 with normal plasma and thus may be confused with inherited deficiency states. More elaborate assays are required to identify this type of inhibitor, which may, for example, produce severe deficiency of prothrombin in some patients with the antiphospholipid syndrome (Chap. 131) and deficiency of von Willebrand factor in some acquired forms of von Willebrand disease (Chap. 126).[19]

PLATELET FUNCTION DISORDERS

Some laboratories nowadays routinely use an automated PFA to detect qualitative defects in primary hemostasis. Use of the RCF activity assay, platelet aggregation, and/or clot retraction are useful for assessing whether the patient has von Willebrand disease or a platelet function disorder (see Fig. 116–2). Chapter 120 contains a flow diagram of the steps required to diagnose the different qualitative disorders of platelet function. Additional platelet function assays and glycoprotein analysis may be required to establish the diagnosis.

REFERENCES

1. Miller CH, Graham JB, Goldin LR, Elston RC: Genetics of classic von Willebrand's disease: II. Optimal assignment of the heterozygous genotype (diagnosis) by discriminant analysis. *Blood* 54:137, 1979.
2. Wahlberg T, Blomback M, Hall P, Axelsson G: Application of indicators, predictors and diagnostic indices in coagulation disorders: I. Evaluation of a self-administered questionnaire with binary questions. *Methods Inf Med* 19:194, 1980.
3. Eikenboom JC, Rosendaal FR, Briet E: Value of the patient interview: All but consensus among haemostasis experts. *Haemostasis* 22:221, 1992.
4. Sramek A, Eikenboom JC, Briet E, et al: Usefulness of patient interview in bleeding disorders. *Arch Intern Med* 155:1409, 1995.
5. Dinehart SM, Henry L: Dietary supplements: Altered coagulation and effects on bruising. *Dermatol Surg* 31:819, 2005.
6. Basila D, Yuan C-S: Effects of dietary supplements on coagulation and platelet function. *Thromb Res* 117:49, 2005.
7. Janssen CAH, Scholten PC, Heintz APM: A simple visual assessment technique to discriminate between menorrhagia and normal menstrual blood loss. *Obstet Gynecol* 85:977, 1995.
8. Kaplinsky C, Kenet G, Seligsohn U, Rechavi G: Association between hyperflexibility of the thumb and an unexplained bleeding tendency: Is it a rule of thumb? *Br J Haematol* 101:260, 1998.
9. Rapaport SI: Preoperative hemostatic evaluation: Which tests, if any? *Blood* 61:229, 1983.
10. Sadler JE: Von Willebrand disease type 1: A diagnosis in search of a disease. *Blood* 101:2089, 2003.
11. Tosetto A, Castaman G, Rodeghiero F: Evidence-based diagnosis of type 1 von Willebrand disease: A Bayes theorem approach. *Blood* 111:3998, 2008.
12. Gastineau DA, Gertz MA, Daniels TM, et al: Inhibitor of the thrombin time in systemic amyloidosis: A common coagulation abnormality. *Blood* 77:2637, 1991.
13. Chee YL, Crawford JC, Watson HG, Greaves M: Guidelines on the assessment of bleeding risk prior to surgery or invasive procedures. *Br J Haematol* 140:496, 2008.
14. Payne BA, Pierre RV: Pseudothrombocytopenia: A laboratory artifact with potentially serious consequences. *Mayo Clin Proc* 59:123, 1984.
15. Clauss A: Gerinnungsphysiologische schnell methodes zur des fibrinogens. *Acta Haematol* 17:327, 1957.
16. Fickenscher K, Aab A, Stuber W: A photometric assay for blood coagulation factor XIII. *Thromb Haemost* 65:535, 1991.
17. McFarlane DE, Stibbe J, Kirby EP, et al: A method for assaying von Willebrand factor (ristocetin cofactor). *Thromb Diath Haemorrh* 34:306, 1975.
18. Kasper CK, Aledort L, Aronson D, et al: Proceedings: A more uniform measurement of factor VIII inhibitors. *Thromb Diath Haemorrh* 34:612, 1975.
19. Inbal A, Bank I, Zivelin A, et al: Acquired von Willebrand disease in a patient with angiodysplasia resulting from immune-mediated clearance of von Willebrand factor. *Br J Haematol* 96:179, 1997.

CHAPTER 117
THROMBOCYTOPENIA

Reyhan Diz-Küçükkaya and José A. López

SUMMARY

Thrombocytopenia is one of the most frequent causes for hematologic consultation in the practice of medicine, and may be life threatening. Although the normal platelet count in humans (150 to 400×10^9/L) far exceeds the minimal level required to avoid pathologic hemorrhage ($<50 \times 10^9$/L), a number of medical conditions either increasing the destruction of platelets or reducing their production, enhance the risk of bleeding. This chapter discusses an approach to the diagnosis of thrombocytopenia, grouping various causes by mechanism of action, and describing our current understanding of the pathogenesis, treatment and prognosis. In the vast majority of patients, a cause for thrombocytopenia can be identified, and effective therapy instituted.

● DEFINITION AND HISTORY

Platelets are anucleate blood cells produced in the marrow by polyploid cells termed megakaryocytes and were described in the 19th century after the application of the improved compound microscope allowed these very small cellules, approximately 2 μM in diameter,

Acronyms and Abbreviations: ACOG, American College of Obstetricians and Gynecologists; ADP, adenosine diphosphate; AFLP, acute fatty liver of pregnancy; AML, acute myelogenous leukemia; APLA, antiphospholipid antibody; APS, antiphospholipid syndrome; ARC, arthrogryposis–renal dysfunction–cholestasis; ASH, American Society of Hematology; ATG, antithymocyte globulin; ATRUS, amegakaryocytic thrombocytopenia with radioulnar synostosis; CAMT, congenital amegakaryocytic thrombocytopenia; CAPTURE, c7E3 Fab Antiplatelet Therapy in Unstable Refractory Angina; CTP, cyclic thrombocytopenia; CVID, common variable immunodeficiency; DIC, disseminated intravascular coagulation; EDTA, ethylenediaminetetraacetic acid; EPIC, Evaluation of 7E3 for the Prevention of Ischemic Complications; EPILOG, Evaluation of Percutaneous Transluminal Coronary Angioplasty to Improve Long-term Outcome of c7E3 GPIIb-IIIa Receptor Blockade; EPISTENT, Evaluation of Platelet IIb/IIIa Inhibitor for Stenting; Flt1, fms-like tyrosine kinase-1; FPD/AML, familial platelet disorder with propensity to acute myeloid malignancy; GP, glycoprotein; HCV, hepatitis C virus; HELLP, hemolysis, elevated liver enzymes, low platelets; HIT, heparin-induced thrombocytopenia; HUS, hemolytic uremic syndrome; HPA, human platelet alloantigen; ICSH, International Council for Standardization in Hematology; IDA, iron-deficiency anemia; IPD, inherited platelet disorder; ITP, immune thrombocytopenia; IVIG, intravenous immunoglobulin; IWG, International Working Group; LTA, light transmission aggregometry; MACE, modified antigen capture enzyme-linked immunosorbent assay; MAIPA, monoclonal antibody-specific immobilization of platelet antigens; MDS, myelodysplastic syndrome; MHC, major histocompatibility complex; NAIT, neonatal alloimmune thrombocytopenia; PAIgG, platelet-associated immunoglobulin G; sFlt1, soluble Flt1; SLE, systemic lupus erythematosus; TAR, thrombocytopenia with absent radii; TPO, thrombopoietin; Treg, T-regulatory; TTP, thrombotic thrombocytopenic purpura; VEGF, vascular endothelial growth factor; VWD, von Willebrand disease; VWF, von Willebrand factor.

to be identified. Many early investigators are associated with the discovery of blood platelets, including Donné, Hayem, Bizzozero, and Osler, but it was James Homer Wright who, in 1906, using his special stain (later called Wright stain), described the morphology of platelets with their central granular area and marginal hyaline zone and established that they were the product of the fragmentation of marrow megakaryocytes. Clot retraction was discovered long before platelets, but Hayem, through a series of studies, showed retraction to be dependent on platelets. During the mid-20th century the aggregation of platelets, their adherence to collagen of damaged tissues, their acceleration of blood coagulation, and their relationship to the bleeding time and the biochemistry underlying several of these processes were described by scientists, among whom were Paul Owren, Kenneth Brinkhaus, Edwin Chargaff, Ernst Lüsher, Marjorie Zucker, and William Duke.

Platelets circulate in close contact with the endothelium, continually monitoring its integrity. When the vessel wall is damaged, platelets bind to subendothelial proteins, initiating the process of primary hemostasis. At sites of blood loss, the platelets aggregate to form a vessel sealing plug to halt bleeding. Activated platelets at sites of injury also provide a surface for assembly of coagulation reactions, resulting in the production of fibrin and consolidation of the thrombus. Both qualitative and quantitative deficiencies of the platelets cause bleeding. Platelets also have important functions in inflammation, tissue remodeling and wound healing.[1]

Approximately 1×10^{11} platelets are produced per day by an adult human, a number that can be increased 20-fold or more, if necessary.[2] One-third of the platelets are stored in the spleen, the remaining two-thirds circulate in blood vessels.[3] Disorders that increase splenic volume cause more platelets to be trapped in the spleen, lowering the concentration of circulating platelets, although alone, this redistribution rarely causes a significant bleeding diathesis.

Under normal conditions, human platelets have a mean life span in the circulation of between 7 and 10 days.[4,5] Patients with thrombocytopenia secondary to platelet destruction have a markedly decreased platelet survival.[6,7] Patients with thrombocytopenia from marrow failure have mildly decreased platelet survival, mostly because the body's fixed daily consumption of platelets accounts for a progressively larger fraction of the reduced total daily production as the platelet count drops.[8] Platelet turnover is a measure of the net effect of platelet production and platelet destruction under steady-state conditions.[7] Several studies using ^{111}In oxine–labeled platelets have established that, under normal conditions, platelet turnover in humans ranges from 40 to 50×10^9/L per day.[7] Although a high platelet turnover is expected in patients with immune thrombocytopenia (ITP), platelet production is not always increased in this disorder.[7] Low platelet production may result from binding of the antiplatelet antibodies to megakaryocytes, inhibiting their maturation or leading to their destruction, causing an inappropriately muted marrow response to the degree of thrombocytopenia.[9]

Every day approximately 10 to 12 percent of circulating platelets are removed by the mononuclear phagocyte system, primarily by macrophages in the spleen and liver. Although the precise mechanisms of platelet clearance are not completely understood, changes that occur as the platelets circulate are thought to lead them to be recognized by macrophages. One of these changes is the progressive loss of sialic acid from platelet surface proteins. Studies in animals and humans with anticancer drugs that inhibit apoptotic pathways have also identified a role for apoptotic proteins in platelet survival and clearance. According to these studies, a classical intrinsic apoptosis pathway regulates the life span of circulating platelets, and antiapoptotic proteins, especially Bcl-$_{XL}$, maintain platelet viability by restraining apoptosis.[10]

THE PLATELET COUNT

The normal platelet count (defined as the values between percentiles 2.5 to 97.5 in normal individuals) is given as 150 to 400 × 10^9/L; classically, thrombocytopenia is defined as a platelet count of less than 150 × 10^9/L. However, a sustained lower platelet count (100 to 150 × 10^9/L) can be seen in otherwise healthy individuals.[11,12] Long-term observation of individuals with platelet counts between 100 and 150 × 10^9/L showed that 88 percent of these individuals had subsequently reached normal platelet counts or remained stable. In those individuals, the probability of developing ITP was 6.9 percent, an autoimmune disease other than ITP 12 percent, and myelodysplastic syndrome (MDS) 2 percent, after 64 months of followup. All patients with MDS in this cohort were found to be older than age 65 years.[13]

THROMBOCYTOPENIA

Thrombocytopenia can be classified as severe (platelet count less than 20 × 10^9/L), moderate (platelet count 20 to 70 × 10^9/L), or mild (above 70 × 10^9/L).[14] Although easy bruising occurs in patients with platelet counts less than 50 × 10^9/L and spontaneous life-threatening bleeding can be expected in patients with platelet counts less than 15 × 10^9/L, bleeding symptomatology is largely determined by comorbid conditions affecting platelets or the coagulation system, including liver cirrhosis, uremia, disseminated intravascular coagulation (DIC), or antiplatelet drug usage.

In clinical practice, platelet counting is automated, and includes several different technologies: impedance, optical, two-dimensional laser, and optical-fluorescence methods. Although automated cell counter technology has progressed considerably during recent decades, the analytic performances of these machines for platelet counts and platelet indices is still not perfect, especially in patients with severe thrombocytopenia and macrothrombocytopenia.[15-17] Each step between the sampling of blood and its analysis is important: the blood sample should be obtained by a clean venipuncture without dilution with other IV solutions or drugs. Blood/anticoagulant ratio should be as recommended. The International Council for Standardization in Hematology (ICSH) recommends use of ethylenediaminetetraacetic acid (EDTA) as the anticoagulant. Adequate mixing of the blood sample with EDTA (the final EDTA concentration should be 1.5 to 2.2 mg/mL) is crucial to prevent clumping of the platelets. Blood samples should be kept at room temperature and analyzed within 6 hours of phlebotomy. If a sample is to be analyzed more than 6 hours after it is drawn, it can be kept at 4°C for 24 hours. The blood count analyzer should be cleaned according to laboratory standards.[17]

Although thrombocytopenia is variably attributed to single factors such as decreased platelet production, increased platelet destruction, or abnormal splenic pooling, combinations of factors are often involved in clinical settings. For instance, the thrombocytopenia seen in patients with viral infection can result from many factors, including platelet destruction (e.g., through an autoimmune mechanism or drug toxicity) or decreased platelet production because of direct megakaryocyte infection by the virus. Table 117–1 lists the multiple causes of thrombocytopenia and classifies them by pathogenesis.

● PSEUDO (SPURIOUS) THROMBOCYTOPENIA

Pseudothrombocytopenia (or spurious thrombocytopenia) is a relatively uncommon phenomenon with multiple causes, including *ex vivo* agglutination of platelets, the presence of abnormally large platelets (improper counting), or improper preparation of blood samples.

The incidence of pseudothrombocytopenia reported in different studies ranges from 0.09 to 0.21 percent, which accounts for 15 to 30 percent of

TABLE 117–1. Classification of Thrombocytopenia

I. Pseudo (spurious) thrombocytopenia
 A. Antibody-induced platelet aggregation
 B. Platelet satellitism
 C. Antiphospholipid antibodies
 D. Glycoprotein IIb/IIIa antagonists
 E. Miscellaneous

II. Thrombocytopenia resulting from impaired platelet production
 A. Inherited platelet disorders
 B. Acquired marrow disorders
  1. Nutritional deficiencies and alcohol-induced thrombocytopenia
  2. Clonal hematological diseases (myelodysplastic syndrome, leukemias, myeloma, lymphoma, paroxysmal nocturnal hemoglobinuria)
  3. Aplastic anemia
  4. Marrow metastasis by solid tumors
  5. Marrow infiltration by infectious agents (HIV, tuberculosis, brucellosis, etc.)
  6. Hemophagocytosis
  7. Immune thrombocytopenia (ITP)
  8. Drug-induced thrombocytopenia
  9. Pregnancy-related thrombocytopenia

III. Thrombocytopenia resulting from increased platelet destruction
 A. Immune thrombocytopenia
  1. Autoimmune thrombocytopenia (primary and secondary ITP)
  2. Alloimmune thrombocytopenia
 B. Thrombotic microangiopathies (TTP, hemolytic uremic syndrome [HUS])
 C. Disseminated intravascular coagulopathy (DIC)
 D. Pregnancy-related thrombocytopenia
 E. Hemangiomas (Kasabach-Merritt phenomenon)
 F. Drug-induced immune thrombocytopenia (quinidine, heparin, abciximab)
 G. Artificial surfaces (hemodialysis, cardiopulmonary bypass, extracorporeal membrane oxygenation)
 H. Type 2B von Willebrand disease

IV. Thrombocytopenia resulting from abnormal distribution of the platelets
 A. Hypersplenism
 B. Hypothermia
 C. Massive blood transfusions
 D. Excessive fluid infusions

V. Miscellaneous Causes
 A. Cyclic thrombocytopenia, acquired pure megakaryocytic thrombocytopenia

all cases of isolated thrombocytopenia.[18-25] Pseudothrombocytopenia has been reported in association with the use of EDTA as an anticoagulant, with platelet cold agglutinins,[26] and with myeloma.[27] A very interesting report demonstrates pseudothrombocytopenia caused by platelet phagocytosis *ex vivo* in the presence of EDTA anticoagulant.[28] An example of *ex vivo* platelet clumping is shown in Chap. 1, Fig. 1–6*H*, accompanied by platelet–neutrophil satellitism (see "Platelet Satellitism" below).

ANTIBODY-INDUCED PLATELET AGGLUTINATION

Platelet agglutination *ex vivo* can be induced by antiplatelet antibodies or by activation of the platelets during collection. The responsible antibodies do not appear to be associated with a pathologic process, as they are found in normal individuals. One hypothesis put forth to explain their presence is that the antibodies are responsible for clearing aged and damaged platelets. Most antibodies implicated in pseudothrombocytopenia recognize platelet membrane glycoproteins that are modified to expose new epitopes when calcium is chelated. Typically, the artifact is most prominent in the presence of EDTA, but other anticoagulants can also cause platelet clumping, including sodium citrate, sodium oxalate, acid citrate dextrose, and heparin. The antibodies usually are of the immunoglobulin (Ig) G type; IgM and IgA antibodies also have been described.[29-31] Most antibodies react at room temperature; thus, the reaction can be prevented by keeping the blood sample at 37°C. In 20 percent of cases, however, the antibodies, usually of the IgM type, are reactive at both 22°C and 37°C.[30] Clumping usually is evident within 60 minutes after the blood is drawn, but may require incubations of 2 to 3 hours. Agglutination can be reproduced by incubating plasma from patients with pseudothrombocytopenia with blood from normal individuals in the presence of EDTA.

In most cases, the antibodies are directed against the integrin $\alpha_{IIb}\beta_3$ (also termed glycoprotein [GP] IIbIIIa), a conclusion supported by the observation that platelets from patients with Glanzmann thrombasthenia, who lack the integrin $\alpha_{IIb}\beta_3$ complex, fail to agglutinate in the presence of patient sera.[32-35] Moreover, pretreatment of fresh blood with anti–integrin $\alpha_{IIb}\beta_3$ dramatically reduces EDTA-induced platelet agglutination.[36] The responsible epitope normally is cryptic and located in the integrin α_{IIb} subunit. Low temperature and calcium chelation combine to change the conformation of integrin $\alpha_{IIb}\beta_3$ and expose the epitope.[33]

PLATELET SATELLITISM

Antibodies directed against integrin $\alpha_{IIb}\beta_3$ may react simultaneously with the leukocyte Fcγ receptor III (FcγRIII) and attach the platelets to neutrophils and monocytes, inducing a phenomenon known as *platelet-leukocyte satellitism*,[32] another form of pseudothrombocytopenia (Fig. 117–1). These antibodies fail to produce satellitism in the presence of platelets from patients with type I Glanzmann thrombasthenia or in the presence of neutrophils from patients with congenital absence of FcγRIII.[32] Typically, the platelets form a rosette around the periphery of leukocytes. Neutrophils are most frequently involved, but the phenomenon also is occasionally observed with monocytes.[37,38] These antibodies also are naturally occurring, and their presence does not clearly correlate with any specific clinical situation, disease, or drug. As with the antibodies that induce only platelet clumping, exposure of a cryptic antigen on EDTA-treated platelets and leukocytes may trigger this phenomenon.

ANTIPHOSPHOLIPID ANTIBODIES

Some antiplatelet antibodies from patients with pseudothrombocytopenia crossreact with negatively charged phospholipids and may exhibit anticardiolipin activity.[30] The sera of these patients lose their ability to clump platelets when adsorbed onto either cardiolipin or activated normal platelets, supporting the hypothesis that antibody subpopulations directed against negatively charged phospholipids can bind to antigens modified by EDTA on the platelet membrane. Another possibility is that the antigens in this case are negatively charged phospholipids on the surface of platelets.

INTEGRIN $\alpha_{IIb}\beta_3$ ANTAGONISTS

Thrombocytopenia has been described in patients suffering from acute coronary syndromes treated with the abciximab and other integrin $\alpha_{IIb}\beta_3$ antagonists.[39-41] Abciximab is associated with both pseudothrombocytopenia and true thrombocytopenia. The mechanism for platelet clumping with abciximab is unknown; the drug itself likely is not crosslinking the platelets because it is monovalent. More likely, other agglutinins bind integrin $\alpha_{IIb}\beta_3$ at new epitopes induced by the combination of abciximab binding and calcium chelation. True abciximab-induced thrombocytopenia occurs in approximately 0.3 to 1 percent of patients treated with the drug.[42] The mechanism is incompletely understood, but likely includes reaction of preformed antibodies with a neoepitope expressed after binding of abciximab to integrin $\alpha_{IIb}\beta_3$ (ligand-induced binding sites) or abciximab-induced platelet activation with subsequent platelet sequestration from the circulation. In some abciximab-treated patients, high antibody titers are detected in the plasma.

The incidence of pseudothrombocytopenia and thrombocytopenia related to abciximab was determined in four large placebo-controlled trials:[40] c7E3 Fab Antiplatelet Therapy in Unstable Refractory Angina (CAPTURE), Evaluation of 7E3 for the Prevention of Ischemic

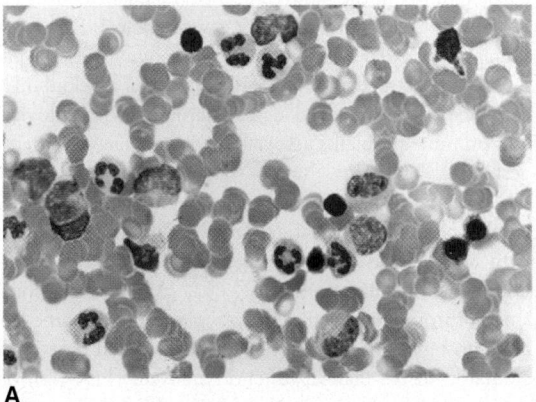
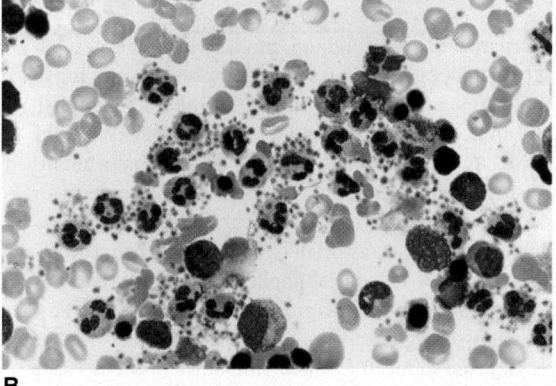

A **B**

Figure 117–1. Platelet satellitism. **A.** Direct (non–anticoagulated) marrow film. No platelet satellitism. **B.** A concentrated marrow film anticoagulated with disodium ethylenediaminetetraacetic acid (Na$_2$EDTA) from same specimen as in **(A)**. Note platelets are adherent to the mature neutrophil surface (satellitism) in the presence of Na$_2$EDTA. The neutrophil precursors do not have surface features that interact with platelets, apparently a feature only present after the final steps in maturation. *(Reproduced with permission from* Lichtman's Atlas of Hematology, *www.accessmedicine.com.)*

Complications (EPIC), Evaluation of Percutaneous Transluminal Coronary Angioplasty to Improve Long-term Outcome of c7E3 GPIIb-IIIa Receptor Blockade (EPILOG), and Evaluation of Platelet IIb/IIIa Inhibitor for Stenting (EPISTENT). In these studies, pseudothrombocytopenia accounted for more than one-third of low platelet counts in patients undergoing coronary interventions and treated with abciximab. These studies demonstrated that pseudothrombocytopenia is a benign laboratory condition not associated with increased bleeding, stroke, transfusion requirements, or the need for repeat revascularization.

MISCELLANEOUS ASSOCIATIONS

Some studies suggest that platelet agglutinins occur more frequently in hospitalized patients and in association with medical conditions such as autoimmune diseases, malignancy, liver disease, and sepsis.[25,43–46] However, others found no association with any particular pathology or with use of specific drugs.[30]

One study showed that antibodies from patients with pseudothrombocytopenia can induce agglutination of donor platelets in the presence of EDTA. This agglutination was prevented by warming the donor platelets to 37°C or by pretreating the platelets with aspirin, prostaglandin E$_1$, apyrase, and monoclonal antibodies against integrin $\alpha_{IIb}\beta_3$ that block the binding site for fibrinogen and von Willebrand factor (VWF), or arg-gly-asp (RGD) peptide, which binds the site on integrin $\alpha_{IIb}\beta_3$ that recognizes cytoadhesive proteins.[33] Whether the same reaction occurs *in vivo* is not known, but in that case the antibodies should have a slow reactivity, or else bleeding would sometimes occur.

MANAGEMENT OF THE PATIENTS WITH PSEUDOTHROMBOCYTOPENIA

An (unexpected) low platelet count reported by automated cell counters should be confirmed by microscopic examination of the blood film. Automated cell counters identify platelets merely based on their small volumes in comparison to those of other blood cells, generally defined as volumes between 2 and 20 fL. Because platelet clumps tend to exceed 20 fL, the clumps may be counted as leukocytes,[18] and even if counted as platelets, several platelets are counted as one. Thus, pseudothrombocytopenia may be accompanied by pseudoleukocytosis.[5,21,24,47] The greater the delay in processing of anticoagulated blood, the greater is the degree of platelet clumping and the greater the potential for artifact.[21] Platelet clumping can be prevented by collecting the sample in EDTA and maintaining its temperature at 37°C. Even with these measures, however, clumping will still occur in approximately 20 percent of cases.[30]

Another alternative is use of sodium citrate, which chelates calcium more weakly than does EDTA but still causes platelet clumping in approximately 10 to 20 percent of cases with EDTA-induced clumping. In some patients, an accurate platelet count can be obtained only by sampling blood directly into ammonium oxalate and manually counting the platelets using a Bruker chamber.[30] Flow cytometry may help for determining exact platelet number by immunostaining of the platelets.

Platelet agglutinins are not associated with bleeding or thrombosis, so they appear to have no clinical implications, except that they may lead to unnecessary therapy because of misdiagnosis. Transplacental transmission of agglutinins has been documented, but the pseudothrombocytopenia induced by these antibodies in the neonate resolves spontaneously.[48,49] No complications have been reported when platelet agglutinins are discovered during pregnancy.[48,50] Transfusion of blood products from patients with pseudothrombocytopenia produces an acceptable corrected count increment in the recipient, again supporting its benign nature.[23] Thus, the clinical importance of

pseudothrombocytopenia concerns conditions with which it is confused rather than any pathology associated with the condition. It is important that this syndrome be recognized promptly to avoid unnecessary diagnostic tests and treatment.

● INHERITED PLATELET DISORDERS

Megakaryopoiesis and thrombopoiesis are regulated by a number of hematopoietic growth factors and transcription factors (Chap. 113). Any genetic defect affecting platelet production, function or morphology may cause inherited platelet disorders (IPDs; Chap. 121). In recent decades, knowledge of normal megakaryocyte and platelet physiology has grown enormously,[51] aided in part by the study of IPDs.[52,53]

IPDs are a very heterogeneous group of disorders. Some disorders, such as Bernard-Soulier syndrome, appear to be restricted to platelets,[54] whereas others appear as a part of a complex pathology, as seen in thrombocytopenia with absent radii (TAR) syndrome (Fig. 117–2). In some IPDs, the platelet count may be normal despite severely impaired platelet function, such as in Glanzmann thrombasthenia. Other disorders are accompanied by abnormal platelet numbers, usually thrombocytopenia. Table 117–2 summarizes the inherited thrombocytopenias.

Severe forms of IPDs that present as a bleeding tendency early in childhood are rare. IPD patients usually present with mucocutaneous bleeding, such as with purpura, epistaxis, and/or gingival bleeding. Menorrhagia and bleeding during pregnancy and labor are common problems in female patients. Spontaneous life-threatening bleeding is rare, including intracranial hemorrhage, massive gastrointestinal or genitourinary bleeding. Recent molecular investigations of IPD patients and their families with bleeding diathesis demonstrated that most IPDs cause mild bleeding tendencies, and IPDs may be more prevalent than previously thought.[55] In these milder cases, a bleeding diathesis may only be diagnosed after an episode of excessive bleeding, such as during surgery or following trauma.

Diagnosis of IPD presents a significant challenge because of the heterogeneity of clinical and laboratory findings of the patients with the same disorder, even in the same family. IPD patients with isolated macrothrombocytopenia share common clinical and basic laboratory features with certain acquired platelet disorders and are sometimes misdiagnosed. It is very important to distinguish IPD patients from those with acquired platelet disorders, such as ITP, to avoid unnecessary or potentially harmful treatments. Helpful in this regard is information obtained during the history, including a family history of bleeding and consanguinity in the family, because the majority of IPDs are inherited as autosomal recessive traits. Because some IPDs are associated with increased risk of developing myeloid malignancies, the patient and family should be asked about a family history of myeloid malignancies. The presence of skeletal, facial, ocular, audiologic, neurologic, renal, cardiac, and immune problems associated with platelet disorders may also suggest IPD.[51,56]

Laboratory evaluation of a potential IPD should start with a careful blood film investigation, which could be helpful for patients with MYH9-related diseases (giant platelets and Döhle-like inclusion bodies within leukocytes; Fig. 117–3), Bernard-Soulier syndrome (macrothrombocytopenia), Gray platelet syndrome (pale platelets), and sitosterolemia (giant platelets surrounded by a circle of vacuoles, stomatocytosis). Platelet function analyzer (PFA-100) occlusion times are usually found to be prolonged. The skin bleeding time is not recommended for screening, because it is invasive and poorly reproducible. Although the PFA-100 test is very sensitive in detecting Bernard-Soulier syndrome and platelet-type von Willebrand disease (VWD), it may be normal in patients with variant forms of these disorders, or patients

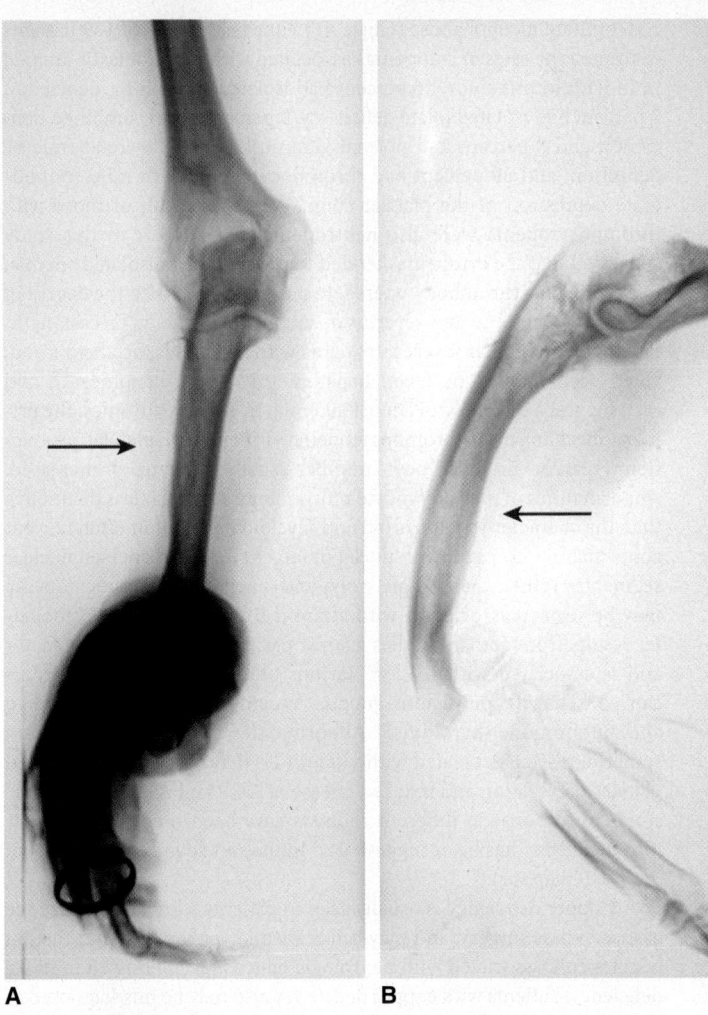

A   B

with storage pool deficiencies.[57] Light transmission aggregometry (LTA) using different concentrations of adenosine diphosphate (ADP), collagen, ristocetin, epinephrine, and arachidonic acid is accepted as a gold standard in diagnosing IPDs, but, again, may be normal in variant forms of IPDs and in some patients with storage pool diseases. Measurement of platelet nucleotide content and release is recommended in patients with platelet granule deficiencies. Flow cytometric analysis is very informative in patients with platelet surface GP deficiencies such as Bernard-Soulier syndrome. Marrow biopsy is needed in patients who have pancytopenia or severe thrombocytopenia, as in Fanconi anemia and congenital amegakaryocytic thrombocytopenia (CAMT), respectively. Unfortunately, these tests may help diagnose only a small portion of the IPD patients. Further tests are only available in specialized centers, and include electron microscopy, Western blotting, and others. Electron microscopy is able to define characteristic ultrastructural abnormalities; Western blotting, enzyme-linked immunosorbent assay (ELISA), or radioimmunoassay can be used for qualitative and quantitative analysis of specific platelet proteins.[51,56] Even with these expensive, complicated, and time-consuming tests, the results are inconclusive in nearly half of patients being evaluated for IPD.[56] Genetic analysis is often able to determine the underlying molecular pathology, but the very large number of candidate genes limits the traditional target gene approach. Within the past decade, next-generation sequencing techniques have not only improved the speed and cost of genetic investigations, but have also begun to generate very interesting data about the genetic causes of IPD.[52,53]

● NUTRITIONAL DEFICIENCIES AND ALCOHOL-INDUCED THROMBOCYTOPENIA

Iron, vitamin B_{12}, and folic acid deficiencies are the nutrient deficiencies most widely recognized to impair blood cell production. Severe nutritional deficiencies primarily cause anemia, rarely causing bicytopenia or pancytopenia. Isolated thrombocytopenia is rare in patients with nutritional deficiencies.

Iron is present in all human cells, and mediates electron transfer reactions. Iron is a key component of hemoglobin, and iron deficiency causes a hypochromic and microcytic anemia (Chap. 42). Iron-deficiency anemia (IDA) generally develops after acute or chronic bleeding, and is usually accompanied by thrombocytosis rather than thrombocytopenia. Thrombocytopenia associated with IDA is relatively rare, reported in only 2.3 percent and 2.4 percent of pediatric and adult IDA patients, respectively.[58,59]

Cobalamin (vitamin B_{12}) and folate are both required for DNA synthesis and repair, but humans can synthesize neither vitamin. Dietary deficiencies, impaired absorption, or inhibition with drugs (as seen in methotrexate therapy) of these vitamins can cause megaloblastic anemia (Chap. 41). Mild thrombocytopenia occurs in approximately 20 percent of patients with megaloblastic anemia resulting from vitamin B_{12} deficiency in the United States.[60] The frequency may be higher in patients with folic acid deficiency because of the high frequency of

TABLE 117–2. Inherited Thrombocytopenia

I. Congenital hypo-/amegakaryocytic thrombocytopenias

  A. Congenital amegakaryocytic thrombocytopenia (CAMT)

  B. Congenital hypo-/amegakaryocytic thrombocytopenia with skeletal abnormalities

    1. Thrombocytopenia with absent radii (TAR) syndrome

    2. Amegakaryocytic thrombocytopenia with radioulnar synostosis (ATRUS)

    3. Fanconi anemia

II. MYH9-related diseases

  A. Macrothrombocytopenia, Döhle-like inclusion bodies in leukocytes; nephritis ± hearing loss ± cataracts

III. Platelet granule deficiencies (storage pool disease)

  A. α-Granule defects

    1. Gray platelet syndrome

    2. Paris-Trousseau syndrome

    3. Quebec platelet syndrome

    4. Arthrogryposis–renal dysfunction–cholestasis (ARC) syndrome

  B. Dense granule defects:

    1. Hermansky-Pudlak syndrome

    2. Chédiak-Higashi syndrome

    3. Griscelli syndrome

  C. α- and dense granule defects

IV. Disorders of platelet surface receptors

  A. Glycoprotein (GP) Ib-IX-V defects

    1. Bernard-Soulier syndrome

    2. Platelet-type von Willebrand disease

    3. Velocardiofacial syndrome

  B. Integrin $\alpha_{IIb}\beta_{IIIa}$ defects: variant forms of Glanzmann thrombasthenia

V. Wiskott-Aldrich syndrome (WAS) protein-related disorders

  A. Classical Wiskott-Aldrich syndrome

  B. X-linked thrombocytopenia

  C. X-linked neutropenia

VI. GATA-1 mutations

  A. X-linked thrombocytopenia

  B. X-linked thrombocytopenia and thalassemia-like phenotype

  C. Congenital erythropoietic porphyria

VII. Ankyrine repeat domain (ANKRD)-26 mutations

  A. Moderate thrombocytopenia with mild bleeding tendency, dysmegakaryopoiesis, increased risk of myeloid malignancies

VIII. RUNX-1 mutations

  A. Familial platelet disorder with propensity to myeloid malignancy (FDP/AML)

IX. Miscellaneous

  A. Sitosterolemia

  B. Montreal platelet syndrome

  C. Others

concomitant alcohol abuse (Chap. 41). One large study of 139 patients examined the rates of cytopenias associated with megaloblastic anemia in India.[61] In this study, 76 percent had isolated vitamin B_{12} deficiency, 7 percent had isolated folate deficiency, 9 percent had a combined deficiency, and 8 percent had normal vitamin levels. All were anemic by definition, and 80 percent had thrombocytopenia with mild to moderate depression of the platelet count. More than half of those with thrombocytopenia were also neutropenic. The authors of this study suggested that the cytopenias tended to progress from isolated anemia, to anemia plus thrombocytopenia, to pancytopenia, with the degree of cytopenia related to the severity of vitamin deficiency. Occasionally, thrombocytopenia is severe in patients with megaloblastic anemia and, when accompanied by fever, hepatomegaly, and splenomegaly, and may suggest a diagnosis of acute leukemia. In these syndromes, the primary mechanism of thrombocytopenia is ineffective platelet production[62]; marrow megakaryocyte number usually is normal or increased. Abnormalities of megakaryocyte morphology are much less distinctive than the characteristic erythroid and myeloid defects, but often nuclear abnormalities are seen, with nuclei of larger size and dispersed nuclear segments, rather than single polyploid nuclei.[63] Thrombocytopenia may be seen in association with vitamin B_{12} deficiency when the latter results from autoantibodies against parietal cells or intrinsic factor and is associated with ITP.[64,65] Various other autoimmune disorders can coexist with pernicious anemia, including autoimmune vitiligo and autoimmune thyroiditis.[66] Abnormalities of platelet function are sometimes seen associated with vitamin B_{12} deficiency.[67,68] Diminished platelet aggregation and reduced release of ADP and ATP from granule stores in response to different agonists have been reported, and vitamin deficiency has been suggested to induce an acquired storage pool disease (Chap. 41).[68]

Copper deficiency is usually seen in patients who have undergone gastric bypass surgery, and may cause anemia, leukopenia, and thrombocytopenia associated with neurologic deficits resembling vitamin B_{12} deficiency. Patients with copper deficiency also may be misdiagnosed as having MDS, because increased ring sideroblasts and dysplastic precursor cells can be seen on marrow smears.[69,70]

Acute and chronic alcohol (ethanol) consumption affects hematopoiesis and blood cell survival both directly and indirectly. Alcohol is one of the leading causes of thrombocytopenia in Western countries. Acute ethanol intoxication in healthy volunteers induces thrombocytopenia.[71] Platelet counts in these cases are usually mildly decreased (generally more than 100×10^9/L); severe thrombocytopenia is quite rare. Acute ethanol-induced thrombocytopenia usually resolves within 5 to 21 days with cessation of ethanol ingestion, sometimes with a transient rebound thrombocytosis that may reach up to $1,000,000 \times 10^9$/L.[72] Although the mechanism of acute alcohol-related thrombocytopenia is not clear, it has been suggested that metabolites of ethanol, especially acetaldehyde, impair the late stages of platelet production and increase platelet destruction.[73] Thus, thrombocytopenia associated with acute alcohol ingestion would be expected to be more frequent in those with poor nutrition (delayed oxidation of acetaldehyde) and those with partial acetaldehyde dehydrogenase defiance. Thrombocytopenia induced by alcohol ingestion is accompanied by a decreased number of marrow megakaryocytes. Vacuolated proerythroblasts and granulocyte precursors are sometimes seen, as are multinuclear erythroblasts and megaloblasts.[74] Vacuolization of the periphery of mature megakaryocytes has been reported.[75] Alcoholism (chronic ethanol consumption, which is defined as consumption of more than 80 g of ethanol per day), on the other hand, may cause thrombocytopenia by other mechanisms, such as alcoholic liver cirrhosis (both splenomegaly and thrombopoietin deficiency), folic acid deficiency, and alcohol-induced marrow suppression.[74–78]

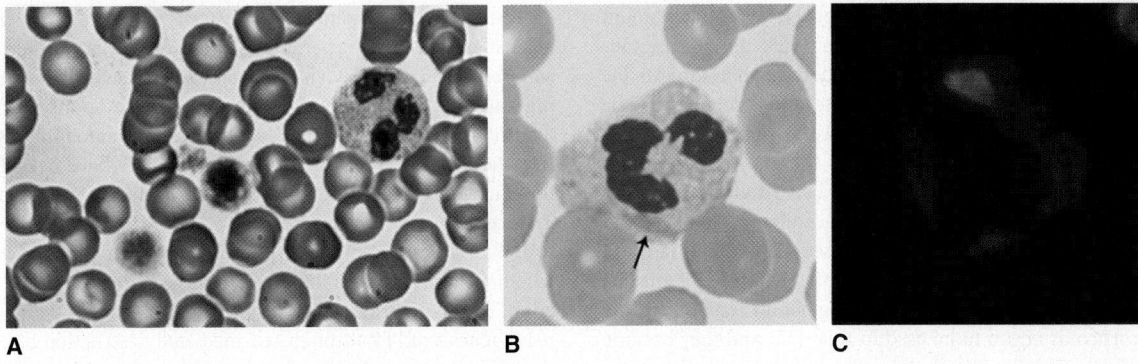

Figure 117–3. MYH9 abnormality. **A.** Blood film. May-Hegglin anomaly. Macrothrombocytes, thrombocytopenia, and light-blue cytoplasmic inclusions in neutrophils. Note two giant platelets approximately the diameter of red cells. The neutrophil has a large gray-blue inclusion in the cytoplasm at the 9 o'clock position. **B.** Blood film. Neutrophil of an individual with a mutation (E1841K) in exon 38 of the MYH9 gene. This mutation results in macrothrombocytopenia and Döhle-body–like inclusions in neutrophils *(arrow)*. **C.** Blood film. Immunofluorescent analysis with antibodies to the A heavy chain of nonmuscle myosin in the neutrophils of the same patient as in **(B)**. The fluorescent body in the neutrophil indicates that the inclusion contains precipitated nonmuscle myosin heavy chains, characteristic of this family of disorders. *(Reproduced with permission from Lichtman's Atlas of Hematology, www.accessmedicine.com. Images B and C kindly were provided for the Atlas by Dr. Shinji Kunishima, the Japanese Red Cross Aichi Blood Center, Nagoya, Japan.)*

ACQUIRED PURE AMEGAKARYOCYTIC THROMBOCYTOPENIA

Thrombocytopenia attributable to pure aplasia or hypoplasia of megakaryocytes is rare.[79] More common are instances in which amegakaryocytic thrombocytopenia anticipates the development of full-blown MDS or aplastic anemia and is associated with subtle abnormalities of other lineages, such as macrocytosis and dyserythropoiesis.[80–84] Most commonly the disorder is caused by autoimmune suppression of megakaryocyte development, either idiopathic,[85] associated with autoimmune disorders such as systemic lupus erythematosus (SLE)[86] and eosinophilic fasciitis, or associated with infections such as hepatitis C.[87] Antibodies against thrombopoietin (TPO)[88] have been described to cause the disorder, as have antibodies against the TPO receptor.[89] Patients may achieve durable remission with therapies designed to blunt the autoimmune response, such as cyclosporine or antithymocyte globulin (ATG).[90]

IMMUNE THROMBOCYTOPENIA

Table 117–3 summarizes the various types of ITP.

PRIMARY IMMUNE THROMBOCYTOPENIA

ITP, formerly known as autoimmune thrombocytopenic purpura, is the most common cause of isolated thrombocytopenia in clinical practice. ITP is characterized by immune-mediated platelet destruction and impaired platelet production. ITP occurs in every age group. Childhood ITP typically is acute in onset, often developing after a viral infection or vaccination. Although thrombocytopenia may be severe, it usually resolves spontaneously, within a few weeks up to 6 months.[91] In contrast to childhood ITP, adult ITP generally is a chronic disease of insidious onset and rarely resolves spontaneously.

"Purpura" was recognized by Hippocrates (c. 460 to c. 370 BC) and Galen (AD 129 to c. 200/c. 216) as a sign associated with fever. Chronic purpura was first described in details by Ibn-i Sina (Avicenna, c. 980 to c. 1037) in his famous book "The Canon of Medicine." In 1705, Werlof suggested that purpura was related to infections and described it as "morbus maculosus haemorrhagicus." Patients with purpura were

diagnosed as having "Werlof disease" for centuries. After the discovery of platelets and their role in hemostasis, the relationship between purpura and low-platelet count was understood.[92]

In 1915, Erich Frank renamed this disorder as "essential thrombocytopenia," and suggested that platelet production from megakaryocytes was impaired because of a toxic substance produced by the spleen.[93] Kaznelson, inspired by Frank's theory, proposed splenectomy for a patient with chronic thrombocytopenic purpura. The treatment was successful, and splenectomy was first-line therapy for ITP until the introduction of glucocorticoids in 1950s.

In the first issue of the journal *Blood* (in 1946) Damashek and Miller reviewed the megakaryocyte count and marrow morphology of patients with "idiopathic thrombocytopenic purpura."[94] They showed that most ITP patients had an increased number of megakaryocytes, but very few of them were producing platelets, so "actual platelet-producing tissue" might be decreased.[94]

TABLE 117–3. Immune-Mediated Thrombocytopenia

I. Auto-antibody-mediated thrombocytopenia
  A. Primary immune thrombocytopenia
  B. Secondary immune thrombocytopenia
    1. Antiphospholipid syndrome, systemic lupus erythematosus, and other connective tissue disorders
    2. Infections: HIV, hepatitis C virus, hepatitis B virus, *Helicobacter pylori*, and others
    3. Vaccination
    4. Drugs and chemical substances
    5. Malignancies including lymphoproliferative disorders
    6. Transplantation
    7. Common variable immune deficiency
II. Alloantibody-mediated thrombocytopenia/platelet destruction
  A. Fetal/neonatal alloimmune thrombocytopenia
  B. Posttransfusion purpura
  C. Platelet alloimmunization after platelet transfusions

Although Marino first showed that antiplatelet antibodies might cause thrombocytopenia in animal studies in 1905, the Harrington-Hollingsworth experiment (1951) was an important milestone in the understanding of autoantibody-directed platelet destruction in the pathophysiology of ITP. In this pioneering work, normal volunteers (including Harrington himself, who received the highest dose) were infused with the plasma from patients with ITP, resulting in severe thrombocytopenia in the recipients, and they postulated that ITP could be caused by antiplatelet antibodies.[95,96] Subsequently, Shulman and coworkers[97] showed that the thrombocytopenic effect of ITP plasma was dose-dependent and associated with the globulin fraction. In the 1950s, glucocorticoids began to be used to treat ITP, and they became first-line therapy for adults. Shortly thereafter other immunosuppressive agents were introduced for the treatment of chronic ITP.[92]

In the early 1970s, two groups showed that platelets from chronic ITP patients had elevated levels of platelet-associated immunoglobulin G (PAIgG).[98,99] In 1982, the first platelet target was identified: autoantibodies from patients with ITP failed to bind platelets deficient in the integrin $\alpha_{IIb}\beta_3$ complex (i.e., from patients with Glanzmann thrombasthenia).[100] In the late 1980s, two specific assays for the target antigens were described: the immunobead assay[101] and the monoclonal antibody-specific immobilization of platelet antigens (MAIPA) assay.[102] These assays showed that the majority of antiplatelet antibodies in patients with ITP are directed against integrin $\alpha_{IIb}\beta_{3(GPIIb-IIIa)}$ (approximately 80 percent), and the remainder are against the GPIb-IX-V complex and other platelet GPs such as GPIV and integrin $\alpha_2\beta_1$ (GPIa-IIa).[103,104] Some sera contain antibodies that recognize several antigens. Most antiplatelet autoantibodies are IgG; the remainder are IgM and IgA. Unfortunately, elevated levels of PAIgG later were found in patients with non-ITP. Therefore, PAIgG could not be used as a specific laboratory test for ITP in the same way that the direct antiglobulin test is used for the diagnosis of autoimmune hemolytic anemia.[105,106] To date there is still no specific laboratory test for ITP, the diagnosis of ITP being based on exclusion of other causes.

Antibody-coated platelets bind tissue macrophages through Fcγ receptors, leading to their destruction primarily in the spleen and, to a lesser extent, in the liver and marrow.[97,107,108] In 1981, Imbach reported successful treatment of pediatric ITP with intravenous immunoglobulin (IVIG) and suggested that the mechanism could involve blockade of macrophage Fc receptors. IVIG became first-line therapy in children, and now is also used in adults when a prompt increase is the platelet count is desired.[109]

Early studies of PAIgG reported that the antibodies in ITP were polyclonal.[110] However, later studies showed that at least some ITP patients had clonal B-cell proliferation, as determined by DNA analysis for immunoglobulin heavy- and light-chain rearrangements and by flow cytometry of B cells from blood and spleen for surface Ig light chains.[111,112] This led to the use in ITP of the chimeric anti-CD20 monoclonal antibody, rituximab, which was designed for the treatment of CD20-positive B-cell lymphomas. The rapid elimination of B cells with rituximab encouraged the use of this agent in the treatment of ITP.

Numerous abnormalities in cell-mediated immunity have been described in patients with ITP, including abnormalities in antigen-presenting cells, T lymphocytes, and cytokine release. Under normal conditions, antigen-presenting cells recognize and process foreign antigens and express the antigens on their surface in association with major histocompatibility complex (MHC) molecules. MHC–antigen complexes activate resting (naïve) CD4+ T cells to differentiate into a variety of phenotypes such as T-helper 1 (Th1) and T-helper 2 (Th2), Th17, and T-regulatory (Treg) cells. Th1 cells are involved in cell-mediated immunity and host defense against intracellular bacteria and protozoa. Th2 cells are involved in humoral immunity and host defense

against extracellular parasites. Th17 cells are involved in host defense against extracellular bacteria and fungi. Treg cells (formerly known as suppressor T cells) play an important role in self-tolerance by inhibiting autoimmune responses. Abnormal T-cell responses drive the differentiation of autoreactive B-cell clones and autoantibody secretion. In patients with ITP, both Th1 and Th17 cells have been found to be upregulated, whereas the number and the suppressor functions of the Treg cells were found to be decreased.[113–115] This imbalance is believed to induce an autoimmune responses against the platelets. It is unclear whether these abnormalities are causative or represent an epiphenomenon.[114,115] In addition, CD8+ cytotoxic T cells might be involved in the pathogenesis of ITP through cell-mediated destruction of platelets and megakaryocytes and through suppression of megakaryocytes, impairing platelet production.[115–117]

Antiplatelet autoantibodies may also activate platelet destruction by activating complement through the classical complement pathway. Increased platelet-associated C3, C4, and C9 have been demonstrated on the platelets from patients with ITP.[118,119] In vitro studies show that, in the presence of antiplatelet antibodies, C3 and C4 can bind platelets, increase the phagocytosis of the platelets by macrophages, and can cause their lysis by stimulating assembly of the membrane attack complex.[120,121]

Early studies demonstrated that platelet survival is shortened in ITP patients and returns to normal after splenectomy-induced remission.[122] Platelet transfusion only transiently increases a patient's platelet count, and the transfused platelets also have a shortened survival, reflecting the fact that the major problem in ITP is platelet destruction. However, later studies showed that platelet life span was not short enough to account for the observed thrombocytopenia on the basis of destruction alone, again suggesting a concomitant defect in platelet production.[123] Potential mechanisms for this observation were provided by later studies that autoantibodies against platelet surface GPs might interfere with the maturation of megakaryocytes, resulting in reduced platelet production, contributing to the severity of thrombocytopenia in some ITP patients.[124] Antibodies that target the GPIb-IX–V complex may induce thrombocytopenia by decreasing platelet production, as GPIb autoantibodies inhibit megakaryopoiesis in vitro,[124] and GPIb monoclonal antibodies inhibit proplatelet formation in vitro.[125]

In 1958, a hematopoietic growth factor regulating platelet production was proposed and named TPO by Kelemen.[126] Although interleukin (IL)-3, IL-6, IL-11, granulocyte-macrophage colony-stimulating factor, and c-KIT ligand increase megakaryocyte or platelet counts in vivo and in vitro, animal studies of these factors proved that they are not the main regulator of megakaryopoiesis.[127] In 1994, TPO was first characterized by five independent groups. TPO binds to its receptor MPL (formerly known as c-MPL), enhances megakaryocyte colony formation, and increases the size, number, and ploidy of megakaryocytes, and platelet production (Chap. 113).[128–130] TPO is synthesized in greatest quantity in the liver but is found in other organs (kidney, muscle, and marrow stromal cells).[128] TPO is also required to maintain the viability of hematopoietic stem cells.[131] The regulation of TPO production is complex. Hepatic production of TPO is both constitutive (in the steady state) and inducible (by inflammation), and the concentration of TPO to which megakaryocytes are exposed is also determined by the platelet concentration. Platelets, bearing TPO receptors, remove the hormone from the circulation, at least partially accounting for the inverse relationship between TPO and platelet levels. TPO levels are markedly elevated in patients with thrombocytopenia associated with megakaryocytic hypoplasia, including disorders such as aplastic anemia or acute leukemia. In most reports, ITP patients have normal or slightly elevated TPO levels whether measured in plasma or serum, but the levels are always lower than the concentrations found in thrombocytopenias resulting from megakaryocytic hypoplasia.[128–130,132,133] Initial studies with recombinant and pegylated TPO molecules showed successful responses in patients with thrombocytopenia, but development of auto-antibodies against these molecules restricted their use in clinical settings. Based on the success of creating erythropoietin receptor agonist peptides, a number of screening efforts were undertaken to design small peptides or organic molecules that might bind to the TPO receptor and stimulate thrombopoiesis. One such molecule contains four copies of a 14-amino-acid peptide grafted onto an Ig Fc domain, forming a "peptibody" termed romiplostim. This agent, which binds to a region of the TPO receptor that overlaps that bound by authentic TPO, was shown to increase platelet counts in patients with ITP who had failed other modalities,[134] and was approved by the FDA for this indication in 2008. Another small organic thrombopoietic molecule, eltrombopag, was developed almost simultaneously[135] and approved in 2008 by FDA for the same indications.[127] This agent activates TPO receptor signaling by binding to the transmembrane domain of the receptor, a site quite distinct from the binding site for TPO and romiplostim. Both TPO-receptor agonists are currently being evaluated for additional clinical indications in clinical trials.[136]

Some patients with ITP appear to display a genetic predisposition. ITP has been documented in monozygotic twins [137] and shown to be highly prevalent in some families.[138] In addition to contributing to the development of ITP, like in other autoimmune disorders heredity may also affect the response to ITP therapy. Human leukocyte antigen (HLA) class I and class II allele frequencies in patients with ITP have been studied by several investigators, with inconsistent results. Some investigators reported an increased frequency of HLA-Aw32, -DRw2, and -DRB1*0410.[108,139–141] Investigation has focused on genetic differences associated with dysregulation of immune tolerance and humoral immunity, but results have been inconclusive. For example, genetic polymorphisms of cytotoxic T-lymphocyte antigen (CTLA)-4, tumor necrosis factor, and Fcγ receptors IIA and IIIA have been suggested to influence the development of ITP and the response to therapy,[141–143] but as yet no strong association has been found.

Accumulating data indicate that the pathophysiology of ITP is more complex than previously thought, with ITP comprising a heterogenous group of disorders with different etiologies and responding to different treatment modalities. The identification of the different subsets of ITP patients will help to better define treatment options.

Definition and Classification

Although ITP has been recognized for centuries, there is as yet no consensus on either the definition or management of the disease. In 1996, the American Society of Hematology (ASH)[144] published practice guidelines for the diagnosis and management of ITP. In 2003, the British Committee for Standards in Haematology published its own guidelines.[145] In spite of these guidelines, the heterogeneity of the definitions and clinical criteria used in different studies has made it difficult to interpret the data regarding the incidence, pathogenesis, and treatment of ITP. In 2008, the International Working Group (IWG) proposed a standardization of terminology, definitions, and outcome criteria for ITP patients.[146] In 2010, an international consensus report on the investigation and management of ITP was published.[147] Shortly thereafter, in 2011, ASH updated its 1996 ITP guidelines.[148]

The IWG definition proposed use of the term "immune thrombocytopenia" instead of "idiopathic thrombocytopenic purpura" as the basis for the ITP acronym, because the immune nature of ITP is clear but most ITP patients do not have purpura. A platelet count of 100×10^9/L was proposed as the threshold level to entertain the diagnosis of ITP, because a sustained lower platelet count (100 to 150×10^9/L) can be seen in otherwise healthy individuals,[11,12] and long-term observation of these

indicate that 88 percent reach normal platelet counts or remain stable.[13] ITP is classified based on the absence or presence of other diseases as "primary" or "secondary." "Primary ITP" denotes the absence of any other identified pathology. All other autoimmune thrombocytopenias are classified as "secondary ITP" (see Table 117–3), and the associated primary disorder is indicated in parenthesis, for example "secondary ITP (SLE-associated)" or "secondary ITP (drug-induced)." Heparin-induced thrombocytopenia (HIT) or alloimmune thrombocytopenias are not classified as ITP, and maintain their standard classifications.[146]

The IWG described three phases of ITP: (1) newly diagnosed ITP (within 3 months of diagnosis); (2) persistent ITP (patients who do not achieve a stable remission between 3 and 12 months after diagnosis); and (3) chronic ITP (continuing for more than 12 months). ITP was formerly classified as mild, moderate, and severe depending on the platelet counts. However, the degree of thrombocytopenia does not always correlate with bleeding. The IWG proposed that the term "severe ITP" only be used for patients with clinically significant bleeding requiring additional therapy regardless of platelet count.[146]

One of the major problems with comparing ITP studies had been the definition of response to therapy. The IWG proposed the following terms and criteria for response to ITP treatment: "complete response, CR" (platelet count exceeding 100×10^9/L and no bleeding symptoms), "response, R" (platelet count higher than 30×10^9/L or at least a twofold increase from the baseline count and no bleeding symptoms), "no response, NR" (platelet count below 30×10^9/L or less than a twofold increase from the baseline count, or presence of bleeding symptoms). "Duration of response" is measured from the time between first measured CR or R to relapse. "Corticosteroid dependence" is defined as the need for ongoing or repeated glucocorticoid use for at least 2 months to maintain CR or R. Patients who relapsed after splenectomy (failure to maintain CR or R) and required therapy are classified as "refractory ITP." "On-demand therapy" is a term used for therapies employed to temporarily increase the platelet count in special situations such as trauma or surgery. "Adjunctive therapies" are treatments that are not designed to increase platelet counts, but that may decrease bleeding symptoms by other means, for example, treatment with oral contraceptives or antifibrinolytic drugs.[146]

Incidence

ITP is relatively common, but demographic studies have yielded a wide range of incidence rates largely because of differences in the age and gender distribution of the populations studied and differences in cut-off platelet counts used to define the disease. ITP can affect males and females of any age. In one detailed study, the reported incidence of ITP was 3.9 per 100,000 per year. Although the overall incidence was higher in women than in men, a male predominance was seen in patients younger than 18 years of age and older than 65 years of age.[149]

Clinical Features

ITP is of acute onset in children, often developing after vaccination or after a viral illness, and resolves spontaneously in 90 percent of cases. In adults, however, ITP usually is a chronic disease. Table 117–4 highlights the differences in ITP in children and adults. Approximately 25 percent of adult ITP patients are diagnosed incidentally on routine complete blood counts. Symptoms and signs of ITP depend not only on the platelet count, but also on the nature of coexisting conditions that can increase the tendency to bleed, such as uremia, trauma, and ingestion of drugs that affect platelet function (Table 117–5). Approximately one-third of patients have platelet counts greater than 30×10^9/L at diagnosis and no significant bleeding.[150] Common bleeding signs include purpura (ecchymoses and petechiae), epistaxis, menorrhagia, and gingival bleeding. Hematuria, hemoptysis, and gastrointestinal bleeding

TABLE 117–4. Clinical Features of Idiopathic Thrombocytopenic Purpura in Children and Adults

	Children	Adults
Occurrence		
Peak age (years)	2–4	15–40
Sex (Female-to-Male)	Equal	1.2–1.7
Presentation		
Onset	Acute (most with symptoms lasting <1 week)	Insidious (most with symptoms lasting >2 months)
Symptoms	Purpura (<10% with severe bleeding)	Purpura (typically bleeding not severe)
Platelet count	Most cases <20,000/μL	Most cases <20,000/μL
Course		
Spontaneous remission	83%	2%
Chronic disease	24%	43%
Response to splenectomy	71%	66%
Eventual complete recovery	89%	64%
Morbidity and mortality		
Cerebral hemorrhage	<1%	3%
Hemorrhagic death	<1%	4%
Mortality of chronic refractory disease	2%	5%

are less common. Intracerebral hemorrhage is rare and generally occurs in patients with platelet counts less than 10×10^9/L and usually is associated with trauma or vascular lesions. The incidence of life-threatening complications is highest in patients older than age 60 years.[150–154] The majority of ITP patients have a good prognosis, the mortality rate being only slightly higher than that of the general population. However, ITP

TABLE 117–5. Situations That Increase the Bleeding Risk in Immune Thrombocytopenia Patients

Drugs: Anticoagulants, antiplatelet drugs, nonsteroidal antiinflammatory drugs, chemotherapy

Gastrointestinal pathologies that may cause bleeding (e.g., active peptic ulcer, inflammatory bowel disease)

Miscellaneous disorders that disturb hemostasis (e.g., congenital bleeding disorders, hepatic cirrhosis, uremia)

Older age (>60 years)

Nutritional factors such as herbal teas, kinin, and tonic water

Previous history of bleeding

Sport and occupational activities that increase bleeding risk

Trauma, surgery, and childbirth

Uncontrolled hypertension

patients who present with severe thrombocytopenia ($<30 \times 10^9$/L) and do not respond to any therapy within 2 years, have a fourfold increased risk of death compared to the general population.[155]

The purpuric lesions seen in ITP are not palpable, do not blanch with pressure, and often develop on distal regions of the extremities and on skin areas exposed to pressure (e.g., around tight belts and stockings and at tourniquet sites). Hemorrhagic bullae, which may develop in the buccal mucosa, generally reflect acute, severe thrombocytopenia. Bleeding after surgery, trauma, or tooth extraction is common.

Besides the physical findings associated with platelet-type bleeding, the history and physical examination are usually unremarkable, except for the possibility of similar symptoms in other family members. Family history is especially important to discriminate familial thrombocytopenic syndromes from ITP. The spleen usually is not enlarged but may be palpable in some patients, a finding considered to occur with the same incidence as in normal adults.[156] Constitutional symptoms, such as fever, significant weight loss, marked splenomegaly, hepatomegaly, and lymphadenopathy provide evidence that the thrombocytopenia has another cause. The presence of skeletal, cardiac, renal abnormalities, hearing loss, albinism. or immune deficiencies in patients with thrombocytopenia should trigger suspicion of IPDs.

Fatigue is one of the common, but often neglected, complaints of patients with primary ITP. In a survey including UK and U.S. ITP cohorts, the prevalence of fatigue was found to be significantly higher in adult primary ITP patients (39 percent and 22 percent for the UK and U.S. cohorts, respectively) compared with healthy controls.[157] Fatigue has also been described in 20 percent of pediatric patients with ITP; fatigue resolved with the elevation of platelet counts.[158] Although glucocorticoids and immunosuppressive agents may induce fatigue, fatigue can occur in untreated ITP patients. The mechanism of fatigue in patients with ITP is unknown.

Patients with ITP are at slightly increased risk of venous and arterial thrombosis.[159] A recent retrospective study evaluating 986 patients with ITP showed the cumulative incidences of venous and arterial thrombosis to be 1.4 percent and 3.2 percent, respectively. This study found that increased thrombotic risk was associated with splenectomy, older age (>60 years), with the presence of more than two thrombotic risk factors at the time of diagnosis, and with glucocorticoid therapy.[160]

Laboratory Features

In ITP patients the blood film usually demonstrates isolated thrombocytopenia without erythrocyte or leukocyte abnormalities. Platelet anisocytosis is a common finding. Mean platelet volume and platelet distribution width are increased. Platelets may be abnormally large or abnormally small. The former reflect accelerated platelet production,[161] and the latter represent platelet fragments associated with platelet destruction.[162] The observation of giant platelets should trigger consideration of IPDs, which often are misdiagnosed as ITP.[163] The bleeding time correlates inversely with platelet count if the count is less than 50×10^9/L, but may be normal in patients with mild or moderate thrombocytopenia,[164] making it an unreliable test for use in such patients. The ultrastructure of ITP platelets viewed by electron microscopy is similar to that of normal platelets.[165]

Hemoglobin concentration and hematocrit are generally normal in patients with ITP. Anemia that is not easily explained (e.g., resulting from iron deficiency in bleeding patients or associated with thalassemia minor in endemic areas) must be investigated further. Autoimmune hemolytic anemia with a positive direct antiglobulin (Coombs) test and reticulocytosis may accompany ITP; this association is termed *Evans syndrome*.[166] Neither erythrocyte poikilocytosis nor schistocytes should be present. Total leukocyte counts and differential are generally normal.

Although atypical lymphocytes and eosinophilia may occur in children with ITP, leukocytosis and leukopenia with immature cells are not consistent with the diagnosis.

Marrow examination, which is not always required to make a diagnosis of ITP in adults, generally reveals a normal or increased number of megakaryocytes of normal morphology, although a decreased number of megakaryocytes does not rule out ITP. Erythropoiesis and myelopoiesis are normal. The international consensus report states that a marrow examination should usually be reserved for patients older than age 60 years, for those with systemic symptoms or other signs, and for those for whom splenectomy is contemplated. Biopsy for morphologic examination should be carried out, along with aspirate for flow cytometric and cytogenetic analysis.[147] The ASH 2011 guidelines, however, conclude that a marrow examination is unnecessary when the presentation is typical, even if the patients are older or being considered for splenectomy.[148]

In ITP patients, initial workup should be targeted to exclude secondary causes of thrombocytopenia (see Table 117–3). Testing for viral etiology (hepatitis C virus [HCV], HIV, and in endemic areas hepatitis B virus [HBV]) and *Helicobacter pylori* is also recommended.[147,148] Quantitative immunoglobulin assessment should be considered for pediatric cases to rule out common variable immunodeficiency (CVID).[147] Mild thrombocytopenia has been reported in patients with hypo- or hyperthyroidism, which returns to normal after appropriate therapy. Thyroid-stimulating hormone (TSH) and antithyroid antibodies may help to evaluate thyroid status in those patients.[147] Other tests to consider include blood group analysis and a pregnancy test for female patients of childbearing age, antiphospholipid antibodies, antinuclear antibody (ANA), viral polymerase chain reaction (PCR) for parvovirus, and cytomegalovirus (CMV). The results of these tests can change the treatment strategy.[147] On the other hand, the ASH 2011 guidelines do not recommend routine testing for antiphospholipid antibodies and ANAs in the initial workup of ITP,[148] unless signs or symptoms of an autoimmune disorder are present in the patient. Other tests, such as TPO levels, reticulated platelets, PAIgG, platelet survival studies, bleeding time, and serum complement levels are not recommended for the diagnosis and management of ITP patients in either of these guidelines.[147,148]

Therapy and Course

What little is known of the natural course of moderate or severe ITP derives from before the glucocorticoid era, and suggests that left untreated, ITP in adults typically is a chronic disease, in contrast to ITP in children. In adults, the rate of spontaneous remission is reported as 9 percent,[167] and can occur even after 3 years in patients who present with severe thrombocytopenia.[168] Although ITP is a benign disease, side effects of the therapies can cause serious morbidity and even mortality. Treatment for patients with ITP should be based on bleeding signs and symptoms and on the presence of factors that increase the bleeding risk (see Table 117–5). Possible side effects of the drugs and other treatments used in ITP should always be considered.

Initial Management

Observation Because a significant portion of ITP patients are diagnosed incidentally in routine evaluation, signs and symptoms of bleeding are important in determining whether any treatment is required. The primary therapeutic goal is not simply to increase the platelet count, but to reach a safe platelet count where the risk of bleeding is minimal. Patients with no bleeding and consistent platelet counts in excess of 30×10^9/L do not require treatment and can be observed periodically. These patients are at low risk for clinically important bleeding. Simple observation is not recommended for patients with platelet counts lower

than 10×10^9/L, in those with platelet counts between 10 and 30×10^9/L and significant mucosal bleeding, or in those with risk factors for bleeding (see Table 117–5).[169] The presence of extensive purpura or hemorrhagic bullae in mucosal tissues (wet purpura) should be regarded as a harbinger of life-threatening bleeding and treated as such. Because ITP patients often have large platelets that may not be recognized by automated cell counters, a blood film should be evaluated before starting therapy in ITP patients with very-low platelet counts who are not bleeding. Identification of secondary ITP cases is very important, and management of these patients should include treatment of the underlying pathology, if possible.

Emergency Treatment of Acute Bleeding Resulting from Severe Thrombocytopenia Bleeding symptoms generally are not severe in adult patients with ITP, even with very-low platelet counts. However, life-threatening bleeding can occur, especially after trauma. Emergency treatment should be instituted in patients with intracranial or gastrointestinal bleeding, massive hematuria or internal hematoma, or those in need of emergency surgical intervention or about to go into labor. Patients who experience significant bleeding should be hospitalized and monitored closely. Recommended treatment includes IVIG and parenteral glucocorticoids in combination. IVIG is given as 1 g/kg per day for 2 days, and high-dose parenteral glucocorticoid therapy includes high-dose prednisone or methylprednisolone (1 g/day for 1 to 3 days). In most patients, IVIG increases the platelet count within 2 to 3 days.[147,148] Although platelet transfusions may not increase the platelet counts because the transfused platelets are destroyed rapidly, they nevertheless may contribute to the formation of platelet plugs at sites of bleeding and improve hemostasis. Platelet transfusion following IVIG infusion may increase the platelet count because IVIG may improve platelet survival.[147,148,170] Aminocaproic acid, which inhibits fibrinolysis, can be used to reduce bleeding[170] and is safe except in the presence of hematuria, in which case it can cause thrombi of the glomeruli, renal pelves, and ureters. This agent does not affect platelet count or function. Aminocaproic acid is usually administered intravenously (initial dose 0.1 g/kg over 30 minutes, then given either by continuous infusion at 0.5 to 1.0 g/h or as an equivalent intermittent dose every 2 to 4 hours). Aminocaproic acid also can be administered orally in a similar dose in emergency situations because it is absorbed very rapidly from the gastrointestinal tract.[147,148] Vincristine can be used in combination with glucocorticoids and IVIG in older patients.[108] Other hemostatic therapies, such as recombinant factor VIIa and fibrinogen infusions, have been reported to be effective in some ITP patients with life-threatening bleeding, but the risk-to-benefit ratio needs to be evaluated in controlled studies.[171,172] Emergency splenectomy has been reported to be successful in refractory ITP with bleeding, but reports of its use in this situation are rare.[173] Because of this, this therapy should only be considered in the most dire circumstances. Although there are some case reports describing successful results with plasmapheresis, this treatment is not recommended in current ITP guidelines.[147,148]

Glucocorticoid Therapy Glucocorticoids are accepted as the standard therapy for initial treatment in adult patients with ITP.[147,148] Glucocorticoids increase the platelet count in several ways, including by inhibiting phagocytosis of antibody-coated platelets by macrophages, decreasing autoantibody production, and improving marrow platelet production.[174,175] These agents also appear to reduce capillary leakage, thereby decreasing blood loss.[176] The major drawback of glucocorticoid therapy is that often the adverse effects of the treatment are worse than the disease itself. Important side effects, which can be severe, include facial swelling (chipmunk or moon facies), weight gain, folliculitis, hyperglycemia, hypertension, cataracts, osteoporosis, aseptic bone necrosis, opportunistic infections, and behavioral disturbances.[177,178]

Still under investigation is which glucocorticoid and dosing regimen is best for raising the platelet count. Prednisolone, dexamethasone and methylprednisolone are all used. Generally, oral prednisone 1 to 2 mg/kg per day (or methylprednisolone at equivalent doses) is preferred as first-line therapy.[147,148] Patients usually respond to prednisone therapy within 3 weeks. In approximately two-thirds of patients, platelet counts increase to greater than 50×10^9/L within 1 week, but decrease again when the prednisone dose is decreased.[152,177] Although no consensus exists regarding the duration of initial therapy, treatment should continue until platelet counts reach a safe range. In patients who respond, the recommendation is to continue glucocorticoid therapy 1 mg/kg per day for a total of 3 weeks before initiating a slow tapering of doses.[148] Sustained remission rates with glucocorticoid therapy are variable, reported rates ranging from 5 to 50 percent.[108,155,177] If the patient does not respond to 3 weeks of prednisone therapy, other therapeutic options should be considered.

In addition to the standard 1 to 2 mg/kg per day dose of prednisone, lower[179,180] and higher doses[181-184] of prednisone, dexamethasone, and methylprednisolone have been investigated, with good results. The major aim of the high-dose glucocorticoid regimes is to reduce duration of therapy, and therefore reduce the side effects of the glucocorticoids. Studies with dexamethasone 40 mg/day for 4 consecutive days for one course, or with the same dose for four courses given every 2 weeks have been reported to produce responses in 50 percent and 89.2 percent of newly diagnosed ITP patients, respectively.[185,186] High-dose methylprednisolone therapy has also been shown to be effective, with an 80 percent response rate.[187] Despite the favorable results of these studies, high-dose glucocorticoid regimens as first-line therapy still have not been validated with randomized controlled trials. ASH 2011 guidelines recommend longer courses of standard doses of glucocorticoids (prednisone 1 to 2 mg/kg per day) as a first-line treatment of ITP.[148]

Splenectomy Splenectomy was demonstrated to be an effective treatment for patients with ITP a century ago[188] and after the glucocorticoid era, it has been used for decades as a standard second-line therapy. The spleen is the major site both for synthesis of antiplatelet antibodies and for destruction of antibody-coated platelets. Splenectomy will decrease antibody production and platelet destruction, and will be effective in patients in whom antibody-mediated platelet destruction rather than platelet production is the major cause of thrombocytopenia. Although splenectomy has been reported to be less preferred in recent ITP cohorts because of the emergence of new therapies such as TPO receptor agonists and rituximab,[189] splenectomy still produces the highest cure rates for ITP patients compared to all other therapies. Approximately 85 percent of patients with persistent or chronic ITP respond well to splenectomy, and 60 to 66 percent of the patients remain in remission after 5 years.[189-191] These high cure rates makes splenectomy an important therapeutic option in the treatment of chronic ITP. The duration of the disease prior to splenectomy does not affect the outcome of the procedure, as it can be effective even years after ITP is diagnosed.[192,193] Splenectomy can be performed during pregnancy (preferably during the second trimester), and does not affect the response rates to other treatments except anti-D therapy in chronic ITP patients. Also, the cost of splenectomy is lower than that of newer treatments such as rituximab and TPO-receptor agonists.[191]

On the other hand, splenectomy is an invasive procedure, causes the permanent loss of an organ, and increases the risk of serious bacterial infection, bleeding and thrombosis. Because ITP can remit spontaneously, splenectomy should be postponed at least 6 to 12 months after diagnosis if possible.[147,148] Splenectomy is not recommended in patients with CVID, with chronic infections such as chronic hepatitis and HIV, or with known thrombophilia.

No validated clinical or laboratory tests exist that can predict whether splenectomy will be effective in elevating platelet counts in ITP patients. Although it has been suggested that ITP patients with predominant splenic sequestration (as determined by radioisotope techniques) have better response rates than patients with predominantly nonsplenic sequestration, these data have not been validated in other studies[189] and the required radioisotope techniques are not widely available.

Over the past decade minimally invasive laparoscopic splenectomy has gained preference over open splenectomy. Modern laparoscopic approaches reduce mortality rates (<1 percent), even in patients with severe thrombocytopenia.[194] The mortality rate increases in older patients, in patients with severe thrombocytopenia, and in the presence of coexisting illnesses.[177,195] Postsplenectomy sepsis is a major cause of morbidity and mortality in ITP. Extended steroid or other immunosuppressive therapy preceding splenectomy may increase the risk of perioperative infection. To minimize the risk of sepsis, patients should be immunized at least 2 weeks before splenectomy with polyvalent pneumococcal vaccine, *Haemophilus influenzae* type B vaccine, and quadrivalent meningococcal polysaccharide vaccine.[196] Interestingly, newer studies of ITP patients undergoing splenectomy show enteric organisms to be responsible for most of the cases of postsplenectomy sepsis, probably because of the widespread vaccination of ITP patients.[191] Splenectomized patients should be informed to be alert for the symptoms and signs of infection and be prepared for an emergency situation. Any fever should be carefully evaluated, and the patient treated with broad-spectrum antibiotics.

Splenectomy also increases the risk of thrombosis in ITP patients. In a large cohort of 9976 ITP patients, in whom 1762 underwent splenectomy; the cumulative incidences of abdominal venous thromboembolism and deep vein thrombosis/pulmonary embolism were increased in splenectomized patients compared to nonsplenectomized patients (1.6 percent vs. 1 percent for abdominal venous thrombosis, 4.3 percent vs. 1.7 percent for deep vein thrombosis–pulmonary embolism, respectively).[197] Several mechanisms may contribute to this enhanced risk for thrombosis, including postsplenectomy thrombocytosis and a failure to clear platelets, other cells and microparticles that express the procoagulant lipid phosphatidylserine. Perioperative measures such as antiembolic stockings and anticoagulant prophylaxis should be considered in those cases.

Both the time required to reach a normal platelet count and the magnitude of platelet recovery are accepted as useful predictors of the long-term efficacy of splenectomy. In most cases, platelet counts recover within 10 days. Patients who attain a normal platelet count within 3 days of splenectomy generally have a good long-term response.[198] In patients refractory to splenectomy, the presence of accessory splenic tissue should be suspected, particularly if the blood film shows no evidence of splenectomy (i.e., pitting and Howell-Jolly bodies are absent in the erythrocytes; Chap. 55). Such patients should be screened with sensitive radionuclide or magnetic resonance scans to identify residual or accessory splenic tissue.

Intravenous Immunoglobulin IVIG was first shown to be effective in childhood ITP in 1981,[109] then later in adult patients.[199] IVIG rapidly increases the platelet count in more than 75 percent of patients with chronic ITP and normalizes the platelet count in approximately 50 percent of the patients.[177,178] The effect of IVIG is similar whether or not the patient has undergone splenectomy and is transient, generally lasting only 3 to 4 weeks. Postulated mechanisms for the action of IVIG include blockade of macrophage Fc receptors, which slows clearance of antibody-coated platelets, antiidiotype neutralization of antiplatelet autoantibodies, cytokine modulation, immunomodulation (increased suppressor T-cell function and decreased autoantibody production), complement neutralization, and dendritic cell priming.[178,200,201] The recommended total dose of IVIG is 2 g/kg administered either as 0.4 g/kg per day on 5 consecutive days or as 1 g/kg per day on 2 consecutive days. If the need to increase the platelet count is urgent, the preferred dosing is 1 g/kg per day for 2 days combined with glucocorticoids.[148] For maintenance therapy, 0.5 to 1.0 g/kg as a single dose may be used, administered every 3 to 4 weeks, or as needed. Although the annual total world consumption of IVIG exceeds 100 tons, the cost of IVIG is still high, and this also limits the use of IVIG in adults.[202] Adverse effects of IVIG therapy include headache, backache, nausea, fever, aseptic meningitis, alloimmune hemolysis, hepatitis, renal failure, pulmonary insufficiency, and thrombosis. Anaphylactic reactions may occur in patients with congenital IgA deficiency.[177] The patient may become refractory to the effect with repeated infusions of IVIG.[203] IVIG is used as a first-line therapy in childhood ITP, because the thrombocytopenia is usually transient. In adult ITP, however, IVIG is usually reserved for patients with life-threatening bleeding, when a prompt increase in platelet count is needed,[147,148] or as first-line therapy when glucocorticoids are contraindicated.[148]

Anti-(Rh)D Anti-(Rh)D is a polyclonal γ-globulin containing high titers of antibodies against the $Rh_o(D)$ antigen of erythrocytes. It is administered intravenously for treatment of ITP. Anti-(Rh)D binds Rh-positive erythrocytes and leads to their destruction in the spleen. Because splenic Fc receptors are blocked, more antibody-coated platelets survive in the circulation.[204,205] Anti-(Rh)D also can also modulate Fcγ receptor expression and regulate the production of various cytokines, including IL-6, IL-10, and tumor necrosis factor-α.[206] A positive direct antiglobulin test, a decrease in serum haptoglobin levels, and mild and transient hemolysis occur in all Rh-positive patients after anti-(Rh)D infusion, generally without requiring a blood transfusion.[205] The rate of serious hemolytic reactions has been estimated as one in 1115 patients; any reaction occurs within 4 hours of administration in almost all cases.[207] Anti-(Rh)D therapy is not effective in patients who have undergone splenectomy or in Rh-negative patients, and is not recommended in patients with a positive direct antiglobulin test.[148]

It is recommended that anti-(Rh)D be given as a single dose of 50 to 100 mcg/kg by intravenous infusion over 3 to 5 minutes.[204,208,209] Adverse effects of anti-(Rh)D therapy resemble those observed with both γ-globulin infusion and autoimmune hemolytic anemia; symptoms include headache, asthenia, chills, fever, abdominal pain, diarrhea, vomiting, dizziness, and myalgia. Patients can experience immediate anaphylactic reactions and both type I (IgE-mediated) and type III (immune complex–mediated) hypersensitivity reactions.[204,205,208,210,211] Although anti-(Rh)D reportedly increases platelet counts within 1 week in more than 70 percent of patients who are Rh-positive and have their spleen,[212] and may obviate the need for splenectomy,[211] a randomized, controlled trial comparing anti-(Rh)D with conventional therapy showed no differences in the rates of spontaneous remission or the need for splenectomy.[209] Anti-(Rh)D is listed in current ASH ITP guidelines as a first-line agent when glucocorticoids are contraindicated.[148] Anti-(Rh)D is currently not available in Europe.

Rituximab B lymphocytes play many roles in the pathophysiology of ITP, including producing antibodies, presenting antigens, and regulating the functions of T cells and dendritic cells. B cells are targeted therapeutically with rituximab, a chimeric monoclonal antibody against CD20, which binds B cells and causes Fc-mediated lysis, thereby depleting these cells from blood, lymph nodes, and marrow. Rituximab rapidly depletes B cells in patients with autoimmune diseases, with the effect usually lasting 6 to 12 months.[114,213–217]

The optimal dosing regimen and duration of therapy have not been determined for patients with ITP. Usual rituximab doses are in the range of 100 to 375 mg/m². Most studies have used weekly infusion for 4 consecutive weeks at, the dose used to treat B-cell lymphoma (375 mg/m²). Studies with low-dose rituximab (100 mg weekly for 4 weeks) showed similar activity to the standard dose.[218] Published studies with rituximab, however, have generally not been controlled and are extremely heterogeneous in terms of rituximab dosing and response criteria. Approximately 40 to 60 percent of the ITP patients demonstrate a response to rituximab at 1 year, and 20 to 25 percent of those have a long-term response (at 5 years).[215,219] Splenectomy does not affect response rates to rituximab therapy.[135,216] In ITP patients who have relapsed more than 1 year after rituximab therapy, retreatment with the drug will induce similar responses in 75 percent of patients who responded initially.[220] In spite of the apparent benefit of rituximab, its use is still considered "off-label" for ITP.

Different patterns of response have been reported in ITP patients treated with rituximab. Although the majority of patients responded within 4 to 6 weeks (early responders), response was delayed for several months in some patients (late responders). In ITP patients who responded to rituximab, the increase in platelet count was associated with reduction in the quantity of platelet-associated autoantibodies. Rituximab also indirectly affects T cells, as depletion of autoreactive B cells prevents T-cell activation. Interestingly, despite the depletion of peripheral B cells, platelet-associated autoantibodies were still found in the plasma of ITP patients who do not respond to rituximab.[221] A study analyzing the spleens of ITP patients who did not respond to rituximab therapy demonstrated the presence in the spleen of long-lived plasma cells that produced antiplatelet antibodies for as long as 6 months after rituximab therapy ended. However, this class of cells was not found in the spleens of patients who had not received rituximab. The authors of this study suggested that depletion of peripheral B cells by rituximab promotes the differentiation of long-lived plasma cells in the spleen of ITP patients, which might be responsible for the persistence of antiplatelet antibodies.[222]

In a meta-analysis of 306 ITP patients treated with rituximab, adverse reactions were reported as mild-to-moderate in 66 patients (21.6 percent) and life-threatening in 10 patients (3.7 percent); nine patients (2.9 percent) died.[215] Although some of these deaths were attributed to ITP-related complications and not to rituximab itself, this mortality rate is higher than expected. Infusion-related reactions in rituximab therapy can be severe, and rarely fatal. Premedication with methylprednisolone is recommend to avoid these reactions.[219] The risk of infection can increase as a result of depletion of B cells, decreased antibody production, and, rarely, neutropenia.[219] Treatment can also reactivate latent viruses, especially hepatitis B. Alteration of T- and B-cell populations, and decreased antibody titers against HBV may stimulate HBV replication, and rarely cause fatal fulminant hepatitis. All patients should be screened for HBV before rituximab therapy.[223] Although preventive lamivudine or entecavir can be used in HBV-positive ITP patients, it is instead recommended that alternative therapies be used.[219] Other viral reactivation syndromes are less common; progressive multifocal leukoencephalopathy (caused by reactivation of polyomavirus JC) is extremely rare.

Thrombopoietin Receptor Agonists The observation that platelet production in patients with ITP is impaired, the massive megakaryopoiesis seen in the marrow of mice and humans treated with recombinant TPO (far greater than seen in patients with ITP), and the unexpectedly normal or only modestly elevated TPO levels in patients with ITP suggested the potential benefit of megakaryocyte-stimulation therapy in patients with refractory ITP. Early use of an altered form of a recombinant TPO molecule to stimulate platelet production in normal platelet donors was halted because of its stimulation of autoantibodies that cleared endogenous TPO. Because of this untoward effect, the use of recombinant TPO was abandoned, and a search for molecules that might bind to and stimulate the TPO receptor ensued. Since then, the TPO receptor agonists romiplostim and eltrombopag have been clinically shown to stimulate platelet production.[224,225]

Romiplostim This drug is a peptibody that carries four copies of a 14-amino-acid TPO-receptor–binding peptide fused to an immunoglobulin scaffold, and binds to the TPO-binding site of the TPO receptor with high affinity. The TPO receptor agonist induces megakaryocyte proliferation and differentiation by activating Janus-type tyrosine kinase (JAK)–signal transducer and activator of transcription (STAT) and mitogen-activated protein (MAP) kinase pathways.[224] The insertion of dimeric peptide into the IgG_1 heavy chain increases the half-life of the molecule.[225] Romiplostim has no homology with endogenous TPO, thus the risk of the development of antibodies against TPO is very low. Romiplostim and TPO may also increase platelet responses to agonists. Weekly subcutaneous injection of romiplostim at doses of 1 to 3 mcg/kg produced a dose-dependent increase in the platelet count, starting from day 5, with peak platelet levels reached by days 12 to 15, and platelet counts returning to baseline by day 28.[131,135,224] Therapy for ITP is usually initiated at a dose of 1 mcg/kg per week, and the dose is then increased by 1 mcg/kg to a maximum of 10 mcg/kg until the patient reaches target platelet counts ($>50 \times 10^9$/L). Higher starting doses up to the maximum dose can be used in emergency situations. If the platelet count does not increase to safe levels after 4 weeks of romiplostim treatment at the maximum dose, the drug should be discontinued. Because platelet responses are highly variable, patients should be evaluated periodically, and the dose adjusted based on the platelet counts. Although discontinuation of romiplostim is recommended when the platelet count exceeds 400×10^9/L, it should be kept in mind that platelet counts can drop to extremely low levels. Close monitoring of the platelet counts is therefore crucial. Romiplostim can be used in patients with hepatic or renal insufficiency, but is not recommended in pregnant patients because it can cross the placenta. Two parallel placebo-controlled trials examined response rates to romiplostim in both splenectomized and nonsplenectomized patients treated for 24 weeks.[134] Durable platelet responses and overall platelet responses were achieved by 38 percent and 79 percent of splenectomized patients, and by 61 percent and 88 percent of nonsplenectomized patients who were given the drug. A newer study evaluating long-term (up to 5 years) results of romiplostim therapy showed that a platelet count of greater than 50×10^9/L was achieved at least once by 95 percent of treated ITP patients.[226]

Eltrombopag This agent is a small (442 Da) nonpeptide molecule that binds to the transmembrane domain of the TPO receptor and triggers megakaryocyte growth and differentiation, increasing platelet production. Eltrombopag has some distinctive features compared to recombinant human thrombopoietin (rhTPO) and romiplostim: Eltrombopag does not compete with TPO binding, and while it induces the phosphorylation of STAT proteins, it does not affect the AKT pathway.[227] Eltrombopag has no effect on platelet activation in response to agonists.[225] In healthy volunteers, daily doses given for 10 days elevated platelet counts beginning at 8 days and peaking at 16 days. Eltrombopag is used orally at daily doses of 25 to 75 mg, and should be given 2 hours before or after meals because food can affect its absorption. Ethnic differences in eltrombopag pharmacokinetics have been described. Lower initial doses and slower titration is preferred in East Asian patients.[228] Divalent cations such as calcium interfere with absorption of the drug, so it should not be taken with dairy products or antacids. Eltrombopag can also interfere with the uptake and metabolism of statins, increasing

their plasma concentrations. Eltrombopag is metabolized in the liver, and causes liver function abnormalities in approximately 13 percent of patients administered the drug. Reduced initial doses are recommended in patients with liver disease.[225] Eltrombopag increases platelet counts (50×10^9/L) in 80 percent of splenectomized and 88 percent of nonsplenectomized chronic ITP patients.[229] A newer study evaluated repeated short-term doses of eltrombopag (50 mg daily for up to 6 weeks followed by up to 4 weeks off therapy over three cycles) and suggested that eltrombopag can be used as on-demand therapy and repeated courses would be effective and safe.[230]

Newer Thrombopoietin Receptor Agonists Other congeners are currently being evaluated. An oral, nonpeptide TPO-receptor agonist, avatrombopag, binds to the transmembrane domain of TPO receptor, and increases platelet counts. Lack of significant food interaction is an important feature of this new drug.[136] Its use is pending FDA approval.

Common side effects of TPO receptor agonists include mild headache, arthralgia, nasopharyngitis, fatigue, diarrhea, and nausea. These side effects are generally mild and usually of insufficient severity to cause the discontinuation of the drugs. Abnormalities of liver function tests (elevated alanine aminotransferase [ALT], aspartate aminotransferase [AST], and bilirubin levels) occur in approximately 2 percent of ITP patients receiving eltrombopag therapy but not with romiplostim.[225] Autoantibodies against romiplostim may develop but rarely have neutralizing activity.

TPO-receptor agonists can induce extreme thrombocytosis, sometimes exceeding 1000×10^9/L. Careful dose titration is very important, because cessation of the TPO-receptor agonists cause rebound thrombocytopenia in approximately 10 percent of ITP patients.[225] Rates of thromboembolic events were reported as 6.5 percent and 4 percent with extended romiplostim and eltrombopag treatment, respectively.[225,230] The authors of these studies concluded that thromboembolic events are not associated with the dose of TPO receptor agonists or platelet counts, and at least one acquired and inherited thrombotic risk factor was present in most of the patients who experienced thrombosis while they were taking TPO-receptor agonists.[226,230] Nevertheless, the frequency of thrombosis in these studies was slightly higher than observed in other ITP studies.[160] Secondary myelofibrosis (increased marrow reticulin) is sometimes associated with therapy with TPO receptor agonists, and is usually reversible. Concerns have also been expressed that these drugs might accelerate the progression of hematologic and solid malignancies. Under normal circumstances, expression of the TPO receptor (mpl) is highly restricted to hematological tissues including marrow, spleen, placenta, brain and fetal liver cells. TPO receptor expression has been demonstrated on the leukemic cells of patients with acute myelogenous leukemia (AML) and MDS, but not in lymphoid malignancies, myeloproliferative neoplasms, or other nonhematologic malignancies.[231] Although romiplostim therapy was discontinued in a study of its use in patients with low-/intermediate-risk MDS and thrombocytopenia because of increased blast and AML rates (interim hazard ratio: 2.51), long-term analysis of the study showed similar survival and AML rates in the romiplostim and control groups.[232] The question of whether use of TPO-receptor agonists increases the risk of leukemia warrants further study.

Azathioprine This purine analogue is converted to 6-mercaptopurine following gastrointestinal absorption and works by suppressing the immune response. At least 4 months of azathioprine therapy at doses ranging from 50 to 250 mg/day are necessary to evaluate therapeutic efficacy. One study reported that azathioprine produced a sustained normalization of the platelet counts in up to 45 percent of patients with refractory ITP.[233] Azathioprine can be used in pregnancy if necessary (see "Thrombocytopenia During Pregnancy" below). As with other immunosuppressive drugs, major adverse effects are marrow suppression and possible increased risk of secondary malignancy.[177,234]

Cyclophosphamide This alkylating drug can be used orally (50 to 200 mg/day) or parenterally (1.0 to 1.5 g/m² IV every 4 weeks) in patients with refractory ITP.[235,236] It increases platelet counts in 60 to 80 percent of patients with ITP, and 20 to 40 percent of those patients will remain in remission for 2 to 3 years[177] after receiving 2 to 3 months of therapy. Its beneficial action is linked to its immunosuppression. The major complications of cyclophosphamide therapy are marrow suppression, hemorrhagic cystitis, infertility, alopecia, and secondary malignancy.

Cyclosporine Cyclosporine is an immunosuppressive drug inhibiting T-cell function, and is primarily used to prevent rejection in patients with organ transplantation. Although cyclosporine may induce a durable remission in patients with ITP when used at relatively low doses (2.5 to 3.0 mg/kg/day),[237] experience with cyclosporine in ITP patients is usually based on small case series. Cyclosporine has several side effects, some potentially serious, including fever, increased risk of opportunistic infections, gingival hyperplasia, diarrhea, peptic ulcer, pancreatitis, renal dysfunction, elevated liver enzymes, hypertension, peripheral neuropathy, convulsions, hirsutism, and increased risk of secondary malignancy.

Danazol This synthetic androgen, with reduced virilizing effects compared to other androgens, has been used to treat patients with refractory ITP. Given at doses of 400 to 800 mg/day for at least 6 months, reported response rates range from 10 to 80 percent.[177,234] Danazol is postulated to decrease Fc receptor numbers on phagocytic cells by antagonizing the effects of estrogens.[153] Danazol should not be given to pregnant women or patients with liver disease. Common side effects of danazol therapy are weight gain, fluid retention, seborrhea, hirsutism, secondary amenorrhea, vocal changes, acne, hepatic toxicity, headache, lethargy, cholesterol spectrum abnormalities (i.e., reduced high-density lipoprotein [HDL] cholesterol) and myalgia. Because liver dysfunction is common with these doses of danazol therapy, liver function should be evaluated monthly.[153,177,234]

Dapsone Dapsone possesses antibacterial and antiinflammatory effects; it is primarily used for leprosy, malaria, and some types of dermatitis. When used at a dose of 75 to 100 mg/day, dapsone may increase platelet counts in patients with persistent, refractory, or chronic ITP.[147,238,239] The median time to response is long, up to 2 months. Partial and CR rates are approximately 50 percent and 20 percent, respectively, but platelet counts return to baseline levels after discontinuation of the therapy.[238,239] The mechanism of dapsone action in ITP is not known. The most important side effects are nausea, headache, skin rashes, hepatitis, cholestasis, dose-dependent hemolysis, and methemoglobinemia. Dapsone should not be given to patients with glucose-6-phosphate dehydrogenase deficiency.

Vinca Alkaloids Both vincristine and vinblastine transiently increase the platelet count in approximately 70 percent of ITP patients within 5 to 21 days, but produce sustained remissions in only 10 percent of treated patients.[108,153,177,234] The recommended dose of vincristine is 1 to 2 mg and of vinblastine is 0.1 mg/kg (maximum: 10 mg), both given by bolus injection at 1-week intervals for a minimum of three courses. It has been proposed that vinca alkaloids bind to platelet microtubules and thereby are transported to the spleen, where they subsequently inhibit the phagocytic functions of splenic macrophages. They may also stimulate megakaryopoiesis. Peripheral neuropathy, neutropenia, jaw pain, alopecia, and constipation are complications of treatment with vinca alkaloids.[234,240–242]

Other Therapies ITP patients with *H. pylori* infection should receive eradication therapy.[148] Many other therapies, including interferon-α,[243] immunoadsorption with staphylococcal protein A,[244] ascorbic acid,[245] colchicine,[246] and plasmapheresis,[247] have been studied for refractory ITP cases, but none has been clearly demonstrated to be effective.

Accessory Therapies Adjunctive therapies include agents designed to reduce bleeding without necessarily affecting the platelet count. Aminocaproic acid or tranexamic acid, both of which inhibit fibrinolysis, can be used for excessive mucosal bleeding. Local bleeding can be controlled by compression and use of gelatin sponges, fibrin sealants, or antifibrinolytic-embedded gauze. Avoiding the use of antiplatelet drugs, contact sports, and activities that increase bleeding risk, and educating patients about maintaining dental hygiene are very important. Menorrhagia is a common problem in patients with chronic ITP; gynecologic evaluation of uterine problems is crucial. Oral contraceptives and hormonal intrauterine devices together with antifibrinolytic drugs may help to reduce excessive menstrual bleeding in these patients.

SECONDARY IMMUNE THROMBOCYTOPENIA

Secondary ITP is defined as immune-mediated platelet destruction in the presence of other conditions, including infections, lymphoproliferative disorders, solid tumors, SLE, or the antiphospholipid syndrome (APS) (Fig. 117–4). ITP can sometimes be the presenting sign of the illness, or may develop during the course of the disease or with certain therapies. Thrombocytopenia in a patient with chronic disease may develop for other reasons, and the diagnosis of immune-mediated platelet destruction may require more detailed tests. Generally,

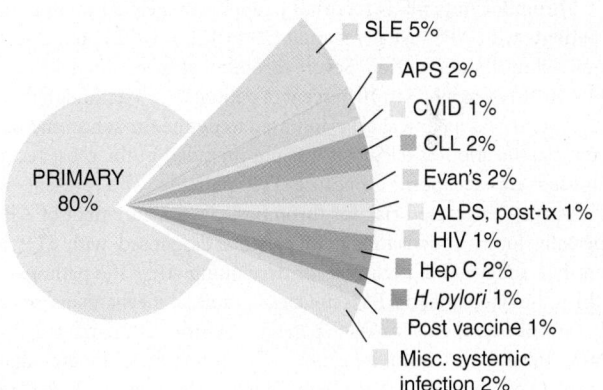

Figure 117–4. Estimated fraction of the various forms of secondary ITP based on clinical experience of the authors. The incidence of *Helicobacter pylori* (HP) ranges from approximately 1 percent in the United States to 60 percent in Italy and Japan. The incidence of the HIV and hepatitis C virus approximates 20 percent in some populations. Miscellaneous causes of immune thrombocytopenia, for example, posttransfusion purpura, myelodysplasia, drugs that lead to the production of autoantibodies, and other conditions, are not discussed further in this chapter. Post marrow or solid-organ transplantation autoimmune lymphoproliferative syndrome (ALPS) occurred in approximately 1 percent of the authors' patients. In the absence of a systematic analysis of the incidence of secondary ITP, the data shown represent the authors' assessment based on our experience and the findings reported in the literature. APS, antiphospholipid syndrome; CLL, chronic lymphocytic leukemia, CVID, common variable immune deficiency; SLE, systemic lupus erythematosus. (*Reproduced with permission from Cines DB, Bussel JB, Liebman HA, Luning Prak ET. The ITP syndrome: Pathogenic and clinical diversity. Blood 113(26):6511–6521, 2009.*)

thrombocytopenia is not severe in patients with secondary ITP, but bleeding risk may be enhanced at a particular platelet count because of the underlying disorder. The treatment strategy should be tailored to the individual patient.

IMMUNE THROMBOCYTOPENIA IN PATIENTS WITH ANTIPHOSPHOLIPID SYNDROME, SYSTEMIC LUPUS ERYTHEMATOSUS AND OTHER CONNECTIVE TISSUE DISORDERS

Thrombocytopenia in the Antiphospholipid Syndrome

APS is characterized by recurrent arterial and/or venous thrombosis and well-defined morbidity during pregnancy in the presence of antiphospholipid antibodies (APLAs) (Chap. 132).[249] APS may affect any organ in the body, including the heart, brain, kidney, skin, lung, and placenta. This syndrome predominantly affects females (female-to-male ratio 5:1), especially during the childbearing years.[250] APLAs (lupus anticoagulant; anticardiolipin antibodies; anti–β_2-GPI antibodies) represent a heterogeneous family of antibodies that react with anionic phospholipids and phospholipid–protein complexes. Despite overwhelming evidence that APLAs are associated with thrombosis, the mechanisms remain uncertain. Many have been proposed, including endothelial cell damage and apoptosis, inhibition of prostacyclin release from endothelial cells, inhibition of the protein C–protein S anticoagulant system, induction of tissue factor, activation of platelets and the complement system, interference with antithrombin, impairment of fibrinolytic activity, and inhibition of annexin V binding to membrane phospholipids, eliminating the antithrombotic effect of annexin V.[251-254] APS is considered one of the most common causes of acquired thrombophilia.[255,256]

Thrombocytopenia is reported in approximately 20 to 40 percent of patients with APS, usually is mild (70 to 120 × 10⁹/L), and does not require clinical intervention. Severe thrombocytopenia (platelet counts <50 × 10⁹/L) occurs in 5 to 10 percent of patients.[257-259] Although thrombocytopenia was a clinical criterion used to define the syndrome in the initial classification of APS,[260] it was not included in the most recently proposed classification.[261] Because ITP patients who present with APLAs are at increased risk for thrombosis,[262] measurement of APLA, especially lupus anticoagulant, in patients diagnosed with ITP may identify a subgroup at high risk for developing APS. The pathogenesis of thrombocytopenia in APS is not clear. Potential mechanisms explaining thrombocytopenia in APS patients include APLA-related direct platelet destruction, immune platelet destruction by antibodies against platelet GPs, complement-mediated platelet destruction, and platelet aggregation and consumption. Evidence indicates APLAs bind platelet membranes and cause platelet destruction, but the link is not definitive. Some investigators suggest that antibodies against platelet GPs, rather than APLAs, are responsible for thrombocytopenia in patients with APS. Antibodies against the integrin $\alpha_{IIb}\beta_3$ or GPIb–IX–V complexes are found in approximately 40 percent of thrombocytopenic patients with APS.[263] Such antibodies do not cross-react with antibodies against phospholipids or β_2-GPI.[264] Immunosuppressive treatment in these patients increases the platelet count and reduces the titers of anti-GP antibodies but not the titers of APLAs.[265] These data suggest that thrombocytopenia is a secondary immune phenomenon that develops concomitantly with APS. Against this conclusion, platelet antigens in thrombocytopenic patients with APS were found to be different from those in ITP and the antibodies to display virtually no reactivity with membrane GPs.[266] CD40 ligand on platelets is another possible antibody target. Anti-CD40 ligand antibodies have been found in patients with APS (13 percent) and ITP (12 percent), but not in healthy controls; and it was suggested

that these antibodies cause thrombocytopenia.[267] Platelet activation, aggregation, and consumption (APS-associated thrombotic microangiopathy) may also contribute to thrombocytopenia.[259] Another issue of clinical importance in evaluating thrombocytopenia associated with APS is the risk for future development of thrombosis. In one study in which APS patients were divided into three groups according to platelet counts as normal, moderately thrombocytopenic (50 to 100 × 10⁹/L), or severely thrombocytopenic (<50 × 10⁹/L), the rates of future thrombosis were 40 percent, 32 percent, and 9 percent, respectively.[268] These data show that moderate thrombocytopenia does not prevent thrombosis in patients with APS. Antithrombotic prophylaxis should be considered in these patients whenever it is possible.[257,268]

Although thrombocytopenia is a common finding in patients with APS, bleeding complications are rare, even with severe thrombocytopenia. Bleeding in an APS patient with moderate thrombocytopenia should trigger evaluation for the presence of antiprothrombin antibodies[269] and other disorders that may affect hemostasis, such as DIC, liver insufficiency, and uremia. Severe thrombocytopenia may require therapy, with treatment strategies similar to those used for patients with ITP. Glucocorticoids are effective in only 15 percent of patients.[257] IVIG and immunosuppressive drugs such as azathioprine and cyclophosphamide can be used in patients with severe bleeding and "catastrophic" APS. In general, splenectomy should be postponed as long as possible, and is only preferred in patients with severe bleeding. Splenectomy may produce sustained remission in approximately two-thirds of patients as in patients with primary ITP.[167,270,271] Because of their increased risk of thrombosis, patients should be prophylactically anticoagulated in the immediate postoperative period. Rituximab has been used to treat refractory thrombocytopenia in patients with APS, with a wide range of results.[272-274] Although there is no consensus on dosing and schedule with rituximab therapy, it is generally administered as in patients with ITP (see ITP therapy in "Therapy and Course" above). TPO receptor agonists may increase thrombosis risk in patients with APS and SLE and these diagnoses in a patient with ITP were accepted as exclusion criteria in some randomized controlled studies of TPO-receptor agonists.[136] Two case reports described acute renal failure (one was a result of thrombotic microangiopathy) after use of eltrombopag.[275,276]

Thrombocytopenia in Patients with Systemic Lupus Erythematosus and Other Connective Tissue Disorders

SLE is a complex autoimmune disease that primarily afflicts women of childbearing age. The autoimmune attack in SLE is not organ specific; it may affect any tissue in the body. The diagnostic criteria for SLE are based on a classification system proposed by the American College of Rheumatology.[277,278] The presence of hematologic findings (leukopenia, thrombocytopenia, or hemolytic anemia) is one of the criteria in the diagnosis and classification of SLE. Thrombocytopenia is common in patients with SLE, occurring in 20 to 40 percent of patients, and may be a presenting symptom.[279] Immunologic destruction of platelets is also seen in several other autoimmune conditions, including polyarteritis nodosa, rheumatoid arthritis, mixed connective tissue disease, and Sjögren syndrome, albeit at much lower rates than in SLE.

The causes of thrombocytopenia in SLE are many and include platelet destruction (ITP, DIC, thrombotic thrombocytopenic purpura [TTP] or hemolytic uremic syndrome [HUS], sepsis, drugs), ineffective hematopoiesis (megaloblastic anemia), abnormal platelet pooling (hypersplenism), marrow hypoplasia (from drugs and infections), and dilutional thrombocytopenia related to therapy. Severe thrombocytopenia is relatively rare, occurring in 5 percent of patients.[279] Although clinically significant bleeding is uncommon even in patients with severe thrombocytopenia, fatal gastrointestinal, cerebral, and pulmonary bleeding have been reported. Among the many potential contributors to thrombocytopenia in SLE patients, platelet destruction by autoantibodies is the major mechanism. Antiplatelet antibodies are present in up to 60 percent of SLE patients.[280,281] The presence of antiplatelet antibodies is correlated with low platelet counts and increased disease severity.[281] Besides the antiplatelet antibodies, APLAs (see "Thrombocytopenia in the Antiphospholipid Syndrome" above) and circulating immune complexes that bind platelets may nonspecifically accelerate platelet destruction.[282] Specific antiplatelet antibodies, especially those against integrin, have an important role in the pathogenesis of thrombocytopenia in SLE patients.[280,281,283] In general, marrow megakaryocytes are normal or increased, and platelet production is not affected in SLE patients with thrombocytopenia. However, decreased numbers of megakaryocytes and even amegakaryocytic thrombocytopenia have been reported.[86,284] High levels of TPO in the plasma, and both anti-TPO and anti-TPO receptor antibodies have been reported in SLE patients,[285,286] the latter associated with a decrease in marrow megakaryocytes and thrombocytopenia.[286] Thrombocytopenia in SLE is associated with serious organ pathology, leading to neuropsychiatric disease,[287] renal disease,[288,289] and APS,[290] and is an independent indicator of poor prognosis.[289,291,292] A study of selected SLE families in which at least one affected member was thrombocytopenic reported genetic linkage to loci at chromosomes 11p13 and 1q22–23.[293] A severe lupus phenotype was much more common in patients with thrombocytopenia and their affected family members than in patients from families with no thrombocytopenic patients. Therefore, thrombocytopenia in a family member may herald severe lupus in familial SLE.

There are no well-established treatment strategies for severe thrombocytopenia in patients with SLE. Because SLE ranges in severity from milder forms with easily controlled symptoms and signs to severe forms that can be fatal, the treatment of severe thrombocytopenia should be tailored to the individual patient. Patients with severe thrombocytopenia are generally treated with glucocorticoids as first-line therapy, but sustained remission is infrequent. Because most patients with severe thrombocytopenia also have nephritis and neurologic symptoms, they receive immunosuppressive therapy either alone or combination with glucocorticoids.[294–297] IVIG is reserved for use in patients with severe bleeding.[298,299] It is well-known that B lymphocytes play an important role in the pathogenesis of SLE. Although lymphopenia is common in patients with active SLE, autoantibody-producing B cells have been shown to be expanded, and B cells were found to be more sensitive to inflammatory cytokines.[300] B-cell targeted therapy—rituximab—is effective in the treatment of refractory SLE patients, especially those with nephritis and severe thrombocytopenia.[300] A retrospective study evaluating the long-term effects of rituximab therapy in 65 patients with refractory ITP associated with SLE and mixed connective tissue disease reported an overall response rate of 80 percent.[301] Although case series indicate that splenectomy yields sustained remission in 61 percent of SLE patients with severe thrombocytopenia[295] and is relatively safe in terms of perioperative complications,[302] splenectomy may increase the risk of thrombotic complications in SLE patients,[303] and may also increase the risk of infection if the patients require further immunosuppressive therapy.

THROMBOCYTOPENIA IN INFECTIOUS DISEASES

The first recorded observation of purpura was made in patients with fever, and purpura was accepted as a sign of severe infections for centuries. Thrombocytopenia can be seen in patients with viral, bacterial, fungal and parasitic infections. Infection can decrease platelet levels in several ways: by decreasing production in the marrow, by increased immune destruction, or by inducing microangiopathy as seen in patients with infection induced DIC or HUS. In addition, drugs used for the treatment of an infection can contribute to thrombocytopenia (see "Drug-Induced Thrombocytopenia" below).

Viral infections are an important cause of secondary ITP. ITP can be seen after a viral infection, especially in children, and usually resolves within 2 to 8 weeks. In patients with viral infections such as rubella, mumps, and infectious mononucleosis, thrombocytopenia can be present with other clinical signs and symptoms. Adult patients with isolated thrombocytopenia with no obvious causes should be screened for HIV, HCV and, in endemic areas, for HBV. Because other clinical symptoms and signs associated with infection with these viruses may not be present initially, and it may not be possible to distinguish these cases from primary ITP.

HIV is a leading cause of isolated thrombocytopenia in Western countries. Thrombocytopenia associated with HIV infection has numerous causes, many of which can be present simultaneously. These include accelerated platelet destruction primarily related to immune complexes, decreased platelet production, especially in advanced disease, splenic sequestration, and, rarely, platelet consumption associated with TTP. Medications, concurrent infections such as hepatitis C, and hematologic malignancies may contribute to the development of thrombocytopenia (Chap. 83).[304–307]

HCV is another important cause of thrombocytopenia in adults. It is a hepatotrophic RNA virus of the Flaviviridae family. HCV infection is chronic in approximately 85 percent of the infected individuals and progresses to cirrhosis in 20 percent of these individuals. The World Health Organization (WHO) estimates that approximately 3 percent of the world's population is infected with HCV, the prevalence ranging from 0.5 to 2 percent in Western countries to 20 percent in some underdeveloped countries.[308] HCV causes thrombocytopenia through different mechanisms, including hypersplenism, decreased TPO level associated with liver insufficiency, the effect of drugs (pegylated interferon [IFN] and ribavirin), and immune-mediated platelet destruction.[309] Immune dysregulation in HCV is associated with several autoimmune disorders, including arthritis, Sjögren syndrome, cryoglobulinemia, and immune cytopenias.[310] As a potential mechanism of immune destruction, one study demonstrated binding of both free and IgG-complexed HCV to platelets.[311] In secondary ITP associated with HCV infection, antiviral therapy with pegylated IFN and ribavirin will decrease viral load and may also treat thrombocytopenia. However, platelet counts can be unaffected or even decrease after these therapies. Severe thrombocytopenia interferes with optimal HCV treatment, and may increase bleeding risk. In this situation, the ASH 2011 guideline recommends IVIG as a first-line therapy, because glucocorticoids may increase viral load.[148] Glucocorticoids and splenectomy both appear to be effective treatments for thrombocytopenia, but their use should be balanced against other considerations after discussion with a hepatologist. TPO receptor agonists may increase the risk of abdominal thrombosis in HCV patients with liver cirrhosis.[312]

The potential role of *H. pylori* in the pathogenesis of chronic ITP is controversial. Japanese and Italian studies showed that eradication of *H. pylori* with antibiotics resulted in marked platelet count increases in patients with ITP. However, this success was not reproduced in American and other European studies.[313] It appears that response rates are higher in countries where *H. pylori* infection is endemic. ITP patients treated for *H. pylori* had higher platelet counts than untreated ITP patients, even if the therapy was unsuccessful in eradicating the infection.[314] It has therefore been speculated that the antibiotic therapy, rather than eradication of *H. pylori*, may be the factor improving platelet counts. However, meta-analysis found that *H. pylori* eradication therapy was much more likely to increase platelet counts in patients with *H. pylori* infection than in uninfected patients,[315] strengthening the case for a causal relationship between infection and thrombocytopenia. On the other hand, eradication was shown to be less effective in patients with severe thrombocytopenia.[309] The recent ASH ITP guideline suggests that ITP patients be screened for *H. pylori* and for eradication therapy to be used if testing is positive.[148]

THROMBOCYTOPENIA DURING PREGNANCY

Thrombocytopenia is the second most common hematologic problem in pregnancy, after anemia. Table 117–6 lists the major causes of thrombocytopenia in pregnancy (Chap. 7). Platelet counts tend to decrease during normal pregnancy, and mild thrombocytopenia (platelet counts ranging from 120 to 150 × 10^9/L) occurs with moderate frequency, especially during the third trimester.[316,317] Bleeding symptoms are generally mild, even in patients with severe thrombocytopenia, probably because of the procoagulant state of pregnancy. Nevertheless, it is important to investigate the cause of thrombocytopenia and exclude the disorders associated with significant morbidity such as eclampsia and hemolysis, elevated liver enzymes, low platelets (HELLP) syndrome (Table 117–6). A medical history should include previous blood counts, history of other diseases, nutritional status, and intake of drugs and herbal supplements. It is important to be alert to constitutional symptoms including fever, and, especially, weight loss; neurologic abnormalities, arthritis, rash, and icterus. Key steps in the evaluation of thrombocytopenia in a pregnant woman include blood pressure measurement, evaluation of coagulation parameters, liver and kidney function tests, and examination of the blood film. Physical examination of the abdomen may be difficult in the third trimester and abdominal ultrasound may be required to detect organomegaly. If there are no suspicious clinical or laboratory findings, marrow aspiration is considered unnecessary.[317,318]

TABLE 117–6. Causes of Thrombocytopenia During Pregnancy

Acute fatty liver of pregnancy

Antiphospholipid syndrome and systemic lupus erythematosus

Marrow disorders (e.g., aplastic anemia, acute leukemia)

Disseminated intravascular coagulation

Drugs (mostly heparins and antibiotics)

Gestational thrombocytopenia

Hemolysis, elevated liver function tests, low platelets (HELLP) syndrome

Hypersplenism

Immune thrombocytopenic purpura

Nutritional deficiencies including folate deficiency

Preeclampsia, eclampsia

Pseudothrombocytopenia

Thrombotic thrombocytopenic purpura–hemolytic uremic syndrome

Viral infections

GESTATIONAL THROMBOCYTOPENIA

Gestational thrombocytopenia is detected in 5 to 7 percent of otherwise healthy pregnant women, accounting for 64 to 80 percent of patients with thrombocytopenia at term.[319–321] Gestational thrombocytopenia is a benign disorder and is not associated with an increased risk of bleeding. Platelet counts are greater than 70 × 10^9/L[316,317,319,320] and return to normal after delivery.

The pathogenesis of gestational thrombocytopenia is unknown. Several mechanisms have been proposed, including hemodilution, a compensated state of subclinical coagulopathy, endothelial cell injury, and immune destruction. Some authors have proposed platelet consumption by the placenta and hormonal depression of megakaryopoiesis as causes of gestational thrombocytopenia, as suggested by the rapid return of the platelet count to normal after delivery and by the transient normalization of the platelet count during pregnancy in some cases of essential thrombocythemia.[321–324] Discriminating gestational thrombocytopenia from ITP can be difficult because ITP is also common in young women, and is often exacerbated by pregnancy. Neither condition can be definitively diagnosed by currently available tests. The diagnosis of ITP is favored if the patient had a previous episode of ITP unassociated with pregnancy or if the thrombocytopenia is severe and associated with bleeding that occurs in the first trimester. In healthy pregnant women, a platelet count greater than 70 × 10^9/L late in pregnancy does not require intensive investigation, because bleeding is not likely in the woman or her newborn child.[325]

IMMUNE THROMBOCYTOPENIA IN PREGNANCY

ITP is responsible for 4 to 5 percent of all cases of pregnancy-associated thrombocytopenia.[319,321] Pregnancy itself may induce ITP, or exacerbate preexisting ITP, but generally the platelet count returns to the prepregnancy level after delivery. Diagnosis of ITP in a pregnant woman requires the exclusion of other causes of thrombocytopenia as in a nonpregnant woman, but also requires the evaluation of other pregnancy-related causes (see Table 117–6). However, the management of ITP during pregnancy is different than in nonpregnant women. First, many of the drugs used to treat ITP may complicate pregnancy-related problems such as gestational diabetes, hypertension, and psychiatric disorders. Second, the fetus can also be affected by ITP and its treatment. Antiplatelet antibodies can cross the placenta, decrease the fetal platelet count, and sometimes cause bleeding.[320] ITP drugs can affect fetal development and growth, a fact to be considered in selecting therapy during pregnancy. And third, all pregnancies will end with delivery of the baby, a process that may happen unexpectedly. Preparation for delivery in a pregnant ITP patient requires close collaboration between the hematologist, the obstetrician, and the neonatologist.

In the management of pregnancy-related ITP, bleeding symptoms and platelet counts should be considered.[147,148] Although previous guidelines have defined threshold platelet levels for treatment during pregnancy and labor, these numbers are arbitrary and not based on randomized controlled studies. Generally, observation without therapy is appropriate if the platelet count is greater than 30 × 10^9/L and the patient has no bleeding symptoms. Therapy is required for a pregnant woman who is bleeding, has a platelet count less than 20 × 10^9/L in any trimester, or has a platelet count of 20 to 30 × 10^9/L in the third trimester.[147,318] Platelet counts should be increased to safe levels (generally >30 × 10^9/L) if invasive procedures are planned. Glucocorticoids are the preferred initial therapy for these patients. Because of their side effects, glucocorticoids should be used at the minimal dose that will keep platelet counts in a safe range. The recommended starting dose of prednisone is 10 mg/day, which can be modified as appropriate.[147,318] Fetal side effects will be minimal with a low-dose glucocorticoid regimen, because approximately 90 percent of the glucocorticoid dose is metabolized in the placenta.[317] IVIG is indicated in pregnant patients who do not respond to or tolerate glucocorticoid treatment, or when it is necessary to rapidly increase the platelet count. A dose of 1 g/kg per day for 2 days, or 400 mg/kg per day for 5 days can be used alone, or combined with low-dose prednisone. If the initial therapy with glucocorticoids and IVIG fails, all second-line therapies generate some concern. Anti-(Rh)D can cause severe hemolytic reactions in both the mother and the fetus, and should be used only in patients refractory to glucocorticoids and IVIG.[148,318] Experience with azathioprine and cyclosporine in pregnancy is largely based on the case series from patients with rheumatologic disorders and solid-organ transplantation. These studies reported that exposure to these drugs during pregnancy was not associated with an increase in the risk of negative pregnancy outcomes and had no significant toxicity to the fetus.[326] Splenectomy can be used in pregnant ITP patients who are unresponsive or intolerant to available drugs and at significant risk of bleeding. If splenectomy is necessary, it is preferable that it be performed during the second trimester.[147,191]

Rituximab is not an optimal drug for use during pregnancy. It can cross the placenta, and transfer from mother to fetus increases with gestational age. The half-life of the drug is also very long; rituximab can be found in blood 6 months after of an infusion. In a review evaluating 231 pregnancies with rituximab exposure reported in the literature, most of the patients had SLE, rheumatoid arthritis. and B-cell lymphoma, with rituximab being used in combination with other drugs. This retrospective study showed low risk of premature births, hematologic abnormalities and birth defects. However, because of the lack of controlled studies, it is recommended that women avoid pregnancy for 1 year after rituximab infusion.[327]

TPO receptor agonists were found to cause fetal loss and reduced fetal body weight in animal studies, and there is no data on humans.[328] Vinca alkaloids, cyclophosphamide, and danazol are not recommended during pregnancy.

The optimal mode of delivery in pregnant ITP patients has not been determined. Because earlier studies reported that thrombocytopenic neonates have an increased risk for intracranial hemorrhage, some physicians recommend delivering the baby by cesarean section in women with ITP to avoid injuries to the fetus during passage through the birth canal.[329] However, because of the rarity of intracerebral hemorrhage, there are no data proving the effectiveness of cesarean delivery in reducing the occurrence of intracerebral hemorrhage in the thrombocytopenic fetus.[322] Measurement of platelet counts in infants before delivery, such as by percutaneous umbilical cord blood sampling or fetal scalp vein sampling after cervical dilatation, is not recommended routinely because the risk of bleeding during these procedures is high.[330–332] The mother's platelet count at delivery does not correlate with the infant's platelet count. In ITP patients who gave birth more than once, however, the first infant's platelet count at birth may be a predictor of severe thrombocytopenia in subsequent pregnancies and may justify further obstetric management.[322,331,333] On the other hand, discordances in degree of thrombocytopenia between dichorionic twins in ITP indicate that fetal factors also are important.[334] In conclusion, there is as yet no definitive method to predict fetal platelet count in pregnant ITP patients, and the method of delivery should be determined by obstetrical evaluation. During vaginal delivery, the target maternal platelet count should be 50×10^9/L or higher. If cesarean section or epidural anesthesia is required, the platelet count should be maintained over 70 to 80×10^9/L.[147,148,318] Glucocorticoids, IVIG and platelet transfusions may help to keep platelet counts in a safe range in these patients. Blood products should be available for possible severe bleeding during labor,

although it is quite rare even in ITP patients with platelet counts lower than 20×10^9/L.

Severe neonatal thrombocytopenia (platelet counts $<20 \times 10^9$/L) occurs in 3 to 5 percent of ITP pregnancies and moderate neonatal thrombocytopenia (platelet counts $<50 \times 10^9$/L) in 9 percent.[330] Severe bleeding occurs in less than 1 percent of the babies. If the newborn is thrombocytopenic, the platelet count should be measured daily for 1 week. IVIG is preferred in neonates with severe thrombocytopenia. Platelet transfusions and glucocorticoids are added if bleeding is life-threatening.

If thrombocytopenia associated with SLE and APS has been complicated with prior pregnancy loss and thromboembolism, pregnant patients should receive antithrombotic prophylaxis with low molecular heparin and/or aspirin if possible. Although there is no defined threshold platelet level for these patients, platelet counts over 50×10^9/L are considered safe for both anticoagulant and antiplatelet therapy.[318]

MICROANGIOPATHIC DISORDERS IN PREGNANCY: PREECLAMPSIA–ECLAMPSIA, HELLP, THROMBOTIC THROMBOCYTOPENIC PURPURA–HEMOLYTIC UREMIC SYNDROME, AND ACUTE FATTY LIVER OF PREGNANCY

Preeclampsia

This condition is a systemic disorder characterized by new onset hypertension after 20 weeks of gestation, and primarily occurs near term. Although proteinuria occurs in the majority of these cases, the American College of Obstetricians and Gynecologists (ACOG) 2012 classification accepts the presence of one of the following in the absence of proteinuria: thrombocytopenia (less than 100×10^9/L), abnormal liver function tests, renal insufficiency, pulmonary edema, or cerebral and visual symptoms. *Eclampsia* is defined by the occurrence of epileptic seizures in a preeclamptic woman during the peripartum period.[335–337] Preeclampsia complicates 5 to 8 percent of all pregnancies, and is a major contributor to maternal and fetal morbidity and mortality (Chap. 7).[335,338] Thrombocytopenia is seen in approximately 50 percent of women with preeclampsia, with the severity of thrombocytopenia correlating with the severity of the preeclampsia.[339]

Attempts to define the pathogenesis of preeclampsia have engendered numerous theories.[340] One clear aspect of the pathogenesis is the requirement for a placenta, given that the condition can be produced in abdominal pregnancies and molar pregnancies.[341] The disease appears to be initiated by defective invasion of the uterine spiral arteries by placental cytotrophoblasts. During normal implantation, these cells convert from epithelial to endothelial morphology, a process called *pseudovasculogenesis*.[342,343] In preeclampsia, this process is defective, resulting in diminished maternal blood flow to the placenta and placental hypoxia. Through unknown mechanisms, the production of membrane and soluble forms of the vascular endothelial growth factor (VEGF) receptor fms-like tyrosine kinase-1 (Flt1) is increased,[344] with resultant increases of soluble Flt1 (sFlt1) in the amniotic fluid[345] and maternal circulation.[346] sFlt1 is the product of an alternately spliced form of the Flt1 messenger RNA that lacks the transmembrane and cytoplasmic domains present in the full-length receptor. A large volume of evidence implicates sFlt1 as playing a key role in the pathogenesis of preeclampsia. By binding to VEGF and the related placental growth factor, sFlt1 blocks their favorable effects on vascular endothelium. Its expression in rats produces a syndrome akin to preeclampsia: hypertension and proteinuria associated with glomerular endotheliosis (occlusion of glomerular capillaries by swollen endothelial cells). Endoglin is another angiogenic receptor expressed on endothelial cells and placental syncytiotrophoblasts, functioning as a coreceptor for the potent angiogenic factor transforming growth factor-β.[347] Expression of its messenger RNA is increased in preeclamptic placenta.[347] The levels of the soluble extracellular domain, produced by proteolysis, are elevated in the blood of preeclamptic patients. In pregnant rats, soluble endoglin works synergistically with sFlt1 to produce vascular damage and a HELLP-like syndrome.[347] These findings strongly suggest that a tonic level of VEGF-like angiogenic factors is required to maintain the normal function of vascular endothelial cells and that this process is dysregulated during preeclampsia/eclampsia.

The connection between preeclampsia and thrombocytopenia is not clear, although many cases have evidence of activation of blood coagulation detected by elevated levels of fibrin-degradation products and thrombin–antithrombin complexes.[321] Low levels of the VWF-cleaving metalloprotease ADAMTS13 (a disintegrin and metalloprotease with a thrombospondin type 1 motif member 13) have also been described,[348] as have elevated levels of VWF, including the hyperadhesive ultralarge forms.[349]

HELLP Syndrome

This syndrome occurs in the peripartum period and is defined by the presence of microangiopathic hemolytic anemia, elevated liver enzymes, and low platelets. In approximately 70 to 80 percent of patients, HELLP occurs in the setting of preeclampsia.[350] Microangiopathic hemolysis results from shearing of the erythrocytes as they pass through arterioles occluded by platelet–fibrin deposits. Adhesion and aggregation of platelets on damaged and activated endothelium presumably accounts for the low platelet count (Chap. 114). HELLP shares a number of features with TTP, including the presence of microangiopathic hemolysis and thrombocytopenia. Involvement of the central nervous system is a more prominent feature of TTP, whereas HELLP more commonly displays severe liver function abnormalities (Chaps. 7, 49, and 124).[351] Because the two syndromes can be confused with one other, one study attempted to distinguish the two by measuring the activity of ADAMTS13, which usually is absent or severely deficient in TTP.[348] The study found that essentially all 17 patients in a cohort with the HELLP syndrome had mild to moderate reductions in the activity of ADAMTS13 in the plasma, and none was severely deficient.

Acute Fatty Liver of Pregnancy

This abnormality is a very severe, but fortunately very rare (1 in 20,000 to 100,000 pregnancies) condition that occurs during the third trimester of pregnancy or early postpartum period. Acute fatty liver of pregnancy (AFLP) is characterized by microvesicular fatty infiltration of liver resulting in hepatic failure and encephalopathy. The "Swansea Criteria" used for the diagnosis of AFLP include encephalopathy, vomiting, abdominal pain, polydipsia/polyuria, elevated transaminases, elevated ammonia, elevated uric acid, elevated bilirubin, leukocytosis, coagulopathy, renal impairment, hypoglycemia, ascites or bright liver on ultrasound evaluation, and microvesicular steatosis on liver biopsy. Six or more of these criteria should be present in a patient who has no obvious reason for hepatic failure. Both maternal and fetal mortality rates are high, ranging from 7 to 18 percent and 9 to 23 percent, respectively.[352]

Delivery of the fetus is the most effective treatment for preeclampsia, HELLP syndrome and AFLP. The platelet count nadir and the peak of serum lactate dehydrogenase may occur postpartum, during the first postpartum day in most patients, but as late as 5 to 7 days in some. For patients with severe thrombocytopenia and microangiopathic hemolytic anemia, plasma exchange may be indicated if the fetus cannot be delivered or if improvement does not follow delivery. This treatment is empirically based on the similarity of the clinical picture to that of TTP. Postpartum day 3 often is considered the limit for supportive therapy

in anticipation of a spontaneous recovery.[348] If thrombocytopenia and hemolysis (as assessed by serum lactate dehydrogenase levels) continue to worsen beyond this time, intervention with plasma exchange is appropriate for the presumed diagnosis of TTP-HUS (Chap. 133). At this point, TTP-HUS cannot be distinguished from atypical preeclampsia/HELLP syndrome, for which plasma exchange treatment may be beneficial.[353] Earlier intervention with plasma exchange is indicated for more severe clinical problems, such as neurologic abnormalities or acute, anuric renal failure. In patients with AFLP, however, liver insufficiency, encephalopathy and coagulopathy may not improve despite immediate delivery and intensive supportive care. These patients may require liver transplantation.[352]

● NEONATAL ALLOIMMUNE THROMBOCYTOPENIA

The platelet count in the fetus reaches normal adult levels ($>150 \times 10^9$/L) after the first trimester, and is maintained throughout gestation. However, thrombocytopenia is more common in preterm infants, of several potential etiologies. Severe thrombocytopenia ($<50 \times 10^9$/L) is an important finding in neonates, and should be carefully managed because of high bleeding risk (Chap. 6).[354]

Fetal–neonatal alloimmune thrombocytopenia (NAIT) is a leading cause of severe thrombocytopenia and life-threatening bleeding in neonates. NAIT is caused by the transplacental transfer of maternal alloantibodies against fetal platelet antigens inherited from the father. NAIT resembles neonatal alloimmune hemolytic anemia (Rh hemolytic disease of the newborn) in many aspects. In both diseases, maternal alloantibodies against fetal blood cell antigens cross the placenta and destroy antigen-positive fetal cells, resulting in significant fetal/neonatal morbidity and mortality. However, unlike neonatal alloimmune hemolytic anemia, which tends to spare the first-born child, the first child is affected in 40 to 60 percent of NAIT cases.[317] Transplacental transfer of antiplatelet antibodies can also occur in babies born from mothers with ITP. Nevertheless, maternal ITP rarely causes serious thrombocytopenia or bleeding in the fetus, whereas thrombocytopenia tends to be more severe and the rate of intracranial hemorrhage is higher (10 to 20 percent) in NAIT.[106] In contrast to maternal ITP, in NAIT the maternal platelet count is normal, a key differential diagnostic finding.

PREVALENCE AND PATHOGENESIS

The estimated frequency of NAIT varies from 1 in 500 to 1 in 2000 livebirths.[355,356] Maternal alloantibodies against human platelet alloantigens (HPAs) are responsible for platelet destruction in NAIT. In populations of European ancestry, the most frequently implicated antigens are HPA-1a or Pl^{A1} (78 percent of cases) and HPA-5b or Br^a (19 percent of cases).[357] These antigens are rare in Asian populations. HPA-4a (80 percent of cases) and HPA-3a (15 percent of cases) are responsible for platelet destruction in the majority of Asian NAIT cases. Besides targeting the HPA system, anti–HLA-2 antibodies have been reported, but whether they are responsible for NAIT is not clear.[355,358,359]

The frequency of NAIT in populations of European ancestry is lower than would be expected given that the prevalence of HPA-1a negativity is 2.5 percent. Only 10 percent of HPA-1a–negative mothers exposed to HPA-1a–positive platelets during pregnancy become immunized. HPA alloimmunization is strongly correlated with the presence of specific class II HLA antigens, with increased risk demonstrated in HPA-1a–negative mothers expressing HLA-B8, HLA-DR3, and HLA-DR52a antigens.[317,360,361] The presence of the HLA-DRB3*0101 allele in HPA-1a–negative women increases the NAIT risk as much as 140-fold.[361]

NAIT tends to be clinically more severe in cases with alloantibodies against HPA-1a.[106] HPA-1 (PlᴬA) antigens are expressed on platelet integrin β_3. Anti–HPA-1a antibodies possibly impair platelet aggregation, which may explain the severity of bleeding symptoms.[362]

CLINICAL FEATURES

IgG alloantibodies can cross the placenta as early as week 14 of pregnancy, and placental passage increases with gestational age.[355] These antibodies bind to fetal platelets and lead to their destruction. In severe cases, intracranial hemorrhage and hydrocephalus may develop and cause fetal death or severe neurologic sequelae. The diagnosis can be difficult in the first affected fetus in a family. Ultrasonography is usually not helpful unless it detects bleeding or hydrocephalus. Unexplained fetal deaths in the maternal history or fetal hydrocephalus or bleeding in previous pregnancies may alert the physician to the possibility of NAIT. Usually the diagnosis of NAIT is possible after birth. NAIT should be suspected in a thrombocytopenic neonate with extensive purpura or visceral hemorrhage but no evidence of sepsis, skeletal anomalies, or other systemic diseases that may cause thrombocytopenia, including maternal ITP. Affected babies may have no signs or symptoms (13 to 59 percent of cases), or they may have signs of bleeding (18 to 65 percent of cases) or intracranial hemorrhage (22 to 23 percent of cases).[363] In a case series of 88 infants with NAIT resulting from anti–HPA-1a antibodies, 90 percent had purpura, 66 percent had hematomas, 30 percent had gastrointestinal bleeding, and 14 percent had intracerebral hemorrhage. Bleeding may be delayed, as the platelet count usually falls further during the first several days of life. Death or neurologic impairment occurs in up to 25 percent of infants. Platelet counts recover to normal in 1 to 2 weeks.[364]

The diagnosis of NAIT usually can be confirmed by tests for circulating maternal alloantibodies against fetal antigens (usually by MAIPA) or modified antigen capture enzyme-linked immunosorbent assay (MACE) or by platelet typing of the parents and neonate by either genotyping or ELISA. These tests may fail to yield the diagnosis because private HPA antigens may be responsible for NAIT.[317,322,357]

MANAGEMENT

Postnatal

In the clinical setting, the confirmation of a diagnosis of NAIT by platelet genotyping, MAIPA, or MACE will require days; thus, an infant born with severe thrombocytopenia with no obvious cause such as sepsis should be regarded as having NAIT. The alternatives in the management of affected neonates are IVIG, glucocorticoids (alone or combined with IVIG), and platelet transfusions. IVIG and/or glucocorticoid therapy may increase platelet counts rapidly, although a substantial increase of platelet counts usually occurs after 24 to 72 hours.[357] In cases with severe bleeding, platelets should be transfused. Transfused platelets should be ABO and (Rh)D compatible and HPA-1a–negative if possible.[365] If such platelet suspensions are not available, transfusion of washed and irradiated maternal platelets to the affected fetus is another alternative.[106] Repeated platelet transfusions may be required.[317] All affected infants should be screened with ultrasound for intracranial hemorrhage.[366]

Prenatal

Pregnant women who had a previous thrombocytopenic infant attributable to NAIT should be carefully monitored in a center with experience with NAIT, because thrombocytopenia will be more severe in a second affected child. Current therapeutic alternatives for antenatal management of NAIT are unsatisfactory. Fetal platelet typing is important, but

available tests usually require invasive procedures such as amniocentesis or fetal blood sampling. Cell-free fetal DNA obtained from maternal blood has been studied for fetal platelet genotyping.[367] However, these tests need validation. The treatment options in high-risk NAIT are weekly IVIG administration to the mother, with or without glucocorticoids, serial in utero platelet transfusions, in utero IVIG administration, and early delivery (after 32 weeks of gestation). Maternal IVIG administration at a dose of 1 g/kg per week with or without glucocorticoids may increase fetal platelet counts,[368] although not all studies support this conclusion.[355,362] IVIG can be administered directly to severely thrombocytopenic fetuses, although this also may fail to raise fetal platelet counts.[369] In patients who do not respond to IVIG and glucocorticoid administration, serial transfusion of matched platelets should be considered. Matched platelet transfusions will only transiently increase the fetal platelet count because the transfused platelets also are targeted by the offending antibodies.[317] Serial platelet transfusions may increase the cumulative risk of hemorrhage and procedure-related hemorrhage and fetal loss.[362] In severely thrombocytopenic fetuses, early delivery by cesarean section may reduce the risk of intracranial hemorrhage.[362] New therapeutic strategies are under investigation, including vaccines and competitive molecules that competitively bind anti–HPA-1a antibodies.[365]

● ABNORMAL PLATELET DISTRIBUTION OR POOLING

SPLENOMEGALY AND HYPERSPLENISM

Splenomegaly may lead to thrombocytopenia by inducing a reversible pooling of up to 90 percent of total body platelets.[370,371] This process can be thought of as an exaggeration of normal splenic pooling, in which approximately one-third of the platelet mass is contained within the spleen at any one time (Chap. 55). The survival of platelets within the spleen can be normal or moderately reduced. Thus, the total blood platelet pool in a patient with splenomegaly could be normal even when the counts measured in venous blood are only 20 percent of normal. Platelet production is usually normal in patients with splenomegaly, as estimated by dividing the total body platelet mass by the platelet life span.[370] This finding provides further evidence that platelet production is more closely tied to total platelet mass than to circulating platelet count.

The most common disorder causing thrombocytopenia because of splenic pooling is chronic liver disease with portal hypertension and congestive splenomegaly. In patients with cirrhosis and portal hypertension, moderate thrombocytopenia is the rule. However, in such cases the thrombocytopenia often results from both splenic pooling and reduced hepatic production of TPO.

Thrombocytopenia associated with splenomegaly is often of no clinical importance and generally does not require therapy. Signs and symptoms are related to the primary disorder, and bleeding manifestations result primarily from coagulation abnormalities caused by the underlying liver disease. This finding is consistent with the relatively moderate degree of thrombocytopenia, the near-normal total body content of platelets,[370] and the ability to mobilize platelets from the spleen to replenish losses.[372] When splenectomy is performed for another reason, however, the platelet count predictably returns to normal or thrombocytosis may even occur.[370] Platelet counts may also return to normal in patients following surgical correction of portal hypertension by portosystemic shunting.[373] Platelet transfusions usually are not needed for splenomegaly-associated thrombocytopenia and rarely produce significant increases in the platelet count because as much as 90 percent of the transfused platelets will be sequestered in the spleen.

HYPERSPLENISM

Hypersplenism is distinguished from uncomplicated splenomegaly in that pooling is accompanied by increased destruction of platelets, leukocytes, and erythrocytes in association with increased marrow precursors of the deficient lines and correction of the cytopenia by splenectomy.[374–377] The clinical manifestations, laboratory findings, and specific treatment are aimed at the underlying disease (Chap. 55).[378]

Imaging studies, such as computed tomographic scans, can be useful for defining the size of the spleen and identifying intrasplenic and extrasplenic disease. Magnetic resonance imaging defines the blood flow pattern, which is especially useful for detecting portal or splenic vein thromboses. Cell survival studies using radiolabeled platelets or red blood cells can be helpful for identifying hypersequestration when weighing the need for splenectomy. Most patients with splenomegaly require therapy for the underlying disease rather than for thrombocytopenia.

● THROMBOCYTOPENIA ASSOCIATED WITH MASSIVE TRANSFUSION

Several definitions are used for massive transfusion including transfusion of one blood volume or more than 10 units of packed red blood cells (RBCs) in 24 hours and transfusion of more than 4 units of packed RBC over 1 hour.[379] Massive transfusion is required in patients with uncontrolled and heavy bleeding. One study of patients requiring massive transfusion demonstrated that mild thrombocytopenia (47 to 100 × 10^9/L) occurred in all patients after transfusion of 15 red cell units, and more severe thrombocytopenia (25 to 61 × 10^9/L) developed after 20 red cell units.[380,381] Several factors contribute to thrombocytopenia in massive transfusion, including direct loss of platelets in the exsanguinated blood, dilution of platelets by the transfused RBCs, DIC triggered by the disease responsible for the blood loss or that develops after trauma, and hypothermia (Chap. 140). Massively transfused patients should be treated with fresh-frozen plasma to replace coagulation factors, and with platelets.[382] The precise ratio of platelets to red cells has not been determined, but studies show that massively transfused trauma patients demonstrated improved survival with increased transfusion of platelet concentrates.[383,384]

● THROMBOCYTOPENIA RESULTING FROM HYPOTHERMIA

Transient thrombocytopenia occurs during hypothermia, in both animals and humans, when the body temperature falls below 25°C.[385] The degree of thrombocytopenia correlates with the degree of the body temperature drop. Thus, thrombocytopenia is less severe in cardiac surgery patients supported by normothermic systemic perfusion (35°C to 37°C) than in those supported by moderately hypothermic systemic perfusion (25°C to 29°C).[386] In this case, the drop in platelet count likely results from splenic and hepatic pooling[387] and from cold activation and clearance of platelets. Cold induces clustering of the GPIb complex and rearrangement of its carbohydrate chains, which then serve as ligands for the macrophage integrin $\alpha_M\beta_2$, which mediates their clearance in hepatic macrophages.[388,389] In hypothermic dogs, radiolabeled platelets are sequestered in the spleen, liver, and other organs; the platelets return to the circulation when normal body temperature is restored.[385,390] The clinical relevance of these observations is illustrated by reports of patients, often elderly, who are hypothermic after periods of unconsciousness in inadequately heated rooms. In one report, a 69-year-old woman had 13 admissions over an 8-year period with repeated hypothermia, her temperature ranging from 31°C to 34°C during the hospitalizations. On each admission she was thrombocytopenic (platelet count 7 to 39 × 10^9/L). With no therapy other than rewarming, platelet counts returned to normal in 4 to 10 days.[391] However, a review of 75 patients admitted with hypothermia (body temperatures 26°C to 35°C) demonstrated that only three patients were thrombocytopenic.[391]

● THROMBOCYTOPENIA RESULTING FROM PLATELET TRAPPING: KASABACH-MERRITT SYNDROME

Kasabach-Merritt syndrome is defined as profound thrombocytopenia related to platelet trapping within a vascular tumor, either a Kaposi-like hemangioendothelioma or a tufted angioma.[392–395] The syndrome presents predominantly during infancy, but several adult cases have been reported.[396] These vascular tumors should be differentiated from vascular malformations such as classic benign hemangiomas. Benign hemangiomas usually are superficial, multiple, not associated with severe thrombocytopenia or DIC (Chap. 130), and usually disappear during childhood. On the other hand, Kaposi-like hemangioendothelioma and tufted angioma are low-grade malignant vascular tumors associated with high morbidity and mortality.

Vascular tumors usually are solitary, can reach 20 cm in diameter, and can be superficial or invade internal organs and the retroperitoneum.[397–399] Superficial tumors can be recognized by the local red to purple discoloration of the skin. The histologic types more frequently associated with Kasabach-Merritt syndrome are Kaposi-like hemangioendothelioma and tufted angiomas or angioblastomas.[392,393,400,401] Kaposi-like hemangioendothelioma is a locally aggressive, low-grade malignant tumor characterized by infiltrating sheets or lobules of poorly formed vascular channels and aberrant lymphatic vessels. These tumors are composed predominantly of plump, round, oval, and/or spindled endothelial cells with hemosiderin deposits.[392] A tufted angioma is a lesion characterized by the presence of vascular tufts and aggregates of round dilated capillaries, lymphangiomatosis, microthrombi, and hemosiderin deposits.[392,393,402,403] Electron microscopic examination shows abnormal endothelial cells with prominent cytoplasmic projections and wide intercellular gaps, fibrin deposition, and platelet aggregates within the vessels.[393] The histology of the tumor is useful for differentiating the vascular tumors associated with Kasabach-Merritt syndrome from benign capillary hemangiomas.[404]

Thrombocytopenia in Kasabach-Merritt syndrome usually is severe and associated with DIC.[405] Contributing factors include "platelet trapping" by abnormally proliferating endothelium within the hemangioma[406,407] and platelet consumption associated with DIC. Platelet trapping has been demonstrated by immunohistochemical staining of the tumors with anti-CD61 antibodies (a marker of platelets and megakaryocytes)[408] and by nuclear studies using ^{51}Cr-labeled platelets[409] and ^{111}In platelet scintigraphy to monitor response to therapy.[410,411] How platelets become trapped is not clear. Initial physical entrapment of the platelets within twisted abnormal vessels may favor their adhesion to abnormal endothelium, which can lead to platelet activation and aggregation followed by activation of the coagulation cascade, fibrin deposition, and formation of microthrombi. Excessive flow and shear rates generated by arteriovenous shunting within the tumor further increase the level of platelet activation. Continuous thrombus formation leads to platelet consumption and activation of the fibrinolytic cascade. Severe thrombocytopenia and DIC result.

The mainstay of treatment is eradication of the tumor. Several specific therapeutic modalities have been proposed, but none has been established as consistently effective.[412] Among the therapies are high-dose glucocorticoids,[412] IFN-α,[412,413] vincristine,[414] cyclophosphamide,[415] combination chemotherapy,[416] and radiation.[417–419] For severe cases, interventions such as arterial embolization,[420,421] surgical resection,[422,423] and pneumatic compression can be attempted.

The mortality rate for advanced Kasabach-Merritt syndrome is approximately 12 percent; the rate is higher when associated with retroperitoneal or intraabdominal tumors. Patients die of complications resulting from DIC, low platelet count, and infections secondary to immunosuppression.

CYCLIC THROMBOCYTOPENIA

Cyclic thrombocytopenia (CTP) is a very rare acquired disorder characterized by a periodic decrease in the platelet count, sometimes followed by rebound thrombocytosis without therapy ($>500 \times 10^9$/L).[424] Fluctuating levels of endogenous TPO, inversely related to the platelet count, was reported in one case.[425] Each thrombocytopenic cycle typically spans a period of 3 to 6 weeks, and women are more often affected than men. The platelet counts may fluctuate across a wide range. In reported cases, the median nadir and peak platelet counts were 10×10^9/L (range: 1 to 90×10^9/L) and 330×10^9/L (range: 72 to 2300×10^9/L), respectively.[426] Rebound thrombocytosis is an important and distinctive feature of CTP. Although some cases are reported as associated with myeloproliferative neoplasms, most CTP cases are idiopathic.[427,428] The pathophysiology is unclear and a number of potential mechanisms have been proposed, including autoimmune platelet destruction, megakaryocytic hypoplasia/aplasia, infections, and hormonal disturbances. Although most premenopausal female CTP patients studied have had low platelet counts during their menstrual periods, hysterectomy with bilateral salpingo-oophorectomy has not been shown to affect the course of the platelet fluctuations.[426]

The clinical presentation of CTP is similar to that of ITP. The bleeding tendency ranges from asymptomatic, to easy bruising, gingival bleeding, recurrent epistaxis, menorrhagia, and hematuria, to more serious bleeding, including gastrointestinal or central nervous system hemorrhage.[426] CTP is rarely considered in the differential diagnosis of thrombocytopenia, so patients are usually diagnosed and treated as having ITP. CTP is a rare disorder, but the diagnosis should be considered in patients with "ITP" who have not responded to therapies such as glucocorticoids, splenectomy, and IVIG, and who have rebound thrombocytosis. Responses have been reported to respond to hormone therapy and cyclosporine. In female patients, oral contraceptives may be useful to prolong the menstrual cycle and cover low-platelet-count days. Antifibrinolytic drugs such as aminocaproic acid or tranexamic acid may also be useful to decrease bleeding symptoms.

DRUG-INDUCED THROMBOCYTOPENIA

Development of thrombocytopenia after quinine was first described by Vipan in 1865, and since then a large number of drugs have been found to cause thrombocytopenia. Drugs should be considered as potentially causative in any thrombocytopenic patient on medication, taking herbal remedies, or using iodinated radiocontrast solutions.[429] Drug-induced thrombocytopenia generally affects only a small percentage of patients taking a particular drug, and is usually not severe, although it can be fatal. Genetic and environmental factors both influence susceptibility to drugs. Discontinuation of the causative drug(s) is the main treatment strategy; glucocorticoids may help in some patients. Drugs may cause thrombocytopenia by different mechanisms. Dose-dependent myelosuppression and immune destruction of the platelets are two well-known causes. One of the most severe and life-threatening forms of drug-induced thrombocytopenia is HIT, an immune-mediated disorder caused by antibodies that recognize a neoepitope in platelet factor 4 that is exposed when platelet factor 4 binds heparin. The result is activation of platelets and the coagulation cascade and, ultimately, venous and arterial thrombosis. HIT affects up to 5 percent of patients exposed to therapeutic doses of unfractionated heparin (Chap. 133). This section discusses drugs, other than heparins, that cause isolated thrombocytopenia by immune platelet destruction; Chap. 34 discusses drug-induced aplastic anemia with thrombocytopenia.

ETIOLOGY

Reviews of drug-induced thrombocytopenia often contain such extensive lists of implicated drugs, many of which are commonly used, that they are not helpful for decisions regarding which therapy to interrupt first. To address the issue of which drugs most likely cause thrombocytopenia, a systematic review of all published case reports defined levels of evidence to document the causal relation between the drug and thrombocytopenia.[430] This review distinguished drugs with definite or probable causal relationships from those for which the evidence was weaker.[430] Table 117–7 lists the drugs for which there is definite evidence of a causal role in producing thrombocytopenia (which includes recurrent thrombocytopenia with rechallenge in the same patient) and drugs for which the causal relation to thrombocytopenia has been validated by at least two reports with probable evidence (thus meeting all of the criteria for definite evidence except for the lack of rechallenge). Quinidine is by far the most commonly cited drug. Other commonly cited drugs are similar to drugs documented in a case-control study.[431] A remarkable observation from the systematic review was how many case reports did not provide sufficient clinical information to allow a determination of even a probable causal relation.[319]

PATHOGENESIS

Thrombocytopenia is usually assumed to result from immune platelet destruction by drug-dependent antibodies.[429] Most of these antibodies bind the platelets only in the presence of the offending drugs. Drugs may trigger different immune mechanisms, as depicted in Table 117–8.

Drugs may bind covalently to membrane proteins, and may induce hapten-dependent antibodies in patients receiving penicillin and cephalosporin. In quinine-induced thrombocytopenia, antibodies bind to membrane proteins only in the presence of soluble drug. In patients receiving tirofiban or eptifibatide, the drug binds to integrin $\alpha_{IIb}\beta_3$, creating a conformation-dependent neoepitope and inducing antibody production. Gold salts and procainamide, however, may induce true autoantibodies, with those induced by gold being unique in targeting platelet GPV.[432] These antibodies can bind and destroy platelets in the absence of the drug. In HIT, heparin–platelet factor 4 complexes induce autoantibodies.

Initial experimental observations suggested that drug–antibody complexes bind to platelets via the platelet Fcγ receptor. This mechanism is confirmed for HIT (see below in this section), but for other drugs, the drug-dependent antibodies appear to bind to platelets via their Fab regions.[433]

The target antigens are the major platelet surface GPs (GPIb-IX-V and integrin $\alpha_{IIb}\beta_3$). Different drugs may provoke drug-dependent antibodies that preferentially react with one of these GPs, or drug-dependent antibodies from a single patient may react with multiple epitopes on both GPs. For example, a study of sera from 15 patients with quinine-induced thrombocytopenia demonstrated that, in the presence of quinine, the antibodies bound to two distinct domains on GPIb-IX, one on GPIbα, and one on GPIX. Some patients had only one of the antibodies; some had both.[434] The same domains on GPIb-IX also appear to be the antigenic targets for quinidine- and ranitidine-dependent

TABLE 117–7. Drugs Causing Thrombocytopenia

CASES: 1

Adefovir dipivoxil (1, 0)	Diflunisal (0, 1)	Isotretinoin (0, 1)	Penicillin (0, 1)
Alatrofloxacin (0, 1)	Digitoxin (0, 1)	Itraconazole (0, 1)	Pentoxifylline (1, 0)
Albendazole (0, 1)	Diltiazem (0, 1)	Lithium (1, 0)	Piperazine (0, 1)
Alprenolol (1, 0)	Doxepin (0, 1)	Lopinavir/ritonavir (1, 0)	Primidone (0, 1)
Amlodipine (0, 1)	Eflornithine (1, 0)	Losartan (0, 1)	Pyrazinamide (0, 1)
Anakinra (0, 1)	Ezetimibe (0, 1)	Mebhydroline (0, 1)	Recombinant hepatitis B
Apalcillin (0, 1)	Famotidine (0, 1)	Meloxicam (0, 1)	vaccine (0, 1)
Aspirin (0, 1)	Felbamate (0, 1)	Meprobamate (0, 1)	Rifampicin (1, 0)
Atorvastatin (1, 0)	Fenoprofen (0, 1)	Mesalamine (1, 0)	Rituximab (1, 0)
Bismuth (0, 1)	Feprazone (0, 1)	Methazolamide (0, 1)	Rofecoxib (0, 1)
Butoconazole (0, 1)	Finasteride (0, 1)	Mexiletine (0, 1)	Rosiglitazone (0, 1)
Cefamandole (0, 1)	Formestane (0, 1)	Minoxidil (1, 0)	Sodium stibogluconate
Cephalothin (1, 0)	G-CSF (filgrastim) (0, 1)	Mirtazapine (0, 1)	(0, 1)
Chlorpheniramine (0, 1)	Haloperidol (1, 0)	Morphine (0, 1)	Sulfadiazine (0, 1)
Chlorpromazine (1, 0)	Inamrinone (1, 0)	Naphazoline (1, 0)	Sulfamethoxazole (0, 1)
Ciprofloxacin (0, 1)	Indomethacin (0, 1)	Nimesulide (0, 1)	Sulfathiazole (1, 0)
Clarithromycin (0, 1)	Infliximab (0, 1)	Nitroglycerin (1, 0)	Suramin (0, 1)
Clopidogrel (0, 1)	Influenza vaccine (0, 1)	Novobiocin (1, 0)	Teicoplanin (1, 0)
Deferoxamine (1, 0)	Interferon 2b (0, 1)	Octreotide (1, 0)	Thiothixene (1, 0)
Desipramine (0, 1)	Iocetamic acid (0, 1)	Oxcarbazepine (0, 1)	Tiagabine (0, 1)
Diazepam (1, 0)	Iopamidol (0, 1)	Oxytetracycline (0, 1)	Tolmetin (1, 0)
Diazoxide (1, 0)	Iron dextran (0, 1)	Penicillamine (0, 1)	Tranilast (0, 1)
Diethylstilbestrol (1, 0)	Isoniazid (1, 0)		

CASES: 2 TO 4

Acetazolamide (1, 2)	Etretinate (0, 2)	Naproxen (0, 4)	Sulindac (0, 2)
Aminoglutethimide (2, 1)	Fluconazole (0, 2)	Oxaliplatin (0, 2)	Sulfamethoxypyridazine
Aminosalicylic acid (2, 1)	Glibenclamide (0, 2)	Oxprenolol (2, 1)	(0, 3)
Amphotericin b (2, 1)	Ibuprofen (0, 2)	Oxyphenbutazone (0, 2)	Sulfasalazine (1, 2)
Ampicillin (0, 2)	Indinavir (3, 0)	Phenytoin (0, 3)	Tamoxifen (2, 1)
Captopril (0, 2)	Interferon (0, 4)	Piperacillin (1, 1)	Terbinafine (0, 2)
Chlordiazepoxide (0, 2)	Iopanoic acid (1, 1)	Roxifiban (0, 2)	Ticlopidine (0, 3)
Chlorothiazide (1, 3)	Levamisole (2, 0)	Simvastatin (0, 2)	Trastuzumab (0, 2)
Digoxin (3, 0)	Meclofenamate (2, 0)	Sulfapyridine (0, 2)	Vancomycin (3, 0)
Ethambutol (1, 1)	Methicillin (2, 0)		

CASES: 5 TO 10

Abciximab c7e3 Fab (1, 6)	Danazol (3, 4)	Hydrochlorothiazide (0, 5)	Procainamide (0, 7)
Amiodarone (2, 0)	Diatrizoate meglumine/	Interferon-α (1, 6)	Ranitidine (0, 5)
Acetaminophen (3, 4)	diatrizoate sodium (3, 2)	Lotrafiban (0, 5)	Rifampin (5, 5)
Carbamazepine (0, 10)	Diclofenac (2, 3)	Methyldopa (3, 3)	Sulfisoxazole (1, 4)
Chlorpropamide (0, 5)	Efalizumab (Raptiva) (0, 6)	Nalidixic acid (1, 5)	Tirofiban (1, 6)
Cimetidine (1, 5)	Eptifibatide (0, 7)		

CASES: >10

Gold (0, 11)	Quinidine (26, 32)	Quinine (14, 9)	Sulfamethoxazole (3, 12)

G-CSF, granulocyte colony-stimulating factor.

Table of drugs that cause thrombocytopenia supported by one or more patient case reports with level I (definite) or level II (probable) clinical evidence. The table is broken down by the total number of single case reports with the individual number of level I cases and level II reports denoted in parentheses, respectively. The full list of articles reviewed, the methodology for establishing levels of evidence, and a complete updated database are available at www.ouhsc.edu/platelets/.

Data from www.ouhsc.edu/platelets/ditp.html.

TABLE 117–8. Mechanisms Underlying Drug-Induced Immune Thrombocytopenia

Classification	Mechanism	Incidence	Example
Hapten-dependent antibody	Hapten links covalently to membrane protein and induces drug-specific immune response	Very rare	Penicillin, possibly some cephalosporin antibiotics
Quinine-type drug	Drug induces antibody that binds to membrane protein in presence of soluble drug	26 cases per 1 million users of quinine per week; probably fewer cases with other drugs	Quinine, sulfonamide antibiotics, nonsteroidal antiinflammatory drugs
Fiban-type drug	Drug reacts with glycoprotein IIb/IIIa to induce a conformational change (neoepitope) recognized by antibody (not yet confirmed)	0.2–0.5%	Tirofiban, eptifibatide
Drug-specific antibody	Antibody recognizes murine component of chimeric Fab fragment specific for platelet membrane glycoprotein IIIa	0.5–1.0% after first exposure; 10–14% after seconds exposure	Abciximab
Autoantibody	Drug induces antibody that reacts with autologous platelets in absence of drug	1% with gold; very rare with procainamide and other drugs	Gold salts, procainamide
Immune complex	Drug binds to platelet factor 4, producing immune complex for which antibody is specific; immune complex activates platelets through Fc receptors	3–6% among patients treated with unfractionated heparin for 7 days; rare with low-molecular-weight heparin	Heparins

Reproduced with permission from Aster RH, Bougie DW. Drug-induced immune thrombocytopenia. *N Engl J Med* 2007 Aug 9;357(6):580–587.

antiplatelet antibodies.[434,435] Definition of the specific epitope involved in patient reactions with drug-dependent antibodies may not only elucidate the mechanism of drug-induced thrombocytopenia but also identify polymorphisms in GPIb-IX that cause sensitivity in producing drug-dependent antiplatelet antibodies. Sulfonamides, quinidine, and quinine are frequent causes of drug-induced thrombocytopenia. Studies of sera from 15 patients with thrombocytopenia caused by sulfamethoxazole or sulfisoxazole demonstrated that the antigenic epitope was part of integrin $\alpha_{IIb}\beta_3$.[436] Some antibodies from patients with quinidine- and quinine-dependent antiplatelet antibodies also react with integrin $\alpha_{IIb}\beta_3$.[437]

In addition to specificity for discrete epitopes on platelet surface GPs, drug-dependent antibodies are highly specific for the structure of the drug. For example, no cross-reactivity occurs between quinidine and quinine-dependent antibodies or between sulfamethoxazole and sulfisoxazole-dependent antibodies, even though both pairs of drugs have similar structures. Therefore, the neoantigens produced by drug binding to platelets create discrete epitopes that are sensitive to minor changes in drug structure.

The implications of this mechanism for platelet destruction are apparent. A patient with prior sensitivity to the drug has preformed antibodies that immediately react with the altered platelets upon repeat drug exposure, as demonstrated. An exception to this situation is the immediate acute thrombocytopenia that may occur with initial administration of antithrombotic agents that bind platelet integrin $\alpha_{IIb}\beta_3$,[42,438] especially abciximab. Abciximab is a humanized monoclonal antibody fragment that lacks the Fc domain, so thrombocytopenia is not caused by phagocytosis of the platelets by macrophages. Patients experiencing thrombocytopenia after receiving integrin $\alpha_{IIb}\beta_3$ inhibitors have been postulated to have preformed antibodies to epitopes exposed on the integrin by drug binding. These could be the same antibodies that cause *in vitro* EDTA-dependent platelet agglutination and pseudothrombocytopenia (see "Pseudo (Spurious) Thrombopenia" above).[33,439,440]

DIAGNOSIS

The diagnosis of drug-induced thrombocytopenia can be made only by recovery from thrombocytopenia upon discontinuation of the drug and can be confirmed if thrombocytopenia recurs with rechallenge by

the drug. Prompt recovery within 5 to 7 days is usual.[430] Gold-induced thrombocytopenia is an exception because gold salts are retained for long periods of time within the body and thrombocytopenia can persist for months, becoming indistinguishable from ITP.[441] Rechallenge with a suspected drug is dangerous, because severe thrombocytopenia can develop rapidly with even very small drug doses. However, when multiple drugs are potentially involved and all are important for management, it may be appropriate to reintroduce them individually, followed by several days of close observation. In general, the smallest possible dose of the drug should be administered. The administration should be performed under direct supervision of the patient, with platelets available for bleeding should it occur. If rechallenge leads to thrombocytopenia, the patient should be advised to wear a Medic Alert bracelet. For common drugs, especially those that can be purchased without a prescription, it may be safer to supervise a rechallenge and unequivocally document risk rather than risk future unintentional use.

Laboratory assays can detect drug-dependent antibodies, and positive results can support a clinical diagnosis. However, the laboratory role remains largely investigational because results are not promptly available when a clinical decision must be made about discontinuing a drug. Furthermore, no laboratory test has been validated that supports continuing a suspected drug with no adverse effects following a negative laboratory test.

Drug-dependent antibodies can be detected by flow cytometric techniques,[436] MAIPA,[442] and solid-phase red cell adherence assays.[443] Strongly positive tests are apparent, but distinction of positive from negative tests is arbitrary and not yet clinically validated. Positive tests for heparin-dependent antibodies have been reported in patients without thrombocytopenia,[444–446] and patients with clinical evidence for drug-induced thrombocytopenia may have negative tests using multiple techniques.[436,447]

CLINICAL AND LABORATORY FEATURES

In patients with newly discovered thrombocytopenia, all medications should be identified. Not only should the history explore use of prescription medications, use of nonprescription drugs should also be queried, including products containing acetaminophen,[430] and drinks that may contain quinine ("tonic water").[448,449] Drug-induced thrombocytopenia is typically severe. Among the 247 case reports with evidence for a definite or probable causal relation of the drug to thrombocytopenia, 23 patients (9 percent) had major bleeding, including two patients who died of bleeding,[430] and 68 patients (28 percent) had overt but minor bleeding; 96 patients (39 percent) had only purpura or trivial bleeding, and the remainder had no bleeding.[430] The time from beginning the drug to the initial occurrence of thrombocytopenia varies from 1 day to 3 years, but the median time is 14 days. With rechallenge, acute thrombocytopenia may occur within minutes but almost always within 3 days.[430] Patients may have other signs and symptoms of drug sensitivity, such as nausea and vomiting, rash, fever, and abnormal liver function tests.[450] Laboratory data may demonstrate leukopenia, indicating that the drug-dependent antibodies target multiple cell types.[450] Patients who have systemic adverse reactions to drugs manifesting as TTP or HUS are described in Chap. 133.

TREATMENT

Withdrawal of the offending drug is the most important therapeutic measure. Prednisone is commonly given because the distinction of drug-induced thrombocytopenia from ITP is almost never clear initially; however, glucocorticoids do not appear to speed recovery.[450] In patients with major bleeding, emergency treatment should be the same as for ITP: platelet transfusions, high doses of parenteral methylprednisolone, and possibly IVIG.[319]

REFERENCES

1. Morrell CN, Aggrey AA, Chapman LM, Modjesks KL: Emerging roles for platelets as immune and inflammatory cells. *Blood* 123:2759–2767, 2014.
2. Kaushansky K: Historical review: Megakaryopoiesis and thrombopoiesis. *Blood* 111:981–986, 2008.
3. Brubaker DB, Marcus C, Holmes E: Intravascular and total body platelet equilibrium in healthy volunteers and in thrombocytopenic patients transfused with single donor platelets. *Am J Hematol* 58:165–176, 1998.
4. Hill-Zobel RL, McCandless B, Kang SA, et al: Organ distribution and fate of human platelets: Studies of asplenic and splenomegalic patients. *Am J Hematol* 23:231–238, 1986.
5. Heyns AD, Lotter MG, Badenhorst PN, et al: Kinetics, distribution and sites of destruction of 111indium-labelled human platelets. *Br J Haematol* 44:269–280, 1980.
6. Heyns AD, Lotter MG, Badenhorst PN, et al: Kinetics and sites of destruction of 111Indium-oxine-labeled platelets in idiopathic thrombocytopenic purpura: A quantitative study. *Am J Hematol* 12:167–177, 1982.
7. Leissinger CA: Platelet kinetics in immune thrombocytopenic purpura and human immunodeficiency virus thrombocytopenia. *Curr Opin Hematol* 8:299–305, 2001.
8. Hanson SR, Slichter SJ: Platelet kinetics in patients with bone marrow hypoplasia: Evidence for a fixed platelet requirement. *Blood* 66:1105–1109, 1985.
9. Pearse BM: Receptors compete for adaptors found in plasma membrane coated pits. *EMBO J* 7:3331–3336, 1988.
10. Kile BT: The role of apoptosis in megakaryocytes and platelets. *Br J Haematol* 165:217–226, 2015.
11. Bain BJ: Ethnic and sex differences in the total and differential white cell count and platelet count. *J Clin Pathol* 49:664–666, 1996.
12. Lozano M, Narvaez J, Faundez A: Platelet count and mean platelet volume in the Spanish population. *Med Clin (Barc)* 110:774–777, 1998.
13. Stasi R, Amadori S, Osborn J, et al: Long-term outcome of otherwise healthy individuals with incidentally discovered borderline thrombocytopenia. *PLoS Med* 3:e24, 2006.
14. Buckley MF, James JW, Brown DE: A novel approach to the assessment of variations in human platelet count. *Thromb Haemost* 83:480–484, 2000.
15. Buttarello M, Plebani M: Automated blood cell counts: State of the art. *Am J Clin Pathol* 130:104–116, 2008.
16. Segal HC, Briggs C, Kunka S: Accuracy of platelet counting haematology analysers in severe thrombocytopenia and potential impact on platelet transfusion. *Br J Haematol* 128:520–525, 2005.
17. Salignac S, Latger-Cannard V, Schlegel N, Lecompte TP: Platelet. *Methods Mol Biol* 992:193–205, 2013.
18. Yoneyama A, Nakahara K: [EDTA-dependent pseudothrombocytopenia—Differentiation from true thrombocytopenia] [in Japanese]. *Nihon Rinsho* 61:569–574, 2003.
19. García Suárez J, Merino JL, Rodriguez M, et al: [Pseudothrombocytopenia: Incidence, causes and methods of detection] [in Spanish]. *Sangre (Barc)* 36:197–200, 1991.
20. Payne BA, Pierre RV: Pseudothrombocytopenia: A laboratory artifact with potentially serious consequences. *Mayo Clin Proc* 59:123–125, 1984.
21. Savage RA: Pseudoleukocytosis due to EDTA-induced platelet clumping. *Am J Clin Pathol* 81:317–322, 1984.
22. Vicari A, Banfi G, Bonini PA: EDTA-dependent pseudothrombocytopaenia: A 12-month epidemiological study. *Scand J Clin Lab Invest* 48:537–542, 1988.
23. Sweeney JD, Holme S, Heaton WA, et al: Pseudothrombocytopenia in plateletpheresis donors. *Transfusion* 35:46–49, 1995.
24. Bartels PC, Schoorl M, Lombarts AJ: Screening for EDTA-dependent deviations in platelet counts and abnormalities in platelet distribution histograms in pseudothrombocytopenia. *Scand J Clin Lab Invest* 57:629–636, 1997.
25. Bragagni G, Bianconcini G, Brogna R, Zoli G: [Pseudothrombocytopenia: Clinical comment on 37 cases] [in Italian]. *Minerva Med* 92:13–17, 2001.
26. Kurata Y, Hayashi S, Jouzaki K, et al: [Four cases of pseudothrombocytopenia due to platelet cold agglutinins] [in Japanese]. *Rinsho Ketsueki* 47:781–786, 2006.
27. Reed BW, Go RS: Pseudothrombocytopenia associated with multiple myeloma. *Mayo Clin Proc* 81:869, 2006.
28. Campbell V, Fosbury E, Bain BJ: Platelet phagocytosis as a cause of pseudothrombocytopenia. *Am J Hematol* 84:362, 2009.
29. Onder O, Weinstein A, Hoyer LW: Pseudothrombocytopenia caused by platelet agglutinins that are reactive in blood anticoagulated with chelating agents. *Blood* 56:177–182, 1980.
30. Bizzaro N: EDTA-dependent pseudothrombocytopenia: A clinical and epidemiological study of 112 cases, with 10-year follow-up. *Am J Hematol* 50:103–109, 1995.
31. Hoyt RH, Durie BG: Pseudothrombocytopenia induced by a monoclonal IgM kappa platelet agglutinin. *Am J Hematol* 31:50–52, 1989.
32. Bizzaro N, Goldschmeding R, von dem Borne AE. Platelet satellitism is Fc gamma RIII (CD16) receptor-mediated. *Am J Clin Pathol* 103:740–744, 1995.
33. Casonato A, Bertomoro A, Pontara E, et al: EDTA dependent pseudothrombocytopenia caused by antibodies against the cytoadhesive receptor of platelet gpIIB-IIIA. *J Clin Pathol* 47:625–630, 1994.
34. Nomura S, Nagata H, Oda K, et al: Effects of EDTA on the membrane glycoproteins IIb-IIIa complex—Analysis using flow cytometry. *Thromb Res* 47:47–58, 1987.
35. Schrezenmeier H, Muller H, Gunsilius E, et al: Anticoagulant-induced pseudothrombocytopenia and pseudoleucocytosis. *Thromb Haemost* 73:506–513, 1995.
36. Ryo R, Sugano W, Goto M, et al: Platelet release reaction during EDTA-induced platelet agglutinations and inhibition of EDTA-induced platelet agglutination by anti-glycoprotein II b/III a complex monoclonal antibody. *Thromb Res* 74:265–272, 1994.
37. Cohen AM, Lewinski UH, Klein B, Djaldetti M: Satellitism of platelets to monocytes. *Acta Haematol* 64:61–64, 1980.
38. Djaldetti M, Fishman P: Satellitism of platelets to monocytes in a patient with hypogammaglobulinaemia. *Scand J Haematol* 21:305–308, 1978.
39. Schell DA, Ganti AK, Levitt R, Potti A: Thrombocytopenia associated with c7E3 Fab (abciximab). *Ann Hematol* 81:76–79, 2002.
40. Sane DC, Damaraju LV, Topol EJ, et al: Occurrence and clinical significance of pseudothrombocytopenia during abciximab therapy. *J Am Coll Cardiol* 36:75–83, 2000.
41. Peters MN, Press CD, Moscona JC: Acute profound thrombocytopenia secondary to local abciximab infusion. *Proc (Bayl Univ Med Cent)* 25:346–348, 2012.
42. Berkowitz SD, Sane DC, Sigmon KN, et al: Occurrence and clinical significance of thrombocytopenia in a population undergoing high-risk percutaneous coronary revascularization. Evaluation of c7E3 for the Prevention of Ischemic Complications (EPIC) Study Group. *J Am Coll Cardiol* 32:311–319, 1998.
43. Berkman N, Michaeli Y, Or R, Eldor A: EDTA-dependent pseudothrombocytopenia: A clinical study of 18 patients and a review of the literature. *Am J Hematol* 36:195–201, 1991.
44. Mori M, Kudo H, Yoshitake S, et al: Transient EDTA-dependent pseudothrombocytopenia in a patient with sepsis. *Intensive Care Med* 26:218–220, 2000.
45. Bizzaro N, Fiorin F: Coexistence of erythrocyte agglutination and EDTA-dependent platelet clumping in a patient with thymoma and plasmocytoma. *Arch Pathol Lab Med* 123:159–162, 1999.
46. Matarazzo M, Conturso V, Di MM, et al: EDTA-dependent pseudothrombocytopenia in a case of liver cirrhosis. *Panminerva Med* 42:155–157, 2000.
47. Recommended methods for radioisotope platelet survival studies: By the panel on Diagnostic Application of Radioisotopes in Hematology, International Committee for Standardization in Hematology. *Blood* 50:1137–1144, 1977.
48. Chiurazzi F, Villa MR, Rotoli B: Transplacental transmission of EDTA-dependent pseudothrombocytopenia. *Haematologica* 84:664, 1999.
49. Kortering JJ, Boersma B, Schoorl M, et al: Pseudothrombocytopenia in a neonate due to mother? *Eur J Pediatr* 172:987–989, 2013.
50. Solanki DL, Blackburn BC: Spurious thrombocytopenia during pregnancy. *Obstet Gynecol* 65:14S–17S, 1985.
51. Diz-Kucukkaya R: Inherited platelet disorders including Glanzmann thrombasthenia and Bernard-Soulier syndrome. *Hematology Am Soc Hematol Educ Program* 2013:275, 2013.
52. Bunimov N, Fuller N, Hayward CP: Genetic loci associated with platelet traits and platelet disorders. *Semin Thromb Hemost* 39:291–305, 2013.
53. Watson SP, Lowe GC, Lordkipanidze M, Morgan NY: Genotyping and phenotyping of platelet function disorders. *J Thromb Haemost* 2013:351–363, 2013.
54. Diz-Kucukkaya R, López JA: Inherited disorders of platelets: Membrane glycoprotein disorders. *Hematol Oncol Clin North Am* 27:613–627, 2013.
55. Gresele P: Diagnosis of inherited platelet function disorders: Guidance from the SSC of the ISTH. *J Thromb Haemost* 13:314–322, 2015.

56. Balduini CL, Pecci A, Noris P: Diagnosis and management of inherited thrombocytopenias. *Semin Thromb Hemost* 39:161–171, 2015.

57. Harrison P, Mackie I, Mumford A, et al: Guidelines for the laboratory investigation of heritable disorders of platelet function. *Br J Haematol* 155:30–44, 2011.

58. Sandoval C, Berger E, Ozkaynak MF: Severe iron deficiency anemia in forty-two pediatric patients. *Pediatr Hematol Oncol* 19:157–161, 2002.

59. Kadikoylu G, Yavasoglu I, Bolaman Z, Senturk T: Platelet parameters in women with iron deficiency anemia. *J Natl Med Assoc* 98:398–402, 2006.

60. Stabler SP, Allen RH, Savage DG, Lindenbaum J: Clinical spectrum and diagnosis of cobalamin deficiency. *Blood* 76:871–881, 1990.

61. Sarode R, Garewal G, Marwaha N, et al: Pancytopenia in nutritional megaloblastic anaemia. A study from north-west India. *Trop Geogr Med* 41:331–336, 1989.

62. Slichter SJ, Harker LA: Thrombocytopenia: Mechanisms and management of defects in platelet production. *Clin Haematol* 7:523–539, 1978.

63. Epstein RD: Cells of the megakaryocyte series in pernicious anemia; in particular, the effect of specific therapy. *Am J Pathol* 25:239–251, 1949.

64. Rabinowitz AP, Sacks Y, Carmel R: Autoimmune cytopenias in pernicious anemia: A report of four cases and review of the literature. *Eur J Haematol* 44:18–23, 1990.

65. Junca J, Flores A, Granada ML, et al: The relationship between idiopathic thrombocytopenic purpura and pernicious anaemia. *Br J Haematol* 111:513–516, 2000.

66. Dittmar M, Kahaly GJ: Polyglandular autoimmune syndromes: Immunogenetics and long-term follow-up. *J Clin Endocrinol Metab* 88:2983–2992, 2003.

67. Ingeberg S, Stoffersen E: Platelet dysfunction in patients with vitamin B_{12} deficiency. *Acta Haematol* 61:75–79, 1979.

68. Terade H, Niikura H, Mori H, et al: [Megaloblastic anemia and platelet function—a qualitative platelet defect in pernicious anemia] [in Japanese]. *Rinsho Ketsueki* 31:254–255, 1990.

69. Green P: Anemias beyond B_{12} and iron deficiency: The buzz about other B's elementary, and nonelementary problems. *Hematology Am Soc Hematol Educ Program* 2012:498, 2012.

70. Agnotti LB, Post GR, Robinson NS, et al: Pancytopenia with myelodysplasia due to copper deficiency. *Pediatr Blood Cancer* 51:693–695, 2008.

71. Ballard HS: The hematological complications of alcoholism. *Alcohol Health Res World* 21:45–52, 2015.

72. Haselager EM, Vreeken J: Rebound thrombocytosis after alcohol abuse: A possible factor in the pathogenesis of thromboembolic disease. *Lancet* 1:774–775, 1977.

73. Ballard HS: The hematological complications of alcoholism. *Alcohol Health Res World* 21:42–52, 2015.

74. Michot F, Gut J: Alcohol-induced bone marrow damage. A bone marrow study in alcohol-dependent individuals. *Acta Haematol* 78:252–257, 1987.

75. Latvala J, Parkkila S, Niemela O: Excess alcohol consumption is common in patients with cytopenia: Studies in blood and bone marrow cells. *Alcohol Clin Exp Res* 28:619–624, 2004.

76. Sullivan LW, Adams WH, Liu YK: Induction of thrombocytopenia by thrombopheresis in man: Patterns of recovery in normal subjects during ethanol ingestion and abstinence. *Blood* 49:197–207, 1977.

77. Smith CM, Tobin JD Jr, Burris SM, White JG: Alcohol consumption in the guinea pig is associated with reduced megakaryocyte deformability and platelet size. *J Lab Clin Med* 120:699–706, 1992.

78. Wolber EM, Jelkmann W: Thrombopoietin: The novel hepatic hormone. *News Physiol Sci* 17:6–10, 2002.

79. Hoffman R: Acquired pure amegakaryocytic thrombocytopenic purpura. *Semin Hematol* 28:303–312, 1991.

80. Antonijevic N, Terzic T, Jovanovic V, et al: [Acquired amegakaryocytic thrombocytopenia: Three case reports and a literature review] [in Serbian]. *Med Pregl* 57:292–297, 2004.

81. Dewulf G, Gouin I, Pautas E, et al: [Myelodisplasic syndromes diagnosed in a geriatric hospital: Morphological profile in 100 patients]. *Ann Biol Clin (Paris)* 62:197–202, 2004.

82. Rochant H: [Myelodysplastic syndromes: Unusual and mild forms] [in French]. *Pathol Biol (Paris)* 45:579–586, 1997.

83. Kini J, Khadilkar UN, Dayal JP: A study of the haematologic spectrum of myelodysplastic syndrome. *Indian J Pathol Microbiol* 44:9–12, 2001.

84. Nand S, Godwin JE: Hypoplastic myelodysplastic syndrome. *Cancer* 62:958–964, 1988.

85. Zafar T, Yasin F, Anwar M, Saleem M: Acquired amegakaryocytic thrombocytopenic purpura (AATP): A hospital based study. *J Pak Med Assoc* 49:114–117, 1999.

86. Nagasawa T, Sakurai T, Kashiwagi H, Abe T: Cell-mediated amegakaryocytic thrombocytopenia associated with systemic lupus erythematosus. *Blood* 67:479–483, 1986.

87. Slater LM, Katz J, Walter B, Armentrout SA: Aplastic anemia occurring as amegakaryocytic thrombocytopenia with and without an inhibitor of granulopoiesis. *Am J Hematol* 18:251–254, 1985.

88. Shiozaki H, Miyawaki S, Kuwaki T, et al: Autoantibodies neutralizing thrombopoietin in a patient with amegakaryocytic thrombocytopenic purpura. *Blood* 95:2187–2188, 2000.

89. Katsumata Y, Suzuki T, Kuwana M, et al: Anti-c-Mpl (thrombopoietin receptor) autoantibody-induced amegakaryocytic thrombocytopenia in a patient with systemic sclerosis. *Arthritis Rheum* 48:1647–1651, 2003.

90. Leach JW, Hussein KK, George JN: Acquired pure megakaryocytic aplasia report of two cases with long-term responses to antithymocyte globulin and cyclosporine. *Am J Hematol* 62:115–117, 1999.

91. Lusher JM, Iyer R: Idiopathic thrombocytopenic purpura in children. *Semin Thromb Hemost* 3:175–199, 1977.

92. Stasi R, Newland AC: ITP: A historical perspective. *Br J Haematol* 153:450, 2011.

93. Frank E: Die essentielle Thrombopenie (Konstitutionelle Purpura-Pseudoha mophilie). *Berl Klin Wochenschr* 52:454, 1915.

94. Dameshek W, Miller EB: The megakaryocytes in idiopathic thrombocytopenic purpura, a form of hypersplenism. *Blood* 1:27–50, 1946.

95. Harrington WJ, Minnich V, Hollingsworth JW, Moore CV: Demonstration of a thrombocytopenic factor in the blood of patients with thrombocytopenic purpura. *J Lab Clin Med* 38:1–10, 1951.

96. Altman LK: Black and blue at the flick of a feather, in *Who goes first?*, pp 273–282. Random House, New York, 1987.

97. Shulman NR, Weinrach RS, Libre EP, Andrews HL: The role of the reticuloendothelial system in the pathogenesis of idiopathic thrombocytopenic purpura. *Trans Assoc Am Physicians* 78:374–390, 1965.

98. McMillan R, Smith RS, Longmire RL, et al: Immunoglobulins associated with human platelets. *Blood* 37:316–322, 1971.

99. Dixon R, Rosse W, Ebbert L: Quantitative determination of antibody in idiopathic thrombocytopenic purpura. Correlation of serum and platelet-bound antibody with clinical response. *N Engl J Med* 292:230–236, 1975.

100. van Leeuwen EF, van der Ven JT, Engelfriet CP, von dem Borne AE: Specificity of autoantibodies in autoimmune thrombocytopenia. *Blood* 59:23–26, 1982.

101. McMillan R, Tani P, Millard F, et al: Platelet-associated and plasma anti-glycoprotein autoantibodies in chronic ITP. *Blood* 70:1040–1045, 1987.

102. Kiefel V, Santoso S, Weisheit M, Mueller-Eckhardt C: Monoclonal antibody–specific immobilization of platelet antigens (MAIPA): A new tool for the identification of platelet-reactive antibodies. *Blood* 70:1722–1726, 1987.

103. Kiefel V, Santoso S, Kaufmann E, Mueller-Eckhardt C: Autoantibodies against platelet glycoprotein Ib/IX: A frequent finding in autoimmune thrombocytopenic purpura. *Br J Haematol* 79:256–262, 1991.

104. He R, Reid DM, Jones CE, Shulman NR: Spectrum of Ig classes, specificities, and titers of serum antiglycoproteins in chronic idiopathic thrombocytopenic purpura. *Blood* 83:1024–1032, 1994.

105. Mueller-Eckhardt C, Mueller-Eckhardt G, Kayser W, et al: Platelet associated IgG, platelet survival, and platelet sequestration in thrombocytopenic states. *Br J Haematol* 52:49–58, 1982.

106. Kelton JG, Powers PJ, Carter CJ: A prospective study of the usefulness of the measurement of platelet-associated IgG for the diagnosis of idiopathic thrombocytopenic purpura. *Blood* 60:1050–1053, 1982.

107. McMillan R: Autoantibodies and autoantigens in chronic immune thrombocytopenic purpura. *Semin Hematol* 37:239–248, 2000.

108. Cines DB, Blanchette VS: Immune thrombocytopenic purpura. *N Engl J Med* 346:995–1008, 2002.

109. Imbach P, Barandun S, d'Apuzzo V, et al: High-dose intravenous gammaglobulin for idiopathic thrombocytopenic purpura in childhood. *Lancet* 1:1228–1231, 1981.

110. Hymes K, Schur PH, Karpatkin S: Heavy-chain subclass of round antiplatelet IgG in autoimmune thrombocytopenic purpura. *Blood* 56:84–87, 1980.

111. van der HD, de Jong D, Limpens J, et al: Clonal B-cell populations in patients with idiopathic thrombocytopenic purpura. *Blood* 76:2321–2326, 1990.

112. Maguire RB, Stroncek DF, Campbell AC: Recurrent pancytopenia, coagulopathy, and renal failure associated with multiple quinine-dependent antibodies. *Ann Intern Med* 119:215–217, 1993.

113. Liu B, Zhao H, Poon MD: Abnormality of CD4(+)CD25(+) regulatory T cells in idiopathic thrombocytopenic purpura. *Eur J Haematol* 78:139–143, 2007.

114. Stasi R, Pagano A, Stipa E, Amadori S: Rituximab chimeric anti-CD20 monoclonal antibody treatment for adults with chronic idiopathic thrombocytopenic purpura. *Blood* 98:952–957, 2001.

115. McKenzie CG, Guo L, Freedman J, Semple JW: Cellular immune dysfunction in immune thrombocytopenia (ITP). *Br J Haematol* 163:10–23, 2013.

116. Zhang F, Chu X, Wang L, et al: Cell-mediated lysis of autologous platelets in chronic idiopathic thrombocytopenic purpura. *Eur J Haematol* 76:427–431, 2006.

117. Li S, Wang L, Zhao C, et al: CD8+ T cells suppress autologous megakaryocyte apoptosis in idiopathic thrombocytopenic purpura. *Br J Haematol* 139:605–611, 2007.

118. Hauch TW, Rosse WF: Platelet-bound complement (C3) in immune thrombocytopenia. *Blood* 50:1129–1136, 1977.

119. Kurata Y, Curd JG, Tamerius JD, McMillan R: Platelet-associated complement in chronic ITP. *Br J Haematol* 60:723–733, 1985.

120. Tsubakio T, Tani P, Curd JG, McMillan R: Complement activation in vitro by antiplatelet antibodies in chronic immune thrombocytopenic purpura. *Br J Haematol* 63:293–300, 1986.

121. Verschoor A, Langer HF: Crosstalk between platelets and the complement system in immune protection and disease. *Thromb Haemost* 110:910–919, 2013.

122. Aster RH, Keene WR: Sites of platelet destruction in idiopathic thrombocytopenic purpura. *Br J Haematol* 16:61–73, 1969.

123. Ballem PJ, Segal GM, Stratton JR, et al: Mechanisms of thrombocytopenia in chronic autoimmune thrombocytopenic purpura. Evidence of both impaired platelet production and increased platelet clearance. *J Clin Invest* 80:33–40, 1987.

124. Chang M, Nakagawa PA, Williams SA, et al: Immune thrombocytopenic purpura (ITP) plasma and purified ITP monoclonal autoantibodies inhibit megakaryocytopoiesis *in vitro*. *Blood* 102:887–895, 2003.

125. Takahashi R, Sekine N, Nakatake T: Influence of monoclonal antiplatelet glycoprotein antibodies on *in vitro* human megakaryocyte colony formation and proplatelet formation. *Blood* 93:1951–1958, 1999.

126. Kelemen E, Cserhati I, Tanos B: Demonstration and some properties of human thrombopoietin in thrombocythaemic sera. *Acta Haematol* 20:350–355, 1958.

127. Kuter DJ: Milestones in understanding platelet production: A historical overview. *Br J Haematol* 165:248–258, 2015.

128. Kaushansky K: Thrombopoietin: The primary regulator of megakaryocyte and platelet production. *Thromb Haemost* 74:521–525, 1995.

129. Chang M, Qian JX, Lee SM, et al: Tissue uptake of circulating thrombopoietin is increased in immune-mediated compared with irradiated thrombocytopenic mice. *Blood* 93:2515–2524, 1999.

130. Kosugi S, Kurata Y, Tomiyama Y, et al: Circulating thrombopoietin level in chronic immune thrombocytopenic purpura. *Br J Haematol* 93:704–706, 1996.

131. Kuter DJ: Thrombopoietin and thrombopoietin mimetics in the treatment of thrombocytopenia. *Annu Rev Med* 60:193–206, 2009.

132. Porcelijn L, Folman CC, Bossers B, et al: The diagnostic value of thrombopoietin level measurements in thrombocytopenia. *Thromb Haemost* 79:1101–1105, 1998.

133. Gouin-Thibault I, Cassinat B, Chomienne C, et al: Is the thrombopoietin assay useful for differential diagnosis of thrombocytopenia? Analysis of a cohort of 160 patients with thrombocytopenia and defined platelet life span. *Clin Chem* 47:1660–1665, 2001.

134. Kuter DJ, Bussel JB, Lyons RM, et al: Efficacy of romiplostim in patients with chronic immune thrombocytopenic purpura: A double-blind randomised controlled trial. *Lancet* 371:395–403, 2008.

135. Psaila B, Bussel JB: Refractory immune thrombocytopenic purpura: Current strategies for investigation and management. *Br J Haematol* 143:16–26, 2008.

136. Bussel JB, Kuter DJ, Aledort LM: A randomized trial of avatrombopag, an investigational thrombopoietin-receptor agonist, in persistent and chronic immune thrombocytopenia. *Blood* 123:3887–3897, 2014.

137. Laster AJ, Conley CL, Kickler TS, et al: Chronic immune thrombocytopenic purpura in monozygotic twins: Genetic factors predisposing to ITP. *N Engl J Med* 307:1495–1498, 1982.

138. Bizzaro N: Familial association of autoimmune thrombocytopenia and hyperthyroidism. *Am J Hematol* 39:294–298, 1992.

139. Karpatkin S, Fotino M, Winchester R: Hereditary autoimmune thrombocytopenic purpura: An immunologic and genetic study. *Ann Intern Med* 94:781–782, 1981.

140. Stanworth SJ, Turner DM, Brown J, et al: Major histocompatibility complex susceptibility genes and immune thrombocytopenic purpura in Caucasian adults. *Hematology* 7:119–121, 2002.

141. Evers KG, Thouet R, Haase W, Kruger J: HLA frequencies and haplotypes in children with idiopathic thrombocytopenic purpura (ITP). *Eur J Pediatr* 129:267–272, 1978.

142. Pavkovic M, Georgievski B, Cevreska L, et al: CTLA-4 exon 1 polymorphism in patients with autoimmune blood disorders. *Am J Hematol* 72:147–149, 2003.

143. Foster CB, Zhu S, Erichsen HC, et al: Polymorphisms in inflammatory cytokines and Fcgamma receptors in childhood chronic immune thrombocytopenic purpura: A pilot study. *Br J Haematol* 113:596–599, 2001.

144. George JN, Woolf SH, Raskob GE, et al: Idiopathic thrombocytopenic purpura: A practice guideline developed by explicit methods for the American Society of Hematology. *Blood* 88:3–40, 1996.

145. Guidelines for the investigation and management of idiopathic thrombocytopenic purpura in adults, children and in pregnancy. *Br J Haematol* 120:574–596, 2003.

146. Rodeghiero F, Stasi R, Gernsheimer T, et al: Standardization of terminology, definitions and outcome criteria in immune thrombocytopenic purpura of adults and children: Report from an international working group. *Blood* 113:2386–2393, 2009.

147. Provan D, Stasi R, Newland AC, et al: International consensus report on the investigation and management of primary immune thrombocytopenia. *Blood* 115:168–186, 2010.

148. Neunert C, Lim W, Crowther M, et al: The American Society of Hematology 2011 evidence-based practice guideline for immune thrombocytopenia. *Blood* 117:4190–4207, 2011.

149. Schoonen WM, Kucera G, Coalson J, et al: Epidemiology of immune thrombocytopenic purpura in the General Practice Research Database. *Br J Haematol* 145:235–244, 2009.

150. Cortelazzo S, Finazzi G, Buelli M, et al: High risk of severe bleeding in aged patients with chronic idiopathic thrombocytopenic purpura. *Blood* 77:31–33, 1991.

151. Frederiksen H, Schmidt K: The incidence of idiopathic thrombocytopenic purpura in adults increases with age. *Blood* 94:909–913, 1999.

152. George JN, el-Harake MA, Raskob GE: Chronic idiopathic thrombocytopenic purpura. *N Engl J Med* 331:1207–1211, 1994.

153. McMillan R: Therapy for adults with refractory chronic immune thrombocytopenic purpura. *Ann Intern Med* 126:307–314, 1997.

154. Schattner E, Bussel J: Mortality in immune thrombocytopenic purpura: Report of seven cases and consideration of prognostic indicators. *Am J Hematol* 46:120–126, 1994.

155. Portielje JE, Ewstentdorp RG, Kluin-Nelemans HC: Morbidity and mortality in adults with idiopathic thrombocytopenic purpura. *Blood* 97:2549–2554, 2001.

156. McIntyre OR, Ebaugh FG Jr: Palpable spleens in college freshmen. *Ann Intern Med* 66:301–306, 1967.

157. Newton JL, Reese JA, Watson SI, et al: Fatigue in adult patients with primary immune thrombocytopenia. *Eur J Haematol* 86:420–429, 2011.

158. Blankenship JC, Tasissa G, O'Shea JC, et al: Effect of glycoprotein IIb/IIIa receptor inhibition on angiographic complications during percutaneous coronary intervention in the ESPRIT trial. *J Am Coll Cardiol* 38:653–658, 2001.

159. Sarpatwari A, Bennett D, Logie JW, et al: Thromboembolic events among adult patients with primary immune thrombocytopenia in the United Kingdom General Practice Research Database. *Haematologica* 95:1167–1175, 2010.

160. Ruggeri M, Tosetto A, Palandri F, et al: Thrombotic risk in patients with primary immune thrombocytopenia is only mildly increased and explained by personal and treatment-related risk factors. *J Thromb Haemost* 12:1266–1273, 2014.

161. Burstein SA, Downs T, Friese P, et al: Thrombocytopoiesis in normal and sublethally irradiated dogs: Response to human interleukin-6. *Blood* 80:420–428, 1992.

162. Khan I, Zucker-Franklin D, Karpatkin S: Microthrombocytosis and platelet fragmentation associated with idiopathic/autoimmune thrombocytopenic purpura. *Br J Haematol* 31:449–460, 1975.

163. Lopez JA, Andrews RK, Afshar-Kharghan V, Berndt MC: Bernard-Soulier syndrome. *Blood* 91:4397–4418, 1998.

164. Rodgers RP, Levin J: A critical reappraisal of the bleeding time. *Semin Thromb Hemost* 16:1–20, 1990.

165. Hughes M, Webert K, Kelton JG: The use of electron microscopy in the investigation of the ultrastructural morphology of immune thrombocytopenic purpura platelets. *Semin Hematol* 37:222–228, 2000.

166. Evans RS, Takahashi K, Duane RT, et al: Primary thrombocytopenic purpura and acquired hemolytic anemia; evidence for a common etiology. AMA. *Arch Intern Med* 87:48–65, 1951.

167. Stasi R, Stipa E, Masi M, et al: Long-term observation of 208 adults with chronic idiopathic thrombocytopenic purpura. *Am J Med* 98:436–442, 1995.

168. Sailer T, Lechner K, Panzer S, et al: The course of severe autoimmune thrombocytopenia in patients not undergoing splenectomy. *Haematologica* 91:1041–1045, 2006.

169. George JN, Raskob GE: Idiopathic thrombocytopenic purpura: Diagnosis and management. *Am J Med Sci* 316:87–93, 1998.

170. Baumann MA, Menitove JE, Aster RH, Anderson T: Urgent treatment of idiopathic thrombocytopenic purpura with single-dose gammaglobulin infusion followed by platelet transfusion. *Ann Intern Med* 104:808–809, 1986.

171. Larsen OH, Stentoft J, Radia D, et al: Combination of recombinant factor VIIa and fibrinogen corrects clot formation in primary immune thrombocytopenia at very low platelet counts. *Br J Haematol* 160:228–236, 2013.

172. Salama A, Rieke M, Kiesewetter H, von Depka H: Experiences with recombinant FVIIa in the emergency treatment of patients with autoimmune thrombocytopenia: A review of the literature. *Ann Hematol* 88:11–15, 2009.

173. Wanachiwanawin W, Piankijagum A, Sindhvananda K, et al: Emergency splenectomy in adult idiopathic thrombocytopenic purpura. A report of seven cases. *Arch Intern Med* 149:217–219, 1989.

174. Gernsheimer T, Stratton J, Ballem PJ, Slichter SJ: Mechanisms of response to treatment in autoimmune thrombocytopenic purpura. *N Engl J Med* 320:974–980, 1989.

175. Bussel JB: Fc receptor blockade and immune thrombocytopenic purpura. *Semin Hematol* 37:261–266, 2000.

176. Kitchens CS: Amelioration of endothelial abnormalities by prednisone in experimental thrombocytopenia in the rabbit. *J Clin Invest* 60:1129–1134, 1977.

177. George JN, Woolf SH, Raskob GE: Idiopathic thrombocytopenic purpura: A guideline for diagnosis and management of children and adults. American Society of Hematology. *Ann Med* 30:38–44, 1998.

178. George JN, Vesely SK: Immune thrombocytopenic purpura—Let the treatment fit the patient. *N Engl J Med* 349:903–905, 2003.

179. Mazzucconi MG, Francesconi M, Fidani P, et al: Treatment of idiopathic thrombocytopenic purpura (ITP): Results of a multicentric protocol. *Haematologica* 70:329–336, 1985.

180. Bellucci S, Charpak Y, Chastang C, Tobelem G: Low doses v conventional doses of corticoids in immune thrombocytopenic purpura (ITP): Results of a randomized clinical trial in 160 children, 223 adults. *Blood* 71:1165–1169, 1988.

181. Ozsoylu S, Irken G, Karabent A: High-dose intravenous methylprednisolone for acute childhood idiopathic thrombocytopenic purpura. *Eur J Haematol* 42:431–435, 1989.

182. Ozsoylu S, Sayli TR, Ozturk G: Oral megadose methylprednisolone versus intravenous immunoglobulin for acute childhood idiopathic thrombocytopenic purpura. *Pediatr Hematol Oncol* 10:317–321, 1993.

183. Albayrak D, Islek I, Kalayci AG, Gurses N: Acute immune thrombocytopenic purpura: A comparative study of very high oral doses of methylprednisolone and intravenously administered immune globulin. *J Pediatr* 125:1004–1007, 1994.

184. Cheng Y, Wong RS, Soo YO, et al: Initial treatment of immune thrombocytopenic purpura with high-dose dexamethasone. *N Engl J Med* 349:831–836, 2003.

185. Stasi R, Brunetti M, Pagano A: Pulsed intravenous high-dose dexamethasone in adults with chronic idiopathic thrombocytopenic purpura. *Blood Cells Mol Dis* 26:582–586, 2000.

186. Mazzucconi MG, Fazi P, Bernasconi S: Therapy with high dose dexamethasone (HD-DXM) in previously untreated patients affected by idiopathic thrombocytopenic purpura: A GIMEMA experience. *Blood* 109:1401–1407, 2007.

187. Alpdogan O, Budak-Alpdogan T, Ratip S: Efficacy of high-dose methylprednisolone as a first-line therapy in adult patients with idiopathic thrombocytopenic purpura. *Br J Haematol* 103:1061–1063, 1998.

188. Bell WR Jr: Long-term outcome of splenectomy for idiopathic thrombocytopenic purpura. *Semin Hematol* 37:22–25, 2000.

189. Kojouri K, Vesely SK, Terrell DR, George JN: Splenectomy for adult patients with idiopathic thrombocytopenic purpura: A systemic review to assess long-term platelet count responses, prediction of response, and surgical complications. *Blood* 104:2623–2635, 2004.

190. Mikhael J, Northridge K, Lindquist K, et al: Short-term and long-term failure of laparoscopic splenectomy in adult immune thrombocytopenic purpura patients: A systematic review. *Am J Hematol* 84:743–748, 2009.

191. Ghanima W, Godeau B, Cines DB, Bussel JB: How I treat immune thrombocytopenia: The choice between splenectomy or a medical therapy as a second-line treatment. *Blood* 120:960–969, 2012.

192. Najean Y, Rain JD, Billotey C: The site of destruction of autologous 111In-labelled platelets and the efficiency of splenectomy in children and adults with idiopathic thrombocytopenic purpura: A study of 578 patients with 268 splenectomies. *Br J Haematol* 97:547–550, 1997.

193. Pizzuto J, Ambriz R: Therapeutic experience on 934 adults with idiopathic thrombocytopenic purpura: Multicentric Trial of the Cooperative Latin American group on Hemostasis and Thrombosis. *Blood* 64:1179–1183, 1984.

194. Dolan JP, Sheppard BC, DeLoughery TG: Splenectomy for immune thrombocytopenic purpura: Surgery for the 21st century. *Am J Hematol* 83:93–96, 2007.

195. Lortan JE: Management of asplenic patients. *Br J Haematol* 84:566–569, 1993.

196. Atkinson WL, Pickering LK, Schwartz B, et al: General recommendations on immunization. Recommendations of the Advisory Committee on Immunization Practices (ACIP) and the American Academy of Family Physicians (AAFP). *MMWR Recomm Rep* 51:1–35, 2002.

197. Boyle S, White RH, Brunson A, Wun T: Splenectomy and the incidence of venous thromboembolism and sepsis in patients with immune thrombocytopenia. *Blood* 121:4782–4790, 2015.

198. Naouri A, Feghali B, Chabal J: Results for splenectomy for idiopathic thrombocytopenic purpura. *Acta Haematol* 89:200–203, 1993.

199. Newland AC, Treleaven JG, Minchinton RM, Waters AH: High-dose intravenous IgG in adults with autoimmune thrombocytopenia. *Lancet* 15:84–87, 1983.

200. Berchtold P, Dale GL, Tani P, McMillan R: Inhibition of autoantibody binding to platelet glycoprotein IIb/IIIa by anti-idiotypic antibodies in intravenous gammaglobulin. *Blood* 74:2414–2417, 1989.

201. Ramamurthi A, Lewis RS: Design of a novel apparatus to study nitric oxide (NO) inhibition of platelet adhesion. *Ann Biomed Eng* 26:1036–1043, 1998.

202. Imbach P: 30 Years of immunomodulation by intravenous immunoglobulin. *Immunotherapy* 4:651–654, 2011.

203. Bussel JB, Pham LC, Aledort L, Nachman R: Maintenance treatment of adults with chronic refractory immune thrombocytopenic purpura using repeated intravenous infusions of gammaglobulin. *Blood* 72:121–127, 1988.

204. Hong F, Ruiz R, Price H, et al: Safety profile of WinRho anti-D. *Semin Hematol* 35:9–13, 1998.

205. Ware RE, Zimmerman SA: Anti-D: Mechanisms of action. *Semin Hematol* 35:14–22, 1998.

206. Crow AR, Lazarus AH: The mechanisms of action of intravenous immunoglobulin and polyclonal anti-d immunoglobulin in the amelioration of immune thrombocytopenic purpura: What do we really know? *Transfus Med Rev* 22:103–116, 2008.

207. Despotovic J, Lambert MP, Herman J: RhIg for the treatment of immuno thrombocytopenia: Consensus and controversy. *Transfusion* 52:1126–1136, 2012.

208. Scaradavou A, Woo B, Woloski BM, et al: Intravenous anti-D treatment of immune thrombocytopenic purpura: Experience in 272 patients. *Blood* 89:2689–2700, 1997.

209. George JN, Raskob GE, Vesely SK, et al: Initial management of immune thrombocytopenic purpura in adults: A randomized controlled trial comparing intermittent anti-D with routine care. *Am J Hematol* 74:161–169, 2003.

210. Johnson GJ: Platelet thromboxane receptors: Biology and function, in *Handbook of Platelet Physiology and Pharmacology*, edited by G Rao, pp 38–79. Kluwer Academic, Boston, 1999.

211. Waintraub SE, Brody JI: Use of anti-D in immune thrombocytopenic purpura as a means to prevent splenectomy: Case reports from two University Hospital Medical Centers. *Semin Hematol* 37:45–49, 2000.

212. Marcus AJ: Transcellular metabolism of eicosanoids. *Prog Hemost Thromb* 8:127–142, 1986.

213. Narang M, Penner JA, Williams D: Refractory autoimmune thrombocytopenic purpura: Responses to treatment with a recombinant antibody to lymphocyte membrane antigen CD20 (rituximab). *Am J Hematol* 74:263–267, 2003.

214. Cooper N, Stasi R, Cunningham-Rundles S, et al: The efficacy and safety of B-cell depletion with anti-CD20 monoclonal antibody in adults with chronic immune thrombocytopenic purpura. *Br J Haematol* 125:232–239, 2004.

215. Arnold DM, Dentali F, Crowther MA, et al: Systematic review: Efficacy and safety of rituximab for adults with idiopathic thrombocytopenic purpura. *Ann Intern Med* 146:25–33, 2007.

216. Garvey B: Rituximab in the treatment of autoimmune haematological disorders. *Br J Haematol* 141:149–169, 2008.

217. Stasi R: Rituximab in autoimmune hematologic disease: Not just a matter of B cells. *Semin Hematol* 47:170–179, 2010.

218. Zaja F, Battista ML, Pirrotta MT: Lower dose rituximab is active in adult patients with idiopathic thrombocytopenic purpura. *Haematologica* 93:930–933, 2008.

219. Godeau B: B-cell depletion in immuno thrombocytopenia. *Semin Hematol* 50:S75–S82, 2013.

220. Hasan A, Michel M, Patel V: Repeated courses of rituximab in chronic ITP: Three different regimens. *Am J Hematol* 84:661–665, 2010.

221. Cooper N, Stasi R, Cunningham-Rundles S: Platelet-associated antibodies, cellular immunity and FCGR3a genotype influence the response to rituximab in immune thrombocytopenia. *Br J Haematol* 158:539–547, 2012.

222. Mahevas M, Patin P, Huetz F: B cell deletion in immuno thrombocytopenia reveals splenic long-lived plasma cells. *J Clin Invest* 123:432–442, 2013.

223. Tsutsumi Y, Yamamoto Y, Shimono Y, et al: Hepatitis B virus reactivation with rituximab-containing regimen. *World J Hepatol* 5:612–620, 2013.

224. Siegal D, Crowther M, Cuker A: Thrombopoietin receptor agonists in primary ITP. *Semin Hematol* 50:S21, 2013.

225. Kuter DJ: The biology of thrombopoietin and thrombopoietin receptor agonists. *Int J Hematol* 98:10–23, 2013.

226. Kuter DJ, Bussel JB, Newland AC: Long-term treatment with romiplostim in patients with chronic immuno thrombocytopenia: Safety and efficacy. *Br J Haematol* 161:411–423, 2013.

227. Erhardt JA, Erickson-Miller CL, Aivado M, et al: Comparative analyses of the small molecule thrombopoietin receptor agonist eltrombopag and thrombopoietin on in vitro platelet function. *Exp Hematol* 37:1030–1037, 2009.

228. Tomiyama Y, Miyakawa Y, Okamoto S: A lower dose of eltrombopag is efficacious in Japanese patients with previously treated chronic immune thrombocytopenia. *J Thromb Haemost* 10:799–806, 2012.

229. Saleh MN, Bussel JB, Cheng G: Safety and efficacy of eltrombopag for the treatment of chronic immuno thrombocytopenia: Result of the long-term, open label EXTEND study. *Blood* 121:537–545, 2013.

230. Bussel JB, Saleh MN, Vasey SY, et al: Repeated short-term use of eltrombopag in patients with chronic immune thrombocytopenia (ITP). *Br J Haematol* 160:538–546, 2013.

231. Columbyova L, Loda M, Scadden DT: Thrombopoietin receptor expression in human cancer cell lines and primary tissues. *Cancer Res* 55:3509–3512, 1995.

232. Giagounidis A, Mufti GJ, Fenaux P: Results of a randomized, double-blind study of romiplostim versus placebo in patients with low/intermediate-1-risk myelodysplastic syndrome and thrombocytopenia. *Cancer* 120:1835–1846, 2014.

233. Quiquandon I, Fenaux P, Caulier MT, et al: Re-evaluation of the role of azathioprine in the treatment of adult chronic idiopathic thrombocytopenic purpura: A report on 53 cases. *Br J Haematol* 74:223–228, 1990.

234. Blanchette V, Freedman J, Garvey B: Management of chronic immune thrombocytopenic purpura in children and adults. *Semin Hematol* 35:36–51, 1998.

235. Verlin M, Laros RK Jr, Penner JA: Treatment of refractory thrombocytopenic purpura with cyclophosphamine. *Am J Hematol* 1:97–104, 1976.

236. Reiner A, Gernsheimer T, Slichter SJ: Pulse cyclophosphamide therapy for refractory autoimmune thrombocytopenic purpura. *Blood* 85:351–358, 1995.

237. Emillia G, Morselli M, Luppi M: Long-term salvage therapy with cyclosporine A in refractory idiopathic thrombocytopenic purpura. *Blood* 99:1482–1485, 2002.

238. Patel AP, Patil AS: Dapsone for immune thrombocytopenic purpura in children and adults. *Platelets* 26:164–167, 2015.

239. Zaja F, Marin L, Chiozzotto M, et al: Dapsone salvage therapy for adults with immune thrombocytopenia relapsed or refractory to steroid and rituximab. *Am J Hematol* 87:321–323, 2012.

240. Ahn YS, Byrnes JJ, Harrington WJ, et al: The treatment of idiopathic thrombocytopenia with vinblastine-loaded platelets. *N Engl J Med* 298:1101–1107, 1978.

241. Jackson CW, Edwards CC: Evidence that stimulation of megakaryocytopoiesis by low dose vincristine results from an effect on platelets. *Br J Haematol* 36:97–105, 1977.

242. Tangun Y, Atamer T: More on vincristine in treatment of ITP. *N Engl J Med* 297:894–895, 1977.

243. Sekreta CM, Baker DE: Interferon alfa therapy in adults with chronic idiopathic thrombocytopenic purpura. *Ann Pharmacother* 30:1176–1179, 1996.

244. Snyder HW Jr, Cochran SK, Balint JP Jr, et al: Experience with protein A-immunoadsorption in treatment-resistant adult immune thrombocytopenic purpura. *Blood* 79:2237–2245, 1992.

245. Emilia G, Messora C, Longo G, Bertesi M: Long-term salvage treatment by cyclosporin in refractory autoimmune haematological disorders. *Br J Haematol* 93:341–344, 1996.

246. Strother SV, Zuckerman KS, LoBuglio AF: Colchicine therapy for refractory idiopathic thrombocytopenic purpura. *Arch Intern Med* 144:2198–2200, 1984.

247. Bussel JB, Saal S, Gordon B: Combined plasma exchange and intravenous gammaglobulin in the treatment of patients with refractory immune thrombocytopenic purpura. *Transfusion* 28:38–41, 1988.

248. Cines DB, Bussel JB, Liebman HA, Luning Prak ET: The ITP syndrome: Pathogenic and clinical diversity. *Blood* 113:6511–6521, 2009.

249. Miyakis S, Lockshin MD, Atsumi T, et al: International consensus statement on an update of the classification criteria for definite antiphospholipid syndrome (APS). *J Thromb Haemost* 4:295–306, 2006.

250. Cervera R, Piette JC, Font J, et al: Antiphospholipid syndrome: Clinical and immunologic manifestations and patterns of disease expression in a cohort of 1,000 patients. *Arthritis Rheum* 46:1019–1027, 2002.

251. Oosting JD, Derksen RH, Bobbink IW, et al: Antiphospholipid antibodies directed against a combination of phospholipids with prothrombin, protein C, or protein S: An explanation for their pathogenic mechanism? *Blood* 81:2618–2625, 1993.

252. D'Cruz D, Hughes G: Antibodies, thrombosis and the endothelium. *Br J Rheumatol* 33:2–4, 1994.

253. Santoro SA: Antiphospholipid antibodies and thrombotic predisposition: Underlying pathogenetic mechanisms. *Blood* 83:2389–2391, 1994.

254. Rand JH, Wu XX: Antibody-mediated interference with annexins in the antiphospholipid syndrome. *Thromb Res* 114:383–389, 2004.

255. Asherson RA, Khamashta MA, Ordi-Ros J, et al: The "primary" antiphospholipid syndrome: Major clinical and serological features. *Medicine (Baltimore)* 68:366–374, 1989.

256. Alarcon-Segovia D, Deleze M, Oria CV, et al: Antiphospholipid antibodies and the anti-phospholipid syndrome in systemic lupus erythematosus. A prospective analysis of 500 consecutive patients. *Medicine (Baltimore)* 68:353–365, 1989.

257. Galli M, Finazzi G, Barbui T: Thrombocytopenia in the antiphospholipid syndrome. *Br J Haematol* 93:1–5, 1996.

258. Cuadrado MJ, Mujic F, Munoz E, et al: Thrombocytopenia in the antiphospholipid syndrome. *Ann Rheum Dis* 56:194–196, 1997.

259. Uthman I, Godeau B, Taher A, Khamashta M: The hematologic manifestations of the antiphospholipid syndrome. *Blood Rev* 22:187–194, 2008.

260. Harris EN: Antiphospholipid antibodies. *Br J Haematol* 74:1–9, 1990.

261. Wilson WA, Gharavi AE, Koike T, et al: International consensus statement on preliminary classification criteria for definite antiphospholipid syndrome: Report of an international workshop. *Arthritis Rheum* 42:1309–1311, 1999.

262. Diz-Kucukkaya R, Hacihanefioglu A, Yenerel M, et al: Antiphospholipid antibodies and antiphospholipid syndrome in patients presenting with immune thrombocytopenic purpura: A prospective cohort study. *Blood* 98:1760–1764, 2001.

263. Galli M, Daldossi M, Barbui T: Anti-glycoprotein Ib/IX and IIb/IIIa antibodies in patients with antiphospholipid antibodies. *Thromb Haemost* 71:571–575, 1994.

264. Lipp E, von Felten A, Sax H, et al: Antibodies against platelet glycoproteins and anti-phospholipid antibodies in autoimmune thrombocytopenia. *Eur J Haematol* 60:283–288, 1998.

265. Stasi R, Stipa E, Masi M, et al: Prevalence and clinical significance of elevated anti-phospholipid antibodies in patients with idiopathic thrombocytopenic purpura. *Blood* 84:4203–4208, 1994.

266. Fabris F, Steffan A, Cordiano I, et al: Specific antiplatelet autoantibodies in patients with antiphospholipid antibodies and thrombocytopenia. *Eur J Haematol* 53:232–236, 1994.

267. Nakamura M, Tanaka Y, Satoh T, et al: Autoantibody to CD40 ligand in systemic lupus erythematosus: Association with thrombocytopenia but not thromboembolism. *Rheumatology (Oxford)* 45:150–156, 2006.

268. Thrombosis and thrombocytopenia in antiphospholipid syndrome (idiopathic and secondary to SLE): First report from the Italian Registry. Italian Registry of Antiphospholipid Antibodies (IR-APA). *Haematologica* 78:313–318, 1993.

269. Bernini JC, Buchanan GR, Ashcraft J: Hypoprothrombinemia and severe hemorrhage associated with a lupus anticoagulant. *J Pediatr* 123:937–939, 1993.

270. Font J, Jimenez S, Cervera R, et al: Splenectomy for refractory Evans' syndrome associated with antiphospholipid antibodies: Report of two cases. *Ann Rheum Dis* 59:920–923, 2000.

271. Hakim AJ, Machin SJ, Isenberg DA: Autoimmune thrombocytopenia in primary antiphospholipid syndrome and systemic lupus erythematosus: The response to splenectomy. *Semin Arthritis Rheum* 28:20–25, 1998.

272. Ames PR, Tommasino C, Fossati G, et al: Limited effect of rituximab on thrombocytopaenia and anticardiolipin antibodies in a patient with primary antiphospholipid syndrome. *Ann Hematol* 86:227–228, 2007.

273. Ahn ER, Lander G, Bidot CJ, et al: Long-term remission from life-threatening hypercoagulable state associated with lupus anticoagulant (LA) following rituximab therapy. *Am J Hematol* 78:127–129, 2005.

274. Kumar D, Roubey RA: Use of rituximab in the antiphospholipid syndrome. *Curr Rheumatol Rep* 12:40–44, 2010.

275. Sperati CL, Streiff MB: Acute renal failure in a patient with antiphospholipid syndrome and immune thrombocytopenic purpura treated with eltrombopag. *Am J Hematol* 85:724–726, 2010.

276. Jansen AJ, Swart RM, te Boekhorst PA. Thrombopoietin receptor agonists for immune thrombocytopenia. *N Engl J Med* 365:2240–2241, 2011.

277. Tan EM, Cohen AS, Fries JF, et al: The 1982 revised criteria for the classification of systemic lupus erythematosus. *Arthritis Rheum* 25:1271–1277, 1982.

278. Hochberg MC: Updating the American College of Rheumatology revised criteria for the classification of systemic lupus erythematosus. *Arthritis Rheum* 40:1725, 1997.

279. Rabinowitz Y, Dameshek W: Systemic lupus erythematosus after "idiopathic" thrombocytopenic purpura: A review. *Ann Intern Med* 52:1–28, 1960.

280. Michel M, Lee K, Piette JC, et al: Platelet autoantibodies and lupus-associated thrombocytopenia. *Br J Haematol* 119:354–358, 2002.

281. Pujol M, Ribera A, Vilardell M, et al: High prevalence of platelet autoantibodies in patients with systemic lupus erythematosus. *Br J Haematol* 89:137–141, 1995.

282. McMillan R: Immune thrombocytopenia. *Clin Haematol* 12:69–88, 1983.

283. Macchi L, Rispal P, Clofent-Sanchez G, et al: Anti-platelet antibodies in patients with systemic lupus erythematosus and the primary antiphospholipid antibody syndrome: Their relationship with the observed thrombocytopenia. *Br J Haematol* 98:336–341, 1997.

284. Griner PF, Hoyer LW: Amegakaryocytic thrombocytopenia in systemic lupus erythematosus. *Arch Intern Med* 125:328–332, 1970.

285. Fureder W, Firbas U, Nichol JL, et al: Serum thrombopoietin levels and anti-thrombopoietin antibodies in systemic lupus erythematosus. *Lupus* 11:221–226, 2002.

286. Kuwana M, Okazaki Y, Kajihara M, et al: Autoantibody to c-Mpl (thrombopoietin receptor) in systemic lupus erythematosus: Relationship to thrombocytopenia with megakaryocytic hypoplasia. *Arthritis Rheum* 46:2148–2159, 2002.

287. Feinglass EJ, Arnett FC, Dorsch CA, et al: Neuropsychiatric manifestations of systemic lupus erythematosus: Diagnosis, clinical spectrum, and relationship to other features of the disease. *Medicine (Baltimore)* 55:323–339, 1976.

288. Miller MH, Urowitz MB, Gladman DD: The significance of thrombocytopenia in systemic lupus erythematosus. *Arthritis Rheum* 26:1181–1186, 1983.

289. Mok CC, Lee KW, Ho CT, et al: A prospective study of survival and prognostic indicators of systemic lupus erythematosus in a southern Chinese population. *Rheumatology (Oxford)* 39:399–406, 2000.

290. Drenkard C, Villa AR, Alarcon-Segovia D, Perez-Vazquez ME: Influence of the antiphospholipid syndrome in the survival of patients with systemic lupus erythematosus. *J Rheumatol* 21:1067–1072, 1994.

291. Reveille JD, Bartolucci A, Alarcon GS: Prognosis in systemic lupus erythematosus. Negative impact of increasing age at onset, black race, and thrombocytopenia, as well as causes of death. *Arthritis Rheum* 33:37–48, 1990.

292. Abu-Shakra M, Urowitz MB, Gladman DD, Gough J: Mortality studies in systemic lupus erythematosus. Results from a single center. II. Predictor variables for mortality. *J Rheumatol* 22:1265–1270, 1995.

293. Scofield RH, Bruner GR, Kelly JA, et al: Thrombocytopenia identifies a severe familial phenotype of systemic lupus erythematosus and reveals genetic linkages at 1q22 and 11p13. *Blood* 101:992–997, 2003.

294. Boumpas DT, Austin HA, III, Fessler BJ, et al: Systemic lupus erythematosus: Emerging concepts. Part 1: Renal, neuropsychiatric, cardiovascular, pulmonary, and hematologic disease. *Ann Intern Med* 122:940–950, 1995.

295. Arnal C, Piette JC, Leone J, et al: Treatment of severe immune thrombocytopenia associated with systemic lupus erythematosus: 59 cases. *J Rheumatol* 29:75–83, 2002.

296. Boumpas DT, Barez S, Klippel JH, Balow JE: Intermittent cyclophosphamide for the treatment of autoimmune thrombocytopenia in systemic lupus erythematosus. *Ann Intern Med* 112:674–677, 1990.

297. Roach BA, Hutchinson GJ: Treatment of refractory, systemic lupus erythematosus-associated thrombocytopenia with intermittent low-dose intravenous cyclophosphamide. *Arthritis Rheum* 36:682–684, 1993.

298. Maier WP, Gordon DS, Howard RF, et al: Intravenous immunoglobulin therapy in systemic lupus erythematosus-associated thrombocytopenia. *Arthritis Rheum* 33:1233–1239, 1990.

299. Cohen MG, Li EK: Limited effects of intravenous IgG in treating systemic lupus erythematosus-associated thrombocytopenia. *Arthritis Rheum* 34:787–788, 1991.

300. Ding C, Foote S, Jones G: B-cell-targeted therapy for systemic lupus erythematosus: An update. *BioDrugs* 22:239–249, 2008.

301. Jovancevic B, Lindholm C, Pullerits R: Anti-B cell therapy against refractory thrombocytopenia in SLE and MCTD patients: Long-term follow up and review of the literature. *Lupus* 22:664–674, 2013.

302. Zhou J, Wu Z, Zhou Z, et al: Efficacy and safety of laparoscopic splenectomy in thrombocytopenia secondary to systemic lupus erythematosus. *Clin Rheumatol* 32:1131–1138, 2013.

303. Delgado AJ, Inanc M, Diz-Kucukkaya R, et al: Thrombocytopenic risk in patients submitted to splenectomy for systemic lupus erythematosus and antiphospholipid syndrome-related thrombocytopenia. *Eur J Intern Med* 15:162–167, 2004.

304. Ciernik IF, Cone RW, Fehr J, Weber R: Impaired liver function and retroviral activity are risk factors contributing to HIV-associated thrombocytopenia. Swiss HIV Cohort Study. *AIDS* 13:1913–1920, 1999.

305. Dominguez A, Gamallo G, Garcia R, et al: Pathophysiology of HIV related thrombocytopenia: An analysis of 41 patients. *J Clin Pathol* 47:999–1003, 1994.

306. Louache F, Vainchenker W: Thrombocytopenia in HIV infection. *Curr Opin Hematol* 1:369–372, 1994.

307. Brook MG, Ayles H, Harrison C, et al: Diagnostic utility of bone marrow sampling in HIV positive patients. *Genitourin Med* 73:117–121, 1997.

308. WHO Global Alert and Response. 2015. http://www.who.int/csr/disease/hepatitis/whocdscsrlyo2003/en/index1.html

309. Stasi R: Therapeutic strategies for hepatitis- and other infection-related immune thrombocytopenias. *Semin Hematol* 46:S15–S25, 2001.

310. Calvaruso V, Craxi A: Immunological alterations in hepatitis C virus infection. *World J Gastroenterol* 19:8916–8923, 2013.

311. Hamaia S, Allain JP: The dynamics of hepatitis C virus binding to platelets and 2 mononuclear cell lines. *Blood* 98:2293–2300, 2001.

312. Cuker A: Toxicities of the thrombopoietic growth factors. *Semin Hematol* 47:289–298, 2010.

313. Jackson S, Beck PL, Pineo GF, Poon MC: *Helicobacter pylori* eradication: Novel therapy for immune thrombocytopenic purpura? A review of the literature. *Am J Hematol* 78:142–150, 2005.

314. Franchini M, Cruciani M, Mengoli C, et al: Effect of *Helicobacter pylori* eradication on platelet count in idiopathic thrombocytopenic purpura: A systematic review and meta-analysis. *J Antimicrob Chemother* 60:237–246, 2007.

315. Arnold DM, Bernotas A, Nazi I, et al: Platelet count response to *H. pylori* treatment in patients with immune thrombocytopenic purpura with and without *H. pylori* infection: A systematic review. *Haematologica* 94:850–856, 2009.

316. Burrows RF, Kelton JG: Incidentally detected thrombocytopenia in healthy mothers and their infants. *N Engl J Med* 319:142–145, 1988.

317. Letsky EA, Greaves M: Guidelines on the investigation and management of thrombocytopenia in pregnancy and neonatal alloimmune thrombocytopenia. Maternal and Neonatal Haemostasis Working Party of the Haemostasis and Thrombosis Task Force of the British Society for Haematology. *Br J Haematol* 95:21–26, 1996.

318. Gernsheimer T, James AH, Stasi R: How I treat thrombocytopenia in pregnancy. *Blood* 121:38–47, 2013.

319. George JN, Saucerman S: Platelet IgG, IgA, IgM, and albumin: Correlation of platelet and plasma concentrations in normal subjects and in patients with ITP or dysproteinemia. *Blood* 72:362–365, 1988.

320. Burrows RF, Kelton JG: Fetal thrombocytopenia and its relation to maternal thrombocytopenia. *N Engl J Med* 329:1463–1466, 1993.
321. McCrae KR, Samuels P, Schreiber AD: Pregnancy-associated thrombocytopenia: Pathogenesis and management. *Blood* 80:2697–2714, 1992.
322. Bussel JB: Immune thrombocytopenia in pregnancy: Autoimmune and alloimmune. *J Reprod Immunol* 37:35–61, 1997.
323. Shehata N, Burrows R, Kelton JG: Gestational thrombocytopenia. *Clin Obstet Gynecol* 42:327–334, 1999.
324. Kaplan C, Forestier F, Dreyfus M, et al: Maternal thrombocytopenia during pregnancy: Diagnosis and etiology. *Semin Thromb Hemost* 21:85–94, 1995.
325. Boehlen F, Hohlfeld P, Extermann P, et al: Platelet count at term pregnancy: A reappraisal of the threshold. *Obstet Gynecol* 95:29–33, 2000.
326. Ostensen M, Forger F: How safe are anti-rheumatic drugs during pregnancy. *Curr Opin Pharmacol* 13:470–475, 2015.
327. Chakravarty EF, Murray ER, Kelman A, Farmer P: Pregnancy outcomes after maternal exposure to rituximab. *Blood* 117:1499–1506, 2011.
328. Cheng G: Eltrombopag a thrombopoietin-receptor agonist in the treatment of adult chronic immune thrombocytopenia: A review of the efficacy and safety profile. *Ther Adv Hematol* 3:155–164, 2012.
329. al-Mofada SM, Osman ME, Kides E, et al: Risk of thrombocytopenia in the infants of mothers with idiopathic thrombocytopenia. *Am J Perinatol* 11:423–426, 1994.
330. Gill KK, Kelton JG: Management of idiopathic thrombocytopenic purpura in pregnancy. *Semin Hematol* 37:275–289, 2000.
331. Webert KE, Mittal R, Sigouin C, et al: A retrospective 11-year analysis of obstetric patients with idiopathic thrombocytopenic purpura. *Blood* 102:4306–4311, 2003.
332. Stamilio DM, Macones GA: Selection of delivery method in pregnancies complicated by autoimmune thrombocytopenia: A decision analysis. *Obstet Gynecol* 94:41–47, 1999.
333. Christiaens GC, Nieuwenhuis HK, Bussel JB: Comparison of platelet counts in first and second newborns of mothers with immune thrombocytopenic purpura. *Obstet Gynecol* 90:546–552, 1997.
334. Moise KJ Jr, Cotton DB: Discordant fetal platelet counts in a twin gestation complicated by idiopathic thrombocytopenic purpura. *Am J Obstet Gynecol* 156:1141–1142, 1987.
335. Mushambi MC, Halligan AW, Williamson K: Recent developments in the pathophysiology and management of pre-eclampsia. *Br J Anaesth* 76:133–148, 1996.
336. Leitch CR, Cameron AD, Walker JJ: The changing pattern of eclampsia over a 60-year period. *Br J Obstet Gynaecol* 104:917–922, 1997.
337. Thomas SV: Neurological aspects of eclampsia. *J Neurol Sci* 155:37–43, 1998.
338. Silver RM, Branch DW, Scott JR: Maternal thrombocytopenia in pregnancy: Time for a reassessment. *Am J Obstet Gynecol* 173:479–482, 1995.
339. McCrae KR: Thrombocytopenia in pregnancy: Differential diagnosis, pathogenesis, and management. *Blood Rev* 17:7–14, 2003.
340. Schlembach D: Pre-eclampsia—Still a disease of theories. *Fukushima J Med Sci* 49:69–115, 2003.
341. Brittain PC, Bayliss P: Partial hydatidiform molar pregnancy presenting with severe preeclampsia prior to twenty weeks gestation: A case report and review of the literature. *Mil Med* 160:42–44, 1995.
342. Luttun A, Carmeliet P: Soluble VEGF receptor Flt1: The elusive preeclampsia factor discovered? *J Clin Invest* 111:600–602, 2003.
343. Torry DS, Hinrichs M, Torry RJ: Determinants of placental vascularity. *Am J Reprod Immunol* 51:257–268, 2004.
344. Maynard SE, Min JY, Merchan J, et al: Excess placental soluble fms-like tyrosine kinase 1 (sFlt1) may contribute to endothelial dysfunction, hypertension, and proteinuria in preeclampsia. *J Clin Invest* 111:649–658, 2003.
345. Vuorela P, Helske S, Hornig C, et al: Amniotic fluid—Soluble vascular endothelial growth factor receptor-1 in preeclampsia. *Obstet Gynecol* 95:353–357, 2000.
346. Zhou Y, McMaster M, Woo K, et al: Vascular endothelial growth factor ligands and receptors that regulate human cytotrophoblast survival are dysregulated in severe preeclampsia and hemolysis, elevated liver enzymes, and low platelets syndrome. *Am J Pathol* 160:1405–1423, 2002.
347. Venkatesha S, Toporsian M, Lam C, et al: Soluble endoglin contributes to the pathogenesis of preeclampsia. *Nat Med* 12:642–649, 2006.
348. Lattuada A, Rossi E, Calzarossa C, et al: Mild to moderate reduction of a von Willebrand factor cleaving protease (ADAMTS-13) in pregnant women with HELLP microangiopathic syndrome. *Haematologica* 88:1029–1034, 2003.
349. Hulstein JJ, van Runnard Heimel PJ, Franx A, et al: Acute activation of the endothelium results in increased levels of active von Willebrand factor in hemolysis, elevated liver enzymes and low platelets (HELLP) syndrome. *J Thromb Haemost* 4:2569–2575, 2006.
350. Abildgaard U, Heimdal K: Pathogenesis of the syndrome of hemolysis, elevated liver enzymes, and low platelet count (HELLP): A review. *Eur J Obstet Gynecol Reprod Biol* 166:117–123, 2013.
351. Egerman RS, Sibai BM: HELLP syndrome. *Clin Obstet Gynecol* 42:381–389, 1999.
352. Hay JE: Liver disease in pregnancy. *Hepatology* 47:1067–1076, 2008.
353. Martin JN Jr, Files JC, Blake PG, et al: Postpartum plasma exchange for atypical preeclampsia-eclampsia as HELLP (hemolysis, elevated liver enzymes, and low platelets) syndrome. *Am J Obstet Gynecol* 172:1107–1125, 1995.
354. Chakravorty S, Roberts I: How I manage neonatal thrombocytopenia. *Br J Haematol* 156:155–162, 2011.
355. Kaplan C: Alloimmune thrombocytopenia of the fetus and the newborn. *Blood Rev* 16:69–72, 2002.
356. Peterson JA, McFarland JG, Curtis BR, Aster RH: Neonatal alloimmune thrombocytopenia: Pathogenesis, diagnosis and management. *Br J Haematol* 161:3–14, 2013.
357. Mueller-Eckhardt C, Kiefel V, Grubert A, et al: 348 Cases of suspected neonatal alloimmune thrombocytopenia. *Lancet* 1:363–366, 1989.
358. Grainger JD, Morrell G, Yates J, Deleacy D: Neonatal alloimmune thrombocytopenia with significant HLA antibodies. *Arch Dis Child Fetal Neonatal Ed* 86:F200–F201, 2002.
359. Chow MP, Sun KJ, Yung CH, et al: Neonatal alloimmune thrombocytopenia due to HLA-A2 antibody. *Acta Haematol* 87:153–155, 1992.
360. Davoren A, McParland P, Crowley J, et al: Antenatal screening for human platelet antigen-1a: Results of a prospective study at a large maternity hospital in Ireland. *BJOG* 110:492–496, 2003.
361. Williamson LM, Hackett G, Rennie J, et al: The natural history of fetomaternal alloimmunization to the platelet-specific antigen HPA-1a (PlA1, Zwa) as determined by antenatal screening. *Blood* 92:2280–2287, 1998.
362. Jolly MC, Letsky EA, Fisk NM: The management of fetal alloimmune thrombocytopenia. *Prenat Diagn* 22:96–98, 2002.
363. Murphy MF, Hambley H, Nicolaides K, Waters AH: Severe fetomaternal alloimmune thrombocytopenia presenting with fetal hydrocephalus. *Prenat Diagn* 16:1152–1155, 1996.
364. Kaplan C, Murphy MF, Kroll H, Waters AH: Feto-maternal alloimmune thrombocytopenia: Antenatal therapy with IvIgG and steroids—More questions than answers. European Working Group on FMAIT. *Br J Haematol* 100:62–65, 1998.
365. Ouwehand WH, Smith G, Ranasinghe E: Management of severe alloimmune thrombocytopenia in the newborn. *Arch Dis Child Fetal Neonatal Ed* 82:F173–F175, 2000.
366. Bertrand G, Kaplan C: How do we treat fetal and neonatal alloimmune thrombocytopenia? *Transfusion* 54:1698–1703, 2014.
367. Le Toriellec E, Chenet C, Kaplan C: Safe fetal platelet genotyping: New developments. *Transfusion* 53:1755–1762, 2013.
368. Porcelijn L, Kanhai HH: Fetal thrombocytopenia. *Curr Opin Obstet Gynecol* 10:117–122, 1998.
369. Weiner E, Zosmer N, Bajoria R, et al: Direct fetal administration of immunoglobulins: Another disappointing therapy in alloimmune thrombocytopenia. *Fetal Diagn Ther* 9:159–164, 1994.
370. Aster RH: Platelet sequestration studies in man. *Br J Haematol* 22:259–263, 1972.
371. Wadenvik H, Denfors I, Kutti J: Splenic blood flow and intrasplenic platelet kinetics in relation to spleen volume. *Br J Haematol* 67:181–185, 1987.
372. Heyns AD, Badenhorst PN, Lotter MG, et al: Kinetics and mobilization from the spleen of indium-111-labeled platelets during platelet apheresis. *Transfusion* 25:215–218, 1985.
373. Lawrence SP, Lezotte DC, Durham JD, et al: Course of thrombocytopenia of chronic liver disease after transjugular intrahepatic portosystemic shunts (TIPS). A retrospective analysis. *Dig Dis Sci* 40:1575–1580, 1995.
374. Peck-Radosavljevic M: Hypersplenism. *Eur J Gastroenterol Hepatol* 13:317–323, 2001.
375. Eichner ER: Splenic function: Normal, too much and too little. *Am J Med* 66:311–320, 1979.
376. Jacob HS: Hypersplenism: Mechanisms and management. *Br J Haematol* 27:1–5, 1974.
377. Cooney DP, Smith BA: The pathophysiology of hypersplenic thrombocytopenia. *Arch Intern Med* 121:332–337, 1968.
378. McCormick PA, Murphy KM: Splenomegaly, hypersplenism and coagulation abnormalities in liver disease. *Bailliures Best Pract Res Clin Gastroenterol* 14:1009–1031, 2000.
379. Sihler KC, Napolitano LM: Massive transfusion: New insights. *Chest* 136:1654–1667, 2009.
380. Hiippala ST, Myllyla GJ, Vahtera EM: Hemostatic factors and replacement of major blood loss with plasma-poor red cell concentrates. *Anesth Analg* 81:360–365, 1995.
381. Leslie SD, Toy PT: Laboratory hemostatic abnormalities in massively transfused patients given red blood cells and crystalloid. *Am J Clin Pathol* 96:770–773, 1991.
382. Hardy JF, de Moerloose P, Samama CM: The coagulopathy of massive transfusion. *Vox Sang* 89:123–127, 2005.
383. Cosgriff N, Moore EE, Sauaia A, et al: Predicting life-threatening coagulopathy in the massively transfused trauma patient: Hypothermia and acidoses revisited. *J Trauma* 42:857–861, 1997.
384. Cinat ME, Wallace WC, Nastanski F, et al: Improved survival following massive transfusion in patients who have undergone trauma. *Arch Surg* 134:964–968, 1999.
385. Villalobos TJ, Adelson E, Riley PA Jr, Crosby WH: A cause of the thrombocytopenia and leukopenia that occur in dogs during deep hypothermia. *J Clin Invest* 37:1–7, 1958.
386. Yau TM, Carson S, Weisel RD, et al: The effect of warm heart surgery on postoperative bleeding. *J Thorac Cardiovasc Surg* 103:1155–1162, 1992.
387. Pina-Cabral JM, Ribeiro-da-Silva A, Almeida-Dias A: Platelet sequestration during hypothermia in dogs treated with sulphinpyrazone and ticlopidine—Reversibility accelerated after intra-abdominal rewarming. *Thromb Haemost* 54:838–841, 1985.
388. Hoffmeister KM, Felbinger TW, Falet H, et al: The clearance mechanism of chilled blood platelets. *Cell* 112:87–97, 2003.
389. Hoffmeister KM, Josefsson EC, Isaac NA, et al: Glycosylation restores survival of chilled blood platelets. *Science* 301:1531–1534, 2003.
390. Reddick RL, Poole BL, Penick GD: Thrombocytopenia of hibernation. Mechanism of induction and recovery. *Lab Invest* 28:270–278, 1973.
391. Chan KM, Beard K: A patient with recurrent hypothermia associated with thrombocytopenia. *Postgrad Med J* 69:227–229, 1993.
392. Enjolras O, Wassef M, Mazoyer E, et al: Infants with Kasabach-Merritt syndrome do not have "true" hemangiomas. *J Pediatr* 130:631–640, 1997.

393. Sarkar M, Mulliken JB, Kozakewich HP, et al: Thrombocytopenic coagulopathy (Kasabach-Merritt phenomenon) is associated with Kaposiform hemangioendothelioma and not with common infantile hemangioma. *Plast Reconstr Surg* 100:1377–1386, 1997.

394. Vin-Christian K, McCalmont TH, Frieden IJ: Kaposiform hemangioendothelioma. An aggressive, locally invasive vascular tumor that can mimic hemangioma of infancy. *Arch Dermatol* 133:1573–1578, 1997.

395. Hall GW: Kasabach-Merritt syndrome: Pathogenesis and management. *Br J Haematol* 112:851–862, 2001.

396. Cooper JG, Edwards SL, Holmes JD: Kaposiform haemangioendothelioma: Case report and review of the literature. *Br J Plast Surg* 55:163–165, 2002.

397. Hoeger PH, Helmke K, Winkler K: Chronic consumption coagulopathy due to an occult splenic haemangioma: Kasabach-Merritt syndrome. *Eur J Pediatr* 154:365–368, 1995.

398. Brasanac D, Janic D, Boricic I, et al: Retroperitoneal kaposiform hemangioendothelioma with tufted angioma-like features in an infant with Kasabach-Merritt syndrome. *Pathol Int* 53:627–631, 2003.

399. Mukhtar IA, Letts M: Hemangioma of the radius associated with Kasabach-Merritt syndrome: Case report and literature review. *J Pediatr Orthop* 24:87–91, 2004.

400. Fukunaga M, Ushigome S, Ishikawa E: Kaposiform haemangioendothelioma associated with Kasabach-Merritt syndrome. *Histopathology* 28:281–284, 1996.

401. Alvarez-Mendoza A, Lourdes TS, Ridaura-Sanz C, Ruiz-Maldonado R: Histopathology of vascular lesions found in Kasabach-Merritt syndrome: Review based on 13 cases. *Pediatr Dev Pathol* 3:556–560, 2000.

402. Jones EW, Orkin M: Tufted angioma (angioblastoma). A benign progressive angioma, not to be confused with Kaposi's sarcoma or low-grade angiosarcoma. *J Am Acad Dermatol* 20:214–225, 1989.

403. Wong SN, Tay YK: Tufted angioma: A report of five cases. *Pediatr Dermatol* 19:388–393, 2002.

404. Mueller BU, Mulliken JB: The infant with a vascular tumor. *Semin Perinatol* 23:332–340, 1999.

405. Mazoyer E, Enjolras O, Laurian C, et al: Coagulation abnormalities associated with extensive venous malformations of the limbs: Differentiation from Kasabach-Merritt syndrome. *Clin Lab Haematol* 24:243–251, 2002.

406. Lyons LL, North PE, Mac-Moune LF, et al: Kaposiform hemangioendothelioma: A study of 33 cases emphasizing its pathologic, immunophenotypic, and biologic uniqueness from juvenile hemangioma. *Am J Surg Pathol* 28:559–568, 2004.

407. Gilon E, Ramot B, Sheba C: Multiple hemangiomata associated with thrombocytopenia: Remarks on the pathogenesis of the thrombocytopenia in this syndrome. *Blood* 14:74–79, 1959.

408. Seo SK, Suh JC, Na GY, et al: Kasabach-Merritt syndrome: Identification of platelet trapping in a tufted angioma by immunohistochemistry technique using monoclonal antibody to CD61. *Pediatr Dermatol* 16:392–394, 1999.

409. Brizel HE, Raccuglia G: Giant hemangioma with thrombocytopenia. Radioisotopic demonstration of platelet sequestration. *Blood* 26:751–764, 1965.

410. Shulkin BL, Argenta LC, Cho KJ, Castle VP: Kasabach-Merritt syndrome: Treatment with epsilon-aminocaproic acid and assessment by indium 111 platelet scintigraphy. *J Pediatr* 117:746–749, 1990.

411. Warrell RP Jr, Kempin SJ, Benua RS, et al: Intratumoral consumption of indium-111 labeled platelets in a patient with hemangiomatosis and intravascular coagulation (Kasabach-Merritt syndrome). *Cancer* 52:2256–2260, 1983.

412. Wananukul S, Nuchprayoon I, Seksarn P: Treatment of Kasabach-Merritt syndrome: A stepwise regimen of prednisolone, dipyridamole, and interferon. *Int J Dermatol* 42:741–748, 2003.

413. MacArthur CJ, Senders CW, Katz J: The use of interferon alfa-2a for life-threatening hemangiomas. *Arch Otolaryngol Head Neck Surg* 121:690–693, 1995.

414. Haisley-Royster C, Enjolras O, Frieden IJ, et al: Kasabach-Merritt phenomenon: A retrospective study of treatment with vincristine. *J Pediatr Hematol Oncol* 24:459–462, 2002.

415. Blei F, Karp N, Rofsky N, et al: Successful multimodal therapy for kaposiform hemangioendothelioma complicated by Kasabach-Merritt phenomenon: Case report and review of the literature. *Pediatr Hematol Oncol* 15:295–305, 1998.

416. Hu B, Lachman R, Phillips J, et al: Kasabach-Merritt syndrome-associated kaposiform hemangioendothelioma successfully treated with cyclophosphamide, vincristine, and actinomycin D. *J Pediatr Hematol Oncol* 20:567–569, 1998.

417. Frevel T, Rabe H, Uckert F, Harms E: Giant cavernous haemangioma with Kasabach-Merritt syndrome: A case report and review. *Eur J Pediatr* 161:243–246, 2002.

418. Atahan IL, Cengiz M, Ozyar E, Gurkaynak M: Radiotherapy in the management of Kasabach-Merritt syndrome: A case report. *Pediatr Hematol Oncol* 18:471–476, 2001.

419. Ogino I, Torikai K, Kobayasi S, et al: Radiation therapy for life- or function-threatening infant hemangioma. *Radiology* 218:834–839, 2001.

420. Billio A, Pescosta N, Rosanelli C, et al: Treatment of Kasabach-Merritt syndrome by embolisation of a giant liver hemangioma. *Am J Hematol* 66:140–141, 2001.

421. Hosono S, Ohno T, Kimoto H, et al: Successful transcutaneous arterial embolization of a giant hemangioma associated with high-output cardiac failure and Kasabach-Merritt syndrome in a neonate: A case report. *J Perinat Med* 27:399–403, 1999.

422. Zukerberg LR, Nickoloff BJ, Weiss SW: Kaposiform hemangioendothelioma of infancy and childhood. An aggressive neoplasm associated with Kasabach-Merritt syndrome and lymphangiomatosis. *Am J Surg Pathol* 17:321–328, 1993.

423. George M, Singhal V, Sharma V, Nopper AJ: Successful surgical excision of a complex vascular lesion in an infant with Kasabach-Merritt syndrome. *Pediatr Dermatol* 19:340–344, 2002.

424. Balduini CL, Stella CC, Rosti V, et al: Acquired cyclic thrombocytopenia-thrombocytosis with periodic defect of platelet function. *Br J Haematol* 85:718–722, 1993.

425. Yujiri T, Tanaka Y, Tanaka M, Tanizawa Y: Fluctuations in thrombopoietin, immature platelet fraction, and glycocalicin levels in a patient with cyclic thrombocytopenia. *Int J Hematol* 90:429–430, 2009.

426. Go RS: Idiopathic cyclic thrombocytopenia. *Blood Rev* 19:53–59, 2005.

427. Steensma DP, Harrison CN, Tefferi A: Hydroxyurea-associated platelet count oscillations in polycythemia vera: A report of four new cases and a review. *Leuk Lymphoma* 42:1243–1253, 2001.

428. Abe Y, Hirase N, Muta K, et al: Adult onset cyclic hematopoiesis in a patient with myelodysplastic syndrome. *Int J Hematol* 71:40–45, 2000.

429. Aster RH, Bougie DW: Drug-induced immune thrombocytopenia. *N Engl J Med* 357:580–587, 2007.

430. George JN, Raskob GE, Shah SR, et al: Drug-induced thrombocytopenia: A systematic review of published case reports. *Ann Intern Med* 129:886–890, 1998.

431. Kaufman DW, Kelly JP, Johannes CB, et al: Acute thrombocytopenic purpura in relation to the use of drugs. *Blood* 82:2714–2718, 1993.

432. Garner SF, Campbell K, Metcalfe P, et al: Glycoprotein V: The predominant target antigen in gold-induced autoimmune thrombocytopenia. *Blood* 100:344–346, 2002.

433. Christie DJ, Mullen PC, Aster RH: Fab-mediated binding of drug-dependent antibodies to platelets in quinidine- and quinine-induced thrombocytopenia. *J Clin Invest* 75:310–314, 1985.

434. Lopez JA, Li CQ, Weisman S, Chambers M: The glycoprotein Ib-IX complex-specific monoclonal antibody SZ1 binds to a conformation-sensitive epitope on glycoprotein IX: Implications for the target antigen of quinine/quinidine-dependent autoantibodies. *Blood* 85:1254–1258, 1995.

435. Chong BH, Du XP, Berndt MC, Horn S, Chesterman CN: Characterization of the binding domains on platelet glycoproteins Ib-IX and IIb/IIIa complexes for the quinine/quinidine-dependent antibodies. *Blood* 77:2190–2199, 1991.

436. Curtis BR, McFarland JG, Wu GG, Visentin GP, Aster RH: Antibodies in sulfonamide-induced immune thrombocytopenia recognize calcium-dependent epitopes on the glycoprotein IIb/IIIa complex. *Blood* 84:176–183, 1994.

437. Visentin GP, Newman PJ, Aster RH: Characteristics of quinine- and quinidine-induced antibodies specific for platelet glycoproteins IIb and IIIa. *Blood* 77:2668–2676, 1991.

438. Berkowitz SD, Harrington RA, Rund MM, Tcheng JE: Acute profound thrombocytopenia after C7E3 Fab (abciximab) therapy. *Circulation* 95:809–813, 1997.

439. Fiorin F, Steffan A, Pradella P, et al: IgG platelet antibodies in EDTA-dependent pseudothrombocytopenia bind to platelet membrane glycoprotein IIb. *Am J Clin Pathol* 110:178–183, 1998.

440. Cancio LC, Cohen DJ: Heparin-induced thrombocytopenia and thrombosis. *J Am Coll Surg* 186:76–91, 1998.

441. Coblyn JS, Weinblatt M, Holdsworth D, Glass D: Gold-induced thrombocytopenia. A clinical and immunogenetic study of twenty-three patients. *Ann Intern Med* 95:178–181, 1981.

442. Nieminen U, Kekomaki R: Quinidine-induced thrombocytopenic purpura: Clinical presentation in relation to drug-dependent and drug-independent platelet antibodies. *Br J Haematol* 80:77–82, 1992.

443. Leach MF, Cooper LK, AuBuchon JP: Detection of drug-dependent, platelet-reactive antibodies by solid-phase red cell adherence assays. *Br J Haematol* 97:755–761, 1997.

444. Visentin GP, Malik M, Cyganiak KA, Aster RH: Patients treated with unfractionated heparin during open heart surgery are at high risk to form antibodies reactive with heparin:platelet factor 4 complexes. *J Lab Clin Med* 128:376–383, 1996.

445. Boon DM, van Vliet HH, Zietse R, Kappers-Klunne MC: The presence of antibodies against a PF4-heparin complex in patients on haemodialysis. *Thromb Haemost* 76:480, 1996.

446. Bauer TL, Arepally G, Konkle BA, et al: Prevalence of heparin-associated antibodies without thrombosis in patients undergoing cardiopulmonary bypass surgery. *Circulation* 95:1242–1246, 1997.

447. Gentilini G, Curtis BR, Aster RH: An antibody from a patient with ranitidine-induced thrombocytopenia recognizes a site on glycoprotein IX that is a favored target for drug-induced antibodies. *Blood* 92:2359–2365, 1998.

448. Belkin GA: Cocktail purpura. An unusual case of quinine sensitivity. *Ann Intern Med* 66:583–586, 1967.

449. Siroty RR: Purpura on the rocks—With a twist. *JAMA* 235:2521–2522, 1976.

450. Pedersen-Bjergaard U, Andersen M, Hansen PB: Drug-induced thrombocytopenia: Clinical data on 309 cases and the effect of corticosteroid therapy. *Eur J Clin Pharmacol* 52:183–189, 1997.

CHAPTER 118
HEPARIN-INDUCED THROMBOCYTOPENIA

Adam Cuker and Mortimer Poncz

SUMMARY

Heparin-induced thrombocytopenia (HIT) is a prothrombotic complication of treatment with heparin. It is associated with mild-to-moderate thrombocytopenia, although the main clinical concern is the high frequency of both arterial and venous thromboembolism, which may be limb- or life-threatening. HIT is an immune complex-based disorder involving platelet factor 4 complexed to negatively charged multimeric molecules, especially surface heparan side chains. It is initiated by exposure to heparin, particularly unfractionated heparin. There is growing understanding of the unusual nature of the underlying immune response in HIT, why certain individuals develop this disorder, and why HIT is prothrombotic. Diagnosis is based upon an assessment of clinical probability and specialized laboratory testing. Management involves immediate cessation of heparin and initiation of parenteral inhibitors of thrombin or factor Xa.

DEFINITION AND HISTORY

Heparin-induced thrombocytopenia (HIT) is a complication of heparin therapy in which there is a fall in platelet count and an unusually high incidence of arterial and/or venous thromboembolic complications in association with heparin therapy.

Although clinical usage of heparin as an anticoagulant began in the late 1950s, it was not until the early 1970s that a small percentage of treated patients were noted to develop a complication consisting of thrombocytopenia with paradoxical, life-threatening thromboemboli (for a historical review see Ref. 1). In the 1980s, it became clear that HIT was caused by immunoglobulin (Ig) G antibodies that activate platelets. It was also recognized that HIT could be divided into two types, the classic immune-mediated prothrombotic disease that is the focus of this chapter (formerly called HIT type II), and a benign nonimmune condition associated with a mild, immediate, and transient drop in platelet count and no increased risk of thrombosis (formerly called HIT type I).[2] In this chapter, "HIT" means the immune-mediated form of the disease.

In the 1970s and 1980s, it became clear that HIT antibodies activated both platelets and endothelial cells.[3,4] Further analysis showed that blocking platelet FcγRIIA inhibited platelet activation by HIT sera *in vitro*,[5] suggesting that platelet activation involved an immune complex. In the early 1990s, this complex was identified as heparin bound to the platelet-specific chemokine, platelet factor 4 (PF4).[6] Over the past 20 years, additional insights into the mechanism(s) underlying this immune complex disorder have emerged that have advanced our understanding of why this disorder is particularly prothrombotic and occurs in a only a small subset of patients. Additionally, advances have been made on the clinical side with respect to prevention, diagnosis, and treatment.

EPIDEMIOLOGY

The frequency of HIT in heparin-treated patients ranges from less than 0.1 percent to 5.0 percent, depending on patient- and heparin-specific risk factors. These include the patient population, gender, nature of the heparin used, and duration of heparin exposure (Table 118–1).

The most important determinant of risk is the patient population. In a meta-analysis of seven prospective studies, the incidence of HIT was greater among surgical than medical patients (odds ratio [OR]: 3.25; 95 percent confidence interval [CI]: 1.98 to 5.35).[7] The incidence of HIT approaches 5 percent in patients who receive unfractionated heparin (UFH) after major orthopedic surgery.[8] Patients undergoing surgery with cardiopulmonary bypass have a very high frequency of anti-PF4/heparin antibody seroconversion (50 to 75 percent by postoperative day 10), but a lesser incidence of HIT (0.5 to 1.0 percent).[8–10] HIT occurs in 0.5 to 1.0 percent of medical patients[7] and in less than 0.1 percent of pregnant women[11,12] and children.[13] In a randomized trial of trauma patients, major trauma was associated with a significantly greater incidence of HIT than minor trauma (2.2 percent vs. 0.0 percent, p = 0.01) despite identical heparin exposure.[14]

Female sex is also a risk factor for HIT. A meta-analysis found an approximately twofold greater risk of HIT in women than men (OR: 2.37; 95 percent CI: 1.37 to 4.09). Analyses of a German database and a randomized trial of UFH versus low-molecular-weight heparin (LMWH) after orthopedic surgery yielded similar findings.[7]

HIT is more common with UFH than LMWH in surgical patients. In a meta-analysis of 15 studies, primarily involving orthopedic surgery patients, the incidence of HIT with UFH and LMWH was 2.6 percent and 0.2 percent, respectively.[15] Data are conflicting on whether the risk of HIT is reduced with LMWH in medical patients.[7,16,17] Fondaparinux, a synthetic pentasaccharide anticoagulant, is associated with a nearly negligible risk of HIT, although several cases of fondaparinux-associated HIT have been reported.[18]

Duration of heparin exposure also influences the risk of HIT. In a meta-analysis of 3529 patients receiving UFH thromboprophylaxis for 6 or more days, the incidence of HIT was 2.6 percent.[15] Review of a hospital database indicated that briefer courses induce a substantially lower incidence of HIT (0.2 percent).[19]

High-quality data on the impact of dose and route of administration of heparin on the risk of HIT are lacking. Some studies suggest a lower rate of HIT with prophylactic dose subcutaneous UFH than therapeutic dose intravenous UFH,[19] but these analyses are confounded by differences in the patients that receive these treatments including the clinical indication for heparin. Rarely, HIT has been reported with very low doses of heparin such as with use of heparin flushes or heparin-bonded catheters.[20,21]

ETIOLOGY AND PATHOGENESIS

The development of HIT antibodies is nonclassical in that these antibodies typically begin as IgG and not IgM,[22] may disappear after a few months, and may not reappear with heparin reexposure.[23] It has been proposed that the initial antigen exposure involves PF4 complexed with

TABLE 118–1. Heparin-Induced Thrombocytopenia Risk Factors

Patient-Specific Factors	Heparin-Specific Factors
Patient population (surgical > medical > obstetric > pediatric)	Type of heparin (unfractionated heparin > low-molecular-weight heparin)
Major trauma > minor trauma	Duration of heparin (~5 days > shorter courses)
Sex (female > male)	

exists as a tetramer. Crystal structure analysis shows that this tetramer is encircled by a ring of positive charge (Fig. 118–2),[26] and heparin is thought to bind to this region.[27] There are two closely spaced HIT antibody recognition domains (Fig. 118–2).[28] These domains are distinct from the heparin-binding domain. About half of patients have antibodies that react with one or the other HIT antigenic domain and one-third of patients do not have antibodies that react to either domain, suggesting that there are other HIT antigenic sites on PF4. Studies of antihuman PF4 monoclonal antibodies suggest that unlike nonpathogenic anti-PF4 antibodies, HIT antibodies markedly increase their binding affinity for PF4 maintained in a tetrameric as opposed to dimeric state.[29] Moreover, tetrameric PF4 and UFH need to be at approximately 1:1 molar ratio for optimal HIT antigenicity.[30,31] At this ratio, ultralarge complexes (>670 kDa) of PF4 and heparin form that appear as visible colloidal complexes, and these are likely to be the antigenic source in HIT.[32,33] At higher or lower ratios, PF4 predominantly forms smaller and less antigenic PF4–heparin complexes. Ultralarge complexes are inefficiently formed with LMWH, offering a potential explanation as to why this class of agents is associated with a lower incidence of HIT compared with UFH. Fondaparinux does not form

bacterial wall (Fig. 118–1) and that antibodies against this complex may be an important antimicrobial defensive mechanism.[24] These antigenic complexes, as well as circulating PF4–heparin complexes, are detected by splenic marginal B cells that subsequently produce pathogenic HIT antibodies.[25]

The nature of the antigenic heparin–PF4 complex has been partially defined. At the concentrations reached at sites of injury, PF4

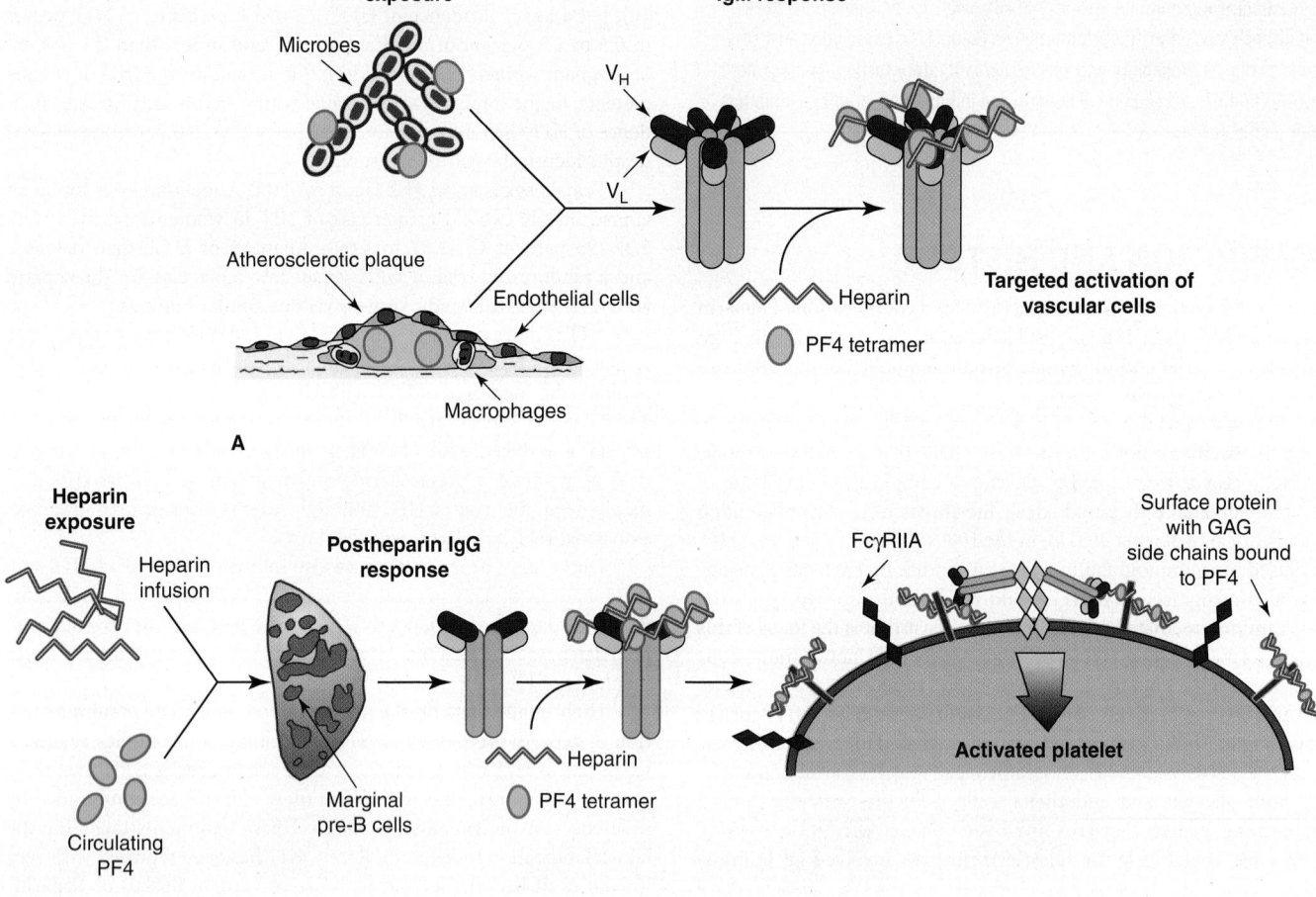

Figure 118–1. Proposed etiology of the immune response in heparin-induced thrombocytopenia (HIT). **A.** Proposed first exposure to HIT antigenic complex either during microbial invasion[24] or within growing atherosclerotic plaques, which are known to contain both platelet factor 4 (PF4) and immune-responsive cells.[49] In both cases, soluble PF4 and negatively charged molecules must be presented to B cells and result in an initial immunoglobulin M—perhaps low affinity—response. **B.** On exposure to heparin, especially unfractionated heparin, complexes form with free PF4 and are presented to splenic marginal B cells,[25] which subsequently produce pathogenic HIT antibodies that bind with high affinity to PF4 complexed to surface GAG complexes.[29] The concentrated binding of HIT antibodies to surface PF4–GAG complexes may enhance FcγRIIA aggregation and subsequent platelet activation.

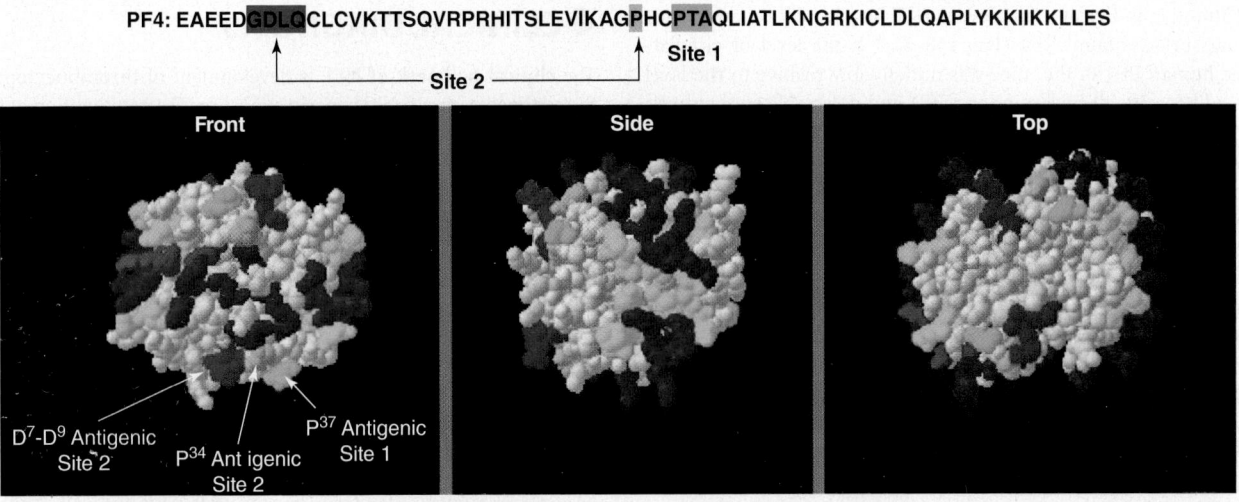

PF4: EAEED**GDLQ**CLCVKTTSQVRPRHITSLEVIKAG**P**HCPTAQLIATLKNGRKICLDLQAPLYKKIIKKLLES

Figure 118–2. Platelet factor 4 (PF4) tetramer structure. At the top is the linear sequence of PF4. The regions that are known to contribute to heparin-induced thrombocytopenia (HIT) antigenicity when PF4 is complexed to heparin are boxed. Below are three views of the PF4 tetramer with the positively charged residues shown in both light and dark blue. Sites at which HIT neoepitopes are exposed on the PF4 tetramer are indicated. *(Adapted with permission from Li ZQ, Liu W, Park KS, et al: Defining a second epitope for heparin-induced thrombocytopenia antibodies using KKO, a murine HIT-like monoclonal antibody. Blood 99(4):1230–1236, 2002.)*

large complexes with PF4, explaining the negligible incidence of HIT with this agent and supporting its potential utility in the prevention or treatment of HIT.

A passive immunization murine model of HIT has been used to demonstrate the following components are necessary to induce both thrombocytopenia and a prothrombotic state in HIT: the presence of human PF4 in platelets, FcγRIIA on the surface of platelets and possibly other vascular cells, and the presence of a pathogenic HIT-like antibody.[34] Heparin has a more complex relationship to the pathogenesis of HIT (Fig. 118-3). In the passive immunization model of HIT,

wherein a pathogenic HIT-like antibody is infused into mice expressing both human PF4 and FcγRIIA, heparin infusion is not needed to cause thrombocytopenia and a prothrombotic state.[35] The explanation for a lack of need to infuse heparin in this model is as follows: One important potential role of heparin in the pathogenesis of HIT is to form soluble, circulating PF4–heparin complexes that induce anti-PF4–heparin antibody production by presentation of the complex to splenic marginal B cells (see Figs. 118–1 and 118–3).[25] Passive immunization with HIT antibodies in these mice obviates the need for delivery of soluble antigenic complexes to the spleen. Another role for infused heparin is

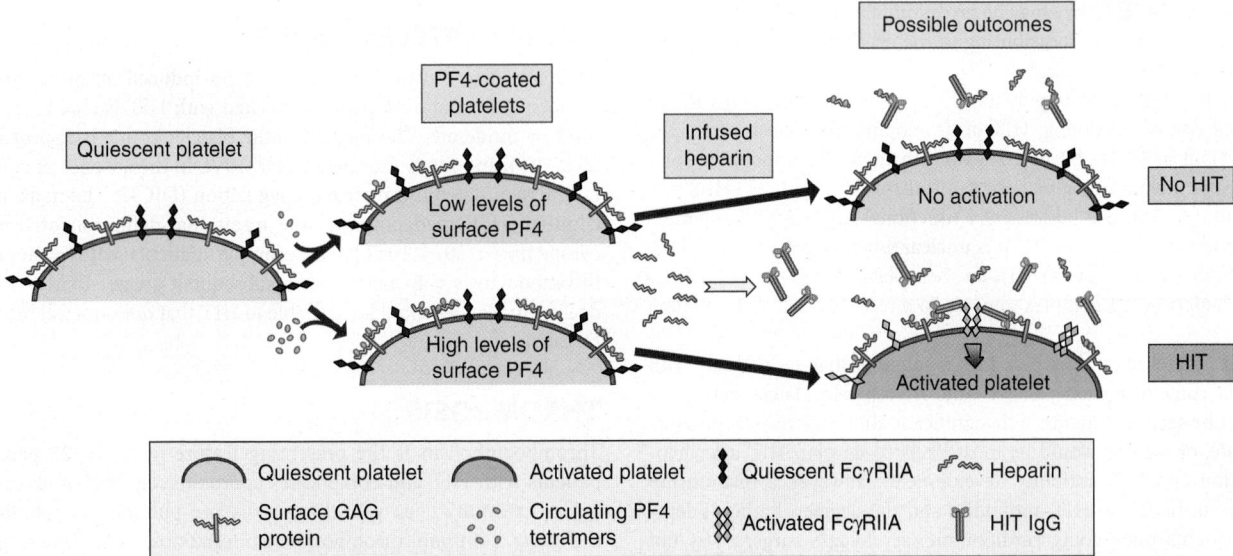

Figure 118–3. The role(s) of heparin in heparin-induced thrombocytopenia (HIT). On the *left* is depicted a quiescent platelet surface with GAG-expressing proteins as well as individual FcγRIIA receptors. Platelet factor 4 (PF4) is normally released by platelets in the steady-state, especially in individuals with underlying inflammation and/or atherosclerosis. Additionally, individuals have a wide range of platelet PF4 content, and this, too, contributes to having individuals with different levels of surface PF4 binding. Heparin infusions leads to HIT immunoglobulin G formation (see Fig. 118-1*B*), but also removes surface-bound PF4. If the individual has little initial surface-bound PF4, the surface of the platelets will be wiped clean of bound PF4 by the infused heparin and not be targeted by the HIT antibodies *(right, top)* so that HIT antibodies circulate but HIT does not develop. If there is significant residual surface-bound PF4 after heparin infusion, HIT antibodies will attach to the cell surface and activate the platelets *(right, bottom)*, potentially leading to HIT.

counterintuitive in that it may prevent HIT by partially or completely removing surface-bound PF4 (Fig. 118–3).[35] If the level of circulating, free human PF4 in the mice was initially low relative to the level of infused heparin, all surface-bound PF4 and detectable surface antigenicity would be removed and the circulating HIT antibodies would have no targets on platelets and other vascular cells (Fig. 118–3). HIT therefore would not develop in spite of the presence of heparin and circulating HIT antibody. On the other hand, if the level of circulating free human PF4 in the mice was initially high relative to the infused heparin, not all surface-bound PF4 would be removed. Circulating HIT antibodies could then target and activate platelets and other vascular cells, leading to thrombocytopenia and thrombosis (Fig. 118–3).

Most patients likely begin with little PF4 bound to surface glycosaminoglycans (GAGs). After therapeutic heparinization, the level of surface PF4 goes down markedly so that the platelets cannot be targeted by anti-PF4–heparin HIT antibodies. However, patients with high levels of surface PF4 and significant surface PF4 antigenic complexes remaining after heparinization may be at risk for binding of pathogenic anti-PF4–heparin HIT antibodies to platelets and other vascular cells. Bound pathogenic antibodies lead to thrombocytopenia by clearance of antibody-coated platelets by the reticuloendothelial system. Bound antibodies also lead to platelet activation through FcγRIIA and the formation of procoagulant platelet microparticles that contribute to thrombosis.[36]

As part of this activation, HIT antibodies also bind to endothelial cells likely via PF4–surface GAG complexes,[4,37] leading to local vascular activation and contributing to further local thrombosis. Additionally, HIT antibodies activate PF4-targeted monocytes[38,39] and neutrophils.[40] Monocyte activation may involve its surface Fcγ receptors[41] with subsequent increased tissue factor expression and other changes consistent with a prothrombotic and inflammatory state. Monocyte and neutrophil GAGs are more complex than GAGs on the surface of platelets, which are mostly chondroitin sulfate[42] and have relatively low affinity for PF4.[43] Monocytes and neutrophils bind PF4 with greater avidity and are more resistant to removal of bound PF4 by circulating heparin than platelets. In HIT, they may be preferentially targeted and activated relative to the platelets, contributing to the prothrombotic state of this immune thrombocytopenia.[44]

Are there any genetic polymorphisms that are associated with an increased risk of developing HIT or developing thrombosis after HIT begins? No clear linkage has been shown with known thrombophilic polymorphisms including Factor V^{Leiden}, Prothrombin^{G20210A}, MTHFR^{C677T}, $\alpha_{IIb}\beta_3$ and $\alpha_I\beta_2$.[45] Studies addressing a functional FcγRIIA$^{R/H131}$ polymorphism had varied outcome.[46,47] It is unclear whether patients with HIT have a higher density of FcγRIIA on their platelets.[48] High IgG affinity for the heparin–PF4 complex appears to affect the risk of developing HIT.

The model shown in Fig. 118–3 suggests that individuals with high PF4 content in their platelets and/or sustained platelet activation as might be seen in patients with significant atherosclerosis, a postsurgery state, or trauma would be most likely to develop HIT after heparinization and HIT antibody development. However, a relationship between formation of HIT antibodies and the degree of atherosclerosis in patients undergoing cardiopulmonary bypass surgery was not noted.[49] If levels of PF4 on the surface of circulating cells determine risk of developing HIT, this would offer a potential method for prescreening patients prior to heparinization and eliminate those at increased risk of HIT or as a useful tool in heparinized patients who develop thrombocytopenia to see whether they potentially can develop HIT. Theoretically, only those heparinized individuals with detectable surface PF4 would be potential candidates for developing HIT if they concurrently develop pathogenic antibodies.

● CLINICAL DIAGNOSIS

The clinical hallmark of HIT is development of thrombocytopenia in the setting of a proximate heparin exposure. The combination of thrombocytopenia and heparin exposure in hospitalized patients is common and has poor specificity for HIT.[50] Therefore, other clinical clues must be sought in estimating the clinical likelihood of HIT. These include timing, degree of platelet count fall, nadir platelet count, presence of thromboembolism or hemorrhage, and the likelihood of other causes of thrombocytopenia.

TIMING

The platelet count in HIT characteristically begins to fall 5 to 10 days after initial heparin exposure.[23] There are three exceptions to this rule: (1) in rapid-onset HIT, patients with recent heparin exposure (within the previous 90 days) and preformed anti-PF4–heparin IgG experience a fall in platelet count immediately upon reexposure; (2) in delayed-onset HIT, clinical manifestations develop a median of 10 to 14 days after heparin is discontinued[51,52]; and (3) a small number of patients with spontaneous HIT have been reported. These patients present with a thrombotic thrombocytopenic disorder reminiscent of HIT in the absence of recognized heparin exposure.[53] Both delayed-onset HIT and spontaneous HIT occur in the absence of circulating heparin and may involve pathogenic HIT antibodies that recognize complexes of PF4 and endogenous GAGs on blood and vascular cells.

DEGREE OF FALL IN PLATELET COUNT

The percentage fall in platelet count is measured from the peak platelet count after initiation of heparin to the nadir platelet count. Most patients with HIT experience a 50 percent or greater fall in platelet count; a more modest decline (30 to 50 percent) occurs in approximately 10 percent of patients.[54]

NADIR PLATELET COUNT

As opposed to most other forms of drug-induced immune thrombocytopenia, thrombocytopenia associated with HIT is characteristically mild or moderate. The median nadir platelet count is approximately $60 \times 10^9/L$ and rarely falls below $20 \times 10^9/L$ in the absence of concomitant disseminated intravascular coagulation (DIC).[54] The nadir platelet count in HIT need not meet the traditional definition of thrombocytopenia ($<150 \times 10^9/L$). For example, patients with postoperative thrombocytosis may experience a subsequent greater than 50 percent decline in platelet count attributable to HIT that does not fall below this threshold.[55]

THROMBOSIS

Thromboembolism is the presenting feature in up to 25 percent of patients with HIT and complicates approximately half of all cases.[56,57] Lower-extremity deep vein thrombosis and pulmonary embolism are the most common thrombotic manifestations, outnumbering arterial events by approximately 2:1.[56] Major venous obstruction can lead to limb gangrene. Catheter-associated upper extremity deep venous thrombosis is common.[58] Arterial thromboembolism most frequently involves the extremities, but may also manifest as stroke or myocardial infarction.[56] Thrombosis of other vascular beds including cerebral sinuses, mesenteric vessels, and adrenal veins is well-documented as is thrombotic occlusion of vascular grafts, fistulas, and extracorporeal circuitry.

HEMORRHAGE

In contrast to most other forms of drug-induced immune thrombocytopenia, spontaneous hemorrhage is rare in HIT, even when thrombocytopenia is severe. In a prospective study, bleeding complications were not increased in HIT patients compared with nonthrombocytopenic controls.[59]

UNUSUAL CLINICAL MANIFESTATIONS

Rare sequelae of HIT include anaphylactoid reactions after intravenous heparin bolus, transient global amnesia, and skin necrosis at subcutaneous heparin injection sites.[60,61] Curiously, these phenomena may occur in the absence of thrombocytopenia. Nonnecrotizing erythematous injection site lesions are generally caused by delayed type IV hypersensitivity rather than HIT.[62]

OTHER CAUSES

The likelihood of other etiologies of thrombocytopenia must be carefully considered in patients with suspected HIT. Common causes of hospital-acquired thrombocytopenia include infection; drugs other than heparin; DIC; dilution; and intravascular devices and extracorporeal circuits such as intraaortic balloon pumps, cardiopulmonary bypass, and extracorporeal membrane oxygenation.[63]

Clinical scoring systems have been developed to permit estimation of the probability of HIT based on the aforementioned features. The most extensively studied of these systems, the 4T score,[64] classifies the probability of HIT as low, intermediate, or high on the basis of four criteria: Thrombocytopenia, Timing, Thrombosis or other sequelae, and the likelihood of other causes of thrombocytopenia (Table 118–2). In a meta-analysis of 13 studies, the negative predictive value of a low probability 4T score was 99.8 percent (95 percent CI: 97.0 to 100.0). The positive predictive value of an intermediate and high probability 4T score was 14 percent (95 percent CI: 9 to 22) and 64 percent (95 percent CI: 40 to 82), respectively.[65] The 4T score is limited by moderate interobserver agreement.[66] An alternative scoring system, the HIT Expert Probability (HEP) Score, exhibited improved reliability and favorable operating characteristics in a retrospective study, but remains to be prospectively validated.[67]

●LABORATORY DIAGNOSIS

In light of the complexity and limited positive predictive value of clinical diagnosis,[65] clinicians rely heavily on laboratory testing to aid in diagnosis. Laboratory assays for HIT fall into two categories: immunoassays and functional assays.

IMMUNOASSAYS

These assays detect the presence of circulating anti-PF4–heparin antibodies, irrespective of whether they are able to activate platelets and cause disease. The prototypical immunoassay is the solid-phase enzyme-linked immunosorbent assay (ELISA), in which dilute patient serum is added to microtiter wells coated with complexes of PF4–heparin (or PF4–polyvinylsulfonate).[6] The polyspecific ELISA detects circulating anti-PF4–heparin IgG, IgM, and IgA. At the manufacturer-recommended cutoff, the sensitivity and specificity of this assay for HIT are 94 to 100 percent and 81 to 93 percent, respectively.[22,68–70]

A key limitation of the polyspecific ELISA is its specificity. False-positive results are common and may result from detection of nonpathogenic anti-PF4–heparin antibodies[69] or antiphospholipid antibodies against either PF4[71] or PF4-bound β_2-glycoprotein I.[72] Specificity may be improved by raising the optical density (OD) cutoff. OD is directly associated with the 4T and HEP scores,[67] the risk of thrombosis,[73] and the likelihood of a positive functional assay.[74] In a Canadian study, only one of 37 patient samples exhibiting a weakly positive OD (0.40 to 0.99) demonstrated heparin-dependent platelet activation compared with 33 out of 37 samples with a strongly positive OD (>2.0).[74] In a recent analysis of 1958 patients, increasing the cutoff from a manufacturer-recommended threshold of 0.4 to 0.8 OD units increased specificity from 85 percent to 93 percent with a slight reduction in sensitivity from 100 percent to 98 percent.[75]

Several modifications have been made to the PF4–heparin ELISA with the goal of improving specificity. Because pathogenic antibodies are primarily of the IgG class, detection systems specific for IgG have been developed. In a pooled analysis of studies comparing the IgG-specific and polyspecific ELISA, the former showed greater specificity (93.5 percent vs. 89.4 percent) at the cost of reduced sensitivity (95.8 percent vs. 98.1 percent).[76] Another modification involves the addition of a high heparin confirmatory step, in which reduction of the OD by 50 percent or more with the addition of excess heparin (100 U/mL) is considered to affirm the presence of heparin-dependent antibodies.[77] This method improves specificity, but false-positives remain common and false-negatives may also occur, particularly at high OD values.[78,79]

Another limitation of the PF4–heparin ELISA is turnaround time. Although the analytical turnaround time of the ELISA is only approximately 2 hours, the assay is most cost-effective when multiple samples are run in batch. Consequently, many laboratories perform the ELISA only once or twice a week, leaving clinicians to make critical initial management decisions without the benefit of laboratory results. This drawback of the ELISA has spawned the development of several rapid immunoassays, which are designed to accommodate single samples and

TABLE 118–2. The 4T Score*			
	Points Per Category		
Clinical Sign	**0**	**1**	**2**
Thrombocytopenia (acute)	Very low nadir (<10 × 10⁹/L) or <30% fall	Low nadir (10–20 × 10⁹/L) or 30–50% fall	Moderate nadir (20–100 × 10⁹/L) or >50% fall
Timing of first event (thrombocytopenia or thrombosis)	≤4 Days (unless prior heparin exposure in last 3 months)	Within 5–10 days (but not well documented) or ≤1 day (with exposure in last 3 months)	Documented occurrence in 5–10 days or ≤1 day with recent prior exposure
Thrombotic-related event	None	Progressive, recurrent, or suspected (unconfirmed) thrombosis; erythematous nonnecrotic skin lesions	New thrombosis (confirmed) or skin necrosis or systemic reaction after heparin bolus
Thrombocytopenia (other causes)	Definite other cause is present	Possible other cause is present	No other strong explanation for thrombocytopenia

*Scores of 0–3, 4–5, and 6–8 are classified as low, intermediate, and high probability, respectively.[64]

TABLE 118–3. Properties of Rapid Platelet Factor 4–Heparin Immunoassays

Assay	Antibody Class Detection	Sensitivity	Specificity	Turnaround Time (Minutes)	Regulatory Approval
Particle gel immunoassay[68,80,81]	IgG	0.91–0.94	0.87–0.95	20	Asia, Canada, Europe
Lateral flow immunoassay[80,82]	IgG	0.98–1.00	0.82–0.93	15	Europe
Latex particle-enhanced immunoturbi-dimetric assay[83,84]	IgG, IgA, IgM	1.00	0.76	13	Europe
Chemiluminescence assay[84-86]	IgG, IgA, IgM	0.98–1.00	0.73–0.82	30	Europe
Chemiluminescence assay[84-86]	IgG	0.96–1.00	0.85–0.97	30	Europe

Ig, immunoglobulin.

yield results in minutes. Table 118–3 summarizes the properties of these rapid assays.[68,80–86] The latex particle-enhanced immunoturbidimetric assay and chemiluminescence assays are instrument-based and must be performed on proprietary analyzers. A rapid particle immunofiltration assay is approved in the Unites States, but published data suggest that it has unacceptable diagnostic accuracy.[87] A modified version of the assay[88] requires further study.

FUNCTIONAL ASSAYS

Functional assays are more specific than commercial immunoassays because they detect only the subset of antibodies capable of inducing platelet activation in a heparin-dependent manner. The prototypical functional assays are the ^{14}C-serotonin release assay (SRA) and the heparin-induced platelet-activation assay (HIPA). In the SRA, various concentrations of heparin and heat-inactivated patient serum are added to washed donor platelets radiolabeled with ^{14}C. A positive test is signified by heparin-dependent release of ^{14}C-serotonin.[89] The HIPA is based on a similar principle, but uses visual assessment of platelet aggregation as an end point.[90] The sensitivity and specificity of the SRA and HIPA are said to exceed 95 percent, but universally accepted reference standards against which to measure their performance do not exist.[63]

Washed platelet functional assays are technically demanding. Both the SRA and HIPA require reactive donor platelets and the SRA requires radioisotope. Because these reagents are impracticable for most clinical laboratories, functional assays are performed at only a small number of reference laboratories around the world. Even among such laboratories, test methodology, result interpretation, and reporting are not well-standardized.[91]

Novel immunoassays and functional assays for HIT designed to overcome the limitations of assays currently in use are in development.[92,93]

●MANAGEMENT

NONHEPARIN ANTICOAGULANTS

Management of HIT requires immediate withdrawal of heparin, including cessation of heparin flushes and removal of heparin-coated catheters. However, discontinuation of heparin alone is insufficient to prevent thromboembolism. Historical studies of untreated patients document a 5 to 10 percent daily risk of thrombosis in the first 48 hours after heparin is stopped and a 30-day cumulative incidence of thrombosis of approximately 50 percent.[57,94] Discontinuation of heparin must therefore be accompanied by initiation of a rapid-acting, parenteral, nonheparin anticoagulant.[95] Table 118–4 summarizes the properties of nonheparin anticoagulants used to treat HIT.

Argatroban and bivalirudin are direct thrombin inhibitors. Argatroban is the only FDA-approved drug for treatment of HIT available in the

United States. Its approval was based on two open-label single-arm studies in which argatroban-treated subjects were compared with untreated historical controls.[96,97] In a pooled analysis of these two studies, argatroban reduced the relative risk of new thrombosis by two-thirds. The incidence of major bleeding was approximately 1 percent per day.[98] An important limitation of these studies was that serologic confirmation of HIT was not required for enrollment. Indeed, 36.4 percent of subjects were found to be anti-PF4–heparin antibody-negative on *post hoc* testing,[99] suggesting that a sizable proportion of the study population did not have HIT.

Bivalirudin is a hirudin analogue. It is approved for patients with and without HIT undergoing percutaneous vascular procedures. It is not approved for treatment of HIT, although it has been used off-label for this indication, particularly in patients with critical illness and multiorgan failure[100] and those undergoing cardiac surgery.[101] Published evidence supporting its use is limited to retrospective single-center cohort studies.[100,102,103]

Two other direct thrombin inhibitors have been studied as treatments for HIT. Lepirudin, a recombinant hirudin, was shown to reduce the risk of thromboembolism compared with untreated historical controls, but is no longer available.[94] A randomized clinical trial of desirudin closed because of poor accrual after only 16 subjects had been randomized.[104]

Danaparoid and fondaparinux are indirect factor Xa inhibitors. Danaparoid is approved for treatment of HIT in multiple jurisdictions, but is no longer marketed in the United States and drug shortages have limited its availability elsewhere. In an open-label randomized trial, 42 patients with HIT complicated by thrombosis were allocated to receive either danaparoid or dextran 70. Significantly more subjects in the danaparoid arm were judged to have complete recovery from thrombosis at hospital discharge (56 percent vs. 14 percent; p = 0.02).[105] *In vitro* crossreactivity of HIT antibodies with danaparoid occurs in some patients, although the clinical relevance of this phenomenon has not been established.[106]

Fondaparinux in not approved for treatment of HIT, nor is it recommended in the 2012 American College of Chest Physicians Guidelines.[95] Its use is supported by several small case series and retrospective cohort studies.[107–110] In a pooled analysis involving 71 patients, no new thrombotic events were reported. Four patients suffered major hemorrhage.[63] A small number of cases of HIT induced or exacerbated by fondaparinux have been reported, although the attribution to fondaparinux in at least some of these cases remains uncertain.[111] Fondaparinux is more convenient to use than other agents given the ease of once-daily administration and a potential lack of need for monitoring (see Table 118–4). This may, in part, account for its increasing use. In a recent multicenter German registry of patients with suspected HIT, a greater proportion of patients were treated with fondaparinux (40 percent) than with danaparoid (23.6 percent) or argatroban (16.4 percent).[112]

Oral direct inhibitors of thrombin (e.g., dabigatran) and factor Xa (e.g., rivaroxaban, apixaban, edoxaban) do not induce platelet

TABLE 118–4. Anticoagulants Used to Treat Heparin-Induced Thrombocytopenia

Drug	Initial Dosing	Monitoring	Clearance (Half-Life)
DIRECT THROMBIN INHIBITORS			
Argatroban	Bolus: None Continuous infusion: Normal organ function → 2 mcg/kg/min Liver dysfunction (total bilirubin >1.5 mg/dL), heart failure, postcardiac surgery, anasarca → 0.5–1.2 mcg/kg/min	Adjust dose to aPTT of 1.5–3.0 × patient baseline	Hepatobiliary (40–50 min)
Bivalirudin	Bolus: None Continuous infusion: Normal organ function → 0.15 mg/kg/h Renal or hepatic insufficiency → consider dose reduction	Adjust dose to aPTT of 1.5–2.5 × patient baseline	Enzymatic and renal (25 min)
INDIRECT FACTOR Xa INHIBITORS			

Danaparoid	Bolus:
	  <60 kg → 1500 U
	  60–75 kg → 2250 U
	  75–90 kg → 3000 U
	  >90 kg → 3750 U
	Accelerated initial infusion:
	  400 U/h × 4 h, then 300 U/h × 4 h
	Maintenance infusion:
	  Normal renal function → 200 U/h
	  Renal insufficiency → 150 U/h
		Adjust to anti–factor Xa of 0.5–0.8 U/mL	Renal (24 h)

Fondaparinux	<50 kg → 5 mg SC daily 50–100 kg → 7.5 mg SC daily >100 kg → 10 mg SC daily Cl_{Cr} 30–50 mL/min → use caution Cl_{Cr} <30 mL/min → contraindicated	None	Renal (17–20 h)

aPTT, activated partial thromboplastin time; Cl_{Cr}, creatinine clearance.

aggregation or PF4 release in the presence of HIT-positive sera *in vitro*[113] and constitute biologically rational approaches to the treatment of HIT. However, clinical evidence is limited to a small number of case reports[114,115] and use of these agents for HIT cannot be recommended outside of a clinical trial. One such trial of rivaroxaban in patients with suspected HIT began enrollment in 2013 and is ongoing.[116]

An important toxicity of anticoagulants used for treatment of HIT is major bleeding, a risk compounded by the absence of effective reversal agents. Novel therapeutic approaches that target pathways proximal to activation of coagulation may provide effective antithrombotic therapy without the degree of bleeding risk associated with anticoagulants. Candidate strategies include a desulfated form of heparin with minimal anticoagulant activity[113] and small molecule PF4 antagonists,[117] which interfere with formation of PF4–heparin complexes; inhibitors of FcγRIIA-mediated platelet activation by HIT immune complexes; and inhibitors of splenic tyrosine kinase and Ca²⁺[118] and diacylglycerol-regulated guanine nucleotide exchange factor I,[119] which disrupt intracellular transduction triggered by immune complex binding.

WHO TO TREAT

Because of the frequency of heparin use and thrombocytopenia among hospitalized patients, the modest specificity of immunologic assays, and clinicians' fears of missing a case of HIT, overdiagnosis and unnecessary treatment with nonheparin anticoagulants of patients without HIT is common.[120] Inappropriate use of these agents is associated with increased costs and bleeding risk.[121] In light of the very-high negative predictive value (99.8 percent) of a low-probability 4T score,[65] a reasonable first step toward reducing unnecessary treatment is to avoid use of nonheparin anticoagulants in patients with a low-probability 4T score. Heparin should be discontinued and a nonheparin anticoagulant initiated in patients with an intermediate- or high-probability 4T score until the results of HIT laboratory testing become available.[65,95,122]

TRANSITIONING TO A VITAMIN K ANTAGONIST

Warfarin and other vitamin K antagonists should not be prescribed as the initial anticoagulant in patients with acute HIT because their use increases the risk of venous limb gangrene as a result of rapid lowering of protein C activity.[123] For patients receiving a vitamin K antagonist at the time HIT is diagnosed, the vitamin K antagonist should be discontinued and its effects reversed with vitamin K. A vitamin K antagonist may be initiated once the platelet count has recovered to a stable plateau. Large loading doses (e.g., warfarin >5 mg/day) should be avoided. The vitamin K antagonist should be overlapped with a parenteral nonheparin anticoagulant for at least 5 days and until the international normalized ratio (INR) has reached its intended target.[63,95] If the patient is being transitioned from argatroban to warfarin, guidelines regarding the appropriate INR target should be followed,[124] because both arga-troban and warfarin increase the INR. This target will vary according to the sensitivity of the prothrombin time reagent to argatroban used in each institution.

DURATION OF ANTICOAGULATION

Patients with HIT-associated thromboembolism are typically treated with therapeutic anticoagulation for 3 to 6 months. The optimal dura-tion of anticoagulation in patients with HIT without thrombosis (i.e., isolated HIT) is unknown. In a historical series of untreated patients with isolated HIT, the cumulative incidence of thromboembolism at 30 days was 53 percent.[57] Most events occurred within 10 days of heparin cessation, corresponding to the platelet recovery phase. It is therefore generally accepted that anticoagulation be continued in patients with isolated HIT until platelet count recovery. Some authorities recommend longer courses (e.g., 4 weeks).[122]

PLATELET TRANSFUSION

There is a long-held concern that platelet transfusion may precipitate thrombosis in HIT by "adding fuel to the fire." Two case series chal-lenge this dogma. Collectively, these series included 41 patients with suspected HIT who underwent platelet transfusion. None developed thrombosis during extended followup.[125,126] Nevertheless, because HIT is characteristically prothrombotic rather than prohemorrhagic, pro-phylactic platelet transfusion is rarely indicated. Transfusion may be considered in the setting of clinically significant bleeding, high bleeding risk, or diagnostic uncertainty.

HEPARIN REEXPOSURE IN PATIENTS WITH A HISTORY OF HEPARIN-INDUCED THROMBOCYTOPENIA

In general, heparin reexposure should be avoided in patients with a his-tory of HIT because of the risk of reoccurrence.[127] An exception to this rule is the use of intraoperative heparin in patients with a history of HIT who are undergoing cardiovascular surgery. The HIT immune response wanes over time. Functional assays become negative at a median of 50 days after heparin cessation, whereas anti-PF4–heparin antibody titers decline more slowly and are no longer detectable in 60 percent of patients by day 100.[23] HIT laboratory testing can be used to deter-mine the safety of heparin reexposure during cardiovascular surgery. Patients with a negative immunologic and functional assay may safely receive UFH during surgery. This was first demonstrated in 10 patients with a history of HIT undergoing cardiac surgery, none of whom devel-oped clinical reoccurrence.[128] In a newer report, 11 of 17 such patients developed recrudescence of anti-PF4–heparin antibodies, but only one developed HIT.[129] Heparin should be strictly avoided in patients with a positive functional assay. If possible, surgery should be delayed in these individuals until functional and immunologic assays become neg-ative. If surgery cannot be delayed, a nonheparin anticoagulant (e.g., bivalirudin) should be used.[101] Appropriate intraoperative anticoag-ulation of patients with a functional assay that has become negative, but an immunologic assay that remains positive is uncertain. The 2012 American College of Chest Physicians Guidelines recommend a non-heparin anticoagulant in this setting.[95] However, intraoperative heparin was used uneventfully in three such patients undergoing urgent heart transplantation.[130] When heparin is administered to patients with HIT, it should be limited to the intraoperative setting. Pre- and postopera-tive exposure should be scrupulously avoided, though patients with a history of HIT who are (inadvertently) reexposed to longer courses of heparin do not always develop recurrent HIT.[129]

In light of its documented efficacy and safety in large coronary angiography trials, bivalirudin is recommended over heparin in patients with a history of HIT who require percutaneous vascular procedures, irrespective of the results of HIT laboratory testing.[95]

HEMODIALYSIS

Although approximately 10 percent of patients on chronic hemodialy-sis develop circulating anti-PF4–heparin antibodies,[131] the incidence of HIT in this population is less than 1 percent.[132] Ongoing heparin expo-sure during dialysis in patients with a history of HIT is contraindicated. Alternative strategies including regional citrate, saline flushing, danap-aroid, argatroban, and vitamin K antagonists use have been reported.[95]

PREGNANCY

HIT is rare (<0.1 percent) in pregnant women exposed to heparin.[11,12] When it does occur, initiation of a nonheparin anticoagulant is war-ranted. The largest published experience is with danaparoid. A ret-rospective cohort of 30 women with acute HIT received danaparoid during pregnancy.[133] Five patients developed thrombosis and three developed major bleeding. Danaparoid does not cross the placenta and there was no measurable anti-Xa activity in the cord blood of six neonates who were tested after delivery. If danaparoid is unavailable, fondaparinux may be considered though evidence supporting its use in pregnant women with HIT is limited to case reports[134,135] and partial transplacental passage has been demonstrated.[136]

REFERENCES

1. Kelton JG, Warkentin TE: Heparin-induced thrombocytopenia: A historical perspec-tive. *Blood* 112;2607, 2008.
2. Chong BH, Berndt MC: Heparin-induced thrombocytopenia. *Blut* 58:53, 1989.
3. Fratantoni JC, Pollet R, Gralnick HR: Heparin-induced thrombocytopenia: Confirma-tion of diagnosis with in vitro methods. *Blood* 45:395, 1975.
4. Cines DB, Tomaski A, Tannenbaum S: Immune endothelial-cell injury in heparin-associated thrombocytopenia. *N Engl J Med* 316:581, 1987.
5. Kelton JG, Sheridan D, Santos A, et al: Heparin-induced thrombocytopenia: Labora-tory studies. *Blood* 72:925, 1988.
6. Amiral J, Bridey F, Dreyfus M, et al: Platelet factor 4 complexed to heparin is the target for antibodies generated in heparin-induced thrombocytopenia. *Thromb Haemost* 68:95, 1992.
7. Warkentin TE, Sheppard JA, Sigouin CS, et al: Gender imbalance and risk factor inter-actions in heparin-induced thrombocytopenia. *Blood* 108:2937, 2006.
8. Warkentin TE, Shepard JA, Horsewood P, et al: Impact of the patient population on the risk for heparin-induced thrombocytopenia. *Blood* 96:1703, 2000.
9. Pouplard C, May MA, Regina S, et al: Changes in platelet count after cardiac surgery can effectively predict the development of pathogenic heparin-dependent antibodies. *Br J Haematol* 128:837, 2005.
10. Selleng S, Malowsky B, Strobel U, et al: Early-onset and persisting thrombocytopenia in post-cardiac surgery patients is rarely due to heparin-induced thrombocytopenia, even when antibody tests are positive. *J Thromb Haemost* 8:30, 2010.
11. Sanson BJ, Lensing AW, Prins MH, et al: Safety of low-molecular-weight heparin in pregnancy: As systematic review. *Thromb Haemost* 81:668, 1999.
12. Fausett MB, Vogtlander M, Lee RM, et al: Heparin-induced thrombocytopenia is rare in pregnancy. *Am J Obstet Gynecol* 185:148, 2001.
13. Avila ML, Shah V, Brandão LR: Systematic review on heparin-induced thrombocytope-nia in children: A call to action. *J Thromb Haemost* 11:660, 2013.
14. Lubenow N, Hinz P, Thomaschewski S, et al: The severity of trauma determines the immune response to PF4/heparin and the frequency of heparin-induced thrombocy-topenia. *Blood* 115:1797, 2010.
15. Martel N, Lee J, Wells PS: Risk for heparin-induced thrombocytopenia with unfrac-tionated and low-molecular-weight heparin thromboprophylaxis: A meta-analysis. *Blood* 106:2710, 2005.
16. Morris TA, Castrejon S, Devendra G, Gamst AC: No difference in risk for thrombocy-topenia during treatment of pulmonary embolism and deep venous thrombosis with either low-molecular-weight heparin or unfractionated heparin: A metaanalysis. *Chest* 132:1131, 2007.
17. Pohl C, Kredteck A, Bastians B, et al: Heparin-induced thrombocytopenia in neuro-logic patients treated with low-molecular-weight heparin. *Neurology* 64:1285, 2005.
18. Warkentin TE: Fondaparinux: Does it cause HIT? Can it treat HIT? *Expert Rev Hematol* 3:567, 2010.

19. Smythe M, Koerber JM, Mattson JC: The incidence of recognized heparin-induced thrombocytopenia in a large, tertiary care teaching hospital. *Chest* 131:1644, 2007.

20. Muslimani AA, Ricaurte B, Daw HA: Immune heparin-induced thrombocytopenia resulting from preceding exposure to heparin catheter flushes. *Am J Hematol* 82:652, 2007.

21. Laster J, Silver D: Heparin-coated catheters and heparin-induced thrombocytopenia. *J Vasc Surg* 7:667, 1988.

22. Juhl D, Eichler P, Lubenow N, et al: Incidence and clinical significance of anti-PF4/heparin antibodies of the IgG, IgM, and IgA class in 755 consecutive patient samples referred for diagnostic testing for heparin-induced thrombocytopenia. *Eur J Haematol* 76:420, 2006.

23. Warkentin TE, Kelton JG: Temporal aspects of heparin-induced thrombocytopenia. *N Engl J Med* 344:1286, 2001.

24. Krauel K, Pötschke C, Weber C, et al: Platelet factor 4 binds to bacteria, [corrected] inducing antibodies cross-reacting with the major antigen in heparin-induced thrombocytopenia. *Blood* 117:1370, 2011.

25. Zheng Y, Yu M, Podd A, et al: Critical role for mouse marginal zone B cells in PF4/heparin antibody production. *Blood* 121:3484, 2013.

26. Zhang X, Chen L, Bancroft DP, et al: Crystal structure of recombinant human platelet factor 4. *Biochemistry* 33:8361, 1994.

27. Stuckey JA, St Charles R, Edwards BF: A model of the platelet factor 4 complex with heparin. *Proteins* 14:277, 1992.

28. Li ZQ, Liu W, Park KS, et al: Defining a second epitope for heparin-induced thrombocytopenia antibodies using KKO, a murine HIT-like monoclonal antibody. *Blood* 99:1230, 2002.

29. Litvinov RI, Yarovoi SV, Rauova L, et al: Distinct specificity and single-molecule kinetics characterize the interaction of pathogenic and non-pathogenic antibodies against platelet factor 4-heparin complexes with platelet factor 4. *J Biol Chem* 288:33060, 2013.

30. Greinacher A, Pötzsch B, Amiral J, et al: Heparin-associated thrombocytopenia: Isolation of the antibody and characterization of a multimolecular PF4-heparin complex as the major antigen. *Thromb Haemost* 71:247, 1994.

31. Horne MK 3rd, Alkins BR: Platelet binding of IgG from patients with heparin-induced thrombocytopenia. *J Lab Clin Med* 127:435, 1996.

32. Rauova L, Poncz M, McKenzie SE, et al: Ultralarge complexes of PF4 and heparin are central to the pathogenesis of heparin-induced thrombocytopenia. *Blood* 105:131, 2005.

33. Suvarna S, Espinasse B, Qi R, et al: Determinants of PF4/heparin immunogenicity. *Blood* 110:4253, 2007.

34. Reilly MP, Taylor SM, Hartman NK, et al: Heparin-induced thrombocytopenia/thrombosis in a transgenic mouse model requires human platelet factor 4 and platelet activation through FcγRIIA. *Blood* 98:2442, 2001.

35. Rauova L, Zhai L, Kowalska MA, et al: Role of platelet surface PF4 antigenic complexes in heparin-induced thrombocytopenia pathogenesis: Diagnostic and therapeutic implications. *Blood* 107:2346, 2006.

36. Warkentin TE, Hayward CP, Boshkov LK, et al: Sera from patients with heparin-induced thrombocytopenia generate platelet-derived microparticles with procoagulant activity: An explanation for the thrombotic complications of heparin-induced thrombocytopenia. *Blood* 84:3691, 1994.

37. Visentin GP, Malik M, Cyganiak KA, Aster RH: Patients treated with unfractionated heparin during open heart surgery are at high risk to form antibodies reactive with heparin:platelet factor 4 complexes. *J Lab Clin Med* 128:376, 1996.

38. Pouplard C, Iochmann S, Renard B, et al: Induction of monocyte tissue factor expression by antibodies to heparin-platelet factor 4 complexes developed in heparin-induced thrombocytopenia. *Blood* 97:3300, 2001.

39. Arepally GM, Mayer IM: Antibodies from patients with heparin-induced thrombocytopenia stimulate monocytic cells to express tissue factor and secret interleukin-8. *Blood* 98:1252, 2001.

40. Xiao Z, Visentin GP, Dayananda KM, Neelaegham S: Immune complexes formed following the binding of anti-platelet factor 4 (CXCL4) antibodies to CXCL4 stimulate human neutrophil activation and cell adhesion. *Blood* 112:1091, 2008.

41. Kasthuri RS, Glover SL, Jonas W, et al: PF4/heparin-antibody complex induces monocyte tissue factor expression and release of tissue factor positive microparticles by activation of FcγRI. *Blood* 119:5285, 2012.

42. Ward JV, Packham MA: Characterization of the sulfated glycosaminoglycans on the surface and in the storage granules of rabbit platelets. *Biochim Biophys Acta* 583:196, 1979.

43. Handin RI, Cohen HJ: Purification and binding properties of human platelet factor four. *J Biol Chem* 251:4273, 1976.

44. Rauova L, Hirsch JD, Greene TK, et al: Monocyte-bound PF4 in the pathogenesis of heparin-induced thrombocytopenia. *Blood* 116:5021, 2010.

45. Carlsson LE, Lubenow N, Blumentritt C, et al: Platelet receptor and clotting factor polymorphisms as genetic risk factors for thromboembolic complications in heparin-induced thrombocytopenia. *Pharmacogenetics* 13:253, 2003.

46. Arepally G, McKenzie SE, Jiang XM, et al: Fc gamma RIIA H/R 131 polymorphism, subclass-specific IgG anti-heparin/platelet factor 4 antibodies and clinical course in patients with heparin-induced thrombocytopenia and thrombosis. *Blood* 89:370, 1997.

47. Carlsson LE, Santoso S, Baurichter G, et al: Heparin-induced thrombocytopenia: New insights into the impact of the FcgammaRIIa-R-H131 polymorphism. *Blood* 92:1526, 1998.

48. Chong BH, Pilgrim RL, Cooley MA, Chesterman CN: Increased expression of platelet IgG Fc receptors in immune heparin-induced thrombocytopenia. *Blood* 81:988, 1993.

49. Cuker A, Rauova L, Bolgiano D, et al: Atherosclerosis is not a risk factor for anti-platelet factor 4/heparin antibody formation after cardiopulmonary bypass surgery. *Thromb Haemost* 111:1191, 2014.

50. Oliveira GB, Crespo EM, Becker RC, et al: Complications After Thrombocytopenia Caused by Heparin (CATCH) Registry Investigators: Incidence and prognostic significance of thrombocytopenia in patients treated with prolonged heparin therapy. *Arch Intern Med* 168:94, 2008.

51. Warkentin TE, Kelton JG: Delayed-onset heparin-induced thrombocytopenia and thrombosis. *Ann Intern Med* 135:502, 2001.

52. Rice L, Attisha WK, Drexler A, Francis JL: Delayed-onset heparin-induced thrombocytopenia. *Ann Intern Med* 136:210, 2002.

53. Warkentin TE, Basciano PA, Knopman J, Bernstein RA: Spontaneous heparin-induced thrombocytopenia syndrome: 2 new cases and a proposal for defining this disorder. *Blood* 123:3651, 2014.

54. Warkentin TE: Clinical presentation of heparin-induced thrombocytopenia. *Semin Hematol* 35:9, 1998.

55. Warkentin TE, Roberts RS, Hirsh J, Kelton JG: An improved definition of immune heparin-induced thrombocytopenia in postoperative orthopedic patients. *Arch Intern Med* 163:2518, 2003.

56. Greinacher A, Farner B, Kroll H, et al: Clinical features of heparin-induced thrombocytopenia including risk factors for thrombosis. A retrospective analysis of 408 patients. *Thromb Haemost* 94:132, 2005.

57. Warkentin TE, Kelton JG: A 14-year study of heparin-induced thrombocytopenia. *Am J Med* 101:502, 1996.

58. Hong AP, Cook DJ, Sigouin CS, Warkentin TE: Central venous catheters and upper-extremity deep-vein thrombosis complicating immune heparin-induced thrombocytopenia. *Blood* 101:3049, 2003.

59. Warkentin TE, Levine MN, Hirsh J, et al: Heparin-induced thrombocytopenia in patients treated with low-molecular-weight heparin or unfractionated heparin. *N Engl J Med* 332:1330, 1995.

60. Warkentin TE, Roberts RS, Hirsh J, Kelton JG: Heparin-induced skin lesions and other unusual sequelae of the heparin-induced thrombocytopenia syndrome: A nested cohort study. *Chest* 127:1857, 2005.

61. Warkentin TE, Greinacher A: Heparin-induced anaphylactic and anaphylactoid reactions: Two distinct but overlapping syndromes. *Expert Opin Drug Saf* 8:129, 2009.

62. Schindewolf M, Kroll H, Ackermann H, et al: Heparin-induced non-necrotizing skin lesions: Rarely associated with heparin-induced thrombocytopenia. *J Thromb Haemost* 8:1486, 2010.

63. Cuker A, Cines DB: How I treat heparin-induced thrombocytopenia. *Blood* 119:2209, 2012.

64. Lo GK, Juhl D, Warkentin TE, et al: Evaluation of pretest clinical score (4 T's) for the diagnosis of heparin-induced thrombocytopenia in two clinical settings. *J Thromb Haemost* 4:759, 2006.

65. Cuker A, Gimotty PA, Crowther MA, Warkentin TE: Predictive value of the 4Ts scoring system for heparin-induced thrombocytopenia: A systematic review and meta-analysis. *Blood* 120:4160, 2012.

66. Nagler M, Fabbro T, Wuillemin WA: Prospective evaluation of the interobserver reliability of the 4Ts score in patients with suspected heparin-induced thrombocytopenia. *J Thromb Haemost* 10:151, 2012.

67. Cuker A, Arepally G, Crowther MA, et al: The HIT Expert Probability (HEP) Score: A novel pre-test probability model for heparin-induced thrombocytopenia based on broad expert opinion. *J Thromb Haemost* 8:2642, 2010.

68. Bakchoul T, Giptner A, Najaoui A, et al: Prospective evaluation of PF4/heparin immunoassays for the diagnosis of heparin-induced thrombocytopenia. *J Thromb Haemost* 7:1260, 2009.

69. Lo GK, Sigouin CS, Warkentin TE: What is the potential for overdiagnosis of heparin-induced thrombocytopenia? *Am J Hematol* 82:1037, 2007.

70. Greinacher A, Juhl D, Strobel U, et al: Heparin-induced thrombocytopenia: A prospective study on the incidence, platelet-activating capacity and clinical significance of antiplatelet factor 4/heparin antibodies of the IgG, IgM, and IgA classes. *J Thromb Haemost* 5:1666, 2007.

71. Pauzner R, Greinacher A, Selleng K, et al: False-positive tests for heparin-induced thrombocytopenia in patients with antiphospholipid syndrome and systemic lupus erythematosus. *J Thromb Haemost* 7:1070, 2009.

72. Sikara MP, Routsias JG, Samiotaki M, et al: β2 Glycoprotein I (β2GPI) binds platelet factor 4 (PF4): Implications for the pathogenesis of antiphospholipid syndrome. *Blood* 115:713, 2010.

73. Zwicker JI, Uhl L, Huang WY, et al: Thrombosis and ELISA optical density values in hospitalized patients with heparin-induced thrombocytopenia. *J Thromb Haemost* 2:2133, 2004.

74. Warkentin TE, Sheppard JI, Moore JC, et al: Quantitative interpretation of optical density measurements using PF4-dependent enzyme-immunoassays. *J Thromb Haemost* 6:1304, 2008.

75. Raschke RA, Curry SC, Warkentin TE, Gerkin RD: Improving clinical interpretation of the anti-platelet factor 4/heparin enzyme-linked immunosorbent assay for the diagnosis of heparin-induced thrombocytopenia through the use of receiver operating characteristic analysis, stratum-specific likelihood ratios, and Bayes theorem. *Chest* 144:1269, 2013.

76. Cuker A, Ortel TL: ASH evidence-based guidelines: Is the IgG-specific anti-PF4/heparin ELISA superior to the polyspecific ELISA in the laboratory diagnosis of HIT? *Hematology Am Soc Hematol Educ Program* 2009:250, 2009.

77. Whitlatch NL, Kong DF, Metjian AD, et al: Validation of the high-dose heparin confirmatory step for the diagnosis of heparin-induced thrombocytopenia. *Blood* 116:1761, 2010.

78. Warkentin TE, Sheppard JI: No significant improvement in diagnostic specificity of an anti-PF4/polyanion immunoassay with use of high heparin confirmatory procedure. *J Thromb Haemost* 4:281, 2006.

79. Selleng S, Schreier N, Wollert HG, Greinacher A: The diagnostic value of the anti-PF4/heparin immunoassay high-dose heparin confirmatory test in cardiac surgery patients. *Anesth Analg* 112:774, 2011.

80. Sachs UJ, von Hesberg J, Santoso S, et al: Evaluation of a new nanoparticle-based lateral-flow immunoassay for the exclusion of heparin-induced thrombocytopenia (HIT). *Thromb Haemost* 106:1197, 2011.

81. Meyer O, Salama A, Pittet N, Schwind P: Rapid detection of heparin-induced platelet antibodies with particle gel immunoassay (ID-HPF4). *Lancet* 354:1525, 1999.

82. Leroux D, Hezard N, Lebreton A, et al: Prospective evaluation of a rapid nanoparticle-based lateral flow immunoassay (STic Expert® HIT) for the diagnosis of heparin-induced thrombocytopenia. *Br J Haematol* 166:774, 2014.

83. Davidson SJ, Ortel TL, Smith LJ: Performance of a new, rapid, automated immunoassay for the detection of anti-platelet factor 4/heparin complex antibodies. *Blood Coagul Fibrinolysis* 22:340, 2011.

84. Althaus K, Hron G, Strobel U, et al: Evaluation of automated immunoassays in the diagnosis of heparin induced thrombocytopenia. *Thromb Res* 131:e85, 2013.

85. Legnani C, Cini M, Pili C, et al: Evaluation of a new automated panel of assays for the detection of anti-PF4/heparin antibodies in patients suspected of having heparin-induced thrombocytopenia. *Thromb Haemost* 104:402, 2010.

86. Van Hoecke F, Devreese K: Evaluation of two new automated chemiluminescent assays (HemosIL® AcuStar HIT-IgG and HemosIL® AcuStar HIT-Ab) for the detection of heparin-induced antibodies in the diagnosis of heparin-induced thrombocytopenia. *Int J Lab Hematol* 34:410, 2012.

87. Warkentin TE, Sheppard JI, Raschke R, Greinacher A: Performance characteristics of a rapid assay for anti-PF4/heparin antibodies: The particle immunofiltration assay. *J Thromb Haemost* 5:2308, 2007.

88. Andrews DM, Cubillos GF, Paulino SK, et al: Prospective evaluation of the particle immunofiltration anti-platelet factor 4 rapid assay in MICU patients with thrombocytopenia. *Crit Care* 17:R143, 2013.

89. Sheridan D, Carter C, Kelton JG: A diagnostic test for heparin-induced thrombocytopenia. *Blood* 67:27, 1986.

90. Greinacher A, Michels I, Kiefel V, Mueller-Eckhardt C: A rapid and sensitive test for diagnosing heparin-associated thrombocytopenia. *Thromb Haemost* 66:734, 1991.

91. Price EA, Hayward CP, Moffat KA, et al: Laboratory testing for heparin-induced thrombocytopenia is inconsistent in North America: A survey of North American specialized coagulation laboratories. *Thromb Haemost* 98:1357, 2007.

92. Cuker A, Rux AH, Hinds JL, et al: Novel diagnostic assays for heparin-induced thrombocytopenia. *Blood* 121:3727, 2013.

93. Nazi I, Arnold DM, Smith JW, et al: FcγRIIa proteolysis as a diagnostic biomarker for heparin-induced thrombocytopenia. *J Thromb Haemost* 11:1146, 2013.

94. Greinacher A, Eichler P, Lubenow N, et al: Heparin-induced thrombocytopenia with thromboembolic complications: Meta-analysis of 2 prospective trials to assess the value of parenteral treatment with lepirudin and its therapeutic aPTT range. *Blood* 96:846, 2000.

95. Linkins LA, Dans AL, Moores LK, et al: American College of Chest Physicians: Treatment and prevention of heparin-induced thrombocytopenia: Antithrombotic Therapy and Prevention of Thrombosis, 9th ed: American College of Chest Physicians Evidence-Based Clinical Practice Guidelines. *Chest* 141:e495S, 2012.

96. Lewis BE, Wallis DE, Berkowitz SD, et al: ARG-911 Study Investigators: Argatroban anticoagulant therapy in patients with heparin-induced thrombocytopenia. *Circulation* 103:1838, 2001.

97. Lewis BE, Wallis DE, Leya F, et al: Argatroban-915 Investigators: Argatroban anticoagulation in patients with heparin-induced thrombocytopenia. *Arch Intern Med* 163:1849, 2003.

98. Lewis BE, Wallis DE, Hursting MJ, et al: Effects of argatroban therapy, demographic variables, and platelet count on thrombotic risks in heparin-induced thrombocytopenia. *Chest* 129:1407, 2006.

99. Walenga JM, Fasanella AR, Iqbal O, Het al: Coagulation laboratory testing in patients treated with argatroban. *Semin Thromb Hemost* 25:61, 1999.

100. Kiser TH, Fish DN: Evaluation of bivalirudin treatment for heparin-induced thrombocytopenia in critically ill patients with hepatic and/or renal dysfunction. *Pharmacotherapy* 26:452, 2006.

101. Koster A, Dyke CM, Aldea G, et al: Bivalirudin during cardiopulmonary bypass in patients with previous or acute heparin-induced thrombocytopenia and heparin antibodies: Results of the CHOOSE-ON trial. *Ann Thorac Surg* 83:572, 2007.

102. Skrupky LP, Smith JR, Deal EN, et al: Comparison of bivalirudin and argatroban for the management of heparin-induced thrombocytopenia. *Pharmacotherapy* 30:1229, 2010.

103. Joseph L, Casanegra AI, Dhariwal M, et al: Bivalirudin for the treatment of patients with confirmed or suspected heparin-induced thrombocytopenia. *J Thromb Haemost* 12:1044, 2014.

104. Boyce SW, Bandyk DF, Bartholomew JR, et al: A randomized, open-label pilot study comparing desirudin and argatroban in patients with suspected heparin-induced thrombocytopenia with or without thrombosis: PREVENT-HIT Study. *Am J Ther* 18:14, 2011.

105. Chong BH, Gallus AS, Cade JF, et al; Australian HIT Study Group: Prospective randomised open-label comparison of danaparoid with dextran 70 in the treatment of heparin-induced thrombocytopaenia with thrombosis: A clinical outcome study. *Thromb Haemost* 86:1170, 2001.

106. Magnani HN, Gallus A: Heparin-induced thrombocytopenia (HIT). A report of 1,478 clinical outcomes of patients treated with danaparoid (Organan) from 1982 to mid-2004. *Thromb Haemost* 95:967, 2006.

107. Blackmer AB, Oertel MD, Valgus JM: Fondaparinux and the management of heparin-induced thrombocytopenia: The journey continues. *Ann Pharmacother* 43:1636, 2009.

108. Grouzi E, Kyriakou E, Panagou I, Spiliotopoulou I: Fondaparinux for the treatment of acute heparin-induced thrombocytopenia: A single-center experience. *Clin Appl Thromb Hemost* 16:663, 2010.

109. Warkentin TE, Pai M, Sheppard JI, et al: Fondaparinux treatment of acute heparin-induced thrombocytopenia confirmed by the serotonin-release assay: A 30-month, 16-patient case series. *J Thromb Haemost* 9:2389, 2011.

110. Goldfarb MJ, Blostein MD: Fondaparinux in acute heparin-induced thrombocytopenia: A case series. *J Thromb Haemost* 9:2501, 2011.

111. Warkentin TE: Fondaparinux: Does it cause HIT? Can it treat HIT? *Expert Rev Hematol* 3:567, 2010.

112. Schindewolf M, Steindl J, Beyer-Westendorf J, et al: Frequent off-label use of fondaparinux in patients with suspected acute heparin-induced thrombocytopenia (HIT)–findings from the GerHIT multi-centre registry study. *Thromb Res* 134:29, 2014.

113. Krauel K, Hackbarth C, Furll B, Greinacher A: Heparin-induced thrombocytopenia: In vivo studies on the interaction of dabigatran, rivaroxaban, and low-sulfated heparin, with platelet factor 4 and anti-PF4/heparin antibodies. *Blood* 119:1248, 2012.

114. Anniccherico FJ, Alonso JL: Dabigatran for heparin-induced thrombocytopenia. *Mayo Clin Proc* 88:1036, 2013.

115. Ng HJ, Than H, Teo EC: First experience with the use of rivaroxaban in the treatment of heparin-induced thrombocytopenia. *Thromb Res* 135:205, 2015.

116. Linkins LA, Warkentin TE, Pai M, et al: Design of the rivaroxaban for heparin-induced thrombocytopenia study. *J Thromb Thrombolysis* 38:485, 2014.

117. Sachias BS, Rux AH, Cines DB, et al: Rational design and characterization of platelet factor 4 antagonists for the study of heparin-induced thrombocytopenia. *Blood* 119:5955, 2012.

118. Reilly MP, Sinha U, André P, et al: PRT-060318, a novel Syk inhibitor, prevents heparin-induced thrombocytopenia and thrombosis in a transgenic mouse model. *Blood* 117:2241, 2011.

119. Stolla M, Stefanini L, André P, et al: CalDAG-GEFI deficiency protects mice in a novel model of Fcγ RIIA-mediated thrombosis and thrombocytopenia. *Blood* 118:1113, 2011.

120. Cuker A: Heparin-induced thrombocytopenia (HIT) in 2011: An epidemic of overdiagnosis. *Thromb Haemost* 106:993, 2011.

121. Smythe MA, Koerber JM, Mehta TP, et al: Assessing the impact of a heparin-induced thrombocytopenia protocol on patient management, outcomes, and costs. *Thromb Haemost* 108:992, 2012.

122. Watson H, Davidson S, Keeling D; Haemostasis and Thrombosis Task Force of the British Committee for Standards in Haematology: Guidelines on the diagnosis and management of heparin-induced thrombocytopenia: Second edition. *Br J Haematol* 159:528, 2012.

123. Warkentin TE, Elavathil LJ, Hayward CP, et al: The pathogenesis of venous limb gangrene associated with heparin-induced thrombocytopenia. *Ann Intern Med* 127:804, 1997.

124. Sheth SB, DiCicco RA, Hursting MJ, et al: Interpreting the International Normalized Ratio (INR) in individuals receiving argatroban and warfarin. *Thromb Haemost* 85:453, 2001.

125. Hopkins CK, Goldfinger D: Platelet transfusions in heparin-induced thrombocytopenia: A report of four cases and review of the literature. *Transfusion* 48:2128, 2008.

126. Refaai MA, Chuang C, Menegus M, et al: Outcomes after platelet transfusion in patients with heparin-induced thrombocytopenia. *J Thromb Haemost* 8:1419, 2010.

127. Gruel Y, Lang M, Darnige L, et al: Fatal effect of re-exposure to heparin after previous heparin-associated thrombocytopenia and thrombosis. *Lancet* 336:1077, 1990.

128. Pötzsch B, Klövekorn WP, Madlener K: Use of heparin during cardiopulmonary bypass in patients with a history of heparin-induced thrombocytopenia. *N Engl J Med* 343:515, 2000.

129. Warkentin TE, Sheppard JA: Serological investigation of patients with a previous history of heparin-induced thrombocytopenia who are reexposed to heparin. *Blood* 123:2485, 2014.

130. Selleng S, Haneya A, Hirt S, et al: Management of anticoagulation in patients with subacute heparin-induced thrombocytopenia scheduled for heart transplantation. *Blood* 112:4024, 2008.

131. Carrier M, Knoll GA, Kovacs MJ, et al: The prevalence of antibodies to the platelet factor 4–heparin complex and associated with access thrombosis in patients on chronic hemodialysis. *Thromb Res* 120:215, 2007.

132. Hutchison CA, Dasgupta I: National survey of heparin-induced thrombocytopenia in the haemodialysis population of the UK population. *Nephrol Dial Transplant* 22:1680, 2007.

133. Magnani HN: An analysis of clinical outcomes of 91 pregnancies in 83 women treated with danaparoid (Organan). *Thromb Res* 125:297, 2010.

134. Hajj-Chahine J, Jayle C, Tomasi J, Corbi P: Successful surgical management of massive pulmonary embolism during the second trimester in a parturient with heparin-induced thrombocytopenia. *Interact Cardiovasc Thorac Surg* 11:679, 2010.

135. Ciurzyński M, Jankowski K, Pietrzak B, et al: Use of fondaparinux in a pregnant woman with pulmonary embolism and heparin-induced thrombocytopenia. *Med Sci Monit* 17:CS56, 2011.

136. Dempfle CE: Minor transplacental passage of fondaparinux *in vivo*. *N Engl J Med* 350:1914, 2004.

CHAPTER 119
REACTIVE THROMBOCYTOSIS

Kenneth Kaushansky

SUMMARY

The three major pathophysiologic causes of thrombocytosis are (1) clonal, including essential (or primary) thrombocythemia and other myeloproliferative neoplasms; (2) familial, including rare cases of nonclonal myeloproliferation resulting from thrombopoietin and thrombopoietin receptor mutations; and (3) reactive, in which thrombocytosis occurs secondary to a variety of acute and chronic clinical conditions. This chapter deals with the latter causes of thrombocytosis.

The upper limit of the normal platelet count in most clinical laboratories is between 350,000/μL (350 × 10^9/L) and 450,000/μL (450 × 10^9/L). In a sample of 10,000 healthy individuals 18 to 65 years of age, 1 percent had platelet counts greater than 400,000/μL. Only in eight of these 99 individuals was thrombocytosis confirmed 6 months to 1 year later.[1] Nevertheless, it is clear that thrombocytosis is a feature of several important disorders, including cancer, and that even a high normal platelet count is associated with morbidity and mortality. In a longitudinal study of healthy Norwegian men, a platelet count in the top quartile of the normal range (from 275 × 10^9/L to 350 × 10^9/L) was associated with a twofold increase in cardiovascular mortality over a 12-year followup.[2] Whether the platelet count per se, or an underlying inflammatory condition resulting in both thrombocytosis and accelerated atherogenesis is responsible for these observations is not certain. The causes of thrombocytosis in which the platelet count exceeds the upper limit can be broadly categorized as (1) clonal, including essential thrombocythemia and other myeloproliferative neoplasms, (2) familial, and (3) reactive, or secondary (see Chap. 85, Table 85–1). This chapter focuses on the causes and molecular mechanisms that underlie reactive, or secondary, thrombocytosis; clonal and familial thrombocytosis are discussed in detail in Chap. 85.

● NORMAL THROMBOPOIESIS

The regulation of platelet production is discussed extensively in Chap. 111, but a brief discussion here provides the appropriate background for discussion of reactive thrombocytosis. Thrombopoietin (TPO), the

ligand for the megakaryocytic growth factor receptor c-Mpl, is the major humoral regulator of megakaryocyte survival, growth, and development, although, curiously, it does not stimulate the final step in thrombopoiesis: platelet release from megakaryocyte proplatelet processes. Although TPO supports the entire continuum of megakaryocyte development from stem cell to mature megakaryocyte,[3] other cytokines including interleukin (IL)-6,[4] IL-3,[5,6] IL-11,[7] leukemia inhibitory factor (LIF),[8,9] fibroblast growth factor (FGF)-4,[10] stromal cell-derived factor (SDF)-1,[10,11] interferon (IFN)-γ,[12] and granulocyte-macrophage colony-stimulating factor (GM-CSF)[13] also affect thrombopoiesis, both in vitro and in vivo. Many of these cytokines act in synergy with other cytokines, including TPO.[11,12,14]

The regulation of thrombopoiesis occurs primarily by humoral mechanisms, with the levels of TPO inversely related to platelet counts.[15,16] In contrast, other cytokines shown to affect megakaryopoiesis in vitro do not vary with platelet levels.[17] Despite these important insights, the regulation of TPO blood levels is complex, and incompletely understood. The liver produces approximately half of all the hormone that circulates, based on platelet production in liver specific knockout mice.[18] However, platelet levels do not affect hepatic TPO production; instead, platelets themselves have an important role in regulating plasma levels, as their receptors for TPO (c-mpl) remove it from plasma.[19] Thus, as the platelet count drops, increased free plasma TPO levels stimulate megakaryopoiesis; conversely, as the platelet count rises, depletion of free plasma TPO decreases platelet production. This modulatory mechanism results in the steady-state level of platelet production. However, marrow stromal cells also produce TPO,[20] and are responsive to platelet products which serve to down-modulate expression of the hormone.[21] A third mechanism by which platelets regulate TPO levels occurs through the Ashwell-Morell hepatocyte receptor, whereby their binding of senescent platelets leads to stimulation of hepatocyte signaling pathways and subsequent expression of TPO.[22]

● ENHANCED THROMBOPOIESIS IN PATHOLOGIC STATES

THROMBOCYTOSIS IN INFLAMMATORY CONDITIONS

Inflammation is the most common cause of secondary thrombocytosis. In one survey, thrombocytosis was believed secondary to one or more inflammatory conditions in nearly 80 percent of all patients with an elevated platelet count. Table 119–1 lists the clinical conditions associated with reactive thrombocytosis. The most common diagnoses in such patients are inflammatory bowel disease and rheumatoid arthritis,[23] although most conditions in which the erythrocyte sedimentation rate or C-reactive protein is elevated have been reported to cause secondary thrombocytosis. Although several cytokines and lymphokines are elevated in the blood of such patients, the most compelling evidence suggests that IL-6 and IFN-γ are responsible for the thrombocytosis seen in patients with inflammation.

Interleukin-6

IL-6 was cloned by several groups of investigators using a number of distinct assays, including antiviral activity, myeloma cell growth, hepatocyte growth, and immunoglobulin secretion.[24] The recombinant protein was later found to affect megakaryocyte growth and differentiation, both in vitro and in vivo.[4,25,26] The IL-6 gene is present on the short arm of human chromosome 7, and encodes a 26-kDa polypeptide produced in almost all tissues from T cells, fibroblasts, macrophages, and stromal cells, and is a key regulator of the inflammatory response.[27]

TABLE 119–1. Major Causes of Thrombocytosis

A. Reactive (secondary) thrombocytosis
  1. Transient reactive processes
  2. Acute blood loss
  3. Recovery ("rebound") from thrombocytopenia
  4. Acute infection, inflammation
  5. Response to exercise
B. Sustained processes
  1. Iron deficiency
  2. Postsplenectomy, asplenic states
  3. Malignancies
  4. Chronic inflammatory and infectious diseases (inflammatory bowel disease, rheumatoid arteritis, tuberculosis, chronic pneumonitis)
  5. Response to drugs (vincristine, epinephrine, all-*trans*-retinoic acid, some antibiotics, cytokines, and growth factors)
  6. Hemolytic anemia

IL-6 production is dependent on the presence of IL-1 and tumor necrosis factor (TNF)-α, cytokines produced by lymphocytes and monocytes in response to phagocytosis of microorganisms, the binding of immune complexes, and several other innate immune stimuli. IL-6 production is regulated primarily by transcriptional enhancement; regulatory elements responsible for IL-6 promoter activation include nuclear factor-κB (NFκB), adapter protein (AP)-1, CCAAT/enhancer binding protein (C/EBP) α and C/EBPβ.

Although not critical for steady-state thrombopoiesis, as the combined genetic elimination of *c-mpl* and the signaling component of the IL-6 receptor (gp130) produces no more severe thrombocytopenia than elimination of *c-mpl* alone,[29] IL-6 contributes to inflammatory thrombopoiesis, primarily by stimulating the hepatic production of TPO.[30] Most studies report that patients with inflammation display an increased level of TPO,[31,32] but TPO is not the only cytokine responsible for this effect,[33] especially when corrected for the thrombocytosis, which would normally act to reduce levels of the hormone. Stimulation of hepatocytes with IL-6 results in enhanced production of TPO mRNA and protein.[34,35]

INTERFERON-γ

A second inflammatory cytokine that contributes to inflammatory thrombopoiesis is IFN-γ. The interferons are proteins first defined by their ability to induce an antiviral state in mammalian cells. Biochemical fractionation revealed three classes of interferons: IFN-α, a family of 17 distinct but highly homologous molecules; IFN-β, a single molecule more distantly related to the various isoforms of IFN-α; and IFN-γ, a unique molecule that shares functional properties but not structure with the others. IFN-γ exerts the most profound hematologic effects of the three classes of protein, including direct suppression of erythroid colony-forming cell growth and the activation of macrophages to secrete a number of inflammatory cytokines; several comprehensive reviews on IFN-γ have been published.[36,37]

IFN-γ is produced by activated T lymphocytes and natural killer (NK) cells in response to T-cell antigen crosslinking and in response to stimulation by the inflammatory mediators TNF-α, IL-12, and IL-15.[38] Prominent hematologic effects include activation of macrophages to assume an inflammatory phenotype (e.g., secretion of TNF-α and enhanced tumor cell killing), upregulation of major histocompatibility

complex (MHC) class I and class II molecules enhancing antigen recognition responses,[37] and inhibition of proliferative responses in stem cells and erythroid progenitors.[39,40] These latter effects accounts for the association of IFN-γ and aplastic anemia[41] are discussed more fully in Chap. 35. However, in stark contrast to the inhibitory effects of IFN-γ on erythropoiesis, the cytokine stimulates megakaryocyte growth and differentiation.[42] This is likely related to its stimulation of signal transducer and activator of transcription (STAT)-1 in megakaryocytes, as transgenic expression of the transcription factor mimics the effect of the cytokine, and corrects the thrombocytopenia seen in a genetic model system.[43] These findings argue that IFN-γ also contributes to the thrombocytosis seen in inflammatory states in humans.

Notwithstanding the above two mechanisms, patients with inflammatory conditions and thrombocytosis might have an additional cause of the elevated platelet count. The evaluation of iron deficiency is often difficult in patients with inflammation, as the most reliable indicator of tissue iron stores, serum ferritin, is an acute-phase reactant, possibly obscuring a diagnosis of iron deficiency in patients with an inflammatory condition. In a recent study of patients with inflammatory bowel disease, thrombocytosis was eliminated in half of the subjects by the administration or iron.[44]

THROMBOCYTOSIS CAUSED BY IRON DEFICIENCY

Although most patients with inflammation-related thrombocytosis display increased production of the hormone, TPO levels in patients with iron deficiency and thrombocytosis are not elevated.[45] In contrast, erythropoietin (EPO) levels are elevated in patients with iron-deficiency anemia, and are thought by some to be the responsible for the thrombocytosis seen in iron deficiency, at least in part. Consistent with this hypothesis, administration of EPO to animals and humans leads to a modest increase in the platelet count.[46] Although some have suggested that this is a result of cross-reactivity of EPO on the TPO receptor,[47] direct EPO- and TPO-receptor binding studies refute this hypothesis.[48] Rather, megakaryocytic progenitors display EPO receptors, and their binding of the hormone leads to many of the same intracellular biochemical signals as induced by TPO (Chap. 17).

However, several lines of evidence indicate that pathophysiologic mechanisms other than anemia must be responsible, at least in part, for the thrombocytosis seen in patients with iron deficiency. For example, many patients with iron-deficiency anemia do not have thrombocytosis.[45] Moreover, EPO levels are elevated in nearly all types of anemia, but iron deficiency is the only type of anemia that is regularly associated with thrombocytosis, other than the anemia of chronic inflammation, in which the inflammatory state that causes the anemia by modulation of hepcidin levels (Chap. 37) also causes thrombocytosis (as discussed in "Thrombocytosis in Inflammatory Conditions" above). Thus, although several lines of evidence suggest that enhanced levels of EPO as a consequence of the anemia associated with iron deficiency contribute to this form of reactive thrombocytosis, elevated EPO levels cannot completely account for it.

THERAPEUTIC ERYTHROPOIETIN AND ENHANCED CARDIOVASCULAR MORTALITY

Several reports have linked the use of large doses of EPO or other erythropoiesis-stimulating agents (ESAs) to enhanced cardiovascular mortality,[49] and in patients with renal insufficiency, to progression to dialysis in patients with renal insufficiency,[50] although not all studies concur with these landmark results.[51] Although also discussed in Chap. 18, this finding is presented here because evidence is accumulating that the rapid expansion of erythropoiesis caused by pharmacologic levels of

EPO often induces functional iron deficiency. If so, because iron deficiency leads to thrombocytosis, the excessive cardiovascular morbidity and mortality associated with the administration of EPO and ESAs to patients is hypothesized to be secondary to the thrombocytosis. Consistent with this view is that even a high normal platelet count was found associated with enhanced cardiovascular morbidity and mortality in a longitudinal study of healthy Norwegian men.[2] In support of this hypothesis (that the excessive cardiovascular morbidity and mortality is secondary to the thrombocytosis) is the finding that patients with renal insufficiency on high therapeutic doses of EPO (>20,000 U/week) and hemoglobin (Hgb) values in excess of 13 g/dL are more likely to develop functional iron deficiency and thrombocytosis, and that those individuals in whom the platelet count exceeds 300,000/μL display a statistically significantly higher 3-year mortality rate.[52] An alternate explanation is that EPO directly increases thrombopoiesis independently of iron deficiency and/or enhances the vascular reactivity of platelets. This hypothesis is based on the finding that megakaryocytes and platelets bear EPO receptors,[53] and that TPO, which stimulates very similar signaling pathways as EPO in receptor-bearing cells (Chap. 17), primes platelets to enhanced aggregation responses to classic platelet agonists.[54] Still other researchers have hypothesized that an alternate form of the EPO receptor, made up of the classic EPO receptor and the β subunit of the GM-CSF, IL-3, and IL-5 receptors, is displayed on vascular endothelial cells,[55] and in that site could mediate enhanced vascular events. Thus, given the widespread use of ESAs in patients with anemia caused by cancer, kidney failure, myelodysplastic syndromes, and many other conditions, verifying these hypotheses or disproving them and establishing new ones appears to be important and a field ripe for new discovery.

CLINICAL FEATURES OF REACTIVE THROMBOCYTOSIS

The clinical features of secondary thrombocytosis are almost always a result of the underlying disorder provoking the reaction, usually an inflammatory condition or iron-deficiency anemia. It is also highly unusual for the thrombocytosis per se to provoke any untoward symptoms. Although pathologic thrombosis is a major feature of primary thrombocythemia (Chap. 85), it is virtually absent in reactive thrombocytosis, unless provoked by other features of the underlying condition (e.g., vasculitis) or completely unrelated conditions in the patient (e.g., atherosclerotic disease). Whether this is because patients with reactive thrombocytosis do not have as high platelet counts, on average, as patients with primary thrombocythemia[56]; or because they have smaller mean platelet volumes[56]; or are a result of the activated signaling characteristic of the platelets or other blood cells in patients with myeloproliferative diseases; or because of the presence of a mutant Janus kinase (JAK) 2,[57] or a constitutively active TPO receptor[58] is uncertain at this time. Nevertheless, because vascular complications of reactive thrombocytosis are so unlikely to be a consequence of the elevated platelet count, treatment of the thrombocytosis per se is not recommended in reactive thrombocytosis except in very unusual circumstances.

REFERENCES

1. Ruggeri M, Tosetto A, Frezzato M, Rodeghiero F: The rate of progression to polycythemia vera or essential thrombocythemia in patients with erythrocytosis or thrombocytosis. *Ann Intern Med* 139:470, 2003.
2. Thaulow E, Erikssen J, Sandvik L, et al: Blood platelet count and function are related to total and cardiovascular death in apparently healthy men. *Circulation* 84:613, 1991.
3. Kaushansky K: The molecular mechanisms that control thrombopoiesis. *J Clin Invest* 115:3339, 2005.
4. Williams N, De Giorgio T, Banu N, et al: Recombinant interleukin 6 stimulates immature megakaryocytes. *Exp Hematol* 18:69, 1990.
5. Yonemura Y, Kawakita M, Masuda T, et al: Synergistic effects of interleukin 3 and interleukin 11 on murine megakaryopoiesis in serum-free culture. *Exp Hematol* 20:1011, 1992.
6. Carrington PA, Hill RJ, Stenberg PE, et al: Multiple *in vivo* effects of interleukin 3 and interleukin 6 on mouse megakaryocytopoiesis. *Blood* 77:34, 1991.
7. Schlerman FJ, Bree AG, Kaviani MD, et al: Thrombopoietic activity of recombinant human interleukin 11 in normal and myelosuppressed nonhuman primates. *Stem Cells* 14:517, 1996.
8. Debili N, Massé J-M, Katz A, et al: Effects of the recombinant hematopoietic growth factors interleukin-3, interleukin-6, stem cell factor, and leukemia inhibitory factor on the megakaryocytic differentiation of CD34+ cells. *Blood* 82:84, 1993.
9. Farese A, Myers LA, MacVittie TJ: Therapeutic efficacy of recombinant leukemia inhibitory factor in a primate model of radiation-induced marrow aplasia. *Blood* 84:3675, 1994.
10. Avecilla ST, Hattori K, Heissig B, et al: Chemokine-mediated interaction of hematopoietic progenitors with the bone marrow vascular niche is required for thrombopoiesis. *Nat Med* 10:64, 2004.
11. Hodohara K, Fujii N, Yamamoto N, Kaushansky K: Stromal cell derived factor 1 acts synergistically with thrombopoietin to enhance the development of megakaryocytic progenitor cells. *Blood* 95:769, 2000.
12. Tsuji-Takayama K, Tahata H, Izumi N, et al: IFN-gamma in combination with IL-3 accelerates platelet recovery in mice with 5-fluorouracil-induced marrow aplasia. *J Interferon Cytokine Res* 16:447, 1996.
13. Kaushansky K, O'Hara PJ, Berkner K, et al: Genomic cloning, characterization, and multilineage expression of human granulocyte-macrophage colony-stimulating factor. *Proc Natl Acad Sci U S A* 83:3101, 1986.
14. Broudy VC, Lin NL, Kaushansky K: Thrombopoietin (c-mpl ligand) acts synergistically with erythropoietin, stem cell factor, and IL-11 to enhance murine megakaryocyte colony growth and increases megakaryocyte ploidy *in vitro*. *Blood* 85:1719, 1995.
15. Kuter DJ, Rosenberg RD: The reciprocal relationship of thrombopoietin (c-Mpl Ligand) to changes in the platelet mass during busulfan-induced thrombocytopenia in the rabbit. *Blood* 85:2720, 1995.
16. Kuter DJ: The physiology of platelet production. *Stem Cells* 14(Suppl 1):88, 1996.
17. Cockrell EM, Gorman J, Hord JD, et al: Endogenous interleukin-11 (IL-11) levels in newly diagnosed children with acquired severe aplastic anemia (SAA). *Cytokine* 28:55, 2004.
18. Qian S, Fu F, Li W, et al: Primary role of the liver in thrombopoietin production shown by tissue-specific knockout. *Blood* 92:2189, 1998.
19. Fielder PJ, Hass P, Nagel M, et al: Human platelets as a model for the binding and degradation of thrombopoietin. *Blood* 89:2782, 1997.
20. Sungaran R, Markovic B, Chong BH: Localization and regulation of thrombopoietin mRNA expression in human kidney, liver, bone marrow and spleen using in situ hybridization. *Blood* 89:101, 1997.
21. McIntosh B, Kaushansky K: Marrow stromal production of thrombopoietin is regulated by transcriptional mechanisms in response to platelet products. *Exp Hematol* 36:799, 2008.
22. Grozovsky R, Begonja AJ, Liu K, et al: The Ashwell-Morell receptor regulates hepatic thrombopoietin production via JAK2-STAT3 signaling. *Nat Med* 21:47, 2015.
23. Griesshammer M, Bangerter M, Sauer T, et al: Aetiology and clinical significance of thrombocytosis: Analysis of 732 patients with an elevated platelet count. *J Intern Med* 245:295, 1999.
24. Kishimoto T: The biology of interleukin-6. *Blood* 74:1, 1989.
25. Asano S, Okano A, Ozawa K, et al: *In vivo* effects of recombinant human interleukin 6 in primates: Stimulated production of platelets. *Blood* 75:1602, 1990.
26. Ishibashi T, Kimura H, Shikama Y, et al: Interleukin-6 is a potent thrombopoietic factor *in vivo* in mice. *Blood* 74:1241, 1989.
27. Naka T, Nishimoto N, Kishimoto T: The paradigm of IL-6: From basic science to medicine. *Arthritis Res* 4(Suppl 3):S233, 2002.
28. Sehgal PB: Regulation of IL6 gene expression. *Res Immunol* 143:724, 1992.
29. Gainsford T, Nandurkar H, Metcalf D, et al: The residual megakaryocyte and platelet production in c-Mpl-deficient mice is not dependent on the actions of interleukin-6, interleukin-11, or leukemia inhibitory factor. *Blood* 95: 528, 2000.
30. Wolber EM, Fandrey J, Frackowski U, Jelkmann W: Hepatic thrombopoietin mRNA is increased in acute inflammation. *Thromb Haemost* 86:1421, 2001.
31. Heits F, Stahl M, Ludwig D, et al: Elevated serum thrombopoietin and interleukin-6 concentrations in thrombocytosis associated with inflammatory bowel disease. *J Interferon Cytokine Res* 19:757, 1999.
32. Ishiguro A, Suzuki Y, Mito M, et al: Elevation of serum thrombopoietin precedes thrombocytosis in acute infections. *Br J Haematol* 116:612, 2002.
33. Ceresa IF, Noris P, Ambaglio C, et al: Thrombopoietin is not uniquely responsible for thrombocytosis in inflammatory disorders. *Platelets* 18:579, 2007.
34. Wolber EM, Jelkmann W: Interleukin-6 increases thrombopoietin production in human hepatoma cells HepG2 and Hep3B. *J Interferon Cytokine Res* 20:499, 2000.
35. Kaser A, Brandacher G, Steurer W, et al: Interleukin-6 stimulates thrombopoiesis through thrombopoietin: Role in inflammatory thrombocytosis. *Blood* 98:2720, 2001.
36. Theofilopoulos AN, Baccala R, Beutler B, Kono DH: Type I interferons (alpha/beta) in immunity and autoimmunity. *Annu Rev Immunol* 23:307, 2005.
37. Young HA, Bream JH: IFN-gamma: Recent advances in understanding regulation of expression, biological functions, and clinical applications. *Curr Top Microbiol Immunol* 316:97, 2007.
38. Schoenborn JR, Wilson CB: Regulation of interferon-gamma during innate and adaptive immune responses. *Adv Immunol* 96:41, 2007.

39. Choi I, Muta K, Wickrema A, et al: Interferon gamma delays apoptosis of mature erythroid progenitor cells in the absence of erythropoietin. *Blood* 95:3742, 2000.

40. Yu JM, Emmons RV, Hanazono Y, et al: Expression of interferon-gamma by stromal cells inhibits murine long-term repopulating hematopoietic stem cell activity. *Exp Hematol* 27:895, 1999.

41. Young NS, Scheinberg P, Calado RT: Aplastic anemia. *Curr Opin Hematol* 15:162, 2008.

42. Tsuji-Takayama K, Tahata H, Harashima A, et al: Interferon-gamma enhances megakaryocyte colony-stimulating activity in murine bone marrow cells. *J Interferon Cytokine Res* 16:701, 1996.

43. Huang Z, Richmond TD, Muntean AG, et al: STAT1 promotes megakaryopoiesis downstream of GATA-1 in mice. *J Clin Invest* 117:3890, 2007.

44. Kulnigg-Dabsch S, Schmid W, Howaldt S, et al. Iron deficiency generates secondary thrombocytosis and platelet activation in IBD: The randomized, controlled thrombo-VIT trial. *Inflamm Bowel Dis* 19:1609, 2013.

45. Akan H, Güven N, Aydogdu I, et al: Thrombopoietic cytokines in patients with iron deficiency anemia with or without thrombocytosis. *Acta Haematol* 103:152, 2000.

46. Loo M, Beguin Y: The effect of recombinant human erythropoietin on platelet counts is strongly modulated by the adequacy of iron supply. *Blood* 93:3286, 1999.

47. Bilic E, Bilic E: Amino acid sequence homology of thrombopoietin and erythropoietin may explain thrombocytosis in children with iron deficiency anemia. *J Pediatr Hematol Oncol* 25:675, 2003.

48. Geddis AE, Kaushansky K: Cross reactivity between erythropoietin and thrombopoietin at the level of Mpl does not account for the thrombocytosis seen in iron deficiency. *J Pediatr Hematol Oncol* 25:919, 2003.

49. Singh AK, Szczech L, Tang KL, et al: Correction of anemia with epoetin alfa in chronic kidney disease. *N Engl J Med* 355:2085, 2006.

50. Drüeke TB, Locatelli F, Clyne N, et al: Normalization of hemoglobin level in patients with chronic kidney disease and anemia. *N Engl J Med* 355:2071, 2006.

51. Rossert J, Levin A, Roger SD, et al: Effect of early correction of anemia on the progression of CKD. *Am J Kidney Dis* 47:738, 2006.

52. Streja E, Kovesdy CP, Greenland S, et al: Erythropoietin, iron depletion, and relative thrombocytosis: A possible explanation for hemoglobin-survival paradox in hemodialysis. *Am J Kidney Dis* 52:727, 2008.

53. Geddis AE, Fox NE, Hitchcock, I: Erythropoietin stimulates thrombopoiesis in the absence of c-Mpl signaling. *Blood* 112(Suppl 1):2451, 2008.

54. Rodríguez-Liñares B, Watson SP: Thrombopoietin potentiates activation of human platelets in association with JAK2 and TYK2 phosphorylation. *Biochem J* 316:93, 1996.

55. Brines M, Grasso G, Fiordaliso F, et al: Erythropoietin mediates tissue protection through an erythropoietin and common beta-subunit heteroreceptor. *Proc Natl Acad Sci U S A* 101:14907, 2004.

56. Osselaer JC, Jamart J, Scheiff JM: Platelet distribution width for differential diagnosis of thrombocytosis. *Clin Chem* 43:1072, 1997.

57. Kaushansky K: On the molecular origins of the chronic myeloproliferative disorders: It all makes sense. *Blood* 105:4187, 2005.

58. Pikman Y, Lee BH, Mercher T, et al: MPLW515L is a novel somatic activating mutation in myelofibrosis with myeloid metaplasia. *PLoS Med* 3:e270, 2006.

CHAPTER 120
HEREDITARY QUALITATIVE PLATELET DISORDERS

A. Koneti Rao and Barry S. Coller

SUMMARY

Abnormalities of platelet function manifest themselves primarily as excessive hemorrhage at mucocutaneous sites, with ecchymoses, petechiae, epistaxis, gingival hemorrhage, and menorrhagia most common. Both quantitative and qualitative platelet abnormalities can produce these symptoms, so it is necessary to exclude thrombocytopenia (Chap. 117) by performing a platelet count. Chapter 121 discusses acquired qualitative platelet abnormalities and this chapter discusses the hereditary qualitative platelet abnormalities.

The hereditary qualitative platelet disorders can be classified according to the major locus of the defect (see Table 120–1 and Fig. 120–1). Thus, abnormalities of platelet glycoproteins, platelet granules, and signal transduction and secretion can all result in hemorrhagic diatheses and prolonged bleeding times. Glanzmann thrombasthenia results from abnormalities in one of two integrin subunits, either α_{IIb} (glycoprotein [GP] IIb) or β_3 (GPIIIa), resulting in loss or dysfunction of the $\alpha_{IIb}\beta_3$ (GPIIb/IIIa) receptor. This results in a profound defect in platelet aggregation and secondary defects in platelet adhesion, secretion, and platelet coagulant activity. Heterozygous gain of function mutations in $\alpha_{IIb}\beta_3$ can result in a syndrome of macrothrombocytopenia. Loss of the platelet GPIb–IX–V complex because of abnormalities in GPIbα, GPIbβ, or GPIX results in the Bernard-Soulier syndrome, which is characterized by giant platelets and modest thrombocytopenia. The major defect is in platelet adhesion because of a decrease in platelet interactions with von Willebrand factor, but abnormalities in $\alpha_{IIb}\beta_3$ activation and thrombin-induced aggregation are also present. A gain of function defect in GPIbα (platelet-type [pseudo-] von Willebrand disease) can produce a hemorrhagic disorder via depletion of high-molecular-weight von Willebrand multimers. Inherited defects in platelet dense or α granules, agonist receptors, or proteins and mechanisms involved in signal transduction and secretion also lead to platelet dysfunction and produce hemorrhagic symptoms.

Abnormalities of platelet coagulant activity, that is, the ability of platelets to facilitate thrombin generation (Chap. 112), can lead to a hemorrhagic diathesis. Impaired platelet function may occur in association with mutations in transcription factors RUNX1, GATA-1, FLI-1, and GFI1B, and these patients have thrombocytopenia as well.

● PLATELET FUNCTION IN HEMOSTASIS

Abnormalities of platelet function manifest themselves primarily as excessive hemorrhage at mucocutaneous sites, with ecchymoses, petechiae, epistaxis, gingival hemorrhage, and menorrhagia being most common. Mild platelet function abnormalities will not cause spontaneous bleeding but may cause (excessive) hemorrhage after trauma or medical interventions. Both quantitative and qualitative platelet abnormalities can produce these symptoms, so it is necessary to exclude thrombocytopenia (Chap. 117) by performing a platelet count. Although no longer performed widely, a prolonged bleeding time in a patient with a normal platelet count is suggestive of a qualitative platelet abnormality. Some patients may have abnormalities in both platelet number and function. Chapter 121 discusses acquired qualitative platelet abnormalities and this chapter discusses hereditary qualitative platelet abnormalities.

Following injury to the blood vessel, platelets adhere to exposed subendothelium by a process that involves, among other events, the interaction of a plasma protein, von Willebrand factor (VWF), and a specific glycoprotein complex on the platelet surface, the glycoprotein (GP) Ib–IX–V complex. Adhesion is followed by recruitment of additional platelets that form clumps (aggregation), which involves binding of fibrinogen to specific platelet surface receptors, a complex comprised of integrin $\alpha_{IIb}\beta_3$ (GPIIb-IIIa). Platelet activation is required for fibrinogen binding; resting platelets do not bind fibrinogen. Activated platelets release the contents of their granules (secretion), including adenosine diphosphate (ADP) and serotonin from the dense granules, which causes the recruitment of additional platelets. Moreover, platelets play a major role in coagulation mechanisms; several key enzymatic reactions occur on the platelet membrane phospholipid surface. A number of physiologic agonists interact with platelet surface receptors to induce responses, including a change in platelet shape from discoid to spherical (shape change), aggregation, secretion, and thromboxane A_2 (TXA_2) production. The binding of agonists to their platelet receptors initiates numerous intracellular events (Chap. 112) including the production or release of several messenger molecules. One pathway leads to the hydrolysis of phosphoinositide (PI) by phospholipase C leading to the formation of diacylglycerol and inositol 1,4,5-triphosphate [IP_3]). These and other mediators induce or modulate the various platelet responses of Ca^{2+} mobilization, protein phosphorylation, aggregation, secretion, and thromboxane production. Numerous other mechanisms, such as activation of tyrosine kinases and phosphatases, are also triggered by platelet activation (Chap. 112). Inherited or acquired defects in the above and other platelet mechanisms may lead to impaired platelet function and a bleeding diathesis.

● CLASSIFICATION OF HEREDITARY QUALITATIVE PLATELET DISORDERS

The hereditary qualitative platelet disorders can be classified according to the major locus of the defect (Table 120–1 and Fig. 120–1). Glanzmann thrombasthenia (GT) is caused by abnormalities in either integrin α_{IIb}

Acronyms and Abbreviations: ADP, adenosine diphosphate; BSS, Bernard-Soulier syndrome; βTG, β-thromboglobulin; BLOC, biogenesis of lysosome-related organelles complex; cAMP, cyclic adenosine monophosphate; EDTA, ethylenediaminetetraacetic acid; GFI1b, growth factor independent 1B; GPS, gray platelet syndrome; GT, Glanzmann thrombasthenia; HLA, human leukocyte antigen; HPS, Hermansky-Pudlak syndrome; Ig, immunoglobulin; LAD, leukocyte adhesion deficiency; MIDAS, metal ion-dependent adhesion site; PAR, protease-activated receptor; PF4, platelet factor 4; PKC; protein kinase C; PLC, phospholipase C; rFVIIa, recombinant factor VIIa; TGF, transforming growth factor; TXA_2, thromboxane A_2; VWD, von Willebrand disease; VWF, von Willebrand factor.

TABLE 120–1. Inherited Disorders of Platelet Function

I. Abnormalities of glycoprotein adhesion receptors

   A. Integrin $\alpha_{IIb}\beta_3$ (Glycoprotein IIb/IIIa; CD41/CD61): Glanzmann thrombasthenia

   B. Glycoproteins Ib (CD42b,c)/IX (CD42a)/V: Bernard-Soulier syndrome

   C. Glycoprotein Ibα (CD42b,c): Platelet-type (Pseudo-) von Willebrand disease

   D. Integrin $\alpha_2\beta_1$ (Glycoprotein Ia/IIa; VLA-2; CD49b/CD29)

   E. CD36 (Glycoprotein IV)

   F. Glycoprotein VI

II. Abnormalities of platelet granules

   A. δ-Storage pool deficiency

   B. Gray platelet syndrome (α-storage pool deficiency)

   C. α,δ-Storage pool deficiency

   D. Quebec platelet disorder

III. Abnormalities of platelet signaling and secretion

   A. Defects in platelet agonist receptors or agonist-specific signal transduction (thromboxane A_2 receptor defect, adenosine diphosphate [ADP] receptor defects [P2Y$_{12}$, P2X$_1$], epinephrine receptor defect, platelet activating factor receptor defect)

   B. Defects in guanosine triphosphate (GTP)–binding proteins (Gαq deficiency, Gαs hyperfunction and genetic variation in extra-large Gαs, Gαi1 deficiency, CaLDAG-GEFI deficiency)

   C. Phospholipase C (PLC)-β_2 deficiency and defects in PLC activation

   D. Defects in protein phosphorylation protein kinase C (PKC)-θ deficiency

   E. Defects in arachidonic acid metabolism and thromboxane production (phospholipase A_2 deficiency cyclooxygenase [prostaglandin H_2 sythase-1 deficiency], thromboxane synthase deficiency)

IV. Abnormalities of platelet coagulant activity (Scott syndrome)

V. Abnormalities of a cytoskeletal structural protein: β_1 tubulin, filamin A

VI. Abnormalities in cytoskeletal linking proteins

   A. Wiskott-Aldrich syndrome protein (WASP)

   B. Kindlin-3: Leukocyte adhesion defect (LAD)-III; LAD-1 variant; integrin activation deficiency disease defect (IADD))

VII. Abnormalities of transcription factors leading to functional defects

   A. RUNX1 (familial platelet dysfunction with predisposition to acute myelogenous leukemia)

   B. GATA-1

   C. FLI1 (dimorphic dysmorphic platelets with giant α granules and thrombocytopenia; Paris-Trousseau/Jacobsen syndrome)

   D. GFI1B

interactions with VWF. A gain-of-function defect in GPIbα (platelet-type [pseudo] von Willebrand disease [VWD]) can also produce a hemorrhagic disorder via depletion of high-molecular-weight VWF multimers. Defects in secretion of granule contents because of deficiencies in the granules or in the mechanisms that mediate secretion results in impaired platelet function. Inherited defects in agonist receptors or proteins or mediators involved in signal transduction or thromboxane synthesis may also produce hemorrhagic symptoms. Abnormalities of platelet coagulant activity, that is, the ability of platelets to facilitate thrombin generation (Chap. 113), and in cytoskeletal-linking proteins, can also lead to a hemorrhagic diathesis. Lastly, it is becoming clear that some patients may have abnormalities multiple aspects of platelet function and number related to a mutation in a hematopoietic transcription factor that regulates gene expression in megakaryocytes and platelets.

● CLINICAL MANIFESTATIONS

Disorders of platelet function are characterized by highly variable mucocutaneous bleeding manifestations and excessive hemorrhage following surgical procedures or trauma. These include ecchymoses, petechiae, epistaxis, gingival bleeding, and menorrhagia. Spontaneous hemarthrosis are distinctly rare, distinguishing them from the hemophilias, and deep hematomas and spontaneous central nervous system bleeding are highly unusual in these patients. Postpartum hemorrhage and postsurgical bleeding may be severe in some patients. In general, most patients with platelet function defects have mild to moderate bleeding manifestations, but may be severe in some entities, such as the GT and the BSS. Individual patients with the same functional defect or even the same genetic defect may also vary in the intensity of bleeding manifestations, suggesting one or more disease-modifying genes exist. Moreover, the severity of bleeding symptoms may vary over the lifetime of the same individual, implying that factors in addition to the platelet defect may be contributing to the bleeding risk. Sometimes, a mild platelet function defect becomes clinically manifest when the patient uses medication interfering with primary hemostasis (e.g., nonsteroidal antiinflammatory drugs [NSAIDs]).

Although normal in many of the inherited platelet function defects, the platelet count may be decreased in some entities, such as the BSS and the gray platelet syndrome (GPS) and in association with mutations in hematopoietic transcription factors. Most patients with platelet function defects, but not all, have a prolonged bleeding time, a test no longer available in most centers because of its inherent inaccuracies. *In vitro* platelet aggregation and secretion studies provide evidence for the dysfunction but are not generally predictive of the severity of clinical manifestations. In some patients, such as those with abnormal platelet coagulant activities, these studies may be normal. Some patients with platelet dysfunction are initially detected through abnormalities on testing with the platelet function analyzer (PFA-100).

● GENERAL APPROACH TO PATIENTS WITH MUCOCUTANEOUS BLEEDING SYMPTOMS FOR ABNORMALITIES IN PLATELET NUMBER OR FUNCTION

Platelet disorders are characterized by alterations in platelet number or function or both. A general approach is shown in Fig. 120-1. A reduced platelet count can occur as an isolated platelet disorder (inherited or acquired) or with evidence of a concomitant defect in platelet function. Platelet size and examination of the blood film may provide insights

(GPIIb) or β_3 (GPIIIa), resulting in loss or dysfunction of the integrin $\alpha_{IIb}\beta_3$ receptor. This results in a profound defect in platelet aggregation and secondary defects in platelet adhesion, secretion, and coagulant activity. Loss of the platelet GPIb–IX–V complex because of abnormalities in GPIbα, GPIbβ, or GPIX results in the Bernard-Soulier syndrome (BSS), which is characterized by giant platelets and thrombocytopenia. The major defect is in platelet adhesion owing to a decrease in platelet

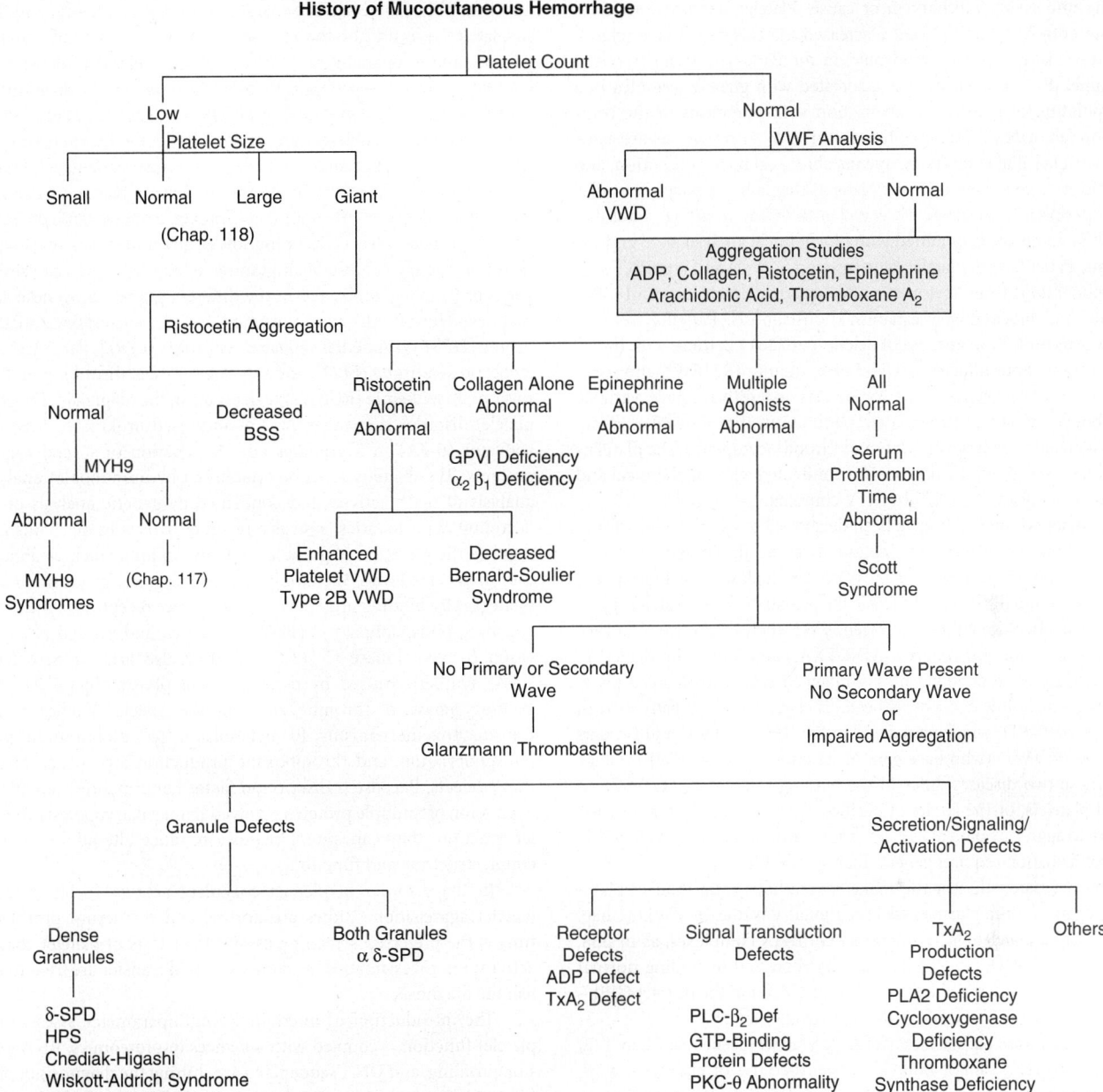

Figure 120–1. Evaluation of patients for inherited abnormalities in platelet number or function. The major and well-recognized entities are shown here. A reduced platelet count occurs in patients with purely quantitative platelet disorders (inherited or acquired) as well as in patients who have inherited qualitative platelet disorders. Chapter 117 discusses inherited thrombocytopenias. Notable among patients with thrombocytopenia and inherited platelet dysfunction is the Bernard-Soulier syndrome (BSS), which is characterized by giant platelets. Patients with the Gray platelet syndrome are characterized by thrombocytopenia and gray appearance of platelets on the blood smear due to paucity of granules. Platelet aggregation studies can provide clues regarding the nature of the underlying platelet abnormality. Decreased response to ristocetin alone with normal responses to other agonists is found in the BSS and von Willebrand disease (VWD; type I and type III). The response to ristocetin is enhanced in VWD type IIB and the platelet-type VWD. Impaired response to collagen or epinephrine alone may suggest a defect in their respective receptors. Patients with adenosine diphosphate (ADP) and thromboxane receptor defects have impaired responses to multiple agonists because of the feedback amplification provided by ADP and thromboxane A_2 (TXA$_2$) when activated by different agonists. Absence of both primary and secondary waves of aggregation in response to all physiologic agonists occurs in Glanzmann thrombasthenia (GT). A heterogeneous group of platelet defects are characterized by a decreased secondary wave of platelet aggregation in response to ADP and epinephrine, and diminished responses to low doses of collagen, TXA$_2$ and thrombin. They can be broadly separated into granule defects (involving dense [δ] or both dense and α granules) and defects in the platelet secretion or release reaction associated with normal dense granule stores. The granule defects may occur in isolation or in association with other syndromes. Secretion abnormalities arise from defects in mechanisms that regulate the release of granule contents, and include defects at the level of platelet receptors (ADP, TXA$_2$), signaling events involving guanosine triphosphate (GTP)–binding proteins that link surface receptors to intracellular enzymes, phospholipase C activation, and protein phosphorylation (protein kinase C [PKC]-θ). They may also arise from defects in TXA$_2$ synthesis because of deficiencies of phospholipase A_2 (PLA2), cyclooxygenase, or thromboxane synthase. Patients with the Scott syndrome are characterized by a normal bleeding time, normal responses in aggregation studies, and a shortened prothrombin time, which reflects the defect in the platelet–coagulant protein interactions. Additional details on the various entities are described in the section "General Approach to Patients with Mucocutaneous Bleeding Symptoms for Abnormalities in Platelet Number or Function." GP, glycoprotein; PLA2, phospholipase A2; PLC, phospholipase C; SPD, storage pool deficiency; u-PA, urokinase plasminogen activator; VWF, von Willebrand factor.

into the underlying mechanism or cause. Platelet size provides clues in some entities (Chap. 117).[1,2] Decreased platelet size is characteristic of the Wiskott-Aldrich syndrome. In the Paris-Trousseau/Jacobsen syndrome, thrombocytopenia is associated with giant α granules in a subpopulation of platelets in association with mutations in the transcription factor *FLI1*. Transcription factor *RUNX1* mutations are associated with familial thrombocytopenia, abnormal platelet function, and predisposition to leukemia. Large platelets that lack the purple granules on the peripheral smear are observed in the GPS (α-storage pool disease). The diagnosis is obtained with biochemical analysis of α-granule contents. Patients with platelet-type (pseudo-) VWD and type 2b VWD have moderate thrombocytopenia and large platelets. Studies of GPIb function and biochemistry establish the diagnosis. Patients who are hemizygous for GPIbβ because of deletion of 22q11.2, those with mutations in transcription factor *GATA-1* or β_1 tubulin (R318W), and some patients who are heterozygous for defects in GPIb/IX have variable thrombocytopenia and large platelets. Mutations that activate $\alpha_{IIb}\beta_3$ are also associated with large platelets and thrombocytopenia. The platelets in BSS are truly giant; the diagnosis is confirmed with biochemical and functional analyses of the GPIb–IX–V complex.

A variety of methods have been developed to assess platelet function and new instrumentation continues to be developed.[3-8] Platelet aggregation studies performed using platelet-rich plasma can loosely separate patients into those with defects in the primary wave of platelet aggregation (dependent on either fibrinogen, VWF, their respective receptors, or agonist receptors for collagen, ADP, TXA$_2$) and those with defects in the secondary wave of aggregation. Enhanced ristocetin-induced platelet aggregation at low doses of ristocetin is characteristic of patients with platelet-type VWD (who have a defect in the GPIb receptor) and patients with type 2b VWD (who have gain-of-function defect in VWF) (Chap. 126). These two diseases differ in the binding of the patient's VWF to normal platelets, or the ability of purified VWF, cryoprecipitate or asialo-VWF to aggregate patient platelets; the diagnosis of platelet-type VWD or its confirmation requires genetic analysis of GPIb.

Neither ristocetin nor the snake venom botrocetin induces platelet aggregation if the plasma lacks functional VWF, as in VWD (Chap. 126), or if the platelets lack functional GPIb–IX complexes, as in BSS. The defect in VWD, but not BSS, can be corrected by adding normal plasma or purified VWF. Direct analysis of VWF and the platelet GPIb–IX complex are used to confirm the diagnosis.

Patients whose plasma lacks fibrinogen (afibrinogenemia; Chap. 125) or whose platelets cannot bind fibrinogen because of abnormal $\alpha_{IIb}\beta_3$ receptors (GT) or inability to activate integrin $\alpha_{IIb}\beta_3$ (leukocyte adhesion deficiency [LAD]-3) as the result of a kindlin-3 abnormality will have no primary wave of platelet aggregation in response to all physiologic agonists, including ADP, epinephrine, collagen, TXA$_2$, and thrombin. Simple coagulation tests (prothrombin time, partial thromboplastin time, and measurement of plasma fibrinogen) and analysis of platelet integrin $\alpha_{IIb}\beta_3$ receptors, and kindlin-3 can differentiate between these two groups. Isolated defects in the primary response to collagen have been observed in patients with abnormalities in platelet integrin $\alpha_2\beta_1$ (GPIa/IIa) or GPVI. Platelet glycoprotein analysis can separate these from each other. Because antibodies to GPVI can result in receptor depletion from circulating platelets, a search for anti-GPVI should be undertaken in patients with reduced platelet GPVI. Defects in ADP, epinephrine, or TXA$_2$ receptors will result in decreased platelet aggregation in response to the specific agonist. However, patients with isolated ADP and TXA$_2$ receptor abnormalities have impaired aggregation in response to other agonists as well because of the feedback potentiation provided by ADP and TXA$_2$.

A very heterogeneous group of platelet defects can result in a decreased secondary wave of platelet aggregation in response to ADP and epinephrine and diminished responses to low doses of collagen

and thrombin. They can be separated into granule defects and defects in platelet secretion or the release reaction. Operationally, these two groups can be separated on the basis of their release of dense granule contents in response to high doses of thrombin. High-dose thrombin activation can overcome most or all of the release reaction (secretion) abnormalities, so platelets from patients with these disorders will release normal amounts of granule contents; in contrast, patients with reduced granule contents have abnormal granule release responses even when using high doses of thrombin. α-Granule contents and dense-body contents can be measured immunologically and biochemically; electron microscopy can establish granule defects. Specific analysis of the genes or proteins implicated in the different granule biogenesis abnormalities (Wiskott-Aldrich syndrome [*WASP*], Hermansky-Pudlak syndrome [*HPS1–9*], Chédiak-Higashi syndrome [*LYST*], Paris-Trousseau/Jacobson syndrome [*FLI1*], and inherited platelet disorder with predisposition to leukemia [*RUNX1*]) can establish the diagnosis. The Quebec platelet disorder is characterized by increased urokinase plasminogen activator (u-PA) in α-granules and degradation of several α-granule proteins. The diagnosis can be established by immunoblot analysis or analysis of u-PA activity and confirmed by genetic analysis of *u-PA*. Secretion abnormalities arise as a result of defects in mechanisms that regulate the secretion of granule contents, and may include abnormalities at various levels, including surface receptors, guanosine triphosphate (GTP)-binding proteins that link surface receptors to intracellular enzymes, phospholipase C (PLC) activation, and protein phosphorylation (protein kinase C [PKC]-θ). They also arise from defects in TXA$_2$ synthesis caused by deficiencies of phospholipase A$_2$ (PLA$_2$), cyclooxygenase, or thromboxane synthase. Specific studies on signal transduction mechanisms, PI metabolism, Ca^{2+} mobilization, protein phosphorylation, and thromboxane production are needed to define these defects. Because transcription factor abnormalities can affect the expression of multiple proteins involved in megakaryopoiesis and platelet function, they can simultaneously produce alterations in platelet count, structure, and function.

In the disorder of platelet coagulant activity (Scott syndrome) platelet aggregation studies are normal and the serum prothrombin time is the preferred screening assay. Other tests of platelet coagulant activity, microvesiculation, and phospholipid transfer are used to establish the diagnosis.

The introduction of microfluidic multiparameter assessments of platelet function,[7,8] coupled with advances in proteomics, RNA expression profiling, and DNA sequencing are shifting the diagnosis of platelet function disorders from a target gene approach to one in which unbiased comprehensive functional and genetic analyses are employed. These methods have identified mutations in *RUNX1* and *FLI-1*[9] in patients with platelet function disorders, in *NBEAL2* in GPS,[10-12] in *TMEM16* in the Scott syndrome,[13] and in *RBM8A* in thrombocytopenia with absent radii (TAR) syndrome.[14,15] Many additional genetic alterations, including ones that affect multiple systems, are likely to be identified in the near future as these techniques are employed more broadly.

● ABNORMALITIES OF ADHESION RECEPTORS

INTEGRIN $\alpha_{IIB}\beta_3$ (GLYCOPROTEIN IIB/IIIA; CD41/CD61)–GLANZMANN THROMBASTHENIA

Definition and History

GT is an inherited hemorrhagic disorder characterized by a severe reduction in, or absence of, platelet aggregation in response to multiple physiologic agonists as a result of qualitative or quantitative abnormalities of platelet integrin α_{IIb} (GPIIb; CD41) and/or integrin β_3 (GPIIIa; CD61).[16]

In 1918, Eduard Glanzmann, a Swiss pediatrician, described a group of patients with hemorrhagic symptoms and a defect in platelet function, namely the ability to retract clots ("weak" platelets or thrombasthenia).[17] Subsequent studies demonstrated that thrombasthenic patients have prolonged bleeding times and that their platelets fail to aggregate in response to physiologic agonists[18-21] and have markedly reduced[18,20-22] platelet fibrinogen. In the mid-1970s, Nurden and Caen[23] and Phillips and colleagues[24] discovered that thrombasthenic platelets are deficient in both integrin α_{IIb} and β_3. Later studies demonstrated that integrin α_{IIb} and β_3 form a calcium-dependent complex in the platelet membrane that functions as a receptor for fibrinogen and other adhesive glycoproteins.[25-28] Cloning and sequencing of the complementary DNAs for integrin α_{IIb}[29] and β_3[30] identified them as separate protein subunits that are members of the integrin receptor superfamily[31] and permitted the molecular biological characterization of patients with the disorder (see database of Glanzmann patients http://med.mssm.edu/glanzmanndb).

Etiology and Pathogenesis

GT is a rare disorder characterized by autosomal recessive inheritance with a worldwide distribution. In regions where consanguineous matings are common, groups of patients with the disorder have been identified, and in several populations founder mutations have been identified by analyzing polymorphisms in the DNA surrounding the affected mutation. These include 42 patients from South India; 39 patients from the Iraqi-Jewish population in Israel; 46 Arab patients from Israel,

Jordan, and Saudi Arabia; 30 patients from Italy; a smaller number of patients from three Gypsy families; and 43 patients from Pakistan.[22,32-40] Perhaps the highest frequency of a GT mutation is found in the Iraqi-Jewish population where the most common mutation causing GT was found in six of 700 individuals.[39]

The platelet integrin $\alpha_{IIb}\beta_3$ receptor is required for platelet aggregation induced by all physiologic agonists (ADP, epinephrine, thrombin, collagen, TXA$_2$) (Chap. 112).[41] Consequently, abnormalities in the receptor result in a failure of platelet plug formation at sites of vascular injury, and excessive bleeding.

The integrin $\alpha_{IIb}\beta_3$ receptor is also responsible for the uptake of fibrinogen from plasma into α granules,[42] hence, patients with GT have markedly reduced platelet fibrinogen.[18,20,21,43,44] Clot retraction requires platelets with intact integrin $\alpha_{IIb}\beta_3$ receptors,[45,46] and is, therefore, usually abnormal in GT.[18]

Defects in either integrin α_{IIb} or β_3 result in the same functional defect because both subunits are required for receptor function (Chap. 112). Biosynthetic studies indicate that integrin α_{IIb} and β_3 form a complex soon after protein synthesis in the rough endoplasmic reticulum[47-49]; subsequent posttranslational processing[50] and transport to the platelet membrane require that the complex be intact (Fig. 120–2).[51,52] Complex formation protects each of the glycoproteins from proteolytic digestion,[47-50] so if either integrin α_{IIb} or β_3 is absent or unable to form a normal complex, the other subunit will be rapidly degraded, most likely through a proteasomal mechanism. Thus, a deficiency in either glycoprotein produces a deficiency in both. Because complex formation and vesicular transport are also required for proteolytic processing of pro-α_{IIb} into its constituent $\alpha_{IIb}\alpha$ and $\alpha_{IIb}\beta$ subunits,[50] if these processes do

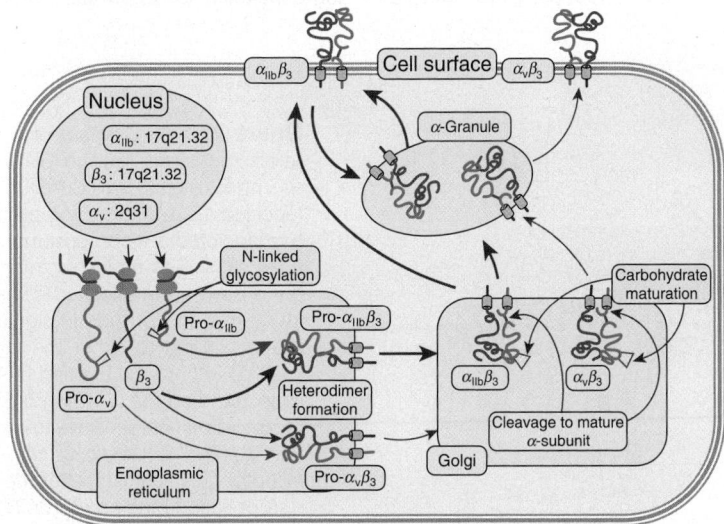

Figure 120–2. Biogenesis of integrin $\alpha_{IIb}\beta_3$ and integrin $\alpha_v\beta_3$ receptors. The nuclear genes for integrins α_{IIb} (chromosome localization 17q21.32; gene designation *ITGA2B*; 30 exons), α_v (2q31; *ITGAV*; 30 exons), and β_3 (17q21.32; *ITGB3*; 14 exons) are transcribed into messenger RNA and translated by ribosomes attached to the membranes of the endoplasmic reticulum (ER). The proteins undergo initial glycosylation and form the integrins $\alpha_{IIb}\beta_3$ and $\alpha_v\beta_3$ heterodimers in the ER. It is presumed that many more integrin $\alpha_{IIb}\beta_3$ complexes form than $\alpha_v\beta_3$ complexes because the final copy number of platelet integrin $\alpha_{IIb}\beta_3$ receptors is approximately 100,000 whereas it is only 50 to 100 for $\alpha_v\beta_3$. This is shown schematically by the differences in the width of the arrows depicting integrin $\alpha_{IIb}\beta_3$ versus $\alpha_v\beta_3$ complex formation. The heteroduplexes are transported to the Golgi where the carbohydrate chains undergo modification to their mature structures and both α_{IIb} and α_v subunits undergo proteolytic cleavage within a disulfide-bonded loop, resulting in two-chain forms of the receptor subunits. Mature integrin $\alpha_{IIb}\beta_3$ receptors are transported to α-granule membranes, where they undergo cycling to and from the plasma membrane. This process results in the internalization of fibrinogen and perhaps other plasma proteins. Integrin $\alpha_v\beta_3$ may be transported directly to the plasma membrane and is transported to α granule membranes. Of the total of approximately 100,000 integrin $\alpha_{IIb}\beta_3$ receptors, approximately two-thirds are on the surface at any given time and the remaining one-third can be brought to the surface by platelet activation. The distribution of integrin $\alpha_v\beta_3$ between the plasma membrane and α granules, and the potential cycling of the receptors between α granules and the plasma membrane have not be defined. *(Used with permission from Dr. W. Beau Mitchell, New York Blood Center, New York, NY.)*

not occur normally, the very small amount of residual integrin α_{IIb} will be pro-α_{IIb}, not mature α_{IIb}.[53] Pro-α_{IIb} has been reported to bind to the membrane-bound endoplasmic reticulum chaperone calnexin, providing a potential mechanism for assessing whether the protein has undergone proper folding (calnexin cycle) and perhaps explaining how the receptor adopts a bent configuration.[54,55]

Integrin β_3 (GPIIIa) can also combine with the integrin α_V (CD51) subunit to form the integrin $\alpha_V\beta_3$ "vitronectin" receptor[30,56,57] (see Fig. 120–2; Chap. 112). This receptor can bind many of the same adhesive glycoproteins as integrin $\alpha_{IIb}\beta_3$, although there are some differences in ligand preference and binding sequences.[57–61] A small number of integrin $\alpha_V\beta_3$ receptors are present on platelets (50 to 100 per platelet)[60,62,63]; osteoclasts, endothelial cells, macrophages, vascular smooth muscle, and uterine cells, among others, also have integrin $\alpha_V\beta_3$ receptors.[64,65] In general, GT patients with defects in integrin β_3 also are deficient in integrin $\alpha_V\beta_3$, whereas patients with defects in integrin α_{IIb} have either normal or increased numbers of platelet integrin $\alpha_V\beta_3$ receptors.[60,63,64,66–68] One exception to this rule is a patient with a defect in β_3 (H280P) that interferes with integrin $\alpha_{IIb}\beta_3$ biogenesis to a much greater extent than integrin $\alpha_V\beta_3$ biogenesis.[69] At present, there is no evidence that patients who lack integrin $\alpha_V\beta_3$ receptors in addition to lacking integrin $\alpha_{IIb}\beta_3$ receptors have a more-severe hemorrhagic diathesis or suffer from any other abnormalities, perhaps because alternative receptors containing integrin α_V associated with other β subunits can substitute for integrin $\alpha_V\beta_3$.[63] Upregulation of integrin $\alpha_2\beta_1$ on osteoclasts of Iraqi-Jewish patients with GT has been reported as a potential compensatory mechanism to explain the lack of bone changes despite the deficiency in osteoclast integrin $\alpha_V\beta_3$.[70]

The molecular biologic abnormalities in more than 100 patients with GT have been identified and they are listed in an internet database that is updated continuously[71] (http://med.mssm.edu/glanzmanndb). Figure 120–3 contains information on mutations of particular interest.

Of note, many of the patients with identified mutations are compound heterozygotes rather than homozygotes, indicating that a sizable number of silent carriers are present in the population. Where consanguinity is common, the disorder is more likely to be caused by a homozygous mutation arising in a founder, but even under these circumstances, more than one mutation may be present. Thus, in the Iraqi-Jewish population, in which consanguinity has been present from 586 BCE to the present, two separate mutations have been identified in more than one family.[39] Most of the missense mutations result in decreased expression of integrin $\alpha_{IIb}\beta_3$ on the surface of platelets. This probably reflects the stringent structural requirements for proper folding and complex formation.

Mutations in Integrin $\alpha_{IIb}\beta_3$ Within the Metal Ion-Dependent Adhesion Site of Integrin β_3 and the Interface with the Integrin α_{IIb} β-Propeller A metal coordination site or MIDAS domain, which is highly conserved in six integrin receptor α-chain subunits and required for ligand-binding, is also present in the β-A (or I-like) domain of the integrin β_3 subunit.[72] Mutagenesis and molecular modeling experiments suggested that a highly conserved DxSxS amino acid sequence[73] motif plus additional coordinating residues are brought together in the three-dimensional structure of the β_3 subunit to form a cation-binding sphere of the MIDAS domain,[74] and this was confirmed by the crystal structures of integrin $\alpha_V\beta_3$ and later integrin $\alpha_{IIb}\beta_3$ (see Chap. 112, Fig. 112–111, and Fig. 120–3).[75,76] Thus, the β_3 MIDAS is composed of Asp[119], Ser[121], Ser[123], Glu[220], and Asp[251]. A region originally termed the ligand-associated metal binding site (LIMBS) in integrin $\alpha_V\beta_3$,[77] but now termed the synergy metal binding site (SyMBS) in integrin $\alpha_{IIb}\beta_3$,[78] binds a Ca^{2+} ion and is required for binding of ligands to the MIDAS. It is composed of atoms from D158, N215, D217, P219, and E220. Integrin β_3 residues 214 and 216 are in close proximity with both the SyMBS residues and the interface with the α_{IIb} subunit. Adjacent to the MIDAS domain is a metal ion site termed the ADMIDAS (adjacent to metal ion-dependent adhesion site), in which calcium is coordinated by

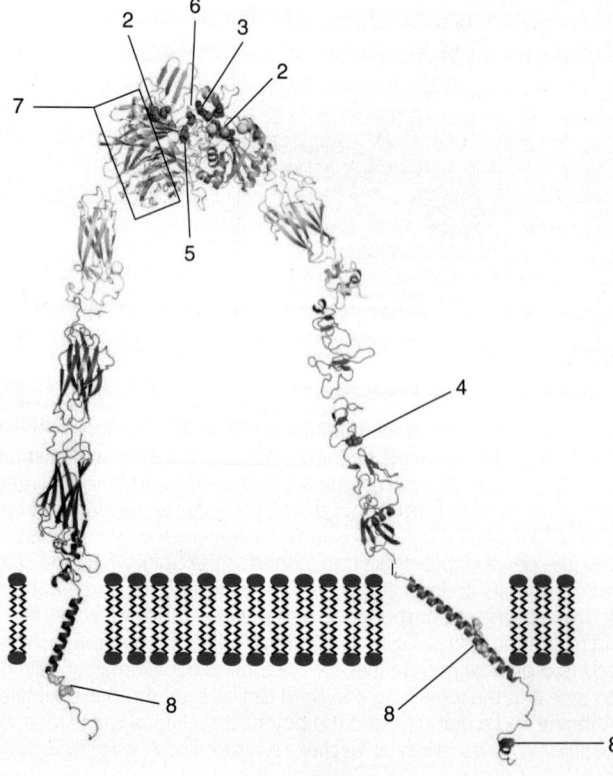

Figure 120–3. Diagram of $\alpha_{IIb}\beta_3$ structure and identification of select mutations causing Glanzmann thrombasthenia. The website http://med.mssm.edu/glanzmanndb contains a full listing of reported Glanzmann thrombasthenia mutations. The $\alpha_{IIb}\beta_3$ structure depicted is a composite of data from crystal and NMR structures, as well as molecular modeling of missing regions. Among the missense mutations identified are ones that (1) interfere with inside-out and outside-in signaling (β_3 S752P); (2) interfere with ligand binding to either the metal ion-dependent adhesion site (MIDAS) in β_3 (β_3 D119Y and D119N) or the α_{IIb} component of the ligand binding site (Y143H, P145L/A, insert R160/T161); (3) result in receptors that are sensitive to dissociation by divalent cation chelation (β_3 R214W, R214Q, R216Q); (4) result in a constitutively active receptor (β_3 C560R); (5) alter the interface between α_{IIb} and β_3 and disrupt ligand binding (β_3 L262Y); (6) result in a β_3 protein that can complex more effectively with αV than α_{IIb} (S162L, R216Q, H280P); or (7) alter the α_{IIb} propeller structure and prevent normal $\alpha_{IIb}\beta_3$ complex formation, processing, and/or transport. The mutations identified by number 8 in α_{IIb} (G991C and R995Q/W) and β_3 (L718P and D723H) are gain-of-function mutations associated with macro/anisothrombocytopenia. *(Reproduced with permission from Dr. Ana Negri based on PDBids 3FCS, 3G9W, 2K9J, 2KNC, and 2KV9 and molecular modeling of the missing segments of the α_{IIb} calf domain, the $\beta3$ hybrid domain, and the link between the $\beta3$ EGF-1 and EGF-2 domains.)*

Ser[123], Asp[126], Asp[127], and Met[335] in unliganded integrin $\alpha_v\beta_3$ and integrin $\alpha_{IIb}\beta_3$, but Asp[251] substitutes for Met[335] in the ligand-bound structures of both integrin $\alpha_v\beta_3$ and integrin $\alpha_{IIb}\beta_3$. The crystal structures also demonstrated that peptide ligands containing the Arg-Gly-Asp (RGD) cell adhesion sequence interact with integrin $\alpha_{IIb}\beta_3$ and integrin $\alpha_v\beta_3$ in part by coordination of the metal ion in the MIDAS by the aspartic acid in the RGD peptide.[77,79] The low-molecular-weight drugs eptifibatide and tirofiban, which block ligand binding to the α_{IIb} subunit, have negatively charged regions that also interact with the MIDAS cation.[76] The fibrinogen γ-chain C-terminal dodecapeptide mediates binding to integrin $\alpha_{IIb}\beta_3$ and a crystal structure of the complex demonstrates that an aspartic acid carboxyl oxygen coordinates the MIDAS cation whereas the carboxy terminal valine interacts with the nearby cation in the ADMIDAS.[76,79] A number of mutations in patients with GT have been identified within the cation-binding sphere of the MIDAS domain (see Fig. 120–3, and Chap. 112, Fig. 112–11). Two mutations D119Y (Cam variant)[80] and D119N (patient NR),[81] are located within the conserved DxSxS amino acid motif and produce severe abnormalities of ligand binding to integrin $\alpha_{IIb}\beta_3$, but do not affect its surface expression. Mutations at residues R214 and R216 result in abnormal integrin $\alpha_{IIb}\beta_3$ receptors that cannot bind ligand and are very sensitive to dissociation by calcium chelation, perhaps because they are at the integrin α_{IIb}–β_3 interface.[32,82–84] Disrupting the SyMBS with a D217V mutation also leads to GT despite the expression of normal amounts of the integrin protein.[85] Further support for the importance of the MIDAS domain, SyMBS, and adjacent residues comes from studies in which the mutations D119N, R214W, D217N, E220Q, and E220K were introduced into Chinese hamster ovary CHO cells *in vitro* and shown to result in functional abnormalities.[86]

The interface between the α_{IIb} β-propeller and the β_3 subunit also involves, in part, the interaction between β_3 R261, contained in a four-amino-acid 3_{10} helix, with a number of hydrophobic residues in the α_{IIb} β-propeller arranged as inner and outer rings, making up a cage.[75] A β_3 subunit L262Y mutation, adjacent to R261 results in disruption of the helix and an unstable integrin $\alpha_{IIb}\beta_3$ complex that is expressed on the surface of platelets but is unable to bind fibrinogen.[87] The platelets of the patient with this mutation were able to bind fibrin and support clot retraction, suggesting different requirements for fibrinogen and fibrin binding.

Mutations in Integrin $\alpha_{IIb}\beta_3$ Within the α_{IIb} β–Propeller Sequence Based on their homology to another integrin α subunit, the aminoterminal 450 amino acids of integrin α_{IIb} and the homologous region in integrin α_v, which contain the minimal ligand-binding sequence,[88] were predicted to fold into seven repeat (blade) β-propellers, containing four cation-binding sites,[89] and this prediction was confirmed by the crystal structures of both α_v and α_{IIb} integrin subunits.[75,76] The upper surface of the propeller interacts with the β_3 subunit β-A (or I-like) domain to form the head of the integrin $\alpha_{IIb}\beta_3$ complex, which is the site of ligand binding. Each repeat (blade) contains four β strands that are connected by loops. The four calcium-binding sites in the α_{IIb} subunit, which are in β-hairpin structures, are located in loops on the undersurface of the propeller. Ligand binding in integrin α_{IIb} has been localized to a hydrophobic (F160, Y190, F231) and negatively charged (D224) pocket that lies adjacent to the MIDAS domain in the β_3 subunit, and is composed of contributions from the loops that link blade 2 to blade 3 (residues 144 to 171), β strand 2 to β strand 3 in blade 3 (residues 186 to 193), and blade 3 to blade 4 (residues 223 to 236). Integrin α_{IIb} contains a unique "cap" subdomain made up of four insertions in β propeller loops (residues 72 to 88, 111 to 126, 147 to 166, 200 to 217) that also plays a role in ligand binding.[76]

GT missense mutations located within the integrin α_{IIb} β-propeller (see Fig. 120–3) primarily affect transport of the integrin $\alpha_{IIb}\beta_3$ complex to the cell surface,[68,90–93] but several missense mutations and an insertion

result in functionally defective receptors. Thus, Y143H affects soluble ligand binding but not adhesion or clot retraction,[94] and P145A, which has been identified in several kindreds,[32,95] and P145L, prevent ligand binding. A two-amino-acid insertion at residues 161 and 162, as well as a T176I missense mutation, also affect ligand binding.[96–98] A L183P mutation, which is near to, but not in the loop containing Y190, affects both receptor expression and function.[99]

Mutations in Integrin $\alpha_{IIb}\beta_3$ That Affect Receptor Activation Several β_3 subunit missense mutations (C560R, V193M) result in the receptor adopting a high-affinity ligand binding state, which is paradoxical as it results in a bleeding diathesis.[100,101] A β_3 subunit S527F mutation in the third I-EGF domain was also associated with a constitutively active receptor, presumably because it prevents the receptor from assuming a bent, inactive conformation.[102] The cytoplasmic domain of the β_3 subunit plays a functional role in integrin activation and the regulation of ligand binding.[103,104] Two GT mutations have been identified in this region. One is an R724X nonsense mutation (patient RM)[105] that results in the deletion of the carboxyterminal 39 residues of integrin β_3 and the other is a β_3 subunit S752P missense mutation (patient P or Paris I).[106–108] This latter patient is unusual in that he had a generally mild history of excessive hemorrhage, but he did have a prolonged bleeding time and his platelets did not aggregate in response to ADP. These mutations do not severely affect surface expression of platelet integrin $\alpha_{IIb}\beta_3$ complexes, but both mutant receptors are unresponsive to agonist stimulation. Mammalian cell expression studies of these mutations show normal adhesion to immobilized fibrinogen, but abnormal cell spreading. Cells expressing the S752P mutant receptors have reduced focal adhesion plaque formation and cells expressing the R724X mutant receptors have undetectable tyrosine phosphorylation of focal adhesion kinase, pp125[FAK]. These mutations provide evidence for the role of the β_3 subunit cytoplasmic tail in inside-out signaling (i.e., platelet signals that lead to integrin $\alpha_{IIb}\beta_3$ adopting a high-affinity ligand-binding conformation) and outside-in signaling (i.e., signaling to the interior of the platelet as a result of integrin $\alpha_{IIb}\beta_3$ binding ligand; see Chap. 112, Figs. 112–3, 112–4, and 112–12).

Variants of Integrin $\alpha_{IIb}\beta_3$ in the Population The application of missense variant whole-exome and whole-genome sequencing to large numbers of individuals has provided valuable information on the frequency of missense variants in the general population and the frequency of the genetic alterations leading to GT. For the most part, the frequency of a variant in a population is a reflection of its impact on reproductive fitness and when it entered the population, with lower frequencies for variants that entered the population more recently. Thus, variants with minor allele frequencies (MAFs) of approximately 0.5 percent or less probably entered the population fewer than 2500 years ago, when the recent explosive growth in human populations began.[109] Data from a study[109A] involving approximately 33,000 alleles from approximately 16,500 people demonstrated the presence of 114 novel missense variant affecting approximately 10 percent of the integrin α_{IIb} amino acids and approximately 9 percent of the β_3 subunit amino acids. Thus, approximately 1.1 percent of the population studied carried at least one missense variant. None of the known GT mutations was observed in any of the alleles studied, indicating that they have MAFs of less than 0.01 percent and thus entered the population very recently. In fact, studies of two GT populations with high intragroup marriages, Palestinian Arabs and French Manouche gypsies, estimated that the GT mutations entered the population approximately 300 to 600 and approximately 300 to 400 years ago, respectively.[110,111] Several novel missense variants identified in this study affected one of the amino acids mutated in patients with GT, and in two cases these variants were shown to profoundly affect expression of the receptor. In one case, a missense variant reduced expression by approximately 50 percent but did not alter function. A series of prediction tools indicated that somewhere between 45 and 74 percent of the 114 novel missense mutations may be deleterious. Thus, perhaps approximately 0.6 percent of individuals in the general population is a silent carrier for a GT variant that profoundly affects structure and/or function. In addition, some of the rare individuals in the healthy population with levels of integrin $\alpha_{IIb}\beta_3$ receptor expression intermediate between those of obligate GT carriers and normal individuals may reflect heterozygosity for "hypomorphic" variants that partially affect receptor expression, but not function.[112]

Clinical Features

Table 120–2 summarizes the clinical manifestations of 177 patients with GT obtained from two reviews.[22,33] Menorrhagia occurs in nearly all female patients. Purpura can be present immediately after birth but often is not dramatic. Petechiae of the face and subconjunctival hemorrhage associated with crying may be the first symptoms in neonates and babies. Spontaneous hemarthroses and central nervous system bleeding are very rare. The hemorrhagic diathesis in patients with GT is notable for its variability and the lack of correlation between the biochemical platelet abnormalities and clinical severity.[22] Even within groups of patients such as the Iraqi Jews, most of whom share the same genetic α_{IIb} or β_3 subunit abnormalities, there is a wide spectrum of clinical severity.[33,39] Moreover, the severity of bleeding symptoms can vary significantly during the lifetime of individual patients. GT does not appear to protect against the development of atherosclerosis as judged by the carotid artery intima-to-media ratio.[113] Carriers of GT are usually asymptomatic or only mildly symptomatic and generally have normal results in platelet function tests.[22,33,112,114,115]

TABLE 120–2. Bleeding in Patients with Glanzmann Thrombasthenia

	No. of Affected Patients	Frequency (%)
SYMPTOMS		
Menorrhagia	54/55	98
Easy bruising, purpura	152/177	86
Epistaxis	129/177	73
Gingival bleeding	97/177	55
Gastrointestinal hemorrhage	22/177	12
Hematuria	10/177	6
Hemarthrosis	5/177	3
Intracranial hemorrhage	3/177	2
Visceral hematoma	1/177	1
SEVERITY		
Requirement for red cell transfusions		
Patients from literature*	32/48	67
Paris patients	54/64	84

*Data are from 177 patients reviewed by George and colleagues[22] of whom 113 were from the literature and 64 were studied in Paris.

Reproduced with permission from Coller BS. Inherited disorders of platelet function. In: Bloom AL, editor. Hemostasis and Thrombosis. UK: Churchill Livingstone p. 721–766, 1992.

Laboratory Features

Table 120–3 provides characteristic laboratory findings in GT. Patients have normal platelet counts and morphology, prolonged bleeding times, decreased or absent clot retraction, and abnormal platelet aggregation responses to physiologic stimuli. The initial slope of high-dose ristocetin-induced aggregation is normal (or near normal), reflecting the normal plasma VWF and the normal platelet GPIb/IX content; at lower doses of ristocetin, however, where GPIb/IX–mediated activation of integrin $\alpha_{IIb}\beta_3$ (Chap. 112) normally contributes to the aggregation response, patients have decreased second wave aggregation.[116] GT platelets undergo normal shape change in response to ADP and thrombin, demonstrating their ability to undergo metabolic and cytoskeletal changes in response to these agents. Similarly, high doses of thrombin and collagen produce normal release of dense body and α-granule contents[18,20,117]; the decreased secretion observed with lower doses of these agents reflect the lack of augmentation of the release reaction normally produced by platelet aggregation.[18,116,118–120]

Platelets in whole blood or platelet-rich plasma adhere to glass because fibrinogen first becomes deposited on the glass and the platelets then adhere to the immobilized fibrinogen.[121,122] Platelets from patients

TABLE 120–3. Laboratory Features of Glanzmann Thrombasthenia

I. Platelet count: Normal

II. Bleeding time: Markedly prolonged

III. Tests of platelet function

  A. Platelet aggregation

    1. Epinephrine—no observable response

    2. ADP and thrombin—shape change, but no aggregation

    3. Collagen—shape change followed by variable increase in light transmission most likely from progressive adhesion to collagen fibers (pseudoaggregation)

    4. Ristocetin—normal initial slope of aggregation; at low doses, inhibition of second wave; at high doses, cyclical aggregation–disaggregation

  B. Aperture closure time (PFA-100): Prolonged

  C. Clot retraction: Absent or reduced

  D. Platelet release reaction: Decreased with epinephrine and low-dose adenosine diphosphate (ADP), thrombin, and collagen; normal with high-dose thrombin and collagen

  E. Interaction with glass (platelet retention test): Absent or reduced

  F. Platelet coagulant activity: Variably abnormal

  G. Microparticle formation: Variably abnormal

  H. *Ex vivo* interaction with deendothelialized blood vessels in flow chambers: Marked abnormality in platelet thrombus formation and defective platelet spreading; decreased platelet adhesion at high shear rates

IV. Tests of $\alpha_{IIb}\beta_3$ and $\alpha_v\beta_3$ receptors: Number and functional integrity

  A. $\alpha_{IIb}\beta_3$ content: Reduced or absent, except in variants

  B. $\alpha_v\beta_3$ content: Reduced or absent in patients with β_3 defects; normal or increased in patients with α_{IIb} defects

  C. Platelet binding of fibrinogen and other adhesive glycoproteins to $\alpha_{IIb}\beta_3$: Reduced or absent

  D. Platelet fibrinogen content: Markedly reduced, except in some variants

with GT fail to adhere to glass,[18,20,121] and this forms the basis of their abnormality in the glass bead retention assay.[123] Platelet coagulant activity has been variably reported as normal or abnormal.[18–21,124–126] A defect in platelet microparticle formation and support of thrombin generation has been identified in some patients,[125–128] but not in all patients.[129] Integrins $\alpha_{IIb}\beta_3$ and $\alpha_V\beta_3$ bind prothrombin, probably accounting for some of the abnormalities identified.[130,131]

In flow-chamber studies, thrombasthenic platelets adhere normally to deendothelialized blood vessels at low and intermediate shear rates, but do not spread normally or form platelet thrombi.[132–134] A defect in adhesion occurs at higher shear rates. A paradoxical increase in fibrin formation on these surfaces has been observed with thrombasthenic platelets, but the explanation for this phenomenon remains unknown.[135] In contrast to normal blood, blood from nearly all patients with GT fails to occlude a 150-μm PFA-100 aperture in collagen-coated membranes under high sheer, either in the presence of ADP or epinephrine.[136,137]

Platelet integrins $\alpha_{IIb}\beta_3$ and $\alpha_V\beta_3$ can be quantitated by several techniques, including, monoclonal antibody binding (using flow cytometry or radiolabeled binding), immunoblotting, and surface-labeling followed by sodium dodecylsulfate polyacrylamide gel electrophoresis (SDS-PAGE). Based on such studies, GT patients are subcategorized by integrin $\alpha_{IIb}\beta_3$ content into those with less than 5 percent of normal (type I), 5 to 20 percent (type II), or 50 percent or more (variants).[22,138] In one review of 64 patients, 78 percent were type I, 14 percent were type II, and 8 percent were variants.[22] This subtyping predated the identification of integrin $\alpha_{IIb}\beta_3$ abnormalities as the cause of GT and was based on functional data; this categorization provides only limited information.

Measuring integrin $\alpha_V\beta_3$ content is technically more demanding than measuring that of integrin $\alpha_{IIb}\beta_3$ because there are only approximately 50 to 100 integrin $\alpha_V\beta_3$ receptors per platelet.[63] The integrin $\alpha_V\beta_3$ level is very useful, however, in making a preliminary assessment of whether the patient has a defect in the α_{IIb} or β_3 subunits, because, in general, patients who lack integrin $\alpha_V\beta_3$ receptors have a defect in the β_3 rather than α_{IIb} subunit.[139] A β_3 subunit missense mutation (H280P) that differentially affected integrin $\alpha_{IIb}\beta_3$ more than $\alpha_V\beta_3$ has, however, been described.[69]

Fibrinogen-binding studies assess the function of the integrin $\alpha_{IIb}\beta_3$ complex.[25] Early studies used radiolabeled fibrinogen to the binding of fibrinogen when the platelets are stimulated with ADP[25] or a similar agonist. Fibrinogen can also be labeled with a fluorescent molecule and then flow cytometry can be used to measure fibrinogen binding. These techniques are most useful in detecting qualitative abnormalities of integrin $\alpha_{IIb}\beta_3$ in patients with variant GT. The binding of a monoclonal antibody (PAC1) to platelets gives similar information because the antibody only binds to the activated form of the integrin.[140]

Carriers of GT have essentially normal platelet function.[34] Their platelets, however, only contain approximately 60 percent of the normal number of integrin $\alpha_{IIb}\beta_3$ receptors; the overlap in values between normal individuals and carriers, however, doesn't permit for unequivocal diagnosis of carriers by this technique.[112] Carrier detection is most accurately performed by DNA analysis.

Platelet fibrinogen is reduced to approximately 10 percent of normal in patients with marked reductions in integrin $\alpha_{IIb}\beta_3$[18,21,43,44] but is variably reduced in patients with significant amounts of integrin $\alpha_{IIb}\beta_3$.[138,141,142]

Therapy and Prognosis

Therapy of GT patients is discussed in the section entitled "Management of Inherited Platelet Function Disorders." Although GT is a severe disease, the prognosis for survival is generally good. In one series, two of 64 patients died of hemorrhage and in another series, three of 43 patients died of hemorrhage.[22,33] A nationwide survey in Japan identified 98 GT

patients in 1976 and 192 in 1991.[143] The mortality rate decreased substantially during this time interval.

$\alpha_{IIb}\beta_3$: **Select Macrothrombocytopenias** Five heterozygous missense mutations in four different amino acids in integrin $\alpha_{IIb}\beta_3$ (α_{IIb} G991C, R995Q, and R995W, and β_3 L718P and D723H), as well as several different deletions, lead to variably mild reductions in both integrin $\alpha_{IIb}\beta_3$ expression and platelet aggregation, as well as constitutively active receptors, in patients with inherited aniso- and macrothrombocytopenia.[144–150] The defects cluster on both sides of the transmembrane domains, and include both members of the α_{IIb} R995-β_3 D723 salt bridge proposed to maintain the receptor in a low affinity state.[151] Proplatelet formation has been reported to be abnormal in several reported cases.

GLYCOPROTEIN Ib (CD42b,c)–IX (CD42a)–V: BERNARD-SOULIER SYNDROME

Definition and History

BSS is an inherited disorder of the platelet GPIb–IX–V complex characterized by thrombocytopenia, giant platelets, and a failure of the platelets to bind GPIb ligands, most importantly, VWF and thrombin.[152–155]

In 1948 Bernard and Soulier described two children from a consanguineous family who had a severe bleeding disorder characterized by mucocutaneous hemorrhage, variable thrombocytopenia, and giant platelets.[156,157] Beginning in the early 1970s, BSS platelets were shown to have a functional defect in VWF-dependent platelet adhesion and agglutination.[158–160] In 1975, Nurden and Caen identified an abnormality in platelet GPIb as the cause of the functional defect.[161] Later studies confirmed the defect in VWF–GPIb interactions[162–164] and identified additional defects in platelet GPV and GPIX.[165,166] Subsequent studies have identified additional ligands for the GPIb–IX complex, including thrombin,[167] P-selectin,[168] leukocyte integrin $\alpha_M\beta_2$,[169] high-molecular-weight kininogen,[170] thrombospondin-1,[171] and coagulation factors XI[172] and XII[173] (Chap. 112), but the precise contributions of these interactions to the disorder are not well defined. Molecular defects in the genes for GPIbα, GPIbβ, and GPIX, but not GPV have been identified in BSS. Mouse models of BSS have been produced by gene targeting of *GPIbα*[174] and *GPIbβ*,[175] and like humans, mice deficient in *GPV* do not demonstrate the typical features of human BSS.[176,177]

Etiology and Pathogenesis

This rare disease, with a prevalence estimated as less than one in 1,000,000, has been reported from countries around the world.[152,154,157,165] Both autosomal recessive ("biallelic") and autosomal dominant ("monoallelic") forms of the disorder have been described, with the biallelic producing the most severe symptoms and the monoallelic causing macrothrombocytopenia and a mild or no bleeding syndrome. Consanguinity is common in the biallelic form, with 85 percent of the reported cases being homozygous for the causative mutation.[154]

Six different features of BSS may contribute to the hemorrhagic diathesis: thrombocytopenia, abnormal platelet adhesive interactions with VWF, abnormal platelet interactions with thrombin, abnormal platelet coagulant activity, abnormal platelet interactions with P-selectin, and abnormal platelet interactions with leukocyte integrin $\alpha_M\beta_2$.

The pathophysiology of the thrombocytopenia is uncertain. Early studies suggested a marked shortening of platelet survival, presumably from the decrease in platelet surface charge resulting from the GPIb defect.[178,179] Later studies using ^{111}In-oxine to label platelets reported more modest or no shortening of platelet survival, indicating that ineffective thrombopoiesis and/or decreased thrombopoiesis may contribute to the thrombocytopenia.[180,181] Morphologic abnormalities have been identified in BSS megakaryocytes and these may contribute to abnormal platelet production.[182] Based on observations in other giant platelet syndromes (Chap. 117), the large size of Bernard-Soulier platelets would tend to diminish the adverse hemostatic effects of the thrombocytopenia because the platelet mass is better preserved. With only rare exceptions,[183] however, the bleeding diathesis with BSS is more severe than expected from the thrombocytopenia, reinforcing the conclusion that a qualitative platelet defect is the predominant problem.[157,184]

The platelet GPIb–IX complex functions as a receptor for VWF (Chaps. 112 and 126).[152,185,186] This interaction is crucial in the adhesion of platelets to subendothelial surfaces, especially under high shear conditions, where VWF acts as a bridge between the subendothelial matrix and the platelet.[133,134] The relative roles of subendothelial VWF, plasma VWF, and platelet VWF have not been completely defined, but they probably all contribute to platelet adhesion.[187] The interaction of VWF with GPIb/IX initiates activation of integrin $\alpha_{IIb}\beta_3$,[188,189] which can also bind to VWF, but at a different site on the molecule.[190] The interaction of GPIb/IX with VWF also directly contributes to platelet–platelet interactions.[191–193]

GPIb/IX–VWF interactions can also occur in platelet suspensions at high shear rates; this can lead to platelet activation, with subsequent aggregation mediated by integrin $\alpha_{IIb}\beta_3$.[187,194–196] Whether sustained shear rates *in vivo* ever reach the levels required to initiate VWF binding, however, is not established.

Abnormalities of the GPIb–IX complex can be a result of genetic defects in *GPIbα, GPIbβ*, or *GPIX*, all of which are required for surface expression. BSS is the most severe form of the disease and is caused by defects in both alleles of one of the proteins as a result of a homozygous mutation, compound heterozygosity, or a combination of hemizygosity of *GPIbβ* because of a microdeletion and a mutation affecting the other *GPIbβ* allele. These abnormalities have been termed the *biallelic forms*.[154] A macrothrombocytopenic syndrome associated with a mild bleeding syndrome has been reported with heterozygous defects in *GPIbα* and *GPIbβ*.[154] Because obligate heterozygotes for the biallelic BSS mutations do not commonly demonstrate macrothrombocytopenia, the heterozygous defects associated with macrothrombocytopenia may exert a dominant negative effect.[154]

The platelets of patients with BSS have a decreased response to platelet activation by thrombin, especially at limiting concentrations of thrombin.[197–199] BSS platelets are deficient in two different proteins that interact with thrombin, namely GPIbα, which binds thrombin,[167] and GPV, which is a thrombin substrate (Chap. 112). The precise nature of the interactions of thrombin with GPIbα and its biologic consequences are still unclear, but binding of thrombin to GPIbα can initiate signaling within the platelet, perhaps directly through GPIbα crosslinking or indirectly by augmenting activation of other thrombin receptors (protease-activated receptors [PARs] 1 and 4) or other thrombin-dependent events at the platelet surface.[167] Paradoxically, mice deficient in GPV actually have increased sensitivity to thrombin activation and variably increased thrombus formation, perhaps because GPV limits access of thrombin to GPIbα.[200,201] Because thrombin is one of the major physiologic activators of platelets, the loss of thrombin binding to GPIbα may contribute to the hemorrhagic diathesis.

Platelets from patients with BSS are defective in supporting thrombin generation as judged by the serum PT,[202] a test performed with whole blood, but in other tests of platelet coagulant activity, BSS platelets support coagulation as well as, or better than, normal platelets.[124,203] Defects in collagen-induced coagulant activity and the association of factors V, VIII, and XI with BSS platelets have been described,[203] but their significance is unclear. Similarly, GPIb/IX has been identified as a binding site for other proteins involved in coagulation, including high-molecular-weight kininogen and factor XII, but the contributions of these interactions to the coagulant abnormality are also uncertain.[170,172,173] Binding of VWF to GPIb/IX has been implicated

in fibrin-dependent, but not fibrin-independent, augmentation of platelet coagulant activity and thus fibrin-dependent coagulant activity is likely to be abnormal in BSS.[126] This finding may partially explain the variability in findings between the serum PT and some of the other assays as fibrin only forms in the serum PT. Abnormal membrane lipids have also been reported.[204]

The mechanism(s) producing the giant platelets in BSS has not been identified, but since giant platelets are found in BSS variants in which GPIb/IX is present, but unable to bind ligand, it has been postulated that the abnormality is a result of the inability of GPIb/IX to bind an unknown marrow ligand.[152] It cannot be because of an inability to bind VWF as, with only rare exceptions,[205] patients lacking VWF do not have large platelets. Moreover, in a mouse model of BSS, restoring a receptor with the GPIb transmembrane and cytoplasmic domains, but not the ligand-binding domain, partially corrected both the thrombocytopenia and large platelet size.[206] A defect in GPIb/IX–mediated signaling has also been proposed to cause the large platelets as a deficiency of PLC has also been described in BSS.[152,207] A mechanical alteration in the plasma membrane of BSS platelets has been identified by micropipette experiments, showing the plasma membrane to be more deformable than normal.[208] Megakaryocytes in BSS have increased ploidy and volume, as well as alterations in the membrane demarcation system, granules, and microtubules.[181,182] Both the increased size and deformability may reflect the loss of the normal interaction of GPIb/IX with the cytoskeleton via actin-binding protein (filamin-1; Chap. 112).

Platelets from patients with BSS are deficient not only in GPIbα, GPIbβ, and GPIX, which are known to be associated as a complex, but also in GPV (Chap. 112).[152,166] All of these proteins share highly conserved leucine-rich regions.[152,187] One possible explanation for the loss of surface expression of all the proteins is that they need to form a complex during biosynthesis in order to be transported to the surface[187]; evidence supports the need for GPIbα, GPIbβ, and GPIX to all be present for optimal surface expression,[209] but data from mice deficient in GPV indicate that this glycoprotein is not required for surface expression of the GPIb–IX complex.[200] GPV may, however, improve the efficiency of expression of the other members of the complex.[210] Moreover, data from the BSS mouse expressing a chimeric GPIbα molecule in which the leucine-rich repeat domain was replaced with the external domain of another receptor indicate that complex formation does not require the GPIbα leucine-rich domain.[206]

At the molecular level, the platelets from different patients with BSS are heterogeneous, with many having no detectable GPIb and others having variable amounts, up to 50 percent of normal.[152,207,211–214] There also is variability in the degree of concordance in the reduction of GPIb and the other deficient proteins.[215,216]

Molecular Defects The molecular biologic basis of BSS has been determined in 161 patients from 132 unrelated families[154] and an online registry of defects is available at http://www.bernardsoulier.org/.[217] An international consortium reported on 211 families with the recessive form of BSS, which they termed "biallelic."[154] In total, 45 different mutations have been reported in *GPIbα*, 52 in *GPIbβ*, and 28 in *GPIX*. No defects in *GPV* have been identified in patients with BSS. The association with consanguineous matings was reinforced as 85 percent of the families had homozygous mutations and 13 percent were compound heterozygotes for defects in one of the genes. None of the variants were identified in several gene variant databases,[154] suggesting that they are all rare and likely entered the population relatively recently. A number of likely founder mutations have been identified in each of the three genes in different populations.[154,218] The ancestry of seven apparently unrelated families with a *GPIbβ* W89D mutation was traced to a common ancestor in 1671 in India.[218] Five mutations in *GPIX* account for 137 of the 184 affected *GPIX* alleles and *GPIX* N61S is found in 64

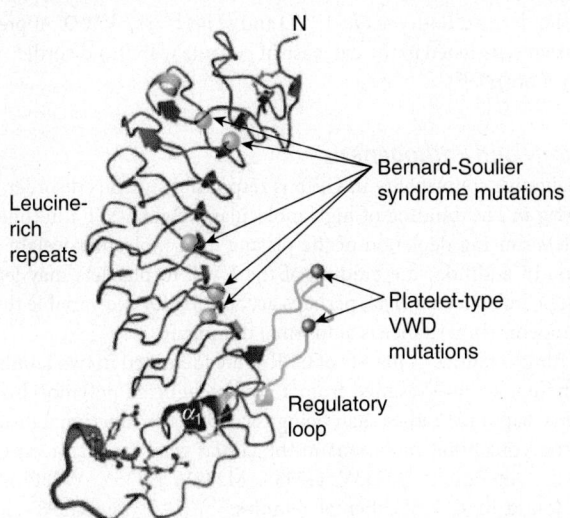

N

Leucine-rich repeats

Bernard-Soulier syndrome mutations

Platelet-type VWD mutations

α₁

Regulatory loop

Figure 120–4. Localization of select missense mutations causing platelet-type von Willebrand disease (VWD) and Bernard-Soulier syndrome (BSS) in the GPIbα N-terminal domain. Ribbon diagram of the topology of GPIbα N-terminal domain viewed from the side. The regulatory loop is colored *blue* with activating platelet-type VWD mutations G233V and M239V indicated as open *black balls*. Five BSS mutations, which cause loss of von Willebrand factor binding, are shown as *blue balls*. L57F and C65R localize to leucine-rich repeat (LRR) 2 with L129P, A156V, and L179del localized to the LRR5, LRR6, and LRR7 β-strands, respectively. The molecular structure of the sulfated tyrosine residues 276, 278, and 279 are shown. (*Adapted with permission from Uff S, Clemetson JM, Harrison T, et al: Crystal structure of the platelet glycoprotein Ib(alpha) N-terminal domain reveals an unmasking mechanism for receptor activation. J BiolChem 277(38):35657–35663, 2002.*)

European families. A number of mutations have been identified to cause the heterozygous monoallelic form, including the *GPIbα* A172V mutation, which has been associated with biallelic and monoallelic forms of the disorder in 42 apparently unrelated families with macrothrombocytopenia in Italy.[154] Many of the defects affect the leucine-rich repeats or the conserved flanking sequences, supporting the importance of these structural elements in the biogenesis and surface expression of the GPIb–IX–V complex (see Chap. 112, Fig. 112–14, and Fig. 120–4). Three patients have been described who are homozygous for a deletion in the last two bases of codon 492 of GPIbα, resulting in a frameshift that alters the membrane spanning region and results in premature termination, and another patient has been described who is heterozygous for this deletion and a missense mutation of GPIbα.[219–222] These defects appear to result in a poorly anchored GPIbα with GPIbα antigen present in plasma. *GPIbβ* mutations have affected the promoter region, at a binding site for the GATA-1 transcription factor,[223] the signal peptide,[224] and the transmembrane and intracellular domains.[225] A homozygous Y88C defect in GPIbβ has been reported to cause BSS in two Japanese families and heterozygotes with this mutation have a giant platelet syndrome.[221,226] Similarly, a patient heterozygous for a GPIbβ R17C mutation also had a giant platelet syndrome.[227] An N45S mutation in GPIX, affecting leucine rich repeat 1, has been reported in at least 12 different white patients, including four patients from a large Swiss family with variable clinical manifestations[228–230] and one Turkish patient.[231]

BSS has been reported in seven patients in association with hemizygous deletion of GPIbβ and several neighboring genes on chromosome 22q11.2, leading to variable manifestations of the DiGeorge syndrome, including cardiac defects, dysmorphic facial features, thymic hypoplasia, and velopharyngeal insufficiency.[154,232–239] Hemizygous mutations

in the remaining *GPIbβ* allele have included P96S and P29L.[236,237] In other studies of patients with the 22q11.2 deletion syndrome, modest reductions in platelet count and increases in platelet volume, as well as reduced platelet agglutination to ristocetin and decreased platelet GPIb/IX expression, have been variably reported, consistent with hemizygosity for *GPIbβ*.[240–244]

A number of monoallelic, heterozygous mutations in the genes of the GPIb–IX complex have been described as causing macrothrombocytopenia, some, but not all, of which have also been implicated in causing the biallelic form either because of homozygosity or compound heterozygosity.[154] These include a heterozygous mutation in the second leucine-rich repeat (L57F)[245] in which the affected patients have moderate bleeding symptoms, moderate thrombocytopenia, and giant platelets. Additional monoallelic mutations of *GPIbα* that appear to produce dominant effects are N41H[246] and Y54D.[247]

The "Bolzano" defect, which involves a mutation in the sixth leucine-rich repeat of GPIbα (A156V), results in a GPIbα molecule that has reduced ability to bind VWF, but can bind thrombin. It has been described in both biallelic and monoallelic forms. Two patients with biallelic forms have been described. In one patient, the Bolzano defect was homozygous, and the patient had a lifelong history of mucocutaneous hemorrhage in association with an approximately 50 percent reduction in GPIb surface expression and total loss of ability to bind VWF.[248] In the other, the Bolzano mutation coexisted with a 12-amino-acid deletion and an amino acid substitution (Q181K).[249] The monoallelic form of the Bolzano defect has been reported in more than 100 patients from 48 pedigrees, primarily from southern Italy.[250] Most patients have no bleeding symptoms, but some have mild to moderate bleeding symptoms. Mild thrombocytopenia, increased mean platelet volume, reduced expression of GPIb/IX/V, and normal or borderline abnormal values for ristocetin-induced platelet aggregation are characteristic of this disorder.

Clinical Features

Epistaxis is the most common symptom of BSS (70 percent); also common are ecchymoses (58 percent), menometrorrhagia (44 percent), gingival hemorrhage (42 percent), and gastrointestinal bleeding (22 percent).[157] The combination of BSS with angiodysplasia can result in particularly severe recurrent hemorrhage.[251–253] Hemorrhagic symptoms that occur with lower frequency include posttraumatic bleeding (13 percent), hematuria (7 percent), cerebral hemorrhage (4 percent), and retinal hemorrhage (2 percent). There is considerable variability in symptoms among patients, even among patients within a single family.[152,254] A review that includes brief descriptions of the clinical features of 55 patients, reported through 1998, has been published.[152]

Laboratory Features

Thrombocytopenia is present in nearly all patients, but is variable in its severity, ranging from approximately 20 × 10⁹ platelets/L to near-normal levels. Platelets are large on smear, with more than one-third usually having diameters greater than 3.5 μm, and some being as large or larger than lymphocytes. By electron microscopy, platelets display only minor variations in vesicular structures and the open canalicular system,[157] but megakaryocytes have more notable abnormalities in their demarcation membranes.[182] The cell membranes of platelets from patients with BSS appear to be more deformable than normal,[208] perhaps because GPIb ordinarily interacts with the platelet cytoskeleton[255] (Chap. 112).

Closure times of the apertures of collagen-coated membranes are markedly prolonged in the presence of ADP or epinephrine (PFA-100).[136] The hallmark findings in the BSS are the failure of platelets to aggregate in response to ristocetin[159] or botrocetin,[162,256] agents that require VWF–GPIb interactions. In VWD, but not BSS, this defect can be corrected by adding normal plasma (or VWF).

Although, the large size of the platelets in BSS and the thrombocytopenia make it technically difficult to perform platelet aggregation studies, in general, aggregation induced by ADP, epinephrine, or collagen is either normal or enhanced.[160,257,258] The aggregation response to thrombin is usually dose-dependent, being essentially normal in response to high doses of thrombin but characterized by a prolonged lag phase and diminished aggregation in response to low doses of thrombin.[197,259]

Platelet Coagulant Activity The coagulant activity of platelets from patients with BSS has been variably reported as reduced, normal, or increased.[124,202,203] The variable presence of fibrin in the different assays used to assess platelet coagulant activity may account for these inconsistent results as GPIb–VWF interactions enhance platelet coagulant activity when fibrin is present, but not when it is absent.[126]

Platelet-Thrombin Interactions Both GPIb and the seven-transmembrane domains PAR-1 and PAR-4 receptors are required for maximal response to thrombin.[167,259] Two different crystal structures of the interactions between thrombin and GPIbα have been reported; in one, two molecules of thrombin bind to each GPIbα molecule, raising the possibility that free thrombin or thrombin adherent to fibrinogen can cluster GPIb–IX–V complexes.[167,260,261] GPV, which is missing from the platelet surface in BSS, is cleaved by thrombin, but the cleavage is neither necessary nor sufficient for thrombin-induced platelet activation.[262,263] In fact, platelets of mice lacking GPV have increased responsiveness to thrombin, perhaps because GPV ordinarily limits access of thrombin to GPIbα or inhibits GPIbα crosslinking.[200,201]

Ex Vivo Interaction with Subendothelial Surfaces Platelets from patients with BSS demonstrate defective adhesion to subendothelial surfaces, especially at shear rates greater than 650 s^{-1}.[133,134,158,264] The results are similar to those in patients with VWD.

Shear-Induced Platelet Aggregation Unlike normal platelets, platelets from patients with BSS are not aggregated by high shear rates.[194,195] The initial interaction in this process appears to be binding of VWF to GPIb,[187] with subsequent activation of integrin $\alpha_{IIb}\beta_3$, perhaps through signaling via the protein 14-3-3ζ associated with the cytoplasmic domain of GPIbα,[196,265] Fcγ receptor IIA, GPVI, and/or the Fc receptor γ chain (Chap. 112).[266–268] Pathologic shear stress has been reported to increase binding of α-actin to GPIb/IX as part of the signaling process.[268–270]

Therapy

The therapy of BSS is described in the section "Management of Inherited Platelet Function Disorders" below. Splenectomy has been performed when the diagnosis of immune thrombocytopenia was mistakenly made, but this usually does not normalize the platelet count or improve the bleeding diathesis.[249]

GPIbα (CD42b,c): PLATELET-TYPE (PSEUDO-) VON WILLEBRAND DISEASE

Definition and History

A heterogeneous group of patients has been described with mild to moderate bleeding symptoms, variably enlarged platelets, variable thrombocytopenia, and diminished plasma high-molecular-weight VWF multimers.[271] The fundamental defect in these patients is thought to be an enhanced interaction between an abnormal platelet GPIb/IX receptor and normal plasma VWF.[272–281] Because these patients have some of the hallmarks of VWD, but the defect is in platelet GPIb/IX, it

has been termed both *pseudo-VWD* and *platelet-type VWD*. At present, 55 patients are listed in the database of patients with this disorder (www.pt-vwd.org).[282,283]

Etiology and Pathogenesis

A qualitative abnormality in GPIb is responsible for this disorder, with ongoing *in vivo* binding of high-molecular-weight VWF multimers to platelets causing depletion of the plasma high-molecular-weight multimers. In addition, the binding of the VWF to platelets may lead to shortened platelet survival, perhaps accounting for the variable thrombocytopenia. Inheritance is autosomal dominant.

Abnormalities in the Mr of GPIb were identified in two families,[277] but these may have resulted from a now-recognized polymorphism in GPIb (Chap. 112) rather than being related to the functional disorder. Heterozygous point mutations in the *GPIbα* gene causing a variety of missense alterations (G233V, G233S, M239V, D235Y, W230L) have been found in several different families.[271,278,284–289] The G238V mutation is the most common among the patients in the database, affecting 31 of 35 patients. All of these mutations are in the R-loop (also termed β-switch) in the carboxyterminal flanking sequence of the leucine-rich repeats, a region implicated in ligand binding (see Fig. 120–4).[152,187,290–293] Molecular modeling suggests that the M239V substitution produces a significant conformational change in the molecule,[294] and this was confirmed by crystallographic analysis.[295] It has been proposed that the platelet-type VWD mutations either destabilize the compact triangular structure of the R-loop by interfering with the D235-K237 salt bridge or stabilizing the extended β-hairpin form of the R-loop, which is better able to engage the VWF A1 domain.[282] A mouse model of the GPIbα G233V mutation recapitulated many of the human manifestations and had an unexpected increase in bone mass.[296] Recombinant GPIbα fragments containing the G233V and M239V mutations demonstrated enhanced interactions with VWF in several different systems, including ones under shear stress.[297,298] An increase in platelet GPIb/IX expression has also been reported.[278,281] An in-frame 27-base-pair (bp) deletion in the macroglycopeptide region of GPIbα has also been reported to cause platelet-type VWD.[279] Because the deletion may lead to the loss of up to four glycosylation sites, it has been proposed that the glycans play a negative regulatory role in ligand binding.[282]

Clinical Features

Patients have variable thrombocytopenia and mild to moderate mucocutaneous hemorrhage. A study of 13 patients with six different mutations using a standardized bleeding assessment tool found a wide range of clinical severity, with approximately 40 percent having a normal bleeding score and the remainder having a wide range of abnormal scores.[271] Bleeding scores did not correlate with age or sex, but did correlate with reductions in both platelet count and ristocetin cofactor activity. All patients had macrothrombocytopenia. Of note, pregnancy may exacerbate the thrombocytopenia and bleeding symptoms.[278]

Laboratory Features and Differential Diagnosis

Mild thrombocytopenia and somewhat enlarged platelets are present in some, but not all, patients. Plasma VWF levels are variably reduced, with a disproportionate reduction in plasma high-molecular-weight multimers. Platelet VWF multimers are normal.

The most characteristic laboratory finding in platelet-type VWD is enhanced platelet aggregation in response to low concentrations of ristocetin[272–276,278,288] or botrocetin.[299] This same abnormality is present in patients with type 2b VWD, as is selective depletion of plasma high-molecular-weight VWF multimers (Chap. 126). In platelet-type VWD, however, the defect is in platelet GPIbα, whereas in type 2b VWD, the defect is in the VWF. In one study comparing platelet-type and type 2b VWD, patients with type 2b VWD had more severe bleeding, especially menorrhagia, and lower platelet counts.[271] Several assays can help differentiate between these abnormalities[274,300–302]: (1) normal VWF (purified or in cryoprecipitate) will aggregate platelets from patients with platelet-type VWD, but not platelets from patients with type 2b VWD; (2) isolated platelets from patients with platelet-type VWD will bind normal VWF at lower concentrations of ristocetin than will normal platelets or platelets from patients with type 2b VWD; (3) plasma VWF from patients with type 2b VWD will bind to normal platelets at lower-than-normal concentrations of ristocetin, whereas higher-than-normal concentrations of ristocetin are required to promote the plasma VWF from patients with platelet-type VWF to bind to normal platelets[301]; and (4) VWF lacking sialic acid residues (asialo-VWF) will agglutinate platelets from patients with platelet-type VWD in the presence of ethylenediaminetetraacetic acid (EDTA).[303] A number of patients with platelet-type VWD were originally diagnosed as having type 2b VWD, leading to the conclusion that platelet-type VWD may be underdiagnosed, and an international registry based study supports this contention.[278,280,304]

Therapy

Because normal VWF (especially the high-molecular-weight forms) can bind excessively to the platelets of patients with platelet-type VWD and potentially lead to rapid platelet clearance from the circulation, increasing the VWF level by any means (desmopressin infusion or VWF replacement with cryoprecipitate or VWF concentrates) poses a potential risk of inducing thrombocytopenia.[300,305] It may be possible to estimate this risk by assessing whether the patient's platelets aggregate *ex vivo* in response to VWF (as in cryoprecipitate).[273] Low-dose cryoprecipitate has successfully supported hemostasis, without inducing thrombocytopenia.[275,305,306] Currently, cryoprecipitate is generally less favored for VWF replacement therapy than plasma-derived factor VIII concentrates such as Humate-P, which is approved in the United States for the therapy of VWD, because the plasma-derived factor VIII concentrates have a reduced risk of viral infection. Consideration should also be given to platelet transfusion in appropriate circumstances. Recombinant factor VIIa infusion may be beneficial and is licensed for this indication in Europe, but this therapy is not yet approved by the FDA; it has the theoretical advantage of avoiding excessive interactions between VWF and the abnormal GPIbα receptor.[307,308]

INTEGRIN $\alpha_2\beta_1$ DEFICIENCY (GLYCOPROTEIN Ia/IIa; VLA-2; CD49B/CD29)

Integrin $\alpha_2\beta_1$ (GPIa/IIa) can mediate platelet adhesion to collagen and platelet activation under certain conditions (Chap. 112). A female patient with excessive posttraumatic bruising and menorrhagia but no epistaxis, gum bleeding, or excessive bleeding after tonsillectomy or appendectomy was described whose platelets selectively failed to aggregate or undergo shape change in response to collagen.[309,310] The bleeding time was markedly prolonged, and the patient's platelets failed to adhere and spread normally on subendothelial surfaces. The patient's platelets only contained approximately 15 to 25 percent of the normal amount of integrin α_2,[309,311] and a reduction in the β_1 subunit was also apparent.[309] It is difficult to draw conclusions about the physiologic role of integrin $\alpha_2\beta_1$ in platelet function from this patient because her $\alpha_2\beta_1$ deficiency was incomplete, her bleeding symptoms were mild and variable, and some of the platelet function abnormalities (e.g., abnormal platelet-collagen interactions in the presence of the divalent chelating agent EDTA) are difficult to ascribe to the deficiency in $\alpha_2\beta_1$.[309,312]

Another patient with integrin α_2 deficiency has been described.[313] She had a history of mucocutaneous and postoperative bleeding. Her bleeding time was prolonged and platelet aggregation in response to collagen was selectively reduced, but not absent. In addition to her α_2 subunit defect, she also had little or no intact thrombospondin, and exogenous thrombospondin corrected the defect in platelet aggregation. The patient's hemorrhagic symptoms and platelet defects disappeared when she entered menopause.

The variation in platelet integrin $\alpha_2\beta_1$ expression in healthy individuals is very wide (10-fold) and platelet levels have been correlated with allelic variants.[314] Reduced $\alpha_2\beta_1$ expression has been associated with alterations in megakaryocyte production and decreased mean platelet volume.[315]

Mice with targeted deletion of integrin $\alpha_2\beta_1$ do not have a hemorrhagic phenotype or prolonged tail bleeding times but they do have reduced platelet adhesion to collagen and reduced thrombus formation after vascular injury[316]; mice with a conditional loss of integrin $\alpha_2\beta_1$ in megakaryocytes and platelets have a decreased mean platelet volume.[315]

CD36 (GPIV; FATTY ACYL TRANSLOCASE [FAT]; SCAVENGER RECEPTOR CLASS B, MEMBER 3 [SCARB3])

CD36 (GPIV) is a highly, but variably expressed platelet glycoprotein that is present on many cell types and documented to participate in long-chain fatty acid transport (Chap. 112). Approximately 3 percent of Japanese, 2 percent of African Americans, and 0.3 percent of whites in the United States have platelets that lack CD36 (GPIV).[317,318] Although CD36 (GPIV) has been implicated in platelet interactions with collagen, thrombospondin, advanced glycation products,[319] and myeloid-related protein (MRP)-14,[320–323] as well as in platelet–monocyte interactions,[324] individuals lacking CD36 (GPIV) do not have a hemorrhagic diathesis. Platelets from these patients can bind thrombospondin via alternative receptors[325] and there are differing data on its role in adhesion to collagen.[326–328] A multiparameter analysis of platelet thrombus formation to different matrix proteins at differing shear rates identified a role for CD36 at low, but not high, shear rates.[8] CD36 (GPIV) has also been implicated as a receptor for oxidized low-density lipoprotein (LDL), and the binding of very-low-density lipoprotein (VLDL) to CD36 (GPIV) has been reported to enhance collagen-induced platelet aggregation and thromboxane production.[329] CD36 (GPIV) platelet expression varies widely among healthy individuals (200 to 14,000 molecules per platelet) and correlates with activation by oxidized LDL and genetic single-nucleotide variants.[330]

Two forms of CD36 (GPIV) deficiency have been described in Japan: type I in which both platelets and monocytes are deficient, and type II in which only platelets are deficient.[331–333] A P90S substitution that also leads to abnormal posttranslational modification is a common abnormality contributing to both type I and type II deficiencies. In the type I form, patients are homozygous for the abnormality, whereas in type II deficiency, patients are doubly heterozygous for the P90S abnormality and an unidentified platelet-specific expression defect.[331,334,335] Other abnormalities that have been associated with type I deficiency include a dinucleotide deletion(539–540) in exon 5, a 161-bp deletion[331–491] corresponding to loss of exon 4, a nucleotide insertion at position 1159 in codon 317 leading to a frameshift and premature stop, and splice-site mutations.[336–338] Other mutations have been identified in other populations.

CD36 (GPIV) deficiency can result in refractoriness to platelet transfusions because of isoimmunization and has been implicated in posttransfusion purpura (Chap. 117),[339] as well as thrombocytopenia caused by the passive transfer of anti-CD36 antibodies.[340]

GLYCOPROTEIN VI DEFICIENCY

GPVI can mediate platelet adhesion to collagen and is important in collagen-induced signal transduction (Chap. 112). Twelve patients with mild to moderate bleeding disorders and variable deficiencies of platelet GPVI or signaling have been described; one had concomitant GPS (α-granule deficiency).[341–350] The others had selective abnormalities in platelet–collagen interactions. Platelet GPVI deficiency associated with an autoantibody to GPVI has been described in several patients, one of whom also had systemic lupus erythematosus and another of whom had coexisting antibodies to integrin $\alpha_{IIb}\beta_3$.[351–353] Antibody to GPVI may be detectable in eluates prepared from patient platelets even when it is not detectable in patient plasma.[354] Acquired forms of GPVI-specific signal transduction have also been described in patients with myelodysplastic syndromes and chronic lymphocytic leukemia.[347] Studies in mice and primates demonstrated that antibodies to GPVI can result in loss of GPVI from the platelet surface through either proteolytic shedding or a cyclic adenosine monophosphate (cAMP)-mediated internalization mechanism, even though the platelets continue to circulate.[346,355] Thus, it is likely that the deficiency of GPVI most commonly results from the autoantibodies.[353] It is unclear whether the patients reported earlier as having GPVI deficiency might also have had an immune basis for their GPVI deficiency.

Three different inherited forms of GPVI deficiency have been described. One patient with a lifelong history of "mild" mucocutaneous, posttraumatic, and postsurgery bleeding had a marked deficiency of platelet membrane GPVI resulting from both a 16-base out-of-frame deletion and a S175N missense mutation.[350] The patient's platelets failed to respond to collagen, convulxin, or collagen-related peptide. Of note, FcRγ expression was normal. Another patient with easy bruising, a prolonged bleeding time, abnormal PFA-100 closure time to collagen/epinephrine, and no platelet aggregation in response to collagen had a combination of a R38C mutation in one allele and a five-nucleotide duplication insertion in the other, leading to a nonsense codon.[356] The R38C mutation led to misfolding of the protein, reduced surface expression, and a qualitative defect in collagen binding. Five subjects from four apparently unrelated families in Chile with variable histories of easy bruising, epistaxis, excessive bleeding after minor trauma, and gingival bleeding were found to have no platelet aggregation in response to collagen, convulxin, or collagen-related peptide.[357] DNA analysis showed a homozygous adenine insertion between bases 711 and 712. Heterozygotes were asymptomatic and had nearly normal platelet function.

● ABNORMALITIES OF PLATELET GRANULES

Platelets contain at least three types of granules: dense or δ granules containing ADP, ATP, calcium, serotonin, and pyrophosphate; α granules containing a variety of proteins, some derived from plasma, others synthesized by the megakaryocyte; and lysosomes containing acid hydrolases. Following platelet activation, the contents of the α and dense granules are secreted. Inability to release these granule contents by virtue of a deficiency of the granules or their contents or in the cellular mechanisms governing the secretory process is associated with impaired platelet function. A heterogeneous group of disorders involving platelet granules has been described. They are broadly categorized into defects affecting dense granules (δ-storage pool deficiency [SPD]), α granules (α-SPD, or GPS), or both dense bodies and α granules ($\alpha\delta$-SPD). Another disorder affecting granules is the Quebec platelet disorder, which affects the α-granules.

δ-STORAGE POOL DEFICIENCY

Definition and History

In 1969, a family with impaired platelet aggregation was described whose platelets displayed decreased levels of ADP.[358] Holmsen and Weiss subsequently established that the defect was a deficiency in the nonmetabolic pool or "storage pool" of ADP present in the dense granules.[359] δ-SPD is a heterogeneous disorder characterized by a bleeding tendency, abnormalities in the second wave of platelet aggregation, and variable deficiencies of platelet dense granule contents.

Etiology and Pathogenesis

Normal platelets contain two pools of adenine nucleotides that exchange very slowly.[360] One pool is a metabolic nongranule pool in which the ratio of ATP to ADP content is 8 to 10:1. The second pool is the "storage pool" present in the dense granules and contains 65 percent of the platelet adenine nucleotides with an ATP-to-ADP ratio of 2:3. It is this storage pool that is deficient in δ-SPD. Dense granules also contain serotonin, which is taken up from plasma at a ratio of approximately 1000:1 via a pH-dependent amine trapping mechanism. Platelet serotonin levels are also decreased in δ-SPD.

δ-SPD can be a primary, inherited platelet disorder or a component of a multisystem (syndromic) disorder, such as the Hermansky-Pudlak syndrome (HPS)[361–365] (variable oculocutaneous albinism, hemorrhagic disorder, and neurologic manifestations), the Chédiak-Higashi syndrome[361,365,366] (partial oculocutaneous albinism, giant lysosomal granules, and frequent pyogenic infections), and the Wiskott-Aldrich syndrome[361,367,368] (see below and Chap. 80). Other diseases associated with δ-SPD are Ehlers-Danlos syndrome,[369] osteogenesis imperfecta,[370] and TAR syndrome.[361,371] The mode of inheritance in δ-SPD is not well defined, but an autosomal dominant pattern for the primary form has been identified in some patients.[372] The inheritance pattern of the syndromic forms follows the autosomal recessive and X-linked patterns characteristic of those disorders. Essential criteria for the diagnosis of HPS are the tyrosinase-positive oculocutaneous albinism and the δ-SPD in platelets.[373] The hallmarks of albinism are diffuse hypopigmentation of skin, iris, hair and retina, although there is phenotypic heterogeneity.

Studies from animal models and, particularly, in patients with the syndromic variants indicate that defects in biogenesis of lysosome-related organelles form the basis of the disorders.[361,374] These organelles share features with lysosomes but have distinct morphology, composition, and functions, and include melanosomes in melanocytes, platelet δ-granules, and Weibel-Palade bodies in endothelial cells.[361,374] In δ-SPD associated with HPS, there may be a total failure of δ-granule formation as judged by electron microscopy of platelets and megakaryocytes[375] and the absence of CD63 (granulophysin; ME491; LIMP-1; LAMP-3), a lysosomal and dense granule membrane protein of Mr 40,000 that is also found in melanosomes.[361,363,376,377] The defect in melanosomes accounts for the oculocutaneous albinism. The defect in lysosomes results in accumulation of ceroid lipofuscin, a lipid-protein complex leading to granulomatous colitis and pulmonary fibrosis, which are variably manifest in these patients. Abnormalities of nine genes have been implicated in causing HPS (Fig. 120–5). Ultrastructural studies in patients with a variety of types of HPS indicate that α granules and other organelles are unaffected.[378] Mutations in HPS-associated genes result in defects in intracellular protein trafficking and in the biogenesis of lysosomes and lysosomes-related organelles.[361] The HPS gene products operate in distinct complexes termed *biogenesis of lysosome-related organelles complexes* (BLOCs), which consist of multiple proteins.[361] HPS is unusually common in patients from northwest Puerto Rico (frequency: 1:1800), and linkage analysis of these patients led to the identification of the abnormality in HPS gene (*HPS1*). The gene encodes a 700-amino-acid protein that participates in the complex of proteins called BLOC-3.[361,363]

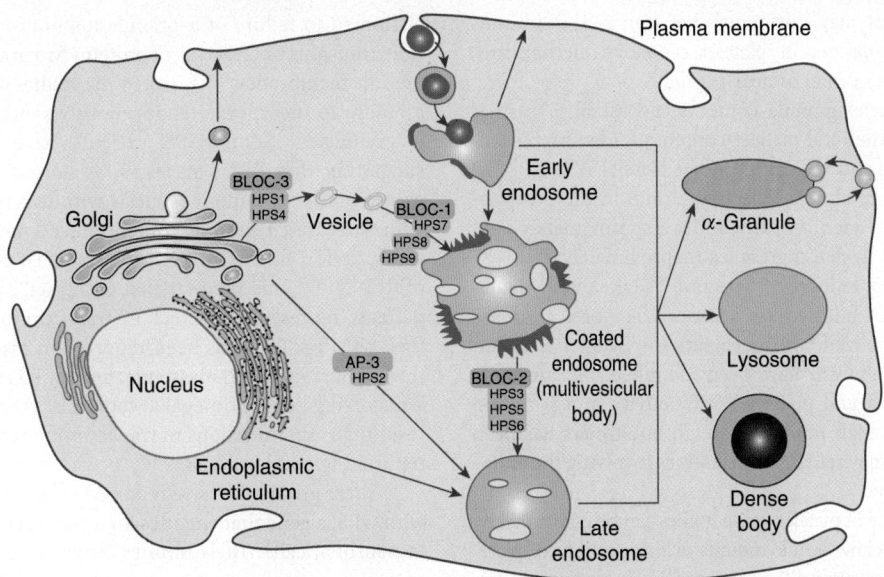

Figure 120–5. Hypothetical model of platelet granule formation and location of defects resulting in Hermansky-Pudlak syndrome (HPS). Early endosomes derive from invaginations from the plasma membrane whereas membrane-bound structures from the Golgi and endoplasmic reticulum contribute to the production of coated endosomes and late endosomes. Three multiprotein complexes termed *biogenesis of lysosome related organelles complexes* (BLOCS) are involved in the transport and interconversion of the different endosomal species. The gene products of HPS1 and HPS4 are involved in BLOC-3, whereas those of HPS3, HPS5, and HPS6 are involved in BLOC-2, and those of HPS7, HPS8, and HPS9 contribute to BLOC-1. HPS2 is a result of mutations in adaptor complex-3 (AP-3). It has not yet been determined which endosomal species contribute to α granules, lysosomes, and dense bodies, but all three organelles are affected in HPS. α Granules are in dynamic exchange with the plasma membrane, selectively taking up fibrinogen via integrin $\alpha_{IIb}\beta_3$ receptors. (*Used with permission of Dr. Marjan Huizing and Dr. William Gahl, National Human Genome Research Institute, National Institutes of Health.*)

The mutation in the Puerto Rican kindreds is a 16-bp duplication in HPS1 exon 15; other mutations of the same gene have been identified in patients from this region and in other ethnic groups.[363,379,380] HPS2 is caused by mutations in the gene *AP3B1 (HPS2)*, which codes for the β_3A subunit of the heterotetrameric adaptor complex-3 (AP-3), which, in turn, facilitates the formation of vesicles of lysosomal lineage from membranes of the *trans*-Golgi network or late endosomes. Patients with mutations in this protein tend to also have neutropenia and childhood infections.[373,381]

Defects in the *HPS3* gene cause a relatively mild form of HPS and pulmonary involvement is usually minimal.[382] *HPS4* encodes a protein that interacts with the *HPS1* protein in the BLOC-3 complex.[383] Patients with mutations in this gene tend to have severe disease, and like patients with defects in *HPS1*, pulmonary involvement is common. The gene products of *HPS5* and *HPS6* interact with the *HPS3* gene product to form BLOC-2.[384,385] Proteins implicated in HPS7 (encoded by *DTNBP1*) and HPS8 (encoded by *BLOC1S3*) are components of BLOC-1.[386,387] Improper trafficking of melanocyte-specific proteins, including tyrosinase, has been found in the melanosomes of patients with *HPS5*.[388] HPS is also associated with mutations in pallidin (*BLOC1S6/PLDN*), a protein of BLOC-1 and labeled as HPS9.[389]

Not all patients with δ-SPD have HPS. Some of the patients described to have δ-SPD have been subsequently shown to have mutations in RUNX1.[358,372,390,391]

In other forms of δ-SPD, data obtained with uranaffin, a dye that specifically stains amine-containing granules, indicate that dense granule membranes are formed but are not properly filled.[392–394] The defects in the different substances contained in dense granules are also heterogeneous, with some patients able to secrete significant amounts of calcium and pyrophosphate even when adenine nucleotide secretion is nearly absent.[392]

Chédiak-Higashi syndrome results from mutation of the *LYST* gene, which encodes a protein of estimated molecular mass of 429 kDa,

predicted from domain analysis to participate in vesicle transport and to interact with microtubules; an *HPS1*-like region is also present.[361,366]

Numerous animal models of human δ-SPD and HPS have been reported and several represent specific counterparts of the human disease. Thus, more than 20 separate inherited mouse defects have been reported to include dense granule deficiencies; of these, pale ear (*ep*) is linked to the mouse equivalent of the *HPS1* gene; pearl (*pe*) to the mouse equivalent of *HSP2* (β_3A subunit of AP-3 complex); cocoa to *HPS3*; light ear (*le*) to *HPS4*; ruby-eye-2 (*ru2*) to *HPS5*; ruby-eye (*ru*) to *HPS6*; sandy (*sdy*) to *HPS7*; and pallid to HPS9 (*PLDN*).[361,395] The beige mouse and rat serve as models for Chédiak-Higashi syndrome.[361]

Clinical Features
Patients with δ-SPD as part of the HPS may have severe, or even lethal, hemorrhage.[363] For all other forms of the disorder, the bleeding tendency is variable, and mild to moderate.

Laboratory Features
When tested with the PFA-100 instrument, both prolonged and normal closure times have been reported, akin to prior findings with bleeding times.[396–399] Interestingly, flow-dependent thrombus formation, assessed using a multisurface and multiparameter flow assay, is reported to be decreased.[8] In platelet aggregation studies, ADP and epinephrine induce a normal primary wave of aggregation, but the secondary wave is variably abnormal. The abnormal platelet response is more easily discernible at low collagen doses than high doses. Secretion of ATP from platelets can be measured by luminescence simultaneously with platelet aggregation using a specially designed instrument.[400] ATP release in response to activation is absent or decreased in δ-SPD patients. Thrombin at high doses causes maximal release of platelet dense body contents, even in patients with secretion abnormalities unrelated to granule deficiency,

and, therefore, this reagent may distinguish between δ-SPD (diminished release) and abnormalities of platelet secretory mechanisms, wherein the release may be normal or near-normal.

Measurement of platelet granule contents can establish further the platelet abnormality. The total platelet content of adenine nucleotides is reduced in δ-SPD, and the ratio of total platelet ATP to ADP is increased because it more closely reflects the ratio in the cytoplasmic, "metabolic" pool of adenine nucleotides (approximately 8:1) than in the "storage" pool in dense granules (approximately 2:3).[360,401] Platelet serotonin is variably reduced.[402] Serotonin is taken up by platelets of patients with δ-SPD, but because it cannot be stored in dense granules, it is rapidly catabolized.[402] Abnormalities in platelet secretion and arachidonic acid metabolism have been identified, but are quite variable.[403] Reduced plasma and platelet VWF activity in association with a decrease in plasma high-molecular-weight multimers has been reported in HPS,[404,405] and may reflect abnormalities involving the endothelial Weibel-Palade bodies.

The decrease or absence of platelet dense bodies can be confirmed by electron microscopy, using either whole mounts or thin sections of platelets fixed in the presence of calcium, although it requires expertise to interpret the results.[5,406] Some patients have abnormal granules. Uranaffin and osmium may help to identify dense granules. The fluorescent amine mepacrine can be used to quantify dense bodies by fluorescent microscopy or by flow cytometry.[407,408] Immunoblot analysis of skin fibroblasts in HPS may facilitate identification of the protein responsible for the defect.[409]

Therapy, Course, and Prognosis

The general principles of patient management are similar to those described for all patients with platelet function defects. Patients with HPS suffer from a number of specific problems related to their albinism, colitis, and pulmonary fibrosis.[373] In particular, they should avoid sun exposure. An antifibrotic agent, pirfenidone, demonstrated modest benefit in the initial study.[410] A second study[411] failed to confirm this and was terminated because of futility.

GRAY PLATELET SYNDROME (α-STORAGE POOL DEFICIENCY)

Definition and History

The GPS is a markedly heterogeneous bleeding disorder characterized by selective deficiency of platelet α-granules and their contents, in combination with thrombocytopenia and large platelet size.[412,413] The name derives from the initial observation by Raccuglia, in 1971,[414] of the gray appearance of platelets with paucity of granules on peripheral blood films from a patient with a life-long bleeding disorder.

Etiology and Pathogenesis

Normal platelets contain approximately 50 spherical or elongated α granules that contain a large number of proteins, some relatively specific for platelets (platelet factor 4 [PF4], β-thromboglobulin [βTG]), others that are also found in plasma, and yet others whose role in platelets is poorly understood.[412,415,416] Plasma proteins present in α granules include fibrinogen, VWF, albumin, coagulation factor V, immunoglobulin (Ig) G, fibronectin, and several protease inhibitors. Some of these proteins, such as VWF are synthesized by megakaryocytes, whereas others, such as albumin and IgG, are incorporated into platelets by endocytosis. The α-granule membrane contains several proteins present in the platelet plasma membrane (integrin $\alpha_{IIb}\beta_3$, GPIb-IX-V) and some specific for α granules (P-selectin and osteonectin).

The molecular mechanisms leading to α-granule deficiency in GPS and the combined αδ-SPD are also heterogeneous; thus, they have been attributed to failure of α-granule maturation during MK differentiation, transport or targeting of proteins to α granules, and/or synthesis of granule membranes.[412,415] Proteomic studies in a GPS patient suggested a failure to incorporate endogenously synthesized MK proteins into α granules.[415] Some GPS patients have elevated plasma PF4[412] suggesting that PF4 synthesis was normal and the primary defect was impaired granule biogenesis with leakage of PF4. Some patients with decreased α-granule contents have a mutation in the gene for the transcription factor RUNX1[372,390] and PF4 is a transcriptional target of RUNX1.[417] This suggests that decreased platelet PF4 levels in these patients represents a defect in transcriptional regulation and synthesis of PF4. GPS has been reported in association with a X-linked thrombocytopenia, thalassemia, and an R216N mutation in GATA-1, a major regulator of megakaryopoiesis.[418] Autosomal dominant GPS resulting from mutations in transcription factor gene *GFI1B* has been reported in two kindreds.[419,420]

Three groups[10–12] have reported mutations in *NBEAL2* in patients with GPS, a gene that encodes for a protein linked to vesicle transport in neuronal cells. These studies implicate defective vesicle transport as a major mechanism in many forms of GPS. Studies in *Nbeal2*-deficient mice provide evidence[421,422] that Nbeal2 is required for α-granule biogenesis, platelet function, and MK survival, development and platelet production—key evidence linking GPS and Nbeal2. These mice were also found to have abnormalities in arterial thrombosis, inflammation, and wound repair. A mutation in the gene encoding the VPS33B protein (a member of the Sec1/Munc18 protein family) involved in vesicle trafficking has also been associated with human α-granule deficiency in the arthrogryposis multiplex congenital, renal dysfunction, and cholestasis (ARC) syndrome.[423] A mutation in *VPS16B* gene has also been linked to α-granule deficiency in the ARC syndrome, and it appears that VPS16B and VPS33B interact with each other.[424] Thus, multiple mechanisms can lead to GPS. The inheritance of α-granule deficiency has been autosomal recessive in most reports, but autosomal dominant and sex-linked cases have also been described.[372,390,412,418]

Clinical Features

GPS patients have a lifelong mild to moderate bleeding diathesis, which is variable in its manifestations.[412]

Laboratory Features

Platelets appear as larger-than-normal, pale, ghost-like, oval forms on blood films and often difficult to identify (Fig. 120–6). Thrombocytopenia is variable but can be moderately severe, with counts below 50,000/μL. Platelet aggregation abnormalities vary considerably.[343,412,413,425–427] ADP- and epinephrine-induced aggregation is normal or nearly normal. Collagen- and thrombin-induced aggregation tend to be more abnormal, but this is not a consistent finding. Concomitant GPVI deficiency was reported in one patient and if the association is more widespread, it may explain the variable abnormalities in collagen-induced aggregation.[343] Studies in one patient showed flow-dependent thrombus formation to be decreased.[8] Additional abnormalities in PI metabolism, protein phosphorylation, calcium mobilization, platelet factor Va, and platelet secretion have been described[428–430] and may contribute to the platelet aggregation abnormalities and clinical symptoms. The failure of exogenous α-granule proteins to fully correct the aggregation defects suggests that these abnormalities may be important in the overall platelet dysfunction in GPS.[425]

Under the electron microscope platelets and megakaryocytes from GPS patients reveal absent or markedly decreased α granules (Fig. 120-6).[412] The platelets are deficient in α-granule proteins: PF4,

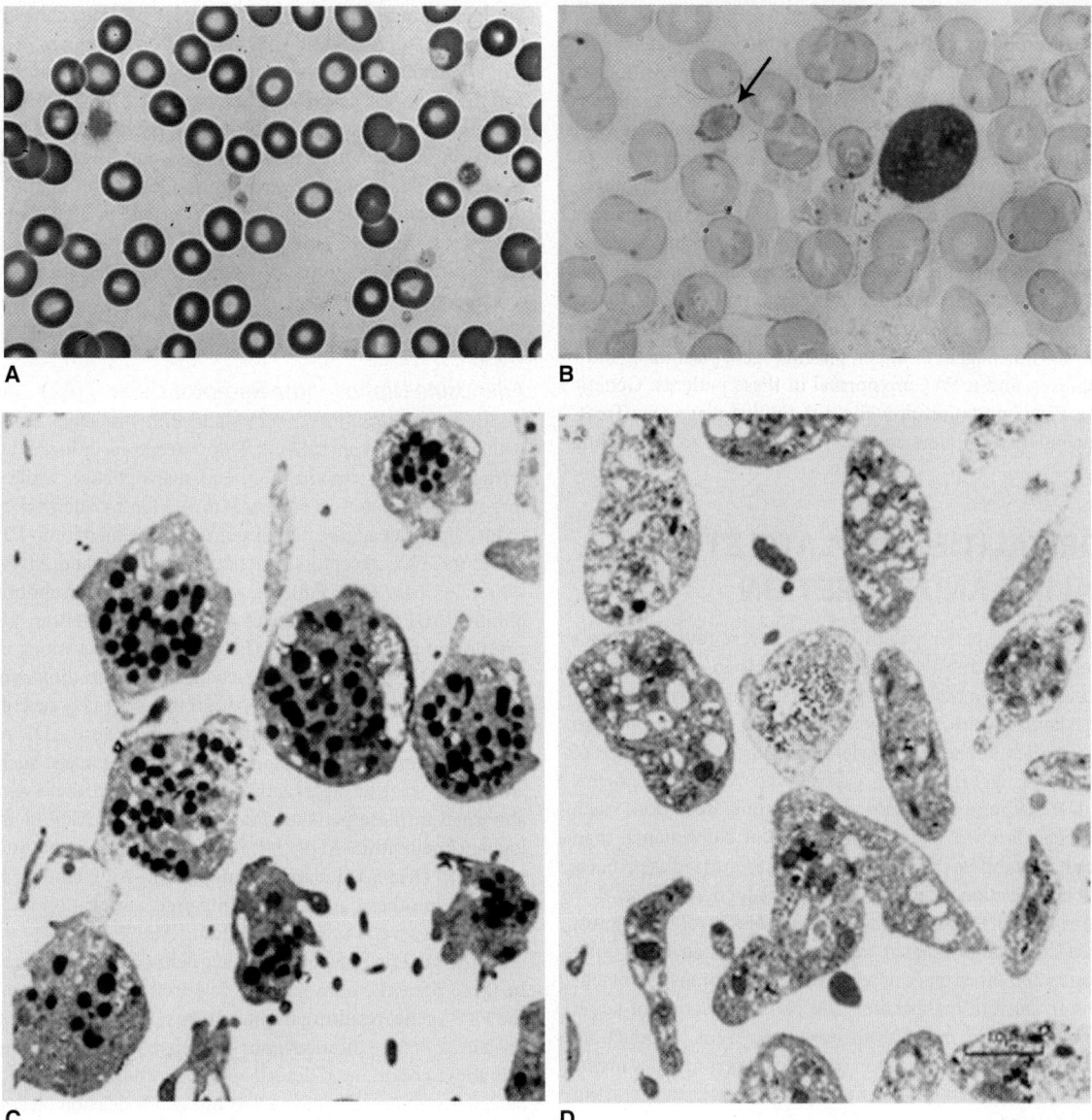

Figure 120–6. Gray platelet syndrome (α-granule deficiency). **A.** Blood film. Note gray-staining of many, but not all, platelets with loss of internal granular structure. Two are megathrombocytes, one platelet being very large, almost the size of a red cell (giant platelet). **B.** Blood film. Treated with periodic acid–Schiff (PAS) stain for carbohydrate. Note large "gray platelet" stained with PAS *(arrow)* and typical PAS staining of neutrophil cytoplasm. **C.** Transmission electron microscopy of normal human platelets with abundant electron-dense α granules. **D.** Transmission electron microscopy of platelets from a patient with gray platelet syndrome. Note profound reduction in electron-dense α granules. *(Reproduced with permission from Lichtman's Atlas of Hematology, www.accessmedicine.com.)*

βTG, VWF, thrombospondin, fibronectin, factor V, high-molecular-weight kininogen, transforming growth factor (TGF)-β_1, and platelet-derived growth factor (PDGF); albumin and IgG may also be decreased. There is increased reticulin in the marrow of some patients with GPS,[431–433] which may be associated with splenomegaly and evidence of extramedullary hematopoiesis.[431,434] The marrow fibrosis has been attributed to elevated marrow levels of PDGF and TGF-β_1 leaked from megakaryocytes.[412] Megakaryocytes show emperipolesis and the capture of neutrophils. P-selectin is a protein present in the α-granule membranes and translocates to platelet surface on platelet activation. The content and surface expression of P-selectin has been reported as normal[412,435] or decreased,[436] which underscores the heterogeneity of the GPS.

α,δ-STORAGE POOL DEFICIENCY

This disorder is characterized by moderate to severe defects in both α and δ granules, with heterogeneous expression in the few patients in whom it has been reported.[372] Clinical and laboratory features are similar to those of δ-SPD. In general, the functional consequences of the defect in dense granules is more severe than the defect in α granules.

QUEBEC PLATELET DISORDER

Quebec platelet disorder (QPD) is an autosomal dominant bleeding disorder associated with reduced platelet counts and decreased α-granule proteins as a result of increased plasmin-mediated degradation of the α-granule proteins.[437,438] Originally described as factor V Quebec, the early description of this disorder included severe bleeding after trauma, mild thrombocytopenia, decreased functional platelet factor V, and normal plasma factor V.[437,439] The bleeding time is normal to mildly prolonged and epinephrine-induced platelet aggregation is selectively decreased. Aggregation response to other agonists is variable. Platelets from patients with QPD display reduced levels of several α-granule proteins (factor V, fibrinogen, VWF, fibronectin, thrombospondin, multimerin, and osteonectin) as a consequence of enhanced proteolysis.[437,440] The excessive plasmin generation inducing the degradation of α-granule proteins results from increased megakaryocyte expression of u-PA because of a tandem duplication mutation of the *cis* regulatory elements of the u-PA gene *(PLAU)*.[441,442] Plasma tests of systemic fibrinolysis (fibrinogen, D-dimer, plasminogen, plasmin-α_2 antiplasmin complexes, and u-PA), are normal in these patients. Genetic testing for the *PLAU* mutation provides a definitive diagnosis. Treatment with fibrinolytic inhibitors appears to be effective in controlling bleeding.[437]

● ABNORMALITIES OF PLATELET SIGNALING AND SECRETION

A sizable percentage of patients with variably severe mucocutaneous bleeding manifestations, mostly mild, have defects in platelet aggregation and secretion. In most of these patients the underlying platelet molecular mechanisms are unknown. The most common pattern on laboratory studies is blunted platelet aggregation and absence of the second wave of aggregation on exposure to ADP, epinephrine, collagen, or U46619, and decreased dense granule secretion. Such patients have been lumped together, more out of convenience than because of an understanding of the mechanisms, categorized as primary secretion defects, activation defects, or signal transduction defects.[443-446] Simplistically, platelet activation is a complex process involving agonist binding to surface receptors; signal transduction through G-protein–coupled receptors and other types of receptors; phosphoinositol metabolism resulting in calcium mobilization and phosphorylation of target proteins; arachidonic acid metabolism leading to TXA$_2$ production; activation of the integrin $\alpha_{IIb}\beta_3$ receptor; and release of granule contents (Chap. 112). Defects involving these and other processes can result in impaired platelet function.

DEFECTS IN PLATELET AGONIST RECEPTORS OR AGONIST-SPECIFIC SIGNAL TRANSDUCTION

Thromboxane A$_2$ Receptor Defect

Platelets contain two different isoforms of the TXA$_2$ receptor. Both forms activate PLC, but they differ in their effects on adenylyl cyclase, with one stimulating and the other inhibiting this enzyme.[447] A mutation in the first cytoplasmic loop of the TXA$_2$ receptor (R601L) has been described as causing an inherited bleeding disorder in several families from Japan.[448,449] The platelets of these patients do not aggregate in response to TXA$_2$ mimetics. The aggregation defect also extends to other agonists, such as ADP, in which TXA$_2$ made by activated platelets and released into the surrounding medium, augments the response. The defect appears to be in signal initiation rather than ligand binding. TXA$_2$-induced activation of PLC (measured as Ca^{2+} mobilization, inositol trisphosphate, and phosphatidic acid formation) is impaired while PLA$_2$ activation and TXA$_2$ production is normal. Of note, the mutation appears to inhibit PLC activation by both receptor isoforms and impairs adenylyl cyclase stimulation by one of the isoforms; it does not, however, affect the inhibition of adenylyl cyclase produced by the

other isoform. Both dominant and recessive inheritance patterns have been reported. The abnormal aggregation responses in heterozygous family members suggests a dominant negative effect of the mutation.[449] Another report[450] describes a heterozygous D304N substitution in the seventh transmembrane region of the TXA$_2$ receptor associated with a bleeding history, a 50 percent reduction in ligand binding and loss of receptor function. A heterozygous TXA$_2$R mutation (V2416) in the third intracellular loop has been reported[7] in a subject without any bleeding symptoms. This subject had impaired aggregation and Ca^{2+} mobilization in response to U46619, normal platelet receptor levels and had aspirin resistance in microfluidic experiments assessing platelet deposition under flow.

Adenosine Diphosphate Receptor Defects (P2Y$_{12}$ and P2X$_1$)

Multiple receptors (P2Y$_{12}$, P2Y$_1$, and P2X$_1$) mediate ADP interactions with platelets (Chap. 112).[451] P2Y$_1$ receptors induce PLC activation, intracellular Ca^{2+} mobilization, and shape change, while P2Y$_{12}$ receptors mediate inhibition of cAMP formation by adenylyl cyclase. ADP-induced platelet aggregation requires activation of both P2Y$_1$ and P2Y$_{12}$ receptors. P2X$_1$ receptors function as an ATP- and ADP-gated cation channel (Chap. 112). Patients with P2Y$_{12}$ receptor abnormalities have blunted ADP-induced platelet aggregation responses, impaired suppression of prostaglandin E$_1$ (PGE$_1$)-induced elevations in cAMP, and normal ADP-stimulated shape change.[452-456] Bleeding symptoms have been variable, with some demonstrating moderately severe hemorrhage in association with surgery and trauma. Because ADP released from platelets potentiates the responses to other agonists, such as collagen and TXA$_2$, platelet aggregation in response to these agonists is also abnormal in these patients. Platelet binding of ADP or the ADP analogue 2-methylthio-ADP[452-454,456] was decreased in all but one patient studied.[457] Decreased platelet 2-methylthio-ADP binding has also been reported in other patients with impaired aggregation and secretion in response to several agonists, including ADP.[459]

The genetic defects have been defined in some of these patients. In three patients, homozygous deletions have been demonstrated in the P2Y$_{12}$ gene, resulting in premature termination and a lack of P2Y$_{12}$ protein.[445,452,456] A homozygous missense mutation in the translation initiation codon was described in another patient,[454] and another patient was reported to have a two-nucleotide deletion (at amino acid 240) in one P2Y$_{12}$ gene allele, resulting in a frameshift and a premature stop codon.[453,460] Although this last patient had one P2Y$_{12}$ allele with a normal coding region, the patient's platelets lacked P2Y$_{12}$ receptors, suggesting repression of the normal allele or an unrelated abnormality in its transcriptional regulation. In contrast, platelets from the patient's daughter had an intermediate number of ADP-binding sites, a normal platelet response to ADP, and one frame-shifted allele and one normal allele, suggesting that the mutant allele does not act in a dominant negative manner.[453] Studies in yet another patient with abnormal ADP-induced aggregation revealed a compound heterozygous state with one allele containing an R256N substitution in the sixth transmembrane domain, and the other allele containing an R265W substitution in the third extracellular loop of the receptor.[457] Platelet binding of ^{33}P-2MeS ADP was normal; neither mutation affected the translocation of the P2Y$_{12}$ receptor to the cell surface, but ADP-induced inhibition of adenylyl cyclase was partially reduced, indicating a functionally abnormal receptor. A heterozygous mutation (K174E) in the second extracellular loop of P2Y$_{12}$ was identified in one patient[455]; this was associated with decreased 2-methylthio-ADP binding. Another heterozygous mutation, P258T in the third extracellular loop has been described in association with a bleeding diathesis.[461] Interestingly, a heterozygous mutation in P2Y$_{12}$ (P341A) has been shown to induce altered interaction with Rab guanosine triphosphatases (GTPases) and endosomal trafficking of the receptor leading to its decreased surface expression.[462]

A defect in the P2X$_1$ purinergic receptor has been described in a 6-year-old patient with bleeding manifestations.[463] The patient had isolated impairment of ADP-induced platelet aggregation and was heterozygous for a deletion of a single leucine in a stretch of four leucine residues[351-354] in the second transmembrane domain of P2X$_1$. The mutant protein apparently caused a dominant negative effect on P2X$_1$-mediated calcium channel activity.

Epinephrine Receptor Defects
Abnormalities of α-adrenergic receptors or α-adrenergic–specific signal transduction have been described in several patients,[464-466] but the relationship to bleeding manifestations remains unclear, particularly because responses to epinephrine are blunted even in some otherwise normal individuals. Responses to epinephrine are blunted in the QPD.[437]

Platelet-Activating Factor Receptor Defect
A defect in the platelet-activating factor receptor or platelet-activating factor-specific signal transduction has been reported.[467]

GUANOSINE TRIPHOSPHATE-BINDING PROTEIN DEFECTS
GTP-binding proteins are a heterotrimeric class of proteins (consisting of α, β, and γ subunits) that link surface receptors and intracellular enzymes (Chap. 112). Abnormalities involving Gαq, Gαi$_1$, and Gαs proteins have been described.

Gaq Deficiency
Gαq plays a major role in mediating platelet responses to activation of G-protein–coupled receptors. One patient has been described with a selective platelet Gαq deficiency in association with a mild bleeding disorder, abnormal platelet aggregation and secretion in response to a number of agonists, and diminished GTPase activity (a reflection of Gα-subunit dysfunction) in response to platelet activation.[468,469] The downstream events from Gαq, including Ca^{2+} mobilization, release of arachidonic acid from phospholipids, and activation of integrin $\alpha_{IIb}\beta_3$ receptors, were impaired. The Gαq coding sequence in this patient was normal, but Gαq mRNA levels were decreased in platelets, suggesting a potential defect in transcriptional regulation of the gene. This abnormality appeared to be selective for platelets as the patient's neutrophils had normal Gαq protein.[470]

Gas Hyperfunction and Genetic Variation in Extra Large Gas
Two unrelated families have been described with inducible hyperactivity of Gαs.[471] These patients had a bleeding diathesis, prolonged bleeding times, variable mental retardation, and mild skeletal malformations. Platelet aggregation responses to physiologic agonists were normal, but the platelets showed increased sensitivity to inhibition by agents (PGE$_1$, prostacyclin [PGI$_2$]) that elevate cAMP. Platelet Gαs, which when activated increases platelet cAMP levels and inhibits platelet aggregation and secretion, was increased in these patients. The Gαs gene (GNAS1) has multiple alternative promoters and isoforms as a result of alternative splicing, including extralarge Gαs (XLαs). XLαs is imprinted and thus normally only expressed from the paternal allele. A heterozygous 36-bp insertion and a 2-bp substitution were identified in exon 1 of the paternal XLαs gene in these patients. Because XLαs is not activated by the usual platelet Gαs-coupled receptors, the mechanisms leading to increased cAMP levels and enhanced expression of Gαs protein is unclear. Of note, 2.2 percent of control subjects also had

the same polymorphism, but only those individuals inheriting it from their father had inducible Gαs hyperfunction and increased platelet Gαs protein.

Platelet Gαs deficiency has also been described in a patient with pseudohypoparathyroidism Ib in association with disturbed imprinting and altered methylation in the GNAS1 gene cluster that encompasses the four GNAS1 splice variants, including the Gαs subunit.[472] The Gαs coding sequence was normal. As expected from the deficiency in Gαs protein, there was decreased platelet cAMP formation upon activation of receptors linked to Gαs. The authors did not indicate whether the patient had a bleeding diathesis.

Gai1 Deficiency
Platelet Gαi1 deficiency has been reported in association with a bleeding disorder and abnormalities in integrin $\alpha_{IIb}\beta_3$ activation, platelet aggregation, and dense granule secretion upon activation with one or more agonists.[473] In keeping with the known function of Gαi in inhibiting the activation of adenylyl cyclase and the subsequent increases in cAMP levels, the patient's platelets failed to inhibit forskolin-stimulated cAMP levels on activation. Platelet Gαi1 protein was decreased by 75 percent, whereas other members of the Gαi family (Gαi2, Gαi3, Gαiz) and Gαq were normal. Although a large subset of patients has been considered as having a defect in Gi signaling,[474] this is based on abnormal responses on platelet aggregation and secretion studies to ADP and epinephrine, and direct evidence at the molecular level to support this conclusion has not been provided.

CalDAG-GEFI Deficiency
Three siblings from first cousin parents and severe mucocutaneous bleeding manifestations, had prolonged bleeding times and reduced platelet aggregation in response to ADP or epinephrine, and to low doses, but not high doses, of a thrombin receptor–activating peptide and collagen.[475] Clot retraction was normal. Whole-exome analysis revealed a homozygous G248W mutation in RAS guanyl-releasing protein-2 (RASGRP2), the gene for the protein calcium- and diacylglycerol (DAG)-regulated guanine exchange factor-1 (CalDAG-GEFI), affecting the CDC25 catalytic domain critical for interacting with GTPases. The platelets demonstrated decreased Rap1 activation and fibrinogen binding and abnormal adhesion and spreading on immobilized fibrinogen and collagen. These results support a model of platelet activation in which CalDAG-GEFI stimulates GTP loading of Rap1 and Rac1 in response to an increase in intracellular Ca^{2+} and the activated Rap1 leads to integrin $\alpha_{IIb}\beta_3$ activation and the activated Rac1 enhances platelet spreading. The heterozygotes were asymptomatic but their platelets had a defective spreading.[475]

PHOSPHOLIPASE C–β_2 DEFICIENCY AND DEFECTS IN PHOSPHOLIPASE C ACTIVATION
Several investigators have described patients with relatively mild bleeding diatheses and impaired platelet aggregation and dense granule secretion, despite normal granule stores and the ability to synthesize TXA$_2$.[445,446,476-478] An early event after stimulating several platelet G-protein–coupled receptors is activation of PLC-β, leading to formation of the intracellular mediators IP$_3$ and DAG (Chap. 112); the former mediates Ca^{2+} mobilization and the latter for PKC-induced protein phosphorylation. Defects in one or more of these responses has been documented in several patients. In one study of eight patients with abnormal platelet aggregation and secretion in response to several different receptor-mediated agonists, Ca^{2+} mobilization and/or pleckstrin phosphorylation was abnormal in seven patients, suggesting that the impaired secretion and aggregation resulted from upstream abnormalities in early signaling events.[478] Specific defects

at the level of PLC-β_2,[479,480] Gαq,[468] and PKC-θ[481] were identified in these eight patients. In another study, eight patients were described who had decreased initial rates and extents of platelet aggregation in response to ADP, epinephrine, and the TXA$_2$ mimetic U44069[476]; subsequent studies in one patient demonstrated impaired phosphatidylinositol hydrolysis, phosphatidic acid formation, and pleckstrin phosphorylation.[482,483]

In two related patients described with PLC-β_2 deficiency, platelet aggregation and secretion were impaired in association with impaired IP$_3$ and DAG formation, calcium mobilization, and pleckstrin phosphorylation following activation with ADP, collagen, platelet-activating factor, or thrombin, indicating a defect in PLC activation.[479] These patients had a mild bleeding disorder. Human platelets contain at least seven PLC isozymes and a selective decrease was observed in only the PLC-β_2 isozyme.[480] The decreased platelet PLC-β_2 protein levels were associated with a normal gene coding sequence but with diminished PLC-β_2 mRNA levels in platelets, but not neutrophils, suggesting a hematopoietic lineage-specific defect in PLC-β_2 gene regulation.[484] Defects in phosphatidylinositol metabolism and protein phosphorylation have been described in other such patients, although the primary protein abnormalities were not defined.[482,483,485–488]

DEFECTS IN PROTEIN PHOSPHORYLATION: PROTEIN KINASE C-Θ DEFICIENCY

PKC isozymes, a family of serine- and threonine-specific protein kinases, phosphorylate a wide array of proteins involved in signal transduction. PKC enzymes regulate several aspects of platelet function, including activation of integrin $\alpha_{IIb}\beta_3$ receptors, platelet aggregation and secretion, and platelet production (Chap. 112). Deficiency of a human platelet PKC isozyme (PKC-θ) has been described in a patient with lifelong mucocutaneous bleeding manifestations, mild thrombocytopenia, and markedly abnormal platelet aggregation (including primary wave) and dense granule secretion in response to multiple agonists.[481,489] Agonist-induced phosphorylation of pleckstrin and myosin light chain were diminished in the patient's platelets. This subject was subsequently shown to have a heterozygous mutation in a transcription factor, RUNX1 (also termed core-binding factor A2, CBFA2, or *AML1*), which has been linked to a familial platelet function defect, associated with thrombocytopenia and predisposition to acute leukemia[481,490] (see "Transcription Factor Mutations and Associated Platelet Dysfunction" below). Platelet expression of myosin light chain (*MYL9*) was also decreased in this patient.[491]

DEFECTS IN ARACHIDONIC ACID METABOLISM AND THROMBOXANE PRODUCTION

Defects in Arachidonic Acid Release from Phospholipids

Release of free arachidonic acid from phospholipids, mediated by cytosolic PLA$_2$, is the initial and rate-limiting step in thromboxane synthesis upon platelet activation. Several patients have been described with abnormalities in the release of arachidonic acid.[469,485,492–494] In general, their platelets aggregated normally in response to arachidonic acid but not to ADP, epinephrine, and/or collagen. In one of these patients this defect was related to an upstream abnormality in Gαq (see "Gαq Deficiency" above).[468] Another patient had the HPS with δ-SPD and abnormal PLA$_2$ activity.[492] An inherited deficiency in cytosolic PLA$_2$ has been reported in a patient with recurrent small intestinal ulceration, markedly decreased eicosanoid synthesis (including in thromboxane, 12-hydroxyeicosatetraenoic acid [12-HETE], and leukotriene B$_4$) and impaired aggregation with ADP and collagen but normal with arachidonic acid.[493] This patient had two heterozygous single-base-pair

mutations in the PLA$_2$ coding region, leading to S111P and R485H substitutions. Another report documents twins with a history of gastrointestinal ulcers, associated with similarly impaired platelet function associated with a homozygous D575H mutation in PLA$_2$ (*PLA2G4A*).[494] These patients had mildly decreased plasma factor XI as well.

Cyclooxygenase (Prostaglandin H$_2$ Synthase-1) Deficiency

Deficient platelet cyclooxygenase (prostaglandin H$_2$ synthase-1) activity leading to impaired platelet function and a mild bleeding disorder has been identified in a number of patients.[495–502] Platelets from such patients cannot make thromboxane from arachidonic acid but can make it from cyclic endoperoxides (prostaglandin G$_2$ and prostaglandin H$_2$). While some patients have had decreased platelet cyclooxygenase protein, others have had evidence of a dysfunctional molecule.[501,502]

Thromboxane Synthase Deficiency

Presumed platelet thromboxane synthase deficiencies have been identified in two families based on the failure of cyclic endoperoxides to be converted into TXA$_2$.[503,504]

⬤ ABNORMALITIES OF PLATELET COAGULANT ACTIVITY (SCOTT SYNDROME)

DEFINITION AND HISTORY

Activated platelets play an essential role in providing the membrane surface on which specific blood coagulation reactions occur leading to thrombin generation.[505,506] Patients whose platelets fail to facilitate thrombin generation are defined as having defects in platelet coagulant activity (PCA) (Chap. 112). Only a few patients have been described with isolated defects in PCA and normal aggregation and secretion responses.[505,507–513] Defects in PCA may also be secondary to abnormalities in platelet aggregation, such as in patients with SPD and thrombasthenia.[505] Patients with isolated abnormalities in PCA are referred to as having the Scott syndrome after the first patient described in 1979 by Weiss and colleagues[505,507–510]

ETIOLOGY AND PATHOGENESIS

The main functional abnormality in the Scott syndrome is the impaired ability of activated platelets to promote coagulation reactions; a second abnormality in these patients is a defect in release of microvesicles on cell activation.[514,515] In resting platelets, membrane phospholipids are asymmetrically distributed, with the aminophospholipids phosphatidylserine (PS) and phosphatidylethanolamine (PE) concentrated in the inner membrane leaflet, and phosphatidylcholine (PC) and sphingomyelin concentrated in the outer leaflet. Cell activation induces phospholipid translocation, with PS moving to the outer leaflet. This process is regulated by several proteins that are descriptively identified by their functions. They include a "flippase" (i.e., an aminophospholipid translocase identified as a P4 adenosine triphosphatase [ATPase]), which promotes inward transport of lipids; a "floppase" that regulates outward phospholipid transport (encoded by gene *ABCC1*); and one or more "scramblase" that promotes bidirectional movement of lipids between the two layers.[506] Surface expression of PS is essential for platelets to accelerate coagulation reactions, in particular, activation of the tenase complex leading to the activation of factor X to Xa and of the prothrombinase complex that converts prothrombin to thrombin (Chaps. 113 and 114). Scott syndrome platelets have a defect in PS translocation resulting in decreased binding of factors Va-Xa and VIIIa-IXa,[505,506] thus leading to impaired blood coagulation. Erythrocytes and lymphocytes also demonstrate similar defects in both microvesicle formation and coagulant activity.[505,512] In a French family with Scott syndrome,[508] the propositus' platelets were found to have a defect in protein tyrosine phosphorylation, suggesting an additional defect in signal transduction.[510]

Apart from the above patients with the Scott syndrome, four patients from three unrelated families have been reported to have abnormal PCA, a bleeding disorder, impaired serum prothrombin consumption, and reduced microparticle formation.[516] However, in contrast to the Scott syndrome, the prothrombinase activity was normal.

The inheritance pattern in the Scott syndrome appears to be autosomal recessive.[505,508] A heterozygous missense mutation has been reported in one patient in the gene *ABCA1*, which encodes the ATP-binding cassette transporter protein implicated in PS translocation; the significance of this remains unclear.[517] Mutations in TMEM16F have been identified in two patients with Scott syndrome. The patient Scott was found to have a homozygous mutation at the splice acceptor site for intron 12 of *TMEM16F*, resulting in a frameshift and premature termination of protein translation.[518] A second patient had compound heterozygosity for a mutation at the donor splice site of intron 6 and a single nucleotide insertion in exon 12, causing a frameshift and premature termination of translation.[13] While these findings constitute strong evidence linking *TMEM16F* mutations to Scott syndrome, they leave open whether TMEM16F is itself the membrane scramblase or a protein that regulates the scramblase.

CLINICAL AND LABORATORY FEATURES

The bleeding symptoms in patients with the Scott syndrome are similar to those with other platelet defects. In contrast to other qualitative platelet abnormalities, the bleeding time in Scott syndrome patients is normal.[508,509,514] The serum PT, which reflects the completeness of clotting of whole blood and consumption of prothrombin, is abnormally, indicating incomplete coagulation.[507-509] More specific assays of "platelet factor 3," the phenomenologic designation of the platelet contribution to accelerating clot formation, are also abnormal.[519]

Patients with the Scott syndrome have normal platelet aggregation and secretion in response to the usually used agonists.[505] The patient Scott[505] also had normal platelet phospholipid content, normal to enhanced platelet adhesion to subendothelium with diminished thrombus formation, diminished factor Va binding to platelets and platelet microparticles, and diminished platelet acceleration of both factor X activation and prothrombin activation. Abnormalities in exposure of negatively charged phospholipids and shedding of microparticles have been consistent findings in all patients described.[506,508-512]

TREATMENT

Platelet or whole blood transfusions have been effective as prophylaxis and as therapy for bleeding episodes.[505,507-509] Prothrombin complex concentrates were effective in the patient Scott,[392] but these preparations may be associated with thrombotic complications.

● ABNORMALITIES OF A CYTOSKELETAL STRUCTURAL PROTEIN: β_1-TUBULIN AND FILAMIN A

Megakaryocytes and platelets express primarily and selectively the β_1 isoform of tubulin. A heterozygous β_1-tubulin Q43P polymorphism was identified in a group of patients with a recessive form of

macrothrombocytopenia; the polymorphism could not account fully for the macrothrombocytopenia because of the difference in inheritance and its presence in approximately 11 percent of the normal population.[520] Individuals heterozygous for the polymorphism had normal platelet counts, relatively high mean platelet volume values, abnormally rounded platelets with abnormal marginal bands of microtubules, and mild abnormalities of platelet aggregation, secretion, and adhesion to collagen. One study found the polymorphism was associated with decreased collagen-induced platelet aggregation and increased risk of intracerebral hemorrhage in men.[521]

Subsequently, two patients with macrothrombocytopenia from a single kindred were reported to be heterozygous for a R318W β_1 tubulin mutation.[522] The mutation is strategically located at the α–β tubulin interface. Of note, the Q43P polymorphism and an R207H substitution were also found in this family, but neither was judged to be responsible for the macrothrombocytopenia.

Filamins are large dimeric actin-binding proteins that stabilize actin filament networks. Filamin A is the predominant platelet filamin. Several patients have been reported with dominant mutations of X-linked *Filamin A (FLNA)* gene associated with thrombocytopenia, and abnormalities in platelet aggregation, secretion, GPVI signaling and thrombus growth on collagen.[522A]

● ABNORMALITIES OF CYTOSKELETAL LINKING PROTEINS

WISKOTT-ALDRICH SYNDROME PROTEIN

The Wiskott-Aldrich syndrome (WAS) is an X-chromosome–linked inherited disorder characterized by small platelets, thrombocytopenia, recurrent infections, eczema, and an increased incidence of autoimmunity and malignancies.[523,524] In addition, a variety of immunologic abnormalities affecting T-lymphocyte function, Ig levels, cellular immunity, and responsiveness to polysaccharide antigens are commonly present. Death from infection, hemorrhage, or malignancy is common before adulthood. Some patients with WAS mutations may have only thrombocytopenia (X-linked thrombocytopenia [XLT]) without other features. WAS is caused by mutations in the WAS gene which encodes the WAS protein (WASP), a multidomain protein that relays signals from the cell surface to the actin skeleton and modulates the latter's reorganization. In platelets, WASP is localized to the cytoskeleton.[524,525] It is phosphorylated on platelet activation by several different protein kinases, including Btk, Grb2, PLC-γ_2, PKC-θ, and SGK1.[524]

Microthrombocytopenia is a consistent feature of WAS and XLT and the major contributor to the bleeding diathesis, which may be life-threatening in some patients because of gastrointestinal hemorrhage or intracranial hemorrhage. Marrow megakaryocytes are normal in number, but platelet formation is abnormal and platelet survival is decreased.[523,524]

Abnormalities in platelet surface glycoprotein sialophorin (CD43, gp115, leukosialin), GPIb, platelet integrin α_2, integrin $\alpha_{IIb}\beta_3$, and GPIV have been reported in some WAS patients.[526,527] Platelets from patients with WAS also have qualitative defects, including SPD[367,368,528] and impaired energy metabolism.[528,529]

Platelet aggregation in WAS has been reported to be reduced, normal, or enhanced.[524,530-533] Interpreting these studies is confounded by the low platelet count, methodological differences, and timing in relation to splenectomy.[524] Despite the role of WASP in cytoskeletal reorganization, shape change and actin polymerization are normal in WAS platelets.[531,534,535]

WASP has been implicated in regulating responses dependent on integrin $\alpha_{IIb}\beta_3$ outside-in signaling.[536] Although Pac-1 binding is normal in WAS platelets, there is decreased spreading on fibrinogen and decreased clot retraction associated with enhanced PS exposure.[536]

Splenectomy usually improves the thrombocytopenia.[523,524] Hematopoietic stem cell transplantation is the accepted curative approach for WAS and can correct all aspects of the disease provided reconstitution is achieved.[523,524] Autologous gene-modified hematopoietic stem cell transplantation is an emerging therapy for WAS patients.[523,524]

● KINDLIN-3 (LEUKOCYTE ADHESION DEFECT-3; LEUKOCYTE ADHESION DEFECT—1 VARIANT; INTEGRIN ACTIVATION DEFICIENCY DISEASE)

DEFINITION AND HISTORY/ETIOLOGY AND PATHOGENESIS

A syndrome with the features of both mild LAD-1 and GT was first described in 1997[537] and termed LAD-1 variant or LAD-3. Since then more than 10 families have been reported, with several from Turkey.[538–541] The etiology is a deficiency or defect in the cytoskeletal linking protein kindlin-3 *(FERMTS3)*. Kindlin-3 is a protein expressed exclusively in hematopoietic cells with homology to talin that also binds to the cytoplasmic domain of the β_3 subunit of integrin $\alpha_{IIb}\beta_3$ (Chap. 112). It has been implicated in the inside-out activation of integrin $\alpha_{IIb}\beta_3$ in mice.[542] It also participates in the activation of leukocyte integrins, which accounts for the defects in immune function. It may also affect red blood cell structure. Defects in *CALDAGGEF1*, the gene for another exchange factor, also cause abnormalities in platelet function and are discussed in the section on Guanosine Triphosphate-Binding Protein Defects.[538,543]

The disorder is characterized by a hemorrhagic diathesis in combination with a variable predisposition to infections and inflammation without pus formation, poor wound healing, delayed umbilical cord stump detachment, and variable osteopetrosis. Intracerebral hemorrhage at birth or soon thereafter has been reported in several of the patients, as well as relatively severe mucosal and gastrointestinal bleeding. Thus, the bleeding diathesis is more severe than is found in patients with GT, perhaps because of additional abnormalities in blood vessels. The need for red blood cell transfusions in infancy has been reported in several patients as a result of blood loss from mucosal surfaces and perhaps red blood cell abnormalities. Leukocytosis, as is found in other LAD syndromes is a constant finding. Normal platelet counts are the usual finding, but thrombocytopenia has been reported. Platelet aggregation studies demonstrate defects similar to those observed in GT.[541–543] Hematopoietic stem cell transplantation has been successful in restoring normal hematopoietic function in patients with life threatening hemorrhagic and infectious complications of the disease.[541]

● TRANSCRIPTION FACTOR MUTATIONS AND ASSOCIATED PLATELET DYSFUNCTION

Transcription factors, and the *cis*-regulatory sequences to which they bind, regulate lineage-specific gene expression. Transcription factors RUNX1, FLI1 (a member of the ETS [E-twenty-six] family), GATA-1, and GFI1B (growth factor independent 1B) are important regulators of hematopoietic lineage differentiation, megakaryopoiesis, and platelet production.[419,420,544] They interact in a combinatorial manner in regulating megakaryocytic genes.[544] A single transcription factor mutation may alter expression of numerous genes, affect diverse cellular mechanisms, and lead to defects in both platelet number and function. Until recently the pursuit of the molecular mechanisms in patients with platelet dysfunction has focused on delineating mutations in the genes encoding postulated candidate proteins. Therefore, the increasing spotlight on transcription factor mutations to explain platelet dysfunction is a paradigm shift.[9,545,545A]

RUNX1 (FAMILIAL PLATELET DISORDER WITH PREDISPOSITION TO ACUTE MYELOGENOUS LEUKEMIA)

An association between inherited platelet dysfunction, thrombocytopenia, and a predisposition to acute myeloid leukemia has been reported in several families in which the platelet abnormalities antedated the leukemia.[390,490,546–551] Inherited mutations in RUNX1 (AML1, CBFA2) is the basis for this constellation, which is inherited as an autosomal dominant trait, because of haploinsufficiency.[490] Patients generally display mild thrombocytopenia from birth and a bleeding disorder disproportionate to the thrombocytopenia. Approximately one-third of patients develop leukemia, with a median age of onset of 33 years.[552]

Platelet abnormalities reported in patients with *RUNX1* mutations include decreased aggregation, secretion, protein phosphorylation (myosin light chain and pleckstrin), production of 12-hydroxyeicosapentaenoic acid; decreased integrin $\alpha_{IIb}\beta_3$ activation upon platelet activation; δ and/or α-granule SPD; and a selective decrease in one PKC isoform (PKC-θ).[372,390,553–555] Of note, several patients described earlier as having SPD (δ or α granules) have been subsequently shown to harbor *RUNX1* mutations.[358,372,390,391] In one patient, platelet albumin and IgG were diminished, suggesting a defect in the uptake and packaging of these proteins into α granules.[481,489]

Most mutations of *RUNX1* have been in the conserved Runt domain,[390] although a mutation in the transactivating domain (Y260X) has been reported.[390] Platelet transcript expression profiling in a patient with *RUNX1* haploinsufficiency revealed downregulation of numerous genes involved in platelet structure and function, including *MYL9* (myosin light chain), *ALOX12* (12-lipoxygenase), *PF4*, and *PRKCQ* (PKC-θ).[491,554–556] *ALOX12*, *PRKCQ*, *PF4*, and *MYL9*[554–556] are direct transcriptional targets of RUNX1. Patients with *RUNX1* haploinsufficiency also have impaired megakaryopoiesis[490] and decreased platelet thrombopoietin receptors (Mpl).[551] Targeted correction of *RUNX1* mutation in induced pluripotent stem cells (iPSCs) developed from skin fibroblasts from two patients resulted in normalization of the defect in megakaryopoiesis.[391] These studies raise the potential for targeted gene therapy for this disorder. Using next-generation sequencing, Stockley and colleagues[9] identified mutations in *RUNX1* and *FLI1*, in six of 13 patients with excessive bleeding, and impaired aggregation and platelet dense granule secretion in response to multiple agonists. Thus, transcription factor mutations are an important mechanism for inherited platelet dysfunction.[545,545A]

GATA-1

GATA-1 is a critical regulator of both megakaryocyte and erythroid development. GATA-1 mutations have been associated with an X-linked syndrome consisting of dyserythropoiesis, anemia, thrombocytopenia, and large platelets[2]; selectively impaired responses to collagen and ristocetin related to abnormalities in GPIbβ[557,558]; diminished platelet Gαs protein and mRNA[557]; and a form of GPS (with R216N mutation).[418]

FLI-1 (DIMORPHIC DYSMORPHIC PLATELETS WITH GIANT A-GRANULES AND THROMBOCYTOPENIA (PARIS-TROUSSEAU/ JACOBSEN SYNDROME])

The Paris-Trousseau syndrome, a variant of Jacobsen syndrome, is a rare autosomal dominant disorder[559-562] characterized by mental retardation, congenital macrothrombocytopenia, giant α granules (1 to 2 μm in diameter) in a subpopulation (1 to 5 percent) of circulating platelets, and marrow dysmegakaryopoiesis in association with deletion of the distal part of either the maternally or paternally derived chromosome 11 (11q23.3–24). Among the genes deleted is the transcription factor FLI1, which is important in megakaryocyte development via its effects on expression of several genes, including *ITGA2, GPIX, GPIbα*, and *c-MPL*.[2] Although platelet survival is normal, there is dramatic expansion of marrow megakaryocytes resulting from arrested megakaryocyte development. Thrombin-induced platelet release of α-granule contents is impaired.[559] Both the inheritance pattern and the dimorphic population of normal and dysmorphic giant α granules are explained by the observation that during a period in early megakaryocyte development, only one of the two FLI1 alleles appears to be expressed in any single megakaryocyte precursor.[561,562]

GFI1B

Two studies[419,420] implicate autosomal dominant mutations in GFI1B with a bleeding disorder and multiple alterations in platelet number and function, and red cell anisopoikilocytosis. In one study,[420] the affected family members had a single nucleotide insertion in exon 7 of GFI1B leading to a frameshift mutation associated with macrothrombocytopenia, impaired platelet aggregation responses, α-granule deficiency, and decreased platelet P-selectin, fibrinogen, GPIbα, and integrin β_3. The second study identified[419] a dominant-negative truncating mutation (c.859C to T) in the zinc finger 5 region of GFI1B in a family originally reported in 1968 with macrothrombocytopenia and platelet dysfunction.[563] The family members had decreased platelet α granules, PF4, βTG, and GP1bα, and deficiency of platelet factor 3. There was myelofibrosis and emperipolesis in the marrow.

MISCELLANEOUS INHERITED DISORDERS ASSOCIATED WITH PLATELET FUNCTION DEFECTS

The TAR syndrome is characterized by a reduction in platelet counts, absence of the radius bone in the forearm, skeletal abnormalities, and decreased marrow megakaryocytes. Dense granule SPD and impaired platelet aggregation and secretion have also been reported in TAR syndrome.[371] Early studies reported that majority of these patients have a deletion on chromosome 1q21.1,[15] and later studies showed that these patients have both a rare null allele of *RBM8A* along with one of two low-frequency single nucleotide polymorphisms (SNPs) in the gene's regulatory regions.[14] *RBM8A* encodes for the Y14 subunit of the exon-junction complex (EJC), which plays an essential in RNA processing.

Platelet function abnormalities have also been reported in inherited connective tissue disorders such as osteogenesis imperfecta, the Ehlers-Danlos syndrome, and the Marfan syndrome[369,370,564,565]; bleeding manifestations are more likely caused by the underlying connective tissue defect than by the platelet dysfunction. Abnormalities in platelet responses and or granules have been reported in patients with

hexokinase deficiency,[566] glucose-6 phosphatase deficiency (glycogen storage disease, type I),[567,568] and the Down syndrome.[569-573] In glucose-6 phosphatase deficiency the platelet abnormalities were reversed following total parenteral nutrition for 10 to 12 days[567,568] indicating that the platelets may be intrinsically normal. The *MYH9*-related disorders (May-Hegglin anomaly) are characterized by giant platelets, thrombocytopenia, and basophilic granulocyte inclusions; some patients with this anomaly have platelet function and ultrastructural abnormalities.[8,574,575] Despite the large platelet size, the surface membrane glycoproteins appear to be normal.[576] Markedly impaired platelet responses to multiple agonists have been reported with partial trisomy 18p associated with three copies of the *PACAP* (pituitary adenylate cyclase-activating polypeptide) gene and elevated plasma levels of *PACAP*, which induces increased platelet cAMP levels via stimulation of Gαs.[577]

Familial hemophagocytic lymphohistiocytosis (FHLH) is a genetic disorder of lymphocyte cytotoxicity associated with mutations in the gene encoding perforin or proteins important for vesicular trafficking and exocytosis. Flow cytometric analyses of the platelets of FHLH type 5 patients, who have MUNC18–2 *(STXBP2)* mutations, revealed that thrombin-induced secretion from both α and δ granules is impaired.[578,579] Platelets from an FHLH type 4 patient with a mutation in syntaxin-11 *(STX11)* also had a defect in agonist-induced secretion associated with normal cargo levels.[580]

MANAGEMENT OF INHERITED PLATELET FUNCTION DISORDERS

Management of patients with inherited platelet function disorders needs to be individualized because of the wide variation in clinical manifestations, even in patients with the same defect. A general approach is described here; additional features specific to some individual entities are provided in their respective descriptions. Management of these patients involves preventive measures and treatment of specific bleeding episodes.[581-583] Dental hygiene is important in minimizing gingival hemorrhage. Antiplatelet agents should be avoided as they increase the bleeding manifestations. Iron and folate supplementation may be needed in patients with chronic hemorrhage. Hepatitis B vaccine should be administered early in life.

PLATELET TRANSFUSIONS AND GENERAL APPROACHES

Transfusion of platelets (Chap. 139) is a time-tested therapy for serious bleeding and as prophylaxis prior to surgery or invasive procedures. In addition to the usual risks associated with transfusions (transmission of infections, allergic reactions, Rh-immunization in Rh-negative individuals, and rarely hemolytic reactions) patients with GT and the BSS may develop specific antibodies against the missing glycoproteins, which may seriously compromise efficacy of future platelet transfusions.[581,582] This occurs particularly in patients whose platelets have no detectable integrin $\alpha_{IIb}\beta_3$.[584] Therefore, platelet transfusions should be kept to a minimum. Transfusions of both platelets and red blood cells should be given with leukocyte depletion filters to decrease the risk of alloimmunization and cytomegalovirus transmission. It is reasonable to use human leukocyte antigen (HLA)-matched and ABO-matched platelets to minimize the risk of alloimmunization and side effects.[581-583]

Treatment with 1-deamino-8-D-arginine vasopressin (DDAVP; desmopressin) may shorten the bleeding time and/or improve hemostasis in some, but not all, patients with platelet function defects.[585-588] Responses to DDAVP appear dependent on the cause of the platelet dysfunction.[585,587,588] Most patients with thrombasthenia do not respond to DDAVP with a shortening of the bleeding time[585,587–589] with exceptions,[590] but it is unknown whether DDAVP improves hemostasis in these patients despite a lack of shortening of the bleeding time. Responses to DDAVP in SPD patients have been variable with a shortening of the bleeding time in some patients[588,591] but not others.[585,587] In uncontrolled studies it has been feasible to manage selected patients with inherited platelet defects undergoing surgical procedures with DDAVP alone.[585,587] However, this approach needs to be individualized based on the nature and location of the surgery and the intensity of the patient's bleeding symptoms, and platelet need to be readily available for transfusion in the event of excess hemorrhage. The abnormal *in vitro* platelet aggregation or secretion responses in patients with platelet defects are usually not corrected by DDAVP.[587,592] It has been proposed that one mechanism by which DDAVP improves platelet function is via increased formation of procoagulant "COAT" platelets induced by combined activation by collagen and thrombin.[592]

Investigators have reported the successful use of recombinant factor VIIa (rFVIIa) in the management of bleeding events in patients with inherited platelet defects, including GT (including patients with antibodies to integrin $\alpha_{IIb}\beta_3$), the BSS and SPD.[581,583,593–596] rFVIIa is thought to increase thrombin generation through both tissue factor dependent and independent mechanisms.

The antifibrinolytic agents epsilon-aminocaproic acid (EACA) and tranexamic acid,[581–583] which may be given orally, intravenously, or topically have been successfully used in patients with coagulation disorders and platelet function abnormalities.[586,597] Antifibrinolytic agents are useful in patients with gingival bleeding, epistaxis, and menorrhagia, and those undergoing dental extractions. A tranexamic acid mouthwash (10 mL of a 5 percent solution used four times daily) has been found effective in controlling gum bleeding and bleeding after tooth extractions.[582] A short 3- to 4-day course of prednisone (20 to 50 mg)[598] has also been used.

Topical agents can also help arrest bleeding and have been used in GT patients. Gelfoam (a form of resolvable, oxidized, regenerated cellulose) soaked in either tranexamic acid or topical thrombin may be effective.[599] Fibrin sealants prepared from a source of fibrinogen and a source of thrombin (exogenous or from the patient's own plasma), with or without antifibrinolytic agents or other components[599] have been used successfully in patients with GT.[600] Some preparations of bovine thrombin induced antibody formation to itself and contaminated factor V and factor XI and have been associated with serious hemorrhage; recombinant human thrombin is now available and appears to have low immunogenicity.[601]

Allogeneic marrow transplantation has successfully in treated patients with GT, BSS,[581] LAD-3,[541] and WAS.[523,524] Progress has been made in gene therapy approaches to correcting the genetic defect in GT in megakaryocytes.[602–604] Several GT animal models are available, including the integrin subunits α_{IIb} and β_3-null mouse models,[605] and dog models involving mutations in the α_{IIb} subunit.[604,606,607] With respect to BSS, in mouse models, lentiviral transduction of hematopoietic stem cells with human GPIbα under the control of the integrin α_{IIb} promoter has been effective in improving hemostasis when transplanted into animals.[289] Thus, as methods of marrow transplantation and gene transfer therapy improve, it will be important to reassess the risk-to-benefit ratios of these therapies for individual patients with GT.

BLEEDING AT SPECIFIC SITES

Control of epistaxis can be particularly difficult in some patients.[608] When topical measures fail, platelet transfusions or factor VIIa should be considered. Nosebleeds occur primarily along the anterior nasal septum at the Kiesselbach area,[608] posterior nosebleeds can occur either

along the septum or the lateral nasal wall. Self-administered home therapy for anterior hemorrhage consists of pinching the outer aspect of the nose against the septum for 15 minutes to tamponade the septal vessels.[608] If this fails, topical application by medical personnel of an anesthetic such as lidocaine in combination with a vasoconstrictor such as phenylephrine or oxymetazoline is commonly effective. Electrical cautery sometimes is effective when chemical cauterization fails. In many cases anterior or posterior packing may be needed for persistent severe epistaxis.

Menarche may be associated with the severe bleeding manifestations and require transfusions in some patients. Antifibrinolytics have been used for menorrhagia; hormonal therapy with progesterone alone or combined progesterone-estrogen is effective in those with persistent hemorrhage.[581,583]

PREGNANCY

Management during pregnancy and delivery requires close interaction between the hematologist and the obstetrician. Most patients with severe bleeding symptoms, particularly those with GT and the BSS, will need platelet transfusions during childbirth and this need may continue for several days after delivery.[581–583] Postpartum bleeding may occur 2 to 4 weeks after delivery in some patients. rFVIIa has been used successfully in women with GT with persistent bleeding despite platelet transfusions, and those with integrin $\alpha_{IIb}\beta_3$ antibodies.[581–583,609,610] Of note, fetal thrombocytopenia and intracranial hemorrhage may occur because of transplacental passage of the antibodies.

SURGERY

Management during surgical procedures needs to be individualized and depends on the bleeding history of the patient, the nature of the surgery, and on information such as alloimmunization and refractoriness to prior transfusions. Therapeutic options include DDAVP, platelet transfusions, rFVIIa and ancillary measures, such as antifibrinolytics, which may be continued for several days postsurgery.[581–583]

REFERENCES

1. Noris P, Biino G, Pecci A, et al: Platelet diameters in inherited thrombocytopenias: Analysis of 376 patients with all known disorders. *Blood* 124:e4–e10, 2014.
2. Kumar R, Kahr WHA: Congenital thrombocytopenia: Clinical manifestations, laboratory abnormalities, and molecular defects of a heterogeneous group of conditions. *Hematol Oncol Clin N Am* 27:465–494, 2013.
3. Harrison P, Lordkipanidze M: Clinical tests of platelet function in AD, editor. *Platelets, Third Edition*, edited by AD Michelson, pp 519–545. Elsevier, San Diego, CA, 2013.
4. Cattaneo M, Hayward CP, Moffat KA, et al: Results of a worldwide survey on the assessment of platelet function by light transmission aggregometry: A report from the platelet physiology subcommittee of the SSC of the ISTH. *J Thromb Haemost* 7:1029, 2009.
5. Hayward CP, Moffat KA, Spitzer E, et al: Results of an external proficiency testing exercise on platelet dense-granule deficiency testing by whole mount electron microscopy. *Am J Clin Pathol* 131:671–675, 2009.
6. Hayward CP, Pai M, Liu Y, et al: Diagnostic utility of light transmission platelet aggregometry: Results from a prospective study of individuals referred for bleeding disorder assessments. *J Thromb Haemost* 7:676–684, 2009.
7. Flamm MH, Colace TV, Chatterjee MS, et al: Multiscale prediction of patient-specific platelet function under flow. *Blood* 120:190–198, 2012.
8. de Witt SM, Swieringa F, Cavill R, et al: Identification of platelet function defects by multi-parameter assessment of thrombus formation. *Nat Commun* 5:4257, 2014.
9. Stockley J, Morgan NV, Bem D, et al: Enrichment of FLI1 and RUNX1 mutations in families with excessive bleeding and platelet dense granule secretion defects. *Blood* 122:4090–4093, 2013.
10. Albers CA, Cvejic A, Favier R, et al: Exome sequencing identifies NBEAL2 as the causative gene for gray platelet syndrome. *Nat Genet* 43:735–737, 2011.
11. Kahr WH, Hinckley J, Li L, et al: Mutations in NBEAL2, encoding a BEACH protein, cause gray platelet syndrome. *Nat Genet* 43:738–740, 2011.
12. Gunay-Aygun M, Falik-Zaccai TC, Vilboux T, et al: NBEAL2 is mutated in gray platelet syndrome and is required for biogenesis of platelet alpha-granules. *Nat Genet* 43:732–734, 2011.

13. Castoldi E, Collins PW, Williamson PL, Bevers EM: Compound heterozygosity for 2 novel TMEM16F mutations in a patient with Scott syndrome. *Blood* 117:4399–4400, 2011.

14. Albers CA, Paul DS, Schulze H, et al: Compound inheritance of a low-frequency regulatory SNP and a rare null mutation in exon-junction complex subunit RBM8A causes TAR syndrome. *Nat Genet* 44:435–439, S1–S2, 2012.

15. Klopocki E, Schulze H, Strauss G, et al: Complex inheritance pattern resembling autosomal recessive inheritance involving a microdeletion in thrombocytopenia-absent radius syndrome. *Am J Hum Genet* 80:232–240, 2007.

16. Nurden P, Nurden AT: Congenital disorders associated with platelet dysfunctions. *Thromb Haemost* 99:253–263, 2008.

17. Glanzmann E: Hereditäre hämmorhagische Thrombasthenie. Ein Beitrag zur Pathologie der Blutplättchen Jahrbuch fur Kinderheilkunde und physische Erziehung 88:113–141, 1918.

18. Caen JP, Castaldi PA, Leclerc JC, et al: Congenital bleeding disorders with long bleeding time and normal platelet count. I. Glanzmann's thrombasthenia. *Am J Med* 41:4, 1966.

19. Hardisty RM, Dormandy KM, Hutton RA: Thrombasthenia: Studies on three cases. *Br J Haematol* 10:371, 1964.

20. Zucker MB, Pert JH, Hilgartner MW: Platelet function in a patient with thrombasthenia. *Blood* 28:524, 1966.

21. Weiss HJ, Kochwa S: Studies of platelet function and proteins in 3 patients with Glanzmann's thrombasthenia. *J Lab Clin Med* 71:153–165, 1968.

22. George JN, Caen JP, Nurden AT: Glanzmann's thrombasthenia: The spectrum of clinical disease. *Blood* 75:1383–1395, 1990.

23. Nurden AT, Caen JP: An abnormal platelet glycoprotein pattern in three cases of Glanzmann's thrombasthenia. *Br J Haematol* 28:253–260, 1974.

24. Phillips DR, Jenkins CS, Luscher EF, Larrieu M: Molecular differences of exposed surface proteins on thrombasthenic platelet plasma membranes. *Nature* 257:599–600, 1975.

25. Peerschke EI: The platelet fibrinogen receptor. *Semin Hematol* 22:241–259, 1985.

26. Bennett JS: The platelet-fibrinogen interaction, in *Platelet Membrane Glycoproteins*, edited by JN George, AT Nurden, DR Phillips, p 193. Plenum, New York, 1985.

27. Phillips DR, Charo IF, Parise LV, Fitzgerald LA: The platelet membrane glycoprotein IIb-IIIa complex. *Blood* 71:831–843, 1988.

28. Plow EF, Ginsberg MH: Cellular adhesion: GPIIb-IIIa as a prototypic adhesion receptor. *Prog Hemost Thromb* 9:117–156, 1989.

29. Poncz M, Eisman R, Heidenreich R, et al: Structure of the platelet membrane glycoprotein IIb. Homology to the alpha subunits of the vitronectin and fibronectin membrane receptors. *J Biol Chem* 262:8476–8482, 1987.

30. Fitzgerald LA, Steiner B, Rall SC, et al: Protein sequence of endothelial glycoprotein IIIa derived from a cDNA clone. Identity with platelet glycoprotein IIIa and similarity to "integrin." *J Biol Chem* 262:3936–3939, 1987.

31. Hynes RO: Integrins: Bidirectional, allosteric signaling machines. *Cell* 110:673–687, 2002.

32. D'Andrea G, Colaizzo D, Vecchione G, et al: Glanzmann's thrombasthenia: Identification of 19 new mutations in 30 patients. *Thromb Haemost* 87:1034–1042, 2002.

33. Seligsohn U, Peretz H, Newman PJ, Coller BS: Glanzmann thrombasthenia in Israel: Clinical, biochemical and molecular genetic characterization, in *Genetic Diversity Among Jews*, edited by B Bonne-Tamir, A Adam, pp 275–282. Oxford University Press, Oxford, 1992.

34. Reichert N, Seligsohn U, Ramot B: Clinical and genetic studies of Glanzmann's thrombasthenia in Israel. *Thromb Diath Haemorrh* 34:806, 1975.

35. Awidi AS: Increased incidence of Glanzmann's thrombasthenia in Jordan as compared with Scandinavia. *Scand J Haematol* 30:218–222, 1983.

36. Khanduri U, Pulimood R, Sudarsanam A, et al: Glanzmann's thrombasthenia. A review and report of 42 cases from South India. *Thromb Haemost* 46:717–721, 1981.

37. Ahmed MA, Al Sohaibani MO, Al Mohaya SA, et al: Inherited bleeding disorders in the Eastern Province of Saudi Arabia. *Acta Haematol* 79:202–206, 1988.

38. Awidi AS: Rare inherited bleeding disorders secondary to coagulation factors in Jordan: A nine-year study. *Acta Haematol* 88:11–13, 1992.

39. Rosenberg N, Yatuv R, Orion Y, et al: Glanzmann thrombasthenia caused by an 11.2-kb deletion in the glycoprotein IIIa (beta3) is a second mutation in Iraqi Jews that stemmed from a distinct founder. *Blood* 89:3654–3662, 1997.

40. Borhany M, Fatima H, Naz A, et al: Pattern of bleeding and response to therapy in Glanzmann thrombasthenia. *Haemophilia* 18:e423–e425, 2012.

41. Coller BS, Shattil SJ: The GPIIb/IIIa (integrin alphaIIbbeta3) odyssey: A technology-driven saga of a receptor with twists, turns, and even a bend. *Blood* 112:3011–3025, 2008.

42. Harrison P: Platelet α-granular fibrinogen. *Platelets* 3:1–10, 1992.

43. Coller BS, Seligsohn U, West SM, et al: Platelet fibrinogen and vitronectin in Glanzmann thrombasthenia: Evidence consistent with specific roles for glycoprotein IIb/IIIA and αVβ3 integrins in platelet protein trafficking. *Blood* 78:2603–2610, 1991.

44. Disdier M, Legrand C, Bouillot C, et al: Quantitation of platelet fibrinogen and thrombospondin in Glanzmann's thrombasthenia by electroimmunoassay. *Thromb Res* 53:521–533, 1989.

45. Cohen I, Gerrard JM, White JG: Ultrastructure of clots during isometric contraction. *J Cell Biol* 91:775, 1982.

46. Gartner TK, Ogilvie ML: Peptides and monoclonal antibodies which bind to platelet glycoproteins IIb and/or IIIa inhibit clot retraction. *Thromb Res* 49:43–53, 1988.

47. Duperray A, Troesch A, Berthier R, et al: Biosynthesis and assembly of platelet GPIIb-IIIa in human megakaryocytes: Evidence that assembly between pro-GPIIb and GPIIIa is a prerequisite for expression of the complex on the cell surface. *Blood* 74:1603–1611, 1989.

48. Bodary SC, Napier MA, McLean JW: Expression of recombinant platelet glycoprotein IIbIIIa results in a functional fibrinogen-binding complex. *J Biol Chem* 264:18859–18862, 1989.

49. O'Toole TE, Loftus JC, Plow EF, et al: Efficient surface expression of platelet GPIIb-IIIa requires both subunits. *Blood* 74:14–18, 1989.

50. Kolodziej MA, Vilaire G, Gonder D, et al: Study of the endoproteolytic cleavage of platelet glycoprotein IIb using oligonucleotide-mediated mutagenesis. *J Biol Chem* 266:23499–23504, 1991.

51. Bennett JS: The molecular biology of platelet membrane proteins. *Semin Hematol* 27:186–204, 1990.

52. Kieffer N, Phillips DR: Platelet membrane glycoproteins: Functions in cellular interactions. *Annu Rev Cell Biol* 6:329–357, 1990.

53. Seligsohn U, Coller BS, Zivelin A, et al: Immunoblot analysis of platelet GPIIb in patients with Glanzmann thrombasthenia in Israel. *Br J Haematol* 72:415–423, 1989.

54. Mitchell WB, Li J, French DL, Coller BS: AlphaIIbbeta3 biogenesis is controlled by engagement of alphaIIb in the calnexin cycle via the N15-linked glycan. *Blood* 107:2713–2719, 2006.

55. Mitchell WB, Li J, Murcia M, et al: Mapping early conformational changes in alphaIIb and beta3 during biogenesis reveals a potential mechanism for alphaIIbbeta3 adopting its bent conformation. *Blood* 109:3725–3732, 2007.

56. Zimrin AB, Eisman R, Vilaire G, et al: Structure of platelet glycoprotein IIIa. A common subunit for two different membrane receptors. *J Clin Invest* 81:1470–1475, 1988.

57. Cheresh DA: Human endothelial cells synthesize and express an Arg-Gly-Asp-directed adhesion receptor involved in attachment to fibrinogen and von Willebrand factor. *Proc Natl Acad Sci U S A* 84:6471–6475, 1987.

58. Smith JW, Cheresh DA: The Arg-Gly-Asp binding domain of the vitronectin receptor. *J Biol Chem* 263:18726–18731, 1988.

59. Cheresh DA, Berliner SA, Vicente V, Ruggeri ZM: Recognition of distinct adhesive sites on fibrinogen by related integrins on platelets and endothelial cells. *Cell* 58:945–953, 1989.

60. Lawler J, Hynes RO: An integrin receptor on normal and thrombasthenic platelets which binds thrombospondin. *Blood* 74:2022–2027, 1989.

61. Yokoyama K, Zhang XP, Medved L, Takada Y: Specific binding of integrin alpha v beta 3 to the fibrinogen gamma and alpha E chain C-terminal domains. *Biochemistry* 38:5872–5877, 1999.

62. Lam SC, Plow EF, D'Souza SE, et al: Isolation and characterization of a platelet membrane protein related to the vitronectin receptor. *J Biol Chem* 264:3742–3749, 1989.

63. Coller BS, Cheresh DA, Asch E, Seligsohn U: Platelet vitronectin receptor expression differentiates Iraqi-Jewish from Arab Patients with Glanzmann thrombasthenia in Israel. *Blood* 77:75–83, 1991.

64. Krissansen GW, Elliott MJ, Lucas CM, et al: Identification of a novel integrin beta subunit expressed on cultured monocytes (macrophages). *J Biol Chem* 265:823, 1990.

65. Byzova TV, Rabbani R, D'Souza SE, Plow EF: Role of integrin alpha(v)beta3 in vascular biology. *Thromb Haemost* 80:726–734, 1998.

66. Newman PJ, Seligsohn U, Lyman S, Coller BS: The molecular genetic basis of Glanzmann thrombasthenia in the Iraqi-Jewish and Arab populations in Israel. *Proc Natl Acad Sci U S A* 88:3160–3164, 1991.

67. Burk CD, Newman PJ, Lyman S, et al: A deletion in the gene for glycoprotein IIb associated with Glanzmann's thrombasthenia. *J Clin Invest* 87:270–276, 1991.

68. Poncz M, Rifat S, Coller BS, et al: Glanzmann thrombasthenia secondary to a Gly273Asp mutation adjacent to the first calcium-binding domain of platelet glycoprotein IIb. *J Clin Invest* 93:172–179, 1994.

69. Tadokoro S, Tomiyama Y, Honda S, et al: Missense mutations in the beta(3) subunit have a different impact on the expression and function between alpha(IIb)beta(3) and alpha(v)beta(3). *Blood* 99:931–938, 2002.

70. Horton MA, Massey HM, Rosenberg N, et al: Upregulation of osteoclast alpha2beta1 integrin compensates for lack of alphavbeta3 vitronectin receptor in Iraqi-Jewish-type Glanzmann thrombasthenia. *Br J Haematol* 122:950–957, 2003.

71. French DL, Coller BS: Hematologically important mutations: Glanzmann thrombasthenia. *Blood Cells Mol Dis* 23:39–51, 1997.

72. Coller BS: aIIbB3: Structure and function. *Thrombos and Haemostas* 13(Suppl 1):S17–S25, 2015.

73. Bajt ML, Loftus JC: Mutation of a ligand binding domain of beta 3 integrin. Integral role of oxygenated residues in alpha IIb beta 3 (GPIIb-IIIa) receptor function. *J Biol Chem* 269:20913–20919, 1994.

74. Lee JO, Rieu P, Arnaout MA, Liddington R: Crystal structure of the A domain from the alpha subunit of integrin CR3 (CD11b/CD18). *Cell* 80:631–638, 1995.

75. Xiong JP, Stehle T, Diefenbach B, et al: Crystal structure of the extracellular segment of integrin alphaVbeta3. *Science* 294:339–345, 2001.

76. Xiao T, Takagi J, Coller BS, et al: Structural basis for allostery in integrins and binding to fibrinogen-mimetic therapeutics. *Nature* 432:59–67, 2004.

77. Xiong JP, Stehle T, Zhang R, et al: Crystal structure of the extracellular segment of integrin alpha Vbeta3 in complex with an Arg-Gly-Asp ligand. *Science* 296:151–155, 2002.

78. Zhu J, Luo BH, Xiao T, et al: Structure of a complete integrin ectodomain in a physiologic resting state and activation and deactivation by applied forces. *Mol Cell* 32:849–861, 2008.

79. Springer TA, Zhu J, Xiao T: Structural basis for distinctive recognition of fibrinogen gammaC peptide by the platelet integrin alphaIIbbeta3. *J Cell Biol* 182:791–800, 2008.

80. Loftus JC, O'Toole TE, Plow EF, et al: A β3 integrin mutation abolishes ligand binding and alters divalent cation-dependent conformation. *Science* 249:915–918, 1990.

81. Ward CM, Chao YL, Kato GJ, et al: Substitution of Asn, but not Tyr, for ASP119 of the β3 integrin subunit preserves fibrin binding and clot retraction. *Blood* 90:26a, 1997.
82. Fournier DJ, Kabral A, Castaldi PA, Berndt MC: A variant of Glanzmann's thrombasthenia characterized by abnormal glycoprotein IIb/IIIa complex formation. *Thromb Haemost* 62:977–983, 1989.
83. Newman PJ, Weyerbusch-Bottum S, Visentin GP, et al: Type II Glanzmann thrombasthenia due to a destabilizing amino acid substitution in platelet membrane glycoprotein IIIa. *Thromb Haemost* 69:1017, 1993.
84. Lanza F, Stierle A, Fournier D, et al: A new variant of Glanzmann's thrombasthenia (Strasbourg I). Platelets with functionally defective glycoprotein IIb-IIIa complexes and a glycoprotein IIIa Arg214Trp mutation. *J Clin Invest* 89:1995–2004, 1992.
85. D'Andrea G, Bafunno V, Del VL, et al: A beta3 Asp217—>Val substitution in a patient with variant Glanzmann Thrombasthenia severely affects integrin alphaIIBbeta3 functions. *Blood Coagul Fibrinolysis*. 19:657–662, 2008.
86. Baker EK, Tozer EC, Pfaff M, et al: A genetic analysis of integrin function: Glanzmann thrombasthenia in vitro. *Proc Natl Acad Sci U S A* 94:1973–1978, 1997.
87. Ward CM, Kestin AS, Newman PJ: A Leu262Pro mutation in the integrin beta(3) subunit results in an alpha(IIb)-beta(3) complex that binds fibrin but not fibrinogen. *Blood* 96:161–169, 2000.
88. Loftus JC, Halloran CE, Ginsberg MH, et al: The amino-terminal one-third of alpha IIb defines the ligand recognition specificity of integrin alpha IIb beta 3. *J Biol Chem* 271:2033–2039, 1996.
89. Springer TA: Folding of the N-terminal, ligand-binding region of integrin α-subunits into a β-propeller domain. *Proc Natl Acad Sci U S A* 94:65–72, 1997.
90. Ruan J, Peyruchaud O, Alberio L, et al: Double heterozygosity of the GPIIb gene in a Swiss patient with Glanzmann's thrombasthenia. *Br J Haematol* 102:918–925, 1998.
91. Wilcox DA, Paddock CM, Lyman S, et al: Glanzmann thrombasthenia resulting from a single amino acid substitution between the second and third calcium-binding domains of GPIIb. Role of the GPIIb amino terminus in integrin subunit association. *J Clin Invest* 95:1553–1560, 1995.
92. Wilcox DA, Wautier JL, Pidard D, Newman PJ: A single amino acid substitution flanking the fourth calcium binding domain of alpha IIb prevents maturation of the alpha IIb beta 3 integrin complex. *J Biol Chem* 269:4450–4457, 1994.
93. Basani RB, Vilaire G, Shattil SJ, et al: Glanzmann thrombasthenia due to a two amino acid deletion in the fourth calcium-binding domain of alpha IIb: Demonstration of the importance of calcium-binding domains in the conformation of alpha IIb beta 3. *Blood* 88:167–173, 1996.
94. Kiyoi T, Tomiyama Y, Honda S, et al: A naturally occurring Tyr143His alpha IIb mutation abolishes alpha IIb beta 3 function for soluble ligands but retains its ability for mediating cell adhesion and clot retraction: Comparison with other mutations causing ligand-binding defects. *Blood* 101:3485–3491, 2003.
95. Basani RB, French DL, Vilaire G, et al: A naturally-occurring mutation near the amino terminus of α_{IIb} defines a new region involved in ligand binding to $\alpha_{IIb}\beta_3$. *Blood* 95: 180–188, 2000.
96. Westrup D, Santoso S, Becker-Hagendorff K, et al: Transfection of GPIIbIle176/IIIa (Frankfurt I) in mammalian cells. *Thromb Haemost* 77:671, 1997.
97. Honda S, Tomiyama Y, Shiraga M, et al: A two-amino acid insertion in the Cys146-Cys167 loop of the α_{IIb} subunit is associated with a variant of Glanzmann thrombasthenia. *J Clin Invest* 102:1183–1192, 1998.
98. Kirchmaier CM, Westrup D, Becker-Hagendorff K, et al: A new variant of Glanzmann thrombasthenia (Frankfurt I). *Thromb Haemost* 73:1058, 1995.
99. Grimaldi CM, Chen F, Wu C, et al: Glycoprotein IIb Leu214Pro mutation produces Glanzmann thrombasthenia with both quantitative and qualitative abnormalities in GPIIb/IIIa. *Blood* 91:1562–1568, 1998.
100. Fullard J, Murphy R, O'Neill S, et al: A Val193Met mutation in GPIIIa results in a GPIIb/IIIa receptor with a constitutively high affinity for a small ligand. *Br J Haematol* 115:131–139, 2001.
101. Ruiz C, Liu CY, Sun QH, et al: A point mutation in the cysteine-rich domain of glycoprotein (GP) IIIa results in the expression of a GPIIb-IIIa (alphaIIbbeta3) integrin receptor locked in a high-affinity state and a Glanzmann thrombasthenia-like phenotype. *Blood* 98:2432–2441, 2001.
102. Vanhoorelbeke K, De Meyer SF, Pareyn I, et al: The novel S527F mutation in the integrin beta3 chain induces a high affinity alphaIIbbeta3 receptor by hindering adoption of the bent conformation. *J Biol Chem* 284:14914–14920, 2009.
103. Chen YP, Djaffar I, Pidard D, et al: Ser-752—>Pro mutation in the cytoplasmic domain of integrin β 3 subunit and defective activation of platelet integrin α IIb β 3 (glycoprotein IIb-IIIa) in a variant of Glanzmann thrombasthenia. *Proc Natl Acad Sci U S A* 89:10169–10173, 1992.
104. Ylanne J, Chen Y, O'Toole TE, et al: Distinct functions of integrin α and β subunit cytoplasmic domains in cell spreading and formation of focal adhesions. *J Cell Biol* 122:223–233, 1993.
105. Wang R, Shattil SJ, Ambruso DR, Newman PJ: Truncation of the cytoplasmic domain of β3 in a variant form of Glanzmann thrombasthenia abrogates signaling through the integrin $\alpha_{IIb}\beta3$ complex. *J Clin Invest* 100:2393–2403, 1997.
106. Chen YP, Djaffar I, Pidard E: Ser752Pro mutation in the cytoplasmic domain of integrin β_3 subunit and defective activation of platelet integrin $\alpha_{IIb}\beta_3$ (glycoprotein IIb-IIIa) in a variant of Glanzmann thrombasthenia. *Proc Natl Acad Sci U S A* 89:10169–10173, 1992.
107. Ylanne J, Huuskonen J, O'Toole TE, et al: Mutation of the cytoplasmic domain of the integrin beta 3 subunit. Differential effects on cell spreading, recruitment to adhesion plaques, endocytosis, and phagocytosis. *J Biol Chem* 270:9550–9557, 1995.
108. Chen YP, O'Toole TE, Ylanne J, et al: A point mutation in the integrin beta 3 cytoplasmic domain (S752—>P) impairs bidirectional signaling through alpha IIb beta 3 (platelet glycoprotein IIb-IIIa). *Blood* 84:1857–1865, 1994.
109. Coventry A, Bull-Otterson LM, Liu X, et al: Deep resequencing reveals excess rare recent variants consistent with explosive population growth. *Nat Commun* 1:131, 2010.
109A. Buitrago L, Rendon A, Liang Y, et al: αIIbβ3 variants defined by next-generation sequencing: Predicting variants likely to cause Glanzmann thrombasthenia. *Proc Natl Acad Sci U S A* E1898–E1907, 2015.
110. Rosenberg N, Hauschner H, Peretz H, et al: A 13-bp deletion in alpha(IIb) gene is a founder mutation that predominates in Palestinian-Arab patients with Glanzmann thrombasthenia. *J Thromb Haemost* 3:2764–2772, 2005.
111. Fiore M, Pillois X, Nurden P, et al: Founder effect and estimation of the age of the French Gypsy mutation associated with Glanzmann thrombasthenia in Manouche families. *Eur J Hum Genet* 19:981–987, 2011.
112. Coller BS, Seligsohn U, Zivelin A, et al: Immunologic and biochemical characterization of homozygous and heterozygous Glanzmann's thrombasthenia in Iraqi-Jewish and Arab populations of Israel: Comparison of techniques for carrier detection. *Br J Haematol* 62:723–735, 1986.
113. Shpilberg O, Rabi I, Schiller K, et al: Patients with Glanzmann thrombasthenia lacking platelet glycoprotein alpha(IIb)beta(3) (GPIIb/IIIa) and alpha(v)beta(3) receptors are not protected from atherosclerosis. *Circulation* 105:1044–1048, 2002.
114. Cronberg S, Nilsson IM, Zetterqvist E: Investigation of a family with members with both severe and mild degree of thrombasthenia. *Acta Paediatr Scand* 56:189–197, 1967.
115. Stormorken H, Gogstad GO, Solum NO, Pande H: Diagnosis of heterozygotes in Glanzmann's thrombasthenia. *Thromb Haemost* 48:217–221, 1982.
116. Coller BS, Peerschke EI, Scudder LE, Sullivan CA: A murine monoclonal antibody that completely blocks the binding of fibrinogen to platelets produces a thrombasthenic-like state in normal platelets and binds to glycoproteins IIb and/or IIIa. *J Clin Invest* 72:325–338, 1983.
117. Malmsten C, Kindahl H, Samuelsson B, et al: Thromboxane synthesis and the platelet release reaction in Bernard- Soulier syndrome, thrombasthenia Glanzmann and Hermansky-Pudlak syndrome. *Br J Haematol* 35:511–520, 1977.
118. Charo IF, Feinman RD, Detwiler TC: Interrelations of platelet aggregation and secretion. *J Clin Invest* 60:866–873, 1977.
119. Heptinstall S, Taylor PM: The effects of citrate and extracellular calcium ions on the platelet release reaction induced by adenosine diphosphate and collagen. *Thromb Haemost* 42:778–793, 1979.
120. Caen JP, Cronberg S, Levy-Toledano S, et al: New data on Glanzmann's thrombasthenia. *Proc Soc Exp Biol Med* 136:1082–1086, 1971.
121. Zucker MB, Vroman L: Platelet adhesion induced by fibrinogen adsorbed onto glass. *Proc Soc Exp Biol Med* 131:318–320, 1969.
122. Stanford MF, Munoz PC, Vroman L: Platelets adhere where flow has left fibrinogen on glass. *Ann N Y Acad Sci* 416:504–512, 1983.
123. Zucker MB, McPherson J: Reactions of platelets near surfaces in vitro: Lessons from the platelet retention test. *Ann N Y Acad Sci* 283:128, 1977.
124. Bevers EM, Comfurius P, Nieuwenhuis HK, et al: Platelet prothrombin converting activity in hereditary disorders of platelet function. *Br J Haematol* 63:335–345, 1986.
125. Reverter JC, Beguin S, Kessels H, et al: Inhibition of platelet-mediated, tissue factor-induced thrombin generation by the mouse/human chimeric 7E3 antibody. Potential implications for the effect of c7E3 Fab treatment on acute thrombosis and "clinical restenosis." *J Clin Invest* 98:863–874, 1996.
126. Beguin S, Kumar R, Keularts I, et al: Fibrin-dependent platelet procoagulant activity requires GPIb receptors and von Willebrand factor. *Blood* 93:564–570, 1999.
127. Gemmell CH, Sefton MV, Yeo EL: Platelet-derived microparticle formation involves glycoprotein IIb- IIIa. Inhibition by RGDS and a Glanzmann's thrombasthenia defect. *J Biol Chem* 268:14586–14589, 1993.
128. Nomura S, Komiyama Y, Matsuura E, et al: Participation of α IIb β 3 in platelet microparticle generation by collagen plus thrombin. *Haemostasis* 26:31–37, 1996.
129. Nomura S, Komiyama Y, Murakami T, et al: Flow cytometric analysis of surface membrane proteins on activated platelets and platelet-derived microparticles from healthy and thrombasthenic individuals. *Int J Hematol* 58:203–212, 1993.
130. Byzova TV, Plow EF: Networking in the hemostatic system. Integrin alphaiibbeta3 binds prothrombin and influences its activation. *J Biol Chem* 272:27183–27188, 1997.
131. Byzova TV, Plow EF: Activation of alphaVbeta3 on vascular cells controls recognition of prothrombin. *J Cell Biol* 143:2081–2092, 1998.
132. Tschopp TB, Weiss HJ, Baumgartner HR: Interaction of thrombasthenic platelets with subendothelium: Normal adhesion, absent aggregation. *Experientia* 31:113–116, 1975.
133. Sakariassen KS, Nievelstein PFEM, Coller BS, Sixma JJ: The role of platelet membrane glycoproteins Ib and IIb-IIIa in platelet adherence to human artery subendothelium. *Br J Haematol* 63:681–691, 1986.
134. Weiss HJ, Turitto VT, Baumgartner HR: Platelet adhesion and thrombus formation on subendothelium in platelets deficient in glycoproteins IIb-IIIa, Ib, and storage granules. *Blood* 67:322, 1986.
135. Weiss HJ, Turitto VT, Baumgartner HR: The role of shear rate and platelets in promoting fibrin formation on rabbit subendothelium: Studies utilizing patients with quantitative and qualitative platelet defects. *J Clin Invest* 78:1072–1082, 1986.
136. Harrison P, Robinson M, Liesner R, et al: The PFA-100: A potential rapid screening tool for the assessment of platelet dysfunction. *Clin Lab Haematol* 24:225–232, 2002.
137. Buyukasik Y, Karakus S, Goker H, et al: Rational use of the PFA-100 device for screening of platelet function disorders and von Willebrand disease. *Blood Coagul Fibrinolysis* 13:349–353, 2002.

138. Lee H, Nurden AT, Thomaidis A, Caen JP: Relationship between fibrinogen binding and platelet glycoprotein deficiencies in Glanzmann's thrombasthenia type I and type II. *Br J Haematol* 48:47, 1981.

139. Coller BS, Seligsohn U, Peretz H, Newman PJ: Glanzmann thrombasthenia: New insights from an historical perspective. *Semin Hematol* 31:301–311, 1994.

140. Shattil SJ, Hoxie JA, Cunningham M, Brass LF: Changes in the platelet membrane glycoprotein IIb.IIIa complex during platelet activation. *J Biol Chem* 260:11107–11114, 1985.

141. Karpatkin M, Howard L, Karpatkin S: Studies of the origin of platelet-associated fibrinogen. *J Lab Clin Med* 104:223–237, 1984.

142. Grimaldi CM, Chen F, Scudder LE, et al: A Cys374Tyr homozygous mutation of platelet glycoprotein IIIa (beta 3) in a Chinese patient with Glanzmann's thrombasthenia. *Blood* 88:1666–1675, 1996.

143. Yasunaga K, Nomura S: Statistical analysis of Glanzmann's thrombasthenia in Japan. *Acta Haematol* 89:165–166, 1993.

144. Kashiwagi H, Kunishima S, Kiyomizu K, et al: Demonstration of novel gain-of-function mutations of alphaIIbbeta3: Association with macrothrombocytopenia and Glanzmann thrombasthenia-like phenotype. *Mol Genet Genomic Med* 1:77–86, 2013.

145. Kunishima S, Kashiwagi H, Otsu M, et al: Heterozygous ITGA2B R995W mutation inducing constitutive activation of the alphaIIbbeta3 receptor affects proplatelet formation and causes congenital macrothrombocytopenia. *Blood* 117:5479–5484, 2011.

146. Ghevaert C, Salsmann A, Watkins NA, et al: A nonsynonymous SNP in the ITGB3 gene disrupts the conserved membrane-proximal cytoplasmic salt bridge in the alphaIIbbeta3 integrin and cosegregates dominantly with abnormal proplatelet formation and macrothrombocytopenia. *Blood* 111:3407–3414, 2008.

147. Nurden AT, Pillois X, Fiore M, et al: Glanzmann thrombasthenia-like syndromes associated with Macrothrombocytopenias and mutations in the genes encoding the alphaIIbbeta3 integrin. *Semin Thromb Hemost* 37:698–706, 2011.

148. Schaffner-Reckinger E, Salsmann A, Debili N, et al: Overexpression of the partially activated alpha(IIb)beta3D723H integrin salt bridge mutant downregulates RhoA activity and induces microtubule-dependent proplatelet-like extensions in Chinese hamster ovary cells. *J Thromb Haemost* 7:1207–1217, 2009.

149. Jayo A, Conde I, Lastres P, et al: L718P mutation in the membrane-proximal cytoplasmic tail of beta 3 promotes abnormal alpha IIb beta 3 clustering and lipid microdomain coalescence, and associates with a thrombasthenia-like phenotype. *Haematologica* 95:1158–1166, 2010.

150. Peyruchaud O, Nurden AT, Milet S, et al: R to Q amino acid substitution in the GFFKR sequence of the cytoplasmic domain of the integrin IIb subunit in a patient with a Glanzmann's thrombasthenia-like syndrome. *Blood* 92:4178–4187, 1998.

151. Hughes PE, Diaz-Gonzalez F, Leong L, et al: Breaking the integrin hinge. A defined structural constraint regulates integrin signaling. *J Biol Chem* 271:6571–6574, 1996.

152. Lopez JA, Andrews RK, Afshar-Kharghan V, Berndt MC: Bernard-Soulier syndrome. *Blood* 91:4397–4418, 1998.

153. Lopez JA, Berndt MC: The GPIb-IX-V complex, in *Platelets*, edited by AD Michelson, p. 85. Academic Press, San Diego, 2002.

154. Savoia A, Kunishima S, De Rocco D, et al: Spectrum of the mutations in Bernard-Soulier syndrome. *Hum Mutat* 35:1033–1045, 2014.

155. Andrews RK, Berndt MC: Bernard-Soulier syndrome: An update. *Semin Thromb Hemost* 39:656–662, 2013.

156. Bernard J, Soulier JP: Sur une nouvelle variete de dystrophie thrombocytaire-hemorragipare congenitale. *Semin Hop Paris.* 24:3217, 1948.

157. Bernard J: History of congenital hemorrhagic thrombocytopathic dystrophy. *Blood Cells* 9:179, 1983.

158. Weiss HJ, Tschopp TB, Baumgartner HR, et al: Decreased adhesion of giant (Bernard-Soulier) platelets to subendothelium. Further implications on the role of the von Willebrand factor in hemostasis. *Am J Med* 57:920–925, 1974.

159. Howard MA, Hutton RA, Hardisty RM: Hereditary giant platelet syndrome: A disorder of a new aspect of platelet function. *Br Med J* 2:586–588, 1973.

160. Bithell TC, Parekh SJ, Strong RR: Platelet-function studies in the Bernard-Soulier syndrome. *Ann N Y Acad Sci* 201:145–160, 1972.

161. Nurden AT, Caen JP: Specific roles for platelet surface glycoproteins in platelet function. *Nature* 255:720–722, 1975.

162. Howard MA, Perkin J, Salem HH, Firkin BG: The agglutination of human platelets by botrocetin: Evidence that botrocetin and ristocetin act at different sites on the factor VIII molecule and platelet membrane. *Br J Haematol* 57:25–35, 1984.

163. Moake JL, Olson JD, Troll JH, et al: Binding of radioiodinated human von Willebrand factor to Bernard- Soulier, thrombasthenic and von Willebrand's disease platelets. *Thromb Res* 19:21–27, 1980.

164. Zucker MB, Kim SJ, McPherson J, Grant RA: Binding of factor VIII to platelets in the presence of ristocetin. *Br J Haematol* 35:535–549, 1977.

165. Berndt MC, Gregory C, Chong BH, et al: Additional glycoprotein defects in Bernard-Soulier's syndrome: Confirmation of genetic basis by parental analysis. *Blood* 62:800–807, 1983.

166. Clemetson KJ, McGregor JL, James E, et al: Characterization of the platelet membrane glycoprotein abnormalities in Bernard-Soulier syndrome and comparison with normal by surface-labeling techniques and high-resolution two-dimensional gel electrophoresis. *J Clin Invest* 70:304–311, 1982.

167. Vanhoorelbeke K, Ulrichts H, Romijn RA, et al: The GPIbalpha-thrombin interaction: Far from crystal clear. *Trends Mol Med* 10:33–39, 2004.

168. Romo GM, Dong JF, Schade AJ, et al: The glycoprotein Ib-IX-V complex is a platelet counterreceptor for P-selectin. *J Exp Med* 190:803–814, 1999.

169. Simon DI, Chen Z, Xu H, et al: Platelet glycoprotein Ibα is a counterreceptor for the leukocyte integrin Mac-1 (CD11b/CD18). *J Exp Med* 192:193–204, 2000.

170. Bradford HN, Dela Cadena RA, Kunapuli SP, et al: Human kininogens regulate thrombin binding to platelets through the glycoprotein Ib-IX-V complex. *Blood* 90:1508–1515, 1997.

171. Jurk K, Clemetson KJ, de Groot PG, et al: Thrombospondin-1 mediates platelet adhesion at high shear via glycoprotein Ib (GPIb): An alternative/backup mechanism to von Willebrand factor. *FASEB J* 17:1490–1492, 2003.

172. Baglia FA, Badellino KO, Li CQ, et al: Factor XI binding to the platelet glycoprotein Ib-IX-V complex promotes factor XI activation by thrombin. *J Biol Chem* 277:1662–1668, 2002.

173. Bradford HN, Pixley RA, Colman RW: Human factor XII binding to the glycoprotein Ib-IX-V complex inhibits thrombin-induced platelet aggregation. *J Biol Chem* 275:22756–22763, 2000.

174. Ware J, Russell S, Ruggeri ZM: Generation and rescue of a murine model of platelet dysfunction: The Bernard-Soulier syndrome. *Proc Natl Acad Sci U S A* 97:2803–2808, 2000.

175. Kato K, Martinez C, Russell S, et al: Genetic deletion of mouse platelet glycoprotein Ibbeta produces a Bernard-Soulier phenotype with increased alpha-granule size. *Blood* 104:2339–2344, 2004.

176. Ramakrishnan V, Reeves PS, DeGuzman F, et al: Increased thrombin responsiveness in platelets from mice lacking glycoprotein V. *Proc Natl Acad Sci U S A* 96:13336–13341, 1999.

177. Nonne C, Hechler B, Cazenave JP, et al: Reassessment of in vivo thrombus formation in glycoprotein V deficient mice backcrossed on a C57Bl/6 strain. *J Thromb Haemost* 6:210–212, 2008.

178. Grottum KA, Solum NO: Congenital thrombocytopenia with giant platelets: A defect in the platelet membrane. *Br J Haematol* 16:277–290, 1969.

179. Greenberg JP, Packham MA, Guccione MA, et al: Survival of rabbit-platelets treated in vitro with chymotrypsin, plasmin, trypsin, and neuraminidase. *Blood* 53:916–927, 1979.

180. Heyns Ad, Badenhorst PN, Wessels P, et al: Kinetics, *in vivo* redistribution and sites of sequestration of indium-111-labelled platelets in giant platelet syndromes. *Br J Haematol* 60:323–330, 1985.

181. Tomer A, Scharf RE, McMillan R, et al: Bernard-Soulier syndrome: Quantitative characterization of megakaryocytes and platelets by flow cytometric and platelet kinetic measurements. *Eur J Haematol* 52:193–200, 1994.

182. Nurden P, Nurden A: Giant platelets, megakaryocytes and the expression of glycoprotein Ib- IX complexes. *C R Acad Sci III* 319:717–726, 1996.

183. Vettore S, Scandellari R, Scapin M, et al: A case of Bernard-Soulier Syndrome due to a homozygous four bases deletion (TGAG) of GPIbalpha gene: Lack of GPIbalpha but absence of bleeding. *Platelets* 19:388–391, 2008.

184. George JN, Nurden AT: Inherited disorders of the platelet membrane: Glanzmann's thrombasthenia and Bernard-Soulier syndrome, in *Hemostasis and Thrombosis: Basic Principles and Clinical Practice*, edited by RW Colman, J Hirsh, VJ Marder, EW Salzman, p 726. Lippincott, Philadelphia, 1987.

185. Ruggeri Z: The platelet glycoprotein Ib-IX complex. *Prog Hemost Thromb* 10:35–68, 1991.

186. Andrews RK, Lopez JA, Berndt MC: The GPIb-IX-V complex, in *Platelets*, 3rd ed, edited by AD Michelson. Academic Press, San Diego, 2013.

187. Roth GJ: Developing relationships: Arterial platelet adhesion, glycoprotein Ib, and leucine-rich glycoproteins. *Blood* 77:5–19, 1991.

188. Yap CL, Hughan SC, Cranmer SL, et al: Synergistic adhesive interactions and signaling mechanisms operating between platelet glycoprotein Ib/IX and integrin alpha IIbbeta 3. Studies in human platelets ans transfected Chinese hamster ovary cells. *J Biol Chem* 275:41377–41388, 2000.

189. Gardiner EE, Arthur JF, Shen Y, et al: GPIbalpha-selective activation of platelets induces platelet signaling events comparable to GPVI activation events. *Platelets* 21:244–252, 2010.

190. Zhou YF, Eng ET, Zhu J, et al: Sequence and structure relationships within von Willebrand factor. *Blood* 120:449–458, 2012.

191. Wu YP, Vink T, Schiphorst M, et al: Platelet thrombus formation on collagen at high shear rates is mediated by von Willebrand factor-glycoprotein Ib interaction and inhibited by von Willebrand factor-glycoprotein IIb/IIIa interaction. *Arterioscler Thromb Vasc Biol* 20:1661–1667, 2000.

192. Kulkarni S, Dopheide SM, Yap CL, et al: A revised model of platelet aggregation. *J Clin Invest* 105:783–791, 2000.

193. Matsui H, Sugimoto M, Mizuno T, et al: Distinct and concerted functions of von Willebrand factor and fibrinogen in mural thrombus growth under high shear flow. *Blood* 100:3604–3610, 2002.

194. Ikeda Y, Handa M, Kawano K, et al: The role of von Willebrand factor and fibrinogen in platelet aggregation under varying shear stress. *J Clin Invest* 87:1234–1240, 1991.

195. Peterson DM, Stathopoulos NA, Giorgio TD, et al: Shear-induced platelet aggregation requires von Willebrand factor and platelet membrane glycoproteins Ib and IIb-IIIa. *Blood* 69:625–628, 1987.

196. Ruggeri ZM: Mechanisms of shear-induced platelet adhesion and aggregation. *Thromb Haemost* 70:119, 1993.

197. Jamieson GA, Okumura T: Reduced thrombin binding and aggregation in Bernard-Soulier platelets. *J Clin Invest* 61:861–864, 1978.

198. Jandrot-Perrus M, Rendu F, Caen JP, et al: The common pathway for alpha- and gamma-thrombin-induced platelet activation is independent of GPIb: A study of Bernard-Soulier platelets. *Br J Haematol* 75:385–392, 1990.

199. Smith PT, Landry ML, Carey H, et al: Papular-purpuric gloves and socks syndrome associated with acute parvovirus B19 infection: Case report and review. *Clin Infect Dis* 27:164–168, 1998.

200. Ramakrishnan V, Reeves PS, DeGuzman F, et al: Increased thrombin responsiveness in platelets from mice lacking glycoprotein V. *Proc Natl Acad Sci U S A* 96:13336–13341, 1999.

201. Ni H, Ramakrishnan V, Ruggeri ZM, et al: Increased thrombogenesis and embolus formation in mice lacking glycoprotein V. *Blood* 98:368–373, 2001.

202. Caen J, Bellucci S: The defective prothrombin consumption in Bernard-Soulier syndrome. Hypotheses from 1948 to 1982. *Blood Cells* 9:389–399, 1983.

203. Walsh PN, Mills DC, Pareti FI, et al: Hereditary giant platelet syndrome. Absence of collagen-induced coagulant activity and deficiency of factor-XI binding to platelets. *Br J Haematol* 29:639–655, 1975.

204. Perret B, Levy-Toledano S, Platavid M: Abnormal phospholipid organization in Bernard-Soulier platelets. *Thromb Res* 31:529, 1983.

205. Nurden P, Nurden AT, La Marca S, et al: Platelet morphological changes in 2 patients with von Willebrand disease type 3 caused by large homozygous deletions of the von Willebrand factor gene. *Haematologica* 94:1627–1629, 2009.

206. Kanaji T, Russell S, Ware J: Amelioration of the macrothrombocytopenia associated with the murine Bernard-Soulier syndrome. *Blood* 100:2102–2107, 2002.

207. McNicol A, Drouin J, Clemetson KJ, Gerrard JM: Phospholipase C activity in platelets from Bernard-Soulier syndrome patients. *Arterioscler Thromb.* 13:1567–1571, 1993.

208. White JG, Burris SM, Hasegawa D, Johnson M: Micropipette aspiration of human blood platelets: A defect in Bernard- Soulier's syndrome. *Blood* 63:1249–1252, 1984.

209. Lopez JA, Leung B, Reynolds CC, et al: Efficient plasma membrane expression of a functional platelet glycoprotein Ib-IX complex requires the presence of its three subunits. *J Biol Chem* 267:12851–12859, 1992.

210. Li CQ, Dong JF, Lanza F, et al: Expression of platelet glycoprotein (GP) V in heterologous cells and evidence for its association with GP Ib alpha in forming a GP Ib-IX-V complex on the cell surface. *J Biol Chem* 270:16302–16307, 1995.

211. Drouin J, McGregor JL, Parmentier S, et al: Residual amounts of glycoprotein Ib concomitant with near-absence of glycoprotein IX in platelets of Bernard-Soulier patients. *Blood* 72:1086–1088, 1988.

212. Stevens MC, Blanchette VS, Freedman MH, et al: A variant form of Bernard-Soulier syndrome: Mild haemostatic defect associated with partial platelet GPIb deficiency. *Clin Lab Haematol* 10:443–451, 1988.

213. Finch CN, Miller JL, Lyle VA, Handin RI: Evidence that an abnormality in the glycoprotein Ib alpha gene is not the cause of abnormal platelet function in a family with classic Bernard-Soulier disease. *Blood* 75:2357–2362, 1990.

214. Poulsen LO, Taaning E: Variation in surface platelet glycoprotein Ib expression in Bernard- Soulier syndrome. *Haemostasis* 20:155–161, 1990.

215. Wright SD, Michaelides K, Johnson DJ, et al: Double heterozygosity for mutations in the platelet glycoprotein IX gene in three siblings with Bernard-Soulier syndrome. *Blood* 81:2339–2347, 1993.

216. Nurden AT, Jallu V, Hourdille P: GP Ib and Bernard-Soulier platelets. *Blood* 73:2225–2227, 1989.

217. Nurden AT, Nurden P: Inherited disorders of platelet function, in *Platelets*, edited by AD Michelson. Academic Press, San Diego, 2007.

218. Lanza F, Baas MJ, Dupuis A, et al: Founder effect for a novel GPIBB mutations in Bernard-Soulier patients from La Reunion island. *J Thromb Haemost* 11:1322 (abstract), 2013.

219. Kenny D, Newman PJ, Morateck PA, Montgomery RR: A dinucleotide deletion results in defective membrane anchoring and circulating soluble glycoprotein Ibalpha in a novel form of Bernard-Soulier syndrome. *Blood* 90:2626–2633, 1997.

220. Holmberg L, Karpman D, Nilsson I, Olofsson T: Bernard-Soulier syndrome Karlstad: Trp 498-Stop mutation resulting in a truncated glycoprotein Ibalpha that contains part of the transmembrane domain. *Br J Haematol* 98:57, 1997.

221. Kunishima S, Lopez JA, Kobayashi S, et al: Missense mutations of the glycoprotein (GP) Ib beta gene impairing the GPIb alpha/beta disulfide linkage in a family with giant platelet disorder. *Blood* 89:2404–2412, 1997.

222. Koskela S, Partanen J, Salmi TT, Kekomaki R: Molecular characterization of two mutations in platelet glycoprotein (GP) Ibalpha in two Finnish Bernard-Soulier syndrome families. *Eur J Haematol* 62:160–168, 1999.

223. Ludlow LB, Schick BP, Budarf ML, et al: Identification of a mutation in a GATA binding site of the platelet glycoprotein Ibbeta promoter resulting in the Bernard-Soulier syndrome. *J Biol Chem* 271:22076–22080, 1996.

224. Strassel C, Alessi MC, Juhan-Vague I, et al: A 13 base pair deletion in the GPIbbeta gene in a second unrelated Bernard-Soulier family due to slipped mispairing between direct repeats. *J Thromb Haemost* 2:1663–1665, 2004.

225. Strassel C, David T, Eckly A, et al: Synthesis of GPIb beta with novel transmembrane and cytoplasmic sequences in a Bernard-Soulier patient resulting in GPIb-defective signaling in CHO cells. *J Thromb Haemost* 4:217–228, 2006.

226. Kurokawa Y, Ishida F, Kamijo T, et al: A missense mutation (Tyr88 to Cys) in the platelet membrane glycoprotein Ibbeta gene affects GPIb/IX complex expression—Bernard-Soulier syndrome in the homozygous form and giant platelets in the heterozygous form. *Thromb Haemost* 86:1249–1256, 2001.

227. Kunishima S, Naoe T, Kamiya T, Saito H: Novel heterozygous missense mutation in the platelet glycoprotein Ib beta gene associated with isolated giant platelet disorder. *Am J Hematol* 68:249–255, 2001.

228. Koskela S, Javela K, Jouppila J, et al: Variant Bernard-Soulier syndrome due to homozygous Asn45Ser mutation in the platelet glycoprotein (GP) IX in seven patients of five unrelated Finnish families. *Eur J Haematol* 62:256–264, 1999.

229. Vanhoorelbeke K, Schlammadinger A, Delville JP, et al: Occurrence of the Asn45Ser mutation in the GPIX gene in a Belgian patient with Bernard Soulier syndrome. *Platelets* 12:114–120, 2001.

230. Zieger B, Jenny A, Tsakiris DA, et al: A large Swiss family with Bernard-Soulier syndrome-Correlation phenotype and genotype. *Hamostaseologie* 29:161–167, 2009.

231. Dagistan N, Kunishima S: First Turkish case of Bernard-Soulier syndrome associated with GPIX N45S. *Acta Haematol* 118:146–148, 2007.

232. Bartsch I, Sandrock K, Lanza F, et al: Deletion of human GP1BB and SEPT5 is associated with Bernard-Soulier syndrome, platelet secretion defect, polymicrogyria, and developmental delay. *Thromb Haemost* 106:475–483, 2011.

233. Kunishima S, Imai T, Kobayashi R, et al: Bernard-Soulier syndrome caused by a hemizygous GPIbbeta mutation and 22q11.2 deletion. *Pediatr Int* 55:434–437, 2013.

234. Budarf ML, Konkle BA, Ludlow LB, et al: Identification of a patient with Bernard-Soulier syndrome and a deletion in the DiGeorge/velo-cardio-facial chromosomal region in 22q11.2. *Hum Mol Genet* 4:763, 1995.

235. Lascone MR, Sacchelli M, Vittorini S, Giusti S: Complex conotruncal heart defect, severe bleeding disorder and 22q11 deletion: A new case of Bernard-Soulier syndrome and of 22q11 deletion syndrome? *Ital Heart J* 2:475–477, 2001.

236. Tang J, Stern-Nezer S, Liu PC, et al: Mutation in the leucine-rich repeat C-flanking region of platelet glycoprotein Ibbeta impairs assembly of von Willebrand factor receptor. *Thromb Haemost* 92:75–88, 2004.

237. Hillmann A, Nurden A, Nurden P, et al: A novel hemizygous Bernard-Soulier Syndrome (BSS) mutation in the amino terminal domain of glycoprotein (GP)Ibbeta—Platelet characterization and transfection studies. *Thromb Haemost* 88:1026–1032, 2002.

238. Nakagawa M, Okuno M, Okamoto N, et al: Bernard-Soulier syndrome associated with 22q11.2 microdeletion. *Am J Med Genet* 99:286–288, 2001.

239. Liang HP, Morel-Kopp MC, Curtin J, et al: Heterozygous loss of platelet glycoprotein (GP) Ib-V-IX variably affects platelet function in velocardiofacial syndrome (VCFS) patients. *Thromb Haemost* 98:1298–1308, 2007.

240. Van Geet C, Devriendt K, Eyskens B, et al: Velocardiofacial syndrome patients with a heterozygous chromosome 22q11 deletion have giant platelets. *Pediatr Res* 44:607–611, 1998.

241. Lawrence S, McDonald-McGinn DM, Zackai E, Sullivan KE: Thrombocytopenia in patients with chromosome 22q11.2 deletion syndrome. *J Pediatr* 143:277–278, 2003.

242. Kato T, Kosaka K, Kimura M, et al: Thrombocytopenia in patients with 22q11.2 deletion syndrome and its association with glycoprotein Ib-beta. *Genet Med* 5:113–119, 2003.

243. Latger-Cannard V, Bensoussan D, Gregoire MJ, et al: Frequency of thrombocytopenia and large platelets correlates neither with conotruncal cardiac anomalies nor immunological features in the chromosome 22q11.2 deletion syndrome. *Eur J Pediatr* 163:327–328, 2004.

244. Ryan AK, Goodship JA, Wilson DI, et al: Spectrum of clinical features associated with interstitial chromosome 22q11 deletions: A European collaborative study. *J Med Genet* 34:798–804, 1997.

245. Miller JL, Lyle VA, Cunningham D: Mutation of leucine-57 to phenylalanine in a platelet glycoprotein Ib alpha leucine tandem repeat occurring in patients with an autosomal dominant variant of Bernard-Soulier disease. *Blood* 79:439–446, 1992.

246. Vettore S, Scandellari R, Moro S, et al: Novel point mutation in a leucine-rich repeat of the GPIbalpha chain of the platelet von Willebrand factor receptor, GPIb/IX/V, resulting in an inherited dominant form of Bernard-Soulier syndrome affecting two unrelated families: The N41H variant. *Haematologica* 93:1743–1747, 2008.

247. Kunishima S, Imai T, Hamaguchi M, Saito H: Novel heterozygous missense mutation in the second leucine rich repeat of GPIbalpha affects GPIb/IX/V expression and results in macrothrombocytopenia in a patient initially misdiagnosed with idiopathic thrombocytopenic purpura. *Eur J Haematol* 76:348–355, 2006.

248. De Marco L, Mazzucato M, Fabris F, et al: Variant Bernard-Soulier syndrome type Bolzano. A congenital bleeding disorder due to a structural and functional abnormality of the platelet glycoprotein Ib-IX complex. *J Clin Invest* 86:25–31, 1990.

249. Margaglione M, D'Andrea G, Grandone E, et al: Compound heterozygosity (554–589 del, C515-T transition) in the platelet glycoprotein Ib alpha gene in a patient with a severe bleeding tendency. *Thromb Haemost* 81:486–492, 1999.

250. Noris P, Perrotta S, Bottega R, et al: Clinical and laboratory features of 103 patients from 42 Italian families with inherited thrombocytopenia derived from the monoallelic Ala156Val mutation of GPIbalpha (Bolzano mutation). *Haematologica* 97:82–88, 2012.

251. Yuksel O, Koklu S, Ucar E, et al: Severe recurrent gastrointestinal bleeding due to angiodysplasia in a Bernard-Soulier patient: An onerous medical concomitance. *Dig Dis Sci* 49:885–887, 2004.

252. Okita R, Hihara J, Konishi K, et al: Intractable gastrointestinal bleeding from angiodysplasia in a patient of Bernard-Soulier syndrome—Report of a case. *Hiroshima J Med Sci* 54:113–115, 2005.

253. Kaya Z, Gursel T, Dalgic B, Aslan D: Gastric angiodysplasia in a child with Bernard-Soulier syndrome: Efficacy of octreotide in long-term management. *Pediatr Hematol Oncol* 22:223–227, 2005.

254. George JN, Reimann TA, Moake JL, et al: Bernard-Soulier disease: A study of four patients and their parents. *Br J Haematol* 48:459, 1981.

255. Fox JE: Linkage of a membrane skeleton to integral membrane glycoproteins in human platelets. Identification of one of the glycoproteins as glycoprotein Ib. *J Clin Invest* 76:1673–1683, 1985.

256. Eaton LA Jr, Read MS, Brinkhous KM: Glycoprotein Ib bioassays. Activity levels in Bernard-Soulier syndrome and in stored blood bank platelets. *Arch Pathol Lab Med* 115:488–493, 1991.

257. Waldenstrom E, Holmberg L, Axelsson U, et al: Bernard-Soulier syndrome in two Swedish families: Effect of DDAVP on bleeding time. *Eur J Haematol* 46:182–187, 1991.

258. Evensen SA, Solum NO, Grottum KA, Hovig T: Familial bleeding disorder with a moderate thrombocytopenia and giant blood platelets. *Scand J Haematol* 13:203–214, 1974.

259. Greco NJ, Tandon NN, Jones GD, et al: Contributions of glycoprotein Ib and the seven transmembrane domain receptor to increases in platelet cytoplasmic [Ca 2+] induced by α-thrombin. *Biochemistry* 35:906–914, 1996.

260. Celikel R, McClintock RA, Roberts JR, et al: Modulation of alpha-thrombin function by distinct interactions with platelet glycoprotein Ibalpha. *Science* 301:218–221, 2003.

261. Dumas JJ, Kumar R, Seehra J, et al: Crystal structure of the GpIbalpha-thrombin complex essential for platelet aggregation. *Science* 301:222–226, 2003.

262. McGowan EB, Ding A, Detwiler TC: Correlation of thrombin-induced glycoprotein V hydrolysis and platelet activation. *J Biol Chem* 258:11243, 1983.

263. Bienz D, Schnippering W, Clemetson KJ: Glycoprotein V is not the thrombin activation receptor on human blood platelets. *Blood* 68:720–725, 1986.

264. Caen JP, Nurden AT, Jeanneau C, et al: Bernard-Soulier syndrome: A new platelet glycoprotein abnormality. Its relationship with platelet adhesion to subendothelium and with the factor VIII von Willebrand protein. *J Lab Clin Med* 87:586–596, 1976.

265. Andrews RK, Harris SJ, McNally T, Berndt MC: Binding of purified 14-3-3 zeta signaling protein to discrete amino acid sequences within the cytoplasmic domain of the platelet membrane glycoprotein Ib-IX-V complex. *Biochemistry* 37:638–647, 1998.

266. Sullam PM, Hyun WC, Szollosi J, et al: Physical proximity and functional interplay of the glycoprotein Ib-IX-V complex and the Fc receptor FcgammaRIIA on the platelet plasma membrane. *J Biol Chem* 273:5331–5336, 1998.

267. Falati S, Edmead CE, Poole AW: Glycoprotein Ib-V-IX, a receptor for von Willebrand factor, couples physically and functionally to the Fc receptor g -chain, Fyn, and Lyn to activate human platelets. *Blood* 94:1648–1656, 1999.

268. Arthur JF, Gardiner EE, Matzaris M, et al: Glycoprotein VI is associated with GPIb-IX-V on the membrane of resting and activated platelets. *Thromb Haemost* 93:716–723, 2005.

269. Feng S, Resendiz JC, Christodoulides N, et al: Pathological shear stress stimulates the tyrosine phosphorylation of alpha-actinin associated with the glycoprotein Ib-IX complex. *Biochemistry* 41:1100–1108, 2002.

270. Aziz KA: An acquired form of Bernard Soulier syndrome associated with acute myeloid leukemia. *Saudi Med J* 26:1095–1098, 2005.

271. Kaur H, Ozelo M, Scovil S, et al: Systematic analysis of bleeding phenotype in PT-VWD compared to type 2B VWD using an electronic bleeding questionnaire. *Clin Appl Thromb Hemost* 20:765–771, 2014.

272. Takahashi H: Studies on the pathophysiology and treatment of von Willebrand's disease. IV. Mechanism of increased ristocetin-induced platelet aggregation in von Willebrand's disease. *Thromb Res* 19:857–867, 1980.

273. Krizek DM, Rick ME, Williams SB, Gralnick HR: Cryoprecipitate transfusion in variant von Willebrand's disease and thrombocytopenia. *Ann Intern Med* 98:484–486, 1983.

274. Weiss HJ, Meyer D, Rabinowitz R, et al: Pseudo-von Willebrand's disease. An intrinsic platelet defect with aggregation by unmodified human factor VIII/von Willebrand factor and enhanced adsorption of its high-molecular-weight multimers. *N Engl J Med* 306:326–333, 1982.

275. Miller JL, Castella A: Platelet-type von Willebrand's disease: Characterization of a new bleeding disorder. *Blood* 60:790–794, 1982.

276. Gralnick HR, Williams SB, Shafer BC, Corash L: Factor VIII/von Willebrand factor binding to von Willebrand's disease platelets. *Blood* 60:328–332, 1982.

277. Takahashi H, Handa M, Watanabe K, et al: Further characterization of platelet-type von Willebrand's disease in Japan. *Blood* 64:1254–1262, 1984.

278. Nurden P, Lanza F, Bonnafous-Faurie C, Nurden A: A second report of platelet-type von Willebrand disease with a Gly233Ser mutation in the GPIBA gene. *Thromb Haemost* 97:319–321, 2007.

279. Othman M, Notley C, Lavender FL, et al: Identification and functional characterization of a novel 27-bp deletion in the macroglycopeptide-coding region of the GPIBA gene resulting in platelet-type von Willebrand disease. *Blood* 105:4330–4336, 2005.

280. Enayat MS, Guilliatt AM, Lester W, et al: Distinguishing between type 2B and pseudo-von Willebrand disease and its clinical importance. *Br J Haematol* 133:664–666, 2006.

281. Bryckaert MC, Pietu G, Ruan C, et al: Abnormality of glycoprotein Ib in two cases of "pseudo"-von Willebrand's disease. *J Lab Clin Med* 106:393–400, 1985.

282. Othman M, Kaur H, Emsley J: Platelet-type von Willebrand disease: New insights into the molecular pathophysiology of a unique platelet defect. *Semin Thromb Hemost* 39:663–673, 2013.

283. Othman M, Emsley J: Platelet-type von Willebrand disease: Toward an improved understanding of the "sticky situation." *Semin Thromb Hemost* 40:146–150, 2014.

284. Miller JL, Cunningham D, Lyle VA, Finch CN: Mutation in the gene encoding the alpha chain of platelet glycoprotein Ib in platelet-type von Willebrand disease. *Proc Natl Acad Sci U S A* 88:4761–4765, 1991.

285. Russell SD, Roth GJ: Pseudo-von Willebrand disease: A mutation in the platelet glycoprotein Ib alpha gene associated with a hyperactive surface receptor. *Blood* 81:1787–1791, 1993.

286. Takahashi H, Murata M, Moriki T, et al: Substitution of Val for Met at residue 239 of platelet glycoprotein Ib alpha in Japanese patients with platelet-type von Willebrand disease. *Blood* 85:727–733, 1995.

287. Kunishima S, Heaton DC, Naoe T, et al: De novo mutation of the platelet glycoprotein Ib alpha gene in a patient with pseudo-von Willebrand disease. *Blood Coagul Fibrinolysis* 8:311–315, 1997.

288. Matsubara Y, Murata M, Sugita K, Ikeda Y: Identification of a novel point mutation in platelet glycoprotein Ibalpha, Gly to Ser at residue 233, in a Japanese family with platelet-type von Willebrand disease. *J Thromb Haemost* 1:2198–2205, 2003.

289. Kanaji S, Fahs SA, Ware J, et al: Non-myeloablative conditioning with busulfan before hematopoietic stem cell transplantation leads to phenotypic correction of murine Bernard-Soulier syndrome. *J Thromb Haemost* 12:1726–1732, 2014.

290. Uff S, Clemetson JM, Harrison T, et al: Crystal structure of the platelet glycoprotein Ib(alpha) N-terminal domain reveals an unmasking mechanism for receptor activation. *J Biol Chem* 277:35657–35663, 2002.

291. Huizinga EG, Tsuji S, Romijn RA, et al: Structures of glycoprotein Ibalpha and its complex with von Willebrand factor A1 domain. *Science* 297:1176–1179, 2002.

292. Enayat S, Ravanbod S, Rassoulzadegan M, et al: A novel D235Y mutation in the GP1BA gene enhances platelet interaction with von Willebrand factor in an Iranian family with platelet-type von Willebrand disease. *Thromb Haemost* 108:946–954, 2012.

293. Woods AI, Sanchez-Luceros A, Bermejo E, et al: Identification of p.W246L as a novel mutation in the GP1BA gene responsible for platelet-type von Willebrand disease. *Semin Thromb Hemost* 40:151–160, 2014.

294. Pincus MR, Carty RP, Miller JL: Structural implications of the substitution of Val for Met at residue 239 in the alpha chain of human platelet glycoprotein Ib. *J Protein Chem* 13:629–633, 1994.

295. Dumas JJ, Kumar R, McDonagh T, et al: Crystal structure of the wild-type von Willebrand factor A1-glycoprotein Ibalpha complex reveals conformation differences with a complex bearing von Willebrand disease mutations. *J Biol Chem* 279:23327–23334, 2004.

296. Suva LJ, Hartman E, Dilley JD, et al: Platelet dysfunction and a high bone mass phenotype in a murine model of platelet-type von Willebrand disease. *Am J Pathol* 172:430–439, 2008.

297. Doggett TA, Girdhar G, Lawshe A, et al: Alterations in the intrinsic properties of the GPIbalpha-VWF tether bond define the kinetics of the platelet-type von Willebrand disease mutation, Gly233Val. *Blood* 102:152–160, 2003.

298. Tait AS, Cranmer SL, Jackson SP, et al: Phenotype changes resulting in high-affinity binding of von Willebrand factor to recombinant glycoprotein Ib-IX: Analysis of the platelet-type von Willebrand disease mutations. *Blood* 98:1812–1818, 2001.

299. Takahashi H, Nagayama R, Hattori A, Shibata A: Botrocetin- and polybrene-induced platelet aggregation in platelet-type von Willebrand disease. *Am J Hematol* 18:179–189, 1985.

300. Miller JL, Kupinski JM, Castella A, Ruggeri ZM: Von Willebrand factor binds to platelets and induces aggregation in platelet-type but not type IIB von Willebrand disease. *J Clin Invest* 72:1532–1542, 1983.

301. Scott JP, Montgomery RR: The rapid differentiation of type IIb von Willebrand's disease from platelet-type (pseudo-) von Willebrand's disease by the "neutral" monoclonal antibody binding assay. *Am J Clin Pathol* 96:723–728, 1991.

302. Miller JL: Sorting out heightened interactions between platelets and von Willebrand factor. "IIB or not IIB?" is becoming an increasingly answerable question in the molecular era. *Am J Clin Pathol* 96:681–683, 1991.

303. Miller JL, Ruggeri ZM, Lyle VA: Unique interactions of asialo von Willebrand factor with platelets in platelet-type von Willebrand disease. *Blood* 70:1804–1809, 1987.

304. Hamilton A, Ozelo M, Leggo J, et al: Frequency of platelet type versus type 2B von Willebrand disease. An international registry-based study. *Thromb Haemost* 105:501–508, 2011.

305. Takahashi H: Replacement therapy in platelet-type von Willebrand disease. *Am J Hematol* 18:351–362, 1985.

306. Miller JL: Platelet-type von Willebrand's disease. *Clin Lab Med* 4:319–331, 1984.

307. Poon MC: Factor VIIa, in *Platelets*, 2nd ed, edited by AD Michelson, p 867. Academic Press, San Diego, 2007.

308. Fressinaud E, Signaud-Fiks M, Le Boterff C, Piot B: Use of recombinant factor VIIa (NovoSevenr) for dental extraction in a patient affected by platelet-type (pseudo-) von Willebrand disease. *Haemophilia* 4:299, 1998.

309. Nieuwenhuis HK, Akkerman JW, Houdijk WP, Sixma JJ. Human blood platelets showing no response to collagen fail to express surface glycoprotein Ia. *Nature* 318:470–472, 1985.

310. Nieuwenhuis HK, Sakariassen KS, Houdijk WP, et al: Deficiency of platelet membrane glycoprotein Ia associated with a decreased platelet adhesion to subendothelium: A defect in platelet spreading. *Blood* 68:692–695, 1986.

311. Beer JH, Nieuwenhuis HK, Sixma JJ, Coller BS: Deficiency of antibody 6F1 binding to the platelets of a patient with an isolated defect in platelet-collagen interaction. *Circulation* 78(Suppl):II-308, 1988.

312. Coller BS, Beer JH, Scudder LE, Steinberg MH: Collagen-platelet interactions: Evidence for a direct interaction of collagen with platelet GPIa/IIa and an indirect interaction with platelet GPIIb/IIIa mediated by adhesive proteins. *Blood* 74:182–192, 1989.

313. Kehrel B, Balleisen L, Kokott R, et al: Deficiency of intact thrombospondin and membrane glycoprotein Ia in platelets with defective collagen-induced aggregation and spontaneous loss of disorder. *Blood* 71:1074–1078, 1988.

314. Kunicki TJ, Williams SA, Nugent DJ: Genetic variants that affect platelet function. *Curr Opin Hematol* 19:371–379, 2012.

315. Habart D, Cheli Y, Nugent DJ, et al: Conditional knockout of integrin alpha2beta1 in murine megakaryocytes leads to reduced mean platelet volume. *PLoS One* 8:e55094, 2013.

316. McCall-Culbreath KD, Zutter MM: Collagen receptor integrins: Rising to the challenge. *Curr Drug Targets* 9:139–149, 2008.

317. Yamamoto N, Ikeda H, Tandon NN, et al: A platelet membrane glycoprotein (GP) deficiency in healthy blood donors: Naka-platelets lack detectable GPIV (CD36). *Blood* 76:1698–1703, 1990.

318. Curtis BR, Aster RH: Incidence of the Nak(a)-negative platelet phenotype in African Americans is similar to that of Asians. *Transfusion* 36:331–334, 1996.

319. Zhu W, Li W, Silverstein RL: Advanced glycation end products induce a prothrombotic phenotype in mice via interaction with platelet CD36. *Blood* 119:6136–6144, 2012.

320. Asch AS, Barnwell J, Silverstein RL, Nachman RL: Isolation of the thrombospondin membrane receptor. *J Clin Invest* 79:1054–1061, 1987.

321. Tandon NN, Kralisz U, Jamieson GA: Identification of glycoprotein IV (CD36) as a primary receptor for platelet-collagen adhesion. *J Biol Chem* 264:7576–7583, 1989.

322. Wang Y, Fang C, Gao H, et al: Platelet-derived S100 family member myeloid-related protein-14 regulates thrombosis. *J Clin Invest* 124:2160–2171, 2014.

323. Matsuno K, Diaz-Ricart M, Montgomery RR, et al: Inhibition of platelet adhesion to collagen by monoclonal anti-CD36 antibodies. *Br J Haematol* 92:960–967, 1996.

324. Silverstein RL, Asch AS, Nachman RL: Glycoprotein IV mediates thrombospondin-dependent platelet-monocyte and platelet-U937 cell adhesion. *J Clin Invest* 84:546–552, 1989.

325. Kehrel B, Kronenberg A, Schwippert B, et al: Thrombospondin binds normally to glycoprotein IIIb deficient platelets. *Biochem Biophys Res Commun* 179:985–991, 1991.

326. Tandon NN, Ockenhouse CF, Greco NJ, Jamieson GA: Adhesive functions of platelets lacking glycoprotein IV (CD36). *Blood* 78:2809–2813, 1991.

327. Saelman EU, Kehrel B, Hese KM, et al: Platelet adhesion to collagen and endothelial cell matrix under flow conditions is not dependent on platelet glycoprotein IV. *Blood* 83:3240–3244, 1994.

328. Kuijpers MJ, de Witt S, Nergiz-Unal R, et al: Supporting roles of platelet thrombospondin-1 and CD36 in thrombus formation on collagen. *Arterioscler Thromb Vasc Biol* 34:1187–1192, 2014.

329. Englyst NA, Taube JM, Aitman TJ, et al: A novel role for CD36 in VLDL-enhanced platelet activation. *Diabetes* 52:1248–1255, 2003.

330. Ghosh A, Murugesan G, Chen K, et al: Platelet CD36 surface expression levels affect functional responses to oxidized LDL and are associated with inheritance of specific genetic polymorphisms. *Blood* 117:6355–6366, 2011.

331. Kashiwagi H, Tomiyama Y, Honda S, et al: Molecular basis of CD36 deficiency. Evidence that a 478C—>T substitution (proline90—>serine) in CD36 cDNA accounts for CD36 deficiency. *J Clin Invest* 95:1040–1046, 1995.

332. Hirano K, Kuwasako T, Nakagawa-Toyama Y, et al: Pathophysiology of human genetic CD36 deficiency. *Trends Cardiovasc Med* 13:136–141, 2003.

333. Febbraio M, Silverstein RL: CD36: Implications in cardiovascular disease. *Int J Biochem Cell Biol* 39:2012–2030, 2007.

334. Kashiwagi H, Tomiyama Y, Kosugi S, et al: Family studies of type II CD36 deficient subjects: Linkage of a CD36 allele to a platelet-specific mRNA expression defect(s) causing type II CD36 deficiency. *Thromb Haemost* 74:758–763, 1995.

335. Ikeda H: Platelet membrane protein CD36. *Hokkaido Igaku Zasshi* 74:99–104, 1999.

336. Kashiwagi H, Tomiyama Y, Kosugi S, et al: Identification of molecular defects in a subject with type I CD36 deficiency. *Blood* 83:3545–3552, 1994.

337. Kashiwagi H, Tomiyama Y, Nozaki S, et al: A single nucleotide insertion in codon 317 of the CD36 gene leads to CD36 deficiency. *Arterioscler Thromb Vasc Biol* 16:1026–1032, 1996.

338. Hanawa H, Watanabe K, Nakamura T, et al: Identification of cryptic splice site, exon skipping, and novel point mutations in type I CD36 deficiency. *J Med Genet* 39:286–291, 2002.

339. Bierling P, Godeau B, Fromont P, et al: Posttransfusion purpura-like syndrome associated with CD36 (Naka) isoimmunization. *Transfusion* 35:777–782, 1995.

340. Morishita K, Wakamoto S, Miyazaki T, et al: Life-threatening adverse reaction followed by thrombocytopenia after passive transfusion of fresh frozen plasma containing anti-CD36 (Nak) isoantibody. *Transfusion (Paris)* 45:803–806, 2005.

341. Moroi M, Jung SM, Okuma M, Shinmyozu K: A patient with platelets deficient in glycoprotein VI that lack both collagen-induced aggregation and adhesion. *J Clin Invest* 84:1440–1445, 1989.

342. Ryo R, Yoshida A, Sugano W, et al: Deficiency of P62, a putative collagen receptor, in platelets from a patient with defective collagen-induced platelet aggregation. *Am J Hematol* 39:25–31, 1992.

343. Nurden P, Jandrot-Perrus M, Combrie R, et al: Severe deficiency of glycoprotein VI in a patient with gray platelet syndrome. *Blood* 104:107–114, 2004.

344. Arai M, Yamamoto N, Moroi M, et al: Platelets with 10% of the normal amount of glycoprotein VI have an impaired response to collagen that results in a mild bleeding tendency. *Br J Haematol* 89:124–130, 1995.

345. Arthur JF, Dunkley S, Andrews RK: Platelet glycoprotein VI-related clinical defects. *Br J Haematol* 139:363–372, 2007.

346. Chu XX, Hou M: [Advances in the studies of platelet glycoprotein VI (GPVI): Review] [in Chinese]. *Zhongguo Shi Yan Xue Ye Xue Za Zhi* 14:1040–1044, 2006.

347. Bellucci S, Huisse MG, Boval B, et al: Defective collagen-induced platelet activation in two patients with malignant haemopathies is related to a defect in the GPVI-coupled signalling pathway. *Thromb Haemost* 93:130–138, 2005.

348. Kojima H, Moroi M, Jung SM, et al: Characterization of a patient with glycoprotein (GP) VI deficiency possessing neither anti-GPVI autoantibody nor genetic aberration. *J Thromb Haemost* 4:2433–2442, 2006.

349. Dunkley S, Arthur JF, Evans S, et al: A familial platelet function disorder associated with abnormal signalling through the glycoprotein VI pathway. *Br J Haematol* 137:569–577, 2007.

350. Hermans C, Wittevrongel C, Thys C, et al: A compound heterozygous mutation in glycoprotein VI in a patient with a bleeding disorder. *J Thromb Haemost* 7:1356–1363, 2009.

351. Sugiyama T, Okuma M, Ushikubi F, et al: A novel platelet aggregating factor found in a patient with defective collagen-induced platelet aggregation and autoimmune thrombocytopenia. *Blood* 69:1712–1720, 1987.

352. Takahashi H, Moroi M: Antibody against platelet membrane glycoprotein VI in a patient with systemic lupus erythematosus. *Am J Hematol* 67:262–267, 2001.

353. Boylan B, Chen H, Rathore V, et al: Anti-GPVI-associated ITP: An acquired platelet disorder caused by autoantibody-mediated clearance of the GPVI/FcRγ-chain complex from the human platelet surface. *Blood* 104:1350–1355, 2004.

354. Akiyama M, Kashiwagi H, Todo K, et al: Presence of platelet-associated anti-GPVI autoantibodies and restoration of GPVI expression in patients with GPVI deficiency. *J Thromb Haemost* 2009.

355. Nieswandt B, Schulte V, Bergmeier W, et al: Long-term antithrombotic protection by in vivo depletion of platelet glycoprotein VI in mice. *J Exp Med* 193:459–469, 2001.

356. Dumont B, Lasne D, Rothschild C, et al: Absence of collagen-induced platelet activation caused by compound heterozygous GPVI mutations. *Blood* 114:1900–1903, 2009.

357. Matus V, Valenzuela G, Saez CG, et al: An adenine insertion in exon 6 of human GP6 generates a truncated protein associated with a bleeding disorder in four Chilean families. *J Thromb Haemost* 11:1751–1759, 2013.

358. Weiss HJ, Chervenick PA, Zalusky R, Factor A: A familial defect in platelet function associated with impaired release of adenosine diphosphate. *N Engl J Med* 281:1264–1270, 1969.

359. Holmsen H, Weiss HJ: Hereditary defect in the platelet release reaction caused by a deficiency in the storage pool of platelet adenine nucleotides. *Br J Haematol* 19:643–649, 1970.

360. Holmsen H: Secretable storage pools in platelets. *Annu Rev Med* 30:119–134, 1979.

361. Huizing M, Helip-Wooley A, Westbroek W, et al: Disorders of lysosome-related organelle biogenesis: Clinical and molecular genetics. *Annu Rev Genomics Hum Genet* 9:359–386, 2008.

362. Hermansky F, Pudlak P: Albinism associated with hemorrhagic diathesis and unusual pigmented reticular cells in the bone marrow: Report of two cases with histochemical studies. *Blood* 14:162, 1959.

363. Gahl WA, Brantly M, Kaiser-Kupfer MI, et al: Genetic defects and clinical characteristics of patients with a form of oculocutaneous albinism (Hermansky-Pudlak syndrome). *N Engl J Med* 338:1258–1264, 1998.

364. Wei ML: Hermansky-Pudlak syndrome: A disease of protein trafficking and organelle function. *Pigment Cell Res* 19:19–42, 2006.

365. Gunay-Aygun M, Huizing M, Gahl WA: Molecular defects that affect platelet dense granules. *Semin Thromb Hemost* 30:537–547, 2004.

366. Shiflett SL, Kaplan J, Ward DM: Chédiak-Higashi syndrome: A rare disorder of lysosomes and lysosome related organelles. *Pigment Cell Res* 15:251–257, 2002.

367. Grottum KA, Hovig T, Holmsen H, et al: Wiskott-Aldrich syndrome: Qualitative platelet defects and short platelet survival. *Br J Haematol* 17:373–388, 1969.

368. Stormorken H, Hellum B, Egeland T, et al: X-linked thrombocytopenia and thrombocytopathia: Attenuated Wiskott- Aldrich syndrome. Functional and morphological studies of platelets and lymphocytes. *Thromb Haemost* 65:300–305, 1991.

369. Onel D, Ulutin SB, Ulutin ON: Platelet defect in a case of Ehlers-Danlos syndrome. *Acta Haematol* 50:238–244, 1973.

370. Hathaway WE, Solomons CC, Ott JE: Platelet function and pyrophosphates in osteogenesis imperfecta. *Blood* 39:500–509, 1972.

371. Day HJ, Holmsen H: Platelet adenine nucleotide "storage pool deficiency" in thrombocytopenia absent radii syndrome. *JAMA* 221:1053, 1972.

372. Weiss HJ, Witte LD, Kaplan KL, et al: Heterogeneity in storage pool deficiency: Studies on granule-bound substances in 18 patients including variants deficient in alpha-granules, platelet factor 4, beta-thromboglobulin, and platelet-derived growth factor. *Blood* 54:1296–1319, 1979.

373. Seward SL Jr, Gahl WA: Hermansky-Pudlak syndrome: Health care throughout life. *Pediatrics* 132:153–160, 2013.

374. Bonifacino JS: Insights into the biogenesis of lysosome-related organelles from the study of the Hermansky-Pudlak syndrome. *Ann N Y Acad Sci* 1038:103–114, 2004.

375. White JG: Inherited abnormalities of the platelet membrane and secretory granules. *Hum Pathol* 18:123–139, 1987.

376. Nishibori M, Cham B, McNicol A, et al: The protein CD63 is in platelet dense granules, is deficient in a patient with Hermansky-Pudlak syndrome, and appears identical to granulophysin. *J Clin Invest* 91:1775–1782, 1993.

377. Huizing M, Boissy RE, Gahl WA: Hermansky-Pudlak syndrome: Vesicle formation from yeast to man. *Pigment Cell Res* 15:405–419, 2002.

378. Huizing M, Parkes JM, Helip-Wooley A, et al: Platelet alpha granules in BLOC-2 and BLOC-3 subtypes of Hermansky-Pudlak syndrome. *Platelets* 18:150–157, 2007.

379. Hermos CR, Huizing M, Kaiser-Kupfer MI, Gahl WA: Hermansky-Pudlak syndrome type 1: Gene organization, novel mutations, and clinical-molecular review of non-Puerto Rican cases. *Hum Mutat* 20:482, 2002.

380. Carmona-Rivera C, Hess RA, O'Brien K, et al: Novel mutations in the HPS1 gene among Puerto Rican patients. *Clin Genet* 79:561–567, 2011.

381. Dell'Angelica EC, Shotelersuk V, Aguilar RC, et al: Altered trafficking of lysosomal proteins in Hermansky-Pudlak syndrome due to mutations in the beta 3A subunit of the AP-3 adaptor. *Mol Cell* 3:11–21, 1999.

382. Huizing M, Anikster Y, Fitzpatrick DL, et al: Hermansky-Pudlak syndrome type 3 in Ashkenazi Jews and other non-Puerto Rican patients with hypopigmentation and platelet storage-pool deficiency. *Am J Hum Genet.* 69:1022–1032, 2001.

383. Anderson PD, Huizing M, Claassen DA, et al: Hermansky-Pudlak syndrome type 4 (HPS-4): Clinical and molecular characteristics. *Hum Genet* 113:10–17, 2003.

384. Huizing M, Helip-Wooley A, Dorward H, et al: Hermansky-Pudlak syndrome: A model for abnormal vesicle formation and trafficking. *Pigment Cell Res* 16:584, 2003.

385. Zhang Q, Zhao B, Li W, et al: Ru2 and Ru encode mouse orthologs of the genes mutated in human Hermansky-Pudlak syndrome types 5 and 6. *Nat Genet* 33:145–153, 2003.

386. Li W, Zhang Q, Oiso N, et al: Hermansky-Pudlak syndrome type 7 (HPS-7) results from mutant dysbindin, a member of the biogenesis of lysosome-related organelles complex 1 (BLOC-1). *Nat Genet* 35:84–89, 2003.

387. Morgan NV, Pasha S, Johnson CA, et al: A germline mutation in BLOC1S3/reduced pigmentation causes a novel variant of Hermansky-Pudlak syndrome (HPS8). *Am J Hum Genet* 78:160–166, 2006.

388. Helip-Wooley A, Westbroek W, Dorward HM, et al: Improper trafficking of melanocyte-specific proteins in Hermansky-Pudlak syndrome type-5. *J Invest Dermatol* 127:1471–1478, 2007.

389. Cullinane AR, Curry JA, Carmona-Rivera C, et al: A BLOC-1 mutation screen reveals that PLDN is mutated in Hermansky-Pudlak Syndrome type 9. *Am J Hum Genet* 88:778–787, 2011.

390. Michaud J, Wu F, Osato M, et al: In vitro analyses of known and novel RUNX1/AML1 mutations in dominant familial platelet disorder with predisposition to acute myelogenous leukemia: Implications for mechanisms of pathogenesis. *Blood* 99:1364–1372, 2002.

391. Connelly JP, Kwon EM, Gao Y, et al: Targeted correction of RUNX1 mutation in FPD patient-specific induced pluripotent stem cells rescues megakaryopoietic defects. *Blood* 124:1926–1930, 2014.

392. Weiss HJ: Inherited disorders of platelet granules and signal transduction, in *Hemostasis and Thrombosis: Basic Principles and Clinical Practice*, 3rd ed, edited by RW Colman, J Hirsh, VJ Marder, M Samama, pp 673–684. Lippincott, Philadelphia, 1993.

393. Payne CM: A qualitative ultrastructural evaluation of the cell organelle specificity of the uranaffin reaction to normal human platelets. *Am J Clin Pathol* 31:62, 1984.

394. Weiss HJ, Lages B, Vicic W, et al: Heterogeneous abnormalities of platelet dense granule ultrastructure in 20 patients with congenital storage pool deficiency. *Br J Haematol* 83:282–295, 1993.

395. Masliah-Planchon J, Darnige L, Bellucci S: Molecular determinants of platelet delta storage pool deficiencies: An update. *Br J Haematol* 160:5–11, 2013.

396. Akkerman JW, Nieuwenhuis HK, Mommersteeg-Leautaud ME, et al: ATP-ADP compartmentation in storage pool deficient platelets: Correlation between granule-bound ADP and the bleeding time. *Br J Haematol* 55:135–143, 1983.

397. Cattaneo M, Lecchi A, Agati B, et al: Evaluation of platelet function with the PFA-100 system in patients with congenital defects of platelet secretion. *Thromb Res* 96:213–217, 1999.

398. Harrison C, Khair K, Baxter B, et al: Hermansky-Pudlak syndrome: Infrequent bleeding and first report of Turkish and Pakistani kindreds. *Arch Dis Child* 86:297–301, 2002.

399. Hayward CP, Harrison P, Cattaneo M, et al: Platelet function analyzer (PFA)-100 closure time in the evaluation of platelet disorders and platelet function. *J Thromb Haemost* 4:312–319, 2006.

400. Cattaneo M: Light transmission aggregometry and ATP release for the diagnostic assessment of platelet function. *Semin Thromb Hemost* 35:158–167, 2009.

401. Akkerman JWN, Nieuwenhuis HK, Mommersteeg-Leautaud ME, et al: ATP-ADP compartmentation in storage pool deficient platelets: Correlation between granule-bound ADP and the bleeding time. *Br J Haematol* 55:135–143, 1983.

402. Weiss HJ, Tschopp TB, Rogers J, Brand H: Studies of platelet 5-hydroxytryptamine (serotonin) in storage pool disease and albinism. *J Clin Invest* 54:421–433, 1974.

403. Weiss HJ, Lages B: Platelet malondialdehyde production and aggregation responses induced by arachidonate, prostaglandin-G2, collagen, and epinephrine in 12 patients with storage pool deficiency. *Blood* 58:27–33, 1981.

404. Witkop CJ Jr, Bowie EJ, Krumwiede MD, et al: Synergistic effect of storage pool deficient platelets and low plasma von Willebrand factor on the severity of the hemorrhagic diathesis in Hermansky-Pudlak syndrome. *Am J Hematol* 44:256–259, 1993.

405. McKeown LP, Hansmann KE, Wilson O, et al: Platelet von Willebrand factor in Hermansky-Pudlak syndrome. *Am J Hematol* 59:115–120, 1998.

406. White JG: Electron opaque structures in human platelets: Which are or are not dense bodies? *Platelets* 19:455–466, 2008.

407. Lorez HP, Richards JG, Da Prada M, et al: Storage pool disease: Comparative fluorescence microscopical, cytochemical and biochemical studies on amine-storing organelles of human blood platelets. *Br J Haematol* 43:297–305, 1979.

408. Gordon N, Thom J, Cole C, Baker R: Rapid detection of hereditary and acquired platelet storage pool deficiency by flow cytometry. *Br J Haematol* 89:117–123, 1995.

409. Nazarian R, Huizing M, Helip-Wooley A, et al: An immunoblotting assay to facilitate the molecular diagnosis of Hermansky-Pudlak syndrome. *Mol Genet Metab* 93:134–144, 2008.

410. Gahl WA, Brantly M, Troendle J, et al: Effect of pirfenidone on the pulmonary fibrosis of Hermansky-Pudlak syndrome. *Mol Genet Metab* 76:234–242, 2002.

411. O'Brien K, Troendle J, Gochuico BR, et al: Pirfenidone for the treatment of Hermansky-Pudlak syndrome pulmonary fibrosis. *Mol Genet Metab* 103:128–134, 2011.

412. Nurden AT, Nurden P: The gray platelet syndrome: Clinical spectrum of the disease. *Blood Rev* 21:21–36, 2007.

413. Nurden AT, Nurden P, Bermejo E, et al: Phenotypic heterogeneity in the Gray platelet syndrome extends to the expression of TREM family member, TLT-1. *Thromb Haemost* 100:45–51, 2008.

414. Raccuglia G: Gray platelet syndrome: A variety of qualitative platelet disorder. *Am J Med* 51:818, 1971.

415. Maynard DM, Heijnen HF, Gahl WA, Gunay-Aygun M: The alpha granule proteome: Novel proteins in normal and ghost granules in gray platelet syndrome. *J Thromb Haemost* 8:1786–1796, 2010.

416. Zufferey A, Schvartz D, Nolli S, et al: Characterization of the platelet granule proteome: Evidence of the presence of MHC1 in alpha-granules. *J Proteomics* 101:130–140, 2014.

417. Aneja K, Jalagadugula G, Mao G, et al: Mechanism of platelet factor 4 (PF4) deficiency with RUNX1 haplodeficiency: RUNX1 is a transcriptional regulator of PF4. *J Thromb Haemost* 9:383–391, 2011.

418. Tubman VN, Levine JE, Campagna DR, et al: X-linked gray platelet syndrome due to a GATA1 Arg216Gln mutation. *Blood* 109:3297–3299, 2007.

419. Monteferrario D, Bolar NA, Marneth AE, et al: A dominant-negative GFI1B mutation in the gray platelet syndrome. *N Engl J Med* 370:245–253, 2014.

420. Stevenson WS, Morel-Kopp MC, Chen Q, et al: GFI1B mutation causes a bleeding disorder with abnormal platelet function. *J Thromb Haemost* 11:2039–2047, 2013.

421. Deppermann C, Cherpokova D, Nurden P, et al: Gray platelet syndrome and defective thrombo-inflammation in Nbeal2-deficient mice. *J Clin Invest* 123:3331–3342, 2013.

422. Kahr WH, Lo RW, Li L, et al: Abnormal megakaryocyte development and platelet function in Nbeal2(−/−) mice. *Blood* 122:3349–3358, 2013.

423. Lo B, Li L, Gissen P, et al: Requirement of VPS33B, a member of the Sec1/Munc18 protein family, in megakaryocyte and platelet alpha-granule biogenesis. *Blood* 106:4159–4166, 2005.

424. Urban D, Li L, Christensen H, et al: The VPS33B binding protein VPS16B is required in megakaryocyte and platelet alpha-granule biogenesis. *Blood* 120:5032–5040, 2012.

425. Srivastava PC, Powling MJ, Nokes TJ, et al: Grey platelet syndrome: Studies on platelet alpha-granules, lysosomes and defective response to thrombin. *Br J Haematol* 65:441–446, 1987.

426. Greenberg-Sepersky SM, Simons ER, White JG: Studies of platelets from patients with the grey platelet syndrome. *Br J Haematol* 59:603–609, 1985.

427. Lages B, Sussman II, Levine SP, et al: Platelet alpha granule deficiency associated with decreased P-selectin and selective impairment of thrombin-induced activation in a new patient with gray platelet syndrome (alpha-storage pool deficiency). *J Lab Clin Med* 129:364–375, 1997.

428. Rendu F, Marche P, Hovig T, et al: Abnormal phosphoinositide metabolism and protein phosphorylation in platelets from a patient with the grey platelet syndrome. *Br J Haematol* 67:199–206, 1987.

429. Baruch D, Lindhout T, Dupuy E, Caen JP: Thrombin-induced platelet factor Va formation in patients with a gray platelet syndrome. *Thromb Haemost* 58:768–771, 1987.

430. Enouf J, Lebret M, Bredoux R, et al: Abnormal calcium transport into microsomes of grey platelet syndrome. *Br J Haematol* 65:437–440, 1987.

431. Jantunen E, Hanninen A, Naukkarinen A, et al: Gray platelet syndrome with splenomegaly and signs of extramedullary hematopoiesis: A case report with review of the literature. *Am J Hematol* 46:218–224, 1994.

432. Caen JP, Deschamps JF, Bodevin E, et al: Megakaryocytes and myelofibrosis in gray platelet syndrome. *Nouv Rev Fr Hematol* 29:109–114, 1987.

433. Coller BS, Hultin MB, Nurden AT: Isolated alpha-granule deficiency (gray platelet syndrome) with slight increase in bone marrow reticulin and possible glycoprotein and/or protease defect. *Thromb Haemost* 50:211, 1983.

434. Falik-Zaccai TC, Anikster Y, Rivera CE, et al: A new genetic isolate of gray platelet syndrome (GPS): Clinical, cellular, and hematologic characteristics. *Mol Genet Metab* 74:303–313, 2001.

435. Lages B, Shattil SJ, Bainton DF, Weiss HJ: Decreased content and surface expression of alpha-granule membrane protein GMP-140 in one of two types of platelet alpha delta storage pool deficiency. *J Clin Invest* 87:919–929, 1991.

436. Lages B, Sussman, II, et al: Platelet alpha granule deficiency associated with decreased P-selectin and selective impairment of thrombin-induced activation in a new patient with gray platelet syndrome (alpha-storage pool deficiency). *J Lab Clin Med* 129:364–375, 1997.

437. Blavignac J, Bunimov N, Rivard GE, Hayward CP: Quebec platelet disorder: Update on pathogenesis, diagnosis, and treatment. *Semin Thromb Hemost* 37:713–720, 2011.

438. Hayward CPM, Rivard GE, Kane WH: An autosomal dominant, qualitative platelet disorder associated with multimerin deficiency, abnormalities in platelet factor V, thrombospondin, von Willebrand factor, and fibrinogen, and an epinephrine aggregation defect. *Blood* 87:4967–4978, 1996.

439. Tracy PB, Giles AR, Mann KG, et al: Factor V (Quebec): A bleeding diathesis associated with a qualitative platelet Factor V deficiency. *J Clin Invest* 74:1221–1228, 1984.

440. Hayward CP, Rivard GE, Kane WH, et al: An autosomal dominant, qualitative platelet disorder associated with multimerin deficiency, abnormalities in platelet factor V, thrombospondin, von Willebrand factor, and fibrinogen and an epinephrine aggregation defect. *Blood* 87:4967–4978, 1996.

441. Veljkovic DK, Rivard GE, Diamandis M, et al: Increased expression of urokinase plasminogen activator in Quebec platelet disorder is linked to megakaryocyte differentiation. *Blood* 113:1535–1542, 2009.

442. Diamandis M, Paterson AD, Rommens JM, et al: Quebec platelet disorder is linked to the urokinase plasminogen activator gene (PLAU) and increases expression of the linked allele in megakaryocytes. *Blood* 113:1543–1546, 2009.

443. Rao AK: Hereditary disorders of platelet secretion and signal transduction, in *Hemostasis and Thrombosis: Basic Principles and Clinical Practice*, 5th ed, edited by RW Colman, VJ Marder, AW Clowes, JN George, SZ Goldhaber, pp 961–974. Lippincott Williams & Wilkins, Philadelphia, 2006.

444. Rao AK, Jalagadugula G, Sun L: Inherited defects in platelet signaling mechanisms. *Semin Thromb Hemost* 30:525–535, 2004.

445. Cattaneo M: Inherited platelet-based bleeding disorders. *J Thromb Haemost* 1: 1628–1636, 2003.

446. Rao AK: Inherited platelet function disorders: Overview and disorders of granules, secretion, and signal transduction. *Hematol Oncol Clin North Am* 27:585–611, 2013.

447. Hirata T, Ushikubi F, Kakizuka A, et al: Two thromboxane A2 receptor isoforms in human platelets. Opposite coupling to adenylyl cyclase with different sensitivity to Arg60 to Leu mutation. *J Clin Invest* 97:949–956, 1996.

448. Hirata T, Kakizuka A, Ushikubi F, et al: Arg60 to Leu mutation of the human thromboxane A2 receptor in a dominantly inherited bleeding disorder. *J Clin Invest* 94: 1662–1667, 1994.

449. Higuchi W, Fuse I, Hattori A, Aizawa Y: Mutations of the platelet thromboxane A2 (TXA2) receptor in patients characterized by the absence of TXA2-induced platelet aggregation despite normal TXA2 binding activity. *Thromb Haemost* 82:1528–1531, 1999.

450. Mumford AD, Dawood BB, Daly ME, et al: A novel thromboxane A2 receptor D304N variant that abrogates ligand binding in a patient with a bleeding diathesis. *Blood* 115:363–369, 2010.

451. Gachet C: P2 receptors, platelet function and pharmacological implications. *Thromb Haemost* 99:466–472, 2008.

452. Cattaneo M, Lecchi A, Randi AM, et al: Identification of a new congenital defect of platelet function characterized by severe impairment of platelet responses to adenosine diphosphate. *Blood* 80:2787–2796, 1992.

453. Nurden P, Savi P, Heilmann E, et al: An inherited bleeding disorder linked to a defective interaction between ADP and its receptor on platelets. Its influence on glycoprotein IIb-IIIa complex function. *J Clin Invest* 95:1612–1622, 1995.

454. Shiraga M, Miyata S, Kato H, et al: Impaired platelet function in a patient with P2Y12 deficiency caused by a mutation in the translation initiation codon. *J Thromb Haemost* 3:2315–2323, 2005.

455. Daly ME, Dawood BB, Lester WA, et al: Identification and characterization of a novel P2Y 12 variant in a patient diagnosed with type 1 von Willebrand disease in the European MCMDM-1VWD study. *Blood* 113:4110–4113, 2009.

456. Cattaneo M: The platelet P2Y12 receptor for adenosine diphosphate: Congenital and drug-induced defects. *Blood* 117: 2102–2012, 2011.

457. Cattaneo M, Zighetti ML, Lombardi R, et al: Molecular bases of defective signal transduction in the platelet P2Y12 receptor of a patient with congenital bleeding. *Proc Natl Acad Sci U S A* 100:1978–1983, 2003.

458. Cattaneo M, Lombardi R, Zighetti ML, et al: Deficiency of (33)P-2MeS-ADP binding sites on platelets with secretion defect, normal granule stores and normal thromboxane A2 production. *Thromb Haemost* 77:986–990, 1997.

459. Cattaneo M, Lecchi A, Lombardi R, et al: Platelets from a patient heterozygous for the defect of P2(CYC) receptors for ADP have a secretion defect despite normal thromboxane A(2) production and normal granule stores: Further evidence that some cases of platelet "primary secretion defect" are heterozygous for a defect of P2(CYC) receptors. *Arterioscler Thromb Vasc Biol* 20:E101–E106, 2000.

460. Hollopeter G, Jantzen HM, Vincent D, et al: Identification of the platelet ADP receptor targeted by antithrombotic drugs. *Nature* 409:202–207, 2001.

461. Remijn JA, Ijsseldijk MJ, Strunk AL, et al: Novel molecular defect in the platelet ADP receptor P2Y12 of a patient with haemorrhagic diathesis. *Clin Chem Lab Med* 45: 187–189, 2007.

462. Cunningham MR, Nisar SP, Cooke AE, et al: Differential endosomal sorting of a novel P2Y12 purinoreceptor mutant. *Traffic* 14:585–598, 2013.

463. Oury C, Toth-Zsamboki E, Van Geet C, et al: A natural dominant negative P2X1 receptor due to deletion of a single amino acid residue. *J Biol Chem* 275:22611–22614, 2000.

464. Scrutton MC, Clare KA, Hutton RA, Bruckdorfer KR: Depressed responsiveness to adrenaline in platelets from apparently normal human donors: A familial trait. *Br J Haematol* 49:303–314, 1981.

465. Rao AK, Willis J, Kowalska MA, et al: Differential requirements for platelet aggregation and inhibition of adenylate cyclase by epinephrine. Studies of a familial platelet alpha 2-adrenergic receptor defect. *Blood* 71:494–501, 1988.

466. Tamponi G, Pannocchia A, Arduino C, et al: Congenital deficiency of alpha-2-adrenoceptors on human platelets: Description of two cases. *Thromb Haemost* 58: 1012–1016, 1987.

467. Pelczar-Wissner CJ, McDonald EG, Sussman II: Absence of platelet activating factor (PAF) mediated platelet aggregation: A new platelet defect. *Am J Hematol* 16:419–422, 1984.

468. Gabbeta J, Yang X, Kowalska MA, et al: Platelet signal transduction defect with Galpha subunit dysfunction and diminished Galphaq in a patient with abnormal platelet responses. *Proc Natl Acad Sci U S A* 94:8750–8755, 1997.

469. Rao AK, Koike K, Willis J, et al: Platelet secretion defect associated with impaired liberation of arachidonic acid and normal hemosyn light chain phosphorylation. *Blood* 64:914–921, 1984.

470. Gabbeta J, Vaidyula VR, Dhanasekaran DN, Rao AK: Human platelet Gaq deficiency is associated with decreased Gaq gene expression in platelets but not neutrophils. *Thromb Haemost* 87:129–133, 2002.

471. Freson K, Hoylaerts MF, Jaeken J, et al: Genetic variation of the extra-large stimulatory G protein alpha-subunit leads to Gs hyperfunction in platelets and is a risk factor for bleeding. *Thromb Haemost* 86:733–738, 2001.

472. Freson K, Thys C, Wittevrongel C, et al: Pseudohypoparathyroidism type Ib with disturbed imprinting in the GNAS1 cluster and Gsalpha deficiency in platelets. *Hum Mol Genet* 11:2741–2750, 2002.

473. Patel YM, Patel K, Rahman S, et al: Evidence for a role for Galphai1 in mediating weak agonist-induced platelet aggregation in human platelets: Reduced Galphai1 expression and defective Gi signaling in the platelets of a patient with a chronic bleeding disorder. *Blood* 101:4828–4835, 2003.

474. Dawood BB, Lowe GC, Lordkipanidze M, et al: Evaluation of participants with suspected heritable platelet function disorders including recommendation and validation of a streamlined agonist panel. *Blood* 120:5041–5049, 2012.

475. Canault M, Ghalloussi D, Grosdidier C, et al: Human CalDAG-GEFI gene (RASGRP2) mutation affects platelet function and causes severe bleeding. *J Exp Med* 211:1349–1362, 2014.

476. Lages B, Weiss HJ: Heterogeneous defects of platelet secretion and responses to weak agonists in patients with bleeding disorders. *Br J Haematol* 68:53–62, 1988.

477. Koike K, Rao AK, Holmsen H, Mueller PS: Platelet secretion defect in patients with the attention deficit disorder and easy bruising. *Blood* 63:427–433, 1984.

478. Yang X, Sun L, Gabbeta J, Rao AK: Platelet activation with combination of ionophore A23187 and a direct protein kinase C activator induces normal secretion in patients with impaired receptor mediated secretion and abnormal signal transduction. *Thromb Res* 88:317–328, 1997.

479. Yang X, Sun L, Ghosh S, Rao AK: Human platelet signaling defect characterized by impaired production of inositol-1,4,5-triphosphate and phosphatidic acid and diminished Pleckstrin phosphorylation: Evidence for defective phospholipase C activation. *Blood* 88:1676–1683, 1996.

480. Lee SB, Rao AK, Lee KH, et al: Decreased expression of phospholipase C-beta 2 isozyme in human platelets with impaired function. *Blood* 88:1684–1691, 1996.

481. Sun L, Mao G, Rao AK: Association of CBFA2 mutation with decreased platelet PKC-theta and impaired receptor-mediated activation of GPIIb-IIIa and pleckstrin phosphorylation: Proteins regulated by CBFA2 play a role in GPIIb-IIIa activation. *Blood* 103:948–954, 2004.

482. Lages B, Weiss HJ: Impairment of phosphatidylinositol metabolism in a patient with a bleeding disorder associated with defects of initial platelet responses. *Thromb Haemost* 59:175–179, 1988.

483. Speiser-Ellerton S, Weiss HJ: Studies on platelet protein phosphorylation in patients with impaired responses to platelet agonists. *J Lab Clin Med* 115:104–111, 1990.

484. Mao GF, Vaidyula VR, Kunapuli SP, Rao AK: Lineage-specific defect in gene expression in human platelet phospholipase C-beta2 deficiency. *Blood* 99:905–911, 2002.

485. Holmsen H, Walsh PN, Koike K, et al: Familial bleeding disorder associated with deficiencies in platelet signal processing and glycoproteins. *Br J Haematol* 67:335–344, 1987.

486. Cartwright I, Hampton KK, Macneil S, et al: A haemorrhagic platelet disorder associated with altered stimulus-response coupling and abnormal membrane phospholipid composition. *Br J Haematol* 88:129–136, 1994.

487. Fuse I, Mito M, Hattori A, et al: Defective signal transduction induced by thromboxane A2 in a patient with a mild bleeding disorder: Impaired phospholipase C activation despite normal phospholipase A2 activation. *Blood* 81:994–1000, 1993.

488. Mitsui T: Defective signal transduction through the thromboxane A2 receptor in a patient with a mild bleeding disorder. Deficiency of the inositol 1,4,5-triphosphate formation despite normal G-protein activation. *Thromb Haemost* 77:991–995, 1997.

489. Gabbeta J, Yang X, Sun L, et al: Abnormal inside-out signal transduction-dependent activation of glycoprotein IIb-IIIa in a patient with impaired pleckstrin phosphorylation. *Blood* 87:1368–1376, 1996.

490. Song WJ, Sullivan MG, Legare RD, et al: Haploinsufficiency of CBFA2 causes familial thrombocytopenia with propensity to develop acute myelogenous leukaemia. *Nat Genet* 23:166–175, 1999.

491. Sun L, Gorospe JR, Hoffman EP, Rao AK: Decreased platelet expression of myosin regulatory light chain polypeptide (MYL9) and other genes with platelet dysfunction and CBFA2/RUNX1 mutation: Insights from platelet expression profiling. *J Thromb Haemost* 5:146–154, 2007.

492. Rendu F, Breton-Gorius J, Trugnan G, et al: Studies on a new variant of the Hermansky-Pudlak syndrome: Qualitative, ultrastructural, and functional abnormalities of the platelet-dense bodies associated with a phospholipase A defect. *Am J Hematol* 4:387–399, 1978.

493. Adler DH, Cogan JD, Phillips JA, et al: Inherited human cPLA(2alpha) deficiency is associated with impaired eicosanoid biosynthesis, small intestinal ulceration, and platelet dysfunction. *J Clin Invest* 2008.

494. Faioni EM, Razzari C, Zulueta A, et al: Bleeding diathesis and gastro-duodenal ulcers in inherited cytosolic phospholipase-A2 alpha deficiency. *Thromb Haemost* 112:1182–1189, 2014.

495. Malmsten C, Hamberg M, Svensson J, Samuelsson B: Physiological role of an endoperoxide in human platelets: Hemostatic defect due to platelet cyclo-oxygenase deficiency. *Proc Natl Acad Sci U S A* 72:1446–1450, 1975.

496. Lagarde M, Byron PA, Vargaftig BB, Dechavanne M: Impairment of platelet thromboxane A2 generation and of the platelet release reaction in two patients with congenital deficiency of platelet cyclo-oxygenase. *Br J Haematol* 38:251–266, 1978.

497. Pareti FI, Mannucci PM, D'Angelo A, et al: Congenital deficiency of thromboxane and prostacyclin. *Lancet* 1:898–901, 1980.

498. Rak K, Boda Z: Haemostatic balance in congenital deficiency of platelet cyclo- oxygenase. *Lancet* 2:44, 1980.

499. Horellou MH, Lecompte T, Lecrubier C, et al: Familial and constitutional bleeding disorder due to platelet cyclo- oxygenase deficiency. *Am J Hematol* 14:1–9, 1983.

500. Rao AK, Koike K, Day HJ, et al: Bleeding disorder associated with albumin-dependent partial deficiency in platelet thromboxane production. Effect of albumin on arachidonate metabolism in platelets. *Am J Clin Pathol* 83:687–696, 1985.

501. Roth GJ, Machuga R: Radioimmune assay of human platelet prostaglandin synthetase. *J Lab Clin Med* 99:187–196, 1982.

502. Matijevic-Aleksic N, McPhedran P, Wu KK: Bleeding disorder due to platelet prostaglandin H synthase-1 (PGHS-1) deficiency. *Br J Haematol* 92:212–217, 1996.

503. Defreyn G, Machin SJ, Carreras LO, et al: Familial bleeding tendency with partial platelet thromboxane synthetase deficiency: Reorientation of cyclic endoperoxide metabolism. *Br J Haematol* 49:29–41, 1981.

504. Mestel F, Oetliker O, Beck E, et al: Severe bleeding associated with defective thromboxane synthetase. *Lancet* 1:157, 1980.

505. Weiss HJ: Impaired platelet procoagulant mechanisms in patients with bleeding disorders. *Semin Thromb Hemost* 35:233–241, 2009.

506. Lhermusier T, Chap H, Payrastre B: Platelet membrane phospholipid asymmetry: From the characterization of a scramblase activity to the identification of an essential protein mutated in Scott syndrome. *J Thromb Haemost* 9:1883–1891, 2011.

507. Weiss HJ, Vicic WJ, Lages BA, Rogers J: Isolated deficiency of platelet procoagulant activity. *Am J Med* 67:206–213, 1979.

508. Toti F, Satta N, Fressinaud E, et al: Scott syndrome, characterized by impaired transmembrane migration of procoagulant phosphatidylserine and hemorrhagic complications, is an inherited disorder. *Blood* 87:1409–1415, 1996.

509. Weiss HJ, Lages B: Platelet prothrombinase activity and intracellular calcium responses in patients with storage pool deficiency, glycoprotein IIb-IIIa deficiency, or impaired platelet coagulant activity—A comparison with Scott syndrome. *Blood* 89:1599–1611, 1997.

510. Dachary-Prigent J, Pasquet JM, Fressinaud E, et al: Aminophospholipid exposure, microvesiculation and abnormal protein tyrosine phosphorylation in the platelets of a patient with Scott syndrome: A study using physiologic agonists and local anaesthetics. *Br J Haematol* 99:959–967, 1997.

511. Zwaal RF, Comfurius P, Bevers EM: Scott syndrome, a bleeding disorder caused by defective scrambling of membrane phospholipids. *Biochim Biophys Acta* 1636:119–128, 2004.

512. Munnix IC, Harmsma M, Giddings JC, et al: Store-mediated calcium entry in the regulation of phosphatidylserine exposure in blood cells from Scott patients. *Thromb Haemost* 89:687–695, 2003.

513. Solum NO: Procoagulant expression in platelets and defects leading to clinical disorders. *Arterioscler Thromb Vasc Biol* 19:2841–2846, 1999.

514. Weiss HJ: Scott syndrome-a disorder of platelet coagulant activity. *Semin Hematol* 31:312–319, 1994.

515. Sims PJ, Wiedmer T, Esmon CT, et.al: Assembly of the platelet prothrombinase complex is linked to vesiculation on the platelet plasma membrane. Studies in Scott syndrome: An isolated defect in platelet procoagulant activity. *J Biol Chem* 264:137–148, 1989.

516. Castaman G, Yu-Feng L, Battistin E, Rodeghiero F: Characterization of a novel bleeding disorder with isolated prolonged bleeding time and deficiency of platelet microvesicle generation. *Br J Haematol* 96:458–463, 1997.

517. Albrecht C, McVey JH, Elliott JI, et al: A novel missense mutation in ABCA1 results in altered protein trafficking and reduced phosphatidylserine translocation in a patient with Scott syndrome. *Blood* 106:542–549, 2005.

518. Suzuki J, Umeda M, Sims PJ, Nagata S: Calcium-dependent phospholipid scrambling by TMEM16F. *Nature* 468:834–838, 2010.

519. Weiss HJ: Platelet aggregation, adhesion and adenosine diphosphate release in thrombopathia (platelet factor 3 deficiency). A comparison with Glanzmann's thrombasthenia and von Willebrand's disease. *Am J Med* 43:570–578, 1967.

520. Freson K, De Vos R, Wittevrongel C, et al: The β_1-tubulin Q43P functional polymorphism reduces the risk of cardiovascular disease in men by modulating platelet function and structure. *Blood* 106:2356–2362, 2005.

521. Navarro-Nunez L, Lozano ML, Rivera J, et al: The association of the beta1-tubulin Q43P polymorphism with intracerebral hemorrhage in men. *Haematologica* 92:513–518, 2007.

522. Kunishima S, Kobayashi R, Itoh TJ, et al: Mutation of the beta1-tubulin gene associated with congenital macrothrombocytopenia affecting microtubule assembly. *Blood* 113:458–461, 2009.

522A.Berrou, E, Adam, F, Lebret, M et al: Heterogeneity of platelet functional alterations in patients with filamin A mutations. *Arterioscler Thromb Vasc Biol* 33: e11–8, 2013.

523. Buchbinder D, Nugent DJ, Fillipovich AH: Wiskott-Aldrich syndrome: Diagnosis, current management, and emerging treatments. *Appl Clin Genet* 7:55–66, 2014.

524. Massaad MJ, Ramesh N, Geha RS: Wiskott-Aldrich syndrome: A comprehensive review. *Ann N Y Acad Sci* 1285:26–43, 2013.

525. Lutskiy MI, Shcherbina A, Bachli ET, et al: WASP localizes to the membrane skeleton of platelets. *Br J Haematol* 139:98–105, 2007.

526. Parkman R, Remold-O'Donnell E, Kenney DM, et al: Surface protein abnormalities in lymphocytes and platelets from patients with Wiskott-Aldrich syndrome. *Lancet* 2:1387–1389, 1981.

527. Semple JW, Siminovitch KA, Mody M, et al: Flow cytometric analysis of platelets from children with the Wiskott-Aldrich syndrome reveals defects in platelet development, activation and structure. *Br J Haematol* 97:747–754, 1997.

528. Baldini MG: Nature of the platelet defect in the Wiskott-Aldrich syndrome. *Ann N Y Acad Sci* 201:437–444, 1972.

529. Verhoeven AJ, van Oostrum IE, van Haarlem H, Akkerman JW: Impaired energy metabolism in platelets from patients with Wiskott-Aldrich syndrome. *Thromb Haemost* 61:10–14, 1989.

530. Marone G, Albini F, di Martino L, et al: The Wiskott-Aldrich syndrome: Studies of platelets, basophils and polymorphonuclear leucocytes. *Br J Haematol* 62:737–745, 1986.

531. Gross BS, Wilde JI, Quek L, et al: Regulation and function of WASp in platelets by the collagen receptor, glycoprotein VI. *Blood* 94:4166–4176, 1999.

532. Shcherbina A, Rosen FS, Remold-O'Donnell E: Pathological events in platelets of Wiskott-Aldrich syndrome patients. *Br J Haematol* 106:875–883, 1999.

533. Tsuboi S, Nonoyama S, Ochs HD: Wiskott-Aldrich syndrome protein is involved in alphaIIb beta3-mediated cell adhesion. *EMBO Rep* 7:506–511, 2006.

534. Rengan R, Ochs HD, Sweet LI, et al: Actin cytoskeletal function is spared, but apoptosis is increased, in WAS patient hematopoietic cells. *Blood* 95:1283–1292, 2000.

535. Falet H, Hoffmeister KM, Neujahr R, Hartwig JH: Normal Arp2/3 complex activation in platelets lacking WASp. *Blood* 100:2113–2122, 2002.

536. Shcherbina A, Cooley J, Lutskiy MI, et al: WASP plays a novel role in regulating platelet responses dependent on alphaIIbbeta3 integrin outside-in signalling. *Br J Haematol* 148:416–427, 2010.

537. Kuijpers TW, van de Vijver E, Weterman MA, et al: LAD-1/variant syndrome is caused by mutations in FERMT3. *Blood* 113:4740–4746, 2009.

538. Harris, ES, Smith, TL, Springett, GM, et al: A Leukocyte adhesion deficiency-I variant syndrome (LAD-Iv, LAD-III): Molecular characterization of the defect in an index family. *Am J Hematol* 87: 311–313, 2012.

539. Mory A, Feigelson SW, Yarali N, et al: Kindlin-3: A new gene involved in the pathogenesis of LAD-III. *Blood* 112:2591, 2008.

540. Svensson L, Howarth K, McDowall A, et al: Leukocyte adhesion deficiency-III is caused by mutations in KINDLIN3 affecting integrin activation. *Nat Med* 15:306–312, 2009.

541. Malinin NL, Zhang L, Choi J, et al: A point mutation in KINDLIN3 ablates activation of three integrin subfamilies in humans. *Nat Med* 15:313–318, 2009.

542. Moser M, Nieswandt B, Ussar S, et al: Kindlin-3 is essential for integrin activation and platelet aggregation. *Nat Med* 14:325–330, 2008.

543. Pasvolsky R, Feigelson SW, Kilic SS, et al: A LAD-III syndrome is associated with defective expression of the Rap-1 activator CalDAG-GEFI in lymphocytes, neutrophils, and platelets. *J Exp Med* 204:1571–1582, 2007.

544. Tijssen MR, Cvejic A, Joshi A, et al: Genome-wide analysis of simultaneous GATA1/2, RUNX1, FLI1, and SCL binding in megakaryocytes identifies hematopoietic regulators. *Dev Cell* 20:597–609, 2011.

545. Rao AK: Spotlight on *FLI1, RUNX1* and platelet dysfunction. *Blood* 122:4004–4006, 2013.

545A.Songdej N, Rao AK: Hematopoietic transcription factor mutations and inherited platelet dysfunction. F1000Prime Reports 7:66, 2015.

546. Gerrard JM, Israels ED, Bisip AJ, et al: Inherited platelet-storage pool deficiency associated with a high incidence of acute myeloid leukaemia. *Br J Haematol* 79:246–255, 1991.

547. Ganly. P, Walker LC, Morris CM: Familial mutations of the transcription factor RUNX1 (AML1, CBFA2) predispose to acute myeloid leukemia. *Leuk Lymphoma* 45:1–10, 2004.

548. Dowton SB, Beardsley D, Jamison D, et al: Studies of a familial platelet disorder. *Blood* 65:557, 1985.

549. Ho CY, Otterud B, Legare RD, et al: Linkage of a familial platelet disorder with a propensity to develop myeloid malignancies to human chromosome 21q22.1–22.2. *Blood* 87:5218–5224, 1996.

550. Arepally G, Rebbeck TR, Song W, et al: Evidence for genetic homogeneity in a familial platelet disorder with predisposition to acute myelogenous leukemia (FPD/AML). *Blood* 92:2600–2602, 1998.

551. Walker LC, Stevens J, Campbell H, et al: A novel inherited mutation of the transcription factor RUNX1 causes thrombocytopenia and may predispose to acute myeloid leukaemia. *Br J Haematol* 117:878–881, 2002.

552. Owen CJ, Toze CL, Koochin A, et al: Five new pedigrees with inherited RUNX1 mutations causing familial platelet disorder with propensity to myeloid malignancy. *Blood* 112:4639–4645, 2008.

553. Sun L, Mao G, Rao AK: Association of CBFA2 mutation with decreased platelet PKC-θ and impaired receptor-mediated activation of GPIIb-IIIa and pleckstrin phosphorylation: Proteins regulated by CBFA2 play a role in GPIIb-IIIa activation. *Blood* 103:948–954, 2004.

554. Rao AK: Inherited platelet function disorders: Overview and disorders of granules, secretion, and signal transduction. *Hematol Oncol Clin North Am* 27:585–611, 2013.

555. Kaur G, Jalagadugula G, Mao G, Rao AK: RUNX1/core binding factor A2 regulates platelet 12-lipoxygenase gene (ALOX12): Studies in human RUNX1 haplodeficiency. *Blood* 115:3128–3135, 2010.

556. Jalagadugula G, Mao G, Kaur G, et al: Regulation of platelet myosin light chain (*MYL9*) by RUNX1: Implications for thrombocytopenia and platelet dysfunction in *RUNX1* haplodeficiency. *Blood* 116:6037–6045, 2010.

557. Freson K, Devriendt K, Matthijs G, et al: Platelet characteristics in patients with X-linked macrothrombocytopenia because of a novel GATA1 mutation. *Blood* 98:85–92, 2001.

558. Hughan SC, Senis Y, Best D, et al: Selective impairment of platelet activation to collagen in the absence of GATA1. *Blood* 105:4369–4376, 2005.

559. Breton-Gorius J, Favier R, Guichard J, et al: A new congenital dysmegakaryopoietic thrombocytopenia (Paris-Trousseau) associated with giant platelet alpha-granules and chromosome 11 deletion at 11q23. *Blood* 85:1805–1814, 1995.

560. Favier R, Jondeau K, Boutard P, et al: Paris-Trousseau syndrome: Clinical, hematological, molecular data of ten new cases. *Thromb Haemost* 90:893–897, 2003.

561. Raslova H, Komura E, Le Couedic JP, et al: FLI1 monoallelic expression combined with its hemizygous loss underlies Paris-Trousseau/Jacobsen thrombopenia. *J Clin Invest* 114:77–84, 2004.

562. Shivdasani RA: Lonely in Paris: When one gene copy isn't enough. *J Clin Invest* 114: 17–19, 2004.

563. Kurstjens R, Bolt C, Vossen M, Haanen C: Familial thrombopathic thrombocytopenia. *Br J Haematol* 15:305–317, 1968.

564. Estes JW: Platelet abnormalities in heritable disorders of connective tissue. *Ann N Y Acad Sci* 201:445–450, 1972.

565. Evensen SA, Myhre L, Stormorken H: Haemostatic studies in osteogenesis imperfecta. *Scand J Haematol* 33:177–179, 1984.

566. Akkerman JWN, Rijksen G, Gorter G, al e. Platelet functions and energy metabolism in a patient with hexokinase deficiency. *Blood* 63:147–153, 1984.

567. Corby DG, Putnam CW, Greene HL: Impaired platelet function in glucose-6-phosphatase deficiency. *J Pediatr* 85:71–76, 1974.

568. Czapek EE, Deykin D, Salzman EW: Platelet dysfunction in glycogen storage disease type I. *Blood* 41:235–247, 1973.

569. Boullin DJ, O'Brien RA: Abnormalities of 5-hydroxytryptamine uptake and binding by blood platelets from children with Down's syndrome. *J Physiol* 212:287–297, 1971.

570. Lott IT, Chase TN, Murphy DL: Down's syndrome: Transport, storage, and metabolism of serotonin in blood platelets. *Pediatr Res* 6:730–735, 1972.

571. McCoy EE, Sneddon JM: Decreased calcium content and 45Ca2+ uptake in Down's syndrome blood platelets. *Pediatr Res* 18:914–916, 1984.

572. More R, Amir N, Meyer S, et al: Platelet abnormalities in Down's syndrome. *Clin Genet* 22:128–136, 1982.

573. Sheppard JR, Schumacher W, White JG, et al: The alpha adrenergic response of Down's syndrome platelets. *J Pharmacol Exp Ther* 225:584–588, 1983.

574. Hamilton RW, Shaikh BS, Ottie JN, et al: Platelet function, ultrastructure, and survival in the May-Hegglin anomaly. *Am J Clin Pathol* 74:663–668, 1980.

575. Lusher JM, Schneider J, Mizukami I, et al: The May-Hegglin anomaly: Platelet function, ultrastructure and chromosome studies. *Blood* 32:950–961, 1968.

576. Coller BS, Zarrabi MH: Platelet membrane studies in the May-Hegglin anomaly. *Blood* 58:279–284, 1981.

577. Freson K, Hashimoto H, Thys C, et al: The pituitary adenylate cyclase-activating polypeptide is a physiological inhibitor of platelet activation. *J Clin Invest* 113:905–912, 2004.

578. Sandrock K, Nakamura L, Vraetz T, et al: Platelet secretion defect in patients with familial hemophagocytic lymphohistiocytosis type 5 (FHL-5). *Blood* 116:6148–6150, 2010.

579. Al Hawas R, Ren Q, Ye S, et al: Munc18b/STXBP2 is required for platelet secretion. *Blood* 120:2493–2500, 2012.

580. Ye S, Karim ZA, Al Hawas R, et al: Syntaxin-11, but not syntaxin-2 or syntaxin-4, is required for platelet secretion. *Blood* 120:2484–2492, 2012.

581. Alamelu J, Liesner R: Modern management of severe platelet function disorders. *Br J Haematol* 149:813–823, 2010.

582. Seligsohn U: Treatment of inherited platelet disorders. *Haemophilia* 18 (Suppl 4:) 161–165, 2012.

583. Bolton-Maggs PH, Chalmers EA, Collins PW, et al: A review of inherited platelet disorders with guidelines for their management on behalf of the UKHCDO. *Br J Haematol* 135:603–633, 2006.

584. Fiore M, Firah N, Pillois X, et al: Natural history of platelet antibody formation against alphaIIbbeta3 in a French cohort of Glanzmann thrombasthenia patients. *Haemophilia* 18:e201–9, 2012.

585. Mannucci PM: Desmopressin (DDAVP) in the treatment of bleeding disorders: The first 20 years. *Blood* 90:2515–2521, 1997.

586. Mannucci PM: Hemostatic Drugs. *N Engl J Med* 339:245–253, 1998.

587. Rao AK, Ghosh S, Sun L, et al: Effect of mechanism of platelet dysfunction on response to DDAVP in patients with congenital platelet function defects. A double-blind placebo-controlled trial. *Thromb Haemost* 74:1071–1078, 1995.

588. Kobrinsky NL, Israels ED, Gerrard JM, et al: Shortening of bleeding time by 1-deamino-8-D-arginine vasopressin in various bleeding disorders. *Lancet* 1:1145–1148, 1984.

589. Schulman S, Johnson H, Egberg N, Blombäck M: DDAVP-induced correction of prolonged bleeding time in patients with congenital platelet function defects. *Thromb Res* 45:165–174, 1987.

590. DiMichele DM, Hathaway WE: Use of DDAVP in inherited and acquired platelet dysfunction. *Am J Hematol* 33:39–45, 1990.

591. Nieuwenhuis HK, Sixma JJ: 1-Desamino-8-D-arginine vasopressin (Desmopressin) shortens the bleeding time in storage pool deficiency. *Ann Intern Med* 108:65–67, 1988.

592. Colucci G, Stutz M, Rochat S, et al: The effect of desmopressin on platelet function: A selective enhancement of procoagulant COAT platelets in patients with primary platelet function defects. *Blood* 123:1905–1916, 2014.

593. Almeida AM, Khair K, Hann I, Liesner R: The use of recombinant factor VIIa in children with inherited platelet function disorders. *Br J Haematol* 121:477–481, 2003.

594. Poon MC, d'Oiron R. Recombinant activated factor VII (NovoSeven) treatment of platelet-related bleeding disorders. International Registry on Recombinant Factor VIIa and Congenital Platelet Disorders Group. *Blood Coagul Fibrinolysis* 11 (Suppl 1:) S55–S68, 2000.

595. Poon MC, Demers C, Jobin F, Wu JW: Recombinant factor VIIa is effective for bleeding and surgery in patients with Glanzmann thrombasthenia. *Blood* 94:3951–3953, 1999.

596. del Pozo Pozo AI, Jimenez-Yuste V, Villar A, et al: Successful thyroidectomy in a patient with Hermansky-Pudlak syndrome treated with recombinant activated factor VII and platelet concentrates. *Blood Coagul Fibrinolysis* 13:551–553, 2002.

597. Sindet-Pedersen S, Ramstrom G, Bernvil S, Blomback M: Hemostatic effect of tranexamic acid mouthwash in anticoagulant-treated patients undergoing oral surgery. *N Engl J Med* 320:840–843, 1989.

598. Mielke CH Jr, Levine PH, Zucker S: Preoperative prednisone therapy in platelet function disorders. *Thromb Res* 21:655–662, 1981.

599. Spotnitz WD, Burks S: Hemostats, sealants, and adhesives: Components of the surgical toolbox. *Transfusion* 48:1502–1516, 2008.

600. Chuansumrit A, Suwannuraks M, Sri-Udomporn N, et al: Recombinant activated factor VII combined with local measures in preventing bleeding from invasive dental procedures in patients with Glanzmann thrombasthenia. *Blood Coagul Fibrinolysis* 14: 187–190, 2003.

601. Singla NK, Foster KN, Alexander WA, Pribble JP: Safety and immunogenicity of recombinant human thrombin: A pooled analysis of results from 10 clinical trials. *Pharmacotherapy* 32:998–1005, 2012.

602. Wilcox DA, Olsen JC, Ishizawa L, et al: Integrin alphaIIb promoter-targeted expression of gene products in megakaryocytes derived from retrovirus-transduced human hematopoietic cells. *Proc Natl Acad Sci U S A* 96:9654–9659, 1999.

603. Wilcox DA, White GC 2nd: Gene therapy for platelet disorders: Studies with Glanzmann's thrombasthenia. *J Thromb Haemost* 1:2300–2311, 2003.

604. Fang J, Jensen ES, Boudreaux MK, et al: Platelet gene therapy improves hemostatic function for integrin alphaIIbbeta3-deficient dogs. *Proc Natl Acad Sci U S A* 108: 9583–9588, 2011.

605. Hodivala-Dilke KM, Tsakiris DA, Rayburn H, et al: Beta3-integrin-deficient mice are a model for Glanzmann thrombasthenia showing placental defects and reduced survival. *J Clin Invest* 103:229–238, 1999.

606. Boudreaux MK, Lipscomb DL: Clinical, biochemical, and molecular aspects of Glanzmann's thrombasthenia in humans and dogs. *Vet Pathol* 38:249–260, 2001.

607. Niemeyer GP, Boudreaux MK, Goodman-Martin SA, et al: Correction of a large animal model of type I Glanzmann's thrombasthenia by nonmyeloablative bone marrow transplantation. *Exp Hematol* 31:1357–1362, 2003.

608. Schlosser RJ: Clinical practice. Epistaxis. *N Engl J Med* 360:784–789, 2009.

609. Siddiq S, Clark A, Mumford A: A systematic review of the management and outcomes of pregnancy in Glanzmann thrombasthenia. *Haemophilia* 17:e858–e869, 2011.

610. Peitsidis P, Datta T, Pafilis I, et al: Bernard Soulier syndrome in pregnancy: A systematic review. *Haemophilia* 16:584–591, 2010.

611. Coller BS: Inherited disorders of platelet function, in *Hemostasis and Thrombosis*, edited by AL Bloom, p. 721–766. Churchill Livingstone, Edinburgh, 1992.

CHAPTER 121
ACQUIRED QUALITATIVE PLATELET DISORDERS

Charles S. Abrams, Sanford J. Shattil, and Joel S. Bennett

be intrinsically abnormal such as the myeloproliferative neoplasms, leukemias, and myelodysplastic syndromes; dysproteinemias in which monoclonal immunoglobulins can impair platelet function; and acquired forms of von Willebrand disease. Of the systemic diseases, renal failure is most prominently associated with abnormal platelet function because of the retention in the circulation of platelet inhibitory compounds. Platelet function may also be abnormal in the presence of antiplatelet antibodies, following cardiopulmonary bypass, and in association with liver disease or disseminated intravascular coagulation.

SUMMARY

Acquired qualitative platelet disorders are frequent causes of abnormal platelet function measured *in vitro*, although by themselves are usually associated with little or no clinical bleeding. However, there are important exceptions. Nevertheless, their major clinical impact becomes apparent in the additional presence of thrombocytopenia, or additional acquired or congenital disorders of hemostasis. Acquired disorders of platelet function can be conveniently classified into those that result from drugs, hematologic diseases, and systemic disorders. Drugs are the most frequent cause of acquired qualitative platelet dysfunction. Aspirin is the most notable drug in this regard because of its frequent use, its irreversible effect on platelet prostaglandin synthesis, and its documented effect on hemostatic competency, although this effect is minimal in normal individuals. Other nonsteroidal antiinflammatory drugs reversibly inhibit platelet prostaglandin synthesis and usually have little effect on hemostasis. The antiplatelet effects of a number of drugs have proven useful in preventing arterial thrombosis, but as would be anticipated, excessive bleeding can be a complication of their use. In addition to aspirin, these drugs include the P2Y$_{12}$ adenosine diphosphate receptor antagonists, clopidogrel, prasugrel and ticagrelor, vorapaxar, an inhibitor of the PAR1 thrombin receptor, and drugs that specifically inhibit adhesive ligand binding to platelet integrin $a_{IIb}\beta_3$ (GPIIb/IIIa). Other drugs used to treat thrombosis, such as heparin and fibrinolytic agents, may also impair platelet function *in vitro* and *ex vivo*, but the clinical significance of these observations is uncertain. High doses of the β-lactam antibiotics can impair platelet function *in vitro*, whereas clinically significant bleeding is unusual in the absence of a coexisting hemostatic defect. Similarly, a number of miscellaneous drugs, including a variety of psychotropic, chemotherapeutic and anesthetic agents, as well as a number of foods and food additives, can affect platelet function *in vitro*, but do not appear to be of clinical significance by themselves. Hematologic diseases associated with abnormal platelet function include marrow processes in which platelets may

Platelet function may be adversely affected by drugs and by hematologic and nonhematologic diseases. Because the use of aspirin and other nonsteroidal antiinflammatory agents is pervasive, acquired platelet dysfunction is much more frequent than inherited platelet dysfunction. Acquired disorders of platelet function can be classified according to the underlying clinical conditions with which they are associated (Table 121–1).

It is important to have a balanced view of the clinical significance of acquired disorders of platelet function. On the one hand, their severity is usually mild. On the other hand, there are important exceptions to this rule, particularly when platelet dysfunction is associated with other hemostatic defects. If a patient does not present with a history of bleeding, it may be difficult to predict the risk of future bleeding. This is not surprising since even patients with thrombocytopenia may experience little or no spontaneous bleeding until their platelet count is less than 10×10^9/L. Furthermore, clinical assessment of these disorders is made problematic by difficulties in standardization and interpretation of laboratory tests of platelet function, including platelet aggregometry. These tests are more useful in diagnosing platelet dysfunction than in predicting the risk of bleeding.[1,2]

DRUGS THAT AFFECT PLATELET FUNCTION

Drugs are the most common cause of platelet dysfunction (Table 121–2). For example, in an analysis of 72 hospitalized patients with a prolonged bleeding time (a test no longer considered reliable), 54 percent were receiving large doses of antibiotics known to prolong the bleeding time and 10 percent were taking aspirin or other nonsteroidal antiinflammatory drugs.[3] Some drugs can prolong the bleeding time and either cause or exacerbate a bleeding diathesis. Other drugs may prolong the bleeding time but not cause bleeding, while many only affect platelet function *ex vivo* or when added to platelets *in vitro*. It is important for the hematologist to understand the clinical significance of these distinctions.

ASPIRIN AND OTHER NONSTEROIDAL ANTIINFLAMMATORY DRUGS

Aspirin

Aspirin irreversibly inactivates the enzyme cyclooxygenase (COX), also known as prostaglandin endoperoxide H synthase, by acetylating a serine residue at position 529.[4] Two isoforms of COX have been identified (COX-1 and COX-2),[5] as well as a splice variant of COX-1, COX-1b (COX-3), whose functional significance is uncertain.[6] COX-1 is constitutively expressed by many tissues, including platelets, the gastric mucosa, and endothelial cells (Chap. 134 discusses the use of aspirin as an antithrombotic agent).[5] COX-2 is undetectable in most tissues, but its synthesis is rapidly induced in cells such as endothelial cells,

TABLE 121–1. Acquired Qualitative Platelet Disorders

Drugs that affect platelet function
- Aspirin and other nonsteroidal antiinflammatory drugs
- P2Y$_{12}$ antagonists (clopidogrel, prasugrel, ticagrelor)
- PAR1 thrombin receptor antagonist (vorapaxar)
- Integrin $\alpha_{IIb}\beta_3$ receptor antagonists (abciximab, eptifibatide, tirofiban)
- Drugs that increase platelet cyclic adenosine monophosphate
- Antibiotics
- Anticoagulants and fibrinolytic agents
- Cardiovascular drugs
- Volume expanders
- Psychotropic agents and anesthetics
- Oncologic drugs
- Foods and food additives

Hematologic disorders associated with abnormal platelet function
- Chronic myeloproliferative neoplasms
- Leukemias and myelodysplastic syndromes
- Dysproteinemias
- Acquired von Willebrand syndrome

Systemic disorders associated with abnormal platelet function
- Uremia
- Antiplatelet antibodies
- Cardiopulmonary bypass
- Liver disease
- Disseminated intravascular coagulation
- Infection with HIV

TABLE 121–2. Drugs That Affect Platelet Function

Nonsteroidal antiinflammatory drugs
- Aspirin, ibuprofen, sulindac, naproxen, meclofenamic acid, mefenamic acid, diflunisal, piroxicam, tolmetin, zomepirac, sulfinpyrazone, indomethacin, phenylbutazone, celecoxib

P2Y$_{12}$ antagonists
- Clopidogrel, prasugrel, ticagrelor

PAR1 receptor antagonist
- Vorapaxar

Integrin $\alpha_{IIb}\beta_3$ antagonists
- Abciximab, eptifibatide, tirofiban

Drugs that affect platelet cyclic adenosine monophosphate levels or function
- Prostacyclin, iloprost, dipyridamole, cilostazol

Antibiotics
- Penicillins
  - Penicillin G, carbenicillin, ticarcillin, methicillin, ampicillin, piperacillin, azlocillin mezlocillin, sulbenicillin, temocillin
- Cephalosporins
  - Cephalothin, moxalactam, cefoxitin, cefotaxime, cefazolin
- Nitrofurantoin
- Miconazole

Anticoagulants, fibrinolytic agents, and antifibrinolytic agents
- Heparin
- Streptokinase, tissue plasminogen activator, urokinase
- ε-aminocaproic acid

Cardiovascular drugs
- Nitroglycerin, isosorbide dinitrate, propranolol, nitroprusside, nifedipine, verapamil, diltiazem, quinidine

Volume expanders
- Dextran, hydroxyethyl starch

Psychotropic drugs and anesthetics
- Psychotropic drugs
  - Imipramine, amitriptyline, nortriptyline, chlorpromazine, promethazine, fluphenazine, trifluoperazine, haloperidol
- Anesthetics
  - Local
    - Dibucaine, tetracaine, Cyclaine, butacaine, nupercaine, procaine, cocaine
  - General
    - Halothane

Oncologic drugs
- Mithramycin, daunorubicin, BCNU, ibrutinib

Miscellaneous drugs
- Ketanserin

Antihistamines
- Diphenhydramine, chlorpheniramine, mepyramine

Radiographic contrast agent
- Iopamidol, iothalamate, ioxaglate, meglumine diatrizoate, sodium diatrizoate

Foods and food additives
- ω-3 Fatty acids, ethanol, Chinese black tree fungus, onion extract ajoene, cumin, turmeric

fibroblasts, and monocytes by growth factors, cytokines, endotoxin, and hormones.[5] Platelets express only COX-1, whereas endothelial cells can express both COX-1 and COX-2.[7,8] In the cardiovascular system, COX products regulate complex interactions between platelets and the vessel wall. The platelet product of COX-1 mediated prostaglandin synthesis, thromboxane A$_2$ (TXA$_2$), produces vasoconstriction and is a receptor-mediated agonist for platelet aggregation and secretion.[4] Thus, inactivation of COX-1 by aspirin prevents platelet synthesis of TXA$_2$, thereby inhibiting platelet responses that depend on this substance. Accordingly, platelet responses to adenosine diphosphate (ADP), epinephrine, low doses of collagen and thrombin, and arachidonic acid are affected (arachidonic acid completely), but there is almost no effect on the responses to higher doses of collagen or thrombin.[9,10] On the other hand, the endothelial cell prostaglandin (PG) product, prostacyclin (PGI$_2$), produces smooth muscle cell relaxation and vasodilation and increases the platelet content of cyclic adenosine monophosphate (AMP), thereby decreasing overall platelet reactivity.[11]

Platelet PG synthesis in an adult is nearly completely inhibited by a single 100-mg dose of aspirin or by 30 mg taken daily for 7 to 10 days.[4] Although single doses of aspirin irreversibly inhibit platelet and endothelial cell COX,[12] they have no lasting effect on PG synthesis by endothelial cells because of the ability of these cells to synthesize additional COX unaffected by aspirin.[13] *In vitro* studies also suggest that the presence of erythrocytes contributes to agonist-stimulated platelet reactivity,[14] an effect that can be inhibited by aspirin at doses greater than those required to inhibit platelet COX-1.[15] A meta-analysis of clinical trials indicates that aspirin doses varying from 50 to 1500 mg daily are equally efficacious in preventing adverse cardiovascular and cerebrovascular events.[16] This has led many to suggest that the lowest effective doses should be prescribed to minimize gastrointestinal toxicity. Nonetheless, even low doses of aspirin can be associated with significant gastrointestinal hemorrhage.[17–19]

Aspirin is one of the relatively few drugs that prolongs the bleeding time in humans and appears to do so by blocking aggregation rather than adhesion. In normal individuals, the effect on the bleeding time is slight (generally no more than 1.2 to 2.0 times the preaspirin bleeding time),[20,21] observed in both males and females, and requires that almost all the COX in the circulating platelets be inhibited.[11] The sensitivity of the bleeding time to aspirin is dependent on such technical variables as the direction of the incision on the forearm and the degree of hydrostatic pressure applied to the arm,[22] and hence the current view that the test is unreliable. The bleeding time may remain prolonged for 1 to 4 days after aspirin has been discontinued, and platelet aggregation tests may remain abnormal for up to a week until platelets affected by aspirin are replaced as the result of thrombopoiesis.[23]

The significance of aspirin ingestion on the hemostatic competency of normal individuals appears to be minimal. Nevertheless, patients taking aspirin chronically report significant increases in bruising, epistaxis, and gastrointestinal blood loss.[17–19] Gastrointestinal blood loss appears to be the result of a direct effect of aspirin on the gastric mucosa.[24,25] Furthermore, there is an increase in the incidence of hemorrhagic stroke when aspirin is used in the primary and secondary prevention of vascular disease, as well as an increase in major gastrointestinal and other extracranial bleeding.[26] Aspirin may also increase bleeding in the mother and the neonate during parturition.[27] In addition, some studies show that aspirin taken preoperatively increases the amount of blood loss following cardiothoracic surgery.[28,29] In contrast, a retrospective analysis has documented the safety of performing epidural and spinal anesthesia in patients who had ingested aspirin.[30] Aspirin may increase the amount of blood loss following general surgery.[31] The significance of aspirin ingestion in this setting was tested in the POISE-2 study[32] in which patients at risk for vascular complications were randomized to aspirin or placebo prior to their noncardiac surgery. Although taking aspirin did not reduce the incidence of cardiovascular events, there was a small increase in hemorrhagic complications. This suggests that discontinuing aspirin prior to surgery is a useful practice, particularly prior to plastic or neurosurgical procedures in which the limits of tolerable bleeding are narrow.[33] On the other hand, patients taking aspirin and other antiplatelet agents for severe cardiovascular disease may be at risk for thrombosis if these medications are discontinued. Thus, the clinician must thoroughly weigh the potential risks and benefits of discontinuing aspirin prior to noncardiac surgery. This is especially true in patients with other hemostatic disorders; for example, aspirin precipitates hemorrhage in individuals with von Willebrand disease, hemophilia A, warfarin ingestion, uremia, and disorders of platelet function.[34–36] Infusion of desmopressin (DDAVP) has been effective in correcting a prolonged bleeding time caused by aspirin.[37,38]

Resistance to the antiplatelet effects of aspirin ("aspirin-resistance") is a controversial topic and whether it exists depends to large extent on whether resistance is considered from a biochemical or clinical perspective.[39] Biochemical resistance to the platelet inhibitory effects of aspirin, that is, the failure to achieve pharmacologic inhibition of TXA_2 production, is uncommon.[39] For example, when healthy subjects were given either standard or enteric-coated aspirin, 49 percent given a single dose of enteric-coated aspirin failed to inhibit TXA_2 synthesis, whereas the failure to inhibit TXA_2 synthesis was never seen in subjects given standard aspirin.[40] Nevertheless, subjects given enteric-coated aspirin eventually responded when taking it daily, implying that although some patients absorb enteric-coated aspirin preparations poorly, they will ultimately absorb sufficient amounts of aspirin to prevent platelet TXA_2 synthesis. Most commonly, aspirin-resistance occurs because patients are non-adherent with aspirin therapy, often because of gastrointestinal toxicity.[41] Clinically, the term aspirin-resistance has been applied to patients who develop cardiovascular events despite taking aspirin. Given that aspirin treatment selectively inhibits platelet synthesis of only one endogenous platelet agonist, TXA_2, it is not surprising that aspirin does not completely abolish platelet-mediated vascular events.

Traditional Nonsteroidal Antiinflammatory Drugs

Unlike aspirin, nonsteroidal antiinflammatory drugs (NSAIDs), such as ibuprofen, naproxen, diclofenac, sulindac, piroxicam, indomethacin, and sulfinpyrazone, *reversibly* inhibit COX enzymes.[42] Although these drugs can cause a transient prolongation of the bleeding time when given in therapeutic doses, this is usually not clinically significant.[43] Population studies have suggested that concurrent treatment with NSAIDs and anticoagulants increases the risk of bleeding complication, but many bleeding events were limited to the gastrointestinal tract where NSAIDs are known to induce gastritis and peptic ulcerations.[44] As evidence of the modest effect of NSAIDs on platelet function, ibuprofen has been given safely to patients with hemophilia A.[45,46] Nonetheless, care must be taken when ibuprofen is given to patients with hemophilia and HIV infection receiving zidovudine because increased bleeding has been reported in this circumstance.[47] Because ibuprofen, and probably other NSAIDs, binds to COX-1, blocking its acetylation by aspirin,[42] coadministration of NSAIDs and aspirin may impair the irreversible, antithrombotic effects of aspirin on platelets.[48] For this reason, patients who require both medications should ingest aspirin at least 2 hours prior to the ingestion of traditional NSAIDs.

Coxibs (COX-2 Inhibitors)

COX-1 is present in the gastric mucosa where its products protect the integrity of the gastric lining cells. In inflammatory cells, COX-2 products such as PGE_2 and PGI_2 elicit an increased sense of pain and perpetuate the inflammatory process.[40] Thus, the coxibs (COX inhibitors), designed to be relatively more specific for COX-2 versus COX-1, were intended to reduce pain and inflammation with fewer gastric side effects than traditional NSAIDs.[40,42] However, clinical trials revealed that coxib administration was associated with cardiovascular toxicity (myocardial infarction, stroke, edema, exacerbation of hypertension), partly because of inhibiting PGI_2 synthesis.[11,49–52] On the basis of these results, rofecoxib and valdecoxib were withdrawn from the market (valdecoxib was also associated with cases of Stevens-Johnson syndrome) and a black box warning regarding serious cardiovascular events was added to prescribing information for celecoxib, the only coxib now available in the United States.[50] Nonetheless, clinical evidence suggests there is no excess cardiovascular risk from daily doses of celecoxib of 200 mg or less.[51] Traditional NSAIDs also inhibit COX-2 to a variable extent and several observational trials have revealed excess cardiovascular events associated with use of these drugs.[50,53–55] Thus, a warning has also been added to their prescribing information. If indicated, analgesics such as acetaminophen, sodium or choline salicylate and narcotics may be substituted for aspirin and NSAIDs for treating musculoskeletal pain.[50] One report suggests that acetaminophen can selectively inhibit COX-2,[56] but the clinical significance of this observation is not clear.

THIENOPYRIDINES

Ticlopidine, clopidogrel, and prasugrel are thienopyridines that are used as antiplatelet agents in arterial diseases (Chap. 134) with results at least comparable to aspirin in the secondary prevention of cerebrovascular and cardiovascular events.[16,57]

Thienopyridines differ from aspirin in their mechanism of anti-platelet activity and their toxicity profile. All three thienopyridines are prodrugs that depend on oxidation by cytochrome P450 (CYP) enzymes in the liver (ticlopidine and clopidogrel) or in liver and intestine (prasugrel) to form the active metabolites that irreversibly inhibit the platelet $P2Y_{12}$ ADP receptor.[58-61] Ticlopidine at 250 mg twice a day, clopidogrel at 75 mg once per day, and prasugrel at 10 mg once a day inhibit platelet aggregation *ex vivo* in humans. The extent of this effect is equivalent to or greater than that of aspirin and the effect of thienopyridines and aspirin appears additive.[62,63] When given at their usual oral doses, the effect of thienopyridines on platelet aggregation and the bleeding time can be seen within hours of the first dose, but are not maximal for 4 to 6 days. A 300-mg loading dose of clopidogrel or 60 mg of prasugrel, followed by their usual daily doses, shortens the time required for their maximal antiplatelet effect to a few hours.[64,65] The common CYP polymorphism CYP2C19 results in lower levels of active clopidogrel and ticlopidine metabolites and has been reported to be associated with decreased platelet inhibition and an elevated risk for major adverse cardiovascular events.[55,66,67] Because the enzyme CYP3A is present in the intestine and can oxidize prasugrel to its pharmacologically active metabolite, intestinal metabolism may account for the rapid appearance and higher levels of the active metabolite in plasma after an oral dose.[61,68-70] Furthermore, prasugrel metabolism and inhibition of platelet function are not affected by CYP2C19 polymorphisms.[61,68-70]

The clinical efficacy of prasugrel has been compared to clopidogrel in patients with acute coronary syndrome scheduled for percutaneous coronary intervention in the Triton-TIMI 38 trial. Patients who received prasugrel had a significantly decreased incidence of ischemic events compared to patients who received clopidogrel (9.9 percent vs. 12.1 percent, p <0.001).[69] However, major bleeding was also significantly increased in patients receiving prasugrel compared to clopidogrel (2.4 percent vs. 1.8 percent, p <0.03). Thus, although prasugrel appeared to be more efficacious than clopidogrel, this benefit was partially offset by a higher rate of hemorrhage.[69]

The platelet inhibitory effects of thienopyridines persist for 4 to 10 days after the drugs have been discontinued, either because of their extended half-life after multiple dosing or their irreversible effect on platelets.[58] Ticlopidine administration is associated with potentially serious hematologic complications, including neutropenia (neutrophils $<1200 \times 10^9$/L in 2.4 percent of individuals)[58,71,72] and, less commonly, aplastic anemia, and thrombocytopenia.[73,74] In addition, at least one in 5000 patients develop a thrombotic thrombocytopenic purpura (TTP)-like syndrome.[75-77] Results from a large clinical trial suggest that hematologic complications may be less common with clopidogrel or prasugrel.[57] Clopidogrel may also be rarely associated with a TTP-like syndrome (one in 270,000),[78] although this rate is close to the TTP incidence in the general population. Because of its toxicity profile, ticlopidine has been replaced by the other thienopyridines in the United States.

Because aspirin and the thienopyridines inhibit platelet function by different mechanisms, their antithrombotic effects may be additive. In theory, this would be beneficial in the treatment of diseases associated with platelet activation such as ischemic heart disease, peripheral vascular disease, and ischemic strokes.[62,79,80] This hypothesis was tested in the CURE trial of patients with acute coronary syndromes.[62] Although clopidogrel plus aspirin decreased the combined incidence of cardiovascular deaths, myocardial infarctions, and strokes from 11.4 percent to 9.3 percent, the benefit was partially offset by an increase in severe bleeding from 2.7 to 3.7 percent. Similarly, in the CHARISMA trial of a broad population of patients at risk for cardiovascular events, there were 94 fewer ischemic events in patients treated with both clopidogrel and aspirin, but this occurred at the expense of 93 more

moderate or severe bleeding events.[81] Furthermore, a meta-analysis of seven randomized controlled trials involving more than 39,000 patients confirmed that intracranial hemorrhage was more frequent in patients who received both clopidogrel plus aspirin compared to clopidogrel alone.[82] Thus, except for special circumstances such as coronary artery stenting, it appears that the added benefit of dual antiplatelet therapy is small and has the added risk of increased bleeding.[83]

OTHER ADENOSINE DIPHOSPHATE RECEPTOR ANTAGONISTS

Ticagrelor, cangrelor, and elinogrel are oral, reversible, nonthienopyridine $P2Y_{12}$ receptor antagonists. Because they are not prodrugs and do not require metabolic activation, the onset of their inhibitory activity is more rapid than that of the thienopyridines. A novel, and as yet unexplained, side effect of treatment with this class of the $P2Y_{12}$ antagonists is the occurrence of dyspnea which can complicate the management of patients with coronary artery disease.[84]

Ticagrelor, the first drug of the class, has been approved for use in acute coronary syndromes. Its efficacy versus clopidogrel was tested in the PLATO trial in which patients with an acute coronary syndrome were randomized to treatment with either ticagrelor or clopidogrel.[85-87] At 1 year, the combined end point of death, myocardial infarction, and stroke was 9.8 percent in patients treated with ticagrelor compared to 11.7 percent in patients treated with clopidogrel.[88] Although stent thrombosis was also decreased in the ticagrelor-treated group, major bleeding not associated with coronary artery bypass surgery was increased in this group. The incidence of fatal intracranial hemorrhage was also greater in the ticagrelor-treated patients, but it was a rare event (0.1 percent of treated patients). In the ATLANTIC trial, patients suffering from an ST-segment elevation myocardial infarction were randomized to receive ticagrelor in the ambulance or in the catheterization laboratory.[89] Although initiating therapy before hospitalization was safe and lowered the incidence of stent thrombosis, there was no overall improvement in preventing major cardiovascular adverse events. Thus, ticagrelor, like prasugrel appears to be more efficacious than clopidogrel at preventing adverse cardiovascular events, but with more hemorrhagic complications.

THROMBIN RECEPTOR ANTAGONISTS

Thrombin is the most potent physiologic platelet agonist. Three G-protein–coupled thrombin receptors have been identified in humans (protease-activated receptors [PARs] 1, 3, and 4).[90] Although human platelets express both PAR-1 and PAR-4, the major platelet thrombin receptor is PAR-1 and can be activated by nanomolar concentrations of thrombin. PAR-4 signaling appears to be unnecessary for platelet activation if PAR-1 signaling is intact.[90] Vorapaxar is a potent, selective, long-acting, oral PAR-1 inhibitor generated from the naturally occurring muscarinic receptor antagonist himbacine.[91] A high-resolution crystal structure of vorapaxar bound to PAR-1 revealed that the binding pocket for the drug is unusual for a peptide-activated G-protein–coupled receptor in that it consists of a superficial tunnel with little of the bound drug surface exposed to aqueous solvent, perhaps accounting for the very slow dissociation rate of vorapaxar from PAR-1.[92]

The efficacy of vorapaxar for the secondary prevention of arterial thrombosis was examined in the phase III TRA 2P–TIMI 50 trial in which patients with a history of myocardial infarction, stroke, or peripheral arterial disease were randomized between vorapaxar and placebo.[93] Most patients were also taking either aspirin or a thienopyridine. Because of a high incidence of intracranial bleeding in the first years of the study, entry criteria were modified to eliminate patients with a history of a stroke. At 3 years, the incidence of the primary end point (cardiovascular death, myocardial infarction, and stroke) was significantly reduced in vorapaxar-treated patients (9.3 percent vs. 11.2 percent, p <0.001). However, moderate to severe bleeding, including intracranial bleeding, was significantly increased in the vorapaxar-treated patients (4.2 percent vs. 2.5 percent, p <0.001). Nonetheless, based on efficacy, vorapaxar received FDA approval in 2014. Atopaxar, a second PAR-1 antagonist, is currently being evaluated in clinical trials.[94] Atopaxar has a shorter half-life than vorapaxar, suggesting that potential bleeding complications might be easier to manage.

INTEGRIN $\alpha_{IIb}\beta_3$ RECEPTOR ANTAGONISTS

Drugs that specifically impair the function of the major platelet integrin $\alpha_{IIb}\beta_3$ (GPIIb/IIIa) have been developed for short-term use as antithrombotic agents in the setting of ischemic coronary artery disease.[95,96] Integrin $\alpha_{IIb}\beta_3$ mediates platelet–platelet cohesion by binding the divalent ligand fibrinogen, thereby crosslinking the integrin on adjacent platelets, causing the formation of platelet aggregates.[97] Thus, integrin $\alpha_{IIb}\beta_3$ is a viable therapeutic target to prevent arterial thrombosis. Abciximab, eptifibatide, and tirofiban are three FDA-approved structurally dissimilar integrin $\alpha_{IIb}\beta_3$ inhibitors that rapidly impair platelet aggregation. Abciximab is a human-murine chimeric Fab fragment, eptifibatide is a cyclic heptapeptide based on the sequence Lys-Gly-Asp (KGD), and tirofiban is an Arg-Gly-Asp (RGD)-based peptidomimetic. All three drugs have demonstrated efficacy in the management of patients with acute coronary syndromes, particularly in the setting of percutaneous coronary interventions (PCI) where iatrogenic artery wall injury occurs.[97]

Inherited integrin $\alpha_{IIb}\beta_3$ abnormalities cause the bleeding disorder Glanzmann thrombasthenia (Chap. 120).[98,99] Thus, it is not surprising that integrin $\alpha_{IIb}\beta_3$ antagonists can predispose to bleeding. In EPIC, a clinical trial of abciximab in patients undergoing PCI, 14 percent of patients given abciximab experienced major bleeding compared to 7 percent of patients given placebo.[100] However, patients were also given aspirin and heparin. When the heparin dose was decreased in the subsequent EPILOG trial, the incidence of major bleeding in patients receiving abciximab decreased to 2.0 percent compared to 3.1 percent in the control group receiving heparin and aspirin alone.[101] Nonetheless, in both EPIC and EPILOG, minor bleeding was significantly more frequent in patients given abciximab and standard-dose heparin compared to patients given standard-dose heparin alone, attesting to the ability of an integrin $\alpha_{IIb}\beta_3$ antagonist to impair normal hemostasis. In the PRISM-PLUS trial of tirofiban and the PURSUIT trial of eptifibatide, major and minor bleeding were slightly more frequent in patients receiving the study drug compared to controls.[102,103] Similarly, patients receiving the oral integrin $\alpha_{IIb}\beta_3$ inhibitors xemilofiban and sibrafiban for 30 and 28 days, respectively, frequently experienced mucocutaneous bleeding similar to that experienced by patients with congenital thrombasthenia.[104,105] Although short-term use of the parenteral integrin $\alpha_{IIb}\beta_3$ antagonists is often beneficial in patients with acute coronary syndrome of following PCI, paradoxically the long-term use of oral integrin $\alpha_{IIb}\beta_3$ inhibitors was associated with an increase in mortality.[106] The cause of this paradoxical effect is not clear, but has been attributed by some to an antagonist-induced conformational change in integrin $\alpha_{IIb}\beta_3$ simulating the effect of physiologic platelet agonists.[107]

The risk of bleeding in patients undergoing PCI in the presence of integrin $\alpha_{IIb}\beta_3$ antagonists can be minimized by using heparin on a weight basis,[101] by avoiding treatment of patients who are receiving warfarin at therapeutic doses, by early vascular sheath removal, and by meticulous care of vascular puncture sites.[108] Platelet transfusions can

rapidly reverse the platelet function defect in patients receiving abciximab, presumably by decreasing the overall extent of integrin blockade. The ability of platelet transfusion to reverse the effects of the other integrin $\alpha_{IIb}\beta_3$ antagonists is less clear, but these drugs have very short half-lives if renal and hepatic function are normal.

Thrombocytopenia occurring within 24 hours of initiating therapy has been observed in small numbers of patients following the administration of all integrin $\alpha_{IIb}\beta_3$ antagonists.[102,105,108,109] In EPIC, the incidence of platelet counts of less than 100×10^9/L and of less than 50×10^9/L in patients receiving abciximab for the first time was 3.9 percent and 0.9 percent, respectively.[109] Thrombocytopenia has also been reported in patients receiving eptifibatide, tirofiban, and a variety of small molecule RGD- and non–RGD-based integrin $\alpha_{IIb}\beta_3$ inhibitors with an incidence of up to 13 percent.[102,105,109–113]

The mechanism responsible for thrombocytopenia following the administration of these drugs is uncertain, but may be related to the presence of preexisting antiintegrin $\alpha_{IIb}\beta_3$ antibodies that recognize epitopes exposed by the antagonist, or, in the case of abciximab, to murine sequences incorporated into the abciximab Fab fragment.[114] The thrombocytopenia usually reverses readily when the drug is stopped, but it may also be reversed by platelet transfusion if clinically indicated.[108] Thrombocytopenia in patients receiving integrin $\alpha_{IIb}\beta_3$ antagonists must be differentiated from pseudothrombocytopenia as a result of drug-induced platelet clumping, from heparin-induced thrombocytopenia in patients receiving heparin concurrently, and from other causes of thrombocytopenia, depending on the clinical circumstances.[115,116] It is important to identify thrombocytopenia early because integrin $\alpha_{IIb}\beta_3$ antagonists are administered as long infusions and the drug should be stopped as soon as true thrombocytopenia has been confirmed. In most cases of profound thrombocytopenia, a platelet count obtained 2 to 4 hours after initiating therapy will provide evidence of a significant decrease in platelet count, although cases of delayed thrombocytopenia have been observed after treatment with abciximab.[114]

DRUGS THAT AFFECT PLATELET CYCLIC NUCLEOTIDE LEVELS OR FUNCTION

The pyrimidopyrimidine derivative, dipyridamole, inhibits platelet cyclic nucleotide phosphodiesterase, resulting in the intraplatelet accumulation of the inhibitory cyclic nucleotide cyclic AMP (cAMP). Dipyridamole may also inhibit the breakdown of cyclic guanosine monophosphate (cGMP), resulting in potentiation of the platelet inhibitory effect of nitric oxide.[117] Although the platelet inhibitory effects of dipyridamole are seen *in vitro*, the clinical utility of dipyridamole has been controversial.[118,119] A meta-analysis failed to demonstrate the clinical benefit of adding dipyridamole to aspirin.[16] However, many older dipyridamole trials used formulations with limited dipyridamole bioavailability.[120] In the European Stroke Prevention Study 2 (ESPS 2), dipyridamole was beneficial in preventing stroke and transient ischemic attack, but there was no difference in mortality between patients taking dipyridamole and placebo or among patients taking dipyridamole plus aspirin compared to either dipyridamole or aspirin alone.[121] The basis for the benefit of dipyridamole in the ESPS 2 trial is unclear, but could be from a higher dipyridamole dosage or to the sustained-release dipyridamole preparation used in the trial.

Intravenous infusions of PGE$_1$, PGI$_2$, or stable PGI$_2$ analogues stimulate platelet adenylyl cyclase, causing an increase in platelet cAMP and a decrease in platelet responsiveness.[122] These agents cause a transient inhibition of platelet shape change, aggregation, and secretion. However, their clinical utility is limited by their short half-life and side effects that include peripheral vasodilation.[123] Cilostazol, a phosphodiesterase III inhibitor has been approved in the United States for the treatment of peripheral vascular disease[124] and may have utility in the prevention of cardiac stent occlusion.[125] Nitric oxide (NO) and organic nitrates such as nitroglycerin inhibit platelet function *in vitro*, probably by activating guanylyl cyclase, thereby increasing cGMP.[126] Their effect on *in vivo* platelet function is uncertain. High concentrations of caffeine and theophylline also inhibit platelet phosphodiesterases *in vitro*.

ANTIBIOTICS

Penicillins contain a β-lactam ring and a unique side chain. Most cause a dose-dependent prolongation of the bleeding time in normal volunteers.[127] Because they reduce platelet aggregation and secretion, as well as ristocetin-induced platelet agglutination, they may affect both platelet adhesion and platelet activation. Tests of platelet aggregation are abnormal in 50 to 75 percent of individuals receiving large doses (at least several grams per day) of carbenicillin, penicillin G, ticarcillin, ampicillin, nafcillin, and azlocillin and in 25 to 50 percent of patients taking piperacillin, azlocillin, or mezlocillin.[127–129] Differences in the antiplatelet effects of these antibiotics probably relate to differences in blood levels and drug potency. Their effect on platelets is maximal after 1 to 3 days of administration and may remain for several days after the antibiotic has been stopped, suggesting that the effect of these antibiotics on platelets *in vivo* is irreversible.

Penicillins can impair the interaction of agonists and von Willebrand factor (VWF) with the platelet membrane.[130] Indeed, when many penicillins are incubated with washed platelets, albeit at concentrations higher than those attained *in vivo*, they inhibit the interaction of VWF and agonists, such as ADP and epinephrine, with their platelet receptors.[131] The relative *in vitro* antiplatelet potency of the penicillins correlates well with their lipid solubility and with the inhibitory potency of the isolated side chains.[132] Moreover, the inhibitory effect of penicillin G on platelet function *in vitro* is potentiated by the presence of probenecid.[133] When platelet function was tested after intravenous administration of penicillin, oxacillin or mezlocillin for 3 to 17 days to patients or normal volunteers, irreversible inhibition of agonist-induced aggregation was noted, along with a 40 percent reduction in low-affinity TXA_2 receptors.[134] Thus, penicillins probably inhibit platelet function by binding to one or more membrane components necessary for adhesive interactions with the vessel wall or for stimulus-response coupling.

Although clinically significant bleeding is associated with the use of carbenicillin, penicillin G, ticarcillin, and nafcillin, it is far less common than prolongation of the bleeding time.[127,135] Patients with coexisting hemostatic defects (e.g., thrombocytopenia, vitamin K deficiency, uremia) may be particularly prone to this complication. On the other hand, high doses of penicillin G did not increase gastrointestinal blood loss in a thrombocytopenic rabbit model.[136] In our experience, bleeding attributable to antibiotic-induced platelet dysfunction is uncommon and unpredictable. Because β-lactam–induced platelet dysfunction resolves with time following cessation of the drug, this class of drugs should only be considered as a cause of bleeding in the appropriate clinical setting. A similar pattern of platelet dysfunction has been reported with some cephalosporins or related antibiotics, but not with others.[127,137,138] Broad-spectrum antibiotics can also cause a bleeding diathesis attributable to killing of gut flora, resulting in vitamin K deficiency. Nitrofurantoin, a structurally unrelated antibiotic, may cause a mild prolongation of the bleeding time and impair platelet aggregation when blood levels of the drug are higher than 20 μM, as may occur in patients with renal insufficiency.[139] Miconazole, an antifungal agent, inhibits human and rabbit platelet COX *in vitro* and rabbit platelet COX after intravenous infusion.[140]

ANTICOAGULANTS, FIBRINOLYTIC AGENTS, ANTIFIBRINOLYTIC AGENTS

Heparin predisposes to bleeding primarily through its anticoagulant effect, but it may also impair platelet function. For example, a bolus injection of heparin (100 U/kg) can cause a significant prolongation of the bleeding time in normal subjects and in patients prior to cardiopulmonary bypass, suggesting that therapeutic doses of heparin may impair platelet function.[126] Heparin likely impairs platelet function by inhibiting the generation and action of the potent platelet agonist thrombin. On the other hand, *in vitro* studies suggest that heparin can enhance platelet aggregation induced by other platelet agonists.[141] Heparin binds to a single class of high-affinity binding sites on resting platelets and to an additional class of lower-affinity binding sites on fully activated platelets.[142] High heparin doses also impair VWF-dependent platelet function, possibly by binding to the heparin-binding domain of VWF.[143] The contributions of these effects on platelet function to the bleeding complications of heparin therapy are uncertain.

Bleeding during fibrinolytic therapy is predominantly a result of the combined effects of structural lesions in blood vessels and the fibrin(ogen)olytic activity of the agent used. However, pharmacologic doses of streptokinase, urokinase, and tissue plasminogen activator (t-PA) can affect platelet function.[144] High concentrations of plasmin *ex vivo* cause platelet aggregation.[145] Moreover, marked increases in the urinary excretion of the TXA_2 metabolite 2,3-dinor-TXB_2 have been detected in patients receiving streptokinase or t-PA for coronary thrombolysis, suggesting that *in vivo* platelet activation had occurred during infusion of the drug.[146,147] Nevertheless, several *in vitro* studies indicate that plasmin generation has an inhibitory effect on platelet function. First, very high levels of fibrin(ogen) degradation products, coupled with very low levels of fibrinogen, may impair platelet aggregation.[148] Second, plasminogen can bind to platelets[149] and after its conversion to plasmin, enzymatically degrade platelet glycoprotein (GP) Ib, impairing the interaction of platelets with VWF.[150,151] Third, plasmin can inhibit platelet arachidonic acid metabolism.[152] Fourth, t-PA promotes the disaggregation of platelet aggregates, presumably by inducing lysis of the fibrinogen that mediates aggregate formation.[153] Finally, after initial activation, platelets incubated with plasmin and recombinant t-PA *in vitro* become refractory to activation by other agonists.[154] Whether any of these *in vitro* and *ex vivo* observations apply to the *in vivo* situation and are clinically significant remains uncertain.[155] The antifibrinolytic drug, ε-aminocaproic acid, can increase the bleeding time when administered for several days at doses 24 g/day or greater.[150]

CARDIOVASCULAR DRUGS

Administration of nitroprusside, which increases platelet cGMP,[156–160] nitroglycerine,[161] and propranolol,[162,163] can decrease platelet aggregation and secretion *ex vivo*. Nitroprusside can increase the bleeding time twofold when administered at infusion rates of 6 to 8 mcg/kg/min.[156,164] Inhalation of NO advocated for the treatment of pulmonary hypertension and the adult respiratory distress syndrome, can impair agonist-induced platelet aggregation *ex vivo*, although the clinical significance of these observations is unclear.[165–167] Calcium channel blockers such as verapamil, nifedipine, and diltiazem inhibit platelet aggregation when added at very high concentrations to washed platelets.[123] This effect is seen primarily with epinephrine-induced aggregation and does not appear to be related to calcium channel blockade.[168] At therapeutic doses, calcium channel blockers do not prolong the bleeding time, although one agent, nisoldipine, has been reported to inhibit agonist-induced calcium transients and platelet aggregation after ten days of oral administration.[169] At high concentrations, the antiarrhythmic drug quinidine has been reported to cause a mild prolongation of the bleeding time and to potentiate the effect of aspirin.[170]

VOLUME EXPANDERS

Dextran is a neutral polysaccharide that is heterogeneous in molecular size. Two preparations with average molecular weights of 40,000 and 70,000 are in clinical use. Although dextran infusions may prolong the bleeding time of normal subjects and patients with von Willebrand disease, this phenomenon has not been observed in most normal subjects.[9,171,172] Infused dextran adsorbs to the platelet surface and can impair platelet aggregation, secretion, and procoagulant activity. The maximal effect of dextran may require several hours, suggesting that larger molecules with a slower rate of clearance are responsible.[9] Curiously, the drug has no effect when added to platelet-rich plasma.[9] Dextran infusion produces a modest reduction in plasma VWF antigen levels and ristocetin cofactor activity.[171] Despite these effects on primary hemostasis, prospective studies indicate that dextran is not associated with significant postoperative bleeding, unless it is administered together with low-dose heparin.[173,174] Hydroxyethyl starch, another volume expander, while generally safe, may prolong the bleeding time and predispose to hemorrhage, particularly if it is administered in doses exceeding 20 mL/kg of a 6-percent solution. Lower doses of hydroxyethyl starch may contribute to bleeding if administered simultaneously with low-dose heparin or if given to patients with preexistent hemostatic defects or after major cardiothoracic surgery.[175-178] Different hydroxyethyl starch preparations vary in the average number of hydroxymethyl groups per glucose unit, and this may affect both intravascular survival and effects on hemostasis.[179,180]

PSYCHOTROPIC DRUGS, ANESTHETICS, AND COCAINE

Platelets from patients taking antidepressants or phenothiazines may exhibit impaired aggregation, but this is not associated with bleeding.[181,182] The effect on aggregation has been attributed to inhibition of intracellular signaling molecules such as protein kinase C (PKC).[183] Selective serotonin reuptake inhibitors such as paroxetine, have been shown to decrease platelet serotonin storage.[184] Fluoxetine does not appear to impair platelet aggregation *in vitro* and has only rarely been associated with clinical bleeding.[185,186] General anesthesia with halothane or propofol may cause a slight prolongation of the bleeding time, most likely the result of an effect on calcium signaling, but this has no adverse effect on surgical hemostasis.[187,188] In addition to an association with thrombocytopenia, cocaine has been reported to either inhibit[189,190] or stimulate platelet activation.[191] It has been suggested that heroin decreases platelet NO production.[192] The clinical relevance of these observations is unknown.

ONCOLOGIC DRUGS

Administering mithramycin to a total dose of 6 to 21 mg decreases platelet aggregation and is associated with mucocutaneous bleeding.[193] An *ex vivo* defect in platelet secretion and secondary aggregation has been reported in patients with solid tumors within 48 hours of receiving infusions of autologous marrow and high-dose chemotherapy consisting of cisplatin, cyclophosphamide, and either *bis*-chloroethylnitrosourea (BCNU) or melphelan.[194] Both daunorubicin and BCNU can inhibit platelet aggregation and secretion when added to platelet-rich plasma, but they have not been shown to cause clinically significant platelet dysfunction.[195-197] Administration of recombinant forms of thrombopoietin to thrombocytopenic patients with cancer results in the production of normally functioning platelets.[198,199] Dasatinib, the broad-spectrum

protein tyrosine kinase inhibitor, impairs collagen-induced platelet activation *in vitro* and increases tail bleeding times in mice, perhaps explaining some bleeding episodes in patients with chronic myelogenous leukemia who have been treated with the drug.[200] Ibrutinib, a Bruton tyrosine kinase (BTK) inhibitor efficacious in a wide variety of lymphoid malignanies,[201,202] is associated with hemorrhagic complications in up to half of patients, with significant hemorrhagic toxicity in 5 percent.[201-203] Exposing platelets to ibrutinib *ex vivo* can produce defective platelet adhesion.[204] Furthermore, humans or mice lacking BTK have impaired *ex vivo* platelet function, although the impairment is quite mild.[205,206] Whether the hemorrhagic toxicity of ibrutinib is caused by platelet BTK inhibition or by an off-target effect remains to be determined.

MISCELLANEOUS AGENTS

The immunosuppressive drug cyclosporine has been reported to enhance ADP-stimulated platelet aggregation *in vitro*.[207] It is unclear whether this contributes to the TTP-like syndrome associated with this drug. Antihistamines,[208] the serotonin antagonist ketanserin,[209] and certain radiographic contrast agents[210,211] can impair platelet aggregation responses *ex vivo* by unknown mechanisms.

FOODS AND FOOD ADDITIVES

Certain foods and food additives affect platelet function *in vitro*, and it is conceivable that some may affect hemostasis, particularly in association with other hemostatic defects. For example, diets rich in fish oils containing ω-3 fatty acids (eicosapentaenoic acid; docosahexaenoic acid) cause a slight prolongation of the bleeding time.[212] These fatty acids act by reducing the platelet content of arachidonic acid and by competing with arachidonic acid for COX.[213,214] Easy bruising noted after eating Chinese food has been attributed to an antiplatelet effect of the black tree fungus.[215] A component of extract of onion can inhibit platelet arachidonic acid metabolism.[216] Ajoene, a component of garlic, is an inhibitor of fibrinogen binding and platelet aggregation.[217] Extracts of two commonly used spices, cumin and turmeric, also inhibit platelet aggregation and eicosanoid biosynthesis.[218]

● HEMATOLOGIC DISORDERS ASSOCIATED WITH ABNORMAL PLATELET FUNCTION

CHRONIC MYELOPROLIFERATIVE NEOPLASMS

Definition and History

Bleeding and thrombosis are significant causes of morbidity and mortality in the chronic myeloproliferative neoplasms, particularly in essential thrombocythemia, polycythemia vera, and primary myelofibrosis.[219-221] Thrombocytosis is a constant finding in essential thrombocythemia, but the differential diagnosis includes these other myeloproliferative neoplasms, including chronic myelogenous leukemia, as well as other diseases associated with reactive thrombosis (Chap. 119).[222,223] Most of the information about platelets, bleeding and thrombosis in the myeloproliferative neoplasms comes from studies of essential thrombocythemia and polycythemia vera.

Etiology and Pathogenesis

Several factors contribute to the hemostatic abnormalities in the myeloproliferative neoplasms: (1) Increased whole-blood viscosity in polycythemia vera: The engorgement of blood vessels associated with polycythemia is a risk factor for thrombosis and bleeding, particularly in postoperative situations.[224–226] (2) Intrinsic defects in platelet function: Many intrinsic platelet function defects have been reported in the myeloproliferative neoplasms, although their precise relationships to clinical bleeding are generally unclear.[227,228] (3) Elevated platelet counts: The contribution of an elevated platelet count, per se, to the risk of hemorrhage and thrombosis in myeloproliferative neoplasms is controversial, as the risk does not extend to patients with reactive thrombocytosis.[229,230] A number of retrospective studies indicate that the risk of abnormal hemostasis cannot be confidently predicted from the degree of thrombocytosis.[227] On the other hand, acquired von Willebrand syndrome, which represents a potential major cause of bleeding in the chronic myeloproliferative neoplasms, is most frequently associated with extreme elevations of the platelet count (e.g., ≥1000 to 1500 × 10^9/L)[231–233]; in some, the VWF abnormality can be corrected, albeit transiently, by infusion of DDAVP or factor VIII/VWF concentrates, while in others it can be partially or completely corrected by cytoreductive therapy.[234] (4) Leukocytosis may represent a risk factor for thrombosis in the myeloproliferative neoplasms.[221,235] In this context, leukocyte and/or endothelial dysfunction may contribute to the thrombotic phenotype in some individuals with polycythemia vera[236,237] or essential thrombocythemia[232] through leukocyte–platelet and leukocyte–endothelial cell interactions.[232,238,239]

Under the light or electron microscope, platelets in these disorders may be larger or smaller than normal, may be abnormally shaped, and may exhibit a reduction in the number of storage granules.[240] In essential thrombocythemia, platelet survival may be modestly reduced.[241] A number of functional and biochemical abnormalities have been described in platelets from patients with myeloproliferative neoplasms. The most frequently encountered functional abnormality is a decrease in platelet aggregation and granule secretion in response to epinephrine, ADP, or collagen.[227] The defect in epinephrine-induced aggregation often includes absence of the primary wave of aggregation, which is unusual in other conditions. This is not simply the result of an elevated platelet count, because it is not encountered in reactive thrombocytosis.[222,242] Thus, loss of platelet responsiveness to epinephrine may help to support the presence of a myeloproliferative neoplasm in otherwise ambiguous cases, although the discovery of genetic abnormalities (e.g., JAK2, thrombopoietin receptor [MPL], calreticulin) is beginning to eliminate all ambiguity in the diagnosis of a myeloproliferative neoplasm (Chaps. 84 to 86).

Reduced platelet aggregation and secretion in the myeloproliferative neoplasms is associated with one or more of the following: decreased agonist-induced release of arachidonic acid from membrane phospholipids[243,244]; reduced conversion of arachidonic acid to PG endoperoxides or lipoxygenase products[245]; reduced platelet responsiveness to TXA_2[246]; decreased numbers of α_2-adrenergic receptors associated with reduced or absent platelet responses to epinephrine[247,248]; deficiency of integrin $\alpha_2\beta_1$, resulting in variable changes in platelet responsiveness to collagen[249]; diminished stimulus–response coupling downstream of several agonists associated with reduced activation of phosphatidylinositide 3′-kinase, Rap1 and integrin $\alpha_{IIb}\beta_3$[250]; and deficiency of dense or α granules.[251,252] Reduction in platelet procoagulant activity has been reported in some patients with myeloproliferative neoplasms and thrombocytosis,[253] as have specific platelet membrane abnormalities, including decreased expression and activation of integrin $\alpha_{IIb}\beta_3$,[254] decreased amounts of the GPIb–V–IX complex, resulting in an acquired form of Bernard-Soulier syndrome[255]; decreased numbers of receptors for PGD_2[256]; increased numbers of FcγRIIa receptors[257]; an increase in GPIV (CD36) with[258,259] or without[260] a corresponding decrease in GPIb; and impaired expression of MPL in polycythemia vera[261] and essential thrombocythemia.[111]

On the other hand, evidence for *in vitro* platelet or coagulation hyperactivity has been reported in the myeloproliferative neoplasms. This includes spontaneous platelet aggregation in a patient with essential thrombocythemia and thrombosis,[262] increased thromboxane biosynthesis by platelets from patients with essential thrombocythemia[263] or polycythemia vera,[264] and increased "procoagulant imbalance" in patients manifested by increased endogenous thrombin potential[265] and increased procoagulant activity in circulating microparticles.[266]

Several features of these protean *in vitro* platelet functional defects require emphasis relative to the clinical setting. First, none are unique to a particular myeloproliferative neoplasm. Second, their relative frequencies have varied widely in reported series. Third, none has been prospectively shown to be predictive of bleeding or thrombosis. Fourth, although the chronic myeloproliferative neoplasms comprise several distinct clinicopathologic entities, they represent clonal abnormalities of hematopoiesis.[267] Consequently, megakaryocytes and their platelet progeny may acquire genetic, biochemical, and structural abnormalities as they develop from clones of abnormal progenitors. Examples of clonal defects in the chronic myeloproliferative neoplasms are acquisition of activating mutations in JAK2 (e.g., V617F in polycythemia vera, essential thrombocythemia, and myelofibrosis; or in exon 12 in polycythemia vera)[268–272] or MPL (W515L/K in essential thrombocythemia and myelofibrosis).[273,274] Mutations in the calreticulin gene have been found in most of the essential thrombocythemia and myelofibrosis patients who lack activating mutations in JAK2 or MPL.[275,276] It is biologically plausible that mutations in these or other leukocyte and platelet proteins might influence hemostatic mechanisms, including the activation state of platelets.[277–279] However, the precise impact of their presence or allele burden on human platelet function and on thrombotic risk is only now beginning to be understood.[232,280] For example, most,[232,268] but not all,[237,281] studies have concluded that the presence of the JAK2 (V617F) mutation or a high JAK2 (V617F) allele burden confers increased thrombotic risk in essential thrombocythemia, the latter in part a result of higher hemoglobin values. On the other hand, essential thrombocythemia or myelofibrosis patients with calreticulin mutations tend to have higher platelet counts, lower hemoglobin and leukocyte values, and fewer thromboses compared to patients with JAK2 mutations.[275,282–285] The same may hold true for rare patients with familial essential thrombocythemia or myelofibrosis and somatically-acquired calreticulin mutations.[282]

Clinical and Laboratory Features

Pathologic bleeding occurs in approximately one-third of patients with myeloproliferative neoplasms and contributes to mortality in 10 percent of those affected patients. Thrombosis also occurs in one-third of patients with myeloproliferative disorders, contributing to mortality in 15 to 40 percent of affected patients.[228,232] Most symptomatic patients experience either bleeding or thrombosis; however, some develop both complications during the course of their disease. Bleeding usually involves the skin or mucous membranes, but may also occur after surgery or trauma. Thrombosis can involve arteries or veins and may occur in unusual locations such as abdominal wall vessels or the hepatic, portal, and mesenteric circulations.[286–291] Indeed, full-blown or latent chronic myeloproliferative neoplasms account for a substantial proportion of patients with splanchnic vein thrombosis.[286,291–294] Individuals with essential thrombocythemia may experience ischemia and necrosis of the fingers and toes from digital artery thrombosis, microvascular occlusion in the coronary circulation, or transient neurologic symptoms, including headaches,[295] because of cerebrovascular occlusion.[296] A syndrome of redness and burning pain in the extremities, termed *erythromelalgia*, is strongly associated with essential thrombocythemia and polycythemia vera and is thought to be partly caused by arteriolar platelet thrombi, although it may also have vasculopathic and neuropathic components.[297,298] It has been difficult to predict the risk of bleeding or thrombosis in an asymptomatic patient,[229] but an increase in leukocyte count[221,232,235] or the number of reticulated platelets in patients with thrombocytosis, thought to reflect an increase in platelet turnover, has been associated with an increased risk for thrombosis.[299] Vascular complications are also more likely to occur in patients older than 60 years of age and, most importantly, in patients with other cardiovascular risk factors, such as diabetes, hypertension, hyperlipidemia and obesity.[221,300-303]

Therapy

Therapy should be risk-adapted and considered for symptomatic patients, for patients with a history of thrombosis or bleeding, for those with standard cardiovascular risk factors, for patients older than 60 years of age, and for individuals about to undergo surgery. Readers are referred to expert recommendations for a summary of the treatment of essential thrombocythemia and polycythemia vera, with particular relevance to risk factors for hemostasis and thrombosis (Chaps. 84 and 85).[221,232,301,303-306] Treatment includes phlebotomy to correct the polycythemia and maintenance of a normal red cell mass, with the goal to achieve a hematocrit of less than 45 percent,[235,307,308] as well as therapy of the underlying disorder.[228,232,309,310] Platelet count reduction to less than 400×10^9/L in patients with thrombocytosis, either by plateletpheresis or cytoreductive agents, has been considered to be a target value associated with clinical improvement in patients with essential thrombocythemia.[228,302,311]

Effective cytoreductive agents include the ribonuclease reductase inhibitor hydroxyurea,[312] interferon-α (most recently the pegylated form of interferon alfa-2a), and anagrelide.[301,311,313,314] In a prospective, randomized trial of 114 "high-risk" individuals with essential thrombocythemia who were either older than 60 years of age or had a previous history of thrombosis, hydroxyurea significantly reduced the incidence of new thrombosis from 24.0 to 3.6 percent.[312] Anagrelide, an imidazoquinazoline derivative, is thought to decrease platelet counts by impairing megakaryocyte maturation.[315] Anagrelide has essentially no effect on red and white cell counts and is not known to be leukemogenic. Nevertheless, 10 to 20 percent of patients experience neurologic, gastrointestinal, and cardiac side effects, in particular fluid retention, often necessitating discontinuation of the drug.[314,316,317] When hydroxyurea and anagrelide were compared head-to-head in a randomized trial of 809 patients with essential thrombocythemia (all of whom were taking aspirin), subjects in the anagrelide group showed an increased rate of arterial thrombosis, major bleeding, and transformation to myelofibrosis relative to the group treated with hydroxyurea; however, the anagrelide group showed a relative decreased rate of venous thrombosis.[318] Progression to myelofibrosis despite treatment with anagrelide has also been observed in a phase II study.[319] However, in a newer, although relatively small, randomized, phase III study of 259 previously untreated high-risk patients with essential thrombocythemia, anagrelide was found to be noninferior to hydroxyurea in the prevention of arterial or venous thrombotic complications.[320] It should be noted that this study used a long-lasting anagrelide drug that is not currently available in the United States. During an episode of acute bleeding in the chronic myeloproliferative neoplasms, DDAVP infusion may temporarily improve hemostasis if the patient has an acquired storage pool defect or acquired von Willebrand syndrome.[252,321] In the case of acquired von Willebrand syndrome, cytoreduction to reduce the platelet count may also ameliorate the process, although this may take time and require more temporizing interventions including DDAVP or factor VIII/VWF concentrates.[234]

Low-dose aspirin (~80 to 100 mg/day) may be useful in patients with essential thrombocythemia and thrombosis, particularly those with erythromelalgia or with digital or cerebrovascular ischemia.[231,232,298,322] However, the evidence to date remains largely anecdotal, and aspirin can exacerbate a bleeding tendency in patients with myeloproliferative neoplasms, particularly in those individuals with acquired von Willebrand syndrome or with World Health Organization (WHO)-defined prefibrotic myelofibrosis masquerading as essential thrombocythemia.[221,301,303,323] Consequently, even though a single, daily, low-dose aspirin is recommended for thromboprophylaxis in essential thrombocythemia, a risk-adapted approach is advised.[221,305] In addition, because platelet volume and turnover may be enhanced in essential thrombocythemia and polycythemia vera, the platelets of some individuals may not achieve total COX-1 inhibition with a single daily dose of aspirin. In such circumstances, 12-hour dosing may be considered, although this protocol has not been formally evaluated in a prospective clinical trial.[324,325]

In a double-blind, placebo-controlled study of 518 patients with polycythemia vera who were judged to have no contraindications to daily low-dose (100 mg) aspirin, subjects in the aspirin arm exhibited a reduced risk of nonfatal arterial and venous cardiovascular end points. Although aspirin was well-tolerated, there was no effect of aspirin on overall and cardiovascular mortality.[326] As has been noted,[307] this study population was heavily pretreated to normalize the platelet count, although some individuals may have had residual elevations in red cell mass. Consequently, the safety and efficacy of aspirin as observed in this study may not be relevant to all patients with polycythemia vera.

Pregnant women with essential thrombocythemia or polycythemia vera pose special challenges because of an apparent increased risk of unsuccessful pregnancy, thrombotic or bleeding complications, and potential teratogenicity of hydroxyurea.[305,327] In essential thrombocythemia, the risk of first trimester miscarriages may be higher among women with the JAK2 (V617F) mutation.[328] Although evidence-based recommendations are not available, Barbui and Finazzi recommend a risk-adapted approach to management in pregnancy. High-risk women are defined as those with previous major bleeding or thrombotic episodes, previous pregnancy complications, or a platelet count greater than 1500×10^9/L.[329] Low-risk individuals are recommended to be maintained at a hematocrit of less than 45 percent and to receive aspirin, 100 mg/day during pregnancy and low-molecular-weight heparin, 4000 U/day for 6 weeks after delivery. Interferon-α, rather than aspirin, is considered if there has been previous major bleeding or if platelets are greater than 1500×10^9/L. High-risk patients are recommended to receive low-molecular-weight heparin throughout pregnancy.

LEUKEMIAS AND MYELODYSPLASTIC SYNDROMES

Clinical and Laboratory Features

The most frequent cause of bleeding in patients with leukemia or a myelodysplastic syndrome is thrombocytopenia. However, abnormal platelet function *in vitro* has been described in acute myelogenous leukemia, and in some patients this may be clinically significant. In acute myelogenous leukemia and its variants, platelets may be larger than normal, abnormally shaped, and exhibit a marked variation in the number of granules. There may be decreased aggregation and serotonin release in response to ADP, epinephrine, or collagen, decreased surface P-selectin expression in response to platelet activation via the PAR-1 thrombin receptor, and decreased platelet procoagulant activity. These functional abnormalities may be caused by either acquired storage pool deficiency or a defect in the process of platelet activation through one or more signaling pathways.[330-334] These defects are intrinsic to the platelet and probably relate to the fact that the megakaryocytes from which platelets were derived originated from a leukemic stem cell. Indeed, in a familial platelet disorder with a predisposition to acute leukemia, platelet dysfunction prior to the development of leukemia occurs, at least in part, because of downregulation of genes such as *NF-E2* or *ALOX12*, themselves target genes of RUNX1, a transcription factor that is germline-mutated in these individuals.[335,336]

As discussed in the section on oncology drugs, drugs used to treat acute leukemias may affect platelet function, at least *in vitro*.[200,337,338] Bleeding in the acute leukemias usually responds to platelet transfusions and to treatment of the underlying disease. Similar *in vitro* platelet abnormalities may be seen in the myelodysplastic syndromes, sometimes accompanied by clinical bleeding disproportionate to that expected for the degree of thrombocytopenia.[330,339–344] In these syndromes, platelets may be less uniformly affected; perhaps because there is a residual population of normal platelets admixed with those from the malignant clone.

Reduced platelet aggregation has been reported in children with acute lymphocytic leukemia.[331] Unless the leukemia is biphenotypic, it is difficult to ascribe the platelet defect to the leukemic process itself. Platelets are normal in children with acute lymphoblastic leukemia in complete remission.[345] Single cases have been reported of patients with acute B-lymphoblastic leukemia[346] or Hodgkin lymphoma[347] whose severe bleeding was attributed, in part, to acquired Glanzmann thrombasthenia associated with antiintegrin $\alpha_{IIb}\beta_3$ antibodies. Hairy cell leukemia is a lymphoproliferative disease in which platelet dysfunction may rarely complicate the clinical picture; bleeding is usually due to thrombocytopenia rather than platelet dysfunction.[348] Some patients may exhibit storage pool deficiency or a defect in the process of platelet activation. These abnormalities have been reported to disappear following splenectomy,[349] which usually corrects the thrombocytopenia as well. Acquired von Willebrand syndrome has been reported in association with hairy cell leukemia.[350]

DYSPROTEINEMIAS

Definition and History

Platelet dysfunction is observed in approximately one-third of patients with Immunoglobulin (Ig) A multiple myeloma or Waldenström macroglobulinemia, 15 percent of patients with IgG myeloma, and in occasional patients with monoclonal gammopathy of undetermined significance (Chap. 106).[351,352] In addition to platelet dysfunction, other causes of bleeding should be considered in these patients, including the hyperviscosity syndrome,[353] thrombocytopenia, complications of amyloidosis such as amyloid angiopathy[354] or acquired factor X deficiency[355,356]), and rarely, a circulating heparin-like anticoagulant[357–359] or systemic fibrino(gen)lysis.[360,361] The monoclonal immunoglobulin may also affect *in vitro* coagulation tests by interfering with fibrin polymerization and with the function of other coagulation proteins. On occasion, paraproteins can impair *in vivo* hemostasis as well.

Etiology and Pathogenesis

The bleeding time may be prolonged in patients with dysproteinemias, even in the absence of clinical bleeding. The platelet defect is caused by the monoclonal protein. It has been suggested that some monoclonal immunoglobulins interact with the platelet surface to interfere nonspecifically with platelet adhesion or stimulus–response coupling. This concept is supported by the observations that platelet dysfunction is more common when the concentration of the paraprotein in plasma or on the platelet membrane is very high[362]; that platelet aggregation, secretion, clot retraction, and platelet procoagulant activity may all be affected; and that normal platelets can acquire these defects when incubated with the purified monoclonal immunoglobulin.[363]

In some cases, specific interactions of the monoclonal protein with platelets or with components of the extracellular matrix have been

described. One reported IgA myeloma protein inhibited the ability of a suspension of aortic connective tissue to aggregate normal platelets.[364] The bleeding time and bleeding diathesis of the patient from whom this myeloma protein was obtained were corrected by removal of the protein by plasmapheresis. In another patient with IgDλ myeloma, λ dimers were found to bind to the A1 domain of VWF, inhibiting shear-induced platelet aggregation.[365] In still another patient, an IgG myeloma protein bound specifically to the platelet integrin β_3 subunit. Both the intact immunoglobulin and its F(ab')2 fragment inhibited the binding of fibrinogen to activated integrin $\alpha_{IIb}\beta_3$, thus inducing a thrombasthenic-like state.[366] A number of patients with myeloma, monoclonal gammopathy of undetermined significance, lymphoma, or chronic lymphocytic leukemia have been reported to have an acquired form of von Willebrand disease in which the level of plasma VWF is reduced or the high-molecular-weight multimers of VWF are selectively reduced.[321,352,367–374]

Therapy

When clinically significant platelet dysfunction occurs in a patient with a dysproteinemia, cytoreductive therapy should be considered as a means to reduce the production and plasma level of the monoclonal immunoglobulin.[351,352] Plasmapheresis can also control bleeding by reducing the level of the abnormal protein and can be lifesaving during acute bleeds.[352,375,376] Cryoprecipitate, DDAVP and/or plasmapheresis may be transiently effective in patients with acquired von Willebrand syndrome.[321,368,377,378] However, high-dose intravenous gamma globulin (IVIG) appears to be particularly effective in individuals with acquired von Willebrand syndrome associated with an IgG monoclonal gammopathy of undetermined significance, although intermittent infusions may be required at approximately 3-week intervals (Chap. 126).[352,369–371,379–381] The reported experience with rituximab for the latter condition is extremely limited, but so far disappointing.[382]

ACQUIRED VON WILLEBRAND SYNDROME

Acquired von Willebrand syndrome is a relatively rare disorder that typically occurs in the setting of an autoimmune or clonal hematologic disease.[231,381,383–385] It is being increasingly recognized in conditions associated with high shear and turbulence in the circulation, such as severe aortic stenosis, hypertrophic obstructive cardiomyopathy and circulatory assist devices.[381,386–390] It also can occur in association with a number of other unrelated medical conditions,[381] including Gaucher disease,[391] hypothyroidism[392,393] and Noonan syndrome.[394] As discussed above, it can represent one cause of bleeding in multiple myeloma,[321,377] Waldenström macroglobulinemia,[395] monoclonal gammopathy of undetermined significance,[370] low grade non-Hodgkin lymphoma,[396,397] chronic lymphocytic leukemia,[398] and chronic myeloproliferative neoplasms, the latter particularly in association with very high platelet counts.[233]

The pathophysiology of acquired von Willebrand syndrome involves a reduction in circulating VWF (and its associated factor VIII molecule), generally because of rapid VWF turnover in the circulation.[381] VWF levels and multimer patterns may simulate type I, II or III von Willebrand disease. In lymphoproliferative disorders, a specific, often nonneutralizing anti-VWF antibody is present,[321,352,377,399] whereas in autoimmune disorders, anti-VWF antibodies are part of a generalized autoimmune response.[400] In other situations, the syndrome may result from increased adsorption of VWF by tumor cells (e.g., Wilms tumor, osteosarcoma[401]) or platelets (myeloproliferative neoplasms),[315,350,402–404] increased VWF proteolysis (e.g., aortic stenosis, ventricular assist devices), or decreased VWF production (hypothyroidism).[381,405,406]

Mucocutaneous bleeding should raise the suspicion of acquired von Willebrand syndrome in patients without a prior personal or family history of bleeding. This is especially important in patients with a known autoimmune, lymphoproliferative, or myeloproliferative disorder.[315,381] Diagnostic evaluation includes measurements of factor VIII activity, VWF antigen, ristocetin cofactor activity, and VWF multimer analysis.[407] The presence of an *in vitro* inhibitor may, or may not, be detected depending on whether the antibody binds to VWF and neutralizes its function or merely leads to accelerated VWF clearance by the reticuloendothelial system.[315] An abnormally high ratio of VWF propeptide to von Willebrand antigen may be present as a result of the rapid clearance of von Willebrand antigen but not VWF.[44]

Given the uncommon prevalence of this syndrome, reports of patient management have been retrospective and largely anecdotal. Treatment should be reserved for patients with active bleeding or those who are likely to bleed if left untreated.[352,381] Infusions of DDAVP[321,398,400] or factor VIII/VWF concentrates[408,409] may be useful, although the rapid clearance of VWF may limit efficacy. Treatment has included glucocorticoids or rituximab in patients with lupus,[231,385,410] and recombinant factor VIIa,[411] or high-dose IVIG.[190,384,412] High-dose IVIG is particularly effective when acquired von Willebrand syndrome is associated with a lymphoproliferative disorder or, as discussed in the section "Dysproteinemias," with an IgG monoclonal gammopathy of undetermined significance. IVIG likely acts by delaying VWF clearance via reticuloendothelial cell blockade, although other mechanisms have been postulated.[297,369,370,379,380,397,413] Treatment of the underlying disease can be effective in some situations[381,414,415] (e.g., hypothyroidism with thyroid replacement,[416,417] Gaucher disease with enzyme replacement therapy,[391] and extreme thrombocytosis with cytoreduction[233,315,323,418]). As with inherited von Willebrand disease, longstanding acquired von Willebrand syndrome can be associated with and complicated by gastrointestinal tract arteriovenous malformations, resulting in severe bleeding.[419] An example of such gastrointestinal bleeding is found in patients with severe aortic stenosis and referred to as Heyde syndrome. In this situation, valve replacement can correct the hemostatic defect.[387,420]

● SYSTEMIC DISORDERS ASSOCIATED WITH ABNORMAL PLATELET FUNCTION

UREMIA

Definition and History

In the predialysis era, hemorrhage occurred in approximately 50 percent of uremic patients and was a cause of death in approximately 30 perccent.[421,422] With the advent of dialysis, the frequency of spontaneous hemorrhage in patients with renal failure has decreased.[422] Experience with percutaneous renal biopsy in several thousand patients with renal disease supports the notion that the hemostatic defect in patients with renal disease is usually mild. Although the incidence of small perirenal hematomas following biopsy may be as high as 85 percent when patients are examined by computerized tomography, gross hematuria is observed in only 5 to 10 percent of cases and is usually transient.[423,424] Severe bleeding following biopsy requiring surgical intervention is even less common and usually can be attributed to factors other than a uremic hemostatic defect, such as needle lacerations of the kidney or spleen, anomalous vessels, heparin anticoagulation, or the presence of amyloid in the kidney.

Etiology and Pathogenesis

The hemostatic defect in uremia has been attributed to defects in platelet function and appears to be multifactorial.[425] One prominent factor is renal failure-associated anemia.[426] A lowered hematocrit *ex vivo*

induces a defect in platelet adhesion that can be corrected by increasing the hematocrit to 30 percent or more.[427] In uremic patients, successful treatment of anemia with red blood cell transfusion or recombinant human erythropoietin (EPO) results in partial or complete correction of prolonged bleeding times when the hematocrit is increased to 27 to 32 percent.[428-431] The effect of anemia on primary hemostasis is not unique to uremia. In normal individuals, the bleeding time correlates with the hematocrit and bleeding times can be prolonged in patients with severe anemia of any etiology.[426] Red cells may have a beneficial effect on hemostasis both because they displace platelets toward the periphery of the column of circulating blood[432] and they may enhance platelet reactivity.[14]

Because correction of anemia does not always return the bleeding time to normal, other factors present in renal failure may perturb platelet function.[427] Ristocetin-induced platelet aggregation, a surrogate for VWF binding to the platelet GPIb–IX–V complex, may be decreased in uremia. However, plasma VWF concentrations are normal or elevated in renal failure[433] and qualitative VWF abnormalities have not been uniformly observed.[434,435] Mixing studies using uremic platelets and normal plasma, and vice versa, do not demonstrate consistent quantitative or qualitative abnormalities in GPIb–IX–V.[434-436] Nonetheless, uremic plasma can inhibit the adhesion of normal platelets to deendothelialized human umbilical artery segments, whereas uremic platelets adhere normally in the presence of normal plasma.[434] Because the defective adhesion appears independent of VWF, an unidentified component of uremic plasma may be responsible for the adhesion defect.[434] Uremic platelets also exhibit markedly reduced spreading on the subendothelium of rabbit vessels, a defect attributed to impaired VWF binding to platelet integrin $\alpha_{IIb}\beta_3$.[437] Because VWF binding to integrin $\alpha_{IIb}\beta_3$ requires platelet stimulation, this observation suggests a uremia-induced defect in platelet signal transduction.

There are a number of reports describing defective agonist-induced platelet activation in uremic patients, including reduced fibrinogen binding, aggregation, and secretion. These abnormalities may be retained after platelets are separated from uremic plasma and in some cases, uremic plasma imparts the defect to normal platelets.[438] Furthermore, the ability of activated platelets to express procoagulant activity is reduced in uremia.[439] These functional defects likely result from uremia-induced abnormalities in platelet biochemistry, including reduced agonist-induced increases in cytoplasmic free calcium,[440] reduced release of arachidonic acid from platelet phospholipids,[421] and reduced conversion of released arachidonic acid to PG endoperoxides and TXA_2.[138,441,442]

A number of dialyzable and nondialyzable substances have been reported to be responsible for the platelet function defects in uremia,[443] but urea itself is not responsible. *Ex vivo* platelet aggregation can be inhibited by small dialyzable substances, such as guanidinosuccinic acid and phenolic acids, as well as by poorly characterized "middle molecules" at concentrations found in uremic plasma.[444,445] Venous and arterial segments from uremic patients have been reported to produce more PGI_2 than segments from normal individuals, an abnormality not corrected by dialysis.[446] Altered NO metabolism has been observed in uremia.[447,448] In a uremic rat model, defective platelet adhesion was normalized by an inhibitor of NO formation,[449] suggesting that increased NO synthesis by endothelial cells or platelets is at least partially responsible for the defective platelet function.[450] Why renal failure increases NO synthesis is not entirely clear, although exposing endothelial cells to guanidinosuccinic acid can mimic the effects of NO, suggesting that retained guanidinosuccinic acid may be the relevant substrate.[451] Uremia has been reported to upregulate the y$^+$L system for L-arginine transport into platelets, enabling platelets to maintain or enhance NO synthesis, even in the face of low circulating L-arginine concentrations.[452,453]

By contrast, some substances found in high concentrations in uremic plasma, such as urea and parathyroid hormone, appear to play no role in platelet dysfunction.[454]

Concurrent medications and thrombocytopenia must always be considered when a patient with renal failure exhibits a bleeding tendency. Aspirin can prolong the bleeding time inordinately in uremia. Unlike aspirin's effect on COX, this effect is transient and correlates with blood levels of aspirin.[34,35] Bleeding may be potentiated by the administration of heparin during hemodialysis; in this situation, the use of an ethylene-vinyl alcohol copolymer hollow fiber dialyzer or intermittent saline infusion and high blood flow rates may eliminate the need for heparin.[455] β-Lactam antibiotics that prolong the bleeding time may have a greater effect in uremic patients and increase the occurrence of bleeding.[456]

Mild thrombocytopenia has been reported in chronic renal failure, particularly in patients on dialysis,[457] as a result of diminished marrow production and decreased platelet survival.[458] Serum thrombopoietin levels in hemodialysis patients are increased,[457,459] perhaps reflecting increased platelet turnover or a decrease in megakaryocyte mass. But when platelet counts are greater than 100×10^9/L, it is necessary to consider whether a systemic disease or medication, such as multiple myeloma, systemic vasculitis, hemolytic uremic syndrome, eclampsia, renal allograft rejection, or heparin, could be responsible for bleeding in a uremic patient.

Clinical and Laboratory Features

Despite dialysis, abnormal platelet function in uremia remains a clinical issue because it may contribute to bleeding following surgery or trauma or in conjunction with anatomic lesions of the gastrointestinal tract.[441,455] The bleeding time has often been used as an indication of hemorrhagic risk in uremia, but critical reviews of the literature indicate that it is not appropriate to use for this purpose.[460,461]

Therapy

Abnormal platelet aggregation is common in uremic patients, but by itself is not an indication for therapeutic intervention.[425] The frequency of excessive bleeding after biopsies or other surgical procedures in uremic patients who have not received specific treatment is not known, but may be uncommon. Thus, if bleeding does complicate a procedure, a thorough search for causes of bleeding other than uremia should be initiated without assuming that uremia is the etiology. However, when therapy for a uremic bleeding diathesis is necessary, the uremic platelet defect can usually be successfully treated.

There are several therapeutic maneuvers that can either partially or completely correct an abnormal bleeding time in uremic patients and anecdotal observations indicate that they may also improve hemostasis. Because prospective studies comparing various treatment regimens have not been performed, the choice of therapy should be based on the severity of the bleeding, the anticipated severity of the hemostatic stress imposed by surgery or trauma, the predicted duration of the therapeutic effect, and the risks of therapy.

The mainstay of therapy is *dialysis*. Intensive dialysis can correct the bleeding diathesis in many patients, but is only partially effective in others.[462] Peritoneal dialysis and hemodialysis are equally effective.[462,463] If a patient undergoing dialysis bleeds, it may be worthwhile to increase the intensity of the dialysis.

In uremic individuals, increasing the hematocrit by transfusion or treatment with recombinant human EPO to 27 to 32 percent is often associated with diminished clinical bleeding.[428–430,464,465] A number of reports suggest that EPO has an effect on platelets independent of an increase in hematocrit,[431] perhaps the result of an increase in the number of young platelets in the circulation.[466]

DDAVP, a vasopressin analogue whose pressor effects are substantially less than its antidiuretic effects, causes the release of VWF from tissue stores, has been reported to shorten the bleeding time in 50 to 75 percent of patients with uremia. In many cases, surgery has been carried out safely after administration of this drug, although no controlled trials have been performed.[467] DDAVP is usually administered intravenously in a dose of 0.3 mcg/kg over 15 to 30 minutes (maximum dose: 20 mcg) but it is also effective at this dose when given subcutaneously.[467] Alternatively, the drug can be given intranasally.[468] Improvement in the bleeding time is seen within 30 to 60 minutes of administration, lasts for approximately 4 hours, and roughly correlates with the rise in the plasma levels of VWF and the appearance in the circulation of high-molecular-weight VWF multimers.[467] In some patients, the drug has been given repeatedly at 12- to 24-hour intervals, although tachyphylaxis can occur.[469]

Side effects of DDAVP have been mild and uncommon and have included a 10 to 15 percent decrease in mean arterial pressure, a 20 to 30 percent increase in pulse rate, facial flushing, water retention, and hyponatremia leading to seizures; the latter is more common after repeated administration and when fluids are given freely.[467] Water retention and hyponatremia have not been observed in patients whose kidneys cannot respond to the hormone. Several uremic and nonuremic individuals with atherosclerosis have been reported to develop stroke or myocardial infarction after DDAVP administration, although such complications appear to be rare.[470,471] If dialysis is not effective, DDAVP is the treatment of choice for uremic bleeding, particularly if only a short-term effect is required.[467]

Conjugated estrogens at a dose of 0.6 mg/kg intravenously for 5 days have also been reported to shorten the bleeding time in most, but not all, uremic individuals, both in uncontrolled studies and in randomized, double-blind studies.[34,472–474] They may also be useful in some patients with uremia who bleed from gastrointestinal telangiectasia.[475] No changes in the plasma levels or multimer distribution of VWF have been noted with this treatment and it has been postulated that the active component in conjugated estrogens, 17β-estradiol, acts through an estrogen receptor mechanism.[476]

Lastly, uncontrolled studies suggest that infusions of cryoprecipitate can shorten the bleeding time in uremic patients and ameliorate bleeding.[243] However, others have reported inconsistent results,[477] and because of concerns of viral contamination, cryoprecipitate is very rarely used for this indication.

ANTIPLATELET ANTIBODIES

Definition and History

Antibody binding to platelets in several pathologic conditions, including immune thrombocytopenia (ITP), systemic lupus erythematosus (SLE), and platelet alloimmunization can cause thrombocytopenia as a result of decreased platelet survival. Less commonly, bleeding times may be shorter than expected for the degree of thrombocytopenia, suggesting enhanced platelet function.[478] On occasion, platelet function is impaired in ITP.[479–483]

Etiology and Pathogenesis

The mechanism by which autoantibodies or alloantibodies impair platelet function is likely antibody binding to specific platelet GPs. Most antiplatelet antibodies are directed against integrin $\alpha_{IIb}\beta_3$,[479–482] but antibodies directed against GPIb–IX–V, integrin $\alpha_2\beta_1$, and GPIV have been detected as well.[484,485] In most instances, the functional consequences of antibody binding are obscured by the presence of thrombocytopenia. However, patients have been reported with normal platelet counts, absent platelet aggregation, autoantibodies against integrin $\alpha_{IIb}\beta_3$, and a bleeding diathesis reminiscent of Glanzmann thrombasthenia.[479–482,486–489] Similarly, autoantibodies against GPIb and integrin $\alpha_2\beta_1$ have been detected that selectively inhibit ristocetin-induced platelet aggregation[490,491] and collagen-induced platelet aggregation,[492,493] respectively. A patient with ITP has also been identified whose anti-GPVI autoantibody produced GPVI shedding from the platelet surface and platelets unresponsive to stimulation by collagen.[494]

Besides interfering with platelet function, some autoantibodies can activate platelets and induce aggregation and secretion *in vitro*. Such antibodies can activate platelets through immune complex binding to platelet Fc receptors, by depositing sublytic quantities of the membrane attack complex of complement (C5b-9) on the cell surface,[495] or by binding to a specific membrane antigen.[246] The prototypic example of this phenomenon is heparin-induced thrombocytopenia in which antibodies bound to neoepitopes exposed on the platelet factor 4 molecule by heparin activate platelets after binding to platelet Fc receptors (Chap. 118).[496]

Clinical Laboratory Features and Therapy

Platelet dysfunction should be suspected in any patient with ITP or SLE who has mucocutaneous bleeding with a platelet count that is not ordinarily associated with bleeding (e.g., equal to or greater than approximately $30 \times 10^9/L$). Likewise, this scenario has been described occasionally in patients with Hodgkin disease,[347,480] non-Hodgkin lymphoma and myeloma,[497,498] and hairy cell leukemia.[499] The clinical spectrum of autoimmune platelet dysfunction may also include some individuals with "easy bruising" and a normal platelet count. These patients may have ITP with "compensated thrombocytolysis," as a substantial proportion have circulating antiplatelet antibodies and large platelets.[500]

Patients with antiplatelet antibodies may exhibit defective platelet function *in vitro*, even if they do not manifest a prolonged bleeding time or excessive bleeding. These deficits include impaired platelet aggregation to ADP, epinephrine, and collagen,[501–504] as well as impaired adhesion to the subendothelial matrix.[20] The most frequently reported abnormalities are absence of platelet aggregation in response to low concentrations of collagen and absence of the second wave of aggregation in response to ADP or epinephrine. This pattern is identical to that seen in individuals with inherited storage pool disease. In fact, both ITP and SLE may be associated with an acquired form of storage pool disease manifested by a reduced platelet content of dense- and α-granule components.[432,505] In one report, platelets in ITP also exhibited an activation defect manifested by impaired conversion of arachidonic acid to TXA_2.[506]

Because antibody-mediated platelet dysfunction and bleeding almost always occur in the setting of ITP, therapeutic efforts should be directed to the treatment of these disorders.

CARDIOPULMONARY BYPASS

Definition and History
Circulating blood through an extracorporeal bypass circuit during cardiac surgery induces a variety of hemostatic defects. The most significant of these are thrombocytopenia, platelet dysfunction, and hyperfibrinolysis.[507–509] At their extreme, these defects can result in substantial postoperative bleeding that may last hours to days after bypass. Approximately 5 percent of patients experience excessive postoperative bleeding after extracorporeal bypass; roughly half of the bleeding is from surgical causes; much of the remainder is caused by qualitative platelet defects and hyperfibrinolysis.

Etiology and Pathogenesis
Thrombocytopenia is a consistent feature of bypass surgery.[126,508] Typically, platelet counts begin to decrease to approximately 50 percent of presurgical levels within the first half hour after the initiation of

bypass, but thrombocytopenia can occur within 5 minutes and often does not nadir for the first few days.[507,509,510] The major factor responsible for thrombocytopenia is hemodilution from priming the pump with colloid or crystalloid solutions, but it is often more profound than can be accounted for by hemodilution alone.[509–511] Platelet adhesion to artificial surfaces in the circuit has been demonstrated by scanning electron microscopy.[512] The mechanism of this interaction is uncertain, but it may be a result of the deposition of fibrinogen on the bypass circuit and platelet adhesion mediated by integrin $\alpha_{IIb}\beta_3$.[513] Less-common causes of thrombocytopenia during bypass are disseminated intravascular coagulation, sequestration of damaged platelets in the liver, and heparin-induced thrombocytopenia.[514] Like antibodies against the complex of platelet factor 4 and heparin that are commonly detected after bypass surgery and can be responsible for heparin-induced thrombocytopenia,[496] antibodies against protamine and protamine/heparin complexes are commonly detected as well.[82,515,516] Such antibodies may contribute to the thrombocytopenia and possibly to thromboembolic events following cardiopulmonary bypass.[517]

Qualitative platelet defects are the primary nonstructural hemostatic defects induced by the bypass circuit[508,518] and are manifest as abnormal *ex vivo* platelet aggregation, decreased ristocetin-induced platelet agglutination, deficiency of platelet α and δ granules, release of soluble CD40 ligand, and the generation of platelet microparticles.[507,509,510,519–522] The severity of these abnormalities correlates with the duration of extracorporeal bypass[523] and they generally resolve within 2 to 24 hours.[508]

Bypass-induced defects in platelet function are likely caused by platelet activation and fragmentation,[521,524] hypothermia, contact with fibrinogen-coated synthetic surfaces, contact with the blood–air interface, cardiotomy suction and retransfusion of cardiotomy suction blood, and platelet exposure thrombin, plasmin, ADP, or complement.[513,519,525–528] Drugs such as heparin, protamine, integrin $\alpha_{IIb}\beta_3$ antagonists, and aspirin, as well as the production of fibrin degradation products, can also impair platelet function.[126,529–531] Controversy exists about the significance of these defects *in vivo*. Some investigators suggest that the entire qualitative platelet defect is a result of the use of heparin during bypass and its inhibitory effect on thrombin activity[529]; however, this would not account for the bleeding diathesis that can exist hours after heparin reversal.

Hyperfibrinolysis may also contribute to the bleeding diathesis associated with cardiopulmonary bypass.[532,533] This is likely from thrombus formation in the pericardial cavity followed by local, and subsequently systemic, fibrinolysis.[532] The relevance of hyperfibrinolysis to postbypass bleeding is bolstered by the efficacy of antifibrinolytic therapy in minimizing cardiopulmonary bypass surgery blood loss.

Therapy
A preoperative evaluation of cardiac surgical candidates should include a history of bleeding in either the patient or family member. Some authors recommend a screening prothrombin time, partial prothrombin time, and bleeding time even in individuals with no history of bleeding.[534] However, the validity of this approach is controversial.[535] Regardless, prophylactic transfusion of allogeneic blood components is not indicated.[508,536,537] Preoperative administration of recombinant human EPO has been reported to reduce the need for allogeneic blood transfusion in undergoing elective open-heart surgery.[538–541] Cell savers are now often used during bypass surgery and the collected washed autologous red blood cells are reinfused after completion of cardiopulmonary bypass. In addition, blood collected from chest tube drainage has been reinfused to minimize allogeneic transfusions.[541] The safety of transfusing large quantities of blood by this technique has not fully been established.[528,542]

A number of maneuvers have been taken to reduce the hemostatic abnormalities associated with cardiac surgery. These include coating the artificial surfaces of cardiopulmonary bypass devices with heparin,[543-547] using centrifugal rather than roller pumps,[548] use of a number of pharmacologic agents,[549] and performing coronary artery surgery without bypass.[301,550] Off-pump coronary artery bypass surgery appears to preserve platelet function, but concerns have been raised about adverse thromboembolic events postsurgery because of the concurrence of normal platelet function, late thrombin generation, and reduced fibrinolysis.[551-553] Several pharmacologic maneuvers have been tried to assist in the management of postoperative bleeding. Postoperative patients with a prolonged bleeding time and excessive blood loss may respond to DDAVP, as evidenced by a shortening of the bleeding time. However, results of trials using this agent have been contradictory, some studies showing a reduced blood loss and most showing no benefit.[554-556] Based on the assumption that platelet activation during bypass could be a major cause of postoperative platelet dysfunction, infusion of platelet activation inhibitors such as PGE_1, PGI_2, or stable PGI_2 analogues have been carried out in animal models and in humans. By increasing platelet cAMP and reducing platelet responsiveness, these agents prevent bypass-induced thrombocytopenia and platelet dysfunction. However, randomized trials using PGI_2 and its analogue, iloprost, have not shown a clear overall benefit, in part because of significant toxicity, including hypotension.[123,557] Recombinant factor VIIa has been recommended to treat uncontrolled postoperative bleeding that has not responded to routine hemostatic therapy.[558] However, the off-label use of recombinant factor VIIa is associated with an increased risk for arterial and venous thromboembolism[559] and a retrospective case-matched review of patients who had received recombinant factor VIIa perioperatively during major cardiac surgery indicated that it was associated with worse survival.[223] Nonetheless, it remains a potentially useful therapeutic consideration in view of the prognosis of uncontrolled postoperative hemorrhage.[560] Based primarily on the cardiovascular complications encountered by patients in two randomized studies of the use of parecoxib/valdecoxib to treat pain after cardiac surgery, the use of coxibs as well as traditional NSAIDs appears contraindicated in this setting.[561,562]

Inhibiting fibrinolysis using ε-aminocaproic acid or tranexamic acid during cardiopulmonary bypass can reduce mediastinal blood loss and transfusion requirements.[549] Aprotinin (Trasylol), a broad-spectrum protease inhibitor, was also used for this purpose, but observational studies,[563-565] as well as a blinded clinical trial,[566] revealed that its use is associated with serious end-organ damage and a higher mortality than the use of ε-aminocaproic acid or no antifibrinolytic agent.

The most important determinant of blood loss following cardiopulmonary surgery is the surgical procedure itself. If excessive nonsurgical postoperative bleeding occurs, one should verify that the patient is no longer hypothermic and that heparin has been fully reversed. At this point, the administration of pharmacologic agents, along with judicious transfusions of platelets, cryoprecipitate, fresh frozen plasma and red blood cells is appropriate.

MISCELLANEOUS DISORDERS

Measurements of hemostatic function are frequently abnormal in patients with end-stage and fulminant liver disease and result from decreased coagulation factor production, fibrinolysis, dysfibrinogenemia, thrombocytopenia as a result of hypersplenism and thrombopoietin deficiency, as well as disseminated intravascular coagulation (DIC).[425,567] However, the clinical consequences of these laboratory abnormalities have been reassessed because they do not take into account that both anti- and prohemostatic pathways are perturbed in liver disease.[568,569] Thus, hemostasis in liver disease is considered to be

"rebalanced," although it remains unstable, with patients prone to both bleeding and thrombosis. Chronic liver disease can be associated with a prolonged bleeding time and reduced platelet aggregation and procoagulant activity,[567,570,571] but there is no evidence for a platelet function defect specific to liver disease.[572] Rather, they are the result of multiple factors, including thrombocytopenia, hypofibrinogenemia, and anemia, none of which imply an intrinsic defect in platelet function.[573] Regardless, the prolonged bleeding in these patients may respond to infusion of DDAVP,[574] but clinical relevance of this observation is uncertain.[575]

Patients with DIC may exhibit reduced platelet aggregation and acquired storage pool deficiency.[576,577] These result from platelet activation in vivo by thrombin or other agonists. Alternatively, elevated levels of fibrin(ogen) degradation products and the low fibrinogen levels that accompany DIC may contribute to the platelet defect. Although purified low-molecular-weight fibrinogen-degradation products can impair platelet aggregation, this effect requires concentrations of degradation products unlikely to occur in vivo.[578] Moreover, it is difficult to assess the significance of platelet dysfunction in most patients with DIC because of the simultaneous presence of thrombocytopenia and other hemostatic defects.

Decreased platelet aggregation and secretion in response to ADP and epinephrine has been reported in Bartter syndrome, a group of rare inherited disorders characterized by severe restrictions of salt reabsorption by the thick ascending limb of Henle, perhaps caused by excessive PGE_2 synthesis.[579-582] However, reviews of series of patients with Bartter syndrome make no mention of hemostatic problems[580] so that the clinical significance of the platelet aggregation abnormalities is doubtful.

In addition to thrombocytopenia, platelet dysfunction has been observed in some patients with hemorrhagic fevers caused by Dengue, Hanta, Lassa, Junín, and Ebola viruses.[583] There are also isolated reports of a slight prolongation of the bleeding time and/or ex vivo platelet function defects in a number of other clinical conditions. These include non-thrombocytopenic purpura with eosinophilia,[584-586] atopic asthma and hay fever,[587] acute respiratory failure,[588] and Wilms tumor elaborating hyaluronic acid.[589] The clinical significance of these associations is not clear.

REFERENCES

1. Hayward CP: Diagnostic evaluation of platelet function disorders. *Blood Rev* 25(4):169–173, 2011.
2. Nurden P, Nurden A, Jandrot-Perrus M: Diagnostic assessment of platelet function, in *Quality in Laboratory Hemostasis and Thrombosis*, edited by S Kitchen, JD Olson, FE Preston, pp 159–173. Blackwell Publishing, London, 2013.
3. Wisloff F, Godal H: Prolonged bleeding time with adequate platelet count in hospital patients. *Scand J Haematol* 27(1):45–50, 1981.
4. Patrono C: Aspirin as an antiplatelet drug. *N Engl J Med* 330(18):1287–1294, 1981.
5. Smith WL, DeWitt DL, Garavito RM: Cyclooxygenases: Structural, cellular, and molecular biology. *Annu Rev Biochem* 69:145–182, 2000.
6. Kis B, Snipes JA, Busija DW: Acetaminophen and the cyclooxygenase-3 puzzle: Sorting out facts, fictions, and uncertainties. *J Pharmacol Exp Ther* 315(1):1–7, 2005.
7. Smith W, Garavito R, DeWitt D: Prostaglandin endoperoxide H synthases (cyclooxygenases)-1 and -2. *Biol Chem* 271:33157, 1996.
8. Chandrasekharan NV, Dai H, Roos KL, et al: COX-3, a cyclooxygenase-1 variant inhibited by acetaminophen and other analgesic/antipyretic drugs: Cloning, structure, and expression. *Proc Natl Acad Sci U S A* 99(21):13926–13931, 2002.
9. Weiss H, Aledort L: Impaired platelet/connective tissue reaction in man after aspirin ingestion. *Lancet* 2:495, 1967.
10. O'Brien JR. Effect of salicylates on human platelets. *Lancet* 1(7557):1431, 1968.
11. Grosser T, Fries S, FitzGerald GA: Biological basis for the cardiovascular consequences of COX-2 inhibition: Therapeutic challenges and opportunities. *J Clin Invest* 116(1):4–15, 2006.
12. Kyrle PA, Eichler HG, Jager U, Lechner K: Inhibition of prostacyclin and thromboxane A2 generation by low-dose aspirin at the site of plug formation in man *in vivo. Circulation* 75(5):1025–1029, 1987.
13. Jaffe EA, Weksler BB: Recovery of endothelial cell prostacyclin production after inhibition by low doses of aspirin. *J Clin Invest* 63(3):532–535, 1979.
14. Marcus AJ, Safier LB: Thromboregulation: Multicellular modulation of platelet reactivity in hemostasis and thrombosis. *FASEB J* 7(6):516–522, 1993.

15. Rich JB: The efficacy and safety of aprotinin use in cardiac surgery. *Ann Thorac Surg* 66(5 Suppl):S6–S11, 1998.

16. Antithrombotic Trialists Collaboration: Collaborative meta-analysis of randomised trials of antiplatelet therapy for prevention of death, myocardial infarction, and stroke in high risk patients. *BMJ* 324(7329):71–86, 2002.

17. Seshasai SR, Wijesuriya S, Sivakumaran R, et al: Effect of aspirin on vascular and non-vascular outcomes: Meta-analysis of randomized controlled trials. *Arch Intern Med* 172(3):209–216, 2012.

18. Raju N, Sobieraj-Teague M, Hirsh J, et al: Effect of aspirin on mortality in the primary prevention of cardiovascular disease. *Am J Med* 124(7):621–629, 2011.

19. Bartolucci AA, Tendera M, Howard G: Meta-analysis of multiple primary prevention trials of cardiovascular events using aspirin. *Am J Cardiol* 107(12):1796–1801, 2011.

20. Kallmann R, Nieuwenhuis HK, de Groot PG, et al: Effects of low doses of aspirin, 10 mg and 30 mg daily, on bleeding time, thromboxane production and 6-keto-PGF1 alpha excretion in healthy subjects. *Thromb Res* 45:355, 1987.

21. Nakajima H, Takami H, Yamagata K, Kariya K, Tamai Y, Nara H: Aspirin effects on colonic mucosal bleeding. *Dis Colon Rectum* 40:1484, 1997.

22. Mielke CH Jr: Aspirin prolongation of the template bleeding time: Influence of venostasis and direction of incision. *Blood* 60(5):1139–1142, 1982.

23. Hirsh J, Salzman EW, Harker L, et al: Aspirin and other platelet active drugs. Relationship among dose, effectiveness, and side effects. *Chest* 95(2 Suppl):12S–18S, 1989.

24. Page IH: Salicylate damage to the gastric mucosal barrier. *N Engl J Med* 276:1307, 1967.

25. Leonards JR, Levy G: The role of dosage form in aspirin-induced gastrointestinal bleeding. *Clin Pharmacol* 8:400, 1969.

26. Baigent C, Blackwell L, Collins R, et al: Aspirin in the primary and secondary prevention of vascular disease: Collaborative meta-analysis of individual participant data from randomised trials. *Lancet* 373(9678):1849–1860, 2009.

27. Stuart MJ, Gross SJ, Elrad H, Graeber JE: Effects of acetylsalicylic-acid ingestion on maternal and neonatal hemostasis. *N Engl J Med* 307(15):909–912, 1982.

28. Ferraris VA, Ferraris SP, Lough FC, Berry WR: Preoperative aspirin ingestion increases operative blood loss after coronary artery bypass grafting. *Ann Thorac Surg* 45(1):71–74, 1988.

29. Sethi GK, Copeland JG, Goldman S, et al: Implications of preoperative administration of aspirin in patients undergoing coronary artery bypass grafting. Department of Veterans Affairs Cooperative Study on Antiplatelet Therapy. *J Am Coll Cardiol* 15(1):15–20, 1990.

30. Horlocker TT, Wedel DJ, Offord KP: Does preoperative antiplatelet therapy increase the risk of hemorrhagic complications associated with regional anesthesia? *Anesth Analg* 70(6):631–634, 1990.

31. Kitchen L, Erichson RB, Sideropoulos H: Effect of drug-induced platelet dysfunction on surgical bleeding. *Am J Surg* 143(2):215–217, 1982.

32. Devereaux PJ, Mrkobrada M, Sessler DI, et al; POISE-2 Investigators: Aspirin in patients undergoing noncardiac surgery. *N Engl J Med* 370(16):1494–1503, 2014.

33. Kennedy BM: Aspirin and surgery—A review. *Ir Med J* 77(11):363–369, 1984.

34. Livio M, Benigni A, Vigano G, et al: Moderate doses of aspirin and risk of bleeding in renal failure. *Lancet* 1(8478):414–416, 1986.

35. Gaspari F, Vigano G, Orisio S, et al: Aspirin prolongs bleeding time in uremia by a mechanism distinct from platelet cyclooxygenase inhibition. *J Clin Invest* 79(6):1788–1797, 1987.

36. Chesebro JH, Fuster V, Elveback LR, et al: Trial of combined warfarin plus dipyridamole or aspirin therapy in prosthetic heart valve replacement: Danger of aspirin compared with dipyridamole. *Am J Cardiol* 51(9):1537–1541, 1983.

37. Kobrinsky NL, Israels ED, Gerrard JM, et al: Shortening of bleeding time by 1-deamino-8-D-arginine vasopressin in various bleeding disorders. *Lancet* 1(8387):1145–1148, 1984.

38. Lethagen S, Rugarn P: The effect of DDAVP and placebo on platelet function and prolonged bleeding time induced by oral acetyl salicylic acid intake in healthy volunteers. *Thromb Haemost* 67(1):185–186, 1992.

39. Kasmeridis C, Apostolakis S, Lip GY: Aspirin and aspirin resistance in coronary artery disease. *Curr Opin Pharmacol* 13(2):242–250, 2013.

40. Grosser T, Fries S, Lawson JA, et al: Drug resistance and pseudoresistance: An unintended consequence of enteric coating aspirin. *Circulation* 127(3):377–385, 2013.

41. Floyd CN, Ferro A: Mechanisms of aspirin resistance. *Pharmacol Ther* 141(1):69–78, 2014.

42. Catella-Lawson F, Reilly MP, Kapoor SC, et al: Cyclooxygenase inhibitors and the antiplatelet effects of aspirin. *N Engl J Med* 345(25):1809–1817, 2001.

43. Mielke CH Jr, Kahn SB, Muschek LD, et al: Effects of zomepirac on hemostasis in healthy adults and on platelet function *in vitro*. *J Clin Pharmacol* 20(5–6 Pt 2):409–417, 1980.

44. Lamberts M, Lip GY, Hansen ML, et al: Relation of nonsteroidal anti-inflammatory drugs to serious bleeding and thromboembolism risk in patients with atrial fibrillation receiving antithrombotic therapy: A nationwide cohort study. *Ann Intern Med* 161(10):690–698, 2014.

45. Thomas P, Hepburn B, Kim HC, Saidi P: Nonsteroidal anti-inflammatory drugs in the treatment of hemophilic arthropathy. *Am J Hematol* 12(2):131–137, 1982.

46. McIntyre BA, Philp RB, Inwood MJ: Effect of ibuprofen on platelet function in normal subjects and hemophiliac patients. *Clin Pharmacol Ther* 24(5):616–621, 1978.

47. Ragni MV, Miller BJ, Whalen R, Ptachcinski R: Bleeding tendency, platelet function, and pharmacokinetics of ibuprofen and zidovudine in HIV(+) hemophilic men. *Am J Hematol* 40(3):176–182, 1992.

48. Li X, Fries S, Li R, et al: Differential impairment of aspirin-dependent platelet cyclooxygenase acetylation by nonsteroidal antiinflammatory drugs. *Proc Natl Acad Sci U S A* 111(47):16830–16835, 2014.

49. Kearney PM, Baigent C, Godwin J, et al: Do selective cyclo-oxygenase-2 inhibitors and traditional non-steroidal anti-inflammatory drugs increase the risk of atherothrombosis? Meta-analysis of randomised trials. *BMJ* 332(7553):1302–1308, 2006.

50. Antman EM, Bennett JS, Daugherty A, et al: Use of nonsteroidal antiinflammatory drugs: An update for clinicians: A scientific statement from the American Heart Association. *Circulation* 115(12):1634–1642, 2007.

51. Solomon SD, Wittes J, Finn PV, et al: Cardiovascular risk of celecoxib in 6 randomized placebo-controlled trials: The cross trial safety analysis. *Circulation* 117(16):2104–2113, 2008.

52. Trelle S, Reichenbach S, Wandel S, et al: Cardiovascular safety of non-steroidal anti-inflammatory drugs: Network meta-analysis. *BMJ* 342:c7086, 2011.

53. McGettigan P, Henry D: Cardiovascular risk and inhibition of cyclooxygenase: A systematic review of the observational studies of selective and nonselective inhibitors of cyclooxygenase 2. *JAMA* 296(13):1633–1644, 2006.

54. Coxib and traditional NSAID Trialists' (CNT) Collaboration, Bhala N, Emberson J, Merhi A, et al: Vascular and upper gastrointestinal effects of non-steroidal anti-inflammatory drugs: Meta-analyses of individual participant data from randomised trials. *Lancet* 382(9894):769–779, 2013.

55. Schmidt M, Christiansen CF, Mehnert F, et al: Non-steroidal anti-inflammatory drug use and risk of atrial fibrillation or flutter: Population based case-control study. *BMJ* 343:d3450, 2011.

56. Hinz B, Cheremina O, Brune K: Acetaminophen (paracetamol) is a selective cyclooxygenase-2 inhibitor in man. *FASEB J* 22(2):383–390, 2008.

57. CAPRIE Steering Committee: A randomised, blinded, trial of clopidogrel versus aspirin in patients at risk of ischaemic events (CAPRIE). CAPRIE Steering Committee. *Lancet* 348(9038):1329–1339, 1996.

58. McTavish D, Faulds D, Goa KL: Ticlopidine. An updated review of its pharmacology and therapeutic use in platelet-dependent disorders. *Drugs* 40(2):238–259, 1990.

59. Geiger J, Brich J, Honig-Liedl P, et al: Specific impairment of human platelet P2Y(AC) ADP receptor-mediated signaling by the antiplatelet drug clopidogrel. *Arterioscler Thromb Vasc Biol* 19(8):2007–2011, 1999.

60. Daniel JL, Dangelmaier C, Jin J, et al: Molecular basis for ADP-induced platelet activation. I. Evidence for three distinct ADP receptors on human platelets. *J Biol Chem* 273(4):2024–2029, 1998.

61. Farid NA, Kurihara A, Wrighton SA: Metabolism and disposition of the thienopyridine antiplatelet drugs ticlopidine, clopidogrel, and prasugrel in humans. *J Clin Pharmacol* 50(2):126–142, 2010.

62. Yusuf S, Zhao F, Mehta SR, et al: Effects of clopidogrel in addition to aspirin in patients with acute coronary syndromes without ST-segment elevation. *N Engl J Med* 345(7):494–502, 2001.

63. De Caterina R, Sicari R, Bernini W, et al: Benefit/risk profile of combined antiplatelet therapy with ticlopidine and aspirin. *Thromb Haemost* 65(5):504–510, 1991.

64. Helft G, Osende JI, Worthley SG, et al: Acute antithrombotic effect of a front-loaded regimen of clopidogrel in patients with atherosclerosis on aspirin. *Arterioscler Thromb Vasc Biol* 20(10):2316–2321, 2000.

65. Parodi G, Valenti R, Bellandi B, et al: Comparison of prasugrel and ticagrelor loading doses in ST-segment elevation myocardial infarction patients: RAPID (Rapid Activity of Platelet Inhibitor Drugs) primary PCI study. *J Am Coll Cardiol* 61(15):1601–1606, 2013.

66. Collet JP, Hulot JS, Pena A, et al: Cytochrome P450 2C19 polymorphism in young patients treated with clopidogrel after myocardial infarction: A cohort study. *Lancet* 373(9660):309–317, 2009.

67. Mega JL, Close SL, Wiviott SD, et al: Cytochrome p-450 polymorphisms and response to clopidogrel. *N Engl J Med* 360(4):354–362, 2009.

68. Jernberg T, Payne CD, Winters KJ, et al: Prasugrel achieves greater inhibition of platelet aggregation and a lower rate of non-responders compared with clopidogrel in aspirin-treated patients with stable coronary artery disease. *Eur Heart J* 27(10):1166–1173, 2006.

69. Brandt JT, Payne CD, Wiviott SD, et al: A comparison of prasugrel and clopidogrel loading doses on platelet function: Magnitude of platelet inhibition is related to active metabolite formation. *Am Heart J* 153(1):66 e9–e16, 2007.

70. Wiviott SD, Braunwald E, McCabe CH,; TRITON-TIMI 38 Investigators: Prasugrel versus clopidogrel in patients with acute coronary syndromes. *N Engl J Med* 357(20):2001–2015, 2007.

71. Hass WK, Easton JD, Adams HP Jr, et al: A randomized trial comparing ticlopidine hydrochloride with aspirin for the prevention of stroke in high-risk patients. Ticlopidine Aspirin Stroke Study Group. *N Engl J Med* 321(8):501–507, 1989.

72. Gent M, Blakely JA, Easton JD, et al: The Canadian American Ticlopidine Study (CATS) in thromboembolic stroke. *Lancet* 1(8649):1215–1220, 1989.

73. Mataix R, Ojeda E, Perez MC, Jimenez S: Ticlopidine and severe aplastic anaemia. *Br J Haematol* 80(1):125–126, 1992.

74. Garnier G, Taillan B, Pesce A, et al: Ticlopidine and severe aplastic anaemia. *Br J Haematol* 81(3):459–460, 1992.

75. Bennett CL, Weinberg PD, Rozenberg-Ben-Dror K, et al: Thrombotic thrombocytopenic purpura associated with ticlopidine. A review of 60 cases. *Ann Intern Med* 128(7):541–544, 1998.

76. Steinhubl SR, Tan WA, Foody JM, Topol EJ: Incidence and clinical course of thrombotic thrombocytopenic purpura due to ticlopidine following coronary stenting. EPISTENT

Investigators. Evaluation of Platelet IIb/IIIa Inhibitor for Stenting. *JAMA* 281(9):806–810, 1999.

77. Chen DK, Kim JS, Sutton DM: Thrombotic thrombocytopenic purpura associated with ticlopidine use: A report of 3 cases and review of the literature. *Arch Intern Med* 159(3):311–314, 1999.

78. Bennett CL, Connors JM, Carwile JM, et al: Thrombotic thrombocytopenic purpura associated with clopidogrel. *N Engl J Med* 342(24):1773–1777, 2000.

79. Leon MB, Baim DS, Popma JJ, et al: A clinical trial comparing three antithrombotic-drug regimens after coronary-artery stenting. Stent Anticoagulation Restenosis Study Investigators. *N Engl J Med* 339(23):1665–1671, 1998.

80. Steinhubl SR, Berger PB, Mann JT 3rd, et al: Early and sustained dual oral antiplatelet therapy following percutaneous coronary intervention: A randomized controlled trial. *JAMA* 288(19):2411–2420, 2002.

81. Bhatt DL, Fox KA, Hacke W, et al: Clopidogrel and aspirin versus aspirin alone for the prevention of atherothrombotic events. *N Engl J Med* 354(16):1706–1717, 2006.

82. Lee GM, Welsby IJ, Phillips-Bute B, et al: High incidence of antibodies to protamine and protamine/heparin complexes in patients undergoing cardiopulmonary bypass. *Blood* 121(15):2828–2835, 2013.

83. Bellemain-Appaix A, O'Connor SA, Silvain J, et al; ACTION Group: Association of clopidogrel pretreatment with mortality, cardiovascular events, and major bleeding among patients undergoing percutaneous coronary intervention: A systematic review and meta-analysis. *JAMA* 308(23):2507–2516, 2012.

84. Parodi G, Storey RF: Dyspnoea management in acute coronary syndrome patients treated with ticagrelor. *Eur Heart J Acute Cardiovasc Care* 2014. [Epub ahead of print]

85. Alexopoulos D, Xanthopoulou I, Gkizas V, et al: Randomized assessment of ticagrelor versus prasugrel antiplatelet effects in patients with ST-segment-elevation myocardial infarction. *Circ Cardiovasc Interv* 5(6):797–804, 2012.

86. Franchi F, Rollini F, Muniz-Lozano A, et al: Cangrelor: A review on pharmacology and clinical trial development. *Expert Rev Cardiovasc Ther* 11(10):1279–1291, 2013.

87. Bhatt DL, Stone GW, Mahaffey KW, et al; CHAMPION PHOENIX Investigators: Effect of platelet inhibition with cangrelor during PCI on ischemic events. *N Engl J Med* 368(14):1303–1313, 2013.

88. Wallentin L, Becker RC, Budaj A, et al: Ticagrelor versus clopidogrel in patients with acute coronary syndromes. *N Engl J Med* 361(11):1045–1057, 2009.

89. Montalescot G, van 't Hof AW, Lapostolle F, et al; ATLANTIC Investigators: Prehospital ticagrelor in ST-segment elevation myocardial infarction. *N Engl J Med* 371(11):1016–1027, 2014.

90. Kahn ML, Nakanishi-Matsui M, Shapiro MJ, et al: Protease-activated receptors 1 and 4 mediate activation of human platelets by thrombin. *J Clin Invest* 103(6):879–887, 1999.

91. Chackalamannil S, Xia Y, Greenlee WJ, et al: Discovery of potent orally active thrombin receptor (protease activated receptor 1) antagonists as novel antithrombotic agents. *J Med Chem* 48(19):5884–5887, 2005.

92. Zhang C, Srinivasan Y, Arlow DH, et al: High-resolution crystal structure of human protease-activated receptor 1. *Nature* 492(7429):387–392, 2012.

93. Morrow DA, Braunwald E, Bonaca MP, et al; TRA 2P-TIMI 50 Steering Committee and Investigators: Vorapaxar in the secondary prevention of atherothrombotic events. *N Engl J Med* 366(15):1404–1413, 2012.

94. Goto S, Ogawa H, Takeuchi M, et al; J-LANCELOT (Japanese-Lesson from Antagonizing the Cellular Effect of Thrombin) Investigators: Double-blind, placebo-controlled Phase II studies of the protease-activated receptor 1 antagonist E5555 (atopaxar) in Japanese patients with acute coronary syndrome or high-risk coronary artery disease. *Eur Heart J* 31(21):2601–2613, 2010.

95. Lefkovits J, Plow EF, Topol EJ: Platelet glycoprotein IIb/IIIa receptors in cardiovascular medicine. *N Engl J Med* 332(23):1553–1559, 1995.

96. Bennett JS, Mousa S: Platelet function inhibitors in the Year 2000. *Thromb Haemost* 85(3):395–400, 2001.

97. Hook KM, Bennett JS: Glycoprotein IIb/IIIa antagonists. *Handb Exp Pharmacol* 2012(210):199–223, 1994.

98. French DL, Seligsohn U: Platelet glycoprotein IIb/IIIa receptors and Glanzmann's thrombasthenia. *Arterioscler Thromb Vasc Biol* 20(3):607–610, 2000.

99. Nurden AT: Inherited abnormalities of platelets. *Thromb Haemost* 82(2):468–480, 1999.

100. Use of a monoclonal antibody directed against the platelet glycoprotein IIb/IIIa receptor in high-risk coronary angioplasty. The EPIC Investigation. *N Engl J Med* 330(14):956–961, 1994.

101. EPILOG Investigators: Platelet glycoprotein IIb/IIIa receptor blockade and low-dose heparin during percutaneous coronary revascularization. *N Engl J Med* 336(24):1689–1696, 1997.

102. Inhibition of the platelet glycoprotein IIb/IIIa receptor with tirofiban in unstable angina and non-Q-wave myocardial infarction. Platelet Receptor Inhibition in Ischemic Syndrome Management in Patients Limited by Unstable Signs and Symptoms (PRISM-PLUS) Study Investigators. *N Engl J Med* 338(21):1488–1497, 1998.

103. Inhibition of platelet glycoprotein IIb/IIIa with eptifibatide in patients with acute coronary syndromes. The PURSUIT Trial Investigators. Platelet Glycoprotein IIb/IIIa in Unstable Angina: Receptor Suppression Using Integrilin Therapy. *N Engl J Med* 339(7):436–443, 1998.

104. Simpfendorfer C, Kottke-Marchant K, Lowrie M, et al: First chronic platelet glycoprotein IIb/IIIa integrin blockade. A randomized, placebo-controlled pilot study of xemilofiban in unstable angina with percutaneous coronary interventions. *Circulation* 96(1):76–81, 1997.

105. Cannon CP, McCabe CH, Borzak S, et al: Randomized trial of an oral platelet glycoprotein IIb/IIIa antagonist, sibrafiban, in patients after an acute coronary syndrome: Results of the TIMI 12 trial. Thrombolysis in Myocardial Infarction. *Circulation* 97(4):340–349, 1998.

106. Bhatt DL, Chew DP, Hirsch AT, et al: Superiority of clopidogrel versus aspirin in patients with prior cardiac surgery. *Circulation* 103(3):363–368, 2001.

107. Bassler N, Loeffler C, Mangin P, et al: A mechanistic model for paradoxical platelet activation by ligand-mimetic alphaIIb beta3 (GPIIb/IIIa) antagonists. *Arterioscler Thromb Vasc Biol* 27(3):e9–e15, 2007.

108. Ferguson JJ, Kereiakes DJ, Adgey AA, et al: Safe use of platelet GP IIb/IIIa inhibitors. *Eur Heart J* 19 Suppl D:D40–D51, 1998.

109. Berkowitz SD, Sane DC, Sigmon KN, et al: Occurrence and clinical significance of thrombocytopenia in a population undergoing high-risk percutaneous coronary revascularization. Evaluation of c7E3 for the Prevention of Ischemic Complications (EPIC) Study Group. *J Am Coll Cardiol* 32(2):311–319, 1998.

110. Giugliano RP, McCabe CH, Sequeira RF, et al: First report of an intravenous and oral glycoprotein IIb/IIIa inhibitor (RPR 109891) in patients with recent acute coronary syndromes: Results of the TIMI 15A and 15B trials. *Am Heart J* 140(1):81–93, 2000.

111. Comparison of sibrafiban with aspirin for prevention of cardiovascular events after acute coronary syndromes: A randomised trial. The SYMPHONY Investigators. Sibrafiban versus Aspirin to Yield Maximum Protection from Ischemic Heart Events Post-acute Coronary Syndromes. *Lancet* 355(9201):337–345, 2000.

112. Hongo RH, Brent BN: Association of eptifibatide and acute profound thrombocytopenia. *Am J Cardiol* 88(4):428–431, 2001.

113. McClure MW, Berkowitz SD, Sparapani R, et al: Clinical significance of thrombocytopenia during a non-ST-elevation acute coronary syndrome. The platelet glycoprotein IIb/IIIa in unstable angina: Receptor suppression using Integrilin therapy (PURSUIT) trial experience. *Circulation* 99(22):2892–2900, 1999.

114. Abrams CS, Cines DB: Platelet glycoprotein IIb/IIIa inhibitors and thrombocytopenia: Possible link between platelet activation, autoimmunity and thrombosis. *Thromb Haemost* 88(6):888–889, 2002.

115. Christopoulos CG, Machin SJ: A new type of pseudothrombocytopenia: EDTA-mediated agglutination of platelets bearing Fab fragments of a chimaeric antibody. *Br J Haematol* 87(3):650–652, 1994.

116. Sane DC, Damaraju LV, Topol EJ, et al: Occurrence and clinical significance of pseudothrombocytopenia during abciximab therapy. *J Am Coll Cardiol* 36(1):75–83, 2000.

117. Ivy DD, Kinsella JP, Ziegler JW, Abman SH: Dipyridamole attenuates rebound pulmonary hypertension after inhaled nitric oxide withdrawal in postoperative congenital heart disease. *J Thorac Cardiovasc Surg* 115(4):875–882, 1998.

118. Gresele P, Arnout J, Deckmyn H, Vermylen J: Mechanism of the antiplatelet action of dipyridamole in whole blood: Modulation of adenosine concentration and activity. *Thromb Haemost* 55(1):12–18, 1986.

119. FitzGerald GA: Dipyridamole. *N Engl J Med* 316:1247, 1987.

120. Reilly M, FitzGerald GA: Gathering intelligence on antiplatelet drugs: The view from 30 000 feet. When combined with other information overviews lead to conviction. *BMJ* 324(7329):59–60, 2002.

121. Diener HC, Cunha L, Forbes C, et al: European Stroke Prevention Study. 2. Dipyridamole and acetylsalicylic acid in the secondary prevention of stroke. *J Neurol Sci* 143(1–2):1–13, 1996.

122. Fisher CA, Kappa JR, Sinha AK, et al: Comparison of equimolar concentrations of iloprost, prostacyclin, and prostaglandin E1 on human platelet function. *J Lab Clin Med* 109(2):184–190, 1987.

123. Fish KJ, Sarnquist FH, van Steennis C, et al: A prospective, randomized study of the effects of prostacyclin on platelets and blood loss during coronary bypass operations. *J Thorac Cardiovasc Surg* 91(3):436–442, 1986.

124. Sorkin EM, Markham A: Cilostazol. *Drugs Aging* 14(1):63–71; discussion 72–73, 1999.

125. Biondi-Zoccai GG, Lotrionte M, Anselmino M, et al: Systematic review and meta-analysis of randomized clinical trials appraising the impact of cilostazol after percutaneous coronary intervention. *Am Heart J* 155(6):1081–1089, 2008.

126. Khuri SF, Valeri CR, Loscalzo J, et al: Heparin causes platelet dysfunction and induces fibrinolysis before cardiopulmonary bypass [see comments]. *Ann Thorac Surg* 60(4):1008–1014, 1995.

127. Sattler FR, Weitekamp MR, Ballard JO: Potential for bleeding with the new beta-lactam antibiotics. *Ann Intern Med* 105(6):924–931, 1986.

128. Pillgram-Larsen J, Wisloff F, Jorgensen JJ, et al: Effect of high-dose ampicillin and cloxacillin on bleeding time and bleeding in open-heart surgery. *Scand J Thorac Cardiovasc Surg* 19(1):45–48, 1985.

129. Fass RJ, Copelan EA, Brandt JT, et al: Platelet-mediated bleeding caused by broad-spectrum penicillins. *J Infect Dis* 155(6):1242–1248, 1987.

130. Cazenave JP, Packham MA, Guccione MA, Mustard JF: Effects of penicillin G on platelet aggregation, release, and adherence to collagen. *Proc Soc Exp Biol Med* 142(1):159–166, 1973.

131. Shattil SJ, Bennett JS, McDonough M, Turnbull J: Carbenicillin and penicillin G inhibit platelet function in vitro by impairing the interaction of agonists with the platelet surface. *J Clin Invest* 65(3):329–337, 1980.

132. Fletcher C, Pearson C, Choi SC, et al: In vitro comparison of antiplatelet effects of beta-lactam penicillins. *J Lab Clin Med* 108(3):217–223, 1986.

133. Packham MA, Rand ML, Perry DW, et al: Probenecid inhibits platelet responses to aggregating agents in vitro and has a synergistic inhibitory effect with penicillin G. *Thromb Haemost* 76(2):239–244, 1996.

134. Burroughs SF, Johnson GJ: Beta-lactam antibiotic-induced platelet dysfunction: Evidence for irreversible inhibition of platelet activation in vitro and in vivo after prolonged exposure to penicillin. *Blood* 75(7):1473–1480, 1990.

135. Sattler FR, Weitekamp MR, Sayegh A, Ballard JO: Impaired hemostasis caused by beta-lactam antibiotics. *Am J Surg* 155(5A):30–39, 1988.

136. Giles AR, Greenwood P, Tinlin S: A platelet release defect induced by aspirin or penicillin G does not increase gastrointestinal blood loss in thrombocytopenic rabbits. *Br J Haematol* 57(1):17–23, 1984.

137. Andrassy K, Koderisch J, Trenk D, et al: Hemostasis in patients with normal and impaired renal function under treatment with cefodizime. *Infection* 15(5):348–350, 1987.

138. Bloom A, Greaves M, Preston FE, Brown CB: Evidence against a platelet cyclooxygenase defect in uraemic subjects on chronic haemodialysis. *Br J Haematol* 62:143, 1986.

139. Rossi EC, Levin NW: Inhibition of primary ADP-induced platelet aggregation in normal subjects after administration of nitrofurantoin (furadantin). *J Clin Invest* 52(10):2457–2467, 1973.

140. Ishikawa S, Manabe S, Wada O: Miconazole inhibition of platelet aggregation by inhibiting cyclooxygenase. *Biochem Pharmacol* 35(11):1787–1792, 1986.

141. Salzman EW, Rosenberg RD, Smith MH, et al: Effect of heparin and heparin fractions on platelet aggregation. *J Clin Invest* 65(1):64–73, 1980.

142. Horne MK 3rd, Chao ES: Heparin binding to resting and activated platelets. *Blood* 74(1):238–243, 1989.

143. Sobel M, McNeill PM, Carlson PL, et al: Heparin inhibition of von Willebrand factor-dependent platelet function in vitro and in vivo. *J Clin Invest* 87(5):1787–1793, 1991.

144. Coller BS: Platelets and thrombolytic therapy. *N Engl J Med* 322(1):33–42, 1990.

145. Niewiarowski S, Senyi AF, Gillies P: Plasmin-induced platelet aggregation and platelet release reaction. Effects on hemostasis. *J Clin Invest* 52(7):1647–1659, 1973.

146. Fitzgerald DJ, Catella F, Roy L, FitzGerald GA: Marked platelet activation in vivo after intravenous streptokinase in patients with acute myocardial infarction. *Circulation* 77(1):142–150, 1988.

147. Kerins DM, Roy L, FitzGerald GA, Fitzgerald DJ: Platelet and vascular function during coronary thrombolysis with tissue-type plasminogen activator. *Circulation* 80(6):1718–1725, 1989.

148. Thorsen LI, Brosstad F, Gogstad G, et al: Competitions between fibrinogen with its degradation products for interactions with the platelet-fibrinogen receptor. *Thromb Res* 44(5):611–623, 1986.

149. Miles LA, Ginsberg MH, White JG, Plow EF: Plasminogen interacts with human platelets through two distinct mechanisms. *J Clin Invest* 77(6):2001–2009, 1986.

150. Adelman B, Michelson AD, Loscalzo J, et al: Plasmin effect on platelet glycoprotein Ib-von Willebrand factor interactions. *Blood* 65(1):32–40, 1985.

151. Stricker RB, Wong D, Shiu DT, et al: Activation of plasminogen by tissue plasminogen activator on normal and thrombasthenic platelets: Effects on surface proteins and platelet aggregation. *Blood* 68(1):275–280, 1986.

152. Schafer AI, Adelman B: Plasmin inhibition of platelet function and of arachidonic acid metabolism. *J Clin Invest* 75(2):456–461, 1985.

153. Loscalzo J, Vaughan DE: Tissue plasminogen activator promotes platelet disaggregation in plasma. *J Clin Invest* 79(6):1749–1755, 1987.

154. Penny WF, Ware JA: Platelet activation and subsequent inhibition by plasmin and recombinant tissue-type plasminogen activator. *Blood* 79(1):91–98, 1992.

155. Winters KJ, Eisenberg PR, Jaffe AS, Santoro SA: Dependence of plasmin-mediated degradation of platelet adhesive receptors on temperature and Ca2+. *Blood* 76(8):1546–1557, 1990.

156. Hines R, Barash PG: Infusion of sodium nitroprusside induces platelet dysfunction *in vitro. Anesthesiology* 70(4):611–615, 1989.

157. Kroll MH, Schafer AI: Biochemical mechanisms of platelet activation. *Blood* 74:1181–1195, 1989.

158. Anfossi G, Russo I, Massucco P, et al: Studies on inhibition of human platelet function by sodium nitroprusside. Kinetic evaluation of the effect on aggregation and cyclic nucleotide content. *Thromb Res* 102(4):319–330, 2001.

159. Bozzo J, Hernandez MR, Galan AM, et al: Antiplatelet effects of sodium nitroprusside in flowing human blood: Studies under normoxic and hypoxic conditions. *Thromb Res* 97(4):217–225, 2000.

160. Jang EK, Azzam JE, Dickinson NT, et al: Roles for both cyclic GMP and cyclic AMP in the inhibition of collagen-induced platelet aggregation by nitroprusside. *Br J Haematol* 117(3):664–675, 2002.

161. Schafer AI, Alexander RW, Handin RI: Inhibition of platelet function by organic nitrate vasodilators. *Blood* 55(4):649–654, 1980.

162. Weksler BB, Gillick M, Pink J: Effect of propranolol on platelet function. *Blood* 49(2):185–196, 1977.

163. Leon R, Tiarks CY, Pechet L: Some observations on the *in vivo* effect of propranolol on platelet aggregation and release. *Am J Hematol* 5(2):117–121, 1978.

164. Hines R: Preservation of platelet function during trimethaphan infusion. *Anesthesiology* 72(5):834–837, 1990.

165. Hogman M, Frostell C, Arnberg H, Hedenstierna G: Bleeding time prolongation and NO inhalation. *Lancet* 341(8861):1664–1665, 1993.

166. Samama CM, Diaby M, Fellahi JL, et al: Inhibition of platelet aggregation by inhaled nitric oxide in patients with acute respiratory distress syndrome. *Anesthesiology* 83(1):56–65, 1995.

167. Gries A, Bode C, Peter K, et al: Inhaled nitric oxide inhibits human platelet aggregation, P-selectin expression, and fibrinogen binding *in vitro* and *in vivo. Circulation* 97(15):1481–1487, 1998.

168. Barnathan ES, Addonizio VP, Shattil SJ: Interaction of verapamil with human platelet alpha-adrenergic receptors. *Am J Physiol* 242(1):H19–H23, 1982.

169. Fujinishi A, Takahara K, Ohba C, et al: Effects of nisoldipine on cytosolic calcium, platelet aggregation, and coagulation/fibrinolysis in patients with coronary artery disease. *Angiology* 48(6):515–521, 1997.

170. Lawson D, Mehta J, Mehta P, et al: Cumulative effects of quinidine and aspirin on bleeding time and platelet a_2-adrenoceptors: Potential mechanism of bleeding diathesis in patients receiving this combination. *J Lab Clin Med* 108:581, 1986.

171. Aberg M, Hedner U, Bergentz SE: Effect of dextran 70 on factor VIII and platelet function in von Willebrand's disease. *Thromb Res* 12(4):629–634, 1978.

172. Mishler JM 4th: Synthetic plasma volume expanders—Their pharmacology, safety and clinical efficacy. *Clin Haematol* 13(1):75–92, 1984.

173. Kelton JG, Hirsh J: Bleeding associated with antithrombotic therapy. *Semin Hematol* 17(4):259–291, 1980.

174. Korttila K, Lauritsalo K, Sarmo A, et al: Suitability of plasma expanders in patients receiving low-dose heparin for prevention of venous thrombosis after surgery. *Acta Anaesthesiol Scand* 27(2):104–107, 1983.

175. Cope JT, Banks D, Mauney MC, et al: Intraoperative hetastarch infusion impairs hemostasis after cardiac operations. *Ann Thorac Surg* 63(1):78–82; discussion 82–83, 1997.

176. Ruttmann TG, James MF, Aronson I: *In vivo* investigation into the effects of haemodilution with hydroxyethyl starch (200/0.5) and normal saline on coagulation. *Br J Anaesth* 80(5):612–616, 1998.

177. Roberts JS, Bratton SL: Colloid volume expanders. Problems, pitfalls and possibilities. *Drugs* 55(5):621–630, 1998.

178. Avorn J, Patel M, Levin R, Winkelmayer WC: Hetastarch and bleeding complications after coronary artery surgery. *Chest* 124(4):1437–1442, 2003.

179. Treib J, Haass A, Pindur G: Coagulation disorders caused by hydroxyethyl starch. *Thromb Haemost* 78(3):974–983, 1997.

180. Scharbert G, Deusch E, Kress HG, et al: Inhibition of platelet function by hydroxyethyl starch solutions in chronic pain patients undergoing peridural anesthesia. *Anesth Analg* 99(3):823–827, 2004.

181. Svehla C, Spankova H, Mlejnkova M: The effect of tricyclic antidepressive drugs on adrenaline and adenosine diphosphate induced platelet aggregation. *J Pharm Pharmacol* 18(9):616–617, 1966.

182. Warlow C, Ogston D, Douglas AS: Platelet function after the administration of chlorpromazine to human subjects. *Haemostasis* 5(1):21–26, 1976.

183. Morishita S, Aoki S, Watanabe S: Different effect of desipramine on protein kinase C in platelets between bipolar and major depressive disorders. *Psychiatry Clin Neurosci* 53(1):11–15, 1999.

184. Hergovich N, Aigner M, Eichler HG, et al: Paroxetine decreases platelet serotonin storage and platelet function in human beings. *Clin Pharmacol Ther* 68(4):435–442, 2000.

185. Alderman CP, Seshadri P, Ben-Tovim DI: Effects of serotonin reuptake inhibitors on hemostasis. *Ann Pharmacother* 30(11):1232–1234, 1996.

186. Pai VB, Kelly MW: Bruising associated with the use of fluoxetine. *Ann Pharmacother* 30(7–8):786–788, 1996.

187. Corbin F, Blaise G, Sauve R: Differential effect of halothane and forskolin on platelet cytosolic Ca2+ mobilization and aggregation. *Anesthesiology* 89(2):401–410, 1998.

188. Aoki H, Mizobe T, Nozuchi S, Hiramatsu N: *In vivo* and *in vitro* studies of the inhibitory effect of propofol on human platelet aggregation. *Anesthesiology* 88(2):362–370, 1998.

189. Heesch CM, Negus BH, Steiner M, Set al: Effects of *in vivo* cocaine administration on human platelet aggregation. *Am J Cardiol* 78(2):237–239, 1996.

190. Jennings LK, White MM, Sauer CM, et al: Cocaine-induced platelet defects. *Stroke* 24(9):1352–1359, 1993.

191. Togna G, Graziani M, Sorrentino C, Caprino L: Prostanoid production in the presence of platelet activation in hypoxic cocaine-treated rats. *Haemostasis* 26(6):311–318, 1996.

192. Batista A, Macedo T, Tavares P, et al: Nitric oxide production and nitric oxide synthase expression in platelets from heroin abusers before and after ultrarapid detoxification. *Ann N Y Acad Sci* 965:479–486, 2002.

193. Ahr DJ, Scialla SJ, Kimball DB Jr: Acquired platelet dysfunction following mithramycin therapy. *Cancer* 41(2):448–454, 1978.

194. Panella TJ, Peters W, White JG, et al: Platelets acquire a secretion defect after high-dose chemotherapy. *Cancer* 65(8):1711–1716, 1990.

195. Pogliani EM, Fantasia R, Lambertenghi-Deliliers G, Cofrancesco E: Daunorubicin and platelet function. *Thromb Haemost* 45(1):38–42, 1981.

196. McKenna R, Ahmad T, Ts'ao CH, Frischer H: Glutathione reductase deficiency and platelet dysfunction induced by 1,3-bis(2-chloroethyl)-1-nitrosourea. *J Lab Clin Med* 102(1):102–115, 1983.

197. Karolak L, Chandra A, Khan W, et al: High-dose chemotherapy-induced platelet defect: Inhibition of platelet signal transduction pathways. *Mol Pharmacol* 43(1):37–44, 1993.

198. O'Malley CJ, Rasko JE, Basser RL, et al: Administration of pegylated recombinant human megakaryocyte growth and development factor to humans stimulates the production of functional platelets that show no evidence of *in vivo* activation. *Blood* 88(9):3288–3298, 1996.

199. Vadhan-Raj S, Murray LJ, Bueso-Ramos C, et al: Stimulation of megakaryocyte and platelet production by a single dose of recombinant human thrombopoietin in patients with cancer. *Ann Intern Med* 126(9):673–681, 1997.

200. Gratacap MP, Martin V, Valera MC, et al: The new tyrosine-kinase inhibitor and anti-cancer drug dasatinib reversibly affects platelet activation *in vitro* and *in vivo. Blood* 114(9):1884–1892, 2009.

201. Byrd JC, Furman RR, Coutre SE, et al: Targeting BTK with ibrutinib in relapsed chronic lymphocytic leukemia. *N Engl J Med* 369(1):32–42, 2013.

202. Wang ML, Rule S, Martin P, et al: Targeting BTK with ibrutinib in relapsed or refractory mantle-cell lymphoma. *N Engl J Med* 369(6):507–516, 2013.

203. Advani RH, Buggy JJ, Sharman JP, et al: Bruton tyrosine kinase inhibitor ibrutinib (PCI-32765) has significant activity in patients with relapsed/refractory B-cell malignancies. *J Clin Oncol* 31(1):88–94, 2013.

204. Levade M, David E, Garcia C, et al: Ibrutinib treatment affects collagen and von Willebrand Factor-dependent platelet functions. *Blood* 124(26):3991–3995, 2014.

205. Quek LS, Bolen J, Watson SP: A role for Bruton's tyrosine kinase (Btk) in platelet activation by collagen. *Curr Biol* 8(20):1137–1140, 1998.

206. Atkinson BT, Ellmeier W, Watson SP: Tec regulates platelet activation by GPVI in the absence of Btk. *Blood* 102(10):3592–3599, 2003.

207. Cohen H, Neild GH, Patel R, et al: Evidence for chronic platelet hyperaggregability and in vivo activation in cyclosporin-treated renal allograft recipients. *Thromb Res* 49(1):91–101, 1988.

208. Thomson C, Forbes CD, Prentice CR: A comparison of the effects of antihistamines on platelet function. *Thromb Diath Haemorrh* 30(3):547–556, 1973.

209. Platelet function during long-term treatment with ketanserin of claudicating patients with peripheral atherosclerosis. A multi-center, double-blind, placebo-controlled trial. The PACK Trial Group. *Thromb Res* 55(1):13–23, 1989.

210. Parvez Z, Moncada R, Fareed J, Messmore HL: Antiplatelet action of intravascular contrast media. Implications in diagnostic procedures. *Invest Radiol* 19(3):208–211, 1984.

211. Rao AK, Rao VM, Willis J, et al: Inhibition of platelet function by contrast media: Iopamidol and ioxaglate versus iothalamate. Work in progress. *Radiology* 156(2):311–313, 1985.

212. Goodnight SH Jr, Harris WS, Connor WE: The effects of dietary omega 3 fatty acids on platelet composition and function in man: A prospective, controlled study. *Blood* 58(5):880–885, 1981.

213. Moncada S, Higgs EA: Arachidonate metabolism in blood cells and the vessel wall. *Clin Haematol* 15(2):273–292, 1986.

214. Leaf A, Weber PC: Cardiovascular effects of n-3 fatty acids. *N Engl J Med* 318(9):549–557, 1988.

215. Hammerschmidt DE: Szechwan purpura. *N Engl J Med* 302(21):1191–1193, 1980.

216. Srivastava KC: Onion exerts antiaggregatory effects by altering arachidonic acid metabolism in platelets. *Prostaglandins Leukot Med* 24(1):43–50, 1986.

217. Apitz-Castro R, Escalante J, Vargas R, Jain MK: Ajoene, the antiplatelet principle of garlic, synergistically potentiates the antiaggregatory action of prostacyclin, forskolin, indomethacin and dipyridamole on human platelets. *Thromb Res* 42(3):303–311, 1986.

218. Srivastava KC: Extracts from two frequently consumed spices—cumin (Cuminum cyminum) and turmeric (Curcuma longa)—inhibit platelet aggregation and alter eicosanoid biosynthesis in human blood platelets. *Prostaglandins Leukot Essent Fatty Acids* 37(1):57–64, 1989.

219. Pearson TC: The risk of thrombosis in essential thrombocythemia and polycythemia vera. *Semin Oncol* 29(3 Suppl 10):16–21, 2002.

220. Kessler CM: Propensity for hemorrhage and thrombosis in chronic myeloproliferative disorders. *Semin Hematol* 41(2 Suppl 3):10–14, 2004.

221. Tefferi A: Polycythemia vera and essential thrombocythemia: 2013 update on diagnosis, risk-stratification, and management. *Am J Hematol* 88(6):507–516, 2013.

222. Schafer AI: Thrombocytosis. *N Engl J Med* 350(12):1211–1219, 2004.

223. Alfirevic A, Duncan A, You J, et al: Recombinant factor VII is associated with worse survival in complex cardiac surgical patients. *Ann Thorac Surg* 98(2):618–624, 2014.

224. Wasserman LR, Gilbert HS: The treatment of polycythemia vera. *Med Clin North Am* 50(6):1501–1518, 1966.

225. Murphy S: Polycythemia vera. *Dis Mon* 38(3):153–212, 1992.

226. Carobbio A, Finazzi G, Antonioli E, et al: Thrombocytosis and leukocytosis interaction in vascular complications of essential thrombocythemia. *Blood* 112(8):3135–3137, 2008.

227. Schafer AI: Essential thrombocythemia. *Prog Hemost Thromb* 10:69–96, 1990.

228. Elliott MA, Tefferi A: Pathogenesis and management of bleeding in essential thrombocythemia and polycythemia vera. *Curr Hematol Rep* 3(5):344–351, 2004.

229. Kessler CM, Klein HG, Havlik RJ: Uncontrolled thrombocytosis in chronic myeloproliferative disorders. *Br J Haematol* 50(1):157–167, 1982.

230. McIntyre KJ, Hoagland HC, Silverstein MN, Petitt RM: Essential thrombocythemia in young adults. *Mayo Clin Proc* 66(2):149–154, 1991.

231. Michiels JJ, Berneman Z, Gadisseur A, et al: Immune-mediated etiology of acquired von Willebrand syndrome in systemic lupus erythematosus and in benign monoclonal gammopathy: Therapeutic implications. *Semin Thromb Hemost* 32(6):577–588, 2006.

232. Carobbio A, Antonioli E, Guglielmelli P, et al: Leukocytosis and risk stratification assessment in essential thrombocythemia. *J Clin Oncol* 26(16):2732–2736, 2008.

233. Budde U, Schaefer G, Mueller N, et al: Acquired von Willebrand's disease in the myeloproliferative syndrome. *Blood* 64(5):981–985, 1984.

234. Tiede A, Rand JH, Budde U, et al: How I treat the acquired von Willebrand syndrome. *Blood* 117(25):6777–6785, 2011.

235. Hernandez-Boluda JC, Gomez M: Target hematologic values in the management of essential thrombocythemia and polycythemia vera. *Eur J Haematol* 94(1):4–11, 2015.

236. Landolfi R, Di Gennaro L, Barbui T, et al: Leukocytosis as a major thrombotic risk factor in patients with polycythemia vera. *Blood* 109(6):2446–2452, 2007.

237. Gangat N, Strand J, Li CY, et al: Leucocytosis in polycythaemia vera predicts both inferior survival and leukaemic transformation. *Br J Haematol* 138(3):354–358, 2007.

238. Villmow T, Kemkes-Matthes B, Matzdorff AC: Markers of platelet activation and platelet-leukocyte interaction in patients with myeloproliferative syndromes. *Thromb Res* 108(2–3):139–145, 2002.

239. Falanga A, Marchetti M, Vignoli A, et al: Leukocyte-platelet interaction in patients with essential thrombocythemia and polycythemia vera. *Exp Hematol* 33(5):523–530, 2005.

240. Maldonado JE, Pintado T, Pierre RV: Dysplastic platelets and circulating megakaryocytes in chronic myeloproliferative diseases. I. The platelets: Ultrastructure and peroxidase reaction. *Blood* 43(6):797–809, 1974.

241. Bautista AP, Buckler PW, Towler HM, et al: Measurement of platelet life-span in normal subjects and patients with myeloproliferative disease with indium oxine labelled platelets. *Br J Haematol* 58(4):679–687, 1984.

242. Ginsberg AD: Platelet function in patients with high platelet counts. *Ann Intern Med* 82:506–511, 1975.

243. Janson PA, Jubelirer SJ, Weinstein MS, Deykin D: Treatment of bleeding tendency in uremia with cryoprecipitate. *N Engl J Med* 303:1318, 1980.

244. Pareti FI, Gugliotta L, Mannucci L, et al: Biochemical and metabolic aspects of platelet dysfunction in chronic myeloproliferative disorders. *Thromb Haemost* 47(2):84–89, 1982.

245. Schafer AI: Deficiency of platelet lipoxygenase activity in myeloproliferative disorders. *N Engl J Med* 306(7):381–386, 1982.

246. Sugiyama T, Okuma M, Ushikubi F, et al: A novel platelet aggregating factor found in a patient with defective collagen-induced platelet aggregation and autoimmune thrombocytopenia. *Blood* 69:1712–1720, 1987.

247. Kaywin P, McDonough M, Insel PA, Shattil SJ: Platelet function in essential thrombocythemia: Decreased epinephrine responsiveness associated with a deficiency of platelet alpha-adrenergic receptors. *N Engl J Med* 299:505–509, 1978.

248. Swart SS, Pearson D, Wood JK, Barnett DB: Functional significance of the platelet alpha2-adrenoceptor: Studies in patients with myeloproliferative disorders. *Thromb Res* 33(5):531–541, 1984.

249. Handa M, Watanabe K, Kawai Y, et al: Platelet unresponsiveness to collagen: Involvement of glycoprotein Ia-IIa (alpha 2 beta 1 integrin) deficiency associated with a myeloproliferative disorder. *Thromb Haemost* 73(3):521–528, 1995.

250. Moore SF, Hunter RW, Harper P, et al: Dysfunction of the PI3 kinase/Rap1/integrin alpha(IIb)beta(3) pathway underlies ex vivo platelet hypoactivity in essential thrombocythemia. *Blood* 121(7):1209–1219, 2013.

251. Malpass TW, Savage B, Hanson SR, et al: Correlation between prolonged bleeding time and depletion of platelet dense granule ADP in patients with myelodysplastic and myeloproliferative disorders. *J Lab Clin Med* 103(6):894–904, 1984.

252. Mohri H: Acquired von Willebrand disease and storage pool disease in chronic myelocytic leukemia. *Am J Hematol* 22(4):391–401, 1986.

253. Walsh PN, Murphy S, Barry WE: The role of platelets in the pathogenesis of thrombosis and hemorrhage in patients with thrombocytosis. *Thromb Haemost* 38(4):1085–1096, 1977.

254. Kaplan R, Gabbeta J, Sun L, et al: Combined defect in membrane expression and activation of platelet GPIIb–IIIa complex without primary sequence abnormalities in myeloproliferative disease. *Br J Haematol* 111(3):954–964, 2000.

255. Berndt MC, Kabral A, Grimsley P, et al: An acquired Bernard-Soulier-like platelet defect associated with juvenile myelodysplastic syndrome. *Br J Haematol* 68(1):97–101, 1988.

256. Cooper B, Schafer AI, Puchalsky D, Handin RI: Platelet resistance to prostaglandin D2 in patients with myeloproliferative disorders. *Blood* 52(3):618–626, 1978.

257. Moore A, Nachman RL: Platelet Fc receptor. Increased expression in myeloproliferative disease. *J Clin Invest* 67(4):1064–1071, 1981.

258. Bolin RB, Okumura T, Jamieson GA: Changes in distribution of platelet membrane glycoproteins in patients with myeloproliferative disorders. *Am J Hematol* 3:63–71, 1977.

259. Eche N, Sie P, Caranobe C, et al: Platelets in myeloproliferative disorders. III: Glycoprotein profile in relation to platelet function and platelet density. *Scand J Haematol* 26(2):123–129, 1981.

260. Thibert V, Bellucci S, Cristofari M, et al: Increased platelet CD36 constitutes a common marker in myeloproliferative disorders. *Br J Haematol* 91(3):618–624, 1995.

261. Moliterno AR, Hankins WD, Spivak JL: Impaired expression of the thrombopoietin receptor by platelets from patients with polycythemia vera. *N Engl J Med* 338(9):572–580, 1998.

262. Humbert M, Nurden P, Bihour C, Pet al: Ultrastructural studies of platelet aggregates from human subjects receiving clopidogrel and from a patient with an inherited defect of an ADP-dependent pathway of platelet activation. *Arterioscler Thromb Vasc Biol* 16(12):1532–1543, 1996.

263. Rocca B, Ciabattoni G, Tartaglione R, et al: Increased thromboxane biosynthesis in essential thrombocythemia. *Thromb Haemost* 74(5):1225–1230, 1995.

264. Landolfi R, Ciabattoni G, Patrignani P, et al: Increased thromboxane biosynthesis in patients with polycythemia vera: Evidence for aspirin-suppressible platelet activation *in vivo*. *Blood* 80(8):1965–1971, 1992.

265. Tripodi A, Chantarangkul V, Gianniello F, et al: Global coagulation in myeloproliferative neoplasms. *Ann Hematol* 92(12):1633–1639, 2013.

266. Marchetti M, Tartari CJ, Russo L, et al: Phospholipid-dependent procoagulant activity is highly expressed by circulating microparticles in patients with essential thrombocythemia. *Am J Hematol* 89(1):68–73, 2014.

267. Cazzola M, Kralovics R: From Janus kinase 2 to calreticulin: The clinically relevant genomic landscape of myeloproliferative neoplasms. *Blood* 123(24):3714–3719, 2014.

268. Baxter EJ, Scott LM, Campbell PJ, et al: Acquired mutation of the tyrosine kinase JAK2 in human myeloproliferative disorders. *Lancet* 365(9464):1054–1061, 2005.

269. Levine RL, Wadleigh M, Cools J, et al: Activating mutation in the tyrosine kinase JAK2 in polycythemia vera, essential thrombocythemia, and myeloid metaplasia with myelofibrosis. *Cancer Cell* 7(4):387–397, 2005.

270. James C, Ugo V, Le Couedic JP, et al: A unique clonal JAK2 mutation leading to constitutive signalling causes polycythaemia vera. *Nature* 434(7037):1144–1148, 2005.

271. Kralovics R, Passamonti F, Buser AS, et al: A gain-of-function mutation of JAK2 in myeloproliferative disorders. *N Engl J Med* 352(17):1779–1790, 2005.

272. Scott LM, Tong W, Levine RL, et al: JAK2 exon 12 mutations in polycythemia vera and idiopathic erythrocytosis. *N Engl J Med* 356(5):459–468, 2007.

273. Pardanani AD, Levine RL, Lasho T, et al: MPL515 mutations in myeloproliferative and other myeloid disorders: A study of 1182 patients. *Blood* 108(10):3472–3476, 2006.

274. Schnittger S, Bacher U, Haferlach C, et al: Characterization of 35 new cases with four different MPLW515 mutations and essential thrombocytosis or primary myelofibrosis. *Haematologica* 94(1):141–144, 2009.

275. Nangalia J, Massie CE, Baxter EJ, et al: Somatic CALR mutations in myeloproliferative neoplasms with nonmutated JAK2. *N Engl J Med* 369(25):2391–2405, 2013.

276. Klampfl T, Gisslinger H, Harutyunyan AS, et al: Somatic mutations of calreticulin in myeloproliferative neoplasms. *N Engl J Med* 369(25):2379–2390, 2013.

277. Arellano-Rodrigo E, Alvarez-Larran A, Reverter JC, et al: Increased platelet and leukocyte activation as contributing mechanisms for thrombosis in essential thrombocythemia and correlation with the JAK2 mutational status. *Haematologica* 91(2):169–175, 2006.

278. Falanga A, Marchetti M, Vignoli A, et al: V617F JAK-2 mutation in patients with essential thrombocythemia: Relation to platelet, granulocyte, and plasma hemostatic and inflammatory molecules. *Exp Hematol* 35(5):702–711, 2007.

279. Robertson B, Urquhart C, Ford I, et al: Platelet and coagulation activation markers in myeloproliferative diseases: Relationships with JAK2 V6I7 F status, clonality, and antiphospholipid antibodies. *J Thromb Haemost* 5(8):1679–1685, 2007.

280. Coucelo M, Caetano G, Sevivas T, et al: JAK2V617F allele burden is associated with thrombotic mechanisms activation in polycythemia vera and essential thrombocythemia patients. *Int J Hematol* 99(1):32–40, 2014.

281. Pemmaraju N, Moliterno AR, Williams DM, et al: The quantitative JAK2 V617F neutrophil allele burden does not correlate with thrombotic risk in essential thrombocytosis. *Leukemia* 21(10):2210–2212, 2007.

282. Rumi E, Harutyunyan AS, Pietra D, et al; Associazione Italiana per la Ricerca sul Cancro Gruppo Italiano Malattie Mieloproliferative I. CALR exon 9 mutations are somatically acquired events in familial cases of essential thrombocythemia or primary myelofibrosis. *Blood* 123(15):2416–2419, 2014.

283. Andrikovics H, Krahling T, Balassa K, et al: Distinct clinical characteristics of myeloproliferative neoplasms with calreticulin mutations. *Haematologica* 99(7):1184–1190, 2014.

284. Tefferi A, Wassie EA, Guglielmelli P, et al: Type 1 versus Type 2 calreticulin mutations in essential thrombocythemia: A collaborative study of 1027 patients. *Am J Hematol* 89(8):E121–E124, 2014.

285. Rotunno G, Mannarelli C, Guglielmelli P et al; Associazione Italiana per la Ricerca sul Cancro Gruppo Italiano Malattie Mieloproliferative I. Impact of calreticulin mutations on clinical and hematological phenotype and outcome in essential thrombocythemia. *Blood* 123(10):1552–1555, 2014.

286. Mitchell MC, Boitnott JK, Kaufman S, et al: Budd-Chiari syndrome: Etiology, diagnosis and management. *Medicine (Baltimore)* 61(4):199–218, 1982.

287. Murphy S: Thrombocytosis and thrombocythaemia. *Clin Haematol* 12(1):89–106, 1983.

288. Schafer AI: Bleeding and thrombosis in the myeloproliferative disorders. *Blood* 64(1):1–12, 1984.

289. Gangat N, Wolanskyj AP, Tefferi A: Abdominal vein thrombosis in essential thrombocythemia: Prevalence, clinical correlates, and prognostic implications. *Eur J Haematol* 77(4):327–333, 2006.

290. Yonal I, Pinarbasi B, Hindilerden F, et al: The clinical significance of JAK2V617F mutation for Philadelphia-negative chronic myeloproliferative neoplasms in patients with splanchnic vein thrombosis. *J Thromb Thrombolysis* 34(3):388–396, 2012.

291. Smalberg JH, Arends LR, Valla DC, et al: Myeloproliferative neoplasms in Budd-Chiari syndrome and portal vein thrombosis: A meta-analysis. *Blood* 120(25):4921–4928, 2012.

292. Valla D, Casadevall N, Huisse MG, et al: Etiology of portal vein thrombosis in adults. A prospective evaluation of primary myeloproliferative disorders. *Gastroenterology* 94(4):1063–1069, 1988.

293. Hoekstra J, Janssen HL: Vascular liver disorders (II): Portal vein thrombosis. *Neth J Med* 67(2):46–53, 2009.

294. Hoekstra J, Janssen HL: Vascular liver disorders (I): Diagnosis, treatment and prognosis of Budd-Chiari syndrome. *Neth J Med* 66(8):334–339, 2008.

295. Frewin R, Dowson A: Headache in essential thrombocythaemia. *Int J Clin Pract* 66(10):976–983, 2012.

296. Singh AK, Wetherley-Mein G: Microvascular occlusive lesions in primary thrombocythaemia. *Br J Haematol* 36(4):553–564, 1977.

297. van Genderen PJ, Terpstra W, Michiels JJ, et al: High-dose intravenous immunoglobulin delays clearance of von Willebrand factor in acquired von Willebrand disease. *Thromb Haemost* 73(5):891–892, 1995.

298. Michiels JJ, Berneman ZN, Schroyens W, Van Vliet HH: Pathophysiology and treatment of platelet-mediated microvascular disturbances, major thrombosis and bleeding complications in essential thrombocythaemia and polycythaemia vera. *Platelets* 15(2):67–84, 2004.

299. Rinder HM, Schuster JE, Rinder CS, et al: Correlation of thrombosis with increased platelet turnover in thrombocytosis. *Blood* 91(4):1288–1294, 1998.

300. Besses C, Cervantes F, Pereira A, et al: Major vascular complications in essential thrombocythemia: A study of the predictive factors in a series of 148 patients. *Leukemia* 13(2):150–154, 1999.

301. Barbui T, Barosi G, Grossi A, et al: Practice guidelines for the therapy of essential thrombocythemia. A statement from the Italian Society of Hematology, the Italian Society of Experimental Hematology and the Italian Group for Bone Marrow Transplantation. *Haematologica* 89(2):215–232, 2004.

302. De Stefano V, Za T, Rossi E, et al: Recurrent thrombosis in patients with polycythemia vera and essential thrombocythemia: Incidence, risk factors, and effect of treatments. *Haematologica* 93(3):372–380, 2008.

303. Finazzi G, Carobbio A, Thiele J, et al: Incidence and risk factors for bleeding in 1104 patients with essential thrombocythemia or prefibrotic myelofibrosis diagnosed according to the 2008 WHO criteria. *Leukemia* 26(4):716–719, 2012.

304. Schafer AI: Molecular basis of the diagnosis and treatment of polycythemia vera and essential thrombocythemia. *Blood* 107(11):4214–4222, 2006.

305. Beer PA, Erber WN, Campbell PJ, Green AR: How I treat essential thrombocythemia. *Blood* 117(5):1472–1482, 2011.

306. Vannucchi AM: How I treat polycythemia vera. *Blood* 124(22):3212–3220, 2014.

307. Spivak J: Daily aspirin—Only half the answer. *N Engl J Med* 350(2):99–101, 2004.

308. Marchioli R, Finazzi G, Specchia G, et al; CYTO-PV Collaborative Group: Cardiovascular events and intensity of treatment in polycythemia vera. *N Engl J Med* 368(1):22–33, 2013.

309. Kaplan ME, Mack K, Goldberg JD, et al: Long-term management of polycythemia vera with hydroxyurea: A progress report. *Semin Hematol* 23(3):167–171, 1986.

310. Gilbert HS: Modern treatment strategies in polycythemia vera. *Semin Hematol* 40(1 Suppl 1):26–29, 2003.

311. Barbui T, Finazzi G: Treatment indications and choice of a platelet-lowering agent in essential thrombocythemia. *Curr Hematol Rep* 2(3):248–256, 2003.

312. Cortelazzo S, Finazzi G, Ruggeri M, et al: Hydroxyurea for patients with essential thrombocythemia and a high risk of thrombosis. *N Engl J Med* 332(17):1132–1136, 1995.

313. Pescatore SL, Lindley C: Anagrelide: A novel agent for the treatment of myeloproliferative disorders. *Expert Opin Pharmacother* 1(3):537–546, 2000.

314. Emadi A, Spivak JL: Anagrelide: 20 years later. *Expert Rev Anticancer Ther* 9(1):37–50, 2009.

315. Solberg LA Jr, Tefferi A, Oles KJ, et al: The effects of anagrelide on human megakaryocytopoiesis. *Br J Haematol* 99(1):174–180, 1997.

316. Fruchtman SM, Petitt RM, Gilbert HS, et al: Anagrelide: Analysis of long-term efficacy, safety and leukemogenic potential in myeloproliferative disorders. *Leuk Res* 29(5):481–491, 2005.

317. Wagstaff AJ, Keating GM: Anagrelide: A review of its use in the management of essential thrombocythaemia. *Drugs* 66(1):111–131, 2006.

318. Campbell PJ, Scott LM, Buck G, et al: Definition of subtypes of essential thrombocythaemia and relation to polycythaemia vera based on JAK2 V617F mutation status: A prospective study. *Lancet* 366(9501):1945–1953, 2005.

319. Hultdin M, Sundstrom G, Wahlin A, et al: Progression of bone marrow fibrosis in patients with essential thrombocythemia and polycythemia vera during anagrelide treatment. *Med Oncol* 24(1):63–70, 2007.

320. Gisslinger H, Gotic M, Holowiecki J, et al; ANAHYDRET Study Group: Anagrelide compared with hydroxyurea in WHO-classified essential thrombocythemia: The ANAHYDRET Study, a randomized controlled trial. *Blood* 121(10):1720–1728, 2013.

321. Mohri H, Noguchi T, Kodama F, et al: Acquired von Willebrand disease due to inhibitor of human myeloma protein specific for von Willebrand factor. *Am J Clin Pathol* 87(5):663–668, 1987.

322. Michiels JJ, Abels J, Steketee J, et al: Erythromelalgia caused by platelet-mediated arteriolar inflammation and thrombosis in thrombocythemia. *Ann Intern Med* 102(4):466–471, 1985.

323. van Genderen PJ, Prins FJ, Lucas IS, et al: Decreased half-life time of plasma von Willebrand factor collagen binding activity in essential thrombocythaemia: Normalization after cytoreduction of the increased platelet count. *Br J Haematol* 99(4):832–836, 1997.

324. Pascale S, Petrucci G, Dragani A, et al: Aspirin-insensitive thromboxane biosynthesis in essential thrombocythemia is explained by accelerated renewal of the drug target. *Blood* 119(15):3595–3603, 2012.

325. Cavalca V, Rocca B, Squellerio I, et al: In vivo prostacyclin biosynthesis and effects of different aspirin regimens in patients with essential thrombocythaemia. *Thromb Haemost* 112(1):118–127, 2014.

326. Landolfi R, Marchioli R, Kutti J, et al: Efficacy and safety of low-dose aspirin in polycythemia vera. *N Engl J Med* 350(2):114–124, 2004.

327. Gangat N, Wolanskyj AP, Schwager S, Tefferi A: Predictors of pregnancy outcome in essential thrombocythemia: A single institution study of 63 pregnancies. *Eur J Haematol* 82(5):350–353, 2009.

328. Passamonti F, Randi ML, Rumi E, et al: Increased risk of pregnancy complications in patients with essential thrombocythemia carrying the JAK2 (617V>F) mutation. *Blood* 110(2):485–489, 2007.

329. Barbui T, Finazzi G: Myeloproliferative disease in pregnancy and other management issues. *Hematology Am Soc Hematol Educ Program* 246–252, 2006.

330. Sultan Y, Caen JP: Platelet dysfunction in preleukemic states and in various types of leukemia. *Ann N Y Acad Sci* 201:300–306, 1972.

331. Cowan DH, Haut MJ: Platelet function in acute leukemia. *J Lab Clin Med* 79(6):893–905, 1972.

332. Cowan DH, Graham RC Jr, Baunach D: The platelet defect in leukemia. Platelet ultrastructure, adenine nucleotide metabolism, and the release reaction. *J Clin Invest* 56(1):188–200, 1975.

333. Foss B, Bruserud O: Platelet functions and clinical effects in acute myelogenous leukemia. *Thromb Haemost* 99(1):27–37, 2008.

334. Leinoe EB, Hoffmann MH, Kjaersgaard E, et al: Prediction of haemorrhage in the early stage of acute myeloid leukaemia by flow cytometric analysis of platelet function. *Br J Haematol* 128(4):526–532, 2005.

335. Glembotsky AC, Bluteau D, Espasandin YR, et al: Mechanisms underlying platelet function defect in a pedigree with familial platelet disorder with a predisposition to acute myelogenous leukemia: Potential role for candidate RUNX1 targets. *J Thromb Haemost* 12(5):761–772, 2014.

336. Kaur G, Jalagadugula G, Mao G, Rao AK: RUNX1/core binding factor A2 regulates platelet 12-lipoxygenase gene (ALOX12): Studies in human RUNX1 haplodeficiency. *Blood* 115(15):3128–3135, 2010.

337. Quintas-Cardama A, Han X, Kantarjian H, Cortes J: Tyrosine kinase inhibitor-induced platelet dysfunction in patients with chronic myeloid leukemia. *Blood* 114(2):261–263, 2009.

338. Neelakantan P, Marin D, Laffan M, et al: Platelet dysfunction associated with ponatinib, a new pan BCR-ABL inhibitor with efficacy for chronic myeloid leukemia resistant to multiple tyrosine kinase inhibitor therapy. *Haematologica* 97(9):1444, 2012.

339. Meschengieser S, Blanco A, Maugeri N, et al: Platelet function and intraplatelet von Willebrand factor antigen and fibrinogen in myelodysplastic syndromes. *Thromb Res* 46(4):601–606, 1987.

340. Zeidman A, Sokolover N, Fradin Z, et al: Platelet function and its clinical significance in the myelodysplastic syndromes. *Hematol J* 5(3):234–238, 2004.

341. Bellucci S, Huisse MG, Boval B, et al: Defective collagen-induced platelet activation in two patients with malignant haemopathies is related to a defect in the GPVI-coupled signalling pathway. *Thromb Haemost* 93(1):130–138, 2005.

342. Girtovitis FI, Ntaios G, Papadopoulos A,: Defective platelet aggregation in myelodysplastic syndromes. *Acta Haematol* 118(2):117–122, 2007.

343. Burbury KL, Seymour JF, Dauer R, Westerman DA: Under-recognition of platelet dysfunction in myelodysplastic syndromes: Are we only seeing the tip of the iceberg? *Leuk Lymphoma* 54(1):11–13, 2013.

344. Frigeni M, Galli M: Childhood myelodysplastic syndrome associated with an acquired Bernard-Soulier-like platelet dysfunction. *Blood* 124(16):2609, 2014.

345. Pui CH, Jackson CW, Chesney C: Normal platelet function after therapy for acute lymphocytic leukemia. *Arch Intern Med* 143(1):73–74, 1983.

346. Andre JM, Galambrun C, Trzeciak MC, et al: Acquired Glanzmann's thrombasthenia associated with acute lymphoblastic leukemia. *J Pediatr Hematol Oncol* 27(10):554–557, 2005.

347. Raman V, Quillen K, Sloan JM: Acquired Glanzmann thrombasthenia associated with Hodgkin lymphoma: Rapid reversal of functional platelet defect with ABVD (Adriamycin/bleomycin/vinblastine/dacarbazine) chemotherapy. *Clin Lymphoma Myeloma Leuk* 14(2):e51–e54, 2014.

348. Westbrook CA, Golde DW: Clinical problems in hairy cell leukemia: Diagnosis and management. *Semin Oncol* 11(4 Suppl 2):514–522, 1984.

349. Rosove MH, Naeim F, Harwig S, Zighelboim J: Severe platelet dysfunction in hairy cell leukemia with improvement after splenectomy. *Blood* 55(6):903–906, 1980.

350. Roussi JH, Houbouyan LL, Alterescu R, et al: Acquired von Willebrand's syndrome associated with hairy cell leukaemia. *Br J Haematol* 46(3):503–506, 1980.

351. Lackner H: Hemostatic abnormalities associated with dysproteinemias. *Semin Hematol* 10(2):125–133, 1973.

352. Coppola A, Tufano A, Di Capua M, Franchini M: Bleeding and thrombosis in multiple myeloma and related plasma cell disorders. *Semin Thromb Hemost* 37(8):929–945, 2011.

353. Perkins HA, MacKenzie MR, Fudenberg HH: Hemostatic defects in dysproteinemias. *Blood* 35(5):695–707, 1970.

354. Rapoport M, Yona R, Kaufman S, et al: Unusual bleeding manifestations of amyloidosis in patients with multiple myeloma. *Clin Lab Haematol* 16(4):349–353, 1994.

355. Furie B, Greene E, Furie BC: Syndrome of acquired factor X deficiency and systemic amyloidosis in vivo studies of the metabolic fate of factor X. *N Engl J Med* 297(2):81–85, 1977.

356. McPherson RA, Onstad JW, Ugoretz RJ, Wolf PL: Coagulopathy in amyloidosis: Combined deficiency of factors IX and X. *Am J Hematol* 3:225–235, 1977.

357. Palmer RN, Rick ME, Rick PD, Zeller JA, Gralnick HR: Circulating heparan sulfate anticoagulant in a patient with a fatal bleeding disorder. *N Engl J Med* 310(26):1696–1699, 1984.

358. Chapman GS, George CB, Danley DL: Heparin-like anticoagulant associated with plasma cell myeloma. *Am J Clin Pathol* 83(6):764–766, 1985.

359. Torjemane L, Guermazi S, Ladeb S, et al: Heparin-like anticoagulant associated with multiple myeloma and neutralized with protamine sulfate. *Blood Coagul Fibrinolysis* 18(3):279–281, 2007.

360. Liebman H, Chinowsky M, Valdin J, et al: Increased fibrinolysis and amyloidosis. *Arch Intern Med* 143(4):678–682, 1983.

361. Meyer K, Williams EC: Fibrinolysis and acquired alpha-2 plasmin inhibitor deficiency in amyloidosis. *Am J Med* 79(3):394–396, 1985.

362. McGrath KM, Stuart JJ, Richards F 2nd: Correlation between serum IgG, platelet membrane IgG, and platelet function in hypergammaglobulinaemic states. *Br J Haematol* 42(4):585–591, 1979.

363. Kasturi J, Saraya AK: Platelet functions in dysproteinaemia. *Acta Haematol* 59(2):104–113, 1978.

364. Vigliano EM, Horowitz HI: Bleeding syndrome in a patient with IgA myeloma: Interaction of protein and connective tissue. *Blood* 29(6):823–836, 1967.

365. Shinagawa A, Kojima H, Berndt MC, et al: Characterization of a myeloma patient with a life-threatening hemorrhagic diathesis: Presence of a lambda dimer protein inhibiting shear-induced platelet aggregation by binding to the A1 domain of von Willebrand factor. *Thromb Haemost* 93(5):889–896, 2005.

366. DiMinno G, Coraggio F, Cerbone AM, et al: A myeloma paraprotein with specificity for platelet glycoprotein IIIa in a patient with a fatal bleeding disorder. *J Clin Invest* 77:157–164, 1986.

367. Mannucci PM, Lombardi R, Bader R, et al: Studies of the pathophysiology of acquired von Willebrand's disease in seven patients with lymphoproliferative disorders or benign monoclonal gammopathies. *Blood* 64(3):614–621, 1984.

368. Takahashi H, Nagayama R, Tanabe Y, et al: DDAVP in acquired von Willebrand syndrome associated with multiple myeloma. *Am J Hematol* 22(4):421–429, 1986.

369. Lamboley V, Zabraniecki L, Sie P, et al: Myeloma and monoclonal gammopathy of uncertain significance associated with acquired von Willebrand's syndrome. Seven new cases with a literature review. *Joint Bone Spine* 69(1):62–67, 2002.

370. Federici AB: Acquired von Willebrand syndrome: Is it an extremely rare disorder or do we see only the tip of the iceberg? *J Thromb Haemost* 6(4):565–568, 2008.

371. Voisin S, Hamidou M, Lefrancois A, et al: Acquired von Willebrand syndrome associated with monoclonal gammopathy: A single-center study of 36 patients. *Medicine (Baltimore)* 90(6):404–411, 2011.

372. Howard CR, Lin TL, Cunningham MT, Lipe BC: IgG kappa monoclonal gammopathy of undetermined significance presenting as acquired type III Von Willebrand syndrome. *Blood Coagul Fibrinolysis* 25(6):631–633, 2014.

373. Coucke L, Marcelis L, Deeren D, et al: Lymphoplasmacytic lymphoma exposed by haemoptysis and acquired von Willebrand syndrome. *Blood Coagul Fibrinolysis* 25(4):395–397, 2014.

374. Scepansky E, Othman M, Smith H: Acquired von Willebrand syndrome with a type 2B phenotype: Diagnostic and therapeutic dilemmas. *Acta Haematol* 131(4):213–217, 2014.

375. Wallace MR, Simon SR, Ershler WB, Burns SL: Hemorrhagic diathesis in multiple myeloma. *Acta Haematol* 72(5):340–342, 1984.

376. Hyman BT, Westrick MA: Multiple myeloma with polyneuropathy and coagulopathy. A case report of the polyneuropathy, organomegaly, endocrinopathy, M-protein, and skin change (POEMS) syndrome. *Arch Intern Med* 146(5):993–994, 1986.

377. Bovill EG, Ershler WB, Golden EA, et al: A human myeloma-produced monoclonal protein directed against the active subpopulation of von Willebrand factor. *Am J Clin Pathol* 85(1):115–123, 1986.

378. Silberstein LE, Abrahm J, Shattil SJ: The efficacy of intensive plasma exchange in acquired von Willebrand's disease. *Transfusion* 27(3):234–237, 1987.

379. Federici AB, Stabile F, Castaman G, et al: Treatment of acquired von Willebrand syndrome in patients with monoclonal gammopathy of uncertain significance: Comparison of three different therapeutic approaches. *Blood* 92(8):2707–2711, 1998.

380. Federici AB: Use of intravenous immunoglobulin in patients with acquired von Willebrand syndrome. *Hum Immunol* 66(4):422–430, 2005.

381. Federici AB, Budde U, Castaman G, et al: Current diagnostic and therapeutic approaches to patients with acquired von Willebrand syndrome: A 2013 update. *Semin Thromb Hemost* 39(2):191–201, 2013.

382. Mazoyer E, Fain O, Dhote R, Laurian Y: Is rituximab effective in acquired von Willebrand syndrome? *Br J Haematol* 144(6):967–968, 2009.

383. Michiels JJ, Budde U, van der Planken M, et al: Acquired von Willebrand syndromes: Clinical features, aetiology, pathophysiology, classification and management. *Best Pract Res Clin Haematol* 14(2):401–436, 2001.

384. Kumar S, Pruthi RK, Nichols WL: Acquired von Willebrand disease. *Mayo Clin Proc* 77(2):181–187, 2002.

385. Hong S, Lee J, Chi H, et al: Systemic lupus erythematosus complicated by acquired von Willebrand's syndrome. *Lupus* 17(9):846–848, 2008.

386. Pruthi RK: Hypertrophic obstructive cardiomyopathy, acquired von Willebrand syndrome, and gastrointestinal bleeding. *Mayo Clin Proc* 86(3):181–182, 2011.

387. Casonato A, Sponga S, Pontara E, et al: Von Willebrand factor abnormalities in aortic valve stenosis: Pathophysiology and impact on bleeding. *Thromb Haemost* 106(1):58–66, 2011.

388. Heilmann C, Geisen U, Beyersdorf F, et al: Acquired von Willebrand syndrome in patients with extracorporeal life support (ECLS). *Intensive Care Med* 38(1):62–68, 2012.

389. Meyer AL, Malehsa D, Budde U, et al: Acquired von Willebrand syndrome in patients with a centrifugal or axial continuous flow left ventricular assist device. *JACC Heart Fail* 2(2):141–145, 2014.

390. Morrison KA, Jorde UP, Garan AR, et al: Acquired von Willebrand disease during CentriMag support is associated with high prevalence of bleeding during support and after transition to heart replacement therapy. *ASAIO J* 60(2):241–242, 2014.

391. Mitrovic M, Elezovic I, Miljic P, Suvajdzic N: Acquired von Willebrand syndrome in patients with Gaucher disease. *Blood Cells Mol Dis* 52(4):205–207, 2014.

392. Federici AB: Acquired von Willebrand syndrome associated with hypothyroidism: A mild bleeding disorder to be further investigated. *Semin Thromb Hemost* 37(1):35–40, 2011.

393. Stuijver DJ, Piantanida E, van Zaane B, et al: Acquired von Willebrand syndrome in patients with overt hypothyroidism: A prospective cohort study. *Haemophilia* 20(3):326–332, 2014.

394. Wiegand G, Hofbeck M, Zenker M, et al: Bleeding diathesis in Noonan syndrome: Is acquired von Willebrand syndrome the clue? *Thromb Res* 130(5):e251–e254, 2012.

395. Mazurier C, Parquet-Gernez A, Descamps J, et al: Acquired von Willebrand's syndrome in the course of Waldenström's disease. *Thromb Haemost* 44(3):115–118, 1980.

396. Handin RI, Martin V, Moloney WC: Antibody-induced von Willebrand's disease: A newly defined inhibitor syndrome. *Blood* 48(3):393–405, 1976.

397. Van Genderen PJ, Papatsonis DN, Michiels JJ, et al: High-dose intravenous gamma-globulin therapy for acquired von Willebrand disease. *Postgrad Med J* 70(830):916–920, 1994.

398. Goudemand J, Samor B, Caron C, et al: Acquired type II von Willebrand's disease: Demonstration of a complexed inhibitor of the von Willebrand factor-platelet interaction and response to treatment. *Br J Haematol* 68(2):227–233, 1988.

399. Mohri H, Hisanaga S, Mishima A, et al: Autoantibody inhibits binding of von Willebrand factor to glycoprotein Ib and collagen in multiple myeloma: Recognition sites present on the A1 loop and A3 domains of von Willebrand factor. *Blood Coagul Fibrinolysis* 9(1):91–97, 1998.

400. Igarashi N, Miura M, Kato E, et al: Acquired von Willebrand's syndrome with lupus-like serology. *Am J Pediatr Hematol Oncol* 11(1):32–35, 1989.

401. Agrawal AK, Golden C, Matsunaga A: Acquired von Willebrand disease in an osteosarcoma patient. *J Pediatr Hematol Oncol* 33(8):622–623, 2011.

402. Scott JP, Montgomery RR, Tubergen DG, Hays T: Acquired von Willebrand's disease in association with Wilms' [sic] tumor: Regression following treatment. *Blood* 58(4):665–669, 1981.

403. Rao KP, Kizer J, Jones TJ, et al: Acquired von Willebrand's syndrome associated with an extranodal pulmonary lymphoma. *Arch Pathol Lab Med* 112(1):47–50, 1988.

404. Baxter PA, Nuchtern JG, Guillerman RP, et al: Acquired von Willebrand syndrome and Wilms tumor: Not always benign. *Pediatr Blood Cancer* 52(3):392–394, 2009.

405. Levesque H, Borg JY, Cailleux N, et al: Acquired von Willebrand's syndrome associated with decrease of plasminogen activator and its inhibitor during hypothyroidism. *Eur J Med* 2(5):287–288, 1993.

406. Aylesworth CA, Smallridge RC, Rick ME, Alving BM: Acquired von Willebrand's disease: A rare manifestation of postpartum thyroiditis. *Am J Hematol* 50(3):217–219, 1995.

407. Tiede A, Priesack J, Werwitzke S, et al: Diagnostic workup of patients with acquired von Willebrand syndrome: A retrospective single-centre cohort study. *J Thromb Haemost* 6(4):569–576, 2008.

408. Joist JH, Cowan JF, Zimmerman TS: Acquired von Willebrand's disease. Evidence for a quantitative and qualitative factor VIII disorder. *N Engl J Med* 298(18):988–991, 1978.

409. Cushing M, Kawaguchi K, Friedman KD, Mark T: Factor VIII/von Willebrand factor concentrate therapy for ventricular assist device-associated acquired von Willebrand disease. *Transfusion* 52(7):1535–1541, 2012.

410. Jimenez AR, Vallejo ES, Cruz MZ, et al: Rituximab effectiveness in a patient with juvenile systemic lupus erythematosus complicated with acquired von Willebrand syndrome. *Lupus* 22(14):1514–1517, 2013.

411. Sucker C, Scharf RE, Zotz RB: Use of recombinant factor VIIa in inherited and acquired von Willebrand disease. *Clin Appl Thromb Hemost* 15(1):27–31, 2009.

412. Macik BG, Gabriel DA, White GC 2nd, et al: The use of high-dose intravenous gamma-globulin in acquired von Willebrand syndrome. *Arch Pathol Lab Med* 112(2):143–146, 1988.

413. Rinder MR, Richard RE, Rinder HM: Acquired von Willebrand's disease: A concise review. *Am J Hematol* 54(2):139–145, 1997.

414. Franchini M, Lippi G: Recent acquisitions in acquired and congenital von Willebrand disorders. *Clin Chim Acta* 377(1–2):62–69, 2007.

415. Biondo F, Matturro A, Santoro C, et al: Remission of acquired von Willebrand syndrome after successful treatment of gastric MALT lymphoma. *Haemophilia* 18(1):e34–e35, 2012.

416. Oliveira MC, Kramer CK, Marroni CP, et al: Acquired factor VIII and von Willebrand factor (aFVIII-VWF) deficiency and hypothyroidism in a case with hypopituitarism. *Clin Appl Thromb Hemost* 16(1):107–109, 2010.

417. Manfredi E, van Zaane B, Gerdes VE, et al: Hypothyroidism and acquired von Willebrand's syndrome: A systematic review. *Haemophilia* 14(3):423–433, 2008.

418. Budde U, Scharf RE, Franke P, et al: Elevated platelet count as a cause of abnormal von Willebrand factor multimer distribution in plasma. *Blood* 82:1749–1757, 1993.

419. Franchini M, Mannucci PM: Von Willebrand disease-associated angiodysplasia: A few answers, still many questions. *Br J Haematol* 161(2):177–182, 2013.

420. Solomon C, Budde U, Schneppenheim S, et al: Acquired type 2A von Willebrand syndrome caused by aortic valve disease corrects during valve surgery. *Br J Anaesth* 106(4):494–500, 2011.

421. Rao AK: Uraemic platelets. *Lancet* 1:913, 1986.

422. Boccardo P, Remuzzi G, Galbusera M: Platelet dysfunction in renal failure. *Semin Thromb Hemost* 30(5):579–589, 2004.

423. Rosenbaum R, Hoffstein PE, Stanley RJ, Klahr S: Use of computerized tomography to diagnose complications of percutaneous renal biopsy. *Kidney Int* 14:87–92, 1978.

424. Diaz-Buxo JA, Donadio JVJ: Complications of percutaneous renal biopsy: An analysis of 1000 consecutive biopsies. *Clin Nephrol* 4:223, 1975.

425. Mannucci PM, Tripodi A: Hemostatic defects in liver and renal dysfunction. *Hematology Am Soc Hematol Educ Program* 168–173, 2012.

426. Valeri CR, Cassidy G, Pivacek LE, et al: Anemia-induced increase in the bleeding time: Implications for treatment of nonsurgical blood loss. *Transfusion* 41(8):977–983, 2001.

427. Castillo R, Lozano T, Escolar G, et al: Defective platelet adhesion on vessel subendothelium in uremic patients. *Blood* 68(2):337–342, 1986.

428. Livio M, Gotti E, Marchesi D, et al: Uraemic bleeding: Role of anaemia and beneficial effect of red cell transfusions. *Lancet* 2(8306):1013–1015, 1982.

429. Fernandez F, Goudable C, Sie P, et al: Low haematocrit and prolonged bleeding time in uraemic patients: Effect of red cell transfusions. *Br J Haematol* 59:139–148, 1985.

430. Moia M, Mannucci PM, Vizzotto L, et al: Improvement in the haemostatic defect of uraemia after treatment with recombinant human erythropoietin. *Lancet* 2:1227–1229, 1987.

431. Tang WW, Stead RA, Goodkin DA: Effects of epoetin alfa on hemostasis in chronic renal failure. *Am J Nephrol* 18:263–273, 1998.

432. Turrito VT, Weiss HJ: Red blood cells: Their dual role in thrombus formation. *Science* 207:541, 1980.

433. Casonato A, Pontara E, Vertolli UP, Steffan A, Durante C, De Marco L, Sartorello F, Girolami A: Plasma and platelet von Willebrand factor abnormalities in patients with uremia: Lack of correlation with uremic bleeding. *Clin Appl Thromb Hemost* 7(2):81–86, 2001.

434. Zwaginga JJ, Ijsseldijk MJ, Beeser-Visser N, et al: High von Willebrand factor concentration compensates a relative adhesion defect in uremic blood. *Blood* 75:1498–1508, 1990.

435. Sloand EM, Sloand JA, Produoz K, et al: Reduction of platelet glycoprotein Ib in uremia. *Br J Haematol* 77:375–381, 1991.

436. Gralnick HR, McKeown LP, Williams SB, et al: Plasma and platelet von Willebrand factor defects in uremia. *Am J Med* 85:806–810, 1988.

437. Escolar G, Cases A, Bastida E, et al: Uremic platelets have a functional defect affecting the interaction of von Willebrand factor with glycoprotein IIb-IIIa. *Blood* 76:1336–1340, 1990.

438. Di Minno G, Cerbone A, Usberti M, et al: Platelet dysfunction in uremia. II. Correction by arachidonic acid of the impaired exposure of fibrinogen receptors by adenosine diphosphate or collagen. *J Lab Clin Med* 108:246–252, 1986.

439. Rabiner SF, Hrodek O: Platelet factor 3 in normal subjects and patients with renal failure. *J Clin Invest* 47(4):901–912, 1968.

440. Ware JA, Clark BA, Smith M, Salzman EW: Abnormalities of cytoplasmic Ca²⁺ in platelets from patients with uremia. *Blood* 73:172–176, 1989.

441. Mannucci PM, Remuzzi G, Pusineri F, et al: Deamino-8-arginine vasopressin shortens the bleeding time in uremia. *N Engl J Med* 308(1):8–12, 1983.

442. Winter M, Frampton G, Bennett A, et al: Synthesis of thromboxane B₂ in uraemia and the effects of dialysis. *Thromb Res* 30:265–272, 1983.

443. Neirynck N, Vanholder R, Schepers E, et al: An update on uremic toxins. *Int Urol Nephrol* 45(1):139–150, 2013.

444. Bazilinski N, Shaykh M, Dunea G, et al: Inhibition of platelet function by uremic middle molecules. *Nephron* 40:423–428, 1985.

445. Remuzzi G, Livio M, Marchiaro G, et al: Bleeding in renal failure: Altered platelet function in chronic uraemia only partially corrected by haemodialysis. *Nephron* 22:347–353, 1978.

446. Livio M, Benigni A, Remuzzi G: Coagulation abnormalities in uremia. *Semin Nephrol* 5:82–90, 1985.

447. Siqueira MA, Brunini TM, Pereira NR, et al: Increased nitric oxide production in platelets from severe chronic renal failure patients. *Can J Physiol Pharmacol* 89(2):97–102, 2011.

448. Meenakshi SR, Agarwal R: Nitric oxide levels in patients with chronic renal disease. Journal of clinical and diagnostic research: *J Clin Diagn Res* 7(7):1288–1290, 2013.

449. Remuzzi G, Perico N, Zoja C, et al: Role of endothelium-derived nitric oxide in the bleeding tendency of uremia. *J Clin Invest* 86(5):1768–1771, 1990.

450. Aiello S, Noris M, Todeschini M, et al: Renal and systemic nitric oxide synthesis in rats with renal mass reduction. *Kidney Int* 52:171–181, 1997.

451. Noris M, Remuzzi G: Uremic bleeding: Closing the circle after 30 years of controversies? *Blood* 94(8):2569–2574, 1999.

452. Mendes Ribeiro AC, Brunini TM, Ellory JC, Mann GE: Abnormalities in L-arginine transport and nitric oxide biosynthesis in chronic renal and heart failure. *Cardiovasc Res* 49(4):697–712, 2001.

453. Brunini TM, Yaqoob MM, Novaes Malagris LE, et al: Increased nitric oxide synthesis in uraemic platelets is dependent on L-arginine transport via system y(+)L. *Pflugers Arch* 445(5):547–550, 2003.

454. Linthorst GE, Avis HJ, Levi M: Uremic thrombocytopathy is not about urea. *J Am Soc Nephrol* 21(5):753–755, 2010.

455. Remuzzi G: Bleeding disorders in uremia: Pathophysiology and treatment. *Adv Nephrol Necker Hosp* 18:171–186, 1989.

456. Andrassy K, Ritz E: Uremia as a cause of bleeding. *Am J Nephrol* 5:313, 1985.

457. Ando M, Iwamoto Y, Suda A, et al: New insights into the thrombopoietic status of patients on dialysis through the evaluation of megakaryocytopoiesis in bone marrow and of endogenous thrombopoietin levels. *Blood* 2001;97(4):915–921, 1989.

458. George CRP, Slichter SJ, Quadracci LJ: A kinetic evaluation of hemostasis in renal disease. *N Engl J Med* 291:1111, 1974.

459. Linthorst GE, Folman CC, van Olden RW, von dem Borne AE. Plasma thrombopoietin levels in patients with chronic renal failure. *Hematol J* 3(1):38–42, 2002.

460. A comparison of two doses of aspirin (30 mg vs. 283 mg a day) in patients after a transient ischemic attack or minor ischemic stroke. The Dutch TIA Trial Study Group. *N Engl J Med* 325(18):1261–1266, 1991.

461. Peterson P, Hayes TE, Arkin CF, et al: The preoperative bleeding time test lacks clinical benefit. *Arch Surg* 133:134–139, 1998.

462. Stewart JH, Castaldi PA: Uraemic bleeding: A reversible platelet defect corrected by dialysis. *Q J Med* 36(143):409–423, 1967.

463. Lindsay RM, Friesen M, Koens F, et al: Platelet function in patients on long-term peritoneal dialysis. *Clin Nephrol* 6:335–339, 1976.

464. Weigert AL, Schafer AI: Uremic bleeding: Pathogenesis and therapy. *Am J Med Sci* 316:94–104, 1998.

465. Vigano G, Benigni A, Mendogni D, et al: Recombinant human erythropoietin to correct uremic bleeding. *Am J Kidney Dis* 18:44–49, 1991.

466. Tassies D, Reventer JC, Cases A, et al: Effect of recombinant human erythropoietin treatment on circulating reticulated platelets in uremic patients: Association with early improvement in platelet function. *Am J Hematol* 59(2):105–109, 1998.

467. Mannucci PM: Desmopressin: A non-transfusional form of treatment for congenital and acquired bleeding disorders. *Blood* 72:1449, 1988.

468. Rose EH, Aledort LM: Nasal spray desmopressin (DDAVP) for mild hemophilia A and von Willebrand disease. *Ann Intern Med* 114:563, 1991.

469. Canavese C, Salomone M, Pacitti A, et al: Reduced response of uraemic bleeding time to repeated doses of desmopressin. *Lancet* 1:867, 1985.

470. Byrnes JJ, Larcada A, Moake JL: Thrombosis following desmopressin for uremic bleeding. *Am J Hematol* 28:63, 1988.

471. Mannucci PM, Lusher JM: Desmopressin and thrombosis. *Lancet* 2(8664):675–676, 1989.

472. Liu YK, Kosfeld RE, Marcum SG: Treatment of uremic bleeding with conjugated estrogen. *Lancet* 2(8408):887–890, 1984.

473. Vigano G, Gaspari F, Locatelli M, et al: Dose-effect and pharmacokinetics of estrogens given to correct bleeding time in uremia. *Kidney Int* 34:853–858, 1988.

474. Heistinger M, Stockenhuber F, Schneider B, et al: Effect of conjugated estrogens on platelet function and prostacyclin generation in CRF. *Kidney Int* 38:1181–1186, 1990.

475. Bronner MH, Pate MD, Cunningham JT, Marsh WH: Estrogen-progesterone therapy for bleeding of gastrointestinal telangiectasias in chronic renal failure. *Ann Intern Med* 105(3):371–374, 1986.

476. Vigano G, Zoja C, Corna D, et al: 17 Beta-estradiol is the most active component of the conjugated estrogen mixture active on uremic bleeding by a receptor mechanism. *Mol Pharmacol* 252(1):344–348, 1990.

477. Triulzi DJ, Blumber N: Variability in response to cryoprecipitate treatment for hemostatic defects in uremia. *Yale J Biol Med* 63:1–7, 1990.

478. Thompson AR, Harker LA: Approach to bleeding disorders, in *Manual of Hemostasis and Thrombosis*, 3rd ed, pp 57–64. FA Davis, Philadelphia, 1983.

479. Bloor AJ, Smith GA, Jaswon M, et al: Acquired thrombasthenia due to GPIIbIIIa platelet autoantibodies in a 4-yr-old child. *Eur J Haematol* 76(1):89–90, 2006.

480. Porcelijn L, Huiskes E, Maatman R, et al: Acquired Glanzmann's thrombasthenia caused by glycoprotein IIb/IIIa autoantibodies of the immunoglobulin G_1 (IgG$_1$), IgG$_2$ or IgG$_4$ subclass: A study in six cases. *Vox Sang* 95(4):324–330, 2008.

481. Blickstein D, Dardik R, Rosenthal E, et al: Acquired thrombasthenia due to inhibitory effect of glycoprotein IIbIIIa autoantibodies. *Isr Med Assoc J* 16(5):307–310, 2014.

482. Solh M, Mescher C, Klappa A, et al: Acquired Glanzmann's thrombasthenia with optimal response to rituximab therapy. *Am J Hematol* 86(8):715–716, 2011.

483. George JN, Woolf SH, Raskob GE, et al: Idiopathic thrombocytopenic purpura: A practice guideline developed by explicit methods for the American Society of Hematology. *Blood* 88(1):3–40, 1996.

484. George JN, El-Harake MA, Raskob GE: Chronic idiopathic thrombocytopenic purpura. *N Engl J Med* 331:1207–1215, 1994.

485. McMillan R: Antiplatelet antibodies in chronic adult immune thrombocytopenic purpura: Assays and epitopes. *J Pediatr Hematol Oncol* 25 Suppl 1:S57–S61, 2003.

486. Meyer M, Kirchmaier CM, Schirmer A, et al: Acquired disorder of platelet function associated with autoantibodies against membrane glycoprotein IIb-IIIa complex-1. Glycoprotein analysis. *Thromb Haemost* 65:491–496, 1991.

487. Balduini CL, Grignani G, Sinigaglia F, et al: Severe platelet dysfunction in a patient with autoantibodies against membrane glycoproteins IIb-IIIa. *Haemostasis* 7:98–104, 1987.

488. Balduini CL, Bertolino G, Noris P, et al: Defect of platelet aggregation and adhesion induced by autoantibodies against platelet glycoprotein IIIa. *Thromb Haemost* 68:208–213, 1992.

489. Fuse I, Higuchi W, Narita M, et al: Overproduction of antiplatelet antibody against glycoprotein IIb after splenectomy in a patient with Evans syndrome resulting in acquired thrombasthenia [see comments]. *Acta Haematol* 99(2):83–88, 1998.

490. Stricker RB, Wong D, Saks SR, et al: Acquired Bernard-Soulier syndrome: Evidence for the role of a 210,000-molecular weight protein in the interaction of platelets with von Willebrand factor. *J Clin Invest* 76:1274–1278, 1985.

491. Devine DV, Currie MS, Rosse WF, Greenberg CS: Pseudo-Bernard-Soulier syndrome: Thrombocytopenia caused by autoantibody to platelet glycoprotein Ib. *Blood* 70:428–431, 1987.

492. Deckmyn H, Zhang J, Van Houtte E, Vermylen J: Production and nucleotide sequence of an inhibitory human IgM autoantibody directed against platelet glycoprotein Ia/IIa. *Blood* 84(6):1968–1974, 1994.

493. Dromigny A, Triadou P, Lesavre P, et al: Lack of platelet response to collagen associated with autoantibodies against glycoprotein (GP) Ia/IIa and Ib/IX leading to the discovery of SLE. *Hematol Cell Ther* 38(4):355–357, 1996.

494. Boylan B, Chen H, Rathore V, et al: Anti-GPVI-associated ITP: An acquired platelet disorder caused by autoantibody-mediated clearance of the GPVI/FcRgamma-chain complex from the human platelet surface. *Blood* 104(5):1350–1355, 2004.

495. Wiedmer T, Ando B, Sims PJ: Complement C5b-9-stimulated platelet secretion is associated with a calcium-initiated activation of cellular protein kinases. *J Biol Chem* 262:13674, 1987.

496. Warkentin TE: Heparin-induced thrombocytopenia: Pathogenesis and management. *Br J Haematol* 121(4):535–555, 2003.

497. Lechner K, Pabinger I, Obermeier HL, Knoebl P: Immune-mediated disorders causing bleeding or thrombosis in lymphoproliferative diseases. *Semin Thromb Hemost* 40(3):359–370, 2014.

498. Giannini S, Mezzasoma AM, Guglielmini G, et al: A new case of acquired Glanzmann's thrombasthenia: Diagnostic value of flow cytometry. *Cytometry B Clin Cytom* 74(3):194–199, 2008.

499. Kannan M, Chatterjee T, Ahmad F, et al: Acquired Glanzmann's thrombasthenia associated with hairy cell leukaemia. *Eur J Clin Invest* 39(12):1110–1111, 2009.

500. Lackner H, Karpatkin S: On the "easy bruising" syndrome with normal platelet count: A study of 75 patients. *Ann Intern Med* 83(2):190–196, 1975.

501. Clancy R, Jenkins E, Firkin B: Qualitative platelet abnormalities in idopathic thrombocytopenic purpura. *N Engl J Med* 286:622, 1972.

502. Heyns DA, Fraser J, Retief FP: Platelet aggregation in chronic idiopathic thrombocytopenic purpura. *J Clin Pathol* 31:1239, 1978.

503. Regan MG, Lackner H, Karpatkin S: Platelet function and coagulation profile in lupus erythematosus. *Am J Med* 81:462, 1974.

504. Dorsch CA, Meyerhoff J: Mechanisms of abnormal platelet aggregation in systemic lupus erythematosus. *Arthritis Rheum* 25:966, 1982.

505. Meyerhoff J, Dorsch CA: Decreased platelet serotonin levels in systemic lupus erythematosus. *Arthritis Rheum* 24:1495, 1981.

506. Stuart MJ, Kelton JG, Allen JB: Abnormal platelet function and arachidonate metabolism in chronic idiopathic thrombocytopenic purpura. *Blood* 58:326, 1981.

507. Harker LA, Malpass TW, Branson HE, et al: Mechanism of abnormal bleeding in patients undergoing cardiopulmonary bypass: Acquired transient platelet dysfunction associated with selective alpha-granule release. *Blood* 56:824–834, 1975, 1980.

508. Woodman RC, Harker LA: Bleeding complications associated with cardiopulmonary bypass. *Blood* 76:1680–1697, 1990.

509. Mammen EF, Koets MH, Washington BC, et al: Hemostasis changes during cardiopulmonary bypass surgery. *Semin Thromb Hemost* 11:281, 1985.

510. Khuri SF, Wolfe JA, Josa M, et al: Hematologic changes during and after cardiopulmonary bypass and their relationship to the bleeding time and nonsurgical blood loss. *J Thorac Cardiovasc Surg* 104:94–107, 1992.

511. Martin JF, Daniel TD, Trowbridge EA: Acute and chronic changes in platelet volume and count after cardiopulmonary bypass induced thrombocytopenia in man. *Thromb Haemost* 57(1):55–58, 1987.

512. Chandler AB, Hutson MS: Platelet plug formation in an extracorporeal unit. *Am J Clin Pathol* 64(1):101–107, 1975.

513. Lindon JN, McManama, Kushner L: Does the conformation of adsorbed fibrinogen dictate platelet interactions with artificial surfaces? *Blood* 68:355, 1986.

514. Singer RL, Mannion JD, Bauer TL, Armenti FR, Edie RN: Complications from heparin-induced thrombocytopenia in patients undergoing cardiopulmonary bypass. *Chest* 104(5):1436–1440, 1993.

515. Pouplard C, Leroux D, Rollin J, et al: Incidence of antibodies to protamine sulfate/heparin complexes incardiac surgery patients and impact on platelet activation and clinical outcome. *Thromb Haemost* 109(6):1141–1147, 2013.

516. Bakchoul T, Zollner H, Amiral J, et al: Anti-protamine-heparin antibodies: Incidence, clinical relevance, and pathogenesis. *Blood* 121(15):2821–2827, 2013.

517. Panzer S, Schiferer A, Steinlechner B, et al: Serological features of antibodies to protamine inducing thrombocytopenia and thrombosis. *Clin Chem Lab Med* 53(2):249–255, 2015.

518. Bick RL: Hemostasis defects associated with cardiac surgery, prosthetic devices, and other extracorporeal circuits. *Semin Thromb Hemost* 11(3):249–280, 1985.

519. Bachmann F, McKenna R, Cole ER, Najafi H: The hemostatic mechanism after open heart surgery. I. Studies on plasma coagulation factors and fibrinolysis in 512 patients after extracorporeal circulation. *J Thorac Cardiovasc Surg* 70:76, 1975.

520. Beurling-Harbury C, Galvan CA: Acquired decrease in platelet secretory ADP associated with increased post-operative bleeding in post-cardiopulmonary bypass patients and in patients with severe valvular heart disease. *Blood* 52:13, 1978.

521. Abrams CS, Ellison N, Budzynski AZ, Shattil S: Direct detection of activated platelets and platelet-derived microparticles in humans. *Blood* 75:128–138, 1990.

522. Nannizzi-Alaimo L, Rubenstein MH, Alves VL, et al: Cardiopulmonary bypass induces release of soluble CD40 ligand. *Circulation* 105(24):2849–2854, 2002.

523. Wahba A, Rothe G, Lodes H, et al: The influence of the duration of cardiopulmonary bypass on coagulation, fibrinolysis and platelet function. *Thorac Cardiovasc Surg* 49(3):153–156, 2001.

524. George JN, Pickett EB, Saucerman S, et al: Platelet surface glycoproteins. Studies on resting and activated platelets and platelet membrane microparticles in normal subjects, and observations in patients during adult respiratory distress syndrome and cardiac surgery. *J Clin Invest* 78(2):340–348, 1986.

525. Gluszko P, Ricinski B, Musial J, et al: Fibrinogen receptors in platelet adhesion to surfaces of extracorporeal circuit. *Am J Physiol* 252:H615, 1987.

526. van den Dengen JJ, Karliczek GF, Brenken U, et al: Clinical study of blood trauma during perfusion with membrane and bubble oxygenators. *J Thorac Cardiovasc Surg* 83(1):108–116, 1982.

527. Edmunds LH Jr, Colman RW: Thrombin during cardiopulmonary bypass. *Ann Thorac Surg* 82(6):2315–2322, 2006.

528. Gabel J, Hakimi CS, Westerberg M, et al: Retransfusion of cardiotomy suction blood impairs haemostasis: *Ex vivo* and *in vivo* studies. *Scand Cardiovasc J* 47(6):368–376, 2013.

529. Kestin AS, Valeri CR, Khuri SF, et al: The platelet function defect of cardiopulmonary bypass. *Blood* 82:107–117, 1993.

530. Weksler BB, Pett SB, Alonso D, et al: Differential inhibition of aspirin of vascular prostaglandin synthesis in atherosclerotic patients. *N Engl J Med* 308:800–805, 1983.

531. Levy JH: Pharmacologic preservation of the hemostatic system during cardiac surgery. *Ann Thorac Surg* 72(5):S1814–S1820, 2001.

532. Tabuchi N, de Haan J, Boonstra PW, van Oeveren W: Activation of fibrinolysis in the pericardial cavity during cardiopulmonary bypass. *J Thorac Cardiovasc Surg* 106(5):828–833, 1993.

533. Hunt BJ, Parratt RN, Segal HC, et al: Activation of coagulation and fibrinolysis during cardiothoracic operations. *Ann Thorac Surg* 65(3):712–718, 1998.

534. Rapaport SI: Preoperative hemostatic evaluation: Which tests, if any? *Blood* 61(2):229–231, 1983.

535. Magovern JA, Sakert T, Benckart DH, et al: A model for predicting transfusion after coronary artery bypass grafting [see comments]. *Ann Thorac Surg* 61(1):27–32, 1996.

536. Simon TA, Akl BF, Murphy W: Controlled trial of routine administration of platelet concentrates in cardiopulmonary bypass surgery. *Ann Thorac Surg* 37:359, 1987.

537. Wasser MN, Houbiers JG, D'Amaro J, et al: The effect of fresh versus stored blood on post-operative bleeding after coronary bypass surgery: A prospective randomized study. *Br J Haematol* 72:81–84, 1989.

538. Sowade O, Warnke H, Scigalla P, et al: Avoidance of allogeneic blood transfusions by treatment with epoetin beta (recombinant human erythropoietin) in patients undergoing open-heart surgery. *Blood* 89(2):411–418, 1997.

539. Shimpo H, Mizumoto T, Onoda K, et al: Erythropoietin in pediatric cardiac surgery: Clinical efficacy and effective dose. *Chest* 111(6):1565–1570, 1997.

540. Schmoeckel M, Nollert G, Mempel M, et al: Effects of recombinant human erythropoietin on autologous blood donation before open heart surgery. *Thorac Cardiovasc Surg* 41(6):364–368, 1993.

541. Axford TC, Dearani JA, Ragno G, et al: Safety and therapeutic effectiveness of reinfused shed blood after open heart surgery [see comments]. *Ann Thorac Surg* 57(3):615–622, 1994.

542. Griffith LD, Billman GF, Daily PO, Lane TA: Apparent coagulopathy caused by infusion of shed mediastinal blood and its prevention by washing of the infusate [see comments]. *Ann Thorac Surg* 47(3):400–406, 1989.

543. Hsu LC: Heparin-coated cardiopulmonary bypass circuits: Current status. *Perfusion* 16(5):417–428, 2001.

544. Spijker HT, Graaff R, Boonstra PW, et al: On the influence of flow conditions and wettability on blood material interactions. *Biomaterials* 24(26):4717–4727, 2003.

545. Lappegard KT, Fung M, Bergseth G, et al: Effect of complement inhibition and heparin coating on artificial surface-induced leukocyte and platelet activation. *Ann Thorac Surg* 77(3):932–941, 2004.

546. Weerwind PW, Caberg NE, Reutelingsperger CP, et al: Exposure of procoagulant phospholipids on the surface of platelets in patients undergoing cardiopulmonary bypass using non-coated and heparin-coated extracorporeal circuits. *Int J Artif Organs* 25(8):770–776, 2002.

547. Johnell M, Elgue G, Larsson R, et al: Coagulation, fibrinolysis, and cell activation in patients and shed mediastinal blood during coronary artery bypass grafting with a new heparin-coated surface. *J Thorac Cardiovasc Surg* 124(2):321–332, 2002.

548. Linneweber J, Chow TW, Kawamura M, et al: *In vitro* comparison of blood pump induced platelet microaggregates between a centrifugal and roller pump during cardiopulmonary bypass. *Int J Artif Organs* 25(6):549–555, 2002.

549. Despotis GJ, Avidan MS, Hogue CW Jr: Mechanisms and attenuation of hemostatic activation during extracorporeal circulation. *Ann Thorac Surg* 72(5):S1821–S1831, 2001.

550. Nuttall GA, Erchul DT, Haight TJ, et al: A comparison of bleeding and transfusion in patients who undergo coronary artery bypass grafting via sternotomy with and without cardiopulmonary bypass. *J Cardiothorac Vasc Anesth* 17(4):447–451, 2003.

551. Mariani MA, Gu YJ, Boonstra PW, et al: Procoagulant activity after off-pump coronary operation: Is the current anticoagulation adequate? *Ann Thorac Surg* 67(5):1370–1375, 1999.

552. Paparella D, Galeone A, Venneri MT, et al: Activation of the coagulation system during coronary artery bypass grafting: Comparison between on-pump and off-pump techniques. *J Thorac Cardiovasc Surg* 131(2):290–297, 2006.

553. Vallely MP, Bannon PG, Bayfield MS, et al: Quantitative and temporal differences in coagulation, fibrinolysis and platelet activation after on-pump and off-pump coronary artery bypass surgery. *Heart Lung Circ* 18(2):123–130, 2009.

554. Hackmann T, Gascoyne R, Naiman SC, et al: A trial of desmopressin to reduce blood loss in uncomplicated cardiac surgery. *N Engl J Med* 321:1437–1444, 1989.

555. Seear MD, Wadsworth LD, Rogers PC, et al: The effect of desmopressin acetate (DDAVP) on postoperative blood loss after cardiac operations in children [see comments]. *J Thorac Cardiovasc Surg* 98(2):217–219, 1989.

556. Wademan BH, Galvin SD: Desmopressin for reducing postoperative blood loss and transfusion requirements following cardiac surgery in adults. *Interact Cardiovasc Thorac Surg* 18(3):360–370, 2014.

557. Walker ID, Davidson JF, Faichney A, et al: A double-blind study of prostacyclin in cardiopulmonary bypass surgery. *Br J Haematol* 49:415–423, 1981.

558. Society of Thoracic Surgeons Blood Conservation Guideline Task F, Ferraris VA, Brown JR, Despotis GJ, et al: 2011 update to the Society of Thoracic Surgeons and the Society of Cardiovascular Anesthesiologists blood conservation clinical practice guidelines. *Ann Thorac Surg* 91(3):944–982, 2011.

559. O'Connell KA, Wood JJ, Wise RP, et al: Thromboembolic adverse events after use of recombinant human coagulation factor VIIa. *JAMA* 295(3):293–298, 2006.

560. Goodnough LT, Levy JH: Off-label use of recombinant human factor VIIa. *Ann Thorac Surg* 98(2):393–395, 2014.

561. Giannini E, Botta F, Borro P, et al: Relationship between thrombopoietin serum levels and liver function in patients with chronic liver disease related to hepatitis C virus infection. *Am J Gastroenterol* 98(11):2516–2520, 2003.

562. Nussmeier NA, Whelton AA, Brown MT, et al: Complications of the COX-2 inhibitors parecoxib and valdecoxib after cardiac surgery. *N Engl J Med* 352(11):1081–1091, 2005.

563. Mangano DT, Tudor IC, Dietzel C: The risk associated with aprotinin in cardiac surgery. *N Engl J Med* 354(4):353–365, 2006.

564. Schneeweiss S, Seeger JD, Landon J, Walker AM: Aprotinin during coronary-artery bypass grafting and risk of death. *N Engl J Med* 358(8):771–783, 2008.

565. Shaw AD, Stafford-Smith M, White WD, et al: The effect of aprotinin on outcome after coronary-artery bypass grafting. *N Engl J Med* 358(8):784–793, 2008.

566. Fergusson DA, Hebert PC, Mazer CD, et al: A comparison of aprotinin and lysine analogues in high-risk cardiac surgery. *N Engl J Med* 358(22):2319–2331, 2008.

567. Amitrano L, Guardascione MA, Brancaccio V, Balzano A: Coagulation disorders in liver disease. *Semin Liver Dis* 22(1):83–96, 2002.

568. Lisman T, Porte RJ: Rebalanced hemostasis in patients with liver disease: Evidence and clinical consequences. *Blood* 116(6):878–885, 2010.

569. Hugenholtz GC, Adelmeijer J, Meijers JC, et al: An unbalance between von Willebrand factor and ADAMTS13 in acute liver failure: Implications for hemostasis and clinical outcome. *Hepatology* 58(2):752–761, 2013.

570. Krauss JS, Jonah MH: Platelet dysfunction (thrombocytopathy) in extra-hepatic biliary obstruction. *South Med J* 75(4):506–507, 1982.

571. Hillbom M, Muuronen A, Neiman J: Liver disease and platelet function in alcoholics. *Br Med J* 295:581, 1987.

572. Stein SF, Harker LA: Kinetic and functional studies of platelets, fibrinogen, and plasminogen in patients with hepatic cirrhosis. *J Lab Clin Med* 99:217, 1982.

573. Violi F, Leo R, Vezza E, et al: Bleeding time in patients with cirrhosis: Relation with degree of liver failure and clotting abnormalities. C.A.L.C. Group. Coagulation Abnormalities in Cirrhosis Study Group. *J Hepatol* 20(4):531–536, 1994.

574. Livio M, Mannucci PM, Vigano G, et al: Conjugated estrogens for the management of bleeding associated with renal failure. *N Engl J Med* 315:731, 1986.

575. Svensson PJ, Bergqvist PB, Juul KV, Berntorp E: Desmopressin in treatment of haematological disorders and in prevention of surgical bleeding. *Blood Rev* 28(3):95–102, 2014.

576. Pareti FI, Capitanio A, Mannucci L: Acquired storage pool disease in platelets during disseminated intravascular coagulation. *Blood* 48:511, 1976.

577. Pareti FI, Capitanio A, Mannucci L, Ponticelli C, Mannucci PM: Acquired dysfunction due to the circulation of "exhausted" platelets. *Am J Med* 69:235–240, 1980.

578. Solum NO, Rigollot C, Budzynski A, Marder VJ: A quantitative evaluation of the inhibition of platelet aggregation by low molecular weight degradation products of fibrinogen. *Br J Haematol* 24:619, 1973.

579. Stoff JS, Stemerman M, Steer M, Salzman E, Brown RS: A defect in platelet aggregation in Bartter's syndrome. *Am J Med* 68:171–180, 1980.

580. van Wersch J, Rodrigues Pereira R: Platelet aggregation in six families with Bartter's syndrome. *Clin Chim Acta* 130:363–368, 1983.

581. Nusing RM, Reinalter SC, Peters M, et al: Pathogenetic role of cyclooxygenase-2 in hyperprostaglandin E syndrome/antenatal Bartter syndrome: Therapeutic use of the cyclooxygenase-2 inhibitor nimesulide. *Clin Pharmacol Ther* 70(4):384–390, 2001.

582. Hebert SC: Bartter syndrome. *Curr Opin Nephrol Hypertens* 12(5):527–532, 2003.

583. Zapata JC, Cox D, Salvato MS: The role of platelets in the pathogenesis of viral hemorrhagic fevers. *PLoS Negl Trop Dis* 8(6):e2858, 2014.

584. Lim SH, Tan CE, Agasthian T, Chew LS: Acquired platelet dysfunction with eosinophilia: Review of seven adult cases. *J Clin Pathol* 42:950–952, 2014, 1989.

585. Poon MC, Ng SC, Coppes MJ: Acquired platelet dysfunction with eosinophilia in white children. *J Pediatr* 126(6):959–961, 1995.

586. Laosombat V, Wongchanchailert M, Sattayasevana B, et al: Acquired platelet dysfunction with eosinophilia in children in the south of Thailand. *Platelets* 12(1):5–14, 2001.

587. Szczeklik A, Milner PC, Birch J, et al: Prolonged bleeding time, reduced platelet aggregation, altered PAF-acether sensitivity and increased platelet mass are a trait of asthma and hay fever. *Thromb Haemost* 56:283–287, 1986.

588. Carvalho AC, Quinn DA, DeMarinis SM, et al: Platelet function in acute respiratory failure. *Am J Hematol* 25:377–388, 1987.

589. Bracey AW, Wu AH, Aceves J, et al: Platelet dysfunction associated with Wilms tumor and hyaluronic acid. *Am J Hematol* 24:247–257, 1987.

CHAPTER 122
THE VASCULAR PURPURAS

Doru T. Alexandrescu and Marcel Levi

SUMMARY

Purpura, the clinical manifestation of blood extravasation into mucosa or skin, results from various conditions, including rheumatologic, infectious, dermatologic, traumatic, and hematologic disorders. This chapter does not detail purpura resulting from quantitative or functional defects in hemostasis and coagulation, such as deficiencies of platelets or coagulation factors; these causes are discussed in other chapters (e.g., thrombocytopenia in Chap. 117; coagulation factor deficiencies in Chaps. 123 and 124).

The differential diagnosis of the disparate causes of noncoagulopathic purpura is best approached by stratifying purpura into three types of lesions: (1) palpable or retiform and noninflammatory, such as hyperglobulinemic purpura of Waldenström; (2) palpable or nonpalpable but inflammatory, such as Henoch-Schönlein purpura; and (3) nonpalpable and noninflammatory, such as senile purpura. By accounting for palpability, presence of inflammation, size, and shape, the differential diagnosis of a particular lesion can be significantly reduced.

DEFINITION AND DIAGNOSTIC APPROACH

Purpura refers to visible hemorrhage into mucous membranes or skin, which corresponds to extravasation of red blood cells around small dermal vessels and chronic hemosiderin deposition.[1] Purpuric lesions, by definition, do not blanch completely upon compression, as opposed to erythema. Blanching is commonly tested by compression of skin lesions with a glass slide, referred to as diascopy (Fig. 122–1). Certain conditions give rise to lesions that mimic purpura with incomplete blanching upon diascopy, but are not purpura because no hemorrhage has occurred. Examples include disorders that impede on the red cell flow, such as tortuous veins.[1]

Assessing lesion palpability is the first step in evaluating purpuric lesions (Fig. 122–2). The causes for palpability are varied and include fibrin deposition, localized edema, significant cellular infiltration, and subcutaneous extravasation of red blood cells.

Inspecting the lesion for inflammatory changes is the next step in evaluating purpuric lesions. The presence of pain, erythema, and palpation for warmth and localized swelling are signs of inflammation and suggest a vasculitis or immune complex disorder.

Acronyms and Abbreviations: ANCA, antineutrophil cytoplasmic antibody; APS, antiphospholipid syndrome; CSS, Churg-Strauss syndrome; DIC, disseminated intravascular coagulation; HCV, hepatitis C virus; HHT, hereditary hemorrhagic telangiectasia; HP, hypergammaglobulinemic purpura; HSP, Henoch-Schönlein purpura; MELAS, mitochondrial encephalopathy, lactic acidosis, stroke-like; SLE, systemic lupus erythematosus; WG, Wegener granulomatosis.

The shape of a purpuric lesion, either round or retiform (branching), is important in assessing the lesion. In the absence of accompanying inflammation, retiform purpuric lesions suggest small vessel occlusion. A retiform, inflammatory purpuric lesion supports the diagnosis of vasculitis as a result of immunoglobulin (Ig) complex formation.[2] Small, focal areas of hemorrhage are referred to as *petechiae* (≤4 mm). Larger lesions are referred to as *intermediate* or *midsize purpura* (>4 mm, <1 cm) or *ecchymosis* (≥1 cm).[3]

Purpuric lesions frequently appear purple; however, they can take on a variety of colors, according to the age of the lesion and the oxygen saturation of the hemoglobin in the extravasated blood. Ecchymosis usually starts as blue or purple, evolves to a greenish brown (a mixture of blue and yellow), and ultimately changes with variable speed to yellow as hemoglobin degrades to bilirubin.[4] These examples of hemorrhage into the dermis must be distinguished from telangiectasia, which are vascular anomalies that blanch with pressure (see Fig. 122–1). Tables 122–1 through 122–3 classify the etiologies for purpura discussed in this chapter.

PALPABLE NONINFLAMMATORY PURPURIC LESIONS

See Table 122–1.

DYSPROTEINEMIAS

Cryoglobulinemia

Cryoglobulinemia refers to the presence in plasma of cold-insoluble immunoglobulins,[5] and is a secondary finding associated with several disease states. Cryoglobulins are commonly present in low concentrations, therefore approximately 90 percent of patients are asymptomatic or have minimal symptoms.[6] Symptoms occur when the abnormal protein precipitates at the temperatures present in superficial venules in the skin and acral parts of the body. Cryoglobulinemia syndromes are divided into three main types based on the immunoglobulin composition of the precipitate. Type I cryoglobulinemia results from the accumulation of monoclonal IgG, IgM, or IgA. It is most commonly seen in association with lymphoproliferative disorders, such as myeloma, Waldenström macroglobulinemia, or lymphoma. Type II, or mixed cryoglobulinemia involves formation of complexes composed of polyclonal IgG with monoclonal immunoglobulins, typically IgM with anti-IgG specificity. Exposure to various exogenous antigens appears to cause polyclonal immunoglobulin production, with activity against bacteria, viruses, and fungi. Mixed cryoglobulinemia is commonly seen secondary to hepatitis C virus (HCV) infection,[7] HIV, collagen vascular disorders, and hematologic neoplasias.[8,9] In mixed cryoglobulinemia secondary to HCV infection, the presence of active cutaneous vasculitis correlates with increased levels of the B-cell–attracting chemokine 1 (CXCL13).[10] This process manifests with petechiae of the legs, palpable purpura, and necrotic skin ulcerations. First-line treatment includes use of interferon-α or other antiviral agents, often with adjunct glucocorticoids or plasmapheresis.[11] Direct treatment of the HCV infection with ribavirin, interferon, or other antiviral therapy, such as the protease inhibitors, ameliorates this associated lymphoproliferative disorder.[12] Deposition of immune complexes on vessel walls leads to tissue damage in the vasculature, nerves, joints, and skin leading to the hallmark findings of mixed cryoglobulinemia: weakness, arthralgia, and purpura. This purpura often is palpable and is accompanied by areas of hemorrhagic necrosis (Fig. 122–3) and occasionally follicular pustular purpura. Other cutaneous manifestations include lower-extremity ulcerations, urticaria, Raynaud phenomena, and subungual purpura (Fig. 122–4). Type III

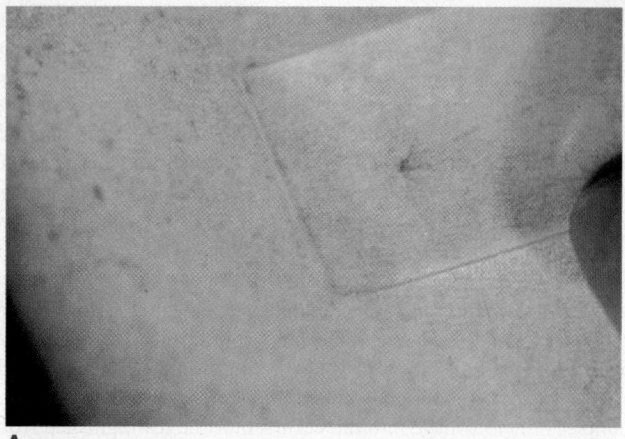

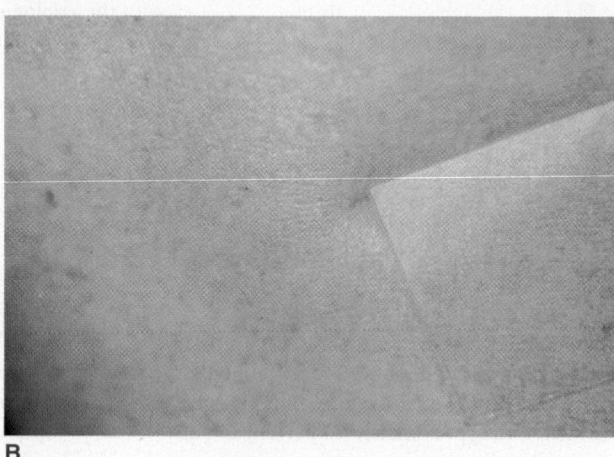

Figure 122–1. A. Spider telangiectasia. **B.** Blanching of spider telangiectasia. Note that spider telangiectasia blanches with diascopy.

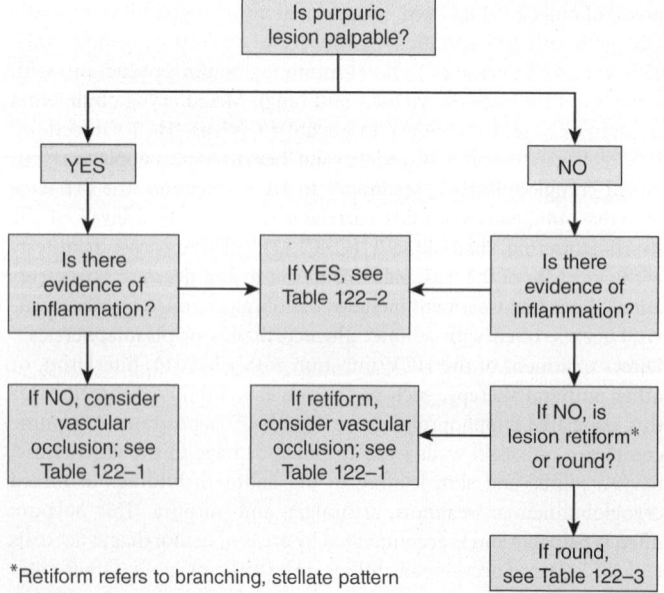

*Retiform refers to branching, stellate pattern

Figure 122–2. Bedside approach to purpuric lesion diagnosis.

TABLE 122–1. Palpable Noninflammatory Purpuric Lesions

A. Dysproteinemias
  1. Cryoglobulinemia (see Figs. 122–3 and 122–4)
  2. Waldenström hyperglobulinemic purpura (see Fig. 122–5)
  3. Light-chain vasculopathy
  4. Cryofibrinogenemia
B. Thrombotic
  1. Heparin necrosis
  2. Warfarin necrosis (see Fig. 122–6)
  3. Protein C and protein S deficiencies
  4. Paroxysmal nocturnal hemoglobinuria
  5. Antiphospholipid syndrome (see Fig. 122–8)
  6. Livedoid vasculitis
C. Embolic
  1. Cholesterol emboli (see Fig. 122–9)
  2. Cutaneous calciphylaxis
  3. Emboli from intracardiac thrombi
D. Arthropod bites

TABLE 122–2. Palpable and Nonpalpable Inflammatory Purpuric Lesions

A. Pyoderma gangrenosum (see Fig. 122–7)
B. Sweet syndrome (see Fig. 122–10)
C. Behçet disease
D. Serum sickness (Fig. 122–11)
E. Henoch-Schönlein purpura (see Fig. 122–12)
F. Infections
G. Erythema multiforme (see Fig. 122–20)
H. Cutaneous polyarteritis nodosum (see Fig. 122–21)
I. Paraneoplastic vasculitis
J. Drug-induced vasculitis
K. Antineutrophilic cytoplasmic antibody–associated vasculitides
  1. Wegener granulomatosis (see Fig. 122–23)
  2. Churg-Strauss

TABLE 122–3. Nonpalpable, Noninflammatory, Round Purpuric Lesions

A. Increased transmural pressure gradient and trauma
B. Drug reactions
C. Coagulation disorders
D. Decreased vessel integrity without trauma
  1. Senile purpura
  2. Excess glucocorticoid (Cushing syndrome, glucocorticoid treatment)
  3. Scurvy—vitamin C deficiency (see Fig. 122–25)
  4. Systemic amyloidosis
  5. Connective tissue disorders (Ehlers-Danlos syndrome, pseudoxanthoma elasticum)
  6. Mitochondrial encephalomyopathy with lactic acidosis and stroke-like syndrome (MELAS)
E. Waldenström hypergammaglobulinemic purpura (see Table 122–1 and Fig. 122–5)
F. Rendu-Osler-Weber disease (see Fig. 122–26)

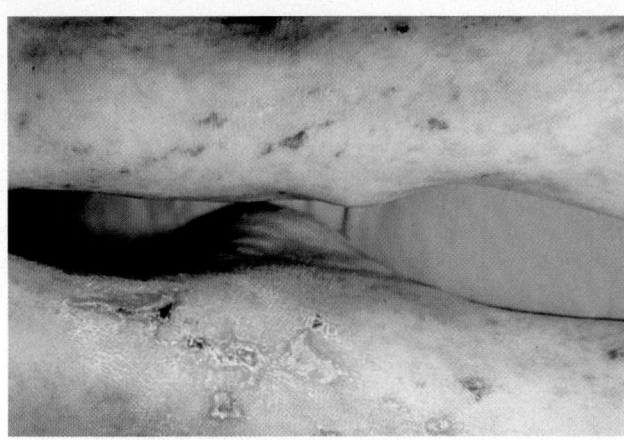

Figure 122–3. Cryoglobulinemia: peripheral purpura.

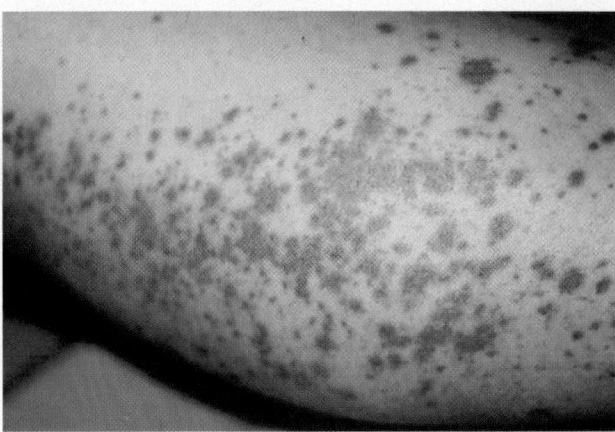

Figure 122–5. Waldenström hyperglobulinemic purpura. Note discrete and coalescing petechiae on lower limb.

cryoglobulinemia associates polyclonal IgG and IgM complexes, also resulting in symptoms of mixed cryoglobulinemia.[6] It is associated with a variety of infections, systemic lupus erythematous (SLE), and poststreptococcal glomerulonephritis.

Waldenström Hyperglobulinemic Purpura

A polyclonal increase of immunoglobulins, most commonly IgG[1], appears to be responsible for the varied cutaneous findings seen in this hypergammaglobulinemic purpura (HP). Waldenström first described a hyperproteinemic syndrome characterized by hypergammaglobulinemia, recurrent purpura, elevated erythrocyte sedimentation rate, and anemia.[13] Most commonly seen in young women, this syndrome is associated with a large number of autoimmune disorders, including rheumatoid arthritis, Sjögren syndrome, SLE, hepatitis C, polymyositis, and sarcoidosis. Discrete to confluent collections of lower limb petechiae are its most common skin findings (Fig. 122–5), but lesions can occur in various body locations.[14] Although lesions are usually self-limited and resolve in 7 to 10 days, recurrence of purpura is common and is associated with exposure to cold temperatures or increases in hydrostatic pressure, such as with the use of tight stockings or prolonged standing.[15] Clinical manifestations consist of palpable purpura or diminutive macular erythematous lesions occurring on the lower legs. A reticulate pattern of purpura has been described.[16] Development of edema and arthralgia has also been described.[17]

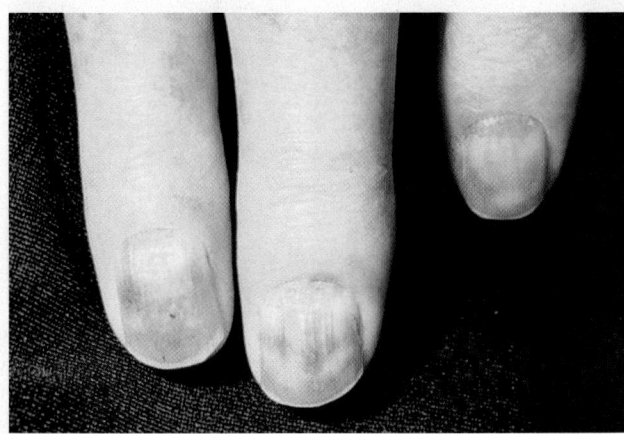

Figure 122–4. Cryoglobulinemia: subungual purpura.

Common histologic findings include perivascular infiltrates, hemorrhage, and vascular necrosis. In addition to a polyclonal increase in either IgA, IgM, or IgG, serology may reveal cryoglobulinemia, rheumatoid factor, or antinuclear antibodies.[18] Imbalances in IgG subclass expression, usually because of a decrease in IgG[2], appear to be associated with recurrent infections.[17] Development of antilymphocyte antibodies results in lymphopenia. Anti-Ro/SSA antibodies occur in up to 78 percent of HP patients, suggesting that screening for anti-Ro/SSA should be considered in cases suspicious for Waldenström.[19]

Light-Chain Vasculopathy

Precipitates of immunoglobulin light chains that form crystalline deposits in the skin cause hemorrhagic palpable purpura. A nonamyloid monoclonal light chain of predominant κ type is involved in two-thirds of the cases.[20,21] Crystalline deposits are present in the skin and other tissues. Although the clinical presentation may mimic a systemic vasculitis, no histologic signs of inflammation are seen. Light-chain vasculopathy with cutaneous findings has also been described in association with multiple myeloma. Intravascular deposition of crystals containing IgG and λ light chains were found on immunohistochemical analysis and manifested with gangrene of the feet and intestinal perforation.[22]

Cryofibrinogenemia

First described by Korst and Kratochvil in 1955, cryofibrinogenemia is a form of serum dysproteinemia characterized by formation of an abnormal cold-precipitable fibrinogen. Cutaneous manifestations include cyanosis, erythema, Raynaud phenomenon, and palpable purpura of the nose, ears, and distal extremities.[23] Tissue ischemia and gangrene may result. Pathogenesis of cryofibrinogenemia may involve an inhibition of normal fibrinolysis produced by a high plasma level of α_1-antitripsin and α_2-macroglobulin proteases.[24] Cryofibrinogenemia is commonly secondary to thromboembolic disorders, metastatic malignancies, infections, and collagen vascular disease.[25] Treatment modalities include avoidance of cold, plasmapheresis, and danazol, an anabolic glucocorticoid, or immunosuppression with glucocorticoids or cytotoxic agents.

THROMBOTIC PURPURA

Heparin Necrosis

Cutaneous reactions to heparin administration vary greatly from a type I urticarial rash to purpuric plaques with cutaneous ulceration or necrosis.[26] The syndrome occurs after both subcutaneous and intravenous

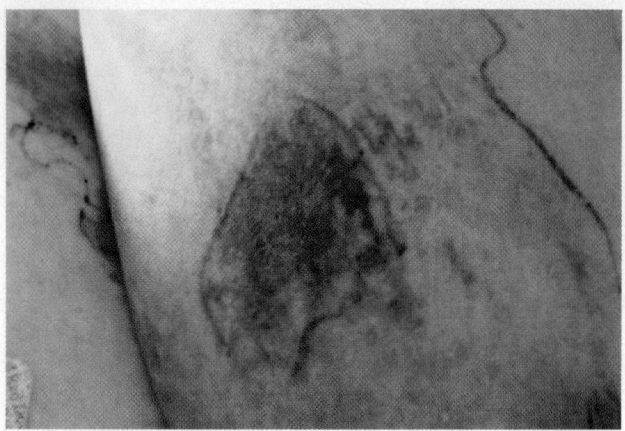

Figure 122–6. Coumadin necrosis. Develops in acral areas and areas of fat deposition such as buttocks or breast. Typically, lesions develop 3 to 10 days after initiation of anticoagulant treatment and are caused by rapid clearing of protein C. The lesions are characterized microscopically by small-vessel thrombosis.

administration of unfractionated heparin, but it has also been rarely described after low-molecular-weight heparin.[27] A delayed-type hypersensitivity reaction to the medication is involved. Skin lesions appear within 1 to 2 weeks after treatment initiation and include necrotic purpuric lesions.[28] Development of cutaneous lesions is closely related to heparin-induced thrombocytopenia (Chap. 118), which involves anti–platelet factor 4 antibody–mediated platelet aggregation with development of thrombosis and microvascular occlusion.[27]

Warfarin Necrosis

The development of painful erythematous plaques and nodules is a potential complication of warfarin therapy (Fig. 122–6). These lesions can rapidly become hemorrhagic and necrotic, leading to large areas of infarct with black eschar formation and subsequent skin sloughing. Purpura, vesicular, maculopapular, or urticarial eruptions can be encountered.[1] Warfarin-induced necrosis has a prevalence between 0.01 and 0.1 percent and presents typically 3 to 10 days after initiation of anticoagulant treatment.[29,30] However, an atypical presentation can occur much later, for example, in a patient with protein S deficiency.[31,32] Although warfarin necrosis tends to develop in areas of greatest fat deposition, such as breasts, thighs, and buttocks, acral areas, including penis, fingers, and toes, can also be involved.[33] Warfarin necrosis results from the rapid decrease of vitamin K–dependent coagulation factors of relatively short half-life, such as proteins C and S, while longer-lasting coagulation factors, such as factor II and factor X, are not yet decreased, resulting in a net procoagulant state. Microvascular occlusion of small dermal and subcutaneous vessels by fibrin deposits is seen on histologic analysis, but true vasculitis is infrequent.[29] Treatment involves prompt cessation of the vitamin K antagonist, along with administration of heparin and vitamin K, and occasionally surgical debridement. Because patients with protein C or S deficiency are at increased susceptibility to warfarin necrosis, heparin should always be administered in these patients prior to initiation of Coumadin.[34]

Proteins C and S Deficiencies

Clinical manifestations of proteins C and S deficiencies include venous thromboembolism, warfarin-induced skin necrosis, and neonatal purpura fulminans (Chap. 129). Congenital and acquired deficiencies in these proteins can lead to palpable necrotic purpura and ecchymosis.[35,36]

Erythematous purpuric lesions associated with homozygous protein C deficiency can develop within hours of birth and can rapidly progress to hemorrhagic necrosis.[37] Acquired deficiencies of protein C are associated with autoantibodies to protein C, antibiotics administration, septic shock, HIV, and liver disease (Chap. 127).[38] Acquired protein S deficiency may occur after varicella infection, when it is associated with the generation of antiprotein S immunoglobulins.[39] Protein repletion with fresh-frozen plasma or protein C concentrate is effective as initial treatment for protein C deficiency to help clear both cutaneous lesions and venous occlusion, while lifelong anticoagulant treatment is used to prevent recurrence.[34,40]

Paroxysmal Nocturnal Hemoglobinuria

Paroxysmal nocturnal hemoglobinuria (Chap. 40) is a hematopoietic clonal disorder resulting in defective production of cell surface-binding proteins.[41] Cutaneous manifestations are secondary to a hypercoagulable state and include palpable purpura, petechiae, ecchymosis, leg ulcers, plaques, necrosis, and hemorrhagic bullae.[42] Parvovirus B19 may play an etiologic role in the development of cutaneous necrosis.[43] An association with pyoderma gangrenosum (Fig. 122–7)[44] and occurrence of purpura fulminans[45] have been described. Histology reveals formation of microvascular fibrin thrombi.[42]

Antiphospholipid Syndrome

Antiphospholipid syndrome (APS) is a disease characterized by hypercoagulability associated with the presence of antibodies against phospholipids, such as anticardiolipin and lupus anticoagulant (Chap. 131).[46] Approximately 40 percent of patients with APS present with cutaneous lesions secondary to both large-vessel and microvascular thrombosis.[47] Skin manifestations include ecchymosis, livedo reticularis and racemosa, leg ulcerations, bullae, splinter hemorrhages, livedoid vasculopathy, superficial venous thrombosis, atrophie blanche, and extensive necrosis (Fig. 122–8).[47,48] Presence of livedo reticularis is frequently the presenting symptom of APS, most commonly when the syndrome is secondary to SLE, and its presence commonly precedes vascular events.[49] Development of acute bullous purpura has been described.[50] Treatment includes anticoagulant agents with immunosuppressant administration for associated thrombocytopenia. Prevention of thromboembolic events with aspirin is of uncertain value.[51]

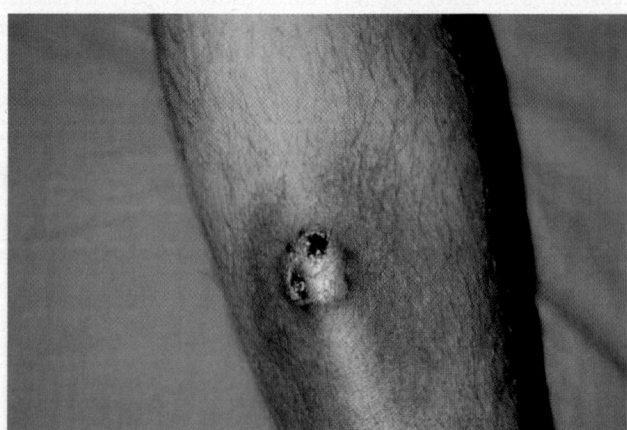

Figure 122–7. Pyoderma gangrenosum. A large number of systemic diseases are associated with pyoderma gangrenosum, including inflammatory bowel diseases, hematologic and solid malignancies, and rheumatologic disorders. Microscopically, the lesions are characterized by central necrotizing, neutrophilic infiltration, and a surrounding perivascular and intramural lymphocytic infiltration.

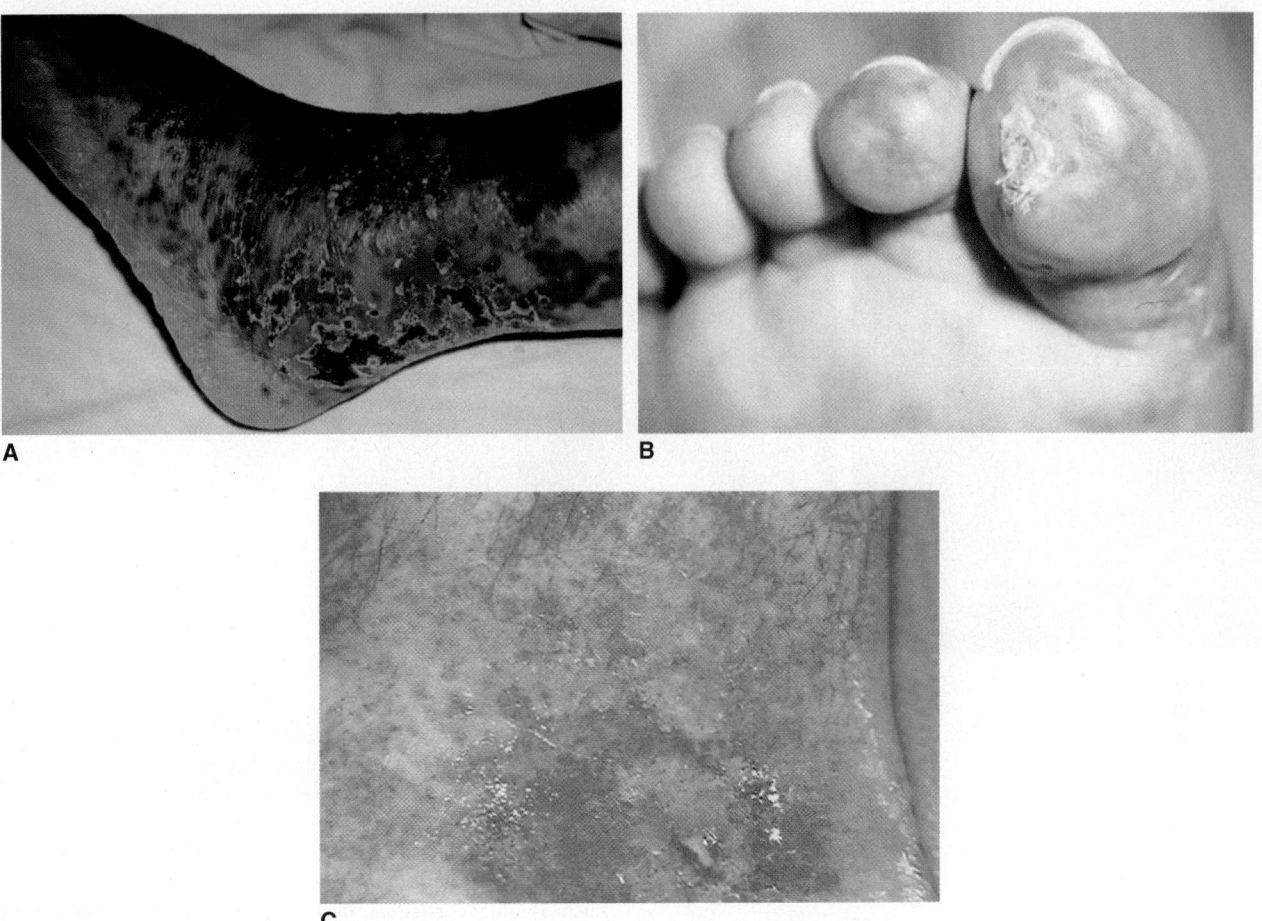

Figure 122–8. A. Antiphospholipid antibody syndrome. A number of skin lesions can be seen, including ecchymosis, livedo reticularis and racemosa, leg ulcerations, bullae, splinter hemorrhages, superficial venous thrombosis, atrophie blanche, and, as shown here, extensive necrosis. **B.** Anticardiolipin antibody. **C.** Lupus anticoagulant.

Livedoid Vasculitis

Livedoid vasculitis (segmental hyalinizing vasculitis) is a chronic recurrent thrombo-occlusive disorder characterized by the initial development of erythematous purpuric lesions with telangiectasis and peripheral petechiae, and lower-extremity ulcerations. Subsequent healing leads to atrophie blanche, a term that refers to the appearance of ivory-white stellate scars commonly surrounded by hyperpigmented areas and telangiectasia. These lesions appear to be caused by small-vessel fibrin thrombi in the middle and lower dermis as a result of a procoagulant tendency.[52] Although most commonly arising without associated cause, livedoid vasculitis is associated with polyarteritis nodosa, APS, and SLE.[53,54] Although not consistently beneficial, common therapies include discontinuation of oral contraceptives, anticoagulation and antiplatelet medications, glucocorticoids, and dapsone. Ketanserin, an S_2 serotoninergic receptor blocker, psoralen plus ultraviolet A therapy, and intravenous immunoglobulins also have been used successfully.[55]

EMBOLIC PURPURA

Cholesterol Crystal Emboli

Also known as atheroemboli, cholesterol crystal emboli are responsible for a syndrome characterized by lower extremity pain and livedo reticularis with preservation of peripheral pulses. Other common cutaneous findings include gangrene, purpura, ulcerations, cyanosis, and nodules (Fig. 122–9).[56] Clinical symptoms include fever, myalgia, and altered mental status. Laboratory features include an elevated erythrocyte sedimentation rate, eosinophilia, and acute renal failure. Onset of symptoms varies from immediate after physical dislodgement of plaque, up to months later when caused by anticoagulant therapy.[1] A blue toe syndrome is, in fact, rare, and most atheroemboli are clinically silent.[57] Atherosclerotic lesions in the descending aorta are the most common source of cholesterol emboli. This explains the propensity for lower-extremity findings during intravascular procedures or initiation of thrombolytic or anticoagulant therapy.[56] Histologic evaluation can offer a definitive diagnosis with findings of intraluminal birefringent cholesterol crystals within blood vessel lumen, in the absence of vasculitis.[58] No effective treatment is available. Nevertheless, supportive care with proper hydration and dialysis may lessen the potential for end-organ damage.

Cutaneous Calciphylaxis

Calciphylaxis (calcific uremic arteriolopathy)[59] is a thrombo-occlusive disorder involving formation of cutaneous, subcutaneous, and vascular calcifications. It is most commonly seen in patients with end-stage renal disease, classically caused by the development of secondary hyperparathyroidism.[60] Approximately 4 percent of hemodialysis-dependent patients suffer from calciphylaxis. Survival is less than 50 percent at 5 years after diagnosis.[61] Other etiologies include primary hyperparathyroidism, malignancy, alcoholic liver disease, and collagen

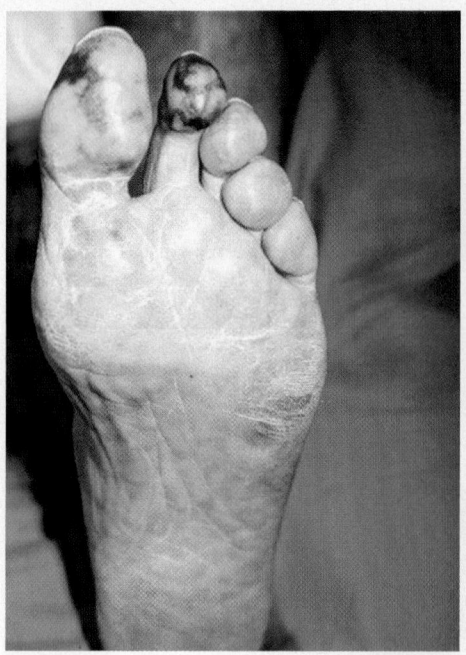 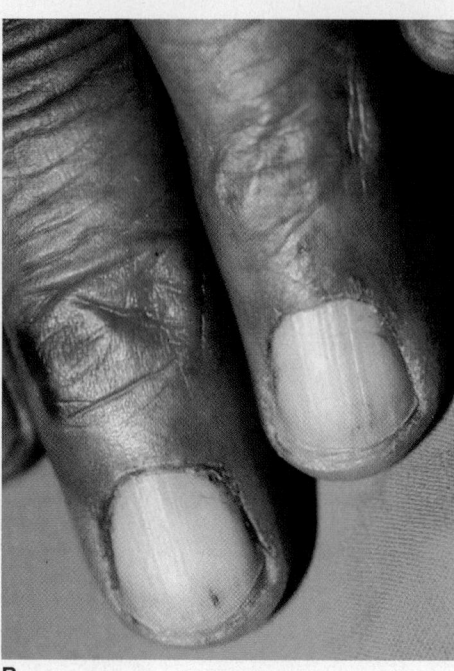

A   B

Figure 122–9. A. Cholesterol emboli. **B.** Rupture of an atherosclerotic plaque can result in showers of microemboli that lodge in distal arterioles, causing splinter hemorrhages.

tissue disorders.[62] Cutaneous lesions present initially as reddish-purple plaques, evolving to tender, gangrenous ulcers or reticular hemorrhagic necrosis. Treatment involves a combination of medical and surgical interventions, such as parathyroidectomy, renal transplantation, wound debridement, and amputation.[61]

Emboli from Intracardiac Thrombi

Acral purpuric lesions secondary to emboli arise from left atrial myxomas or right atrial clots through paradoxical embolization.[63] These purpuric lesions include palpable purpura, livedo reticularis, erythematous macules and papules, cyanosis, petechiae, splinter hemorrhages, ulcerations, and cutaneous necrosis. Cyanosis, livedo reticularis, and lower-extremity ulcerations can also be seen.[64]

ARTHROPOD BITES

Purpuric lesions are not uncommon after arthropod bites. Bites from bed bugs, *Cimex lectularius*, can give rise to localized purpuric macules or papules, while bites from kissing bugs, *Reduviidae*, often manifest as urticaria with hemorrhagic bulla.[65] Cutaneous findings after envenomation from a brown recluse spider, *Loxosceles reclusa*, include purpuric necrosis with surrounding erythema evolving to ulcer formation.

● PALPABLE AND NONPALPABLE INFLAMMATORY PURPURIC LESIONS

See Table 122–2.

PYODERMA GANGRENOSUM

Pyoderma gangrenosum is an idiopathic inflammatory skin condition characterized by early follicular erythematous papules and pustules or tender, fluctuant nodules with surrounding erythema that spread peripherally and ulcerate, surrounded by a violaceous rim (see Fig. 122–7).[66] In 50 percent of cases of pyoderma gangrenosum, there is an associated disorder, such as inflammatory bowel disorders (classically ulcerative colitis), arthritis, hematologic disorders,

and solid tumors.[67] All four main clinical variants (ulcerative, pustular, bullous, and vegetative) share the histopathologic finding of a sterile abscess with central necrotizing neutrophilic infiltration, and a surrounding perivascular and intramural lymphocytic infiltration. First-line treatment involves wound care and immunosuppressants, such as glucocorticoids, cyclosporine, dapsone, azathioprine, and infliximab.[68]

SWEET SYNDROME

Also referred to as acute, febrile neutrophilic dermatosis, Sweet syndrome is characterized by the acute manifestation of painful erythematous and violaceous papules, nodules, and plaques accompanied by fever and elevated neutrophil count (Fig. 122–10).[69] These papules, which most commonly appear on face, neck, and upper extremities, present a central yellowish discoloration and tend to coalesce, forming well-circumscribed, irregularly bordered plaques. Other organs can be involved, including the central nervous system, kidneys, lungs,

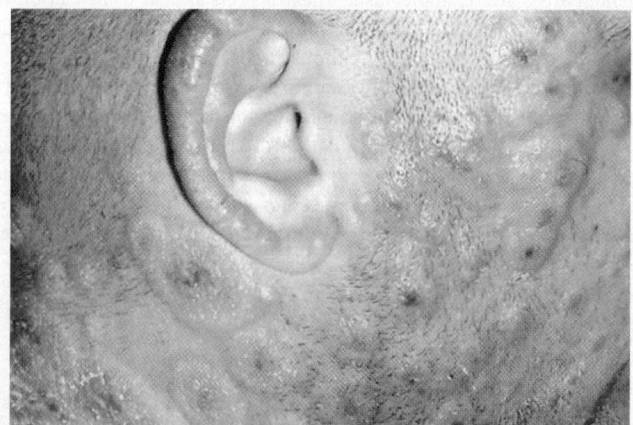

Figure 122–10. Sweet syndrome. The lesions are characterized by nonvasculitic neutrophilic infiltration, commonly on the face.

and bones.[70] Classically more prominent in middle-aged women, this syndrome associates a complex cytokine dysregulation. Other manifestations include respiratory and urinary infections and autoimmune disorders (including rheumatoid arthritis), SLE, inflammatory bowel disease). Histologic analysis shows a distinct nonvasculitic neutrophilic infiltrate in the superficial dermis with dermal edema. Systemic glucocorticoid treatment is the standard treatment, while clofazimine, dapsone, colchicine, indomethacin, and cyclosporine have also been used successfully.[71]

BEHÇET DISEASE

Besides its classification as a neutrophilic dermatosis, Behçet disease is also an inflammatory disorder that affects multiple organ systems. Clinical features include chronic and relapsing cutaneous manifestations, such as palpable purpura, infiltrative erythema, and papulopustular lesions, as well as oral mucosal and genital ulcers, arthralgias, and gastrointestinal and central nervous system involvement.[72] Genetic studies show an association between Behçet disease and human leukocyte antigen B51.[73] Histologic features include leukocytoclastic or lymphocytic vasculitis, hence its previous classification as a vasculitis. Antitumor necrosis factor-α directed therapies (infliximab, etanercept), interferon-α, immunosuppressive and immunomodulatory agents such as thalidomide, intravenous immunoglobulin, and even stem cell transplantation are used in Behçet disease.[74,75]

SERUM SICKNESS

Serum sickness reflects the clinical manifestations of immune complex formation and deposition. Cutaneous lesions such as urticarial and morbilliform eruptions predominate, though palpable purpura and erythema multiforme can also be encountered. Serum sickness associated with infection or medical therapy can result in specific characteristic lesions. The use of antithymocyte globulin for marrow failure, for instance, results in 75 percent of patients developing serpiginous bands of erythema and purpura on the sides of their hands and feet (Fig. 122–11).[76] These characteristic lesions consistently appear 1 to 2 days prior to the onset of systemic symptoms of serum sickness, which include fever and malaise. Analysis of biopsies by direct immunofluorescence reveals deposition of IgM, IgE, IgA, and C3. This deposition appears to activate neutrophils leading to release of lysosomal enzymes and the development of dermal vasculitis.[77]

HENOCH-SCHÖNLEIN PURPURA

Henoch-Schönlein purpura (HSP), is a predominantly pediatric vasculitic syndrome characterized by the acute onset of abdominal pain and lower-extremity eruption of diffuse urticarial plaques and palpable purpura. It was first described in 1801 by Dr. William Heberden.[78] HSP predominantly affects patients 2 to 20 years of age, 90 percent of patients being younger than 10 years old.[79] Several environmental triggers precede HSP onset, such as viral (upper respiratory infections, hepatitis B virus, HCV, parvovirus B19, and HIV) and bacterial (*Streptococcus* spp., *Staphylococcus aureus*, and *Salmonella* spp.) infections in children. Adult disease may be precipitated by medications (nonsteroidal antiinflammatory drugs [NSAIDs], angiotensin-converting enzyme inhibitors, and antibiotics), food allergies, vaccinations, and insect bites.[80] The pathogenesis of HSP leukocytoclastic vasculitis is complex. It appears to involve IgA$_1$ immune complex and complement deposition on vessel walls. Elevated values of thrombomodulin, tissue plasminogen activator, and plasminogen activator inhibitor-1 appear to correlate with endothelial injury and fibrinolytic activity in the acute phase of HSP.[81]

Cutaneous eruptions often begin acutely as urticarial papules and plaques evolving to petechiae, ecchymoses, and palpable and nonpalpable purpura over the lower extremities and buttocks (Fig. 122–12). Palpable purpura is a universal finding, being present in one series in 98.6 percent of patients.[82] Clinically, lesions may take the form of retiform or patterned purpura, presence of a retiform edge of various inflammatory lesions, or skin necrosis.[83] Other common manifestations include localized subcutaneous edema, glomerulonephritis, arthritis, and (severe) abdominal pain.

In spite of its chronic relapsing pattern, the long-term evolution is benign in the majority of patients.[82] The self-limited course of HSP may be contributed by an enhanced apoptosis of immune cells, which diminishes the severity of the acute inflammatory response.[84] Consequently, treatment is frequently supportive. Immunosuppressive drugs, including glucocorticoids, are typically reserved for cases with renal involvement.[78]

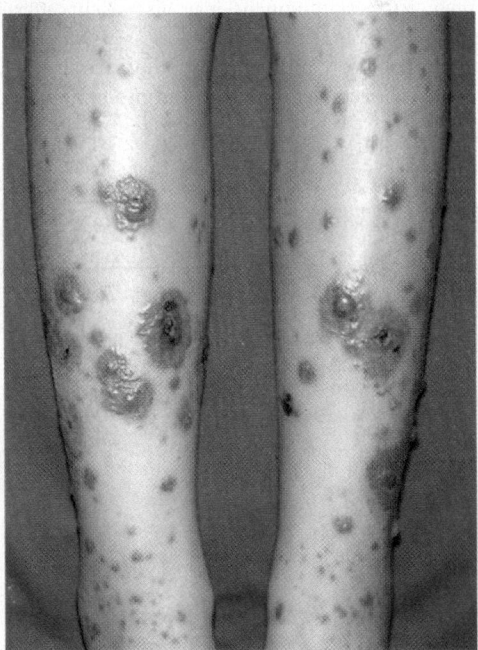

Figure 122–12. Henoch-Schönlein purpura. Urticarial papules and plaques can evolve into palpable purpura. The lesions are characterized by leukocytoclastic vasculitis.

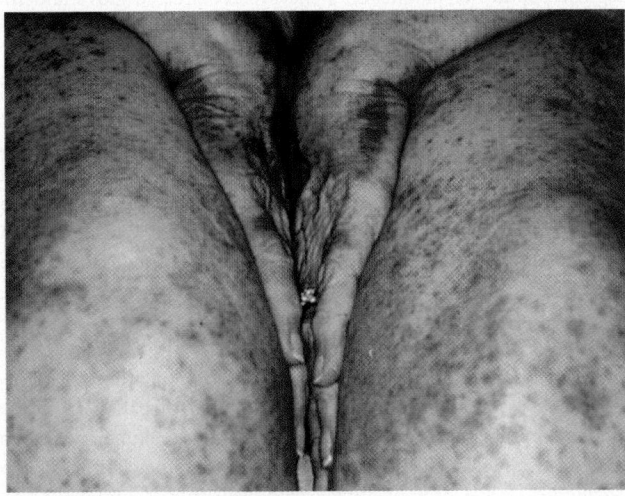

Figure 122–11. Serum sickness caused by antithymocyte globulin. The lesions consist of immunoglobulins and neutrophils.

Persistent purpura, severe abdominal symptoms, and diminished plasma coagulation factor XIII activity are predictive of renal involvement, requiring initiation of glucocorticoids.[85]

INFECTIONS

Careful analysis of skin lesions of infectious etiology can provide important hints toward identifying the responsible pathogen. Purpura can arise through a variety of pathophysiologic mechanisms associated with infection: (1) vascular effects of toxins, (2) septic emboli, (3) direct invasion of vessels with subsequent vascular occlusion, and (4) immune complex formation.[86] Although the morphology of such purpuric lesions may be nonspecific, many pathogens lead to characteristic findings.

Bacterial

Gram-positive and Gram-negative infections may give rise to a large array of purpuric patterns depending on organism virulence and patient immune status. Skin lesions range from simple macules and papules to bullae, ulcers, and necrosis.

Purpura fulminans, a hemorrhagic infarction syndrome consisting of disseminated intravascular coagulation (DIC), acral purpura, and shock may manifest in the setting of bacterial sepsis with encapsulated organisms (Chap. 129).[87] Most commonly seen in immunocompromised hosts, purpura fulminans can also be produced by bacterial pathogens in immunocompetent patients.[88] This syndrome can be associated with asplenism or functional hyposplenism.[89] Although most patients are younger than the age of 10 years, adults can also be affected.[90] Retiform purpuric lesions result from fibrin-induced microvascular occlusion, and commonly have a rapid evolution toward necrosis and eschar formation. Adult patients with purpura fulminans as a result of meningococcemia have significantly depressed proteins C and S levels, which may explain the tendency toward fibrin deposition and development of cutaneous ischemic lesions, such as symmetrical peripheral gangrene.[91] Facial purpura and livedo reticularis may be seen during fulminant pneumococcal infection in asplenic patients.[92] Postinfectious purpura fulminans may also occur after infections with streptococci or varicella zoster,[39] and was associated with development of anti–protein S antibodies. Another characteristic lesion is the development of ecthyma gangrenosum in immunocompromised hosts (Fig. 122–13).

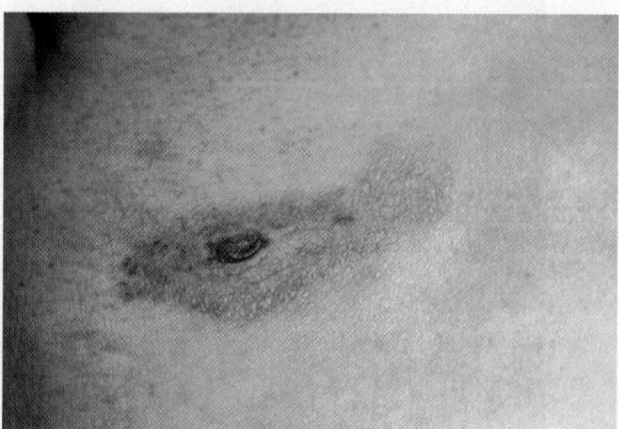

Figure 122–13. Ecthyma gangrenosum. Associated with Gram-negative sepsis, disseminated fungal infection, or other serious infectious diseases, these hemorrhagic bullae evolve from erythematosus plaques, both of which are shown here.

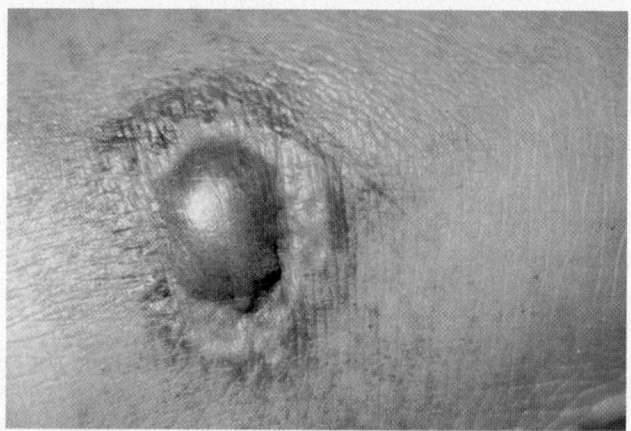

Figure 122–14. Lyme disease. Erythema migrans with a central hemorrhagic bulla is the characteristic lesion.

In children, more than 20 percent of cases admitted to the hospital with petechiae and fever were found to have invasive bacterial infections (*Neisseria meningitidis, Haemophilus influenzae* type B, and *Streptococcus pneumoniae*), and approximately 7 percent of cases were diagnosed with meningiococcemia.[93] Sepsis secondary to *N. meningitidis* can produce a characteristic pattern of purpuric lesions. Erythematous papules can quickly progress to numerous petechiae combined with violaceous reticular purpuric lesions.[94] A retiform aspect can be seen during progression of the infection to purpura fulminans. The finding of petechiae on a patient with symptoms and signs of bacterial meningitis is predictive of meningococcal meningitis.[95]

Borrelia burgdorferi infection gives rise to erythema migrans, the characteristic lesion of Lyme disease. Skin lesion is classically a nonpruritic annular erythematous expanding plaque, occasionally including a central hemorrhagic bullae (Fig. 122–14). Other reported cutaneous findings associated with this infection include papular urticaria, Henoch-Schönlein–like purpura, and morphea.[96]

Viral

Purpuric lesions can also be a manifestation of a viral infection. For example, the adenoviruses and enteroviruses have been associated with fever and petechiae in children.[97] Similarly, parvovirus B19 can produce a syndrome of petechiae or purpuric papules progressing to confluent purpuric papules or plaques in a sharply demarcated glove-and-sock distribution.[98] In addition to the cutaneous findings, the "gloves-and-socks syndrome" is characterized by fever and occasionally leukopenia, and can also be produced by the measles virus.[99] Purpura in the axilla and chest also has been described during parvovirus B19 infection (Fig. 122–15).[100] Histopathologic analysis of these purpuric lesions show an evolution from superficial perivascular lymphocytic infiltrate to a dermatitis accompanied by necrotic keratinocytes and hemorrhage.[101] *Hantavirus* causes a syndrome of hemorrhagic fever and renal failure accompanied by headache, cutaneous and mucosal petechiae, and purpuric lesions.[102]

Fungal

Fungal infections in the immunocompromised population are a growing medical issue, given the increasing number of patients receiving immunosuppressants for organ transplantation or malignancy. Disseminated or locally invasive infections can give rise to petechiae and hemorrhagic necrosis. Common fungal pathogens in disseminated disease includes *Candida* (Fig. 122–16), *Aspergillus* (Fig. 122–17), *Histoplasma*, and *Fusarium*.[103] Disseminated candidiasis can manifest as ecthyma

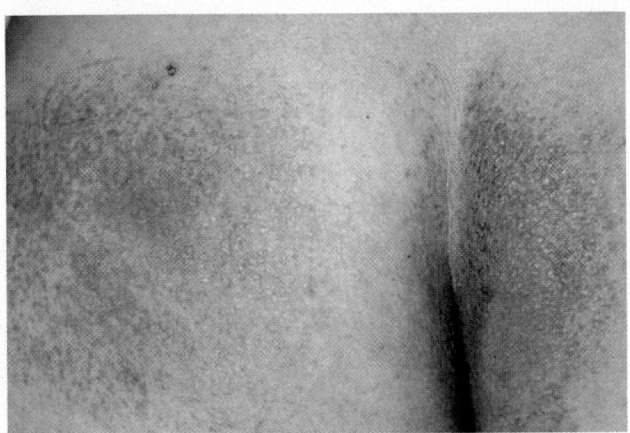

Figure 122–15. Parvovirus B19 erythema and petechiae. The classic slapped-cheek rash on the face can appear on other areas of the body, sometimes punctuated with petechiae of unclear etiology.

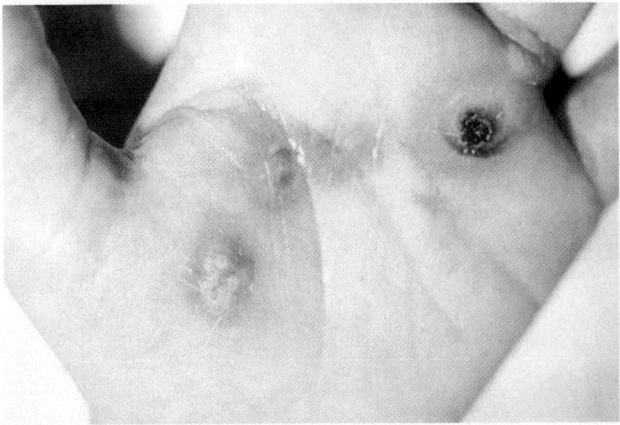

Figure 122–17. Aspergillosis: primary cutaneous inoculation from contaminated armboard.

gangrenosum in immunocompromised patients, suggesting consideration for a skin biopsy.[104] Cutaneous aspergillosis can also occur in immunocompetent individuals, and manifest as eruptive maculopapules, necrotizing plaques, or subcutaneous granulomas.[105]

Parasitic

Immunocompromised patients are at risk of developing purpuric lesions secondary to parasitic infections, such as *Pneumocystis jiroveci*. Disseminated strongyloidiasis is characterized by larva currens, a serpiginous urticarial eruption caused by the migration of filiform larvae through the dermis.[106] Other cutaneous lesions include generalized petechiae and widespread reticular purpura of the arms, legs, and abdomen (Fig. 122–18), with a characteristic *thumbprint* periumbilical distribution.[107]

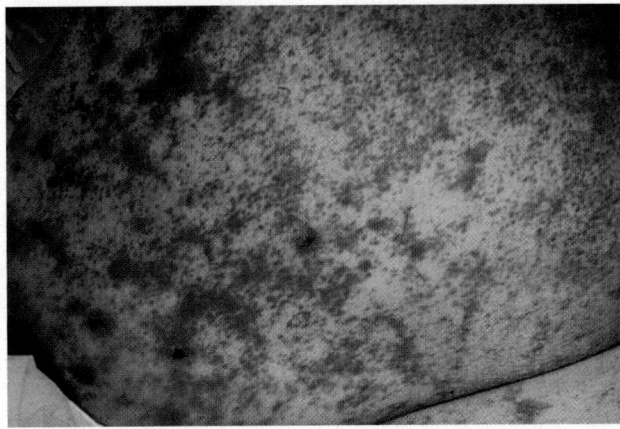

Figure 122–18. Disseminated strongyloidiasis.

Rickettsial

Infections caused by *Rickettsia* species can also lead to purpuric lesions as a result of their direct invasion of endothelial cells. This is followed by medial and intimal necrosis with subsequent thrombosis and hemorrhage.[86] Cutaneous lesions in Rocky Mountain spotted fever range from petechiae to acral purpuric lesions and hemorrhagic necrosis (Fig. 122–19). Maculopapular and vesicular rashes along with

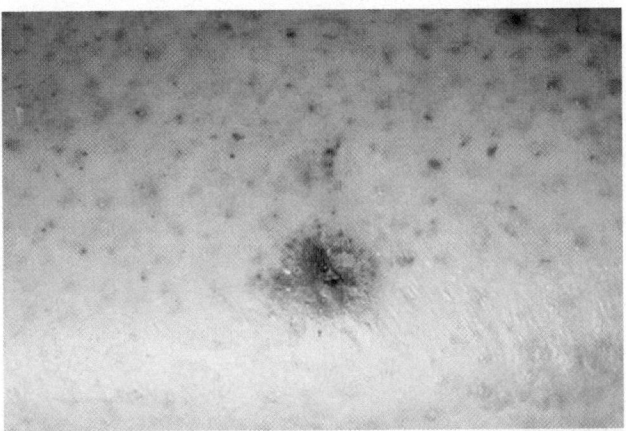

Figure 122–16. Disseminated candidiasis. Purpuric nodules in a patient with acute myelogenous leukemia. Ecthyma gangrenosum can also occur in this disease.

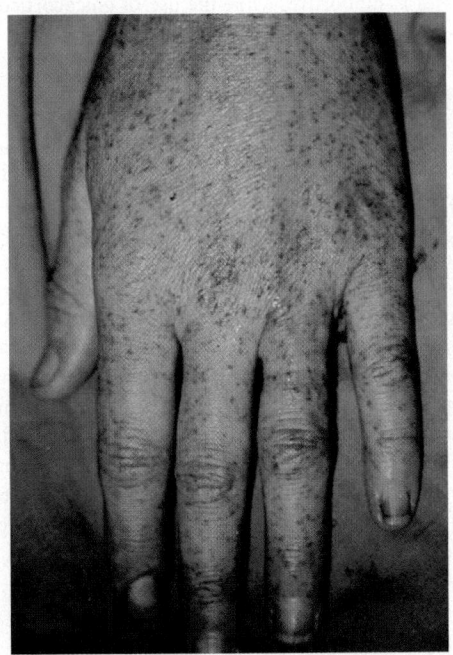

Figure 122–19. Rocky Mountain spotted fever. This rickettsial disorder can present with petechiae on the dorsum of the hand.

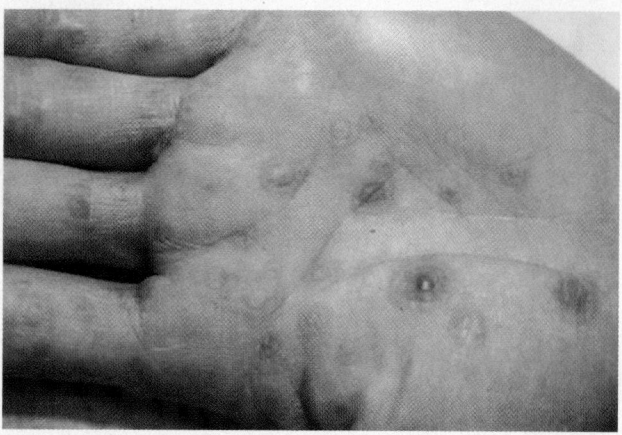

Figure 122–20. Erythema multiforme. This hypersensitivity reaction, usually to one of various drugs, characteristically presents with targetoid lesions.

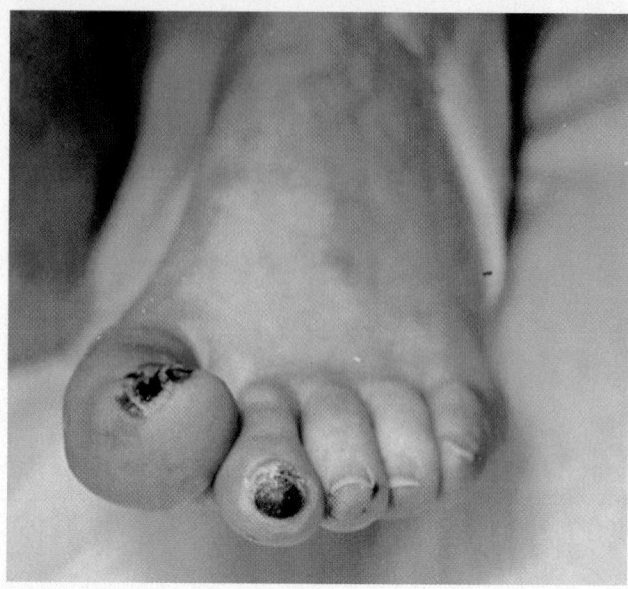

Figure 122–21. Polyarteritis nodosa. Acral purpura accompanying tender erythematous nodules.

lower-extremity eschars produced by *Rickettsia africae* may also occur in travelers to sub-Saharan Africa.[108]

ERYTHEMA MULTIFORME

Erythema multiforme (EM) is a cutaneous disorder characterized by the development of crops of well-demarcated, erythematous target lesions with central clearing,[109] most commonly representing a hypersensitivity reaction triggered by infection or drug exposure (Fig. 122–20). The severity of this disorder ranges from mild (EM minor), to severe (EM major or Stevens-Johnson syndrome). EM has been reported to be triggered by a number of viruses (most commonly herpes simplex, but also adenovirus, cytomegalovirus, and HIV),[110,111] and medications (sulfonamides, penicillins, bupropion, phenylbutazone, phenytoin, NSAIDs, adalimumab).[112] A cellular allergic reaction coupled with impaired histamine metabolism because of a decrease in histamine-*N*-methyltransferase activity may be causative.[113] Treatment for mild cases is supportive, while the use of glucocorticoids is warranted in severe cases.

CUTANEOUS POLYARTERITIS NODOSA

Classic polyarteritis nodosa represents a systemic small- and medium-size vessel vasculitis most commonly involving the skin, heart, liver, and kidneys. A relatively benign cutaneous form exists that lacks significant systemic involvement[114] and consistently involves the deep dermis and panniculus.[115] Lesions develop as tender erythematous nodules[116] with occasional retiform purpura and livedo reticularis localized to the upper and lower extremities, but the trunk, neck, and face can also be involved (Fig. 122–21). The duration of lesions varies from days to a few months.[115] Histologic analysis of involved skin shows deep dermal artery necrosis with infiltration of neutrophils and eosinophils, and fibrin deposition. Treatment typically involves the use of NSAIDs and glucocorticoids, alone or in combination. Some cases of cutaneous polyarteritis nodosa are reported to have progressed on long-term followup,[117] hence the need for close monitoring of patients diagnosed with an apparently benign, cutaneous form of disease.[118]

PARANEOPLASTIC VASCULITIS

Most common vasculitis associated with neoplasia are cutaneous leukocytoclastic vasculitis, paraneoplastic vasculitis, and HSP.[119,120]

Paraneoplastic vasculitis is most commonly associated with hematologic neoplasia,[121] and is commonly a result of paraproteinemia. However, an association with carcinomas of the lung, colon, breast, and cervix has been observed.[122-124] Solid tumors predominate in certain types of paraneoplastic vasculitis, such as the HSP.[125] Cutaneous manifestations include petechiae, urticaria, and palpable purpura, and are often intensely pruritic. In hematologic disorders, these lesions often precede the development of malignancy by an average of 10 months.[126] Histologic examination shows necrotizing leukocytoclastic vasculitis with neutrophilic infiltration.

DRUG-INDUCED VASCULITIS

A long list of drugs are reported to cause a vasculitis resulting in erythematous purpuric lesions. One-fifth of all cutaneous vasculitis are produced by drugs, including allopurinol, cefaclor, colony-stimulating factors, D-penicillamine, furosemide (Fig. 122–22), hydralazine, isotretinoin, methotrexate, phenytoin, minocycline, and propylthiouracil.[127]

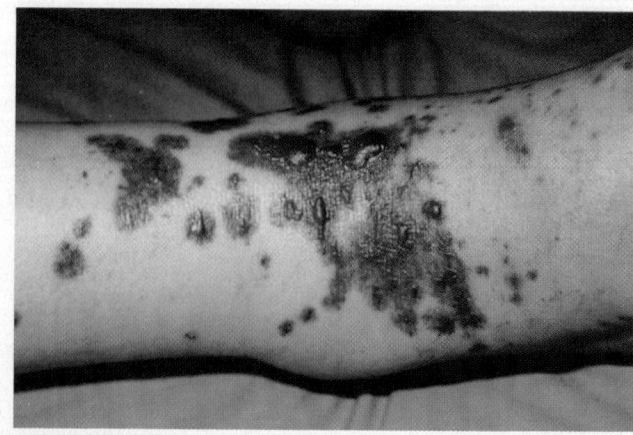

Figure 122–22. Leukocytoclastic vasculitis secondary to furosemide.

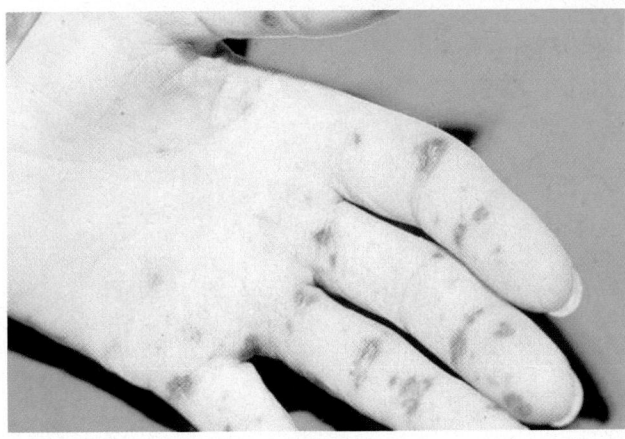

Figure 122–23. Wegener granulomatosis.

ANTINEUTROPHIL CYTOPLASMIC ANTIBODY–ASSOCIATED VASCULITIS

Wegener Granulomatosis

This small- to medium-vessel vasculitis most commonly affects upper and lower respiratory tracts and kidneys and is strongly associated with the development of circulating antineutrophil cytoplasmic antibodies (ANCAs).[128] Skin involvement has been reported in 35 to 50 percent of cases.[129] Cutaneous manifestations include a combination of palpable purpura, oral ulcers, and erythematous cutaneous and subcutaneous nodules (Fig. 122–23).[130] Necrotizing vasculitis, palisading granulomas, and granulomatous vasculitis are characteristic histologic findings.[131]

Churg-Strauss Syndrome

Churg-Strauss syndrome (CSS) is characterized by granulomatous inflammation in the lungs associated with asthma and eosinophilia.[132] Cutaneous findings such as ulcers, papules, palpable purpura, cutaneous nodules, and infarcts of fingers and toes are encountered in 50 to 80 percent of cases.[130] CSS limited to the skin was described.[133] Eosinophilia accompanies elevated IgE levels and a positive perinuclear ANCA. Granulomatous inflammation and necrotizing vasculitis of small- to medium-size blood vessels are present histologically.[131]

● NONPALPABLE, NONINFLAMMATORY, ROUND PURPURIC LESIONS

See Table 122–3.

INCREASED TRANSMURAL PRESSURE GRADIENT AND TRAUMA

Acute increases in vascular transmural pressure gradients lead to extravasation of red blood cells resulting in nonpalpable, noninflammatory petechial and larger purpuric lesions. Examples include postictal purpura,[134] weightlifting,[135] postemesis facial purpura,[136] prolonged Valsalva, and childbirth. Acute decreases in extravascular negative pressure, referred to as suction purpura from gas mask, kissing, or cupping, can also increase this gradient, resulting in well-circumscribed lesions in the shape of the causative device.[137] The development of petechiae in mountain climbers, is presumably caused by significantly reduced atmospheric pressures at high elevations.[138] Lower-extremity venous incompetence, predominantly at the medial ankle, can result in macules or patches of yellowish-brown purpura.

Focal ecchymosis and other purpuric lesions can manifest as a result of trauma. Characteristic patterns of purpuric lesions are commonly used in forensic science. Traumatic asphyxia, for instance, is characterized by cervicofacial cyanosis and swelling, petechiae, and subconjunctival hemorrhage.[139] Factitious purpura, often related to deliberate suction purpura, should be considered in the differential for purpura.[140] Other physical causes of purpura consist of physical remedies, such as spooning (Quat Sha) or coin rubbing (Cao Gio). Exercise-induced purpura results in purpuric, erythematous, or urticarial lesions distributed on the lower legs.[141]

THROMBOCYTOPENIAS

Disseminated Intravascular Coagulation

DIC is defined as widespread, amplified and uncontrolled intravascular coagulation with a range of causes including sepsis, trauma, and malignancy.[142] Petechiae and purpuric plaques result from thrombocytopenia, and are common manifestations of DIC (Chap. 129).

Immune Thrombocytopenia Purpura

Immune (or idiopathic) thrombocytopenia purpura is an acquired disease characterized by autoantibody-mediated platelet destruction commonly resulting in purpuric lesions of the skin and mucosa as well as other sites of abnormal bleeding (Chap 117).[143]

Thrombotic Thrombocytopenia Purpura

Thrombotic thrombocytopenia purpura is characterized by nonimmune platelet consumption, microvascular hemolysis, and organ damage. It is associated with a deficiency in the von Willebrand factor cleaving protease, ADAMTS-13 (a disintegrin and metalloproteinase with thrombospondin domain 13; Chap. 132).[144] Petechiae and purpuric plaques may occur.

DRUG REACTIONS

A large number of medications are reported to result in vasculitic and nonvasculitic purpuric eruptions.[145] Nevertheless, *any* drug on the medication list of a patient with a purpuric lesion (within 2 weeks of starting a new drug or a few days if prior sensitization is suspected) may be involved.[146]

COAGULATION DISORDERS

A large number of disorders manifest with thrombocytopenia or impaired thrombocyte function, that result in increased bruising. Also, impaired fibrin formation, resulting from coagulation factor deficiencies, the use of anticoagulants, vitamin K deficiency, or poor hepatic function may cause bruising and hematomas.

DECREASED VESSEL INTEGRITY WITHOUT TRAUMA

Senile Purpura

Synonymous with actinic purpura, senile purpura refers to the easy bruising seen in the aged and sun-damaged skin, commonly appearing on the dorsal aspect of the hands and forearms (Fig. 122–24). One proposed etiology is the degeneration of skin extracellular matrix components that leaves dermal capillaries unsupported and vulnerable to shearing injuries,[147] but zinc deficiency is also suspected.[148]

Excess Glucocorticoid

The presence of excess endogenous (Cushing syndrome) or exogenous (iatrogenic) glucocorticoid use can result in dermal thinning and

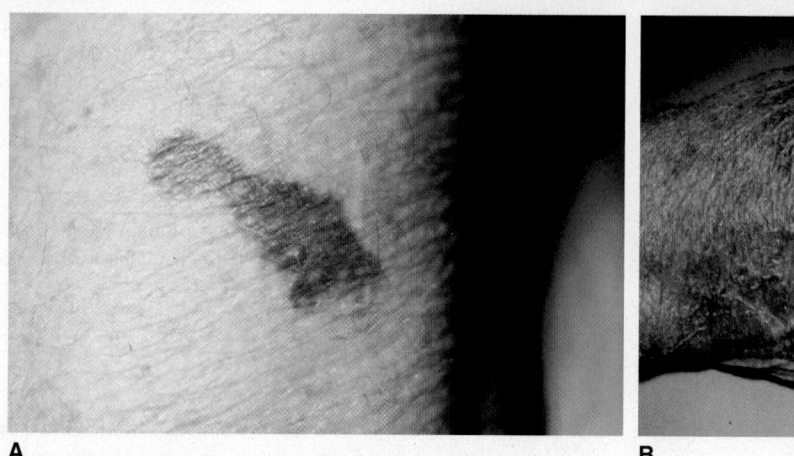

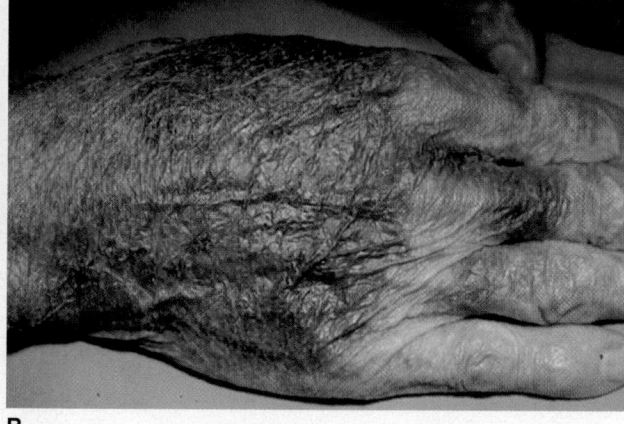

A   **B**

Figure 122–24. Senile purpura. Note accompanying skin atrophy.

vessel fragility. Consequently, bright red, nonpalpable purpuric lesions tend to arise after slight or even undetected trauma and manifest in a linear or geometric pattern.[149]

Scurvy—Vitamin C Deficiency

Vitamin C (ascorbic acid) deficiency occurs because of reduced dietary intake or absorption. A consequent disruption in normal collagen production results in blood vessel fragility leading to petechiae, perifollicular hemorrhage, and larger purpuric plaques, most commonly on the lower extremities (Fig. 122–25).[150] Thus, scurvy is usually a clinical diagnosis. Cutaneous features can also include follicular hyperkeratotic papules, poor wound healing, and bent or corkscrew-shaped body hairs.[151] Vitamin C supplementation is rapidly effective.

Systemic Amyloidosis

Systemic amyloidosis is characterized by a clonal proliferation of plasma cells with consequent immunoglobulin light-chain deposition in vital organs. Microscopic 8 to 10 nm protofilaments aggregate to form fibrils.[152] It can present as a primary disorder or secondarily to multiple myeloma (Chaps. 107 and 108). Characteristic features are periorbital "pinch purpura," "raccoon eyes," and macroglosia.[153]

Waxy, purpuric cutaneous and mucocutaneous lesions manifest when light-chain aggregates deposit in dermal blood vessels. Although rare, palmodigital purpura has been reported as the sole cutaneous finding in a case of myeloma-associated systemic amyloidosis.[154] A distinct

localized form, primary cutaneous amyloidosis, is caused by local dermal infiltration of plasma cells.[155]

CONNECTIVE TISSUE DISORDERS

Ehlers-Danlos Syndrome

A rare autosomal dominant syndrome, Ehlers-Danlos syndrome is a consequence of a mutation in collagen synthesis, tenascin X, or lysyl hydroxylase, and others. This leads to loss of skin elasticity, delayed wound healing, easy bruising, joint hypermobility, and systemic organ and tissue fragility.[156] Cutaneous findings include thin skin and a tendency to develop nonpalpable purpuric lesions.[157]

Pseudoxanthoma Elasticum

Pseudoxanthoma elasticum is genetic disorder characterized by mineralization and fragmentation of elastin in the skin, retina, and blood vessels.[158] This autosomally inherited disease is associated with a mutation in the *ABCC6* gene, an ATP-binding cassette transporter, which may play an important role in connective tissue turnover.[159] Cutaneous lesions include small white or yellow papules classically appearing on the neck in a "gooseflesh" aspect,[160] but systemic hemorrhagic events are also encountered.

Melas Syndrome

Nonpalpable purpuric lesions can occur on the palms and soles in *m*itochondrial *e*ncephalomyopathy with *l*actic *a*cidosis and *s*troke-like episodes (MELAS) syndrome.[161] MELAS syndrome, one of a family of mitochondrial encephalomyopathies, has been associated with a mutation in a mitochondrial transfer RNA (tRNA) or the reduced form of nicotinamide adenine dinucleotide (NADH) dehydrogenase complex I.[162] Skin manifestations can also include hypertrichosis, ichthyosis, and vitiligo.[163]

RENDU-OSLER-WEBER DISEASE (HEREDITARY HEMORRHAGIC TELANGIECTASIA)

Rendu-Osler-Weber disease is an autosomal dominant hereditary disorder characterized by local angiodysplasia, mostly present in the skin, mucous membranes, and often in organs such as the lungs, liver, and brain.[164] It may lead to nose bleeding, acute and chronic digestive tract bleeding, and various problems resulting from the involvement of other organs. Vascular malformations may present as telangiectasias

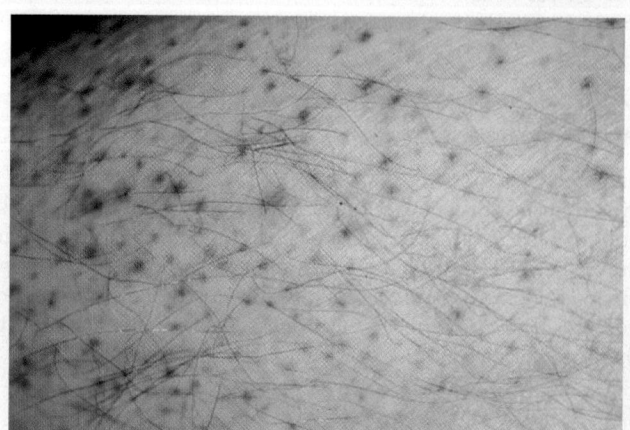

Figure 122–25. Parafollicular purpura characteristic of scurvy.

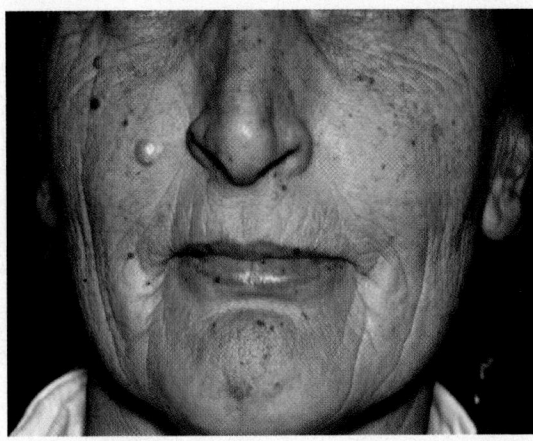

Figure 122–26. Rendu-Osler-Weber disease (hereditary hemorrhagic telangiectasia).

(small vascular malformations) in the skin (Fig. 122–26). Subcutaneous bleeding may occur as well, presenting as non-palpable purpuric lesions. Angiodysplasia in Rendu-Osler-Weber disease is caused by a defect in angiogenesis. Five genetic types of hereditary hemorrhagic telangiectasia (HHT) are recognized. More than 80 percent of all cases of HHT are caused by mutations in either *ENG (endoglin, HHT1)* or ALK1 *(ACVRL1, HHT2).*[165] Treatment of the disease is symptomatic, for example, by iron administration when iron-deficiency anemia occurs, or by laser treatment of small (bleeding) malformations in mucous membranes or embolization of larger arteriovenous malformations.

REFERENCES

1. Carlson JA, Chen KR: Cutaneous pseudovasculitis. *Am J Dermatopathol* 29:44, 2007.
2. Piette WW: The differential diagnosis of purpura from a morphologic perspective. *Adv Dermatol* 9:3, discussion 24, 1994.
3. Piette WW: Hematologic diseases, in *Fitzpatrick's Dermatology in General Medicine*, 6th ed, edited by IM Freedburg, AZ Eisen, K Wolff, KF Austen, LA Goldsmith, SI Katz, p 1523. McGraw-Hill, New York, 2003.
4. Stephenson T: Ageing of bruising in children. *J R Soc Med* 90:312, 1997.
5. Winfield JB: Cryoglobulinemia. *Hum Pathol* 14:350, 1983.
6. Galossi A, Guarisco R, Bellis L, Puoti C: Extrahepatic manifestations of chronic HCV infection. *J Gastrointestin Liver Dis* 16:65, 2007.
7. Agnello V, Romain PL: Mixed cryoglobulinemia secondary to hepatitis C virus infection. *Rheum Dis Clin North Am* 22:1, 1996.
8. Braun GS, Horster S, Wagner KS, et al: Cryoglobulinaemic vasculitis: Classification and clinical and therapeutic aspects. *Postgrad Med J* 83:87, 2007.
9. Sansonno D, Dammacco F: Hepatitis C virus, cryoglobulinaemia, and vasculitis: Immune complex relations. *Lancet Infect Dis* 5:227, 2005.
10. Sansonno D, Tucci FA, Troiani L, et al: Increased serum levels of the chemokine CXCL13 and up-regulation of its gene expression are distinctive features of HCV-related cryoglobulinemia and correlate with active cutaneous vasculitis. *Blood* 112:1620, 2008.
11. Fabrizi F, Dixit V, Messa P: Antiviral therapy of symptomatic HCV-associated mixed cryoglobulinemia: Meta-analysis of clinical studies. *J Med Virol* 85:1019, 2013.
12. Casato M, Mecucci C, Agnello V, et al: Regression of lymphoproliferative disorder after treatment for hepatitis C virus infection in a patient with partial trisomy 3, Bcl-2 overexpression, and type II cryoglobulinemia. *Blood* 99:2259, 2002.
13. Waldenström J: Clinical methods for determination of hyperproteinemia and their practical value for diagnosis. *Nord Med* 20:2288, 1943.
14. Finder KA, McCollough ML, Dixon SL, et al: Hypergammaglobulinemic purpura of Waldenstrom. *J Am Acad Dermatol* 23:669, 1990.
15. Malaviya AN, Kaushik P, Budhiraja S, et al: Hypergammaglobulinemic purpura of Waldenström: Report of 3 cases with a short review. *Clin Exp Rheumatol* 18:518, 2000.
16. Tan E, Ng SK, Tan SH, Wong GC: Hypergammaglobulinaemic purpura presenting as reticulate purpura. *Clin Exp Dermatol* 24:469, 1999.
17. Al-Mayouf SM, Ghonaium A, Bahabri S: Hypergammaglobulinaemic purpura associated with IgG subclass imbalance and recurrent infection. *Clin Rheumatol* 19:499, 2000.
18. Oosterkamp HM, van der Pijl H, Derksen J, et al: Arthritis and hypergammaglobulinemic purpura in hypersensitivity pneumonitis. *Am J Med* 100:478, 1996.
19. Miyagawa S, Fukumoto T, Kanauchi M, et al: Hypergammaglobulinaemic purpura of Waldenstrom and Ro/SSA autoantibodies. *Br J Dermatol* 134:919, 1996.
20. Pozzi C, D'Amico M, Fogazzi GB, et al: Light chain deposition disease with renal involvement: Clinical characteristics and prognostic factors. *Am J Kidney Dis* 42:1154, 2003.
21. Stone GC, Wall BA, Oppliger IR, et al: A vasculopathy with deposition of lambda light chain crystals. *Ann Intern Med* 110:275, 1989.
22. Usuda H, Emura I, Naito M: Crystal globulin-induced vasculopathy accompanying ischemic intestinal lesions of a patient with myeloma. *Pathol Int* 46:165, 1996.
23. Sankarasubbaiyan S, Scott G, Holley JL: Cryofibrinogenaemia: An addition to the differential diagnosis of calciphylaxis in end-stage renal disease. *Am J Kidney Dis* 32:494, 1998.
24. Amdo TD, Welker JA. An approach to the diagnosis and treatment of cryofibrinogenemia. *Am J Med* 116:332, 2004.
25. Blain H, Cacoub P, Musset L, et al: Cryofibrinogenaemia: A study of 49 patients. *Clin Exp Immunol* 120:253, 2000.
26. Wutschert R, Piletta P, Bounameaux H: Adverse skin reactions to low molecular weight heparins: Frequency, management and prevention. *Drug Saf* 20:515, 1999.
27. Moore A, Lau E, Yang C, et al: Dalteparin-induced skin necrosis in a patient with metastatic lung adenocarcinoma. *Am J Clin Oncol* 30:329, 2007.
28. Chong BH: Heparin-induced thrombocytopenia. *J Thromb Haemost* 1:1471, 2003.
29. Chan YC, Valenti D, Mansfield AO, Stansby G: Warfarin induced skin necrosis. *Br J Surg* 87:266, 2000.
30. Harenberg J, Hoffmann U, Huhle G, et al: Cutaneous reactions to anticoagulants. Recognition and management. *Am J Clin Dermatol* 2:69, 2001.
31. Scarff CE, Baker C, Hill P, Foley P: Late-onset warfarin necrosis. *Australas J Dermatol* 43:202, 2002.
32. Ward CT, Chavalitanonda N: Atypical warfarin-induced skin necrosis. *Pharmacotherapy* 26:1175, 2006.
33. Stone MS, Rosen T: Acral purpura: An unusual sign of coumarin necrosis. *J Am Acad Dermatol* 14:797, 1986.
34. Segel GB, Francis CA: Anticoagulant proteins in childhood venous and arterial thrombosis: A review. *Blood Cells Mol Dis* 26:540, 2000.
35. Marlar RA, Neumann A: Neonatal purpura fulminans due to homozygous protein C or protein S deficiencies. *Semin Thromb Hemost* 16:299,1990.
36. Kemahli S, Alhenc-Gelas M, Gandrille S, et al: Homozygous protein C deficiency with a double variant His 202 to Tyr and Ala 346 to Thr. *Blood Coagul Fibrinolysis* 9:351, 1998.
37. Ezer U, Misirlioglu ED, Colba V, et al: Neonatal purpura fulminans due to homozygous protein C deficiency. *Pediatr Hematol Oncol* 18:453, 2001.
38. Gruber A, Blasko G, Sas G: Functional deficiency of protein C and skin necrosis in multiple myeloma. *Thromb Res* 42:579, 1986.
39. van Ommen CH, van Wijnen M, de Groot FG, et al: Postvaricella purpura fulminans caused by acquired protein s deficiency resulting from antiprotein s antibodies: Search for the epitopes. *J Pediatr Hematol Oncol* 24:413, 2002.
40. De Stefano V, Mastrangelo S, Schwarz HP, et al: Replacement therapy with a purified protein C concentrate during initiation of oral anticoagulation in severe protein C congenital deficiency. *Thromb Haemost* 70:247, 1993.
41. Hillman RS, Ault, KA: The dysplastic and sideroblastic anemias, in *Hematology in Clinical Practice*, 2nd ed, edited by J Morgan, P Hanley, p 151. McGraw-Hill, New York, 1998.
42. White JM, Watson K, Arya R, Du Vivier AW: Haemorrhagic bullae in a case of paroxysmal nocturnal haemoglobinuria. *Clin Exp Dermatol* 28:504, 2003.
43. Cholez C, Schmutz JL, Hulin C, et al: Cutaneous necrosis during paroxysmal nocturnal haemoglobinuria: Role of parvovirus B19? *J Eur Acad Dermatol Venereol* 19:381, 2005.
44. Goulden V, Bond L, Highet A: Pyoderma gangrenosum associated with paroxysmal nocturnal haemoglobinuria. *Clin Exp Dermatol* 19:271, 1994.
45. Watt SG, Winhoven S, Hay CR, Lucas GS: Purpura fulminans in paroxysmal nocturnal haemoglobinuria. *Br J Haematol* 137:271, 2007.
46. Blume JE, Miller CC: Antiphospholipid syndrome: A review and update for the dermatologist. *Cutis* 78:409, 2006.
47. DiFrancesco LM, Burkart P, Hoehn JG: A cutaneous manifestation of antiphospholipid antibody syndrome. *Ann Plast Surg* 51:517, 2003.
48. Weinstein S, Piette W: Cutaneous manifestations of antiphospholipid antibody syndrome. *Hematol Oncol Clin North Am* 22:67, 2008.
49. Uthman IW, Khamashta MA: Livedo racemosa: A striking dermatological sign for the antiphospholipid syndrome. *J Rheumatol* 33:2379, 2006.
50. Martin L, Armingaud P, Georgescu V, et al: Acute bullous purpura associated with hyperhomocysteinemia and antiphospholipid antibodies. *J Am Acad Dermatol* 49:S161, 2003.
51. Hereng T, Lambert M, Hachulla E, et al: Influence of aspirin on the clinical outcomes of 103 anti-phospholipid antibodies-positive patients. *Lupus* 17:11, 2008.
52. Hairston BR, Davis MD, Pittelkow MR, Ahmed I: Livedoid vasculopathy: Further evidence for procoagulant pathogenesis. *Arch Dermatol* 142:1413, 2006.
53. Mimouni D, Ng PP, Rencic A, et al: Cutaneous polyarteritis nodosa in patients presenting with atrophie blanche. *Br J Dermatol* 148:789, 2003.
54. Acland KM, Darvay A, Wakelin SH, Russell-Jones R: Livedoid vasculitis: A manifestation of the antiphospholipid syndrome? *Br J Dermatol* 140:131, 1999.
55. Ravat FE, Evans AV, Russell-Jones R: Response of livedoid vasculitis to intravenous immunoglobulin. *Br J Dermatol* 147:166, 2002.
56. Donohue KG, Saap L, Falanga V: Cholesterol crystal embolization: An atherosclerotic disease with frequent and varied cutaneous manifestations. *J Eur Acad Dermatol Venereol* 17:504, 2003.

57. Jucgla A, Moreso F, Muniesa C, et al: Cholesterol embolism: Still an unrecognized entity with a high mortality rate. *J Am Acad Dermatol* 55:786, 2006.
58. Meyrier A: Cholesterol crystal embolism: Diagnosis and treatment. *Kidney Int* 69:1308, 2006.
59. Floege J: When man turns to stone: Extraosseous calcification in uremic patients. *Kidney Int* 65:2447, 2004.
60. Parker RW, Mouton CP, Young DW, Espino DV: Early recognition and treatment of calciphylaxis. *South Med J* 96:53, 2003.
61. Hayashi M: Calciphylaxis: Diagnosis and clinical features. *Clin Exp Nephrol* 17:498, 2013.
62. Nigwekar SU, Wolf M, Sterns RH, Hix JK: Calciphylaxis from nonuremic causes: A systematic review. *Clin J Am Soc Nephrol* 3:1139, 2008.
63. Alexandrescu DT, Wiernik PH: Cutaneous manifestations of a catheter-related thrombus. *Arch Dermatol* 141:1049, 2005.
64. García-F-Villalta MJ, Sanz-Sánchez T, Aragüés M, et al: Cutaneous embolization of cardiac myxoma. *Br J Dermatol* 147:379, 2002.
65. Zhu YI, Stiller MJ: Arthropods and skin diseases. *Int J Dermatol* 41:533, 2002.
66. Shankar S, Sterling JC, Rytina E: Pustular pyoderma gangrenosum. *Clin Exp Dermatol* 28:600, 2003.
67. Crowson AN, Mihm MC Jr, Magro C: Pyoderma gangrenosum: A review. *J Cutan Pathol* 30:97, 2003.
68. Gettler S, Rothe M, Grin C, Grant-Kels J: Optimal treatment of pyoderma gangrenosum. *Am J Clin Dermatol* 4:597, 2003.
69. Cohen PR, Kurzrock R: Sweet's syndrome: A neutrophilic dermatosis classically associated with acute onset and fever. *Clin Dermatol* 18:265, 2000.
70. Nobeyama Y, Kamide R: Sweet's syndrome with neurologic manifestation: Case report and literature review. *Int J Dermatol* 42:438, 2003.
71. Cohen PR, Kurzrock R: Sweet's syndrome: A review of current treatment options. *Am J Clin Dermatol* 3:117, 2002.
72. Chen KR, Kawahara Y, Miyakawa S, Nishikawa T: Cutaneous vasculitis in Behçet disease: A clinical and histopathologic study of 20 patients. *J Am Acad Dermatol* 36:689, 1997.
73. Yurdakul S, Hamuryudan V, Yazici H: Behçet syndrome. *Curr Opin Rheumatol* 16:38, 2004.
74. Olivieri I, Latanza L, Siringo S, et al: Successful treatment of severe Behçet's disease with infliximab in an Italian Olympic athlete. *J Rheumatol* 35:930, 2008.
75. Curigliano V, Giovinale M, Fonnesu C, et al: Efficacy of etanercept in the treatment of a patient with Behçet's disease. *Clin Rheumatol* 27:933, 2008.
76. Bielory L, Gascon P, Lawley TJ, et al: Human serum sickness: A prospective analysis of 35 patients treated with equine anti-thymocyte globulin for bone marrow failure. *Medicine (Baltimore)* 67:40, 1988.
77. Jegasothy BV: Immune complexes in the reactive inflammatory vascular dermatoses. *Dermatol Clin* 3:185, 1985.
78. Ballinger S: Henoch-Schönlein purpura. *Curr Opin Rheumatol* 15:591, 2003.
79. Saulsbury FT: Henoch-Schönlein purpura. *Curr Opin Rheumatol* 13:35, 2001.
80. Eftychiou C, Samarkos M, Golfinopoulou S, et al: Henoch-Schönlein purpura associated with methicillin-resistant *Staphylococcus aureus* infection. *Am J Med* 119:85, 2006.
81. Besbas N, Saatci U, Ruacan S, et al: The role of cytokines in Henoch-Schönlein purpura. *Scand J Rheumatol* 26:456, 1997.
82. Fretzayas A, Sionti I, Moustaki M, et al: Henoch-Schönlein purpura: A long-term prospective study in Greek children. *J Clin Rheumatol* 14:324, 2008.
83. Carlson JA, Chen KR: Cutaneous vasculitis update: Small vessel neutrophilic vasculitis syndromes. *Am J Dermatopathol* 28:486, 2006.
84. Ozaltin F, Besbas N, Uckan D, et al: The role of apoptosis in childhood Henoch-Schönlein purpura. *Clin Rheumatol* 22:265, 2003.
85. Kaku Y, Nohara K, Honda S: Renal involvement in Henoch-Schönlein purpura: A multivariate analysis of prognostic factors. *Kidney Int* 53:1755, 1998.
86. Kingston ME, Mackey D: Skin clues in the diagnosis of life-threatening infections. *Rev Infect Dis* 8:1, 1986.
87. Childers BJ, Cobanov B: Acute infectious purpura fulminans: A 15-year retrospective review of 28 consecutive cases. *Am Surg* 69:86, 2003.
88. Cnota JF, Barton LL, Rhee KH: Purpura fulminans associated with *Streptococcus pneumoniae* infection in a child. *Pediatr Emerg Care* 15:187, 1999.
89. Ward KM, Celebi JT, Gmyrek R, Grossman ME: Acute infectious purpura fulminans associated with asplenism or hyposplenism. *J Am Acad Dermatol* 47:493, 2002.
90. Betrosian AP, Berlet T, Agarwal B: Purpura fulminans in sepsis. *Am J Med Sci* 332:339, 2006.
91. Rintala E, Kauppila M, Seppala OP, et al: Protein C substitution in sepsis-associated purpura fulminans. *Crit Care Med* 28:2373, 2000.
92. Rusonis PA, Robinson HN, Lamberg SI: Livedo reticularis and purpura: Presenting features in fulminant pneumococcal septicemia in an asplenic patient. *J Am Acad Dermatol* 15:1120, 1986.
93. Baker RC, Seguin JH, Leslie N, et al: Fever and petechiae in children. *Pediatrics* 84:1051, 1989.
94. Baselga E, Drolet BA, Esterly NB: Purpura in infants and children. *J Am Acad Dermatol* 37:673, quiz 706, 1997.
95. Mancebo J, Domingo P, Blanch L, et al: The predictive value of petechiae in adults with bacterial meningitis. *JAMA* 256:2820, 1986.
96. Berger BW: Dermatologic manifestations of Lyme disease. *Rev Infect Dis* 11(Suppl 6):S1475, 1989.
97. Nielsen HE, Andersen EA, Andersen J, et al: Diagnostic assessment of haemorrhagic rash and fever. *Arch Dis Child* 85:160, 2001.
98. McNeely M, Friedman J, Pope E: Generalized petechial eruption induced by parvovirus B19 infection. *J Am Acad Dermatol* 52:S109, 2005.
99. Perez-Ferriols A, Martinez-Aparicio A, Aliaga-Boniche A: Papular-purpuric "gloves and socks" syndrome caused by measles virus. *J Am Acad Dermatol* 30:291, 1994.
100. Shiraishi H, Umetsu K, Yamamoto H, et al: Human parvovirus (HPV/B19) infection with purpura. *Microbiol Immunol* 33:369, 1989.
101. Smith SB, Libow LF, Elston DM, et al: Gloves and socks syndrome: Early and late histopathologic features. *J Am Acad Dermatol* 47:749, 2002.
102. Bruno P, Hassell LH, Brown J, et al: The protean manifestations of hemorrhagic fever with renal syndrome. A retrospective review of 26 cases from Korea. *Ann Intern Med* 113:385, 1990.
103. Helm TN, Longworth DL, Hall GS, et al: Case report and review of resolved fusariosis. *J Am Acad Dermatol* 23:393, 1990.
104. Fine JD, Miller JA, Harrist TJ, Haynes HA: Cutaneous lesions in disseminated candidiasis mimicking ecthyma gangrenosum. *Am J Med* 70: 1133, 1981.
105. Galimberti R, Kowalczuk A, Hidalgo Parra I, et al: Cutaneous aspergillosis: A report of six cases. *Br J Dermatol* 139:522, 1998.
106. von Kuster LC, Genta RM: Cutaneous manifestations of strongyloidiasis. *Arch Dermatol* 124:1826, 1988.
107. Ly MN, Bethel SL, Usmani AS, et al: Cutaneous *Strongyloides stercoralis* infection: An unusual presentation. *J Am Acad Dermatol* 49:S157, 2003.
108. Jensenius M, Fournier PE, Kelly P, et al: African tick bite fever. *Lancet Infect Dis* 3:557, 2003.
109. Lamoreux MR, Sternbach MR, Hsu WT: Erythema multiforme. *Am Fam Physician* 74:1883, 2006.
110. Ng PP, Sun YJ, Tan HH, Tan SH: Detection of herpes simplex virus genomic DNA in various subsets of erythema multiforme by polymerase chain reaction. *Dermatology* 207:349, 2003.
111. Schechner AJ, Pinson AG: Acute human immunodeficiency virus infection presenting with erythema multiforme. *Am J Emerg Med* 22:330, 2004.
112. Yang YH, Tsai MJ, Tsau YK, et al: Clinical observations of erythema multiforme in children. *Acta Paediatr Taiwan* 40:107, 1999.
113. Imamura S, Horio T, Yanase K, et al: Erythema multiforme: Pathomechanism of papular erythema and target lesion. *J Dermatol* 19:524, 1992.
114. Siberry GK, Cohen BA, Johnson B: Cutaneous polyarteritis nodosa. Reports of two cases in children and review of the literature. *Arch Dermatol* 130:884, 1994.
115. Díaz-Pérez JL, De Lagrán ZM, Díaz-Ramón JL, Winkelmann RK: Cutaneous polyarteritis nodosa. *Semin Cutan Med Surg* 26:77, 2007.
116. Kluger N, Pagnoux C, Guillevin L, et al: Comparison of cutaneous manifestations in systemic polyarteritis nodosa and microscopic polyangiitis. *Br J Dermatol* 159:615, 2008.
117. Minkowitz G, Smoller BR, McNutt NS: Benign cutaneous polyarteritis nodosa. Relationship to systemic polyarteritis nodosa and to hepatitis B infection. *Arch Dermatol* 127:1520, 1991.
118. Chen KR: Cutaneous polyarteritis nodosa: A clinical and histopathological study of 20 cases. *J Dermatol* 16:429, 1989.
119. Diez-Porres L, Rios-Blanco JJ, Robles-Marhuenda A, et al: ANCA-associated vasculitis as paraneoplastic syndrome with colon cancer: A case report. *Lupus* 14:632, 2005.
120. Ayob S, McDonagh AJ: Paraneoplastic leucocytoclastic vasculitis heralding a solid-organ tumour. *Clin Exp Dermatol* 40:206, 2015.
121. Farrell AM, Stern SC, El-Ghariani K, et al: Splenic lymphoma with villous lymphocytes presenting as leucocytoclastic vasculitis. *Clin Exp Dermatol* 24:19, 1999.
122. Carlson JA, Ng BT, Chen KR: Cutaneous vasculitis update: Diagnostic criteria, classification, epidemiology, etiology, pathogenesis, evaluation and prognosis. *Am J Dermatopathol* 27:504, 2005.
122. Ponge T, Boutoille D, Moreau A, et al: Systemic vasculitis in a patient with small-cell neuroendocrine bronchial cancer. *Eur Respir J* 12:1228, 1998.
123. Pertuiset E, Lioté F, Launay-Russ E, et al: Adult Henoch-Schönlein purpura associated with malignancy. *Semin Arthritis Rheum* 29:360, 2000.
124. Nakajima H, Ikeda M, Yamamoto Y, Kodama H: Large annular purpura and paraneoplastic purpura in a patient with Sjögren's syndrome and cervical cancer. *J Dermatol* 27:40, 2000.
125. El Tal AK, Tannous Z: Cutaneous vascular disorders associated with internal malignancy. *Dermatol Clin* 26:45, 2008.
126. Greer JM, Longley S, Edwards NL, et al: Vasculitis associated with malignancy. Experience with 13 patients and literature review. *Medicine (Baltimore)* 67:220, 1988.
127. Radić M, Martinović Kaliterna D, Radić J: Drug-induced vasculitis: A clinical and pathological review. *Neth J Med* 70:12, 2012.
128. Seo P, Stone JH: The antineutrophil cytoplasmic antibody-associated vasculitides. *Am J Med* 117:39, 2004.
129. Daoud MS, Gibson LE, DeRemee RA, et al: Cutaneous Wegener's granulomatosis: Clinical, histopathologic, and immunopathologic features of thirty patients. *J Am Acad Dermatol* 31:605, 1994.
130. Puéchal X: Antineutrophil cytoplasmic antibody-associated vasculitides. *Joint Bone Spine* 74:427, 2007.
131. Csernok E, Gross WL: Primary vasculitides and vasculitis confined to skin: Clinical features and new pathogenic aspects. *Arch Dermatol Res* 292:427, 2000.
132. Keogh KA, Specks U: Churg-Strauss syndrome. *Semin Respir Crit Care Med* 27:148, 2006.

133. Khan NA, Shenoy PK, McClymont L, Palmer TJ: Exophthalmos and facial swelling: A case of limited Churg-Strauss syndrome. *J Laryngol Otol* 110:578, 1996.

134. Reis JJ, Kaplan PW: Postictal hemifacial purpura. *Seizure* 7:337, 1998.

135. Pierson JC, Suh PS: Powerlifter's purpura: A Valsalva-associated phenomenon. *Cutis* 70:93, 2002.

136. Alcalay J, Ingber A, Sandbank M: Mask phenomenon: Postemesis facial purpura. *Cutis* 38:28, 1986.

137. Metzker A, Merlob P: Suction purpura. *Arch Dermatol* 128:822, 1992.

138. Forster PJ: Microvascular fragility at high altitude. *Br Med J (Clin Res Ed)* 296:1004, 1988.

139. Kondo T, Betz P, Eisenmenger W: Retrospective study on skin reddenings and petechiae in the eyelids and the conjunctivae in forensic physical examinations. *Int J Legal Med* 110:204, 1997.

140. Urkin J, Katz M: Suction purpura. *Isr Med Assoc J* 2:711, 2000.

141. Ramelet AA: Exercise-induced purpura. *Dermatology* 208:293, 2004.

142. Levi M, ten Cate H: Disseminated intravascular coagulation. *N Engl J Med* 341:586, 2001.

143. Beardsley DS: Pathophysiology of immune thrombocytopenic purpura. *Blood Rev* 16:13, 2002.

144. Tsai HM: Advances in the pathogenesis, diagnosis, and treatment of thrombotic thrombocytopenic purpura. *J Am Soc Nephrol* 14:1072, 2003.

145. Bruinsma W: The file of side effects to the skin: A guide to drug eruptions. *Semin Dermatol* 8:141, 1989.

146. Stern, RS, Shear, NH: Cutaneous reactions to drugs and biological modifiers, in *Cutaneous Medicine and Surgery*, vol 1, edited by KA Arndt, PE LeBoit, JK Robinson, BU Wintroub, p 412. WB Saunders, Philadelphia, 1996.

147. Feinstein RJ, Halprin KM, Penneys NS, et al: Senile purpura. *Arch Dermatol* 108:229, 1973.

148. Haboubi NY, Haboubi NA, Gyde OH, et al: Zinc deficiency in senile purpura. *J Clin Pathol* 38:1189, 1985.

149. Del Rosso J, Friedlander SF: Corticosteroids: Options in the era of steroid-sparing therapy. *J Am Acad Dermatol* 53:S50, 2005.

150. Nguyen RT, Cowley DM, Muir JB: Scurvy: A cutaneous clinical diagnosis. *Australas J Dermatol* 44:48, 2003.

151. Olmedo JM, Yiannias JA, Windgassen EB, Gornet MK: Scurvy: A disease almost forgotten. *Int J Dermatol* 45:909, 2006.

152. Goldsbury C, Green J: Time-lapse atomic force microscopy in the characterization of amyloid-like fibril assembly and oligomeric intermediates. *Methods Mol Biol* 299:103, 2005.

153. Eder L, Bitterman H: Image in clinical medicine. Amyloid purpura. *N Engl J Med* 356:2406, 2007.

154. Vella FS, Simone B, Antonaci S: Palmodigital purpura as the only skin abnormality in myeloma-associated systemic amyloidosis. *Br J Haematol* 120:917, 2003.

155. Breathnach SM: Amyloid and amyloidosis. *J Am Acad Dermatol* 18:1, 1988.

156. Fernandes NF, Schwartz RA: A "hyperextensive" review of Ehlers-Danlos syndrome. *Cutis* 82:242, 2008.

157. Germain DP: Clinical and genetic features of vascular Ehlers-Danlos syndrome. *Ann Vasc Surg* 16:391, 2002.

158. Bercovitch L, Terry P: Pseudoxanthoma elasticum 2004. *J Am Acad Dermatol* 51:S13, 2004.

159. Hu X, Plomp AS, Van Soest S, et al: Pseudoxanthoma elasticum: A clinical, histopathological, and molecular update. *Surv Ophthalmol* 48:424, 2003.

160. Laube S, Moss C: Pseudoxanthoma elasticum. *Arch Dis Child* 90:754, 2005.

161. Horiguchi Y, Fujii T, Imamura S: Purpuric cutaneous manifestations in mitochondrial encephalomyopathy. *J Dermatol* 18:295, 1991.

162. Kubota Y, Ishii T, Sugihara H, et al: Skin manifestations of a patient with mitochondrial encephalomyopathy with lactic acidosis and strokelike episodes (MELAS syndrome). *J Am Acad Dermatol* 41:469, 1999.

163. Sproule DM, Kaufmann P: Mitochondrial encephalopathy, lactic acidosis, and strokelike episodes: Basic concepts, clinical phenotype, and therapeutic management of MELAS syndrome. *Ann N Y Acad Sci* 1142:133, 2008.

164. Dupuis-Girod S, Bailly S, Plauchu H: Hereditary hemorrhagic telangiectasia (HHT): From molecular biology to patient care. *J Thromb Haemost* 8:1447, 2010.

168. Duffau P, Lazarro E, Viallard JF: Hereditary hemorrhagic telangiectasia. *Rev Med Interne* 35:21, 2014.

CHAPTER 123
HEMOPHILIA A AND HEMOPHILIA B

Miguel A. Escobar and Nigel S. Key

SUMMARY

Hemophilias A and B are the only two bleeding disorders inherited in a sex-linked fashion. The gene for both disorders is on the long arm of the X-chromosome. Both disorders appear as otherwise clinically indistinguishable hemorrhagic diseases of mild, moderate, or life-threatening severity. In the most-severe form, both hemophilias A and B are characterized by multiple bleeding episodes into joints and other tissues leading to chronic crippling hemarthropathy and internal organ hemorrhage unless treated early or prophylactically with factor VIII or IX concentrates, respectively. Even though phenotypically similar, both diseases are genetically heterogeneous with more than 1000 mutations leading to the absence of or dysfunctional factor VIII or IX molecules that do not support normal thrombin generation nor adequate fibrin clot formation.

Despite similarities in hemorrhagic symptoms, there are major differences between hemophilias A and B. Hemophilia A is about five times more common than hemophilia B, and is caused by defects in the factor VIII gene, a large 186-kb gene with 26 exons. A common mutation results from inversion and crossing over of intron 22 during meiosis. This mutation leads to severe hemophilia, and because no factor VIII protein is made, these patients are prone to developing antibody inhibitors to therapeutically administered factor VIII that neutralize its coagulant function, making adequate therapy problematic. Approximately 20 percent of severely affected hemophilia A patients develop such inhibitors, whereas only 3 percent or fewer of severely affected hemophilia B patients develop inhibitors against factor IX. About one-third of the mutations in hemophilias A and B arise de novo at CpG "hotspots." These mutations are apt to occur in the germ cells of a maternal grandfather whose daughters will be carriers and whose grandsons will have a 50 percent chance of having hemophilia.

Replacement therapy is available for both hemophilia A and hemophilia B patients. Safe, effective, and highly purified factor VIII and factor IX concentrates derived from plasma or made by recombinant technology are available for prophylactic therapy to prevent bleeding episodes or prompt treatment of hemorrhagic events. Prophylaxis is the treatment of choice and can prevent disabling joint disease and other hemorrhagic events such that patients can expect a relatively normal life span provided that adequate replacement therapy is available. For patients with inhibitors, factor VIIa and factor VIII inhibitor bypassing activity can be used to "bypass" the factor VIII or factor IX deficiency. Both disorders are good candidates for gene therapy that may eventually lead to their cure.

Acronyms and Abbreviations: AAV, adeno-associated virus; aPTT, activated partial thromboplastin time; BT, bleeding time; BU, Bethesda unit; CGA, cytosine, guanine, adenine; CJD, Creutzfeldt-Jakob disease; COX, cyclooxygenase; CRM, cross-reacting material; CT, computerized tomography; DDAVP, 1-desamino-8-D-arginine vasopressin, desmopressin; DVT, deep vein thrombosis; EACA, ε-aminocaproic acid; FEIBA, factor VIII inhibitor bypassing activity; GLA, γ-carboxyglutamic acid; Ig, immunoglobulin; PT, prothrombin time; PTC, plasma thromboplastin component (factor IX); RFLP, restriction fragment length polymorphism; TCT, thrombin clotting time; VWD, von Willebrand disease; VWF, von Willebrand factor.

● HEMOPHILIA A (CLASSIC HEMOPHILIA, FACTOR VIII DEFICIENCY)

DEFINITION AND HISTORY

Hemophilia A is an X-linked hereditary disorder caused by defective synthesis of factor VIII. Hemophilia A is less common than von Willebrand disease (VWD; Chap. 126), but it is more common than other inherited clotting factor abnormalities. The estimated incidence of hemophilia A is one in every 5000 to 7000 live male births. It occurs in all ethnic groups in all parts of the world.[1]

Sex-linked hemophilia was recognized at least as early as the 2nd century, when a rabbi correctly deduced that sons of hemophilic carriers were at risk for bleeding following circumcision.[2] In the 19th century, several authors noted the sex-linked inheritance pattern of the disease and ascribed the hemorrhagic episodes to delayed blood coagulation. Morawitz[3] developed the classic theory of blood coagulation, which recognized two major reactions: (1) conversion of prothrombin to thrombin by a tissue substance that Morawitz termed thrombokinase, and (2) conversion of fibrinogen to fibrin by thrombin. In 1911, Addis[4] demonstrated that thrombin formed more slowly in hemophilic blood than in normal blood and that the defect could be corrected by small amounts of normal plasma. However, he incorrectly theorized that hemophilia resulted from prothrombin deficiency. As protein purification techniques improved throughout the 1930s and 1940s, thrombokinase was resolved into several distinct components. Brinkhous[5] demonstrated that the prothrombin content of hemophilic plasma was normal and that the basic defect in hemophilia was the delayed conversion of prothrombin to thrombin. The defect could be corrected by a fraction of normal plasma containing the antihemophilic factor, later named factor VIII. In 1947, Pavlovsky[6] observed that when blood from one patient with hemophilia was transfused into another patient with a similar clinical phenotype, the prolonged clotting time in the recipient was corrected. At the time, Pavlovsky did not recognize that he was dealing with two different types of hemophilia. This fact was recognized by Aggeler and coworkers[7] in 1952, when they described a patient deficient in "plasma thromboplastin component", a blood clotting factor different from factor VIII. A deficiency of "plasma thromboplastin component," later termed factor IX, was identified as the cause of hemophilia B. A month later, Biggs and colleagues described a similar patient whose surname was Christmas, thus the synonym "Christmas disease."[8] Hemophilias A and B are the only two hereditary clotting factor defects inherited in a sex-linked pattern, and they are clinically indistinguishable, although data suggest that on the whole, hemophilia B may be less severe than hemophilia A.[9] However, in an individual patient, the disorders cannot be distinguished without a specific assay for factor VIII or IX.

In 1964, a proposal to organize the growing number of coagulation factors into a cascade or waterfall mechanism was put forth by Davie and Ratnoff and by Macfarlane.[10,11] In this scheme, each zymogen clotting factor was sequentially activated to a protease that subsequently activated the next zymogen until thrombin ultimately was produced. In this scheme, factors VIII and IX were considered to be proenzymes. Later, however, factor VIII, when activated by thrombin, was shown not to be a proenzyme but rather an essential cofactor for factor IXa. The waterfall hypothesis has been modified so that the primary role of the tissue factor–factor VII complex in the initiation of coagulation is emphasized (Chap. 113).[12]

ETIOLOGY AND PATHOGENESIS

Hemophilia A is a heterogeneous disorder resulting from defects in the factor VIII gene that leads to absent or reduced circulating levels of functional factor VIII. The reduced activity can result from a decreased amount of factor VIII protein, the presence of a functionally abnormal protein, or a combination of both. For factor VIII to be an effective cofactor for factor IXa, it must first be activated by thrombin, a reaction that results in the formation of a heterotrimer composed of the A_1, A_2, A_3, C_1, and C_2 domains of factor VIII in a complex with calcium (Chap. 113).[13] Activated factor VIII (factor VIIIa) and activated factor IX (factor IXa) associate on the surface of activated platelets, forming a functional factor X-activating complex ("tenase" or "Xase").[14] In the presence of factor VIIIa, the rate of factor X activation by factor IXa is dramatically enhanced. That hemophilia A and hemophilia B have similar clinical manifestations is not surprising, because both factor VIIIa and factor IXa are required to form the Xase complex. The lack of either activated protein leads to a similar lack of platelet surface Xase activity with subsequent decreased thrombin generation. In patients with hemophilia, clot formation is delayed because of the decreased thrombin generation. The clot that is formed is friable, easily dislodged, and highly susceptible to fibrinolysis, all of which lead to excessive bleeding and poor wound healing.[15]

GENETICS

Hemophilia A results when mutations occur in the factor VIII gene located on the long arm of the X-chromosome (X-q28). The disease occurs almost exclusively in males. Figure 123–1 shows the inheritance pattern of hemophilia A and hemophilia B. All the sons of affected hemophilic males are normal, whereas all the daughters are obligatory carriers of the factor VIII defect. Sons of carriers have a 50 percent chance of being affected, whereas daughters of carriers have a 50 percent chance of being carriers themselves.

	Hemophilic male X^h	Hemophilic male Y
Normal female X	XX^h (Carrier female)	XY (Normal male)
Normal female X	XX^h (Carrier female)	XY (Normal male)

	Normal male X	Normal male Y
Carrier female X^h	XX^h (Carrier female)	X^hY (Hemophilic male)
Carrier female X	XX (Normal female)	XY (Normal male)

Figure 123–1. Inheritance pattern of hemophilia. All daughters of a hemophilic male are carriers of hemophilia, whereas all sons are normal. Daughters of carriers have a 50 percent chance of being a carrier, whereas sons of carriers have a 50 percent chance of having hemophilia. X, normal; X^h, abnormal X chromosome with the hemophilic gene; X^hY, hemophilic male; XX, normal female; XX^h, carrier female; XY, normal male; Y, normal.

The factor VIII gene is very large, approximately 186 kb, with approximately 9 kb of exons. The gene contains 26 exons and 25 introns.[16] Based on the sequence of the factor VIII gene in normal individuals and patients with hemophilia A, numerous specific mutations have been described[16,17]; as of 2015, more than 2000 specific variants in the factor VIII gene resulting in classic hemophilia have been described.[17]

Hemophilia A can result from multiple alterations in the factor VIII gene. These include gene rearrangements; missense mutations, in which a single base substitution leads to an amino acid change in the molecule; nonsense mutations, which result in a stop codon; abnormal splicing of the gene; deletions of all or portions of the gene; and insertions of genetic elements.[18] The genetic defects leading to hemophilia have been reviewed.[17]

One of the most common mutations, accounting for 40 to 50 percent of severe hemophilia A patients, is a unique "combined gene inversion and crossing over" that disrupts the factor VIII gene.[19,20] Figures 123–2 and 123–3 schematically depict the factor VIII gene and the mechanism of the "inversion–crossing over."[21] Within intron 22 are two other genes: (1) *F8A*(a_1), which is transcribed in the 5′ direction, and (2) *F8B*, which is transcribed in the 3′ direction of the factor VIII gene. The hatched boxes in Figure 123–3 show two other extragenic homologous sequences (a_2,a_3) 5′ to the *F8A* gene that lies within intron 22 (a_1). The presence of extragenic *F8A* sequences 5′ to the *F8A* gene within intron 22 is central to the inversion and translocation of part of the factor VIII gene from exon 1 to exon 22. The mechanism is homologous recombination between the *F8A* sequence that lies within intron 22 and one of the homologous extragenic sequences of the *F8A* gene 5′ to the factor VIII gene. During meiosis, crossing over of homologous sequences occurs between the *F8A* gene lying within intron 22 and one of the extragenic homologous *F8A* sequences 5′ to intron 22. Thus, the transcription of the complete factor VIII sequence is interrupted (Fig. 123–3). Figure 123–3 shows a common inversion and crossing over, but homologous recombinations can occur with either of the extragenic genes. Approximately 2 to 5 percent of the severe cases of hemophilia A carry the intron 1 inversion resulting in the separation of the F8 promoter-exon 1 sequence from the remainder of the *F8* gene.[22] The "inversion–crossing over" mutations result in severe hemophilia, and approximately 20 percent of these patients are susceptible to developing antibody inhibitors that neutralize factor VIII coagulant function.

Of the different insertions in the factor VIII gene that have been reported, a few are long interspersed elements (LINEs) that are transposon sequences; that is, sequences that have been inserted frequently throughout the genome.[23] Most of these insertions result in severe hemophilia.

In many cases of hemophilia, there is no family history of the disease, and at least 30 percent of the cases of hemophilia are a result of spontaneous *(de novo)* mutations. Most of these occur at CpG dinucleotides in the factor VIII gene.[23] *De novo* occurrences of hemophilia usually result from a mutation in the gamete of a normal male; for example, a mutation in the germ cell of a maternal grandfather will give rise to the hemophilia gene in his daughters such that his grandsons may have hemophilia.[18] Codons for the amino acid arginine (CGA [cytosine, guanine, adenine]) are frequently affected by mutations at CG doublets. A C→T transition often results in a stop codon with synthesis of a truncated factor VIII molecule and usually is associated with severe hemophilia A. However, a G→A transition results in a missense mutation, which often leads to a dysfunctional factor VIII molecule that may be associated with mild, moderate, or severe hemophilia. Some missense

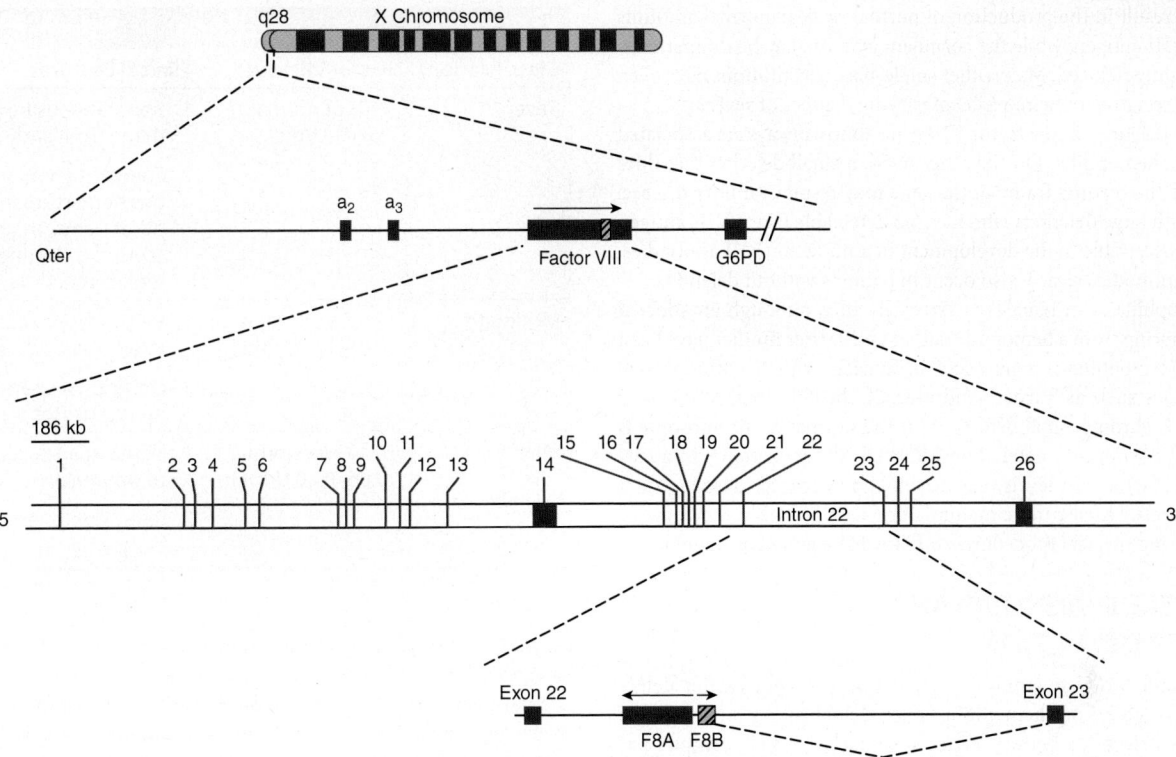

Figure 123–2. Schematic of the factor VIII gene *(FVIII)*. The *FVIII* gene is located at q28 on the long arm of the X chromosome. The region of the *FVIII* gene is enlarged on the *second line*. Note that two genes, designated a₂ and a₃, are 5′ to the *FVIII* gene. The *hatched area* indicated on *FVIII* corresponds to intron 22 shown on the *third line*. Within intron 22 *(fourth line)* are two nested genes, one designated *F8A*, which is transcribed in a direction opposite to that of the whole *FVIII* and is homologous to the a₂ and a₃ genes shown on *line 2*. G6PD, glucose-6-phosphate dehydrogenase. *(Reproduced with permission from Scriver CR, Beaudet AL, Sly WS et al: Metabolic and Molecular Basis of Inherited Diseases, 8th ed. McGraw-Hill, New York, 1995.)*

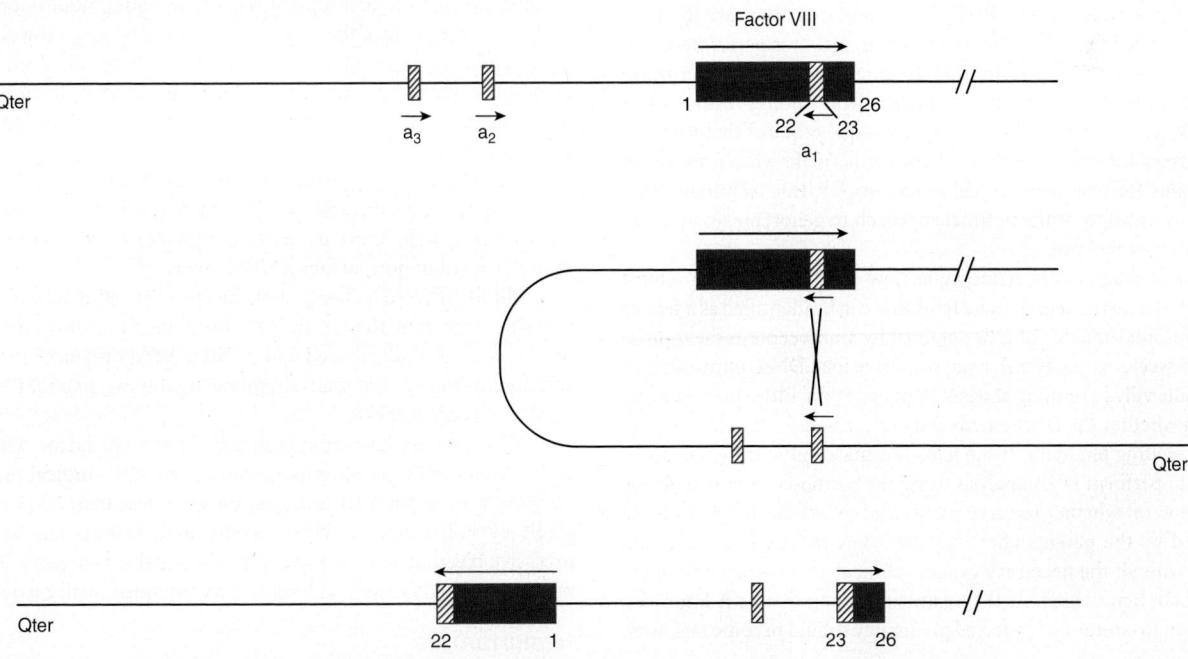

Figure 123–3. Schematic of inversion and crossing over at intron 22. Inversion and crossing-over of the a₃ gene with its homologous sequence a₁ nested within intron 22 are shown. *Middle panel:* When crossing over of the a₁ gene nested within intron 22 and the a₃ gene extragenic to *FVIII* occurs, a portion of *FVIII* is transcribed in a reverse manner from exon 1 through exon 22. Homologous recombination with the extragenic a₂ gene is also possible. In some individuals there are two a₂ or a₃ extragenic sequences giving rise to four possible types of the "inversion–crossing over" mechanism. *(Reproduced with permission from Antonarakis SE, Kazazian HH, Tuddenham EG: Molecular etiology of factor VIII deficiency in hemophilia A. Hum Mutat 1995;5(1):1–22.)*

mutations result in the production of normal or near-normal amounts of factor VIII antigen, while the coagulant activity may be dramatically or only slightly reduced. Many other single-base substitutions have been described, resulting in hemophilia of varying degrees of severity.

Large deletions in the factor VIII gene almost always are associated with severe hemophilia. On the other hand, a small deletion that does not change the reading frame of the gene may result in milder disease. Patients with large deletions who have no detectable factor VIII antigen are more susceptible to the development of anti–factor VIII antibodies, although antibodies clearly also occur in patients without deletions.[16,23]

Hemophilia A in females is extremely rare, although an affected female offspring from a hemophilic father and carrier mother have been reported. Hemophilia A may occur in females with X chromosomal abnormalities such as Turner syndrome, X chromosomal mosaicism, and other X chromosomal defects.[23,24] If the normal X chromosome is inactivated disproportionately ("imbalanced X inactivation") in a carrier female, factor VIII levels may be sufficiently low to cause bleeding manifestations. Usually these manifestations are mild, but they may be serious during surgical procedures or following significant trauma.

PRENATAL DIAGNOSIS AND CARRIER DETECTION

A careful and complete family history is important for carrier detection.[25] All daughters of a hemophilic father are obligatory carriers of the hemophilic defect. If a known carrier has a daughter, that daughter has a 50 percent chance of being a carrier.

Carrier detection is important when a daughter of a known carrier or a female offspring of a hemophilic patient wishes to become pregnant. At times, the history of hemophilia in the family is in a distant blood relative, and the gene for hemophilia may skip several generations. The current standard for identifying carrier status is through direct gene sequencing. Carriers who harbor the intron 22 inversion or intron 1 inversion can be identified using the Southern blot technique and polymerase chain reaction, respectively.[22,25] If these mutations are found to be absent, sequencing of the complete coding region is performed.[26]

Use of markers for restriction fragment length polymorphism (RFLP) is simpler than direct sequencing of the coding region of the factor VIII gene, but use of the RFLP technique requires that the pedigree analyses include at least one hemophilic male whose mother is heterozygous for one or more RFLP markers.[27,28] This technique is no longer considered to be the optimal approach in genotyping of affected males or carrier females.

Prenatal diagnosis of hemophilia now can be performed almost routinely.[29] If a carrier female has a fetus that can be identified as a female by chromosomal analysis of cells obtained by amniocentesis (at approximately 16 weeks of gestation), analysis of free fetal DNA, ultrasound or by chorionic villus sampling at week 10 of gestation, little concern exists regarding whether the female fetus is a carrier because carriers usually have no bleeding tendency. If the fetus is a male, sufficient cells can be obtained to perform DNA analysis using the methods described above. The decision on whether to carry an affected male fetus to term should be decided by the parents after they are appropriately counseled and provided with all the necessary genetic, clinical, and therapeutic information about hemophilia. As the treatment for hemophilia A improves, the decision to continue an affected pregnancy should become far easier.

CLINICAL FEATURES

Hemophilia A is characterized by excessive bleeding into various tissues of the body, including soft-tissue hematomas and hemarthroses that can lead to severe crippling hemarthropathy. Recurrent hemarthroses are characteristic of the disease. The disease has been broadly classified

TABLE 123–1. Clinical Classification of Hemophilia		
Classification	**Factor VIII Level**	**Clinical Features**
Severe	≤1% of normal (≤0.01 U/mL)	1. Spontaneous hemorrhage from early infancy 2. Frequent spontaneous hemarthroses and other hemorrhages, requiring clotting factor replacement
Moderate	1–5% of normal (0.01–0.05 U/mL)	1. Hemorrhage secondary to trauma or surgery 2. Occasional spontaneous hemarthroses
Mild	6–40% of normal (0.06–0.40 U/mL)	1. Hemorrhage secondary to trauma or surgery 2. Rare spontaneous hemorrhage

as mild, moderate, and severe, although overlap exists between these categories. Table 123–1 shows a classification based on the severity of clinical manifestations. A range of plasma factor VIII concentrations in percentages of normal and in units per milliliter is given for each category. Approximately 10 percent of individuals with factor VIII levels compatible with severe hemophilia may exhibit milder symptoms.[30] Among other explanations, this phenotypic heterogeneity could be a result of coinheritance of thrombophilic mutations, such as the factor V Leiden mutation (R506Q).[31] Severely affected patients (<1 percent factor VIII) frequently experience "spontaneous" bleeding without known trauma other than that associated with the usual day-to-day activities. Without effective treatment, recurrent hemarthroses, resulting in chronic hemophilic arthropathy, occur by young adulthood and are highly characteristic of the severe form of the disorder. However, bleeding episodes are intermittent, and some patients do not bleed for weeks or months. Except for intracranial bleeding, sudden death because of hemorrhage is rare in societies where clotting factor concentrates are freely available.

Moderately affected patients with hemophilia may have occasional hematomas. Hemarthroses, usually associated with a known trauma, may occur as well. These patients have greater than 1 percent but less than 5 percent of normal factor VIII activity.

Mildly affected patients with hemophilia, who have factor VIII levels between 6 to 40 percent, have infrequent bleeding episodes. The disease may go undiagnosed and be discovered only because of excessive hemorrhage postoperatively, following trauma, or after the toss and tumble of contact sports.

Most carriers have approximately 50 percent factor VIII activity and experience no bleeding symptoms, even with surgical procedures. Carriers with factor VIII levels significantly less than 50 percent, as a result of imbalanced X chromosome inactivation, may experience excessive bleeding after trauma (e.g., childbirth or surgery). Therefore, measurement of factor VIII level is recommended in all carriers.

Hemarthroses

Bleeding into joints accounts for approximately 75 percent of bleeding episodes in severely affected patients with hemophilia A.[32,33] The normal synovium has few cells, but numerous capillaries beneath the synovial layer can be damaged by the mechanical trauma associated with daily use of joints. The joints most frequently involved, in decreasing order of frequency are knees, elbows, ankles, shoulders, wrists, and hips.

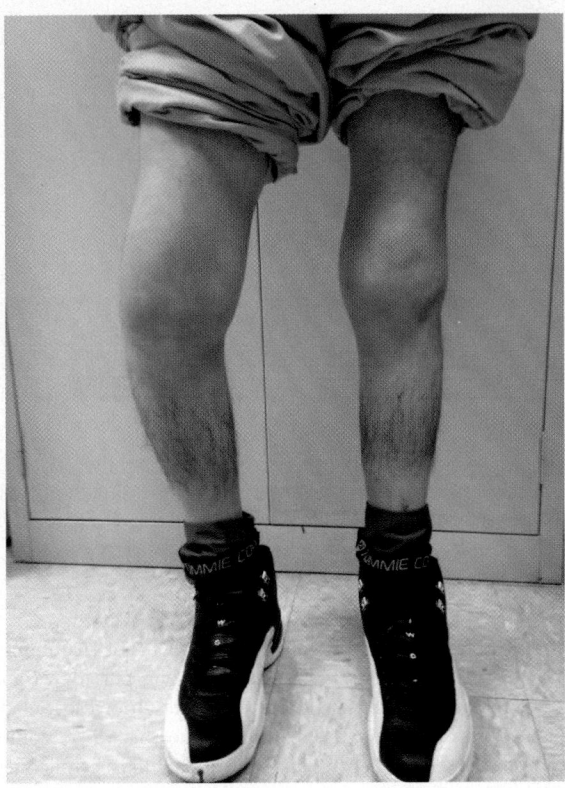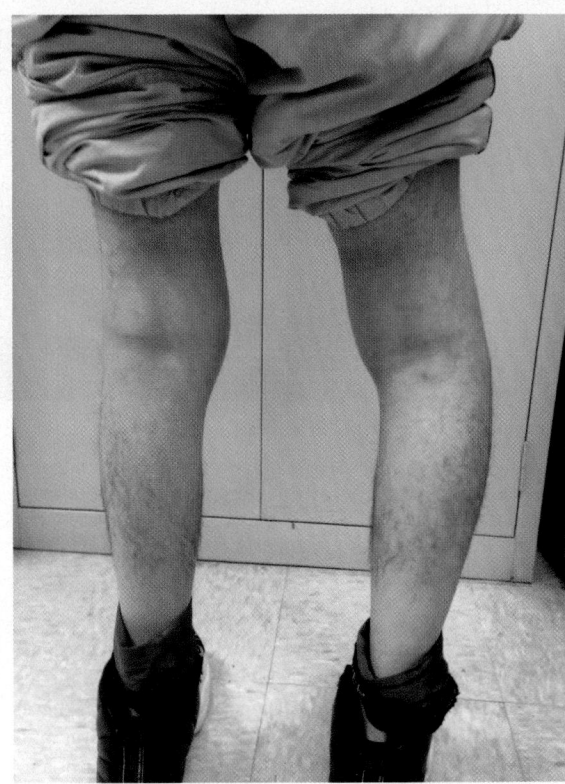

Figure 123–4. Hemophilic arthropathy. The chronic effects of repeated hemorrhage into the knees of a severely affected hemophilic patient are seen. Note contractures, and deformity with atrophy of muscle tissue.

Hinge joints are much more likely to be involved than are ball-and-socket joints. Hemarthroses usually occur when an affected child begins to walk.

Hemarthroses are heralded by an aura of mild discomfort that, over a period of minutes to hours, becomes progressively painful. The joint usually swells, becomes warm, and exhibits limited motion. Occasionally, the patient experiences a mild fever. Significant and sustained fever, however, suggests an infected joint. When joint bleeding does not respond to replacement therapy, one should suspect the presence of an inhibitor of factor VIII or an infected joint. Bleeding into the knee joint is more easily detected by physical findings than is bleeding into either the elbow or shoulder. When bleeding stops, the blood resorbs, and the symptoms gradually subside over a period of several days. If hemarthroses are treated early, pain usually subsides in 6 to 8 hours and disappears in 12 to 24 hours. However, repeated hemorrhage into the joints eventually results in extensive destruction of articular cartilage, synovial hyperplasia, and other reactive changes in the adjacent bone and tissues. Iron deposits from residual blood is a major factor in the pathogenesis of hemophilic arthropathy.[33] Acute bleeding into a chronically affected joint may be difficult to distinguish from the pain of degenerative arthritis.

A major complication of repeated hemarthroses is joint deformity complicated by muscle atrophy and soft-tissue contractures (Fig. 123–4). Figure 123–5 shows the various radiologic stages of progressive destruction of joint cartilage and adjacent bone. Osteoporosis and cystic areas in the subchondral bone may develop, and progressive loss of joint space occurs. Figure 123–6 shows a magnetic resonance image (MRI) of a normal knee in comparison to a knee from an individual with severe hemophilia with arthropathy. Figure 123–7 depicts bleeding into a hemophilic ankle.

Repeated bleeding into a joint results in synovial hypertrophy and inflammation. The synovium is thickened and folded, leading to limited joint motion. The result is a tendency for repeated hemorrhages leading to a so-called target joint.[32] Indeed, a target joint is defined by the occurrence of three or more spontaneous bleeds within a 6-month period. The joints most often involved are the knees, ankles, and elbows, which become chronically swollen. Chronic synovitis may persist for months or years unless the condition is adequately treated.

Infection of hemophilic joints is not common but must be suspected in all patients with fever, leukocytosis, or other systemic manifestations. Rapid diagnosis is mandatory, because infection of such joints leads to rapid loss of joint architecture and function. A painful and swollen joint may require aspiration, which should be performed by experienced personnel using meticulous aseptic techniques and appropriate factor replacement therapy prior to aspiration.

Hematomas

Soft-tissue hematomas are also characteristic of hemophilia A. Hemorrhage into subcutaneous connective tissues or into muscles may occur with or without a known trauma. Hematomas, once formed, may stabilize and slowly resorb. However, in moderately and severely affected patients, hematomas have a tendency to enlarge progressively and to dissect in all directions, unless appropriately treated. Rarely, retroperitoneal hematomas, after beginning in the iliopsoas muscle, can dissect superiorly through the diaphragm, into the chest, and sometimes even into the soft tissues of the neck, compromising the airway. A retroperitoneal hematoma is more likely to compromise renal function by causing ureteral obstruction. Figure 123–8 shows the computed tomography (CT) scan of a patient with a retroperitoneal hemorrhage. Other hematomas expand locally and may compress adjacent organs, blood

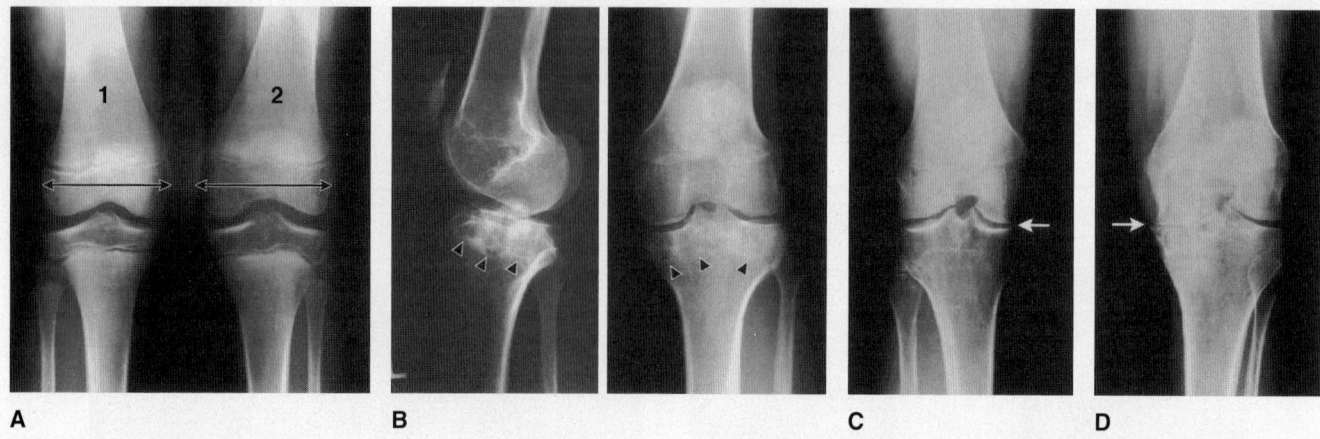

Figure 123–5. Various radiologic stages of hemophilic arthropathy. Stages 0 (normal joint) and 1 (fluid in the joint) are not shown. **A.** Stage 2. Some osteoporosis and epiphyseal overgrowth are present in knee 2. Epiphysis is wider in knee 2 than in knee 1 *(arrows)*. **B.** Stage 3. Subchondral bone cysts *(arrowheads)*. Joint spaces exhibit irregularities. **C.** Stage 4. Prominent bone cysts with marked narrowing of joint space *(arrow)*. **D.** Stage 5. Obliteration of joint space with epiphyseal overgrowth *(arrow)*.

vessels, and nerves. A rare, and often fatal, complication of an abdominal hematoma is perforation and drainage into the colon. Subcutaneous hematomas may dissect into muscle. Pharyngeal and retropharyngeal hematomas, sometimes complicating simple colds, may enlarge and obstruct the airway. Hemorrhage in or around the airway is a potentially life-threatening situation that requires prompt administration of factor VIII.

Hemorrhages occur into muscle in the following order of frequency: calf, thigh, buttocks, and forearm. Recurrent or unresolved hematomas may lead to muscle contractures, nerve palsies, and muscle

atrophy. Bleeding into the tongue (Fig. 123–9) or frenulum is particularly frequent in young children and usually is caused by trauma.

Bleeding into fascia and muscle can result in a so-called compartment syndrome. This results when hemorrhage in a confined space compresses the arterial vasculature resulting in ischemic muscle injury. Compartment syndrome tends to occur in the distal part of the extremities, particularly in the flexor muscles, and sometimes requires urgent fasciotomy under cover of clotting factor replacement therapy. Bleeding into the myocardium or erect penis is very unusual, perhaps explained by the high concentration of tissue factor in these tissues.

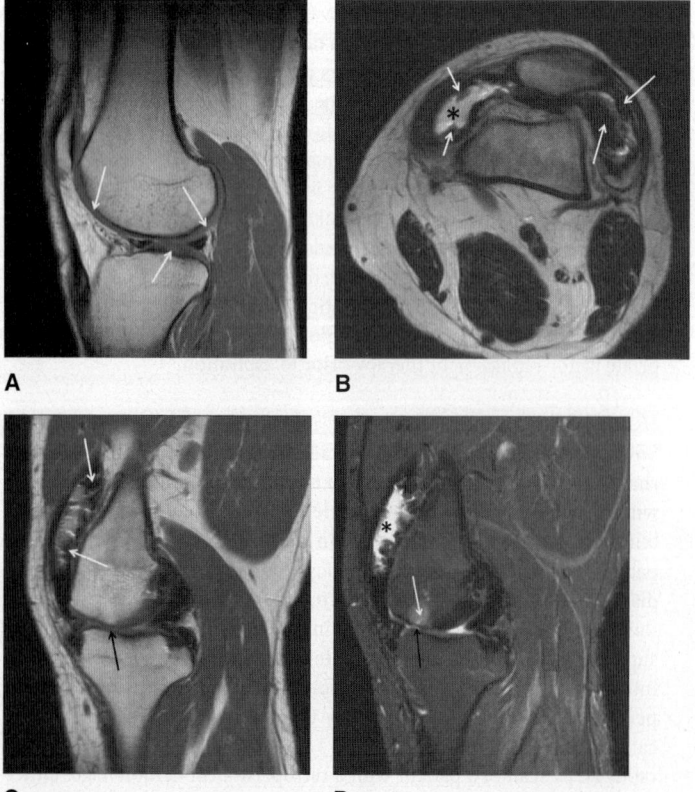

Figure 123–6. Magnetic resonance imaging (MRI) of normal and hemophilic knees. **A.** MRI of normal knee. **B.** A transverse T2-weighted spin-echo image of the knee shows an effusion *(*)* and multiple foci of hemosiderin deposition *(arrows)* along the synovium lining the suprapatellar bursa. **C.** A sagittal T2-weighted spin-echo image of the knee shows dark foci of synovial hemosiderin deposition *(white arrows)* accompanied by narrowing of the femorotibial joint *(black arrow)*. **D.** A sagittal STIR (short tau inversion recovery) image of the knee (in the same patient as **B**) demonstrates an effusion in the suprapatellar bursa *(asterisks)*. The irregular, lumpy surface of the bursa represents thickened, hemosiderin-laden synovium. Femorotibial joint narrowing *(black arrow)* is associated with edema in the subchondral bone of the femoral condyle *(white arrow)*. *(Used with permission of Dr. Jordan Renner, University of North Carolina.)*

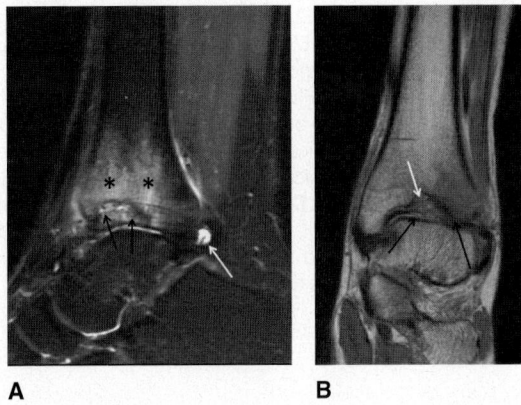

A   **B**

Figure 123–7. A. A sagittal STIR (short tau inversion recovery) image of an ankle shows an effusion *(white arrow)*. Edema in the distal tibia *(asterisks)* surrounds a debris-filled defect in the subchondral bone of the distal tibia *(black arrows)*. **B.** A coronal proton density of the ankle in the same patient as in **A** shows the defect in the subchondral bone of the distal tibia *(white arrow)*. Mild narrowing of the tibiotalar joint *(black arrows)* is more apparent laterally.

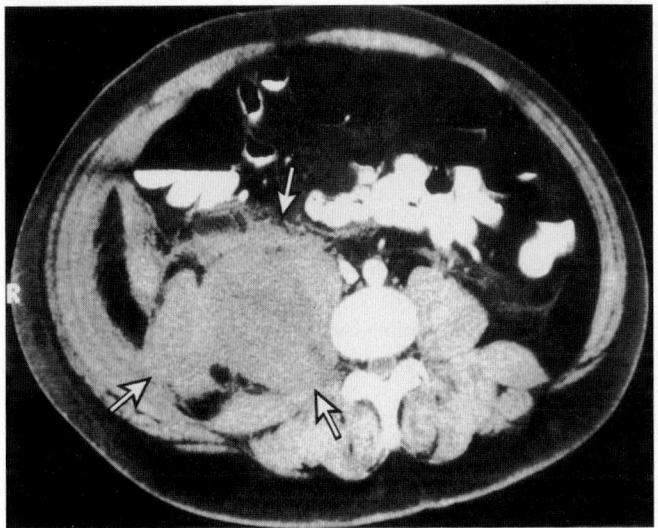

Figure 123–8. Computed tomography scan of a retroperitoneal hematoma in a patient with severe hemophilia A. Extent of the hematoma is indicated by the *arrows*.

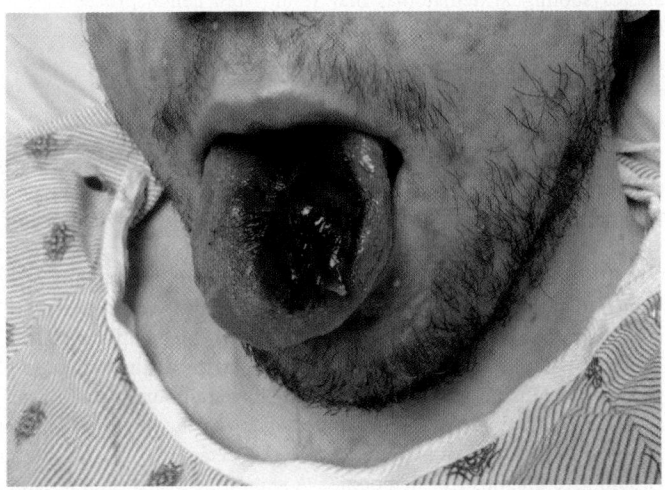

Figure 123–9. Photograph of a tongue hematoma caused by trauma.

Pseudotumors (Blood Cysts)

Pseudotumors are blood cysts that occur in soft tissues or bone. They are rare but dangerous complications of hemophilia (Fig. 123–10).[34] They are classified into three types. One type is a simple cyst that is confined by tendinous attachments within the fascial envelope of a muscle. The second type initially develops as a simple cyst in soft tissues such as a tendon, but it interferes with the vascular supply to the adjacent bone and periosteum, resulting in cyst formation and resorption of bone. The third type is thought to result from subperiosteal bleeding that separates the periosteum from the bony cortex. Most pseudotumors are not associated with pain unless rapid growth or nerve compression occurs. As the volume of the cyst increases, the cyst compresses and destroys the adjacent muscle, nerve, and/or bone or expands around structures like ureters causing renal failure. Pseudotumors usually contain either serosanguineous fluid or a viscous brownish material surrounded by a fibrous membrane (Fig. 123–10). Pseudotumors have a tendency to expand over several years and eventually become multiloculated. Some reach enormous size and involve so many structures that make them inoperable. Erosion through surrounding tissues and penetration into viscera or through the skin can occur, usually as a late event. Sinus tracts from the pseudotumor predispose to infection and septicemia. Pseudotumors often develop in the lower half of the body, usually in the thigh, buttock, or pelvis, but they can occur anywhere, including the temporal bone. CT or MRI is useful for diagnosis. Needle biopsies of pseudotumors should be avoided because of the risk of infection and hemorrhage. A reliable treatment is operative removal of the entire mass because the pseudotumor likely will reform if it is not completely removed. Embolization, percutaneous drainage, and radiotherapy of a pseudotumor have been reported and may be of value in hemophiliacs with inhibitors when surgery is not possible.[35] Surgical treatment of patients with large pseudotumors should be done in a hemophilia treatment center with a specialized multidisciplinary team of experts.[36]

Hematuria

Many severely affected patients with hemophilia experience episodes of spontaneous and asymptomatic hematuria. The urine may be brown or red, depending upon the rate of bleeding. Most bleeding arises from the renal pelvis, usually from one kidney but occasionally from both. Appropriate studies to exclude a structural lesion in the kidneys should be performed. Administration of factor replacement and hydration is usually sufficient to arrest the bleeding. Antifibrinolytic agents, such as aminocaproic acid and tranexamic acid should be avoided in individuals with hematuria because of the risk of forming clots and producing obstructing clots in the ureter.

Neurologic Complications

Intracranial bleeding is one of the most dangerous hemorrhagic events in hemophilic patients.[37] Currently, bleeding into the brain is a leading cause of death in hemophilic patients. Hemorrhage into the central nervous system may be "spontaneous" but usually follows trauma, which may be trivial. Symptoms often occur soon after trauma, but sometimes are delayed. For example, symptoms of a subdural hematoma may be delayed for days or several weeks. Hemorrhage into the brain parenchyma or a subdural or epidural hematoma should always be suspected in hemophilic patients with unusual headaches. When intracranial bleeding is suspected, the patient should be treated immediately with factor VIII and diagnostic procedures, such as CT scans or MRI studies should be delayed until after treatment is initiated. Although lumbar puncture has been performed safely in severe hemophilic patients without replacement therapy, replacing factor VIII to a level of approximately 50 percent of normal prior to the procedure is advisable.

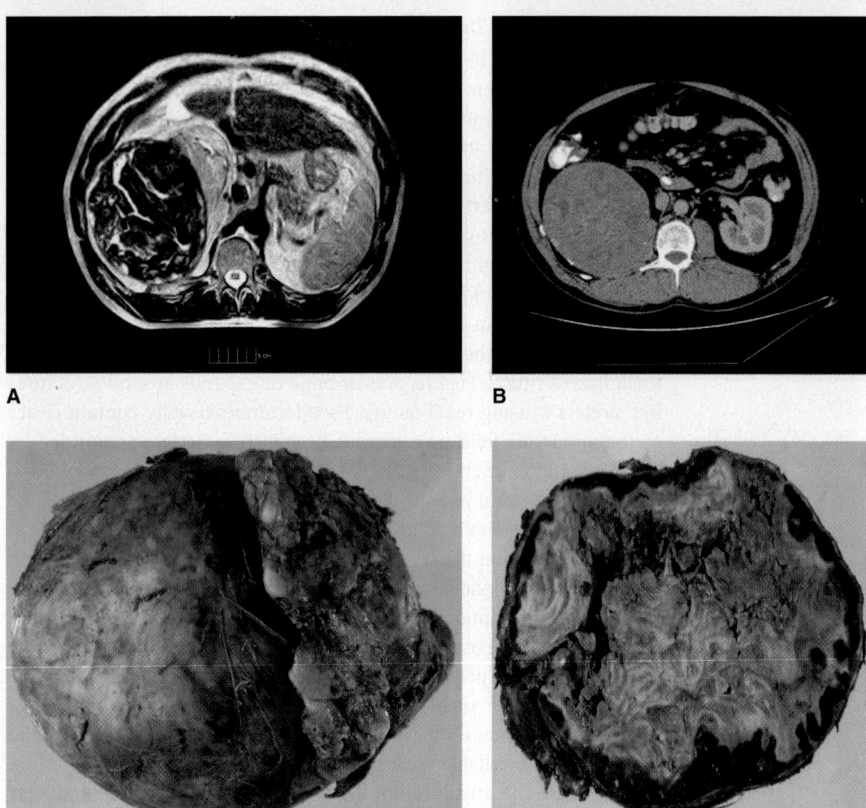

Figure 123–10. Retroperitoneal pseudotumor. **A** and **B.** Magnetic resonance imaging and computed tomography scan of pseudotumor arising from the iliopsoas muscle compressing the kidney and other adjacent structures. Loculations and calcifications can be seen. **C.** Gross specimen after surgical removal, weighting approximately 6 pounds. **D.** Cross-section of pseudotumor shows peripheral red hemorrhage, centrally caseified blood and necrosis. Note the thick capsule that surrounds the tumor.

Hemorrhage into the spinal canal is an uncommon neurologic complication in hemophilia, mostly related to trauma that can result in paraplegia. Bleeding may occur within the spinal cord itself, but epidural bleeding compressing the cord is more common.

Peripheral nerve compression is a frequent complication of muscle hematomas, particularly in the extremities. Compression of the femoral nerve by a hematoma in the iliopsoas muscle can result in sensory loss over the lateral and anterior thigh, weakness and atrophy of the quadriceps, and loss of the patellar reflex. The ulnar nerve is the next most frequently involved peripheral nerve. Bleeding may occur in any muscle and may compress local neural blood supply. This situation can be followed by permanent neuromuscular defects and multiple contractures.

Mucous Membrane Hemorrhage

Mucous membrane bleeding is common in hemophilia. Epistaxis and hemoptysis, often resulting from allergic reactions or trauma, can be associated with local structural lesions involving the upper and/or lower respiratory tract. Treatment of epistaxis by cautery or nasal packing sometimes is followed by recurrent bleeding because of sloughing of the cauterized area or dislodging of a poorly formed clot when the packing is removed. Gastrointestinal hemorrhage has a 1.3 percent annual incidence and is mostly associated with older age and complications of advanced liver disease. Ingestion of antiinflammatory drugs for relief of pain of hemophilic arthropathy is a frequent cause of upper gastrointestinal hemorrhage, and a history of ingestion of aspirin and other antiinflammatory drugs should be specifically addressed (and proscribed) when assessing the etiology of such bleeding.[38]

Dental and Surgical Bleeding

Hemophilic patients are treated with clotting factor preoperatively and postoperatively to prevent bleeding. Mildly or sometimes moderately affected patients may go unrecognized until surgery results in excessive bleeding at the surgical site. Bleeding may be delayed for several hours or, occasionally, for several days. Surgery in such patients is characterized by delayed wound healing because of poor clot formation.[15] Prolonged bleeding and subsequent infection of the wound hematoma may further complicate healing. Appropriate factor VIII replacement therapy, sometimes supplemented by anti-fibrinolytic agents, can prevent intraoperative and postoperative hemorrhages.

Dental extraction is the most frequent surgical procedure performed on hemophilic patients. Loss of deciduous teeth seldom causes excessive bleeding, but extraction of permanent teeth may result in excessive hemorrhage that can persist intermittently for several days to weeks unless appropriate treatment is administered. In the untreated patient with severe hemophilia, life-threatening, dissecting pharyngeal and/or sublingual hematomas may result from dental procedures or from administration of regional block anesthesia.

LABORATORY FEATURES

Patients with severe hemophilia A have a prolonged activated partial thromboplastin time (aPTT). The prothrombin time (PT) and thrombin clotting time (TCT) are normal. Different combinations of aPTT reagents and instrumentation exhibit varying sensitivities to factor VIII levels. In mild hemophilia, the aPTT may be only slightly prolonged or at the upper limit of normal, especially if factor VIII activity is 20 percent or greater. The aPTT is corrected when hemophilic plasma is mixed with an equal volume of normal plasma. If the hemophilic plasma contains an anti-factor VIII inhibitor antibody, the aPTT on a similar mixture is prolonged, but incubation of the mixture for 1 or 2 hours at 37°C is sometimes required to detect the prolongation. A definitive diagnosis of hemophilia A should be based on a specific assay for factor VIII activity.

Functional factor VIII coagulant activity is measured by one-stage clotting assays based on the aPTT. Chromogenic assays for factor VIII activity also are used widely, but do not always agree with one-stage assays.[39] Although infrequently measured in practice, factor VIII antigen is measured by immunologic assays, which detect normal and most abnormal factor VIII molecules. If the factor VIII antigen level is normal but the clotting activity is reduced, the patient has a dysfunctional factor VIII molecule. Such patients have antigen-positive hemophilia, also referred to as cross-reacting material (CRM)-positive.[40] Patients in whom both the factor VIII antigen level and activity are nearly undetectable are said to be CRM-negative.

DIFFERENTIAL DIAGNOSIS

VWD sometimes is confused with hemophilia A. The basic defect in VWD is reduced activity of von Willebrand factor (VWF), which acts as a carrier of factor VIII *in vivo* (Chap. 126). Thus, in VWD, factor VIII levels are reduced, although considerable variability exists. Although factor VIII is synthesized normally in patients with VWD, the half-life of factor VIII is markedly shortened because the VWF "carrier" molecule is decreased or absent. Other abnormalities in VWD that distinguish VWD from hemophilia A are decreased VWF antigen level, and decreased VWF activity, often measured using the ristocetin cofactor activity assay and a prolonged closure time using the platelet function analyzer PFA-100. In type III VWD, factor VIII levels may be very low (<5 percent of normal), making it difficult to distinguish from classical hemophilia. The lack of a sex-linked pattern of inheritance in the family will help in the differential diagnosis.

Another variant of VWD that is particularly difficult to distinguish from hemophilia A is VWD-Normandy, in which VWF multimers are normal but plasma factor VIII levels are low.[41] Several mutations causing VWD-Normandy have been described, but all of them result in decreased binding of factor VIII to VWF.[42] The result is shortening of the intravascular survival of factor VIII and thus reduced factor VIII activity. The Normandy variant of VWD should be suspected in patients with mild hemophilia A who do not exhibit a sex-linked recessive inheritance pattern.

Hemophilia A must be distinguished from other hereditary blood clotting factor deficiencies that exhibit a prolonged aPTT, including deficiencies of factors IX, XI, and XII, prekallikrein, and high-molecular-weight kininogen. Only deficiencies of factors VIII and IX cause chronic crippling hemarthroses with a family history suggestive of an X-linked bleeding disorder. Only specific assays can distinguish hemophilia A from factor IX deficiency (hemophilia B). Factor XI deficiency occurs in males and females and is a milder hemorrhagic disorder compared to severe hemophilia A or B. Factor XI deficiency can be confused with mild hemophilia A or B on screening laboratory tests, but specific assays distinguish them. Deficiencies of factor XII, prekallikrein, and high-molecular-weight kininogen can be distinguished from hemophilia because they are not associated with bleeding. Mild hemophilia A, with factor VIII levels of approximately 10 to 20 percent of normal, must be distinguished from combined deficiency of factors V and VIII.[43,44] Both the PT and aPTT are moderately prolonged in the combined disorder.[44]

THERAPY

General

General principles applicable to therapy for hemophilia A include avoidance of aspirin, nonsteroidal antiinflammatory drugs, and other agents that interfere with platelet aggregation. Acetaminophen or relatively specific cyclooxygenase (COX)-2 inhibitors such as celecoxib have been recommended, but these drugs can be harmful when taken in excessive doses or for prolonged periods. Patients should be advised of the numerous nonprescription analgesics and herbals that contain aspirin or other antiplatelet agents. Addictive narcotic agents should be used with great caution and only when clearly indicated, because drug dependency can be a major problem for patients with hemophilia. In general, intramuscular injections should be avoided unless the patient receives adequate replacement therapy. In the absence of prophylactic therapy, patients with hemophilia A must be treated as early as possible to avoid bleeding complications. Surgical procedures in hemophilic patients should be scheduled early in the week to avoid "weekend crises." Ample supplies of factor VIII should be available in the blood bank or pharmacy to ensure rapid access to treatment when needed. All hemophilic patients should have access to home treatment and periodic examinations at a comprehensive hemophilia treatment center. Prophylactic therapy is recommended in all severely affected patients, and it should be initiated before the onset of recurrent hemarthroses (primary prophylaxis) or as directed. Secondary prophylaxis for an established "target" joint may be necessary.[45]

Factor VIII Replacement Therapy

Hemorrhagic episodes in patients with hemophilia A can be managed by replacing factor VIII. Several products are available for use in raising factor VIII to hemostatic levels (Table 123–2). Fresh-frozen plasma and

TABLE 123–2. Currently Available Factor VIII Products[a]		
	Origin	**Viral Inactivation**
Intermediate purity		
Humate P[b]	Plasma	Pasteurization[c]
High purity		
Koate DVI[b]	Plasma	Solvent-detergent[d], heat treated[i]
Alphanate[b]	Plasma	Solvent-detergent, heat treated[i]
Ultrapure[e]		
Hemofil M	Plasma	Solvent-detergent[d]
Monoclate P	Plasma	Pasteurization[c]
Recombinant		
Advate[h]	CHO cells[f]	Solvent-detergent[d]
Recombinate[e]	CHO cells[f]	
Kogenate FS[e]	BHK cells[g]	Solvent-detergent
Helixate FS[e]	BHK cells[g]	Solvent-detergent
Xyntha[h]	CHO cells[f]	Solvent-detergent, nanofiltration
Eloctate*[h]	HEK cells[j]	Solvent-detergent

*Extended half-life FVIII product.
[a]Additional concentrates are available in Europe.
[b]Contains von Willebrand factor (VWF).
[c]Pasteurization at 60°C for 10 hours.
[d]Solvent-detergent: tri-n-butyl phosphate (TNBP) + polysorbate 80.
[e]Human albumin added; insignificant VWF.
[f]Chinese hamster ovarian cells.
[g]Baby hamster kidney cells.
[h]Not exposed to human or animal protein during manufacture.
[i]Heat treated at 80°C for 72 hours.
[j]Human embryonic kidney cells.

cryoprecipitate both contain factor VIII and once were the only products available for treatment. A disadvantage of plasma is that large volumes must be infused to achieve and maintain even minimal factor VIII levels. The highest factor VIII level that can be achieved with plasma is approximately 20 percent of normal, which is not always attainable or sufficient for hemostasis. Cryoprecipitate, containing approximately 80 U of factor VIII in 10 mL of solution, can be used to attain normal factor VIII levels, but individual bags of cryoprecipitate must be pooled; the factor VIII dose can only be estimated; and the product must be stored frozen. Several commercial lyophilized factor VIII concentrates, using cryoprecipitate of pooled normal human plasmas as starting material (2000 to 20,000 donors), are available and do not have the disadvantages of plasma and cryoprecipitate (Table 123–2). Factor VIII concentrates have been sterilized by heating in solution, by superheating to 80°C after lyophilization, and by exposure to organic solvent-detergents that inactivate lipid-enveloped viruses, including HIV and hepatitides B and C viruses, but do not inactivate parvovirus or hepatitis A.[46,47] Parvovirus infection does not occur frequently in hemophilia A patients because parvovirus is transmitted by cellular elements of the blood. Nevertheless, seroconversion to B19 parvovirus has been observed in patients receiving plasma-derived concentrates undergoing solvent-detergent extraction or pasteurization.

Some of these products contain significant amounts of VWF (see Table 123–2). Plasma-derived factor VIII concentrates prepared by monoclonal antibody techniques, and subjected to viral inactivation techniques, are highly purified and, barring breakdown in manufacturing procedures, are considered to be safe in terms of transmission of viral diseases.

Factor VIII produced by recombinant DNA techniques is available, safe, and effective. There are new "third-generation" factor VIII products that are manufactured without exposure to animal or human protein. Although all factor VIII products, both recombinant and plasma-derived, are currently safe and effective, some physicians and patients prefer products that are not exposed to human or animal proteins during the manufacturing process.

The dose of factor VIII can be determined as follows. If 1 U of factor VIII per milliliter of plasma is considered 100 percent of normal, the dose required to raise the level to a given value depends upon the patient's plasma volume (approximately 5 percent of body weight in kilograms) and the level to which factor VIII is to be raised. Thus, the plasma volume of a 70 kg adult is approximately equivalent to 3500 mL (5 percent × 70 kg = 3.5 kg = 3500 g, approximately equivalent to 3500 mL). To achieve normal factor VIII levels of 1 U/mL (100 percent), 3500 U of factor VIII should be given. This scenario assumes a 100 percent recovery of the administered dose. Recovery has approached 100 percent in studies, but depends upon the method of assay and the factor VIII standard used for comparison.[48] After the initial dose of factor VIII, further doses of factor VIII are based on a half-life of 8 to 12 hours. Thus, after a loading dose of 3500 U of factor VIII, a dose of 1750 U could be given in 12 hours. However, for practical purposes, the dose of factor VIII is based on the knowledge that 1 U of factor VIII per kilogram of body weight raises the circulating factor VIII level by approximately 0.02 U/mL. Thus, to raise the factor VIII level to 100 percent, that is, 1 U/mL, the dose of factor VIII required is approximately 50 U per kilogram of body weight, assuming the patient's baseline factor VIII level is less than 1 percent of normal. The site and severity of hemorrhage determine the frequency and dose of factor VIII to be infused.

Table 123–3 summarizes the recommended doses of factor VIII for various types of hemorrhage.[48] These doses are not based on rigorous randomized studies, and recommendations vary among hemophilia centers. Given the high cost of factor VIII, some physicians prefer to use lower doses.

Factor VIII can be given as a constant infusion to hospitalized patients. Following a loading dose to raise factor VIII to the desired level, 150 to 300 U of factor VIII per hour can be infused. Factor VIII levels can be conveniently monitored in blood obtained from veins other than the vein into which factor VIII was infused intravenously.[49] In selected patients, factor VIII can be given outside the hospital in a continuous infusion using pump devices.[50]

DDAVP (Desmopressin)

During the 1970s, 1-desamino-8-D-arginine vasopressin (DDAVP; desmopressin) was found to cause a transient increase in factor VIII in normal subjects and in patients with mild to moderate hemophilia. After a dose of DDAVP (0.3 mcg per kilogram body weight), given intravenously or subcutaneously, factor VIII levels increase two- to

TABLE 123–3. Doses of Factor VIII for Treatment of Hemorrhage*

Site of Hemorrhage	Desired Factor VIII Level (% of Normal)	Factor VIII Dose† (U/kg Body Weight)	Frequency of Dose‡ (Every No. of Hours)	Duration (Days)
Hemarthroses	30–50	~25	12–24	1–2
Superficial intramuscular hematoma	30–50	~25	12–24	1–2
Gastrointestinal tract	50–100	50	12	7–10
Epistaxis	30–50	~25	12	Until resolved
Oral mucosa	30–50	~25	12	Until resolved
Hematuria	30–100	~25–50	12	Until resolved
Central nervous system	50–100	50	12	At least 7–10 days
Retropharyngeal	50–100	50	12	At least 7–10 days
Retroperitoneal	50–100	50	12	At least 7–10 days

*Mild or moderately affected patients may respond to 1-deamino-8-D-arginine vasopressin (DDAVP), which should be used in lieu of blood or blood products whenever possible.

†Factor VIII may be administered in a continuous infusion if the patient is hospitalized. After initial bolus, approximately 2 to 5 U/kg/h of factor VIII usually are sufficient in an average-size adult. Bolus doses are given every 12 to 24 hours.

‡The frequency of dosing and duration of therapy can be adjusted, depending on the severity and duration of the patient's bleeding episode.

threefold above baseline in most, but not all, mildly or moderately affected hemophilia A patients. Patients with severe hemophilia A do not respond to DDAVP.[51] A concentrated intranasal spray of DDAVP also can be used (150 mcg in each nostril for adults and 150 mcg in one nostril for children weighing less than 50 kg). The degree of response to the drug should always be determined in patients before a bleeding episode, because occasionally mildly or moderately affected patients do not respond. The peak response to DDAVP usually occurs 30 to 60 minutes after dosing. In patients with mild or moderate hemophilia A and in carriers whose baseline factor VIII levels are less than 0.5 U/mL, DDAVP may be used in lieu of blood products. The mechanism by which DDAVP increases factor VIII is unknown.

Repeated administration of DDAVP results in a diminished response to the agent (tachyphylaxis). In many patients, the response to the second DDAVP dose averages 30 percent less than the response to the first dose, and the response rate may be even less after additional doses.[52] DDAVP is a potent antidiuretic. As a result, hyponatremia has been reported in some patients whose water intake exceeds approximately 1 L per 24 hours after dosing. There is no convincing evidence to indicate that DDAVP administration is associated with thrombosis in hemophilic patients.

Antifibrinolytic Agents

Antifibrinolytic agents, such as ε-aminocaproic acid (EACA) and tranexamic acid, have been used to enhance hemostasis in patients with hemophilia A.[53,54] Fibrinolytic inhibitors may be given as adjunctive therapy for bleeding from mucous membranes and are particularly valuable as adjunctive therapy for dental procedures. The usual oral dose of tranexamic acid for adults is 1 g four times per day. EACA can be given as a loading dose of 4 to 5 g followed by 1 g/h by continuous IV infusion in adults. Another regimen of EACA is 4 g every 4 to 6 hours orally for 2 to 8 days, depending upon the severity of the bleeding episode. Antifibrinolytic therapy is contraindicated in the presence of hematuria because clots resistant to lysis may obstruct the ureters.

Fibrin Glue

Fibrin glue, otherwise known as fibrin tissue adhesive, has been used as adjunctive therapy to factor VIII in hemophilic patients.[55] Briefly, fibrin glue contains fibrinogen, thrombin, and factor XIII. Fibrinolytic inhibitors are added to some commercial products. The fibrinogen–factor XIII mixture is placed on the injury site and clotted with a human thrombin solution containing calcium. As a result, the fibrin clot is crosslinked and anchored to tissue. It is especially useful for hemostasis in patients undergoing dental surgery who receive a preextraction bolus of factor VIII followed by application of fibrin glue to the tooth socket. Fibrin glue also has been used as adjunctive therapy to factor VIII following orthopedic procedures and circumcision. It is very valuable for controlling bleeding when applied to the bed of a surgical wound following removal of large pseudotumors. Some hemophilia centers prepare their own "homemade" fibrin glue using cryoprecipitate as a source of fibrinogen and factor XIII.

Treatment of Minor or Moderate Hemorrhage

On occasion, superficial cuts and abrasions are managed with local measures, that is, application of pressure sometimes suffices to control bleeding, although oozing may continue intermittently for several hours. Topical thrombin is of little value in this type of bleeding. In general, cautery should be avoided because bleeding may restart when the cauterized area is sloughed.

When replacement therapy for epistaxis is needed, the factor VIII level should be raised to approximately 30 to 50 percent of normal. For treatment of hematuria, patients should be instructed to drink large quantities of fluids. If hematuria is mild, uncomplicated, and painless, factor VIII replacement may not be necessary unless the hematuria persists. Gross or protracted hematuria requires replacement therapy. In these patients, factor VIII levels of at least 50 percent of normal or higher are needed, probably because urine is rich in urokinase that rapidly lyses clots.

Hemophilic patients requiring endoscopic procedures first should be treated with factor VIII to raise levels to at least 0.5 U/mL before the procedure. Only one dose may be necessary if endoscopy is uncomplicated. In cases of biopsies, severe abrasions or perforations following endoscopy, factor VIII replacement should be continued until healing of the lesion is complete. For expanding soft-tissue hematomas, factor VIII therapy should be started immediately and maintained until the hematoma begins to resolve. With effective therapy, the patient usually experiences rapid relief from pain. For treatment of acute hemarthroses, prompt administration of factor VIII decreases the occurrence of extensive degenerative joint changes, deformity, and muscle wasting. For chronic synovitis and for bleeding into "target" joints, daily administration of factor VIII to raise levels to 100 percent of normal for 6 to 8 weeks ("secondary prophylaxis") is usually indicated.

Treatment of Major Nonsurgical Hemorrhages

Any hemorrhage in a patient with hemophilia A may become major, but the following hemorrhages are common and frequently life-threatening: retropharyngeal, retroperitoneal, and central nervous system bleeding, whether subdural, subarachnoid, or into the brain parenchyma.[56]

For treatment of retropharyngeal bleeding, particularly that associated with a sensation of tightness in the throat, pain in the neck, dysphagia, or difficulty breathing, patients should receive factor VIII immediately in doses sufficient to raise factor VIII levels to normal (1.0 U/mL). Near-normal levels should be maintained until bleeding ceases and the hematoma begins to resolve. For retroperitoneal hemorrhage, early treatment is required, and therapy should be continued for 7 to 10 days; otherwise, bleeding may recur upon resumption of activity.

Immediate administration of factor VIII, sufficient to raise the level to normal, should be started upon the first sign of an intracranial hemorrhage or following a history of head trauma. Even asymptomatic patients with a history of head trauma should receive at least one dose of factor VIII as a prophylactic measure, and this dose should be given before diagnostic procedures such as a CT scan. Treatment of a known intracranial hemorrhage should be maintained for a minimum of 7 to 10 days, and the circulating factor VIII level should be kept normal throughout this period. Prolonged secondary prophylaxis is often indicated following an intracerebral hemorrhage, particularly in patients with HIV disease, who seem to have a high recurrence rate. Evacuation of subdural hematomas and surgical removal of hematomas involving the brain parenchyma can be performed, depending upon location. Despite aggressive replacement therapy, however, mortality from central nervous system bleeding is high.

Replacement of Factor VIII for Surgical Procedures

For major surgical procedures, factor VIII should be raised to normal levels before operation and maintained for 7 to 10 days or until healing is complete. Treatment can be started a few hours before surgery and continued intraoperatively using a continuous infusion or boluses every 8 to 12 hours. Postoperatively, factor VIII levels should be monitored at least one or two times per day to ensure that adequate levels are maintained. Because factor VIII may be "consumed" during surgery, factor VIII levels should be monitored intraoperatively and doses of factor VIII higher than normal may be required. Bone and joint surgery may require longer periods of factor VIII coverage. Replacement of knee, hip, ankle, and elbow joints may be required for intractable pain associated with loss of function, and several weeks of replacement therapy may be needed postoperatively.[57]

Home Therapy

Home therapy using available factor VIII concentrates was introduced in the United States in 1977 and was a major advance in the treatment of all forms of hemophilia.[58,59] Current practice for home therapy is to treat patients at home using a regular prophylactic regimen. Patients, age 6 years and older, can be taught to treat themselves with factor VIII. The training of patients and their families for home therapy is best accomplished in a regional comprehensive hemophilia diagnostic and treatment center or an affiliate of one of these centers. Patients are given an adequate quantity of factor concentrates and the supplies required for intravenous administration. Prompt treatment of hemarthroses and hematomas made possible by home therapy has markedly improved the morbidity and mortality associated with hemophilia. In addition, the quality of life of hemophilia A patients has improved dramatically.[59,60]

Prophylactic Therapy

The advent of stable and safe factor VIII concentrates has made prophylactic therapy for hemophilia A in severely affected patients feasible. Such therapy is now the treatment of choice for all severely affected hemophilia patients (unfortunately, such treatment is not available or affordable for all patients). Administration of 25 to 40 U of factor VIII per kilogram of body weight three times per week or every other day markedly decreases the frequency of hemophilic arthropathy and other long-term effects of hemorrhagic episodes.[60-62] Primary prophylaxis is usually initiated before the age of 2 years or after the first joint bleed, which is usually when the child begins to walk. Central venous catheters may be required sometimes for very young children; however, they are associated with a risk of infections and thrombosis.[63] Secondary prophylaxis is started after the onset of hemarthrosis and can be used for short periods of time or to manage target joints. The consumption of factor concentrate is higher when patients are on prophylaxis when compared to on-demand but analysis of the economic impact of prophylactic therapy, weighing the benefits against the high costs of factor VIII concentrates, suggests the clinical benefit of prophylaxis is warranted, as evidenced by significant improvement in the clinical condition of patients and improvement in the quality of life.[62,64]

COURSE AND PROGNOSIS

After the advent of factor VIII concentrates in the 1960s, the morbidity and mortality from bleeding in hemophilia were significantly reduced, and by the late 1970s the life expectancy of hemophilia A patients began to approach that of normal individuals in those populations. However, use of replacement therapy has not been without significant complications. Prior to 1985, common and serious adverse side effects of treatment included chronic liver disease resulting from hepatitides B and C and, from about 1978, infection with HIV.[65] Factor VIII concentrates were prepared from many thousands of donors, making contamination of factor VIII concentrates by bloodborne viruses highly likely. With the introduction of heat- or solvent-detergent–treated concentrates in 1985, contamination of blood products with these viruses has been eliminated for all practical purposes. However, AIDS became a leading cause of death in older patients with hemophilia.[65] Chronic liver disease in hemophilia A patients resulting from transfusion-related hepatitides B and C may be accelerated by HIV infection and by the associated hepatotoxicity of antiviral drug therapy.[66] Fortunately, patients treated prophylactically after 1985 can expect almost normal life spans free of the complications of hepatitis, AIDS, and other currently recognized bloodborne viral diseases. However, the development of inhibitor

antibodies against factor VIII has been, and continues to be, one of the more serious complications of replacement therapy.

Factor VIII Inhibitors

Other than the transmission of viral diseases by factor VIII infusions, the main complication of hemophilia A replacement therapy is the development of specific inhibitor antibodies that neutralize factor VIII.[67] The reported prevalence of anti–factor VIII inhibitors in severe hemophilia A patients is variable, ranging from 3.6 percent to 27 percent. In the white population the estimated prevalence is approximately 13 percent, compared to 27 percent and 25 percent in the black and Hispanic population, respectively.[68] The risk of inhibitor development is higher in patients with large deletions and nonsense mutations when compared to small deletions/insertions and missense mutations. Frequent testing for inhibitors in previously untreated patients receiving newer highly purified factor VIII products from plasma or by recombinant technology revealed the frequent occurrence of transient inhibitors to factor VIII, many of which were of low titer and did not necessitate cessation of treatment with the same product. Although still controversial, some believe that the risk of inhibitors does not appear to be higher with the use of highly purified products than the risk reported in earlier studies using products of intermediate purity that contain VWF.[69-74] Some studies have reported that VWF is immunomodulatory, so that products containing VWF may be less likely to induce inhibitors compared to highly purified products. One outbreak of inhibitors in Europe appeared to be related to the neoantigenicity of an intermediate-purity plasma-derived factor VIII concentrate. Fortunately, inhibitors disappeared from affected patients when use of the product was stopped.[75]

Table 123–4 lists the risk factors that have been associated with the development of inhibitors. They arise most frequently in severely affected patients, following treatment at an early age. Many have gross gene rearrangements or the intron 22 inversion abnormality of the factor VIII gene.

Factor VIII inhibitors are antibodies, most often of the immunoglobulin (Ig) G class and frequently restricted to the IgG_4 subclass.[67] Antibodies against the A_2 and C domains of factor VIII are most common. These antibodies interfere with the interactions of factor VIII with other hemostatic components.[67,76]

Early diagnosis of factor VIII inhibitors is essential. Although the presence of an inhibitor can be suspected on clinical grounds, as when a patient does not respond to conventional doses of factor VIII,

TABLE 123–4. Risk Factors for Development of Anti–Factor VIII Antibodies in Hemophilia A Patients

Disease severity: 80% of hemophilia A patients with inhibitors have <1% factor VIII activity

Early exposure to factor VIII concentrates: majority of high-titer inhibitors develop after <90 days of exposure to factor VIII

Genetic factors
1. Family history of inhibitor development
2. Ethnic background: Blacks > Hispanics > whites
3. Molecular defects: inversion and crossing over defect in intron 22, gene deletions, and nonsense point mutations resulting in patients without factor VIII antigen

Method of purification of factor VIII concentrate

Adapted and modified from Roberts HR: Inhibitors and their management, in *Hemophilia & Other Bleeding Disorders*, edited by Rizza, G Lowe, p 371. WB Saunders, New York, 1997.

laboratory diagnosis is required for confirmation. Factor VIII inhibitors are time and temperature dependent *in vitro*. The prolonged aPTT of the plasma of a patient without an inhibitor is corrected when mixed 1:1 with normal plasma even after incubation at 37°C for 1 to 2 hours. In contrast, the aPTT of a 1:1 mixture of plasma from a patient with an inhibitor and normal plasma is significantly prolonged after incubation at 37°C for 1 to 2 hours. Specific diagnosis rests upon demonstrating that an appropriate dilution of the patient's plasma, when added to normal plasma, specifically neutralizes factor VIII and not other blood clotting factors that influence the aPTT (i.e., factors IX, XI, XII, prekallikrein, high-molecular-weight kininogen). The demonstration that the inhibitor is specific for factor VIII distinguishes it from inhibitors of other clotting factors, for example, the lupus anticoagulant, and nonspecific inhibitors. A common assay used for inhibitor detection and quantification is the Bethesda assay.[77] In the Bethesda assay, the patient's plasma is diluted such that, when the plasma is mixed with an equal volume of normal pooled human plasma and incubated for 2 hours at 37°C, the factor VIII activity in the mixture is decreased by 50 percent. A modification of the Bethesda assay is the Nijmegen assay, in which buffer is used instead of factor VIII–deficient plasma. This method has shown to be more dependable at detecting low concentration of inhibitors.[78]

Several approaches to treatment of factor VIII inhibitors are available (Table 123–5). Use of these treatments requires knowledge of whether the patient with an inhibitor is a "high" or "low" responder and whether the bleeding episode requiring treatment is minor or major.[67]

High-Responder Patients   Approximately 60 percent of patients who have inhibitors are high responders. High responders are defined as patients whose inhibitor titer is higher than 5 Bethesda units (BU) at baseline or whose initial inhibitor titer is less than 5 BU but rises to greater than 5 BU after administration of factor VIII. Thus, high responders who are not treated with factor VIII for long periods may have a sustained high level of inhibitor, or they may have a very low to undetectable level of inhibitor until they are challenged with factor VIII.

Major bleeding episodes in a high-responder patient whose initial inhibitor titer is less than 5 BU can be treated with human factor VIII concentrate (see Table 123–5). When the initial titer is low, sufficient factor VIII can be administered in high doses to neutralize the inhibitor and attain adequate factor VIII levels for hemostasis. Although factor VIII inhibitor bypassing agents can be used (see below), they are not as reliable as factor VIII in achieving hemostasis, and their effect cannot be adequately monitored with specific laboratory tests. If factor VIII is used, a loading dose of 10,000 to 15,000 U may be required, followed by up to 1000 U of factor VIII per hour, depending upon the factor VIII level. One can expect an anamnestic response approximately 5 days after administration of factor VIII.

In high-responder patients whose initial inhibitor titer is less than 5 BU and who experience a minor bleeding episode, the agent of choice is a factor VIII inhibitor bypassing agent. Recombinant factor VIIa in

doses of 90 to 120 mcg per kilogram of body weight or higher every 2 to 3 hours is safe and effective in most hemorrhagic episodes.[79] The dosing frequency is based on a factor VIIa plasma half-life of approximately 2 to 3 hours. The mechanisms of action of factor VIIa have been investigated using *in vitro* techniques. After coagulation is initiated by the tissue factor–factor VIIa pathway, factor VIIa at recommended doses is hypothesized to activate factor X on the surface of activated platelets, even in the absence of additional tissue factor activity.[80] Factor Xa then can associate with factor Va and convert prothrombin to thrombin. Because activated platelets are localized to the site of vessel injury, thrombin generation by factor VIIa is localized to the site of bleeding. This process may account for the reported safety of factor VIIa.[80] Factor VIII inhibitor bypassing activity (FEIBA), a plasma-derived agent, has also been used successfully to treat bleeding episodes in inhibitor patients and is both safe and effective[81] given at a recommended dose of 50 to 100 U per kilogram body weight every 8 to 12 hours (not to exceed 200 U per kilogram per day).

High-responder patients whose initial inhibitor titer is greater than 5 BU usually do not respond to even very high doses of human factor VIII. Thus, recombinant factor VIIa or FEIBA should be used.[81] If these agents are not available, nonactivated prothrombin complex concentrates or plasma exchange with high dose replacement factor VIII can be considered.

Low-Responder Patients   Low-responder patients are arbitrarily defined as patients whose inhibitor titer is less than 5 BU even after a challenge with factor VIII. For major bleeding episodes, high doses of human factor VIII can be used as recommended above. For minor bleeds, recombinant factor VIIa or FEIBA are recommended because some "low" responders may convert to high responders when they are challenged repeatedly with factor VIII.

Nonactivated or activated prothrombin complex concentrates both contain variable amounts of activated factors, including factors VIIa, IXa, and Xa. The activated products have higher concentrations of activated factors than do nonactivated products. FEIBA contains a complex of prothrombin and factor Xa that can bind to membrane surfaces and enhance thrombin generation in the absence of factors VIII or IX.[80,81]

Surgery in Inhibitor Patients   The question of whether major surgery can be performed in patients with hemophilia A or B with inhibitors arises now that joint replacement is possible.[82] Knee, ankle, hip, and elbow replacements have been carried out successfully in patients with inhibitor antibodies using bypassing agents. Basically, the patient is given a loading dose of factor VIIa followed by bolus doses of factor VIIa and use of fibrin sealant and antifibrinolytic therapy until healing is complete. FEIBA has also been successfully used in surgery in hemophilic patients with inhibitors.[83]

Immune Tolerance   Removal of the antibody is the definitive goal of inhibitor management. Plasmapheresis, adsorption of the antibody on an affinity column during plasma exchange, and administration of

TABLE 123–5. Treatment of Inhibitors in Hemophilia A Patients

Type of Patient	Initial Titer	Minor Hemorrhage*	Major Hemorrhage*
High responder	<5 BU	Recombinant factor VIIa; FEIBA	Factor VIII[†]; recombinant factor VIIa; FEIBA
High responder	>5 BU	Recombinant factor VIIa; FEIBA	Recombinant factor VIIa; FEIBA; plasma exchange
Low responder	<5 BU	Recombinant factor VIIa; FEIBA	High-dose factor VIII; recombinant factor VIIa; FEIBA

BU, Bethesda unit; FEIBA, factor VIII inhibitor bypassing activity.

*Choice of agents for treatment of major and minor hemorrhage are listed. Some physicians will choose the first product listed as the agent of choice, but the choice varies among physicians.

[†]High dose of factor VIII may overcome an initial low-titer inhibitor, although an anamnestic response can be expected in high responders.

Data from Hoffman M, Dargaud Y: Mechanisms and monitoring of bypassing agent therapy. *J Thromb Haemost* 10(8):1478–1485, 2012.

TABLE 123–6. Examples of Tolerance Protocols for Hemophilia A Inhibitor Patients with Good-Risk Factors

Immune Tolerance Protocols	Dose	Time to Negative Inhibitor
High-dose regimen	200 U/kg factor VIII per day	4.6 months
Low-dose regimen	50 U/kg factor VIII three times per week	9.2 months

Data from DiMichele DM: Immune tolerance in haemophilia: The long journey to the fork in the road. *Heamophilia* 159(2):123–134, 2012.

intravenous γ-globulin have been used in patients with an inhibitor. The Malmö protocol uses nearly all of these approaches in combination, including extracorporeal adsorption of antibody to a Sepharose A column, administration of cyclophosphamide, daily administration of factor VIII, and intravenous γ-globulin.[84]

The most promising approach to eradication of an inhibitor is use of immune tolerance regimens. The basis of this approach is administration of frequent (daily or thrice weekly) doses of factor VIII until the inhibitor titer is undetectable.[85] Low- and high-dose regimens have been described (Table 123–6). Predictors of success have been described in clinical studies in patients with high titer inhibitors and include young age at detection of inhibitor; inhibitor titer less than 10 BU before starting immune tolerance induction (ITI); peak titer less than 100 BU after starting ITI; historical peak titer less than 200 BU; age less than 5 years old between diagnosis and start of ITI; and genotype (small deletions and insertions, and missense mutations). Factor VIII inhibitor bypassing agents are used for prevention and treatment of acute bleeds that occur during immune tolerance induction.

Other approaches to treatment of factor VIII inhibitors include immunosuppressive drugs, like cyclosporine and rituximab.[85–87] However, these drugs, although occasionally successful, seem to be more effective in patients with acquired hemophilia resulting from autoantibodies against factor VIII.

Infectious Complications

Hepatitis Almost all multitransfused patients with hemophilia treated before 1985 were infected with one or more viruses that caused hepatitis. Although many infected patients did not suffer acute symptoms, at least 50 percent developed chronic persistent or chronic active hepatitis that in many cases, resulted in cirrhosis. Hepatitis C and B viruses are commonly associated with chronic liver disease. Many adult hemophilia patients treated with concentrates before 1985 have circulating antibodies to hepatitis B surface antigen, and hepatitis C. Hepatitis C infection progresses more rapidly in the presence of HIV infection. Until recently, therapy with pegylated interferon, and ribavirin reduced viral load and improve survival of many affected patients; however, newer approaches using serine protease inhibitors and nucleotide polymerase inhibitors has led to a high rate of sustained virologic responses.[88] All patients with hemophilia should be vaccinated against hepatitis A and hepatitis B.

Human Immunodeficiency Virus Many of the older, severely affected hemophilia A patients who were treated before 1985 have antibodies to HIV, indicating infection with the virus. The incidence of HIV antibodies in mildly affected patients is much lower and correlates with treatment with factor VIII concentrates before viral inactivation procedures were used. In one study, 14 percent of patients treated only with cryoprecipitate from 1979 to 1985 were infected with HIV, whereas 88 percent of patients treated with factor VIII concentrates became infected.[89] Screening of donor populations and new techniques

for preparing factor VIII concentrates since 1985 have eliminated the risk of HIV transmission.

Risk of Viral Disease Transmission By New Factor VIII Products All available factor VIII concentrates, both plasma-derived and recombinant products, are considered safe and effective with almost no risk of transmitting currently known viral diseases. However, occasional exceptions have been observed. For example, solvent-detergent treatment does not inactivate viruses without lipid envelopes, including the hepatitis A virus and parvovirus. As a result, outbreaks of hepatitis A have been reported in patients receiving some solvent detergent–treated products. These outbreaks of viral diseases usually have been related to breakdowns in the manufacturing process.

Prions Prions are infectious particles consisting of proteinaceous material devoid of a nucleic acid genome.[90] They are thought to be variant forms of a normal protein with an altered conformation. The "infectious" nature of prions may result from their ability to bind to other proteins and induce similar conformational changes in them such that new "infectious" particles can be generated. Prions are responsible for several neurodegenerative disorders, including Creutzfeldt-Jakob disease (CJD) in humans, scrapie in sheep, and spongiform encephalopathy in cows. Prions are resistant to most currently available viral inactivation techniques. Removal of prion particles using iodine column chromatography has been claimed.[91] Although prion diseases generally are transmitted by ingestion of infected neural tissues, a new variant of CJD appears to occur in people who have eaten beef from cows infected with a form of prion causing bovine spongiform encephalopathy. This form of CJD has been reported mainly in the United Kingdom and in certain other European countries and has been related to the bovine disease.[92] For example, prions have been found in tonsillar tissue of patients with new-variant CJD, heightening concern about whether prions of this type might be transmitted by blood products.[93] Conclusive data about possible prion infection of hemophilic patients are lacking, so continued vigilance is necessary.

● HEMOPHILIA B (FACTOR IX DEFICIENCY, CHRISTMAS FACTOR DEFICIENCY)

ETIOLOGY AND PATHOGENESIS

Hemophilia B occurs in one of every 25,000 to 30,000 live male births. As with hemophilia A, hemophilia B is found in all ethnic groups and has no geographic predilection.

Factor IX is a vitamin K-dependent, single-chain glycoprotein consisting of 415 amino acids. It is activated by the factor VIIa–tissue factor complex, or factor XIa, forming the active enzyme factor IXa (Chap. 113). Once activated, factor IXa activates factor X in the presence of factor VIIIa, phospholipid (activated platelets), and calcium. Factor VIIIa is a necessary cofactor for activity of factor IXa. Therefore, deficiency of either factor IX or VIII leads to a similar lack of factor X-activating activity on the platelet surface. Factor Xa converts prothrombin to thrombin in the presence of factor Va, activated platelets, and calcium. Hemophilia B can result from either the absence or the dysfunction of factor IX molecules. Clinical severity of hemophilia B is roughly correlated with factor IX functional activity.

GENETICS AND MOLECULAR BIOLOGY

The factor IX gene is located on the long arm of the X chromosome. It is approximately 33 kb long, which is much smaller than the gene for factor VIII.[94] Because it is less complex, the factor IX gene has been studied in greater detail than the factor VIII gene. Figure 123–11 is a schematic of the gene and the protein product. The protein consists of a signal

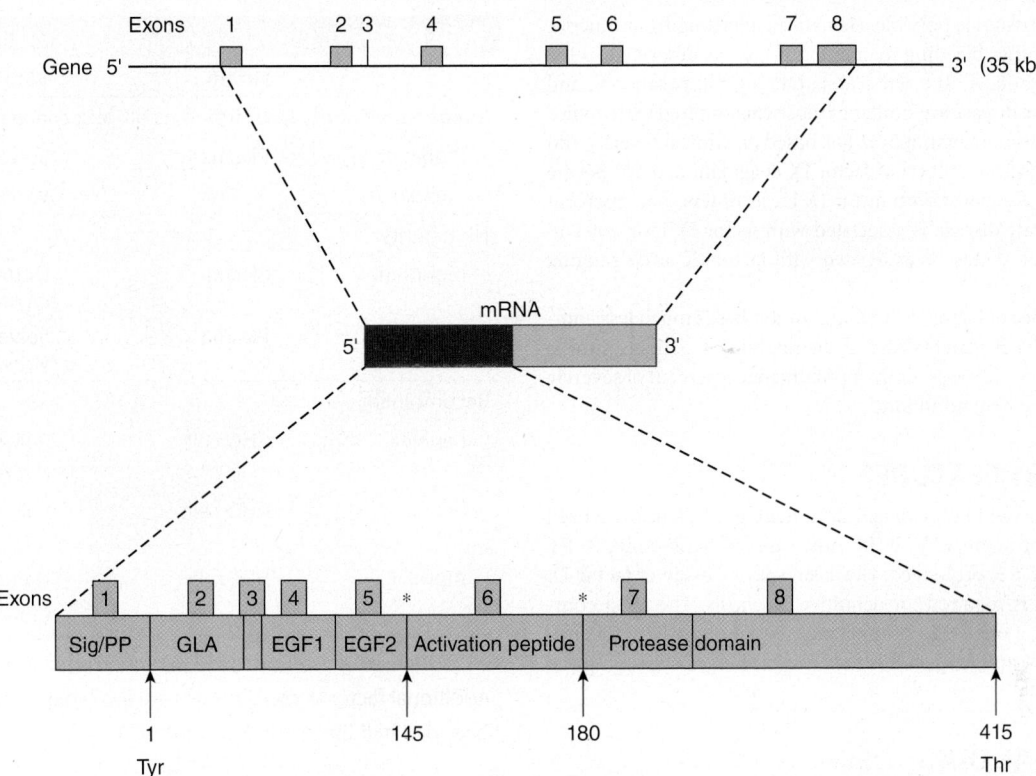

Figure 123–11. Schematic of the factor IX gene, the messenger RNA, and the protein. Exons are depicted by the tan boxes. The light 3′ portion of the mRNA is untranslated. The diagram of the protein shows the domains and the exons that encode each portion of the protein. The cleavage sites of factor XIa or factor VIIa–tissue factor complex are indicated by *asterisks*.

peptide that targets the protein for secretion from the hepatocyte to the circulation. The propeptide is necessary for posttranslational modification of 12 aminoterminal glutamic acid residues by an intracellular vitamin K-dependent carboxylase. The propeptide is cleaved from the mature protein before it enters the circulation. The aminoterminus of factor IX contains 12 γ-carboxyglutamic acid (GLA) residues necessary for calcium-dependent lipid binding. The activation peptide is cleaved from the zymogen form of factor IX by either factor VIIa/tissue factor or factor XIa, resulting in the two-chain active enzyme, factor IXaβ. The catalytic triad (His 221, Asp 229, ser 365) resides on the heavy chain (Chap. 113).[94]

There are more than 1000 distinct mutations or deletions in the factor IX gene reported in the factor IX database, including more than 900 distinct amino acid substitutions and numerous complete gene deletions.[95,96] More than 30 percent of factor IX mutations occur at CpG dinucleotides. These mutations often involve critical Arg residues that result in a dysfunctional molecule.[96–99] Many mutations have been reported in more than one kindred, and some of these mutations derive from the same "founder."[100] As predicted by genetic theory of X chromosome-linked recessive disorders, approximately one-third of mutations resulting in hemophilia B arise *de novo*.

Mutations in regulatory regions of the factor IX gene have been identified. Particularly interesting examples are mutations in the 5′ promoter region that lead to the hemophilia B Leyden phenotype.[101] This disorder is characterized by very low levels of factor IX antigen and activity at birth and during early childhood. The factor IX levels gradually rise to 60 percent of normal or greater following puberty, possibly caused by the age-related stability element/age-related increase element mediated genetic mechanism.[102] Several different mutations in the promoter region of the factor IX gene disrupt binding of transcription factors, resulting in reduced transcription of the factor IX gene.[101,103]

The hormonal changes occurring at puberty apparently can overcome the transcription defect and maintain hemostatic levels of factor IX.

Hemophilia B inheritance is similar to that of hemophilia A. All daughters of affected males are obligate carriers, whereas all sons are normal. Female carriers may have factor IX levels ranging from less than 10 to 100 percent of normal, but the mean level is approximately 50 percent. Carriers of hemophilia B usually are asymptomatic, except in cases of extreme X chromosome inactivation, X mosaicism, Turner syndrome, or testicular feminization.[104] When the level of factor IX activity is less than 25 percent of normal, abnormal bleeding may occur, especially after trauma and surgery.

Carrier Detection and Prenatal Diagnosis

Factor IX genotyping is achieved by direct sequencing. Prenatal diagnosis may be accomplished by analysis of DNA obtained by chorionic villus sampling as early as 8 to 10 weeks after conception.[105] This procedure also can be performed on fetal cells obtained by amniocentesis and is more accurate than fetal blood sampling for factor IX activity and factor IX antigen. Large deletions are relatively rare in severe hemophilia B, but are associated with a higher risk of factor IX inhibitors when present.

CLINICAL FEATURES

Bleeding episodes in patients with hemophilia B are clinically indistinguishable from patients with hemophilia A, although as stated elsewhere, the hemophilia B population as a whole seem to have fewer and less-severe complications than severely affected hemophilia A patients[9] (see "Clinical Features" under "Hemophilia A" above). When patients are inadequately treated, repeated hemarthroses leading to chronic, crippling hemarthropathy occur. Hematoma formation with dissection into surrounding tissues is possible. Hematuria, bleeding from mucous membranes, and other bleeding manifestations are as described in the section on hemophilia A. The physical, psychological, vocational, and social aspects of the disease are similar to those encountered with hemophilia A. Classification of hemophilia B is based on clinical severity and roughly correlates with the level of factor IX coagulant activity. Severe disease usually is associated with factor IX levels of less than 1percent of normal; moderate disease is associated with factor IX levels of 1 to 5 percent; and mild disease is associated with factor IX levels ranging from 5 to 40 percent.

The occurrence of factor IX inhibitor antibodies is much less common in hemophilia B patients than in hemophilia A patients, and is very rare in nonsevere disease. Only approximately 3 percent of severely affected patients develop inhibitors.

LABORATORY FEATURES

The screening tests used in the diagnosis of hemophilia A also are used in the diagnosis of hemophilia B. In most cases of hemophilia B, PT is normal and aPTT is prolonged. However, specific assay of factor IX coagulant activity is required for definitive diagnosis. The most commonly used test is a one-stage clotting assay based on aPTT. Determination of factor IX antigen levels is valuable in further classifying the disorder.

DIFFERENTIAL DIAGNOSIS

Hemophilia B must be distinguished from hemophilia A. Both forms are inherited as X-linked recessive disorders, and both have almost identical hemorrhagic and clinical manifestations. The only method for differentiating hemophilia B from hemophilia A is performing specific assays for factors VIII and IX on the patient's plasma.

Inherited and acquired deficiencies of other vitamin K–dependent factors, liver disease, and warfarin overdose must be distinguished from hemophilia B. In these cases, not only factor IX but all other vitamin K–dependent clotting factors, including prothrombin, factor VII, and factor X, are decreased. Acquired antibodies specific for factor IX occur in nonhemophilic patients but are very rare.

THERAPY

Factor IX Replacement

The basic treatment of hemophilia B is replacement of factor IX. Several products are available for use (Table 123–7). The older factor IX–containing products often are referred to as prothrombin complex concentrates. These products, which are prepared from large pools of human plasma (several thousand donors), contain not only factor IX but also prothrombin, factors VII and X, and proteins C and S. In addition, the products may contain small amounts of activated factors, such as factors VIIa, IXa, and Xa. Some of these products are associated with thromboembolic events, presumably resulting from contamination with the activated components. Deep venous thrombosis (DVT) and disseminated intravascular coagulation have been reported in some patients who receive large doses of prothrombin complex concentrates, but these complications seem to occur less frequently with currently available purified factor IX products than with earlier preparations. Prothrombin complex concentrates are no longer the optimal choice for replacement therapy in hemophilia B, even though they are much less expensive than the highly purified factor IX concentrates. When prothrombin complex concentrates are used for replacement therapy, factor IX levels greater than 50 percent of normal should not be exceeded in order to minimize the risk of thrombosis. Use of these products in factor IX–deficient patients with liver dysfunction may be hazardous because the activated

TABLE 123–7. Currently Available Factor IX Products*

	Origin	Viral Inactivation
Intermediate purity (prothrombin complex concentrates)		
Profilnine SD	Plasma	Solvent-detergent
Bebulin VH	Plasma	Vapor heating
High purity		
Mononine	Plasma	Ultrafiltration; chemical
AlphaNine	Plasma	Solvent-detergent; virus filtered
Recombinant		
BeneFIX	CHO cells	Solvent-detergent Nanofiltration
Rixubis	CHO cells	Solvent-detergent Nanofiltration
Alprolix†	HEK cells	Nanofiltration Chromatography

CHO, Chinese hamster ovary; HEK, human embryo kidney.
*Additional factor IX concentrates are available in Europe.
†Extended half-life factor IX product.

factors contaminating these preparations may not be cleared efficiently by a diseased liver, and thrombosis might be induced.

Table 123–7 lists the highly purified factor IX products. Some products are prepared from human plasma; at present, three products are produced by recombinant DNA technology. Although all available factor IX concentrates are considered safe and effective, the recombinant product undergoes a final viral inactivation step. In addition, the recombinant products are not exposed to human albumin or bovine serum during preparation. Thus, even the theoretical risk of transmission of prion diseases is averted with this preparation. Some clinicians consider the recombinant product to be the agent of choice, although it has a major drawback in that the intravascular recovery of factor IX generally is lower than the recovery of highly purified factor IX product prepared from plasma.[106] The recombinant factor IX products are not thought to be thrombogenic. New factor IX products have been recently approved and others undergoing clinical trials or currently being developed, some of them with extended half-life (see Table 123–7).[107] Different technologies have been applied to extend the half-life of factor IX including Fc-fusion, recombinant albumin fusion and PEGylation (glycoPEGylation), so one can expect the number of available factor IX products to increase in the near future.

Dosing of Factor IX

The dose calculations for all factor IX products are different from those used in hemophilia A because intravascular recovery of factor IX is only approximately 50 percent, and the recovery is even lower with the recombinant product. The reason for this finding is unclear, but as factor IX binds to type IV collagen, a component of the vascular wall, infused factor IX adsorption may contribute to the reduced recovery.[108] The dose of factor IX can be estimated by assuming that 1 U of factor IX per kilogram body weight increases circulating factor IX by 1 percent of normal or 0.01 U/mL.[109] Thus, to achieve 100 percent of normal (using only highly purified factor IX products) in a severely affected patient, 100 U of factor IX per kilogram body weight should be given as a bolus, followed by half this amount every 12 to 18 hours. Dosing should be monitored by assays of factor IX before and after bolus administration. Factor IX also can be administered as a constant infusion in hospitalized patients after the bolus administration. The dose of factor IX to be infused per hour can be estimated based on a factor IX half-life of 18 to 24 hours. Thus, in a 60-kg adult who receives highly purified factor IX, 6000 U of the factor should raise the factor IX level to approximately 100 percent of normal. Over the next 12 to 18 hours, the level decreases by approximately 50 percent. Thus, the patient needs approximately 3000 U of factor IX during that period or 250 U of factor IX per hour as an infusion.[109] These calculations are only estimates of average responses, so factor IX dosing should be monitored by factor IX assays and the dose adjusted appropriately. Prophylactic therapy for hemophilia B also can be attempted in individuals selected in the same manner as that described for hemophilia A patients. The prophylactic dose of factor IX is 25 to 40 U/kg of body weight two times per week or 50 to 100 U/kg every 7 to 10 days if using extended half-life products.

Although currently available factor IX concentrates are safe in terms of transmission of HIV and hepatitides B and C viruses, patients treated prior to 1985 may have been infected with these agents.

COURSE AND PROGNOSIS

Unless treated properly, severe hemophilia B is fraught with the same complications of recurrent hemorrhages as hemophilia A. Thus, hemarthroses and chronic hemophilic arthropathy are common in inadequately treated patients. In addition to joint deformities, chronic active hepatitis is common in patients treated before 1985. Approximately 50 percent of older and severely affected patients now are HIV-positive. Patients treated after 1985, when HIV testing became available, are not likely to have contracted HIV.

Patients with severe hemophilia B may develop inhibitory antibodies against factor IX, making treatment very difficult.[110,111] Approximately 3 percent of patients with severe hemophilia B develop specific inhibitor antibodies, frequently restricted in immunoglobulin composition to the IgG_4 subclass and κ light chains.[111] Most inhibitors can be detected when the aPTT of a mixture of normal plasma and the patient's plasma is prolonged. In contrast to the inhibitors in hemophilia A patients, inhibitor antibodies against factor IX are not time and temperature dependent; thus, incubating the mixtures for 2 hours at 37°C usually is unnecessary. Inhibitors to factor IX can be quantitated by modifying the Bethesda method for detecting factor VIII inhibitors. Many patients with inhibitors have mutations that result in the absence of circulating factor IX antigen, most commonly because of deletions and nonsense mutations.

TREATMENT OF PATIENTS WITH FACTOR IX INHIBITOR ANTIBODIES

When the inhibitor titer is less than 5 BU/mL, the factor IX inhibitor possibly can be neutralized using large doses of highly purified factor IX concentrates. However, when the inhibitor titer is greater than 5 BU/mL, acute bleeding in patients should be treated with the same agents used to bypass factor VIII inhibitors (see Table 123–5). Recombinant factor VIIa in doses of 90 to 120 mcg per kilogram body weight administered intravenously every 2 to 3 hours can be used. Alternatively, FEIBA at a dose of 50 to 100 U per kilogram body weight every 8 to 12 hours (not to exceed 200 U/kg per day) or nonactivated prothrombin complex concentrates can be used.

Induction of immune tolerance can be attempted in hemophilia B patients using daily infusions of purified factor IX preparations. However, significant adverse reactions, including anaphylaxis and nephrotic syndrome, have been reported in severely affected patients

with inhibitors.[112] Of the reported cases, many patients were younger than 12 years of age, and suffered from severe hemophilia B as a result of large deletions of the factor IX gene. The nephrotic syndrome may be transient and remit upon cessation of factor IX replacement. The pathogenesis of the nephrotic syndrome is not known. Patients with hemophilia B and factor IX antibodies who experience anaphylaxis with factor IX infusions and have hemorrhage should be treated with factor VIIa concentrates because both unactivated prothrombin complex concentrates and FEIBA contain factor IX.[112]

Curative Approaches for Hemophilia: Liver Transplantation and Gene Therapy

Normal livers have been transplanted successfully into patients with hemophilia A or B, with resulting cure of the hemophilic condition.[113,114] The procedure is most often performed for end-stage chronic viral hepatitis that afflicts many older hemophilic patients. However, given the obvious limitations of this approach, it cannot be considered a viable treatment option to treat hemophilia per se.

On the other hand, gene replacement therapy for hemophilia offers an ideal theoretical approach for prophylactic therapy or even for a definitive cure. Proof of concept of gene therapy as a viable long-term option for the treatment of hemophilia B has been established, as discussed below. Currently, however, the challenges associated with gene transfer of the much larger *FVIII* gene have slowed down progress in the development of gene therapy for hemophilia A, although these limitations are being addressed.

There are several approaches by which the defective gene encoding factor VIII or factor IX can be introduced into a congenitally deficient host (Chap. 29). Viruses have evolved to introduce genetic material into target cells, and are usually employed as the vector, or "Trojan Horse" to allow transfection or transduction of the genetic information.[115,116] Several potential vectors have been used in clinical gene therapy studies for hemophilia and other single gene disorders over the past 2 decades, including adenoviruses, recombinant adeno-associated viral vectors (rAAVs), and retroviral vectors, which include the lentiviral vectors based on HIV-1. At present, rAAVs are favored by the majority of ongoing trials in hemophilia, although preexisting immunity to some of these naturally occurring serotypes, which limits their use, is quite prevalent (up to 40 percent) in human populations. Although concerns exist about oncogenic genotoxicity (also known as insertional mutagenesis) associated with the earlier generation lentiviral vectors, they also have theoretical benefits; specifically, they are capable of infecting both dividing and nondividing cells with resultant persistent expression after integration into the host cell genome. In addition, they avoid the vector-mediated cytotoxicity (such as hepatic transaminitis) and immunologic reactions associated with rAAV.[117]

Certain vectors (such as rAAV) can be injected intravenously—usually on a single occasion—with resultant tropism of the vector and its payload to the liver. Previously, gene transfer via multiple intramuscular injections was also evaluated, and while not unduly toxic, sustained levels of factor IX greater than 1 percent were not maintained long-term. These "in vivo" gene transfer protocols vary from "ex vivo" gene therapy, in which a specific type of cell is targeted before being reintroduced into the host. Target cells used for gene transfer in hemophilia have included human fibroblasts, hematopoietic stem cells, and platelets.

Despite a number of early phase clinical trials over 20+ years, it was not until 2011 that the first report of predictable and consistent maintenance of factor IX levels (in the range of 1 to 6 percent of normal) was achieved in six subjects with hemophilia B. The bleeding frequency and clotting factor usage was reduced by 90 percent in these patients. This experience, from the groups at University College London and St. Jude's Research Hospital in Memphis, Tennessee, was updated with a followup of up to 3 years in the original cohort of six patients, together with an additional four treated individuals.[118] The protocol consisted of a single intravenous injection of a self-complementary rAAV-8; at the highest vector doses used, biochemical transaminitis occurred in some of the patients. This hepatotoxicity was mediated by a host cytotoxic T-lymphocyte response to viral capsid antigens expressed on transfected hepatocytes. Fortunately, however, there was a consistently beneficial and prompt response to modest doses of oral prednisolone.

This milestone study has prompted a resurgent interest in gene therapy for hemophilia, with several phase I studies now underway. Remaining challenges include the use of purer vector preparations (with fewer empty capsids) and strategies to circumvent the natural immunity to AAV.[116] These modifications should permit this approach to be applicable in a greater proportion of patients, and result in even higher long-term expression of factor IX.

Finally, utilization of the same approach to hemophilia A is limited by the inefficient expression of factor VIII, as well as the large size of the coding sequence, even in the absence of the B domain. However, the use of B-domain-deleted codon optimized factor VIII molecules has produced encouraging results in animal models of gene therapy. It is hoped that these preclinical data translate into persistent factor VIII expression levels in patients with hemophilia A. It remains to be seen how often inhibitors to factor VIII occur in these patients.

● SPECIAL PROBLEMS ASSOCIATED WITH HEMOPHILIAS A AND B

Unusual problems are occasionally encountered in both hemophilia A and B. Some of these are discussed in a brief publication.[119] For example, scuba diving can be dangerous in severely affected hemophiliacs and should be avoided. Hemophilic patients requiring laser treatment for visual problems may not require replacement therapy provided that a surgical incision is not required during such therapy. Carriers of either hemophilia A or B may have bleeding problems during delivery or surgery and will require replacement therapy. Carriers whose fetuses have hemophilia may require cesarean section if vaginal delivery is found to be difficult. Forceps and mechanical devices should be avoided during delivery of infants who are hemophilic. Some patients with hemophilia may also have another familial bleeding disorder, such as VWD.

Hemophilic patients that survived the HIV epidemic are aging and are developing comorbidities similar to nonhemophilia males, including hypertension, cardiovascular disease, renal failure, and dyslipidemias. The deficiency of either factor VIII or IX seems to provide some protection against thrombosis.[120] However, myocardial infarction has been reported in hemophilic patients even without treatment.[121] DVT has also been reported following replacement therapy in both hemophilia A and hemophilia B. Acute DVT can be treated with heparin for 7 to 10 days as long as the patient receives factor replacement therapy. Thereafter, anticoagulation is not recommended. Thromboembolic episodes in hemophilia B are much less common since the advent of highly purified factor IX products.

The management of cardiovascular disease in the hemophilia population is a challenge.[122,123] The use of antiplatelet therapy seems safe in mild and moderate individuals; for the severely deficient patient, however, prophylaxis with factor VIII or factor IX should be used. For anticoagulation with heparin or vitamin K antagonists, factor trough levels above 0.25 U/L are recommended. For the management of acute coronary syndromes and arrhythmias requiring intervention, replacement with adequate factor concentrate should be done without exceeding levels above 80 to100 percent of normal. Radial artery access rather than femoral and bare metal stents are preferred over drug-eluting stents.

Individuals requiring valve replacement should receive a biologic rather than a mechanical valve when possible.

Hemophilia patients who have atrial fibrillation should undergo cardioversion when possible. If cardioversion is not successful, some physicians recommend treatment with aspirin but anticoagulants should be used with caution taking into consideration the severity of the hemophilia and the risk of stroke.

REFERENCES

1. Brinkhous KM: A short history of hemophilia, with some comments on the word "hemophilia," in *Handbook of Hemophilia*, edited by KM Brinkhous, HC Hemker, p 3. Elsevier, New York, 1975.
2. Katznelson JL: Hemophilia, with special reference to the Talmud. *Harofe Haivri Heb Med J* 1:165, 1958.
3. Morawitz P: Die Chemie der Blutgerinnung. *Ergeb Physiol* 4:307, 1905.
4. Addis T: The pathogenesis of hereditary haemophilia. *J Pathol Bacteriol* 15:427, 1911.
5. Brinkhous KM: A study of the clotting defect in hemophilia. The delayed formation of thrombin. *Am J Med Sci* 198:509, 1939.
6. Pavlovsky A: Contribution to the pathogenesis of hemophilia. *Blood* 2:185, 1947.
7. Aggeler PM, White SG, Glendenning MB: Plasma thromboplastin component (PTC) deficiency: A new disease resembling hemophilia. *Proc Soc Exp Biol Med* 79:692, 1952.
8. Biggs R, Douglas AS, Macfarlane AG, et al: Christmas disease: A condition previously mistaken for hemophilia. *Br Med J* 2:1378, 1952.
9. Escobar M, Sallah S: Hemophilia A and hemophilia B: Focus on arthropathy and variables affecting bleeding and prophylaxis. *J Thromb Haemost* 11:1449, 2013.
10. Davie EW, Ratnoff OD: Waterfall sequence for intrinsic blood clotting. *Science* 145:1310, 1964.
11. Macfarlane RG: An enzyme cascade in the blood clotting mechanism, and its function as a biological amplifier. *Nature* 202:498, 1964.
12. Broze GR Jr: Tissue factor pathway inhibitor and the revised theory of coagulation. *Annu Rev Med* 46:103, 1995.
13. Fay PJ: Reconstitution of human factor VIII from isolated subunits. *Arch Biochem Biophys* 262:525, 1988.
14. Roberts HR: Contributions to the evolution of knowledge about hereditary hemorrhagic disorders. *Cell Mol Life Sci* 64:517, 2007.
15. Hoffman M, Hargen A, Lewkowski A, et al: Cutaneous wound healing is impaired in hemophilia B. *Blood* 108:3053, 2006.
16. Tuddenham EG: Factor VIII, in *Molecular Basis of Thrombosis and Hemostasis*, edited by KA High, HR Roberts, p 167. Marcel Dekker, New York, 1995.
17. Factor VIII variant database. Available at: http://www.factorviii-db.org
18. Tuddenham EG, Cooper DN, Gitschier J, et al: Haemophilia A: Database of nucleotide substitutions, deletions, insertions and rearrangements of the factor VIII gene. *Nucleic Acids Res* 22:4851, 1996.
19. Antonarakis SE, Rossiter JP, Young M, et al: Factor VIII gene inversions in severe hemophilia A: Results of an international consortium study. *Blood* 86:2206, 1995.
20. Higuchi M, Kazazian HH Jr, Kasch L, et al: Molecular characterization of severe hemophilia A suggests that about half the mutations are not within the coding regions and splice junctions of the factor VIII gene. *Proc Natl Acad Sci U S A* 88:7405, 1991.
21. Gitschier J, Kogan S, Diamond C, Levinson B: Genetic basis of hemophilia A. *Thromb Haemost* 66:37, 1991.
22. Bagnall RD, Waseem N, Green PM, Giannelli F: Recurrent inversion breaking intron 1 of the factor VIII gene is a frequent cause of severe hemophilia A. *Blood* 99:168, 2002.
23. Kazazian HH, Wong C, Youssoufian H, et al: Hemophilia A resulting from de novo insertion of L1 sequences represents a novel mechanism for mutation in man. *Nature* 332:164, 1998.
24. Mori PG, Pasino M, Vadala CR, et al: Haemophilia "A" in a 46Xi(Xq) female. *Br J Haematol* 43:143, 1979.
25. Lakich D, Kazazian HH, Antonarakis SE, Gitschier J: Inversions disrupting the factor VIII gene are a common cause of severe hemophilia A. *Nat Genet* 5:236, 1993.
26. Peake IR, Lillicrap DP, Boulyjenkov V, et al: Report of a joint WHO/WFH meeting on control of haemophilia: Carrier detection and prenatal diagnosis. *Blood Coagul Fibrinolysis* 4:313, 1993.
27. Ljung RC: Prenatal diagnosis of haemophilia. *Haemophilia* 5:84, 1999.
28. Poon MC, Hoar DI, Low S, et al: Hemophilia A carrier detection by restriction fragment length polymorphism analysis and discriminant analysis based on ELISA of factor VIII and vWf. *J Lab Clin Med* 119:751, 1992.
29. Chi C, Lee CA, Shiltagh N, et al: Pregnancy in carriers of hemophilia. *Haemophilia* 14:56, 2008.
30. Brummel-Ziedins KE, Orfeo T, Rosendaal FR, et al: Empirical and theoretical phenotypic discrimination. Phenotypic discrimination models. *J Thromb Haemost* 7(1):181, 2009.
31. Nichols WC, Amano K, Cacheris PM, et al: Moderation of hemophilia A phenotype by the factor V R506Q mutation. *Blood* 88:1183, 1996.
32. Gilbert MS: Musculoskeletal complications of haemophilia: The joint. *Haemophilia* 6:34, 2000.
33. Jansen NA, Rosendaal G, Lafeber FP: Understanding haemophilic arthropathy: An exploration of current issues. *Br J Haematol* 143:632, 2008.

34. Rodriguez Merchan EC: The hemophilic pseudotumour. *Int Orthop* 19:255, 1995.

35. Caviglia H, Candela M, Landro ME, et al: Haemophilia pseudotumours in patients with inhibitors. *Haemophilia* 2015. [Epub ahead of print]

36. Hein M, Martinowitz U: Pseudotumors in patients with hemophilia, in *Textbook of Hemophilia*, 3rd ed, edited by CA Lee, EE Berntorp, WK Hoots, p 233. Wiley Blackwell, Hoboken, NJ, 2014.

37. Zanon E, Iorio A, Rocino A, et al: Intracraneal haemorrhage in the Italian population of haemophilia patients with and without inhibitors. *Heamophilia* 18:39, 2012.

38. Eyster ME, Asaad SM, Gold BD, et al: Upper gastrointestinal bleeding in haemophiliacs: Incidence and relation to use of non-steroidal anti-inflammatory drugs. *Haemophilia* 13:279, 2007.

39. Moser KA, Funk DM: Chromogenic factor VIII activity assay. *Am J Hematol* 89:781, 2014.

40. McGinniss MJ, Kazazian HH Jr, Hoyer LW, et al: Spectrum of mutations in CRM-positive and CRM-reduced hemophilia A. *Genomics* 15:392, 1993.

41. Tully EA, Gaucher C, Jorieux S, et al: Expression of von Willebrand factor "Normandy." An autosomal mutation that mimics hemophilia A. *Proc Natl Acad Sci U S A* 88:6377, 1991.

42. Michiels JJ, Gadisseur A, Vangenegten I, et al: Recessive von Willebrand disease type 2 Normandy: Variable expression of mild hemophilia and VWD type 1. *Acta Haematol* 121:119, 2009.

43. Seligsohn U, Zwang E, Zivelin A: Combined factor V and factor VIII deficiency among non-Ashkenazi Jews. *N Engl J Med* 307:1191, 1982.

44. Ginsberg D: Identifying novel genetic determinants of hemostatic balance. *J Thromb Haemost* 8:1561, 2005.

45. Srivastava A, Brewer AK, Mauser-Bunschoten EP, et al: Guidelines for the management of hemophilia. *Haemophilia* 19:e1, 2013.

46. Santagostino E, Mannucci PM, Gringeri A, et al: Transmission of parvovirus B19 by coagulation factor concentrates exposed to 100 degrees C of heat after lyophilization. *Transfusion* 37:517, 1997.

47. Robertson BH, Alter MJ, Bell BP, et al: Hepatitis A virus sequence detected in clotting factor concentrates associated with disease transmission. *Biologicals* 26:95, 1998.

48. Escobar MA: Treatment on demand—*In vivo* dose finding studies. *Haemophilia* 9:360, 2003.

49. McMillan CW, Webster WP, Roberts HR, Blythe WB: Continuous intravenous infusion of factor VIII in classic hemophilia. *Br J Haematol* 18:659, 1972.

50. Schulman S: Continuous infusion. *Haemophilia* 9:368, 2003.

51. Rodeghiero F, Castaman G, Di Bona E, Ruggeri M: Consistency of responses to repeated DDAVP infusions in patients with von Willebrand's disease and hemophilia A. *Blood* 74:1997, 1989.

52. Mannucci PM, Bettega D, Cattaneo M: Patterns of development of tachyphylaxis in patients with haemophilia and von Willebrand disease after repeated doses of desmopressin (DDAVP). *Br J Haematol* 82:87, 1992.

53. Coppola A, Windyga J, Tufano A, et al: Treatment for preventing bleeding in people with haemophilia or other congenital bleeding disorders undergoing surgery. *Cochrane Database Syst Rev* 2:CD009961, 2015.

54. Ghosh K, Shetty S, Jijina F, Mohanty D: Role of epsilon amino caproic acid in the management of haemophilic patients with inhibitors. *Haemophilia* 10:58, 2004.

55. Martinowitz U, Saltz R: Fibrin sealant. *Curr Opin Hematol* 3:395, 1996.

56. Revel-Vilk S, Golomb MR, Achonu C, et al: Effect of intracranial bleeds on the health and quality of life of boys with hemophilia. *J Pediatr* 144: 490, 2004.

57. Rodriguez-Merchan EC: Orthopaedic surgery in persons with hemophilia. *Thromb Haemost* 89:34, 2003.

58. Rabiner SF, Telfer MC: Home transfusion for patients with hemophilia A. *N Engl J Med* 283:1011, 1977.

59. Teitel JM, Barnard D, Israels S, et al: Home management of haemophilia. *Haemophilia* 10:118, 2004.

60. Manco-Johnson MJ, Riske B, Kasper CK: Advances in care of children with hemophilia. *Semin Thromb Hemost* 29:585, 2003.

61. Nilsson IM, Berntorp E, Lofqvist T, Pettersson H: Twenty-five years' experience of prophylactic treatment in severe haemophilia A and B. *J Intern Med* 232:25, 1992.

62. Manco-Johnson MJ, Abshire TC, Shapiro AD et al: Prophylaxis versus episodic treatment to prevent joint disease in boys with severe hemophilia. *N Engl J Med* 357:535, 2007.

63. Price VE, Carcao M, Connolly B, et al: A prospective, longitudinal study of central venous catheter-related deep venous thrombosis in boys with hemophilia. *J Thromb Haemost* 2:737, 2004.

64. Globe DR, Curtis RG, Koerper MA: Utilization of care in haemophilia: A resource-based method for cost analysis from the Haemophilia Utilization Group Study (HUGS). *Haemophilia* 10(Suppl 1):63, 2004.

65. Levetow LB, Sox HC, Stoto MA: *HIV and the Blood Supply: An Analysis of Crisis Decision Making, Institute of Medicine*, p 1. National Academy Press, Washington, DC, 1994.

66. Santagostino E, De Filippi F, Rumi MG, et al: Sustained suppression of hepatitis C virus by high doses of interferon and ribavirin in adult hemophilic patients. *Transfusion* 44:790, 2004.

67. Lollar P: Pathogenic antibodies to coagulation factors: I. Factor VIII and factor IX. *J Thromb Haemost* 2:1082, 2004.

68. Iorio A: Epidemiology of inhibitors in hemophilia, in *Textbook of Hemophilia*, 3rd ed, edited by CA Lee, EE Berntorp, WK Hoots, p 53. Wiley Blackwell, Hoboken, NJ, 2014.

69. Hoots WK, Lusher J: High-titer inhibitor development in hemophilia A: Lack of product specificity. *J Thromb Haemost* 2:358, 2004.

70. Gouw SC, van den Berg HM, le Cessie S, van der Bom JG: Treatment characteristics and the risk of inhibitor development: A multicenter cohort study among previously untreated patients with severe hemophilia A. *Blood* 109:4648, 2007.

71. Gouw SC, van der Bom JG, Auerswald G, et al: Recombinant versus plasma-derived factor VIII products and the development of inhibitors in previously untreated patients with severe hemophilia A: The CANAL cohort study. *Blood* 109:4693, 2007.

72. Gouw SC, van der Bom JG, Ljung R et al: Factor VIII products and inhibitor development in severe hemophilia A. *N Engl J Med* 17:231, 2013.

73. Iorio A, Halimeh S Holzhauer S, et al: Rate of inhibitor development in previously untreated hemophilia A patients treated with plasma-derived or recombinant VIII concentrates: A systematic review. *J Thromb Haemost* 8:1256, 2010.

74. Gouw SC, van der Berg HM, Oldenberg et al: F8 gene mutation type and inhibitor development in patients with severe hemophilia A: Systematic review and meta-analysis. *Blood* 119:2922, 2012.

75. Peerlinck K, Arnout J, Gilles JH, et al: A higher than expected incidence of factor VIII inhibitors in multitransfused haemophilia A patients treated with an intermittent purity pasteurized factor VIII concentrate. *Thromb Haemost* 69:115, 1993.

76. Parker ET, Healey JF, Barrow RT, et al: Reduction of the inhibitory antibody response to human factor VIII in hemophilia A mice by mutagenesis of the A2 domain B cell epitope. *Blood* 104:704, 2004.

77. Kasper CK: Laboratory tests for factor VIII inhibitors, their variation, significance and interpretation. *Blood Coagul Fibrinolysis* 2:S7, 1991.

78. Verbruggen B, Novakova I, Wessels H, et al: The Nijmegen modification of the Bethesda assay for factor VIII:C inhibitors: Improved specificity and reliability and specificity. *Thromb Haemost* 73:247, 1995.

79. Ananyeva NM, Lee TK, Jain N, et al: Inhibitors in hemophilia A: Advances in elucidation of inhibitory mechanisms and in inhibitor management with bypassing agents. *Semin Thromb Hemost* 35:735, 2009.

80. Monroe DM, Roberts HR: Mechanism of action of high-dose factor VIIa: Points of agreement and disagreement. *Arterioscler Thromb Vasc Biol* 23:8, 2003.

81. Hoffman M, Dargaud Y: Mechanisms and monitoring of bypassing agent therapy. *J Thromb Haemost* 10:1478, 2012.

82. Escobar M, Maahs J, Hellman E, et al: Multidisciplinary management of patients with haemophilia with inhibitors undergoing surgery in the United States: Perspectives and best practices derived from experienced treatment centers. *Haemophilia* 18:971, 2012.

83. Rangarajan S, Austin S, Goddard NJ, et al: Consensus recommendations for the use of FEIBA in hemophilia A patients with inhibitors undergoing elective orthopedic and non-orthopedic surgery. *Haemophilia* 19:294, 2013.

84. DiMichele DM: Immune tolerance in haemophilia: The long journey to the fork in the road. *Haemophilia* 159:123, 2012.

85. DiMichele DM, Hoots WK, Pipe SW, et al: International workshop on immune tolerance induction: Consensus recommendations. *Haemophilia* 13:1, 2007.

86. Kempton CL, Meeks SL. Toward optimal therapy for inhibitors in hemophilia. *Blood* 124:3365, 2014.

87. Collins PN, Mathias M, Hanley J, et al: Rituximab and immune tolerance in severe hemophilia A: A consecutive national cohort. *J Thromb Haemost* 7:787, 2009.

88. Kohli A, Shaffer A, Sherman A, et al: Treatment of hepatitis C: A systematic review. *JAMA* 312:631, 2014.

89. Gjerset GF, Clements MJ, Counts RB, et al: Treatment type and amount influenced human immunodeficiency virus seroprevalence of patients with congenital bleeding disorders. *Blood* 78:1623, 1991.

90. Aguzzi A, Nuvolone M, Zhu C: The immunobiology of prion diseases. *Nat Rev Immunol* 13:888, 2013.

91. Shanbrom E, Owens W: Cascade iodination: A novel method to enhance the safety and efficacy of therapeutic proteins. *J Thromb Haemost* 2:836, 2004.

92. Ironside JW: Variant Creutzfeldt-Jakob disease. *Folia Neuropathol* 50:50, 2012.

93. Dolan G: Clinical implications of emerging pathogens in haemophilia: The variant Creutzfeldt-Jakob disease experience. *Haemophilia* 12:16, 2006.

94. Kurachi K, Davie EW: Isolation and characterization of a cDNA coding for factor IX. *Proc Natl Acad Sci U S A* 79:6461, 1982.

95. Rallapalli PM, Kemball-Cook G, Tuddenham EG, et al: An interactive mutation database for human coagulation factor IX provides novel insights into the phenotypes and genetics of hemophilia B. *J Thromb Haemost* 11:1329, 2013.

96. F9 Mutation database available at http://www.factorix.org

97. Monroe DM, McCord DM, Huang MN, et al: Functional consequences of an arginine 180 to glutamine mutation in factor IX Hilo. *Blood* 73:1540, 1989.

98. Bertina RM, van der Linden IK, Mannucci PM, et al: Mutations in hemophilia Bm occur at the Arg180-Val activation site or in the catalytic domain of factor IX. *J Biol Chem* 265:10876, 1990.

99. Bottema CD, Ketterling RP, Ii S, et al: Missense mutations and evolutionary conservation of amino acids: Evidence that many of the amino acids in factor IX function as "spacer" elements. *Am J Hum Genet* 49:820, 1991.

100. Ketterling RP, Bottema CD, Phillips JA III, Sommer SS: Evidence that descendants of three founders constitute about 25% of hemophilia B in the United States. *Genomics* 10:1093, 1991.

101. Briet E, Bertina RM, van Tilburg NH, Veltkamp JJ: Hemophilia B Leyden: A sex-linked hereditary disorder that improves after puberty. *N Engl J Med* 306:788, 1982.

102. Kurachi S, Huo JS, Ameri A, et al: An age-related homeostasis mechanism is essential for spontaneous amelioration of hemophilia B Leyden. *Proc Natl Acad Sci U S A* 106:7921, 2009.

103. Reijnen MJ, Sladek FM, Bertina RM, Reitsma PH: Disruption of a binding site for hepatocyte nuclear factor 4 results in hemophilia B Leyden. *Proc Natl Acad Sci U S A* 89:6300, 1992.

104. Lusher JM, McMillan CW: Severe factor VIII and factor IX deficiency in females. *Am J Med* 65:637, 1978.

105. Goodeve AC: Laboratory methods for the genetic diagnosis of bleeding disorders. *Clin Lab Haematol* 20:3, 1998.

106. White GC, Bebe A, Nielsen B: Recombinant factor IX. *Thromb Haemost* 78:261, 1997.

107. Escobar MA: Advances in the treatment of inherited coagulation disorders. *Haemophilia* 19:648, 2013.

108. Wolberg AS, Stafford DW, Erie DA: Human factor IX binds to specific sites on the collagenous domain of collagen IV. *J Biol Chem* 272:16717, 1997.

109. Kim HC, McMillan CW, White GC, et al: Purified factor IX using monoclonal immunoaffinity technique: Clinical trials in hemophilia B and comparison to prothrombin complex concentrates. *Blood* 79:568, 1992.

110. Puetz J, Soucie JM, Kempton CL, et al: Prevalent inhibitors in haemophilia B subjects enrolled in the Universal Data Collection database. *Haemophilia* 20:25, 2014.

111. High KA: Factor IX: Molecular structure, epitopes, and mutations associated with inhibitor formation, in *Inhibitors to Coagulation Factors*, edited by LM Aledort, LW Hoyer, JM Lusher, HM Reisner, CG White, p 79. Plenum, New York, 1995.

112. Warrier I, Ewenstein BM, Koerper MA, et al: Factor IX inhibitors and anaphylaxis in hemophilia B. *J Pediatr Hematol Oncol* 19:23, 1997.

113. Bontempo FA, Lewis JH, Gorenc TJ, et al: Liver transplantation in hemophilia A. *Blood* 69:1721, 1987.

114. Wilde J, Teixeira P, Bramhall SR, et al: Liver transplantation in haemophilia. *Br J Haematol* 117:952, 2002.

115. High KA, Nathwani A, Spencer T, Lillicrap D: Current status of haemophilia gene therapy. *Haemophilia* 20:43, 2014.

116. Monahan PE, Gui T: Gene therapy for hemophilia: Advancing beyond the first clinical success. *Curr Opin Hematol* 20:410, 2013.

117. Chuah MK, Evens H, VandenDriessche T: Gene therapy for hemophilia. *J Thromb Haemost* 11:99, 2013.

118. Nathwani AC, Reiss UM, Tuddenham EG, at al: Long-term safety and efficacy of factor IX gene therapy in hemophilia B. *N Engl J Med* 371:1994, 2014.

119. Ma A, Roberts HR, Escobar MA, editors: *Haemophilia and Haemostasis: A Case-Based Approach to Management*, 2nd ed. Blackwell, Oxford, 2012.

120. Girolami A, Ruzzon E, Fabris F, et al: Myocardial infarction and other arterial occlusions in hemophilia A patients. A cardiological evaluation of all 42 cases reported in the literature. *Acta Haemotol* 116:120, 2006.

121. Kulkarni R, Soucie JM, Evatt BL: Prevalence and risk factors for heart disease among males with hemophilia. *Am J Hematol* 79:36, 2005.

122. Mannucci PM, Schutgens RE, Santagostino E, et al: How I treat age-related morbidities in elderly persons with hemophilia. *Blood* 114:5256, 2009.

123. Tuinenburg A, Damen SAj, Ypma PF, et al: Cardiac catheterization and intervention in haemophilia patients: Prospective evaluation of the 2009 institutional guideline. *Haemophilia* 19:370, 2013.

CHAPTER 124

INHERITED DEFICIENCIES OF COAGULATION FACTORS II, V, V+VIII, VII, X, XI, AND XIII

Flora Peyvandi and Marzia Menegatti*

SUMMARY

Rare bleeding disorders (RBDs), accounting for the 3 to 5 percent of patients with abnormal hemostasis, include the nonhemophilia inherited deficiencies of the coagulation factor II (prothrombin), factor V, combined factor V/VIII, factor VII, factor X, factor XI, factor XIII, and fibrinogen. The prevalence of RBDs is variable, both the relative frequency among the different factors and frequency in different regions of the world. The genetic transmission of these disorders is usually autosomal recessive. Bleeding manifestations caused by these inherited deficiencies are of variable severity and usually related to the extent of the decreased activity of the particular coagulation factor. Usually, only homozygous and compound heterozygous patients are symptomatic, although occasionally heterozygotes display a bleeding tendency. On the whole, the most typical symptom, common to all RBDs, is the occurrence of mucosal bleeding, while life-endangering bleeding, such as the central nervous system or umbilical cord bleeding, are more frequent only in the some deficiencies, such as afibrinogenemia and severe factor XIII and factor X deficiencies, characterized by very low or undetectable coagulant activity. Treatment of patients affected with the various coagulation factor deficiencies could be (1) on demand for spontaneous bleeding episodes, (2) after surgical procedures, and (3) for prevention (prophylaxis). Because of the rarity of these disorders and the technical limitations of laboratory testing and the lack of specific concentrates, a unified, evidence-based therapeutic approach to many such patients is not always clear. To overcome these limitations, new strategies, such as the creation of global partnerships and networking between treatment centers, have been developed to increase our knowledge and create platforms for researchers and clinicians to exchange information.

Acronyms and Abbreviations: aPTT, activated partial thromboplastin time; COPII, coat protein complex II; EGF, epidermal growth factor; ELISA, enzyme-linked immunosorbent assay; ERGIC, endoplasmic reticulum–Golgi intermediate compartment; FFP, fresh-frozen plasma; GGCX, γ-glutamyl carboxylase; Gla, γ-carboxyglutamic acid; LMAN, mannose-binding lectin; MCFD, multiple combined-factor deficiency; PAR, protease-activated receptor; PCC, prothrombin complex concentrate; PPH, postpartum hemorrhage; PT, prothrombin time; TAFI, thrombin-activatable fibrinolysis inhibitor; TF, tissue factor; TT, thrombin time; VKORC1, vitamin K epoxide reductase–oxidase complex.

*The authors would like to thank Dr. U. Selighson and Dr. O. Salomon who wrote the chapter "Inherited Deficiencies of Coagulation Factors II, V, VII, X, XI, and XIII and Combined Deficiencies of Factors V and VIII and of the Vitamin K–Dependent Factors" contained in the previous edition of this book.

Rare congenital deficiencies of plasma proteins involved in blood coagulation, such as fibrinogen, prothrombin, and factors V, V+VIII, VII, X, XI, and XIII, generally lead to lifelong bleeding disorders. These disorders have been described in most populations with an incidence varying from one case in 500,000 for factor VII deficiency, to one case in 2 to 3 million for prothrombin and factor XIII deficiency.[1,2] However, their relative frequency varies among populations, being higher in regions where consanguineous or endogamous marriages are common, partly as a result of increased high frequencies of specific mutant genes in these inbred populations.[3-8] Two large surveys were made by the World Federation of Hemophilia (WFH; www.wfh.org) and the European Network of the Rare Bleeding Disorders (EN-RBD; www.rbdd.eu), with the aim of collecting epidemiologic data and providing information to hemophilia organizations and treatment centers to reduce and prevent complications of bleeding. Data collected by these surveys showed that factor VII and factor XI deficiencies are the most prevalent rare bleeding disorders (RBDs), each accounting for approximately one-third of all RBDs, while the rarest disorders are factor II (prothrombin) deficiency and combined deficiency of factors V and VIII (Table 124–1). The severity of bleeding manifestations in affected patients is variable. The most typical symptom, common to all RBDs, is bleeding from the mucosal tracts or at the site of invasive procedures; life- and limb-endangering symptoms, such as umbilical cord and central nervous system bleeding, recurrent hemarthroses, and soft tissue hematomas, occur with higher frequency only in some severe deficiencies.[9-15] Although heterozygotes for the coagulation factor deficiencies usually do not manifest a bleeding tendency, some cases of postdelivery and post–dental-extraction bleeding in heterozygotes for factor X deficiency have been reported.[16]

LABORATORY DIAGNOSIS

The complexity of blood coagulation and the large number of proteins and nonprotein substances involved necessitate that a global test be used to simply and reproducibly assess its function: the screening tests such as prothrombin time (PT) and activated partial thromboplastin time (aPTT) are the first step in evaluating patients reporting a clinical and family history of bleeding. The PT interrogates the extrinsic coagulation pathway, its prolongation is indicative of the deficiency of factor VII; a normal aPTT is highly dependent on the intrinsic coagulation pathway, so that its prolongation is indicative of deficiencies of factors XI, VIII, IX, and XII. However, all patients homozygous or compound heterozygous for factor XI deficiency have aPTT values longer than 2 SD above the normal mean,[17] while heterozygotes substantially overlap the normal range.[17,18] Consequently, screening of patients for a hemostatic abnormality prior to surgery (which is recommended for Jewish patients because of the high prevalence of factor XI deficiency) identifies patients with severe factor XI deficiency. The prolongation of both the PT and aPTT indicates the lack of a factor belonging to the common pathway, including prothrombin, factor V or factor X. However, patients with factor X deficiency harboring mutations that cause a defect only in the tissue factor (TF) pathway will only display a prolonged PT and their aPTT will be normal. Other patients who carry mutations that only affect the intrinsic pathway activity of factor X, will exhibit a normal PT and prolonged aPTT.[19] Abnormal results of either of these screening tests should be followed by mixing studies where equal amounts of patient plasma and normal plasma are mixed and retested; the relevant test time is normalized in patients with factor deficiencies, but is not corrected or only minimally corrected in patients with factor inhibitors. In case of correction, specific coagulation assays are then performed to make the diagnosis of the specific factor deficiency. To evaluate fibrinogen deficiency, all coagulation tests that depend on the formation of fibrin as the end point are necessary; hence,

TABLE 124–1. Worldwide Distribution of Rare Bleeding Disorders Derived from the World Federation of Haemophilia and the European Network of the Rare Bleeding Disorders Surveys

Deficiency	WFH Survey (%)	EN-RBD Database (%)
Fibrinogen	7	8
Factor II	1	1
Factor V	9	10
Factor V + Factor VIII	3	3
Factor VII	36	39
Factor X	8	8
Factor XI	30	24
Factor XIII	6	7

EN-RBD, European Network of the Rare Bleeding Disorders (www .rbdd.eu); WFH, World Federation of Haemophilia (www.wfh.org).

beside PT and aPTT, thrombin time (TT) has to be also performed. In factor XIII deficiency, PT and aPTT are normal. Diagnosis of factor XIII deficiency is established by demonstrating increased clot solubility in 5 M urea, dilute monochloroacetic acid, or acetic acid. However, this method, quantitative and not yet standardized, detects only severe factor XIII deficiency (with activity <5 percent), thus leading to a possible underdiagnosis of factor XIII deficiency. The factor XIII deficiency diagnosis protocol requires a number of assays, which test for both activity as well as antigen levels. In the case of estimation of factor XIII activity using quantitative (e.g., photometric assays, which measure the ammonia released during a transglutaminase reaction) or incorporation assays (dansylcadaverine-casein assay which measures the level of incorporation of a labeled amine into a protein substrate) during transglutaminase mediated cross linking,[20] the plasma blanking procedure is mandatory to avoid the factor XIIIa-independent ammonia release that could lead to incorrect results in the low-activity range (below 5 to 10 percent).[21,22] Factor XIII A-subunit antigen can be measured by enzyme-linked immunosorbent assay (ELISA).[23] Factor antigen assays are not strictly necessary for diagnosis and treatment but are necessary to distinguish type I from type II deficiencies that become very important in fibrinogen or prothrombin deficiency, where normal antigen levels and reduced coagulant activity (dysfibrinogenemia and dysprothrombinemia) are associated with higher risk of thrombosis. Hereditary factor V deficiency is also a peculiar case that can be confused with combined deficiency of factor V + factor VIII because the two entities have similar manifestations, and are characterized by prolonged PT and aPTT. Consequently, assays of factor V and factor VIII are mandatory for making the distinction.

CLASSIFICATION

The development of guidelines for classification of RBDs has been historically hampered by a lack of sufficient knowledge about epidemiology and clinical outcomes, the difficulty in recognizing affected patients and collecting longitudinal clinical data, the limits of laboratory assays, and a lack of consensus concerning the criteria by which these disorders are classified. Classification of RBDs based on the residual level of plasma coagulant activity of the missing factor has considered for many years all RBDs as a single entity and a mild, moderate, or severe classification as in hemophilia was adopted (except for some disorders

such as afibrinogenemia and factor XIII deficiency). In 2012, the Rare Bleeding Disorders Working Group, under the umbrella of the Factor VIII & Factor IX Scientific and Standardisation Committee (SSC) of the International Society on Thrombosis and Haemostasis (ISTH), analyzed the results of data coming from four registries (EN-RBD, the United Kingdom Haemophilia Centre Doctors' Organization registry, the North American Rare Bleeding Disorders Registry, and the Indian registry) for a total of 4359 patients. Despite the large number of patients evaluated in this overview (both from the literature and the aforementioned registries), there is a large heterogeneity in the preassigned severity definitions for both coagulant activity and bleeding symptoms.[24] At the same time the EN-RBD, based on a cross-sectional study using data from 489 patients and involving 13 European treatment centers, for the first time evaluated the correlation between the coagulant residual plasma activity level and clinical bleeding severity in each RBD. Clinical bleeding episodes were classified into four categories of severity based on the location and the potential clinical impact, as well as the trigger of bleeding (spontaneous, after trauma or drug induced). By means of linear regression analysis, this study found a strong association between coagulant activity level and clinical bleeding severity for fibrinogen, combined factors V + VIII, X and XIII deficiencies. A weak association with clinical bleeding severity was present for factors V and VII deficiencies, while coagulation activity level of factor XI did not predict clinical bleeding severity. From the same study it also clear that the minimum level to ensure complete absence of clinical symptoms is different for each disorder, leading to the conclusion that RBDs should not be considered as a single class of disorders, but instead studies should focus on the evaluation of specific aspects of each single RBD and different from hemophilia.[25]

MOLECULAR ANALYSIS

The molecular diagnosis of RBDs is based on the mutation search in the genes encoding the corresponding coagulation factor. Exceptions are the combined deficiency of coagulation factors V+VIII, caused by mutations in genes encoding proteins involved in the factor V and factor VIII intracellular transport (multiple combined-factor deficiency [MCFD] 2 and mannose-binding lectin [LMAN] 1) and the combined deficiency of vitamin K–dependent proteins (prothrombin and factors VII, IX, and X), caused by mutations in genes that encode enzymes involved in posttranslational modifications[26] and in vitamin K metabolism (γ-glutamyl carboxylase [GGCX] and vitamin K epoxide reductase–oxidase complex [VKORC1]).[27] Coagulant factors genes are located on different chromosomes except for the genes of factor VII (*F7*), factor X (*F10*), fibrinogen (*FGA, FGB, FGG*), and factor XI (*F11*) (Table 124–2). In particular *F10* lays only 2.8 kb downstream of the *F7* thus the combined deficiency of the two factors can be also the result of chromosomal abnormalities of the long arm of chromosome 13.[28] The strategy for molecular analysis is generally based on polymerase chain reaction amplification followed by Sanger sequencing of all exons, flanking intronic sequence and 5′ and 3′ untranslated regions. In contrast with hemophilia A, caused in approximately half of the patients by an inversion mutation involving introns 1 or 22 of the factor VIII gene, RBDs are often caused by mutations unique for each kindred and scattered throughout the genes. Information on already identified mutations causing RBDs is traceable from the mutation database on the ISTH website (http://www.isth.org/?MutationsRareBleedin). Missense mutations are the most frequent gene abnormalities, representing 50 to 80 percent of all identified mutations, except for LMAN1 variants where the most frequent mutations are insertions/deletions (50 percent). Insertion/deletion mutations represent 20 to 30 percent of the gene variations of the fibrinogen, factor V (*F5*), MCFD2, and factor XIII (*F13A*)

TABLE 124–2. General Genetic Features of Coagulation Factors

Deficiency	Gene	Chromosome	Reference
Factor II	F2	11p11–q12	58
Factor V	F5	1q21–25	84
Factors V + VIII	LMAN1	8q21.3–q22	112, 113, 126
	MCFD2	2p21–p16.3	26
Factor VII	F7	13q34	30, 151
Factor X	F10	13q34–qter	192
Factor XI*	F11	4q34–35	235, 236
Factor XIII	F13A	6p24–p25	293, 294
	F13B	1q31–q32.1	296, 297

*F11 gene is located on the same chromosome of fibrinogen genes (fibrinogen deficiency is not discussed in this chapter)

genes, and less than 15 percent of the remaining coagulation factor gene mutations. Splicing and nonsense mutations comprise 5 to 15 percent of all identified mutations in all coagulation factors, with a maximum rate of 20 percent in the LMAN1 gene. Variants located in the 3′ and 5′ untranslated regions of the genes are the least-frequent types of mutation (<5 percent) found only at the fibrinogen, factor VII, factor XI, and factor XIII loci. The combined presence of more than one recessively transmitted coagulation factor defect may also rarely occur resulting in combined deficiency of factors VII and X[31–33] and combined deficiency of factors VII and V, VIII, X, or XI.[34] Despite significant advances in our knowledge of the genetic basis of the RBDs, in 5 to 10 percent of patients affected with severe clotting factor deficiencies, no genetic defect can be found. In these patients, the use of next-generation sequencing might help to identify novel pathways in coagulation disorders.

TREATMENT

Treatment of RBDs is a difficult task because the absence of longitudinal clinical data and the limitations of available laboratory assays make it difficult to develop evidenced-based guidelines for the diagnosis and treatment of RBDs. A patient's personal and family history of bleeding are important guides for management. Dosages and frequency of treatment depend on the minimal hemostatic level of the deficient factor, its plasma half-life (see Table 124–3) and the type of bleeding episode. At variance with patients affected with hemophilia A or B who have vastly improved the quality of life from advances in the manufacture of safe and effective products,[35] patients with RBDs have seen less progress. The main treatments in RBDs are represented by replacement therapy of the deficient coagulation factor and nontransfusional adjuvant therapies (antifibrinolytic amino acids, estrogen/progestin). Fresh-frozen plasma (FFP) and cryoprecipitate are the backbone of RBD treatment, particularly in those countries with low economic resources. However, specific plasma-derived concentrates are currently available only for fibrinogen and factors VII, XI, and XIII, and they are licensed only in some European countries; replacement therapy of coagulation factors may require the prescription of unlicensed products that are not readily available.

Prothrombin and factor X deficiencies are often treated with prothrombin complex concentrates (PCCs), which often also contain uncontrolled amounts of factor II, factor VII, and factor X. Products to cover the need for a dedicated therapy of patients with factor V deficiency and to facilitate the prophylaxis scheme in patients with factor X deficiency are of recent production. Finally, only two recombinant products are currently available for treatment of RBDs: recombinant

factor VIIa (rFVIIa; see factor VII deficiency paragraph) and rFXIII (see "Factor XIII Deficiency" below). Although there are a number of reports available in the literature reporting on treatment on demand and by prophylaxis in RBDs,[36,37] no clear cut guidelines are yet available apart from those of the United Kingdom Haemophilia Centre Doctors' Organization.[38] Table 124–3 shows available treatment for each deficiency and suggested dosages.

WOMEN WITH RARE BLEEDING DISORDERS

Women with RBDs require specific attention and care because in addition to experiencing the common associated bleeding symptoms, they may also experience bleeding complications from regular hemostatic challenges during menstruation, pregnancy, and childbirth, as well as from other gynecologic conditions, such as hemorrhagic ovarian cysts, endometriosis, hyperplasia, polyps, and fibroids. Menorrhagia, defined as blood loss of more than 80 mL per menstruation, is reported to be one of the most important symptoms in women with RBDs.[39,40] Menstruation may be quite problematic for women with coagulation disorders who have excessive blood loss, which can have a major impact on their quality of life and employment.

Pregnancy and childbirth pose particular clinical challenges to women with RBDs, as apart from factor XI deficiency, detailed information about these issues and their management are very scarce and limited to just a few case reports.[41,42] Pregnancy is accompanied by increased concentrations of fibrinogen, factor VII, factor VIII, factor X, and von Willebrand factor, particularly marked in the third trimester.[43–47] In contrast, prothrombin, factor V, factor IX, and factor XIII are relatively unchanged.[43] All of these changes contribute to the hypercoagulable state of pregnancy and, in women with RBDs, contribute to improved hemostasis. Despite improved hemostasis, however, women with factor deficiencies do not achieve the same factor levels as those of women without factor deficiencies,[39] increasing the possibility of pregnancy loss or bleeding complications, especially if the defect is severe.

PROTHROMBIN DEFICIENCY

DEFINITION

Inherited prothrombin deficiency is one of the rarest coagulation factor deficiencies. It presents in two forms: type I, true deficiency (hypoprothrombinemia), and type II, in which a dysfunctional prothrombin

TABLE 124–3. Treatment of Inherited Coagulation Disorders

Deficient Factor	Plasma Half-Life	Recommended Trough Levels	On-Demand Dosages	Recommended Trough Levels After Publication of the EN-RBD Results to Maintain Patient Asymptomatic
Fibrinogen	2–4 days	0.5–1.0 g/L	Cryoprecipitate (5–10 bags)	1 g/L
			SD-treated plasma (15–30 mL/kg)	
			Fibrinogen concentrate (50–100 mg/kg)	
Prothrombin	3–4 days	20–30%	SD-treated plasma (15–20 mL/kg)	>10%
			PCC (20–30 units/kg) with dosing based on labeled factor IX units	
Factor V	36 hours	10–20%	SD-treated plasma (15–20 mL/kg)	10%
Factors V and VIII	Factor V 36 hours Factor VIII 10–14 hours	10–15%	As for factor V	40%
Factor VII	4–6 hours	10–15%	Factor VII concentrate (30–40 mL/kg)	>20%
			PCC (20–30 units/kg)	
			rFVIIa (15–30 mcg/kg every 4–6 hours)	
Factor X	40–60 hours	10–20%	SD-treated plasma (10–20 mL/kg)	>40%
			PCC (20–30 units/kg)	
			Factor X/factor IX concentrate (10–20 units/kg)	
Factor XI	50 hours	15–20%	SD-treated plasma (15–20 mL/kg)	15–20%
			Factor XI concentrate (15–20 units/kg)	
Factor XIII	9–12 days	2–5%	Cryoprecipitate (2–3 bags)	30%
			SD-treated plasma (3 mL/kg)	
			Factor XIII concentrate (50 units/kg for high hemorrhagic events)	

PCC, prothrombin complex concentrate; rFVIIa, recombinant factor VIIa; SD, solvent-detergent.

is produced (dysprothrombinemia). These autosomal recessive disorders are genetically heterogeneous, and characterized by a mild to moderate bleeding tendency. Both types of prothrombin deficiency impair the generation or function of thrombin, the central enzyme of the blood coagulation system.

PROTEIN

Prothrombin, approximate Mr 72,000, is structurally homologous with other members of the vitamin K–dependent proteins, factors VII, IX, and X, proteins C, S, and Z, and bone γ-carboxyglutamic acid (Gla) protein. Prothrombin is synthesized in the liver as a prepropeptide of 622 amino acids and its plasma concentration is 100 to 150 mcg/mL. The circulating protein in its mature form is a single chain glycoprotein of 579 residues, composed of the Gla domain (residues 1 to 37) and the catalytic domain (residues 272 to 579), where a light A chain is disulfide-bonded to the heavy B chain containing the catalytic triad. In the zymogen molecule there are several exodomains, such as two kringle domains—kringle 1 domain (F1; residues 38 to 155), kringle 2 domain (F2; residues 156 to 271)—and the prepropeptide regions.[48,49] The prepropeptide domain is responsible for protein processing, targeting, and carboxylation, and it is removed prior to secretion from the cell. The Gla domain constitutes the aminoterminus of the mature prothrombin molecule and contains the 10 glutamic acid residues that are posttranslationally modified through action of vitamin K–dependent

carboxylase to Gla. As a result of this modification, prothrombin acquires the capacity to bind calcium and membranes containing acidic phospholipids. The kringle domain contains two extensively folded, disulfide-bonded "kringle" motifs. They are present in diverse proteins and are thought to mediate protein–protein interactions. For example, the second kringle mediates interaction of prothrombin with activated factor V.[50] Notably, previous data shows that the kringle 2 domain, generated from the precursor prothrombin that is endogenously expressed in human, mouse, and rat brains, including in dopaminergic neurons in the nervous system,[51,52] is able to activate *in vitro* microglia cells and may be involved in the neuropathologic processes of dopaminergic neuronal death occurring in Parkinson disease.[52] However, the real clinical significance of these *in vitro* findings is still to be unraveled. The catalytic domain contains the enzyme active site, which is responsible for fibrinogen cleavage. The residues characteristic for the serine protease family, His363, Asp419, and Ser525, constitute a charge relay system responsible for bond cleavage. The crystal structure of prothrombin has not been determined, but the crystal structure of human α-thrombin complexed with *D-Phe-Pro-Arg chloromethylketone* (an inhibitor that is a transition state analogue covalently bound to the enzyme) has been determined.[53]

Prothrombin plays a central role in coagulation, functioning in both TF and contact activation pathways. Prothrombin is converted to its proteolytically active form thrombin by the prothrombinase complex consisting of activated factor X, factor Va, and phospholipid surface of platelets and other cells. Two forms of thrombin are generated: meizothrombin, if prothrombin is cleaved at residue 320, and α-thrombin, if cleavage occurs first at residue 271, removing prothrombin fragment 1.2, and subsequently cleaved at residue 320. The α-thrombin A-chain (residues 272 to 320) formed by factor Xa cleavage is encoded by exons 8 and 9. The B-chain (residues 321 to 579) containing the catalytic site and regulatory elements is encoded by exons 9 to 14. Thrombin is a multifunctional serine protease. In addition to converting fibrinogen to fibrin, thrombin also exerts functions in the coagulation cascade, consisting of both pro- and anticoagulant effects[54] and activates platelets by cleavage of the protease-activated receptor (PAR)-1 and PAR-4, initiating signals leading to platelet adhesion and aggregation.[55,56] Thrombin also stimulates wound healing through its action as a growth factor and its proangiogenic activity.[57]

GENETICS

The prothrombin gene is located on the short (p) arm of chromosome 11.[58] It is 20-kb long and consists of 14 exons separated by 13 introns. Fifty-four mutations that cause prothrombin deficiency have been identified, of which 42 are missense, three nonsense, seven deletions/insertions, and two splicing mutations (see mutation database on the ISTH website, http://www.isth.org/?MutationsRareBleedin and Ref. 9). Type II deficiency (dysprothrombinemias) results from missense mutations that are located throughout the gene. As expected, many mutations are in the catalytic domain, imparting catalytic dysfunction on thrombin. Other mutations give rise to abnormally slow activation of prothrombin. Only about 10 mutations were identified in patients with type I deficiency, of which five were present in homozygotes. Globally, there is a clear prevalence of patients with a Latin/Hispanic origin, as nearly 70 percent of all patients with thrombin gene defects come from such areas (Barcelona, Padua, Segovia, and Puerto Rico).[9]

A number of polymorphisms have been identified in the prothrombin gene. One of these polymorphisms, a G>A change at nucleotide 20210 in the 3′ untranslated region of the prothrombin gene, is associated with increased plasma levels of prothrombin and an increased tendency to venous thrombosis (Chap. 130).[59]

CLINICAL MANIFESTATIONS

According to a recent classification by the SSC of the ISTH, prothrombin deficiency may be classified as severe, moderate, and mild corresponding to blood levels of less than 5 percent, 5 to 10 percent, and greater than 10 percent, respectively.[24] In severely prothrombin-deficient patients, bleeding may be marked, including spontaneous hemarthroses; less-severe patients may show mild to moderate mucocutaneous and soft-tissue bleeding that usually correlates with the degree of functional prothrombin deficiency. Heterozygous subjects, having plasma prothrombin levels between 30 and 60 percent of normal, are usually asymptomatic; however, occasionally, excessive bleeding after moderate-intensity trauma, tooth extractions, or after surgical procedures may occur. Patients with dysprothrombinemias show a variable bleeding tendency that is usually less severe than in type I deficiency. Women with prothrombin deficiency may suffer from menorrhagia. Because of the extreme rarity of such deficiency, reports on event during pregnancy/delivery are very scarce, being only one describing in four of eight pregnancies in a hypoprothrombinemic woman.[60] In the same report, one postpartum hemorrhage (PPH) episode on the four-term pregnancies was reported, despite administration of clotting factor concentrate[60]; however, this data was not confirmed by a following Iranian series, including a total of 14 patients with the same deficiency (coagulant activity levels 4 to 10 percent).[61]

Undetectable plasma prothrombin probably is incompatible with life, as inferred from the partial embryonic and neonatal lethality of prothrombin knockout mice, which do not survive to adulthood.[62,63]

THERAPY

Replacement therapy is needed only in severe patients, in case of bleeding or to ensure adequate prophylaxis before surgical procedures. In severe clinical settings, higher levels of prothrombin may be achieved with FFP, or with PCCs, which avoids the risk of volume overload sometimes associated with the use of FFP.[64] However, PCCs contain other vitamin K–dependent coagulation factors (VII, IX, and X) and small amounts of their activated forms, which could potentially induce thrombotic complications; those containing an amount of factor VII below 10 percent are commonly known as three-factor PCCs. These concentrates are heated or treated with solvent–detergent, processes that remove HIV, hepatitis B, hepatitis C, and other viruses, but which do not remove parvovirus B19 or hepatitis A virus[65–67]; the latter viruses can be effectively removed by dry heat and nanofiltration.[68] However, transmission of other possible bloodborne agents, such as prions causing Creutzfeldt-Jakob disease and its new variant, have not been totally eliminated. Bruises and mild superficial bleeding generally do not require replacement therapy. Antifibrinolytic agents (tranexamic acid and gabexate mesylate) have also been used for minor surgical procedures. The oral contraceptives have been shown to exert beneficial effects on menometrorrhagia in women characterized by prothrombin coagulant levels less than 3 percent.[9] Thromboprophylaxis in dysprothrombinemic patients considered at high risk for a thrombotic event (e.g., orthopedic surgery) is a controversial issue. It is likely that administering low-molecular-weight heparin prophylactically to surgical patients at the same doses and schedules as those recommended for nondefect patients having similar procedures may be a valuable and safe procedure after correction of factor II deficiency by FFP or PCC infusion.

● FACTOR V DEFICIENCY

DEFINITION AND HISTORY

Hereditary factor V deficiency was initially termed parahemophilia because of its similarities with classical hemophilia.[69] In most of the affected individuals the phenotype is characterized by the concomitant deficiency of factor V activity and antigen (type I deficiency); however, approximately 25 percent of the patients have normal antigen levels (type II deficiency), thus indicating the presence of a dysfunctional protein.[70]

PROTEIN

Factor V is synthesized by the liver[71] and its plasma concentration is approximately 20 nM (7 mcg/mL).[72–74] Factor V is a high-molecular-weight (Mr ~330,000), single-chain, large glycoprotein that consists of 2196 amino acids that bears significant, regional sequence homology to factor VIII. Analysis of the approximately 7-kb factor V complementary DNA showed that the protein is organized according to the following domain structure: A_1-A_2-B-A_3-C_1-C_2. The A and C domains have approximately 40 percent homology with analogous domains in factor VIII.[74,75] The large B domain shows no homology with the corresponding B domain of factor VIII. Factor V is converted to its activated form following several proteolytic cleavages by thrombin[76] or factor Xa.[77] These cleavages remove the B domain and yield factor Va, which consists of a heavy chain (A_1-A_2 domains) associated by Ca^{2+} with a light chain (A_3-C_1-C_2 domains). The light chain contains the binding sites for membrane phospholipids, prothrombin, and activated protein C; both light and heavy chains probably are necessary for factor Xa binding. Assembly of factors Va and Xa on the phospholipid membrane of platelets in the presence of calcium ions forms the prothrombinase complex, which catalyzes the conversion of prothrombin to thrombin. The contribution of factor Xa in the absence of factor Va to overall thrombin generation is relatively minor. Importantly, incorporation of the cofactor into the macromolecular enzyme complex enhances prothrombin activation by several orders of magnitude.[78]

In addition to hepatocytes, the primary site of factor V secretion, approximately 20 percent of the protein in whole blood is localized in the α granules of platelets, where it is complexed with an extremely large protein, multimerin.[79] Megakaryocytes do not synthesize factor V; rather, endocytosis of plasma-derived factor V accounts for the platelet factor V pool.[80] Following endocytosis factor V is modified intracellularly; these changes to platelet factor V appear to provide the cofactor with unique physical and functional characteristics, which render it more procoagulant compared with its plasma counterpart.[81] Platelet degranulation and release of platelet factor V at the site of vascular injury is thought to be a critical contributor to the local factor V concentration. Furthermore, there is some evidence that, because platelet factor V is locally released in high concentrations, it is less susceptible to inhibition and may function normally in hemostasis. Factor Va is inactivated by activated protein C through limited proteolysis at Arg506, Arg306, and Arg679 in the presence of protein S, calcium ions, and either platelet or endothelial cell membrane phospholipids.[82] Partial protection from this cleavage is provided by factor Xa when bound to factor Va on the surface of platelets.[83]

GENETICS

The factor V gene maps to chromosome 1q21–25.[84] It is greater than 80 kb in length and the coding sequence is divided into 25 exons, ranging in size from 72 to 2820 base pairs (bp), and 24 introns, varying between 0.4 kb and 11 kb.[85] The sequence encoding the large B domain is contained within exon 13.

A total of 132 distinct mutations of the factor V gene have been identified, of which 64 are missense, 36 are insertions/deletions, 17 are nonsense, 15 are splice site mutations, and one is a deletion of the whole gene (see http://www.isth.org/?MutationsRareBleedin and Ref. 10). Most mutations cause truncations and are localized throughout the gene. Several mutations have interesting features. One, a Tyr1702Cys transition, was identified in eight unrelated families, of whom six were Italian. The frequency of this mutant allele in Italy is 0.002.[86] Another mutation, an Ala221Val (New Brunswick) alteration, characterized in the homozygous state by activity and antigen levels of 29 and 39 percent of normal, respectively displays decreased stability of the expressed protein and was the first genetic defect reported to be associated with type II deficiency.[87] Additional mutations exhibit decreased secretion of the protein from producing cells.[88,89] Remarkably, the Gln773ter and Arg1133ter mutations and a 4-bp deletion mutation, all present in exon 13 and predicted to result in partial truncation of the B-domain and complete truncation of the A3-, C1-, and C2-domains, cause no bleeding or only a mild bleeding tendency in affected patients having factor V antigen and activity levels 1 percent of normal.[90–92]

Factor V Leiden (Arg506Gln) is a highly prevalent (up to 5 percent in some populations) polymorphism in the factor V gene that decreases the efficiency of factor Va inactivation by activated protein C.[93] Patients with factor V Leiden are at increased risk of unprovoked thrombosis,

with homozygotes at greater risk than heterozygotes. The *trans* association of factor V Leiden and a mutation in factor V that causes factor V deficiency results in a prothrombotic state comparable to factor V Leiden homozygosity. This is sometimes termed "pseudohomozygous" activated protein C resistance and does not cause bleeding despite low factor V antigen levels.[94] Among several polymorphisms detected in the factor V gene, His1299Arg in exon 13 is particularly interesting because it is associated with a reduced plasma factor V level and mild activated protein C resistance.[95] His1299Arg co-segregates with several other polymorphisms encoding several amino acid changes, together named R2 haplotype.[96] In two heterozygotes for factor V Arg506Gln mutation who presented with venous thrombosis, reduced factor V activity resulting from the His1299Arg polymorphism harbored by the non-Leiden chromosome, imparted a pseudohomozygous phenotype for activated protein C resistance.[97] Additional polymorphisms or mutations in the factor V gene have been observed to increase the risk of venous thrombosis.[98]

In addition, there are at least two examples in which platelet factor V is reduced. In the Quebec platelet disorder, initially described as an autosomal dominant disorder with severe bleeding manifestations, platelet factor V levels are reduced because of enhanced proteolysis resulting from overexpression of urokinase-type plasminogen activator,[99] as they are in factor V New York.[100]

CLINICAL MANIFESTATIONS

Factor V deficiency is inherited as an autosomal recessive trait. Heterozygotes, whose plasma factor V activity ranges between 25 and 60 percent of normal, usually are asymptomatic, although an American registry recorded mild bleeding in 50 percent of the cases.[101] According to a recent classification by the SSC of the ISTH, factor V deficiency may be classified as severe, moderate, and mild when factor V levels are undetectable, less than 10 percent, and 10 percent or greater, respectively.[24]

Common manifestations include ecchymoses, epistaxis, gingival bleeding, hemorrhage following minor lacerations, and menorrhagia.[101–103] Severe deficiency typically presents at birth or in early childhood, but depending on factor levels some patients remain asymptomatic. Bleeding from other sites is less common, but instances of hemarthroses unrelated to trauma and intracerebral hemorrhage have been reported.[102] Trauma, dental extractions, and surgery confer a high risk of excessive bleeding.

PPH occurs in more than 50 percent of pregnancies in women with factor V deficiency,[104,105] especially those with low factor V activity levels. Venous and arterial thromboses have been described in patients with factor V levels ranging between 2 and 14 percent of normal.[106] Factor V deficiency deprives activated protein C of one of its essential substrates, thereby downregulating the inhibitory function of the protein C system.

Development of a functional factor V inhibitor after receiving plasma transfusions was reported in only two patients with hereditary deficiency; the inhibitor disappeared in one patient, but a low titer of the inhibitor persisted in the other patient.[107,108] Factor V is indispensable for life, as was demonstrated by experimental knockout mice lacking the factor V gene, which die either in utero at embryonic day 9 or 10 because of defects in yolk-sac vasculature and somite formation; the remaining half develop to term but die of massive hemorrhage within hours of birth.[109] The expression of a minimal factor V activity because of the introduction of a liver-specific transgene, below the sensitivity threshold of the detection assay (<0.1 percent), leads to the survival of mice.[110]

THERAPY

Patients with epistaxis and gingival bleeding may respond to tranexamic acid (1 g four times daily), and local hemostatic measures may suffice for minor lacerations. Menorrhagia can also be managed directly using oral contraceptives, progestin-containing intrauterine devices, endometrial ablation, or hysterectomy. If these measures fail, severe spontaneous bleeding occurs, or surgery is performed, treatment option is limited to FFP replacement as no specific factor V concentrate is yet available on the market and factor V is not present in cryoprecipitate or PCCs. However, a new factor V concentrate has been developed for clinical use in patients deficient in factor V and preclinical studies are currently being performed for the orphan drug designation application to the European Medicine Agency (EMA) and the Food and Drug Administration (FDA) so as to make it available on the market as soon as possible.

● COMBINED DEFICIENCY OF FACTORS V AND VIII

DEFINITION AND HISTORY

Combined deficiency of factors V and VIII (F5F8D) is completely separate from factor V deficiency and factor VIII deficiency. The latter two are transmitted with different patterns of inheritance (autosomal recessive for factor V, X-linked for factor VIII) and involve proteins encoded by two different genes (*F5* gene and *F8* gene). F5F8D was first described in 1954[111]; however, the molecular mechanism of the association of the combined factor deficiency was not understood until late 1990s,[112,113] when null mutations in the endoplasmic reticulum–Golgi intermediate compartment (*ERGIC*)-53 gene, now called the *LMAN1* gene, were determined to be causative. In 2003, a second locus associated with the deficiency in approximately 15 percent of affected families with no mutation in LMAN1 was identified[26]: the *MCFD2* gene encoding for a cofactor for LMAN1. Even if a debate were carried out on the possible existence of other loci involved in the intracellular transport of factors V and VIII and associated with the disease, until now previous biochemical studies failed to identify additional components of the LMAN1–MCFD2 receptor complex,[114] supporting the idea that F5F8D might be limited to the *LMAN1* and *MCFD2* genes.[115] The disorder has been detected in many populations, but a relatively high frequency occurs among Tunisian and Middle Eastern Jews residing in Israel[116] and among Iranians.[117]

PROTEIN

Factors V and VIII are essential coagulation factors that circulate in plasma as precursors. Upon limited proteolysis by thrombin or factor Xa and in concert with negatively charged phospholipid surfaces, factors VIIIa and Va exhibit profound cofactor activities for activation of factor X by factor IXa and for activation of prothrombin by factor Xa, respectively. Inactivation of factors Va and VIIIa is accomplished by activated protein C in the presence of protein S and phospholipids through several proteolytic cleavages at distinct sites. Factor V and factor VIII have similar domain organizations with partial homology (see "Factor V Deficiency" above).

The pathogenesis of combined deficiency of factors V and VIII puzzled investigators for more than 40 years. The enigma was resolved by the finding that the disease stems from the deficiency of either one of two interacting proteins, LMAN1 and MCFD2, which play a role in the intracellular transport of factors V and VIII. LMAN1 is a 53-kDa type 1 transmembrane nonglycosylated protein with homology to leguminous lectin proteins.[118] It displays different oligomerization states—monomer, dimer, and hexamer—which have been implicated in its exit/retention within the endoplasmic reticulum (ER), and is thought to bind correctly folded glycosylated cargo proteins, including factors V and VIII in the ER, recruiting the cargo for package into coat protein complex II (COPII)–coated vesicles and to transport them first to the ERGIC and then to the Golgi. MCFD2 is a small (146 residues) soluble protein of 16 kDa with a signal sequence mediating translocation into the ER and two EF-hand motifs that may bind Ca^{2+} ions in the C-terminal region.[119] MCFD2 forms a Ca^{2+}-dependent 1:1 stoichiometric complex with LMAN1, which works as a cargo receptor for efficient ER–Golgi transfer of coagulation factors V and VIII during their secretion. Although several proteins have been identified as cargo of LMAN1 (factor V, factor VIII, cathepsin C, cathepsin Z, nicastrin, and α_1-antitrypsin),[120-123] MCFD2 is only known to be required for transport of the blood coagulation factors, suggesting a possible role for MCFD2 as a specific recruitment factor for this subset of LMAN1 cargo proteins.[124] The three-dimensional structure of the complex between MCFD2 and the carbohydrate recognition domain (CRD) of LMAN1 was determined and a model of functional coordination between the two proteins was proposed: MCFD2 is converted into the active form upon complex formation with LMAN1, thereby becoming able to capture polypeptide segments of factors V and VIII. The coagulation factors bind the LMAN1 oligomer in the ER, but are released upon arrival in the acidic post-ER compartments because the sugar-binding of ERGIC-53 is pH-dependent.[125]

GENETICS

Homozygosity mapping and positional cloning in nine unrelated Jewish families demonstrated that the *LMAN1*, composed of 13 exons, localizes on the long arm of chromosome 18.[112,113,126] Using a similar approach in other families with the combined factors V and VIII deficiency identified the short *MCFD2*, made up of four exons on the short arm of chromosome 2.[26] Thirty-four mutations identified in *LMAN1* predicted either a truncated protein product or no protein at all, being more than 90 percent deletion/insertion, null, or splicing mutations. In contrast, of the 22 mutations identified in the *MCFD2*, 11 are missense and 11 are null mutations. Missense mutations are located at the EF-2 domains, giving rise to defective binding to LMAN1.[127] A distinct founder haplotype was found in patients belonging to six unrelated families of Tunisian-Jewish origin bearing a donor splice-site mutation in intron 9 of *LMAN1*.[112,127] All six families originated from an ancient Jewish community that has resided on the island of Djerba for more than 2 millennia. A survey of this community, which presently lives in Israel, disclosed that the mutation is prevalent at an allele frequency of 0.0107.[128] Another founder effect for a G insertion in exon 1 of *LMAN1* was observed in eight unrelated Jewish families of Middle Eastern origin.[112,127] A Met to Thr mutation in *LMAN1* has been detected in several unrelated Italian families, implying another founder effect.[127]

CLINICAL MANIFESTATIONS

Symptoms of F5F8D are generally mild. Comparison of relatively large cohorts of F5F8D in India, Iran, and Israel indicates that bleeding from trauma/surgery is the most frequently reported clinical manifestation.[116,117,129,130] This observation likely reflects the fact that often F5F8D is brought to the attention of physicians following excessive bleeding during and after trauma, surgery, and labor. Homozygous patients exhibit spontaneous and posttraumatic bleeding. Menorrhagia, epistaxis, easy bruising, hemarthrosis and gingival hemorrhage are commonly observed, and is unrelated to trauma in approximately 20 percent of cases.[117,131] Hematuria, GI, and spontaneous CNS bleeding is less common.[117] There is insufficient data on the incidence of bleeding during pregnancy and PPH in women with combined factor V+VIII.

Heterozygotes exhibit slight but significantly reduced mean levels of factors V and VIII.[116] In a literature survey of 161 heterozygotes, 22 reported having significant bleeding manifestations.[132] However, no correlation between the factor V or factor VIII levels and bleeding tendency was noted.[25]

LMAN1 gene knockout mice duplicate the F5F8-deficient phenotype in humans, albeit with a milder presentation, resulting from a lesser reduction in plasma levels of factors V and VIII.[133] The partial perinatal lethality observed in LMAN1-deficient mice on some genetic backgrounds was unexpected and has been explained as the result of a further drop in the level of LMAN1-dependent protein(s) below a critical threshold, or because of a strain-specific difference in another cargo receptor whose function overlaps with LMAN1.

THERAPY

Because of the mild-to-moderate bleeding symptoms, treatment is on demand, depending on the severity of bleeding. According to a recent result from the EN-RBD project, however, the level of F5F8 to ensure the absence of bleeding symptoms should be greater than 40 percent.[25] The recommended therapy includes FFP, which provides factor V, and factor VIII concentrate, which compensates for the shorter half-life of plasma factor VIII. An antifibrinolytic agent such as tranexamic acid or ε-aminocaproic acid can be helpful in patients exhibiting menorrhagia, epistaxis, or gingival bleeding. DDAVP (1-deamino-8-D-arginine vasopressin, desmopressin) could be administered for less-severe bleeding. Patients with severe bleeding episodes or patients undergoing surgical procedures, including dental extractions, should receive FFP as replacement for factor V and cryoprecipitate or factor VIII concentrate as a source of factor VIII. DDAVP can be used to increase factor VIII level, but this treatment sometimes fails.[134]

● FACTOR VII DEFICIENCY

DEFINITION AND HISTORY

Factor VII was first identified as serum prothrombin conversion accelerator or proconvertin and its hereditary deficiency described by Alexander and colleagues in 1951.[135] Among the rare clotting factor deficiencies, the relative frequency of factor VII deficiency is high (see Table 124–1).[101,102] A presumptive diagnosis can be easily made because, except for very rare cases of factor X deficiency only affecting the TF pathway of coagulation (see "Laboratory Diagnosis" below), factor VII deficiency is the only coagulation disorder that produces a prolonged PT and a normal aPTT.

PROTEIN

Human factor VII is a single-chain glycoprotein (Mr ~50,000) that is secreted from the liver parenchymal cells as a zymogen. The mature protein consists of 406 amino acids organized in three main domains: a Gla domain at the N-terminus containing 10 Gla residues, an epidermal growth factor (EGF) domain in the center, and a serine protease domain at the C-terminus.[136] Factor VII zymogen circulates in blood at an extremely low concentration (~500 ng/mL)[137] and has the shortest half-life of all coagulation factors (4 to 6 hours; see Table 124–3). Factor VII is converted to the activated form, factor VIIa, by cleavage of an Arg152-Ile153 bond, resulting in a two-chain molecule held together by a disulfide bond. Factor VII can be converted to factor VIIa by factor Xa,[138] factor IXa,[139] factor XIIa,[140] thrombin,[138] and factor VIIa in the presence of TF, in an autoactivation reaction.[141] Binding of factor VII to TF strikingly enhances these reactions.[142–146]

The initial generation of thrombin that heralds blood coagulation occurs when blood is exposed to TF present in the subendothelium in tissues, or on the surface of stimulated monocytes or microparticles. The exposed TF forms a complex with circulating factor VIIa and supports the initiation of coagulation by converting factors IX and X into their active forms (factor IXa and factor Xa).[147,148] Following the generation of trace amounts of factor VIIa there is a feedback amplification of the signal, as factor VII bound to TF: factor VIIa is both self-activated, and activated by factor IXa and factor Xa. Hence, the TF–factor VIIa complex has two roles: to increase the conversion of factor VII to factor VIIa and to increase the proteolytic activity of factor VIIa toward its substrates, factors IX and X. Factors IXa and Xa may remain associated with cells that display the TF, or disseminate in the blood and bind to the surface of activated platelets, which form the initial platelet plug.[149]

GENETICS

The factor VII gene (*F7*) spans approximately 12.8 kb[150] and is located on chromosome 13q34,[30,151] 2.8 kb upstream from the factor X gene.[152] The gene contains a prepro leader sequence and eight exons that encode the mature protein. Promoter and silencer elements of the 5′ flanking region have been characterized.[153,154] The disorder manifests in homozygotes or compound heterozygotes, some of which are also homozygotes for polymorphisms associated with reduced factor VII levels.[155,156]

More than 240 mutations have been reported (see http://www.isth.org/?MutationsRareBleedin and Ref. 12). The mutations are distributed throughout the gene, and most are missense mutations (62.2 percent); other type of mutations are equally present (ranging from approximately 6.2 percent of mutations in 3′-5′ untranslated region [UTR] to 12.3 percent of deletions/insertions [del/ins]). Most mutations causing factor VII deficiency have been observed in individual patients. However, one missense mutation (Ala244Val) was detected in 102 (84 percent) of 121 independent mutant alleles discerned in 88 unrelated patients in Israel.[157] Most subjects were of Iranian and Moroccan-Jewish origin and shared an identical haplotype, consistent with a founder effect. In the general Iranian-Jewish and Moroccan-Jewish populations, the prevalence of the Ala244Val allele are 0.023 and 0.025, respectively.[156] Several additional clusters of patients with a specific mutation were reported: (1) Ala294Val, with or without a deletion of nt C, at position 11128, prevails in patients from Poland and Germany but has also been identified in other Europeans[158,159]; (2) 12 unrelated families from Norway who carry Gln100Arg[160]; (3) IVS75G>A, which was detected in six unrelated patients from the Lazio region in Italy, all of whom bear the same haplotype, suggesting a founder effect[161]; and (4) Gly331Ser, which was identified in 10 Italian and four German patients on one haplotype.[162] The widely distributed and common Arg304Gln mutation probably is a recurrent mutation.[163]

Three polymorphisms in the factor VII gene are also associated with reduced plasma levels of the factor. The first polymorphism, an Arg353Gln substitution, results in impaired secretion of factor VII from cells[164] and gives rise to a 20- to 25-percent decrease in plasma factor VII level in heterozygotes and a 40- to 50-percent decrease in homozygotes.[165,166] The second polymorphism associated with a diminished factor VII level is a decanucleotide insertion upstream from the 5′ end of the gene at −323, which confers a 33 percent decrease in the promoter activity.[154] A third polymorphism associated with factor VII level is a hypervariable region 4 polymorphism (HVR4) in intron 7.[167] The variable number of tandem repeats (five to eight copies of 37 bp) apparently influences the splicing efficiency. The effect of the variable repeats on factor VII level is less conspicuous than the decanucleotide insertion at the promoter region and the Arg353Gln polymorphism.

CLINICAL FEATURES

Bleeding manifestations occur in homozygotes and in compound heterozygotes for factor VII deficiency. However, a typical feature of this disease is its clinical heterogeneity: some patients do not bleed at all after major hemostatic challenge, while others with similar levels report frequent bleeding episodes. Life- or limb-endangering bleeding manifestations are relatively rare, the most frequent symptoms being epistaxis and menorrhagia. However, CNS bleeding was also reported to have high incidence (16 percent) in a series of 75 infants,[168] the authors concluding that the greatest risk factor for this development was trauma related to the birth process. In addition, heterozygotes who have partial factor VII deficiency may present with bleeding; a recent survey of 499 heterozygotes revealed that 19 percent reported pathologic bleeding.[155] Dental extractions, tonsillectomy, and surgical procedures involving the urogenital tracts frequently are accompanied by bleeding when no prior therapy is instituted. Normal pregnancy is accompanied by increased concentrations of fibrinogen and factor VII, nonetheless, cases of miscarriages and PPH, albeit at relatively low rates, have been observed in patients with factor VII deficiency.[169,170]

Thrombotic episodes have also been reported in 3 to 4 percent of patients with factor VII deficiency, particularly in the presence of surgery and replacement treatment, but spontaneous thrombosis may also occur. A survey of 514 cases with severe or partial factor VII deficiency recorded seven patients with venous thrombosis and one patient with arterial thrombosis.[171] Most of the cases presented with associated risk factors, mainly surgery, prolonged immobilization, and treatment with PCCs.[172]

When factor VII is completely lacking, as in knockout mice, there is no embryonic lethality; however, fatal hemorrhage occurs perinatally.[173,174]

THERAPY

As for all the other congenital bleeding disorders, replacement therapy is essential in patients who present with severe hemorrhage, such as hemarthrosis or intracerebral bleeding, surgical hemostasis, and for individuals with a bleeding history. Factor replacement therapy may also be used for prophylaxis in children with severe factor VII deficiency.[175] The EN-RBD study suggests a trough factor VII activity level of 25 percent is needed for patients to remain asymptomatic[25]; prophylactic treatment is usually recommended for patients with major bleeding episodes such as CNS and gastrointestinal bleeding and hemarthroses. A number of replacement therapeutic options have been administered to patients with factor VII deficiency, including FFP, PCCs, plasma-derived factor VII concentrates (volume overload should be expected if plasma is used as the replacement material) and rFVIIa. rFVIIa has been successful in managing patients with hemarthroses and during surgery,[176,177] and is the only treatment supported by substantial literature[12,176] (see Table 124–3). PCCs containing activated clotting factors can be used, but they confer a risk of thrombosis,[175] while specific factor VII concentrates have been used successfully in series of patients.[175] The treatment of factor VII deficiency is sometimes challenging, because of the short *in vivo* half-life of factor VII, its low recovery, and its rapid clearance, which is more evident in children.[178] Because of these features, replacement regimens require frequent dosing. A significant rise in the factor VII level is observed during pregnancy in women with mild/moderate forms of factor VII deficiency (heterozygotes), but not in women with severe deficiency.[179–182] Therefore, in women with mild/moderate

deficiency, replacement therapy may not be required during labor and delivery, while it would be required in women with low factor VII coagulant activity levels or a positive bleeding history who are more likely to be at risk of PPH.[181,183–185] A recent review of the literature noted that hemorrhage rates were equivalent in women with and without prophylaxis, thus concluding that use of hemostatic prophylaxis should not be considered mandatory, but as part of an individualized discussion taking into consideration response to previous hemostatic challenges and mode of delivery.[186] Replacement therapy is unnecessary for minor bleeding episodes. Local hemostasis for skin lacerations and administration of an antifibrinolytic agent for menorrhagia, epistaxis, and gingival hemorrhage usually are sufficient to arrest bleeding. Asymptomatic patients undergoing minimally invasive surgery, such as dental procedures, can be successfully treated with tranexamic acid given both orally or intravenously at the usual dosages.

● FACTOR X DEFICIENCY

DEFINITION AND HISTORY

Inherited factor X deficiency was identified by two independent groups, each of which described a patient with a bleeding diathesis that could not be attributed to deficiencies in other known coagulation factors. The factor in both patients was subsequently named factor X.[187–189]

PROTEIN

Factor X is mainly synthesized by the liver as a 488-amino-acid protein and circulates in plasma at a concentration of 8 to 10 mcg/mL.[190] Its primary structure is homologous to that of other vitamin K–dependent proteins, such as prothrombin, factor VII, factor IX, protein C, and protein S.[191] The first 40-amino-acid residues, the prepropeptide, contain the hydrophobic signal sequences targeting the protein for secretion.[192] The Gla domain forms the N-terminus of the mature protein and contains 11 Gla residues that are responsible for calcium and phospholipid binding.[193] Adjacent to the Gla domain is a short aromatic amino acid stack of predominantly hydrophobic amino acids, followed by the EGF domain, believed to mediate protein–protein interactions. The heavily glycosylated 52-amino-acid activation peptide of factor X separates the EGF domain from the C-terminal catalytic domain. Factor X undergoes proteolytic processing in the ER so that circulating factor is a two-chain, disulfide-linked protein consisting of a 17-kDa light chain made up of the Gla and EGF domains and a 40-kDa heavy chain made up of the activation and catalytic domains.[194] The heavy chain contains the activation peptide (residues 143 to 195) and the catalytic serine protease domain, structurally homologous to that of other coagulation serine proteases containing the catalytic site formed by residues His236, Asp282, and Ser379. The 52-residue activation peptide is released after factor X is converted to its active form factor Xa by the cleavage between residues Arg194 and Ile195. Physiologically factor X is activated by TF/factor VIIa (extrinsic pathway) and factor IXa/factor VIIIa (intrinsic pathway),[195] but it can also be activated *in vitro* by Russel viper venom.[196] In turn, factor Xa catalyses thrombin formation. In presence of factor Va, Ca^{2+}, and phospholipid membrane, factor Xa forms the prothrombinase complex that accelerates to 280,000-fold thrombin formation.[197]

GENETICS

The factor X gene spans approximately 25 kb and is made up of eight exons.[192] The factor X gene shows significant homology with the genes of other vitamin K–dependent serine proteases, which suggests all of these multidomain genes evolved from a common ancestral gene.[198]

The currently described 105 mutations that cause factor X deficiency include large deletions, small frameshift deletions, nonsense mutation, and missense mutations; the missense mutations group is the largest (80 percent), while mutations in the 3'- and 5'-UTRs are completely absent (see http://www.isth.org/?MutationsRareBleedin and Ref. 13). Activation through the TF pathway may be affected when the mutations are located, for example, in the Gla domain, as in Glu7Gly (St. Louis II) or Glu19Ala.[19,199,200] Activation through factor IXa is affected by, for example, Thr318Met (Roma).[201] Activation of factor X through Russell viper venom is almost intact in the Pro343Ser (Friuli) mutation.[202] Two interesting clusters of unrelated families were described in Algeria, with Phe31Ser mutation,[203] and in the border region between Turkey and Iran, with the Gly222Asp mutation.[204]

CLINICAL MANIFESTATIONS

The clinical manifestations of factor X deficiency are related to the functional levels of the protein. According to the recent results of the EN-RBD study, strong associations between clinical bleeding severity and coagulation factor activity level were shown in factor X deficiency; consequently, patients with factor X activity levels less than 10 percent of normal have a higher occurrence of spontaneous major bleeding.[25] Bleeding occurs primarily into joints and soft tissues, from the umbilical cord and mucous membranes.[205] The bleeding tendency may appear at any age, although patients with factor X activity less than 2 percent present early in life with, for instance, umbilical-stump or CNS hemorrhage.[13,205,206]

In an analysis of 102 patients from Europe and Latin America, three mutations were associated with intracerebral hemorrhage (Gly380Arg, IVS7–1G>A, and Tyr163delAT) and Gly−20Arg mutation was associated with severe hemarthrosis.[205] The most common bleeding symptom reported at all levels of severity of the deficiency is epistaxis. Patients with severe deficiencies commonly experience hemarthrosis and hematomas, but gastrointestinal and umbilical cord bleeding, hematuria, and CNS bleeding also occur. In a small group of patients with factor X deficiency, one-third of heterozygous patients who had dental extraction, surgery, or delivery without prophylactic replacement therapy showed postoperative bleeding which required treatment.[16] Menorrhagia is a common symptom affecting women with all degrees of severity and PPH was also reported in 4 of 14 pregnancies.[207] Two successful pregnancies out of four pregnancies were reported in a woman only when receiving regular prophylaxis; the other two pregnancies, without regular prophylaxis, resulted in preterm labor (both babies died in the neonatal period).[208] Other case reports, however, have described successful term pregnancies in women with severe factor X deficiency without antenatal prophylaxis.[207,209] Knockout mice show partial embryonic lethality (E11.5–E12.5); complete absence of factor X is incompatible with murine survival to adulthood, but minimal factor X activity (range: 1 to 3 percent) is sufficient to rescue the lethal phenotype.[210–212]

THERAPY

Therapy for inherited factor X deficiency usually is administration of heated and solvent-detergent–treated PCCs containing factor X, in addition to factors II, VII, and IX. Use of these concentrates carries a low risk of transmission of bloodborne viruses. However, a risk of thrombosis, including venous thromboembolism, diffuse intravascular coagulation, and myocardial infarction has been reported.

For soft-tissue, mucous membrane, and joint hemorrhage, the aim of treatment should be maintaining a factor X level that is at least 10 to 20 percent of normal. For more serious hemorrhage, a factor X level

that is greater than 40 percent of normal should be the goal.[25] In patients with particularly severe bleeding manifestations, prophylactic therapy should be considered. FFP also can be used to treat patients with factor X deficiency, however, the administration of FFP can be associated with complications, particularly in children and elderly patients with cardiac disease, because of fluid overload.[38] The arrival on the market of a new freeze-dried human factor X concentrate has facilitated prophylaxis in patients with factor X deficiency (Factor X P Behring)[213]; however, factor X P Behring also contains factor IX, although in a known amount. A clinical trial investigating the pharmacokinetics of a new high-purity factor X concentrate has been completed (ClinicalTrials.gov identifier: 00930176).

● FACTOR XI DEFICIENCY

DEFINITION AND HISTORY

Factor XI deficiency initially was described as a "new hemophilia" in two sisters and their maternal uncle by Rosenthal and colleagues in 1953.[214] Because it manifested in both sexes—two sisters and their maternal uncle—the clinical features were not consistent with hemophilia A or B and was called hemophilia C.[215] The deficiency was erroneously thought to be transmitted as an autosomal dominant disorder with variable expressivity. Later studies clearly established that, in most cases, the mode of transmission of factor XI deficiency is autosomal recessive.[215] Affected subjects have been described in most populations, but the disorder is common in Jews, particularly those of Ashkenazi origin.[216]

Factor XI deficiency as a result of a dysfunctional protein is rare, as only a few patients with deficiency of factor XI activity and seemingly normal antigen levels have been described thus far.[217–220]

PROTEIN

Factor XI is a glycoprotein that consists of two identical 80-kDa polypeptide chains linked by a disulfide bond.[221] Each subunit contains 607 amino acids with a serine protease domain at the C-terminus and four tandem repeats of 90 or 91 amino acids, designated "apple domains," at the N-terminus. The described crystal structure of factor XI dimer[222] defined the interface of the monomers in apple 4 domains in which three residues—Leu284, Ile290, and Tyr329—are essential for noncovalent binding between the monomers. This binding enables the formation of a disulfide bond between Cys321 residues in the fourth apple domain of each monomer.[223,224]

Although factor XI is synthesized by the liver, very low levels of factor XI transcript can also be detected in megakaryocytes and platelets, renal tubules, and pancreatic islet cells.[225] Factor XI circulates in blood as an equimolar complex with high-molecular-weight kininogen (HK)[226] at a concentration of 3 to 7 mcg/mL. The importance of the factor XI–HK interaction is not fully understood. Activation of factor XI involves cleavage of an Arg369-Ile370 bond, yielding a heavy chain containing the four apple domains linked by a disulfide bond to a light chain that contains the catalytic domain.[221] The physiologic activator of factor XI during hemostasis has long been debated. The original scheme of the coagulation cascade—according to which factor XI is activated by factor XIIa through the intrinsic pathway (the "contact phase")—was challenged by the observation that deficiencies of factor XII as well as of the other contact factors (HK and prekallikrein) are not associated with a bleeding diathesis.[14]

The major activator of factor XI in vivo is thrombin.[227,228] Factor XI binds through its apple 3 domain to lipid rafts on platelets containing glycoprotein Ib–IX–V complex. This glycoprotein complex also binds thrombin; thus, both substrate and enzyme are colocalized at the same site.[229] Factor XI activation also can occur on the fibrin surface after a clot forms.[230] Factor XIa, once generated, activates factor IX by limited proteolysis of two peptide bonds in the presence of calcium ions.[231] The presence of factor XI contributes to the activation of thrombin-activatable fibrinolysis inhibitor (TAFI), that once activated, removes terminal lysine residues from fibrin, which impairs binding of certain forms of plasminogen to fibrin and disrupts tissue plasminogen activator-induced plasmin generation in the blood clot.[232] Large amounts of thrombin are necessary for TAFI activation, but the reaction is substantially augmented when thrombin is bound to thrombomodulin.[233] It follows that impaired generation of thrombin, for example, in inherited deficiency of factor VIII, IX, or XI, not only delays clot formation but also enhances premature lysis of clots.[234] These data fit well with clinical observations in factor XI–deficient patients who are particularly susceptible to bleeding following injury at sites exhibiting local fibrinolytic activity.[18]

GENETICS

The 23-kb gene encoding for factor XI consists of 15 exons and 14 introns and is located on chromosome 4q34–35.[235,236]

Three mutations, designated types I, II, and III, were first described in six Ashkenazi-Jewish patients with severe factor XI deficiency.[237] The types II and III, a change in exon 5 at Glu117 leading to a stop codon and a change in exon 9 that results in a substitution of Phe283 by Leu, respectively, account for 95 percent of cases in Ashkenazi Jewish patients.[237] Most patients with factor XI deficiency are Jewish.[18,216,238] A recent study indicated that both type II and type III mutations are also prevalent in the Italian population, although at a much lower rate.[239] In patients belonging to different ethnic groups, a significantly higher level of allelic heterogeneity has been reported. Remarkable exceptions are represented by some "closed populations" harboring mutations compatible with a founder effect: Cys38Arg in French Basques,[240] Gln88Stop in French families from Nantes,[219] Cys128Stop in Britons,[6] Ile436Lys in Northeastern Italy,[241] and Q263X in Korean patients.[242]

As of this writing, 220 mutations have been reported in non-Jewish and Jewish patients of various origins, including 154 missense, 23 nonsense, and 23 del/ins mutations, with the remaining being splice site (18 mutations) and 5′- and 3′-UTR (2 mutations). Inheritance of factor XI deficiency is usually autosomal recessive, as other RBDs, although some missense mutations exert a dominant negative effect through heterodimer formation between the mutant and wild-type polypeptides, resulting in a pattern of dominant transmission.[243]

CLINICAL FEATURES

Factor XI deficiency is the only RBD in which the EN-RBD study showed no association between clinical bleeding severity and coagulation factor activity level.[25] This disorder manifests as a mild to moderate bleeding manifestations and most bleeding episodes of patients with severe FXI deficiency are injury-related. Most bleeding manifestations of patients with severe FXI deficiency are injury-related. Some patients with severe factor XI deficiency may not bleed at all following trauma.[244] The phenotype of bleeding is not correlated with the genotype but frequently with site of injury.[18,238,244] Surgical procedures involving tissues with high fibrinolytic activity (urinary tract, tonsils, nose, tooth sockets) frequently are associated with excessive bleeding in patients with severe factor XI deficiency, irrespective of the genotype.[245]

Most women with severe factor XI deficiency are asymptomatic or minimally so. During 93 deliveries (85 vaginal, eight cesarean), 43 of 62 women did not experience PPH despite no prophylactic treatment,[41] which was confirmed not to be mandatory for these women, by a subsequent study of 33 women who had approximately 70 uneventful pregnancies out of 105 pregnancies. In the subsequent study, only three women had factor XI activity less than 15 IU/dL, and none of them had PPH.[42]

Whether heterozygotes exhibit a bleeding tendency (except for those bearing mutations causing a dominant negative effect) is controversial because there are reports on both heterozygotes with no bleeding complications following a variety of surgical procedures, and reports that 20 to 48 percent of heterozygotes do bleed.[215,238,243,246,247]

In regard to venous thrombosis, it was reported that in five patients, two developed pulmonary embolism following infusion of factor XI concentrate[248–250] and a third patient developed thrombus in the inferior vena cava following cryptococcal infection. In contrast, severe factor XI deficiency was shown to confer protection against ischemic stroke.[251]

Mice homozygous for a knockout factor XI allele show a tendency for slightly prolonged tail transection bleeding times and are protected from vessel-occluding fibrin formation after transient ischemic brain injury.[252,253]

THERAPY

Available treatments for patients with the severe form of factor XI deficiency are FFP and factor XI concentrate. Factor XI concentrates currently available (Bio Products Laboratory, United Kingdom, and LFB Biomedicaments, France) are associated with thrombosis even after adding heparin to the antithrombin in the Bio Products Laboratory product, and antithrombin and heparin to the C1 esterase in the LFB Biomedicaments product.[14,254] Therefore, it is advisable to monitor patients for clinical and laboratory signs of coagulation activation, in particular in elderly patients, in those with cardiovasclar disease and in those undergoing surgery with thrombotic potential, especially when factor XI concentrate[255] or rFVIIa is considered.[256,257] In addition, the presence of an inhibitor, particularly in patients with less than 1 percent of factor XI activity and previously exposed to plasma, factor XI concentrates, or immunoglobulins, should be evaluated. Low doses of rFVIIa along with tranexamic acid seem promising in the treatment of patients with inhibitors. When procedures are planned at tissues exhibiting fibrinolytic activity, which is associated with higher risk of bleeding in comparison to sites without fibrinolytic activity, the use of antifibrinolytic agents alone or in combination with other treatments is recommended. Patients undergoing dental extractions do not require replacement therapy. No plasma replacement therapy is necessary during or after labor unless excessive bleeding occurs. Patients with factor XI deficiency and inhibitor do not bleed spontaneously. Acquired inhibitors that neutralize the activity of factor XI have been described in patients with severe factor XI deficiency and baseline activity of less than 1 IU/dL after being exposed to plasma,[258] after injections of Rh immunoglobulin and without previous exposure to blood products,[259] or after exposure to factor XI concentrates. Use of PCCs[262,263] and rFVIIa[178] have been successful for major surgical procedures, and an *in vitro* study revealed that abnormal thrombin generation in the plasma of patients with an inhibitor was corrected by adding moderate amounts of rFVIIa.[262]

● FACTOR XIII DEFICIENCY

DEFINITION AND HISTORY

The first clinical report of factor XIII deficiency was in 1960[265]; since then, more than 500 cases of factor XIII deficiency have been identified worldwide, with an incidence of one individual in 1 to 3 million population.[22,264] Congenital factor XIII deficiency is characterized by severe delayed spontaneous bleeding and recurrent abortion with normal coagulation screening tests.

PROTEIN

Factor XIII (fibrin-stabilizing factor) is a plasma transglutaminase that crosslinks γ-glutamyl–ε-lysine residues of fibrinogen chains, thereby stabilizing the fibrin clot. Plasma factor XIII is an Mr 340,000 heterotetramer composed of two catalytic A subunits and two carrier B subunits linked by noncovalent bonds. The average concentration of the A_2B_2 tetramer in plasma is approximately 22 mcg/mL, and its half-life is 9 to 14 days.[265] Intracellularly, factor XIII is found as a homodimer composed of two A subunits (A_2).[266,267] Factor XIII-A subunit is mainly synthesized in macrophages and megakaryocytes.[266,267] Because factor XIII-A subunit lacks a signal sequence, it cannot be released by the classic secretory pathway through the Golgi apparatus. Conceivably, factor XIII-A subunit is released into the circulation from cells as a consequence of cell injury.[268] Structurally, each A monomeric subunit (Mr ~82,000) is composed of an activation peptide, that is removed by thrombin cleavage of an Arg37-Gly38 bond in the presence of calcium ions, and four distinct domains: β-sandwich, central core, barrel 1, and barrel 2 regions. The central core domain contains a catalytic triad (common to the transglutaminase family) formed through hydrogen bond interactions between Cys314, His373, and Asp396.[269–271] It is structurally homologous with the α chain of tissue transglutaminase,[272] the α chain of keratinocyte transglutaminase,[273] and band 4.2 of erythrocytes,[274] although the latter lacks transglutaminase activity.

The site of synthesis for factor XIII-B subunit has been suggested to be the liver.[275] The B subunit (Mr 76,500) is composed of 10 tandem repeats of complement control protein (CCP) modules designated as Sushi domains, which are also observed in proteins of the complement system.[276,277] The two B subunits of factor XIII function as carrier proteins for the A subunits,[278,279] stabilizing them in the circulation and regulating the calcium-dependent activation of factor XIII.

On activation by thrombin and Ca^{2+} the A and B subunits dissociate. Proteolytic activation by thrombin involves the cleavage of a N-terminal 37-residue activation peptide. The cleavage and the calcium binding both serve to induce structural changes that open up the catalytic triad to substrate access.[280] This process is accelerated by fibrin.[281–283] The clot stabilizing effect of factor XIII is achieved by the crosslinking of fibrinogen chains, between the γ-carbonyl group of glutamine and the ε-amino group of lysine. In fibrin, this amide bond is located between Aα-chain sequences and between γ-chain sequences[284–288]; factor XIIIA also crosslinks α_2 antiplasmin to the α-chain fibrin,[289] thereby increasing the resistance of fibrin to plasmin degradation, and crosslinks fibronectin to the α-chain of fibrin,[290] thereby affecting the mechanical properties of the clot and increasing cell adhesion.[291]

In addition to fibrinogen and α_2-antiplasmin, factor XIII has many other substrates, including fibronectin, vitronectin, collagen, factor V, von Willebrand factor, α_2-antiplasmin, actin, myosin, vinculin, thrombospondin, plasminogen-activating inhibitor (PAI), TAFI 2, and AT1 receptor dimers of monocytes, implicating multiple and different roles for factor XIII in various systems other than coagulation.[292]

GENETICS

The gene for the factor XIII A-subunit is located on chromosome 6p24-p25.[293,294] It spans more than 170 kb and is composed of 15 exons.[295] The B-subunit gene is located on chromosome 1q31-q32.1.[296,297] The gene for the B subunit spans 28 kb and is composed of 12 exons.[297]

One hundred and twenty-one mutations causing factor XIII A-subunit deficiency have been reported as of this writing, of which only one maps to the promoter region, 57 are missense, 11 are nonsense, 17 are splice-site, and 35 are del/ins mutants (http://www.isth.org/?MutationsRareBleedin and Ref. 298). A homozygous four-bases

insertion in exon 14 (c.2116insAAGA) introducing a frameshift that after seven altered amino acids results a stop codon and a protein with AQ3 truncated second β-barrel domain (p.Pro675TyrfsX7)[299] has been reported to cause an extremely rare type II variant. The mutant protein lost its activity, but the plasma factor XIII antigen level was at the lower limit of the reference interval. This finding suggests that the C-terminal part of β-barrel 2 is essential for the expression of factor XIII activity.

Splice-site mutation in intron 5 (IVS5–1 G>A) seems to be the most common mutation as it has already been reported in six unrelated families from six different European countries, whereas the Arg660Pro was found in Palestinian Arabs, consistently with founder effects.[264,300] It is likely that the Arg661stop mutation in Finnish patients and the Arg-77Cys mutation in Swiss patients are also a result of founder effects, although both are at CpG dinucleotides and therefore can be considered recurrent mutations.[264,301,302] Another mutation, Ser295Arg, was identified in six Pakistani families and may also stem from a common founder, but this remains to be established.[303] Six nonsynonymous/coding polymorphisms in the factor XIIIA1 *(F13A1)* gene,[25] Val34Leu in exon 2, Tyr204Phe in exon 5, Pro(CCA)331(CCC)Pro in exon 8, Glu(GAA)567Glu(GAG) and Pro564Leu in exon 12, and Val650Ile and Glu651Gln in exon 14 have been analyzed in an association study. The study showed that only the Val34Leu is a true functional polymorphism and the rest are in linkage disequilibrium with this polymorphism. In this study, only haplotypes containing the "34L" allele affected factor XIII function.[298,304] However, a larger number of synonymous/noncoding polymorphisms (>500) are known for the *F13A1* gene.[304] Only 16 different mutations have been reported so far for the *FXIIIB* gene.[298]

CLINICAL MANIFESTATIONS

Factor XIII deficiency causes formation of blood clots that are unstable and susceptible to fibrinolytic degradation by plasmin. As a result, affected individuals have an increased tendency to bleed and rebleeding. Delayed umbilical cord bleeding reported in 80 percent of patients with factor XIII deficiency can be considered as diagnostic symptom of the deficiency. CNS bleeding is reported in approximately 30 percent of cases,[305,306] making primary prophylaxis mandatory in patients affected with severe factor XIII deficiency. Ecchymoses, intramuscular and subcutaneous hematomas, oral cavity, mouth and gingival bleeding, and prolonged bleeding following trauma are also characteristic symptoms.[305]

Delayed wound healing occurs in approximately 15 percent of patients deficient in factor XIII. The exact mechanism by which factor XIII, or factor XIIIa, exerts its beneficial effect on wound healing is unknown. A proangiogenic effect of factor XIIIa was described, suggesting that decreased vascularization of wounds results in improper repair.[306]

In a review of the literature on 121 women with factor XIII deficiency, menorrhagia and ovulation bleeding were found to be common gynecologic problems, affecting 26 and 8 percent of women, respectively.[307] Of 192 pregnancies, 127 (66 percent) resulted in a miscarriage and 65 (34 percent) reached viability stage, whereas of 136 pregnancies without prophylactic therapy, 124 (91 percent) resulted in a miscarriage and 12 (9 percent) progressed to viability stage. In affected women, formation of the cytotrophoblastic shell is impaired.[308] Conceivably, factor XIII A-subunit deficiency at the implantation site abrogates fibrin/fibronectin crosslinking, which is essential for attachment of the placenta to the uterus.[309]

Placental abruption, preterm delivery, and PPH could be also problem if not adequately treated.[309]

No large clinical reports on heterozygous patients with factor XIII deficiency are available, thus not allowing to draw evidence-based conclusion on the prevalence of clinical symptoms in this group of patients. Recently, a subset of 28 heterozygotes for factor XIII deficiency among 350 carriers of an autosomal recessive inherited coagulation disorders show an association with prolonged or massive bleeding after minor trauma.[310] However, these data need to be confirmed in other cohorts of patients.

Factor XIII A-subunit knockout mice manifest no excess embryonic lethality or bleeding into the thoracic cavity, peritoneum, or skin, compatible with survival to adulthood. However, the survival rate of knockout males was markedly lower than that of the wild-types.[311] Female factor XIII knockout mice show intrauterine bleeding during pregnancy, similar to women with severe factor XIII A-subunit deficiency who experience the same problem, as well as recurrent abortions. Factor XIIIB knockout mice show a prolonged bleeding time at variance with patients with a complete factor XIII B-subunit deficiency, who report only mild bleeding symptoms and display normal bleeding times.[312,313]

THERAPY

According to the EN-RBD results, blood levels of factor XIII that are 30 percent of normal are necessary to assure an asymptomatic state. This goal may be reached via a number of options. Many case reports show improved bleeding symptoms in patients on prophylactic therapy.[314] Plasma replacement therapy is highly satisfactory because of the long half-life of factor XIII (9 to 12 days). Plasma-derived, virus-inactivated concentrates of factor XIII are available[315] and are the treatment of choice. The development of adverse events after treatment is rare. The most dreaded adverse event is the development of inhibitors, although its incidence is rare.[316] A RBD registry created in North America discovered that 3 percent of factor XIII-deficient patients who received FFP or factor XIII concentrate treatment developed inhibitors.[102] A new rFXIIIA$_2$ concentrate has become available and a phase III clinical trial (ClinicalTrials.gov identifier: 00713648) has been completed, establishing that rFXIII is safe and effective in preventing bleeding episodes in patients with congenital factor XIII A-subunit deficiency. The rFXIII was recently approved for the treatment of factor XIIIA deficiency in Australia, Canada, the European Union, Switzerland, and the United States.[317]

● ACQUIRED DEFICIENCIES

Acquired coagulation factor deficiencies may occur in patients with liver disease, amyloidosis (specifically factor X),[318,319] autoimmune disorders, patients on oral anticoagulant therapy, and, rarely, in patients who develop nonneutralizing antibodies that remove the protein from the circulation. Such antibodies directed against prothrombin[320] and factor VII[321] have been described in patients with lupus anticoagulants. Rare instances of an acquired factor V inhibitor as a result of exposure to bovine thrombin preparations and drugs, or because of an unknown cause, should also be considered.[322] Acquired isolated factor X deficiency with severe bleeding manifestations occurs rarely because of the formation of specific antibodies with no underlying autoimmune disorder[323] or in association with upper respiratory tract infections, burns, and leprosy.[324-326] Inhibitors of factor X with no known precipitating factors have also been described.[327] Acquired factor XIII deficiency with significant reductions in factor XIII levels (down to as low as 20 percent of normal) as a result of decreased synthesis or increased consumption, has been reported in several medical conditions, including

pulmonary embolism, Crohn disease, ulcerative colitis, Henoch-Schönlein purpura, liver cirrhosis, and sepsis. There are several case reports of an autoimmune bleeding disorder, designated as autoimmune/acquired hemorrhaphilia, being caused by anti–factor XIII inhibitors.[328] The anti–factor XIII inhibitors tend to be more severe than regular hemorrhagic-acquired factor XIII deficiency and requires both immunosuppressive therapy to eradicate autoantibodies and factor XIII replacement therapy to stop the bleeding.[329]

REFERENCES

1. Tuddenham EGD, Cooper DN: *The Molecular Genetics of Haemostasis and Its Inherited Disorders.* Oxford University Press, New York, 1994.
2. Peyvandi F, Palla R, Menegatti M, Mannucci PM: Introduction. Rare bleeding disorders: General aspects of clinical features, diagnosis, and management. *Semin Thromb Hemost* 35:349, 2009.
3. Borhany M, Pahore Z, Ul Qadr Z, et al: Bleeding disorders in the tribe: Result of consanguineous in breeding. *Orphanet J Rare Dis* 5:23, 2010.
4. Jaouad IC, Elalaoui SC, Sbiti A, et al: Consanguineous marriages in Morocco and the consequence for the incidence of autosomal recessive disorders. *J Biosoc Sci* 41:575, 2009.
5. Saadat M, Ansari-Lari M, Farhud DD: Consanguineous marriage in Iran. *Ann Hum Biol* 31:263, 2004.
6. Peretz H, Mulai A, Usher S, et al: The two common mutations causing factor XI deficiency in Jews stem from distinct founders: One of ancient Middle Eastern origin and another of more recent European origin. *Blood* 90:2654, 1997.
7. Karimi M, Haghpanah S, Amirhakimi A, et al: Spectrum of inherited bleeding disorders in southern Iran, before and after the establishment of comprehensive coagulation laboratory. *Blood Coagul Fibrinolysis* 20:642, 2009.
8. Viswabandya A, Baidya S, Nair SC, et al: Correlating clinical manifestations with factor levels in rare bleeding disorders: A report from Southern India. *Haemophilia* 18:e195, 2012.
9. Lancellotti S, Basso M, De Cristofaro R: Congenital prothrombin deficiency: An update. *Semin Thromb Hemost* 39:596, 2013.
10. Thalji N, Camire RM: Parahemophilia: New insights into factor V deficiency. *Semin Thromb Hemost* 39:607, 2013.
11. Zheng C, Zhang B: Combined deficiency of coagulation factors V and VIII: An update. *Semin Thromb Hemost* 39:613, 2013.
12. Mariani G, Bernardi F: Factor VII Deficiency. *Semin Thromb Hemost* 35:400, 2009.
13. Menegatti M, Peyvandi F: Factor X deficiency. *Semin Thromb Hemost* 35:407, 2009.
14. Duga S, Salomon O: Congenital factor XI deficiency: An update. *Semin Thromb Hemost* 39:621, 2013.
15. Schroeder V, Kohler HP: Factor XIII deficiency: An update. *Semin Thromb Hemost* 39:632, 2013.
16. Karimi M, Menegatti M, Afrasiabi A, et al: Phenotype and genotype report on homozygous and heterozygous patients with congenital factor X deficiency. *Haematologica* 93:934, 2008.
17. Seligsohn U, Modan M: Definition of the population at risk of bleeding due to factor XI deficiency in Ashkenazic Jews and the value of activated partial thromboplastin time in its detection. *Isr J Med Sci* 17:413, 1981.
18. Asakai R, Chung DW, Davie EW, Seligsohn U: Factor XI deficiency in Ashkenazi Jews in Israel. *N Engl J Med* 325:153, 1991.
19. Girolami A, Scarparo P, Scandellari R, Allemand E: Congenital factor X deficiencies with a defect only or predominantly in the extrinsic or in the intrinsic system: A critical evaluation. *Am J Hematol* 83:668, 2008.
20. Katona E, Penzes K, Molnar E, Muszbek L: Measurement of factor XIII activity in plasma. *Clin Chem Lab Med* 50:1191, 2012.
21. Kohler HP, Ichinose A, Seitz R, et al: Diagnosis and classification of factor XIII deficiencies. *J Thromb Haemost* 9:1404, 2011.
22. Muszbek L, Bagoly Z, Cairo A, Peyvandi F: Novel aspects of factor XIII deficiency. *Curr Opin Hematol* 18:366, 2011.
23. Katona E, Haramura G, Karpati L, et al: A simple, quick one-step ELISA assay for the determination of complex plasma factor XIII (A2B2). *Thromb Haemost* 83:268, 2000.
24. Peyvandi F, Di Michele D, Bolton-Maggs PHB, et al: Classification of rare bleeding disorders (RBDs) based on the association between coagulant factor activity and clinical bleeding severity. *J Thromb Haemost* 10:1938, 2012.
25. Peyvandi F, Palla R, Menegatti M, et al: Coagulation factor activity and clinical bleeding severity in rare bleeding disorders: Results from the European Network of Rare Bleeding Disorders. *J Thromb Haemost* 10:615, 2012.
26. Zhang B, Cunningham MA, Nichols WC, et al: Bleeding due to disruption of a cargo-specific ER-to-Golgi transport complex. *Nat Genet* 34:220, 2003.
27. Sadler JE. Medicine: K is for koagulation. *Nature* 427:493, 2004.
28. Pfeiffer RA, Ott R, Gilgenkrantz S, Alexandre P: Deficiency of coagulation factors VII and X with deletion of a chromosome 13 (q34). Evidence from two cases with 46,XY,t(13;Y)(q11;q34). *Hum Genet* 62:358, 1982.

29. Scambler PJ, Williamson R: The structural gene for human coagulation factor X is located on chromosome 13q34. *Cytogenet Cell Genet* 39:231, 1985.

30. Gilgenkrantz S, Briquel M-E, Andre E, et al: Structural genes of coagulation factors VII and X located on 13q34. *Ann Genet* 29:32, 1986.

31. Boxus G, Slacmeulder M, Ninane J: Combined hereditary deficiency in factors VII and X revealed by a prolonged partial thromboplastin time. *Arch Pediatr* 4:44, 1997.

32. Menegatti M, Karimi M, Garagiola I, et al: A rare inherited coagulation disorder: Combined homozygous factor VII and factor X deficiency. *Am J Hematol* 77:90, 2004.

33. Girolami A, Ruzzon E, Tezza F, et al: Congenital FX deficiency combined with other clotting defects or with other abnormalities: A critical evaluation of the literature. *Haemophilia* 14:323, 2008.

34. Girolami A, Ruzzon E, Tezza F, et al: Congenital combined defects of factor VII: A critical review. *Acta Haematol* 117:51, 2007.

35. Carr ME Jr: Future directions in hemostasis: Normalizing the lives of patients with hemophilia. *Thromb Res* 125(Suppl 1):S78, 2010.

36. Hunt BJ: Bleeding and coagulopathies in critical care. *N Engl J Med* 370:847, 2014.

37. Kadir RA, Davies J, Winikoff R, et al: Pregnancy complications and obstetric care in women with inherited bleeding disorders. *Haemophilia* 19(Suppl 4):1, 2013.

38. Bolton-Maggs PH, Perry DJ, Chalmers EA, et al: The rare coagulation disorders: Review with guidelines for management from the United Kingdom Haemophilia Centre Doctors' Organization. *Haemophilia* 10:593, 2004.

39. James AH: More than menorrhagia: A review of the obstetric and gynaecological manifestations of bleeding disorders. *Haemophilia* 11:295, 2005.

40. Kadir RA, Economides DL, Sabin CA, et al: Frequency of inherited bleeding disorders in women with menorrhagia. *Lancet* 351:485, 1998.

41. Salomon O, Steinberg DM, Tamarin I, et al: Plasma replacement therapy during labor is not mandatory for women with severe factor XI deficiency. *Blood Coagul Fibrinolysis* 16:37, 2005.

42. Myers B, Pavord S, Kean L, et al: Pregnancy outcome in factor XI deficiency: Incidence of miscarriage, antenatal and postnatal haemorrhage in 33 women with factor XI deficiency. *BJOG* 114:643, 2007.

43. Stirling Y, Woolf L, North WR, et al: Haemostasis in normal pregnancy. *Thromb Haemost* 52:176, 1984.

44. Sanchez-Luceros A, Meschengieser SS, Marchese C, et al: Factor VIII and von Willebrand factor changes during normal pregnancy and puerperium. *Blood Coagul Fibrinolysis* 14:647, 2003.

45. Wickstrom K, Edelstam G, Lowbeer CH, et al: Reference intervals for plasma levels of fibronectin, von Willebrand factor, free protein S and antithrombin during third-trimester pregnancy. *Scand J Clin Lab Invest* 64:31, 2004.

46. Bremme KA: Haemostatic changes in pregnancy. *Best Pract Res Clin Haematol* 16:153, 2003.

47. Hellgren M, Blomback M: Studies on blood coagulation and fibrinolysis in pregnancy, during delivery and in the puerperium. Normal condition. *Gynecol Obstet Invest* 12:141, 1981.

48. Lanchantin GF, Hart DW, Friedmann JA, et al: Amino acid composition of human plasma prothrombin. *J Biol Chem* 243:5479, 1968.

49. Degen SJ, MacGillivray RT, Davie EW: Characterization of the complementary deoxyribonucleic acid and gene coding for human prothrombin. *Biochemistry* 22:2087, 1983.

50. Kotkow KJ, Deitcher SR, Furie B, Furie BC: The second kringle domain of prothrombin promotes factor Va-mediated prothrombin activation by prothrombinase. *J Biol Chem* 270:4551, 1995.

51. Dihanich M, Kaser M, Reinhard E, et al: Prothrombin mRNA is expressed by cells of the nervous system. *Neuron* 6:575, 1991.

52. Kim SR, Chung ES, Bok E, et al: Prothrombin kringle-2 induces death of mesencephalic dopaminergic neurons in vivo and in vitro via microglial activation. *J Neurosci Res* 88:1537, 2010.

53. Bode W, Mayr I, Baumann U, et al: The refined 1.9 A crystal structure of human α-thrombin interaction with D-Phe-Pro-Arg chloromethylketone and significance of the Tyr-Pro-Pro-Trp insertion segment. *EMBO J* 8:3467, 1989.

54. Esmon CT: Regulation of blood coagulation. *Biochim Biophys Acta* 1477:349, 2000.

55. Lee H, Hamilton JR: Physiology, pharmacology, and therapeutic potential of protease-activated receptors in vascular disease. *Pharmacol Ther* 134:246, 2012.

56. Coughlin SR: Protease-activated receptors in hemostasis, thrombosis and vascular biology. *J Thromb Haemost* 3:1800, 2005.

57. Lane DA, Phillipu H, Huntington JA: Directing thrombin. *Blood* 106:2605, 2005.

58. Royle NJ, Irwin DM, Koschnsky ML, et al: Human genes encoding prothrombin and ceruloplasmin map to 11p11-q12, and 3q21-24, respectively. *Somat Cell Mol Genet* 13:285, 1987.

59. Poort SR, Rosendaal FR, Reitsma PH, Bertina RM: A common genetic variation in the 3'-untranslated region of the prothrombin gene is associated with elevated plasma prothrombin levels and an increase in venous thrombosis. *Blood* 88:3698, 1996.

60. Catanzarite VA, Novotny WF, Cousins LM, Schneider JM: Pregnancies in a patient with congenital absence of prothrombin activity: Case report. *Am J Perinatol* 14:135, 1997.

61. Peyvandi F, Mannucci PM: Rare coagulation disorders. *Thromb Haemost* 82:1207, 1999.

62. Sun WY, Witte DP, Degen JL, et al: Prothrombin deficiency results in embryonic and neonatal lethality in mice. *Proc Natl Acad Sci U S A* 95:7597, 1998.

63. Xue J, Wu Q, Westfield LA, et al: Incomplete embryonic lethality and fatal neonatal hemorrhage caused by prothrombin deficiency in mice. *Proc Natl Acad Sci U S A* 95:7603, 1998.

64. Lechler E: Use of prothrombin complex concentrates for prophylaxis and treatment of bleeding episodes in patients with hereditary deficiency of prothrombin, factor VII, factor X, protein C, protein S, or protein Z. *Thromb Res* 95(Suppl 1):S39, 1999.

65. Mannucci PM: Outbreak of hepatitis A among Italian patients with haemophilia. *Lancet* 339:819, 1992.

66. Gerritzen A, Schneweis KE, Brackmann HH, et al: Acute hepatitis A in haemophilias. *Lancet* 340:1231, 1992.

67. Ragni MV, Koch WC, Jorda JA: Parvovirus B19, infection in patients with hemophilia. *Transfusion* 36:238, 1996.

68. Jorquera JI: Safety procedures of coagulation factors. *Haemophilia* 13(Suppl 5):41, 2007.

69. Owren PA: Parahemophilia: Hemorrhagic diathesis due to absence of a previously unknown factor. *Lancet* 1:446, 1947.

70. Chiu HC, Whitaker E, Colman RW: Heterogeneity of human factor V deficiency. Evidence for the existence of an antigen-positive variant. *J Clin Invest* 72:493, 1983.

71. Wilson DB, Salem HH, Mruk JS, et al: Biosynthesis of coagulation factor V by human hepatocellular carcinoma cell line. *J Clin Invest* 73:654, 1983.

72. Mazzorana M, Baffet G, Kneip B, et al: Expression of coagulation factor V gene by normal adult human hepatocytes in primary culture. *Br J Haematol* 78:229, 1991.

73. Tracy PB, Eide LL, Bowie EJW, Mann KG: Radioimmunoassay of factor V in human plasma and platelets. *Blood* 60:59, 1982.

74. Mann KG, Kalafatis M: Factor V: A combination of Dr Jekyll and Mr Hyde. *Blood* 101:20, 2003.

75. Camire RM, Bos MHA: The molecular basis of factor V and VIII procofactor activation. *J Thromb Haemost* 7:1951, 2009.

76. Suzuki K, Dahlback B, Stenflo J: Thrombin-catalyzed activation of human coagulation factor V. *J Biol Chem* 257:6556, 1982.

77. Foster WB, Nesheim ME, Mann KG: The factor Xa-catalyzed activation of factor V. *J Biol Chem* 258:13970, 1983.

78. Mann KG, Nesheim ME, Church WR, et al: Surface-dependent reactions of the vitamin K-dependent enzyme complexes. *Blood* 76:1, 1990.

79. Hayward CP, Furmaniak-Kazmierczak E, Cieutat AM, et al: Factor V is complexed with multimerin in resting platelet lysates and colocalizes with multimerin in platelet alpha-granules. *J Biol Chem* 270:19217, 1995.

80. Camire RM, Pollak ES, Kaushansky K, Tracy PB: Secretable human platelet-derived factor V originates from the plasma pool. *Blood* 92:3035, 1998.

81. Gould WR, Silveira JR, Tracy PB: Unique in vivo modifications of coagulation factor V produce a physically and functionally distinct platelet-derived cofactor: Characterization of purified platelet-derived factor V/Va. *J Biol Chem* 279:2383, 2004.

82. Suzuki K, Stenflo J, Dahlback B, et al: Inactivation of human coagulation factor V by activated protein C. *J Biol Chem* 258:1914, 1983.

83. Nesheim ME, Canfield WM, Kisiel W, et al: Studies of the capacity of factor Xa to protect factor Va from inactivation by activated protein C. *J Biol Chem* 257:1443, 1982.

84. Wang H, Riddell DC, Guinto ER, et al: Localization of the gene encoding human factor V to chromosome 1q21-25. *Genomics* 2:324, 1988.

85. Cripe LD, Moore KD, Kane WH: Structure of the gene for human coagulation factor V. *Biochemistry* 31:3777, 1992.

86. Castoldi E, Lunghi B, Mingozzi F, et al: A missense mutation (Y1702C) in the coagulation factor V gene is a frequent cause of factor V deficiency in the Italian population. *Haematologica* 86:629, 2001.

87. Steen M, Miteva M, Villoutreix BO, et al: Factor V New Brunswick: Ala221Val associated with FV deficiency reproduced in vitro and functionally characterized. *Blood* 102:1316, 2003.

88. Duga S, Montefusco MC, Asselta R, et al: Arg2074Cys missense mutation in the C2 domain of factor V causing moderately severe factor V deficiency: Molecular characterization by expression of the recombinant protein. *Blood* 101:173, 2003.

89. Montefusco MC, Duga S, Asselta R, et al: Clinical and molecular characterization of 6 patients affected by severe deficiency of coagulation factor V: Broadening of the mutational spectrum of factor V gene and in vitro analysis of the newly identified missense mutations. *Blood* 102:3210, 2003.

90. Van Wijk R, Nieuwenhuis K, van den Berg M, et al: Five novel mutations in the gene for human blood coagulation factor V associated with type I factor V deficiency. *Blood* 98:358, 2001.

91. Van Wijk R, Montefusco MC, Duga S, et al: Coexistence of a novel homozygous nonsense mutation in exon 13, of the factor V gene with the homozygous Leiden mutation in two unrelated patients with severe factor V deficiency. *Br J Haematol* 114:871, 2001.

92. Guasch JF, Cannegieter S, Reitsma PH, et al: Severe coagulation factor V deficiency caused by a 4 bp deletion in the factor V gene. *Br J Haematol* 101:32, 1998.

93. Dahlbäck B, Villoutreix BO: Molecular recognition in the protein C anticoagulant pathway. *J Thromb Haemost* 1:1525, 2003.

94. Simioni P, Scudeller A, Radossi P, et al: "Pseudo homozygous" activated protein C resistance due to double heterozygous factor V defects (factor V Leiden mutation and type I quantitative factor V defect) associated with thrombosis: Report of two cases belonging to two unrelated kindreds. *Thromb Haemost* 75:422, 1996.

95. Lunghi B, Iacoviello L, Gemmati D, et al: Detection of new polymorphic markers in the factor V gene: Association with factor V levels in plasma. *Thromb Haemost* 75:45, 1996.

96. Yamazaki T, Nicolaes GA, Sorensen KW, et al: Molecular basis of quantitative factor V deficiency associated with factor V R2 haplotype. *Blood* 100:2515, 2002.

97. Castaman G, Lunghi B, Missiaglia E, et al: Phenotypic homozygous activated protein C resistance associated with compound heterozygosity for Arg506Gln (factor V Leiden) and His1299Arg substitutions in factor V. *Br J Haematol* 99:257, 1997.

98. Vos HL: Inherited defects of coagulation Factor V: The thrombotic side. *J Thromb Haemost* 4:35, 2006.

99. Blavignac J, Bunimov N, Rivard GE, Hayward CP: Quebec platelet disorder: Update on pathogenesis, diagnosis, and treatment. *Semin Thromb Hemost* 37:713, 2011.

100. Weiss HJ, Lages B, Zheng S, Hayward CP: Platelet factor V New York: A defect in factor V distinct from that in factor V Quebec resulting in impaired prothrombinase generation. *Am J Hematol* 66:130, 2001.

101. Acharya SS, Coughlin A, Dimichele DM: Rare Bleeding Disorder Registry: Deficiencies of factors II V, VII X, XIII, fibrinogen and dysfibrinogenemias. *J Thromb Haemost* 2:248, 2004.

102. Peyvandi F, Duga S, Akhavan S, Mannucci PM: Rare coagulation deficiencies. *Haemophilia* 8:308, 2002.

103. Asselta R, Tenchini ML, Duga S: Inherited defects of coagulation factor V: The hemorrhagic side. *J Thromb Haemost* 4:26, 2006.

104. Girolami A, Scandellari R, Lombardi AM, et al: Pregnancy and oral contraceptives in factor V deficiency: A study of 22, patients (five homozygotes and 17 heterozygotes) and review of the literature. *Haemophilia* 11:26, 2005.

105. Noia G, De Carolis S, De Stefano V, et al: Factor V deficiency in pregnancy complicated by Rh immunization and placenta previa. A case report and review of the literature. *Acta Obstet Gynecol Scand* 76:890, 1997.

106. Girolami A, Ruzzon E, Tezza F: Arterial and venous thrombosis in rare congenital bleeding disorders: A critical review. *Haemophilia* 12:345, 2006.

107. Fratantoni JC, Hilgartner M, Nachman RL: Nature of the defect in congenital factor V deficiency: Study in a patient with an acquired circulating anticoagulant. *Blood* 39:751, 1972.

108. Mazzucconi MG, Solinas S, Chistolini A, et al: Inhibitor to factor V in severe factor V congenital deficiency: A case report. *Nouv Rev Fr Hematol* 27:303, 1985.

109. Cui J, O'Shea KS, Purkayastha A, et al: Fatal haemorrhage and incomplete block to embryogenesis in mice lacking coagulation factor V. *Nature* 384:66, 1996.

110. Yang TL, Cui J, Taylor JM, et al: Rescue of fatal neonatal hemorrhage in factor V deficient mice by low transgene expression. *Thromb Haemost* 83:70, 2000.

111. Oeri J, Matter M, Isenschmid H, et al: Congenital factor V deficiency (parahemophilia) with true hemophilia in two brothers. *Bibl Paediatr* 58:575, 1954.

112. Nichols WC, Seligsohn U, Zivelin A, et al: Linkage of combined factors V and VIII deficiency to chromosome 18q by homozygosity mapping. *J Clin Invest* 99:596, 1997.

113. Nichols WC, Seligsohn U, Zivelin A, et al: Mutations in the ER–Golgi intermediate compartment protein ERGIC-53 cause combined deficiency of coagulation factors V and VIII. *Cell* 93:61, 1998.

114. Zhang B, Kaufman RJ, Ginsburg D: LMAN1 and MCFD2 form a cargo receptor complex and interact with coagulation factor VIII in the early secretory pathway. *J Biol Chem* 280:25881, 2005.

115. Zhang B, McGee B, Yamaoka JS, et al: Combined deficiency of factor V and factor VIII is due to mutations in either LMAN1 or MCFD2. *Blood* 107:903, 2006.

116. Seligsohn U, Zivelin A, Zwang E: Combined factor V and factor VIII deficiency among non-Ashkenazi Jews. *N Engl J Med* 307:1191, 1982.

117. Peyvandi F, Tuddenham EG, Akhtari AM, et al: Bleeding symptoms in 27 Iranian patients with the combined deficiency of factor V and factor VIII. *Br J Haematol* 100:773, 1998.

118. Itin C, Roche AC, Monsigny M, et al: ERGIC-53 is a functional mannose-selective and calcium-dependent human homologue of leguminous lectins. *J Cell Biol* 107:483, 1996.

119. Guy JE, Wigren E, Svärd M, et al: New insights into multiple coagulation factor deficiency from the solution structure of human MCFD2. *J Mol Biol* 381:941, 2008.

120. Appenzeller C, Andersson H, Kappeler F, et al: The lectin ERGIC-53 is a cargo transport receptor for glycoproteins. *Nat Cell Biol* 1:330, 1999.

121. Vollenweider F, Kappeler F, Itin C, et al: Mistargeting of the lectin ERGIC-53 to the endoplasmic reticulum of HeLa cells impairs the secretion of a lysosomal enzyme. *J Cell Biol* 142:377, 1998.

122. Nyfeler B, Reiterer V, Wendeler MW, et al: Identification of ERGIC-53 as an intracellular transport receptor of alpha1-antitrypsin. *J Cell Biol* 180:705, 2008.

123. Morais VA, Brito C, Pijak DS, et al: N-glycosylation of human nicastrin is required for interaction with the lectins from the secretory pathway calnexin and ERGIC-53. *Biochim Biophys Acta* 1762:802, 2006.

124. Nyfeler B, Zhang B, Ginsburg D, et al: Cargo selectivity of the ERGIC-53/MCFD2 transport receptor complex. *Traffic* 7:1473, 2006.

125. Nishio M, Kamiya Y, Mizushima T, et al: Structural basis for the cooperative interplay between the two causative gene products of combined factor V and factor VIII deficiency. *Proc Natl Acad Sci U S A* 107:4034, 2010.

126. Neerman-Arbez M, Antonarakis SE, Blouin JL, et al: The locus for combined factor V-factor VIII deficiency (F5F8D) maps to 18q21, between D18S849, and D18S1103. *Am J Hum Genet* 61:143, 1997.

127. Zhang B, Spreafico M, Zheng C, et al: Genotype-phenotype correlation in combined deficiency of factor V and factor VIII. *Blood* 111:5592, 2008.

128. Segal A, Zivelin A, Rosenberg N, et al: A mutation in LMAN 1, (ERGIC-53) causing combined factor V and factor VIII deficiency is prevalent in Jews originating from the island of Djerba in Tunisia. *Blood Coagul Fibrinolysis* 15:99, 2004.

129. Viswabandya A, Baidya S, Nair SC, et al: Clinical manifestations of combined factor V and VIII deficiency: A series of 37 cases from a single center in India. *Am J Hematol* 85:538, 2010.

130. Mansouritorgabeh H, Rezaieyazdi Z, Pourfathollah AA, et al: Haemorrhagic symptoms in patients with combined factors V and VIII deficiency in north-eastern Iran. *Haemophilia* 10:271, 2004.

131. Seligsohn U: Combined factor V and factor VIII deficiency, in *Factor VIII: Von Willebrand Factor*, vol 2, edited by J Seghatchian, GT Savidge, p 89. CRC Press, Boca Raton, FL, 1989.

132. Fischer RR, Giddings JC, Roisenberg I: Hereditary combined deficiency of clotting factors V and VIII with involvement of von Willebrand factor. *Clin Lab Haematol* 10:53, 1988.

133. Zhang B, Zheng C, Zhu M, et al: Mice deficient in LMAN1 exhibit FV and FVIII deficiencies and liver accumulation of α_1-antitrypsin. *Blood* 118:3384, 2011.

134. Sallah AS, Angchaisuksiri P, Roberts HR: Use of plasma exchange in hereditary deficiency of factor V and factor VIII. *Am J Hematol* 52:229, 1996.

135. Alexander B, Goldstein R, Landwehr G, Cook CD: Congenital SPCA deficiency: A hitherto unrecognized coagulation defect with hemorrhage rectified by serum and serum fractions. *J Clin Invest* 30:596, 1951.

136. Hagen FS, Gray CL, O'Hara P, et al: Characterization of a cDNA coding for human factor VII. *Proc Natl Acad Sci U S A* 83:2412, 1986.

137. Fair DS: Quantitation of factor VII in the plasma of normal and warfarin-treated individuals by radioimmunoassay. *Blood* 62:784, 1983.

138. Radcliffe R, Nemerson Y: Activation and control of factor VII by activated factor X and thrombin: Isolation and characterization of a single chain form of factor VII. *J Biol Chem* 250:388, 1975.

139. Seligsohn U, Osterud B, Brown SF, et al: Activation of human factor VII in plasma and in purified systems: Roles of activated factor IX, kallikrein, and activated factor XII. *J Clin Invest* 64:1056, 1979.

140. Radcliffe R, Bagdasarian A, Colman R, Nemerson Y: Activation of bovine factor VII by Hageman factor fragments. *Blood* 50:611, 1977.

141. Nakagaki T, Foster DC, Berkner KL, Kisiel W: Initiation of the extrinsic pathway of blood coagulation: Evidence for the tissue factor dependent autoactivation of human coagulation factor VII. *Biochemistry* 30:10819, 1991.

142. Rapaport SI, Rao LV: The tissue factor pathway: How it has become a "prima ballerina." *Thromb Haemost* 74:7, 1995.

143. Banner DW, D'Arcy A, Chene C, et al: The crystal structure of the complex of blood coagulation factor VIIa with soluble tissue factor. *Nature* 380:41, 1996.

144. Cooper DN, Millar DS, Wacey A, et al: Inherited factor VII deficiency: Molecular genetics and pathophysiology. *Thromb Haemost* 78:151, 1997.

145. Edgington TS, Dickinson CD, Ruf W: The structural basis of function of the TF-VIIa complex in the cellular initiation of coagulation. *Thromb Haemost* 78:401, 1997.

146. Morrissey JH, Neuenschwander PF, Huang Q, et al: Factor VIIa–tissue factor: Functional importance of protein-membrane interactions. *Thromb Haemost* 78:112, 1997.

147. Kirchhofer D, Nemerson Y: Initiation of blood coagulation: The tissue factor/factor VIIa complex. *Curr Opin Biotechnol* 7:386, 1996.

148. Mann KG, van't Veer C, Cawthern K, et al: The role of the tissue factor pathway in initiation of coagulation. *Blood Coagul Fibrinolysis* 9:S3, 1998.

149. Hoffman M, Monroe DM, Roberts HR: Cellular interactions in hemostasis. *Haemostasis* 1:12, 1996.

150. O'Hara PJ, Grant FJ, Haldeman BA, et al: Nucleotide sequence of the gene coding for human factor VII, a vitamin K-dependent protein participating in blood coagulation. *Proc Natl Acad Sci U S A* 84:5158, 1987.

151. Ott R, Pfeiffer RA: Evidence that activities of coagulation factors VII and X are linked to chromosome 13, (q34). *Hum Hered* 34:123, 1984.

152. Miao CH, Leytus SP, Chung DW, Davie EW: Liver-specific expression of the gene coding for human factor X, a blood coagulation factor. *J Biol Chem* 267:7395, 1992.

153. Greenberg D, Miao CH, Ho WT, et al: Liver-specific expression of the human factor VII gene. *Proc Natl Acad Sci U S A* 92:12347, 1995.

154. Pollak ES, Hung HL, Godin W, et al: Functional characterization of the human factor VII 5′-flanking region. *J Biol Chem* 271:1738, 1996.

155. Herrmann FH, Wulff K, Auerswald G, et al: Factor VII deficiency: Clinical manifestation of 717, subjects from Europe and Latin America with mutations in the factor 7, gene. *Haemophilia* 15:267, 2008.

156. Tamary H, Fromovich Y, Shalmon L, et al: Ala244Val is a common, probably ancient mutation causing factor VII deficiency in Moroccan and Iranian Jews. *Thromb Haemost* 76:283, 1996.

157. Fromovich-Amit Y, Zivelin A, Rosenberg N, et al: Characterization of mutations causing factor VII deficiency in 61, unrelated Israeli patients. *J Thromb Haemost* 2:1774, 2004.

158. Wulff K, Herrmann FH: Twenty-two novel mutations of the factor VII gene in factor VII deficiency. *Hum Mutat* 15:489, 2000.

159. Giansily-Blaizot M, Aguilar-Martinez P, Biron-Andreani C, et al: Analysis of the genotypes and phenotypes of 37, unrelated patients with inherited factor VII deficiency. *Eur J Hum Genet* 9:105, 2001.

160. Chaing S, Clarke B, Sridhara S, et al: Severe factor VII deficiency caused by mutations abolishing the cleavage site for activation and altering binding to tissue factor. *Blood* 83:3524, 1994.

161. Bernardi F, Patracchini P, Gemmati D, et al: Molecular analysis of factor VII deficiency in Italy: A frequent mutation (FVII Lazio) in a repeated intronic region. *Hum Genet* 92:446, 1993.

162. Etro D, Pinotti M, Wulff K, et al: The Gly331Ser mutation in factor VII in Europe and the Middle East. *Haematologica* 88:1434, 2003.

163. Bernardi F, Liney DL, Patracchini P, et al: Molecular defects in CRM+ factor VII deficiencies: Modeling of missense mutations in the catalytic domain of FVII. *Br J Haematol* 86:610, 1994.

164. Hunault M, Arbini AA, Lopaciuk S, et al: The Arg353,Gln polymorphism reduces the level of coagulation factor VII: In vivo and in vitro studies. *Arterioscler Thromb Vasc Biol* 17:2825, 1997.

165. Green F, Kelleher C, Wilkes H, et al: A common genetic polymorphism associated with lower coagulation factor VII levels in healthy individuals. *Arterioscler Thromb* 11:540, 1991.

166. Bernardi F, Marchetti G, Pinotti M, et al: Factor VII gene polymorphisms contribute about one-third of the factor VII level variation in plasma. *Arterioscler Thromb Vasc Biol* 16:72, 1996.

167. Marchetti G, Gemmati D, Patracchini P, et al: PCR detection of a repeat polymorphism within the F7, gene. *Nucleic Acids Res* 19:4570, 1991.

168. Ragni MV, Lewis JH, Spero JA, Hasiba U: Factor VII deficiency. *Am J Hematol* 10:79-88, 1981.

169. Kulkarni AA, Lee CA, Kadir RA: Pregnancy in women with congenital factor VII deficiency. *Haemophilia* 12:413, 2006.

170. Rizk DE, Castella A, Shaheen H, Deb P: Factor VII deficiency detected in pregnancy: A case report. *Am J Perinatol* 16:223, 1999.

171. Mariani G, Herrmann FH, Schulman S, et al: Thrombosis in inherited factor VII deficiency. *J Thromb Haemost* 1:2153, 2003.

172. Girolami A, Berti de Marinis G, Vettore S, Girolami B: Congenital FVII Deficiency and Pulmonary Embolism: A Critical Appraisal of All Reported Cases. *Clin Appl Thromb Hemost* 19:55, 2013.

173. Rosen ED, Chan JC, Idusogie E, et al: Mice lacking factor VII develop normally but suffer fatal perinatal bleeding. *Nature* 390:290, 1997.

174. Chan JC, Carmeliet P, Moons L, et al: Factor VII deficiency rescues the intrauterine lethality in mice associated with a tissue factor pathway inhibitor deficit. *J Clin Invest* 103:475, 1999.

175. Napolitano M, Giansily-Blaizot M, Dolce A, et al: Prophylaxis in congenital factor VII deficiency: Indications, efficacy and safety. Results from the Seven Treatment Evaluation Registry (STER). *Haematologica* 98:538, 2013.

176. Mariani G, Konkle BA, Ingerslev J: Congenital factor VII deficiency: Therapy with recombinant activated factor VII—A critical appraisal. *Haemophilia* 12:19, 2006.

177. Tcheng WY, Donkin J, Konzal S, Wong WY: Recombinant factor VIIa in a patient with severe congenital factor VII deficiency. *Haemophilia* 10:295, 2004.

178. Berrettini M, Mariani G, Schiavoni M, et al: Pharmacokinetic evaluation of recombinant, activated factor VII in patients with inherited factor VII deficiency. *Haematologica* 86:640, 2001.

179. Robertson LE, Wasserstrum N, Banez E, et al: Hereditary factor VII deficiency in pregnancy: Peripartum treatment with factor VII concentrate. *Am J Hematol* 40:38, 1992.

180. Aynaoğlu G, Durdağ GD, Ozmen B, Söylemez F: Successful treatment of hereditary factor VII deficiency presented for the first time with epistaxis in pregnancy: A case report. *J Matern Fetal Neonatal Med* 23:1053, 2010.

181. Braun MW, Triplett DA: Case report: Factor VII deficiency in an obstetrical patient. *J Indiana State Med Assoc* 72:900, 1979.

182. Fadel HE, Krauss JS: Factor VII deficiency and pregnancy. *Obstet Gynecol* 73:453, 1989.

183. Eskandari N, Feldman N, Greenspoon JS: Factor VII deficiency in pregnancy treated with recombinant factor VIIa. *Obstet Gynecol* 99:935, 2002.

184. Jimenez-Yuste V, Villar A, Morado M, et al: Continuous infusion of recombinant activated factor VII during caesarean section delivery in a patient with congenital factor VII deficiency. *Haemophilia* 6:588, 2000.

185. Pike GN1, Bolton-Maggs PH. Factor deficiencies in pregnancy. *Hematol Oncol Clin North Am* 25:359, 2011.

186. Baumann kreuziger LM, Morton CT, Reding MT: Is prophylaxis required for delivery in women with factor VII deficiency? *Haemophilia* 19,827, 2013.

187. Duckert F, Fluckinger P, Matter M, Koller F: Clotting factor X. Physiologic and physicochemical properties. *Proc Soc Exp Biol Med* 90:17, 1955.

188. Telfer TP, Denson KW, Wright DR: A "new" coagulation defect. *Br J Haematol* 2:308, 1956.

189. Hougie C, Barrow EM, Graham JB: Stuart clotting defect. I. Segregation of an hereditary hemorrhagic state from the heterogeneous group heretofore called "stable factor" (SPCA, proconvertin, factor VII) deficiency. *J Clin Invest* 36:485, 1957.

190. Bajaj SP, Mann KG: Simultaneous purification of bovine prothrombin and factor X. Activation of prothrombin by trypsin-activated factor X. *J Biol Chem* 248:7729, 1973.

191. Ichinose A, Takeya H, Espling E, et al: Amino acid sequence of human protein Z, a vitamin K-dependent plasma glycoprotein. *Biochem Biophys Res Commun* 172:1139, 1990.

192. Leytus SP, Foster DC, Kurachi K, Davie EW: Gene for human factor X: A blood coagulation factor whose gene organization is essentially identical with that of factor IX and protein C. *Biochemistry* 25:5098, 1986.

193. McMullen BA, Fujikawa K, Kisiel W, et al: Complete amino acid sequence of the light chain of human blood coagulation factor X: Evidence for identification of residue 63, as beta-hydroxyaspartic acid. *Biochemistry* 22:2875, 1983.

194. Jackson CM: Characterization of two glycoprotein variants of bovine factor X and demonstration that the factor X zymogen contains two polypeptide chains. *Biochemistry* 11:4873, 1972.

195. Fujikawa K, Coan MH, Legaz ME, Davie EW: The mechanism of activation of bovine factor X (Stuart factor) by intrinsic and extrinsic pathways. *Biochemistry* 13:5290, 1974.

196. Kisiel W, Hermodson MA, Davie EW: Factor X activating enzyme from Russell's viper venom: Isolation and characterization. *Biochemistry* 15:4901, 1976.

197. Furie B, Furie BC: The molecular basis of blood coagulation. *Cell* 53:505, 1988.

198. Neurath H: Evolution of proteolytic enzymes. *Science* 224:350, 1984.

199. Rudolph AE, Mullane MP, Porche-Sorbet R, et al: Factor X St. Louis II. Identification of a glycine substitution at residue 7, and characterization of the recombinant protein. *J Biol Chem* 271:28601, 1996.

200. Pinotti M, Marchetti G, Baroni M, et al: Reduced activation of the Gla19Ala FX variant via the extrinsic coagulation pathway results in symptomatic CRMred FX deficiency. *Thromb Haemost* 88:236, 2002.

201. De Stefano V, Leone G, Ferrelli R, et al: Factor X Roma: A congenital factor X variant defective at different degrees in the intrinsic and the extrinsic activation. *Br J Haematol* 69:387, 1988.

202. James HL, Girolami A, Fair DS: Molecular defect in coagulation factor X Friuli results from a substitution of serine for proline at position 343. *Blood* 77:317, 1991.

203. Akhavan S, Chafa O, Obame FN, et al: Recurrence of a Phe31Ser mutation in the Gla domain of blood coagulation factor X, in unrelated Algerian families: A founder effect? *Eur J Haematol* 78:405, 2007.

204. Menegatti M, Vangone A, Palla R, et al: A recurrent Gly43Asp substitution in coagulation Factor X rigidifies its catalytic pocket and impairs catalytic activity and intracellular trafficking. *Thromb Res* 133:481, 2014.

205. Herrmann FH, Auerswald G, Ruiz-Saez A, et al: Factor X deficiency: Clinical manifestation of 102 subjects from Europe and Latin America with mutations in the factor 10 gene. *Haemophilia* 12:479, 2006.

206. Peyvandi F, Mannucci PM, Lak M, et al: Congenital Factor X deficiency: Spectrum of bleeding symptoms in 32 Iranian patients. *Br J Haematol* 102:626, 1998.

207. Romagnolo C, Burati S, Ciaffoni S, et al: Severe factor X deficiency in pregnancy: Case report and review of the literature. *Haemophilia* 10:665, 2004.

208. Kumar M, Mehta P: Congenital coagulopathies and pregnancy: Report of four pregnancies in a factor X-deficient woman. *Am J Hematol* 46:241, 1994.

209. Larrain C: Congenital blood coagulation factor X deficiency. Successful result of the use prothrombin concentrated complex in the control of caesarean section hemorrhage in 2 pregnancies. *Rev Med Chil* 122:1178, 1994.

210. Dewerchin M, Liang Z, Moons L, et al: Blood coagulation factor X deficiency causes partial embryonic lethality and fatal neonatal bleeding in mice. *Thromb Haemost* 83:185, 2000.

211. Rosen ED, Cornelissen I, Liang Z, et al: In utero transplantation of wild-type fetal liver cells rescues factor X-deficient mice from fatal neonatal bleeding diatheses. *J Thromb Haemost* 1:19, 2003.

212. Tai SJ, Herzog RW, Margaritis P, et al: A viable mouse model of factor X deficiency provides evidence for maternal transfer of factor X. *J Thromb Haemost* 6:339, 2008.

213. Karimi M, Vafafar A, Haghpanah S, et al: Efficacy of prophylaxis and genotype-phenotype correlation in patients with severe Factor X deficiency in Iran. *Haemophilia* 18:211, 2012.

214. Rosenthal RL, Dreskin OH, Rosenthal N: A new hemophilia like disease caused by deficiency of a third plasma thromboplastin factor. *Proc Soc Exp Biol Med* 82:171, 1953.

215. Rapaport SI, Proctor RR, Patch NJ, Yettra M: The mode of inheritance of PTA deficiency: Evidence for the existence of major PTA deficiency and minor PTA deficiency. *Blood* 18:149, 1961.

216. Seligsohn U: High gene frequency of factor XI (PTA) deficiency in Ashkenazi-Jews. *Blood* 51:1223, 1978.

217. Mannhalter C, Hellstern P, Deutsch E: Identification of a defective factor XI cross-reacting material in a factor XI-deficient patient. *Blood* 70:31, 1987.

218. Zivelin A, Ogawa T, Bulvik S, et al: Severe factor XI deficiency caused by a Gly555 to Glu mutation (factor XI-Glu555): A cross-reactive material positive variant defective in factor IX activation. *J Thromb Haemost* 2:1782, 2004.

219. Quelin F, Trossaert M, Sigaud M, et al: Molecular basis of severe factor XI deficiency in seven families from the west of France. Seven novel mutations, including an ancient Q88X mutation. *J Thromb Haemost* 2:71, 2004.

220. Martincic D, Zimmerman SA, Ware RE, et al: Identification of mutations and polymorphisms in the factor XI genes of an African-American family by dideoxy fingerprinting. *Blood* 92:3309, 1998.

221. McMullen BA, Fujikawa K, Davie EW: Location of the disulfide bonds in human coagulation factor XI: The presence of tandem apple domains. *Biochemistry* 30:2056, 1991.

222. Papagrigoriou E, McEwan PA, Walsh PN, Emsley J: Crystal structure of the factor XI zymogen reveals a pathway for transactivation. *Nat Struct Mol Biol* 13:557, 2006.

223. Zucker M, Zivelin A, Landau M, et al: Three residues at the interface of factor XI monomers augment covalent dimerization of factor XI. *J Thromb Haemost* 7:970, 2009.

224. Wu W, Sinha D, Shikov S, et al: Factor XI homodimer structure is essential for normal proteolytic activation by factor XIIa, thrombin, and factor XIa. *J Biol Chem* 283:18655, 2008.

225. Cheng Q, Kantz J, Poffenberger G, et al: Factor XI protein in human pancreas and kidney. *Thromb Haemost* 100:158, 2008.

226. Thompson RE, Mandle R Jr, Kaplan AP: Association of factor XI and high molecular weight kininogen in human plasma. *J Clin Invest* 60:1376, 1997.

227. Gailani D, Broze GJ Jr: Factor XI activation in a revised model of blood coagulation. *Science* 253:909, 1991.
228. Naito K, Fujikawa K: Activation of human blood coagulation factor XI independent of factor XII: Factor XI is activated by thrombin and factor XIa in the presence of negatively charged surfaces. *J Biol Chem* 266:7353, 1991.
229. Baglia FA, Shrimpton CN, Lopez JA, Walsh PN: The glycoprotein Ib-IX-V complex mediates localization of factor XI to lipid rafts on the platelet membrane. *J Biol Chem* 278:21744, 2003.
230. Von dem Borne PA, Meijers JC, Bouma BN: Effect of heparin on the activation of factor XI by fibrin-bound thrombin. *Thromb Haemost* 76:347, 1996.
231. Osterud B, Bouma BN, Griffin JH: Human blood coagulation factor IX: Purification, properties, and mechanism of activation by activated factor XI. *J Biol Chem* 253:5946, 1978.
232. Bouma BN, Meijers JC: Thrombin-activatable fibrinolysis inhibitor (TAFI, plasma procarboxypeptidase B, procarboxypeptidase R, procarboxypeptidase U). *J Thromb Haemost* 1:1566, 2003.
233. Bajzar L, Morser J, Nesheim M: TAFI, or plasma procarboxypeptidase B, couples the coagulation and fibrinolytic cascades through the thrombin-thrombomodulin complex. *J Biol Chem* 271:16603, 1996.
234. Broze GJ Jr, Higuchi DA: Coagulation-dependent inhibition of fibrinolysis: Role of carboxypeptidase-U and the premature lysis of clots from hemophilic plasma. *Blood* 88:3815, 1996.
235. Asakai R, Davie EW, Chung DW: Organization of the gene for human factor XI. *Biochemistry* 26:7221, 1987.
236. Kato A, Asakai R, Davie EW, Aoki N: Factor XI gene (F11) is located on the distal end of the long arm of human chromosome 4. *Cytogenet Cell Genet* 52:77, 1989.
237. Asakai R, Chung DW, Ratnoff OD, Davie EW: Factor XI (plasma thromboplastin antecedent) deficiency in Ashkenazi Jews is a bleeding disorder that can result from three types of point mutations. *Proc Natl Acad Sci U S A* 86:7667, 1989.
238. Bolton-Maggs PH, Young Wan-Yin B, McCraw AH, et al: Inheritance and bleeding in factor XI deficiency. *Br J Haematol* 69:521, 1988.
239. Zadra G, Asselta R, Tenchini ML, et al: Simultaneous genotyping of coagulation factor XI type II and type III mutations by multiplex real-time polymerase chain reaction to determine their prevalence in healthy and factor XI-deficient Italians. *Haematologica* 93:715, 2008.
240. Zivelin A, Bauduer F, Ducout L, et al: Factor XI deficiency in French Basques is caused predominantly by an ancestral Cys38Arg mutation in the factor XI gene. *Blood* 99:2448, 2002.
241. Girolami A, Scarparo P, Bonamigo E, et al: A cluster of factor XI-deficient patients due to a new mutation (Ile 436 Lys) in northeastern Italy. *Eur J Haematol* 88:229, 2012.
242. Kim I, Song J, Lyu CJ, et al: Population-specific spectrum of the F11 mutations in Koreans: Evidence for a founder effect. *Clin Genet* 82:180, 2012.
243. Kravtsov DV, Wu W, Meijers JC, et al: Dominant factor XI deficiency caused by mutations in the factor XI catalytic domain. *Blood* 104:128, 2004.
244. Bolton-Maggs PH, Patterson DA, Wensley RT, Tuddenham EG: Definition of the bleeding tendency in factor XI-deficient kindreds: A clinical and laboratory study. *Thromb Haemost* 73:194, 1995.
245. Salomon O, Steinberg DM, Seligsohn U: Variable bleeding manifestations characterize different types of surgery in patients with severe factor XI deficiency enabling parsimonious use of replacement therapy. *Haemophilia* 12:490, 2006.
246. Sidi A, Seligsohn U, Jonas P, Many M: Factor XI deficiency: Detection and management during urological surgery. *J Urol* 119:528, 1978.
247. Brenner B, Laor A, Lupo H, et al: Bleeding predictors in factor-XI deficient patients. *Blood Coagul Fibrinolysis* 8:511, 1997.
248. Bolton-Maggs PH, Peretz H, Butler R, et al: A common ancestral mutation (C128X) occurring in 11 non-Jewish families from the UK with factor XI deficiency. *J Thromb Haemost* 2:918, 2004.
249. Brodsky JB, Burgess GE III: Pulmonary embolism with factor XI deficiency. *JAMA* 234:1156, 1975.
250. Evans G, Pasi KJ, Mehta A, et al: Recurrent venous thromboembolic disease and factor XI concentrate in a patient with severe factor XI deficiency, chronic myelomonocytic leukaemia, factor V Leiden and heterozygous plasminogen deficiency. *Blood Coagul Fibrinolysis* 8:437, 1997.
251. Salomon O, Steinberg DM, Koren-Morag N, et al: Reduced incidence of ischemic stroke in patients with severe factor XI deficiency. *Blood* 111:4113, 2008.
252. Luo D, Szaba FM, Kummer LW, et al: Factor XI deficient mice display reduced inflammation, coagulopathy, and bacterial growth during listeriosis. *Infect Immun* 80:91, 2012.
253. Gailani D, Lasky NM, Broze GJ Jr: A murine model of factor XI deficiency. *Blood Coagul Fibrinolysis* 8:134, 1997.
254. James P, Salomon O, Mikovic D, Peyvandi F: Rare bleeding disorders-bleeding assessment tools, laboratory aspects and phenotype and therapy of FXI deficiency. *Haemophilia* 20(Suppl 4):71, 2014.
255. Mannucci PM, Bauer KA, Santagostino E, et al: Activation of the coagulation cascade after infusion of a factor XI concentrate in congenitally deficient patients. *Blood* 84:1314, 1994.
256. O'Connell NM, Riddell AF, Pascoe G, et al: Recombinant factor VIIa to prevent surgical bleeding in factor XI deficiency. *Haemophilia* 14:775, 2008.
257. Schulman S, Németh: An illustrative case and a review on the dosing of recombinant factor VIIa in congenital factor XI deficiency. *Haemophilia* 12:223, 2006.
258. Salomon O, Zivelin A, Livnat T, et al: Prevalence, causes, and characterization of factor XI inhibitors in patients with inherited factor XI deficiency. *Blood* 101:4783, 2003.
259. Zucker M, Zivelin A, Teitel J, Seligsohn U: Induction of an inhibitor antibody to factor XI in a patient with severe inherited factor XI deficiency by Rh immune globulin. *Blood* 111:1306, 2008.
260. Stern DM, Nossel HL, Owen J: Acquired antibody to factor XI in a patient with congenital factor XI deficiency. *J Clin Invest* 69:1270, 1982.
261. Connelly NR, Brull SJ: Anesthetic management of a patient with factor XI deficiency and factor XI inhibitor undergoing a cesarean section. *Anesth Analg* 76:1365, 1993.
262. Livnat T, Zivelin A, Martinowitz U, et al: Prerequisites for recombinant factor VIIa-induced thrombin generation in plasmas deficient in factors VIII, IX or XI. *J Thromb Haemost* 4:192, 2006.
263. Duckert F, Jung E, Sherling DH: An undescribed congenital haemorrhagic diathesis probably due to fibrin stabilizing factor deficiency. *Thromb Diath Haemorrh* 5:179, 1960.
264. Ivaskevicius V, Seitz R, Kohler HP et al: International registry on factor XIII deficiency: A basis formed mostly on European data. *Thromb Haemost* 97:914, 2007.
265. Muszbek L, Adany R, Mikkola H: Novel aspects of blood coagulation factor XIII: I. Structure, distribution, activation, and function. *Crit Rev Clin Lab Sci* 33:357, 1996.
266. Schwartz ML, Pizzo SV, Hill RL, McKee PA: Human factor XIII from plasma and platelets. Molecular weights, subunit structures, proteolytic activation, and cross-linking of fibrinogen and fibrin. *J Biol Chem* 248:1395, 1973.
267. Muszbek L, Ariens RA, Ichinose A, ISTH SSC Subcommittee On Factor X: Factor XIII: Recommended terms and abbreviations. *J Thromb Haemost* 5:181, 2007.
268. Weiss MS, Metzner HJ, Hilgenfeld R: Two nonproline cis peptide bonds may be important for factor XIII function. *FEBS Lett* 423:291, 1998.
269. Yee VC, Pedersen LC, Le Trong I, et al: Three-dimensional structure of a transglutaminase: Human blood coagulation factor XIII. *Proc Natl Acad Sci U S A* 91:7296, 1994.
270. Lorand L, Graham RM: Transglutaminases: Crosslinking enzymes with pleiotropic functions. *Nat Rev Mol Cell Biol* 4:140, 2003.
271. Yee VC, Le Trong I, Bishop PD, et al: Structure and function studies of factor XIIIa by X-ray crystallography. *Semin Thromb Hemost* 22:377, 1996.
272. Gentile V, Saydak M, Chiocca EA, et al: Isolation and characterization of cDNA clones to mouse macrophage and human endothelial cell tissue transglutaminases. *J Biol Chem* 266:478, 1991.
273. Phillips MA, Stewart BE, Qin Q, et al: Primary structure of keratinocyte transglutaminase. *Proc Natl Acad Sci U S A* 87:9333, 1990.
274. Sung LA, Chien S, Chang LS, et al: Molecular cloning of human protein 4.2: A major component of the erythrocyte membrane. *Proc Natl Acad Sci U S A* 87:955, 1990.
275. Ichinose A, McMullen BA, Fujikawa K, Davie EW: Amino acid sequence of the b subunit of human factor XIII, a protein composed of ten repetitive segments. *Biochemistry* 25:4633, 1986.
276. Souri M, Kaetsu H, Ichinose A: Sushi domains in the B subunit of factor XIII responsible for oligomer assembly. *Biochemistry* 47:8656, 2008.
277. Lorand L, Gray AJ, Brown K, et al: Dissociation of the subunit structure of fibrin stabilizing factor during activation of the zymogen. *Biochem Biophys Res Commun* 56:914, 1974.
278. Mary A, Achyuthan KE, Greenberg CS: B-chains prevent the proteolytic inactivation of the a-chains of plasma factor XIII. *Biochim Biophys Acta* 966:328, 1988.
279. Biswas A, Ivaskevicius V, Thomas A, Oldenburg J: Coagulation factor XIII deficiency. *Hamostaseologie* 34:160, 2014.
280. Komaromi I, Bagoly Z, Muszbek L: Factor XIII: Novel structural and functional aspects. *J Thromb Haemost* 9:9, 2011.
281. Kohler HP: Interaction between FXIII and fibrinogen. *Blood* 121:1934, 2013.
282. Smith KA, Adamson PJ, Pease RJ et al: Interactions between factor XIII and the alpha C region of fibrinogen. *Blood* 2011; 117: 3460–3468.
283. Ariens RA, Lai TS, Weisel JW, et al: Role of factor XIII in fibrin clot formation and effects of genetic polymorphisms. *Blood* 100:743, 2002.
284. Varadi A, Scheraga HA: Localization of segments essential for polymerization and for calcium binding in the gamma-chain of human fibrinogen. *Biochemistry* 25:519, 1986.
285. Smith KA, Adamson PJ, Pease RJ et al: Interactions between factor XIII and the alpha C region of fibrinogen. *Blood* 117:3460, 2011.
286. Smith KA, Pease RJ, Avery CA et al: The activation peptide cleft exposed by thrombin cleavage of FXIII-A(2) contains a recognition site for the fibrinogen alpha chain. *Blood* 121:2117, 2013.
287. Doolittle RF, Hong S, Wilcox D: Evolution of the fibrinogen gamma' chain: Implications for the binding of factor XIII, thrombin and platelets. *J Thromb Haemost* 7:1431, 2009.
288. Sakata Y, Aoki N: Cross-linking of alpha 2-plasmin inhibitor to fibrin by fibrin-stabilizing factor. *J Clin Invest* 65:290, 1980.
289. Mosher DF, Schad PE, Vann JM: Cross-linking of collagen and fibronectin by factor XIIIa: Localization of participating glutaminyl residues to a tryptic fragment of fibronectin. *J Biol Chem* 255:1181, 1980.
290. Fraser SR, Booth NA, Mutch NJ: The antifibrinolytic function of factor XIII is exclusively expressed through alpha(2)-antiplasmin cross-linking. *Blood* 117:6371, 2011.
291. Van Giezen JJ, Minkema J, Bouma BN, Jansen JW: Cross-linking of alpha 2-antiplasmin to fibrin is a key factor in regulating blood clot lysis: Species differences. *Blood Coagul Fibrinolysis* 4:869, 1993.
292. Richardson VR, Cordell P, Standeven KF, Carter AM: Substrates of factor XIII-A: Roles in thrombosis and wound healing. *Clin Sci (Lond)* 124:123, 2013.

293. Board PG, Webb GC, McKee J, Ichinose A: Localization of the coagulation factor XIII A subunit gene (F13A) to chromosome bands 6p24-p25. *Cytogenet Cell Genet* 48:25, 1988.

294. Weisberg LJ, Shiu DT, Greenberg CS, et al: Localization of the gene for coagulation factor XIII a-chain to chromosome 6, and identification of sites of synthesis. *J Clin Invest* 79:649, 1987.

295. Ichinose A, Davie EW: Characterization of the gene for the a subunit of human factor XIII (plasma transglutaminase), a blood coagulation factor. *Proc Natl Acad Sci U S A* 85:5829, 1988.

296. Webb GC, Coggan M, Ichinose A, Board PG: Localization of the coagulation factor XIII B subunit gene (F13B) to chromosome bands 1q31–32.1, and restriction fragment length polymorphism at the locus. *Hum Genet* 81:157, 1989.

297. Bottenus RE, Ichinose A, Davie EW: Nucleotide sequence of the gene for the b subunit of human factor XIII. *Biochemistry* 29:11195, 1990.

298. Biswas A, Ivaskevicius V, Seitz R, et al: An update of the mutation profile of Factor 13A and B genes. *Blood Rev* 25:193, 2011.

299. Morange P, Trigui N, Frere C, et al: Molecular characterization of a novel mutation in the factor XIII a subunit gene associated with a severe defect: Importance of prophylactic substitution. *Blood Coagul Fibrinolysis* 20:605, 2009.

300. Inbal A, Yee VC, Kornbrot N, et al: Factor XIII deficiency due to a Leu660Pro mutation in the factor XIII subunit-A gene in three unrelated Palestinian Arab families. *Thromb Haemost* 77:1062, 1997.

301. Mikkola H, Syrjala M, Rasi V, et al: Deficiency in the A-subunit of coagulation factor XIII: Two novel point mutations demonstrate different effects on transcript level. *Blood* 84:517, 1994.

302. Schroeder V, Durrer D, Meili E, et al: Congenital factor XIII deficiency in Switzerland: From the worldwide first case in 1960, to its molecular characterisation in 2005. *Swiss Med Wkly* 137:272, 2007.

303. Aslam S, Standen GR, Khurshid M, Bilwani F: Molecular analysis of six factor XIII-A-deficient families in Southern Pakistan. *Br J Haematol* 109:463, 2000.

304. Hsieha L, Nugent D: Rare factor deficiencies. *Curr Opin Hematol* 19:380, 2012.

305. Karimi M, Bereczky Z, Cohan N, Muszbek L: Factor XIII deficiency. *Semin Thromb Hemost* 35:426, 2009.

306. Dardik R, Loscalzo J, Inbal A: Factor XIII (FXIII) and angiogenesis. *J Thromb Haemost* 4:19, 2006.

307. Sharief LAT, Kadir RA: Congenital factor XIII deficiency in women: A systematic review of literature. *Haemophilia* 19:e349, 2013.

308. Asahina T, Kobayashi T, Okada Y, et al: Maternal blood coagulation factor XIII is associated with the development of cytotrophoblastic shell. *Placenta* 21:388, 2000.

309. Inbal A, Muszbek L: Coagulation factor deficiencies and pregnancy loss. *Semin Thromb Hemost* 29:171, 2003.

310. Mahmoodi M, Peyvandi F, Afrasiabi A, et al: Bleeding symptoms in heterozygous carriers of inherited coagulation disorders in southern Iran. *Blood Coagul Fibrinolysis* 22:396, 2011.

311. Koseki-Kuno S, Yamakawa M, Dickneite G, Ichinose A: Factor XIII A subunit-deficient mice developed severe uterine bleeding events and; subsequent spontaneous miscarriages. *Blood* 102:4410, 2003.

312. Lauer P, Metzner HJ, Zettlmeissl G, et al: Targeted inactivation of the mouse locus encoding coagulation factor XIIIA: Hemostatic abnormalities in mutant mice and characterization of the coagulation deficit. *Thromb Haemost* 88:967, 2002.

313. Souri M, Koseki-Kuno S, Takeda N, et al: Male specific cardiac pathologies in mice lacking either the A or B subunit of factor XIII. *Thromb Haemost* 99:401, 2008.

314. Dreyfus M, Barrois D, Borg JY, et al: Successful long-term replacement therapy with FXIII concentrate (Fibrogammin1 P) for severe congenital factor XIII deficiency: A prospective multicentre study. *J Thromb Haemost* 9:1264, 2011.

315. Gootenberg JE: Factor concentrates for the treatment of factor XIII deficiency. *Curr Opin Hematol* 5:372, 1998.

316. Odame JE, Chan AK, Wu JK, Breakey VR: Factor XIII deficiency management: A review of the literature. *Blood Coagul Fibrinolysis* 25:199, 2014.

317. Dorey E: First recombinant Factor XIII approved. *Nat Biotechnol* 32:210, 2014.

318. Furie B, Voo L, McAdam KP, Furie BC: Mechanism of factor X deficiency in systemic amyloidosis. *N Engl J Med* 304:827, 1981.

319. Fair DS, Edgington TS: Heterogeneity of hereditary and acquired factor X deficiencies by combined immunochemical and functional analyses. *Br J Haematol* 59:235, 1985.

320. Bajaj SP, Rapaport SI, Fierer DS, et al: A mechanism for the hypoprothrombinemia of the acquired hypoprothrombinemia-lupus anticoagulant syndrome. *Blood* 61:684, 1983.

321. Lim S, Zuha R, Burt T, et al: Life-threatening bleeding in a patient with a lupus inhibitor and probable acquired factor VII deficiency. *Blood Coagul Fibrinolysis* 17:867, 2006.

322. Wiwanitkit V: Spectrum of bleeding in acquired factor V inhibitor: A summary of 33 cases. *Clin Appl Thromb Hemost* 12:485, 2006.

323. Rao LV, Zivelin A, Iturbe I, Rapaport SI: Antibody-induced acute factor X deficiency: Clinical manifestations and properties of the antibody. *Thromb Haemost* 72:363, 1994.

324. Mulhare PE, Tracy PB, Golden EA, et al: A case of acquired factor X deficiency with in vivo and in vitro evidence of inhibitor activity directed against factor X. *Am J Clin Pathol* 96:196, 1991.

325. Matsunaga AT, Shafer FE: An acquired inhibitor to factor X in a pediatric patient with extensive burns. *J Pediatr Hematol Oncol* 18:223, 1996.

326. Gallais V, Bredoux H, leRoux G, Laroche L: Acquired and transient factor X deficiency associated with sodium valproate treatment. *Eur J Haematol* 57:330, 1996.

327. Lankiewicz MW, Bell WR: A unique circulating inhibitor with specificity for coagulation factor X. *Am J Med* 93:343, 1992.

328. Ichinose A, Souri M: Japanese Collaborative Research Group on Acquired Haemorrhaphilia Due to Factor XIII Deficiency: As many as 12 cases with haemorrhagic acquired factor XIII deficiency due to its inhibitors were recently found in Japan. *Thromb Haemost* 105:925, 2011.

329. Ichinose A: Factor XIII as a key molecule at the intersection of coagulation and fibrinolysis as well as inflammation and infection control. *Int J Hematol* 95:362, 2012.

CHAPTER 125
HEREDITARY FIBRINOGEN ABNORMALITIES

Marguerite Neerman-Arbez and Philippe de Moerloose*

SUMMARY

Hereditary fibrinogen abnormalities make up two classes of plasma fibrinogen defects: (1) type I, afibrinogenemia or hypofibrinogenemia, in which there are low or absent plasma fibrinogen antigen levels (quantitative fibrinogen deficiencies), and (2) type II, dysfibrinogenemia or hypodysfibrinogenemia, in which there are normal or reduced antigen levels associated with disproportionately low functional activity (qualitative fibrinogen deficiencies). In afibrinogenemia, most mutations of the three encoding genes of fibrinogen chains are null. In some cases, missense or late-truncating nonsense mutations allow synthesis of the corresponding fibrinogen chain, but intracellular fibrinogen assembly and/or secretion is impaired. In certain hypofibrinogenemic cases, the mutant fibrinogen molecules are produced and retained in the rough endoplasmic reticulum of hepatocytes in the form of inclusion bodies, causing endoplasmic reticulum storage disease. Afibrinogenemia is associated with mild to severe bleeding, whereas hypofibrinogenemia is often asymptomatic. Thromboembolism may also occur and affected women may suffer from recurrent pregnancy loss. Hereditary dysfibrinogenemias are characterized by biosynthesis of a structurally abnormal fibrinogen molecule that exhibits reduced functional properties. Dysfibrinogenemia is commonly associated with bleeding, thrombosis, or both thrombosis and bleeding, but in many patients it is asymptomatic. Hypodysfibrinogenemia is a subcategory of this disorder. Certain mutations involving the C-terminus of the fibrinogen α chain are associated with amyloidosis, in which an abnormal fragment from the fibrinogen α C domain is deposited in the kidneys. The cause for thrombophilia in type II fibrinogen abnormalities often is uncertain but may involve defective calcium binding, impaired tissue-type plasminogen activator-mediated fibrinolysis, resistance to fibrinolysis, or reduced thrombin binding to fibrin. Replacement therapy with fibrinogen concentrates has proven to be useful for management of fibrinogen disorders but should be adapted to each patient, based on the personal and family history.

Acronyms and Abbreviations: FFP, fresh-frozen plasma; *FGA*, fibrinogen Aα-chain gene; *FGB*, fibrinogen Bβ-chain gene; *FGG*, fibrinogen γ-chain gene; FpA, fibrinopeptide A; FpB, fibrinopeptide B; LMWH, low-molecular-weight heparin; PCR: polymerase chain reaction; TAFI, thrombin-activatable fibrinolysis inhibitor; t-PA, tissue-type plasminogen activator.

*The authors thank Dr. Alessandro Casini for helpful comments and suggestions.

Several detailed and thoroughly annotated reviews of mutations causing inherited fibrinogen disorders have been published[1-3] and the previous version of this chapter published in the eighth edition[4] contained tables compiling causative mutations identified before 2009. In addition, a registry for hereditary fibrinogen abnormalities[5] can be accessed at http://www.geht.org/databaseang/fibrinogen/ that lists variants reported in publications, conference abstracts, and submitted online, with original references. This chapter discusses the major molecular mechanisms leading to disease, as well as the laboratory and clinical aspects of fibrinogen disorders and their treatment, without listing all fibrinogen gene anomalies.

● INTRODUCTION

Fibrinogen plays a major role in hemostasis as the precursor molecule for the insoluble fibrin clot (Fig. 125–1). In addition fibrinogen participates in numerous other biologic processes, such as inflammation, wound healing, and angiogenesis. Fibrinogen binds plasminogen, α-antiplasmin, fibronectin, and factor XIII, among other proteins. It also binds to platelets and supports platelet aggregation. After fibrinogen is converted to fibrin by thrombin, it provides nonsubstrate binding sites for thrombin; consequently, fibrinogen is sometimes termed *antithrombin I*.[6] Fibrinogen also binds to vascular endothelial and other cells, plasma or tissue matrix components such as fibronectin and glycosaminoglycans, and peptide growth factors. Fibrin provides a template for assembly and activation of the fibrinolytic system components and is the major substrate for the enzyme plasmin (Chap. 135). Both fibrinogen and fibrin serve as substrates for plasma factor XIIIa that catalyzes covalent crosslinking/ligation.

● STRUCTURE AND SYNTHESIS

Fibrinogen is a 340-kDa glycoprotein synthesized in hepatocytes[7] that circulates in plasma at a concentration of 1.5 to 3.5 mg/mL (~4 to 10 μM). Each fibrinogen molecule is approximately 45 nm in length. The core structure consists of two outer D regions (or D domains) and a central E region (or E domain) connected through coiled-coil connectors (Fig. 125–2).[8] The molecule exhibits a twofold axis of symmetry perpendicular to the long axis, consisting of two sets of three polypeptide chains (Aα, Bβ, γ) that are joined in their aminoterminal regions by disulfide bridges to form the E region. The outer D regions contain the globular C terminal domains of the Bβ chain (βC) and γ chain (γC). The βC and γC domains, which are highly conserved in vertebrates, are members of the FreD (fibrinogen-related domain) family of proteins. Unlike the βC and γC domains, the C-terminal domains of the Aα chain (αC) are intrinsically unfolded and flexible and tend to be noncovalently tethered in the vicinity of the central E region (Fig. 125–2). The three genes encoding fibrinogen Bβ *(FGB)*, Aα *(FGA)*, and γ *(FGG)*, ordered from centromere to telomere, are clustered in a region of approximately 50 kb on human chromosome 4.[9] *FGA* and *FGG* are transcribed from the reverse strand, in the opposite direction to *FGB*. Alternative splicing[10] results in two isoforms for the fibrinogen α chain: the common Aα chain, encoded by exons 1 to 5, and an extended Aα-E isoform, encoded by exons 1 to 6 which represents only 1 to 2 percent of transcripts. Alternative splicing for *FGG* also produces two transcripts: the major mRNA species contains all 10 exons and encodes the common γ chain (or γA), while the minor product (γ′) does not splice out intron 9 and the corresponding open reading frame replaces the four codons of exon 10 with 20 alternative codons. *FGB* encodes a single 1.9-kb transcript with a 1.5-kb coding sequence. Each gene is separately transcribed and translated to produce nascent polypeptides of 644 amino acids (Aα), 491 amino acids (Bβ), and 437 amino acids (γ).

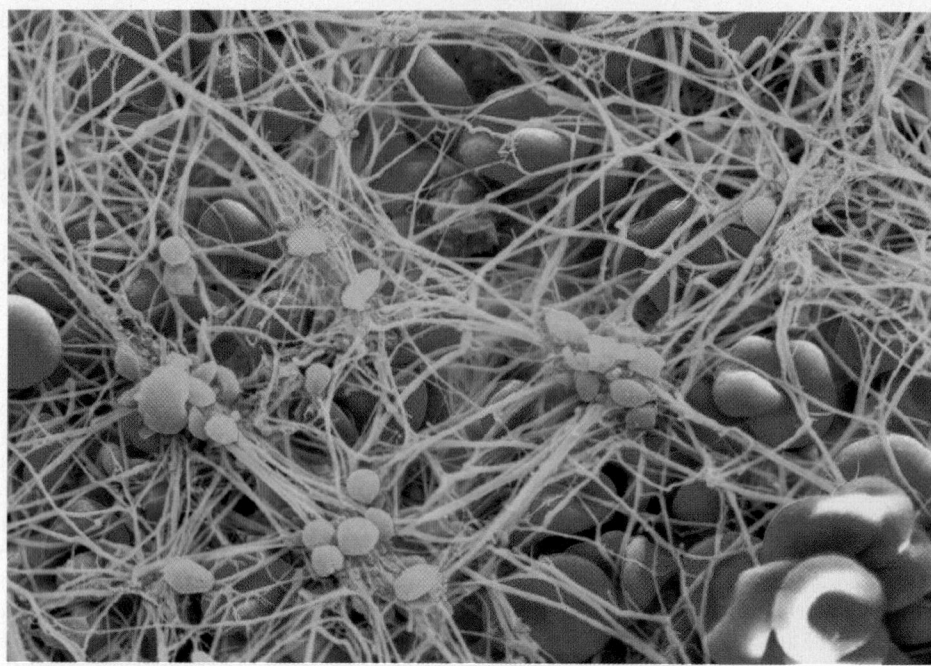

Figure 125–1. Colorized scanning electron micrograph of a whole blood clot. The fibrin mesh is shown in green, and trapped platelets and erythrocytes are colored violet and red, respectively. *(Used with permission of Yuri Veklich and John W. Weisel, University of Pennsylvania School of Medicine.)*

During translocation of the single chains into the lumen of the endoplasmic reticulum (ER), a signal peptide is cotranslationally cleaved from each chain. The resulting chains have 625 amino acids (Aα), 461 amino acids (Bβ), and 411 amino acids (γ). Assembly proceeds in the ER with the formation of an Aα-γ or Bβ-γ intermediate. The addition of either a Bβ or Aα chain gives rise to a [AαB$\beta\gamma$] half-molecule, which dimerizes to form the functional hexamer.[11] The protein undergoes several posttranslational modifications in the Golgi complex, including maturation of N-linked oligosaccharides, phosphorylation, hydroxylation, and sulfation.[12]

Following assembly, which is completed within minutes, the mature molecule is constitutively secreted into the circulation, where it exhibits a half-life of approximately 4 days.[13] In addition to plasma fibrinogen, blood contains an internalized intracellular fibrinogen pool that is stored within platelet α granules. Both megakaryocytes and platelets are capable of internalizing plasma fibrinogen via the fibrinogen integrin $\alpha_{IIb}\beta_3$ receptor,[14] which binds to a C-terminal platelet recognition sequence that is present on γA chains but is absent from γ' chains. Consequently, internalized platelet fibrinogen molecules contain only γA chains.[15]

FIBRINOGEN CONVERSION TO FIBRIN AND NETWORK ASSEMBLY

Fibrin polymerization consists of several consecutive reactions, each affecting the ultimate structure and properties of the fibrin scaffold, which, in turn, determines the development and outcome of numerous diseases including coagulopathies and thrombosis.[16,17] Conversion of fibrinogen to a fibrin clot[18] occurs in three distinct phases: (1) enzymatic cleavage by thrombin to produce fibrin monomers; (2) self-assembly of fibrin units to form an organized polymeric structure; and (3) covalent crosslinking of fibrin by factor XIIIa. In the first phase of conversion to

fibrin, cleavage of fibrinogen at AαR35/G36 (R16/G17)* and later Bβ R44/G45 (R14/G15) results in release of fibrinopeptides A (FpA) and B (FpB), respectively, thus exposing "A" knobs and "B" knobs (Fig. 125–3). The "A" knob located at the new aminoterminal end of the fibrin α chain starts with the GPRV amino acid sequence. The "A" knob in fibrin interacts with the constitutive complementary association site known as hole "a" in another molecule to initiate the fibrin assembly process. Hole "a" is encompassed by residues 363 to 405 (337 to 379) of the γ chain.

A knob-hole a (A:a) interaction results in formation of double-stranded fibrils in which fibrin molecules become aligned in an end-to-middle, staggered overlapping arrangement (see Fig. 125–3).[16–18] Fibrils subsequently undergo branching by lateral fibril associations in which two fibrils converge to form a four-stranded "bilateral" fibril junction. Progressive lateral associations among fibrils result in larger fibril bundles or fibers. A second type of junction, termed *equilateral branching*, is formed by three fibrils converging to form a three-member junction.[19] Both types of branch junctions provide scaffolding for the clot network, the ultimate

---

*The recommendation of the Human Genome Variation Society (HGVS) is to number amino acid residues from the initiator Met, with the protein reference sequences representing the primary translation product, not the processed, mature, protein. This is the standard nomenclature used by geneticists. For fibrinogen, however, as for many other secreted proteins, such as the coagulation factors, this is not the nomenclature used in earlier publications (historically fibrinogen residues are numbered according to the secreted product lacking the signal peptide). In this text both nomenclatures are used: amino acid residues and substitutions are described first according to HGVS guidelines followed in brackets by the corresponding amino acid in the mature chain lacking the signal peptide. To convert from the HGVS nomenclature to the mature protein nomenclature, subtract 19 for Aα, 30 for Bβ, or 26 for γ. A one-letter abbreviation for amino acids is used in this chapter. A, alanine; C, cysteine; D, aspartic acid; E, glutamic acid; F, phenylalanine; G, glycine; H, histidine; I, isoleucine; K, lysine; L, leucine; M, methionine; N, asparagine; P, proline; Q, glutamine; R, arginine; S, serine; T, threonine; V, valine; W, tryptophan; Y, tyrosine.

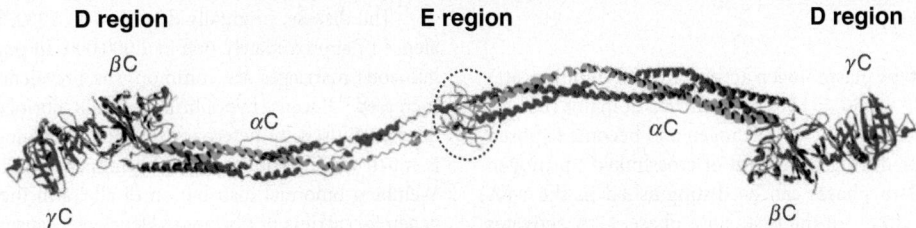

Figure 125–2. Ribbon representation of native chicken fibrinogen[22] modified from PDB file 1M1J (www.pdb.org/pdb/). α Chains are in green, β chains are in purple, and γ chains are in blue. The globular C-terminal domains of the Bβ and γ chains forming the D regions are shown, as well as the central E region, which contains the N-terminal portions of all three chains. Unlike the βC and γC domains, the C-terminal domains of the Aα chain (αC) are flexible and tend to be noncovalently tethered in the vicinity of the central E region.

structure of which is governed by several variables, including salt concentration, pH, fibrinogen concentration and thrombin concentration.[16,17,20]

Fibrinopeptide B (FpB) release occurs more slowly than fibrinopeptide A (FpA) release and exposes another polymerization site known as the "B" knob beginning with the amino acid sequence GHRP. GHRP interacts with a constitutive hole "b" in the β chain encompassed by residues 427 to 462 (397 to 432). FpB cleavage is accelerated by fibrin polymerization, whereas FpA cleavage is independent of fibrin polymerization. B:b interactions are not required for lateral fibril associations, but they contribute to lateral association by inducing rearrangements in βC that allow βC:βC contacts to occur.[21,22]

The flexible αC domains also participate in fibrin polymerization.[23] Fibrin clots made from plasma fibrinogen molecules lacking more than 100 C-terminal residues from the αC domain display prolonged thrombin times, reduced turbidity, and produce thinner fibers, indicating that αC domains participate in lateral fibril associations. In addition, αC domains become dissociated as a result of FpB cleavage. This allows αC domains to participate in noncovalent interactions with other αC domains, thereby promoting lateral fibril associations and fibrin network assembly. Finally, additional self-associating sites in the D region participate in fibrin assembly. These are the D:D sites and $γ_{XL}$ sites that promote end-to-end alignment of assembling fibrin units and factor XIIIa crosslinking, respectively.[24,25]

CROSSLINKING BY FACTOR XIII

The clot formed by fibrin polymerization requires further stabilization to increase its mechanical strength and resist immediate degradation by the fibrinolytic pathway. Factor XIIIa (a heterotetramer FXIII-A2B2) is a transglutaminase that stabilizes the elongating protofibril by crosslinking adjacent γ chains through the formation of ε-(γ-glutamyl) lysine isopeptide bonds.[26] These occur between lysine 432 (406) of one γ chain and glutamine 424 (398) or 425 (399) of another chain. Crosslinking increases the resistance of the clot to deformation. The same process occurs, but at lower rate, between α chains and also between α chains and γ chains. In the presence of factor XIIIa, α-antiplasmin becomes covalently bound to the distal α chains of fibrin or fibrinogen.[26] The factor XIII binding site for fibrin has been characterized: residues in the Aα-C domain, that is, 408 to 421 (389 to 402) bind a cleft in FXIII-A2 that is exposed only after cleavage of the activation peptide by thrombin.[27] Fibronectin is also incorporated into the fibrin clot. This occurs by noncovalent interactions between the two proteins through specific binding sites, followed by their covalent crosslinking with factor XIIIa.[28] Fibronectin incorporation appears to affect the adhesion and migration of cells at sites of fibrin deposition, thereby contributing to wound healing and other cell-dependent processes.

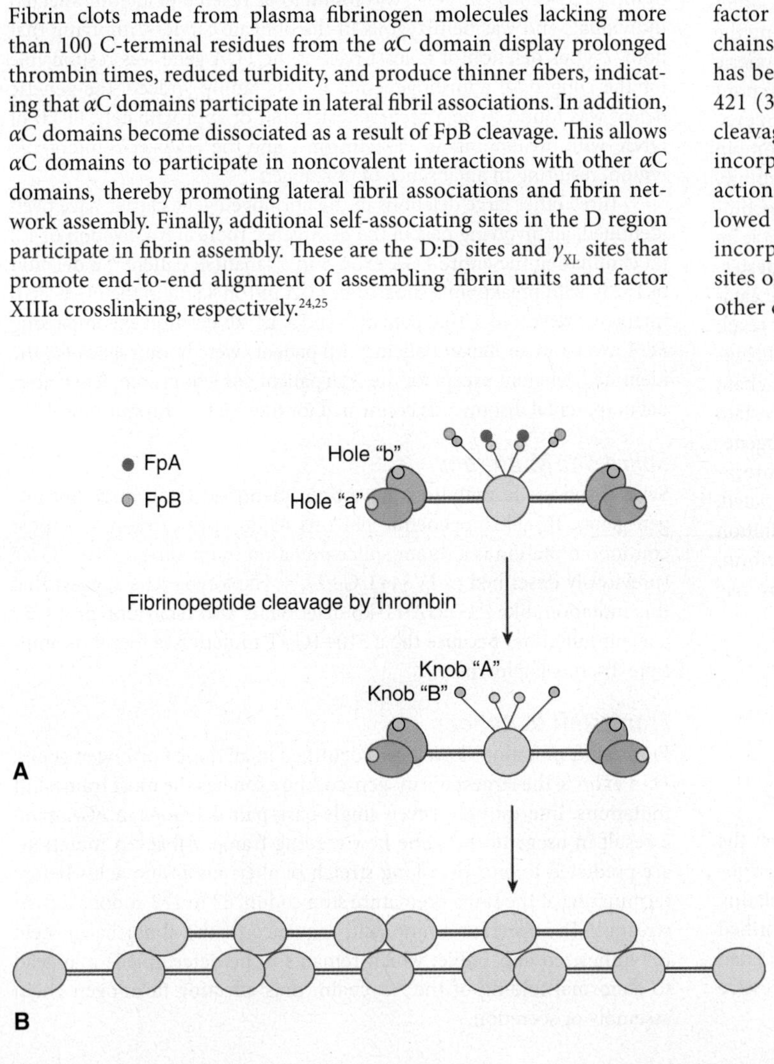

- ● FpA
- ○ FpB

Hole "b"

Hole "a"

Fibrinopeptide cleavage by thrombin

Knob "A"
Knob "B"

A

B

Figure 125–3. First steps of fibrinogen conversion to fibrin and fibrin assembly. **A.** Schematic of fibrinogen showing fibrinopeptides A (FpA) and B (FpB), the constitutive holes "a" and "b" in the globular C-terminal domains of the γ chains and β chains, respectively, and the "A" and "B" knobs, which are exposed only after FpA and FpB cleavage by thrombin. Here the globular βC and γC domains are shown separately, βC in purple, γC in blue as in Fig. 125–2. **B.** Self-assembly of fibrin units to form an organized polymeric structure. Here, for simplicity, the D regions are represented as a single globular unit.

FIBRINOLYSIS

Plasminogen and tissue-type plasminogen activator (t-PA) binding sites in the D regions (i.e., γ 337 to 350) (312 to 324), and αC domains (i.e., Aα 167 to 179) (148 to 160), are cryptic in fibrinogen and become exposed during fibrin assembly or during formation of crosslinked fibrinogen fibrils (Chap. 135).[29-30] Two phases can be distinguished in the t-PA induced lysis of a fibrin clot.[31] In the first, slow, phase, t-PA activates plasminogen on the intact fibrin surface. The generation of C-terminal lysine residues in partially degraded fibrin (by plasmin) in the second phase of clot lysis may result in accumulation of plasminogen at the clot surface and a concomitant increase in lysis rate. Thrombin-activatable fibrinolysis inhibitor (TAFI) removes C-terminal lysine residues, resulting in a strongly reduced binding of plasminogen and in an inhibition of the second phase of clot lysis by a reduction of the activation of plasminogen on the fibrin surface. TAFI, as well as α-antiplasmin, lipoprotein(a), and histidine-rich glycoprotein, bind to fibrin and all have an inhibitory effect on fibrinolysis through various mechanisms.

ANTITHROMBIN ACTIVITY OF FIBRIN

Thrombin binds to its substrate, fibrinogen, through a fibrinogen recognition site in thrombin, referred to as exosite 1. The fibrin clot itself also exhibits significant thrombin-binding potential; this nonsubstrate binding potential of fibrin for thrombin is referred to as antithrombin activity I.[6] This activity is defined by two classes of nonsubstrate thrombin-binding sites in fibrin, one of "low-affinity" in the E-region and the other of "high-affinity" in D regions of fibrin(ogen) molecules containing the variant γ' chain. Altogether, heterodimeric γA/γ' and homodimeric molecules γ'/γ' chains make up 8 to 15 percent of the total γ-chain population.[10] Low-affinity thrombin-binding activity reflects thrombin exosite 1 binding in the E region of fibrin, whereas high-affinity thrombin binding to γ' chains takes place through exosite 2. The binding affinity of thrombin for γ'-containing fibrin molecules is increased by concomitant fibrin binding to thrombin exosite 1. Antithrombin I (fibrin) is an important inhibitor of thrombin generation that functions by sequestering thrombin in the forming fibrin clot, and also by reducing the catalytic activity of fibrin-bound thrombin. Vascular thrombosis may result from absence of antithrombin I (as in afibrinogenemia; see "Afibrinogenemia and Hypofibrinogenemia" below), reduced plasma γ'-chain content,[32] or defective thrombin binding to fibrin as found in certain dysfibrinogenemias (see "Dysfibrinogenemia and Hypodysfibrinogenemia" below). In contrast, an increased susceptibility to arterial thrombosis has been reported when γ'-chain levels are significantly elevated. Moreover, thrombin bound to γ_A/γ'-fibrin is protected from inhibition by antithrombin to a greater extent than thrombin bound to γ_A/γ_A-fibrin. Thus, γ_A/γ'-fibrin serves as a reservoir of active thrombin, which may contribute to the prothrombotic nature of thrombi.[33]

AFIBRINOGENEMIA AND HYPOFIBRINOGENEMIA

DEFINITION, HISTORY, AND EPIDEMIOLOGY

Type I disorders (afibrinogenemia and hypofibrinogenemia) affect the quantity of fibrinogen in circulation. Type II disorders (dysfibrinogenemia and hypodysfibrinogenemia) affect the quality of circulating fibrinogen.[1] While the first dysfibrinogenemia mutation was identified as early as 1968,[34] the molecular basis of afibrinogenemia was elucidated much later.[35] This disorder is characterized by autosomal recessive inheritance and the complete absence of fibrinogen in plasma.

The disease, originally described in 1920,[36] has an estimated prevalence of approximately one in 1,000,000. In populations where consanguineous marriages are common, the prevalence of afibrinogenemia, is increased.[37] Because hypofibrinogenemia (fibrinogen levels below 1.5 g L^{-1}) is often caused by heterozygosity for a fibrinogen gene mutation, this is much more frequent than afibrinogenemia. If one applies the Hardy Weinberg binomial distribution of alleles in the population to afibrinogenemia, carriers of fibrinogen deficiency causing mutations could be as frequent as 1 in 500.

ETIOLOGY AND PATHOGENESIS

Since the identification of the first causative mutation for congenital afibrinogenemia in 1999,[35] approximately 100 distinct mutations, the majority in *FGA*, have been identified in patients with afibrinogenemia (in homozygosity or in compound heterozygosity) or in hypofibrinogenemia. Causative mutations can be divided into two main classes: null mutations with no protein production at all and mutations producing abnormal protein chains which are retained inside the cell.[1]

Large Deletions

The first causative mutation for afibrinogenemia was identified in a nonconsanguineous Swiss family with two pairs of afibrinogenemic brothers.[35] In a first step toward establishing whether or not the disease was linked to the fibrinogen gene cluster on chromosome 4, haplotype data were obtained for five microsatellite markers surrounding this locus. One of these, FGAi3, a (TCTT)n polymorphic marker located in intron 3 of the *FGA* gene, was found to be deleted in all four affected individuals and was hemizygous in the obligate carriers, implying that homozygous deletion of at least part of the *FGA* gene was responsible for the congenital afibrinogenemia in this family. Indeed, the genetic defect was found to be a recurrent deletion of approximately 11 kb of DNA, with breakpoints in *FGA* intron 1 and the *FGA–FGB* intergenic region, resulting in an absence of fibrinogen.

Three other large deletions in the fibrinogen gene cluster have been identified, all involving part of the *FGA* gene. These are: a deletion of 1.2 kb eliminating the entire *FGA* exon 4 in a Japanese patient[38]; a deletion of 15 kb, with breakpoints situated in *FGA* intron 4 and in the *FGA–FGB* intergenic region in a Thai patient[39]; and a 4.1-kb deletion encompassing *FGA* exon 1 in an Italian patient.[40] All patients were homozygous for the identified deletions except for the Thai patient, for whom complete maternal uniparental disomy was confirmed for the deleted chromosome 4.[39]

Splice-Site Mutations

Several splice-site mutations have been identified in all three fibrinogen genes. In afibrinogenemic patients of European origin, the most common mutation is a donor splice mutation in intron 4, c.510+1G→T (previously described as IVS4+1 G→T).[1,41] Haplotype data suggest that this mutation, like the *FGA* 11-kb deletion, is also recurrent, or a very ancient mutation, because the c.510+1G→T mutation is found on multiple discrete haplotypes.

Frameshift Mutations

Frameshift mutations have been identified in all three fibrinogen genes. *FGA* exon 5, the largest fibrinogen-coding exon has the most frameshift mutations. Interestingly, seven single base-pair deletions in *FGA* exon 5 result in usage of the same new reading frame. All seven mutations are predicted to encode a long stretch of aberrant amino acids before terminating at the same premature stop codon, 69 to 158 codons downstream.[42] The aberrant amino acid sequence (if the abnormal protein is synthesized and stable, which remains to be determined) may lead to abnormal folding of the Aα chain, thus affecting fibrinogen chain assembly or secretion.

Nonsense Mutations

Many nonsense mutations accounting for afibrinogenemia and hypofibrinogenemia have been identified. Of the nine nonsense mutations identified in *FGB*, four are located in *FGB* exon 8.[43] In particular, two *FGB* nonsense mutations—W467X (W437X) and W470X (W440X)—are localized very close to the β-chain C-terminus and are expected to cause the synthesis of βC chains truncated of only 25 and 22 residues, respectively.[44,45] Expression studies in transfected COS cells performed for both mutations showed that the mutations allowed individual chain synthesis and intracellular assembly of the hexamer but impaired secretion, suggesting that an intact *FGB* C-terminal domain is necessary for fibrinogen secretion into the circulation.[46]

Missense Mutations

Null mutations, that is, large deletions, frameshift, early truncating nonsense, and splice-site mutations account for the majority of afibrinogenemia alleles, as expected. Missense mutations leading to complete fibrinogen deficiency are therefore particularly interesting, revealing the functional importance of individual residues or three-dimensional structures. Missense mutations are clustered in the highly conserved C-terminal globular domains of the γ and Bβ chains.[1,43] Expression studies in transfected cells for five *FGB* missense mutations, all identified in homozygosity or compound heterozygosity in afibrinogenemic patients, showed that these mutations, like the late-truncating nonsense mutations discussed previously, allowed individual chain synthesis and intracellular assembly of the hexamer but again impaired secretion.[47–50] Further characterization of the *FGB* G444S (G414S) mutant using immunostaining for fibrinogen and visualization by confocal microscopy revealed that the secretion-impaired mutant was retained in the ER proving the existence of an efficient quality control mechanism for fibrinogen secretion.[46]

Several missense mutations have been identified in *FGG* in heterozygosity in patients with hypofibrinogenemia. For the majority of these mutations, analysis of patient plasma fibrinogen by mass spectrometry confirmed absence of the mutant γ chain in the circulation. Others have been studied at the functional level in transfected cells: fibrinogen Matsumoto IV C179R (C153R) was found to impair intracellular hexamer assembly,[51] whereas fibrinogen Bratislava W253C (W227C) was found to impair fibrinogen secretion.[52]

Mutations Causing Hepatic Endoplasmic Reticulum Retention and Hypofibrinogenemia

In the majority of patients with afibrinogenemia or hypofibrinogenemia there is no evidence of intracellular accumulation of the mutant fibrinogen chain. This implies the existence of an efficient degradation pathway for fibrinogen mutants that allow individual chain synthesis and assembly but not secretion. Four mutations, all in *FGG*, are known to cause hypofibrinogenemia accompanied by hepatic storage disease. These are three missense mutations (fibrinogen Brescia, Aguadilla, and Al duPont,[53–55] and a 15-bp deletion at the end of *FGG* exon 8 (fibrinogen Angers),[56] which creates a new *FGG* exon 8–intron 8 junction and donor splice site. All four mutations cause fibrinogen deficiency in the heterozygous state because of the absence of the mutant γ chain in patient plasma, but also progressive liver disease associated with hepatocellular cytoplasmic inclusions. The molecular mechanism by which these mutations, localized in the five-stranded β-sheet of γC and hole "a," which are crucial for fibrin polymerization, leads to impaired secretion, retention in the ER, and formation of aggregates remains to be determined.

CLINICAL FEATURES

Afibrinogenemia

Bleeding because of afibrinogenemia usually manifests in the neonatal period, with 85 percent of cases presenting umbilical cord bleeding, but a later age of onset is not unusual. Bleeding may occur in the skin, gastrointestinal tract, genitourinary tract, or the central nervous system with intracranial hemorrhage being the major cause of death. Joint bleeding, which is common in patients with severe hemophilia, is less frequent: in a series of 72 patients with severe fibrinogen deficiency, hemarthrosis was observed in 25 percent of cases.[57] There is an intriguing susceptibility of spontaneous rupture of the spleen in afibrinogenemic patients. Bone cysts have also been described as a rare complication of afibrinogenemia and appear to benefit from prophylactic therapy with fibrinogen concentrate.[58]

Menstruating women may experience menometrorrhagia but some have normal menses. First trimester abortion is usual in afibrinogenemic women. The importance of fibrinogen in pregnancy was demonstrated in studies with fibrinogen knockout mice that cannot carry fetuses to term.[59] Women may also have antepartum and postpartum hemorrhage. Hemoperitoneum after rupture of the corpus luteum has also been observed.

Paradoxically both arterial and venous thromboembolic complications are observed in afibrinogenemic patients. These complications can occur in the presence of concomitant risk factors such as a coinherited thrombophilic risk factor or after replacement therapy. However, in many patients, no known risk factors are present. Many hypotheses have been put forward to explain this predisposition to thrombosis. One explanation is that even in the absence of fibrinogen platelet aggregation is possible because of the action of von Willebrand factor and, in contrast to patients with severe hemophilia, afibrinogenemic patients are able to generate thrombin, both in the initial phase of limited production and also in the secondary burst of thrombin generation. In some patients, an increase of prothrombin activation fragments or thrombin–antithrombin complexes has been observed, which may reflect enhanced thrombin generation.[60] These abnormal levels can be normalized by fibrinogen infusions.

As previously mentioned, fibrin also acts as antithrombin I by both sequestering and downregulating thrombin activity.[6] Thrombin which is not trapped by the clot is available for platelet activation and smooth muscle cell migration and proliferation, particularly in the arterial vessel wall. Thrombus formation is maintained in fibrinogen-deficient mice,[61] and in fibrinogen-deficient zebrafish,[62] but the thrombus is unstable and has a tendency to embolize. Similarly, the absence of fibrinogen in human plasma results in large but loosely packed thrombi under flow conditions.[63]

Hypofibrinogenemia

Hypofibrinogenemia patients are very often heterozygous carriers of afibrinogenemia mutations.[1] These patients are usually asymptomatic with fibrinogen levels of approximately 1.0 g L^{-1}, levels which are in theory high enough to protect against bleeding and maintain pregnancy. However they can bleed when exposed to trauma, or if they have a second associated hemostatic abnormality. Hypofibrinogenemic women may also suffer from pregnancy loss.

LABORATORY FEATURES

The clinical diagnosis is established by functional and immunologic measurements of fibrinogen concentration backed by genetic analyses.

Phenotype Analysis

Absence of immunoreactive fibrinogen is essential for the diagnosis of congenital afibrinogenemia. All coagulation tests that depend on the formation of fibrin as the end point—that is, prothrombin time (PT), partial thromboplastin time (PTT), or thrombin time (TT)—are infinitely prolonged. Plasma activity of all other clotting factors is usually normal. Some abnormalities in platelet functions tests can be observed which can be reversed upon addition of fibrinogen. Because fibrinogen is one of the main determinants of erythrocyte sedimentation, it is not surprising that afibrinogenemic patients have very low erythrocyte sedimentation rates. When skin testing is performed for delayed hypersensitivity, there is no induration because of the lack of fibrin deposition.

Hypofibrinogenemia is defined as a proportional decrease of functional and immunoreactive fibrinogen. Coagulation tests depending on the formation of fibrin as well as the assays used are variably prolonged, the most sensitive assay being the TT.

Genotype Analysis

The large number of mutations identified in patients with afibrinogenemia allows the design of an efficient flow-chart for mutation detection in new cases.[64] Two common mutations are found in individuals of European origin, both in *FGA*: the c.510+1G→T intron 4 donor splice-site mutation and the *FGA* 11-kb deletion, both found on multiple haplotypes. In all new patients of European origin, the *FGA* c.510+1G→T should be the first mutation to be screened. Southern blot or polymerase chain reaction (PCR) analysis of the *FGA* 11-kb deletion should also be performed, because it is the second most common mutation in patients of European origin and because of the risk of diagnostic error: a nonconsanguineous patient who appears to be homozygous for a mutation in *FGA* exons 2 to 6 may in reality be a heterozygous carrier of the large 11-kb deletion.[65] Given the high frequency of mutations in *FGA*, the other *FGA* exons (starting with exon 5) should then be studied for mutations before screening *FGB* (starting with exon 8) and *FGG* (starting with exons 7 and 8). The same strategy can also be applied to afibrinogenemic patients of non-European origin for whom recurrent mutations have yet to be identified. If the patient comes from a geographical region or population in which a mutation has already been identified, that mutation should be the first to be screened for. Screening of patients with hypofibrinogenemia can follow the same strategy apart from patients with ER fibrinogen-positive liver inclusions, for which four mutations in *FGG* are known so far to cause hepatic storage disease.

Prenatal diagnosis has been performed in a few cases.[66] This is important for families with afibrinogenemia and access to adequate treatment because the prenatal diagnosis of an affected infant allows initiation of treatment immediately after birth before the first bleeding manifestation.

Genotype–Phenotype Correlations: Potential Importance of Global Assays

Current diagnostic tests are appropriate for establishing the diagnosis but clearly additional tests are required for a more accurate prediction of the clinical phenotype of a patient and consequently the appropriate treatment. Indeed, although in afibrinogenemia all patients have unmeasurable functional fibrinogen, the severity of bleeding is highly variable amongst patients, even amongst those with the same genotype. Similarly, there is no clear relationship between the molecular defect and the risk of thrombosis.

One possible explanation for the observed variability of clinical manifestations is the existence of modifier genes/alleles: some variants may increase the severity of bleeding while others may ameliorate the phenotype. Such modifiers have yet to be identified. However, the common thrombophilias (e.g., factor V Leiden) most certainly play a role in decreasing the severity of bleeding. The existence of modifying genes/polymorphisms is also strongly suspected in the previously discussed cases of hypofibrinogenemia associated with fibrinogen inclusion bodies in hepatocytes. Indeed, all individuals heterozygous for one of the four *FGG* causative mutations have hypofibrinogenemia, but not all have fibrinogen aggregates and associated liver disease.

Global assays, such as thromboelastography and thrombin generation test, may provide a complementary and in some cases a better evaluation of an individual's hemostatic state. Such global assays could be useful for the design of individual therapeutic strategies.[67]

DIFFERENTIAL DIAGNOSIS

Inherited afibrinogenemia and hypofibrinogenemia have to be distinguished from acquired disorders. These include disseminated intravascular coagulation, primary fibrinolysis, liver disease, and can be caused by certain drugs (e.g., thrombolytic agents and L-asparaginase). In addition, one should be aware that artifactually low levels of fibrinogen can be observed with samples that have clotted as a result of improper collection. In most cases, the clinical context as well as the association with other laboratory abnormalities will allow differentiation of inherited from acquired disorders. Identification of a causative mutation in one of the three fibrinogen genes will confirm the diagnosis.

THERAPY

Available Treatments and Modalities

Replacement therapy is effective in treating bleeding episodes in congenital fibrinogen disorders. Depending on the country of residence, patients receive fresh-frozen plasma (FFP), cryoprecipitate, or fibrinogen concentrates.[64] Fibrinogen concentrate preparations include safety steps for inactivation or removal of viruses, which make them safer than cryoprecipitate or FFP. Furthermore, more precise dosing can be accomplished with fibrinogen concentrates because their potency is known, in contrast to FFP or cryoprecipitates.

The conventional treatment is on demand, in which fibrinogen is administered as soon as possible after onset of bleeding. Another approach is primary prophylaxis that includes administration of fibrinogen concentrates from an early age to prevent bleeding and, in the case of pregnancy, to prevent miscarriage. Effective long-term secondary prophylaxis with administration of fibrinogen every 7 to 14 days (particularly after central nervous system bleeds) has been advocated. The frequency and dose of fibrinogen concentrates should be adjusted to maintain a level above 0.5 g L^{-1}.[64]

The United Kingdom guidelines on therapeutic products for coagulation disorders[68] provide recommendations about the best treatment options (dosage, management of bleeding, surgery and pregnancy as well as prophylaxis). According to these guidelines, in case of bleeding fibrinogen levels should be increased to 1.0 g L^{-1} and maintained above this threshold until hemostasis is secured, and above 0.5 g L^{-1} until wound healing is complete. To increase the fibrinogen concentration of 1 g L^{-1}, a dose of approximately 50 mg/kg is required. The doses and duration of treatment also vary depending on the type of injury or operative procedure and on the patient's personal and familial history of bleeding and thrombosis.

Women with congenital afibrinogenemia are able to conceive and embryonic implantation is normal, but the pregnancy usually results in spontaneous abortion at 5 to 8 weeks of gestation unless fibrinogen replacement is given.[69] Maintaining the fibrinogen level above 0.6 g L^{-1} and if possible higher than 1.0 g L^{-1} is recommended. Lower fibrinogen concentrations (<0.4 g L^{-1}) have proven adequate to maintain pregnancy but not to avoid hemorrhagic complications. Continuous infusion of fibrinogen concentrate should be performed during labor to maintain fibrinogen higher than 1.5 g L^{-1} (ideally greater than 2.0 g L^{-1}).[70] Thromboembolic events can occur, particularly with the use of cryoprecipitates that contain appreciable quantities of factor VIII and von Willebrand factor in addition to fibrinogen.

In addition to fibrinogen substitution, antifibrinolytic agents may be given, particularly to treat mucosal bleeding or to prevent bleeding following procedures such as dental extraction. Fibrin glue is useful to treat superficial wounds or following dental extractions. Oral contraceptive preparations are useful in case of menorrhagia. Oral iron preparations can be given in cases with associated iron-deficiency anemia. Routine vaccination against hepatitis, as well as a regular surveillance for both the disease and treatment-related complications in a comprehensive care setting, is highly recommended.[64]

Finally, orthotopic liver transplantation is a possible rescue treatment for failure of fibrinogen replacement therapy. This procedure successfully restored normal hemostasis in an afibrinogenemic patient with severe Budd-Chiari syndrome and inferior cava vein thrombosis[71] and in one of the four afibrinogenemic patients homozygous for the 11-kb *FGA* mutation.[35,72]

Complications of Therapy

In many countries only FFP or cryoprecipitate are available, which is problematic because the viral inactivation process is in general not as efficient as it is for fibrinogen concentrates (although emerging non-viral pathogens such as the prion responsible for variant Creutzfeldt-Jacob disease must be considered, even for concentrates). Even if viral inactivation steps are performed, these preparations (particularly FFP) can induce volume overload. There is also a risk of transfusion-related acute lung injury, because of the presence of cytotoxic antibodies in the infused plasma.

Acquired inhibitors to fibrinogen after replacement therapy have been reported in only two cases. It is not clear why afibrinogenemic patients do not develop inhibitors more frequently. One explanation for some cases is that minute amounts of fibrinogen, which can only be detected by highly sensitive immunoassays, are present in the circulation.

One of the major complications in afibrinogenemic patients is thrombosis, which can occur spontaneously following blood component therapy. Some clinicians give small doses of heparin or low-molecular-weight heparin (LMWH) during administration of fibrinogen. Before surgery, patients with a thrombotic phenotype should be treated with compression stockings and LMWH. Successful use of lepirudin has been reported for an afibrinogenemic patient who suffered recurrent arterial thrombosis despite treatment with heparin and aspirin.[73] Thromboembolic complications are difficult to manage because both anticoagulants and fibrinogen preparations have to be administered.

New Preparations

The increasing need for fibrinogen preparations in congenital but also in acquired deficiencies has stimulated some companies to improve existing preparations or to develop new ones. A recombinant fibrinogen molecule is also under development.[74]

● DYSFIBRINOGENEMIA AND HYPODYSFIBRINOGENEMIA

DEFINITION, HISTORY, AND EPIDEMIOLOGY

The second class of hereditary fibrinogen abnormalities comprises the type II disorders, that is, dysfibrinogenemia and hypodysfibrinogenemia. Dysfibrinogenemia is defined by the presence of normal levels of functionally abnormal plasma fibrinogen. Hypodysfibrinogenemia is defined by low levels of a dysfunctional protein. As in afibrinogenemia and hypofibrinogenemia, both are heterogeneous disorders caused by

many different mutations in the three fibrinogen-encoding genes. Dysfibrinogenemias and hypodysfibrinogenemias are autosomal dominant disorders. Most affected patients are heterozygous for missense mutations in the coding region of one of the three fibrinogen genes. Because the secreted fibrinogen hexamer contains two copies of each of the three fibrinogen chains, and the resulting fibrin network contains multiple copies of the molecule, heterozygosity for one mutant allele is sufficient to impair the structure and function of the fibrin clot (Fig. 125–4).

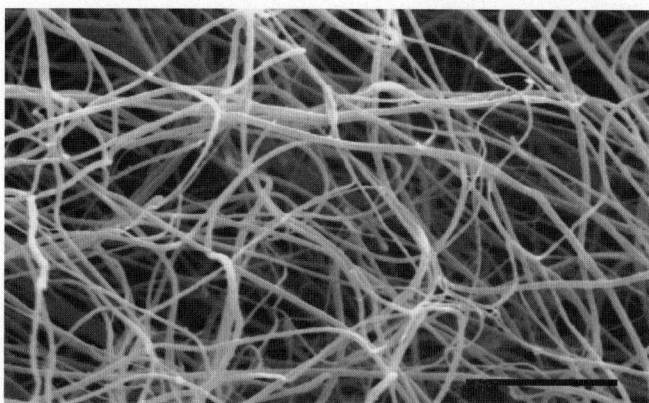
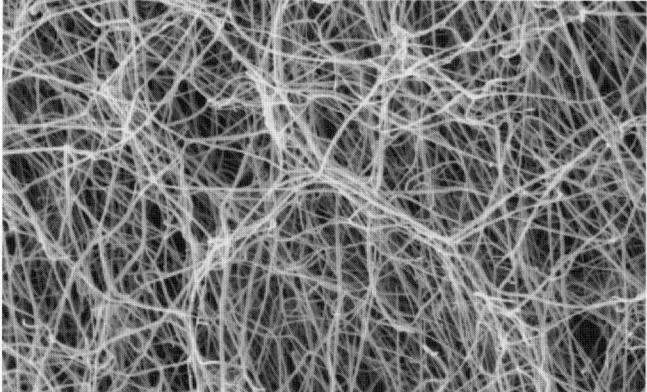
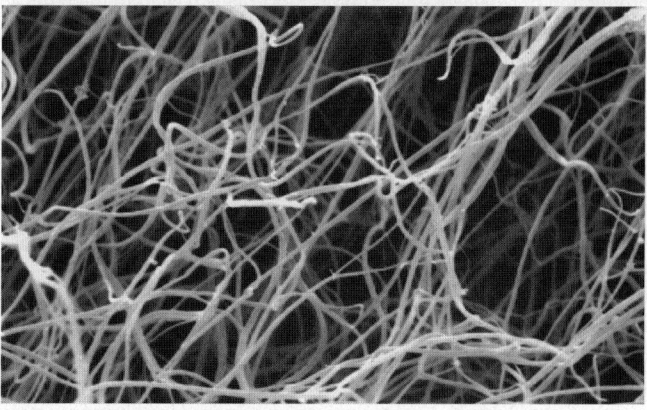

Figure 125–4. Scanning electron micrographs showing structural variations in clots formed from dysfibrinogens. **Top.** Control clot from normal purified fibrinogen clotted with thrombin showing relatively uniform distribution of fibers forming a branched network. **Middle.** Clot from fibrinogen Caracas I[96] showing very thin fibers, indicating a defect in lateral aggregation. **Bottom.** Clot from fibrinogen Caracas VI[97] showing a nonuniform distribution of thin and thick fibers in the clot, with bundles of fibers, larger pores, and more fiber ends than control clots. Magnification bar: 5 μm. *(Used with permission of John W. Weisel and Rita Marchi.)*

As of this writing, more than 100 distinct mutations have been identified in patients with dysfibrinogenemia and hypodysfibrinogenemia. The described mutants are very often named after the city of origin of the family or the city of the laboratory characterizing the mutation. Many cases are asymptomatic and are only identified as a result of routine coagulation screening. Indeed, a compilation of approximately 250 cases revealed that 55 percent of patients were asymptomatic, 25 percent had a history of bleeding, and 20 percent, a tendency toward thrombosis.[75] However, our retrospective multicentric study of the long-term outcomes of 101 genotyped patients suggests that bleeding and thrombotic events are more frequent.[76]

ETIOLOGY AND PATHOGENESIS

Dysfibrinogenemic abnormalities usually are reflected in one or more phases of the fibrinogen-fibrin conversion and fibrin assembly process, notably impaired release of fibrinopeptides and defective fibrin polymerization or factor XIIIa–mediated crosslinking.[77,78] Other abnormalities involve abnormal tissue deposition such as in renal amyloidosis,[79] defective fibrinolysis,[80] abnormal interactions with platelets,[77,80] and defective calcium binding.[81]

Mutations Resulting in Abnormal "A" Knobs or Deficient Fibrinopeptide Release

Fibrinogen Detroit was the first abnormal fibrinogen in which the specific mutation was identified at the protein level.[34] This *FGA* R38S (R19S) mutation is located in the "A" knob (i.e., GPRV) resulting in impaired fibrin polymerization and a bleeding tendency. Other substitutions involving residue R38 (R19) have been found to be associated with bleeding in some cases, for example, Munich I, R38N (R19N), and Mannheim I, R38G (R19G), and with thrombosis in other cases, for example, Aarhus and Kumamoto, which are also a result of R38G (R19G). The mechanism for thrombophilia remains unclear, but coexisting risk factors may contribute to the clinical manifestations. Furthermore, the inability of a mutant fibrin to effectively bind and sequester thrombin may play a role in such a clinical presentation. Bleeding that occurs under conditions involving defective fibrinopeptide release or production of a defective "A" knob is most likely related to the reduced polymerization potential of the mutant fibrins that are produced, with resulting defective clot formation.[82]

Missense mutations at residue *FGA* R35 (R16) which is part of the thrombin cleavage site in the fibrinogen α chain appear to be the most common causative mutations accounting for dysfibrinogenemia, based on information compiled in the GEHT registry for hereditary fibrinogen abnormalities.[5] The R35 (R16) residue can be mutated to either H (CGT→CAT) or C (CGT→TGT) leading to delayed or absent FpA release, respectively, and subsequent delayed polymerization. A prolonged reptilase time is observed for both variants. Most patients do not have a bleeding tendency. Some patients have been found to be homozygous for these mutations or phenotypically homozygous,[65] as a result of compound heterozygosity for an R35 (R16) missense mutation and the large 11-kb *FGA* deletion first characterized in afibrinogenemia. In these cases, a mild bleeding tendency is observed.

Missense mutations in *FGB* affecting FpB release have been identified,[83] but are much less common than those affecting FpA release.

Mutations Leading to Polymerization Defects in the D Region

Sites in the D region important for fibrin polymerization are affected in many dysfibrinogenemias. Mutations affecting hole "a" in the γ chain are numerous, while no naturally occurring mutation involving hole "b" in the Bβ chain has been described, compatible with the view that A:a

interactions are the driving force of fibrin polymerization.[16] The interface for the end-to-end D:D site in the γ chain lies between R301 (R275) and S326 (S300), with T306 (T280) contacting R301 (R275) at the D:D interface. Mutations at the R301 (R275) residue to C (CGT→TGT) or H (CGT→CAT) are the second most common cause of dysfibrinogenemia, accounting for around 10 percent of fibrinogen variants.[5] Impaired polymerization has been observed for all substitutions at this position. Most of these cases are asymptomatic, but some patients heterozygous for R301C (R275C) have thrombophilia, sometimes in association with an additional thrombotic risk factor such as factor V Leiden.[84]

Mutations Accounting for Hypodysfibrinogenemia

Hypodysfibrinogenemia which is defined by low levels of a dysfunctional protein can be caused by different molecular mechanisms. One mechanism is heterozygosity for a single mutation that leads to synthesis of an abnormal fibrinogen chain which is secreted less efficiently than normal fibrinogen, for example, fibrinogen Kyoto IV.[85] Another mechanism is the presence of two different mutations with one mutation responsible for the fibrinogen deficiency (the "hypo phenotype") and one mutation responsible for the abnormal function of the molecule (the "dys phenotype"). For example, in fibrinogen Keokuk,[86] there is compound heterozygosity for the common afibrinogenemia splice-site mutation c.510G→T and a premature truncating nonsense mutation in *FGA* Q347X (Q328X). Another example is fibrinogen Leipzig II in which the common hypofibrinogenemia mutation *FGG* A108G (A82G) and *FGG* G377S (G351S) are located on the same allele.[87] Homozygosity for a single mutation, which allows reduced secretion of a functionally impaired molecule, has been described in fibrinogens Otago[88] and Marburg.[89] Finally, maternal uniparental disomy for a nonsense mutation in *FGB*, W323X (W293X), was found to be the cause of severe hypodysfibrinogenemia in a Chinese patient.[90]

CLINICAL FEATURES

Patients with inherited dysfibrinogenemia are frequently asymptomatic and can be discovered incidentally because of abnormal coagulation tests. A compilation of more than 260 cases of dysfibrinogenemia revealed that 55 percent of the patients had no clinical complications while 25 percent exhibited bleeding, and 20 percent had a tendency to thrombosis, mainly venous.[75] However, when 2376 patients with deep vein thrombosis were screened for thrombophilia, the prevalence of dysfibrinogenemia was very low (0.8 percent) and hence testing for dysfibrinogenemia in patients with deep vein thrombosis is not recommended.[91] Patients with dysfibrinogenemia associated with hemorrhage bleed most often after trauma, surgery, or during the puerperium.[76] Thrombosis may also occur during pregnancy and in the postpartum period. Women with dysfibrinogenemia can also suffer from spontaneous abortions. The problems during and after pregnancy are not necessarily correlated to the fibrinogen concentration.

Some mutations in the Aα chain of fibrinogen are associated with a particular form of hereditary amyloidosis.[79,92] The E545V (E526V) amino acid substitution is the most common of these mutations.[92] The abnormal fibrinogen fragments form amyloid fibrils and the extracellular deposition of these fibrils leads to renal failure. Chronic renal dialysis is performed for managing renal failure. Renal transplantation can be envisaged as an alternative to chronic dialysis. However, continuous fibrinogen-related amyloid deposition ultimately results in allograft destruction. Combined liver and kidney transplantation prevents further amyloid deposition in the renal allograft and elsewhere but is associated with additional perioperative and subsequent risks.

LABORATORY FEATURES

Phenotype Analysis

Initial screening tests for fibrinogen dysfunction should include fibrinogen concentration, measured functionally and immunochemically, TT, and reptilase time. Dysfibrinogenemia is diagnosed by a discrepancy between clottable and immunoreactive fibrinogen. However, even in specialized laboratories, this diagnosis can be difficult because the sensitivity of the tests depends on the specific mutation, reagents, and techniques.[93,94]

In classical dysfibrinogenemias, the functional assay of fibrinogen yields low levels compared with the immunologic assays, but levels are sometimes concordant and the functional level may even be normal (as well as TT). The determination of the precise nature of a fibrinogen defect has to be performed in highly specialized laboratories since it involves purification of fibrinogen, measurement of the rate of fibrinopeptide cleavage, analysis of fibrin monomer polymerization, and fibrinolysis. Thromboelastography, commonly used for decision making for fibrinolytic and anticoagulant therapy, may be particularly useful for investigation of dysfibrinogenemia. The thromboelastography signal is fibrin dependant, its amplitude is enhanced by platelets and reflects the stretch and recovery of the clot during its formation.[95]

Genotype Analysis

The gold standard for the diagnosis of dysfibrinogenemia is the characterization of the molecular defect. However, although advances in DNA analysis have made mutation detection easier, it is not always clear whether the identified mutation is the cause of the presenting phenotype. Family studies showing segregation of the mutation with the phenotype, exclusion that the DNA alteration is a common polymorphism in the general population, and structural correlations are necessary for establishing the link between the DNA alteration and the disorder. As previously mentioned, two mutations "hotspots" are of prime interest in screening for dysfibrinogenemia mutations: residue R35 (R16) situated in *FGA* exon 2, and residue R301 (R275) in *FGG* exon 8. Other causative mutations are common in the surrounding residues. Thus, it is recommended to initially screen *FGA* exon 2 and *FGG* exon 8 in cases of dysfibrinogenemia. In our recent study of 101 dysfibrinogenemia cases,[76] 87 percent of the causative mutations were located in these two exons. Here, mutations of *FGG* R301 (R275) were more common than mutations of FGA R35 (R16), 52 percent and 23 percent, respectively.

Genotype–Phenotype Correlations

As previously discussed, the clinical manifestations of dysfibrinogenemia are highly variable and may relate in some cases to differences in clot strength, structure and stability.[1,17] In a few cases, mutations are predictive of the clinical phenotype, such as the R573C (R554C) substitution in the Aα chain (e.g., fibrinogens Chapel Hill III, Paris V, and Dusart) that predisposes patients to thrombosis. Impaired fibrinolysis exhibited by this dysfibrinogen appears to be responsible for the thrombotic complications. Other examples associated with thrombosis include dysfibrinogens Barcelona III, Haifa I, or Bergamo II as a result of the common γ R301H (R275H) mutation and Cedar Rapids I caused by γ R301C (R275C). However, in fibrinogen Cedar Rapids I, only patients heterozygous for both factor V Leiden and the *FGG* R301C (R275C) substitutions were symptomatic, suggesting that this mutation causes thrombosis when associated with another defect. On the other hand, several mutations in the aminoterminal region of the Aα chain, such as fibrinogen Detroit R38S (R19S) and Mannheim I R38G (R19G), are associated with bleeding.

DIFFERENTIAL DIAGNOSIS

Inherited dysfibrinogenemia has to be distinguished from acquired dysfibrinogenemia. Liver diseases (e.g., cirrhosis, chronic active liver disease, hepatoma, liver failure) are the main causes of acquired dysfibrinogenemia. L-Asparaginase treatment also may result in the production of abnormal fibrinogen. In addition, there are a few case reports of acquired dysfibrinogenemia secondary to pancreatitis, paraneoplastic syndrome, and renal carcinoma. The acquired dysfibrinogenemias represent a heterogeneous group of disorders with multiple pathogenetic mechanisms, the most clearly defined fibrinogen abnormalities being an increase in carbohydrate content in patients with liver disease. These abnormal fibrinogens are usually characterized by prolonged thrombin and reptilase times, by abnormal fibrin monomer polymerization but with normal fibrinopeptide release. Fibrinogen concentration is variable.

In some cases no underlying disease is found, and to determine whether a fibrinogen abnormality is congenital or acquired may be difficult. The demonstration of the same fibrinogen abnormality in another family member is a strong argument for a congenital disorder. When measured in newborns, fibrinogen levels should be interpreted with caution because neonatal fibrinogen has an altered content of carbohydrate that can mimic dysfibrinogenemia in certain laboratory tests.

Rare cases of circulating autoantibodies to fibrinogen, for example in systemic lupus erythematosus and in patients receiving surgical sealants containing bovine fibrinogen, have also been reported.

THERAPY

Any treatment considered in patients with dysfibrinogenemia should be based on the personal and family history. Indeed, as already discussed, subjects with hereditary dysfibrinogenemias may be asymptomatic throughout their whole life or may suffer from bleeding and/or thrombotic complications.[1,75,76] In patients who bleed, functional levels of fibrinogen should be raised above 1.0 g L^{-1} and maintained above this threshold until hemostasis is secured and above 0.5 g L^{-1} until wound healing is complete. Topical fibrin glue or antifibrinolytic agents may be used for superficial bleeds. In pregnant women with a bleeding phenotype, the recommendations for afibrinogenemia and hypofibrinogenemia can be followed. With a personal or familial history of thrombosis, thromboprophylaxis and antithrombotic treatments may be proposed after a careful analysis of each particular situation. Long-term management strategies for thrombophilic dysfibrinogenemia are the same as the strategies for patients with recurrent thromboembolism and may include long-term anticoagulant therapy.

REFERENCES

1. de Moerloose P, Casini A, Neerman-Arbez M: Congenital fibrinogen disorders: An update. *Semin Thromb Hemost* 39:585, 2013.
2. Asselta R, Duga S, Tenchini ML: The molecular basis of quantitative fibrinogen disorders. *J Thromb Haemost* 4:2115, 2006.
3. Galanakis DK: Afibrinogenemias and dysfibrinogenemias, in *Hemostasis and Thrombosis: Basic Principles and Clinical Practice*, 6th ed, edited by JS Bennett, WC Aird, VJ Marder, S Schulman, GC White. Lippincott Williams and Wilkins, Baltimore, 2012.
4. Neerman-Arbez M, de Moerloose P: Hereditary fibrinogen abnormalities, in *Williams Hematology*, 8th ed, edited by M Lichtman, E Beutler, TJ Kipps, U Seligsohn, K Kaushansky, J Prchal, p 2051. McGraw-Hill, New York, 2010.
5. Hanss M, Biot F: A database for human fibrinogen variants. *Ann N Y Acad Sci* 936:89, 2001.
6. Mosesson MW: Update on antithrombin I (fibrin). *Thromb Haemost* 98:105, 2007.
7. Tennent GA, Brennan SO, Stangou AJ, et al: Human plasma fibrinogen is synthesized in the liver. *Blood* 109:1971, 2007.
8. Medved L, Weisel JW: Recommendations for nomenclature on fibrinogen and fibrin. *J Thromb Haemost* 7:355, 2009.
9. Kant J, Fornace AJ Jr, Saxe D, et al: Organization and evolution of the human fibrinogen locus on chromosome four. *Proc Natl Acad Sci U S A* 82:2344, 1985.

10. de Maat M, Verschuur M: Fibrinogen heterogeneity: Inherited and noninherited. *Curr Opin Hematol* 12:377, 2005.

11. Huang S, Mulvihill ER, Farrell DH, et al: Biosynthesis of human fibrinogen. Subunit interactions and potential intermediates in the assembly. *J Biol Chem* 268:8919, 1993.

12. Henschen-Edman AH: On the identification of beneficial and detrimental molecular forms of fibrinogen. *Haemostasis* 29:179, 1999.

13. Collen D, Tytgat GN, Claeys H, Piessens R: Metabolism and distribution of fibrinogen I. *Br J Haematol* 22:681, 1972.

14. Handagama P, Scarborough RM, Shuman MA, Bainton DF: Endocytosis of fibrinogen into megakaryocytes and platelet alpha-granules is mediated by alpha IIb beta 3 (glycoprotein IIb-IIIa). *Blood* 82:135, 1993.

15. Francis CW, Nachman RL, Marder VJ: Plasma and platelet fibrinogen differ in gamma chain content. *Thromb Haemost* 51:84, 1984.

16. Weisel JW, Litvinov RI: Mechanisms of fibrin polymerization and clinical implications. *Blood* 121:1712, 2013.

17. Ariëns RA: Fibrin(ogen) and thrombotic disease. *J Thromb Haemost* 11 Suppl 1:294, 2013.

18. Mosesson MW: The structure and biological features of fibrinogen and fibrin. *Ann N Y Acad Sci* 936:11, 2001.

19. Mosesson MW, DiOrio JP, Siebenlist KR, et al: Evidence for a second type of fibril branch point in fibrin polymer networks, the trimolecular junction. *Blood* 82:1517, 1993.

20. Lord ST: Fibrinogen and fibrin: Scaffold proteins in hemostasis. *Curr Opin Hematol* 14:236, 2007.

21. Medved LV, Litvinovich SV, Ugarova TP, et al: Localization of a fibrin polymerization site complimentary to Gly-His-Arg sequence. *FEBS Lett* 320:239, 1993.

22. Yang Z, Mochalkin I, Doolittle RF: A model of fibrin formation based on crystal structures of fibrinogen and fibrin fragments complexed with synthetic peptides. *Proc Natl Acad Sci U S A* 97:14156, 2000.

23. Weisel JW, Medved LV: The structure and function of the alpha C domains of fibrinogen. *Ann N Y Acad Sci* 936:312, 2001.

24. Mosesson MW, Siebenlist KR, Hainfeld JF, Wall JS: The covalent structure of factor XIIIa crosslinked fibrinogen fibrils. *J Struct Biol* 115:88, 1995.

25. Siebenlist KR, Meh D, Mosesson MW: Protransglutaminase (factor XIII) mediated crosslinking of fibrinogen and fibrin. *Thromb Haemost* 86:1221, 2001.

26. Mosesson MW, Siebenlist KR, Hernandez I, et al: Evidence that alpha2-antiplasmin becomes covalently ligated to plasma fibrinogen in the circulation: A new role for plasma factor XIII in fibrinolysis regulation. *J Thromb Haemost* 6:1565, 2008.

27. Smith KA, Pease RJ, Avery CA, et al: The activation peptide cleft exposed by thrombin cleavage of FXIII-A(2) contains a recognition site for the fibrinogen α chain. *Blood* 121:2117, 2013.

28. Makogonenko E, Ingham KC, Medved L: Interaction of the fibronectin COOH-terminal Fib-2 regions with fibrin: Further characterization and localization of the Fib-2-binding sites. *Biochemistry* 46:5418, 2006.

29. Mosesson MW, Siebenlist KR, Voskuilen M, Nieuwenhuizen W: Evaluation of the factors contributing to fibrin-dependent plasminogen activation. *Thromb Haemost* 79:796, 1998.

30. Medved L, Niewenhuizen W: Molecular mechanisms of initiation of fibrinolysis by fibrin. *Thromb Haemost* 89:409, 2003.

31. Rijken DC, Lijnen HR: New insights into the molecular mechanisms of the fibrinolytic system. *J Thromb Haemost* 7:4, 2009.

32. Uitte de Willige S, de Visser MC, Houwing-Duistermaat JJ, et al: Genetic variation in the fibrinogen gamma gene increases the risk for deep venous thrombosis by reducing plasma fibrinogen gamma' levels. *Blood* 106:4176, 2005.

33. Fredenburgh JC, Stafford AR, Leslie BA, Weitz JI: Bivalent binding to to gammaA/gamma'-fibrin engages both exosites of thrombin and protects it from inhibition by the antithrombin-heparin complex. *J Biol Chem* 283:2470, 2008.

34. Blomback M, Blomback B, Mammen EF, Prasad AS: Fibrinogen Detroit—A molecular defect in the N-terminal disulphide knot of human fibrinogen? *Nature* 218:134, 1968.

35. Neerman-Arbez M, Honsberger A, Antonarakis SE, Morris MA: Deletion of the fibrinogen alpha-chain gene (FGA) causes congenital afibrinogenemia. *J Clin Invest* 103:215, 1999.

36. Rabe F, Salomon E: Ueber-faserstoffmangel im Blute bei einem Falle von Hämophilie. *Arch Intern Med* 95:2, 1920.

37. Peyvandi F, Mannucci PM: Rare coagulation disorders. *Thromb Haemost* 82:1207, 1999.

38. Watanabe K, Shibuya A, Ishii E, et al: Identification of simultaneous mutation of fibrinogen alpha chain and protein C genes in a Japanese kindred. *Br J Haematol* 120:101, 2003.

39. Spena S, Duga S, Asselta R, et al: Congenital afibrinogenaemia caused by uniparental isodisomy of chromosome 4 containing a novel 15-kb deletion involving fibrinogen Aalpha-chain gene. *Eur J Hum Genet* 12:891, 2004.

40. Monaldini L, Asselta R, Duga S, et al: Mutational screening of six afibrinogenemic patients: Identification and characterization of four novel molecular defects. *Thromb Haemost* 97:546, 2007.

41. Neerman-Arbez M, de Moerloose P: Mutations in the fibrinogen gene cluster accounting for congenital afibrinogenemia: An update and report of 10 novel mutations. *Hum Mutat* 28:540, 2006.

42. Robert-Ebadi H, de Moerloose P, El Khorassani M, et al: A novel frameshift mutation in FGA accounting for congenital afibrinogenemia predicted to encode an aberrant peptide terminating 158 amino acids downstream. *Blood Coagul Fibrinolysis* 20:385, 2009.

43. Casini A, Lukowski S, Quintard VL, et al: FGB mutations leading to congenital quantitative fibrinogen deficiencies: An update and report of four novel mutations. *Thromb Res* 133:868, 2014.

44. Homer VM, Brennan SO, Ockelford P, George PM: Novel fibrinogen truncation with deletion of Bbeta chain residues 440–461 causes hypofibrinogenaemia. *Thromb Haemost* 88:427, 2002.

45. Neerman-Arbez M, Vu D, Abu-Libdeh B, et al: Prenatal diagnosis for congenital afibrinogenemia caused by a novel nonsense mutation in the FGB gene in a Palestinian family. *Blood* 101:3492, 2003.

46. Vu D, Di Sanza C, Caille D, et al: Quality control of fibrinogen secretion in the molecular pathogenesis of congenital afibrinogenemia. *Hum Mol Genet* 14:3271, 2005.

47. Duga S, Asselta R, Santagostino E, et al: Missense mutations in the human beta fibrinogen gene cause congenital afibrinogenemia by impairing fibrinogen secretion. *Blood* 95:1336, 2000.

48. Vu D, Bolton-Maggs PH, Parr JR, et al: Congenital afibrinogenemia: Identification and expression of a missense mutation in FGB impairing fibrinogen secretion. *Blood* 102:4413, 2003.

49. Spena S, Asselta R, Duga S, et al: Congenital afibrinogenemia: Intracellular retention of fibrinogen due to a novel W437G mutation in the fibrinogen Bbeta-chain gene. *Biochim Biophys Acta* 1639:87, 2003.

50. Monaldini L, Asselta R, Duga S, et al: Fibrinogen Mumbai: Intracellular retention due to a novel G434D mutation in the Bbeta-chain gene. *Haematologica* 91:628, 2006.

51. Terasawa F, Okumura N, Kitano K, et al: Hypofibrinogenemia associated with a heterozygous missense mutation gamma153Cys to Arg (Matsumoto IV): In vitro expression demonstrates defective secretion of the variant fibrinogen. *Blood* 94:4122, 1999.

52. Vu D, de Moerloose P, Batorova A, et al: Hypofibrinogenaemia caused by a novel FGG missense mutation (W253C) in the gamma chain globular domain impairing fibrinogen secretion. *J Med Genet* 42:e57, 2005.

53. Brennan SO, Wyatt J, Medicina D, et al: Fibrinogen Brescia: Hepatic endoplasmic reticulum storage and hypofibrinogenemia because of a gamma284 Gly→Arg mutation. *Am J Pathol* 157:189, 2000.

54. Brennan SO, Maghzal G, Shneider BL, et al: Novel fibrinogen gamma375 Arg→Trp mutation (fibrinogen Aguadilla) causes hepatic endoplasmic reticulum storage and hypofibrinogenemia. *Hepatology* 36:652, 2002.

55. Brennan SO, Davis RL, Conard K, et al: Novel fibrinogen mutation γ314Thr→Pro (fibrinogen AI duPont) associated with hepatic fibrinogen storage disease and hypofibrinogenaemia. *Liver Int* 30:1541, 2010.

56. Dib N, Quelin F, Ternisien C, et al: Fibrinogen Angers with a new deletion gamma GVYYQ 346–350 causes hypofibrinogenemia with hepatic storage. *J Thromb Haemost* 5:1999, 2007.

57. Peyvandi F, Kaufman RJ, Seligsohn U, et al: Rare bleeding disorders. *Haemophilia* 12(Suppl 3):137, 2006.

58. Van Meegeren ME, de Rooy JW, Schreuder HW, Brons PP: Bone cysts in patients with afibrinogenaemia: a literature review and two new cases. *Haemophilia* 20:244, 2014.

59. Iwaki T, Sandoval-Cooper MJ, Paiva M, et al: Fibrinogen stabilizes placental-maternal attachment during embryonic development in the mouse. *Am J Pathol* 160:1021, 2002.

60. Korte W, Feldges A: Increased prothrombin activation in a patient with congenital afibrinogenemia is reversible by fibrinogen substitution. *Clin Investig* 72:396, 1994.

61. Ni H, Denis CV, Subbarao S, et al: Persistence of platelet thrombus formation in arterioles of mice lacking both von Willebrand factor and fibrinogen. *J Clin Invest* 106:385, 2000.

62. Fish RJ, Di Sanza C, Neerman-Arbez M. Targeted mutation of zebrafish FGA models human congenital afibrinogenemia. *Blood* 123:2278, 2014.

63. Remjin JA, Wu Y-P, Ijsseldijk W, et al: Absence of fibrinogen in afibrinogenemia results in large but loosely packed thrombi under flow conditions. *Thromb Haemost* 85:736, 2001.

64. de Moerloose P, Neerman-Arbez M: Treatment of congenital fibrinogen disorders. *Expert Opin Biol Ther* 8:979, 2008.

65. Galanakis DK, Neerman-Arbez M, Scheiner T, et al: Homophenotypic A-alpha R16H fibrinogen (Kingsport): Uniquely altered polymerization associated with slower fibrinopeptide A than fibrinopeptide B release. *Blood Coagul Fibrinolysis* 18:731, 2007.

66. Neerman-Arbez M, Vu D, Abu-Libdeh B, et al: Prenatal diagnosis for congenital afibrinogenemia caused by a novel nonsense mutation in the FGB gene in a Palestinian family. *Blood* 101:3492, 2003.

67. Kalina U, Stöhr HA, Bickhard H, et al: Rotational thromboelastography for monitoring of fibrinogen concentrate therapy in fibrinogen deficiency. *Blood Coagul Fibrinolysis* 19:777, 2008.

68. Bolton-Maggs PH, Perry DJ, Chalmers EA, et al: The rare coagulation disorders—Review with guidelines for management from the United Haemophilia Centre Doctor's Organisation. *Haemophilia* 10:593, 2004.

69. Grech H, Majumdar G, Lawrie AS, Savidge GF: Pregnancy in congenital afibrinogenaemia: Report of a successful case and review of the literature. *Br J Haematol* 78:571, 1991.

70. Kobayashi T, Kanayama N, Tokunaga N, et al: Prenatal and peripartum management of congenital afibrinogenaemia. *Br J Haematol* 109:364, 2000.

71. Fuchs RJ, Levin J, Tadel M, Merritt W: Perioperative coagulation management in a patient with afibrinogenemia undergoing liver transplantation. *Liver Transpl* 13:752, 2007.

72. Stroka D, Keogh A, Vu D et al: In vitro rescue of FGA deletion by lentiviral transduction of afibrinogenemic patient's hepatocytes. *J Thromb Haemost* 12:1874, 2014.

73. Schuepbach RA, Meili EO, Schneider E, et al: Lepirudin therapy for thrombotic complications in congenital afibrinogenaemia. *Thromb Haemost* 91:1044, 2004.

74. Radulovic V, Baghaei F, Blixter IF, et al: Comparable effect of recombinant and plasma-derived human fibrinogen concentrate on ex vivo clot formation after cardiac surgery. *J Thromb Haemost* 10:1696, 2012.

75. Haverkate F, Samama M: Familial dysfibrinogenemia and thrombophilia. Report on a study of the SSC Subcommittee on Fibrinogen. *Thromb Haemost* 73:151, 1995.

76. Casini A, Blondon M, Lebreton A, et al: Natural history of patients with congenital dysfibrinogenemia. *Blood* 125:553, 2015.

77. Rosenberg JB, Newman PJ, Mosesson MW, et al: Paris I dysfibrinogenemia: A point mutation in intron 8 results in insertion of a 15 amino acid sequence in the fibrinogen gamma-chain. *Thromb Haemost* 69:217, 1993.

78. Hamano A, Mimuro J, Aoshima M, et al: Thrombophilic dysfibrinogen Tokyo V with the amino acid substitution of gammaAla327Thr: Formation of fragile but fibrinolysis-resistant fibrin clots and its relevance to arterial thromboembolism. *Blood* 103:3045, 2004.

79. Uemichi T, Liepnieks JJ, Benson MD: Hereditary renal amyloidosis with a novel variant fibrinogen. *J Clin Invest* 93:731, 1994.

80. Miesbach W, Scharrer I, Henschen A, et al: Inherited dysfibrinogenemia: Clinical phenotypes associated with five different fibrinogen structure defects. *Blood Coagul Fibrinolysis* 21:35–40, 2010.

81. Koopman J, Haverkate F, Briet E, Lord ST: A congenitally abnormal fibrinogen (Vlissingen) with a 6-base deletion in the gamma-chain gene, causing defective calcium binding and impaired fibrin polymerization. *J Biol Chem* 266:13456, 1991.

82. Casini A, De Maistre E, Casini-Stuppi V, et al: Fibrinogen Geneva II: A new congenitally abnormal fibrinogen alpha chain (Gly17Asp) with a review of similar mutations resulting in abnormal knob A. *Blood Coagul Fibrinolysis* 25:280, 2014.

83. Hirota-Kawadobora M, Terasawa F, Yonekawa O, et al: Fibrinogens Kosai and Ogasa: Bbeta15Gly→Cys (GGT→TGT) substitution associated with impairment of fibrinopeptide B release and lateral aggregation. *J Thromb Haemost* 1:275, 2003.

84. Siebenlist KR, Mosesson MW, Meh DA, et al: Coexisting dysfibrinogenemia (gammaR275C) and factor V Leiden deficiency associated with thromboembolic disease (fibrinogen Cedar Rapids). *Blood Coagul Fibrinolysis* 11:293, 2000.

85. Okumura N, Terasawa F, Hirota-Kawadobora M, et al: A novel variant fibrinogen, deletion of Bbeta111Ser in coiled-coil region, affecting fibrin lateral aggregation. *Clin Chim Acta* 365:160, 2006.

86. Lefebvre P, Velasco PT, Dear A, et al: Severe hypodysfibrinogenemia in compound heterozygotes of the fibrinogen AalphaIVS4 + 1G→T mutation and an AalphaGln328 truncation (fibrinogen Keokuk). *Blood* 103:2571, 2004.

87. Meyer M, Dietzel H, Kaetzel R, et al: Fibrinogen Leipzig II (gamma351Gly→Ser and gamma82Ala→Gly): Hypodysfibrinogenaemia due to two independent amino acid substitutions within the same polypeptide chain. *Thromb Haemost* 98:903, 2007.

88. Ridgway HJ, Brennan SO, Faed JM, George PM: Fibrinogen Otago: A major alpha chain truncation associated with severe hypofibrinogenaemia and recurrent miscarriage. *Br J Haematol* 98:632, 1997.

89. Koopman J, Haverkate F, Grimbergen J, et al: Fibrinogen Marburg: A homozygous case of dysfibrinogenemia, lacking amino acids A alpha 461–610 (Lys 461 AAA→stop TAA). *Blood* 80:1972, 1992.

90. Ding Q, Ouyang Q, Xi X, et al: Maternal chromosome 4 heterodisomy/isodisomy and Bβ chain Trp323X mutation resulting in severe hypodysfibrinogenaemia. *Thromb Haemost* 108:654, 2012.

91. Hayes T: Dysfibrinogenemia and thrombosis. *Arch Pathol Lab Med* 126:1387, 2002.

92. Uemichi T, Liepnieks JJ, Benson MD: Hereditary renal amyloidosis with a novel variant fibrinogen. *J Clin Invest* 93:731, 1994.

93. Shapiro SE, Phillips E, Manning RA, et al: Clinical phenotype, laboratory features and genotype of 35 patients with heritable dysfibrinogenaemia. *Br J Haematol* 160:220, 2013.

94. Miesbach W, Schenk J, Alesci S, Lindhoff-Last E: Comparison of the fibrinogen Clauss assay and the fibrinogen PT derived method in patients with dysfibrinogenemia. *Thromb Res* 126:e428, 2010.

95. Galanakis DK, Neerman-Arbez M, Brennan S, et al: Thromboelastographic phenotypes of fibrinogen and its variants: Clinical and non-clinical implications. *Thromb Res* 133:1115, 2014.

96. Marchi R, Meyer M, de Bosch N, et al: Biophysical characterization of fibrinogen Caracas I with an Aalpha-chain truncation at Aalpha-466 Ser: Identification of the mutation and biophysical characterization of properties of clots from plasma and purified fibrinogen. *Blood Coagul Fibrinolysis* 15:285, 2004.

97. Marchi RC, Meyer MH, de Bosch NB, et al: A novel mutation (deletion of Aalpha-Asn 80) in an abnormal fibrinogen: Fibrinogen Caracas VI. Consequences of disruption of the coiled-coil for the polymerization of fibrin: Peculiar clot structure and diminished stiffness of the clot. *Blood Coagul Fibrinolysis* 15:559, 2004.

CHAPTER 126
VON WILLEBRAND DISEASE

Jill Johnsen and David Ginsburg

SUMMARY

von Willebrand factor (VWF) is a central component of hemostasis, serving both as an adhesive link between platelets and the injured blood vessel wall and as a carrier for clotting factor VIII (FVIII). Abnormalities in VWF function result in von Willebrand disease (VWD), the most common inherited bleeding disorder in humans. The overall prevalence of VWD has been estimated to be as high as 1 percent of the general population, although the prevalence of clinically significant disease is probably closer to 1:1000. VWD is associated with either quantitative deficiency (type 1 and type 3) or qualitative abnormalities of VWF (type 2). The uncommon type 3 variant is the most severe form of VWD and is characterized by very low or undetectable levels of VWF, a severe bleeding diathesis, and a generally autosomal recessive pattern of inheritance. Type 1 VWD, the most common variant, is characterized by VWF that is normal in structure and function but decreased in quantity (in the range of 20 to 50 percent of normal). In type 2 VWD, the VWF is abnormal in structure and/or function. Type 2A VWD is associated with selective loss of the largest and most functionally active VWF multimers. Type 2A is further subdivided into group 1, as a result of mutations that interfere with biosynthesis and secretion, and group 2, in which the mutant VWF exhibits an increased sensitivity to proteolysis in plasma. Type 2B VWD is caused by mutations clustered within the VWF A1 domain, in a segment critical for binding to the platelet glycoprotein Ib receptor. These mutations produce a "gain of function" resulting in spontaneous VWF binding to platelets and clearance of the resulting platelet complexes, leading to thrombocytopenia and loss of the most active (large) VWF multimers. Type 2N VWD is characterized by mutations within the FVIII binding domain of VWF, leading to disproportionately decreased factor VIII and a disorder resembling mild to moderate hemophilia A, but with autosomal rather than X-linked inheritance. Type 1 VWD can often be effectively managed by treatment with DDAVP (1-deamino-8-D-arginine vasopressin, desmopressin), which produces a two- to threefold increase in plasma VWF level due to release from endothelial storage sites in the vessel wall. Response to DDAVP is generally poor in type 3 and some type 2 VWD variants. These disorders often require treatment with factor replacement in the form of VWF/FVIII concentrates containing large quantities of intact VWF multimers.

Acronyms and Abbreviations: ADAMTS13, a disintegrin and metalloprotease with thrombospondin type 1 motifs; aPTT, activated partial thromboplastin time; DDAVP, 1-desamino-8-D-arginine vasopressin or desmopressin; ER, endoplasmic reticulum; GP, glycoprotein; HHT, hereditary hemorrhagic telangiectasia; PCR, polymerase chain reaction; RIPA, ristocetin-induced platelet aggregation; VWD, von Willebrand disease; VWF, von Willebrand factor.

● DEFINITION AND HISTORY

In 1926, Eric von Willebrand described a bleeding disorder in 24 of 66 members of a family from the Åland Islands.[1] Both sexes were afflicted, and the bleeding time was prolonged despite normal platelet counts and normal clot retraction. von Willebrand distinguished this condition from the other hemostatic diseases known at the time and recognized its genetic basis, calling the disorder "hereditary pseudohemophilia," but incorrectly characterizing the inheritance as X-linked dominant. von Willebrand's confusion about the inheritance pattern was probably the result of, at least in part, the greater recognition of bleeding symptoms in women because of the hemostatic stresses of menstruation and parturition. The proband in the original family, Hjördis, was 5 years old at the time of von Willebrand's initial evaluation and ultimately died at age 13 years during her fourth menstrual cycle. Four of Hjördis' sisters died between the ages of 2 and 4 years, and deaths in the family were also noted during childbirth.

An apparently similar disorder was independently reported in the United States by Minot and others in 1928. The original family in the Åland Islands was reexamined by von Willebrand and Jürgens in 1933, leading to the conclusion that the defect in this disorder was caused by an impairment of platelet function. It was not until 1953 that Alexander and Goldstein demonstrated reduced levels of coagulation factor VIII (FVIII) in von Willebrand disease (VWD) patients, along with prolonged bleeding time. This observation was confirmed by others, including studies of the original von Willebrand pedigree by Nilsson and coworkers. In the late 1950s, Nilsson and coworkers demonstrated that a fraction of plasma referred to as "I-0" could correct the FVIII deficiency and normalize the bleeding time, indicating that the defect in VWD was a result of the deficiency of a plasma factor rather than an intrinsic platelet abnormality. Infusion of fraction I-0 promptly increased the FVIII level in a hemophilic patient, while in VWD the FVIII level rose gradually, peaking at 5 to 8 hours. Fraction I-0 prepared from a hemophilia A patient was also shown to correct the defect in VWD, demonstrating that these disorders were caused by deficiencies of distinct plasma factors (reviewed in Refs. 2 and 3).

It was not until 1971 that Zimmerman, Ratnoff, and Powell prepared the first antibodies against what was thought to be a highly purified form of FVIII.[4] This FVIII-related antigen was found to be normal in hemophilia A patients but decreased in VWD. This puzzle was finally resolved with the demonstration that von Willebrand factor (VWF) and FVIII are closely associated, with more than 98 percent of the mass of the complex made up of VWF (see section The Function of von Willebrand Factor below). Thus, antibodies raised against this complex predominantly recognize VWF. The first direct assay of VWF function was based on the observation that the antibiotic ristocetin induced thrombocytopenia and the demonstration by Howard and Firkin[5] that ristocetin-induced platelet aggregation (RIPA) was absent in some VWD patients. Weiss and coworkers[6] used this observation to develop a quantitative assay for VWF function that remains a mainstay of laboratory evaluation for VWD to this day. In 1973, several groups succeeded in dissociating VWF from FVIII procoagulant activity.[7,8]

Final proof that VWF and FVIII are independent proteins encoded by distinct genes came with the complementary DNA (cDNA) cloning of the two molecules in 1984 and 1985.[9-14] These discoveries also marked the beginning of the molecular genetic era for the study of VWF and FVIII, leading to the identification of gene mutations in many patients with hemophilia and VWD, as well as considerable insight into the structure and function of these related proteins.

Table 126–1 summarizes the current nomenclature and terminology for FVIII and VWF. VWD is a heterogeneous disorder with more

TABLE 126–1. von Willebrand Factor and Factor VIII Terminology

Factor VIII

Antihemophilic factor, the protein that is reduced in plasma of patients with classic hemophilia A and most von Willebrand disease (VWD) and is measured in standard coagulation assays

Factor VIII activity (factor VIII:C)

The coagulant property of the factor VIII protein (this term is sometimes used interchangeably with factor VIII)

Factor VIII antigen (VIII:Ag)

The antigenic determinant(s) on factor VIII measured by immunoassays, which may employ polyclonal or monoclonal antibodies

von Willebrand factor (VWF)

The large multimeric glycoprotein that is necessary for normal platelet adhesion, a normal bleeding time, and stabilizing factor VIII

von Willebrand factor antigen (VWF:Ag)

The antigenic determinant(s) on VWF measured by immunoassays, which may employ polyclonal or monoclonal antibodies; *inaccurate designations of historical interest only* include factor VIII-related antigen (VIIIR:Ag), factor VIII antigen, AHF antigen, and AHF-like antigen

Ristocetin cofactor activity (VWF:RCo)

The property of VWF that supports ristocetin-induced agglutination of washed or fixed normal platelets

von Willebrand factor collagen-binding activity (VWF:CB)

The property of VWF that supports binding to collagen, measured by enzyme-linked immunosorbent assay (ELISA)

than 20 variants described. The previous complex and confusing classification has been consolidated and simplified into six distinct types,[15] as summarized in Table 126–2. Type 3 VWD is associated with very low or undetectable levels of VWF and severe bleeding. Type 1 VWD is characterized by concordant reductions in FVIII activity, VWF antigen, and ristocetin cofactor activity, generally to the range of 20 to 30 percent of normal, but sometimes up to 50 percent of normal, in association with a normal VWF multimer distribution. Type 2 VWD is heterogeneous and further divided into four subtypes (2A, 2B, 2M, and 2N) by the nature of the VWF qualitative dysfunction. Type 2A VWD results from abnormal VWF secretion or proteolysis and is characterized by a disproportionately low level of ristocetin cofactor activity relative to VWF antigen and absence of large and intermediate-sized multimers. Type 2B VWD results from an abnormal VWF molecule with increased affinity for platelet glycoprotein Ib (GPIb), and can also be associated with reduced high-molecular-weight VWF multimers and thrombocytopenia. Functional abnormalities in VWF can also result in defective interactions with platelets, as in type 2M VWD, or decreased FVIII binding to VWF, designated type 2N VWD and characterized by mild to moderate FVIII deficiency. Many other subtypes have been reported, including platelet-type (pseudo-) VWD, which is actually an intrinsic platelet disorder caused by mutations in GPIb (Chap. 120). Finally, acquired forms of VWD also occur, such as in patients with antibodies to VWF or thrombocytosis secondary to myeloproliferative neoplasms, resulting in accelerated loss of circulating VWF.

ETIOLOGY AND PATHOGENESIS

VWF is synthesized exclusively in endothelial cells and megakaryocytes. The VWF monomer is assembled into higher-order multimers, a structure required for optimal adhesive function, and performs two major functions in hemostasis. First, VWF serves as the initial critical bridge between circulating platelets and the injured blood vessel wall, accounting for the apparent defect in platelet function and prolonged bleeding times historically observed in VWD patients. Second, VWF serves as the carrier in plasma for FVIII, ensuring its stability and localizing it to the initial platelet plug for participation in thrombin generation and fibrin clot formation (Chap. 113). This tight, noncovalent interaction between VWF and FVIII accounts for the copurification of these two molecules and the resulting initial confusion as to the origin of hemophilia and VWD. FVIII is encoded by the *F8* gene on the X chromosome (Chaps. 113 and 123), while VWF is encoded by the *VWF* gene on human chromosome 12.

THE VON WILLEBRAND FACTOR GENE AND COMPLEMENTARY DNA

The VWF cDNA was initially cloned from endothelial cells,[11–14] and the corresponding gene mapped to the short arm of chromosome 12 (12p13.3).[11] The VWF mRNA is approximately 9 kb in length, encoding a primary translation product of 2813 amino acid residues with an estimated Mr of 310,000. Comparison of the primary peptide sequence obtained from plasma VWF[16] with the VWF cDNA sequence established the prepropolypeptide nature of VWF.[17] Prepropolypeptide VWF is composed of a 22-amino-acid signal peptide, a 741-amino-acid precursor polypeptide known as the VWF propeptide (VWFpp), and the mature subunit.[11,17–20] Cleavage of the 741-amino-acid propeptide from the amino terminus produces the mature VWF monomer subunit of 2050 amino acids (Fig. 126–1).

Analysis of the VWF sequence identifies four distinct types of repeated domains: three A domains, three B domains, two C domains, and four D domains,[18,21] within which appear additional repeating motifs (schematic in Ref. 22). The first pair of D domains is tandemly arranged in the VWFpp, followed by a partial and full D domain at the N terminus of the mature subunit. The final complete D domain is separated by a segment of more than 600 amino acids containing the triplicated A domains. The repeated domain structure of VWF suggests that the gene may have evolved via a complex series of partial duplications, although exon structure is not highly conserved between homologous domains.

Comparison of the VWF amino acid sequence to other proteins identifies a superfamily of related proteins that share sequence similarity with the VWF A domains.[23] The common theme among these potentially evolutionarily related genes is a role in extracellular matrix or adhesive function. Consistent with this notion, VWF functional domains for binding to the platelet receptor GPIb and specific ligands within the extracellular matrix have been localized to the VWF A repeats. A potential relationship between the VWF C domains and portions of thrombospondin and procollagen has also been proposed.[24]

The *VWF* gene spans 178 kb and is divided into 52 exons.[25] Exons range in size from 40 bases to 1.4 kb (exon 28). Exon 28 is unusually large, encoding the entire A1 and A2 domains and containing most of the known type 2A and all of the type 2B VWD mutations. The concentration of these defects within one exon has facilitated the identification of human mutations responsible for these VWD variants (see "Molecular Genetics of von Willebrand Disease," below). A partial, nonfunctional duplication of the *VWF* gene, termed a pseudogene, is located on human chromosome 22.[26] The pseudogene, known as *VWFP1*, duplicates the

TABLE 126-2. Classification of von Willebrand Disease

Type	Molecular Characteristics	Inheritance	Frequency	Factor VIII Activity	VWF Antigen	Ristocetin Cofactor Activity	RIPA	Plasma VWF Multimer Structure
Type 1	Partial quantitative VWF deficiency	Autosomal dominant, incomplete penetrance	1–30:1000; most common VWD variant (>70% of VWD)	Decreased	Decreased	Decreased	Decreased or normal	Normal distribution (mutant subunits permitted)
Type 3	Severe quantitative reduction or absence of VWF	Autosomal recessive (or codominant)	1–5:1,000,000	Markedly decreased	Very low or absent	Very low or absent	Absent	Usually absent
Type 2A	Qualitative VWF defect; loss of large VWF multimers, decreased VWF-dependent platelet adhesion	Usually autosomal dominant	~10–15% of clinically significant VWD	Decreased to normal	Usually low	Markedly decreased	Decreased	Largest and intermediate multimers absent
Type 2B	Qualitative VWF defect; increased VWF–platelet interaction (GPIb)	Autosomal dominant	Uncommon variant (<5% of clinical VWD)	Decreased to normal	Usually low	Decreased to normal	Increased to low concentrations of ristocetin	Largest multimers reduced/absent
Type 2M	Qualitative VWF defect; decreased VWF-platelet interaction, no loss of large VWF multimers	Usually autosomal dominant	Rare (case reports)	Variably decreased	Variably decreased	Decreased	Variably decreased	Normal and occasionally ultralarge forms
Type 2N	Qualitative VWF defect; decreased VWF-factor VIII binding capacity	Autosomal recessive	Uncommon; heterozygotes may be prevalent in some populations	Decreased	Normal	Normal	Normal	Normal
Platelet-type (pseudo-)	Platelet defect; decreased platelet-VWF interactions	Autosomal dominant	Rare	Decreased to normal	Decreased to normal	Decreased	Increased to low concentrations of ristocetin	Largest multimers absent

GPIb, glycoprotein Ib; RIPA, ristocetin-induced platelet aggregation; VWD, von Willebrand disease; VWF, von Willebrand factor.

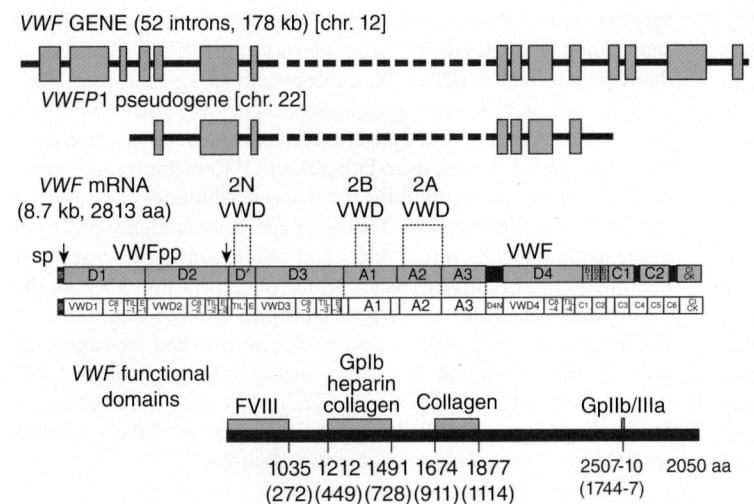

VWF GENE (52 introns, 178 kb) [chr. 12]

VWFP1 pseudogene [chr. 22]

VWF mRNA (8.7 kb, 2813 aa)

VWF functional domains

Figure 126–1. Schematic of the human *VWF* gene, mRNA, and protein. The *VWF* gene and *VWFP1* pseudogene are depicted at the top, with boxes representing exons and the solid black line representing introns. Schematics of the VWF mRNA encoding the full prepro-VWF subunit are depicted in the middle as bar and lettered boxes. The upper schematic denotes commonly annotated regions of internally repeated sequences; the lower schematic illustrates the multiple repeating motifs of VWF. The locations of signal peptide (sp) and VWF propeptide (VWFpp) cleavage sites are indicated by *arrowheads*. The approximate localizations for known VWF functional domains within the mature VWF subunit are indicated at the bottom. Numbers underneath the domains refer to amino acid residues numbered from the ATG start site; numbers in parentheses indicate the amino acid residue position in the mature VWF subunit. aa, Amino acids; chr, chromosome. *(Adapted with permission from Ginsburg D, Bowie EJW. Molecular genetics of von Willebrand disease. Blood 79(10):2507–2519, 1992.)*

middle portion of the *VWF* structural gene, spanning exons 23 to 34 and the intervening noncoding sequences. *VWFP1* is approximately 97 percent identical in sequence to the authentic *VWF* gene, indicating that it is of fairly recent evolutionary origin.[27] Gene conversion involving the *VWFP1* pseudogene, possibly through recombination with the large homologous exon 28 sequence, has been proposed as a mechanism for introducing mutations into the *VWF* gene.[28–31]

VWF is synthesized exclusively in megakaryocytes and endothelial cells and, as a result, has frequently been used as a specific histochemical marker to identify cells of endothelial cell origin. Although generally assumed to mark all endothelial cells, VWF is expressed at widely varying levels among endothelial cells, depending on the size and location of the associated blood vessel.[32,33] A careful survey in the mouse identified wide differences in the level of VWF mRNA, with 5 to 50 times higher concentrations in the lung and brain, particularly in small vessels, than in comparable vessels in the liver and kidney. In general, the higher levels of VWF mRNA and antigen were found in the endothelial cells of large vessels rather than in microvasculature, and in venous rather than arterial endothelial cells.[33]

Specific DNA sequences within or near the proximal promoter of the *VWF* gene appear to be required for endothelial-specific gene expression,[34–39] although it is likely that additional important regulatory elements exist outside of this region, some of which may lie at a great distance.[40] VWF is expressed in most, but not all, endothelial cells,[41] and this vascular-bed specific gene expression program is likely a result of the concerted action of multiple regulatory elements. Endothelial *VWF* gene expression also appears to be upregulated by exposure to shear stress. The length of a polymorphic GT repeat in the proximal *VWF* promoter correlates with the magnitude of this response, and several other more distal DNA sequences are predicted to be involved in a shear stress response.[42] However, this GT repeat does not appear to influence circulating VWF levels.[43]

VON WILLEBRAND FACTOR BIOSYNTHESIS

The processing steps involved in the biosynthesis of VWF are similar in megakaryocytes and endothelial cells (reviewed in Refs. 46 and 47). VWF is first synthesized as a large precursor monomer polypeptide, depicted schematically in Fig. 126–1. VWF is unusually rich in cysteine, which accounts for 8.3 percent of its amino acid content. All cysteines in the mature VWF molecule are thought to be involved in disulfide bonds,[48] although these bonds may be exposed in circulating mature VWF by shear stress.[49] Pro-VWF monomers are assembled into dimers through disulfide bonds at both C termini, and only dimers are exported from the endoplasmic reticulum (ER).[48,50,51]

Glycosylation begins in the ER, with 12 potential *N*-linked glycosylation sites present on the mature subunit and three on the propeptide. Extensive additional posttranslational modification of VWF occurs in the Golgi apparatus, including the addition of multiple *O*-linked carbohydrate structures, sulfation, and multimerization through the formation of disulfide bonds at the N termini of adjacent dimers. It is unusual for a protein to undergo extensive disulfide bond formation at this late stage, and this process appears to be catalyzed by disulfide isomerase activity present within the VWFpp.[52] Mutations at either of two specific cysteines within the propeptide that are thought to be critical for disulfide isomerase activity, or a shift in the spacing between them, results in loss of multimer formation.[52] An intermediate species with disulfide bonds between the propeptide and VWF D'D3 domain appears briefly in either the late ER or early Golgi,[53] which may position these domains for subsequent multimerization. The multimerization process appears to require the slightly acidic environment of the distal Golgi.[54] The VWFpp self-associates and may also serve to align VWF

subunits for multimer assembly.[55] However, the propeptide facilitates multimer assembly even when coexpressed as a separate molecule from the mature VWF monomer.[56,57]

Propeptide cleavage occurs late in VWF synthesis or just prior to secretion. Cleavage occurs adjacent to two basic amino acids, Lys-Arg at positions –2 and –1. An Arg at position –4 is also required for recognition by the intracellular protease responsible for propeptide cleavage.[58] Multimerization and propeptide cleavage are not linked to each other. The multimers secreted by cultured endothelial cells contain both pro-VWF and mature subunits,[59,60] and recombinant VWF with a point mutation inhibiting propeptide cleavage is still assembled into normal multimer structures.[61] Although propeptide cleavage appears to occur primarily intracellularly, cleavage may also occur after secretion.

VWF is stored in tubular structures within the α-granules of platelets and within the Weibel-Palade bodies in endothelial cells[62,63] (reviewed in Ref. 64). These large VWF structures form by tubular packing of the VWF N-terminal domains within the secretory granules.[65] Weibel-Palade bodies are derived from the Golgi apparatus and are found in most endothelial cells, although the number varies considerably between endothelial cell beds. It has been shown that VWF and FVIII colocalize in storage granules. Although VWF is not required to traffic FVIII to platelets,[66] VWF appears to play a role in trafficking FVIII to Weibel-Palade bodies in endothelial cells.[67,68] Weibel-Palade bodies mature as they move to the periphery of the cell in an ordered process dependent on Rab proteins and Rab effector proteins, which act as chaperones and organizers of the various stages of Weibel-Palade body maturity and subsequent exocytosis (reviewed in Ref. 69). The transmembrane glycoprotein P-selectin is also found in the membranes of both the α-granule and the Weibel-Palade body.[70] The VWF D'D3 domain has been shown *in vitro* to associate with P-selectin and to be necessary for the recruitment of P-selectin to Weibel-Palade bodies.[71] There appears to be heterogeneity within Weibel-Palade body populations both in relative content of VWF and P-selectin and in response to regulated secretion by different stimuli.[72] In addition to VWF and P-selectin, the Weibel-Palade body also contains tissue-type plasminogen activator (t-PA), a thrombolytic secreted protein that also may be released distinctly from VWF,[73] and several other proteins that are known to participate in inflammation or angiogenesis (for a complete list of Weibel-Palade contents see Ref. 74).

VWF is secreted from endothelial cells continuously via constitutive and constitutive-like (or basal) pathways and upon stimulated release of storage granules via a classic regulated pathway.[46,75] Regulated secretion of VWF from its storage site in the Weibel-Palade body is triggered by a number of secretagogues, including thrombin,[76] fibrin,[77] histamine,[78] the C5b-9 complement complex,[79] and several inflammatory cytokines.[80] Recent *in vitro* data suggests that there may also be suppression of regulated VWF secretion by statins.[81,82] The secretagogue desmopressin acetate (DDAVP), a vasopressin analogue, is used clinically for its capacity to cause a marked release of VWF and FVIII *in vivo* by acting through type 2 vasopressin receptors to induce secretion from the Weibel-Palade bodies in endothelial cells.[83] Constitutive-like secretion of VWF occurs evenly at the luminal and abluminal surface, while regulated secretion from the Weibel-Palade body is highly polarized in the luminal direction (Fig. 126–2).[75,84] While constitutively secreted multimers are of relatively small size, the multimers stored within the Weibel-Palade body are the largest, most biologically potent form.[85,86] The VWF stored in platelet α-granules is also enriched for large multimers.[87] The N-terminal D domains appear to be required for VWF storage, with deletion of any of the individual domains resulting in constitutive secretion.[88,89] It also appears that cleavage of the VWFpp is required for efficient formation of storage granules.[90]

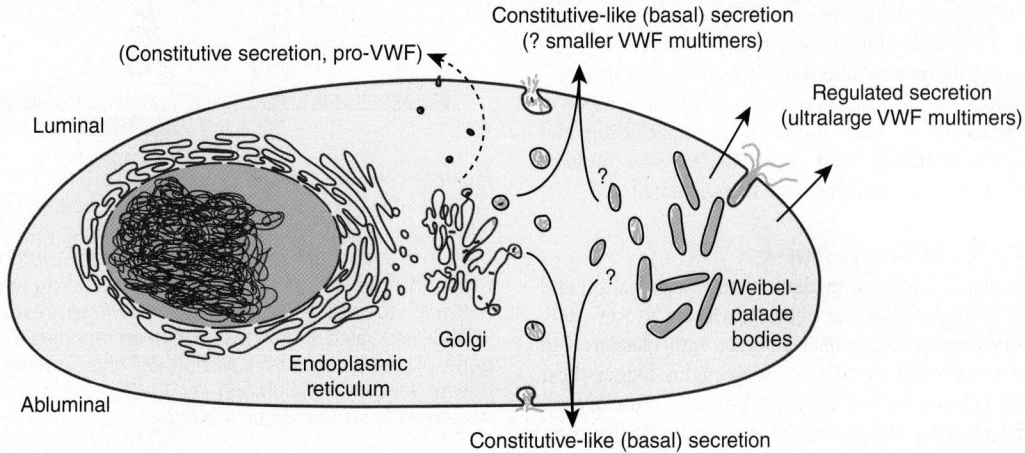

Figure 126–2. Schematic of von Willebrand factor (VWF) processing and secretion from endothelial cells. VWF dimers are formed in the endoplasmic reticulum, where VWF begins to be glycosylated. VWF dimers are transported to the Golgi, where the VWF undergoes further glycosylation and sulfation. Multimerization begins in the Golgi and continues within the secretory granules (Weibel-Palade bodies). A small amount of immature VWF is released constitutively (i.e., without regulation or storage) from endothelial cells as dimers or very small multimers. VWF is also released continuously from both the luminal and abluminal endothelial cell surfaces by constitutive-like (or basal) secretion. This VWF has been processed in the Golgi and may be transiently stored in an intermediate secretory granule or Weibel-Palade bodies. Mature VWF is packaged and stored as ultralarge multimers in Weibel-Palade bodies. This ultralarge VWF is released from the luminal surface of stimulated endothelial cells by regulated secretion. Once in circulation, VWF multimers undergo proteolysis by ADAMTS13 (a disintegrin and metalloprotease with a thrombospondin type 1 motif member 13) under moderate to high shear conditions. *(Adapted with permission from Johnsen J, Lopez JA. VWF secretion: What's in a name? Blood 112(4):926–927, 2008.)*

The concentration of VWF in plasma is approximately 10 mcg/mL, with approximately 15 percent of circulating VWF localized to the platelet compartment.[91] Marrow transplants between normal and VWD pigs demonstrate that platelet VWF is derived entirely from synthesis within marrow megakaryocytes and does not contribute to the normal plasma VWF pool.[92-94] These studies also demonstrate that both the plasma and the platelet VWF pools are required for full hemostasis, although the plasma pool appears to be more critical.

Plasma VWF is further processed in the circulation through cleavage by a specific protease, ADAMTS13 (*a d*isintegrin *a*nd *m*etalloprotease with *t*hrombospondin type 1 motifs–13), resulting in reduction in the size of the largest multimers (reviewed in Ref. 95). After regulated secretion *in vitro*, ultralarge VWF multimers may anchor to the endothelial cell surface via P-selectin[96,97] resulting in shear stress and VWF cleavage by ADAMTS13. The major proteolytic cleavage site maps to the peptide bond between Tyr1605 and Met1606 in the VWF A2 domain,[98] and recombinant VWF missing the A2 domain is resistant to proteolysis.[99] VWF carrying a subgroup of type 2A VWD mutations exhibits increased susceptibility to cleavage by this protease,[100] and this is the proposed mechanism for the selective loss of large VWF multimers in this group of patients (see "Molecular Genetics of von Willebrand Disease," below). Increased VWF susceptibility to proteolysis by ADAMTS13 has also been described in a subset of type 1 VWD patients, but the clinical significance of this is unclear as increased proteolysis appears to only occur under certain conditions.[101] Decreased ADAMTS13 activity, either because of congenital deficiency or acquired inhibitors, plays a central role in the pathophysiology of thrombotic thrombocytopenic purpura (Chap. 132).

THE FUNCTION OF VON WILLEBRAND FACTOR

VWF is a large multivalent adhesive protein that plays an important role in platelet attachment to subendothelial surfaces, platelet aggregation at sites of vessel injury, and stabilization of coagulation FVIII in the circulation. Not only is the interaction of VWF and FVIII important for

the protection of FVIII from inactivation or degradation, FVIII bound to VWF may localize to cells and/or sites where it can more readily participate in the promotion of blood coagulation and/or thrombus formation.

VWF is required for the adhesion of platelets to the subendothelium, particularly at moderate to high shear force. VWF performs this bridging function by binding to two platelet receptors, GPIb and GPIIb/IIIa, as well as to specific ligands within the exposed subendothelium at sites of vascular injury (reviewed in Ref. 103). Binding of VWF to its platelet receptors generally does not occur in the circulation under normal conditions. However, the interaction of VWF with exposed ligands in the vessel wall, combined with high shear stress conditions, facilitates VWF binding to platelet GPIb and subsequent platelet adhesion and activation. Activation of platelets leads to the exposure of the GPIIb/IIIa complex, an integrin receptor that can bind to fibrinogen, VWF, and other ligands, to form the platelet–platelet bridges required for thrombus propagation. Platelet adhesion to VWF immobilized at a site of injury appears to be a two-step process, with the initial tethering of the rapidly moving platelet dependent on the VWF–GPIb interaction and subsequent firm adhesion occurring through GPIIb/IIIa after platelet activation.[104] VWF may also play a role in inflammation by directly interacting with leukocytes,[105] but the clinical significance of this observation is not clear.

Von Willebrand Factor Binding to the Vessel Wall

VWF binds to the vessel wall at sites of vascular endothelial injury (reviewed in Ref. 106). VWF binds to several different types of collagens, including types I through VI. Distinct binding domains for the fibrillar collagens, types I and III, have been localized to specific segments within the VWF A1 and A3 repeats (see Fig. 126–1),[107,108] and a potential third domain has been identified in the VWFpp.[109] Studies of recombinant VWF suggest that the A3 collagen-binding domain may be the most important.[110,111] VWF has also been shown to bind to the nonfibrillar collagen type VI, which is resistant to collagenase[112] and colocalizes with VWF in the subendothelium.[113] Type VI collagen supports the binding of VWF under high shear through cooperative interactions between binding domains within the VWF A1 and A3 repeat.[114] Although VWF binding has also been demonstrated to a number of other potential components of the subendothelium, including glycosaminoglycans,[115,116] sulfatides,[117] and VWF itself,[118] the biologic significance of these interactions remains to be demonstrated.

Von Willebrand Factor Binding to Platelets

VWF interacts with platelets both to mediate platelet aggregation and platelet localization to sites of vascular injury (reviewed in Ref. 106). Circulating VWF does not spontaneously interact with platelets, but once bound to an injured vessel wall VWF is subjected to higher shear stresses and a platelet-binding site in the VWF A1 domain is uncovered. VWF interacts with a receptor complex on the surface of platelets composed of the disulfide-linked GPIbα and GPIbβ chains noncovalently associated with GPIX and GPV. The binding site for VWF is within a 293-amino-acid segment at the N-terminus of GPIb and requires sulfation of several key tyrosine residues for optimal binding.[119] The GPIb binding domain within VWF lies within the A1 segment, within the disulfide loop formed between the cysteine residues at 1272 (amino acid 509 in mature VWF) and 1458 (695) (see Fig. 126–1).[120,121] GPIb binding to the A1 domain enhances proteolysis of recombinant VWF fragments by ADAMTS13 and suggests a feedback mechanism for limiting thrombus propagation *in vivo*.[122] Scanning mutagenesis studies of recombinant VWF characterized a number of amino acid residues within the VWF A1 domain that are critical for binding to GPIb and for interaction with botrocetin.[123] Several mutations were also identified that increase platelet binding, an effect similar to that of mutations associated with type 2B VWD (see "Molecular Genetics of von Willebrand Disease," below). These natural and synthetic mutations cluster in a small area on the surface of the VWF A1 domain structure, as revealed by x-ray crystallographic studies.[124] The complexity of the VWF A1–GPIb interaction is evidenced by the ability of gain-of-function and loss-of-function VWF A1 mutants to counterbalance each other in mice.[125] The structure of the A1 domain closely resembles that of other previously studied A domains, including the VWF A3 domain.[126-128] The structure of GPIb in complex with the VWF A1 domain provides insight into the structural basis for the gain of function mutations associated with type 2B VWD.[129] The abundant plasma protein β$_2$-glycoprotein I can bind the VWF A1 domain when VWF is structurally open to GPIbα binding. This may result in biologically relevant inhibition of the VWF-platelet interaction, as inhibitory anti–β$_2$-glycoprotein I autoantibodies found in some patients with antiphospholipid antibody syndrome are associated with thrombosis.[130]

Ristocetin binds to both VWF and platelets, but the mechanism by which it enhances the VWF/GPIb interaction is still poorly understood.[131,132] The snake venom botrocetin appears to induce GPIb binding through a different alteration in the VWF A1 domain and is also used to study this interaction.[128] Heparin binds the VWF A1 domain within the loop formed by the disulfide bond formed between the residues Cys1272 and Cys1458,[133] where it appears to competitively inhibit VWF binding to GPIb[134,135] and enhance VWF proteolysis by ADAMTS13 *in vitro*.[136] Although it has been suggested that this may account for hemorrhage not predicted by conventional heparin monitoring, the clinical significance of the VWF-heparin interaction is not clear.

The arg-gly-asp-ser (RGDS) sequence at amino acids 2507 to 2510 of the mature VWF subunit serves as the binding site within VWF for GPIIb/IIIa. The GPIIb/IIIa complex, also known as integrin α$_{IIb}$β$_3$, is a member of the integrin family of cell surface receptors. GPIIb/IIIa undergoes a conformational change to a high-affinity ligand-binding

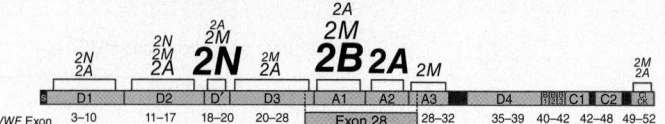

Figure 126–3. von Willebrand disease (VWD) mutations. The von Willebrand factor domain locations of all reported mutations associated with type 2A, 2B, 2M, and 2N VWD. Lettering size represents the proportion of total mutations reported within the designated VWF domain for that subtype, with larger letters indicating more mutations. Shown below are the relative positions of the VWF gene exons. Type 1 and type 3 VWD associated mutations have been reported throughout the *VWF* gene. *(Mutation data from Nichols WC and Ginsburg D: von Willebrand disease.* Medicine (Baltimore) *76(1):1–20, 1997 and the VWD mutation database at www.vwf.group.shef.ac.uk.)*

state following platelet activation which, in addition to VWF, can bind a number of other adhesive proteins, including fibrinogen. Although VWF is present in blood at much lower concentrations than is fibrinogen, evidence suggests that VWF may be a critical ligand. VWF participates in platelet tethering and adhesion to fibrin under flow conditions,[104,137] where the C1C2 domains of VWF are required for fibrin binding.[138] An RGD sequence is also present in the VWFpp, although its functional significance is unknown.

The Interaction of von Willebrand Factor with Factor VIII

The noncovalent interaction between FVIII and VWF is required for the stability of FVIII in the circulation, as is evident from the FVIII levels of less than 10 percent that are observed in most severe VWD patients. Although each VWF subunit appears to carry a binding site for FVIII, the stoichiometry for the VWF–FVIII complex found in normal plasma is approximately one to two FVIII molecules per 100 VWF monomers.[139] FVIII bound to VWF is also protected from proteolytic degradation by activated protein C (reviewed in Ref. 140). FVIII also appears to increase the susceptibility of VWF to proteolysis by ADAMTS13 under shear conditions.[141]

The FVIII binding domain within VWF has been localized to the first 272 N-terminal amino acids of the mature subunit.[142] In mice, expression of the VWF D'-D3 domains alone has been shown to be sufficient to stabilize FVIII levels.[143] Antibody studies suggest a particularly critical role for amino acids 841 to 859.[144,145] The mutations identified in patients with type 2N VWD, in which VWF binding to FVIII is specifically affected (see "Molecular Genetics of von Willebrand Disease," below), are all clustered in this region, including the most common type 2N mutation Arg854Gln.[146] The corresponding binding site for VWF on FVIII includes an acidic region at the N-terminus of the light chain (residues 1669 to 1689)[147] and requires sulfation of Tyr1680 for optimal binding.[148] Overlay of VWD 2N mutations with the crystal structure of the VWF A1–FVIII domains shows the 2N mutations clustered in a dynamic VWF TIL' domain (shown in Fig. 126–3), implicating a need for flexibility in this domain for normal FVIII binding.[149] Thrombin cleavage after Arg1689 in FVIII activates and releases FVIII from VWF. Thus, VWF may serve to efficiently deliver FVIII to the sites of clot formation, where it can complex with factor IXa on the platelet surface.

MOLECULAR GENETICS OF VON WILLEBRAND DISEASE

VWD is an extremely heterogeneous and complex disorder, with more than 20 distinct subtypes reported (referenced in Ref. 150). A large number of mutations within the *VWF* gene have been identified (see Fig. 126–3). However, because of both the genetic complexity of VWD and the practical considerations of *VWF* gene sequencing in most clinical settings, a *VWF* gene mutation is not required for the diagnosis of VWD.[151] A list is maintained by a consortium of VWD investigators and can be accessed through the Internet at http://www.vwf.group.shef .ac.uk/. These findings form the basis for the simplified classification of VWD outlined in Table 126–2[151] and used throughout this chapter. Types 1 and 3 VWD are defined as pure quantitative deficiencies of VWF that are either partial (type 1) or complete (type 3). Type 2 VWD is characterized by qualitative abnormalities of VWF structure and/or function. The quantity of VWF found in type 2 VWD may be normal, but it is usually mildly to moderately decreased (see Table 126–2).

The diagnosis of VWD, particularly type 1 VWD, can be confounded by the incomplete penetrance of the disease and the wide range of VWF levels in normal populations (see "Laboratory Features" below). Nonpathogenic variation can impact laboratory assays *in vitro*, as is the case with Asp1472His, which alters VWF-ristocetin interactions but has no impact on hemostasis *in vivo*.[152] Ethnicity should also be considered. European ancestries were overrepresented in the studies which informed laboratory cutoffs, while African Americans exhibit generally higher VWF and FVIII levels. Additionally, there are numerous *VWF* gene "mutations" previously thought to be causative of VWD which are now known to be common in African Americans[153,154] who have normal VWF and FVIII levels,[153] including the Asp1472His variant.[155]

Type 1 von Willebrand Disease

Type 1 VWD is the most common form, accounting for approximately 70 percent of patients with the disease. Type 1 VWD is generally autosomal dominant in inheritance and is associated with coordinate reductions in FVIII, ristocetin cofactor activity, and VWF antigen with maintenance of the full complement of multimers (Fig. 126–4).

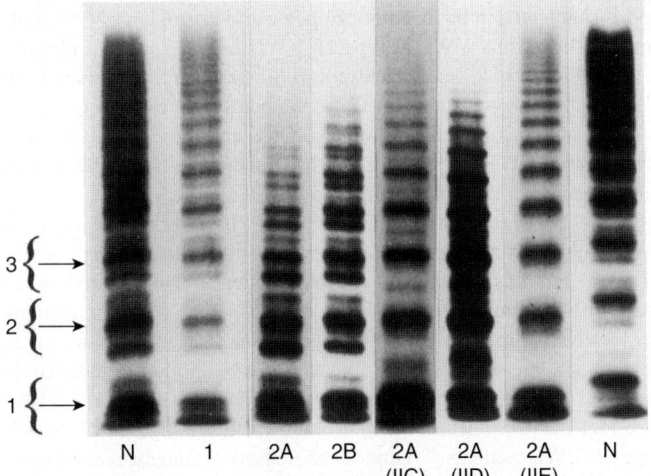

Figure 126–4. Agarose gel electrophoresis of plasma von Willebrand factor (VWF). VWF multimers from plasma of patients with various subtypes of von Willebrand disease (VWD) are shown. The brackets to the left encompass three individual multimer subunits, including the main band and its associate satellite bands. *N* indicates normal control lanes. Lanes 5 through 7 are rare variants of type 2A VWD. The former designations for these variants are indicated in parentheses below the lanes (IIC through E). *(Adapted with permission from Zimmerman TS, Dent JA, Ruggeri ZM, Nannini LH: Subunit composition of plasma von Willebrand factor. Cleavage is present in normal individuals, increased in IIA and IIB von Willebrand disease, but minimal in variants with aberrant structure of individual oligomers (types IIC, IID, and IIE). J Clin Invest 1986 Mar;77(3):947–951.)*

Subgroups within type 1 VWD have been proposed based on the relative levels of VWF present in the plasma and platelet pools,[156-159] but with the exception in some circumstances for an accelerated VWF clearance phenotype (unofficially termed VWF type 1C[160]), subtype distinctions in type 1 VWD are not generally used in clinical practice.

Type 1 VWF was previously assumed to simply represent the heterozygous form of type 3 VWD. However, in a large Canadian study, 48 percent of heterozygous carriers of type 3 VWD gene mutations carried a diagnosis of type 1 VWD, while the remainder were asymptomatic.[161] Furthermore, in two large studies of type 1 VWD families, numerous putative *VWF* mutations were identified, but very few were predictive of *VWF* null alleles.[31,162] Thus, some, but probably not all (see section Clinical Features below), type 1 VWD is the result of defects within the *VWF* gene. Studies of type 1 VWD mutations in patients, *in vitro*, and in animal models have characterized diverse mechanisms underlying type 1 VWD, including decreased VWF production,[163] retention of VWF in the ER,[164,165] impaired VWF secretion,[165,166] and decreased VWF survival.[163,166,167] Mutations that give rise to defective VWF subunits that interfere in a dominant negative way with the normal allele may be particularly likely to cause symptomatic VWD in the heterozygote.[168] For example, mutations at several cysteine residues in the VWF D3 domain and in the VWFpp of patients with moderately severe type 1 VWD. VWF carrying one of these mutations is retained in the ER, where it is proposed to exert a dominant negative effect on VWF derived from the normal allele via heterodimerization and degradation.[169,170]

To date, most mutation studies and genetic linkage analysis of type 1 VWD have been consistent with defects within the *VWF* gene. Although no single mutation can explain the majority of type 1 VWD, common *VWF* founder mutations can occur within populations, such as Tyr1584Cys identified in 14 percent of Canadian type 1 VWD patients, and possibly a similar proportion of patients in Europe.[162,171] The Tyr1584Cys mutation is associated with decreased VWF survival, likely a result of increased susceptibility to proteolysis by ADAMTS13.[172-175] These large multicenter studies of type 1 VWD families found candidate *VWF* mutations in 63 to 70 percent of families with type 1 VWD, leaving 37 to 40 percent of type 1 VWD index cases without a putative mutation in *VWF*.[162,171] Cases with *VWF* gene mutations tend to be more severe and highly heritable, while cases without an identifiable *VWF* mutation generally have higher VWF antigen (VWF:Ag) levels (>30 IU/dL).[31] In a large, multicenter European study of 150 type 1 VWD families, about one-third of cases historically diagnosed to have type 1 VWD were found to have abnormal multimers, and of these nearly all (95 percent) had a putative *VWF* gene mutation and significantly lower VWF:Ag, VWF ristocetin cofactor activity (VWF:RCo), assay of FVIII activity (FVIII:C), and VWF collagen-binding assay (VWF:CB) levels. Conversely, index cases with normal multimers had higher laboratory VWF values and fewer identifiable *VWF* mutations (55 percent), suggesting that the pathogenic mechanism(s) underlying this cohort of "true" type 1 VWD patients is more genetically complex.[162] Given the complex biosynthesis and processing of VWF, defects at a number of other loci could also be expected to result in quantitative VWF abnormalities (reviewed in Ref. 176). This concept is supported by families with type 1 VWD in which bleeding histories and low ristocetin cofactor activities do not always cosegregate with genetic markers at the VWF locus,[31,177] while one or more genetic factors outside the *VWF* locus may be associated with the variation in bleeding severity observed within VWD pedigrees.[178,179] It is interesting to note that a spontaneous mouse model of type 1 VWD exhibits up to 20-fold reductions in plasma VWF as a result of an unusual mutation in a glycosyltransferase gene, leading to aberrant posttranslational processing of VWF and accelerated clearance from plasma.[180] Similar mechanisms affecting VWF survival, perhaps combined with altered proteolysis,[181-183] may explain the observed modifying effect of the ABO blood group glyco-syltransferases on plasma VWF survival.[184] Additional genetic factors have been implicated to influence VWF via altered survival, including the clearance receptors CLEC4M and LRP1 (CD91) (reviewed in Ref. 185). The biologic consequences of VWF modifiers identified in normal populations are unclear, and studies are needed to determine their significance in VWD.

Type 3 von Willebrand Disease

Patients with type 3 VWD account for 1 to 5 percent of clinically significant VWD, have very low or undetectable levels of plasma and platelet VWF:Ag and VWF:RCo, and generally present early in life with severe bleeding.[186] FVIII coagulant activity is markedly reduced but usually detectable at levels of 3 to 10 percent of normal. Type 3 VWD has generally been considered an autosomal recessive disorder, but in a recent Canadian study of 100 individuals in 34 families, 48 percent of "carriers" had a diagnosis of type 1 VWD,[161] suggesting the dominant type 1 VWD pattern of inheritance is common in type 3 VWD families.

Mutations associated with type 3 VWD have been reported throughout the *VWF* gene (http://www.vwf.group.shef.ac.uk/). Gross *VWF* gene deletion detectable by Southern blot[26,187-190] or multiple ligation-probe amplification[161,191] is the molecular mechanism for type 3 VWD in only a small subset of families. However, large deletions may confer an increased risk for the development of alloantibodies against VWF.[26,189] A similar correlation between gene deletion and risk for alloantibody formation has been observed in hemophilia (Chap. 123). Comparative analysis of VWF genomic DNA and platelet VWF mRNA has identified nondeletion defects resulting in complete loss of VWF mRNA expression as a molecular mechanism in some patients with type 3 VWD.[192,193] A number of nonsense and frameshift mutations that would be predicted to result in loss of VWF protein expression or in expression of a markedly truncated or disrupted protein have been identified in some type 3 VWD families.[168,194-196] A frameshift mutation in exon 18 appears to be a particularly common cause of type 3 VWD in the Swedish population and has been shown to be the defect responsible for VWD in the original Åland Island pedigree.[197,198] This mutation results in a stable mRNA encoding a truncated protein that is rapidly degraded in the cell.[199] This mutation also appears to be common among type 3 VWD patients in Germany,[200] but not in the United States.[201]

Type 2A von Willebrand Disease

Type 2A is the most common qualitative variant of VWD and is generally associated with autosomal dominant inheritance and selective loss of the large and intermediate VWF multimers from plasma (see Fig. 126–4). A 176-kDa proteolytic fragment present in normal individuals is markedly increased in quantity in many type 2A VWD patients. This fragment is consistent with proteolytic cleavage of the peptide bond between Tyr1605 and Met1606.[98,202] Based on this observation, initial DNA sequence analysis in patients centered on VWF exon 28, in the region encoding this segment of the VWF protein, leading to the identification of the first point mutations responsible for VWD.[203] Since that time, a large number of mutations have been identified, accounting for the majority of type 2A VWD patients.[194] Many of these mutations are clustered within a 134-amino-acid segment of the VWF A2 domain (between Gly1505 and Glu1638; see Fig. 126–3), and the most common, Arg1597Trp, appears to account for about one-third of type 2A VWD patients.[194,195,204]

Type 2A VWD mutations have been grouped by two distinct molecular mechanisms. In the first subset, classified as group 1, the type 2A VWD mutation has been commonly considered a defect in intracellular transport, with retention of mutant VWF in the ER. In addition to retention or degradation of mutant VWF in the ER, type 2A mutations

can also disrupt intracellular processing and secretion via defective multimerization and/or loss of regulated storage.[205] In the second subset, or group 2, mutant VWF is normally processed and secreted *in vitro*, and thus loss of multimers *in vivo* is presumed to occur based on increased susceptibility to proteolysis in plasma[98,206-209] at the Tyr1605-Met1606 site cleaved by ADAMTS13.[101,210] The susceptibility of type 2A VWD mutations to proteolysis by ADAMTS13 *in vitro* supports accelerated proteolysis as a mechanism for the loss of high-molecular-weight VWF multimers in these patients.[204]

The multimer structure of platelet VWF correlates well with the underlying type 2A mechanisms. Group 1 patients show loss of large VWF multimers within platelets as a result of defective synthesis, while group 2 patients have normal VWF multimers within the protected environment of the α granule.[206] These observations confirm the earlier subclassification of type 2A VWD based on platelet multimers.[156] Subclassification into group 1 or 2 might be expected to predict response to DDAVP therapy, although this remains to be demonstrated.

In addition to the major classes of type 2A VWD described above, a number of rare variants historically classified as types IIC to IIH, type IB, and "platelet discordant" are included in the more general type 2A category. Most of these rare variants were distinguished on the basis of subtle differences in the multimer pattern (see Fig. 126–4; multimer changes relative to the location of type 2 mutations is reviewed in Ref. 211). The IIC variant is usually inherited as an autosomal recessive trait and is associated with loss of large multimers and a prominent dimer band. Several mutations have been identified in the VWFpp of these patients,[212-214] presumably interfering with multimer assembly and/or trafficking to storage granules. A mutation at the C terminus of VWF, interfering with dimer formation, was described in a patient with the IID variant.[215] Most of the other reported variants of type 2A VWD are quite rare, often limited to single case reports.

Type 2B von Willebrand Disease

Type 2B VWD is usually inherited as an autosomal dominant disorder and is characterized by thrombocytopenia and loss of large VWF multimers. The plasma VWF in type 2B VWD binds to normal platelets in the presence of lower concentrations of ristocetin than does normal VWF and can aggregate platelets spontaneously. Accelerated clearance of the resulting complexes between platelets and the large, most adhesive forms of VWF accounts for the thrombocytopenia and the characteristic multimer pattern (see Fig. 126–4).

The peculiar functional abnormality characteristic of type 2B VWD suggested a molecular defect within the GPIb binding domain of VWF. For this reason, initial DNA sequence analysis focused on the corresponding portion of VWF exon 28.[216,217] Type 2B mutations are located within the VWF A1 domain at one surface of the described crystallographic structure.[124,129] The four most common mutations are clustered within a 36-amino-acid stretch between Arg1306 and Arg1341 (see Fig. 126–3); together, these account for more than 80 percent of type 2B VWD patients.[195] Functional analysis of mutant recombinant VWF[218-222] confirms that these single-amino-acid substitutions are sufficient to account for increased GPIb binding and the resulting characteristic type 2B VWD phenotype. Structural studies of type 2B VWD mutations show that these residues interact with the leucine rich repeats of GPIb thought to be critical to the VWF A1–GPIb interactions under shear.[223] Type 2B mutations have now been modeled extensively in mice, all of which exhibited accelerated VWF clearance, as expected.[224] Type 2B VWD mice also had short-lived platelets, with evidence of macrophage-mediated platelet clearance.[225] In these models, platelets were observed to be coated by type 2B VWF,[225] a phenomenon that may contribute to a previously unsuspected acquired platelet function defect.[226] Interestingly, mice with the same type 2B mutations exhibit variable loss of large multimers[224] and varying degrees of thrombocytopenia,[227] similar to the variation observed in human pedigrees. Individual type 2B patients can also exhibit varying multimer structure and platelet counts over time. For example, two siblings with the Arg1306Trp mutation and abnormal multimers intermittently regained normal VWF multimer distribution during periods of thrombocytopenia.[228]

Families have been described that exhibit enhanced VWF binding to GPIb but a normal distribution of VWF multimers. These variants, previously referred to as type I New York, type I Malmö, and type I Sydney, are now all designated as type 2B VWD. Type I New York and type I Malmö are caused by the same *VWF* mutation, Pro1266Leu. This mutation is located within the cluster of type 2B mutations in the VWF A1 domain and results in a similar increase in platelet GPIb binding.[229]

Type 2N von Willebrand Disease

As described in Chap. 123, hemophilia A results from defects in the FVIII gene and is inherited in an X-linked recessive manner. Distinct from hemophilia A, families have been reported in which the inheritance of low FVIII appeared to be autosomal, based on the occurrence of affected females or direct transmission from an affected father.[230,231] Several cases of an apparent autosomal recessive decrease in FVIII were shown to be caused by decreased VWF binding of FVIII,[232–234] now referred to as VWD type 2N, after the Normandy province of origin of the first patient. DNA sequence analysis has identified more than 37 distinct mutations[235] associated with this disorder, most located at the VWF N terminus (see Fig. 126–3) (curated in the Scientific and Standardisation Committee of the International Society on Thrombosis and Haemostasis VWF Database, http://www.vwf.group.shef.ac.uk/). One of these mutations, Arg854Gln, appears to be particularly common, may contribute to variability in the severity of type 1 VWD in some cases,[236] and may also cause a VWF secretion defect.[237] Rare cases of misdiagnosis of type 2N have led to treatment with recombinant FVIII for presumed hemophilia A, with poor responses and adverse clinical outcomes.[238]

Type 2M von Willebrand Disease

This category was classically reserved for rare VWD variants in which a defect in VWF platelet-dependent function leads to significant bleeding but VWF multimer structure is not affected (although some have subtle multimer abnormalities). Most contemporary type 2M variants are indeed associated with absent ristocetin cofactor activity but normal platelet binding with other agonists. A total of 28 type 2M VWD mutations have been described,[235] including a number of other families with normal VWF multimers and disproportionately decreased ristocetin cofactor activity,[239,240] families with a combination of defects in VWF:CB and VWF–GPIb interactions of varying severities,[241,242] and mutations with isolated defects in VWF:CB with normal VWF:RCo activity.[235] Several families have also been described with a VWD variant (VWD Vicenza) characterized by larger-than-normal VWF multimers and classified as either type 1 or type 2M VWD.[243] Genetic linkage analysis indicates that the Vicenza defect lies within the VWF gene,[244] and mutations within the VWF gene have been reported to be associated with VWD Vicenza.[245] The underlying molecular mechanism responsible for the VWD Vicenza phenotype remains controversial,[246] although recent kinetic modeling suggests that altered VWF survival alone could account for the VWF perturbations observed in this disorder.[247]

● CLINICAL FEATURES

INHERITANCE

Type 1 VWD is generally transmitted as an autosomal dominant disorder, and accounts for approximately 70 percent of clinically significant VWD. However, disease expressivity is variable, and penetrance is incomplete.[168] Laboratory values and clinical symptoms can vary considerably, even within the same individual, and establishing a definite diagnosis of VWD is often difficult. In two large families with type 1 VWD, only 65 percent of individuals with both an affected parent and an affected descendent had significant clinical symptoms.[249] For comparison, 23 percent of the unrelated spouses of the patients, who presumably did not have a bleeding disorder, were judged to have a positive bleeding history.

A number of factors have long been known to modify VWF levels, including ABO blood group, secretor blood group, estrogens, thyroid hormones, age, and stress.[250–252] ABO blood group is the best characterized of these factors. Genome-wide linkage has repeatedly confirmed strong linkage between the ABO locus and VWF levels (reviewed in Ref. 253). Mean VWF:Ag levels are approximately 75 percent for type O individuals and 123 percent for type AB individuals when compared to a pool of normal donor plasmas. Thus, it may be difficult to differentiate between a low-normal VWF value and mild type 1 VWD in blood group O individuals. In recent years, additional modifiers of VWF have been identified in large genetic association studies,[254,255] including genes associated with VWF intracellular trafficking (*STXBP5*[256,257]) and VWF clearance (*CLEC4M*[258]). Additionally, a genome-wide association study identified a novel genetic locus on chromosome 2 contributing to variation in plasma VWF.[259] The variable expressivity and incomplete penetrance of type 1 VWD and overlap in VWF levels between mild type 1 VWD and normal populations has complicated the determination of accurate incidence figures for VWD, with estimates ranging from as high as 1 percent[260,261] to as low as 2 to 10 per 100,000 population.[262]

In general, the type 2 VWD variants, which comprise 20 to 30 percent of all VWD diagnoses,[263] are more uniformly penetrant. Type 2A and type 2B VWD account for the vast majority of patients with qualitative VWF abnormalities. Types 2A, 2B, and 2M are generally autosomal dominant in inheritance, although Type 2N and other rare cases of apparent recessive inheritance have been reported.

Estimates of prevalence for severe (type 3) VWD range from 0.5 to 5.3 per 1,000,000 population.[264–266] Although this variant is frequently defined as autosomal recessive in inheritance, this is not a consistent finding. As described above, one or both parents of a severe VWD patient can be clinically asymptomatic and have entirely normal laboratory test results, although in many families one or both parents appear to be affected with classic type 1 VWD. Thus, in some families, severe VWD may represent the homozygous form of type 1 VWD. In this model, the apparent recessive inheritance in a subset of families could simply be the result of the incomplete penetrance of type 1 VWD. Alternatively, there may be a fundamental difference in the molecular mechanisms responsible for type 1 and type 3 VWD.[168]

Compound heterozygosity (the presence of more than one *VWF* gene mutation) can occur, and the clinical presentation in such cases can depend on the interaction between the different mutant VWF proteins. Compound heterozygosity can impact response to therapy because of a complex VWD phenotype and has implications for genetic counseling. If compound heterozygosity is deduced from the family history and/or laboratory studies or discovered during genetic testing, the most recent update to the VWD nomenclature represents both types separated by a slash (/), such as VWD type 2B/2N.[151]

CLINICAL SYMPTOMS

Mucocutaneous bleeding is the most common symptom in patients with type 1 VWD.[249] It is important to note that more than 20 percent of normal individuals may give a positive bleeding history.[267] Bleeding assessment scores have evolved over many years,[268] leading the International Society on Thrombosis and Haemostasis to propose a unified

Bleeding Assessment Test[269] for research purposes. Although high bleeding scores are suggestive of a bleeding diathesis and can predict future bleeding,[270] no bleeding questionnaire as yet is clearly diagnostic for VWD. These observations, together with the limited sensitivity and specificity of the currently available laboratory tests (see below), makes the diagnosis of mild VWD quite difficult and probably contributes to the wide range of prevalence figures for type 1 VWD currently in the literature. A National Heart Lung and Blood Institute Expert Panel has proposed clinical guidelines for evaluating patients to determine whether laboratory testing for VWD or other bleeding disorders is warranted.[150]

Epistaxis occurs in approximately 60 percent of type 1 VWD patients, 40 percent have easy bruising and hematomas, 35 percent have menorrhagia, and 35 percent have gingival bleeding. Gastrointestinal bleeding occurs in approximately 10 percent of patients.[150] An apparent association between hereditary hemorrhagic telangiectasia (HHT) and VWD has been reported in several families. The causative genes in HHT were identified and are located on chromosomes 9q33–34, and 12q13[271] (Chap. 122), distinct from the VWF gene on chromosome 12p13. However, because inheriting VWD is likely to increase the severity of bleeding from HHT, the diagnosis is more likely to be made in patients inheriting both defects.[272] Mucocutaneous bleeding is common after trauma, with approximately 50 percent of patients reporting bleeding after dental extraction, approximately 35 percent after trauma or wounds, 25 percent postpartum, and 20 percent postoperatively. Hemarthroses in patients with moderate disease are extremely rare and are generally only encountered after major trauma. The bleeding symptoms can be quite variable among patients within the same family and even in the same patient over time. An individual may experience postpartum bleeding with one pregnancy but not with others, and clinical symptoms in mildly to moderately affected type 1 individuals often ameliorate by the second or third decade of life. Aside from an infrequent type 3 patient, death from bleeding rarely occurs in VWD.

Thrombocytopenia is a common feature of type 2B VWD and is not seen in any other form of VWD. Most patients only experience thrombocytopenia at times of increased VWF production or secretion, such as during physical effort, in pregnancy, in newborn infants, postoperatively, or if an infection develops. The platelet count rarely drops to levels thought to contribute to clinical bleeding.[273,274] Infants with type 2B VWD may present with neonatal thrombocytopenia, which could be confused with neonatal alloimmune thrombocytopenia, neonatal sepsis, or congenital thrombocytopenia.

Patients who are homozygous or compound heterozygous for type 2N VWD generally have normal levels of VWF:Ag and VWF:RCo and normal VWF platelet adhesive function. However, FVIII levels are moderately decreased, resulting in a mild to moderate hemophilia-like phenotype.[146] In contrast to patients with classic hemophilia A (FVIII deficiency), these patients do not respond to infusion of purified FVIII and should be treated with VWF-containing concentrates.[275] Heterozygotes for this disorder may have mildly decreased FVIII levels but are generally asymptomatic. Although type 2N VWD appears to be considerably less common than classic hemophilia A, it should be considered in the differential diagnosis of FVIII deficiency, particularly if any features suggest an autosomal pattern of inheritance. Although the FVIII level rarely drops below 5 percent, type 2N VWD mutation can be associated with FVIII levels as low as 1 percent, when co-inherited with a type 3 VWD allele.[276] The latter observation further suggests that a diagnosis of type 2N VWD should also be considered in patients with marked reductions of FVIII.

Patients with type 3 VWD can suffer from severe clinical bleeding and experience hemarthroses and muscle hematomas, as in severe hemophilia A (Chap. 123). After infusion of VWF-containing plasma fractions, some of these patients develop anti-VWF antibodies that neutralize VWF (reviewed in Ref. 277).

Other heritable coagulopathies can coexist with VWF deficiency. An evaluation for other factor deficiencies or platelet disorders should be considered in patients that have a suggestive family history, a bleeding phenotype out or proportion or inconsistent with an expected VWD pattern, or a poor response to therapy. In VWD patients with combination coagulopathies, treatment of both disorders may be necessary to achieve a good clinical result.[278]

●LABORATORY FEATURES

In the initial laboratory evaluation of patients suspected by history of having VWD, the following tests are routinely performed: assay of FVIII:C, VWF:Ag, and VWF:RCo. Other tests that are commonly used include RIPA, VWF:CB, and VWF multimer analysis. Routine coagulation studies, such as prothrombin time (PT) or activated partial-thromboplastin time (aPTT), are generally not useful in the evaluation of VWD. However, the aPTT can be prolonged in subjects with VWF deficiency,[279] or in patients with homozygous type 2N VWD, because of the reduction in FVIII level. The wide range of normal and the considerable overlap with the levels observed in type 1 VWD make borderline levels difficult to interpret. A variety of concurrent diseases and drugs may modify the results of individual tests. Many conditions, such as recent exercise, age, pregnancy, time of the menstrual cycle, estrogen therapy, hypo- or hyperthyroidism, diabetes, uremia, liver disease, infection, myeloproliferative neoplasms, or malignancy can affect the FVIII activity, VWF:Ag, and ristocetin cofactor activity levels. These values can be regarded as acute-phase reactants, and even minor illnesses can increase the levels in a VWD patient to normal. Appropriate processing of laboratory specimens is also critical as VWF parameters can be artifactually skewed (either high or low) by phlebotomy conditions or specimen handling (reviewed in Ref. 150). Even controlling for many of these factors, the coefficients of variation of repeated VWF:Ag and ristocetin cofactor assays in a single person are quite large,[280] and can be influenced by numerous factors including diurnal variation.[281] For this reason, repeated measurements are usually necessary, and the diagnosis of VWD or its exclusion should generally not be based on a single set of laboratory values.

The laboratory diagnosis of type 1 VWD can be confounded by the wide range of VWF levels in "normals" and borderline laboratory results. An alternative strategy is to classify some patients for whom the diagnosis of VWD is ambiguous as "low VWF," recognizing that these patients may have an increased risk of bleeding without labeling them as type 1 VWD.[282,283] In response to this need to distinguish those patients with VWD from nonbleeding individuals with moderately low levels of VWF (30 to 50 IU/dL), a threshold of less than 30 IU/dL has been recommended.[150] In clinical practice there remains wide variation in the assignment of normal VWF ranges and in the interpretation of laboratory results to make a VWD diagnoses.[284–286]

FACTOR VIII

FVIII levels in VWD patients are generally coordinately decreased along with plasma VWF, although skewing of FVIII-to-VWF ratios can be observed.[287] Levels in type 3 VWD generally range from 3 to 10 percent. In contrast, the levels in type 1 and the type 2 VWD variants (other than 2N) are variable and usually only mildly or moderately decreased. The FVIII level in type 2N VWD is more severely decreased, but rarely to less than 5 percent.

VON WILLEBRAND FACTOR ANTIGEN

Plasma VWF:Ag is usually quantitated by electroimmunoassay or an enzyme-linked immunosorbent assay (ELISA) technique. In type 1 VWD, the VWF:Ag assay usually parallels VWF:RCo, but it has lower specificity and sensitivity than the VWF:RCo assay. In patients with type 2 VWD, the VWF:Ag is variably decreased but can be normal (see Table 126–2).

RISTOCETIN COFACTOR ACTIVITY

The standard measure of VWF activity, the VWF:RCo quantitates the ability of plasma VWF to agglutinate platelets via platelet membrane GPIbα in the presence of ristocetin.[288] In the most common method, normal platelets washed free of plasma VWF are used either as fresh platelets or after formaldehyde fixation. This assay has long been reported to be the most sensitive and specific single test for the detection of VWD.[289] Numerous alternative methods have been proposed as adjuncts or replacements of the standard platelet-based ristocetin cofactor activity assay. However, none as yet can serve as a surrogate for VWF:RCo (reviewed in Ref. 290).

Ristocetin cofactor activity is generally decreased coordinately with VWF:Ag and FVIII in type 1 VWD patients. In type 2 VWD variants, ristocetin cofactor activity can be disproportionately decreased, as is usually the case in type 2A variants (and sometimes type 2B), because of the greater dependence of the ristocetin-mediated platelet–VWF interaction on the presence of larger VWF multimers, and in type 2M, because of decreased VWF-platelet interactions (see Table 126–2). Thus, the VWF:RCo-to-VWF:Ag ratio has been proposed as a means to distinguish between type 1 and type 2 VWD, with a ratio of VWF:RCo-to-VWF:Ag of less than 0.7 being indicative of a qualitative (type 2) VWF defect.[151] However, in patients with very low VWF:Ag levels this ratio may not be reliable because of the limits of sensitivity of most VWF:RCo assays. The VWF:RCo assay is uninformative in the presence of the VWF Asp1472His variant, which interferes with the VWF–ristocetin interaction *in vitro*.[155]

RISTOCETIN-INDUCED PLATELET AGGLUTINATION

Similar to the ristocetin cofactor assay above, the RIPA assay also measures platelet agglutination caused by ristocetin-mediated VWF binding to platelet membrane GPIbα. In the case of RIPA, ristocetin is added directly to patient platelet-rich plasma and platelet aggregation is measured. Hyperresponsiveness to RIPA results either from a type 2B VWD mutation or an intrinsic defect in the platelet (platelet-type or pseudo-VWD). In these disorders, patient platelet-rich plasma agglutinates spontaneously or at low ristocetin concentrations of only 0.2 to 0.7 mg/mL. At these concentrations, normal platelet-rich plasma does not agglutinate. Type 2B and platelet-type VWD can be distinguished by RIPA experiments performed with separated patient platelets or plasma mixed with the corresponding component from a normal individual or paraformaldehyde-fixed platelets. The RIPA is generally reduced in most other subtypes of VWD (see Table 126–2).

MULTIMER ANALYSIS

Analysis of plasma VWF multimers is critical for the proper diagnosis and subclassification of VWD (see Fig. 126–4). This is generally accomplished by agarose gel electrophoresis of plasma VWF to separate VWF multimers on the basis of molecular size, with the largest multimers migrating more slowly than the intermediate or smaller multimers. The multimers may be visualized by autoradiography after incubation with ^{125}I-monospecific antihuman VWF antibody or, more commonly, by nonradioactive immunologic techniques. The normal multimeric distribution is an orderly ladder of major protein bands of increasing molecular weight, going from the smallest to the largest VWF multimers (see Fig. 126–4). Each normal multimer has a fine structure consisting of one major component and two to four satellite bands.[291] Type 2B and most of the type 2A variants were initially distinguished from each other on the basis of subtle variations in the satellite band pattern. In a large European multicenter type 1 VWD study, careful analysis of VWF multimers in subjects historically diagnosed as type 1 VWD, including patients diagnosed at experienced centers, found one-third of "type 1" VWD patients had subtly abnormal multimers.[292] Although this previously would have required reclassification of these patients as type 2 VWD, the most recent update on the classification of VWD by the International Society on Thrombosis and Haemostasis Subcommittee on von Willebrand Factor expanded the category of type 1 VWD to permit subtle VWF multimer abnormalities.[151] The authors of the European type 1 VWD study note that having samples from the index case, affected family members, and unaffected family members on one gel made qualitative defects more readily detectable, and that intermediate-resolution multimer gels were superior to low-resolution multimer gels in detecting abnormalities in this population. Use of VWF tests sensitive to VWF multimer structure have been proposed by some experts as proxies for VWF multimer testing, such the VWF:RCo-to-VWF:Ag ratio (VWF RCo:Ag ratio) or VWF:CB assay.[293] In studies comparing these approaches as surrogates for VWF multimer assays, the (VWF RCo:Ag ratio) ratio was found to be less sensitive than multimer gel techniques in identifying qualitative VWF defects,[292] while VWF:CB an detect some type 2M VWD patients who have normal VWF multimers.[294,295] These observations support a continued important role for VWF multimer analysis in the laboratory evaluation of VWD.

ADDITIONAL LABORATORY TESTS

As a result of the variable sensitivity and specificity of laboratory testing for VWD, additional diagnostic studies may be useful in the classification of VWD patients. The VWF:CB measures VWF binding to collagen (type I, type III, type VI, or mixed) by ELISA. As above, assays based upon VWF:CB can complement the VWF:RCo in detecting type 2 VWD variants,[296–299] and an abnormal VWF:CB-to-VWF:Ag ratio (VWF CB:Ag ratio) is suggestive of a qualitative VWF defect.[151] Abnormalities in VWF:CB can reflect loss of high-molecular-weight multimers and/or the discrete loss of collagen binding caused by a type 2M mutation. Use of VWF:CB assays is expanding in clinical practice, with select sites including this test routinely in initial VWD diagnostic laboratory testing.

Another group of tests are included in the term VWF "activity" (VWF:Act). These tests seek to assess VWF-GPIb binding capacity independent of ristocetin, usually by using antibodies to the VWF A1 domain in ELISAs. These tests are easily confused with the VWF:RCo, which has also been referred to as "VWF activity." None of these tests measures activity; rather both VWF:RCo and VWF:Act are sensitive to VWF conformation. The VWF:Act does not always provide the same results as VWF:RCo, particularly with regards to type 2M VWD, and is not considered a substitute for the VWF:RCo (reviewed in Ref. 290).

When type 2N VWD is suspected, VWF:FVIII binding capacity can be measured.[234] Specific assays of FVIII binding to VWF (VWF:FVIIIB) have been developed and can be used to confirm the diagnosis of type 2N VWD.[300,301] Type 2N carriers do not always exhibit a decrease in VWF:FVIIIB, but a decreased VWF:FVIIIB-to-VWF:Ag ratio may correlate with heterozygosity for a type 2N *VWF* mutation.[302] Although this assay is widely used in European hemostasis laboratories, its availability in the United States is currently limited to a few specialized reference laboratories.

An assay measuring the VWFpp can be used to calculate the VWFpp:antigen ratio (VWFpp:Ag ratio) to detect a subset of VWD patients with decreased VWF survival. Good correlation has been reported between subjects with significantly shortened VWF half-life after DDAVP challenge and an increased VWFpp:Ag ratio.[287,303,304] This assay is currently available in a few reference laboratories. A normal platelet VWF:Ag in the setting of decreased plasma VWF laboratory parameters also suggests an accelerated clearance phenotype such as that seen in VWD type Vicenza,[305] but platelet VWF:Ag testing also is not widely available in clinical laboratories.

A number of other assays for VWF activity have been developed. The PFA-100 system, which measures platelet binding under high shear,[306,307] is controversial in the diagnosis or monitoring of VWD. Although the PFA-100 is usually abnormal in type 2 VWD and in more severe type 1 and type 3 VWD cases, milder type 1 VWD and some type 2 VWD patients can have normal results.[150] Other VWF assays can measure binding of an antibody to the GPIb binding site on VWF as a proposed screening test for VWD.[308–311] Additional assays can measure platelet agglutination induced by botrocetin (which is no longer commercially available) and other snake venom proteins.[312] In the National Heart Lung and Blood Institute Expert Panel guidelines (http://www.nhlbi.nih.gov/files/docs/guidelines/vwd.pdf), none of these tests are recommended for screening for VWD.[150]

With advances in understanding the molecular genetics of VWD, it is now possible to precisely diagnose and subclassify many variants of VWD on the basis of DNA mutations (reviewed in Ref. 313). DNA testing, particularly for type 2 VWD mutations which cluster within specific regions of the *VWF* gene (see Fig. 126–3), can be used to confirm the diagnosis and is available in specialized reference laboratories. The analysis of type 3 and type 1 VWD is more complex, as the currently known mutations are scattered throughout the gene[235] and account only for a subset of patients.

The bleeding time is mentioned here for historical purposes only, as it was used as a screening test for VWD and other abnormalities of platelet function. Bleeding time varied considerably with the experience of the operator and a variety of other factors, did not prolong with FVIII deficiency, and correlated poorly with bleeding risk. Thus, the bleeding time is no longer recommended in the evaluation of VWD.[150]

PRENATAL TESTING

Given the mild clinical phenotype of most patients with the common variants of VWD, prenatal diagnosis for the purpose of deciding on terminating a pregnancy is rarely performed. However, type 3 VWD patients often have a profound bleeding disorder, similar to or more severe than classic hemophilia, and some families may request prenatal diagnosis. In those cases of VWD in which the precise mutation is known, DNA diagnosis can be performed rapidly and accurately by polymerase chain reaction (PCR) from amniotic fluid or chorionic villus biopsies (reviewed in Ref. 313) and would be expected to be compatible with new noninvasive prenatal testing methods.[314] In those cases where the mutation is unknown, diagnosis can still be attempted by genetic linkage analysis using the large panel of known polymorphisms within the VWF gene.[313] Although all cases of VWD analyzed to date appear to be linked to the VWF gene, the possibility of locus heterogeneity (i.e., a similar phenotype caused by a mutation in a gene other than VWF) should be considered.[315] As with all DNA testing, if prenatal testing is

being considered, genetic counseling should be provided before the decision to test is made as well as following the procedure.

DIFFERENTIAL DIAGNOSIS

PLATELET-TYPE (PSEUDO-) VON WILLEBRAND DISEASE

Platelet-type (pseudo-) VWD is a platelet defect that phenotypically mimics VWD (Chap. 120). Patients have mucocutaneous bleeding, plasma VWF often lacks the largest multimers, RIPA is enhanced at low concentrations of ristocetin, and thrombocytopenia of variable degree is often present. Molecular analysis has identified missense mutations within the GPIbα gene as the molecular basis for pseudo-VWD. These mutations are located within the segment of GPIb that encodes the VWF binding domain and appear to induce the conformational change complementary to that produced in VWF by type 2B VWD mutations (reviewed in Ref. 316).

The specialized RIPA test should be performed at low ristocetin concentrations to distinguish type 2B and platelet type VWD from type 2A VWD. In this test, purified normal plasma VWF or cryoprecipitate added to platelet preparations from patients with platelet-type VWD causes platelet aggregation, distinguishing this disorder from type 2B VWD where patient platelets aggregate only at higher ristocetin concentrations. In addition, type 2B VWD plasma transfers the enhanced RIPA to normal platelets, whereas plasma from patients with platelet-type VWD interacts normally with control platelets.

ACQUIRED VON WILLEBRAND SYNDROME

Acquired VWD, or acquired von Willebrand syndrome (AVWS), is a relatively rare acquired bleeding disorder that usually presents as a late-onset bleeding diathesis in a patient with no prior bleeding history and a negative family history of bleeding (reviewed in Ref. 317). Decreased levels of FVIII, VWF:Ag, and VWF:RCo are common, and VWF multimers can be abnormal. AVWS is usually associated with another underlying disorder and has been reported to occur in patients with myeloproliferative neoplasms,[318] amyloidosis,[319] benign or malignant B-cell disorders,[320] hypothyroidism,[321] autoimmune disorders,[322] several solid tumors (particularly Wilms tumor),[323] cardiac or vascular defects (such as aortic stenosis),[324] ventricular assist devices,[325] or in association with several drugs, including ciprofloxacin and valproic acid.[326,327]

The mechanisms that cause AVWS can generally be attributed to an associated medical condition. A variety of B-cell disorders have been associated with the development of anti-VWF autoantibodies. In most cases the AVWS appears to be due to rapid clearance of VWF induced by the circulating inhibitor, although these antibodies may also interfere with VWF function. Hypothyroidism results in decreased VWF synthesis.[321] In some cases of malignancy, AVWS is thought to be due to selective adsorption of VWF to the tumor cells or in myeloproliferative neoplasms, clearance/alterations of VWF by the high circulating platelet mass. AVWS associated with valvular heart disease, ventricular assist devices, or certain drugs, VWF may be lost by accelerated destruction or proteolysis under shear.[325–327]

Although the VWF multimers in AVWS usually exhibit a type 2A pattern with relative depletion of the large multimer forms, AVWS can manifest as a wide range of VWD phenotypes.[322,328] Distinguishing AVWS from genetic VWD can be difficult, as testing for the associated autoantibodies is generally not available in the clinical setting. The diagnosis often rests on the late onset of the disease, the absence of a family history, and the identification of an associated underlying disorder.

Management of AVWS is generally aimed at treating the underlying disorder. VWF levels and bleeding symptoms often improve with successful treatment of hypothyroidism or an associated malignancy. Refractory patients have been treated with glucocorticoids, plasma exchange, intravenous gamma globulin, rituximab, DDAVP, and VWF-containing FVIII concentrates.[317,329]

THERAPY, COURSE, AND PROGNOSIS

The mainstays of therapy for VWD are DDAVP, which induces secretion of both VWF and FVIII (reviewed in Ref. 330), and replacement therapy with VWF-containing plasma concentrates. The choice of treatment in any given patient depends upon the type and severity of VWD, the clinical setting, and the type of hemostatic challenge that must be met. Type 1 patients are most often treated with DDAVP alone, types 2A and 2B with a combination of DDAVP and a VWF-containing FVIII product, and type 2N and type 3 patients with VWF-containing concentrates.[150] A previous history of trauma or surgery and the success of previous treatment are important parameters to include in assessing the risk of bleeding. Prophylaxis is used in anticipation of hemostatic challenges,[150] such as dental extractions, and is efficacious in preventing recurrent bleeding in severe VWD patients.[331] Although in general there is a correlation between normal hemostasis and correction of VWF and FVIII activity, this does not occur in all cases.

DESMOPRESSIN

DDAVP is an analogue of antidiuretic hormone that acts through type 2 vasopressin receptors to induce secretion of FVIII and VWF, likely via cyclic adenosine monophosphate–mediated secretion from the Weibel-Palade bodies in endothelial cells.[83] When DDAVP is administered to healthy subjects, it causes sustained increases of FVIII and ristocetin cofactor activity for approximately 4 hours.[332] Patients with type 1 VWD treated with DDAVP release unusually high-molecular-weight VWF multimers into the circulation for 1 to 3 hours after the infusion.[332,333] Therapy with DDAVP often increases the FVIII activity, VWF:Ag, and ristocetin cofactor activity to two to five times the basal level.

DDAVP has become a mainstay for the treatment of mild hemophilia and VWD[334] because it is relatively inexpensive, widely available, and avoids the risks of plasma-derived products. Approximately 80 percent of type 1 VWD patients have excellent responses to DDAVP, although this figure may be substantially lower depending on the criteria for diagnosis and response.[335] It is regularly used in the setting of mild to moderate bleeding and for prophylaxis of patients undergoing surgical procedures. DDAVP is administered at a dose of 0.3mcg/kg continuous intravenous infusion over 30 minutes. DDAVP is also available for subcutaneous injection (at the same 0.3mcg/kg dose) and in intranasal form (at a fixed dose of 300mcg for adults and 150mcg for children), which appears to be similar in efficacy to intravenous administration,[336,337] although the response may be more variable.

The response to DDAVP in any given individual with VWD is generally reproducible and predicts response to future doses as long as the follow doses are at least 2 to 4 days later. In one study, 22 type 1 VWD patients showed a departure of less than 20 percent from the mean FVIII peak level calculated from two separate infusions. In addition, the consistency of response in one patient reliably predicted the future response of that patient and other affected family members.[338] In a study of 77 type 1 VWD patients, DDAVP response was associated both with *VWF* mutation and baseline multimeric pattern, although subtle abnormalities in VWF multimers did not preclude a patient response to DDAVP. Interestingly, patients with the same *VWF* mutation did not necessarily exhibit the same degree of responsiveness to DDAVP, implying the influence of other factors in the magnitude of DDAVP effect.[339] For patients requiring repeated infusions of DDAVP, the FVIII activity and VWF responses may not be of the same magnitude as after the first infusion. Although this decay in response has considerable individual variability, after one infusion of DDAVP per day for 4 days it was found that the responses on days 2 to 4 were reduced approximately 30 percent compared to day 1.[336–338,340]

Therefore, in patients for whom DDAVP is potentially the treatment of choice, a test dose should be given at the planned therapeutic dose and route in advance of the first required course of treatment with measurements of before and after VWF and FVIII:C levels to ensure an adequate therapeutic response. Sampling additional time points after DDAVP infusion should be considered as some type 1 and type 2 VWD patients have a significantly shortened VWF half-life and it may be more appropriate to treat with VWF replacement therapy in clinical scenarios requiring more durable therapy to maintain hemostasis. For patients with type 1 VWD who are undergoing surgical procedures, DDAVP can be administered 1 hour before surgery and approximately every 12 hours thereafter for up to two to four doses before loss of clinically significant response. Patients should be monitored for response of FVIII and ristocetin cofactor activity and side effects, particularly hyponatremia (and then should be water restricted), when DDAVP is administered at frequent intervals. VWF-containing FVIII concentrates should be available for infusion as backup.

Approximately 20 to 25 percent of patients with VWD do not respond adequately to DDAVP. Type 2 VWD patients are less likely to have a response than type 1 patients,[341,335] and virtually no patients with type 3 VWD respond. The response to DDAVP of patients with type 2A VWD is variable. Although most patients respond only transiently, some patients exhibit complete hemostatic correction after DDAVP infusion.[342,343] It has been hypothesized that the differences in DDAVP efficacy among type 2A patients may correspond to the type of mutation, with better responses predicted in patients with group 2 mutations. A prospective study of the biologic response to DDAVP in well-characterized VWD patients included type 2A VWD patients with both group 1 and group 2 defects. Although patients with group 2 mutations had greater improvements in VWF:RCo and shortening of bleeding times than patients with group 1 defects, neither groups could be classified as responders.[341]

Common side effects of DDAVP administration are mild cutaneous vasodilation resulting in a feeling of heat, facial flushing, tachycardia, tingling, and headaches. The potential for dilutional hyponatremia, especially in elderly and very young patients and with repeat dosing, requires appropriate attention to fluid restriction, as it may result in seizures. There have been isolated reports of acute arterial thrombosis associated with administration of DDAVP, but the risk appears to be very low when judged against the total number of patients treated. DDAVP is contraindicated in patients with unstable coronary artery disease because of increased risk of thrombotic events, such as myocardial infarction.[344] Patients receiving DDAVP at closely spaced intervals of less than 24 to 48 hours can develop tachyphylaxis.[340]

Many experts consider DDAVP to be contraindicated in the treatment of type 2B VWD, as the high-molecular-weight VWF released from storage sites has an increased affinity for binding to GPIb and might be expected to induce spontaneous platelet aggregation and worsening thrombocytopenia.[229] However, there are reports of DDAVP used successfully in type 2B VWD patients, with an associated shortening of bleeding times and variable thrombocytopenia.[345,346] Although type 2N patients can exhibit increased FVIII:C levels after DDAVP, in some cases the FVIII:C levels rapidly decline, likely a result of the absence of stabilizing normal VWF, attenuating clinical efficacy. Type 2M patients generally do not have a satisfactory response to DDAVP.[341,347]

VON WILLEBRAND FACTOR REPLACEMENT THERAPY

It is important to determine the response to DDAVP for each individual so as to avoid the unnecessary use of plasma products. For type 3 VWD patients and other patients unresponsive to DDAVP, the use of selected virus-inactivated, VWF-containing FVIII concentrates is generally safe and effective.[150] Humate-P, Alphanate, Wilate, and Koate are all acceptable commercial VWF-containing plasma concentrates that have been evaluated in VWD replacement therapy in clinical studies, and other VWF-containing FVIII concentrates may also be effective. A plasma-free recombinant VWF–recombinant FVIII combination (rVW-F-rFVIII) shows promise in clinical trials and may become available in the near future.[348] Cryoprecipitate was useful in the past, but because it is not generally treated to inactivate bloodborne pathogens, is less targeted to correcting the VWD hemostatic defect, and its administration is associated with a large volume load, it is less desirable. It is important to note that most standard FVIII concentrates and all recombinant FVIII products are not effective in VWD because they lack clinically significant quantities of VWF. Although such products can substantially increase circulating FVIII:C, the infused factor is short-lived in the circulation in the absence of stabilizing VWF.[349] Only preparations that contain large quantities of VWF with well-preserved multimer structure are suitable for use in VWD patients.

In practice, VWD replacement therapy dosing and timing has been largely empiric. Recommendations for therapy have been outlined based upon the degree and nature of hemorrhage and experience in clinical practice.[150] The objective is to elevate FVIII:C and VWF:RCo until bleeding stops and healing is complete. In general, replacement goals of FVIII:C and VWF:RCo should be initial replacement to greater than 100 IU/dL and maintenance of greater than 50 IU/dL for 7 to 14 days for major trauma, surgery, or central nervous system hemorrhage; greater than 30 to 50 IU/dL for 3 to 5 days for minor surgery or bleeding; greater than 50 IU/dL for delivery and continued for at least 3 to 5 days in the postpartum period; greater than 30 to 50 IU/dL for 1 to 5 days for dental extractions and minor surgery; and greater than 20 to 50 IU/dL for mucous membrane bleeding or menorrhagia. Laboratory monitoring of posttreatment FVIII:C and VWF levels is important in guiding therapy and avoidance of supratherapeutic replacement doses (>200 IU/dL VWF:RCo, >250 IU/dL FVIII), which are associated with an increased risk of thrombosis.[150,350,351] Although thrombosis is rare overall, VWD patients on prolonged therapy or with central access catheters appear to be at higher risk.[352]

In patients who have concomitant thrombocytopenia associated with or in addition to VWD, it may be necessary to transfuse platelets in addition to factor concentrates. If clinical bleeding continues, additional replacement therapy must be given and searches undertaken for other hemostatic defects. Type 3 VWD patients receiving multiple transfusions can develop antibodies directed against VWF (reviewed in Ref. 277). Continued replacement with VWF-containing concentrates is contraindicated because of the risk of anaphylaxis. A variety of approaches to the management of VWD inhibitors, similar to the treatment of FVIII inhibitors in hemophilia A (Chap. 123), have been attempted. Immunosuppression, recombinant FVIII, and recombinant factor VIIa have been reported to be useful in patients with type 3 VWD who have developed anti-VWF antibodies.

OTHER NONREPLACEMENT THERAPIES

Fibrinolytic inhibitors, such as ε-aminocaproic acid or tranexamic acid, have been used effectively in some VWD patients. Antifibrinolytics are commonly used alone or in conjunction with DDAVP or a plasma-derived VWF replacement product in patients with gynecologic bleeding, mucous membrane bleeding, or undergoing dental procedures.[150] Fibrinolytic inhibitors can be delivered systemically or topically and are generally well tolerated, but rarely can cause nausea or diarrhea and are contraindicated in patients with gross hematuria.

Estrogens or oral contraceptives have been used empirically in treating menorrhagia. In addition to their effects on the ovaries and uterus, some estrogens can increase plasma VWF levels. Patients with VWD frequently normalize their levels of FVIII, VWF:Ag, and VWF:RCo during pregnancy (Chap. 8). Postpartum hemorrhage within the first few days after parturition may be related to the relatively rapid return of FVIII and VWF activities to prepregnancy levels, and postpartum hemorrhage in all forms of VWD may occur as long as 1 month postpartum. In pregnant patients with type 1 VWD, the FVIII and ristocetin cofactor activities usually rise above 50 percent. These patients usually do not require any specific therapy at the time of parturition. In contrast, individuals who have 30 percent or less FVIII or variant forms of VWD are more likely to require prophylactic therapy before delivery. In a recent study, women receiving treatment for VWD postpartum were unexpectedly found not to have corrected to target levels.[353] Therefore, laboratory testing is recommended at term and should be considered in the postpartum period in patients at risk for immediate and/or delayed bleeding complications or receiving therapy.

Recombinant activated factor VII (rFVIIa, or NovoSeven) has also been successfully used in VWD patients with severe hemorrhage refractory to VWF replacement therapy and in bleeding patients with anti-VWF antibodies (reviewed in Ref. 354). In the case of minor accessible bleeding, topical drugs such as fibrin sealants or topical bovine thrombin may also be considered when standard VWD therapies fail to provide adequate local hemostasis.[150]

REFERENCES

1. von Willebrand EA: Hereditär Pseudohemofili. *Fin Lakaresallsk Handl* 67:7–112, 1926.
2. Hoyer LW: Von Willebrand's disease. *Prog Hemost Thromb* 3:231–287, 1976.
3. Nilsson IM: Von Willebrand's disease—Fifty years old. *Acta Med Scand* 201:497–508, 1977.
4. Zimmerman TS, Ratnoff OD, Powell AE: Immunologic differentiation of classic hemophilia (Factor VIII deficiency) and von Willebrand disease. *J Clin Invest* 50:244–254, 1971.
5. Howard MA, Firkin BG: Ristocetin—A new tool in the investigation of platelet aggregation. *Thromb Diath Haemorrh* 76:362–369, 1971.
6. Weiss HJ, Rogers J, Brand H: Defective ristocetin-induced platelet aggregation in von Willebrand's disease and its correction by Factor VIII. *J Clin Invest* 52:2697–2707, 1973.
7. Weiss HJ, Hoyer LW: Von Willebrand factor: Dissociation from antihemophilic factor procoagulant activity. *Science* 182:1149–1151, 1973.
8. Zimmerman TS, Edgington TS: Factor VIII coagulant activity and factor VIII-like antigen: Independent molecular entities. *J Exp Med* 138:1015–1020, 1973.
9. Gitschier J, Wood WI, Goralka TM, et al: Characterization of the human factor VIII gene. *Nature* 312:326–330, 1984.
10. Toole JJ, Knopf JL, Wozney JM, et al: Molecular cloning of a cDNA encoding human antihaemophilic factor. *Nature* 312:342–347, 1984.
11. Ginsburg D, Handin RI, Bonthron DT, et al: Human von Willebrand factor (vWF): Isolation of complementary DNA (cDNA) clones and chromosomal localization. *Science* 228:1401–1406, 1985.
12. Lynch DC, Zimmerman TS, Collins CJ, et al: Molecular cloning of cDNA for human von Willebrand factor: Authentication by a new method. *Cell* 41:49–56, 1985.
13. Sadler JE, Shelton-Inloes BB, Sorace JM, et al: Cloning and characterization of two cDNAs coding for human von Willebrand factor. *Proc Natl Acad Sci U S A* 82:6394–6398, 1985.
14. Verweij CL, de Vries CJM, Distel B, et al: Construction of cDNA coding for human von Willebrand factor using antibody probes for colony-screening and mapping of the chromosomal gene. *Nucleic Acids Res* 13:4699–4717, 1985.
15. Sadler JE, Budde U, Eikenboom JC, et al: Update on the pathophysiology and classification of von Willebrand disease: A report of the Subcommittee on von Willebrand Factor. *J Thromb Haemost Thromb Haemost* 4:2103–2114, 2006.
16. Titani K, Kumar S, Takio K, et al: Amino acid sequence of human von Willebrand factor. *Biochemistry* 25:3171–3184, 1986.
17. Fay PJ, Kawai Y, Wagner DD, et al: Propolypeptide of von Willebrand factor circulates in blood and is identical to von Willebrand antigen II. *Science* 232:995–998, 1986.

18. Bonthron DT, Handin RI, Kaufman RJ, et al: Structure of pre-pro-von Willebrand factor and its expression in heterologous cells. *Nature* 324:270–273, 1986.
19. Bonthron DT, Orr EC, Mitsock LM, et al: Nucleotide sequence of pre-pro-von Willebrand factor cDNA. *Nucleic Acids Res* 14:7125–7127, 1986.
20. Shelton-Inloes BB, Broze GJ Jr, Miletich JP, Sadler JE: Evolution of human von Willebrand Factor: CDNA sequence polymorphisms, repeated domains, and relationship to von Willebrand antigen II. *Biochem Biophys Res Commun* 144:657–665, 1987.
21. Shelton-Inloes BB, Titani K, Sadler JE: CDNA sequences for human von Willebrand Factor reveal five types of repeated domains and five possible protein sequence polymorphisms. *Biochemistry* 25:3164–3171, 1986.
22. Springer TA: Von Willebrand factor, Jedi knight of the bloodstream. *Blood* 124:1412–1425, 2014.
23. Colombatti A, Bonaldo P: The superfamily of proteins with von Willebrand factor type A-like domains: One theme common to components of extracellular matrix, hemostasis, cellular adhesion, and defense mechanisms. *Blood* 77:2305–2315, 1991.
24. Hunt LT, Barker WC: Von Willebrand factor shares a distinctive cysteine-rich domain with thrombospondin and procollagen. *Biochem Biophys Res Commun* 144:876–882, 1987.
25. Mancuso DJ, Tuley EA, Westfield LA, et al: Structure of the gene for human von Willebrand factor. *J Biol Chem* 264:19514–19527, 1989.
26. Shelton-Inloes BB, Chehab FF, Mannucci PM, et al: Gene deletions correlate with the development of alloantibodies in von Willebrand disease. *J Clin Invest* 79:1459–1465, 1987.
27. Mancuso DJ, Tuley EA, Westfield LA, et al: Human von Willebrand factor gene and pseudogene: Structural analysis and differentiation by polymerase chain reaction. *Biochemistry* 30:253–269, 1991.
28. Zhang ZP, Blomback M, Nyman D, Anvret M: Mutations of von Willebrand factor gene in families with von Willebrand disease in the Aland Islands. *Proc Natl Acad Sci U S A* 90:7937–7940, 1993.
29. Eikenboom JC, Vink T, Briet E, et al: Multiple substitutions in the von Willebrand factor gene that mimic the pseudogene sequence. *Proc Natl Acad Sci U S A* 91:2221–2224, 1994.
30. Eikenboom JC, Castaman G, Vos HL, et al: Characterization of the genetic defects in recessive type 1 and type 3 von Willebrand disease patients of Italian origin. *Thromb Haemost* 79:709–717, 1998.
31. James PD, Notley C, Hegadorn C, et al: The mutational spectrum of type 1 von Willebrand disease: Results from a Canadian cohort study. *Blood* 109:145–154, 2007.
32. Rand JH, Badimon L, Gordon RE, et al: Distribution of von Willebrand factor in porcine intima varies with blood vessel type and location. *Arteriosclerosis* 7:287–291, 1987.
33. Yamamoto K, de Waard V, Fearns C, Loskutoff DJ: Tissue distribution and regulation of murine von Willebrand factor gene expression *in vivo*. *Blood* 92:2791–2801, 1998.
34. Jahroudi N, Lynch DC: Endothelial-cell-specific regulation of von Willebrand factor gene expression. *Mol Cell Biol* 14:999–1008, 1994.
35. Harvey PJ, Keightley AM, Lam YM, et al: A single nucleotide polymorphism at nucleotide -1793 in the von Willebrand factor (VWF) regulatory region is associated with plasma VWF:Ag levels. *Br J Haematol* 109:349–353, 2000.
36. Guan J, Guillot PV, Aird WC: Characterization of the mouse von Willebrand factor promoter. *Blood* 94:3405–3412, 1999.
37. Hough C, Cuthbert CD, Notley C, et al: Cell type-specific regulation of von Willebrand factor expression by the E4BP4 transcriptional repressor. *Blood* 105:1531–1539, 2005.
38. Kleinschmidt AM, Nassiri M, Stitt MS, et al: Sequences in intron 51 of the von Willebrand factor gene target promoter activation to a subset of lung endothelial cells in transgenic mice. *J Biol Chem* 283:2741–2750, 2008.
39. Aird WC, Jahroudi N, Weiler-Guettler H, et al: Human von Willebrand factor gene sequences target expression to a subpopulation of endothelial cells in transgenic mice. *Proc Natl Acad Sci U S A* 92:4567–4571, 1995.
40. Bernat JA, Crawford GE, Ogurtsov AY, et al: Distant conserved sequences flanking endothelial-specific promoters contain specific DNase-hypersensitive sites and over-represented motifs. *Hum Mol Genet* 15:2098–2105, 2006.
41. Pusztaszeri MP, Seelentag W, Bosman FT: Immunohistochemical expression of endothelial markers CD31, CD34, von Willebrand factor, and Fli-1 in normal human tissues. *J Histochem Cytochem* 54:385–395, 2006.
42. Hough C, Cameron CL, Notley CR, et al: Influence of a GT repeat element on shear stress responsiveness of the VWF gene promoter. *J Thromb Haemost* 6:1183–1190, 2008.
43. Daidone V, Cattini MG, Pontara E, et al: Microsatellite (GT)(n) repeats and SNPs in the von Willebrand factor gene promoter do not influence circulating von Willebrand factor levels under normal conditions. *Thromb Haemost* 101:298–304, 2009.
44. Zhou YF, Eng ET, Zhu J, et al: Sequence and structure relationships within von Willebrand factor. *Blood* 120:449–458, 2012.
45. Ginsburg D, Bowie EJ: Molecular genetics of von Willebrand disease. *Blood* 79:2507–2519, 1992.
46. Wagner DD: Cell biology of von Willebrand factor. *Annu Rev Cell Biol* 6:217–246, 1990.
47. de Wit TR, van Mourik JA: Biosynthesis, processing and secretion of von Willebrand factor: Biological implications. *Best Pract Res Clin Haematol* 14:241–255, 2001.
48. Marti T, Rosselet SJ, Titani K, Walsh KA: Identification of disulfide-bridged substructures within human von Willebrand factor. *Biochemistry* 26:8099–8109, 1987.
49. Choi H, Aboulfatova K, Pownall HJ, et al: Shear-induced disulfide bond formation regulates adhesion activity of von Willebrand factor. *J Biol Chem* 282:35604–35611, 2007.
50. Wagner DD, Lawrence SO, Ohlsson-Wilhelm BM, et al: Topology and order of formation of interchain disulfide bonds in von Willebrand factor. *Blood* 69:27–32, 1987.
51. Voorberg J, Fontijn R, Calafat J, et al: Assembly and routing of von Willebrand factor variants: The requirements for disulfide-linked dimerization reside within the carboxy-terminal 151 amino acids. *J Cell Biol* 113:195–205, 1991.
52. Mayadas TN, Wagner DD: Vicinal cysteines play a role in von Willebrand factor multimer assembly. *Proc Natl Acad Sci U S A* 89:3531–3535, 1992.
53. Purvis AR, Sadler JE: A covalent oxidoreductase intermediate in propeptide-dependent von Willebrand factor multimerization. *J Biol Chem* 279:49982–49988, 2004.
54. Mayadas TN, Wagner DD: *In vitro* multimerization of von Willebrand factor is triggered by low pH: Importance of the propolypeptide and free sulfhydryls. *J Biol Chem* 264:13497–13503, 1989.
55. Wagner DD, Fay PJ, Sporn LA, et al: Divergent fates of von Willebrand factor and its propolypeptide (von Willebrand antigen II) after secretion from endothelial cells. *Proc Natl Acad Sci U S A* 84:1955–1959, 1987.
56. Verweij CL, Hart M, Pannekoek H: Expression of variant von Willebrand factor (vWF) cDNA in heterologous cells: Requirement of the pro-polypeptide in vWF multimer formation. *EMBO J* 6:2885–2890, 1987.
57. Wise RJ, Pittman DD, Handin RI, et al: The propeptide of von Willebrand factor independently mediates the assembly of von Willebrand multimers. *Cell* 52:229–236, 1988.
58. Rehemtulla A, Kaufman RJ: Preferred sequence requirements for cleavage of pro-von Willebrand propeptide-processing enzymes. *Blood* 79:2349–2355, 1992.
59. Wagner DD, Marder VJ: Biosynthesis of von Willebrand protein by human endothelial cells: Processing steps and their intracellular localization. *J Cell Biol* 99:2123–2130, 1984.
60. Lynch DC, Zimmerman TS, Ling EH, Browning PJ: An explanation for minor multimer species in endothelial cell-synthesized von Willebrand factor. *J Clin Invest* 77:2048–2051, 1986.
61. Verweij CL, Hart M, Pannekoek H: Proteolytic cleavage of the precursor of von Willebrand Factor is not essential for multimer formation. *J Biol Chem* 263:7921–7924, 1988.
62. Weibel ER, Palade GE: New cytoplasmic components in arterial endothelia. *J Biol Chem* 23:101–112, 1964.
63. Wagner DD, Olmsted JB, Marder VJ: Immunolocalization of von Willebrand protein in Weibel-Palade bodies of human endothelial cells. *J Cell Biol* 95:355–360, 1982.
64. Metcalf DJ, Nightingale TD, Zenner HL, et al: Formation and function of Weibel-Palade bodies. *J Cell Sci* 121:19–27, 2008.
65. Huang RH, Wang Y, Roth R, et al: Assembly of Weibel-Palade body-like tubules from N-terminal domains of von Willebrand factor. *Proc Natl Acad Sci U S A* 105:482–487, 2008.
66. Yarovoi H, Nurden AT, Montgomery RR, et al: Intracellular interaction of von Willebrand factor and factor VIII depends on cellular context: Lessons from platelet-expressed factor VIII. *Blood* 105:4674–4676, 2005.
67. Rosenberg JB, Foster PA, Kaufman RJ, et al: Intracellular trafficking of factor VIII to von Willebrand factor storage granules. *J Clin Invest* 101:613–624, 1998.
68. van den Biggelaar M, Bierings R, Storm G, et al: Requirements for cellular co-trafficking of factor VIII and von Willebrand factor to Weibel-Palade bodies. *J Thromb Haemost* 5:2235–2242, 2007.
69. Nightingale T, Cutler D: The secretion of von Willebrand factor from endothelial cells; an increasingly complicated story. *J Thromb Haemost* 11(Suppl 1):192–201, 2013.
70. Bonfanti R, Furie BC, Furie B, Wagner DD: PADGEM (GMP140) is a component of Weibel-Palade bodies of human endothelial cells. *Blood* 73:1109–1112, 1989.
71. Michaux G, Pullen TJ, Haberichter SL, Cutler DF: P-selectin binds to the D'-D3 domains of von Willebrand factor in Weibel-Palade bodies. *Blood* 107:3922–3924, 2006.
72. Cleator JH, Zhu WQ, Vaughan DE, Hamm HE: Differential regulation of endothelial exocytosis of P-selectin and von Willebrand factor by protease-activated receptors and cAMP. *Blood* 107:2736–2744, 2006.
73. Knop M, Aareskjold E, Bode G, Gerke V: Rab3D and annexin A2 play a role in regulated secretion of vWF, but not tPA, from endothelial cells. *EMBO J* 23:2982–2992, 2004.
74. Rondaij MG, Bierings R, Kragt A, et al: Dynamics and plasticity of Weibel-Palade bodies in endothelial cells. *Arterioscler Thromb Vasc Biol* 26:1002–1007, 2006.
75. Giblin JP, Hewlett LJ, Hannah MJ: Basal secretion of von Willebrand factor from human endothelial cells. *Blood* 112:957–964, 2008.
76. Levine JD, Harlan JM, Harker LA, et al: Thrombin-mediated release of factor VIII antigen from human umbilical vein endothelial cells in culture. *Blood* 60:531–534, 1982.
77. Ribes JA, Francis CW, Wagner DD: Fibrin induces release of von Willebrand factor from endothelial cells. *J Clin Invest* 79:117–123, 1987.
78. Hamilton KK, Sims PJ: Changes in cytosolic Ca²⁺ associated with von Willebrand factor release in human endothelial cells exposed to histamine. Study of microcarrier cell monolayers using the fluorescent probe indo-1. *J Clin Invest* 79:600–608, 1987.
79. Hattori R, Hamilton KK, McEver RP, Sims PJ: Complement proteins C5b-9 induce secretion of high molecular weight multimers of endothelial von Willebrand factor and translocation of granule membrane protein GMP-140 to the cell surface. *J Biol Chem* 264:9053–9060, 1989.
80. Bernardo A, Ball C, Nolasco L, et al: Effects of inflammatory cytokines on the release and cleavage of the endothelial cell-derived ultralarge von Willebrand factor multimers under flow. *Blood* 104:100–106, 2004.
81. Fish RJ, Yang H, Viglino C, et al: Fluvastatin inhibits regulated secretion of endothelial cell von Willebrand factor in response to diverse secretagogues. *Biochem J* 405:597–604, 2007.
82. Yamakuchi M, Greer JJ, Cameron SJ, et al: HMG-CoA reductase inhibitors inhibit endothelial exocytosis and decrease myocardial infarct size. *Circ Res* 96:1185–1192, 2005.

83. Kaufmann JE, Oksche A, Wollheim CB, et al: Vasopressin-induced von Willebrand factor secretion from endothelial cells involves V2 receptors and cAMP. *J Clin Invest* 106:107–116, 2000.

84. Sporn LA, Marder VJ, Wagner DD: Differing polarity of the constitutive and regulated secretory pathways for von Willebrand factor in endothelial cells. *J Cell Biol* 108:1283–1289, 1989.

85. Ewenstein BM, Warhol MJ, Handin RI, Pober JS: Composition of the von Willebrand factor storage organelle (Weibel-Palade body) isolated from cultured human umbilical vein endothelial cells. *J Cell Biol* 104:1423–1433, 1987.

86. Sporn LA, Marder VJ, Wagner DD: Inducible secretion of large, biologically potent von Willebrand factor multimers. *Cell* 46:185–190, 1986.

87. Fernandez MF, Ginsberg MH, Ruggeri ZM, et al: Multimeric structure of platelet factor VIII/von Willebrand factor: The presence of larger multimers and their reassociation with thrombin-stimulated platelets. *Blood* 60:1132–1138, 1982.

88. Wagner DD, Saffaripour S, Bonfanti R, et al: Induction of specific storage organelles by von Willebrand factor propolypeptide. *Cell* 64:403–413, 1991.

89. Voorberg J, Fontijn R, Calafat J, et al: Biogenesis of von Willebrand factor-containing organelles in heterologous transfected CV-1 cells. *EMBO J* 12:749–758, 1993.

90. Journet AM, Saffaripour S, Cramer EM, et al: von Willebrand factor storage requires intact prosequence cleavage site. *Eur J Cell Biol* 60:31–41, 1993.

91. Nachman RL, Jaffe EA: Subcellular platelet factor VIII antigen and von Willebrand factor. *J Exp Med* 141:1101–1113, 1975.

92. Bowie EJW, Solberg LA Jr, Fass DN, et al: Transplantation of normal bone marrow into a pig with severe von Willebrand's disease. *J Clin Invest* 78:26–30, 1986.

93. Nichols TC, Samama CM, Bellinger DA, et al: Function of von Willebrand factor after crossed bone marrow transplantation between normal and von Willebrand disease pigs: Effect on arterial thrombosis in chimeras. *Proc Natl Acad Sci U S A* 92:2455–2459, 1995.

94. André P, Brouland JP, Roussi J, et al: Role of plasma and platelet von Willebrand factor in arterial thrombogenesis and hemostasis in the pig. *Exp Hematol* 26:620–626, 1998.

95. Bowen DJ, Collins PW: Insights into von Willebrand factor proteolysis: Clinical implications. *Br J Haematol* 133:457–467, 2006.

96. Padilla A, Moake JL, Bernardo A, et al: P-selectin anchors newly released ultralarge von Willebrand factor multimers to the endothelial cell surface. *Blood* 103:2150–2156, 2004.

97. Lopez JA, Dong JF: Shear stress and the role of high molecular weight von Willebrand factor multimers in thrombus formation. *Blood Coagul Fibrinolysis* 16 Suppl 1:S11–S16, 2005.

98. Dent JA, Berkowitz SD, Ware J, et al: Identification of a cleavage site directing the immunochemical detection of molecular abnormalities in type IIA von Willebrand factor. *Proc Natl Acad Sci U S A* 87:6306–6310, 1990.

99. Lankhof H, Damas C, Schiphorst ME, et al: von Willebrand factor without the A2 domain is resistant to proteolysis. *Thromb Haemost* 77:1008–1013, 1997.

100. Tsai H-M, Sussman II, Ginsburg D, et al: Proteolytic cleavage of recombinant type 2A von Willebrand factor mutants R834W and R834Q: Inhibition by doxycycline and by monoclonal antibody VP-1. *Blood* 89:1954–1962, 1997.

101. Bowen DJ, Collins PW: An amino acid polymorphism in von Willebrand factor correlates with increased susceptibility to proteolysis by ADAMTS13. *Blood* 103:941–947, 2004.

102. Johnsen J, Lopez JA: VWF secretion: What's in a name? *Blood* 112:926–927, 2008.

103. Reininger AJ: Function of von Willebrand factor in haemostasis and thrombosis. *Haemophilia* 14 Suppl 5:11–26, 2008.

104. Savage B, Almus-Jacobs F, Ruggeri ZM: Specific synergy of multiple substrate-receptor interactions in platelet thrombus formation under flow. *Cell* 94:657–666, 1998.

105. Pendu R, Terraube V, Christophe OD, et al: P-selectin glycoprotein ligand 1 and beta2-integrins cooperate in the adhesion of leukocytes to von Willebrand factor. *Blood* 108:3746–3752, 2006.

106. Ruggeri ZM, Ware J, Ginsburg D: Von Willebrand factor, in *Thrombosis and Hemorrhage*, edited by J Loscalzo, AI Schafer, pp 246–265. Lippincott Williams & Wilkins, Philadelphia, 2003.

107. Kalafatis M, Takahashi Y, Girma J-P, Meyer D: Localization of a collagen-interactive domain of human von Willebrand factor between amino acid residues Gly 911 and Glu 1365. *Blood* 70:1577–1583, 1987.

108. Pareti FI, Niiya K, McPherson JM, Ruggeri ZM: Isolation and characterization of two domains of human von Willebrand Factor that interact with fibrillar collagen types I and III. *J Biol Chem* 262:13835–13841, 1987.

109. Takagi J, Sekiya F, Kasahara K, et al: Inhibition of platelet-collagen interaction by propolypeptide of von Willebrand factor. *J Biol Chem* 264:6017–6020, 1989.

110. Cruz MA, Yuan H, Lee JR, et al: Interaction of the von Willebrand factor (vWF) with collagen. Localization of the primary collagen-binding site by analysis of recombinant vWF A domain polypeptides. *J Biol Chem* 270:10822–10827, 1995.

111. Lankhof H, Van Hoeij M, Schiphorst ME, et al: A3 domain is essential for interaction of von Willebrand factor with collagen type III. *Thromb Haemost* 75:950–958, 1996.

112. Rand JH, Patel ND, Schwartz E, et al: 150-kD von Willebrand factor binding protein extracted from human vascular subendothelium is Type VI collagen. *J Clin Invest* 88:253–259, 1991.

113. Rand JH, Wu X-X, Potter BJ, et al: Co-localization of von Willebrand factor and type VI collagen in human vascular subendothelium. *Am J Pathol* 142:843–850, 1993.

114. Mazzucato M, Spessotto P, Masotti A, et al: Identification of domains responsible for von Willebrand factor type VI collagen interaction mediating platelet adhesion under high flow. *J Biol Chem* 274:3033–3041, 1999.

115. Fretto LJ, Fowler WE, McCaslin DR, et al: Substructure of human von Willebrand factor: Proteolysis by V8 and characterization of two functional domains. *J Biol Chem* 261:15679–15689, 1986.

116. Fujimura Y, Titani K, Holland LZ, et al: A heparin-binding domain of human von Willebrand factor. Characterization and localization to a tryptic fragment extending from amino acid residue Val[449] to Lys[728]. *J Biol Chem* 262:1734–1739, 1987.

117. Christophe O, Obert B, Meyer D, Girma J-P: The binding domain of von Willebrand factor to sulfatides is distinct from those interacting with glycoprotein Ib, heparin, collagen and residues between amino acid residues Leu 512 and Lys 673. *Blood* 78:2310–2317, 1991.

118. Yuan H, Deng N, Zhang S, et al: The unfolded von Willebrand factor response in bloodstream: The self-association perspective. *J Hematol Oncol* 5:65, 2012.

119. Marchese P, Murata M, Mazzucato M, et al: Identification of three tyrosine residues of glycoprotein IBα with distinct roles in von Willebrand factor and α-thrombin binding. *J Biol Chem* 270:9571–9578, 1995.

120. Fujimura Y, Titani K, Holland LZ, et al: von Willebrand factor: A reduced and alkylated 52/48-kDa fragment beginning at amino acid residue 449 contains the domain interacting with platelet glycoprotein Ib. *J Biol Chem* 261:381–385, 1986.

121. Mohri H, Fujimura Y, Shima M, et al: Structure of the von Willebrand factor domain interacting with glycoprotein Ib. *J Biol Chem* 263:17901–17904, 1988.

122. Nishio K, Anderson PJ, Zheng XL, Sadler JE: Binding of platelet glycoprotein Ibalpha to von Willebrand factor domain A1 stimulates the cleavage of the adjacent domain A2 by ADAMTS13. *Proc Natl Acad Sci U S A* 101:10578–10583, 2004.

123. Matsushita T, Sadler JE: Identification of amino acid residues essential for von Willebrand factor binding to platelet glycoprotein Ib. Charged-to-alanine scanning mutagenesis of the A1 domain of human von Willebrand factor. *J Biol Chem* 270:13406–13414, 1995.

124. Emsley J, Cruz M, Handin RI, Liddington R: Crystal structure of the von Willebrand factor A1 domain and implications for the binding of platelet glycoprotein Ib. *J Biol Chem* 273:10396–10401, 1998.

125. Chen J, Zhou H, Diacovo A, et al: Exploiting the kinetic interplay between GPIbα-VWF binding interfaces to regulate hemostasis and thrombosis. *Blood* 124:3799–3807, 2014.

126. Bienkowska J, Cruz M, Atiemo A, et al: The von Willebrand factor A3 domain does not contain a metal ion-dependent adhesion site motif. *J Biol Chem* 272:25162–25167, 1997.

127. Huizinga EG, van der Plas RM, Kroon J, et al: Crystal structure of the A3 domain of human von Willebrand factor: Implications for collagen binding. *Structure* 5:1147–1156, 1997.

128. Fukuda K, Doggett TA, Bankston LA, et al: Structural basis of von Willebrand factor activation by the snake toxin botrocetin. *Structure* 10:943–950, 2002.

129. Huizinga EG, Tsuji S, Romijn RA, et al: Structures of glycoprotein Ibalpha and its complex with von Willebrand factor A1 domain. *Science* 297:1176–1179, 2002.

130. Hulstein JJ, Lenting PJ, de Laat B, et al: beta2-Glycoprotein I inhibits von Willebrand factor dependent platelet adhesion and aggregation. *Blood* 110:1483–1491, 2007.

131. Scott JP, Montgomery RR, Retzinger GS: Dimeric ristocetin flocculates proteins, binds to platelets, and mediates von Willebrand factor-dependent agglutination of platelets. *J Biol Chem* 266:8149–8155, 1991.

132. Berndt MC, Du XP, Booth WJ: Ristocetin-dependent reconstitution of binding of von Willebrand factor to purified human platelet membrane glycoprotein Ib-IX complex. *Biochemistry* 27:633–640, 1988.

133. Adachi T, Matsushita T, Dong Z, et al: Identification of amino acid residues essential for heparin binding by the A1 domain of human von Willebrand factor. *Biochem Biophys Res Commun* 339:1178–1183, 2006.

134. Sobel M, McNeill PM, Carlson PL, et al: Heparin inhibition of von Willebrand factor-dependent platelet function *in vitro* and *in vivo*. *J Clin Invest* 87:1787–1793, 1991.

135. Sobel M, Bird KE, Tyler-Cross R, et al: Heparins designed to specifically inhibit platelet interactions with von Willebrand factor. *Circulation* 93:992–999, 1996.

136. Nishio K, Anderson PJ, Zheng XL, Sadler JE: Binding of platelet glycoprotein Ibalpha to von Willebrand factor domain A1 stimulates the cleavage of the adjacent domain A2 by ADAMTS13. *Proc Natl Acad Sci U S A* 101:10578–10583, 2004.

137. Keuren JF, Baruch D, Legendre P, et al: von Willebrand factor C1C2 domain is involved in platelet adhesion to polymerized fibrin at high shear rate. *Blood* 103:1741–1746, 2004.

138. Keuren JF, Baruch D, Legendre P, et al: von Willebrand factor C1C2 domain is involved in platelet adhesion to polymerized fibrin at high shear rate. *Blood* 103:1741–1746, 2004.

139. Vlot AJ, Koppelman SJ, van den Berg MH, et al: The affinity and stoichiometry of binding of human factor VIII to von Willebrand factor. *Blood* 85:3150–3157, 1995.

140. Terraube V, O'Donnell JS, Jenkins PV: Factor VIII and von Willebrand factor interaction: Biological, clinical and therapeutic importance. *Haemophilia* 16:3–13, 2010.

141. Cao W, Krishnaswamy S, Camire RM, et al: Factor VIII accelerates proteolytic cleavage of von Willebrand factor by ADAMTS13. *Proc Natl Acad Sci U S A* 105:7416–7421, 2008.

142. Foster PA, Fulcher CA, Marti T, et al: A major factor VIII binding domain resides within the amino-terminal 272 amino acid residues of von Willebrand factor. *J Biol Chem* 262:8443–8446, 1987.

143. Yee A, Gildersleeve RD, Gu S, et al: A von Willebrand factor fragment containing the D'D3 domains is sufficient to stabilize coagulation factor VIII in mice. *Blood* 124:445–452, 2014.

144. Bahou WF, Ginsburg D, Sikkink R, et al: A monoclonal antibody to von Willebrand factor (vWF) inhibits factor VIII binding. Localization of its antigenic determinant to a nonadecapeptide at the amino terminus of the mature vWF polypeptide. *J Clin Invest* 84:56–61, 1989.

145. Ginsburg D, Bockenstedt PL, Allen EA, et al: Fine mapping of monoclonal antibody epitopes on human von Willebrand factor using a recombinant peptide library. *Thromb Haemost* 67:166–171, 1992.

146. Mazurier C: Von Willebrand disease masquerading as haemophilia A. *Thromb Haemost* 67:391–396, 1992.

147. Lollar P, Hill-Eubanks DC, Parker CG: Association of the factor VIII light chain with von Willebrand Factor. *J Biol Chem* 263:10451–10455, 1988.

148. Leyte A, van Schijndel HB, Niehrs C, et al: Sulfation of Tyr[1680] of human blood coagulation factor VIII is essential for the interaction of factor VIII with von Willebrand factor. *J Biol Chem* 266:740–746, 1991.

149. Shiltagh N, Kirkpatrick J, Cabrita LD, et al: Solution structure of the major factor VIII binding region on von Willebrand factor. *Blood* 123:4143–4151, 2014.

150. National Heart Lung and Blood Institute (NHLBI): *The Diagnosis, Evaluation, and Management of von Willebrand Disease*. National Institutes of Health, Bethesda, MD, 2007.

151. Sadler JE, Budde U, Eikenboom JC, et al: Update on the pathophysiology and classification of von Willebrand disease: A report of the Subcommittee on von Willebrand Factor. *J Thromb Haemost* 4:2103–2114, 2006.

152. Flood VH, Friedman KD, Gill JC, et al: No increase in bleeding identified in type 1 VWD subjects with D1472H sequence variation. *Blood* 121:3742–3744, 2013.

153. Johnsen JM, Auer PL, Morrison AC, et al: Common and rare von Willebrand factor (VWF) coding variants, VWF levels, and factor VIII levels in African Americans: The NHLBI Exome Sequencing Project. *Blood* 122:590–597, 2013.

154. Wang QY, Song J, Gibbs RA, et al: Characterizing polymorphisms and allelic diversity of von Willebrand factor gene in the 1000 Genomes. *J Thromb Haemost* 11:261–269, 2013.

155. Flood VH, Gill JC, Morateck PA, et al: Common VWF exon 28 polymorphisms in African Americans affecting the VWF activity assay by ristocetin cofactor. *Blood* 116:280–286, 2010.

156. Weiss HJ, Piétu G, Rabinowitz R, et al: Heterogeneous abnormalities in the multimeric structure, antigenic properties, and plasma-platelet content of factor VIII/von Willebrand factor in subtypes of classic (type I) and variant (type IIA) von Willebrand's disease. *J Lab Clin Med* 101:411–425, 1983.

157. Hoyer LW, Rizza CR, Tuddenham EG, et al: Von Willebrand factor multimer patterns in von Willebrand's disease. *Br J Haematol* 55:493–507, 1983.

158. Mannucci PM, Lombardi R, Bader R, et al: Heterogeneity of type I von Willebrand disease: Evidence for a subgroup with an abnormal von Willebrand factor. *Blood* 66:796–802, 1985.

159. Mannucci PM: Platelet von Willebrand factor in inherited and acquired bleeding disorders. *Proc Natl Acad Sci U S A* 92:2428–2432, 1995.

160. Haberichter SL, Balistreri M, Christopherson P, et al: Assay of the von Willebrand factor (VWF) propeptide to identify patients with type 1 von Willebrand disease with decreased VWF survival. *Blood* 108:3344–3351, 2006.

161. Bowman M, Tuttle A, Notley C, et al: The genetics of Canadian type 3 von Willebrand disease: Further evidence for co-dominant inheritance of mutant alleles. *J Thromb Haemost* 9:1752–1760, 2011.

162. Goodeve A, Eikenboom J, Castaman G, et al: Phenotype and genotype of a cohort of families historically diagnosed with type 1 von Willebrand disease in the European study, Molecular and Clinical Markers for the Diagnosis and Management of Type 1 von Willebrand Disease (MCMDM-1VWD). *Blood* 109:112–121, 2007.

163. Robertson JD, Yenson PR, Rand ML, et al: Expanded phenotype-genotype correlations in a pediatric population with type 1 von Willebrand disease. *J Thromb Haemost* 9:1752–1760, 2011.

164. Eikenboom J, Hilbert L, Ribba AS, et al: Expression of 14 von Willebrand factor mutations identified in patients with type 1 von Willebrand disease from the MCMDM-1VWD study. *J Thromb Haemost* 7:1304–1312, 2009.

165. Wang JW, Valentijn KM, de Boer HC, et al: Intracellular storage and regulated secretion of von Willebrand factor in quantitative von Willebrand disease. *J Biol Chem* 286:24180–24188, 2011.

166. Pruss CM, Golder M, Bryant A, et al: Pathologic mechanisms of type 1 VWD mutations R1205H and Y1584C through in vitro and in vivo mouse models. *Blood* 117:4358–4366, 2011.

167. Millar CM, Riddell AF, Brown SA, et al: Survival of von Willebrand factor released following DDAVP in a type 1 von Willebrand disease cohort: Influence of glycosylation, proteolysis and gene mutations. *Thromb Haemost* 99:916–924, 2008.

168. Mohlke KL, Ginsburg D: Von Willebrand disease and quantitative deficiency of von Willebrand factor. *J Lab Clin Med* 130:252–261, 1997.

169. Eikenboom JC, Matsushita T, Reitsma PH, et al: Dominant type 1 von Willebrand disease caused by mutated cysteine residues in the D3 domain of von Willebrand factor. *Blood* 88:2433–2441, 1996.

170. Bodo I, Katsumi A, Tuley EA, et al: Type 1 von Willebrand disease mutation Cys-1149Arg causes intracellular retention and degradation of heterodimers: A possible general mechanism for dominant mutations of oligomeric proteins. *Blood* 98:2973–2979, 2001.

171. O'Brien LA, James PD, Othman M, et al: Founder von Willebrand factor haplotype associated with type 1 von Willebrand disease. *Blood* 102:549–557, 2003.

172. Bowen D: Type 1 von Willebrand disease: A possible novel mechanism. *Blood Coagul Fibrinolysis* 15 Suppl 1:S21–S23, 2004.

173. Bowen DJ, Collins PW, Lester W, et al: The prevalence of the cysteine1584 variant of von Willebrand factor is increased in type 1 von Willebrand disease: Co-segregation with increased susceptibility to ADAMTS13 proteolysis but not clinical phenotype. *Br J Haematol* 128:830–836, 2005.

174. Davies JA, Collins PW, Hathaway LS, Bowen DJ: Von Willebrand factor: Evidence for variable clearance *in vivo* according to Y/C1584 phenotype and ABO blood group. *J Thromb Haemost* 6:97–103, 2008.

175. Keeney S, Grundy P, Collins PW, Bowen DJ: C1584 in von Willebrand factor is necessary for enhanced proteolysis by ADAMTS13 in vitro. *Haemophilia* 13:405–408, 2007.

176. Desch KC, Ozel AB, Siemieniak D, et al: Linkage analysis identifies a locus for plasma von Willebrand factor undetected by genome-wide association. *Proc Natl Acad Sci U S A* 110:588–593, 2013.

177. Castaman G, Eikenboom JC, Bertina RM, Rodeghiero F: Inconsistency of association between type 1 von Willebrand disease phenotype and genotype in families identified in an epidemiological investigation. *Thromb Haemost* 82:1065–1070, 1999.

178. Kunicki TJ, Federici AB, Salomon DR, et al: An association of candidate gene haplotypes and bleeding severity in von Willebrand disease (VWD) type 1 pedigrees. *Blood* 104:2359–2367, 2004.

179. Kunicki TJ, Baronciani L, Canciani MT, et al: An association of candidate gene haplotypes and bleeding severity in von Willebrand disease type 2A, 2B, and 2M pedigrees. *J Thromb Haemost* 4:137–147, 2006.

180. Mohlke KL, Purkayastha AA, Westrick RJ, et al: *Mvwf*, a dominant modifier of murine von Willebrand factor, results from altered lineage-specific expression of a glycosyltransferase. *Cell* 96:111–120, 1999.

181. McKinnon TA, Chion AC, Millington AJ, et al: N-linked glycosylation of VWF modulates its interaction with ADAMTS13. *Blood* 111:3042–3049, 2008.

182. O'Donnell JS, McKinnon TA, Crawley JT, et al: Bombay phenotype is associated with reduced plasma-VWF levels and an increased susceptibility to ADAMTS13 proteolysis. *Blood* 106:1988–1991, 2005.

183. Bowen DJ: An influence of ABO blood group on the rate of proteolysis of von Willebrand factor by ADAMTS13. *J Thromb Haemost* 1:33–40, 2003.

184. Gallinaro L, Cattini MG, Sztukowska M, et al: A shorter von Willebrand factor survival in O blood group subjects explains how ABO determinants influence plasma von Willebrand factor. *Blood* 111:3540–3545, 2008.

185. Casari C, Lenting PJ, Wohner N, et al: Clearance of von Willebrand factor. *J Thromb Haemost* 11 Suppl 1:202–211, 2013.

186. Zimmerman TS, Abildgaard CF, Meyer D: The factor VIII abnormality in severe von Willebrand's disease. *N Engl J Med* 301:1307–1310, 1979.

187. Ngo KY, Glotz VT, Koziol JA, et al: Homozygous and heterozygous deletions of the von Willebrand factor gene in patients and carriers of severe von Willebrand Disease. *Proc Natl Acad Sci U S A* 85:2753–2757, 1988.

188. Peake IR, Liddell MB, Moodie P, et al: Severe type III von Willebrand's disease caused by deletion of exon 42 of the von Willebrand factor gene: Family studies that identify carriers of the condition and a compound heterozygous individual. *Blood* 75:654–661, 1990.

189. Mancuso DJ, Tuley EA, Castillo R, et al: Characterization of partial gene deletions in type III von Willebrand disease with alloantibody inhibitors. *Thromb Haemost* 72:180–185, 1994.

190. Xie F, Wang X, Cooper DN, et al: A novel Alu-mediated 61-kb deletion of the von Willebrand factor (VWF) gene whose breakpoints co-locate with putative matrix attachment regions. *Blood Cells Mol Dis* 36:385–391, 2006.

191. Cabrera N, Casaña P, Cid AR, et al: First application of MLPA method in severe von Willebrand disease. Confirmation of a new large VWF gene deletion and identification of heterozygous carriers. *Br J Haematol* 152:240–242, 2011.

192. Nichols WC, Lyons SE, Harrison JS, et al: Severe von Willebrand disease due to a defect at the level of von Willebrand factor mRNA expression: Detection by exonic PCR-restriction fragment length polymorphism analysis. *Proc Natl Acad Sci U S A* 88:3857–3861, 1991.

193. Eikenboom JC, Ploos van Amstel HK, Reitsma PH, Briët E: Mutations in severe, type III von Willebrand's disease in the Dutch population: Candidate missense and nonsense mutations associated with reduced levels of von Willebrand factor messenger RNA. *Thromb Haemost* 68:448–454, 1992.

194. Nichols WC, Ginsburg D: Von Willebrand disease. *Medicine (Baltimore)* 76:1–20, 1997.

195. Ginsburg D, Sadler JE: Von Willebrand disease: A database of point mutations, insertions, and deletions. *Thromb Haemost* 69:177–184, 1993.

196. Eikenboom JC, Castaman G, Vos HL, et al: Characterization of the genetic defects in recessive type 1 and type 3 von Willebrand disease patients of Italian origin. *Thromb Haemost* 79:709–717, 1998.

197. Zhang ZP, Falk G, Blombäck M, et al: A single cytosine deletion in exon 18 of the von Willebrand factor gene is the most common mutation in Swedish vWD type III patients. *Hum Mol Genet* 1:767–768, 1992.

198. Zhang ZP, Blombäck M, Nyman D, Anvret M: Mutations of von Willebrand factor gene in families with von Willebrand disease in the Åland Islands. *Proc Natl Acad Sci U S A* 90:7937–7940, 1993.

199. Mohlke KL, Ginsburg D: Von Willebrand disease and quantitative deficiency of von Willebrand factor. *J Lab Clin Med* 130:252–261, 1997.

200. Schneppenheim R, Krey S, Bergmann F, et al: Genetic heterogeneity of severe von Willebrand disease type III in the German population. *Hum Genet* 94:640–652, 1994.

201. Mohlke KL, Ginsburg D: Von Willebrand disease and quantitative deficiency of von Willebrand factor. *J Lab Clin Med* 130:252–261, 1997.

202. Berkowitz SD, Dent JA, Roberts J, et al: Epitope mapping of the von Willebrand factor subunit distinguishes fragments present in normal and type IIA von Willebrand Disease from those generated by plasmin. *J Clin Invest* 79:524–531, 1987.

203. Ginsburg D, Konkle BA, Gill JC, et al: Molecular basis of human von Willebrand disease: Analysis of platelet von Willebrand factor mRNA. *Proc Natl Acad Sci U S A* 86:3723–3727, 1989.
204. Hassenpflug WA, Budde U, Obser T, et al: Impact of mutations in the von Willebrand factor A2 domain on ADAMTS13-dependent proteolysis. *Blood* 107:2339–2345, 2006.
205. Jacobi PM, Gill JC, Flood VH, et al: Intersection of mechanisms of type 2A VWD through defects in VWF multimerization, secretion, ADAMTS-13 susceptibility, and regulated storage. *Blood* 119:4543–4553, 2012.
206. Lyons SE, Bruck ME, Bowie EJ, Ginsburg D: Impaired intracellular transport produced by a subset of type IIA von Willebrand disease mutations. *J Biol Chem* 267:4424–4430, 1992.
207. Dent JA, Galbusera M, Ruggeri ZM: Heterogeneity of plasma von Willebrand factor multimers resulting from proteolysis of the constituent subunit. *J Clin Invest* 88:774–782, 1991.
208. Gralnick HR, Williams SB, McKeown LP, et al: *In vitro* correction of the abnormal multimeric structure of von Willebrand factor in Type IIA von Willebrand's disease. *Proc Natl Acad Sci U S A* 82:5968–5972, 1985.
209. Kunicki TJ, Montgomery RR, Schullek J: Cleavage of human von Willebrand factor by platelet calcium-activated protease. *Blood* 65:352–356, 1985.
210. Chung DW, Fujikawa K: Processing of von Willebrand Factor by ADAMTS-13. *Biochemistry* 41:11065–11070, 2003.
211. Budde U: Diagnosis of von Willebrand disease subtypes: Implications for treatment. *Haemophilia* 14:27–38, 2008.
212. Schneppenheim R, Thomas KB, Krey S, et al: Identification of a candidate missense mutation in a family with von Willebrand disease type IIC. *Hum Genet* 95:681–686, 1995.
213. Gaucher C, Diéval J, Mazurier C: Characterization of von Willebrand factor gene defects in two unrelated patients with type IIC von Willebrand disease. *Blood* 84:1024–1030, 1994.
214. Haberichter SL, Budde U, Obser T, et al: The mutation N528S in the von Willebrand factor (VWF) propeptide causes defective multimerization and storage of VWF. *Blood* 115:4580–4587, 2010.
215. Schneppenheim R, Brassard J, Krey S, et al: Defective dimerization of von Willebrand factor subunits due to a Cys -> Arg mutation in type IID von Willebrand disease. *Proc Natl Acad Sci U S A* 93:3581–3586, 1996.
216. Cooney KA, Nichols WC, Bruck ME, et al: The molecular defect in type IIB von Willebrand disease. Identification of four potential missense mutations within the putative GpIb binding domain. *J Clin Invest* 87:1227–1233, 1991.
217. Ribba AS, Lavergne JM, Bahnak BR, et al: Duplication of a methionine within the glycoprotein Ib binding domain of von Willebrand factor detected by denaturing gradient gel electrophoresis in a patient with type IIB von Willebrand disease. *Blood* 78:1738–1743, 1991.
218. Cooney KA, Ginsburg D: Comparative analysis of type 2B von Willebrand disease mutations: Implications for the mechanism of von Willebrand factor to binding platelets. *Blood* 87:2322–2328, 1996.
219. Cooney KA, Lyons SE, Ginsburg D: Functional analysis of a type IIB von Willebrand disease missense mutation: Increased binding of large von Willebrand factor multimers to platelets. *Proc Natl Acad Sci U S A* 89:2869–2872, 1992.
220. Ware J, Dent JA, Azuma H, et al: Identification of a point mutation in type IIB von Willebrand disease illustrating the regulation of von Willebrand factor affinity for the platelet membrane glycoprotein Ib-IX receptor. *Proc Natl Acad Sci U S A* 88:2946–2950, 1991.
221. Kroner PA, Kluessendorf ML, Scott JP, Montgomery RR: Expressed full-length von Willebrand factor containing missense mutations linked to type IIB von Willebrand disease shows enhanced binding to platelets. *Blood* 79:2048–2055, 1992.
222. Randi AM, Jorieux S, Tuley EA, et al: Recombinant von Willebrand factor Arg578->Gln: A type IIB von Willebrand disease mutation affects binding to glycoprotein Ib but not to collagen or heparin. *J Biol Chem* 267:21187–21192, 1992.
223. Blenner MA, Dong X, Springer TA: Structural basis of regulation of von Willebrand factor binding to glycoprotein Ib. *J Biol Chem* 289:5565–5579, 2014.
224. Rayes J, Hollestelle MJ, Legendre P, et al: Mutation and ADAMTS13-dependent modulation of disease severity in a mouse model for von Willebrand disease type 2B. *Blood* 115:4870–4877, 2010.
225. Casari C, Du V, Wu YP, et al: Accelerated uptake of VWF/platelet complexes in macrophages contributes to VWD type 2B-associated thrombocytopenia. *Blood* 122:2893–2902, 2013.
226. Casari C, Berrou E, Lebret M, et al: von Willebrand factor mutation promotes thrombocytopathy by inhibiting integrin alphaIIbbeta3. *J Clin Invest* 123:5071–5081, 2013.
227. Golder M, Pruss CM, Hegadorn C, et al: Mutation-specific hemostatic variability in mice expressing common type 2B von Willebrand disease substitutions. *Blood* 115:4862–4869, 2010.
228. Ozeki M, Kunishima S, Kasahara K, et al: A family having type 2B von Willebrand disease with an R1306W mutation: Severe thrombocytopenia leads to the normalization of high molecular weight multimers. *Thromb Res* 125:e17–e22, 2010.
229. Holmberg L, Dent JA, Schneppenheim R, et al: von Willebrand factor mutation enhancing interaction with platelets in patients with normal multimeric structure. *J Clin Invest* 91:2169–2177, 1993.
230. Veltkamp JJ, van Tilburg NH: Autosomal haemophilia: A variant of von Willebrand's disease. *Br J Haematol* 26:141–152, 1974.
231. Graham JB, Barrow ES, Roberts HR, et al: Dominant inheritance of hemophilia A in three generations of women. *Blood* 46:175–188, 1975.
232. Mazurier C, Gaucher C, Jorieux S, et al: Evidence for a von Willebrand factor defect in factor VIII binding in three members of a family previously misdiagnosed mild haemophilia A and haemophilia A carriers: Consequences for therapy and genetic counselling. *Br J Haematol* 76:372–379, 1990.
233. Mazurier C, Diéval J, Jorieux S, et al: A new von Willebrand Factor (vWF) defect in a patient with factor VIII (FVIII) deficiency but with normal levels and multimeric patterns of both plasma and platelet vWF. Characterization of abnormal vWF/FVIII interaction. *Blood* 75:20–26, 1990.
234. Nishino M, Girma J-P, Rothschild C, et al: New variant of von Willebrand disease with defective binding to factor VIII. *Blood* 74:1591–1599, 1989.
235. Hampshire DJ, Goodeve AC: The international society on thrombosis and haematosis von Willebrand disease database: An update. *Semin Thromb Hemost* 37:470–479, 2011.
236. Eikenboom JC, Reitsma PH, Peerlinck KM, Briët E: Recessive inheritance of von Willebrand's disease type I. *Lancet* 341:982–986, 1993.
237. Castaman G, Giacomelli SH, Jacobi P, et al: Homozygous type 2N R854W von Willebrand factor is poorly secreted and causes a severe von Willebrand disease phenotype. *J Thromb Haemost* 8:2011–2016, 2010.
238. Gupta M, Lillicrap D, Stain AM, Friedman KD, Carcao MD: Therapeutic consequences for misdiagnosis of type 2N von Willebrand disease. *Pediatr Blood Cancer* 57:1081–1083, 2011.
239. Nichols WC, Cooney KA, Ginsburg D, Ruggeri ZM: Von Willebrand disease, in *Thrombosis and Hemorrhage*, edited by J Loscalzo, AI Schafer, pp 539–559. Lipincott Williams & Wilkins, Philadelphia, 2003.
240. Meyer D, Fressinaud E, Gaucher C, et al: Gene defects in 150 unrelated French cases with type 2 von Willebrand disease: From the patient to the gene. *Thromb Haemost* 78:451–456, 1997.
241. McKinnon TA, Nowak AA, Cutler J, et al: Characterisation of von Willebrand factor A1 domain mutants I1416N and I1416T: Correlation of clinical phenotype with flow-based platelet adhesion. *J Thromb Haemost* 10:1409–1416, 2012.
242. Larsen DM, Haberichter SL, Gill JC, et al: Variability in platelet- and collagen-binding defects in type 2M von Willebrand disease. *Haemophilia* 19:590–594, 2013.
243. Mannucci PM, Lombardi R, Castaman G, et al: von Willebrand disease "Vicenza" with larger-than-normal (supranormal) von Willebrand factor multimers. *Blood* 71:65–70, 1988.
244. Randi AM, Sacchi E, Castaman GC, et al: The genetic defect of type I von Willebrand disease "Vicenza" is linked to the von Willebrand factor gene. *Thromb Haemost* 69:173–176, 1993.
245. Casonato A, Pontara E, Sartorello F, et al: Reduced von Willebrand factor survival in type Vicenza von Willebrand disease. *Blood* 99:180–184, 2002.
246. Castaman G, Rodeghiero F, Mannucci PM: The elusive pathogenesis of von Willebrand disease Vicenza. *Blood* 99:4243–4244, 2002.
247. Gezsi A, Budde U, Deak I, et al: Accelerated clearance alone explains ultra-large multimers in von Willebrand disease Vicenza. *J Thromb Haemost* 8:1273–1280, 2010.
248. Berkowitz SD, Ruggeri ZM, Zimmerman TS: Von Willebrand disease, in *Coagulation and Bleeding Disorders. The Role of Factor VIII and von Willebrand Factor*, edited by TS Zimmerman, ZM Ruggeri, pp 215–259. Marcel Dekker, New York, 1989.
249. Miller CH, Graham JB, Goldin LR, Elston RC: Genetics of classic von Willebrand's disease. I. Phenotypic variation within families. *Blood* 54:117–145, 1979.
250. Gill JC, Endres-Brooks J, Bauer PJ, et al: The effect of ABO blood group on the diagnosis of von Willebrand disease. *Blood* 69:1691–1695, 1987.
251. Orstavik KH, Kornstad L, Reisner H, Berg K: Possible effect of secretor locus on plasma concentration of Factor VIII and von Willebrand factor. *Blood* 73:990–993, 1989.
252. O'Donnell J, Boulton FE, Manning RA, Laffan MA: Genotype at the secretor blood group locus is a determinant of plasma von Willebrand factor level. *Br J Haematol* 116:350–356, 2002.
253. Franchini M, Crestani S, Frattini F, et al: ABO blood group and von Willebrand factor: Biological implications. *Clin Chem Lab Med* 52:1273–1276, 2014.
254. Antoni G, Oudot-Mellakh T, Dimitromanolakis A, et al: Combined analysis of three genome-wide association studies on vWF and FVIII plasma levels. *BMC Med Genet* 12:102, 2011.
255. Smith NL, Chen MH, Dehghan A, et al: Novel associations of multiple genetic loci with plasma levels of factor VII, factor VIII, and von Willebrand factor: The CHARGE (Cohorts for Heart and Aging Research in Genome Epidemiology) Consortium. *Circulation* 121:1382–1392, 2010.
256. Zhu Q, Yamakuchi M, Ture S, et al: Syntaxin-binding protein STXBP5 inhibits endothelial exocytosis and promotes platelet secretion. *J Clin Invest* 124:4503–4516, 2014.
257. Ye S, Huang Y, Joshi S, et al: Platelet secretion and hemostasis require syntaxin-binding protein STXBP5. *J Clin Invest* 124:4517–4528, 2014.
258. Rydz N, Swystun LL, Notley C, et al: The C-type lectin receptor CLEC4M binds, internalizes, and clears von Willebrand factor and contributes to the variation in plasma von Willebrand factor levels. *Blood* 121:5228–5237, 2013.
259. Desch KC, Ozel AB, Siemieniak D, et al: Linkage analysis identifies a locus for plasma von Willebrand factor undetected by genome-wide association. *Proc Natl Acad Sci U S A* 110:588–593, 2013.
260. Werner EJ, Broxson EH, Tucker EL, et al: Prevalence of von Willebrand disease in children: A multiethnic study. *J Pediatr* 123:893–898, 1993.
261. Rodeghiero F, Castaman G, Dini E: Epidemiological investigation of the prevalence of von Willebrand's disease. *Blood* 69:454–459, 1987.

262. Sadler JE: Von Willebrand disease type 1: A diagnosis in search of a disease. *Blood* 101:2089–2093, 2003.

263. Lillicrap D: Von Willebrand disease: Advances in pathogenetic understanding, diagnosis, and therapy. *Blood* 122:3735–3740, 2013.

264. Weiss HJ, Ball AP, Mannucci PM: Incidence of severe von Willebrand's disease. *N Engl J Med* 307:127, 1982.

265. Berliner SA, Seligsohn U, Zivelin A, et al: A relatively high frequency of severe (type III) von Willebrand's disease in Israel. *Br J Haematol* 62:535–543, 1986.

266. Mannucci PM, Bloom AL, Larrieu MJ, et al: Atherosclerosis and von Willebrand factor. I. Prevalence of severe von Willebrand's disease in western Europe and Israel. *Br J Haematol* 57:163–169, 1984.

267. Nosek-Cenkowska B, Cheang MS, Pizzi NJ, et al: Bleeding/bruising symptomatology in children with and without bleeding disorders. *Thromb Haemost* 65:237–241, 1991.

268. Rydz N, James PD: The evolution and value of bleeding assessment tools. *J Thromb Haemost* 10:2223–2229, 2012.

269. Elbatarny M, Mollah S, Grabell J, et al: Normal range of bleeding scores for the ISTH-BAT: Adult and pediatric data from the merging project. *Haemophilia* 20:831–835, 2014.

270. Federici AB, Bucciarelli P, Castaman G, et al: The bleeding score predicts clinical outcomes and replacement therapy in adults with von Willebrand disease. *Blood* 123:4037–4044, 2014.

271. van den Driesche S, Mummery CL, Westermann CJ: Hereditary hemorrhagic telangiectasia: An update on transforming growth factor beta signaling in vasculogenesis and angiogenesis. *Cardiovasc Res* 58:20–31, 2003.

272. Iannuzzi MC, Hidaka N, Boehnke ML, et al: Analysis of the relationship of von Willebrand disease (vWD) and hereditary hemorrhagic telangiectasia and identification of a potential type IIA vWD mutation (IIe865 to Thr). *Am J Hum Genet* 48:757–763, 1991.

273. Rick ME, Williams SB, Sacher RA, McKeown LP: Thrombocytopenia associated with pregnancy in a patient with type IIB von Willebrand's disease. *Blood* 69:786–789, 1987.

274. Mazurier C, Parquet-Gernez A, Goudemand J, et al: Investigation of a large kindred with type IIB von Willebrand's disease, dominant inheritance and age-dependent thrombocytopenia. *Br J Haematol* 69:499–505, 1988.

275. Gupta M, Lillicrap D, Stain AM, et al: Therapeutic consequences for misdiagnosis of type 2N von Willebrand disease. *Pediatr Blood Cancer* 57:1081–1083, 2011.

276. Schneppenheim R, Budde U, Krey S, et al: Results of a screening for von Willebrand disease type 2N in patients with suspected haemophilia A or von Willebrand disease type 1. *Thromb Haemost* 76:598–602, 1996.

277. James PD, Lillicrap D, Mannucci PM: Alloantibodies in von Willebrand disease. *Blood* 122:636–640, 2013.

278. Asatiani E, Kessler CM: Multiple congenital coagulopathies co-expressed with von Willebrand's disease: The experience of Hemophilia Region III Treatment Centers over 25 years and review of the literature. *Haemophilia* 13:685–696, 2007.

279. Lippi G, Franchini M, Poli G, et al: Is the activated partial thromboplastin time suitable to screen for von Willebrand factor deficiencies? *Blood Coagul Fibrinolysis* 18:361–364, 2007.

280. Abildgaard CF, Suzuki Z, Harrison J, et al: Serial studies in von Willebrand's disease: Variability versus "variants." *Blood* 56:712–716, 1980.

281. Timm A, Fahrenkrug J, Jorgensen HL, et al: Diurnal variation of von Willebrand factor in plasma: The Bispebjerg study of diurnal variations. *Eur J Haematol* 93:48–53, 2014.

282. Sadler JE: Von Willebrand disease type 1: A diagnosis in search of a disease. *Blood* 101:2089–2093, 2003.

283. Sadler JE: New concepts in von Willebrand disease. *Annu Rev Med* 56:173–191, 2005.

284. Quiroga T, Goycoolea M, Belmont S, et al: Quantitative impact of using different criteria for the laboratory diagnosis of type 1 von Willebrand disease. *J Thromb Haemost* 12:1238–1243, 2014.

285. Hayward CP, Moffat KA, Plumhoff E, Van Cott EM: Approaches to investigating common bleeding disorders: An evaluation of North American coagulation laboratory practices. *Am J Hematol* 87 Suppl 1:S45–S50, 2012.

286. Favaloro EJ, Bonar R, Chapman K, et al: Differential sensitivity of von Willebrand factor (VWF) "activity" assays to large and small VWF molecular weight forms: A cross-laboratory study comparing ristocetin cofactor, collagen-binding and mAb-based assays. *J Thromb Haemost* 10:1043–1054, 2012.

287. Eikenboom J, Federici AB, Dirven RJ, et al: VWF propeptide and ratios between VWF, VWF propeptide, and FVIII in the characterization of type 1 von Willebrand disease. *Blood* 121:2336–2339, 2013.

288. Weiss HJ, Hoyer LW, Rickles FR, et al: Quantitative assay of a plasma factor deficient in von Willebrand's disease that is necessary for platelet aggregation. *J Clin Invest* 52:2708–2716, 1973.

289. Rodeghiero F, Castaman G, Tosetto A: Von Willebrand factor antigen is less sensitive than ristocetin cofactor for the diagnosis of type I von Willebrand disease-results based on an epidemiological investigation. *Thromb Haemost* 64:349–352, 1990.

290. Favaloro EJ: Diagnosis and classification of von Willebrand disease: A review of the differential utility of various functional von Willebrand factor assays. *Blood Coagul Fibrinolysis* 22:553–564, 2011.

291. Ruggeri ZM, Zimmerman TS: The complex multimeric composition of factor VIII/von Willebrand factor. *Blood* 57:1140–1143, 1981.

292. Budde U, Schneppenheim R, Eikenboom J, et al: Detailed von Willebrand factor multimer analysis in patients with von Willebrand disease in the European study, molecular and clinical markers for the diagnosis and management of type 1 von Willebrand disease (MCMDM-1VWD). *J Thromb Haemost* 6:762–771, 2008.

293. Flood VH, Gill JC, Friedman KD, et al: Collagen binding provides a sensitive screen for variant von Willebrand disease. *Clin Chem* 59:684–691, 2013.

294. Flood VH, Lederman CA, Wren JS, et al: Absent collagen binding in a VWF A3 domain mutant: Utility of the VWF:CB in diagnosis of VWD. *J Thromb Haemost* 8:1431–1433, 2010.

295. Flood VH, Gill JC, Christopherson PA, et al: Critical von Willebrand factor A1 domain residues influence type VI collagen binding. *J Thromb Haemost* 10:1417–1424, 2012.

296. Favaloro EJ, Dean M, Grispo L, et al: Von Willebrand's disease: Use of collagen binding assay provides potential improvement to laboratory monitoring of desmopressin (DDAVP) therapy. *Am J Hematol* 45:205–211, 1994.

297. Riddell AF, Jenkins PV, Nitu-Whalley IC, et al: Use of the collagen-binding assay for von Willebrand factor in the analysis of type 2M von Willebrand disease: A comparison with the ristocetin cofactor assay. *Br J Haematol* 116:187–192, 2002.

298. Popov J, Zhukov O, Ruden S, et al: Performance and clinical utility of a commercial von Willebrand factor collagen binding assay for laboratory diagnosis of von Willebrand disease. *Clin Chem* 52:1965–1967, 2006.

299. Meiring M, Badenhorst PN, Kelderman M: Performance and utility of a cost-effective collagen-binding assay for the laboratory diagnosis of Von Willebrand disease. *Clin Chem Lab Med* 45:1068–1072, 2007.

300. Mazurier C, Meyer D: Factor VIII binding assay of von Willebrand factor and the diagnosis of type 2N von Willebrand disease-results of an international survey. On behalf of the Subcommittee on von Willebrand Factor of the Scientific and Standardization Committee of the ISTH. *Thromb Haemost* 76:270–274, 1996.

301. Zhukov O, Popov J, Ramos R, et al: Measurement of von Willebrand factor-FVIII binding activity in patients with suspected von Willebrand disease type 2N: Application of an ELISA-based assay in a reference laboratory. *Haemophilia* 15:788–796, 2009.

302. Casonato A, Pontara E, Sartorello F, et al: Identifying carriers of type 2N von Willebrand disease: Procedures and significance. *Clin Appl Thromb Hemost* 13:194–200, 2007.

303. Haberichter SL, Balistreri M, Christopherson P, et al: Assay of the von Willebrand factor (VWF) propeptide to identify patients with type 1 von Willebrand disease with decreased VWF survival. *Blood* 108:3344–3351, 2006.

304. Haberichter SL, Castaman G, Budde U, et al: Identification of type 1 von Willebrand disease patients with reduced von Willebrand factor survival by assay of the VWF propeptide in the European study: Molecular and clinical markers for the diagnosis and management of type 1 VWD (MCMDM-1VWD). *Blood* 111:4979–4985, 2008.

305. Casonato A, Pontara E, Sartorello F, et al: Identifying type Vicenza von Willebrand disease. *J Lab Clin Med* 147:96–102, 2006.

306. Fressinaud E, Veyradier A, Truchaud F, et al: Screening for von Willebrand disease with a new analyzer using high shear stress: A study of 60 cases. *Blood* 91:1325–1331, 1998.

307. Cattaneo M, Federici AB, Lecchi A, et al: Evaluation of the PFA-100 system in the diagnosis and therapeutic monitoring of patients with von Willebrand disease. *Thromb Haemost* 82:35–39, 1999.

308. De Vleeschauwer A, Devreese K: Comparison of a new automated von Willebrand factor activity assay with an aggregation von Willebrand ristocetin cofactor activity assay for the diagnosis of von Willebrand disease. *Blood Coagul Fibrinolysis* 17:353–358, 2006.

309. Salem RO, Van Cott EM: A new automated screening assay for the diagnosis of von Willebrand disease. *Am J Clin Pathol* 127:730–735, 2007.

310. Sucker C, Senft B, Scharf RE, Zotz RB: Determination of von Willebrand factor activity: Evaluation of the HaemosIL assay in comparison with established procedures. *Clin Appl Thromb Hemost* 12:305–310, 2006.

311. Pinol M, Sales M, Costa M, et al: Evaluation of a new turbidimetric assay for von Willebrand factor activity useful in the general screening of von Willebrand disease. *Haematologica* 92:712–713, 2007.

312. Fujimura Y, Kawasaki T, Titani K: Snake venom proteins modulating the interaction between von Willebrand factor and platelet glycoprotein Ib. *Thromb Haemost* 76:633–639, 1996.

313. Keeney S, Bowen D, Cumming A, et al: The molecular analysis of von Willebrand disease: A guideline from the UK Haemophilia Centre Doctors' Organisation Haemophilia Genetics Laboratory Network. *Haemophilia* 14:1099–1111, 2008.

314. Snyder MW, Simmons LE, Kitzman JO, et al: Noninvasive fetal genome sequencing: A primer. *Prenat Diagn* 33:547–554, 2013.

315. James PD, Lillicrap D: The molecular characterization of von Willebrand disease: Good in parts. *Br J Haematol* 161:166–176, 2013.

316. Othman M, Kaur H, Emsley J: Platelet-type von Willebrand disease: New insights into the molecular pathophysiology of a unique platelet defect. *Semin Thromb Hemost* 39:663–673, 2013.

317. Federici AB, Budde U, Castaman G, et al: Current diagnostic and therapeutic approaches to patients with acquired von Willebrand syndrome: A 2013 update. *Semin Thromb Hemost* 39:191–201, 2013.

318. Budde U, Schaefer G, Mueller N, et al: Acquired von Willebrand's disease in the myeloproliferative syndrome. *Blood* 64:981–985, 1984.

319. Kos CA, Ward JE, Malek K, et al: Association of acquired von Willebrand syndrome with AL amyloidosis. *Am J Hematol* 82:363–367, 2007.

320. Mannucci PM, Lombardi R, Bader R, et al: Studies of the pathophysiology of acquired von Willebrand's disease in seven patients with lymphoproliferative disorders or benign monoclonal gammopathies. *Blood* 64:614–621, 1984.

321. Rogers JS, Shane SR, Jencks FS: Factor VIII activity and thyroid function. *Ann Intern Med Intern Med* 97:713–716, 1982.

322. Viallard JF, Pellegrin JL, Vergnes C, et al: Three cases of acquired von Willebrand disease associated with systemic lupus erythematosus. *Br J Haematol* 105:532–537, 1999.

323. Scott JP, Montgomery RR, Tubergen DG, Hays T: Acquired von Willebrand's disease in association with Wilm's tumor: Regression following treatment. *Blood* 58:665–669, 1981.

324. Warkentin TE, Moore JC, Morgan DG: Aortic stenosis and bleeding gastrointestinal angiodysplasia: Is acquired von Willebrand's disease the link? *Lancet* 340:35–37, 1992.

325. Geisen U, Heilmann C, Beyersdorf F, et al: Non-surgical bleeding in patients with ventricular assist devices could be explained by acquired von Willebrand disease. *Eur J Cardiothorac Surg* 33:679–684, 2008.

326. Castaman G, Lattuada A, Mannucci PM, Rodeghiero F: Characterization of two cases of acquired transitory von Willebrand syndrome with ciprofloxacin: Evidence for heightened proteolysis of von Willebrand factor. *Am J Hematol* 49:83–86, 1995.

327. Tefferi A, Nichols WL: Acquired von Willebrand disease: Concise review of occurrence, diagnosis, pathogenesis, and treatment. *Am J Med* 103:536–540, 1997.

328. Kumar S, Pruthi RK, Nichols WL: Acquired von Willebrand disease. *Mayo Clin Proc* 77:181–187, 2002.

329. Kanakry JA, Gladstone DE: Maintaining hemostasis in acquired von Willebrand syndrome: A review of intravenous immunoglobulin and the importance of rituximab dose scheduling. *Transfusion* 53:1730–1735, 2013.

330. Svensson PJ, Bergqvist PB, Juul KV, Berntorp E: Desmopressin in treatment of haematological disorders and in prevention of surgical bleeding. *Blood Rev* 28:95–102, 2014.

331. Abshire TC, Federici AB, Alvarez MT, et al: Prophylaxis in severe forms of von Willebrand's disease: Results from the von Willebrand Disease Prophylaxis Network (VWD PN). *Haemophilia* 19:76–81, 2013.

332. Mannucci PM, Ruggeri ZM, Pareti FI, Capitanio A: 1-Deamino-8-d-arginine vasopressin: A new pharmacological approach to the management of haemophilia and von Willebrands' diseases. *Lancet* 1:869–872, 1977.

333. Ruggeri ZM, Mannucci PM, Lombardi R, Federici AB, Zimmerman TS: Multimeric composition of factor VIII/von Willebrand Factor following administration of DDAVP: Implications for pathophysiology and therapy of von Willebrand's disease subtypes. *Blood* 59:1272–1278, 1982.

334. Mannucci PM: Desmopressin (DDAVP) in the treatment of bleeding disorders: The first 20 years. *Blood* 90:2515–2521, 1997.

335. Federici AB, Mazurier C, Berntorp E, et al: Biologic response to desmopressin in patients with severe type 1 and type 2 von Willebrand disease: Results of a multicenter European study. *Blood* 103:2032–2038, 2004.

336. Lethagen S, Harris AS, Nilsson IM: Intranasal desmopressin (DDAVP) by spray in mild hemophilia A and von Willebrand's disease type I. *Blut* 60:187–191, 1990.

337. Rose EH, Aledort LM: Nasal spray desmopressin (DDAVP) for mild hemophilia A and von Willebrand disease. *Ann Intern Med Intern Med* 114:563–568, 1991.

338. Rodeghiero F, Castaman G, Di Bona E, Ruggeri M: Consistency of responses to repeated DDAVP infusions in patients with von Willebrand's disease and hemophilia A. *Blood* 74:1997–2000, 1989.

339. Castaman G, Lethagen S, Federici AB, et al: Response to desmopressin is influenced by the genotype and phenotype in type 1 von Willebrand disease (VWD): Results from the European Study MCMDM-1VWD. *Blood* 111:3531–3539, 2008.

340. Mannucci PM, Bettega D, Cattaneo M: Patterns of development of tachyphylaxis in patients with haemophilia and von Willebrand disease after repeated doses of desmopressin (DDAVP). *Br J Haematol* 82:87–93, 1992.

341. Federici AB, Mazurier C, Berntorp E, et al: Biologic response to desmopressin in patients with severe type 1 and type 2 von Willebrand disease: Results of a multicenter European study. *Blood* 103:2032–2038, 2004.

342. de la Fuente B, Kasper CK, Rickles FR, Hoyer LW: Response of patients with mild and moderate hemophilia A and von Willebrand's disease to treatment with desmopressin. *Ann Intern Med* 103:6–14, 1985.

343. Gralnick HR, Williams SB, McKeown LP, et al: DDAVP in type IIa von Willebrand's disease. *Blood* 67:465–468, 1986.

344. Mannucci PM: Treatment of von Willebrand's disease. *N Engl J Med* 351:683–694, 2004.

345. Casonato A, Sartori MT, De Marco L, Girolami A: 1-Desamino-8-D-arginine vasopressin (DDAVP) infusion in type IIB von Willebrand's disease: Shortening of bleeding time and induction of a variable pseudothrombocytopenia. *Thromb Haemost* 64: 117–120, 1990.

346. McKeown LP, Connaghan G, Wilson O, et al: 1-Desamino-8-arginine-vasopressin corrects the hemostatic defects in type 2B von Willebrand's disease. *Am J Hematol* 51: 158–163, 1996.

347. Mazurier C, Gaucher C, Jorieux S, Goudemand M: Biological effect of desmopressin in eight patients with type 2N ("Normandy") von Willebrand disease. Collaborative Group. *Br J Haematol* 88:849–854, 1994.

348. Mannucci PM, Kempton C, Millar C, et al: Pharmacokinetics and safety of a novel recombinant human von Willebrand factor manufactured with a plasma-free method: A prospective clinical trial. *Blood* 122:648–657, 2013.

349. Morfini M, Mannucci PM, Tenconi PM, et al: Pharmacokinetics of monoclonally-purified and recombinant factor VIII in patients with severe von Willebrand disease. *Thromb Haemost* 70:270–272, 1993.

350. Makris M, Colvin B, Gupta V, et al: Venous thrombosis following the use of intermediate purity FVIII concentrate to treat patients with von Willebrand's disease. *Thromb Haemost* 88:387–388, 2002.

351. Mannucci PM, Chediak J, Hanna W, et al: Treatment of von Willebrand disease with a high-purity factor VIII/von Willebrand factor concentrate: A prospective, multicenter study. *Blood* 99:450–456, 2002.

352. Coppola A, Franchini M, Makris M, et al: Thrombotic adverse events to coagulation factor concentrates for treatment of patients with haemophilia and von Willebrand disease: A systematic review of prospective studies. *Haemophilia* 18:e173–e187, 2012.

353. James AH, Konkle BA, Kouides P, et al: Postpartum von Willebrand factor levels in women with and without von Willebrand disease and implications for prophylaxis. *Haemophilia* 21:81–87, 2015.

354. Sucker C, Scharf RE, Zotz RB: Use of recombinant factor VIIa in inherited and acquired von Willebrand disease. *Clin Appl Thromb Hemost* 15:27–31, 2009.

CHAPTER 127
ANTIBODY-MEDIATED COAGULATION FACTOR DEFICIENCIES

Sean R. Stowell, John S. (Pete) Lollar, and Shannon L. Meeks

SUMMARY

Clinically significant autoantibodies to coagulation factors deficiencies are uncommon, but can produce life-threatening bleeding and death. The most commonly targeted coagulation factor in autoimmunity is factor VIII. Acquired hemophilia A, which results from these antibodies, can either be idiopathic or associated with older age, other autoimmune disorders, malignancy, the postpartum period, and the use of drugs such as penicillin and sulfonamides. Bleeding in acquired hemophilia A is treated with factor VIII bypassing agents. The underlying autoimmune disorder frequently responds to immunosuppressive medication. Antiprothrombin antibodies usually are found in patients with lupus anticoagulant and are associated with bleeding. Antibodies of von Willebrand factor are found in patients with type 3 von Willebrand disease in response to infusion of plasma concentrates containing von Willebrand factor. Antibodies to factor V can occur as autoantibodies or as cross-reacting antibovine factor V antibodies that develop after exposure to bovine thrombin products that are contaminated with factor V. Pathogenic autoantibodies also have been described that target thrombin, factor IX, factor XI, factor XIII, protein C, protein S, and the endothelial cell protein C receptor.

DEFINITION AND HISTORY

Antibodies directed against coagulation factors can develop as an acquired, autoimmune phenomenon. These "circulating anticoagulants" or "inhibitors" were recognized as early as 1906 as a cause of an acquired bleeding disorder.[1] The most common coagulation factor targeted in autoimmunity is factor VIII. The key feature that distinguishes antibody-mediated from other acquired coagulation factor deficiencies, such as impaired synthesis (e.g., a result of vitamin K deficiency) or increased consumption (e.g., in disseminated intravascular coagulation), is the ability of the patient's plasma to inhibit the coagulation of normal plasma. Inhibitors also can develop in response to replacement therapy in patients with congenital coagulation factor deficiencies as discussed in Chap. 123.

ACQUIRED HEMOPHILIA A

DEFINITIONS AND EPIDEMIOLOGY

The incidence of autoantibodies to factor VIII, which is the most commonly targeted coagulation factor in autoimmunity, is 1.4 per million people per year.[2-4] The associated clinical condition is called acquired hemophilia A. Approximately 40 to 50 percent of acquired hemophilia A patients have underlying conditions, including other autoimmune disorders (e.g., rheumatoid arthritis and systemic lupus erythematosus), malignancy, pregnancy, or a history consistent with a drug reaction.[5] The remaining idiopathic cases most commonly occur in elderly patients of either sex with the median age at diagnosis being in the mid-70s.

MECHANISMS OF ANTIBODY DEVELOPMENT

Even though adaptive immunity provides a unique ability to recognize a nearly infinite range of antigenic determinants, mechanisms of immunologic tolerance exist that reduce the probability of autoimmunity.[6] Self non-self discrimination provides the key foundation upon which immune activity can be specifically directed toward potential pathogens.[6] However, self non-self discrimination alone does not possess the capacity to distinguish innocuous antigens from antigens associated with a real threat of infection.[7] As a result, an elaborate network of innate immune factors also exist that recognize potential danger in the form of cellular injury or conserved determinants on pathogens themselves, often referred to as damage-associated molecular patterns (DAMPs) and pathogen-associated molecular patterns (PAMPs), respectively.[7,8] Activation of immune cell function following exposure to PAMPs or DAMPs provide the necessary signals required for an efficient immunologic response to foreign antigen.[7-9]

The development of anti–factor VIII antibodies following factor VIII infusion in individuals with hemophilia A provides a classic example of the deleterious outcome of alloantibody formation following exposure to alloantigen. In this scenario, the factor VIII protein is foreign to the patients; consequently, central tolerance to the factor VIII protein does not occur. In contrast, acquired hemophilia results from loss of previous tolerance to a self antigen.[10-12]

For alloantibody development in patients with hemophilia A, individual variability in factor VIII levels accounts for some of the divergent level of tolerance to factor VIII observed. However, some individuals with undetectable levels of factor VIII antigen fail to generate factor VIII inhibitors, regardless of factor VIII exposure. Although these individuals would not be predicted to be tolerized to factor VIII, 70 to 80 percent of patients with baseline factor VIII levels of less than 1 percent do not develop an immune response to repeated dosing and are considered tolerized.[13-16] For the 20 to 30 percent of patients who develop inhibitors there are both genetic and nongenetic risk factors for inhibitor development. Patients with a positive family history of inhibitors, those who have large factor VIII gene deletions, and nonwhites have a higher risk of inhibitor development.[17-20] The non–factor VIII genes—interleukin-10, tumor necrosis factor-α, and cytotoxic T-lymphocyte antigen 4–318 allele—are associated with inhibitor development.[17-20] Nongenetic risk factors, such as infusing factor at the time of a "danger" signal (e.g., a surgical procedure), intense factor exposure, and prophylaxis versus no prophylaxis, also are associated with inhibitor development.[16] Patients who receive factor at the time of a "danger" signal may experience sufficient tissue injury to provide the necessary immune activation through DAMPs. Furthermore, it remains possible that low grade and potentially clinically undetectable infection may provide low levels of PAMPs that could likewise stimulate anti–factor VIII antibodies following factor VIII exposure. However, while PAMPs and/or DAMPs may provide the important immune activation signals,[21,22] several studies using animal models suggest that significant factor VIII antibody development can occur in the absence of known tissue injury or DAMP exposure.[23] Consistent with this, immune activation can occur in the apparent absence of DAMPs or PAMPs toward several model antigens.[24] Unique B-cell populations, especially those in the spleen, can rapidly respond to bloodborne antigens in the absence of any identifiable PAMPs or tissue injury, suggesting that these cells may be uniquely poised to respond to factor VIII.[25] Consistent with this, in experimental models, splenectomy can significantly inhibit factor VIII inhibitor development following factor VIII exposure,[26,27] suggesting that several of these unique B-cell populations may be involved in the development of factor VIII antibodies irrespective of DAMP or PAMP exposure.[25,26]

Although examples of antigens inducing B-cell activation in the absence of known DAMPs or PAMPs exist, most of these antigens require crosslinking of cell-surface B-cell receptors for efficient activation and therefore reflect highly repetitive antigenic structures.[28] In contrast, factor VIII represents a soluble antigen with little inherent predicted crosslinking ability. Most soluble antigen of this type actually induce tolerance following injection, likely because of the inability of soluble monovalent antigens to adequately crosslink and thereby stimulate B-cell receptors. Although factor VIII can exist in a soluble, monovalent form, it remains possible that factor VIII may form complexes with higher-molecular-weight species and thus form a network of factor VIII antigens that may serve as a suitable substrate for efficient B-cell receptor crosslinking and subsequent activation. Consistent with this, induction of tolerance to factor VIII by exposure to high levels of factor VIII may partially reflect a saturation of sites for factor VIII complex formation,[29] which may, in turn, result in B-cell exposure to high levels of soluble, monovalent factor VIII. However, if this occurs, studies suggest that it likely takes place independent of interactions with von Willebrand factor, the primary binding partner of factor VIII, or its own coagulant activity.[30] Clearly, there is much more to learn regarding the immunologic factors responsible for factor VIII inhibitor development.

In contrast to generating alloantibodies following factor VIII infusion, some patients generate autoantibodies against factor VIII, which can result in acquired factor VIII deficiency. As coagulation typically occurs at sites of inflammation and injury where DAMPs presumably are generated, tolerance to factor VIII may unfortunately be lost in these settings. Additionally, nonproteolytic and proteolytic degradation of coagulation proteins potentially could present neoepitopes. However, the fact that the development of acquired factor VIII deficiency is rare (1.4 per million population) provides a testimony to the ability of the immune system to discriminate efficiently between infectious non-self from noninfectious self.[12] Essentially, nothing is known about the breakdown of tolerance in patients that develop autoantibodies to coagulation factors.

MOLECULAR PATHOLOGY

Factor VIII inhibitors in congenital and acquired hemophilia nearly always consist of a polyclonal immunoglobulin (Ig) G population. Although IgG$_4$ accounts for only 5 percent of the total IgG in normal plasma, it usually is a major, but not the sole, component of the anti–factor VIII antibody population.[31] IgG$_4$ antibodies do not fix complement, which has been cited as a reason that immune complex disease is not observed in factor VIII inhibitor patients. However, it is more likely that factor VIII simply is not present in sufficient quantity to form enough immune complex deposition to mediate tissue damage.

Factor VIII contains a sequence of domains designated A1-A2-B-ap-A3-C1-C2 (Chap. 123). During the activation of factor VIII by thrombin, the B and ap domains are released, producing an A1/A2/A3-C1-C2 activated factor VIII heterotrimer.[32] Anti–factor VIII

antibodies in both congenital and acquired hemophilia A inhibitor are primarily directed to the A2 and C2 domains, although antibodies to all domains have been described.[33-35] The similarity in the properties of antibodies in congenital and acquired hemophilia, which represent very different immunologic settings, suggests that intrinsic structural features in the factor VIII molecule are an important determinant driving the immune response. Epitope spreading from a single "problem" epitope, which has been implicated in some autoantibody phenomena,[36] does not appear to be a property of factor VIII inhibitors because anti–C2 antibodies can occur in the absence of anti–A2 antibodies and *vice versa*.

The only known biologic function of factor VIII is to become proteolytically activated and participate as a cofactor for factor IXa during intrinsic pathway factor X activation on phospholipid membranes. Theoretically, antibodies could inhibit factor VIII procoagulant function in several ways, including blocking the binding of factor VIIIa to factor IXa, factor X, or phospholipid, or by interfering with the proteolytic activation of factor VIII. Some anti-A2 antibodies map to a region bounded by Arg484-Ile508[37] and inhibit activated factor VIII by blocking its ability to bind factor X.[38] Anti-C2 antibodies bind to the NH$_2$-terminal half of the C2 domain.[39] Anti-C2 antibodies have been identified that inhibit the binding of activated factor VIII to phospholipid membranes,[40] which is critical for its interaction with the platelet surfaces. However, the C2 domain also apparently contributes to the binding of factor VIII to its activators, thrombin and factor Xa.[41-43] Consistent with this, anti-C2 inhibitors have been identified that block factor VIII activation.[41,44]

Factor VIII inhibitors also have been identified in approximately 20 percent of normal healthy donors.[45] These inhibitors inhibit factor VIII activity in pooled normal plasma, but not autologous plasma, indicating that they are not autoantibodies, but rather alloantibodies directed against an unidentified polymorphism. Anti–factor VIII IgG also has been identified in all normal plasmas tested by affinity chromatography on immobilized factor VIII.[46] The increased sensitivity of the method is a consequence of its ability to resolve anti–factor VIII antibodies from anti–anti–factor VIII idiotypic antibodies that also are present. Idiotypic regulation has been proposed as a mechanism for controlling autoantibody activity *in vivo*.[47]

CLINICAL FEATURES

Acquired hemophilia A patients usually present with spontaneous bleeding, which often is severe and life- or limb-threatening, although large cohort studies have shown that approximately 30 percent of patients do not require hemostatic management.[2,48] Patients with acquired hemophilia are more likely to have a severe bleeding diathesis than congenital hemophilia A inhibitor patients.[49] Additionally, in contrast to patients with congenital hemophilia A, hemarthrosis in these patients is rare. The reasons for these differences is puzzling, especially in light of the fact that the properties of factor VIII inhibitors in the two patient populations is similar. As noted above, inhibitors can block factor VIII function in several ways. Conceivably, unidentified mechanistic differences in inhibitor action account for the difference in clinical severity. Factor VIII inhibitors sometimes resolve spontaneously. However, it is not possible to predict in which subset of patients this will occur.

LABORATORY FEATURES AND DIFFERENTIAL DIAGNOSIS

The new onset of an acquired bleeding disorder should immediately lead to screening tests that include an activated partial thromboplastin time (aPTT), a prothrombin time, and a platelet count. Patients with acquired hemophilia A have a prolonged aPTT resulting from decreased or absent factor VIII activity in the intrinsic pathway of blood coagulation. The autoantibody inhibits the factor VIII in the plasma from normal individuals, which forms the basis of mixing study that is used to screen for inhibitors. The presence of a prolonged aPTT in a mixing study establishes the diagnosis of a circulating anticoagulant. Specific factor assays then are performed to determine whether a specific coagulation factor inhibitor or a lupus anticoagulant is present. The activity of other intrinsic pathway coagulation factors may be decreased in the presence of high titer factor VIII inhibitors. However, the levels of these factors normalize at increasing dilutions of patient plasma, whereas factor VIII activity remains decreased.

Once the identity of an inhibitor has been established, its titer is determined using the Bethesda assay.[50] Inhibitors frequently take minutes to hours to maximally inhibit factor VIII. Therefore, dilutions of patient plasma are preincubated with normal plasma for 2 hours at 37°C. The inhibitor titer is defined as the dilution of patient plasma that produces 50 percent inhibition of the factor VIII activity and is expressed in Bethesda units per milliliter (BU/mL). Inhibitors are classified informally as low titer or high titer when the titers are less than 5 BU/mL or greater than 5 to 10 BU/mL, respectively. The Bethesda assay has been modified by the addition of 0.1 M imidazole, pH 7.4, and by diluting test plasma into factor VIII–deficient plasma during the preincubation phase to prevent assay variation resulting from pH changes and adsorptive losses of factor VIII.[51] This "Nijmegen" modification of the Bethesda assay decreases false-positive low-titer inhibitors.[52] Patients with acquired hemophilia often have measurable residual factor VIII activity. This activity may cause an underestimate of the inhibitory titer. Preanalytical heat treatment has been proposed as a simple way to denature factor VIII to allow for more accurate determination of titer in both patients with acquired hemophilia A and patients with congenital hemophilia A who may have infused factor VIII.[53,54]

Factor VIII inhibitors are classified based on the kinetics and extent of inactivation of factor VIII in plasma.[55] Type I inhibitors follow second-order kinetics and inactivate factor VIII completely, which would be expected for a simple bimolecular antigen-antibody reaction. Type II inhibitors inactivate factor VIII incompletely and display more complex kinetics of inhibition. Hemophilia A inhibitor patients and acquired hemophilia A patients tend to have type I and type II inhibitors, respectively.[56] However, the borderline between type I and type II inhibitors is not always clear and the distinction is not useful clinically. Additionally in a recent observational study of patients with acquired hemophilia in the United Kingdom, factor VIII levels and inhibitor titers at presentation were not predictive of the severity of bleeding events. The median factor VIII level and inhibitory titers were nearly identical for patients with fatal bleeding events compared to those who did not require treatment for their bleeding symptoms.[2]

TREATMENT

The severe bleeding that often is the presenting feature of this disorder requires urgent action to establish a diagnosis and initiate therapeutic measures. Ideally, this is carried out in a setting where factor VIII inhibitors can be identified and quantitated and where there is subspecialty expertise in the management of bleeding disorders. Invasive procedures should be performed only if absolutely necessary and venipuncture should be kept to a minimum given the risk of significant bleeding.[57]

Treatment of patients with acquired hemophilia A depends on the inhibitor titer. Although no prospective trials are available, clinical experience indicates that patients with a factor VIII inhibitor titer of less than 5 BU/mL often are treated successfully with sufficient doses of recombinant or plasma-derived factor VIII to neutralize the inhibitor. Patients with titers between 5 and 10 BU/mL also may respond to factor VIII,

whereas those with titers greater than 10 BU/mL generally do not respond. Formulas exist to calculate the amount of factor VIII needed to treat a patient, but these are rough estimates at best. The efficacy of factor VIII concentrates was lower than that of bypassing agents in a large registry study, which was likely secondary to challenges in appropriately dosing the factor VIII concentrate.[48]

Desmopressin can be administered by intravenous, subcutaneous, or intranasal routes and results in an increase in plasma von Willebrand factor levels and factor VIII activity.[58] Its potential use is in patients with baseline factor VIII levels greater than 5 IU/dL and minor bleeding. However, like factor VIII concentrates, response is not predictable and close monitoring of hemostatic efficacy and factor VIII levels is needed.

Factor VIII bypassing agents, which drive the coagulation mechanism through the extrinsic pathway, are the mainstays of management of patients with a high titer of an inhibitor. Two agents, recombinant activated factor VII (rFVIIa; NovoSeven RT) and plasma-derived anti-inhibitor coagulant complex (AICC; FEIBA VH Immuno, also called activated prothrombin complex concentrate [aPCC]) are commercially available and approved by the U.S. Food and Drug Administration for treatment of acquired hemophilia A. Although no comparative trials have been done, analysis of the European Acquired Haemophilia (EACH2) Registry showed similar hemostatic efficacy between rFVIIa and aPCC at approximately 90 percent.[48] Similar hemostatic efficacy between rFVIIa and aPCC has been seen in the treatment of congenital hemophilia A with inhibitors.[59] The recommended dose range of rFVIIa for the treatment of patients with acquired hemophilia is 70 to 90 mcg/kg repeated every 2 to 3 hours until hemostasis is achieved. aPCC is given at doses of 50 to 100 U/kg every 8 to 12 hours, but should not exceed 200 U/kg per day. Lower doses (50 to 75 U/kg) are used for mild bleeding, whereas higher doses (100 U/kg) are given for severe limb or life-threatening bleeding. Treatment should be continued until there are clear signs of clinical improvement.

Although there are similar rates of efficacy between the two available bypassing agents, not all patients respond. Additionally, there are no widely accepted methods available for predicting response to therapy or monitoring patients on therapy. The use of thromboelastography and the thrombin generation assays as a predictor of response to therapy in congenital hemophilia A and inhibitors has been reported but large clinical studies linking clinical data to outcome are lacking, leaving clinical response as the only available monitoring option.[60]

The major serious adverse event associated with bypassing agents is thrombosis. The EACH2 Registry reported similar rates in patients treated with rFVIIa or aPCC.[48] However, the risk of thrombosis is considered low when used for approved indications at the recommended doses. The incidence of thrombosis in patients with acquired hemophilia A treated with bypassing agents appears higher than that for patients with congenital hemophilia. This is probably because of cardiovascular risk factors in the acquired hemophilia population given their age and associated medical conditions. Escalating doses of either bypassing agent or combination of the two agents should be done with caution, especially in older patients.

Factor VIII inhibitors usually cross-react poorly with porcine factor VIII.[61] A commercial plasma-derived porcine factor VIII concentrate was useful in the treatment of factor VIII inhibitor patients for approximately 20 years,[62] but was discontinued in 2004 because of viral contamination of the product. Porcine factor VIII has the advantage of potentially being guided by laboratory monitoring of recovery of factor VIII activity in plasma. However, the development of antiporcine factor VIII antibodies may preclude its long-term use. A phase II/III clinical trial of a recombinant porcine factor VIII product has been completed in patients with acquired hemophilia A[63] and a phase II trial has been completed in congenital hemophilia inhibitor patients.[64]

Although acquired inhibitors may remit spontaneously, fatal bleeding may occur up to several months after the initial diagnosis, even in patients who present with mild bleeding. Therefore, immunosuppressive therapy at the time of diagnosis to eradicate the inhibitor is recommended.[57] A variety of immunosuppressive agents have been used, including cyclophosphamide, azathioprine, cyclosporine, intravenous immunoglobulin, and rituximab. Immune tolerance induction using human factor VIII similar to what is done for patients with congenital hemophilia A and inhibitors has been used successfully. Additionally, plasmapheresis and immunoadsorption of the inhibitory antibody have been used.

First-line immunosuppressive regimens at many centers consist of glucocorticoids alone or glucocorticoids combined with cyclophosphamide.[65] No appropriately powered randomized studies have been performed, so the information available is from a single small randomized study, case reports, national surveys, and large registry data. The single randomized trial of 31 patients comparing prednisone and cyclophosphamide showed no difference in the treatment arms. A national registry study also showed no difference with 76 percent of patients achieving complete remission in the steroid arm and 78 percent in the steroids plus cytotoxic agent arm.[66] The EACH2 Registry has the largest reported experience with 331 patients and reported a higher rate of stable complete remission at 70 percent for patients treated with steroids and cyclophosphamide compared with 48 percent for steroids alone and 59 percent for rituximab containing regimens. Extensive analysis to control for potential confounding factors in this non-randomized study confirmed that stable complete remission was more likely with a steroid and cyclophosphamide than steroids alone (odds ratio of 3.25). The median time to remission was 5 weeks in patients treated with steroids alone or steroids and cyclophosphamide and 10 weeks in patients treated with rituximab. There have been no studies that have shown a difference in long-term outcomes including survival and sustained remission.[57,67]

The rarity of this disease, the severity of bleeding at onset, and the delay in diagnosis of these patients has all contributed to the lack of controlled trials. Given the lack of controlled trial clinical management decisions are guided from the limited data available and clinical judgment.

● ACQUIRED ANTIBODIES TO OTHER COAGULATION FACTORS

ANTI–FACTOR V AND ANTITHROMBIN ANTIBODIES

Thrombin and factor V inhibitors are discussed together because of their frequent coexistence in immune responses to commercial products that contain thrombin. Thrombin products have been used widely in surgical and endoscopic procedures. It has been estimated that more than 500,000 patients are treated annually with products containing thrombin.[68] Thrombin is used either alone or as a component of fibrin sealants, which consist of fibrinogen and thrombin preparations that are mixed together at the wound site to form a topical fibrin clot.[69] Additionally, factor XIII sometimes is added to crosslink and stabilize the clot.

Fibrin sealants contain thrombin and fibrinogen derived from human plasma, whereas stand-alone thrombin products are prepared from bovine plasma. Both types of products are heavily contaminated with other plasma proteins, including factor V and prothrombin.[70,71] Almost all patients exposed to bovine proteins develop a detectable immune response. In half of these patients antibovine antibodies

cross-react with human thrombin, factor V, or prothrombin.[68] Usually, these antibodies are subclinical.[72] However, mild to life-threatening hemorrhage can occur, especially if the titer of anti–human factor V antibodies is high. The risk of bleeding is higher in patients who receive bovine thrombin products more than once because of the development of a secondary immune response.

There have been no clinical trials comparing the safety and efficacy of fibrin sealants to stand-alone thrombin products. Because fibrin sealants are composed mainly of human proteins, they may be less immunogenic. However, anti–factor V antibodies have been reported in a patient receiving fibrin sealant.[73] There currently is no stand-alone human thrombin product. It seems likely that the development of highly purified plasma-derived or recombinant products containing human thrombin in the presence or absence of human fibrinogen would decrease the incidence of antithrombin and anti–factor V antibodies.[70]

Autoantibodies to thrombin are rare. However, the mechanisms of action of antithrombin antibodies have been studied extensively because of the wealth of information about thrombin structure and function.[74-77] In contrast, approximately half of the 105 cases of inhibitory anti–factor V antibodies reported and reviewed between 1955 and 1997 appeared to be autoantibodies not associated with the exposure to bovine thrombin products.[72] β-Lactam antibiotics also are associated with anti–factor V autoantibodies and may partly explain the increased incidence with surgery. In approximately 20 percent of cases of autoantibody formation, no underlying disease was identified. Anti–factor V autoantibodies have been identified rarely in patients with autoimmune diseases, solid tumors, and monoclonal gammopathies. In addition to autoantibody formation, alloantibodies to factor V have developed in patients with severe factor V deficiency in response to replacement therapy with fresh-frozen plasma.

Patients with inhibitory antibodies to factor V have prolonged prothrombin and aPTT, low factor V levels, and a normal thrombin time. The diagnosis of a factor V inhibitor is based on the specific loss of factor V coagulant activity when patient and normal plasma are mixed in a coagulation assay. The antibody titer can be defined as in the factor VIII Bethesda assay as the dilution of test plasma that produces 50 percent inhibition of factor V activity.

Not all patients with factor V inhibitors have hemorrhagic manifestations. Factor V inhibitors anecdotally produce a less serious bleeding disorder than factor VIII inhibitors. The relationship between inhibitor titer and bleeding has not been studied. The reported incidence of bleeding has been higher in patients with autoantibodies to factor V compared to anti–factor V antibodies in patients receiving bovine thrombin. However, this may reflect a bias resulting from the reason the patient sought medical attention.

Factor V contains an A1-A2-B-A3-C1-C2 domain structure that is homologous to factor VIII. Also, like factor VIII, the N-terminal half of the factor V C2 domain contains a phospholipid-binding site[78] that is necessary for normal procoagulant function[79] and is targeted by factor V inhibitors.[80,81]

ANTIPROTHROMBIN ANTIBODIES

Antiprothrombin antibodies are most commonly associated with the antiphospholipid syndrome. The antiphospholipid syndrome is caused by lupus anticoagulants, which are defined as antibodies that produce phospholipid-dependent prolongation of *in vitro* coagulation assays. Anionic phospholipids participate as cofactors for the lupus anticoagulant binding to protein antigens, primarily β_2-glycoprotein I[82] and prothrombin.[83] The antibody–antigen complexes compete for the binding of coagulation factors to the phospholipid present in coagulation assays and produce the lupus anticoagulant phenomenon.

The role of prothrombin in the generation of lupus anticoagulant activity initially was suggested from studies of a bleeding patient with severe hypoprothrombinemia. However, in the absence of hypoprothrombinemia, lupus anticoagulants do not produce a bleeding diathesis and bleeding in patients with lupus anticoagulants is uncommon.[84] Antiprothrombin antibodies are associated with an increased incidence of thrombosis in these patients.[85] In patients with antiprothrombin antibodies and hypoprothrombinemia, precipitating, noninhibitory antibodies are present and prothrombin antigen levels are low, indicating that the hypoprothrombinemia is the result of rapid clearance of antigen–antibody complexes.[86] However, most patients with lupus anticoagulants have demonstrable antiprothrombin antibodies but do not have hypoprothrombinemia.[87] Thus, antibody-mediated hypoprothrombinemia appears to represent a relatively uncommon evolution of the autoimmune response to prothrombin in patients with lupus anticoagulants.

ANTIBODIES TO COMPONENTS OF THE PROTEIN C SYSTEM

An acquired inhibitor to protein C associated with a fatal thrombotic disorder has been reported,[88] but evidently is rare. In contrast, there is a relatively high prevalence of pathogenic anti-protein S antibodies. Inhibitory antibodies to protein S were detected in five of 15 patients with acquired protein S deficiency.[89] Anti–protein S antibodies, but not antibodies to cardiolipin, β_2-glycoprotein I, prothrombin, or protein C, appear to be a risk factor for acquired activated protein C (APC) resistance, defined as APC resistance in the absence of the factor V Leiden mutation, and for deep venous thrombosis.[90] Additionally, antibodies to the endothelial cell protein receptor have been identified that are associated with fetal death in patients with the antiphospholipid syndrome.[91]

ACQUIRED ANTIBODIES TO OTHER COAGULATION FACTORS

Clinically significant antibodies to coagulation factors other than factor VIII, factor V, and prothrombin that produce acquired bleeding disorders are sufficiently rare that they merit case reports, which are only incompletely listed here. In contrast to acquired hemophilia A, acquired hemophilia B is extremely rare.[92,93] Patients with antifibrinogen antibodies have been identified either who are asymptomatic with abnormal laboratory values[94] or who have abnormal bleeding.[95] Patients with abnormal bleeding associated with acquired inhibitors to factor VII,[96] factor X,[97] factor XI,[98] or factor XIII[98–107] also have been described. The development of alloantibodies against von Willebrand factor occurs in patients with type 3 von Willebrand disease in response to treatment with plasma concentrates that contain von Willebrand factor.[108] Acquired von Willebrand disease can be caused by adsorption of von Willebrand factor to tumor cells, loss of high-molecular-weight von Willebrand factor multimers at as well as by autoantibodies to von Willebrand factor.[109]

REFERENCES

1. Margolius A Jr, Jackson DP, Ratnoff OD: Circulating anticoagulants: A study of 40 cases and a review of the literature. *Medicine (Baltimore)* 40:145–202, 1961.
2. Collins PW, Hirsch S, Baglin TP, et al: Acquired hemophilia A in the United Kingdom: A 2-year national surveillance study by the United Kingdom Haemophilia Centre Doctors' Organisation. *Blood* 109(5):1870–1877, 2007.
3. Borg JY, Guillet B, Le Cam-Duchez V, et al: Outcome of acquired haemophilia in France: The prospective SACHA (Surveillance des Auto antiCorps au cours de l'Hemophilie Acquise) registry. *Haemophilia* 19(4):564–570, 2013.
4. Knoebl P, Marco P, Baudo F, et al: Demographic and clinical data in acquired hemophilia A: Results from the European Acquired Haemophilia Registry (EACH2). *J Thromb Haemost* 10(4):622–631, 2012.
5. Green D, Lechner K: A survey of 215 non-hemophilic patients with inhibitors to Factor VIII. *Thromb Haemost* 45(3):200–203, 1981.
6. Hogquist KA, Baldwin TA, Jameson SC: Central tolerance: Learning self-control in the thymus. *Nat Rev Immunol* 5(10):772–782, 2005.
7. Janeway CA Jr, Medzhitov R: Innate immune recognition. *Annu Rev Immunol* 20: 197–216, 2002.
8. Matzinger P: Tolerance, danger, and the extended family. *Annu Rev Immunol* 12: 991–1045, 1994.
9. Rubtsov AV, Swanson CL, Troy S, et al: TLR agonists promote marginal zone B cell activation and facilitate T-dependent IgM responses. *J Immunol* 180(6):3882–3888, 2008.
10. Lollar P: Pathogenic antibodies to coagulation factors. Part one: Factor VIII and factor IX. *J Thromb Haemost* 2(7):1082–1095, 2004.
11. Dunn AL, Abshire TC: Current issues in prophylactic therapy for persons with hemophilia. *Acta Haematol* 115(3–4):162–171, 2006.
12. Franchini M, Lippi G: Acquired factor VIII inhibitors. *Blood* 112(2):250–255, 2008.
13. White GC 2nd, Kempton CL, Grimsley A, et al: Cellular immune responses in hemophilia: Why do inhibitors develop in some, but not all hemophiliacs? *J Thromb Haemost* 3(8):1676–1681, 2005.
14. Lorenzo JI, Lopez A, Altisent C, Aznar JA: Incidence of factor VIII inhibitors in severe haemophilia: The importance of patient age. *Br J Haematol* 113(3):600–603, 2001.
15. Lusher JM, Arkin S, Abildgaard CF, Schwartz RS: Recombinant factor VIII for the treatment of previously untreated patients with hemophilia A. Safety, efficacy, and development of inhibitors. Kogenate Previously Untreated Patient Study Group. *N Engl J Med* 328(7):453–459, 1993.
16. Gouw SC, van der Bom JG, Marijke van den Berg H: Treatment-related risk factors of inhibitor development in previously untreated patients with hemophilia A: The CANAL cohort study. *Blood* 109(11):4648–4654, 2007.
17. Astermark J, Berntorp E, White GC, et al: The Malmo International Brother Study (MIBS): Further support for genetic predisposition to inhibitor development in hemophilia patients. *Haemophilia* 7(3):267–272, 2001.
18. Astermark J, Oldenburg J, Escobar M, et al: The Malmo International Brother Study (MIBS). Genetic defects and inhibitor development in siblings with severe hemophilia A [see comment]. *Haematologica* 90(7):924–931, 2005.
19. Goodeve A: The incidence of inhibitor development according to specific mutations—and treatment? [review] [8 refs]. *Blood Coagul Fibrinolysis* 14 Suppl 1:S17–S21, 2003.
20. Oldenburg J, Schroder J, Brackmann HH, et al: Environmental and genetic factors influencing inhibitor development [review] [44 refs]. *Semin Hematol* 41(1 Suppl 1): 82–88, 2004.
21. Hendrickson JE, Desmarets M, Deshpande SS, et al: Recipient inflammation affects the frequency and magnitude of immunization to transfused red blood cells. *Transfusion* 46(9):1526–1536, 2006.
22. Hendrickson JE, Chadwick TE, Roback JD, et al: Inflammation enhances consumption and presentation of transfused RBC antigens by dendritic cells. *Blood* 110(7): 2736–2743, 2007.
23. Meeks SL, Healey JF, Parker ET, et al: Antihuman factor VIII C2 domain antibodies in hemophilia A mice recognize a functionally complex continuous spectrum of epitopes dominated by inhibitors of factor VIII activation. *Blood* 110(13):4234–4242, 2007.
24. Stowell SR, Henry KL, Smith NH, et al: Alloantibodies to a paternally derived RBC KEL antigen lead to hemolytic disease of the fetus/newborn in a murine model. *Blood* 122(8):1494–1504, 2013.
25. Martin F, Kearney JF: Marginal-zone B cells. *Nat Rev Immunol* 2(5):323–335, 2002.
26. Navarrete A, Dasgupta S, Delignat S, et al: Splenic marginal zone antigen-presenting cells are critical for the primary allo-immune response to therapeutic factor VIII in hemophilia A. *J Thromb Haemost* 7(11):1816–1823, 2009.
27. Zhang AH, Skupsky J, Scott DW: Effect of B-cell depletion using anti-CD20 therapy on inhibitory antibody formation to human FVIII in hemophilia A mice. *Blood* 117(7):2223–2226, 2011.
28. Bachmann MF, Rohrer UH, Kundig TM, et al: The influence of antigen organization on B cell responsiveness. *Science* 262(5138):1448–1451, 1993.
29. Kempton CL, White GC 2nd: How we treat a hemophilia A patient with a factor VIII inhibitor. *Blood* 113(1):11–17, 2009.
30. Meeks SL, Cox CL, Healey JF, et al: A major determinant of the immunogenicity of factor VIII in a murine model is independent of its procoagulant function. *Blood* 120(12):2512–2520, 2012.
31. Hoyer LW, Gawryl MS, de la Fuente B: Immunochemical characterization of factor VIII inhibitors. *Prog Clin Biol Res* 150:73–85, 1984.
32. Lollar P, Parker CG: Subunit structure of thrombin-activated porcine factor VIII. *Biochemistry* 28(2):666–674, 1989.
33. Fulcher CA, de Graaf Mahoney S, Roberts JR, et al: Localization of human factor FVIII inhibitor epitopes to two polypeptide fragments. *Proc Natl Acad Sci U S A* 82(22): 7728–7732, 1985.
34. Prescott R, Nakai H, Saenko EL, et al: The inhibitor antibody response is more complex in hemophilia A patients than in most nonhemophiliacs with factor VIII autoantibodies. Recombinate and Kogenate Study Groups. *Blood* 89(10):3663–3671, 1997.
35. Scandella D, Mattingly M, de Graaf S, Fulcher CA: Localization of epitopes for human factor VIII inhibitor antibodies by immunoblotting and antibody neutralization. *Blood* 74(5):1618–1626, 1989.
36. James JA, Harley JB: B-cell epitope spreading in autoimmunity. *Immunol Rev* 164: 185–200, 1998.

37. Healey JF, Barrow RT, Tamim HM, et al: Residues Glu2181-Val2243 contain a major determinant of the inhibitory epitope in the C2 domain of human factor VIII. *Blood* 92(10):3701–3709, 1998.

38. Lollar P, Parker ET, Curtis JE, et al: Inhibition of human factor VIIIa by anti-A2 subunit antibodies. *J Clin Invest* 93(6):2497–2504, 1994.

39. Healey JF, Lubin IM, Nakai H, et al: Residues 484–508 contain a major determinant of the inhibitory epitope in the A2 domain of human factor VIII. *J Biol Chem* 270(24):14505–14509, 1995.

40. Arai M, Scandella D, Hoyer LW: Molecular basis of factor VIII inhibition by human antibodies. Antibodies that bind to the factor VIII light chain prevent the interaction of factor VIII with phospholipid. *J Clin Invest* 83(6):1978–1984, 1989.

41. Nogami K, Shima M, Hosokawa K, et al: Factor VIII C2 domain contains the thrombin-binding site responsible for thrombin-catalyzed cleavage at Arg1689. *J Biol Chem* 275(33):25774–25780, 2000.

42. Nogami K, Shima M, Hosokawa K, et al: Role of factor VIII C2 domain in factor VIII binding to factor Xa. *J Biol Chem* 274(43):31000–31007, 1999.

43. Saenko EL, Shima M, Rajalakshmi KJ, Scandella D: A role for the C2 domain of factor VIII in binding to von Willebrand factor. *J Biol Chem* 269(15):11601–11605, 1994.

44. Meeks SL, Healey JF, Parker ET, et al: Nonclassical anti-C2 domain antibodies are present in patients with factor VIII inhibitors. *Blood* 112(4):1151–1153, 2008.

45. Algiman M, Dietrich G, Nydegger UE, et al: Natural antibodies to factor VIII (anti-hemophilic factor) in healthy individuals. *Proc Natl Acad Sci U S A* 89(9):3795–3799, 1992.

46. Gilles JG, Saint-Remy JM: Healthy subjects produce both anti-factor VIII and specific anti-idiotypic antibodies. *J Clin Invest* 94(4):1496–1505, 1994.

47. Guilbert B, Dighiero G, Avrameas S: Naturally occurring antibodies against nine common antigens in human sera. I. Detection, isolation and characterization. *J Immunol* 128(6):2779–2787, 1982.

48. Baudo F, Collins P, Huth-Kuhne A, et al: Management of bleeding in acquired hemophilia A: Results from the European Acquired Hemophilia (EACH2) Registry. *Blood* 120(1):39–46, 2012.

49. Ludlam CA, Morrison AE, Kessler C: Treatment of acquired hemophilia. *Semin Hematol* 31(2 Suppl 4):16–19, 1994.

50. Kasper CK, Aledort L, Aronson D, et al: Proceedings: A more uniform measurement of factor VIII inhibitors. *Thromb Diath Haemorrh* 34(2):612, 1975.

51. Verbruggen B, Novakova I, Wessels H, et al: The Nijmegen modification of the Bethesda assay for factor VIII:C inhibitors: Improved specificity and reliability. *Thromb Haemost* 73(2):247–251, 1995.

52. Giles AR, Verbruggen B, Rivard GE, et al: A detailed comparison of the performance of the standard versus the Nijmegen modification of the Bethesda assay in detecting factor VIII:C inhibitors in the haemophilia A population of Canada. Association of Hemophilia Centre Directors of Canada. Factor VIII/IX Subcommittee of Scientific and Standardization Committee of International Society on Thrombosis and Haemostasis. *Thromb Haemost* 79(4):872–875, 1998.

53. Batty P, Platton S, Bowles L, et al: Pre-analytical heat treatment and a FVIII ELISA improve factor VIII antibody detection in acquired haemophilia A. *Br J Haematol* 166(6):953–956, 2014.

54. Soucie JM, Miller CH, Kelly FM, et al: A study of prospective surveillance for inhibitors among persons with haemophilia in the United States. *Haemophilia* 20(2):230–237, 2014.

55. Biggs R, Austen DE, Denson KW, et al: The mode of action of antibodies which destroy factor VIII. II. Antibodies which give complex concentration graphs. *Br J Haematol* 23(2):137–155, 1972.

56. Hoyer LW, Scandella D: Factor VIII inhibitors: Structure and function in autoantibody and hemophilia A patients. *Semin Hematol* 31(2 Suppl 4):1–5, 1994.

57. Collins PW, Chalmers E, Hart DP, et al: Diagnosis and treatment of factor VIII and IX inhibitors in congenital haemophilia: (4th edition). UK Haemophilia Centre Doctors Organization. *Br J Haematol* 160(2):153–170, 2013.

58. Franchini M, Lippi G: The use of desmopressin in acquired haemophilia A: A systematic review. *Blood Transfus* 9(4):377–382, 2011.

59. Astermark J, Donfield SM, DiMichele DM, et al: A randomized comparison of bypassing agents in hemophilia complicated by an inhibitor: The FEIBA NovoSeven Comparative (FENOC) Study. *Blood* 109(2):546–551, 2007.

60. Young G, Sorensen B, Dargaud Y, et al: Thrombin generation and whole blood viscoelastic assays in the management of hemophilia: Current state of art and future perspectives. *Blood* 121(11):1944–1950, 2013.

61. Brettler DB, Forsberg AD, Levine PH, et al: The use of porcine factor VIII concentrate (Hyate:C) in the treatment of patients with inhibitor antibodies to factor VIII. A multicenter US experience. *Arch Intern Med* 149(6):1381–1385, 1989.

62. Hay CR: Porcine factor VIII: Past, present and future. *Haematologica* 85(10 Suppl):21–24; discussion 24–25, 2000.

63. Kruse-Jarres R, St-Louis J, Greist A, et al: Efficacy and safety of OBI-1, an antihaemophilic factor VIII (recombinant), porcine sequence, in subjects with acquired haemophilia A. *Haemophilia* 21(2):162–170,2015.

64. Kempton CL, Abshire TC, Deveras RA, et al: Pharmacokinetics and safety of OBI-1, a recombinant B domain-deleted porcine factor VIII, in subjects with haemophilia A. *Haemophilia* 18(5):798–804, 2012.

65. Collins P, Baudo F, Huth-Kuhne A, et al: Consensus recommendations for the diagnosis and treatment of acquired hemophilia A. *BMC Res Notes* 3:161, 2010.

66. Green D, Rademaker AW, Briet E: A prospective, randomized trial of prednisone and cyclophosphamide in the treatment of patients with factor VIII autoantibodies. *Thromb Haemost* 70(5):753–757, 1993.

67. Collins P, Baudo F, Knoebl P, et al: Immunosuppression for acquired hemophilia A: Results from the European Acquired Haemophilia Registry (EACH2). *Blood* 120(1):47–55, 2012.

68. Schoenecker JG, Johnson RK, Lesher AP, et al: Exposure of mice to topical bovine thrombin induces systemic autoimmunity. *Am J Pathol* 159(5):1957–1969, 2001.

69. Ortel TL, Charles LA, Keller FG, et al: Topical thrombin and acquired coagulation factor inhibitors: Clinical spectrum and laboratory diagnosis. *Am J Hematol* 45(2):128–135, 1994.

70. Schoenecker JG, Johnson RK, Fields RC, et al: Relative purity of thrombin-based hemostatic agents used in surgery. *J Am Coll Surg* 197(4):580–590, 2003.

71. Zehnder JL, Leung LL: Development of antibodies to thrombin and factor V with recurrent bleeding in a patient exposed to topical bovine thrombin. *Blood* 76(10):2011–2016, 1990.

72. Knobl P, Lechner K: Acquired factor V inhibitors. *Baillieres Clin Haematol* 11(2):305–318, 1998.

73. Caers J, Reekmans A, Jochmans K, et al: Factor V inhibitor after injection of human thrombin (tissucol) into a bleeding peptic ulcer. *Endoscopy* 35(6):542–544, 2003.

74. Arnaud E, Lafay M, Gaussem P, et al: An autoantibody directed against human thrombin anion-binding exosite in a patient with arterial thrombosis: Effects on platelets, endothelial cells, and protein C activation. *Blood* 84(6):1843–1850, 1994.

75. La Spada AR, Skalhegg BS, Henderson R, et al: Brief report: Fatal hemorrhage in a patient with an acquired inhibitor of human thrombin. *N Engl J Med* 333(8):494–497, 1995.

76. Lian F, He L, Colwell NS, et al: Anticoagulant activities of a monoclonal antibody that binds to exosite II of thrombin. *Biochemistry* 40(29):8508–8513, 2001.

77. Sie P, Bezeaud A, Dupouy D, et al: An acquired antithrombin autoantibody directed toward the catalytic center of the enzyme. *J Clin Invest* 88(1):290–296, 1991.

78. Macedo-Ribeiro S, Bode W, Huber R, et al: Crystal structures of the membrane-binding C2 domain of human coagulation factor V. *Nature* 402(6760):434–439, 1999.

79. Ortel TL, Devore-Carter D, Quinn-Allen M, Kane WH: Deletion analysis of recombinant human factor V. Evidence for a phosphatidylserine binding site in the second C-type domain. *J Biol Chem* 267(6):4189–4198, 1992.

80. Izumi T, Kim SW, Greist A, et al: Fine mapping of inhibitory anti-factor V antibodies using factor V C2 domain mutants. Identification of two antigenic epitopes involved in phospholipid binding. *Thromb Haemost* 85(6):1048–1054, 2001.

81. Ortel TL, Moore KD, Quinn-Allen MA, et al: Inhibitory anti-factor V antibodies bind to the factor V C2 domain and are associated with hemorrhagic manifestations. *Blood* 91(11):4188–4196, 1998.

82. McNeil HP, Simpson RJ, Chesterman CN, Krilis SA: Anti-phospholipid antibodies are directed against a complex antigen that includes a lipid-binding inhibitor of coagulation: Beta 2-glycoprotein I (apolipoprotein H). *Proc Natl Acad Sci U S A* 87(11):4120–4124, 1990.

83. Fleck RA, Rapaport SI, Rao LV: Anti-prothrombin antibodies and the lupus anticoagulant. *Blood* 72(2):512–519, 1988.

84. Feinstein DI, Rapaport SI: Acquired inhibitors of blood coagulation. *Prog Hemost Thromb* 1:75–95, 1972.

85. Lakos G, Kiss E, Regeczy N, et al: Antiprothrombin and antiannexin V antibodies imply risk of thrombosis in patients with systemic autoimmune diseases. *J Rheumatol* 27(4):924–929, 2000.

86. Bajaj SP, Rapaport SI, Fierer DS, et al: A mechanism for the hypoprothrombinemia of the acquired hypoprothrombinemia-lupus anticoagulant syndrome. *Blood* 61(4):684–692, 1983.

87. Edson JR, Vogt JM, Hasegawa DK: Abnormal prothrombin crossed-immunoelectrophoresis in patients with lupus inhibitors. *Blood* 64(4):807–816, 1984.

88. Mitchell CA, Rowell JA, Hau L, et al: A fatal thrombotic disorder associated with an acquired inhibitor of protein C. *N Engl J Med* 317(26):1638–1642, 1987.

89. Sorice M, Arcieri P, Griggi T, et al: Inhibition of protein S by autoantibodies in patients with acquired protein S deficiency. *Thromb Haemost* 75(3):555–559, 1996.

90. Nojima J, Kuratsune H, Suehisa E, et al: Acquired activated protein C resistance associated with anti-protein S antibody as a strong risk factor for DVT in non-SLE patients. *Thromb Haemost* 88(5):716–722, 2002.

91. Hurtado V, Montes R, Gris JC, et al: Autoantibodies against EPCR are found in antiphospholipid syndrome and are a risk factor for fetal death. *Blood* 104(5):1369–1374, 2004.

92. Boggio LN, Green D: Acquired hemophilia. *Rev Clin Exp Hematol* 5(4):389–404; quiz following 431, 2001.

93. Krishnamurthy P, Hawche C, Evans G, Winter M: A rare case of an acquired inhibitor to factor IX. *Haemophilia* 17(4):712–713, 2011.

94. Nawarawong W, Wyshock E, Meloni FJ, et al: The rate of fibrinopeptide B release modulates the rate of clot formation: A study with an acquired inhibitor to fibrinopeptide B release. *Br J Haematol* 79(2):296–301, 1991.

95. Ruiz-Arguelles A: Spontaneous reversal of acquired autoimmune dysfibrinogenemia probably due to an antiidiotypic antibody directed to an interspecies cross-reactive idiotype expressed on antifibrinogen antibodies. *J Clin Invest* 82(3):958–963, 1988.

96. Aguilar C, Lucia JF, Hernandez P: A case of an inhibitor autoantibody to coagulation factor VII. *Haemophilia* 9(1):119–120, 2003.

97. Rao LV, Zivelin A, Iturbe I, Rapaport SI: Antibody-induced acute factor X deficiency: Clinical manifestations and properties of the antibody. *Thromb Haemost* 72(3):363–371, 1994.

98. Goodrick MJ, Prentice AG, Copplestone JA, et al: Acquired factor XI inhibitor in chronic lymphocytic leukaemia. *J Clin Pathol* 45(4):352–353, 1992.

99. Ajzner E, Schlammadinger A, Kerenyi A, et al: Severe bleeding complications caused by an autoantibody against the B subunit of plasma factor XIII: A novel form of acquired factor XIII deficiency. *Blood* 113(3):723–725, 2009.

100. Daly HM, Carson PJ, Smith JK: Intracerebral haemorrhage due to acquired factor XIII inhibitor—Successful response to factor XIII concentrate. *Blood Coagul Fibrinolysis* 2(4):507–514, 1991.

101. Fukue H, Anderson K, McPhedran P, et al: A unique factor XIII inhibitor to a fibrin-binding site on factor XIIIA. *Blood* 79(1):65–74, 1992.

102. Krumdieck R, Shaw DR, Huang ST, et al: Hemorrhagic disorder due to an isoniazid-associated acquired factor XIII inhibitor in a patient with Waldenstrom's macroglobulinemia. *Am J Med* 90(5):639–645, 1991.

103. Lopaciuk S, Bykowska K, McDonagh JM, et al: Difference between type I autoimmune inhibitors of fibrin stabilization in two patients with severe hemorrhagic disorder. *J Clin Invest* 61(5):1196–1203, 1978.

104. Lorand L, Maldonado N, Fradera J, et al: Haemorrhagic syndrome of autoimmune origin with a specific inhibitor against fibrin stabilizing factor (factor XIII). *Br J Haematol* 23(1):17–27, 1972.

105. Lorand L, Velasco PT, Murthy SN, et al: Autoimmune antibody in a hemorrhagic patient interacts with thrombin-activated factor XIII in a unique manner. *Blood* 93(3):909–917, 1999.

106. Lorand L, Velasco PT, Rinne JR, et al: Autoimmune antibody (IgG Kansas) against the fibrin stabilizing factor (factor XIII) system. *Proc Natl Acad Sci U S A* 85(1):232–236, 1988.

107. Tosetto A, Rodeghiero F, Gatto E, et al: An acquired hemorrhagic disorder of fibrin crosslinking due to IgG antibodies to FXIII, successfully treated with FXIII replacement and cyclophosphamide. *Am J Hematol* 48(1):34–39, 1995.

108. James PD, Lillicrap D, Mannucci PM: Alloantibodies in von Willebrand disease. *Blood* 122(5):636–640, 2013.

109. Federici AB: Acquired von Willebrand syndrome: Is it an extremely rare disorder or do we see only the tip of the iceberg? *J Thromb Haemost* 6(4):565–568, 2008.

CHAPTER 128

HEMOSTATIC ALTERATIONS IN LIVER DISEASE AND LIVER TRANSPLANTATION

Frank W.G. Leebeek and Ton Lisman

SUMMARY

In patients with acute liver failure or chronic liver disease, many changes in the hemostatic system occur. The liver is the site of synthesis of nearly all coagulation factors, both pro- and anticoagulant proteins. A reduced synthesis function of the liver will lead to reduced levels of these factors in circulation. In addition, the liver is involved in the clearance of many activated coagulation factors and protein-inhibitor complexes from the circulation, which, in turn, can lead to activation of the coagulation system if liver function is impaired. Furthermore, the liver is involved in the synthesis and clearance of pro- and antifibrinolytic proteins, which may lead to a shift in the balance of the fibrinolytic system. Also primary hemostasis might be affected in liver disease because of thrombocytopenia and impaired platelet function, which is frequently encountered in these patients. It is evident that patients with liver disease have frequent bleeding episodes, mainly in the gastrointestinal tract, such as variceal bleeding. It has been a longstanding dogma that patients with liver disease are at a high risk of bleeding caused by the above mentioned hemostatic changes. However, in recent years this cause of the bleeding tendency has been questioned because of the concomitant reductions of pro- and anticoagulant factors and pro- and antifibrinolytic factors. More recent studies using more sophisticated coagulation tests showed that thrombin generation is normal in patients with chronic liver failure and that some may even have a prothrombotic phenotype. This led to the development of a model of a rebalanced hemostatic system in these patients, which may have immediate implications for treatment. Hematologists and other clinicians taking care of patients with acute liver failure of chronic liver disease, such as cirrhosis, are still faced with the questions whether these patients need correction of the changes in hemostasis before interventions such as paracentesis, biopsies, dental care, and surgery. It was generally believed that replacement therapy with frozen plasma or prothrombin complex concentrate was indicated. However, based on these new findings, physicians should now be more restrictive in the use of hemostatic agents and blood products in these patients both in liver disease and during liver transplantation.

Acronyms and Abbreviations: ADAMTS13, a disintegrin-like and metalloprotease with thrombospondin domain 13; aPTT, activated partial thromboplastin time; DDAVP, 1-deamino-8-D-arginine vasopressin; DIC, disseminated intravascular coagulation; FFP, fresh-frozen plasma; HAT, hepatic artery thrombosis; INR, international normalized ratio; ISI, international sensitivity index; MELD, model of end-stage liver disease; PAI-1, plasminogen activator inhibitor 1; PFA, platelet function analyzer; PT, prothrombin time; PVT, portal vein thrombosis; TAFI, thrombin-activatable fibrinolysis inhibitor; t-PA, tissue-type plasminogen activator; VWF, von Willebrand factor.

The liver plays a central role in the hemostatic system. Liver parenchymal cells are the site of synthesis of most coagulation factors (except factor VIII), the natural inhibitors of coagulation, including protein C, protein S, and antithrombin, and essential components of the fibrinolytic system, such as plasminogen, α_2-antiplasmin, and thrombin activatable fibrinolysis inhibitor (TAFI). The liver also regulates hemostasis and fibrinolysis by clearing activated coagulation factors and coagulation factor-inhibitor complexes from the circulation. In addition, changes in primary hemostasis mediated by platelets, von Willebrand factor (VWF) and ADAMTS13 (a disintegrin-like and metalloprotease with thrombospondin type 1 repeats) may occur. Therefore, when acute or chronic liver dysfunction is present in patients with liver disease, complicated hemostatic derangement may occur, which can lead to bleeding, thrombosis, or neither bleeding nor thrombosis.

● HEMOSTATIC ALTERATIONS IN CHRONIC LIVER DISEASE

PRIMARY HEMOSTASIS

More than 75 percent of patients with chronic liver disease, especially in moderate to severe cirrhosis (Child B and C) have reduced levels of platelets (<150,000/μL) and 13 percent have platelet counts between 50,000 and 75,000/μL.[1] This may be caused by splenomegaly resulting in sequestration of platelets in the spleen, reduced synthesis of thrombopoietin by the diseased liver, or consumption coagulopathy.[2–5] In addition, it has been suggested that autoantibodies against platelets may reduce the half-life of platelets in cirrhosis.[6] Primary hemostasis may also be defective by a reduced platelet function. In vitro platelet aggregation studies in response to various agonists is frequently diminished in patients with liver disease. Defective platelet function may result from impaired signal transduction, acquired storage pool deficiency, proteolysis of platelet membrane proteins, and increased production of the endothelial-derived platelet inhibitors, nitric oxide and prostacyclin. (reviewed in Ref. 7). A reduced hematocrit may contribute to defective platelet–vessel wall interaction. Platelet adhesion defects were also found under conditions of flow, but were in some studies attributed to thrombocytopenia and a low hematocrit.[8–10] Platelet procoagulant activity measured by a thrombin generation assay using platelet-rich plasma was similar in patients and healthy controls, which casts additional doubt on the extent of the functional defects of platelets in patients with liver disease.[11]

VWF antigen levels are strongly elevated in patients with liver disease. It has been suggested that this is the result from endothelial damage possibly mediated by endotoxemia (bacterial infection).[12,13] VWF mRNA and protein expression in the liver itself are substantially increased in cirrhosis, but VWF ristocetin cofactor activity is variable.[10,14–16] The high levels of VWF may ameliorate the hemostatic defect caused by thrombocytopenia and platelet function defects.[13] In a flow-based model, platelet adhesion to collagen was normalized in thrombocytopenia because of the high levels of VWF in cirrhotic plasma. In patients with liver disease the regulation of VWF multimer size and activity can be impaired because of reduced synthesis of the VWF-cleaving protease ADAMTS13 by stellate cells in the liver.[17] Several studies showed, however, that the most active high-molecular-weight multimers of VWF are diminished in plasma of patients with cirrhosis, which may be mediated by plasmin or other proteases.[18,19] Classical tests of primary hemostasis, such as bleeding time, which is becoming obsolete as a result of its assay-variability and inability to predict bleeding, may still be abnormal in patients with liver disease. Also newer global tests of primary hemostasis, such as platelet function analyzer (PFA), show prolonged closure times with various agonists, but its value in prediction of bleeding in liver disease is unknown.[20]

SECONDARY HEMOSTASIS: COAGULATION AND ANTICOAGULATION

The liver is the site of synthesis of most procoagulant proteins. As a result, decreased levels of coagulation factors II, V, VII, IX, X, and XI are commonly observed in patients with liver failure.[21] In contrast, factor VIII levels are increased, which may be related to the elevated level of its carrier protein VWF and to decreased clearance of factor VIII from the circulation by the liver low-density lipoprotein-related receptor.[14] Factor VIII is synthesized primarily in hepatic sinusoidal endothelial cells, whose function is preserved in liver disease.[14,22] Acquired vitamin K–dependent carboxylation deficiency may lead qualitative defects in coagulation factors. Because of vitamin K deficiency or decreased production of gamma-glutamyl carboxylase, circulating vitamin K–dependent coagulation factors II, VII, IX, and X may be deficient in γ-carboxylated glutamic acid residues in their GLA domains, giving rise to impaired function of these factors.[23] On the other hand, levels of anticoagulant protein C, protein S, antithrombin, heparin cofactor II, and α_2-macroglobulin are also decreased in patients with liver disease.[24] Fibrinogen levels are frequently in the normal range in patients with chronic liver disease, but may be decreased in patients with decompensated cirrhosis or acute liver failure.[25] A qualitative defect in fibrinogen may be found in patients with liver disease.[26] Screening tests of coagulation, such as the prothrombin time (PT) or activated partial thromboplastin time (aPTT), are frequently prolonged in patients with chronic liver disease. These results have been traditionally interpreted to reflect a hypocoagulable state. The PT and aPTT are sensitive to levels of procoagulant proteins in plasma, but not to the natural anticoagulants, proteins C, protein S, and antithrombin. The use of a more sophisticated test of coagulation, such as total thrombin generation test, illustrates the limitation of the PT and aPTT. In a thrombin-generation test measuring the total amount of thrombin generated during coagulation, decreased total thrombin generation is measured in patients with cirrhosis compared to controls.[11,27,28] Yet, when measured in the presence of thrombomodulin to enable protein C activation and thereby also taking into account the contribution of the main inhibitor of coagulation protein C, thrombin generation was indistinguishable from controls, despite abnormal conventional coagulation tests. Others found normal thrombin generation without addition of thrombomodulin and even increased thrombin generation with addition of thrombomodulin.[29,30] These results suggest that thrombin generation *in vivo* can be normal in patients with liver failure, and that a prolonged PT does not per se indicate a bleeding risk. These findings indicate that a concomitant decrease of pro-and anticoagulant factors result in a rebalanced hemostatic system.[31]

Despite the limitations of the use of the PT in patients with liver disease the international normalized ratio (INR), which is a derivative of the PT, is still used in prognostic scores for patients with acute or chronic liver disease. The model of end-stage liver disease (MELD) score is used to prioritize patients for liver transplantation. The INR was originally developed and validated only to monitor anticoagulant therapy with vitamin K antagonists. The interlaboratory variation of the INR in patients with liver disease is substantial, and its use results in significant differences in MELD scores when a single patient sample is tested in different laboratories using various PT reagents.[32,33] The use of alternative international sensitivity index (ISI) values obtained by calibration against plasma samples from patients with liver disease was shown to decrease this variability.[34,35]

FIBRINOLYSIS

Except for tissue-type plasminogen activator (t-PA) and plasminogen-activator inhibitor (PAI)-1, all proteins involved in fibrinolysis, both

pro- and antifibrinolytic, are synthesized by the liver.[36] Therefore, chronic liver disease leads to decreased plasma levels of plasminogen, α_2-antiplasmin, TAFI, and factor XIII. Plasma levels of t-PA are elevated as a result of increased secretion from endothelial cells and/or reduced clearance by the diseased liver. Plasma levels of PAI-1 also are increased but not to the same extent as t-PA, which may lead to a shift in balance in the fibrinolytic system.[37] It has long been assumed that most patients with chronic liver disease had accelerated fibrinolysis. This was based on *in vitro* assays, including various clot lysis assays and on measurements of increased fibrin(ogen) degradation products, D-dimer and plasmin–antiplasmin complexes (reviewed in Ref. 36). However, more recent studies found no evidence of hyperfibrinolysis in the majority of patients with cirrhosis despite decreased levels of TAFI and elevated D-dimer levels.[38,39] This conclusion was recently challenged by a study that used two assays to detect fibrinolysis in patients with various degrees of severity of cirrhosis. In both tests approximately 40 percent of patients had evidence of hyperfibrinolysis, and in 60 percent of the patients, one of the tests revealed an increased fibrinolytic capacity, especially in those with severe liver dysfunction.[40] Hyperfibrinolysis in patients with cirrhosis may also occur secondary to low-grade disseminated intravascular coagulation (DIC) induced by endotoxemia and is manifested by concomitant increased levels of prothrombin fragment 1+2, fibrinopeptide A, D-dimer, thrombin–antithrombin complex, and plasmin–antiplasmin complex.[41] However, it has been argued that the increased levels of these markers may result from their decreased clearance by the liver rather than from DIC. In patients with liver disease who presented with gastrointestinal bleeding or soft-tissue bleeding after trauma, *in vitro* signs of increased fibrinolysis have been reported.[42,43]

⬤ A REBALANCED HEMOSTATIC SYSTEM IN CHRONIC LIVER DISEASE

It has been a longstanding dogma that patients with liver disease are at a high risk of bleeding due to reduction of synthesis of coagulation factors and other changes in hemostasis. More recent studies using more sophisticated coagulation tests have shown that thrombin generation is normal in patients with chronic liver failure and that some may even have a prothrombotic phenotype.[24,27,44] Because both procoagulant and anticoagulant proteins decline in patients with chronic liver diseases, it has been postulated that the hemostatic system is rebalanced (Table 128-1).[24,31,45] In addition reductions of platelet number and impairment of platelet function is counteracted by high levels of VWF and in many patients the decline in profibrinolytic factors is balanced by the reduction of inhibitors of fibrinolysis.[13,38] This led to the model of a rebalanced hemostatic system in these patients, which has important implications for treatment.[24,31] This model also explains why most patients with liver disease usually do not exhibit severe bleeding manifestations—neither during minor invasive procedures, such as biopsies and paracentesis, nor during major surgeries, including liver transplantation.[46,47] Furthermore, patients with liver disease may even have increased risk of venous thromboembolism, not only liver-specific thrombosis, but also deep vein thrombosis.[48–50] The hemostatic balance in patients with liver disease is, however, quite delicate and vulnerable to be tipped toward bleeding or thrombosis. So far it is impossible to identify which patients are more prone to bleeding or to thrombosis based on current laboratory assays. The complex changes in hemostasis encountered in patients with liver disease are depicted in Table 128-1. The delicate hemostatic balance in patients with liver disease may be changed by comorbidities, such as bacterial infections and renal failure frequently observed in these patients. It is of major importance to treat these comorbidities so as to reduce the risk of bleeding and thrombosis.[51]

TABLE 128–1. Changes in the Hemostatic System in Patients with Liver Disease That Contribute to Bleeding (Left) or Contribute to Thrombosis (Right)

Changes That Impair Hemostasis	Changes That Promote Hemostasis
PRIMARY HEMOSTASIS	
Thrombocytopenia	Elevated levels of VWF
Platelet function defects	Decreased levels of ADAMTS13
Enhanced production of nitric oxide and prostacyclin	
SECONDARY HEMOSTASIS	
Low levels of factors II, V, VII, IX, X, and XI	Elevated levels of factor VIII
Vitamin K Deficiency	Decreased levels of protein C, protein S, antithrombin, a_2-macroglobulin, and heparin cofactor II
Dysfibrinogenemia	
FIBRINOLYSIS	
Low levels of a_2-antiplasmin, factor XIII, and TAFI	Low levels of plasminogen
	Increase in PAI-1 levels
Elevated t-PA levels	

ADAMTS13, a disintegrin-like and metalloprotease with thrombospondin domain 13; PAI-I, plasminogen activator inhibitor 1; TAFI, thrombin-activatable fibrinolysis inhibitor; t-PA, tissue-type plasminogen activator; VWF, von Willebrand factor.

HEMOSTATIC ALTERATIONS IN ACUTE LIVER FAILURE

Patients presenting with acute liver failure, for instance in acetaminophen intoxication, have profound changes in the hemostatic system. A severe decrease of coagulation factors is observed, with strongly increased INR.[52] However, an intact thrombin generation has been observed in acute liver failure patients and hardly any changes were observed using thromboelastography.[53,54] In contrast to chronic liver disease, patients with acute liver failure frequently have normal platelet counts. Highly elevated levels of VWF are observed and strongly decreased levels of ADAMTS13. This imbalance may lead to a prothrombotic state.[55] In patients with acute liver failure, there is an increased level of PAI-1, and reduced levels of plasminogen which is consistent with a hypofibrinolytic state.[53,56] A strong increase of procoagulant microparticles has been observed in acute liver failure.[57] Spontaneous bleeding is not frequently encountered in patients with acute liver failure.[58]

HEMOSTATIC ALTERATIONS DURING LIVER TRANSPLANTATION

Liver transplantation performed in patients in acute or chronic liver failure has always been complicated by significant and sometimes life-threatening bleeding problems requiring massive use of coagulation factors and erythrocyte transfusion.[59] Therefore blood products were also transfused before and during transplantation to correct the hemostatic dysfunction. Improved surgical techniques and anesthesiologic care have led to a remarkable reduction of blood loss during liver transplantation. Currently, no blood transfusion is given in up to 50 to 80 percent of patients undergoing a liver transplantation, depending on the center.[60,61] This improvement is also because of a better understanding of the coagulation profile during the various stages of the surgical intervention. During the first stage of liver transplantation, the removal of the diseased liver, no significant worsening of the preoperative hemostatic status occurs.[62] After removal of the diseased liver, the so-called anhepatic stage, significant hemostatic changes occur. Because activated coagulation factors are not cleared from the circulation, DIC can develop, with consumption of platelets and coagulation factors and secondary hyperfibrinolysis. Moreover, hyperfibrinolysis may also occur as a result of defective clearance of t-PA.[63] The most severe hemostatic changes during liver transplantation occur immediately after reperfusion of the donor liver. Platelets are trapped in the graft, giving rise to an aggravation of thrombocytopenia and causing damage to the graft by induction of endothelial cell apoptosis.[64] Release of tissue factor and t-PA from the reperfused graft causes DIC with primary or secondary fibrinolysis.[63] Moreover, the graft also releases heparin-like substances that can inhibit coagulation.[65] In addition, other factors such as hypothermia, metabolic acidosis, and hemodilution adversely affect hemostasis during this phase.

During transplantation, the balance between VWF and ADAMTS13 changes because levels of VWF remain high, the functional properties of VWF improve, and the levels of ADAMTS13 decline, which may partially compensate for the hemostatic dysfunction.[66] The platelet count and hemostatic proteins are at their nadir after reperfusion and rise gradually during the early postoperative period. However, the levels of procoagulant factors rise more rapidly than the levels of anticoagulant factors, which results in a temporary hypercoagulable state.[67] A transiently increased level of PAI-1 immediately after surgery can result in a hypofibrinolytic state that may aggravate the hypercoagulable status.

CLINICAL PROBLEMS ENCOUNTERED IN PATIENTS WITH LIVER DISEASE

BLEEDING IN PATIENTS WITH LIVER DISEASE

Although sophisticated hemostatic tests have now shown that disorders of primary hemostasis, a hypocoagulable status, and hyperfibrinolysis are generally not encountered or are only seen in a minority of patients with chronic liver disease, bleeding still may occur in these patients.[24] This is because individual patients still may have a compromised hemostatic function or because patients bleed for nonhemostatic reasons.[68] The most severe bleeding manifestation in patients with liver disease is bleeding from ruptured esophageal varices. This results from local vascular abnormalities and portal hypertension and not from deranged hemostasis. Occasionally, impaired hemostasis does cause easy bruising, purpura, epistaxis, gingival bleeding, menorrhagia and gastrointestinal bleeding. Also in acute liver failure bleeding has frequently been reported in the past, but more recent studies clearly indicate that spontaneous bleeding occurs rarely.[58]

HEMOSTATIC MANAGEMENT OF PATIENTS WITH LIVER DISEASE

Hemostatic Management of Bleeding Episodes

Variceal bleeding in patients with liver disease should be immediately managed by local interventions, such as endoscopy and rubber band ligation or even shunt (transjugulair intrahepatic portosystemic shunt [TIPS]) placement.[69] Fluid resuscitation should be given in case of hypotension and restricted blood transfusion in case of severe drop of hemoglobin level.[70] Because there is no evidence that changes in hemostasis are associated with the risk of variceal bleeding, treatment with coagulation factor concentrates is not indicated.

Infusion of plasma may even lead to more bleeding as a result of an increase of portal pressure.[71,72] Upper gastrointestinal bleeding from peptic ulcer disease also occurs frequently in patients with liver disease. Infusion of recombinant factor VIIa did not result in reduction of blood loss or mortality in randomized clinical studies in patients with upper gastrointestinal bleeding and is not indicated.[72] Recently the use of hemostatic powder was used in patients who did not respond to other measures and was successfully used in some cases, but its value should be tested in larger randomized studies before it will be registered and can be recommended in this setting.[73,74] The most important intervention is to prevent variceal bleeding by prophylactic measures, such as rubber band ligation.

Minor bleeding, including bruising, purpura and gingival bleeding occur more frequently in patients with liver disease, but do not always need treatment, or can be managed by local measures. Mucocutaneous bleeding, such as epistaxis, can be treated with fibrinolysis inhibitors, for instance tranexamic acid, and menorrhagia by oral contraceptives. In case of bleeding in patients with severe thrombocytopenia (<50,000/μL) platelet transfusion should be given, as would also be indicated in patients without underlying liver disease.

Hemostatic Management Before Interventions and Surgical Procedures

Traditional guidelines have advised not to perform invasive procedures in patients with liver disease when routine hemostatic tests are abnormal unless they are corrected by blood products or pharmacologic prohemostatic agents. The rationale for such a prophylactic approach has been questioned for several reasons. First and most important because abnormal coagulation tests in patients with liver disease are not necessarily associated with a bleeding risk.[24] As mentioned before, these results have been traditionally interpreted to reflect a hypocoagulable state, but appeared to have no impact on the bleeding risk after invasive procedures.[75-77] For instance, in a large prospective study there was no evidence that prolongation of the INR was associated with bleeding after large-volume paracentesis in patients with liver disease and ascites.[75] Furthermore normalization of traditional coagulation tests is rarely achieved by infusion of plasma products and the efficacy of prophylactic treatment has not been proven.[78,79] In addition, transfusion of blood products carry a substantial risk of allergic reactions, volume overload and potential transmission of pathogens.[80] Consequently, the current guideline of the American Association for the Study of Liver Diseases (AASLD) do not recommend the routine use of fresh-frozen plasma (FFP) transfusion for prophylactic correction of an abnormal PT before interventions, such as liver biopsy,[81] whereas other guidelines advise the use of FFP with low grade of evidence.[82] Vitamin K is generally recommended in patients with liver disease and prolonged INR, however its clinical benefit has been questioned.[83]

Thrombocytopenia in patients with cirrhosis is often mild and does not cause spontaneous bleeding or bleeding following minimally invasive procedures. There is little evidence that tests showing platelet dysfunction, including prolonged bleeding time or closure time measured with the PFA-100 predict bleeding in patients with cirrhosis. Nevertheless, an early study showed that a prolonged bleeding time was associated with a fivefold increase in the risk of bleeding after liver biopsy.[84] Although shortening of the bleeding time was achieved by administration of 1-deamino-8-D-arginine vasopressin (DDAVP) in patients with liver disease,[85] no effect of DDAVP was observed in patients with bleeding from esophageal varices or on the blood loss in patients undergoing hepatectomy[86] or liver transplantation.[87] Although this has not been addressed in many studies yet, it has been shown that bleeding complications during interventional procedures are associated with a low preprocedural platelet count.[88,89] If platelet counts are below

50×10^9/L, platelet transfusion is recommended before any intervention, as in other patients without underlying liver disease.[90] In case of neurosurgical interventions platelets should be transfused up to a level of 100×10^9/L.[91] A novel strategy to improve primary hemostasis in patients with hepatitis C is the administration of a thrombopoietin analogue (Eltrombopag). In the ELEVATE study, a short course of Eltrombopag was used to elevate the platelet count prior to invasive procedures. Use of Eltrombopag was associated with a higher rate of thrombosis, but no difference in bleeding was observed in this study, which may be related to the highly elevated VWF levels in patients with liver disease.[92,93] Eltrombopag is not indicated for the treatment of thrombocytopenia in patients with chronic liver disease before surgical interventions.

In individuals with generalized mucosal bleeding symptoms, which may be indicative of disorders of primary hemostasis or hyperfibrinolysis, treatment with fibrinolysis inhibitors such as tranexamic acid after the procedure should be considered.[68,89] Tranexamic acid is also advised in case of dental extractions because of the high fibrinolytic activity in the oral mucosa.

The use of fibrin sealant has been studied to reduce blood loss in patient undergoing liver surgery. Although these products reduce the time to hemostasis when applied on the transected liver surface, no improvement in postoperative complications was observed. Therefore its value in these settings has not yet been established.[94]

Hemostatic Management During Liver Transplantation

For many years excessive blood loss during liver transplantation has been recognized as an important cause of morbidity and mortality; consequently, transfusion of a combination of blood products has been advocated for correction of the hemostatic derangements.[59] Experiments in experimental animal models have shown that the quality of the graft determines the extent of hemostatic changes following reperfusion.[59a] Indeed, blood loss following graft reperfusion is substantially increased in recipients of "extended criteria" donor livers (i.e., grafts with poorer quality because of, e.g., elevated donor age or prolonged cold ischemia times).[59b]

Because prophylactic transfusion of blood products may be associated with serious side effects, many centers have discontinued to attempt to improve hemostatic functions by administration of blood products prior to liver transplantation.[60] Liver transplantation procedures can now be performed without a requirement for transfusion of blood products in a substantial proportion of patients. One study reported that 79 percent of patients could be transplanted without the use of any blood product, provided the patient's central venous pressure was controlled through restriction of volume replacement, and by using intraoperative phlebotomy during the transplantation.[61] Increased experience and improvements in surgical technique, anesthesiologic care, and better graft preservation methods have contributed to a steady decrease in blood transfusion requirements. When uncontrolled bleeding does occur, packed red cells, platelets, FFP, or fibrinogen concentrate can be transfused guided by laboratory values or thromboelastography.[95] Hyperfibrinolysis is thought to contribute significantly to impaired hemostasis during the anhepatic and reperfusion phases.[63] Use of synthetic antifibrinolytic agents, such as tranexamic acid (a lysine analogue) and aprotinin (a serine protease inhibitor) have reduced red cell and plasma transfusion.[96,97] Aprotinin was taken off the market in 2008 because of severe adverse events and mortality in patients undergoing cardiac surgery.[98]

THROMBOSIS IN PATIENTS WITH LIVER DISEASE

Deep Vein Thrombosis and Pulmonary Embolism

The reappraisal of changes in the hemostatic system in patients with liver disease has indicated that the coagulopathy of liver disease may not only reflect a reduced bleeding risk, but may even lead to a prothrombotic state.[99] Studies indicate that deep vein thrombosis and pulmonary embolism can occur in patients with cirrhosis.[48,100] A large nationwide population-based case-control study in Denmark indicated that patients with liver disease have a substantially increased risk for venous thromboembolism compared to controls with an odds ratio of 1.7 for patients with cirrhosis, and an odds ratio of 1.9 for patients with other liver diseases.[48] Between 0.5 and 1.8 percent of all hospitalized patients with cirrhosis developed venous thrombosis. Therefore liver disease should not be considered a contraindication for thromboprophylaxis with low-molecular-weight heparin (LMWH). Thromboprophylaxis is warranted in patients that are immobilized or undergo surgery and in hospitalized patients with active cancer. Treatment of venous thromboembolism in patients with liver disease is difficult, because of a higher risk of bleeding associated with anticoagulant treatment than in healthy individuals, although recent data suggest that therapeutic dose LMWH is safe.[101–104] This, again, indicates that the balanced hemostatic system in patients with cirrhosis involves a narrow safety margin. Furthermore, the choice of anticoagulant may be difficult. LMWH or unfractionated heparin may be difficult to monitor as a result of low levels of antithrombin. Anti–factor Xa measurement seems to be unreliable in patients with liver disease because of analytical problems.[102,105] Also monitoring of treatment with vitamin K antagonists is difficult and may not be reliable based on the preexistent prolongation of the PT as a result of the underlying disease.[44] Considering the lack of studies, it is advised however to maintain the INR between 2.0 and 3.0.[24]

Portal Vein Thrombosis

Patients with advanced liver disease may develop thrombosis in the portal and mesenteric veins. These complications are not only related to decreased levels of the natural inhibitors of coagulation, antithrombin, protein C, and protein S, but occur also more often in individuals carrying common inherited thrombophilia's such as factor V Leiden mutation and prothrombin G20210A variant.[106,107] A decreased blood flow in the splanchnic venous circulation because of portal hypertension has also been indicated as a risk factor for portal vein thrombosis (PVT). The prevalence of PVT in patients with cirrhosis increases with the progression of the disease, being less than 1 percent in patients with compensated cirrhosis, and 8 to 25 percent in liver transplantation candidates.[44,108] Prophylactic treatment of patients with cirrhosis with low-dose of LMWH reduced the risk of PVT and even increased survival.[101] The optimal treatment of PVT in cirrhosis patients remains to be established. Although randomized trials are still lacking, treatment with anticoagulants, such as LMWH of vitamin K antagonists may prevent progression of thrombosis and may achieve recanalization in patients with PVT with or without cirrhosis.[109,110] However not all patients with cirrhosis and PVT will benefit and an individualized approach seems warranted.[111] Recently the new direct oral anticoagulants have been approved for use in patients with venous thrombosis. Their use is not yet recommended in patients with liver disease, but recently some case reports have been published in patients with splanchnic vein thrombosis.[112]

Thrombosis Following Liver Transplantation

Following liver transplantation, both immediate and delayed thrombotic complications frequently occur.[113] Hepatic artery thrombosis (HAT) occurs in 1.6 to 8.9 percent of patients and may lead to graft failure, requiring retransplantation.[114,115] Thrombosis of the portal vein or inferior caval vein are much less common.[116] Although HAT has been considered a surgical complication, recent evidence suggests that excessive coagulation activation or inherited thrombophilia also may contribute to HAT.[117] Postoperative use of anticoagulants has been limited

in liver transplant recipients as a result of the perceived bleeding risk. However, thrombotic complications do occur, and liver-related thrombosis in particular, such as HAT and PVT, are of concern as they often lead to graft loss. A single, uncontrolled retrospective study showed aspirin to substantially reduce the risk of posttransplantation HAT, without increase of bleeding.[118] Pulmonary emboli and intracardiac thrombosis may occur during liver transplantation, indicating that the hemostatic system may also tip toward thrombus formation during this procedure.[119] Whether or not other anticoagulants will prevent postoperative thrombosis remains to be established.

Role of Coagulation in Fibrosis of the Liver

Thrombin, the key mediator of coagulation, also has several cellular effects mediated by protease-activated receptors (PARs). These PARs are expressed on hepatic stellate cells (HSCs), which are mediators of liver fibrosis. Thrombin generation leads to activation of HSCs and fibrogenesis.[120] Indeed, patients with prothrombotic phenotypes, such as carriers of the factor V Leiden mutation of antithrombin-deficient individuals were shown to have enhanced progression of liver fibrosis in viral hepatitis.[121,122] In line with these observations, fibrogenesis may be reduced by using anticoagulant treatment, however this has to be established in clinical studies.[44]

REFERENCES

1. Afdhal N, McHutchison J, Brown R, et al: Thrombocytopenia associated with chronic liver disease. *J Hepatol* 48(6):1000–1007, 2008.
2. Aster RH: Pooling of platelets in the spleen: Role in the pathogenesis of "hypersplenic" thrombocytopenia. *J Clin Invest* 45(5):645–657, 1966.
3. Schmidt KG, Rasmussen JW, Bekker C, Madsen PE: Kinetics and in vivo distribution of 111-In-labelled autologous platelets in chronic hepatic disease: Mechanisms of thrombocytopenia. *Scand J Haematol* 34(1):39–46, 1985.
4. Goulis J, Chau TN, Jordan S, et al: Thrombopoietin concentrations are low in patients with cirrhosis and thrombocytopenia and are restored after orthotopic liver transplantation. *Gut* 44(5):754–758, 1999.
5. Ben-Ari Z, Osman E, Hutton RA, Burroughs AK: Disseminated intravascular coagulation in liver cirrhosis: Fact or fiction? *Am J Gastroenterol* 94(10):2977–2982, 1999.
6. Kajihara M, Kato S, Okazaki Y, et al: A role of autoantibody-mediated platelet destruction in thrombocytopenia in patients with cirrhosis. *Hepatology* 37(6):1267–1276, 2003.
7. Witters P, Freson K, Verslype C, et al: Review article: Blood platelet number and function in chronic liver disease and cirrhosis. *Aliment Pharmacol Ther* 27(11):1017–1029, 2008.
8. Ordinas A, Escolar G, Cirera I, et al: Existence of a platelet-adhesion defect in patients with cirrhosis independent of hematocrit: Studies under flow conditions. *Hepatology* 24(5):1137–1142, 1996.
9. Lisman T, Adelmeijer J, de Groot PG, et al: No evidence for an intrinsic platelet defect in patients with liver cirrhosis—Studies under flow conditions. *J Thromb Haemost* 4(9):2070–2072, 2006.
10. Escolar G, Cases A, Vinas M, et al: Evaluation of acquired platelet dysfunctions in uremic and cirrhotic patients using the platelet function analyzer (PFA-100): Influence of hematocrit elevation. *Haematologica* 84(7):614–619, 1999.
11. Tripodi A, Primignani M, Chantarangkul V, et al: Thrombin generation in patients with cirrhosis: The role of platelets. *Hepatology* 44(2):440–445, 2006.
12. Ferro D, Quintarelli C, Lattuada A, et al: High plasma levels of von Willebrand factor as a marker of endothelial perturbation in cirrhosis: Relationship to endotoxemia. *Hepatology.* 23(6):1377–1383, 1996.
13. Lisman T, Bongers TN, Adelmeijer J, et al: Elevated levels of von Willebrand Factor in cirrhosis support platelet adhesion despite reduced functional capacity. *Hepatology.* 44(1):53–61, 2006.
14. Hollestelle MJ, Thinnes T, Crain K, et al: Tissue distribution of factor VIII gene expression in vivo—A closer look. *Thromb Haemost* 86(3):855–861, 2001.
15. Beer JH, Clerici N, Baillod P, et al: Quantitative and qualitative analysis of platelet GPIb and von Willebrand factor in liver cirrhosis. *Thromb Haemost* 73(4):601–609, 1995.
16. Hollestelle MJ, Geertzen HG, Straatsburg IH, et al: Factor VIII expression in liver disease. *Thromb Haemost* 91(2):267–275, 2004.
17. Mannucci PM, Canciani MT, Forza I, et al: Changes in health and disease of the metalloprotease that cleaves von Willebrand factor. *Blood* 98(9):2730–2735, 2001.
18. Federici AB, Berkowitz SD, Lattuada A, Mannucci PM: Degradation of von Willebrand factor in patients with acquired clinical conditions in which there is heightened proteolysis. *Blood* 81(3):720–725, 1993.
19. Tersteeg C, de Maat S, De Meyer SF, et al: Plasmin cleavage of von Willebrand factor as an emergency bypass for ADAMTS13 deficiency in thrombotic microangiopathy. *Circulation* 129(12):1320–1331, 2014.

20. Hugenholtz GG, Porte RJ, Lisman T: The platelet and platelet function testing in liver disease. *Clin Liver Dis* 13(1):11–20, 2009.

21. Kerr R, Newsome P, Germain L, et al: Effects of acute liver injury on blood coagulation. *J Thromb Haemost* 1(4):754–759, 2003.

22. Fahs SA, Hille MT, Shi Q, Weiler H, Montgomery RR: A conditional knockout mouse model reveals endothelial cells as the principal and possibly exclusive source of plasma factor VIII. *Blood* 123(24):3706–3713, 2014.

23. Blanchard RA, Furie BC, Jorgensen M, et al: Acquired vitamin K-dependent carboxylation deficiency in liver disease. *N Engl J Med* 305(5):242–248, 1981.

24. Tripodi A, Mannucci PM: The coagulopathy of chronic liver disease. *N Engl J Med* 365(2):147–156, 2011.

25. de Maat MP, Nieuwenhuizen W, Knot EA, et al: Measuring plasma fibrinogen levels in patients with liver cirrhosis. The occurrence of proteolytic fibrin(ogen) degradation products and their influence on several fibrinogen assays. *Thromb Res* 78(4):353–362, 1995.

26. Francis JL, Armstrong DJ: Acquired dysfibrinogenaemia in liver disease. *J Clin Pathol* 35(6):667–672, 1982.

27. Tripodi A, Salerno F, Chantarangkul V, et al: Evidence of normal thrombin generation in cirrhosis despite abnormal conventional coagulation tests. *Hepatology* 41(3):553–558, 2005.

28. Lisman T, Bakhtiari K, Pereboom IT, et al: Normal to increased thrombin generation in patients undergoing liver transplantation despite prolonged conventional coagulation tests. *J Hepatol* 52(3):355–361, 2010.

29. Gatt A, Riddell A, Calvaruso V, et al: Enhanced thrombin generation in patients with cirrhosis-induced coagulopathy. *J Thromb Haemost* 8(9):1994–2000, 2010.

30. Potze W, Arshad F, Adelmeijer J, et al: Differential in vitro inhibition of thrombin generation by anticoagulant drugs in plasma from patients with cirrhosis. *PloS One* 9(2):e88390, 2014.

31. Lisman T, Porte RJ: Rebalanced hemostasis in patients with liver disease: Evidence and clinical consequences. *Blood* 116(6):878–885, 2010.

32. Trotter JF, Brimhall B, Arjal R, Phillips C: Specific laboratory methodologies achieve higher model for endstage liver disease (MELD) scores for patients listed for liver transplantation. *Liver Transpl* 10(8):995–1000, 2004.

33. Lisman T, van Leeuwen Y, Adelmeijer J, et al: Interlaboratory variability in assessment of the model of end-stage liver disease score. *Liver Int* 28(10):1344–1351, 2008.

34. Tripodi A, Chantarangkul V, Primignani M, et al: The international normalized ratio calibrated for cirrhosis (INR[liver]) normalizes prothrombin time results for model for end-stage liver disease calculation. *Hepatology* 46(2):520–527, 2007.

35. Bellest L, Eschwege V, Poupon R, et al: A modified international normalized ratio as an effective way of prothrombin time standardization in hepatology. *Hepatology* 46(2):528–534, 2007.

36. Leebeek FW: *Hyperfibrinolysis in Liver Disease.* CRC Press, Boca Raton, FL, 1996.

37. Leebeek FW, Kluft C, Knot EA, et al: A shift in balance between profibrinolytic and antifibrinolytic factors causes enhanced fibrinolysis in cirrhosis. *Gastroenterology* 101(5):1382–1390, 1991.

38. Lisman T, Leebeek FW, Mosnier LO, et al: Thrombin-activatable fibrinolysis inhibitor deficiency in cirrhosis is not associated with increased plasma fibrinolysis. *Gastroenterology* 121(1):131–139, 2001.

39. Stravitz RT: Potential applications of thromboelastography in patients with acute and chronic liver disease. *Nat Rev Gastroenterol Hepatol* 8(8):513–520, 2012.

40. Rijken DC, Kock EL, Guimaraes AH, et al: Evidence for an enhanced fibrinolytic capacity in cirrhosis as measured with two different global fibrinolysis tests. *J Thromb Haemost* 10(10):2116–2122, 2012.

41. Violi F, Ferro D, Basili S, et al: Association between low-grade disseminated intravascular coagulation and endotoxemia in patients with liver cirrhosis. *Gastroenterology* 109(2):531–539, 1995.

42. Francis RB Jr, Feinstein DI: Clinical significance of accelerated fibrinolysis in liver disease. *Haemostasis* 14(6):460–465, 1984.

43. Violi F, Ferro D, Basili S, et al: Hyperfibrinolysis increases the risk of gastrointestinal hemorrhage in patients with advanced cirrhosis. *Hepatology* 15(4):672–676, 1992.

44. Tripodi A, Anstee QM, Sogaard KK, et al: Hypercoagulability in cirrhosis: Causes and consequences. *J Thromb Haemost* 9(9):1713–1723, 2011.

45. Lisman T, Caldwell SH, Leebeek FW, Porte RJ: Is chronic liver disease associated with a bleeding diathesis? *J Thromb Haemost* 4(9):2059–2060, 2006.

46. Massicotte L, Lenis S, Thibeault L, et al: Effect of low central venous pressure and phlebotomy on blood product transfusion requirements during liver transplantations. *Liver Transpl* 12(1):117–123, 2006.

47. De Gottardi A, Thevenot T, Spahr L, et al: Risk of complications after abdominal paracentesis in cirrhotic patients: A prospective study. *Clin Gastroenterol Hepatol* 7(8):906–909, 2009.

48. Sogaard KK, Horvath-Puho E, Gronbaek H, et al: Risk of venous thromboembolism in patients with liver disease: A nationwide population-based case-control study. *Am J Gastroenterol* 104(1):96–101, 2009.

49. Northup PG, McMahon MM, Ruhl AP, et al: Coagulopathy does not fully protect hospitalized cirrhosis patients from peripheral venous thromboembolism. *Am J Gastroenterol* 101(7):1524–1528; quiz 1680, 2006.

50. Gulley D, Teal E, Suvannasankha A, et al: Deep vein thrombosis and pulmonary embolism in cirrhosis patients. *Dig Dis Sci* 53(11):3012–3017, 2008.

51. Vivas S, Rodriguez M, Palacio MA, et al: Presence of bacterial infection in bleeding cirrhotic patients is independently associated with early mortality and failure to control bleeding. *Dig Dis Sci* 46(12):2752–2757, 2001.

52. Munoz SJ, Rajender Reddy K, Lee W; Acute Liver Failure Study Group: The coagulopathy of acute liver failure and implications for intracranial pressure monitoring. *Neurocrit Care* 9(1):103–107, 2008.

53. Lisman T, Bakhtiari K, Adelmeijer J, et al: Intact thrombin generation and decreased fibrinolytic capacity in patients with acute liver injury or acute liver failure. *J Thromb Haemost* 10(7):1312–1319, 2012.

54. Stravitz RT, Lisman T, Luketic VA, et al: Minimal effects of acute liver injury/acute liver failure on hemostasis as assessed by thromboelastography. *J Hepatol* 56(1):129–136, 2012.

55. Hugenholtz GC, Adelmeijer J, Meijers JC, et al: An unbalance between von Willebrand factor and ADAMTS13 in acute liver failure: Implications for hemostasis and clinical outcome. *Hepatology* 58(2):752–761, 2013.

56. Pernambuco JR, Langley PG, Hughes RD, et al: Activation of the fibrinolytic system in patients with fulminant liver failure. *Hepatology* 18(6):1350–1356, 1993.

57. Stravitz RT, Bowling R, Bradford RL, et al: Role of procoagulant microparticles in mediating complications and outcome of acute liver injury/acute liver failure. *Hepatology* 58(1):304–313, 2013.

58. Munoz SJ, Stravitz RT, Gabriel DA: Coagulopathy of acute liver failure. *Clin Liver Dis* 13(1):95–107, 2009.

59. Porte RJ, Knot EA, Bontempo FA: Hemostasis in liver transplantation. *Gastroenterology* 97(2):488–501, 1989.

59a. Bakker CM, Blankensteijn JD, Schlejen P, et al: The effects of long-term graft preservation on intraoperative hemostatic changes in liver transplantation. A comparison between orthotopic and heterotopic transplantation in the pig. *HPB Surg* 7(4):265–80, 1994.

59b. de Boer MT, Westerkamp A, van den Berg AP, et al: Impact of extended criteria donor grafts on post-reperfusion transfusion requirements in liver transplantation; abstract *Liver Transpl* 15(7):S128–S129, 2009.

60. de Boer MT, Molenaar IQ, Hendriks HG, et al: Minimizing blood loss in liver transplantation: Progress through research and evolution of techniques. *Dig Surg* 22(4):265–275, 2005.

61. Massicotte L, Denault AY, Beaulieu D, et al: Transfusion rate for 500 consecutive liver transplantations: Experience of one liver transplantation center. *Transplantation* 93(12):1276–1281, 2012.

62. Kang YG, Martin DJ, Marquez J, et al: Intraoperative changes in blood coagulation and thrombelastographic monitoring in liver transplantation. *Anesth Analg* 64(9):888–896, 1985.

63. Porte RJ, Bontempo FA, Knot EA, et al: Systemic effects of tissue plasminogen activator-associated fibrinolysis and its relation to thrombin generation in orthotopic liver transplantation. *Transplantation* 47(6):978–984, 1989.

64. Sindram D, Porte RJ, Hoffman MR, et al: Platelets induce sinusoidal endothelial cell apoptosis upon reperfusion of the cold ischemic rat liver. *Gastroenterology* 118(1):183–191, 2000.

65. Agarwal S, Senzolo M, Melikian C, et al: The prevalence of a heparin-like effect shown on the thromboelastograph in patients undergoing liver transplantation. *Liver Transpl* 14(6):855–860, 2008.

66. Pereboom IT, Adelmeijer J, van Leeuwen Y, et al: Development of a severe von Willebrand factor/ADAMTS13 dysbalance during orthotopic liver transplantation. *Am J Transplant* 9(5):1189–1196, 2009.

67. Stahl RL, Duncan A, Hooks MA, et al: A hypercoagulable state follows orthotopic liver transplantation. *Hepatology* 12(3 Pt 1):553–558, 1990.

68. Boks AL, Brommer EJ, Schalm SW, Van Vliet HH: Hemostasis and fibrinolysis in severe liver failure and their relation to hemorrhage. *Hepatology* 6(1):79–86, 1986.

69. Garcia-Tsao G, Bosch J: Management of varices and variceal hemorrhage in cirrhosis. *N Engl J Med* 362(9):823–832, 2010.

70. Villanueva C, Colomo A, Bosch A, et al: Transfusion strategies for acute upper gastrointestinal bleeding. *N Engl J Med* 368(1):11–21, 2013.

71. Castaneda B, Debernardi-Venon W, Bandi JC, et al: The role of portal pressure in the severity of bleeding in portal hypertensive rats. *Hepatology* 31(3):581–586, 2000.

72. Marti-Carvajal AJ, Karakitsiou DE, Salanti G: Human recombinant activated factor VII for upper gastrointestinal bleeding in patients with liver diseases. *Cochrane Database Syst Rev* 3:CD004887, 2012.

73. Holster IL, Poley JW, Kuipers EJ, Tjwa ET: Controlling gastric variceal bleeding with endoscopically applied hemostatic powder (Hemospray). *J Hepatol* 57(6):1397–1398, 2012.

74. Sung JJ, Luo D, Wu JC, et al: Early clinical experience of the safety and effectiveness of Hemospray in achieving hemostasis in patients with acute peptic ulcer bleeding. *Endoscopy* 43(4):291–295, 2011.

75. De Gottardi A, Thevenot T, Spahr L, et al: Risk of complications after abdominal paracentesis in cirrhotic patients: A prospective study. *Clin Gastroenterol Hepatol* 7(8):906–909, 2009.

76. Piccinino F, Sagnelli E, Pasquale G, Giusti G: Complications following percutaneous liver biopsy. A multicentre retrospective study on 68,276 biopsies. *J Hepatol* 2(2):165–173, 1986.

77. Segal JB, Dzik WH, Transfusion Medicine/Hemostasis Clinical Trials Network: Paucity of studies to support that abnormal coagulation test results predict bleeding in the setting of invasive procedures: An evidence-based review. *Transfusion* 45(9):1413–1425, 2005.

78. Youssef WI, Salazar F, Dasarathy S, et al: Role of fresh frozen plasma infusion in correction of coagulopathy of chronic liver disease: A dual phase study. *Am J Gastroenterol* 98(6):1391–1394, 2003.

79. Gazzard BG, Henderson JM, Williams R: The use of fresh frozen plasma or a concentrate of factor IX as replacement therapy before liver biopsy. *Gut* 16(8):621–625, 1975.

80. Alter HJ, Klein HG: The hazards of blood transfusion in historical perspective. *Blood* 112(7):2617–2626, 2008.

81. Rockey DC, Caldwell SH, Goodman ZD, et al: American Association for the Study of Liver Diseases: Liver biopsy. *Hepatology* 49(3):1017–1044, 2009.

82. Liumbruno G, Bennardello F, Lattanzio A, et al: Recommendations for the transfusion of plasma and platelets. *Blood Transfus* 7(2):132–150, 2009.

83. Saja MF, Abdo AA, Sanai FM, et al: The coagulopathy of liver disease: Does vitamin K help? *Blood Coagul Fibrinolysis* 24(1):10–17, 2013.

84. Boberg KM, Brosstad F, Egeland T, et al: Is a prolonged bleeding time associated with an increased risk of hemorrhage after liver biopsy? *Thromb Haemost* 81(3):378–381, 1999.

85. Agnelli G, Parise P, Levi M, et al: Effects of desmopressin on hemostasis in patients with liver cirrhosis. *Haemostasis* 25(5):241–247, 1995.

86. Wong AY, Irwin MG, Hui TW, et al: Desmopressin does not decrease blood loss and transfusion requirements in patients undergoing hepatectomy. *Can J Anaesth* 50(1):14–20, 2003.

87. de Franchis R, Arcidiacono PG, Carpinelli L, et al: Randomized controlled trial of desmopressin plus terlipressin vs. terlipressin alone for the treatment of acute variceal hemorrhage in cirrhotic patients: A multicenter, double-blind study. New Italian Endoscopic Club. *Hepatology* 18(5):1102–1107, 1993.

88. Sharma P, McDonald GB, Banaji M: The risk of bleeding after percutaneous liver biopsy: Relation to platelet count. *J Clin Gastroenterol* 4(5):451–453, 1982.

89. Lisman T, Caldwell SH, Burroughs AK, et al: Hemostasis and thrombosis in patients with liver disease: The ups and downs. *J Hepatol* 53(2):362–371, 2010.

90. Violi F, Basili S, Raparelli V, et al: Patients with liver cirrhosis suffer from primary haemostatic defects? Fact or fiction? *J Hepatol* 55(6):1415–1427, 2011.

91. Slichter SJ: Evidence-based platelet transfusion guidelines. *Hematology Am Soc Hematol Educ Program* 2007:172–178.

92. Afdhal NH, Giannini EG, Tayyab G, et al: Eltrombopag before procedures in patients with cirrhosis and thrombocytopenia. *N Engl J Med* 367(8):716–724, 2012.

93. Lisman T, Porte RJ: Eltrombopag before procedures in patients with cirrhosis and thrombocytopenia. *N Engl J Med* 367(21):2055–2056, 2012.

94. de Boer MT, Boonstra EA, Lisman T, Porte RJ: Role of fibrin sealants in liver surgery. *Dig Surg* 29(1):54–61, 2012.

95. Wang SC, Shieh JF, Chang KY, et al: Thromboelastography-guided transfusion decreases intraoperative blood transfusion during orthotopic liver transplantation: Randomized clinical trial. *Transplant Proc* 42(7):2590–2593, 2010.

96. Porte RJ, Molenaar IQ, Begliomini B, et al: Aprotinin and transfusion requirements in orthotopic liver transplantation: A multicentre randomised double-blind study. EMSALT Study Group. *Lancet* 355(9212):1303–1309, 2000.

97. Boylan JF, Klinck JR, Sandler AN, et al: Tranexamic acid reduces blood loss, transfusion requirements, and coagulation factor use in primary orthotopic liver transplantation. *Anesthesiology* 85(5):1043–1048; discussion 30A–31A, 1996.

98. Fergusson DA, Hebert PC, Mazer CD, et al: A comparison of aprotinin and lysine analogues in high-risk cardiac surgery. *N Engl J Med* 358(22):2319–2331, 1996.

99. Tripodi A, Anstee QM, Sogaard KK, et al: Hypercoagulability in cirrhosis: Causes and consequences. *J Thromb Haemost* 9(9):1713–1723, 2011.

100. Northup PG, Sundaram V, Fallon MB, et al: Hypercoagulation and thrombophilia in liver disease. *J Thromb Haemost* 6(1):2–9, 2008.

101. Villa E, Camma C, Marietta M, et al: Enoxaparin prevents portal vein thrombosis and liver decompensation in patients with advanced cirrhosis. *Gastroenterology* 143(5):1253–1260, 2012.

102. Bechmann LP, Sichau M, Wichert M, et al: Low-molecular-weight heparin in patients with advanced cirrhosis. *Liver Int* 31(1):75–82, 2011.

103. Cerini F, Garcia-Pagán JC: Tromboprophylaxis with heparin in hospitalized patients with cirrhosis: Friend or foe. *Liver Int* 34(7):971–973, 2014.

104. Intagliata NM, Henry ZH, Shah N, et al: Prophylactic anticoagulation for venous thromboembolism in hospitalized cirrhosis patients is not associated with high rates of gastrointestinal bleeding. *Liver Int* 34(1):26–32, 2014.

105. Potze W, Arshad F, Adelmeijer J, et al: Routine coagulation assays underestimate levels of antithrombin-dependent drugs but not of direct anticoagulant drugs in plasma from patients with cirrhosis. *Br J Haematol* 163(5):666–673, 2013.

106. Amitrano L, Brancaccio V, Guardascione MA, et al: Inherited coagulation disorders in cirrhotic patients with portal vein thrombosis. *Hepatology* 31(2):345–348, 2000.

107. Zocco MA, Di Stasio E, De Cristofaro R, et al: Thrombotic risk factors in patients with liver cirrhosis: Correlation with MELD scoring system and portal vein thrombosis development. *J Hepatol* 51(4):682–689, 2009.

108. Okuda K, Ohnishi K, Kimura K, et al: Incidence of portal vein thrombosis in liver cirrhosis. An angiographic study in 708 patients. *Gastroenterology* 89(2):279–286, 1985.

109. Senzolo M, M Sartori T, Rossetto V, et al: Prospective evaluation of anticoagulation and transjugular intrahepatic portosistemic shunt for the management of portal vein thrombosis in cirrhosis. *Liver Int* 32(6):919–927, 2012.

110. Plessier A, Darwish-Murad S, Hernandez-Guerra M, et al: Acute portal vein thrombosis unrelated to cirrhosis: A prospective multicenter follow-up study. *Hepatology* 51(1):210–218, 2010.

111. Confer BD, Hanouneh I, Gomes M, Alraies MC: Q: Is anticoagulation appropriate for all patients with portal vein thrombosis? *Cleve Clin J Med* 80(10):611–613, 2013.

112. Intagliata N, Maitland H, Northup P, Caldwell S: Treating thrombosis in cirrhosis patients with new oral agents: Ready or not? *Hepatology* 61(2):738–739, 2015.

113. Washington K: Update on post-liver transplantation infections, malignancies, and surgical complications. *Adv Anat Pathol* 12(4):221–226, 2005.

114. Silva MA, Jambulingam PS, Gunson BK, et al: Hepatic artery thrombosis following orthotopic liver transplantation: A 10-year experience from a single centre in the United Kingdom. *Liver Transpl* 12(1):146–151, 2006.

115. Bekker J, Ploem S, de Jong KP: Early hepatic artery thrombosis after liver transplantation: A systematic review of the incidence, outcome and risk factors. *Am J Transplant* 9(4):746–757, 2009.

116. Quiroga S, Sebastia MC, Margarit C, et al: Complications of orthotopic liver transplantation: Spectrum of findings with helical CT. *Radiographics* 21(5):1085–1102, 2001.

117. Hirshfield G, Collier JD, Brown K, et al: Donor factor V Leiden mutation and vascular thrombosis following liver transplantation. *Liver Transpl Surg* 4(1):58–61, 1998.

118. Vivarelli M, La Barba G, Cucchetti A, et al: Can antiplatelet prophylaxis reduce the incidence of hepatic artery thrombosis after liver transplantation? *Liver Transpl* 13(5):651–654, 2007.

119. Warnaar N, Molenaar IQ, Colquhoun SD, et al: Intraoperative pulmonary embolism and intracardiac thrombosis complicating liver transplantation: A systematic review. *J Thromb Haemost* 6(2):297–302, 2008.

120. Jairath V, Burroughs AK: Anticoagulation in patients with liver cirrhosis: Complication or therapeutic opportunity? *Gut* 62(4):479–482, 2013.

121. Wright M, Goldin R, Hellier S, et al: Factor V Leiden polymorphism and the rate of fibrosis development in chronic hepatitis C virus infection. *Gut* 52(8):1206–1210, 2003.

122. Papatheodoridis GV, Papakonstantinou E, Andrioti E, et al: Thrombotic risk factors and extent of liver fibrosis in chronic viral hepatitis. *Gut* 52(3):404–409, 2003.

CHAPTER 129
DISSEMINATED INTRAVASCULAR COAGULATION

Marcel Levi and Uri Seligsohn

SUMMARY

When procoagulants are produced or introduced into the blood and overcome the anticoagulant mechanisms of coagulation, intravascular thrombin is generated systemically, which can lead to disseminated intravascular coagulation (DIC). The clinical manifestations of intravascular coagulation include (1) multiorgan dysfunction caused by microthrombi; (2) bleeding caused by consumption of platelets, fibrinogen, and other coagulation factors; and (3) secondary fibrinolysis. Exposure of blood to tissue factor is the most common trigger. This event can occur when mononuclear cells and endothelial cells are induced to generate and express tissue factor during the systemic inflammatory response syndrome (e.g., Gram-negative and Gram-positive infections, fungemia, burns, severe trauma), or when contact is established between blood and tissue factor constitutively present on membranes of cells foreign to blood (e.g., malignant, placental, brain, adventitial cells, or traumatized tissues). Laboratory features include thrombocytopenia, reduced levels of fibrinogen and other coagulation factors (leading to prolonged partial thromboplastin, prothrombin, and thrombin times), and elevated levels of D-dimer and fibrin(ogen) degradation products. Several underlying disorders affect these hemostatic parameters and can lead to a false-positive diagnosis of DIC (e.g., liver disease–related coagulation abnormalities and thrombocytopenia) or to a false-negative diagnosis (e.g., pregnancy-related high fibrinogen levels). Reexamining these variables every 6 to 8 hours may permit a specific diagnosis. Early detection, vigorous treatment of the underlying disorder, and support of vital functions are essential for survival of affected patients. Blood component therapy is effective in patients who bleed excessively, whereas heparin administration is indicated in a limited number of circumstances. Intravascular coagulation and the underlying disorders causing it contribute to a high rate of mortality. The severity of the organ dysfunction and extent of hemostatic failure, as well as increasing patient age, have been associated with a grave prognosis.

Acronyms and Abbreviations: APACHE, acute physiology and chronic health evaluation; APC, activated protein C; APL, acute promyelocytic leukemia; aPTT, activated partial thromboplastin time; ARDS, adult respiratory distress syndrome; AT, antithrombin; DIC, disseminated intravascular coagulation; EPCR, endothelial protein C receptor; FDP, fibrinogen degradation product; HELLP, hemolysis, elevated liver enzymes, low platelet count; IL, interleukin; LCAD, long-chain acyl-coenzyme A dehydrogenase; LPS, lipopolysaccharide; PAI, plasminogen-activator inhibitor; PAR, protease-activated receptor; TAFI, thrombin-activatable fibrinolysis inhibitor; TAT, thrombin–antithrombin; TF, tissue factor; TFPI, tissue factor pathway inhibitor; TNF, tumor necrosis factor; t-PA, tissue-type plasminogen activator.

DEFINITION AND HISTORY

Disseminated intravascular coagulation (DIC) is a clinicopathologic syndrome in which widespread intravascular coagulation occurs as a result of exposure or production of procoagulants insufficiently balanced by natural anticoagulant mechanisms and endogenous fibrinolysis. Perturbation of the endothelium in the microcirculation along with stimulated inflammatory cells and release of inflammatory mediators play a key role in this mechanism. DIC may cause tissue ischemia from occlusive microthrombi, and bleeding from the consumption of platelets and coagulation factors and, in some cases, an excessive fibrinolytic response. DIC complicates a variety of disorders, and the complexity of its pathophysiology has made it the subject of a voluminous literature.[1-7]

In 1834, Dupuy reported that injection of brain material into animals caused widespread clots in blood vessels, thus providing the first description of DIC.[8] In 1865, Trousseau described the tendency to thrombosis, sometimes disseminated, in cachectic patients with malignancies.[9] In 1873, Naunyn showed that disseminated thrombosis could be evoked by intravenous injection of dissolved red cells, and Wooldridge demonstrated that the procoagulant involved was a substance contained in the stroma of the red cells.[10-12]

In 1955, Ratnoff and associates described the hemostatic abnormalities, which we would currently classify as DIC, that occur in women with fetal death or amniotic fluid embolism.[13] The mechanism by which DIC can lead to bleeding was clarified only in 1961, when Lasch and coworkers introduced the concept of consumption coagulopathy, and McKay established that DIC is a pathogenetic feature of a variety of diseases.[1,14] Sizable series of cases were first described in the late 1960s, following the introduction of defined laboratory criteria for DIC.[15] Yet despite the vast experience that has been accumulated, DIC still constitutes a major clinicopathologic and therapeutic challenge.

PATHOLOGY

Diffuse multiorgan bleeding, hemorrhagic necrosis, microthrombi in small blood vessels, and thrombi in medium and large blood vessels are common findings at autopsy, although patients who had unequivocal clinical and laboratory signs of DIC may not have had confirming postmortem findings.[16,17] Conversely, some patients in whom clinical and laboratory signs were not consistent with DIC had typical autopsy findings.[18,19] This occasional lack of correlation among clinical, laboratory, and pathologic findings is partly a result of extensive postmortem changes in the blood, for example, excessive fibrinolysis, but remains unexplained in most instances.[17] Organs most frequently involved by diffuse microthrombi are the lungs and kidneys, followed by the brain, heart, liver, spleen, adrenal glands, pancreas, and gut. Specific immunohistologic techniques and ultrastructural analysis have revealed that most thrombi consist of fibrin monomers or polymers in combination with platelets. In addition, involvement of activated mononuclear cells and other signs of inflammatory activation are frequently present.[20] In cases of long-lasting DIC, organization and endothelialization of the microthrombi are often observed. Acute tubular necrosis is more frequent than renal cortical necrosis.[16]

A significant proportion of patients with chronic DIC have nonbacterial thrombotic endocarditis involving mainly the mitral and aortic valves.[19] Moreover, in a retrospective pathologic study, approximately 50 percent of patients with nonbacterial thrombotic endocarditis had DIC.[18] These heart lesions can be a source of arterial embolization, leading to infarction of the brain, kidneys, and myocardium.

PATHOGENESIS

INFLAMMATION AND ENDOTHELIUM IN DISSEMINATED INTRAVASCULAR COAGULATION

Various triggers cause an hemostatic imbalance that gives rise to a pro-coagulant state (Fig. 129–1). The most important mediators responsible for this imbalance are cytokines.[21] There is an extensive crosstalk between coagulation and inflammatory systems, whereby inflammation leads to activation of coagulation, and coagulation stimulates inflammatory activity.[22] These interactions are highlighted in sepsis-induced systemic activation of coagulation and inflammation that lead to specific organ dysfunctions.[23] The endothelium of the capillary bed is the most important interface in which the interaction between inflammation and coagulation takes place. Endothelial cells may be a source of tissue factor and can thereby be involved in the initiation of coagulation activation. All physiologic anticoagulant systems and various adhesion molecules that may modulate both inflammation and coagulation are connected to the endothelium. In sepsis, endothelial glycosaminoglycans present in the glycocalyx are downregulated by proinflammatory cytokines, thereby impairing the functions of antithrombin (AT), tissue factor pathway inhibitor (TFPI), leukocyte adhesion, and leukocyte transmigration. Because the glycocalyx also plays a role in other endothelial functions, including maintenance of the vascular barrier function, nitric oxide–mediated vasodilation, and antioxidant activity, all these processes can be impaired in DIC (see "Role of Oxidative Stress and Vasoactive Molecules" below).[24,25] Moreover, specific disruption of the glycocalyx results in thrombin generation and platelet adhesion within a few minutes.[26,27]

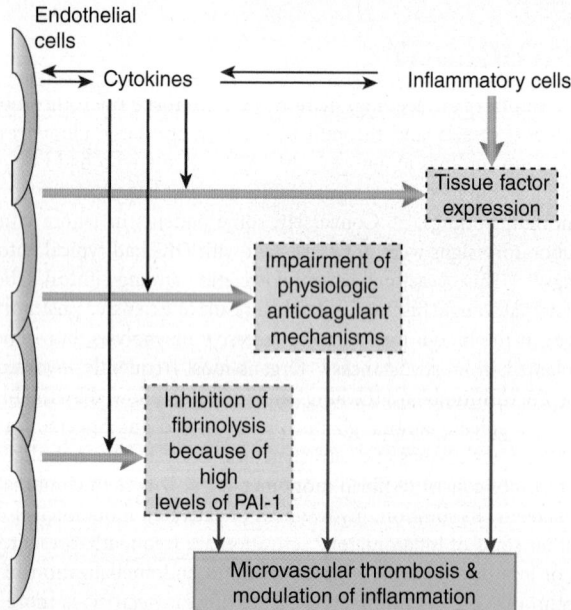

Figure 129–1. Schematic presentation of pathogenetic pathways involved in the activation of coagulation in disseminated intravascular coagulation (DIC). In DIC, both perturbed endothelial cells and activated mononuclear cells may produce proinflammatory cytokines that mediate coagulation activation. Activation of coagulation is initiated by tissue factor expression on activated mononuclear cells and endothelial cells. In addition, downregulation of physiologic anticoagulant mechanisms and inhibition of fibrinolysis by endothelial cells further promote intravascular fibrin deposition. PAI-1, plasminogen-activator inhibitor type 1.

Endothelial perturbation constitutes a *sine qua non* for most patients with DIC. Following injury or infection, the integrity of the endothelium is compromised, mononuclear cells are activated by cytokine and hormonal signals, additional cytokines and surface receptors are upregulated, procoagulant proteins and platelets are activated, the endothelium changes from an anticoagulant to procoagulant surface, and fibrinolysis is impeded. This sequence of events is typical for the *systemic inflammatory response syndrome* and can lead to microvascular thrombosis with ensuing multiorgan dysfunction and eventually to multiorgan failure.

ROLE OF CYTOKINES AND TISSUE FACTOR

Tissue factor (TF) plays a central role in the initiation of inflammation-induced coagulation in DIC.[28] Blocking TF activity completely inhibits inflammation-induced thrombin generation in experimental models of endotoxemia or bacteremia.[29,30] Most cells constitutively expressing TF are found in tissues not in direct contact with blood, such as the adventitial layer of larger blood vessels. TF becomes exposed to blood upon disruption of the vascular integrity, or when cells present in the circulation, such as monocytes, are triggered to express TF. The *in vivo* expression of TF is dependent on interleukin (IL)-6 generation; inhibition of IL-6, unlike inhibition of other proinflammatory cytokines, completely abrogates TF-dependent thrombin generation in experimental endotoxemia.[21,31] In severe sepsis, monocytes, stimulated by proinflammatory cytokines, express TF, which leads to systemic activation of coagulation.[32] Even in experimental low-dose endotoxemia in healthy subjects, a 125-fold increase in TF mRNA levels in blood monocytes can be detected.[33] A potential alternative source of TF may be endothelial cells, polymorphonuclear cells, and other cell types. It is hypothesized that TF from these sources is shuttled between cells through microparticles derived from activated mononuclear cells.[34] However, it is unlikely that cells other than monocytes synthesize TF in substantial quantities.[32,35] Tumor necrosis factor (TNF)-α and IL-1, also generated during inflammation, impair the physiologic anticoagulant pathways.[31,36,37]

AMPLIFYING ROLE OF THROMBIN AND PLATELETS

The TF–factor VIIa complex catalyzes the conversion of factor X to Xa, and factor Xa, in turn, forms the prothrombinase complex with factor Va, prothrombin (factor II), and calcium ions, thereby generating thrombin, and converting fibrinogen into fibrin. The TF–factor VIIa complex can also activate factor IX, and factor IXa forms the tenase complex with activated factor VIII and calcium ions, generating additional factor Xa, thereby forming an essential amplification loop of thrombin generation. The assembly of the prothrombinase and tenase complexes are markedly facilitated if a suitable phospholipid surface is available, such as the membrane of activated platelets. In the setting of inflammation-induced activation of coagulation, platelets can be activated directly by endotoxin or by proinflammatory mediators, such as the membrane of platelet-activating factor. Thrombin itself is one of the strongest platelet activators (Chap. 115).

Activation of platelets may also accelerate fibrin formation by another mechanism. The expression of TF on monocytes is markedly stimulated by the presence of platelets and granulocytes in a P-selectin–dependent reaction.[38] This effect may be the result of nuclear factor kappa B (NF-κB) activation induced by binding of activated platelets to neutrophils and mononuclear cells.[39] This cellular interaction also markedly enhances the production of IL-1β, IL-8, monocyte chemotactic protein (MCP)-1, and TNF-α.[40]

Thrombin generated by the TF pathway amplifies both clotting and inflammation through the following activities: (1) it activates platelets, giving rise to platelet aggregation and augmenting platelet functions in coagulation; (2) it activates factors VIII, V, and XI, yielding further thrombin generation; (3) it activates proinflammatory factors via protease-activated receptors (PARs); (4) it activates factor XIII to factor XIIIa, which crosslinks fibrin clots; (5) it activates thrombin-activatable fibrinolysis inhibitor (TAFI), making clots resistant to fibrinolysis; and (6) it increases expression of adhesion molecules, such as L-selectin, thereby promoting the inflammatory effects of leukocytes.[41]

Paradoxically, at low concentrations, thrombin exhibits both antiinflammatory and anticoagulant effects because it binds to thrombomodulin and activates protein C to the activated form, which, in turn, downregulates inflammation and serves as an "off switch" for further thrombin generation (Chap. 116).

ROLE OF COAGULATION PROTEASES IN UPREGULATING INFLAMMATION

Coagulation proteases and protease inhibitors not only interact with coagulation proteins, but also with specific cell receptors to induce signaling pathways. In particular, protease interactions that affect inflammatory processes may be important in critically ill patients. Coagulation of whole blood *in vitro* results in a detectable expression of IL-1β mRNA in blood cells,[42] and thrombin markedly enhances endotoxin-induced IL-1 activity in culture supernatants of guinea pig macrophages.[43] Similarly, clotted blood produces IL-8 *in vitro.*[44]

Factor Xa, thrombin, and fibrin can also activate endothelial cells, eliciting the synthesis of IL-6 and IL-8.[45,46] Coagulation proteases such as thrombin, factor Xa, and factor VIIa–TF complex induce inflammatory upregulation via leukocyte, endothelial cell, and platelet PAR-1, PAR-2, PAR-3, and PAR-4, which are located on leukocytes, endothelial cells, and platelets.[47] PARs have an extracellular domain, seven transmembrane domains, and an intracellular domain that is coupled to specific G-proteins that transmit signaling. PAR-1, PAR-3, and PAR-4 are

activated by thrombin through cleavage of a specific aminoterminus bond creating a tethered ligand that activates the receptor. PAR-2 can be cleaved by factor Xa–TF–factor VIIa complex and by other proteases.[48] Activated PARs then lead through mitogen-activated protein kinase and NF-κB signaling pathways to cell motility, shape change, proliferation, endogenous secretagogue release, and apoptosis. The activated protein C (APC)–endothelial protein C receptor complex (see "Role of Natural Anticoagulant Pathways" below) appears to be the "off switch" for PAR activation by the proteases. These counterbalances determine the magnitude of coagulation and inflammation upregulation by PARs. For example, factor VIIa–TF binding to PAR-2 in the lungs is proinflammatory and appears to play a role in acute respiratory distress syndrome (ARDS), raising the possibility that TFPI might be therapeutic in this circumstance.[49] This finding is consistent with data from animal studies demonstrating that TFPI can protect baboons from a LD100 of *Escherichia coli*, likely by impeding factor VIIa–TF activation of PAR-2 and thereby attenuating release of IL-6 and other proinflammatory agents.

ROLE OF FIBRINOGEN AND FIBRIN

Fibrinogen and fibrin directly influence the production of proinflammatory cytokines and chemokines (including TNF-α, IL-1β, and MCP-1) by mononuclear cells and endothelial cells.[50] Fibrinogen-deficient mice display inhibition of macrophage adhesion and less thrombin-mediated cytokine production *in vivo*. The effects of fibrinogen on mononuclear cells seem to be mediated by toll-like receptor-4, which is also the receptor of endotoxin.

ROLE OF NATURAL ANTICOAGULANT PATHWAYS

Procoagulant activity is regulated by three important anticoagulant pathways: AT, the protein C system, and TFPI. In DIC, the function of all three pathways can be impaired (Fig. 129–2).[51]

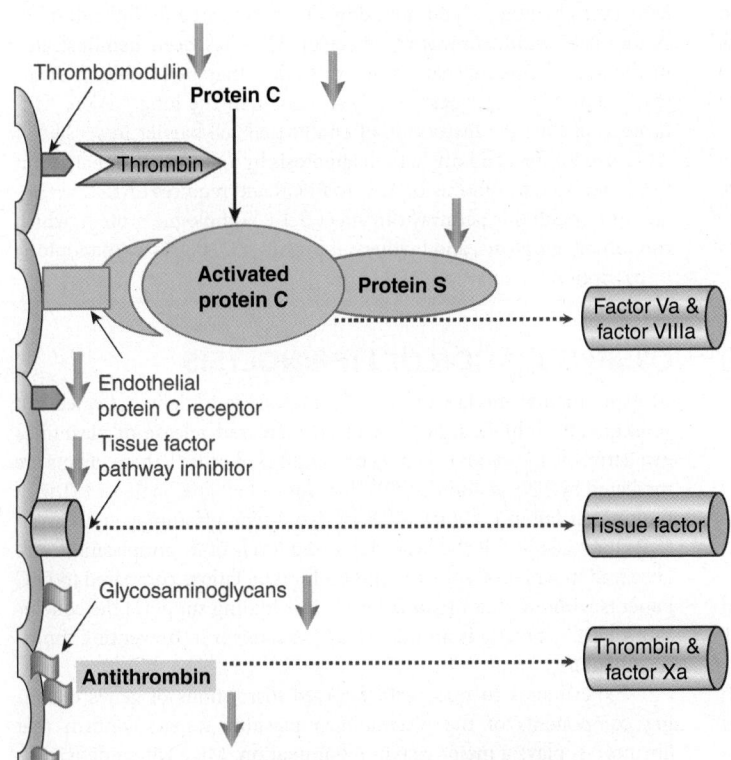

Figure 129–2. Schematic of the three important physiologic anticoagulant mechanisms and their point of impact in the coagulation system. In sepsis, these mechanisms are impaired by various mechanisms *(green arrows)*. The protein C system is dysfunctional as a result of low levels of zymogen protein C, downregulation of thrombomodulin and the endothelial protein C receptor, and low levels of free protein S because of acute phase-induced high levels of its binding protein (i.e., C4b-binding protein). There is a relative insufficiency of the endothelial cell-associated tissue factor pathway inhibitor. The antithrombin system is defective because of low levels of antithrombin and impaired glycosaminoglycan expression on perturbed endothelial cells.

The serine protease inhibitor AT is the main inhibitor of thrombin and factor Xa. Without heparin, AT neutralizes coagulation enzymes in a slow, progressive manner.[52] Heparin induces conformational changes in AT that result in at least a 1000-fold enhancement of AT activity. Thus, the clinical efficacy of heparin is attributed to its interaction with AT. Endogenous glycosaminoglycans, such as heparan sulfate, also promote on the vessel wall AT-mediated inhibition of thrombin and other coagulation enzymes. During severe inflammatory responses, AT levels are markedly decreased because of impaired synthesis, degradation by elastase from activated neutrophils, and consumption as a consequence of ongoing thrombin generation.[53] Proinflammatory cytokines also cause reduced synthesis of glycosaminoglycans on the endothelial surface, thereby reducing AT function.[54]

APC appears to play a central role in the pathogenesis of sepsis and associated organ dysfunction.[55] There is ample evidence that decreased function of the protein C pathway contributes to the derangement of coagulation in sepsis.[49,56] The circulating zymogen protein C is activated by thrombin when it is bound to thrombomodulin at the endothelial cell surface.[57] APC acts with its cofactor protein S and degrades the essential cofactors Va and VIIIa, and hence, is an effective anticoagulant. The endothelial protein C receptor (EPCR) accelerates the activation of protein C several-fold, and also serves as a receptor for APC, thereby augmenting APC's anticoagulant and antiinflammatory activities.[58]

In patients with severe inflammation, the protein C pathway malfunctions at virtually all levels. Plasma levels of the zymogen protein C are decreased because of impaired synthesis, consumption, and degradation by proteolytic enzymes, such as neutrophil elastase.[59–61] Furthermore, a significant downregulation of thrombomodulin, caused by proinflammatory cytokines such as TNF-α and IL-1, results in diminished protein C activation.[62,63] Low levels of free protein S may further compromise the function of the protein C system. In plasma, 60 percent of protein S is complexed with a complement regulatory protein, C4b-binding protein (C4bBP), and exhibits no activity. The remaining protein S in plasma is free and functional. It was suggested that increased plasma levels of C4bBP caused by the acute phase reaction in inflammatory diseases results in a relative protein S deficiency, which further contributes to a procoagulant state during sepsis. Indeed, infusion of C4bBP in combination with a sublethal dose of E. coli into baboons resulted in a lethal response with severe organ damage because of DIC.[64]

In sepsis, the EPCR is downregulated, which further impairs the function of the protein C pathway.[65] Sepsis can also cause resistance toward APC because of a substantial increase in factor VIII levels.[66]

A third inhibitory mechanism of thrombin generation involves TFPI, the main inhibitor of the TF–factor VIIa complex and factor Xa. The role of TFPI in the regulation of inflammation-induced coagulation activation is not completely clear. Administration of recombinant TFPI blocks inflammation-induced thrombin generation in humans, and pharmacologic doses of TFPI prevent mortality during systemic infection and inflammation in experimental animals suggesting that TFPI can modulate TF-mediated coagulation.[67,68]

NATURAL ANTICOAGULANTS AND INFLAMMATION

AT possesses antiinflammatory properties, many of which are mediated by its actions in the coagulation cascade.[69] By inhibiting thrombin, AT blunts activation of many inflammatory mediators released by platelets and endothelial cells that recruit and activate leukocytes.[70] At high concentrations, AT also possesses potent antiinflammatory properties that are independent of its anticoagulant activity.[70] Another effect of AT is the induction of prostacyclin release from endothelial cells.[71–73]

Prostacyclin inhibits platelet activation and aggregation, blocks neutrophil tethering to blood vessels, and decreases endothelial cell production of various cytokines and chemokines.[74]

AT also interacts directly with leukocytes and lymphocytes. It binds to receptors, such as syndecan-4, on the cell surfaces of neutrophils, monocytes, and lymphocytes, thereby blocking the adhesion of these cells to endothelial cells, their activation and migration. This effect, in turn, ameliorates the severity of capillary leakage and subsequent organ damage.

The protein C system also has an important function in modulating inflammation.[75,76] Blocking the protein C pathway in septic baboons exacerbates the inflammatory response, and in contrast, administration of APC ameliorates the inflammatory activation upon the intravenous infusion of E. coli.[77] Support for the notion that APC has antiinflammatory properties comes from in vitro observations, demonstrating an APC binding site on monocytes, that may mediate downstream inflammatory processes,[78,79] and from experiments showing that APC can block NF-κB nuclear translocation, which is a prerequisite for increased proinflammatory cytokine levels and adhesion molecules.[80] These in vitro findings are supported by in vivo studies in mice with targeted disruption of the protein C gene. In these mice with genetic deficiencies of protein C, endotoxemia was associated with a more marked increase in proinflammatory cytokines and other inflammatory responses as compared with wild-type mice.[81,82]

It is likely that the antiinflammatory effects of APC are mediated by the EPCR.[75] Binding of APC to EPCR influences gene expression profiles of cells by inhibiting NF-κB nuclear translocation.[79,80] The EPCR-APC complex itself can translocate from the plasma membrane into the cell nucleus, which may be another mechanism of modulating gene expression, although the relative contribution of this nuclear translocation and cell surface signaling is uncertain.[56] Like APC, EPCR itself may have antiinflammatory properties. Blocking the EPCR with a specific monoclonal antibody aggravates both the coagulation and the inflammatory response to E. coli infusion.[65]

Apart from the effect on cytokine levels, APC causes diminished leucocyte chemotaxis and adhesion to the activated endothelium.[83–85] A localized antiinflammatory effect of APC has been demonstrated in the lung.[86] One mechanism for this effect may be inhibition of the expression of platelet-derived growth factor in the lung.[87] Also, APC protects against the disruption of endothelial cell barrier in sepsis.[88–90] APC also inhibits endothelial cell apoptosis by a mechanism that seems to be mediated by binding of APC to EPCR and requires PAR-1.[91,92] Signaling through this pathway can affect Bcl-2 homologue protein, which can inhibit apoptosis, and further suppresses p53, that is a proapoptotic transcription factor.[93,94]

DYSREGULATION OF FIBRINOLYSIS

In experimental models of DIC, fibrinolysis is initially activated but subsequently inhibited, because of an increased release of plasminogen activator inhibitor-I (PAI-1) by endothelial cells.[95] These effects are mediated by TNF-α and IL-1.[96,97] In a study of 69 DIC patients (31 with multiorgan failure), higher levels of tissue-type plasminogen activator (t-PA) antigen and PAI-1 with depressed levels of α_2-antiplasmin were observed in patients with DIC and multiorgan failure compared to DIC patients without multiorgan failure.[98] This finding supports the conclusion that fibrinolysis is an important mechanism in preventing multiorgan failure.

Experiments in mice with targeted disruptions of genes encoding components of the plasminogen–plasmin system confirm that fibrinolysis plays a major role in inflammation. Mice with a deficiency of plasminogen activators have more extensive fibrin deposition in organs when challenged with endotoxin, whereas PAI-1 knockout mice, in contrast to wild-type controls, have no microvascular thrombosis upon endotoxin administration.[99]

TAFI, like PAI-1, may play a role in impeding fibrinolysis and in augmenting formation of microvascular thrombi. Studies in a DIC cohort demonstrated very low levels of TAFI proportionate to thrombin generation in such patients, particularly in those with infection-associated DIC.[100] Hence, TAFI may contribute (along with PAI-1) to microvascular thrombosis-induced ischemia in organs resulting in multiorgan dysfunction.

ROLE OF OXIDATIVE STRESS AND VASOACTIVE MOLECULES

Superoxides and hydroxyl radicals are generated during sepsis and other organ injury states that predispose to DIC. Each is a proinflammatory agent that may lead to recruitment of neutrophils, formation of chemotactic factors, lipid peroxidation, and stimulation of NF-κB, which induces cytokine upregulation.[101] In addition, formation of peroxynitrite by these radicals exacerbates inflammation by (1) deactivating superoxide dismutase, which ordinarily would eliminate these superoxides and other radicals, and (2) exerting damaging effects on deoxyribonucleic acid, nicotinamide adenine dinucleotide, and ATP. For example, evidence indicates that the poor response to pressors in shock-like states associated with DIC may be directly related to their deactivation by superoxides.

Adding further insult, high levels of superoxide impair vascular response to nitrous oxide, thereby creating an imbalance in the signaling to vascular cells. Because of the strategic importance of an intact endothelium for attenuating any microangiopathic process, the most devastating effect of excessive generation of superoxides and associated free radicals may be their role in inducing endothelial apoptosis, which exacerbates capillary leak.[101]

Vasoactive substances play a critical role in the evolution of DIC. The vasodilatory agent nitric oxide (NO) and the vasoconstrictor endothelin have been measured in experimental rat models of DIC induced by both TF infusion and lipopolysaccharide (LPS) infusion.[102] LPS infusion increased both NO and endothelin remarkably, whereas TF infusion increased NO more than did LPS but did not stimulate endothelin significantly. The differential stimuli–response mechanisms may explain why LPS-induced DIC so prominently displays tissue infarction leading to multiorgan dysfunction (e.g., sepsis) compared to DIC that is predominately induced by TF exposure (e.g., head trauma).

METABOLIC MODULATION OF COAGULATION IN DISSEMINATED INTRAVASCULAR COAGULATION

Because there is a tight relationship between plasma lipoproteins and coagulation, it has been suggested that lipoprotein metabolism modulates coagulation in DIC.[103] In vitro experiments showed that plasma large very-low-density lipoprotein, small very-low-density lipoprotein, intermediate-density lipoprotein, and low-density lipoprotein stimulate activation of coagulation by supporting factor VII activation or by stimulating monocytes to express TF.[104] Lipid infusion potentiates in animals endotoxin-induced coagulation activation, as indicated by increased plasma levels of prothrombin fragments 1 and 2, thrombin–AT III complex, and PAI-1.[105] High-density lipoprotein (HDL) exerts opposite effects. Administration of recombinant HDL (rHDL) ameliorates the inflammatory response, inhibits coagulation, and augments fibrinolysis,[106] as reflected by reduced thrombin generation and increased levels of t-PA antigen following administration of endotoxin.

Endogenous lipid levels may have similar effects. Human subjects with low endogenous HDL-cholesterol plasma levels injected with small doses of endotoxin had a more pronounced increase in markers of coagulation activation in comparison with subjects with high endogenous HDL levels.[107] Also, patients heterozygous for familial hypercholesterolemia whose low-density lipoproteins level is increased were more prone to activation of coagulation upon an inflammatory stimulus.[108]

Hyperglycemia and hyperinsulinemia, as seen in type 2 diabetes mellitus and the associated metabolic syndrome, affect hemostasis.[109-111] In these circumstances, there is a marked decrease of endogenous fibrinolysis because of increased upregulation of plasma levels of PAI-1. Also, a modulatory effect of glucose/insulin on coagulation in an inflammatory setting has been described. Inflammation-induced TF gene expression was elevated in the brain, lung, kidney, heart, liver, and adipose tissues of diabetic mice compared with controls. Administration of insulin to lean mice induced enhanced inflammation-driven TF mRNA in the kidney, brain, lung, and adipose tissue.[112] In a hyperglycemic normoinsulinemic study in healthy subjects, there was an increased sensitivity toward endotoxin exhibited by upregulation of TF expression.[113] Strict glucose regulation in critically ill patients improves survival and reduces morbidity that is probably related to a better control of the derangement of coagulation and a faster resolution of coagulation abnormalities.[103]

CONSUMPTION OF HEMOSTATIC FACTORS

The widespread generation of thrombin in DIC induces deposition of fibrin, which leads to the consumption of substantial amounts of platelets, fibrinogen, factors V and VIII, protein C, AT, and components of the fibrinolytic system. This situation results in massive depletion of these components that is further aggravated because of their decreased synthesis by the liver, which frequently is affected in DIC. Depending on the magnitude and nature of component depletion, bleeding, enhanced thrombosis, or both can result. Bleeding can be promoted by fibrinolysis-derived fibrin degradation products (FDPs) that exhibit anticoagulant and antiplatelet aggregation effects (see Fig. 129–1). Microangiopathic hemolytic anemia also occurs as a result of blood cells passing through vessels that are partially occluded by thrombi.

● CLINICAL FEATURES

Numerous disorders can provoke DIC, but only a few constitute major causes, as can be inferred from retrospective clinical studies (Table 129–1).[114] Infectious diseases and malignant disorders together account for approximately two-thirds of DIC cases in the major series (Table 129–2). Trauma was a major cause of DIC in some series, probably reflecting the specialized nature of the clinical practice in those centers.[115]

Clinical manifestations are attributable to DIC, the underlying disease, or both (Table 129–3). Bleeding manifestations were common in all series of DIC cases, but considerable variation existed in the relative frequency of shock and of dysfunction of the liver, kidney, lungs, and central nervous system. These variations probably reflect the different nature of the underlying disorders in the respective series.

BLEEDING

Acute DIC frequently is heralded by hemorrhage into the skin at multiple sites.[115] Petechiae, ecchymoses, and oozing from venipunctures, arterial lines, catheters, and injured tissues are common. Bleeding also may occur on mucosal surfaces. Hemorrhage may be life-threatening, with massive bleeding into the gastrointestinal tract, lungs, central nervous system, or orbit. Patients with chronic DIC usually exhibit only minor skin and mucosal bleeding.

TABLE 129–1. Clinical Conditions That May Be Complicated By Disseminated Intravascular Coagulation

Infectious diseases

   Purpura fulminans

Malignancy

   Solid tumors

   Leukemias

Trauma

   Brain injury

   Burns

Liver diseases

Heat stroke

Severe allergic/toxic reactions

   Snake bites

Vascular abnormalities/Hemangiomas

   Kasabach-Merritt syndrome

   Other vascular malformations

   Aortic aneurysms

Severe immunologic reactions (e.g., transfusion reaction)

Obstetrical conditions

   Abruptio placentae

   Amniotic fluid embolism

   Preeclampsia/eclampsia

   HELLP (hemolysis, elevated liver enzymes, and low platelet count) syndrome

   Sepsis during pregnancy

   Acute fatty liver

THROMBOSIS AND THROMBOEMBOLISM

Extensive organ dysfunction can result from microvascular thrombi or from venous and/or arterial thromboembolism (Table 129–4). For example, involvement of the skin can cause hemorrhagic bullae, acral necrosis, and gangrene. Thrombosis of major veins and arteries and pulmonary embolism occur but are rare. Cerebral embolism can complicate nonbacterial thrombotic endocarditis in patients with chronic DIC.

SHOCK

Both the diseases underlying DIC and the DIC itself can cause shock. For example, septicemia and excessive blood loss because of trauma or obstetric complications by themselves can cause shock. Whatever the cause of shock, its advent in cases with DIC is a serious adverse event.

RENAL DYSFUNCTION

Renal cortical ischemia induced by microthrombosis of afferent glomerular arterioles and acute tubular necrosis related to hypotension are the major causes of renal dysfunction in DIC. Oliguria, anuria, azotemia, and hematuria were observed in 25 to 67 percent of cases in all series (see Table 129–3).

LIVER DYSFUNCTION

Hepatocellular dysfunction sufficient to cause jaundice has been reported in 20 to 50 percent of patients with DIC.[4,115] Infectious diseases and prolonged hypotension contribute to hepatic dysfunction.

CENTRAL NERVOUS SYSTEM DYSFUNCTION

Microthrombi, macrothrombi, emboli, and hemorrhage in the cerebral vasculature all have been held responsible for the nonspecific neurologic symptoms and signs displayed by patients with DIC.[116] These manifestations include coma, delirium, transient focal neurologic symptoms, and signs of meningeal irritation. Careful exclusion of causes other than DIC is essential.

PULMONARY DYSFUNCTION

Symptoms and signs of respiratory dysfunction in DIC range from transient hypoxemia in mild cases to pulmonary hemorrhage and ARDS in severe cases.[117–119] Pulmonary hemorrhage is heralded by hemoptysis, dyspnea, and chest pain. Physical examination reveals rales, wheezing, and occasionally a pleural friction rub. Chest imaging shows diffuse infiltration resulting from excessive intraalveolar hemorrhage. ARDS is characterized by tachypnea, auscultatory silence, hypoxemia, low lung compliance, normal wedge pressure, and "white lungs" on chest images.[120] It stems from severe damage to the pulmonary vascular endothelium, which permits egress of blood components into the pulmonary interstitium and alveoli. This situation leads to intraalveolar hyaline membrane formation and severe respiratory insufficiency. ARDS can be caused by septic shock, severe trauma, fat embolism, amniotic fluid

TABLE 129–2. Relative Frequency (%) of Major Underlying Diseases in Case Series of Patients with Disseminated Intravascular Coagulation

Study	Number of Patients	Infectious Disease	Trauma and Major Surgery	Malignant Disease	Liver Disease	Obstetric Complications	Miscellaneous Diseases
Minna et al.[347]	60	41	30	2	5	2	20
Siegal et al.[115]	118	40	24	7	4	4	21
Spero et al.[122]	346	26	19	24	8	0	23
Matsuda et al.[348]	503	15	2	61	6	4	12
Kobayash et al.[139]	345	16	—	55	4	5	20
Larcan et al.[349]	361	15	14	6	3	38	24

TABLE 129–3. Frequency (%) and Type of Organ Dysfunction or Other Clinical Manifestations in Case Series of Patients with Disseminated Intravascular Coagulation

Study	Number of Patients	Bleeding	Thrombo-embolism	Renal Failure	Liver Failure	Respiratory Failure	CNS Manifestation	Shock	Acral Cyanosis[*]
Minna et al.[347]	60	87	22	67	NR	78	65	NR	14
Al-Mondhiry et al.[116]	89	76	23	39	NR	NR	11	NR	0
Siegal et al.[115]	118	64	8	25	22	16	2	14	0
Matsuda et al.[348]	47	87	47	40	NR	38	NR	NR	NR
Spero et al.[122]	346	77	NR	NR	NR	NR	NR	NR	NR
Larcan et al.[349]	361	73	11	61	57	37	13	55	13

NR, not reported.

*Including necrotizing purpura and acral gangrene.

embolism, and heat stroke, all of which can also incite DIC. Yet only a fraction of patients with ARDS exhibit signs of DIC. When DIC and ARDS are simultaneously triggered, each aggravates the other. Regardless of the mechanism, ARDS is a serious complication in patients with DIC.

MORTALITY

Both DIC and its underlying disorders contribute to the high mortality rate. Mortality correlates independently with the extent of organ dysfunction,[115] the degree of hemostatic failure,[121] and increasing age.[122] Mortality rates in major series of patients with DIC ranged from 31 to 86 percent,[121-124] whether or not heparin was administered. Of note, there is a clear correlation between the severity of DIC and the mortality rate.[121,123,124] In patients with sepsis, the presence of DIC is one of the strongest predictors of 28-day mortality.[124]

● LABORATORY FEATURES AND DIAGNOSIS

No single laboratory test is sensitive or specific enough to allow a definite diagnosis of DIC (Table 129–5). However, some sophisticated laboratory tests, for example, thrombin–AT complex, prothrombin fragment 1.2, are sensitive to ongoing activation of coagulation pathways. Determination of soluble fibrin in plasma is one of the best parameters for detection of ongoing DIC[125-128]; when the concentration is above a defined threshold, a diagnosis of DIC is likely.[129,130] Most of the other parameters show a sensitivity of 90 to 100 percent for the diagnosis of DIC but have a rather low specificity,[131] and a wide discordance among various assays.[132] FDPs may be detected by specific enzyme-linked immunosorbent assays or by latex agglutination assays, allowing rapid and bedside determination.[133] None of the available assays discriminates

TABLE 129–4. Organ Dysfunction Associated with Severe Disseminated Intravascular Coagulation

Organ	Manifestation
Skin	Purpura, bleeding from injury sites, hemorrhagic bullae, focal necrosis, acral gangrene
Cardiovascular	Shock, acidosis, myocardial infarction, cerebrovascular events, thromboembolism in all types and caliber blood vessels
Renal	Acute renal insufficiency (acute tubular necrosis), oliguria, hematuria, renal cortical necrosis
Liver	Hepatic failure, jaundice
Lungs	Adult respiratory distress syndrome, hypoxemia, edema, hemorrhage
Gastrointestinal	Bleeding, mucosal necrosis and ulceration, intestinal ischemia
Central nervous system	Coma, convulsions, focal lesions, bleeding
Adrenals	Adrenal insufficiency (hemorrhagic necrosis)

TABLE 129–5. Routine Laboratory Value Abnormalities in Disseminated Intravascular Coagulation

Test	Abnormality	Causes Other Than DIC Contributing to Test Result
Platelet count	Decreased	Sepsis, impaired production, major blood loss, hypersplenism
Prothrombin time	Prolonged	Vitamin K deficiency, liver failure, major blood loss
aPTT	Prolonged	Liver failure, heparin treatment, major blood loss
Fibrin degradation products	Elevated	Surgery, trauma, infection, hematoma
Protease inhibitors (e.g., protein C, AT, protein S)	Decreased	Liver failure, capillary leakage

aPTT, activated partial thromboplastin time, AT, antithrombin; DIC, disseminated intravascular coagulation.

between degradation products of crosslinked fibrin and fibrinogen, a situation that may cause spuriously high results.[134,135] The specificity of high levels of FDPs is therefore limited and many other conditions, such as trauma, recent surgery, inflammation or venous thromboembolism, are associated with elevated FDPs.

Newly developed tests are aimed at the detection of neoantigens on degraded crosslinked fibrin, one of which detects an epitope related to plasmin-degraded crosslinked γ-chain, associated with D-dimer formation. These tests better differentiate degradation of crosslinked fibrin from fibrinogen or fibrinogen degradation products.[136] D-dimer level is substantially elevated in patients with DIC, but this poorly distinguishes patients with DIC from patients with venous thromboembolism, recent surgery, or inflammatory conditions.[133,137]

In routine practice, simple laboratory tests in conjunction with clinical considerations are used for establishing the diagnosis of DIC. The simple tests include platelet count, prothrombin time, fibrinogen level, and fibrin-related markers, such as FDP or D-dimer. Caution should be exercised when using these laboratory parameters in the algorithms described below, because an underlying disease by itself can cause an abnormality. For example, impairment of hemostasis and/or thrombocytopenia unrelated to DIC can arise from hepatic disease and from marrow involvement by leukemia. Impaired hemostasis also may occur normally in the neonatal period. Conversely, the elevated levels of some hemostatic components that are normally observed during pregnancy may obscure the presence of DIC. These limitations in laboratory diagnosis of DIC can be overcome by repeated testing, thereby following the dynamics of the process.

A scoring system utilizing the simple laboratory tests has been developed by the subcommittee on DIC of the International Society on Thrombosis and Haemostasis,[138] and Table 129-6 summarizes a five-step diagnostic algorithm to calculate a DIC score. Tentatively, a score of 5 or more is compatible with DIC, whereas a score of less than 5 may

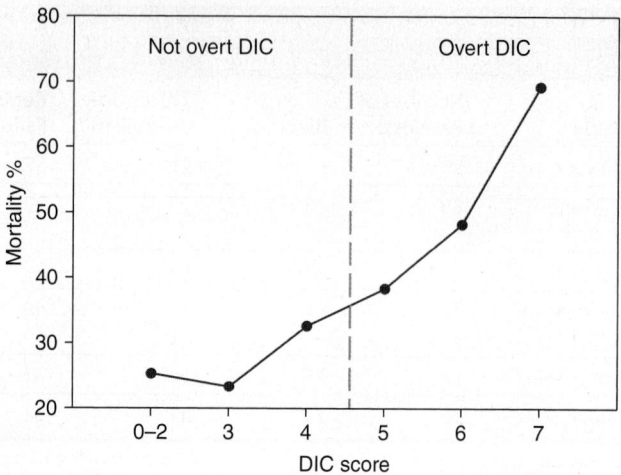

Figure 129-3. Number of points on the International Society of Thrombosis and Haemostasis disseminated intravascular coagulation (DIC) score and 28-day mortality in patients with severe sepsis. Data were derived from the placebo group (n = 840) in the Prowess trial on the efficacy of activated protein C in sepsis.

be indicative but is *not* affirmative for nonovert DIC. By using receiver-operating characteristics curves, an optimal cutoff for a quantitative D-dimer assay was determined, thereby optimizing sensitivity and the negative predictive value of the system.[131] Prospective studies show that the sensitivity of the DIC score is 93 percent, and the specificity is 98 percent.[123] The severity of DIC according to this scoring system is related to the mortality in patients with sepsis (Fig. 129-3).[124] Linking prognostic determinants from critical care measurement scores such as acute physiology and chronic health evaluation (APACHE-II) to DIC scores is an important means to assess prognosis in critically ill patients. In addition, certain biochemical indicators of organ dysfunction may imply a DIC risk. For example, serial assessment of arterial lactate has proved to be a reliable prognostic indicator of DIC development among patients with the systemic inflammatory response syndrome.[139]

Criteria for less-overt DIC have been more difficult to establish.[138,140] In the algorithm for nonovert DIC, the global coagulation tests are scored as with the overt DIC algorithm; however, when scoring by the algorithm is being serially repeated, improvement in any laboratory test confers a negative score (rather than a zero or neutral score). This "trend" scoring allows longitudinal assessment of the patient's microangiopathy and, when therapy has been instituted, inference on whether the therapy has improved the course of the disease.[121,141] Measurements of several markers for assessing the risk of progression from nonovert to overt DIC and prediction of multiorgan dysfunction are potentially valuable and in the future can be accommodated in the nonovert DIC score. For example, impaired fibrinolysis may play a particularly important role in multiorgan dysfunction resulting from DIC of sepsis.[142] Therefore, assaying PAI-1, plasmin–antiplasmin complexes, or TAFI in septic patients may be important. Another highly sensitive early marker of impending DIC is a monoclonal antibody against APC that identifies a calcium ion-dependent epitope involved in factor Va inactivation.[143] Whether serial measurement of von Willebrand factor-cleaving protease also will identify individuals at risk early in their disease course, or will help differentiate individuals with microangiopathy who are not prone to progress, needs further data.[144,145]

Techniques, such as rotational thrombelastography (ROTEM) enable bedside performance of this test and has again become popular recently in acute care settings.[146] The theoretical advantage of

TABLE 129-6. Diagnostic Algorithm for the Diagnosis of Overt Disseminated Intravascular Coagulation*

1. Presence of an underlying disorder known to be associated with DIC (see Table 129–2)   ❏

   (no = 0, yes = 2)

2. Score global coagulation test results   ❏

   Platelet count (>100 = 0; <100 = 1; <50= 2)

   Level of fibrin markers (soluble fibrin monomers/fibrin degradation products)   ❏

   (no increase: 0; moderate increase: 2; strong increase: 3)

   Prolonged prothrombin time   ❏

   (<3 s= 0; >3 s but <6 s= 1; >6 s = 2)

   Fibrinogen level   ❏

   (>1.0 g/L = 0; <1.0 g/L = 1)

3. Calculate score   ❏

4. If ≥5: compatible with overt DIC; repeat scoring daily

   If <5: suggestive (not affirmative) for nonovert DIC; repeat next 1–2 days

DIC, disseminated intravascular coagulation.

*According to the Scientific Standardization Committee of the International Society of Thrombosis and Haemostasis.[138]

Data from Taylor FBJ, Toh CH, Hoots WK, et al: Towards definition, clinical and laboratory criteria, and a scoring system for disseminated intravascular coagulation. *Thromb Haemost* 86(5):1327–1330, 2001.

thrombelastography (TEG) over conventional coagulation assays is that is provides an idea of platelet function as well as fibrinolytic activity. Hyper- and hypocoagulability as demonstrated with TEG was shown to correlate with clinically relevant morbidity and mortality in several studies, although its superiority over conventional tests has not unequivocally been established.[147] Even though there are no systematic studies on the diagnostic accuracy of TEG for the diagnosis of DIC, the test may be useful for assessing the global status of the coagulation system in critically ill patients.[148]

● SPECIFIC UNDERLYING DISORDERS

INFECTIOUS DISEASES

Bacterial infections are among the most common causes of DIC.[5,149] Certain patients are particularly vulnerable to infection-induced DIC, such as immune-compromised hosts, asplenic patients whose ability to clear bacteria, particularly pneumococci and meningococci, is impaired, and newborns whose coagulation inhibitory systems are immature. Infections are frequently superimposed on trauma and malignancies, which themselves are potential triggers of DIC. In addition, infections can aggravate bleeding and thrombosis by directly inducing thrombocytopenia, hepatic dysfunction, and shock associated with diminished blood flow in the microcirculation.[150] Clinically overt DIC may occur in 30 to 50 percent of patients with Gram-negative sepsis.[151,152] DIC is similarly common in patients with Gram-positive sepsis.[153,154] Extreme examples of sepsis-related DIC are (1) group A streptococcus toxic shock syndrome, characterized by deep tissue infection, vascular collapse, vascular leakage, and multiorgan dysfunction; a streptococcal M protein forms complexes with fibrinogen, and these complexes bind to β_2 integrins of neutrophils leading to their activation[155]; and (2) meningococcemia, a fulminant Gram-negative infection characterized by extensive hemorrhagic necrosis, DIC, and shock. The extent of hemostatic derangement in patients with meningococcemia correlates with prognosis.[156,157] More frequent Gram-negative infections associated with DIC are caused by *Pseudomonas aeruginosa*, *E. coli*, and *Proteus vulgaris*. Patients affected by such bacteremias may have only laboratory signs of activated coagulation or may present with severe DIC, especially when shock develops.[158,159]

Severe secondary deficiency of a disintegrin-like metalloprotease with thrombospondin type 1 repeats (ADAMTS13), the von Willebrand cleaving protease, occurs in patients with sepsis-induced DIC and is associated with a high incidence of acute renal failure.[160]

Among the Gram-positive infections, *Staphylococcus aureus* bacteremia can cause DIC accompanied by renal cortical and dermal necrosis. The mechanism by which DIC is elicited may be related to an α-toxin that activates platelets and induces IL-1 secretion by macrophages.[161] *Streptococcus pneumoniae* infection is associated with the Waterhouse-Friderichsen syndrome,[162] particularly in asplenic patients. Initiation of DIC in these conditions is ascribed to the capsular antigen of the bacterium and to antigen–antibody complex formation.[163] Other Gram-positive bacteria that can cause DIC are the anaerobic clostridia. Clostridial bacteremia is a highly lethal disease characterized by septic shock, DIC, renal failure, and hemolytic anemia.[164]

Activation of the coagulation system has also been documented for nonbacterial pathogens, that is, viruses (causing hemorrhagic fevers),[164,165] protozoa (Malaria),[166,167] and fungi.[168] Common viral infections, such as influenza, varicella, rubella, and rubeola, rarely are associated with DIC.[169] However, purpura fulminans associated with DIC has been reported in patients with infections and either hereditary thrombophilias,[170,171] or acquired antibodies to protein S.[172] Other viral infections can cause "hemorrhagic fevers" characterized by fever,

hypotension, bleeding, and renal failure. Laboratory evidence of DIC can accompany Korean, rift valley, and dengue-related hemorrhagic fevers.[173-175] Release of TF from cells in which viruses replicate[28] and increased levels of proinflammatory cytokines have been suggested as mechanisms for initiation of the TF pathway in these conditions.[163]

PURPURA FULMINANS

Purpura fulminans is a severe, often lethal form of DIC in which extensive areas of the skin over the extremities and buttocks undergo hemorrhagic necrosis.[176] The disease affects infants and children predominantly, and occasionally adults.[177,178] Diffuse microthrombi in small blood vessels, necrosis, and occasionally vasculitis are present in biopsies of skin lesions. Onset can be within 2 to 4 weeks of a mild infection such as scarlet fever, varicella, or rubella, or can occur during an acute viral or bacterial infection in patients with acquired or hereditary thrombophilias affecting the protein C inhibitory pathway.[156,177] Homozygous protein C deficiency presents in neonates soon after birth as purpura fulminans, with or without extensive thrombosis.[179,180] Patients affected by purpura fulminans are acutely ill with fever, hypotension, and hemorrhage from multiple sites; they frequently have typical laboratory signs of DIC.[177] Excision of necrotic skin areas and grafting are indispensable at a later stage.

SOLID TUMORS

Trousseau was the first to describe the propensity to thrombosis of patients with cancer and cachexia, and evidence for malignancy-related primary fibrinolysis and/or DIC was provided 75 years ago.[9,181,182]

In 182 patients with malignant disorders, excessive bleeding was recorded in 75 cases, venous thrombosis in 123, migratory thrombophlebitis in 96, arterial thrombosis in 45, and arterial embolism resulting from nonbacterial thrombotic endocarditis in 31.[183] Multifocal hemorrhagic infarctions of the brain, caused by fibrin microemboli and manifested as disorders of consciousness, have been described. Patients with solid tumors and DIC are more prone to thrombosis than to bleeding, whereas patients with leukemia and DIC are more prone to hemorrhage. The incidence of DIC in consecutive patients with solid tumors was 7 percent.[184]

Solid-tumor cells can express different procoagulant molecules including TF, which forms a complex with factor VII(a) to activate factors IX and X, and a cancer procoagulant, a cysteine protease with factor X activating properties.[185,186] In breast cancer, TF is expressed by vascular endothelial cells as well as the tumor cells.[187,188] TF also appears to be involved in tumor metastasis and angiogenesis.[189-191] Cancer procoagulant is an endopeptidase that can be found in extracts of neoplastic cells but also in the plasma of patients with solid tumors.[192,193] The exact role of cancer procoagulant in the pathogenesis of cancer-related DIC is unclear.

Interactions of P- and L-selectins with mucin from mucinous adenocarcinoma can induce formation of platelet microthrombi and probably constitute a third mechanism of cancer-related thrombosis.[194] Depending on the rate and quantity of exposure or influx of shed vesicles from tumors containing TF, a nonovert or overt DIC develops.[39,195,196] For instance, a patient may be asymptomatic or present with venous thromboembolism if the tumor cells expose or release TF slowly or intermittently and the ensuing utilization of fibrinogen and platelets is compensated by increased production of these components. Conversely, massive thrombosis or severe bleeding may supervene in a patient whose circulation is deluged by TF.[184,186]

Another mechanism by which tumor cells may contribute to the pathogenesis of DIC is by expressing fibrinolytic proteins.[197,198] Despite the ability of many malignant cells to express urokinase-type plasminogen activator and t-PA, most tumors induce a hypofibrinolytic state. Because DIC is commonly characterized by a shutdown of the fibrinolytic system, mostly because of high levels of PAI-1, this may represent an alternative mechanism for the development of DIC in cancer.

Virtually all pathways that contribute to the occurrence of DIC are driven by cytokines. IL-6 has been identified as one of the most important proinflammatory cytokines that is able to induce TF expression on cells.[21,199] Indeed, inhibition of IL-6 results in an inhibition of endotoxin-stimulated activation of coagulation. In contrast, changes in fibrinolysis and microvascular physiologic anticoagulant pathways are mostly dependent on TNF-α.[200–202] Other cytokines that participate in the systemic activation of coagulation are IL-1β and IL-8, whereas antiinflammatory cytokines, such as IL-10, are able to inhibit DIC.[203–205] Because many types of tumors have the ability to synthesize and release cytokines or to stimulate other cells to activate the cytokine network, it is likely that cytokine-dependent modulation of coagulation and fibrinolysis plays a role in cancer-related DIC.

Patients with solid tumors are vulnerable to risk factors and additional triggers of DIC that can aggravate thromboembolism and bleeding.[182] Risk factors include advanced age, stage of the disease, and use of chemotherapy or antiestrogen therapy.[197] Triggers include septicemia, immobilization, and involvement of the liver by metastases that impede the function of the liver in controlling DIC. Microangiopathic hemolytic anemia frequently is induced by DIC in patients with malignancies and is particularly severe in patients with widespread intravascular metastases of mucin-secreting adenocarcinomas.[206]

LEUKEMIAS

Numerous reports on DIC and fibrinolysis complicating the course of acute leukemias have been published. In 161 consecutive patients who presented with acute myeloid leukemia, DIC was diagnosed in 52 (32 percent).[207] In acute lymphoblastic leukemia, DIC was diagnosed in 15 to 20 percent.[208] Some reports indicate that the incidence of DIC in acute leukemia patients might further increase during remission induction with chemotherapy.[209] In patients with acute promyelocytic leukemia (APL), DIC is present in more than 90 percent of patients at the time of diagnosis or after initiation of remission induction.[210,211]

The pathogenesis of hemostatic disturbance in APL is related to properties of the malignant cells and their interaction with the host's endothelial cells.[192,208] APL cells express TF and the cancer procoagulant that can initiate coagulation, and they release IL-1β and TNF-α, which downregulate endothelial thrombomodulin, thereby compromising the protein C anticoagulant pathway. APL cells also express increased amounts of annexin II, which mediates augmented conversion of plasminogen to plasmin (Chap. 135). The overall results of these processes are DIC and hyperfibrinolysis, followed by major bleeding that can lead to death.[212] All-*trans*-retinoic acid, used for induction and maintenance therapy of APL, inhibits *in vitro* and *in vivo* the deleterious effect of APL cells and has led to a reduced frequency of early hemorrhagic death; however, all-*trans*-retinoic acid may induce thrombotic complications.[192,213]

TRAUMA

When DIC complicates trauma, it usually occurs in severely injured patients. Extensive exposure of TF to the blood circulation and hemorrhagic shock probably are the most immediate triggers of DIC in such instances, although direct proof of this mechanism is lacking. An alternative hypothesis is that cytokines play a pivotal role in the occurrence of DIC in trauma patients. In fact, the changes in cytokine levels are virtually identical in trauma patients and septic patients.[214] The levels of TNF-α, IL-1β, PAI-1, circulating TF, plasma elastase derived from neutrophils, and soluble thrombomodulin all can be elevated in patients with signs of DIC, predicting multiorgan dysfunction (ARDS included) and death.[215,216] Careful monitoring of laboratory signs of DIC, reduced fibrinolytic activity, and perhaps low AT levels also are useful for predicting the outcome of such patients.[217]

DIC can be aggravated in patients with severe trauma who require massive blood replacement because stored blood components are diluted and do not contain sufficient amounts of viable platelets and factors V and VIII. Moreover, in such patients, there is an activation of fibrinolysis that further aggravate bleeding in combination with acidosis, and hypotension.[218–221] Infection commonly occurs in such patients and may contribute to the DIC.

The time interval between trauma and medical intervention correlates with the development and magnitude of DIC. Experience during wars proved that fast evacuation and prompt medical care reduce the risk of DIC.[222–224]

BRAIN INJURY

Brain injury can be associated with DIC, most likely because the injury exposes the abundant TF of brain to blood. Specimens of contused brain, obtained during surgery in patients with head injury and of liver, lungs, kidneys, and pancreas obtained during autopsy, revealed microthrombi in arterioles and venules.[225,226] In adults and children with head injuries, a high rate of mortality occurred when DIC was present.[227] A laboratory DIC score has predictive value for prognosis in patients with head injuries, thereby supplementing the Glasgow coma score.[228] Bleeding in patients with DIC that is related to brain injury can be managed by replacement therapy.

BURNS

TF exposed to blood at sites of burned tissue, the systemic inflammatory response syndrome induced by the burn, and the common presence of superimposed infections, all can trigger DIC.[229] Bleeding, laboratory tests indicative of DIC, and vascular microthrombi in biopsies of undamaged skin have been described in patients with extensive burns.[230] Kinetic studies with labeled fibrinogen and labeled platelets disclosed that, in addition to systemic consumption of hemostatic factors, significant local consumption occurs in burned areas.[231] Laboratory signs of DIC are associated with organ failure; the extent of protein C and AT deficiencies correlates with a poor outcome.[230] A clinicopathologic study of 139 patients who died during treatment for a severe burn disclosed that 18 percent had cerebral infarctions caused by septic arterial occlusions or DIC and approximately 4 percent had intracranial hemorrhage.[232]

LIVER DISEASES

Very complicated derangements of hemostasis occur in patients with severe liver disease and during liver transplantation (Chap. 129). Synthesis of most coagulation factors and natural anticoagulants (protein C, protein S, and AT) and of the main components of the fibrinolytic system (plasminogen, TAFI, and α_2-antiplasmin) is reduced. The capacity of the liver to clear the circulation of activated factors IX, X, and XI, and of t-PA is decreased. Moreover, thrombocytopenia is common as a result of hypersplenism and decreased production of thrombopoietin by the liver. The similarities between the hemostatic defects observed in patients with liver disease and in patients with DIC are striking and have evoked an ongoing controversy as to whether or not DIC contributes to hemostatic derangements associated with liver disease.[233]

Several laboratory and clinical observations support the hypothesis that DIC accompanies hepatic disorders. They include a shortened half-life of radiolabeled fibrinogen and prolongation of fibrinogen half-life by administration of heparin[234,235]; failure of replacement therapy to significantly increase the levels of hemostatic factors (suggesting continuous consumption); and increased blood levels of D-dimer, thrombin–AT (TAT) complexes, and fibrinopeptide A, all consistent with ongoing thrombin generation.[236–238]

Other observations and considerations argue against the hypothesis that DIC accompanies liver diseases. They include (1) a very low incidence (2.2 percent) of microthrombosis in the tissues of patients who die of liver disease and (2) causes other than, or inconsistent with, DIC for the deranged findings in liver disease.[237] Examples of alternative explanations include the following: (1) a prolonged thrombin time may result from acquired dysfibrinogenemia[239]; (2) low levels of coagulation factors and inhibitors may result from reduced synthesis[240]; (3) increased FDP levels may be a consequence of primary fibrinogenolysis induced by reduced synthesis of α_2-antiplasmin and PAI-1 and by decreased clearance of t-PA; (4) factor VIII levels are commonly increased rather than decreased[241]; (5) the kinetic data show that the apparently excessive consumption of fibrinogen can be explained by loss of fibrinogen into extravascular spaces[242]; and (6) fibrinogen and plasminogen do not appear to be removed rapidly when labeled endogenously by ^{75}Se-selenomethionine.[243]

A third hypothesis maintains that patients with liver disease usually do not present with DIC but are extremely sensitive to the various triggers of DIC because of their impeded capacity to clear procoagulants and to synthesize essential components of the coagulation, inhibitory, and fibrinolytic systems. Patients with primary or metastatic liver disease who undergo a peritoneovenous shunt operation for severe ascites are more likely to develop DIC than are patients with ascites who undergo the same procedure because of other causes.[244]

What, then, should be the approach to patients with liver disease and bleeding without an apparent local cause? First, possible underlying causes of DIC should be considered and identified, and then a hemostatic profile should be examined at frequent intervals so as to detect any dynamic changes that may be helpful in recognizing DIC. The sensitive assays that reflect thrombin generation (TAT complex and prothrombin fragments 1.2) or concomitant thrombin and plasmin generation (D-dimer), as well as finding a normal or decreased level of factor VIII may help establish the diagnosis of DIC in a patient with liver disease.[245]

HEAT STROKE

In 1841, James Wellstead published his book *Travels to the City of the Caliphs* (currently known as Baghdad) and vividly described that on an extremely hot day in the Persian Gulf the decks of the ship *Liverpool* resembled a slaughterhouse, so numerous were the bleeding patients.[246] This is probably one of the first written reports on the occurrence of DIC in humans who suffer from heatstroke.[229] Heat stroke is a syndrome characterized by a rise in body temperature to higher than 42°C, which follows collapse of the thermoregulatory mechanism. The following predisposing factors have been identified: high environmental temperature, strenuous physical activity, infection, dehydration, and lack of acclimatization.[247,248] Extensive hemorrhage, unclottable blood, and venous engorgement were found as early as 1838 in postmortem examinations of patients who died of heat stroke.[246] Investigations confirm that a severe hemorrhagic diathesis and multiple organ failure often accompany heat stroke.[229,249–251] Diffuse fibrin deposition and hemorrhagic infarctions are found in fatal human cases. DIC associated with profound fibrin(ogen)olysis is evident in patients with heat stroke. The possible triggers of DIC in patients with heat stroke include endothelial cell damage and TF released from heat-damaged tissues.[249]

In a series of 18 critically ill patients from Paris with heat stroke during the 2003 heat wave in Western Europe that caused numerous deaths in France alone,[251] patients had very high levels of IL-6 and IL-8. In addition, there was a striking activation of white blood cells, as demonstrated by β_2-integrin upregulation and increased production of reactive oxygen species. All patients also had evidence of a significant systemic activation of coagulation and DIC was present in approximately 35 percent of patients. There was a marked correlation between the extent of inflammation and coagulation activation and the clinical severity of the heat stroke.

The severity of the syndrome and the stage of its development affect the type and magnitude of hemostatic alterations. Thus, in a study of 56 patients, three groups were discernible: nonbleeders, bleeders without DIC but with slight consumption of hemostatic factors, and bleeders with typical signs of DIC.[252] Prompt cooling and support of vital functions have substantially reduced the high mortality that was commonly observed in early studies.

SNAKE BITES

Several species of snakes belonging to the Viperidae family produce venoms that have a wide range of activities affecting hemostasis. Prominent among these species are the *Vipera*, *Echis* (*E. carinatus* or *E. coloratus*), *Aspis*, *Crotalus*, *Bothrops*, and *Agkistrodon*. Venoms of these snakes contain enzymes or peptides that exert the following activities[253–255]: (1) thrombin-like activity, cleaving fibrinopeptide A from the Aα chain of fibrinogen (*Agkistrodon rhodostoma*); (2) activation of prothrombin even in the absence of calcium ions (*E. carinatus*); (3) activation of factors X and V (Russell viper venom); (4) fibrinogenolytic activity (*Agkistrodon acutus*); (5) induction of thrombocytopenia by platelet aggregation; (6) inhibition of platelet aggregation by the low-molecular-weight arginine-glycine-aspartic acid–containing peptides from a variety of snake species; (7) activation of protein C; and (8) activities causing damage to endothelial cells, leading to bleeding, tissue ischemia, and edema. Interestingly, victims of snake bites rarely experience excessive bleeding or thromboembolism, in spite of the serious derangements in hemostatic tests and findings that are sometimes consistent with DIC.[256–258]

The major symptoms and signs related to envenomation are vomiting, diarrhea, apprehension, hypotension, local swelling, ischemia, and necrosis. Consequently, treatment for victims of snake bites consists of immediate immobilization, administration of antivenom and fluids, and other general measures to preserve vital functions. Local incisions, cooling, and application of tourniquet should be avoided.[253]

HEMANGIOMAS

In 1940, Kasabach and Merritt described the association between giant hemangioma and a bleeding tendency occurring mainly in infants. The pathogenesis and management of this syndrome have been reviewed.[259] Studies using radiolabeled fibrinogen and platelets provided evidence that within the hemangioma, consumption of platelets and fibrinogen occurs because of localized intravascular clotting and excessive fibrinogenolysis.[260,261] Conceivably, concomitant local activation of the coagulation pathway and release of large amounts of t-PA by the abnormal endothelium lining the tumor vessels occur. Microangiopathic hemolytic anemia and laboratory signs of DIC and fibrinolysis have been demonstrated in patients with giant hemangiomas.[262] Accelerated growth of these hemangiomas in infants is associated with augmented consumption of hemostatic factors, and can be effectively treated with glucocorticoids. Radiotherapy and interferon-α are also effective, but should only be used in life-threatening circumstances after failure of glucocorticoid therapy because of severe adverse events.[263] Spontaneous mild to moderate bleeding manifestations have been observed, but severe bleeding generally occurs only after surgery or trauma.

Extensive vascular malformation may persist and cause pain, probably resulting from thrombosis, and bleeding following trauma, which is related to the localized or generalized consumption of clotting factors and platelets and hyperfibrinolysis.[264] Graded permanent elastic compression, when possible, and low-molecular-weight heparin constitute the only effective treatment in such cases.

AORTIC ANEURYSM

An association between aortic aneurysm and DIC is well documented.[265,266] In a series of patients with aortic aneurysm, 40 percent had elevated levels of FDPs, but only 4 percent had significant bleeding and laboratory evidence of DIC.[265] Several factors predispose patients with aortic aneurysms to the development of DIC: a large surface area, dissection, and expansion of the aneurysm.[267] Clinical and laboratory signs of DIC should be carefully sought in patients with an aortic aneurysm because bleeding may seriously complicate surgical repair of the aneurysm.[267,268] The initiation of localized and generalized intravascular coagulation can be ascribed to activation of the TF pathway by the abundant amounts of TF present in atherosclerotic plaques.[269] When patients present with significant bleeding or when surgery is planned, hemostatic defects should be sought and ongoing coagulation activation may be corrected by (low-molecular-weight) heparin.[270] Stent-grafting, which is a common procedure for repair of aortic aneurysms, was complicated by DIC and death in two patients, of whom one had cirrhosis and the other underwent a lengthy procedure.[271] However, a study of 31 such patients failed to detect DIC following stent-grafting of thoracic aneurysms.[272]

TRANSFUSION REACTION

DIC accompanies incompatible blood transfusion, in which massive hemolysis is commonly associated with excessive bleeding with widespread thrombosis in fatal cases (Chap. 138). The trigger of DIC in these cases cannot be simply ascribed to the release of red cell stroma, as patients with massive oxidative hemolysis because of glucose-6-phosphate dehydrogenase deficiency do not develop DIC.[273] Rather, extensive antigen–antibody reaction appears to cause DIC as a result of release of elastase and TNF-α from neutrophils, and activation of monocytes that release TNF-α express TF and complement, with assembly of the membrane attack complex inflicting damage to endothelial cells.[274,275]

DISSEMINATED INTRAVASCULAR COAGULATION DURING PREGNANCY

Pregnancy predisposes patients to DIC for at least four reasons: (1) pregnancy itself produces a hypercoagulable state, manifested by evidence of low-grade thrombin generation, with elevated levels of fibrin monomer complexes and fibrinopeptide A; (2) during labor, leakage of TF from placental tissue into the maternal circulation causes a hypercoagulable state; (3) pregnancy is associated with reduced fibrinolytic activity because of increased plasma levels of PAI-1; and (4) pregnancy is associated with a decline in the plasma level of protein S. DIC may be difficult to diagnose during pregnancy because of the high initial levels of coagulation factors such as fibrinogen, factor VIII, and factor VII.[276,277] Progressive reductions in these factors, however, can confirm or exclude the diagnosis of DIC in suspected cases. Thrombocytopenia may be particularly helpful in determining whether DIC is present, provided other causes of thrombocytopenia are excluded.[278]

Abruptio Placentae

The dramatic clinical presentation of abruptio placentae was first reported by DeLee in 1901,[279] but the immediate cause of sudden rupture of uterine spiral arteries and detachment of the placenta is still unknown. Placental abruption is a leading cause of perinatal death.[280] Older multiparous women or patients with one of the hypertensive disorders of pregnancy are thought to be at highest risk. The severe hemostatic failure accompanying abruptio placentae is the result of acute DIC emanating from the introduction of large amounts of TF into the blood circulation from the damaged placenta and uterus.[281] Amniotic fluid is able to activate coagulation *in vitro*, and the degree of placental separation correlates with the extent of DIC, suggesting that leakage of thromboplastin-like material from the placental system is responsible for the occurrence of DIC. Abruptio placentae occurs in 0.2 to 0.4 percent of pregnancies,[282] but only 10 percent of these cases are associated with DIC.[278] Different grades of severity are found among those who develop DIC, with only the more severe forms resulting in shock and fetal death. Rapid volume replenishment and evacuation of the uterus is the treatment of choice.[280] Transfusion of cryoprecipitate, fresh-frozen plasma, and platelets should be given when profuse bleeding occurs. However, in the absence of severe bleeding, administration of blood components may not be necessary because depleted coagulation factors increase rapidly following delivery. Heparin or antifibrinolytic agents are not indicated.

Amniotic Fluid Embolism

This rare catastrophic disorder, described by Steiner and Lushbaugh in 1941, occurs only in one in 8000 to one in 80,000 deliveries.[283] A maternal mortality rate of 86 percent was reported in a 1979 review of 272 cases, but in a later population-based study, the maternal mortality (26.4 percent) was significantly lower.[284,285] Patients predisposed to amniotic fluid embolism are multiparous women whose pregnancies are postmature with large fetuses and women undergoing a tumultuous labor after pharmacologic or surgical induction. Apparently, amniotic fluid is introduced into the maternal circulation through tears in the chorioamniotic membranes, rupture of the uterus, and injury of uterine veins.[284] The trigger of DIC probably is TF present in amniotic fluid.[286,287] The mechanical obstruction of pulmonary blood vessels by fetal debris, meconium, and other particulate matter in the amniotic fluid enhances local fibrin–platelet thrombus formation and fibrinolysis. The extensive occlusion of the pulmonary arteries and an acute anaphylactoid response reminiscent of severe systemic inflammatory response syndrome provoke sudden dyspnea, cyanosis, acute cor pulmonale, left ventricular dysfunction, shock, and convulsions. These symptoms are followed within minutes to several hours by severe bleeding in 37 percent of patients.[284] Hemorrhage is particularly severe from the atonic uterus, puncture sites, gastrointestinal tract, and other organs. The best prospect for decreasing mortality lies in early termination of parturition in patients at high risk and prevention of hypertonic and tetanic uterine contractions during labor. When the syndrome is recognized, immediate termination of pregnancy under pulmonary and cardiovascular support is essential.

Preeclampsia and Eclampsia

Thrombocytopenia described in early reports of eclampsia and widespread deposition of fibrin in blood vessels observed in fatal cases were interpreted as evidence of DIC triggered by placental TF exposure to the circulation.[1] A critical analysis of the literature concluded that the thrombocytopenia in these patients stems from endothelial injury rather than DIC.[288] However, other investigators provided evidence for significant DIC in preeclampsia and eclampsia.[289,290] Moreover, in a large series of patients, a good correlation was noted between the clinical severity and abnormalities in platelet counts and FDPs.[291] Also consistent with DIC were results of assays of sensitive parameters of thrombin generation and activation of fibrinolysis, such as TAT complexes, D-dimer, and fibrinopeptide Bβ1–42. Despite these observations, administration of heparin to patients with preeclampsia and eclampsia has not resulted in convincing benefits.[292]

HELLP Syndrome

The syndrome of hemolysis (H), elevated liver enzymes (EL), low platelet count (LP), and severe epigastric pain is a complication of pregnancy-induced hypertension.[293] Seventy percent of the cases occur during the third trimester of pregnancy and 30 percent occur during the postpartum period.[294] HELLP syndrome occurs more often in whites, multipara, and women older than 35 years.[292] Liver biopsy findings of fibrin deposition in hepatic blood vessels and laboratory tests consistent with DIC in a significant proportion of patients imply that DIC plays a role in the pathogenesis of the syndrome.[294–296] Hepatic imaging in 33 patients revealed subcapsular hematomas in 13 and intraparenchymal hemorrhage in 6.[297] What actually triggers DIC in these cases is not known but has been related to endothelial dysfunction.[292] Multiple organ dysfunctions manifested by acute renal failure, ascites, pulmonary edema, and severe hemorrhage resulting from DIC may develop, leading to significant maternal and perinatal mortality rates. Management of patients with HELLP syndrome consists of supportive care, careful monitoring, and blood component replacement therapy. With few exceptions, immediate delivery, not necessarily by cesarian section, is indicated. HELLP syndrome tends to recur in subsequent gestations.[298]

Sepsis During Pregnancy

Gram-negative bacteria, group A streptococci, and *Clostridium perfringens* are among the more common causes of sepsis during pregnancy. These infections are frequently associated with fulminant DIC. The pathogens gain entry into the circulation during abortion, via amnionitis that may follow invasive procedures or rupture of membranes, by endometritis developing during labor, and by way of the urinary tract. Approximately 40 percent of bacteremic patients experience shock, which is associated with significant mortality.[299] In addition, a high rate of bleeding and organ dysfunction affects the kidneys, lungs, and central nervous system.

Treatment of all cases of sepsis-related DIC should include antibiotics, support of vital functions, and surgical intervention to remove any local nidus of infection. Abortion or hysterectomy may be considered.

Dead Fetus Syndrome

Several weeks after intrauterine fetal death, approximately one-third of patients may exhibit laboratory signs of DIC, occasionally accompanied by bleeding.[278,300] Apparently, TF from the retained dead fetus or placenta slowly enters the maternal circulation and initiates DIC, which sometimes is accompanied by significant fibrinolysis.[13] This complication currently is rarely observed because labor is induced promptly after the diagnosis of fetal death is made. However, if labor induction is unavoidably delayed, serial blood coagulation tests should be performed.

The entity of fetal death and DIC can occur following the demise of one of multiple gestations. If it occurs at term, therapy is started as discussed. If it occurs prior to fetal maturity, prolonged administration of heparin can be useful. Interestingly, when selective termination of the life of an anomalous fetus is performed in women with multiple pregnancies, hemostatic abnormalities develop in only approximately 3 percent of cases.[301]

Acute Fatty Liver

Acute fatty liver of pregnancy is a rare disorder that occurs during the third trimester of pregnancy.[302] It can lead to hepatic failure, encephalopathy, and death of the mother and fetus.[303–306] In 15 to 20 percent of cases, acute fatty liver of pregnancy is associated with fetal homozygosity or compound heterozygosity for long-chain acyl-coenzyme A dehydrogenase (LCAD) deficiency.[307] Infants born with LCAD deficiency

fail to thrive and are prone to liver failure and death. LCAD is one of four enzymes taking part in β-oxidation of fatty acids in mitochondria. When it is deficient, accumulation of medium- and long-chain fatty acid occurs. One predominant mutation (G1528C) accounts for 65 to 90 percent of cases with the deficiency. The precise mechanism by which LCAD deficiency in the fetus causes the severe liver disease in the heterozygous mother is unclear. The acute fatty liver disease of pregnancy is characterized by severe liver dysfunction, renal failure, hypertension, and signs of DIC.[304,308] The typical histologic feature is microvesicular fatty infiltration of the liver. Exceedingly low levels of AT and other laboratory signs of DIC were observed in a series of 28 patients, but no definite clinical benefit from AT concentrate infusion was achieved.[308] The primary therapy for these patients is early delivery and supportive care, which yield a maternal survival of 90 percent and perinatal survival of more than 85 percent.[304,309] Pancreatitis is a potentially lethal complication of acute fatty liver of pregnancy.[310]

NEWBORNS

Newborns have a limited capacity to cope with triggers of DIC for several reasons: (1) their ability to clear soluble fibrin and activated factors is reduced; (2) their fibrinolytic potential is decreased because of a low plasminogen level; and (3) their capacity to synthesize coagulation factors and inhibitors is limited.[311,312] Criteria for diagnosis of DIC in newborns are different from those for diagnosis in adults.[313] Important to consider are the physiologic hemostatic findings common at this age, which include low levels of the vitamin K–dependent factors, reduced AT and protein C levels, and prolonged thrombin time. The laboratory evidence of DIC in the newborn is based on the progressive decline of hemostatic parameters, thrombocytopenia, and reduced levels of fibrinogen, factor V, and factor VIII.[311,314,315]

DIC occurs in sick neonates and particularly in those who are premature. More than one underlying cause usually can be identified in newborns with DIC. The most frequent underlying conditions are sepsis, hyaline membrane disease (respiratory distress syndrome), asphyxia, necrotizing enterocolitis, intravascular hemolysis, abruptio placentae, and eclampsia.[312,316]

Bleeding from multiple sites is the most common manifestation of DIC in newborns, with intracranial hemorrhage being the most life-threatening condition. No clinical manifestations of DIC are apparent in approximately 20 percent of neonates,[314] so a high index of suspicion in patients at risk is essential.

●THERAPY

Controlled studies of patients with DIC are difficult to perform in view of the variabilities in DIC triggers, clinical presentations, and grades of severity. Figure 129–4 shows general guidelines for management of patients with DIC, but decisions regarding treatment must be individualized after careful consideration of all clinically important aspects.

TREATMENT OF UNDERLYING DISORDERS AND VITAL SUPPORT

The survival of patients with DIC depends on vigorous treatment of the underlying disorder to alleviate or remove the inciting injurious cause. For sepsis-induced DIC, treatment includes aggressive use of intravenous organism-directed antibiotics and source control (e.g., by surgery or drainage). Other examples of vigorous treatment of underlying conditions are cancer surgery or chemotherapy, uterus evacuation or even hysterectomy in patients with abruptio placentae, resection of aortic aneurysm, and debridement of crushed tissues.

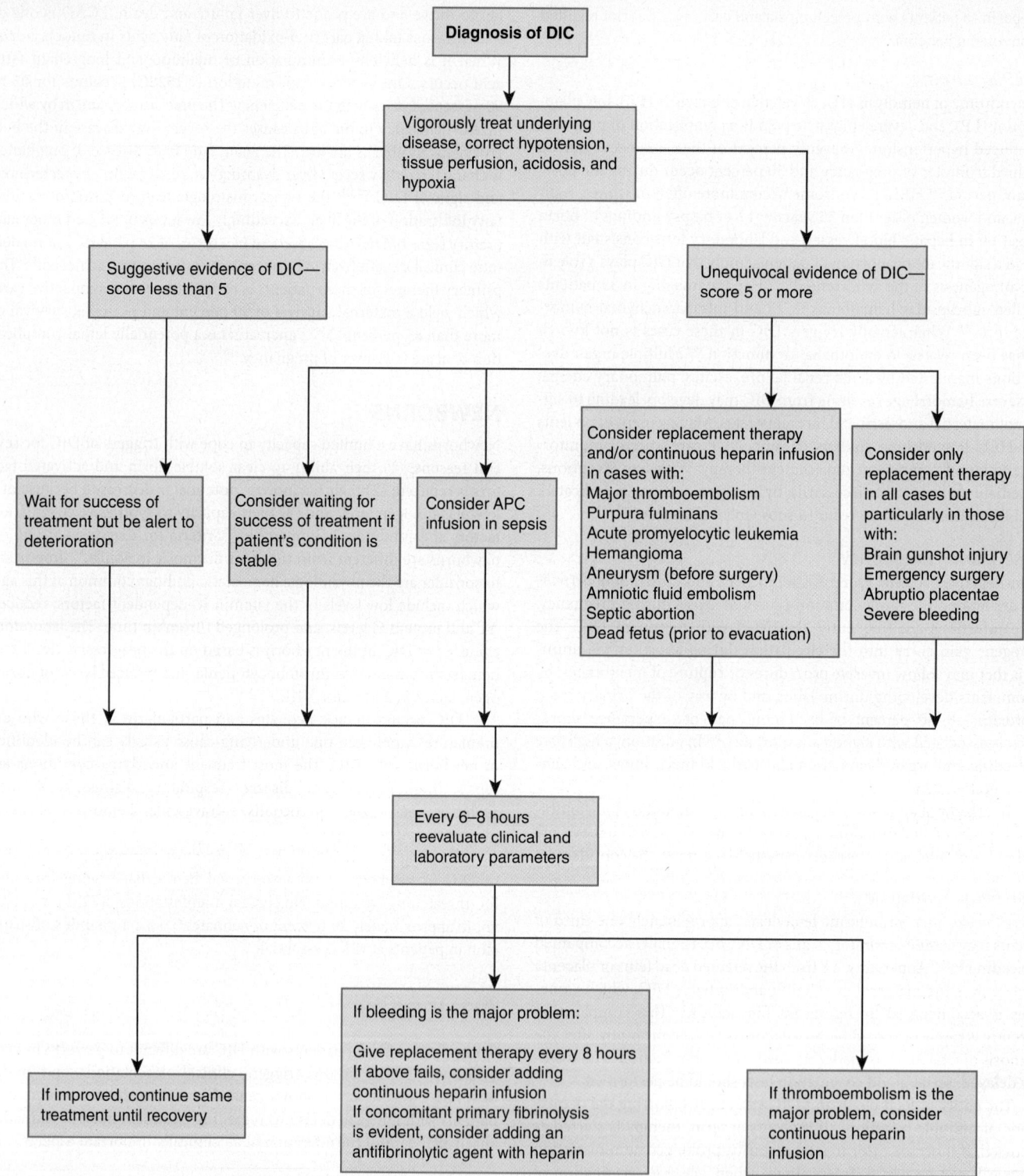

Figure 129–4. General guidelines for initial treatment and follow up of patients with disseminated intravascular coagulation (DIC). The success of management is related to taking rapid, vigorous measures against the underlying disease, support of vital functions, close clinical observation, thoughtful consideration in each individual patient, availability of 24-hour coagulation laboratory services, and an adequate supply of platelet concentrate, cryoprecipitate, fresh-frozen plasma, and packed red cells for replacement therapy. Heparin, when indicated, should be administered by continuous infusion. The basis and limitations of each of the outlined recommendations are detailed throughout the text. APC, activated protein C.

Intensive support of vital functions is required. Volume replacement and correction of hypotension, acidosis, and oxygenation may improve blood flow and oxygen delivery to the microcirculation. Careful monitoring of pulmonary, cardiac, and renal function enables prompt institution of supportive measures, such as use of a respirator for respiratory support, inotropic and vasoactive drugs for improvement of organ perfusion, renal function, and maintenance of electrolyte balance.

BLOOD COMPONENT THERAPY

Treatment of the underlying disease and vital support are necessary but usually insufficient to treat DIC or forestall progression of nonovert DIC to overt DIC. Additional supportive treatment directly aimed at the coagulation system may be required. These interventions include replacing the coagulation factors, natural anticoagulant, fibrinolytic proteins, and platelets that are actively consumed during DIC.[317]

Low levels of platelets and coagulation factors may increase the risk of bleeding. However, plasma or platelet substitution therapy should not be instituted on the basis of laboratory results alone; it is indicated only in patients with active bleeding and in those requiring an invasive procedure or are at risk for bleeding complications.[318,319] The suggestion that administration of blood components might "add fuel to the fire" has never been proven in clinical or experimental studies. The presumed efficacy of treatment with plasma, fibrinogen concentrate, cryoprecipitate, or platelets is not based on randomized controlled trials but appears to be rational therapy in bleeding patients or in patients at risk of bleeding who have a significant depletion of these hemostatic factors.[319] One of the major challenges of infusion of fresh-frozen plasma in these dire circumstances is the propensity of the added volume, which is necessary to correct the coagulation defect, to exacerbate capillary leak. This situation can increase the risk of inducing or worsening pulmonary edema and, by extension, predispose to ARDS, and induce ascites. Coagulation factor concentrates, such as prothrombin complex concentrate, may partially overcome this obstacle, but do not contain essential factors, such as factor V. Moreover, caution is advocated with the use of prothrombin complex concentrates in DIC, as it may worsen the coagulopathy because of traces of activated factors that are present in these concentrates. Specific deficiencies of coagulation factors, such as fibrinogen, may be corrected by administration of purified coagulation factor concentrates.

Platelet transfusion is often required in patients with DIC to prevent bleeding into already ischemic or damaged organs (particularly the central nervous system). The threshold platelet count that should prompt transfusion is patient and disease specific. Cryoprecipitate can be used to rapidly raise the fibrinogen and factor VIII levels, particularly when bleeding is part of the DIC and fibrinogen level is less than 1 g/L. Cryoprecipitate has at least four to five times the mass of fibrinogen per milliliter of infusate compared to fresh-frozen plasma. Fresh-frozen plasma contains fibrinogen in sufficient amounts for treatment of patients with mild to moderate hypofibrinogenemia.

Replacement therapy for thrombocytopenia should consist of 5 to 10 units of platelet concentrate or single-donor apheresis-derived platelets to raise the platelet count to 20 to 30 × 10⁹/L, and in patients who need an invasive procedure, to 50 × 10⁹/L.

RESTORATION OF PHYSIOLOGIC ANTICOAGULANT PATHWAYS

Because the levels of the physiologic anticoagulants are reduced in patients with DIC, restoration of these inhibitors may be a rational approach.[49,320] Based on successful preclinical studies, the use of AT concentrates and heparin in patients with DIC has been examined mainly in randomized controlled trials, that included patients with sepsis, septic shock, or both. All trials have shown some beneficial effect in terms of improvement of laboratory parameters, shortening of the duration of DIC, or even improvement in organ function.[6,321,322] In several small clinical trials, use of very high doses of AT concentrate showed a modest reduction in mortality, but without being statistically significant.[323–325] A large-scale, multicenter, randomized controlled trial also showed no significant reduction in mortality of patients with sepsis.[326] Interestingly, post hoc subgroup analyses of the latter study indicated some benefit in patients who did not receive concomitant heparin, but this observation needs validation. In a small randomized trial in patients with burns and DIC, AT administration decreased mortality, reduced multiple organ failure, and improved coagulation parameters compared to placebo-control patients.[327]

Because a decreased function of the protein C system contributes to the pathogenesis of DIC, therapy by an APC concentrate was predicted to be beneficial.[328] Indeed, a dose-ranging controlled trial using continuous infusion of recombinant human APC disclosed that a dose of 24 mcg/kg per hour was optimal, judged by a decrease of D-dimer level in plasma.[329] A subsequent phase III trial of APC concentrate in patients with sepsis was prematurely stopped because of efficacy in reducing mortality in these patients.[330] All-cause mortality at 28 days after inclusion was 24.7 percent in the APC group versus 30.8 percent in the control group (a 19.4 percent relative risk reduction). Amelioration of coagulation abnormalities and less organ failure were noted in patients who received the concentrate.[331] However, meta-analyses of subsequent trials concluded that the basis for treatment with APC, even in patients with a high disease severity, was not very strong.[332,333] A recently completed placebo-controlled trial in patients with severe sepsis and septic shock was prematurely stopped because of the lack of any significant benefit of APC.[334] Subsequently, the manufacturer of APC has decided to withdraw the product from the market, which has resulted in a revision of current guidelines for treatment of DIC.[335]

HEPARIN ADMINISTRATION AND OTHER ANTICOAGULANTS

Although the question of heparin therapy in patients with DIC has been studied by several investigators, this therapy remains controversial. Experimental studies show that heparin can at least partly inhibit the activation of coagulation in DIC.[336,337] However, a beneficial effect of heparin on clinically important outcome events in patients with DIC has not been demonstrated in controlled clinical trials.[338] Also, the safety of heparin treatment is debatable in DIC patients who are prone to bleeding. A large trial in patients with severe sepsis showed a slight, but nonsignificant benefit, of low-dose heparin on 28-day mortality in patients with severe sepsis.[339]

Notwithstanding these considerations, administration of heparin is beneficial in some categories of chronic DIC, such as metastatic carcinomas, purpura fulminans, and aortic aneurysm (prior to resection). Heparin also is indicated for treating thromboembolic complications in large vessels and before surgery in patients with chronic DIC (see Fig. 129–4). Heparin administration may be helpful in patients with acute DIC when intensive blood component replacement fails to improve excessive bleeding or when thrombosis threatens to cause irreversible tissue injury (e.g., acute cortical necrosis of the kidney or digital gangrene).

Heparin should be used cautiously in all these conditions. In patients with chronic DIC because of metastatic carcinoma or aortic aneurysm, continuous infusion of heparin 500 to 750 U/h without a bolus injection may be sufficient. If no response is obtained within 24 hours, escalating dosages can be used. In hyperacute DIC cases, such as mismatched transfusion, amniotic fluid embolism, septic abortion, and purpura fulminans, intravenous bolus injection of 5000 to 10,000 U heparin may be given simultaneously with replacement therapy with blood products. Some experts would not administer a bolus dose of heparin even under these circumstances. Continuous infusion of 500 to 1000 U/h heparin may be necessary to maintain the benefit until the underlying disease responds to treatment.[339]

Theoretically, the most logical anticoagulant agent to use in DIC is directed against TF activity. Potential agents include recombinant TFPI, inactivated factor VIIa, and recombinant nematode anticoagulant protein c2 (NAPc2), a potent and specific inhibitor of the ternary complex of TF–factor VIIa and factor Xa.[340] Phase II trials of recombinant TFPI in patients with sepsis showed promising results,[341] but a phase III trial did not show an overall survival benefit in patients who were treated with TFPI.[341,342]

Recombinant human soluble thrombomodulin binds to thrombin to form a complex that inactivates thrombin's coagulant activity and activates protein C, and thus, is a potential drug for the treatment of patients with DIC. In a phase III randomized double-blind clinical trial in patients with DIC, administration of the soluble thrombomodulin had a significantly better effect on bleeding manifestations and coagulation parameters than heparin.[343] Ongoing trials with soluble thrombomodulin focus on DIC, organ failure, and mortality rate.

INHIBITORS OF FIBRINOLYSIS

Patients with DIC should not be treated with antifibrinolytic agents such as ε-aminocaproic acid or tranexamic acid because these drugs block fibrinolysis that preserves tissue perfusion in patients with DIC. Use of these agents in patients with DIC has been complicated by severe thrombosis.[344,345]

A different situation prevails in patients with DIC accompanied by primary fibrino(geno)lysis, as in some cases of APL, giant hemangioma, heat stroke, amniotic fluid embolism, some forms of liver disease, and metastatic carcinoma of the prostate. In these conditions, the use of fibrinolytic inhibitors can be considered,[346] provided (1) the patient is bleeding profusely and has not responded to replacement therapy and (2) excessive fibrino(geno)lysis is observed, that is, rapid whole blood clot lysis or a very short euglobulin lysis time. In such circumstances, use of antifibrinolytic agents should be preceded by replacement of depleted blood components and continuous heparin infusion (see Fig. 129–4).

REFERENCES

1. McKay DG: *Disseminated Intravascular Coagulation: an Intermediary Mechanism of Disease.* Hoeber Medical, New York, 1965.
2. Mammen EF: Disseminated intravascular coagulation (DIC). *Clin Lab Sci* 13:239, 2000.
3. Colman RW, Robboy SJ, Minna JD: Disseminated intravascular coagulation: A reappraisal. *Annu Rev Med* 30:359, 1979.
4. Seligsohn U: Disseminated intravascular coagulation, in *Blood: Principles and Practice of Hematology*, edited by RI Handin, SE Lux, TP Stossel, p 1289. J.B. Lippincott, Philadelphia, 2000.
5. Levi M, ten Cate H: Disseminated intravascular coagulation. *N Engl J Med* 341:586, 1999.
6. Levi M, ten Cate H, van der Poll T: Disseminated intravascular coagulation: State of the art. *Thromb Haemost* 82:695, 1999.
7. Levi M: Disseminated intravascular coagulation. *Crit Care Med* 29:2191, 2007.
8. Dupuy M: Injections de matière cérébrale dans les veines. *Gaz Med (Paris)* 2:524, 1834.
9. Trousseau A: Phlegmasia alba dolens. *Clin Med Hotel Dieu Paris* 695, 1865.
10. Naunyn C: Untersuchungen uber Blutgerinnung im lebenden tiere und ihre Folgen. *Arch Exp Pathol Pharmacol* 1873.
11. Woolridge LC: Note on the relation of the red cell corpuscles to coagulation. *Practitioner* 187, 1886.
12. Woolridge LC: Ueber intravasculare gerinnungen. *Arch Ant Physiol Abt (Leipzig)* 397, 1886.
13. Ratnoff OD, Pritchard JA, Colopy JE: Hemorrhagic states during pregnancy. *N Engl J Med* 253:63, 1955.
14. Lasch HG, Heene DL, Huth K, et al: Pathophysiology, clinical manifestations and therapy of consumption-coagulopathy ("Verbrauchskoagulopathie"). *Am J Cardiol* 20:381, 1967.
15. Merskey C, Johnson AJ, Kleiner GJ, et al: The defibrination syndrome: Clinical features and laboratory diagnosis. *Br J Haematol* 13:528, 1967.
16. Robboy SJ, Major MC, Colman RW, et al: Pathology of disseminated intravascular coagulation (DIC). Analysis of 26 cases. *Hum Pathol* 3:327, 1972.
17. Wilde JT, Roberts KM, Greaves M, et al: Association between necropsy evidence of disseminated intravascular coagulation and coagulation variables before death in patients in intensive care units. *J Clin Pathol* 41:138, 1988.
18. Kim HS, Suzuki M, Lie JT, et al: Clinically unsuspected disseminated intravascular coagulation (DIC): An autopsy survey. *Am J Clin Pathol* 66:31, 1976.
19. Watanabe T, Imamura T, Nakagaki K, et al: Disseminated intravascular coagulation in autopsy cases. Its incidence and clinicopathologic significance. *Pathol Res Pract* 165:311, 1979.
20. Shimamura K, Oka K, Nakazawa M, et al: Distribution patterns of microthrombi in disseminated intravascular coagulation. *Arch Pathol Lab Med* 107:543, 1983.
21. Levi M, van der Poll T, ten Cate H, et al: The cytokine-mediated imbalance between coagulant and anticoagulant mechanisms in sepsis and endotoxaemia. *Eur J Clin Invest* 27:3, 1997.
22. Levi M, van der Poll T, Buller HR: The bidirectional relationship between coagulation and inflammation. *Circulation* 109:2698, 2004.
23. Aird WC: Vascular bed-specific hemostasis: Role of endothelium in sepsis pathogenesis. *Crit Care Med* 29:S28, 2001.
24. Weinbaum S, Zhang X, Han Y, et al: Mechanotransduction and flow across the endothelial glycocalyx. *Proc Natl Acad Sci U S A* 100:7988, 2003.
25. Maczewski M, Duda M, Pawlak W, et al: Endothelial protection from reperfusion injury by ischemic preconditioning and diazoxide involves a SOD-like anti-O_2-mechanism. *J Physiol Pharmacol* 55:537, 2004.
26. Vink H, Constantinescu AA, Spaan JA: Oxidized lipoproteins degrade the endothelial surface layer: Implications for platelet-endothelial cell adhesion. *Circulation* 101:1500, 2000.
27. Nieuwdorp M, van Haeften TW, Gouverneur MC, et al: Loss of endothelial glycocalyx during acute hyperglycemia coincides with endothelial dysfunction and coagulation activation *in vivo*. *Diabetes* 55:480, 2006.
28. Levi M, van der Poll T, ten Cate H: Tissue factor in infection and severe inflammation. *Semin Thromb Hemost* 32:33, 2006.
29. Taylor FBJ, Chang A, Ruf W, et al: Lethal *E. coli* septic shock is prevented by blocking tissue factor with monoclonal antibody. *Circ Shock* 33:127, 1991.
30. Levi M, ten Cate H, Bauer KA, et al: Inhibition of endotoxin-induced activation of coagulation and fibrinolysis by pentoxifylline or by a monoclonal anti-tissue factor antibody in chimpanzees. *J Clin Invest* 93:114, 1994.
31. van der Poll T, Levi M, Hack CE, et al: Elimination of interleukin 6 attenuates coagulation activation in experimental endotoxemia in chimpanzees. *J Exp Med* 179:1253, 1994.
32. Osterud B, Rao LV, Olsen JO: Induction of tissue factor expression in whole blood—Lack of evidence for the presence of tissue factor expression on granulocytes. *Thromb Haemost* 83:861, 2000.
33. Franco RF, de Jonge E, Dekkers PE, et al: The *in vivo* kinetics of tissue factor messenger RNA expression during human endotoxemia: Relationship with activation of coagulation. *Blood* 96:554, 2000.
34. Rauch U, Bonderman D, Bohrmann B, et al: Transfer of tissue factor from leukocytes to platelets is mediated by CD15 and tissue factor. *Blood* 96:170, 2000.
35. Osterud B, Bjorklid E: Sources of tissue factor. *Semin Thromb Hemost* 32:11, 2006.
36. van Deventer SJ, Buller HR, ten Cate JW, et al: Experimental endotoxemia in humans: Analysis of cytokine release and coagulation, fibrinolytic, and complement pathways. *Blood* 76:2520, 1990.
37. Boermeester MA, van Leeuwen P, Coyle SM, et al: Interleukin-1 blockade attenuates mediator release and dysregulation of the hemostatic mechanism during human sepsis. *Arch Surg* 130:739, 1995.
38. Osterud B: Tissue factor expression by monocytes: Regulation and pathophysiological roles. *Blood Coagul Fibrinolysis* 9 Suppl 1:S9, 1998.
39. Furie B, Furie BC: Role of platelet P-selectin and microparticle PSGL-1 in thrombus formation. *Trends Mol Med* 10:171, 2004.
40. Neumann FJ, Marx N, Gawaz M, et al: Induction of cytokine expression in leukocytes by binding of thrombin-stimulated platelets. *Circulation* 95:2387, 1997.
41. Esmon CT: Protein C anticoagulant pathway and its role in controlling microvascular thrombosis and inflammation. *Crit Care Med* 29:S48, 2001.
42. Mileno MD, Margolis NH, Clark BD, et al: Coagulation of whole blood stimulates interleukin-1 beta gene expression. *J Infect Dis* 172:308, 1995.
43. Jones A, Geczy CL: Thrombin and factor Xa enhance the production of interleukin-1. *Immunology* 71:236, 1990.
44. Johnson K, Choi Y, DeGroot E, et al: Potential mechanisms for a proinflammatory vascular cytokine response to coagulation activation. *J Immunol* 160:5130, 1998.
45. Sower LE, Froelich CJ, Carney DH, et al: Thrombin induces IL-6 production in fibroblasts and epithelial cells. Evidence for the involvement of the seven-transmembrane domain (STD) receptor for alpha-thrombin. *J Immunol* 155:895, 1995.
46. van der Poll T, de Jonge E, Levi M: Regulatory role of cytokines in disseminated intravascular coagulation. *Semin Thromb Hemost* 27:639, 2001.
47. Coughlin SR: Thrombin signalling and protease-activated receptors. *Nature* 407:258, 2000.

48. Versteeg HH, Peppelenbosch MP, Spek CA: The pleiotropic effects of tissue factor: A possible role for factor VIIa-induced intracellular signalling? *Thromb Haemost* 86:1353, 2001.

49. Levi M, de Jonge E, van der Poll T: Rationale for restoration of physiological anticoagulant pathways in patients with sepsis and disseminated intravascular coagulation. *Crit Care Med* 29:S90, 2001.

50. Szaba FM, Smiley ST: Roles for thrombin and fibrin(ogen) in cytokine/chemokine production and macrophage adhesion *in vivo*. *Blood* 99:1053, 2002.

51. Levi M, van der Poll T: The role of natural anticoagulants in the pathogenesis and management of systemic activation of coagulation and inflammation in critically ill patients. *Semin Thromb Hemost* 34:459, 2008.

52. Levi M: Antithrombin in sepsis revisited. *Crit Care* 9:624, 2005.

53. Levi M, van der Poll T: Two-way interactions between inflammation and coagulation. *Trends Cardiovasc Med* 15:254, 2005.

54. Kobayashi M, Shimada K, Ozawa T: Human recombinant interleukin-1 beta- and tumor necrosis factor alpha-mediated suppression of heparin-like compounds on cultured porcine aortic endothelial cells. *J Cell Physiol* 144:383, 1990.

55. Levi M, van der Poll T: Recombinant human activated protein C: Current insights into its mechanism of action. *Crit Care* 11 Suppl 5:S3, 2007.

56. Esmon CT: Role of coagulation inhibitors in inflammation. *Thromb Haemost* 86:51, 2001.

57. Esmon CT: The regulation of natural anticoagulant pathways. *Science* 235:1348, 1987.

58. Esmon CT: The endothelial cell protein C receptor. *Thromb Haemost* 83:639, 2000.

59. Mesters RM, Helterbrand J, Utterback BG, et al: Prognostic value of protein C concentrations in neutropenic patients at high risk of severe septic complications. *Crit Care Med* 28:2209, 2000.

60. Vary TC, Kimball SR: Regulation of hepatic protein synthesis in chronic inflammation and sepsis. *Am J Physiol* 262:C445, 1992.

61. Eckle I, Seitz R, Egbring R, et al: Protein C degradation *in vitro* by neutrophil elastase. *Biol Chem Hoppe Seyler* 372:1007, 1991.

62. Nawroth PP, Stern DM: Modulation of endothelial cell hemostatic properties by tumor necrosis factor. *J Exp Med* 163:740, 1986.

63. Faust SN, Levin M, Harrison OB, et al: Dysfunction of endothelial protein C activation in severe meningococcal sepsis. *N Engl J Med* 345:408, 2001.

64. Taylor FB Jr, Dahlback B, Chang AC, et al: Role of free protein S and C4b binding protein in regulating the coagulant response to *Escherichia coli*. *Blood* 86:2642, 1995.

65. Taylor FB Jr, Stearns-Kurosawa DJ, Kurosawa S, et al: The endothelial cell protein C receptor aids in host defense against *Escherichia coli* sepsis. *Blood* 95:1680, 2000.

66. De Pont AC, Bakhtiari K, Hutten BA, et al: Endotoxaemia induces resistance to activated protein C in healthy humans. *Br J Haematol* 134:213, 2006.

67. de Jonge E, Dekkers PE, Creasey AA, et al: Tissue factor pathway inhibitor (TFPI) dose-dependently inhibits coagulation activation without influencing the fibrinolytic and cytokine response during human endotoxemia. *Blood* 95:1124, 2000.

68. Creasey AA, Chang AC, Feigen L, et al: Tissue factor pathway inhibitor reduces mortality from *Escherichia coli* septic shock. *J Clin Invest* 91:2850, 1993.

69. Roemisch J, Gray E, Hoffmann JN, et al: Antithrombin: A new look at the actions of a serine protease inhibitor. *Blood Coagul Fibrinolysis* 13:657, 2002.

70. Opal SM: Interactions between coagulation and inflammation. *Scand J Infect Dis* 35:545, 2003.

71. Harada N, Okajima K, Kushimoto S, et al: Antithrombin reduces ischemia/reperfusion injury of rat liver by increasing the hepatic level of prostacyclin. *Blood* 93:157, 1999.

72. Horie S, Ishii H, Kazama M: Heparin-like glycosaminoglycan is a receptor for antithrombin III-dependent but not for thrombin-dependent prostacyclin production in human endothelial cells. *Thromb Res* 59:895, 1990.

73. Mizutani A, Okajima K, Uchiba M, et al: Antithrombin reduces ischemia/reperfusion-induced renal injury in rats by inhibiting leukocyte activation through promotion of prostacyclin production. *Blood* 101:3029, 2003.

74. Uchiba M, Okajima K, Murakami K: Effects of various doses of antithrombin III on endotoxin-induced endothelial cell injury and coagulation abnormalities in rats. *Thromb Res* 89:233, 1998.

75. Esmon CT: New mechanisms for vascular control of inflammation mediated by natural anticoagulant proteins. *J Exp Med* 196:561, 2002.

76. Okajima K: Regulation of inflammatory responses by natural anticoagulants. *Immunol Rev* 184:258, 2001.

77. Taylor FB Jr, Chang A, Esmon CT, et al: Protein C prevents the coagulopathic and lethal effects of *Escherichia coli* infusion in the baboon. *J Clin Invest* 79:918, 1987.

78. Hancock WW, Tsuchida A, Hau H, et al: The anticoagulants protein C and protein S display potent antiinflammatory and immunosuppressive effects relevant to transplant biology and therapy. *Transplant Proc* 24:2302, 1992.

79. Hancock WW, Grey ST, Hau L, et al: Binding of activated protein C to a specific receptor on human mononuclear phagocytes inhibits intracellular calcium signaling and monocyte-dependent proliferative responses. *Transplantation* 60:1525, 1995.

80. White B, Schmidt M, Murphy C, et al: Activated protein C inhibits lipopolysaccharide-induced nuclear translocation of nuclear factor kappaB (NF-kappaB) and tumour necrosis factor alpha (TNF-alpha) production in the THP-1 monocytic cell line. *Br J Haematol* 110:130, 2000.

81. Levi M, Dorffler-Melly J, Reitsma PH, et al: Aggravation of endotoxin-induced disseminated intravascular coagulation and cytokine activation in heterozygous protein C deficient mice. *Blood* 101:4823, 2003.

82. Lay AJ, Donahue D, Tsai MJ, et al: Acute inflammation is exacerbated in mice genetically predisposed to a severe protein C deficiency. *Blood* 109:1984, 2007.

83. Feistritzer C, Sturn DH, Kaneider NC, et al: Endothelial protein C receptor-dependent inhibition of human eosinophil chemotaxis by protein C. *J Allergy Clin Immunol* 112:375, 2003.

84. Sturn DH, Kaneider NC, Feistritzer C, et al: Expression and function of the endothelial protein C receptor in human neutrophils. *Blood* 102:1499, 2003.

85. Hoffmann JN, Vollmar B, Laschke MW, et al: Microhemodynamic and cellular mechanisms of activated protein C action during endotoxemia. *Crit Care Med* 32:1011, 2004.

86. Nick JA, Coldren CD, Geraci MW, et al: Recombinant human activated protein C reduces human endotoxin-induced pulmonary inflammation via inhibition of neutrophil chemotaxis. *Blood* 104:3878, 2004.

87. Shimizu S, Gabazza EC, Taguchi O, et al: Activated protein C inhibits the expression of platelet-derived growth factor in the lung. *Am J Respir Crit Care Med* 167:1416, 2003.

88. Zeng W, Matter WF, Yan SB, et al: Effect of drotrecogin alfa (activated) on human endothelial cell permeability and Rho kinase signaling. *Crit Care Med* 32:S302, 2004.

89. Feistritzer C, Riewald M: Endothelial barrier protection by activated protein C through PAR1-dependent sphingosine 1-phosphate receptor-1 cross activation. *Blood* 105:3178, 2005.

90. Finigan JH, Dudek SM, Singleton PA, et al: Activated protein C mediates novel lung endothelial barrier enhancement: Role of sphingosine 1-phosphate receptor transactivation. *J Biol Chem* 280:17286, 2005.

91. Cheng T, Liu D, Griffin JH, et al: Activated protein C blocks p53-mediated apoptosis in ischemic human brain endothelium and is neuroprotective. *Nat Med* 9:338, 2003.

92. Riewald M, Petrovan RJ, Donner A, et al: Activation of endothelial cell protease activated receptor 1 by the protein C pathway. *Science* 296:1880, 2002.

93. Mosnier LO, Griffin JH: Inhibition of staurosporine-induced apoptosis of endothelial cells by activated protein C requires protease activated receptor-1 and endothelial cell protein C receptor. *Biochem J* 373:65, 2003.

94. Mosnier LO, Zlokovic BV, Griffin JH: The cytoprotective protein C pathway. *Blood* 109:3161, 2007.

95. Biemond BJ, Levi M, ten Cate H, et al: Plasminogen activator and plasminogen activator inhibitor I release during experimental endotoxaemia in chimpanzees: Effect of interventions in the cytokine and coagulation cascades. *Clin Sci* 88:587, 1995.

96. Schleef RR, Bevilacqua MP, Sawdey M, et al: Cytokine activation of vascular endothelium. Effects on tissue-type plasminogen activator and type 1 plasminogen activator inhibitor. *J Biol Chem* 263:5797, 1988.

97. van Hinsbergh VW, Kooistra T, van den Berg EA, et al: Tumor necrosis factor increases the production of plasminogen activator inhibitor in human endothelial cells *in vitro* and in rats *in vivo*. *Blood* 72:1467, 1988.

98. Asakura H, Ontachi Y, Mizutani T: An enhanced fibrinolysis prevents the development of multiple organ failure in disseminated intravascular coagulation in spite of much activation of blood coagulation. *Crit Care Med* 29:1164, 2001.

99. Yamamoto K, Loskutoff DJ: Fibrin deposition in tissues from endotoxin-treated mice correlates with decreases in the expression of urokinase-type but not tissue-type plasminogen activator. *J Clin Invest* 97:2440, 1996.

100. Nesheim M, Wang W, Boffa M, et al: Thrombin, thrombomodulin and TAFI in the molecular link between coagulation and fibrinolysis. *Thromb Haemost* 78:386, 1997.

101. Salvemini D, Cuzzocrea S: Oxidative stress in septic shock and disseminated intravascular coagulation. *Free Radic Biol Med* 33:1173, 2002.

102. Asakura H, Okudaira M, Yoshida T: Induction of vasoactive substances differs in LPS-induced and TF-induced DIC models in rats. *Thromb Haemost* 88:663, 2002.

103. Levi M, Nieuwdorp M, van der Poll T, et al: Metabolic modulation of inflammation-induced activation of coagulation. *Semin Thromb Hemost* 34:26, 2008.

104. Kjalke M, Silveira A, Hamsten A, et al: Plasma lipoproteins enhance tissue factor-independent factor VII activation. *Arterioscler Thromb Vasc Biol* 20:1835, 2000.

105. van der Poll T, Coyle SM, Levi M, et al: Fat emulsion infusion potentiates coagulation activation during human endotoxemia. *Thromb Haemost* 75:83, 1996.

106. Pajkrt D, Lerch PG, van der Poll T, et al: Differential effects of reconstituted high-density lipoprotein on coagulation, fibrinolysis and platelet activation during human endotoxemia. *Thromb Haemost* 77:303, 1997.

107. Birjmohun RS, van Leuven SI, Levels JH, et al: High-density lipoprotein attenuates inflammation and coagulation response on endotoxin challenge in humans. *Arterioscler Thromb Vasc Biol* 27:1153, 2007.

108. Bisoendial RJ, Kastelein JJ, Peters SL, et al: Effects of CRP infusion on endothelial function and coagulation in normocholesterolemic and hypercholesterolemic subjects. *J Lipid Res* 48:952, 2007.

109. Grant PJ: Diabetes mellitus as a prothrombotic condition. *J Intern Med* 262:157, 2007.

110. Juhan-Vague I, Roul C, Alessi MC, et al: Increased plasminogen activator inhibitor activity in non insulin dependent diabetic patients—Relationship with plasma insulin. *Thromb Haemost* 61:370, 1989.

111. Mansfield MW, Stickland MH, Grant PJ: PAI-1 concentrations in first-degree relatives of patients with non-insulin-dependent diabetes: Metabolic and genetic associations. *Thromb Haemost* 77:357, 1997.

112. Samad F, Pandey M, Loskutoff DJ: Regulation of tissue factor gene expression in obesity. *Blood* 98:3353, 2001.

113. Stegenga ME, van der Crabben SN, Levi M, et al: Hyperglycemia enhances coagulation and reduces neutrophil degranulation, whereas hyperinsulinemia inhibits fibrinolysis during human endotoxemia. *Blood* 112:82, 2008.

114. Levi M: Current understanding of disseminated intravascular coagulation. *Br J Haematol* 124:567, 2004.
115. Siegal T, Seligsohn U, Aghai E, et al: Clinical and laboratory aspects of disseminated intravascular coagulation (DIC): A study of 118 cases. *Thromb Haemost* 39:122, 1978.
116. Al-Mondhiry H: Disseminated intravascular coagulation: Experience in a major cancer center. *Thromb Diath Haemorrh* 34:181, 1975.
117. Hofstra JJ, Haitsma JJ, Juffermans NP, et al: Role of broncho-alveolar hemostasis in the pathogenesis of acute lung injury. *Semin Thromb Hemost* 34:475, 2008.
118. Rinaldo JE, Rogers RM: Adult respiratory distress syndrome [editorial]. *N Engl J Med* 315:578, 1986.
119. Katsumura Y, Ohtsubo K: Incidence of pulmonary thromboembolism, infarction and hemorrhage in disseminated intravascular coagulation. *Thorax* 50:160, 1995.
120. Kollef MH, Schuster DP: The acute respiratory distress syndrome. *N Engl J Med* 332:27, 1995.
121. Dhainaut JF, Shorr AF, Macias WL, et al: Dynamic evolution of coagulopathy in the first day of severe sepsis: Relationship with mortality and organ failure. *Crit Care Med* 33:341, 2005.
122. Spero JA, Lewis JH, Hasiba U: Disseminated intravascular coagulation. Findings in 346 patients. *Thromb Haemost* 43:28, 1980.
123. Bakhtiari K, Meijers JC, de Jonge E, et al: Prospective validation of the international society of thrombosis and haemostasis scoring system for disseminated intravascular coagulation. *Crit Care Med* 32:2416, 2004.
124. Dhainaut JF, Yan SB, Joyce DE, et al: Treatment effects of drotrecogin alfa (activated) in patients with severe sepsis with or without overt disseminated intravascular coagulation. *J Thromb Haemost* 2:1924, 2004.
125. Dempfle CE, Pfitzner SA, Dollman M, et al: Comparison of immunological and functional assays for measurement of soluble fibrin. *Thromb Haemost* 74:673, 1995.
126. Bredbacka S, Blomback M, Wiman B, et al: Laboratory methods for detecting disseminated intravascular coagulation (DIC): New aspects. *Acta Anaesthesiol Scand* 37:125, 1993.
127. Bredbacka S, Blomback M, Wiman B: Soluble fibrin: A predictor for the development and outcome of multiple organ failure. *Am J Hematol* 46:289, 1994.
128. McCarron BI, Marder VJ, Kanouse JJ, et al: A soluble fibrin standard: Comparable dose-response with immunologic and functional assays. *Thromb Haemost* 82:145, 1999.
129. Shorr AF, Thomas SJ, Alkins SA, et al: D-dimer correlates with proinflammatory cytokine levels and outcomes in critically ill patients. *Chest* 121:1262, 2002.
130. Dempfle CE: The use of soluble fibrin in evaluating the acute and chronic hypercoagulable state. *Thromb Haemost* 82:673, 1999.
131. Horan JT, Francis CW: Fibrin degradation products, fibrin monomer and soluble fibrin in disseminated intravascular coagulation. *Semin Thromb Hemost* 27:657, 2001.
132. McCarron BI, Marder VJ, Francis CW: Reactivity of soluble fibrin assays with plasmic degradation products of fibrin and in patients receiving fibrinolytic therapy. *Thromb Haemost* 82:1722, 1999.
133. Carr JM, McKinney M, McDonagh J: Diagnosis of disseminated intravascular coagulation. Role of D-dimer. *Am J Clin Pathol* 91:280, 1989.
134. Boisclair MD, Ireland H, Lane DA: Assessment of hypercoagulable states by measurement of activation fragments and peptides. *Blood Rev* 4:25, 1990.
135. Prisco D, Paniccia R, Bonechi F, et al: Evaluation of new methods for the selective measurement of fibrin and fibrinogen degradation products. *Thromb Res* 56:547, 1989.
136. Shorr AF, Trotta RF, Alkins SA, et al: D-dimer assay predicts mortality in critically ill patients without disseminated intravascular coagulation or venous thromboembolic disease. *Intensive Care Med* 25:207, 1999.
137. Greenberg CS, Devine DV, McCrae KM: Measurement of plasma fibrin D-dimer levels with the use of a monoclonal antibody coupled to latex beads. *Am J Clin Pathol* 87:94, 1987.
138. Taylor FB Jr, Toh CH, Hoots WK, et al: Towards definition, clinical and laboratory criteria, and a scoring system for disseminated intravascular coagulation. *Thromb Haemost* 86:1327, 2001.
139. Kobayashi S, Gando S, Morimoto Y: Serial measurement of arterial lactate concentrations as a prognostic indicator in relation to the incidence of disseminated intravascular coagulation in patients with systemic inflammatory response syndrome. *Surg Today* 31:853, 2001.
140. Wada H, Gabazza EC, Asakura H, et al: Comparison of diagnostic criteria for disseminated intravascular coagulation (DIC): Diagnostic criteria of the International Society of Thrombosis and Hemostasis and of the Japanese Ministry of Health and Welfare for overt DIC: *Am J Hematol* 74:17, 2003.
141. Kinasewitz GT, Zein JG, Lee GL, et al: Prognostic value of a simple evolving DIC score in patients with severe sepsis. *Crit Care Med* 33:2214, 2005.
142. Levi M, van der Poll T, de Jonge E, et al: Relative insufficiency of fibrinolysis in disseminated intravascular coagulation. *Sepsis* 3:103, 2000.
143. Liaw PC, Ferrell G, Esmon CT. A monoclonal antibody against activated protein C allows rapid detection of activated protein C in plasma and reveals a calcium ion dependent epitope involved in factor Va inactivation. *J Thromb Haemost* 1:662, 2003.
144. Moore JC, Hayward CP, Warkentin TE, et al: Decreased von Willebrand factor protease activity associated with thrombocytopenic disorders. *Blood* 98:1842, 2001.
145. Levi M, Lowenberg EC: Thrombocytopenia in critically ill patients. *Semin Thromb Hemost* 34:417, 2008.
146. Dempfle CE, Borggrefe M: Point of care coagulation tests in critically ill patients. *Semin Thromb Hemost* 34:445, 2008.
147. Collins PW, Macchiavello LI, Lewis SJ, et al: Global tests of haemostasis in critically ill patients with severe sepsis syndrome compared to controls. *Br J Haematol* 135:220-, 2006.
148. Toh CH, Hoots WK: The scoring system of the Scientific and Standardisation Committee on Disseminated Intravascular Coagulation of the International Society on Thrombosis and Haemostasis: A 5-year overview. *J Thromb Haemost* 5:604, 2007.
149. Bone RC: Modulators of coagulation. A critical appraisal of their role in sepsis. *Arch Intern Med* 152:1381, 1992.
150. Keller TT, Mairuhu AT, de Kruif MD, et al: Infections and endothelial cells. *Cardiovasc Res* 60:40, 2003.
151. Gando S, Nanzaki S, Sasaki S, et al: Activation of the extrinsic coagulation pathway in patients with severe sepsis and septic shock. *Crit Care Med* 26:2005, 1998.
152. Wiersinga WJ, Meijers JC, Levi M, et al: Activation of coagulation with concurrent impairment of anticoagulant mechanisms correlates with a poor outcome in severe melioidosis. *J Thromb Haemost* 6:32, 2008.
153. Bone RC: Gram-positive organisms and sepsis. *Arch Intern Med* 154:26, 1994.
154. Levi M, van der Poll T: Coagulation in sepsis: All bugs bite equally. *Crit Care* 8:99, 2004.
155. Herwald H, Cramer H, Morgelin M: M-protein, a classical bacterial virulence determinant forms complexes with fibrinogen that induce vascular leakage. *Cell* 116:367, 2004.
156. Fijnvandraat K, Derkx B, Peters M, et al: Coagulation activation and tissue necrosis in meningococcal septic shock: Severely reduced protein C levels predict a high mortality. *Thromb Haemost* 73:15, 1995.
157. Hazelzet JA, Risseeuw-Appel IM, Kornelisse RF, et al: Age-related differences in outcome and severity of DIC in children with septic shock and purpura. *Thromb Haemost* 76:932, 1996.
158. Levi M, Opal SM: Coagulation abnormalities in critically ill patients. *Crit Care* 10:222, 2006.
159. Levi M: Hemostasis and thrombosis in critically ill patients. *Semin Thromb Hemost* 34:415, 2008.
160. Ono T, Mimuro J, Madoiwa S, et al: Severe secondary deficiency of von Willebrand factor-cleaving protease (ADAMTS13) in patients with sepsis-induced disseminated intravascular coagulation: Its correlation with development of renal failure. *Blood* 107:528, 2006.
161. Bhakdi S, Muhly M, Mannhardt U: Staphylococcal alpha toxin promotes blood coagulation via attack on human platelets. *J Exp Med* 168:527, 1988.
162. Ratnoff OD, Nebehay WG: Multiple coagulative defects in a patient with the Waterhouse-Friderichsen syndrome. *Ann Intern Med* 56:627, 1962.
163. van Gorp E, Suharti C, ten Cate H, et al: Review: Infectious diseases and coagulation disorders. *J Infect Dis* 180:176, 1999.
164. Levi M, Keller TT, van Gorp E, et al: Infection and inflammation and the coagulation system. *Cardiovasc Res* 60:26, 2003.
165. Heller MV, Marta RF, Sturk A, et al: Early markers of blood coagulation and fibrinolysis activation in Argentine hemorrhagic fever. *Thromb Haemost* 73:368, 1995.
166. Clemens R, Pramoolsinsap C, Lorenz R, et al: Activation of the coagulation cascade in severe falciparum malaria through the intrinsic pathway. *Br J Haematol* 87:100, 1994.
167. Mohanty D, Ghosh K, Nandwani SK, et al: Fibrinolysis, inhibitors of blood coagulation, and monocyte derived coagulant activity in acute malaria. *Am J Hematol* 54:23, 1997.
168. Fera G, Semeraro N, De MV, et al: Disseminated intravascular coagulation associated with disseminated cryptococcosis in a patient with acquired immunodeficiency syndrome. *Infection* 21:171, 1993.
169. Cosgriff TM: Viruses and haemostasis. *Rev Infect Dis* 11:672, 1989.
170. Inbal A, Kenet G, Zivelin A, et al: Purpura fulminans induced by disseminated intravascular coagulation following infection in 2 unrelated children with double heterozygosity for factor V Leiden and protein S deficiency. *Thromb Haemost* 77:1086, 1997.
171. Hofstra JJ, Schouten M, Levi M: Thrombophilia and outcome in severe infection and sepsis. *Semin Thromb Hemost* 33:604, 2007.
172. Levin M, Eley BS, Louis J: Postinfectious purpura fulminans caused by an autoantibody directed against protein S. *J Pediatr* 127:355, 1995.
173. Bhamarapravati N: Hemostatic defects in dengue hemorrhagic fever. *Rev Infect Dis* 11 Suppl 4:S826, 1989.
174. Suvatte V: Dengue hemorrhagic fever: Hematological abnormalities and pathogenesis. *J Med Assoc Thai* 61 Suppl 3:53, 1978.
175. Linder M, Muller-Berghaus G, Lasch HG, et al: Virus infection and blood coagulation. *Thromb Diath Haemorrh* 23:1, 1970.
176. Carpenter CT, Kaiser AB: Purpura fulminans in pneumococcal sepsis: Case report and review. *Scand J Infect Dis* 29:479, 1997.
177. Gerson WT, Dickerman JD, Bovill EG, et al: Severe acquired protein C deficiency in purpura fulminans associated with disseminated intravascular coagulation: Treatment with protein C concentrate. *Pediatrics* 91:418, 1993.
178. Tishler M, Abramov AL, Seligsohn U, et al: Purpura fulminans in an adult. *Isr J Med Sci* 22:820, 1986.
179. Bramson HE, Katz J, Marble R, et al: Inherited protein C deficiency and a coumarin responsive chronic relapsing purpura fulminans in a newborn infant. *Lancet* 2:1156, 1983.
180. Seligsohn U, Berger A, Abend M: Homozygous protein C deficiency manifested by massive venous thrombosis in the newborn. *N Engl J Med* 310:559, 1984.
181. Goad KE, Gralnick HR: Coagulation disorders in cancer. *Hematol Oncol Clin North Am* 10:457, 1996.
182. Levi M: Cancer and DIC: *Haemostasis* 31 Suppl 1:47, 2001.

183. Sack GH Jr, Levin J, Bell WR: Trousseau's syndrome and other manifestations of chronic disseminated coagulopathy in patients with neoplasms: Clinical, pathophysiologic, and therapeutic features. *Medicine (Baltimore)* 56:1, 1977.

184. Sallah S, Wan JY, Nguyen NP, et al: Disseminated intravascular coagulation in solid tumors: Clinical and pathological study. *Thromb Haemost* 86:828, 2001.

185. Donati MB: Cancer and thrombosis: From Phlegmasia alba dolens to transgenic mice. *Thromb Haemost* 74:278, 1995.

186. Levi M: Cancer and thrombosis. *Clin Adv Hematol Oncol* 1:668, 2003.

187. Contrino J, Hair G, Kreutzer DL, et al: *In situ* detection of tissue factor in vascular endothelial cells: Correlation with the malignant phenotype of human breast disease. *Nat Med* 2:209, 1996.

188. Rickles FR, Brenner B: Tissue factor and cancer. *Semin Thromb Hemost* 34:143, 2008.

189. Bromberg ME, Konigsberg WH, Madison JF, et al: Tissue factor promotes melanoma metastasis by a pathway independent of blood coagulation. *Proc Natl Acad Sci U S A* 92:8205, 1995.

190. Zhang Y, Deng Y, Luther T, et al: Tissue factor controls the balance of angiogenic and antiangiogenic properties of tumor cells in mice. *J Clin Invest* 94:1320, 1994.

191. Nadir Y, Vlodavsky I, Brenner B: Heparanase, tissue factor, and cancer. *Semin Thromb Hemost* 34:187, 2008.

192. Falanga A, Consonni R, Marchetti M, et al: Cancer procoagulant and tissue factor are differently modulated by all-trans-retinoic acid in acute promyelocytic leukemia cells. *Blood* 92:143, 1998.

193. Levi M: Disseminated intravascular coagulation in cancer patients. *Best Pract Res Clin Haematol* 22:129, 2009.

194. Wahrenbrock M, Borsig L, Le Duc M: Selectin-mucin interactions as a probable molecular explanation for the association of Trousseau syndrome with mucinous adenocarcinoma. *J Clin Invest* 112:853, 2003.

195. Dvorak HF, Quay SC, Orenstein NS: Tumor shedding and coagulation. *Science* 212:923, 1981.

196. Zwicker JI: Tissue factor-bearing microparticles and cancer. *Semin Thromb Hemost* 34:195, 2008.

197. Nijziel MR, van OR, Hillen HF, et al: From Trousseau to angiogenesis: The link between the haemostatic system and cancer. *Neth J Med* 64:403, 2006.

198. Rickles FR, Falanga A: Molecular basis for the relationship between thrombosis and cancer. *Thromb Res* 102:V215, 2001.

199. Stouthard JM, Levi M, Hack CE, et al: Interleukin-6 stimulates coagulation, not fibrinolysis, in humans. *Thromb Haemost* 76:738, 1996.

200. van der Poll T, Coyle SM, Levi M, et al: Effect of a recombinant dimeric tumor necrosis factor receptor on inflammatory responses to intravenous endotoxin in normal humans. *Blood* 89:3727, 1997.

201. van der Poll T, Levi M, ten Cate H, et al: The role of tumor necrosis factor in systemic inflammatory responses in primate endotoxemia. *Prog Clin Biol Res* 388:425, 1994.

202. van der Poll T, Levi M, van Deventer SJ, et al: Differential effects of anti-tumor necrosis factor monoclonal antibodies on systemic inflammatory responses in experimental endotoxemia in chimpanzees. *Blood* 83:446, 1994.

203. Sewnath ME, Olszyna DP, Birjmohun R, et al: IL-10-deficient mice demonstrate multiple organ failure and increased mortality during *Escherichia coli* peritonitis despite an accelerated bacterial clearance. *J Immunol* 166:6323, 2001.

204. van der Poll T, Jansen J, Levi M, et al: Interleukin 10 release during endotoxaemia in chimpanzees: Role of platelet-activating factor and interleukin 6. *Scand J Immunol* 43:122, 1996.

205. van der Poll T, Jansen PM, Montegut WJ, et al: Effects of IL-10 on systemic inflammatory responses during sublethal primate endotoxemia. *J Immunol* 158:1971, 1997.

206. Seligsohn U, Weber H, Yoran C: Microangiopathic hemolytic anemia and defibrination syndrome in metastatic carcinoma of the stomach. *Isr J Med Sci* 4:69, 1968.

207. Uchiumi H, Matsushima T, Yamane A, et al: Prevalence and clinical characteristics of acute myeloid leukemia associated with disseminated intravascular coagulation. *Int J Hematol* 86:137, 2007.

208. Barbui T, Falanga A: Disseminated intravascular coagulation in acute leukemia. *Semin Thromb Hemost* 27:593, 2001.

209. Sarris AH, Kempin S, Berman E, et al: High incidence of disseminated intravascular coagulation during remission induction of adult patients with acute lymphoblastic leukemia. *Blood* 79:1305, 1992.

210. Avvisati G, ten Cate JW, Sturk A, et al: Acquired alpha-2-antiplasmin deficiency in acute promyelocytic leukaemia. *Br J Haematol* 70:43, 1988.

211. Falanga A: Mechanisms of hypercoagulation in malignancy and during chemotherapy. *Haemostasis* 28 Suppl 3:50, 1998.

212. Stein E, McMahon B, Kwaan H, et al: The coagulopathy of acute promyelocytic leukaemia revisited. *Best Pract Res Clin Haematol* 22:153, 2009.

213. Barbui T, Finazzi G, Falanga A: The impact of all-*trans*-retinoic acid on the coagulopathy of acute promyelocytic leukemia. *Blood* 91:3093, 1998.

214. Gando S, Nakanishi Y, Tedo I: Cytokines and plasminogen activator inhibitor-1 in posttrauma disseminated intravascular coagulation: Relationship to multiple organ dysfunction syndrome. *Crit Care Med* 23:1835, 1995.

215. Gando S: Disseminated intravascular coagulation in trauma patients. *Semin Thromb Hemost* 27:585, 2001.

216. Gando S: Tissue factor in trauma and organ dysfunction. *Semin Thromb Hemost* 32:48, 2006.

217. Owings JT, Gosselin RC, Anderson JT, et al: Practical utility of the D-dimer assay for excluding thromboembolism in severely injured trauma patients. *J Trauma* 51:425, 2001.

218. Attar S, Boyd D, Layne E, et al: Alterations in coagulation and fibrinolytic mechanisms in acute trauma. *J Trauma* 9:939, 1969.

219. Cosgriff N, Moore EE, Sauaia A, et al: Predicting life-threatening coagulopathy in the massively transfused trauma patient: Hypothermia and acidoses revisited. *J Trauma* 42:857, 1997.

220. Hess JR, Holcomb JB: Transfusion practice in military trauma. *Transfus Med* 18:143, 2008.

221. Armand R, Hess JR: Treating coagulopathy in trauma patients. *Transfus Med Rev* 17:223, 2003.

222. Simmons RL, Collins JA, Heisterkamp CA, et al: Coagulation disorders in combat casualties. I: Acute changes after wounding. II: Effects of massive transfusion. 3. Post-resuscitative changes. *Ann Surg* 169:455, 1969.

223. Gomez R, Murray CK, Hospenthal DR, et al: Causes of mortality by autopsy findings of combat casualties and civilian patients admitted to a burn unit. *J Am Coll Surg* 208:348, 2009.

224. Niles SE, McLaughlin DF, Perkins JG, et al: Increased mortality associated with the early coagulopathy of trauma in combat casualties. *J Trauma* 64:1459, 2008.

225. Kaufman HH, Hui KS, Mattson JC, et al: Clinicopathological correlations of disseminated intravascular coagulation in patients with head injury. *Neurosurgery* 15:34, 1984.

226. Stein SC, Chen XH, Sinson GP, et al: Intravascular coagulation: A major secondary insult in nonfatal traumatic brain injury. *J Neurosurg* 97:1373, 2002.

227. Olson JD, Kaufman HH, Moake J, et al: The incidence and significance of hemostatic abnormalities in patients with head injuries. *Neurosurgery* 24:825, 1989.

228. Selladurai BM, Vickneswaran M, Duraisamy S, et al: Coagulopathy in acute head injury—A study of its role as a prognostic indicator. *Br J Neurosurg* 11:398, 1997.

229. Levi M: Burning issues surrounding inflammation and coagulation in heatstroke. *Crit Care Med* 56:2455, 2008.

230. Garcia-Avello A, Lorente JA, Cesar-Perez J, et al: Degree of hypercoagulability and hyperfibrinolysis is related to organ failure and prognosis after burn trauma. *Thromb Res* 89:59, 1998.

231. Simon TL, Curreri PW, Harker LA: Kinetic characterization of hemostasis in thermal injury. *J Lab Clin Med* 89:702, 1977.

232. Winkelman MD, Galloway PG: Central nervous system complications of thermal burns. A postmortem study of 139 patients. *Medicine (Baltimore)* 71:271, 1992.

233. Carr ME Jr: Disseminated intravascular coagulation: Pathogenesis, diagnosis, and therapy. *J Emerg Med* 5:311, 1987.

234. Tytgat GN, Collen D, Verstraete M: Metabolism of fibrinogen in cirrhosis of the liver. *J Clin Invest* 50:169, 1971.

235. Coleman M, Finlayson N, Bettigole RE, et al: Fibrinogen survival in cirrhosis: Improvement by "low dose" heparin. *Ann Intern Med* 83:79, 1975.

236. Coccheri S, Mannucci PM, Palareti G, et al: Significance of plasma fibrinopeptide A and high molecular weight fibrinogen in patients with liver cirrhosis. *Br J Haematol* 52:503, 1982.

237. Oka K, Tanaka K: Intravascular coagulation in autopsy cases with liver diseases. *Thromb Haemost* 42:564, 1979.

238. Paramo JA, Rifon J, Fernandez J, et al: Thrombin activation and increased fibrinolysis in patients with chronic liver disease. *Blood Coagul Fibrinolysis* 2:227, 1991.

239. Palascak JE, Martinez J: Dysfibrinogenemia associated with liver disease. *J Clin Invest* 60:89, 1977.

240. Ben-Ari Z, Osman E, Hutton RA, et al: Disseminated intravascular coagulation in liver cirrhosis: Fact or fiction? [See comments.] *Am J Gastroenterol* 94:2977, 1999.

241. Hollestelle MJ, Geertzen HG, Straatsburg IH, et al: Factor VIII expression in liver disease. *Thromb Haemost* 91:267, 2004.

242. Straub PW: Diffuse intravascular coagulation in liver disease? *Semin Thromb Hemost* 4:29, 1977.

243. Canoso RT, Hutton RA, Deykin D: The hemostatic defect of chronic liver disease. Kinetic studies using 75Se-selenomethionine. *Gastroenterology* 76:540, 1979.

244. Tempero MA, Davis RB, Reed E, et al: Thrombocytopenia and laboratory evidence of disseminated intravascular coagulation after shunts for ascites in malignant disease. *Cancer* 55:2718, 1985.

245. Bakker CM, Knot EA, Stibbe J, et al: Disseminated intravascular coagulation in liver cirrhosis. *J Hepatol* 15:330, 1992.

246. Wakefield EG, Hall WW: Heat injuries: A preparatory study for experimental heatstroke. *JAMA* 89:92, 1927.

247. Chao TC, Sinniah R, Pakiam JE: Acute heat stroke deaths. *Pathology* 13:145, 1981.

248. Bouchama A, Knochel JP: Heat stroke. *N Engl J Med* 346:1978, 2002.

249. Bouchama A, Hammami MM, Haq A, et al: Evidence for endothelial cell activation/injury in heatstroke. *Crit Care Med* 24:1173, 1996.

250. Gauss P, Meyer KA: Heat stroke: Report of one hundred and fifty-eight cases from Cook County Hospital, Chicago. *Am J Med Sci* 154:554, 1917.

251. Huisse MG, Pease S, Hurtado-Nedelec M, et al: Leucocyte activation: The link between inflammation and coagulation during heatstroke. A study of patients during the 2003 heat wave in Paris. *Crit Care Med* 36:2288, 2008.

252. Mustafa KY, Omer O, Khogali M, et al: Blood coagulation and fibrinolysis in heat stroke. *Br J Haematol* 61:517, 1985.

253. Seegers WH, Ouyang C: Snake venoms and blood coagulation, in *Snake Venoms*, edited by L Chen-Yuan L, p 684. Springer Verlag, Berlin, 1979.

254. Huang TF, Holt JC, Lukasiewicz H, et al: Trigramin. A low molecular weight peptide inhibiting fibrinogen interaction with platelet receptors expressed on glycoprotein IIb-IIIa complex. *J Biol Chem* 262:16157, 1987.

255. Klein JD, Walker FJ: Purification of a protein C activator from the venom of the southern copperhead snake (*Agkistrodon contortrix contortrix*). *Biochemistry* 25:4175, 1986.

256. Weiss HJ, Phillips LL, Hopewell WS, et al: Heparin therapy in a patient bitten by a saw-scaled viper (*Echis carinatus*), a snake whose venom activates prothrombin. *Am J Med* 54:653, 1973.

257. Schulchynska-Castel H, Dvilansky A, Keynan A: eEchis colorata bites: Clinical evaluation of 42 patients. A retrospective study. *Isr J Med Sci* 22:880, 1986.

258. Fainaru M, Eisenberg S, Manny N, et al: The natural course of defibrination syndrome caused by *Echis colorata* venom in man. *Thromb Diath Haemorrh* 31:420, 1974.

259. Hall GW: Kasabach-Merritt syndrome: Pathogenesis and management. *Br J Haematol* 112:851, 2001.

260. Straub PW, Kessler S, Schreiber A, et al: Chronic intravascular coagulation in Kasabach-Merritt syndrome. Preferential accumulation of fibrinogen ¹³¹I in a giant hemangioma. *Arch Intern Med* 129:475, 1972.

261. Warrell RPJ, Kempin SJ, Benua RS, et al: Intratumoral consumption of indium-111 labeled platelets in a patient with hemangiomatosis and intravascular coagulation (Kasabach-Merritt syndrome). *Cancer* 52:2256, 1983.

262. Propp RP, Scharfman WB: Hemangioma-thrombocytopenia syndrome associated with microangiopathic hemolytic anemia. *Blood* 28:623, 1966.

263. Hesselmann S, Micke O, Marquardt T, et al: Case report: Kasabach-Merritt syndrome: A review of the therapeutic options and case report of successful treatment with radiotherapy and interferon alpha. *Br J Radiol* 75:180, 2002.

264. Mazoyer E, Enjolras O, Laurian C, et al: Coagulation abnormalities associated with extensive venous malformations of the limbs: Differentiation from Kasabach-Merritt syndrome. *Clin Lab Haematol* 24:243, 2002.

265. Fisher DF Jr, Yawn DH, Crawford ES: Preoperative disseminated intravascular coagulation associated with aortic aneurysms: A prospective study of 76 cases. *Arch Surg* 118:1252, 1983.

266. Bieger R, Vreeken J, Stibbe J, et al: Arterial aneurysm as a cause of consumption coagulopathy. *N Engl J Med* 285:152, 1971.

267. ten Cate JW, Timmers H, Becker AE: Coagulopathy in ruptured or dissecting aortic aneurysms. *Am J Med* 59:171, 1975.

268. Mulcare RJ, Royster TS, Phillips LL: Intravascular coagulation in surgical procedures on the abdominal aorta. *Surg Gynecol Obstet* 143:730, 1976.

269. Wilcox JN, Smith KM, Schwartz SM, et al: Localization of tissue factor in the normal vessel wall and in the atherosclerotic plaque. *Proc Natl Acad Sci U S A* 86:2839, 1989.

270. Cummins D, Segal H, Hunt BJ, et al: Chronic disseminated intravascular coagulation after surgery for abdominal aortic aneurysm: Clinical and haemostatic response to dalteparin. *Br J Haematol* 113:658, 2001.

271. Cross KS, Bouchier-Hayes D, Leahy AL: Consumptive coagulopathy following endovascular stent repair of abdominal aortic aneurysm. *Eur J Vasc Endovasc Surg* 19:94, 2000.

272. Shimazaki T, Ishimaru S, Kawaguchi S, et al: Blood coagulation and fibrinolytic response after endovascular stent grafting of thoracic aorta. *J Vasc Surg* 37:1213, 2003.

273. Mannucci PM, Lobina GF, Caocci L, et al: Effect on blood coagulation of massive intravascular haemolysis. *Blood* 33:207, 1969.

274. Butler J, Parker D, Pillai R, et al: Systemic release of neutrophil elastase and tumour necrosis factor alpha following ABO incompatible blood transfusion. *Br J Haematol* 79:525, 1991.

275. Hamilton KK, Hattori R, Esmon CT, et al: Complement proteins C5b-9 induce vesiculation of the endothelial plasma membrane and expose catalytic surface for assembly of the prothrombinase enzyme complex. *J Biol Chem* 265:3809, 1990.

276. Weiner CP: The obstetric patient and disseminated intravascular coagulation. *Clin Perinatol* 13:705, 1986.

277. Bonnar J: Massive obstetric haemorrhage. *Best Pract Res Clin Obstet Gynaecol* 14:1, 2000.

278. Letsky EA: Disseminated intravascular coagulation. *Best Pract Res Clin Obstet Gynaecol* 15:623, 2001.

279. DeLee JB: Acase of fatal hemorrhagic diathesis with premature detachment of the placenta. *Am J Obstet Gynecol* 44:785, 1901.

280. Eskes TK: Abruptio placentae. A "classic" dedicated to Elizabeth Ramsey. *Eur J Obstet Gynecol Reprod Biol* 75:63, 1997.

281. Kuczynski J, Uszynski W, Zekanowska E, et al: Tissue factor (TF) and tissue factor pathway inhibitor (TFPI) in the placenta and myometrium. *Eur J Obstet Gynecol Reprod Biol* 105:15, 2002.

282. Pritchard JA, Brekken AL: Clinical and laboratory studies on severe abruptio placentae. *Am J Obstet Gynecol* 97:681, 1967.

283. Steiner PE, Lushbaugh CC: Maternal pulmonary embolism by amniotic fluid as a cause of obstetric shock and unexpected deaths in obstetrics. *JAMA* 117:1245, 1941.

284. Morgan M: Amniotic fluid embolism. *Anaesthesia* 34:20, 1979.

285. Gilbert WM, Danielsen B: Amniotic fluid embolism: Decreased mortality in a population-based study. *Obstet Gynecol* 93:973, 1999.

286. Uszynski M, Zekanowska E, Uszynski W, et al: Tissue factor (TF) and tissue factor pathway inhibitor (TFPI) in amniotic fluid and blood plasma: Implications for the mechanism of amniotic fluid embolism. *Eur J Obstet Gynecol Reprod Biol* 95:163, 2001.

287. Boer K, den Hartog I, Meijers JC, et al: Tissue factor-dependent blood coagulation is enhanced following delivery irrespective of the mode of delivery. *J Thromb Haemost* 5:2415, 2007.

288. Gibson B, Hunter D, Neame PB, et al: Thrombocytopenia in preeclampsia and eclampsia. *Semin Thromb Hemost* 8:234, 1982.

289. O'Riordan MN, Higgins JR: Haemostasis in normal and abnormal pregnancy. *Best Pract Res Clin Obstet Gynaecol* 17:385, 2003.

290. Levi M: Disseminated intravascular coagulation (DIC) in pregnancy and the peri-partum period. *Thromb Res* 123 Suppl 2:S63, 2009.

291. Giles C: Intravascular coagulation in gestational hypertension and pre-eclampsia: The value of haematological screening tests. *Clin Lab Haematol* 4:351, 1982.

292. Norwitz ER, Hsu CD, Repke JT: Acute complications of preeclampsia. *Clin Obstet Gynecol* 45:308, 2002.

293. Weinstein L: Syndrome of hemolysis, elevated liver enzymes, and low platelet count: A severe consequence of hypertension in pregnancy. *Am J Obstet Gynecol* 142:159, 1982.

294. Sibai BM, Ramadan MK, Usta I, et al: Maternal morbidity and mortality in 442 pregnancies with hemolysis, elevated liver enzymes, and low platelets (HELLP syndrome). *Am J Obstet Gynecol* 169:1000, 1993.

295. Aarnoudse JG, Houthoff HJ, Weits J, et al: A syndrome of liver damage and intravascular coagulation in the last trimester of normotensive pregnancy. A clinical and histo-pathological study. *Br J Obstet Gynaecol* 93:145, 1986.

296. Audibert F, Friedman SA, Frangieh AY, et al: Clinical utility of strict diagnostic criteria for the HELLP (hemolysis, elevated liver enzymes, and low platelets) syndrome. *Am J Obstet Gynecol* 175:460, 1996.

297. Barton JR, Sibai BM: Hepatic imaging in HELLP syndrome (hemolysis, elevated liver enzymes and low platelet count. *Am J Obstet Gynecol* 174:1820, 1996.

298. Sullivan CA, Magann EF, Perry KG Jr, et al: The recurrence risk of the syndrome of hemolysis, elevated liver enzymes, and low platelets (HELLP) in subsequent gestations. *Am J Obstet Gynecol* 171:940, 1994.

299. Lee W, Clark SL, Cotton DB, et al: Septic shock during pregnancy. *Am J Obstet Gynecol* 159:410, 1988.

300. Romero R, Copel JA, Hobbins JC: Intrauterine fetal demise and hemostatic failure: The fetal death syndrome. *Clin Obstet Gynecol* 28:24, 1985.

301. Berkowitz RL, Stone JL, Eddleman KA: One hundred consecutive cases of selective termination of an abnormal fetus in a multifetal gestation. *Obstet Gynecol* 90:606, 1997.

302. Hay JE: Liver disease in pregnancy. *Hepatology* 47:1067, 2008.

303. Bacq Y, Riely CA: Acute fatty liver of pregnancy: The hepatologist's view. *Gastroenterologist* 1:257, 1993.

304. Usta IM, Barton JR, Amon EA, et al: Acute fatty liver of pregnancy: An experience in the diagnosis and management of fourteen cases. *Am J Obstet Gynecol* 171:1342, 1994.

305. Pereira SP, O'Donohue J, Wendon J, et al: Maternal and perinatal outcome in severe pregnancy-related liver disease. *Hepatology* 26:1258, 1997.

306. Rahman TM, Wendon J: Severe hepatic dysfunction in pregnancy. *Q J Med* 95:343, 2002.

307. Ibdah JA, Yang Z, Bennett MJ: Liver disease in pregnancy and fetal fatty acid oxidation defects. *Mol Genet Metab* 71:182, 2000.

308. Castro MA, Goodwin TM, Shaw KJ, et al: Disseminated intravascular coagulation and antithrombin III depression in acute fatty liver of pregnancy. *Am J Obstet Gynecol* 174:211, 1996.

309. Watson WJ, Seeds JW: Acute fatty liver of pregnancy. *Obstet Gynecol Surv* 45:585, 1990.

310. Moldenhauer JS, O'brien JM, Barton JR, et al: Acute fatty liver of pregnancy associated with pancreatitis: A life-threatening complication. *Am J Obstet Gynecol* 190:502, 2004.

311. Hathaway WE, Mull MM, Pechet GS: Disseminated intravascular coagulation in the newborn. *Pediatrics* 43:233, 1969.

312. Corrigan JJ Jr: Activation of coagulation and disseminated intravascular coagulation in the newborn. *Am J Pediatr Hematol Oncol* 1:245, 1979.

313. Williams MD, Chalmers EA, Gibson BE: The investigation and management of neonatal haemostasis and thrombosis. *Br J Haematol* 119:295, 2002.

314. Buchanan GR: Coagulation disorders in the neonate. *Pediatr Clin North Am* 33:203, 1986.

315. Stanworth SJ, Bennett C: How to tackle bleeding and thrombosis in the newborn. *Early Hum Dev* 84:507, 2008.

316. Corrigan JJ Jr, Ray WL, May N: Changes in the blood coagulation system associated with septicemia. *N Engl J Med* 279:851, 1968.

317. Levi M, de Jonge E, van der Poll T: New treatment strategies for disseminated intravascular coagulation based on current understanding of the pathophysiology. *Ann Med* 36:41, 2004.

318. Alving BM, Spivak JL, DeLoughery TG: Consultative hematology: Hemostasis and transfusion issues in surgery and critical care medicine, in *The American Society of Hematology Education Program Book*, edited by JR McArthur, GP Schechter, SL Schrier, p 320. American Society of Hematology, Washington DC, 1998.

319. de Jonge E, Levi M, Stoutenbeek CP, et al: Current drug treatment strategies for disseminated intravascular coagulation. *Drugs* 55:767, 1998.

320. de Jonge E, van der Poll T, Kesecioglu J, et al: Anticoagulant factor concentrates in disseminated intravascular coagulation: Rationale for use and clinical experience. *Semin Thromb Hemost* 27:667, 2001.

321. Abraham E: Coagulation abnormalities in acute lung injury and sepsis. *Am J Respir Cell Mol Biol* 22:401, 2000.

322. Levi M, Schouten M, van der Poll T: Sepsis, coagulation, and antithrombin: Old lessons and new insights. *Semin Thromb Hemost* 34:742, 2008.

323. Fourrier F, Chopin C, Huart JJ, et al: Double-blind, placebo-controlled trial of antithrombin III concentrates in septic shock with disseminated intravascular coagulation. *Chest* 104:882, 1993.

324. Eisele B, Lamy M, Thijs LG, et al: Antithrombin III in patients with severe sepsis. A randomized, placebo-controlled, double-blind multicenter trial plus a meta-analysis on

all randomized, placebo-controlled, double-blind trials with antithrombin III in severe sepsis. *Intensive Care Med* 24:663, 1998.

325. Baudo F, Caimi TM, de CF, et al: Antithrombin III (ATIII) replacement therapy in patients with sepsis and/or postsurgical complications: A controlled double-blind, randomized, multicenter study. *Intensive Care Med* 24:336, 1998.

326. Warren BL, Eid A, Singer P, et al: Caring for the critically ill patient. High-dose antithrombin III in severe sepsis: A randomized controlled trial. *JAMA* 286:1869, 2001.

327. Lavrentieva A, Kontakiotis T, Bitzani M, et al: The efficacy of antithrombin administration in the acute phase of burn injury. *Thromb Haemost* 100:286, 2008.

328. Levi M: Activated protein C in sepsis: A critical review. *Curr Opin Hematol* 15:481, 2008.

329. Bernard GR, Ely EW, Wright TJ, et al: Safety and dose relationship of recombinant human activated protein C for coagulopathy in severe sepsis. *Crit Care Med* 29:2051, 2001.

330. Bernard GR, Vincent JL, Laterre PF, et al: Efficacy and safety of recombinant human activated protein C for severe sepsis. *N Engl J Med* 344:699, 2001.

331. Vincent JL, Angus DC, Artigas A, et al: Effects of drotrecogin alfa (activated) on organ dysfunction in the PROWESS trial. *Crit Care Med* 31:834, 2003.

332. Abraham E, Laterre PF, Garg R, et al: Drotrecogin alfa (activated) for adults with severe sepsis and a low risk of death. *N Engl J Med* 353:1332, 2005.

333. Laterre PF: Clinical trials in severe sepsis with drotrecogin alfa (activated). *Crit Care* 11 Suppl 5:S5, 2007.

334. Ranieri VM, Thompson BT, Barie PS, et al: Drotrecogin alfa (activated) in adults with septic shock. *N Engl J Med* 366:2055-, 2012.

335. Thachil J, Toh CH, Levi M, Watson HG: The withdrawal of activated protein C from the use in patients with severe sepsis and DIC [amendment to the BCSH guideline on disseminated intravascular coagulation]. *Br J Haematol* 157:493, 2012.

336. du Toit H, Coetzee AR, Chalton DO: Heparin treatment in thrombin-induced disseminated intravascular coagulation in the baboon. *Crit Care Med* 19:1195, 1991.

337. Pernerstorfer T, Hollenstein U, Hansen JB, et al: Lepirudin blunts endotoxin-induced coagulation activation. *Blood* 95:1729, 2000.

338. Feinstein DI: Diagnosis and management of disseminated intravascular coagulation: The role of heparin therapy. *Blood* 60:284, 1982.

339. Levi M, Levy M, Williams MD, et al: Prophylactic heparin in patients with severe sepsis treated with drotrecogin alfa (activated). *Am J Respir Crit Care Med* 176:483, 2007.

340. Vlasuk GP, Bergum PW, Bradbury AE, et al: Clinical evaluation of rNAPc2, an inhibitor of the fVIIa/tissue factor coagulation complex. *Am J Cardiol* 80:66S, 1997.

341. Abraham E, Reinhart K, Svoboda P, et al: Assessment of the safety of recombinant tissue factor pathway inhibitor in patients with severe sepsis: A multicenter, randomized, placebo-controlled, single-blind, dose escalation study. *Crit Care Med* 29:2081, 2001.

342. Abraham E, Reinhart K, Opal S, et al: Efficacy and safety of tifacogin (recombinant tissue factor pathway inhibitor) in severe sepsis: A randomized controlled trial. *JAMA* 290:238, 2003.

343. Saito H, Maruyama I, Shimazaki S, et al: Efficacy and safety of recombinant human soluble thrombomodulin (ART-123) in disseminated intravascular coagulation: Results of a phase III, randomized, double-blind clinical trial. *J Thromb Haemost* 5:31, 2007.

344. Gralnick HR, Greipp P: Thrombosis with epsilon aminocaproic acid therapy. *Am J Clin Pathol* 56:151, 1971.

345. Naeye RL: Thrombotic state after a hemorrhagic diathesis, a possible complication of therapy with epsilon-aminocaproic acid. *Blood* 19:694, 1962.

346. Mannucci PM, Levi M: Prevention and treatment of major blood loss. *N Engl J Med* 356:2301, 2007.

347. Minna JD, Robboy SJ, Colman RW: *Disseminated Intravascular Coagulation in Man*. Charles C Thomas, Springfield, IL, 1974.

348. Matsuda M, Aoki N: Statistics on underlying and causative diseases of DIC in Japan, in *Disseminated Intravascular Coagulation*, edited by T Abe, M Yamanake, p 15. Karger, Basel, 1983.

349. Larcan A, Lambert H, Gerard A: *Consumption Coagulopathies*. Masson, New York, 1987.

CHAPTER 130
HEREDITARY THROMBOPHILIA

Saskia Middeldorp and Michiel Coppens

SUMMARY

Thrombophilia refers to laboratory abnormalities that increase the risk of venous thromboembolism (VTE). Over the last several decades numerous factors have been identified. The most prevalent examples of hereditary forms of thrombophilia include the factor V Leiden and prothrombin G20210A mutations; deficiencies of the natural anticoagulants antithrombin, protein C, and protein S; persistently elevated levels of coagulation factor VIII; and mild hyperhomocysteinemia. Taken together, some form of hereditary thrombophilia can be identified in more than 50 percent of patients with VTE who are without obvious reasons for VTE, such as trauma or prolonged stasis. Moreover, hereditary thrombophilia has been associated with arterial cardiovascular disease and obstetric complications such as (recurrent) pregnancy loss and preeclampsia. The high yield of thrombophilia testing has led to widespread testing for these abnormalities in patients. Nevertheless, thrombophilia testing remains a topic of ongoing debate, mostly because of the lack of therapeutic consequences. While hereditary thrombophilia is a clear risk factor for a first VTE, the risk for recurrent episodes is hardly increased compared with nonaffected patients and prolonged anticoagulation is not warranted unless VTE is recurrent. A similar lack of therapeutic consequences applies to patients with arterial cardiovascular disease and women with obstetric complications. Thrombophilia testing in asymptomatic relatives of patients with VTE may be useful in families with antithrombin, protein C, or protein S deficiency, or for siblings of patients who are homozygous for factor V Leiden, and is limited to women who intend to become pregnant or who would like to use oral contraceptives. Careful counseling with knowledge of absolute risks helps patients to making an informed decision in which their own preferences can be taken into account.

To our knowledge, the term *thrombophilia* was first used by Nygaard and Brown in 1937, when they described sudden occlusion of large arteries, sometimes with coexistent venous thrombosis.[1] In 1956, Jordan and Nandorff extensively reviewed their own and previously published cases on the familial tendency in thromboembolic disease.[2] The term *thrombophilia* was then used to describe patients with prominent manifestations of venous thromboembolism (VTE; venous thrombosis in any site or pulmonary embolism) such as recurrent spontaneous VTE, VTE at young age, a strong family history of VTE, or thrombosis in an unusual site, such as the splanchnic veins or cerebral sinuses. Currently, the term *thrombophilia* is generally used for laboratory abnormalities, usually in the coagulation system, which increase the risk of VTE. Thrombophilia can be either acquired or hereditary. An example of acquired thrombophilia is the antiphospholipid syndrome, which is characterized by a tendency toward venous or arterial thrombosis or pregnancy complications, in combination with persistent lupus anticoagulant or antibodies to cardiolipin or β_2-glycoprotein-1 (Chap. 131). Furthermore, there are many acquired and transient conditions that lead to a prothrombotic state, including cancer, surgery, strict immobilization, pregnancy and the postpartum period, and the use of estrogen-containing medication, such as oral contraceptives and hormone replacement therapy.

Patients with hereditary thrombophilia have an increased risk of developing VTE and just like in patients without thrombophilia, approximately half of patients will develop their first episode in relation to an acquired prothrombotic risk factor. Moreover, despite young age being a criterion for thrombophilia and the mean age at time of a first thrombosis being approximately 10 years lower than in the general population, the majority of patients with thrombophilia will have the first episode later in life.[3] The theoretical concept is that patients with thrombophilia have an intrinsic prothrombotic state, which in itself is insufficient to cause thrombosis, but may lead to an event when superimposed upon (clinical) risk factors, including increasing age.[3]

The role of hereditary thrombophilia in arterial cardiovascular disease has been extensively studied.[4,5] Most of those studies did not demonstrate significant associations between hereditary thrombophilia and arterial disease with the exception of patients with events before the age of 55 years.[5] Moreover, the relative risk increase was very modest (odds ratios [OR] of 1.1 to 1.8) in studies that did find significant associations, indicating that hereditary thrombophilia is not a major risk factor for arterial cardiovascular disease.[4]

Like the acquired antiphospholipid syndrome, most hereditary thrombophilias are also modestly associated with pregnancy related disorders such as (recurrent) miscarriage, stillbirth, intrauterine growth retardation, preeclampsia and the hemolysis, elevated liver enzymes, and low platelets (HELLP) syndrome of pregnancy, although for later pregnancy complications this association is controversial.[6–8]

In the past decades, hereditary thrombophilia has evolved from a very rare genetic disorder to a prevalent trait. This evolution is a direct consequence of increasing insight into the blood coagulation system, as well as advanced genetic research tools that allowed the search for abnormalities in candidate coagulation proteins and their encoding genes. At present, some form of thrombophilia can be identified in about half of the patients presenting with VTE. Likely inspired by the high yield of thrombophilia testing, testing has increased tremendously for various indications,[9] but whether the results of such tests help in the clinical management of patients has still not been settled.[10,11] This chapter provides an overview of the most important hereditary thrombophilias and of the history of thrombophilia research. It reviews the risks associated with the most commonly tested thrombophilias and provides guidance on the indications and potential implications of the results of thrombophilia testing in various patient groups.

Acronyms and Abbreviations: 95% CI, 95% confidence interval; APC, activated protein C; ASA, acetylsalicylic acid; HELLP, hemolysis, elevated liver enzymes, low platelets; LMWH, low-molecular-weight heparin; MTHFR, methylenetetrahydrofolate reductase; OR, odds ratio; VKA, vitamin K antagonist; VTE, venous thromboembolism; VWF, von Willebrand factor.

HISTORY, CLASSIFICATION, PATHOPHYSIOLOGY, AND PREVALENCE OF THROMBOPHILIA

HISTORY OF THROMBOPHILIA RESEARCH

Research into thrombophilia began with the investigation of candidate coagulation proteins and their genes in highly thrombophilic families and linking abnormalities with the clinical phenotype within these families. As a next step, findings were confirmed in case-control studies, which yielded risk increases compared to controls, often derived from the general population. For clinicians and patients however, absolute risk estimates were needed to guide decisions regarding prevention or treatment. These were sought again in family studies of consecutive probands with a specific thrombophilic defect. The major progress in genetic and bioinformatics techniques now allows investigation in populations of patients with VTE, as well as in thrombophilic families.[12-14]

In 1965, deficiency of the natural anticoagulant antithrombin became the first hereditary thrombophilia when Egeberg reported a Norwegian family with a remarkable tendency to VTE.[15] Deficiencies of the other anticoagulant proteins, that is, protein C and protein S, were discovered as hereditary risk factors for VTE in the early 1980s.[16,17] By that time, genes could be cloned and numerous mutations in the genes encoding antithrombin, protein C, and protein S had been identified as underlying causes of low plasma levels of the anticoagulant proteins.[18-20] Another decade later, in 1993, Dahlbäck and colleagues described the phenomenon of activated protein C (APC) resistance, a poor anticoagulant response to APC, in a Swedish family with an increased tendency to develop VTE.[21] The genetic basis for this APC resistance was discovered independently in several laboratories in 1995 and is caused by a single point mutation in the factor V gene which was termed *factor V Leiden*.[22-25] In 1996, genetic analysis of prothrombin revealed a G-to-A transition at position 20210 that was more common in patients with VTE and a strong family history of this disease than in healthy controls without VTE.[26] In the 1970s, it was found that individuals with non–O blood group have an increased risk of VTE.[27] Individuals with non–O blood group have higher levels of von Willebrand factor (VWF) and factor VIII than people with blood group O, which was the presumed mechanism of increased risk. In 1995, data from the Leiden Thrombophilia Study, a case-control study of patients with VTE and matched healthy controls, demonstrated that increased factor VIII (FVIII) activity, but not VWF activity, was independently associated with an increased risk of VTE.[28] Homocysteine is an intermediary amino acid formed by the conversion of methionine to cysteine. Homocystinuria or severe hyperhomocysteinemia is a rare autosomal recessive disorder characterized by severe elevations in plasma and urine homocysteine concentrations. This disease is characterized by developmental delay, osteoporosis, ocular abnormalities, and severe occlusive vascular disease. About half of the vascular complications are of venous origin.[29] Mild hyperhomocysteinemia was therefore studied as a risk factor for VTE in the 1990s and homocysteine levels exceeding the 95th percentile of the normal population were confirmed to be a risk factor for VTE.[30]

Since then, numerous genetic variants that increase the risk of VTE to a more or lesser extent have been identified and are variably included in diagnostic panels of thrombophilia testing.[31] Essentially, the majority of hereditary thrombophilias exert their effect either by upregulation of procoagulant clotting factors, or by downregulation of anticoagulant factors (Fig. 130–1). An overview of the common hereditary thrombophilias that increase the risk at least twofold, and their prevalence in patients with VTE and in the general population is presented in Table 130–1. For these more common thrombophilias a large

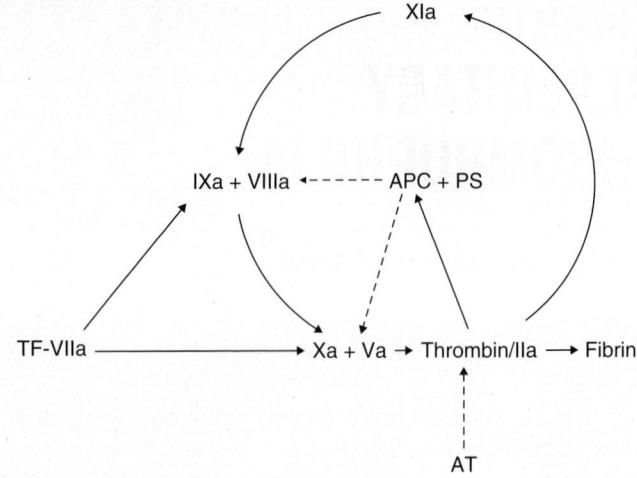

Figure 130–1. Regulation of blood coagulation. Coagulation is initiated by a tissue factor (TF)–factor VIIa complex that can activate factor IX or factor X. At high TF concentrations, factor X is activated primarily by the TF-VIIa complex, whereas at low TF concentrations, the contribution of the factor IXa–factor VIIIa complex to the activation of factor X becomes more pronounced. Coagulation is maintained through the activation by thrombin of factor XI. The coagulation system is regulated by the protein C pathway. Thrombin activates protein C. Together with protein S, activated protein C (APC) is capable of inactivating factors Va and VIIIa, which results in a downregulation of thrombin generation and consequently in an upregulation of the fibrinolytic system. The activity of thrombin is controlled by the inhibitor antithrombin. The *solid arrows* indicate activation and the *broken arrows* inhibition.

number of clinical studies provided reliable estimates of the relative and absolute risk for VTE.

CLASSIFICATION, PATHOPHYSIOLOGY AND PREVALENCE OF COMMON HEREDITARY THROMBOPHILIA

Deficiencies of the Natural Anticoagulants Antithrombin, Protein C, and Protein S

Deficiencies of the natural anticoagulants antithrombin, protein C, and protein S, were among the first established hereditary thrombophilias. For antithrombin and protein C, two types of deficiencies are distinguished. In type I deficiency, levels of both antigen and activity are

TABLE 130–1. Prevalence of Common Hereditary Thrombophilia

	General Population	Patients with VTE
Antithrombin, protein S, or protein C deficiency	1%[42-44]	7%[41]
Factor V Leiden	Whites 4–7%[46,118]	21%[22]
	Nonwhites 0–1%	
Prothrombin G20210A	Whites 2–3%[56,119]	6%
	Nonwhites 0–1%	
Elevated FVIII:c levels	11%[28]	25%[28]
Mild hyperhomocysteinemia	5%[30]	10%[30]

FVIII, factor VIII; VTE, venous thromboembolism.

reduced and in type II, antigen levels are normal, but one or more functional defects in the molecule lead to a decreased activity. Type II antithrombin deficiencies are further subdivided according to the site of the defect in antithrombin. The defect is located in the thrombin binding domain (i.e., the reactive site) in type IIa deficiency, in the heparin binding domain in type IIb deficiency, and type IIc deficiency comprises a pleiotropic group of mutations.[32] Interestingly, patients with type IIb deficiency seem to have a significantly lower risk of VTE than other types.[32] Protein S circulates in two forms: free protein S (approximately 40 to 50 percent) which functions as a cofactor for APC, and protein S bound to complement component C4b-binding protein. In type I deficiency, total and free antigen levels and activity are all reduced, in type II deficiency, total and free antigen are normal, but activity is reduced, and in type III deficiency, activity and free antigen are reduced, while total antigen is low to normal. Type I and type III are probably phenotypical variants of the same disease as family members with the same DNA mutation can present with either type I or type III deficiency.[33] Whether this classification into various subtypes is truly clinically relevant for any of the deficiencies of the natural anticoagulants is largely unknown. Moreover, most laboratory panels now only test the activity of antithrombin, protein C, or protein S, and thereby do not distinguish between different types of deficiencies. Homozygous antithrombin deficiency is extremely rare and the only reported cases involve type IIb deficiencies.[34] Homozygous type I deficiency has never been described in humans and is believed to be incompatible with life. Complete antithrombin deficiency in knockout mice leads to embryonic death.[35] Homozygous protein C and protein S deficiencies are also very rare and these are associated with neonatal purpura fulminans and massive thrombosis.[36,37] In a similar fashion, warfarin-induced skin necrosis has been described in patients with heterozygous protein C or S deficiencies after initiation of vitamin K antagonists (VKAs).[38,39] The concept is that after VKA initiation vitamin K–dependent protein C and S levels drop sooner than levels of factors II, IX, and X, thereby temporarily causing a paradoxal procoagulant state.[40] This is, however, a rare clinical complication, possibly resulting from concomitant treatment with (low-molecular-weight) heparin in the acute phase of VTE. Deficiencies can be caused by a large number of mutations, that are recorded in occasionally updated databases.[18–20] Overall, deficiencies of the natural

anticoagulants are rare (see Table 130–1). In cohorts of consecutive patients with VTE, the prevalence of a deficiency of one of the natural anticoagulants is below 10 percent.[41] In the general population, the prevalence of the deficiencies combined is approximately 1 percent.[42–44]

Factor V Leiden/Factor V G1691A

In 1993, Dahlbäck and colleagues first described APC resistance in a Swedish family with a high tendency of VTE.[21] In the original paper, Dahlbäck proposed that APC resistance was best explained by an hereditary deficiency of a previously unrecognized cofactor to APC, after having ruled out several possible mechanisms, including deficiencies of protein S and protein C, or linkage with polymorphisms in the FVIII or VWF genes. He then showed that this "cofactor" was identical to coagulation factor V.[21] Soon thereafter, several laboratories independently from each other reported the underlying genetic defect, a single G-to-A substitution in the gene of factor V at nucleotide position 1691, resulting in an amino acid change from Arginine (Arg) to Glutamine (Gln) at position 506, the first cleavage site of factor Va for APC[22–25] (Fig. 130–2). The mutation was named factor V Leiden after the city in the Netherlands in which the group with the first publication was located.[22] The proteolytic inactivation of activated factor V (FVa) is approximately 10 times slower for Gln506-FVa compared with Arg506-FVa, which explains the partial, but not full, resistance to APC.[45] Factor V Leiden is the most common hereditary thrombophilia. In unselected consecutive patients with VTE, the prevalence is 20 to 25 percent.[22] The prevalence in the general population varies considerably between different ethnic groups. Factor V Leiden is very rare among Asians and Africans but has a high prevalence (approximately 5 percent) among whites (see Table 130–1).[46] Within Europe, the prevalence is higher in the north than in the south.[46] This implies a founder effect that suggests that the mutation occurred after the separation of non-Africans from Africans and after the divergence of whites and Asians. Studies using linkage disequilibria between factor V Leiden and specific markers indicate that the mutation occurred around 21,000 years ago.[47] The high prevalence of factor V Leiden suggests an evolutionary benefit.[48] The presumed mechanism is reduced peripartum and menstrual blood loss in affected female carriers.[49,50] More recently, factor V Leiden was associated with increased sperm counts and a shorter conception time in affected male

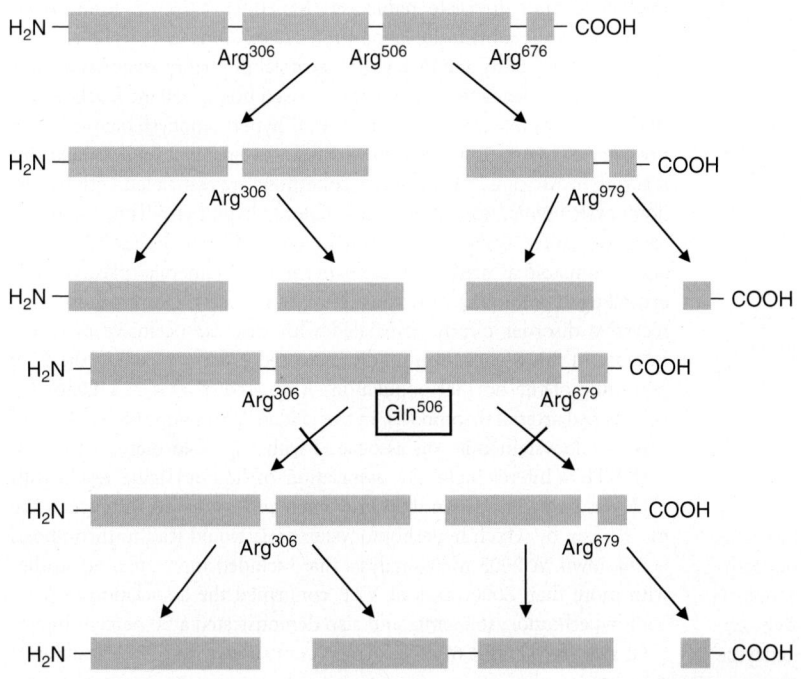

Figure 130–2. Pathophysiology of the factor V Leiden mutation. **A.** Activated protein C inactivates factor Va by cleaving the protein at the Arginine (Arg)[506] cleavage site. **B.** In carriers of the factor V Leiden mutation, a point mutation in the gene coding for factor V, causes replacement of the amino acid Arginine by Glutamine (Gln) at position 506 of the protein, making factor Va resistant to inactivation by activated protein C (i.e., APC resistance).

and female carriers, suggesting another evolutionary benefit.[51-53] The mechanism for this increased fertility is unknown.

Prothrombin G20210A

The prothrombin G20210A mutation was discovered in 1996 by genetic analysis of the prothrombin gene in families with a strong tendency of VTE and confirmed in a case-control study of patients with VTE.[26] The mutation is located in the 3′-untranslated region of the prothrombin gene and augments translation and stability of prothrombin messenger RNA.[54] This leads to an average 32 percent higher blood levels of the zymogen prothrombin that is structurally identical to the protein produced by patients with the wild-type gene.[26] In unselected patients with VTE, the prevalence of prothrombin G20210A is approximately 6 percent.[55] Like factor V Leiden, the prothrombin G20210A mutation is found largely in whites and genetic linkage disequilibrium studies date the mutation back to 24,000 years ago.[47,56] Within Europe, the prevalence of the mutation increases from 3 to 5 percent in Southern Europe and the Middle East to 1 to 2 percent in Northern Europe, which opposes the observed geographical gradient of factor V Leiden.[56]

Increased Levels of Factor VIII

Most of coagulation FVIII circulates in complex with VWF. Therefore, determinants of VWF, including ABO-blood group and endothelial stimulation, indirectly also determine FVIII levels.[57] Furthermore, many other factors have been associated with high FVIII levels, including increasing age, high body mass index, diabetes mellitus, and hypertriglyceridemia.[57] High FVIII levels are part of acute phase reactions and sustained increases are observed during pregnancy, surgery, chronic inflammation, malignancy, liver disease, hyperthyroidism, renal disease. In most of these conditions, there is a concordant increase of FVIII and VWF levels.[57] Apart from ABO blood group, the genetic causes of high FVIII levels are largely unknown. Nevertheless, persistence over time and familial clustering of high FVIII levels in patients with VTE implies that genetic factors are prevalent. In a family study of consecutive patients with persistently elevated levels of FVIII of at least 150 percent and venous or arterial thrombosis, the prevalence of high FVIII in first degree family members was 40 percent, which is almost in the range to what one would expect from an autosomal dominant inheritance.[58] Despite the uncertainty about the mechanisms of high FVIII levels, the association between high FVIII levels and venous thrombosis is well established. The very clear dose-dependent relationship between FVIII levels and the risk of VTE suggests that elevated FVIII is causative for thrombosis.[28] Interestingly, increased FVIII levels in patients with VTE are usually not influenced by acute-phase reactions.[57] The prevalence of elevated FVIII levels is high: 25 percent of patients with a first episode of deep-vein thrombosis and 11 percent of healthy control subjects have FVIII levels of 150 percent or higher.[28] Hence, an increased level of FVIII is the most common familial, albeit not monogenetic, thrombophilia with an estimated population attributable risk of 15 percent.[57] Whether measurement of FVIII levels should be part of a hereditary thrombophilia panel is debatable as FVIII levels may be transiently increased by a multitude of external factors including the acute VTE episode itself (Table 130–2). This leads to a significant proportion of "false-positive" test results, a necessity for repeat testing, and potentially unnecessary concern among tested patients.

Mild Hyperhomocysteinemia

Homocysteine is an intermediate in the metabolism of the amino acids methionine and cysteine and participates in several metabolic pathways. Some of the enzymes involved in homocysteine metabolism are dependent on vitamin B_6, folic acid, and vitamin B_{12}, and deficiencies lead to hyperhomocysteinemia. A polymorphism in the enzyme

TABLE 130–2. Acquired Conditions That Can Yield False-Positive Thrombophilia Test Results

Test	Acquired Conditions That Can Cause Abnormal Test Results
Increased activated protein C (APC) resistance	Pregnancy, use of oral contraceptives, stroke, presence of lupus anticoagulant, increased factor VIII levels, autoantibodies against APC
Factor V Leiden	—
Prothrombin G20210A	—
Hyperhomocysteinemia	Deficiencies of folate (vitamin B_{11}), vitamin B_{12}, or vitamin B_6, old age, renal failure, excessive consumption of coffee, smoking
Increased factor VIII levels	Pregnancy, use of oral contraceptives, exercise, stress, older age, acute phase response, liver disease, hyperthyroidism, cancer
Decreased level of protein C	Liver disease, use of vitamin K antagonist (VKA), vitamin K deficiency, childhood, disseminated intravascular coagulation, presence of autoantibodies against protein C
Decreased level of free protein S	Liver disease, use of VKA, vitamin K deficiency, pregnancy, use of oral contraceptives, nephrotic syndrome, childhood, presence of autoantibodies against protein S, disseminated intravascular coagulation
Decreased level of antithrombin	Use of heparin, thrombosis, disseminated intravascular coagulation, liver disease, nephrotic syndrome

methylenetetrahydrofolate reductase (MTHFR), c.C677T, leads to an alanine to valine substitution at position 222 resulting in a variant enzyme with reduced activity and increased thermolability. Homozygosity for this polymorphism leads to 24 percent increased homocysteine levels and is the most common genetic cause of mild hyperhomocysteinemia.[59] The prevalence is 10 to 20 percent in whites and 10 percent in Orientals, but it is rare in Africans.[60] Many other conditions are associated with hyperhomocysteinemia, including renal failure, hypothyroidism, smoking, excessive coffee consumption, inflammatory bowel disease, psoriasis, and rheumatoid arthritis.[61] Severe hyperhomocysteinemia (plasma levels exceeding 100 μmol/L), also named homocystinuria, is a rare autosomal recessive disorder clearly associated with vascular occlusive disease.[29] Because of this association, mildly increased levels (exceeding the 95th percentile of the normal population) were studied as a risk factor for venous and arterial thrombosis. In the Leiden Thrombophilia Study mild hyperhomocysteinemia was associated with a 2.5-fold increased risk of first VTE.[30] Interestingly, the association of homocysteine levels with VTE was stronger in men than in women and increased with age.[30] The mechanism by which hyperhomocysteinemia would lead to thrombosis is unknown. A 2005 meta-analysis that included more than 50 studies with more than 8000 cases of VTE confirmed the association of VTE with hyperhomocysteinemia and also demonstrated a 20 percent higher VTE risk in MTHFR 677TT carriers compared with 677CC carriers.[62]

The association between homocysteine levels is again under scrutiny in newer studies. The single largest case-control study of more than 4000 patients with a first VTE found no association between MTHFR 677TT and VTE.[63] Furthermore, a family study of probands with mild hyperhomocysteinemia and venous or arterial thrombosis found that the association between homocysteine and VTE disappeared after adjustment for FVIII levels.[64] Finally, homocysteine lowering by B vitamins did not reduce the incidence of recurrent events both in patients with VTE as well as in patients with arterial cardiovascular disease.[65,66] As a result of these studies, homocysteine testing (either its levels of polymorphisms) as part of a thrombophilia panel has been largely abandoned.

PITFALLS IN LABORATORY TESTING FOR HEREDITARY THROMBOPHILIA

Testing for hereditary thrombophilia is performed in many patients, or family members of patients, with various thromboembolic diseases or pregnancy complications.[9] However, it is important to realize that many acquired, often transient, conditions may affect the test results. Most known is the use of VKAs, which reduces the levels of anticoagulant factors protein C and protein S, which can thereby mimic severe deficiencies. Another example is pregnancy that reduces free protein S levels and increases APC resistance and FVIII levels.[67] However, other factors can also affect test results and should be considered in the interpretation of results or, better yet, in the timing of testing. Table 130–2 presents an overview of acquired conditions that can yield false-positive thrombophilia tests. For deficiencies of the natural anticoagulants as well as for elevated FVIII levels, repeated testing should be performed to exclude spuriously abnormal tests. Genetic testing for deficiencies of the natural anticoagulants is not performed because of the large number of known mutations. The hereditary nature of deficiencies must be established by confirming the abnormality in a first-degree family member.

● HEREDITARY THROMBOPHILIA AND THE RISK OF DISEASE

VENOUS THROMBOEMBOLISM

The relative risk of a first episode of VTE in individuals with a form of common hereditary thrombophilia ranges from 2 to 11 (Table 130–3). These figures were derived from family and population-based cohort or case-control studies.[11] Individuals homozygous for the prothrombin G20210A or factor V Leiden mutations are at higher risk for VTE than

heterozygotes. Likewise, patients with combined thrombophilic disorders have a higher risk of VTE than those with a single defect.[11] One can estimate the absolute risk of VTE by multiplying the relative risk with the absolute incidence in cohorts from the general population, in which the risk of first VTE is approximately 0.2 to 0.3 per 100 person-years.[68] Because this may however lead to imprecise estimates, it is preferable to use absolute risk estimates derived from cohort studies. Retrospective cohort studies may produce less-reliable incidence estimates because retrospective studies carry the risk of (unconscious) selection of patients and data and the clinical diagnosis of VTE may not have been confirmed by objective tests. Prospective cohort studies of asymptomatic carriers of hereditary thrombophilic defects are probably better suited to estimate the true incidence of thrombosis in thrombophilic patients. It is important to note that cohort studies have been mainly performed in relatives of (consecutive) patients with a particular thrombophilic defect. Absolute risk estimates from family studies are higher than from population based studies. Even in the absence of any hereditary thrombophilia, the risk of VTE is still twofold increased in first degree family members of patients with VTE.[69] This suggests cosegregation of other, unmeasured or unknown thrombophilias. Table 130–4 presents absolute risk estimates for a first-episode VTE for asymptomatic carriers with a family history of VTE. These risk estimates can be used to counsel both affected and unaffected family members about their risk of VTE. These studies also provide absolute risk estimates for VTE associated with exogenous additional risk factors such as surgery, trauma or immobilization, and pregnancy or use of hormonal contraception (Table 130–4). These incidences are derived from retrospective family studies, as prospective studies are limited by shorter followup duration and reduced power.

Thrombophilia and the Risk of Recurrent Venous Thromboembolism

Regardless of thrombophilia, the absolute risk of a recurrent episode is much higher than the risk of a first episode of VTE. The most important determinant of recurrence is the presence of transient clinical risk factors during the time of the first episode.[70] After an unprovoked first episode of VTE, the risk of recurrence is approximately 10 percent in the first year after cessation of anticoagulation and approximately 5 percent per year thereafter.[70] The risk is lower after VTE that was associated with a transient risk factor, with an incidence in the first 2 years of 0.7 percent per year for surgery-provoked VTE and 4.2 percent per year for VTE provoked by estrogen use, pregnancy, temporary immobilization, or trauma.[70] Other determinants for recurrence are male sex, proximal

TABLE 130–3. Relative Risk Estimates for Common Hereditary Thrombophilias and Venous or Arterial Thrombosis and Pregnancy Complications

| | Relative Risk | | | |
	First VTE	Recurrent VTE	Arterial Thrombosis	Pregnancy Complications
Antithrombin deficiency	5–10	1.9–2.6	No association	1.3–3.6
Protein C deficiency	4–6.5	1.4–1.8	No consistent association	1.3–3.6
Protein S deficiency	1–10	1.0–1.4	No consistent association	1.3–3.6
Factor V Leiden	3–5	1.4	1.3	1.0–2.6
Prothrombin G20210A	2–3	1.4	0.9	0.9–1.3
Persistently elevated FVIII	2–11	6–11	–	4.0
Mild hyperhomocysteinemia	2.5–2.6	2.6–3.1	–	No consistent association

FVIII, factor VIII; VTE, venous thromboembolism.
Risk estimated are derived from studies reviewed in detail elsewhere.[11]

TABLE 130–4. Absolute Incidences for a First Episode of Venous Thromboembolism in Asymptomatic Family Members of Consecutive Patients with Venous Thromboembolism

	Incidence Any VTE (% Per Year)	Surgery, Trauma, Immobilization (% Per Episode)	Pregnancy (% Per Pregnancy Including Postpartum Period)	Oral Contraceptive Use (% Per Year of Use)
Antithrombin, protein C, or protein S deficiency[120]				
Affected family members	1.0 (0.7–1.4)	8.1 (4.5–13.2)	4.1 (1.7–8.3)	4.3 (1.4–9.7)
Unaffected family members	0.1 (0.0–0.2)	0.9 (0.3–3.2)	0.5 (0.0–2.8)	0.7 (0.0–3.3)
Factor V Leiden[121]				
Affected family members	0.5 (0.3–0.6)	1.8 (0.7–4.0)	2.1 (0.7–4.9)*	0.5 (0.1–1.4)
Unaffected family members	0.1 (0.0–0.2)	0.7 (0.1–2.7)	0.0 (0.0–1.9)†	0.2 (0.0–0.8)
Prothrombin G20210A*[122,123]				
Affected family members	0.4 (0.1–1.1)	2.0 (0.8–4.2)	2.8 (1.0–6.0)	0.2 (0.0–0.9)
Unaffected family members	0.1 (0.0–0.7)	2.4 (1.0–4.9)	1.2 (0.1–4.2)	0.3 (0.0–1.1)
Persistently elevated FVIII[58,81]				
Affected family members	2.3 (1.2–4.2)	1.2 (0.4–2.8)	1.3 (0.4–3.4)	0.6 (0.2–1.5)
Unaffected family members	0.5 (0.1–1.2)	1.5 (0.6–3.1)	0.0 (0.0–1.1)†	0.3 (0.1–0.8)
Mild hyperhomocysteinemia[124,125]				
Affected family members	0.2 (0.1–0.3)	0.6 (0.2–2.3)	1.9 (0.7–4.7)	0.4 (0.1–1.0)
Unaffected family members	0.1 (0.1–0.2)	1.7 (0.8–3.5)	0.7 (0.2–2.6)	0.0 (0.0–0.3)†

FVIII, factor VIII; VTE, venous thromboembolism.

*Does not apply to homozygous carriers; see Table 130–5.

†The population risk of pregnancy-related VTE is 0.2% per pregnancy.[103]

(vs. distal) deep venous thrombosis (DVT), and elevated D-dimer levels after stopping anticoagulation.[70]

Although individuals with hereditary thrombophilia have a higher risk of developing a first episode of VTE, the risk increases for recurrent events in patients with prior VTE are much lower. Numerous case-control studies in VTE patients with a specific thrombophilia with nonthrombophilic VTE patients as controls yield relative risks of 1.5 to 2.0 for most hereditary thrombophilias.[71-76] Patients develop VTE when the combination of individual susceptibility (including hereditary thrombophilia) and acquired, sometimes transient, risk factors are sufficient to cause VTE. This individual susceptibility is constant throughout life. Therefore, patients with a previous episode of VTE have proven to have sufficient individual susceptibility, irrespective of hereditary thrombophilia being part of that susceptibility. This explains why the risk for recurrence is at best only marginally increased for carriers of hereditary thrombophilia.[77]

ARTERIAL THROMBOEMBOLIC DISEASE

The increased risk of VTE in patients with hereditary thrombophilia has led to many studies investigating the association of thrombophilia with arterial thromboembolic disease. Factor V Leiden and prothrombin G20210A are the most extensively studied as risk factors for arterial disease. The largest meta-analysis of case-control studies of patients with myocardial infarction found an OR of 1.17 (95% confidence interval [95% CI] 1.08 to 1.28) for factor V Leiden (60 studies with 42,390 patients) and 1.31 (95% CI 1.12 to 1.52) for prothrombin G20210A (40 studies with 26,087 patients).[4] The association between these mutations and myocardial infarction is stronger when analyses are limited to patients with myocardial infarction below the age of 55 years with ORs of 1.34 (95% CI 0.94 to 1.91) for factor V Leiden and 1.86 (95% CI

1.00 to 3.51) for prothrombin G20210A.[5] Meta-analyses of studies in patients with ischemic stroke have shown similar modest risk increases in patients with factor V Leiden or prothrombin G20210A.[78]

Deficiencies of the natural anticoagulants are less prevalent than factor V Leiden and prothrombin G20210A and as a result, the association with arterial thromboembolic disease has not been extensively studied. Although various case reports of patients with antithrombin, protein C, or protein S deficiency have been published, most case-control studies have failed to demonstrate a significant association with myocardial infarction and ischemic stroke.[79] A retrospective cohort study of 552 first-degree family members of patients with venous or arterial thrombosis and a deficiency of either antithrombin, protein C or protein S found no increased risk of arterial cardiovascular disease in affected family members older than age 55 years.[80] However, in persons younger than age 55 years, protein C and protein S were associated with a five- to ninefold increased risk, whereas antithrombin deficiency did not confer an increased risk.[80]

Several case-control studies have found associations with elevated FVIII levels and myocardial infarction.[57] Furthermore, prospective cohort studies of healthy individuals have demonstrated marginally increased risks of myocardial infarction and stroke in patients with elevated FVIII levels (ORs between 1.0 and 1.4).[57] In a prospective family study of asymptomatic first-degree family members of patients with elevated FVIII and either VTE or premature arterial thrombosis, the risk of arterial thromboembolism was increased 4.5-fold compared with family members with normal FVIII levels.[81] However, elevated FVIII levels are associated with several well-known risk factors for arterial cardiovascular disease, including obesity, high glucose levels, increasing age, chronic inflammatory diseases, and renal disease.[57] It is possible that studies evaluating the association between elevated FVIII and arterial thromboembolic disease have not been able to sufficiently adjust for known and unknown confounders. Moreover, acute myocardial infarction and ischemic stroke may cause acute-phase reactions that transiently increase FVIII levels, hampering interpretation of case-control or retrospective cohort studies. However, patients with hemophilia A, a genetic cause of decreased FVIII levels, have an approximate 80 percent lower risk of death from ischemic heart disease, indicating a potential causal relation between FVIII levels and arterial thrombosis.[82]

Mild hyperhomocysteinemia and MTHFR 677TT have been extensively studied in relation to arterial thromboembolic disease. A meta-analysis of studies that included more than 5000 patients with ischemic heart disease and more than 1000 patients with ischemic stroke demonstrated a significant correlation between homocysteine level and the risk of arterial thrombosis.[83] The risk increase in was higher in retrospective studies than in prospective studies in which homocysteine levels are measured before the thrombotic episodes. This could, in part, be explained by the observed association between hyperhomocysteinemia and other well-known risk factors for arterial cardiovascular disease, including smoking, chronic inflammatory disorders, and renal failure.[61] Like with elevated FVIII levels, it is uncertain whether studies that investigate the relation between homocysteine and arterial cardiovascular disease have been able to sufficiently adjust for confounding variables. The association between MTHFR 677TT and ischemic heart disease has shown mixed results with no association in studies in North American patients and a modest 16 percent risk increase in studies in European patients.[84] It was initially hypothesized that this difference is attributable to a lower dietary folate intake in Europe. However, this hypothesis conflicts with the results of trials in patients with vascular disease in whom homocysteine lowering with folic acid and B vitamins did not reduce the risk of recurrent episodes.[66]

PREGNANCY COMPLICATIONS

Although many studies have observed a relationship between hereditary thrombophilia and pregnancy complications, including recurrent miscarriage, late pregnancy loss, preeclampsia, intrauterine growth restriction, and placental abruption, this should be regarded as controversial. Most associations are modest in strength and vary with type of thrombophilia and type of pregnancy complication.[8,85,86] Furthermore, the most recent and larger prospective cohort studies found lower ORs for hereditary thrombophilia than older and smaller case-control studies, which may point to a bias in the observed associations.[8,87,88] The mechanisms of how thrombophilia would lead to pregnancy complications remain largely unknown. It is unlikely that mere hypercoagulability with thrombosis of placental vasculature is the pathophysiologic substrate for an association with thrombophilia. Animal and *in vitro* studies have implicated a role for both procoagulant and inflammatory pathways in pregnancy failure and interesting effects of acetylsalicylic acid (ASA) and heparin.[89] For instance, in a murine high-risk pregnancy model, heparin rescued factor V Leiden–associated placental failure, but this was independent of anticoagulation.[90]

● CLINICAL IMPLICATIONS OF THROMBOPHILIA INCLUDING TESTING

GENERAL CONSIDERATIONS OF THROMBOPHILIA TESTING

Several arguments against testing for thrombophilia should be considered.[10] First, an obvious disadvantage of testing for thrombophilia is the high cost. Although two studies concluded that testing for thrombophilia

in some scenarios could be cost-effective, the underlying assumptions from inconsistent observational studies seriously hamper their interpretation.[91,92] Second, although the psychological impact and consequences of knowing that one is a carrier of a (genetic) thrombophilic defect are considered limited, a qualitative study described several negative effects of both psychological and social origins.[93,94] Difficulties in obtaining life or disability insurance are frequently encountered by individuals who are known carriers of thrombophilia, regardless of whether they are symptomatic or asymptomatic.[93] Third, the most compelling argument against testing is the potential false reassurance that may arise from a negative thrombophilia test for individuals who come from families with a thrombotic tendency. For example, Table 130–4 indicates that in these families, women without thrombophilia have a markedly increased risk of oral contraceptive-related VTE compared to pill users from the general population (0.7 percent in women with a natural anticoagulant deficiency versus 0.04 percent per year of use), reflecting a selection of families with a strong thrombotic tendency in which yet unknown thrombophilias have co-segregated.

The following paragraphs discuss the potential scenarios for thrombophilia testing in more detail.

TESTING FOR THROMBOPHILIA TO MODIFY THE RISK OF A FIRST VENOUS THROMBOEMBOLISM

Having a family history of VTE is a poor predictor of the presence of thrombophilia.[69,95] Still, a potential advantage of testing patients with VTE for thrombophilia may be the identification of asymptomatic family members in order to take preventive measures if tested positive, and to withhold such measures if relatives have tested negative. An important requisite is that a test result indeed dichotomizes carriers and non-carriers in terms of their risk for a first episode of VTE.

Based on the absolute risks for a first episode of VTE (see Table 130–4), it is clear that the 1 to 3 percent annual major bleeding risk associated with continuous oral anticoagulant treatment outweighs the risk of VTE.[96,97] Table 130–4 also shows that during high-risk situations such as surgery, immobilization, trauma, pregnancy, and the postpartum period, and during the use of oral contraceptives, the absolute risk is generally low, with the exception of women with a natural anticoagulant deficiency who use oral contraceptives or are pregnant.

Estimates of the effect of avoidance of oral contraceptives on the number of prevented episodes of VTE by means of thrombophilia testing can be calculated for women who have a positive first-degree relative with VTE in whom the thrombophilic defect is known.[98] To avoid one VTE event, 28 women with antithrombin, protein C or protein S deficiency, and a positive family history for VTE would need to refrain from oral contraceptives, and to identify these women, 56 female relatives would need to be tested.[98] For factor V Leiden or the prothrombin 20210A mutation, approximately 333 women would need to avoid oral contraceptives and 666 female relatives would need to be tested. Although the number of tested women for the natural deficiencies seems quite acceptable, the major argument against this scenario is that a normal level of antithrombin, protein C, or protein S in women from these families does not exclude a strongly increased risk of VTE during oral contraceptive use, as compared to the general population (see Table 130–4). The same, but to a lesser extent, is true for women from thrombophilic families who do not carry either the factor V Leiden or prothrombin mutation, but here also the number needed to screen is unacceptably high.

Table 130–5 indicates the estimated number needed to test to initiate prophylactic measurements around pregnancy, again applicable

TABLE 130–5. Estimated Number of Asymptomatic Thrombophilic Women Who Should Use Low-Molecular-Weight Heparin Prophylaxis During Pregnancy and/or the Postpartum Period to Prevent Pregnancy-Related Venous Thromboembolism, and Estimated Number Needed to Test

Thrombophilia	Risk of VTE Per Pregnancy*, %	Risk Difference Per 100 Women	Number Using Prophylaxis to Prevent 1 VTE[†]	Number of Female Relatives to Be Tested
Antithrombin, protein C, or protein S deficiency				
Deficient relatives	4.1[‡]	3.6	28	56
Nondeficient relatives	0.5[‡]			
Factor V Leiden or prothrombin 20210A mutation, heterozygous				
Relatives with the mutation	2.0[‡]	1.5	66	132
Relatives without the mutation	0.5[‡]			
Factor V Leiden or prothrombin 20210A mutation, homozygous				
Homozygous relatives	16.0	15.5	6	24
Relatives without the mutation	0.5[§]			

VTE, venous thromboembolism.

*Antepartum and postpartum combined.

[†]These estimates apply to women with a positive family history of VTE and assume an unrealistic 100% efficacy of prophylaxis with low-molecular-weight heparin.

[‡]Based on family studies as outlined in Table 130–4.

[§]Summary estimate of the data as outlined in Table 130–4, combined for factor V Leiden and prothrombin mutation.

to women from thrombophilic families. Only for women with antithrombin, protein C, or protein S deficiency, or those who are homozygous for factor V Leiden (Table 130–5), the risks of 4 and 16 percent respectively during pregnancy and the postpartum period may outweigh the nuisance of daily subcutaneous low-molecular-weight heparin (LMWH) injections with frequently occurring skin reactions, and the very small risk for severe complications of anticoagulant therapy during pregnancy.[99–102] Furthermore, the numbers in Table 130–5 underestimate the number of women that need to use prophylaxis (and be tested prior to this decision) in order to avoid pregnancy-related VTE, because a 100 percent efficacy of prophylaxis is assumed in these calculations. Whether the absolute risks of pregnancy-related VTE justifies prophylaxis for 8 months during pregnancy, or the shorter postpartum period of 6 weeks is a matter of the physicians' and patients' preference.[102] The risk of pregnancy-related VTE in women from these families who do not have the hereditary thrombophilic defect is approximately 0.5 percent, compared to 0.2 percent in the general population.[103] Hence, withholding prophylaxis to women from thrombophilic families who do not have the defect is supported by evidence from well-designed studies of individuals in the same clinical context.

THROMBOPHILIA TESTING IN PATIENTS WITH VENOUS THROMBOEMBOLISM

Thrombophilia testing is most often considered in patients with VTE, particularly if they are young, have recurrent episodes, have thrombosis at unusual sites, or have a positive family history for the disease. However, although such a strategy may lead to an increased yield of testing, the main question is whether a positive test result should alter management. As previously discussed, thrombophilia is a very poor predictor of recurrent VTE, and whether the very modest risk increase warrants prolongation of the duration of anticoagulation, particularly after

provoked VTE, is a matter of debate.[70,104] Furthermore, given the rarity of homozygous or double heterozygous thrombophilias in unselected patients with VTE, the efficiency of testing is obviously very low.[10,105] A randomized controlled trial of testing for thrombophilia in patients with a first episode of VTE would provide the ultimate evidence to decide whether this is justified, but no such trials have been successfully performed.[106] To investigate whether testing for thrombophilia reduced the risk of recurrent VTE, 197 patients who had had a recurrent event were compared to 324 patients who did not have a recurrence.[107] The OR for recurrence was 1.2 (95% CI 0.9 to 1.8) for tested versus nontested patients, indicating that testing, with real life clinical decisions based on the outcome of testing, did not reduce the risk of recurrent VTE in patients after a first episode.

THROMBOPHILIA TESTING IN PATIENTS WITH ARTERIAL CARDIOVASCULAR DISEASE

The association between hereditary thrombophilia and arterial cardiovascular disease is questionable, or at least much weaker than for VTE. The association is stronger in patients with events before the age of 55 years. As a result, thrombophilia test panels are often ordered in with arterial cardiovascular disease. In a survey among Dutch physicians that ordered thrombophilia tests in 2000 consecutive patients in 2003 and 2004, arterial cardiovascular disease, mainly ischemic stroke, was the indication for testing in 23 percent of patients.[9] Interestingly, only 54 percent of those patients were younger than 50 years of age. Testing for hereditary thrombophilia in patients with (premature) arterial cardiovascular disease could only be justified if the test results would mandate different secondary prevention. However, more vigorous secondary prevention such as long-term dual antiplatelet therapy or oral anticoagulation instead of ASA monotherapy is not beneficial for most patients with arterial cardiovascular events, mainly because of the increased risk of bleeding. Whether such a strategy is beneficial for patients with hereditary thrombophilia has never been tested, but is very unlikely given the very modest risk increases associated with hereditary thrombophilia. Therefore, testing in this setting is not justified.

THROMBOPHILIA TESTING IN WOMEN WITH PREGNANCY COMPLICATIONS

Thrombophilia testing in women with pregnancy complications would be indicated if a test result would alter management. However, to date, testing for hereditary thrombophilia in this setting cannot be justified[10,102] for the following reasons. For women at moderate to high risk of preeclampsia, ASA provides a modest benefit in reducing the risk of preeclampsia, but this is regardless of the presence of hereditary thrombophilia.[102,108] Whether anticoagulant treatment with heparin or LMWH improves the chance of a successful pregnancy outcome in women with pregnancy complications is presently unknown as results from randomized clinical trials are extremely inconsistent.[109–113] It is also uncertain whether presence of hereditary thrombophilia is a prerequisite for an assumed beneficial effect, if any. Only three randomized controlled trials have been exclusively dedicated to women with hereditary thrombophilia and recurrent miscarriage, a single fetal loss, or late pregnancy complications. The first trial found promising results in women with heterozygous factor V Leiden mutation, prothrombin G20210A mutation, or protein S deficiency and a single previous pregnancy loss after 10 weeks gestation.[114] Women who were allocated to enoxaparin had a much higher chance of a livebirth than those allocated to ASA (86 percent and 29 percent, respectively; OR 15.5; 95% CI 7 to 34), but several methodologic issues were raised, and the results of this single study have not been confirmed by other trials.[102,115] Second, in the FRUIT trial, women with hereditary thrombophilia and a history of preeclampsia or intrauterine growth restriction requiring delivery before 34 weeks of gestation, were randomized between dalteparin with ASA and ASA alone.[116] The primary outcome (recurrence of a hypertensive disorder, e.g., preeclampsia, HELLP, or eclampsia) did not differ between the two groups, but none of the women in the LMWH/ASA group developed recurrent hypertensive disorders prior to 34 weeks gestational age, whereas six women in the ASA-only group delivered before 34 weeks because of recurrent hypertensive disorders (risk difference 8.7 percent; 95% CI 1.9 to 15.5 percent). Finally, the TIPPS study included thrombophilic women at high risk for pregnancy complications or at increased risk of VTE and randomized them between dalteparin and no dalteparin.[113] The primary composite outcome (severe or early onset preeclampsia, small-for-gestational-age infant, pregnancy loss, or VTE) did not differ between the groups. Hence, to date, there is no evidence from sufficiently powered and adequately designed clinical trials that justify use of heparin to improve pregnancy outcome in women with hereditary thrombophilia, and heparin should only be given in the context of a clinical trial.[117]

● CONCLUSIONS

The knowledge about the hereditary contribution to the etiology of VTE has increased tremendously over the past decades. Still, testing for thrombophilia serves only a limited purpose and should not be performed on a routine basis. Thrombophilia testing in asymptomatic relatives may be useful in families with antithrombin, protein C, or protein S deficiency, or for siblings of patients who are homozygous for factor V Leiden, and is limited to women who intend to become pregnant or who would like to use oral contraceptives. Careful counseling with knowledge of absolute risks helps patients make an informed decision in which their own preferences can be taken into account, and in which

the clinician should be cautious to not provide false reassurance in case of a negative test result. Observational studies show that patients who have had VTE and have thrombophilia are at most at a slightly increased risk for reoccurrence. Other determinants, including circumstances during the first VTE, elevated D-dimer levels, and male sex, are better predictors of recurrent VTE.[70] Furthermore, no beneficial effect on the risk of recurrent VTE was observed in patients who had been tested for inherited thrombophilia. In the absence of trials that compared routine and prolonged anticoagulant treatment in patients testing positive for thrombophilia, testing for such defects to prolong anticoagulant therapy cannot be justified. Finally, there is at present no reason to test patients with arterial cardiovascular disease, or women with recurrent miscarriage or late pregnancy complications for hereditary thrombophilia, in the absence of evidence-based guidelines for changes in management.

REFERENCES

1. Nygaard KK, Brown GE: Essential thrombophilia: Report of five cases. *Arch Intern Med* 59:82, 1937.
2. Jordan FLJ, Nandorff A: The familial tendency in thrombo-embolic disease. *Acta Med Scand* 156:267, 1956.
3. Rosendaal FR: Venous thrombosis: A multicausal disease. *Lancet* 353:1167, 1999.
4. Ye Z, Liu EH, Higgins JR, et al: Seven haemostatic gene polymorphisms in coronary disease: Meta-analysis of 66,155 cases and 91,307 controls. *Lancet* 367:651, 2006.
5. Boekholdt SM, Bijsterveld NR, Moons AH, et al: Genetic variation in coagulation and fibrinolytic proteins and their relation with acute myocardial infarction: A systematic review. *Circulation* 104:3063, 2001.
6. Lin J, August P: Genetic thrombophilias and preeclampsia: A meta-analysis. *Obstet Gynecol* 105:182, 2005.
7. Rey E, Kahn SR, David M, Shrier I: Thrombophilic disorders and fetal loss: A meta-analysis. *Lancet* 361:901, 2003.
8. Rodger MA, Walker MC, Smith GN, et al: Is thrombophilia associated with placenta-mediated pregnancy complications? A prospective cohort study. *J Thromb Haemost* 12:469, 2014.
9. Coppens M, van Mourik JA, Eckmann CM, et al: Current practice of testing for hereditary thrombophilia in The Netherlands. *J Thromb Haemost* 5:1979, 2007.
10. Baglin T, Gray E, Greaves M, et al: Clinical guidelines for testing for heritable thrombophilia. *Br J Haematol* 149:209, 2010.
11. Middeldorp S, van Hylckama Vlieg A: Does thrombophilia testing help in the clinical management of patients? *Br J Haematol* 143:321, 2008.
12. Bezemer ID, Bare LA, Doggen CJ, et al: Gene variants associated with deep vein thrombosis. *JAMA* 299:1306, 2008.
13. Gohil R, Peck G, Sharma P: The genetics of venous thromboembolism. A meta-analysis involving approximately 120,000 cases and 180,000 controls. *Thromb Haemost* 102:360, 2009.
14. Lotta LA, Wang M, Yu J, et al: Identification of genetic risk variants for deep vein thrombosis by multiplexed next-generation sequencing of 186 hemostatic/pro-inflammatory genes. *BMC Med Genomics* 5:7, 2012.
15. Egeberg O: Inherited antithrombin III deficiency causing thrombophilia. *Thromb Diath Haemorrh* 13:516, 1965.
16. Comp PC, Esmon CT: Recurrent venous thromboembolism in patients with a partial deficiency of protein S. *N Engl J Med* 311:1525, 1984.
17. Griffin JH, Evatt B, Zimmerman TS, et al: Deficiency of protein C in congenital thrombotic disease. *J Clin Invest* 68:1370, 1981.
18. Gandrille S, Borgel D, Sala N, et al: Protein S deficiency: A database of mutations—Summary of the first update. *Thromb Haemost* 84:918, 2000.
19. Lane DA, Bayston T, Olds RJ, et al: Antithrombin mutation database: 2nd (1997) update. For the Plasma Coagulation Inhibitors Subcommittee of the Scientific and Standardization Committee of the International Society on Thrombosis and Haemostasis. *Thromb Haemost* 77:197, 1997.
20. Reitsma PH, Bernardi F, Doig RG, et al: Protein C deficiency: A database of mutations, 1995 update. On behalf of the Subcommittee on Plasma Coagulation Inhibitors of the Scientific and Standardization Committee of the ISTH. *Thromb Haemost* 73:876, 1995.
21. Dahlbäck B, Carlsson M, Svensson PJ: Familial thrombophilia due to a previously unrecognized mechanism characterized by poor anticoagulant response to activated protein C: Prediction of a cofactor to activated protein C. *Proc Natl Acad Sci U S A* 90:1004, 1993.
22. Bertina RM, Koeleman BP, Koster T, et al: Mutation in blood coagulation factor V associated with resistance to activated protein C. *Nature* 369:64, 1994.
23. Greengard JS, Sun X, Xu X, et al: Activated protein C resistance caused by Arg506Gln mutation in factor Va. *Lancet* 343:1361, 1994.
24. Voorberg J, Roelse J, Koopman R, et al: Association of idiopathic venous thromboembolism with single point-mutation at Arg506 of factor V. *Lancet* 343:1535, 1994.
25. Zoller B, Dahlback B: Linkage between inherited resistance to activated protein C and factor V gene mutation in venous thrombosis. *Lancet* 343:1536, 1994.

26. Poort SR, Rosendaal FR, Reitsma PH, Bertina RM: A common genetic variation in the 3'-untranslated region of the prothrombin gene is associated with elevated plasma prothrombin levels and an increase in venous thrombosis. *Blood* 88:3698, 1996.

27. Talbot S, Wakley EJ, Ryrie D, Langman MJ: ABO blood-groups and venous thrombo-embolic disease. *Lancet* 1:1257, 1970.

28. Koster T, Blann AD, Briet E, et al: Role of clotting factor VIII in effect of von Willebrand factor on occurrence of deep-vein thrombosis. *Lancet* 345:152, 1995.

29. Mudd SH, Skovby F, Levy HL, et al: The natural history of homocystinuria due to cystathionine beta-synthase deficiency. *Am J Hum Genet* 37:1, 1985.

30. den Heijer M, Koster T, Blom HJ, et al: Hyperhomocysteinemia as a risk factor for deep-vein thrombosis. *N Engl J Med* 334:759, 1996.

31. Reitsma PH, Rosendaal FR: Past and future of genetic research in thrombosis. *J Thromb Haemost* 5(Suppl 1):264, 2007.

32. Finazzi G, Caccia R, Barbui T: Different prevalence of thromboembolism in the sub-types of congenital antithrombin III deficiency: Review of 404 cases. *Thromb Haemost* 58:1094, 1987.

33. Zoller B, Garcia de FP, Dahlback B: Evaluation of the relationship between protein S and C4b-binding protein isoforms in hereditary protein S deficiency demonstrating type I and type III deficiencies to be phenotypic variants of the same genetic disease. *Blood* 85:3524, 1995.

34. Okajima K, Ueyama H, Hashimoto Y, et al: Homozygous variant of antithrombin III that lacks affinity for heparin, AT III Kumamoto. *Thromb Haemost* 61:20, 1989.

35. Ishiguro K, Kojima T, Kadomatsu K, et al: Complete antithrombin deficiency in mice results in embryonic lethality. *J Clin Invest* 106:873, 2000.

36. Seligsohn U, Berger A, Abend M, et al: Homozygous protein C deficiency manifested by massive venous thrombosis in the newborn. *N Engl J Med* 310:559, 1984.

37. Mahasandana C, Suvatte V, Marlar RA, et al: Neonatal purpura fulminans associated with homozygous protein S deficiency. *Lancet* 335:61, 1990.

38. McGehee WG, Klotz TA, Epstein DJ, Rapaport SI: Coumarin necrosis associated with hereditary protein C deficiency. *Ann Intern Med* 101:59, 1984.

39. Grimaudo V, Gueissaz F, Hauert J, et al: Necrosis of skin induced by coumarin in a patient deficient in protein S. *BMJ* 298:233, 1989.

40. Weiss P, Soff GA, Halkin H, Seligsohn U: Decline of proteins C and S and factors II, VII, IX and X during the initiation of warfarin therapy. *Thromb Res* 45:783, 1987.

41. Heijboer H, Brandjes DP, Buller HR, et al: Deficiencies of coagulation-inhibiting and fibrinolytic proteins in outpatients with deep-vein thrombosis. *N Engl J Med* 323:1512, 1990.

42. Miletich J, Sherman L, Broze G Jr: Absence of thrombosis in subjects with heterozygous protein C deficiency. *N Engl J Med* 317:991, 1987.

43. Tait RC, Walker ID, Perry DJ, et al: Prevalence of antithrombin deficiency in the healthy population. *Br J Haematol* 87:106, 1994.

44. Tait RC, Walker ID, Reitsma PH, et al: Prevalence of protein C deficiency in the healthy population. *Thromb Haemost* 73:87, 1995.

45. Rosing J, Hoekema L, Nicolaes GA, et al: Effects of protein S and factor Xa on peptide bond cleavages during inactivation of factor Va and factor VaR506Q by activated protein C. *J Biol Chem* 270:27852, 1995.

46. Rees DC, Cox M, Clegg JB: World distribution of factor V Leiden. *Lancet* 346:1133, 1995.

47. Zivelin A, Mor-Cohen R, Kovalsky V, et al: Prothrombin 20210G>A is an ancestral prothrombotic mutation that occurred in whites approximately 24,000 years ago. *Blood* 107:4666, 2006.

48. Van Mens TE, Levi M, Middeldorp S: Evolution of factor V Leiden. *Thromb Haemost* 110:23, 2013.

49. Lindqvist PG, Svensson PJ, Dahlback B, Marsal K: Factor V Q506 mutation (activated protein C resistance) associated with reduced intrapartum blood loss—A possible evolutionary selection mechanism. *Thromb Haemost* 79:69, 1998.

50. Lindqvist PG, Zoller B, Dahlback B: Improved hemoglobin status and reduced menstrual blood loss among female carriers of factor V Leiden—An evolutionary advantage? *Thromb Haemost* 86:1122, 2001.

51. Cohn DM, Repping S, Buller HR, et al: Increased sperm count may account for high population frequency of factor V Leiden. *J Thromb Haemost* 8:513, 2010.

52. van Dunne FM, Doggen CJ, Heemskerk M, et al: Factor V Leiden mutation in relation to fecundity and miscarriage in women with venous thrombosis. *Hum Reprod* 20:802, 2005.

53. Kaandorp SP, Van Mens TE, Middeldorp S, et al: Time to conception and time to live birth in women with unexplained recurrent miscarriage. *Hum Reprod* 29:1146, 2014.

54. Carter AM, Sachchithananthan M, Stasinopoulos S, et al: Prothrombin G20210A is a bifunctional gene polymorphism. *Thromb Haemost* 87:846, 2002.

55. Cumming AM, Keeney S, Salden A, et al: The prothrombin gene G20210A variant: Prevalence in a U.K. anticoagulant clinic population. *Br J Haematol* 98:353, 1997.

56. Rosendaal FR, Doggen CJ, Zivelin A, et al: Geographic distribution of the 20210 G to A prothrombin variant. *Thromb Haemost* 79:706, 1998.

57. Kamphuisen PW, Eikenboom JC, Bertina RM: Elevated factor VIII levels and the risk of thrombosis. *Arterioscler Thromb Vasc Biol* 21:731, 2001.

58. Bank I, Libourel EJ, Middeldorp S, et al: Elevated levels of FVIII:c within families are associated with an increased risk for venous and arterial thrombosis. *J Thromb Haemost* 3:79, 2005.

59. Jacques PF, Bostom AG, Williams RR, et al: Relation between folate status, a common mutation in methylenetetrahydrofolate reductase, and plasma homocysteine concentrations. *Circulation* 93:7, 1996.

60. Rosenberg N, Murata M, Ikeda Y, et al: The frequent 5,10-methylenetetrahydrofolate reductase C677T polymorphism is associated with a common haplotype in whites, Japanese, and Africans. *Am J Hum Genet* 70:758, 2002.

61. Key NS, McGlennen RC: Hyperhomocyst(e)inemia and thrombophilia. *Arch Pathol Lab Med* 126:1367, 2002.

62. den Heijer M, Lewington S, Clarke R: Homocysteine, MTHFR and risk of venous thrombosis: A meta-analysis of published epidemiological studies. *J Thromb Haemost* 3:292, 2005.

63. Bezemer ID, Doggen CJ, Vos HL, Rosendaal FR: No association between the common MTHFR 677C->T polymorphism and venous thrombosis: Results from the MEGA study. *Arch Intern Med* 167:497, 2007.

64. Lijfering W, Coppens M, Veeger NJ, et al: Hyperhomocysteinemia is not a risk factor for venous and arterial thrombosis, and is associated with elevated factor VIII levels. *Thromb Res* 123:244, 2008.

65. den Heijer M, Willems HP, Blom HJ, et al: Homocysteine lowering by B vitamins and the secondary prevention of deep-vein thrombosis and pulmonary embolism. A randomized, placebo-controlled, double blind trial. *Blood* 109:139, 2007.

66. Lonn E, Yusuf S, Arnold MJ, et al: Homocysteine lowering with folic acid and B vitamins in vascular disease. *N Engl J Med* 354:1567, 2006.

67. Barco S, Nijkeuter M, Middeldorp S: Pregnancy and venous thromboembolism. *Semin Thromb Hemost* 39:549, 2013.

68. Naess IA, Christiansen SC, Romundstad P, et al: Incidence and mortality of venous thrombosis: A population-based study. *J Thromb Haemost* 5:692, 2007.

69. Bezemer ID, van der Meer FJ, Eikenboom JC, et al: The value of family history as a risk indicator for venous thrombosis. *Arch Intern Med* 169:610, 2008.

70. de Jong PG, Coppens M, Middeldorp S: Duration of anticoagulant therapy for venous thromboembolism: Balancing benefits and harms on the long term. *Br J Haematol* 158:433, 2012.

71. Baglin T, Luddington R, Brown K, Baglin C: Incidence of recurrent venous thromboembolism in relation to clinical and thrombophilic risk factors: Prospective cohort study. *Lancet* 362:523, 2003.

72. Brouwer JL, Lijfering WM, Ten Kate MK, et al: High long-term absolute risk of recurrent venous thromboembolism in patients with hereditary deficiencies of protein S, protein C or antithrombin. *Thromb Haemost* 101:93, 2009.

73. Segal JB, Brotman DJ, Necochea AJ, et al: Predictive Value of Factor V Leiden and Prothrombin G20210A in Adults With Venous Thromboembolism and in Family Members of Those With a Mutation: A Systematic Review. *JAMA* 301:2472, 2009.

74. Lijfering WM, Middeldorp S, Veeger NJ, et al: Risk of recurrent venous thrombosis in homozygous carriers, and double heterozygous carriers of factor V Leiden and prothrombin G20210A. *Circulation* 121:1706, 2010.

75. van den Belt AG, Sanson BJ, Simioni P, et al: Recurrence of venous thromboembolism in patients with familial thrombophilia. *Arch Intern Med* 157:2227, 1997.

76. Vossen CY, Walker ID, Svensson P, et al: Recurrence rate after a first venous thrombosis in patients with familial thrombophilia. *Arterioscler Thromb Vasc Biol* 25:1992, 2005.

77. Cannegieter SC, van Hylckama Vlieg A. Venous thrombosis: Understanding the paradoxes of recurrence. *J Thromb Haemost* 11(Suppl 1):161, 2013.

78. Casas JP, Hingorani AD, Bautista LE, Sharma P: Meta-analysis of genetic studies in ischemic stroke: Thirty-two genes involving approximately 18,000 cases and 58,000 controls. *Arch Neurol* 61:1652, 2004.

79. Boekholdt SM, Kramer MH: Arterial thrombosis and the role of thrombophilia. *Semin Thromb Hemost* 33:588, 2007.

80. Mahmoodi BK, Brouwer JL, Veeger NJ, van der Meer J: Hereditary deficiency of protein C or protein S confers increased risk of arterial thromboembolic events at a young age: Results from a large family cohort study. *Circulation* 118:1659, 2008.

81. Bank I, Van de Poel MH, Coppens M, et al: Absolute annual incidences of first events of venous thromboembolism and arterial vascular events in individuals with elevated FVIII:c: A prospective family cohort study. *Thromb Haemost* 98:1040, 2007.

82. Rosendaal FR, Varekamp I, Smit C, et al: Mortality and causes of death in Dutch haemophiliacs, 1973–86. *Br J Haematol* 71:71, 1989.

83. Homocysteine Studies Collaboration: Homocysteine and risk of ischemic heart disease and stroke: A meta-analysis. *JAMA* 288:2015, 2002.

84. Klerk M, Verhoef P, Clarke R, et al: MTHFR 677C—>T polymorphism and risk of coronary heart disease: A meta-analysis. *JAMA* 288:2023, 2002.

85. Robertson L, Wu O, Langhorne P, et al: Thrombophilia in pregnancy: A systematic review. *Br J Haematol* 132:171, 2006.

86. Opatrny L, David M, Kahn SR, et al: Association between antiphospholipid antibodies and recurrent fetal loss in women without autoimmunie disease: A metaanalysis. *J Rheumatol* 33:2214, 2006.

87. Clark P, Walker ID, Govan L, et al: The GOAL study: A prospective examination of the impact of factor V Leiden and ABO(H) blood groups on haemorrhagic and thrombotic pregnancy outcomes. *Br J Haematol* 140:236, 2008.

88. Kahn SR, Platt R, McNamara H, et al: Inherited thrombophilia and preeclampsia within a multicenter cohort: The Montreal Preeclampsia Study. *Am J Obstet Gynecol* 200:151, 2009.

89. Bose P, Black S, Kadyrov M, et al: Heparin and aspirin attenuate placental apoptosis in vitro: Implications for early pregnancy failure. *Am J Obstet Gynecol* 192:23, 2005.

90. An J, Waitara MS, Bordas M, et al: Heparin rescues factor V Leiden-associated placental failure independent of anticoagulation in a murine high-risk pregnancy model. *Blood* 121:2127, 2013.

91. Marchetti M, Pistorio A, Barosi G: Extended anticoagulation for prevention of recurrent venous thromboembolism in carriers of factor V Leiden: Cost-effectiveness analysis. *Thromb Haemost* 84:752, 2000.

92. Wu O, Robertson L, Twaddle S, et al: Screening for thrombophilia in high-risk situations: Systematic review and cost-effectiveness analysis. The Thrombosis: Risk and

Economic Assessment of Thrombophilia Screening (TREATS) study. *Health Technol Assess* 10:1, 2006.

93. Bank I, Scavenius MP, Buller HR, Middeldorp S: Social aspects of genetic testing for factor V Leiden mutation in healthy individuals and their importance for daily practice. *Thromb Res* 113:7, 2004.

94. Cohn DM, Vansenne F, Kaptein AA, et al: The psychological impact of testing for thrombophilia: A systematic review. *J Thromb Haemost* 6:1099, 2008.

95. van Sluis GL, Sohne M, El Kheir DY, et al: Family history and inherited thrombophilia. *J Thromb Haemost* 4:2182, 2006.

96. Ruff CT, Giugliano RP, Braunwald E, et al: Comparison of the efficacy and safety of new oral anticoagulants with warfarin in patients with atrial fibrillation: A meta-analysis of randomised trials. *Lancet* 383:955, 2014.

97. van Es N, Coppens M, Schulman S, et al: Direct oral anticoagulants compared with vitamin K antagonists for acute symptomatic venous thromboembolism: Evidence from phase 3 trials. *Blood* 124:1968, 2014.

98. Bleker SM, Coppens M, Middeldorp S: Sex, thrombosis and inherited thrombophilia. *Blood Rev* 28:123, 2014.

99. Bank I, Libourel EJ, Middeldorp S, et al: High rate of skin complications due to low-molecular-weight heparins in pregnant women. *J Thromb Haemost* 1:859, 2003.

100. Deruelle P, Denervaud M, Hachulla E, et al: Use of low-molecular-weight heparin from the first trimester of pregnancy: A retrospective study of 111 consecutive pregnancies. *Eur J Obstet Gynecol Reprod Biol* 127:73, 2006.

101. Schindewolf M, Gobst C, Kroll H, et al: High incidence of heparin-induced allergic delayed-type hypersensitivity reactions in pregnancy. *J Allergy Clin Immunol* 132:131, 2013.

102. Bates SM, Greer IA, Middeldorp S, et al: VTE, thrombophilia, antithrombotic therapy, and pregnancy: Antithrombotic Therapy and Prevention of Thrombosis, 9th ed: American College of Chest Physicians Evidence-Based Clinical Practice Guidelines. *Chest* 141 (Suppl 2):e691S, 2012.

103. Heit JA, Kobbervig CE, James AH, et al: Trends in the incidence of venous thromboembolism during pregnancy or postpartum: A 30-year population-based study. *Ann Intern Med* 143:697, 2005.

104. Middeldorp S: Duration of anticoagulation for venous thromboembolism. *BMJ* 342:d2758, 2011.

105. Evaluation of Genomic Applications in Practice and Prevention (EGAPP) Working Group: Recommendations from the EGAPP Working Group: Routine testing for factor V Leiden (R506Q) and prothrombin (20210G>A) mutations in adults with a history of idiopathic venous thromboembolism and their adult family members. *Genet Med* 13:67, 2011.

106. Cohn DM, Vansenne F, de Borgie CA, Middeldorp S: Thrombophilia testing for prevention of recurrent venous thromboembolism. *Cochrane Database Syst Rev* 12:CD007069, 2009.

107. Coppens M, Reijnders JH, Middeldorp S, et al: Testing for inherited thrombophilia does not reduce recurrence of venous thrombosis. *J Thromb Haemost* 6:1474, 2008.

108. Henderson JT, Whitlock EP, O'Connor E, et al: Low-dose aspirin for prevention of morbidity and mortality from preeclampsia: A systematic evidence review for the U.S. Preventive Services Task Force. *Ann Intern Med* 160:695, 2014.

109. Middeldorp S: Thrombophilia and pregnancy complications: Cause or association? *J Thromb Haemost* 5:276, 2007.

110. Rodger MA, Paidas MJ, Mclintock C, et al: Inherited thrombophilia and pregnancy complications revisited: Association not proven causal and antithrombotic prophylaxis is experimental. *Obstet Gynecol* 112:320, 2008.

111. de Jong PG, Goddijn M, Middeldorp S: Antithrombotic therapy for pregnancy loss. *Hum Reprod Update* 19:674, 2013.

112. de Jong PG, Kaandorp SP, Di Nisio M, et al: Aspirin or anticoagulants for treating recurrent miscarriage in women without antiphospholipid syndrome. *Cochrane Database Syst Rev* 7:CD004734, 2014.

113. Rodger MA, Hague WM, Kingdom J, et al: Antepartum dalteparin versus no antepartum dalteparin for the prevention of pregnancy complications in pregnant women with thrombophilia (TIPPS): A multinational open-label randomised trial. *Lancet* 384:1673, 2014.

114. Gris JC, Mercier E, Quere I, et al: Low-molecular-weight heparin versus low-dose aspirin in women with one fetal loss and a constitutional thrombophilic disorder. *Blood* 103:3695, 2004.

115. Rodger M: Important publication missing key information. *Blood* 104:3413, 2004.

116. de Vries JI, van Pampus MG, Hague WM, et al: Low-molecular-weight heparin added to aspirin in the prevention of recurrent early-onset preeclampsia in women with inheritable thrombophilia: The FRUIT-RCT. *J Thromb Haemost* 10:64, 2012.

117. Middeldorp S: Thrombosis in women: What are the knowledge gaps in 2013? *J Thromb Haemost* 11(Suppl 1):180, 2013.

118. Ridker PM, Miletich JP, Hennekens CH, Buring JE: Ethnic distribution of factor V Leiden in 4047 men and women. Implications for venous thromboembolism screening. *JAMA* 277:1305, 1997.

119. Dilley A, Austin H, Hooper WC, et al: Prevalence of the prothrombin 20210 G-to-A variant in blacks: Infants, patients with venous thrombosis, patients with myocardial infarction, and control subjects. *J Lab Clin Med* 132:452, 1998.

120. Simioni P, Sanson BJ, Prandoni P, et al: The incidence of venous thromboembolism in families with inherited thrombophilia. *Thromb Haemost* 81:198, 1999.

121. Middeldorp S, Henkens CMA, Koopman MM, et al: The incidence of venous thromboembolism in family members of patients with factor V Leiden mutation and venous thrombosis. *Ann Intern Med* 128:15, 1998.

122. Bank I, Libourel EJ, Middeldorp S, et al: Prothrombin 20210A mutation: A mild risk factor for venous thromboembolism but not for arterial thrombotic disease and pregnancy-related complications in a family study. *Arch Intern Med* 164:1932, 2004.

123. Coppens M, van der Poel MH, Bank I, et al: A prospective cohort study on the absolute incidence of venous thromboembolism and arterial cardiovascular disease in asymptomatic carriers of the prothrombin 20210A mutation. *Blood* 108:2604, 2006.

124. Lijfering W, Coppens M, van der Poel MH, et al: The risk of venous and arterial thrombosis in hyperhomocysteinemia is low and mainly depends on concomitant thrombophilic defects. *Thromb Haemost* 98:457, 2007.

125. Van de Poel MH, Coppens M, Middeldorp S, et al: Absolute risk of venous and arterial thromboembolism associated with mild hyperhomocysteinemia. results from a retrospective family cohort study. *J Thromb Haemost* 3 (Suppl 1):P0481, 2005.

CHAPTER 131
THE ANTIPHOSPHOLIPID SYNDROME

Jacob H. Rand and Lucia Wolgast

SUMMARY

The antiphospholipid (aPL) syndrome (APS) is an acquired thrombophilic disorder in which patients have vascular thrombosis and/or pregnancy complications attributable to placental insufficiency, accompanied by laboratory evidence for the presence of antiphospholipid antibodies in blood. The disorder is referred to as *primary APS* when it occurs in the absence of systemic lupus erythematosus (SLE), and *secondary APS* in its presence. Any portion of the circulatory tree can be affected, although the most frequently affected vessels are the deep veins of the lower extremities. Abnormalities that have been reported in association with the syndrome include virtually all other autoimmune disorders, immune thrombocytopenia, acquired platelet function abnormalities, hypoprothrombinemia, acquired inhibitors of coagulation factors, livedo reticularis, heart valve abnormalities, atherosclerosis, pulmonary hypertension, and migraine. Rare patients have a catastrophic form of APS (CAPS) in which there is disseminated thrombosis in large- and small-vessel thrombi, often after a triggering event such as infection or surgery, and often with multiorgan ischemia and infarction.

APS is a misnomer, the main antigenic targets for thrombogenic aPL antibodies are epitopes on phospholipid-binding proteins, the most important of which appears to be β_2-glycoprotein I (β_2GPI). The syndrome is identified by persistent abnormalities of laboratory tests for antibodies against these phospholipid–protein cofactor complexes, detected by immunoassays and by coagulation assays (also known as "lupus anticoagulant assays") that, paradoxically, report the inhibition of phospholipid-dependent coagulation reactions. Long-term warfarin anticoagulant therapy is the usual treatment for thrombosis in patients with APS, although there is some controversy about whether treatment of patients with APS stroke might be better treated with aspirin. Patients with recurrent spontaneous pregnancy losses and APS generally are treated with aspirin and heparin for prophylaxis against deep vein thrombosis

during their pregnancies and the postpartum period. CAPS patients have a high mortality and, in addition to anticoagulants, often require plasmapheresis and immunosuppressive agents. Patients without clinical manifestations of APS or a history of SLE should generally not undergo diagnostic screening for aPL antibodies and, if tested and found to be positive, should not be committed to antithrombotic therapy solely on the basis of laboratory abnormalities.

DEFINITION AND HISTORY

The antiphospholipid (aPL) antibody syndrome (APS) is a disorder in which vascular thrombosis or pregnancy complications attributable to placental insufficiency occur in patients with laboratory evidence for antibodies directed against proteins that bind to phospholipids. The syndrome was first proposed to be a distinct entity, "the anticardiolipin (aCL) syndrome," in 1985[1] and soon was renamed APS.[2] While precise data are not available, the syndrome is thought to affect approximately 10 percent of patients with venous thrombosis,[3,4] and approximately 20 percent of women with three unexplained fetal losses before 12 weeks of gestation, or at least one intrauterine fetal death after 12 weeks of gestation.[5]

The term "aPL antibodies" can refer to (1) antibodies that recognize protein-phospholipid complexes as in cofactor-dependent aCL assays, (2) antibodies that recognize the proteins directly as in anti-$\beta_2$glycoprotein I assays (anti-β_2GPI), (3) an abnormal coagulation test in several assays that report inhibition of phospholipid-dependent coagulation reactions, collectively as termed *lupus anticoagulant* (LA) tests, and (4) antibodies that recognize phospholipid directly as in syphilis and are not associated with the APS disease entity.

A brief review of the history of APS[6-8] helps explain the confusing terminology (Table 131–1); the reader is referred to references 6 to 8 for more detailed accounts. In retrospect, the first assay for aPL autoantibodies was Moore and Mohr's report of the "biologic false-positive" serologic tests for syphilis (BFP syphilis test) in 1952[9]; this abnormality came to be associated with systemic lupus erythematosus (SLE).[10] The contemporaneous introduction, of the activated partial thromboplastin time (aPTT), which used cephalin, a phospholipid extract of animal brains, as the "partial thromboplastin" (distinct from the "complete thromboplastin," tissue factor, and phospholipid),[11] led to the recognition of a unique type of anticoagulant in patients with SLE, that was frequently associated with BFP syphilis tests.[12] Because the of its initial association with SLE this phenomenon was misnamed LA.[13] It became recognized that the LA was purely an *in vitro* phenomenon that was not limited to SLE and that was not associated with bleeding complications unless another hemostatic defect was present.[6] Furthermore, the LA came to be associated with recurrent pregnancy losses[14,15] and with thrombotic and embolic manifestations.[16] The development, in 1983, of the aCL antibody assay, that measured antibodies against the anionic phospholipid, cardiolipin (diphosphatidylglycerol), the primary antigen in the syphilis test reagent,[17] was the advance that led to the identification of a new syndrome. Within a few years, it became recognized that aPL antibodies did not bind phospholipids directly but instead were directed against proteins that bound to the phospholipid, primarily β_2GPI (see "Pathogenesis" below). This information became important in helping to unravel the mechanisms for APS and in advancing diagnostic testing toward the goal of distinguishing between the syndrome and incidental false-positive tests. Table 131–2 describes the current consensus investigational criteria for diagnosing APS.[18]

Most patients with elevated aPL antibodies do not have the syndrome; elevated aPL antibody levels can occur in patients with several

Acronyms and Abbreviations: aCL, anticardiolipin; APC, activated protein C; aPL, antiphospholipid; APS, antiphospholipid syndrome; aPTT, activated partial thromboplastin time; ARDS, acute respiratory distress syndrome; ASIA, autoimmune/autoinflammatory syndrome induced by adjuvants; AVWS, acquired von Willebrand syndrome; BFP syphilis test, biologic false-positive serologic test for syphilis; β_2GPI, β_2-glycoprotein I; CAPS, catastrophic APS; CMV, cytomegalovirus; dRVVT, dilute Russell viper venom time; ELISA, enzyme-linked immunosorbent assay; HCQ, hydroxychloroquine; Ig, immunoglobulin; IL, interleukin; LA, lupus anticoagulant; LDL, low-density lipoprotein; LMWH, low-molecular-weight heparin; MAPK, mitogen-activated protein kinase; NOACs, new oral anticoagulants; RVV, Russell viper venom; SCR, short consensus repeat; SLE, systemic lupus erythematosus; TLR, toll-like receptor; TM, thrombomodulin; t-PA, tissue-type plasminogen activator; UFH, unfractionated heparin; VWF, von Willebrand factor.

TABLE 131–1. Paths of Development of Antiphospholipid Assays: Historical Summary

Immunoassay Path	Coagulation Path
1950s: Syphilis testing	1950s: Partial thromboplastin time inhibitor
	1970s: Lupus anticoagulant (LA)
1980s: Antiphospholipid (aPL) antibody enzyme-linked immunosorbent assay (ELISA; e.g., anticardiolipin [aCL] immunoassays)	1980s: Recognition that LAs are inhibitors of phospholipid-dependent coagulation reactions
1990s: Anticofactor ELISA (anti-β_2-glycoprotein I [β_2GPI], antiprothrombin, etc.)	
2005: Demonstration that antibodies against domain I of β_2GPI are associated with increased risk of thrombosis	2004: Demonstration that resistance to the anticoagulant effect of annexin A5 correlates with thrombosis in antiphospholipid syndrome

types of infections that induce formation of antibodies recognizing anionic phospholipids directly, patients taking medications such as chlorpromazine or procainamide, and even in normal healthy individuals. Testing of patients who have neither clinical manifestations of the disorder or SLE for aPL antibodies should be discouraged because it incurs the risk of inappropriate diagnostic and treatment decisions.

TABLE 131–2. Sydney Investigational Criteria for Diagnosis of Antiphospholipid Syndrome

Clinical

• Vascular thrombosis (one or more episodes of arterial, venous, or small vessel thrombosis). For histopathologic diagnosis, there should <u>not</u> be evidence of inflammation in the vessel wall.

• Pregnancy morbidities attributable to placental insufficiency, including three or more otherwise unexplained recurrent spontaneous miscarriages, before 10 weeks of gestation. Also, one or more fetal losses after the 10th week of gestation, stillbirth, episode of preeclampsia, preterm labor, placental abruption, intrauterine growth restriction or oligohydramnios that are otherwise unexplained.

Laboratory

• aCL or anti-β_2GPI IgG and/or IgM antibody present in medium or high titer on two or more occasions, at least 12 weeks apart, measured by standard ELISAs.

• Lupus anticoagulant in plasma, on two or more occasions, at least 12 weeks apart detected according to the guidelines of the International Society of Thrombosis and Hemostasis Scientific Standardization Committee on Lupus Anticoagulants and Phospholipid-Dependent Antibodies.

• "Definite APS" is considered to be present if at least one of the clinical criteria and one of the laboratory criteria are met.

aCL, anticardiolipin; aPL, antiphospholipid; β_2GPI, β_2-glycoprotein I; ELISA, enzyme-linked immunosorbent assay; Ig, immunoglobulin. Data from Miyakis S, Lockshin MD, Atsumi T et al: International consensus statement on an update of the classification criteria for definite antiphospholipid syndrome (APS). *J Thromb Haemost* 4:295–306, 206.

● ETIOLOGY AND PATHOGENESIS

ETIOLOGY

As with most autoimmune conditions, the etiology of APS is not understood. It has been demonstrated that even normal healthy individuals have memory B cells that produce aPL antibodies. In a study of patients with infectious mononucleosis, 10 to 60 percent of immunoglobulin (Ig) M aPL-producing cells expressed CD27, the marker of memory B cells.[19] The affinity of aPL antibodies for their target becomes increased by the inclusion of amino acids lysine, arginine, and asparagine within the complementary determining regions of the heavy and light chains.[20]

Although antibodies against anionic phospholipid moieties arise during the course of infections such as syphilis and Lyme disease, those are distinct from antibodies generated by patients with the syndrome because they generally recognize phospholipid epitopes directly (also referred to as "cofactor independent") and are not associated with the clinical manifestations of the syndrome. There are intriguing hints for molecular mimicry mechanisms and that infection and vaccination-induced APS could be related to autoimmune/autoinflammatory syndrome induced by adjuvants (ASIA).[21] aPL antibodies have been reported in patients who developed thrombosis after varicella infection,[8,22,23] and in patients with hepatitis C.[24,25] aPL antibodies were reported in a patient with cytomegalovirus (CMV) infection, mesenteric and femoropopliteal thrombosis.[26,27] β_2GPI cofactor-dependent antibodies against cardiolipin, phosphatidyl serine, and phosphatidyl ethanolamine have been identified in sera from patients with parvovirus B19.[28] Bacterial infections are a predisposing risk factor for the catastrophic form of APS (CAPS).[29] A high proportion of HIV-1 patients have aPL antibodies; more than 40 percent in one study, in which 18 percent had aCL and 30 percent had anti-β_2GPI (mostly of the IgA isotype),[30]; however, positivity for these antibodies was not associated with thrombosis. A link has been proposed between the cardiac valvular disease in acute rheumatic fever and the presence of aPL antibodies.[31] aCL antibodies having β_2GPI dependence and LA activity have been generated in rabbits immunized with lipid A and lipoteichoic acid, suggesting that some bacteria can contribute to the production of pathogenic aPL antibodies.[32] It has also been proposed that cellular apoptosis, with the resulting exposure of anionic phospholipids on cell surfaces, may trigger the generation of aPL antibodies.[33–35] Molecular mimicry between β_2GPI-related synthetic peptides and structures within bacteria, viruses, and tetanus toxoid[36] have been demonstrated in an experimental model for APS.[37] Mice immunized with a CMV-derived peptide developed aPL antibodies and thrombosis, and showed evidence for endothelial cell activation.[38]

Reports of familial clustering of raised aPL antibody levels[39] indicate that genetic susceptibility can play a role in their development. In one study of 84 APS patients, more than 35 percent had at least one relative, and more than 20 percent had two or more relatives, with evidence of at least one clinical feature of APS, such as thrombosis or recurrent fetal loss.[40]

PATHOGENESIS

Experimental Evidence That Antiphospholipid Antibodies Are Pathogenic

It has been clearly established in a number of experimental animal models for APS that aPL antibodies play a causal role in the development of thrombosis and pregnancy loss.[41–45] Although it is reasonable to assume that the same holds for the human disorder, the epitopic specificities of the autoantibodies that cause disease and the mechanisms by which they produce clinical manifestations require further elucidation.

Antigenic Specificities

Antibodies against phospholipid that arise during the immunologic response to syphilis and other infections (with the notable exception of leprosy[46]) recognize anionic phospholipid epitopes directly,[47] whereas pathogenic aPL antibodies recognize phospholipid-binding proteins, primarily β_2GPI.[48,49]

β_2GPI (also named apolipoprotein H), a member of the complement control protein or short consensus repeat superfamily,[50] is a highly glycosylated single-chain plasma protein composed of 326 amino acids, with a molecular weight of approximately 50 kDa (Fig. 131–1). β_2GPI has five short consensus repeat (SCR) stretches of approximately 60 amino acids[45] (also referred to as complement control protein [CCP] repeats). Epitopic specificities for individual domains may have pathogenic and prognostic significance (see "Immunoassays" below).[51–54]

The affinity of β_2GPI for anionic phospholipids derives from cationic residues from its aminoterminus that have affinity for anionic polar heads of phospholipids and a hydrophobic loop which inserts into the lipid bilayer. β_2GPI has five domains for which antibodies have been identified. IgG antibodies against an epitope comprising Gly40-Arg43 in the domain I of β_2GPI have been reported to have a stronger correlation with thrombosis than antibodies against other epitopes.[51] Recent data support the concept that β_2GPI undergoes conformational changes that may be important for the APS disease process. By transmission electron microscopy, unbound β_2GPI appears to be in a closed conformation because of the affinity of a portion of carboxyterminal domain V for the protein's amninoterminal domain I, where the phospholipid binding site is located near the carboxy-terminus of SCR domain V (see Fig. 131–1).[55] The binding of β_2GPI to anionic phospholipid membranes, requires a conformational change which exposes an epitope in domain I that had been cryptic in the unbound conformation (see Fig. 131–1).[55]

Although β_2GPI bind to phospholipids, its role in aPL-mediated cell signaling (described in the section Proposed Pathogenic Mechanisms), is mediated via binding to toll-like receptors (TLRs) and not by direct binding to the lipid bilayer.

While the *in vivo* biologic function(s) of the protein has (have) not been defined, several interesting properties have been demonstrated. The molecule binds to apoptotic cells,[56] and may play a role in their phagocytosis and clearance.[57] β_2GPI binds to oxidized low-density lipoprotein (LDL) and may play a role in its clearance.[58] β_2GPI binds to lipopolysaccharide and the scavenged complex is taken up by monocytes/macrophages.[59] β_2GPI reduces platelet adhesion to collagen in flow chambers by interfering with the platelet–von Willebrand factor (VWF) interaction by binding to its A2 domain, thereby interfering with its binding to the platelet glycoprotein Ib complex.[60] β_2GPI may also promote fibrinolysis as a cofactor for tissue-type plasminogen activator (t-PA) via its SCR domain V, which increases fibrinolytic activity.[61] The protein may have a further effect on fibrinolysis by binding to endothelial cells via annexin A2, a protein that also serves as a receptor for plasminogen and t-PA.[62] Homozygous β_2GPI-null mice have not been demonstrated to display a thrombotic phenotype.[63] However, the protein may play a role—though not a critical one—in the reproductive process, as there was a reduction in the number of viable implantation sites in β_2GPI-null mice and reduced fetal weight and fetal-to-placental weight ratio in late gestation, suggesting compromised placental function.[64]

In addition to β_2GPI, a number of other antigenic targets have been identified for aPL, including, but not limited to, prothrombin, coagulation factor V, protein C, protein S, annexin A2, annexin A5, high- and low-molecular-weight kininogens, and factors VII/VIIa and vimentin–cardiolipin complex.[65–68]

Proposed Pathogenic Mechanisms

Table 131–3 and Fig. 131–2 summarize several of the main current hypotheses for pathogenic mechanisms in APS. The mechanisms of the human APS disease process have been difficult to elucidation, mainly for two reasons: (1) The phenotypes of vascular thrombosis and pregnancy morbidity are not unique to APS, so it is difficult to ascertain whether the candidate mechanism is playing a causal role or is incidental. (2) Antibodies isolated from APS patients recognize a multiplicity of antigenic determinants[69,70] that can have a broad range of effects, so it is difficult to determine which specificities and effects are responsible for disease manifestations in humans.

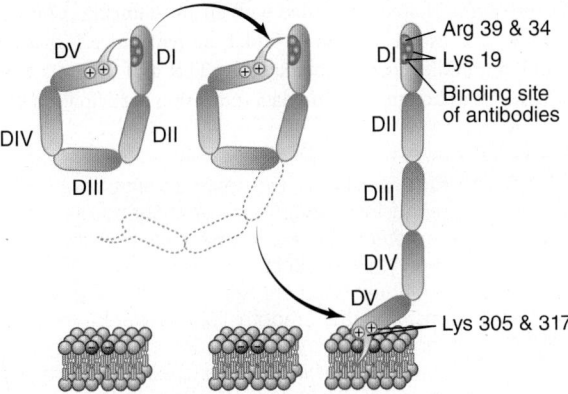

Figure 131–1. Schematic of the conformational states of β_2GPI. The unbound protein is in a closed conformation in which the epitope on domain I (DI) is shielded by a portion of domain V (DV). Binding to phospholipid membranes via a "barb," consisting of a hydrophobic loop formed by Ser311 to Lys317, near the carboxyterminus of DV, requires the protein to open and exposes an immunogenic epitope near the aminoterminal portion of the molecule. *(Reproduced with permission from Rand JH A snappy new concept for APS. Blood 2010 Aug 26;116(8):1193–1194.)*

TABLE 131–3. Proposed Pathogenic Mechanisms for Antiphospholipid Syndrome

I. Disruption of endothelial surface and annexin A5 anticoagulant shield

II. Enhanced cell signaling
   A. Mediated by antibodies against annexin A2
   B. Mediated by antibodies to ApoE2R
   C. Induction of endothelial surface proadhesive molecules
   D. Induction of tissue factor expression on monocytes and endothelial cells
   E. Complement-mediated signaling and injury

III. Impeding of fibrinolysis and endogenous anticoagulation
   A. Interference with plasminogen and tissue plasminogen activator
   B. Interference with components of the protein C activation pathway

IV. Activation of platelets
   A. Interference with β_2-glycoprotein I dampening of von Willebrand factor–mediated platelet adhesion

V. Other mechanisms
   A. Mammalian target of rapamycin complex pathway–mediated vasculopathy

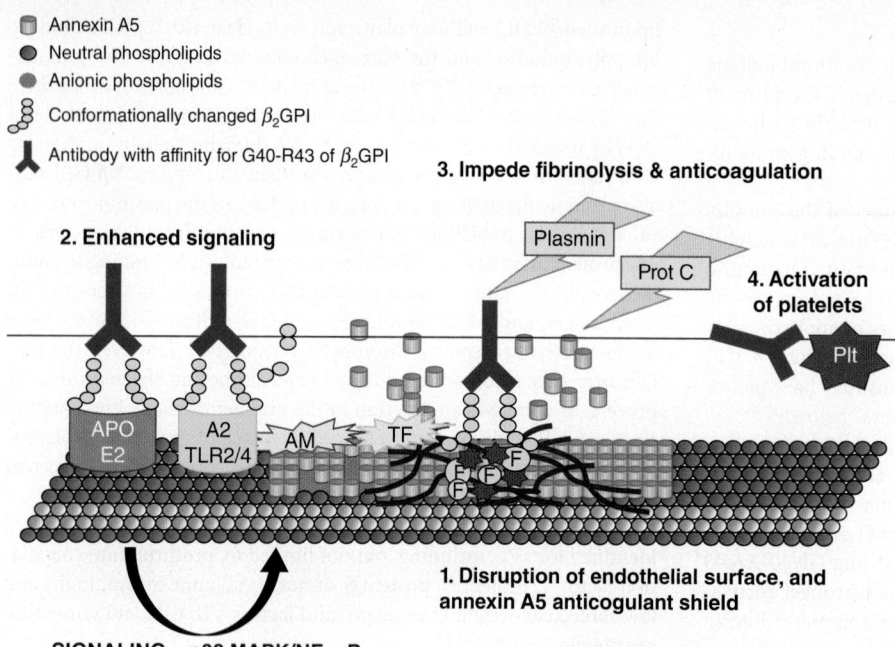

Figure 131-2. Multiple pathogenic mechanisms of aPL antibodies. (1) On a disrupted endothelial surface, anti-β_2GPI–β_2GPI complexes bind through the cationic domain V of β_2GPI to anionic structures, such as heparan sulfate to provide a prothrombotic surface. (2) In addition, anti-β_2GPI–β_2GPI complexes activate endothelial cell receptors such as ApoE2, TLR2/TLR4 and annexin A2 to promote downstream signaling pathways involving p38 mitogen-activated protein kinase (p38 MAPK) and nuclear factor-κB (NF-κB), leading to the upregulation of tissue factor (TF) and adhesion molecules (AM) and a proinflammatory/prothrombotic phenotype. (3) Anti-β_2GPI–β_2GPI complexes also impede fibrinolysis and anticoagulation by impeding plasmin, annexin A5 anticoagulant activity, and the protein C (Prot C) pathways. (4) Anti-β_2GPI–β_2GPI complexes bind to directly to activate platelets (Plt) and promote aggregation.

Disruption of the Endothelial Surface and Annexin A5 Anticoagulant Shield Annexin A5 is a potent anticoagulant protein with high affinity for phospholipid membranes that contain anionic phospholipids, specifically phosphatidyl serine.[71] Annexin A5 forms two-dimensional crystals over the phospholipid bilayers that shield them from binding coagulation factors[72] and it has been proposed that the protein may play a thrombomodulatory role on the surfaces of cells lining the placental and systemic vasculatures. Annexin A5 is highly expressed on the apical membranes of placental syncytiotrophoblasts, the location where maternal blood interfaces with fetal cells.[73] Pregnant annexin A5-null mice develop placental infarctions of fetuses and yield reduced litter sizes.[74] Pregnant mice treated with anti–annexin A5 antibodies developed placental necrosis, fibrosis, and pregnancy loss.[75] Dissociation of annexin A5 from the surface of human placental trophoblasts and human umbilical vein endothelial cells accelerates the coagulation of plasma exposed to those cells.[76] Annexin A5 binds to the surfaces of endothelial cells and inhibits thrombin formation.[77]

aPL antibody–antigen complexes disrupt the crystallization of annexin A5 and displace the protein from phospholipid membrane surfaces (Fig. 131–3).[78–81] In contrast to the LA phenomenon, aPL antibodies

accelerate coagulation reactions in systems that include annexin A5.[78,82–85] IgG fractions from APS patients reduce the quantity of annexin A5 on cultured placental trophoblasts[76,86] and endothelial cells[76,87] and accelerate the coagulation of plasma exposed to these cells.[76] This effect of aPL antibodies on annexin A5 binding has been correlated with IgG antibodies that recognize a specific epitope—domain I of β_2GPI in patients with APS who have thrombosis[52] and spontaneous pregnancy losses. Figure 131–2 includes a model for this mechanism.

Binding to Endothelial Surface Receptors Enhances Cell Signaling aPL antibodies can bind, injure, and activate cultured vascular endothelial cells.[88–91] Cultured endothelial cells incubated with aPL antibodies with specificity for cell surface β_2GPI express increased levels of cell adhesion molecules[92] triggered by their binding to cell surface β_2GPI.[93] Annexin A2 serves as a receptor for β_2GPI,[62] and anti-β_2GPI antibodies may thereby stimulate expression of tissue factor on endothelial cells.[94] In animal models, the signaling effects of aPL antibodies were significantly reduced in mice treated with an anti-annexin A2 monoclonal antibody and also in annexin A2-null transgenic mice.[95] These effects of the aPL antibodies may be mediated by TLR-4 of the innate immunity system,[96,97] although there are data indicating participation of other

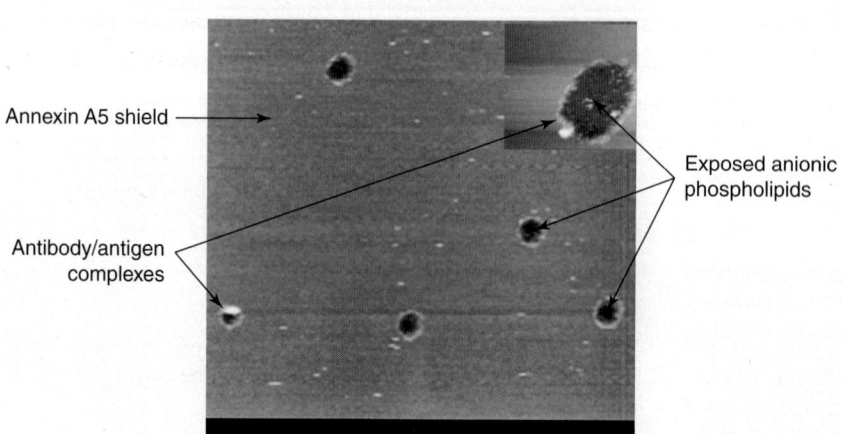

Figure 131-3. Disruption of annexin A5 shield by monoclonal antiphospholipid antibodies and β_2-glycoprotein I (β_2GPI). Atomic force microscopy picture showing the effect of a monoclonal aPL antibody on a preformed annexin A5 crystal. The figure demonstrates the smooth lipid bilayer covered by the annexin A5 crystals, disrupted by antibody–β_2GPI complexes (white circles) and exposing anionic phospholipids (black holes) to coagulation factors and accelerated coagulation. (Modifed with permission from Rand JH, Wu XX, Quinn AS, et al: Human monoclonal antiphospholipid antibodies disrupt the annexin A5 anticoagulant crystal shield on phospholipid bilayers: evidence from atomic force microscopy and functional assay. Am J Pathol 163(3):1193–1200, 2003.)

TLRs, particularly TLR-2.[98] This binding results in downstream signaling that involves TRAF6 (tumor necrosis factor receptor-associated factor 6) and MyD88 (myeloid differentiation factor 88).[99] Increased expression of tissue factor is mediated by p38 mitogen-activated protein kinase (MAPK).[100]

Binding of autoantibodies to annexin A2 may also promote thrombosis by inhibiting fibrinolysis. APS patients have increased titers of antibodies against annexin A2, an endothelial surface receptor for t-PA, and plasminogen.[101] The blocking of annexin A2 by aPL antibodies impedes plasmin generation in a t-PA–dependent generation assay, and inhibits cell surface plasmin generation on human umbilical vein endothelial cells.[94] Several additional mechanisms have been identified by which aPL antibodies can interfere with fibrinolysis. β_2GPI is a cofactor for t-PA–mediated activation of plasminogen, and aPL antibodies against β_2GPI interfere with its binding to t-PA, thereby downregulating plasminogen activation.[61] Finally, fibrinolysis may also be impaired by autoantibodies directed against the catalytic site of plasmin or t-PA,[102,103] by an increased level of plasminogen activator inhibitor-1,[104] and by inhibition of autoactivation of factor XII with ensuing reductions of kallikrein and urokinase.[105]

Apolipoprotein E receptor 2 (apoER2), a member of the LDL-receptor family is found on endothelial surfaces,[106] monocytes,[107] and platelets, and may also serve as receptor for anti-β_2GPI–β_2GPI complexes where it can also trigger the phosphatidylinositol 3′-kinase (PI3K)/Akt pathway[108] and increase tissue factor and cell adhesion molecule expression. IgG-mediated dimerization of β_2GPI and binding to ApoER2′ increases the sensitivity of platelets to agonists of aggregation.[109]

Complement-Mediated Injury Complement activation may play a role in the APS disease process. The IgG$_2$ subtype of aPL most closely correlates with thrombosis.[110,111] Blockade of complement activation using a C3 convertase inhibitor or genetic deletion of C3 protected mice from pregnancy complications induced by aPL antibodies.[112–114] These effects involve the aPL-stimulated expression of tissue factor by myeloid cells,[115] and to involve proteinase-activated G-protein–coupled receptor (PAR)-2 signaling,[116] indicating that complement activation can be pathogenic via both direct injury and downstream signaling.

Induction of Tissue Factor Activity in Leukocytes aPL antibodies can promote tissue factor expression by leukocytes.[115,117–119] The specific binding site on these cells has not been elucidated.

Inhibition of Fibrinolysis and Endogenous Anticoagulation aPL antibodies can interfere with fibrinolysis in several ways. Antibodies against annexin A2, an endothelial surface receptor for t-PA and plasminogen, can interfere with binding of plasminogen and t-PA and thereby reduce plasmin formation and fibrinolysis.[94,101,103] Monoclonal aPL antibodies derived from APS patients can directly inhibit plasmin's enzymatic activity.[102] β_2GPI is a cofactor for t-PA–mediated activation of plasminogen,[120] and anti-β_2GPI can interfere with this activity. Also, it has been reported that women with APS have significantly increased levels of circulating plasminogen activator inhibitor-1 (PAI-1), implying impaired fibrinolysis.[104]

Interference with Components of the Protein C Activation Pathway The protein C pathway (Chaps. 114 and 139) is initiated by thrombin binding to thrombomodulin (TM), which activates protein C bound to the endothelial protein C receptor (EPCR). Activated protein C (APC), together with free protein S, then proteolyses coagulation factors Va and VIIIa. APC also modulates signaling events by interfering with PAR-1 signalling.[121,122] aPL antibodies can interfere with the activation of protein C by TM–thrombin and with the activity of APC, as well as protect factors Va and VIIIa from proteolysis by APC.[65] Acquired APC resistance has been described in APS plasmas[123] and has been correlated with anti-β_2GPI domain I antibodies,[124] a risk factor for

thrombosis. The presence of antibodies against EPCR in APS patients was proposed to be a risk factor for fetal death.[125]

Antiphospholipid Antibodies Activate Platelets An experimental animal model that includes *in vivo* imaging has provided data indicating that aPL-induced thrombosis is a consequence of platelet activation that then promotes endothelial activation and fibrin formation.[126] aPL antibodies can induce platelet aggregation,[127] an effect that might be promoted via signaling through apoER2 receptors; the β_2GPI binding site for apoER2 on platelets was localized to its domain V.[128] As described above (see "Antigenic Specificities"), β_2GPI also has a dampening effect on platelet adhesion by interfering with the platelet–VWF interaction, and consequently aPL antibodies, by interfering with this β_2GPI-mediated dampening, can increase platelet adhesion in flow systems.[60]

Other Mechanisms APS patients have been shown to have autoantibodies against tissue factor pathway inhibitor.[129] Some aPL antibodies cross-react with heparin and heparinoid molecules, which are highly polyanionic, and hence, inhibit their contribution to antithrombin activity.[69] aPL antibodies show cross-reactivity against oxidized LDL[130] and are associated with an increased risk of atherosclerosis.[131] Antibodies against β_2GPI-oxidized LDL complexes have been proposed to be atherogenic by reducing their clearance.[132] Finally, in addition to promoting thrombosis, aPL antibodies may contribute to other vascular lesions by stimulating the mammalian target of rapamycin complex (mTORC) pathway (Fig. 131–4).[133]

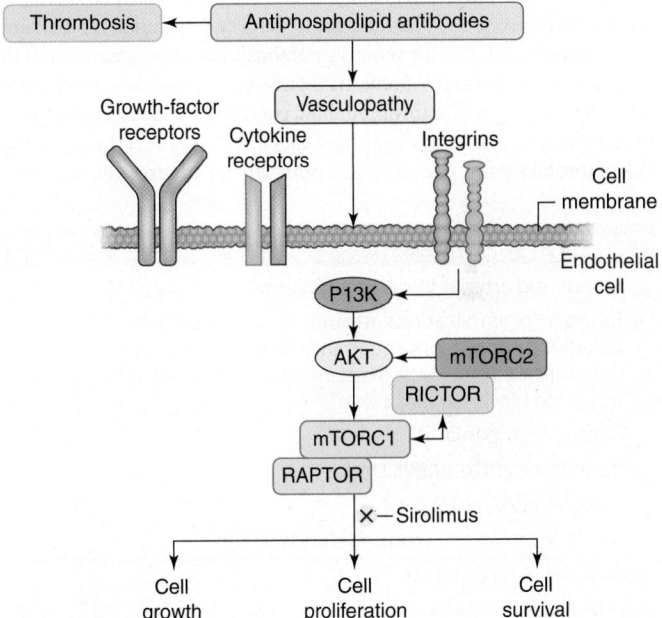

Figure 131–4. Pathogenesis of vasculopathy in the antiphospholipid syndrome. In addition to promoting thrombosis, antiphospholipid antibodies also trigger vasculopathy by binding to vascular endothelial cells and activating the mammalian target of rapamycin (mTOR) signaling pathway. Extracellular and intracellular signals through the phosphatidylinositide 3′-kinase (PI3K)-AKT pathway activate mTOR pathway which regulates cell growth, proliferation and survival. The mTOR enzyme is a component of two complexes, mammalian target of rapamycin complex (mTORC) 1 and mTORC2. The activity of mTORC1 is regulated by a subunit of the regulatory-associated protein of mTORC1 (RAPTOR), whereas the activity of mTORC2 is regulated by a subunit of the rapamycin-insensitive companion of mTOR (RICTOR). (*Modifed with permission from Eikelbloom JW, Weitz JI: The mTORC pathway in the antiphospholipid syndrome.* N Engl J Med 371(4):369–371, 2014.)

●CLINICAL FEATURES

Table 131–4 summarizes the clinical features of APS. Patients generally present with thrombotic manifestations, that is, evidence for vasoocclusion or end-organ ischemia or infarction, and/or pregnancy losses and complications attributable to placental insufficiency. The usual age at presentation with thrombosis is approximately 35 to 45 years. Except for patients with SLE, men and women are equally susceptible to thrombotic manifestations. No differences have been observed between the arterial and venous distributions of thromboses of primary and secondary APS patients.[134]

SYSTEMIC VASCULAR THROMBOSIS

Patients can present with spontaneous venous and/or arterial thrombosis or embolism in any site; however, about half of all patients have deep vein thrombosis of the lower extremities.[135,136] Other sites of venous thromboembolic events include pulmonary embolism, thoracic veins (superior vena cava, subclavian vein, or jugular vein), and abdominal or pelvic veins.[136] Approximately one-fourth of patients present with arterial thromboses; the remainder present with concurrent arterial and venous thrombosis.[136] Patients may also present with stroke, cerebral venous thrombosis, upper-extremity venous thrombosis,[135] myocardial infarction, adrenal infarction, acalculous gallbladder infarction, aortic thrombosis with renal infarction,[120] and mesenteric artery thrombosis.[137,138] Thrombosis may occur spontaneously or in the presence of some other risk factor such as estrogen replacement therapy, oral contraceptives,[134,139] vascular stasis, surgery, or trauma. Women are at particularly high risk for venous thrombosis during pregnancy and in the postpartum period.[134] Some APS patients with venous thrombosis have concurrent genetic thrombophilic conditions such as the factor V Leiden variant, and it has been postulated that this may increase the risk of thrombosis.[140-143] Concurrent positivity for all three aPL antibody

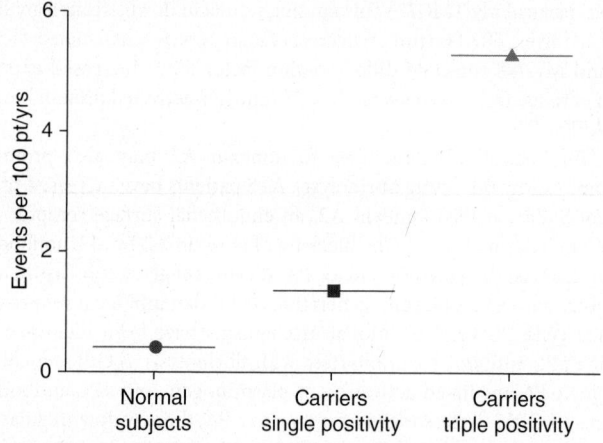

Figure 131–5. Average annual rates of first cardiovascular events (including venous thromboembolism) among antiphospholipid (aPL) antibody–negative and aPL antibody-positive populations. Concurrent positivity for all three aPL antibody assays—that is, "triple positivity" for the aCL antibody assay, anti-β_2GPI antibody assay, and the lupus anticoagulant assay—is a highly significant risk factor for a first thrombotic event. (*Modified with permission from Pengo V, Ruffatti A, Legnani C et al: Incidence of a first thromboembolic event in asymptomatic carriers of high-risk antiphospholipid antibody profile: A multicenter prospective study. Blood 118(17):4714–4718, 2011.*)

assays—that is, the aCL antibody assay, anti-β_2GPI antibody assay, and the LA assay—appears to be a highly significant risk factor for having an initial thrombotic event (Fig. 131–5).[144] If this finding is confirmed, it could identify a group of patients who might warrant consideration for prophylactic treatment. A history of having had a thromboembolic event is probably the most significant risk factor for recurrence of venous thromboembolism in APS, with a reported frequency that reached approximately 30 percent in patients followed for 4 years after the first episode.[145] The risk of recurrent thromboembolism correlates with the titer of antibodies,[145,146] and with the presence of LA. In addition, it appears that the presence of anti-β_2GPI domain I antibodies significantly increase the risk of thrombosis, compared to patients who have antibodies that are not domain I dependent and LA that is not domain I dependent.[51]

SYSTEMIC LUPUS ERYTHEMATOSUS AND OTHER AUTOIMMUNE CONDITIONS

APS patients frequently present with other autoimmune conditions. A significant proportion of SLE patients have elevated aPL antibodies, with estimates ranging between 12 and 30 percent for aCL antibodies and 15 and 34 percent for LA antibodies.[147] APS has been associated with the concurrence of other autoimmune conditions including, but not limited to, rheumatoid arthritis,[148] Sjögren syndrome,[149] myasthenia gravis,[150] Budd-Chiari syndrome in the setting of SLE,[151] Graves disease,[152] autoimmune hemolytic anemia, progressive systemic sclerosis,[153] Evans syndrome,[154] Takayasu arteritis,[155] polyarteritis nodosa,[156] and immune thrombocytopenia (see section Thrombocytopenia below and also Chap. 117).

STROKE AND OTHER NEUROLOGIC CONDITIONS

The most common neurologic manifestations of APS are stroke or transient ischemic attacks (TIAs), which were the initial presentation of up to 30 percent of adults with APS in a large European cohort.[157] In the European Catastrophic Antiphospholipid Antibody Syndrome (CAPS)

TABLE 131–4. Clinical Manifestations Associated with APS

- Venous and arterial thromboembolism*
- Pregnancy complications attributable to placental insufficiency, including spontaneous pregnancy losses as detailed in Table 132–3, intrauterine growth restriction, preeclampsia, preterm labor, and placental abruption*
- Thrombocytopenia
- Thrombotic and embolic stroke*
- Cerebral vein thrombosis*
- Livedo reticularis, necrotizing skin vasculitis
- Coronary artery disease
- Valvular heart disease
- Kidney disease
- Pulmonary hypertension
- Acute respiratory distress syndrome
- Atherosclerosis and peripheral artery disease
- Nonthrombotic retinal disease
- Adrenal failure, hemorrhagic adrenal infarction*
- Budd-Chiari syndrome, mesenteric and portal vein obstructions, hepatic infarction, esophageal necrosis, gastric and colonic ulceration, gallbladder necrosis*
- Catastrophic antiphospholipid syndrome with thrombotic microangiopathy*

*Manifestations that qualify as consensus criteria for diagnosis of antiphospholipid syndrome.[18]

Registry, cerebral manifestations occurred in 62 percent of patients and caused 13 percent of deaths.[158] Recurrent strokes are more likely in patients with APS and other risk factors for cerebrovascular disease, such as cigarette smoking, hypertension hyperlipidemia, oral contraceptive use, and SLE.[159,160]

Most APS patients with stroke have arterial thromboembolic occlusive events that are clinically indistinguishable from the more common arteriosclerotic strokes. APS should be suspected in young patients with TIAs or stroke, particularly when the more typical risk factors for cerebrovascular disease are absent.[161] Cerebral venous thrombosis is less common in APS patients and presents at a younger age, and is more extensive than in non-APS patients with the disorder.[162] In one series of 40 cases of cerebral venous thrombosis, three patients (8 percent) had elevated aPL antibody levels.[163] Superior sagittal sinus thrombosis has been reported with primary APS.[164]

There is controversy about whether migraines in patients with aPL antibodies should be regarded as thromboocclusive events.[165] Other neurologic abnormalities reported to be associated with aPL antibodies include seizures/epilepsy,[166] chorea, Guillain-Barré syndrome, transient global amnesia, dementia, diabetic peripheral neuropathy, and orthostatic hypotension.[167] Recurrent acute transverse myelopathy has been described with APS.[168-172] However, in one study of 315 SLE patients, including 10 with a history of transverse myelopathy, that disorder was not associated with aPL antibodies.[173] Multiple sclerosis patients have a high incidence of elevated aCL antibody levels (in one series, 9 percent had IgG antibodies and 44 percent had IgM antibodies),[174] however, no clinical distinctions were found between aPL-positive and aPL-negative patients and the antibodies do not appear to be associated with thrombosis. Patients with psychotic disorders have an increased prevalence of LA and aCL antibodies, even in the absence of treatment with antipsychotic drugs.[175]

CATASTROPHIC ANTIPHOSPHOLIPID SYNDROME

CAPS is a relatively infrequent but devastating presentation of APS, is characterized by severe widespread vascular occlusions.[176] Diagnostic criteria for CAPS include evidence of involvement of at least three organs, systems, and/or tissues; development of manifestations simultaneously or in less than 1 week; histopathologic confirmation of small-vessel occlusion; and laboratory confirmation of the presence of aPL antibodies.[177] According to the CAPS Registry, a web-based database of 433 patients with CAPS (https://ontocrf.costaisa.com/en/web/caps/), the majority of CAPS patients are female (69 percent), in their late thirties (mean age of 38.5 years), but the condition can present at any age (range: 0 to 85 years). In half of the CAPS cases, the patients' catastrophic event was their first APS manifestation. Precipitating factors of CAPS include infections, drugs (sulfur-containing diuretics, captopril, and oral contraceptives), surgical procedures, and cessation of prior anticoagulant therapy. In 26.9 percent of cases, the patients also had SLE. The most frequently affected organ was the kidney (73 percent of episodes), followed by lungs (58.9 percent), the brain (55.9 percent), the heart (49.7 percent), and the skin (45.4 percent). Other organs were also affected, including the peripheral vessels, intestines, spleen, adrenal glands, pancreas, retina, and marrow. Patients present with evidence for severe multiorgan ischemia/infarction, often with concurrent disseminated microvascular thrombosis. Patients with CAPS can present with renal insufficiency, respiratory failure resulting from acute respiratory distress syndrome (ARDS) and pulmonary emboli, cerebral manifestations such as encephalopathy, stroke and seizures, cardiac problems such as heart failure, myocardial infarction and valvular defects, and skin complications such as livedo reticularis and skin necrosis.[178] Most

patients show histologic evidence of microangiopathy mainly affecting small vessels of the kidneys, lungs, brain, heart, and liver. Only a minority of patients experience large-vessel occlusions. Laboratory evidence for disseminated intravascular coagulation is frequently present. An LA is present in 81.7 percent of patients, and the aCL IgG is the most common positive aPL antibody.[178] Improved treatment has reduced mortality from approximately 50 percent to approximately 20 percent.[176] Relapse is rare in survivors. The only identified predictive factor for adverse outcome is underlying SLE.[179]

PREGNANCY LOSSES, OBSTETRIC COMPLICATIONS, AND INFERTILITY

At this time, aPL screening of otherwise asymptomatic with no history of prior complications obstetrical patients is not warranted because of the high frequency of false-positive tests; most studies have estimated the prevalence of aPL antibodies among general obstetric populations to be approximately 5 percent or less and most of these aPL-positive patients are not clinically affected.[180]

Among obstetric patients with recurrent fetal losses, approximately 16 to 38 percent have aPL antibodies. In addition, pregnant women with elevated aPL antibodies had significantly more obstetric complications, including preeclampsia, abruption placentae, miscarriage, prematurity, intrauterine fetal demise, intrauterine growth restriction, and oligohydraminos, than aPL antibody-negative pregnant women.[181-183] In approximately half of patients, the pregnancy losses occur in the first trimester. Other patients present with later losses, most in the second trimester, but some even later, including stillbirth. Pregnancy complications attributable to APS include three or more recurrent spontaneous first trimester miscarriages, one or more fetal losses during the second trimester, stillbirth, episode of preeclampsia, preterm labor, placental abruption, intrauterine growth restriction, and oligohydramnion.[184-186] Pregnant patients with APS are also more prone to developing deep vein thrombosis during pregnancy or the puerperium. Rarely, pregnant patients develop CAPS.[187,188] The best predictor for pregnancy loss in a patient who tests positive for aPL antibodies has been demonstrated to simply be a previous history of pregnancy loss, complications, or thrombosis.[146,189] A recent study reported that any aPL antibody-positive women with an unexplained early loss prior to 10 weeks have a higher risk of complications in their second pregnancy[190] but the degree of laboratory abnormalities were not associated with increased risk. Positivity by more than one assay appears to correlate with increased pregnancy morbidities.[182,191] Histologic abnormalities were found in many, but not all, placentas of aPL patients.[192] Studies of placental pathology in patients with aPL antibodies, but without a prior history of fetal loss, showed that approximately half had evidence of uteroplacental vascular pathology, approximately half had evidence of thrombotic occlusion, and approximately one-third had chronic villitis and/or decidual plasma cell infiltrates.[193,194]

Overall, it appears that the presence of aPL antibodies does not affect the success rate of implantation. Although one group has reported data that indicated that women with recurrent implantation failure were more likely to have positive assays for aPL antibodies compared to fertile negative controls,[195] a review of 29 studies showed mixed results.[196] Many of the studies were noted to have limitations, including problems with study design and statistical power. The current consensus is that aPL antibodies are not a cause of infertility.[197] Recently, the 14th International Congress on Antiphospholipid Antibodies Task Force also concluded that "there are no data to support the inclusion of infertility as criteria for APS and investigation of APS in patients with infertility should not be done in routine clinical practice, being reserved only for research purposes."[196]

CUTANEOUS MANIFESTATIONS

The cutaneous manifestations of APS may comprise the first signs of APS in some patients.[198,199] Livedo reticularis is relatively common, occurring in 24 percent of a series of 1000 aPL patients,[200] and occasionally presents in a necrosing form.[201] Noninflammatory vascular thrombosis is the most frequent histopathologic feature. Necrotizing vasculitis, livedoid vasculitis, thrombophlebitis, cutaneous ulceration and necrosis, erythematous macules, purpura, ecchymoses, painful skin nodules, and subungual splinter hemorrhages, anetoderma (macular atrophy), discoid lupus erythematosus, and cutaneous T-cell lymphoma have all been reported.

CORONARY ARTERY DISEASE

aPL antibodies are associated with increased susceptibility to coronary artery disease,[202] particularly premature atherosclerosis.[203,204] APS should be considered in patients who lack the usual risk factors for coronary artery disease and in patients with evidence for thrombotic or embolic coronary artery occlusion that lack angiographic evidence of atherosclerotic disease. aPL antibodies appear to be a risk factor for adverse outcomes following all coronary revascularization procedures,[202] and for restenosis after percutaneous transluminal coronary angioplasty.[205,206] An ultrasound study of carotid arteries provided evidence supporting an association of aPL antibodies with premature atherosclerosis; relatively young primary APS patients (mean age: 37 ± 11 years) had significantly increased intimal medial thickness compared to control non-APS groups.[207]

VALVULAR HEART DISEASE

Approximately 35 percent of patients with primary APS have cardiac valvular abnormalities detected by echocardiography.[208] In one study, approximately 20 percent of cardiac patients with valvular heart disease had evidence for aPL antibodies compared with approximately 10 percent of matched control subjects.[209] Valvulopathy includes leaflet thickening, vegetations, regurgitation, and stenosis.[210] The mitral valve is mainly affected, followed by the aortic valve.[211] Histologically, APS valvular lesions consist mainly of superficial or intravalvular fibrin deposits in association with variable degrees of vascular proliferation, fibroblast influx, fibrosis, and calcification. These can result in valve thickening, fusion, and rigidity, and lead to functional abnormalities.[212] Deposits of immunoglobulins, including aCL antibodies, and of complement components are commonly found in the affected valves.[213]

PERIPHERAL VASCULAR DISEASE

Approximately one-third of patients with peripheral arterial disease undergoing bypass grafting procedures had elevated aPL antibody levels (mostly aCL antibodies).[214] Intraarterial thromboembolic events are common at presentation of these patients and may complicate surgical management. However, these patients did not have an increased risk for reocclusion, a finding that was attributable to the use of anticoagulant therapy.

PULMONARY MANIFESTATIONS

Patients with APS may present with *in situ* thrombosis in pulmonary vessels. aPL antibodies are associated with pulmonary hypertension.[215] In one prospective trial of 38 consecutive patients with precapillary pulmonary hypertension, approximately 30 percent had aPL antibodies with various phospholipid specificities.[216] An interinstitutional study of 687 patients with chronic thromboembolic pulmonary hypertension reported that aPL antibodies were a significant risk factor.[217] The

majority of patients with CAPS (see "Catastrophic Antiphospholipid Syndrome" above) have dyspnea, and most of these individuals have ARDS.[218]

ABDOMINAL MANIFESTATIONS

The liver is the most frequently affected abdominal organ in APS, with occlusion of hepatic vessels, including those supplying the biliary tree.[219] aPL antibody levels frequently are elevated in patients with chronic liver disease of various causes. In one prospective study of patients with liver disease, approximately half of patients with alcoholic liver disease and one-third of patients with chronic hepatitis C virus had elevated aPL antibody levels. The frequency was even higher in patients with more severe cirrhosis.[220] A review reported that approximately 20 percent of patients with chronic hepatitis B and hepatitis C had aPL antibodies, most of which were cofactor independent.[221] Some patients with hepatitis C present with true autoimmune aPL antibodies, the most common features reported being intraabdominal thrombosis and myocardial infarction.[222]

Reported gastrointestinal manifestations of APS also include esophageal necrosis with perforation, intestinal ischemia and infarction, pancreatitis, and colonic ulceration. Primary biliary cirrhosis,[223] acute acalculous cholecystitis with gallbladder necrosis,[224,225] and giant gastric ulceration are associated with APS.[226] APS has been reported in patients with mesenteric inflammatory venoocclusive disease[227] and in patients with mesenteric and portal venous obstruction.[228]

THROMBOCYTOPENIA

Approximately 20 to 40 percent of patients with APS have varying degrees of thrombocytopenia. The decrease in platelet count is generally mild or moderate and is rarely significant enough to cause bleeding complications or affect anticoagulant therapy.[229,230] The majority of patients with APS and thrombocytopenia have antibodies against $\alpha_{IIb}\beta_3$ integrin and/or glycoprotein Ib-IX complex.[231] Patients presenting with immune thrombocytopenic purpura frequently have elevated aPL antibodies, and these patients are more prone to thrombosis.[232] aPL antibodies and antibodies against platelet membrane glycoprotein were present simultaneously in approximately 70 percent of patients with immune-mediated thrombocytopenia.[233] Thrombocytopenia itself is not protective against thrombosis in these patients. In a prospective cohort study, 5-year thrombosis-free survival of aPL-positive and aPL-negative immune thrombocytopenic purpura patients were 39 percent and 98 percent, respectively.[234]

BLEEDING

The presence of a concurrent hemostasis defect needs to be considered when patients with APS exhibit a bleeding tendency (Table 131–5). Acquired hypoprothrombinemia with severe bleeding has been reported.[235,236] This diagnosis may be missed when coagulation abnormalities are attributed only to the LA effect, so a specific assay

TABLE 131–5. Causes of Bleeding in Antiphospholipid Syndrome

- Hypoprothrombinemia
- Thrombocytopenia
- Acquired platelet function abnormality
- Acquired inhibitor to specific coagulation factor, e.g., factor VIII
- Acquired von Willebrand syndrome

for prothrombin should be performed when the prothrombin time is prolonged. Other causes of bleeding in APS include acquired thrombocytopathies, thrombocytopenia (see "Thrombocytopenia," above), acquired inhibitors against specific coagulation factors, such as factor VIII, and the acquired von Willebrand syndrome (AVWS).

RETINAL ABNORMALITIES

The diagnosis of aPL antibody retinopathy should be suspected in patients with diffuse retinal vasoocclusion, particularly when characterized by involvement of arteries and veins, neovascularization at presentation, and symptoms of systemic rheumatologic disease.[237] aPL antibodies were present in 5 to 33 percent of patients with retinal vein occlusion.[238,239] Cilioretinal artery occlusion,[240] optic neuropathy,[241] and severe vasoocclusive retinopathy[242] have been described with APS.

KIDNEY DISEASES

APS may affect the renal system. Patients may present with renal artery stenosis and/or thrombosis, renal infarction, renal vein thrombosis, and glomerulonephritis that is distinct from vasoocclusive disease.[200,243] An entity named "APS nephropathy" has been described, which consists of a vasoocclusive disease of small-size intrarenal vessels.[244] This nephropathy features fibrous intimal hyperplasia, focal cortical atrophy, and thrombotic microangiopathy. A review of 29 consecutive renal biopsies from patients with primary APS, performed at two institutions over 22 years, described 20 cases of APS nephropathy and nine cases with other distinct pathologic features.[243] These features included membranous nephropathy, minimal change disease/focal segmental glomerulonephritis, mesangial C3 nephropathy, and pauci-immune crescentic glomerulonephritis.

ANTIPHOSPHOLIPID SYNDROME AND AIDS

Although patients with HIV-1 infection frequently have elevated aPL antibody levels, they do not often have thrombotic manifestations. A review indicated that approximately 50 percent of HIV-1 patients test positive for aPL antibodies, most of which are not cofactor dependent.[221] HIV-infected patients with manifestations of APS have also presented with avascular bone and cutaneous necrosis.[222]

ANTIPHOSPHOLIPID SYNDROME IN CHILDREN

Increasingly, APS has become recognized in children,[245] in whom diverse clinical features are common. The results of a European registry have been reported.[246] Review of 121 cases indicated that although the thrombotic manifestations were similar to adults with APS, there was a difference between children with primary APS and the secondary APS; the children with primary APS were younger and had a higher frequency of arterial thrombotic events, whereas the children with secondary APS patients had a higher frequency of venous thrombotic events associated with hematologic and skin manifestations. CAPS has been reported in children, but is rare.[247,248]

Thrombosis is rare in newborns delivered from mothers with APS, and only a few cases are reported, mostly associated with other prothrombotic factors.[249] aPL antibodies have been found in up to 30 percent of offspring of mothers with APS.[250]

In a recent European prospective study, 17 percent of neonates born to APS mothers were premature; however, no specific complications were found during the 5-year followup.[251] The study did show a higher rate of neurodevelopmental abnormalities with learning disabilities similar to two retrospective reports where learning disabilities without other neurodevelopmental abnormalities were present in 15 to 20 percent of cases.[252,253]

OTHER MANIFESTATIONS

Acute adrenal failure secondary to bilateral infarction of the adrenal glands has been reported as the first manifestation of primary APS.[254] Adrenal hemorrhage has been reported.[255] aPL antibodies have been associated with marrow necrosis.[256]

● LABORATORY FEATURES

Diagnosis of APS requires the demonstration of antibodies against phospholipids and/or relevant protein cofactors (Table 131–6). The current tests for APS recommended by the most recent consensus on investigational criteria[18] and the Scientific Standardization Committee of the International Society of Thrombosis and Hemostasis are aCL, anti-β_2GPI (IgG and IgM), and LA.[257] The laboratory diagnosis of APS frequently is problematic, with limitations that have been detailed.[258,259] aCL IgG and IgM assays are the most sensitive, but the least specific. Anti-β_2GPI IgG and IgM assays are more specific but less sensitive. LA assays, of which the dilute Russell viper venom time (dRVVT) is the most common, generally tend to be the least sensitive but the most specific. The current recommended tests are less than ideal because they are empirically derived tests and do not yet measure antibodies directed against disease specific epitopes or functional parameters that correlate with disease mechanisms. Despite these limitations, positivity for all three criteria assays ("triple positivity") has been correlated with an increased risk for a future thrombotic event (see Fig. 131–5).[144] Investigational criteria have been developed to identify patients with

TABLE 131–6. Diagnostic Tests for Antiphospholipid Syndrome

Immunoassays

Anticardiolipin IgG and IgM antibodies*

Anti-β_2GPI IgG and IgM antibodies*

Serologic test for syphilis ("biologic false-positive")

Antiphosphatidyl serine antibodies

Antiprothrombin antibodies

Coagulation Tests†

Dilute Russell viper venom time with mixing incubations and neutralization with excess phospholipid

aPTT with mixing incubation and neutralization with excess phospholipids

aPL-sensitive and -insensitive reagents and platelet neutralization procedure

Kaolin clotting time

Dilute prothrombin time (a.k.a tissue thromboplastin inhibition test)

Hexagonal phase array test

Textarin/ecarin test

aPL, antiphospholipid; APS, antiphospholipid syndrome; aPTT, activated partial thromboplastin time; β_2GPI, β_2-glycoprotein I; Ig, immunoglobulin; LA, lupus anticoagulant.

*Recommended by the International Society on Thrombosis and Haemostasis (ISTH) Scientific and Standardisation Committee (SSC) Subcommittee on Lupus Anticoagulants and Antiphospholipid Antibodies.[258]

†The committee recommended that two coagulation assays be performed if LA or APS are suspected, preferably the dilute Russell viper venom time (dRVVT) and aPTT.

the "definite" autoimmune APS (see Table 131–3).[18] Because no single test is sufficient for diagnosing the disorder, a panel of tests, including antibodies against cardiolipin, and β_2GPI, and coagulation tests for LA should be performed when APS is suspected.[257] The investigational criteria require that positive results have to be obtained on two or more occasions at least 12 weeks apart to qualify for diagnosis.

IMMUNOASSAYS

Anticardiolipin Antibody Assays

Most patients with APS are identified by elevated levels of aCL antibodies, a test with high sensitivity but poor specificity. The prevalence of positive tests in the asymptomatic healthy population has generally ranged from approximately 3 to 10 percent. In a prospective study of 2132 consecutive Spanish patients with venous thromboembolism, 4.1 percent had elevated levels of aCL antibodies (i.e., about the same prevalence as in the asymptomatic healthy population),[260] but in a group of healthy young women in another study, the prevalence of elevated levels of aCL was 18.2 percent.[261] Many individuals have antibody levels that are elevated in response to infections that are not associated with thrombotic complications. Patients with syphilis, Lyme disease, and other infections may be misdiagnosed with APS based on elevated aCL antibody levels when concurrent stroke or arterial thrombosis is present, so these conditions must always be ruled out in susceptible patients. In a systematic literature review, 15 of 28 studies showed significant associations between aCL antibodies and thrombosis.[262] In all cases, a correlation existed between high antibody titers and a high risk of thrombosis. Elevated levels of aCL antibodies, whether high or low titer, were significantly associated with both myocardial infarction and cerebral stroke. Only high-titer aCL antibodies significantly increased the risk of deep vein thrombosis. During a 10-year followup of patients with elevated levels of aCL antibodies, approximately 50 percent of patients who presented with the antibodies but without clinical manifestations of the syndrome subsequently developed the APS.[263] The presence of elevated titers of aCL antibodies 6 months after an episode of venous thromboembolism is a predictor for increased risk of recurrence and of death.[145] Women with aCL IgM antibodies, or with an aCL IgG antibody titer less than 20 IgG-binding units, and without a positive LA do not appear to be at risk for APS.[264] In contrast, women with an aCL IgG titer greater than 20 binding units or a positive LA were more likely to develop complications.[264] With respect to pregnancy losses, a meta-analysis of 25 studies on aPL antibodies in women with recurrent fetal losses showed a significant correlation with increased aCL IgG, and particularly with the LA.[262]

With respect to stroke, elevated levels of aCL antibodies of IgG or IgM isotype were reported to be significant risk factors.[265] aPL antibodies also are an independent risk factor for stroke in young women.[266]

Approximately 20 percent of patients taking procainamide have moderate to high levels of aCL antibodies.[267] In these patients, the antibodies are associated with anti-β_2GPI specificity. There have been case reports of associated thrombosis.[268] Treatment with chlorpromazine has been associated with the development of aCL antibodies,[269] although more recent data indicate that aPL antibodies are frequently elevated in patients with severe psychiatric disorders whether or not they are treated with antipsychotic medications.[270]

Anti-β_2 Glycoprotein I Antibody Assays

β_2GPI is believed to be the major protein cofactor for aPL antibodies. Enzyme-linked immunosorbent assays (ELISAs) for anti-β_2GPI antibodies are considered to be more specific but less sensitive to APS than to aCL assays.[271] In a systematic literature review, 34 of 60 studies showed significant associations between anti-β_2GPI antibodies and

thrombosis.[262] None of the studies were prospective. Of the 10 studies that included multivariate analysis, only two confirmed that anti-β_2GPI IgG antibodies were independent risk factors for venous thrombosis. Anti-β_2GPI antibodies were more often associated with venous than arterial thrombosis. Anti-β_2GPI IgA antibodies were significantly associated with thrombosis.

Although these antibodies usually are present in conjunction with abnormal aCL and antiphosphatidyl serine antibodies, some patients with APS present solely with antibodies to β_2GPI.[272,273] Despite their higher specificity for APS (98 percent), β_2GPI antibodies alone cannot be relied upon for the diagnosis because of their low sensitivity (40 to 50 percent).[274,275] Also, interlaboratory variability is a significant problem with anti-β_2GPI antibody assays.[276]

Epitope-specific anti-β_2GPI antibodies, not yet in general use, may offer a better predictive value for diagnosis and prognosis of APS. A recent analysis of 198 samples from patients with a variety of autoimmune conditions revealed that the 52 patients with anti-β_2GPI IgG antibodies could be divided into those that recognize domain I alone and those with reactivity for all domains[51]; the former were positive for LA and were associated with an increased risk for thrombosis. As mentioned earlier, positivity for this assay has been correlated with positivity for a functional coagulation assay that measures resistance to annexin A5 anticoagulant activity.[52]

Assays for Antibodies Against Prothrombin and Phosphatidyl Serine

Prothrombin is considered the second major cofactor for aPL antibodies. In a systematic literature review, 17 of 46 studies showed significant associations between antiprothrombin antibodies and thrombosis.[262] Of the eight studies that included multivariate analysis, two confirmed that antiprothrombin antibodies were independent risk factors for thrombosis, and three other studies showed that antiprothrombin antibodies added to the risk borne by LA or aCL antibodies. A recent study indicated that the sensitivity of antiprothrombin immunoassays in the primary aPL syndrome is too low to warrant inclusion in recommendations for APS testing.[277]

Tests for antibodies against phosphatidyl serine have been hypothesized to be more relevant than antibodies against cardiolipin, because the latter are present in intracellular membranes, whereas phosphatidyl serine is exposed on syncytialized cells, on apoptotic cells, and on activated platelets. Antibodies against phosphatidyl serine were reported to correlate more specifically with APS than aCL antibodies, particularly in arterial thrombosis.[278,279] However, antiphosphatidyl serine antibody tests are not included as an international consensus criterion.[257]

Newer studies indicate that assays for detecting autoantibodies that recognize prothrombin complexed to the anionic phospholipid, phosphatidyl serine, may have improved utility for diagnosing APS by identifying patients suspected for the disorder but with negative results in the conventional assays; in one series of 728 patients who were suspected of having APS but tested negative by conventional assays, 41 were found to be positive for anti–prothrombin/phosphatidyl serine.[280] It has also been suggested that positivity for these assays may correlate with positivity for LA assays.[281]

Assays for Antibodies Against Other Phospholipids

Some investigators have advocated testing for antibodies against a panel of phospholipids other than cardiolipin,[282-285] but others have disagreed.[286] Although one review has indicated that measurement for antiphosphatidyl ethanolamine antibodies may identify some patients whose conventional tests are negative for aPL antibodies,[287] the current consensus holds that no benefit has been demonstrated for tests for antibodies against panels of different phospholipids.[257]

COAGULATION TESTS

Lupus Anticoagulants

One of the most intriguing aspects of APS is the LA phenomenon.[288,289] The various LA tests all report the inhibition of phospholipid-dependent blood coagulation reactions,[6] but by different detection methods. These include modifications of the aPTT test with LA-sensitive and LA-insensitive reagents, the kaolin clotting time, the dRVVT, the tissue thromboplastin inhibition time, the hexagonal phase array test, and the platelet neutralization procedure. Readers who are interested in the latest consensus recommendations on details of the procedures are directed to reference 257.

The results of LA tests can be so variable that even specialized laboratories will disagree as to the results of LA tests. For example, three surveys in the United Kingdom have shown that although most laboratories agreed on identification of plasmas containing strong positive LA activity, they frequently have disagreed about samples with a weak LA activity.[286]

Despite these limitations, the presence of a positive LA appears to be the strongest predictive diagnostic test for future thrombosis. In a meta-analysis of the risk for aPL-associated venous thromboembolism in individuals with aPL antibodies without an underlying autoimmune disease or previous thrombosis, the mean odds ratios were 1.6 for aCL antibodies, 3.2 for high titers of aCL, and 11.0 for LA.[290] In a systematic literature review, 12 of 12 studies showed significant associations between LA and thrombosis, with odds ratios from 5.7 to 9.4.[262] LA increased the risks of arterial and venous events to the same extent. Positivity for both LA and aCL, but not for aCL alone, predicted a higher risk of recurrent thromboocclusive events in patients with first ischemic stroke.[135] In a prospective study of pregnant women, the PROMISSE study (Predictors of Pregnancy Outcome: Biomarkers in Antiphospholipid Antibody Syndrome and Systemic Lupus Erythematosus study), LA was the primary predictor of adverse pregnancy outcome after 12 weeks' gestation in aPL-associated pregnancies.; aCL antibody and anti-β_2GPI, did not predict adverse pregnancy outcome if LA was not also present.[291]

In patients with SLE as well, the presence of LA activity is more predictive and more specific for the occurrence of thrombosis or pregnancy loss than aCL assays.[292] This was also found in a meta-analysis of women without autoimmune conditions who had recurrent pregnancy losses.[293]

Dilute Russell Viper Venom Time

dRVVT is considered to be one of the most sensitive of the LA tests. The assay uses Russell viper venom (RVV) in a system containing limiting quantities of diluted rabbit brain phospholipid. RVV directly activates coagulation factor X, leading to formation of fibrin clot. LA prolongs dRVVT by interfering with assembly of the prothrombinase complex; however, the prolongation is reversed by adding excess phospholipid to the reaction (sometimes referred to a "confirmatory test"). To ensure that prolongation of the clotting time is not a result of a factor deficiency, the procedure includes mixture of patient and control plasmas. Anticoagulant therapy with heparin, warfarin, or direct thrombin inhibitors can yield falsely abnormal test results.

Activated Partial Thromboplastin Time Tests

Prolongation of the aPTT detects some LAs, and prolonged aPTTs in otherwise healthy individuals are most frequently caused by LAs.[294] The various commercial aPTT reagents vary widely with regard to sensitivity to LA, so it is important to know the characteristics of the particular reagent(s) that is (are) being used. When the aPTT of a particular plasma sample is prolonged and not correctable by immediate mixture with normal plasma, the presence of an LA should be suspected, especially if the patient does not have bleeding symptoms. The LA needs to be differentiated from inhibitors of specific coagulation factors and from anticoagulants such as heparin. Besides specific assays to exclude the latter two possibilities, the clinician should check whether the aPTT normalizes when an LA-insensitive aPTT reagent is used or when the assay is performed using frozen washed platelets as the source of phospholipid, a procedure referred to as the platelet neutralization procedure. The effects of incubation with normal plasma may be helpful in differentiating LAs from coagulation factor inhibitors. aPTTs performed on mixtures of normal plasma and plasma containing a factor VIII inhibitor usually show no prolongation immediately after mixing but marked prolongation following incubation for 1 to 2 hours at 37°C, whereas LA-containing plasmas usually prolong the aPTT immediately after mixing with normal plasma and show no further prolongation with incubation. The clinician should be aware that both types of anticoagulants, LA and specific coagulation factor inhibitors, may coexist in rare patients and yield confusing laboratory results. Specific coagulation factor inhibitor assays and using an aPTT reagent that is insensitive to LA are helpful for clarifying most of these cases. LAs may result in artifactual decreases in contact activation pathway coagulation factor assays, because these assays are based on aPTT. Consequently, these patients are sometimes misdiagnosed as having multiple coagulation factor deficiencies. This problem can be handled by repeating the coagulation factor assays following dilution of the plasma samples; this usually results in complete or partial normalization of coagulation factor levels with progressive dilution. The use of an aPTT reagent that is insensitive to LA for specific factor assays is another way to solve this problem.

Other Methods for Detecting Lupus Anticoagulant

The dilute prothrombin time (dPT) (also known as the tissue thromboplastin inhibition test [TTIT]) is essentially a prothrombin time assay done with diluted tissue factor–phospholipid complex. It can be performed with standard or recombinant tissue factor.[295,296] The results are expressed as a ratio of the patient-to-control clotting times.

The kaolin clotting time (KCT) depends on the ability of aPL antibodies to block the coagulant activity of trace amounts of phospholipid present in centrifuged plasma. Some authors maintain that the KCT–LA test reflects dependence on prothrombin as a cofactor and is less likely to be associated with thrombosis than the dRVVT, which appears to be more dependent on β_2GPI.[297,298] The hexagonal phase array test is based on a prior idea that aPL antibodies recognize phosphatidyl ethanolamine directly in the hexagonal phase array configuration but not in the lamellar phase. Although this assay remains in use, the correction of the prolonged clotting time with hexagonal phase phosphatidyl ethanolamine is probably similar to the confirmatory step used in the other LA assays, that is, a result of the excess of phospholipid in the reaction.

The textarin/ecarin test depends on the difference in phospholipid dependence of coagulation mechanisms triggered by two snake venoms: textarin, which activates prothrombin via a phospholipid-dependent pathway, and ecarin, which activates prothrombin directly without phospholipid.[296]

Annexin A5 Resistance Assay

In addition to the various LA tests, there is a coagulation test that reports on a thrombogenic mechanism—resistance to annexin A5 anticoagulant activity.[80] This assay has been correlated with an immunoassay for IgG antibodies against domain I of β_2GPI.[52] The assay has two stages: a first, in which a tissue factor-phospholipid suspension is exposed to test plasma, and a second, in which the washed suspension is used to coagulate pooled normal plasma in the presence and absence of annexin A5. Patients with annexin A5 resistance show a less-than-expected annexin

A5 anticoagulant effect, reported as a reduction in the annexin A5 anticoagulant ratio. In contrast to the lupus "anticoagulant" effect, this assay measures and reports a procoagulant effect for the antibodies.[70] (*Disclosure: One of the authors (J.H.R.) is inventor of this assay, U.S. Patents #6284475 and #7252959.*)

DIFFERENTIAL DIAGNOSIS

Chapters 133 and 134 address the general subject of vascular thrombosis and its differential diagnosis. When vascular occlusion occurs in the setting of a known autoimmune disorder such as SLE, the possibility of a vasculitis, rather than a thrombotic condition, should be considered. Patients with CAPS may, at first, appear to have other multisystem vasoocclusive disorders, such as thrombotic thrombocytopenic purpura or disseminated vasculitis, and may also manifest laboratory findings of disseminated intravascular coagulation.

The differential diagnosis of a prolonged aPTT includes hereditary and acquired coagulation factor deficiencies, inhibitors to coagulation proteins (e.g., acquired hemophilia A; Chap. 128), and the presence, or use, of anticoagulants. The diagnosis of LA is substantiated through plasma mixing studies and specific factor assays. A positive immunoassay for aPL—that is, aCL and/or anti-β_2GPI antibodies—helps confirm the diagnosis.

When an elevated level aPL antibody level is detected, the clinician must exclude the possibility of an infectious etiology for the antibodies; these occur frequently in syphilis, Lyme disease, HIV-1, and hepatitis C. Occasional patients may have artifactually elevated antibodies from increased polyclonal immunoglobulin levels.[299] In such cases, diagnosis is aided by specific tests for suspected infection, quantitative measurement of serum immunoglobulins, and subtraction of background controls using uncoated microtiter wells. Antipsychotic or other medications should be excluded as causative agents.

PREGNANCY COMPLICATIONS

A systematic review of treatments given to maintain pregnancy in women with prior miscarriages and APS concluded that combined unfractionated heparin and aspirin may reduce pregnancy loss by 54 percent compared to aspirin alone.[300] Three trials of aspirin alone showed no significant reduction in pregnancy loss[300]; intravenous immunoglobulin, whether in combination with or without unfractionated heparin (UFH) and aspirin, was associated with an increased risk of pregnancy loss or premature birth when compared to UFH or low-molecular-weight heparin (LMWH) combined with aspirin.

Taking together the available data, women with a history of three or more spontaneous pregnancy losses and evidence of aPL antibodies should be treated with a combination of low-dose aspirin (75 to 81 mg/day) and prophylactic doses of UFH (i.e., 5000 U every 12 hours subcutaneously). Treatment should be started as soon as pregnancy is documented and continued until delivery so as to reduce the rate of late complications.[183,301] In especially high-risk situations, induction of early delivery may be necessary. Unfractionated heparin at the prophylactic dosage of 5000 U q12h subcutaneously should be started approximately 4 to 6 hours after delivery, if significant bleeding has ceased, and continued at least until the patient is fully ambulatory. Many physicians recommend continuing prophylactic therapy for 6 weeks after delivery even if the patients have not experienced thrombosis. For patients who experienced thromboembolism, prophylaxis by heparin or oral anticoagulant therapy is warranted for at least 6 weeks after delivery.

Although treatment with LMWH has become widely used for recurrent fetal loss as a replacement for prophylactic dose UFH, a prospective randomized controlled trial has questioned the benefit of LMWH treatment versus aspirin therapy. In the LMWH/aspirin group 35/47 (77.8%) had a livebirth, and in the aspirin group 34/43 (79.1 percent) had a livebirth (p = 0.7).[302]

The presence of positive aPL laboratory assays alone is not an indication for treatment in pregnant women without a history of spontaneous pregnancy losses, other attributable pregnancy complications, thrombosis, or SLE. Therefore, the inclusion of aPL tests in routine prenatal testing panels should be discouraged.

Although prednisone was reported to possibly improve the outcome of pregnancy in women with APS, those benefits are associated with significant toxicity.[303] Glucocorticoids or intravenous IgG should be considered only for patients who are refractory to anticoagulant therapy, who have a severe immune thrombocytopenia or a significant contraindication to heparin therapy. Treatment with the combination of prednisone and heparin is associated with an increased risk of osteopenia and vertebral fractures.[304]

THERAPY, COURSE, AND PROGNOSIS

There is general agreement that APS patients with recurrent spontaneous thrombosis require long-term, and perhaps lifelong, anticoagulant therapy and APS patients with recurrent spontaneous pregnancy losses require antithrombotic therapy for most of the gestational period. There are differences of opinion among experts regarding the approaches to treatment of patients with a single thrombotic event, patients with a history of thrombotic events in the distant past (>5 years), patients with stroke, and patients with thrombotic events that were associated with a provocative factor such as trauma, surgery, stasis, pregnancy, and estrogens.

THROMBOSIS

The accumulated evidence from randomized controlled trials indicates that patients with APS and thrombosis should be treated with warfarin for the long-term, and maintained at a therapeutic international normalized ratio (INR) of 2.0 to 3.0.[305] Patients with arterial thrombosis may require a higher anticoagulant intensity as a retrospective study showed that a higher intensity (INR >3.0) was necessary for preventing recurrences in this group of patients, but this issue is controversial.[306] Two other studies reported no benefit for high-intensity warfarin but the number of patients with arterial thrombosis was not high.[299,305] The issue of appropriate antithrombotic treatment of aPL-associated stroke is even more controversial. One major study concluded that there was no benefit for warfarin anticoagulation compared to aspirin therapy.[307]

For patients treated acutely with intravenous UFH, care must be taken to determine whether the patient has a preexisting LA that can interfere with aPTT monitoring of heparin levels. This problem can be circumvented by using an LA-insensitive aPTT reagent or be avoided by treatment, where appropriate, with a LMWH.

An important practical consequence of the LA effect is that prothrombin time and INR results can be artifactually elevated in some patients with APS and LAs treated with warfarin anticoagulant therapy.[308] A multicenter study reported that all but one of the commercial thromboplastins in use at nine centers provided acceptable INR values for APS patients with LA.[309] New thromboplastins should be checked for their responsiveness to LA prior to their use in monitoring oral anticoagulant treatment in patients with APS. Chromogenic factor X (CFX) assays can be used as an alternative to INR for APS patients, especially in patients with a prolonged baseline prothrombin time prior to initiating warfarin therapy, those who are persistently positive for LA and those patients who continue to have recurrent venous thromboembolism

(VTE).[310] Therapeutic CFX values range from 20 to 40 percent; thus, a CFX of 40 percent would approximate an INR of 2.0, and a CFX of 20 percent would approximate an INR of 3.0.

New oral anticoagulants (NOACs), either direct factor Xa or thrombin inhibitors, are effective for treatment of VTE.[311] However, their use specifically in APS patients has not been thoroughly evaluated. In two recent case studies, NOACs have failed to prevent thrombosis in APS patients. Of six APS patients studied, five suffered recurrent VTE and one suffered a recurrent TIA after transitioning to NOACs.[312,313] At the time of writing, a prospective randomized controlled trial of warfarin versus rivaroxaban named "RAPS" (Rivaroxaban in Antiphospholipid Syndrome) is ongoing in patients with thrombotic APS (study ISRCTN68222801). Until the trial is concluded (expected completion in 2015), caution should be applied in using NOACs for APS patients.

Fibrinolytic treatment has been reported for patients with primary APS and extensive thrombosis of the common femoral and iliac veins extending to the lower vena cava,[314] acute ischemic stroke,[315] and acute myocardial infarction.[316]

The antimalarial drug hydroxychloroquine (HCQ) is associated with reduced risk of thrombosis in patients with APS[271–273,317–319] and SLE.[319–321] The potential effectiveness of this treatment has been supported by an animal model for aPL thrombosis[322] and by a recent report that HCQ directly disrupts aPL IgG–β_2GPI complexes,[323] and also reverses the aPL antibody-mediated disruption of annexin A5 binding on phospholipid bilayers[324] and on human placental syncitiotrophoblasts.[325] In a longitudinal cohort study consisting of 272 patients with the APS and 152 taking HCQ (17 of 272 patients on warfarin, 203 were on prednisolone, 112 on azathioprine, 38 on aspirin) investigators found fewer thrombotic complications for patients on HCQ (odds ratio [OR] 0.17, 95% confidence interval [CI] 0.07 to 0.44; p <0.0001).[326] In asymptomatic aPL antibody-positive patients with SLE, primary prophylaxis with aspirin and HCQ appeared to reduce the frequency of thrombotic events.[327] A published prospective, nonrandomized study compared oral anticoagulant plus HCQ versus oral anticoagulant alone. In this study, 30 percent (6/20) of patients had a thrombotic event if they were on oral anticoagulant alone, despite therapeutic range INR, versus no thrombotic events in the oral anticoagulant plus HCQ group (0/20). This study, however, was limited given the small number of patients studied and short followup.[328] Recently, the natural 4-aminoquinolone, quinine, was shown in vitro to disrupt the immune complexes bound to phospholipid layers.[329] However, both HCQ and quinine will require clinical testing in appropriately designed clinical trials. A prospective randomized controlled trial comparing HCQ to placebo in aPL-positive patients without a prior history for thrombosis is currently in progress.

Other proposed treatments for APS include statins, rituximab and vitamin D. Statins have immunomodulatory, antiinflammatory and antithrombotic properties that may benefit APS patients. In recent studies, APS patients treated with statins demonstrated downregulation of tissue factor and reduced proinflammatory/prothrombotic markers such as interleukin-1β, vascular endothelial growth factor, tumor necrosis factor α, interferon-inducible protein 10, and soluble CD40L.[330,331] It has been suggested that a B-cell inhibitor such rituximab may be useful in reducing aPL antibody titers in APS patients. The Rituximab in Antiphospholipid Syndrome (RITAPS) trial did not show reduction in aPL antibody profiles by rituximab; however, rituximab may be effective in controlling noncriteria manifestations of APS.[332] Because low vitamin D levels correlate with arterial and venous thrombosis as well as noncriteria APS manifestations,[333–335] it is recommended that vitamin D deficiency (<10 to 20 ng/mL) and insufficiency (<30 ng/mL) be corrected in aPL antibody-positive patients.[336]

Conventional anticoagulant therapy is usually not sufficient for treatment of CAPS; these patients require aggressive treatment because of the high mortality.[176] Treatment for CAPS is directed toward the thrombotic events and suppression of the cytokine cascade. This includes anticoagulation with heparin and immunosuppressive therapy in the form of high-dose glucocorticoids. A triple therapy strategy of anticoagulation, glucocorticoids, and either intravenous immunoglobulin or plasma exchange or both has improved outcomes. Cyclophosphamide is recommended for patients with CAPS and inflammatory features of SLE or high-titer aPL antibodies. Rituximab may be useful in refractory or relapsing cases of CAPS.[178]

PREGNANCY COMPLICATIONS

The current approach to treating pregnant women with APS and recurrent pregnancy losses or the other aPL antibody–associated complications of pregnancy includes daily low-dose aspirin (75 to 81 mg/day) and either UFH or LMWH.[300,337,338] Although clinical studies have shown efficacy with UFH, most clinicians treat with LMWH because it has a better pharmacokinetic profile and a lower risk of heparin-induced thrombocytopenia and osteopenia. Heparin is then withheld when labor begins or 24 hours prior to a cesarean section. Anticoagulation is resumed 6 weeks postpartum because of the increased risk of VTE in this time period.[301] Interestingly, the current standard of care for pregnant APS patients is based on two randomized controlled trials conducted prior to 2000 that included only 150 patients. Newer trials show conflicting results, with some showing no difference in prevention of pregnancy loss in APS patients receiving aspirin alone versus aspirin and LMWH,[302] and others showing a small benefit.[339] With this management, the likelihood of a good pregnancy outcome in women with APS has been estimated to be approximately 75 to 80 percent.

Other treatment modalities such as glucocorticoids or intravenous IgG (IVIG) should be considered only for patients who are refractory to anticoagulant therapy, who have a severe immune thrombocytopenia, or who have a significant contraindication to heparin therapy. The addition of glucocorticoids has shown no clear benefits and has been associated with premature rupture of membranes or preeclampsia; however, a newer study showed that for patients with refractory APS, the addition of low-dose prednisolone (10 mg) from time of a positive pregnancy test up to 14 weeks' gestation may help to increase livebirth rates.[340] Although the addition of IVIG has not been shown to be superior to heparin and aspirin in large multicenter clinical trials,[341] it has shown some efficacy in patients with refractory APS in small case studies.[342,343]

REFERENCES

1. Hughes GR: The anticardiolipin syndrome. *Clin Exp Rheumatol* 3:285–286, 1985.
2. Harris EN, Hughes GRV, Gharavi AE: The antiphospholipid antibody syndrome. *J Rheumatol Suppl* 13:210, 1987.
3. Simioni P, Prandoni P, Zanon E, et al: Deep venous thrombosis and lupus anticoagulant. A case-control study. *Thromb Haemost* 76:187–189, 1996.
4. Ginsberg JS, Wells PS, Brill-Edwards P, et al: Antiphospholipid antibodies and venous thromboembolism. *Blood* 86:3685–3691, 1995.
5. Out HJ, Bruinse HW, Christiaens GC, et al: Prevalence of antiphospholipid antibodies in patients with fetal loss. *Ann Rheum Dis* 50:553–557, 1991.
6. Shapiro SS, Thiagarajan P: Lupus anticoagulants. *Prog Hemost Thromb* 6:263–285, 1982.
7. Shapiro SS: Lupus anticoagulants and anticardiolipin antibodies: Personal reminiscences, a little history, and some random thoughts. *J Thromb Haemost* 3:831–833, 2005.
8. Asherson RA: The primary, secondary, catastrophic, and seronegative variants of the antiphospholipid syndrome: A personal history long in the making. *Semin Thromb Hemost* 34:227–235, 2008.
9. Moore JE, Mohr CF: Biologically false positive serological tests for syphilis: Type, incidence, and cause. *JAMA* 150:467–473, 1952.
10. Moore JE, Lutz WB: Natural history of systemic lupus erythematosus: Approach to its study through chronic biologic false positive reactors. *J Chronic Dis* 1:297–316, 1955.
11. Bell WN, Alton HG: A brain extract as a substitute for platelet suspensions in the thromboplastin generation test. *Nature* 174:880–881, 1955.
12. Conley CL, Hartmann RC: A hemorrhagic disorder caused by circulating anticoagulant in patients with disseminated lupus erythematousus. *J Clin Invest* 31:621, 1952.

13. Feinstein DI, Rapaport SI: Acquired inhibitors of blood coagulation, in *Progress in Hemostasis and Thrombosis*, edited by TH Spaet pp 75–95. Grune & Stratton, New York, 1972.

14. Beaumont JL: Acquired hemorrhagic syndrome caused by a circulating anticoagulant; inhibition of the thromboplastic function of the blood platelets; description of a specific test. *Sang* 25:1–15, 1954.

15. Nilsson IM, Astedt B, Hedner U, Berezin D: Intrauterine death and circulating anticoagulant ("antithromboplastin"). *Acta Med Scand* 197:153–159, 1975.

16. Bowie EJ, Thompson JH Jr, Pascuzzi CA, Owen GA Jr: Thrombosis in systemic erythematosus despite circulating anticoagulants. *J Clin Invest* 62:416–430, 1963.

17. Harris EN, Gharavi AE, Boey ML, et al: Anticardiolipin antibodies: Detection by radioimmunoassay and association with thrombosis in systemic lupus erythematosus. *Lancet* 2:1211–1214, 1983.

18. Miyakis S, Lockshin MD, Atsumi T, et al: International consensus statement on an update of the classification criteria for definite antiphospholipid syndrome (APS). *J Thromb Haemost* 4:295–306, 2006.

19. Lieby P, Soley A, Knapp AM, et al: Memory B cells producing somatically mutated antiphospholipid antibodies are present in healthy individuals. *Blood* 102:2459–2465, 2003.

20. Giles I, Lambrianides A, Rahman A: Examining the non-linear relationship between monoclonal antiphospholipid antibody sequence, structure and function. *Lupus* 17:895–903, 2008.

21. Cruz-Tapias P, Blank M, Anaya JM, Shoenfeld Y: Infections and vaccines in the etiology of antiphospholipid syndrome. *Curr Opin Rheumatol* 24:389–393, 2012.

22. Barcat D, Constans J, Seigneur M, et al: Deep venous thrombosis in an adult with varicella. *Rev Med Interne* 19:509–511, 1998.

23. Peyton BD, Cutler BS, Stewart FM: Spontaneous tibial artery thrombosis associated with varicella pneumonia and free protein S deficiency. *J Vasc Surg* 27:563–567, 1998.

24. Prieto J, Yuste JR, Beloqui O, et al: Anticardiolipin antibodies in chronic hepatitis C: Implication of hepatitis C virus as the cause of the antiphospholipid syndrome [see comments]. *Hepatology* 23:199–204, 1996.

25. Cojocaru IM, Cojocaru M, Iacob SA: High prevalence of anticardiolipin antibodies in patients with asymptomatic hepatitis C virus infection associated acute ischemic stroke. *Rom J Intern Med* 43:89–95, 2005.

26. Labarca JA, Rabaggliati RM, Radrigan FJ, et al: Antiphospholipid syndrome associated with cytomegalovirus infection: Case report and review. *Clin Infect Dis* 24:197–200, 1997.

27. Delbos V, Abgueguen P, Chennebault JM, et al: Acute cytomegalovirus infection and venous thrombosis: Role of antiphospholipid antibodies. *J Infect* 54:e47–e50, 2007.

28. Loizou S, Cazabon JK, Walport MJ, et al: Similarities of specificity and cofactor dependence in serum antiphospholipid antibodies from patients with human parvovirus B19 infection and from those with systemic lupus erythematosus. *Arthritis Rheum* 40:103–108, 1997.

29. Martin E, Winn R, Nugent K: Catastrophic antiphospholipid syndrome in a community-acquired methicillin-resistant *Staphylococcus aureus* infection: A review of pathogenesis with a case for molecular mimicry. *Autoimmun Rev* 10:181–188, 2011.

30. Galrao L, Brites C, Atta ML, et al: Antiphospholipid antibodies in HIV-positive patients. *Clin Rheumatol* 26:1825–1830, 2007.

31. Blank M, Aron-Maor A, Shoenfeld Y: From rheumatic fever to Libman-Sacks endocarditis: Is there any possible pathogenetic link? *Lupus* 14:697–701, 2005.

32. Gotoh M, Matsuda J: Induction of anticardiolipin antibody and/or lupus anticoagulant in rabbits by immunization with lipoteichoic acid, lipopolysaccharide and lipid A. *Lupus* 5:593–597, 1996.

33. Eschwege V, Freyssinet JM: The possible contribution of cell apoptosis and necrosis to the generation of phospholipid-binding antibodies. *Ann Med Interne (Paris)* 147(Suppl 1):33–35, 1996.

34. Price BE, Rauch J, Shia MA, et al: Anti-phospholipid autoantibodies bind to apoptotic, but not viable, thymocytes in a beta 2-glycoprotein I-dependent manner. *J Immunol* 157:2201–2208, 1996.

35. Pittoni V, Isenberg D: Apoptosis and antiphospholipid antibodies. *Semin Arthritis Rheum* 28:163–178, 1998.

36. Inic-Kanada A, Stojanovic M, Zivkovic I, et al: Murine monoclonal antibody 26 raised against tetanus toxoid cross-reacts with beta2-glycoprotein I: Its characteristics and role in molecular mimicry. *Am J Reprod Immunol* 61:39–51, 2009.

37. Blank M, Asherson RA, Cervera R, Shoenfeld Y: Antiphospholipid syndrome infectious origin. *J Clin Immunol* 24:12–23, 2004.

38. Gharavi AE, Pierangeli SS, Espinola RG, et al: Antiphospholipid antibodies induced in mice by immunization with a cytomegalovirus-derived peptide cause thrombosis and activation of endothelial cells in vivo. *Arthritis Rheum* 46:545–552, 2002.

39. Hellan M, Kuhnel E, Speiser W, et al: Familial lupus anticoagulant: A case report and review of the literature. *Blood Coagul Fibrinolysis* 9:195–200, 1998.

40. Weber M, Hayem G, DeBandt M, et al: The family history of patients with primary or secondary antiphospholipid syndrome (APS). *Lupus* 9:258–263, 2000.

41. Garcia CO, Kanbour-Shakir A, Tang H, et al: Induction of experimental antiphospholipid antibody syndrome in PL/J mice following immunization with beta 2 GPI. *Am J Reprod Immunol* 37:118–124, 1997.

42. Holers VM, Girardi G, Mo L, et al: Complement C3 activation is required for antiphospholipid antibody-induced fetal loss. *J Exp Med* 195:211–220, 2002.

43. Pierangeli SS, Liu X, Espinola R, et al: Functional analyses of patient-derived IgG monoclonal anticardiolipin antibodies using in vivo thrombosis and in vivo microcirculation models. *Thromb Haemost* 84:388–395, 2000.

44. Jankowski M, Vreys I, Wittevrongel C, et al: Thrombogenicity of beta 2-glycoprotein I-dependent antiphospholipid antibodies in a photochemically induced thrombosis model in the hamster. *Blood* 101:157–162, 2003.

45. Arad A, Proulle V, Furie RA, et al: Beta(2)-Glycoprotein-1 autoantibodies from patients with antiphospholipid syndrome are sufficient to potentiate arterial thrombus formation in a mouse model. *Blood* 117:3453–3459, 2011.

46. Loizou S, Singh S, Wypkema E, Asherson RA: Anticardiolipin, anti-beta(2)-glycoprotein I and antiprothrombin antibodies in black South African patients with infectious disease. *Ann Rheum Dis* 62:1106–1111, 2003.

47. Roubey RA, Pratt CW, Buyon JP, Winfield JB: Lupus anticoagulant activity of autoimmune antiphospholipid antibodies is dependent upon beta 2-glycoprotein I. *J Clin Invest* 90:1100–1104, 1992.

48. Galli M, Comfurius P, Maassen C, et al: Anticardiolipin antibodies (ACA) directed not to cardiolipin but to a plasma protein cofactor. *Lancet* 335:1544–1547, 1990.

49. McNeil HP, Simpson RJ, Chesterman CN, Krilis SA: Anti-phospholipid antibodies are directed against a complex antigen that includes a lipid-binding inhibitor of coagulation: Beta 2-glycoprotein I (apolipoprotein H). *Proc Natl Acad Sci U S A* 87:4120–4124, 1990.

50. Goldsmith GH, Pierangeli SS, Branch DW, et al: Inhibition of prothrombin activation by antiphospholipid antibodies and beta 2-glycoprotein 1. *Br J Haematol* 87:548–554, 1994.

51. de Laat HB, Derksen RH, Urbanus RT, de Groot PG: IgG antibodies that recognize epitope Gly40-Arg43 in domain I of beta 2-glycoprotein I cause LAC, and their presence correlates strongly with thrombosis. *Blood* 105:1540–1545, 2005.

52. de Laat B, Wu XX, van Lummel M, et al: Correlation between antiphospholipid antibodies that recognize domain i of β_2-glycoprotein I and a reduction in the anticoagulant activity of annexin A5. *Blood* 109:1490–1494, 2007.

53. Hunt BJ, Wu XX, de Laat B, et al: Association of anti-β_2GPI domain I IgG and resistance to annexin A5 with obstetrical antiphospholipid syndrome: Evidence for a specific mechanism in a patient subset. *ASH Annual Meeting Abstracts* 112:3821, 2008.

54. Hunt BJ, Wu XX, de LB, et al: Resistance to annexin A5 anticoagulant activity in women with histories for obstetric antiphospholipid syndrome. *Am J Obstet Gynecol* 205:485.e17–485.e23, 2011.

55. Agar C, van Os GM, Mörgelin M, et al: Beta-2-glycoprotein I can exist in 2 conformations: Implications for our understanding of the antiphospholipid syndrome. *Blood* 116:1336–1343, 2010.

56. Balasubramanian K, Maiti SN, Schroit AJ: Recruitment of beta-2-glycoprotein 1 to cell surfaces in extrinsic and intrinsic apoptosis. *Apoptosis* 10:439–446, 2005.

57. Maiti SN, Balasubramanian K, Ramoth JA, Schroit AJ: Beta-2-glycoprotein 1-dependent macrophage uptake of apoptotic cells. Binding to lipoprotein receptor-related protein receptor family members. *J Biol Chem* 283:3761–3766, 2008.

58. Matsuura E, Kobayashi K, Matsunami Y, Lopez LR: The immunology of atherothrombosis in the antiphospholipid syndrome: Antigen presentation and lipid intracellular accumulation. *Autoimmun Rev* 8:500–505, 2009.

59. Agar C, de Groot PG, Morgelin M, et al: Beta2-glycoprotein I: A novel component of innate immunity. *Blood* 117:6939–6947, 2011.

60. Hulstein JJ, Lenting PJ, de Laat B, et al: Beta2-Glycoprotein I inhibits von Willebrand factor dependent platelet adhesion and aggregation. *Blood* 110:1483–1491, 2007.

61. Bu C, Gao L, Xie W, et al: Beta2-glycoprotein i is a cofactor for tissue plasminogen activator-mediated plasminogen activation. *Arthritis Rheum* 60:559–568, 2009.

62. Ma K, Simantov R, Zhang JC, et al: High affinity binding of beta 2-glycoprotein I to human endothelial cells is mediated by annexin II. *J Biol Chem* 275:15541–15548, 2000.

63. Sheng Y, Reddel SW, Herzog H, et al: Impaired thrombin generation in beta 2-glycoprotein I null mice. *J Biol Chem* 276:13817–13821, 2001.

64. Robertson SA, Roberts CT, van Beijering E, et al: Effect of beta2-glycoprotein I null mutation on reproduction outcome and antiphospholipid antibody mediated pregnancy pathology in mice. *Mol Hum Reprod* 10:409–416, 2004.

65. de-Groot PG, Horbach DA, Derksen RH: Protein C and other cofactors involved in the binding of antiphospholipid antibodies: Relation to the pathogenesis of thrombosis. *Lupus* 5:488–493, 1996.

66. Atsumi T, Khamashta MA, Amengual O, et al: Binding of anticardiolipin antibodies to protein C via beta2-glycoprotein I (beta2-GPI): A possible mechanism in the inhibitory effect of antiphospholipid antibodies on the protein C system. *Clin Exp Immunol* 112:325–333, 1998.

67. Bidot CJ, Jy W, Horstman LL, et al: Factor VII/VIIa: A new antigen in the anti-phospholipid antibody syndrome. *Br J Haematol* 120:618–626, 2003.

68. Ortona E, Capozzi A, Colasanti T, et al: Vimentin/cardiolipin complex as a new antigenic target of the antiphospholipid syndrome. *Blood* 116:2960–2967, 2010.

69. Shibata S, Harpel PC, Gharavi A, et al: Autoantibodies to heparin from patients with antiphospholipid antibody syndrome inhibit formation of antithrombin III-thrombin complexes. *Blood* 83:2532–2540, 1994.

70. Lieby P, Soley A, Levallois H, et al: The clonal analysis of anticardiolipin antibodies in a single patient with primary antiphospholipid syndrome reveals an extreme antibody heterogeneity. *Blood* 97:3820–3828, 2001.

71. Andree HAM, Hermens WT, Hemker HC, Willems GM: Displacement of factor Va by annexin V, in Phospholipid Binding and Anticoagulant Action of Annexin V, edited by HAM Andree, pp 73–85. Universitaire Pers Maastricht, Maastricht, The Netherlands, 1992.

72. Reviakine I, Bergsma-Schutter W, Brisson A: Growth of protein 2-D crystals on supported planar lipid bilayers imaged in situ by AFM. *J Struct Biol* 121:356–361, 1998.

73. Krikun G, Lockwood CJ, Wu XX, et al: The expression of the placental anticoagulant protein, annexin V, by villous trophoblasts: Immunolocalization and in vitro regulation. *Placenta* 15:601–612, 1994.

74. Ueki H, Mizushina T, Laoharatchatathanin T, et al: Loss of maternal annexin A5 increases the likelihood of placental platelet thrombosis and foetal loss. *Sci Rep* 2:827, 2012.

75. Wang X, Campos B, Kaetzel MA, Dedman JR: Annexin V is critical in the maintenance of murine placental integrity. *Am J Obstet Gynecol* 180:1008–1016, 1999.

76. Rand JH, Wu XX, Andree HA, et al: Pregnancy loss in the antiphospholipid-antibody syndrome—A possible thrombogenic mechanism. *N Engl J Med* 337:154–160, 1997.

77. van Heerde WL, Poort S, van 't Veer C, et al: Binding of recombinant annexin V to endothelial cells: Effect of annexin V binding on endothelial-cell-mediated thrombin formation. *Biochem J* 302:305–312, 1994.

78. Rand JH, Wu XX, Andree HAM, et al: Antiphospholipid antibodies accelerate plasma coagulation by inhibiting annexin-V binding to phospholipids: A "lupus procoagulant" phenomenon. *Blood* 92:1652–1660, 1998.

79. Rand JH, Wu XX, Quinn AS, et al: Human monoclonal antiphospholipid antibodies disrupt the annexin A5 anticoagulant crystal shield on phospholipid bilayers: Evidence from atomic force microscopy and functional assay. *Am J Pathol* 163:1193–1200, 2003.

80. Rand JH, Wu XX, Lapinski R, et al: Detection of antibody-mediated reduction of annexin A5 anticoagulant activity in plasmas of patients with the antiphospholipid syndrome. *Blood* 104:2783–2790, 2004.

81. Wu XX, Pierangeli SS, Rand JH: Resistance to annexin A5 binding and anticoagulant activity in plasmas from patients with the antiphospholipid syndrome but not with syphilis. *J Thromb Haemost* 4:271–273, 2006.

82. Hanly JG, Smith SA: Anti-beta2-glycoprotein I (GPI) autoantibodies, annexin V binding and the anti-phospholipid syndrome. *Clin Exp Immunol* 120:537–543, 2000.

83. Tomer A: Antiphospholipid antibody syndrome: Rapid, sensitive, and specific flow cytometric assay for determination of anti-platelet phospholipid autoantibodies. *J Lab Clin Med* 139:147–154, 2002.

84. Tomer A, Bar-Lev S, Fleisher S, et al: Antiphospholipid antibody syndrome: The flow cytometric annexin A5 competition assay as a diagnostic tool. *Br J Haematol* 139:113–120, 2007.

85. Gaspersic N, Ambrozic A, Bozic B, et al: Annexin A5 binding to giant phospholipid vesicles is differentially affected by anti-beta2-glycoprotein I and anti-annexin A5 antibodies. *Rheumatology* 46:81–86, 2007.

86. Rand JH, Wu XX, Guller S, et al: Reduction of annexin-V (placental anticoagulant protein-I) on placental villi of women with antiphospholipid antibodies and recurrent spontaneous abortion. *Am J Obstet Gynecol* 171:1566–1572, 1994.

87. Cederholm A, Svenungsson E, Jensen-Urstad K, et al: Decreased binding of annexin V to endothelial cells: A potential mechanism in atherothrombosis of patients with systemic lupus erythematosus. *Arterioscler Thromb Vasc Biol* 25:198–203, 2005.

88. Dueymes M, Levy Y, Ziporen L, et al: Do some antiphospholipid antibodies target endothelial cells? *Ann Med Interne (Paris)* 147(Suppl 1):22–23, 1996.

89. Del-Papa N, Raschi E, Catelli L, et al: Endothelial cells as a target for antiphospholipid antibodies: Role of anti-beta 2 glycoprotein I antibodies. *Am J Reprod Immunol* 38:212–217, 1997.

90. Matsuda J, Gotoh M, Gohchi K, et al: Anti-endothelial cell antibodies to the endothelial hybridoma cell line (EAhy926) in systemic lupus erythematosus patients with antiphospholipid antibodies. *Br J Haematol* 97:227–232, 1997.

91. Navarro M, Cervera R, Teixido M, et al: Antibodies to endothelial cells and to beta 2-glycoprotein I in the antiphospholipid syndrome: Prevalence and isotype distribution. *Br J Rheumatol* 35:523–528, 1996.

92. Simantov R, Lo SK, Gharavi A, et al: Antiphospholipid antibodies activate vascular endothelial cells. *Lupus* 5:440–441, 1996.

93. Meroni PL, Papa ND, Beltrami B, et al: Modulation of endothelial cell function by anti-phospholipid antibodies. *Lupus* 5:448–450, 1996.

94. Cockrell E, Espinola RG, McCrae KR: Annexin A2: Biology and relevance to the anti-phospholipid syndrome. *Lupus* 17:943–951, 2008.

95. Romay-Penabad Z, Montiel-Manzano MG, Shilagard T, et al: Annexin A2 is involved in antiphospholipid antibody-mediated pathogenic effects in vitro and in vivo. *Blood* 114:3074–3083, 2009.

96. Raschi E, Borghi MO, Grossi C, et al: Toll-like receptors: Another player in the pathogenesis of the anti-phospholipid syndrome. *Lupus* 17:937–942, 2008.

97. Xie H, Sheng L, Zhou H, Yan J: The role of TLR4 in pathophysiology of antiphospholipid syndrome-associated thrombosis and pregnancy morbidity. *Br J Haematol* 164:165–176, 2014.

98. Brandt KJ, Fickentscher C, Boehlen F, et al: NF-kappaB is activated from endosomal compartments in antiphospholipid antibodies-treated human monocytes. *J Thromb Haemost* 12:779–791, 2014.

99. Raschi E, Testoni C, Bosisio D, et al: Role of the MyD88 transduction signaling pathway in endothelial activation by antiphospholipid antibodies. *Blood* 101:3495–3500, 2003.

100. Vega-Ostertag ME, Ferrara DE, Romay-Penabad Z, et al: Role of p38 mitogen-activated protein kinase in antiphospholipid antibody-mediated thrombosis and endothelial cell activation. *J Thromb Haemost* 5:1828–1834, 2007.

101. Cesarman-Maus G, Rios-Luna NP, Deora AB, et al: Autoantibodies against the fibrinolytic receptor, annexin 2, in antiphospholipid syndrome. *Blood* 107:4375–4382, 2006.

102. Chen PP, Yang CD, Ede K, et al: Some antiphospholipid antibodies bind to hemostasis and fibrinolysis proteases and promote thrombosis. *Lupus* 17:916–921, 2008.

103. Cugno M, Cabibbe M, Galli M, et al: Antibodies to tissue-type plasminogen activator (tPA) in patients with antiphospholipid syndrome: Evidence of interaction between the antibodies and the catalytic domain of tPA in 2 patients. *Blood* 103:2121–2126, 2004.

104. Ames PR, Tommasino C, Iannaccone L, et al: Coagulation activation and fibrinolytic imbalance in subjects with idiopathic antiphospholipid antibodies—A crucial role for acquired free protein S deficiency. *Thromb Haemost* 76:190–194, 1996.

105. Schousboe I, Rasmussen MS: Synchronized inhibition of the phospholipid mediated autoactivation of factor XII in plasma by beta 2-glycoprotein I and anti-beta 2-glycoprotein I. *Thromb Haemost* 73:798–804, 1995.

106. Sacre SM, Stannard AK, Owen JS: Apolipoprotein E (apoE) isoforms differentially induce nitric oxide production in endothelial cells. *FEBS Lett* 540:181–187, 2003.

107. Yang XV, Banerjee Y, Fernandez JA, et al: Activated protein C ligation of ApoER2 (LRP8) causes Dab1-dependent signaling in U937 cells. *Proc Natl Acad Sci U S A* 106:274–279, 2009.

108. Shi T, Giannakopoulos B, Yan X, et al: Anti-beta2-glycoprotein I antibodies in complex with beta2-glycoprotein I can activate platelets in a dysregulated manner via glycoprotein Ib-IX-V. *Arthritis Rheum* 54:2558–2567, 2006.

109. Lutters BC, Derksen RH, Tekelenburg WL, et al: Dimers of beta 2-glycoprotein I increase platelet deposition to collagen via interaction with phospholipids and the apolipoprotein E receptor 2′. *J Biol Chem* 278:33831–33838, 2003.

110. Graham A, Ford I, Morrison R, et al: Anti-endothelial antibodies interfere in apoptotic cell clearance and promote thrombosis in patients with antiphospholipid syndrome. *J Immunol* 182:1756–1762, 2009.

111. Sammaritano LR: Significance of aPL IgG subclasses. *Lupus* 5:436–439, 1996.

112. Salmon JE, Girardi G, Holers VM: Complement activation as a mediator of antiphospholipid antibody induced pregnancy loss and thrombosis. *Ann Rheum Dis* 61(Suppl 2):ii46–ii50, 2002.

113. Salmon JE, Girardi G: The role of complement in the antiphospholipid syndrome. *Curr Dir Autoimmun* 7:133–148, 2004.

114. Girardi G, Redecha P, Salmon JE: Heparin prevents antiphospholipid antibody-induced fetal loss by inhibiting complement activation. *Nat Med* 10:1222–1226, 2004.

115. Redecha P, Tilley R, Tencati M, et al: Tissue factor: A link between C5a and neutrophil activation in antiphospholipid antibody induced fetal injury. *Blood* 110:2423–2431, 2007.

116. Redecha P, Franzke CW, Ruf W, et al: Neutrophil activation by the tissue factor/Factor VIIa/PAR2 axis mediates fetal death in a mouse model of antiphospholipid syndrome. *J Clin Invest* 118:3453–3461, 2008.

117. Zhou H, Wolberg AS, Roubey RA: Characterization of monocyte tissue factor activity induced by IgG antiphospholipid antibodies and inhibition by dilazep. *Blood* 104:2353–2358, 2004.

118. Roubey RA: New approaches to prevention of thrombosis in the antiphospholipid syndrome: Hopes, trials, and tribulations. *Arthritis Rheum* 48:3004–3008, 2003.

119. Martini F, Farsi A, Gori AM, et al: Antiphospholipid antibodies (aPL) increase the potential monocyte procoagulant activity in patients with systemic lupus erythematosus. *Lupus* 5:206–211, 1996.

120. Bu C, Gao L, Xie W, et al: Beta2-glycoprotein i is a cofactor for tissue plasminogen activator-mediated plasminogen activation. *Arthritis Rheum* 60:559–568, 2009.

121. Riewald M, Ruf W: Protease-activated receptor-1 signaling by activated protein C in cytokine-perturbed endothelial cells is distinct from thrombin signaling. *J Biol Chem* 280:19808–19814, 2005.

122. Niessen F, Furlan-Freguia C, Fernandez JA, et al: Endogenous EPCR/aPC-PAR1 signaling prevents inflammation-induced vascular leakage and lethality. *Blood* 113:2859–2866, 2009.

123. Nojima J, Kuratsune H, Suehisa E, et al: Acquired activated protein C resistance associated with IgG antibodies against beta2-glycoprotein I and prothrombin as a strong risk factor for venous thromboembolism. *Clin Chem* 51:545–552, 2005.

124. de Laat B, Eckmann CM, van SM, et al: Correlation between the potency of a beta2-glycoprotein I-dependent lupus anticoagulant and the level of resistance to activated protein C. *Blood Coagul Fibrinolysis* 19:757–764, 2008.

125. Hurtado V, Montes R, Gris JC, et al: Autoantibodies against EPCR are found in antiphospholipid syndrome and are a risk factor for fetal death. *Blood* 104:1369–1374, 2004.

126. Proulle V, Furie RA, Merrill-Skoloff G, Furie BC: Platelets are required for enhanced activation of the endothelium and fibrinogen in a mouse thrombosis model of APS. *Blood* 124:611–622, 2014.

127. Lin YL, Wang CT: Activation of human platelets by the rabbit anticardiolipin antibodies. *Blood* 80:3135–3143, 1992.

128. van Lummel M, Pennings MT, Derksen RH, et al: The binding site in (beta)2-glycoprotein I for ApoER2′ on platelets is located in domain V. *J Biol Chem* 280:36729–36736, 2005.

129. Forastiero RR, Martinuzzo ME, Broze GJ: High titers of autoantibodies to tissue factor pathway inhibitor are associated with the antiphospholipid syndrome. *J Thromb Haemost* 1:718–724, 2003.

130. Witztum JL, Horkko S: The role of oxidized LDL in atherogenesis: Immunological response and anti-phospholipid antibodies. *Ann N Y Acad Sci* 811:88–96, 1997.

131. Vaarala O: Antiphospholipid antibodies and atherosclerosis. *Lupus* 5:442–447, 1996.

132. Lopez LR, Kobayashi K, Matsunami Y, Matsuura E: Immunogenic oxidized low-density lipoprotein/beta2-glycoprotein i complexes in the diagnostic management of atherosclerosis. *Clin Rev Allergy Immunol* 37:12–19, 2009.

133. Canaud G, Bienaime F, Tabarin F, et al: Inhibition of the mTORC pathway in the antiphospholipid syndrome. *N Engl J Med* 371:303–312, 2014.

134. Krnic BS, O'Connor CR, Looney SW, et al: A retrospective review of 61 patients with antiphospholipid syndrome. Analysis of factors influencing recurrent thrombosis. *Arch Intern Med* 157:2101–2108, 1997.

135. Martinelli I, Cattaneo M, Panzeri D, et al: Risk factors for deep venous thrombosis of the upper extremities. *Ann Intern Med* 126:707–711, 1997.

136. Provenzale JM, Ortel TL, Allen NB: Systemic thrombosis in patients with antiphospholipid antibodies: Lesion distribution and imaging findings. *AJR Am J Roentgenol* 170:285–290, 1998.

137. Poux JM, Boudet R, Lacroix P, et al: Renal infarction and thrombosis of the infrarenal aorta in a 35-year-old man with primary antiphospholipid syndrome. *Am J Kidney Dis* 27:721–725, 1996.

138. Kojima E, Naito K, Iwai M, et al: Antiphospholipid syndrome complicated by thrombosis of the superior mesenteric artery, co-existence of smooth muscle hyperplasia. *Intern Med* 36:528–531, 1997.

139. Girolami A, Zanon E, Zanardi S, et al: Thromboembolic disease developing during oral contraceptive therapy in young females with antiphospholipid antibodies. *Blood Coagul Fibrinolysis* 7:497–501, 1996.

140. Montaruli B, Borchiellini A, Tamponi G, et al: Factor V Arg506—>Gln mutation in patients with antiphospholipid antibodies. *Lupus* 5:303–306, 1996.

141. Simantov R, Lo SK, Salmon JE, et al: Factor V Leiden increases the risk of thrombosis in patients with antiphospholipid antibodies. *Thromb Res* 84:361–365, 1996.

142. Schutt M, Kluter H, Hagedorn GM, et al: Familial coexistence of primary antiphospholipid syndrome and factor V Leiden. *Lupus* 7:176–182, 1998.

143. Brenner B, Vulfsons SL, Lanir N, Nahir M: Coexistence of familial antiphospholipid syndrome and factor V Leiden: Impact on thrombotic diathesis. *Br J Haematol* 94:166–167, 1996.

144. Pengo V, Ruffatti A, Legnani C, et al: Incidence of a first thromboembolic event in asymptomatic carriers of high-risk antiphospholipid antibody profile: A multicenter prospective study. *Blood* 118:4714–4718, 2011.

145. Schulman S, Svenungsson E, Granqvist S: Anticardiolipin antibodies predict early recurrence of thromboembolism and death among patients with venous thromboembolism following anticoagulant therapy. Duration of Anticoagulation Study Group. *Am J Med* 104:332–338, 1998.

146. Finazzi G, Brancaccio V, Moia M, et al: Natural history and risk factors for thrombosis in 360 patients with antiphospholipid antibodies: A four-year prospective study from the Italian Registry. *Am J Med* 100:530–536, 1996.

147. Gezer S: Antiphospholipid syndrome. *Dis Mon* 49:696–741, 2003.

148. Gladd DA, Olech E: Antiphospholipid antibodies in rheumatoid arthritis: Identifying the dominoes. *Curr Rheumatol Rep* 11:43–51, 2009.

149. Fauchais AL, Lambert M, Launay D, et al: Antiphospholipid antibodies in primary Sjogren's syndrome: Prevalence and clinical significance in a series of 74 patients. *Lupus* 13:245–248, 2004.

150. Shoenfeld Y, Meroni PL: The beta-2-glycoprotein I and antiphospholipid antibodies. *Clin Exp Rheumatol* 10:205–209, 1992.

151. Yun YY, Yoh KA, Yang HI, et al: A case of Budd-Chiari syndrome with high antiphospholipid antibody in a patient with systemic lupus erythematosus. *Korean J Intern Med* 11:82–86, 1996.

152. Hofbauer LC, Spitzweg C, Heufelder AE: Graves' disease associated with the primary antiphospholipid syndrome. *J Rheumatol* 23:1435–1437, 1996.

153. Chun WH, Bang D, Lee SK: Antiphospholipid syndrome associated with progressive systemic sclerosis. *J Dermatol* 23:347–351, 1996.

154. Frolow M, Jankowski M, Swadzba J, Musial J: Evan's syndrome with antiphospholipid-protein antibodies. *Pol Merkur Lekarski* 1:344–345, 1996.

155. Yokoi K, Hosoi E, Akaike M, et al: Takayasu's arteritis associated with antiphospholipid antibodies. Report of two cases. *Angiology* 47:315–319, 1996.

156. Dasgupta B, Almond MK, Tanqueray A: Polyarteritis nodosa and the antiphospholipid syndrome. *Br J Rheumatol* 36:1210–1212, 1997.

157. Cervera R, Boffa MC, Khamashta MA, Hughes GR: The Euro-Phospholipid project: Epidemiology of the antiphospholipid syndrome in Europe. *Lupus* 18:889–893, 2009.

158. Bucciarelli S, Espinosa G, Cervera R: The CAPS Registry: Morbidity and mortality of the catastrophic antiphospholipid syndrome. *Lupus* 18:905–912, 2009.

159. Urbanus RT, Siegerink B, Roest M, et al: Antiphospholipid antibodies and risk of myocardial infarction and ischaemic stroke in young women in the RATIO study: A case-control study. *Lancet Neurol* 8:998–1005, 2009.

160. Levine SR, Deegan MJ, Futrell N, Welch KM: Cerebrovascular and neurologic disease associated with antiphospholipid antibodies: 48 cases. *Neurology* 40:1181–1189, 1990.

161. Weingarten K, Filippi C, Barbut D, Zimmerman RD: The neuroimaging features of the cardiolipin antibody syndrome. *Clin Imaging* 21:6–12, 1997.

162. Carhuapoma JR, Mitsias P, Levine SR: Cerebral venous thrombosis and anticardiolipin antibodies. *Stroke* 28:2363–2369, 1997.

163. Deschiens MA, Conard J, Horellou MH, et al: Coagulation studies, factor V Leiden, and anticardiolipin antibodies in 40 cases of cerebral venous thrombosis. *Stroke* 27:1724–1730, 1996.

164. Nagai S, Horie Y, Akai T, et al: Superior sagittal sinus thrombosis associated with primary antiphospholipid syndrome—Case report. *Neurol Med Chir (Tokyo)* 38:34–39, 1998.

165. Tanasescu R, Nicolau A, Caraiola S, et al: Antiphospholipid antibodies and migraine: A retrospective study of 428 patients with inflammatory connective tissue diseases. *Rom J Intern Med* 45:355–363, 2007.

166. Ong MS, Kohane IS, Cai T, et al: Population-level evidence for an autoimmune etiology of epilepsy. *JAMA Neurol* 71:569–574, 2014.

167. Brey RL, Escalante A: Neurological manifestations of antiphospholipid antibody syndrome. *Lupus* 7(Suppl 2):S67–S74, 1998.

168. Matsushita T, Kanda F, Yamada H, Chihara K: Recurrent acute transverse myelopathy: An 83-year-old man with antiphospholipid syndrome. *Rinsho Shinkeigaku* 37:987–991, 1997.

169. Ruiz AG, Guzman RJ, Flores FJ, Garay MJ: Refractory hiccough heralding transverse myelitis in the primary antiphospholipid syndrome. *Lupus* 7:49–50, 1998.

170. Takamura Y, Morimoto S, Tanooka A, Yoshikawa J: Transverse myelitis in a patient with primary antiphospholipid syndrome—A case report. *No To Shinkei* 48:851–855, 1996.

171. Campi A, Filippi M, Comi G, Scotti G: Recurrent acute transverse myelopathy associated with anticardiolipin antibodies. *AJNR Am J Neuroradiol* 19:781–786, 1998.

172. Smyth AE, Bruce IN, McMillan SA, Bell AL: Transverse myelitis: A complication of systemic lupus erythematosus that is associated with the antiphospholipid syndrome. *Ulster Med J* 65:91–94, 1996.

173. Mok CC, Lau CS, Chan EY, Wong RW: Acute transverse myelopathy in systemic lupus erythematosus: Clinical presentation, treatment, and outcome. *J Rheumatol* 25:467–473, 1998.

174. Sugiyama Y, Yamamoto T: Characterization of serum anti-phospholipid antibodies in patients with multiple sclerosis. *Tohoku J Exp Med* 178:203–215, 1996.

175. Schwartz M, Rochas M, Weller B, et al: High association of anticardiolipin antibodies with psychosis. *J Clin Psychiatry* 59:20–23, 1998.

176. Espinosa G, Bucciarelli S, Asherson RA, Cervera R: Morbidity and mortality in the catastrophic antiphospholipid syndrome: Pathophysiology, causes of death, and prognostic factors. *Semin Thromb Hemost* 34:290–294, 2008.

177. Erkan D, Cervera R, Asherson RA: Catastrophic antiphospholipid syndrome: Where do we stand? *Arthritis Rheum* 48:3320–3327, 2003.

178. Cervera R, Rodriguez-Pinto I, Colafrancesco S, et al: 14th International Congress on Antiphospholipid Antibodies Task Force report on catastrophic antiphospholipid syndrome. *Autoimmun Rev* 13:699–707, 2014.

179. Bucciarelli S, Espinosa G, Cervera R, et al: Mortality in the catastrophic antiphospholipid syndrome: Causes of death and prognostic factors in a series of 250 patients. *Arthritis Rheum* 54:2568–2576, 2006.

180. Lockshin MD: Pregnancy loss and antiphospholipid antibodies. *Lupus* 7(Suppl 2):S86–S89, 1998.

181. Saha SP, Bhattacharjee N, Ganguli RP, et al: Prevalence and significance of antiphospholipid antibodies in selected at-risk obstetrics cases: A comparative prospective study. *J Obstet Gynaecol* 29:614–618, 2009.

182. Ruffatti A, Calligaro A, Hoxha A, et al: Laboratory and clinical features of pregnant women with antiphospholipid syndrome and neonatal outcome. *Arthritis Care Res (Hoboken)* 62:302–307, 2010.

183. Rai R: Obstetric management of antiphospholipid syndrome. *J Autoimmun* 15:203–207, 2000.

184. Rai R, Regan L: Obstetric complications of antiphospholipid antibodies. *Curr Opin Obstet Gynecol* 9:387–390, 1997.

185. Saha SP, Bhattacharjee N, Ganguli RP, et al: Prevalence and significance of antiphospholipid antibodies in selected at-risk obstetrics cases: A comparative prospective study. *J Obstet Gynaecol* 29:614–618, 2009.

186. Ruffatti A, Calligaro A, Hoxha A, et al: Laboratory and clinical features of pregnant women with antiphospholipid syndrome and neonatal outcome. *Arthritis Care Res (Hoboken)* 62:302–307, 2010.

187. Ornstein MH, Rand JH: An association between refractory HELLP syndrome and antiphospholipid antibodies during pregnancy; a report of 2 cases. *J Rheumatol* 21:1360–1364, 1994.

188. Neuwelt CM, Daikh DI, Linfoot JA, et al: Catastrophic antiphospholipid syndrome: Response to repeated plasmapheresis over three years. *Arthritis Rheum* 40:1534–1539, 1997.

189. Ramsey-Goldman R, Kutzer JE, Kuller LH, et al: Pregnancy outcome and anti-cardiolipin antibody in women with systemic lupus erythematosus. *Am J Epidemiol* 138:1057–1069, 1993.

190. Chauleur C, Galanaud JP, Alonso S, et al: Observational study of pregnant women with a previous spontaneous abortion before the 10th gestation week with and without antiphospholipid antibodies. *J Thromb Haemost* 8:699–706, 2010.

191. Bergrem A, Jacobsen EM, Skjeldestad FE, et al: The association of antiphospholipid antibodies with pregnancy-related first time venous thrombosis—A population-based case-control study. *Thromb Res* 125:e222–e227, 2010.

192. Locatelli A, Patane L, Ghidini A, et al: Pathology findings in preterm placentas of women with autoantibodies: A case-control study. *J Matern Fetal Neonatal Med* 11:339–344, 2002.

193. Salafia CM, Cowchock FS: Placental pathology and antiphospholipid antibodies: A descriptive study. *Am J Perinatol* 14:435–441, 1997.

194. Salafia CM, Parke AL: Placental pathology in systemic lupus erythematosus and phospholipid antibody syndrome. *Rheum Dis Clin North Am* 23:85–97, 1997.

195. Sauer R, Roussev R, Jeyendran RS, Coulam CB: Prevalence of antiphospholipid antibodies among women experiencing unexplained infertility and recurrent implantation failure. *Fertil Steril* 93:2441–2443, 2010.

196. de Jesus GR, Rodrigues G, de Jesus NR, Levy RA: Pregnancy morbidity in antiphospholipid syndrome: What is the impact of treatment? *Curr Rheumatol Rep* 16:403, 2014.

197. Practice Committee of American Society for Reproductive Medicine. Anti-phospholipid antibodies do not affect IVF success. *Fertil Steril* 90(5 Suppl):S172–S173, 2008.

198. Kriseman YL, Nash JW, Hsu S: Criteria for the diagnosis of antiphospholipid syndrome in patients presenting with dermatologic symptoms. *J Am Acad Dermatol* 57:112–115, 2007.

199. Gibson GE, Su WP, Pittelkow MR: Antiphospholipid syndrome and the skin. *J Am Acad Dermatol* 36:970–982, 1997.

200. Asherson RA, Cervera R: The antiphospholipid syndrome: Multiple faces beyond the classical presentation. *Autoimmun Rev* 2:140–151, 2003.

201. Aronoff DM, Callen JP: Necrosing livedo reticularis in a patient with recurrent pulmonary hemorrhage. *J Am Acad Dermatol* 37:300–302, 1997.

202. Greco TP, Conti-Kelly AM, Matsuura E, et al: Antiphospholipid antibodies in patients with coronary artery disease: New cardiac risk factors? *Ann N Y Acad Sci* 1108:466–474, 2007.

203. Vaarala O: Antiphospholipid antibodies and myocardial infarction. *Lupus* 7(Suppl 2): S132–S134, 1998.

204. Sherer Y, Shoenfeld Y: Antiphospholipid antibodies: Are they pro-atherogenic or an epiphenomenon of atherosclerosis? *Immunobiology* 207:13–16, 2003.

205. Ludia C, Domenico P, Monia C, et al: Antiphospholipid antibodies: A new risk factor for restenosis after percutaneous transluminal coronary angioplasty? *Autoimmunity* 27:141–148, 1998.

206. Chambers-JD J, Haire HD, Deligonul U: Multiple early percutaneous transluminal coronary angioplasty failures related to lupus anticoagulant. *Am Heart J* 132:189–190, 1996.

207. Ames PR, Antinolfi I, Scenna G, et al: Atherosclerosis in thrombotic primary antiphospholipid syndrome. *J Thromb Haemost* 7:537–542, 2009.

208. Niaz A, Butany J: Antiphospholipid antibody syndrome with involvement of a bioprosthetic heart valve. *Can J Cardiol* 14:951–954, 1998.

209. Bouillanne O, Millaire A, de Groote P, et al: Prevalence and clinical significance of antiphospholipid antibodies in heart valve disease: A case-control study. *Am Heart J* 132:790–795, 1996.

210. Nesher G, Ilany J, Rosenmann D, Abraham AS: Valvular dysfunction in antiphospholipid syndrome: Prevalence, clinical features, and treatment. *Semin Arthritis Rheum* 27:27–35, 1997.

211. Hojnik M, George J, Ziporen L, Shoenfeld Y: Heart valve involvement (Libman-Sacks endocarditis) in the antiphospholipid syndrome. *Circulation* 93:1579–1587, 1996.

212. Bulckaen HG, Puisieux FL, Bulckaen ED, et al: Antiphospholipid antibodies and the risk of thromboembolic events in valvular heart disease. *Mayo Clin Proc* 78:294–298, 2003.

213. Ziporen L, Goldberg I, Arad M, et al: Libman-Sacks endocarditis in the antiphospholipid syndrome: Immunopathologic findings in deformed heart valves. *Lupus* 5:196–205, 1996.

214. Lee RW, Taylor-LM J, Landry GJ, et al: Prospective comparison of infrainguinal bypass grafting in patients with and without antiphospholipid antibodies. *J Vasc Surg* 24:524–531, 1996.

215. Porres-Aguilar M, Pena-Ruiz MA, Burgos JD, et al: Chronic thromboembolic pulmonary hypertension as an uncommon presentation of primary antiphospholipid syndrome. *J Natl Med Assoc* 100:734–736, 2008.

216. Karmochkine M, Cacoub P, Dorent R, et al: High prevalence of antiphospholipid antibodies in precapillary pulmonary hypertension. *J Rheumatol* 23:286–290, 1996.

217. Bonderman D, Wilkens H, Wakounig S, et al: Risk factors for chronic thromboembolic pulmonary hypertension. *Eur Respir J* 33:325–331, 2009.

218. Asherson RA: The catastrophic antiphospholipid syndrome, 1998. A review of the clinical features, possible pathogenesis and treatment. *Lupus* 7(Suppl 2):S55–S62, 1998.

219. Uthman I, Khamashta M: The abdominal manifestations of the antiphospholipid syndrome. *Rheumatology (Oxford)* 46:1641–1647, 2007.

220. Biron C, Andreani H, Blanc P, et al: Prevalence of antiphospholipid antibodies in patients with chronic liver disease related to alcohol or hepatitis C virus: Correlation with liver injury. *J Lab Clin Med* 131:243–250, 1998.

221. Sene D, Piette JC, Cacoub P: Antiphospholipid antibodies, antiphospholipid syndrome and infections. *Autoimmun Rev* 7:272–277, 2008.

222. Ramos-Casals M, Cervera R, Lagrutta M, et al: Clinical features related to antiphospholipid syndrome in patients with chronic viral infections (hepatitis C virus/HIV infection): Description of 82 cases. *Clin Infect Dis* 38:1009–1016, 2004.

223. Hoffman M, Burke M, Fried M, et al: Primary biliary cirrhosis associated with antiphospholipid syndrome. *Isr J Med Sci* 33:681–686, 1997.

224. Date K, Shirai Y, Hatakeyama K: Antiphospholipid antibody syndrome presenting as acute acalculous cholecystitis. *Am J Gastroenterol* 92:2127–2128, 1997.

225. Dessailloud R, Papo T, Vaneecloo S, et al: Acalculous ischemic gallbladder necrosis in the catastrophic antiphospholipid syndrome. *Arthritis Rheum* 41:1318–1320, 1998.

226. Kalman DR, Khan A, Romain PL, Nompleggi DJ: Giant gastric ulceration associated with antiphospholipid antibody syndrome. *Am J Gastroenterol* 91:1244–1247, 1996.

227. Gul A, Inanc M, Ocal L, et al: Primary antiphospholipid syndrome associated with mesenteric inflammatory veno-occlusive disease. *Clin Rheumatol* 15:207–210, 1996.

228. Lee HJ, Park JW, Chang JC: Mesenteric and portal venous obstruction associated with primary antiphospholipid antibody syndrome. *J Gastroenterol Hepatol* 12:822–826, 1997.

229. Galli M, Finazzi G, Barbui T: Thrombocytopenia in the antiphospholipid syndrome. *Br J Haematol* 93:1–5, 1996.

230. Cuadrado MJ, Mujic F, Munoz E, Khamashta MA, Hughes GR: Thrombocytopenia in the antiphospholipid syndrome. *Ann Rheum Dis* 56:194–196, 1997.

231. Macchi L, Rispal P, Clofent SG, et al: Anti-platelet antibodies in patients with systemic lupus erythematosus and the primary antiphospholipid antibody syndrome: Their relationship with the observed thrombocytopenia. *Br J Haematol* 98:336–341, 1997.

232. Pierrot-Deseilligny DC, Michel M, Khellaf M, et al: Antiphospholipid antibodies in adults with immune thrombocytopenic purpura. *Br J Haematol* 142:638–643, 2008.

233. Lipp E, von-Felten A, Sax H, Muller D, Berchtold P: Antibodies against platelet glycoproteins and antiphospholipid antibodies in autoimmune thrombocytopenia. *Eur J Haematol* 60:283–288, 1998.

234. Diz-Kucukkaya R, Hacihanefioglu A, Yenerel M, et al: Antiphospholipid antibodies and antiphospholipid syndrome in patients presenting with immune thrombocytopenic purpura: A prospective cohort study. *Blood* 98:1760–1764, 2001.

235. Vivaldi P, Rossetti G, Galli M, Finazzi G: Severe bleeding due to acquired hypoprothrombinemia-lupus anticoagulant syndrome. Case report and review of literature. *Haematologica* 82:345–347, 1997.

236. Hudson N, Duffy CM, Rauch J, Paquin JD, Esdaile JM: Catastrophic haemorrhage in a case of paediatric primary antiphospholipid syndrome and factor II deficiency. *Lupus* 6:68–71, 1997.

237. Dunn JP, Noorily SW, Petri M, et al: Antiphospholipid antibodies and retinal vascular disease. *Lupus* 5:313–322, 1996.

238. Coniglio M, Platania A, Di Nucci GD, et al: Antiphospholipid-protein antibodies are not an uncommon feature in retinal venous occlusions. *Thromb Res* 83:183–188, 1996.

239. Glacet BA, Bayani N, Chretien P, et al: Antiphospholipid antibodies in retinal vascular occlusions. A prospective study of 75 patients. *Arch Ophthalmol* 112:790–795, 1994.

240. Dori D, Gelfand YA, Brenner B, Miller B: Cilioretinal artery occlusion: An ocular complication of primary antiphospholipid syndrome. *Retina* 17:555–557, 1997.

241. Reino S, Munoz RF, Cervera R, et al: Optic neuropathy in the "primary" antiphospholipid syndrome: Report of a case and review of the literature. *Clin Rheumatol* 16:629–631, 1997.

242. Au A, O'Day J: Review of severe vaso-occlusive retinopathy in systemic lupus erythematosus and the antiphospholipid syndrome: Associations, visual outcomes, complications and treatment. *Clin Experiment Ophthalmol* 32:87–100, 2004.

243. Fakhouri F, Noel LH, Zuber J, et al: The expanding spectrum of renal diseases associated with antiphospholipid syndrome. *Am J Kidney Dis* 41:1205–1211, 2003.

244. Nochy D, Daugas E, Droz D, et al: The intrarenal vascular lesions associated with primary antiphospholipid syndrome. *J Am Soc Nephrol* 10:507–518, 1999.

245. Breda L, Nozzi M, De SS, Chiarelli F: Laboratory tests in the diagnosis and follow-up of pediatric rheumatic diseases: An update. *Semin Arthritis Rheum* 40:53–72, 2010.

246. Avcin T, Cimaz R, Silverman ED, et al: Pediatric antiphospholipid syndrome: Clinical and immunologic features of 121 patients in an international registry. *Pediatrics* 122:e1100–e1107, 2008.

247. Falcini F, Taccetti G, Ermini M, Trapani S, Matucci CM: Catastrophic antiphospholipid antibody syndrome in pediatric systemic lupus erythematosus. *J Rheumatol* 24: 389–392, 1997.

248. Ol'binskaia LI, Poptsov VN, Gofman AM: [Hemodynamic changes in patients with myocardial infarct complicated by acute left ventricular failure during combined nitroglycerin and dobutamine therapy] [in Russian]. *Kardiologiia* 31:49–51, 1991.

249. Boffa MC, Lachassinne E: Infant perinatal thrombosis and antiphospholipid antibodies: A review. *Lupus* 16:634–641, 2007.

250. Motta M, Chirico G, Rebaioli CB, et al: Anticardiolipin and anti-beta2 glycoprotein I antibodies in infants born to mothers with antiphospholipid antibody-positive autoimmune disease: A follow-up study. *Am J Perinatol* 23:247–251, 2006.

251. Mekinian A, Lachassinne E, Nicaise-Roland P, et al: European registry of babies born to mothers with antiphospholipid syndrome. *Ann Rheum Dis* 72:217–222, 2013.

252. Brewster JA, Shaw NJ, Farquharson RG: Neonatal and pediatric outcome of infants born to mothers with antiphospholipid syndrome. *J Perinat Med* 27:183–187, 1999.

253. Nacinovich R, Galli J, Bomba M, et al: Neuropsychological development of children born to patients with antiphospholipid syndrome. *Arthritis Rheum* 59:345–351, 2008.

254. Marie I, Levesque H, Heron F, et al: Acute adrenal failure secondary to bilateral infarction of the adrenal glands as the first manifestation of primary antiphospholipid antibody syndrome. *Ann Rheum Dis* 56:567–568, 1997.

255. Espinosa G, Santos E, Cervera R, et al: Adrenal involvement in the antiphospholipid syndrome: Clinical and immunologic characteristics of 86 patients. *Medicine (Baltimore)* 82:106–118, 2003.

256. Paydas S, Kocak R, Zorludemir S, Baslamisli F: Bone marrow necrosis in antiphospholipid syndrome. *J Clin Pathol* 50:261–262, 1997.

257. Pengo V, Tripodi A, Reber G, et al: Update of the guidelines for measuring the presence of Lupus Anticoagulant. *J Thromb Haemost* 7:1737–1740, 2009.

258. de Groot PG, Derksen RH, de LB: Twenty-two years of failure to set up undisputed assays to detect patients with the antiphospholipid syndrome. *Semin Thromb Hemost* 34:347–355, 2008.

259. Favaloro EJ: Variability and diagnostic utility of antiphospholipid antibodies including lupus anticoagulants. *Int J Lab Hematol* 35:269–274, 2013.

260. Mateo J, Oliver A, Borrell M, et al: Laboratory evaluation and clinical characteristics of 2,132 consecutive unselected patients with venous thromboembolism—results of the Spanish Multicentric Study on Thrombophilia (EMET-Study). *Thromb Haemost* 77:444–451, 1997.

261. Naarendorp M, Spiera H: Sudden sensorineural hearing loss in patients with systemic lupus erythematosus or lupus-like syndromes and antiphospholipid antibodies. *J Rheumatol* 25:589–592, 1998.

262. Galli M, Luciani D, Bertolini G, Barbui T: Anti-beta 2-glycoprotein I, antiprothrombin antibodies, and the risk of thrombosis in the antiphospholipid syndrome. *Blood* 102:2717–2723, 2003.

263. Shah NM, Khamashta MA, Atsumi T, Hughes GR: Outcome of patients with anticardiolipin antibodies: A 10 year follow-up of 52 patients. *Lupus* 7:3–6, 1998.

264. Silver RM, Porter TF, van Leeuween I, et al: Anticardiolipin antibodies: Clinical consequences of "low titers." *Obstet Gynecol* 87:494–500, 1996.

265. Tuhrim S, Rand JH, Wu XX, et al: Elevated anticardiolipin antibody titer is a stroke risk factor in a multiethnic population independent of isotype or degree of positivity. *Stroke* 30:1561–1565, 1999.

266. Brey RL, Stallworth CL, McGlasson DL, et al: Antiphospholipid antibodies and stroke in young women. *Stroke* 33:2396–2400, 2002.

267. Merrill JT, Shen C, Gugnani M, et al: High prevalence of antiphospholipid antibodies in patients taking procainamide. *J Rheumatol* 24:1083–1088, 1997.

268. El-Rayes BF, Edelstein M: Unusual case of antiphospholipid antibody syndrome presenting with extensive cutaneous infarcts in a patient on long-term procainamide therapy. *Am J Hematol* 72:154, 2003.

269. Karmochkine M, Piette JC, Mazoyer E, et al: Antiphospholipid antibodies: Cause of thrombosis or an epiphenomenon? *Presse Med* 24:267–270, 1995.

270. Delluc A, Rousseau A, Le GM, et al: Prevalence of antiphospholipid antibodies in psychiatric patients users and non-users of antipsychotics. *Br J Haematol* 164:272–279, 2014.

271. Amengual O, Atsumi T, Khamashta MA, et al: Specificity of ELISA for antibody to beta 2-glycoprotein I in patients with antiphospholipid syndrome. *Br J Rheumatol* 35:1239–1243, 1996.

272. Alarcon-Segovia D, Mestanza M, Cabiedes J, Cabral AR: The antiphospholipid/cofactor syndromes. II. A variant in patients with systemic lupus erythematosus with antibodies to beta 2-glycoprotein I but no antibodies detectable in standard antiphospholipid assays. *J Rheumatol* 24:1545–1551, 1997.

273. Cabral AR, Amigo MC, Cabiedes J, Alarcon-Segovia D: The antiphospholipid/cofactor syndromes: A primary variant with antibodies to beta 2-glycoprotein I but no antibodies detectable in standard antiphospholipid assays. *Am J Med* 101:472–481, 1996.

274. Sanmarco M, Soler C, Christides C, et al: Prevalence and clinical significance of IgG isotype anti-beta 2-glycoprotein I antibodies in antiphospholipid syndrome: A comparative study with anticardiolipin antibodies. *J Lab Clin Med* 129:499–506, 1997.

275. Day HM, Thiagarajan P, Ahn C, et al: Autoantibodies to beta2-glycoprotein I in systemic lupus erythematosus and primary antiphospholipid antibody syndrome: Clinical correlations in comparison with other antiphospholipid antibody tests. *J Rheumatol* 25:667–674, 1998.

276. Reber G, Schousboe I, Tincani A, et al: Inter-laboratory variability of anti-beta2-glycoprotein I measurement. A collaborative study in the frame of the European Forum on Antiphospholipid Antibodies Standardization Group. *Thromb Haemost* 88:66–73, 2002.

277. Hoxha A, Ruffatti A, Pittoni M, et al: The clinical significance of autoantibodies directed against prothrombin in primary antiphospholipid syndrome. *Clin Chim Acta* 413:911–913, 2012.

278. Lopez LR, Dier KJ, Lopez D, et al: Anti-beta 2-glycoprotein I and antiphosphatidylserine antibodies are predictors of arterial thrombosis in patients with antiphospholipid syndrome. *Am J Clin Pathol* 121:142–149, 2004.

279. Audrain MA, El-Kouri D, Hamidou MA, et al: Value of autoantibodies to beta(2)-glycoprotein 1 in the diagnosis of antiphospholipid syndrome. *Rheumatology (Oxford)* 41:550–553, 2002.

280. Sanfelippo MJ, Joshi A, Schwartz S, et al: Antibodies to phosphatidylserine/prothrombin complex in suspected antiphospholipid syndrome in the absence of antibodies to cardiolipin or beta-2-glycoprotein I. *Lupus* 22:1349–1352, 2013.

281. Sciascia S, Khamashta MA, Bertolaccini ML: New tests to detect antiphospholipid antibodies: Antiprothrombin (aPT) and anti-phosphatidylserine/prothrombin (aPS/PT) antibodies. *Curr Rheumatol Rep* 16:415, 2014.

282. Berard M, Chantome R, Marcelli A, Boffa MC: Antiphosphatidylethanolamine antibodies as the only antiphospholipid antibodies. I. Association with thrombosis and vascular cutaneous diseases. *J Rheumatol* 23:1369–1374, 1996.

283. Rauch J, Janoff AS: Antibodies against phospholipids other than cardiolipin: Potential roles for both phospholipid and protein. *Lupus* 5:498–502, 1996.

284. Yetman DL, Kutteh WH: Antiphospholipid antibody panels and recurrent pregnancy loss: Prevalence of anticardiolipin antibodies compared with other antiphospholipid antibodies. *Fertil Steril* 66:540–546, 1996.

285. de Maistre E, Gobert B, Bene MC, et al: Comparative assessment of phospholipid-binding antibodies indicates limited overlapping. *J Clin Lab Anal* 10:6–12, 1996.

286. Branch DW, Silver R, Pierangeli S, et al: Antiphospholipid antibodies other than lupus anticoagulant and anticardiolipin antibodies in women with recurrent pregnancy loss, fertile controls, and antiphospholipid syndrome. *Obstet Gynecol* 89:549–555, 1997.

287. Staub HL, Bertolaccini ML, Khamashta MA: Anti-phosphatidylethanolamine antibody, thromboembolic events and the antiphospholipid syndrome. *Autoimmun Rev* 12:230–234, 2012.

288. Shapiro SS: The lupus anticoagulant/antiphospholipid syndrome. *Annu Rev Med* 47:533–553, 1996.

289. Triplett DA: Antiphospholipid-protein antibodies: Clinical use of laboratory test results (identification, predictive value, treatment). *Haemostasis* 26 Suppl 4:358–367, 1996.

290. Nojima J, Suehisa E, Akita N, et al: Risk of arterial thrombosis in patients with anticardiolipin antibodies and lupus anticoagulant. *Br J Haematol* 96:447–450, 1997.

291. Lockshin MD, Kim M, Laskin CA, et al: Prediction of adverse pregnancy outcome by the presence of lupus anticoagulant, but not anticardiolipin antibody, in patients with antiphospholipid antibodies. *Arthritis Rheum* 64:2311–2318, 2012.

292. Somers E, Magder LS, Petri M: Antiphospholipid antibodies and incidence of venous thrombosis in a cohort of patients with systemic lupus erythematosus. *J Rheumatol* 29:2531–2536, 2002.

293. Opatrny L, David M, Kahn SR, Shrier I, Rey E: Association between antiphospholipid antibodies and recurrent fetal loss in women without autoimmune disease: A metaanalysis. *J Rheumatol* 33:2214–2221, 2006.

294. Kitchens CS: Prolonged activated partial thromboplastin time of unknown etiology: A prospective study of 100 consecutive cases referred for consultation. *Am J Hematol* 27:38–45, 1988.

295. Liu HW, Wong KL, Lin CK, et al: The reappraisal of dilute tissue thromboplastin inhibition test in the diagnosis of lupus anticoagulant. *Br J Haematol* 72:229–234, 1989.

296. Forastiero RR, Cerrato GS, Carreras LO: Evaluation of recently described tests for detection of the lupus anticoagulant. *Thromb Haemost* 72:728–733, 1994.

297. Galli M, Barbui T: Prothrombin as cofactor for antiphospholipids. *Lupus* 7(Suppl 2): S37–S40, 1998.

298. Galli M, Finazzi G, Bevers EM, Barbui T: Kaolin clotting time and dilute Russell's viper venom time distinguish between prothrombin-dependent and beta 2-glycoprotein I-dependent antiphospholipid antibodies. *Blood* 86:617–623, 1995.

299. Lenzi R, Rand JH, Spiera H: Anticardiolipin antibodies in pregnant patients with systemic lupus erythematosus. *N Engl J Med* 314:1392–1393, 1986.

300. Empson M, Lassere M, Craig J, Scott J: Prevention of recurrent miscarriage for women with antiphospholipid antibody or lupus anticoagulant. *Cochrane Database Syst Rev* 2:CD002859, 2005.

301. Galli M, Barbui T: Antiphospholipid antibodies and pregnancy. *Best Pract Res Clin Haematol* 16:211–225, 2003.

302. Laskin CA, Spitzer KA, Clark CA, et al: Low molecular weight heparin and aspirin for recurrent pregnancy loss: Results from the randomized, controlled HepASA trial. *J Rheumatol* 36:279–287, 2009.

303. Cowchock S, Reece EA: Do low-risk pregnant women with antiphospholipid antibodies need to be treated? Organizing Group of the Antiphospholipid Antibody Treatment Trial. *Am J Obstet Gynecol* 176:1099–1100, 1997.

304. Cowchock S: Treatment of antiphospholipid syndrome in pregnancy. *Lupus* 7(Suppl 2): S95–S97, 1998.

305. Lim W, Crowther MA, Eikelboom JW: Management of antiphospholipid antibody syndrome: A systematic review. *JAMA* 295:1050–1057, 2006.

306. Khamashta MA, Cuadrado MJ, Mujic F, et al: The management of thrombosis in the antiphospholipid-antibody syndrome. *N Engl J Med* 332:993–997, 1995.

307. Levine SR, Brey RL, Tilley BC, et al: Antiphospholipid antibodies and subsequent thrombo-occlusive events in patients with ischemic stroke. *JAMA* 291:576–584, 2004.

308. Moll S, Ortel TL: Monitoring warfarin therapy in patients with lupus anticoagulants. *Ann Intern Med* 127:177–185, 1997.

309. Tripodi A, Chantarangkul V, Clerici M, et al: Laboratory control of oral anticoagulant treatment by the INR system in patients with the antiphospholipid syndrome and lupus anticoagulant. Results of a collaborative study involving nine commercial thromboplastins. *Br J Haematol* 115:672–678, 2001.

310. Crowl A, Schullo-Feulner A, Moon JY: A review of warfarin monitoring in antiphospholipid syndrome and lupus anticoagulant. *Ann Pharmacother* 48:1479–1483, 2014.

311. Agnelli G, Becattini C, Franco L: New oral anticoagulants for the treatment of venous thromboembolism. *Best Pract Res Clin Haematol* 26:151–161, 2013.

312. Schaefer JK, McBane RD, Black DF, et al: Failure of dabigatran and rivaroxaban to prevent thromboembolism in antiphospholipid syndrome: A case series of three patients. *Thromb Haemost* 112: 947–950, 2014.

313. Win K, Rodgers GM: New oral anticoagulants may not be effective to prevent venous thromboembolism in patients with antiphospholipid syndrome. *Am J Hematol* 89:1017, 2014.

314. Camps GM, Guil M, Sanchez LJ, et al: Fibrinolytic treatment in primary antiphospholipid syndrome. *Lupus* 5:627–629, 1996.

315. Julkunen H, Hedman C, Kauppi M: Thrombolysis for acute ischemic stroke in the primary antiphospholipid syndrome. *J Rheumatol* 24:181–183, 1997.

316. Ho YL, Chen MF, Wu CC, et al: Successful treatment of acute myocardial infarction by thrombolytic therapy in a patient with primary antiphospholipid antibody syndrome. *Cardiology* 87:354–357, 1996.

317. Wallace DJ: The use of chloroquine and hydroxychloroquine for non-infectious conditions other than rheumatoid arthritis or lupus: A critical review. *Lupus* 5(Suppl 1): S59–S64, 1996.

318. Erkan D, Yazici Y, Peterson MG, Sammaritano L, Lockshin MD: A cross-sectional study of clinical thrombotic risk factors and preventive treatments in antiphospholipid syndrome. *Rheumatology (Oxford)* 41:924–929, 2002.

319. Tektonidou MG, Laskari K, Panagiotakos DB, Moutsopoulos HM: Risk factors for thrombosis and primary thrombosis prevention in patients with systemic lupus erythematosus with or without antiphospholipid antibodies. *Arthritis Rheum* 61:29–36, 2009.

320. Petri M: Thrombosis and systemic lupus erythematosus: The Hopkins Lupus Cohort perspective. *Scand J Rheumatol* 25:191–193, 1996.

321. Kaiser R, Cleveland CM, Criswell LA: Risk and protective factors for thrombosis in systemic lupus erythematosus: Results from a large, multi-ethnic cohort. *Ann Rheum Dis* 68:238–241, 2009.

322. Edwards MH, Pierangeli S, Liu X, et al: Hydroxychloroquine reverses thrombogenic properties of antiphospholipid antibodies in mice. *Circulation* 96:4380–4384, 1997.

323. Rand JH, Wu XX, Quinn AS, et al: Hydroxychloroquine directly reduces the binding of antiphospholipid antibody-beta2-glycoprotein I complexes to phospholipid bilayers. *Blood* 112:1687–1695, 2008.

324. Rand JH, Wu XX, Quinn AS, et al: Hydroxychloroquine reverses a procoagulant mechanism for antiphospholipid syndrome: Evidence for a novel effect for an old antimalarial drug. *Blood* 115:2292–2299, 2010.

325. Wu XX, Guller S, Rand JH: Hydroxychloroquine reduces binding of antiphospholipid antibodies to syncytiotrophoblasts and restores annexin A5 expression. *Am J Obstet Gynecol* 205:576.e7–576.e14, 2011.

326. Mok MY, Chan EY, Fong DY, et al: Antiphospholipid antibody profiles and their clinical associations in Chinese patients with systemic lupus erythematosus. *J Rheumatol* 32:622–628, 2005.

327. Wahl DG, Bounameaux H, de MP, Sarasin FP: Prophylactic antithrombotic therapy for patients with systemic lupus erythematosus with or without antiphospholipid antibodies: Do the benefits outweigh the risks? A decision analysis. *Arch Intern Med* 160:2042–2048, 2000.

328. Schmidt-Tanguy A, Voswinkel J, Henrion D, et al: Antithrombotic effects of hydroxychloroquine in primary antiphospholipid syndrome patients. *J Thromb Haemost* 11:1927–1929, 2013.

329. Bezati E, Wu XX, Quinn A, et al: A new trick for an ancient drug: Quinine dissociates antiphospholipid immune complexes. *Lupus* 24:32–41, 2014.

330. Lopez-Pedrera C, Ruiz-Limon P, Aguirre MA, et al: Global effects of fluvastatin on the prothrombotic status of patients with antiphopholipid syndrome. *Ann Rheum Dis* 70:675–682, 2011.

331. Erkan D, Willis R, Murthy VL, et al: A prospective open-label pilot study of fluvastatin on proinflammatory and prothrombotic biomarkers in antiphospholipid antibody positive patients. *Ann Rheum Dis* 73:1176–1180, 2014.

332. Erkan D, Vega J, Ramon G, et al: A pilot open-label phase II trial of rituximab for non-criteria manifestations of antiphospholipid syndrome. *Arthritis Rheum* 65:464–471, 2013.

333. Agmon-Levin N, Blank M, Zandman-Goddard G, et al: Vitamin D: An instrumental factor in the anti-phospholipid syndrome by inhibition of tissue factor expression. *Ann Rheum Dis* 70:145–150, 2011.

334. Andreoli L, Piantoni S, Dall'Ara F, et al: Vitamin D and antiphospholipid syndrome. *Lupus* 21:736–740, 2012.

335. Piantoni S, Andreoli L, Allegri F, et al: Low levels of vitamin D are common in primary antiphospholipid syndrome with thrombotic disease. *Reumatismo* 64:307–313, 2012.

336. Erkan D, Aguiar CL, Andrade D, et al: 14th International Congress on Antiphospholipid Antibodies: Task force report on antiphospholipid syndrome treatment trends. *Autoimmun Rev* 13:685–696, 2014.

337. Kutteh WH: Antiphospholipid antibody-associated recurrent pregnancy loss: Treatment with heparin and low-dose aspirin is superior to low-dose aspirin alone. *Am J Obstet Gynecol* 174:1584–1589, 1996.

338. Rai R, Cohen H, Dave M, Regan L: Randomised controlled trial of aspirin and aspirin plus heparin in pregnant women with recurrent miscarriage associated with phospholipid antibodies (or antiphospholipid antibodies) [see comments]. *BMJ* 314:253–257, 1997.

339. Cohn DM, Goddijn M, Middeldorp S, et al: Recurrent miscarriage and antiphospholipid antibodies: Prognosis of subsequent pregnancy. *J Thromb Haemost* 8:2208–2213, 2010.

340. Bramham K, Thomas M, Nelson-Piercy C, et al: First trimester low-dose prednisolone in refractory antiphospholipid antibody-related pregnancy loss. *Blood* 117:6948–6951, 2011.

341. Dendrinos S, Sakkas E, Makrakis E: Low-molecular-weight heparin versus intravenous immunoglobulin for recurrent abortion associated with antiphospholipid antibody syndrome. *Int J Gynaecol Obstet* 104:223–225, 2009.

342. Sherer Y, Levy Y, Shoenfeld Y: Intravenous immunoglobulin therapy of antiphospholipid syndrome. *Rheumatology* 39:421–426, 2000.

343. Branch DW, Peaceman AM, Druzin M, et al: A multicenter, placebo-controlled pilot study of intravenous immune globulin treatment of antiphospholipid syndrome during pregnancy. The Pregnancy Loss Study Group. *Am J Obstet Gynecol* 182:122–127, 2000.

CHAPTER 132
THROMBOTIC MICROANGIOPATHIES

J. Evan Sadler

SUMMARY

Thrombotic microangiopathy is a general term for the combination of microangiopathic hemolytic anemia and thrombocytopenia, often accompanied by signs and symptoms consistent with disseminated microvascular thrombosis. Thrombotic thrombocytopenic purpura (TTP) refers to thrombotic microangiopathy, without an obvious predisposing condition, and without oliguric renal failure. TTP is caused by autoantibodies to ADAMTS13 (a disintegrin and metalloprotease with a thrombospondin type 1 motif member 13), a plasma metalloprotease that normally cleaves von Willebrand factor (VWF) and regulates VWF-dependent platelet aggregation. Inherited deficiency of ADAMTS13 causes congenital TTP, which typically responds to plasma infusion. Most patients with acquired TTP respond to plasma exchange, although many have relapsing disease. Hemolytic uremic syndrome (HUS) refers to thrombotic microangiopathy that usually causes oliguric or anuric renal failure. Ingestion of *Shiga* toxin-producing *Escherichia coli* can cause the most common or "typical" form of HUS that is usually preceded by bloody diarrhea. Inherited or acquired defects in the regulation of the alternative complement pathway cause HUS referred to as "atypical" because it occurs without a prodrome of bloody diarrhea. Secondary thrombotic microangiopathy can occur in association with metastatic cancer, infections, organ transplantation, and certain drugs. These variants of thrombotic microangiopathy differ in pathogenesis and prognosis, but can be difficult to distinguish because their clinical features often overlap.

● THROMBOTIC THROMBOCYTOPENIC PURPURA

DEFINITION AND HISTORY

Thrombotic thrombocytopenic purpura (TTP) refers to thrombotic microangiopathy without another apparent cause and without acute renal failure, although mild or modest renal insufficiency may be seen.

Acronyms and Abbreviations: ADAMTS, a disintegrin and metalloprotease with thrombospondin repeats; aHUS, atypical hemolytic uremic syndrome; ANA, anti-nuclear antibody; APS, antiphospholipid syndrome; aPTT, activated partial thromboplastin time; CFH, complement factor H; CFHR, complement factor H-related protein; DDAVP, desmopressin; DGKE, diacylglycerol kinase ε; Gb3, globotriaosylceramide 3; HELLP, hemolysis, elevated liver enzymes, low platelet count; HIT, heparin-induced thrombocytopenia; HUS, hemolytic uremic syndrome; LDH, lactate dehydrogenase; MCP, membrane cofactor protein; MMACHC, methylmalonic aciduria and homocystinuria type C protein; PT, prothrombin time; SLE, systemic lupus erythematosus; STEC, *Shiga* toxin-producing *Escherichia coli*; Stx, *Shiga* toxin; TM, thrombomodulin (gene name *THBD*); TTP, thrombotic thrombocytopenic purpura; VEGF, vascular endothelial growth factor; VWF, von Willebrand factor.

Tissue injury can affect almost any organ but often results in neurologic damage. TTP is associated with autoantibodies against the plasma metalloprotease ADAMTS13 (a member of the "a disintegrin and metalloprotease with thrombospondin repeats" family) that reduce plasma ADAMTS13 activity to less than 10 percent of normal.

Eli Moschcowitz reported the first detailed description of TTP in 1924.[1] The patient was a 16-year-old girl with fever, severe anemia, leukocytosis, petechiae, and hemiparesis. Her renal function was not impaired, but the urine contained albumin, hyaline casts, and granular casts. She became comatose and died 2 weeks after her first symptoms. At autopsy, hyaline thrombi were found diffusely in terminal arterioles and capillaries, particularly of the heart and kidney. For many years, patients with similar findings were said to have Moschcowitz disease. The name *TTP* was proposed in 1947[2] and widely adopted thereafter.

In 1966, a review of 272 published cases defined the major clinical features of TTP.[3] Most patients were females between the ages of 10 and 39 years. The symptoms and physical findings included thrombocytopenia, hemolytic anemia with numerous fragmented red cells or schistocytes, neurologic findings, renal damage, and fever. Mortality exceeded 90 percent; the average hospital stay was only 14 days before death, and 80 percent of patients lived fewer than 90 days after the onset of symptoms. However, dramatic recoveries occurred in some cases following splenectomy.

This grim prognosis was recorded before a report in 1976 that whole blood exchange transfusions induced prompt remissions in eight of 14 patients.[4] Similar responses were described after plasmapheresis with plasma replacement.[5] One remarkable case report showed that plasmapheresis was effective if the replacement fluid was plasma or cryoprecipitate-depleted plasma, but ineffective if the replacement fluid contained just albumin.[6] Furthermore, simple plasma infusions without plasmapheresis could induce sustained remissions, suggesting that replacement of a missing plasma factor sometimes was sufficient to ameliorate TTP.[6]

These reports led to the widespread adoption of plasma therapy for TTP, and two studies published in 1991 provided compelling evidence for its efficacy. Plasma infusion was associated with 91 percent survival in 108 patients, an impressive improvement over historical experience.[7] The same year, a prospective randomized comparison of plasma exchange and plasma infusion in 102 patients with TTP was reported.[8] Long-term survival was 78 percent for the plasma exchange group and 63 percent for the plasma infusion group, a significant difference in favor of plasma exchange.

A link between TTP and von Willebrand factor (VWF) was proposed in 1982, based on studies of four patients with chronic relapsing TTP.[9] Their plasma VWF multimers were much larger than those of healthy controls and similar in size to the VWF multimers secreted by endothelial cells. Patients with TTP were proposed to lack a depolymerase activity, perhaps a protease or a reductase, that shortens newly secreted VWF multimers *in vivo* and produces the multimer distribution of normal plasma. The absence of this depolymerase would cause the persistence of "unusually large" VWF, which promotes intravascular platelet aggregation, thrombocytopenia, and microvascular thrombosis. Plasma exchange therapy could provide the missing depolymerase activity, or remove other factors that provoke clinical relapses.

A candidate depolymerase was identified in 1996, when a metalloprotease in plasma was shown to cleave VWF multimers subjected to high fluid shear stress or to mild protein denaturants.[10,11] Soon thereafter, children with congenital TTP were shown to have inherited deficiency of this metalloprotease,[12] and adults with acquired TTP were shown to have autoantibody inhibitors of the enzyme.[13,14] The VWF cleaving protease was purified,[15,16] cloned,[17,18] and named ADAMTS13, a new member of the ADAMTS family of metalloproteases. Simultaneously, the *ADAMTS13* locus was identified by linkage analysis in families affected by congenital TTP and causative *ADAMTS13* mutations were characterized.[19]

ETIOLOGY AND PATHOGENESIS

TTP is caused by unregulated VWF-dependent platelet thrombosis. Large VWF multimers mediate platelet adhesion at sites of vascular injury by binding to connective tissue and to glycoprotein Ib (GPIb) on the platelet surface (Chap. 120). The VWF subunit from which multimers are constructed has a modular structure consisting of five types of conserved structural motifs (Fig. 132–1). VWF multimers bind to collagen through domain A3, and to platelet GPIb through domain A1. When platelets bind to VWF under conditions of high fluid shear stress, the VWF multimer is stretched and the Tyr^{1605}-Met^{1606} bond within domain A2 becomes accessible to ADAMTS13, which cleaves it and thereby can release any adherent platelets. ADAMTS13 deficiency prevents this feedback inhibition of platelet adhesion and leads to widespread microvascular thrombosis. ADAMTS13 levels greater than 10 percent appear sufficient to prevent thrombotic microangiopathy.

ADAMTS13 deficiency in TTP is caused by polyclonal autoantibodies against ADAMTS13, usually immunoglobulin (Ig) G but occasionally IgA or IgM.[13,14] These antibodies almost always bind the ADAMTS13 spacer domain, and often bind to the CUB domains and first thrombospondin-1 repeat; they bind less frequently to other thrombospondin-1 repeats, the metalloprotease domain, or the propeptide.[20-22] Most patients have autoantibodies that inhibit ADAMTS13 activity. The rest have noninhibitory antibodies that are likely to mediate clearance of ADAMTS13 from the circulation.[23]

EPIDEMIOLOGY

The annual incidence of TTP reportedly is two to six per million population in the United States and approximately 2.2 per million in the United Kingdom.[24,25] Seasonal or geographical trends have not been observed consistently. The demographics of TTP are similar to those of systemic lupus erythematosus (SLE). TTP is relatively uncommon before age 20 years, with a peak incidence between ages 30 and 50 years.[24,25] Across many reports the female-to-male ratio averages approximately 2:1, but female preponderance is more pronounced below age 50 years and the ratio approaches equality above age 60 years.[24,25] Other risk factors for TTP include African ancestry[26,27] and obesity.[27,28] Women have a tendency to present during late pregnancy or peripartum (reviewed in Refs. 29 and 30). HLA-DRB1*11 is overrepresented severalfold in whites with TTP.[31,32]

CLINICAL FEATURES

The onset of TTP can be dramatically acute or insidious, developing over weeks. Approximately one-third of patients have symptoms of hemolytic anemia.[3,29] Thrombocytopenia typically causes petechiae or purpura; oral, gastrointestinal or genitourinary bleeding is less common but can be severe. Many patients describe an antecedent upper respiratory tract infection or flu-like illness. Abdominal pain and tenderness are common. Nausea, vomiting, and diarrhea may occur, but bloody diarrhea is uncommon.

Systemic microvascular thrombosis typically affect the kidney, heart, brain, pancreas, adrenals, skin, spleen, marrow, and most other tissues except the lungs, which are spared. Renal involvement is common, but acute renal failure occurs in fewer than 10 percent of cases.[26,27,29] Neurologic findings can be transient or persistent and may include headache, visual disturbances, vertigo, personality change, confusion, lethargy, syncope, coma, seizures, aphasia, hemiparesis, and other focal sensory or motor deficits.[3,29] The frequency of neurologic findings or fever has decreased from more than 90 percent to approximately 50 percent over the past 40 years,[3,8,26,27,29] probably because these features no longer are recognized as necessary to diagnose TTP.

The symptoms of TTP sometimes can be quite atypical, either at first presentation or upon relapse. Thrombocytopenia without hemolytic anemia may herald the onset of disease. In rare instances, visual disturbances, pancreatitis, stroke, or other thrombosis may

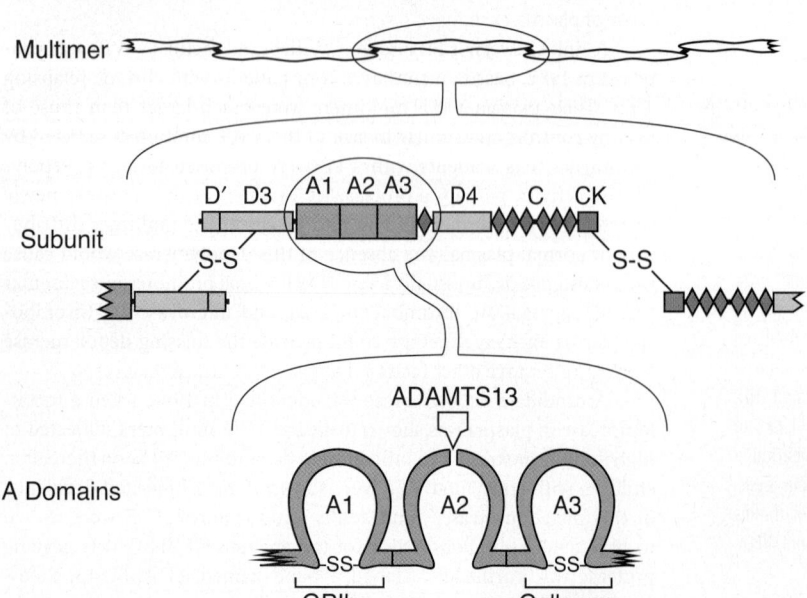

Figure 132–1. Structure of von Willebrand factor (VWF). Multimeric VWF *(top)* is composed of identical subunits with four kinds of structural motifs, including three A domains, six C domains and a homologous D4N domain, two complete and one partial D domains, and a cystine knot (CK) domain. Subunits *(middle)* are linked into multimers by disulfide bonds between C-terminal CK domains and N-terminal D3 domains. Domain A1 *(bottom)* binds platelet glycoprotein Ibα (GPIbα), domain A3 binds collagen in extracellular matrix, and domain A2 contains a Tyr-Met bond that is susceptible to cleavage by ADAMTS13 (a disintegrin and metalloprotease with a thrombospondin type 1 motif member 13).

precede overt thrombotic microangiopathy by days to months.[33–36] Macrovascular venous or arterial thrombosis occurs in up to one-half of patients.[37]

Cardiac involvement may cause chest pain, myocardial infarction, congestive heart failure or arrhythmias.[29,38,39] Direct pulmonary involvement is uncommon but severe acute respiratory distress syndrome may occur, possibly secondary to cardiac failure.[29] Gastrointestinal symptoms are common and can include abdominal pain, nausea, vomiting, and diarrhea.[3,29] Physical examination may suggest acute pancreatitis or mesenteric ischemia. Infrequent findings include Raynaud phenomenon, arthralgia, myalgia, and retinal hemorrhage or detachment.[3,29]

LABORATORY FEATURES

The symptoms and signs of TTP are nonspecific. The diagnosis depends on laboratory testing to document microangiopathic hemolytic anemia and thrombocytopenia, without another predisposing cause. Anemia is almost universal with a mean hemoglobin of approximately 8 g/dL.[27,40] Thrombocytopenia typically is severe, with a mean platelet count of approximately 20×10^9/L.[26,27,40] Hemolysis is indicated by an elevated reticulocyte count and serum lactate dehydrogenase (LDH), undetectable serum haptoglobin, and increased total and unconjugated bilirubin. Coombs test is almost always negative.[7,8] Renal microvascular injury is common with microhematuria, granular or red cell casts, and proteinuria, but the serum creatinine is often normal and seldom greater than 2 mg/dL.[7,8,27,40] Approximately 50 percent of patients have a positive anti-nuclear antibody (ANA) test.[40]

Almost all patients have normal values for plasma fibrinogen, prothrombin time (PT) and activated partial thromboplastin time (aPTT),[7,8] reflecting a minor role of blood coagulation in TTP. Evidence of myocardial damage is common, with elevated troponin levels.[38,39]

The characteristic morphological feature of TTP on the blood film is a marked increase in schistocytes. Schistocytes are helmet cells, or small irregular triangular or crescent shaped cells with pointed projections, that lack central pallor (Chap. 2).[41] Patients with TTP often have markedly increased schistocytes; in a study of six patients, schistocytes comprised a mean of 8.3 percent of all red cells with a range of 1 percent to 18.4 percent.[42] Spherocytes also may be seen.

ADAMTS13 activity is characteristically less than 10 percent and this degree of acquired ADAMTS13 deficiency appears to be specific for TTP.[13,14,43,44] If adult patients with thrombotic microangiopathy are selected with no plausible secondary cause, no diarrheal prodrome, and no features suggestive of hemolytic uremic syndrome (HUS) (e.g., oliguria, severe hypertension, dialysis, serum creatinine >3.5 mg/dL), then at least 80 percent of those selected have ADAMTS13 activity less than 10 percent of normal. The majority of patients with severe ADAMTS13 deficiency have autoantibody inhibitors[13,14,26,45] and almost all patients have autoantibodies that bind ADAMTS13 by enzyme-linked immunosorbent assay (ELISA).

Depending on the clinical context, laboratory tests should be considered to detect conditions that may cause thrombotic microangiopathy by mechanisms other than ADAMTS13 deficiency such as pregnancy, cobalamin deficiency, SLE and other autoimmune diseases, antiphospholipid syndrome (APS), HIV, and *Shiga* toxin–producing organisms.

The histologic appearance of microvascular lesions in TTP is consistent with a pathophysiologic role of VWF-dependent platelet thrombosis. Amorphous thrombi and subendothelial hyaline deposits may be found in the small arterioles and capillaries of any organ, but are particularly common (in order of decreasing severity) in the myocardium, pancreas, kidney, adrenal gland and brain. The liver and lung are relatively spared. The lesions consist mainly of platelets and VWF, with little fibrin and few inflammatory cells. They often include focal endothelial cell proliferation.[46,47]

DIFFERENTIAL DIAGNOSIS

The diagnosis of TTP should be entertained for any patient with microangiopathic hemolytic anemia and thrombocytopenia, without evidence for disseminated intravascular coagulation, and without features associated with *Shiga* toxin–producing *Escherichia coli* (STEC)-HUS such as a prodromal diarrheal illness and acute oliguric or anuric renal failure. These criteria can only be approximate, however, because many diseases associated with secondary thrombotic microangiopathy can produce overlapping clinical and laboratory findings. As a consequence, making a diagnosis of TTP can be a challenge and a wide differential diagnosis often must be considered (Table 132–1).

Schistocytes occur in a variety of conditions besides TTP, although the level seldom enters the 1 to 18 percent range typical of TTP. For example, schistocytes were seen in the blood film of 58 percent of healthy controls, with a mean of 0.05 percent and a range of 0 to 0.27 percent of all red cells.[42] Up to 0.6 percent schistocytes were observed in patients with chronic renal failure, preeclampsia, or properly functioning

TABLE 132–1. Classification and Differential Diagnosis of Thrombotic Microangiopathy

Thrombotic Thrombocytopenic Purpura (TTP)
   Autoimmune, with antibodies against ADAMTS13

Congenital Thrombotic Thrombocytopenic Purpura (Upshaw-Schulman Syndrome)
   Inherited ADAMTS13 deficiency, with mutations in *ADAMTS13*

Shiga Toxin-Producing Escherichia Coli Hemolytic Uremic Syndrome (STEC-HUS)

Atypical Hemolytic Uremic Syndrome (aHUS)
   Alternative complement pathway defects
   Diacylglycerol kinase ε (DGKE) defects

Secondary Thrombotic Microangiopathy
   Disseminated intravascular coagulation
   Infections (viral, bacterial, fungal)
      Streptococcus pneumoniae
   Tissue transplant-associated
      Chemotherapy or radiation injury
      Tissue rejection
      Graft-versus-host disease
   Cancer
   Pregnancy associated (preeclampsia, eclampsia, HELLP [hemolysis, elevated liver enzymes, low platelet count] syndrome)
   Autoimmune disorders
      Systemic lupus erythematosus and other vasculitides
      Antiphospholipid syndrome
   Drugs (commonly implicated)
      Immune (quinine, ticlopidine)
      Toxic (cyclosporine, tacrolimus, mitomycin C, gemcitabine)
   Cobalamin metabolic defects
   Malignant hypertension
   Mechanical hemolysis (e.g., malfunctioning aortic or mitral valve prosthesis)

prosthetic heart valves.[42] Severe hemolysis and marked schistocytosis occur in patients with defective mechanical heart valves. Patients receiving marrow allografts or autografts for a variety of indications had a mean of 0.7 percent schistocytes 6 weeks after transplantation, with a range of 0 to approximately 4 percent schistocytes.[48,49] Approximately 10 percent of patients had at least 1.3 percent schistocytes, placing them at risk for a diagnosis of thrombotic microangiopathy.[49]

ADAMTS13 levels are normal to moderately decreased in newborns, during pregnancy, after surgery, and in chronic liver cirrhosis, chronic renal insufficiency, acute inflammatory states, and a variety of thrombocytopenic disorders other than TTP.[44,50] Severe sepsis may sometimes cause acquired severe ADAMTS13 deficiency, although the incidence and clinical significance of the finding remain uncertain.[51] Some patients with acute viral hepatitis, severe liver cirrhosis[52] or venoocclusive disease after stem cell transplantation[53] have had severe ADAMTS13 deficiency (<10 percent) at least transiently, which is consistent with the synthesis of ADAMTS13 in liver.[17–19]

THERAPY

Plasma Exchange

The mainstay of therapy for TTP is plasma exchange, which removes antibody inhibitors of ADAMTS13 and replenishes the enzyme. After diagnosing TTP, or determining that the diagnosis is sufficiently likely to justify treatment, plasma exchange therapy should be started as soon as feasible. Studies establishing the value of plasma therapy have excluded secondary thrombotic microangiopathy,[7,8] so the efficacy of plasma exchange has been demonstrated directly only for TTP. The optimal dose of plasma is not known, but a common practice is to perform plasma exchange once daily at a volume of 40 or 60 mL/kg, equivalent to 1.0 or 1.5 plasma volumes. For refractory disease, the intensity of plasma exchange can be increased to 1 plasma volume twice daily.[54] Prompt treatment is important and if plasma exchange must be delayed more than a few hours, plasma should be given by simple infusion at 20 to 40 mL/kg total dose per day, consistent with the patient's ability to tolerate the fluid load.[55]

The replacement fluid should contain ADAMTS13. Satisfactory results have been obtained with fresh-frozen plasma,[7,8] plasma cryosupernatant,[56–58] and various pathogen-inactivated plasma products.[59] The incidence of allergic reactions and transfusion-associated lung injury may be lower with solvent/detergent-treated plasma than with fresh-frozen plasma,[60] but the incidence of thrombosis may be increased with some preparations.[59,61] Cryosupernatant is depleted in the largest VWF multimers but has normal ADAMTS13 levels,[62] which could make cryosupernatant particularly suitable for the treatment of TTP. Nevertheless, small randomized trials suggest that cryosupernatant is not superior to fresh-frozen plasma for the initial treatment of TTP.[56,57] Methylene blue-treated plasma may be less effective than fresh-frozen plasma,[59,63] despite having a similar concentration of ADAMTS13.[59]

Plasma exchange should be continued daily until the patient has a treatment response as shown by a platelet count greater than 150×10^9/L for at least 2 days.[55] Whether plasma exchange then should be simply stopped or tapered is not known. A typical strategy is to reduce the frequency of plasma exchange to every other day (or twice per week) for several days. If the disease remains quiescent, then treatment can be stopped and the patient monitored closely for recurrence. Alternatively, plasma exchange can be stopped abruptly with monitoring for recurrent thrombocytopenia over several days.

Glucocorticoids

TTP is an autoimmune disease and the use of glucocorticoids is logical, although a beneficial effect has not been demonstrated conclusively.

Common practice is to give prednisone or equivalent at a total daily dose of 1 mg/kg, in one or two doses, for the duration of plasma exchange, followed by tapering. An alternative regimen is methylprednisolone 1 g intravenously daily for 3 days.[55]

Antiplatelet Agents

The use of antiplatelet agents in TTP is controversial. Aspirin and dipyridamole often are combined with plasma exchange but have not been shown conclusively to modify the course of TTP.[8,64] Low-dose aspirin (e.g., 80 mg/day) has been suggested for thromboprophylaxis, once the platelet count exceeds 50×10^9/L.[55]

Platelet Transfusion

Transfusion of platelets may correlate with acute deterioration and death in TTP.[7,29,65,66] Therefore, platelet transfusions are relatively contraindicated and should be reserved for the treatment of life-threatening hemorrhage, preferably after plasma exchange treatment has been initiated. Platelets generally need not be given prophylactically before establishing venous access for plasma exchange.[67,68] Platelets have been transfused before emergency surgery, immediately after preparation by intensive plasma exchange.[65]

Rituximab

TTP that is refractory to plasma exchange usually responds to rituximab (e.g., 375 mg/m² weekly for 4 doses). At least 80 percent of patients have complete responses within 1 to 3 weeks of starting treatment,[69] including a normal ADAMTS13 level and disappearance of anti-ADAMTS13 antibodies (if present). Relapses occur in a minority of patients after successful treatment, usually after intervals of 6 months to 4 years, and most such patients respond to retreatment.

Acute reactions to rituximab are controlled by premedication with glucocorticoids, antihistamines, and analgesics. Because rituximab is removed by plasma exchange, it should be administered immediately after plasma exchange to maximize the interval until the next plasma exchange.

Rituximab has been given together with plasma exchange at the time of initial diagnosis, which may shorten the time to treatment response and reduce the incidence of relapse.[55,69,70] Rituximab also has been administered preemptively to patients with persistent or recurrent severe ADAMTS13 deficiency after achieving remission of TTP, and this approach may prevent subsequent relapses.[70,71]

In some settings, rare but serious complications associated with rituximab have included bronchospasm, hypotension, serum sickness, susceptibility to infections, and progressive multifocal leukoencephalopathy.[72] Such events have been very rare for patients with autoimmune diseases like TTP.[73,74]

Patients who have not been vaccinated for hepatitis B should be screened for hepatitis B infection before receiving rituximab. Those with evidence of past infection should be considered for antiviral prophylaxis as well as monitoring for hepatic injury and viral reactivation for 6 to 12 months after treatment.[74]

Splenectomy

Splenectomy can result in lasting remissions or reduce the frequency of relapses for some patients with TTP that is refractory to plasma exchange or immunosuppressive therapy, presumably by removing a major site of anti-ADAMTS13 antibody production.[75,76] Laparoscopic splenectomy can be performed safely in most patients regardless of platelet count.[77]

Other Treatments

Anecdotal experience suggests that vincristine may be beneficial for refractory TTP, although its efficacy is difficult to assess. Dosing schedules have included 2 mg intravenously on day 1 followed by 1 mg on days 4 and 7,[78] or 2 mg intravenously per week for 2 to 14 weeks.[79] Prostacyclin analogues[80,81] or high-dose intravenous immunoglobulins[82,83] have been used without convincing evidence of efficacy.

Although cyclosporine can cause secondary thrombotic microangiopathy, apparent responses, with normalization of ADAMTS13 activity, have been observed with cyclosporine 2 to 3 mg/kg daily in two divided doses as an adjunct to plasma exchange.[84]

Other treatments have included oral or intravenous cyclophosphamide, oral azathioprine,[55] bortezomib,[85] mycophenolate,[86] N-acetylcysteine,[87] combination chemotherapy with cyclophosphamide, doxorubicin, vincristine, and prednisone,[88] and autologous stem cell transplantation.[89] Agents that prevent the binding of VWF to platelets are under development and may prove useful for the treatment of TTP.[90,91]

Supportive Therapy

Daily laboratory monitoring should include complete blood count with platelet count, LDH, electrolytes, blood urea nitrogen and creatinine. Because of the high incidence of cardiac damage,[29] continuous electrocardiographic monitoring and periodic assessment of cardiac enzymes should be considered. Patients should receive supplemental folic acid and vaccination for hepatitis B.[55] Allergic reactions, metabolic alkalosis, and hypocalcemia associated with plasma exchange should be prevented or treated by appropriate adjustments in therapy.

After the platelet count increases to above 50×10^9/L, prophylaxis for venous thromboembolism may be instituted with low-molecular-weight heparin[61] and low-dose aspirin.[55]

COURSE AND PROGNOSIS

The platelet count normalizes after a median of 11 plasma exchanges, with a wide range of four to 55 sessions.[92] Normalization of serum LDH lags behind the platelet count by approximately 9 days and persistent elevation of LDH does not correlate with the risk of exacerbation or relapse.[93]

Exacerbations are defined as TTP recurring within 30 days after a treatment response and 25 to 50 percent of patients have an acute exacerbation within 2 weeks that requires further treatment with plasma exchange. Some have repeated exacerbations over several months.[94] A durable treatment response, lasting more than 30 days, is achieved eventually in approximately 80 percent of patients.[92]

Relapses, defined as recurrences more than 30 days after a complete response, occur in up to one-third of patients within 2 years after treatment with plasma exchange and glucocorticoids alone. Most relapses occur during the first year, but have occurred 13 years or more after diagnosis.[26,94] Evaluation for relapsing TTP should be considered for any symptom compatible with thrombotic microangiopathy, especially in association with a common trigger of relapse such as infection, surgery, or pregnancy.[34,95] Relapsing patients typically respond to plasma exchange. Relapses in TTP are associated with severe ADAMTS13 deficiency and detectable ADAMTS13 autoantibody inhibitors. Conversely, patients without severe ADAMTS13 deficiency at diagnosis rarely relapse (approximately 9 percent across several studies) (reviewed in Ref. 96).

Serious catheter-related complications of plasma exchange therapy occur in approximately 26 percent of patients with TTP and include pneumothorax and hemorrhage, cardiac perforation, venous thrombosis, catheter thrombosis, and bacterial or fungal infections.[97]

Hives or pruritic reactions to fresh-frozen plasma occur in one-to two-thirds of patients but usually can be managed by premedication with antihistamines. High-volume plasma exchange causes metabolic

alkalosis and hypocalcemia, and may cause unintentional platelet removal. Serious complications attributable to plasma are less common, occurring in approximately 4 percent of patients, and include bronchospasm, anaphylaxis, hypotension, hypoxia, and serum sickness.[97]

The mortality rate for TTP treated with plasma exchange ranges from 10 to 20 percent. Most deaths occur within a few days after presentation, and almost all occur within the first month.[7,8,26,94]

Late sequelae of TTP may include long-term deficits in quality of life and cognition in many patients,[98,99] severe persistent neurologic deficits in 5 to 13 percent,[100] chronic renal insufficiency in up to 25 percent,[100] and dialysis dependent renal failure in 3 to 8 percent of patients.[100,101]

● CONGENITAL THROMBOTIC THROMBOCYTOPENIC PURPURA

DEFINITION AND HISTORY

Congenital TTP, or Upshaw-Schulman syndrome, refers to TTP that is caused by inherited deficiency of ADAMTS13.

Schulman and colleagues[102] and Upshaw[103] first described a congenital disorder resembling TTP characterized by autosomal recessive inheritance and chronic relapsing thrombotic microangiopathy from infancy. Congenital TTP, or Upshaw-Schulman syndrome, shared many features with acquired TTP in adults, including the consistent response to plasma.[103]

ETIOLOGY AND PATHOGENESIS

Congenital TTP is caused by homozygosity or compound heterozygosity for inactivating mutations in the *ADAMTS13* gene[19] on chromosome 9q34 (reviewed in Ref. 104). The mutations usually impair the synthesis or secretion of ADAMTS13. As yet no evidence convincingly indicates locus heterogeneity in congenital TTP.

EPIDEMIOLOGY

Congenital TTP is autosomal recessive and affects the genders almost equally.[105] The prevalence of congenital TTP is approximately one per million population in Japan[106] and appears to be similar elsewhere. Congenital TTP accounts for a few percent of patients presenting with TTP.

CLINICAL FEATURES

The clinical features of congenital TTP are similar to those of acquired TTP, except for age of onset. Most children with congenital ADAMTS13 deficiency have neonatal jaundice and hemolysis but no evidence of ABO blood group or Rh incompatibility. Approximately half of the children continue to have a chronic relapsing course from infancy. The remaining children usually develop symptoms in their late teens or early twenties. In either case, acute exacerbations often are triggered by infections, otitis media, surgery, or other inflammatory stress.[105,107] Patients may suffer an acute attack after receiving desmopressin (DDAVP), which stimulates the release of VWF from endothelial cell stores; one such patient was receiving a low dose of intranasal DDAVP for enuresis.[108] As in acquired TTP, most patients with congenital TTP have some renal involvement with proteinuria, hematuria, or a mildly elevated serum creatinine during acute attacks. Chronic renal failure can occur, usually after a prolonged course of relapsing disease.[107]

Females often present during their first pregnancy, possibly because VWF levels are increased late in pregnancy. If untreated, pregnancies usually end in spontaneous abortion, stillbirth or premature delivery.

TTP usually occurs in the third trimester or postpartum, whereas fetal loss is most common in the second trimester.[109]

LABORATORY FEATURES

Severe congenital ADAMTS13 deficiency (<5 percent) is characteristic of congenital TTP. Alloantibodies to ADAMTS13 as a consequence of treatment with plasma are extremely rare in congenital TTP; only one such patient has been reported.[110] Other laboratory findings in congenital TTP are similar to those in acquired TTP. The histologic features of congenital TTP are similar to those of acquired TTP.[111]

DIFFERENTIAL DIAGNOSIS

For patients presenting during early childhood, other causes of thrombotic microangiopathy to consider include STEC-HUS, atypical HUS and secondary thrombotic microangiopathy associated with disorders that are characteristic of childhood. For adolescents and adults, the differential diagnosis is the same as for acquired TTP (see Table 132–1).

Testing of stool and urine for STEC should be considered for all patients with thrombotic microangiopathy because a significant fraction of patients with STEC infection never have bloody diarrhea.

THERAPY

Congenital TTP can be treated with periodic infusions of fresh-frozen plasma or an equivalent virucidally treated product, if available. The half-life of ADAMTS13 is 2 to 3 days[112] and the level of ADAMTS13 required to avoid symptoms is approximately 5 percent of normal; 5 to 20 mL/kg of plasma every 2 to 3 weeks usually is sufficient to maintain ADAMTS13 at a greater than 5 percent level and prevent symptoms.[105,107] Patients with severe allergic reactions to plasma have been treated successfully with plasma-derived factor VIII/VWF concentrates that contain significant amounts of ADAMTS13.[55]

Pregnancy Management

Fetal loss and premature birth can be prevented by plasma infusions 10 mL/kg every 2 weeks beginning at 8 weeks of gestation, increasing to weekly in the second trimester. Any sign of thrombotic microangiopathy is an indication to increase the volume or frequency of plasma infusion. Plasma exchange may be necessary to avoid fluid overload.[55,109]

COURSE AND PROGNOSIS

The severity of congenital TTP varies considerably and correlates to some extent with the underlying genotype and residual plasma ADAMTS13 activity. Patients with ADAMTS13 activity of less than 2.5 percent of normal tend to have their first TTP episode in childhood, have more than one episode of TTP per year, and require regular plasma prophylaxis. Conversely, patients with ADAMTS13 activity of 2.5 to 6.0 percent tend to present in adulthood and have infrequent episodes of disease.[113,114] Some of these patients have prolonged symptom-free intervals and can be treated on demand. However, inadequately treated patients are at risk for developing chronic renal failure and stroke.[55]

● *SHIGA* TOXIN *ESCHERICHIA COLI*–ASSOCIATED HEMOLYTIC UREMIC SYNDROME

DEFINITION AND HISTORY

HUS refers to thrombotic microangiopathy that mainly affects the kidney and usually causes oliguric or anuric renal failure. Ingestion of STEC causes HUS (STEC-HUS) that is usually is associated with a prodrome of diarrhea. Other names in the literature for STEC-HUS include diarrhea-associated HUS (D+HUS) and "typical" HUS.

In 1955, the term *HUS* was proposed for thrombotic microangiopathy occurring in children and associated with acute anuric renal failure, which is uncommon in TTP.[115] HUS was often preceded by a diarrheal illness and, unlike TTP in adults, the prognosis was relatively favorable. Most patients survived and recovered normal renal function with only supportive care.[116] Although cases were known to cluster in endemic areas, the cause of HUS was unknown until 1983, when *E. coli* O157:H7 was shown to express a *Shiga*-like toxin and cause epidemic hemorrhagic colitis that could evolve into HUS.[117–119]

ETIOLOGY AND PATHOGENESIS

STEC may make two types of *Shiga* toxin (Stx) that are similar in structure and function to ricin. Stx1 is identical to *Shigella dysenteriae* serotype 1 toxin. Stx2 is approximately 50 percent identical in sequence to Stx1 and occurs in several closely related forms. Both toxins consist of pentameric B subunits that bind globotriaosylceramide (Gb3) on cell surfaces and a single A subunit that is responsible for cytotoxicity. Pathogenic *E. coli* almost always express a variant of Stx2 and approximately two-thirds express Stx1.[120]

When STEC colonize the gut they damage the epithelium and secrete Stx that is delivered to target organs through the blood, probably by neutrophils. Stx bound to Gb3 on cell surfaces is endocytosed and transported in a retrograde fashion through the secretory pathway to the endoplasmic reticulum, where the A subunit is translocated into the cytoplasm. The A subunit is an *N*-glycosidase that removes a specific base from the large ribosomal subunit, which inhibits protein synthesis and activates a response pathway that leads to apoptosis. The observed predilection for renal injury is a result of the relatively high expression of Gb3 on renal tubular epithelial, mesangial, and glomerular endothelial cells.

EPIDEMIOLOGY

STEC-HUS can occur at any age but affects mainly children younger than age 5 years and is rare before age 6 months. The disease occurs sporadically and in epidemics, associated with ingestion of foods or other materials contaminated with Stx-producing bacteria. *E. coli* O157:H7 accounts for at least 80 percent of cases in many series, but STEC-HUS can be caused by other toxin-bearing *E. coli* serotypes[121,122] or by *S. dysenteriae* type 1. Most cases occur in summer and autumn in rural environments. The incidence is approximately 10 to 30 per million children per year, but depends on the risk of exposure, which varies considerably with the time of year, location, and other factors. STEC-HUS is a common cause of chronic renal failure in children.[120]

CLINICAL FEATURES

Patients develop abdominal pain, tenderness and diarrhea between 2 and 12 days after ingesting STEC, with a mean incubation period of 3 to 7 days and a median of 3 days. The diarrhea usually becomes bloody within 1 to 3 days, at which time patients are typically afebrile. Nausea and vomiting are common. The abdominal pain is greater than is typical for other causes of gastroenteritis, and defecation is often painful. Most patients recover spontaneously within a few days. Of children younger than 10 years of age with bloody diarrhea and *E. coli* O157:H7 infection, approximately 15 percent will develop STEC-HUS with the acute onset of microangiopathic hemolytic anemia, thrombocytopenia, and renal injury an average of 7 days (range: 5 to 13 days) after the start of diarrhea.[120]

LABORATORY FEATURES

Aside from signs of dehydration or electrolyte imbalances from diarrhea or vomiting, laboratory testing may be unremarkable before bloody diarrhea develops. Thrombocytopenia and hemolysis with associated laboratory abnormalities develop after bloody diarrhea and usually before renal failure. The platelet count falls to an average of 40×10^9/L. Renal signs may include a rising creatinine, proteinuria, hematuria, hypertension, and oliguria or anuria. Usually the PT and aPTT are normal or minimally prolonged, plasma fibrinogen is normal or elevated, and fibrin degradation products may be moderately elevated.[120,123] ADAMTS13 levels are normal.[124,125]

Stool should be cultured on selective media for *E. coli* O157:H7 and tested for Stxs to detect non–O157 strains. STEC in the stool are found in at least 90 percent of patients during the first 6 days but in less than 30 percent of patients at later times. Fecal leukocytes are not always present and generally are not abundant.[120]

Serologic testing for antibodies to STEC surface antigens at diagnosis and after 2 weeks can facilitate the diagnosis of STEC-HUS if stool cultures are not informative. Titers rise after infection and persist for 8 to 12 weeks.

STEC-HUS mainly affects the renal cortex, which often shows extensive necrosis. Lesions occur less frequently in the pancreas, brain, adrenal glands, and myocardium. The thrombi of HUS typically involve glomerular capillaries and arterioles and are composed mainly of fibrin and red cells with few platelets.[47,126]

DIFFERENTIAL DIAGNOSIS

Unlike STEC-HUS, bloody diarrhea caused by *Salmonella*, *Shigella*, or *Clostridium difficile* is likely to be accompanied by fever and prostration. Coinfection with STEC and *C. difficile* can occur. Otherwise the differential diagnosis of apparent STEC-HUS includes unusual presentations of other causes of thrombotic microangiopathy (see Table 132–1).

THERAPY

Patients with acute bloody diarrhea should be admitted to the hospital for diagnosis and management of presumed STEC infection as well as infection control. Early intravenous hydration to maintain renal perfusion protects against the development of HUS.[120] Most patients require red cell transfusions. Daily monitoring of hemoglobin, platelet count, electrolytes, blood urea nitrogen (BUN), and creatinine is important.

The risks and benefits of antibiotic use in STEC-HUS may depend on the stage of illness. Antibiotics should not be used early in the course of acute diarrheal illness caused by *E. coli* O157:H7 because antibiotics increase the risk of HUS.[127] However, retrospective analysis of a 2011 outbreak of *E. coli* O104:H4 infection suggests that treatment with multiple antibiotics after the development of HUS may have reduced the incidence of seizures and death.[128]

Antimotility agents and narcotics increase the risk of HUS and neurologic complications. Nonsteroidal antiinflammatory drugs and antihypertensives that reduce renal perfusion such as angiotensin-converting enzyme inhibitors and angiotensin receptor blockers should be avoided. No convincing data indicate that antiplatelet agents, anticoagulants, plasma exchange, glucocorticoids, rituximab, or an inhibitor of the terminal components of complement, eculizumab, add benefit to supportive therapy and dialysis, for children or adults.[58,120,128]

COURSE AND PROGNOSIS

Patients often have a degree of diffuse vascular injury and may become edematous with intravenous hydration. Consequently more sodium than expected may be required for adequate volume replacement, and monitoring for fluid overload and hypertension is essential. A rising platelet count signals the end of the period of risk for developing HUS. For patients with HUS, hemolysis can persist as the HUS resolves and require additional red cell transfusions.

Extrarenal involvement is common, although the incidence of specific complications varies widely. Depending on the outbreak, central nervous system involvement (seizures, coma, or stroke) occurs in 10 to 65 percent of cases and is more common in older patients. Cardiac dysfunction is associated with ischemia or congestive heart failure. Patients may require mechanical ventilation for seizures, coma, pulmonary edema, or pneumonia. Gastrointestinal involvement can include hemorrhagic colitis, necrosis, perforation, peritonitis, pancreatitis, diabetes mellitus, and rectal prolapse.[120,128,129]

The incidence of death and end-stage renal failure also varies widely, but correlates with the need for initial dialysis and central nervous system involvement. In a meta-analysis of more than 3400 patients with STEC-HUS, an average of 9 percent died and 3 percent developed permanent end-stage renal failure 1 or more years later. Another 25 percent had persistent hypertension, proteinuria, or chronic renal insufficiency.[130]

Inability to detect STEC may not strongly affect the clinical course. In a study of 268 patients with HUS, 59 percent had prodromal diarrhea plus bacteriologic or serologic evidence of infection by STEC; 21 percent had only diarrhea, and 10 percent had only positive bacteriologic or serologic studies. All three groups had similar outcomes: approximately 1 percent died and 73 percent recovered normal renal function. In contrast, the 11 percent of patients with neither diarrhea nor documented STEC infection had a significantly worse outcome; 10 percent died and only 34 percent recovered normal renal function.[121] Most of these latter patients probably had "atypical hemolytic uremic syndrome (aHUS)," which has a distinct cause and prognosis.

● ATYPICAL HEMOLYTIC UREMIC SYNDROME

DEFINITION AND HISTORY

Diarrhea-negative or *aHUS* is not associated with diarrhea or Stx-producing organisms and occurs in patients without an obvious predisposing condition.

Reporting on patients seen in southern Africa in 1965, Barnard and Kibel first distinguished typical diarrhea-associated HUS from "atypical" patients who did not have diarrhea.[131] In the 1970s, Kaplan proposed that recurrent familial cases of HUS represented a distinct genetic illness.[132,133] By 1993, aHUS was an accepted diagnosis of uncertain cause,[134] although increased consumption of complement C3 and deficiency of factor H had been described in some patients.[135] In 1998, Warwicker and colleagues showed that mutations in complement factor H (CFH) caused familial HUS,[136] and mutations in other proteins of the alternative complement pathway quickly followed. These results provided a rationale for treating aHUS with inhibitors of complement activation, which has proved very effective.[137]

ETIOLOGY AND PATHOGENESIS

The alternative complement pathway drives the pathogenesis of aHUS. Complement component C3 is spontaneously converted to C3b at a low rate and deposited on cell surfaces. Under normal circumstances this C3b is promptly cleaved and inactivated by the serine protease factor I, and this reaction is accelerated by factor H or membrane

TABLE 132–2. Complement Defects in Atypical Hemolytic Uremic Syndrome

Gene or Subgroup	Prevalence in aHUS	Low C3	Progression to End-Stage Renal Disease	Death
CFH	25–30%	50–60%	50–60%	5–20%
CFI	4–10%	20–50%	~60%	0–10%
MCP	7–10%	6–30%	6–35%	0%
CFB	<1.5%	≤100%	~50%	0%
C3	4–8%	70–80%	55–70%	0%
THBD (TM)*	<5%	~50%	~50%	~30%
Anti–complement factor H antibody	3–7%	~40%	30–60%	0%
No mutation	30–50%	~20%	~40%	3–7%

Based on outcomes after 5 years from the International Registry of Recurrent and Familial HUS/TTP[138] and after 3 years from the French Study Group for aHUS.[139]

THBD is the gene for thrombomodulin.

cofactor protein (MCP, CD46). These cofactors are structurally and functionally similar, but factor H is a plasma protein whereas MCP is a transmembrane protein found on the surface of almost all cells. If not restrained by these inhibitors, C3b interacts with factor B to form a potent C3 convertase that amplifies the deposition of C3b, which attracts phagocytes and promotes membrane attack complex formation on renal glomerular and arteriolar endothelium and basement membrane. The resultant vascular damage causes thrombotic microangiopathy.

Heterozygous mutations in alternative complement pathway proteins have been identified in 60 to 70 percent of patients with aHUS (Table 132–2). These include loss-of-function mutations in factor H, MCP, factor I, complement factor H-related proteins 1 and 3 (CFHR1, CFHR3), and thrombomodulin (TM); and gain-of-function mutations in factor B and C3. In addition, autoantibodies to factor H have been identified in some patients with aHUS, often in association with mutations in CFHR1 and CFHR3. Patients sometimes have mutations at more than one locus, or a combination of autoantibodies to CFH and mutations.[138,139]

Homozygous or compound heterozygous mutations in diacylglycerol kinase ε (DGKE) cause aHUS with high penetrance that presents before 1 year of age with hypertension, hematuria, and proteinuria. How DGKE mutations cause aHUS is not established. DGKE mutations may account for a few percent of aHUS.[140]

EPIDEMIOLOGY

Atypical HUS affects approximately 5 percent as many children as develop STEC-HUS, with an estimated incidence of two per million population per year.[141] Approximately one-half of patients are younger than age 18 years. Approximately 60 percent of affected children have their first episode of aHUS before age 2 years, and 25 percent before age 6 months. In contrast, STEC-HUS is rare before age 6 months. Most adults have their first episode of aHUS between ages 20 and 40 years. Childhood aHUS affects males and females equally, whereas onset in adults disproportionately affects females mainly because of disease triggered by pregnancy. Analysis of relatives of probands shows that the penetrance

of aHUS may be approximately 50 percent for mutations in any of the predisposing genes.[138,139]

CLINICAL FEATURES

Approximately 20 percent of patients have a subacute or chronic course of mild anemia, variable thrombocytopenia and relatively normal renal function. However, patients usually present acutely with thrombotic microangiopathy and renal failure, sometimes with progressive hypertension. Most patients report a possible triggering event such as a viral or bacterial upper respiratory infection, gastroenteritis, or pregnancy. aHUS is not classically preceded by bloody or painful diarrhea.[138,139]

Women with pregnancy-associated aHUS usually present postpartum. Most of the rest develop symptoms in the third trimester, sometimes complicated by fetal loss and preeclampsia.[142]

Extrarenal symptoms occur in 10 to 20 percent of patients. Central nervous system involvement is most common. Myocardial infarction, pancreatitis, and necrosis of skin or digits have been reported. Extrarenal involvement is relatively uncommon for aHUS caused by MCP mutations.[138,139]

LABORATORY FEATURES

Patients have the laboratory findings characteristic of microangiopathic hemolysis, as observed for TTP and STEC-HUS. The mean platelet count in aHUS is 40 × 10⁹/L, typically higher than in TTP. Serum creatinine can be markedly elevated, with microhematuria and proteinuria if the patient is not anuric.

Complement C4 is usually normal and C3 may be low, consistent with activation of the alternative complement pathway, but the likelihood of a low C3 level varies considerably and depends on the involved locus (see Table 132–2). Approximately 3 to 7 percent of patients have autoantibodies against CFH that can be detected by ELISA. In favorable cases, flow cytometry on peripheral blood leukocytes can identify cell-surface MCP deficiency for patients with *MCP* mutations. Assays of CFH and CFI may be useful to identify specific deficiencies, but patients are usually heterozygous and mutations at these loci may not clearly decrease the factor levels.[138,139]

DNA sequencing should be considered to detect mutations in *CFH, CFI, MCP, C3, CFB* and *TM* before renal transplantation because the risk of relapse and need for subsequent prophylaxis depends on the affected locus. Candidate mutations in one of these loci or antibodies to CFH can be found in approximately 70 percent of patients with aHUS. Sequencing of *DGKE* should be considered for patients presenting before age 1 year.

As in STEC-HUS, renal lesions in aHUS are rich in fibrin but poor in platelets or VWF.

DIFFERENTIAL DIAGNOSIS

Signs and symptoms consistent with aHUS may occur in TTP or STEC-HUS, and distinguishing among these entities is important because they are treated differently. Correct diagnosis is not always straightforward. For example, MCP mutations may cause thrombotic microangiopathy without renal insufficiency that resolves coincidentally during a course of plasma exchange and therefore resembles TTP except for normal ADAMTS13 activity.[143] Infection with STEC may be difficult to document, and some patients with STEC-HUS do not have a diarrheal prodrome.[121]

Secondary causes of thrombotic microangiopathy should be considered (see Table 132–1). For children, conditions that usually present in that age group deserve special attention such as *Streptococcus pneumoniae* infections and inherited cobalamin defects.

THERAPY

Plasma Exchange

For patients without a previous diagnosis of aHUS, plasma exchange should be started at 1 to 2 volumes daily for adults or 50 to 100 mL/kg for children.[141] Plasma exchange can induce responses at least transiently for patients with deficiency of plasma complement proteins or autoantibodies to CFH but not for deficiency of the membrane protein MCP. If an isolated *MCP* mutation is identified, plasma exchange can be stopped.

Eculizumab

After excluding severe ADAMTS13 deficiency, STEC and secondary causes of thrombotic microangiopathy, plasma exchange can be stopped and eculizumab started for presumptive aHUS at 900 mg intravenously every week for 4 weeks, followed by 1200 mg in week 5 and every other week thereafter, in many cases indefinitely. For patients younger than 18 years of age, doses are adjusted based on body weight. Supplementary doses are recommended during plasma exchange or infusion,[137] but concurrent plasma exchange and eculizumab is not beneficial and should be avoided.

Adverse reactions to eculizumab during the treatment of aHUS have included infections, fever, hypertension, headache, diarrhea, abdominal pain, nausea, and vomiting. Adverse reactions are common but seldom require discontinuation of therapy.

Ideally, patients should be vaccinated against *Neisseria meningitides* at least 2 weeks before treatment. If timely vaccination is not possible or the available vaccine does not cover prevalent strains, then antibiotic prophylaxis should be considered. Children also should be vaccinated for *S. pneumoniae* and *Haemophilus influenzae* type b.

Rituximab

Rituximab and glucocorticoids can be added to eculizumab for treatment of aHUS caused by autoantibodies to CFH. If the autoantibodies are eradicated, then eculizumab can be discontinued.

Renal Transplantation

Patients with end-stage renal disease that does not improve on eculizumab may be treated by renal transplantation. Living related donors generally are not used because the donated kidney may be at risk for aHUS and the donor may have the same risk factors as the recipient and develop aHUS after donation.

Mutation screening should be performed before transplantation to guide subsequent therapy. Unless patients are treated preemptively with eculizumab, aHUS recurs predictably in transplanted kidneys. Isolated MCP deficiency is an exception because normal membrane-bound MCP in the transplanted kidney protects it from complement attack. HUS has not recurred after renal transplantation in children with *DGKE* mutations.[141,144]

Liver transplantation or combined liver-kidney transplantation can cure aHUS caused by deficiency of plasma complement proteins that are synthesized in the liver. However, the risk and complications of liver transplantation can be avoided by prophylactic treatment with eculizumab after renal transplantation.[141,144]

COURSE AND PROGNOSIS

Treatment of aHUS with just plasma exchange and supportive care is associated with up to 8 percent mortality during the first episode of disease and rapid progression to end stage renal failure in many survivors. Mortality at 1 year appears substantially higher for children but progression to end-stage renal failure is more common for adults. MCP mutations are associated with a less-aggressive clinical course: patients may improve during plasma exchange but have similar outcomes without

plasma exchange, with 90 percent alive and dialysis free after several years (see Table 132–2).[138,139]

Treatment with eculizumab is associated with sustained resolution of thrombotic microangiopathy, improvement in renal function and prevention of relapses. The platelet count normalizes in approximately 50 percent of patients by day 7 and in 80 to 90 percent of patients by week 26. Earlier initiation of eculizumab is associated with greater improvement in renal function.[137]

Most patients are likely to need lifelong treatment to prevent recurrent thrombotic microangiopathy and progressive renal failure. Some patients with aHUS and no remaining renal function may still benefit from eculizumab to prevent the progression of neurologic or other extrarenal injury. Patients with MCP mutations can have a relatively mild course with normal renal function and long intervals between exacerbations; they may not need chronic prophylaxis with eculizumab.[138,139]

DGKE mutations are associated with the development of nephrotic syndrome,[140] which is otherwise uncommon in aHUS. Case reports suggest that aHUS caused by *DGKE* mutations is associated with complement activation and can respond to plasma therapy.[145,146] The efficacy of eculizumab is not known. HUS has not recurred after renal transplantation in children with DGKE mutations.[140,145,146]

● SECONDARY THROMBOTIC MICROANGIOPATHY

Secondary thrombotic microangiopathy occurs in patients with predisposing medical conditions such as metastatic cancer, malignant hypertension, systemic infection, solid-organ or hematopoietic stem cell transplantation, vasculitis, catastrophic APS, radiation exposure, chemotherapy, certain other drugs, inherited or acquired metabolic disorders, and various causes of disseminated intravascular coagulation. Endothelial injury may be a common cause, although the mechanism of disease varies and in most cases is not understood.

The clinical features of secondary thrombotic microangiopathy usually are dominated by the predisposing illness, and the most important clinical intervention is correcting the underlying "primary" condition. The clinical history and laboratory testing can identify most causes of secondary thrombotic microangiopathy. Severe ADAMTS13 deficiency almost never occurs in secondary thrombotic microangiopathy, and treatment with plasma exchange, rituximab, or eculizumab is not known to be beneficial.

DISSEMINATED INTRAVASCULAR COAGULATION

Conditions resulting in disseminated intravascular coagulation sometimes cause microangiopathic changes and thrombocytopenia with little change in blood coagulation tests, which can suggest a diagnosis of TTP.

INFECTIONS

Infections may trigger disease in patients with severe ADAMTS13 deficiency, but infections typically cause secondary thrombotic microangiopathy by other mechanisms. Secondary thrombotic microangiopathy caused by infections may respond to antimicrobial or antiviral therapy, but not to plasma exchange.

Thrombotic microangiopathy, often with acute renal failure, is a rare complication of invasive infections with *S. pneumoniae* in children. A surveillance study in Atlanta, Georgia, identified HUS in 0.6 percent of pneumococcal infections in children younger than 2 years of age.[147] Patients usually have complicated pneumococcal pneumonia or meningitis, with normal plasma fibrinogen and normal or minimally prolonged PT and aPTT. The pathophysiology is thought to involve bacterial neuraminidase, made by *S. pneumoniae* and some other organisms, which removes sialic acid residues from cell surface glycoproteins and exposes Thomsen-Friedenreich antigen (T antigen). T antigen is recognized by naturally occurring antibodies that fix complement, causing hemolysis and damaging the renal microvasculature. Because donor blood usually contains high levels of antibodies against T antigen, red cells and platelets should be washed before transfusion, and plasma should not be used as a replacement fluid. Exchange transfusion has been proposed to stop hemolysis by replacing T-antigen–bearing red blood cells and removing circulating neuraminidase, but the efficacy of this treatment is uncertain.[148]

TISSUE TRANSPLANTS

Recipients of solid-organ transplants can develop thrombotic microangiopathy, often dominated by renal involvement associated with immunosuppression by cyclosporine or tacrolimus.[149] These drugs appear to damage renal endothelial cells directly and can cause neurotoxicity, adding another feature suggestive of TTP. Similarly, hematopoietic stem cell transplant recipients may develop thrombotic microangiopathy associated with high-dose chemotherapy or radiation, immunosuppressive drugs, graft-versus-host disease, or infections. ADAMTS13 levels are normal[150] and plasma therapy is ineffective.[151]

CANCER

Thrombotic microangiopathy occurs in a small fraction of patients with cancer, most commonly with adenocarcinoma of the pancreas, lung, prostate, stomach, colon, ovary, breast, or unknown primary site that usually is widely metastatic. These cancers also are associated with Trousseau syndrome or paraneoplastic hypercoagulability and thrombosis. Patients often have variable prolongation of the PT and aPTT and increased fibrin degradation products. The thrombosis of Trousseau syndrome may respond to anticoagulation with heparin but not warfarin.[152,153] Abundant schistocytes also have been described in acute erythroleukemia.[154] Plasma exchange is ineffective.[26,27,153]

PREGNANCY-ASSOCIATED THROMBOTIC MICROANGIOPATHY

The differential diagnosis of thrombotic microangiopathy in pregnancy includes preeclampsia, eclampsia, HELLP syndrome (hemolysis, elevated liver enzymes, low platelet count), acute fatty liver of pregnancy, abruptio placenta, amniotic fluid embolism, and retained products of conception (Chap. 129). Severe ADAMTS13 deficiency has not been observed in these conditions.[155] Pregnancy also can trigger disease in patients with congenital or acquired ADAMTS13 deficiency or defects in the alternative complement pathway.

AUTOIMMUNE DISORDERS

Autoimmune thrombocytopenia may be confused with TTP if other causes of microangiopathic hemolytic anemia are present. Asymptomatic thrombocytopenia also may sometimes be the only finding in TTP. Patients have been described in whom TTP and autoimmune thrombocytopenia appeared to occur simultaneously or sequentially.[156] Evan syndrome (autoimmune hemolytic anemia with autoimmune thrombocytopenia) usually can be distinguished from TTP by a positive Coombs test and the prominence of spherocytes relative to schistocytes in the blood film. Heparin-induced thrombocytopenia (HIT) may sometimes resemble TTP (Chap. 118).

SLE can cause autoimmune hemolysis and thrombocytopenia, and lupus vasculitis can cause microangiopathic changes, renal insufficiency, and neurologic defects consistent with TTP. Vasculitis associated with other autoimmune disorders can pose a similar diagnostic problem. Although ADAMTS13 deficiency is uncommon among patients with SLE,[157] in rare cases they develop autoimmune ADAMTS13 deficiency and TTP that responds to plasma exchange.[158] Conversely, patients with TTP and autoantibodies against ADAMTS13 may have other markers of autoimmune disease, including ANA or anti-DNA antibodies, polyarthritis, discoid lupus, or ulcerative colitis.[101,159]

Thrombotic microangiopathy can develop in patients with APS, with or without concurrent SLE.

Thrombotic microangiopathy occurs in patients with progressive systemic sclerosis, particularly in association with acute scleroderma renal crisis and malignant hypertension. Treatment with angiotensin-converting enzyme inhibitors may be effective.[160]

DRUG-INDUCED THROMBOTIC MICROANGIOPATHY

Nearly 80 drugs are associated with thrombotic microangiopathy, and evidence supports a definite or probable causal association for approximately 44 of them. Three drugs (quinine, cyclosporine, tacrolimus) account for 60 percent of the patient reports with definite evidence.[161] Some agents cause disease by an immune mechanism and others by direct toxicity; a few drugs reportedly act by either mechanism. With the exception of ticlopidine-induced disease, plasma exchange appears to be ineffective or possibly harmful for drug-induced thrombotic microangiopathy.[162]

Immune Mechanisms

Quinine is the most common cause of drug-induced thrombotic microangiopathy. Most patients are women. Severe thrombotic microangiopathy occurs suddenly within several hours after ingestion of a quinine tablet or a beverage containing it such as tonic water, with fever, abdominal and back pain, nausea, vomiting, diarrhea, rash, and oliguric renal failure. Neurologic changes are common.[163] ADAMTS13 levels are normal.[164] The mechanism involves a broad range of quinine-dependent antibodies against platelets, endothelium, and other cells. Most patients recover with normal renal function over several weeks, although some develop end stage renal disease.

The antiplatelet drug ticlopidine is unusual because it induces autoantibody inhibitors of ADAMTS13, effectively causing TTP that responds to plasma exchange.[165] The related thienopyridine drugs clopidogrel, prasugrel and ticagrelor do not appear to cause thrombotic microangiopathy by this mechanism.

Direct Toxicity

Cyclosporine and tacrolimus are structurally distinct immunosuppressive drugs that indirectly inhibit calcineurin and suppress T-cell activation. Both agents cause dose-dependent nephrotoxicity, neurotoxicity, and thrombotic microangiopathy.[166-168] The renal damage is thought to involve toxic effects on endothelium.[166] Thrombotic microangiopathy can develop during the first few weeks of treatment, although graft rejection, graft-versus-host disease, or systemic infections can cause similar microangiopathic changes. The thrombotic microangiopathy often remits with dose reduction or substitution of other immunosuppressive drugs and may not recur if therapy with cyclosporine or tacrolimus is reinstituted.

Mitomycin C is an alkylating agent that is used for anal carcinoma and for some adenocarcinomas. It appears to cause dose-dependent nephrotoxicity, with renal failure occurring in approximately 16 percent of patients who receive a cumulative dose of at least 50 mg.[169] About half of the patients with renal toxicity also develop thrombotic microangiopathy, usually 4 to 8 weeks after the latest dose. Mitomycin C-induced thrombotic microangiopathy does not respond to plasma exchange and has a high mortality rate of approximately 70 percent within 4 months of onset.[170]

Gemcitabine is a nucleoside analogue often used for carcinoma of the pancreas, bladder, or lung. Thrombotic microangiopathy with renal failure occurs with an incidence of approximately 0.3 percent.[171] The median time to develop thrombotic microangiopathy is 7 months with a median cumulative dose of 22 g/m², although the range of doses is broad and very low doses have been associated with thrombotic microangiopathy.[172] Death or disability usually results from cancer progression or renal failure, not from extrarenal manifestations of thrombotic microangiopathy.

Drugs that inhibit vascular endothelial growth factor (VEGF) signaling like sunitinib and bevacizumab are associated with proteinuria, hypertension, and mild thrombotic microangiopathy that usually improve when the drug is discontinued. Inhibition of VEGF produced within the kidney appears to damage glomerular endothelium.[173] In some cases disease has responded to an angiotensin receptor blocker, allowing continued treatment with the VEGF inhibitor.[174]

COBALAMIN METABOLIC DEFECTS

Cobalamin C deficiency is a rare autosomal recessive condition caused by mutations in the *MMACHC* (methylmalonic aciduria and homocystinuria type C protein) gene. Clinical features may include developmental delay, ataxia, seizures, cognitive impairment, pulmonary hypertension, thrombotic microangiopathy and renal failure. Symptoms usually appear during infancy but can occur later in childhood or rarely in adulthood. Laboratory studies show elevated plasma methylmalonic acid and homocysteine, low plasma methionine, and normal or elevated plasma vitamin B_{12}. Treatment with high-dose hydroxycobalamin and betaine may reverse or prevent HUS.[175]

The abnormal red cell and platelet morphology in adults with severe vitamin B_{12} deficiency rarely may suggest thrombotic microangiopathy.

MALIGNANT HYPERTENSION

Malignant hypertension is associated with microangiopathic hemolytic anemia, thrombocytopenia, neurological symptoms and renal insufficiency.[176]

MECHANICAL HEMOLYSIS

A malfunctioning aortic or mitral valve prosthesis may sufficiently increase the fluid shear stress experienced by the blood to cause significant hemolysis, with schistocytes and thrombocytopenia, suggesting a diagnosis of thrombotic microangiopathy.[41,42] Such patients also are likely to have acquired von Willebrand syndrome.

REFERENCES

1. Moschcowitz E: Hyaline thrombosis of the terminal arterioles and capillaries: A hitherto undescribed disease. *Proc N Y Pathol Soc* 24:21, 1924.
2. Singer K, Bornstein FP, Wile SA: Thrombotic thrombocytopenic purpura. Hemorrhagic diathesis with generalized platelet thromboses. *Blood* 2:542, 1947.
3. Amorosi EL, Ultmann JE: Thrombotic thrombocytopenic purpura: Report of 16 cases and review of the literature. *Medicine (Baltimore)* 45:139, 1966.
4. Bukowski RM, Hewlett JS, Harris JW, et al: Exchange transfusions in the treatment of thrombotic thrombocytopenic purpura. *Semin Hematol* 13:219, 1976.
5. Bukowski RM, King JW, Hewlett JS: Plasmapheresis in the treatment of thrombotic thrombocytopenic purpura. *Blood* 50:413, 1977.
6. Byrnes JJ, Khurana M: Treatment of thrombotic thrombocytopenic purpura with plasma. *N Engl J Med* 297:1386, 1977.
7. Bell WR, Braine HG, Ness PM, Kickler TS: Improved survival in thrombotic thrombocytopenic purpura-hemolytic uremic syndrome. Clinical experience in 108 patients. *N Engl J Med* 325:398, 1991.
8. Rock GA, Shumak KH, Buskard NA, et al: Comparison of plasma exchange with plasma infusion in the treatment of thrombotic thrombocytopenic purpura. Canadian Apheresis Study Group. *N Engl J Med* 325:393, 1991.
9. Moake JL, Rudy CK, Troll JH, et al: Unusually large plasma factor VIII:von Willebrand factor multimers in chronic relapsing thrombotic thrombocytopenic purpura. *N Engl J Med* 307:1432, 1982.
10. Furlan M, Robles R, Lämmle B: Partial purification and characterization of a protease from human plasma cleaving von Willebrand factor to fragments produced by *in vivo* proteolysis. *Blood* 87:4223, 1996.
11. Tsai H-M: Physiologic cleavage of von Willebrand factor by a plasma protease is dependent on its conformation and requires calcium ion. *Blood* 87:4235, 1996.
12. Furlan M, Robles R, Solenthaler M, et al: Deficient activity of von Willebrand factor-cleaving protease in chronic relapsing thrombotic thrombocytopenic purpura. *Blood* 89:3097, 1997.
13. Furlan M, Robles R, Galbusera M, et al: Von Willebrand factor-cleaving protease in thrombotic thrombocytopenic purpura and the hemolytic-uremic syndrome. *N Engl J Med* 339:1578, 1998.
14. Tsai HM, Lian EC: Antibodies to von Willebrand factor-cleaving protease in acute thrombotic thrombocytopenic purpura. *N Engl J Med* 339:1585, 1998.
15. Fujikawa K, Suzuki H, McMullen B, Chung D: Purification of human von Willebrand factor-cleaving protease and its identification as a new member of the metalloproteinase family. *Blood* 98:1662, 2001.
16. Gerritsen HE, Robles R, Lammle B, Furlan M: Partial amino acid sequence of purified von Willebrand factor-cleaving protease. *Blood* 98:1654, 2001.
17. Zheng X, Chung D, Takayama TK, et al: Structure of von Willebrand factor-cleaving protease (ADAMTS13), a metalloprotease involved in thrombotic thrombocytopenic purpura. *J Biol Chem* 276:41059, 2001.
18. Soejima K, Mimura N, Hirashima M, et al: A novel human metalloprotease synthesized in the liver and secreted into the blood: Possibly, the von Willebrand factor-cleaving protease? *J Biochem* 130:475, 2001.
19. Levy GG, Nichols WC, Lian EC, et al: Mutations in a member of the ADAMTS gene family cause thrombotic thrombocytopenic purpura. *Nature* 413:488, 2001.
20. Klaus C, Plaimauer B, Studt JD, et al: Epitope mapping of ADAMTS13 autoantibodies in acquired thrombotic thrombocytopenic purpura. *Blood* 103:4514, 2004.
21. Luken BM, Turenhout EA, Hulstein JJ, et al: The spacer domain of ADAMTS13 contains a major binding site for antibodies in patients with thrombotic thrombocytopenic purpura. *Thromb Haemost* 93:267, 2005.
22. Zheng XL, Wu HM, Shang D, et al: Multiple domains of ADAMTS13 are targeted by autoantibodies against ADAMTS13 in patients with acquired idiopathic thrombotic thrombocytopenic purpura. *Haematologica* 95:1555, 2010.
23. Scheiflinger F, Knobl P, Trattner B, et al: Nonneutralizing IgM and IgG antibodies to von Willebrand factor-cleaving protease (ADAMTS-13) in a patient with thrombotic thrombocytopenic purpura. *Blood* 102:3241, 2003.
24. Miller DP, Kaye JA, Shea K, et al: Incidence of thrombotic thrombocytopenic purpura/hemolytic uremic syndrome. *Epidemiology* 15:208, 2004.
25. Terrell DR, Williams LA, Vesely SK, et al: The incidence of thrombotic thrombocytopenic purpura-hemolytic uremic syndrome: All patients, idiopathic patients, and patients with severe ADAMTS-13 deficiency. *J Thromb Haemost* 3:1432, 2005.
26. Zheng XL, Kaufman RM, Goodnough LT, Sadler JE: Effect of plasma exchange on plasma ADAMTS13 metalloprotease activity, inhibitor level, and clinical outcome in patients with idiopathic and nonidiopathic thrombotic thrombocytopenic purpura. *Blood* 103:4043, 2004.
27. Kremer Hovinga JA, Vesely SK, Terrell DR, et al: Survival and relapse in patients with thrombotic thrombocytopenic purpura. *Blood* 115:1500, 2010.
28. Nicol KK, Shelton BJ, Knovich MA, Owen J: Overweight individuals are at increased risk for thrombotic thrombocytopenic purpura. *Am J Hematol* 74:170, 2003.
29. Ridolfi RL, Bell WR: Thrombotic thrombocytopenic purpura. Report of 25 cases and review of the literature. *Medicine (Baltimore)* 60:413, 1981.
30. McMinn JR, George JN: Evaluation of women with clinically suspected thrombotic thrombocytopenic purpura-hemolytic uremic syndrome during pregnancy. *J Clin Apher* 16:202, 2001.
31. Coppo P, Busson M, Veyradier A, et al: HLA-DRB1*11: A strong risk factor for acquired severe ADAMTS13 deficiency-related idiopathic thrombotic thrombocytopenic purpura in Caucasians. *J Thromb Haemost* 8:856, 2010.
32. Scully M, Brown J, Patel R, et al: Human leukocyte antigen association in idiopathic thrombotic thrombocytopenic purpura: Evidence for an immunogenetic link. *J Thromb Haemost* 8:257, 2010.
33. O'Brien TE, Crum ED: Atypical presentations of thrombotic thrombocytopenic purpura. *Int J Hematol* 76:471, 2002.
34. Sarode R: Atypical presentations of thrombotic thrombocytopenic purpura: A review. *J Clin Apher* 24:47, 2009.
35. Imanirad I, Rajasekhar A, Zumberg M: A case series of atypical presentations of thrombotic thrombocytopenic purpura. *J Clin Apher* 27:221, 2012.
36. Htun KT, Davis AK: Neurological symptoms as the sole presentation of relapsed thrombotic thrombocytopenic purpura without microangiopathic haemolytic anaemia. *Thromb Haemost* 112:838, 2014.

37. Camous L, Veyradier A, Darmon M, et al: Macrovascular thrombosis in critically ill patients with thrombotic micro-angiopathies. *Intern Emerg Med* 9:267, 2014.

38. Hawkins BM, Abu-Fadel M, Vesely SK, George JN: Clinical cardiac involvement in thrombotic thrombocytopenic purpura: A systematic review. *Transfusion* 48:382, 2008.

39. Hughes C, McEwan JR, Longair I, et al: Cardiac involvement in acute thrombotic thrombocytopenic purpura: Association with troponin T and IgG antibodies to ADAMTS 13. *J Thromb Haemost* 7:529, 2009.

40. Benhamou Y, Assie C, Boelle PY, et al: Development and validation of a predictive model for death in acquired severe ADAMTS13 deficiency-associated idiopathic thrombotic thrombocytopenic purpura: The French TMA Reference Center experience. *Haematologica* 97:1181, 2012.

41. Zini G, d'Onofrio G, Briggs C, et al: ICSH recommendations for identification, diagnostic value, and quantitation of schistocytes. *Int J Lab Hematol* 34:107, 2012.

42. Burns ER, Lou Y, Pathak A: Morphologic diagnosis of thrombotic thrombocytopenic purpura. *Am J Hematol* 75:18, 2004.

43. Veyradier A, Obert B, Houllier A, et al: Specific von Willebrand factor-cleaving protease in thrombotic microangiopathies: A study of 111 cases. *Blood* 98:1765, 2001.

44. Bianchi V, Robles R, Alberio L, et al: Von Willebrand factor-cleaving protease (ADAMTS13) in thrombocytopenic disorders: A severely deficient activity is specific for thrombotic thrombocytopenic purpura. *Blood* 100:710, 2002.

45. Tsai HM: Is severe deficiency of ADAMTS-13 specific for thrombotic thrombocytopenic purpura? Yes. *J Thromb Haemost* 1:625, 2003.

46. Asada Y, Sumiyoshi A, Hayashi T, et al: Immunohistochemistry of vascular lesion in thrombotic thrombocytopenic purpura, with special reference to factor VIII related antigen. *Thromb Res* 38:469, 1985.

47. Hosler GA, Cusumano AM, Hutchins GM: Thrombotic thrombocytopenic purpura and hemolytic uremic syndrome are distinct pathologic entities. A review of 56 autopsy cases. *Arch Pathol Lab Med* 127:834, 2003.

48. Zomas A, Saso R, Powles R, et al: Red cell fragmentation (schistocytosis) after bone marrow transplantation. *Bone Marrow Transplant* 22:777, 1998.

49. Kanamori H, Takaishi Y, Takabayashi M, et al: Clinical significance of fragmented red cells after allogeneic bone marrow transplantation. *Int J Hematol* 77:180, 2003.

50. Mannucci PM, Canciani MT, Forza I, et al: Changes in health and disease of the metalloprotease that cleaves von Willebrand factor. *Blood* 98:2730, 2001.

51. Kremer Hovinga JA, Zeerleder S, Kessler P, et al: ADAMTS-13, von Willebrand factor and related parameters in severe sepsis and septic shock. *J Thromb Haemost* 5:2284, 2007.

52. Uemura M, Fujimura Y, Matsumoto M, et al: Comprehensive analysis of ADAMTS13 in patients with liver cirrhosis. *Thromb Haemost* 99:1019, 2008.

53. Park YD, Yoshioka A, Kawa K, et al: Impaired activity of plasma von Willebrand factor-cleaving protease may predict the occurrence of hepatic veno-occlusive disease after stem cell transplantation. *Bone Marrow Transplant* 29:789, 2002.

54. Nguyen L, Li X, Duvall D, et al: Twice-daily plasma exchange for patients with refractory thrombotic thrombocytopenic purpura: The experience of the Oklahoma Registry, 1989 through 2006. *Transfusion* 48:349, 2008.

55. Scully M, Hunt BJ, Benjamin S, et al: Guidelines on the diagnosis and management of thrombotic thrombocytopenic purpura and other thrombotic microangiopathies. *Br J Haematol* 158:323, 2012.

56. Zeigler ZR, Shadduck RK, Gryn JF, et al: Cryoprecipitate poor plasma does not improve early response in primary adult thrombotic thrombocytopenic purpura (TTP). *J Clin Apher* 16:19, 2001.

57. Rock G, Anderson D, Clark W, et al: Does cryosupernatant plasma improve outcome in thrombotic thrombocytopenic purpura? No answer yet. *Br J Haematol* 129:79, 2005.

58. Michael M, Elliott EJ, Craig JC, et al: Interventions for hemolytic uremic syndrome and thrombotic thrombocytopenic purpura: A systematic review of randomized controlled trials. *Am J Kidney Dis* 53:259, 2009.

59. Prowse C: Properties of pathogen-inactivated plasma components. *Transfus Med Rev* 23:124, 2009.

60. McCarthy LJ: Evidence-based medicine for apheresis: An ongoing challenge. *Ther Apher Dial* 8:112, 2004.

61. Yarranton H, Cohen H, Pavord SR, et al: Venous thromboembolism associated with the management of acute thrombotic thrombocytopenic purpura. *Br J Haematol* 121:778, 2003.

62. Allford SL, Harrison P, Lawrie AS, et al: Von Willebrand factor—Cleaving protease activity in congenital thrombotic thrombocytopenic purpura. *Br J Haematol* 111:1215, 2000.

63. del Rio-Garma J, Alvarez-Larran A, Martinez C, et al: Methylene blue-photoinactivated plasma versus quarantine fresh frozen plasma in thrombotic thrombocytopenic purpura: A multicentric, prospective cohort study. *Br J Haematol* 143:39, 2008.

64. Bobbio-Pallavicini E, Gugliotta L, Centurioni R, et al: Antiplatelet agents in thrombotic thrombocytopenic purpura (TTP). Results of a randomized multicenter trial by the Italian Cooperative Group for TTP. *Haematologica* 82:429, 1997.

65. Coppo P, Lassoued K, Mariette X, et al: Effectiveness of platelet transfusions after plasma exchange in adult thrombotic thrombocytopenic purpura: A report of two cases. *Am J Hematol* 68:198, 2001.

66. Goel R, Ness PM, Takemoto CM, et al: Platelet transfusions in platelet consumptive disorders are associated with arterial thrombosis and in-hospital mortality. *Blood* 125:1470, 2015.

67. Doerfler ME, Kaufman B, Goldenberg AS: Central venous catheter placement in patients with disorders of hemostasis. *Chest* 110:185, 1996.

68. Rizvi MA, Vesely SK, George JN, et al: Complications of plasma exchange in 71 consecutive patients treated for clinically suspected thrombotic thrombocytopenic purpura-hemolytic-uremic syndrome. *Transfusion* 40:896, 2000.

69. Lim W, Vesely SK, George JN: The role of rituximab in the management of patients with acquired thrombotic thrombocytopenic purpura. *Blood* 125:1526, 2015.

70. Westwood JP, Webster H, McGuckin S, et al: Rituximab for thrombotic thrombocytopenic purpura: Benefit of early administration during acute episodes and use of prophylaxis to prevent relapse. *J Thromb Haemost* 11:481, 2013.

71. Hie M, Gay J, Galicier L, et al: Preemptive rituximab infusions after remission efficiently prevent relapses in acquired thrombotic thrombocytopenic purpura. *Blood* 124:204, 2014.

72. Carson KR, Evens AM, Richey EA, et al: Progressive multifocal leukoencephalopathy after rituximab therapy in HIV-negative patients: A report of 57 cases from the Research on Adverse Drug Event and Reports project. *Blood* 113:4834, 2009.

73. Bharat A, Xie F, Baddley JW, et al: Incidence and risk factors for progressive multifocal leukoencephalopathy among patients with selected rheumatic diseases. *Arthritis Care Res (Hoboken)* 64:612, 2012.

74. Lunel-Fabiani F, Masson C, Ducancelle A: Systemic diseases and biotherapies: Understanding, evaluating, and preventing the risk of hepatitis B reactivation. *Joint Bone Spine* 81:478, 2014.

75. Aqui NA, Stein SH, Konkle BA, et al: Role of splenectomy in patients with refractory or relapsed thrombotic thrombocytopenic purpura. *J Clin Apher* 18:51, 2003.

76. Kappers-Klunne MC, Wijermans P, Fijnheer R, et al: Splenectomy for the treatment of thrombotic thrombocytopenic purpura. *Br J Haematol* 130:768, 2005.

77. Katkhouda N, Hurwitz MB, Rivera RT, et al: Laparoscopic splenectomy: Outcome and efficacy in 103 consecutive patients. *Ann Surg* 228:568, 1998.

78. Ferrara F, Annunziata M, Pollio F, et al: Vincristine as treatment for recurrent episodes of thrombotic thrombocytopenic purpura. *Ann Hematol* 81:7, 2002.

79. Bobbio-Pallavicini E, Porta C, Centurioni R, et al: Vincristine sulfate for the treatment of thrombotic thrombocytopenic purpura refractory to plasma-exchange. The Italian Cooperative Group for TTP. *Eur J Haematol* 52:222, 1994.

80. Bobbio-Pallavicini E, Porta C, Tacconi F, et al: Intravenous prostacyclin (as epoprostenol) infusion in thrombotic thrombocytopenic purpura. Four case reports and review of the literature. Italian Cooperative Group for Thrombotic Thrombocytopenic Purpura. *Haematologica* 79:429, 1994.

81. Sagripanti A, Carpi A, Rosaia B, et al: Iloprost in the treatment of thrombotic microangiopathy: Report of thirteen cases. *Biomed Pharmacother* 50:350, 1996.

82. Dervenoulas J, Tsirigotis P, Bollas G, et al: Efficacy of intravenous immunoglobulin in the treatment of thrombotic thrombocytopaenic purpura. A study of 44 cases. *Acta Haematol* 105:204, 2001.

83. Anderson D, Ali K, Blanchette V, et al: Guidelines on the use of intravenous immune globulin for hematologic conditions. *Transfus Med Rev* 21:S9, 2007.

84. Cataland SR, Jin M, Lin S, et al: Cyclosporin and plasma exchange in thrombotic thrombocytopenic purpura: Long-term follow-up with serial analysis of ADAMTS13 activity. *Br J Haematol* 139:486, 2007.

85. Shortt J, Oh DH, Opat SS: ADAMTS13 antibody depletion by bortezomib in thrombotic thrombocytopenic purpura. *N Engl J Med* 368:90, 2013.

86. Ahmad HN, Thomas-Dewing RR, Hunt BJ: Mycophenolate mofetil in a case of relapsed, refractory thrombotic thrombocytopenic purpura. *Eur J Haematol* 78:449, 2007.

87. Li GW, Rambally S, Kamboj J, et al: Treatment of refractory thrombotic thrombocytopenic purpura with N-acetylcysteine: A case report. *Transfusion* 54:1221, 2014.

88. Spiekermann K, Wormann B, Rumpf KW, Hiddemann W: Combination chemotherapy with CHOP for recurrent thrombotic thrombocytopenic purpura. *Br J Haematol* 97:544, 1997.

89. Passweg JR, Rabusin M, Musso M, et al: Haematopoetic stem cell transplantation for refractory autoimmune cytopenia. *Br J Haematol* 125:749, 2004.

90. Callewaert F, Roodt J, Ulrichts H, et al: Evaluation of efficacy and safety of the anti-VWF Nanobody ALX-0681 in a preclinical baboon model of acquired thrombotic thrombocytopenic purpura. *Blood* 120:3603, 2012.

91. Cataland SR, Peyvandi F, Mannucci PM, et al: Initial experience from a double-blind, placebo-controlled, clinical outcome study of ARC1779 in patients with thrombotic thrombocytopenic purpura. *Am J Hematol* 87:430, 2012.

92. O'Brien KL, Price TH, Howell C, Delaney M: The use of 50% albumin/plasma replacement fluid in therapeutic plasma exchange for thrombotic thrombocytopenic purpura. *J Clin Apher* 28:416, 2013.

93. Zhan H, Streiff MB, King KE, Segal JB: Thrombotic thrombocytopenic purpura at the Johns Hopkins Hospital from 1992 to 2008: Clinical outcomes and risk factors for relapse. *Transfusion* 50:868, 2010.

94. Bandarenko N, Brecher ME: United States Thrombotic Thrombocytopenic Purpura Apheresis Study Group (US TTP ASG): Multicenter survey and retrospective analysis of current efficacy of therapeutic plasma exchange. *J Clin Apher* 13:133, 1998.

95. Tsai H-M, Shulman K: Rituximab induces remission of cerebral ischemia caused by thrombotic thrombocytopenic purpura. *Eur J Haematol* 70:183, 2003.

96. Sadler JE: Von Willebrand factor, ADAMTS13, and thrombotic thrombocytopenic purpura. *Blood* 112:11, 2008.

97. McClain RS, Terrell DR, Vesely SK, George JN: Plasma exchange complications in patients treated for thrombotic thrombocytopenia purpura-hemolytic uremic syndrome: 2011 to 2014. *Transfusion* 54:3257, 2014.

98. Kennedy AS, Lewis QF, Scott JG, et al: Cognitive deficits after recovery from thrombotic thrombocytopenic purpura. *Transfusion* 49:1092, 2009.

99. Lewis QF, Lanneau MS, Mathias SD, et al: Long-term deficits in health-related quality of life after recovery from thrombotic thrombocytopenic purpura. *Transfusion* 49:118, 2009.

100. Hayward CP, Sutton DM, Carter WH Jr, et al: Treatment outcomes in patients with adult thrombotic thrombocytopenic purpura-hemolytic uremic syndrome. *Arch Intern Med* 154:982, 1994.

101. Coppo P, Bengoufa D, Veyradier A, et al: Severe ADAMTS13 deficiency in adult idiopathic thrombotic microangiopathies defines a subset of patients characterized by various autoimmune manifestations, lower platelet count, and mild renal involvement. *Medicine (Baltimore)* 83:233, 2004.

102. Schulman I, Pierce M, Lukens A, Currimbhoy Z: Studies on thrombopoiesis. I. A factor in normal human plasma required for platelet production; chronic thrombocytopenia due to its deficiency. *Blood* 16:943, 1960.

103. Upshaw JD Jr: Congenital deficiency of a factor in normal plasma that reverses microangiopathic hemolysis and thrombocytopenia. *N Engl J Med* 298:1350, 1978.

104. Zheng XL, Sadler JE: Pathogenesis of thrombotic microangiopathies. *Annu Rev Pathol* 3:249, 2008.

105. Furlan M, Lämmle B: Aetiology and pathogenesis of thrombotic thrombocytopenic purpura and haemolytic uraemic syndrome: The role of von Willebrand factor-cleaving protease. *Best Pract Res Clin Haematol* 14:437, 2001.

106. Miyata T, Kokame K, Matsumoto M, Fujimura Y: ADAMTS13 activity and genetic mutations in Japan. *Hamostaseologie* 33:131, 2013.

107. Loirat C, Girma JP, Desconclois C, et al: Thrombotic thrombocytopenic purpura related to severe ADAMTS13 deficiency in children. *Pediatr Nephrol* 24:19, 2009.

108. Veyradier A, Meyer D, Loirat C: Desmopressin, an unexpected link between nocturnal enuresis and inherited thrombotic thrombocytopenic purpura (Upshaw-Schulman syndrome). *J Thromb Haemost* 4:700, 2006.

109. Scully M, Thomas M, Underwood M, et al: Thrombotic thrombocytopenic purpura and pregnancy: Presentation, management, and subsequent pregnancy outcomes. *Blood* 124:211, 2014.

110. Raval JS, Padmanabhan A, Kremer Hovinga JA, Kiss JE: Development of a clinically significant ADAMTS13 inhibitor in a patient with hereditary thrombotic thrombocytopenic purpura. *Am J Hematol* 90:E22, 2015.

111. Wallace DC, Lovric A, Clubb JS, Carseldine DB: Thrombotic thrombocytopenic purpura in four siblings. *Am J Med* 58:724, 1975.

112. Furlan M, Robles R, Morselli B, et al: Recovery and half-life of von Willebrand factor-cleaving protease after plasma therapy in patients with thrombotic thrombocytopenic purpura. *Thromb Haemost* 81:8, 1999.

113. Lotta LA, Wu HM, Mackie IJ, et al: Residual plasmatic activity of ADAMTS13 is correlated with phenotype severity in congenital thrombotic thrombocytopenic purpura. *Blood* 120:440, 2012.

114. Camilleri RS, Scully M, Thomas M, et al: A phenotype-genotype correlation of ADAMTS13 mutations in congenital thrombotic thrombocytopenic purpura patients treated in the United Kingdom. *J Thromb Haemost* 10:1792, 2012.

115. Gasser C, Gautier E, Steck A, et al: Hämolytisch-urämische Syndrome: Bilaterale Nierenrindennekrosen bei akuten erworbenen hämolytischen Anämien. *Schweiz Med Wochenschr* 85:905, 1955.

116. Kibel MA, Barnard PJ: The haemolytic-uraemic syndrome: A survey in Southern Africa. *S Afr Med J* 42:692, 1968.

117. Karmali MA, Steele BT, Petric M, Lim C: Sporadic cases of haemolytic-uraemic syndrome associated with faecal cytotoxin and cytotoxin-producing *Escherichia coli* in stools. *Lancet* 1:619, 1983.

118. O'Brien AO, Lively TA, Chen ME, et al: *Escherichia coli* O157:H7 strains associated with haemorrhagic colitis in the United States produce a Shigella dysenteriae 1 (SHIGA) like cytotoxin. *Lancet* 1:702, 1983.

119. Riley LW, Remis RS, Helgerson SD, et al: Hemorrhagic colitis associated with a rare *Escherichia coli* serotype. *N Engl J Med* 308:681, 1983.

120. Tarr PI, Gordon CA, Chandler WL: Shiga-toxin-producing *Escherichia coli* and haemolytic uraemic syndrome. *Lancet* 365:1073, 2005.

121. Gianviti A, Tozzi AE, De Petris L, et al: Risk factors for poor renal prognosis in children with hemolytic uremic syndrome. *Pediatr Nephrol* 18:1229, 2003.

122. Frank C, Werber D, Cramer JP, et al: Epidemic profile of Shiga-toxin-producing *Escherichia coli* O104:H4 outbreak in Germany. *N Engl J Med* 365:1771, 2011.

123. Proesmans W: The role of coagulation and fibrinolysis in the pathogenesis of diarrhea-associated hemolytic uremic syndrome. *Semin Thromb Hemost* 27:201, 2001.

124. Tsai HM, Chandler WL, Sarode R, et al: Von Willebrand factor and von Willebrand factor-cleaving metalloprotease activity in *Escherichia coli* O157:H7-associated hemolytic uremic syndrome. *Pediatr Res* 49:653, 2001.

125. Hunt BJ, Lämmle B, Nevard CH, et al: Von Willebrand factor-cleaving protease in childhood diarrhoea-associated haemolytic uraemic syndrome. *Thromb Haemost* 85:975, 2001.

126. Inward CD, Howie AJ, Fitzpatrick MM, et al: Renal histopathology in fatal cases of diarrhoea-associated haemolytic uraemic syndrome. British Association for Paediatric Nephrology. *Pediatr Nephrol* 11:556, 1997.

127. Wong CS, Mooney JC, Brandt JR, et al: Risk factors for the hemolytic uremic syndrome in children infected with *Escherichia coli* O157:H7: A multivariable analysis. *Clin Infect Dis* 55:33, 2012.

128. Menne J, Nitschke M, Stingele R, et al: Validation of treatment strategies for enterohaemorrhagic *Escherichia coli* O104:H4 induced haemolytic uraemic syndrome: Case-control study. *BMJ* 345:e4565, 2012.

129. Braune SA, Wichmann D, von Heinz MC, et al: Clinical features of critically ill patients with Shiga toxin-induced hemolytic uremic syndrome. *Crit Care Med* 41:1702, 2013.

130. Garg AX, Suri RS, Barrowman N, et al: Long-term renal prognosis of diarrhea-associated hemolytic uremic syndrome: A systematic review, meta-analysis, and meta-regression. *JAMA* 290:1360, 2003.

131. Barnard PJ, Kibel M: The haemolytic-uraemic syndrome of infancy and childhood. A report of eleven cases. *Cent Afr J Med* 11:31, 1965.

132. Kaplan BS, Chesney RW, Drummond KN: Hemolytic uremic syndrome in families. *N Engl J Med* 292:1090, 1975.

133. Kaplan BS: Hemolytic uremic syndrome with recurrent episodes: An important subset. *Clin Nephrol* 8:495, 1977.

134. Fitzpatrick MM, Walters MD, Trompeter RS, et al: Atypical (non-diarrhea-associated) hemolytic-uremic syndrome in childhood. *J Pediatr* 122:532, 1993.

135. Thompson RA, Winterborn MH: Hypocomplementaemia due to a genetic deficiency of beta 1H globulin. *Clin Exp Immunol* 46:110, 1981.

136. Warwicker P, Goodship TH, Donne RL, et al: Genetic studies into inherited and sporadic hemolytic uremic syndrome. *Kidney Int* 53:836, 1998.

137. Legendre CM, Licht C, Muus P, et al: Terminal complement inhibitor eculizumab in atypical hemolytic-uremic syndrome. *N Engl J Med* 368:2169, 2013.

138. Noris M, Caprioli J, Bresin E, et al: Relative role of genetic complement abnormalities in sporadic and familial aHUS and their impact on clinical phenotype. *Clin J Am Soc Nephrol* 5:1844, 2010.

139. Fremeaux-Bacchi V, Fakhouri F, Garnier A, et al: Genetics and outcome of atypical hemolytic uremic syndrome: A nationwide French series comparing children and adults. *Clin J Am Soc Nephrol* 8:554, 2013.

140. Lemaire M, Fremeaux-Bacchi V, Schaefer F, et al: Recessive mutations in DGKE cause atypical hemolytic uremic syndrome. *Nat Genet* 45:531, 2013.

141. Taylor CM, Machin S, Wigmore SJ, et al: Clinical practice guidelines for the management of atypical haemolytic uraemic syndrome in the United Kingdom. *Br J Haematol* 148:37, 2010.

142. Fakhouri F, Roumenina L, Provot F, et al: Pregnancy-associated hemolytic uremic syndrome revisited in the era of complement gene mutations. *J Am Soc Nephrol* 21:859, 2010.

143. Rossio R, Lotta LA, Pontiggia S, et al: A novel CD46 mutation in a patient with microangiopathy clinically resembling thrombotic thrombocytopenic purpura and normal ADAMTS13 activity. *Haematologica* 100:e87, 2015.

144. Noris M, Remuzzi G: Managing and preventing atypical hemolytic uremic syndrome recurrence after kidney transplantation. *Curr Opin Nephrol Hypertens* 22:704, 2013.

145. Sanchez Chinchilla D, Pinto S, Hoppe B, et al: Complement mutations in diacylglycerol kinase-epsilon-associated atypical hemolytic uremic syndrome. *Clin J Am Soc Nephrol* 9:1611, 2014.

146. Westland R, Bodria M, Carrea A, et al: Phenotypic expansion of DGKE-associated diseases. *J Am Soc Nephrol* 25:1408, 2014.

147. Cabrera GR, Fortenberry JD, Warshaw BL, et al: Hemolytic uremic syndrome associated with invasive Streptococcus pneumoniae infection. *Pediatrics* 101:699, 1998.

148. Copelovitch L, Kaplan BS: Streptococcus pneumoniae-associated hemolytic uremic syndrome. *Pediatr Nephrol* 23:1951, 2008.

149. Singh N, Gayowski T, Marino IR: Hemolytic uremic syndrome in solid-organ transplant recipients. *Transpl Int* 9:68, 1996.

150. Arai S, Allan C, Streiff M, et al: Von Willebrand factor-cleaving protease activity and proteolysis of von Willebrand factor in bone marrow transplant-associated thrombotic microangiopathy. *Hematol J* 2:292, 2001.

151. Ho VT, Cutler C, Carter S, et al: Blood and marrow transplant clinical trials network toxicity committee consensus summary: Thrombotic microangiopathy after hematopoietic stem cell transplantation. *Biol Blood Marrow Transplant* 11:571, 2005.

152. Sack GH Jr, Levin J, Bell WR: Trousseau's syndrome and other manifestations of chronic disseminated coagulopathy in patients with neoplasms: Clinical, pathophysiologic, and therapeutic features. *Medicine (Baltimore)* 56:1, 1977.

153. Elliott MA, Letendre L, Gastineau DA, et al: Cancer-associated microangiopathic hemolytic anemia with thrombocytopenia: An important diagnostic consideration. *Eur J Haematol* 85:43, 2010.

154. Domingo-Claros A, Larriba I, Rozman M, et al: Acute erythroid neoplastic proliferations. A biological study based on 62 patients. *Haematologica* 87:148, 2002.

155. Lattuada A, Rossi E, Calzarossa C, et al: Mild to moderate reduction of a von Willebrand factor cleaving protease (ADAMTS-13) in pregnant women with HELLP microangiopathic syndrome. *Haematologica* 88:1029, 2003.

156. Baron BW, Martin MS, Sucharetza BS, et al: Four patients with both thrombotic thrombocytopenic purpura and autoimmune thrombocytopenic purpura: The concept of a mixed immune thrombocytopenia syndrome and indications for plasma exchange. *J Clin Apher* 16:179, 2001.

157. Mannucci PM, Vanoli M, Forza I, et al: Von Willebrand factor cleaving protease (ADAMTS-13) in 123 patients with connective tissue diseases (systemic lupus erythematosus and systemic sclerosis). *Haematologica* 88:914, 2003.

158. Güngör T, Furlan M, Lämmle B, et al: Acquired deficiency of von Willebrand factor-cleaving protease in a patient suffering from acute systemic lupus erythematosus. *Rheumatology (Oxford)* 40:940, 2001.

159. Ahmed S, Siddiqui AK, Chandrasekaran V: Correlation of thrombotic thrombocytopenic purpura disease activity with von Willebrand factor-cleaving protease level in ulcerative colitis. *Am J Med* 116:786, 2004.

160. Steen VD: Scleroderma renal crisis. *Rheum Dis Clin North Am* 29:315, 2003.

161. Al-Nouri ZL, Reese JA, Terrell DR, et al: Drug-induced thrombotic microangiopathy: A systematic review of published reports. *Blood* 125:616, 2015.

162. Schwartz J, Winters JL, Padmanabhan A, et al: Guidelines on the use of therapeutic apheresis in clinical practice-evidence-based approach from the Writing Committee of the American Society for Apheresis: The sixth special issue. *J Clin Apher* 28:145, 2013.

163. Kojouri K, Vesely SK, George JN: Quinine-associated thrombotic thrombocytopenic purpura-hemolytic uremic syndrome: Frequency, clinical features, and long-term outcomes. *Ann Intern Med* 135:1047, 2001.

164. Dlott JS, Danielson CF, Blue-Hnidy DE, McCarthy LJ: Drug-induced thrombotic thrombocytopenic purpura/hemolytic uremic syndrome: A concise review. *Ther Apher Dial* 8:102, 2004.

165. Bennett CL, Kim B, Zakarija A, et al: Two mechanistic pathways for thienopyridine-associated thrombotic thrombocytopenic purpura: A report from the SERF-TTP Research Group and the RADAR Project. *J Am Coll Cardiol* 50:1138, 2007.

166. Remuzzi G, Bertani T: Renal vascular and thrombotic effects of cyclosporine. *Am J Kidney Dis* 13:261, 1989.

167. Bechstein WO: Neurotoxicity of calcineurin inhibitors: Impact and clinical management. *Transpl Int* 13:313, 2000.

168. Scott LJ, McKeage K, Keam SJ, Plosker GL: Tacrolimus: A further update of its use in the management of organ transplantation. *Drugs* 63:1247, 2003.

169. Valavaara R, Nordman E: Renal complications of mitomycin C therapy with special reference to the total dose. *Cancer* 55:47, 1985.

170. Lesesne JB, Rothschild N, Erickson B, et al: Cancer-associated hemolytic-uremic syndrome: Analysis of 85 cases from a national registry. *J Clin Oncol* 7:781, 1989.

171. Humphreys BD, Sharman JP, Henderson JM, et al: Gemcitabine-associated thrombotic microangiopathy. *Cancer* 100:2664, 2004.

172. Glezerman I, Kris MG, Miller V, et al: Gemcitabine nephrotoxicity and hemolytic uremic syndrome: Report of 29 cases from a single institution. *Clin Nephrol* 71:130, 2009.

173. Eremina V, Jefferson JA, Kowalewska J, et al: VEGF inhibition and renal thrombotic microangiopathy. *N Engl J Med* 358:1129, 2008.

174. Bollee G, Patey N, Cazajous G, et al: Thrombotic microangiopathy secondary to VEGF pathway inhibition by sunitinib. *Nephrol Dial Transplant* 24:682, 2009.

175. Carrillo-Carrasco N, Chandler RJ, Venditti CP: Combined methylmalonic acidemia and homocystinuria, cblC type. I. Clinical presentations, diagnosis and management. *J Inherit Metab Dis* 35:91, 2012.

176. van den Born BJ, van der Hoeven NV, Groot E, et al: Association between thrombotic microangiopathy and reduced ADAMTS13 activity in malignant hypertension. *Hypertension* 51:862, 2008.

CHAPTER 133
VENOUS THROMBOSIS

Gary E. Raskob, Russell D. Hull, and Harry R. Buller

SUMMARY

Venous thromboembolism, consisting of deep vein thrombosis and/or pulmonary embolism, is a common disorder with an estimated 900,000 patients each year in the United States and more than 1 million each year in the European Union. Approximately one-third of these cases are fatal pulmonary emboli, and the remaining two-thirds are nonfatal episodes of symptomatic deep vein thrombosis or pulmonary embolism. The majority of fatal events occur as sudden death, underscoring the importance of prevention as the critical strategy for reducing death from pulmonary embolism. Of the nonfatal cases, approximately 60 percent present clinically as deep vein thrombosis and 40 percent present as pulmonary embolism. Most clinically important pulmonary emboli arise from proximal deep vein thrombosis of the leg (popliteal, femoral, or iliac vein thrombosis). Upper-extremity deep vein thrombosis also may lead to clinically important pulmonary embolism. The clinical features of deep vein thrombosis and pulmonary embolism are nonspecific. Objective diagnostic testing is required to confirm or exclude the presence of venous thromboembolism. A validated assay for plasma D-dimer, if available, provides a simple, rapid, and cost-effective first-line exclusion test in patients with low, unlikely, or intermediate clinical probability. Compression ultrasonography is highly sensitive and specific for clinically important deep vein thrombosis and is the primary imaging test for symptomatic patients. Compression ultrasonography of the proximal veins performed at presentation, and if normal, repeated once 5 to 7 days later, can safely exclude clinically important deep vein thrombosis. In centers with the expertise, a single comprehensive evaluation of the proximal and calf veins with duplex ultrasonography is sufficient. In patients with suspected pulmonary embolism, computed tomographic angiography, with or without additional testing using computed tomographic venography or compression ultrasonography of the legs, provides a definitive basis to give or withhold antithrombotic therapy in 90 percent of patients. Anticoagulant therapy is the preferred treatment for most patients with acute venous thromboembolism. Initial treatment with heparin or low-molecular-weight heparin, followed by long-term treatment with an oral vitamin K antagonist such as warfarin, is highly effective for preventing recurrent venous thromboembolism, and has been the traditional standard care. More recently, the direct oral anticoagulants including the thrombin inhibitor dabigatran, and the factor Xa inhibitors rivaroxaban, apixaban, and edoxaban, have been established to be as effective and safer than traditional standard anticoagulant therapy. Rivaroxaban and apixaban can be used as a single drug approach. Dabigatran and edoxaban are preceded by at least 5 days of heparin or low-molecular-weight heparin treatment. The direct oral anticoagulants are preferred over the vitamin K antagonists in most new patients commencing anticoagulant therapy. In cancer patients with venous thromboembolism, treatment with low-molecular-weight heparin for at least 6 months is the recommended approach. Thrombolytic therapy is indicated for patients with pulmonary embolism who present with hypotension or shock, and in selected patients who have impaired right ventricular function who are at high risk of hemodynamic collapse. Insertion of a vena cava filter is indicated for patients who have an absolute contraindication to anticoagulant therapy or who have recurrent venous thromboembolism despite adequate anticoagulant treatment. Anticoagulant treatment should be continued for at least 3 months in all patients, and 3 months is a sufficient duration for patients with first episode of venous thromboembolism secondary to a reversible risk factor. Indefinite anticoagulant therapy should be considered for patients with unprovoked (idiopathic) venous thromboembolism, and those with recurrent venous thromboembolism.

● DEFINITION AND EPIDEMIOLOGY

Venous thrombosis commonly develops in the deep veins of the leg or the arm or in the superficial veins of these extremities. Venous thrombosis of superficial veins is a relatively benign disorder unless extension into the deep venous system occurs. Confusingly, one of the major deep veins in the leg is called the superficial femoral vein. Thrombosis involving the deep veins of the leg is divided into two prognostic categories: (1) calf vein thrombosis, in which thrombi remain confined to the deep calf veins, and (2) proximal vein thrombosis, in which thrombosis involves the popliteal, femoral, or iliac veins.[1]

Pulmonary emboli originate from thrombi in the deep veins of the leg in 90 percent or more of patients. Other less common sources of pulmonary embolism (PE) include the deep pelvic veins, renal veins, inferior vena cava, right side of the heart, and axillary veins. Most clinically important pulmonary emboli arise from proximal deep vein thrombosis (DVT) of the leg. Upper-extremity DVT also may lead to important PE.[2] DVT and/or PE are referred to collectively as *venous thromboembolism (VTE)*.

VTE is a common disorder.[3] The estimated annual incidence of clinically evident VTE ranges between 0.75 and 2.7 per 1000 population based on studies done in North America, Western Europe, Australia, and Argentina.[3] The literature indicates a strong and consistent association of increasing incidence of VTE with increasing age. The annual incidence increased to between 2 and 7 per 1000 population among those 70 years of age, and to between 3 and 12 per 1000 population among those 80 years of age or older.[3] Although the incidence is lower in individuals of Chinese and Korean ethnicity,[3] their disease burden is not low because of population aging. The high incidence of VTE in the elderly likely reflects the high prevalence of comorbid acquired risk factors in these patients, especially malignancy, heart failure, and surgery or hospitalization for medical illness, which account for the majority of the population-attributable risk of VTE in older individuals.

VTE causes a major burden of disease across low-, middle-, and high-income countries. VTE associated with hospitalization was the leading cause of premature death and years lived with disability in low- and middle-income countries, and second in high-income countries, and responsible for more premature death and disability than nosocomial pneumonia, catheter-related bloodstream infections, and adverse drug events.[3]

Acronyms and Abbreviations: aPTT, activated partial thromboplastin time; CDT, catheter-directed thrombolysis; CT, computed tomography; CTA, computed tomographic angiography; CTV, computed tomographic venography; DOAC, direct-acting oral anticoagulant; DVT, deep vein thrombosis; ELISA, enzyme-linked immunosorbent assay; INR, international normalized ratio; LMW, low molecular weight; PE, pulmonary embolism; PIOPED, Prospective Investigation of Pulmonary Embolism Diagnosis; VTE, venous thromboembolism.

The direct ascertainment of deaths from VTE is difficult because of the low rate of autopsy in most countries, and because autopsy studies have consistently demonstrated that PE is often not diagnosed antemortem. The strongest evidence comes from the study by Cohen and colleagues, who used an incidence-based model in six European countries to estimate that there were 534,454 deaths related to VTE across the European Union in 2004.[4] A similar approach applied to the data from the United States suggested approximately 300,000 deaths from VTE each year.[5] The majority of deaths from VTE occur as sudden death, underscoring the critical role of prevention for reducing death from VTE.

Effective prophylaxis against VTE is available for most high-risk patients. Use of prophylaxis is more effective for preventing death and morbidity from VTE than is treatment of the established disease. Evidence-based recommendations for prevention are available.[6–9] Multifaceted interventions with alerts, such as computerized reminders or stickers on patient charts, are effective for increasing the prescription of appropriate thromboprophylaxis in hospitalized adult medical or surgical patients.[10] There is also evidence that inclusion of VTE risk assessment at the time of hospital admission and the provision of appropriate prophylaxis is effective for reducing VTE-related death and readmission with nonfatal VTE.[11,12]

Historically, the majority of the disease burden from VTE occurred in hospitalized patients. The burden of illness from VTE has shifted to the community setting such that most patients now present as outpatients to their primary care physician or to the emergency department. The main reason for this shift is the greatly reduced length of hospital stay for most surgical procedures or medical conditions, such that patients are discharged from the hospital either before the period of risk of VTE has ended or who have subclinical venous thrombi that subsequently evolve to symptomatic DVT or PE. The shift in burden of illness from the hospital to the community setting has led to an emphasis on effective and safe methods for outpatient prophylaxis, diagnosis and treatment.

ETIOLOGY AND PATHOGENESIS

Venous thrombi are composed mainly of fibrin and red blood cells, with variable numbers of platelets and leukocytes. The formation, growth, and breakdown of venous thromboemboli reflect a balance between thrombogenic stimuli and protective mechanisms. The thrombogenic stimuli first identified by Virchow in the 19th century are (1) venous stasis, (2) activation of blood coagulation, and (3) vascular damage. The protective mechanisms are (1) inactivation of activated coagulation factors by circulating inhibitors (e.g., antithrombin and activated protein C), (2) clearance of activated coagulation factors and soluble fibrin polymer complexes by mononuclear phagocytes and the liver, and (3) lysis of fibrin by fibrinolytic enzymes derived from plasma and endothelial cells.

PE occurs in at least 50 percent of patients with documented proximal vein thrombosis.[1] Many of these emboli are asymptomatic. The clinical importance of PE depends on the size of the embolus and the patient's cardiorespiratory reserve. Usually only part of the thrombus embolizes, and 30 to 70 percent of patients with PE detected by angiography also have identifiable DVT of the legs.[13,14] DVT and PE are not separate disorders but a continuous syndrome of VTE in which the initial clinical presentation may be symptoms of either DVT or PE. Therefore, strategies for diagnosis of VTE include both tests for detection of PE (e.g., computed tomography [CT] or lung scanning)[13–16] and tests for DVT of the legs (e.g., ultrasonography)[17–19] (see "Objective Testing for Pulmonary Embolism" and "Objective Testing for Deep Vein Thrombosis" below).

TABLE 133–1. Risk Factors for Thromboembolism*

Acquired	Hereditary Thrombophilias*
Advancing age (age >40 years)	Activated protein C resistance
History of prior thromboembolic event	Prothrombin G20210A
Recent surgery	Antithrombin deficiency
Recent trauma	Protein C deficiency
Prolonged immobilization	Protein S deficiency
Certain forms of cancer	Dysfibrinogenemia
Congestive heart failure	
Recent myocardial infarction	
Paralysis of legs	
Use of female hormones	
Pregnancy or postpartum period	
Varicose veins	
Obesity	
Antiphospholipid antibody syndrome**	
Hyperhomocysteinemia	

*See also Chap. 130
**See also Chap. 131

Acquired and inherited risk factors for VTE have been identified[20–23] and are shown in Table 133–1 (Chap. 130). Aging is the dominant risk factor for VTE (population attributable risk >90 percent).[23] Comorbidities, such as malignancy and heart failure, contribute to a higher population-attributable risk in older patients (≥65 years).[23] The risk of VTE increases when more than one risk factor is present.[24]

Activated protein C resistance is the most common hereditary abnormality predisposing to VTE. The defect results from substitution of glutamine for arginine at residue 506 in the factor V molecule, making factor Va resistant to proteolysis by activated protein C. The gene mutation is commonly designated *factor V Leiden* and follows autosomal dominant inheritance. Patients who are homozygous for the factor V Leiden mutation have a markedly increased risk of VTE and present with clinical thromboembolism at a younger age (median age: 31 years) than those who are heterozygous (median age: 46 years).[20,22] Factor V Leiden is present in approximately 5 percent of the normal population of European descent, 16 percent of patients with a first episode of DVT, and up to 35 percent of patients with unprovoked (idiopathic) DVT.[20,22,25] Prothrombin G20210A is another common gene mutation that predisposes to VTE. It is present in approximately 2 to 3 percent of apparently healthy individuals and in 7 percent of those with DVT.[22] An inherited abnormality cannot be detected in up to 40 to 50 percent of patients with unprovoked DVT, suggesting that as yet undefined gene mutations are present that have an etiologic role (Chap. 130).

CLINICAL FEATURES

VENOUS THROMBOSIS

The clinical features of DVT include leg pain, tenderness, and swelling, a palpable cord representing a thrombosed vessel, discoloration, venous distention, prominence of the superficial veins, and cyanosis.

The clinical diagnosis of DVT is highly nonspecific because each of the symptoms or signs can be caused by nonthrombotic disorders. The rare exception is the patient with phlegmasia cerulea dolens (occlusion of the whole venous circulation, extreme swelling of the leg, and compromised arterial flow), in whom the diagnosis of massive iliofemoral thrombosis is obvious. This syndrome occurs in less than 1 percent of patients with symptomatic venous thrombosis. In most patients, the symptoms and signs are nonspecific. In 50 to 85 percent of patients, the clinical suspicion of DVT is not confirmed by objective testing.[17-19] Patients with minor symptoms and signs may have extensive deep venous thrombi. Conversely, patients with florid leg pain and swelling, suggesting extensive DVT, may have negative results by objective testing.

Although the clinical diagnosis is nonspecific, prospective studies have established that patients can be categorized as low, moderate, or high probability for DVT using a clinical prediction rule that incorporates signs, symptoms, and risk factors. A systematic review[26] of the studies found that the prevalence of DVT in the low, moderate, and high probability categories, respectively, was 5 percent (95 percent confidence interval [95% CI]: 4 to 8 percent), 17 percent (95% CI: 13 to 23 percent), and 53 percent (95% CI: 44 to 61 percent). The prevalence in the pretest category of "low probability" is not sufficiently low to withhold further diagnostic testing and treatment, and the prevalence in the "high probability" category is not sufficiently high to give anticoagulant therapy without performing further diagnostic testing. Consequently, the key role for clinical pretest categorization is for use within integrated diagnostic strategies employing measurement of D-dimer and venous imaging.

PULMONARY EMBOLISM

The clinical features of acute PE include the following symptoms and signs that may overlap: (1) transient dyspnea and tachypnea in the absence of other clinical features; (2) pleuritic chest pain, cough, hemoptysis, pleural effusion, and pulmonary infiltrates noted on chest radiogram caused by pulmonary infarction or congestive atelectasis (also known as *ischemic pneumonitis* or *incomplete infarction*); (3) severe dyspnea and tachypnea and right-side heart failure; (4) cardiovascular collapse with hypotension, syncope, and coma (usually associated with massive PE); and (5) several less common and nonspecific clinical presentations, including unexplained tachycardia or arrhythmia, resistant cardiac failure, wheezing, cough, fever, anxiety/apprehension, and confusion. All of these clinical features are nonspecific and can be caused by a variety of cardiorespiratory disorders. Patients can be assigned to categories of pretest probability using implicit clinical judgement, or clinical decision rules such as the Geneva score or approach of Wells.[27-30] However, the prevalences of PE in these categories are not sufficiently low or high to withhold further investigation altogether, and the measurement of D-dimer and/or diagnostic imaging is mandatory to exclude or confirm the presence of PE. The assessment of clinical pretest probability is an important first step in integrated diagnostic strategies that employ, for example, D-dimer, computed tomographic angiography (CTA), and objective testing for DVT.[27-30]

● LABORATORY FEATURES

VTE is associated with nonspecific laboratory changes that constitute the acute-phase response to tissue injury. This response includes elevated levels of fibrinogen and factor VIII, increases in leukocyte and platelet counts, and systemic activation of blood coagulation, fibrin formation, and fibrin breakdown, with increases in plasma concentrations of prothrombin fragment 1.2, fibrinopeptide A, complexes of thrombin–antithrombin, and fibrin degradation products. All of these

changes are nonspecific and may occur as a result of surgery, trauma, infection, inflammation, or infarction. None of the above reported laboratory changes can be used to establish the diagnosis of VTE or predict its development with high probability. The fibrin breakdown fragment D-dimer can be measured by an enzyme-linked immunosorbent assay (ELISA) or by a latex agglutination assay. Some of these assays have a rapid turnaround time and some are quantitative. A negative D-dimer result is useful for excluding the diagnosis in many patients with suspected DVT or suspected PE (see "Objective Testing for Deep Vein Thrombosis" and "Objective Testing for Pulmonary Embolism" below).[16,27,28,31] A positive result is highly nonspecific.

● DIFFERENTIAL DIAGNOSIS OF DEEP VEIN THROMBOSIS

The differential diagnosis in patients with clinically suspected DVT includes muscle strain or tear, direct twisting injury to the leg, lymphangitis or lymphatic obstruction, venous reflux, popliteal cyst, cellulitis, leg swelling in a paralyzed limb, and abnormality of the knee joint. An alternate diagnosis frequently is not evident at presentation, so excluding DVT is not possible without objective testing. The cause of symptoms often can be determined by careful followup once DVT has been excluded by objective testing. In approximately 25 percent of patients, however, the cause of pain, tenderness, and swelling remains uncertain even after careful followup.[19]

● OBJECTIVE TESTING FOR DEEP VEIN THROMBOSIS

D-DIMER ASSAY

Measurement of plasma D-dimer has been extensively evaluated as an exclusion test in patients with clinically suspected DVT.[31] The different D-dimer assays (ELISA, quantitative rapid ELISA, latex agglutination, and whole-blood agglutination) have different sensitivities, specificities, and likelihood ratios for DVT. ELISA and quantitative rapid ELISA have high sensitivity (96 percent) and negative likelihood ratios of approximately 0.10 for DVT in symptomatic patients. Thus, for excluding DVT in symptomatic patients with a low or intermediate clinical pretest probability, a negative D-dimer result by a quantitative rapid ELISA technique is as diagnostically useful as a negative result by duplex ultrasonography.[31] Measurement of D-dimer using an appropriate assay method can also be combined with ultrasonography imaging. If the two tests are negative at presentation, repeat ultrasonography imaging is unecessary.[32] Use of the D-dimer test for patient care decisions depends on the local availability of an appropriate assay that has high sensitivity and has been validated by clinical outcome studies. The use of age-adjusted D-dimer cut-off levels for a negative result enhance the clinical utility of the test. Figure 133–1 shows a practical approach for the diagnosis of suspected DVT.

IMAGING TESTS

The objective diagnostic imaging tests that have a role in patients with clinically suspected DVT are ultrasonography and venography. Both of these tests have been validated by properly designed clinical trials, including prospective studies with long-term followup that have established the safety of withholding anticoagulant treatment in patients with negative test results.[17-19,33] Ultrasonography is the preferred imaging test for most patients. The role of venography is for selected patients,

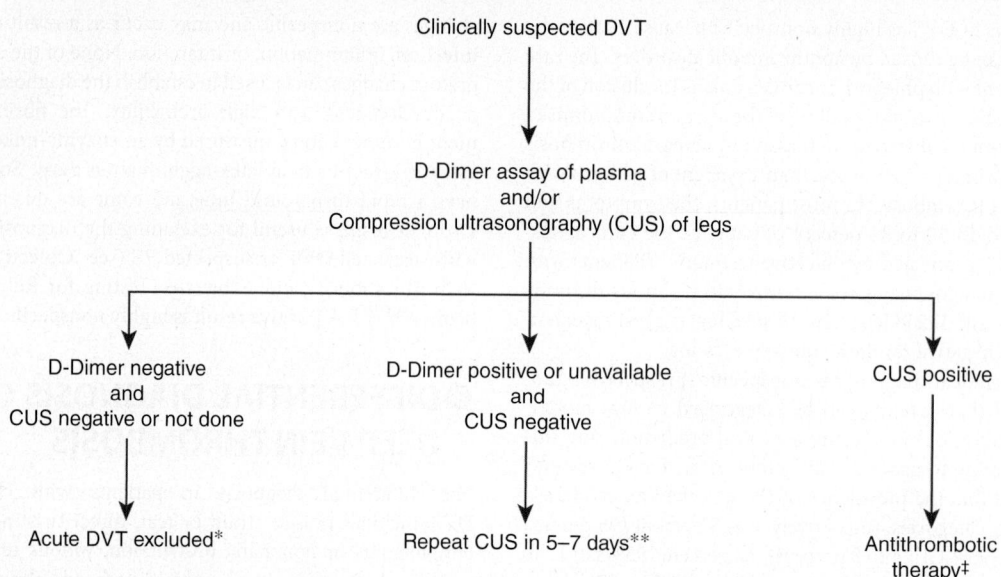

Figure 133–1. Diagnosis of patients with suspected first episode of deep vein thrombosis (DVT). *Negative D-dimer can be used to exclude acute DVT, without the need for further diagnostic testing with compression ultrasonography (CUS), if the patient has low, unlikely, moderate, or intermediate clinical probability.[26,31] Ultrasonography should be performed in patients with a high clinical probability. A negative D-dimer can also be used with a negative CUS at presentation to exclude acute DVT without the need for a repeat CUS.[32,34] **CUS is performed with imaging of the common femoral vein in the groin and of the popliteal vein in the popliteal fossa extending distally 10 cm from midpatella. A repeat CUS is required in 5 to 7 days to detect extending calf vein thrombi.[17] In centers with the expertise, a single negative result of full-leg duplex ultrasonography (CUS plus flow evaluation) is sufficient to exclude acute DVT.[18,34] ‡CUS that indicates noncompressibility of deep vein segments is highly predictive of DVT (>95%) and provides an indication for antithrombotic therapy in most patients. If CUS is positive at a single site isolated in the groin, additional testing with venography, computed tomography, or magnetic resonance imaging should be performed because of the potential for false-positive CUS results from disorders producing vein compression in the groin (e.g., tumor mass).

such as those in whom ultrasonography is unavailable or inconclusive. Ultrasonography using vein compression is effective for identifying patients with proximal vein thrombosis. Compression ultrasonography of the proximal veins performed at presentation (and, if normal, repeated once 5 to 7 days later) is a safe approach in symptomatic patients.[17] In centers with experienced ultrasonography staff, a single comprehensive evaluation of the proximal and calf veins with duplex ultrasonography is sufficient and, if negative, a repeat test is not required.[18] A randomized trial supports the equivalence of a comprehensive whole-leg color-coded Doppler ultrasonography approach to that of an approach using combined D-dimer testing and repeated ultrasonography for the management of suspected DVT.[34]

The positive predictive value of a positive ultrasonography result isolated to the calf veins may vary among centers based on expertise and thrombosis prevalence. Therefore, the number of repeat ultrasonography evaluations avoided by evaluating the calf veins may be partially offset by an increased number of patients with positive ultrasonography results confined to the calf, for whom additional diagnostic testing and/or anticoagulant treatment is required. Most patients with a negative ultrasonographic result at presentation require a followup visit to establish the alternate diagnosis and to guide further care, so the return visit for repeat ultrasonography at 5 to 7 days may have added practical value.[17]

Diagnosis of acute recurrent DVT is particularly challenging because recurrent symptoms such as pain and swelling are common in patients with DVT despite adequate anticoagulant therapy, and because both ultrasonography and venography have limitations for excluding the presence of acute recurrent DVT.[35] Compression ultrasonography may remain abnormal for 1 year in 50 percent of patients, and for even longer in some patients,[36] because of persistent noncompressibility of the vein caused by fibrous organization of the original thrombus.

Venography is of limited value for excluding the diagnosis of recurrent DVT because of obliteration or recanalization of the previously affected venous segments or nonfilled venous segments. Thus, measurement of plasma D-dimer may be particularly useful as an exclusion test in patients with suspected acute recurrent DVT. However, use of D-dimer must be evaluated separately in this patient group because many patients with a past history of VTE are receiving long-term oral anticoagulant therapy, which has the potential to cause a false-negative D-dimer result. Promising initial results were obtained in one study,[37] but further studies in larger numbers of patients are needed before using a negative D-dimer alone to exclude acute recurrent DVT can be routinely recommended.

● DIFFERENTIAL DIAGNOSIS OF PULMONARY EMBOLISM

The differential diagnosis in patients with suspected PE includes cardiopulmonary disorders for each of the modes of presentation (see "Pulmonary Embolism" above). For the presentation of dyspnea and tachypnea, they include atelectasis, pneumonia, pleuritis, pneumothorax, acute pulmonary edema, bronchitis, bronchiolitis, and acute bronchial obstruction. For pulmonary infarction exhibited by pleuritic chest pain or hemoptysis, they include pneumonia, pneumothorax, pericarditis, pulmonary or bronchial neoplasm, bronchiectasis, acute bronchitis, tuberculosis, diaphragmatic inflammation, myositis, muscle strain, and rib fracture. For the clinical presentation of right-side heart failure, they include myocardial infarction, myocarditis, and cardiac tamponade. For cardiovascular collapse, they include myocardial infarction, acute massive hemorrhage, Gram-negative septicemia, cardiac tamponade, and spontaneous pneumothorax.

OBJECTIVE TESTING FOR PULMONARY EMBOLISM

The objective diagnostic imaging tests include CT, CTA, radionuclide lung scanning, selective pulmonary arteriography, and objective testing for DVT. Measurement of plasma D-dimer is useful as an exclusion test in patients with an unlikely or intermediate clinical probability.

D-DIMER ASSAY

The assay for plasma D-dimer is useful as an exclusion test, provided an appropriately validated test is available. A negative result by the rapid quantitative ELISA for D-dimer has a negative likelihood ratio similar to that of a normal perfusion scan.[31] A positive D-dimer result is not useful diagnostically. Several management studies have found that PE can be excluded without performing imaging studies in patients with a low, intermediate, or unlikely clinical probability.[38] When combined with pretest clinical probability assessment, the use of an age-adjusted D-dimer cutoff value instead of a fixed D-dimer cutoff of 500 mcg/mL, improves the utility of the test, and enables more patients to have the diagnosis of PE safely excluded.[39]

COMPUTED TOMOGRAPHY IMAGING AND ANGIOGRAPHY

CT imaging is the primary imaging test for the diagnosis of PE in most centers. Single-detector spiral CT is highly sensitive for large emboli (segmental or larger arteries), but is much less sensitive for emboli in subsegmental pulmonary arteries[16,40]; such emboli may be clinically important in patients with severely impaired cardiorespiratory reserve. Therefore, a negative result by single-detector spiral CT should not be used alone to exclude the diagnosis of PE. A filling defect of a segmental or larger artery on single-detector spiral CT is associated with a high probability (>90 percent) of PE.[40]

The development of multidetector row CT, together with the use of contrast enhancement, has established CT as the preferred diagnostic imaging test in most patients.[41–43] Contrast-enhanced CTA has the advantage of providing clear results (positive or negative), with a low rate of nondiagnostic test results, good characterization of nonvascular structures for alternate or associated diagnoses, and the ability to simultaneously evaluate the deep venous system of the legs (computed tomographic venography [CTV]).

The accuracy and clinical utility of multidetector CTA and combined CTA-CTV were evaluated in the Prospective Investigation of Pulmonary Embolism Diagnosis (PIOPED) II study.[43] Among 824 patients with a reference diagnosis and a completed CT study, CTA was inconclusive in 51 (6 percent) because of poor image quality. The sensitivity of CTA was 83 percent and the specificity was 96 percent. CTA-CTV was inconclusive in 87 (11 percent) of 824 patients because the image quality of either CTA or CTV was poor. Multidetector CTA-CTV had a higher sensitivity (90 percent) than CTA alone (83 percent), with similar specificity (~95 percent for both testing techniques). Positive results on CTA in combination with a high probability or intermediate probability of PE by the clinical assessment, or normal findings on CTA with a low clinical probability had a predictive value (positive or negative) of 92 to 96 percent.[43] Such values are consistent with those generally considered adequate to confirm or rule out the diagnosis of PE. Additional testing is necessary when the clinical probability is discordant with CTA or CTA-CTV imaging results.[43]

Figure 133–2 summarizes the approach to diagnosis of suspected PE using CTA or CTA-CTV as the primary imaging test. A high-quality image by CTA is sufficient to establish or exclude the diagnosis of PE

with high predictive value in most patients, and withholding anticoagulant therapy based on a negative CTA alone is associated with a low rate of subsequent VTE on followup.[44] Objective testing for DVT is useful in patients in whom the CTA image is of poor quality or inconclusive, and in patients who also have symptoms suggesting DVT. CTV has the advantage of being easily performed at the time of CTA, but incurs the risk of added radiation exposure for the patient. Compression ultrasonography can also be used, and avoids added radiation exposure and can be performed serially if needed.

RADIONUCLIDE LUNG SCANNING

Radionuclide lung scanning continues to have a role in the diagnosis of suspected PE A normal perfusion lung scan excludes the diagnosis of clinically important PE.[15,45] A normal perfusion lung scan is found in approximately 10 percent of all patients with suspected PE seen at academic health centers or tertiary referral centers. A high-probability lung scan result (i.e., large perfusion defects with ventilation mismatch) has a positive predictive value for PE of 85 percent and provides a diagnostic end point to give antithrombotic treatment in most patients.[15,46,47] A high-probability lung scan is found in approximately 10 to 15 percent of symptomatic patients. For patients with a history of PE, careful comparison of the lung scan results to the most recent lung scan is required to ensure the perfusion defects are new. Further diagnostic testing is indicated for patients with a high-probability lung scan who have a "low" pretest clinical suspicion, and in those who are at high risk for major bleeding, to reduce the likelihood of a false-positive diagnosis.

The major limitation of lung scanning is that the results are inconclusive in most patients, even when considered together with the pretest clinical probability.[15] The nondiagnostic lung scan patterns are found in approximately 70 percent of all patients with suspected PE.[13,15,47] These lung scan results have historically been called "low probability" (matching ventilation–perfusion abnormalities or small perfusion defects), "intermediate probability," or "indeterminate" (because the perfusion defects correspond to an area of abnormality on chest radiograph). Further diagnostic testing is required in most of these patients because, regardless of the pretest clinical suspicion, the posttest probabilities of PE associated with these lung scan results are neither sufficiently high to give antithrombotic treatment nor sufficiently low to withhold therapy. The uncommon exception is the patient with a low clinical suspicion and a so-called low-probability lung scan result. However, even in these patients, objective testing for DVT with ultrasonography and/or measurement of plasma D-dimer is without risk for the patient and may provide added diagnostic value (see "Objective Testing for Deep Vein Thrombosis" below). A randomized trial has established that CTA is not inferior to using ventilation–perfusion lung scanning for excluding the diagnosis of PE when either test is used in an algorithm together with venous ultrasonography of the legs.[48]

In centers where CTA is available, the major role for lung scanning is in select patients; for example, in younger women to reduce radiation exposure to the breast. Lung scanning can be useful in such patients who are less likely to have comorbid cardiorespiratory disorders and therefore a higher proportion of diagnostic scan results (normal or high probability).

MAGNETIC RESONANCE ANGIOGRAPHY

The accuracy of magnetic resonance angiography for diagnosing PE, with or without the addition of magnetic resonance venography, was evaluated in the PIOPED III study.[49] This was a prospective study of 371 adults with suspected PE recruited from seven hospitals and their emergency services. Magnetic resonance angiography was technically inadequate in 25 percent of patients (92 of 371); this rate ranged from

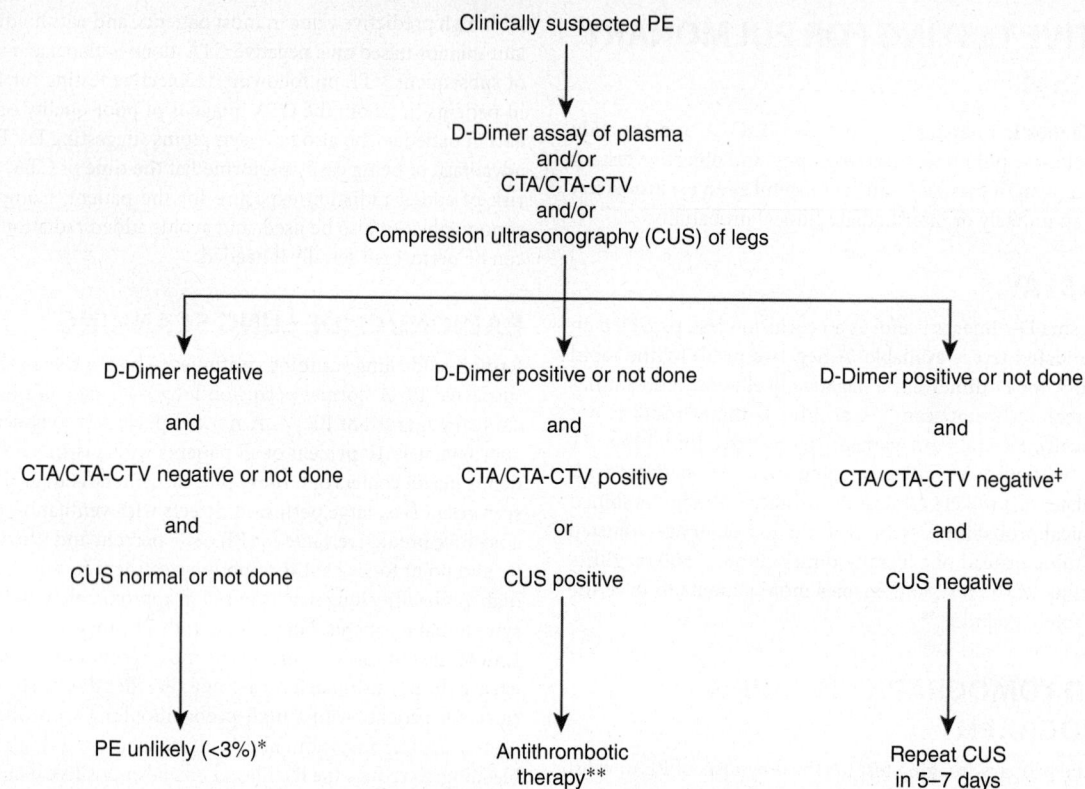

Figure 133–2. Integrated strategy for diagnosis of patients with suspected pulmonary embolism (PE) using computed tomographic angiography (CTA) as the primary imaging test. *Negative D-dimer alone can be used as an exclusion test with high negative predictive value (>96%) in patients with low or moderate probability by the clinical assessment.[27,30,31] Patients with a high clinical probability should undergo imaging with CTA or combined CTA-computed tomographic venography (CTV). **Positive results on CTA or combined CTA-CTV, in patients with a high or moderate probability of pulmonary embolism by the clinical assessment, have positive predictive value of 90% or more for venous thromboembolism. Similarly, abnormal results by compression ultrasonography (CUS) of the proximal deep veins of the legs have high positive predictive value for proximal vein thrombosis and provide an indication to give antithrombotic therapy. If the patient has a low probability by the clinical assessment, positive results by CTA or CTA-CTV in the main or lobar pulmonary arteries are still highly predictive (97%) for the presence of pulmonary embolism[43]; further testing is recommended for patients with low clinical probability and positive CTA results only of segmental or subsegmental arteries, and the options include pulmonary arteriography or serial CUS. ‡Negative results by CTA or by combined CTA-CTV have high negative predictive value (96%) in patients with low probability by the clinical assessment.[43] For patients with moderate clinical probability, the negative predictive value for combined CTA-CTV is also high (92%), but slightly lower for CTA alone (89%)[43]; in CTA-alone group, and in patients with a high probability by the clinical assessment, serial CUS or pulmonary arteriography are recommended options.

11 percent to 52 percent among the centers. If a technically adequate image was obtained, magnetic resonance angiography had a sensitivity of 78 percent and a specificity of 99 percent, and combined magnetic resonance angiography and venography had a sensitivity of 92 percent and a specificity of 96 percent. However, 52 percent of patients (194 of 370) had technically inadequate results with the combined approach.[49] Based on these findings, magnetic resonance angiography has a very limited role in the diagnosis of PE. In centers that routinely perform it well with a high rate of technically adequate images, magnetic resonance angiography and venography may be useful for patients in whom CTA or lung scanning are contraindicated.

PULMONARY ANGIOGRAPHY

Pulmonary angiography using selective catheterization of the pulmonary arteries is a relatively safe technique for patients who do not have pulmonary hypertension or cardiac failure.[13,15] If the expertise is available, pulmonary angiography should be used when other approaches are inconclusive and when definitive knowledge about the presence or absence of PE is required, because the risk of angiography in properly

selected patients is less than the risk of unnecessary anticoagulant therapy.

OBJECTIVE TESTING FOR DEEP VEIN THROMBOSIS

Objective testing for DVT is useful in patients with suspected PE, particularly those with nondiagnostic lung scan results[33,47] or inconclusive CT results.[50] Detection of proximal vein thrombosis by objective testing provides an indication for anticoagulant treatment, regardless of the presence or absence of PE, and prevents the need for further testing. However, a negative result by objective testing for DVT does not exclude the presence of PE.[13,14] If the patient has adequate cardiorespiratory reserve, then serial ultrasonography testing for proximal vein thrombosis can be used as an alternative to pulmonary angiography in patients with nondiagnostic lung scan or inconclusive CT results, and withholding anticoagulant therapy is safe if repeated ultrasonography testing of the legs is negative.[33,47,50] The rationale is that the clinical objective in such patients is to prevent recurrent PE, which is unlikely in the absence of proximal vein thrombosis. Selective pulmonary angiography should be done among patients with features suggesting a possible alternate source of embolism to proximal DVT of the leg (e.g., upper-extremity thrombosis, renal vein thrombosis, pelvic vein thrombosis, or right-heart thrombus).

● THERAPY, COURSE, AND PROGNOSIS

CLINICAL COURSE OF VENOUS THROMBOEMBOLISM

Proximal Vein Thrombosis

Proximal vein thrombosis is a serious and potentially lethal condition. Untreated proximal vein thrombosis is associated with a 10 percent rate of fatal PE. Inadequately treated proximal vein thrombosis results in a 20 to 50 percent risk of recurrent VTE events.[51] Prospective studies of patients with clinically suspected DVT or PE indicate that new VTE events on followup are uncommon (≤2 percent) among patients in whom proximal vein thrombosis is absent by objective testing.[17,32,33,47,50] The aggregate data from diagnostic and treatment studies indicate that the presence of proximal vein thrombosis is the key prognostic marker for recurrent VTE.

Calf Vein Thrombosis

Thrombosis that remains confined to the calf veins is associated with low risk (≤1 percent) of clinically important PE. Extension of thrombosis into the popliteal vein or more proximally occurs in 15 to 25 percent of patients with untreated calf vein thrombosis.[1] Patients with documented calf vein thrombosis should either receive anticoagulant treatment to prevent extension or undergo monitoring for proximal extension using serial ultrasonography.

Postthrombotic Syndrome

The postthrombotic syndrome is a frequent complication of DVT.[52] Patients with the postthrombotic syndrome complain of pain, heaviness, swelling, cramps, and itching or tingling of the affected leg. Ulceration may occur. The symptoms usually are aggravated by standing or walking and improve with rest and elevation of the leg. A prospective study documented a 25 percent incidence of moderate-to-severe postthrombotic symptoms 2 years after the initial diagnosis of proximal vein thrombosis in patients who were treated with initial heparin and oral anticoagulants for 3 months.[53] The study also demonstrated that ipsilateral recurrent venous thrombosis is strongly associated with subsequent development of moderate or severe postthrombotic symptoms. Thus, prevention of ipsilateral recurrent DVT likely reduces the incidence of the postthrombotic syndrome. Application of a properly fitted graded compression stocking, as soon after diagnosis as the patient's symptoms will allow, can improve edema and pain in the acute stage of DVT and may also help control or relieve symptoms in patients who develop the postthrombotic syndrome. Conflicting findings have been found in randomized trials of graded compression stockings for preventing the development of the postthrombotic syndrome.[54,55]

Chronic Thromboembolic Pulmonary Hypertension

Chronic thromboembolic pulmonary hypertension is a serious complication of PE. Historically, thromboembolic pulmonary hypertension was believed to be relatively rare and to occur only several years after the diagnosis of PE. A prospective cohort study provides important information on the incidence and timing of thromboembolic pulmonary hypertension.[56] The results indicate that thromboembolic pulmonary hypertension is more common and occurs earlier than previously thought. On prospective followup of 223 patients with documented PE, the cumulative incidence of chronic thromboembolic pulmonary

hypertension was 3.8 percent at 2 years after diagnosis, despite state-of-the-art treatment for PE. The strongest independent risk factors were a history of PE (odds ratio: 19) and idiopathic PE at presentation (odds ratio: 5.7).[56]

OBJECTIVES AND PRINCIPLES OF ANTITHROMBOTIC TREATMENT

The objectives of treatment in patients with established VTE are to (1) prevent death from PE, and (2) prevent morbidity from recurrent DVT or PE, especially the postthrombotic syndrome and chronic pulmonary hypertension.

For most patients, these objectives are achieved by providing adequate anticoagulant treatment. Thrombolytic therapy is indicated in selected patients (see "Thrombolytic Therapy" below). Use of an inferior vena cava filter is indicated to prevent death from PE in patients in whom anticoagulant treatment is absolutely contraindicated and in other selected patients (see "Anticoagulant Therapy" below). These recommendations and those below are linked to the strength of the evidence from clinical trials and evidence-based guidelines.[9,30,57,58]

ANTICOAGULANT THERAPY

Anticoagulant therapy is the treatment of choice for most patients with proximal vein thrombosis or PE.[9,57,58] Patients with proximal DVT require both adequate initial anticoagulant treatment with heparin or low-molecular-weight (LMW) heparin and adequate long-term anticoagulant therapy to prevent recurrent VTE.[51,59,60] Anticoagulant therapy for at least 3 months is required to prevent a high frequency (15 to 25 percent) of symptomatic extension of thrombosis and/or recurrent venous thromboembolic events.[51,60,61] Adequate anticoagulant treatment reduces the incidence of recurrence during the first 3 months after diagnosis to 5 percent or less.[51,59-61]

The absolute contraindications to anticoagulant treatment include intracranial bleeding, severe active bleeding, recent brain, eye, or spinal cord surgery, and malignant hypertension. Relative contraindications include recent major surgery, recent cerebrovascular accident, active gastrointestinal tract bleeding, severe hypertension, severe renal or hepatic failure, and severe thrombocytopenia (platelets $<50 \times 10^9/L$).

Parenteral Anticoagulants

Heparin and Low-Molecular-Weight Heparin Initial therapy with continuous intravenous heparin was the standard approach to treatment of VTE during the 1970s and 1980s. During the 1990s, LMW heparin given by subcutaneous injection once or twice daily was evaluated by clinical trials and shown to be as effective and safe as continuous intravenous heparin for the initial treatment of patients with proximal DVT and submassive PE.[57,58,62] The advantage of LMW heparin is that it does not require anticoagulant monitoring. LMW heparin given subcutaneously once or twice daily is preferred over intravenous unfractionated heparin for the initial treatment of most patients with either DVT or PE.[57,58] LMW heparin enables outpatient therapy for many patients with uncomplicated DVT and selected patients with PE. Intravenous unfractionated heparin remains a useful approach for initial anticoagulant therapy in patients with severe renal failure. Initial treatment with LMW heparin or unfractionated heparin should be continued for at least 5 days. Table 133–2 lists the specific LMW heparin regimens for the treatment of VTE.

If unfractionated heparin is used for initial therapy, it is important to achieve an adequate anticoagulant effect, defined as an activated partial thromboplastin time (aPTT) above the lower limit of therapeutic range within the first 24 hours.[63,64] Failure to achieve an adequate aPTT effect

TABLE 133–2. Anticoagulant Drug Regimens for Treatment of Venous Thromboembolism

Drug	Regimen
LOW-MOLECULAR-WEIGHT HEPARINS	
Enoxaparin	1.0 mg/kg BID*
Dalteparin	200 IU/kg once daily[†]
Tinzaparin	175 IU/kg once daily[‡]
Nadroparin	6150 IU BID for 50–70 kg
	4100 IU BID if patient weighs <50 kg
	9200 IU BID if patient weighs >70 kg
Reviparin	4200 IU BID for 46–60 kg
	3500 IU BID if patient weighs 35–45 kg
	6300 IU BID if patient weighs >60 kg
INDIRECT FACTOR Xa INHIBITOR	
Fondaparinux	7.5 mg once daily if patient weight 50–100 kg
	5.0 mg once daily if patient weight <50 kg
	10.0 mg once daily if patient weight >100 kg
DIRECT ORAL ANTICOAGULANTS	
Dabigatran	150 mg BID after 5 days of parenteral low-molecular-weight heparin or heparin
Rivaroxaban	15 mg BID for 21 days, then 20 mg once daily
	Taken with food
Apixaban	10 mg BID for 7 days, then 5 mg BID
	After 6 months, 2.5 mg BID for extended therapy
Edoxaban	60 mg once daily after 5 days of parenteral low-molecular-weight heparin or heparin[§]

*A once-daily regimen of 1.5 mg/kg can be used but probably is less effective in patients with cancer.

[†]After 1 month, can be followed by 150 IU/kg once daily as an alternative to an oral vitamin K antagonist for long-term treatment.

[‡]This regimen can also be used for long-term treatment as an alternative to an oral vitamin K antagonist.

[§]30 mg once daily if patient's creatinine clearance is 30–50 mL/min or weight is ≤60 kg or if patient is taking strong P-glycoprotein inhibitor drugs.

early during therapy is associated with a high incidence (25 percent) of recurrent VTE.[63] Two-thirds of the recurrent events occur between 2 and 12 weeks after the initial diagnosis despite treatment with oral anticoagulants, and the initial management with either unfractionated heparin or LMW heparin is critical to the patient's long-term outcome.[63,64]

Fondaparinux The synthetic pentasaccharide fondaparinux, which is an indirect inhibitor of factor Xa, has been evaluated by large randomized clinical trials.[65,66] These studies indicate fondaparinux is as effective and safe as LMW heparin for treatment of established DVT and as effective and safe as intravenous heparin for treatment of symptomatic PE. Fondaparinux is given subcutaneously once daily at a dose of 7.5 mg for patients weighing between 50 and 100 kg (85 percent of all patients evaluated in the clinical trials), 5 mg for patients weighing less than 50 kg, and 10 mg for patients weighing more than 100 kg.[65,66]

Oral Anticoagulants

Vitamin K Antagonists Oral anticoagulant treatment using a vitamin K antagonist (e.g., sodium warfarin) has been the standard approach for long-term treatment in most patients for more than 60 years. Treatment

with a vitamin K antagonist is started with initial heparin or LMW heparin therapy and overlapped for 4 to 5 days.

The preferred intensity of the anticoagulant effect of treatment with a vitamin K antagonist has been established by clinical trials.[69–72] The dose of vitamin K antagonist should be adjusted to maintain the international normalized ratio (INR) between 2.0 and 3.0. High-intensity vitamin K antagonist treatment (INR 3.0 to 4.0) should not be used because it has not improved effectiveness in patients with the antiphospholipid syndrome and recurrent thrombosis[71] and has caused more bleeding.[72] Low-intensity therapy (INR 1.5 to 1.9) is not recommended because it is less effective than standard-intensity treatment (INR 2.0 to 3.0) and does not reduce bleeding complications.[70]

Long-term treatment with LMW heparin is indicated for select patients in whom vitamin K antagonists are contraindicated (e.g., pregnant women), and in patients with concurrent cancer for whom LMW heparin regimens are more effective. [67,68]

Direct Oral Anticoagulants Oral anticoagulants that bind directly to the target coagulation enzyme of either thrombin or factor Xa have been evaluated in phase III clinical trials for the treatment of patients with VTE (Chap. 25).[73–78] The advantages of these drugs are: (1) they can be administered orally once or twice daily without the need for anticoagulant monitoring and dose titration; (2) they have fewer clinically relevant drug interactions; (3) because of a fast onset of anticoagulant action, similar to that of LMW heparin, they can simplify treatment for many patients by replacing the standard approach of a parenteral drug (heparin, LMW heparin or fondaparinux) followed by an oral vitamin K antagonist with a single drug given for both initial and long-term therapy; and (4) they result in less clinically important bleeding. Table 133-2 lists the direct-acting oral anticoagulant (DOAC) regimens that have been evaluated by clinical trials for the treatment of established VTE.

Six phase III clinical trials evaluating the DOACs for the treatment of acute VTE have been completed and published.[73–78] Table 133–3 outlines the design features of these trials and the efficacy and bleeding results. Each of these trials met the prespecified criteria for noninferiority of the efficacy of the DOAC for preventing recurrent VTE.

The six trials included more than 27,000 patients with acute VTE, and meta-analyses of these studies has been done.[79] The meta-analyses provide added clinically useful information regarding specific major bleeding outcomes (intracranial bleeding and fatal bleeding), and regarding the risk-to-benefit profile in key patient subgroups commonly encountered by the clinician. These subgroups are patients presenting with symptomatic PE or symptomatic DVT, the elderly (age ≥75 years), the obese, patients with moderate renal impairment (creatinine clearance 30 to 49 mL/min), and patients with cancer. The DOACs were associated with clinically important reductions in major bleeding (relative risk [RR] 0.61), intracranial bleeding (RR 0.37), and fatal bleeding (RR 0.36).[79] For each of these outcomes, the results are consistent among the trials; none of the trials have a point estimate for these outcomes in favor of the vitamin K antagonists (supplementary data online[79]). The number of patients who would need to be treated with a DOAC rather than a vitamin K antagonist to avoid one event of intracranial bleeding is 588, and for fatal bleeding is 1250. In view of the large number of VTE patients each year, and the devastating nature of these bleeding events, these are important impacts on population health. The results of cost-effectiveness studies have shown the DOACs to be cost-effective.

Regarding the key patient subgroups evaluated, the noninferior efficacy of the DOACs was consistent across all subgroups, with possibly superior efficacy in the elderly and in cancer patients.[79] The safety advantage of reduced major bleeding was also consistent across the subgroups, except possibly in cancer patients, in whom the pooled estimate of a 33 percent risk reduction did not achieve statistical significance.

TABLE 133–3. Clinical trials of direct oral anticoagulants for treatment of venous thromboembolism.

	Hokusai-VTE[78]	AMPLIFY[77]	EINSTEIN-DVT[75]	EINSTEIN-PE[76]	RE-COVER II[74]	RE-COVER I[73]
Drug	Edoxaban	Apixaban	Rivaroxaban	Rivaroxaban	Dabigatran	Dabigatran
Study design	Double-blind	Double-blind	Open label	Open label	Double-blind	Double blind
Heparin lead-in	At least 5 days	None	None	None	At least 5 days	At least 5 days
Regimen	60 mg QD 30 mg QD if CrCl 30–50 mL/min, bw ≤60 kg or P-gp inhibitors	10 mg BID × 7 days then 5 mg BID	15 mg BID × 21 days then 20 mg QD	15 mg BID × 21 days then 20 mg QD	150 mg BID	150 mg BID
Sample size	8292	5400	3449	4832	2568	2564
Treatment duration	Flexible: 3–12 months	6 months	Prespecified: 3, 6, or 12 months	Prespecified: 3, 6, or 12 months	6 months	6 months
Recurrent VTE	Edoxaban 3.2%* LMW(Hep)/warfarin 3.5%* P <0.001 noninferiority	Apixaban 2.3% Enoxaparin/warfarin 2.7% P <0.001 noninferiority	Rivaroxaban 2.1% Enoxaparin/VKA 3.0%** P <0.001 noninferiority	Rivaroxaban 2.1% Enoxaparin/VKA 1.8% P = 0.003 noninferiority	Dabigatran 2.4% Warfarin 2.1% P <0.001 noninferiority	Dabigatran 2.3% Warfarin 2.2% P <0.001 noninferiority
Major bleeding	Edoxaban 1.4% LMW(Hep)/warfarin 1.6%	Apixaban 0.6% Enoxaparin/warfarin 1.8% P <0.001 superiority	Rivaroxaban 0.8% Enoxaparin/VKA 1.2%	Rivaroxaban 1.1% Enoxaparin/VKA 2.2% P = 0.003 superiority	Dabigatran 1.6% Warfarin 1.9%	Dabigatran 1.2% Warfarin 1.7%
CRNM bleeding	Edoxaban 7.2% LMW(Hep)/warfarin 8.9% P = 0.004 superiority	Apixaban 3.8% Enoxaparin/warfarin 8.0% P <0.001 superiority	Rivaroxaban 7.3% Enoxaparin/VKA 7.0%	Rivaroxaban 9.5% Enoxaparin/VKA 9.8%	Dabigatran 5.6%§ Warfarin 8.8%§ P = 0.002 superiority	Dabigatran 5.0%§ Warfarin 7.9%§ P <0.05 superiority

bw, Body weight; CrCl, creatinine clearance; CRNM, clinically relevant non-major bleeding; Hep, heparin; LMW, low molecular weight; P-gp, P glycoprotein; VKA, vitamin K antagonist; VTE, venous thromboembolism.

*During overall study period. On-treatment rates were 1.6% for edoxaban and 1.9% for heparin/warfarin. The analysis for all the other studies used rates on treatment.

**Either warfarin or acenocoumarol was used for the vitamin K antagonist therapy.

§Rates are for the composite of major and clinically relevant nonmajor bleeding.

Adapted with permission from Raskob G, Büller H, Prins M, et al: Edoxaban for the long-term treatment of venous thromboembolism: Rationale and design of the Hokusai-venous thromboembolism study—Methodological implications for clinical trials. *J Thromb Haemost* 11(7): 1287–1294, 2013.

The DOACs are preferred over vitamin K antagonists in most new patients commencing anticoagulant treatment for VTE. The exceptions are patients with severe renal impairment (creatinine clearance <30 mL/min), because they were not included in the clinical trials, and cancer patients, because only relatively small numbers of selected cancer patients were included, and because clinical trials comparing DOACs to the currently recommended standard therapy with LMW heparin have not been performed. For patients already taking long-term vitamin K antagonist therapy who are well controlled with a high proportion of time in therapeutic range, and for whom regular anticoagulant monitoring is not a burden, switching treatment to a DOAC is not indicated unless a clinical reason develops.

Some practical issues remain incompletely resolved. Rivaroxaban and apixaban can be used as a single-drug approach, whereas dabigatran and edoxaban are preceded by at least 5 days of heparin or LMW heparin treatment. Whether DOAC monotherapy is sufficient for the full spectrum of VTE severity, or whether "lead-in" heparin treatment is preferred in some patients, such as those with PE who have right ventricular dysfunction,[78] remains uncertain. The DOACs currently lack a specific reversal agent. In general, this should not be a reason to withhold from most patients the benefit of significantly reduced risks of major bleeding, intracranial bleeding and fatal bleeding with the DOACs. For the near term, vitamin K antagonists may be preferred in patients in whom prompt and measurable reversal of the anticoagulant effect will be required because of planned surgery or invasive procedures. Multiple rapid reversal agents for the DOACs are currently in development. Because the DOACs do not require laboratory monitoring, patients receiving DOACs may have less-frequent contact with their physician or anticoagulation clinic, and nonadherence to the prescribed therapy may not be detected as readily. Physicians and health systems should employ evidence-based strategies to enhance adherence and should evaluate patients at intervals to assess if ongoing anticoagulant therapy is appropriate and adhered to. The effectiveness and safety of the DOACs compared with LMW heparin treatment in cancer patients with VTE has not been evaluated, and LMW heparin remains indicated for these patients.

Duration of Anticoagulant Therapy

Anticoagulant treatment should be continued for at least 3 months in all patients with VTE.[9,57,58,80] Stopping treatment at 4 to 6 weeks resulted in an increased incidence of recurrent VTE during the following 6 months (absolute risk increase: 8 percent).[57, 80–82] In contrast, treatment for 3 to 6 months resulted in a low rate of recurrence during the following 1 to 2 years (annual incidence 3 percent).[80–82]

The decision to stop anticoagulant therapy, or continue treatment after 3 months is influenced mainly by the patient's clinical presentation of thromboembolism as either "provoked," which refers to VTE occurring in association with known risk factors, or "unprovoked," in which identifiable risk factors for VTE are absent. Approximately 20 to 40 percent of all symptomatic patients present as unprovoked VTE.

In patients with a first episode of DVT or PE provoked by a reversible risk factor (e.g., surgery), treatment for 3 months is usually sufficient if the risk factor(s) is no longer present. If the risk factor(s) persist, for example prolonged immobility or cancer, treatment should be continued until the risk factor is reversed. It has been a customary practice to treat patients with PE for 6 months rather than 3 months, but the clinical trials indicate there is little to no added benefit of doing so, with a small but additional risk of bleeding.[80] Thus, for patients with DVT or PE provoked by a risk factor that has reversed, 3 months is sufficient and recommended over longer therapy.[57]

Patients with a first episode of unprovoked VTE should be considered for indefinite anticoagulant therapy.[57,58] The term "indefinite" refers to continued treatment without a scheduled stopping date; treatment may be stopped in the future if the patient's risk-to-benefit profile or preference for continued treatment changes. The decision to stop or continue anticoagulation after 3 months in patients with a first episode of unprovoked VTE should take into consideration the risk of recurrent VTE, the risk of bleeding, and patient preference. If indefinite anticoagulant treatment is chosen, the risks and benefits of continuing such treatment should be reassessed at periodic intervals.[57]

There has been significant research to develop strategies to aid the clinician in assessing the risk of recurrent VTE in patients with unprovoked VTE. The presence of residual DVT assessed by compression ultrasonography,[83] elevated levels of plasma D-dimer after discontinuing anticoagulant treatment,[84] and male gender[85] are associated with an increased incidence of recurrent thromboembolism. The challenge, however, has been to identify the subgroup of patients with a sufficiently low annual risk of recurrence to warrant stopping anticoagulant therapy. Palaretti and colleagues evaluated an approach for patients with a first episode of unprovoked VTE or VTE associated with a minor risk factor (e.g., estrogens, pregnancy, or travel related thrombosis) which combined evaluation of the presence or absence of residual thrombosis by ultrasonography with serial D-dimer measurement to guide the decision to stop or continue anticoagulant therapy.[86] Patients in whom residual vein thrombosis was absent after 3 months of treatment, or in those with residual vein thrombosis who had been treated for at least 1 year, and who had serially negative D-dimer measurements for 3 months after stopping vitamin K antagonist treatment, had an annual rate of recurrent VTE of 3 percent during followup off anticoagulant therapy; this compared to 0.7 percent per year in 373 patients who resumed anticoagulation because of an elevated D-dimer measurement, and 8.8 percent per year among the 109 patients with elevated D-dimer who did not continue anticoagulant therapy.[86] An annual risk of recurrent VTE of 3 percent may be low enough to discontinue therapy in patients in

whom the annual risk of bleeding, especially major bleeding, is similar or higher. However, if the risk of major bleeding is low, for example 1 percent per year or lower, then the annual risk of recurrent VTE of 3 percent may not be sufficiently low to stop anticoagulation, especially if the patient's preference is on avoiding further recurrent VTE events.

A variety of thrombophilic conditions have been identified and can be evaluated in the laboratory. These include deficiencies of the naturally occurring inhibitors of coagulation such as antithrombin, protein C, and protein S; specific gene mutations including factor V Leiden and prothrombin 20210A; elevated levels of coagulation factor VIII; and the presence of antiphospholipid antibodies (Chap. 131). The role of the presence or absence of thrombophilia in guiding decisions about duration of therapy has been controversial and is incompletely resolved. Indefinite anticoagulant treatment should be considered in patients with a first episode of VTE and antiphospholipid antibodies or the presence of one or a combination of the more potent thrombophilias (deficiency of antithrombin, protein C or protein S, homozygous factor V Leiden, or prothrombin 20210A gene mutation, or one of these with a family history of VTE). Again, patient preference is important to the decision.

The DOACs have been evaluated by randomized trials for the extended treatment of patients with VTE who have completed an initial course of 6 months of anticoagulant therapy.[75,87–89] Most of the patients in these trials had unprovoked VTE at their initial presentation and all had clinical equipoise about the benefit to risk tradeoff of receiving extended anticoagulant therapy. The results of the trials are consistent. The DOACs produced 80 percent or greater reductions in the annual incidence of recurrent VTE of 7 to 9 percent per year in patients receiving placebo to approximately 2 percent per year in those given DOACs.[75,87–89] The rates of major bleeding were 0.1 to 0.7 percent. Clinically relevant nonmajor bleeding occurred in 3 to 4 percent of patients.[75,87–89] In the AMPLIFY Extension trial,[89] the rate of major bleeding for the 2.5 mg apixaban regimen was 0.2 percent per year, compared with 0.5 percent for placebo. The low rates of major bleeding, coupled with the advantage of not requiring laboratory monitoring of the anticoagulant effect, will likely tip the balance in favor of extended treatment for more patients with unprovoked VTE.

Aspirin has also been evaluated for the extended treatment of patients with a first episode of unprovoked VTE who have received a course of 6 months or more of anticoagulant therapy.[90,91] Aspirin produced a statistically significant 42 percent RR reduction in recurrent VTE in one study (from 11.2 percent to 6.6 percent per year),[90] and a nonsignificant (p = 0.09) 26 percent RR reduction in the second study (from 6.5 percent to 4.8 percent per year).[91] The rates of major bleeding for aspirin (0.5 to 0.6 percent per year) were similar to placebo. Although intuitive to the clinician, there is no data to indicate that aspirin causes less major bleeding than the DOACs, although it is likely that the efficacy for preventing recurrent VTE is significantly less (only about half as effective as the DOACs).

Oral anticoagulant treatment should be given indefinitely for most patients with a second episode of unprovoked VTE,[57,58,92] because stopping treatment at 3 to 6 months in these patients results in a high incidence (21 percent) of recurrent VTE during the following 4 years.[92] The risk of recurrent thromboembolism during 4-year followup was reduced by 87 percent (from 21 percent to 3 percent) by continuing anticoagulant treatment[92]; this benefit is partially offset by the risk of bleeding.

Anticoagulant Therapy of Venous Thromboembolism in Cancer Patients

Use of LMW heparin for long-term treatment of VTE has been evaluated in clinical trials.[67,68] The studies indicate that long-term treatment with subcutaneous LMW heparin for 3 to 6 months is at least as effective as, and in cancer patients is more effective than, an oral vitamin K antagonist adjusted to maintain the INR between 2.0 and 3.0.

Therefore, patients with VTE associated with concurrent cancer should be treated with LMW heparin for the first 3 to 6 months of long-term treatment.[9,57,58] The patients then should receive anticoagulation indefinitely or until the cancer resolves. The regimens of LMW heparin that are established as effective for long-term treatment are dalteparin 200 U/kg once daily for 1 month, followed by 150 U/kg daily thereafter, or tinzaparin 175 U/kg once daily.

Anticoagulant Therapy During Pregnancy

LMW heparin or adjusted-dose subcutaneous heparin are the options for anticoagulant therapy of pregnant patients with VTE.[94-96] LMW heparin is preferred because it has the safety advantages of causing less thrombocytopenia and probably less osteoporosis than unfractionated heparin An additional advantage is that LMW heparin is effective when given once daily, whereas unfractionated heparin requires twice-daily injection. A study indicates no major change in the peak anti–factor Xa levels over the course of pregnancy in most patients treated with a once-daily therapeutic LMW heparin regimen (tinzaparin 175 U/kg).[96] Measurement of the anti–factor Xa level may provide reassurance that major drug accumulation is not occurring. However, the appropriate dose adjustments in response to a decreased anti–factor Xa level are uncertain. The DOACs have not been evaluated in pregnant patients. Evidence-based guidelines for antithrombotic therapy during pregnancy are available.[94]

Side Effects of Anticoagulant Therapy

Bleeding Bleeding is the most common side effect of anticoagulant therapy. Bleeding can be classified as major or clinically relevant nonmajor according to standardized international criteria. *Major bleeding* is defined as clinically overt bleeding resulting in a decline of hemoglobin of at least 2 g/dL, transfusion of at least 2 U of packed red cells, or bleeding that is retroperitoneal or intracranial, or occurs into other critical spaces. The rates of major bleeding in contemporary clinical trials of initial therapy with intravenous heparin, LMW heparin, or fondaparinux are 1 to 2 percent.[65,66,73-78] Patients at increased risk of major bleeding are those who have undergone surgery or experienced trauma within the previous 14 days; those with a history of gastrointestinal or intracranial bleeding, peptic ulcer disease, or genitourinary bleeding; and those with miscellaneous conditions predisposing to bleeding, such as thrombocytopenia, liver disease, and multiple invasive lines.

Major bleeding occurs in approximately 1 to 2 percent of patients during the first 3 months of oral anticoagulant treatment using a vitamin K antagonist and in 1 to 3 percent per year of treatment thereafter.[97] A meta-analysis suggests the clinical impact of major bleeding during long-term oral vitamin K antagonist treatment is greater than widely appreciated.[97] The estimated case fatality rate for this major bleeding is 13 percent, and the rate of intracranial bleeding was 1.15 per 100 patient-years. These risks are important considerations in the decision about extended or indefinite anticoagulant therapy in patients with VTE. As noted above, clinical trials of the DOACs and meta-analysis indicate clinically important lower rates of bleeding, including major, intracranial, and fatal bleeding than the vitamin K antagonists.[73-79]

Heparin-Induced Thrombocytopenia (See also Chap. 118.) Heparin or LMW heparin may cause thrombocytopenia. In large clinical studies of acute VTE treatment, thrombocytopenia occurred in less than 1 percent of more than 2000 patients treated with unfractionated heparin or LMW heparin.[66] Nevertheless, heparin-induced thrombocytopenia can be a serious complication when accompanied by extension or recurrence of VTE or the development of arterial thrombosis. Such complications may precede or coincide with the fall in platelet count and are associated with a high rate of limb loss and a high mortality. Heparin in all forms should be discontinued when the diagnosis of heparin-induced thrombocytopenia is made on clinical grounds, and treatment with an alternative anticoagulant, such as danaparoid, bivalirudin, or argatroban, should be initiated. The DOACs have potential to be useful for anticoagulant therapy in patients with heparin-induced thrombocytopenia, but their use has not been evaluated by clinical trials in this patient group.

Heparin-Induced Osteoporosis Osteoporosis may occur as a result of long-term treatment with heparin or LMW heparin (usually after more than 3 months). The earliest clinical manifestation of heparin-associated osteoporosis usually is nonspecific low back pain primarily involving the vertebrae or the ribs. Patients also may present with spontaneous fractures. Up to one-third of patients treated with long-term heparin may have subclinical reduction in bone density. Whether these patients are predisposed to future fractures is not known. The incidence of symptomatic osteoporosis in clinical trials of LMW heparin treatment for 3 to 6 months was very low and are not increased compared to warfarin treatment. Patients with osteoporosis or fractures often had other risk factors such as bone metastases.

Other Side Effects of Heparin Heparin or LMW heparin may cause elevated liver transaminase levels. These elevations are of unknown clinical significance and usually return to normal after the heparin or LMW heparin is discontinued. Awareness of this biochemical effect is important so as to avoid unnecessary interruption of heparin therapy and unnecessary liver biopsies in patients who may develop elevated transaminase levels during heparin or LMW heparin therapy. Additional rare side effects of heparin include hypersensitivity and skin reactions, such as skin necrosis, alopecia, and hyperkalemia occurring as a result of hypoaldosteronism.

THROMBOLYTIC THERAPY

Thrombolytic therapy is indicated for patients with PE who present with hypotension or shock, and for select patients with PE who have evidence of right ventricular dysfunction and are at high risk of hemodynamic collapse.[30] Thrombolytic therapy provides more rapid lysis of pulmonary emboli and more rapid restoration of right ventricular function and pulmonary perfusion than does anticoagulant treatment.[30,98,99] Effective regimens are 100 mg of recombinant tissue plasminogen activator by intravenous infusion over 2 hours (50 mg/h), or 30 to 50 mg (depending on body weight) of tenecteplase given as a single bolus injection.[98,99] Heparin then is given by continuous infusion once the thrombin time or aPTT is less than twice the control value.[98,99] The starting infusion dose is 1000 U/h. Chapters 25 and 135 provide further details of thrombolytic therapy.

The recently reported PEITHO trial[99] evaluated the effectiveness and safety of thrombolysis with tenecteplase followed by anticoagulant therapy compared with anticoagulant therapy alone in 1006 patients with PE and evidence of both right ventricular dysfunction by echocardiography or CT scan, and evidence of myocardial injury by the results of troponin I or troponin T measurement. The primary outcome of death or hemodynamic compensation (or collapse) within 7 days occurred in 13 of 506 patients (2.6 percent) given thrombolysis, compared with 28 of 499 (5.6 percent) receiving anticoagulant therapy alone (p = 0.02).[99] Stroke occurred in 12 patients (2.4 percent) in the thrombolysis group, compared with one (0.2 percent) in the anticoagulant alone group (p = 0.003). Extracranial bleeding occurred in 32 patients (6.3 percent) given thrombolysis, and in six patients (1.2 percent) receiving anticoagulant therapy alone (p <0.001). At day 7, death had occurred in six patients (1.2 percent) given thrombolysis and in nine patients (1.8 percent) given anticoagulant therapy alone; the corresponding rates at day 30 were 2.4 percent and 3.2 percent, respectively.[99] The findings indicate thrombolytic therapy prevented hemodynamic decompensation, but increased the risk of major bleeding and stroke. The study was not large enough to resolve the key question of whether thrombolysis will improve survival. At present, the risk of thrombolysis outweighs the benefit for most patients with PE who do not have hypotension but who do have evidence of right ventricular dysfunction. Further trials are needed in this group of patients.

The role of thrombolytic therapy in patients with DVT is limited. Thrombolytic therapy may be indicated in patients with acute massive proximal vein thrombosis (phlegmasia cerulea dolens with impending venous gangrene) or in occasional patients with extensive iliofemoral vein thrombosis who have severe symptoms because of venous outflow obstruction. Thrombolytic therapy can be given by systemic infusion or catheter-directed infusion. Catheter-directed thrombolysis (CDT) is probably effective for reducing the incidence of the postphlebitic syndrome.[100] Although it was hoped that the catheter-directed approach might be associated with a lower risk of major bleeding, particularly intracranial bleeding, than systemic injection, comparative effectiveness research data suggest the risks of bleeding still outweigh the benefits of this approach.[101] From a national database of more than 90,000 patients with a principal diagnosis of proximal DVT or thrombosis involving the vena cava, the outcomes of the 3600 patients who received CDT with a similar number of propensity-matched patients treated with anticoagulation alone were compared. The CDT patients were more likely to have intracranial bleeding (0.9 percent vs. 0.3 percent), and transfusion (11.1 percent vs. 6.5 percent), and more likely to have filter placement (34.8 percent vs. 15.6 percent) and to experience PE (17.9 percent vs. 11.4 percent).[101] The important message from this analysis of CDT use in practice is that the rate of intracranial bleeding is appreciable (0.9 percent) and not sufficiently low to recommend the use of CDT for DVT, other than exceptional circumstances such as threatened limb viability.

INFERIOR VENA CAVA FILTER

Insertion of an inferior vena cava filter is indicated for patients with acute VTE and an absolute contraindication to anticoagulant therapy and also indicated for the rare patients who have objectively documented recurrent VTE during adequate anticoagulant therapy.

Insertion of a vena cava filter is effective for preventing PE. However, use of a permanent filter results in an increased incidence of recurrent DVT 1 to 2 years after insertion (increase in cumulative incidence at 2 years increases from 12 percent to 21 percent).[102] Therefore, if the indication for filter placement is transient, such as a contraindication to anticoagulation as the result of a temporary high risk of bleeding, a retrievable vena cava filter should be used. A retrievable filter can then be removed in the several weeks to months later, once the filter is no longer required. If a permanent filter is placed, long-term anticoagulant treatment should be given as soon as safely possible to prevent morbidity from recurrent DVT.

REFERENCES

1. Moser KM, Lemoine JR: Is embolic risk conditioned by localization of deep venous thrombosis? *Ann Intern Med* 94:439, 1981.
2. Prandoni P, Polistena P, Bernardi E, et al: Upper-extremity deep vein thrombosis. Risk factors, diagnosis, and complications. *Arch Intern Med* 157:57, 1997.
3. ISTH Steering Committee for World Thrombosis Day: Thrombosis: A major contributor to the global disease burden. *J Thromb Haemost* 12:1580, 2014.
4. Cohen AT, Agnelli G, Anderson FA, et al: VTE Impact Assessment Group in Europe (VITAE): Venous thromboembolism (VTE) in Europe. The number of VTE events and associated morbidity and mortality. *Thromb Haemost* 98:756, 2007.
5. Heit J, Cohen A, Anderson FJ: Estimated annual number of incident and recurrent, fatal and non-fatal venous thromboembolism (VTE) events in the US. *Blood* 106:267A, 2005.
6. Kahn S, Lim W, Dunn AS, et al: American College of Chest Physicians: Prevention of VTE in nonsurgical patients: Antithrombotic Therapy and Prevention of Thrombosis, 9th ed: American College of Chest Physicians Evidence-based Clinical Practice Guidelines. *Chest* 141(2 Suppl):e195S, 2012.
7. Gould MK, Garcia DA, Wren SM, et al: American College of Chest Physicians: Prevention of VTE in nonorthopedic surgical patients: Antithrombotic Therapy and Prevention of Thrombosis, 9th ed: American College of Chest Physicians Evidence-based Clinical Practice Guidelines. *Chest* 141(2 Suppl):e227S, 2012.
8. Falck-Yitter Y, Francis CW, Johanson NA, et al: American College of Chest Physicians. Prevention of VTE in orthopedic surgery patients: Antithrombotic Therapy and Prevention of Thrombosis, 9th ed: American College of Chest Physicians Evidence-based Clinical Practice Guidelines. *Chest* 141(2 Suppl):e278S, 2012.
9. Nicolaides AN, Fareed J, Kakkar AK, et al: Prevention and treatment of venous thromboembolism—International consensus statement. *Int Angiol* 32:111, 2013.
10. Kahn SR, Morrison DR, Cohen JM, et al: Interventions for implementation of thromboprophylaxis in hospitalized medical and surgical patients at risk for venous thromboembolism. *Cochrane Database Syst Rev* 7:CD008201, 2013.
11. Lester W, Freemantle N, Begaj I, et al: Fatal venous thromboembolism associated with hospital admission: A cohort study to assess the impact of a national risk assessment target. *Heart* 99:1734, 2013.
12. Catterick D, Hunt BJ: Impact of the national thromboembolism risk assessment tool in secondary care in England: Retrospective population-based database study. *Blood Coagul Fibrinolysis* 25:571, 2014.
13. Hull R, Hirsh J, Carter C, et al: Diagnostic value of ventilation-perfusion lung scanning in patients with suspected pulmonary embolism. *Chest* 88:819, 1985.
14. Turkstra F, Kuijer P, van Beck EJ, et al: Diagnostic utility of ultrasonography of leg veins in patients suspected of having pulmonary embolism. *Ann Intern Med* 126:775, 1997.
15. PIOPED Investigators: Value of the ventilation/perfusion scan in acute pulmonary embolism: Results of the Prospective Investigation of Pulmonary Embolism Diagnosis (PIOPED). *JAMA* 263:2753, 1990.
16. Kruip M, Leclercq M, van der Heul C, et al: Diagnostic strategies for excluding pulmonary embolism in clinical outcome studies. A systematic review. *Ann Intern Med* 138:941, 2003.
17. Birdwell BG, Raskob GE, Whitsett TL, et al: The clinical validity of normal compression ultrasonography in outpatients suspected of having deep venous thrombosis. *Ann Intern Med* 128:1, 1998.
18. Stevens S, Elliott CG, Chan K, et al: Withholding anticoagulation after a negative result on Duplex ultrasonography for suspected symptomatic deep venous thrombosis. *Ann Intern Med* 140:985, 2004.
19. Hull R, Hirsh J, Sackett DL, et al: Clinical validity of a negative venogram in patients with clinically suspected venous thrombosis. *Circulation* 64:622, 1981.
20. Rosendaal FR: Risk factors for venous thrombosis: Prevalence, risk and interaction. *Semin Hematol* 34:171, 1997.
21. Heit JA, O'Fallon WM, Peterson TM, et al: Relative impact of risk factors for deep vein thrombosis and pulmonary embolism: A population-based study. *Arch Intern Med* 162:1245, 2002.
22. Bezemer ID, Bare LA, Doggen CJ, et al: Gene variants associated with deep vein thrombosis. *JAMA* 299:1306, 2008.
23. Engbers MJ, Van Hylckama Vlieg A, Rosendaal F: Venous thrombosis in the elderly: Incidence, risk factors, and risk groups. *J Thromb Haemost* 8:2105, 2010.
24. Hull R, Merali T, Mills A, et al: Venous thromboembolism in elderly high-risk medical patients: Time course of events and influence of risk factors. *Clin Appl Thromb Hemost* 19:357, 2013.
25. Simioni P, Prandoni P, Lensing AW, et al: The risk of recurrent venous thromboembolism in patients with an Arg506Gln mutation in the gene for factor V (factor V Leiden). *N Engl J Med* 336:399, 1997.
26. Wells PS, Owen C, Doucette S, et al: Does this patient have deep vein thrombosis? *JAMA* 295:199, 2006.
27. Stein PD, Woodard PK, Weg JG, et al: Diagnostic pathways in acute pulmonary embolism: Recommendations of the PIOPED II Investigators. *Am J Med* 119:1048, 2006.
28. Qaseem A, Snow V, Barry P, et al: Current diagnosis of venous thromboembolism in primary care: A clinical practice guideline from the American Academy of Family Physicians and the American College of Physicians. *Ann Fam Med* 5:57, 2007.
29. Mos IC, Douma RA, Erkens PM et al: Diagnostic outcome management study in patients with clinically suspected recurrent pulmonary embolism with a structured algorithm. *Thromb Res* 133:1039, 2014.
30. Konstantinides SV, Torbicki A, Agnelli G, et al: Task Force for the Diagnosis and Management of Acute Pulmonary Embolism of the European Society of Cardiology (ESC) endorsed by the European respiratory Society (ERS): 2014 ESC Guidelines on the diagnosis and management of acute pulmonary embolism. *Eur Heart J* 35:3033, 2014.
31. Stein P, Hull RD, Patel K, et al: D-dimer for the exclusion of acute venous thrombosis and pulmonary embolism. A systematic review. *Ann Intern Med* 140:589, 2004.
32. Bernardi E, Prandoni P, Lensing AW, et al: D-dimer testing as an adjunct to ultrasonography in patients with clinically suspected deep-vein thrombosis: Prospective cohort study. *BMJ* 317:1037, 1998.
33. Kearon C, Ginsberg J, Hirsh J: The role of venous ultrasonography in the diagnosis of suspected deep vein thrombosis and pulmonary embolism. *Ann Intern Med* 129:1044, 1998.
34. Bernardi E, Camporese G, Buller HR, et al: Serial 2-point ultrasonography plus D-dimer vs whole-leg color-coded Doppler ultrasonography for diagnosing suspected symptomatic deep vein thrombosis: A randomized controlled trial. *JAMA* 300:1653, 2008.
35. Hull RD, Carter CJ, Jay RM, et al: The diagnosis of acute, recurrent deep-vein thrombosis: A diagnostic challenge. *Circulation* 67:901, 1983.
36. Prandoni P, Cogo A, Bernardi E, et al: A simple ultrasound approach for detection of recurrent proximal-vein thrombosis vein diameter. *Circulation* 88:1730, 1993.
37. Rathbun S, Whitsett T, Raskob G: Negative D-dimer to exclude recurrent deep-vein thrombosis in symptomatic patients. *Ann Intern Med* 141:839, 2004.
38. Ten Cate-Hoek AJ, Prins MH: Management studies using a combination of D-dimer test result and clinical probability to rule out venous thromboembolism: A systematic review. *J Thromb Haemost* 3:2465, 2005.

39. Righini M, Van Es J, Den Exter PL, et al: Age-adjusted D-dimer cutoff levels to rule out pulmonary embolism: The ADJUST-PE study. *JAMA* 311:1117, 2014.

40. Rathbun S, Whitsett T, Raskob G: Sensitivity and specificity of helical computed tomography in the diagnosis of pulmonary embolism: A systematic review. *Ann Intern Med* 132:227, 2000.

41. Patel S, Kazerooni EA, Cascade PN: Pulmonary embolism: Optimization of small pulmonary artery visualization at multi-detector row CT. *Radiology* 227:455, 2003.

42. Perrier A, Roy PM, Sanchez O, et al: Multi-detector row computed tomography in suspected pulmonary embolism. *N Engl J Med* 352:1760, 2005.

43. Stein PD, Fowler SE, Goodman LR, et al: Multi-detector computed tomography for acute pulmonary embolism. *N Engl J Med* 354:2317, 2006.

44. van Belle A, Büller HR, Huisman MV, et al: Effectiveness of managing suspected pulmonary embolism using an algorithm combining clinical probability, D-dimer testing, and computed tomography. *JAMA* 295:172, 2006.

45. Hull R, Raskob G, Coates G, Panju A: Clinical validity of a normal perfusion lung scan in patients with suspected pulmonary embolism. *Chest* 97:23, 1990.

46. Miniati M, Prediletto A, Fornichi B, et al: Accuracy of clinical assessment in the diagnosis of pulmonary embolism. *Am J Respir Crit Care Med* 159:864, 1999.

47. Hull RD, Raskob GE, Ginsberg JS, et al: A noninvasive strategy for the treatment of patients with suspected pulmonary embolism. *Arch Intern Med* 154:289, 1994.

48. Anderson DR, Kahn SR, Rodger MA, et al: Computed tomographic pulmonary angiography vs ventilation-perfusion lung scanning in patients with suspected pulmonary embolism: A randomized controlled trial. *JAMA* 298:2743, 2007.

49. Stein PD, Chenevert TL, Fowler SE, et al: Gadolinium-enhanced magnetic resonance angiography for pulmonary embolism: A multicenter prospective study (PIOPED III). *Ann Intern Med* 152:434, 2010.

50. van Strijen M, de Monye W, Schiereck J, et al: Single-detector helical computed tomography as the primary diagnostic test in suspected pulmonary embolism: A multicenter clinical management study of 510 patients. *Ann Intern Med* 138:307, 2003.

51. Hull R, Delmore T, Genton E, et al: Warfarin sodium versus low-dose heparin in the long-term treatment of venous thrombosis. *N Engl J Med* 301:855, 1979.

52. Prandoni P, Kahn S: Post-thrombotic syndrome: Prevalence, prognostication and need for progress. *Br J Haematol* 145:286, 2009.

53. Prandoni P, Lensing AWA, Cogo A, et al: The long-term clinical course of acute deep venous thrombosis. *Ann Intern Med* 125:1, 1996.

54. Prandoni P, Lensing AW, Prins MH, et al: Below knee elastic compression stockings to prevent the post-thrombotic syndrome: A randomized controlled trial. *Ann Intern Med* 141:249, 2004.

55. Kahn SR, Shapiro S, Wells PS, et al: SOX Trial Investigators: Compression stockings to prevent post-thrombotic syndrome: A randomized placebo-controlled trial. *Lancet* 383:880, 2014.

56. Pengo V, Lensing A, Prins M, et al: Incidence of chronic thromboembolic pulmonary hypertension after pulmonary embolism. *N Engl J Med* 350:2257, 2004.

57. Kearon C, Akl EA, Comerota A, et al: Antithrombotic therapy for VTE disease. Antithrombotic Therapy and Prevention of Thrombosis, 9th ed: American College of Chest Physicians Evidence-based Clinical Practice Guidelines. *Chest* 141 (2 Suppl):E419S, 2012.

58. Wells PS, Forgie MA, Rodger MA: Treatment of venous thromboembolism. *JAMA* 311:717, 2014.

59. Hull R, Raskob G, Hirsh J, et al: Continuous intravenous heparin compared with intermittent subcutaneous heparin in the initial treatment of proximal vein thrombosis. *N Engl J Med* 315:1109, 1986.

60. Brandjes D, Heijboer H, Buller H, et al: Acenocoumarol and heparin compared with acenocoumarol alone in the initial treatment of proximal-vein thrombosis. *N Engl J Med* 327:1485, 1992.

61. Lagerstedt C, Olsson C, Fagher B, et al: Need for long-term anticoagulant treatment in symptomatic calf-vein thrombosis. *Lancet* 2:515, 1986.

62. Quinlan D, McQuillan A, Eikelboom J: Low-molecular-weight heparin compared with intravenous unfractionated heparin for treatment of pulmonary embolism. *Ann Intern Med* 140:175, 2004.

63. Hull RD, Raskob GE, Brant RF, et al: Relation between the time to achieve the lower limit of the APTT therapeutic range and recurrent venous thromboembolism during heparin treatment for deep vein thrombosis. *Arch Intern Med* 157:2562, 1997.

64. Hull RD, Raskob GE, Brant RF, et al: The importance of initial heparin treatment on long-term clinical outcomes of antithrombotic therapy: The emerging theme of delayed recurrence. *Arch Intern Med* 157:2317, 1997.

65. Buller H, Davidson B, Decousus H, et al: Fondaparinux or enoxaparin for the initial treatment of symptomatic deep venous thrombosis. A randomized trial. *Ann Intern Med* 140:867, 2004.

66. Matisse Investigators: Subcutaneous fondaparinux versus intravenous unfractionated heparin in the initial treatment of pulmonary embolism. *N Engl J Med* 349:1695, 2003.

67. Lee A, Levine M, Baker R, et al: Low-molecular-weight heparin versus Coumadin for the prevention of recurrent venous thromboembolism in patients with cancer. *N Engl J Med* 349:146, 2003.

68. Hull R, Pineo G, Brant R, et al: Long-term low-molecular-weight heparin versus usual care in proximal-vein thrombosis patients with cancer. *Am J Med* 119:1062, 2006.

69. Ridker P, Goldhaber S, Danielson E, et al: Long-term low-intensity warfarin therapy for the prevention of recurrent venous thromboembolism. *N Engl J Med* 348:1425, 2003.

70. Kearon C, Ginsberg J, Kovacs M, et al: Comparison of low-intensity warfarin therapy with conventional intensity warfarin therapy for long-term prevention of recurrent venous thromboembolism. *N Engl J Med* 349:631, 2003.

71. Crowther M, Ginsberg J, Julian J, et al: A comparison of two intensities of warfarin for the prevention of recurrent thrombosis in patients with the antiphospholipid antibody syndrome. *N Engl J Med* 349:1133, 2003.

72. Hull R, Hirsh J, Jay R, et al: Different intensities of oral anticoagulant therapy in the treatment of proximal-vein thrombosis. *N Engl J Med* 307:1676, 1982.

73. Schulman S, Kearon C, Kakkar A, et al: Dabigatran versus warfarin in the treatment of acute venous thromboembolism. *N Engl J Med* 361:2342, 2009.

74. Schulman S, Kakkar AK, Goldhaber SZ, et al: Treatment of acute venous thromboembolism with dabigatran or warfarin and pooled analysis. *Circulation* 129:764, 2014.

75. EINSTEIN Investigators, Bauersachs R, Berkowitz SD, et al: Oral rivaroxaban for symptomatic venous thromboembolism. *N Engl J Med* 363:2499, 2010.

76. EINSTEIN-PE Investigators, Büller HR, Prins MH, et al: Oral rivaroxaban for the treatment of symptomatic pulmonary embolism. *N Engl J Med* 366:1287, 2012.

77. Agnelli G, Buller H, Cohen A, et al: Oral apixaban for the treatment of acute venous thromboembolism. *N Engl J Med* 369:799, 2013.

78. Hokusai-VTE Investigators, Büller HR, Décousus H, et al: Edoxaban versus warfarin for the treatment of symptomatic venous thromboembolism. *N Engl J Med* 369:1406, 2013.

79. van Es N, Coppens M, Schulman S, et al: Direct oral anticoagulants compared with vitamin K antagonists for acute symptomatic venous thromboembolism: Evidence from phase 3 trials. *Blood* 124:1968, 2014.

80. Kearon C, Akl E: Duration of anticoagulant therapy for deep vein thrombosis and pulmonary embolism. *Blood* 123:1794, 2014.

81. Schulman S, Rhedin A-S, Lindmarker P, et al: A comparison of six weeks with six months of oral anticoagulant therapy after a first episode of venous thromboembolism. *N Engl J Med* 332:1661, 1995.

82. Levine M, Hirsh J, Gent M, et al: Optimal duration of oral anticoagulant therapy: A randomized trial comparing four weeks with three months of warfarin in patients with proximal deep-vein thrombosis. *Thromb Haemost* 74:606, 1995.

83. Prandoni P, Lensing A, Prins M, et al: Residual venous thrombosis as a predictive factor of recurrent venous thromboembolism. *Ann Intern Med* 137:955, 2002.

84. Palareti G, Cosmi B, Vigano D'Angelo S, et al: D-dimer testing to determine the duration of anticoagulant therapy. *N Engl J Med* 355:1780, 2006.

85. Kyrle P, Minar E, Bialonczyk, et al: The risk of recurrent venous thromboembolism in men and women. *N Engl J Med* 350:2558, 2004.

86. Palareti G, Cosmi B, Legnani C et al: D-dimer to guide the duration of anticoagulation in patients with venous thromboembolism: A management study. *Blood* 124:196, 2014.

87. Connors JM. Extended treatment of venous thromboembolism. *N Engl J Med* 368; 767–769, 2013.

88. Schulman S, Kearon C, Kakkar A, et al: Extended use of dabigatran, warfarin, or placebo in venous thromboembolism. *N Engl J Med* 368:709, 2013.

89. Agnelli G, Buller H, Cohen A, et al: Apixaban for extended treatment of venous thromboembolism. *N Engl J Med* 368:699, 2013.

90. Becattini C, Agnelli G, Schenone A, et al: Aspirin for preventing the recurrence of venous thromboembolism. *N Engl J Med* 366:1959, 2012.

91. Brighton T, Eikelboom J, Mann K, et al: Low-dose aspirin for preventing recurrent venous thromboembolism. *N Engl J Med* 367:1979, 2012.

92. Schulman S, Granqvist S, Holmström M, et al: The duration of oral anticoagulant therapy after a second episode of venous thromboembolism. *N Engl J Med* 336:393, 1997.

93. Hull R, Pineo G, Brant R, et al: Self-managed long-term low-molecular-weight heparin therapy: The balance of benefits and harms. *Am J Med* 120:72, 2007.

94. Bates S, Greer IA, Middledorp S, et al: VTE, thrombophilia, antithrombotic therapy, and pregnancy: Antithrombotic Therapy and Prevention of Thrombosis, 9th ed: American College of Chest Physicians Evidence-Based Clinical Practice Guidelines. *Chest* 141 (2 Suppl):E691S, 2012.

95. Pettila V, Kaaja R, Leinonen P, et al: Thromboprophylaxis with low molecular weight heparin (dalteparin) in pregnancy. *Thromb Res* 96:275, 1999.

96. Smith M, Norris L, Steer P, et al: Tinzaparin sodium for thrombosis treatment and prevention during pregnancy. *Am J Obstet Gynecol* 190:495, 2004.

97. Linkins L, Choi P, Douketis J: Clinical impact of bleeding in patients taking oral anticoagulant therapy for venous thromboembolism. A meta-analysis. *Ann Intern Med* 139:893, 2003.

98. Goldhaber SZ, Haire WD, Feldstein ML, et al: Alteplase versus heparin in acute pulmonary embolism: Randomized trial assessing right-ventricular function and pulmonary perfusion. *Lancet* 341:507, 1993.

99. Meyer G, Vicaut E, Danays T et al: Fibrinolysis for patients with intermediate-risk pulmonary embolism. *N Engl J Med* 370:1402, 2014.

100. Enden T, Haig Y, Klow NE et al: CaVenT Study Group: Long-term outcome after additional catheter-directed thrombolysis versus standard treatment for acute iliofemoral deep vein thrombosis (the CaVenT study): A randomized controlled trial. *Lancet* 379:31, 2012.

101. Bashir R, Zack CJ, Zhao H, et al: Comparative outcomes of catheter-directed thrombolysis plus anticoagulation vs anticoagulation alone to treat lower-extremity proximal deep vein thrombosis. *JAMA Intern Med* 174:1494, 2014.

102. Decousus H, Leizorovicz A, Parent F, et al: A clinical trial of vena caval filters in the prevention of pulmonary embolism in patients with proximal deep-vein thrombosis. *N Engl J Med* 338:409, 1998.

CHAPTER 134

ATHEROTHROMBOSIS: DISEASE INITIATION, PROGRESSION, AND TREATMENT

Emile R. Mohler III and Andrew I. Schafer

SUMMARY

The consequences of atherosclerotic vascular disease are the leading cause of morbidity and mortality in the developed countries of the world and are rapidly approaching that status in the developing world. This chapter reviews the pathologic mechanisms of atherosclerotic disease development and progression, and details the interaction of these processes with the coagulation system. The earliest morphologically visible lesion of arterial atherosclerosis, the fatty streak, already is an advanced metabolic and immunologic locus that manifests as abnormalities of vascular tone, inflammation, cellular growth, and endothelial cell dysfunction. After years to decades, the lesions advance to form plaques that grow and eventually either impinge on the arterial lumen or rupture. Rupture of a vulnerable plaque is a catastrophic event that, through activation of both platelets and the coagulation cascade, triggers thrombosis, which leads to complete occlusion, and unless collateral circulation has already been established, results in tissue ischemia. Based on an increased understanding of the pathogenesis and consequences of atheromatous plaque development and progression, medical management of atherothrombotic syndromes has improved and is reviewed for the coronary, cerebrovascular, and peripheral arteries.

Acronyms and Abbreviations: ACC, American College of Cardiology; ACCP, American College of Chest Physicians; ACS, acute coronary syndrome; AHA, American Heart Association; apo, apolipoprotein; aPTT, activated partial thromboplastin time; CABG, coronary artery bypass graft; CAD, coronary artery disease; CAPRIE, Clopidogrel Versus Aspirin in Patients at Risk of Ischaemic Events; CCL, CC chemokine ligand; CK, creatine kinase; CVD, cardiovascular disease; ECG, electrocardiogram; eNOS, endothelial nitric oxide synthase; EPC, endothelial progenitor cell; EV, extracellular vesicle; HAART, highly active antiretroviral therapy; HDL, high-density lipoprotein; hsCRP, high-sensitivity C-reactive protein; IFN, interferon; Ig, immunoglobulin; IL, interleukin; LDL, low-density lipoprotein; Lp-PLA$_2$, lipoprotein phospholipase A$_2$; MCP, monocyte chemoattractant protein; MHC, major histocompatibility complex; MI, myocardial infarction; NO, nitric oxide; NOX, nicotinamide adenine dinucleotide phosphate oxidase; NSTEMI, non–ST-segment elevation myocardial infarction; PAD, peripheral arterial disease; PAI, plasminogen-activator inhibitor; PCI, percutaneous coronary intervention; SLE, systemic lupus erythematosus; SNP, single nucleotide polymorphisms; TF, tissue factor; TFPI, tissue factor pathway inhibitor; TGF, transforming growth factor; Th, T helper; t-PA, tissue-type plasminogen activator; VCAM, vascular cell adhesion molecule; VLDL, very-low-density lipoprotein; VWF, von Willebrand factor.

● ATHEROSCLEROSIS

Atherothrombosis describes a disease process that begins with atherosclerosis and predisposes to thrombosis in the artery. In the 1850s, Virchow[1] described atherosclerosis as an inflammatory and prothrombotic process. Rokitansky, and later Duguid, posited that atherosclerotic lesions are initiated by incorporation of platelet lipids into the vessel wall ("encrustation") following thrombosis. It was subsequently demonstrated that insudation of plasma lipoproteins is responsible for most of the lipid content of the atherosclerotic lesions. In 1913, Anitschkow noted atherosclerosis developing in rabbits fed a relatively high cholesterol diet. Although the involvement of inflammation in atherosclerosis has been known for more than 100 years, the molecular mechanisms of atherosclerotic disease initiation and progression have become clearer only in the recent past.[2] It is now understood that the classical disagreement between the "lipid" hypothesis and the "inflammation" hypothesis of atherogenesis can be reconciled because there is direct linkage between cholesterol deposition and arterial inflammation in the process.[3,4]

Lipid accumulation in the arterial intima, termed a *fatty streak*, can occur in adolescents and may progress in paroxysmal fashion to a hemodynamically significant lesion causing arterial insufficiency. Autopsy studies of young soldiers and young trauma victims indicated that occult coronary atherosclerotic plaques are commonly present in healthy individuals in their teens and twenties.[5,6] In addition, intracoronary ultrasonograph studies demonstrated the presence of coronary atherosclerosis in 37 percent of healthy heart donors age 20 to 29 years, 60 percent of those age 30 to 39 years, and 85 percent of those older than age 50 years.[7] Several theories are espoused for this propitious condition. One well-recognized theory is the *response to injury hypothesis* whereby the inciting event that predisposes to atherosclerosis is injury to the endothelial lining of the artery. This hypothesis was formulated in animal studies that showed vessel narrowing and intimal thickening after endothelial denudation with angioplasty.[8,9] However, human pathologic studies of early atherosclerotic plaques indicate that endothelium is structurally present but is dysfunctional. The dysfunctional state of endothelium induces abnormalities in vascular tone, inflammation, growth, and thrombosis. Atherosclerotic risk factors contribute to endothelial dysfunction and promote atherosclerosis. This section describes the mechanisms responsible for endothelial dysfunction and the impact of atherosclerotic risk factors.

ATHEROSCLEROTIC RISK FACTORS

Increasing age, male gender, and heredity are the major atherosclerotic cardiovascular disease risk factors that cannot be modified (Table 134–1). Abnormal lipids, smoking, improperly controlled hypertension, improperly controlled diabetes mellitus, abdominal obesity, physical inactivity, and psychosocial factors are established risk factors that can be modified, accounting for most of the risk of myocardial infarction worldwide in both sexes and at all ages.[10]

In addition to these traditional risk factors, newer risk factors have been recognized.[11] With the use of highly active antiretroviral therapy (HAART), HIV-infected patients have demonstrated a dramatic overall increase in life expectancy.[12] At the same time, HAART-treated HIV patients also have an increased risk of developing premature cardiovascular disease over time. Both HIV viral proteins and the antiretroviral drugs themselves cause endothelial dysfunction. They activate cell signaling cascades, induce oxidative stress, disturb mitochondrial function, alter gene expression, and impair lipid metabolism in vascular cells, macrophages, and adipocytes.[13,14]

TABLE 134–1. Cardiovascular Risk Factors That Cause Impaired Endothelium-Dependent Vasodilation

Smoking
Dyslipidemia
Hypertension
Diabetes mellitus
Hyperhomocysteinemia

Cardiovascular morbidity and mortality is also recognized to be exceedingly high in patients with chronic renal failure.[15,16] Increased risk of premature atherosclerotic cardiovascular disease in patients on chronic hemodialysis has been known for many years, but recent studies point to an increased risk even at early stages of chronic kidney diseases. Low glomerular filtration rates and/or proteinuria are independently associated with increased rates of cardiovascular disease.[17] Other factors, such as sympathetic overactivity,[18] are likely to contribute to the pathophysiology of cardiac risk in these patients. Among other emerging risk factors is obstructive sleep apnea, in which treatment may improve cardiovascular outcomes.[19]

ENDOTHELIAL DYSFUNCTION

Cardiovascular risk factors and abnormal blood rheology are thought to result in endothelial dysfunction that predisposes the aorta and arteries to atherosclerotic plaque development, sparing the arterioles and capillaries (Fig. 134–1). *Endothelial dysfunction* is a term that encompasses perturbations in the diverse physiologic functions of normal arteries, including regulation of vascular tone, inflammation, growth, and preservation of blood fluidity. Lipid accumulation[20] and endothelial

dysfunction are intimately connected and seminal to the initiation and progression of atherosclerosis. Endothelial dysfunction occurs early in the development of plaque and is systemic in nature, afflicting vessels throughout the arterial circulation without gross evidence of atherosclerotic plaque formation. Emerging data indicate that proatherosclerotic genes are upregulated and antiatherosclerotic genes are downregulated in areas of turbulent blood flow, as seen at branch points of arteries,[21] resulting in vascular adhesion molecule expression and recruitment of monocytes.[22] The atherosclerotic plaque initially may expand outward rather than inward into the vessel wall, making some significant lesions difficult to visualize by angiography. The components of the mature atherosclerotic lesion include smooth muscle cells, macrophages, T lymphocytes, and calcification, in addition to accumulation of lipoproteins.[23] Neutrophils and mast cells also are implicated in the atherosclerotic process.[22] Later in the process, increased activity of matrix metalloproteinases in the atherosclerotic cap predisposes to plaque rupture or ulceration, resulting in tissue factor (TF) exposure and platelet adhesion, culminating in thrombus formation.[24] The thrombus may undergo endogenous fibrinolysis with plaque healing or become occlusive and produce organ damage (e.g., myocardial infarction [MI]). In severe lesions, lamellar bone, presumably from endochondral calcification, may appear.[25] There is evolving evidence that extracellular vesicles (EVs), also known as microparticles, are involved in the atherosclerotic process.[26] The following sections describe in detail the major manifestations of endothelial dysfunction that occur early in the atherosclerotic process.

Abnormal Vascular Tone

The importance of the endothelium in maintaining vascular tone was first recognized when endothelial cells of rabbit aorta were inadvertently removed and resulted in paradoxical vasoconstriction after administration of acetylcholine.[27] The major endothelium-dependent vasodilator normally produced was found to be nitric oxide (NO), a free

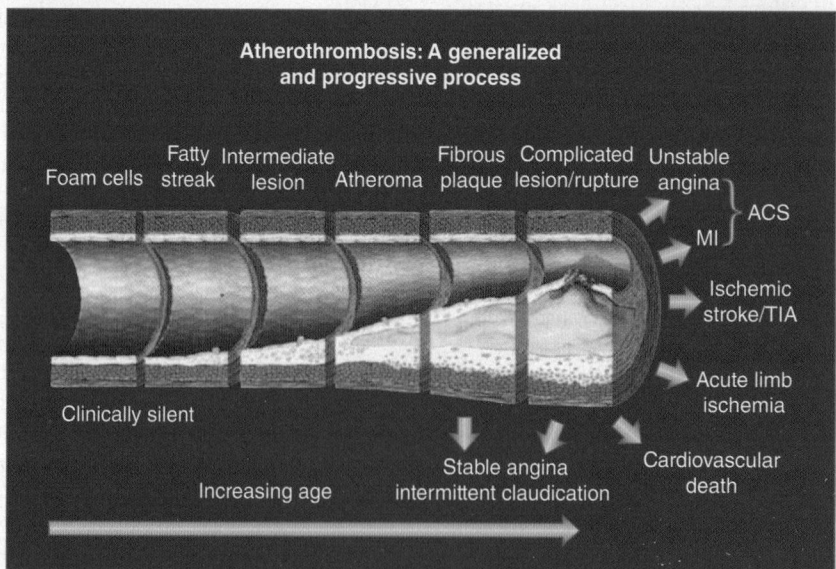

Figure 134–1. Schematic showing the life span of the atherosclerotic plaque, beginning with the fatty streak and resulting in a thrombotic event. Cardiovascular risk factors and disturbed blood flow at branch points of vessels are thought to cause endothelial dysfunction that results in atherosclerotic plaque development in the aorta and conduit arteries. Early lipid accumulation in the intimal layer is called the *fatty streak*. A series of stimuli, including lipid peroxidation, are thought to signal adhesion molecule expression on the endothelium, which results in monocyte adhesion and diapedesis into the intimal space. The monocytes develop into macrophages and become sessile with accumulation of lipid (foam cells). Smooth muscle cells, primarily from the media, enter the plaque and participate in cap formation. The plaque accumulates hydroxyapatite mineral and forms calcific deposits. Matrix metalloproteinases also accumulate in the lesion and may predispose to plaque rupture or ulceration resulting in tissue factor exposure and thrombus formation. Risk factor modification favors a more stable plaque, which may have relatively less lipid accumulation and more sclerotic tissue than an unstable plaque. Severe lesions may even develop lamellar bone. ACS, acute coronary syndrome; MI, myocardial infarction; TIA, transient ischemic attack.

radical gas with multiple physiologic properties,[28] including inhibition of platelet aggregation and inflammation and stimulation of angiogenesis. Numerous studies indicate that the endothelium does not vasodilate appropriately in the setting of traditional and emerging cardiovascular risk factors. Cardiovascular risk factors are thought to reduce NO availability through a variety of mechanisms, including increased oxidative stress, through generation of reactive oxygen species, and in so doing create an environment conducive to development of atherosclerosis.[29] Major sources of reactive oxygen species are nicotinamide adenine dinucleotide phosphate (NADPH) oxidases (NOXs). The catalytic subunits of the NOXs are the NOX proteins and are found in atherosclerotic lesions.[30] A reduction in NO synthesis is thought to occur because of decreased availability of tetrahydrobiopterin, an essential cofactor for synthesis of NO.[31] Administration of sepiapterin, a substrate for tetrahydrobiopterin, improves endothelial dysfunction.[32] Also, recent evidence indicates that the transcription factor p53 and the adaptor protein Shc both play essential roles in impairing endothelium-dependent vascular relaxation.[33] High cholesterol levels are thought to produce oxygen free radicals that may inactivate NO. NO synthases are the enzymes responsible for converting L-arginine to NO (Fig. 134–2) (Chap. 115). The enzyme may be perturbed by modified low-density lipoprotein (LDL), resulting in decreased NO production. Supplementation of the diet with L-arginine leads to improvement in endothelial-dependent vasodilation.[34] Elevated levels of asymmetric dimethylarginine, an endogenous competitive inhibitor of NO synthase, found in patients with hypercholesterolemia and diabetes, also may result in decreased NO availability.[35] Oxidized LDL is thought to increase the elaboration of asymmetric dimethylarginine by endothelial cells and decrease its degradation by the enzyme dimethylarginine dimethylaminohydrolase.[36] Administration of acetylcholine to patients with elevated serum LDL[37] and relatively low high-density lipoprotein (HDL)[38] may result in abnormal vasoconstriction, which can be reversed with nitroglycerin (an endothelium-independent vasodilator).[39] Intravenous infusion of HDL improves endothelial-mediated vasodilation through improved

NO availability.[40] The decreased vasodilatory capacity because of dyslipidemia may facilitate the development of coronary ischemia.

Impaired endothelial vasodilation is noted with advanced aging,[41] when the hands are exposed acutely to cold, and during mental stress. The impairment may be mediated by increased production of endothelin, a potent vasoconstrictor.[42] Sex differences are also seen in endothelial function as women in middle age tend to have more endothelial vasodilation than men at any age.[43] Proinflammatory cytokines may induce formation of endothelial-derived EVs making them a surrogate marker for endothelial dysfunction[44] and a biomarker for cardiovascular events.[45] Infection with concomitant inflammation is associated with impaired endothelial vasodilation. For example, repeated infection with *Chlamydia pneumoniae* results in endothelial dysfunction via impaired NO availability.[46] The combination of coronary artery disease and elevated serum levels of high-sensitivity C-reactive protein (hsCRP) is an independent predictor of abnormal endothelial vasoreactivity.[47] External radiation therapy also results in endothelial dysfunction and may explain the increased risk of atherosclerosis in patients receiving mantle irradiation for Hodgkin lymphoma.[48]

Endothelial Inflammation

The endothelium does not routinely interact with inflammatory cells but is poised to express adhesion molecules after stimulation with inflammatory mediators. An inflammatory response is thought to begin in the vessel wall after "invasion" of pathogenic lipoproteins.[49] The presence of lipoproteins, especially oxidized LDL, results in expression of adhesion molecules such as vascular cell adhesion molecule (VCAM)-1 on the luminal surface of endothelial cells, leading to adherence of monocytes (Fig. 134–3).[50] Endothelial cell expression of adhesion molecules and accumulation of monocytes can be regarded as endothelial dysfunction because these events may occur in the absence of morphologic changes in the vessel wall. Inflammation may develop without the demonstrable presence of an external microbial pathogen. It is now recognized that diseases with inflammatory component such as psoriasis and systemic lupus erythematosus (SLE) confer an increased risk for atherosclerosis and MI.[51] The complex interactions of inflammation and the endothelium on the initiation and progression of atherosclerosis are reviewed in more detail in "Inflammation and Atherosclerosis" below.

Abnormal Control of Vascular Growth: Smooth Muscle Cells and Extracellular Matrix

Normal endothelium inhibits vascular smooth muscle cell proliferation.[52] The specific function of vascular smooth muscle cells in atherosclerosis is unclear. However, evidence indicates that, in early atherosclerosis, vascular smooth muscle cells contribute to the development of atheroma through production of proinflammatory mediators such as CC chemokine ligand (CCL)2 (previously termed *monocyte chemoattractant protein*, or MCP-1) and VCAMs. Although smooth muscle cells primarily play a role in modulating vascular tone, they also are involved in the control of extracellular matrix formation and degradation through matrix modulators such as proteases, protease inhibitors, matrix proteins, and integrins (Fig. 134–4).

The importance of vascular smooth muscle cells in controlling the synthesis of matrix molecules is evident at the clinical level. They provide a thick, fibrous cap that promotes stability and inhibits plaque rupture and ulceration. Factor VII–activating protease, thought to play a role in coagulation and fibrinolysis, is also a potent inhibitor of vascular smooth muscle cell proliferation, and migration *in vitro* and local application of factor VII–activating protease (but not Marburg I variant) in animal models reduces neointima formation.[53] Furthermore, it has been localized to unstable atherosclerotic plaques and may contribute to plaque instability.

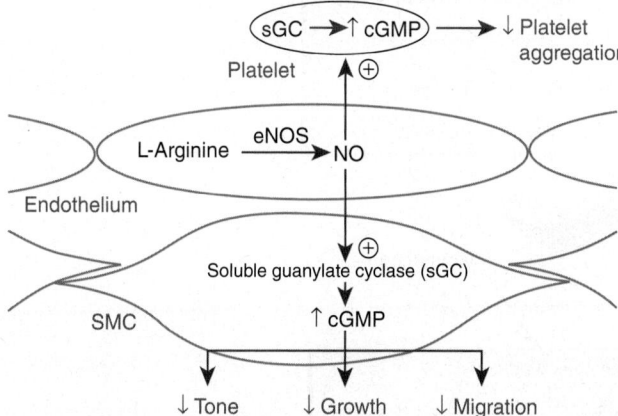

Figure 134–2. Vascular tone depends on endothelial production and release of various vasoconstricting and vasodilating substances. The endothelial-derived vasodilators include nitric oxide (NO) and prostacyclin. NO is generated from the amino acid L-arginine by constitutive endothelial NO synthase (eNOS, or NOSIII). The enzyme is stimulated by blood flow across the endothelial surface (shear stress) or by chemical mediators, such as acetylcholine, which stimulate receptors on the endothelial surface. NO diffuses to the underlying smooth muscle cells (SMCs), where it stimulates guanylate cyclase to generate cyclic guanosine V monophosphate (cGMP), which causes smooth muscle relaxation and vasodilation. It also diffuses into blood, where it increases intraplatelet cGMP and thereby inhibits platelet adhesion and aggregation.

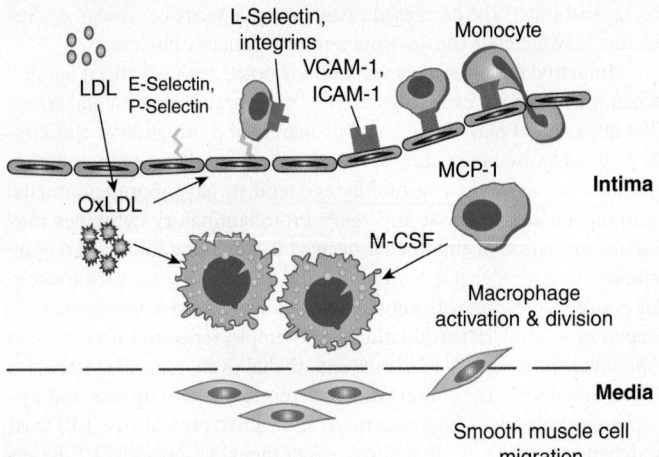

Figure 134–3. Atherosclerotic lesion initiation is stimulated by oxidized low-density lipoprotein (OxLDL). Induction of inflammatory gene products in vascular cells is activated by the transcription factor nuclear factor-κB, which results in increased expression of cellular adhesion molecules. The adhesion molecules have specific functions for endothelial leukocyte interaction. The selectins tether and trap monocytes and other leukocytes. Vascular cell adhesion molecule-1 (VCAM-1) and intracellular adhesion molecule-1 (ICAM-1) mediate firm attachment of these leukocytes to the endothelial layer. OxLDL also augments expression of monocyte chemoattractant protein-1 (MCP-1 or CCL2) and macrophage colony-stimulating factor (M-CSF). MCP-1 mediates the attraction of monocytes and leukocytes and facilitates diapedesis through the endothelium into the intima. M-CSF is an important cytokine for the transformation of monocytes to macrophage foam cells. Macrophages express scavenger receptors and internalize oxidized low-density lipoprotein (LDL) during their transformation into foam cells. Smooth muscle cells migrate from the media into the intima and participate in the formation of a fibrous atheroma. (*Adapted with permission from S Kinlay, AP Selwyn, P Libby: Inflammation, the endothelium, and the acute coronary syndromes. J Cardiovasc Pharmacol 32[Suppl 3]:S62, 1998.*)

Evidence indicates that vascular smooth muscle cells that undergo apoptosis, especially at the shoulder region of the plaque, may create a more unstable cap.[54] Both intact vascular smooth muscle cells and fibroblasts are thought to stabilize plaques through modulation of extracellular calcification and formation of a fibrocalcific plaque.

Vascular smooth muscle cells arise primarily from the medial layer and are considered monoclonal in origin.[55] Evidence also indicates that vascular smooth muscle cells may originate from the adventitia.[56] The rate and timing of smooth muscle cell replication is unclear. It may occur at a constant low rate throughout the development of the atherosclerotic lesion or episodically at a higher rate. Animal studies indicate that new intimal cells may originate from outside the vessel wall from subpopulations of marrow- and non–marrow-derived circulating cells.[57] Smooth muscle progenitor cells circulating in blood may contribute to the arterial remodeling that occurs after angioplasty and after bypass graft surgery.[58]

Vascular proliferation and inflammation are linked processes. Inflammation-induced impaired NO bioactivity contributes to vascular smooth muscle proliferation.[2] Overexpression of NO synthase results in reduction of atherosclerotic or restenotic lesion formation in rabbits through both inhibition of vascular smooth muscle cell proliferation and inhibition of adhesion and chemoattractant molecule expression, with subsequent reduction of vascular mononuclear cell infiltration.[59] Thus, the vascular smooth muscle cell participates in the atherosclerotic process by affecting lipoprotein retention, modulating inflammation, and controlling plaque stability through formation of the fibrous cap. Several vascular disorders involve vascular smooth muscle proliferation as the primary pathophysiologic mechanism, including in-stent restenosis, transplant vasculopathy, and vein bypass graft failure.[60] The control of smooth muscle proliferation is thought to involve NR4A nuclear receptors that are expressed in atherosclerotic lesion macrophages, smooth muscle cells, and endothelial cells, and are induced by atherogenic stimuli. Inhibition of the transcriptional activity of the NR4A nuclear receptors results in enhanced smooth muscle proliferation.[61]

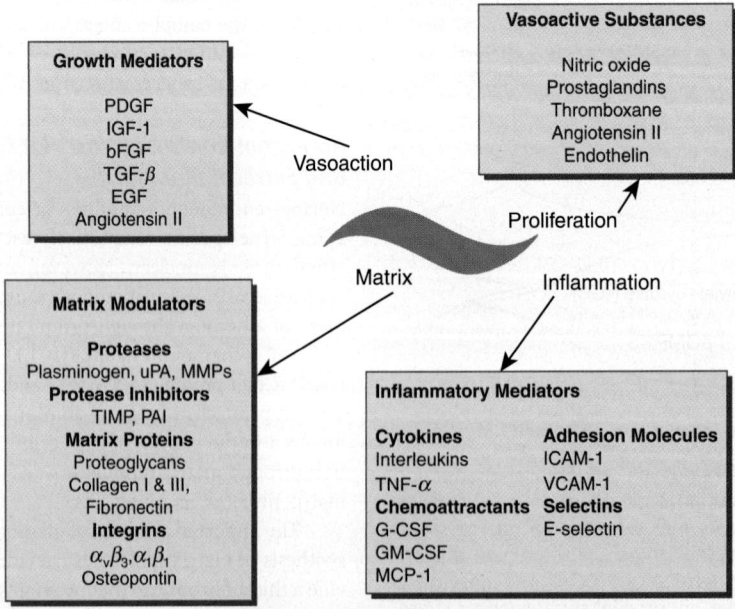

Figure 134–4. Vascular smooth muscle cells mediate vascular proliferation, inflammation, matrix composition, and contraction. Many of these mediators have multiple functions. For example, angiotensin is a vasoconstrictor, but it also stimulates proliferation and inflammation. This is only a partial list of mediators secreted by vascular smooth muscle cells. bFGF, Basic fibroblast growth factor; EGF, epidermal growth factor; G-CSF, granulocyte colony-stimulating factor; GM-CSF, granulocyte-monocyte colony-stimulating factor; ICAM, intracellular adhesion molecule; IGF, insulin-like growth factor; MCP, monocyte chemoattractant protein; MMPs, matrix metalloproteinases; PAI, plasminogen-activator inhibitor; PDGF, platelet-derived growth factor; TGF-β, transforming growth factor-β; TIMP, tissue inhibitor of metalloproteinases; TNF, tumor necrosis factor; uPA, urokinase-type plasminogen activator; VCAM, vascular cell adhesion molecule. (*Adapted with permission from Dzau VJ, Braun-Dullaeus RC, Sedding DG: Vascular proliferation and atherosclerosis: New perspectives and therapeutic strategies. Nat Med 8(11):1249–1256, 2002.*)

The NR4A nuclear receptors are also expressed in vein segments exposed to arterial pressure and it is postulated that they are responsible for an inhibitory feedback mechanism that occurs in activated vascular cells. Drug-eluting vascular stents that release agents such as sirolimus and paclitaxel interfere with the cell cycle and inhibit restenosis in part via decreased smooth muscle cell proliferation.[62]

Abnormal Endothelial Control of Blood Fluidity

Endothelial cells normally elaborate a number of antithrombotic substances. Some of these substances are released into blood whereas others are properties of the unactivated endothelial cell surface. These antiplatelet, anticoagulant, and profibrinolytic activities of endothelium, some of which also possess vasodilatory properties (e.g., prostacyclin, NO), act in concert to promote blood fluidity under normal circumstances. Acute activation or chronic dysfunction of endothelial cells alters the hemostatic balance, transforming them from predominantly antithrombotic to prothrombotic cells.[63]

To this end, endothelial cells modulate the activities of thrombin in health and disease. In the presence of intact and normally functioning endothelium, the prothrombotic actions of thrombin are quenched and the antithrombotic actions of the enzyme predominate. Thrombin binds to thrombomodulin, an integral membrane protein expressed by endothelial cells, and activates protein C (accelerated in the presence of endothelial protein C receptor, another endothelial cell protein) (Chap. 116). Activated protein C, in concert with its cofactor, protein S, has anticoagulant and profibrinolytic actions. It degrades by proteolytic digestion factors Va and VIIIa, and inactivates plasminogen-activator inhibitor (PAI)-1. Simultaneously, by binding to thrombomodulin, enzymatically active procoagulant thrombin is removed from the circulation, thereby limiting its availability to catalyze fibrin formation. Endothelial dysfunction causes loss of thrombomodulin activity from the vascular surface. In fact, increased circulating plasma levels of free (truncated) thrombomodulin represent a marker of endothelial damage. In addition to the role of thrombomodulin in clearance of circulating thrombin, the procoagulant activity of thrombin is normally blocked by endothelial cells through the action of antithrombin, which binds to heparin-like glycosaminoglycans on their luminal surface, thereby catalyzing the inactivation of thrombin by antithrombin. Like thrombomodulin, this thrombin-neutralizing action of endothelial heparan sulfate glycosaminoglycans is lost with endothelial dysfunction.

Endothelial cells do not normally express TF, but they do so upon activation by inflammatory cytokines or exposure to endothelium-activating levels of homocysteine or free thrombin. The procoagulant effects of expression of TF by dysfunctional endothelial cells are potentially compounded by the loss of TF pathway inhibitor (TFPI), which normally is synthesized by endothelial cells. Studies show that monocyte-derived EVs (or microparticles) express TF and platelet-derived EVs express phosphatidylserine and thus support coagulation complex formation.[64] There is also evidence that P-selectin on platelets binds to P-selection protein ligand-1 on EVs.[65]

Normal endothelium is profibrinolytic. It synthesizes and releases tissue-type plasminogen activator (t-PA); it possesses binding sites for t-PA and plasminogen to provide a surface for the concentrated assembly of the fibrinolytic complex and thereby enhance local plasmin generation; and it fails to produce significant amounts of PAI-1. This profibrinolytic state is converted to an antifibrinolytic state in the presence of endothelial dysfunction. In activated or dysfunctional endothelium, PAI-1 gene expression and PAI-1 secretion are induced; simultaneously, the profibrinolytic properties of normal endothelium are lost (Chap. 135).

The antithrombotic profile of normal endothelium also manifests through the elaboration of several antiplatelet substances. NO is constitutively released into blood by normal endothelial cells and inhibits platelet adhesion and aggregation by stimulating platelet soluble guanylyl cyclase and raising intraplatelet levels of cyclic guanosine monophosphate (see Fig. 134–2).[66] Physiologic flow and shear forces maintain the activity of endothelial (endothelium-derived) NO synthase (eNOS)[67] under normal circumstances. Vascular cell-derived carbon monoxide, a product of heme catabolism by heme oxygenase, may have similar antiplatelet activity.[68,69] Prostacyclin (prostaglandin I_2) likewise is released basally by normal endothelial cells and inhibits platelet aggregation by inducing platelet adenylyl cyclase and raising intraplatelet levels of cyclic adenosine monophosphate.[70]

NO, carbon monoxide, and prostaglandin I_2 are labile autacoids, acting only in the immediate vicinity of their release into blood from endothelial cells. An endothelial surface ecto-adenosine diphosphatase (CD39) also blocks platelet activity by metabolizing and disposing of platelet agonist adenosine diphosphate (ADP).[71] In endothelial dysfunction, these various antiplatelet activities are lost, and endothelial release of von Willebrand factor (VWF) is increased, which promotes platelet adhesion. In the case of NO, oxidative stress in the microenvironment of endothelial dysfunction actually "uncouples" eNOS activity[68,72] to preferentially generate superoxide over NO. Oxygen free radicals bind any remaining available NO to produce the toxic product peroxynitrite. Bioactive NO is further reduced in endothelial dysfunction by the presence of asymmetric dimethylarginine, which competes to block eNOS and limit NO production.[67,73]

Progenitor Cells and Atherosclerosis

Endothelial progenitor cells (EPCs) are heterogenous in origin and participate in endothelial cell regeneration and neovascularization of ischemic tissue. The mobilization of EPCs from the marrow is stimulated by hypoxia, cytokines such as vascular endothelial growth factor, hormones such as erythropoietin, and statin drugs, whereas mobilization is inhibited in the diabetic state.[74] The role of EPCs in atherosclerosis is unclear as there are conflicting data.[22] A study in apolipoprotein (apo) E−/− mice showed that there is rapid turnover of endothelial cells in atherosclerosis-prone areas and marrow derived EPCs are recruited to sites of atheroprogression.[75]

INFLAMMATION AND ATHEROSCLEROSIS

Innate Immunity and Atherosclerosis

The endothelial response to injury manifests as a chronic inflammatory response that involves both innate and adaptive immunity.[76] Innate immunity provides the first line of defense for the host and involves several cell types, most importantly macrophages and dendritic cells, which express a limited number of highly conserved sensing molecules such as scavenger receptors and toll-like receptors.[76,77] Microbial infection can be detected by pathogen-associated molecular patterns, which are present in bacteria, viruses, and yeasts, but not in mammalian cells, and are recognized by the toll-like receptors.[78] Ligation of a pathogen or other substances containing pathogen-associated molecular patterns (such as lipopolysaccharides, aldehyde-derivatized proteins, mannans, teichoic acids) elicits endocytosis or activation of endothelial cells (e.g., through nuclear factor-κB) that results in an inflammatory response (Chaps. 17 and 18).[77,79] Proinflammatory cytokines, such as tumor necrosis factor, nuclear factor-κB and interleukin (IL)-1, magnify the innate inflammatory response.

Innate defense involves soluble factors, such as complement, which is involved in atherosclerotic lesion formation. hsCRP has been found to be an important and independent predictor for cardiovascular events.[80] Natural antibodies that are generated in the absence of known antigen stimulation, mainly immunoglobulin (Ig) M, provide an immediate response against bacteria and viruses but also may be involved in atherosclerosis. For example, innate B lymphocytes, the so-called

B1 cells, express a restricted set of germline–encoded antigen receptors that may bind oxidized LDL.

Adaptive Immunity and Atherosclerosis

Compared to innate immunity, adaptive immunity is slower but more precise (Chap. 77).[76] T cells can be activated by dendritic cells and macrophages, whereas most antigens cannot stimulate B cells without assistance from CD4+ T cells, which recognize the peptide–major histocompatibility complex (MHC) complexes on B cells. By genetic recombination, the number of T-cell and B-cell receptors that can be formed is almost unlimited and far exceed the number of pattern recognition receptors used by the innate immune system. Most CD4+ cells are cytokine-secreting T-helper (Th) cells and express $\alpha\beta$–T-cell receptors, which interact with MHC class II molecules. A smaller number of Th cells express $\gamma\delta$–T-cell receptors, which interact with the nonpolymorphic, nonclassic MHC molecules, CD1, which present certain antigens (particularly lipids and glycolipids). Th cells are classified according to the cytokines they secrete. Th1 cells secrete interferon (IFN)-γ and IL-2 and promote cell-mediated immunity (Chap. 78). Th2 cells secrete IL-4, IL-5, IL-10, and IL-13, and help B cells produce antibodies. CD8+ T cells are primarily cytotoxic killer cells, although they can secrete cytokines, such as tumor necrosis factor-α, IFN-γ, and lymphotoxin. Some thymus-independent antigens can activate these cells without the help of T cells. Oxidized LDL is considered such an antigen because it expresses multiple copies of oxidation-specific epitopes on a single LDL particle.

Adhesion Molecules and Atherosclerosis

Monocyte recruitment to inflammatory foci initially involves the expression of endothelial cell selectins, which mediate monocyte rolling on the endothelium (see Fig. 134–3). The rolling phenomenon is followed by a firmer attachment to endothelial cells mediated by integrins. Perhaps the most important of these is VCAM-1, which is upregulated in cultured endothelial cells in the presence of oxidized LDL. The appearance of this molecule before the development of grossly visible atherosclerotic lesions supports oxidized LDL as an initial recruiter of macrophages. The finding of reduced atherosclerosis in VCAM-1–deficient mice further supports the important role of macrophages and VCAM-1 in the pathogenesis of atherosclerosis.[81,82] Other adhesion molecules, such as P-selectin and intracellular cell adhesion molecule-1, also may be involved in monocyte adhesion at sites of lesion formation.[83] The entry of monocytes into the vascular intima leads to their differentiation into resident macrophages. Here they take up cholesterol that has also accumulated in the vascular intima, thereby becoming cholesterol-engorged foam cells.[84] It has been demonstrated that the accumulation of macrophage foam cells in established atherosclerotic lesions actually originates mainly from the proliferation of macrophages within the lesion rather than from the recruitment of circulating monocytes.[85] Platelet-derived EVs contain and deliver the chemokine "regulated upon activation, normal T-cell expressed and secreted" (RANTES) to activate endothelium in atherosclerosis to promote attraction of monocytes.[86]

Lipoprotein Phospholipase A₂ and Atherosclerosis

Lipoprotein phospholipase A_2 (Lp-PLA$_2$) is an inflammatory enzyme belonging to the large family of phospholipases that are capable of hydrolyzing the sn-2 ester bond of phospholipids of cell membranes and lipoproteins.[87] This enzyme, produced by macrophages, circulates bound to LDL and in the intimal space of the artery can produce oxidized fatty acids and lysophosphatidyl choline. These molecules have a range of potentially atherogenic effects, including chemoattraction of monocytes, increased expression of adhesion molecules, and

inhibition of endothelial NO production.[88] Although originally designated as platelet-activating factor acetylhydrolase because of its ability to degrade platelet-activating factor, the clinical importance of this effect is not thought significant. Numerous epidemiologic studies show that Lp-PLA$_2$ is a significant biomarker associated with cardiovascular events. The selective inhibition of Lp-PLA$_2$ with the drug darapladib reduced development of advanced coronary atherosclerosis in diabetic and hypercholesterolemic swine.[89] A phase 2 clinical study of patients with cardiovascular disease showed that sustained inhibition of plasma Lp-PLA$_2$ activity with background of intensive atorvastatin therapy resulted in reduction in IL-6 and hsCRP after 12 weeks of darapladib 160 mg, suggesting a possible reduction in inflammatory burden.[90] However, a prospective double-blind phase III trial of 15,828 patients, darapladib did not reduce the composite end point of cardiovascular death, MI, or stroke. There was a significant reduction in major coronary events and total coronary events.[91]

Immune Cells and Atherosclerosis

Macrophages are essential for the clearance of modified lipoproteins and the efflux of lipoprotein-derived cholesterol to HDL receptors for reverse cholesterol transport, the process by which HDL removes cholesterol from cells. Multiple lines of evidence indicate that macrophages promote lesion initiation and progression. For example, hypercholesterolemic mice become markedly resistant to atherosclerosis if they are bred to macrophage-deficient animals.[92]

The earliest grossly visible sign of atherosclerosis is the fatty streak, which is composed mainly of macrophage foam cells containing relatively large amounts of cholesterol. Foam cells also can derive from smooth muscle cells, as these cells can express scavenger receptors when appropriately activated.[93,94] Formation of the fatty streak is thought to begin with adherence of circulating monocytes to activated endothelial cells at sites in the arterial system prone to atherosclerotic disease, such as at branch points in vessels. Multiple chemoattractant molecules have been identified in these nascent lesions, which recruit monocytes and induce their diapedesis into the subendothelial space where they further differentiate into macrophages. As noted above, however, more recent evidence indicates that microenvironment-supported macrophage proliferation *in situ* within the atherosclerotic lesion is likewise a key event in atherogenesis.[84]

The chemoattractant CCL2 (MCP-1) facilitates recruitment of monocytes to atherosclerotic lesions, as noted in studies of mouse models of atherosclerosis, such as apoE−/− or LDL receptor (LDLR−/−)–deficient mice fed a Western-style diet. When these mice are crossed to the model lacking CCL2, or its receptor CCR-2, lesion development decreases significantly.[95–97]

Macrophages and T cells were once thought to be the only inflammatory cells to significantly promote angiogenesis. More recent data showing that neutrophils are found at sites of plaque rupture or erosion and in thrombus from patients with acute coronary artery syndromes indicate that they also have an important role in atherothrombosis.[18] Mast cells have been found in the adventitia of lesions and in areas of plaque hemorrhage; they have been implicated in macrophage apoptosis, increased vascular permeability, degradation of HDL and reduced cholesterol efflux.[22] Neutrophils and mast cells are recruited to atherosclerotic lesions in response to CXC-chemokine receptor 2 (CXCR2) signals. The mobilization of neutrophils to atherosclerotic lesions is inhibited by CXC-chemokine receptor 4 (CXCR4) and its ligand CXC-chemokine ligand 12 (CXCRL12; also known as stromal-derived factor (SDF) 1. A subset of CD31+ T cells, so called T$_{ang}$ cells, was shown to promote endothelial repair and revascularization, and to be inversely correlated with age and cardiovascular disease (CVD) risk in patients undergoing coronary angiography.[98]

Lipid Peroxidation and Atherosclerosis

Macrophages control the amount of cholesterol loading by downregulating the native LDL receptor. Therefore, knowing how cholesterol is taken up into macrophages is important. Cell culture experiments revealed a "foam cell paradox," in which macrophages engulf only modified lipids. Treatment of native LDL with copper or acetic anhydride (causing acetylation) led to increased LDL uptake through use of the scavenger receptor, leading to the formation of lipid-laden macrophages. These experiments led to the peroxidation theory of atherosclerosis,[94] whereby LDL modification is an essential step in the development of foam cells. Although the precise mechanisms responsible for LDL oxidation remain unclear, enzymes including myeloperoxidase, inducible NO synthase, and NADPH oxidases are involved in the process.[99,100] Of note, macrophages express each of these enzymes, which normally are used as antimicrobial reactive oxygen species essential for innate immunity.[101] Thus, accumulation of cholesterol in the macrophage occurs via scavenger (not LDL) receptors of oxidized (and not native) LDL. Myeloperoxidase is an enzyme thought to cause lipid peroxidation in the intimal space and circulating levels are associated with adverse clinical outcomes in the setting of acute coronary syndromes and predictive of major adverse cardiovascular events.[99]

Scavenger Receptors and Atherosclerosis

Conserved pattern recognition receptors expressed by macrophages include scavenger receptors A and B1 and CD36, all of which internalize oxidized LDL.[102,103] Macrophages express various genes in response to oxidized LDL, including peroxisome proliferator-activated receptor-γ and adenosine triphosphate–binding cassette transporter A1, which profoundly influence macrophage-mediated inflammation and atherosclerotic activity.

Cell culture studies indicate that scavenger receptor A recognizes acetylated LDL but, unlike the LDL receptor, is not downregulated in response to increased cholesterol content and thus likely accounts for foam cell formation.[104] However, no evidence indicates that acetyl LDL is generated *in vivo*, indicating other modifications of LDL, such as oxidation, may be required for foam cell formation.[105,106] Another scavenger receptor presumed to be involved in the atherosclerotic process is CD36, a receptor that avidly binds oxidized LDL.

Circulating IgG and IgM antibodies against products of lipid peroxidation are present in the plasma of animals and humans.[107] These antibodies closely correlate with measures of lipid peroxidation and with atherosclerotic progression and regression in murine models.[108] Immunization of hypercholesterolemic rabbits and mice with products of oxidized LDL, such as malonyldialdehyde LDL or copper-oxidized LDL, inhibits the progression of atherosclerotic lesion formation.[109-112] These experiments have been interpreted to indicate that an immunologic response to oxidized LDL components can alter the atherosclerotic process.

Leukocyte-derived 5-lipoxygenase also contributes to atherosclerosis susceptibility in mice.[113] Animal studies indicate the importance of lipoxygenases in atherosclerosis as disruption of the 12,15-lipoxygenase gene diminishes atherosclerosis in apoE-deficient mice, and overexpression of 15-lipoxygenase in vascular endothelium accelerates early atherosclerosis in LDL receptor-deficient mice.[114,115] This enzyme is under study as a potential target to inhibit the atherosclerotic process.[116]

Gut Microbiome There are newer data indicating that intestinal microbes are involved in cardiometabolic diseases.[117] Systemic inflammation is activated is the setting of chronic bacterial translocation (secondary to increased intestinal permeability) leading to macrophage influx into adipose tissue resulting in insulin resistance and nonalcoholic fatty liver disease. The increased inflammation may also be secondary to trimethylamine-*N*-oxide via influx of macrophages and cholesterol accumulation via upregulation of macrophage scavenger receptors and reduction in reverse cholesterol transport. Thus, gut microbiota may accelerate atherosclerosis risk.

Accumulation of Low-Density Lipoprotein in the Vascular Wall

Three potential factors lead to accumulation of LDL in the vascular wall: increased permeability of the endothelium, prolonged retention of lipoproteins in the intima, and slow removal of lipoproteins from the vessel wall.[118] Rabbits fed a high-cholesterol diet develop aortic wall lesions at specific lesion-susceptible sites; however, endothelial permeability is not increased at those sites, indicating that LDL is selectively retained in these regions.[119,120] Retention of LDL molecules likely results from their adherence to proteoglycans in the vessel wall.[121] LDL genetically engineered to not bind to proteoglycans is hypothesized to be less atherogenic than native LDL.[20]

Oxidized LDL and its products, oxidized phospholipids and oxysterols, have other properties that make them potentially proatherogenic.[122] These properties include proinflammatory characteristics, such as chemotactic signaling for monocytes, smooth muscle cells, and T lymphocytes (but not for B lymphocytes or neutrophils, neither of which is found in lesions) and increased expression of VCAM-1 on, and stimulation of CCL2 release from, endothelial cells.[123] Oxidized LDL also may contribute to instability of the atherosclerotic plaque via induction of type 1 metalloproteinase expression and increase in TF activity.[124] For oxidized LDL to be a ligand for the scavenger receptor, extensive degradation of the polyunsaturated fatty acid in the sn-2 position of phospholipids by oxidation is essential.

To test the oxidized LDL hypothesis, several clinical studies have been conducted using antioxidant vitamins, most commonly vitamin E; however, most of the completed studies gave negative results.[125,126] At the present time, treatment with vitamin E does not appear to be beneficial in preventing cardiovascular events.

High-Density Lipoprotein and Atherosclerosis

A low level of HDL cholesterol is a strong predictor of adverse cardiovascular events, presumably because the low level is associated with insufficient reverse cholesterol transport. Animal studies using liver-directed gene transfer of human apoA–apoI resulted in significant promotion of reverse cholesterol transport and regression of preexisting atherosclerotic lesions in LDL receptor-deficient mice.[127,128] The HDL level may not be as important as amount of reverse cholesterol transport. For example, the capacity of HDL to accept cholesterol from macrophages is predictive of atherosclerotic burden.[129] However, HDL has additional antiatherogenic properties that may confer protection against atherosclerosis.[130] For example, HDL is protective against oxidation of LDL, at least in part because of paraoxonase, an enzyme physically associated with HDL that degrades organophosphates.[131] Paraoxonase polymorphisms are associated with increased risk of CVD, also indicating that oxidized LDL is an important factor in atherosclerotic development.[132]

Research studies currently are evaluating novel ways to increase HDL levels or to use apoA–apoI variants and mimetics that hopefully will cause regression of atherosclerosis. So far, initial clinical studies were not successful. Cholesteryl ester transfer protein promotes the transfer of cholesteryl esters from antiatherogenic HDLs to proatherogenic apoB-containing lipoproteins, including very-low-density lipoproteins (VLDLs), VLDL remnants, intermediate-density lipoproteins, and LDLs. A deficiency of this molecule results in increased HDL levels and decreased LDL levels, a lipid profile that is antiatherogenic. A large clinical study in humans showed that inhibition of the transfer protein with torcetrapib increased HDL levels but was associated with increased mortality and hypertension.[133] It is supposed that the increase in mortality was a result of an off-target effect of the drug increasing blood pressure and not because of cholesterol ester transfer protein inhibition. Clinical trials evaluating the effect of other inhibitors of cholesteryl ester transfer protein on atherosclerosis and cardiovascular events have not shown clinical efficacy thus far. Along similar lines, delivery of a mutant form of apoA1 (apoA1 Milano) resulted in regression of plaque size as measured by intravascular ultrasound in a small phase II clinical trial.[134] However, studies evaluating the effect of apoA1 mimetics on atherosclerosis also are have not shown compelling data regarding reducing plaque size or cardiovascular events.[135]

CD40, CD40 Ligand, and Atherosclerosis

Studies indicate that human atherosclerotic lesions express the immune mediator CD40 and its soluble ligand, sCD40L. Increasing evidence indicates that the CD40–sCD40L signaling pathway plays a central role in several inflammatory processes, including atherosclerosis and graft rejection following transplantation.[136] Interruption of CD40 signaling in hyperlipidemic mice reduces the size of aortic atherosclerotic lesions and their lipid, macrophage, and T-lymphocyte content.[137] Atorvastatin, lovastatin, pravastatin, and simvastatin reduce IFN-γ–induced CD40 expression in a dose-dependent manner. Activation of atheroma-associated cells with human recombinant sCD40L is reduced when cells are treated with statins. In addition, retrospective *ex vivo* immunostaining of human carotid atherosclerotic lesions of patients treated with simvastatin for more than 3 months revealed less CD40 expression and atheroma-associated cells compared with patients who were not treated with the drug. A reduction in sCD40L is associated with pravastatin or cerivastatin therapy.[138] These findings support the notion that statins are antiinflammatory, in addition to their cholesterol-lowering effects.

Transforming Growth Factor-β and Atherosclerosis

Transforming growth factor (TGF)-β is a cytokine secreted by macrophages, smooth muscle cells, and the Th3 subset of Th cells that has multiple regulatory functions. TGF-β is speculated to contribute to plaque stabilization because it stimulates collagen synthesis and is fibrogenic. One study found that inhibition of TGF-β signaling by neutralizing antibodies led to a larger plaque size with an unstable phenotype.[139] Further studies are needed to clarify the role of TGF-β in atherosclerotic plaque initiation and growth.

ABO Blood Type and Cardiovascular Risk The ABO blood group is determined from presence of A and B antigens on the surface of the red blood cells and is thought to confer cardiovascular risk.[140] These antigens are also expressed on the surface of platelets and the endothelium and consist of terminal carbohydrate molecules which are synthesized by the sequential action of the ABO glycosyltransferases. Genetic studies showed that carriers of single nucleotide polymorphisms (SNPs) that mark non-O blood group types have higher levels of plasma VWF when compared to O individuals. Epidemiologic and genetic studies show that the non-O blood group is associated with adverse cardiovascular events. One study demonstrated that the SNP rs514659 was associated with coronary artery diseases (CADs) when complicated by MI but not with CAD without MI, suggesting that the primary relationship of ABO to clinical CAD is through modulation of coronary thrombosis or plaque rupture in patients with established coronary atherosclerosis rather than through primary promotion of atherosclerosis per se.

Infection and Atherosclerosis

Several infectious agents have been implicated as pathogens in atherosclerosis.[141] A well-studied infectious pathogen is *C. pneumoniae*. Animals infected with this agent develop atherosclerosis, and patients

with CVD have higher titers of antibodies against this pathogen. Viruses, such as herpes simplex and cytomegalovirus, also are implicated in human atherosclerotic lesion formation. Gingivitis as a consequence of poor dental hygiene or smoking may lead to cellular immune activation and provoke atherosclerosis by cytokines or antibodies.[142] Endogenous proteins, such as heat shock proteins, also are implicated in atherosclerosis. One study showed that progression of carotid disease correlated with antibodies against heat shock proteins 65 and 60.[143]

Splenectomy and Atherosclerosis

The relationship between the immune system and atherosclerosis is complex, as evident from an animal study that showed that splenectomy of cholesterol-fed apoE−/− mice led to significantly increased atherosclerosis.[144] This proatherogenic effect was rescued by transfer of either purified B cells or T cells from the spleens of atherosclerotic apoE−/− donors. A long-term study of soldiers who underwent splenectomy after trauma found the soldiers had a twofold increased incidence of CAD, providing evidence that the spleen has antiatherogenic activity.[145] Further studies are needed to determine if splenectomy significantly impacts the atherosclerotic process, and if so, by what mechanism.

Genetics and Myocardial Infarction

Atherosclerotic disease is a complex human trait involving multiple genes and environmental factors. Through the study of linkage analysis of families and sibling pairs as well as candidate genes and genome-wide association studies, the genetic predisposition to MI is starting to be understood.[146] The clinical importance of this knowledge is the potential identification of markers of disease for risk prediction and potential intervention to lower the risk of atherosclerotic-based cardiovascular events.

The use of genome-wide linkage analyses of families or sib-pairs has identified chromosomal loci linked to or genetic variations in the arachidonic 5-lipoxygenase-activating protein gene (*ALOX5AP*)[147] and leukotriene A$_4$ hydrolase gene (*LTA$_4$H*).[148] The genes are both involved in inflammation-related pathway of leukotriene B$_4$ production. Interestingly, a small molecule inhibitor of ALOX5AP was shown to reduce leukotriene production and plasma levels of C-reactive protein.

Several association studies of unrelated individuals have identified genetic variations that confer susceptibility to atherosclerotic disease and cardiovascular events. Studies using genome-wide linkage analysis identified four SNPs on chromosome 9p21.3 that were associated with MI in white cohorts.[146,149] Other genetic polymorphisms also contribute to increased risk of CVD through a variety of mechanisms.[150]

ATHEROSCLEROTIC PLAQUE

Plaque Classification

The American Heart Association classification of atherosclerotic plaques into types I through VIII is based on lesion composition and structure (Fig. 134–5).[23] Types I through III atherosclerotic plaques have foam cells organized in a fatty streak, ranging from those not visible on close examination (type I) to those that are apparent on examination (type III). Types I through III lesions are small and clinically silent, whereas types IV through VI lesions may obstruct the lumen and produce a clinical event. Type IV lesions contain a confluent pool of lipid and in most patients do not cause anginal symptoms because of the ability of the artery to remodel outward. Type V lesions contain a fibromuscular cap resulting from replacement of tissue disrupted by accumulated lipid and hematoma or organized thrombotic deposits. Type VI lesions involve thrombosis that may be either mural or obstructive. Of note, a type IV lesion may develop type VI changes without ever passing through a type V change and accumulating significant fibrous tissue. Plaques that are

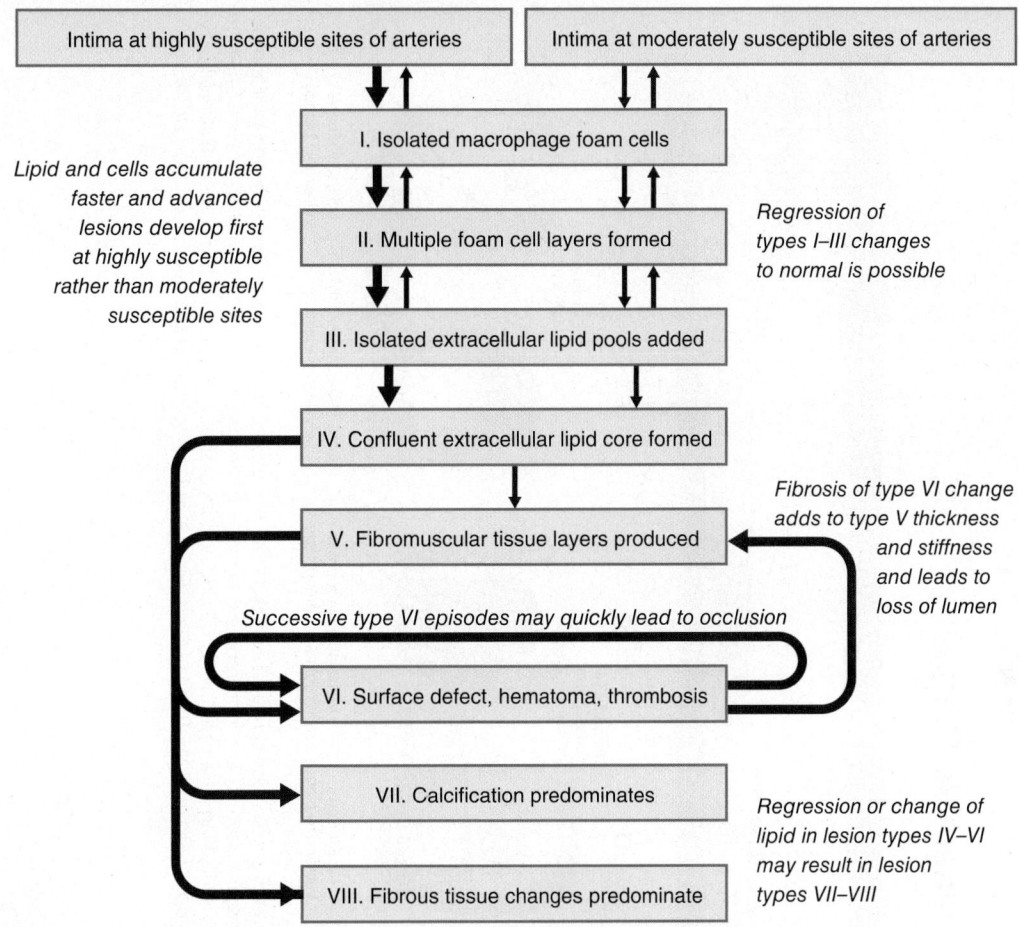

Figure 134–5. Flow diagram in *center column* indicates pathways in evolution and progression of human atherosclerotic lesions. *Roman numerals* indicate histologically characteristic types of lesions. The direction of *arrows* indicates sequence in which characteristic morphologies may change. From type I to type IV, changes in lesion morphology occur primarily because of increasing accumulation of lipid. The *loop* between types V and VI illustrates how lesions increase in surfaces. Thrombotic deposits may develop repeatedly over varied time spans in the same location and may be the principal mechanism for gradual occlusion of medium-sized arteries.

complex and primarily composed of calcium are type VII lesions or, if fibrous tissue predominates, are type VIII lesions.

Vulnerable Plaque and the Vulnerable Patient

The pathologic mechanisms responsible for converting chronic coronary atherosclerosis to an acute coronary event result, in part, from *plaque disruption*, a term that was synonymously used with *plaque rupture*.[151,152] The term *vulnerable plaque* was used by Muller and colleagues[153,154] to describe rupture-prone plaques as the underlying cause of most clinical coronary events. The current definition for "vulnerable plaque" includes all thrombosis-prone plaques and those with a high probability of undergoing rapid progression, thus becoming culprit plaques (Fig. 134–6).[155] Criteria for development of the vulnerable plaque have been proposed based on histopathologic study of culprit plaques (Table 134–2).[155] The major criteria involve the presence of active inflammation, a thin cap with large lipid core, endothelial denudation with superficial platelet aggregation, a fissured plaque, and stenosis greater than 90 percent. The minor criteria for a vulnerable plaque include superficial calcified nodule, glistening yellow plaque, intraplaque hemorrhage, endothelial dysfunction, and outward (positive) remodeling. Some studies indicate plaques that are heavily calcified and without a significant lipid core are more stable.[25,48]

An important concept concerning plaque remodeling is that atherosclerotic plaques commonly grow outward (positive remodeling) before a luminal stenosis occurs. Therefore, a contrast dye coronary angiogram may underestimate the plaque burden in the vessel. Arterial thrombosis may result from plaque hemorrhage (majority of events) or occur in an area of endothelial denudation (30 to 40 percent) without breach of the intimal space.[156] Thrombosis has also been reported in plaques that have a superficial calcified nodule protruding into the lumen.[156] Most atherosclerotic plaques that underlie a fatal or nonfatal MI are, as shown by angiography, less than 70 percent stenosed.[157] Some patients have more than one vulnerable plaque, which underscores the importance of medical therapy in addition to coronary revascularization.[158] Several technologies are currently being tested to identify the location of the vulnerable plaque.[159] Hopefully these developing technologies will shed more light on the natural history of the vulnerable plaque and afford the ability to conduct studies using local or regional antiatherosclerotic therapy.

Because of the dynamic interaction of atherosclerotic plaque with circulating blood, the term *cardiovascular vulnerable patient* has been proposed to define subjects susceptible to an acute coronary syndrome (ACS) or sudden cardiac death based on atherosclerotic plaque or blood or myocardial vulnerability.[160] The vulnerable (thrombogenic) blood includes serum markers of atherosclerosis and inflammation, such as hsCRP, inflammatory cytokines (e.g., IL-6, sCD40L), EVs, and hypercoagulable factors. The blood markers of vulnerability that reflect the hypercoagulable state include those of the fibrinolytic system and platelets (Table 134–3).[161] Patients may have an MI because of a nonfatal or fatal arrhythmia as a result of coronary atherosclerosis or other

Different Types of Vulnerable Plaque

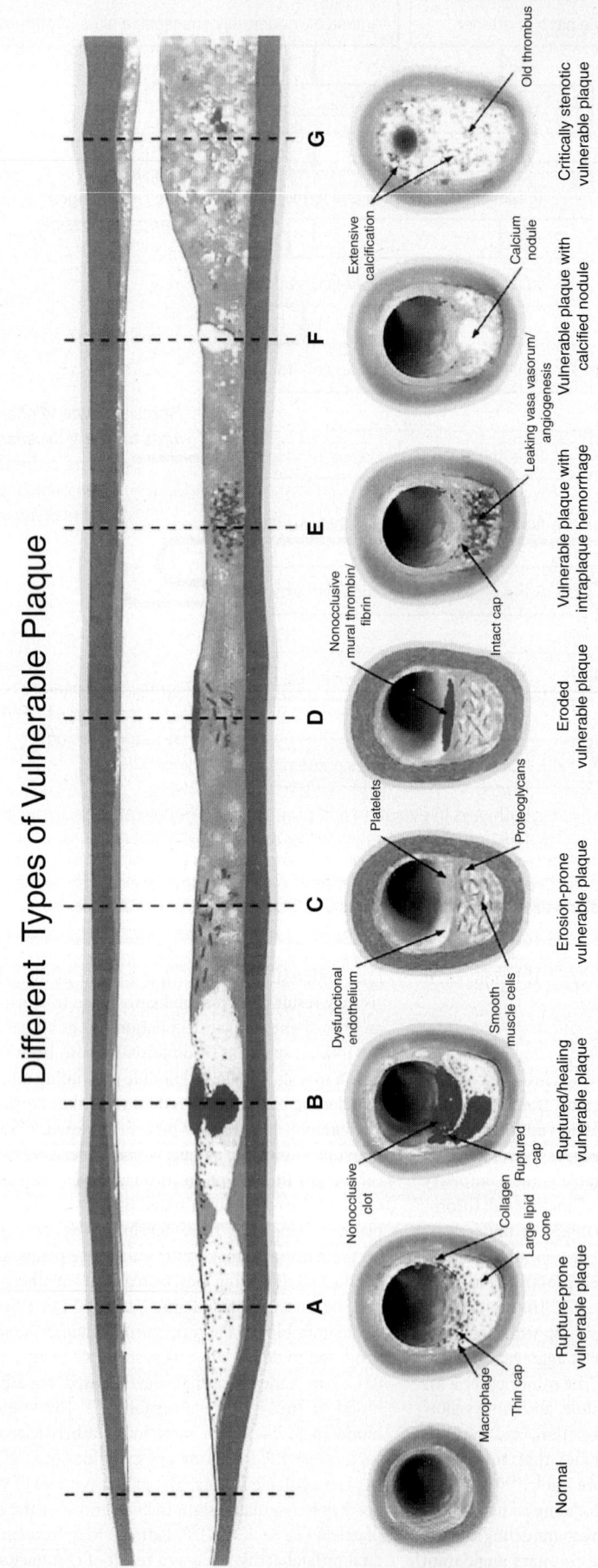

Figure 134–6. Different types of vulnerable plaque as underlying cause of acute coronary events and sudden cardiac death. **A.** Rupture-prone plaque with large lipid core and thin fibrous cap infiltrated by macrophages. **B.** Ruptured plaque with subocclusive thrombus and early organization. **C.** Erosion-prone plaque with proteoglycan matrix in a smooth muscle cell–rich plaque. **D.** Eroded plaque with subocclusive thrombus. **E.** Intraplaque hemorrhage secondary to leaking vasa vasorum. **F.** Calcific nodule protruding into the vessel lumen. **G.** Chronically stenotic plaque with severe calcification, old thrombus, and eccentric lumen. *(Reproduced with permission from Naghavi M, Libby P, Falk E et al: From vulnerable plaque to vulnerable patient: A call for new definitions and risk assessment strategies: Part I. Circulation 108(14):1664–1672, 2003.)*

TABLE 134–2. Criteria for Defining the Vulnerable Plaque, Based on the Study of Culprit Plaques

MAJOR CRITERIA

Active Inflammation (monocyte/macrophage and sometimes T-cell infiltration)

Thin cap with large lipid core

Endothelial denudation with superficial platelet aggregation

Fissured plaque

Stenosis >90%

MINOR CRITERIA

Superficial calcified nodule

Glistening yellow

Intraplaque hemorrhage

Endothelial dysfunction

Outward (positive) remodeling

Reproduced with permission from Naghavi M, Libby P, Falk E, et al: From vulnerable plaque to vulnerable patient: A call for new definitions and risk assessment strategies: Part I. *Circulation* 2003 Oct 7;108(14):1664-1672.

nonatherosclerotic disease, such as hypertrophic cardiomyopathy or right ventricular dysplasia. Thus, a vulnerable patient should be considered from the standpoint of the combined presence of a vulnerable atherosclerotic plaque, vulnerable blood (prone to thrombosis), and/or vulnerable myocardium (prone to life-threatening arrhythmia).

Arterial Thrombosis

Atherothrombosis refers to the occurrence of thrombosis upon atherosclerotic lesions,[161] the typical setting for arterial thrombosis. It represents the acute event that converts chronic atherosclerosis—a silent, asymptomatic, progressive disease—into symptomatic, life-threatening

TABLE 134–3. Blood Hypercoagulability Factors That May Contribute to Patient Vulnerability to Coronary Heart Disease Events

1. Markers of blood hypercoagulability

    Decreased anticoagulation factors (e.g., proteins C and S and antithrombin)

    Prothrombotic gene polymorphisms (e.g., factor V Leiden, G20210A prothrombin mutation)

    Increased coagulation factors (e.g., fibrinogen, factor VII, factor VIII, von Willebrand factor)

2. Increased platelet activation (e.g., gene polymorphisms of platelet integrin $α_{IIb}β_3$, integrin $α_2β_1$, glycoprotein Ib/IX)

3. Decreased endogenous fibrinolysis activity (e.g., reduced tissue-type plasminogen activator, increased plasminogen-activator inhibitor (PAI)-1, certain PAI-1 polymorphisms)

4. Other thrombogenic factors (e.g., anticardiolipin antibodies, thrombocytosis, sickle cell disease, polycythemia, diabetes mellitus, hyperhomocysteinemia, hypercholesterolemia)

5. Increased viscosity

6. Transient hypercoagulability (e.g., smoking, dehydration, infection, adrenergic surge, cocaine, estrogens, postprandial)

Data from Naghavi M, Libby P, Falk E, et al: From vulnerable plaque to vulnerable patient: A call for new definitions and risk assessment strategies: Part I. *Circulation* 2003 Oct 7;108(14):1664-1672.

TABLE 134–4. Pathophysiologic Differences Between Arterial and Venous Thrombi

	Arterial Thrombosis	Venous Thrombosis
Underlying vasculature	Abnormal • Atherosclerosis • Vasculitis • Trauma	Normal
Thrombus pathology	Occlusive or nonocclusive (mural thrombi in large arteries)	Occlusive
	"White thrombus" composed mainly of platelets	"Red thrombus" composed mainly of fibrin, red cells
Pathophysiology	Local shear stress and thrombogenic vascular surface	Stasis and hypercoagulability

clinical complications, including acute MI, stroke, and critical limb ischemia. The previous section described in detail the current concepts of the consecutive stages of atherosclerotic lesion development.

However, thrombosis is not simply the final occlusive event. It also contributes to atherosclerosis lesion development. Intraplaque hemorrhage and *in situ* thrombosis localizes thrombin activity within plaques. Thus, atheroma evolution is not only a proliferative process but also involves thrombosis.[162]

Pathobiology of Arterial Thrombi

Fundamental pathologic and pathophysiologic distinctions exist between arterial and venous thrombi (Table 134–4). Arterial thrombi usually are occlusive in smaller arteries and arterioles. Nonocclusive mural thrombi often occur in the lumina of the heart chambers and large arteries, such as the aorta and the iliac and common carotid arteries. In any arterial vessel, however, thrombi develop almost invariably upon preexisting abnormal intimal surfaces, which typically are atherosclerotic lesions. Less commonly, arterial thrombosis is superimposed on other forms of vascular disease, such as vasculitis or traumatic injury.[163] Thus, in the high-flow and high-pressure arterial system, thrombi form in response to increased local shear forces and exposure of thrombogenic substances on damaged vascular surfaces. Arterial thrombi, referred to as *white thrombi*, are composed mainly of platelets and relatively little fibrin or red cells. Leukocytes are likewise actively recruited into growing, platelet-rich arterial thrombi.[164]

Thus, at sites of atherosclerotic plaque rupture, circulating platelets are activated not only by thrombogenic substances exposed to them by a disrupted plaque but also directly by the locally increased shear forces the platelets encounter.[85] At any given point in the circulation, shear rates are maximal adjacent to the vessel wall (measured as "wall shear rates"), and they are minimal in the center of the vessel lumen where velocity of flowing blood is the greatest. Normally, wall shear rates are in the range of 300 to 800 s^{-1} in large arteries, and they increase to about 500 to 1600 s^{-1} in arterioles of the microcirculation. However, in pathologically stenotic vessels the wall shear rates can reach 10,000 s^{-1} or even higher. Increased shear stress in the microenvironment of an atherosclerotic plaque is usually compounded by turbulent blood flow. These locally abnormal hemodynamic forces can directly activate platelets as they pass through the region. Disturbed flow can simultaneously cause localized endothelial dysfunction.[165]

High shear stresses, especially in the presence of marked shear gradients around stenotic sites, are sufficient to cause the release of VWF from endothelial cells, and promote the unfolding and binding of VWF to its receptors on platelet surface glycoprotein (GP) Ib-V-IX. This interaction, which does not occur in the normal circulation, mediates the adhesion of platelets to the intimal surface and triggers GPIb-V-IX–dependent platelet thrombus formation. The mechanisms of arterial thrombogenesis are further elaborated below in the section on "Platelet Activation."

In contrast, wall shear rates are much lower in the venous circulation where the hemodynamic forces are insufficient to directly activate platelets.[166] Venous thrombi are almost always occlusive and may form virtual casts of the vessel in which they arise. Unlike the setting for arterial thrombi, gross vascular damage generally is not found at sites of venous thrombosis. Any ultrastructural abnormalities of adjacent endothelium likely are the consequences rather than the causes of thrombus formation. Therefore, in the low-flow and low-pressure venous system, reduced blood flow (stasis) and systemic activation of the coagulation cascade play the primary pathophysiologic roles. Venous thrombi are composed predominantly of red cells enmeshed in fibrin and contain relatively few platelets; hence, they have been described pathologically as *red thrombi*.

The generalizations described are consistent with the following clinical observations: (1) hereditary hypercoagulable states (also called "thrombophilias"), characterized by chronic hyperactivity of the coagulation system, are primarily associated with venous rather than arterial thrombosis; and (2) anticoagulants that prevent fibrin formation (e.g., heparin, warfarin) are generally used to prevent venous thrombosis, whereas antiplatelet agents (e.g., aspirin) are more effective in preventing arterial thrombosis. The differences between arterial and venous thrombosis are not, however, absolute because both types of thrombi are composed of different amounts of platelets, fibrin, and leukocytes. In addition, all thrombi continually undergo propagation, organization, embolization, lysis, and rethrombosis, and this dynamic remodeling results in their constantly changing compositions.

Site-Specific Arterial Thrombosis

The model of atherothrombosis described is best characterized in coronary arteries. This pathophysiology may not be entirely applicable to arterial thrombosis at other sites. It cannot be assumed that the local determinants of thrombosis that are operative in the coronary arteries are identical to those encountered in the cerebrovascular and peripheral arterial circulations. Basic regional differences may involve (1) distribution and composition of atherosclerotic lesions, (2) variable local rheology, and (3) underlying vascular cell heterogeneity.

Atherosclerosis is highly localized within the systemic vasculature. Lesion formation particularly affects the carotid artery bifurcation, coronary arteries (especially the left coronary artery bifurcation), abdominal aorta (especially its posterior wall downstream of the renal arteries, but with little disease usually present in the upstream thoracic aorta), and profunda femoral arteries. These lesion-prone sites in the arterial circulation correspond to regions where wall shear stress is very low and may even oscillate between positive and negative directions (i.e., reversal of flow) during the cardiac cycle. A strong correlation exists between local hemodynamic conditions of low shear stress and the development of atherosclerotic plaque formation and intimal thickening.[167-169] However, as arteries become progressively diseased and as stenoses develop at these sites, local hemodynamics change. Stenotic flows are characterized by sharp increases in shear rate that achieve their peak just upstream of the stenosis throat, with development of intensive turbulence downstream of the stenosis. The mechanisms of platelet activation and accumulation that initiate arterial thrombosis at these high-shear sites are further described in "Platelet Activation" below.

Striking heterogeneity is seen in the composition of atherothrombotic plaques, even within the same individual. In addition to plaque composition, the basic structural differences between specific arteries contribute to differences in thrombogenic substrates that are exposed upon arterial injury. For example, carotid and iliac arteries contain relatively more elastic fibers and proportionately fewer smooth muscle cells than coronary arteries.[170] Furthermore, ACSs typically result from disruption of only modestly stenotic, lipid-rich plaques, whereas disruption-prone, high-risk plaques in the carotid arteries usually are severely stenotic. Thus, a proposed more appropriate term is *high-risk plaque* rather than *vulnerable plaque* (which connotes its composition) to define a disruption-prone or thrombosis-prone plaque in different parts of the circulation.[171]

The pathophysiology of arterial thrombosis at different sites in the circulation may also be determined in part by vascular bed-specific heterogeneity of endothelial and smooth muscle cells. Endothelial cell-derived anticoagulant and procoagulant activities are differentially expressed throughout the vascular tree. Endothelial cell heterogeneity throughout the circulation is a function of varying organ- and tissue-specific microenvironments, hemodynamic forces, and site-specific changes in epigenetic footprinting. The heterogeneity of endothelial cells and the vascular bed-specific signaling pathways that control endothelial gene expression have been considered to play an important role in the localization of arterial thrombosis.[172] Heterogeneity of vascular smooth muscle cells likewise exists throughout the arterial tree. They vary in embryonic origin, sources of progenitors, and lineage. With subsequent development, they acquire various phenotypes that can be traced to preferential sites within vessel walls.[173]

Less is known about the pathophysiology of cerebrovascular thrombosis, and even less about peripheral arterial thrombosis, than about coronary artery thrombosis. Future research in these areas should permit the development of more rational antithrombotic strategies in noncoronary artery thrombosis.

Overview of Arterial Thrombotic Process

Arterial thrombosis typically occurs in the presence of underlying atherosclerosis (hence the term "atherothrombosis"). Less frequently, however, it may also occur in nonatherosclerotic arteries, such as in the setting of vasculitis.

Atherothrombosis Disruption of an atherosclerotic plaque triggers an explosive cascade of events that results in the formation of a platelet-rich thrombus at the site of arterial injury.[57] Focal loss of the antithrombotic and the vasodilatory properties of endothelium is compounded by plaque rupture or erosion. These events induce the local activation of platelets and the coagulation system by exposure of blood to previously encrypted thrombogenic substances (e.g., subendothelial cells, such as smooth muscle cells and fibroblasts; subendothelial structures, such as collagen; and subendothelial prothrombotic substances, such as TF, from all of which flowing blood is normally insulated by the barrier of a healthy endothelial monolayer). The local milieu for thrombus formation is aggravated by focal vasoconstriction, rapidly increased shear forces, and platelet-mediated recruitment of leukocytes. Platelet and coagulation activation are inseparable, reciprocally self-amplifying processes. Activation of platelets generates procoagulant properties on their cell surfaces. Combined with non–platelet-dependent local activators of the coagulation cascade, platelet activation culminates in the formation of thrombin, which itself is a potent stimulus for further platelet activation. Superimposed on these local determinants of arterial thrombosis, the thrombotic process may be modulated by systemic, circulating factors. The factors include the systemic state of activation of platelets and coagulation, which may be governed by acquired or genetic factors and by hormonal influences (e.g., adrenergic state).

Arterial thrombi generally are localized to the site of acute vascular injury. They are prevented from extending beyond this site by the restoration of hemostatic balance that promotes blood fluidity along healthy endothelial surfaces immediately adjacent to the site of injury. Thrombus propagation may occur, however, through a bloodborne pool of thrombogenic substances that originate at the site of vascular injury and thrombosis. These substances can be in the form of platelets, leukocytes, red cells, sloughed endothelial cells, other cellular microparticles, and circulating active TF derived from leukocytes activated within the thrombus.[174,175] In fact, cellular microparticles[176] constitute the main reservoir of bloodborne TF, the principal initiator of coagulation.

Thrombus persistence within an artery depends on the local balance between prothrombotic, antithrombotic, and fibrinolytic factors. Ulcerated and thrombotic atherosclerotic plaques, particularly in the aorta, tend to persist or recur.[177] Atherosclerotic plaques of the aortic arch have been detected in almost one-third of patients with cryptogenic stroke. Although aortic arch atheroma are more frequent and more severe causes of cryptogenic stroke in individuals older than 55 years of age, patent foramen ovale (and presumably paradoxical embolism) are more strongly associated with cryptogenic stroke in those younger than 55 years of age.[178]

Advances in the development of coronary stents have created a new form of arterial thrombosis that usually can only be prevented by administration of two different platelet inhibitors (e.g., aspirin in combination with a thienopyridine derivative, such as clopidogrel or prasugrel). Although drug-eluting stents that deliver sirolimus or paclitaxel have been successful in reducing the problem of restenosis that is caused by smooth muscle cell proliferation and intimal hyperplasia following the coronary intervention, they have actually increased the occurrence of "late stent thrombosis" compared to bare metal stents. This form of arterial thrombosis, which typically occurs after discontinuation of (dual) antiplatelet therapy, is probably caused by eluting drugs interfering with endothelialization of the stent surface.[179]

Thrombosis in Nonatherosclerotic Arteries Thrombosis may occur in arteries that are affected by vasculitis.[180] As both SLE and atherosclerosis are immune-driven processes, it is to be expected that some patients with active SLE are more susceptible to accelerated atherosclerosis (and related atherothrombosis) resulting from autoantibody-mediated proatherogenic mechanisms.[181,182] However, even in the absence of underlying atherosclerosis, various types of arterial thrombosis can complicate active vasculitis. For example, patients with SLE may have MI with angiographically normal coronary arteries. Giant cell arteritis, which characteristically targets the extracranial carotid and vertebral arteries, leads to inflammation and necrosis of the arterial wall and subsequent arterial occlusions in a distribution that is quite different from that of atherosclerosis. Takayasu arteritis has an unusual predilection for the aortic arch and its branches, leading to panarteritis, medial layer enlargement with luminal narrowing, and sometimes thrombotic occlusion. Other types of vasculitis and autoimmune processes that may cause arterial thrombosis include polyarteritis nodosa, Behçet disease, and antiphospholipid antibody syndrome.

Arterial thrombosis in the absence of atherosclerosis is also seen with immune- and nonimmune disorders of platelets and/or the vascular endothelium, such as heparin-induced thrombocytopenia (with arterial thrombosis most commonly occurring in the aorta, iliofemoral arteries, as well as in cerebral and coronary arteries),[183] and in the myeloproliferative neoplasms (e.g., essential thrombocythemia, polycythemia vera; Chaps. 84 to 86).[184-186]

Platelet Activation

Disruption of an advanced atherosclerotic plaque results in abrupt exposure of highly thrombogenic material to flowing blood. This process leads locally to both thrombin generation and platelet activation, which operate simultaneously in a mutually self-amplifying process.

As noted above in the section on "Pathobiology of Arterial Thrombi," plaque rupture and the development of new intimal surface irregularities also suddenly alter local rheologic characteristics, increasing local shear rates. Increased shear stress resulting from sudden changes in degree of stenosis following rupture is compounded by increased focal vasoconstriction induced by thrombin, thromboxane A_2, and other vasoactive substances released in the milieu of acute injury.

At high shear rates (>1000 s^{-1}), platelets must be initially tethered to the vascular surface through a shear-activated interaction between the platelet membrane GPIbα (of the GPIb–IX–V complex) and its adhesive ligand, VWF.[187-189] Platelet adhesion also involves collagen binding to platelet collagen receptors (integrin $\alpha_2\beta_1$ and GPVI). Other matrix constituents that become exposed to platelets and serve as adhesive ligands include fibronectin, laminin, fibrinogen, and fibrin. These initial adhesive interactions induce intracellular signaling pathways that activate platelets. High shear stress also activates platelets both directly,[190] as noted previously, and by lowering the threshold of platelet activation by chemical agonists to which platelets are simultaneously exposed in the microenvironment of the arterial thrombus.[191] Thus, following adhesion, platelets are explosively activated by several interacting pathways: (1) intracellular signaling initiated by the adhesion event itself, (2) direct action of locally increased shear stress, and (3) agonists released (e.g., ADP, thromboxane A_2) and generated (e.g., thrombin) at the site of vascular injury.

Finally, the occlusive arterial platelet thrombus is created by the aggregation of platelets. This process is mediated by several alternative ligands (VWF, fibrinogen, fibronectin) that bind to their activated receptors in the platelet integrin $\alpha_{IIb}\beta_3$ complex. Stability of the platelet aggregate is conferred by additional ligand–receptor interactions, including CD40L binding to integrin $\alpha_{IIb}\beta_3$.[192] Platelet thrombus stabilization is designed to counteract shear forces that promote not only the formation of arterial thrombi but also their embolization.

The importance of the inflammatory component of arterial thrombosis,[164] which is characterized by complex interactions among leukocytes, endothelial cells, and platelets, is increasingly being recognized. Activated platelets recruit leukocytes to the site of vascular damage, promoting their adhesion to endothelium and their activation on endothelium-bound chemokines. In fact, the presence of leukocytosis in myeloproliferative neoplasms is a better predictor of pathologic thrombosis than the platelet count.

Tissue Factor and Phospholipids

Tissue factor is a cell-surface–bound transmembrane protein that normally is not exposed to circulating blood. When expressed, TF initiates coagulation by binding to factor VIIa and activates factors IX and X, thereby triggering the common pathway of coagulation and the formation of thrombin. Strong evidence indicates that TF is the principal thrombogenic factor in the lipid-rich core of atherosclerotic plaques. While much of this TF is associated with monocytes/macrophages and vascular smooth muscle cells, more recent studies suggest that TF-positive microparticles are the most abundant sources of TF in atherosclerotic plaques. The main inhibitor of TF-mediated coagulation is TFPI. In atherosclerotic plaques TFPI colocalizes with TF and therefore may play an atheroprotective role.[162,193]

Upon rupture of the atherosclerotic plaque, exposure of vascular TF to flowing blood initiates the coagulation cascade. Coagulation reactions are accelerated on the surfaces of activated platelets, microparticles, and on other activated cells in the microenvironment of vascular injury. The surfaces of these activated cells express anionic phospholipids, particularly phosphatidylserine. Apoptotic cells, with which advanced lesions are enriched, likewise translocate phospholipids from the inner to the outer leaflet of the cell membrane.[194] Plasma lipoproteins can provide a phospholipid surface for the assembly of enzymatic complexes of the coagulation cascade; in particular, oxidized LDL, LDL, and VLDL have procoagulant effects.[195,196] In contrast, HDL has multiple antithrombotic actions, including suppression of the coagulation cascade, stimulation of fibrinolysis, and stimulation of endothelial cell release of prostacyclin and NO, which are inhibitors of platelet activation.[197]

Arterial thrombosis is triggered by the acute exposure of circulating blood to TF and anionic phospholipids, leading to explosive thrombin formation. Thrombin, a potent platelet agonist, further fuels the platelet activation process described in the previous section. These reactions create a self-amplifying process that is tightly localized to the site of vascular injury. The arterial thrombus is further contained to this site by the restoration of normal, antithrombotic endothelium in adjacent areas of the vessel wall.

Systemic Factors

As described above in "Overview of Arterial Thrombotic Process," the pathophysiology of arterial thrombosis is primarily determined by local, "solid-state" factors that operate in concert in the immediate microenvironment of acute vascular injury, typically disruption of an atherosclerotic plaque. However, interindividual differences in systemic, circulating factors can modify susceptibility to the focal formation of an arterial thrombus.[198] Systemic determinants of blood thrombogenicity (i.e., hypercoagulability) can enhance the local risk of arterial thrombosis. There is increasing evidence for an association between venous and arterial thrombosis, with several studies now showing that patients with venous thromboembolism (deep vein thrombosis and/or pulmonary embolism) are at increased risk of having coexisting asymptomatic atherosclerosis or subsequent symptomatic atherothrombotic events. Conversely, patients with clinically overt atherosclerotic CVD are at increased risk of venous thromboembolism.[199-201] In addition to certain thrombophilic abnormalities, such as antiphospholipid antibody syndrome, hyperhomocysteinemia, and the myeloproliferative neoplasms, which are known to predispose individuals to both venous and arterial thromboembolism, some traditional cardiovascular risk factors (e.g., advanced age, obesity, metabolic syndrome, abnormal lipid profiles, immobility, estrogens) also appear to be independent risk factors for venous thromboembolism.[39,202-204]

Genetic determinants of the coagulation system may exert modifying effects on susceptibility to arterial thrombosis. The known hypercoagulable states that predispose to venous thrombosis (e.g., factor V Leiden, prothrombin gene mutation, antithrombin deficiency, protein C and protein S deficiencies) generally are weakly[205] or not at all associated with increased risk of arterial thrombosis. However, decreased mortality from ischemic heart disease has been noted in patients with hemophilia A or B and even in carriers of hemophilia.[206] This finding most likely results from reduced arterial thrombotic tendency in these individuals because early atherogenesis itself does not appear to be significantly affected by the coexistence of hemophilia.[207] Conversely, some epidemiologic studies have correlated elevated levels of fibrinogen and some other coagulation factors with both subclinical atherosclerosis and clinical cardiovascular events,[208,209] although cause-and-effect relationships between elevated levels of hemostatic factors and cardiovascular risk have not been established.

Several lines of evidence suggest that genetic determinants of increased platelet reactivity likewise enhance focal determinants of arterial thrombosis. Animal models of atherosclerosis in pigs and mice with von Willebrand disease suggest that an extremely low or absent VWF level exerts a protective effect on the development and distribution of atherosclerotic lesions,[210,211] although these observations are inconclusive. Whether or not von Willebrand disease protects against development of human atherosclerosis remains in dispute.

Platelet membrane glycoproteins are highly polymorphic and can be recognized as alloantigens or autoantigens. Polymorphisms in platelet membrane glycoprotein receptors have been considered to increase platelet reactivity, thereby potentially contributing to susceptibility to arterial thrombosis.[212,213] The first such genetic variation reported involves the HPA-1a/HPA-1b polymorphism, which results in a Leu33Pro substitution in the β_3 subunit of the platelet integrin $\alpha_{IIb}\beta_3$ complex. The 33Pro (HPA-1b) allele was found to be associated with risk of MI in young individuals.[214] Most, but not all, subsequent studies have agreed that the HPA-1b allele represents an inherited risk factor for ACS.[213] Other platelet receptor polymorphisms that have been inconclusively linked to risk of CVD include three different polymorphisms of the integrin α_{IIb} (HPA-3), GPIb gene, and a polymorphism of the collagen receptor integrin $\alpha_2\beta_1$. However, as is the case for the soluble hemostatic factors, lack of a clear relationship among genotype, phenotype, and clinical manifestations has failed to establish convincing cause-and-effect relationships for any of these genetic variations.

Although none of these individual hemostatic proteins or platelet polymorphisms plays a clear, dominant role in the pathophysiology of arterial thrombosis, future application of platelet proteomics[215] and genomics are likely to reveal new disorders of platelet activation associated with arterial thrombosis.

High blood levels of catecholamines likely contribute systemically to localized arterial thrombus formation. Catecholamines may be increased by physical or emotional stress or by cigarette smoking, thereby triggering acute cardiovascular events in these settings. In addition to their vasoactive actions, catecholamines are direct platelet agonists and enhance shear stress-induced platelet activation.[191,216]

Changes in lipid metabolism may exert systemic prothrombotic actions. The thrombogenicity of lipoprotein(a) has been attributed to its structural similarity to plasminogen, leading to reduced plasmin formation and impaired thrombolysis.[163] Elevated LDL cholesterol can contribute to blood hypercoagulability.[217] The prothrombotic state of diabetes involves multiple mechanisms, including platelet hyperreactivity and increased leukocyte procoagulant activity.[177]

● ISCHEMIC VASCULAR DISEASE

MYOCARDIAL INFARCTION

MI is a term that reflects necrosis of cardiac myocytes caused by prolonged ischemia. In the past, MI was defined by the combination of two of three characteristics: typical symptoms (i.e., chest discomfort), a rise in serum enzymatic markers derived from myocardial cells, and a typical electrocardiographic pattern involving the development of Q waves. The advent of sensitive and specific serologic biomarkers and precise imaging techniques has led to the development of revised criteria for MI.[218] For example, patients can be diagnosed with a "ST-segment elevation MI"[219] or "non–Q-wave or non–ST-segment elevation" MI (NSTEMI)[220] if certain criteria are met. The criteria agreed upon by the American College of Cardiology for acute, evolving, or recent MI[218] are as follows:

1. Typical rise and gradual fall (troponin) or more rapid rise and fall (creatinine kinase-MB isoform) or biochemical markers of myocardial necrosis with at least one of the following: (A) ischemic symptoms; (B) development of pathologic Q waves on the electrocardiogram (ECG); (C) electrocardiographic changes indicative of ischemia (ST segment elevation or depression); or (D) coronary artery intervention (e.g., coronary angioplasty).
2. Pathologic findings of an acute MI.

The criteria for established MI[218] (i.e., event that occurred in the past) is any one of the following:

1. Development of new pathologic Q waves on serial ECGs. The patient may or may not remember previous symptoms. Biochemical markers of myocardial necrosis may have normalized, depending on the length of time since the infarct developed.
2. Pathologic findings of a healed or healing MI.

Clinical Features of Acute Coronary Syndromes

Stable angina pectoris is ischemic discomfort symptomatology caused by a narrowed coronary artery that does not allow sufficient oxygen delivery to meet the metabolic demands of the myocardium. *Unstable angina* is defined clinically as a change in the pattern of stable angina to more frequent or more severe symptoms, uninterrupted angina symptoms for 20 minutes or more, or the development of angina at rest. The term *acute coronary syndrome* has evolved as a useful description of the spectrum of patients presenting with angina pectoris caused by unstable angina through MI.[220] The underlying pathologic mechanism for the development of ACS is usually a vulnerable atherosclerotic plaque with either plaque rupture or plaque ulceration leading to thrombosis. Unstable angina and NSTEMI are differentiated by pathologic elevation in the levels of cardiac biomarkers that confirm MI.

Angina pectoris can be associated with other symptoms, such as diaphoresis, dizziness, nausea, clamminess, and fatigue. Some patients with ACS present with atypical symptoms rather than chest pain. The presentation may be dyspnea alone, nausea and/or vomiting, palpitations/syncope, or cardiac arrest. Rarely, patients with diabetes mellitus and other patients have a "silent MI" diagnosed incidentally on ECG or cardiac imaging study.

The initial ECG is often not diagnostic in patients with ACS. In one clinical study, the ECG was not diagnostic in approximately 45 percent and was normal in 20 percent of patients who subsequently were shown to have experienced an acute MI.[221] ST-segment elevation and Q waves are consistent with ST-segment elevation myocardial infarction (STEMI), but other conditions, such as acute pericarditis with early repolarization variant and hypertrophic cardiomyopathy with Q waves, may mimic the ECG manifestations of STEMI.

Laboratory Features of Acute Myocardial Infarction

A variety of serum biomarkers are used to evaluate patients with suspected acute MI. The three most commonly used tests are (1) troponin I and troponin T, (2) creatine kinase (CK) and its isoform CK-myocardial band (MB), and (3) myoglobin. An elevated serum concentration of one or more of the three biomarkers is seen in almost all patients with acute MI. The preferred biomarkers are the troponins because the troponin assays are more specific than the other tests.

Therapy for Acute Coronary Syndromes

Therapy for Acute Myocardial Infarction The initial management of patients with STEMI depends upon prompt recognition and therapy to reduce morbidity and mortality. A carefully coordinated plan of care is essential for optimal results in patients with STEMI, given that multiple therapies usually are initiated simultaneously. The goals of therapy are to reduce ischemic pain, stabilize hemodynamic status, and quickly establish myocardial reperfusion. The American College of Cardiology (ACC)/American Heart Association (AHA) guidelines for management of patients with acute MI are available at the ACC website.[222]

Antiplatelet Agents Unless contraindicated, all patients with acute MI should be given antiplatelet therapy. The Antiplatelet Trialists' Collaboration indicated a 30 percent reduction in vascular events with

an absolute benefit of 38 vascular events prevented per 1000 patients at 1 month with antiplatelet therapy.[220] Aspirin 325 mg/day or a $P2Y_{12}$-receptor antagonist such as clopidogrel is commonly used in the setting of MI. Vorapaxar, a protease-activated receptor-1 (PAR-1) antagonist, is indicated for the reduction of thrombotic events in patients with a history of MI or with peripheral artery disease (PAD).[223] Contraindications to antiplatelet therapy include active bleeding, coagulopathy, and severe, untreated hypertension (a relative contraindication). The combination of dipyridamole and aspirin has not been proven to provide incremental clinical benefit over aspirin alone.

β-Adrenergic Blockade The control of heart rate with β-adrenergic blocker agents has been efficacious in the setting of acute MI or unstable angina.[222] According to guidelines, oral β-blocker should be initiated during the first 24 hours of care of STEMI. Intravenous administration of β-blockers should be given only to selected, hemodynamically stable patients according to guidelines.

Management of Chest Pain A cornerstone of ischemic pain management has been intravenous nitroglycerin (beginning at 5 to 10 mcg/min) in combination with morphine sulfate if necessary. Nitroglycerin also may improve hypertension and symptoms of heart failure, if present. Intravenous nitroglycerin therapy has not been proven to improve mortality and usually is discontinued within 24 to 48 hours of presentation.[222] Patients who have taken drugs (e.g., sildenafil) for erectile dysfunction within the preceding 24 hours are at increased risk for vasodilation and hypotension, so caution is advised in these patients when intravenous nitroglycerin is given.

Reperfusion Therapy The overriding goal of treatment of STEMI is restoration of myocardial blood flow and salvage of myocardial tissue. A decision should be made immediately whether the patient will undergo a primary (direct) percutaneous coronary intervention (PCI) or receive a fibrinolytic agent. The currently preferred approach is PCI, but the relative advantages and limitations of each therapy should be considered. The most important factor to consider is whether PCI is immediately available. Several randomized trials indicate enhanced survival with PCI compared to fibrinolysis, with a lower rate of intracranial hemorrhage and recurrent MI.[224,225] Transfer to a center that can provide PCI, if necessary, should be accomplished in less than 2 hours.[226]

Fibrinolytic therapy should be given immediately if PCI cannot be performed promptly.[219] Prior to fibrinolysis, the patient should be initially assessed for possible contraindications, which include active bleeding, history of cerebrovascular disease, intracranial neoplasm, drug allergy, and trauma. A systolic blood pressure greater than 175 torr is a relative contraindication but should not prohibit therapy, especially if the pressure can be rapidly controlled. Many different fibrinolytic regimens with different dosing schemes are available. Streptokinase was the first thrombolytic agent tested but has proved less effective than alteplase.[227] In addition, streptokinase is antigenic and can cause an allergic reaction, particularly with repeat administration. Other thrombolytic agents, such as tenecteplase and reteplase, have reportedly similar results compared to alteplase.[228] Tenecteplase is popular on hospital formularies because of its relatively easy single-bolus administration and reported lower rate of noncerebral bleeding.[229]

Anticoagulation Heparin, both unfractionated and low molecular weight, is commonly used in patients with STEMI.[219] The exact role of heparin therapy with different fibrinolytic agents is evolving. Patients who undergo primary PCI usually are given unfractionated heparin 7500 U subcutaneously twice daily or low-molecular-weight heparin, for example, enoxaparin, 1 mg/kg twice daily unless contraindications are evident. For patients receiving intravenous unfractionated heparin, the recommended dose is an initial 60 to 70 U/kg bolus (maximum: 5000 U) followed by 12 to 15 U/kg per hour (maximum: 1000 U/h) as continuous infusion with monitoring of the activated partial thromboplastin time (aPTT) measured at 6 hours. The heparin dose is adjusted to maintain an aPTT between 50 and 75 seconds.

Current guidelines recommend maintaining the aPTT at 50 to 75 seconds for short-term use. Heparin should be continued beyond this period only in the case of high risk of systemic or venous thromboembolism. Patients can be switched to a subcutaneously administered heparin or converted to oral warfarin during the high-risk period. The anticoagulant drugs unfractionated heparin, enoxaparin, fondaparinux, and bivalirudin are all excreted by the kidneys; consequently, although the first dose is usually safe, longer-term therapy should be guided by assessment of creatinine clearance.[230] The Coumadin-Aspirin Reinfarction Study (CARS) did not show a significant benefit with the combination of low-dose warfarin (1 or 3 mg) and aspirin 80 mg daily compared to aspirin 160 mg daily monotherapy on cardiovascular morbidity in patients who had an MI.[231]

Statins All patients with MI should be started on a 3-hydroxy-3-methylglutaryl-coenzyme A reductase inhibitor (statin) unless the MI was caused by a nonatherosclerotic process such as coronary vasospasm, vasculitis, or embolus. Numerous studies indicate that statins reduce the risk of subsequent MI by approximately 30 to 50 percent.[232] Current evidence suggests that a serum LDL level less than 80 mg/dL with statin treatment is more efficacious in retarding atherosclerotic disease progression than a serum LDL level of 100 mg/dL or above.[233] Other nonstatin drugs, such as ezetimibe, PCSK9 inhibitors, and microsomal triglyceride transfer protein inhibitors, also reduce cholesterol levels but relative reduction in cardiovascular events compared to statins is not yet clear.

Therapy for Unstable Angina Pectoris and Non–ST-Elevation Myocardial Infarction The distinction between unstable angina and NSTEMI initially may be difficult because levels of troponins and/or CK-MB may not be elevated until hours after presentation. Similar to STEMI, the initial treatment of unstable angina and NSTEMI includes supplemental oxygen, pain control, and bed rest.[230] Nitrates, given either intravenously or subcutaneously, are the treatment of choice for angina pectoris. Oral β-blockers also are routinely given to patients with unstable angina to relieve symptoms of angina and to reduce the risk of progression to MI.

Treatment of unstable angina and NSTEMI involves administration of an antiplatelet agent and anticoagulation.[230] Fibrinolytic therapy is not beneficial in patients with unstable angina, and its use is associated with unacceptably high bleeding risk. Antiplatelet treatment, most commonly aspirin at a dose of 325 mg daily, was shown in the Antithrombotic Trialists' Collaboration to reduce the combined end point of subsequent nonfatal MI, nonfatal stroke, or vascular death (8.0 percent vs. 13.3 percent) in patients with non–ST-segment elevation ACS.[234] Clinical trials involving patients with non–ST-segment elevation ACS have demonstrated significantly reduced cardiovascular events and mortality with aspirin administration, mostly at a lower dose of 80 to 100 mg orally once per day.[235–237] Some patients do not benefit from aspirin, and this finding has generated an interest as to whether these patients are "aspirin resistant." Nonrandomized studies indicate that aspirin resistance may occur, but because of the limitations of these studies, the definition and prognostic significance of this phenomenon are uncertain.[238]

The thienopyridine clopidogrel (75 mg/day) is effective in reducing the risk of MI and mortality in patients with unstable angina.[220] The combination of aspirin and clopidogrel has been tested in patients with NSTEMI and unstable angina. The combination of these antiplatelet agents resulted in improved survival and decreased progression to MI.[239] The patients with non–ST-segment elevation ACS who underwent PCI benefited the most from the combination of aspirin

and clopidogrel.[240] However, the combination was associated with an increase in major bleeding and reoperation for bleeding in patients who underwent coronary artery bypass grafting (CABG). Therefore, a 5-day, but preferably a 7-day, period off clopidogrel is recommended before CABG.[241]

A meta-analysis of randomized clinical trials found that intravenous platelet integrin IIb/IIIa inhibitors substantially benefited patients with non–ST-segment elevation ACS undergoing coronary intervention.[242] The integrin $\alpha_{IIb}\beta_{IIIa}$ receptor antagonist abciximab (ReoPro) is a monoclonal antibody fragment that reduces short-term and long-term clinical events in patients with ACS undergoing angioplasty with or without stent placement. Other platelet integrin $\alpha_{IIb}\beta_{IIIa}$ antagonists, such as tirofiban and Integrilin, also are effective and safe in treating unstable angina when combined with heparin anticoagulation.[243] Guidelines from an ACC/AHA task force recommend administration of an integrin $\alpha_{IIb}\beta_{IIIa}$ inhibitor, in addition to aspirin and heparin, for patients with unstable angina/NSTEMI undergoing planned PCI.[220]

Unfractionated heparin reduces the rate of MI and death, and relieves anginal pain, when used in combination with an antiplatelet agent.[220] Intravenous heparin usually is given as a 5000-U bolus followed by continuous infusion. Low-molecular-weight heparins can be substituted for unfractionated heparin. Some studies have shown superior efficacy of low-molecular-weight heparins, but other studies have not indicated a significant difference. Direct thrombin inhibitors, such as hirudin and bivalirudin, have been shown to reduce the rate of death, nonfatal MI, and refractory angina compared to heparin.[244,245] The American College of Chest Physicians (ACCP) recommends lepirudin (recombinant hirudin), argatroban, bivalirudin, or danaparoid in patients with a history of heparin-associated thrombocytopenia,[246] although some of these agents are no longer available in the United States.

Therapy for Stable Angina Pectoris Patients with stable angina pectoris can be treated with either medical management or revascularization.[247] Limited clinical trial data comparing revascularization, either percutaneous or surgical, to medical therapy are available. The older trials evaluating percutaneous and surgical revascularization were limited by several factors: antiplatelet treatment, angiotensin-converting enzyme inhibitors, and aggressive lipid lowering with statins were not given as background medical therapy of angina. Given these limitations, determining whether revascularization is better than medical management for long-term care of patients with stable angina in modern practice is difficult.

Both PCI and coronary bypass surgery significantly reduce angina. The Coronary Artery Surgery Study (CASS) showed more patients remained symptom-free after CABG compared to medical therapy 5 years after the procedure.[248] At 10 years, however, no significant difference in symptoms was observed. Clinical trials showed significant improvement in angina with PCI compared to medical therapy; however, patients who underwent the former had similar rates of death and MI as those undergoing medical therapy and were less likely to have angina and more likely to have undergone a coronary bypass graft.[249]

Restenosis is a complex process involving inflammation, cellular proliferation, thrombosis, and matrix deposition. Restenosis occurring after PCI may result in flow-limiting luminal narrowing in 20 to 30 percent of therapeutically dilated vessels.[250] Numerous pharmacologic agents, including heparin,[251] have been given in an attempt to reduce the restenosis rate but have met with limited or no success. Intraarterial radiation (brachytherapy) reduces the restenosis rate but is cumbersome to perform because of radiation safety issues and has fallen out of favor. Drug-eluting arterial stents, including the immunosuppressive macrocyclic lactone rapamycin (sirolimus)[252] and the chemotherapeutic agent paclitaxel (Taxol),[253] significantly reduce the rate of restenosis. Because drug-eluting stents were not available at the time of the previous clinical trials, extrapolating the benefits of PCI versus CABG or over medical therapy is difficult. The medical management of patients with stable angina pectoris should include antiplatelet therapy, statin drug treatment, a β-blocker, an angiotensin-converting enzyme inhibitor, and a long-acting nitrate.

PERIPHERAL ARTERY DISEASE

PAD is a term that encompasses any arterial disease of the lower extremities, upper extremities, and iliac vessels. It most commonly results from atherosclerosis. Patients who have atherosclerotic disease that compromises blood flow to the extremities may present with exertional pain in a muscle group, called *claudication* (derived from the Latin *claudicare* meaning "to limp"). Claudication is an intermittent but reproducible discomfort of a defined group of muscles that is induced by exercise and relieved with rest.[254] Acute limb ischemia is a relatively rare problem in patients with PAD. In general, it is caused by *in situ* thrombosis or an embolic event from arrhythmias, such as atrial fibrillation, or after manipulation of an artery or aorta with a catheter. Approximately 4 percent of patients with claudication progress to *critical limb ischemia*, which is defined as rest pain and/or foot ulceration that heralds impending tissue loss.

The 5-year mortality rate is estimated to be 30 percent in patients with lower-extremity PAD.[255] Approximately 75 percent of mortality results from a cardiovascular event, such as MI or stroke.[255] The ankle-brachial index is a noninvasive measure of limb vascular pressure in the lower extremities and has been noted in several studies to be predictive of cardiovascular events.[254] However, a decreased index is not just a predictor; it also is a physical finding that indicates significant atherosclerotic plaque burden is present. Other noninvasive imaging studies for PAD include the combination of segmental pressures and pulse volume recordings, duplex Doppler ultrasound, computed tomographic angiography and magnetic resonance imaging.[256,257]

Medical therapy for patients with PAD includes risk-factor modification, antiplatelet therapy, and treatment of claudication symptoms with exercise rehabilitation and possible pharmacologic agents. The risk factors for development of peripheral atherosclerosis include cigarette smoking, diabetes mellitus, hypertension, and dyslipidemia.[258] Aggressive management of risk factors for PAD is recommended to prevent disease progression.[259] Treatment with antiplatelet agents reduces the risk of cardiovascular events, such as MI and stroke, in patients with PAD.[255] The Antithrombotic Trialists' Collaboration evaluated 9214 patients with PAD enrolled in 42 trials and found that use of antiplatelet drugs, such as aspirin 75 to 325 mg/day, resulted in a proportional reduction of 23 percent in serious vascular events.[234] Evaluation of patients with PAD in the Physicians' Health Study found that aspirin 325 mg every other day decreased the need for peripheral artery surgery.[260] However, no difference between the aspirin and placebo groups with regard to development of claudication was observed. Several studies have evaluated the ADP receptor blockers ticlopidine and clopidogrel. Clopidogrel was evaluated in 19,185 patients in the Clopidogrel Versus Aspirin in Patients at Risk of Ischaemic Events (CAPRIE) study.[261] A dose of clopidogrel 75 mg/day had a modest but significant advantage over aspirin 325 mg/day in preventing stroke, MI, and peripheral vascular disease. Subgroup analysis revealed that the patients with PAD benefited the most with clopidogrel treatment. One study evaluating the effect of aspirin, 100 mg, compared to placebo in asymptomatic patients with diabetes mellitus and PAD found no benefit in reducing cardiovascular events.[262] The PAR-1 antagonist,

vorapaxar, is approved to prevent cardiovascular events in patients with PAD.[223] The clinical consensus is that antiplatelet therapy should be offered to all patients with PAD unless contraindicated by allergy or comorbidities.[263]

The options for treating claudication symptoms include exercise rehabilitation, pharmacologic agents, and a revascularization procedure. Several studies indicate exercise rehabilitation improves the symptoms of claudication, and a supervised program is better than an unstructured program, and comparable to percutaneous revascularization.[264,265] Two drugs are approved by the FDA for treatment of claudication symptoms: pentoxifylline, a methylxanthine derivative that may improve abnormal red cell deformability and reduce blood viscosity, and cilostazol, a type III phosphodiesterase inhibitor with antiplatelet and vasodilating properties. Cilostazol is generally considered more effective than pentoxifylline for improving walking distance in patients with claudication.[266] The addition of cilostazol to either aspirin or clopidogrel does not increase the bleeding risk.[267] A revascularization procedure in patients with stable, intermittent claudication generally is reserved for those with severe lifestyle-limiting symptoms or manifestation of critical limb ischemia.

CEREBROVASCULAR DISEASE

The etiology of ischemic stroke is multifactorial and can be categorized into embolic, small-vessel disease, large-vessel disease, and cryptogenic. Carotid artery disease accounts for approximately 30 percent of strokes. Major risk factors for developing carotid artery atherosclerosis are hypertension, diabetes, smoking, and dyslipidemia.[268] Emerging risk factors for stroke include hyperhomocysteinemia and an elevated plasma level of lipoprotein(a). An elevated hsCRP level is a risk factor associated with ischemic stroke in both men and women. However, at this time hsCRP is not routinely measured as an additional marker for increased risk of stroke. Similar to CAD and PAD, control of atherosclerotic risk factors is essential in the primary prevention of stroke in patients with evidence of carotid atherosclerosis and for those who have undergone carotid endarterectomy.[269,270]

Carotid endarterectomy is indicated for patients with symptoms and a greater than 50 percent stenosis[271] or for patients who are asymptomatic with a greater than 60 to 99 percent stenosis of the common carotid or internal carotid arteries.[272] Carotid stent with embolic protection is a therapy used for treatment of carotid atherosclerosis in selective patients.[273]

Two antiplatelet drug regimens are approved for prevention of stroke: clopidogrel (Plavix) and the combination of aspirin 25 mg and dipyridamole 200 mg daily. Approval of clopidogrel is based on the CAPRIE study, which showed a reduction in the combined end point of stroke, MI, and death in patients treated with clopidogrel 75 mg/day compared to those treated with aspirin 325 mg/day.[261] The FDA indication for dipyridamole/aspirin is primarily based on the European Stroke Protection Study 2, which noted a reduction in stroke with the combination of dipyridamole 200 mg and aspirin 25 mg given together (Aggrenox) twice per day.[274] The Prevention Regimen for Effectively Avoiding Second Strokes (PRoFESS) trial was a secondary stroke–prevention trial comparing the combination of aspirin and extended-release dipyridamole (Aggrenox) versus clopidogrel (Plavix) in preventing stroke recurrence after a first event. The difference between the agents was not statistically significant for the primary outcome of recurrent stroke.[275] Fish oil (omega-3 fatty acids) lowers triglycerides and VLDLs and may reduce serum viscosity by lowering fibrinogen. Some studies suggest that fish oil consumption lowers the risk of ischemic stroke. The effect of fish oils on carotid atherosclerosis is unknown.[276]

● ATHEROEMBOLISM

Atheromatous embolism refers to the dislodgment into the bloodstream of arterial plaque material, including cholesterol crystals ("cholesterol embolism") from ulcerated vascular plaques. The cholesterol embolization syndrome involves systemic microembolism to the end arteries of almost any circulatory bed. Atheroembolism most characteristically originates from lesions in the abdominal aorta and ileofemoral arteries. Cholesterol emboli that lodge in an arteriole incite an acute inflammatory response, followed by a foreign-body reaction, intravascular thrombus formation, endothelial proliferation, and eventually fibrosis. These processes generally result in ischemia that sometimes leads to infarction and necrosis.[277] Mortality rate of clinically diagnosed atheroembolism can be as high as 80 percent, depending on the anatomic location and size of the vascular beds involved.[278]

Patients with atheroembolism, including the cholesterol embolization syndrome, generally have advanced atherosclerosis, often complicated by a history of hypertension, diabetes mellitus, renal failure, or aortic aneurysms. Atherosclerotic plaques can disrupt and embolize spontaneously; however, the clinical syndrome typically is triggered by vascular intervention, including vascular surgery, catheterization, angioplasty, endarterectomy, or angiography. Anticoagulation or thrombolytic therapy may be risk factors with atheroembolism.[278] Clinical presentation depends on the sites of embolization. When these sites involve the distal extremity microcirculation, the "blue toe syndrome" may develop. The syndrome presents with the acute appearance of painful and tender discoloration or mottled blue and patchy appearance of one or more toes that may progress to ulceration and gangrene. Other common cutaneous manifestations are livedo reticularis involving the legs, buttocks, or abdomen, painful nodules, and purpura. Cerebrovascular embolism can cause transient neurologic abnormalities. Cholesterol emboli lodged in retinal arterial bifurcations can be visualized by ophthalmoscopy as bright, refractile, yellow rectangular crystals. Visceral organs most commonly affected by atheroembolism include the kidneys, sometimes causing renal failure, and the gastrointestinal tract, where abdominal pain, ischemic colitis, and bleeding may ensue.

Diagnosis is based on clinical presentation associated with imaging evidence of atherosclerosis of the arterial supply of affected organs.[278] Transient eosinophilia occurs in most cases.[279] Treatment of atheroembolism should include surgical removal or bypass of the source of emboli. No medical treatment modalities have been established to be effective. Anticoagulation or fibrinolytic therapy may increase the risk of further atheroembolism.

REFERENCES

1. Virchow R: *Cellular Pathology: As Based upon Physiological and Pathological Histology.* New York: Dover, 1863.
2. Ross R: Atherosclerosis-an inflammatory disease. *N Engl J Med* 340:115–126, 1999.
3. Ridker PM: Inflammation, C-reactive protein, and cardiovascular disease: Moving past the marker versus mediator debate. *Circ Res* 114:594–595, 2014.
4. Duewell P, Kono H, Rayner KJ, et al: NLRP3 inflammasomes are required for atherogenesis and activated by cholesterol crystals. *Nature* 464:1357–1361, 2010.
5. Enos WF, Holmes RH, Beyer J: Coronary disease among United States soldiers killed in action in Korea; preliminary report. *J Am Med Assoc* 152:1090–1093, 1953.
6. Joseph A, Ackerman D, Talley JD, et al: Manifestations of coronary atherosclerosis in young trauma victims—an autopsy study. *J Am Coll Cardiol* 22:459–467, 1993.
7. Tuzcu EM, Kapadia SR, Tutar E, et al: High prevalence of coronary atherosclerosis in asymptomatic teenagers and young adults: Evidence from intravascular ultrasound. *Circulation* 103:2705–2710, 2001.
8. Ross R, Glomset JA: The pathogenesis of atherosclerosis (first of two parts). *N Engl J Med* 295:369–377, 1976.
9. Ross R, Glomset JA: The pathogenesis of atherosclerosis (second of two parts). *N Engl J Med* 295:420–425, 1976.
10. Yusuf S, Hawken S, Ounpuu S, et al: Effect of potentially modifiable risk factors associated with myocardial infarction in 52 countries (the INTERHEART study): Case-control study. *Lancet* 364:937–952, 2004.
11. Mallika V, Goswami B, Rajappa M: Atherosclerosis pathophysiology and the role of novel risk factors: A clinicobiochemical perspective. *Angiology* 58:513–522, 2007.
12. Hemkens LG, Bucher HC: HIV infection and cardiovascular disease. *Eur Heart J* 35:1373–1381, 2014.
13. Kline ER, Sutliff RL: The roles of HIV-1 proteins and antiretroviral drug therapy in HIV-1-associated endothelial dysfunction. *J Investig Med* 56:752–769, 2008.
14. Calza L, Manfredi R, Pocaterra D, Chiodo F: Risk of premature atherosclerosis and ischemic heart disease associated with HIV infection and antiretroviral therapy. *J Infect* 57:16–32, 2008.
15. de Zeeuw D. Renal disease: A common and a silent killer. *Nat Clin Pract Cardiovasc Med* 5 Suppl 1:S27–S35, 2008.
16. Budoff MJ, Rader DJ, Reilly MP, et al: Relationship of estimated GFR and coronary artery calcification in the CRIC (Chronic Renal Insufficiency Cohort) Study. *Am J Kidney Dis* 58:519–526, 2011.
17. Said S, Hernandez GT: The link between chronic kidney disease and cardiovascular disease. *J Nephropathol* 3:99–104, 2014.
18. Vonend O, Rump LC, Ritz E: Sympathetic overactivity—The Cinderella of cardiovascular risk factors in dialysis patients. *Semin Dial* 21:326–330, 2008.
19. Bradley TD, Floras JS: Obstructive sleep apnoea and its cardiovascular consequences. *Lancet* 373:82–93, 2009.
20. Skalen K, Gustafsson M, Rydberg EK, et al: Subendothelial retention of atherogenic lipoproteins in early atherosclerosis. *Nature* 417:750–754, 2002.
21. Passerini AG, Polacek DC, Shi C, et al: Coexisting proinflammatory and antioxidative endothelial transcription profiles in a disturbed flow region of the adult porcine aorta. *Proc Natl Acad Sci U S A* 101:2482–2487, 2004.
22. Weber C, Zernecke A, Libby P: The multifaceted contributions of leukocyte subsets to atherosclerosis: Lessons from mouse models. *Nat Rev Immunol* 8:802–815, 2008.
23. Stary HC, Chandler AB, Dinsmore RE, et al: A definition of advanced types of atherosclerotic lesions and a histological classification of atherosclerosis. A report from the Committee on Vascular Lesions of the Council on Arteriosclerosis, American Heart Association. *Circulation* 92:1355–1374, 1995.
24. Johnson JL: Matrix metalloproteinases: Influence on smooth muscle cells and atherosclerotic plaque stability. *Expert Rev Cardiovasc Ther* 5:265–282, 2007.
25. Hunt JL, Fairman R, Mitchell ME, et al: Bone formation in carotid plaques: A clinicopathological study. *Stroke* 33:1214–1219, 2002.
26. Curtis AM, Edelberg J, Jonas R, et al: Endothelial microparticles: Sophisticated vesicles modulating vascular function. *Vasc Med* 18:204–214, 2013.
27. Furchgott RF, Zawadzki JV: The obligatory role of endothelial cells in the relaxation of arterial smooth muscle by acetylcholine. *Nature* 288:373–376, 1980.
28. Loscalzo J: The identification of nitric oxide as endothelium-derived relaxing factor. *Circ Res* 113:100–103, 2013.
29. Lubos E, Handy DE, Loscalzo J: Role of oxidative stress and nitric oxide in atherothrombosis. *Front Biosci* 13:5323–5344, 2008.
30. Guzik TJ, Chen W, Gongora MC, et al: Calcium-dependent NOX5 nicotinamide adenine dinucleotide phosphate oxidase contributes to vascular oxidative stress in human coronary artery disease. *J Am Coll Cardiol* 52:1803–1809, 2008.
31. De Pascali F, Hemann C, Samons K, et al: Hypoxia and reoxygenation induce endothelial nitric oxide synthase uncoupling in endothelial cells through tetrahydrobiopterin depletion and S-glutathionylation. *Biochemistry* 53:3679–3688, 2014.
32. Tiefenbacher CP, Bleeke T, Vahl C, et al: Endothelial dysfunction of coronary resistance arteries is improved by tetrahydrobiopterin in atherosclerosis. *Circulation* 102:2172–2179, 2000.
33. Kim CS, Jung SB, Naqvi A, et al: P53 impairs endothelium-dependent vasomotor function through transcriptional upregulation of p66shc. *Circ Res* 103:1441–1450, 2008.
34. Creager MA, Gallagher SJ, Girerd XJ, et al: L-Arginine improves endothelium-dependent vasodilation in hypercholesterolemic humans. *J Clin Invest* 90:1248–1253, 1992.
35. Chen S, Li N, Deb-Chatterji M, et al: Asymmetric dimethylarginine as marker and mediator in ischemic stroke. *Int J Mol Sci* 13:15983–16004, 2012.
36. Niu PP, Cao Y, Gong T, et al: Hypermethylation of DDAH2 promoter contributes to the dysfunction of endothelial progenitor cells in coronary artery disease patients. *J Transl Med* 12:170, 2014.
37. Ludmer PL, Selwyn AP, Shook TL, et al: Paradoxical vasoconstriction induced by acetylcholine in atherosclerotic coronary arteries. *N Engl J Med* 315:1046–1051, 1986.
38. Kuhn FE, Mohler ER, Satler LF, et al: Effects of high-density lipoprotein on acetylcholine-induced coronary vasoreactivity. *Am J Cardiol* 68:1425–1430, 1991.
39. Kuhn FE, Mohler ER 3rd, Rackley CE: Cholesterol and lipoproteins: Beyond atherogenesis. *Clin Cardiol* 15:883–890, 1992.
40. Luscher TF, Landmesser U, von Eckardstein A, Fogelman AM: High-density lipoprotein: Vascular protective effects, dysfunction, and potential as therapeutic target. *Circ Res* 114:171–182, 2014.
41. Oakley R, Tharakan B: Vascular hyperpermeability and aging. *Aging Dis* 5:114–125, 2014.
42. van den Heuvel M, Sorop O, Koopmans SJ, et al: Coronary microvascular dysfunction in a porcine model of early atherosclerosis and diabetes. *Am J Physiol Heart Circ Physiol* 302:H85–H94, 2012.
43. Mohler ER 3rd, O'Hare K, Darze ES, et al: Cardiovascular function in normotensive offspring of persons with essential hypertension and black race. *J Clin Hypertens (Greenwich)* 9:506–512, 2007.
44. Yong PJ, Koh CH, Shim WS: Endothelial microparticles: Missing link in endothelial dysfunction? *Eur J Prev Cardiol* 20:496–512, 2013.

45. Nozaki T, Sugiyama S, Koga H, et al: Significance of a multiple biomarkers strategy including endothelial dysfunction to improve risk stratification for cardiovascular events in patients at high risk for coronary heart disease. *J Am Coll Cardiol* 54:601–608, 2009.

46. Liuba P, Karnani P, Pesonen E, et al: Endothelial dysfunction after repeated *Chlamydia pneumoniae* infection in apolipoprotein E-knockout mice. *Circulation* 102:1039–1044, 2000.

47. Fichtlscherer S, Rosenberger G, Walter DH, et al: Elevated C-reactive protein levels and impaired endothelial vasoreactivity in patients with coronary artery disease. *Circulation* 102:1000–1006, 2000.

48. Beckman JA, Ganz J, Creager MA, et al: Relationship of clinical presentation and calcification of culprit coronary artery stenoses. *Arterioscler Thromb Vasc Biol* 21:1618–1622, 2001.

49. Libby P, Ridker PM, Maseri A: Inflammation and atherosclerosis. *Circulation* 105:1135–1143, 2002.

50. Moore KJ, Sheedy FJ, Fisher EA: Macrophages in atherosclerosis: A dynamic balance. *Nat Rev Immunol* 13:709–721, 2013.

51. Takeshita J, Mohler ER, Krishnamoorthy P, et al: Endothelial cell-, platelet-, and monocyte/macrophage-derived microparticles are elevated in psoriasis beyond cardiometabolic risk factors. *J Am Heart Assoc* 3:e000507, 2014.

52. Lim S, Park S: Role of vascular smooth muscle cell in the inflammation of atherosclerosis. *BMB Rep* 47:1–7, 2014.

53. Kanse SM, Parahuleva M, Muhl L, et al: Factor VII-activating protease (FSAP): Vascular functions and role in atherosclerosis. *Thromb Haemost* 99:286–289, 2008.

54. Fuster V: Lewis A. Conner Memorial Lecture. Mechanisms leading to myocardial infarction: Insights from studies of vascular biology. *Circulation* 90:2126–2146, 1994.

55. Schwartz SM, Murry CE: Proliferation and the monoclonal origins of atherosclerotic lesions. *Annu Rev Med* 49:437–460, 1998.

56. Scott NA, Cipolla GD, Ross CE, et al: Identification of a potential role for the adventitia in vascular lesion formation after balloon overstretch injury of porcine coronary arteries. *Circulation* 93:2178–2187, 1996.

57. Sakakura K, Nakano M, Otsuka F, et al: Pathophysiology of atherosclerosis plaque progression. *Heart Lung Circ* 22:399–411, 2013.

58. Majesky MW, Dong XR, Regan JN, Hoglund VJ: Vascular smooth muscle progenitor cells: Building and repairing blood vessels. *Circ Res* 108:365–377, 2011.

59. Der Leyen HE, Gibbons GH, Morishita R, et al: Gene therapy inhibiting neointimal vascular lesion: In vivo transfer of endothelial cell nitric oxide synthase gene. *Proc Natl Acad Sci U S A* 92:1137–1141, 1995.

60. Dzau VJ, Braun-Dullaeus RC, Sedding DG: Vascular proliferation and atherosclerosis: New perspectives and therapeutic strategies. *Nat Med* 8:1249–1256, 2002.

61. Bonta PI, Pols TW, de Vries CJ: NR4A nuclear receptors in atherosclerosis and vein-graft disease. *Trends Cardiovasc Med* 17:105–111, 2007.

62. Lemos PA, Lee CH, Degertekin M, et al: Early outcome after sirolimus-eluting stent implantation in patients with acute coronary syndromes: Insights from the Rapamycin-Eluting Stent Evaluated At Rotterdam Cardiology Hospital (RESEARCH) registry. *J Am Coll Cardiol* 41:2093–2099, 2003.

63. Sagripanti A, Carpi A: Antithrombotic and prothrombotic activities of the vascular endothelium. *Biomed Pharmacother* 54:107–111, 2000.

64. van Der Meijden PE, van Schilfgaarde M, van Oerle R, Renne T, et al: Platelet- and erythrocyte-derived microparticles trigger thrombin generation via factor XIIa. *J Thromb Haemost* 10:1355–1362, 2012.

65. Falati S, Liu Q, Gross P, et al: Accumulation of tissue factor into developing thrombi in vivo is dependent upon microparticle P-selectin glycoprotein ligand 1 and platelet P-selectin. *J Exp Med* 197:1585–1598, 2003.

66. Feil R, Lohmann SM, de Jonge H, et al: Cyclic GMP-dependent protein kinases and the cardiovascular system: Insights from genetically modified mice. *Circ Res* 93:907–916, 2003.

67. Gonzalez MA, Selwyn AP: Endothelial function, inflammation, and prognosis in cardiovascular disease. *Am J Med* 115 Suppl 8A:99S–106S, 2003.

68. Anderson TJ: Nitric oxide, atherosclerosis and the clinical relevance of endothelial dysfunction. *Heart Fail Rev* 8:71–86, 2003.

69. Tulis DA, Durante W, Liu X, et al: Adenovirus-mediated heme oxygenase-1 gene delivery inhibits injury-induced vascular neointima formation. *Circulation* 104:2710–2715, 2001.

70. Sachais BS: Platelet-endothelial interactions in atherosclerosis. *Curr Atheroscler Rep* 3:412–416, 2001.

71. Marcus AJ, Broekman MJ, Drosopoulos JH, et al: Metabolic control of excessive extracellular nucleotide accumulation by CD39/ecto-nucleotidase-1: Implications for ischemic vascular diseases. *J Pharmacol Exp Ther* 305:9–16, 2003.

72. Landmesser U, Merten R, Spiekermann S, et al: Vascular extracellular superoxide dismutase activity in patients with coronary artery disease: Relation to endothelium-dependent vasodilation. *Circulation* 101:2264–2270, 2000.

73. Cooke JP: Does ADMA cause endothelial dysfunction? *Arterioscler Thromb Vasc Biol* 20:2032–2037, 2000.

74. Mohler ER 3rd, Shi Y, Moore J, et al: Diabetes reduces bone marrow and circulating porcine endothelial progenitor cells, an effect ameliorated by atorvastatin and independent of cholesterol. *Cytometry A* 75:75–82, 2009.

75. Foteinos G, Hu Y, Xiao Q, et al: Rapid endothelial turnover in atherosclerosis-prone areas coincides with stem cell repair in apolipoprotein E-deficient mice. *Circulation* 117:1856–1863, 2008.

76. Binder CJ, Chang MK, Shaw PX, et al: Innate and acquired immunity in atherogenesis. *Nat Med* 8:1218–1226, 2002.

77. Medzhitov R: Toll-like receptors and innate immunity. *Nat Rev Immunol* 1:135–145, 2001.

78. Erridge C: The roles of pathogen-associated molecular patterns in atherosclerosis. *Trends Cardiovasc Med* 18:52–56, 2008.

79. Medzhitov R, Janeway CA Jr: Decoding the patterns of self and nonself by the innate immune system. *Science* 296:298–300, 2002.

80. Ridker PM: Clinical application of C-reactive protein for cardiovascular disease detection and prevention. *Circulation* 107:363–369, 2003.

81. Dansky HM, Barlow CB, Lominska C, et al: Adhesion of monocytes to arterial endothelium and initiation of atherosclerosis are critically dependent on vascular cell adhesion molecule-1 gene dosage. *Arterioscler Thromb Vasc Biol* 21:1662–1667, 2001.

82. Cybulsky MI, Iiyama K, Li H, et al: A major role for VCAM-1, but not ICAM-1, in early atherosclerosis. *J Clin Invest* 107:1255–1262, 2001.

83. Collins RG, Velji R, Guevara NV, et al: P-Selectin or intercellular adhesion molecule (ICAM)-1 deficiency substantially protects against atherosclerosis in apolipoprotein E-deficient mice. *J Exp Med* 191:189–194, 2000.

84. Parks BW, Lusis AJ: Macrophage accumulation in atherosclerosis. *N Engl J Med* 369:2352–2353, 2013.

85. Robbins CS, Hilgendorf I, Weber GF, et al: Local proliferation dominates lesional macrophage accumulation in atherosclerosis. *Nat Med* 19:1166–1172, 2013.

86. Weber C, Noels H: Atherosclerosis: Current pathogenesis and therapeutic options. *Nat Med* 17:1410–1422, 2011.

87. Zalewski A, Macphee C, Nelson JJ: Lipoprotein-associated phospholipase A2: A potential therapeutic target for atherosclerosis. *Curr Drug Targets Cardiovasc Haematol Disord* 5:527–532, 2005.

88. Shi Y, Zhang P, Zhang L, et al: Role of lipoprotein-associated phospholipase A(2) in leukocyte activation and inflammatory responses. *Atherosclerosis* 191:54–62, 2006.

89. Wilensky RL, Shi Y, Mohler ER 3rd, et al: Inhibition of lipoprotein-associated phospholipase A2 reduces complex coronary atherosclerotic plaque development. *Nat Med* 14:1059–1066, 2008.

90. Mohler ER 3rd, Ballantyne CM, Davidson MH, et al: The effect of darapladib on plasma lipoprotein-associated phospholipase A2 activity and cardiovascular biomarkers in patients with stable coronary heart disease or coronary heart disease risk equivalent: The results of a multicenter, randomized, double-blind, placebo-controlled study. *J Am Coll Cardiol* 51:1632–1641, 2008.

91. Investigators S, White HD, Held C, et al: Darapladib for preventing ischemic events in stable coronary heart disease. *N Engl J Med* 370:1702–1711, 2014.

92. Smith JD, Trogan E, Ginsberg M, et al: Decreased atherosclerosis in mice deficient in both macrophage colony-stimulating factor (op) and apolipoprotein E. *Proc Natl Acad Sci U S A* 92:8264–8268, 1995.

93. Endemann G, Stanton LW, Madden KS, et al: CD36 is a receptor for oxidized low density lipoprotein. *J Biol Chem* 268:11811–11816, 1993.

94. Steinberg D, Parthasarathy S, Carew TE, et al: Beyond cholesterol: Modifications of low-density lipoprotein that increase its atherogenicity. *N Engl J Med* 320:915–924, 1989.

95. Boring L, Gosling J, Cleary M, Charo IF: Decreased lesion formation in CCR2–/– mice reveals a role for chemokines in the initiation of atherosclerosis. *Nature* 394:894–897, 1998.

96. Gu L, Okada Y, Clinton SK, et al: Absence of monocyte chemoattractant protein-1 reduces atherosclerosis in low density lipoprotein receptor-deficient mice. *Mol Cell* 2:275–281, 1998.

97. Gosling J, Slaymaker S, Gu L, et al: MCP-1 deficiency reduces susceptibility to atherosclerosis in mice that overexpress human apolipoprotein B. *J Clin Invest* 103:773–778, 1999.

98. Hur J, Yang HM, Yoon CH, et al: Identification of a novel role of T cells in postnatal vasculogenesis: Characterization of endothelial progenitor cell colonies. *Circulation* 116:1671–1682, 2007.

99. Tang WH, Wu Y, Nicholls SJ, Hazen SL: Plasma myeloperoxidase predicts incident cardiovascular risks in stable patients undergoing medical management for coronary artery disease. *Clin Chem* 57:33–39, 2011.

100. Sugiyama S, Okada Y, Sukhova GK, et al: Macrophage myeloperoxidase regulation by granulocyte macrophage colony-stimulating factor in human atherosclerosis and implications in acute coronary syndromes. *Am J Pathol* 158:879–891, 2001.

101. Babior BM: Phagocytes and oxidative stress. *Am J Med* 109:33–44, 2000.

102. Suzuki H, Kurihara Y, Takeya M, et al: A role for macrophage scavenger receptors in atherosclerosis and susceptibility to infection. *Nature* 386:292–296, 1997.

103. Febbraio M, Podrez EA, Smith JD, et al: Targeted disruption of the class B scavenger receptor CD36 protects against atherosclerotic lesion development in mice. *J Clin Invest* 105:1049–1056, 2000.

104. Kodama T, Reddy P, Kishimoto C, Krieger M: Purification and characterization of a bovine acetyl low density lipoprotein receptor. *Proc Natl Acad Sci U S A* 85:9238–9242, 1988.

105. Henriksen T, Mahoney EM, Steinberg D: Enhanced macrophage degradation of low density lipoprotein previously incubated with cultured endothelial cells: Recognition by receptors for acetylated low density lipoproteins. *Proc Natl Acad Sci U S A* 78:6499–6503, 1981.

106. Steinbrecher UP, Parthasarathy S, Leake DS, Witztum JL, Steinberg D: Modification of low density lipoprotein by endothelial cells involves lipid peroxidation and degradation of low density lipoprotein phospholipids. *Proc Natl Acad Sci U S A* 81:3883–3887, 1984.

107. Shaw PX, Horkko S, Chang MK, et al: Natural antibodies with the T15 idiotype may act in atherosclerosis, apoptotic clearance, and protective immunity. *J Clin Invest* 105:1731–1740, 2000.

108. Tsimikas S, Palinski W, Witztum JL: Circulating autoantibodies to oxidized LDL correlate with arterial accumulation and depletion of oxidized LDL in LDL receptor-deficient mice. *Arterioscler Thromb Vasc Biol* 21:95–100, 2001.

109. Palinski W, Ord VA, Plump AS, et al: ApoE-deficient mice are a model of lipoprotein oxidation in atherogenesis. Demonstration of oxidation-specific epitopes in lesions and high titers of autoantibodies to malondialdehyde-lysine in serum. *Arterioscler Thromb* 14:605–616, 1994.

110. Ameli S, Hultgardh-Nilsson A, Regnstrom J, et al: Effect of immunization with homologous LDL and oxidized LDL on early atherosclerosis in hypercholesterolemic rabbits. *Arterioscler Thromb Vasc Biol* 16:1074–1079, 1996.

111. Freigang S, Horkko S, Miller E, et al: Immunization of LDL receptor-deficient mice with homologous malondialdehyde-modified and native LDL reduces progression of atherosclerosis by mechanisms other than induction of high titers of antibodies to oxidative neoepitopes. *Arterioscler Thromb Vasc Biol* 18:1972–1982, 1998.

112. Zhou X, Caligiuri G, Hamsten A, et al: LDL immunization induces T-cell-dependent antibody formation and protection against atherosclerosis. *Arterioscler Thromb Vasc Biol* 21:108–114, 2001.

113. Mehrabian M, Allayee H, Wong J, et al: Identification of 5-lipoxygenase as a major gene contributing to atherosclerosis susceptibility in mice. *Circ Res* 91:120–126, 2002.

114. Cyrus T, Witztum JL, Rader DJ, et al: Disruption of the 12/15-lipoxygenase gene diminishes atherosclerosis in apo E-deficient mice. *J Clin Invest* 103:1597–1604, 1999.

115. Harats D, Shaish A, George J, et al: Overexpression of 15-lipoxygenase in vascular endothelium accelerates early atherosclerosis in LDL receptor-deficient mice. *Arterioscler Thromb Vasc Biol* 20:2100–2105, 2000.

116. Whatling C, McPheat W, Herslof M: The potential link between atherosclerosis and the 5-lipoxygenase pathway: Investigational agents with new implications for the cardiovascular field. *Expert Opin Investig Drugs* 16:1879–1893, 2007.

117. Vinje S, Stroes E, Nieuwdorp M, Hazen SL: The gut microbiome as novel cardiometabolic target: The time has come! *Eur Heart J* 35:883–887, 2014.

118. Williams KJ, Feig JE, Fisher EA: Cellular and molecular mechanisms for rapid regression of atherosclerosis: From bench top to potentially achievable clinical goal. *Curr Opin Lipidol* 18:443–450, 2007.

119. Schwenke DC: Comparison of aorta and pulmonary artery: I. Early cholesterol accumulation and relative susceptibility to atheromatous lesions. *Circ Res* 81:338–345, 1997.

120. Schwenke DC: Comparison of aorta and pulmonary artery: II. LDL transport and metabolism correlate with susceptibility to atherosclerosis. *Circ Res* 81:346–354, 1997.

121. Camejo G, Hurt-Camejo E, Wiklund O, Bondjers G: Association of apo B lipoproteins with arterial proteoglycans: Pathological significance and molecular basis. *Atherosclerosis* 139:205–222, 1998.

122. Navab M, Hama SY, Reddy ST, et al: Oxidized lipids as mediators of coronary heart disease. *Curr Opin Lipidol* 13:363–372, 2002.

123. Rajavashisth TB, Andalibi A, Territo MC, et al: Induction of endothelial cell expression of granulocyte and macrophage colony-stimulating factors by modified low-density lipoproteins. *Nature* 344:254–257, 1990.

124. Steinberg D: Atherogenesis in perspective: Hypercholesterolemia and inflammation as partners in crime. *Nat Med* 8:1211–1217, 2002.

125. MRC/BHF Heart Protection Study of antioxidant vitamin supplementation in 20,536 high-risk individuals: A randomised placebo-controlled trial. *Lancet* 360:23–33, 2002.

126. Brown BG, Zhao XQ, Chait A, et al: Simvastatin and niacin, antioxidant vitamins, or the combination for the prevention of coronary disease. *N Engl J Med* 345:1583–1592, 2001.

127. Tangirala RK, Tsukamoto K, Chun SH, et al: Regression of atherosclerosis induced by liver-directed gene transfer of apolipoprotein A-I in mice. *Circulation* 100:1816–1822, 1999.

128. Zhang Y, Zanotti I, Reilly MP, et al: Overexpression of apolipoprotein A-I promotes reverse transport of cholesterol from macrophages to feces in vivo. *Circulation* 108:661–663, 2003.

129. Khera AV, Cuchel M, de la Llera-Moya M, et al: Cholesterol efflux capacity, high-density lipoprotein function, and atherosclerosis. *N Engl J Med* 364:127–135, 2011.

130. Mineo C, Deguchi H, Griffin JH, Shaul PW: Endothelial and antithrombotic actions of HDL. *Circ Res* 98:1352–1364, 2006.

131. Shih DM, Gu L, Xia YR, et al: Mice lacking serum paraoxonase are susceptible to organophosphate toxicity and atherosclerosis. *Nature* 394:284–287, 1998.

132. Haraguchi Y, Toh R, Hasokawa M, et al: Serum myeloperoxidase/paraoxonase 1 ratio as potential indicator of dysfunctional high-density lipoprotein and risk stratification in coronary artery disease. *Atherosclerosis* 234:288–294, 2014.

133. Barter PJ, Caulfield M, Eriksson M, et al: Effects of torcetrapib in patients at high risk for coronary events. *N Engl J Med* 357:2109–2122, 2007.

134. Nissen SE, Tsunoda T, Tuzcu EM, et al: Effect of recombinant ApoA-I Milano on coronary atherosclerosis in patients with acute coronary syndromes: A randomized controlled trial. *JAMA* 290:2292–2300, 2003.

135. Van Lenten BJ, Navab M, Anantharamaiah GM, et al: Multiple indications for anti-inflammatory apolipoprotein mimetic peptides. *Curr Opin Investig Drugs* 9:1157–1162, 2008.

136. Rizvi M, Pathak D, Freedman JE, Chakrabarti S: CD40-CD40 ligand interactions in oxidative stress, inflammation and vascular disease. *Trends Mol Med* 14:530–538, 2008.

137. Zhang B, Wu T, Chen M, et al: The CD40/CD40L system: A new therapeutic target for disease. *Immunol Lett* 153:58–61, 2013.

138. Cipollone F, Mezzetti A, Porreca E, et al: Association between enhanced soluble CD40L and prothrombotic state in hypercholesterolemia effects of statin therapy. *Circulation* 106:399–402, 2002.

139. Mallat Z, Gojova A, Marchiol-Fournigault C, et al: Inhibition of transforming growth factor-beta signaling accelerates atherosclerosis and induces an unstable plaque phenotype in mice. *Circ Res* 89:930–934, 2001.

140. Zhang H, Mooney CJ, Reilly MP: ABO blood groups and cardiovascular diseases. *Int J Vasc Med* 2012:641917, 2012.

141. Gurfinkel E, Lernoud V: The role of infection and immunity in atherosclerosis. *Expert Rev Cardiovasc Ther* 4:131–137, 2006.

142. Ford PJ, Yamazaki K, Seymour GJ: Cardiovascular and oral disease interactions: What is the evidence? *Prim Dent Care* 14:59–66, 2007.

143. Mayr M, Kiechl S, Willeit J, et al: Infections, immunity, and atherosclerosis: Associations of antibodies to *Chlamydia pneumoniae*, *Helicobacter pylori*, and cytomegalovirus with immune reactions to heat-shock protein 60 and carotid or femoral atherosclerosis. *Circulation* 102:833–839, 2000.

144. Caligiuri G, Nicoletti A, Poirier B, Hansson GK: Protective immunity against atherosclerosis carried by B cells of hypercholesterolemic mice. *J Clin Invest* 109:745–753, 2002.

145. Robinette CD, Fraumeni JF Jr: Splenectomy and subsequent mortality in veterans of the 1939–45 war. *Lancet* 2:127–129, 1977.

146. Yamada Y, Ichihara S, Nishida T: Molecular genetics of myocardial infarction. *Genomic Med* 2:7–22, 2008.

147. Helgadottir A, Manolescu A, Thorleifsson G, et al: The gene encoding 5-lipoxygenase activating protein confers risk of myocardial infarction and stroke. *Nat Genet* 36:233–239, 2004.

148. Topol EJ, Smith J, Plow EF, Wang QK: Genetic susceptibility to myocardial infarction and coronary artery disease. *Hum Mol Genet* 15 Spec No 2:R117–R123, 2006.

149. Helgadottir A, Thorleifsson G, Manolescu A, et al: A common variant on chromosome 9p21 affects the risk of myocardial infarction. *Science* 316:1491–1493, 2007.

150. Roberts R: Genetics of coronary artery disease. *Circ Res* 114:1890–1903, 2014.

151. Falk E: Plaque rupture with severe pre-existing stenosis precipitating coronary thrombosis. Characteristics of coronary atherosclerotic plaques underlying fatal occlusive thrombi. *Br Heart J* 50:127–134, 1983.

152. Davies MJ, Thomas AC: Plaque fissuring—The cause of acute myocardial infarction, sudden ischaemic death, and crescendo angina. *Br Heart J* 53:363–373, 1985.

153. Muller JE: Circadian variation and triggering of acute coronary events. *Am Heart J* 137:S1–S8.

154. Muller JE, Abela GS, Nesto RW, Tofler GH: Triggers, acute risk factors and vulnerable plaques: The lexicon of a new frontier. *J Am Coll Cardiol* 23:809–813, 1999, 1994.

155. Naghavi M, Libby P, Falk E, et al: From vulnerable plaque to vulnerable patient: A call for new definitions and risk assessment strategies: Part I. *Circulation* 108:1664–1672, 2003.

156. Virmani R, Kolodgie FD, Burke AP, et al: Lessons from sudden coronary death: A comprehensive morphological classification scheme for atherosclerotic lesions. *Arterioscler Thromb Vasc Biol* 20:1262–1275, 2000.

157. Casscells W, Naghavi M, Willerson JT: Vulnerable atherosclerotic plaque: A multifocal disease. *Circulation* 107:2072–2075, 2003.

158. Uchida Y, Nakamura F, Tomaru T, et al: Prediction of acute coronary syndromes by percutaneous coronary angioscopy in patients with stable angina. *Am Heart J* 130:195–203, 1995.

159. Ambrose JA: In search of the "vulnerable plaque": Can it be localized and will focal regional therapy ever be an option for cardiac prevention? *J Am Coll Cardiol* 51:1539–1542, 2008.

160. Naghavi M, Libby P, Falk E, et al: From vulnerable plaque to vulnerable patient: A call for new definitions and risk assessment strategies: Part II. *Circulation* 108:1772–1778, 2003.

161. Davi G, Patrono C: Platelet activation and atherothrombosis. *N Engl J Med* 357:2482–2494, 2007.

162. Owens AP 3rd, Mackman N: Role of tissue factor in atherothrombosis. *Curr Atheroscler Rep* 14:394–401, 2012.

163. Frostegard J: Systemic lupus erythematosus and cardiovascular disease. *Lupus* 17:364–367, 2008.

164. Rohla M, Weiss TW: Metabolic syndrome, inflammation and atherothrombosis. *Hamostaseologie* 33:283–294, 2013.

165. Heo KS, Fujiwara K, Abe J: Shear stress and atherosclerosis. *Mol Cells* 37:435–440, 2014.

166. Cosemans JM, Angelillo-Scherrer A, Mattheij NJ, Heemskerk JW: The effects of arterial flow on platelet activation, thrombus growth, and stabilization. *Cardiovasc Res* 99:342–352, 2013.

167. Aird WC: Vascular bed-specific thrombosis. *J Thromb Haemost* 5 Suppl 1:283–291, 2007.

168. Chien S: Effects of disturbed flow on endothelial cells. *Ann Biomed Eng* 36:554–562, 2008.

169. Helderman F, Segers D, de Crom R, et al: Effect of shear stress on vascular inflammation and plaque development. *Curr Opin Lipidol* 18:527–533, 2007.

170. Badimon JJ, Ortiz AF, Meyer B, et al: Different response to balloon angioplasty of carotid and coronary arteries: Effects on acute platelet deposition and intimal thickening. *Atherosclerosis* 140:307–314, 1998.

171. Halvorsen B, Otterdal K, Dahl TB, et al: Atherosclerotic plaque stability—What determines the fate of a plaque? *Prog Cardiovasc Dis* 51:183–194, 2008.

172. Regan ER, Aird WC: Dynamical systems approach to endothelial heterogeneity. *Circ Res* 111:110–130, 2012.

173. Cheung C, Bernardo AS, Pedersen RA, Sinha S: Directed differentiation of embryonic origin-specific vascular smooth muscle subtypes from human pluripotent stem cells. *Nat Protoc* 9:929–938, 2014.

174. Lechner D, Weltermann A: Circulating tissue factor-exposing microparticles. *Thromb Res* 122 Suppl 1:S47–S54, 2008.

175. George FD: Microparticles in vascular diseases. *Thromb Res* 122 Suppl 1:S55–S9, 2008.

176. Lacroix R, Dubois C, Leroyer AS, et al: Revisited role of microparticles in arterial and venous thrombosis. *J Thromb Haemost* 11 Suppl 1:24–35, 2013.

177. Rauch U, Osende JI, Fuster V, et al: Thrombus formation on atherosclerotic plaques: Pathogenesis and clinical consequences. *Ann Intern Med* 134:224–238, 2001.

178. Ma B, Liu G, Chen X, et al: Risk of stroke in patients with patent foramen ovale: An updated meta-analysis of observational studies. *J Stroke Cerebrovasc Dis* 23:1207–1215, 2014.

179. Nallu K, Yang DC, Swaminathan RV, et al: Innovations in drug-eluting stents. *Panminerva Med* 55:345–352, 2013.

180. Springer J, Villa-Forte A: Thrombosis in vasculitis. *Curr Opin Rheumatol* 25:19–25, 2013.

181. Matsuura E, Kobayashi K, Lopez LR: Preventing autoimmune and infection triggered atherosclerosis for an enduring healthful lifestyle. *Autoimmun Rev* 7:214–222, 2008.

182. Mok CC: Accelerated atherosclerosis, arterial thromboembolism, and preventive strategies in systemic lupus erythematosus. *Scand J Rheumatol* 35:85–95, 2006.

183. Dasararaju R, Singh N, Mehta A: Heparin induced thrombocytopenia: Review. *Expert Rev Hematol* 6:419–428, 2013.

184. Barbui T, Finazzi G, Falanga A: Myeloproliferative neoplasms and thrombosis. *Blood* 122:2176–2184, 2013.

185. Casini A, Fontana P, Lecompte TP: Thrombotic complications of myeloproliferative neoplasms: Risk assessment and risk-guided management. *J Thromb Haemost* 11:1215–1227, 2013.

186. Finazzi G, De Stefano V, Barbui T: Are MPNs vascular diseases? *Curr Hematol Malig Rep* 8:307–316, 2013.

187. De Ceunynck K, De Meyer SF, Vanhoorelbeke K: Unwinding the von Willebrand factor strings puzzle. *Blood* 121:270–277, 2013.

188. Nightingale T, Cutler D: The secretion of von Willebrand factor from endothelial cells; an increasingly complicated story. *J Thromb Haemost* 11 Suppl 1:192–201, 2013.

189. Wong AK: Platelet biology: The role of shear. *Expert Rev Hematol* 6:205–212, 2013.

190. Kulkarni S, Dopheide SM, Yap CL, et al: A revised model of platelet aggregation. *J Clin Invest* 105:783–791, 2000.

191. Wagner CT, Kroll MH, Chow TW, et al: Epinephrine and shear stress synergistically induce platelet aggregation via a mechanism that partially bypasses VWF-GP IB interactions. *Biorheology* 33:209–229, 1996.

192. Andre P, Prasad KS, Denis CV, et al: CD40L stabilizes arterial thrombi by a beta3 integrin-dependent mechanism. *Nat Med* 8:247–252, 2002.

193. Winckers K, ten Cate H, Hackeng TM: The role of tissue factor pathway inhibitor in atherosclerosis and arterial thrombosis. *Blood Rev* 27:119–132, 2013.

194. Tedgui A, Mallat Z: Apoptosis as a determinant of atherothrombosis. *Thromb Haemost* 86:420–426, 2001.

195. Shah PK: Inflammation and plaque vulnerability. *Cardiovasc Drugs Ther* 23:31–40, 2009.

196. Kuge Y, Kume N, Ishino S, et al: Prominent lectin-like oxidized low density lipoprotein (LDL) receptor-1 (LOX-1) expression in atherosclerotic lesions is associated with tissue factor expression and apoptosis in hypercholesterolemic rabbits. *Biol Pharm Bull* 31:1475–1482, 2008.

197. van der Stoep M, Korporaal SJ, Van Eck M: High-density lipoprotein as a modulator of platelet and coagulation responses. *Cardiovasc Res* 103:362–371, 2014.

198. Endler G, Mannhalter C: Polymorphisms in coagulation factor genes and their impact on arterial and venous thrombosis. *Clin Chim Acta* 330:31–55, 2003.

199. Prandoni P, Bilora F, Marchiori A, et al: An association between atherosclerosis and venous thrombosis. *N Engl J Med* 348:1435–1441, 2003.

200. Franchini M, Mannucci PM: Association between venous and arterial thrombosis: Clinical implications. *Eur J Intern Med* 23:333–337, 2012.

201. Lind C, Flinterman LE, Enga KF, et al: Impact of incident venous thromboembolism on risk of arterial thrombotic diseases. *Circulation* 129:855–863, 2014.

202. Celermajer DS, Sorensen KE, Spiegelhalter DJ, et al: Aging is associated with endothelial dysfunction in healthy men years before the age-related decline in women. *J Am Coll Cardiol* 24:471–476, 1994.

203. Franchini M, Targher G, Montagnana M, Lippi G: The metabolic syndrome and the risk of arterial and venous thrombosis. *Thromb Res* 122:727–735, 2008.

204. Lowe GD: Common risk factors for both arterial and venous thrombosis. *Br J Haematol* 140:488–495, 2008.

205. Ye Z, Liu EH, Higgins JP, et al: Seven haemostatic gene polymorphisms in coronary disease: Meta-analysis of 66,155 cases and 91,307 controls. *Lancet* 367:651–658, 2006.

206. Kamphuisen PW, ten Cate H: Cardiovascular risk in patients with hemophilia. *Blood* 123:1297–1301, 2014.

207. Sramek A, Reiber JH, Gerrits WB, Rosendaal FR: Decreased coagulability has no clinically relevant effect on atherogenesis: Observations in individuals with a hereditary bleeding tendency. *Circulation* 104:762–767, 2001.

208. Haverkate F: Levels of haemostatic factors, arteriosclerosis and cardiovascular disease. *Vascul Pharmacol* 39:109–112, 2002.

209. Kannel WB: Overview of hemostatic factors involved in atherosclerotic cardiovascular disease. *Lipids* 40:1215–1220, 2005.

210. Montoro-Garcia S, Shantsila E, Lip GY: Potential value of targeting von Willebrand factor in atherosclerotic cardiovascular disease. *Expert Opin Ther Targets* 18:43–53, 2014.

211. van Galen KP, Tuinenburg A, Smeets EM, Schutgens RE: Von Willebrand factor deficiency and atherosclerosis. *Blood Rev* 26:189–196, 2012.

212. Williams MS, Bray PF: Genetics of arterial prothrombotic risk states. *Exp Biol Med (Maywood)* 226:409–419, 2001.

213. Lekakis J, Bisti S, Tsougos E, et al: Platelet glycoprotein IIb HPA-3 polymorphism and acute coronary syndromes. *Int J Cardiol* 127:46–50, 2008.

214. Weiss EJ, Bray PF, Tayback M, et al: A polymorphism of a platelet glycoprotein receptor as an inherited risk factor for coronary thrombosis. *N Engl J Med* 334:1090–1094, 1996.

215. Burkhart JM, Gambaryan S, Watson SP, et al: What can proteomics tell us about platelets? *Circ Res* 114:1204–1219, 2014.

216. Berger JS, Becker RC, Kuhn C, et al: Hyperreactive platelet phenotypes: Relationship to altered serotonin transporter number, transport kinetics and intrinsic response to adrenergic co-stimulation. *Thromb Haemost* 109:85–92, 2013.

217. Rauch U, Osende JI, Chesebro JH, et al: Statins and cardiovascular diseases: The multiple effects of lipid-lowering therapy by statins. *Atherosclerosis* 153:181–189, 2000.

218. Alpert JS, Thygesen K, Antman E, Bassand JP: Myocardial infarction redefined—A consensus document of The Joint European Society of Cardiology/American College of Cardiology Committee for the redefinition of myocardial infarction. *J Am Coll Cardiol* 36:959–969, 2000.

219. O'Gara PT, Kushner FG, Ascheim DD, et al: 2013 ACCF/AHA guideline for the management of ST-elevation myocardial infarction: Executive summary: A report of the American College of Cardiology Foundation/American Heart Association Task Force on Practice Guidelines: Developed in collaboration with the American College of Emergency Physicians and Society for Cardiovascular Angiography and Interventions. *Catheter Cardiovasc Interv* 82:E1–E27, 2013.

220. Wright RS, Anderson JL, Adams CD, et al: 2011 ACCF/AHA focused update incorporated into the ACC/AHA 2007 Guidelines for the Management of Patients with Unstable Angina/Non-ST-Elevation Myocardial Infarction: A report of the American College of Cardiology Foundation/American Heart Association Task Force on Practice Guidelines developed in collaboration with the American Academy of Family Physicians, Society for Cardiovascular Angiography and Interventions, and the Society of Thoracic Surgeons. *J Am Coll Cardiol* 57:e215–e367, 2011.

221. Pope JH, Ruthazer R, Beshansky JR, et al: Clinical Features of Emergency Department Patients Presenting with Symptoms Suggestive of Acute Cardiac Ischemia: A Multicenter Study. *J Thromb Thrombolysis* 6:63–74, 1998.

222. American College of Emergency Physicians, Society for Cardiovascular Angiography and Interventions, et al: 2013 ACCF/AHA guideline for the management of ST-elevation myocardial infarction: A report of the American College of Cardiology Foundation/American Heart Association Task Force on Practice Guidelines. *J Am Coll Cardiol* 61:e78–e140, 2013.

223. Morrow DA, Braunwald E, Bonaca MP, et al: Vorapaxar in the secondary prevention of atherothrombotic events. *N Engl J Med* 366:1404–1413, 2012.

224. Grines CL, Browne KF, Marco J, et al: A comparison of immediate angioplasty with thrombolytic therapy for acute myocardial infarction. The Primary Angioplasty in Myocardial Infarction Study Group. *N Engl J Med* 328:673–679, 1993.

225. Le May MR, Davies RF, Labinaz M, et al: Hospitalization costs of primary stenting versus thrombolysis in acute myocardial infarction: Cost analysis of the Canadian STAT Study. *Circulation* 108:2624–2630, 2003.

226. Pollack CV Jr, Braunwald E: 2007 Update to the ACC/AHA guidelines for the management of patients with unstable angina and non-ST-segment elevation myocardial infarction: Implications for emergency department practice. *Ann Emerg Med* 51:591–606, 2007.

227. Califf RM, White HD, Van de Werf F, et al: One-year results from the Global Utilization of Streptokinase and TPA for Occluded Coronary Arteries (GUSTO-I) trial. GUSTO-I Investigators. *Circulation* 94:1233–1238, 1996.

228. Llevadot J, Giugliano RP, Antman EM: Bolus fibrinolytic therapy in acute myocardial infarction. *JAMA* 286:442–449, 2001.

229. Brieger DB, Mak KH, White HD, et al: Benefit of early sustained reperfusion in patients with prior myocardial infarction (the GUSTO-I trial). Global Utilization of Streptokinase and TPA for occluded arteries. *Am J Cardiol* 81:282–287, 1998.

230. Pollack CV Jr, Antman EM, Hollander JE: 2007 Focused update to the ACC/AHA guidelines for the management of patients with ST-segment elevation myocardial infarction: Implications for emergency department practice. *Ann Emerg Med* 52:344–355.e1, 2008.

231. Randomised double-blind trial of fixed low-dose warfarin with aspirin after myocardial infarction. Coumadin Aspirin Reinfarction Study (CARS) Investigators. *Lancet* 350:389–396, 1997.

232. Stone NJ, Robinson JG, Lichtenstein AH, et al: 2013 ACC/AHA guideline on the treatment of blood cholesterol to reduce atherosclerotic cardiovascular risk in adults: A report of the American College of Cardiology/American Heart Association Task Force on Practice Guidelines. *J Am Coll Cardiol* 63:2889–2934, 2014.

233. Cannon CP, Murphy SA, Braunwald E: Intensive lipid lowering with atorvastatin in coronary disease. *N Engl J Med* 353:93–96; author reply 93–96, 2005.

234. Antithrombotic Trialists' Collaboration: Collaborative meta-analysis of randomised trials of antiplatelet therapy for prevention of death, myocardial infarction, and stroke in high risk patients. *BMJ* 324:71–86, 2002.

235. Lewis HD Jr, Davis JW, Archibald DG, et al: Protective effects of aspirin against acute myocardial infarction and death in men with unstable angina. Results of a Veterans Administration Cooperative Study. *N Engl J Med* 309:396–403, 1983.

236. Cairns JA, Gent M, Singer J, et al: Aspirin, sulfinpyrazone, or both in unstable angina. Results of a Canadian multicenter trial. *N Engl J Med* 313:1369–1375, 1985.

237. Boersma E, Harrington RA, Moliterno DJ, et al: Platelet glycoprotein IIb/IIIa inhibitors in acute coronary syndromes. *Lancet* 360:342–343, 2002.

238. Gaglia MA Jr, Clavijo L: Cardiovascular pharmacology core reviews: Aspirin. *J Cardiovasc Pharmacol Ther* 18:505–513, 2013.

239. Yusuf S, Zhao F, Mehta SR, et al: Effects of clopidogrel in addition to aspirin in patients with acute coronary syndromes without ST-segment elevation. *N Engl J Med* 345:494–502, 2001.

240. Mehta SR: Aspirin and clopidogrel in patients with ACS undergoing PCI: CURE and PCI-CURE. *J Invasive Cardiol* 15 Suppl B:17B–20B, 2003.

241. Hongo RH, Ley J, Dick SE, Yee RR: The effect of clopidogrel in combination with aspirin when given before coronary artery bypass grafting. *J Am Coll Cardiol* 40:231–237, 2002.

242. Antoniucci D, Migliorini A, Parodi G, et al: Abciximab-supported infarct artery stent implantation for acute myocardial infarction and long-term survival: A prospective, multicenter, randomized trial comparing infarct artery stenting plus abciximab with stenting alone. *Circulation* 109:1704–1706, 2004.

243. Nguyen CM, Harrington RA: Glycoprotein IIb/IIIa receptor antagonists: A comparative review of their use in percutaneous coronary intervention. *Am J Cardiovasc Drugs* 3:423–436, 2003.

244. Direct thrombin inhibitors in acute coronary syndromes: Principal results of a meta-analysis based on individual patients' data. *Lancet* 359:294–302, 2002.

245. Lincoff AM, Kleiman NS, Kereiakes DJ, et al: Long-term efficacy of bivalirudin and provisional glycoprotein IIb/IIIa blockade vs heparin and planned glycoprotein IIb/IIIa blockade during percutaneous coronary revascularization: REPLACE-2 randomized trial. *JAMA* 292:696–703, 2004.

246. Linkins LA, Dans AL, Moores LK, et al: Treatment and prevention of heparin-induced thrombocytopenia: Antithrombotic Therapy and Prevention of Thrombosis, 9th ed: American College of Chest Physicians Evidence-Based Clinical Practice Guidelines. *Chest* 141:e495S–530S, 2012.

247. Fraker TD Jr, Fihn SD; Chronic Stable Angina Writing Committee, et al: 2007 chronic angina focused update of the ACC/AHA 2002 guidelines for the management of patients with chronic stable angina: A report of the American College of Cardiology/American Heart Association Task Force on Practice Guidelines Writing Group to develop the focused update of the 2002 guidelines for the management of patients with chronic stable angina. *J Am Coll Cardiol* 50:2264–2274, 2007.

248. Kaiser GC, Davis KB, Fisher LD, et al: Survival following coronary artery bypass grafting in patients with severe angina pectoris (CASS). An observational study. *J Thorac Cardiovasc Surg* 89:513–524, 1985.

249. Shaw LJ, Berman DS, Maron DJ, et al: Optimal medical therapy with or without percutaneous coronary intervention to reduce ischemic burden: Results from the Clinical Outcomes Utilizing Revascularization and Aggressive Drug Evaluation (COURAGE) trial nuclear substudy. *Circulation* 117:1283–1291, 2008.

250. Mintz GS, Kimura T, Nobuyoshi M, Leon MB: Intravascular ultrasound assessment of the relation between early and late changes in arterial area and neointimal hyperplasia after percutaneous transluminal coronary angioplasty and directional coronary atherectomy. *Am J Cardiol* 83:1518–1523, 1999.

251. Wilensky RL, Tanguay JF, Ito S, et al: Heparin Infusion Prior to Stenting (HIPS) trial: Final results of a prospective, randomized, controlled trial evaluating the effects of local vascular delivery on intimal hyperplasia. *Am Heart J* 139:1061–1070, 2000.

252. Morice MC, Serruys PW, Sousa JE, et al: A randomized comparison of a sirolimus-eluting stent with a standard stent for coronary revascularization. *N Engl J Med* 346:1773–1780, 2002.

253. Simonton CA, Brodie B, Cheek B, et al: Comparative clinical outcomes of paclitaxel- and sirolimus-eluting stents: Results from a large prospective multicenter registry—STENT Group. *J Am Coll Cardiol* 50:1214–1222, 2007.

254. Mohler ER 3rd: Peripheral arterial disease: Identification and implications. *Arch Intern Med* 163:2306–2314, 2003.

255. Rooke TW, Hirsch AT, Misra S, et al: 2011 ACCF/AHA Focused update of the guideline for the management of patients with peripheral artery disease (updating the 2005 guideline): A report of the American College of Cardiology Foundation/American Heart Association Task Force on Practice Guidelines. *J Am Coll Cardiol* 58:2020–2045, 2011.

256. Norgren L, Hiatt WR, Dormandy JA, et al: Inter-Society Consensus for the Management of Peripheral Arterial Disease (TASC II). *Eur J Vasc Endovasc Surg* 33 Suppl 1:S1–S75, 2007.

257. Goyen M, Edelman M, Perreault P, et al: MR angiography of aortoiliac occlusive disease: A phase III study of the safety and effectiveness of the blood-pool contrast agent MS-325. *Radiology* 236:825–833, 2005.

258. Mohler ER 3rd. Therapy insight: Peripheral arterial disease and diabetes—From pathogenesis to treatment guidelines. *Nat Clin Pract Cardiovasc Med* 4:151–162, 2007.

259. Mohler ER, Jaff MR: *Peripheral Arterial Disease*. American College of Physicians, Philadelphia, 2008.

260. Goldhaber SZ, Manson JE, Stampfer MJ, et al: Low-dose aspirin and subsequent peripheral arterial surgery in the Physicians' Health Study. *Lancet* 340:143–145, 1992.

261. CAPRIE Steering Committee: A randomised, blinded, trial of clopidogrel versus aspirin in patients at risk of ischaemic events (CAPRIE). *Lancet* 348:1329–1339, 1996.

262. Belch J, MacCuish A, Campbell I, et al: The prevention of progression of arterial disease and diabetes (POPADAD) trial: Factorial randomised placebo controlled trial of aspirin and antioxidants in patients with diabetes and asymptomatic peripheral arterial disease. *BMJ* 337:a1840, 2008.

263. Mohler E 3rd, Giri J: Management of peripheral arterial disease patients: Comparing the ACC/AHA and TASC-II guidelines. *Curr Med Res Opin* 24:2509–2522, 2008.

264. Gardner AW, Poehlman ET: Exercise rehabilitation programs for the treatment of claudication pain. A meta-analysis. *JAMA* 274:975–980, 1995.

265. Murphy TP, Cutlip DE, Regensteiner JG, et al: Supervised exercise versus primary stenting for claudication resulting from aortoiliac peripheral artery disease: Six-month outcomes from the claudication: Exercise versus endoluminal revascularization (CLEVER) study. *Circulation* 125:130–139, 2012.

266. Reilly MP, Mohler ER 3rd: Cilostazol: Treatment of intermittent claudication. *Ann Pharmacother* 35:48–56, 2001.

267. Wilhite DB, Comerota AJ, Schmieder FA, et al: Managing PAD with multiple platelet inhibitors: The effect of combination therapy on bleeding time. *J Vasc Surg* 38:710–713, 2003.

268. Bogousslavsky J, Kaste M, Skyhoj OT, et al: Risk factors and stroke prevention. European Stroke Initiative (EUSI). *Cerebrovasc Dis* 10 Suppl 3:12–21, 2000.

269. Mohler ER 3rd, Delanty N, Rader DJ, Raps EC: Statins and cerebrovascular disease: Plaque attack to prevent brain attack. *Vasc Med* 4:269–272, 1999.

270. Mohler ER 3rd: Carotid stenting for atherothrombosis. *Heart* 93:1147–1151, 2007.

271. Rerkasem K, Rothwell PM: Carotid endarterectomy for symptomatic carotid stenosis. *Cochrane Database Syst Rev* (4):CD001081, 2011.

272. Halliday A, Harrison M, Hayter E, et al: 10-year stroke prevention after successful carotid endarterectomy for asymptomatic stenosis (ACST-1): A multicentre randomised trial. *Lancet* 376:1074–1084, 2010.

273. American College of Cardiology Foundation; American Society of Interventional & Therapeutic Neuroradiology; Society for Cardiovascular Angiography and Interventions, et al: ACCF/SCAI/SVMB/SIR/ASITN 2007 clinical expert consensus document on carotid stenting: A report of the American College of Cardiology Foundation Task Force on Clinical Expert Consensus Documents (ACCF/SCAI/SVMB/SIR/ASITN Clinical Expert Consensus Document Committee on Carotid Stenting). *J Am Coll Cardiol* 49:126–170, 2007.

274. Diener HC, Cunha L, Forbes C, et al: European Stroke Prevention Study. 2. Dipyridamole and acetylsalicylic acid in the secondary prevention of stroke. *J Neurol Sci* 143:1–13, 1996.

275. Sacco RL, Diener HC, Yusuf S, et al: Aspirin and extended-release dipyridamole versus clopidogrel for recurrent stroke. *N Engl J Med* 359:1238–1251, 2008.

276. Chowdhury R, Stevens S, Gorman D, et al: Association between fish consumption, long chain omega 3 fatty acids, and risk of cerebrovascular disease: Systematic review and meta-analysis. *BMJ* 345:e6698.

277. Scolari F, Ravani P, Gaggi R, et al: The challenge of diagnosing atheroembolic renal disease: Clinical features and prognostic factors. *Circulation* 116:298–304, 2012, 2007.

278. Voetsch B, Afshar-Kharghan V, Loscalzo J, Schafer AI: Less common thrombotic and embolic disorders, in *Thrombosis and Hemorrhage*, edited by Loscalzo J and Schafer AI, pp 707–762. Lippincott Williams & Wilkins, Philadelphia, 2003.

279. Quinones A, Saric M: The cholesterol emboli syndrome in atherosclerosis. *Curr Atheroscler Rep* 15:315, 2013.

CHAPTER 135
FIBRINOLYSIS AND THROMBOLYSIS

Katherine A. Hajjar and Jia Ruan

SUMMARY

Improved understanding of the molecular mechanisms of fibrinolysis has led to major advances in fibrinolytic and antifibrinolytic therapy. Characterization of the genes for all the major fibrinolytic proteins has revealed the structure of the relevant serine proteases, their inhibitors, and their receptors. The development of genetically engineered animals deficient in one or more fibrinolytic protein(s) has revealed both expected and unexpected functions. In addition, we now have a catalog of acquired and inherited disorders reflective of either fibrinolytic deficiency with thrombosis or fibrinolytic excess with hemorrhage. These advances have led to development of more effective and safer protocols for both pro- and antifibrinolytic therapy in a variety of circumstances.

● BASIC CONCEPTS OF FIBRINOLYSIS

In response to vascular injury, fibrin, the insoluble end product of the action of thrombin on fibrinogen, is deposited in blood vessels, thus stemming the flow of blood. Once the vessel has healed, the fibrinolytic system is activated, converting fibrin to its soluble degradation products through the action of the serine protease, plasmin (Fig. 135–1A). Fibrinolysis is subject to precise control because of the actions of multiple activators, inhibitors, and cofactors.[1] In addition, receptors expressed by endothelial, monocytoid, and myeloid cells provide specialized, protected environments where plasmin can be generated without compromise by circulating inhibitors (Fig. 135–1B).[2,3] Beyond its more traditional role in fibrin degradation, the fibrinolytic system also supports a variety of tissue remodeling mechanisms. This chapter reviews the fundamental features of plasmin generation, considers the major clinical syndromes resulting from abnormalities in fibrinolysis, and discusses approaches to fibrinolytic and antifibrinolytic therapy.

● COMPONENTS OF THE FIBRINOLYTIC SYSTEM

PLASMINOGEN

Synthesized primarily in the liver,[4,5] plasminogen is a Mr approximately 92,000 single–chain proenzyme that circulates in plasma at a concentration of approximately 1.5 μM[6] (Table 135–1). The plasma half-life of

Acronyms and Abbreviations: a_2-PI, alpha-2 plasmin inhibitor; APL, acute promyelocytic leukemia; IL, interleukin; MMP, matrix metalloproteinase; Plg, plasminogen; PAI, plasminogen activator inhibitor; TAFI, thrombin-activatable fibrinolysis inhibitor; TGF-β, transforming growth factor beta; t-PA, tissue-type plasminogen activator; u-PA, urokinase-type plasminogen activator; uPAR, urokinase-type plasminogen activator receptor.

plasminogen in adults is approximately 2 days.[7] Its 791 amino acids are crosslinked by 24 disulfide bridges, 16 of which give rise to five homologous triple loop structures called "kringles" (Fig. 135–2).[8] The first (K1) and fourth (K4) of these 80–amino-acid, Mr approximately 10,000 structures impart high- and low-affinity lysine binding, respectively.[9] The lysine–binding domains of plasminogen appear to mediate its specific interactions with fibrin, cell surface receptors, and other proteins, including its circulating inhibitor α_2–plasmin inhibitor (α_2-PI).[10–14]

Posttranslational modification of plasminogen results in two glycosylation variants (forms 1 and 2; see Table 135–1).[15–17] O–linked oligosaccharide, consisting of sialic acid, galactose, and galactosamine resident on Thr345, is common to both forms. Only form 2, however, contains N–linked oligosaccharide on Asn 288 that is comprised of sialic acid, galactose, glucosamine, and mannose. The carbohydrate portion of plasminogen appears to regulate its affinity for cellular receptors, and may also specify its physiologic degradation pathway.

Activation of plasminogen results from cleavage of a single Arg–Val peptide bond at position 560–561,[6] giving rise to the active protease, plasmin (see Table 135–1). Plasmin contains a typical serine protease catalytic triad (His 602, Asp 645, and Ser 740), but exhibits broad substrate specificity when compared to other proteases of this class.[18] The circulating form of plasminogen, aminoterminal glutamic acid plasminogen (Glu–Plg), can be converted by limited proteolysis to several modified forms known collectively as Lys–Plg.[19,20] Hydrolysis of the Lys77–Lys78 peptide bond gives rise to a conformationally modified form of the zymogen that more readily binds fibrin, displays two- to threefold higher avidity for cellular receptors, and is activated 10 to 20 times more rapidly than Glu-Plg[11,21,22] Lys–Plg does not normally circulate in plasma,[21] but has been identified on cell surfaces.[23,24]

Spanning 52.5 kb of DNA on chromosome 6q26–27, the Plg gene consists of 19 exons[25,26] and directs expression of a 2.7-kb mRNA[8] (see Fig. 135–2). The 5′ upstream region of the Plg gene contains two regulatory elements common to genes for acute–phase reactants (CTGGGA) and six interleukin (IL)-6 response elements.[26] Plg gene activity, moreover, is stimulated by the acute-phase-mediator IL-6 both in vitro and in vivo.[27] The gene is closely linked and structurally related to that of apolipoprotein(a), an apoprotein associated with the highly atherogenic low density lipoprotein–like particle lipoprotein(a),[28] and more distantly related to other kringle-containing proteins such as tissue-type plasminogen activator (t-PA), urokinase-type plasminogen activator (u-PA), macrophage-stimulating protein, and hepatocyte growth factor.[29–34]

The Physiologic Functions of Plasmin(ogen)

Mice made completely deficient in Plg through gene targeting undergo normal embryogenesis and development, are fertile, and survive to adulthood (Table 135–2).[35,36] These animals display runting and ligneous conjunctivitis,[37] and harbor spontaneous thrombi in the liver, stomach, colon, rectum, lung, and pancreas, as well as fibrin deposition in the liver and ulcerative lesions in the gastrointestinal tract and rectum. These results suggested that Plg is not strictly required for normal development, but does play a central role in fibrin homeostasis. In humans, Plg deficiency presents most often with ligneous mucositis as a result of fibrin deposition, and is rarely a cause of macrovascular thrombosis (see Fibrinolytic Deficiency and Thrombosis below).

PLASMINOGEN ACTIVATORS

Tissue-Type Plasminogen Activator

One of two major endogenous Plg activators, t-PA consists of 527 amino acids comprising a glycoprotein of Mr approximately 72,000 (see Table 135–1).[38] t-PA contains five structural domains including a fibronectin–like "finger," an epidermal growth factor–like domain, two

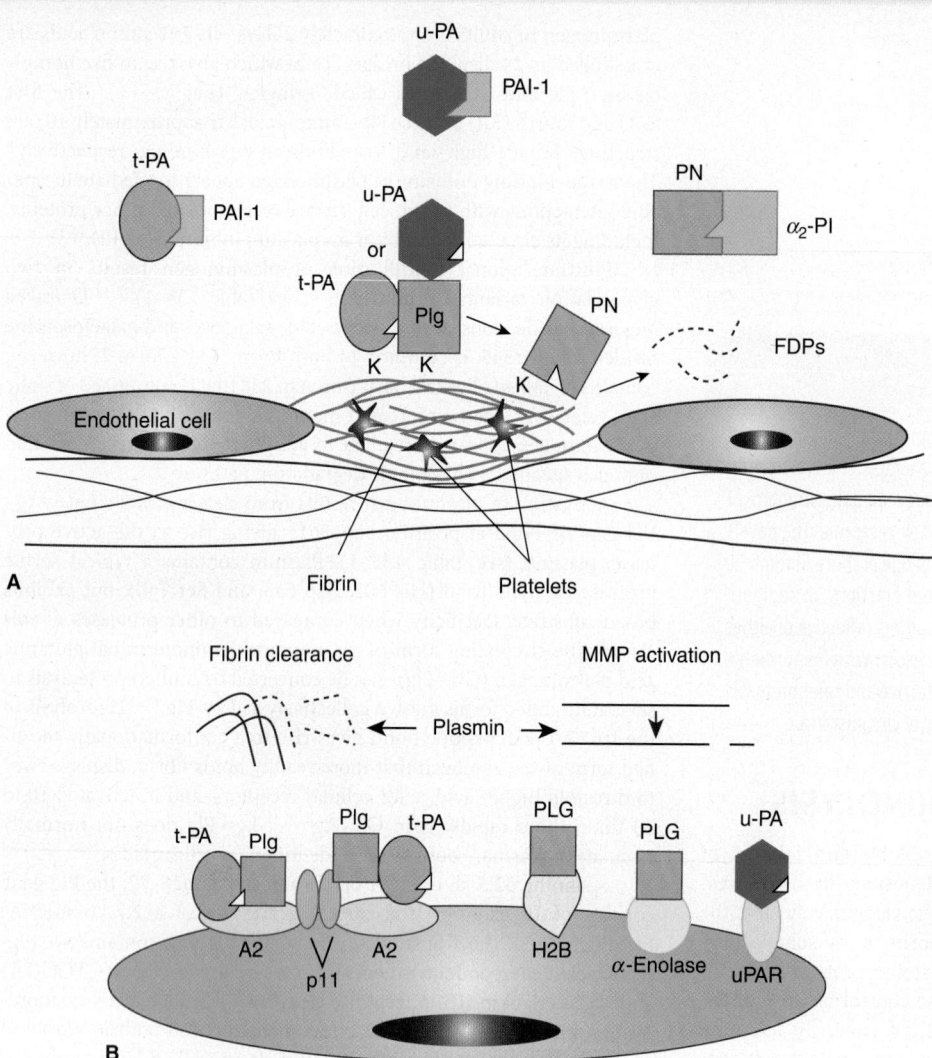

Figure 135–1. Overview of the fibrinolytic system. **A**. Fibrin–based plasminogen activation. The zymogen plasminogen (Plg) is converted to the active serine protease, plasmin (PN), through the action of tissue plasminogen activator (t-PA) or urokinase (u-PA). The activity of t-PA is greatly enhanced by its assembly with Plg through lysine residues (K) on a fibrin–containing thrombus. u-PA acts independently of fibrin. Both t-PA and u-PA can be inhibited by plasminogen activator inhibitor–1 (PAI-1), the main physiologic regulator of plasminogen activator activity. By binding to fibrin, PN is protected from its major inhibitor, a_2–plasmin inhibitor (a_2–PI). Fibrin-bound plasmin degrades crosslinked fibrin, giving rise to soluble fibrin degradation products (FDPs). **B**. Cell surface plasminogen activation. Although many cell types express receptors for Plg, urokinase, and t-PA, only the endothelial cell is depicted here. The annexin A2 heterotetramer, consisting of two copies each of annexin A2 (A2) and protein p11 (p11), binds both t-PA and Plg, thereby augmenting the efficiency of plasmin generation on endothelial cells. Plg may also bind to other endothelial cell receptors, including histone H2B (H2B), a-enolase, and may be activated by u-PA bound to its receptor, uPAR, to effect plasmin generation.

TABLE 135–1. Fibrinolytic Proteins			
A. MAJOR PROTEASES			
Property	Plasminogen	t-PA	u-PA
Molecular mass	92,000	72,000	54,000
Amino acids	791	527	411
Chromosome	6	8	10
Site of synthesis	Liver	Endothelium	Endothelium, kidney
Plasma concentration			
nM	1500	0.075	0.150
mcg/mL	140	0.005	0.008
Plasma half-life	48 h	5 min	8 min
N-glycosylation (%)	2	13	7
Form 1	–	Asn117, Asn184, Asn448	Asn302
Form 2	Asn288	Asn117, –, Asn448	–
O-Glycosylation			
a-Fucose	–	Thr61	Thr18
Complex	Thr345	–	–

(continued)

TABLE 135–1. Fibrinolytic Proteins *(Continued)*

Two-chain cleavage site	Arg560-Val561	Arg275-Ile276	Lys158-Ile159
Heavy chain domains			
Finger	No	Yes	No
Growth factor	No	Yes	Yes
Kringles (no.)	5	2	1
Light-chain catalytic triad	His602, Asp645, Ser740	His322, Asp371, Ser478	His204, Asp255, Ser356

B. MAJOR SERPIN INHIBITORS

Property	α_2-PI	PAI-1	PAI-2
Molecular mass	70,000	52,000	60,000 (glycosylated) 47,000 (nonglycosylated)
Amino acids	452	402	393
Chromosome	18	7	18
Sites of synthesis	Kidney, liver	Endothelium	Placenta
		Monocytes/macrophages	Monocytes/macrophages
		Hepatocytes	Tumor cells
		Adipocytes	
Plasma concentration			
nM	900	0.1–0.4	ND
mcg/mL	50	0.02	ND
Serpin reactive site	Arg364–Met365	Arg346–Met347	Arg358–Thr359
Specificity	Plasmin	u-PA = t-PA	u-PA > t-PA

C. MAJOR ACTIVATION RECEPTORS

Property	uPAR	Annexin A2	p11	Plg-R$_{KT}$	Histone 2B
Molecular mass	55,000–60,000	36,000	11,000	17,000	17,000
Amino acids	313	339	4544	147	126
Chromosome	19	15	12	9	6
Source	Endothelial cells	Endothelial cells	Endothelial cells	–	Endothelial cells
	Monocytes	Monocytes	Monocytes	Monocytes	Monocytes
	Macrophages	Macrophages	Macrophages	Macrophages	Macrophages
	Fibroblasts	Myeloid cells	Myeloid cells	Myeloid cells	Neutrophils
	Tumor cells	Tumor cells	Tumor cells	Tumor cells	
Ligand(s)	u-PA	t-PA, Plg	Plg	Plg	

α_2-PI, α_2-plasmin inhibitor; ND, not determined; PAI-1, plasminogen activator inhibitor type 1; PAI-2, plasminogen activator inhibitor type 2; Plg, plasminogen; Plg-R$_{KT}$, plasminogen receptor with terminal lysine; PN, plasmin; t-PA, tissue-type plasminogen activator; u-PA, urokinase plasminogen activator; uPAR, urokinase plasminogen activator receptor.

"kringle" structures homologous to those of Plg, and a serine protease domain (see Fig. 135–2). Cleavage of the Arg275–Ile276 peptide bond by plasmin converts t-PA to a disulfide–linked, two–chain form.[38] Although single–chain t-PA is less active than two–chain t-PA in the fluid phase, both forms demonstrate equivalent activity when fibrin–bound.[39]

The two glycosylation forms of t-PA are distinguishable by the presence (type 1) or absence (type 2) of a complex *N–linked* oligosaccharide moiety on Asn184 (see Table 135–1).[40,41] Both types, however, contain high mannose carbohydrate on Asn 117, complex oligosaccharide on Asn448, and an *O–linked* α–fucose residue on Thr61.[42] The carbohydrate moieties of t-PA may modulate its functional activity, regulate its binding to cell surface receptors, and specify its degradation pathways.

Located on chromosome 8p12–q11.2, the gene for human t-PA is encoded by 14 exons spanning a total of 36.6 kb (see Fig. 135–2).[43-45] Although exon 1 encodes a 58-nucleotide mRNA leader sequence, each of the structural domains of t-PA is encoded by one or two of the remaining 13 exons. This arrangement suggests that the t-PA gene arose by an evolutionary process called "exon shuffling," whereby functionally

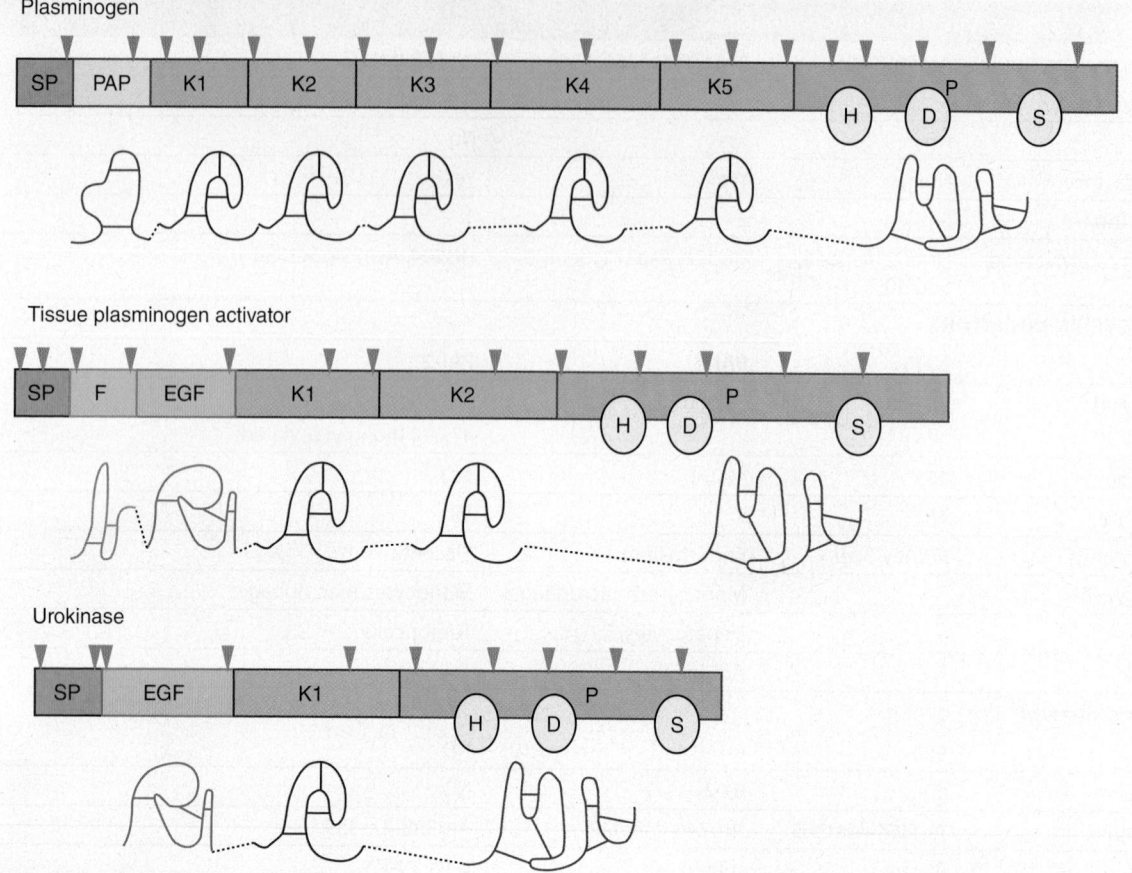

Figure 135–2. Alignment of the intron–exon structure of plasminogen, tissue plasminogen activator, and urokinase genes showing functional protein domains. Protein domains are labeled signal peptide (SP), preactivation peptide (PAP), "kringle" domains (K), fibronectin–like "finger" (F), epidermal growth factor–like domain (EGF), and protease (P). The position of catalytic triad amino acids histidine (H), aspartic acid (D), and serine (S) are shown within individual protease domains. The positions of individual introns relative to amino acid encoding exons are indicated with inverted triangles.

related genes evolved through rearrangement of exons encoding autonomous domains. Consistent with this hypothesis, deletion of exons encoding the fibronectin–like finger or kringle 2, but not kringle 1, domains of t-PA results in expression of mutants resistant to the cofactor activity of fibrin, while catalytic activity in the absence of fibrin remains intact.[46]

The proximal promoter of the human t-PA gene contains binding sequences for potentially important transcriptional factors including AP1, NF1, SP1, and AP2,[47,48] as well as a potential cyclic adenosine monophosphate (cAMP)–responsive element (CRE).[49] *In vitro*, many agents have been shown to exert small effects on the expression of t-PA mRNA, but relatively few enhance t-PA synthesis without augmenting plasminogen activator inhibitor (PAI)–1 synthesis as well. Agents that regulate t-PA gene expression independently of PAI–1 include histamine, butyrate, retinoids, arterial levels of shear stress, and dexamethasone.[50–55] Forskolin, which increases intracellular cAMP levels, has been reported to decrease synthesis of both t-PA and PAI–1.[48,56]

In the vascular system, t-PA is synthesized and secreted primarily by endothelial cells belonging to a restricted set of blood vessels. In rodents, t-PA expression appears in 7- to 30-μm diameter precapillary arterioles in the lung, postcapillary venules, and vasa vasorum; much less expression is seen in endothelial cells of the femoral artery, femoral vein, carotid artery, or aorta.[57] In the mouse lung, bronchial arteriolar endothelial cells express t-PA antigen, especially at branch points, while pulmonary blood vessels are uniformly negative.[51,58–60] t-PA has

also been detected in sympathetic neurons associated with the blood vessel wall.[61] Release of t-PA is governed by a variety of stimuli such as thrombin, histamine, bradykinin, epinephrine, acetylcholine, arginine vasopressin, gonadotropins, exercise, venous occlusion, and shear stress.[50,51,62,63] Its circulating half-life is exceedingly short (~5 minutes). Alone, t-PA is actually a poor activator of Plg, but, in the presence of fibrin, the catalytic efficiency of t-PA–dependent plasmin generation (k_{cat}/K_m) increases by at least two orders of magnitude.[22] This is the result of a dramatic increase in affinity (decreased K_m) between t-PA and its substrate Plg in the presence of fibrin. Although it is also expressed by extravascular cells, t-PA appears to represent the major intravascular activator of Plg.[18]

Urokinase

The second endogenous Plg activator, single–chain u-PA or prourokinase, is a Mr approximately 54,000 glycoprotein consisting of 411 amino acids (see Table 135–1). u-PA possesses an epidermal growth factor–like domain, a single Plg-like "kringle," and a classical catalytic triad (His204, Asp255, Ser356) within its serine protease domain (see Fig. 135–2).[64] Cleavage of the Lys158–Ile159 peptide bond by plasmin or kallikrein converts single-chain u-PA to a disulfide–linked two-chain derivative.[65] Located on chromosome 10, the human u-PA gene is encoded by 11 exons spanning 6.4 kb, and expressed by activated endothelial cells, macrophages, renal epithelial cells, and some tumor cells.[66,67] Its intron–exon structure is closely related to that of the t-PA

TABLE 135-2. Mouse Gene Deletion Models Relevant to Fibrinolysis

Genotype	Some Phenotypic Features	References
Plasminogen		
Plg–/–	Spontaneous thrombosis, runting, premature death	35, 36
	Fibrin in liver, lungs, stomach; gastric ulcers	35, 36
	Impaired wound healing	243, 244
	Ligneous mucositis	37
	Impaired monocyte recruitment	245
	Impaired neointima formation after electrical injury	246
	Impaired dissemination of *Borrelia burgdorferi*	247
Plasminogen Activators		
t-PA–/–	Reduced lysis of fibrin clot	84
	Increased endotoxin-induced thrombosis	84
u-PA–/–	Occasional fibrin in liver/intestine	84
	Rectal prolapse, ulcers of eyelids, face, ears	84
	Reduced macrophage degradation of fibrin	84
	Increased endotoxin-induced thrombosis	84
u-PA–/– t-PA–/–	Reduced growth, fertility, and life span; cachexia	84
	Fibrin deposits in liver, gonads, lungs	84
	Ulcers in intestine, skin, ears; rectal prolapse	84
	Impaired clot lysis	84
Inhibitors		
α_2PI–/–	Reduced fibrin deposition following endotoxin	90
	Enhanced lysis of injected plasma clots	90
PAI-1–/–	Mildly increased lysis of fibrin clot	123
	Resistance to endotoxin-induced thrombosis	124
TAFI–/–	Increased clot lysis	140, 142
	Reduced injury-related venous thrombosis	141
Receptors		
uPAR–/–	Normal development and fertility	163
	Normal clot lysis	164
Annexin A2–/–	Fibrin deposition in microvasculature	205
	Impaired clearance of arterial thrombi	205
	Impaired postnatal neoangiogenesis	198, 205, 270
S100A10–/–	Reduced baseline fibrin deposition	199

gene. u-PA expression appears to be induced during neoplastic transformation, possibly through the action of transcription factors AP1 and AP2.[68] Other *in vitro* u-PA inducers include hormones, angiogenic growth factors, and cAMP,[55] as well as tumor necrosis factor and transforming growth factor-β (TGF-β).[69–71]

Two–chain u-PA occurs in both high– (Mr 54,000) and low-molecular-weight (Mr 33,000) forms that differ by the presence or absence, respectively, of a 135–residue aminoterminal fragment released by plasmin cleavage between Lys135 and Lys136.[72,73] Although both forms are capable of activating Plg, only the high-molecular-weight form binds to the u-PA receptor (see Urokinase Plasminogen Activator Receptors below). u-PA has much lower affinity for fibrin than t-PA, and is an effective Plg activator both in the presence and in the absence of fibrin.[74,75]

Accessory Plasminogen Activators and Fibrinolysins

Under certain conditions, proteases traditionally classified within the intrinsic arm of the coagulation cascade have been shown to be capable of activating Plg directly. These include kallikrein, factor XIa, and factor XIIa.[76–78] These proteases, however, normally account for no more than 15 percent of total plasmin generating activity in plasma.[79] In addition, the membrane type 1 matrix metalloproteinase (MT1- MMP) appears to exert fibrinolytic activity in the absence of Plg, and may explain the unexpectedly mild phenotype observed in Plg-deficient mice.[80]

Physiologic Function of the Plasminogen Activators

Because there are no clinical examples of complete deficiency of t-PA or u-PA in humans, except for patients with deficient release in the setting of chronic renal disease and hypertension,[81–83] the most compelling data regarding the physiologic functions of t-PA and u-PA come from gene disruption analysis in mice.[84] Both u-PA and t-PA null deletion mice exhibit normal fertility and embryonic development. However, u-PA–/– mice develop rectal prolapse, nonhealing ulcerations of the face and eyelids, and occasional fibrin deposition in tissues. Although they show normal lysis rates of pulmonary clots injected via the jugular vein, endotoxin–induced microvascular thrombus formation is significantly enhanced. t-PA–deficient mice also display a normal spontaneous phenotype, but have a decreased rate of lysis of artificially induced pulmonary thrombi, as well as enhanced thrombus formation, in response to injection of endotoxin. Like Plg–/– mice, mice doubly deficient in t-PA and u-PA (t-PA–/–; u-PA–/–) exhibit rectal prolapse, nonhealing ulceration, runting, and cachexia, with extensive fibrin deposition in liver, intestine, gonads, and lung. Not surprisingly, clot lysis is also markedly impaired.

INHIBITORS OF FIBRINOLYSIS

Plasmin Inhibitors

The action of plasmin is negatively modulated by a family of serine protease inhibitors, called serpins (see Table 135–1).[85] Serpins form an irreversible complex with the active site serine of their target protease following proteolytic cleavage of the inhibitor by the target protease. Within such a complex, both protease and inhibitor lose their activity.

A single–chain glycoprotein of Mr approximately 70,000, α_2-PI is synthesized primarily in the liver, circulates in plasma at relatively high concentrations (~0.9 μM), and enjoys a plasma half–life of 2.4 days (see Table 135–1).[86] This serpin contains approximately 13 percent carbohydrate by mass and consists of 452 amino acids with two disulfide bridges.[87] In humans, the gene is located on chromosome 18 and contains 10 exons distributed over 16 kb of DNA.[88] The promoter region of the α_2-PI gene contains a hepatitis B–like enhancer element that directs tissue–specific expression in the liver.[87] α_2-PI is also a constituent of platelet α granules.[89] Plasmin released into flowing blood or in the vicinity of a platelet–rich thrombus, is immediately neutralized upon forming an irreversible 1:1 stoichiometric, lysine-binding site–dependent complex with α_2-PI. Interaction with plasmin is accompanied by cleavage of the Arg364–Met365 peptide bond, and the resulting covalent complexes are cleared in the liver. Mice globally deficient in α_2-PI display reduced fibrin deposition, following treatment with endotoxin and enhanced lysis of injected plasma clots, but no spontaneous bleeding (see Table 35–2).[90]

Several additional proteins can act as plasmin inhibitors (see Table 135–1). α_2–Macroglobulin is a Mr 725,000 dimeric protein synthesized by endothelial cells and macrophages, and found in platelet α granules. This nonserpin inhibits plasmin with approximately 10 percent of the efficiency exhibited by α_2–PI by forming noncovalent complexes with several distinct serine proteases.[91] C_1-esterase inhibitor can inhibit t-PA in plasma[92] and protease nexin may function as a noncirculating cell surface inhibitor of trypsin, thrombin, factor Xa, urokinase, or plasmin, resulting in protease–inhibitor complexes that are endocytosed via a specific nexin receptor.[93,94] The purpose of these multiple plasmin inhibitors is to guard against premature plasmin activation and subsequent degradation of fibrinogen, until intravascular fibrin begins to appear/.

Plasminogen Activator Inhibitors

Plasminogen Activator Inhibitor-1 Of the two major Plg activator inhibitors, PAI-1 is the most ubiquitous (see Table 135–1).[95] This Mr approximately 52,000 single–chain, cysteine–less glycoprotein is released by endothelial cells, monocytes, macrophages, hepatocytes, adipocytes, and platelets.[96-98] Release of PAI-1 is stimulated by many cytokines, growth factors, and lipoproteins common to the global inflammatory response.[69,70,99,100,101] The PAI-1 gene consists of nine exons, spanning 12.2 kb on chromosome 7q21.3–q22.[102] The serpin-reactive site is located at Arg346–Met347, and activity of this labile serpin is stabilized upon complex formation with vitronectin, a component of plasma and pericellular matrix.[103-105]

Regulation of PAI-1 gene expression is complex.[106,107] The upstream regulatory region of the human PAI-1 gene contains a strong endothelial cell/fibroblast-specific element[108,109] a glucocorticoid–responsive enhancer,[109] and TGF-β responsive elements.[110] TGF-β is known to stimulate fos and jun, the two components of the AP1 complex, and an AP1 binding site (GGAGTCA) is located upstream of the PAI-1 cap site.[111] Agents shown to enhance expression of PAI-1 at the message level, the protein level, or both, without affecting t-PA synthesis, include the inflammatory cytokines lipopolysaccharide, IL-1, tumor necrosis factor-α,[69,70,99,112,113] TGF-β and basic fibroblast growth factor,[71,99,110,114] very-low-density lipoprotein and lipoprotein(a),[115,116] angiotensin II,[117] thrombin,[118,119] and phorbol esters.[120] In addition, endothelial cell PAI-1 is downregulated by forskolin[56] and by endothelial cell growth factor in the presence of heparin.[121]

PAI-1 is the most important and rapidly acting physiologic inhibitor of both t-PA and u-PA. Transgenic mice that overexpress PAI-1 exhibit thrombotic occlusion of tail veins and swelling of hind limbs within 2 weeks of birth.[122] Mice deficient in PAI-1, on the other hand, exhibit normal fertility, viability, tissue histology, and development, and are resistant to endotoxin-induced thrombosis, but show no evidence of overt hemorrhage (see Table 135–2).[123,124] These observations contrast with the moderately severe bleeding disorder observed in a human patient with complete PAI-1 deficiency.[125]

Plasminogen Activator Inhibitor-2 Originally purified from human placenta, PAI-2 is a 393-amino-acid member of the serpin family whose reactive site is the Arg358–Thr359 peptide bond[126] (see Table 135–1). The gene encoding PAI-2 is located on chromosome 18q21-23, spans 16.5 kb, and contains eight exons.[127] PAI-2 exists as both a Mr 47,000 nonglycosylated intracellular form and an Mr 60,000 glycosylated form secreted by leukocytes and fibrosarcoma cells. Functionally, PAI-2 inhibits both two–chain t-PA and two–chain u-PA with comparable efficiency (second order rate constants 10^5 $M^{-1}s^{-1}$). However, it is less effective toward single-chain t-PA (second order rate constant 10^3 $M^{-1}s^{-1}$), and does not inhibit prourokinase.

Significant levels of PAI–2 are found in human plasma primarily during pregnancy. The gene's 5′–untranslated region contains a potent silencer, the PAUSE-1 element, which may be responsible for its low level of expression in nonpregnant individuals.[127,128] The 3′–downstream sequences include the TTATTTAT motif which has been identified with inflammatory mediators.[129,130] In macrophages *in vitro*, secretion of PAI-2 is enhanced by endotoxin and phorbol esters[130,131] and dexamethasone decreases PAI-2 expression in HT–1080 cells.[55]

Thrombin-Activatable Fibrinolysis Inhibitor

Thrombin-activatable fibrinolysis inhibitor (TAFI) is a plasma carboxypeptidase with specificity for carboxy terminal arginine and lysine residues.[132] The action of TAFI eliminates binding sites for Plg and t-PA on fibrin.[133] This single-chain Mr 60,000 polypeptide circulates in plasma at concentrations of approximately 75 nM, and undergoes limited proteolysis in the presence of thrombin, which leads to its activation.[134-136] The profibrinolytic effect of activated protein C in plasma is a result of its ability to inactivate coagulation factors Va and VIIIa, which reduces activation of thrombin, the primary activator of TAFI.[132] The profibrinolytic effect of activated protein C in an *in vitro* plasma-based system was TAFI-dependent,[137] and, in a system of purified components, TAFI has been shown to downregulate t-PA–induced fibrinolysis half-maximally at a concentration of approximately 1 nM, which is 2 percent of its concentration in plasma.[138] Inhibition of either the intrinsic pathway of coagulation or TAFI itself results in a doubling of endogenous clot lysis in an *in vivo* rabbit jugular vein model of thrombolysis.[139,140] TAFI-deficient mice display increased lysis of plasma clots and reduced injury-induced venous thrombosis (see Table 135–2).[141,142] In plasma, TAFI may regulate Plg binding to both cell surface receptors and to fibrin.[143]

CELLULAR RECEPTORS

A large number of structurally diverse fibrinolytic "activation" and "clearance" receptors have been described. Here, we focus on endothelial cell activation receptors that are likely to contribute to homeostatic control of plasmin activity (see Table 135–1).[2] Clearance receptors eliminate plasmin and Plg activators from the blood or focal microenvironments.

Activation Receptors

Plasminogen Receptors Proposed Plg receptors include α–enolase, glycoprotein IIb/IIIa complex, the Heymann nephritis antigen, amphoterin, the annexin A2/S100A10 complex, histone H2B, and plasminogen receptor-KT (Plg-R_{KT})[2,3]; these are expressed on a wide spectrum of cells, including monocytoid cells, platelets, renal epithelial cells, neuroblastoma cells, endothelial cells, and tumor cells.[144-151] Typically, Plg receptors interact with the kringle structures of Plg through carboxyl–terminal lysine residues that are either present on the native protein, or generated by limited proteolysis.[144]

Urokinase Plasminogen Activator Receptor The u-PA receptor (uPAR) is expressed on monocytes, macrophages, fibroblasts, endothelial cells, and many tumor cells (see Table 135–1).[152,153] uPAR complementary DNA (cDNA) was cloned and sequenced from a human fibroblast cDNA library[154] and encodes a protein of 313 amino acids with a 21–residue signal peptide. The gene consists of seven exons distributed over 23 kb of genomic DNA, and places this glycoprotein within the Ly-1/elapid venom toxin superfamily of cysteine rich proteins.[155,156]

uPAR is anchored to the plasma membrane through glycosylphosphatidylinositol linkages.[157] u-PA bound to its receptor maintains its activity and susceptibility to the physiologic inhibitor, PAI–1.[158] Formation of u-PA–PAI-1 complexes hastens clearance of u-PA by hepatic or monocytoid cells.[158–161]

Although originally thought to function only as a means of localizing Plg activation to the cell surface, uPAR now appears to play a central role in cellular signaling and adhesion events.[152,162] The uPAR-deficient mouse has normal development and fertility, and unimpaired fibrin clot lysis (see Table 135–2).[163,164] uPAR binds the adhesive glycoprotein vitronectin at a site distinct from the u-PA binding domain[165,166] and u-PA transfected renal epithelial cells acquire enhanced adhesion to vitronectin while they lose their adhesion to fibronectin.[167] uPAR, furthermore, colocalizes with integrins in focal contacts and at the leading edge of migrating cells,[168] and also associates with caveolin, a major component of caveolae, structures abundant in endothelial cells and thought to participate in signaling events.[169–171] In addition, cleaved and soluble forms of uPAR have recently been detected in the sera of patients with cancer, and these modified forms are thought to regulate the activity of several receptors involved in inflammatory and angiogenic responses.[153]

The Annexin A2-S100a10 System Annexin A2, a Mr 36,000, 339-amino-acid member of the annexin superfamily of calcium-dependent, phospholipid-binding proteins, forms a heterotetramer with the S100 family protein, S100A10 (see Table 135–1).[172–174] It is highly conserved, and abundantly expressed on endothelial cells,[175–178] monocyte/macrophages,[179,180] early myeloid cells,[181] developing neuronal cells,[182] and some tumor cells.[183–185] All of the more than 60 annexin family members have in common a conserved membrane-binding C-terminal "core" region and a more variable N-terminal "tail."[186] The human annexin A2 gene consists of 13 exons distributed over 40 kb of genomic DNA on chromosome 15 (15q21).[187]

Annexin A2 is unique among fibrinolytic receptors in that it possesses binding affinity for both Plg (Kd 114 nM)[148] and t-PA (Kd 30 nM), but not u-PA.[149] In a fluid phase system of purified proteins, native human annexin A2 stimulates the catalytic efficiency of t-PA–dependent Plg activation by 60-fold.[188] This effect is completely inhibited in the presence of lysine analogues or upon treatment of annexin A2 with carboxypeptidase B, an agent that removes basic carboxyl-terminal amino acids. Although it lacks a classical signal peptide, annexin A2 is constitutively translocated to the endothelial cell surface within 16 hours of its biosynthesis. This translocation event can be stimulated either by thrombin or by heat stress, in a process that requires phosphorylation of annexin A2 at Tyr23, the action of a Src family kinase, and the presence of the annexin A2 binding protein p11 (S100A10).[189]

At the cell surface, A2 binds phospholipid via core repeat 2, which contains the linear amino acid sequence KGLGT and downstream aspartate residue (Asp 161); together these moieties constitute a classical "annexin" motif.[190] The annexin A2 heterotetramer, which consists of two A2 monomers and two protein p11 subunits and constitutes the cell surface form of A2, appears to have even greater stimulatory effects on t-PA–dependent plasmin generation.[177] Interestingly, A2 regulates endogenous levels of protein p11 in the endothelial cell by masking a polyubiquitination site on p11, which otherwise directs p11 to the proteasome where it is rapidly degraded.[191]

Plg and t-PA appear to bind to distinct domains. Lys307 appears to be crucial for the effective interaction of Plg with annexin A2, and may be revealed upon limited proteolysis of the parent protein.[188] The atherogenic low-density lipoprotein (LDL)-like particle, lipoprotein(a), competes with Plg for binding to annexin A2 in vitro,[192] thereby reducing cell surface plasmin generation. t-PA binding to annexin A2 requires a domain consisting of residues 8 to 13 (LCKLSL) within the receptor's amino terminal "tail" domain.[193] This region is a target for homocysteine

(HC), a thiol-containing amino acid that accumulates in association with nutritional deficiencies of vitamin B$_6$, vitamin B$_{12}$, or folic acid, or in inherited abnormalities of cystathionine β-synthase, methylenetetrahydrofolate reductase, or methionine synthase,[194] and is associated with atherothrombotic disease.[195,196] In vitro, HC impairs t-PA–dependent plasmin generation at the endothelial cell surface by approximately 50 percent[197] by forming a covalent derivative with Cys,[197] and mice with diet-induced hyperhomocysteinemia have deficient annexin A2 function[198] The half-maximal dose of HC for inhibition of t-PA binding to annexin A2 is approximately 11 μM HC, a value close to the upper limit of normal for HC in plasma (12 μM).

The important role of S100A10 in fibrin balance has recently been underscored. S100A10–/– mice display increased deposition of fibrin in the vasculature and reduced clearance of batroxobin-induced vascular thrombi, and S100A10-deficient endothelial cells demonstrate a 40 percent reduction in Plg binding and plasmin generation in vitro (see Table 135–2).[199] S100A10 also appears to contribute to Plg-dependent macrophage invasion in vitro by enhancing plasmin-dependent activation of matrix metalloporetinase-9.[200]

Several studies suggest a physiologic role for the annexin A2 system in fibrin homeostasis. First, blast cells from human patients with acute promyelocytic leukemia overexpress annexin A2 in proportion to their degree of hyperfibrinolytic coagulopathy[181]; S100A10 also appears to be upregulated by the PML-RAR-α oncoprotein,[201] and both annexin A2 and S100A10 are downregulated by treatment with all-trans-retinoic acid. Second, in rats, arterial thrombosis can be significantly attenuated by pretreatment with intravenous annexin A2.[202] Third, the prevalence of high-titer anti–annexin A2 antibodies correlates with a history of severe thrombosis in humans with antiphospholipid syndrome and in a cohort of individuals with cerebral venous thrombosis.[203,204] Finally, mice with total deficiency of annexin A2 display impaired clearance of artificial arterial thrombi, fibrin deposition in the microvasculature, and angiogenic defects in a variety of tissues (see Table 135–2).[205]

Clearance Receptors

Clearance of serpin-enzyme complexes, such as t-PA–PAI–1 and u-PA–PAI-1, occurs mainly in the liver, and is mediated by a large two–chain receptor called the LDL receptor–related protein 1 (LRP1).[206,207] LRP1 binds a large number of serpin-protease complexes and other ligands, indicating a multifunctional role in mammalian physiology. An additional Mr 39,000 "receptor associated protein" copurifies with LRP1 and appears to regulate the binding and uptake of LRP1 ligands.[208] Interestingly, LRP1 "knockout" embryos undergo developmental arrest by 13.5 days after conception, suggesting that regulation of serine protease activity may be crucial for early embryogenesis.[209,210] Although PAI–1-independent clearance pathways for t-PA have been proposed involving the mannose receptor,[211] or an α–fucose–specific receptor,[212] in vivo studies in mice suggest that LRP1 and the mannose receptor play a dominant role in t-PA clearance.[213]

● THE FIBRINOLYTIC ACTIONS OF PLASMIN

DEGRADATION OF FIBRINOGEN AND FIBRIN

Fibrinogen

Plasmin releases carboxyl–terminal Aα and N–terminal fibrinopeptide B moieties from fibrinogen (Fig. 135–3). This reaction is distinct from the proteolytic cleavage of fibrinogen by thrombin, which releases fibrinopeptide A, exposing the Gly–Pro–Arg tripeptide sequence and allowing fibrinogen to polymerize and form insoluble fibrin.[214] Plasmin cleavage of fibrinogen (Mr 340,000) initially produces

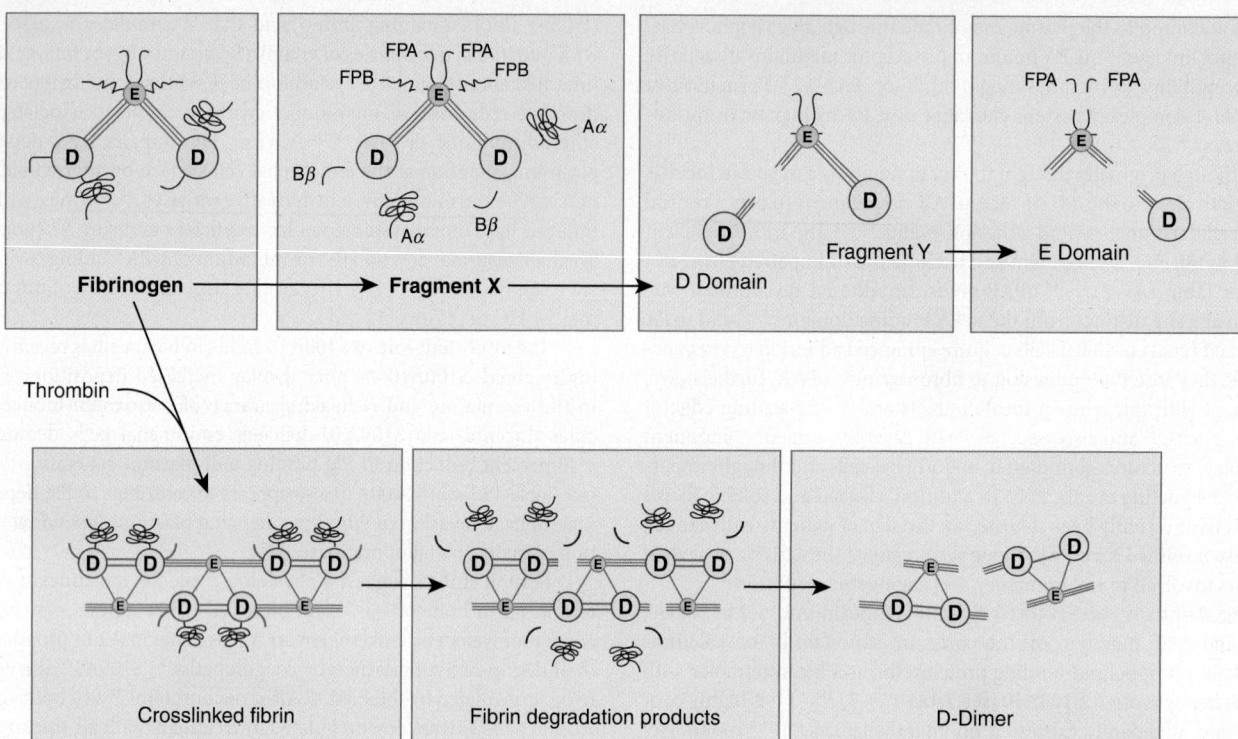

Figure 135–3. Degradation of fibrinogen and crosslinked fibrin by plasmin. **Top panel:** On fibrinogen, plasmin initially cleaves the C-terminal regions of the α and β chains within the D domain, releasing the Aα and Bβ fragments. In addition, a fragment containing fibrinopeptide B (FPB) from the N-terminal region of the β chain is released giving rise to the intermediate fragment known as "fragment X." Subsequently, plasmin cleaves the three connecting polypeptide chains connecting D and E domains, giving rise to fragments D, E, and Y. **Bottom panel:** Upon polymerizatoin by thrombin, fibrinogen forms fibrin. When degrading crosslinked fibrin, plasmin initially cleaves the C-terminal region of the α and β chains within the D domain. Subsequently, some of the connecting regions between the D and E domains are severed. Fibrin is ultimately solubilized upon hydrolysis of additional peptide bonds within the central portions of the coiled–coil connectors, giving rise to fibrin degradation products such as D-dimer. *(Reproduced with permission Nathan DG, Orkin SH, Ginsburg D, et al:* Hematology of Infancy and Childhood. *6th edition. Philadelphia, PA: WB Saunders; 2003.)*

carboxyl–terminal fragments from the α chain within the D domain of fibrinogen (Aα fragment).[205–208,215–218] Simultaneously, but more slowly, the N–terminal segments of the β chains are cleaved, releasing a peptide containing fibrinopeptide B. The resulting Mr approximately 250,000 molecule is termed fragment X and represents a clottable form of fibrinogen. Additional cleavage events may release the Bβ fragment from the β chain's carboxyl–terminus, and, in a series of subsequent reactions, plasmin cleaves the three polypeptide chains that connect the D and E domains giving rise to free D domain (Mr ~100,000) plus the binodular D–E fragment known as fragment Y (Mr ~150,000). Finally, domains D and E are separated from each other, and some of the N–terminal fibrinopeptide A sites on domain E are also modified. Although fragment X can be converted to fibrin by thrombin, the fragments Y, D, and E are all nonclottable, and, in fact, may inhibit polymerization of fibrinogen.[219]

Fibrin

Plasmin degradation of fibrin leads to a distinct set of molecular products (see Fig. 135–3).[220] Species similar to fragments Y, D, and E, but lacking fibrinopeptide sites, are released from noncrosslinked fibrin. If fibrin has been extensively crosslinked by factor XIII, however, the resulting D fragments are crosslinked to an E domain fragment. Assay of crosslinked D–dimer fragments is hemployed clinically to identify disseminated intravascular coagulation–like states associated with excessive plasmin–mediated fibrinolysis. Several biologic activities, including inhibition of platelet function,[221] potentiation of the hypotensive effects

of bradykinin,[222] chemotaxis,[223] and immune modulation,[224] have been ascribed to fibrin breakdown products.

TISSUE-TYPE PLASMINOGEN ACTIVATOR – MEDIATED PLASMINOGEN ACTIVATION

With or without fibrin, t-PA–mediated activation of Plg follows Michaelis–Menten kinetics.[22] In the absence of fibrin, t-PA is a weak activator of Plg. However, in the presence of fibrin, the catalytic efficiency (k_{cat}/K_m) of t-PA–dependent Plg activation is enhanced by approximately 500-fold. This is the basis for its specificity as a lytic agent in the treatment of thrombosis. The affinity between t-PA and Plg in the absence of fibrin is low (K_m 65 μM), but increases significantly in its presence (K_m 0.16 μM), even though the catalytic rate constant remains essentially unchanged (kcat ~0.05 sec^{-1}). When plasmin forms on the fibrin surface, both its lysine binding sites and its active site are occupied. Thus, it is relatively protected from its physiologic inhibitor, α_2-PI.[225]

The interaction of t-PA with fibrin is probably initiated by its "finger" domain. However, once fibrin is modified by plasmin, carboxy-terminal lysine residues are generated, and these become binding sites for "kringle" 2 of t-PA and "kringles" 1 and 4 of Plg.[226] Therefore, fibrin accelerates its own destruction by (1) enhancing the catalytic efficiency of plasmin formation by t-PA, (2) protecting plasmin from its physiologic inhibitor, α_2-PI, and (3) providing new binding sites for Plg and t-PA once its degradation has begun.

UROKINASE-TYPE PLASMINOGEN ACTIVATOR– MEDIATED PLASMIN GENERATION

For the activation of Glu–Plg by u-PA in a fibrin–free system, reported Michaelis constants (K_m) vary from 1.4 to 200 μM, while catalytic rate constants (kcat) range from 0.26 to 1.48 sec^{-1}.[1] Interestingly, activation of Glu–Plg by two–chain u-PA is increased in the presence of fibrin by approximately 10–fold even though u-PA does not bind to fibrin.[227] In contrast, single-chain u-PA has considerable fibrin–specificity. This may reflect neutralization by fibrin of components in plasma that impair Plg[74] also reflect a conformational change in Plg upon binding to fibrin.[228] It is important to recognize, however, that the intrinsic Plg activating potential of single-chain u-PA is less than 1 percent of that of two-chain u-PA. Two–chain u-PA has been used effectively as a thrombolytic agent for many years.[229]

● THE NONFIBRINOLYTIC ACTIONS OF PLASMIN

PLASMIN AS A TISSUE REMODELER

A large number of *in vitro* studies suggest a role for plasmin in tissue remodeling. Basement membrane proteins such as thrombospondin,[230] laminin,[231] fibronectin,[232] and fibrinogen,[233] are readily degraded by plasmin *in vitro,* suggesting possible roles in inflammation,[234] tumor cell invasion,[235] embryogenesis,[236] ovulation,[237] neurodevelopment,[238,239] and prohormone activation.[240,241] Plasmin also activates MMPs 3 and 13 in the mouse, thereby facilitating the degradation of matrix proteins such as the collagens, laminin, fibronectin, vitronectin, elastin, aggrecan, and tenascin C.[242] On the other hand, activation of other MMPs apparently proceeds in the absence of Plg, possibly providing the basis for the mild phenotype observed in Plg-null homozygote animals.[80]

Roles for plasmin in tissue remodeling and host defense mechanisms are further supported by *in vivo* observations in Plg-deficient mice (see Table 135–2). Impaired wound healing is observed in the Plg "knockout,"[243] and is reversed upon simultaneous deletion of fibrinogen.[244] Plg-deficient mice also display diminished recruitment of monocytes in response to intraperitoneal thioglycolate,[245] and impaired neointima formation following electrical injury to blood vessels.[246] In studies involving *Borrelia burgdorferi,* the agent of Lyme disease, dissemination of the spirochete within its arthropod vector *Ixodes dammini* is absolutely dependent upon host Plg even though the deer tick contains no fibrin.[247] Furthermore, kainate-induced excitotoxicity and attendant neuronal cell dropout in the hippocampus is not observed in Plg knockout mice but does occur in fibrinogen-deficient animals.[248] The latter two studies may define new roles for plasmin, which appear to be unrelated to degradation of fibrin.

In the lung, the fibrinolytic system mediates lung matrix remodeling, through mechanisms that appear to be independent of fibrin degradation.[249] In mice, deficiency of fibrinogen has no effect on the development of bleomycin-induced pulmonary fibrosis.[250] Mice lacking either PAI-1 or TAFI are protected from lung fibrosis in the same model,[251–253] whereas inducible expression of u-PA within alveoli abrogates the fibrotic response.[254]

Plasmin may play a role in the activation of growth factors. TGF-β is a Mr 25,000 homodimeric polypeptide that regulates vascular cell responses and epithelial-mesenchymal transformation in development and in tissue fibrosis.[255,256] In culture, cell–associated plasmin appears to convert latent TGF-β to its physiologically relevant active state. Inhibition of wound healing in this system was dependent upon active TGF-β, and activation of this agent could be blocked in the presence of plasmin inhibitors such as aprotinin or α_2-PI. Activation of TGF-β by plasmin

may reflect alteration of its tertiary structure upon cleavage of an aminoterminal glycopeptide.[257] Once activated by plasmin, TGF-β can stimulate production of PAI-1, thus impairing further activation of Plg.

The role of the fibrinolytic system in vascular remodeling during atherosclerosis appears to be complex.[258] In the evolution of an injury to the endothelial cell lining of blood vessels, deposition of intravascular fibrin and organization of a thrombus occurs.[259] As the injury resolves, fibrin participates in plaque growth and luminal narrowing. Evidence of the importance of fibrinolytic balance in this process is that, in the absence of PAI-1, there is less neointima formation and reduced luminal stenosis, possibly because of more rapid resolution of fibrin.[260] In areas of the vasculature where injury is not associated with fibrin deposition, however, absence of PAI-1 may lead to enhanced lesion formation, as cells that invade the developing plaque may require plasmin activity for their directed migration.[261]

FIBRINOLYSIS AND ANGIOGENESIS

Although the fibrinolytic system has generally been assumed to be proangiogenic by virtue of its ability to promote "tunneling" of endothelial cells through fibrin-containing matrices, its effect, in actuality, appears to be context specific.[262,263] PAI-1 deficiency in mice, for example, seems to prevent tumor vascularization in a malignant keratinocyte model.[264] The same mice are also resistant to laser-induced neovascularization of the choroid.[265,266] The paradoxical proangiogenic effect of PAI-1 in some settings may relate to its ability to protect endothelial cells from apoptosis mediated by FasL, which is activated by plasmin.[267]

In the mouse cornea, absence of t-PA, u-PA, or TAFI, had no effect on neovascularization, whereas loss of Plg, PAI-1, or annexin A2 significantly diminished this response.[205,268] Within the atherosclerotic plaque, moreover, expression of a truncated form of PAI-1 (rPAI-1$_{23}$) was antiangiogenic, inhibiting the proliferation of vasa vasorum, and reducing overall plaque area and plaque cholesterol in the descending aorta.[269] As a gene product that is transcriptionally upregulated by hypoxia, annexin A2 is required for the normal corneal angiogenic response to growth factor stimulation, and also for hypoxia-induced retinal angiogenesis.[198,205,270]

● DISORDERS OF PLASMIN GENERATION

FIBRINOLYTIC DEFICIENCY AND THROMBOSIS

Although partial human Plg deficiency was first described in a young man with a history of venous thrombosis and pulmonary embolism,[271] there is currently little evidence that hypoplasminogenemia alone is a significant cause of deep venous thrombosis.[272] In a study of 23 consecutive patients with thrombophilia, the prevalence of Plg deficiency was only 1.9 percent.[273] Approximately half of these individuals had other risk factors such as deficiency of antithrombin, protein C, or protein S, or resistance to activated protein C. Among 93 patients with type I Plg deficiency, the prevalence of thrombosis was 24 percent, or 9 percent when the propositi were excluded.[274] Two additional epidemiologic studies concluded, moreover, that isolated hypoplasminogenemia is not a risk factor for thrombosis.[275,276]

Although there are no reported cases of complete absence of Plg in humans, a large number of Plg polymorphisms and dysplasminogenemias have been reported.[272] Congenital Plg deficiency has been classified into two types: in type I the concentration of immunoreactive Plg is reduced in parallel with functional activity,[277] whereas in type II (dysplasminogenemia), immunoreactive protein is normal while functional activity is reduced.[278] Patients with type I Plg deficiency are most likely to present with ligneous conjunctivitis, which resolves completely upon infusion of Lys-Plg.[279,280] In a study of a Japanese cohort, approximately 27 percent of individuals with type II deficiency had a clinical history of thrombosis, but it is not clear whether there were other explanations for thrombophilia in these individuals.[281] Acquired Plg deficiency may occur in liver disease, sepsis, and Argentine hemorrhagic fever due to decreased synthesis and/or increased catabolism,[282] but associated thrombosis may be due to abnormalities in other hemostatic factors in these very ill patients. Similarly, there are no reported cases of complete t-PA or u-PA deficiency in humans, and no mutations or polymorphisms in these genes have so far been clinically linked to thrombophilia. Defects in Plg activator release, as well as increased inhibition of t-PA by PAI-1, have been reported in associated with thrombosis,[283,284] and with chronic renal disease and hypertension.[81,83]

Global deficiency in fibrinolytic function, moreover, is associated with increased risk for venous thrombosis, as well as first myocardial infarction in young men.[285,286] Increased circulating PAI-1 appears to represent an independent risk factor for vascular reocclusion in young survivors of myocardial infarction.[287] In addition, increased levels of PAI-1 have been associated with deep vein thrombosis in patients undergoing hip replacement surgery[288] and in individuals with insulin resistance.[289] Although a 4G versus 5G polymorphism in the PAI-1 promoter has been reported, the 4G form being associated with higher PAI-1 plasma levels, it is not yet established as to whether this allele correlates with elevated thrombotic risk.[290,291] With regard to such studies, one should bear in mind that PAI-1 is itself an acute phase reactant, and thus may not be directly responsible for the observed prothrombotic tendency.[292]

ENHANCED FIBRINOLYSIS AND BLEEDING

Enhanced fibrinolysis resulting from congenital or acquired loss of fibrinolytic inhibitor activity may be associated with a bleeding diathesis.[293] Patients with congenital deficiency of α_2-PI may present with a severe hemorrhagic disorder as a result of impaired inactivation of plasmin and premature lysis of the hemostatic plug.[294] Acquired α_2-PI deficiency may be seen in patients with severe liver disease from decreased synthesis, disseminated intravascular coagulation from consumption, nephrotic syndrome from urinary losses, or during thrombolytic therapy, which induces excessive utilization of the inhibitor.[294] TAFI levels are markedly reduced in liver cirrhosis, correlating with enhanced plasma fibrinolysis, and serving as an independent predictor of mortality.[295]

Patients with acute promyelocytic leukemia demonstrate excessive expression of annexin A2 on their developmentally arrested promyelocytes. Bleeding in this disorder is accompanied by evidence of high levels of plasmin generation and depletion of α_2-PI. Bleeding resolves upon initiation of all-*trans*-retinoic acid therapy, which eliminates expression of promyelocyte annexin A2, probably through a transcriptional mechanism.[181] In this setting, A2 acts most likely in concert with S100A10, which is also upregulated in an acute promyelocytic leukemia (APL) cell line.[201,296]

Complete loss of PAI-1 expression resulting in hemorrhage in a 9-year-old child was associated with severe hemorrhage in the setting of trauma or surgery.[297] This autosomal recessive trait reflected a frameshift mutation within exon 4 that induced a premature stop codon. This case demonstrates that PAI-1 is a central regulator of fibrinolysis in humans.

DEVELOPMENTAL REGULATION OF THE FIBRINOLYTIC SYSTEM

In the resting, nonstressed state, the plasmin–generating potential in the newborn is significantly less than that of the adult.[298,299] Although

the amino acid composition and apparent molecular mass of neonatal Plg are indistinguishable from those of the adult protein,[300,301] plasma concentrations of Plg in the neonate are approximately 50 to 75 percent of those observed in adults.[300,302,303] On the other hand, levels of histidine-rich glycoprotein, a carrier protein that may limit Plg's interaction with fibrin, are also reduced by 50 to 80 percent in healthy, term newborns.[304] Neonatal Plg is heavily glycosylated, less readily activated by t-PA, and only weakly bound to the endothelial cell surface.[301] Throughout childhood, global plasma fibrinolytic activity and plasmin generation are decreased in comparison to adults, and this relative deficiency may contribute to the high frequency of thrombosis associated with central venous line placement, Kawasaki disease, and Henoch-Schönlein purpura in this age group.[305]

Although t-PA antigen and activity levels are reduced by 50 to 75 percent compared with adult values throughout childhood,[303] stressed infants, such as those with severe congenital heart disease or respiratory distress syndrome, may have t-PA antigen levels that are increased by up to eightfold because of the t-PA release response.[306,307] In contrast, the principal plasmin inhibitors undergo only minimal change from birth to adulthood.[302,308–310] Thus, reduced fibrinolytic activity may contribute to the thrombogenic state commonly observed in the newborn,[311] but this predilection may be reversed under conditions of physiologic stress.

FIBRINOLYTIC ACTIVITY DURING PREGNANCY AND PUERPERIUM

Pregnancy is a hypofibrinolytic state.[312–314] Both Plg and fibrinogen levels in plasma increase by 50 to 60 percent in the third trimester. However, overall fibrinolytic activity, as reflected in euglobulin lysis activity, is reduced, and increased fibrin deposition is suggested by increasing D-dimer levels throughout pregnancy.[315] Between the 20th week of pregnancy and term, PAI-1 levels increase to three times their normal level, while PAI-2 levels rise to 25 times their level in early pregnancy.[312] Less dramatic increases in both u-PA and t-PA levels are also observed. Within 1 hour of delivery, however, concentrations of both PAI-1 and PAI-2 begin to decrease, and return to normal within 3 to 5 days.[312]

In preeclampsia, the hemostatic and fibrinolytic imbalances seen in pregnancy are further exaggerated.[316] Circulating PAI-1 levels exceed those in normal pregnancy, and fibrin deposition is seen in the glomerular capillaries and spiral arteries of the placenta. Interestingly, levels of PAI-2, a marker of placental function, are reduced during preeclampsia compared with normal pregnancy, and this decrease correlates with intrauterine growth retardation of the fetus. Elevated TAFI levels may be a cause of fibrin deposition and occlusion of placental vessels in preeclampsia.[317]

● FIBRINOLYTIC THERAPY

The goal of thrombolytic therapy is rapid restoration of flow to an occluded vessel achieved by accelerating fibrinolytic proteolysis of the thrombus.[318] The fibrinolytic system functions physiologically to remove fibrin deposits through the action of plasmin, but this is often too slow to prevent tissue injury following acute vascular occlusion. Because arterial thrombosis immediately renders distal tissue ischemic with rapid onset of dysfunction and necrosis, a critical problem is minimizing time to restoration of flow. Thrombolytic therapy should be viewed as one part of an overall antithrombotic plan that frequently includes anticoagulants, antiplatelet agents, and mechanical approaches, all designed to rapidly restore flow, prevent reocclusion, and promote healing. Here we review thrombolytic approaches to stroke and peripheral vascular disease. Thrombolytic therapy for deep vein thrombosis, pulmonary embolism, and myocardial infarction are discussed elsewhere.

PRINCIPLES OF THERAPY

The basic principle of all fibrinolytic therapy is administration of sufficient Plg activator to achieve a high local concentration at the site of the thrombus, thereby accelerating conversion of Plg to plasmin, and increasing the rate of fibrin dissolution. However, if large amounts of Plg activator overwhelm the natural regulatory systems, plasmin may be formed in the blood, resulting in degradation of susceptible proteins, the "lytic state."[319] In addition, if high concentrations of activator reach fibrin deposits at sites of injury, bleeding, often exacerbated by plasmic proteolysis of other proteins in the blood may ensue.

Several therapeutic agents, from both recombinant and natural sources, are available and approved for thrombolytic use (Table 135–3). The degree of "fibrin specificity," is critical in determining the intensity of action at the site of a thrombus. The plasma half-life of most agents is short, ranging, for example, from 5 to 70 minutes for t-PA and anistreplase, respectively. Decisions to administer by bolus versus continuous infusion, as well as the duration of therapy, are determined by the agent's half-life and the condition being treated. Regarding site of delivery, systemic therapy via peripheral vein is simpler and does not require specialized facilities, but results in greater systemic complications. Regional delivery with a catheter placed close to the proximal end of the thrombus can provide a high local concentration with a smaller total dose, thereby increasing the local effect and limiting systemic exposure. Fibrinolytic therapy is often administered in combination with an anticoagulant to block fibrin formation and with an antiplatelet agent to limit continued platelet deposition. Anticoagulant therapy is routinely continued after completion of fibrinolytic therapy to prevent reocclusion. In addition, mechanical approaches such as percutaneous coronary intervention often play a vital role in removing the underlying cause of thrombosis.

The activation of plasmin has effects beyond the thrombus, including a reduction in fibrinogen, increase in fibrinogen degradation products, and depletion of Plg and α_2-plasmin inhibitor. Screening coagulation tests, including the activated partial thromboplastin time (aPTT), prothrombin time (PT), and thrombin clotting time, will be prolonged depending on the intensity of the lytic state. Tests reflecting Plg activation, such as the euglobulin clot lysis time, will be abnormal. Platelet membrane proteins may also be degraded, resulting in abnormal platelet function.[320–322] Overall, these effects contribute to a hypocoagulable lytic state that may be beneficial for vessel patency, but may also exacerbate a bleeding complication. High doses of a nonspecific activator, such as streptokinase, will cause a more marked lytic state, compared to that seen with a fibrin-specific agent such as reteplase.

Patient selection for fibrinolytic therapy depends on careful consideration of risks and benefits (Table 135–4). For patients with acute myocardial infarction or stroke there is a higher tolerance of bleeding complications, because lytic therapy can be lifesaving and limit disability. Timing of treatment is also critical, with greater benefit achieved with earlier administration. Whereas fibrinolytic therapy for acute pulmonary embolism may be lifesaving, the potential benefits for venous disease are less clear and more likely to be associated with bleeding problems.

THROMBOLYTIC THERAPY FOR STROKE

Stroke is the third leading cause of death, and the leading cause of serious disability in the United States.[323] Its incidence has been declining in

TABLE 135–3. Comparison of Plasminogen Activators

Agent (Regimen)	Source (Approved)	Antigenic	Half-Life (min)
Streptokinase (infusion)	Streptococcus (Y)	Yes	20
Urokinase (infusion)	Cell culture; recombinant (Y)	No	15
Alteplase (t-PA) (infusion)	Recombinant (Y)	No	5
Anistreplase (bolus)	Streptococcus + plasma product (Y)	No	70
Reteplase (double bolus)	Recombinant (Y)	No	15
Saruplase (scu-PA) (infusion)	Recombinant (N)	No	5
Staphylokinase (infusion)	Recombinant (N)	Yes	
Tenecteplase (bolus)	Recombinant (Y)	No	15

N, no; scu-PA, single chain urokinase-type plasminogen activator; t-PA, tissue-type plasminogen activator; Y, yes.

TABLE 135–4. Selection of Patients for Thrombolytic Therapy

Treat those most likely to respond and benefit
  Acute MI: Within 12 hours of onset; consider percutaneous intervention
  Stroke: Ischemic stroke within 4.5 hours of symptom onset
  Peripheral arterial obstruction
    Acute occlusions
    Distal obstruction not correctable by surgery
  Deep vein thrombosis
    Large proximal thrombi with symptoms for less than 7 days (Chap. 134)
  Pulmonary embolism
    Massive or submassive embolism, especially with hemodynamic compromise
Avoid bleeding complications
  Major contraindications
    Risk of intracranial bleeding
    Recent head trauma or central nervous system surgery
    History of stroke or subarachnoid bleed
    Intracranial metastatic disease
  Risk of major bleeding
    Active gastrointestinal or genitourinary bleeding
    Major surgery or trauma within 7 days
    Dissecting aneurysm
  Relative contraindications
    Remote history of gastrointestinal bleeding
    Remote history of genitourinary bleeding
    Remote history of peptic ulcer
    Other lesion with potential for bleeding
    Recent minor surgery or trauma
    Severe, uncontrolled hypertension
    Coexisting hemostatic abnormalities
    Pregnancy

recent years due to control of risk factors, but total numbers are increasing as a consequence of aging of the population. Although aspirin and anticoagulants may be useful in prevention, thrombolytic therapy is the only available intervention during the acute stage.

The appropriate use of thrombolytic therapy for stroke is based on an understanding of its pathogenesis. Ischemic stroke is most commonly caused by rupture of an atherosclerotic plaque within a large or medium-sized artery in the neck or cranium. In addition, transient ischemic attacks (TIAs) and strokes involving small arteries can result from embolization of platelet-fibrin thrombi that form on atherosclerotic vessels in the neck and ascending aorta, or from embolization of thrombi that form in the heart in association with atrial fibrillation, valve dysfunction, artificial valves, or endocardial thrombi. Up to 30 percent of strokes have no defined etiology.

Current approaches to thrombolytic therapy for stroke are based on imaging to define the etiology, results of clinical trials, and the experience with thrombolysis for acute myocardial infarction. Modern computed tomography (CT) imaging and magnetic resonance imaging (MRI) can identify ischemic areas and localize areas of hemorrhage quite early. Additionally, arteriography can identify obstructed vessels and follow the course of recanalization during thrombolytic therapy. Clinical studies have generally followed the successful designs used for myocardial infarction that demonstrated the critical pathologic role of the occluded vessel, the importance of early recanalization in preserving myocardium, and the impressive decrease in morbidity and mortality resulting from early reperfusion. They have also characterized the bleeding risk.

The experience with thrombolytic treatment for stroke also highlights important differences from myocardial infarction. The arterial anatomy of the brain is more complex, the time from onset of ischemia to irreversible necrosis is shorter, the risk and consequences of bleeding are greater, and there is more variability in the thrombo(embolic) occluding lesion. Further, the occlusive platelet-fibrin thrombus that precipitates a myocardial infarction is quite small, whereas the occlusive lesion causing ischemic stroke may be a large *in situ* thrombus, small platelet-fibrin embolus, or large embolus of varying age and composition originating from the left atrium. Thrombolysis has had a smaller impact for stroke than it has for myocardial infarction, based largely on these differences.

Early Thrombolytic Studies

The current therapeutic approach began with small, open-label studies that used intravenous or intraarterial streptokinase, urokinase, and t-PA to determine dose, recanalization rate, hemorrhagic potential, and clinical predictors of response.[324-339] These studies demonstrated that recanalization could be achieved, that early treatment was essential, and that the rate of intracranial hemorrhage and hemorrhagic transformation within the ischemic area was high. Phase II studies defined the optimum dosage and time window for intravenous t-PA and served as the basis for larger phase III trials that led to the current t-PA-based approach to thrombolytic therapy for stroke (Table 135–5). At present, the only FDA-approved therapy for acute stroke is intravenous alteplase (recombinant t-PA) given within 3 hours of symptom onset.

Tissue Plasminogen Activator Therapy

The National Institute of Neurological Disorders and Stroke (NINDS) Study was a two-part randomized, double-blind, placebo-controlled study[340] to test whether t-PA improved clinical outcome at 24 hours and 3 months. All patients were treated within 3 hours of symptom onset with a total dose of 0.9 mg/kg of t-PA. The combined results showed a

TABLE 135–5. Major Fibrinolytic Therapy Trials in Stroke

Study	No. of Patients	Time	Drug	Thrombolytic Dose*[†]	Main Efficacy Result
NINDS	624	≤3 h	t-PA, IV	0.9 mg/kg	Reduced disability at 3 months
ECASS I	620	≤6 h	t-PA, IV	1.1 mg/kg	No significant difference
ECASS II	800	≤6 h	t-PA, IV	0.9 mg/kg	No significant difference
ECASS III	821	3–4.5 h	t-PA, IV	0.9 mg/kg	Improved outcome at 3 months
ATLANTIS	613	≤6 h[‡]	t-PA, IV	0.9 mg/kg	No significant difference
SITS-ISTR[#]	11,865 vs. 664	≤3 vs. 3–4.5 h	t-PA, IV	0.9 mg/kg	No significant difference
ASK	340	≤4 h	SK, IV	1.5 million units	Increased morbidity and mortality
MAST-I	622	≤6 h	SK, IV[¶]	1.5 million units	Increased mortality
MAST-II	310	≤6 h	SK, IV[§]	1.5 million units	Increased mortality
PROACT II	180	≤6 h	pro-UK,[‖] IA	9 mg	Improved 3-month outcome
MELT	114	≤6 h	u-PA, IA	variable[<]	No significant difference in favorable outcome; significant difference in excellent functional outcome

ASK, Australian Streptokinase; ATLANTIS, Alteplase Thrombolysis for Acute Noninterventional Therapy in Ischemic Stroke; ECASS, European Cooperative Acute Stroke Study; IA, intraarterial; MAST, Multicentre Acute Stroke Trial; MELT, The Middle Cerebral Artery Embolism Local Fibrinolytic Intervention Trial; NINDS, National Institute of Neurological Disorders and Stroke; Pro-UK, pro-urokinase; PROACT II, Prolyse in Acute Cerebral Thromboembolism II; SITS-ISTR, Safe Implementation of Treatments in Stroke—International Stroke Thrombolysis Registry; SK, streptokinase; t-PA, tissue-type plasminogen activator; u-PA, urokinase plasminogen activator.

*All placebo controlled.

[†]All given over 1 h except PROACT II, which was 2 h.

[‡]547/613 within 3–5 h.

[#]Observational study without placebo arm.

[¶]2 × 2 factorial design with acetylsalicylic acid (ASA) 300 mg/day.

[§]Acetylsalicylic acid (ASA) 100 mg/day.

[‖]Pro-UK and placebo group also received heparin.

[<]Mean doses of u-PA in patients with good and poor outcome were 555,000 IU and 789,000 IU.

30 percent improvement in clinical outcomes at 3 months and the benefit persisted at 12 months, despite a 10-fold increase in early symptomatic intracranial hemorrhage. At 3 months, there was no difference in mortality between the groups. This study formed the basis of the approval by the FDA of intravenous t-PA for stroke in 1996.

Early randomized trials of IV t-PA did not show clear benefit for patients treated beyond 3 hours after stroke onset. In the European Cooperative Acute Stroke Study (ECASS) Study, subjects with moderate to severe symptoms were randomized to placebo or t-PA within 6 hours of symptom onset[341]; results showed no significant difference in either the primary end point of functional status at 90 days or in 30-day mortality. In the ECASS II, in which patients were randomized and stratified for presentation up to 3 hours after symptom onset or between 3 and 6 hours, there was no significant benefit of thrombolytic therapy using the primary end point of functional capacity of 90 days.[342] The Alteplase Thrombolysis for Acute Noninterventional Therapy in Ischemic Stroke (ATLANTIS) Study evaluated the safety of recombinant t-PA (rt-PA) in a double-blind, placebo controlled study with administration of drug between 3 and 5 hours after symptom onset,[343] and the primary end point of excellent neurological recovery was observed in 32 percent of placebo and 34 percent of rt-PA–treated patients. Early symptomatic intracranial hemorrhage occurred in 1.1 percent of control and 7.0 percent of rt-PA–treated patients. There was a nonsignificant trend toward increased mortality with rt-PA treatment at 90 days (6.9 percent vs. 11.0 percent, p = 0.09). A meta-analysis pooling data from NINDS, ATLANTIS, and ECASS II patients who received either alteplase or placebo within 6 hours showed that the odds of a favorable 3-month outcome decreased as the interval from stroke onset to the start of alteplase treatment increased. Furthermore, the study alluded to the potential benefit of extending the treatment window to 4.5 hours with favorable but decreasing odds ratio for alteplase treatment beyond 3 hours.[344]

The benefit of IV t-PA for treatment beyond the 3-hour window was established by the ECASS III trial.[345] This study showed that IV t-PA treatment initiated at 3 to 4.5 hours after ischemic stroke onset led to a modest improvement in the 3-month outcome. More patients had a favorable outcome with t-PA than with placebo (52.4 percent vs. 45.2 percent; odds ratio: 1.34; 95 percent CI 1.02 to 1.76). While the incidence of intracranial hemorrhage was higher with t-PA treatment (2.4 percent vs. 0.2 percent; p = 0.008), there was no difference in mortality between the two groups.

The effect of alteplase given beyond 3 hours after stroke on infarct growth and reperfusion was studied in the Echoplanar Imaging Thrombolytic Evaluation Trial (EPITHET) trial.[346] Alteplase was shown to be significantly associated with increased reperfusion in patients who had mismatch at baseline (p = 0.001), better neurologic outcome (p <0.0001), and better functional outcome (p = 0.010). The observational Safe Implementation of Treatment in Stroke International Stroke Thrombolysis Register (SITS-ISTR) study further supported the safety of administering IV t-PA between 3 and 4.5 hours after acute ischemic stroke.[347,348] Compared to patients treated within less than 3 hours (n = 11,865), those treated at 3 to 4.5 hours (n = 664) had similar rates of independence, symptomatic intracranial hemorrhage, and mortality. An updated pooled analysis of ECASS, ATLANTIS, NINDS, and EPITHET trials continues to demonstrate that patients with ischemic stroke, selected by clinical symptoms and CT, benefit from intravenous alteplase when treated no later than 4.5 hours.[349]

Streptokinase Therapy

Streptokinase has been evaluated in three large stroke trials. The Australian Streptokinase (ASK) study showed an increase in death rate at 90 days in streptokinase-treated patients, and the study was prematurely terminated.[350] The Multicentre Acute Stroke Trial–Italy (MAST-I) study examined benefits and risks of streptokinase treatment with or without aspirin in patients with acute ischemic stroke who presented within 6 hours of symptom onset.[351] An interim analysis resulted in early termination because streptokinase treatment was associated with a 2.7-fold increase in fatality at 10 days among patients receiving both streptokinase and aspirin. In the Multicenter Acute Stroke Trial-Europe (MAST-E) trial, the mortality rate at 10 days was higher in patients who received streptokinase (34.0 percent) compared with placebo (18.2 percent, p <0.02) primarily because of hemorrhagic transformation of infarcts.[352]

Tenecteplase Therapy

Tenecteplase is a genetically modified and genetically engineered recombinant t-PA; it has a higher fibrin specificity and greater resistance to inactivation by its endogenous inhibitor (PAI-1) compared to native t-PA. In a phase IIB study, there were no significant differences in intracranial bleeding or other serious adverse events in patients receiving alteplase versus tenecteplase.[353] However, the two tenecteplase groups had greater reperfusion (p = 0.004) and clinical improvement (p <0.001) at 24 hours compared with the alteplase group. The study outcome supports ongoing phase II–III trials of tenecteplase versus alteplase in the time window that is currently approved for stroke thrombolysis (NCT01472926 and NCT01949948).

Intraarterial Thrombolysis

Intraarterial administration allows delivery of a high concentration of a Plg activator in proximity to the thrombus, more accurate anatomic diagnosis, the ability to observe the course of recanalization, and lower total doses of drug that might reduce intracranial hemorrhage. On the other hand, this approach requires specialized facilities and experienced personnel to perform arteriography and selective catheterization, which may delay treatment. Several small open-label trials observed a high rate of recanalization and apparent clinical benefit with intraarterial therapy using urokinase, streptokinase or t-PA, but hemorrhagic transformation was a frequent problem.[327,331,334,337,354-360]

The Prolyse in Acute Cerebral Thromboembolism (PROACT) and PROACT II trials evaluated recombinant human prourokinase by catheter-directed intraarterial administration.[361,362] In the PROACT trial, a significantly higher recanalization rate was observed with prourokinase treatment with no increase in intracranial hemorrhage. This led to the larger PROACT II trial, which revealed a significantly higher recanalization rate with prourokinase (66 percent vs. 18 percent, p <0.001), and superior functional improvement at 90 days.[363,364] Symptomatic intracranial hemorrhage occurred in 10 percent of patients treated with prourokinase and 2 percent of controls. Although promising, these results did not lead to FDA approval of intraarterial prourokinase for treatment of stroke.

A third study, the Middle Cerebral Artery Embolism Local Fibrinolytic Intervention Trial (MELT), was underpowered because of premature study closure.[365] A favorable, but not statistically significant, outcome at 90 days was more likely with intraarterial urokinase compared with placebo. The proportion of patients with an excellent functional outcome was significantly better in the intraarterial urokinase group (42 percent vs. 23 percent, p = 0.045). Intracerebral hemorrhage within 24 hours of treatment occurred in 9 percent and 2 percent, respectively (p = 0.206). This study suggested that intraarterial fibrinolysis has the potential to increase the likelihood of excellent functional outcome in appropriate clinical settings.

Overall, these studies show that treatment of acute stroke with thrombolytic therapy can lead to recanalization of the occluded artery and improvement in clinical outcomes. The need for early treatment, which improves outcome, is currently the single largest limitation to greater application of thrombolytic therapy for stroke, and less than 5 percent of stroke patients currently receive t-PA treatment, indicating the need for focused community educational efforts.[366-368] Randomized studies with rt-PA have shown that intravenous thrombolytic therapy can be safely extended to 4.5 hours after symptom onset in selected patients, whereas streptokinase was associated with an unacceptably high rate of intracranial hemorrhage.[344,345,347] In addition, intracranial hemorrhage can be reduced by identifying patients at greatest risk using MRI diffusion–perfusion mismatch to identify reversible ischemia.[346,369-371] The combination of potent antiplatelet therapy using a glycoprotein IIb/IIIa antagonist with a lower dose of a thrombolytic agent may improve results.[372-377]

In summary, current recommendations limit thrombolytic therapy for stroke to patients presenting within 3 hours of symptom onset.[378-380] The approved therapy is with 0.9 mg/kg (maximum: 90 mg) of t-PA administered intravenously with 10 percent as an initial bolus and the remainder infused over 60 minutes. The best results are obtained in patients who meet strict eligibility requirements (Table 135-6). Patients should be closely monitored for bleeding complications, especially intracranial hemorrhage, and careful attention should be paid to blood pressure and other comorbidities.

PERIPHERAL VASCULAR DISEASE

Acute peripheral arterial occlusion presents with the sudden onset of new, severe leg symptoms or acute worsening of chronic ischemia, and often involves embolic or thrombotic occlusion of leg arteries. The goals of treatment are to preserve limb function through restoration of flow.

TABLE 135–6. Guidelines for Tissue-Type Plasminogen Activator Therapy in Stroke

Eligibility

Time from symptom onset to therapy ≤3 hours

Results from European Cooperative Acute Stroke Study (ECASS) III trial suggest treatment within 4.5 h of onset is beneficial

Exclusions

Prior intracranial hemorrhage

Major surgery within 14 days

Gastrointestinal or urinary tract bleeding with 21 days

Arterial puncture in noncompressible site

Recent lumbar puncture

Intracranial surgery, serious head trauma, or prior stroke within 3 months

Minor neurologic deficit

Seizure at time of stroke onset

Clinical findings of subarachnoid hemorrhage

Active bleeding

Persistent systolic blood pressure (BP) >185 and/or diastolic BP >110 or requiring aggressive treatment

Arteriovenous malformation or aneurysm

Evidence of hemorrhage on computed tomography scan

Platelets <100,000/μL

International normalized ratio >1.5 on warfarin

Elevated partial thromboplastin time on heparin

Blood glucose <40 or >400 mg/dL

ECASS III additionally excluded patients >80 years old, patients with a combination of previous stroke and diabetes mellitus, and patients with an National Institutes of Health Stroke Scale score of >25.

Anticoagulation is useful to prevent thrombus extension, while thrombolytic therapy or surgery can restore perfusion.

Early approaches to acute peripheral arterial occlusion involved streptokinase. Several small studies demonstrated reperfusion in approximately 40 percent of patients, with greatest success when occlusions were recent; bleeding complications occurred in up to one-third of subjects.[381] Following the report in 1974 by Dotter[382] of successful thrombolysis in peripheral arterial occlusion using locally administered thrombolysis, practice moved progressively to the nearly exclusive use of local intraarterially administered treatment. Advantages include delivery of a high concentration of drug directly to the site of thrombosis, the ability to follow the course of treatment using the treatment catheter, and identification of local vascular lesions requiring endovascular or surgical treatment after recanalization.

Treatment involves arterial access from a remote site followed by fluoroscopic guidance of the catheter to administer drug directly into the thrombus. Therapy is delivered by continuous infusion over hours to days and requires close monitoring and a large dose of thrombolytic agent. Successful reperfusion occurs in approximately three-quarters of cases.[383] Ouriel and colleagues[384] reported that thrombolytic therapy resulted in a 70 percent recanalization rate, and a frequency of limb salvage that mirrored that of operative intervention. There was, however, a survival advantage in patients receiving primary thrombolytic therapy resulting primarily from a decrease in the occurrence of in-hospital complications. The Surgery versus Thrombolysis for Ischemia of the Lower Extremity (STILE) trial, which compared the optimal surgical procedure to catheter directed thrombolysis with either t-PA or urokinase, was terminated prematurely because of ongoing or recurrent ischemia at 30 days in surgically treated patients.[385] More than half of patients receiving thrombolysis had a decrease in the magnitude of the surgical procedure eventually required, with significant reductions in the 1-year rate of major amputation. In addition, there was no difference in outcome with t-PA versus urokinase.

The Thrombolysis or Peripheral Arterial Surgery (TOPAS) I study compared recombinant urokinase or surgery for initial therapy of acute lower-extremity ischemia of less than 14 days duration.[386] The 1-year mortality and amputation-free survival were similar in the urokinase and surgery groups. There was a significant reduction in the frequency and magnitude of surgical interventions eventually required in patients randomized to initial thrombolysis. The larger TOPAS II study showed recanalization in 80 percent of patients who received urokinase.[387] Amputation-free survival at 1 year was not significantly different between the surgical and thrombolysis groups, 70 percent and 65 percent, respectively. Major hemorrhagic complications were significantly more frequent with urokinase (13 percent) compared to 6 percent with surgery (p = 0.005).

In other studies, reteplase appears to be equally effective as t-PA or urokinase with comparable recanalization rates, and clinical outcomes and bleeding complications.[388,389] Prourokinase also gave similar overall results to urokinase in a phase II study.[390] In an open-label trial, staphylokinase, a highly fibrin-specific Plg activator, resulted in revascularization in 83 percent of subjects with occluded arteries.[391] Occasional allergic reactions occurred, and severe bleeding complications were comparable to those with other agents. The addition of abciximab, a glycoprotein IIb/IIIa, inhibitor, to urokinase resulted in more rapid clot like lysis in a randomized study,[392] and good results were also reported with reteplase and abciximab.[393] Intraoperative thrombolysis during thromboembolectomy has been used successfully to improve clearance of distal thromboemboli with or without adjunctive mechanical thrombectomy.[394-398]

Thrombolysis should be viewed as one part of a combined, comprehensive management approach to peripheral arterial occlusion.

Key points include early, accurate angiographic diagnosis, appropriate intrathrombic catheter positioning, and, in some cases, definitive endovascular or surgical procedures.[399-402] Evidence favors mechanical thromboembolectomy as adjunctive therapy for acute limb ischemia resulting from peripheral arterial occlusion.[403]

OTHER INDICATIONS

Thrombolytic therapy has been useful in treating acute venous and arterial occlusions in a wide variety of sites. Reports document successful treatment of intraabdominal thrombosis including Budd-Chiari Syndrome,[404] portal vein thrombosis,[405-407] and mesenteric vein thrombosis.[407-409] Thrombolytic agents are frequently used to open thrombosed central venous catheters,[410-413] as well as access devices for hemodialysis.[414-418]

MANAGEMENT OF BLEEDING COMPLICATIONS

Bleeding complications are more frequent with fibrinolytic than with anticoagulant therapy and require rapid diagnosis and management. The most serious complication, intracranial hemorrhage, occurs in approximately 1 percent of patients and is associated with a high mortality and serious disability in survivors. Risk factors for intracranial hemorrhage, including prior stroke, serious head trauma, intracranial surgery, tumor or vascular disease such as aneurysms or arteriovenous malformation and uncontrolled hypertension, are strong contraindications to fibrinolytic therapy.[419] Bleeding is most common at sites of invasive vascular procedures or preexisting gastrointestinal or genitourinary lesions, and should not interrupt therapy if it can be managed with local pressure or other simple measures.

Treatment of bleeding involves local measures as well as correction of the systemic hypocoagulable state resulting from proteolysis of plasma proteins and platelets (Table 135-7).[420] The fibrinolytic agent should be discontinued, and most will be cleared rapidly, because of the short half-life. For serious bleeding, an antifibrinolytic agent such as epsilon aminocaproic acid can be administered, but will be effective only if the fibrinolytic agent remains in the blood. Replacement of fibrinogen and other hemostatic proteins can be accomplished with cryoprecipitate and fresh frozen plasma, respectively; treatment should be monitored with repeated coagulation tests. Administration of platelet concentrates may also be useful because fibrinolytic therapy results in

TABLE 135-7. Treatment of Fibrinolytic Bleeding

If intracranial bleeding is suspected, obtain imaging, consult neurosurgery, and correct hemostasis as below.

For major bleeding:

Send diagnostic test: activated partial thromboplastin time (aPTT), platelet count, and fibrinogen.

Attend to local hemostatic problems. Apply pressure if bleeding related to arterial puncture. Proceed with general supportive measures, including intravenous fluid hydration and transfusion of packed red cells if indicated. Proceed with diagnostic evaluation for gastrointestinal or genitourinary tract bleeding.

Correct abnormal hemostasis:

Prevent further fibrinolysis: stop fibrinolytic therapy; consider ε-aminocaproic acid or tranexamic acid.

Replacement therapy to repair hemostasis defect induced by fibrinolytic therapy: give cryoprecipitate 5–10 U and 2 U fresh-frozen plasma; consider platelet transfusion.

Correct other hemostatic defects: stop anticoagulant and antiplatelet agents; consider protamine to reverse heparin.

TABLE 135-8. Principal Uses of Antifibrinolytic Agents

Condition	Comment
SYSTEMIC FIBRINOLYSIS	
α_2-Plasmin inhibitor or plasminogen activating inhibitor (PAI)-1 deficiency	Rare inherited disorders
Acute promyelocytic leukemia	Must distinguish fibrinolysis from disseminated intravascular coagulation (DIC)
Cirrhosis and liver transplantation	Occasional cases of cirrhosis; common in anhepatic phase of liver transplantation
Malignancy	Occasional cases of prostate and other carcinomas
DIC	Must be used with caution; thrombosis can result
Cardiopulmonary bypass	Decreases blood loss and transfusion needs
Fibrinolytic therapy	Can be used in treating bleeding complications
Localized fibrinolysis	
Hemophilia and von Willebrand disease	Decreases bleeding after dental extractions and possibly other procedures
Prostatectomy	Can decrease postoperative bleeding
Kasabach-Merritt syndrome	May shrink hemangioma
Menorrhagia	Often decreases bleeding

platelet dysfunction from proteolysis of surface proteins. Heparin can be reversed by administration of protamine sulfate, and 1-deamino-8-D-arginine vasopressin (DDAVP) may have some value in reversing platelet dysfunction.

ANTIFIBRINOLYTIC THERAPY

Pharmacologic agents can be used to inhibit fibrinolytic bleeding, but care must be exercised given the risk of thrombosis (Table 135-8). For example, in patients with consumption coagulopathies there may be excessive activation of both the coagulation and fibrinolytic systems, resulting in clinical manifestations of both bleeding and thrombosis. In this situation, inhibiting fibrinolysis to treat bleeding can precipitate or worsen thrombosis.

ANTIFIBRINOLYTIC AGENTS

Both ε-aminocaproic acid and tranexamic acid are synthetic lysine analogues. These agents inhibit fibrinolysis by competitively blocking binding of Plg to lysine residues on fibrin.[421-424] Both can be administered orally or intravenously, have rapid absorption after oral administration and are excreted primarily through the kidneys. Only ε-aminocaproic acid is approved for use in the United States, with the exception that tranexamic acid can be used for treatment of menorrhagia. Pharmacologically, tranexamic acid is approximately 10-fold more potent than ε-aminocaproic acid because of its higher binding affinity. Both drugs have a short half-life of 2 to 4 hours and must, therefore, be administered frequently. ε-Aminocaproic acid can be administered intravenously with a loading dose of approximately 100 mg/kg over 30 to

60 minutes followed by a continuous infusion of up to 1 g/h, or the dose can be divided for intermittent administration. For oral treatment, the same loading dose can be administered followed by a maximum dose of 24 g/day in divided doses given every 1 to 6 hours as indicated. The use of tranexamic acid follows similar principles. The intravenous dose is 10 mg/kg followed by 10 mg/kg every 2 to 6 hours as needed. It can also be administered orally in a dose of 25 mg/kg given three or four times daily. Both ε-aminocaproic acid and tranexamic acid are generally well tolerated, but patients must be observed for possible thrombotic complications. Additionally, thrombotic ureteral obstruction can occur in patients with upper urinary tract bleeding, and such patients should be treated only after careful consideration. The risks of ureteral obstruction can be decreased by insuring high urine flow. Thrombotic complications can occur in patients with hypercoagulability, and thrombotic events can be precipitated or worsened in patients with disseminated intravascular coagulation (DIC). Myonecrosis is a rare complication. Minor complications, including rash, abdominal discomfort, nausea, and vomiting, are reported.

Aprotinin is a naturally occurring, broad-spectrum, proteinase inhibitor derived from bovine lung.[425-427] It has both antiinflammatory and antifibrinolytic properties. Until recently, aprotinin was used in the United States for reducing perioperative blood loss and blood transfusions in patients undergoing cardiopulmonary bypass. However, its use is associated with an increased risk of postoperative renal dysfunction, cardiac and cerebral events,[428,429] and of increased short- and long-term mortality in patients who received aprotinin compared to ε-aminocaproic acid, tranexamic acid, or placebo. In a retrospective analysis of electronic records from 33,517 aprotinin recipients and 44,682 ε-aminocaproic acid recipients, the unadjusted risk of death within the first 7 days after coronary artery bypass graft was 4.5 percent for aprotinin recipients compared to 2.5 percent for ε-aminocaproic acid recipients. The relative risk of death was significantly increased in the aprotinin group (relative risk: 1.64; 95 percent CI 1.50 to 1.78).[430] Another retrospective study found that use of aprotinin was associated with both a significantly increased mortality risk at 1 year, and a larger risk-adjusted increase in serum creatinine ($p < 0.001$).[431] The prospective Blood Conservation Using Antifibrinolytics in a Randomized Controlled Trial (BART), which was designed to randomize a total of 3000 patients to either aprotinin, aminocaproic acid or tranexamic acid to further assess the safety of aprotinin, was terminated early because of a significantly higher death rate from any cause at 30 days in the aprotinin recipients.[432] Based on these studies, aprotinin was removed from U.S. market in May 2008, and its access is limited to investigational use.

Excessive systemic fibrinolytic activation can lead to bleeding and may result in a shortened euglobulin clot lysis time, decreased Plg, decreased α_2-plasmin inhibitor, increased plasmin-antiplasmin complexes, decreased fibrinogen and increased fibrinogen degradation products. Screening tests including the PT and aPTT may be prolonged. It may be difficult to distinguish between abnormal hemostasis caused by DIC versus systemic fibrinolysis. Useful features include a more prominent decrease in fibrinogen and increase in fibrinogen degradation products and relatively less thrombocytopenia, and elevation of D-dimer with primary fibrinolysis. Homozygous deficiencies of either α_2-plasmin inhibitor or of PAI-1 can cause a lifelong bleeding disorder and have been treated effectively with antifibrinolytic agents.[297,433-436]

APL is often associated with a severe bleeding disorder that may have elements of both DIC and systemic fibrinolysis in addition to thrombocytopenia. Administration of ε-aminocaproic acid to inhibit fibrinolysis can be useful, but must be given with care to avoid thrombosis.[437-440] In severe liver disease, fibrinolysis caused by reduced inhibitor synthesis can contribute to bleeding and may occasionally be the primary abnormality.[441-443] During orthotopic liver transplantation, accelerated fibrinolysis often contributes to bleeding, particularly during the anhepatic phase. Treatment with antifibrinolytic agents can improve bleeding complications and decrease blood loss.[444-447]

Primary fibrinolysis with bleeding may rarely occur with some malignant tumors including prostatic carcinoma,[444-453] and also with heat stroke.[454] Fibrinolytic activation routinely occurs as a compensatory mechanism in consumption coagulopathy. If fibrinolytic activation is prominent in DIC and other measures do not control bleeding, use of antifibrinolytic therapy can be helpful, but must be used with caution, to avoid exacerbation of underlying thrombotic events.

The contact system is activated during cardiopulmonary bypass, resulting in alterations in the coagulation, fibrinolytic and complement systems[455,456] and both postoperative bleeding and the need for large transfusion volumes can be a major problems. Several trials of antifibrinolytic therapy have established that total blood loss and transfusion requirements can be reduced, with aminocaproic acid and tranexamic acid often used for this purpose.[450,451,457-460] Antifibrinolytic therapy can also be useful in treating bleeding associated with some snakebites and following administration of fibrinolytic therapy.

In hemophilia or von Willebrand disease, bleeding associated with a local lesion such as dental extraction may also respond to antifibrinolytic therapy. Both the oral and urinary mucosas are rich in fibrinolytic activity, and inhibition of normal fibrinolysis can prevent local bleeding, such as after prostatectomy.[461-463] Similarly, endometrial fibrinolysis contributes to menstrual bleeding, and antifibrinolytic therapy can be useful in treating menorrhagia.[464,465] Antifibrinolytic therapy may also be useful in rare cases of Kasabach-Merritt syndrome in which a giant hemangioma is associated with consumption coagulopathy.[466,467] Antifibrinolytic therapy has been used in treating gastrointestinal or genitourinary bleeding in patients with severe thrombocytopenia, ulcerative colitis, hereditary hemorrhagic telangiectasia, traumatic hyphema, following tonsillectomy, and with subarachnoid hemorrhage. However, caution is advised in the latter condition, as rebleeding may be decreased with antifibrinolytic therapy, but vasospasm and distal ischemia may worsen.[467]

REFERENCES

1. Hajjar KA: The molecular basis of fibrinolysis, in *Nathan and Oski's Hematology of Infancy and Childhood*. 7th ed, edited by SH Orkin, DG Nathan, D Ginsburg, AT Look, DE Fisher, SE Lux, pp 1–15. Elsevier, Philadelphia, 2014.
2. Hajjar KA: Cellular receptors in the regulation of plasmin generation. *Thromb Haemost* 74:294–301, 1995.
3. Plow EF, Doeuvre L, Das R: So many plasminogen receptors: Why? *J Biomed Biotechnol* 2012:1–6, 2012.
4. Raum D, Marcus D, Alper CA, et al: Synthesis of human plasminogen by the liver. *Science* 208:1036–1037, 1980.
5. Bohmfalk J, Fuller G: Plasminogen is synthesized by primary cultures of rat hepatocytes. *Science* 209:408–410, 1980.
6. Castellino FJ: Biochemistry of human plasminogen. *Semin Thromb Hemost* 10:18–23, 1984.
7. Collen D, Tytgat G, Claeys H, et al: Metabolism of plasminogen in healthy subjects: Effect of tranexamic acid. *J Clin Invest* 51:1310–1318, 1972.
8. Forsgren M, Raden B, Israelsson M, et al: Molecular cloning and characterization of a full-length cDNA clone for human plasminogen. *FEBS Lett* 213:254–260, 1987.
9. Miles LA, Dahlberg CM, Plow EF: The cell-binding domains of plasminogen and their function in plasma. *J Biol Chem* 263:11928–11934, 1988.
10. Markus G, De Pasquale JL, Wissler FC: Quantitative determination of the binding of epsilon-aminocaproic acid to native plasminogen. *J Biol Chem* 253:727–732, 1978.
11. Markus G, Priore RL, Wissler FC: The binding of tranexamic acid to native (glu) and modified (lys) human plasminogen and its effect on conformation. *J Biol Chem* 254:1211–1216, 1979.
12. Hajjar KA, Harpel PC, Jaffe EA, Nachman RL: Binding of plasminogen to cultured human endothelial cells. *J Biol Chem* 261:11656–11662, 1986.
13. Miles LA, Plow EF: Cellular regulation of fibrinolysis. *Thromb Haemost* 66:32–36, 1991.
14. Rakoczi I, Wiman B, Collen D: On the biologic significance of the specific interaction between fibrin, plasminogen, and antiplasmin. *Biochim Biophys Acta* 540:295–300, 1978.
15. Hayes ML, Castellino FJ: Carbohydrate of the human plasminogen variants. I. Carbohydrate composition, glycopeptide isolation, and characterization. *J Biol Chem* 254:8768–8771, 1979.

16. Hayes ML, Castellino FJ: Carbohydrate composition of the human plasminogen variants. II. Structure of the asparagine-linked oligosaccharide unit. *J Biol Chem* 254:8772–8776, 1979.

17. Hayes ML, Castellino FJ: Carbohydrate of the human plasminogen variants. III. Structure of the O-glycosidically-linked oligosaccharide unit. *J Biol Chem* 254:8777–8780, 1979.

18. Saksela O: Plasminogen activation and regulation of proteolysis. *Biochim Biophys Acta* 823:35–65, 1985.

19. Wallen P, Wiman B: Characterization of human plasminogen. I. On the relationship between different molecular forms of plasminogen demonstrated in plasma and found in purified preparations. *Biochim Biophys Acta* 221:20–30, 1970.

20. Wallen P, Wiman B: Characterization of human plasminogen. II. Separation and partial characterization of different molecular forms of human plasminogen. *Biochim Biophys Acta* 157:122–134, 1972.

21. Holvoet P, Lijnen HR, Collen D: A monoclonal antibody specific for lys-plasminogen. *J Biol Chem* 260:12106–12111, 1985.

22. Hoylaerts M, Rijken DC, Lijnen HR, Collen D: Kinetics of the activation of plasminogen by human tissue plasminogen activator: Role of fibrin. *J Biol Chem* 257:2912–2929, 1982.

23. Hajjar KA, Nachman RL: Endothelial cell-mediated conversion of glu-plasminogen to lys-plasminogen: Further evidence for assembly of the fibrinolytic system on the endothelial cell surface. *J Clin Invest* 82:1769–1778, 1988.

24. Silverstein RL, Friedlander RJ, Nicholas RL, Nachman RL: Binding of lys-plasminogen to monocytes and macrophages. *J Clin Invest* 82:1948–1955, 1988.

25. Murray JC, Buetow KH, Donovan M, et al: Linkage disequilibrium of plasminogen polymorphisms and assignment of the gene to human chromosome 6q26–6q27. *Am J Hum Genet* 40:338–350, 1987.

26. Petersen TE, Martzen MR, Ichinose A, Davie EW: Characterization of the gene for human⁺ plasminogen, a key proenzyme in the fibrinolytic system. *J Biol Chem* 265:6104–6111, 1990.

27. Jenkins GR, Seiffert D, Parmer RJ, Miles LA: Regulation of plasminogen gene expression by interleukin-6. *Blood* 89:2394–2403, 1997.

28. McLean JW, Tomlinson JE, Kuang WJ, et al: cDNA sequence of human apolipoprotein(a) is homologous to plasminogen. *Nature* 330:132–137, 1987.

29. Nakamura T, Nishizawa T, Hagiya M, et al: Molecular cloning and expression of human hepatocyte growth factor. *Nature* 342:440–443, 1989.

30. Weissbach L, Treadwell BV: A plasminogen-related gene is expressed in cancer cells. *Biochem Biophys Res Commun* 186:1108–1114, 1992.

31. Yoshimura T, Yuhki N, Wang MH, et al: Cloning, sequencing, and expression of human macrophage stimulating protein (MSP, MST 1) confirms MSP as a member of the family of kringle proteins and locates the MSP gene on chromosome 3. *J Biol Chem* 268:15461–15468, 1993.

32. Byrne CD, Schwartz K, Meer K, et al: The human apolipoprotein(a)/plasminogen gene cluster contains a novel homologue transcribed in liver. *Arterioscler Thromb* 14:534–541, 1994.

33. Ichinose A: Multiple members of the plasminogen-apolipoprotein(a) gene family associated with thrombosis. *Biochemistry* 31:3113–3118, 1992.

34. Shanmukhappa K, Matte U, Degen JL, Bezerra JA: Plasmin-mediated proteolysis is required for hepatocyte growth factor activation during liver repair. *J Biol Chem* 284:12917–12923, 2009.

35. Bugge TH, Flick MJ, Daugherty CC, Degen JL: Plasminogen deficiency causes severe thrombosis but is compatible with development and reproduction. *Genes Dev* 9:794–807, 1995.

36. Ploplis VA, Carmeliet P, Vazirzadeh S, et al: Effects of disruption of the plasminogen gene on thrombosis, growth, and health in mice. *Circulation* 92:2585–2593, 1995.

37. Drew AF, Kaufman AH, Kombrinck KW, et al: Ligneous conjunctivitis in plasminogen-deficient mice. *Blood* 91:1616–1624, 1998.

38. Pennica D, Holmes WE, Kohr WJ, et al: Cloning and expression of human tissue-type plasminogen activator cDNA in *E. coli. Nature* 301:214–221, 1983.

39. Tate KM, Higgins DL, Holmes WE, et al: Functional role of proteolytic cleavage at arginine-275 of human tissue plasminogen activator as assessed by site-directed mutagenesis. *Biochemistry* 26:338–343, 1987.

40. Pohl G, Kenne L, Nilsson B, Einarsson M: Isolation and characterization of three different carbohydrate chains from melanoma tissue plasminogen activator. *Eur J Biochem* 170:69–75, 1987.

41. Spellman MW, Basa LJ, Leonard CK, Chakel JA: Carbohydrate structures of tissue plasminogen activator expressed in Chinese hamster ovary cells. *J Biol Chem* 264:14100–14111, 1989.

42. Harris RJ, Leonard CK, Guzzetta AW: Tissue plasminogen activator has an *O*-linked fucose attached to threonine-61 in the epidermal growth factor domain. *Biochemistry* 30:2311–2314, 1991.

43. Ny T, Elgh F, Lund B: Structure of the human tissue-type plasminogen activator gene: Correlation of intron and exon structures to functional and structural domains. *Proc Natl Acad Sci U S A* 81:5355–5359, 1984.

44. Browne MJ, Tyrrell AWR, Chapman CG, et al: Isolation of a human tissue-type plasminogen activator genomic clone and its expression in mouse L cells. *Gene* 33:279–284, 1985.

45. Degen SJF, Rajput B, Reich E: The human tissue plasminogen activator gene. *J Biol Chem* 261:6872–6885, 1986.

46. Van Zonnefeld AJ, Veerman H, Pannekoek H: Autonomous functions of structural domains on human tissue-type plasminogen activator. *Proc Natl Acad Sci U S A* 83:4670–4674, 1986.

47. Feng P, Ohlsson M, Ny T: The structure of the TATA-less rat tissue-type plasminogen activator gene. *J Biol Chem* 265:2022–2027, 1990.

48. Kooistra T, Bosma PJ, Toet K, et al: Role of protein kinase C and cyclic adenosine monophosphate in the regulation of tissue-type plasminogen activator, plasminogen activator inhibitor-1, and platelet-derived growth factor mRNA levels in human endothelial cells. Possible involvement of proto-oncogenes c-jun and c-fos. *Arterioscler Thromb* 11:1042–1052, 1991.

49. Medcalf RL, Ruegg M, Schleuning WD: A DNA motif related to the cAMP-responsive element and an exon-located activator protein-2 binding site in the human tissue-type plasminogen activator gene promoter cooperate in basal expression and convey activation by phorbol ester and cAMP. *J Biol Chem* 265:14618–14626, 1990.

50. Kooistra T, Van den Berg J, Tons A, et al: Butyrate stimulates tissue type plasminogen activator synthesis in cultured human endothelial cells. *Biochem J* 247:605–612, 1987.

51. Diamond SL, Eskin SG, McIntire LV: Fluid flow stimulates tissue plasminogen activator secretion by cultured human endothelial cells. *Science* 243:1483–1485, 1989.

52. Hanss M, Collen D: Secretion of tissue-type plasminogen activator and plasminogen activator inhibitor by cultured human endothelial cells: Modulation by thrombin, endotoxin, and histamine. *J Lab Clin Med* 109:97–104, 1987.

53. Thompson EA, Nelles L, Collen D: Effect of retinoic acid on the synthesis of tissue-type plasminogen activator and plasminogen activator inhibitor 1 in human endothelial cells. *Eur J Biochem* 201:627–632, 1991.

54. Kooistra T, Opdenberg JP, Toet K, et al: Stimulation of tissue-type plasminogen activator synthesis by retinoids in cultured human endothelial cells and rat tissue *in vivo*. *Thromb Haemost* 65:565–572, 1991.

55. Medcalf RL, Van den Berg E, Schleuning WD: Glucocorticoid-modulated gene expression of tissue- and urinary-tyype plasminogen activator and plasminogen activator inhibitor-1 and 2. *J Cell Biol* 106:971–978, 1988.

56. Santell L, Levin EG: Cyclic AMP potentiates phorbol ester stimulation of tissue plasminogen activator release and inhibits secretion of plasminogen activator inhibitor-1 from human endothelial cells. *J Biol Chem* 263:16802–16808, 1988.

57. Levin EG, del Zoppo GJ: Localization of tissue plasminogen activator in the endothelium of a limited number of vessels. *Am J Pathol* 144:855–861, 1994.

58. Levin EG, Santell L, Osborn KG: The expression of endothelial tissue plasminogen activator in vivo: A function defined by vessel size and anatomic location. *J Cell Sci* 110:139–148, 1997.

59. Levin EG, Osborn KG, Schleuning WD: Vessel-specific gene expression in the lung: Tissue plasmingen activator is limited to bronchial arteries and pulmonary vessels of discrete size. *Chest* 114:68S, 1998.

60. Diamond SL, Sharefkin JB, Dieffenbach C, et al: Tissue plasminogen activator messenger RNA levels increase in cultured human endothelial cells exposed to laminar shear stress. *J Cell Physiol* 143:364–371, 1990.

61. O'Rourke J, Jiang X, Hao Z, et al: Distribution of sympathetic tissue plasminogen activator (tPA) to a distant microvasculature. *J Neurosci* 79:727–733, 2005.

62. Dichek D, Quertermous T: Thrombin regulation of mRNA levels of tissue plasminogen activator inhibitor-1 in cultured human umbilical vein endothelial cells. *Blood* 74:222–228, 1989.

63. Levin EG, Marotti KR, Santell L: Protein kinase C and the stimulation of tissue plasminogen activator release from human endothelial cells. *J Biol Chem* 264:16030–16036, 1989.

64. Kasai S, Arimura H, Nishida M, Suyama T: Primary structure of single-chain prourokinase. *J Biol Chem* 260:12382–12389, 1985.

65. Gunzler WA, Steffens GJ, Otting F, et al: Structural relationship between high and low molecular mass urokinase. *Hoppe Seylers Z Physiol Chem* 363:133–141, 1982.

66. Riccio A, Grimaldi G, Verde P, Sebastio G, Boast S, Blasi F: The human urokinase-plasminogen activator gene and its promoter. *Nucleic Acids Res* 13:2759–2771, 1985.

67. Holmes WE, Pennica D, Blaber M, et al: Cloning and expression of the gene for pro-urokinase in *Escherichia coli*. *Nat Biotechnol* 3:923, 1985.

68. Schmitt M, Wilhelm O, Janicke F, et al: Urokinase-type plasminogen activator (uPA) and its receptor (CD87): A new target in tumor invasion and metastasis. *J Obstet Gynaecol* 21:151–165, 1995.

69. Van Hinsbergh VW, Kooistra T, Van den Berg EA, et al: Tumor necrosis factor increases the production of plasminogen activator inhibitor in human endothelial cells *in vitro* and in rats *in vivo*. *Blood* 72:1467–1473, 1988.

70. Medina R, Socher SH, Han JH, Friedman PA: Interleukin-1, endotoxin, or tumor necrosis factor/cachectin enhance the level of plasminogen activator inhibitor messenger RNA in bovine aortic endothelial cells. *Thromb Res* 54:41–52, 1989.

71. Gerwin BI, Keski-Oja J, Seddon M, et al: TGF beta 1 modulation of urokinase and PAI-1 expression in human bronchial epithelial cells. *Am J Pathol* 259:262–269, 1990.

72. Stump DC, Lijnen HR, Collen D: Purification and characterization of a novel low molecular weight form of single-chain urokinase-type plasminogen activator. *J Biol Chem* 261:17120–17126, 1986.

73. Steffens GJ, Gunzler WA, Olting F, et al: The complete amino acid sequence of low molecular mass urokinase from human urine. *Hoppe Seylers Z Physiol Chem* 363:1043–1058, 1982.

74. Lijnen HR, Zamarron C, Blaber M, et al: Activation of plasminogen by prourokinase: I. Mechanism. *J Biol Chem* 261:1253–1258, 1986.

75. Gurewich V, Pannell R, Louie S, et al: Effective and fibrin-specific clot lysis by a zymogen precursor from urokinase (pro-urokinase). A study in vitro and in two animal species. *J Clin Invest* 73:1731–1739, 1984.

76. Colman RW: Activation of plasminogen by human plasma kallikrein. *Biochem Biophys Res Commun* 35:273–279, 1968.

77. Mandle RJ, Kaplan AP: Hageman factor-dependent fibrinolysis: Generation of fibrinolytic activity by the interaction of human activated factor XI and plasminogen. *Blood* 54:850–862, 1979.

78. Goldsmith GH, Saito H, Ratnoff OD: The activation of plasminogen by Hageman factor (factor XII) and Hageman factor fragments. *J Clin Invest* 62:54–60, 1978.

79. Ouimet H, Loscalzo J, Schafer AI: Fibrinolysis, in *Thrombosis and Hemorrhage*, vol 1, edited by J Loscalzo and AI Schafer, p 127. Blackwell Scientific, Boston, 1994.

80. Hiraoka N, Allen E, Apel IJ, et al: Matrix metalloproteinases regulate neovascularization by acting as pericellular fibrinolysins. *Cell* 95:365–377, 1998.

81. Hrafnkelsdottir T, Ottosson P, Gudnason T, et al: Impaired endothelial release of tissue-type plasminogen activator in patients with chronic kidney disease and hypertension. *Hypertension* 44:300–304, 2004.

82. Patrassi GM, Sartori MT, Viero ML, et al: Venous thrombosis and tissue plasminogen activator release deficiency: A family study. *Blood Coagul Fibrinolysis* 2:231–235, 1991.

83. Sjogren LS, Doroudi R, Gan L, et al: Elevated intraluminal pressure inhibits vascular tissue plasminogen activator secretion and downregulates its gene expression. *Hypertension* 35:1002–1008, 2000.

84. Carmeliet P, Schoonjans L, Kieckens L, et al: Physiological consequences of loss of plasminogen activator gene function in mice. *Nature* 368:419–424, 1994.

85. Rau JC, Beaulieu LM, Huntington JA, Church FC: Serpins in thrombosis, hemostasis and fibrinolysis. *J Thromb Haemost* 5:102–115, 2007.

86. Aoki N: The past, present and future of plasmin inhibitor. *Thromb Res* 116:455–464, 2005.

87. Holmes WE, Nelles L, Lijnen HR: Primary structure of human alpha2-antiplasmin, a serine protease inhibitor (serpin). *J Biol Chem* 262:1659–1664, 1987.

88. Hirosawa S, Nakamura Y, Miura O, et al: Organization of the human alpha2-antiplasmin inhibitor gene. *Proc Natl Acad Sci U S A* 85:6836–6840, 1988.

89. Plow EF, Collen D: The presence and release of alpha-2-antiplasmin from human platelets. *Blood* 58:1069–1074, 1981.

90. Lijnen HR, Okada K, Matsuo O, et al: Alpha2-Antiplasmin gene deficiency in mice is associated with enhanced fibrinolytic potential without overt bleeding. *Blood* 93:2274–2281, 1999.

91. Aoki N, Moroi M, Tachiya K: Effects of alpha-2-plasmin inhibitor on fibrin clot lysis. Its comparison with alpha-2-macroglobulin. *Thromb Haemost* 39:22–31, 1978.

92. Huisman LG, Van Griensven JM, Kluft C: On the role of C1-inhibitor as inhibitor of tissue-type plasminogen activator in human plasma. *Thromb Haemost* 73:466–471, 1995.

93. Scott RW, Bergman BL, Bajpai A, et al: Protease nexin: Properties and a modified purification procedure. *J Biol Chem* 260:7029–7034, 1985.

94. Cunningham DD, Van Nostrand WE, Farrell DH, Campbell CH: Interactions of serine proteases with cultured fibroblasts. *J Cell Biochem* 32:281–291, 1986.

95. Sprengers ED, Kluft D: Plasminogen activator inhibitors. *Blood* 69:381–387, 1987.

96. Ny T, Sawdey M, Lawrence D, et al: Cloning and sequence of a cDNA coding for the human beta-migrating endothelial-cell-type plasminogen activator inhibitor. *Proc Natl Acad Sci U S A* 83:6776–6780, 1986.

97. Kruithof EK: Plasminogen activator inhibitor type 1: Biochemical, biological, and clinical aspects. *Fibrinolysis* 2:59–70, 1988.

98. Samad F, Yamamoto K, Loskutoff DJ: Distribution and regulation of plasminogen activator inhibitor-1 in murine adipose tissue *in vivo*. *J Clin Invest* 97:37–46, 1996.

99. Sawdey M, Podor TJ, Loskutoff DJ: Regulation of type-1 plasminogen activator inhibitor gene expression in cultured bovine aortic endothelial cells. *J Biol Chem* 264:10396–10401, 1989.

100. Van den Berg EA, Sprengers ED, Jaye M, et al: Regulation of plasminogen activator inhibitor-1 mRNA in human endothelial cells. *Thromb Haemost* 60:63–67, 1988.

101. Van Hinsbergh VW, Van den Berg EA, Fiers W, Dooijewaard G: Tumor necrosis factor induces the production of urokinase-type plasminogen activator by human endothelial cells. *Blood* 75:1991–1998, 1990.

102. Loskutoff DJ, Linders M, Keijer J, et al: Structure of the human plasminogen activator inhibitor-1 gene: Non-random distribution of introns. *Biochemistry* 26:3763–3768, 1987.

103. Mottonen J, Strand A, Symersky J, et al: Structural basis of latency in plasminogen activator inhibitor-1. *Nature* 355:270–273, 1992.

104. Declerck PJ, De Mol M, Alessi MC, et al: Purification and characterization of a plasminogen activator inhibitor-1 binding protein from human plasma. Identification as multimeric form of S protein (vitronectin). *J Biol Chem* 263:15454–15461, 1988.

105. Dupont DM, Madsen JB, Kristensen T, et al: Biochemical properties of plasminogen activator inhibitor-1. *Front Biosci* 14:1337–1361, 2009.

106. Kruithof EK: Regulation of plasminogen activator inhibitor type 1 gene expression by inflammatory mediators and statins. *Thromb Haemost* 100:969–975, 2008.

107. Nagamine Y: Transcriptional regulation of the plasminogen activator inhibitor type 1— With an emphasis on negative regulation. *Thromb Haemost* 100:1007–1013, 2008.

108. Bosma PJ, Van den Berg EA, Kooistra T, et al: Human plasminogen activator inhibitor-1 gene: Promoter and structural nucleotide sequences. *J Biol Chem* 263:9129–9141, 1988.

109. Van Zonnefeld AJ, Curriden SA, Loskutoff DJ: Type 1 plasminogen activator inhibitor gene: Functional analysis and glucocorticoid regulation of its promoter. *Proc Natl Acad Sci U S A* 85:5525–5529, 1988.

110. Westerhausen DR, Hopkins WE, Billadello JJ: Multiple transforming growth factor beta-inducible elements regulate expression of the plasminogen activator inhibitor type-1 gene in HepG2 cells. *J Biol Chem* 266:1092–1100, 1991.

111. Keeton MR, Curriden SA, Van Zonneveld AJ, Loskutoff DJ: Identification of regulatory sequences in the type 1 plasminogen activator inhibitor gene responsive to transforming growth factor. *J Biol Chem* 266:23048–23052, 1991.

112. Van Hinsbergh VW, Bauer KA, Kooistra T, et al: Progress of fibrinolysis during tumor necrosis factor infusions in humans. Concomitant increase in tissue-type plasminogen activator, plasminogen activator inhibitor type-1, and fibrin(ogen) degradation products. *Blood* 76:2284–2289, 1990.

113. Schleef RR, Bevilacqua MP, Sawdey M, et al: Cytokine activation of vascular endothelium: Effects on tissue-type plasminogen activator and type 1 plasminogen activator inhibitor. *J Biol Chem* 263:5797–5803, 1988.

114. Craik CS, Rutter WJ, Fletternick R: Splice junctions: Association with variation in protein structure. *Science* 220:1125–1129, 1983.

115. Stiko-Rahm A, Wiman B, Hamsten A, Nilsson J: Secretion of plasminogen activator inhibitor-1 from cultured human umbilical vein endothelial cells is induced by very low density lipoprotein. *Arteriosclerosis* 10:1067–1073, 1990.

116. Etingin OR, Hajjar DP, Hajjar KA, et al: Lipoprotein(a) regulates plasminogen activator inhibitor-1 expression in endothelial cells. *J Biol Chem* 266:2459–2465, 1990.

117. Vaughan DE, Lazos SA, Tong K: Angiotensin II regulates the expression of plasminogen activator inhibitor-1 in cultured endothelial cells. A potential link between the renin-angiotensin system and thrombosis. *J Clin Invest* 95:995–1001, 1995.

118. Gelehrter TD, Scyncer-Laszuk R. Thrombin induction of plasminogen activator-inhibitor synthesis in vitro. *J Clin Invest* 77:165–169, 1986.

119. Van Hinsbergh VW, Sprengers ED, Kooistra T: Effect of thrombin on the production of plasminogen activators and PA inhibitor-1 by human foreskin microvascular endothelial cells. *Thromb Haemost* 57:148–153, 1987.

120. Scarpati EM, Sadler JE: Regulation of endothelial cell coagulant properties. Modulation of tissue factor, plasminogen activator inhibitors, and thrombomodulin by phorbol 12-myristate 13-acetate and tumor necrosis factor. *J Biol Chem* 264:20705–20713, 1989.

121. Konkle BA, Kollros PR, Kelly MD: Heparin-binding growth factor-1 modulation of plasminogen activator inhibitor-1 expression. *J Biol Chem* 265:21867–21873, 1990.

122. Erickson LA, Fici GJ, Lund JE, et al: Development of venous occlusions in transgenic mice for the plasminogen activator inhibitor-1 gene. *Nature* 346:74–76, 1990.

123. Carmeliet P, Kieckens L, Schoonjans L, et al: Plasminogen activator inhibitor-1 gene-deficient mice: I. Generation by homologous recombination and characterization. *J Clin Invest* 92:2746–2755, 1993.

124. Carmeliet P, Stassen JM, Schoonjans L, et al: Plasminogen activator inhibitor-1 gene-deficient mice. II. Effects on hemostasis, thrombosis, and thrombolysis. *J Clin Invest* 92:2756–2760, 1993.

125. Fay WP, Shapiro AD, Shih JL, et al: Complete deficiency of plasminogen activator inhibitor type 1 due to a frame-shift mutation. *N Engl J Med* 327:1729–1733, 1992.

126. Ye RD, Wun TC, Sadler JE: CDNA cloning and expression in Escherichia coli of a plasminogen activator inhibitor from human placenta. *J Biol Chem* 262:3718–3725, 1987.

127. Ye RD, Aherns SM, Le Beau MM, et al: Structure of the gene for human plasminogen activator inhibitor-2. The nearest mammalian homologue of chicken ovalbumin. *J Biol Chem* 264:5495–5502, 1989.

128. Ogbourne SM, Antalis TM: Characterization of PAUSE-1, a powerful silencer in the human plasminogen activator inhibitor type 2 gene promoter. *Nucleic Acids Res* 29:3919–3927, 2001.

129. Antalis TM, Clok MA, Barnes T, et al: Cloning and expression of a cDNA coding for a human monocyte-derived plasminogen activator inhibitor. *Proc Natl Acad Sci U S A* 85:985–989, 1988.

130. Schleuning WD, Medcalf RL, Hession C, et al: Plasminogen activator inhibitor 2: Regulation of gene transcription during phorbol ester-mediated differentiation of U-937 human histiocytic lymphoma cells. *Mol Cell Biol* 7:4564–4567, 1987.

131. Chapman HA, Stone OL: A fibrinolytic inhibitor of human alveolar macrophages. Induction with endotoxin. *Am Rev Respir Dis* 132:569–575, 1985.

132. Nesheim M, Wang W, Boffa M, et al: Thrombin, thrombomodulin and TAFI in the molecular link between coagulation and fibrinolysis. *Thromb Haemost* 78:386–391, 1997.

133. Mosnier LO, Bouma BN: Regulation of fibrinolysis by thrombin activatable fibrinolysis inhibitor, an unstable carboxypeptidase B that unites the pathways of coagulation and fibrinolysis. *Arterioscler Thromb Vasc Biol* 26:2445–2453, 2006.

134. Bajzar L, Manuel R, Nesheim M: Purification and characterization of TAFI, a thrombin activatable fibrinolysis inhibitor. *J Biol Chem* 270:14477–14484, 1995.

135. Eaton DL, Malloy BE, Tsai SP, et al: Isolation, molecular cloning, and partial characterization of a novel carboxypeptidase B from plasma. *J Biol Chem* 269:21833–21834, 1991.

136. Wang W, Hendriks DF, Scharpe SS: Carboxypeptidase U, a plasma carboxypeptidase with high affinity for plasminogen. *J Biol Chem* 269:15937–15944, 1994.

137. Bajzar L, Nesheim ME, Tracy PB: The profibrinolytic effect of activated protein C in clots formed from plasma is TAFI-dependent. *Blood* 88:2093–2100, 1996.

138. Bajzar L, Morser J, Nesheim M: TAFI, or plasma procarboxypeptidase B, couples the coagulation and fibrinolytic cascades through the thrombin-thrombomodulin complex. *J Biol Chem* 271:16603–16608, 1996.

139. Minnema MC, Friederich PW, Levi M, et al: Enhancement of rabbit jugular vein thrombolysis by neutralization of factor XI: *In vivo* evidence for a role of factor XI as an antifibrinolytic factor. *J Clin Invest* 101:10–14, 1998.

140. Nagashima M, Yin ZF, Zhao L, et al: Thrombin-activatable fibrinolysis inhibitor (TAFI) deficiency is compatible with murine life. *J Clin Invest* 109(101):110, 2002.

141. Wang X, Smith PL, Hsu MY, et al: Deficiency in thrombin-activatable fibrinolysis inhibitor (TAFI) protected mice from ferric chloride-induced vena cava thrombosis. *J Thromb Thrombolysis* 23:41–49, 2007.

142. Mao SS, Holahan MA, Bailey C, et al: Demonstration of enhanced endogenous fibrinolysis in thrombin activatable fibrinolysis inhibitor-deficient mice. *Blood Coagul Fibrinolysis* 16:407–415, 2005.

143. Redlitz A, Tan AK, Eaton D, Plow EF: Plasma carboxypeptidases as regulators of the plasminogen system. *J Clin Invest* 96:2534–2538, 1995.

144. Miles LA, Dahlberg CM, Plescia J, et al: Role of cell surface lysines in plasminogen binding to cells: Identification of alpha-enolase as a candidate plasminogen receptor. *Biochemistry* 30:1682–1691, 1991.

145. Miles LA, Ginsberg MA, White JG, Plow EF: Plasminogen interacts with platelets through two distinct mechanisms. *J Clin Invest* 77:2001–2009, 1986.

146. Kanalas JJ, Makker SP: Identification of the rat Heymann nephritis autoantigen (GP330) as a receptor site for plasminogen. *J Biol Chem* 266:10825–10829, 1991.

147. Barnathan ES, Kuo A, Van der Keyl H, et al: Tissue-type plasminogen activator binding to human endothelial cells: Evidence for two distinct binding sites. *J Biol Chem* 263:7792–7799, 1988.

148. Hajjar KA: The endothelial cell tissue plasminogen activator receptor: Specific interaction with plasminogen. *J Biol Chem* 266:21962–21970, 1991.

149. Hajjar KA, Hamel NM: Identification and characterization of human endothelial cell membrane binding sites for tissue plasminogen activator and urokinase. *J Biol Chem* 265:2908–2916, 1990.

150. Das R, Burke T, Plow EF: Histone H2B as a functionally important plasminogen receptor on macrophages. *Blood* 110:3763–3772, 2007.

151. Lighvani S, Baik N, Diggs JE, et al: Regulation of macrophage migration by a novel plasminogen receptor Plg-R$_{KT}$. *Blood* 118:5622–5630, 2011.

152. D'Alessio S, Blasi F: The urokinase receptor as an entertainer of signal transduction. *Front Biosci* 14:4575–4587, 2009.

153. Montuori N, Ragno P: Multiple activities of a multifaceted receptor: Roles of cleaved and soluble uPAR. *Front Biosci* 14:2492–2503, 2009.

154. Roldan AL, Cubellis MV, Masucci MT, et al: Cloning and expression of the receptor for human urokinase plasminogen activator, a central molecule in cell surface, plasmin-dependent proteolysis. *EMBO J* 9:467–474, 1990.

155. Casey JR, Petranka JG, Kottra J, et al: The structure of the urokinase-type plasminogen activator receptor gene. *Blood* 84:1151–1156, 1994.

156. Behrendt N, Ronne E, Ploug M, et al: The human receptor for urokinase plasminogen receptor. *J Biol Chem* 265:6453–6460, 1990.

157. Ploug M, Ronne E, Behrendt N, et al: Cellular receptor for urokinase plasminogen activator. Carboxyl-terminal processing and membrane anchoring by glycosylphosphatidylinositol. *J Biol Chem* 266:1926–1933, 1991.

158. Cubellis MV, Andreasson P, Ragno P, et al: Accessibility of receptor-bound urokinase to type-1 plasminogen activator inhibitor. *Proc Natl Acad Sci U S A* 86:4828–4832, 1989.

159. Ellis V, Wun TC, Behrendt N, et al: Inhibition of receptor-bound urokinase by plasminogen activator inhibitor. *J Biol Chem* 265:9904–9908, 1990.

160. Cubellis MV, Wun TC, Blasi F: Receptor-mediated internalization and degradation of urokinase is caused by its specific inhibitor PAI-1. *EMBO J* 9:1079–1085, 1990.

161. Ellis V, Behrendt N, Dano K: Plasminogen activation by receptor-bound urokinase. *J Biol Chem* 266:12752–12758, 1991.

162. Kugler MC, Wei Y, Chapman HA: Urokinase receptor and integrin interactions. *Curr Pharm Des* 9:1565–1574, 2003.

163. Bugge TH, Suh TT, Flick MJ, et al: The receptor for urokinase-type plasminogen activator is not essential for mouse development or fertility. *J Biol Chem* 270:16886–16894, 1995.

164. Dewerchin M, Van Nuffelen A, Wallays G, et al: Generation and characterization of urokinase receptor-deficient mice. *J Clin Invest* 97:870–878, 1996.

165. Waltz DA, Chapman HA: Reversible cellular adhesion to vitronectin linked to urokinase receptor occupancy. *J Biol Chem* 269:14746–14750, 1994.

166. Wei Y, Waltz DA, Rao N, et al: Identification of the urokinase receptor as an adhesion receptor for vitronectin. *J Biol Chem* 269:32380–32388, 1994.

167. Wei Y, Lukashev M, Simon DI, et al: Regulation of integrin function by the urokinase receptor. *Science* 273:1551–1555, 1996.

168. Xue W, Kindzelskii AL, Todd RF, Petty HR: Physical association of complement receptor type 3 and urokinase-type plasminogen activator in neutrophil membranes. *J Immunol* 152:4630–4640, 1994.

169. Stahl A, Mueller BM: The urokinase-type plasminogen activator receptor, a GPI-linked protein, is localized in caveolae. *J Cell Biol* 129:335–344, 1995.

170. Anderson RG: Caveolae: Where incoming and outgoing messengers meet. *Proc Natl Acad Sci U S A* 90:10909–10913, 1993.

171. Okamoto T, Schlegel A, Scherer PE, Lisanti MP: Caveolins, a family of scaffolding proteins for organizing "preassembled signaling complexes" at the plasma membrane. *J Biol Chem* 273:5419–5422, 1998.

172. Gerke V, Creutz CE, Moss SE: Annexins: Linking Ca++ signalling to membrane dynamics. *Nat Rev Mol Cell Biol* 6(6):449–461, 2005.

173. Flood EC, Hajjar KA: The annexin A2 system and vascular homeostasis. *Vascul Pharmacol* 54:59–67, 2011.

174. Luo M, Hajjar KA: Annexin A2 system in human biology: Cell surface and beyond. *Semin Thromb Hemost* 39(4):338–346, 2013.

175. Chung CY, Erickson HP: Cell surface annexin II is a high affinity receptor for the alternatively spliced segment of tenascin-C. *J Cell Biol* 126:539–548, 1994.

176. Wright JF, Kurosky A, Wasi S: An endothelial cell-surface form of annexin II binds human cytomegalovirus. *Biochem Biophys Res Commun* 198:983–989, 1994.

177. Kassam G, Choi KS, Ghuman J, et al: The role of annexin II tetramer in the activation of plasminogen. *J Biol Chem* 273:4790–4799, 1998.

178. Siever DA, Erickson HP: Extracellular annexin II. *Int J Biochem Cell Biol* 29:1219–1223, 1997.

179. Falcone DJ, Borth W, Faisal Khan KM, Hajjar KA: Plasminogen-mediated matrix invasion and degradation by macrophages is dependent on surface expression of annexin II. *Blood* 97:777–784, 2001.

180. Brownstein C, Deora AB, Jacovina AT, et al: Annexin II mediates plasminogen-dependent matrix invasion by human monocytes: Enhanced expression by macrophages. *Blood* 103:317–324, 2004.

181. Menell JS, Cesarman GM, Jacovina AT, et al: Annexin II and bleeding in acute promyelocytic leukemia. *N Engl J Med* 340:994–1004, 1999.

182. Lee TH, Rhim. T, Kim SS: Prothrombin kringle 2 domain has a growth inhibitory activity against basic fibroblast growth factor-stimulated capillary endothelial cells. *J Biol Chem* 273:28805–28812, 1998.

183. Tressler RJ, Updyke TV, Yeatman TJ, Nicolson GL: Extracellular annexin is associated with divalent cation-dependent tumor cell adhesion of metastatic RAW 117 large-cell lymphoma cells. *J Cell Biochem* 53:265–276, 1993.

184. Yeatman TJ, Updyke TV, Kaetzel MA, et al: Expression of annexins on the surfaces of non-metastatic human and rodent tumor cells. *Clin Exp Metastasis* 11:37–44, 1993.

185. Tressler RJ, Nicolson GL: Butanol-extractable and detergent-solubilized cell surface components from murine large nucle cell lymphoma cells associated with adhesion to organ microvessel endothelial cells. *J Cell Biochem* 48:162–171, 1992.

186. Swairjo MA, Seaton BA: Annexin structure and membrane interactions: A molecular perspective. *Annu Rev Biophys Biomol Struct* 23:193–213, 1994.

187. Spano F, Raugei G, Palla E, et al: Characterization of the human lipocortin-2-encoding multigene family: Its structure suggests the existence of a short amino acid unit undergoing duplication. *Gene* 95:243–251, 1990.

188. Cesarman GM, Guevara CA, Hajjar KA: An endothelial cell receptor for plasminogen/tissue plasminogen activator: II. Annexin II-mediated enhancement of t-PA-dependent plasminogen activation. *J Biol Chem* 269:21198–21203, 1994.

189. Deora AB, Kreitzer G, Jacovina AT, Hajjar KA: An annexin 2 phosphorylation switch mediates its p11-dependent translocation to the cell surface. *J Biol Chem* 279:43411–43418, 2004.

190. Hajjar KA, Guevara CA, Lev E, et al: Interaction of the fibrinolytic receptor, annexin II, with the endothelial cell surface: Essential role of endonexin repeat 2. *J Biol Chem* 271:21652–21659, 1996.

191. He K, Deora AB, Xiong H, et al: Endothelial cell annexin A2 regulates polyubiquitination and degradation of its binding partner, S100A10/p11. *J Biol Chem* 283:19192–19200, 2008.

192. Hajjar KA, Gavish D, Breslow J, Nachman RL: Lipoprotein(a) modulation of endothelial cell surface fibrinolysis and its potential role in atherosclerosis. *Nature* 339:303–305, 1989.

193. Hajjar KA, Mauri L, Jacovina AT, et al: Tissue plasminogen activator binding to the annexin II tail domain: Direct modulation by homocysteine. *J Biol Chem* 273:9987–9993, 1998.

194. Kraus JP: Molecular basis of phenotype expression in homocystinuria. *J Inherit Metab Dis* 17:383–390, 1994.

195. Boushey CJ, Beresford SA, Omenn GS, Motulsky AG: A quantitative assessment of plasma homocysteine as a risk factor for vascular disease. *JAMA* 274:1049–1057, 1995.

196. Refsum H, Ueland PM, Nygard O, Vollset SE: Homocysteine and cardiovascular disease. *Annu Rev Med* 49:31–62, 1998.

197. Hajjar KA: Homocysteine-induced modulation of tissue plasminogen activator binding to its endothelial cell membrane receptor. *J Clin Invest* 91:2873–2879, 1993.

198. Jacovina AT, Deora AB, Ling Q, et al: Homocysteine inhibits neoangiogenesis in mice through blockade of annexin A2-dependent fibrinolysis. *J Clin Invest* 119:3384–3394, 2009.

199. Surette AP, Madureira PA, Phipps KD, et al: Regulation of fibrinolysis by S100A10 *in vivo*. *Blood* 118:3172–3181, 2011.

200. O'Connell PA, Surette AP, Liwski RS, et al: S100A10 regulates plasminogen-dependent macrophage invasion. *Blood* 116:1136–1146, 2010.

201. O'Connell PA, Madureira PA, Berman JN, et al: Regulation of S100A10 by the PML-RARalpha oncoprotein. *Blood* 117:4095–4105, 2011.

202. Ishii H, Yoshida M, Hiraoka M, et al: Recombinant annexin II modulates impaired fibrinolytic activity *in vitro* and in rat carotid artery. *Circ Res* 89:1240–1245, 2001.

203. Cesarman-Maus G, Cantu-Brito C, Barinagarrementeria F, et al: Autoantibodies against the fibrinolytic receptor, annexin A2, in cerebral venous thrombosis. *Stroke* 42:501–503, 2011.

204. Cesarman-Maus G, Rios-Luna NP, Deora AB, et al: Autoantibodies against the fibrinolytic receptor, annexin 2, in antiphospholipid syndrome. *Blood* 107:4375–4382, 2006.

205. Ling Q, Jacovina AT, Deora A, et al: Annexin II is a key regulator of fibrin homeostasis and neoangiogenesis. *J Clin Invest* 113:38–48, 2004.

206. Bu G, Warshawsky I, Schwartz AL: Cellular receptors for the plasminogen activators. *Blood* 83:3427–3436, 1994.

207. Lillis AP, Van Duyn LB, Murphy-Ullrich J, Strickland DK: LDL receptor-related protein 1: Unique tissue-specific functions revealed by selective gene knockout studies. *Physiol Rev* 88:887–918, 2008.

208. Herz J, Goldstein JL, Strickland DK, et al: 39 kDa protein modulates binding of ligands to low density lipoprotein receptor-related protein/alpha-2-macroglobulin receptor. *J Biol Chem* 266:21232–21238, 1991.

209. Herz J, Clouthier DE, Hammer RE: LDL receptor-related protein internalizes and degrades uPA-PAI-1 complexes and is essential for embryo implantation. *Cell* 71:411–421, 1992.

210. Herz J, Clouthier DE, Hammer RE: Correction: LDL receptor-related protein internalizes and degrades uPA-PAI-1 complexes and is essential for embryo implantation. *Cell* 73:428, 1993.

211. Otter M, Barrett-Bergshoeff MM, Rijken DC: Binding of tissue type plasminogen activator by the mannose receptor. *J Biol Chem* 266:13931–13935, 1991.
212. Hajjar KA, Reynolds CM: Alpha-fucose-mediated binding and degradation of tissue plasminogen activator by HepG2 cells. *J Clin Invest* 93:703–710, 1994.
213. Narita M, Bu G, Herz J, Schwartz AL: Two receptor systems are involved in the plasma clearance of tissue-type plasminogen activator (t-PA) *in vivo. J Clin Invest* 96:1164–1168, 1995.
214. Bailey K, Bettelheim FR, Lorand L, Middlebrook WR: Action of thrombin in the clotting of fibrinogen. *Nature* 167:233–234, 1951.
215. Doolittle RF, Stamatoyannopoulos G, Nienhuis AW, et al: The molecular biology of fibrin, in *The Molecular Basis of Blood Diseases*, vol 2, edited by G Stamatoyannopoulos, pp 701–723. WB Saunders, Philadelphia, 1994.
216. Marder VJ, Budzinski AZ: Data for defining fibrinogen and its plasmic degradation products. *Thromb Diath Haemorrh* 33:199–207, 1975.
217. Furlan M, Kemp G, Beck EA: Plasmic degradation of fibrinogen. *Biochim Biophys Acta* 400:95–111, 1975.
218. Gaffney PJ, Dobos P: A structural aspect of human fibrinogen suggested by its plasmin degradation. *FEBS Lett* 15:13–16, 1971.
219. Latallo ZS, Flether AP, Alkjaersig N, Sherry S: Inhibition of fibrin polymerization by fibrinogen proteolysis products. *Am J Physiol* 202:681–686, 1962.
220. Pizzo SV, Schwartz ML, Hill RL, McKee PA: The effect of plasmin on the subunit structure of human fibrin. *J Biol Chem* 248:4574–4583, 1973.
221. Culasso DE, Donati MB, DeGaetano G, et al: Inhibition of human platelet aggregation by plasmin digests of human and bovine preparations: Role of contaminating factor VIII-related material. *Blood* 44:169–175, 1974.
222. Buluk K, Malofiejew M: The pharmacologic properties of fibrinogen degradation products. *Br J Pharmacol* 35(1):79–89, 1969.
223. Richardson DL, Pepper DS, Kay AB: Chemotaxis for human monocytes by fibrinogen degradation products. *Br J Haematol* 32(4):507–513, 1976.
224. Girmann G, Pees H, Schwarze G, Scheulen PG: Immunosuppression by micromolecular fibrin-fibrinogen degradation products in cancer. *Nature* 259:399–391, 1976.
225. Wiman B, Collen D: On the kinetics of the reaction between human antiplasmin and plasmin. *Eur J Biochem* 84:573–578, 1978.
226. Van Zonnefeld AJ, Veerman H, Pannekoek H: On the interaction of the finger and the kringle-2 domain of tissue-type plasminogen activator with fibrin: Inhibition of kringle-1 binding to fibrin by epsilon-aminocaproic acid. *J Biol Chem* 261:14214–14218, 1986.
227. Camiolo SM, Thorsen S, Astrup T: Fibrinogenolysis and fibrinolysis with tissue plasminogen activator, urokinase, streptokinase-activated human globulin and plasmin. *Proc Soc Exp Biol Med* 138:277–280, 1971.
228. Pannell R, Black J, Gurewich V: Complementary modes of action of tissue-type plasminogen activator and pro-urokinase by which their synergistic effect on clot lysis may be explained. *J Clin Invest* 81:853–859, 1988.
229. Bell W: Fibrinolytic therapy: Indications and management, in *Hematology: Basic Principles and Practice*, vol 2, edited by R Hoffman, EJ Benz, SJ Shattil, B Furie, HJ Cohen, LE Silberstein, pp 1814–1829. Churchill Livingstone, New York, 1995.
230. Coligan JE, Slayter HS: Structure of thrombospondin. *J Biol Chem* 259:3944–3948, 1984.
231. Ott U, Odermatt E, Engel J, et al: Protease resistance and conformation of laminin. *Eur J Biochem* 123:63–72, 1982.
232. Aplin JD, Hughes RC: Complex carbohydrates of the extracellular matrix structures, interactions, and biologic roles. *Biochim Biophys Acta* 694:375–418, 1982.
233. Marder VJ, Sherry S: Thrombolytic therapy: Current status. *N Engl J Med* 318:1512–1520, 1988.
234. Unkeless JC, Gordon S, Reich E: Secretion of plasminogen activator by stimulated macrophages. *J Exp Med* 139:834–850, 1974.
235. Ossowski L, Reich E: Antibodies to plasminogen activator inhibit human tumor metastasis. *Cell* 35:611–619, 1983.
236. Strickland S, Reich E, Sherman MI: Plasminogen activator in early embryogenesis: Enzyme production by trophoblast and parietal endoderm. *Cell* 9:231–240, 1976.
237. Strickland SE, Beers WH: Studies on the role of plasminogen activator in ovulation. *J Biol Chem* 254:5694–5702, 1976.
238. Moonen G, Grau-Wagemans MP, Selak I: Plasminogen activator-plasmin system and neuronal migration. *Nature* 298:753–755, 1982.
239. Pittman RN, Ivins JK, Buettner HM: Neuronal plasminogen activators: Cell surface binding sites and involvement in neurite outgrowth. *J Neurosci* 9:4269–4286, 1989.
240. Virji MA, Vassalli JD, Estensen R, Reich E: Plasminogen activator of islets of Langerhans: Modulation by glucose and correlation with insulin production. *Proc Natl Acad Sci U S A* 77:875–879, 1980.
241. Russell J, Schneider AB, Katzhendler J, et al: Modification of human placental lactogen with plasmin. *J Biol Chem* 254:2296–2302, 1979.
242. Loskutoff DJ, Quigley JP: PAI-1, fibrosis, and the elusive provisional fibrin matrix. *J Clin Invest* 106:1441–1443, 2000.
243. Romer J, Bugge TH, Pyke C, et al: Impaired wound healing in mice with a disrupted plasminogen gene. *Nat Med* 2:287–292, 1996.
244. Bugge TH, Kombrinck KW, Flick MJ, et al: Loss of fibrinogen rescues mice from the pleiotropic effects of plasminogen deficiency. *Cell* 87:709–719, 1996.
245. Ploplis VA, French EL, Carmeliet P, et al: Plasminogen deficiency differentially affects recruitment of inflammatory cell populations in mice. *Blood* 91:2005–2009, 1998.
246. Carmeliet P, Moons L, Ploplis VA, et al: Impaired arterial neointima formation in mice with disruption of the plasminogen gene. *J Clin Invest* 99:200–208, 1997.
247. Coleman JL, Gebbia JA, Piesman J, et al: Plasminogen is required for efficient dissemination of B. burfdoreri in ticks and for enhancement of spirochetemia in mice. *Cell* 89:1111–1119, 1997.
248. Chen ZL, Strickland SE: Neuronal death in the hippocampus is promoted by plasmin-catalyzed degradation of laminin. *Cell* 91:917–925, 1997.
249. Chapman HA: Disorders of lung matrix remodeling. *J Clin Invest* 113:148–157, 2004.
250. Hattori N, Degen JL, Sisson TH, et al: Bleomycin-induced pulmonary fibrosis in fibrinogen-null mice. *J Clin Invest* 106:1341–1350, 2000.
251. Eitzman DT, McCoy RD, Zheng X, et al: Bleomycin-induced pulmonary fibrosis in transgenic mice that either lack or overexpress the murine plasminogen activator inhibitor-1 gene. *J Clin Invest* 97:232–237, 1996.
252. Olman MA, Mackman N, Gladson CL, et al: Changes in procoagulant and fibrinolytic gene expression during bleomycin-induced lung injury in the mouse. *J Clin Invest* 96:1621–1630, 1995.
253. Fujimoto H, Gabazza EC, Taguchi O, et al: Thrombin-activatable fibrinolysis inhibitor deficiency attenuates bleomycin-induced lung fibrosis. *Am J Pathol* 168:1086–1096, 2006.
254. Sisson TH, Hanson KE, Subbotina N, et al: Inducible lung-specific urokinase expression reduces fibrosis and mortality after lung injury in mice. *Am J Physiol Lung Cell Mol Physiol* 283:L1023–L1032, 2002.
255. Krishnan S, Deora AB, Annes JP, et al: Annexin II-mediated plasmin generation activates TGF-beta3 during epithelial-mesenchymal transformation in the developing avian heart. *Dev Biol* 265:140–154, 2004.
256. Sporn MB, Roberts AB, Wakefield LM, Assoian RK: Transforming growth factor-beta: Biological function and chemical structure. *Science* 233:532–534, 1986.
257. Lyons RM, Gentry LE, Purchio AF, Moses HL: Mechanism of activation of latent recombinant transforming growth factor beta1 by plasmin. *J Cell Biol* 110:1361–1367, 1990.
258. Konstantinides S, Schafer K, Loskutoff DJ: Do PAI-1 and vitronectin promote or inhibit neointima formation? *Arterioscler Thromb Vasc Biol* 22:1943–1945, 2002.
259. Ross R: Atherosclerosis: An inflammatory disease. *N Engl J Med* 340:115–126, 1999.
260. Konstantinides S, Schafer K, Thinnes T, Loskutoff DJ: Plasminogen activator inhibitor-1 and its cofactor vitronectin stabilize arterial thrombi following vascular injury in mice. *Circulation* 103:576–583, 2001.
261. Peng L, Bhatia N, Parker AC, et al: Endogenous vitronectin and plasminogen activator inhibitor-1 promote neointima formation in murine carotid arteries. *Arterioscler Thromb Vasc Biol* 22:934–939, 2002.
262. Engelse MA, Hanemaaijer R, Koolwijk P, Van Hinsbergh VW: The fibrinolytic system and matrix metalloproteinases in angiogenesis and tumor progression. *Semin Thromb Hemost* 30:71–82, 2004.
263. Hajjar KA, Deora AB: New concepts in fibrinolysis and angiogenesis. *Curr Atheroscler Rep* 2:417–421, 2000.
264. Bajou K, Noel A, Gerard RD, et al: Absence of host plasminogen activator inhibitor 1 prevents cancer invasion and vascularization. *Nat Med* 4:923–928, 1998.
265. Rakic JM, Lambert V, Munaut C, et al: Mice without uPA, tPA, or plasminogen genes are resistant to experimental choroidal neovascularization. *Invest Ophthalmol Vis Sci* 44:1732–1739, 2003.
266. Lambert V, Munaut C, Noel A, et al: Influence of plasminogen activator inhibitor type 1 on choroidal neovascularization. *FASEB J* 15:1021–1027, 2001.
267. Bajou K, Peng H, Laug WE, et al: Plasminogen activator inhibitor-1 protects endothelial cells from FasL-mediated apoptosis. *Cancer Cell* 14:324–334, 2008.
268. Vogten JM, Reijerkerk A, Meijers JC, et al: The role of the fibrinolytic system in corneal angiogenesis. *Angiogenesis* 6:311–316, 2003.
269. Drinane M, Mollmark J, Zagorchev L, et al: The antiangiogenic activity of rPAI-1 23 inhibits vasa vasorum and growth of atherosclerotic plaque. *Circ Res* 104:337–345, 2009.
270. Huang B, Deora AB, He K, et al: Hypoxia-inducible factor-1 drives annexin A2 system-mediated perivascular fibrin clearance in oxygen-induced retinopathy in mice. *Blood* 118:2918–2929, 2011.
271. Aoki N, Moroi M, Sakata Y, et al: Abnormal plasminogen: A hereditary molecular abnormality found in a patient with recurrent thrombosis. *J Clin Invest* 61:1186–1195, 1978.
272. Schuster V, Hugle B, Tefs K: Plasminogen deficiency. *J Thromb Haemost* 5:2315–2322, 2007.
273. Demarmels Biasiutti F, Sulzer I, Stucki B, et al: Is plasminogen deficiency a thrombotic risk factor? A study on 23 thrombophilic patients and their family members. *Thromb Haemost* 80:167–170, 1998.
274. Sartori MT, Patrassi GM, Theodoridis P, et al: Heterozygous type I plasminogen deficiency is associated with an increased risk for thrombosis: A statistical analysis of 20 kindreds. *Blood Coagul Fibrinolysis* 5:889–893, 1994.
275. Shigekiyo T, Uno Y, Tomonari A, et al: Type I congenital plasminogen deficiency is not a risk factor for thrombosis. *Thromb Haemost* 67:189–192, 1992.
276. Tait RC, Walker ID, Conkie JA, et al: Isolated familial plasminogen deficiency may not be a risk factor for thrombosis. *Thromb Haemost* 76:1004–1008, 1996.
277. Azuma H, Mima N, Shirakawa M, et al: Molecular pathogenesis of type I congenital plasminogen deficiency: Expression of recombinant human mutant plasminogens in mammalian cells. *Blood* 89:183–190, 1997.
278. Ichinose A, Espling ES, Takamatsu J, et al: Two types of abnormal genes for plasminogen in families with a predisposition for thrombosis. *Proc Natl Acad Sci U S A* 88:115–119, 1991.

279. Schott D, Dempfle CE, Beck P, et al: Therapy with a purified plasminogen concentrate in an infant with ligneous conjunctivitis and homozygous plasminogen deficiency. *N Engl J Med* 339:1679–1686, 1998.

280. Robbins KC: Dysplasminogenemia. *Prog Cardiovasc Dis* 34:295–308, 1992.

281. Tsutsumi S, Saito T, Sakata T, et al: Genetic diagnosis of dysplasminogenemia: Detection of an Ala601-Thr mutation in 118 out of 125 families and identification of a new Asp676-Asn mutation. *Thromb Haemost* 76:135–138, 1996.

282. Lijnen HR, Collen D: Congenital and acquired deficiencies of components of the fibrinolytic system and their relationship to bleeding or thrombosis. *Fibrinolysis* 3:67–77, 1989.

283. Rakoczi I, Chamone D, Collen D, Verstraete M: Prediction of postoperative leg vein thrombosis in gynaecological patients. *Lancet* 1:509–510, 1978.

284. Nilsson IM, Ljungner H, Tengborn L: Two different mechanisms in patients with venous thrombosis and defective fibrinolysis: Low concentrations of plasminogen activator or increased concentration of plasminogen activator inhibitor. *Br Med J* 290:1453–1456, 1985.

285. Meltzer ME, Doggen CJ, De Groot PG, et al: The impact of the fibrinolytic system on the risk of venous and arterial thrombosis. *Semin Thromb Hemost* 35:469–477, 2009.

286. Meltzer ME, Doggen CJ, De Groot PG, et al: Reduced plasma fibrinolytic capacity as a potential risk factor for a first myocardial infarction in young men. *Br J Haematol* 145:121–127, 2009.

287. Hamsten A, Wiman B, De Faire U, Blomback M: Increased plasma levels of a rapid inhibitor of tissue plasminogen activator in young survivors of myocardial infarction. *N Engl J Med* 313:1557–1563, 1985.

288. Paramo JA, Alfaro MJ, Rocha E: Postoperative changes in the plasmatic levels of tissue-type plasminogen activator and its fast-acting inhibitor: Relationship to deep vein thrombosis and influence of prophylaxis. *Thromb Haemost* 54:713–716, 1985.

289. Juhan-Vague I, Roul C, Alessi MC, et al: Increased plasminogen activator inhibitor activity in non-insulin dependent diabetic patients: Relationship with plasma insulin. *Thromb Haemost* 61:370–373, 1989.

290. Francis CW: Plasminogen activator inhibitor-1 levels and polymorphisms: Association with venous thromboembolism. *Arch Pathol Lab Med* 126:1401–1404, 2002.

291. Tsantes AE, Nikolopoulos GK, Bagos PG, et al: The effect of the plasminogen activator inhibitor-1 4G/5G polymorphism on the thrombotic risk. *Thromb Res* 122:736–742, 2008.

292. Juhan-Vague I, Alessi MC, Joly P, et al: Plasma plasminogen activator inhibitor-1 in angina pectoris: Influence of plasma insulin and acute-phase response. *Arteriosclerosis* 9:362–367, 1989.

293. Stump DC, Taylor FB, Nesheim ME, et al: Pathologic fibrinolysis as a cause of clinical bleeding. *Semin Thromb Hemost* 16:260–273, 1990.

294. Saito H: Alpha-2-plasmin inhibitor and its deficiency states. *J Lab Clin Med* 112:671–678, 1988.

295. Gresele P, Binetti BM, Branca G, et al: TAFI deficiency in liver cirrhosis: Relation with plasma fibrinolysis and survival. *Thromb Res* 121:763–768, 2008.

296. Stein E, McMahon B, Kwaan H, et al: The coagulopathy of acute promyelocytic leukaemia revisited. *Best Pract Res Clin Haematol* 22:152–163, 2009.

297. Fay WP, Shapiro AD, Shih JL, et al: Brief report: Complete deficiency of plasminogen-activator inhibitor type 1 due to a frame-shift mutation. *N Engl J Med* 327:1729–1733, 1992.

298. Suarez CR, Walenga J, Mangogna LC, Fareed J: Neonatal and maternal fibrinolysis: Activation at time of birth. *Am J Hematol* 19:365–372, 1985.

299. Albisetti M: The fibrinolytic system in children. *Semin Thromb Hemost* 29(4):339–348, 2003.

300. Summaria L: Comparison of human normal, full-term, fetal and adult plasminogen by physical and clinical analyses. *Haemostasis* 19:266–273, 1989.

301. Edelberg JM, Enghild JJ, Pizzo SV, Gonzales-Gronow M: Neonatal plasminogen displays altered cell surface binding and activation kinetics: Correlation with increased glycosylation of the protein. *J Clin Invest* 86:107–112, 1990.

302. Andrew M, Brooker L, Leaker M, et al: Fibrin clot lysis by thrombolytic agents is impaired in newborns due to a low plasminogen concentration. *Thromb Haemost* 68:325–330, 1992.

303. Corrigan JJ, Sleeth JJ, Jeter MA, Lox CD: Newborn's fibrinolytic mechanism: Components and plasmin generation. *Am J Hematol* 32:273–278, 1989.

304. Corrigan JJ, Jeter MA: Histidine-rich glycoprotein and plasminogen plasma levels in term and preterm newborns. *Am J Dis Child* 144:825–828, 1990.

305. Parmar N, Albisetti M, Berry LR, Chan AK: The fibrinolytic system in newborns and children. *Clin Lab* 52:115–124, 2006.

306. Corrigan JJ, Jeter MA: Tissue-type plasminogen activator, plasminogen activator inhibitor, and histidine-rich glycoprotein in stressed human newborns. *Pediatrics* 89:43–46, 1992.

307. Brus F, Van Oeveren W, Okkern A, Oetomo SB: Activation of the plasma clotting, fibrinolytic, and kinin-kallikrein system in preterm infants with severe idiopathic respiratory distress syndrome. *Pediatr Res* 36:647–653, 1994.

308. Cederholm-Williams SA, Spencer JA, Wilkerson AR: Plasma levels of selected haemostatic factors in newborn babies. *Thromb Res* 23:555–558, 1981.

309. Andrew M, Paes B, Milner R, et al: Development of the human coagulation system in the full-term infant. *Blood* 70:165–172, 1987.

310. Andrew M, Massicotte-Nolan PM, Karpatkin M: Plasma protease inhibitors in premature infants: Influence of gestational age, postnatal age, and health status. *Proc Soc Exp Biol Med* 173:495–500, 1983.

311. Corrigan JJ: Thrombosis and thromboembolism, in *Hemorrhagic and Thrombotic Disease in Childhood and Adolescence*, pp 147–176. Churchill Livingstone, New York, 1985.

312. Bonnar J, Daly L, Sheppard BL: Changes in the fibrinolytic system during pregnancy. *Semin Thromb Hemost* 16:221–229, 1990.

313. Brenner B: Haemostatic changes in pregnancy. *Thromb Res* 114:409–414, 2004.

314. Bremme KA: Haemostatic changes in pregnancy. *Best Pract Res Clin Haematol* 16:153–168, 2003.

315. Hellgren M: Hemostasis during pregnancy and puerperium. *Haemostasis* 26:244–247, 1996.

316. Schjetlein R, Haugen G, Wisloff F: Markers of intravascular coagulation and fibrinolysis in preeclampsia: Association with intrauterine growth retardation. *Acta Obstet Gynecol Scand* 76:541–546, 1997.

317. SantAna Dusse LM, Cooper AJ, Lwaleed BA: Thrombin activatable fibrinolysis inhibitor (TAFI): A role in pre-eclampsia? *Clin Chim Acta* 378:1–6, 2007.

318. Hajjar KA, Francis CW: Fibrinolysis and thrombolysis, *Williams Hematology*, 7th ed, edited by K Kaushansky, MA Lichtman, E Beutler, TJ Kipps, U Seligsohn, JT Prchal, pp 2089–2115. McGraw-Hill, New York, 2006.

319. Sherry S, Fletcher AP, Alkjaersig N: Fibrinolysis and fibrinolytic activity in man. *Physiol Rev* 39:343–382, 1959.

320. Adelman B, Michelson AD, Loscalzo J, et al: Plasmin effect on platelet glycoprotein Ib-von Willebrand factor interactions. *Blood* 65:32–40, 1985.

321. Loscalzo J, Vaughan DE: Tissue plasminogen activator promotes platelet disaggregation in plasma. *J Clin Invest* 79:1749–1755, 1987.

322. Rudd MA, George D, Amarante P, et al: Temporal effects of thrombolytic agents on platelet function in vivo and their modulation by prostaglandins. *Circ Res* 67:1175–1181, 1990.

323. Go AS, Mozaffarian D, Roger VL, et al: Executive summary: Heart disease and stroke statistics—2014 update: A report from the American Heart Association. *Circulation* 129:399–410, 2014.

324. Abe T, Kazama M, Naito I, et al: Clinical evaluation for efficacy of tissue culture urokinase (TCUK) on cerebral thrombosis by means of multicenter double blind study. *Blood Vessels* 12:321–341, 1981.

325. Abe T, Kazama M, Naito I, et al: Clinical effect of urokinase (60,000 units/day) on cerebral infarction comparative study by means of multiple center double blind test. *Blood Vessels* 12:342–358, 1981.

326. Atarashi J, Otomo E, Araki G, et al: Clinical utility of urokinase in the treatment of acute stage of cerebral thrombosis: Multi-center double-blind study in comparison with placebo. *Clin Eval* 13:659–709, 1985.

327. del Zoppo GJ, Ferbert A, Otis S, et al: Local intra-arterial fibrinolytic therapy in acute carotid territory stroke. A pilot study. *Stroke* 19:307–313, 1988.

328. Fletcher AP, Alkjaersig N, Lewis M, et al: A pilot study of urokinase therapy in cerebral infarction. *Stroke* 7:135–142, 1976.

329. Hacke W, Zeumer H, Ferbert A, et al: Intra-arterial thrombolytic therapy improves outcome in patients with acute vertebrobasilar occlusive disease. *Stroke* 19:1216–1222, 1988.

330. Hanaway J, Torack R, Fletcher AP, Landau WM: Intracranial bleeding associated with urokinase therapy for acute ischemic hemispheral stroke. *Stroke* 7:143–146, 1976.

331. Matsumoto K, Satoh K: *Topical Intraarterial Urokinase Infusion for Acute Stroke*. Springer-Verlag, Heidelberg, 1991.

332. Meyer JS, Gilroy J, Barnhart MI, Johnson JF: Therapeutic thrombolysis in cerebral thromboembolism. Double-blind evaluation of intravenous plasmin therapy in carotid and middle cerebral arterial occlusion. *Neurology* 13:927–937, 1963.

333. Meyer JS, Gilroy J, Barnhart MI, Johnson JF: Anticoagulants plus streptokinase therapy in progressive stroke. *JAMA* 189:373, 1964.

334. Mori E, Tabuchi M, Yoshida T, Yamadori A: Intracarotid urokinase with thromboembolic occlusion of the middle cerebral artery. *Stroke* 19:802–812, 1988.

335. Mori E: *Fibrinolytic Recanalization Therapy in Acute Cerebrovascular Thromboembolism*. Springer-Verlag, Heidelberg, 1991.

336. Otomo E, Araki G, Itoh E, et al: Clinical efficacy of urokinase in the treatment of cerebral thrombosis. *Clin Eval* 13:711–751, 1985.

337. Theron J, Courtheoux P, Casasco A, et al: Local intraarterial fibrinolysis in the carotid territory. *AJNR Am J Neuroradiol* 10:753–765, 1989.

338. Zeumer H, Freitag HJ, Grzyska U, Neunzig HP: Local intra-arterial fibrinolysis in acute vertebrobasilar occlusion. Technical developments and recent results. *Neuroradiology* 31(4):336–340, 1989.

339. Zeumer H, Freitag HJ, Zanella F, et al: Local intra-arterial fibrinolytic therapy in patients with stroke: Urokinase versus recombinant tissue plasminogen activator (r-TPA). *Neuroradiology* 35:159–162, 1993.

340. Tissue plasminogen activator for acute ischemic stroke. The National Institute of Neurological Disorders and Stroke rt-PA Stroke Study Group. *N Engl J Med* 333:1581–1587, 1995.

341. Hacke W, Kaste M, Fieschi C, et al: Intravenous thrombolysis with recombinant tissue plasminogen activator for acute hemispheric stroke. The European Cooperative Acute Stroke Study (ECASS). *JAMA* 274(13):1017–1025, 1995.

342. Hacke W, Kaste M, Fieschi C, et al: Randomised double-blind placebo-controlled trial of thrombolytic therapy with intravenous alteplase in acute ischaemic stroke (ECASS II). Second European-Australasian Acute Stroke Study Investigators. *Lancet* 352:1245–1251, 1998.

343. Clark WM, Wissman S, Albers GW, et al: Recombinant tissue-type plasminogen activator (Alteplase) for ischemic stroke 3 to 5 hours after symptom onset. The ATLANTIS Study: A randomized controlled trial. Alteplase Thrombolysis for Acute Noninterventional Therapy in Ischemic Stroke. *JAMA* 282:2019–2026, 1999.

344. Hacke W, Donnan G, Fieschi C, et al: Association of outcome with early stroke treatment: Pooled analysis of ATLANTIS, ECASS, and NINDS rt-PA stroke trials. *Lancet* 363:768–774, 2004.

345. Hacke W, Kaste M, Bluhmki E, et al: Thrombolysis with alteplase 3 to 4.5 hours after acute ischemic stroke. *N Engl J Med* 359:1317–1329, 2008.

346. Davis SM, Donnan GA, Parsons MW, et al: Effects of alteplase beyond 3 h after stroke in the Echoplanar Imaging Thrombolytic Evaluation Trial (EPITHET): A placebo-controlled randomised trial. *Lancet Neurol* 7:299–309, 2008.

347. Wahlgren N, Ahmed N, Davalos A, et al: Thrombolysis with alteplase 3–4.5 h after acute ischaemic stroke (SITS-ISTR): An observational study. *Lancet* 372:1303–1309, 2008.

348. Ahmed N, Wahlgren N, Grond M, et al: Implementation and outcome of thrombolysis with alteplase 3–4.5 h after an acute stroke: An updated analysis from SITS-ISTR. *Lancet Neurol* 9:866–874, 2010.

349. Lees KR, Bluhmki E, von Kummer R, et al: Time to treatment with intravenous alteplase and outcome in stroke: An updated pooled analysis of ECASS, ATLANTIS, NINDS, and EPITHET trials. *Lancet* 375:1695–1703, 2010.

350. Donnan GA, Davis SM, Chambers BR, et al: Streptokinase for acute ischemic stroke with relationship to time of administration: Australian Streptokinase (ASK) Trial Study Group. *JAMA* 276(12):961–966, 1996.

351. Randomised controlled trial of streptokinase, aspirin, and combination of both in treatment of acute ischaemic stroke. Multicentre Acute Stroke Trial–Italy (MAST-I) Group. *Lancet* 346:1509–1514, 1995.

352. Thrombolytic therapy with streptokinase in acute ischemic stroke. The Multicenter Acute Stroke Trial—Europe Study Group. *N Engl J Med* 335:145–150, 1996.

353. Parsons M, Spratt N, Bivard A, et al: A randomized trial of tenecteplase versus alteplase for acute ischemic stroke. *N Engl J Med* 366:1099–1107, 2012.

354. Barnwell SL, Clark WM, Nguyen TT, et al: Safety and efficacy of delayed intraarterial urokinase therapy with mechanical clot disruption for thromboembolic stroke. *AJNR Am J Neuroradiol* 15:1817–1822, 1994.

355. Barr JD, Mathis JM, Wildenhain SL, et al: Acute stroke intervention with intraarterial urokinase infusion. *J Vasc Interv Radiol* 5(5):705–713, 1994.

356. Casto L, Caverni L, Camerlingo M, et al: Intra-arterial thrombolysis in acute ischaemic stroke: Experience with a superselective catheter embedded in the clot. *J Neurol Neurosurg Psychiatry* 60:667–670, 1996.

357. Jansen O, von Kummer R, Forsting M, et al: Thrombolytic therapy in acute occlusion of the intracranial internal carotid artery bifurcation. *AJNR Am J Neuroradiol* 16:1977–1986, 1995.

358. Nesbit GM, Clark WM, O'Neill OR, Barnwell SL: Intracranial intraarterial thrombolysis facilitated by microcatheter navigation through an occluded cervical internal carotid artery. *J Neurosurg* 84:387–392, 1996.

359. Tarr R, Taylor CL, Selman WR, et al: Good clinical outcome in a patient with a large CT scan hypodensity treated with intra-arterial urokinase after an embolic stroke. *Neurology* 47:1076–1078, 1996.

360. Janjua N, Brisman JL: Endovascular treatment of acute ischaemic stroke. *Lancet Neurol* 6:1086–1093, 2007.

361. Liu M, Wardlaw J: Thrombolysis (different doses, routes of administration and agents) for acute ischaemic stroke. *Cochrane Database Syst Rev* (2):CD000514, 2000.

362. Wardlaw JM, Del Zoppo G, Yamaguchi T, Berge E: Thrombolysis for acute ischaemic stroke. *Cochrane Database Syst Rev* (3):CD000213, 2003.

363. del Zoppo GJ, Higashida RT, Furlan AJ, et al: PROACT: A phase II randomized trial of recombinant pro-urokinase by direct arterial delivery in acute middle cerebral artery stroke. PROACT Investigators. Prolyse in Acute Cerebral Thromboembolism. *Stroke* 29:4–11, 1998.

364. Furlan A, Higashida R, Wechsler L, et al: Intra-arterial prourokinase for acute ischemic stroke. The PROACT II study: A randomized controlled trial. Prolyse in Acute Cerebral Thromboembolism. *JAMA* 282:2003–2011, 1999.

365. Ogawa A, Mori E, Minematsu K, et al: Randomized trial of intraarterial infusion of urokinase within 6 hours of middle cerebral artery stroke: The middle cerebral artery embolism local fibrinolytic intervention trial (MELT) Japan. *Stroke* 38:2633–2639, 2007.

366. Broderick JP: William M. Feinberg Lecture: Stroke therapy in the year 2025: Burden, breakthroughs, and barriers to progress. *Stroke* 35:205–211, 2004.

367. Kleindorfer D, Khoury J, Alwell K, et al: Eligibility for rt-PA in acute ischemic stroke: A population-based study. *Stroke* 34:281, 2003.

368. Kothari RU, Pancioli A, Liu T, Brott T, Broderick J: Cincinnati Prehospital Stroke Scale: Reproducibility and validity. *Ann Emerg Med* 33:373–378, 1999.

369. Albers GW, Thijs VN, Wechsler L, et al: Magnetic resonance imaging profiles predict clinical responses to early reperfusion: The diffusion and perfusion imaging evaluation for understanding stroke evolution (DEFUSE) study. *Ann Neurol* 60:508–517, 2006.

370. Furlan A, Eyding D, Albers GW, et al: Dose Escalation of Desmoteplase for Acute Ischemic Stroke (DEDAS): Evidence of safety and efficacy 3 to 9 hours after stroke onset. *Stroke* 37:1227–1231, 2006.

371. Hacke W, Albers G, Al-Rawi Y, et al: The Desmoteplase on Acute Ischemic Stroke Trial (DIAS): A phase II MRI-based 9-hour window acute stroke thrombolysis trial with intravenous desmoteplase. *Stroke* 36:66–73, 2005.

372. Abciximab in Ischemic Stroke Investigators: Abciximab in acute ischemic stroke: A randomized, double-blind, placebo-controlled, dose-escalation study. *Stroke* 31(3):601–609, 2000.

373. Qureshi AI, Suri MF, Khan J, et al: Abciximab as an adjunct to high-risk carotid or vertebrobasilar angioplasty: Preliminary experience. *Neurosurgery* 46:1316–1324, 2000.

374. Qureshi AI, Ali Z, Suri MF, et al: Intra-arterial third-generation recombinant tissue plasminogen activator (reteplase) for acute ischemic stroke. *Neurosurgery* 49:41–48, 2001.

375. Seitz RJ, Hamzavi M, Junghans U, et al: Thrombolysis with recombinant tissue plasminogen activator and tirofiban in stroke: Preliminary observations. *Stroke* 34:1932–1935, 2003.

376. Seitz RJ, Meisel S, Moll M, et al: The effect of combined thrombolysis with rtPA and tirofiban on ischemic brain lesions. *Neurology* 62:2110–2112, 2004.

377. Straub S, Junghans U, Jocanovic V, et al: Systemic thrombolysis with recombinant tissue plasminogen activator and tirofiban in acute middle cerebral artery occlusion. *Stroke* 35:705–709, 2004.

378. Adams HP Jr, Adams RJ, Brott T, et al: Guidelines for the early management of patients with ischemic stroke: A scientific statement from the Stroke Council of the American Stroke Association. *Stroke* 34:1056–1083, 2003.

379. Broderick JP, Hacke W: Treatment of acute ischemic stroke: Part I: Recanalization strategies. *Circulation* 106:1563–1569, 2002.

380. Kaste M, Thomassen L, Grond M, et al: Thrombolysis for acute ischemic stroke: A consensus statement of the 3rd Karolinska Stroke Update, October 30–31, 2000. *Stroke* 32:2717–2718, 2001.

381. Brogden RN, Speight TM, Avery GS: Streptokinase: A review of its clinical pharmacology, mechanism of action and therapeutic uses. *Drugs* 5:357–445, 1973.

382. Dotter CT, Rosch J, Seaman AJ: Selective clot lysis with low-dose streptokinase. *Radiology* 111:31–37, 1974.

383. Ouriel K: Current status of thrombolysis for peripheral arterial occlusive disease. *Ann Vasc Surg* 16:797–804, 2002.

384. Ouriel K, Shortell CK, DeWeese JA, et al: A comparison of thrombolytic therapy with operative revascularization in the initial treatment of acute peripheral arterial ischemia. *J Vasc Surg* 19:1021–1030, 1994.

385. Results of a prospective randomized trial evaluating surgery versus thrombolysis for ischemia of the lower extremity. The STILE trial. *Ann Surg* 220:251–266, 1994.

386. Ouriel K, Veith FJ, Sasahara AA: Thrombolysis or peripheral arterial surgery: Phase I results. TOPAS Investigators. *J Vasc Surg* 23:64–73, 1996.

387. Ouriel K, Veith FJ, Sasahara AA: A comparison of recombinant urokinase with vascular surgery as initial treatment for acute arterial occlusion of the legs. Thrombolysis or Peripheral Arterial Surgery (TOPAS) Investigators. *N Engl J Med* 338:1105–1111, 1998.

388. Castaneda F, Swischuk JL, Li R, et al: Declining-dose study of reteplase treatment for lower extremity arterial occlusions. *J Vasc Interv Radiol* 13:1093–1098, 2002.

389. Ouriel K, Katzen B, Mewissen M, et al: Reteplase in the treatment of peripheral arterial and venous occlusions: A pilot study. *J Vasc Interv Radiol* 11:849–854, 2000.

390. Ouriel K, Kandarpa K, Schuerr DM, et al: Prourokinase versus urokinase for recanalization of peripheral occlusions, safety and efficacy: The PURPOSE trial. *J Vasc Interv Radiol* 10:1083–1091, 1999.

391. Heymans S, Vanderschueren S, Verhaeghe R, et al: Outcome and one year follow-up of intra-arterial staphylokinase in 191 patients with peripheral arterial occlusion. *Thromb Haemost* 83:666–671, 2000.

392. Duda SH, Tepe G, Luz O, et al: Peripheral artery occlusion: Treatment with abciximab plus urokinase versus with urokinase alone—A randomized pilot trial (the PROMPT Study). Platelet Receptor Antibodies in Order to Manage Peripheral Artery Thrombosis. *Radiology* 221:689–696, 2001.

393. Drescher P, McGuckin J, Rilling WS, Crain MR: Catheter-directed thrombolytic therapy in peripheral artery occlusions: Combining reteplase and abciximab. *AJR Am J Roentgenol* 180:1385–1391, 2003.

394. Cohen LH, Kaplan M, Bernhard VM: Intraoperative streptokinase. An adjunct to mechanical thrombectomy in the management of acute ischemia. *Arch Surg* 121:708–715, 1986.

395. Comerota AJ, White JV, Grosh JD: Intraoperative intra-arterial thrombolytic therapy for salvage of limbs in patients with distal arterial thrombosis. *Surg Gynecol Obstet* 169:283–289, 1989.

396. Parent FN, Bernhard VM, Pabst TS, et al: Fibrinolytic treatment of residual thrombus after catheter embolectomy for severe lower limb ischemia. *J Vasc Surg* 9:153–160, 1989.

397. Quinones-Baldrich WJ, Zierler RE, Hiatt JC: Intraoperative fibrinolytic therapy: An adjunct to catheter thromboembolectomy. *J Vasc Surg* 2:319–326, 1985.

398. Vedantham S, Vesely TM, Parti N, et al: Lower extremity venous thrombolysis with adjunctive mechanical thrombectomy. *J Vasc Interv Radiol* 13:1001–1008, 2002.

399. Berridge DC, Kessel D, Robertson I: Surgery versus thrombolysis for acute limb ischaemia: Initial management. *Cochrane Database Syst Rev* (3):CD002784, 2002.

400. Kessel D, Berridge D, Robertson I: Infusion techniques for peripheral arterial thrombolysis. *Cochrane Database Syst Rev* 1:CD000985, 2004.

401. Thrombolysis in the management of lower limb peripheral arterial occlusion—A consensus document. Working Party on Thrombolysis in the Management of Limb Ischemia. *Am J Cardiol* 81:207–218, 1998.

402. Hirsch AT, Haskal ZJ, Hertzer NR, et al: ACC/AHA 2005 practice guidelines for the management of patients with peripheral arterial disease (lower extremity, renal, mesenteric, and abdominal aortic): A collaborative report. *Circulation* 113:e463–e654, 2006.

403. Alonso-Coello P, Bellmunt S, McGorrian C, et al: Antithrombotic therapy in peripheral artery disease: Antithrombotic Therapy and Prevention of Thrombosis, 9th ed: American College of Chest Physicians Evidence-Based Clinical Practice Guidelines. *Chest* 141:e669S–e690S, 2012.

404. Menon KV, Shah V, Kamath PS: The Budd-Chiari syndrome. *N Engl J Med* 350(6):578–585, 2004.

405. Aytekin C, Boyvat F, Kurt A, et al: Catheter-directed thrombolysis with transjugular access in portal vein thrombosis secondary to pancreatitis. *Eur J Radiol* 39:80–82, 2001.

406. Ciccarelli O, Goffette P, Laterre PF, et al: Transjugular intrahepatic portosystemic shunt approach and local thrombolysis for treatment of early posttransplant portal vein thrombosis. *Transplantation* 72:159–161, 2001.

407. Tateishi A, Mitsui H, Oki T, et al: Extensive mesenteric vein and portal vein thrombosis successfully treated by thrombolysis and anticoagulation. *J Gastroenterol Hepatol* 16:1429–1433, 2001.

408. Calin GA, Calin S, Ionescu R, et al: Successful local fibrinolytic treatment and balloon angioplasty in superior mesenteric arterial embolism: A case report and literature review. *Hepatogastroenterology* 50:732–734, 2003.

409. Savassi-Rocha PR, Veloso LF: Treatment of superior mesenteric artery embolism with a fibrinolytic agent: Case report and literature review. *Hepatogastroenterology* 49:1307–1310, 2002.

410. Haire WD, Atkinson JB, Stephens LC, Kotulak GD: Urokinase versus recombinant tissue plasminogen activator in thrombosed central venous catheters: A double-blinded, randomized trial. *Thromb Haemost* 72:543–547, 1994.

411. Semba CP, Deitcher SR, Li X, et al: Treatment of occluded central venous catheters with alteplase: Results in 1,064 patients. *J Vasc Interv Radiol* 13:1199–1205, 2002.

412. Shen V, Li X, Murdock M, et al: Recombinant tissue plasminogen activator (alteplase) for restoration of function to occluded central venous catheters in pediatric patients. *J Pediatr Hematol Oncol* 25:38–45, 2003.

413. Timoney JP, Malkin MG, Leone DM, et al: Safe and cost effective use of alteplase for the clearance of occluded central venous access devices. *J Clin Oncol* 20:1918–1922, 2002.

414. Cooper SG: Original report. Pulse-spray thrombolysis of thrombosed hemodialysis grafts with tissue plasminogen activator. *AJR Am J Roentgenol* 180:1063–1066, 2003.

415. Cynamon J, Pierpont CE: Thrombolysis for the treatment of thrombosed hemodialysis access grafts. *Rev Cardiovasc Med* 3 Suppl 2:84–91, 2002.

416. Daeihagh P, Jordan J, Chen J, Rocco M: Efficacy of tissue plasminogen activator administration on patency of hemodialysis access catheters. *Am J Kidney Dis* 36:75–79, 2000.

417. Hilleman DE, Dunlay RW, Packard KA: Reteplase for dysfunctional hemodialysis catheter clearance. *Pharmacotherapy* 23:137–141, 2003.

418. Shrivastava D, Lundin AP, Dosunmu B, et al: Salvage of clotted jugular vein hemodialysis catheters. *Nephron* 68:77–79, 1994.

419. Sobel BE: Intracranial bleeding, fibrinolysis, and anticoagulation. Causal connections and clinical implications. *Circulation* 90:2147–2152, 1994.

420. Sane DC, Califf RM, Topol EJ, et al: Bleeding during thrombolytic therapy for acute myocardial infarction: Mechanisms and management. *Ann Intern Med* 111:1010–1022, 1989.

421. Alkjaersig N, Fletcher AP, Sherry S: Xi-aminocaproic acid: An inhibitor of plasminogen activation. *J Biol Chem* 234:832–837, 1959.

422. Andersson L, Nilsson IM, Nilehn JE, et al: Experimental and clinical studies on AMCA, the antifibrinolytically active isomer of p-aminomethyl cyclohexane carboxylic acid. *Scand J Haematol* 2:230–247, 1965.

423. Brockway WJ, Castellino FJ: The mechanism of the inhibition of plasmin by xi-aminocaproic acid. *J Biol Chem* :246:4641–4647, 1971.

424. McNicol GP, Fletcher AP, Alkjaersig N, et al: The absorption, distribution and excretion of xi-aminocaproic acid following oral or intravenous administration to man. *J Lab Clin Med* 59:15, 1962.

425. Huber R, Kukla D, Ruhlmann A, Steigemann W: Pancreatic trypsin inhibitor (Kunitz). I. Structure and function. *Cold Spring Harb Symp Quant Biol* 36:141–148, 1971, 1972.

426. Ruhlmann A, Kukla D, Schwager P, et al: Structure of the complex formed by bovine trypsin and bovine pancreatic trypsin inhibitor. Crystal structure determination and stereochemistry of the contact region. *J Mol Biol* 77:417–436, 1973.

427. Wiman B: On the reaction of plasmin or plasmin-streptokinase complex with aprotinin or alpha 2-antiplasmin. *Thromb Res* 17:143–152, 1980.

428. Mangano DT, Tudor IC, Dietzel C: The risk associated with aprotinin in cardiac surgery. *N Engl J Med* 354:353–365, 2006.

429. Mouton R, Finch D, Davis I, Zacharowski K: Effect of aprotinin on renal dysfunction. *Lancet* 372:1543–1544, 2008.

430. Schneeweiss S, Seeger JD, Landon J, Walker AM: Aprotinin during coronary-artery bypass grafting and risk of death. *N Engl J Med* 358:771–783, 2008.

431. Shaw AD, Stafford-Smith M, White WD, et al: The effect of aprotinin on outcome after coronary-artery bypass grafting. *N Engl J Med* 358:784–793, 2008.

432. Fergusson DA, Hebert PC, Mazer CD, et al: A comparison of aprotinin and lysine analogues in high-risk cardiac surgery. *N Engl J Med* 358:2319–2331, 2008.

433. Aoki N, Moro M, Matsuda M, Tachiya K: The behavior of alpha-2 plasmin inhibitor in fibrinolytic states. *J Clin Invest* 60:361–369, 1977.

434. Aoki N, Sakata Y, Matsuda M, Tateno K: Fibrinolytic states in a patient with congenital deficiency of alpha 1-plasmin inhibitor. *Blood* 55:483–488, 1980.

435. Dieval J, Nguyen G, Gross S, et al: A lifelong bleeding disorder associated with a deficiency of plasminogen activator inhibitor type 1. *Blood* 77(3):528–532, 1991.

436. Lee MH, Vosburgh E, Anderson K, McDonagh J: Deficiency of plasma plasminogen activator inhibitor 1 results in hyperfibrinolytic bleeding. *Blood* 81:2357–2362, 1993.

437. Avvisati G, Ten Cate JW, Sturke A, et al: Acquired alpha-2-antiplasmin deficiency in acute promyelocytic leukemia. *Br J Haematol* 70:43–48, 1988.

438. Avvisati G, Ten Cate JW, Buller HR, Mandelli F: Tranexamic acid for control of haemorrhage in acute promyelocytic leukemia. *Lancet* 1989;ii:122–124.

439. Rodeghiero F, Avvisati G, Castaman G, et al: Early deaths and anti-hemorrhagic treatments in acute promyelocytic leukemia. A GIMEMA retrospective study in 268 consecutive patients. *Blood* 75:2112–2117, 1990.

440. Schwartz BS, Williams EC, Conlan MG, Mosher DF: Epsilon-aminocaproic acid in the treatment of patients with acute promyelocytic leukemia and acquired alpha-2-plasmin inhibitor deficiency. *Ann Intern Med* 105:873–877, 1986.

441. Booth NA, Anderson JA, Bennett B: Plasminogen activators in alcoholic cirrhosis: Demonstration of increased tissue type and urokinase type activator. *J Clin Pathol* 37:772–777, 1984.

442. Hayashi T, Kamogawa A, Ro S, et al: Plasma from patients with cirrhosis increases tissue plasminogen activator release from vascular endothelial cells *in vitro. Liver* 18:186–190, 1998.

443. Violi F, Basili V, Ferro D: Association between high values of D-dimer and tissue-plasminogen activator activity and first gastrointestinal bleeding in cirrhotic patients. *Thromb Haemost* 76:177, 1996.

444. Boylan JF, Klinck JR, Sandler AN, et al: Tranexamic acid reduces blood loss, transfusion requirements, and coagulation factor use in primary orthotopic liver transplantation. *Anesthesiology* 85:1043–1048, 1996.

445. Kaspar M, Ramsay MA, Nguyen AT, et al: Continuous small-dose tranexamic acid reduces fibrinolysis but not transfusion requirements during orthotopic liver transplantation. *Anesth Analg* 85:281–285, 1997.

446. Segal HC, Hunt BJ, Cottam S, et al: Fibrinolytic activity during orthotopic liver transplantation with and without aprotinin. *Transplantation* 58:1356–1360, 1994.

447. Soilleux H, Gillon MC, Mirand A, et al: Comparative effects of small and large aprotinin doses on bleeding during orthotopic liver transplantation. *Anesth Analg* 80:349–352, 1995.

448. Al-Mondhiry H, Manni A, Owen J, Gordon R: Hemostatic effects of hormonal stimulation in patients with metastatic prostate cancer. *Am J Hematol* 28:141–145, 1988.

449. Bennett B, Croll AM, Robbie LA, Herriot R: Tumour cell u-PA as a cause of fibrinolytic bleeding in metastatic disease. *Br J Haematol* 99:570–574, 1997.

450. Mannucci PM, Cugno M, Bottasso B, et al: Changes in fibrinolysis in patients with localized tumors. *Eur J Cancer* 26:83–87, 1990.

451. Meijer K, Smid WM, Geerards S, van der Meer J: Hyperfibrinogenolysis in disseminated adenocarcinoma. *Blood Coagul Fibrinolysis* 9:279–283, 1998.

452. Webber MM, Waghray A: Urokinase-mediated extracellular matrix degradation by human prostatic carcinoma cells and its inhibition by retinoic acid. *Clin Cancer Res* 1:755–761, 1995.

453. Zacharski LR, Memoli VA, Ornstein DL, et al: Tumor cell procoagulant and urokinase expression in carcinoma of the ovary. *J Natl Cancer Inst* 85:1225–1230, 1993.

454. Bouchama A, Bridey F, Hammami MM, et al: Activation of coagulation and fibrinolysis in heatstroke. *Thromb Haemost* 76:909–915, 1996.

455. Harker LA: Bleeding after cardiopulmonary bypass. *N Engl J Med* 314:1446–1448, 1986.

456. Williams GD, Bratton SL, Nielsen NJ, Ramamoorthy C: Fibrinolysis in pediatric patients undergoing cardiopulmonary bypass. *J Cardiothorac Vasc Anesth* 12:633–638, 1998.

457. Horrow JC, Hlavacek J, Strong MD, et al: Prophylactic tranexamic acid decreases bleeding after cardiac operations. *J Thorac Cardiovasc Surg* 99:70–74, 1990.

458. Horrow JC, Van Riper DF, Strong MD, et al: Hemostatic effects of tranexamic acid and desmopressin during cardiac surgery. *Circulation* 84:2063–2070, 1991.

459. Munoz JJ, Birkmeyer NJ, Birkmeyer JD, et al: Is epsilon-aminocaproic acid as effective as aprotinin in reducing bleeding with cardiac surgery?: A meta-analysis. *Circulation* 99:81–89, 1999.

460. Soslau G, Horrow J, Brodsky I: Effect of tranexamic acid on platelet ADP during extracorporeal circulation. *Am J Hematol* 38:113–119, 1991.

461. Blomback M, Johansson G, Johnsson H, et al: Surgery in patients with von Willebrand's disease. *Br J Surg* 76:398–400, 1989.

462. Hedlund PO: Antifibrinolytic therapy with Cyklokapron in connection with prostatectomy. A double blind study. *Scand J Urol Nephrol* 3:177–182, 1969.

463. Sindet-Pedersen S, Stenbjerg S: Effect of local antifibrinolytic treatment with tranexamic acid in hemophiliacs undergoing oral surgery. *J Oral Maxillofac Surg* 44:703–707, 1986.

464. Callender ST, Warner GT, Cope E: Treatment of menorrhagia with tranexamic acid. A double-blind trial. *Br Med J* 4:214–216, 1970.

465. Ong YL, Hull DR, Mayne EE: Menorrhagia in von Willebrand disease successfully treated with single daily dose tranexamic acid. *Haemophilia* 4:63–65, 1998.

466. Ortel TL, Onorato JJ, Bedrosian CL, Kaufman RE: Antifibrinolytic therapy in the management of the Kasabach Merritt syndrome. *Am J Hematol* 29:44–48, 1988.

467. Stahl RL, Henderson JM, Hooks MA, et al: Therapy of the Kasabach-Merritt syndrome with cryoprecipitate plus intra-arterial thrombin and aminocaproic acid. *Am J Hematol* 36:272–274, 1991.

PART XIII Transfusion Medicine

136. Erythrocyte Antigens and
     Antibodies 2329

137. Human Leukocyte and Platelet
     Antigens 2353

138. Blood Procurement and Red Cell
     Transfusion. 2365

139. Preservation and Clinical Use of
     Platelets. 2381

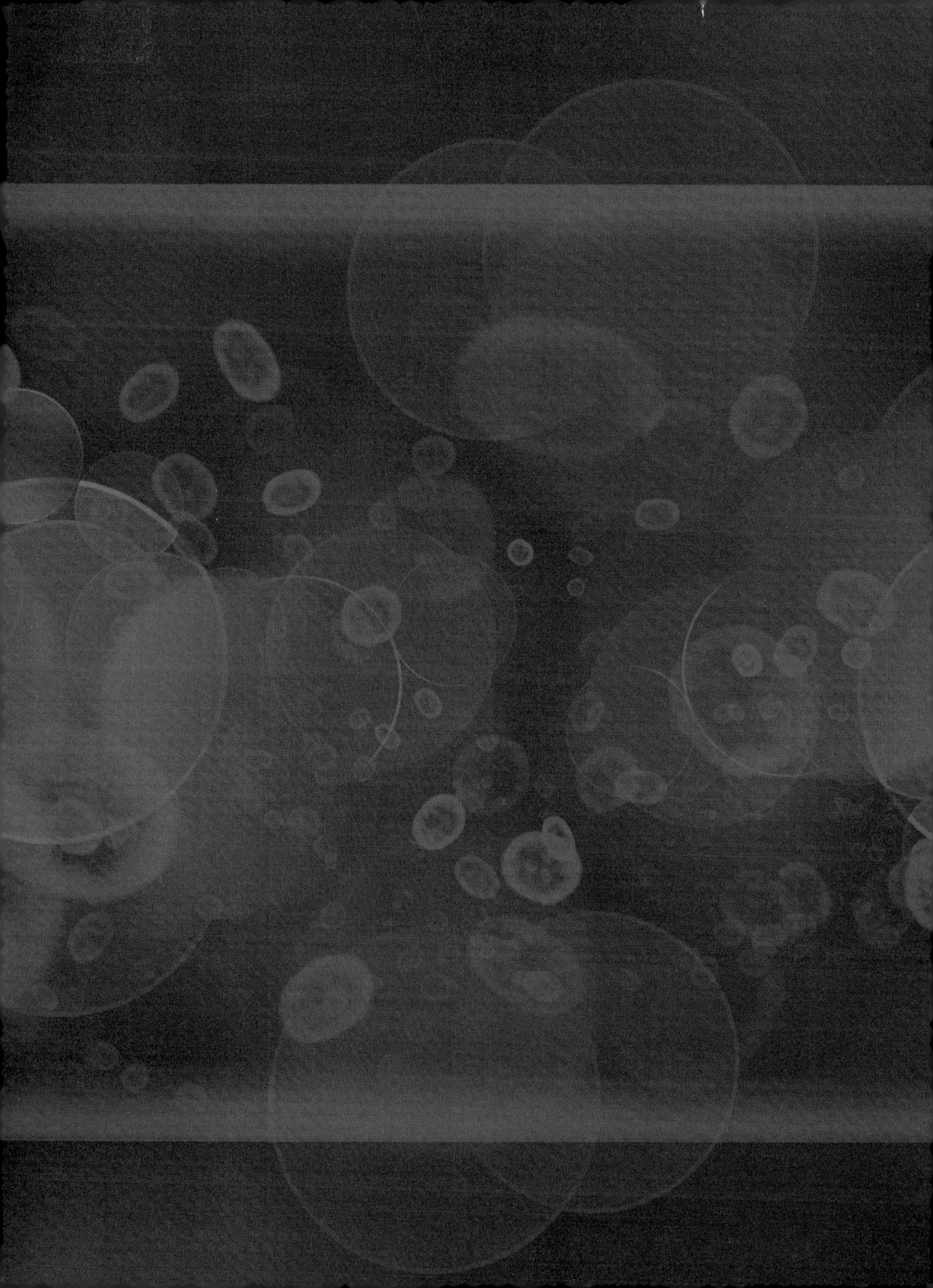

CHAPTER 136
ERYTHROCYTE ANTIGENS AND ANTIBODIES

Marion E. Reid and Christine Lomas-Francis

SUMMARY

Blood group antigens are structures on the outer surface of human red blood cells (RBCs) that can be recognized by the immune system of individuals who lack that particular structure. Identification of RBC antigens and antibodies has been the basis of pretransfusion compatibility testing and the safe transfusion practices used today and also can provide insights into understanding the etiology of hemolytic disease of the fetus and the newborn. Biochemical and molecular studies have led to definition of the biologic functions of molecules expressing blood group antigens. These molecules play a critical role in susceptibility to infection by malarial parasites, some viruses, and bacteria. Alteration of RBC antigen expression is associated with many molecular backgrounds and some play a role in the clinical manifestations of certain diseases. Erythrocytes, far from being inert containers of hemoglobin, are active in a variety of physiologic processes.

● DEFINITIONS AND HISTORY

A *blood group system* consists of a group of antigens encoded by alleles at a single gene locus or at gene loci so closely linked that crossing over does not occur or is very rare. An *antigen collection* consists of antigens that are phenotypically, biochemically, or genetically related, but the genes encoding them have not been identified.[1] Placement of a blood group antigen into a system or collection begins with the discovery of an antibody, usually in the serum of a multiparous woman or a multiply transfused recipient, with a unique pattern of reactivity. The antibody can be used to study basic biochemical properties of the corresponding antigen, to enable recognition of the pattern of inheritance of the antigen in families and in populations, to identify red blood cells (RBCs) that lack the antigen, and to search for an antithetical antigen. Identified characteristics, such as prevalence of positive reactions or sensitivity or resistance to specific enzymes, are compared to antigens in known systems and collections. A newly recognized antigen is also evaluated using biochemical and molecular genetic methods. Orphan antigens of low or high prevalence are placed in "holding tanks" until the gene that encodes them is established.

The majority of genes encoding blood group antigens have been cloned and sequenced,[2] and the molecular bases of most blood group antigens have been determined.[3-6] Details on the alleles associated with blood group antigens and phenotypes can be obtained from the National Center for Biotechnology Information (NCBI) "dbRBC" website: http://www.ncbi.nlm.nih.gov/gv/mhc/xslcgi.cgi?cmd=bgmut/home and from the International Society of Blood transfusion (ISBT) website: www.isbt-web.org.

RBC antigens are inherited carbohydrate or protein structures located on the outside surface of the RBC membrane (Fig. 136–1). Although most of the protein blood group antigens are carried on integral transmembrane proteins (either single-pass type I or type II, or multipass; Fig. 136–1), a few are carried on glycosylphosphatidylinositol (GPI)-linked proteins or adsorbed from plasma. Some carbohydrate antigens are attached to proteins or lipids and some require a combination of a specific portion of protein and carbohydrate. Blood group antigens have revealed that certain transmembrane proteins interact with other transmembrane proteins (e.g., band 3 and glycophorin A [GPA]; Kell and Kx; Rh and RhAG), with lipids (e.g., Rh), or with proteins in the membrane skeleton (e.g., band 3 and ankyrin, glycophorin C [GPC], and protein 4.1 and p55). Many of the proteins carrying blood group antigens reside in the erythrocyte membrane as complexes.[7-10] Many components carrying blood group antigens have been assigned cluster of differentiation (CD) numbers (Table 136–1). In human blood grouping, agglutination of RBCs usually serves as the detectable end point, but it can also be hemolysis.[11] Our ability to detect and identify blood group antigens and antibodies has contributed significantly to current safe blood transfusion practice, reducing death from hemolytic disease of the fetus and newborn (HDFN) from 40 percent to less than 2 percent, and supporting patients receiving chemotherapy or organ transplantation.

The naming of blood group antigens usually does not follow the classic convention wherein dominant traits are given capital letters and recessive traits are designated with lowercase letters. For example, in the ABO blood group system, A and B are codominant and the recessive O phenotype is encoded by a gene designated *O*, whereas in the MNS system the genes *S* and *s* are codominant. To standardize terminology used to describe RBC blood groups, the ISBT Working Party for Terminology for Red Cell Surface Antigens recommended using the traditional name for an antigen for verbal communication and a numerical system in computer databases (see Blood Group Terminology website at www.isbt-web.org). The working party has placed blood group antigens into four categories: (1) genetically discrete blood group systems; (2) serologically, biochemically, or genetically related antigens in blood group collections; (3) series of low-incidence antigens; and (4) series of high-incidence antigens. Each system and collection has been given a number and letter designation, and each antigen within the system is numbered sequentially in order of discovery. At the time of going to press (2015), 35 blood group systems and 6 antigen collections are defined (see Table 136–1; www.isbt-web.org).[1,5,6,12-14] Over time, notations devised to describe blood group antigens have changed. A single letter (e.g., A, D, K), a symbol with a superscript (e.g., Fy^a, Jk^b, Lu^a), a symbol with a number (e.g., Fy3, Lu4, K12), and three to four letters (e.g., Vel, JMH, ELO, FPPT) are all used, sometimes within the same blood group system. The ISBT Working Party name has changed to ISBT Working Party on Red Cell Immunogenetics and Blood Group Terminology, which reflects that DNA testing is now often used to predict a blood group.

Acronyms and Abbreviations: AET, 2-aminoethylisothiouronium bromide; CD, cluster of differentiation; DTT, dithiothreitol; GPA, glycophorin A; GPB, glycophorin B; GPC, glycophorin C; GPD, glycophorin D; GPI, glycosylphosphatidylinositol; HDFN, hemolytic disease of the fetus and newborn; HEMPAS, hereditary erythroblastic multinuclearity with a positive acidified serum test; Ig, immunoglobulin; ISBT, International Society of Blood Transfusion; LAD, leukocyte adhesion deficiency; 2-ME, 2-mercaptoethanol; PNH, paroxysmal nocturnal hemoglobinuria; RBC, red blood cell.

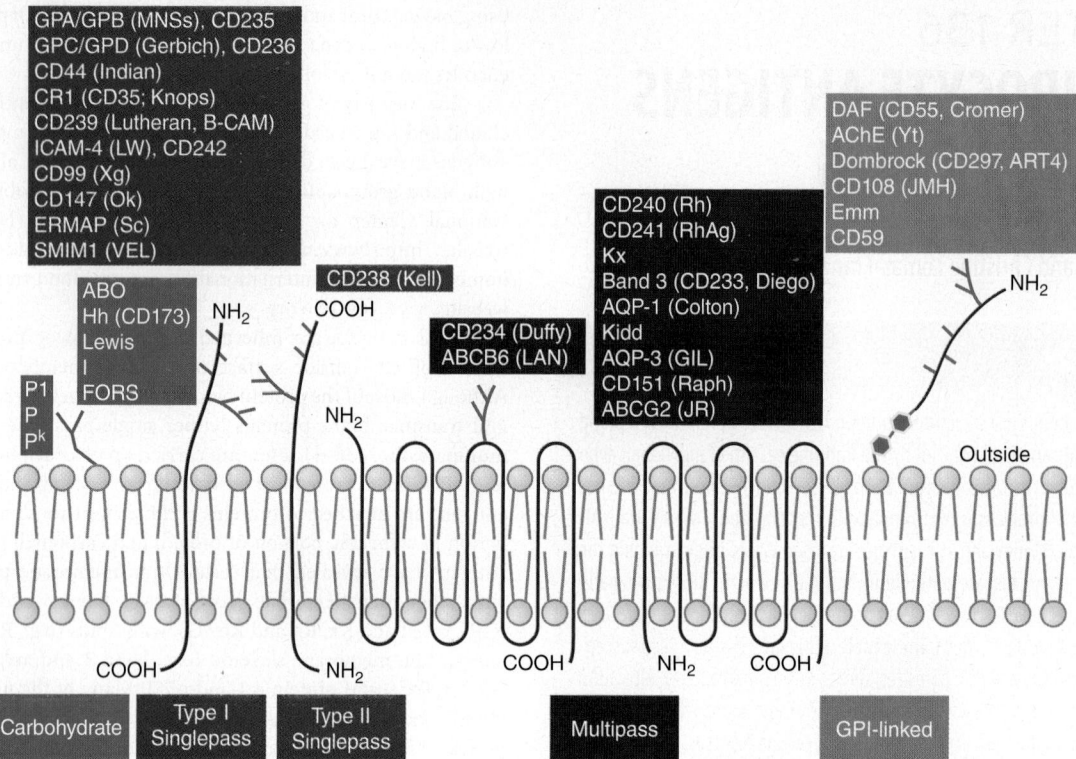

Figure 136–1. Membrane structures carrying blood group activity.

BLOOD GROUP SYSTEMS

Tables 136–1 and 136–2 summarize the characteristics of common blood group antigens. The following sources provide more detail: Issitt and Anstee,[5] Reid, Lomas-Francis and Olsson,[6] Reid and Lomas-Francis,[15] Mollison and colleagues,[16] Daniels,[4] and Fung and associates.[11] In the interest of space, reviews or books are referenced in place of original reports.

ABO BLOOD GROUP SYSTEM

The ABO blood group system was the first system described and remains the most significant in transfusion medicine. A mismatch of ABO may be fatal, whereas a mismatch of other blood groups initially mostly is harmless. This situation occurs because anti-A and anti-B antibodies usually are present in the blood of adults lacking the corresponding antigen. These antibodies are stimulated by the ubiquitous distribution of the antigen that forms part of the membrane structure of many bacteria, plants, and animals. For this reason, all donor blood for transfusion is tested and labeled with the ABO group. The four main phenotypes are A, B, AB, and O, the latter indicating a lack of A and B antigens. The sugars defining A and B antigens are added to carbohydrate chains carrying the H antigen (fucose), which is "hidden" by the A (GalNAc) or B (Gal) sugar. Thus, group A or B erythrocytes appear to have less H antigen than group O cells. Nonetheless, H is found on all human erythrocytes except those from rare individuals of the O_h (Bombay) phenotype.

Anti-A or anti-B immunoglobulins can cause intravascular hemolysis when ABO-incompatible RBCs are transfused. Because A and B antigens also are expressed on most tissue cells, ABO compatibility is a significant consideration in solid-organ transplantation. However, ABO incompatibility only rarely causes severe HDFN because antibodies directed against A and B antigens are predominantly immunoglobulin (Ig) M, which do not cross the placenta, in addition, A and B antigens are not fully developed on RBCs from a fetus (Chap. 55).

Although the ABO blood group system has only four phenotypes, hundreds of alleles have been identified by DNA analyses. The ABO gene was cloned in 1990 following purification of A transferase.[17,18] A and B transferases have only four amino acid differences in the catalytic domain, two of which (Leu266Met and Gly268Ala) are primarily responsible for substrate specificity.[19] The group O phenotype results from nucleotide changes in A and/or B alleles that cause loss of glycosyltransferase activity. The most common group O (O_1) results from a single nucleotide deletion near the 5′ end of the gene that causes a frameshift and early termination with no active enzyme production.[20] The *ABO* gene has seven exons, and A or B subgroups (with only few exceptions) result from a variety of nucleotide changes in exon 7 that cause alterations in the catalytic domain of the glycosyltransferase (reviewed by Chester and Olsson[21]). The rare B(A), A(B), and *cis*-AB phenotypes expressing both A and B antigens result from variant glycosyltransferases that have a combination of A- and B-specific residues.[21] Numerous common and rare ABO alleles have been reported, and current information is available on websites: http://www.ncbi.nlm.nih.gov/gv/mhc/xslcgi.cgi?cmd=bgmut/home and www.isbt-web.org. In addition to nucleotide changes, recombinations and gene rearrangements can result in hybrid alleles that encode for unexpected transferase activity. This situation makes typing of ABO by DNA analysis difficult to interpret.[22] The function of the ABO system is not known, although several disease associations are well established.[23]

Rh BLOOD GROUP SYSTEM

The Rh (*not* Rhesus) system is the second most important blood group system in transfusion medicine because antigen-positive RBCs frequently immunize antigen-negative individuals through transfusion and pregnancy.

Inheritance of Rh antigens is determined by a complex of two closely linked genes: one encodes the protein carrying D antigen (RhD); the other encodes the protein carrying C or c and E or e antigens (RhCE).

TABLE 136–1. Characteristics of International Society of Blood Transfusion Defined Blood Group Systems and Antigen Collections

Conventional Name	ISBT Symbol (No.)	Chromosome Location	ISBT Gene Name (ISGN If Different)	Associated Antigens [Null Phenotype]	Function of RBC Membrane Component (CD No.)	Disease Association
BLOOD GROUP SYSTEMS						
ABO	ABO (001)	9q34.2	*ABO*	A, B, A, B, A1 [group O]	Glycocalyx	Altered expression in some hematologic disorders
MNS	MNS (002)	4q31.21	*MNS (GYPA, GYPB)*	M, N, S, s, U, and 43 more [En(a–); U–; M^kM^k]	Binds microbe glycocalyx, complement regulation, chaperone for band 3 (CD235)	Decreased *Plasmodium falciparum* invasion, may be receptor for *Escherichia coli*
P1PK	P1PK (003)	22q13.2	*P1 (A4GALT)*	P1, P^k, NOR	Glycocalyx	
Rh	RH (004)	1p36.11	*RHD, RHCE (RH)*	D, C, E, c, e, and 49 more [Rh_{null}]	Possibly transports CO_2 or NH_3 (CD240)	Hemolytic anemia, hereditary stomatocytosis, hematologic malignancies
Lutheran	LU (005)	19q13.32	*LU*	Lu^a, Lu^b, Lu3, and 18 more [recessive Lu(a–b–)]	Binds laminin (CD239)	Increased expressions possibly involved in vasoocclusion in sickle cell disease
Kell	KEL (006)	7q34	*KEL*	K, k, Kp^a, Kp^b, Js^a, Js^b, and 29 more [K_0 or K_{null}]	Cleaves big endothelin-3 to ET-3, a potent vasoconstrictor (CD238)	
Lewis	LE (007)	19p13.3	*LE (FUT3)*	Le^a, Le^b, and 4 more [Le(a–b–)]	Glycocalyx, Le^b is receptor for *Helicobacter pylori*	Increased expression in fucosidosis, Lewis antibodies may be important in graft rejection
Duffy	FY (008)	1q23.2	*FY (DARC)*	Fy^a, Fy^b, Fy3, Fy5, Fy6 [Fy(a–b–)]	Chemokine, *Plasmodium vivax* receptor (CD234)	Resistance to *P. vivax* invasion
Kidd	JK (009)	18q12.3	*JK(HUT11, SLC14AI)*	Jk^a, Jk^b, Jk3 [Jk(a–b–)]	Urea transporter	Impaired urea transport, urine-concentrating defect
Diego	DI (010)	17q21.31	*DI (SLC4A1; AE1)*	Di^a, Di^b, Wr^a, Wr^b, and 18 more	Anion exchanger (CD233), Band 3 cytoskeletal protein	Southeast Asian ovalocytosis, hereditary spherocytosis, renal tubular acidosis
Yt	YT(011)	7q22.1	*Yt (ACHE)*	Yt^a, Yt^b	Acetylcholinesterase	Absent from PNH III RBCs
Xg	XG (012)	Xp22.33	*XG (XG, MIC2)*	Xg^a, CD99	Adhesion molecules (CD99)	
Scianna	SC (013)	1p34.2	*SC (ERMAP)*	Sc1, Sc2, Sc3, and 4 more [SC: –1, –2, –3]	Possible adhesion	
Dombrock	DO (014)	12p12.3	*DO (ART4)*	Do^a, Do^b, Gy^a, Hy, Jo^a and 3 more [Gy(a–)]	Enzymatic (CD297)	Absent from PNH III RBCs
Colton	CO (015)	7p14.3	*CO (AQP1)*	Co^a, Co^b, Co3, Co4 [Co(a–b–)]	Water transport	Monosomy 7, inability to maximally concentrate urine, congenital dyserythropoietic anemia
Landsteiner-Wiener	LW (016)	19p13.2	*LW (ICAM4)*	LW^a, LW^{ab}, LW^b [LW(a–b–)]	Binds CD11/CD18, ligand for integrins (CD242)	Depressed in pregnancy and some malignant diseases
Chido/Rogers	CH/RG (017)	6p21.32	*C4A,C4B*	CH1, RGl, and 7 more	Complement components	Certain phenotypes have increased susceptibility to certain autoimmune conditions and infections

(continued)

TABLE 136–1. Characteristics of International Society of Blood Transfusion Defined Blood Group Systems and Antigen Collections (Continued)

Conventional Name	ISBT Symbol (No.)	Chromosome Location	ISBT Gene Name (ISGN If Different)	Associated Antigens [Null Phenotype]	Function of RBC Membrane Component (CD No.)	Disease Association
H	H (018)	19q13.33	H (FUT1)	H [Bombay, O$_h$]	Glycocalyx (CD 173)	Decreased in some tumor cells, increased in hematopoietic stress
Kx	XK (019)	Xp21.1	XK	Kx [McLeod]	Possible neurotransmitter, function in RBCs not known	Acanthocytosis, muscular dystrophy, hemolytic anemia; McLeod syndrome sometimes associated with CGD, peripheral neuropathy, cardiomyopathy seizures, a late-onset dementia, and behavioral changes
Gerbich	GE (020)	2q14.3	GE (GYPC)	Ge2, Ge3, Ge4, and 8 more [Leach phenotype]	Membrane attachment; interacts with 4.1R and p55 (CD236)	Hereditary elliptocytosis, hemolytic anemia, decreased 4.1R and p55
Cromer	CROM (021)	1q32.2	CROM (CD55; DAF)	Cr^a, Tc^a, Tc^b, Tc^c, Dr^a, and 13 more [Inab phenotype]	Complement regulation, binds C3b, disassembles C3/C5 convertase (CD55)	Absent from PNH III RBCs, Dr^a is the receptor for uropathogenic E. coli
Knops	KN (022)	1q32.2	KN (CR1)	Kn^a, Kn^b, McC^a, Sl^a, Yk^a, and 4 more [Helgeson phenotype]	Complement regulation, binds C3b and C4b, mediates phagocytosis (CD35)	Antigens depressed in certain autoimmune and malignant conditions
Indian	IN (023)	11p13	IN (CD44)	In^a, In^b, INFI, INJA	Binds hyaluronic acid, mediates adhesion of leukocytes (CD44)	Depressed in pregnancy, congenital dyserythropoietic anemia
Ok	OK (024)	19p13.3	OK (BSG)	Ok^a, OKGV, OKVM	Possible adhesion (CD147)	
Raph	RAPH (025)	11p15.5	MER2 (CD151)	MER2 [RAPH$_{null}$]	Adhesion molecule involved in kidney function (CD151)	Renal disease, associated with pretibial epidermolysis bullosa and sensorineural deafness
John Milton Hagen	JMH (026)	15q24.1	JMH (SEMA7A)	JMH, and 5 more	Adhesion molecule, function in RBCs not known (CD108)	Absent from PNH III RBCs
I	I (027)	6p24.2	GCNT2	I [I–; i adult]	Glycocalyx	Congenital cataracts in Asians
GLOB	Globoside (028)	3q26.1	P (β3GALNT1)	P, PX2 [P–]	Glycocalyx	Receptor E. coli and parvovirus B19
Gil	GIL (029)	9p13.3	GIL (AQP3)	GIL [GIL–]	Glycerol/water/urea transporter	
Rh-associated glycoprotein	RHAG (030)	6p21.3	RHAG	Duclos, and 3 more	Possibly transports CO_2, or NH_3 (CD241)	Hemolytic anemia, hereditary stomatocytosis
FORS	FORS (031)	9q34.2	GBGT1	FORS1	Glycocalyx	
JR	JR (032)	4q22.1	JR, ABCG2	Jr^a [Jr(a–)]	ATP-dependent transporter	
Lan	LAN (033)	2q36	LAN, ABCB6	Lan [Lan–]	ATP-dependent transporter	

(continued)

TABLE 136–1. Characteristics of International Society of Blood Transfusion Defined Blood Group Systems and Antigen Collections (Continued)

Conventional Name	ISBT Symbol (No.)	Chromosome Location	ISBT Gene Name (ISGN If Different)	Associated Antigens [Null Phenotype]	Function of RBC Membrane Component (CD No.)	Disease Association
Vel	VEL (034)	1p36.32	*VEL, SMIM1*	Vel [Vel-]		CD59
CD59	CD59 (035)	1p13.33	*CD59*	CD59.1 [CD59-]	Complement regulation (CD59)	Absent from PNH III RBCs
Antigen Collections						
Cost	COST (205)	—	—	Cs^a, Cs^b		
Ii	I (207)	—	—	i		
Er	ER (208)	—	—	Er^a, Er^b, Er3		
	GLOB (209)	—	—	LKE,		
	Unnamed: (210)	—	—	Le^c, Le^d		
	MN CHO (213)	—	—	Hu, M$_1$, Tm, Can, Sext, Sj		
Low-incidence series	— (700)	—	—	17		
High-incidence series	— (901)	—	—	At^a, Emm, AnWj, Sd^a, PEL, ABTI, MAM		

CGD, chronic granulomatous disease; ISGN, International Society for Gene Nomenclature; PNH, paroxysmal nocturnal hemoglobinuria; RBC, red blood cell.

Data from Daniels GL, Anstee DJ, Cartron J-P, et al: Blood group terminology 1995. ISBT working party on terminology for red cell surface antigens. *Vox Sang* 69:265, 1995; Issitt PD, Anstee DJ: *Applied Blood Group Serology*, 4th ed. Montgomery Scientific, Durham, NC, 1998; Reid ME, Lomas-Francis C, Olsson ML: *Blood Group Antigen FactsBook*, 3rd. Academic Press, San Diego, 2012; Reid ME, Lomas-Francis C: *Blood Group Antigens & Antibodies: A Guide to Clinical Relevance & Technical Tips*. Star Bright Books, New York, 2007; www.isbt-web.org.

TABLE 136–2. Summary of Common Blood Group Systems or Collections and Their Antigens

Blood Group (Year Reported)	Common Phenotypes	Frequency White/ Black (%)	No. Antigen Copies on Adult RBC × 10^3	Dosage (See Text)	Cord Cell Expression	Biochemistry	Antigen Distribution in Blood, Fluids, and Tissues	Comments
ABO (1900)	A B AB	40/27 11/20 4/4	AB: ~800–1000	A/B: not evident	Weak: ~1/3 adult expression	Carbohydrate on types 1, 2, 3, and 4 precursor chains	RBC, lymphs, plts	Most significant antigens in transfusion and transplantation
H (1948)	O	45/29	H: ~1700	H expression depends on ABO: O>A$_2$>B> A$_2$B>A$_1$>A$_1$B	Weak Main RBC carrier: bands 3 and 4.5	Attached to lipids in plasma and protein in secretions	Plasma, secretions; broad tissue distribution; most epithelial/endothelial cells	Weak subgroups result from variant transferases
Rh (1939)	R$_1$ Dce r ce R$_2$ DcE R$_0$ Dce r'Ce r''cE	42/17 37/26 14/11 4/44 2/2 1/0	D on R$_2$R$_2$: 15–33 R$_1$R$_1$: 14–19 R$_0$r: 12–20 R$_1$r: 9–14 c on cc: 70–85	D: not evident C and c: yes E and e: yes	Normal adult	Multipass, nonglycosylated protein: 30–32 kDa; 417 aa C: serine 103/c: proline 103 E: proline 226/e: alanine 226	Erythroid specific Possible cation transport Possible role in RBC membrane integrity	D most significant antigen after A and B Three causes for weak D expression (see text) Nulls: amorphic type and regulator type

(continued)

TABLE 136–2. Summary of Common Blood Group Systems or Collections and Their Antigens (Continued)

Blood Group (Year Reported)	Common Phenotypes	Frequency White/Black (%)	No. Antigen Copies on Adult RBC × 10³	Dosage (See Text)	Cord Cell Expression	Biochemistry	Antigen Distribution in Blood, Fluids, and Tissues	Comments
	R$_z$ DCE	<1	Cc: 37–53			Forms "Rh complex" with LW, GPB, and Rh-related glycoprotein (chromosome 6)		
	r^y CE	<1	e on ee: 18–24					
			Ee: 13–14					
Lewis (1946)	Le(a+b–)	22/23	Le^a: ~3	Not evident	Weak: adult expression at age 2 years	Carbohydrate on type 1 precursor chains only	Plasma and secretion antigen; on RBC, lymphs, plts only by adsorption of plasma antigen	Le antigens depend on *Le/Se* interaction; *Le/Se* = Le(a–b+), ABH secretor; *lele/sese* = Le(a+b–), ABH nonsecretor; *lele* = Le(a–b–), Sese status not apparent
	Le(a–b+)	72/55						
	Le(a–b–)	6/22				Attached to lipids in plasma and protein in secretions		
	Le(a+b+)	Rare in European populations; found in Australasian populations; 10 in Japanese						Le(a–b+) express some Le^a, do not make anti-Le^a. Women test Le(a–b–) during pregnancy
I (1956)	I adult(↑↑↓i)	Common	I: ~500	Not evident	Strong i; weak I. Adult expressions at age 2 years	Carbohydrate on ABH active chains; lipid on RBC; protein in plasma	Broad tissue distribution; RBCs, plts, lymphs, granules, monos; also in plasma, secretions (e.g., milk, saliva, urine)	I and i expression are inversely proportional but not products of alleles
	i cord (↓I↑i)	Common						
	i adult (↓I↑↑i)	<1:10,000						
P1PK and GLOB								
P1 (1927)	P$_1$:	79/94	P1: ~500	Not evident, but inherited variations exist; e.g., P1 may be normal, strong, or weak	Weak: adult expression by 7 years	Carbohydrate on RBC and plasma glycolipids; not in secretions	RBC, lymphs, plts, monos, fibroblasts, uroepithelial cells	P1-like antigen is associated with pigeon and earthworm protein and parasitic infections
GLOB (1951)	P$_2$:	21/6	Globoside: ~15,000					
	p: P^k–P–P1–	Rare						
MNS	M+N–	28/26	GPA: ~800	Yes	Normal adult	Single-pass sialoglycoprotein type 1	RBCs plus renal capillary epithelial/endothelium	GPA and GPB carry multiple antigens and many hybrids of GPA–GPB
	M+N+	50/44	GPB: ~200					
(M: 1927)	M–N+	22/30				GPA: 43 kDa, 131 aa, carries MN		Can have absence of GPA, GPB, or both
(S: 1947)	S+s–	11/3						
	S+s+	44/28				GPB: 25 kDa, 72 aa, carries SsU; part of Rh complex		
	S–s+	45/69						
	S–s–U–	0/<1						
Kell (1946)	K–k+	91/98	Kell: 2–6	Yes	Normal adult	Single-pass glycoprotein type II highly folded: 93kDa, 732 aa	Kell: RBC plus marrow and fetal liver tissue; not on brain, kidney, adult liver	System of high- and low-frequency antigens

(continued)

TABLE 136–2. Summary of Common Blood Group Systems or Collections and Their Antigens (Continued)

Blood Group (Year Reported)	Common Phenotypes	Frequency White/Black (%)	No. Antigen Copies on Adult RBC × 10³	Dosage (See Text)	Cord Cell Expression	Biochemistry	Antigen Distribution in Blood, Fluids, and Tissues	Comments
Kpᵃ/Jsᵃ: (1957)	K+k+ K+k– Kp(a–b+) Kp(a+b+) Kp(a+b–) Js(a–b+) Js(a+b+) Js(a+b–)	8.8/2 0.2/rare 97.7/100 2.3/rare Rare/0 100/80 Rare/19 0/1				K/k Met 193 Thr Kpᵃ/Kpᵇ: Trp 281 Arg Jsᵃ/Jsᵇ: Pro 597 Leu	Kx: RBC plus skeletal/heart muscle, neurologic tissues	Common phenotype: k, Kpᵇ, Jsᵇ Kell antigen expression depends on both Kell and Xk genes K$_{null}$ lacks Kell antigens, has Kx Kx$_{null}$ lacks Kx, has poor Kell antigen expression (McLeod phenotype) Other causes of poor Kell expression: *cis* Kpᵃ, Ge–, K$_{mod}$, autoantibody
Duffy (1950)	Fy(a+b–) Fy(a+b+) Fy(a–b+) Fy(a–b–)	17/9 49/1 34/22 Rare/68	Fyᵃ: 6–13	Yes, but not always evident because of *Fy* gene	Normal: adult levels at 12 weeks	Multipass glycoprotein: 35–45 kDa, 338 aa Fyᵃ/Fyᵇ Gly 42Asp	RBC plus brain, colon, lung, spleen, thyroid, thymus, kidney, endothelium; not in liver or placenta tissue	Fy(a–b–) blacks do not express Fyᵇ on their RBC, but express it on other tissues and seldom make anti-Fyᵇ
Kidd (1951)	Jk(a+b–) Jk(a+b+) Jk(a–b+) Jk(a–b–)	28/57 49/34 23/9 <1% Polynesians	Jkᵃ: ~14	Yes	Normal adult	Multipass protein: ~43 kDa, 391 aa 1 potential *N*-glycan Jkᵃ/Jkᵇ: Asp284 Asn	RBC specific	Important cause of DHTR Nulls are unable to fully concentrate urine; dominant inhibitor *In(Jk)* has weak Jk antigen
Lutheran (1951)	Lu(a+b–) Lu(a+b+) Lu(a–b+) Lu(a–b–)	0.15/– 7.5/0 92.3/– Very rare	Luᵇ: 1.5–4	Yes, but family variations exist	Weak: adult level at 15 years	Single-pass glycoprotein type I: 85 kDa, 597 aa 78 kDa 5 Ig superfamily domains: two variable, three constant B-CAM Luᵃ/Luᵇ: His77Arg	RBC plus brain, heart, kidney, lung, pancreas, placenta, skeletal muscle	System of high- and low-frequency antigens Dominant inhibitor *In(Lu)* and X-linked inhibitor *(XS2)* cause greatly reduced Lu expression First known autosomal linkage to *Se*

aa, amino acids; B-CAM, B-cell adhesion molecule; DHTR, delayed hemolytic transfusion reactions; GPA, glycophorin A; GPB, glycophorin B; granulos, granulocytes; Ig, immunoglobulin; ISBT, International Society of Blood Transfusion; lymphs, lymphocytes; monos, monocytes; plts, platelets; RBC, red blood cell.

RBCs from Rh-positive people have both RhD and RhCE, whereas Rh-negative RBCs have only RhCE. In the Rh system, eight common antigen combinations or haplotypes are possible: Dce (R_0, Rh_0), DCe (R_1, Rh_1), DcE (R_2, Rh_2), DCE (R_z, Rh_z), ce (r, rh), Ce (r', rh'), cE (r", rh"), and CE (r^y, rh^y). The letter "d" is commonly used to designate the lack of D, but there is no d antigen or anti-d.

Several nomenclatures can be used to describe Rh genes and antigens. The Fisher-Race nomenclature, which uses CDE terminology, is more commonly used for antigens; the Wiener nomenclature, which uses Rh/rh (or R/r) designations, is favored for haplotypes and gene complexes; and the Rosenfield and Rubinstein nomenclature, which uses numerical designations, was introduced to allow interpretation without bias.[24]

The Rh blood group system has over 50 antigens (the ABO system has 4). By far the most important and immunogenic antigen is D (Rh_0 in Wiener terminology, referring to Wiener's discovery that a rhesus monkey injected with human RBCs would produce antibody that agglutinated the RBCs of 85 percent of white New Yorkers). For most clinical purposes, testing individuals for the D antigen and classifying them as D+ (or Rh-positive), or D– (or Rh-negative) is sufficient. Approximately 85 percent of the white population is Rh-positive, and 15 percent is Rh-negative. Most Rh-negative recipients produce anti-D if they receive Rh-positive blood. Anti-D can cause hemolysis in adults following an Rh-mismatched transfusion and in the newborn (HDFN) if antibodies were made by the mother from a prior transfusion or pregnancy. Thus, donors and recipients are routinely typed and matched for D. The risk of anti-D sensitization by transfusion is essentially eliminated by matching. The risk of anti-D sensitization in pregnancy is minimized by passive immunization of mothers at risk against D.

The antigens C, c, E, and e are less immunogenic and become important in patient care only after the corresponding antibody develops or when the basic Rh haplotype must be determined. The remaining 45+ antigens are other Rh protein epitopes whose corresponding antibodies are seldom encountered. Some are encoded by variant Rh alleles and appear as antithetical antigens to C, c, E, or e, or as related "extra" antigens. Others are referred to as *compound* antigens or *cis* gene products. For example, the protein produced by *RHCE*ce* encodes c and e antigens, and the compound f (or ce) antigen. Other compound antigens include Ce (rh_i), cE and CE. Still other Rh antigens are related to the complex "mosaic" nature of D and e, and less commonly C, c and E antigens. If immunized, individuals who lack a part of an antigen and who make antibody to the portion they lack, can present with a challenging serologic picture. For example, the D+ person who lacks part of the D antigen and makes an antibody to the missing portion appears to make alloanti-D because normal D+ RBCs carry all D epitopes.[25]

Some, but not all, individuals who lack part of the D antigen (partial D) have weak expression of D on their red cells that is detected only by the antiglobulin test. Having a *RHCE*C* gene in trans position to a *RHD* gene (e.g., *Dce/Ce* or *DCe/Ce* genotypes) also can weaken expression of D in some individuals. A third type of weak D expression results from inheriting a *RHD* gene that encodes all epitopes of D, but in less-than-normal quantity.

DNA analyses have revealed the molecular basis underlying antigens and phenotypes. A list of the alleles that have been described to date is available at: http://www.ncbi.nlm.nih.gov/gv/mhc/xslcgi.cgi?cmd=bgmut/home and www.isbt-web.org. Rh blood group orthologs are present in nonhuman primates and other species on the evolutionary tree.[26] The RhD and RhCE proteins complex with the Rh-associated glycoprotein (RhAG) in the membrane. RhAG acts as a transporter of gases, most likely for ammonium, nitrous oxide, CO_2 and/or O_2 but confirmation is needed as to which it is.

OTHER BLOOD GROUP SYSTEMS

In terms of transfusion and HDFN, the other blood group systems and their antigens become clinically relevant only when antibody develops. Transfusion service laboratories identify (*antibody identification*) the specificity and characterize the reactivity of antibodies detected in routine testing (*antibody screening*). Once this information is known, the blood bank assesses the clinical significance of the antibody and selects the most appropriate blood for transfusion. Tables 136–1 and 136–2 summarize the number of antigens in each blood group system and other relevant information. A detailed description of all the blood group antigens is beyond the scope of this chapter. Because the molecular bases of most blood group antigens and phenotypes are known,[6] DNA analysis can be used to predict the type of transfused patients and to identify the fetus at risk for HDFN.[27]

● GENERAL IMMUNOLOGY OF BLOOD GROUP ANTIGENS

An *antigen* is a substance that can evoke an immune response when introduced into an immunocompetent host and react with the antibody produced from that immune response. An antigen can have several *epitopes*, which together are called an *antigenic determinant*, each of which is capable of eliciting an antibody response.

The ability of an antigen to stimulate an immune response is called *immunogenicity*, and its ability to react with an antibody is called *antigenicity*. These primary characteristics are affected by antigen size, shape, rigidity, and the number and location of the determinants on the red cell membrane.

IMMUNOGENICITY

Immunogenicity depends on many antigen characteristics, not just the number of antigen sites. Relative immunogenicity is estimated by comparing the actual observed incidence of an antibody to the calculated likelihood of a possible immunizing event. After A and B, the D antigen is most immunogenic (early work suggested that approximately 80 percent of Rh-negative individuals produce anti-D after receiving a single Rh-positive RBC component but more recent studies indicate it is more like 20 to 30 percent[4]), followed by K, which stimulates anti-K in approximately 10 percent of cases.[16] The antigens c and E are one-third as immunogenic; Fy^a is one-twenty-fifth as potent; and Jk^a is one-fiftieth to one-one hundredth times as potent as K.[28] It should be noted that immunogenicity does not always correlate with the hemolytic potential of an antibody specificity; for example, K is more immunogenic than Jk^a but anti-Jk^a is more likely to cause hemolysis.

● ANTIGEN EXPRESSION

NUMBER OF ANTIGEN SITES

The number of antigen sites per RBC has been estimated by measuring the uptake of ^{125}I-labeled antibody or of ferritin-conjugated anti-IgG. Numbers vary widely among blood group systems from a few hundred to over a million (see Table 136–2). Also, estimates for any given antigen can vary greatly.

ANTIGEN DEVELOPMENT ON FETAL ERYTHROCYTES

Most RBC antigens can be detected early in fetal development (A, B, and H antigens can be detected at 5 to 6 weeks' gestation), but not all are fully developed at birth. A, B, H, I, P1, Lu^a, Lu^b, Yt^a, Xg^a, Vel, Bg,

Do^a, Do^b, and Kn^a antigen expression is considerably weaker on cord RBCs than on RBCs from adults. Le^a, sometimes Le^b, Ch/Rg, AnWj, and Sd^a, are not readily detectable, although 50 percent of cord samples type Le(a+) with more sensitive test methods. Full expression of A, B, H, I, and Lewis antigens usually is present by age 3 years, whereas full expression of P1 and Lutheran antigens may not occur until age 7 years.

VARIATION IN ANTIGEN EXPRESSION

RBCs from individuals who are homozygous for an allele typically have a greater number of antigen sites than do RBCs from individuals who are heterozygous. Consequently, their RBCs can react more strongly with antibody. This difference in expression and antigen–antibody reactivity because of zygosity is known as *dosage*. For example, RBCs from a homozygous *MM* individual carry a double dose of M antigen and react more strongly with anti-M than do RBCs from a *MN* heterozygous individual carrying only a single dose of M. Antithetical antigens C/c, E/e, M/N, S/s, and Jk^a/Jk^b commonly show dosage effect. Dosage is less obvious with D, K/k, and Lu^a/Lu^b antigens. It typically is more apparent within a family than between families. Dosage within the Duffy system also may not be serologically obvious because Fy(a+b–) or Fy(a–b+) phenotypes are seen in either homozygous (*Fy^{a}Fy^a* or *Fy^{b}Fy^b*) or hemizygous (*Fy^{a}Fy* or *Fy^{b}Fy*) individuals.

Some blood group antigens are inherited as closely linked genes or haplotypes. Haplotype pairings and gene interaction (either *cis* or *trans*) also can affect phenotypic expression. For example, the pairing of *RHCE*C* in *trans* position to *RHD* can result in weak expression of D (see "Rh Blood Group System" above), whereas *RHCE*E* in *cis* position with *RHD* is associated with strong expression of D. Among the common phenotypes, R$_2$R$_2$ RBCs carry the strongest expression of D. In the Kell system, Kp^a is associated with weakened expression of *in cis* k and Js^b antigens.

Still other antigens are affected by regulator genes.[29] The dominant type of the Lu(a–b–) phenotype [In(Lu)] results from heterozygosity for an allele of the *KLF1* gene, the gene that encodes erythroid Krüppel-like factor (EKLF). The dominant inhibitor gene *KLF1* suppresses expression of Lutheran, P1, i, and many other antigens.[30] The dominant inhibitor *In(Jk)* suppresses expression of Jk^a and Jk^b antigens.[31] Rare variants of the *RHAG* gene depress or prevent expression of the Rh antigens (see "Rh$_{null}$ Syndrome" below).

● BIOCHEMISTRY OF ERYTHROCYTE ANTIGENS

An antibody typically recognizes an epitope consisting of four to five amino acids on linear proteins or one to seven sugars. Alternatively, the antibody-binding site may encompass a more complex three-dimensional structure with branches or folds, and recognition may depend on both amino acids and sugars. Tables 136–2 and 136–3 and Fig. 136–1 summarize blood group biochemistry and antigen structure.[4,6,16]

CARBOHYDRATE ANTIGENS

Polysaccharides with blood group activity are made by sequential addition of specific sugars (or sugar derivatives) to specific precursors in specific linkages by specific transferases. Sugars commonly involved are galactose (Gal), *N*-acetyl-D-galactosamine (GalNAc), *N*-acetylglucosamine (Glc-NAc), fucose (Fuc), and *N*-acetylneuraminic acid (NeuAc).

Antigens in ABO, LE, P1PK, and GLOB blood group systems depend on an immunodominant sugar, usually terminally located, the polysaccharide to which the sugar is attached, and the type of linkage involved. I/i specificity is defined by a series of sugars on the inner portion of ABH saccharide chains. The presence of at least two repeating Gal(β1–4)GlcNAc(β1–3)Gal units in a linear structure defines i activity. I activity involves these same sugars in branched form (see Table 136–3). The gene for I (*GCNT2*) encodes the transferase responsible for branching (β(1–6) glucosaminyltransferase). During the first years of a child's life, linear chains are modified into branched chains, resulting in the appearance of I antigens.[32] The I antigen is reduced on RBCs from fetuses and infants. A rare i phenotype occurs in adults (see "I-Negative Phenotype [i Adult]" below).

Polysaccharide chains are attached to glycoproteins in secretions (on type 2 chains), to glycolipids in plasma (on type 1 chains), and to both on the RBC membrane. Approximately 70 percent of A, B, H, and I antigens on the RBC membrane are carried on glycoproteins, primarily on the anion transporter, but also on the glucose transporter, the RhAG, and others. Approximately 10 percent of these antigens are on NeuAc-rich glycoproteins, 5 percent on simple glycolipids, and the remainder on polyglycosylceramide.[16] P1, P^k, and P antigens are found on glycolipids both on the membrane and in plasma.[33]

Lewis antigens are unique because they occur only on type 1 polysaccharide chains, which are found in plasma and secretions but not made by RBCs. Hence, they exist on RBCs only by adsorption of Lewis substance from plasma. The Le (or *FUT3*) gene encodes an α(1–4)fucosyltransferase. Whether the resulting antigen is Le^a or Le^b depends on the secretor gene Se (or *FUT2*), which encodes an α(1–2) fucosyltransferase.

PROTEIN ANTIGENS

Protein structures that carry blood group antigens can be grouped into three categories: (1) those that make a single pass through the erythrocyte membrane, (2) those that make multiple passes through the membrane, and (3) those that are attached to the membrane through a covalent linkage to lipid (GPI-linked; see Fig. 136–1).

Single-pass proteins include GPA with M and N antigens, glycophorin B (GPB) with S, s, and U antigens, GPC and glycophorin D (GPD) with Gerbich antigens, and the Lutheran, LW, Indian, Knops, Xg, Ok, and Scianna proteins (see Fig. 136–1). These proteins have an extracellular amino-terminus and an intracellular carboxyl-terminus (referred to as *type I*). In contrast, the Kell glycoprotein has an extracellular carboxyl-terminus and an intracellular amino-terminus (referred to as *type II*).

Most proteins that carry blood group antigens and make multiple passes through the erythrocyte membrane have both carboxyl- and amino-terminal ends that are intracellular, are hydrophobic, and have a transport function. Rh, RhAG, Diego, Colton, Kidd, Kx, GIL, and Raph proteins are included in this category. Duffy and Lan are multipass proteins, but they have an extracellular amino-terminus. Duffy has homology with a family of cytokine receptors and the Lan protein belongs to the family of ATP-binding cassettes.[4,6,34]

Lipid-linked proteins have their carboxyl-terminus attached to the lipid GPI and are said to be GPI-linked or anchored. Cromer, Yt, Dombrock, and JMH proteins belong to this category. GPI-linked proteins are of special interest to hematologists because defective synthesis of the GPI anchor is responsible for paroxysmal nocturnal hemoglobinuria (PNH).[35] Thus, PNH-III RBCs lack all proteins attached by a GPI anchor, including those carrying blood groups (Chap. 40).

TABLE 136–3. Biochemistry of Common Carbohydrates and Antigens on Glycophorin A and Glycophorin B

Specificity	Structure	Gene for Bolded Determinant
i	$-$**Gal**$(\beta1\rightarrow4)$**GlcNAc**$(\beta1\rightarrow3)$**Gal**$(\beta1\rightarrow4)$**GLcNAc**$(\beta1\rightarrow3)$Gal$-$R$-$	
I	$-$Gal$(\beta1\rightarrow4)$**GlcNAc**$(\beta1\rightarrow6)$	
	$\quad\quad\quad\quad\quad$**Gal**$(\beta1\rightarrow4)$**GlcNAc**$(\beta1\rightarrow3)Gal-$R	GCNT2
	$-$Gal$(\beta1\rightarrow4)$GlcNAc$(\beta1\rightarrow3)$	
H	Gal$(\beta1\rightarrow4$ or $\beta1\rightarrow3)$GlcNAc$(\beta1\rightarrow3)$Gal$-$R	H (FUTI)
	Fuc$(\alpha1\rightarrow2)$	
A	**GalNAc**$(\alpha1\rightarrow3)$Gal$(\beta1\rightarrow4$ or $\beta1\rightarrow3)$GlcNAc$(\beta1\rightarrow3)$Gal$-$R	A
	Fuc$(\alpha1\rightarrow2)$	
B	**Gal**$(\alpha1\rightarrow3)$Gal$(\beta1\rightarrow4$ or $\beta1\rightarrow3)$GlcNAc$(\beta1\rightarrow3)$Gal$-$R	B
	Fuc$(\alpha1\rightarrow2)$	
Le^a	Gal$(\beta1\rightarrow3)$GlcNAc$(\beta1\rightarrow3)$Gal$-$R	LE (FUT3)
	Fuc$(\alpha1\rightarrow4)$	
Le^b	Gal$(\beta1\rightarrow3)$GlcNAc$(\beta1\rightarrow3)$Gal$-$R	SE (FUT2)
	Fuc$(\alpha1\rightarrow2)$**Fuc**$(\alpha1\rightarrow4)$	
P	Gal$(\alpha1\rightarrow4)$Gal$(\beta1\rightarrow4)$Glc$-$Cer	Pk*
P	**GalNAc**$(\beta1\rightarrow3)$Gal$(\alpha1\rightarrow4)$Gal$(\beta1\rightarrow4)$Glc$-$Cer	β3GALNT1
P$_1$	**Gal**$(\alpha1\rightarrow4)$Gal$(\beta1\rightarrow4)$GlcNAc$(\beta1\rightarrow3)$Gal$(\alpha1\rightarrow4)$Gal$(\beta1\rightarrow4)$Glc$-$Cer	P1
M	$\quad\nabla\quad\nabla\quad\nabla$ **Ser**$-$Ser$-$Thr$-$Thr$-$**Gly**$-$(GPA chain: 131 amino acids)	GYPA(M)
N	$\quad\nabla\quad\nabla\quad\nabla$ **Leu**$-$Ser$-$Thr$-$Thr$-$**GluA**$-$(GPA chain: 131 amino acids)	GYPA(N)
S	$\quad\nabla\quad\nabla\quad\nabla$ Leu$-$Ser$-$Thr$-$Thr$-$GluA$-$**Met48**$-$(GPB chain: 72 amino acids)	GPYB(S)
S	$\quad\nabla\quad\nabla\quad\nabla$ Leu$-$Ser$-$Thr$-$Thr$-$GluA$-$**Thr48**$-$(GPB chain: 72 amino acids)	GPYB(s)

GPA, glycophorin A; GPB, glycophorin B; R, primary glycolipid attachment Glc-Ger, primary glycoprotein attachment GlcNAc-Asp; ∇, Immunodominant sugars and amino acids are indicated in bold.

*Proposed gene.

$-$Gal$-$GalNAc$-$NeuNAc

NeuNac

EFFECT OF ENZYMES AND OTHER CHEMICALS ON ERYTHROCYTE ANTIGENS

Expression of an RBC antigen is determined by its exposure as a result of its position on the cell surface and its biochemical structure. Expression can be modified with treatment of RBCs by enzymes and other chemicals. These reagents are used to help identify complex mixtures of antibodies and to help characterize antibody specificity when identity is not readily apparent.

Proteolytic enzymes, such as ficin, papain, bromelin, trypsin, and α-chymotrypsin, cleave proteins from the erythrocyte membrane at specific amino acids. Enzyme treatment of RBCs cleaves certain protein antigens and allows carbohydrate and other resistant protein antigens to react more strongly with their antibody. The reactivity of antibodies with antigens in ABO, I, P1PK, LE, RH, and JK systems is enhanced after enzyme treatment of the RBCs, whereas reactivity of antibodies to M, N, Fy^a, Fy^b, and many minor antigens (Xg^a, Ch, Rg, JMH, In^b, Ge2, Ge4, Pr, Tn, and some examples of Yt^a) is reduced or eliminated. S and s are variably affected by enzyme treatment, and Kell and Scianna antigens are relatively unaffected.[4–6]

Reagents that reduce disulfide bonds, such as 2-mercaptoethanol (2-ME), dithiothreitol (DTT), and 2-aminoethylisothiouronium bromide (AET), denature Kell blood group antigens but enhance Kx. Reducing reagents also denature antigens in LW, SC, IN, JMH, and YT systems and weaken antigens in LU, DO, CROM, KN, and RAPH systems and the AnWj antigen.[4–6]

Acid treatment of RBCs (ethylenediaminetetraacetic acid [EDTA]/glycine/acid reagent), which is frequently used to remove IgG from RBCs, can weaken or completely denature antigens in the KEL blood group system. Chloroquine treatment of erythrocytes (also sometimes used to remove IgG from RBCs) at room temperature has little effect on most antigens. However, treatment for 30 minutes at 37°C can weaken expression of many antigens, including Fy^b, Lu^b, Yt^a, JMH, and those in the RH, DO, and KN systems.

GENETICS OF ERYTHROCYTE ANTIGENS

Protein antigens are direct gene products: The gene encodes a protein that expresses one or more antigens. Carbohydrate antigens, made by transferase action, are indirect gene products. Most blood group genes are located on autosomes; only two, *Xg* and *XK*, are located on the X chromosome (see Table 136–1 for locations of genes on chromosomes).

Most genes that encode blood groups have two or more alleles. Individuals who inherit two identical alleles are homozygous and make a double dose of a single gene product, whereas those who inherit two different alleles are heterozygous and make single dose of each of two gene products. Males are hemizygous for the genes located on their single X chromosome and make a single gene product. In contrast, females produce a double dose of the *Xg* and *XK* gene products, as X-chromosome inactivation does not involve Xg^a or Kx antigens.[36]

ALLELES

Alleles encoding blood group antigens commonly arise from only a single or a few nucleotide changes. For example, A and B alleles differ by only seven DNA base substitutions, which result in four amino acid substitutions in their respective transferases.[4–6] The common O allele is similar to *A* except for a single base deletion at nucleotide 261 that shifts the reading frame during RNA translation. The resulting protein is truncated and has no transferase activity. Another variant O allele encodes a transferase identical to that of B except it has arginine instead of alanine at amino acid position 268, which blocks the enzyme activity. A comprehensive listing of blood group alleles is available at the following websites: http://www.ncbi.nlm.nih.gov/gv/mhc/xslcgi.cgi?cmd=bgmut/home and www.isbt-web.org.

GENE COMPLEXES

Some blood group genes are complexes of several closely linked genes or loci that evolved through duplication of an ancestral gene. The antigens they encode are inherited as a haplotype with no or few crossovers. Blood group examples include the Rh system with genes *RHD* and *RHCE*, and the MNS system with genes *GYPA*, *GYPB*, and *GYPE*.

RHD and *RHCE* show remarkable homology between them and with *RHAG*, which encodes the RhAG. *GYPA* and *GYPB* probably arose by duplication of an ancestral GYPA gene encoding the N antigen.[37] The most common MNS complex is Ns, followed by Ms, MS, and NS.

In both RH and MNS systems, other antigens arose by further nucleotide changes, deletions, or rearrangements within the gene complex. Unequal pairing of *GYPA* and *GYPB* during meiosis, with subsequent recombination, resulted in several hybrids, such as *GYP(A-B)* (called Lepore type, by analogy with a similar hemoglobin hybrid), which encodes a protein with the amino-terminal end of GPA but the carboxyl-terminal end of GPB. Anti–Lepore-type hybrids, *GYP(B-A)* (amino-terminal end of GPB and carboxyl-terminal end of GPA), and other rearrangements (e.g., *GYP[B-A-B]* and *GYP[A-B-A]*) are known. Within the Rh complex, numerous hybrids of *RH(D-CE-D)* and *RH(CE-D-CE)* have been identified. Such hybrids can result in altered antigen expression and new antigens.[4–6]

Kell and Lutheran proteins are single-gene products that carry multiple antigens. The most common alleles in humans are *kKp^{b}Js^{b}K*[11] and *Lu^{b}Lu^{6}Lu^{8}Au^a*. Antigens of lower prevalence (K, Kp^a/Kp^c, or Js^a, and Lu^a, Lu9, Lu14, or Au^b) arise from separate nucleotide changes.

SILENT ALLELES

Some blood group alleles are amorphs, or silent; that is, they do not produce a recognizable antigen, although they may encode a product that is simply not detected with standard test methods. As discussed with regard to the ABO system, A and B genes produce transferases that add GalNAc or Gal, respectively, to the same precursors, but O produces no active enzyme. *AB* individuals express both A and B antigen, but *AA* and *AO* individuals express A, and *BB* and *BO* individuals express B. Amorphic alleles are recognized only in a homozygous state, and the result is a "null" phenotype. Null phenotypes exist in most blood group systems (see Table 136–1). Group O is the most common, followed by Fy(a–b–) and Le(a–b–) in Africans. Other null phenotypes are rare.

The Fy(a–b–) phenotype is especially interesting. Fy(a–b–) Africans have *Fy^b* genes that express normal Fy^b glycoprotein on tissue cells but not on RBCs. A nucleotide change that disrupts the GATA-1 binding site for RBC transcription is present in these individuals,[38] which helps explain why many Fy(a–b–) Africans do not make anti-Fy^b despite exposure to antigen-positive RBCs from transfusion.

GENE FREQUENCIES

Gene and phenotype frequencies vary widely with race and geographical boundaries.[6,11,16,39] This information is useful when estimating the availability of compatible blood and the probability of HDFN.

RED CELL ANTIGENS IN HEALTH AND DISEASE

EXPRESSION OF RED CELL ANTIGENS IN OTHER BODY TISSUES AND FLUIDS

Antigens in the RH and JK blood group systems are present only on RBCs and have not been detected on platelets, lymphocytes, or granulocytes or in plasma, other body tissues, or secretions (saliva, milk, amniotic fluid).[4-6,16] Antigens in MNS, LU, KEL, and FY systems are found on RBCs and other body tissues (see Table 136–2).

ABH antigens have broad tissue distribution. In embryos, A, B, and H antigens are detectable on all endothelial cells and all epithelial cells except those of the central nervous system. Antigens in ABO, P1PK, LE, H, and I systems are in plasma and on platelets and lymphocytes. Granulocytes carry I antigen but no ABH. ABH on platelets and lymphocytes may be acquired at least in part by adsorption from plasma. Lewis antigen is acquired by RBCs by adsorption. Secretions (saliva, milk, sweat, semen, and urine, but not cerebral spinal fluid) contain soluble A, B, H, I, and Le[a] and Le[b] antigens but no P1PK or GLOB system antigens. Sd[a] antigen is found in most body secretions, with the greatest concentration in urine.[5,16]

ASSOCIATIONS OF RED CELL ANTIGENS WITH DISEASE

ANTIGENS ASSOCIATED WITH POSSIBLE SUSCEPTIBILITY TO DISEASE

Some blood groups are statistically associated with medical conditions or disease (Table 136–4).[4-6,16] For example, blood group A is more common in persons with cancer of the salivary glands, stomach, colon, or ovary and with thrombosis (because of higher levels of coagulation factors VIII, V, and IX). Blood group O is more common in patients with duodenal and gastric ulcers, rheumatoid arthritis, and von Willebrand disease.

Associations with infection arise when microorganisms carry structures homologous with blood group activity. The presence of blood group antibody and/or soluble blood group antigen in secretions may help confer protection. Having anti-B may offer protection against *Salmonella*, *Shigella*, *Neisseria gonorrhoeae*, and some *Escherichia coli* infections. An association exists between nonsecretion of ABH antigen and susceptibility to *Candida albicans*, *Neisseria meningitidis*, *Streptococcus pneumoniae*, and *Haemophilus influenzae*.[6]

A number of disease associations with globoside have been identified. *Streptococcus suis*, which can cause meningitis and septicemia in humans, binds exclusively to P[k] antigen. A class of toxins secreted by *Shigella dysenteriae*, *Vibrio cholerae*, and *Vibrio parahaemolyticus* have binding specificity for Gal(α1–4)-Gal(β1–4). In addition, globoside is the receptor of human parvovirus B19. Some strains of *E. coli* use the disaccharide receptor Gal(α1–4)-Galβ on uroepithelial cells to gain entry to the urinary tract receptors associated with P1, P[k], and P antigens.[5,33] People with the rare p phenotype lack this disaccharide and are not susceptible to acute pyelonephritis from such *E. coli* strains nor to infection by human parvovirus B19.

PHENOTYPES ASSOCIATED WITH DISEASE RESISTANCE

Erythrocytes lacking Fy[a] and Fy[b] antigens are not infected by the malarial parasite *Plasmodium vivax* or by the simian malarial parasite *Plasmodium knowlesi*. These parasites attach to the Fy(a–b–) RBC membrane, but penetration does not take place. The Fy6 antigen is the critical receptor for *P. vivax* attachment.[5] *Plasmodium falciparum* attaches to RBC glycophorins and their *O*-linked oligosaccharides (carrying NeuAc). RBCs with the following phenotypes have a decreased rate of infection: M–N– (GPA-deficient), S–s–U– (GPB-deficient), Ge– (Leach type or GPC/GPD-deficient), and Cad-positive and Tn-positive RBCs (which have abnormal *O*-linked sugars).

DISEASES ASSOCIATED WITH ALTERED ANTIGEN EXPRESSION

Antigen expression can be altered with inherited or acquired disease. Inherited changes are fixed and consistent; acquired changes can disappear with remission or recovery. In some diseases, antigen expression weakens; in others, antigen expression increases or new antigens appear.

Weakened ABH expression on RBCs has been noted in acute myeloid leukemias and may result from reduced transferase activity.[5,16] Normal antigen expression returns with disease remission. Transient weakened expression of target antigen also occurs in some cases of autoimmune hemolytic anemia. Weak Rh, Kell, Kidd, LW and AnWj blood group activity has been reported with concurrent autoantibody.[5,16,40]

Increased expression of i on RBCs is associated with inherited disorders, such as thalassemia, sickle cell disease, Diamond-Blackfan syndrome, and hereditary erythroblastic multinuclearity with a positive acidified serum test (HEMPAS). Increased i expression also is noted with acquired conditions that decrease the red cell maturation time in the marrow, such as myeloblastic or sideroblastic myeloblastic erythropoiesis, refractory anemia, and excessive phlebotomy.[16,23] Expression of the *de novo* antigen Tn is caused by a galactosyltransferase deficiency acquired by somatic mutation in a population of stem cells. The antigen is present on RBCs, platelets, and granulocytes arising from these stem cells. This condition (seen as persistent mixed-field agglutination because of the presence of both normal and abnormal cells) causes other RBC changes, such as depressed MN expression, enhanced H, and reduced NeuAc content. Tn antigen exposure is associated with myelodysplastic syndrome and acute myelomonocytic leukemia.[16] Other antigens (T, Tk) occur as a result of infection when microbes produce enzymes that remove some sugars (NeuAc) and expose new ones. Group A individuals can appear to acquire a B antigen when bacterial deacetylase removes the acetyl group on GalNAc.[4,16] This phenomenon is associated with severe infection, gastrointestinal lesions, and malignancies.

RBCs may acquire blood group activity when they adsorb material from certain microorganisms. Group B activity has been associated with *E. coli*[86] and *Proteus vulgaris* infection, and K antigen with *Enterococcus faecium*. Acquired Jk[b]-like activity has been associated with *E. faecium* and *Micrococcus* infections, although the mechanism is not clear.[41]

DISEASES ASSOCIATED WITH ABSENT ANTIGENS OR NULL PHENOTYPES

Rh_null Syndrome

The Rh_null phenotype is associated with hereditary stomatocytosis, hemolytic anemia (usually mild and well compensated), and a lack of proteins carrying Rh antigens. The Rh protein resides in the RBC membrane, interacts with other membrane proteins and possibly the membrane skeleton, and may help regulate or organize the lipids within the red cell membrane bilayer.[9,10] Hence, it is an important determinant of membrane shape and expression of other antigens. Rh_null cells have depressed expression or absence of S, s, U, LW, and Fy5 antigens.

Most Rh_null red cells are stomatocytes or occasionally spherocytes and demonstrate increased osmotic fragility, increased potassium

TABLE 136–4. Blood Group Antigens and Antibodies Associated with Disease

PHENOTYPES ASSOCIATED WITH DISEASE SUSCEPTIBILITY

Group A	Carcinoma of the salivary glands, stomach, colon, rectum, ovary, uterus, cervix, bladder (T1 and T2 tumors); idiopathic thrombocytopenic purpura, coronary thrombosis, thrombosis (oral contraceptives), pernicious anemia, giardiasis, meningococcal meningitis infections
Group B	*Escherichia coli* urinary tract infection, gonorrhea
Group O	Duodenal and gastric ulcers, rheumatoid arthritis, von Willebrand disease, typhoid, paratyphoid, cholera
ABH nonsecretors	Duodenal ulcers, spondyloarthropathies; increased susceptibility to *Candida albicans, Neisseria meningitidis, Streptococcus pneumoniae, Haemophilus influenzae*
Le(a–b–)	Sjögren syndrome
Group O, Le(a–b+)	*Helicobacter pylori*
Globoside	Parvovirus

PHENOTYPES ASSOCIATED WITH DISEASE RESISTANCE

p (PP1 P^k–)	Pyelonephritogenic infections of *E. coli*, parvovirus B
Fy(a–b–)	*Plasmodium vivax, Plasmodium knowlesi*
Tn–, Cad–, En(a–), U–, Ge–	*Plasmodium falciparum*

DISEASES ASSOCIATED WITH ALTERED ANTIGEN EXPRESSION

Weakened AB	Leukemia, myelodysplastic syndrome, Hodgkin lymphoma and non-Hodgkin lymphomas, aplastic anemia, bacterial infections
Weakened MN	Bacterial infections, myelodysplastic syndrome, leukemia (Tn, T, Tk activation)
Enhanced i	Thalassemia, sickle cell disease, HEMPAS, Diamond-Blackfan anemia, myeloblastic or sideroblastic erythropoiesis, refractory anemia
Acquired A (Tn)	Myelodysplastic syndrome, acute myelogenous leukemia
Acquired B	Bacterial infections, gastrointestinal lesions or malignancies
Acquired T, Tk	Bacterial infections
Acquired K antigens	*Enterococcus faecium*
Acquired Jk^b antigen	*E. faecium* or *Micrococcus* infection
Absent Cromer, Yt, Dombrock, JMH, Emm antigens	Paroxysmal nocturnal hemoglobinuria
Weakened target antigens (Rh, Kell, Kidd, LW)	Autoimmune hemolytic anemia
LW	Hodgkin disease, lymphoma, leukemia, sarcoma
Weakened I, Rh, S, s, U, Kp^b, Jk^a, Xg^a, or En^a	Stomatocytic hereditary elliptocytosis

DISEASES ASSOCIATED WITH NULL PHENOTYPES

Rh$_{null}$ (D–C–E–c–e–)	Hereditary stomatocytosis, mild hemolytic anemia
McLeod phenotype (Kx–)	Hereditary acanthocytosis, mild hemolytic anemia, see text
GE$_{null}$ (Leach type)	Hereditary elliptocytosis, mild hemolytic anemia
Bombay (O$_h$)	Leukocyte adhesion deficiency II (some)
I– (i Adult)	Congenital cataracts in Asians (some)
CO$_{null}$	Inability to maximally concentrate urine
RAPH$_{null}$	Kidney disease

DISEASES ASSOCIATED WITH ANTIBODY PRODUCTION

Anti-I, -IH, -i, -H, -Pr	Cold agglutinin disease
Anti-"Rh," -"Kell," -U, -Wr^b	Warm autoimmune hemolytic anemia
Anti-I	*Mycoplasma pneumoniae*, chronic lymphocytic leukemia, Hodgkin lymphoma and non-Hodgkin lymphomas
Anti-i	Infectious mononucleosis, reticuloendothelial diseases

(continued)

TABLE 136–4. Blood Group Antigens and Antibodies Associated with Disease (Continued)

Anti-I^T	Hodgkin lymphoma and non-Hodgkin lymphomas
Anti-K	Enterocolitis, bacterial infections (*E. coli* 0125:B15, *Campylobacter jejuni*, *E. coli*)
Anti-P1	Parasitic infections: hydatid cyst disease, liver flukes
Anti-PP1P^k	Early spontaneous abortions
Anti-P	Paroxysmal cold hemoglobinuria, early spontaneous abortions, lymphoma
Anti-NF	Renal dialysis (formaldehyde exposure)
Anti-Forssman	Neoplastic disorders
Anti-Rx	Virally induced hemolysis
Decreased anti-A or -B	Agammaglobulinemia or hypogammaglobulinemia
"NULL" PHENOTYPES ASSOCIATED WITH BIOLOGIC DIFFERENCES BUT NO OR MILD DISEASE	
Group O	Lack GalNAc or Gal on terminal Gal
Bombay	Lack Fuc on terminal Gal
Le(a–b–)	Lack Fuc on terminal GlcNAc
M–N– or En(a–)	Lack or have altered GPA
S–s–U–	Lack or have altered GPB
Wr(a–b–)	Lack or have altered GPA
M^k phenotype	Lack GPA and GPB
K$_0$	Lack Kell glycoprotein
Jk(a–b–)	Lack or have altered Jk protein, reduced ability to concentrate urine
Lu(a–b–)	Lack or have reduced or altered Lu glycoprotein; RBC may show poikilocytosis, potassium loss, increased hemolysis during storage
LW(a–b–)	Lack or have altered LW glycoprotein
Do(a–b–), Gy(a–)	Lack a GPI-linked protein (Do glycoprotein)
SC:–1,–2,–3	Lack or have altered Sc glycoprotein

Fuc, fucose; GlcNAc, *N*-acetylglucosamine; GPA, glycophorin A; GPB, glycophorin B; GPI, glycosylphosphatidylinositol; HEMPAS, hereditary erythroblastic multinuclearity with positive acidified serum lysis test.

Data from Issitt PD, Anstee DJ: *Applied Blood Group Serology*, 4th ed. Montgomery Scientific, Durham, NC, 1998; Daniels G: *Human Blood Groups*, 3rd. Blackwell Science, Oxford, 2013; Reid ME, Lomas-Francis C, Olsson ML: *Blood Group Antigen FactsBook*, 3rd. Academic Press, San Diego, 2012; Reid ME, Lomas-Francis C: *Blood Group Antigens & Antibodies: A Guide to Clinical Relevance & Technical Tips*. Star Bright Books, New York, 2007.

permeability, and higher potassium pump activity. They have reduced cation and water content and a relative deficiency of membrane cholesterol. Although these abnormalities are assumed to contribute to shortened *in vivo* survival, Rh$_{null}$ RBCs survive normally in splenectomized patients, suggesting their removal is related more to splenic clearance because of shape rather than some other intrinsic factor.

Two genetic mechanisms account for the Rh$_{null}$ phenotype. Persons with the amorphic type are homozygous for the silent *RHCE* gene on a deleted *RHD* background. Individuals with the more common regulator type of Rh$_{null}$ have normal RH genes but an altered (silenced) *RHAG* gene. RhAG is required for expression of Rh antigens. Individuals with the Rh$_{mod}$ phenotype have similar membrane and clinical anomalies associated with Rh$_{null}$ syndrome but demonstrate some Rh antigen expression. The reduced expression of Rh antigens results from the presence of an altered form of RhAG.[24,26,42]

McLeod Phenotype

Numerous males (but no females) with the McLeod phenotype have been identified. These individuals have acanthocytosis, decreased RBC survival, very weak expression of Kell blood group antigens, lack of Kx antigen on RBCs, and a well-compensated hemolytic anemia.[43]

Kx antigen is carried on the Xk protein encoded by the XK gene on the X chromosome, which interacts with the RBC membrane skeleton and helps stabilize the membrane. The absence of Kx is associated with a lipid deficiency in the membrane bilayer that may be critical to the Kell glycoprotein and general RBC discoid shape. RBCs with the McLeod phenotype show a defect in water transport, increased mobility of phosphatidylcholine across the membrane, and increased phosphorylation of protein band 3 and β-spectrin.[43]

After age 40 years, patients with the McLeod phenotype develop a slowly progressive form of muscular dystrophy that is associated with areflexia, choreiform movements, and cardiomegaly, leading to cardiomyopathy. They have elevated levels of serum creatine kinase and carbonic anhydrase III. Some patients with the McLeod phenotype and X-linked chronic granulomatous disease (CGD) have a deletion of both the XK and Phox-91 genes (Chap. 66). The McLeod phenotype results from deletions or nucleotide changes in the XK gene.[44]

Gerbich-Negative Phenotype

The *GYPC* on chromosome 2 encodes two proteins: GPC, with antigens Ge3 and Ge4 (the Ge2 portion is "hidden" by the Ge4-bearing terminal end), and its shorter partner GPD, with antigens Ge2 (now exposed) and Ge3. GPC and GPD interact with membrane skeleton proteins 4.1

and p55, which are involved in cell deformability and membrane stability. Gerbich-negative RBCs of the Leach type (Ge:−2, −3, −4) lack both GPC and GPD, have reduced protein 4.1, and elliptocytosis but exhibit normal survival *in vivo*.[6,10]

Bombay (O$_h$) Phenotype

Rare people lack A, B, and H antigens and have naturally occurring anti-A, anti-B, and anti-H in their plasma. Such people are said to have the Bombay (O$_h$) phenotype. In rare people with the Le(a−b−) Bombay phenotype, the gene that encodes the Fuc transporter is silenced. As a consequence, all cells lack Fuc. Without Fuc, neutrophils lack sialyl Le^X and thus cannot roll and ingest bacteria. These patients have a high white blood cell count and severe recurrent infections. The condition is called *leukocyte adhesion deficiency II* (LADII) or congenital disorder of glycosylation II (CDG II).[45,46]

I-Negative Phenotype (i Adult)

The gene encoding the I-branching β-1,6-N-acetylglucosaminyltransferase *(GCNT2)* has three alternative forms of exon 1, with common exons 2 and 3. Mutations in exon 2 or 3 silence *GCNT2* and give rise to the form of I-negative phenotype associated with congenital cataracts in Asians.[47,48] Mutations in exon 1C *(IGnTC or IGnT3)* silence the gene in RBCs but not in other tissues, and lead to the I-negative phenotype (i adult) without cataracts.[49]

CO$_{null}$ Phenotype

Antigens of the Colton blood group system are carried on the water transporter (aquaporin [AQP1]). Although an absence of this protein from the RBC membrane was thought to be incompatible with life, in reality these rare individuals have been shown only to be unable to maximally concentrate urine.[50]

RAPH$_{null}$ Phenotype

The MER2 antigen in the RAPH blood group system is carried on CD151. Rare individuals who lack CD151 have chronic renal failure, skin ulcers, and deafness.[51]

Other Null Phenotypes

Patients with null phenotypes can develop RBC antibodies that make it difficult to find compatible blood to avoid the otherwise serious hemolytic transfusion reactions. For example, people with the Bombay phenotype (O$_h$ or H$_{null}$) demonstrate no red cell abnormality but make potent hemolytic anti-H as well as anti-A and anti-B. These antibodies are incompatible with all RBCs except those from other persons with the Bombay phenotype. Likewise, p individuals (PP1P^k-negative) or P^k individuals (P-negative) can make hemolytic antibodies to the antigens they lack. Anti-PP1P^k and anti-P also are associated with spontaneous abortions in the first trimester.[16] Women with such antibodies (notably IgG anti-P), even those with a history of spontaneous abortions, have delivered viable infants after plasmapheresis.[52]

Null phenotypes in the MNSs and Lutheran systems are interesting because several types of null phenotypes are known. Within the MNSs blood group system, people may lack GPA (En[a−] or MN-negative), GPB (SsU-negative), or both (M^{k}M^k phenotype). The rare Lu(a−b−) phenotype is caused by a dominant inhibitor called *In(Lu)*, by homozygous pairing of the silent allele *Lu*, or by a recessive sex-linked inhibitor *XS2*.[5,16] Only the *LuLu*-type null (recessive Lu[a−b−]) is associated with antibody production because the inhibitor type nulls produce small amounts of Lutheran antigen. *In(Lu)* type, Lu(a−b−) RBCs have low expression of CD44 and AnWj, and have varying degrees of poikilocytosis and acanthocytosis. RBCs of this type tend to hemolyze more

quickly during storage, even though they demonstrate normal osmotic fragility.[53] Inactivating nucleotide changes in *KLF1*, which encodes an altered transcription factor, cause the InLu phenotype.[30]

The Jk(a−b−) phenotype is caused by the silent alleles *JkJk* or the dominant inhibitor *In(Jk)*. RBCs having the Jk(a−b−) phenotype resist lysis in 2*M* urea,[54] a reagent commonly used in automated platelet counting systems; resulting in erroneously high platelet counts. No significant clinical abnormalities have been identified to date, although Jk(a−b−) individuals have reduced ability to concentrate urine.[55]

The following diagnoses are made easily by simply typing the RBCs with appropriate antisera: Rh syndrome, McLeod syndrome, and LAD II.

● ERYTHROCYTE ANTIBODIES

IMMUNOLOGY OF RED CELL ANTIBODIES

Blood group antibodies are classified as *alloantibodies* if they only react with antigens present on the RBCs of other people and as *autoantibodies* if they react with *self-antigens* present on the patient's own RBC. Alloantibodies also can be classified according to their mode of sensitization as *naturally occurring* (no apparent sensitization) or *immune* (following sensitization). Table 136–5 summarizes the common anti-erythrocyte antibodies.[4,6,15,16]

IMMUNOGLOBULIN CLASSES ASSOCIATED WITH BLOOD GROUP ACTIVITY

Immunoglobulin G

IgG is the predominant antibody made in an immune response and constitutes approximately 80 percent of total serum Ig (Chap. 75). These antibodies, when specific for RBC antigens, can attach to or induce hemolysis of transfused antigen-positive RBCs. Receptors on macrophages in the liver and spleen allow the macrophages to remove IgG-coated RBCs from the circulation. IgG blood group antibodies also are capable of fixing complement, although some subclasses do so less efficiently than others: IgG$_3$ > IgG$_1$ > IgG$_2$ > IgG$_4$. How well an IgG erythrocyte antibody binds complement, depends on the surface density and location of the recognized antigen. This situation occurs because C1q, the initiator of the classic complement cascade, requires binding of at least two IgG molecules to the RBC within a span of 20 to 30 nm to initiate the complement cascade.[16] For example, IgG anti-D rarely binds complement, presumably because most D sites are spaced too far apart.[16] Most IgG blood group antibodies do not agglutinate saline-suspended RBCs, presumably because the IgG molecule is too small to span the distance between RBCs, although some exceptions are known (i.e., potent IgG examples of anti-A, anti-B, anti-M, and anti-K). Some IgG anti-D can directly agglutinate RBCs with the D-phenotype. Most IgG antibodies sensitize RBCs at 37°C and are detected with an antiglobulin reagent.[11]

Immunoglobulin M

IgM is a pentamer of five basic units (having μ heavy chains plus a short J, or joining, chain) and makes up only approximately 4 percent of total serum Ig (Chap. 75). IgM is the first class of Ig produced by the fetus and is the predominant antibody in a primary immune response, but it does not cross the placenta. Because of their pentameric structure, even low-affinity IgM blood group antibodies can agglutinate RBCs and activate complement. Both hemolyzing and agglutinating abilities of IgM molecules are destroyed by reducing reagents, such as 2-ME and DTT. IgM antibodies of low affinity may agglutinate RBCs only at temperatures below 37°C. Such antibodies still may fix complement onto the

TABLE 136–5. Summary of Selected Erythrocyte Antibodies

Blood Group	Antibody	Ig Class		Serologic Activity			Activates Complement	Implicated in		Antigen Frequency (%)		Comments
		IgM	IgG	RT	37°C AHG	ENZ/DTT		HTR	HDFN	Whites	Blacks	
ABO	A	Most	Some	Most	Most	I/nc	Yes	Yes	Mild	40	27	A/B: very clinically significant, sometimes IgA
	B	Most	Some	Most	Most	I/nc	Yes	Yes	Mild	11	20	
	A1	Most	Rare	Most	Rare	I/nc	Rare	Rare	No	30	—	A1: usually not clinically significant
	H	Most	Rare	Most	Rare	I/nc	Rare	Rare	—	>99.9	—	H: usually weak autoantibody, but strong alloantibody in O_h
Rh	D	Some	Most	Some	Most	I/nc	No	Yes	Mild to Sev	85	92	D: most common immune antibody
	C	Few	Most	—	Most	I/nc	No	Yes	Mild to Sev	70	33	C: often found with D
	E	Some	Most	Some	Most	I/nc	No	Yes	Mild	30	21	E/C or E/c: often found together
	c	—	Most	—	Most	I/nc	No	Yes	Mild to Sev	80	97	All alloantibodies: clinically significant
	e	—	Most	—	Most	I/nc	No	Yes	Mild	98	99	Autoantibodies commonly directed against Rh protein
	f (ce)	—	Most	—	Most	I/nc	No	Yes	Mild	64	—	
	C^w	Some	Most	—	Most	I/nc	No	Yes	Mild to Mod	1	—	
	VS/V	—	Most	—	Most	I/nc	No	Yes	No	<1	30	
Lewis	Le^a	Most	Rare	Most	Some	I/nc	Yes	Rare	No	22	23	Common in pregnancy
	Le^b	Most	Rare	Most	Some	I/nc	Yes	No	No	72	55	Not clinically significant; Le(a−b−) individuals commonly make anti-Le^a but can simultaneously make anti-Le^a and anti-Le^b
Ii	I	Most	—	Most	Some	I/nc	Yes	Rare	No	>99.9	>99.9	I: common autoantibody, rare significant alloantibody
	i	Most	—	Most	Some	I/nc	Yes	No	Rare (mild)	100	100	i: rare autoantibody
P1PK	P1	Most	Rare	Most	Some	I/nc	Few	Rare	No	79	94	P1: usually not clinically significant
GLOB	P	Most	Few	Most	Some	I/nc	Yes	Yes	No–Mild	>99.9	>99.9	P: Donath-Landsteiner antibody in PCH
	PP1P^k	Most	Few	Most	Some	I/nc	Yes	Yes	No–Sev	>99.9	>99.9	
MNSs	M	Some	Some	Most	Few	D/nc	No	Rare	Rare	78	70	M: common, usually not clinically significant
	N	Some	Some	Most	Rare	D/nc	No	Rare	(Rare)	72	74	N: rare, usually not clinically significant
	S	Some	Some	Some	Most	V/nc	Some	Yes	Mild – Sev	55	31	
	s	Few	Most	Few	Most	V/nc	Rare	Yes	No – Sev	89	97	
	U	—	Most	—	Most	nc/nc	Rare	Yes	Mild–Sev	100	99.7	SsU: clinically significant autoantibody specificities reported

(continued)

System	Antigen					Dosage			HDN	%	%	Comments
Kell	K	Some	Most	Few	Most	nc/D	Rare	Yes	Mild–Sev	9	2	K: very common immune antibody
	k	–	Most	Rare	Most	nc/D	No	Yes	Mild–Sev	99.9	—	
	Kp^a	–	Most	Rare	Most	nc/D	No	Yes	Mild–Sev	2.3	—	
	Kp^b	–	Most	Rare	Most	nc/D	No	Yes	Mild–Mod	>99.9	100	Autoantibodies reported
	Js^a	–	Most	Rare	Rare	nc/D	No	Yes	Mild–Sev	—	20	
	Js^b	–	Most	–	Most	nc/D	No	Yes	Mild–Sev	>99.9	99	
Duffy	Fy^a	–	Most	Rare	Most	D/nc	Rare	Yes	Mild–Sev	66	10	Fy^a: common immune antibody
	Fy^b	–	Most	Rare	Most	D/nc	Rare	Yes	Mild	83	23	
Kidd	Jk^a	Few	Most	Rare	Most	I/nc	Yes	Yes	Mild–Mod	77	92	Jk^a: associated with delayed HTR; hemolytic; disappears quickly from serum
	Jk^b	Few	Most	Rare	Most	I/nc	Yes	Yes	No–Mild	72	41	
Lutheran	Lu^a	Some	Few	Most	Few	nc(V)/D	No	No	No–Mild	7.7	—	Mild RBC destruction
	Lu^b	Some	Some	Few	Most	nc(V)/D	No	Yes	Mild	99.9	—	Lu glycoprotein on placental tissue may adsorb maternal Lu antibodies
Xg	Xg^a	Some	Most	Rare	Most	D/nc	Some	No	No	64(m) 89(f)	—	Xg^a: poor immunogen
Yt	Yt^a	–	Most	–	Most	D(V)/D(V)	No	No–Mod	No	99.7	—	Yt: some antibody examples clinically significant, others not
	Yt^b	–	Most	–	Most	D(V)/D	No	No	No	8	—	
Ch/Rg	Ch	Rare	Most	Most	Most	D/nc	No	No	No	96	—	Ch/Rg: associated with C4 complement, clinically insignificant antibodies
	Rg	–	Most	–	Most	D/nc	No	No	No	98	—	
Colton	Co^a	–	Most	Some	Most	nc/nc	Some	No–Mod	Mild–Sev	99.9	—	
	Co^b	–	Most	Some	Most	nc/nc	Rare	No–Mod	Mild	10	—	
Cromer	General group	–	Most	–	Most	nc/V	No	No–Mild	No	>99.9	>99.9	
Diego	Di^a	–	Most	Some	Some	nc/nc	Rare	Yes	Mild–Sev	Rare	—	Di^a: antigen found in South American Indians and Asians
	Di^b	–	Most	–	Most	nc/nc	No	No–Mod	Mild	100	—	
Dombrock	Do^a	–	Most	–	Most	nc/D(V)	No	Yes	+DAT	67	—	Do^a Do^b: poor immunogens
	Do^b	–	Most	–	Most	nc/D(V)	No	Yes	+DAT	83	—	

(continued)

TABLE 136–5. Summary of Selected Antierythrocyte Antibodies (Continued)

Blood Group	Antibody	Ig Class		Serologic Activity			Activates Complement	Implicated in		Antigen Frequency (%)		Comments
		IgM	IgG	RT	37°C AHG	ENZ/DTT		HTR	HDFN	Whites	Blacks	
	Hy	–	Most	–	Most	nc(l)/D(V)	No	No–Mod	+DAT	>99	–	Hy– and Jo(a–): found only in blacks Gy(a–) (Do$_{null}$) found in eastern Europeans and Japanese
	Gy^a	–	Most	–	Most	nc(l)/D(V)	No	No–Moderate	+DAT	>99	–	
	Jo^a	–	Most	–	Most	nc(l)/D(V)	No	No–Mod	No	>99	–	
Gerbich	General group	–	Most	–	Most	D/nc	Yes	No–Mod	(+DAT)	>99.9	>99.9	Ge: located on glycophorins C and D
Indian	In^a	–	Most	–	Most	D/D	No	Yes	(+DAT)	<0.1	<0.1	In: located on CD44 adhesion protein
	In^b	–	Most	–	Most	D/D	No	No–Sev	(+DAT)	99	96	
Knops	Kn^a	–	Most	–	Most	D/D/V	No	No	No	98	99	Knops antigens associated with CR1 (complement) receptor, clinically insignificant antibodies
	McC^a	–	Most	–	Most	D/D	No	No	No	98	94	
	Yk^a	–	Most	–	Most	D/D	No	No	No	92	98	
Scianna	Sc1	–	Most	–	Most	nc/nc	Yes	No	+DAT	>99.9	–	Sc1: some antibodies react in serum but not plasma
	Sc2	–	Most	–	Most	nc/–V	No	No	+DAT	1	–	
	Sc3	–	Most	–	Most	nc(l)/nc	No	No–Mild	Mild	>99.9	–	
JMH	JMH	–	Most	–	Most	D/D	No	No	No	>99.9	>99.9	JMH: carrier protein CDw108

D, destroyed; DTT, dithiothreitol; ENZ, enzyme (papain/ficin); I, increased; nc, no change; V, variable.

RBC membrane *in vivo*, at the lower temperatures in the extremities, and activate the complement cascade in the core of the body. Because such IgM antibodies dissociate from RBCs at higher temperatures, their reactivity may be detected in routine antiglobulin tests (using polyspecific antiglobulin) by virtue of the complement components that remain bound to the red cell membrane.[11,16]

Immunoglobulin A

IgA is the primary Ig in body secretions, where it exists predominantly as a dimer with a secretory component (Chap. 75). IgA does not cross the placenta or fix complement, but aggregated IgA can activate the alternative pathway of complement, and IgA can trigger cell-mediated events. Multimeric IgA antibodies in serum are seen as hemagglutinins in blood bank tests and most often are associated with anti-A or anti-B.

IMMUNOGLOBULIN IN THE FETUS AND NEWBORN

Initially, the fetus acquires low levels of maternal IgG, probably by diffusion across the placenta. These levels rise significantly between 20 and 33 weeks' gestation as a selective transport system matures and maternal IgG is actively transported across the placenta. Thus, almost all blood group antibodies detected in the fetus and newborn originate from the mother and disappear within the first few months of life.

Actual fetal antibody production begins shortly before birth with low levels of IgM, followed by IgG and IgA several weeks after birth. Anti-A and anti-B usually are readily detected by age 2 to 6 months.

Because of this late immune response in the newborn and because maternal antibody is so predominant at birth, blood bank standards permit abbreviated testing on neonates younger than 4 months.[56] If available, the mother's serum is used (and preferred) for identifying antibodies in a newborn and for crossmatching RBC components.

NATURALLY OCCURRING ANTIBODIES

Naturally Occurring Antibodies in Development

An antibody is said to be *naturally occurring* when it is found in the serum of an individual who has not been exposed to the antigen through transfusion or pregnancy. These antibodies most likely are heteroagglutinins produced in response to substances in the environment that are similar to those on RBC antigens.

Evidence supporting this concept has come from studies on the formation of anti-B in chickens.[57] Chicks raised in a normal environment made anti-B within the first 30 days of life, whereas chicks raised in a germ-free environment did not make anti-B by day 60. Naturally occurring anti-A and anti-B in humans, also called *isoagglutinins*, can increase in titer following ingestion or inhalation of suitable bacteria.[58]

However, a great many antigens that likely are not present in the environment have been associated with naturally occurring antibodies, so the stimulus for naturally occurring antibodies is not clearly known.

Blood Group Associations and Presence of Naturally Occurring Antibodies

Naturally occurring alloantibodies are commonly associated with the carbohydrate antigens of the ABO, LE, and P1PK blood group systems. Anti-A and anti-B are expected in people who lack the corresponding antigens, as are antibodies specific for H, PP1P^k, or P antigens. Naturally occurring antibodies reactive with A1, Le^a, Le^b, or P1 determinants also are seen frequently. Carbohydrate antigens, especially those with repetitive epitopes, can stimulate B cells to make specific antibody without the aid of helper T cells. Such thymus-independent immune responses typically result in antigen-specific antibodies of the IgM class.

Within other systems,[16] anti-Sd^a, anti-Vw, and anti-Wr^a are found in up to 2 percent of normal people. Other, less-common antibody specificities in approximate order of descending occurrence are anti-M, -S, -N, -Ge, -K, -Lu^a, -Di^a, and -Xg^a. Rh antigens are thought to reside only on RBCs, but apparent naturally occurring anti-D has been reported in 0.15 percent of Rh-negative donors and anti-E in more than 0.1 percent of Rh-positive donors when more sensitive enzyme detection methods are used. Examples of naturally occurring anti-C, anti-C^W, and anti-C^X also have been described.[4–6]

Some naturally occurring antibodies exist as autoagglutinins (e.g., anti-H and anti-I). Patients with autoimmune hemolytic anemia can produce many antibodies to low-prevalence antigens with no specific stimulus, in addition to autoantibody.[5,6,16,40]

Characteristics of Naturally Occurring Alloantibodies

Most naturally occurring antibodies are IgM, but some have an IgG component and a few are predominantly IgG. Some anti-A or anti-B may even be of the IgA class. Antibodies that cause direct agglutination of saline-suspended RBCs most commonly are of the IgM class. However, even IgG antibodies may cause agglutination of RBCs when they bind antigens that are present at high density on the RBC membrane, such as the ABO or MN antigens. With the exception of anti-A and anti-B, most common naturally occurring antibodies do not react at body temperature and are considered clinically insignificant. However, if they are found to react at 37°C, providing crossmatch-compatible blood for transfusion is prudent.

ANTIBODIES GENERATED IN RESPONSE TO IMMUNIZATION: IMMUNE ANTIBODIES

Blood Group Associations and Occurrence of Immune Antibodies

Immune antibodies are produced following exposure to foreign RBC antigens through pregnancy or transfusion. The primary immune response is seen several weeks to several months after the first exposure to antigen. IgM usually is associated with early primary responses, but whether it is always the first antibody class made is unclear. In most individuals, IgG soon predominates. This process is characteristic of a thymus-dependent immune response, where T cells help induce B cells to undergo isotype switching from IgM to IgG.

In a secondary or anamnestic response, antibody concentration starts to increase several days to several weeks following exposure, and IgG may rise to very high levels. Some IgG antibodies remain detectable for decades after a stimulus. Others, especially Kidd antibodies, can disappear after several months and are more commonly associated with delayed hemolytic transfusion reactions.[5,6,16]

Immune antibodies are found more commonly in individuals who have been multiply transfused than in multiparous women. This situation occurs because in pregnancy the immunizing dose of red cells often is too small to elicit a primary response and the foreign antigens are limited to those of the father.[16]

Anti-D used to be the most common immune antibody, but with the advent of Rh matching of donors and recipients in the late 1940s and use of RhIg prophylaxis since the 1970s, its incidence has sharply decreased. Anti-D is present in 0.27 to 0.56 percent of transfusion recipients, 0.10 to 0.20 percent of pregnant women, and 0.16 to 0.25 percent of healthy blood donors.[16]

In contrast, the occurrence of immune antibodies other than anti-D has increased. Specificities other than anti-D have been reported in approximately 0.6 percent of transfusion recipients, 0.14 percent of pregnant women, and 0.19 percent of healthy blood donors. Pooled data from three 5-year periods and approximately 300,000 patients suggest the absolute occurrence of Rh antibodies other than anti-D is 0.22 percent, other than anti-K is 0.19 percent, other than anti-Fy^a is 0.05 percent, and other than anti-Jk^a is 0.04 percent.[16] The rate of allo-immunization in patients with sickle cell anemia was 18.6 percent in one survey, and 55 percent of the immunized patients made more than one antibody. The most common specificities were anti-C, anti-E, and anti-K.[16]

Characteristics of Immune Antibodies

Immune antibodies most often are IgG but may be IgM and sometimes are IgA. Most immune antibodies react at body temperature and are considered clinically significant, except those directed against Bg, Knops, Cs^a, JMH, and sometimes Yt^a and Lutheran antigens.

● CLINICAL SIGNIFICANCE OF ERYTHROCYTE ANTIBODIES

Information about the clinical significance of alloantibodies is available at www.nybloodcenter.org.[59,60]

HEMOLYTIC TRANSFUSION REACTIONS

Clinically significant antibodies are capable of destroying transfused RBCs. The severity of the reaction varies with antigen density and antibody characteristics.

Antibodies commonly associated with intravascular hemolysis include anti-A, anti-B, anti-Jk^a, and anti-Jk^b. ABO incompatibility is the most potent cause of immediate hemolytic reactions because A and B antigens are strongly expressed on RBCs and the antibodies so efficiently bind complement. Kidd antibodies are associated more often with delayed hemolytic reactions because they typically are difficult to detect and can disappear quickly from the circulation. IgG anti-Jk^a appears to bind complement only when traces of IgM anti-Jk^a are present.[16] Anti-PP1P^k, anti-Vel, and anti-Le^a have been associated with hemolysis, but such examples are rare.

Extravascular hemolysis occurs with IgG$_1$ and IgG$_3$ antibodies that react at body temperature; that is, immune antibodies reactive with Rh, Kidd, Kell, Duffy, or Ss antigens. These antibodies make up the bulk of clinically significant antibodies. Antibodies not expected to cause RBC destruction are those that react only at temperatures below 37°C and IgG antibodies of the IgG$_2$ or IgG$_4$ subclass.[16]

HEMOLYTIC DISEASE OF THE FETUS AND NEWBORN

HDFN is caused by blood group incompatibility between a sensitized mother and her antigen-positive fetus (Chap. 55). The antibodies most significant in HDFN are those that cross the placenta (IgG$_1$ and IgG$_3$), react at body temperature to cause red cell destruction, and are directed against well-developed RBC antigens. ABO incompatibility most commonly is seen, but ABO HDFN is clinically mild, presumably because the antigens are not fully expressed at birth. Antibodies directed against the D antigen can cause severe HDFN, and fetal health should be carefully monitored when anti-D titers are greater than 16. The severity of HDFN is less predictable with other blood group antibodies and can vary from mild to severe. For example, anti-K and anti-Ge3 not only causes red cell hemolysis but also may suppress erythropoiesis.[4,6]

AUTOIMMUNE HEMOLYTIC ANEMIA

Autoimmune hemolytic anemia is caused by the production of "warm-" or "cold-" reactive autoantibodies directed against RBC

antigens (Chap. 54).[40] Production can be triggered by disease, viral infection, or drugs; from breakdown in immune system tolerance to self-antigens; or from exposure to foreign antigens that induce antibodies that crossreact with self-RBC antigens. Autologous specificity is not always obvious because antigen expression can be depressed when autoantibody is present.[40]

Warm autoantibodies react best at 37°C and are primarily IgG (rarely IgM or IgA). Most are directed against the Rh protein, but Wr^b, Kell, Kidd, and U blood group specificities have been reported.[40]

Cold-reactive autoantibodies are primarily IgM. They react best at temperatures below 25°C but can agglutinate RBCs or activate complement at or near 37°C, causing hemolysis or vascular occlusion upon exposure to cold.[16] Patients with cold agglutinin disease often have C3d on their RBCs, which can provide some protection from hemolysis. Most cold-reactive autoantibodies have anti-I activity. Reactivity with i, H, Pr, P, or other antigenic specificities is much less common.

The biphasic cold-reactive IgG antibody associated with paroxysmal cold hemoglobinuria ("Donath-Landsteiner" antibody) typically reacts with the high-prevalence antigen P (GLOB). It attaches to RBCs in the cold and very efficiently activates complement before it dissociates at warmer temperatures.

DISEASES ASSOCIATED WITH ANTIBODY PRODUCTION

Table 136–4 lists diseases associated with specific antibody production. These antibodies cause autoimmune hemolytic anemia only if the patient carries the corresponding antigen.

● SEROLOGIC DETECTION OF ERYTHROCYTE ANTIGENS AND ANTIBODIES

ABO

ABO grouping is the single most important test performed in the transfusion service because it is the fundamental basis for determining blood compatibility. ABO grouping is determined by testing RBCs with licensed antisera to identify the A or B antigens they carry (forward, or cell, grouping) and by testing the corresponding serum or plasma with known A and B cells to identify the antibodies present (reverse, or serum, grouping). Positive reactions are seen as hemagglutination or hemolysis, and the results of one test should confirm the results of the other.

If results are discrepant or reactions are weaker than expected, the cause must be investigated before the ABO group can be interpreted with confidence. Discrepancies can be related to RBC anomalies, serum anomalies, or both, and they may be associated with disease.[5,11,16] Table 136–6 lists common causes, excluding clerical and technical error. If the ABO group of a patient cannot be determined, group O blood can be used for transfusion.

Rh

The D type is the next most important test performed for blood compatibility. Individuals whose RBCs type D+ are called *Rh-positive*, and those who type D– are called *Rh-negative*, provided controls are acceptable. Blood donors who type D– using standard typing sera are tested further for weak D expression using more sensitive methods, such as an indirect antiglobulin test. Donors with weak D antigen are considered

TABLE 136–6. Common Causes of Abo Discrepancies

RED CELLS MAY APPEAR TO HAVE

Weak or missing antigens	Weak subgroup of A or B antigen
	Excess soluble A or B antigen in plasma
	Disease-associated loss (leukemia)
	ABO nonidentical marrow transplantation
	ABO nonidentical red blood cell (RBC) transfusions
Extra antigens	Positive direct antiglobulin test
	Antibody to reagent additive or dye
	Rouleaux or cold agglutinin on cells
	Disease-associated acquisition (polyagglutination)

SERUM MAY APPEAR TO HAVE

Weak or missing antibody	Age related (newborns or the very elderly)
	Disease-associated immunosuppression
	Congenital hypogammaglobulinemia
	ABO nonidentical marrow transplantation
Extra antibody	Alloantibodies (A₁, Leᵃ, Leᵇ, P₁, M, N)
	Autoantibodies (I, i, H, Pr, P)
	Rouleaux
	Antibodies to additives in reagent RBCs
	Passive antibody acquisition from transfusion or from passenger lymphocytes in organ transplantation

Rh-positive. Testing for weak D is optional for transfusion recipients and pregnant women.[56]

EXTENDED ANTIGEN PHENOTYPING

Reagent antisera to detect other common antigens (e.g., CcEe, MNSs, Kk, FyᵃFyᵇ, JkᵃJkᵇ) are available and used when identification of the red cell phenotype is essential to antibody identification, blood compatibility, determination of zygosity, or paternity or forensic issues. Extended phenotyping is especially important to patients who are at high risk for alloimmunization from chronic blood transfusion, for example, those with sickle cell anemia or thalassemia. Ideally, an extended RBC phenotype of patients who are likely to be chronically transfused should be determined prior to initiation of transfusion therapy. Prediction of a blood group antigen can be made by testing DNA of a patient, even in the presence of transfused RBCs.[27]

ANTIBODY SCREEN

The antibody screen, or indirect antiglobulin test, detects "atypical" or "unexpected" antibodies in the serum (i.e., other than anti-A and anti-B) using group O reagent red cells that are known to carry various combinations of antigens. The methods used must be able to detect clinically significant antibodies. Typically, serum or plasma and screening cells are incubated at 37°C with an additive to potentiate antibody–antigen reactions, then an indirect antiglobulin test is performed. Hemagglutination or hemolysis at any point is a positive reaction, indicating the presence of naturally occurring or immune alloantibody or autoantibody. The antibody screen will not detect all atypical antibodies in serum, such as antibodies to low-prevalence antigens not present on screening cells and antibodies that are not apparent at 37°C and in the antiglobulin phase.

DIRECT ANTIGLOBULIN TEST

The direct antiglobulin test (often referred to as the direct Coombs test, a term discouraged by Robin Coombs because he said that Race and Mourant were also key to the description of the test) detects antibody or complement bound to RBCs *in vivo*. Red cells are washed free of serum and then mixed with an antiglobulin reagent that agglutinates RBCs coated with IgG or the C3 component of complement.

Positive direct antiglobulin test results are associated with the following: (1) transfusion reactions, in which recipient alloantibody coats transfused donor RBCs or transfused donor antibody coats recipient RBCs; (2) HDFN, in which maternal antibody crosses the placenta and coats fetal RBCs; (3) autoimmune hemolytic anemias, in which autoantibody coats the patient's own RBCs; (4) drug or drug–antibody complex interactions with RBCs that sometimes lead to hemolysis; (5) passenger lymphocyte syndrome, in which transient antibody produced by passenger lymphocytes from a transplanted organ coats recipient RBCs; and (6) hypergammaglobulinemia, in which Ig nonspecifically adsorb onto circulating RBCs.

A positive direct antiglobulin test result does not always indicate decreased red cell survival. As many as 10 percent of hospital patients and 0.1 percent of blood donors have a positive direct antiglobulin test result with no clinical indication of hemolysis.[11]

COMPATIBILITY TESTING

Compatibility testing refers to a set of donor and recipient tests that are performed prior to red cell transfusion. The collecting facility tests donors for ABO, Rh, and unexpected antibody. However, transfusing hospitals retest the ABO (and D on Rh-negative units) to verify the accuracy of the blood label.[56] Routine recipient testing includes an ABO, D, and antibody screening on a blood sample collected within 3 days of the intended transfusion. Results are checked against historical records to verify ABO, D, and antibody status.[56]

If the recipient has a negative antibody screening test result and no history of clinically significant antibodies, a serologic immediate spin crossmatch between recipient serum and donor red cells or a "computer crossmatch" (wherein computer software compares the ABO test results of both donor and recipient) is required to confirm ABO compatibility.[11]

If clinically significant antibodies are detected in a recipient's serum or previously were identified, red cell components should test negative for the corresponding antigens and be crossmatch compatible at 37°C by the antiglobulin test. The chance of finding compatible units usually reflects the antigen prevalence in the population, that is, 91 percent of units should be compatible with a patient making anti-K because 9 percent of the population is K+. This reasoning will not be valid if the local donor population varies significantly from the general population. When more than one antibody is present, the probability of finding compatible blood is the product of the prevalence (probability) of each independent antigen tested. For example, only 21 percent of units will be compatible for the recipient having both anti-K and anti-Jkᵃ: (0.91 for K–) × (0.23 for Jk[a–]) = 0.21.

When multiple clinically significant antibodies or an antibody directed against a high-prevalence antigen are present, finding compatible RBC components can be extremely difficult. Such antibody producers should be encouraged to give autologous donations prior to their elective blood needs. If the patient is not a candidate for autologous donation, compatible units may be found by testing the patient's siblings or by asking regional blood suppliers to check their rare donor inventories and files. Such procurement requires additional time.

TABLE 136–7. ABO-Rh Compatibility Guidelines

	Antigen on Red Cells	Antibody in Serum	Compatible Blood Groups	
			Donor Red Cells	Donor Plasma
If recipient blood group is				
A	A	Anti-B	A, O	A, AB
B	B	Anti-A	B, O	B, AB
O	O	Anti-A, anti-B	O	O, A, B, AB
AB	A, B	None	AB, A, B, O	AB
Rh-positive	D	None	Rh-positive, Rh-negative	Rh not considered
Rh-negative	None	Anti-D only if immunized	Rh-negative	Rh not considered

Whole blood must be identical to recipient's blood group. Red blood cell (RBC) products must be compatible with recipient's serum. Plasma products should be compatible with recipient's RBCs. Platelet and cryoprecipitate products should be compatible with recipient's RBCs, but any ABO group can be given if compatible products are not available.

Repeat donor testing and crossmatching are not performed for plasma and platelet components, but the recipient's ABO and Rh phenotypes must be known for appropriate selection of components. Table 136–7 gives general ABO-D compatibility guidelines.

ANTIBODY IDENTIFICATION

All unexpected antibodies should be investigated. Those detected in serum or plasma as an ABO discrepancy, a positive antibody screening result, or an incompatible crossmatch are identified using a panel of eight to 16 different group O red cells that have been typed for antigens corresponding to clinically significant antibodies. Serum reactions with these RBCs are compared to their antigen typing to determine specificity.[11] For example, an antibody that reacts with all K+ RBCs but not with K– cells most likely is anti-K.

A control of autologous RBCs and serum is tested concurrently with panel RBCs. Absence of reactivity with autologous cells implies the antibody is an alloantibody, whereas a positive result suggests autoantibody or a positive direct antiglobulin test result. Once antibody specificity is identified, the patient's RBCs are tested for the corresponding antigen. If the alloantibody is anti-K, the cells should type K–. Such antigen typing helps to confirm serum findings.

When antibody is detected both on red cells (a positive direct antiglobulin test result) and in serum, only the antibody in serum is identified unless a review of the medical, pregnancy and transfusion history offers evidence that the antibodies might be different. When antibody is detected only on RBCs and *in vivo* hemolysis is suspected, the antibody can be eluted from the patient's RBCs and tested against panel RBCs to identify the specificity.

REFERENCES

1. Lewis M, Anstee DJ, Bird GWG, et al: Blood group terminology 1990. ISBT working party on terminology for red cell surface antigens. *Vox Sang* 58:152, 1990.
2. Lögdberg L, Reid ME, Zelinsky T: Human blood group genes 2010: Chromosomal locations and cloning strategies revisited. *Transfus Med Rev* 25:36, 2011.
3. Cartron JP, Bailly P, Le Van Kim C, et al: Insights into the structure and function of membrane polypeptides carrying blood group antigens. *Vox Sang* 74(Suppl 2):29, 1998.
4. Daniels G: *Human Blood Groups*, 3rd ed. Blackwell Science, Oxford, 2013.
5. Issitt PD, Anstee DJ: *Applied Blood Group Serology*, 4th ed. Montgomery Scientific, Durham, NC, 1998.
6. Reid ME, Lomas-Francis C, Olsson ML: *Blood Group Antigen FactsBook*, 3rd ed. Academic Press, San Diego, 2012.
7. Telen MJ: Erythrocyte blood group antigens: Not so simple after all. *Blood* 85:299, 1995.
8. Cartron JP, Colin Y: Structural and functional diversity of blood group antigens. *Transfus Clin Biol* 8:163, 2001.
9. Bruce LJ, Ghosh S, King MJ, et al: Absence of CD47 in protein 4.2-deficient hereditary spherocytosis in man: An interaction between the Rh complex and the band 3 complex. *Blood* 100:1878, 2002.
10. Reid ME, Mohandas N: Red blood cell blood group antigens: Structure and function. *Semin Hematol* 41:93, 2004.
11. Fung MK, Grossman BJ, Hillyer C, et al, editors: *Technical Manual*, 18th ed. American Association of Blood Banks, Bethesda, MD, 2014.
12. Storry JR, Castilho L, Daniels G, et al: International Society of Blood Transfusion Working Party on Red Cell Immunogenetics and Terminology: Cancun report (2012). *Vox Sang* 107:90, 2014.
13. Daniels GL, Anstee DJ, Cartron J-P, et al: Blood group terminology 1995. ISBT working party on terminology for red cell surface antigens. *Vox Sang* 69:265, 1995.
14. Garratty G, Dzik WH, Issitt PD, et al: Terminology for blood group antigens and genes: Historical origins and guidelines in the new millennium. *Transfusion* 40:477, 2000.
15. Reid ME, Lomas-Francis C: *Blood Group Antigens & Antibodies: A Guide to Clinical Relevance & Technical Tips.* Star Bright Books, New York, 2007.
16. Klein HG, Anstee DJ: *Mollison's Blood Transfusion in Clinical Medicine*, 11th ed. Wiley-Blackwell, Oxford, 2006.
17. Clausen H, White T, Takio K, et al: Isolation to homogeneity and partial characterization of a histo-blood group A defined Fuca1—>2Gala1—>3-N-acetylglucosaminyl-transferase from human lung tissue. *J Biol Chem* 265:1139, 1990.
18. Yamamoto F, Marken J, Tsuji T, et al: Cloning and characterization of DNA complementary to human UDP-GalNAc: Fuca1—>2Gala1—>3GalNAc transferase (histo-blood group A transferase) mRNA. *J Biol Chem* 265:1146, 1990.
19. Yamamoto F, Hakomori S: Sugar-nucleotide donor specificity of histo-blood group A and B transferases is based on amino acid substitutions. *J Biol Chem* 265:19257, 1990.
20. Yamamoto F, Clausen H, White T, et al: Molecular genetic basis of the histo-blood group ABO system. *Nature* 345:229, 1990.
21. Chester MA, Olsson ML: The ABO blood group gene: A locus of considerable genetic diversity. *Transfus Med Rev* 15:177, 2001.
22. Olsson ML, Chester MA: Polymorphism and recombination events at the *ABO* locus: A major challenge for genomic ABO blood grouping strategies. *Transfus Med* 11:295, 2001.
23. Garratty G: Association of blood groups and disease: Do blood group antigens and antibodies have a biological role? *Hist Philos Life Sci* 18:321, 1996.
24. Avent ND, Reid ME: The Rh blood group system: A review. *Blood* 95:375, 2000.
25. Tippett P, Lomas-Francis C, Wallace M: The Rh antigen D: Partial D antigens and associated low incidence antigens. *Vox Sang* 70:123, 1996.
26. Huang C-H, Liu PZ, Cheng JG: Molecular biology and genetics of the Rh blood group system. *Semin Hematol* 37:150, 2000.
27. Reid ME: Applications of DNA-based assays in blood group antigen and antibody identification. *Transfusion* 43:1748, 2003.
28. Giblett ER: A critique of the theoretical hazard of inter vs. intra-racial transfusion. *Transfusion* 1:233, 1961.
29. Tippett P: Regulator genes affecting red cell antigens [review]. *Transfus Med Rev* 4:56, 1990.
30. Singleton BK, Burton NM, Green C, et al: Mutations in EKLF/KLF1 form the molecular basis of the rare blood group In(Lu) phenotype. *Blood* 112:2081, 2008.
31. Okubo Y, Yamaguchi H, Nagao N, et al: Heterogeneity of the phenotype Jk(a–b–) found in Japanese. *Transfusion* 26:237, 1986.
32. Hakomori S: Blood group ABH and Ii antigens of human erythrocytes: Chemistry, polymorphism, and their developmental change. *Semin Hematol* 18:39, 1981.
33. Spitalnik PF, Spitalnik SL: The P blood group system: Biochemical, serological, and clinical aspects. *Transfus Med Rev* 9:110, 1995.
34. Pogo AO, Chaudhuri A: The Duffy protein: A malarial and chemokine receptor. *Semin Hematol* 37:122, 2000.
35. Araten DJ, Swirsky D, Karadimitris A, et al: Cytogenetic and morphological abnormalities in paroxysmal nocturnal haemoglobinuria. *Br J Haematol* 115:360, 2001.
36. Tippett P, Ellis NA: The Xg blood group system: A review. *Transfus Med Rev* 12:233, 1998.
37. Cartron J-P, Rahuel C: Human erythrocyte glycophorins: Protein and gene structure analyses. *Transfus Med Rev* 6:63, 1992.
38. Tournamille C, Colin Y, Cartron JP, Le Van Kim C: Disruption of a GATA motif in the *Duffy* gene promoter abolishes erythroid gene expression in Duffy-negative individuals. *Nat Genet* 10:224, 1995.
39. Mourant AE, Kopec AC, Domaniewska-Sobczak K: *Distribution of the Human Blood Groups and Other Polymorphisms*, 2nd ed. Oxford University Press, London, 1976.
40. Petz LD, Garratty G: *Acquired Immune Hemolytic Anemias*, 2nd ed. Churchill Livingstone, New York, 2003.
41. Moulds JM, Moulds JJ: Blood group associations with parasites, bacteria, and viruses. *Transfus Med Rev* 14:302, 2000.

42. Cartron JP: Molecular basis of red cell protein antigen deficiencies. *Vox Sang* 78:7, 2000.

43. Lee S, Russo D, Redman CM: The Kell blood group system: Kell and XK membrane proteins. *Semin Hematol* 37:113, 2000.

44. Danek A, Rubio JP, Rampoldi L, et al: McLeod neuroacanthocytosis: Genotype and phenotype. *Ann Neurol* 50:755, 2001.

45. Luhn K, Wild MK, Eckhardt M, et al: The gene defective in leukocyte adhesion deficiency II encodes a putative GDP-fucose transporter. *Nat Genet* 28:69, 2001.

46. Etzioni A, Tonetti M: Leukocyte adhesion deficiency II-from A to almost Z. *Immunol Rev* 178:138, 2000.

47. Yu L-C, Twu Y-C, Chang C-Y, Lin M: Molecular basis of the adult i phenotype and the gene responsible for the expression of the human blood group I antigen. *Blood* 98:3840, 2001.

48. Inaba N, Hiruma T, Togayachi A, et al: A novel I-branching beta-1,6-N-acetylglucosaminyltransferase involved in human blood group I antigen expression. *Blood* 101:2870, 2003.

49. Yu LC, Twu YC, Chou ML, et al: The molecular genetics of the human I locus and molecular background explaining the partial association of the adult i phenotype with congenital cataracts. *Blood* 101:2081, 2003.

50. Agre P, King LS, Yasui M, et al: Aquaporin water channels—From atomic structure to clinical medicine. *J Physiol* 542:3, 2002.

51. Crew VK, Burton N, Kagan A, et al: CD151, the first member of the tetraspanin (TM4) superfamily detected on erythrocytes, is essential for the correct assembly of human basement membranes in kidney and skin. *Blood* 104:2217, 2004.

52. Rock JA, Shirey RS, Braine HG, et al: Plasmapheresis for the treatment of repeated early pregnancy wastage associated with anti-P. *Obstet Gynecol* 66:57S, 1985.

53. Udden MM, Umeda M, Hirano Y, Marcus DM: New abnormalities in the morphology, cell surface receptors, and electrolyte metabolism of In(Lu) erythrocytes. *Blood* 69:52, 1987.

54. Heaton DC, McLoughlin K: Jk(a–b–) red blood cells resist urea lysis. *Transfusion* 22:70, 1982.

55. Sands JM: Molecular mechanisms of urea transport. *J Membr Biol* 191:149, 2003.

56. Standards Committee of American Association of Blood Banks: *Standards for Blood Banks and Transfusion Services*, 29th ed. American Associations of Blood Banks, Bethesda, MD, 2014.

57. Springer GF, Horton RE, Forbes M: Origin of anti-human blood group B agglutinins in white leghorn chicks. *J Exp Med* 110:221, 1959.

58. Springer GF, Horton RE: Blood group isoantibody stimulation in man by feeding blood group-active bacteria. *J Clin Invest* 48:1280, 1969.

59. Reid ME, Øyen R, Marsh WL: Summary of the clinical significance of blood group alloantibodies. *Semin Hematol* 37:197, 2000.

60. Poole J, Daniels G: Blood group antibodies and their significance in transfusion medicine. *Transfus Med Rev* 21:58, 2007.

CHAPTER 137
HUMAN LEUKOCYTE AND PLATELET ANTIGENS

Myra Coppage, David Stroncek, Janice McFarland, and Neil Blumberg

SUMMARY

The human leukocyte antigens (HLAs) are highly polymorphic glycoproteins encoded by the major histocompatibility complex on chromosome 6. Their biologic function is presentation of antigenic peptides to T lymphocytes, and there are two major classes: class I (A, B, and C loci) and class II (DR, DQ, and DP loci). Class I antigens are present on almost all nucleated cells, whereas class II antigens are primarily expressed on B cells and other antigen-presenting cells such as dendritic cells, endothelial cells, and monocytes. These antigens play key roles in hematopoietic cell transplantation acceptance/rejection and allosensitization to nonleukoreduced blood transfusions leading to platelet transfusion refractoriness, with lesser, but distinct roles in solid-organ transplantation. Other clinically important lineage-specific white cell antigens include those on neutrophils, which are much less polymorphic and less commonly a cause of clinical problems than the HLA system. Antibody to neutrophil antigens plays a role in autoimmune neutropenia, and reactions such as transfusion-related acute lung injury. Platelets also possess a relatively limited number of polymorphic antigens that are involved in clinical problems such as posttransfusion purpura and platelet transfusion refractoriness, and neonatal problems such as alloimmune thrombocytopenia.

● HUMAN LEUKOCYTE ANTIGENS (MAJOR HISTOCOMPATIBILITY COMPLEX)

DEFINITION

The human leukocyte antigens (HLAs) are highly polymorphic glycoproteins encoded by a region of genes known as the major histocompatibility complex (MHC) located on chromosome 6p21 and covering a region of approximately 7.6 Mbp.[1,2] After ABO antigens, HLA antigens are the major barrier to transplantation. Their biologic function is to present antigenic peptides to T lymphocytes. The MHC codes for several groups of antigens. The best understood are the highly polymorphic, classical class I (HLA-A, HLA-B, and HLA-C) and class II (HLA-DR, HLA-DQ, and HLA-DP) antigens. Class I antigens are ubiquitous and present on most nucleated somatic cells. Class II antigens exhibit more

restricted distribution, with varying levels of expression on B cells, dendritic cells, monocytes, macrophages, and endothelial cells. However, class II antigens can be induced on many cell types through activation.[3] The nonclassical class Ib antigens HLA-E, HLA-F, and HLA-G, and the MHC class I chain-related antigens are much less polymorphic, their function less understood, and their tissue expression more limited. In addition the MHC region codes for a number of pseudogenes. This chapter focuses on the classic class I and II molecules because of their importance in transfusion and transplantation.

The two major classes of HLA antigens are homologous. However, there are areas of high variability (polymorphism) that distinguish individual HLA molecules (alleles) and confer antigen specificity. HLA antigens are codominantly expressed so that each individual expresses two antigens at each locus (A, B, DR, etc.). As of July 2014, many thousands of HLA alleles had been characterized.[5] Table 137–1 lists the number of known HLA alleles at each locus.

GENETICS OF THE MAJOR HISTOCOMPATIBILITY COMPLEX

The first sequence map of the MHC encompassed approximately 3.6 Mbp on chromosome 6p21 and was divided into three regions: class I, class II, and class III genes.[2] Newer analysis confirming high linkage disequilibrium and conserved synteny led to the concept of an extended MHC (xMHC), and a new map was produced in 2004.[6] The xMHC occupies approximately 7.6 Mbp, and is composed of five subregions, which include the classical classes I, II, and III genes. Class II genes are the most centromeric and occupy approximately 1 Mbp of DNA. The genes are ordered sequentially beginning with HLA-DP genes followed by HLA-DM, TAP, HLA-DQ and lastly the HLA-DR genes. The class III genes occupy space between the class I and class II genes. The class III genes include genes that encode other proteins that participate in immune response such as complement, heat shock proteins, tumor necrosis factor, and other lymphocyte antigens. Telomeric are the class I genes sequentially as MICA, MICB, HLA-B, HLA-C, HLA-E, HLA-A, HLA-F, and HLA-G. Extended class I genes include histone clusters and zinc finger genes. Figure 137–1B is a representative map of the MHC.

STRUCTURE AND FUNCTION

Class I Antigens

The HLA-A, -B, and -C molecules are transmembrane glycoproteins with an Mr 56,000.[7] Each is a heterodimer composed of one α heavy chain (Mr 45,000) noncovalently bound to β_2-microglobulin (Mr 11,000). The α heavy chain is the polymorphic glycoprotein encoded by the MHC genes. The extracellular region of the α chain consists of three domains (α_1, α_2, α_3) based on folding and disulfide bonding (see Fig. 137–1A). Antigenicity resides in the α_1 and α_2 domains, the areas of highest polymorphism. These two chains form a platform composed of a single β-pleated sheet "floor" topped by two α helices with a cleft or groove between them. The structure is supported by the third, α_3, domain of the heavy chain in conjunction with β_2-microglobulin, which stabilizes the molecule on the cell surface. Class I HLA molecules present peptide fragments from endogenously derived proteins (e.g., viral infection, intracellular bacteria, or transformation) to CD8+ T cells. The highly polymorphic groove permits presentation of highly variable peptides of nine amino acids average length. Class I HLA-A, -B, and -C antigens are found on most nucleated somatic cells.[8] Platelets express HLA-A antigens, but lack some HLA-B and most HLA-C antigens.[9]

Class II Antigens

The class II antigens are also transmembrane glycoproteins formed by two noncovalently bound chains.[12] Both the α heavy chain (Mr 34,000)

TABLE 137–1. Number of Known Alleles for Each Human Leukocyte Antigen Locus as of July 2014

HLA CLASS I						
Gene	A	B	C	E	F	G
Alleles	2884	3590	2375	15	22	50
HLA CLASS II						
Gene	DRA	DRB	DQA	DQB	DPA	DPB
Alleles	7	1642	52	664	38	422
NON-HLA						
Gene	MICA	MICB	TAP1	TAP2		
Alleles	100	40	12	12		

HLA, human leukocyte antigen (HLA).

Data from Robinson J, Waller MJ, Parham P, et al: IMGT/HLA and IMGT/MHC: Sequence databases for the study of the major histocompatibility complex. *Nucleic Acids Res* 31(1):311–314, 2003.

and the light β chain (Mr 29,000) are encoded in the MHC region. Class II molecules, like class I, consist of an extracellular hydrophilic NH_2–terminal region, a hydrophobic transmembrane region, and an intracellular COOH– terminus region. Unlike class I antigens, the extracellular regions of each chain contain only two domains. The two domains of the α chain are designated α_1 and α_2, and the two domains of the β-chain are called β_1 and β_2. The α chain of HLA-DR is constant for all HLA-DR molecules, whereas the β chain is polymorphic and determines specificity of the molecule. Both α and β chains of HLA-DQ and -DP are polymorphic, although the β chain is more so than the α chain. In all class II antigens the β_1 domain represents the most polymorphic region. The structure of HLA-DR is essentially similar to the structure of class I molecules. Class II antigens present peptides from exogenous sources, such as bacterial pathogens, to CD4+ cells. The binding groove is more open than that of class I, and peptides of longer length (11 to 18 amino

acids) are accommodated.[13,14] Class II antigens have a more restricted tissue distribution, being found primarily on B lymphocytes and other antigen-presenting cells such as dendritic cells, monocytes, and macrophages. They may also be expressed on activated endothelial cells and T lymphocytes.[12]

The extraordinarily polymorphic nature of HLA has probably evolved because of the need to present a very large array of different antigenic peptides in host defense. Antigen processing and presentation is a tightly regulated process, especially among the professional antigen-presenting cells such as dendritic cells. A number of alternative mechanisms have been demonstrated *in vitro*, such as cross-presentation, whereby dendritic cells transfer antigen derived from endocytic sources to the class I pathway, but are poorly understood.[15] One promising area of research is the ability of HLA molecules to present antigenic peptides derived from tumors. Such peptides could arise via point mutation, or reactivation of a normally silent gene that produces a peptide that can bind to HLA and induce a T-cell immune response. Several such peptides (melanoma-associated gene [MAGE] antigens) have been identified for melanoma.[16]

NOMENCLATURE

Distinguishing polymorphic variations among HLA antigens is clinically important in stem cell transplantation. Terminology used to describe accepted HLA alleles or antigens is standardized by the World Health Organization (WHO), Nomenclature Committee for Factors of the HLA System, which issues biannual reports and monthly updates.[4] In addition, an HLA dictionary defining HLA antigens, their assigned nomenclature, and serologic equivalents is published periodically.[5] The nomenclature committee approved major changes to the system that were implemented in 2010.[17] The revisions were designed to accommodate the unexpected number of new sequenced alleles. Under this system, colons are used as delimiters to separate fields. The first field signifies the allele family that often corresponds to the serological antigen. The second field denotes the alleles, assigned in order of determination. The third field is used for defining synonymous nucleotide substitutions.

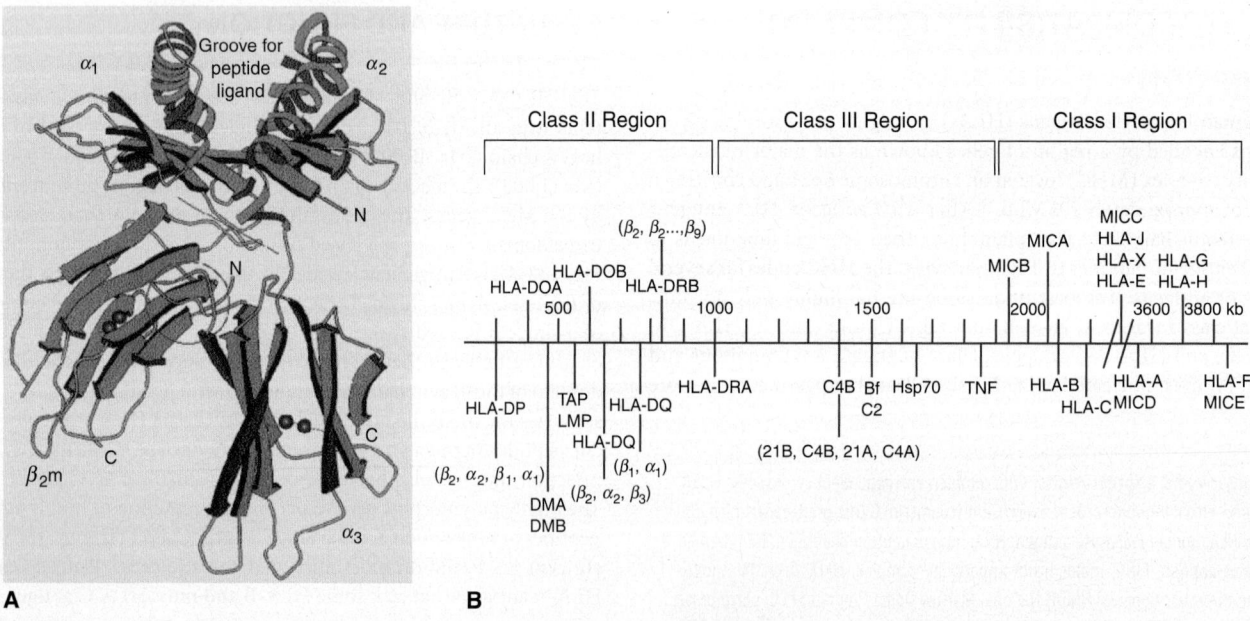

Figure 137–1. A. Schematic of the HLA-A2 molecule. The peptide groove is formed by the *a* helices and β-pleated sheet floor. The groove holds processed peptide antigen. The peptide and the polymorphic *a* helices interact with the T-cell receptor. **B.** Representative diagram of the genes of the MHC on chromosome 6. (*A, reproduced with permission from Bjorkman PJ, Saper MA, Samraoui B, et al: The foreign antigen binding site and T cell recognition regions of class I histocompatibility antigens.* Nature *329(6139):512–518, 1987. B, adapted with permission from Campbell RD, Trowsdale J: Map of the human MHC,* Immunol Today *14(7):349–352, 1993.*)

The last field defines alleles that differ by sequence polymorphisms in introns or in the 5′ or 3′ untranslated regions that flank the exons and introns. In addition, there are suffixes that are used to describe expression status. Null alleles (not expressed) are identified by the suffix "N." Low surface expression is represented by "L." Secreted molecules not present at the surface are assigned "S."

INHERITANCE OF MAJOR HISTOCOMPATIBILITY COMPLEX ANTIGENS

The genes of the MHC demonstrate more polymorphism than any other genetic system; that is, many alleles exist for each locus. Each individual, however, has one allele for each locus per chromosome, and therefore, encodes two HLA antigens per locus. The identification of each HLA antigen of an individual is called a *phenotype*. Because HLA genes are closely linked, recombination within the MHC is rare (≤1%), and a complete set of HLA genes usually is inherited from each parent as a unit. The genes inherited from each parent are referred to as a *haplotype*. Maternal and paternal haplotypes can be identified through family studies. Identification of both haplotypes of an individual provides the *genotype*. Family studies consist of typing for the HLA-A, HLA-B, HLA-C, HLA-DR, and HLA-DQ antigens to identify haplotypes and to rule out genetic recombination within the MHC. Because HLA genes are inherited together on a single chromosome, four combinations of maternal and paternal haplotypes are possible provided no recombination occurs (Fig. 137–2).

Linkage Disequilibrium

Because the MHC is so highly polymorphic, the probability that any two unrelated individuals are HLA identical is extremely low. However, the system exhibits a phenomenon known as *linkage disequilibrium*. That is, HLA alleles are inherited together on the same chromosome more often than would be predicted if HLA loci were in equilibrium. At equilibrium, the frequency of an allele at one locus is independent of the frequencies of alleles at linked loci. For example, the gene frequency of HLA-A1 is 0.145 and that of HLA-B8 is 0.1 in North American whites. Given no preferential association between A1 and B8, then the haplotype frequency would be 0.0145 (0.145 × 0.1). However, population studies demonstrate that the actual frequency of the HLA-A1, B8 haplotype is 0.0726.[18] The degree of linkage disequilibrium is defined as the observed frequency minus its expected frequency, 0.0581 in this example. Although particular alleles found in linkage disequilibria differ for various racial groups, all racial groups display significant disequilibria. Different races and ethnic groups can vary greatly in the frequency with which HLA antigens are found.[19]

HUMAN LEUKOCYTE ANTIGEN TYPING

Tissue typing for HLA antigens can be performed by various methods using serologic, cellular, and molecular technologies. The most frequent procedures used in the clinical setting are serologic and molecular. Cellular assays such as the mixed lymphocyte reaction and the primed lymphocyte test were common prior to the widespread adoption of DNA methods. Compared to DNA techniques, cellular methods are labor-intensive and require the use of radioisotopes; they are mainly used in research laboratories.

Serology

The microlymphocytotoxicity complement-dependent cytotoxicity (CDC) test has been a fundamental procedure for defining HLA antigens for more than 30 years,[20] although it has been supplanted by molecular typing methods. In this assay, a suspension of lymphocytes is incubated with human alloantisera or monoclonal antibody in a microtiter tray.[21] Rabbit serum is added as a source of complement. Cell death is induced when antibody binds to antigen on the cell surface and the complement cascade activated. Death is visualized microscopically by the uptake of vital dye or by immunofluorescence. Panels used to determine a patient's HLA type consist of two to four antisera that recognize the same specificity, which requires approximately 150 different reagents for class I antigens and 80 to 150 for class II antigens. Antisera are usually obtained from multiparous women, multiply transfused patients, and from patients who have rejected allografts. Monoclonal antibodies are also commercially available for many HLA specificities. Serology for class II (DR and DQ) antigens requires enrichment for B lymphocytes, which can be accomplished with antibody or immunomagnetic bead reagents.

Molecular Human Leukocyte Antigen Typing

The development of the polymerase chain reaction (PCR)[22] revolutionized the approach to HLA typing. Several DNA-based methods are commonly accepted for HLA typing. These include sequence-based typing, sequence-specific primer (SSP) amplification[23] and sequence-specific oligonucleotide (SSO) probe hybridization. All of these methods involve amplification of genomic DNA from selected portions of HLA genes with oligonucleotide primer pairs. Generally exons 2 and 3 of class I and exon 2 of class II genes are amplified. These exons encode most of the polymorphisms of the classes I and II molecules. Molecular HLA typing is primarily of clinical interest in marrow/blood stem cell transplantation.

The advent of "next-generation sequencing" (NGS) strategies has proven useful to high-throughput sequencing of HLA genes. NGS methods also overcome limitations of Sanger-based methods, including combination ambiguities that result from heterozygous samples in diploid genomes or between alleles where sequence varies outside the target region (i.e., exons 2 and 3). NGS methods are described as

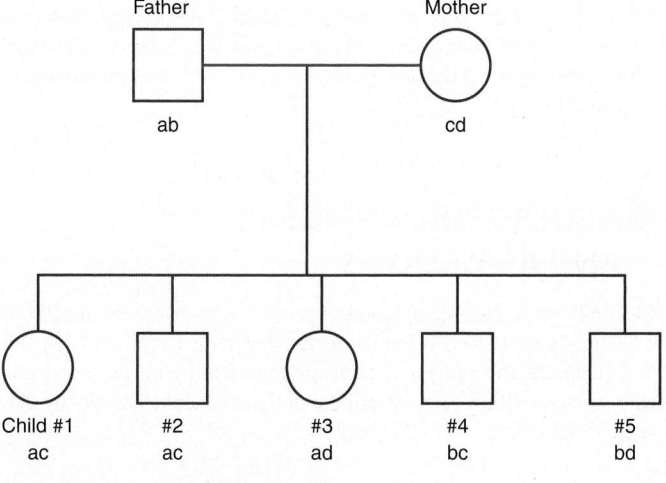

Figure 137–2. Pedigree representing inheritance of HLA antigens. Each of the four parental haplotypes is coded by a letter: *a* and *b* represent paternal haplotypes; *c* and *d* represent maternal haplotypes. Each child inherits one paternal and one maternal haplotype such that four combinations are possible.

Code:	Haplotype:					
a	A1,	B8,	Cw1,	DR17,	DR52,	DQ2
b	A2,	B44,	Cw2,	DR11,	DR52,	DQ7
c	A3,	B7,	Cw3,	DR15,	DR51,	DQ6
d	A11,	B55,	Cw3,	DR4,	DR53,	DQ8

massively parallel allowing for many overlapping reads of the same sequence area. Multiple platforms using different chemistries are available; bioinformatics expertise is required to analyze the extensive data provided by these methods.

Detection of Antibodies to Human Leukocyte Antigen Molecules

In addition to typing for HLA antigens, most laboratories also use technology to detect antibodies to HLA antigens. This is very important for solid-organ transplantation where the presence of anti-HLA antibodies can cause irreversible rejection upon transplantation. It is of less concern for marrow/stem cell transplantation where donors and recipients are generally matched for HLA antigens. The microcytotoxicity serologic test is still in use, but solid phase assays have become standard practice as they are more sensitive than the CDC method. These assays include enzyme-linked immunosorbent assay (ELISA) and microbead-based flow assays such as FlowPRA and Luminex assays. These tests require HLA antigen, in either recombinant or native form, bound to a solid surface such as a microsphere and used to capture alloantibody in patient serum. Analysis of the reaction patterns yields information about the breadth of alloimmunization, or PRA (panel reactive antibody), and the specificity of the reactions. Prior to most solid-organ transplants, a donor-specific crossmatch is also performed to ensure that the recipient does not have anti-HLA antibodies against donor HLA antigens. Crossmatches are performed by microlymphocytotoxicity (CDC), flow cytometry, and by solid-phase (ELISA and microbead) assays. Labs are now adopting the "virtual" crossmatch using data from the sensitive microbead assays to predict crossmatch outcome. For low-risk cases this allows a transplant to proceed without waiting for a physical crossmatch and shortens cold ischemic time for an organ.[24]

CLINICAL APPLICATIONS

The HLA antigens coded by the MHC play a central role in transplantation, regulation of immune responses, and susceptibility to a variety of diseases. The most common application, however, is the field of transplantation. In renal and stem cell transplantation, allografts from HLA-identical sibling donors have significantly greater survival than grafts from nonmatched family or unrelated donors.

For solid-organ transplantation, a living donor is not always available or feasible (e.g., for heart transplantation). HLA typing for matching of kidneys and pancreas is performed at the HLA-A, HLA-B, and HLA-DR loci at low resolution (serologic or antigen level by DNA). In the early years of renal transplantation a high degree of match was sought between recipients and donors. However, as more potent immunotherapies have developed, the level and use of HLA matching has declined. HLA matching is not prospectively performed for hepatic or cardiac transplantation. Detection of alloantibody by screening techniques and the donor specific crossmatch is of prime importance for kidney and heart transplants where its existence could cause a hyperacute rejection and graft failure. The role of alloantibody is less clear in the immediate posttransplantation period, but may be detrimental to long-term survival.[25] In the last several years, several "paired donor exchanges" have arisen to assist recipients who have incompatible, but willing living donors. These programs, such as the National Kidney Registry allow donor-recipient pairs to swap within or between transplantation centers. Chains of up to 30 cross-country swaps in the United States have facilitated more than 1200 transplantations since its inception.

Marrow or stem cell transplantation entails problems other than allograft survival. In these therapies an immunocompetent graft is transplanted to an immunocompromised/immunoablated host.

The graft may recognize the host tissue as foreign and mount an immune response resulting graft-versus-host disease (GVHD). With HLA-identical sibling donors, disease-free survival of greater than 80 percent can be achieved for some hematopoietic malignancies.[26,27] However, fewer than 30 percent of individuals have an HLA-identical sibling. For these patients, alternative donors, such as phenotypically matched unrelated volunteers and partially matched family members, may be considered. However, the risks and incidence of graft failure and GVHD are higher than seen with HLA-identical siblings, and increase with the level of HLA disparity. HLA typing for stem cell transplants is generally performed by molecular methods. For those with a family donor, low-resolution typing may be sufficient to identify a match. However for unrelated or haploidentical family donors, high-resolution (allele-level) typing for HLA-A, HLA-B, HLA-C, HLA-DR, and HLA-DQ should be performed, and is required by the national registry program (National Marrow Donor Program [NMDP]).[26] HLA alloantibody is becoming common, especially when incompletely matched donors are used.

Patients requiring platelet transfusions may be broadly sensitized to HLA-A, and -B (i.e., have high PRA) through prior transfusions (particularly nonleukoreduced) or pregnancies. HLA antibody screening to select nonreactive donors and/or HLA donor platelet matching may enable these refractory patients to achieve improved platelet transfusion count increments.

HLA typing at one or a few antigens or alleles may also be performed to support diagnosis of diseases associated with specific HLA antigens. The most common of these is the association between HLA-B27 and ankylosing spondylitis[28] and HLA-DQ2's association with narcolepsy.[29] HLA typing may also be performed to determine eligibility for vaccine trials that use peptides and HLA.[30,31] HLA antigens also are implicated in drug hypersensitivity. For example, HLA-B*5701 is associated with hypersensitivity to the drug for treatment of the human immunodeficiency virus, abacavir.[32]

HLA tetramers may be used to monitor the efficacy of HLA-based peptide vaccines. Recombinant HLA molecules are loaded with the peptide vaccine and linked via a fluoresceinated streptavidin molecule. They are incubated with patient blood lymphocytes. Effector T cells specific for the peptide-HLA will be bound by the tetramer and monitored by flow cytometry.

● NEUTROPHIL ANTIGENS AND ANTIBODIES

Clinically significant alloantigens expressed only or predominantly by neutrophils are known as human neutrophil antigens (HNAs).[33] In this nomenclature, the antigen systems are indicated by integers, and specific antigens within each system are designated alphabetically by date of publication (Table 137–2).

THE HNA-1 ANTIGEN SYSTEM

HNA-1 Antigens

The neutrophil-specific HNA-1 antigen system is made up of the four antigens alleles, HNA-1a, -1b, -1c and -1d (see Table 137–2).[34] HNA-1 antigens are located on the low-affinity Fcγ receptor IIIb (FcγRIIIb), CD16, and are expressed only on neutrophils.[35-38] FcγRIIIb and HNA-1 antigens are expressed on all segmented neutrophils, on approximately one-half of neutrophilic metamyelocytes, and on approximately 10 percent of neutrophilic myelocytes.[39] Soluble FcγRIIIb is present in plasma and has the same HNA-1 polymorphisms found on neutrophils.[40]

TABLE 137-2. Human Neutrophil Antigens

System	Alleles	Location of Antigens	Genes
HNA-1	HNA-1a, -1b, -1c, and 1d	FcγRIIIb	*FCGR3B*01, FCGR3B*02,* and *FCGR3B*03*
HNA-2	HNA-2	NB1gp	*CD177*
HNA-3	HNA-3a	Choline transporter-like protein-2 (CTL2)	*SLC44A2*01*
HNA-4	HNA-4a	α_M integrin, C3bi-receptor (CR3)(CD11b)	*ITGAM*01*
HNA-5	HNA-5a	αL integrin, LFA-1(CD11a)	*ITGAL*01*

Molecular Biology

FcγRIIIb and the HNA-1 antigens are encoded by the *FCGR3B* gene located on chromosome 1q23–24. *FCGR3B* is highly homologous to *FCGR3A*, which encodes FcγRIIIa. In addition to the polymorphic *FCGRB3B* nucleotides only four others differ between *FCGR3B* and *FCGR3A*. The most important difference between the two genes is a C-to-T change at 733 in *FCGR3B* that creates a stop codon. As a result, *FCGR3A* has 21 more amino acids than *FCGR3B* and *FCGR3B* is a glycosylphosphatidylinositol (GPI)-anchored rather than a transmembrane glycoprotein (GP).

The four HNA-1 system antigens are encoded by three alleles. The *FCGR3B*01* allele differs from *FCGR3B*02* by only five nucleotides in the coding region, at positions 141, 147, 227, 277, and 349.[35–38] Four of the nucleotide changes result in changes in amino acid sequence between the HNA-1a and HNA-1b forms of FcγRIIIb. The glycosylation pattern of FcγRIIIb differs between the two antigens because of two nucleotide changes at bases 227 and 277. The HNA-1b form of FcγRIIIb has six *N*-linked glycosylation sites and the HNA-1a form has four glycosylation sites.

The *FCGR3B*03* allele is identical to *FCGR3B*02* except for a C-to-A substitution at nucleotide 266 resulting in an alanine to aspartate change at amino acid 78 of FcγRIIIb.[34] In many cases, *FCGR3B*03* exists on the same chromosome with a second or duplicate *FCGR3B* gene.[41,42] *FCGR3B*03* encodes both HNA-1b and HNA-1c. *FCGR3B*02* also encodes HNA-1d which is characterized by the FcγRIIIb sequence Ala78–Asn82.[43]

The antigen frequencies of three of the alleles vary widely among different racial groups. Among whites, HNA-1b is the most common antigen (Table 137–3),[44–46,48–50] but in Japanese and Chinese populations HNA-1a is most common.[44,46,48,49,51] The frequency of the gene encoding HNA-1c antigen also varies among racial groups. HNA-1c is expressed by neutrophils in 4 to 5 percent of whites, 25 to 38 percent of African Americans, and 10 percent of Brazilians.[52,53] The antigen frequency of HNA-1d should be nearly the same as that of HNA-1b, but it has not yet been investigated.

Several other sequence variations in FCGR3B have been described.[46] Most of these chimeric alleles have single-base substitutions involving one of the five single nucleotide polymorphisms (SNPs) that distinguish *FCGR3B*1* and *FCGR3B*2*. *FCGR3B* alleles that most closely resembled *FCGR3B*2* were found more often in African Americans than in whites or Japanese.[46,47]

Genetic deficiencies of neutrophil FcγRIIIb and HNA-1 antigens have also been reported. Among whites the incidence of individuals homozygous for *FCGR3B* deletion is approximately 0.1 percent.[52,54,55] However, among Africans and African Americans the incidence is much higher. In one study, 3 of 126 Africans were found to be *FCGR3B* deficient,[48] and in another study, 1 of 53 were found to be *FCGR3B* deficient.[46]

Function of HNA-1 Antigens

Polymorphisms in FcγRIIIb have some effect on neutrophil function. Neutrophils that are homozygous for HNA-1b have a lower affinity for immunoglobulin (Ig) G_3 than those homozygous for HNA-1a.[56] Neutrophils from those who are homozygous for HNA-1b phagocytize erythrocytes sensitized with IgG_1 and IgG_3 anti-Rh monoclonal antibodies and bacteria opsonized with IgG_1 at a lower level than neutrophils homozygous for HNA-1a.[57,58]

THE HNA-2 ANTIGEN SYSTEM

The HNA-2 Antigen

HNA-2 is an isoantigen without allelic variation. HNA-2 is expressed only on neutrophils, neutrophilic metamyelocytes, and myelocytes.[39,59] It's unique in that it is expressed on subpopulations of neutrophils. The mean size of the HNA-2-positive subpopulation of neutrophils is 45 to

TABLE 137-3. Human Neutrophil Antigen Frequencies

System	Alleles	Antigen Frequencies			
		Europeans/ North Americans	Africans and African Americans	Asians	Brazilians/ Argentineans
HNA-1	HNA-1a	58%	59–67%	91%	68%
	HNA-1b	88%	71–88%	54%	76%
	HNA-1c	5%	25–38%	<1%	5–10%
	HNA-1d	NA	NA	NA	NA
HNA-2	HNA-2	95–97%	95%	89–99%	NA
HNA-3	HNA-3a	89–92%	NA	NA	NA
HNA-4	HNA-4a	99%	NA	99%	97%
HNA-5	HNA-5a	85%	88%	81–96%	78–92%

NA, not available.

65 percent[60-62] and is dependent on gender. The size of the HNA-2 positive subpopulation of neutrophils from women is approximately 60 percent, compared with approximately 50 percent for men.[62,63] Neutrophil expression of HNA-2 is greater in pregnant women than in healthy female blood donors.[64]

HNA-2 Molecular Biology

The glycoprotein carrying HNA-2, NB1 glycoprotein, is located on neutrophil plasma membranes and secondary granules[60,64] and is a GPI-anchored glycoprotein.[60] The gene encoding NB1 glycoprotein, *CD177*, is located on chromosome 19q13.31[65,66] and belongs to the *Ly-6* snake toxin superfamily. Other genes in this family include urokinase-type plasminogen activator receptor (CD87) and decay accelerating factor (CD59).

HNA-2 is expressed on neutrophils by approximately 95 to 97 percent of whites, 95 percent of African Americans, and 89 to 99 percent of Japanese.[62,67,68] SNPs have been identified in *CD177*. These SNPs have been associated with the size of the HNA-2–positive population of neutrophils, but not the HNA-2–negative phenotype.[69] The HNA-2–negative neutrophil phenotype is the result of a *CD177* transcription defect.[70]

Role of NB1 Glycoprotein in Neutrophil Function

NB1 glycoprotein binds to platelet endothelial cell adhesion molecule-1 (PECAM-1, CD31) and functions as a cell adhesion molecule.[71] PECAM-1 is expressed on both neutrophils and endothelial cells and PECAM-1–PECAM-1 interactions are important in the migration of neutrophils through endothelial cells. Interactions between NB1 glycoprotein and PECAM-1 are also involved with neutrophil–endothelial cell interactions, and mediate neutrophil transendothelial cell migration.[71] However, women who produce HNA-2 specific alloantibodies and who lack NB1 glycoprotein are healthy.

CD177 mRNA is overexpressed by neutrophils from patients with polycythemia rubra vera and essential thrombocytosis, but the expression of HNA-2 is not.[72,73] The increased expression of CD177 mRNA in neutrophils from these patients may be secondary to the constitutive activation of Janus kinase 2 (JAK2) by JAK2 V617F.

THE HNA-3 ANTIGEN SYSTEM

The HNA-3 antigen system has one antigen, HNA-3a, that was previously known as 5b. HNA-3a is expressed by neutrophils, lymphocytes, platelets, endothelial cells, kidney, spleen, and placental cells. HNA-3a has an antigen frequency of 89 to 92 percent and is located on a 70- to 95-kDa neutrophil glycoprotein.[74] HNA-3a is a result of a single nucleotide change in choline transporter-like protein-2 gene (*SLC44A2*) at nucleotide 455, which results in an amino acid change at position 152.[75,76] Several cases of transfusion-related acute lung injury (TRALI) have been associated with transfusion of plasma containing anti–HNA-3a.[77-79]

THE HNA-4 AND HNA-5 ANTIGEN SYSTEMS

The HNA-4 and HNA-5 antigens are located on the β_2 integrins. Each antigen system contains only a single antigen, HNA-4a and HNA-5a, respectively. The HNA-4a antigen was previously known as Mart(a). HNA-4a was defined by an antibody in the sera of three nontransfused multiparous blood donors. This antigen has an autosomal dominant inheritance and an antigen frequency of 99 percent in whites[80] and Asians,[81] and 97 percent in Brazilians.[82] HNA-4a is located on the α_M chain (CD11b) of the C3bi receptor (CR3) and is caused by a single nucleotide substitution of G-to-A at position 302[83] that results in an Arg-to-His polymorphism at amino acid 61. The significance of the antibody is not known, and none of the infants of the three multiparous

women with anti–HNA-4a showed evidence of neonatal alloimmune neutropenia.

A second polymorphism of the β_2 integrins, HNA-5a, was first described as Ond(a). A chronically transfused man with aplastic anemia became alloimmunized to HNA-5a. HNA-5a was found to be expressed on the α_L integrin unit, leukocyte function antigen-1 (CD11a), and is a result of a G-to-C single nucleotide substitution at position 2446 that results in a change of Arg to Thr at amino acid 766.[87] The antigen frequency of HNA-5a is 78 to 96 percent.[81,82,84]

ANTIBODIES TO NEUTROPHIL ANTIGENS

Alloimmune Neonatal Neutropenia

Neutrophil antibody tests are performed by agglutination or fluorescent techniques, and these are not widely available because clinical syndromes caused by these antibodies are uncommon. A commercial solid-phase assay that allows for the detection of antibodies directed to HNA-1, HNA-2, HNA-3, HNA-4, and HNA-5 antigens is now available.[85] During pregnancy, mothers can become alloimmunized to fetal neutrophil antigens. Maternal IgG directed to neutrophils can cross the placenta and destroy the neonate's neutrophils. Maternal alloimmunization to neutrophil antigens can affect the first child. Most neonates experience isolated neutropenia, but the cytopenias are self-limiting and resolve as the antibody is cleared. Antibodies to neutrophil-specific antigens HNA-1a, HNA-1b, and HNA-2 most commonly cause neonatal alloimmune neutropenia.[74,86] Mothers with FcγRIIIb deficiency have also produced antibodies to FcγRIIIb, causing neonatal neutropenia.[55,74,86]

Most often the neutropenia is detected in the first week of life when the neonate becomes febrile or develops an infection and a neutrophil count is done. Typically, the counts are 0.1 to 0.2×10^9/L. Total white blood cell count, platelet count, and hemoglobin are usually normal, but eosinophilia or monocytosis may be present. The clinical course is quite variable. An occasional infant is asymptomatic, but almost all affected children have an infection. The duration of the neutropenia may be as short as a few days or as long as 28 weeks.[86] The mean duration of neutropenia is approximately 11 weeks.[86] Intravenous immunoglobulin (IVIG) and granulocyte colony-stimulating factor (G-CSF) have a limited role in the treatment of neonatal alloimmune neutropenia.[86]

Autoimmune Neutropenia of Childhood

Autoimmune neutropenia is well described in children.[87-90] Typically, the onset of the autoimmune neutropenia of children begins at 8 months of age, but children between 1 and 36 months of age can be affected. Most studies have found that neutrophil counts recover spontaneously by the age of 5 years, with a median duration of neutropenia of 13 to 20 months.[87-90] In most cases, children presented with severe neutropenia, having neutrophil counts less than 0.5×10^9/L. Monocytosis has been reported to occur in up to 38 percent of patients. Marrow biopsies in affected patients usually show normal to hypercellular marrow with a decreased number of mature neutrophils.

Antibodies to neutrophils can be detected in up to 98 percent of affected patients. If an antibody specificity is identified, the antibodies are almost always specific to epitopes located on FcγRIIIb. The antibodies are directed to HNA-1a in 10 to 46 percent of patients, to HNA-1b in 2 to 3 percent of patients, and rarely to FcγRIIIb epitopes expressed by neutrophils from all donors.[88-89] Autoimmune neutropenia has been treated with glucocorticoids, IVIG, and G-CSF.[88]

Transfusion Reactions

Antibodies to neutrophil and HLA antigens in transfused blood can cause febrile nonhemolytic reactions. Febrile nonhemolytic transfusion reactions occur within a few hours of a transfusion and can be associated with chills and rigors. These reactions are a result of neutrophil antibodies in the transfusion recipient binding to leukocytes in the transfused blood component. Febrile transfusion reactions can be prevented in recipients of platelet and red blood cell component transfusions by the use of leukocyte-reduced blood components.

A more serious type of neutrophil antibody-mediated transfusion reaction is TRALI. TRALI is often caused by the transfusion of neutrophil antibodies in the plasma portion of a blood component. TRALI occurs within 6 hours of a transfusion when hypoxia and noncardiogenic pulmonary edema occur, as measured by a fall in hemoglobin oxygen saturation to less than 90 percent or a partial pressure of arterial oxygen (PaO$_2$)-to-fraction of inspired oxygen (FIO$_2$) ratio (PaO$_2$:FIO$_2$) of less than 300 torr.[91]

Many case reports have associated TRALI with the inadvertent transfusion of neutrophil antibodies. Investigations of transfusion recipients of blood components from donors with neutrophil antibodies who have been implicated in cases of TRALI suggest that a large proportion of neutrophil antibodies can cause TRALI and less-severe pulmonary transfusion reactions.[78,92–94] A prospective case study with controls and a prospective nested case-control study have confirmed that the transfusion of blood products containing antibodies directed to neutrophil antigen are an important cause of TRALI.[95,96]

Antibodies to HNA-2 and -3a have most frequently been implicated in lung injury. Animal models also show that the transfusion of anti–HNA-2 and anti–HNA-3a can cause acute lung injury.[97–99]

● HUMAN PLATELET ANTIGENS

Platelets express a variety of immunogenic markers on the cell surface. Some of these antigens are shared with other cell types as in the case of HLAs or blood group (ABO) antigens, whereas others are specific to platelets. Some of these platelet-specific markers can be recognized by autoantibodies[100–103] or by antibodies induced by certain drugs,[104–106] and still others by antibodies made by pregnant women or recipients of blood transfusions.

PLATELET ALLOANTIGENS

Platelet alloantigens are associated with polymorphisms of platelet surface GPs and can induce production of alloantibodies when individuals lacking a particular polymorphism are exposed via pregnancy or transfusion.[107] Immune responses to platelet alloantigens are involved in the pathogenesis of several clinical syndromes, including fetal or neonatal alloimmune thrombocytopenia (FNAIT), posttransfusion purpura (PTP), and occasionally in unresponsiveness to platelet transfusion.[108] Alloimmune thrombocytopenia can also be an unusual complication of solid-organ transplantation in which donor lymphocytes make alloantibodies specific for the platelets produced by the recipient of an organ allograft.[109]

PLATELET ISOANTIGENS

A condition similar to alloimmune platelet destruction occurs in patients who lack part or all of a particular platelet GP because of defective alleles of the GP-encoding genes. Such patients can make isoantibodies against platelets of virtually all donors that bear the platelet GP. For example, patients with Bernard-Soulier syndrome, who lack platelet GPIb-V-IX (CD 42a-c), or patients with Glanzmann thrombasthenia, who lack expression of GPIIb (CD41) and GPIIIa (CD61), can be induced to make broadly reactive antiplatelet isoantibodies.[110–113]

Platelet GPIV (CD36) is expressed on various human cells including platelets, macrophages, capillary endothelium, erythroblasts, and adipocytes.[114,115] Some apparently normal individuals lack CD36 on their platelets (type II deficiency) or platelets and monocytes (type I deficiency).[116] CD36 deficiency is common in Asians (3 to 11 percent)[117] and Africans (3 to 6 percent),[118] but is rare in white populations (0.1 percent).[118] CD36 deficiency may confer protection from malaria and has been shown to be a receptor for red cells infected with *Plasmodium falciparum*. However, one report suggests CD36 deficiency may actually *increase the risk* for more severe forms of malarial infection.[119] The role of CD36 deficiency as either a protective or aggravating factor in malarial infection remains controversial.[120,121] Type I CD36-deficient individuals can become immunized via transfusion or pregnancy and make isoantibodies against CD36 that have been implicated in cases of FNAIT, PTP, and platelet transfusion refractoriness.[117,122–125]

PLATELET ANTIGENS: GENETICS AND STRUCTURE

Platelet-specific alloantigens result from genetic polymorphism in genes encoding platelet surface proteins.[126] These *allo*antigens were first defined by antiplatelet antibodies discovered in the sera of multiparous females who gave birth to thrombocytopenic infants (FNAIT) or in patients who developed PTP. Many of these alloantibodies were subsequently found to recognize allotypic determinants of platelet-associated membrane GPs, such as GPIIb/IIIa (CD41/CD61). Almost all of these determinants are generated by single-amino-acid substitutions encoded by SNPs in the GP genes (Table 137–4).[127] In some cases, differential glycosylation may contribute to or influence the expression of certain human platelet antigen (HPA) epitopes, such as those associated with HPA-3.[128,129] In any case, these amino acid substitutions generally do not appear to affect platelet function *in vitro*. However, the genetic polymorphism in platelet GPs may be associated with more subtle differences in platelet physiology that can contribute to the relative risk for thrombosis and/or atherosclerosis.[130–135]

To date, 33 HPA expressed on six different platelet GPs: GPIIb (CD41), GPIIIa (CD61), GPIbα (CD42b), GPIbβ (CD42c), GPIa (CD49b), and CD109 have been described including localization to platelet surface GPs, quantification of their density on the platelet surface, and determination of DNA polymorphisms in genes encoding for them (see Table 137–4).[127,136] For a current list see http://www.ebi.ac.uk/ipd/hpa/table1.html and http://www.ebi.ac.uk/ipd/hpa/table2.html.[127] Thirteen antigens are clustered into one triallelic[137] (HPA-1) and five biallelic groups (HPA-2, HPA-3, HPA-4, HPA-5, HPA-15). HPA for which antibodies against only one of the alleles have been detected are labeled with a "w" for workshop, for example, HPA-8bw. To date, 20 such low-frequency single-allele HPAs have been discovered, essentially all involved in FNAIT cases.[138]

Although the frequencies of HPAs have been most extensively studied in white populations, it should be noted that they have been determined for other racial and ethnic groups as well and in some cases vary significantly from white frequencies. For example, HPA-1b is expressed on the platelets of approximately 15 percent of persons of European ancestry but of less than 1 percent of persons of Asian ancestry. For more information re HPA frequencies in different populations, readers are directed to: http://www.ebi.ac.uk/ipd/hpa/freqs_1.html[127]

NOMENCLATURE

A nomenclature for human platelet alloantigens has been adopted to replace the old complex "classic" nomenclatures that previously were developed independently in laboratories throughout the world (see

TABLE 137–4. Human Platelet Alloantigens[127,136,163]*

Alloantigens	Other Names	Phenotypic Frequency (Whites)	Glycoprotein Location/ Amino Acid Substitution	Encoding Gene/ Nucleotide Change
HPA1a	PlA, Zw	72% a/a	GPIIIa	*ITGB3*
HPA1b		26% a/b	L33P	T176C
HPA-1c		2% b/b	L33V	C175G
		<1% a/c		
HPA2a	Ko, Sib	85% a/a	GPIbα	*GPIBA*
HPA2b		14% a/b	T145M	C482T
		1% b/b		
HPA3a	Bak, Lek	37% a/a	GPIIb	*ITGA2B*
HPA3b		48% a/b	I843S	T2621G
		15% b/b		
HPA4a	Pen, Yuk	>99.9% a/a	GPIIIa	*ITGB3*
HPA4b		<0.1% a/b	R143Q	G506A
		<0.1% b/b		
HPA-5a (Brb)	Br, Hc, Zav	80% a/a	GPIa	*ITGA2*
HPA-5b (Bra)		19% a/b	E505K	G1600A
		1% b/b		
HPA-6bw	Caa, Tu	<1%	GPIIIa R489Q	*ITGB3* G1544A
HPA-7bw	Mob	<1%	GPIIa P407A	*ITGB3* C1297G
HPA-8bw	Sra	<0.1%	GPIIIa R636C	*ITGB3* C1984T
HPA-9bw	Maxa	<1%	GPIIb V837M	*ITGA2B* G2602A
HPA-10bw	Laa	1%	GPIIIa R62Q	*ITGB3* G263A
HPA-11bw	Groa	<0.5%	GPIIIa R633H	*ITGB3* G1976A
HPA-12bw	Iya	1%	GPIbβ G15E	*GPIBB* G119A
HPA-13bw	Sita	<1%	GPIa T799M	*ITGA2* C2483T
HPA-14bw	Oea	1%	GPIIIa K611del	*ITGB3* 1909_1911delAAG
HPA-15a	Gov	35% a/a	CD109	*CD109*
HPA-15b		42% a/b	S682Y	C2108A
		23% b/b		
HPA-16bw	Duva	<1%	GPIIIa T140I	*ITGB3* C497T
HPA-17bw	Vaa	<1%	GPIIIa T195M	*ITGB3* C662T
HPA-18bw		<1%	GPIa Q716H	*ITGA2* G2235T
HPA-19bw		<1%	GPIIIa K137Q	*ITGB3* A487C

(continued)

TABLE 137–4. Human Platelet Alloantigens[127,136,163]* (continued)

Alloantigens	Other Names	Phenotypic Frequency (Whites)	Glycoprotein Location/ Amino Acid Substitution	Encoding Gene/ Nucleotide Change
HPA-20bw		<1%	GPIIb T619M	*ITGA2B* C1949T
HPA-21bw		<1%	GPIIIa E628K	*ITGB3* G1960A
HPA-22bw		<1%	GPIIb K164T	*ITGA2B* A584C
HPA-23bw		<1%	GPIIIa R622W	*ITGB3* C1942T
HPA-24bw		<1%	GPIIb S472N	*ITGA2B* G1508A
HPA-25bw		<1%	GPIa T1087M	*ITGA2* C3347T
HPA-26bw		<1%	GPIIIa K580N	*ITGB3* G1818T
HPA-27bw		<1%	GPIIb L841M	*ITGA2B* C2614A
HPA-28bw		<1%	GPIIb V740L	*ITGA2B* G2311T
NA†	Naka	<1% 97% (African) 96% (Asian)	CD36 (GPIV)	T:G1 264 C:T 478

*Phenotypic frequencies for the antigens shown are for the white population only. Significant differences in gene frequencies may be found in African and Asian populations.

†Sensitization to CD36 (GPIV) is an example of isoimmunization. Anti-CD36 antibodies have been implicated in cases of neonatal alloimmune thrombocytopenia (NAIT) and posttransfusion purpura (PTP) and thus are included in the list of platelet alloantigens that are associated with these disorders.

Table 137–4). In most cases, an HPA site has two alleles, designated by the suffix *a* or *b*. These alleles are expressed by platelets codominantly. The *a* allele represents the more prevalent form of the protein, while the *b* allele represents the less-common form. There is one example of a triallelic HPA system, HPA-1, with the *c* allele being least prevalent.[137] A number of HPA alleles, for example, HPA-6b, HPA-7b, HPA-8b, and HPA-10b, are present at gene frequencies of less than 0.1 percent and were recognized in the sera of mothers of thrombocytopenic babies (FNAIT) in a single or only a very few families. Their putative high-frequency alternative alleles or the *a* form of the HPAs have not yet been identified serologically, probably because of the extremely low frequency of individuals who are homozygous for the rare alleles and who could therefore be sensitized to the high-frequency alternative allele. When such low-frequency markers are detected in only one family, they are referred to as *private* alleles. When more than one family is discovered to have such low-frequency markers and the families are unrelated, the alleles are then designated as *rare*. Such extremely rare or private alleles are unlikely to be present in the blood donor population. For this reason, these markers are unlikely to account for cases of PTP, but can be found in isolated cases of FNAIT in selected families. Alleles present at gene frequencies greater than 2 percent within the population are designated as *public* alleles. These alleles are more likely to encode alloantigens involved in PTP. Similarly, sensitization to HPA alleles with frequencies less than 50 percent are unlikely to account for platelet

transfusion refractoriness by themselves, as it would be expected that randomly selected platelet products would have been collected from a donor population with a similar frequency of these more common antigens.

TESTING FOR PLATELET-SPECIFIC ANTIGENS AND ANTIBODIES

Three types of platelet antibody detection methods have been developed. The earliest were phase I assays that involved mixing of patient serum with normal platelets and used platelet function-dependent end points such as α-granule release, aggregation, or agglutination. The serotonin release assay, used for the laboratory diagnosis of heparin-induced thrombocytopenia, and in which radiolabeled serotonin, a dense-granule constituent, is measured, is the only major phase I assay remaining in wide use today.[139] Other phase I assays were largely succeeded by phase II tests that detect either surface or total platelet-associated immunoglobulin on patient platelets or on normal platelets after sensitization with patient serum. An example of a phase II assay in wide use today is the solid-phase red cell adherence test, used for platelet crossmatching.[140] Phase III assays have been developed in which the binding of antibodies to isolated platelet surface GPs is detected. These assays are used to detect alloantibodies in the evaluation of suspected FNAIT and PTP cases as well as autoantibodies in some cases of idiopathic thrombocytopenic purpura.[141] Phase III assays have an advantage over both phase I and phase II tests in that they detect antibodies that bind to platelet GPs, and not to non–platelet-specific epitopes, such as class I HLA. Examples of phase III assays are the monoclonal antibody immobilization of platelet antigens assay (MAIPA)[142] and the modified antigen capture ELISA (MACE).[143]

Although most of the platelet antibody detection methods can be employed to determine platelet alloantigen types of individuals, because of limited access to rare typing sera and the need to establish platelet typing in patients with very few platelets, they have been largely supplanted by molecular typing using methods based on PCR. Molecular typing is now available for all of the platelet alloantigens that have been elucidated at the gene level.[144–150]

CLINICAL IMPORTANCE

Antibodies recognizing platelet-specific alloantigens have been discovered in three clinical situations: mothers who give birth to infants with FNAIT; patients who develop dramatic thrombocytopenia after blood transfusion (PTP); and patients who have received multiple transfusions. Chapter 117 discusses the clinical syndromes of FNAIT.

Although antibodies to class I HLA antigens are the principal cause of immunologic platelet transfusion refractoriness (discussed in Chap. 139), occasionally patients receiving multiple platelet transfusions will develop antibodies to platelet specific alloantigens. Many of the best-documented platelet-specific antibodies detected in such patients are directed against platelet antigens whose phenotypic frequencies are less than 30 percent in the blood-donor population.[151–154] Therefore, it is difficult to attribute refractory responses in random-donor and/or HLA-matched platelet transfusions to these antibodies alone. Indeed, the majority of refractory patients with platelet-specific antibodies also have HLA antibodies. Alloimmunization to high-frequency platelet-specific antigens would be expected to present a major challenge in finding compatible platelets to support a patient requiring multiple platelet transfusions. Fortunately, these cases are extremely rare.[152,154] If platelet transfusion refractoriness does develop because of platelet-specific antibodies, compatible platelet products may be identified by using either platelet crossmatching or by accessing family member or other HPA-typed donors who are compatible with the patient's antibodies.[155,156] Platelet GP reactivity in transfusion recipients that lacks specificity usually does not influence transfusion responses.[151,157–159]

Antibodies against some HPA-allelic determinants can inhibit platelet function. Anti–HPA-1 alloantibodies, for example, can inhibit clot retraction and platelet aggregation, presumably because they block the binding of GPIIb/IIIa ($\alpha_{IIb}\beta_3$) (CD41/CD61) to fibrinogen. Moreover, anti–HPA-4 alloantibodies can completely inhibit aggregation of HPA-4 platelets that are homozygous for the allele recognized by the alloantibodies because the epitope is in close proximity to the RGD (arginine-glycine-aspartic acid peptide sequence)-binding domain of the $\alpha_{IIb}\beta_3$ integrin.[160,161] On the other hand, other anti–HPA-alloantibodies, such as those specific for HPA-3, may not significantly interfere with platelet function but nonetheless can cause Fc-mediated platelet destruction and immune thrombocytopenia.[162]

REFERENCES

1. Breuning MH, van den Berg-Loonen EM, Bernini LF, et al: Localization of HLA on the short arm of chromosome 6. *Hum Genet* 37:131, 1977.
2. Complete sequence and gene map of a human major histocompatibility complex. The MHC sequencing consortium. *Nature* 401:921, 1999.
3. Berrih S, Arenzana-Seisdedos F, Cohen S, et al: Interferon-gamma modulates HLA class II antigen expression on cultured human thymic epithelial cells. *J Immunol* 135:1165, 1985.
4. Robinson J, Waller MJ, Parham P, et al: IMGT/HLA and IMGT/MHC: Sequence databases for the study of the major histocompatibility complex. *Nucleic Acids Res* 31:311, 2003.
5. Holdsworth R, Hurley CK, Marsh SG, et al: The HLA dictionary 2008: A summary of HLA-A, -B, -C, DRB1/3/4/5, and DQB1 alleles and their association with serologically defined HLA-A, -B, -C, -DR, -DQ antigens. *Tissue Antigens* 73:95, 2009.
6. Horton R, Wilming L, Rand V, et al: Gene map of the extended human MHC. *Nat Rev Genet* 5:889, 2004.
7. Thorsby E: Structure and function of HLA molecules. *Transplant Proc* 19:29, 1987.
8. Le Bouteiller P: HLA class I chromosomal region, genes, and products: Facts and questions. *Crit Rev Immunol* 14:89, 1994.
9. Mueller-Eckhardt G, Hauck M, Kayser W, Mueller-Eckhardt C: HLA-C antigens on platelets. *Tissue Antigens* 16:91, 1980.
10. Bjorkman PJ, Saper MA, Samraoui B, et al: The foreign antigen binding site and T cell recognition regions of class I histocompatibility antigens. *Nature* 329:512, 1987.
11. Campbell RD, Trowsdale J: Map of the human MHC. *Immunol Today* 14:349, 1993.
12. Trowsdale J: Genetics and polymorphism: Class II antigens. *Br Med Bull* 43:15, 1987.
13. Germain RN, Margulies DH: The biochemistry and cell biology of antigen processing and presentation. *Annu Rev Immunol* 11:403, 1993.
14. Yewdell JW, Bennink JR: The binary logic of antigen processing and presentation to T cells. *Cell* 62:203, 1990.
15. Vyas JM, Van der Veen AG, Ploegh HL: The known unknowns of antigen processing and presentation. *Nat Rev Immunol* 8:607, 2008.
16. Boon T, Coulie PG, Van den Eynde BJ, van der Bruggen P: Human T cell responses against melanoma. *Annu Rev Immunol* 24:175, 2006.
17. Marsh SG; WHO Nomenclature Committee for Factors of the HLA System: Nomenclature for factors of the HLA system, update April 2010. *Tissue Antigens* 76: 501, 2010.
18. Cao K, Hollenbach J, Shi X, et al: Analysis of the frequencies of HLA-A, B, and C alleles and haplotypes in the five major ethnic groups of the United States reveals high levels of diversity in these loci and contrasting distribution patterns in these populations. *Hum Immunol* 62:1009, 2001.
19. Maiers M, Gragert L, Klitz W: High-resolution HLA alleles and haplotypes in the United States population. *Hum Immunol* 68:779, 2007.
20. Terasaki PI, Park MS, Bernoco D, Iwaki Y: Serology of HLA. *Transplant Proc* 13:900, 1981.
21. Terasaki PI, McClelland JD: Microdroplet assay of human serum cytotoxins. *Nature* 204:998, 1964.
22. Saiki RK, Gelfand DH, Stoffel S, et al: Primer-directed enzymatic amplification of DNA with a thermostable DNA polymerase. *Science* 239:487, 1988.
23. Schaffer M, Olerup O: HLA-AB typing by polymerase-chain reaction with sequence-specific primers: More accurate, less errors, and increased resolution compared to serological typing. *Tissue Antigens* 58:299, 2001.
24. Tait BD, Süsal C, Gebel HM, et al: Consensus guidelines on the testing and clinical management issues associated with HLA and non-HLA antibodies in transplantation. *Transplantation* 95:19, 2013.
25. O'Leary JG, Michelle Shiller S, Bellamy C, et al: Acute liver allograft antibody-mediated rejection: An inter-institutional study of significant histopathological features. *Liver Transpl* 20:1244, 2014.
26. Flomenberg N, Baxter-Lowe LA, Confer D, et al: Impact of HLA class I and class II high-resolution matching on outcomes of unrelated donor bone marrow transplantation: HLA-C mismatching is associated with a strong adverse effect on transplantation outcome. *Blood* 104:1923, 2004.
27. Petersdorf EW, Gooley T, Malkki M, Horowitz M: Clinical significance of donor-recipient HLA matching on survival after myeloablative hematopoietic cell transplantation from unrelated donors. *Tissue Antigens* 69 Suppl 1:25, 2007.
28. Bowness P: HLA and the spondyloarthropathies, in *HLA in Health and Disease*, 2nd ed, edited by A Warrens, R Lechler, p 187. Academic Press, London, 2000.
29. Sollid L, Spurkland A, Thorsby T: HLA and gastrointestinal diseases, in *HLA in Health and Disease*, 2nd ed, edited by A Warrens, R Lechler, p 249. Academic Press, London, 2000.
30. Riley JP, Rosenberg SA, Parkhurst MR: Identification of a new shared HLA-A2.1 restricted epitope from the melanoma antigen tyrosinase. *J Immunother* 24:212, 2001.
31. Rezvani K, Yong AS, Mielke S, et al: Leukemia-associated antigen-specific T-cell responses following combined PR1 and WT1 peptide vaccination in patients with myeloid malignancies. *Blood* 111:236, 2008.
32. Abel S, Paturel L, Cabie A: Abacavir hypersensitivity. *N Engl J Med* 358:2515, 2008.
33. Bux J: Nomenclature of neutrophil alloantigens. ISBT Working Party on Platelet and Neutrophil Serology, Neutrophil Antigen Working Party. International Society of Blood Transfusion. *Transfusion* 39:662, 1999.
34. Bux J, Stein EL, Bierling P, et al: Characterization of a new alloantigen (SH) on the human neutrophil Fc gamma receptor IIIb. *Blood* 89:1027, 1997.
35. Trounstine ML, Peltz GA, Yssel H, et al: Reactivity of cloned, expressed human Fc gamma RIII isoforms with monoclonal antibodies which distinguish cell-type-specific and allelic forms of Fc gamma RIII. *Int Immunol* 2:303, 1990.
36. Ory PA, Clark MR, Kwoh EE, et al: Sequences of complementary DNAs that encode the NA1 and NA2 forms of Fc receptor III on human neutrophils. *J Clin Invest* 84:1688, 1989.
37. Ravetch JV, Perussia B: Alternative membrane forms of Fc gamma RIII(CD16) on human natural killer cells and neutrophils. Cell type-specific expression of two genes that differ in single nucleotide substitutions. *J Exp Med* 170:481, 1989.
38. Huizinga TW, Kleijer M, Tetteroo PA, et al: Biallelic neutrophil Na-antigen system is associated with a polymorphism on the phospho-inositol-linked Fc gamma receptor III (CD16). *Blood* 75:213, 1990.
39. Stroncek DF, Shankar R, Litz C, Clement L: The expression of the NB1 antigen on myeloid precursors and neutrophils from children and umbilical cords. *Transfus Med* 8:119, 1998.

40. Huizinga TW, de Haas M, Kleijer M, et al: Soluble Fc gamma receptor III in human plasma originates from release by neutrophils. *J Clin Invest* 86:416, 1990.
41. Koene HR, Kleijer M, Roos D, et al: Fc gamma RIIIB gene duplication: Evidence for presence and expression of three distinct Fc gamma RIIIB genes in NA(1+,2+)SH(+) individuals. *Blood* 91:673, 1998.
42. Steffensen R, Gulen T, Varming K, Jersild C: FcgammaRIIIB polymorphism: Evidence that NA1/NA2 and SH are located in two closely linked loci and that the SH allele is linked to the NA1 allele in the Danish population. *Transfusion* 39:593, 1999.
43. Reil A, Sachs UJ, Siahanidou T, Flesch BK, Bux J. HNA-1d: a new human neutrophil antigen located on Fcγ receptor IIIb associated with neonatal immune neutropenia. *Transfusion* 53:2145, 2013.
44. Hessner MJ, Curtis BR, Endean DJ, Aster RH: Determination of neutrophil antigen gene frequencies in five ethnic groups by polymerase chain reaction with sequence-specific primers. *Transfusion* 36:895, 1996.
45. Bux J, Stein EL, Santoso S, Mueller-Eckhardt C: NA gene frequencies in the German population, determined by polymerase chain reaction with sequence-specific primers. *Transfusion* 35:54, 1995.
46. Matsuo K, Procter J, Stroncek D: Variations in genes encoding neutrophil antigens NA1 and NA2. *Transfusion* 40:645, 2000.
47. Covas DT, Kashima S, Guerreiro JF, et al: Variation in the FcgammaR3B gene among distinct Brazilian populations. *Tissue Antigens* 65:178, 2005.
48. Lin M, Chen CC, Wang CL, Lee HL: Frequencies of neutrophil-specific antigens among Chinese in Taiwan. *Vox Sang* 66:247, 1994.
49. Ohto H, Matsuo Y: Neutrophil-specific antigens and gene frequencies in Japanese. *Transfusion* 29:654, 1989.
50. de La Vega Elena CD, Nogues N, Fernandez MA, et al: HNA-1a, HNA-1b and HNA-1c gene frequencies in Argentineans. *Tissue Antigens* 71:475, 2008.
51. Abid S, Zili M, Bouzid L, et al: Gene frequencies of human neutrophil antigens in the Tunisian blood donors and Berbers. *Tissue Antigens* 58:90, 2001.
52. Kissel K, Hofmann C, Gittinger FS, et al: HNA-1a, HNA-1b, and HNA-1c (NA1, NA2, SH) frequencies in African and American Blacks and in Chinese. *Tissue Antigens* 56:143, 2000.
53. Kuwano ST, Bordin JO, Chiba AK, et al: Allelic polymorphisms of human Fcgamma receptor IIa and Fcgamma receptor IIIb among distinct groups in Brazil. *Transfusion* 40:1388, 2000.
54. Muniz-Diaz E, Madoz P, de la Calle MO, Puig L: The polymorphonuclear neutrophil Fc gamma RIIIb deficiency is more frequent than hitherto assumed. *Blood* 86:3999, 1995.
55. Fromont P, Bettaieb A, Skouri H, et al: Frequency of the polymorphonuclear neutrophil Fc gamma receptor III deficiency in the French population and its involvement in the development of neonatal alloimmune neutropenia. *Blood* 79:2131, 1992.
56. Nagarajan S, Chesla S, Cobern L, et al: Ligand binding and phagocytosis by CD16 (Fc gamma receptor III) isoforms. Phagocytic signaling by associated zeta and gamma subunits in Chinese hamster ovary cells. *J Biol Chem* 270:25762, 1995.
57. Salmon JE, Edberg JC, Kimberly RP: Fc gamma receptor III on human neutrophils. Allelic variants have functionally distinct capacities. *J Clin Invest* 85:1287, 1990.
58. Bredius RG, Fijen CA, de Haas M, et al: Role of neutrophil Fc gamma RIIa (CD32) and Fc gamma RIIIb (CD16) polymorphic forms in phagocytosis of human IgG1- and IgG3-opsonized bacteria and erythrocytes. *Immunology* 83:624, 1994.
59. Clement LT, Lehmeyer JE, Gartland GL: Identification of neutrophil subpopulations with monoclonal antibodies. *Blood* 61:326, 1983.
60. Goldschmeding R, van Dalen CM, Faber N, et al: Further characterization of the NB1 antigen as a variably expressed 56–62 kD GPI-linked glycoprotein of plasma membranes and specific granules of neutrophils. *Br J Haematol* 81:336, 1992.
61. Stroncek DF, Shankar RA, Noren PA, et al: Analysis of the expression of NB1 antigen using two monoclonal antibodies. *Transfusion* 36:168, 1996.
62. Matsuo K, Lin A, Procter JL, et al: Variations in the expression of neutrophil antigen NB1. *Transfusion* 40:654, 2000.
63. Caruccio L, Bettinotti M, Matsuo K, et al: Expression of human neutrophil antigen-2a (NB1) is increased in pregnancy. *Transfusion* 43:357, 2003.
64. Stroncek DF, Skubitz KM, McCullough JJ: Biochemical characterization of the neutrophil-specific antigen NB1. *Blood* 75:744, 1990.
65. Kissel K, Santoso S, Hofmann C, et al: Molecular basis of the neutrophil glycoprotein NB1 (CD177) involved in the pathogenesis of immune neutropenias and transfusion reactions. *Eur J Immunol* 31:1301, 2001.
66. Caruccio L, Bettinotti M, Director-Myska AE, et al: The gene overexpressed in polycythemia rubra vera, PRV-1, and the gene encoding a neutrophil alloantigen, NB1, are alleles of a single gene, CD177, in chromosome band 19q13.31. *Transfusion* 46:441, 2006.
67. Taniguchi K, Kobayashi M, Harada H, et al: Human neutrophil antigen-2a expression on neutrophils from healthy adults in western Japan. *Transfusion* 42:651, 2002.
68. Bierling P, Poulet E, Fromont P, et al: Neutrophil-specific antigen and gene frequencies in the French population. *Transfusion* 30:848, 1990.
69. Caruccio L, Walkovich K, Bettinotti M, et al: CD177 polymorphisms: Correlation between high-frequency single nucleotide polymorphisms and neutrophil surface protein expression. *Transfusion* 44:77, 2004.
70. Kissel K, Scheffler S, Kerowgan M, Bux J: Molecular basis of NB1 (HNA-2a, CD177) deficiency. *Blood* 99:4231, 2002.
71. Sachs UJ, Andrei-Selmer CL, Maniar A, et al: The neutrophil specific antigen CD177 is a counter-receptor for endothelial PECAM-1 (CD31). *J Biol Chem* 282:23603, 2007.
72. Temerinac S, Klippel S, Strunck E, et al: Cloning of PRV-1, a novel member of the uPAR receptor superfamily, which is overexpressed in polycythemia rubra vera. *Blood* 95:2569, 2000.
73. Klippel S, Strunck E, Busse CE, et al: Biochemical characterization of PRV-1, a novel hematopoietic cell surface receptor, which is overexpressed in polycythemia rubra vera. *Blood* 100:2441, 2002.
74. de Haas M, Muniz-Diaz E, Alonso LG, et al: Neutrophil antigen 5b is carried by a protein, migrating from 70 to 95 kDa, and may be involved in neonatal alloimmune neutropenia. *Transfusion* 40:222, 2000.
75. Greinacher A, Wesche J, Hammer E, et al: Characterization of the human neutrophil alloantigen-3a. *Nat Med* 16:45, 2010.
76. Curtis BR, Cox NJ, Sullivan MJ, et al: The neutrophil alloantigen HNA-3a (5b) is located on choline transporter-like protein 2 and appears to be encoded by an R>Q154 amino acid substitution. *Blood* 115:2073, 2010.
77. Nordhagen R, Conradi M, Dromtorp SM: Pulmonary reaction associated with transfusion of plasma containing anti-5b. *Vox Sang* 51:102, 1986.
78. Kopko PM, Marshall CS, MacKenzie MR, et al: Transfusion-related acute lung injury: Report of a clinical look-back investigation. *JAMA* 287:1968, 2002.
79. Reil A, Keller-Stanislawski B, Gunay S, Bux J: Specificities of leucocyte alloantibodies in transfusion-related acute lung injury and results of leucocyte antibody screening of blood donors. *Vox Sang* 95:313, 2008.
80. Clague HD, Fung YL, Minchinton RM: Human neutrophil antigen-4a gene frequencies in an Australian population, determined by a new polymerase chain reaction method using sequence-specific primers. *Transfus Med* 13:149, 2003.
81. Han TH, Han KS: Gene frequencies of human neutrophil antigens 4a and 5a in the Korean population. *Korean J Lab Med* 26:114, 2006.
82. Cardone JD, Bordin JO, Chiba AK, et al: Gene frequencies of the HNA-4a and -5a neutrophil antigens in Brazilian persons and a new polymerase chain reaction-restriction fragment length polymorphism method for HNA-5a genotyping. *Transfusion* 46:1515, 2006.
83. Simsek S, van der Schoot CE, Daams M, et al: Molecular characterization of antigenic polymorphisms (Ond(a) and Mart(a)) of the beta 2 family recognized by human leukocyte alloantisera. *Blood* 88:1350, 1996.
84. Sachs UJ, Reil A, Bauer C, et al: Genotyping of human neutrophil antigen-5a (Ond). *Transfus Med* 15:115, 2005.
85. Fromont P, Prié N, Simon P, et al: Granulocyte antibody screening: evaluation of a bead-based assay in comparison with classical methods. *Transfusion* 50:2643, 2010.
86. Bux J, Jung KD, Kauth T, Mueller-Eckhardt C: Serological and clinical aspects of neutrophil antibodies leading to alloimmune neonatal neutropenia. *Transfus Med* 2:143, 1992.
87. Bux J, Behrens G, Jaeger G, Welte K: Diagnosis and clinical course of autoimmune neutropenia in infancy: Analysis of 240 cases. *Blood* 91:181, 1998.
88. Bruin MC, dem Borne AE, Tamminga RY, et al: Neutrophil antibody specificity in different types of childhood autoimmune neutropenia. *Blood* 94:1797, 1999.
89. Lalezari P, Khorshidi M, Petrosova M: Autoimmune neutropenia of infancy. *J Pediatr* 109:764, 1986.
90. Conway LT, Clay ME, Kline WE, et al: Natural history of primary autoimmune neutropenia in infancy. *Pediatrics* 79:728, 1987.
91. Toy P, Popovsky MA, Abraham E, et al: Transfusion-related acute lung injury: Definition and review. *Crit Care Med* 33:721, 2005.
92. Davoren A, Curtis BR, Shulman IA, et al: TRALI due to neutrophil-agglutinating human neutrophil antigen-3a (5b) alloantibodies in donor plasma: A report of 2 fatalities. *Transfusion* 43:641, 2003.
93. Muniz M, Sheldon S, Schuller RM, et al: Patient-specific transfusion-related acute lung injury. *Vox Sang* 94:70, 2008.
94. Fadeyi EA, Los Angeles MM, Wayne AS, et al: The transfusion of neutrophil-specific antibodies causes leukopenia and a broad spectrum of pulmonary reactions. *Transfusion* 47:545, 2007.
95. Toy P, Gajic O, Bacchetti P, et al: TRALI Study Group: Transfusion-related acute lung injury: incidence and risk factors. *Blood* 119:1757, 2012.
96. Gajic O, Rana R, Winters JL, et al: Transfusion-related acute lung injury in the critically ill: Prospective nested case-control study. *Am J Respir Crit Care Med* 176:886, 2007.
97. Seeger W, Schneider U, Kreusler B, et al: Reproduction of transfusion-related acute lung injury in an *ex vivo* lung model. *Blood* 76:1438, 1990.
98. Sachs UJ, Hattar K, Weissmann N, et al: Antibody-induced neutrophil activation as a trigger for transfusion-related acute lung injury in an *ex vivo* rat lung model. *Blood* 107:1217, 2006.
99. Silliman CC, Curtis BR, Kopko PM, et al: Donor antibodies to HNA-3a implicated in TRALI reactions prime neutrophils and cause PMN-mediated damage to human pulmonary microvascular endothelial cells in a two-event in vitro model. *Blood* 109:1752, 2007.
100. McMillan R: The pathogenesis of chronic immune thrombocytopenic purpura. *Semin Hematol* 44(4 Suppl 5): S3, 2007.
101. McMillan R: Antiplatelet antibodies in chronic adult immune thrombocytopenic purpura: Assays and epitopes. *J Pediatr Hematol Oncol* 25 Suppl 1:S57, 2003.
102. Wadenvik H, Stockelberg D, Hou M: Platelet proteins as autoantibody targets in idiopathic thrombocytopenic purpura. *Acta Paediatr Suppl* 424:26, 1998.
103. Beardsley DS, Ertem M: Platelet autoantibodies in immune thrombocytopenic purpura. *Transfus Sci* 19:237, 1998.
104. Bougie DW, Wilker PR, Wuitschick ED, et al: Acute thrombocytopenia after treatment with tirofiban or eptifibatide is associated with antibodies specific for ligand-occupied GPIIb/IIIa. *Blood* 100:2071, 2002.
105. Gentilini G, Curtis BR, Aster RH: An antibody from a patient with ranitidine-induced thrombocytopenia recognizes a site on glycoprotein IX that is a favored target for drug-induced antibodies. *Blood* 92:2359, 1998.

106. Peterson JA, Nyree CE, Newman PJ, Aster RH: A site involving the "hybrid" and PSI homology domains of GPIIIa (beta 3-integrin subunit) is a common target for antibodies associated with quinine-induced immune thrombocytopenia. *Blood* 101:937, 2003.

107. McFarland JG: Platelet and granulocyte antigens and antibodies, in *Technical Manual* edited by JD Roback, p. 525. American Association of Blood Banks, Bethesda, MD, 2008.

108. Warkentin TE, Smith JW: The alloimmune thrombocytopenic syndromes. *Transfus Med Rev* 11:296, 1997.

109. West KA, Anderson DR, McAlister VC, et al: Alloimmune thrombocytopenia after organ transplantation. *N Engl J Med* 341:1504, 1999.

110. Li C, Pasquale DN, Roth GJ: Bernard-Soulier syndrome with severe bleeding: Absent platelet glycoprotein Ib alpha due to a homozygous one-base deletion. *Thromb Haemost* 76:670, 1996.

111. Conte R, Cirillo D, Ricci F, et al: Platelet transfusion in a patient affected by Glanzmann's thrombasthenia with antibodies against GPIIb-IIIa. *Haematologica* 82:73, 1997.

112. Skouri H, Bettaieb A, Fromont P, et al: Platelet and granulocyte alloimmunisation in multitransfused Tunisian patients. *Eur J Haematol* 75:248, 2005.

113. Kashyap R, Kriplani A, Saxena R, et al: Pregnancy in a patient of Glanzmann's thrombasthenia with antiplatelet antibodies. *J Obstet Gynaecol Res* 23:247, 1997.

114. Greenwalt DE, Lipsky RH, Ockenhouse CF, et al: Membrane glycoprotein CD36: A review of its roles in adherence, signal transduction, and transfusion medicine. *Blood* 80:1105, 1992.

115. Yanai H, Chiba H, Morimoto M, et al: Human CD36 deficiency is associated with elevation in low-density lipoprotein-cholesterol. *Am J Med Genet* 93:299, 2000.

116. Yanai H, Chiba H, Fujiwara H, et al: Phenotype-genotype correlation in CD36 deficiency types I and II. *Thromb Haemost* 84:436, 2000.

117. Ikeda H, Mitani T, Ohnuma M, et al: A new platelet-specific antigen, Naka, involved in the refractoriness of HLA-matched platelet transfusion. *Vox Sang* 57:213, 1989.

118. Curtis BR, Aster RH: Incidence of the Nak(a)-negative platelet phenotype in African Americans is similar to that of Asians. *Transfusion* 36:331, 1996.

119. Aitman TJ, Cooper LD, Norsworthy PJ, et al: Malaria susceptibility and CD36 mutation. *Nature* 405:1015, 2000.

120. Kajeguka D, Mwanziva C, Daou M, et al: CD36 c.1264 T>G null mutation impairs acquisition of IgG antibodies to *Plasmodium falciparum* MSP1$_{19}$ antigen and is associated with higher malaria incidences in Tanzanian children. *Scand J Immunol* 75:355, 2012.

121. Chilongola J, Balthazary S, Mpina M, et al: CD36 deficiency protects against malarial anaemia in children by reducing Plasmodium falciparum-infected red blood cell adherence to vascular endothelium. *Trop Med Int Health* 14:810, 2009.

122. Bierling P, Godeau B, Fromont P, et al: Posttransfusion purpura-like syndrome associated with CD36 (Naka) isoimmunization. *Transfusion* 35:777, 1995.

123. Kankirawatana S, Kupatawintu P, Juji T, et al: Neonatal alloimmune thrombocytopenia due to anti-Nak(a). *Transfusion* 41:375, 2001.

124. Curtis BR, Ali S, Glazier AM, et al: Isoimmunization against CD36 (glycoprotein IV): description of four cases of neonatal isoimmune thrombocytopenia and brief review of the literature. *Transfusion* 42:1173, 2002.

125. Saw CL, Szykoluk H, Curtis BR, et al: Two cases of platelet transfusion refractoriness associated with anti-CD36. *Transfusion* 50:2638, 2010.

126. Newman PJ, Valentin N: Human platelet alloantigens: recent findings, new perspectives. *Thromb Haemost* 74:234, 1995.

127. European Molecular Biology Laboratory EBI. 2014. http://www.ebi.ac.uk/ipd/hpa/freqs_1.html (last accessed August, 2015).

128. Lyman S, Aster RH, Visentin GP, Newman PJ: Polymorphism of human platelet membrane glycoprotein IIb associated with the Baka/Bakb alloantigen system. *Blood* 75:2343, 1990.

129. Harrison CR, Curtis BR, McFarland JG, et al: Severe neonatal alloimmune thrombocytopenia caused by antibodies to human platelet antigen 3a (Baka) detectable only in whole platelet assays. *Transfusion* 43:1398, 2003.

130. Bray PF: Integrin polymorphisms as risk factors for thrombosis. *Thromb Haemost* 82:337, 1999.

131. Goldschmidt-Clermont PJ, Roos CM, Cooke GE: Platelet PlA2 polymorphism and thromboembolic events: from inherited risk to pharmacogenetics. *J Thromb Thrombolysis* 8:89, 1999.

132. Harris K, Nguyen P, Van Cott EM: Platelet PlA2 Polymorphism and the risk for thrombosis in heparin-induced thrombocytopenia. *Am J Clin Pathol* 129:282, 2008.

133. Ollikainen E, Mikkelsson J, Perola M, et al: Platelet membrane collagen receptor glycoprotein VI polymorphism is associated with coronary thrombosis and fatal myocardial infarction in middle-aged men. *Atherosclerosis* 176:95, 2004.

134. Martinelli N, Trabetti E, Pinotti M, et al: Combined effect of hemostatic gene polymorphisms and the risk of myocardial infarction in patients with advanced coronary atherosclerosis. *PLoS One* 3:e1523, 2008.

135. Pellitero S, Reverter JL, Tassies D, et al: Polymorphisms in platelet glycoproteins Ia and IIIa are associated with arterial thrombosis and carotid atherosclerosis in type 2 diabetes. *Thromb Haemost* 103:630, 2008.

136. Curtis BR, McFarland JG: Human platelet antigens—2013. *Vox Sang* 106:93, 2014.

137. Santoso S, Kroll H, Andrei-Selmer CL, et al: A naturally occurring LeuVal mutation in beta3-integrin impairs the HPA-1a epitope: the third allele of HPA-1. *Transfusion* 46:790, 2006.

138. Peterson JA, Gitter M, Bougie DW, et al: Low-frequency human platelet antigens as triggers for neonatal alloimmune thrombocytopenia. *Transfusion* 54:1286, 2014.

139. Sheridan D, Carter C, Kelton JG: A diagnostic test for heparin-induced thrombocytopenia. *Blood* 67:27, 1986.

140. Rachel JM, Summers TC, Sinor LT, Plapp FV: Use of a solid phase red blood cell adherence method for pretransfusion platelet compatibility testing. *Am J Clin Pathol* 90:63, 1988.

141. Davoren A, Bussel J, Curtis BR, et al: Prospective evaluation of a new platelet glycoprotein (GP)-specific assay (PakAuto) in the diagnosis of autoimmune thrombocytopenia (AITP). *Am J Hematol* 78:193, 2005.

142. Kiefel V, Santoso S, Weisheit M, Mueller-Eckhardt C: Monoclonal antibody-specific immobilization of platelet antigens (MAIPA): A new tool for the identification of platelet-reactive antibodies. *Blood* 70:1722, 1987.

143. Visentin GP, Wolfmeyer K, Newman PJ, Aster RH: Detection of drug-dependent, platelet-reactive antibodies by antigen-capture ELISA and flow cytometry. *Transfusion* 30:694, 1990.

144. Panzer S: Report on the Tenth International Platelet Genotyping and Serology Workshop on behalf of the International Society of Blood Transfusion. *Vox Sang* 80:72, 2001.

145. Simsek S, Faber NM, Bleeker PM, et al: Determination of human platelet antigen frequencies in the Dutch population by immunophenotyping and DNA (allele-specific restriction enzyme) analysis. *Blood* 81:835, 1993.

146. McFarland JG, Aster RH, Bussel JB, et al: Prenatal diagnosis of neonatal alloimmune thrombocytopenia using allele-specific oligonucleotide probes. *Blood* 78:2276, 1991.

147. Curtis B, McFarland J: Detection and identification of platelet antibodies and antigens in the clinical laboratory. *Immunohematology* 25:125, 2009.

148. Curtis BR: Genotyping for human platelet alloantigen polymorphisms: applications in the diagnosis of alloimmune platelet disorders. *Semin Thromb Hemost* 34:539, 2008.

149. Skogen B, Bellissimo DB, Hessner MJ, et al: Rapid determination of platelet alloantigen genotypes by polymerase chain reaction using allele-specific primers. *Transfusion* 34:955, 1994.

150. Hurd CM, Cavanagh G, Schuh A, et al: Genotyping for platelet-specific antigens: techniques for the detection of single nucleotide polymorphisms. *Vox Sang* 83:1, 2002.

151. Leukocyte reduction and ultraviolet B irradiation of platelets to prevent alloimmunization and refractoriness to platelet transfusions. The Trial to Reduce Alloimmunization to Platelets Study Group. *N Engl J Med* 337:1861, 1997.

152. Taaning E, Simonsen AC, Hjelms E, et al: Platelet alloimmunization after transfusion. A prospective study in 117 heart surgery patients. *Vox Sang* 72:238, 1997.

153. Kiefel V, Konig C, Kroll H, Santoso S: Platelet alloantibodies in transfused patients. *Transfusion* 41:766, 2001.

154. Langenscheidt F, Kiefel V, Santoso S, Mueller-Eckhardt C: Platelet transfusion refractoriness associated with two rare platelet-specific alloantibodies (anti-Baka and anti-PlA2) and multiple HLA antibodies. *Transfusion* 28:597, 1988.

155. Kekomaki S, Volin L, Koistinen P, et al: Successful treatment of platelet transfusion refractoriness: the use of platelet transfusions matched for both human leucocyte antigens (HLA) and human platelet alloantigens (HPA) in alloimmunized patients with leukaemia. *Eur J Haematol* 60:112, 1998.

156. Verran J, Grey D, Bennett J, et al: HPA-1, 3, 5 genotyping to establish a typed platelet donor panel. *Pathology* 32:89, 2000.

157. Godeau B, Fromont P, Seror T, et al: Platelet alloimmunization after multiple transfusions: a prospective study of 50 patients. *Br J Haematol* 81:395, 1992.

158. Novotny VM: Prevention and management of platelet transfusion refractoriness. *Vox Sang* 76:1, 1999.

159. Meenaghan M, Judson PA, Yousaf K, et al: Antibodies to platelet glycoprotein V in polytransfused patients with haematological disease. *Vox Sang* 64:167, 1993.

160. Wang R, Furihata K, McFarland JG, et al: An amino acid polymorphism within the RGD binding domain of platelet membrane glycoprotein IIIa is responsible for the formation of the Pena/Penb alloantigen system. *J Clin Invest* 90:2038, 1992.

161. Furihata K, Nugent DJ, Bissonette A, et al: On the association of the platelet-specific alloantigen, Pena, with glycoprotein IIIa. Evidence for heterogeneity of glycoprotein IIIa. *J Clin Invest* 80:1624, 1987.

162. Glade-Bender J, McFarland JG, Kaplan C, et al: Anti-HPA-3A induces severe neonatal alloimmune thrombocytopenia. *J Pediatr* 138:862, 2001.

163. Santoso S: Human platelet alloantigens. *Transfus Apher Sci* 28:227, 2003.

CHAPTER 138
BLOOD PROCUREMENT AND RED CELL TRANSFUSION

Jeffrey McCullough, Majed A. Refaai, and Claudia S. Cohn

SUMMARY

Blood procurement is a vital national priority that is met in the United States by volunteer donors and a pluralistic blood collection program that includes the American Red Cross, independent community blood centers, and hospitals. More than 15 million units of whole blood are collected from approximately 10 million donors annually. Recruitment of donors is preceded by a medical history and limited physical examination. The donated blood is subjected to tests of blood type, red cell antibodies, and infectious agents that may be transmitted by blood transfusion. In some cases, collection of red cells, platelets, leukocytes, or plasma is achieved by hemapheresis. Plasma for the subsequent manufacture of derivatives such as albumin and intravenous immunoglobulin is obtained from paid donors by for-profit organizations different from those that collect whole blood and prepare blood components. The meticulous attention to donor risk characteristics and the use of sensitive assays to detect infectious agents that may be transmitted by blood have greatly improved the safety of blood.

It is widely accepted that red blood cell (RBC) transfusions save lives and prevent ischemia-related morbidity in severely hemorrhaging patients and those with acute anemia (hemoglobin [Hgb] less than 6 g/dL). When a patient's Hgb level exceeds 10 g/dL, oxygen delivery and consumption do not necessarily increase with RBC transfusions. For patients in the 6 to 10 g/dL Hgb "gray zone," the benefit of a transfusion depends upon a patient's clinical status and should be weighed against the inherent risks of allogeneic blood.

These risks include adverse reactions, which occur in up to 3 percent of transfusions. Transfusion-related acute lung injury is the number one cause of transfusion-related fatalities, and new pathogens causing transfusion-transmitted infections continue to pose a threat to the blood supply. Transfusion-associated circulatory overload is often not recognized, but is associated with increased morbidity and prolonged lengths of stay.

As the aging population grows in the United States, the demand for blood will increase, even as the donor population declines. Patient blood management efforts are growing in popularity as hospitals grapple with the risks and costs associated with transfusion. The implementation of evidence-based practice is the best way to benefit patients and minimize the risks of transfusion.

● OVERVIEW OF THE BLOOD BANKING SYSTEM IN THE UNITED STATES

The United States has a pluralistic system of blood collection rather than the single national system that exists in other developed countries. In the United States during 2011, approximately 15,721,000 units of blood were available for use (Table 138–1). This was a 9 percent decrease from 2008. Approximately 94 percent of the blood was collected in regional blood centers and hospitals collected 7 percent.[1] Less than 1percent of the units donated in the United States were autologous donations or directed donations, that is, blood given by family or friends for a specific patient. Both autologous and directed donations decreased substantially from 2008.[1] Of red cells collected, 97.7 percent of allogeneic, 59.0 percent of autologous, and 72.0 percent of directed donor red cells were transfused to the intended recipient.

All whole blood for transfusion in the United States is donated by unpaid volunteers; however, costs are incurred in the collection, testing, production, and distribution of blood components. Blood banks pass on these costs to hospitals. Some areas of the United States are able to collect more blood than is needed locally and other areas are unable to collect enough blood to meet their local needs. Several inventory-sharing systems are used to move blood around the United States so as to alleviate the shortages.

Blood is considered a drug and all aspects of the selection of donors, collection, processing, testing, preservation, and dispensing are regulated by the FDA. The FDA requirements define the procedures, record-keeping, staff proficiency, specific testing, and donor medical requirements that blood banks must follow. Blood banks meet these requirements using the FDA-defined good manufacturing practices that are similar to those used by pharmaceutical manufacturers.[2] Additional standards are formulated by the American Association of Blood Banks (AABB), a voluntary organization that accredits blood banks.

● INTERNATIONAL PRACTICES

Approximately 107 million units of blood are collected annually worldwide. Considerable differences in the availability of blood and blood components throughout the world are related to the extent of development in the country and the country's healthcare system.[3] The amount of blood collected in relation to the population ranges from 50 donations per 1000 population in industrialized countries to five to 15 per 1000 population in developing countries and one to five per 1000

Acronyms and Abbreviations: 2,3-BPG, 2,3-bisphophosglyceric acid,; AABB, American Association of Blood Banks; AHTR, acute hemolytic transfusion reaction; APACHE II, Acute Physiology and Chronic Health Evaluation II; ATR, allergic transfusion reaction; BCSH, British Committee for Standards in Haematology; BNP, B-type natriuretic peptide; CI, confidence interval; CMV, cytomegalovirus; CPD, citrate, phosphate, and dextrose; DAT, direct antiglobulin test; DHTR, delayed hemolytic transfusion reaction; ESA, erythropoiesis-stimulating agents; FNHTR, febrile non-hemolytic transfusion reactions; FOCUS trial, Transfusion Trigger Trial for Functional Outcomes in Cardiovascular Patients Undergoing Surgical Hip Fracture Repair; G-CSF, granulocyte colony-stimulating factor; GVHD, graft-versus-host disease; Hct, hematocrit; Hgb, hemoglobin; HLA, human leukocyte antigen; HNA, human neutrophil antigen; HPC-A, hematopoietic progenitor cells obtained by apheresis; HPC-C, hematopoietic progenitor cells obtained from umbilical cords; HSCT, hematopoietic stem cell transplant; IL, interleukin; LDH, lactate dehydrogenase; MOD, multiple-organ dysfunction; MODS, multiple-organ dysfunction syndrome; NATP, neonatal alloimmune thrombocytopenic purpura; NT-proBNP, N-terminal pro-BNP; PAS, platelets stored in additive solution; PBM, patient blood management; PEPFAR, President's Emergency Plan for AIDS Relief; PINT, Premature Infants in Need of Transfusion; PLS, passenger lymphocyte syndrome; PRCA, pure red cell aplasia; RBC, red blood cell; SCD, sickle cell disease; TACO, transfusion-associated circulatory overload; TA-GVHD, transfusion-associated graft-versus-host disease; TNF-α, tumor necrosis factor-alpha; TRACS, Transfusion Requirements After Cardiac Surgery; TRALI, transfusion-related acute lung injury; TRICC, Transfusion Requirements in Critical Care; TRIPICU, Transfusion Strategies for Patients in Pediatric Intensive Care Units.

population in the least-developed countries.[3] Thus, industrialized countries utilize transfused blood products far more commonly. In developed countries, especially Western Europe and parts of Asia, a governmental agency usually oversees the blood collection activities, although the extent to which the government sets requirements and monitors or inspects the blood collection system varies. In developed countries, the basic processes of donor medical screening, blood collection, laboratory testing, and preparation of blood components are similar to the system found in the United States. In virtually all developed countries, blood is donated by volunteers because paid donors are associated with a higher risk of disease transmission.[4] The basic blood components—red cells, platelets, and plasma—usually are available and apheresis instruments are used to collect platelets. Plasma derivatives such as albumin, coagulation factor VIII, other plasma protein concentrates (coagulation factors or inhibitors, or complement factor-1 inhibitor) and immune globulins are available.

However, in the developing world the blood supply is very limited and components are often not available. Patients may be required to arrange for the blood they need so donors may be friends or family members of patients or even individuals who have been paid by the patient's family to donate the blood needed. Donor screening may not be as extensive, transmissible disease testing may be lacking, and equipment may be reused. These difficulties may be compounded by the presence of endemic transfusion-transmissible diseases for which screening is difficult or expensive and thus not performed as extensively as in more developed countries. Great strides have been made during the last decade primarily from the U.S.-funded President's Emergency Plan for AIDS Relief (PEPFAR) program.[5] Thus, the availability of blood and its components around the world varies widely, from inadequate supplies and uncertain safety to sophisticated supply systems and component availability equal to or surpassing those of the United States.

PROCUREMENT OF PLASMA DERIVATIVES

The plasma industry is separate from the blood banking system described above. Plasma can be subjected to a fractionation process to produce several medically valuable products referred to as *plasma derivatives*. Plasma fractionation is performed in manufacturing plants in batches of up to 10,000 L involving the pooling of plasma from a large number of donors. Plasma for manufacture or fractionation into derivatives can be obtained from units of whole blood, but this amount of plasma is inadequate to meet the needs for plasma derivatives. Consequently, large amounts of plasma are obtained by plasmapheresis in which only the plasma and not red cells or platelets are retained from the donor. Individuals can donate plasma up to two times per week and usually are paid because of the more extensive time commitment. This plasma collection system usually is operated by for-profit organizations and functions separately from the system for whole-blood donation.

Approximately 29 million liters of plasma were collected in the United States in 2013. Twenty-six plasma derivatives are approved for licensure by the FDA. Disruption in the sources of plasma or in one manufacturer's plant can have serious consequences and create shortages of certain derivatives.

The remainder of this chapter describes the blood collection system operated by voluntary community organizations to provide cellular and whole-blood–derived components.

RECRUITMENT OF BLOOD DONORS

Although most Americans will require a blood transfusion at some time in their lives, only about one-third of the U.S. population is eligible to donate blood,[6] and only a small portion of those actually donate. Blood donors are more likely than the general population to be male, age 30 to 50 years, white, employed, and have more education and higher income.[7] It is generally believed that the most effective way to get someone to donate blood is to ask him or her personally. Factors such as the convenience of donation, peer pressure, receipt of blood by a family member, and perceived community needs are important factors that are superimposed onto the individual's basic social commitments.

WHOLE-BLOOD DONOR SCREENING

The approach to the selection of blood donors is designed to (1) ensure the safety of the donor and (2) obtain a high-quality blood component that is as safe as possible for the recipient. Some specific steps that are taken to ensure that blood is as safe as possible are the use of only volunteer blood donors; questioning of donors about their general health before their donation is scheduled; obtaining a medical history, including specific risk factors, before donation; conducting a brief physical examination before donation; laboratory testing of donated blood; checking the donor's identity against a donor deferral registry; and providing a method by which the donor can confidentially designate the unit as unsuitable for transfusion after the donation is completed.

HEALTH HISTORY, PHYSICAL EXAMINATION, AND LABORATORY EXAMINATION OF THE BLOOD

The health history is usually done by a computer-assisted self-interview. The questions designed to protect the safety of the donor include

TABLE 138–1. United States Blood Supply System in 2011*

	Number	Percent
Total units whole blood	15,721,000	100
Blood centers	14,686,000	93
Hospitals	1,036,0000	7
Red blood cell transfusions	13,785,000	100
Allogeneic	13,785,000	99
Autologous	65,000	<1
Directed	37,000	<1
Platelets–total dose	1,738,000	100
SDP collected	2,516,000	92
WB platelet concentrates	1,110,000	8
Total platelets transfused*	9,875,000	
Fresh-frozen plasma	5,926,000	—
Fresh-frozen plasma transfused	4,089,000	—
Cryoprecipitate	1,690,000	
Cryoprecipitate transfused	890,000	

SDP, single-donor platelet concentrate prepared by plateletpheresis. One SDP is equivalent to five platelet concentrates; WB, whole-blood derived platelet concentrate. Usually five units are pooled to obtain a therapeutic dose.

Data from Whitaker BI, Henry, RA, World Health Organization: National blood transfusion services [on the Internet]. www.who.int/bloodsafety/transfusion_services/en/. Accessed September 1, 2009.

whether the donor is under the care of a physician or has a history of cardiovascular or lung disease, seizures, present or recent pregnancy, recent donation of blood or plasma, recent major illness or surgery, unexplained weight loss, unusual bleeding, or is taking medication(s). Some medications may make the donor unsuitable because of the condition requiring the medication, whereas other medications may be potentially harmful to the recipient. Questions designed to protect the safety of the recipient include those related to the donor's general health, history of receipt of growth hormone, and occurrence of or exposure to patients with hepatitis or other liver disease, or a previous diagnosis of HIV or AIDS (or symptoms of AIDS), Chagas disease, or babesiosis. A history also is obtained regarding the injection of drugs; receipt of coagulation factor concentrates; blood transfusion; tattoos; acupuncture; body piercing; receipt of an organ or tissue transplant; recent travel to areas endemic for malaria; recent immunizations; ingestion of medications (especially aspirin); presence of a major illness or surgery; and previous notice of a positive test for a transmissible disease. In addition, several questions are related to AIDS risk behavior, including whether the potential donor has had sex with anyone with AIDS, given or received money or drugs for sex, (for males) had sex with another male, or (for females) had sex with a male who has had sex with another male.

The physical examination includes determination of the temperature, pulse, blood pressure, weight, and blood hemoglobin (Hgb) concentration. The donor's general appearance is assessed for any signs of illness or the influence of drugs or alcohol. The skin at the venipuncture site is examined for signs of intravenous drug abuse, and local lesions that would make disinfecting the skin difficult and thus lead to contamination of the blood unit during venipuncture.

COLLECTION OF WHOLE BLOOD

BLOOD CONTAINERS

Blood must be collected into single-use, sterile, FDA-licensed containers. The containers are made of plasticized material that is biocompatible with blood cells and allows diffusion of gases so as to provide optimal cell preservation. These blood containers are combinations of bags and integral tubing that allow separation of the whole blood into its components in a closed system, thus minimizing the chance of bacterial contamination while making storage of the components for days or weeks possible. Plasticizers from the bags accumulate in red cell components during storage and can be found in tissues of multitransfused patients but also in healthy nontransfused individuals. Although no evidence indicates that transfusion of this material causes clinical problems, containers without plasticizers are now used in some countries.

VENIPUNCTURE AND BLOOD COLLECTION

The blood should be drawn from an area free of skin lesions and the phlebotomy site should be decontaminated. The site is scrubbed with a soap solution, followed by the application of tincture of iodine or iodophor complex solution. The venipuncture is done with a needle that should be used only once in order to prevent contamination. The blood must flow freely and be mixed with anticoagulant frequently as the blood fills the container to prevent the development of small clots. The actual time for collection of 450 to 500 mL usually is approximately 7 minutes and almost always is less than 10 minutes. During blood donation, cardiac output falls slightly but heart rate changes little. A slight decrease in systolic pressure results with a rise in peripheral resistance and diastolic blood pressure.

Usually 500 mL is collected. The blood is mixed with 63 to 70 mL of anticoagulant composed of citrate, phosphate, and dextrose (CPD).

The amount of blood withdrawn must be within prescribed limits so as to maintain the proper ratio with the anticoagulant; otherwise, the blood cells may be damaged and/or anticoagulation may be unsatisfactory.

An untoward reaction occurs after approximately 2 to 5 percent of blood donations, but, fortunately, most of the reactions are not serious. Donors who have reactions are more likely to be younger, unmarried, have a higher predonation heart rate and lower diastolic blood pressure, lower weight, female, and first-time or infrequent donors. Donors who experience a reaction are less likely to donate in the future.

The most common reactions to blood donation are weakness, cool skin, and diaphoresis.[8] More extensive, but still moderate, reactions are dizziness, pallor, hypertension, and bradycardia.[9] Bradycardia usually is considered a sign of a vasovagal reaction rather than hypotensive or cardiovascular shock, where tachycardia would be expected. In a more severe form, a vasovagal reaction may progress to loss of consciousness, convulsions, and involuntary passage of urine or stool. Other reactions include nausea and vomiting; hyperventilation, sometimes leading to twitching or muscle spasms; hematoma at the venipuncture site; convulsions; and serious cardiac difficulties. Such serious reactions are rare. Injury of the brachial nerve and resulting pain and/or paresthesia may occur as a result of needle puncture of the nerve or compression from a hematoma.

Donors are advised to drink extra fluids to replace lost blood volume and to avoid strenuous exercise for the remainder of the day of donation. The latter advice is given to prevent fainting and to minimize the possibility of hematoma development at the venipuncture site. Some donors are subject to lightheadedness or even fainting if they change position quickly. Therefore, donors are advised not to return to work for the remainder of the day if they have an occupation where fainting would be hazardous to themselves or others.

SPECIAL BLOOD DONATIONS

AUTOLOGOUS DONOR BLOOD

Autologous blood for transfusion can be obtained by preoperative donation, acute normovolemic hemodilution, intraoperative salvage, and postoperative salvage, but only preoperative donation is discussed here. Most commonly, this situation occurs with elective surgery. Autologous blood accounts for a very low level (<1 percent) of the United States' blood supply.[1]

If patient candidates for autologous blood donation meet the usual FDA criteria for blood donation, their blood can be used for other patients if the original autologous donor has no need for the blood. However, this practice is not allowed by AABB standards and is usually not relevant because most patients do not meet the FDA donation criteria. If the autologous donor does not meet the FDA criteria for blood donation, the blood must be specially labeled, segregated during storage, and discarded if it is not used by that specific patient. Thus, the autologous blood donation should be collected only for procedures with a substantial likelihood that the blood will be used. Without this type of planning, a very high rate of wastage of autologous blood is observed, estimated at 59 percent in 2011.[1] Thus, the cost of autologous blood is high.

No age or weight restrictions exist for autologous donation. Pregnant women can donate, but this practice is not recommended routinely because these patients rarely require transfusion. The autologous donor's Hgb may be lower (11 g/dL) than that required for routine donors (12.5 g/dL), although usually only 2 to 4 units of blood can be obtained before the Hgb falls below 11 g/dL. Autologous blood donors can be given erythropoietin and iron to increase the number of units of blood they can donate,[10,11] although this strategy has not been shown to reduce the need for allogeneic donor blood. Reactions in autologous donors are similar to allogeneic donors and are related to first-time donation, female gender, lower age, and lower weight.

Autologous blood must be typed for ABO and Rh antigens. If the unit is to be shipped to another facility for transfusion, it must be tested for transmissible diseases similar to allogeneic blood. If any of the transmissible disease tests are positive, the unit must be labeled with a biohazard label.

DIRECTED DONOR BLOOD

Directed donors are friends or relatives who wish to give blood for a specific patient because the patient hopes those donors will be safer than the regular blood supply. However, directed donors do not have a lower incidence of transmissible disease markers[12] and thus do not support a realistic rationale for these donations. Because the blood becomes part of the community's general blood supply if it is not used for the originally intended patient, directed donors must meet all the usual FDA requirements for routine blood donation.

PATIENT-SPECIFIC DONATION

In a few situations, appropriate transfusion therapy involves collecting blood from a particular donor for a particular patient. Examples are donor-specific transfusions prior to kidney transplantation, maternal platelets for a fetus projected to have neonatal alloimmune thrombocytopenic purpura (NATP), or family members of a patient with a rare blood type. Usually, these donors must meet all the usual FDA requirements, except that they may donate as often as every 3 days so long as the Hgb remains above the normal donor minimum of 12.5 g/dL. An exception is donation of maternal platelets for a neonate with NATP. Patient-specific donated units must undergo all routine laboratory testing.

THERAPEUTIC BLEEDING

Blood can be collected as part of the therapy of diseases such as polycythemia vera or primary hemochromatosis. Usually such blood is not used for transfusion because the donors do not meet the FDA standards for donor health. As the genetic basis of hemochromatosis has become better understood, blood removed from these patients appears to be safe and red cells from patients with hemochromatosis are normal during blood bank storage,[13] and although a blood collection program can operate successfully, this has not gained general acceptance.

● COLLECTION AND PRODUCTION OF BLOOD COMPONENTS BY APHERESIS

Blood components can be obtained by apheresis rather than prepared from whole blood. In apheresis, the donor's anticoagulated whole blood is passed through an instrument in which they use centrifugation to separate the blood components. Red cells, platelets, granulocytes, blood stem cells, mononuclear cells, and plasma can be obtained by apheresis.

PLATELETPHERESIS

In the United States, approximately 92 percent of platelet concentrates are produced by plateletpheresis (see Table 138–1). Plateletpheresis requires approximately 90 minutes, during which approximately 4000 to 5000 mL of the donor's blood is processed through the blood cell separator. The process results in a platelet concentrate with a volume of approximately 200 mL and containing approximately 4.0×10^{11} platelets and less than 0.5 mL red cells. Currently manufactured blood cell separators produce a platelet concentrate that contains less than 5×10^6

leukocytes and thus can be considered leukocyte reduced. Following plateletpheresis, the donor's platelet count declines by approximately 30 percent but returns to preplateletpheresis levels in approximately 4 days.

COLLECTION OF RED CELLS BY APHERESIS

Chronic shortages of group O red cells stimulated interest in the use of apheresis for collecting the equivalent of 2 units of red cells from some donors, especially group O.[14] In 2011, 1,978,000 units of red cells were collected by apheresis.[1] The collection procedure is similar to other apheresis procedures, except that red cells are retained rather than returned to the donor. The red cells usually have a very high hematocrit (Hct) as they are removed from the instrument, but an additive solution is incorporated and the red cells can be stored for the usual 42 days. Red cells obtained by apheresis have the same characteristics as those produced from whole blood. Because 2 U of red cells are removed, donors may donate only every 4 months.

LEUKAPHERESIS

Leukapheresis has been used to produce a granulocyte concentrate for transfusion therapy of infections unresponsive to antibiotics. Because the efficiency of granulocyte extraction from whole blood is less than for platelets, the leukapheresis procedure involves processing 6500 to 8000 mL of donor blood for approximately 3 hours. To increase the separation of granulocytes from other blood components, hydroxyethyl starch is added to the blood-cell–separator flow system. In addition, glucocorticoids and granulocyte colony-stimulating factor (G-CSF) have been administered to granulocyte donors to increase the granulocyte count and the granulocyte yield.[15]

PLASMAPHERESIS

Plasmapheresis is used to obtain plasma for manufacture of derivatives but not plasma for transfusion. Plasmapheresis usually can be performed in approximately 30 minutes and produces up to 750 mL of plasma. Because few red cells are removed, the procedure can be repeated up to two times per week, so theoretically a donor could provide a large amount of plasma. Because of the nature and possible frequency of plasma donation, special donor criteria apply.

● SELECTION OF APHERESIS DONORS

The selection of donors for apheresis uses the same criteria as for whole-blood donation with some additional donor requirements. No more than 15 percent of the donor's blood should be extracorporeal during apheresis; thus, the donor's size is considered when making decisions about specific apheresis procedures or instruments to be used. The platelet count must be monitored for frequent donors. Because a plateletpheresis concentrate would be the sole source of platelets for the transfusion, the donor must not have taken aspirin for at least 3 days.

The amount of blood components removed from apheresis donors must be monitored. Not more than 200 mL of red cells per 2 months or approximately 1500 mL of plasma per week can be removed. The laboratory testing of donors and apheresis components for transmissible diseases is the same as for whole-blood donation. Thus, the likelihood of disease transmission from apheresis components is the same as from whole blood.

● REACTIONS IN APHERESIS DONORS

Apheresis donors can experience the same kind of reactions as whole-blood donors. In addition, apheresis donors experience a higher incidence of paresthesias, probably because of the infusion of citrate (that may affect calcium levels) used to anticoagulate the donor's blood while it is in the cell separator. This type of reaction is managed by slowing the blood flow rate through the instrument, which slows the rate of citrate infusion. In leukapheresis, donors can be given glucocorticoid and/or G-CSF to increase the granulocyte count, and the sedimenting agent hydroxyethyl starch is used in the cell separator to improve the granulocyte yield. When G-CSF and glucocorticoids are used, approximately 60 percent of donors experience side effects, usually myalgia, arthralgia, headache, or flu-like symptoms.[15] The major side effect of hydroxyethyl starch is blood volume expansion manifested by headache and/or hypertension.

LABORATORY TESTING OF DONATED BLOOD

Each unit of whole blood or each apheresis component undergoes a standard battery of tests, including those for blood type, red cell antibodies (including ABO, Rh, minor antigens), and transmissible diseases (Table 138–2). Additional tests, such as those for cytomegalovirus (CMV) antibodies, may be done. During the last few years, testing for West Nile virus and *Trypanosoma cruzi* have been added. Babesia is another transfusion transmissible disease[16] for which a donor screening test has been developed. It is not clear whether routine testing will be introduced.

SAFETY OF THE BLOOD SUPPLY

Ironically, the improvements in blood safety have occurred at a time of the public's increased fear of transfusion and the more cautious use of blood components by physicians. Each step in the overall process of

TABLE 138–2. Laboratory Tests for Transmissible Agents of Donated Blood

Agent	Disease
Treponema	Syphilis
Hepatitis B$_s$ antigen	Hepatitis B
Hepatitis B$_c$ antibody	Hepatitis B
Hepatitis B virus nucleic acids	Hepatitis B
Hepatitis C antibody	Hepatitis C
Hepatitis C nucleic acids	Hepatitis C
HIV-1 and HIV-2 antibody	AIDS
HIV nucleic acids	AIDS
West Nile virus nucleic acids	West Nile infection
Bacteria*	Sepsis
HTLV-I antibody	Leukemia
	Lymphoma
	Tropical paresis
HTLV-II antibody	Disease unknown
Trypanosoma cruzi†	Chagas disease
West Nile virus	Viral infection
CMV‡	CMV disease

CMV, cytomegalovirus; HTLV, human T-cell lymphotropic virus.

*Only platelet concentrates tested.

†Only first time donors are tested.

‡Of use for immunodeficient recipients.

donor evaluation and testing adds to blood safety in important ways, and the medical history is important as illustrated by the 90 percent reduction in HIV infectivity from the use of donor-selection criteria identifying HIV risk behavior.[17] Tests for transmissible diseases further reduce the proportion of infectious donors.[18] Donor deferral registries detect individuals who previously were deferred as blood donors but who for various reasons attempt to donate again. Currently, the risk of acquiring a transfusion-transmitted disease ranges from one per 150,000/unit for hepatitis B to one per 2,135,000/unit for HIV (Table 138–3). Thus, although the blood supply is safer than ever, transfusion is not risk free and should be undertaken only after careful consideration of the patient's clinical situation and specific blood component needs.

RED CELL TRANSFUSIONS

Red blood cell (RBC) transfusions are indicated to increase oxygen carrying capacity in anemic patients. While oxygen extraction and delivery may be measured using invasive procedures, these methods are not available in most clinical settings. As a result, the decision to transfuse RBCs is often based on Hgb or Hct value(s).

Transfusing RBCs to a critically anemic patient will increase the oxygen-carrying capacity; however, the utility of RBC transfusions in an asymptomatic patient with a Hgb between 6 and 10 g/dL is less clear. Most of the large, prospective, randomized controlled studies looking at RBC usage and transfusion triggers did not specifically address the question of increased oxygen-carrying capacity at various Hgb/Hct levels. Instead they used the more practical markers of mortality, end-organ dysfunction, or adverse events to determine the efficacy and safety of restrictive (low Hgb threshold) versus liberal (higher Hgb threshold) transfusion strategies.

RED BLOOD CELL TRANSFUSION THRESHOLDS

The Transfusion Requirements in Critical Care (TRICC) trial was the first adequately powered study to compare a restrictive and liberal strategy for RBC transfusions in critically ill patients.[19] A total of 838 ICU patients were randomized into two groups: a liberal arm, which maintained Hgb concentrations between 10 and 12 g/dL and gave transfusions when the Hgb concentration fell below 10 g/dL; and a restrictive arm, which maintained Hgb levels between 7 and 9 g/dL and used a Hgb value of 7 g/dL as the trigger for transfusion. The exclusion criteria included age younger than 16 years; active blood loss at the time of enrollment; admission after a routine cardiac procedure; chronic anemia; imminent death; and others. Thirty-day mortality from all causes was the primary outcome measure. Secondary outcomes included 60-day mortality, death during hospitalization, and multiple-organ dysfunction (MOD). The severity of a patient's illness was classified using the Acute Physiology and Chronic Health Evaluation II (APACHE II) scores. This and other patient characteristics were statistically similar in the two study arms. This study was designed as an equivalency trial, and overall found similar results in the two groups for 30-day mortality (18.7 vs. 23.3 percent; p = 0.11), as well as for the secondary outcomes. Thirty-day mortality rates among patients in the restrictive transfusion arm who were less acutely ill (APACHE II ≤20) (8.7 vs. 16.1 percent; p = 0.03), or were younger than 55 years old (5.7 vs. 13.0 percent; p = 0.02). The restrictive group also received fewer transfusions (54 percent) than the liberal group. The authors concluded that "a restrictive strategy is as least as effective as and possibly superior to a liberal transfusion strategy in critically ill patients...."

Studies conducted after the TRICC trial have used various categories of high-risk patients to better define RBC transfusion thresholds in these populations (Table 138–4). Studies have focused on patients

TABLE 138–3. Incidence of Transfusion-Transmitted Diseases

	Data from Strong and Katz (2002)[75]	Data from Dodd, Notari, and Stramer (2002)[18]	Data from Tabor (2002)[77]	Total U.S. Cases*
Hepatitis C	1/1,200,000	1/1,935,000	1/625,000	8
Hepatitis B	1/150,000	—	1/150,000	80[†]
HTLV-I/HTLV-II	1/641,000	—	—	20[†]
HIV	1/1,400,000	1/2,135,000	1/769,230	7

HTLV, human T-cell lymphotropic virus.
*Calculated based on transfusion of 15,000,000 U of blood annually and Dodd[76] incidence figures.
[†]Calculations based on data from Strong and Katz.[75]

with upper gastrointestinal bleeding, cardiovascular risk factors, orthopedic surgery patients and other populations that usually require a large number of RBC transfusions. All studies followed the basic structure of the TRICC trial, randomizing patients into a restrictive versus liberal arm. Most studies also used mortality or end-organ dysfunction as end points.

A total of 899 patients with an upper gastrointestinal bleed were randomized so that the restrictive arm had a transfusion threshold of 7 g/dL versus a Hgb level of 9 g/dL for the liberal arm.[20] Death from any cause within the first 45 days was the primary outcome, and the rate of further bleeding and in-hospital complications were used as secondary outcomes. The two patient groups had similar characteristics, including equivalent numbers and grades of cirrhosis. The results of this study also favored a restrictive transfusion strategy. The probability of survival at 6 weeks was higher in the restrictive strategy group (p = 0.02) and the risk of further bleeding was lower (p = 0.01). Overall adverse events were also lower in the restrictive group when compared to the liberal transfusion arm (p = 0.02). The rate of survival was slightly higher in the restrictive group compared to the liberal group for patients with peptic ulcers (hazard ratio, 0.70; 95 percent confidence interval [CI], 0.26 to 1.25); and was significantly higher in patients with cirrhosis and Child-Pugh class A or B disease (hazard ratio, 0.30; 95 percent CI, 0.11 to 0.85). No difference was found for cirrhosis patients and Child-Pugh class C disease (hazard ratio 1.04; 95 percent CI, 0.45 to 2.37). As with the TRICC study, a highly significant difference in transfusion rates was reported. In the restrictive arm, 51 percent of patients did not receive a transfusion, compared to 15 percent of patients in the liberal arm who

did not receive RBC transfusions (p <0.001). These two major trials demonstrated that a 7 g/dL Hgb threshold was safe for a variety of critically ill patients.

RED BLOOD CELL TRANSFUSIONS FOR CARDIOVASCULAR PATIENTS

Moderate anemia may lead to increased rates of myocardial ischemia and infarction in patients with cardiovascular risk factors. Several studies were designed to test whether lower transfusion thresholds were deleterious in this patient population. A subgroup analysis of the TRICC trial found that patients with cardiovascular disease had similar outcomes in the restrictive and liberal cohorts; however, the rate of patients suffering from acute pulmonary edema was significantly higher in the liberal transfusion arm.[21]

The Transfusion Trigger Trial for Functional Outcomes in Cardiovascular Patients Undergoing Surgical Hip Fracture Repair (FOCUS trial) compared the transfusion thresholds of 10 g/dL versus less than 8 g/dL in patients who were status post–hip fracture repair and had cardiovascular risk factors.[22] The trial enrolled 2016 patients older than 50 years of age who were randomized into the restrictive or liberal transfusion threshold group. The primary outcome was death or an inability to walk across a room without human assistance on 60-day followup. Secondary outcomes included in-hospital myocardial infarction, unstable angina, or death for any reason. The liberal transfusion strategy, when compared with the restrictive strategy, did not reduce rates of death or inability to walk independently at 60-day followup or reduce in-hospital

TABLE 138–4. Major Randomized Controlled Trials for Safe Hemoglobin Thresholds in Adults

Trial	Patient Population	Number Enrolled	Hgb/Hct Thresholds (Rest/Lib)	Primary End Point	Conclusions
TRICC[93]	ICU	838	7/10 g/dL	30-Day all-cause mortality	Restrictive strategy as effective and possibly superior to liberal strategy
FOCUS[97]	History or risk factor for CV disease following hip fracture surgery	2016	8/10 g/dL	60-Day all-cause mortality or inability to walk 10 ft	Liberal strategy did not reduce death rates or inability to walk
TRACS[98]	Cardiac surgery	502	24/30 percent	30-Day all-cause mortality and severe morbidity	Restrictive strategy was noninferior to liberal strategy
Upper GI bleed[94]	Severe acute upper GI bleed	921	7/9 g/dL	45-Day all-cause mortality	Restrictive strategy improved outcomes compared with liberal

CV, cardiovascular; FOCUS, Functional Outcomes in Cardiovascular Patients Undergoing Surgical Hip Fracture Repair; GI, gastrointestinal; Hct, hematocrit; Hgb, hemoglobin; TRACS, Transfusion Requirements After Cardiac Surgery; TRICC, Transfusion Requirements in Critical Care.

morbidity in elderly patients at high cardiovascular risk. The rates of in-hospital complications were similar in the two groups.

The Transfusion Requirements After Cardiac Surgery (TRACS) trial randomized patients who underwent cardiac surgery with cardiopulmonary bypass into a liberal (Hct ≥30 percent) or restrictive (Hct ≥24 percent) strategy for RBC transfusions.[23] This noninferiority study found similar rates of 30-day all-cause mortality and severe morbidity. The number of transfused RBC units was found to be an independent risk factor for complications or death at 30 days.

Taken together, the evidence points to a Hgb threshold of 8 g/dL as a safe level to maintain most patients with a history of cardiovascular disease. Patients with acute coronary syndrome continue to be an important exception for which current data is insufficient to support any guidance.

RED BLOOD CELL TRANSFUSIONS FOR ORTHOPEDIC PATIENTS

The FOCUS trial, discussed above (see "Red Blood Cell Transfusions for Cardiovascular Patients"), specifically identified patients with cardiovascular risk factors undergoing hip repair.[22] Other studies with orthopedic patients looked at more general outcome measures such as ability to ambulate after hip surgery. One prospective study found a significant association between anemia and a decreased ability to walk independently before the anemia was corrected.[24] However, a second prospective study found no differences in postoperative functional mobility or length of stay when comparing patients maintained on restrictive (8 g/dL) or liberal (10 g/dL) transfusion strategies.[25] However, the liberal transfusion group had few cardiovascular complications and lower mortality when compared to the restrictive group. The authors concluded that a liberal transfusion strategy does not increase ambulation scores but that a restrictive strategy should be treated with caution in elderly high-risk hip fracture patients.

The population in the FOCUS trial was elderly, high-risk cardiovascular patients; the finding of an 8 g/dL Hgb threshold for RBC transfusions may not be generalizable to the remaining lower-risk orthopedic patient population. However, until adequately powered studies are conducted in these populations, applying the 8 g/dL trigger is the safest approach for lower risk patients. While a Hgb of 8 g/dL is safe for orthopedic patients, the quality-of-life studies indicate that a higher Hgb allows for faster recovery.

RED BLOOD CELL TRANSFUSIONS FOR NEUROLOGICALLY IMPAIRED PATIENTS

No large scale, prospective randomized trial has been done regarding the safety and efficacy of transfusion practice in neurocritically ill patients. The lack of large studies led to a systematic review of six studies that had a combined total of 537 patients.[26] The Hgb triggers in these studies ranged from 7 to 10 g/dL in restrictive groups, to 9.3 to 11.5 g/dL in higher Hgb groups. While some studies reported shorter lengths of stay in the lower Hgb groups, the systematic review found insufficient evidence to guide transfusion practice in neurocritically ill patients.

RED BLOOD CELL TRANSFUSIONS FOR PEDIATRIC PATIENTS

Clinical trials of transfusion triggers for pediatric patients fall into two basic categories: general studies of critically ill pediatric patients and studies focused on high-risk neonates. The Transfusion Strategies for Patients in Pediatric Intensive Care Units (TRIPICU) trial and its affiliated subanalyses represent the major data set covering the pediatric

population ranging from 3 days old to 14 years of age.[27] The trial enrolled 626 patients who had Hgb less than or equal to 9.5 during their first 7 days in the pediatric ICU. The restrictive arm used a Hgb threshold of 7 g/dL, versus the liberal threshold of 9.5 g/dL. The restrictive group received significantly fewer transfusions yet multiple-organ dysfunction syndrome (MODS) and mortality were almost identified in the two arms of the study. Thus, for critically ill children, a Hgb threshold of 7 g/dL could decrease transfusion requirements without increasing adverse outcomes.

Three subgroup analyses were conducted with the TRIPICU data. One study analyzed postoperative patients,[28] the second looked at pediatric patients after cardiac surgery,[29] and the third examined patients with sepsis.[30] All three found no significant differences between new or progressive MODS or 28-day mortality in the restrictive and liberal groups. However, all three studies suffered from small sample size and could not draw strong conclusions because of insufficient power.

Trials in the neonate population have focused on premature babies and infants of very low birth weight. Unlike the clinical trials in adults, where the results of all studies found that a restrictive transfusion approach was as good as, or possibly superior to a liberal transfusion strategy, the results from clinical trials in neonates were mixed. One trial enrolled 100 preterm infants with birth weights between 500 and 1300 g.[31] The transfusion thresholds in the restrictive and liberal arms were dependent upon the infant's age and respiratory status and varied from 22 to 34 percent in the low group to 30 to 46 percent in the high group. In each age group the transfusion threshold levels decreased with improving clinical status, as indicated by the level of respiratory support required. In either arm of the study, additional RBC transfusions could be given at the discretion of the attending neonatologist based on a set of predetermined circumstances. Infants in the restrictive arm of the study were more likely to have intraparenchymal brain hemorrhage or periventricular leukomalacia and also had more frequent episodes of mild and severe apnea. The liberal arm received more RBC transfusions; however, donor exposure was similar in both groups. The authors concluded that a restrictive transfusion practice may be harmful to preterm infants.

The largest trial of transfusion practice in preterm infants was the Premature Infants in Need of Transfusion (PINT) study.[32] This randomized trial asked whether extremely-low-birth-weight infants transfused at different Hgb thresholds had different rates of survival or morbidity at discharge. A total of 451 infants, each weighing less than 1000 g at birth, were randomized into a low or high Hgb threshold group. The thresholds ranged from 6.8 g/dL to 11.5 g/dL in the low group and 7.7 g/dL to 13.5 g/dL in the high group. The actual threshold was determined by a combination of age and presence or absence of respiratory support. There was no statistically significant difference between the two groups in terms of death before home discharge or survival with severe morbidity. In addition, fewer infants received one or more transfusions in the low threshold group. The authors concluded that maintaining extremely-low-birth-weight infants at a higher Hgb threshold conferred no benefit.

A Cochrane review of transfusion in neonates concluded that a restrictive approach resulted in a modest reduction in exposure to transfusion, but did not appear to have a significant impact on death or major morbidities (Table 138–5).[33]

⬤ HEMOGLOBINOPATHIES

SICKLE CELL DISEASE

Transfusion therapy is indicated for sickle cell patients suffering from stroke, acute chest syndrome, acute exacerbations of anemia, and other complications. Regular transfusions also significantly reduce

TABLE 138–5. Major Randomized Controlled Trials for Safe Hemoglobin Thresholds in Children

Trial	Patient Population	Number Enrolled	Hgb/Hct	Primary End Point	Conclusions
TRIPICU[27]	PICU (age from 3 days old to 14 years of age)	626	7/9.5	New or progressive multiple-organ dysfunction syndrome	In stable, critically ill children, a Hgb threshold of 7 g/dL can decrease transfusions without increasing adverse outcomes
PINT[32]	ELBW	451	6.8–11.5 g/dL (low) 7.7–13.5 g/dL (high)	Death before home discharge or survival with severe retinopathy, bronchopulmonary dysplasia or brain injury	In ELBW, maintaining a higher Hgb results in more transfusions but confers little evidence of benefit

ELBW, extremely-low-birth-weight infants; Hct, hematocrit; Hgb, hemoglobin; PICU, pediatric intensive care units; PINT, Premature Infants in Need of Transfusion; TRIPICU, Transfusion Strategies for Patients in Pediatric Intensive Care Units.

the recurrence of cerebral infarcts in children with sickle cell disease (SCD).[34] Transfusions are usually not necessary to correct baseline anemia or alleviate vasoocclusive crises. Because transfusion also creates complications, such as iron overload, transfusion reactions, alloimmunization, and delayed hemolytic transfusion reactions, clinicians should take particular care when considering transfusions for sickle cell patients.

Chronic transfusion can lead to a high rate of RBC alloimmunization in patients with SCD. Rates ranged from 18 to 47 percent, which is significantly higher than found in the general U.S. population (0.5 to 1.5 percent),[35] or the highly transfused hematology-oncology population (9 to 15 percent). The reasons for this high rate include number of transfusions, age at first transfusion, the inflammatory milieu created by SCD,[36] and the different RBC antigens present in donors of mostly European descent versus sickle cell patients of African ancestry.

The multiple antibodies specific for RBC antigens can cause delayed hemolytic transfusion reactions (DHTRs).[37] DHTRs may be difficult to recognize, because some occur without any detectable antibody present, and with a negative direct antiglobulin test (DAT).[38] In addition, some DHTRs occur without obvious clinical signs of hemolysis.[37] Severe cases of DHTR result in the hyperhemolysis syndrome, defined by a drop in the patient's Hgb to a level lower than the pretransfusion value. This steep decline in Hgb suggests hemolysis of autologous cells, as well as the transfused allogeneic RBCs.

Transfusion services may attempt to ameliorate the alloimmunization rate by prophylactically matching donor and patient for Rh (antigens D, C, c, E, e) and Kell antigens. A few will also provide an extended phenotype match for the common Kidd, Duffy and S antigens. Both strategies reduce alloimmunization, yet even with matched transfusions, SCD patients continue to form RBC antibodies at rates up to 58 percent of chronically transfused and 15 percent of episodically transfused SCD patients.[37] Most of these antibodies were made against Rh antigens, and more than half occurred in patients who received RBCs phenotypically matched for the corresponding Rh antigen. The likely explanation for this seeming paradox is that SCD patients have variant *RH* genes. In fact, high resolution *RH* genotyping showed variant alleles in 87 percent of the subjects.[37,39]

THALASSEMIA

Thalassemia major patients are chronically transfusion dependent. Over time, this will lead to iron overload, and can result in RBC alloimmunization. No clinical trial has been staged to find the optimal transfusion threshold for patients with thalassemia; however, the consequences of anemia can be severe and must be balanced with the risks of

transfusion. Transfusing to maintain a Hgb of 10 g/dL is considered sufficient to suppress erythropoiesis, thereby averting the bone deformities and other sequelae of this disease; however, some transfusion regimens call for a pretransfusion minimum of greater than 10 g/dL, with a post-transfusion goal of more than 15 g/dL. Thalassemia intermedia patients have more varied transfusion requirements, in keeping with the wide clinical presentation of this disease. If transfusion therapy is clinically indicated, the transfusion recommendations are similar to those for thalassemia major (Chap. 48).

HEMATOPOIETIC STEM CELL TRANSPLANT

TRANSFUSION SUPPORT

The duration and specificity of transfusion support for hematopoietic stem cell transplantation (HSCT) patients depends upon the disease, the source of the stem cells, the preparative regimen applied prior to transplant, and patient factors during the post-transplant recovery period. Human leukocyte antigen (HLA) matching remains an important predictor of success with HSCT. As a result, the ABO barrier is often crossed when searching for the best HLA match between donor and patient. Crossing the ABO barrier has little or no effect upon overall outcomes; however, transfusion difficulties can arise due to antigenic incompatibility between the transplanted cells and the patient.

Transfusion support can be divided into the pre- and posttransplantation periods. Prior to an HSCT, an immunocompetent patient (e.g., aplastic anemia, hemoglobinopathies) is capable of mounting an immune response to transfusions, leading to alloimmunization against HLA antigens present on the surface of leukocytes. Leukoreduction reduces alloimmunization rates, but sufficient white blood cells remain in the unit for alloimmunization to occur. Antibodies against HLA contribute to delayed engraftment and graft rejection in some patient populations.[40] As a result, pretransplantation transfusions in immunocompetent patients should be avoided, as they are associated with increased graft failure rates.[41,42] RBC transfusions can be minimized by using a Hgb trigger of 8 g/dL for stable patients.[43]

Patients who are immunocompromised, either because of their disease, or from chemotherapy, are less likely to become immunized to foreign antigens. Nonetheless, using leukoreduced products to minimize the risk of alloimmunization is still recommended. Extra care must also be taken if the stem cell donation comes from a blood relative. In this situation family members should not give directed blood donations prior to transplantation, as this may lead to alloimmunization against major and/or minor HLA antigens that are present in the transplant organ. In addition, all RBC and platelet transfusions should be irradiated as the risk for transfusion-associated graft-versus-host disease (TA-GVHD) is high in HSCT patients (see section Transfusion-Associated-Graft-versus-Host Disease below for more in-depth discussion of TA-GVHD).

RBC engraftment is difficult to assess, but may be defined by the appearance of 1 percent reticulocytes in the peripheral blood, or as the day of the last RBC transfusion, with no transfusion given in the following 30 days. In general, engraftment time is shortest when hematopoietic progenitor cells are obtained by apheresis (HPC-A), and greatest when hematopoietic progenitor cells are obtained from umbilical cords (HPC-C) are used; however, considerable patient-to-patient variability exists. Prolonged engraftment directly translates into higher transfusion rates for RBCs and platelets.

When an ABO incompatible transplant is used, group O red cells are used to avoid incompatibility issues. The ABO type of plasma products may be different from the red cell type (Table 138–6). Once the patient begins to produce "donor-type" erythrocytes, their blood type should be reassessed. The decision to switch a patient's blood type is highly variable across institutions. In our hospital, when a patient is RBC transfusion independent for 100 days, and no incompatible isohemagglutinins against the new RBC phenotype can be detected in two consecutive blood samples, the patient's native blood type is switched to the donor type for future transfusions.

TRANSFUSION-RELATED COMPLICATIONS

There are transfusion-related complications that are specific to, or more frequently seen, in the HSCT population. Some of these complications arise when lymphocytes within the transplant are activated against the

TABLE 138–6. Component Type Selection for Hematopoietic Stem Cell Transplantations That Cross the ABO Barrier

Mismatch	Transplant		Transfuse	
	Donor Type	Recipient Type	Red Blood Cell	Platelets*/ Plasma
Major mismatch	A	O	O	A, AB
	B	O	O	B, AB
	AB	O	O	AB
	AB	A	A, O	AB
	AB	B	B, O	AB
Minor mismatch	O	A	O	A, AB
	O	B	O	B, AB
	O	AB	O	AB
	A	AB	A, O	AB
	B	AB	B, O	AB
Bidirectional mismatch	A	B	O	AB
	B	A	O	AB

*Platelets stored in additive solution reduce the volume of incompatible plasma transfused.

Modified with permission from Cohn CS: Transfusion support issues in hematopoietic stem cell transplantation. *Cancer Control* 22(1): 52–59, 2015.

recipient; these include TA-GVHD and passenger lymphocyte syndrome (PLS). Another complication, pure red cell aplasia (PRCA), occurs when the patient's residual antibodies attack the transplanted red cells. Standard transfusion reactions, such as allergic or febrile nonhemolytic reactions, are frequently seen in this heavily transfused patient population; however, these "standard" transfusion reactions are discussed more fully later in this chapter in the section Adverse Effects of Red Cell Transfusions.

Major and Minor ABO Mismatches

Complications from ABO incompatibility depend upon whether a major or minor ABO mismatch is present (see Table 138–6). A major mismatch occurs when the transplant contains RBCs that are incompatible with the recipient's plasma. Conversely, a minor mismatch is present when the donor plasma contains isohemagglutinins against the recipient's RBCs. Bidirectional transplants (e.g., group A transplant into group B recipient) carry both major and minor mismatches.

Major ABO Mismatch When a major ABO mismatched transplant is given, immediate hemolysis may occur during the infusion. This complication is more commonly seen when the HSCT is derived from marrow, because more red cells are present; however, RBC depletion techniques have effectively eliminated this complication. Because HPC-A units contain a minimal volume of RBCs (8 to 15 mL), clinically significant cases of immediate hemolysis have not been identified.[44] Most HPC-C units are RBC-depleted prior to cryopreservation, and the residual erythrocytes lyse during cryopreservation, therefore immediate hemolysis is not a problem with cord blood transplants.

Preformed antibodies against non-ABO RBC antigens can remain in a recipient's peripheral circulation for many weeks after transplantation. These antibodies may cause lysis when engrafted cells begin to produce new RBC. Also chimeric patients may develop antibodies against ABO or non-ABO RBC antigens, resulting in delayed hemolysis. When recipients have isohemagglutinins specific for the ABO type of the transplant, delayed erythrocyte engraftment and PRCA may ensue. This is seen most frequently when group O patients receive a group A transplant, or with bidirectional mismatches. PRCA develops when anti-ABO antibodies destroy erythrocyte progenitor cells in the marrow.

Minor Mismatches When lymphocytes within the HSCT recognize the recipient RBCs as foreign, antibodies may be produced that are specific for ABO or minor RBC antigens. This PLS usually presents 7 to 14 days after the transplant with the abrupt onset of hemolysis. The hemolysis ranges from mild to severe, and may be intra- or extravascular, depending upon the nature of the antibody involved. These "passenger lymphocytes" are reported most frequently in transplants that use a group O donor with a group A recipient.[45] Antibodies against minor RBC antigens are less frequently reported, and cause less-severe hemolysis.[45]

In cases involving the ABO system, the Hgb level may drop precipitously. The laboratory signs of intravascular hemolysis, that is, hemoglobinemia, hemoglobinuria and an elevated lactate dehydrogenase (LDH) should be used to follow the course of disease. In most cases a DAT will be positive, unless all antibody bound cells have already been lysed. The hemolysis can persist as long as incompatible RBCs are present, but usually subsides within 5 to 10 days.[45]

Nonmyeloablative conditioning regimens carry a greater risk for PLS than when full ablation is used. Because HPC-A preparations carry a greater lymphocyte load when compared to hematopoietic cell concentrate-marrow (HPC-M) and hematopoietic cell concentrate-cord (HPC-C) collections, recipients of peripheral blood stem cells are at an increased risk of developing PLS. The authors are not aware of a case of PLS that has been reported with an umbilical cord stem cell transplant.

Maintaining graft-versus-host disease (GVHD) prophylaxis with only a T-cell inhibitor, such as cyclosporine, without an accompanying B-cell inhibitor, is also considered a risk factor.

Transfusion-Transmitted Cytomegalovirus

CMV infection continues to be a serious complication following HSCTs. Most CMV infections are likely the result of reactivation of virus from a previous infection rather than acquisition of a new strain. However, in CMV-antibody–negative patients there is a risk of developing a transfusion-transmitted *de novo* CMV infection. To reduce this risk, one may use CMV-antibody-negative blood, or leukocyte-reduced components. A large controlled trial and a meta-analysis from 2007 showed that leukocyte-reduced components are as effective as antibody-negative components in preventing transfusion-transmitted CMV.[46,47] Two additional studies support the safety of using only leukoreduced blood in preventing transfusion transmission of CMV.[48,49] Both studies found 0 percent risk of transfusion-transmitted CMV infection. Nonetheless, the overall risk of transfusion transmission of CMV in leukoreduced components is not zero. CMV DNA was found in 44 percent of newly seropositive blood donors, and the overall prevalence of CMV DNA was 0.13 percent in nearly 32,000 donations.[50] While blood products could be obtained from donors with a longstanding history of CMV-positive serology, a more practical approach is to screen donated blood for CMV DNA or immunoglobulin (Ig) M antibodies, although we believe that the use of leukoreduced blood components is adequate.

Transfusion-Associated Graft-Versus-Host Disease

All HSCT patients should receive irradiated components from the time of initiation of conditioning chemotherapy, and for at least 1 year following transplantation to prevent TA-GVHD. However, many centers continue to provide irradiated products for the life of the patient. The British Committee for Standards in Haematology (BCSH) recommends that allogeneic transplant recipients should receive irradiated components for 6 months posttransplantation, or until the patient's lymphocyte count is greater than 1×10^9/L; however, if chronic GVHD is present, then irradiated products should be given indefinitely.[51] Autologous transplant patients should begin receiving irradiated components from the time of initiation of conditioning chemotherapy, but can revert to nonirradiated components 3 months after the transplantation. If autologous transplant patients received total-body irradiation, then the BCSH recommends extending the use of irradiated products for 6 months after the transplantation.

● SOLID-ORGAN TRANSPLANT

Patients awaiting a solid-organ transplant should have minimal exposure to allogeneic blood products to reduce the risk of alloimmunization. Leukoreduced components contain sufficient white blood cells to immunize a patient against class I and class II HLA molecules. The risk of sensitization from a blood transfusion ranges from 2 to 21 percent.[52] Sensitization may increase the extent of alloimmunization, which contributes to delays in finding a compatible organ for transplantation. In fact, patients who have been transfused have an 11 percent reduction in the likelihood of ever receiving a renal transplant.[52] Attempts to reduce alloimmunization by matching blood donors and patients[53] or matching for the DR locus have shown no consistent reduction.[54] Using a Hgb of 7 g/dL as a safe threshold for transfusions can minimize exposure. In some patients the use of erythropoiesis-stimulating agents (ESA) may help decrease the number of RBC transfusions; however, ESAs are contraindicated in patients with a history of malignancy or stroke.

● ADVERSE EFFECTS OF RED CELL TRANSFUSIONS

The precise risk of an adverse reaction is difficult to estimate; many reactions may be wrongly attributed to the patient's underlying illness, and approximately half of all transfusions are given to anesthetized patients in the operating rooms where reactions may be blunted or more difficult to recognize. The incidence of some adverse reactions has fallen in the past decade due to changes in component handling. Adverse reactions may occur soon after a transfusion begins, as seen with acute hemolytic reactions or acute lung injury, or within days to weeks of a transfusion, as seen with delayed hemolytic reactions.[55] Fortunately, the majority of acute transfusion reactions are mild and manageable. Many of the reported transfusion-related fatalities involve human errors which may be as much as 1:18,000 transfusions.

IMMEDIATE TRANSFUSION REACTIONS

In general, immediate transfusion reactions are more dangerous than delayed reactions. Severe complications, including death, can on rare occasions develop within a few minutes of initiating transfusion. Close attention and early vital sign assessments are recommended at the beginning and within 15 minutes of starting a transfusion.

Acute Hemolytic Transfusion Reactions

Acute hemolytic transfusion reactions (AHTRs) are almost always caused by the immune-mediated destruction of ABO-incompatible transfused blood. ABO incompatible transfusions are estimated to occur in one in 38,000 to one in 70,000 RBC transfusions.[56] Isohemagglutinins can activate the complement and coagulation systems. C3a and C5a can activate white blood cells to release inflammatory cytokines (interleukin [IL]-1, IL-6, IL-8, and tumor necrosis factor-alpha [TNF-α]), contributing to fever, hypotension, wheezing, chest pain, nausea, and vomiting.[57] The presence of antigen-antibody complexes and activated complement on donor RBCs may lead to bradykinin generation. This can increase capillary permeability and arteriolar dilatation causing a fall in systemic blood pressure. Activation of factor XII may initiate the coagulation cascade with formation of thrombin and lead to disseminated intravascular coagulation. Renal failure may also develop as a result of ischemia, hypotension, antigen-antibody complex deposition, and thrombosis. Although rare, AHTRs can also be seen because of other blood group antibodies, particularly those in the Kidd blood group system.

Clinical Presentation The most common presenting symptom is fever with or without chills or rigors. In mild cases, this may be accompanied with abdominal, chest, flank, or back pain, whereas dyspnea, hypotension, hemoglobinuria, and eventually shock can be seen in severe cases. Bleeding, caused by the consumptive coagulopathy, can occur. Hematuria can be the first sign of intravascular hemolysis, particularly in anesthetized or unconscious patients. The severity of AHTR is extremely variable and usually depends on the rate and total volume of blood administered. Approximately 47 percent of the recipients of ABO incompatible blood show no effects, even after receiving a whole unit, 41 percent show symptoms of AHTR, and mortality is approximately 2 percent.[55,56]

Laboratory Evaluation Laboratory evaluation involves checking for technical and identification errors, examine a posttransfusion specimen for hemolysis, and perform a DAT to detect antibody-coated red cells. If AHTR is strongly suspected, repeat ABO and Rh typing of the patient and the transfused blood and repeat antibody screen and crossmatch may be helpful. A negative DAT occurs in rare cases when all transfused RBCs are lysed.

Management Immediate discontinuation of transfusion should always be the first step in any transfusion reaction. Maintaining vascular access with slow infusion of normal saline, monitoring vital signs, and assessing urine output are key early steps. A blood specimen should be collected immediately for laboratory evaluation. The component bag should be returned to the blood bank. If severe hemolysis has occurred, therapy focuses on management of hypotension, coagulation disorders, and renal function. A urine output of approximately 100 mL/h for 24 hours should be maintained in adults without contraindications. In simple cases, normal saline infusion may be sufficient; however, diuretics may be necessary in some cases. Intravenous administration of furosemide (40 to 80 mg) promotes diuresis and improves blood flow to the renal cortex. In severe cases of hypotension, intravenous dopamine, which dilates renal vasculature and increases cardiac output, can be used. Patients with coagulopathy and active bleeding may require administration of platelets, fresh-frozen plasma, or cryoprecipitate.

Prevention The most common basis for AHTRs is a clerical error resulting from mistakes in identifying the patient, labeling the pretransfusions sample, or identifying the correct red cell unit for the patient.[56–58]

Febrile Nonhemolytic Transfusion Reactions

A febrile nonhemolytic transfusion reaction (FNHTR) is defined, arbitrarily, as a temperature increase of 1°C or more during or up to 4 hours after transfusion. Other possible symptoms include increases in respiratory rate, anxiety, and, more unusually, nausea or vomiting.

FNHTRs are one of the most commonly encountered transfusion reactions occurring in approximately 0.12 to 0.5 percent of RBC units transfused, and are more likely to occur following transfusion of platelets than RBCs. Leukocyte reduction decreases the incidence of FNHTRs with both whole-blood derived and apheresis platelets.

Clinical Presentation Fever is triggered by the action of cytokines (e.g., IL-1, IL-6, TNF-α). This may be the result of activation of donor leukocytes by anti-HLA or other antibodies in the recipient, activation of recipient leukocyte and endothelial cells by transfused donor leukocytes or plasma constituents, or by the passive transfer of cytokines or CD40 ligand (CD154) that accumulated in the unit during storage.

Fever should not be solely attributed to FNHTR until other potential life-threatening transfusion reactions or patient-related factors have been excluded. Past transfusion reaction history should be reviewed to determine if additional measures should be implemented for future transfusions.

Laboratory Evaluation The laboratory investigation should concentrate on ruling out a septic transfusion reaction. A Gram stain is not a highly sensitive technique in this setting, but may be used to rule-in bacterial contamination. Rapid qualitative immunoassay tests (e.g., Verax or BacTx) are highly sensitive for most commonly encountered bacterial contaminants and may be used in lieu of Gram stain to screen implicated platelet units. In cases with a high index of suspicion, the unit should be cultured. If all results are negative and the patient's presentation is consistent with a mild FNHTR, no additional testing is required.

Management FNHTRs are typically benign, and usually resolve completely within 1 to 2 hours after the transfusion is discontinued. The remainder of the transfused unit and a posttransfusion blood sample from the patient should be sent to the laboratory for investigation. Antipyretics may be administered to shorten the duration of the fever and provide analgesia. Acetaminophen 325 to 650 mg orally for adults or 10 to 15 mg/kg/dose orally for children is effective for this purpose.

Transfusing leukoreduced RBCs and/or platelets stored in additive solution will significantly reduce the risk of FNHTRs.[59] Premedication with antipyretics (acetaminophen) is not helpful.[60,61]

Allergic Transfusion Reactions

These are a common adverse reaction of transfusion therapy, ranging from mild forms characterized by localized pruritus and/or urticaria, to severe anaphylactic or anaphylactoid reactions. The mild forms of allergic transfusion reaction (ATR) occur in 1 to 3 percent of transfusions of plasma-rich components (i.e., platelets/fresh-frozen plasma) and in 0.1 to 0.3 percent for red cells. Severe anaphylactic reactions are much less frequent and estimated at one in 20,000 to 50,000 transfusions.[7]

The majority of ATRs are immediate (type 1) hypersensitivity reactions, mediated by preformed IgE antibodies binding to soluble proteins present within donor plasma.[62] Severe anaphylactic reactions may occur after transfusion of blood products to IgA-deficient patients who have anti-IgA antibodies. Most patients labeled as IgA deficient still have low levels of the immunoglobulin (2 to 4 mg/dL) and will not produce anti-IgA antibodies. The rare patient with complete IgA deficiency (<0.05 mg/dL) may develop anti-IgA antibodies and thus might experience anaphylaxis with transfusion. Anaphylactoid reactions are similar to anaphylaxis but clinically less severe and caused by non–IgE-mediated activation of mast cells.

Clinical Presentation ATRs usually begin during or within an hour of starting a transfusion, but may not become evident until several hours later. Common findings include urticaria, rash, pruritus, and flushing. More severe reactions occur sooner and may include angioedema, chest tightness, dyspnea, cyanosis, hoarseness, stridor, or wheezing. In addition, gastrointestinal symptoms such as abdominal pain, nausea, vomiting, and diarrhea may also occur. Unlike other acute transfusion reactions, fever is usually absent. Anaphylaxis occurs immediately after starting the transfusion. Symptoms can include bronchospasm, angioedema, respiratory distress, nausea, vomiting, abdominal cramps, diarrhea, shock, and loss of consciousness.

Laboratory Evaluation There is no need for laboratory investigation with simple urticarial and/or localized pruritus. However, the incident should be reported to the blood bank to update the patient's record for any future transfusions. In anaphylactic reactions, the patient should be tested for complete IgA deficiency; however, a history of anaphylactic reactions mandate use of washed red cells and platelets and avoidance of plasma transfusions regardless of the results of these tests.

Management Most ATRs are mild, self-limited and respond well to transfusion discontinuation and, if indicated, administration of antihistamine (diphenhydramine hydrochloride, usually orally). In cases limited to urticaria, the transfusion may be resumed immediately after symptoms resolve. However, transfusion should never be resumed when there is a severe reaction. In acute anaphylaxis, fluid resuscitation may be needed to maintain blood pressure followed by administration of subcutaneous or intramuscular epinephrine (0.3 mL of 1:1000 dilution), as well as airway management and intensive care. In case of shock, a higher concentration of intravenous epinephrine (3 to 5 mL of a 1:10,000 dilution) can be administered. Steroids are usually not helpful in acute crises.

Prevention Patients with a history of mild ATRs should not be premedicated with an antihistamine, as this does not reduce the overall risk of ATRs.[61] Platelets stored in additive solution may be used to reduce the risk of a reaction. In IgA-deficient patients with a history of anaphylaxis to transfusion, components from IgA-deficient donors are sometimes available.[59]

Transfusion-Related Acute Lung Injury

Transfusion-related acute lung injury (TRALI) is a syndrome of acute hypoxia attributable to noncardiogenic pulmonary edema that occurs within 6 hours of a transfusion.[63,64] TRALI has been the leading cause of transfusion-related fatalities for several years.

There are two main hypotheses regarding the capillary leak seen in TRALI. The two-hit hypothesis states that underlying patient factors act as a necessary first hit, leading to adherence of primed neutrophils to the pulmonary endothelium. The second hit is caused by mediators within the transfused component, which activate pulmonary neutrophils, which, in turn, damage the endothelium.[64] The mediators are often antibodies specific for either class II HLA or for human neutrophil antigens (HNAs). There are also cases in which no antibody was detected, which are thought to be a result of proinflammatory mediators, bioactive lipids, and CD40 ligand that accumulate in the blood product during storage.[65] Despite reports of a direct correlation between storage time of cellular blood components and TRALI, this mechanism remains controversial.

Specific patient factors (first hits) that are associated with a greater risk of TRALI include patients on mechanical ventilation, sepsis, chronic alcohol abuse, severe liver disease, hematologic malignancy, and others. It is not known whether the risk is determined by the patient's condition, or by a greater transfusion requirement. The two-hit hypothesis accounts for critically ill patients who develop TRALI; however, there are reports of TRALI in reasonably healthy patients. This observation led to the threshold model of TRALI.[66] In this paradigm, a threshold, or tipping point, must be surpassed to induce TRALI. A healthy patient may develop TRALI when transfused with a high titer of antibody. Conversely, a critically ill patient with primed neutrophils can be tipped into TRALI with a lower titer of antibody.

Clinical Presentation and Differential Diagnosis It is often impossible to fully distinguish TRALI from other causes of respiratory distress. The typical presentation of TRALI is the sudden development of dyspnea, severe hypoxemia (O_2 saturation <90 percent in room air) hypotension, and fever that develop within 6 hours of transfusion and usually resolves with supportive care within 48 to 96 hours. Although hypotension is considered one of the important signs in diagnosing TRALI, hypertension can occur in some cases.

In addition to new or worsening oxygen desaturation, TRALI is characterized by chest x-ray findings of bilateral diffuse patchy pulmonary densities without cardiac enlargement. TRALI can be ruled out as the sole cause of pulmonary failure by the presence of rales and jugular venous distention on physical exam and/or dilated pulmonary arteries on chest x-ray, which are evidence of congestive heart failure with or without transfusion-associated circulatory overload (TACO). Transient leukopenia, which follows the reaction within few hours, can also distinguish TRALI from TACO.

Management Supportive care is the mainstay of therapy in TRALI, including oxygen supplementation and aggressive respiratory support plus intravenous fluid and vasopressors for hypotension, if indicated. It has been suggested that diuretics, which are indicated in TACO management, are not efficacious and should be avoided in TRALI. Glucocorticoids may provide benefit.

Prevention HLA alloimmunization has been directly correlated with the number of times a woman is pregnant and plasma from multiparous women has been implicated as a risk factor in TRALI. To reduce this risk, blood banks attempt to collect plasma from males, nulliparous females, and/or females tested and found to be negative for HLA antibodies. After blood collection centers implemented TRALI mitigation strategies, the incidence of TRALI dropped from an estimate of one in 4000 transfusions, to approximately one in 12,000.[67] Nonetheless, TRALI continues to be the leading cause of transfusion-related fatalities.

Pooled plasma may also be used for TRALI mitigation because antibody titers drop due to dilution. No cases of TRALI resulting from transfusion of pooled solvent detergent treated plasma have been reported.[68,69]

Transfusion-Associated Circulatory Overload

TACO occurs when patients are unable to effectively process the expansion in intravascular volume from a blood transfusion. Circulatory overload may be the consequence of the infusions rates, the volume of infused blood product, and/or an underlying cardiac, renal, and/or pulmonary pathology. The fluid volume transfused may be less important than the infusion flow rate and the patient's ability to process the fluid.

The incidence of TACO is difficult to ascertain, as there are inconsistent case definitions, passive reporting systems and poor clinical recognition. Approximately 1 percent of orthopedic patients developed TACO postoperatively, compared to 6 percent of patients in an ICU setting.[70] Reports of TACO have surged as awareness has increased. Active surveillance also increases the number of cases. In one institution the historical prevalence rate from 6 years of passive reporting was one in 1566 from plasma transfusions. After 1 month of active surveillance the prevalence rate jumped to one in 68.[71]

TACO is seen more in younger and advanced age patients.[72] Additional risk factors include female sex, a history of congestive heart failure, hemodialysis, mechanical ventilation, recent vasopressors, and positive fluid balance.[73]

Clinical Presentation Symptoms of TACO may include dyspnea, orthopnea, cough, headache, and hypoxemia, which are not specific. However, signs such as rales, hypertension, and jugular vein distention may differentiate TACO from TRALI. These signs and symptoms usually present within 2 hours of the onset of transfusion, but may be up to 6 hours or even 24 hours after the onset of transfusion.

Laboratory Evaluation Oxygen saturation may decrease along with the partial pressure of oxygen in the arterial blood. New bilateral infiltrates on chest x-ray is characteristic for TACO; however, it is also seen in TRALI. Elevated levels of B-type natriuretic peptide (BNP) and N-terminal pro-BNP (NT-proBNP) are both useful markers for TACO, but NT-proBNP may be more useful as it has a longer *in vivo* and *in vitro* half-life. Unfortunately neither peptide was found to be useful in distinguishing TACO from TRALI in critically ill patients.[74]

Management Once TACO is suspected, intravenous fluids should be restricted, followed by the administration of supplemental oxygen and a diuretic, if not contraindicated. Placing the patient in a sitting position can also be helpful. In severe cases, mechanical ventilation may be required.

If a patient is at risk for TACO and blood transfusion is imperative, blood should be administered slowly at a rate of 1 to 4 mL/kg/h. Most blood banks can also reduce the transfusion volume by splitting the blood product into smaller volumes if the transfusion is going to last longer than 4 hours. Close monitoring of the patient's vital signs throughout the transfusion may also help in decreasing the development of TACO.

Transfusion-Related Sepsis

Transfusion-related sepsis when it occurs is usually from platelet units that are stored at room temperature. Red cells, stored at refrigerator temperatures, are very rarely contaminated by unusual cold-growing organisms (e.g., *Yersinia, Serratia, Pseudomonas*). The rate of fatal transfusion-transmitted bacteremia from red cells has been estimated to be 0.13 per million units transfused in the United States.[75]

Clinical Presentation The infusion of large numbers of Gram-negative microorganisms may lead to fever (>38.5°C), rigors, marked hypotension, abdominal pain, vomiting, diarrhea, and the development of profound shock. Gram-positive contaminants may cause fever and rigors, but are not associated with the severe symptoms produced by Gram-negative toxins.

Laboratory Evaluation Rapid diagnosis usually may be made via Gram stain of the residual donor blood; however, a culture of the transfused component is necessary.

Management Septic shock from transfusion of contaminated blood should be managed as for septic shock from other causes and is not discussed further here.

DELAYED TRANSFUSION REACTIONS

Delayed Hemolytic Transfusion Reactions

DHTRs occur when a previously immunized patient receives red cells containing the corresponding antigen but are compatible in the cross-match because of a low titer of circulating alloantibody. DHTRs occur in 0.2 to 2.6 percent of patients. It is vanishingly rare in infants younger than 4 months of age, and more common in chronically transfused patients.

Approximately 30 to 40 percent of alloantibodies become undetectable months to years after their initial identification. However, a patient previously immunized by transfusion or pregnancy may develop a secondary immune response after reexposure to a blood group antigen. Decreasing Hct or failure to see the typical 1 g/dL Hgb/3 percent Hct increment following transfusion may be noted within several days to weeks of a blood transfusion, as well as an unexplained fever. Hemolysis from DHTR is typically extravascular, without dramatic clinical symptoms and signs, although some classes of IgG bind complement and will cause intravascular hemolysis. Hemolysis in DHTRs is usually mild and gradual, however, when antibodies are produced against antigens in the Kidd blood system, the hemolysis may be rapid, intravascular, and may be severe.

The usual evidence of hemolysis is seen. The appearance of spherocytes and reticulocytes on peripheral blood film, increases in total and unconjugated bilirubin, and increased LDH. The DAT is usually positive but may be negative if all the transfused RBCs have been eliminated from the circulation. The antibody screen is usually positive and the antibody can be identified. No specific management is usually needed as these reactions are usually subtle and clinically silent. In cases of intravascular hemolysis, clinical support measures are similar to those described for an acute hemolytic transfusion reaction. If transfusion is necessary donor red cells negative for the offending antigen may be selected.

Posttransfusion Purpura

Posttransfusion purpura is a rare immune-mediated disorder that is discussed in greater detail in Chap. 139.

IRON OVERLOAD

One of the most common complications of chronic RBCs transfusion is iron overload, which is further discussed in the chapters on congenital hemoglobinopathies (Chaps. 48 and 49).

TRANSFUSION-ASSOCIATED GRAFT-VERSUS-HOST DISEASE

Most cases of TA-GVHD are associated with HSCT. TA-GVHD is a very rare complication that occurs when a susceptible patient is exposed to viable lymphocytes introduced in a blood transfusion. This can occur when transfusions from close relatives or other unintentionally genetically matched donors are administered to severely immunocompromised recipients. The immunocompromised recipient is incapable of "rejecting" or mounting an attack against the lymphocytes in the transfused blood. In addition, cases of TA-GVHD have been reported in recipients with an intact immune system.[76,77]

TA-GVHD may present with maculopapular rash, fever, watery diarrhea, liver dysfunction, and marrow failure within 8 to 10 days of transfusion. The mortality rate in is approximately 90 percent and the downhill course often rapid.

RBC, platelet, and granulocyte units all contain some lymphocytes and therefore carry a risk of TA-GVHD; plasma and cryoprecipitate are acellular and therefore pose no risk. To prevent TA-GVHD, lymphocytes within a blood component must be eliminated or disabled. Leukoreduction is not sufficient, as it reduces, but does not completely eliminate white blood cells. Frozen units may also carry a risk, as the lymphocytes may survive. Gamma and X-ray irradiation of components are effective prophylaxis for TA-GVHD.[78] A dose of at least 2500 centigray to the center of a cellular blood component and 1500 centigray throughout the unit leaves lymphocytes intact but unable to proliferate. This simple precaution prevents TA-GVHD.

Irradiation at the indicated dose appears to damage the red cell membrane. The damage does not affect the oxygen carrying capacity of the erythrocyte, but does allow potassium to leak from the cell. The level of extracellular potassium has been shown to increase with storage time. As a result, red cells may be stored for only 28 days after irradiation.

POTENTIAL EFFECT OF AGE OF RED CELLS ON TRANSFUSION OUTCOME

In the United States, RBC may be stored in additive solution for up to 42 days. The criteria used to determine storage limits are based on *in vivo* recovery and *in vitro* hemolysis data. During storage, RBC units develop a progressive "storage lesion." Some of these changes include an increase in free Hgb which acts as a nitric oxide scavenger; a reduction in 2,3-bisphophosglyceric acid (2,3-BPG), which leads to increased oxygen affinity/decreased oxygen delivery; an increase in hydrogen ions in the supernatant causing a drop in the pH; an increase in microvesicles in the supernatant, creating a procoagulant effect and reduced RBC membrane deformability. Each of these changes is a dynamic process, with some occurring on the first day of blood storage, and others taking days or weeks to be evident. Aspects of the storage lesion have been demonstrated *in vivo* using healthy volunteers who are transfused with autologous units that are stored for widely divergent time periods. In three of these controlled experiments, no differences were found in pulmonary function,[79] nitric oxide-mediated hyperemic response to ischemia,[80] or cognitive function.[81] A fourth volunteer study found significant differences with *in vivo* iron-related parameters and signs of hemolysis when fresh and older units were compared.[82]

The clinical relevance of these *in vitro* and *in vivo* studies is not clear. Some of the *in vitro* findings are reversed within 24 to 48 hours of transfusion, and no adverse effects were reported in the volunteers used for the *in vivo* studies; however, they were healthy and may be more able to withstand insults to their system. Multiple retrospective and prospective studies have looked for an association between the storage age of a RBC unit and clinical outcomes. In one study,[83] in more than 5000 cardiac surgery patients receiving more than 18,000 units of RBCs, patients receiving blood that was stored for longer than 2 weeks were at a significantly higher risk of postoperative complications as well as short-term and long-term survival. Subsequently, a large number of retrospective studies and a smaller number of prospective studies were performed. A recent review summarizing the findings of 32 studies reported that 18 found a detrimental effect from prolonged RBC storage, while 14 studies did not.[84,85] It is notable that the four prospective randomized trials included in the review found no significant ill effect. A meta-analysis of 21 studies, either observational studies or randomized controlled trials, found that use of older stored blood is associated with a significantly increased risk of death.[85]

The question of higher risk from transfusion of older units continues to be studied in multiple, large prospective clinical trials. These studies are being conducted with ICU and cardiac surgery patients, among others. Until the results of these studies are available, no changes to practice should be made based on the available data.

● PATIENT BLOOD MANAGEMENT

Patient blood management (PBM) is an evidence-based, systematic and multifaceted approach to optimizing the care of patients who might need transfusion. The risks associated with unnecessary transfusions, coupled with the rising cost of blood have helped fuel the growth of PBM efforts. PBM was recently adopted by the World Health Organization as the new standard of care, and the AABB has issued guidelines and other tools designed to help hospitals implement a PBM program. A comprehensive PBM program includes (1) hospital-wide guidelines for evidence-based use of blood components, (2) early assessment and correction of preoperative anemia, and (3) application of a variety of techniques to minimize perioperative blood loss.

Guidelines for transfusion have been published by multiple medical professional societies, and can serve as a useful starting point for hospitals; however, the evidence for Hgb thresholds was developed in selected patient populations and does not always apply in all clinical situations. Combining evidence with a clinical assessment is necessary when deciding if a transfusion is indicated. Adding decision support tools into computerized physician order entry systems can remind clinicians of guidelines and safety considerations when ordering blood.[86] These systems have been shown to reduce blood use and decrease costs associated with transfusions.[87] Auditing transfusion orders may reveal patterns of blood utilization that can be corrected with education.

Preoperative anemia is associated with adverse outcomes in surgery.[88-90] Anemia levels act as an inverted sliding scale, with higher mortality seen in patients with lower preoperative Hgb. The effect of blood loss on mortality was also more pronounced in patients with lower versus higher preoperative Hgb values. When preexisting comorbidities and other confounders were considered, preoperative anemia continued to be independently associated with adverse outcomes after cardiac and noncardiac surgery. Even relatively mild preoperative anemia was shown to be an independent risk factor for higher early mortality in cardiac surgeries,[89] and for 30-day morbidity and mortality in patients undergoing major noncardiac surgery.[90]

Given the risks of preoperative anemia, both patients and hospitals may benefit from a preoperative anemia assessment program for all surgical patients. When possible, this assessment should be undertaken 28 days before surgery, to correct anemia with oral iron when possible, and IV iron or erythropoietin when necessary and not contraindicated. Hematologists should be consulted for cases of refractory anemia.

Perioperative blood management is the third pillar of a strong PBM program. Blood sparing surgical techniques and anesthesiology-based blood conservation tools should be used whenever possible. Minimizing perioperative blood loss reduces the need for RBC transfusion and the length of hospital stay.[91] Together the combination of a restrictive transfusion strategy, preoperative anemia correction and perioperative blood management has been shown to reduce RBC transfusions, decrease adverse events and reduce hospital costs.[91]

REFERENCES

1. Whitaker BI, Henry RA: *2011 National Blood Collection and Utilization Survey Report*. United States Department of Health and Human Services, Rockville, MD, 2011.
2. McCullough J: The nation's changing blood supply system. *JAMA* 269:2239, 1993.
3. World Health Organization: Blood transfusion safety: Blood system strengthening. http://www.who.int/bloodsafety/transfusion_services/en/
4. Eastlund T: Monetary blood donation incentives and the risk of transfusion-transmitted infection. *Transfusion* 38:874, 1998.
5. Dybul M: Partnerships for blood safety in Africa: The US President's emergency plan for AIDS relief. *Transfusion* 48:1044, 2008.
6. Riley W, Schwei M, McCullough J: The United States' potential blood donor pool: Estimating the prevalence of donor exclusion factors on the pool of potential donors. *Transfusion* 47:1180, 2007.
7. McCullough J: *Transfusion Medicine*, 3rd ed. Wiley-Blackwell, Oxford, UK, 2011.
8. Eder AF, Dy BA, Kennedy JM, et al: The American Red Cross donor hemovigilance program: Complications of blood donation reported in 2006. *Transfusion* 48:1809, 2008.
9. Goldman M, Osmond L, Yi QL, et al: Frequency and risk factors for donor reactions in an anonymous blood donor survey. *Transfusion* 53:1979, 2013.
10. Goodnough LT, Rednick S, Price TH, et al: Increased preoperative collection of autologous blood with recombinant human erythropoietin therapy. *N Engl J Med* 321:1163, 1989.
11. Spivak JL: Recombinant human erythropoietin and its role in transfusion medicine. *Transfusion* 34:1, 1994.
12. Williams AE, Kleinman S, Gilcher RO, et al: The prevalence of infectious disease markers in directed versus homologous blood donations [abstract]. *Transfusion* 32:45S, 1992.
13. Luten M, Roerdinkholder-Stoelwinder B, Rombout-Sestrienkova E, et al: Red cell concentrates of hemochromatosis patients comply with the storage guidelines for transfusion purposes. *Transfusion* 48:436, 2008.
14. Shi PA, Ness PM: Two-unit red cell apheresis and its potential advantages over traditional whole-blood donation. *Transfusion* 39:219, 1999.
15. McCullough J, Clay M, Herr G, et al: Effects of granulocyte colony stimulating factor (G-CSF) on potential normal granulocyte donors. *Transfusion* 39:1136, 1999.
16. Herwaldt BL, Linden JV, Bosserman E, et al: Transfusion-associated babesiosis in the United States: a description of cases. *Ann Intern Med* 155:509, 2011.
17. Busch MP, Young MJ, Samson SM, et al: Risk of human immunodeficiency virus (HIV) transmission by blood transfusions before the implementation of HIV-1 antibody screening. *Transfusion* 31:4, 1991.
18. Dodd RY, Notari EP, Stramer SL: Current prevalence and incidence of infectious disease markers and estimated window-period risk in the American Red Cross blood donor population. *Transfusion* 42:975, 2002.
19. Hebert PC, Wells G, Blajchman MA, et al: A multicenter, randomized, controlled clinical trial of transfusion requirements in critical care. *N Engl J Med* 340(6):409, 1999.
20. Villanueva C, Colomo A, Bosch A, et al: Transfusion strategies for acute upper gastrointestinal bleeding. *N Engl J Med* 368(1):11, 2013.
21. Hebert PC, Yetisir E, Martin C, et al: Is a low transfusion threshold safe in critically ill patients with cardiovascular diseases? *Crit Care Med* 29(2):227, 2001.
22. Carson JL, Terrin ML, Noveck H, et al: Liberal or restrictive transfusion in high-risk patients after hip surgery. *N Engl J Med* 365(26):2453, 2011.
23. Hajjar LA, Vincent JL, Galas FR, et al: Transfusion requirements after cardiac surgery: The TRACS randomized controlled trial. *JAMA* 304(14):1559, 2010.
24. Foss NB, Kristensen MT, Kehlet H: Anaemia impedes functional mobility after hip fracture surgery. *Age Ageing* 37(2):173, 2008.
25. Foss NB, Kristensen MT, Jensen PS, et al: The effects of liberal versus restrictive transfusion thresholds on ambulation after hip fracture surgery. *Transfusion* 49(2):227, 2009.
26. Desjardins P, Turgeon AF, Tremblay MH, et al: Hemoglobin levels and transfusions in neurocritically ill patients: A systematic review of comparative studies. *Crit Care* 16(2):R54, 2012.
27. Lacroix J, Hebert PC, Hutchison JS, et al: Transfusion strategies for patients in pediatric intensive care units. *N Engl J Med* 356(16):1609, 2007.
28. Rouette J, Trottier H, Ducruet T, et al: Red blood cell transfusion threshold in postsurgical pediatric intensive care patients: A randomized clinical trial. *Ann Surg* 251(3):421, 2010.
29. Willems A, Harrington K, Lacroix J, et al: Comparison of two red-cell transfusion strategies after pediatric cardiac surgery: A subgroup analysis. *Crit Care Med* 38(2):649, 2010.
30. Karam O, Tucci M, Ducruet T, et al: Red blood cell transfusion thresholds in pediatric patients with sepsis. *Pediatr Crit Care Med* 12(5):512, 2011.
31. Bell EF, Strauss RG, Widness JA, et al: Randomized trial of liberal versus restrictive guidelines for red blood cell transfusion in preterm infants. *Pediatrics* 115(6):1685, 2005.
32. Kirpalani H, Whyte RK, Andersen C, et al: The premature infants in need of transfusion (PINT) study: A randomized, controlled trial of a restrictive (low) versus liberal (high) transfusion threshold for extremely low birth weight infants. *J Pediatr* 149(3):301, 2006.
33. Whyte R, Kirpalani H: Low versus high haemoglobin concentration threshold for blood transfusion for preventing morbidity and mortality in very low birth weight infants. *Cochrane Database Syst Rev* (11):CD000512, 2011.
34. DeBaun MR, Gordon M, McKinstry RC, et al: Controlled trial of transfusions for silent cerebral infarcts in sickle cell anemia. *N Engl J Med* 371:699, 2014.
35. Lasalle-Williams M, Nuss R, Le T, et al: Extended red blood cell antigen matching for transfusions in sickle cell disease: A review of a 14-year experience from a single center (CME). *Transfusion* 51(8):1732, 2011.
36. Hendrickson JE, Desmarets M, Deshpande SS, et al: Recipient inflammation affects the frequency and magnitude of immunization to transfused red blood cells. *Transfusion* 46(9):1526, 2006.
37. Chou ST, Jackson T, Vege S, et al: High prevalence of red blood cell alloimmunization in sickle cell disease despite transfusion from Rh-matched minority donors. *Blood* 122(6):1062, 2013.
38. de Montalembert M, Dumont MD, Heilbronner C, et al: Delayed hemolytic transfusion reaction in children with sickle cell disease. *Haematologica* 96(6):801, 2011.

39. Reid ME, Halter Hipsky C, Hue-Roye K, Hoppe C: Genomic analyses of RH alleles to improve transfusion therapy in patients with sickle cell disease. *Blood Cells Mol Dis* 52(4):195, 2014.

40. Storb R, Prentice RL, Thomas ED: Marrow transplantation for treatment of aplastic anemia. an analysis of factors associated with graft rejection. *N Engl J Med* 296(2):61, 1977.

41. Champlin RE, Horowitz MM, van Bekkum DW, et al: Graft failure following bone marrow transplantation for severe aplastic anemia: Risk factors and treatment results. *Blood* 73(2):606, 1989.

42. Patel SR, Zimring JC: Transfusion-induced bone marrow transplant rejection due to minor histocompatibility antigens. *Transfus Med Rev* 27(4):241, 2013.

43. Webert KE, Cook RJ, Couban S, et al: A multicenter pilot-randomized controlled trial of the feasibility of an augmented red blood cell transfusion strategy for patients treated with induction chemotherapy for acute leukemia or stem cell transplantation. *Transfusion* 48(1):81, 2008.

44. Rowley SD: Hematopoietic stem cell transplantation between red cell incompatible donor-recipient pairs. *Bone Marrow Transplant* 28(4):315, 2001.

45. Petz LD: Immune hemolysis associated with transplantation. *Semin Hematol* 42(3):145, 2005.

46. Vamvakas EC: White-blood-cell-containing allogeneic blood transfusion and postoperative infection or mortality: An updated meta-analysis. *Vox Sang* 92(3):224, 2007.

47. Bowden RA, Slichter SJ, Sayers M, et al: A comparison of filtered leukocyte-reduced and cytomegalovirus (CMV) seronegative blood products for the prevention of transfusion-associated CMV infection after marrow transplant. *Blood* 86(9):3598, 1995.

48. Nash T, Hoffmann S, Butch S, et al: Safety of leukoreduced, cytomegalovirus (CMV)-untested components in CMV-negative allogeneic human progenitor cell transplant recipients. *Transfusion* 52(10):2270, 2012.

49. Thiele T, Kruger W, Zimmermann K, et al: Transmission of cytomegalovirus (CMV) infection by leukoreduced blood products not tested for CMV antibodies: A single-center prospective study in high-risk patients undergoing allogeneic hematopoietic stem cell transplantation (CME). *Transfusion* 51(12):2620, 2011.

50. Ziemann M, Krueger S, Maier AB, et al: High prevalence of cytomegalovirus DNA in plasma samples of blood donors in connection with seroconversion. *Transfusion* 47(11):1972, 2007.

51. Treleaven J, Gennery A, Marsh J, et al: Guidelines on the use of irradiated blood components prepared by the british committee for standards in haematology blood transfusion task force. *Br J Haematol* 152(1):35, 2011.

52. Obrador GT, Macdougall IC: Effect of red cell transfusions on future kidney transplantation. *Clin J Am Soc Nephrol* 8(5):852, 2013.

53. Reed A, Pirsch J, Armbrust MJ, et al: Multivariate analysis of donor-specific versus random transfusion protocols in haploidentical living-related transplants. *Transplantation* 51(2):382, 1991.

54. Christiaans MH, van Hooff JP, Nieman F, van den Berg-Loonen EM: HLA-DR matched transfusions: Development of donor-specific T- and B-cell antibodies and renal allograft outcome. *Transplantation* 67(7):1029, 1999.

55. Pineda AA, Brzica SM Jr, Taswell HF: Hemolytic transfusion reaction. recent experience in a large blood bank. *Mayo Clin Proc* 53(6):378, 1978.

56. Linden JV, Wagner K, Voytovich AE, Sheehan J: Transfusion errors in New York State: An analysis of 10 years' experience. *Transfusion* 40(10):1207, 2000.

57. Davenport RD: The role of cytokines in hemolytic transfusion reactions. *Immunol Invest* 24(1-2):319, 1995.

58. Sazama K. Reports of 355 transfusion-associated deaths: 1976 through 1985. *Transfusion* 30(7):583, 1990.

59. Cohn CS, Stubbs J, Schwartz J, et al: A comparison of adverse reaction rates for PAS C versus plasma platelet units. *Transfusion* 54(8):1927, 2014.

60. Marti-Carvajal AJ, Sola I, Gonzalez LE, et al: Pharmacological interventions for the prevention of allergic and febrile non-haemolytic transfusion reactions. *Cochrane Database Syst Rev* (6):CD007539, 2010.

61. Tobian AA, King KE, Ness PM: Prevention of febrile nonhemolytic and allergic transfusion reactions with pretransfusion medication: Is this evidence-based medicine? *Transfusion* 48(11):2274, 2008.

62. Savage WJ, Tobian AA, Savage JH, et al: Scratching the surface of allergic transfusion reactions. *Transfusion* 53(6):1361, 2013.

63. Goldman M, Webert KE, Arnold DM, et al: Proceedings of a consensus conference: Towards an understanding of TRALI. *Transfus Med Rev* 19(1):2, 2005.

64. Marik PE, Corwin HL: Acute lung injury following blood transfusion: Expanding the definition. *Crit Care Med* 36(11):3080, 2008.

65. Silliman CC, Voelkel NF, Allard JD, et al: Plasma and lipids from stored packed red blood cells cause acute lung injury in an animal model. *J Clin Invest* 101(7):1458, 1998.

66. Bux J, Sachs UJ: The pathogenesis of transfusion-related acute lung injury (TRALI). *Br J Haematol* 136(6):788, 2007.

67. Eder AF, Dy BA, Perez JM, Rambaud M, Benjamin RJ: The residual risk of transfusion-related acute lung injury at the American Red Cross (2008–2011): Limitations of a predominantly male-donor plasma mitigation strategy. *Transfusion* 53(7):1442, 2013.

68. Report of the US Department of Health and Human Services: *The 2010 National Blood Collection and Utilization Survey Report.* US Department of Health and Human Services, Washington, DC, 2011.

69. Flesland O: A comparison of complication rates based on published haemovigilance data. *Intensive Care Med* 33 Suppl 1:S17, 2007.

70. Popovsky MA, Audet AM, Andrzejewski C Jr: Transfusion-associated circulatory overload in orthopedic surgery patients: A multi-institutional study. *Immunohematology* 12(2):87, 1996.

71. Narick C, Triulzi DJ, Yazer MH: Transfusion-associated circulatory overload after plasma transfusion. *Transfusion* 52(1):160, 2012.

72. Robillard P, Nawej K, Chapdelaine A: Transfusion-associated circulatory overload (TACO): Current leading cause of transfusion-associated fatalities reported to the Quebec hemovigilance system. *Transfus Med* 19:280, 2009.

73. Li G, Rachmale S, Kojicic M, et al: Incidence and transfusion risk factors for transfusion-associated circulatory overload among medical intensive care unit patients. *Transfusion* 51(2):338, 2011.

74. Li G, Daniels CE, Kojicic M, et al: The accuracy of natriuretic peptides (brain natriuretic peptide and N-terminal pro-brain natriuretic) in the differentiation between transfusion-related acute lung injury and transfusion-related circulatory overload in the critically ill. *Transfusion* 49(1):13, 2009.

75. Kuehnert MJ, Roth VR, Haley NR, et al: Transfusion-transmitted bacterial infection in the United States, 1998 through 2000. *Transfusion* 41(12):1493, 2001.

76. Triulzi D, Duquesnoy R, Nichols L, et al: Fatal transfusion-associated graft-versus-host disease in an immunocompetent recipient of a volunteer unit of red cells. *Transfusion* 46(6):885, 2006.

77. Petz LD, Calhoun L, Yam P, et al: Transfusion-associated graft-versus-host disease in immunocompetent patients: Report of a fatal case associated with transfusion of blood from a second-degree relative, and a survey of predisposing factors. *Transfusion* 33(9):742, 1993.

78. Moroff G, Luban NL: The irradiation of blood and blood components to prevent graft-versus-host disease: Technical issues and guidelines. *Transfus Med Rev* 11(1):15, 1997.

79. Weiskopf RB, Feiner J, Toy P, et al: Fresh and stored red blood cell transfusion equivalently induce subclinical pulmonary gas exchange deficit in normal humans. *Anesth Analg* 114(3):511, 2012.

80. Berra L, Coppadoro A, Yu B, et al: Transfusion of stored autologous blood does not alter reactive hyperemia index in healthy volunteers. *Anesthesiology* 117(1):56, 2012.

81. Weiskopf RB, Feiner J, Hopf H, et al: Fresh blood and aged stored blood are equally efficacious in immediately reversing anemia-induced brain oxygenation deficits in humans. *Anesthesiology* 104(5):911, 2006.

82. Hod EA, Brittenham GM, Billote GB, et al: Transfusion of human volunteers with older, stored red blood cells produces extravascular hemolysis and circulating non-transferrin-bound iron. *Blood* 118(25):6675, 2011.

83. Koch CG, Li L, Sessler DI, et al: Duration of red-cell storage and complications after cardiac surgery. *N Engl J Med* 358(12):1229, 2008.

84. Aubron C, Nichol A, Cooper DJ, Bellomo R: Age of red blood cells and transfusion in critically ill patients. *Ann Intensive Care* 3:1, 2013.

85. Wang D, Sun J, Solomon SB, Klein HG, Natanson C: Transfusion of older stored blood and risk of death: A meta-analysis. *Transfusion* 52(6):1184, 2012.

86. Fernandez Perez ER, Winters JL, Gajic O: The addition of decision support into computerized physician order entry reduces red blood cell transfusion resource utilization in the intensive care unit. *Am J Hematol* 82(7):631, 2007.

87. Cohn CS, Welbig J, Bowman R, et al: A data-driven approach to patient blood management. *Transfusion* 54(2):316, 2014.

88. Carson JL, Duff A, Poses RM, et al: Effect of anaemia and cardiovascular disease on surgical mortality and morbidity. *Lancet* 348(9034):1055, 1996.

89. van Straten AH, Hamad MA, van Zundert AJ, et al: Preoperative hemoglobin level as a predictor of survival after coronary artery bypass grafting: A comparison with the matched general population. *Circulation* 120(2):118, 2009.

90. Musallam KM, Tamim HM, Richards T, et al: Preoperative anaemia and postoperative outcomes in non-cardiac surgery: A retrospective cohort study. *Lancet* 378(9800):1396, 2011.

91. Spahn DR. Anemia and patient blood management in hip and knee surgery: A systematic review of the literature. *Anesthesiology* 113(2):482, 2010.

CHAPTER 139
PRESERVATION AND CLINICAL USE OF PLATELETS

Terry Gernsheimer and Sherrill Slichter

SUMMARY

The numbers of platelet transfusions administered in the United States increased dramatically during the 1980s, and has continued to grow as increasingly aggressive medical and surgical treatments have been developed and become more widely available. In particular, the growth of more intensive treatments for hematologic and other malignancies has spurred demands for platelet transfusion support and put pressure on platelet inventories nationwide.

The response to a platelet transfusion is affected by platelet recovery and platelet survival and includes the random loss of platelets in maintaining endothelial integrity. In a normal individual, weighing 70 kg, approximately 4.8×10^{10} platelets per day will be consumed maintaining the endothelium, less than the number of platelets in a single concentrate. However, many clinical conditions can adversely affect platelet recovery and platelet survival in the circulation. Prophylactic platelet transfusion is an important part of supportive care of patients with hypoproliferative thrombocytopenia because of hematologic malignancy and the effects of its treatment with cytotoxic drugs. A morning blood platelet count of less than 10×10^9/L appears to be an appropriate threshold for prophylactic transfusion. Although higher thresholds may be indicated for patients at high risk or who have active bleeding, little or no data support specific platelet count goals and a transfusion plan should be guided by the clinical setting. Larger doses of platelets do not confer additional protection against bleeding in this patient population, although they do result in higher increments and a longer interval until the next platelet transfusion, a potential benefit in the outpatient setting. The platelet count at which an invasive procedure or major surgery can be safely performed is not supported by randomized control studies and practice has been governed by retrospective data and case reports. Most minor invasive procedures and even major surgery can be safely performed at platelet counts of 20 to 50×10^9/L whereas high-risk procedures or severe bleeding may require platelet counts above 100×10^9/L. Patients may become refractory to platelet transfusion and fail to respond for many reasons. Patients alloimmunized to platelets may respond to platelet transfusions from class I human leukocyte antigen (HLA)-matched donors.

Platelets can be collected by apheresis or obtained from whole blood and pooled for transfusion. Both preparations have comparable effectiveness in the prevention of bleeding in patients with hematologic malignancy. Platelets should remain at room temperature and so are approved for only 5 days of storage because of risks of bacterial contamination and may lose viability within days after that. Leukocyte reduction of platelet components, either upon apheresis collection or by filtration, reduces HLA alloimmunization, prevents cytomegalovirus transmission by transfusion, and reduces febrile transfusion reactions. Pathogen reduction of platelets prevents replication of RNA and DNA in contaminating organisms and leukocytes and may prevent alloimmunization and decrease transfusion reactions. Prospective clinical trials are needed to better define indications for platelet transfusion and improve upon the effectiveness of transfusion therapy.

CLINICAL PLATELET TRANSFUSION THERAPY

The number of platelet units transfused in the United States increased by 33 percent between the years 1997 and 2008 (data available at the time of this writing).[1] Of more than 2,000,000 doses of platelets transfused in the United States in 2008, hematology-oncology patients used 32 percent, compared to the next highest usage of 15 percent in general medicine and 12 percent in cardiac surgery patients. Platelet transfusion therapy is associated with multiple adverse effects, including transfusion reactions, infection, alloimmunization, and immune modulation. The cost of platelets, their short storage time, and inventory pressures have made appropriate use of platelet transfusions a high priority for the management of thrombocytopenic patients to either prevent or control bleeding. Improved methods of collecting, processing, and storing platelets will be paramount in maintaining platelet inventories in the coming decade.

EXPECTED RESPONSE TO A PROPHYLACTIC PLATELET TRANSFUSION

The expected response to a prophylactic platelet transfusion in nonrefractory thrombocytopenic patients is assessed by two parameters: (1) the number of platelets that circulate immediately after transfusion, as measured by platelet recovery; and (2) the survival time of the transfused platelet as measured by days-to-next-transfusion. Platelets circulate for a shorter time in thrombocytopenic patients (≤ 5 days) compared with normal subjects (8 to 10 days).[2] This can be explained by the two mechanisms by which platelets are lost from circulation: (1) senescence, whereby platelets are removed by the mononuclear phagocyte system, and (2) random, whereby platelets are consumed during hemostasis to provide endothelial support.[3] The random loss has been estimated to be 7.1×10^9 platelets/L per day. Thus, the more thrombocytopenic a patient is, the higher the percentage of their circulating platelets that will be removed randomly versus lost by senescence (Fig. 139–1A). At a platelet count of 300×10^9/L, approximately 15 percent of the platelets will be randomly removed—a fraction too small to influence the overall platelet survival. However, in a patient with a platelet count of 50×10^9/L, approximately 60 percent of the platelets will be

Acronyms and Abbreviations: AML, acute myeloid leukemia; AP, apheresis platelet; BC, buffy coat; CCI, corrected count increment; GVHD, graft-versus-host disease; HIT, heparin-induced thrombocytopenia; HLA, human leukocyte antigen; HSCT, hematopoietic stem cell transplant; ITP, immune thrombocytopenia; LP, lumbar puncture; PLADO, Platelet Dose study; PRP, platelet-rich plasma; PROPPR, Pragmatic Randomized Optimal Platelet and Plasma Ratios study; rdWBP, random-donor whole-blood platelet; TOPPS, Therapeutic or Prophylactic Platelet Transfusion Study; TPO, thrombopoietin; TTP, thrombotic thrombocytopenic purpura; TRAP, Trial to Reduce Alloimmunization to Platelets; WHO, World Health Organization.

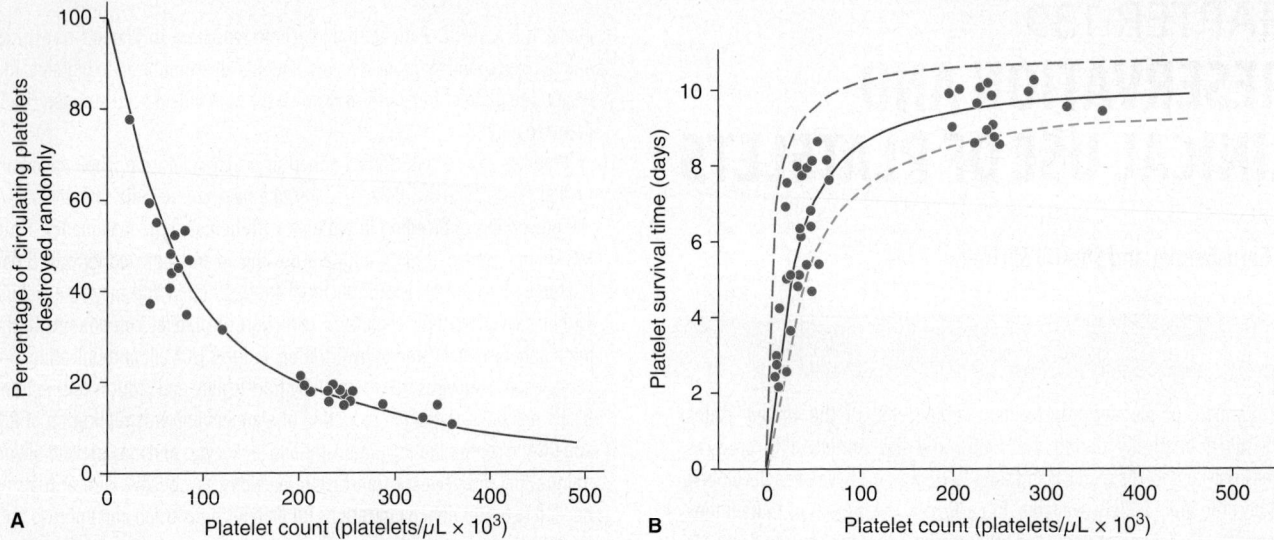

Figure 139–1. A. Relationship between platelet count and random platelet destruction. Studies were performed on healthy volunteers receiving autologous radiolabeled platelets as well as on patients receiving allogeneic platelet transfusions. Data points were obtained by dividing the fixed number of platelets lost per day by the number of circulating platelets lost from turnover.[3] **B.** Relationship between platelet count and radiolabeled platelet survival measurements in healthy and thrombocytopenic patients. The curve (*solid line*) was obtained from an equation predicting the dependence of platelet life span on platelet count, assuming a fixed platelet requirement. The data show a high correlation of a finite rate of random platelet destruction per day with a fixed life span of the platelets.[3]

used for endothelial support, and this will have a significant impact on reducing platelet survival time. This random platelet loss at low platelet counts results in a direct relationship between platelet count and platelet survival at platelet counts of less than 100×10^9/L (Fig. 139–1B).

The number of platelets needed daily to support the random loss of platelets in maintaining endothelial integrity can be calculated. For example, a man weighing 70 kg with an estimated blood volume of 5 L would need 7.1×10^9 platelets/L per day, thus 3.6×10^{10} platelets per day. To account for the platelets pooled in the spleen, an additional 30 percent should be added giving a daily requirement of 4.8×10^{10} platelets for endothelial support. As one random donor platelet concentrate contains on average 8.3×10^{10} platelets, the daily requirement for endothelial support should be easily maintained with the transfusion of only one platelet concentrate per day. A somewhat higher number of platelet concentrates may be needed for patients who are also consuming transfused platelets based on clinical conditions such as sepsis, extensive tumor burden, and others.

PATIENTS WITH HEMATOLOGIC MALIGNANCY

Bleeding Risks

Prior to the availability of platelets for transfusion, observational studies found the incidence of spontaneous bleeding increases at platelets counts of 100×10^9/L or less in children with acute leukemia,[4] but minor and major bleeding began to increase (>1 percent chance of observable bleeding per patient-day) when the platelet count fell below 50×10^9/L. Major bleeding was only observed below 20×10^9/L, and on only 3 percent of days. Major bleeding was much more common below a platelet count of 5×10^9/L, as high as 33 percent as the count fell toward zero. Notably, many of the patients observed in this study were treated with aspirin for pain and fever resulting in some degree of platelet dysfunction that likely increased their bleeding risk. More recent observations suggest that the amount of bleeding is not dependent on the platelet count as long as it is above 5×10^9/L.[2,5] Life-threatening bleeding rarely

occurs above platelet counts of 5×10^9/L to 10×10^9/L without disruption of the vessel wall. In the Platelet Dose (PLADO) study, bleeding occurred on 17 percent of the study days at platelet counts between 6×10^9/L and 85×10^9/L and increased to 25 percent when counts fell below 6×10^9/L.[6] These data are remarkably consistent with the increase in bleeding time when platelet counts fall below 100×10^9/L,[7] although the bleeding time is not an accurate enough test to be relied upon clinically. There was also a marked increase in bleeding at platelet counts below 5×10^9/L as determined by stool blood loss measurements.[2]

Most recent large platelet transfusion trials have used the World Health Organization (WHO) bleeding scale or some modification of this scale to standardize the incidence and severity of bleeding in thrombocytopenic patients (Table 139–1).[8] Grade 1 bleeding is noticeable but without clinical significance. Grade 2 bleeding, which requires some minor intervention to control bleeding, is an observable and reliable measurement for monitoring bleeding risk in platelet transfusion trials. It occurs frequently enough to be a useful end point for comparison of bleeding incidence and severity with different platelet transfusion strategies. In two large platelet transfusion trials, the incidence of Grade 2 bleeding in patients being treated for hematologic malignancies with chemotherapy was between 38 and 73 percent.[6,9] In patients undergoing autologous hematopoietic stem cell transplantation (HSCT), bleeding rates were 45 percent and 57 percent; however, it was much higher (79 percent) in patients undergoing allogeneic HSCT. The 79 percent bleeding rate in allogeneic HSCT patients is likely because of their intensive conditioning therapies and the occurrence of graft-versus-host disease (GVHD).

In a study of 1244 hematology-oncology patients, the 198 pediatric patients had a significantly higher overall risk of Grade 2 or higher bleeding than did adults (86 percent, 88 percent, and 77 percent for patients ages 0 to 5 years, 6 to 12 years, and 13 to 18 years, respectively, vs. 67 percent for adults).[10] Children also experienced more days with Grade 2 or higher bleeding (median: 3 days in each pediatric group vs. 1 day in adults; p <0.001). The pediatric patients were at higher risk of

TABLE 139–1. General Criteria for World Health Organization Bleeding Grade Categories Including Grade 2a Modification

Grade 1	Grade 2	Grade 3	Grade 4
Minor bleeding	Bleeding requires intervention or treatment, e.g., nasal packing, bladder irrigation, platelet transfusion or medications, to treat bleeding Grade 2a: Grade 2 bleeding excluding skin manifestations	Bleeding requires red cell transfusion related to treatment of bleeding *or* Significant intervention to treat bleeding, e.g., endoscopy or surgery	Bleeding that is fatal or life-threatening

bleeding over a wide range of platelet counts, indicating that their excess bleeding risk may be a result of factors other than just platelets.

Platelet Transfusion Therapy in the Patient with Hematologic Malignancy

Hematologic malignancies accounted for approximately 9 percent of all new cancers reported in the United States in 2012.[11] More aggressive therapies have led to increased 5-year survival rates, but also resulted in substantial increases in the demand for platelet transfusions to support extended periods of marrow failure. The disturbance of endothelial integrity that frequently occurs with these therapies[12] and the associated inflammation can induce hemorrhage in periods of thrombocytopenia.[13] Mucositis, GVHD, infection, and organ dysfunction can all increase daily platelet consumption and negatively affect posttransfusion platelet increments and life span. Multiple strategies have been evaluated for maximizing the hemostatic effect of platelets while minimizing platelet use. Prospective randomized controlled trials have evaluated the relative safety of different platelet count thresholds for transfusion, whether platelets should be transfused prophylactically or can be administered therapeutically at the first sign of bleeding, and optimal platelet dose for platelet transfusion.

Platelet Transfusion Threshold

Prophylactic platelet transfusions were shown to decrease the incidence of bleeding into vital organs noted at autopsy of leukemia patients as early as 1966,[14] and have become an integral part of treatment regimens for hematologic malignancy. However, maintaining platelet counts may be difficult owing to very short platelet survivals in severely thrombocytopenic patients.[2,6,15] Several prospective randomized platelet transfusion trials have shown no differences in spontaneous bleeding events when patients are transfused at platelet counts below 10×10^9/L versus 20×10^9/L[16–18] or even versus 30×10^9/L,[19] and a threshold for transfusion as low as 5×10^9/L may be safe.[20] In one study, 85 patients with acute leukemia were randomized to receive prophylactic platelet transfusions when their platelet count fell to 20×10^9/L, 10×10^9/L, or 5×10^9/L.[20] An aliquot of each patient's red cells were labeled with radioactive ^{51}chromium and daily stool collections were performed to quantify the amount of gastrointestinal mucosal bleeding. There were no differences in stool blood loss, red blood cell transfusion rates, or incidence of bleeding events among the three study arms. However, there was a significant decrease in both the frequency and number of platelet transfusions required among patients randomized to the lower

transfusion threshold compared to the higher transfusion thresholds. A platelet transfusion threshold of less than 10×10^9/L in stable patients has been recommended by both the American Association of Blood Banks (AABB)[21] and Sanquin Blood Supply in 2014.[22] Patients with active infection, fever, or who are bleeding may require higher transfusion thresholds.[23]

Prophylactic Versus Therapeutic Platelet Transfusions

WHO Grade 4 bleeding that causes life threatening hemorrhage or death is a rare occurence.[6,9] Several prospective trials have evaluated the potential bleeding risk of withholding platelet transfusions until WHO Grade 2 bleeding occurs with the assumption that Grade 4 bleeding would very rarely take place before Grade 2 bleeding was observed. A trial comparing a therapeutic-only transfusion strategy versus prophylactic platelet transfusion given routinely for a morning platelet count of less than 10×10^9/L in 396 patients who were undergoing intensive chemotherapy for acute myeloid leukemia (AML) (n = 190) or autologous HSCT patients (n = 201) monitored patients for bleeding according to the WHO bleeding scale.[24] Despite randomization to the therapeutic-only transfusion arm, 30 percent of patients were transfused with platelets prophylactically and 22 percent for extended petechiae or bruising. The primary end point (number of platelet transfusions) was 33.5 percent higher in the prophylactic transfusion group. However, Grade 4 bleeding occurred in 14 patients with AML in the therapeutic-only transfusion arm, two of which were fatal cerebral hemorrhages. No Grade 4 bleeding occurred in patients undergoing autologous HSCT. In the Therapeutic or Prophylactic Platelet Study (TOPPS), 600 patients with acute leukemia, lymphoma, or myeloma undergoing chemotherapy alone (n = 98), autologous HSCT (n = 411) or reduced-intensity allogeneic HSCT (n = 74) were randomized to a therapeutic-only or prophylactic transfusion strategy.[9] Patients in the therapeutic-only transfusion arm had a significantly shorter time to their first Grade 2 or greater bleeding event, and they also experienced more bleeding overall. Although both of these studies showed a decrease in the number of platelet transfusions administered in the therapeutic-only arms compared to the prophylactic transfusion arms, and there were no differences in the number of red cell transfusions, this strategy cannot be considered safe in the majority of patients undergoing HSCT or induction chemotherapy for acute leukemia.

Platelet Dose

It has been estimated that 4.8×10^{10} platelets are used daily to maintain endothelial integrity in an individual weighing 70 kg with an estimated blood volume of 5 L.[3] As long as this minimal number of platelets is provided, higher platelet doses do not appear to decrease the incidence of bleeding in patients with hematologic malignancy. The PLADO trial studied more than 1200 patients with hematologic malignancies who were receiving prophylactic platelet transfusions at a threshold of less than 10×10^9/L during chemotherapy or HSCT.[6] Patients were randomized to one of three platelet doses; the accepted current standard dose of 2.2×10^{11} platelets/m^2 (expected to be equivalent to four to six pooled platelet concentrates or one apheresis platelet [AP] collection in most adults), a low dose of 1.1×10^{11}/m^2 (half of standard), or a high dose of 4.4×10^{11}/m^2 (twice standard). WHO Grade 2 bleeding was common in all patients and similar at all doses. Seventy percent of patients had at least one episode of Grade 2 or greater bleeding with no significant differences among the dose groups (71 percent, 69 percent, and 70 percent, respectively). Grade 3 bleeding occurred in 8 percent of patients and Grade 4 in only 2 percent with no differences among the groups. Only one hemorrhagic death occurred, in a patient in the high-dose group. By treatment category, 79 percent of patients undergoing allogeneic HSCT had at least one episode of Grade 2 or greater bleeding compared to 73 percent of patients undergoing chemotherapy for hematologic malignancy, and 57 percent of autologous or syngeneic HSCT patients. There were no differences in bleeding risk based on transfused platelet dose among any of these patient categories. Lower platelet doses required fewer number of platelets overall, but more frequent transfusions to maintain a platelet threshold of 10×10^9/L. However, as the cost of platelet therapy is predominantly related to the number of transfused platelets rather than the frequency of administration, low-dose therapy may be the most cost-effective strategy, at least during hospitalization.[25] Platelet transfusion intervals were significantly longer in the higher-dose groups, resulting in fewer transfusion events, which may make higher-dose transfusions the preferred strategy for outpatients.

EFFECT OF THROMBOPOIETIN MIMETICS ON PLATELET TRANSFUSION REQUIREMENTS

Only mild shortening of the period of thrombocytopenia in patients undergoing chemotherapy for hematologic malignancy has been observed with the use of thrombopoietin mimetic agents. Treatment with romiplostim, a thrombopoietin (TPO) receptor agonist, in patients with low-risk/intermediate-1–risk myelodysplastic syndrome increased platelet counts and decreased the number of bleeding events and platelet transfusions. Although the study drug was discontinued because of an initial concern of risk of progression to AML, survival and AML rates were similar in patients receiving romiplostim and a placebo.[26] At this time, TPO receptor agonists cannot be routinely recommended as an adjunct to or replacement for platelet transfusions in patients with hypoproliferative thrombocytopenia, but clinical trials are ongoing.

PLATELET TRANSFUSION THRESHOLDS FOR INVASIVE PROCEDURES

Little data exist to guide platelet transfusions in patients who are undergoing invasive procedures.[27] Most recommendations are based on reports of "no harm" observed in groups of patients undergoing planned procedures. Some implications can be drawn from bleeding time measurements performed at various platelet counts (Fig. 139–2).[7] At platelet

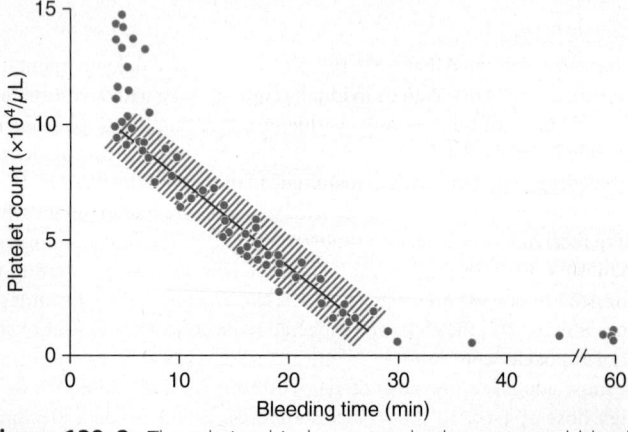

Figure 139–2. The relationship between platelet count and bleeding time. With normal platelet function, bleeding time above a platelet count of greater than 100×10^9/L is maintained at approximately 5 minutes. Bleeding time has an inverse relationship with platelet count below a platelet count of 100×10^9/L, prolonging as the platelet count decreases. *(Reproduced with permission from Harker LA, Slichter SJ: The bleeding time as a screening test for evaluation of platelet function. N Engl J Med 27;287(4):155–159. 1972.)*

counts of 100×10^9/L or greater, the bleeding time averages approximately 5 minutes. At platelet counts of less than 100×10^9/L, there is an inverse relationship between platelet count and bleeding time; that is, as the platelet count decreases, the bleeding time increases.[7] Figure 139–2 provides a graphical comparison of bleeding times at different platelet counts but does not predict the risk of bleeding at surgery. Neither platelet counts nor bleeding times are exact measurements, and small differences in platelet counts are unlikely to make a significant difference in the time it takes for bleeding to cease. The need for a prophylactic platelet transfusion for an invasive procedure must consider platelet count, platelet function, and endothelial integrity, as well as the consequences of prolonged bleeding. Procedures that would result in significant harm with even small amounts of bleeding (e.g., neurosurgical procedures) should probably be performed at higher platelet counts ($\geq 100 \times 10^9$/L), although most procedures can safely be performed at lower platelet levels. Abnormal coagulation parameters, drugs or diseases (e.g., uremia) that inhibit platelet function should be corrected as much as possible before any procedure. Although international guidelines exist for platelet counts at which a procedure can be safely performed, evidence for these recommendations are generally weak and of low quality.[22,27]

Platelet Transfusion for Minor Invasive Procedures

Central Venous Catheter Placement Observational studies of central venous catheter placement have reported low bleeding rates of 0 to 9 percent. The largest study included the placement of 604 nontunneled catheters in 193 consecutive patients and found only patients with preprocedure platelet counts below 20×10^9/L were at increased risk of bleeding compared to those with counts above 100×10^9/L.[28] Ninety-six percent of bleeding events were Grade 1, and the remaining were Grade 2, requiring only local compression for bleeding cessation. A study of 3170 tunneled catheter placements under ultrasound guidance reported no bleeding complications in 344 patients with platelet counts less than 50×10^9/L, nor in the 42 patients with even lower platelet counts of 25×10^9/L or less.[29]

Lumbar Puncture Lumbar puncture (LP) can often be safely performed at platelet counts below 20×10^9/L. A study of 5223 LPs performed in 956 pediatric leukemic patients reported that 941 procedures were done at or below 50×10^9/L, with 199 done below 21×10^9/L, with no bleeding complications.[30] Even in those patients who had a traumatic LP (>500 red blood cells/high power field), which occurred in 10.5 percent of the patients, there were no adverse clinical outcomes. In a study in 66 adults with acute leukemia undergoing 195 LPs, there were no bleeding complications in the 40 LPs performed at platelet counts of 31 to 50 × 10^9/L nor in the 35 LPs performed at platelet counts of 20 to 30 × 10^9/L.[31]

Major Invasive Procedures

High-level evidence is again lacking for determining a safe platelet count for major invasive procedures. At this time there are no data to support increased perioperative bleeding risk in patients with platelet counts below 50×10^9/L who are undergoing major surgery.[32] However, the presence of other hemostatic abnormalities, especially platelet dysfunction, should be considered. Although there is no evidence to support platelet transfusion in the nonbleeding cardiac surgery patient, a bleeding patient post–cardiopulmonary bypass may benefit from platelet transfusion, even in the setting of a normal platelet count as a result of the detrimental effect of bypass on platelet function.[33] The patient undergoing major neuraxial surgery may require higher platelet counts perioperatively to minimize increased accumulation of blood in an enclosed space. Although no specific evidence supports the practice other than normalization of the bleeding time, a platelet count of 100×10^9/L is generally accepted as appropriate for major neurosurgical procedures.[21,22]

The Thrombocytopenic Patient on Anticoagulation Therapy

Anticoagulation itself does not slow the formation of the primary platelet plug, although a decrease in thrombin generation would slow activation of more platelets and clot stabilization. It is not known whether higher counts are more appropriate for patients on anticoagulation, and if so what the appropriate level would be. Although platelet counts of 40 to 50×10^9/L are often considered to be a safe level for patients anticoagulated with warfarin or heparin therapy,[22] there have been no trials to evaluate whether lower counts would be as safe.

Platelet Transfusion Thresholds for Bleeding A paucity of evidence exists on the target platelet count in bleeding patients. The site of bleeding and other hemostatic abnormalities or drugs that might result in a bleeding tendency should be considered and corrected as needed. A target platelet count of 100×10^9/L should be used in life threatening bleeding such as intracerebral bleeding or diffuse alveolar hemorrhage to minimize compromise of healthy tissue. For diffuse microvascular bleeding, a platelet count of 100×10^9/L is also usually recommended,[22,34] but difficulties of obtaining timely results during massive hemorrhage make the feasibility of this approach unrealistic in the field and in many trauma centers. Retrospective analysis of combat casualties requiring massive transfusion (>10 units in 24 hours) found a transfusion ratio of one AP platelet component to every 8 units of red blood cells to be associated with significantly improved survival at 24 hours and 30 days in combat casualties requiring a massive transfusion (MT) within 24 hours of injury.[35] Equal ratios of plasma, platelets, and red blood cells, is an essential element of the United States Department of Defense "Damage Control Resuscitation" clinical practice guideline for control of massive hemorrhage adopted in 2006.[36] In the Pragmatic Randomized Optimal Platelet and Plasma Ratios (PROPPR) study,[37] 680 patients at level 1 trauma centers requiring massive transfusion were randomized to one of two standard transfusion ratio interventions: 1:1:1 or 1:1:2 (plasma: platelets: red cells), the equivalent of one AP platelet to every 6 or 12 units of red blood cells. Both 24-hour and 30-day mortality were significantly improved when the numbers of platelets and plasma transfusions were increased to a 1:1 ratio with red blood cell transfusions.[38]

The Bleeding Patient on Platelet Inhibitor Therapy

Although aspirin inhibits the production of thromboxane A_2, an effect that lasts for days after ingestion, the drug itself has a relatively short half-life of 2 to 3 hours, whereas other nonsteroidal antiplatelet agents have effects that last less than 24 hours.[39] Thienopyridine-class antiplatelet agents such as clopidogrel have much longer half-lives, as do the active metabolites of these drugs, and may continue to affect platelets for more than a week. Although it is common practice to transfuse platelets to patients treated with these drugs if they suffer serious or life-threatening bleeding, there are no data that have established the effectiveness of platelet transfusions in these patients.

MANAGEMENT OF PATIENTS REFRACTORY TO PLATELET TRANSFUSIONS

The incremental increase in platelet count following a platelet transfusion is dependent upon the platelet dose (number) and the patient's blood volume (which is, in turn, dependent on their body size). The corrected count increment (CCI), generally measured 30 minutes to 1 hour following a platelet transfusion, takes into account both patient size and the dose of platelets transfused and can be calculated by the formula:

$$CCI = \frac{(\text{Posttransfusion Platelet Count} - \text{Pretransfusion Platelet Count})}{\text{Number of Platelets Transfused } (\times 10^{11})}$$

Patients who have a CCI of less than 5×10^9/L on at least two consecutive occasions are considered to be "refractory" to platelet transfusions. As the platelet count of the product is not usually available to the clinician, two sequential 1-hour platelet increments of 11×10^9/L or less may also be used to indicate refractoriness.[40] Platelet refractoriness can be classified as immune or nonimmunologically mediated with the latter being the most common cause of platelet refractoriness.[41] Unfortunately, many patients concurrently experience both types of platelet refractoriness. In the Trial to Reduce Alloimmunization to Platelets (TRAP)[42] that involved 533 patients given 6379 transfusions, the factors that most likely resulted in platelet refractoriness, in order of frequency, were: developing lymphocytotoxic antibodies; being female with two or more pregnancies or male; heparin administration; fever; bleeding; transfusion of γ-irradiated platelets; and receiving an increasing number of platelet transfusions. In addition, platelets express ABO antigen on their surface and occasionally patients with high anti-A agglutinin titers may benefit from ABO-matched platelets.[43] Similar factors are associated with poor platelet responses in many other platelet transfusion studies.[23,44,45]

Active bleeding or denuded endothelium may cause increased platelet consumption so that the incremental increase in platelet count is decreased. Patients with reduced responses to transfused platelets due to increased platelet consumption may benefit from more frequent transfusions. The use of very frequent or continuous ("drip") platelet transfusions in patients with life-threatening bleeding is sometimes undertaken,[46] although no trials of this mode of therapy have been performed.

Patients who have been previously transfused or pregnant may fail to increase their platelet count following transfusion as a consequence of human leukocyte antigen (HLA) antibodies directed against the class I HLA antigens on the platelet surface. Transfusion of leukocyte reduced cellular blood components can reduce the rate of formation of these antibodies.[42] A minority of patients will develop or recall these antibodies and have only minimal or no increase in the platelet count following transfusion. There are a number of methods for HLA antibody testing, either by cell-based or solid-phase assays. Testing can be used to screen for antibodies and to identify antibody specificity to aid in donor selection.[47] The results of these assays are expressed as a percentage of the test cells or beads that bind patient antibodies. Patients with poor responses to platelet transfusions because of HLA antibodies may benefit from HLA-matched platelets, identifying the specificity of the patient's antibodies and avoiding any incompatible antigens or using platelet crossmatching assays to select compatible donors.[43,48,49]

In patients with marked splenomegaly, large doses of platelets may increase the total body platelet mass and increase the platelet count. Platelets are released from the spleen upon injection of epinephrine,[50] suggesting that under times of stress these sequestered platelets may become available for hemostasis. Homologous platelets transfused to patients with immune thrombocytopenia survive only a few hours in the majority of patients studied.[51] Therefore, transfusion of platelets to patients with immune thrombocytopenia is appropriate only for life- or organ-threatening bleeding.[47] Platelet transfusion was associated with an increased risk of arterial thrombosis in patients with thrombotic thrombocytopenic purpura (TTP) and heparin-induced thrombocytopenia (HIT), but not in patients with immune thrombocytopenia (ITP).[52]

Use of Antifibrinolytic Therapy

Tranexamic acid and aminocaproic acid improve bleeding and decrease platelet use in patients with thrombocytopenia associated with hematologic malignancy.[53] The use of antifibrinolytic therapy with tranexamic acid or -ε-aminocaproic acid has been suggested to augment other measures to decrease or prevent bleeding in patients who continue to bleed in spite of platelet transfusions.

●PLATELET PRODUCTS AVAILABLE FOR TRANSFUSION

Platelets are obtained by two different methods: platelet concentrates from whole blood or apheresis platelets. The FDA requires at least 5.5×10^{10} platelets/concentrate and 3.0×10^{11} platelets/apheresis collection.

PLATELET CONCENTRATES FROM WHOLE BLOOD

Platelet concentrates can be prepared from units of whole blood using two different methods as outlined in Fig. 139–3. These are referred to as the platelet-rich plasma (PRP) method, which is used exclusively in the United States,[54] and the buffy coat (BC) method,[55] which is predominantly used in Europe and Canada. Comparative studies show no difference in the quality of these platelet concentrates when they are stored for up to 7 days.[56,57] That there are no differences in these products was confirmed in a controlled trial in which the same normal subjects donated whole blood on two occasions.[58] A buffy-coat platelet concentrate or a PRP platelet concentrate was randomly assigned to be prepared from either the first or second whole-blood donation. After storage for 7 days, the platelets were radiolabeled and transfused back into their normal donor. Recovery differences averaged 3.7 ± 2.4 percent ($\pm$ SE, p = 0.15) and survival differences 0.48 ± 0.56 days (p = 0.41).

APHERESIS PLATELETS

The major advantage of AP platelets is that enough platelets can be collected from a single donor to constitute a transfusion dose. In contrast, to obtain an equivalent number of platelets requires pooling four or five whole-blood–derived platelet concentrates.

The reduction in donor exposures by using AP platelets has the potential advantages of reducing transfusion-transmitted infections and the incidence of platelet alloimmunization. However, the current tests for detecting viral transmission by transfusion have reduced the infectious risk/donor exposure to very low levels.[59] The bacterial risk associated with platelet transfusions is high because platelets are stored at 22°C. Some studies suggest a reduction in bacterial transmission by transfusion with the use of single-donor platelets.[60] However, both the American College of Pathologists and the AABB mandate testing of all platelet products for bacteria,[61] which should reduce this potential advantage of single-donor platelets. Currently, the requirement for bacterial testing has increased the use of APs because the costs for culture-based testing of an apheresis unit versus testing each platelet concentrate that would be used in a pool has provided a significant cost advantage for APs. As platelet concentrates are less expensive to produce, this current cost advantage of APs will likely shift to pooled random donor platelets with more widespread use of prestorage pooling of platelet concentrates allowing bacterial testing of the pool.[62] Certainly, there were no differences in posttransfusion platelet responses between patients given either pre- or poststorage pooled platelet concentrates.[63] Although transfusion reactions may occur less frequently with APs, leukoreduction appears to mitigate this advantage over pooled platelets.[64] In addition, the use of leukoreduced pooled random donor platelets does not appear to lead to increased alloimmunization rates or broaden the specificity of any preexisting or developing antibodies compared to leukoreduced single-donor platelets.[42]

COMPARATIVE EFFECTIVENESS OF PLATELET-RICH PLASMA PLATELET CONCENTRATES VERSUS APHERESIS PLATELETS, ABO MATCHING, STORAGE DURATION, AND ADVERSE EVENTS

Transfusion Responses

Many clinicians consider that platelets obtained by AP give superior posttransfusion platelet responses compared to PRP pooled random-donor whole-blood platelets (rdWBPs). The large

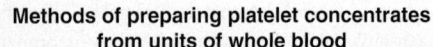

Methods of preparing platelet concentrates from units of whole blood

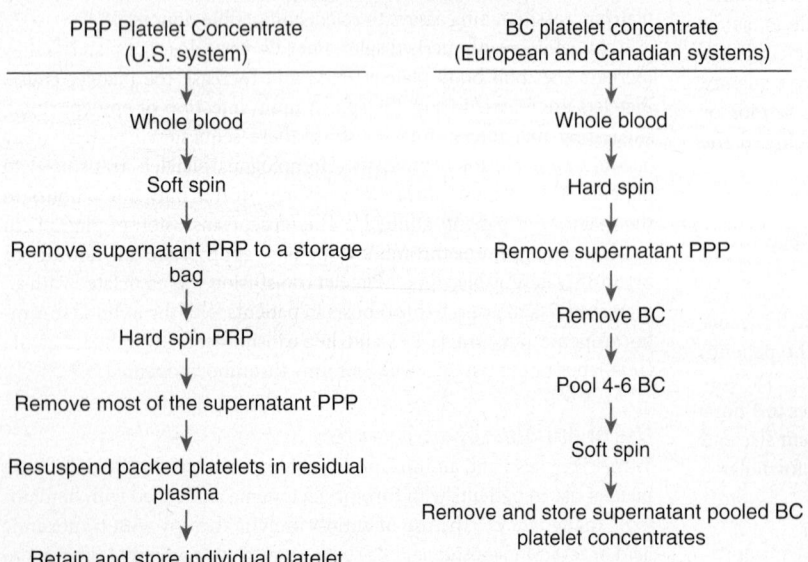

PRP Platelet Concentrate (U.S. system)

↓

Whole blood

↓

Soft spin

↓

Remove supernatant PRP to a storage bag

↓

Hard spin PRP

↓

Remove most of the supernatant PPP

↓

Resuspend packed platelets in residual plasma

↓

Retain and store individual platelet concentrates or store pre-storage pooled platelet concentrates

BC platelet concentrate (European and Canadian systems)

↓

Whole blood

↓

Hard spin

↓

Remove supernatant PPP

↓

Remove BC

↓

Pool 4-6 BC

↓

Soft spin

↓

Remove and store supernatant pooled BC platelet concentrates

Figure 139–3. Preparation of platelet concentrates from whole blood. Two methods of preparing platelet concentrates from whole blood have been developed. The main differences are related to the centrifugation steps that are used when proceeding from whole blood to a platelet concentrate. Specific details of the methods are described in Slichter and Harker[54] for platelet-rich plasma (PRP) method platelet concentrates and Pietersz, Loos, and Reesink[55] for buffy coat (BC) method platelet concentrates. PPP, platelet-poor plasma.

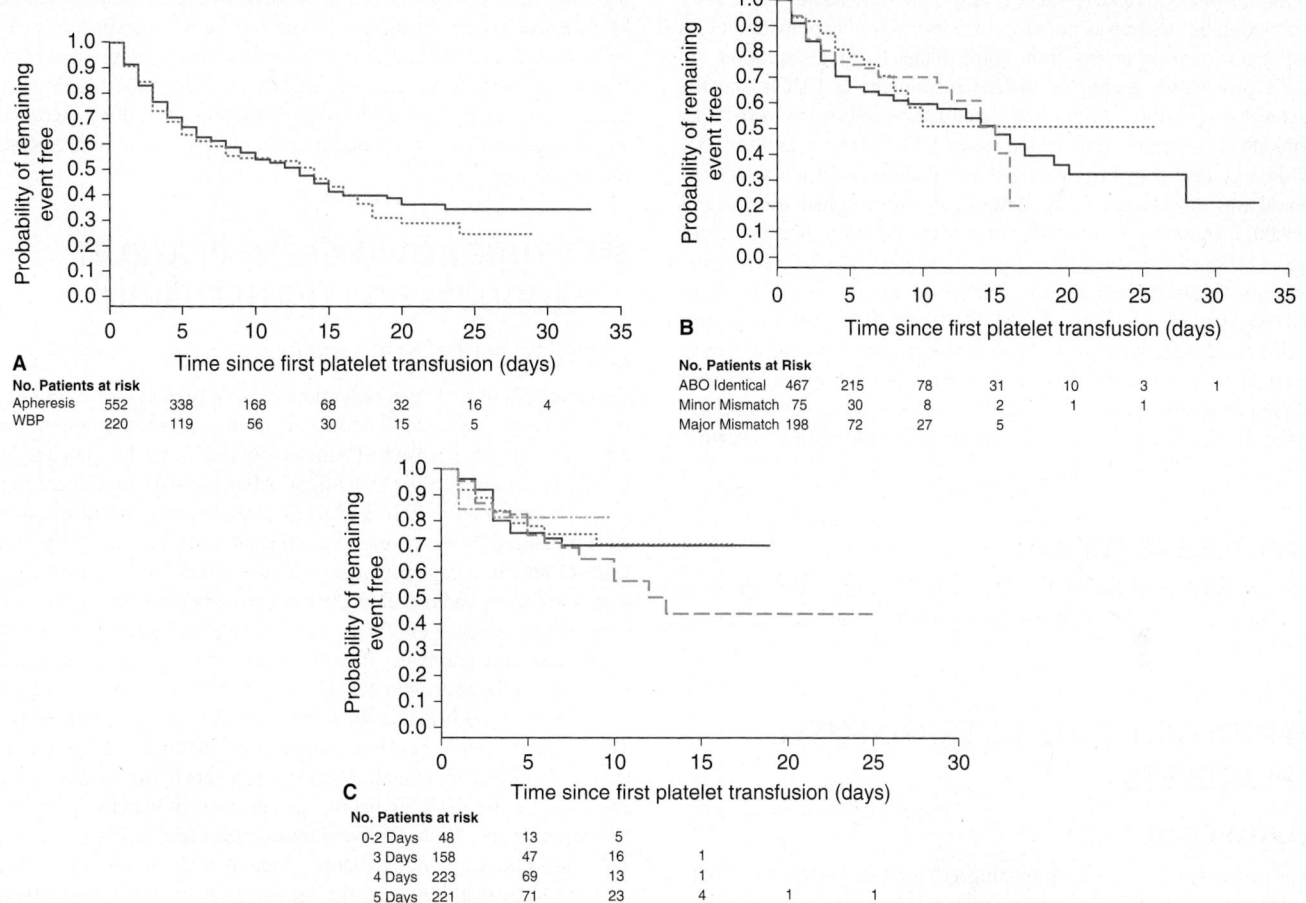

Figure 139–4. Kaplan-Meier plots of time from platelet transfusion to first Grade 2 or higher bleeding for each platelet characteristic. **A.** Time from first platelet transfusion to first Grade 2 or higher bleeding by source of platelets. Time to bleeding was censored at the first date that any of the following occurred: transfusion of a platelet unit with a different source from the patient's initial platelet transfusion; missing data on whether Grade 2 or higher bleeding occurred; or end of study. Platelet source was not a significant predictor of time to Grade 2 or higher bleeding (p = 0.44). Apheresis platelets (_) and random-donor whole-blood platelets (rdWBPs) (..). **B.** Time from first platelet transfusion to first Grade 2 or higher bleeding by ABO matching status from the patient's initial platelet transfusion or missing data on ABO matching status; missing data on whether Grade 2 or higher bleeding occurred; or end of study. Divergence of the curves after 15 days is probably the result of the small number of patients still at risk by that time. ABO matching status was not a significant predictor of time to Grade 2 or higher bleeding (p = 0.33). ABO identical platelets (_), ABO minor mismatched platelets (..), and major ABO mismatched platelets (_). **C.** Time from first platelet transfusion to first Grade 2 or higher bleeding, by platelet storage duration, among patients whose first platelet transfusion was stored for 0 to 5 days. Time to bleeding was censored at the first date that any of the following occurred: transfusion of a platelet unit with a different storage duration from the patient's initial platelet transfusion; transfusion of a platelet unit with missing data on storage duration; transfusion of pooled rdWBPs of different storage durations; missing data on whether Grade 2 or higher bleeding occurred; or end of study. Divergence of the curves after 10 days is probably the result of the small number of patients still at risk by that time. Duration of platelet storage was not a significant predictor of time to Grade 2 or higher bleeding (p = 0.87). Platelet storage times: 0 to 2 days (..), 3 days (..), 4 days (_), and 5 days (_). *(Reproduced with permission from Triulzi DJ, Assmann SF, Strauss RG, et al: The impact of platelet transfusion characteristics on posttransfusion platelet increments and clinical bleeding in patients with hypo-proliferative thrombocytopenia. Blood 7;119(23):5553–5562, 2012.)*

multiinstitutional PLADO trial provides new information on the relative merits of the two products.[6] The PLADO trial involved 1272 platelet-transfused patients who received 8994 platelet transfusions of which 6031 were given prophylactically. The patients were observed for 24,309 days. Subsets of this database were used to analyze bleeding outcomes, posttransfusion increments, and CCI within 4 and 24 hours posttransfusion, and transfusion intervals based on blood product transfused, ABO matching between donor and recipient, and duration of platelet storage.[65]

Time to Bleeding

Importantly, in the PLADO trial neither differences in platelet product, ABO matching, nor in storage duration affected time to bleeding (Fig. 139–4).[65]

PLATELET INCREMENTS, CORRECTED COUNT INCREMENTS, AND TRANSFUSION INTERVAL

In the PLADO trial, the absolute increments for rdWBPs at 4 hours posttransfusion were on average 3.5×10^9/L lower than APs (p = 0.002), and CCIs were 1400 less (p = 0.01), with no differences for these parameters at 24 hours.[65] Major ABO-incompatible (donor red cell A or B antigens incompatible with recipient's anti-A or anti-B antibodies), but not ABO-minor (donor's anti-A or anti-B antibodies incompatible with recipient's red cell A or B antigens), transfusions were associated with lower increments of 2.2×10^9/L (p = 0.0001) and lower CCIs of 1.4×10^9/L (p <0.0001) at 4 hours posttransfusion, respectively, compared to ABO-identical transfusions. Similarly, at 24 hours post-transfusion, major ABO-mismatched transfusions had lower platelet increments of 2.6×10^9/L (p <0.001) and CCIs were less by 1.8×10^9/L (p <0.0001), but there was no effect of minor ABO incompatibility on these measurements at any time point. Platelet storage duration did show a progressive decline in platelet increments and CCIs, but the effect was very modest. Importantly, transfusion intervals showed only trivial effects based on transfusion type (AP or rdWBP) and only for low-dose platelet transfusions (1.1×10^{11} platelets/m²) (p = 0.02), the interval was 3.9 hours less for ABO-major-mismatched transfusions (p <0.001), and there was no effect of storage duration. Because of the large number of transfusions, some of the differences between platelet products, ABO matching, and storage duration were highly statistically significant. However, for the two most important parameters for clinicians (e.g., bleeding risk and interval between transfusions), there were no important differences based on product transfused, ABO matching, and storage duration of 5 or fewer days.[65] Even differences in platelet increments and CCIs were modest, as confirmed by previous meta-analysis.[66–68]

ADVERSE EVENTS

Additional analysis of the PLADO data base showed no differences in any adverse event based on platelet source, ABO matching, or storage duration.[69]

● MODIFICATIONS TO TRANSFUSED PLATELETS

LEUKOREDUCTION

There are clear indications for providing leukoreduced platelet products: (1) reduction of platelet alloimmunization,[42] (2) prevention of cytomegalovirus transmission by transfusion,[70] and (3) reduction in febrile transfusion reactions.[71] In addition, some studies suggest that white cells that contaminate platelet and red cell transfusions may contribute to immunomodulatory effects of transfusion, such as an increased incidence of postoperative infections and metastasis formation in cancer patients.[72] However, controversy still surrounds whether transfusions have immunomodulatory effects.[73]

γ-IRRADIATION

γ-Irradiation of platelets is indicated to prevent transfusion-related GVHD, which is uniformly fatal.[74] γ-Irradiation with the usual dose of 25 Gy in one study did not affect either posttransfusion platelet survival or function.[75] However, in a transfusion study in thrombocytopenic patients, γ-irradiation decreased 1-hour posttransfusion increments by 2.8×10^9/L and showed an increased hazard ratio of 1.45 for the development of platelet refractoriness.[76] Furthermore, additional observations from the TRAP demonstrated that γ-irradiation prolonged the duration of HLA alloantibodies in patients who developed these antibodies during the course of their transfusions.[77] Therefore, indiscriminate use of γ-irradiation should be avoided. Situations in which γ-irradiation should be performed are: (1) patients receiving allogeneic HSCT and (2) patients who are severely immunocompromised, usually because of their disease or its treatment (e.g., patients who have Hodgkin or other lymphomas).[73]

VOLUME REDUCTION

For some patients who are receiving large volumes of fluids where consideration of intravenous line availability is an issue, who are volume overloaded, or for infants/young children where an adult volume may be excessive, volume reduction of platelets before transfusion is a consideration. For most children, volume reduction is often unnecessary.[78] Whenever platelets are concentrated by centrifugation, there is likely to be some damage to the platelets, re-suspension is often incomplete, and, therefore, this extra processing should only be done if necessary for patient care.[79]

● FUTURE ADVANCES IN PLATELET PRODUCTS FOR TRANSFUSION

PATHOGEN REDUCTION

Two methods of pathogen reduction[80,81] have been evaluated in clinical trials. Both systems involve adding an agent—either amotosalen (Intercept system)[80] or riboflavin (Mirasol system)[81]—to the platelets prior to exposure to ultraviolet (UV) light. After UV exposure, these agents prevent replication of RNA and DNA in pathogenic organisms, as well as eliminating the function of contaminating leukocytes.[82,83] Both the Mirasol and Intercept methods produce a reduction in posttransfusion autologous radiolabeled platelet recoveries and survivals[84,85] that is related to the dose of UV used in the pathogen-reduction process.[86] Recoveries and survivals of 5-day stored pathogen-treated platelets were reduced by approximately 15 to 25 percent, compared to similarly stored nontreated platelets from the same subjects (p <0.05 to <0.01). The Intercept system has been evaluated in a 645-patient U.S. randomized trial comparing treated to control platelets.[87] This technology was approved by the FDA for pathogen reduction of platelet components on December 19, 2014. A limited randomized trial in France involving 110 thrombocytopenic patients documented hemostatic efficacy of Mirasol-treated platelets and similar rates of red cell and platelet utilization but lower CCIs for patients who received treated compared to control platelets.[88] However, there were no adverse events following transfusion of the treated platelets, and more studies will likely be needed for FDA approval. Both technologies have received regulatory approval for their use in Europe.

Several centers in Europe that have incorporated pathogen reduction technology have eliminated γ-irradiation of platelets to prevent transfusion-associated GVHD. Inactivating leukocytes may also decrease transfusion-related adverse events such as fever, chills, and allergic reactions associated with cytokine release from residual white cells during platelet storage, and it may also reduce rates of platelet alloimmunization. All of these benefits will mean safer, more cost-effective platelets for transfusion.

EXTENDED PLATELET STORAGE

The major risk of extended platelet storage at 22°C is bacterial overgrowth usually as a consequence of inadequate sterilization of the venipuncture site. Most bacteria have been demonstrated to grow to confluence by 3 to 5 days.[89] Therefore, once platelets have been stored beyond 5 days, there is little increased risk from bacterial overgrowth. The only remaining issue to allow extended platelet storage will likely be having either a sensitive and specific point of release bacterial assay or incorporating a prestorage pathogen reduction process.

The FDA has suggested a hierarchical system for evaluating stored platelets prior to licensing[90] proceeding from a variety of *in vitro* assays, to radiolabeled autologous platelet recovery and survival measurements in normal subjects, and, finally, depending on the magnitude of the differences in the new product compared to products that are currently licensed, to transfusion trials in thrombocytopenic patients

TABLE 139–2. Extended Platelet Storage in Plasma

Platelet Product	N	Storage Time (Days)	PLATELET Recovery (%) Fresh	Stored	% of Fresh	PLATELET Survival (Days) Fresh	Stored	% of Fresh	Reference
PRP-PC†	10	6	61 ± 2	46 ± 4	78 ± 11*	8.1 ± 0.5	5.7 ± 0.5	64 ± 22*	42
	12	7	60 ± 3	43 ± 4	72 ± 11*	8.7 ± 0.5	4.1 ± 0.4	51 ± 16	42
BC-PC‡	10	6	67 ± 14	54 ± 13	80 ± 9*	8.1 ± 1.3	5.4 ± 1.3	67 ± 10*	43
	10	7	63 ± 17	50 ± 14	79 ± 6*	8.2 ± 0.8	4.8 ± 1.1	59 ± 16	43
Haemonetics Apheresis‡	20	8	66 ± 16	50 ± 15	81 ± 21*	8.5 ± 1.6	5.6 ± 1.6	67 ± 17*	44

*Percent of fresh platelet recoveries and survivals that meet FDA poststorage platelet viability criteria.

†Data reported as average ±1 SE.

‡Data reported as average ±1 SD.

to document efficacy (predominantly hemostatic) and safety. Previously, most platelets have not been stored beyond 7 days.[57,91] We have completed a series of studies based on autologous radiolabeled platelet recovery and survival measurements in normal subjects to determine how long PRP or BC platelet concentrates or AP platelets can be stored in either plasma or a platelet additive solution (Plasmalyte) while still meeting FDA poststorage platelet viability guidelines; that is, the 95 percent lower confidence limits for each donor's stored radiolabeled autologous platelet recoveries should be 66 percent of the same donor's fresh radiolabeled recoveries, and survivals should be 58 percent of fresh. As shown in Table 139–2, both plasma-stored PRP and BC platelet concentrates met FDA recoveries and survivals for 6 days of storage but only recoveries for 7 days of storage with no differences between the two types of platelet concentrates.[92,93] In contrast, Haemonetics plasma stored AP could meet both FDA's platelet recovery and survival criteria for 8 says of storage, but, by 9 days, low pH values resulted in loss of platelet viability.[94] Although concurrent data with the same donor's

fresh platelets were not obtained, AP had poststorage platelet viability that was not significantly different than Haemonetics platelets when both products were stored for 1 to 9 days.[95]

When platelets are stored in a platelet additive solution (Plasmalyte), the longest storage times that were achieved were the same as in plasma; that is, 6 days (Table 139–3).[93] However, Haemonetics platelets could be stored for 13 days. The significance of these data are (1) the life span of the platelet is not intrinsic to the cell as after 13 days of storage platelet survivals still averaged 4.6 ± 0.3 days, and (2) platelet viability is better maintained in vitro than in vivo as normal subjects in vivo fresh autologous platelet survivals are only 8 to 10 days.[96] This may be because platelets in vivo have a work-related function that shortens their life span compared to in vitro storage. In addition, our studies may suggest much longer storage times are possible in platelet additive solution than plasma, the same bags that are acceptable for storing platelets in plasma may not allow long-term platelet storage in this solution, and the method of platelet collection significantly affects storage duration.[96]

TABLE 139–3. Extended Platelet Storage in Plasmalyte

Platelet Product	N	Storage Time (Days)	Plasmalyte Concentration (%)	PLATELET Recovery (%) Fresh§	Stored	% of Fresh	PLATELET Survival (Days) Fresh	Stored	% of Fresh	Ref.
PRP-PC‡	10	6	65 ± 3	68 ± 12	55 ± 11	82 ± 6*	8.1 ± 1.4	5.0 ± 1.4	62 ± 17	43
BC-PC‡	10	6	67 ± 5	61 ± 13	49 ± 12	80 ± 10*	8.0 ± 1.5	5.5 ± 1.2	70 ± 14*	43
	5	7	65 ± 7	74 ± 3	58 ± 3	79 ± 5*	7.3 ± 1.8	4.1 ± 1.6	55 ± 10	43
Haemonetics Apheresis†,‡	4	9	79 ± 3	67 ± 4	55 ± 5	82 ± 10*	7.6 ± 1.1	6.6 ± 0.6	93 ± 19*	46
	10	13	81 ± 1	67 ± 4	49 ± 3	73 ± 4*	7.0 ± 0.6	4.6 ± 0.3	69 ± 6	46
	10	14	82 ± 1	65 ± 4	43 ± 3	67 ± 4	7.4 ± 0.6	4.2 ± 0.5	57 ± 4	46
Trima Apheresis†	8	9	83 ± 1	54 ± 4	44 ± 4	78 ± 5*	7.7 ± 0.4	5.0 ± 0.2	59 ± 2	46

*Percent of fresh platelet recoveries and survivals that meet FDA poststorage platelet viability criteria.

†Data reported as average ±1 SE.

‡Data reported as average ±1 SD.

§Data reported as "fresh results" are for platelets that have been stored for 1 day.

REFERENCES

1. Report of the US Department of Health and Human Services: *The 2009 National Blood Collection and Utilization Survey Report.* US Department of Health and Human Services, Office of the Assistant Secretary for Health, Washington, DC, 2011.
2. Slichter SJ, Harker LA: Thrombocytopenia: Mechanisms and management of defects in platelet production. *Clin Haematol* 7:523, 1978.
3. Hanson SR, Slichter SJ: Platelet kinetics in patients with bone marrow hypoplasia: Evidence for a fixed platelet requirement. *Blood* 66:1105. 1985.
4. Gaydos LA, Freireich EJ, Mantel N: The quantitative relation between platelet count and hemorrhage in patients with acute leukemia. *N Engl J Med* 266:905, 1962.
5. Gmür J, Burger J, Schanz U, et al: Safety of stringent prophylactic platelet transfusion policy for patients with acute leukaemia. *Lancet* 338:1223, 1991.
6. Slichter SJ, Kaufman RM, Assman SF, et al: Dose of prophylactic platelet transfusions and prevention of hemorrhage. *N Engl J Med* 362:600, 2010.
7. Harker LA, Slichter SJ: The bleeding time as a screening test for evaluation of platelet function. *N Engl J Med* 287:155, 1972.
8. Miller AB, Hoogstraten B, Staquet M, Winkler A: Reporting results of cancer treatment. *Cancer* 47:207, 1981.
9. Stanworth SJ, Estcourt L, Powter G, et al: A no-prophylaxis platelet-transfusion strategy for hematologic cancers. *N Engl J Med* 368:1771, 2013.
10. Josephson CD, Granger S, Assmann SF, et al: Bleeding risks are higher in children versus adults given prophylactic platelet transfusions for treatment-induced hypoproliferative thrombocytopenia. *Blood* 120:748, 2012.
11. American Cancer Society: *Cancer Facts & Figures 2012.* American Cancer Society, Atlanta, GA, 2012.
12. Palomo M, Diaz-Ricart M, Carbo C, et al: Endothelial dysfunction after hematopoietic stem cell transplantation: Role of the conditioning regimen and the type of transplantation. *Biol Blood Marrow Transplant* 16:985, 2010.
13. Goerge T, Ho-Tin-Noe B, Carbo C, et al: Inflammation induces hemorrhage in thrombocytopenia. *Blood* 111:4958, 2008.
14. Han T, Stutzman L, Cohen E, Kim U: Effect of platelet transfusion on hemorrhage in patients with acute leukemia. An autopsy study. *Cancer* 19:1937, 1966.
15. Hanson SR, Slichter SJ: Platelet kinetics in patients with bone marrow hypoplasia: Evidence for a fixed platelet requirement. *Blood* 66:1105, 1985.
16. Rebulla P, Finazzi G, Marangoni F, et al:: The threshold for prophylactic platelet transfusions in adults with acute myeloid leukemia. Gruppo Italiano Malatie Ematologiche Maligne dell'Adulto. *N Engl J Med* 337:1870, 1997.
17. Wandt H, Frank M, Ehninger G, et al: Safety and cost effectiveness of a 10 × 10(9)/L rigger for prophylactic platelet transfusions compared with the traditional 20 × 10(9)/L trigger: A prospective comparative trial in 105 patients with acute myeloid leukemia. *Blood* 91:3601, 1998.
18. Heckman KD, Weiner GJ, Davis CS, et al: Randomized study of prophylactic platelet transfusion threshold during induction therapy for adult acute leukemia: 10,000/microL versus 20,000/microL. *J Clin Oncol* 15:1143, 1997.
19. Diedrich B, Remberger M, Shanwell A, et al: A prospective randomized trial of a prophylactic platelet transfusion trigger of 10 × 10(9) per L versus 30 × 10(9) per L in allogeneic hematopoietic progenitor cell transplant recipients. *Transfusion* 45:1064, 2005.
20. Slichter SJ, Le Blanc R, Jones MK, et al: Quantitative analysis of bleeding risk in cancer patients prophylactically transfused at platelet counts of 5,000 10,000 or 20,000 plts/µl. *Blood* 94:376a, 1999.
21. Kaufman RM, Djulbegovic B, Gernsheimer T, et al: Platelet Transfusion: A clinical practice guideline from the AABB. *Ann Intern Med* 162:205, 2015.
22. Haas FJ, van Rhenen DJ, de Vries RR, et al; National Users' Board Sanquin Blood Supply: *Blood Transfusion Guideline.* 2011. http://www.sanquin.nl/repository/documenten/en/prod-en-dienst/287294/blood-transfusion-guideline.pdf.
23. Norol F, Kuentz M, Cordonnier C, et al: Influence of clinical status on the efficacy of stored platelet transfusion. *Rev Fr Transfus Hemobiol* 36:427, 1993.
24. Wandt H, Schaefer-Eckart K, Wendelin K, et al: Therapeutic platelet transfusion versus routine prophylactic transfusion in patients with haematological malignancies: An open-label, multicentre, randomised study. *Lancet* 380:1309, 2012.
25. Riley W, Smalley B, Pulkrabek S, et al: Using lean techniques to define the platelet transfusion process and cost effectiveness to evaluate platelet dose transfusion strategies. *Transfusion* 52:1957, 2012.
26. Giagounidis A, Mufti GJ, Fenaux P, et al: Results of a randomized, double-blind study of romiplostim versus placebo in patients with low/intermediate-1-risk myelodysplastic syndrome and thrombocytopenia. *Cancer* 120:1838, 2014.
27. Kumar A, Mhaskar R, Grossman BJ, et al: Platelet transfusion: A systematic review of the clinical evidence. *Transfusion* 55:1116, 2015.
28. Zeidler K, Arn K, Senn O, et al:. Optimal preprocedural platelet transfusion threshold for central venous catheter insertions in patients with thrombocytopenia. *Transfusion* 51:2269, 2011.
29. Haas B, Chittams JL, Trerotola S: Large-bore tunneled central venous catheter insertion in patients with coagulopathy. *J Vasc Interv Radiol* 21:212, 2010.
30. Howard SC, Gajjar A, Ribeiro, et al: Safety of lumbar puncture for children with acute lymphoblastic leukemia and thrombocytopenia. *JAMA* 284:2222, 2000.
31. Vavricka SR, Walter RB, Irani S, et al: Safety of lumbar puncture for adults with acute leukemia and restrictive prophylactic platelet transfusion. *Ann Hematol* 82:570, 2003.
32. Bishop JF, Schiffer CA, Aisner J, et al: Surgery in acute leukemia: A review of 167 operations in thrombocytopenic patients. *Am J Hematol* 26:147, 1987.
33. Harker LA, Malpass TW, Branson HE, et al: Mechanism of abnormal bleeding in patients undergoing cardiopulmonary bypass: Acquired transient platelet dysfunction associated with selective alpha-granule release. *Blood* 56:824, 1980.
34. Cooper ES, Bracey AW, Horvath AE, et al: Practice parameter for the use of fresh-frozen plasma, cryoprecipitate, and platelets. *JAMA* 271:777, 1994.
35. Perkins JG, Cap PA, Spinella PC, et al: An evaluation of the impact of apheresis platelets used in the setting of massively transfused trauma patients. *J Trauma* 66:S77, 2009.
36. Simmons JW, White CE, Eastridge BJ, et al: Impact of policy change on US Army combat transfusion practices. *J Trauma* 69 Suppl 1:S75, 2010.
37. Baraniuk S, Tilley BC, del Junco DJ, et al: Pragmatic Randomized Optimal Platelet and Plasma Ratios (PROPPR) Trial: Design, rationale and implementation. *Injury* 45:1287, 2014.
38. Holcomb JB, Tilley BC, Baraniuk S, et al for the PROPPR Study Group: Transfusion of plasma, platelets, and red blood cells in a 1:1:1 vs. a 1:1:2 ratio and mortality in patients with severe trauma: The PROPPR Randomized Clinical Trial. *JAMA* 313:483, 2015.
39. Kocsis JJ, Hernandovich J, Silver MJ, et al: Duration of inhibition of platelet prostaglandin formation and aggregation by ingested aspirin or indomethacin. *Prostaglandins* 3:141, 1973.
40. Davis KB, Slichter SJ, Corash L: Corrected count increment and percent platelet recovery as measures of posttransfusion platelet response: Problems and a solution. *Transfusion* 39: 586, 1999.
41. Doughty HA, Murphy MF, Metcalfe P, et al: Relative importance of immune and non-immune causes of platelet refractoriness. *Vox Sang* 66: 200, 1994.
42. Leukocyte reduction and ultraviolet B irradiation of platelets to prevent alloimmunization and refractoriness to platelet transfusions. The Trial to Reduce Alloimmunization To Platelets Study Group. *N Engl J Med* 337:1861, 1997.
43. Heal JM, Blumberg N, Masel D: An evaluation of crossmatching, HLA, and ABO matching for platelet transfusions to refractory patients. *Blood* 70:23,1987.
44. Bishop JF, McGrath K, Wolf MM, et al: Clinical factors influencing the efficacy of pooled platelet transfusions. *Blood* 71:383. 1988.
45. Klumpp TR, Herman JH, Innis S, et al: *Bone Marrow Transplant* 17:1035, 1996.
46. Salama A, Kiesewetter, Kalus U, et al: Massive platelet transfusion is a rapidly effective emergency treatment in patients with refractory autoimmune thrombocytopenia. *Thromb Haemost* 100:762, 2008.
47. Peña JR, Saidman SL: Anti-HLA antibody testing in hematology patients. *Am J Hematol* 90:361, 2015.
48. Pavenski K, Rebulla P, Duquesnoy R, et al: International Collaboration for Guideline Development, Implementation, and Evaluation for Transfusion Therapies (ICTMG) Collaborators: Efficacy of HLA-matched platelet transfusions for patients with hypoproliferative thrombocytopenia: A systematic review. *Transfusion* 53:2230, 2013.
49. Vassallo RR, Fung M, Rebulla P, et al for the International Collaboration for Guideline Development, Implementation and Evaluation for Transfusion Therapies: Utility of cross-matched platelet transfusions in patients with hypoproliferative thrombocytopenia: A systematic review. *Transfusion* 54:1180, 2014.
50. Aster RH: Pooling of platelets in the spleen: Role in the pathogenesis of "hypersplenic" thrombocytopenia. *J Clin Invest* 45:645, 1966.
51. Ballem PJ, Segal GM, Stratton JR: Mechanisms of thrombocytopenia in chronic autoimmune thrombocytopenic purpura. Evidence of both impaired platelet production and increased platelet clearance. *J Clin Invest* 80:33, 1987.
52. Goel R, Ness PM, Takemoto, et al: Platelet transfusions in platelet consumptive disorders are associated with arterial thrombosis and in-hospital mortality. *Blood* 125:1470, 2015.
53. Jain S, Gernsheimer T, Slichter S: A retrospective analysis of epsilon-amino-caproic acid therapy in hypoproliferative thrombocytopenia. *European Hematology Association Annual Meetings,* P1040, unpublished 2013.
54. Slichter SJ, Harker LA: Preparation and storage of platelet concentrates. I. Factors influencing the harvest of viable platelets from whole blood. *Br J Haematol* 34:395, 1976.
55. Pietersz RN, Loos JA, Reesink HW: Platelet concentrates stored in plasma for 72 hours at 22°C prepared from buffy coats of citrate-phosphate-dextrose blood collected in a quadruple-bag saline-adenine-glucose-mannitol system. *Vox Sang* 49:81, 1985.
56. Keegan T, Heaton A, Holme S, et al: Paired comparison of platelet concentrates prepared from platelet-rich plasma and buffy coats using a new technique with ¹¹¹In and ⁵¹Cr. *Transfusion* 32:113, 1992.
57. Cardigan R, Williamson LM: The quality of platelets after storage for 7 days. *Transfus Med* 13:173, 2003.
58. Dumont LJ, Dumont DF, Unger ZM, et al for the BEST Collaborative: A randomized controlled trial comparing autologous radiolabeled *in vivo* platelet recoveries and survivals of 7-day stored platelet-rich plasma and buffy coat platelets from the same subjects. *Transfusion* 51:1241, 2011.
59. Schreiber GB, Busch MP, Kleinman SH, Korelitz JJ: The risk of transfusion-transmitted viral infections. The Retrovirus Epidemiology Donor Study. *N Engl J Med* 334:1685, 1996.
60. Ness P, Braine H, King K, et al: Single-donor platelets reduce the risk of septic platelet transfusion reactions. *Transfusion* 41:857, 2001.
61. Fridey JL, editor: *Standards for Blood Banks and Transfusion Services,* 22nd ed, p 13. American Association of Blood Banks, Bethesda, MD, 2003.
62. Chambers LA, Herman JH: Considerations in the selection of a platelet component: Apheresis versus whole blood-derived. *Transfus Med Rev* 13:311, 1999.
63. Heddle NM, Cook RJ, Blajchman MA, et al: Assessing the effectiveness of whole blood-derived platelets stored as a pool: A randomized block noninferiority trial. *Transfusion* 45:896, 2005.

64. Heddle NM, Arnold DM, Boye D, et al: Comparing the efficacy and safety of apheresis and whole blood derived platelet transfusions: A systematic review. *Transfusion* 48:1447, 2008.

65. Triulzi DJ, Assmann SF, Strauss RG, et al: The impact of platelet transfusion characteristics on posttransfusion platelet increments and clinical bleeding in patients with hypo-proliferative thrombocytopenia. *Blood* 119:5553, 2012.

66. Heddle NM, Arnold DM, Boye D, et al: Comparing the efficacy and safety of apheresis and whole blood-derived platelet transfusions: A systematic review. *Transfusion* 48:1447, 2008.

67. Shehata NS, Tinmouth A, Naglie G, et al: ABO-identical versus nonidentical platelet transfusion: A systematic review. *Transfusion* 49:2442, 2009.

68. Pavenski K, Warkentin TE, Shen H, et al: Posttransfusion platelet count increments after ABO-compatible versus ABO-incompatible platelet transfusions in noncancer patients: An observational study. *Transfusion* 50:1552, 2010.

69. Kaufman RM, Assmann SF, Triulzi DJ, et al: Transfusion-related adverse events in the Platelet Dose study. *Transfusion* 55:144, 2015.

70. Bowden RA, Slichter SJ, Sayers M, et al: A comparison of filtered leukocyte-reduced and cytomegalovirus (CMV) seronegative blood products for the prevention of transfusion-associated CMV infection after marrow transplantation. *Blood* 86:3598, 1995.

71. Heddle NM, Blajchman MA, Meyer RM, et al: A randomized controlled trial comparing the frequency of acute reactions to plasma-removed platelets and prestorage WBC-reduced platelets. *Transfusion* 42:556, 2002.

72. Dzik S, AuBuchon J, Jeffries L, et al: Leukocyte reduction of blood components: Public policy and new technology. *Transfus Med Rev* 14:34, 2000.

73. Vamvakas EC, Blajchman MA: Deleterious clinical effects of transfusion-associated immunomodulation: Fact or fiction? *Blood* 97:1180, 2001.

74. Leitman SF: Use of blood cell irradiation in the prevention of posttransfusion graft-versus-host disease. *Transfus Sci* 10:219, 1989.

75. Moroff G, George VM, Siegel AM, Luban NL: The influence of irradiation on stored platelets. *Transfusion* 26:453, 1986.

76. Slichter SJ, Davis K, Enright H, et al: Factors affecting post-transfusion platelet increments, platelet refractoriness, and platelet transfusion intervals in thrombocytopenic patients. *Blood* 105:4106, 2005.

77. Slichter SJ, Bolgiano D, Kao KJ, et al: Persistence of lymphocytotoxic antibodies in patients in the Trial to Reduce Alloimmunization to Platelets: Implications for using modified blood products. *Transfus Med Rev* 25:102, 2011.

78. Saxonhouse M, Slayton W, Sola MC: Platelet transfusions in the infant and child, in *Handbook of Pediatric Transfusion Medicine*, edited by CD Hillyer, NL Luban, RG Strauss, p 253. Elsevier Academic Press, San Diego, CA, 2004.

79. Schoenfeld H, Muhm M, Doepfmer UR, et al: The functional integrity of platelets in volume-reduced platelet concentrates. *Anesth Analg* 100:78, 2005.

80. Lin L, Cook DN, Wiesehahn GP, et al: Photochemical inactivation of viruses and bacteria in platelet concentrates by use of a novel psoralen and long-wavelength ultraviolet light. *Transfusion* 37:423, 1997.

81. Ruane PH, Edrich R, Gampp D, et al: Photochemical inactivation of selected viruses and bacteria in platelet concentrates using riboflavin and light. *Transfusion* 44:877, 2004.

82. Fast LD, DiLeone G, Li J, Goodrich R: Functional inactivation of white blood cells by Mirasol treatment. *Transfusion* 46:642, 2006.

83. Grass JA, Wafa T, Reames A, et al: Prevention of transfusion-associated graft-versus-host disease by photochemical treatment. *Blood* 93:3140, 1999.

84. AuBuchon JP, Herschel L, Roger J, et al: Efficacy of apheresis platelets treated with riboflavin and ultraviolet light for pathogen reduction. *Transfusion* 45:1335, 2005.

85. Snyder E, Raife T, Lin L, et al: Recovery and life span of 111indium-radiolabeled platelets treated with pathogen inactivation with amotosalen HCl (S-59) and ultraviolet A light. *Transfusion* 44:1732, 2004.

86. Goodrich RP, Li J, Pieters H, et al: Correlation of *in vitro* platelet quality measurements with *in vivo* platelet viability in human subjects. *Vox Sang* 90:279, 2006.

87. McCullough J, Vesole DH, Benjamin RJ, et al: Therapeutic efficacy and safety of platelets treated with a photochemical process for pathogen inactivation: The SPRINT trial. *Blood* 104:1534, 2004.

88. Ostrowski SR, Bochsen L, Windelov NA, et al: Hemostatic function of buffy coat platelets in additive solution treated with pathogen reduction technology. *Transfusion* 51:344, 2011.

89. Wagner SJ, Moroff G, Katz AJ, Friedman LI: Comparison of bacterial growth in single and pooled platelet concentrates after deliberate inoculation and storage. *Transfusion* 35:298, 1995.

90. Vostal JG: Efficacy evaluation of current and future platelet transfusion products. *J Trauma* 60(Suppl):S78, 2006.

91. Slichter SJ: Platelet transfusion: Future directions. *Vox Sang* 87(Suppl 2):S47, 2004.

92. Slichter SJ, Bolgiano D, Corson J, et al: Extended storage of platelet-rich plasma prepared platelet concentrates in plasma or plasmalyte. *Transfusion* 50:2199, 2010.

93. Slichter SJ, Bolgiano D, Corson J, et al: Extended storage of buffy coat platelet concentrates in plasma or plasmalyte. *Transfusion* 54:2283, 2014.

94. Slichter SJ, Bolgiano D, Jones MK, et al: Viability and function of 8-day stored apheresis platelets. *Transfusion* 46:1763, 2006.

95. Slichter SJ, Bolgiano D, Corson J, et al: Extended storage of autologous apheresis platelets in plasma. *Vox Sang* 104:324, 2013.

96. Slichter SJ, Corson J, Jones MK, et al: Exploratory studies of extended storage of apheresis platelets in a platelet additive solution (PAS). *Blood* 123:271, 2014.

INDEX

Page numbers in **bold** indicate a major discussion of the topic. Page numbers followed by *f* and *t* indicate the location of figures and tables, respectively.

A

AA4, 260
AA amyloidosis, 1773, 1774*t*
AAV (adeno-associated viral) vectors, 438–439, 442, 2129
ABCB7, 918
ABCD1, 439
Abciximab, **405–406**
  clinical uses, 404*t*, 405–406, 2077
  dosage, 404*t*
  mechanism of action, 404*t*
  for peripheral vascular disease, 2316
  pseudothrombocytopenia and, 1995–1996
  thrombocytopenia and, 2077
  for unstable angina, 2296
Abdominal pain/fullness
  in acute intermittent porphyria, 902
  in chronic myelogenous leukemia, 1445
  in enteropathy-associated T-cell lymphoma, 1699
  in follicular lymphoma, 1641
  history of, 5
  in polycythemia vera, 1293
Abelson oncogene. *See ABL1*
Abetalipoproteinemia (Bassen-Kornzweig syndrome), 670*f*, **681**
Aβ peptide, 1848
ABL1. See also BCR-ABL1
  in B-cell acute lymphoblastic leukemia, 232*t*
  in chronic myelogenous leukemia, 176, 1438, 1441–1442, 1442*f*, 1456–1457, 1457*t*
ABL2, 232*t*
ABO blood group, **2330**
  antibodies, 2341*t*, 2344*t*, 2350*t*
  antigens, 2331*t*, 2337, 2339, 2340, 2350*t*
  cardiovascular risk and, 2288
  characteristics, 2331*t*, 2333*t*
  compatibility guidelines, 2350*t*
  discrepancies, 2349*t*
  disease association, 2331*t*, 2341*t*
  frequency, 2333*t*
  Fy(a–b–) phenotype, 2339
  genetics, 2339

  mismatch in hematopoietic cell transplantation, 2373–2374, 2373*t*
  phenotypes, 2333*t*
  serologic detection, 2348, 2349*t*
  von Willebrand factor levels and, 2171
ABO hemolytic disease, 851, 852*t*, 856*f*. *See also* Alloimmune hemolytic disease of the fetus and newborn (HDFN)
ABO-Rh compatibility guidelines, 2350*t*
Abortion, spontaneous, 1988, 2239
Abraxane, 326
Abruptio placentae, 2210
Absolute anemia, 506, 507*t*. *See also* Anemia
ABT-199 (venetoclax)
  for chronic lymphocytic leukemia, 1539
  for mantle cell lymphoma, 1660*t*
ABT-737, 1403
ABVD regimen, for Hodgkin lymphoma
  in advanced disease, 1614
  clinical trials, 1611, 1615*t*
  complications, 1617–1618
  dose, route, and schedule, 1612*t*
  history, 1604, 1611
  in HIV-associated disease, 1247–1248
  in limited-stage disease, 1611, 1613
  in nodular lymphocyte-predominant disease, 1616
  with radiation therapy, 1248, 1613, 1614
  in unfavorable limited-stage disease, 1613
Acanthocytes, 21*f*, 472*f*, 472*t*, 474*f*, **475**, 671*f*, 680
Acanthocytosis, **680–681**
Accelerated phase, of chronic myelogenous leukemia. *See* Chronic myelogenous (myeloid) leukemia (CML), accelerated phase and blast crisis
Accessory spleen, 88
Aceruloplasminemia, 640
Acetaminophen, 767, 2375
Acetylcholinesterase, 692*t*, 701*t*
Acetyl-coenzyme A (CoA), 193, 193*f*, 196
Acid-sphingomyelinase deficiency. *See* Niemann-Pick disease
Aclarubicin, for acute myelogenous leukemia, 1395

aCML (atypical chronic myelogenous leukemia), 1279
Acquired hemophilia A, 2145, **2183–2186**
Acquired immunodeficiency syndrome. *See* AIDS
Acquired prothrombin complex deficiency, 109
Acquired pure amegakaryocytic thrombocytopenia, 1999
Acquired von Willebrand syndrome (AVWS), **2082–2083**, 2174–2175
Acral cyanosis, 2205*t*
Acrocentric centromere, 175*t*
Acrocyanosis, 829
ACS (acute coronary syndrome), 2295. *See also* Myocardial infarction (MI)
ACTG1, 234*t*, 1737
Actin, 663*t*, 667, 1832*t*, 1838–1839, 1839*f*, 1840–1841
α-Actinin, 1832*t*
Activated B-cell-like diffuse large B-cell lymphoma, 234–235*t*, 1495*t*, 1626, 1627*t*
Activated partial thromboplastin time (aPTT)
  in antiphospholipid syndrome, 2243
  in disseminated intravascular coagulation, 2205*t*
  in hemophilia A, 2120
  in hemostatic disorders, 1988, 1989*f*
  in heparin monitoring, 397
Activated protein C (APC), 1949–1950, 1950*f*, **1954**
  activities, 1954–1955
  anticoagulant cofactors, 1918*t*, 1923, 1955–1956, 2202
  direct cellular activities, 1923, 1956–1958, 1957*f*
  endothelial protein C receptor and, 1953
  inhibition, 1958
  neuroprotective effects, 1956
  protein S and, 1926
  sepsis and, 1956, 2202
  structure, 1923
  therapeutic forms, 1952
Activated protein C (APC) concentrate, 2213

Activated protein C (APC) resistance, 1955, 2222, 2224t, 2268. *See also* Factor V Leiden/factor V G1691A

Activated prothrombin complex concentrate, 2185

Activation-induced deaminase (AID), 1169, 1213, 1214t, 1215, 1710

Activator protein 1 (AP1), 1606

Activator protein 3 (AP3) complex, 1843

Activin A, 1713, 1738

Acute basophilic leukemia, 1389t, **1393**

Acute chest syndrome, 768–769, 769f

Acute coronary syndrome (ACS), 2295. *See also* Myocardial infarction (MI)

Acute eosinophilic leukemia, 955t, 1389t, **1392**

Acute erythroid leukemia, 608, 1382f, 1389t, **1390**

Acute fatty liver of pregnancy, 2012, 2211

Acute graft-versus-host disease. *See* Graft-versus-host disease (GVHD)

Acute hemolytic transfusion reaction, 2374–2375

Acute infection lymphocytosis, 1202, 1203f

Acute inflammation. *See* Inflammatory response, acute

Acute intermittent porphyria (AIP), 889, **900–904**
  clinical features, 890t, 902
  definition and history, 900–901
  diagnosis, 903–904
  drugs and, 901, 902t
  enzymes affected by, 890t, 891f
  laboratory features, 891t, 903f
  pathogenesis of clinical findings, 901–902
  pathophysiology, 901
  precipitating factors, 901
  therapy, 904

Acute iron poisoning, 638–639

Acute liver failure, 2193. *See also* Hepatic disease/dysfunction

Acute lymphoblastic (lymphocytic) leukemia (ALL), **1505–1521**
  aplastic anemia and, 520
  B-cell. *See* B-cell acute lymphoblastic leukemia (B-ALL)
  cell metabolism in, 197–198
  chronic myelogenous leukemia transformation to, 1465–1466
  clinical features, **1508–1509**, 1509t
    physical findings, 1509, 1509f
    signs and symptoms, 1508–1509
  course and prognosis, **1518–1521**
    event-free survival, 1505–1506, 1506f, 1513t
    indicators of, 183, 1520–1521, 1521t

relapse, 1518
  treatment sequelae, 1519–1520
definition and history, 1505–1506
development *in utero*, 1507
differential diagnosis, 1513–1514
disseminated intravascular coagulation and, 2208
early T-cell precursor, 1512, 1512t
etiology and pathogenesis, **1506–1508**
  cell-cycle defects, 217
  chromosomal abnormalities, 177f, **183**, 184t, **186**, 186f, 1508t, 1513t
  gene mutations, 166, 1506–1507, 1507–1508, 1508t, 1513t. *See also ETV6-RUNX1*, in acute lymphoblastic leukemia
  incidence, 1506, 1506f
  risk factors, 1506–1507
flow cytometry, 36f
laboratory features, **1509–1513**, 1510t
  blood, 1509–1510, 1509t
  cerebrospinal fluid examination, 1510, 1510t
  chest radiography, 1509f, 1510
  genetic classification, 1512–1513, 1513t
  immunologic classification, 1511–1512, 1512t
  marrow, 1510–1511, 1510t
  morphologic and cytochemical analysis, 1511, 1511f
  Philadelphia chromosome-negative, 364
  Philadelphia chromosome-positive, 183, 364, 1517, 1521
  platelet function and, 2082
  T-cell. *See* T-cell acute lymphoblastic leukemia (T-ALL)
therapy, **1514–1518**
  central nervous system, 1517
  continuation, 1516–1517
  hematopoietic cell transplantation, 364, 1517–1518
  history of, 197
  intensification (consolidation), 1516
  investigational therapies, 415
  remission induction, 1515
  supportive care, 1514–1515
  targeted, 1518
  transient myeloproliferative disorder and, 1385–1386

Acute mast cell leukemia, 1389t, **1393**
Acute megakaryoblastic (megakaryocytic) leukemia, 1382f, 1389t, **1392**
Acute megaloblastic anemia, **604–605**
Acute monocytic leukemia, 181, 1096, 1382f, 1388t, **1391–1392**
Acute mountain sickness, 881

Acute myeloblastic leukemia, 1382f, **1387**, 1388t
Acute myelofibrosis, 1392
Acute myelogenous (myeloid) leukemia (AML), **1373–1415**
  cell metabolism in, 197–198
  classification, 1279–1280, 1380, 1380t
  clinical features, **1380–1381**
    extramedullary tumors, 1285
    hyperleukocytic syndromes, 1285–1286, 1286t, 1384
    marrow necrosis, 1287, 1385
    metabolic signs, 1286–1287
    myeloid sarcoma, 1379
    procoagulant and fibrinolytic activator release, 1285
    signs and symptoms, 1380
    specific organ system involvement, 1379–1380
    splenomegaly, 1287
    systemic symptoms, 1286
  clonal myeloid disease transition and, 1280–1281
  course and prognosis, **1411–1415**
    clonal remissions, 1411–1412
    detection of minimal residual disease, 1412–1415
    factors influencing, 1412, 1413–1414t
    genetic abnormalities and, 220–221t, 363, 1411t
    long-term survival, 1412, 1412t
    after relapse, 363–364
    remission-relapse pattern, 1284, 1284f
    spontaneous remissions, 1412
    treatment results, 1411–1412
  definition and history, 1373–1374
  differential diagnosis, **1393**
  disseminated intravascular coagulation and, 2208
  epidemiology, 1379–1380
  essential thrombocythemia and, 1310
  etiology and pathogenesis, **1374–1380**
    chromosomal abnormalities, **180–182**, **225**, **1383**
      in chromosomes 5 and 7, 1383, 1384t
      deletions, 177f, 179t, 1384t
      frequency, 182f
      inversions, 179t, 180–181, 220t, 1384t
      prognosis and, 1280, 1413–1414t
      t(8;21), 180, 220t, 1383, 1384t, 1415
      t(15;17), 181, 220t, 1280, 1383, 1384t, 1415
      t(16;16), 180–181, 220t
      translocations, 177f, 179t, 1280, 1384t, 2388
      translocations involving 11q, 181, 220t

trisomy 8, 1384*t*

trisomy 11, 181

chromosome markers, 1377

deregulated signaling pathways, 1379

environmental factors, 1320, 1374

evolution from a chronic myeloid

neoplasm, 1373–1374

gene markers, 1376–1377

gene mutations, **181–182, 1377–1379,**

1378*t*

ASXL1, 226*t*

CEBPA, 181, 181*t*, 182, 226*t*, 363,

1378*t*, 1379

DNMT3A, 226*t*, 1377–1378, 1378*t*

FLT3, 181, 181*t*, 198, 226*t*, 363, 1377,

1378*t*, 1383, 1415

frequency, 181*t*, 1308*f*

hematopoietic cell transplantation

response and, 363

IDH1/2, 226*t*, 1378*t*, 1379

KIT, 181, 181*t*, 227*t*, 1376

MLL-PTD, 226*t*, 1378*t*

NPM1, 181, 226*t*, 363, 1377, 1378*t*

NRAS, 227*t*, 1376, 1378*t*, 1386

PHF6, 227*t*

prognosis and, 181, 1413–1414*t*

RUNX1 (AML1), 181*t*, 226*t*, 237,

1351, 1376, 1378, 1378*t*, 1384*t*,

1415, 2060

somatic, 1376

TET2, 226*t*, 1378–1379, 1378*t*

TP53, 227*t*

WT1, 227*t*, 1378*t*, 1379

mode of inheritance, 1379

molecular pathogenesis, 1376

predisposing diseases, 1374*t*, 1375

familial platelet disorder with

predisposition to, 2060

hybrid, 1386

hypoplastic, 1384

immunologic phenotypes, 1380*t*

laboratory features, **1381–1387**

basophilia, 972, 972*t*

blood, 1381, 1382*f*

cytogenetic abnormalities, 1383,

1384*t*

eosinophilia, 955*t*

hyperleukocytosis, 1384

hypoplastic leukemia, 1384

lymphocytosis, 1204

marrow, 1381–1383, 1382*f*

plasma chemical, 1383

mediastinal germ cell tumors and,

1377–1388

mixed, 1386

monocytosis and, 1096

morphological variants, 1282–1283, 1283*f*,

1387–1393, 1388–1389*t*

acute basophilic leukemia, **1393**

acute eosinophilic leukemia, 955*t*, **1392**

acute erythroid leukemia, 608, 1382*f*,

1390

acute mast cell leukemia, **1393**

acute megakaryoblastic

(megakaryocytic) leukemia, 1382*f*,

1392

acute monocytic leukemia, 181, 1096,

1382*f*, **1391–1392**

acute myeloblastic leukemia, 1382*f*, **1387**

acute myelomonocytic leukemia, 180,

1382*f*, 1387, **1390**

acute promyelocytic leukemia. *See* Acute

promyelocytic leukemia (APL)

myelodysplastic syndromes and, 178, 181

neonatal myeloproliferative syndromes

and, **1385–1386**

oligoblastic, 1384–1385

pathogenesis, 1281–1282, 1281*f*

Philadelphia-chromosome–positive, 1385,

1407

during pregnancy, 124

progenitor cell leukemia and, 1283

secondary, 1407

therapy-related, 177*f*, 179*t*, **182–183,** 182*f*,

1520

treatment, **1393–1411**

decision to treat, 1393–1394

leukocytapheresis, 433

nonhematopoietic adverse effects,

1410–1411

overview, 1393

patient preparation, 1394

postremission therapy, **1398–1401**

autologous stem cell infusion, 1399

cytotoxic therapy, 1398–1399

donor leukocyte infusion, 1400–1401

hematopoietic cell transplantation,

363–364, 1398, 1399–1400

recurrent leukemia in donor cells,

1401

in relapsed or refractory disease

antiangiogenesis agents/agents

that inhibit microenvironmental

interactions, 1404

CD33 antibodies, 1403

chemotherapy, 1401, 1402*t*

cyclin-dependent kinase inhibitors,

218

DOT1L inhibitors, 1403

epigenetic modulation, 1403

hematopoietic cell transplantation,

363–364, 1400, 1402

histone deacetylase inhibitors, 219,

240

immunotherapy and antisense DNA

approaches, 1404

modulation of drug resistance, 1404

therapies targeted to signal

transduction mediators, 1403–1404

Wee1 inhibitors, 219

remission-induction therapy,

1394–1398

cytotoxic regimens, 1394–1396, 1395*t*

principles, 1394

special considerations, 1396–1398

special considerations

in acute promyelocytic leukemia,

1404–1407, 1405*t*

in children, 1409–1410

in older patients, 1408–1409

in Ph-chromosome-positive AML,

1407

in pregnant patients, 1409

in secondary acute myelogenous

leukemia, 1407

Acute myelomonocytic leukemia (AMML),

180, 1382*f*, 1387, 1388*t*, **1390**

Acute myocardial infarction. *See* Myocardial

infarction (MI)

Acute-phase response, 284–285

Acute porphyrias, 889

Acute promyelocytic leukemia (APL),

1390–1391

chromosomal abnormalities, 177*f*, 181,

1390–1391

clinical features, 1388*t*, 1390

disseminated intravascular coagulation

and, 2208

epidemiology, 1390

laboratory features, 1382*f*, 1388*t*, 1391

long-term survival, 1412

treatment, 1391, **1404–1407,** 2317*t*, 2318

Acute respiratory distress syndrome (ARDS),

2201, 2204–2205, 2208

ACVRP regimen, for diffuse large B-cell

lymphoma, 1628

ACY-1215, 1754

Acyclovir

as empiric therapy for infections, 386, 387*t*

for Epstein-Barr virus infection, 1269

for HSV infection, 370

megaloblastic anemia and, 606*t*

prophylactic, 369, 389

ADA. *See* Adenosine deaminase (ADA)

ADAM17 (TACE), 1144, 1874

ADAMTS-13 (ADAMTS13)

acquired deficiency, 2256

congenital deficiency, 2257–2258

ADAMTS-13 (ADAMTS13) (*Cont.*):
  in disseminated intravascular coagulation, 2207
  in liver disease, 2191, 2193
  preeclampsia and, 2012
  in thrombotic microangiopathies, 1252
  in thrombotic thrombocytopenia purpura, 428, 2107, 2253–2255
  von Willebrand factor and, 1874, 1879, 1979, 2012, 2167, 2167*f*, 2254*f*
Adaptive immunity
  activation, **303–304**
  atherosclerosis and, 2286
  dendritic cells and, 307–308, 308*t*
  vs. innate immunity, **293**, 294*t*
  natural killer cells and, 1191
Adaptive tolerance, 308
Adaptor proteins, 251–252, 1833*t*
ADCC (antibody-dependent cellular cytotoxicity), 344–345, 1645
Addison disease, 559–560
Adducins, 663*t*, 667, 668*f*, 1833*t*, 1837, 1840
Adenine nucleotides, metabolic and storage pools of, 1843
Adenine phosphoribosyl transferase, 701*t*
Adeno-associated viral (AAV) vectors, 438–439, 442, 2129
Adenosine deaminase (ADA), 692*t*, 699, 700*t*, 701*t*, 705–706
Adenosine deaminase (ADA) deficiency, 439, 1214*t*, 1217, 1218
Adenosine diphosphate. *See* ADP (adenosine diphosphate)
Adenosine monophosphate kinase (AMPK), 194–195
Adenosine signaling, in sickle cell disease, 765–766
Adenosine triphosphate. *See* ATP (adenosine triphosphate)
Adenosylcobalamin, 589, 589*f*, 592, 592*f*
Adenoviral vectors, 438
Adenovirus infection. *See also* Viral infections
  in immunocompromised host, 384
  T-cell therapy for, 412
Adenylate kinase (AK), 692*t*, 699, 700*t*, 705
Adenylate kinase 2 deficiency, 1217
Adhesion molecules
  atherosclerosis and, 2286
  in cell signaling, **250**
  eosinophil, 948–949, 949*t*
  leukocyte, 280–283, 282*f*, 282*t*
  leukocyte–endothelial cell, 1977–1978, 1977*t*
  monocytes and macrophages, 1059, 1060*t*

  neutrophil, 934*t*, 1006
  in thrombotic milieu, 1978, 1979*t*
Adipocytes, marrow, 59, 59*f*
Adiponectin, in myeloma, 1709
Adipose tissue
  eosinophils and, 952
  hematopoiesis and, 44
  macrophage phenotypes in, 1078
Adoptive cellular therapy. *See* Immune cell therapy
Adoptive immune therapy, 353
ADP (δ-aminolevulinate dehydratase porphyria), 890*t*, 891*f*, 891*t*, 894, 900
ADP (adenosine diphosphate)
  activation of Akt by, 1882
  in glucose metabolism, 692
  oxidation of red cells with, 499
  platelet response to, 2074
  receptors for, 1874–1876
ADP receptor blockers, **405**, 2076
ADP receptor defects (P2Y$_{12}$ and P2X$_1$), 2056–2057
Adrenal disease/dysfunction
  anemia and, 559–560
  in antiphospholipid syndrome, 2241
  in disseminated intravascular coagulation, 2205*t*
  primary lymphomas, 1583
Adrenoleukodystrophy, X-linked, 439
Adriamycin. *See also* ABVD regimen; BEACOPP regimen
  for acute lymphoblastic leukemia, 1516
Adult Langerhans cell histiocytosis, **1108–1109**. *See also* Langerhans cell histiocytosis
Adult T-cell leukemia/lymphoma (ATL/ATLL)
  chromosomal abnormalities, 185*t*, 186*f*
  clinical features, 1700
  definition, 1700
  epidemiology, 1573, 1694*t*, 1700
  laboratory features, 1498*t*, 1700
  prognosis, 1700–1701
  treatment, 1701
Adventitial reticular cells, marrow, 57–59, 57*f*, 58*f*
AE1 (anion exchanger), 663*t*, 664
Aes-103, for sickle cell disease, 777*t*
AF4 proteins, 169
AF9 proteins, 169
Afamelanotide, for erythropoietic protoporphyria, 899
Afibrinogenemia/hypofibrinogenemia, **2154–2157**
  clinical features, 2155

  definition, history, and epidemiology, 2134*t*, 2154
  differential diagnosis, 2156
  etiology and pathogenesis, 2154–2155
  laboratory features, 2155–2156
  in pregnancy, 2156
  therapy, 2136*t*, 2156–2157
African Americans
  cardiac amyloidosis and, 1778
  monoclonal gammopathy and, 1722
  myeloma and, 1734
  sickle cell disease and, 763
African iron overload, 640, 641, 643
Age
  acute lymphoblastic leukemia incidence and, 1506, 1506*f*
  acute lymphoblastic leukemia prognosis and, 1520–1521, 1521*t*
  chronic myelogenous leukemia incidence and, 1438, 1439*f*
  endothelial vasodilation and, 2283
  hairy cell leukemia incidence and, 1554
  hematopoietic cell transplantation and, **361–362**
  Hodgkin lymphoma incidence and, 1604, 1604*f*
  immune function and, **135–136**, 136*f*
  leukocyte count and, 17
  lymphoma incidence and, 1570, 1570*f*
  mononucleosis symptoms and, 1263*t*
  myelodysplastic syndrome incidence and, 1344, 1344*f*
  neutrophil concentration and, 991
  primary myelofibrosis incidence and, 1319
  reference ranges and, 19
Agent Orange, 1528
Agglutinins, direct (saline), 823
Aggressive systemic mastocytosis, 973. *See also* Systemic mastocytosis
AGI-6780, 1403
Aging. *See also* Newborns/infants; Older persons
  acute myelogenous leukemia and, 1375, 1375*f*, 1412, 1412*t*
  cellular senescence, 132
  hematopoietic microenvironment and, 267
  median life span vs. maximum survival, 131
  neutrophil motility and, 1026
  organismal, 132
  theories, **130–131**, 130*t*
AGM (aorta-gonad-mesonephros) region, 54, 100*f*, 101, 257–258, 1149–1150
Agranulocytosis, 991, 1097. *See also* Neutropenia
Agrin, 62

AH50, 1232

aHUS (atypical hemolytic uremic syndrome), **2259–2261**, 2259t

AI. *See* Anemia of inflammation (AI)

AICAR, 585, 590

AICC (anti-inhibitor coagulant complex), 2185

AID (activation-induced deaminase), 1169, 1213, 1214t, 1215, 1710

AIDS (acquired immunodeficiency syndrome). *See also* Human immunodeficiency virus (HIV) infection

   acute myelogenous leukemia and, 1375

   cobalamin deficiency and, 601–602

   diagnosis, 1240–1242, 1241t

   malignancies associated with. *See* Human immunodeficiency virus (HIV)–associated malignancies

   natural killer cells and, 1192

   opportunistic infections in, 1240–1241, 1241t

AIDS-defining conditions, 1240–1241, 1241t, 1243, 1243t, 1244f

AIP. *See* Acute intermittent porphyria (AIP)

AIRE, 1181, 1219, 1224

Airway hyperreactivity

   eosinophilia and, 954

   sickle cell disease and, 769

AITL (angioimmunoblastic T-cell lymphoma), 1498t, 1598, 1694, 1694t, **1697–1698**

Ajoene, 2079

AK (adenylate kinase), 692t, 699, 700t, 705

AK1, 699

A knobs, fibrin, 2152, 2153f, 2158

AKT, 209, 1666

Akt (protein kinase B), 208f, 209, 251, 1882

AKT inhibitors, 1403

ALA (δ-aminolevulinic acid), 889, 891f, 893f

ALAD (δ-aminolevulinate dehydratase), 894

ALA (δ-aminolevulinic acid) dehydrase, 701t

AL amyloidosis. *See* Immunoglobulin light-chain (AL) amyloidosis

ALAS (δ-aminolevulinate synthase), 892–894, 917–918

ALAS1, 892–894, 896, 901

ALAS2, 892–894, 896, 918

ALAS2, 894, 916, 920

ALCL. *See* Anaplastic large cell lymphoma (ALCL)

Alcohol abuse

   acquired stomatocytosis in, 684

   hematologic effects, 654–655

   lymphocytopenia in, 1206

   neutrophil motility and, 1026

   porphyria cutanea tarda and, 906

   thrombocytopenia in, 1998

ALDOA, 695

Aldolase

   activity, 692t

   deficiency, 700t, 704

   in glucose metabolism, 695

Aldosteronism, 560

Alefacept, for acquired aplastic anemia, 527

Alemtuzumab, **345**

   adverse effects, 343t, 1535, 1695

   for autoimmune hemolytic anemia, 839

   for B-cell prolymphocytic leukemia, 1542

   for chronic lymphocytic leukemia, 1535

   dose, 343t

   for mycosis fungoides, 1687

   for myelodysplastic syndromes, 1359

   for peripheral T-cell lymphoma, 1695

   for pure red cell aplasia, 544

   for reduced intensity conditioning, 1115

   for T-cell large granular lymphocytic leukemia, 1567

ALG (antilymphocyte serum), 522

Alglucerase, for Gaucher disease, 1127

ALK, 188, 1576

ALK-1, 1688

ALK-positive large B-cell lymphoma, 1496t, 1598–1599

ALK-positive/negative anaplastic large cell lymphoma. *See* Anaplastic large cell lymphoma (ALCL)

Alkylating drugs, **329–331**. *See also specific drugs*

   adverse effects, 330–331

   for chronic lymphocytic leukemia, 1534

   high-dose, 331, 331t

   mechanism of action, 329, 330f

   pharmacology, 329–330

   resistance to, 319t

   secondary acute myelogenous leukemia and, 1407

ALL. *See* Acute lymphoblastic (lymphocytic) leukemia (ALL)

Allele-specific oligonucleotide polymerase chain reaction (ASO-PCR), 1716

Allelic exclusion, 1168

Allergic disorders

   basophils and mast cells in, 969

   eosinophilia in, 955t

Allergic irritability, 303

Allergic transfusion reaction, 2375

Alloantibodies, 2343

Allogeneic hematopoietic stem cell transplantation. *See* Hematopoietic cell transplantation (HCT), allogeneic

Alloimmune hemolytic anemia, 836

Alloimmune hemolytic disease of the fetus and newborn (HDFN), **847–859**

   antenatal monitoring, 853f

      amniotic fluid spectrophotometry in, 854

      fetal blood sampling, 854

      maternal immunohematologic testing, 852–853

      paternal zygosity/fetal blood type, 852

      ultrasonography, 854, 855f

   clinical features, **848–849**

   definition and history, 847, 2329

   differential diagnosis, 849

   epidemiology, 847–848, 848t

   obstetric history and, 849

   outcome, 858

   pathophysiology

      ABO hemolytic disease, 851, 852t, 2330, 2348

      Kell hemolytic disease, 851

      minor RBC antigens, 851

      RhD hemolytic disease, 849–850, 851f, 852t, 2348

   prevention, **858–859**, 859f, 2339

   therapy, **854–858**

      delivery, 855

      erythropoietin, 859

      exchange transfusion, 856–857

      immediate postnatal, 856

      intrauterine transfusion, 854–855

      IVIG, 858–859

      neonatal monitoring, 855–856, 856f

      phototherapy, 857

Alloimmune neonatal neutropenia, 995, 2358

Allopurinol, 322

   for acute lymphoblastic leukemia, 1505, 1514

   for hyperuricemia, 1394, 1450, 1514

Allotypes, immunoglobulin, 1170–1171

All-*trans*-retinoic acid. *See* ATRA (all-*trans*-retinoic acid)

Alopecia, 632, 1223

ALOX5AP, 2288

ALOX12, 2060

α2a adrenergic receptors, 1876

αβ heterodimers, 1175, 1176f

$\alpha_1\beta_1$ interface, mutations in, 781

αβ T-cell receptor, 1177

α-chain (AM) allotypes, 1170

α chemokines, 288, 288t

αδ-storage pool deficiency, 2055

α-enolase, 696

α-globin chains

   β-thalassemias and, 742

   hemoglobin, 728, 760–761

α-globin chains (*Cont.*):
    in hemoglobin H disease, 1353
    variants, 751, 778
α-globin gene cluster, 728–729, 729*f*
α granules, 1818, 1819*f*, 1843–1845, 1844*f*,
        1846–1847*t*, 1848, 2166
α-heavy-chain disease, **1806–1809**
    chromosomal abnormalities, 1808
    clinical features, 1806–1807
    course and prognosis, 1809
    definition and history, 1806
    differential diagnosis, 1808
    epidemiology, 1806
    etiology and pathogenesis, 1806
    gene mutations, 1807, 1807*f*
    laboratory features, 1807–1808, 1807*f*
    therapy, 1808–1809
α helix, disruption of, 781
α integrins. *See under* Integrin
α-storage pool deficiency (gray platelet
        syndrome), 1850, 1853,
        2054–2055, 2055*f*
α-thalassemia–myelodysplastic syndrome,
        1353
α-thalassemias
    α⁰
        deletion forms, 748
        epidemiology/population genetics, 727,
            727*f*
        laboratory features, 747–748
        molecular basis, 736–737, 737*t*, 738*f*
    α⁺
        epidemiology/population genetics, 727,
            727*f*
        laboratory features, 747
        molecular basis, 737–738, 737*t*, 738*f*
    with α- and β-chain hemoglobin variants,
        731
    clinical features, **745**
    deletional, 771
    differential diagnosis, 748, 749*f*
    epidemiology/population genetics,
        727–728, 727*f*
    haplotype interactions, 739
    hemoglobin Bart's hydrops fetalis
            syndrome. *See* Hemoglobin Bart's
            hydrops fetalis syndrome
    hemoglobin H disease. *See* Hemoglobin H
            disease
    hemoglobin variants causing, 778*t*
    leukemia and, 739
    mental retardation and, 739, 745
    minor, 636
    molecular basis, **736–739**, 737*t*,
            739*f*
    myelodysplasia and, 739

pathophysiology. *See* Thalassemias,
        pathophysiology
    in pregnancy, 126
    unusual forms, 739
ALPS (autoimmune lymphoproliferative
        syndrome), 210, **1224**, 1575*t*
Alteplase, **403**
    for myocardial infarction, 2295
    for stroke, 2314, 2314*t*, 2315
Alternative pathway of complement, 572,
        572*f*
Alum, 422
Alvocidib, for chronic lymphocytic leukemia,
        218
Alzheimer disease, 1848
AM (α-chain) allotypes, 1170
Ambroxol, 1128
Amenorrhea, history of, 5
Amifostine, for acute myelogenous leukemia,
        1404
Amikacin, 386, 387*t*
Amino acids
    deletions, unstable hemoglobins and, 781
    in neutrophils, 935, 935*t*
Aminocaproic acid. *See* ε-aminocaproic acid
        (EACA)
Aminoglycosides, 384
δ-Aminolevulinate dehydratase (ALAD), 894
δ-Aminolevulinate dehydratase porphyria
        (ADP), 890*t*, 891*t*, 894, 900
δ-Aminolevulinate hydrolase, 894
δ-Aminolevulinate synthase (ALAS),
        892–894
5-Aminolevulinic acid (ALA), 1686
δ-Aminolevulinic acid (ALA), 889, 891*f*, 893*f*
δ-Aminolevulinic acid (ALA) dehydrase,
        701*t*
Aminopeptidase N. *See* CD13
Aminopterin (4-aminopteroylglutamic acid)
    for acute lymphoblastic leukemia, 1505
    mechanism of action, 197
    megaloblastic anemia and, 605, 606*t*
Aminopyrine, 996
AML. *See* Acute myelogenous (myeloid)
        leukemia (AML)
AML1. See RUNX1 (AML1)
AML1-ETO, 225, 240
AMLI-3, 926
AMML (acute myelomonocytic leukemia),
        180, 1382*f*, 1387, 1388*t*, **1390**
AMN (amnionless), 591, 605
Amniotic fluid embolism, 2210
Amniotic fluid spectrophotometry, 854
Amotosalen, 2388
AMP deaminase, 701*t*
Amphotericin B, 385, 387*t*

AMPK (adenosine monophosphate kinase),
        194–195
Amsacrine
    for acute myelogenous leukemia, 1395
    secondary acute myelogenous leukemia
        and, 1407
Amyloid, 1773
Amyloid light-chain amyloidosis. *See*
        Immunoglobulin light-chain (AL)
        amyloidosis
Amyloidoses
    AA (secondary), 1773, 1774*t*, 1776
    classification, 1773, 1774*t*
    in familial Mediterranean fever, 1006, 1773
    immunoglobulin light-chain. *See*
        Immunoglobulin light-chain (AL)
        amyloidosis
    inherited forms, 1773, 1774*t*, 1776,
        1777–1778
    systemic, 2108
Amyloid precursor protein (APP), 1848
Anagrelide
    adverse effects, 1314, 2081
    for chronic myeloproliferative disorders,
        2081
    for cytoreduction in chronic myelogenous
        leukemia, 1450–1451
    for essential thrombocythemia, 1313*t*,
        1314, 1314*t*, 2081
    for polycythemia vera, 1298*t*, 1300
Anakinra, for Erdheim-Chester disease, 1111
Anal cancer, 1243
Anaphylactic reactions, 2375
Anaphylatoxin, 932
Anaplastic large cell lymphoma (ALCL)
    ALK-negative, 1694*t*, 1695*t*, 1698, 1699
    ALK-positive, **1637**, 1694*t*, 1695*t*,
        1698–1699
    breast implant–associated, 1698
    chromosomal abnormalities, 185*t*, 188,
        224*t*, 1499*t*, 1576–1577
    clinical features, 1698
    definition, 1698
    epidemiology, 1694*t*, 1698
    gene mutations, 1499*t*
    laboratory features, 1499*t*, 1598–1599,
        1599*f*, 1600*f*, 1699–1700
    primary cutaneous. *See* Primary cutaneous
        anaplastic large cell lymphoma
    prognosis, 1695*t*, 1699
    treatment, 1694–1696, 1695*t*, 1696*t*, 1699
ANCAs (antineutrophil cytoplasmic
        antibodies), 959–960, 2107
Ancylostomiasis, 957*t*
Anderson disease, 567
Androgens

adverse effects, 579
for anemia of primary myelofibrosis, 1328
for aplastic anemia, 526
deficiency, anemia and, 560
erythropoietic effects, 560, 879, 880*f*
for Fanconi anemia, 529
for paroxysmal nocturnal hemoglobinuria, 578–579
Anemia, **503–506**
in acute lymphoblastic leukemia, 1509
in acute myelogenous leukemia, 1381
in alcoholism, 654–655
aplastic. *See* Aplastic anemia
from blood donation, 629–630
of chronic disease, 549. *See also* Anemia of inflammation (AI)
of chronic kidney disease. *See* Anemia of chronic kidney disease
of chronic liver disease, 636
classification, **506**, 507–508*t*
clonal, 1277
congenital dyserythropoietic. *See* Congenital dyserythropoietic anemias (CDAs)
consultative approach to, 42
cow's milk, 630
of critical illness, 549
differential diagnosis, 42
dilution, 554, 742
of endocrine disorders, **559–561**
factitious, 630
Fanconi. *See* Fanconi anemia
hemolytic. *See* Hemolytic anemia
of hemolytic disease, 637
in HIV infection. *See* Human immunodeficiency virus (HIV) infection, anemia in
in Hodgkin lymphoma, 1610
hypoplastic, 637
of hypothyroidism, **559**, 637
iatrogenic, 629
of inflammation. *See* Anemia of inflammation (AI)
iron-deficiency. *See* Iron deficiency
with marrow infiltration. *See* Marrow, infiltration
from metastatic invasion of marrow, 553–554
newborn, 103, 849
pathophysiology and manifestations, **503–506**
cardiac output, 505
oxygen transport, 503–505, 504*f*, 505*f*
pulmonary function, 505
red cell production, 505–506, 505*f*
tissue hypoxia, 506

pernicious. *See* Pernicious anemia (PA)
in pregnancy, **120**
preoperative, 2378
prevalence of, 134, 134*t*
in primary myelofibrosis, 1328
of protein deficiency (kwashiorkor), **654**
sideroblastic. *See* Sideroblastic anemias
of starvation, **654**
trace metal deficiency, 653–654
unexplained, 134, 136
vitamin-deficiency, **651–653**. *See also* specific vitamins
Anemia of chronic kidney disease
clinical features, 552
epidemiology, 550
iron deficiency and, 637
laboratory features, 552
pathophysiology, 549, 550*f*
therapy, course, and prognosis, 554*t*, 555
Anemia of inflammation (AI), **549–555**
clinical features, 552
conditions associated with, 550*t*
definition and history, 549
differential diagnosis, 553–554
epidemiology, 550
etiology and pathogenesis, **550–552**, 551*f*
vs. iron deficiency, 636
laboratory features, 552–553, 553*f*, 553*t*
therapy, course, and prognosis, **554–555**, 554*t*
Anesthesia
for marrow aspiration, 28
platelet function and, 2079
in sickle cell disease, 773
Aneuploidy, 175*t*
Aneurysm, formation of, 1975, 1975*f*
Angina pectoris, 5, 2295–2297
Angiogenesis, 279
fibrinolysis and, 2311
in myelodysplastic syndromes, 1353
in primary myelofibrosis, 1321
regulation by hypoxia, 504*f*
Angiogenin, 1449
Angiography, for pulmonary embolism, 2271–2272, 2272*f*
Angioimmunoblastic T-cell lymphoma (AITL), 1498*t*, 1598, 1694–1695, 1694*t*, 1695*t*, **1697–1698**
Angioma, tufted, 2014
Angiotensin II, 1879
Anhydrotic ectodermal dysplasia with immunodeficiency caused by NEMO mutations, 1215
Anidulafungin, 385, 388*t*, 389
Animal models
eosinophilic disease, 951

hemochromatosis, 642–643
knockout, 153
transgenic, 153
Anion exchanger (AE1), 663*t*, 664
Anisocytosis, 21
Anistreplase, 2313, 2313*t*
*ANK1*i, 666
Ankyrin, 663*t*, 666, 666*f*, 670*t*, 671–672
Annexin A2, 1973*f*, 1974, 1976, 2237, 2305*t*, 2309
Annexin A5 anticoagulant shield, 2236, 2236*f*
Annexin A5 resistance assay, 2243–2244
Anorexia, history of, 5
Anorexia nervosa, 654
Anosmia, history of, 5
Anthracyclines, **327–328**. *See also* specific drugs
for acute lymphoblastic leukemia, 1515
for acute myelogenous leukemia, 1394–1396, 1395*t*
adverse effects, 327–328, 1520
for anaplastic large cell lymphoma, 1699
for intravascular large B-cell lymphoma, 1635–1636
for mantle cell lymphoma, 1655
mechanism of action, 327
pharmacology, 327–328
for primary cutaneous diffuse large B-cell lymphoma, leg type, 1637
resistance to, 319*t*
Antiangiogenesis agents, for acute myelogenous leukemia, 1404
Antiannexin A2 antibodies, 1976
Anti-B$_2$ glycoprotein antibody assays, 2242
Antibiotics. *See also* specific drugs
for α-heavy-chain disease, 1808
anthracycline. *See* Anthracyclines
platelet effects, 2078
Antibodies
dendritic cells and, 309
erythrocyte. *See* Erythrocyte antibodies
to human leukocyte antigens, 2356
to neutrophil antigens, 2358–2359
to platelet antigens, 2361–2362
reaginic, 1162
Antibody-dependent cellular cytotoxicity (ADCC), 344–345, 1645
Antibody identification, 2336
Antibody screening, 2336, 2349.
See also Erythrocyte antibodies
Anticardiolipin antibody, 2101*f*
Anticardiolipin antibody assays, 2242
Anti-CCR4 monoclonal antibody.
See Mogamulizumab
Anti-CD20 monoclonal antibody.
See Rituximab

Anti-CD52 monoclonal antibody.
  See Alemtuzumab
Anticoagulants/anticoagulation.
  See Antithrombotic therapy
Anticodon, 147
Anticonvulsants, megaloblastic anemia and,
  606t
Anti-D alloimmunization, 850, 1253–1254
Antidepressants, platelet function and, 2079
Antierythrocyte antibodies. *See* Erythrocyte
  antibodies
Antifibrinolytic therapy, **2317–2318**
  agents
    aprotinin, 2318
    ε-aminocaproic acid (EACA).
      See ε-aminocaproic acid (EACA)
    tranexamic acid. *See* Tranexamic acid
  for bleeding not response to platelet
    transfusion, 2385
  for combined deficiency of factors V and
    VIII, 2140
  for disseminated intravascular coagulation,
    2214
  for hemophilia A, 2123
  indications, 2317t
  platelet function and, 2078
Antigen collection, 2329
Antigenicity, 2336
Antigen-presenting cells. *See* Dendritic cells
  (DCs)
Antigens
  cross-presentation, 308
  for cytomegalovirus-specific T cells,
    409–410
  defined, 2336
  discovery of, for cancer vaccine therapy,
    421, 422t
  erythrocyte. *See* Erythrocyte antigens
  for leukemia-specific T cells, 413
  leukocyte. *See* Human leukocyte antigen
    (HLA)
  for melanoma-specific T cells, 412
  minor histocompatibility, 413–414
  neutrophil. *See* Human neutrophil antigens
    (HNAs)
  platelet. *See* Human platelet antigens
    (HPAs)
  self-, 2343
  tumor, categories of, 412t
  uptake and processing in dendritic cells,
    308–309
Antihemophilic factor. *See* Factor VIII
Antihistamines
  for allergic transfusion reactions, 2375
  for mastocytosis, 976
  platelet function and, 2079

Anti-IL-5 monoclonal antibody, 959, 1470
Anti-IL-6 monoclonal antibody. *See*
  Siltuximab
Anti-IL-6 receptor monoclonal antibody.
  See Tocilizumab
Anti-inhibitor coagulant complex (AICC),
  2185
Anti-integrin α$_{IIb}$β$_3$, 1995
Antilymphocyte serum (ALG), 522
Antineoplastic drugs/chemotherapy,
  315–346. *See also specific drugs*
  acute myelogenous leukemia and, 1374,
    1374t
  agents of diverse mechanisms, **331–333**
    L-asparaginase. *See* L-Asparaginase
    bleomycin. *See* Bleomycin
  alkylating drugs. *See* Alkylating drugs
  antitubulins, 325–326
    taxanes, 326
    vinca alkaloids. *See* Vinblastine;
      Vincristine
  aplastic anemia and, 517t, 519
  basic principles, **316–318**
  cell cycle-specific agents, **318–325**
    5-azacytidine. *See* 5-Azacytidine
    cladribine. *See* Cladribine
    clofarabine. *See* Clofarabine
    cyclin-dependent kinase inhibitors, 218
    cytarabine. *See* Cytarabine (ara-C)
    fludarabine phosphate. *See* Fludarabine
      phosphate
    gemcitabine. *See* Gemcitabine
    hydroxyurea. *See* Hydroxyurea
    methotrexate. *See* Methotrexate
    nelarabine, 323f, **325**, 1518
    pentostatin. *See* Pentostatin
      (deoxycoformycin)
    purine analogues. *See* Purine analogues
  cell kinetics and, **317**
  combination chemotherapy, **317**
  differentiating agents, **335–336**
    arsenic trioxide. *See* Arsenic trioxide
    retinoids, 335. *See also* ATRA
      (all-*trans*-retinoic acid)
  dose modification for renal or hepatic
    dysfunction, 316, 316t
  epigenetic agents, **336–338**
    demethylating agents, 336. *See also*
      5-Azacytidine; Decitabine
    future targets, **337–338**, 337f
    histone deacetylase inhibitors, 240,
      336–337. *See also* Romidepsin;
      Vorinostat
  high-dose regimens with stem cell support,
    331, 331t, 332t
  history, 315–316

immunomodulatory drugs, **333–335**, 333f
  lenalidomide. *See* Lenalidomide
  pomalidomide. *See* Pomalidomide
  thalidomide. *See* Thalidomide
molecularly targeted small molecules,
  338–343, 339t, 340f
  ibrutinib. *See* Ibrutinib
  janus kinase inhibitors, **341–342**
  proteasome inhibitors, **342–343**. *See also*
    Bortezomib; Carfilzomib
  tyrosine kinase inhibitors. *See* Tyrosine
    kinase inhibitors
monoclonal antibodies. *See* Monoclonal
  antibodies
platelet function and, 2079
resistance to, 318, 319t
topoisomerase inhibitors, **326–329**
  anthracycline antibiotics, 327–328. *See
    also* Daunorubicin; Doxorubicin;
    Epirubicin; Idarubicin;
    Mitoxantrone
  camptothecins, 326–327
  epipodophyllotoxins, 328–329. *See also*
    Etoposide; Teniposide
for transplantation preparation, **360–361**
Antineutrophil cytoplasmic antibodies
  (ANCAs), 959–960, 2107
Antioxidant protein 2 (AOP2), 790
Antioxidants, porphyria cutanea tarda and,
  907
Anti-PF4–heparin antibodies, 2029–2030,
  2030t. *See also* Heparin-induced
    thrombocytopenia (HIT)
Antiphosphatidyl serine antibody assay, 2242
Antiphospholipid antibodies, 1995,
  2233–2235, 2236f, 2237
Antiphospholipid syndrome (APS),
  2233–2245
  antiannexin A2 antibodies in, 1976
  catastrophic, 2239, 2245
  in children, 2241
  clinical features, 2100, 2101f, 2234t,
    2238–2241, 2238f, 2238t, 2240t
  definition and history, 2233–2234
  differential diagnosis, 2244
  etiology, 2234
  immune thrombocytopenia in, 2008
  laboratory features, 2234t, **2241–2244**,
    2241t
  pathogenesis, **2234–2237**, 2235f, 2235t,
    2236f, 2237f
  in pregnancy, 2239, 2244, 2245
  therapy, course, and prognosis, 2234–2245
Antiplatelet antibodies, **2084–2085**
Antiplatelet drugs, 394t, **403–406**, 404t. *See
  also specific drugs*

ADP receptor blockers, 405

$\alpha_{IIb}\beta_3$ blockers, 405–406

cyclic adenosine monophosphate modulators, 404–405

cyclooxygenase inhibitors, 403–404

for essential thrombocythemia, 1313

for myocardial infarction, 2295–2296

for peripheral artery disease, 2297

platelet transfusion and, 2385

thrombin receptor blockers, 406

for thrombotic thrombocytopenic purpura, 2256

Anti-protein S antibodies, 2187

Antiprothrombin antibodies, 2186–2187

Antiretroviral therapy (ART)

chemotherapy drugs and, 1249

for HIV infection

adverse effects, 1242, 2281

effectiveness, 1242

with Hodgkin lymphoma, 1249

initiation, 1242, 1242t

maternal ingestion, effects on fetus and newborn, 112t

Anti-(Rh)D, 2005, 2011

Antisense DNA, 153

Antisense RNA, 153

Antiswitching therapies, for sickle cell disease, 774–775, 774t

Antithrombin (AT), **1959–1960**

antibodies, 2186

characteristics, 1916t, 1936

in disseminated intravascular coagulation, 2202

functions, 1936–1937, 1936f, 1968, 2202

gene structure and variations, 1937, 1959

mutations, 1959

as protease inhibitor, 1919, 1919t, 1958–1959

structure, 1936, 1952t

synthesis, 1958

Antithrombin (AT) concentrate, 2213

Antithrombin (AT) deficiency

acquired causes, 2224t

clinical implications of testing for, 2228t

epidemiology, 2222t

etiology and pathogenesis, 1937, 1959, 2222–2223

heparin resistance in, 397

venous thromboembolism risk and, 2225t, 2226t

Antithrombin I. See Fibrinogen

Antithrombin III. See Antithrombin (AT)

Antithrombotic therapy, **393–406**

adverse effects, 2277

antiplatelet drugs. See Antiplatelet drugs in cancer, 2276–2277

contraindications, 2273

direct thrombin inhibitors, 2031t. See also Argatroban; Bivalirudin

fibrinolytic therapy. See Fibrinolytic therapy

heparin. See Heparin

indirect factor Xa inhibitors. See Danaparoid; Fondaparinux

low-molecular-weight heparin. See Low-molecular-weight heparin (LMWH)

for myocardial infarction, 2295–2296

overview, 393

platelet function and, 2078

platelet transfusion and, 2385

in pregnancy, 580, 2277

targeted oral anticoagulants. See Apixaban; Dabigatran; Edoxaban; Rivaroxaban

types and function, 394t

for venous thromboembolism. See Venous thrombosis/thromboembolism, therapy

vitamin K antagonists. See Warfarin

Antithymocyte globulin (ATG)

for aplastic anemia, 523, 524t, 525f, 525t, 527

for graft-versus-host disease prophylaxis, 371

for hemophagocytic lymphohistiocytosis, 1115

for myelodysplastic syndromes, 1359

for pure red cell aplasia, 544

Antitubulins, 325–326

Antitumor necrosis factor (TNF)-α therapy, 285, 1071, 1359

AOP2 (antioxidant protein 2), 790

Aorta-gonad-mesonephros (AGM) region, 54, 100f, 101, 257–258, 1149–1150

Aortic aneurysms, 2210

AP1 (activator protein 1), 1606

AP3 (activator protein 3) complex, 1843

AP-3 endosomal protein, 1229

AP1903, 440, 440f

Apaf1, 205

APC. See Activated protein C (APC)

APC, 1346

APECED (autoimmune polyendocrinopathy-candidiasis ectodermal dystrophy), 87, 1181, **1224**

Apheresis

for blood component collection and production, 2368–2369, 2386

definition and history, 427

extracorporeal photochemotherapy, 429t, 433, 1687

leukocytapheresis. See Leukocytapheresis

plasma exchange. See Plasma exchange

red cell depletion. See Erythrocytapheresis

red cell exchange. See Red cell exchange

thrombocytapheresis, 433

Apixaban, **402**

adverse effects, 2275t

clinical studies, 401t

mechanism of action, 1922

for venous thromboembolism, 2274–2275, 2274t, 2275t

APL. See Acute promyelocytic leukemia (APL)

Aplastic anemia, **513–527**

acute myelogenous leukemia and, 1375

clinical features, 519

clonal myeloid diseases and, 521

course and prognosis, 527

definition, 513

degree of severity, 513, 514t

differential diagnosis, 520–521, 637, 1513

epidemiology, 513–514

etiology and pathogenesis, **514–519**, 514t, 516f

autoimmune disorders in, 518

autoreactive cytotoxic T lymphocytes in, 515, 516f

drug-related, 515–516

iatrogenic, 518–519

pregnancy-related, 518

stromal microenvironment and growth factors in, 519

telomere shortening in, 515

toxic chemicals in, 516–518

viral, 518

hereditary

dyskeratosis congenita, **530–532**, 531f, 531t

Fanconi anemia. See Fanconi anemia

rare syndromes, 530t, 532

Shwachman-Diamond syndrome, **532**, 993–994, 1026

history, 513

laboratory features, 519–520, 519t, 520f

monocytopenia in, 1098

paroxysmal nocturnal hemoglobinuria and, 521

Ph chromosome–positive clonal myeloid diseases and, 1450

treatment, **521–527**

androgens, 526

approach to, 521–522, 521t, 525f

cytokines, 526

hematopoietic cell transplantation, 522–523

immunosuppressive therapy, 523–526, 524t, 525t

Aplastic anemia, treatment (*Cont.*):
  investigative, 527
  rituximab, 526
  splenectomy, 527
  supportive care, 522
Aplastic crisis
  in hereditary spherocytosis, 674
  in sickle cell disease, 767
Apo-1. *See* Fas (CD95)
Apoferritin, 618
Apoferritin mRNA, 624*f*, 625*f*
Apolipoprotein A (ApoA), 1976
Apolipoprotein A1 (ApoA1), 2288
Apolipoprotein E receptor 2 (apoER2), 2237
Apolipoprotein H. *See* β2Glycoprotein (GP)I
      (apolipoprotein H)
Apoptosis
  BCR-ABL and, 1444
  caspases in, 203–205, 204*f*
  definition, 203
  of eosinophils, 951
  genotoxic stress and, 209
  hematologic diseases and, 209–211
  of hematopoietic stem cells, 74–75
  macrophages in, 1060–1061, 1061*f*
  of neutrophils, 285, 992
  signal transduction pathways and,
      208–209, 208*f*
  suppressors, 205–208
Apoptosome, 205
Apoptotic cells, 23
APP (amyloid precursor protein), 1848
APRIL, 309
Aprotinin, 2318
APS. *See* Antiphospholipid syndrome (APS)
aPTT. *See* Activated partial thromboplastin
      time (aPTT)
Arabidopsis thaliana, 293
Arabinosyl cytosine. *See* Cytarabine (ara-C)
Ara-C. *See* Cytarabine (ara-C)
Arachidonic acid, 288, 1854, 1857*f*, 1874
Arachidonic acid metabolism, 1016, 2058
Arachidonic acid metabolites, 284*t*, 286*t*,
      1876–1877
Arasulfatase A, 439
ARDS (acute respiratory distress syndrome),
      2201, 2204–2205, 2208
Arf, 1883
Argatroban, **399**
  clinical uses, 399
  for heparin-induced thrombocytopenia,
      2030, 2031*t*
  pharmacology, 399
  for unstable angina, 2296
Arginase-1, 1013*t*, 1014
Arginine, for sickle cell disease, 777*t*

L-Arginine, 286
Arginine butyrate, 775
ARID1A, 235*t*, 1788
ARID1B, 1788
Arp2/3 complex, 1841
Arry-614, 1360
ARSA, 439
Arsenic, megaloblastic anemia and, 606*t*
Arsenic hydride, 52., 810
Arsenic trioxide, **335–336**
  for acute myelogenous leukemia, 1404
  for acute promyelocytic leukemia, 1404,
      1405*t*, 1406
  for myelodysplastic syndromes, 1360
Arsine gas, 810
Artemis, 1166*f*, 1167, 1214*t*
Arterial thrombosis
  in antiphospholipid syndrome, 2238
  in chronic myeloproliferative neoplasms,
      2080–2081
  consultative approach to, 47
  in disseminated intravascular coagulation,
      2204
  in heparin-induced thrombocytopenia,
      2028
  in hereditary thrombophilia, 2226–2227
  in nonatherosclerotic arteries, 2293
  pathobiology, 2291–2292, 2291*t*
  pathogenesis, 2292–2293
  platelet activation in, 2245
  site-specific characteristics, 2292
  systemic factors, 2246
  thrombophilia testing in, 2228–2229
  tissue factor and phospholipids in,
      2245–2246
  vs. venous thrombosis, 2291*t*
  vorapaxar for prevention of, 2076–2077
Arthralgia, history of, 6
Arthritis
  in acute myelogenous leukemia, 1381
  history of, 6
  rheumatoid. *See* Rheumatoid arthritis
  septic, 771
Arthropathy
  in hemochromatosis, 643
  in hemophilia, 2117, 2117*f*, 2118*f*
Arthropod bites, 2102
Ascariasis, 957*t*
Ascorbic acid. *See* Vitamin C (ascorbic acid)
ASCT2 (SLC1A5), 197, 198
ASO-PCR (allele-specific oligonucleotide
      polymerase chain reaction), 1716
L-Asparaginase, **332–333**
  for acute lymphoblastic leukemia, 1515,
      1516, 1517
  adverse effects, 333, 1519*t*, 1520

  formulations, 1515
  mechanism of action, 197, 198, 332–333
  for NK/T-cell lymphoma, 1702
ASPEN syndrome, 770
Aspergillus infections
  as cause of hemolytic anemia, 820
  in chronic granulomatous disease, 1030,
      1032
  cutaneous, 2104–2105, 2105*f*
  after hematopoietic cell transplantation,
      369
  in immunocompromised host, 383
  prevention, 389
Aspirin
  for antiphospholipid syndrome in
      pregnancy, 2245
  avoidance in hemophilia A, 2121
  for chronic myeloproliferative disorders,
      2081
  clinical uses, 404, 404*t*
  dosage, 404*t*
  for essential thrombocythemia, 1313, 2081
  hemolytic anemia and, 708
  hemostatic effects, 2075
  maternal ingestion
    effect on fetus and newborn, 112, 112*t*
    platelet aggregation in newborn and,
      107
  mechanism of action, 404, 404*t*, 2073–2074
  myeloma incidence and, 1709
  for myocardial infarction, 2295–2296
  for peripheral arterial disease, 2297
  platelet effects, 2073–2075
  for polycythemia vera, 1300, 2081
  resistance, 2075
  for stroke prevention, 2297
  for thrombotic thrombocytopenic
      purpura, 2256
  for venous thromboembolism, 2276
Asplenia, 868
Asthma
  eosinophils and, 954, 955*t*
  mast cells in, 969
  sickle cell disease and, 769
ASXL1, 226*t*, 227*t*, 229*t*, 1346*t*, 1351
AT. *See* Antithrombin (AT)
AT1-type receptors, 1879
Ataxia-pancytopenia, 530*t*
Ataxia-telangiectasia, **1226–1227**
  acute lymphoblastic leukemia and, 1507
  clinical features, 1215*t*, 1226–1227
  gene mutations, 1227, 1575*t*
  laboratory features, 1214*t*
  lymphomas and, 1575*t*
  pathophysiology, 1226
  treatment, 1227

Ataxia-telangiectasia-like disorder, **1227**
Ataxia-telangiectasia mutated and
    rad3-related (ATR) kinase, 532
Atazanavir, 1249
ATG. *See* Antithymocyte globulin (ATG)
Atheroembolism, 2101, 2102*f*, **2298**
Atheromatous embolism, 2298
Atherosclerosis, **2281–2291**
    in antiphospholipid syndrome, 2237,
        2237*f*, 2240
    carotid artery, 2297
    endothelial dysfunction in, 2282–2285
        blood fluidity and, 2285
        inflammation, 2282*f*
        progenitor cells and, 2285
        vascular growth and, 2283–2285, 2284*f*
        vascular tone and, 2282–2283, 2282*f*
    inflammation and, 2285–2288
        adaptive immunity, 2286
        adhesion molecules, 2286
        CD40 and CD40 ligand, 2288
        genetics, 2288
        high-density lipoprotein levels,
            2287–2288
        immune cells, 2286
        infection, 2288
        innate immunity, 2285–2286
        lipid peroxidation, 2287
        lipoprotein phospholipase A$_2$, 2286
        low-density lipoprotein in vascular wall,
            2287
        scavenger receptors, 2287
        splenectomy, 2288
        transforming growth factor-β, 2288
    monocytes/macrophages in, 1079
    plaque in
        atherothrombi formation and. *See*
            Arterial thrombosis
        classification, 2288–2289, 2289*f*
        formation, 1975*f*
        life span, 2282*f*
        vulnerable, 2289–2291, 2290*f*,
            2291*t*
    risk factors, 2281–2282, 2282*t*
Atherothrombosis
    arterial thrombosis and. *See* Arterial
        thrombosis
    definition, 2291
    gene variants, 1850, 1850*f*
ATL/ATLL. *See* Adult T-cell leukemia/
    lymphoma (ATL/ATLL)
ATM
    in acute lymphoblastic leukemia, 1507
    in ataxia-telangiectasia, 1227
    in chronic lymphocytic leukemia, 187,
        231*t*, 1529

    in lymphomas, 187
    in mantle cell lymphoma, 187, 236*t*, 1654
Atovaquone
    for babesiosis, 819
    as empiric therapy for infections, 386
    prophylactic, 389
ATP (adenosine triphosphate)
    in glucose metabolism, 192, 692
    in platelet metabolism, 1839–1840
    receptors for, 1874
ATP-dependent chromatin remodeling
        complexes (*remodelers*), 166–168,
        166*f*
ATP diphosphohydrolase. *See* CD39
ATRA (all-*trans*-retinoic acid), **335**
    for acute myelogenous leukemia, 1396,
        1404, 1409
    for acute promyelocytic leukemia, 1391,
        1404–1406, 1405*t*
        in pregnancy, 124
    dose and action mechanism, 1404–1405
    for Langerhans cell histiocytosis, 1107
    resistance to, 197
    toxic effects, 1405
ATRX, 1346*t*, 1353
Atypical chronic myelogenous leukemia
        (aCML), 1279, 1473
Atypical hemolytic uremic syndrome
        (aHUS), 1932, 1953, **2259–2261**,
        2259*t*
Atypical myeloproliferative disease, 1473
Auer rods, 23, 1390
Aurora kinase inhibitors, 1403
Autoantibodies
    development, 2183–2184
    induction, 825*f*, 830*t*, 831
    red cell, 2343. *See also* Erythrocyte
        antibodies
Autoimmune diseases
    antiphospholipid syndrome and, 2238
    aplastic anemia and, 518
    cobalamin deficiency and, 600
    hyposplenism and, 868
    lymphocytopenia and, 1206
    myeloma and, 1734
    primary immunodeficiency
        disorders presenting as. *See*
        Immunodeficiency diseases,
        primary, presenting as autoimmune
        diseases
    thrombotic microangiopathy and, 2262
Autoimmune hemolytic anemia, **823–840**
    in chronic lymphocytic leukemia, 824, 827,
        831, 839, 840, 1541
    classification, 824–825, 824*t*
    cold-antibody

    classification, 824, 824*t*
    clinical features, 831–832
    course and prognosis, 840
    epidemiology, 825, 827
    etiology, 828
    laboratory features, 832–833, 833*f*, 834*t*
    pathogenesis, 829, 2348
    serologic features, 835–836
    therapy, 839
    course and prognosis, 840
    definition and history, 823–824
    differential diagnosis, 836–837
    direct antiglobulin test findings in, 823,
        833, 834*t*
    drug-induced. *See* Hemolytic anemia,
        drug-induced immune
    laboratory features, 832–834, 833*f*
    primary/idiopathic, 824, 827
    secondary, 824, 827
    therapy, **837**
    warm-antibody
        classification, 824, 824*t*
        clinical features, 832
        course and prognosis, 840
        epidemiology, 825
        etiology, 827–828
        laboratory features, 832–834, 833*f*,
            834*t*
        pathogenesis, 828–829, 2348
        serologic features, 834–835, 834*f*
        therapy, 838–839
        thrombocytopenia with. *See* Evans
            syndrome
Autoimmune lymphoproliferative syndrome
        (ALPS), 210, **1224**, 1575*t*
Autoimmune neutropenia, 995, 996*f*, 2358
Autoimmune polyendocrinopathy-
        candidiasis ectodermal dystrophy
        (APECED), 87, 1181, **1224**
Autoimmune thrombocytopenic purpura. *See*
        Immune thrombocytopenia (ITP)
Autoimmunity
    forward feedback loops and, **304**
    lymphomas and, 1574–1575
Autologous blood donations, 2367–2368
Autologous hematopoietic stem cell
        transplantation. *See* Hematopoietic
        cell transplantation (HCT),
        autologous
Autologous stem cell infusion
    for acute myelogenous leukemia, 1399,
        1408
    for chronic myelogenous leukemia, 1460
    for myelodysplastic syndromes, 1362
Autophagy, 487, 1062, 1065*f*
Autosomal dominant inheritance, 148, 148*f*

Autosomal recessive agammaglobulinemia, **1212–1213**, 1214*t*

Autosomal recessive hyper-IgE syndrome. *See* Hyperimmunoglobulin E syndrome (HIES)

Autosomal recessive hyper-IgM syndrome. *See* Hyperimmunoglobulin M syndromes

Autosomal recessive inheritance, 149, 149*f*

Autosomal recessive megaloblastic anemia (MGA1), 605

Avascular necrosis, 771, 771*f*

Avatrombopag, for immune thrombocytopenia, 526

5-Azacytidine, **322**
    for acute myelogenous leukemia, 1403
    for chronic myelomonocytic leukemia, 1469
    mechanism of action, 239, 1360
    for myelodysplastic syndromes, 336, 1360, 1361
    for sickle cell disease, 774*t*, 775

5-Aza-2′-deoxycytidine. *See* Decitabine

6-Azantidine, megaloblastic anemia and, 606*t*

Azathioprine, 322
    for autoimmune hemolytic anemia, 839
    for immune thrombocytopenia, 2006–2007
    megaloblastic anemia and, 606*t*
    for pure red cell aplasia, 544

Azidothymidine, anemia induced by, 561

Azithromycin, for babesiosis, 819

AZT. *See* Zidovudine (AZT)

Aztreonam, 387*t*

Azurocidin (heparin-binding protein), 1012*t*, 1013

Azurophil granules
    in acute myeloblastic leukemia, 1387
    formation, 1009, 1010*f*
    heterogeneity, 1009
    laboratory features, 926, 928*f*
    physical-chemical and functional properties, 1011–1013, 1012*t*

B

B-1 B cells, 1141, 1151

B-2 B cells, 1151

B19 parvovirus infection. *See* Parvovirus B19 infection

BA2. *See* CD9

Babesia, 819–820

Babesiosis, 429*t*, 432, 817*f*, **818–819**

Bacillus cereus, 809

Back disorders, history of, 6

Bacterial infections. *See also specific bacteria*
    antiphospholipid antibodies and, 2234
    disseminated intravascular coagulation and, 2207

empiric therapy, 384–385, 387*t*
    in febrile nonhemolytic transfusion reaction, 2375
    after hematopoietic cell transplantation, 369
    in immunocompromised host, **383**
    from platelet products, 2386, 2388
    prevention, 388–389
    purpura and, 2104, 2104*f*
    TLR-signaling defects with increased susceptibility to, 1230

Bacterial permeability-increasing protein (BPI), 106–107, 1011, 1012*t*, 1013

Bactericidal activity, in newborn, 106–107

Baculovirus inhibitor of apoptosis repeat (BIR) domains, 207, 298

BAF (BRG/BAF-associated factors) complex, 166, 166*f*

BAFF (B-cell activation factor), 309, 1713

Bak, 204*f*, 206

BAK, 1528

B-ALL. *See* B-cell acute lymphoblastic leukemia (B-ALL)

Band 3, **664**, 664*f*, 670*t*, 672

Band 3 clustering models, 498

Band cells, marrow, 34

Banded chromosome, 175*t*

Band form, marrow, 32*t*

Band neutrophils
    development, 926*f*, 939
    kinetics, 941*t*
    structure, 20*f*, 926–927, 927*f*

Bands, 22

Baroreflex, 91

Barr bodies, 150, 150*f*

Bartonella infection (bartonellosis, Oroya fever), **818**, 997

Bartter syndrome, 2086

Basal coagulation, 1942

Basket cells, 23

Basophilia, 971–972
    in clonal myeloid diseases, 971–972, 972*t*
    consultative approach to, 44
    in inflammatory and immunologic responses, 971
    punctate, 468

Basophilic erythroblasts, 34, 463*f*, 464, 464*f*

Basophilic leukemia, 971–972, 972*t*

Basophilic megaloblasts, 595*f*

Basophilic stippling, 467*f*, 468

Basophilopenia, **971**

Basophils
    alterations in numbers, 970–972, 971*t*, 972*t*
    biologic functions, **969–970**

in chronic myelogenous leukemia, 1445
    development, 926*f*
    distinguishing features, **966**, 966*f*
    heterogeneity, 966–967
    mast cells and, **967–968**
    mediators, 967*t*, 968
    natural history, 967*t*
    in newborn, 105*t*
    reference ranges, 15*t*, 970
    role in IgE-associated immune response, 968–969
    structure, 20*f*, 23, 929*f*, **930–931**, 930*f*, 931*f*, **968**
    surface membrane structures, 967*t*

Bassen-Kornzweig syndrome (abetalipoproteinemia), 670*f*, **681**

Bax, 204*f*, 206

BAX, 951

BAX, 210

B-cell activation factor (BAFF), 309, 1713

B-cell acute lymphoblastic leukemia (B-ALL). *See also* Acute lymphoblastic (lymphocytic) leukemia (ALL)
    chromosomal abnormalities, 186*f*, 221–222*t*, 1494*t*
    vs. chronic lymphocytic leukemia, 1543
    differential diagnosis, 1674
    gene mutations, 232–233*t*, 1494*t*
    immunologic subtypes, 1512*t*
    laboratory features, 1511, 1511*f*, 1512*t*
    Philadelphia chromosome-like, 177*f*, 186, 232–233*t*
    precursor (immature), 183, 184*t*, 186*f*, 1515–1517, 1521*t*
    prognosis, 1520
    therapy, 1514, 1515

B-cell antigen-receptor vaccines, **423**

B-cell antigens, 1141, 1141*f*

B-cell linker protein (BLNK), 1144, 1163

B-cell lymphoblastic lymphoma. *See* B-cell acute lymphoblastic leukemia (B-ALL)

B-cell maturation antigen (BCMA), 1606

B-cell neoplasms. *See also specific types*
    development stages, 1591*f*
    immature/precursor, 1494*t*, 1592
    leukemias, 1494*t*
    lymphomas
        chromosomal abnormalities, 184*t*, 186*f*, 1494–1497*t*
        chronic lymphocytic leukemia and, 1542
        classification, 1493, 1494–1497*t*
        clinical features, 1501–1502
        extranodal involvement, 1502

B-cell precursor acute lymphoblastic leukemia, 1512*t*

B-cell progenitors, **270**
B-cell prolymphocytic lymphoma, 1542
B-cell receptors (BCRs), 1151, 1528–1529
B cells. *See also* Lymphocytes
  in chronic inflammation, 291
  development, 61, 1151, 1155, 1589–1590,
    1589f, 1707–1708
  differentiation, 1169, 1172
  disorders, 1195, 1196t, 1215
  fetal, 101, 1151
  function, in neonate, 108–109
  immunoglobulins and activation of, 1163
  in lymph nodes, 93
  memory, 1172
  monocytoid, 1595
  neoplasms. *See* B-cell neoplasms
  persistent polyclonal lymphocytosis,
    1200–1202, 1201f
  receptor diversity, 1177
  in spleen, 90, 90f
BCL2 (BCL-2)
  in apoptosis, 209–210
  in chronic lymphocytic leukemia, 1529
  in diffuse large B-cell lymphoma, 187,
    1596, 1626, 1627t, 1632
  in "double-hit" lymphoma, 1674
  in follicular lymphoma, 187, 236t, 1576,
    1576f, 1594, 1642
  in memory B cells, 1172
  in Waldenström macroglobulinemia, 1785
BCL2A1, 414
Bcl-2 family, **205–206**
  in apoptosis, 206, 208–209, 208f, 237
  in caspase activation, 204t
  in chronic lymphocytic leukemia, 1528,
    1539
  in diffuse large B-cell lymphoma, 198
  interactions, 206f
  in leukemic stem cells, 198
  in life span of hematopoietic stem cells,
    206
  in mitochondrial metabolism, 198
  in myeloma, 1711
  p53 inhibition, 209
  structure, 206
  as therapeutic target, 1539
Bcl-2 homologue protein, 2202
BCL6
  in anaplastic large cell lymphoma, 1699
  in diffuse large B-cell lymphoma, 187,
    235t, 1625–1626, 1632
  in follicular lymphoma, 1642, 1644
  memory B cells and, 1172
BCL7A, 166
BCL9, 1736
BCL11A, 484

BCL11A, 736
Bcl11b, 1156
BCL11B, 166
Bcl-W, 206
BCL-X, 210
Bcl-X$_L$, 206, 483
BCL-XL, 1172
BCMA (B-cell maturation antigen), 1606
BCNU (bischloroethylnitrosourea). *See*
    Carmustine (BCNU)
BCR, 176, 1441–1442, 1442f, 1666, 1710
BCR-ABL1
  in acute lymphoblastic leukemia, 183, 221t,
    1508, 1513t, 1521, 1521t
  in acute myelogenous leukemia, 1384t
  apoptosis and, 1444
  cell adhesion and, 1440–1441
  in chronic myelogenous leukemia
    apoptosis and, 1444
    cell adhesion and, 1440–1441
    CML stem cell formation and, 1439
    detection, 176f
    disease progression and, 1464–1465
    in healthy subjects, 1443
    imatinib resistance and, 178, 230t, 1439
    inhibition of, 176
    molecular pathology, 1441–1442, 1441f,
      1442f
    progenitors, 1440
    prognosis and, 221t, 230t
    signal transduction and, 1443–1444,
      1444f
  in clonal myeloid disorders, 1278
  detection, 1447–1448
  in healthy subjects, 1443
  molecular pathology, 1441–1442, 1442f
  p210$^{BCR-ABL}$ fusion protein, 1442–1443
  signal transduction and, 1443–1444, 1444f
BCR-ABL1–negative cells, 1439, 1440
BCR-ABL1–positive cells, 1439, 1440
BCR-ABL1–positive thrombocythemia, 1449
bcr-abl fusion protein, 230
BCR-ABL kinase, 318
BCR-ABL peptide vaccine, 423
BCR-ABL–positive thrombocythemia, 1449
BCR-ABL tyrosine kinase inhibitors. *See*
    Tyrosine kinase inhibitors
BCR breakpoints, 1442–1443, 1442f
BCR rearrangement, 1447
BCRs (B-cell receptors), 1151, 1528–1529
BEACOPP regimen, for Hodgkin lymphoma
  in advanced disease, 1613–1614
  adverse effects/complications, 1614, 1617
  clinical trials, 1614, 1615t
  dose, route, and schedule, 1612t
  in favorable limited-stage disease, 1613

  history, 1611
  in HIV-associated disease, 1248
  with radiation therapy, 1613
  in unfavorable limited-stage disease, 1613
BEAM regimen
  for diffuse large B-cell lymphoma, 1632
  for Hodgkin lymphoma, 1616
Becaplermin, 1848
Beclin, 206
Bee stings, 809, 970
Behçet disease, 2103
Belching, history of, 5
Belinostat, 1696, 1696t
Bence Jones proteinuria, 1721, 1725, 1810
Bendamustine
  adverse effects, 1534
  for chronic lymphocytic leukemia, 1534,
    1537
  for follicular lymphoma, 1644, 1645t, 1647,
    1649
  for mantle cell lymphoma, 1656, 1659t
  for myeloma, 1755
  pharmacology, 330
Benign monoclonal gammopathy. *See*
    Essential monoclonal gammopathy
Benzene exposure
  acute myelogenous leukemia and, 1319, 1374
  aplastic anemia and, 516–517
  myelodysplastic syndromes and, 1342,
    1345
  primary myelofibrosis and, 1319
Benzocaine, toxic methemoglobinemia and,
    789
Berger disease, 1161
Bernard-Soulier syndrome (glycoprotein
    Ib-IX-V defect), **2048–2050**
  clinical features, 2049
  definition and history, 2047
  etiology and pathogenesis, 2047–2048
  laboratory features, 1839–1840, 1996
  molecular defects, 2048–2049, 2049f
  platelet defects, 1839, 1867, 1868, 1877,
    2048, 2359
  therapy, 1840
Berry cell. *See* Echinocytes
β-adrenergic blockers, 2295, 2296
β-adrenergic receptors, 1059
β-carotene, 899
β chemokines, 288t
β-globin, 893
β-globin chains, 728
  β-thalassemia and, 749–750
  developmental switches in synthesis, 730
  vs. γ-globin chains, 760
  structure, 760–761, 760f
  variants, 733, 751

β-globin gene cluster
  β-thalassemia mutations unlinked to, 733
  δβthalassemia-like disorders resulting
      from mutations in, 734–735
  dominantly inherited β-thalassemia and,
      732
  regulation, 730
  sickle cell disease and, 762, 763
  structure, 729, 729f
β-globin synthesis, 730
β-integrins. See under Integrin
β-thalassemias
  β+, 726
  β⁰, 726
  β-globin chain variants and, 733, 749–750
  clinical features, **743–745**
  differential diagnosis, **748**, 749f
  dominantly inherited, 732–733
  epidemiology/population genetics,
      727–728
  forms, 726
  gene therapy, 441, 441f
  hemoglobin A₂ levels in, 750–751
  hemoglobin variants causing, 778t
  inclusion body, 732
  intermedia, 744–745, 744t, 746f
  laboratory features, **745–747**, 746f
  major, 725, 743–744, 744f, 745–746
  minor, 636, 745, 746–747, 746f
  molecular basis, **730–733**, 731f, 731t, 732f
  pathophysiology. See Thalassemias,
      pathophysiology
  in pregnancy, 126
  prevention, 753–754
  prognosis, 753
  silent, 733, 750
  treatment, 441, 441f, **751–753**, 2372
  variant forms, 733, 751
BET (bromodomain and extraterminal)-
      family, 169
BET (bromodomain and extraterminal)
      inhibitors, 170, 338
Bevacizumab
  adverse effects, 2263
  for myeloma, 346t
Bexarotene, 1685–1686, 1702
BFP (biologic false-positive) syphilis test,
      2233
BFU-E. See Burst-forming unit-erythroid
      (BFU-E)
BH3 domain, 206
Bicytopenia, 1277
Bid, 204f, 206
Bilineal (biphenotypic) leukemia, 1386
Bilirubin, destruction of hemoglobin and
      excretion of, 499–500

Biliverdin, 499
Bim, 206, 1672
Binet clinical staging system, 1533t
Bing-Neel syndrome, 1791
Biogenesis of lysosome-related organelles
      complexes (BLOCs), 1843, 2053,
      2053f
Biologic false-positive (BFP) syphilis test,
      2233
Biopterin, 585
Biotin method, for red cell life span
      measurement, 496
Birbeck granules, 310, 1101
BIRC3, 231t, 233t, 236t, 1664t
BIR (baculovirus inhibitor of apoptosis
      repeat) domains, 207, 298
Bischloroethylnitrosourea (BCNU). See
      Carmustine (BCNU)
Bispecific antibodies, 344
1,3-Bisphosphoglycerate (1,3-BPG), 692, 695
2,3-Bisphosphoglycerate (2,3-BPG)
  in glucose metabolism, 692–693, 695
  hemoglobin M and, 792
  hemoglobin oxygen affinity and, 504, 760,
      760f, 2377
Bisphosphoglycerate mutase
      (bisphosphoglyceromutase)
  abnormalities, 701t
  actions, 692t
  in glucose metabolism, 695
Bisphosphoglycerate mutase deficiency, 695,
      705, 876
Bisphosphonates
  adverse effects, 1756, 1757
  for bone disease in primary myelofibrosis,
      1330
  mechanism of action, 1738
  for myeloma, 1738, 1756
  for osteoporosis in mastocytosis, 977
Bivalirudin, **399**
  clinical uses, 399
  for heparin-induced thrombocytopenia,
      2030, 2031t
  pharmacology, 399
  for unstable angina, 2296
BL. See Burkitt lymphoma (BL)
Blackfan-Diamond anemia, **539–540**
Black tree fungus, 2079
Blackwater fever, 817. See also Malaria
Bladder, primary lymphomas in, 1582
Bladder dysfunction, history of, 5
Blast crisis, of chronic myelogenous
      leukemia. See Chronic
      myelogenous (myeloid) leukemia
      (CML), accelerated phase and blast
      crisis

Bleeding
  anticoagulant therapy and, 2277
  antifibrinolytic therapy for, 2318
  in antiphospholipid syndrome, 2240–2241,
      2240t
  APC concentrate and, 2213
  in cardiac surgery, 2085–2086
  categories, 2382–2383, 2383t
  chronic, 553
  in chronic myeloproliferative neoplasms,
      2080–2081
  consultative approach to, 46
  dental. See Dental bleeding/extractions
  disorders. See Hemostasis, disorders
  in disseminated intravascular coagulation,
      2203–2204, 2205t
  enhanced fibrinolysis and, 2312
  in essential thrombocythemia, 1308–1309
  in fibrinolytic therapy, 2317, 2317t
  gingival, 5, 8, 1987
  in Glanzmann thrombasthenia, 2046,
      2046t
  in hemophilia, 2118, 2120, 2121–2122,
      2122t, 2123
  history, 1985–1986
  iatrogenic, 629
  in immune thrombocytopenia, 2001–2002,
      2002t, 2003
  iron deficiency and. See Iron deficiency
  in liver disease and liver transplantation,
      2192–2193, 2193t
  major, 2277, 2382, 2382t
  in myeloma, 1740–1741
  newborn, 111
  platelet count and risk of, 2382–2383
  platelet transfusion threshold for, 2385. See
      also Platelet transfusion
  in polycythemia vera, 1293
  in pregnancy, **120–122**
  retinal, 8
  sources of, 628–630, 628t
  in thrombocythemic syndromes, 1286
Bleeding time
  in newborn, 107
  in von Willebrand disease, 2174
Bleomycin, **331–332**. See also ABVD
      regimen; BEACOPP regimen;
      Stanford V regimen
  adverse effects, 331–332
  for α-heavy-chain disease, 1808
  for mycosis fungoides, 1687
  pharmacology, 331
  resistance to, 319t
Blimp-1 (B-lymphocyte-induced maturation
      protein-1), 1171–1172, 1710, 1710f
Blinatumomab, 1536, 1539

Blind loop syndrome, 601, 604
BLM, 1227
BLNK (B-cell linker protein), 1144, 1163
BLOCs (biogenesis of lysosome-related
  organelles complexes), 1843, 2053,
  2053*f*
Blood
  basophil count, 970
  control of fluidity of, 2285
  dendritic cell count, 1098
  eosinophil count, 953–954
  examination, **11–23**. *See also specific blood
    cells*
    automated analyses, 11–12, 12*f*, 13*f*
    morphological, **20**, 20*f*, 21*f*, 22*f*
    reference ranges/normal values, 14*t*,
      18–19, 18*t*, 19*f*
  heterogeneity of monocytes in, 1079*f*
  neutrophil kinetics, 941–942, 942*t*
  as source of hematopoietic stem cells for
    transplantation, **355–356**
  umbilical cord, **357**
  viscosity of
    hematocrit and, 506, 508*f*
    in newborns, 103–104
Blood banking system (blood procurement/
  screening), **2365–2369**
  autologous donor blood, 2367–2368
  blood containers, 2367
  collection by apheresis, **2368–2369**
  directed donor blood, 2368
  donor recruitment, 2366
  donor screening, 2366–2367
  international practices, 2365–2366
  laboratory testing in, 2349, 2369, 2369*t*
  patient-specific donation, 2368
  procurement of plasma derivatives, 2366
  safety of, 2369, 2369*t*, 2370*t*
  storage times, 2377
  therapeutic bleeding, 2368
  U.S. system, 2365, 2366*t*
  venipuncture and blood collection, 2367
Blood blisters, 1987
Blood count
  in essential thrombocythemia, 1310
  in Gaucher disease, 1125
  in primary myelofibrosis, 1325–1326
Blood cysts (pseudotumors), 2119, 2120*f*
Blood dendritic cells, 1092, 1098
Blood donation, iron deficiency and, 629–630
Blood films/findings, 20–23, 22*f*
  in acute infection lymphocytosis, 1203*f*
  in acute lymphoblastic leukemia, 1511,
    1511*f*
  in acute myelogenous leukemia, 1381,
    1382*f*

  in alloimmune hemolytic disease of the
    fetus and newborn, 856*f*
  in autoimmune hemolytic anemia, 833*f*
  in babesiosis, 817*f*
  in β-thalassemia, 746*f*
  in chronic lymphocytic leukemia,
    1530–1531, 1530*f*
  in chronic myelogenous leukemia,
    1445–1446, 1446*f*
  in *C. perfringens* septicemia, 817*f*
  in Epstein-Barr virus mononucleosis,
    1264*f*
  in erythrocyte membrane disorders, 670*f*
  in hemoglobin H disease, 747*f*
  in hemolytic anemia, 810*f*
  in hereditary elliptocytosis, 670*f*, 679
  in hereditary pyropoikilocytosis, 677*f*,
    679
  in hereditary spherocytosis, 670*f*, 675
  in hereditary stomatocytosis, 670*f*
  in iron deficiency, 633*f*
  lymphocytes, 1138*f*
  in malaria, 817*f*
  monocytes, 1047*f*
  in mycosis fungoides, 1683, 1683*f*
  in myelodysplastic syndromes, 1350*f*
  in myeloma, 1743*f*
  in pernicious anemia, 594*f*
  in persistent polyclonal lymphocytosis of B
    lymphocytes, 1201*f*
  plasma cells, 1138*f*
  postsplenectomy, 869*f*
  in primary myelofibrosis, 1323*f*
  in sickle cell disease, 775*f*, 779*f*
  in structural hemoglobinopathies, 779*f*
  in thalassemia intermedia, 746*f*
  in Waldenström macroglobulinemia,
    1786*f*, 1791
Blood group systems, **2329–2336**, 2330*t*,
    2331–2333*t*. *See also* Erythrocyte
    antibodies; Erythrocyte antigens;
    specific blood groups
  definitions and history, 2329
  disease and, 2340
  genetics, 2339
  immune antibodies and, 2347–2348
  naturally occurring antibodies and,
    2347
  serologic detection, 2348–2350
Blood islands, 257
Blood loss. *See* Bleeding
Blood volume
  in pregnancy, 119
  regulation, 91
Bloom syndrome, **1227**, 1507, 1575*t*
Blue toe syndrome, 2298

B-lymphocyte-induced maturation protein-1
    (Blimp-1), 1171–1172, 1710, 1710*f*
B lymphocytes. *See* B cells
BMP. *See* Bone morphogenetic protein
    (BMP)
Bohr effect, 504
Bolzano effect, 2049
Bombay (Oh) phenotype, 2341*t*, 2343
Bone
  giant cell tumor, 1110
  infarction, 771
  primary lymphomas in, 1583
Bone cells, marrow, 59–60
Bone lesions/pain
  in acute myelogenous leukemia, 1381,
    1385
  in Gaucher disease, 1124, 1125*f*, 1127
  in hairy cell leukemia, 1555
  history of, 6
  in Langerhans cell histiocytosis, 1104,
    1105, 1105*f*, 1106
  in myeloma, 1713, 1737–1738, 1738*f*, 1745,
    1756
  in primary myelofibrosis, 1325, 1325*t*
Bone morphogenetic protein (BMP)
  in early stem cell development, 54
  in fibroplasia, 1322
Bone morphogenetic protein (BMP)-4
  upregulation, 54
Bone morphogenetic protein (BMP)-6, in
    iron homeostasis, 621*t*
Bone morphogenetic protein (BMP) receptor
    subunit, 42., 621*t*
Bone morphogenetic protein (BMP)
    subfamilies, 249
Borderline lesions, in cutaneous T-cell
    lymphoma, 1688
Bordetella pertussis infections, 1137, 1138*f*,
    1139, 1202
Borrelia burgdorferi, 1574, 1664, 2104, 2311
Bortezomib, **342–343**, 342*f*
  for acute myelogenous leukemia, 1396,
    1403
  adverse effects, 343, 1740, 1746, 1757, 1794
  for AL amyloidosis, 1761, 1781
  for autoimmune hemolytic anemia, 839
  for gastric MALT lymphoma, 1666*t*
  for mantle cell lymphoma, 1657*t*, 1658,
    1659*t*, 1660*t*
  mechanism of action, 241, 1193
  for myelodysplastic syndromes, 1360
  for myeloma, 1750, 1751, 1752, 1752*t*,
    1753*t*, 1754
  for primary effusion lymphoma, 1247
  for Waldenström macroglobulinemia,
    1794, 1795

Bosutinib
adverse effects, 339t, 341, 1451t
for chronic myelogenous leukemia, 339t, 1451t, 1454, 1457–1458, 1466
comparison with other tyrosine kinase inhibitors, 1451t
drug interactions, 339t, 1451t
pharmacology, 339t
structure, 340f
Botrocetin, 1867, 1868
Boyadjiev-Jabs syndrome, 567
1,3-BPG (1,3-Bisphosphoglycerate), 692, 695
2,3-BPG. See 2,3-Bisphosphoglycerate (2,3-BPG)
BPGM, 695
BPI (bacterial permeability-increasing protein), 106–107, 1011, 1012t, 1013
Bradykinin, 286t, 289, 2374
Bradyrhizobium enterica, 357
BRAF, 232t, 233t, 1103, 1108, 1111, 1737, 1759
BRAF inhibitors
for hairy cell leukemia, 1559
for Langerhans cell histiocytosis, 1107
BRAF V600E, 1554
Brain injury/tumors. See Neurologic disease/symptoms
BRCA2, 529
BRCC3, 1346t
Breakpoint, 175t
Breast, primary lymphomas in, 1583
Breast cancer
disseminated intravascular coagulation in, 2207
Hodgkin lymphoma treatment and, 1617–1618
secondary acute myelogenous leukemia and, 1407
Breast implants, 1698
Brentuximab vedotin, 346
for anaplastic large cell lymphoma, 1699
for CD30+ lymphoproliferative disorders, 1687
dose and toxicity, 343t, 1687
for Hodgkin lymphoma, 1248, 1614, 1616
for mycosis fungoides, 1687
for peripheral T-cell lymphoma, 1696, 1696t
for primary effusion lymphoma, 1247
BRG/BAF-associated factors (BAF) complex, 166, 166f
Brill-Symmers disease, 1569
Bromodomain and extraterminal (BET)-family, 169

Bromodomain and extraterminal (BET) inhibitors, 170, 338
Bronzed diabetes, 639. See also Hemochromatosis
Brown recluse spider bites, 836
Brucella/brucellosis, 1062, 1268
Bruising, 6, 1987
Bruton tyrosine kinase (BTK), 1144, 1212, 1529, 1712, 1713, 1787
Bruton tyrosine kinase (BTK) inhibitors, 342. See also Ibrutinib
BTCC-1. See CD9
BTK, 235t, 993
BTRC, 1711
Budd-Chiari syndrome, 575t, 581, 1293
Buffy-coat method, 2386, 2386f
Burkholderia cepacia, 1030, 1033
Burkitt lymphoma (BL), 1671–1676
cell metabolism in, 199
clinical features, 1672
course and prognosis, 1676
definition and history, 1671
differential diagnosis, 1674
epidemiology, 1570, 1671
etiology and pathogenesis
chromosomal abnormalities, 184t, 186f, 187, 1496t, 1576, 1596, 1672
Epstein-Barr virus infection and malaria, 1265, 1573, 1672
gene mutations, 1496t, 1672
HIV-associated, 187, 1244f, 1245, 1247, 1672, 1676
laboratory features
blood and marrow, 1673, 1673f
cytogenetics, 1674
Epstein-Barr virus studies, 1674
histopathology, 1496t, 1596, 1597f, 1598, 1673–1674, 1673f
immunophenotype, 1674
staging, 1577f, 1673t
therapy, 1675, 1675t
tumor lysis syndrome in, 1675
Burns
disseminated intravascular coagulation and, 2208
hemolysis and, 809, 810f
Burr cells. See Echinocytes
Burst-forming unit-erythroid (BFU-E)
in aplastic anemia and, 514
development, 63, 461, 462
in erythropoiesis, 480, 480f, 483f
progenitors, 270
in yolk sac and fetus, 100, 100f
Burst-forming unit-erythroid (BFU-E)
precursors, polycythemia vera and, 1292

Busulfan
adverse effects, 330
for chronic myelogenous leukemia, 1459
for essential thrombocythemia, 1313t, 1314
high-dose, before hematopoietic cell transplantation, 331t, 332, 360, 1399
mechanism of action, 329
for polycythemia vera, 1298t, 1299

C
C1 (C$_1$) esterase inhibitor, 290, 839, 1845, 2308
C1q receptors, 284, 1873
C3. See CD11b
C3, 2259t
C3a, 290, 1932, 2374
C3AR1, 1643
C3b, 290, 1017, 2260, 2374
C3b-coated erythrocytes, 829
C3bi, 829, 831
C3 convertases, 289f, 290
C3 receptors, 1015
C4, 2000
C4b-binding protein, 1958, 2202
C5a, 283, 942, 1932, 1972
C5a receptor, 1015
C5 convertases, 289f, 290
C9, 2000
C15ORF41, 565
Cabot rings, 467f, 468, 594
Cachexin/cachectin. See Tumor necrosis factor (TNF)-α
Cadherins, 68
CAFC (cobblestone area-forming cell), 260
Café-au-lait spots, 529, 1471
CAGE questions, 6
Calciphylaxis, cutaneous, 2101–2102
Calcium, in platelet activation, 1836, 1837f, 1881–1882
Calcium channel blockers, 2078
Calcium-dependent proteases (Calpains), 1842, 1848, 1883
Calcium (Ca^{2+}) entry channel deficiency, 1221
CALDAGGEF1, 2060
CalDAG-GEF1 deficiency, 2057
Caldesmon, in platelet cytoskeleton, 1832t
Calf vein thrombosis, 2273
CALLA. See CD10 (CALLA)
Calmodulin, 1833t
CALR, 229t, 1278, 1307, 1308f, 1310, 1321
Calreticulin, 1836
cAMP (cyclic adenosine monophosphate), 404–405
CAMP (hCAP-18, LL-37), 1012t, 1013

Camptotheca acuminata, 326
Camptothecins, 319*t*, **326–328**
Campylobacter, 820, 1212, 1216, 1574, 1664
Campylobacter jejuni, 1790
CAMT (congenital amegakaryocytic
    thrombocytopenia), 530*t*, 532,
    1822
Canale-Smith syndrome. *See* Autoimmune
    lymphoproliferative syndrome
    (ALPS)
cANCA (cytoplasmic antineutrophil
    cytoplasmic antibody), 1013
Cancer. *See also individual types*
    ataxia-telangiectasia and, 1226–1227
    cellular senescence and, 132
    chemotherapy. *See* Antineoplastic drugs/
        chemotherapy
    disseminated intravascular coagulation in,
        803–804, 2207–2208
    HIV-associated. *See* Human
        immunodeficiency virus
        (HIV)–associated malignancies
    immune cell therapy. *See* Immune cell
        therapy (adoptive cellular therapy),
        of malignancy
    lymphocytosis and, 1204
    marrow infiltration in, 658, 659*f*
    microangiopathic hemolytic anemia and,
        803–804, 803*t*
    monocytosis and, 1097
    neutrophilia and, 1001
    next-generation sequencing analysis,
        160–161
    thrombotic microangiopathy in, 2262
    vaccine therapy for. *See* Vaccine therapy
    venous thromboembolism in, 2276–2277
Candida infections
    acute myelogenous leukemia treatment
        and, 1410
    in chronic granulomatous disease, 1021
    disseminated, 2104–2105, 2105*f*
    after hematopoietic cell transplantation,
        1182
    in hyperimmunoglobulin E syndrome,
        1026, 1225
    in immunocompromised host, 383
    in Langerhans cell histiocytosis, 1104
    in leukocyte adhesion deficiency, 1023
    in newborn, 106
    pattern-recognition signaling defects with
        increased susceptibility to, 1230
    prevention, 389
    red cell antigens and susceptibility to, 2340
    in specific granule deficiency, 1021
    Th17 T cells and, 369
    treatment, 385

Cangrelor, 404*t*, 405, 2076
CANNTG (consensus E-box motifs), 262
Cao Gio, 2107
CAPS (catastrophic antiphospholipid
    syndrome), 2239, 2245
CapZ, 1833*t*, 1839*f*, 1840
CAR (chimeric antigen receptor), 415–416,
    415*f*, 438, 442, 454, 1193
Carbamazepine, megaloblastic anemia and,
    606*t*
Carbohydrates
    antigens, 2337, 2338*f*
    in erythrocytes, 471*t*
    loading, for acute intermittent porphyria,
        904
    metabolism in neutrophils, 932
Carbonic anhydrase I, 701*t*
Carbonic anhydrase II, 701*t*
Carbon monoxide (CO), in red cell life span
    measurement, 496
Carbon monoxide poisoning
    clinical and laboratory features, 795
    epidemiology, 795
    etiology and pathogenesis, 795
    therapy, course, and prognosis, 795–796
Carbonyl iron, 638
Carboplatin
    adverse effects, 330
    for diffuse large B-cell lymphoma, 1629*t*,
        1631
    high-dose, 331*t*, 332*t*
    for Hodgkin lymphoma, 1616
    pharmacology, 330
Carboxyhemoglobin, **795–796**
Carbromal, 830
CARD (caspase activation and recruitment
    domain), 205, 298–299, 1025, 1054,
    1230
CARD9, 1230
CARD11, 233*t*, 235*t*, 236*t*
Cardiacos negros, 871
Cardiac output, anemia and, 505
CARDIF. *See* Mitochondrial antiviral
    signaling protein (MAVS)
Cardiolipin, 1955
Cardiopulmonary bypass, 2085–2086, 2318,
    2384
Cardiovascular disease. *See also* Vascular
    disease/injury
    in acute myelogenous leukemia, 1381,
        1410
    in AL amyloidosis, 1760, 1761, 1775,
        1775*t*, 1777–1779, 1778*f*, 1780*f*,
        1781
    anthracycline-induced, 1520
    in antiphospholipid syndrome, 2240

erythrocytosis and, 871, 872, 876, 881
fibrinolytic system in, 1974–1976, 1974*t*,
    1975*f*
heart valve hemolysis, **804–806**, 805*t*, 806*f*
hemochromatosis and, 642
in hemolytic uremic syndrome, 2259
in hemophilia, 2130
hereditary thrombophilia and, 2226–2227
history of, 5
Hodgkin lymphoma treatment and, 1618
monocytes/macrophages in, 1079
myocardial infarction. *See* Myocardial
    infarction (MI)
neutrophilia and, 1001
primary lymphoma, 1581
red cell transfusion in, 6–7, 2370*t*
regenerative therapies for, 450
risk factors, 2281–2282, 2282*t*, 2288
in sickle cell disease, 769
thrombophilia testing in, 2228–2229
in thrombotic thrombocytopenic purpura,
    2255
vulnerability to, 2289–2291, 2290*f*, 2291*t*.
    See also Atherosclerosis
Carfilzomib, **342–343**, 342*f*
    mechanism of action, 241
    for myeloma, 1750–1751, 1753*t*, 1754
    for Waldenström macroglobulinemia, 1794
Carmustine (BCNU)
    aplastic anemia and, 516
    for diffuse large B-cell lymphoma, 1632
    doses and toxicities, 331, 332*t*, 368
    in hematopoietic cell transplantation
        conditioning, 360
    for Hodgkin lymphoma, 1616
    for mycosis fungoides, 1685
    platelet function and, 2079
Carotid endarterectomy, 2297
Carrier, 147
Carrión disease, 818
CAR-T (chimeric antigen receptor T) cells,
    1539
Cartilage hair hypoplasia, 993, **1226**
Caspase activation and recruitment domain
    (CARD), 205, 298–299, 1025, 1054,
    1065*f*, 1230
Caspases
    activation, 204–205, 204*f*, 1065*f*
    in apoptosis, 203–204
    in lymphoma, 210
    in T-cell therapy, 416
Caspofungin, 385, 388*t*, 389
Castleman disease, **1249–1250**, 1496*t*, 1573
Catalase, 286
    abnormalities, 701*t*
    activity, 692*t*

Catastrophic antiphospholipid syndrome (CAPS), 2239, 2245
Cathelicidins, 1014
Cathepsin B, 523
Cathepsin C (dipeptidyl peptidase 1), 1013
Cathepsin G, 283, 1012*t*, 1013, 1856
Catheter-directed thrombolysis, 2278
Cationic proteins, 284*t*
Cat-scratch fever, 818, 1268
CBF, 1376, 1377
CBL, 228*t*, 229*t*, 1352
CBL/CBLB, 1346*t*
CBV regimen, for Hodgkin lymphoma, 1616
CC chemokines, 288, 288*t*
ccff-DNA (circulating cell-free fetal DNA), 852
CCL2 (monocyte chemoattractant protein, MCP-1)
   in atherosclerosis, 2283, 2284*f*, 2286, 2287
   basophils and, 288*t*
   in chronic myelogenous leukemia, 1440
   monocyte activity and, 288, 288*t*, 2286
CCL5 (RANTES), 1607, 1852*f*, 1855, 2286
CCL17, 1607
CCL22, 1607
CCND1, 187, 234*t*, 236*t*
CCND2, 1632
CCND3, 1672
CCR. *See under* Chemokine receptor
CCyR (complete cytogenic response), 1452*t*
CD1, 308–309, 1177
CD1a–e, 308–309
CD2 (LFA-2), **1185**, 1185*f*
CD3, 1142, 1143, 1176*f*
CD3γ chain, 1178
CD3δ chain, 1178
CD3ε chain, 1178
CD4
   function, 1179
   in HIV infection, 1240
   in lymphocytes, 1142, 1143
   in monocytes and macrophages, 1056–1057
   in peripheral T-cell lymphoma, 1697
   in precursor thymocytes, 1179
   structure, 1052*f*, 1179
CD4+CD25+ regulatory T (T$_{REG}$) cells
   in aplastic anemia, 515
   in chronic lymphocytic leukemia, 1528
   eosinophils and, 950
   functions, **1180–1182**
   in immune thrombocytopenia, 2000
CD4+ T cells (helper T cells), 409
   antigens, 1142*t*
   depletion, idiopathic, 1206
   epitopes, vaccine therapy and, 421

   in HIV infection, 1240
   in Hodgkin lymphoma, 1607
   in immune cell therapy, 409, 411
   immune response and, 423*t*
   minor histocompatibility antigens and, 413–414
   subsets, 1180–1182, 1181*f*
      CD4+CD25+ T cells. *See* CD4+CD25+ regulatory T (T$_{REG}$) cells
      T$_{FH}$ cells, 1182
      Th1 and Th2 cells, 1180
      Th9 cells, 1182
      Th17 cells, 1182
CD5
   in diffuse large B-cell lymphoma, 1627
   in mantle cell lymphoma, 1593, 1653
   in prolymphocytes, 1542
   in thymocytes, 1141
   in Waldenström macroglobulinemia, 1785, 1791
CD5+ B cells, 1141, 1495*t*
CD7, 1153
CD7, 1643
CD8
   function, 1179
   in natural killer cells, 1142
   in peripheral T-cell lymphoma, 1697
   in precursor thymocytes, 1179
   structure, 1179
CD8B1, 1643
CD8+CD28- T-cell population, in aplastic anemia, 515
CD8+ T cells (cytotoxic T lymphocytes, CTLs)
   activation, 308
   antigens, 1142*t*
   in cellular therapy, **409–410**, 412
   cytoplasmic granules in, 1145
   defects in, 1227–1228
   epitopes, vaccine therapy and, 421
   function, 1179–1180
   in HIV infection, 1240
   immune response and, 423*t*
   in lymphocyte activation, 1139
   minor histocompatibility antigens and, 413–414
   in mycosis fungoides, 1682*f*
   in spleen, 863
   in T-cell large granular lymphocytic leukemia, 1563, 1565*f*
CD9, 1393, 1836, 1871
CD10 (CALLA)
   in angioimmunoblastic T-cell lymphoma, 1698
   in diffuse large B-cell lymphoma, 1627
   ectoenzyme activity, 1143, 1144*t*

   in follicular lymphoma, 1642
   lymphoid progenitors and, 1153
   in Waldenström macroglobulinemia, 1785, 1791
CD11a (LFA-1)
   in diffuse large B-cell lymphoma, 1627
   expression, 1056
   human neutrophil antigens and, 2358
   in inflammation, 1977*t*
   in monocytes, 1056, 1078
   in myeloma, 1712
   structure, 1056
CD11a/CD18, 282, 1083
CD11b (C3)
   in acute basophilic leukemia, 1393
   in acute myelogenous leukemia, 1380*t*, 1383
   antibodies, 1056
   in antiphospholipid syndrome, 2237
   in atypical hemolytic uremic syndrome, 2259–2260
   in B-cell development, 1151
   in cell signaling, 1015
   expression, 1056
   in immune thrombocytopenia, 2000
   in leukocyte adhesion deficiency, 1023
   in monocytes, 1054, 1056
   in neutrophils, 1024, 2358
CD11b/CD18 (Mac-1, Mo1, CR3, α$_M$β$_2$)
   in eosinophils, 948
   human neutrophil antigens and, 2357*t*, 2358
   in inflammation, 282, 283
   in leukocyte–platelet and endothelial cell–platelet interactions, 1977*t*, 1978–1979, 1979*t*
   in monocytes/macrophages, 1052*f*, 1053*f*, 1059, 1083
   in neutrophils, 1007, 1013*t*
CD11c, 1056, 1383
CD11c+, 1082
CD11c/CD18, 282–283
CD11/CD18, 1015, 1021–1022, 1023*f*
CD13
   in acute lymphoblastic leukemia, 1512
   in acute myelogenous leukemia, 1380*t*, 1383
   leukemoid reaction and, 986
   in lymphocytes, 1144*t*
   in monocytes, 271
CD14
   in acute monocytic leukemia, 1391
   in acute myelogenous leukemia, 1380*t*, 1383
   in innate immunity, 294*t*, 296*f*
   in lymphoid progenitors, 1153

in monocytes, 1046, 1052, 1052f, 1054, 1056, 1095, 1097
CD15
  in acute lymphoblastic leukemia, 1512
  in acute myelogenous leukemia, 1380t, 1383
  in Hodgkin lymphoma, 1599, 1609, 1610
  leukemoid reaction and, 986
CD16. See Fcγ receptor III (FcγRIII, CD16)
CD16/CD18, 1627
CD18, 950, 1083, 1184
CD19
  in B cells, 1141
  in Burkitt lymphoma, 1674
  in chronic lymphocytic leukemia, 1528, 1530, 1539
  in diffuse large B-cell lymphoma, 1627
  in follicular lymphoma, 1642, 1644
  in mantle cell lymphoma, 1653
  natural killer cell tumor killing and, 1193
  in primary mediastinal large B-cell lymphoma, 1634
  as T-cell therapy target, 415–416
  in Waldenström macroglobulinemia, 1785
CD20
  in B cells, 1141
  in Burkitt lymphoma, 1674
  in chronic lymphocytic leukemia, 1528
  in diffuse large B-cell lymphoma, 1627
  in extranodal marginal zone lymphoma, 1665
  in follicular lymphoma, 1576f, 1642, 1645, 1647
  in Hodgkin lymphoma, 1599, 1609, 1610, 1617
  leukemia cell expression, 1518
  in mantle cell lymphoma, 1653
  in primary mediastinal large B-cell lymphoma, 1634
  in pure red cell aplasia, 543
  at target of rituximab, 1141
  in Waldenström macroglobulinemia, 1785
CD20+ cells, in Hodgkin lymphoma, 1609
CD20-targeting antibodies. See Obinutuzumab; Ofatumumab; Rituximab
CD21, 1573, 1665
CD22, 1141, 1163, 1555
  in Burkitt lymphoma, 1674
  in diffuse large B-cell lymphoma, 1627
  in follicular lymphoma, 1642, 1647
  in primary mediastinal large B-cell lymphoma, 1634
  in Waldenström macroglobulinemia, 1785

CD23
  in chronic lymphocytic leukemia, 1531, 1532t, 1542
  in mantle cell lymphoma, 1593
  in Waldenström macroglobulinemia, 1785, 1791
CD24, 1856
CD25 (IL-2Rα), 1700
CD25 deficiency, 1223
CD25-targeted therapy. See Denileukin diftitox
CD26, 1143, 1144t, 1682
CD27, 1172, 1528, 1785, 1788, 2234
CD27 deficiency, 1220
CD28, 415–416, 1183, 1184, 1185f
CD30
  in anaplastic large cell lymphoma, 1698
  in cutaneous lymphoproliferative disorders, 1688, 1689f
  in Hodgkin lymphoma, 1599, 1607, 1609, 1610, 1617
  in primary effusion lymphoma, 1247
  in primary mediastinal large B-cell lymphoma, 1634
  as therapeutic target. See Bortezomib; Brentuximab vedotin
CD31. See Platelet-endothelial cell adhesion molecule-1 (PECAM-1, CD31)
CD32. See Fcγ receptor IIA (FcγRIIA, CD32)
CD33
  in acute lymphoblastic leukemia, 1512
  in acute myelogenous leukemia, 271, 1380t, 1383
  lymphoid progenitors and, 1154
  structure, 1052f
CD33 antibodies. See Gemtuzumab ozogamicin
CD34
  in aorta-gonad-mesonephros region, 258
  in hematopoietic stem cells, 260
  in inflammatory response, 1977
  in leukocyte adhesion, 283
  lymphoid progenitors and, 1153
  in stem cell adhesion and homing, 66
CD34+ cells
  in acute myelogenous leukemia, 1376
  in aplastic anemia, 515, 516f
  in chronic myelogenous leukemia, 1444–1445
  cultures, 463
  in hematopoietic cell transplantation, 356
  in lymphopoiesis, 1150
  in myeloma, 1714
  in primary myelofibrosis, 1321, 1326
CD35, 1009, 1054, 1665
CD36. See Glycoprotein (GP)IV (CD36, FAT, SCARB3)

CD38, 68, 1141, 1144t, 1531t, 1532
CD39, 1144t, 1834, 1885–1886
CD39 (ecto-ATP/Dase-1/CD39), 1967, 1968, 1969f, 1971, 1972f
CD40
  atherosclerosis and, 2288
  in dendritic cells, 309
  in heavy-chain class switching, 1168
  in Hodgkin lymphoma, 1599, 1607
  in inflammatory response, 1978
  mutations, autosomal recessive hyper-IgM with, 1213
  in myelodysplastic syndromes, 1352
  in platelets, 1872–1873
CD40 ligand (CD40L, CD154)
  in atherosclerosis, 2288
  in heavy-chain class switching, 1168
  in hyperimmunoglobulin M syndromes, 1213, 1214t
  in immune thrombocytopenia, 2008
  in myelodysplastic syndromes, 1352
  platelet activation and, 2293
  in platelets, 1856, 1872–1873
  in red cell transfusion, 2375, 2376
  structure, 1872
  in T cells, 93
CD41/CD61. See Integrin $\alpha_{IIb}\beta_3$
CD42. See Glycoprotein (GP)Ib/IX/V complex (CD42)
CD42a. See Glycoprotein (GP)IX (CD42a)
CD42b,c. See Glycoprotein (GP)Ibα (CD42b,c)
CD43, 1653, 1873
CD44
  in B-1 B cells, 1141
  chronic myelogenous leukemia and, 1440
  deficiency, 498
  in diffuse large B-cell lymphoma, 1627
  dyserythropoietic anemia and, 568
  hematopoietic stem cell trafficking and, 355
  in marrow cells, 62, 266–267
  memory T cells and, 1183
  in myeloma, 1737
CD45, 1599
CD45 (T200), 1183, 1247
CD45RA, 1153, 1183
CD45RB, 1183
CD45RO, 1183
CD45RO+ cells, 411, 411f
CD47, 1845, 1879
CD48, 949
CD49b/CD29. See Integrin $\alpha_2\beta_1$
CD49d, 1532, 1532t
CD49e/CD29. See Integrin $\alpha_5\beta_1$

CD49f/CD29. *See* Integrin $\alpha_6\beta_1$

CD 50, 1184

CD51/CD61. *See* Integrin $\alpha_v\beta_3$

CD 52, 1535

CD 52-targeting antibody. *See* Alemtuzumab

CD54. *See* ICAM-1 (CD54)

CD55, 572, 1053f, 1871

CD56 (NCAM), 1142, 1189, 1699, 1726, 1737

CD56^{bright} NK cells, 93, 1189

CD57 (LEU7), 1528

CD58 (LFA-3), 1184, 1185, 1978

CD59, 572, 1053f, 1285, 1871, 2358

CD59 blood group, 2333t

CD61, 1184

CD62E. *See* E-selectin

CD62L. *See* L-selectin

CD62L+ cells (memory stem cells), 411

CD62P. *See* P-selectin

CD63, 1009, 1011, 1013, 1836, 1871

CD64. *See* Fcγ receptor I (FCγRI, CD64)

CD65, 1380t, 1383, 1512

CD66, 1014

CD68, 1013

CD69, 948

CD70, 1788

CD72, 1163

CD73, 1144t, 1834, 1971, 1972f

CD79, 1785

CD79a (Ig-α)

  in Burkitt lymphoma, 1674

  in diffuse large B-cell lymphoma, 1627

  in extranodal marginal zone lymphoma, 1665

  in follicular lymphoma, 1642

  immunoglobulin M and, 1162, 1162f

  in precursor B cells, 1168

  in primary mediastinal large B-cell lymphoma, 1634

CD79B, 233t, 236t

CD79b (Ig-β), 1162, 1162f, 1168

CD80, 1183, 1184, 1185f

CD86

  in dendritic cell maturation, 309

  in T-cell interactions, 1183, 1184, 1185f

CD87, 2358

CD89, 1008

CD90, 260

CD94, 1190

CD95. *See* Fas (CD95)

CD97, 1059

CD99, 1977t, 1978

CD102. *See* ICAM-2 (CD102)

CD106. *See* Vascular cell adhesion molecule (VCAM)-1

CD107a (LAMP-1), 1873

CD107b (LAMP-2), 1873

CD109, 1871

CD110. *See* Thrombopoietin (TPO) receptor (c-mpl, CD110)

CD117, 260, 974, 1380t, 1393

CD123, 1393

CD133, 260

CD135 (Flt3), 309

CD138 (syndecan 1), 1141, 1712, 1714, 1737

CD142. *See* Tissue factor (TF)

CD143, 1144t

CD144, 68

CD148, 1172

CD151, 1871

CD152 (CTLA-4), 424, 1184

CD154. *See* CD40 ligand (CD40L, CD154)

CD156a, 1144t

CD156b, 1144t

CD157, 1144t

CD163, 499, 1061, 1080

CD164, 260

CD178, 1564

CD200, 1084

CD-209 (DC-SIGN), 308, 1057t, 1082

CD224, 1144t

CD244, 949

CD247, 1177

CD278 (iCOS), 1184

CD279 (PDCD1), 1184

2-CDA. *See* Cladribine

CDAN1, 565

CDAs. *See* Congenital dyserythropoietic anemias (CDAs)

Cdc42, 309, 1841, 1883

CDDO-Me, 1403

CDK4, 1653

CDKIs (cyclin-dependent kinase inhibitors), 217–218, 1539

CDKN1B, 234t

CDKN2 (*p16*), 232t, 236t, 1654, 1734

CDKN2A/B, 177f, 1508

CDKN2c, 234t

cdks. *See under* Cyclin-dependent kinase (cdk)

CDRs (complementarity determining region), 1170

CDw32 (FcγRII), 953

ceAML (clonally evolved acute myelogenous leukemia), 1281

C/EBPA (*CEBPA*, *CEPBα*)

  in acute myelogenous leukemia, 181, 181t, 182, 226t, 363, 1378t, 1379

  in myelodysplastic syndromes, 181t, 1345, 1351

CEBPB, 1699

C/EBP homologous protein (CHOP), 204f, 205, 208f

C/EBPε, 926, 1011

Cefepime, 384, 385, 387t

Ceftaroline, 384

Ceftazidime, 384, 385, 387t

Ceftobiprole, 385

Celecoxib, 2075, 2121

Celiac disease, 597, 630, 1575

Cell adhesion, 65–68, 67t

  BCR-ABL1 and, 1440–1441

  in sickle cell disease, 764–765

Cell cycle

  cancer chemotherapy and, **317**

  regulation, 213–241, 214f

    checkpoints, **218–219**

    cyclins and cyclin-dependent kinases, **213–218**, 215t, 217f

    histone deacetylases, **239–240**, 239t, 240f

    oncogenes, **219–222**

    proteasome, **240–241**

    tumor-suppressor genes, **237–239**

Cell cycle-active antineoplastic agents, **329–331**

Cell dehydration, in sickle cell disease, 764

Cell fusion, 269

Cell growth and metabolism

  gene expression and, 196

  in hematopoietic stem cells, 196–197, 197f

  homeostasis, 191

  in leukemias, 197–198, 199f

  in lymphomas, 199–200

  in myeloma, 200–201

  signaling and nutrients, 191–192

  signal transduction and, 193–196, 194f, 195f

Cell homing, **68–71**

Cell-mediated cytotoxicity, 1190–1191, 1190f

Cell proliferation gene signature, 1654

Cell signaling. *See* Signal transduction pathways

Cell-surface proteins, 487

Cellular immunity, newborn, 108

Cellular senescence, **132**

Cellular therapy. *See* Immune cell therapy (adoptive cellular therapy)

Central nervous system. *See also* Neurologic disease/symptoms

  leukemia, 1510, 1515, 1516, 1518

  macrophages, 1083

  microglia, 1083

  primary lymphoma, 1244f, 1246, 1579

Central venous catheter placement, bleeding risk and, 2384

Centromere, 175t

CEP. *See* Congenital erythropoietic porphyria (CEP)

CEPBA, 1280, 1377, 1378*t*, 1379, 1383
Cephalosporins, 830
Cerebral thrombosis, 1519–1520, 1520*f*
Cerebrovascular disease. *See* Stroke
Ceruloplasmin, 621*t*
Cervix, primary lymphomas in, 1582
CFB, 2259*t*
CFC (colony-forming cell), 269
CFH, 2259*t*
CFI, 2259*t*
CFU (colony-forming unit), 269
CFU-E. *See* Colony-forming unit-erythroid
    (CFU-E)
CFU-GEMM (colony-forming unit-
    granulocyte-erythroid-monocyte
    macrophage), 100
CFU-GM (colony-forming unit-granulocyte-
    monocyte), 100, 263
CH50, 1232
Chaenocephalus aceratus, 479
"Chaperone therapy," 1128
Charcot-Leyden crystal (CLC) protein, 929,
    947, 953
CHARGE syndrome, 1223
CHD7, 1222
CHD (chromodomain)-family remodelers,
    166, 166*f*
Chédiak-Higashi syndrome, **1018–1020**
    abnormal granules in, 22*f*, 23, 1843
    clinical features, 994, 1018, 1019*t*, 1229
    definition and history, 1018
    differential diagnosis, 1020
    epidemiology, 1018
    etiology and pathogenesis, 1018, 1019*t*,
        1229
    laboratory features, 994, 1018
    macrophage defects in, 1091
    natural killer cells and, 1192
    neutrophil abnormalities in, 984*t*, 986,
        1019*t*
    therapy, 1020, 1229
Chelation therapy. *See* Iron chelation therapy
Chemicals
    hemolytic anemia caused by, **809–811**
    history of exposure to, **6–7**
    porphyrias caused by, **907**
Chemokine ligands, 70*t*
Chemokine receptor (CCR) 1, 1878
Chemokine receptor (CCR) 2, 1052*f*, 2286
Chemokine receptor (CCR) 3, 950, 1878
Chemokine receptor (CCR) 4, 1878
Chemokine receptor (CCR) 5, 440, 454, 1057,
    1240
Chemokine receptor (CCR) 7, 1183, 1699,
    1710
Chemokine receptors (CCRs), 70*t*

eosinophil, 950–951, 951*t*
monocytes, 1057–1058, 1058*t*, 1080*t*
Chemokines
    cellular homing and, 68–71, 70*t*
    extracellular matrix, 62*t*
    in extracellular matrix, 60–61
    inactivation and sequestration, 285
    in innate immune response, 303
    in regulation of inflammation, 286*t*,
        287–288, 288*t*
Chemotactic receptors, on neutrophils, 934*t*
Chemotaxis
    leukocyte, 283–284
    monocytes and macrophages, 1059, 1060*t*
    neutrophil, 1005
    in newborns, 106
Chemotherapy. *See* Antineoplastic drugs/
    chemotherapy
Chest
    examination, 8
    history of disorders of, 5
    pain, 5, 2295. *See also* Myocardial
        infarction (MI)
    primary lymphomas in, 1581
Chickenpox, 835
Chido/Rogers blood group, 2331*t*
Children
    acute lymphoblastic leukemia in
        chromosomal abnormalities, 1508*t*,
            1513*t*
        clinical features, 1509*t*
        development *in utero*, 1507
        differential diagnosis, 1513–1514
        gene mutations, 1508*t*, 1513*t*
        incidence, 1506, 1526*f*
        laboratory features, 1509–1510, 1510*t*
        survival, 1506*f*, 1513*t*
        treatment, 1505, 1515, 1516
    acute myelogenous leukemia in, 1380,
        1409–1410
    antiphospholipid syndrome in, 2241
    autoimmune neutropenia in, 2358
    bleeding risk in, 2382–2383
    chronic myelogenous leukemia in, 1445
    immune thrombocytopenia in, 2001, 2002*t*
    iron deficiency in, 632
    juvenile myelomonocytic leukemia in,
        1096, 1468*t*, **1470–1471**
    juvenile xanthogranuloma in, 1101, 1102*t*,
        1111–1112
    Langerhans cell histiocytosis in. *See*
        Langerhans cell histiocytosis
    lymphocyte subsets, 109*t*
    megaloblastic anemia in, **605, 607**
    paroxysmal nocturnal hemoglobinuria in,
        580

red cell transfusion in, 2371
reference ranges for blood examination,
    15*t*
Chills, history of, 4
Chimeric antigen receptor T (CAR-T) cells,
    1539
Chimeric antigen receptor (CAR), 415–416,
    415*f*, 438, 442, 454, 1193, 1404
Chimeric proteins, 173
Chitotriosidase, 1126
Chk1 inhibitors, 219
Chlamydia pneumoniae, 2283
Chlamydophila psittaci infection, lymphomas
    and, 1574, 1579, 1664
Chlorambucil
    adverse effects, 1534
    for autoimmune hemolytic anemia, 839
    for chronic lymphocytic leukemia, 1534,
        1536
    for follicular lymphoma, 1644, 1645*t*
    for γ-heavy-chain disease, 1806
    for mantle cell lymphoma, 1657*t*
    mechanism of action, 329
    for mycosis fungoides, 1687
    for polycythemia vera, 1298*t*
    for Waldenström macroglobulinemia, 1793
N-Chloramines, 284*t*
Chloramphenicol
    aplastic anemia and, 515
    for bartonellosis, 818
    hemolytic anemia and, 708
Chlorates, erythrocyte damage from, 810
Chlordane, aplastic anemia and, 517
Chlorguanide, megaloblastic anemia and,
    606*t*
2-Chloro-2′-fluoro-arabinosyladenine. *See*
    Clofarabine
2-Chlorodeoxyadenosine. *See* Cladribine
Chloroma. *See* Myeloid (granulocytic)
    sarcoma
Chloroquine, for porphyria cutanea tarda,
    908
Chlorosis, 628
Cholesterol crystal emboli, 2101, 2102*f*, 2298
CHOP (C/EBP homologous protein), 204*f*,
    205, 208*f*
CHOP regimen. *See also* R-CHOP regimen
    for anaplastic large cell lymphoma, 1699
    for diffuse large B-cell lymphoma,
        1628–1630, 1628*t*, 1629*t*
    for enteropathy-associated T-cell
        lymphoma, 1699
    for gastric MALT lymphoma, 1666
    for HIV-associated lymphoma, 1245
    for mantle cell lymphoma, 1655, 1657*t*
    for NK/T-cell lymphoma, 1702

CHOP regimen (*Cont.*):
  for peripheral T-cell lymphoma, 1694–1696, 1695*t*, 1697
  poor clinical response to, 200
  for posttransplant lymphoproliferative disorders, 1636
  for primary mediastinal large B-cell lymphoma, 1635
  for T-cell-histiocyte-rich large B-cell lymphoma, 1637
  for Waldenström macroglobulinemia, 1794–1795
Chorea-acanthocytosis syndrome, **681**
CHR (complete hematologic response), 1452*t*
Ch/Rg blood group, 2345*t*
Christmas disease/Christmas factor deficiency. *See* Hemophilia B
Christmas factor. *See* Factor IX
Chromatin
  in blood cell differentiation, 166–167
  gain-of-function mutations, 170
  genome access and, 166, 166*f*
  loss-of-function mutations, 170
  next-generation sequencing–based studies, 161–162
  transcription factors and, 165–166, 168, 169*f*
Chromium, in red cell labeling, 488, 495–496, 497
Chromodomain (CHD)-family remodelers, 166, 166*f*
Chromosomal abnormalities
  analytic techniques, 174–176, 176*f*
  in hematologic and lymphoid malignancies, **176–188**, 179–180*t*, 184–185*t*, 219, 220–225*t*, 225, 230. *See also specific diseases*
  nomenclature, 174, 175*t*
Chromosomal instability syndromes. *See* Immunodeficiency diseases, chromosomal instability syndromes associated with
Chronic basophilic leukemia, 1279, 1468*t*, 1470
Chronic cyclic neutropenia, 983, 985
Chronic eosinophilic leukemia, **1469–1470**. *See also* Hypereosinophilic syndromes
  clinical features, 1469
  course and prognosis, 1470
  differential diagnosis, 1469–1470
  etiology and pathogenesis, 1279, 1468*t*
  history and definition, 1469
  laboratory features, 1467, 1469–1470
  therapy, 977, 1470

Chronic graft-versus-host disease. *See* Graft-versus-host disease (GVHD)
Chronic granulomatous disease
  clinical features, 1030–1031, 1031*t*
  definition and history, 1027
  diagnostic classification, 1028*t*
  differential diagnosis, 1032
  epidemiology, 1027
  etiology and pathogenesis, 1027
    genetic alterations affecting cytochrome b, 1029
    genetic alterations affecting cytosolic proteins, 1029
    NADPH-oxidase function, 1027–1029, 1028*f*
    predisposition to infection, 1029–1030, 1030*f*, 1031*t*
  laboratory features, 1031–1032
  neutrophil abnormalities in, 984*t*, 986
  therapy, course, prognosis, 1032
Chronic idiopathic neutropenia, 983, 985, 987
Chronic inflammation, **290–291**
Chronic kidney disease, anemia of. *See* Anemia of chronic kidney disease
Chronic lymphocytic leukemia (CLL)
  chronic myelogenous leukemia and, 1449
  clinical features, 1530
  complications
    autoimmune hemolytic anemia, 824, 827, 831, 839, 840, 1541
    immune thrombocytopenic purpura, 1541–1542
    infectious, 1541
    pure red cell aplasia, 1542
    Richter syndrome, 1542
    secondary cancer risk, 1541
    small lymphocytic lymphoma, 1543
  definition, 1527
  differential diagnosis, 1200, 1543, 1655
  epidemiology, 1527
  etiology and pathogenesis
    B-cell receptor pathway, 1528–1529
    chromosomal abnormalities, 185*t*, **187**, 210, 223*t*, 1494*t*, 1529
    disease biology, 1528
    environmental factors, 1528
    gene mutations, 231–232*t*, 1349, 1494*t*, 1528, 1592
    immune dysregulation, 1528, 1592
  laboratory findings
    blood, 1494*t*, 1530–1531, 1531*f*
    histopathology, 1592–1593, 1592*f*
    marrow, 36*f*, 37
  monoclonal B-cell lymphocytosis and, 1200, 1542–1543

  prognosis
    CD38 expression and, 1532
    CD49d expression and, 1532
    cytogenetics and, 1531, 1531*t*
    gene mutations and, 187, 223*t*
    immunoglobulin heavy-chain variable mutations and, 1531, 1531*t*
    markers, 1532, 1532*t*
    ZAP-70 and, 1531–1532
  staging, 1532–1533, 1533*t*
  treatment, **1533–1540**
    alkylating agents, 1534
    antibody therapy, 1535–1536
    assessment of response, 1540
    B-cell receptor kinase inhibitors, 1538
    blinatumomab, 1539
    chemoimmunotherapy, 1537
    chimeric antigen receptor-T cells, 415, 1539
    combination chemotherapy, 1534–1535
    cyclin-dependent kinase inhibitors, 218, 1539
    gene therapy, 438, 442
    glucocorticoids, 1536–1537
    hematopoietic cell transplantation, 1539
    ibrutinib, 342
    initial, 1540
    lenalidomide, 1538–1539
    leukapheresis, 1540
    minimal residual disease evaluation, 1540
    nucleoside analogues, 1534
    radiation therapy, 1540
    for relapsed disease, 1540
    splenectomy, 1539
    venetoclax, 1539
Chronic lymphoproliferative disorders of NK cells (CLPD-NK)
  clinical features, 1566
  definition and history, 1563
  etiology and pathogenesis, 1563–1564
  gene mutations, 1564
  immunophenotypic features, 1565
Chronic mountain sickness, 875
Chronic myelogenous (myeloid) leukemia (CML), **1437–1473**
  accelerated phase and blast crisis
    clinical features, 1465
    course and prognosis, 1467
    cytogenetics, 1466
    definition, 1464
    extramedullary blast crisis, 1465
    laboratory features, 1465
    marrow blast crisis, 1465–1466
    pathogenesis, 1464–1465
    treatment, 1466–1467

atypical, 1279
clinical features, 1445
  BCR-ABL1–positive thrombocythemia,
    1449
  in children, 1445
  concurrence of lymphoid malignancies,
    1449
  extramedullary tumors, 1285
  hyperleukocytic syndromes, 1285–1286,
    1286t, 1449
  marrow necrosis, 1287
  metabolic signs, 1286–1287
  signs and symptoms, 1445
  splenomegaly, 1287, 1445
  systemic symptoms, 1286
  thrombocytosis, 1311–1312
course and prognosis, 1462–1464, 1462t
definition and history, 1437–1438
differential diagnosis, 1327, **1449–1450**
epidemiology, 1438, 1439f
etiology and pathogenesis, **1438–1445**
  BCR-ABL1. See BCR-ABL1, in chronic
    myelogenous leukemia
  chromosomal abnormalities, **176–178**,
    177f, 179t, 221t, 225, 230, 1278
  chronic myelogenous leukemia stem
    cell, 1439
  coexistence of normal stem cells, 1440
  environmental leukemogens, 1438
  gene mutations, 230t
  molecular pathology, 1441–1443, 1441f,
    1442f
  origin from mutant hematopoietic stem
    cell, 1438–1439
  Ph chromosome, 1440
  pluripotential stem cell lesion, 1439–1440
  progenitor cell characteristics,
    1440–1441
  telomere length, 1444–1445
laboratory features, **1445–1449**
  basophilia, 971, 972t
  blood, 1445–1446, 1445f, 1446f, 1447t
  chemical abnormalities, 1449–1450
  cytogenetics, 1447, 1448f
  eosinophilia, 955t, 1445
  marrow, 1446–1447, 1446f
  molecular probes, 1448–1449
  monocytosis, 1096
  progenitor cell growth, 1447
minimal residual disease detection,
  1463–1464
minor-BCR breakpoint-positive, 1449
neutrophilic, 1449
pathogenesis, 1282
Ph-chromosome–positive acute
  myelogenous leukemia and, 1385

phenotypic expression, 1283–1284
progression, 1280–1281, 1464
related diseases without BCR
    rearrangement, **1467–1473**, 1468t
  atypical myeloproliferative disease,
    1468t, 1472–1473
  BCR rearrangement-negative
    phenotypically typical chronic
    myelogenous leukemia, 1472–1473
  chronic basophilic leukemia, 1279, 1470
  chronic eosinophilic leukemia. See
    Chronic eosinophilic leukemia
  chronic myelomonocytic leukemia. See
    Chronic myelomonocytic leukemia
    (CMML)
  chronic neutrophilic leukemia, 1279,
    1450, **1471–1472**
  juvenile myelomonocytic leukemia,
    1096, **1470–1471**
therapy
  in accelerated and blast crisis, 1466–1467
  busulfan, 1459
  cytarabine, 1459
  donor leukocyte infusion for
    posttransplantation relapse, 1462
  hematopoietic cell transplantation,
    1460–1461, 1466–1467
  high-dose chemotherapy with
    autologous stem cell infusion, 1460
  hydroxyurea, 1459
  for hyperuricemia, 1450
  for initial cytoreduction, 1450–1451
  interferon-α, 1459
  potential agents, 1459
  during pregnancy, 1459–1460
  radiation therapy, 1459
  splenectomy, 1459, 1467
  tyrosine kinase inhibitors
    in accelerated phase and blast crisis,
      1466
    adherence to therapy, 1456
    bosutinib, 339t, 1457–1458
    comparison, 339t, 1451t
    dasatinib, 176, 319t, 1453–1454, 1457
    discontinuation of, 1460
    disease progress and monitoring
      during treatment, 1458–1459
    effect on rate of progression, 1464
    after hematopoietic cell
      transplantation, 1461–1462
    imatinib, 176, 319t, 1451–1453, 1452t
    nilotinib, 176, 339t, 1454, 1457
    pharmacology, 338–341
    ponatinib, 339t, 1458
    resistance to. See Tyrosine kinase
      inhibitors, resistance to

    response to, 1452t, 1454–1456, 1455t,
      1463
    secondary chromosomal changes
      with, 1456
    selection for initial therapy in chronic
      phase, 1454
    vaccine, 423
  transformation to acute lymphoblastic
    leukemia, 1465–1466
Chronic myelogenous (myeloid) leukemia
  (CML) stem cell, 1439
Chronic myelomonocytic leukemia (CMML)
  chromosomal abnormalities, 180t
  clinical features, 1467–1468, 1468t
  differential diagnosis, 1450
  epidemiology, 1467
  gene mutations, 170, 1351, 1468t
  monocytosis in, 1096
Chronic natural killer cell lymphocytosis,
  1197
Chronic neutrophilic leukemia, 1279, 1450,
  1468t, **1471–1472**
Chronic thromboembolic pulmonary
  hypertension, 2273
CHS1, 1018
Churg-Strauss syndrome. See Eosinophilic
    granulomatosis with polyangiitis
    (EGPA)
Chuvash polycythemia
  clinical features, 510, 880
  course and prognosis, 884
  epidemiology, 873
  etiology and pathogenesis, 876–877,
    877f
  laboratory features, 881–882
  VHL mutations and, 510, 876–877, 877f,
    878f, 882t
CID. See Combined immunodeficiencies
    (CID)
Cigarette smoking
  acute myelogenous leukemia and, 1374
  adult Langerhans cell histiocytosis and,
    1108, 1109
  lymphoma and, 1573
  myelodysplastic syndromes and, 1342
  neutrophilia and, 1001
  persistent polyclonal lymphocytosis of
    B lymphocytes and, 1200
  polycythemia and, 872, 876, 876t
  porphyria cutanea tarda and, 906
Cilostazol
  antiplatelet effects, 404
  clinical uses, 404t, 405
  dosage, 404t
  for peripheral arterial disease, 2297
  platelet effects, 2077–2078

Cimetidine
  for acute intermittent porphyria, 904
  aplastic anemia and, 516
  for toxic methemoglobinemia, 793
Ciprofloxacin, 387t, 388
Circulating cell-free fetal DNA (ccff-DNA), 852
Circulatory overload, transfusion-associated, 2376
Circumcision, 1988
CIS3 (SOCS3), 485, 486f
Cisplatin, 331, 331t. *See also* ESHAP regimen
  for diffuse large B-cell lymphoma, 1629t, 1631
  for Hodgkin lymphoma, 1616
  platelet function and, 2079
  secondary acute myelogenous leukemia and, 1407
Citrovorum factor, 584
c-Kit, 258, 264–265
c-Kit ligand. *See* Stem cell factor (SCF)
CKS1B, 1712, 1736
CLA-1 (scavenger receptor-B1, SCARB1), 1872
Cladribine, **324**
  for acute myelogenous leukemia, 1395t, 1396, 1402t
  for adult Langerhans cell histiocytosis, 1108–1109
  for autoimmune hemolytic anemia, 839
  autoimmune hemolytic anemia and, 831
  for chronic lymphocytic leukemia, 1534, 1535
  for Erdheim-Chester disease, 1111
  for follicular lymphoma, 1645t
  for gastric MALT lymphoma, 1666
  for hairy cell leukemia, 1553, 1557, 1559t
  with IFN-α, for mastocytosis, 977
  for juvenile xanthogranuloma, 1112
  for Langerhans cell histiocytosis, 1106, 1107
  for pure red cell aplasia, 544
  resistance to, 319t
  structure, 323f
  for Waldenström macroglobulinemia, 1793, 1794–1795
Classic von Hippel-Lindau syndrome, 877–878
Class switching, heavy-chain, 1168–1169
Class switch recombination (CSR), 1213
Claudication, 2297
CLC (Charcot-Leyden crystal) protein, 929, 947, 953
Clearance receptors, 2309
CLEC-2, 1857, 1871
Clindamycin, for babesiosis, 819

CLL. *See* Chronic lymphocytic leukemia (CLL)
Clofarabine, 322, **324–325**
  for acute myelogenous leukemia, 1402t
  for Langerhans cell histiocytosis, 1107
  for myelodysplastic syndromes, 1362
  resistance, 319t
  structure, 323f
Clonal disorders. *See* Chromosomal abnormalities
Clonal hematopoiesis, 1284
Clonal hemopathy, in myelofibrosis, 1328
Clonality assay, 883–884
Clonally evolved acute myelogenous leukemia (ceAML), 1281
Clonal myeloid disorders, **1275–1287**, 1276t. *See also specific disorders*
  aplastic anemia and, 521
  basophilia in, 971–972, 972t
  clinical manifestations, **1284–1287**
    blood cell deficiency, excess, or dysfunction, 1284–1285
    extramedullary tumors, 1285
    factitious laboratory results, 1287
    hyperleukocytic syndromes, 1285–1286, 1286t
    marrow necrosis, 1287
    metabolic signs, 1286–1287
    organ involvement, 1287
    procoagulant and fibrinolytic activator release, 1285
    splenomegaly, 1287
    systemic symptoms, 1286
    thrombocythemic syndromes, 1286
  interplay of clonal and polyclonal hematopoiesis in, 1284
  minimal-deviation, 1276t, **1277–1278**
  moderate-deviation, 1276t, **1278–1279**
  moderately severe-deviation, 1276t, **1279**
  pathogenesis, **1281–1282**, 1281f
  Ph chromosome–positive, 1450
  phenotype, **1282–1283**, 1282f, 1283f
  pluripotential stem cell pool and, 1283
  quantitativeness, 1283–1284
  severe-deviation, 1276t, **1279–1280**
  transitions among, **1280–1281**
Clone, 175t
Cloning, DNA, 152
Clonogenic myeloerythroid progenitors, 1154
Clopidogrel, **405**
  antiplatelet effects, 405, 2076
  clinical uses, 404t, 405
  dosage, 404t
  for essential thrombocythemia, 1313
  for peripheral arterial disease, 2297
  platelet transfusion and, 2385

  for stroke prevention, 2076, 2297
  for unstable angina, 2296
Clostridial bacteremia, 2207
Clostridium difficile, 384, 388, 1182
Clostridium perfringens, 817f, 2211
Clostridium perfringens septicemia, **819**
Closure time, in newborn, 107
Clot retraction, 1842
CLP (common lymphoid progenitor), **269–270**, 1151
CLPD-NK. *See* Chronic lymphoproliferative disorders of NK cells (CLPD-NK)
CLRs (C-type lectin receptors), 1008, 1870–1871
Clustered, regularly interspaced, short palindromic repeats (CRISPR), 444
Cluster of differentiation. *See under* CD
CML. *See* Chronic myelogenous (myeloid) leukemia (CML)
CMML. *See* Chronic myelomonocytic leukemia (CMML)
C-MOPP regimen, for diffuse large B-cell lymphoma, 1628–1629
CMP (common myeloid progenitor), **270–271**, 1151
c-mpl. See Thrombopoietin (TPO) receptor (c-mpl, CD110)
CMR (complete molecular response), 1452t
CMV infection. *See* Cytomegalovirus (CMV) infection
CMV mononucleosis. *See* Cytomegalovirus (CMV) mononucleosis
CMX-001, 369
c-Myc, 237
c-MYC, 230t, 235t, 1626
CNVs (copy number variants), 147
CoA (acetyl-coenzyme A), 193, 193f, 196
CoA (succinyl coenzyme A), 892, 893f
Coagulation. *See also* Hemostasis
  activation of, in sickle cell disease, 765
  control of, **1949–1961**, 2222f. *See also* Coagulation factors
    activated protein C. *See* Activated protein C (APC)
    activated protein C–independent activity of protein S, 1958
    coagulation pathways. *See* Coagulation, pathways
    heparin cofactor II, 1960
    hereditary deficiencies associated with, 1951
    inhibition of activated protein C, 1958
    protease inhibitors, 1958–1959
    protein C pathway. *See* Protein C pathway

protein Z-dependent protease inhibitor, 1960

tissue factor pathway inhibitor. *See* Tissue factor pathway inhibitor (TFPI)

in inflammation, 286t, 290

metabolic modulation of, 2203

monocytes and macrophages in, 1059

in neonate, **109–111**, 110t, 111t

in older adults, 137

pathways. *See also* Coagulation factors

basal coagulation/anticoagulation and, 1942

cascade model, 1938–1939

cell-based model, 1940, 1940f

endothelial cells in, 1941–1942, 1941f

fibrinolysis in, 1942

immune cells in, 1940–1941, 1941f

plasma protease inhibitors in, 1942

platelet activation in, 1842, 1940, 1940f

protein C pathway and, 1949–1951, 1950f

revised model, 1939–1940, 1939f

Coagulation factors

aging and, 135

cell-associated

endothelial protein C receptor. *See* Endothelial protein C receptor (EPCR)

thrombomodulin. *See* Thrombomodulin (TM)

tissue factor. *See* Tissue factor (TF)

contact system

factor XII. *See* Factor XII

high-molecular-weight kininogen, 1916t, 1929

prekallikrein, 1929

deficiencies. *See also specific factors*

acquired, 2145

antibody-mediated, **2183–2187**

assays, 1990

diagnosis, 1988, 1989f

in hepatic disease, 2192

inherited. *See* Rare bleeding disorders (RBDs)

in pregnancy, 121

in disseminated intravascular coagulation, 2203

factor XI. *See* Factor XI

fibrin network

factor XIII. *See* Factor XIII

fibrinogen. *See* Fibrinogen

thrombin-activatable fibrinolysis inhibitor. *See* Thrombin-activatable fibrinolysis inhibitor (TAFI)

in inflammation, 2201

inhibitors, 1991

antithrombin. *See* Antithrombin (AT)

protein Z, 1938, 1952t

protein Z-dependent protease inhibitor, 1916t, 1938, 1952t, **1960**

tissue factor pathway inhibitor. *See* Tissue factor pathway inhibitor (TFPI)

procoagulant factors

factor V. *See* Factor V

factor VII. *See* Factor VIII

soluble cofactors

protein S. *See* Protein S

von Willebrand factor. *See* Von Willebrand factor (VWF)

vitamin K–dependent zymogens, 1915–1918, 1916t, 1917f, 1918f, 1918t

factor VII. *See* Factor VII

factor IX. *See* Factor IX

factor X. *See* Factor X

protein C. *See* Protein C

prothrombin. *See* Prothrombin (factor II)

Cobalamin, **588–593**

cell uptake, 592

chemistry, 588f, 589f

daily requirements, 589

intestinal absorption, 583, **591–592**, 591t

metabolism, inborn errors of, **607**, 607t

oral, 604

plasma haptocorrin and, 592–593

role in metabolism, 583, 589–590, 589f

serum assay, 593

sources, 589

Cobalamin-binding proteins

childhood megaloblastic anemia and defects in, 605, 607

levels in disease, 593t

Cobalamin C deficiency, 2263

Cobalamin deficiency, **599–604**. *See also* Pernicious anemia (PA)

clinical features, **602–603**, 602f

etiology and pathogenesis, 583, 596t, **599–602**

AIDS, 601–602

blind loop syndrome, 601

in children, 605, 607

defective intrinsic factor secretion. *See* Pernicious anemia (PA)

dietary deficiency, 602

fish tapeworm, 601

gastrectomy syndromes, 601

intestinal disorders, 601

pancreatic disease, 602

Zollinger-Ellison syndrome, 601

folate deficiency and, 590–591, 590f

laboratory features, **603**, 994

neural tube defects and, 598

neurologic effects, 602

pregnancy and, 120

subtle, 602–603

therapy, course, and prognosis, **603–604**, 604f

thrombocytopenia and, 1997–1998

Cobalophilin. *See* Haptocorrins

Cobblestone area-forming cell (CAFC), 260

Cocaine, 2079

Coccidioides infection, 384, 385

Codanin-1, 565

Codocytes (target cells), 21, 21f, 473f, 473t, 474f, **475**

CODOX-M/IVAC regimen, for Burkitt lymphoma, 1245, 1675, 1675t

Coenzymes, in erythrocytes, 470t

Cofilin, 1833t

COH1, 994

Cohen syndrome, 994

Cohort methods, for red cell life span measurement, 495, 496f

Coin rubbing, purpura and, 2107

Colchicine

for familial Mediterranean fever, 1025–1026

megaloblastic anemia and, 606t

Cold agglutinin disease, 823–824, 837, 840, 1790. *See also* Autoimmune hemolytic anemia, cold-antibody

Cold agglutinins, 828, 829

Cold-antibody hemolytic anemia. *See* Autoimmune hemolytic anemia, cold-antibody

Collagen, 63

interactions, 1846t

platelet activation and, 1879–1881

structure, 1846t

type III, 267, 1446, 1846t

types I, V, VI, 267, 1846t

Collagenases, 283

Collagen receptor. *See* Integrin $\alpha_2\beta_1$

Collagen-related peptide (CRP), 1851

Colon

cancer, folic acid deficiency and, 599

primary lymphomas in, 1581

Colony-forming cell (CFC), 269

Colony-forming unit (CFU), 269

Colony-forming unit-erythroid (CFU-E)

development, 462

in erythropoiesis, 480f, 481, 483f

progenitors, 270

Colony-forming unit–granulocyte-erythroid-monocyte macrophage (CFU-GEMM), 100

Colony-forming unit-granulocyte-monocyte (CFU-GM), 100, 263
  in aplastic anemia, 515
Colony-stimulating factor (CSF), 105, 939–940
Colony-stimulating factor (CSF)-1, 1287
Colton blood group/antigens, 2331t, 2345t
Combined immunodeficiencies (CID)
  Ca²⁺ entry channel defects, 1221
  CD27 deficiency, 1220
  clinical features, 1213t
  coronin-1A deficiency, 1220
  CTPS1 deficiency, 1220–1221
  dedicator of cytokinesis 9 deficiency, 1221–1222
  defects of T-cell–receptor signaling, 1220
  magnesium transporter 1 defects, 1221
  major histocompatibility complex class I deficiency, 1221
  major histocompatibility complex class II deficiency, 1221
  with multiple intestinal atresia, 1222
  Omenn syndrome, 1166, **1219–1220**
  severe. *See* Severe combined immunodeficiency (SCID)
  T-cell immunodeficiencies with impaired NF-κB activation, 1220
  with venoocclusive disease, 1222
Combined system disease, 602, 602f
COMMD7, 1853
Common lymphoid progenitor (CLP), **269–270**, 1151
Common myeloid progenitor (CMP), **270–271**, 1151
Common variable immunodeficiency (CVID), 993, 1214t, **1216**, 1575t
Compartment syndrome, 2118
Compatibility testing, 2349–2350, 2350t
Competitive repopulation, 259
Complement
  in antiphospholipid syndrome, 2237
  defects, in atypical hemolytic uremic syndrome, 2259–2260, 2259t
  in paroxysmal nocturnal hemoglobinuria, 572, 573f
Complementarity determining region (CDRs), 1170
Complementary DNA (cDNA)
  in Fanconi anemia, 530
  libraries, 421
  von Willebrand factor, 2164
Complement (C3)-coated red cells, 499
Complement fixation, 829
Complement receptor 1, 815, 1054
Complement receptor 3. *See* CD11b
Complement receptors, 1053f, 1054

Complement system
  deficiencies, 1213t, 1232
  in inflammation, 286t, 289–290, 289f
Complete cytogenic response (CCyR), 1452t
Complete hematologic response (CHR), 1452t
Complete molecular response (CMR), 1452t
Computed tomography (CT), in pulmonary embolism, 2271, 2272f
Concentrate film, 29
Conditional ablation, suicide genes for, 416
Confusion, history of, 5
Congenital adrenal hyperplasia, 560
Congenital alopecia and absence of thymus, 1223
Congenital amegakaryocytic thrombocytopenia (CAMT), 530t, 532, 1822
Congenital disorder of glycosylation II. *See* Leukocyte adhesion deficiency type 2 (LAD-2)
Congenital dyserythropoietic anemias, 608
Congenital dyserythropoietic anemias (CDAs), **563–569**
  atypical, 568, 568t
  definition and history, 563
  differential diagnosis, 563, 564f, 568–569, 637
  epidemiology, 563–564
  type I
    clinical features, 564–565, 566f
    genetics, 565–566
    laboratory features, 565, 565f
    therapy, course, and prognosis, 566
  type II
    clinical and laboratory features, 566–567
    genetics, 567
    therapy, course, and prognosis, 567–568
  type III, 568
Congenital erythropoietic porphyria (CEP), 889, **896–897**
  clinical features, 890t, 896f, 897
  definition and history, 890, 896
  diagnosis, 897
  enzymes affected by, 890t
  laboratory features, 891t
  pathogenesis of clinical findings, 897
  pathophysiology, 896
  therapy, 897
Congenital Heinz body hemolytic anemia, **781–782**
Congenital immunodeficiency diseases. *See* Immunodeficiency diseases
Congenital leukemia, 1386
Congenital neutropenia, 992–993, 993f

Congenital thrombotic thrombocytopenic purpura (Upshaw-Schulman syndrome), 2257–2258
Congestive heart failure, history of, 5
Congo red stain, 1773, 1776, 1776f
Conjugated estrogens, for uremia, 2084
Connective tissue tumors, polycythemia with, 879
Consciousness, history of impairment of, 5
Consensus E-box motifs (CANNTG), 262
Constant region, 1175
Constipation, history of, 5
Co_null phenotype, 2343
Cooley anemia, 743. *See also* β-thalassemias
Coombs (direct antiglobulin) test, 823, 833, 834t, 2349, 2372
COPP-ABVD regimen, for Hodgkin lymphoma, 1612t, 1614
Copper, 652t, 811
Copper deficiency, **653**
  neutropenia and, 995
  sideroblastic anemia and, 919–920
COPP regimen
  for diffuse large B-cell lymphoma, 1628–1629
  for Hodgkin lymphoma, 1612t
Coproporphyrinogen oxidase (CPO), 895
Coproporphyrinogens, 891f, 891t, 893f
Copy-number neutral LOH, 174, 177f
Copy number variants (CNVs), 147
Cord blood, 102, **357**, 358
Cord colitis, 357
Cordocentesis, 854
Coronary artery bypass grafting, 2296
Coronary artery disease, 1850, 2240. *See also* Cardiovascular disease
Coronary stents, 2293
Coronin-1A deficiency, 1220
Cor pulmonale, 882
Corrected count increment (CCI), 2385, 2387–2388
Corrinoids, 588
Corrin ring, 588, 588f, 589f
Corynebacterium diphtheriae pharyngitis, 1268
Cost antigens, 2333t
Cough, history of, 5
Coumadin. *See* Warfarin
Coumarin, 393
Cow's milk anemia, 630
COX. *See under* Cyclooxygenase (COX)
CPB2, 1935–1936
Cpg islands, 168
CPO, 905
CPO (coproporphyrinogen oxidase), 895
CPX-351, for myelodysplastic syndromes, 1361

CR1, 1053*f*

CR3. *See* CD11b/CD18

CR4, 1053*f*

C-reactive protein
in Castleman disease, 1250
high-sensitivity, 2283
in pregnancy, 119–120
in primary myelofibrosis, 1325
in reactive thrombocytosis, 2035
in sickle cell disease, 765

CRE-BBP, 235*t*

CREBBP, 1644

C-REL, 209

Crenated cell. *See* Echinocytes

Crenolanib, 1403

CRIs (cross-reactive idiotypes), 1170

CRISPR (clustered, regularly interspaced, short palindromic repeats), 444

Critical limb ischemia, 2297

Crizotinib
for anaplastic large cell lymphoma, 1699
for peripheral T-cell lymphoma, 1696

CRKL, 1443–1444

CRLF2, 232*t*, 1508

Crohn disease, 1229

Cromer blood group/antigens, 2332*t*, 2337, 2345*t*

Crossover, genetic, 151, 151*f*

Cross-presentation, 308

Cross-reacting material (CRM), in hemophilia, 2121

Cross-reactive idiotypes (CRIs), 1170

Crosstalk, 253

CRP (collagen-related peptide), 1851

CRS (cytokine release syndrome), 415–416, 1539

Cryofibrinogenemia, 2099

Cryoglobulinemia, 428, 429*t*, 1789, 1790*f*, 2097, 2099*f*

Cryohydrocytosis, 682*t*, **684**

Cryoprecipitate
for afibrinogenemia, 2156
for bleeding, 2317, 2317*t*
for disseminated intravascular coagulation, 2213
for hemophilia A, 2122

Cryptococcus infection, 384

Cryptosporidium, 1017, 1213

Crypts, 94

CSF (colony-stimulating factor), 105, 939–940

CSF-1 (colony-stimulating factor-1), 1287

CSF1R, 232*t*

CSF3R, 228*t*, 1468*t*, 1472

CSR (class switch recombination), 1213

CT (computed tomography), in pulmonary embolism, 2271, 2272*f*

CTAP-III, 1844–1845

CTCL. *See* Cutaneous T-cell lymphoma (CTCL)

CTLA-4 (cytotoxic T-lymphocyte antigen-4, CD152), 424, 1184, 1224

CTLs. *See* CD8+ T cells

CTP (cyclic thrombocytopenia), 2015

CTPS1, 1220–1221

CTPS1 (cytidine 5-triphosphate synthase 1) deficiency, 1220–1221

C-type lectin receptors (CLRs), 1008, 1870–1871

CUBAM complex, 591

Cubilin, 591–592

Cumin, 2079

Cushing disease, 1986

Cushing syndrome, 543, 544, 560, 1987, 2108

Cutaneous calciphylaxis, 2101–2102

Cutaneous disorders. *See* Skin disorders

Cutaneous mastocytosis, 973*t*

Cutaneous polyarteritis nodosa, 2106, 2106*f*

Cutaneous T-cell lymphoma (CTCL). *See also* Mycosis fungoides (MF)
chromosomal abnormalities, 1498*t*
classification, 1680*t*, 1684*t*
definition and history, 1679
differential diagnosis, 1683–1684, 1688
erythrodermic subset, 1683, 1684*t*
etiology and pathogenesis, 1680
lymphomatoid papulosis, 1499*t*, **1688–1689**, 1688*t*
primary cutaneous anaplastic large cell lymphoma, 1499*t*, **1688**, 1688*f*

CUX1, 1347

CVID (common variable immunodeficiency), 993, 1214*t*, **1216**, 1575*t*

CVP regimen, for follicular lymphoma, 1646*f*, 1646*t*

CXC chemokines, 288, 288*t*

CXCL4 (platelet factor 4)
in gray platelet syndrome, 2054
in heparin-induced thrombocytopenia, 2026–2028, 2026*f*
in inflammation, 1856
in platelet signaling, 1878
structure, 2027*f*
target cells, 288*t*
in α granules, 1844

CXCL12 (stromal cell-derived factor-1), **265–266**, 1823
in chronic lymphocytic leukemia, 1528
in hematopoiesis, 259

in hematopoietic stem cell homing, 355, 356
in megakaryopoiesis, 1817
stem cell function and, 261
in WHIM syndrome, 994

CXCL12-abundant reticular cells, 264

CXCL12 (SDF-1)/CXCR4, 1712–1713, 1737

CXCL13, 1698, 2097

CXCR1, 1878

CXCR2, 2286

CXCR4 (CXCR-4)
antagonists, 1404
in atherosclerosis, 2286
in chronic lymphocytic leukemia, 1528
in hematopoietic stem cell homing, 355
in HIV infection, 1240
in megakaryopoiesis, 1823
in platelets, 1878
in WHIM syndrome, 994

CXCR4 promoter, 1321

CXCR4^{WHIM}, 1787–1788, 1787*f*

CXCR5, 1710

CXCR12, 2286

Cyanide, cobalamin and, 590

Cyanocobalamin (vitamin B$_{12}$), 588, 588*f*, 589, 592*f*. *See also* Cobalamin

Cyanosis
definition and history, 789
differential diagnosis, 794–795
etiology, 789
history of, 6
in methemoglobinemia, 792
in polycythemia, 508
in sulfhemoglobinemia, 794

CYBA (p22^{phox}), 1013*t*, 1027, 1028*t*, 1029

CYBB (gp91^{phox}), 1013*t*, 1028*t*, 1029

Cyclic adenosine monophosphate (cAMP), 404–405

Cyclic neutropenia, 983, 985, 994, 1097

Cyclic thrombocytopenia (CTP), 2015

Cyclin A, 213, 215, 215*t*

Cyclin B, 213, 215, 215*t*

Cyclin box, 214–215

Cyclin D, 215–216, 215*t*, 1710

Cyclin D1
in essential monoclonal gammopathy, 1736*t*
in mantle cell lymphoma, 1593–1594, 1593*f*, 1653
in myeloma, 1735, 1736*t*

Cyclin D2, 1735

Cyclin D3, 1735

Cyclin-dependent kinase (cdk), **213–218**
functions, 213, 215–217, 215*t*
pharmacologic inhibition, 218
substrates and inhibitors, 217–218, 217*f*

Cyclin-dependent kinase 4 inhibitors gene, 1465

Cyclin-dependent kinase 7 (cdk7), 216

Cyclin-dependent kinase 8 (cdk8), 216

Cyclin-dependent kinase 9 (cdk9), 216

Cyclin-dependent kinase 10 (cdk10), 216

Cyclin-dependent kinase 11 (cdk11), 216–217

Cyclin-dependent kinase inhibitors (CDKIs), 217–218, 1539

Cyclin E, 215

Cyclins, **213–216**, 214*f*, 215*t*

Cyclooxygenase (COX)-1, 403, 1857*f*, 1876, 1969–1970, 2073–2074

Cyclooxygenase (COX)-1b, 2073

Cyclooxygenase (COX)-1 inhibitors, 404

Cyclooxygenase (COX)-2, 404, 1876, 1970, 2073–2074

Cyclooxygenase (COX)-2 inhibitors, 2075, 2121

Cyclooxygenase (prostaglandin H$_2$ synthase-1) deficiency, 2058

Cyclophosphamide. *See also* BEACOPP regimen; CHOP regimen; CODOX-M/IVAC regimen; COPP regimen; EPOCH regimen; HyperCVAD regimen
for acute lymphoblastic leukemia, 1515, 1516
adverse effects, 331, 368, 1407, 1519*t*
for AL amyloidosis, 1761, 1780–1781
for α-heavy-chain disease, 1808
for antiphospholipid syndrome, 2245
for aplastic anemia, 526, 527
for autoimmune hemolytic anemia, 839
for Burkitt lymphoma, 1675, 1675*t*, 1676
for chronic lymphocytic leukemia, 1534, 1535, 1537
for diffuse large B-cell lymphoma, 1629*t*
for follicular lymphoma, 1645*t*, 1646
for γ-heavy-chain disease, 1806
before hematopoietic cell transplantation, 360
high-dose, before hematopoietic cell transplantation, 331*t*, 332*t*, 360
for Hodgkin lymphoma, 1616
for immune thrombocytopenia, 2007
for large granular lymphocytic leukemia, 1567
mechanism of action, 329
for μ-heavy-chain disease, 1810
for mycosis fungoides, 1687
pharmacology, 330
platelet function and, 2079
posttransplantation, 357
for pure red cell aplasia, 544

in reduced-intensity conditioning, 360
for Waldenström macroglobulinemia, 1794–1795

Cycloserine, megaloblastic anemia and, 606*t*

Cyclosporine
adverse effects, 2262
for aplastic anemia, 523–524, 525*f*, 525*t*, 527
for autoimmune hemolytic anemia, 840, 1541
for Diamond-Blackfan anemia, 540
for drug resistance in acute myelogenous leukemia, 1404
for familial hemophagocytic lymphohistiocytosis, 1228
for hemophagocytic lymphohistiocytosis, 1115
for immune thrombocytopenia, 2007
for IPEX syndrome, 1223
for large granular lymphocytic leukemia, 1567
for myelodysplastic syndromes, 1359
for primary myelofibrosis, 1329
for pure red cell aplasia, 544
in reduced-intensity conditioning, 360
for thrombotic thrombocytopenic purpura, 2257

CYLD (CYLD), 233*t*, 1711, 1737

CYP2C9, 395

CYP2C19, 1850, 2076

CYP enzymes
acute intermittent porphyria and, 901
porphyria cutanea tarda and, 906

Cysteine aspartyl-specific proteases. *See* Caspases

Cytarabine (ara-C), **321–322**. *See also* CODOX-M/IVAC regimen; ESHAP regimen
for acute lymphoblastic leukemia, 1515
or acute lymphoblastic leukemia, 1516
for acute myelogenous leukemia, 1394–1396, 1395*t*, 1398–1399, 1402*t*
in children, 1409
high-dose vs. standard-dose, 1396
in older patients, 1408
in pregnant patients, 1409
for acute promyelocytic leukemia, 1404, 1405*t*
for adult Langerhans cell histiocytosis, 1108–1109
adverse effects, 322, 1519*t*
for chronic lymphocytic leukemia, 1534
for chronic myelogenous leukemia, 1459
for chronic myelomonocytic leukemia, 1469

in combination chemotherapy, 327
for diffuse large B-cell lymphoma, 1628, 1629*t*, 1631
high-dose, 331*t*
for Hodgkin lymphoma, 1616
for juvenile myelomonocytic leukemia, 1471
for Langerhans cell histiocytosis, 1106, 1107
for mantle cell lymphoma, 1656, 1658*t*, 1659*t*
mechanism of action, 321
megaloblastic anemia and, 606*t*
for myelodysplastic syndromes, 1358–1359, 1361
pharmacology, 321–322
for primary myelofibrosis, 1330
resistance to, 319*t*
for transient myeloproliferative disorder, 1386

Cytidine 5-triphosphate synthase 1 (CTPS1) deficiency, 1220–1221

Cytochrome b, 621*t*, 1013*t*, 1014, 1029

Cytochrome b_5 deficiency, 790

Cytochrome b_5 reductase, 701*t*

Cytochrome b_5 reductase deficiency. *See also* Methemoglobinemia
clinical features, 793
epidemiology, 789
etiology and pathogenesis, 789–790
heterozygosity for, 790
laboratory features, 792
treatment, 793

Cytochrome c (Cyt-c), 204*f*, 205

Cytogenetics, **173–188**. *See also* Chromosomal abnormalities
in aplastic anemia, 520
cell preparation methods, **173–174**
chromosome nomenclature, 174, 175*t*
metaphase, 1711–1712

Cytokine release syndrome (CRS), 415–416, 1539

Cytokines. *See also specific cytokines*
for aplastic anemia, 526
in apoptosis regulation, 209
in B-cell precursor development, 270
in disseminated intravascular coagulation, 2200
in erythropoietic precursor development, 550
in extracellular matrix, 61–62, 62*t*
for Fanconi anemia, 529
in hematopoietic stem cell regulation, **264–265**, 264*t*
in innate immune response, **303**
in lymphopoiesis regulation, 1154

in macrophage activation, 1085–1086, 1085f
in megakaryopoiesis, 1817, 1821
natural killer cells and, 1191
in neonatal phagocytic function, 107
in regulation of inflammation, 286t, 287–288
stem cell factor. *See* Stem cell factor (SCF)
in transfusion reactions, 2374, 2375
for vaccine therapy enhancement, 422
Cytolytic T cells, 1139
Cytomegalovirus (CMV) infection
antiphospholipid antibodies and, 2234
complications, 1266t
differential diagnosis, 1269
epidemiology, 1261–1262
after hematopoietic cell transplantation, 369–370, 2374
in immunocompromised host, 385, 1267–1268
preventive therapy, 389, 1268, 2374
T-cell therapy, **409–411**, 410f, 411f
in transplant recipients, 1267–1268
Cytomegalovirus (CMV) mononucleosis, **1266–1268**
clinical manifestations, 1263t, 1267
complications, 1267
epidemiology, 1266
history, 1266
laboratory features, 1267, 1267t
treatment, 1269
Cytopenias, 1277, 1610
Cytoplasmic antineutrophil cytoplasmic antibody (cANCA), 1013
Cytoplasmic granules, 1145, 1511, 1511f
Cytoreductive therapy, for essential thrombocythemia, 1313–1314, 1313t
Cytosine arabinoside. *See* Cytarabine (ara-C)
Cytosine methylation, 162
Cytotoxicity disorders. *See* Immunodeficiency diseases, cytotoxicity disorders
Cytotoxic T cells. *See* CD8+ T cells (cytotoxic T lymphocytes, CTLs)
Cytotoxic T-lymphocyte antigen (CTLA)-4, 424, 1184, 1224

D
D6, 285
D409H, 1123, 1123t
Dabigatran, **399**, **401**
adverse effects, 2275t
clinical studies, 400t
mechanism of action, 1919

for venous thromboembolism, 2274–2275, 2274t, 2275t
Dacarbazine. *See also* ABVD regimen
for malignant histiocytic diseases, 1110
mechanism of action, 329
Dacetuzumab, for myeloma, 346t
Daclizumab, for pure red cell aplasia, 544
Dacryocytes (teardrop cells), 21f, 473f, 473t, 474f
Dactylitis, 771
DAF (decay accelerating factor), 572
DAG (diacylglycerol), 935, 1016, 1849
DAH (diffuse alveolar hemorrhage), 368
DAI (DNA-dependent activator of IRFs), 302f, 303
Dalbavancin, 385
Dalteparin, for venous thromboembolism, 2274t
Damaged ("smudge," "basket") cells, 23
Danaparoid, **398**
for heparin-induced thrombocytopenia, 2030, 2031t
for unstable angina, 2296
Danazol
for autoimmune hemolytic anemia, 839
for immune thrombocytopenia, 2007
for paroxysmal nocturnal hemoglobinuria, 579
D antigen, 2330, 2336
DAP (γ-D-glutamyl diaminopimelic acid), 299, 301f
DAP12, 1190
DAPK, 1528
Dapsone
adverse effects, 2007
G6PD deficiency and, 708t, 712, 1252
for immune thrombocytopenia, 2007
prophylactic, 389
toxic methemoglobinemia and, 790t, 793
Dapsone-trimethoprim, 386
Daptomycin, 384, 385, 388t
Darapladib, for atherosclerosis, 2286
Daratumumab, for myeloma, 345, 345f, 346t, 1754–1755
Darbepoetin, 554. *See also* Erythropoiesis-stimulating agents (ESAs)
DARC (Duffy antigen receptor for chemokines), 285
Darling-Roughton effect, 795
Dasatinib, **338–341**
for acute lymphoblastic leukemia, 1518
for acute myelogenous leukemia, 1403
adverse effects, 339t, 341, 1203, 1451t, 1453–1454
for chronic myelogenous leukemia, 176, 339t, 1451t, 1453–1454, 1457, 1466

comparison with other tyrosine kinase inhibitors, 1451t
drug interactions, 339t, 1451t
for mastocytosis, 977
pharmacology, 338, 339t, 340–341, 1454
resistance to, 319t
structure, 340f
Daunomycin, for acute myelogenous leukemia in children, 1409
Daunorubicin, **327–328**
for acute lymphoblastic leukemia, 1515, 1516
for acute myelogenous leukemia, 1395, 1395t, 1408
for acute promyelocytic leukemia, 1404, 1405t
adverse effects, 328, 1519t
DCs. *See* Dendritic cells (DC)
DC-SIGN (CD-209), 308, 1057t, 1082
DDAVP. *See* Desmopressin (DDAVP)
D-dimer levels
aging and, 135, 137
in deep vein thrombosis, 2269
in disseminated intravascular coagulation, 2206
in pulmonary embolism, 2271
DDT, 517
Dead fetus syndrome, 2211
Death domain (DD), 205, 249
Death effector domains (DEDs), 205, 207f
Death-inducing signaling complex (DISC), 205
DEC205, 310
DEC205/CD205 lectin receptor, 308, 310
Decay accelerating factor (DAF), 572
Decitabine, **322**
for acute myelogenous leukemia, 1403
mechanism of action, 239, 1360–1361
for myelodysplastic syndromes, 239, 336, 1360–1361
for sickle cell disease, 774t, 775
Dectin-1
in fungal infection susceptibility, 1057t, 1230
in innate immunity, 295, 1084
toll-like receptors and, 1054, 1055f, 1057t
Dedicator of cytokinesis 8 (DOCK) deficiency, 1215t, 1221–1222
DEDs (death effector domains), 205, 207f
Deep vein thrombosis (DVT).
See also Venous thrombosis/thromboembolism
in antiphospholipid syndrome, 2238
complications, 2269
definition and epidemiology, 2267
differential diagnosis, 2269, 2270f

Deep vein thrombosis (DVT) (*Cont.*):
  etiology and pathogenesis, 2268
  objective testing for, 2269–2270, 2272–2273
  therapy. *See* Venous thrombosis/thromboembolism, therapy
Defensins, 107, 1009–1010, 1011, 1012*t*, 1013
Deferasirox, for iron chelation therapy, 644, 752, 776, 1358
Deferiprone, for iron chelation therapy, 644, 752, 776
Deferoxamine, for iron chelation therapy, 751–752, 1358
Deferoxamine mesylate, 5
Defibrotide, 368
Deformin, 818
Degranulation, 948
Degranulation abnormalities
  Chédiak-Higashi syndrome. *See* Chédiak-Higashi syndrome
  specific granule deficiency, 1019*t*, 1020–1021
Dehydrated stomatocytosis. *See* Hereditary xerocytosis
Delayed hemolytic transfusion reaction (DHTR), 2372, 2377
Deletions, chromosomal, 175*t*
δβ-thalassemias, 726
  (^Aγδβ)^0, 733, 733*t*
  clinical features, 743
  (δβ)^+, 733–734, 735*f*, 748
  (δβ)^0, 733, 748
  epidemiology/population genetics, 727–728
  laboratory features, 750*f*
  molecular basis, 733–734, 733*t*, 734*f*, 735*f*
  nondeletion, 734–735
Delta ligand, 1824
δ-storage pool deficiency, **2052–2054**
δ-thalassemias, 726, 736, 751
Demargination (pseudoneutrophilia), 999–1000
Dematin, 663*t*
Demethylating agents, 239, **336**. *See also* 5-Azacytidine; Decitabine
Dendritic cells (DCs)
  antigen uptake and processing in, 308–309
  blood, 1092, 1098
  in cellular therapy, 413
  classification, 309–310
  development, 309, 1151
  differentiation, 1076*f*
  functions, **307–308**, 308*t*
  in immunotherapy, 310
  in Langerhans cell histiocytosis, 1103
  in malignant histiocytosis, 1101

  markers, 1080*t*
  progenitors, 310
  for vaccine delivery, 422
Dendritic cell sarcomas, 1110
Denileukin diftitox
  adverse effects, 1687
  for mature T-cell lymphomas, 1695
  mechanism of action, 346
  for mycosis fungoides, 1687
  for subcutaneous panniculitis-like T-cell lymphoma, 1702
Denosumab, for myeloma, 1737
Dense granules, platelet, 1843
Dense tubular system (DTS), 1836
Dental bleeding/extractions
  antibiotic prophylaxis, 869
  antifibrinolytic therapy for, 2317*t*
  fibrin glue for, 2157
  gingival bleeding, 5, 8, 1987
  in hemophilia, 2120
  in hemostatic disorders, 1987, 1988
2'-Deoxycoformycin. *See* Pentostatin (deoxycoformycin)
Deoxyhemoglobin, 761, 761*f*
Deoxynucleotide synthesis, 587*f*
Deoxypyridinoline (DPD), 1738
Deoxyuridine (dU) suppression test, 594, 598, 603
Depsipeptide, 335, 1403
Desferrioxamine, 639, 644, 751, 776
Desirudin, 2030
Desmopressin (DDAVP)
  adverse effects, 2175
  for bleeding
    in chronic myeloproliferative neoplasms, 2081
    in fibrinolytic therapy, 2317
    in inherited platelet disorders, 2061–2062
    postsurgical, 2086
    in uremia, 2084
  for combined deficiency of factors V and VIII, 2140
  for hemophilia A, 2122–2123, 2185
  release of von Willebrand factor and factor VIII and, 2166
  for von Willebrand disease, 2175
    contraindication during pregnancy, 121
Deviation, 1275
Dexamethasone. *See also* HyperCVAD regimen
  for acute lymphoblastic leukemia, 1515, 1516, 1517
  adverse effects, 1519*t*
  for AL amyloidosis, 1779–1781
  for α-heavy-chain disease, 1808

  for Burkitt lymphoma, 1676
  for chronic lymphocytic leukemia, 1537
  for diffuse large B-cell lymphoma, 1629*t*
  for familial hemophagocytic lymphohistiocytosis, 1228
  for follicular lymphoma, 1645*t*
  for hemophagocytic lymphohistiocytosis, 1115
  for Hodgkin lymphoma, 1616
  for immune thrombocytopenia, 2004
  for myeloma, 1750–1751, 1753*t*
  for Waldenström macroglobulinemia, 1794–1795
Dexrazoxane, cardioprotective effects, 1396, 1520
Dextran, 2079
DGKE/*DGKE*, 2260, 2261
DGKH, 233*t*
DHAP regimen
  for diffuse large B-cell lymphoma, 1629*t*, 1631
  for Hodgkin lymphoma, 1616
  for peripheral T-cell lymphoma, 1696
DHFR (dihydrofolate reductase), 318, 584
DHFR (dihydrofolate reductase) deficiency, 608
DHTR (delayed hemolytic transfusion reaction), 2372
Diabetes insipidus (DI)
  in acute myelogenous leukemia, 1384
  in Langerhans cell histiocytosis, 1104–1105
Diabetes mellitus, hemostasis and, 2203
Diacylglycerol (DAG), 935, 1016, 1849
Dialysis, 2083–2084
Diamond-Blackfan anemia (inherited pure red cell anemia), **539–540**, 994
Diamond-Blackfan syndrome, 2340
Diapedesis, 1059
Diaphragmatic hernia, blood loss from, 629
Diarrhea, history of, 5
Diazoxide, maternal ingestion of, effect on fetus and newborn, 112, 112*t*
DIC. *See* Disseminated intravascular coagulation (DIC)
Dickkopf-1 (DKK1), 1713, 1737, 1738, 1739*f*
Diclofenac, 2075
Didanosine, 1249
Diego blood group/antigens, 2331*t*, 2337, 2345*t*
Dietary restriction, aging and, 131–132
Diferric transferrin pool, 491
Differential count
  in children, 15*t*
  in newborn, 105, 105*t*

Differentiating agents, **335–336**. *See also*
Arsenic trioxide; ATRA
(all-*trans*-retinoic acid)
Differentiation syndrome (retinoic acid
syndrome), 1405
Diffuse alveolar hemorrhage (DAH), 368
Diffuse large B-cell lymphoma (DLBCL),
1625–1637
activated B-cell-like, 234–235t, 1495t,
1626, 1627t, 1632, 1634f
autoimmune disorders and, 1574–1575
cell metabolism in, 199
central nervous system, 1579
clinical features, 1626
course and prognosis, **1632–1633**, 1632t,
1633f, 1633t, 1634f
definition and history, 1625
differential diagnosis, 1627, 1674
endocrine glands, 1583
epidemiology, 1571, 1625
etiology and pathogenesis, **1625–1626**
chromosomal abnormalities, 184t, 187,
224t, 225t, 1495–1496t, 1625–1626
gene expression, 1595–1596, 1596f,
1626, 1632
gene mutations, 234–235t, 1626
BCL2, 209, 234t, 1596, 1626, 1627t
BCL6, 235t, 1625
CD79B, 235t
C-REL, 209
EZH2, 170, 234t, 1626, 1627t
GNA12/13, 1627t
IRF (MUM1), 235t
MEF2B, 1627t
MYC, 235t, 1596, 1626, 1627t
MYD88, 235t
PRDM1, 1171
PTEN, 234t
TNFAIP3, 235t
TNFRSF14, 1627t
germinal center B-cell-like, 234–235t,
1495t, 1626, 1627t, 1632, 1634f
hepatitis and, 1573
histologic/morphologic variants,
1495–1497t, 1572t, 1595–1596,
1595f
HIV-associated, 187, 1243–1245, 1244f,
1247, 1571
laboratory features
blood and marrow, 1627
cell immunophenotype, 1627
histopathology, 1495–1497t,
1595–1596, 1595f, 1627
mediastinal, 1596, 1596f, 1597f
molecular subtypes, 1495–1496t
OSPHOS group, 200

paranasal sinuses, 1581
therapy, **1627–1632**
in advanced stage diffuse disease,
1628–1630, 1629t
general considerations, 1627
hematopoietic cell transplantation,
1631–1632
in limited stage diffuse (stages I and II)
disease, 1627–1628, 1628t
during pregnancy, 1634
radioimmunotherapy, 1632
in recurrent and refractory disease,
1631–1632
variants and subtypes, 1626t
anaplastic. *See* Anaplastic large cell
lymphoma (ALCL)
intravascular large B-cell lymphoma,
1496t, 1626, **1635–1636**
lymphomatoid granulomatosis,
1635
posttransplant lymphoproliferative
disorders, 1265–1266, 1500t, 1574,
1636
primary cutaneous diffuse large B-cell
lymphoma, leg type, **1637**
primary mediastinal large B-cell
lymphoma. *See* Primary
mediastinal large B-cell lymphoma
primary testicular lymphoma, 1246,
1581–1582, 1582f, **1634**
T-cell-histiocyte-rich large B-cell
lymphoma, **1636–1637**
Diffuse reticuloendotheliosis. *See* Langerhans
cell histiocytosis
DiGeorge syndrome (22q 11.2 deletion
syndrome), 86–87, 1214t, **1222**
Di Guglielmo syndrome, 1342
Dihydrofolate (FH$_2$), 584
Dihydrofolate reductase (DHFR), 318, 584
Dihydrofolate reductase (DHFR) deficiency,
608
Dihydroxyacetone/Lawsone, 899
Dihydroxyacetone phosphate, 695
Dilute prothrombin time, 2243
Dilute Russell viper venom time (dRVVT),
2241, 2243
Dilution anemia, 554, 742
5,6-Dimethylbenzimidazolyl group, 588
Dimethylglycine dehydrogenase, 588
Dimethyltriazenoimidazole carboxamide
(DTIC), 329, 330
Dimorphic anemia, 637
Dimorphic dysmorphic platelets with giant
A-granules and thrombocytopenia,
2061
Dinaciclib

for chronic lymphocytic leukemia, 326,
1539
for myeloma, 218
Dipeptidyl peptidase 1 (cathepsin C), 1013
Diphyllobothrium latum, 41, 601
Diploid, 175t
Dipyridamole
for acute myocardial infarction, 2295
antiplatelet effects, 404–405, 2077
clinical uses, 404t
dosages, 404t
for stroke prevention, 404–405, 2297
Direct (saline) agglutinins, 823
Direct antiglobulin (Coombs) test, 823, 833,
834t, 2349, 2372
Directed donation (directed donor blood),
2368
Direct film, 29
Direct glycolytic pathway, 692–694, 693f
Direct thrombin inhibitors. *See* Argatroban;
Bivalirudin
DIS3, 1736t, 1737, 1759
DISC (death-inducing signaling complex),
205
Discocyte, 472f, 472t, 474f
Discoid platelets, 1835f
Disodium cromoglycate, for mastocytosis,
976
Disseminated candidiasis, 2104–2105, 2105f.
See also Candida infections
Disseminated intravascular coagulation
(DIC), **2199–2214**
clinical features, 2107, **2203–2205**, 2204t,
2205t, 2261
definition and history, 2199
vs. HELLP syndrome, 802
laboratory features and diagnosis,
2205–2207, 2205t, 2206f, 2206t
in liver transplantation, 2193
mortality, 2205
in newborns, 2211
pathogenesis, **2200–2203**
anticoagulant pathways, 2201–2202,
2201f
coagulation proteases in upregulating
inflammation, 2201
cytokines and tissue factor, 2200
fibrinogen and fibrin, 2201
fibrinolysis dysregulation, 2202–2203
hemostatic factor consumption, 2203
inflammation and endothelium, 2200,
2200f
metabolic modulation of coagulation,
2203
natural anticoagulants and
inflammation, 2202

Disseminated intravascular coagulation (DIC), pathogenesis (*Cont.*):
  oxidative stress and vasoactive molecules, 2203
  thrombin and platelets, 2200–2201
 pathology, 2199
 platelet dysfunction in, 2086
 during pregnancy, 120–121, **2210–2211**
 therapy, 2210–2214, 2212f, 2317t, 2318
 underlying diseases, **2207–2210**
  aortic aneurysm, 2210
  brain injury, 2208
  burns, 2208
  heat stroke, 2209
  hemangiomas, 2209–2210
  hepatic disease, 2193, 2208–2209
  infectious diseases, 2207
  leukemias, 2208
  purpura fulminans, 2207
  snake bites, 2209
  solid tumors, 803–804, 2207–2208
  transfusion reaction, 2210
  trauma, 2208
Disulfide bonds, of heavy and light chains, 1159
Divalent metal transporter (DMT)-1, 619, 623, 623f
Divalent metal transporter (DMT)-1 mutations, 642
DIVA regimen, 1408
DKC1, 530–531
DKK1 (Dickkopf-1), 1713, 1737, 1738, 1739f
DLBCL. *See* Diffuse large B-cell lymphoma (DLBCL)
DLI (donor lymphocyte infusions), 359, 373, 1400–1401, 1462
DNA
 antisense, 153
 cloning, 152
 complementary. *See* Complementary DNA (cDNA)
 functions, 145–146
 hydroxymethylation, 162
 methylation, 162
 replication, megaloblastic anemia and, 593
 sequencing, 152, 155. *See also* Next-generation sequencing
 structure, 145, 146f
 synthesis, 587f
DNA damage checkpoint, 213
DNA-dependent activator of IRFs (DAI), 302f, 303
DNA ligase IV, 1167
DNA ligase IV deficiency, 530t
DNA methylation/demethylation, 168–170, 1349

DNA methyltransferases (DNMTs), 168, 336
DNA polymerase, 146
DNA protein kinase, 1166f, 1167
DNA repair theory, 130
DNMT3a, 170
DNMT3A
 in acute myelogenous leukemia, 226t, 1376, 1377–1378, 1378t
 in clonal myeloid disorders, 1280
 in myelodysplastic syndromes, 227t, 1346t, 1348, 1349, 1350–1351
 in Ph-chromosome negative myeloproliferative neoplasms, 229t
DOCK (dedicator of cytokinesis 8) deficiency, 1215t, 1221–1222
Docosahexaenoic acid, 2079
Döhle bodies, 22f, 23
Dombrock blood group/antigens, 2331t, 2337, 2345–2346t
Dominance, 147, 148
Donath-Landsteiner antibody, 824, 829, 835
Donath-Landsteiner autoantibody, 823
Donath-Landsteiner hemolytic anemia, 824, 824t
Donor cells, recurrent leukemia in, 1401
Donor lymphocyte infusions (DLI), 359, 373, 1400–1401, 1462
Doripenem, 384, 387t
Dosage compensation, 150
DOT1, 169
DOT1L, 225
DOT1L inhibitors, 170, 337, 1403
Double-helix model, 145, 146f
Double-hit lymphoma, 1502, 1596, 1633, 1674
Double-stranded RNA (dsRNA), 295, 298, 301
Downeast anemia, 704
Down syndrome. *See* Trisomy 21
Doxorubicin, **327–328**. *See also* ABVD regimen; BEACOPP regimen; CHOP regimen; CODOX-M/IVAC regimen; EPOCH regimen; HyperCVAD regimen; Stanford V regimen
 for acute lymphoblastic leukemia, 1515, 1516
 for acute myelogenous leukemia
  in children, 1409
  in pregnant patients, 1409
 adverse effects, 328, 1519t
 for α-heavy-chain disease, 1808
 for Burkitt lymphoma, 1676
 for diffuse large B-cell lymphoma, 1629t
 for Hodgkin lymphoma, 1616

 for malignant histiocytic diseases, 1110
 for mantle cell lymphoma, 1657t
 for μ-heavy-chain disease, 1810
 for mycosis fungoides, 1687
 for myeloma, 1750, 1752t, 1753t, 1755
 secondary acute myelogenous leukemia and, 183, 1407
 thalidomide and, 334
DPD (deoxypyridinoline), 1738
DP proteins, 238
DRAP-27. *See* CD9
D region, polymerization defects in, 2158
Drepanocytes (sickle cells), 473f, 473t, 474f, **475**
Driver mutations, 1348
Drosophila Imd pathway, 303
Drosophila melanogaster, 293
Drugs. *See also* Antineoplastic drugs/chemotherapy; *specific drugs*
 aplastic anemia induced by, 515–516, 517t
 erythema multiforme induced by, 2106, 2106f
 hemolysis induced by, 553, 706–707
 hemolytic anemia induced by, 708, 708t, 710, 810t
 lymphocytopenia induced by, 1205–1206, 1205t
 lymphocytosis induced by, 1203–1204
 marrow suppression induced by, 553
 maternal, effects on fetus and newborn, **112**, 112t
 megaloblastic anemia caused by, 596t, **605**, 606t
 methemoglobinemia induced by, 789, 790t, 792, 793
 neutropenia induced by, 985, 992, 996–997, 998t
 neutrophilia induced by, 1001
 neutrophil motility impairment and, 1026
 platelet disorders induced by, **2073–2079**, 2074t
 purpuras induced by, 2107
 red cell aplasia induced by, 543
 sulfhemoglobinemia induced by, 793
 thrombocytopenia induced by, 2015–2018, 2016t, 2017t
 thrombotic microangiopathy induced by, 428, 431, 2262–2263
 vasculitis induced by, 2106, 2106f
Drug use/abuse, history of, **6**
Drüsenfieber, 1261
dRVVT (dilute Russell viper venom time), 2241, 2243
Dryness of the mouth, history of, 5
dsRNA (double-stranded RNA), 295, 298, 301

DTIC (dimethyltriazenoimidazole carboxamide), 329
DTS (dense tubular system), 1836
Dubowitz syndrome, 530t
Duffy antigen receptor for chemokines (DARC), 285
Duffy blood group, 104, 2331t, 2335t, 2337, 2345t
Duncan syndrome, 1266
Duodenal cytochrome b, 621t
DUSP22 (DUSP22), 1696, 1699
dU (deoxyuridine) suppression test, 594, 598, 603
Dutcher-Fahey bodies, 1791
DVT. *See* Deep vein thrombosis (DVT)
Dyserythropoiesis, 473, 563. *See also* Congenital dyserythropoietic anemias (CDAs)
Dysfibrinogenemia/hypodysfibrinogenemia, **2157–2159**
  acquired, 2159
  clinical features, 2158
  definition, history, and epidemiology, 2157–2158, 2157f
  differential diagnosis, 2159
  etiology and pathogenesis, 2158
  laboratory features, 2159
  in pregnancy, 2159
  therapy, 2159
Dyshemoglobins/dyshemoglobinemias, 789
  carboxyhemoglobin, **795–796**
  low-oxygen-affinity hemoglobins, **794–795**, 794t
  methemoglobinemia. *See* Methemoglobinemia
  nitric oxide hemoglobins, **796–797**, 796f, 797f
  sulfhemoglobin, **793–794**
Dyskeratosis congenita, **530–532**, 531f, 531t
Dyskerin, 530–531, 531f
Dysmorphia of neoplasia, 1342
Dysphagia, 5, 632
Dysplasia, 1343
Dyspnea, 5
Dysproteinemias
  cryofibrinogenemia, 2099
  cryoglobulinemia, 2097, 2099f
  light-chain vasculopathy, 2099
  platelet dysfunction in, 2082
  Waldenström hyperglobulinemic purpura, 2099, 2099f

E
E2A, 270, 1155
E2A-HLF, 1510
E2A-PBX1 (*TCF3-PBX1*), 1507, 1516

E2F transcription factor, 217
EACA. *See* ε-aminocaproic acid (EACA)
Early T-cell precursor acute lymphoblastic leukemia, 1512, 1512t
Ears, history of disorders of, 5
Eastern Cooperative Oncology Group Performance Status, 3, 4t
EATL (enteropathy-associated T-cell lymphoma), 1694t, **1699–1700**
EBF, 1155
EBF1, 236t, 1644
EBIs (erythroblastic islands), 64, **462–463**, 462f
E box-binding proteins, 195, 270
EBV infections. *See* Epstein-Barr virus (EBV) infections
EBVP regimen, for Hodgkin lymphoma, 1611
E-cadherin, 657
Ecchymoses, 6, 8, 1987
Echinocandins, 385, 389
Echinococcus, 957t
Echinocytes, 21f, 472f, 472t, 474f, 671f, 680
Eclampsia, 122, **801–802**, 2011, 2210–2211
ECMs (extracellular matrix proteins), 61–62
ECP (eosinophil cationic protein), 929, 931, 953
Ecto-ATP/Dase-1. *See* CD39 (ecto-ATP/Dase-1/CD39)
Ectoenzymes, 1143–1144, 1144t
Eculizumab
  for atypical hemolytic uremic syndrome, 2261
  contraindication during pregnancy, 580
  for hemolytic anemia, 839
  mechanism of action, 572f, 836
  meningococcal infections and, 578, 581
  for paroxysmal nocturnal hemoglobinuria, 576t, **578**, 580, 581
Edema, history of, 6
EDN (eosinophil-derived neurotoxin), 931, 953
Edoxaban, **402**
  clinical studies, 401t
  mechanism of action, 1922
  for venous thromboembolism, 2274–2275, 2274t, 2275t
EDRF (endothelium-derived relaxing factor). *See* Nitric oxide (NO)
EDTA (ethylenediaminetetraacetic acid), 1994, 1995, 2339
EEC (endogenous erythroid colonies), 1292
EGF (epidermal growth factor), 1848
EGF-TM7 (epidermal growth factor-seven transmembrane), 1059
EGLN1, 875, 878

EGPA (eosinophilic granulomatosis with polyangiitis), 959–960, 2107
EGR1, 234t, 1737
EGR2, 231t
Ehlers-Danlos syndrome, 1986, 1987, 2061, 2108
Eicosanoid metabolism, 1856, 1857f
Eicosanoid pathway, **1969–1970**
Eicosanoids, 1967, 1968t
Eicosapentaenoic acid, 2079
Eisenmenger syndrome, erythrocytosis of, 872, 876, 881
EKLF (erythroid Kruppel-like factor), 484
ELANE, 983, 993, 994
Elastase, 283, 1012t, 1013
Electron beam therapy, 1686
Electron transport chain (ETC), 196
Eliglustat tartrate, 1128
Elinogrel, 2076
Elliptocytes (ovalocytes), **473**, 474f
  abnormal, 671f, 679. *See also* Hereditary elliptocytosis (HE)
  characteristics, 472t
  disease states associated with, 472t
Elongin-C, 487
Elotuzumab
  mechanism of action, 1755
  for myeloma, 345, 345f, 346t, 1754t, 1755
Eltrombopag
  adverse effects, 2006
  for aplastic anemia, 526
  for hypersplenism, 867
  for immune thrombocytopenia, 2006
  for myelodysplastic syndromes, 1358
  for platelet count elevation before surgery, 2194
EM (erythema multiforme), 2106, 2106f
Embden-Meyerhof (glycolytic) pathway, 692–694, 693f, 932, 933t
Emberger syndrome, 1098, 1351, 1379
Embolism/emboli
  amniotic fluid, 2210
  atheromatous, 2298
  cholesterol, 2101, 2102f
  from intracardiac thrombi, 2102
  pulmonary. *See* Pulmonary embolism
Embryogenesis, stem cell development and, 54
Embryonic erythropoiesis, 480
Embryonic stem cells (ESCs), 448–449, 450
EMMPRIN, 1869
Emp, 481
EMR1 (F4/80), 1079–1080, 1081f, 1082
EMR2, 1059, 1080, 1081f
EMZL. *See* Extranodal marginal zone lymphoma of MALT type

Endocrine disorders
 anemia in, 553, **559–561**
 in Langerhans cell histiocytosis, 1104–1105
 polycythemia and, 872, 879
 primary lymphomas, 1583
Endocytosis
 of extracellular heme and hemoglobin, 499, 500*f*
 pathways, 1061, 1062*f*
 of transferrin, 622–623, 623*f*
Endogenous erythroid colonies (EEC), 1292
Endogenous pyrogen. *See* Interleukin (IL)-1β
Endoglin, 801–802, 1449
Endoglycan, 68
Endokinins A and B, 1878
Endomitosis, 1816–1817, 1816*f*, 1817–1818
Endomucin, 68
Endomyocardial biopsy, 1778, 1778*f*
Endoplasmic reticulum, 204*f*, 205, 1171
Endoplasmic reticulum-Golgi intermediate compartment protein (ERGIC)-53, 1171
Endothelial cells
 antiphospholipid antibodies and, 2236–2237
 on blood/marrow films, 22*f*, 23
 in coagulation, 1941, 1941*f*
 in disseminated intravascular coagulation, 2200, 2200*f*
 fibrinolytic proteins production by, 1973–1974, 1973*f*
 heterogeneity, 1967
 leukocyte interactions with, 1977–1978, 1977*t*, 1979
 marrow, 56–57
 platelet interactions with, 1969*f*, 1978–1979
 thromboregulatory molecules production by, 1967–1968, 1968*f*, 1968*t*
 von Willebrand factor in, 1969*f*
Endothelial dysfunction. *See* Atherosclerosis, endothelial dysfunction in
Endothelial nitric oxide synthase (eNOS), 2283*f*, 2285
Endothelial progenitor cells (EPCs), 2285
Endothelial protein C receptor (EPCR), **1953–1954**
 activated protein C and, 1972
 characteristics, 1916*t*, 1932
 functions, 1932, 1949, 1952*t*, 1968
 gene structure and variations, 1932
 in inflammation, 2202
 protein C activation and, 1932, 1954
 in sepsis, 2202
 structure, 1932, 1951*f*, 1952*t*, 1972

Endothelins, 1968*t*
Endothelium-derived relaxing factor (EDRF). *See* Nitric oxide (NO)
Endotoxin, 294. *See also* Lipopolysaccharide (LPS)
Endotoxin tolerance, 298
Energy clutch, 692
Energy metabolism, regulation by hypoxia, 504*f*
Enhancer of zest homologue 2 (EZH2), 170
Enhancer of zest homologue 2 (EZH2) inhibitors, 337–338
Enolase, 692*t*, 695–696, 701*t*
eNOS (endothelial nitric oxide synthase), 2283*f*, 2285
Enoxaparin, 2274*t*, 2295
Enterococcus faecium, 2340
Enterococcus infections, 383, 385. *See also* Bacterial infections
Enteropathy-associated T-cell lymphoma (EATL), 1694*t*, 1695*t*, **1699–1700**
Entinostat
 for breast cancer, 240
 for myelodysplastic syndromes, 1361
Enzyme replacement therapy, for Gaucher disease, 1127–1128, 1128*f*
Enzymes
 erythrocyte, disorders of. *See* Erythrocyte enzyme disorders
 folate-dependent, 584–585
 in heme biosynthesis, 891*f*, 893*f*
 leukocyte, 1049*t*
 lymphocyte membrane, 1143–1144, 1144*t*
 macrophage, 1066*t*
 neutrophil granules, 930*t*
 in neutrophils, 933*t*
Eosinophil cationic protein (ECP), 929, 931, 953
Eosinophil-derived neurotoxin (EDN), 931, 953
Eosinophil granules, 20*f*, 952–953
Eosinophilia
 in asthma, 954, 955*t*
 causes, 954, 955–956*t*
 in chronic eosinophilic leukemia, 1469
 consultative approach to, 44
 differential diagnosis, 1470
 in gastrointestinal disorders, 955*t*, 956
 in parasitic disease, 956–957, 957*t*
 in skin disorders, 954, 955*t*, 956*t*
Eosinophilic bronchitis, 954
Eosinophilic fasciitis, 518, 960
Eosinophilic granuloma. *See* Langerhans cell histiocytosis
Eosinophilic granulomatosis with polyangiitis (EGPA), 959–960, 2107

Eosinophilorrhachia, 960
Eosinophil peroxidase, 929, 948, 952
Eosinophils
 in asthma, 954, 955*t*
 in chronic inflammation, 291
 in chronic myelogenous leukemia, 1445
 development, 926*f*
 disorders, **953–960**
  animal models, 951
  eosinophilia. *See* Eosinophilia
  hypereosinophilia. *See* Hypereosinophilic syndromes
 functions, **952–953**, 954
  eosinophilic granule proteins, 952–953
  immunoregulation, 952
  inactivation of helminths, 952
  mediator release, 952
 in gastrointestinal disease, 956
 granules, 928–929, 929*f*, 931, 931*f*
 heterogeneity, 950
 hypodense, 950
 inflammation and, 279
 measurement in blood, 953–954
 in newborn, 105*t*
 in parasitic disease, 952, 956–957, 957*t*
 production, 949–950
 receptors, 948–949, 949*t*
 reference ranges in children, 15*t*
 secretion and activation, 953
 in skin conditions, 954, 955*t*
 structure, 20*f*, 23, 928–929, 931, 931*f*, 947–948, 948*f*
 trafficking and tissue accumulation, 950–951
Eosinophiluria, 960
Eotaxin, 291, 950
EP300, 1644
EPAS1, 875, 878, 880
EPCR. *See* Endothelial protein C receptor (EPCR)
EPCs (endothelial progenitor cells), 2285
EPCs (epithelial progenitor cells), 450, 451
Eph kinases, 1871–1872
Ephrin ligands, 1871–1872
Epidermal growth factor (EGF), 1848
Epidermal growth factor-seven transmembrane (EGF-TM7), 1059
Epidermodysplasia verruciformis, 1230
Epigenetic modulation
 for acute myelogenous leukemia, 1403
 for polycythemia vera, 1300
Epigenetic regulation, 213
Epigenetics, 151, **165–170**
 chromatin factors in. *See* Chromatin
 definition and overview, 165
 DNA methylation/demethylation, 168–170

fusion proteins, 169–170, 1016–1017
histone modification, **167–168**, 167*f*
trained immunity, 168
Epinephrine
    for allergic transfusion reactions, 2375
    for evaluation of neutrophil reserves, 943
    for mastocytosis, 976
    neutrophilia and, 1001
    neutrophil motility and, 1026
    in platelet activation, 1876
Epinephrine receptor defects, 2057
Epipodophyllotoxins, 328–329. *See also*
        Etoposide; Teniposide
Epirubicin, **327–328**
    adverse effects, 328, 1519*t*
    for enteropathy-associated T-cell
        lymphoma, 1700
    for Hodgkin lymphoma, 1611
Epistaxis
    in Bernard-Soulier syndrome, 2049
    etiology, 1987
    in factor V deficiency, 2139
    in hemophilia, 2120, 2122*t*, 2123
    history of, 5
    therapy, 2062
    in von Willebrand disease, 2172
Epithelial progenitor cells (EPCs), 450, 451
Epitopes, 2336
EPO. *See* Erythropoietin (EPO)
EPO, 485
EPOCH regimen
    for diffuse large B-cell lymphoma, 1629*t*,
        1630
    for HIV-associated lymphoma, 1243–1245,
        1247
    for primary mediastinal large B-cell
        lymphoma, 1634
EPO-EPOR signaling, 484–485, 486*f*
Epoetin, 554. *See also* Erythropoiesis-
        stimulating agents (ESAs)
EPOR. *See* Erythropoietin receptor (EPOR)
EPOR, 232*t*, 485, 873, 873*t*
EPP. *See* Erythropoietic protoporphyria
        (EPP)
ε-aminocaproic acid (EACA)
    adverse effects, 2318
    for bleeding in thrombocytopenia, 2003,
        2007
    for bleeding not response to platelet
        transfusion, 2385
    in cardiopulmonary bypass, 2086
    for combined deficiency of factors V and
        VIII, 2140
    for disseminated intravascular coagulation,
        2214
    for hemophilia A, 2123

for inherited platelet disorders, 2062
    mechanism of action, 2317
    pharmacology, 2317–2318
    for von Willebrand disease, 2176
εγδβ-thalassemia, 735, 745, 751
εωδβ-thalassemia, 726
Epstein-Barr virus (EBV) infections
    aplastic anemia and, 518
    Burkitt lymphoma and, 1265, 1573, 1672,
        1674
    differential diagnosis, 1269, 1513
    epidemiology, 1261–1262
    future therapeutic approaches, 1266
    Hodgkin lymphoma and, 1604, 1605
    infectious mononucleosis. *See* Epstein-Barr
        virus (EBV) mononucleosis
    lymphomas and, 1573, 1576, 1599
    neoplastic potential, 1265–1266, 1266*t*
    posttransplant lymphoproliferative
        disorders and, 1636
    primary CNS lymphoma and, 1246
    T-cell–receptor signaling defects and, 1220
    T-cell therapy, **411–412**
    in X-linked lymphoproliferative disease,
        1228–1229, 1266
Epstein-Barr virus (EBV) mononucleosis
    clinical manifestations, 1262–1263, 1263*t*
    complications, 1263*t*, 1265
    course and prognosis, 1265
    epidemiology, 1263
    laboratory features, 1264–1265, 1264*f*,
        1267*t*
    secondary leukocytosis in, 1202
    treatment, 1269
    virology and pathogenesis, 1262
Eptifibatide, **405**
    for acute coronary syndrome, 2077
    clinical uses, 404*t*, 405
    dosage, 404*t*
    mechanism of action, 405, 2045, 2077
    for sickle cell disease, 777*t*
    thrombocytopenia and, 2015, 2077
EPX (eosinophil-derived neurotoxin), 931,
        953
EPZ-5676, 1403
Equilateral branching, 2153
Er antigens, 2333*t*
Erdheim-Chester disease, 1101, 1102*t*,
        1110–1111
ERGIC (endoplasmic reticulum-Golgi
        intermediate compartment
        protein)-53, 1171
ERK (extracellular signal-regulated kinase),
        298, 1103
ERK1, 1529
Erlenmeyer flask deformity, 1124, 1125*f*

Error catastrophe theory, 130
Ertapenem, 384, 387*t*
Erwinia chrysanthemi, 332
Erwinia chrysanthemi-derived asparaginase,
        1515
Erythema multiforme (EM), 2106, 2106*f*
Erythremic myelosis, 1390
Erythroblastic islands (EBIs), 64, **462–463**,
        462*f*
Erythroblasts
    basophilic, 463*f*, 464, 464*f*
    differentiation, 64
    enucleation, 481–482
    iron in, 623–624
    marrow, 32*t*, 34
    maturation, 465–467, 466*f*, 467*f*
    normal, 465
    numbers, 481, 482*t*
    orthochromic, 463*f*, 465, 465*f*
    pathologic, 465, 466*f*
    polychromatophilic, 463*f*, 464–465, 465*f*
    precursors, 463–465, 463*f*, 464*f*
    primitive, 100, 100*f*
    proerythroblasts, 463–464, 463*f*, 464*f*
    progenitors, 64, 463
    release, 72
    reticulocytes. *See* Reticulocytes
Erythrocytapheresis
    adverse effects, 433
    for hereditary hemochromatosis, 432
    indications for, 429*t*, 430*t*
    for polycythemia vera, 432
    principles, 432
Erythrocyte antibodies, **2343–2350**,
        2344–2346*t*
    in autoimmune hemolytic anemia. *See*
        Autoimmune hemolytic anemia
    fetal production, 2347
    in hemolytic disease of the fetus and
        newborn, 2348. *See also* Hemolytic
        disease of the fetus and newborn
    immunoglobulin A, 2347
    immunoglobulin G, 2343
    immunoglobulin M, 2343, 2347
    immunology, 2343
    naturally occurring, 2347
    in response to immunization, 2347–2348
    serologic detection, 2350
    in transfusion reactions, 2348. *See also*
        Transfusion reactions
Erythrocyte antigens, **2327–2350**. *See also*
        Blood group systems
    antibodies to. *See* Erythrocyte antibodies
    biochemistry, 2337, 2338*f*
    carbohydrate, 2337
    collections, 2333*t*

Erythrocyte antigens (*Cont.*):
 diseases associated with, 2340, 2341–2342t, 2342–2343
 enzymes/chemicals affecting, 2339
 expression, 104, 2336–2337, 2340
 genetics, 2339
 immunogenicity, 2336
 protein, 2337
 serologic detection, 2348–2350, 2349t, 2350t
Erythrocyte binding-like antigen, 815
Erythrocyte enzyme disorders, **689–712**.
  See also specific enzymes
 clinical features, **708–710**, 876
 course and prognosis, **712**
 definition and history, **689–690**
 differential diagnosis, **711**
 epidemiology, **690**, 690f
 etiology and pathogenesis, **691–699**, 876
 genetics, **699–708**
 laboratory features, **710–711**
 therapy, **711–712**
Erythrocyte membrane, **661–669**, 662f
 altered surface properties, 499
 damage to, 809
 deformability, 668
 ion transport and exchange channels, 668, 669f
 lipids, 662
 in newborn, 104–105
 organization, **667–668**
 permeability, 669, 669f
 proteins. *See* Membrane proteins
 stability, 668
Erythrocyte membrane disorders, 21f
 acanthocytosis, **680–681**
 cryohydrocytosis, 682t, **684**
 familial deficiency of high-density lipoproteins, **684**
 hereditary elliptocytosis. *See* Hereditary elliptocytosis (HE)
 hereditary pyropoikilocytosis. *See* Hereditary pyropoikilocytosis (HPP)
 hereditary spherocytosis. *See* Hereditary spherocytosis (HS)
 laboratory features, 670f, 671f
 neuroacanthocytosis. *See* Neuroacanthocytosis
 protein defects, 670t
 Rh-deficiency syndrome, **684**
 Southeast Asian ovalocytosis, **680**
 stomatocytosis. *See* Stomatocytosis
Erythrocytes
 aged, 134, 471, 473, **497–498**
 antibodies. *See* Erythrocyte antibodies
 antigens. *See* Erythrocyte antigens

automated analysis, 13–16
collection by apheresis, 2368
composition, 469
 carbohydrates, organic acids, and metabolites, 471t
 coenzyme and vitamins, 470t
 electrolytes, 471t
 nucleotides, 470t
 phospholipids, 469t
 protein and water content, 469t
concentration of, in clonal hematopoietic disorders, 1284–1285
deformability, 469–471, 499
destroyed, fate of, **499–500**, 500f
destruction/turnover, **495–500**. *See also* Hemolysis
 in anemia of inflammation, 550
 in situ localization of, **496–498**, 497f
 measurement of, **495–496**, 496f
 mechanisms of, **498–499**, 619
 senescence and, 497–498
disorders
 anemia. *See* Anemia
 from chemical or physical agents, **809–811**
 enzyme. *See* Erythrocyte enzyme disorders
 fragmentation. *See* Hemolytic anemia, fragmentation
 membrane. *See* Erythrocyte membrane disorders
 paroxysmal nocturnal hemoglobinuria. *See* Paroxysmal nocturnal hemoglobinuria (PNH)
 polycythemia (erythrocytosis). *See* Polycythemia
fetal, antigen development on, 2337–2338
hemoglobin and, **479–480**
inclusions, 467–468, 468f
iron deficiency and, 633, 633f, 634f
life span, 495
marrow, 34
mass measurement, **488–489**, 882, 1295
membrane. *See* Erythrocyte membrane
metabolism, **691–699**
 antioxidant enzymes, 698–699
 glucose
  enzymes, 692t, 694–697
  pathways, 692–694, 693f
 glutathione, 698
 nucleotide, 699
morphology, 21, **21**
 in marrow infiltration, 658, 659f
 pathophysiology of, 472–473t, 473, 475
 structure and shape, 468–469, 468f
neonatal, **102–105**, 103t

functions of, 104–105
 life span, 104
 nucleated, 47–48
 organelle removal in, 478
 pocked (pitted), 468
 in polycythemia vera, 1295
 precursor cell kinetics, 75t
 precursors, 463–465, 463f, 464f, 465f
 production. *See* Erythropoiesis
 progenitors, 463
 splenic clearance/sequestration, 90–91
 viscosity, 668
Erythrocyte zinc protoporphyrin, 635
Erythrocytosis. *See* Polycythemia (erythrocytosis)
Erythroderma, history of, 6
Erythroid cells
 heme synthesis in, 895–896
 marrow, 34
Erythroid colony cultures
 in polycythemia diagnosis, 882
 in polycythemia vera, 1296
Erythroid Kruppel-like factor (EKLF), 484
Erythroid/megakaryopoietic progenitors, 271
Erythroid progenitors, **271**, **463**
Erythroleukemia, 1390
Erythromelalgia, 1293, 1294f, 1308, 2080
Erythron, 461. *See also* Erythrocytes
Erythrophagocytosis, 619, 1050f
Erythropoiesis, 508f
 androgens and, 560
 anemia and, 505–506
 in anemia of inflammation, 551–552
 effective, **489–490**
 embryonic and fetal, 480
 erythroblast enucleation in, 481–482
 ferrokinetics, **490–491**, 490f, 491t
 hepcidin regulation by, 622
 history of, 479
 ineffective, **490**
  as cause of iron overload, 641
 lead and, 811
 measurements, **489–491**
 megaloblastic anemia and, 597
 microRNAs in, 487–488
 neonatal, **102–105**
 phylogeny, 479–480
 precursor cells in, **481**, 482f, 482t, 483f
 progenitor cells in, 32.**2–3**, 480f
 regulation, **482–487**, 504f
  deterministic model of lineage commitment, 483, 483f
  erythropoietin in, 484
  erythropoietin receptor in, 484–485, 486f
  hypoxia-inducible factors in, 486–487, 486f

insulin-like growth factor in, 487
molecular mechanisms in, 484, 485f
stochastic model of erythroid
differentiation, 483–484
total, **490**
Erythropoiesis-stimulating agents (ESAs)
for alloimmune hemolytic disease of the
fetus and newborn, 858
for anemia in HIV infection, 1252
for anemia of chronic kidney disease, 554t,
555
for anemia of inflammation, 554, 554t
for anemia of primary myelofibrosis, 1328
cardiovascular mortality and, 2036–2037
for hypersplenism, 867
for myelodysplastic syndromes, 1357–1358
self-administration, 872
Erythropoietic porphyrias. See Porphyrias
Erythropoietic protoporphyria (EPP)
clinical features, 890t, 898–899, 898t
definition and history, 897
diagnosis, 899
enzymes affected by, 890t, 891f
laboratory features, 891t
pathogenesis of clinical findings, 898
pathophysiology, 897–898
therapy, 899–900
Erythropoietin (EPO), 264t
activation of JAK, 252
anemia and, 505–506
anemia and increases in, 505f
for anemia of primary myelofibrosis, 1328
in erythropoiesis, **484**
history of, 479
inappropriate tissue elaboration of, 872
levels
congenital polycythemias and, 878
in HIV infection, 1251
in iron-deficiency anemia, 2036
in older persons, 134
in polycythemia, 882–883
in polycythemia vera, 1296
in pregnancy, 119
nonerythroid effects, 486
physiologic anemia of newborn and, 103
resistance to and deficiency of, 550–551
response to anemia, 247
restriction of, as result of iron
unavailability, 551–552, 551f
therapeutic. See Erythropoiesis-stimulating
agents (ESAs)
thrombopoietin and, 265
Erythropoietin receptor (EPOR). See also
EPOR
in erythropoiesis, 481, **484–485**, 486f
structure and function, **247–248**

Escherichia coli-derived asparaginase,
332–333, 1515
Escherichia coli infections. See also Bacterial
infections
in chronic granulomatous disease, 1030
disseminated intravascular coagulation
and, 2207
hemolytic anemia and, 819
hemolytic uremic syndrome and, 2258–2259
in immunocompromised host, 383
neutropenia and, 985
neutrophil abnormalities and, 986
in newborn, 106
red cell antigens and resistance to, 2340
ESCs (embryonic stem cells), 448–449, 450
E-selectin (CD62E)
activities, 66, 68
counterreceptor, 282t
distribution, 67t, 282t
expression, 281, 1870
hematopoietic stem cell trafficking and,
355
in inflammatory response, 1977t, 1978
ligands, 67t
natural killer cells and, 1193
neutrophils and, 1006, 1007f
ESHAP regimen
for diffuse large B-cell lymphoma, 1629t,
1631
for HIV-associated lymphoma, 1245
E-SLAM approach, 260
Essential monoclonal gammopathy, **1721–1727**
classification, 1722t
clinical features, **1723–1725**
blood cells and marrow, 1723
coinciding disorders, 1724–1725, 1725t
cytogenetic analysis, 1723
functional impairment from
monoclonal protein, 1723–1724,
1723t
monoclonal protein, 1723
neuropathies, 1724
consultative approach to, 48–49
course and prognosis, 1726–1727
definition and history, 1721
differential diagnosis, 1726t
epidemiology, 1721–1722
etiology and pathogenesis, 1497t, 1708,
1722–1723, 1736t
in Gaucher disease, 1126
hyperviscosity in, 428
laboratory features, 1497t, **1725–1726**
myeloma and, 1722, 1734, 1734f
platelet dysfunction in, 2082
therapy, 429t, 1727
Essential thrombocythemia (ET), **1307–1315**

clinical features, 1286, **1308–1310**,
2079–2080
complications, 1315t
course and prognosis, 1278t, **1315**
definition and history, 1307
diagnostic criteria, 1311t
differential diagnosis, **1310–1313**, 1311f
blastic phase disease, 1313
chronic myelogenous leukemia,
1311–1312, 1449–1450
familial thrombocytosis, 1310, 1312t
myelodysplasia, 1312
myelofibrosis and accelerated phase
disease, 1312–1313
polycythemia vera, 1311, 1312, 1312f,
1313f
primary myelofibrosis, 1311
epidemiology, 1307
etiology, 1307, 2079–2080
gene mutations, 228–229t, 1278, 1308f,
1310, 1851
laboratory features, 1309f, **1310**
leukemic transformation in, 1280–1281,
1310
myelofibrotic transformation in, 1309
pathogenesis, 1278, 1307–1308, 1308f
platelet abnormalities in, 2080
in pregnancy, **124–125**, 1314–1315, 2081
surgery and, 1315
therapy, 341–342, **1313–1315**, 1313t,
1314t, 2081
Essential thrombocytopenia, 1999. See also
Immune thrombocytopenia (ITP)
Estren-Dameshek syndrome, 529
Estrogens
acute intermittent porphyria and, 901, 902t
erythropoietic effects, 560
porphyria cutanea tarda and, 906
for von Willebrand disease, 2176
ET. See Essential thrombocythemia (ET)
Etanercept
for diffuse alveolar hemorrhage, 368
for myelodysplastic syndromes, 1359
for primary myelofibrosis, 1329
secondary acute myelogenous leukemia
and, 1407
ETC (electron transport chain), 196
Ethambutol, for tuberculosis, 386
Ethanol abuse. See Alcohol abuse
Ethylenediaminetetraacetic acid (EDTA),
1994, 1995, 2339
ETO, 225, 237
Etoposide, **328–329**. See also BEACOPP
regimen; CODOX-M/IVAC
regimen; EPOCH regimen; ESHAP
regimen; Stanford V regimen

Etoposide (*Cont.*):
  for acute lymphoblastic leukemia, 1515
  for acute myelogenous leukemia, 1402*t*
    in children, 1409
    in older patients, 1408
  adverse effects, 329, 1519*t*, 1520, 1534
  for α-heavy-chain disease, 1808
  for Burkitt lymphoma, 1676
  for chronic lymphocytic leukemia, 1534
  for diffuse large B-cell lymphoma, 1628,
    1629*t*, 1630, 1631
  for enteropathy-associated T-cell
    lymphoma, 1700
  for familial hemophagocytic
    lymphohistiocytosis, 1228
  for hemophagocytic lymphohistiocytosis,
    1115
  high-dose, 331*t*, 332*t*
  for Hodgkin lymphoma, 1616
  for myelodysplastic syndromes, 1362
  for peripheral T-cell lymphoma, 1695–
    1696, 1697
  resistance to, 319*t*
  secondary acute myelogenous leukemia
    and, 183, 1407
ETV6 (TEL), 228*t*, 230, 1346*t*, 1351
ETV6-RUNX1, in acute lymphoblastic
    leukemia
  acquired, 1507
  detection, 1512
  Down syndrome and, 1507
  features associated with, 1512, 1513*t*
  frequency, 1508*t*
  immunologic classification and, 1512
  prognosis and, 183, 1513*t*, 1518, 1520–
    1521, 1521*t*
  treatment response and, 1516
  in utero development, 1508
Evans syndrome
  course and prognosis, 840
  laboratory features, 43, 832, 1804, 2002
Evelyn-Malloy method, 792
Everolimus
  adverse effects, 1796
  for mantle cell lymphoma, 1660*t*
  for Waldenström macroglobulinemia,
    1795–1796
Exchange transfusion
  for alloimmune hemolytic disease of the
    fetus and newborn, 856–857
  for sickle cell disease, 776
Excoriation, 8
Exercise-induced purpura, 2107
Exercise tolerance, iron deficiency and, 631
Exfoliative dermatitis, 598
Exons, 147

Exosomes, platelet, 1848
Expressivity, 149
Extracellular matrix
    marrow, **61–64**, 62*t*
    vascular growth and, 2283–2284, 2284*f*
Extracellular matrix glycoproteins, 266
Extracellular matrix proteins (ECMs), 61–62
Extracellular signal-regulated kinase (ERK),
    298, 1103
Extracorporeal photochemotherapy/
    photopheresis, 429*t*, 433, 1687
Extramedullary blast crisis, 1465
Extramedullary disease, in myeloma, 1746
Extramedullary hematopoiesis, 1323, 1324
Extramedullary marrow crisis, 1465–1466
Extramedullary tumors, 1285, 1324
Extranodal histiocytic sarcoma, 1110
Extranodal lymphoma, 1502. *See also*
    Primary extranodal lymphoma
Extranodal marginal zone lymphoma of
    MALT type, **1663–1666**
  chromosomal abnormalities
    gains, 1664*t*
    losses, 1664*t*
    t(11;18), 184*t*, 224*t*, 1664, 1664*t*
    translocations, 184*t*, 187–188, 210, 224*t*,
      1495*t*, 1577, 1664, 1664*t*
    trisomy 3, 187–188
  clinical features, 1664–1665
  course and prognosis, 1666
  definition, 1663
  differential diagnosis, 1665
  epidemiology, 1663
  etiology and pathogenesis, 1574, 1663–
    1664
  gastric, 1581, 1664–1666, 1666*f*, 1666*t*
  laboratory features, 1495*t*, 1595, 1595*f*,
    1665, 1665*f*
  staging, 1665
  therapy, 1665–1666
Extranodal natural killer (NK)/T-cell
    lymphoma, nasal type, 1498*t*,
    1500*t*, 1573, **1701–1702**
Extraosseous plasmacytoma, 1497*t*
Extremities, 6, 9
Extrinsic pathway inhibitor. *See* Tissue factor
    pathway inhibitor (TFPI)
Exudates, eye, 8
Eye disorders. *See* Ocular disorders
Eye examination, 8
EZH2
  in chronic myelomonocytic leukemia,
    1468
  in diffuse large B-cell lymphoma, 234*t*,
    1626, 1627*t*
  in follicular lymphoma, 235*t*

    gain of function mutations, 170
    in mantle cell lymphoma, 170
    in myelodysplastic syndromes, 228*t*, 1346*t*,
      1347, 1351
    in Ph-chromosome negative
      myeloproliferative neoplasms, 229*t*
EZH2 (enhancer of zest homologue 2), 170
EZH2 (enhancer of zest homologue 2)
    inhibitors, 337–338
Ezrin, 1006

F

F1P1L1-PDGFR-α, 1279
F2, 1920, 1920*f*, 2135*t*
F4/80 (EMR1), 1079–1080, 1081*f*, 1082
F5, 1925, 1925*f*, 2135*t*, 2138
F7, 1920, 1921*f*, 2135*t*, 2140
F8 (FVIII), 1926, 1926*f*, 2114
F8A, 2114
F8B, 2114
F9, 1921, 1921*f*
F10, 1922, 1922*f*, 2135*t*, 2141–2142
F11, 1929, 1929*f*, 2135*t*, 2143
F13A, 2135*t*, 2144
F13A1, 1935, 1935*f*, 2144
F13B, 2135*t*, 2144
FA/BRCA pathway, in Fanconi anemia, 527,
    529*f*
F-actin, 481
Factitious anemia, 630
Factitious purpura, 2107
Factor II. *See* Prothrombin (factor II)
Factor V
  activated protein C and, 1954, 1955–1956
  activation, 1924–1925, 1949, 1950
  antibodies, 2186
  characteristics, 1916*t*, 1924, 2137
  gene structure and variations, 1925, 1925*f*,
    2138
  in platelets, 1845, 1856, 1924, 2137
  structure, 1924, 1924*f*, 2137–2138
Factor V deficiency (parahemophilia),
    2137–2139
  clinical features, 2137
  definition and history, 2137
  gene mutations, 1925, 2135*t*, 2137
  incidence, 2134*t*
  therapy, 2136*t*, 2138
Factor(s) V and VIII deficiency, 2134*t*, 2135*t*,
    2136*t*, **2139–2140**
Factor V1, 1955
Factor V2, 1955
Factor Va
  activated protein C and, 1924–1925, 1955
  platelet microparticles and, 1854
  protein S and, 1949

prothrombin activation and, 1854
structure, 1924
variability in cleavage, 1924, 1955–1956
Factor V Leiden/factor V G1691A
activated protein C resistance and, 1955, 2222
arterial thromboembolic disease risk and, 2226–2227
clinical features, 2138
clinical implications of testing for, 2227–2228, 2228t
fetal loss and, 122
pathophysiology, 2223, 2223f
prevalence, 2138, 2222t, 2223
venous thromboembolism risk and, 2222, 2225, 2225t, 2226t, 2268
Factor VII, **1920–1921**
activation, 1920, 2140
characteristics, 1916t, 2140
gene structure and variations, 1920–1921, 1921f
structure, 1917f, 1920, 2140
Factor VII deficiency, **2140–2141**
clinical features, 2141
definition and history, 2140
diagnosis, 1988, 1989f
gene mutations, 2135t, 2140–2141
incidence, 1920–1921, 2133, 2134t
therapy, 2136t, 2141
Factor VIIa
cofactor and substrates, 1918t
in control of coagulation, 1950, 1959f, 1960
functions, 1920, 1930
structure, 1920, 1920f
in thrombin generation, 1940, 1940f
Factor VIIa replacement
in cardiac surgery, 2086
for factor VII deficiency, 2141
for hemophilia A, 2125, 2125t, 2185
Factor VII-activating protease, 2283
Factor VIII
activated protein C and, 1955
activation, 1926
antibodies, 2183–2184
characteristics, 1916t, 1925
defined, 2164t
functions, 2183–2184
gene structure and variations, 1926, 1926f
in hepatic disease, 2192
interaction with von Willebrand factor, 2168
platelet microparticles and, 1854
structure, 1925–1926
synthesis, 1925, 1925f
terminology, 2164t
thrombin and, 1949

von Willebrand disease and, 2163, 2172
Factor VIII, increased levels
acquired causes, 2224t
epidemiology, 2222t, 2224
etiology and pathogenesis, 1926
history, 2222
myocardial infarction risk and, 2226–2227
pathophysiology, 2224
venous thromboembolism risk and, 2224, 2225–2226, 2225t, 2226t
von Willebrand factor and, 2224
Factor VIII deficiency
acquired, 2145, **2183–2186**
combined with factor V deficiency, 2134t, 2135t, 2136t, **2139–2140**
diagnosis, 1988, 1989f
inherited. See Hemophilia A (classic hemophilia, factor VIII deficiency)
Factor VIII inhibitor antibodies, **2124–2126**
diagnosis, 2124–2125
molecular pathology, 2184
prevalence, 2124
risk factors, 2124, 2124t
treatment, 2125–2126, 2125t, 2126t, 2185
Factor VIII replacement
for acquired hemophilia A, 2185
for anti-factor VIII inhibitor antibodies, 2125–2126, 2125t
disease transmission risk with, 2126
for factor VIII deficiency, 2136t, 2145
for hemophilia A, 2121–2122, 2121t, 2122t
for inherited platelet disorders, 2062
Factor VIIIa
activation, 1854
functions, 1926
in hemophilia, 2114
protein S and, 1949
structure, 1926
as substrate for activated protein C, 1955
variability in cleavage, 1955–1956
Factor IX, **1921–1922**
activation, 1921
characteristics, 1916t, 1921
gene structure and variations, 1921–1922, 1921f
increased levels, 1922
structure, 1917f, 1921
Factor IX deficiency. See Hemophilia B
Factor IX replacement, 2128–2129, 2128t
Factor IX inhibitor antibodies, 2129
Factor IXa
characteristics, 1918t, 1921
factor VIII and, 2184
generation, 1921
in hemophilia, 2114

platelet microparticles and, 1854
prothrombin activation and, 1854
Factor X, **1922–1923**
activation, 1854, 1922, 2141
characteristics, 1916t, 1922
gene structure and variations, 1922–1923, 1922f, 2141–2142
structure, 1854, 1917f, 1922, 2141
Factor X deficiency, **2141–2142**
acquired, 2145
clinical features, 2142
definition and history, 2141
diagnosis, 1988, 1989f
gene mutations, 1922, 2135t, 2141–2142
incidence, 1922, 2134t
therapy, 2136t, 2142
Factor Xa
activity, 1922
characteristics, 1918t
indirect inhibitors. See Danaparoid; Fondaparinux
in inflammation, 2201
inhibitors, 1922, 1959f, 1960
protein S and, 1949
structure, 1922
thrombin and, 1854, 1940, 1940f
Factor XI, **1928–1929**
acquired antibodies to, 2187
activation, 1929, 1949, 2142–2143
characteristics, 1916t, 2142–2143
gene structure and variations, 1928f, 1929
structure, 1927f, 1928–1929, 2142
Factor XI deficiency, **2142–2143**
clinical features, 2142
definition and history, 2142
diagnosis, 1988, 1989f
differential diagnosis, 2121
epidemiology, 1929
gene mutations, 1929, 2135t, 2143
incidence, 2133, 2134t
therapy, 2143
Factor XII, **1929–1930**
in acute hemolytic transfusion reactions, 2374
characteristics, 1916t
kinin system and, 289
structure, 1927f, 1929
Factor XII deficiency, 1988, 2121
Factor XIII
acquired inhibitors to, 2187
activation, 1934–1935, 1934f, 2144
characteristics, 1916t, 1933–1934, 2144
crosslinking by, 2153
gene structure and variations, 1935, 1935f, 2144
in platelets, 1848

Factor XIII (*Cont.*):
  structure, 1934, 2144
  synthesis, 2144
Factor XIIIa, 2153
Factor XIII deficiency, **2143–2145**
  clinical features, 2144–2145
  definition and history, 2144
  gene mutations, 1935, 2135*t*, 2144
  incidence, 2133, 2134*t*
  therapy, 2136*t*, 2145
Factor H, 2260
FADD (fas-associated death domain), 204*f*,
      205, 249, 302, 302*f*
Faggot cells, 1390
FAK (focal adhesion kinase), 266, 1841
FAM46C, 233*t*, 1736, 1736*t*, 1737, 1759
Famciclovir, 386, 387*t*
Familial deficiency of high-density
      lipoproteins, **684**
Familial hemophagocytic
      lymphohistiocytosis (FHL), **1228**,
      1849, 2061
Familial Mediterranean fever, **1024–1026**
Familial neutropenia, 994
Familial platelet disorder with predisposition
      to acute myelogenous leukemia,
      2060
Familial thrombocytosis, 1310
Family history, 7
FANC, 1346*t*
Fanconi anemia, **527–530**
  clinical features, 529
  clonal myeloid disorders and, 1345
  definition and history, 527
  differential diagnosis, 529
  epidemiology, 527
  etiology and pathogenesis, 527–528, 528*f*,
      529*f*
  gene mutations, 527–528, 528*t*
  gene therapy, 442
  laboratory features, 529
  therapy and course, 529–530
Fanconi genes, 442, 527, 528*f*, 528*t*
FAO (fatty acid oxidation), 198, 200
Farnesyltransferase inhibitors, for acute
      myelogenous leukemia, 1403
Fas (CD95), 210, 1224, 1564, 1873
Fas-associated death domain (FADD), 204*f*,
      205, 249, 302, 302*f*
Fasciitis, eosinophilic, 960
Fascioliasis, 957*t*
FAS-dependent pathway, in aplastic anemia,
      515
Fas/Fas ligand system, 210, 1873
FAT (fatty acyl translocase). *See* Glycoprotein
      (GP)IV

FAT3, 1737
Fat aspiration, subcutaneous, 1776, 1776*f*
Fatigue, history of, 4
Fatty acid oxidation (FAO), 198, 200
Fatty acyl translocase (FAT). *See*
      Glycoprotein (GP)IV
Fatty marrow, 28
Fatty streak, 2286
Favism, 707, 709
FBXW7, 231*t*, 1521
FcαR, 1161
Fcγ receptor I (FCγR1, CD64), 948, 1053,
      1095, 1383
Fcγ receptor IIA (FcγRIIA, CD32)
  in acute myelomonocytic leukemia, 1380*t*
  in heparin-induced thrombocytopenia,
      2027, 2027*f*
  in monocytes/macrophages, 1053
  in neutrophils, 1008, 1015–1016
  in phospholipid metabolism, 1016
  in platelets, 1856, 1869–1870
Fcγ receptor III (FcγRIII, CD16)
  CD14 and, 1056
  in monocytes, 1052
    in eosinophils, 949, 949*t*, 953
    expression, 1053
    in monocytes, 1095
    in natural killer cells, 1142, 1190
    in neutrophils, 1008, 1015–1016
    rituximab response and, 1794
    structure, 1053, 1053*f*
Fcγ receptors, 308, 953, 1009, 1063*f*, 2000
FcγRII (CDw32), 953
F cells, 730
Fcε receptor I (FcεRi), 968, 969, 1870
FcγRIIIb, 2357
FCGR1A, 1643
FCGR3A, 2357
FCGR3B, 2357
Fc receptors, 284, 1008, 1015–1016, 1053*f*,
      1058*t*
Fc receptor γ (FcRγ)-chain, 1869, 1879–1880,
      1880*f*
FcRI, in newborns, 107
FDG-PET
  in diffuse large B-cell lymphoma staging,
      1633
  in Hodgkin lymphoma staging, 1608,
      1608*f*, 1611, 1613, 1617
  in myeloma staging, 1715, 1749–1750,
      1750*f*
Febrile nonhemolytic transfusion reaction
      (FNHTR), 2375
FECH, 897–898
FECH (ferrochelatase, heme synthetase),
      893*f*, 895, 917

Felty syndrome, 996, 1203, 1565
FERMTS3, 2060
Ferric iron, 619
Ferritin, **617–618**
  in anemia of inflammation, 552, 553*f*, 553*t*
  in hemophagocytic lymphohistiocytosis,
      1115
  in iron deficiency, 552, 553*f*, 553*t*, 634–635
  in iron homeostasis, 623, 624*f*
  mitochondrial, 624, 919
Ferritin H chain, 621*t*
Ferrochelatase (FECH, heme synthetase),
      893*f*, 895, 917
Ferrokinetics, **490–491**, 490*f*, 491*t*
Ferroportin (SLC40A1, SLC11A3), 620, 621*t*,
      642
Ferroprotoporphyrin IX. *See* Heme
Ferruginous micelles, 466*f*, 468
Fetal blood, **102**
Fetal DNA, circulating cell-free, 852
Fetal erythrocytes, 2336–2337
Fetal hemoglobin. *See* Hemoglobin F
Fetal loss, 122–123
Fetus
  alloimmune hemolytic disease of. *See*
      Alloimmune hemolytic disease of
      the fetus and newborn (HDFN)
  blood sampling, 854
  erythropoiesis in, 480
  hematolymphopoiesis in, **99–102**, 100*f*,
      101*t*, 102*f*
  immunoglobulin in, 2347
  intrauterine transfusion, 854–855
Fever
  following recovery from chemotherapy,
      386, 388
  history of, 3–4
FGA, 2151, 2154–2155, 2156, 2158, 2159
FGB, 2151, 2156, 2158
FGFR1, 958, 1279
FGFR3, 233*t*, 1735, 1736
FGG, 2151, 2155, 2158, 2159
FGL2 (fibrinogen-like protein 2), 1182
FH (fumarate hydratase), 193
FH$_2$ (dihydrofolate), 584
FH$_2$ (dihydrofolate) reductase, 584
FH$_4$ (tetrahydrofolate acid), 584, 586*f*
FHL (familial hemophagocytic
      lymphohistiocytosis), **1228**, 1849,
      2061
Fibrin
  antithrombin activity, 2154
  degradation, 2303, 2310, 2310*f*. *See also*
      Fibrinolysis
  in disseminated intravascular coagulation,
      2201

fibrinogen conversion to, 2152–2153, 2154f
formation, 2200
functions, 1933
in inflammation, 2201
polymerization, 1933, 1933f
Fibrin degradation products, 2205–2206, 2205t
Fibrin glue/sealant
  for hemophilia A, 2123
  for inherited platelet disorders, 2062
  for superficial bleeds in fibrinogen abnormalities, 2159
  for superficial wounds/dental extractions, 2157
Fibrinogen
  activation, 1933, 1933f
  characteristics, 1916t, 1932
  conversion to fibrin and network assembly, 2152–2153, 2153f
  crosslinking by factor XIII, 2153
  degradation, 2309–2310, 2310f
  in disseminated intravascular coagulation, 2201
  in fibrinolysis, 2154
  functions, 1933, 1979t
  gene structure and variations, 1933, 1934f, 2151, 2154–2155
  hereditary abnormalities
    afibrinogenemia/hypofibrinogenemia. See Afibrinogenemia/ hypofibrinogenemia
    dysfibrinogenemia/ hypodysfibrinogenemia. See Dysfibrinogenemia/ hypodysfibrinogenemia
  integrin $\alpha_{IIb}\beta_3$ and, 1854
  interactions, 1846t
  in platelets, 1845
  structure, 1846t, 1932, 1933f, 2151, 2152f
  synthesis, 2152
Fibrinogen concentrates, 2136t, 2156–2157
Fibrinogen-like protein 2 (FGL2), 1182
Fibrinogen receptor. See Integrin $\alpha_{IIb}\beta_3$
Fibrinolysins, 2307
Fibrinolysis
  angiogenesis and, 2311
  in antiphospholipid syndrome, 2237
  basic concepts, 2303, 2304f
  cellular receptors, 2308–2309
  in coagulation, 1942
  deficiency, thrombosis and, 2310–2311
  developmental regulation, 2312
  in disseminated intravascular coagulation, 2202–2203
  enhanced, 2312
  in hepatic disease, 2192

inhibitors, 2307–2308. See also Antifibrinolytic therapy
  plasminogen activator inhibitors. See Plasminogen activator inhibitor (PAI)-1
  serpins, 1145, 1958, 2304t, 2307–2308
  thrombin-activatable fibrinolysis inhibitor. See Thrombin-activatable fibrinolysis inhibitor (TAFI)
  phases, 2154
  plasmin in. See Plasmin
  plasminogen activators in. See Plasminogen activators
  plasminogen in, 2303, 2303, 2304–2305t, 2304f, 2304t
  in pregnancy, 2312
  vascular, 1972–1976
    endothelial cells in, 1973–1974, 1973f
    in vascular disease, 1975–1976, 1975f
    in vascular injury, 1974–1975, 1974t
Fibrinolytic activators, 1285
Fibrinolytic proteins, 1973–1974, 1973f, 2304–2305t
Fibrinolytic therapy, 393, 402–403, 2312–2317
  agents for
    alteplase. See Alteplase
    comparison, 2313t
    reteplase, 403, 2313t
    streptokinase. See Streptokinase
    tenecteplase. See Tenecteplase
    tissue-type plasminogen activator, 403, 2277
  bleeding complications, 2304t, 2317t
  for myocardial infarction, 2295
  patient selection, 2313t
  for peripheral vascular disease, 2316–2317
  platelet effects, 1855t, 2078
  principles of, 2313
  for stroke. See Stroke, fibrinolytic therapy for
  for venous thromboembolism, 2277–2278
Fibrinopeptide release, 2153, 2158
Fibrin tissue adhesive, for hemophilia A, 2123
Fibroblast-growth factor-4, 1817
Fibroblasts, 264
Fibronectin, 62–63
  in hematopoietic stem cells, 261, 266
  in inflammation, 283
  interactions, 1846t
  macrophages and, 1054
  in newborn, 106
  in platelets, 1845, 1865
  structure, 1846t
Fibronectin receptor. See Integrin $\alpha_5\beta_1$

Fibroplasia, 1322–1323, 1322t
Fibrosis, marrow, 32
Fibulins, 64
Ficolin-1, 1013t, 1014
Filamin, 1838–1839, 1838f, 1848
Filamin A, 1832t, 1837, 1838, 2059
Filamin B, 1832t, 1838
Filanesib, for myeloma, 1756
Filariasis, 957t
Filgrastim, for supportive therapy, 1243, 1247. See also Granulocyte colony-stimulating factor (G-CSF)
Fimbrin (L-plastin), 1833t
FIPILI-PDGFR-α (FIFPLI-PDGFRA), 977, 1469, 1470
FISH (fluorescence in situ hybridization), 175t, 176, 176f, 1711
Fish oils, 2079
Fish tapeworm, 601, 604
5q-minus syndrome, 1312, 1347, 1347f
FIX, 441–442
FKBP51, 1322
FKHD (forkhead transcription factors), 209
FL. See Flt3 ligand (FL)
FLAER (fluorescently labeled inactive variant of protein aerolysin), 37–38
FLAG-Ida regimen, for myelodysplastic syndromes, 1361
Flavopiridol
  for acute myelogenous leukemia, 218
  for chronic lymphocytic leukemia, 1539
FLCs (free light chains), 1708, 1714, 1741, 1742f, 1775, 1781. See also Immunoglobulin (Ig) light chains
FLI1, 2060, 2061
c-FLIP, 207
Flippases, 662, 742
FLIP proteins, 207
FLJ9586. See TSSC6
FLJ17158. See TSSC6
FLK-1, 258
Floppases, 662
Flow cytometry, 35–37, 36f, 1715, 1716
Floxuridine, megaloblastic anemia and, 606t
Flt1 (fms-like tyrosine kinase-1), 2011
FLT3, 1155
FLT3
  in acute myelogenous leukemia, 181, 181t, 198, 226t, 363, 1377, 1378t, 1383, 1415
  in acute promyelocytic leukemia, 1391
  in B-cell acute lymphoblastic leukemia, 232t
  detecting mutations in, 163, 1415
Flt3 (CD135), 309

FLT3 inhibitors, for acute myelogenous leukemia, 1403

Flt3 ligand (FL)
 hematopoiesis and, 258*f*, **265**
 in megakaryopoiesis, 1822

Fluconazole
 as empiric therapy for infections, 385, 387*t*
 prophylactic, 369, 389

Fludarabine phosphate (fludarabine), 322, **324**
 for acute myelogenous leukemia, 1396, 1402*t*
 adverse effects, 1534
 autoimmune hemolytic anemia and, 831
 for chronic lymphocytic leukemia, 1534, 1535, 1537
 for follicular lymphoma, 1645*t*, 1647
 for γ-heavy-chain disease, 1806
 before hematopoietic cell transplantation, 360
 for μ-heavy-chain disease, 1810
 for mycosis fungoides, 1687
 for pure red cell aplasia, 544
 resistance to, 319*t*
 structure, 323*f*
 for Waldenström macroglobulinemia, 1793, 1795

Fluorescence in situ hybridization (FISH), 175*t*, **176**, 176*f*, 1711

Fluorescent polymerase chain reaction (F-PCR), 1716

5-Fluorouracil
 megaloblastic anemia and, 606*t*
 resistance to, 319*t*

Fluoxetine, platelet effects, 2079

Fluoxymesterone, for anemia of primary myelofibrosis, 1328

Flushing, skin, 6

Fms-like tyrosine kinase-1 (Flt1), 2011

FN1, 1632

FND regimen, for follicular lymphoma, 1645*t*

FNHTR (febrile nonhemolytic transfusion reaction), 2375

Foam cells, 1129, 1129*f*

Focal adhesion kinase (FAK), 266, 1841

FOG (friend of GATA), 271, 483–484

Folate, **583–588**
 blood levels, 588, 652*t*
 chemistry, 584, 585*f*
 daily requirements, 584
 excretion, 588
 inborn errors of metabolism, **607–608**
 metabolism, **584–586**, 586*f*, 586*t*, 588
 in neutrophils, 935
 physiology, 586–587, 587*f*
 sources, 584

Folate-binding proteins, of serum and milk, 588

Folate deficiency, **597–599**
 clinical features, 598
 cobalamin deficiency and, 590–591, 590*f*
 colon cancer and, 599
 differential diagnosis, **598**
 etiology and pathogenesis, 583, **597–598**
 HELLP syndrome and, 599
 laboratory features, **598**
 neural tube defects and, 598
 nonhematologic effects, 598
 in pregnancy, 120, 597–598
 therapy, course, and prognosis, **599**
 thrombocytopenia and, 1997
 vascular disease and, 598–599

Folate-dependent enzymes, 584–585

Folate hydrolase (glutamate carboxypeptidase II), 586–587

Folate supplementation, 584
 for autoimmune hemolytic anemia, 839
 for paroxysmal nocturnal hemoglobinuria, 579
 in pregnancy, 120, 584
 for sideroblastic anemia, 920
 for thalassemias, 753

Folic acid (pteroylglutamic acid), 584, 585*f*, 935. *See also* Folate

Folic acid coenzymes, 584, 586*t*

Folinic acid, 584

Follicular dendritic cell tumors, 1110

Follicular hyperplasia, 1589*f*

Follicular lymphoma, **1641–1650**
 chromosomal abnormalities, 187, 224*t*, 1495*t*, 1576, 1642–1643, 1642*f*
 clinical features, 1641
 course and prognosis, 1649–1650, 1650*f*
 definition and history, 1641
 differential diagnosis, 1655, 1667, 1668
 epidemiology, 1571, 1573, 1641
 extranodal, 1579
 gene mutations, 170, 235–236*t*, 1495*t*, 1594, 1643–1644
 grades, 1594, 1594*f*, 1641, 1642*f*
 laboratory features, 1495*t*, 1576*f*, 1594–1595, 1594*f*, 1641–1643
 prognostic factors, 1643–1644, 1643*f*
 staging, 1643
 therapy
  of advanced stage disease, **1644–1648**
   combination chemotherapy, 1645*t*
   hematopoietic cell transplantation, 1648, 1648*f*
   idiotype vaccines, 1648
   interferon-α, 1647–1648
   maintenance rituximab, 1647

   monoclonal antibodies, 1645–1646
   observation alone, 1644
   radioimmunotherapy, 1647
   rituximab plus chemotherapy, 1645*t*, 1646–1647, 1646*f*, 1646*t*
   single agent chemotherapy, 1644, 1645*t*
  of limited stage I-II disease, 1644
  pragmatic approach to, 1649
  of transformed disease, 1648–1649
  vaccine, 423
 transformed, 1648–1649, 1649*f*

Follicular small-cleaved-cell lymphoma, 1594

Follicular small noncleaved cell lymphoma, 184*t*

Folylpolyglutamates, 585–586

Folylpoly-γ-glutamyl synthase (FPGS), 585–586

Fondaparinux, **398–399**
 for acute myocardial infarction, 2296
 clinical uses, 399
 for heparin-induced thrombocytopenia, 2030, 2031*t*
 mechanism of action, 398, 1922
 pharmacology, 398
 for venous thromboembolism, 2274, 2274*t*

Food/food additives, platelet function and, 2079

Forkhead box P3 (FOXP3), 1181, 1223

Forkhead transcription factors (FKHD), 209

Formaldehyde, 810

Formate starvation hypothesis, 590*f*, 591

Formyl peptide receptor, 1014–1015

FORS blood group, 2332*t*

Foscarnet, 386, 387*t*

Founder effects, 690

4T score, 2029, 2029*t*

FOXN1, 1223

FOXO-1, 894

FOXP3 (forkhead box P3), 1181, 1223

F-PCR (fluorescent polymerase chain reaction), 1716

FPGS (folylpoly-γ-glutamyl synthase), 585–586

Fractalkine, 62*t*, 69

Fragment X, of fibrinogen, 2310, 2310*f*

Frameshift mutations, 146

Francisella tularensis, 1064*f*

Free light chains (FLCs), 1708, 1714, 1741, 1742*f*, 1775, 1781. *See also* Immunoglobulin (Ig) light chains

Free radical hypothesis of aging, 130*t*, 131

Fresh-frozen plasma
 for afibrinogenemia, 2156
 for congenital thrombotic thrombocytopenic purpura, 2258

for disseminated intravascular coagulation, 2213
Friend of GATA (FOG), 271, 483–484
Frizzled related protein-2 (FRP-2), 1738, 1739*f*
Fructose-1,6-biphosphate, 192
Fructose-1,6-diphosphate, 694, 695
Fructose-6-diphosphate, 696, 696*f*
Fructose-6-phosphate, 192, 694
Fumarate hydratase (FH), 193
Functional decline, coagulation and, 135
Fungal infections
    in chronic lymphocytic leukemia, 1541
    empiric therapy, 385–388, 387–388*t*
    after hematopoietic cell transplantation, 369
    in immunocompromised host, **383**
    pattern-recognition signaling pathways with increased susceptibility to, 1230
    prevention, 389
    purpura and, 2104–2105, 2105*f*
Furosemide
    for acute hemolytic transfusion reactions, 2375
    vasculitis induced by, 2106, 2106*f*
Fusion proteins, 169–170, 1016–1017
FUT, 2337
FVIII, 442
Fy(a-b-) phenotype, 2339

G
G_1/S checkpoint, 219
G_2/M checkpoint, 219
G6PC3, 993
G6PD. *See under* Glucose-6-phosphate dehydrogenase
G20210A, 1920
GAGs (glycosaminoglycans), 69, 2027*f*, 2028
Gaisböck syndrome, 872
Galactokinase, 692*t*, 701*t*
Galactose-1-P-uridyltransferase, 701*t*
Galactose-4-epimerase, 692*t*
Galectin-1, 1182
Gallbladder disease
    in hereditary spherocytosis, 674
    primary lymphomas, 1581
    in sickle cell disease, 772
Gαi, 1875
Gαi₁ deficiency, 2057
Gαq deficiency, 2057
Gαs, genetic variation in extra large, 2057
Gαs hyperfunction, 2057
Gαz, 1876
GALT (gut-associated lymphoid tissue), 93–94, 94*f*

γ-carboxyl glutamic acid (Gla) domain, 1915–1918, 1917*f*, 1918*f*, 1919*f*
γδ heterodimers, 1175–1176
γδ T cells, 1142, 1142*t*
γδ T-cell receptors, 1177, 1565, 2286
γ-globin chains, 728
    β-thalassemias and production of, 742
    developmental changes in synthesis of, 730
    fetal hemoglobin, 760
    thalassemias and, 740
γ-heavy-chain disease, **1803–1806**, 1804*t*, 1805*f*
γ-retroviral vectors, 439
Ganciclovir
    adverse effects, 1252, 1269
    for CMV infection, 369, 1269
    as empiric therapy for infections, 386, 387*t*
    prophylactic, 389
    suicide gene activation by, 440
Gas 6 (growth arrest-specific 6) protein, 484, 1845
Gastrectomy, 601, 604, 1665
Gastritis, 629
Gastrointestinal tract
    absorption
        of cobalamin, **591–592**
        of folate, 586–587, 587*f*
        of iron, 552
    macrophages in, 1082
    microbiome, 2287
    mucosa, iron transport across, 619, 620*f*
    in pernicious anemia, 583, 600–601, 601*f*
Gastrointestinal tract bleeding
    anemia from, 553
    in hemophilia, 2120
    history of, 5
    iron deficiency and, 628–629, 628*t*
    in polycythemia vera, 1293
    red cell transfusion for, 2370, 2370*t*
Gastrointestinal tract disorders
    in acute myelogenous leukemia, 1380–1381, 1387
    in AL amyloidosis, 1760
    in α-heavy-chain disease, 1806, 1808
    in antiphospholipid syndrome, 2240
    cobalamin deficiency and, 601
    eosinophils and, 955*t*, 956
    folic acid deficiency and, 597
    gastric MALT lymphoma, 1664–1666, 1665*f*, 1666*t*
    in hemolytic uremic syndrome, 2258
    history of, 5
    immunoproliferative small intestinal disease, 1663, 1665, 1808, 1809
    inflammatory bowel disease, 1229
    in Langerhans cell histiocytosis, 1105

in mantle cell lymphoma, 1593, 1593*f*, 1654
    monocytosis and, 1097
    pernicious anemia and, 600
    primary lymphomas, 1581
    in thrombotic thrombocytopenic purpura, 2255
    in Waldenström macroglobulinemia, 1791
GATA-1
    ALAS expression and, 893
    in biosynthesis of neutrophil granules, 1011
    eosinophils and, 949
    in erythropoiesis, 483
    erythropoietin secretion and, 550
    in hematopoiesis, 271, 2060
    in hematopoietic tissue, 730
    in megakaryopoiesis, 1817, 1818, 1820
    neutrophil granules and, 926
    in primary myelofibrosis, 1320
    PU.1 and, 268
GATA-1, 539, 568, 2060
GATA2, 258, 262, 483–484, 949, 1215*t*, 1231, 1606
GATA2, 1089, 1098, 1345, 1346*t*, 1351–1352, 1379
GATA-3, 1156, 1180, 1181*f*
GATA transcription factor family, 262
Gating strategies, 36
Gaucher cells, 1126–1127, 1126*f*
Gaucher disease, **1121–1128**
    clinical features, 1123–1125, 1123*t*, 1125*f*
    course and prognosis, 1128
    differential diagnosis, 1127
    epidemiology, 1121–1122
    etiology and pathogenesis, 1122, 1122*f*
    gammopathy in, 1725
    genetic basis, 1122–1123
    heterozygote detection, 1127
    history and definition, 1121
    laboratory features, 635, 1124*f*, 1125–1127, 1126*f*
    pathophysiology, 1091
    therapy, 1127–1128, 1128*f*
    types, 1123, 1123*t*
"Gaucheroma," 1124, 1124*f*
GCL (glutamate cysteine ligase) deficiency, 705
GCNT2, 2337
G-CSF. *See* Granulocyte colony-stimulating factor (G-CSF)
GDF15, 567
GEF (guanine-nucleotide exchange factor), 1063*f*
Gelatinase, 1012*t*, 1014
Gelatinase granules, 1009

Gelatinous transformation, of marrow, 33
Gelfoam, 2062
Gelsolin, 1832*t*, 1840
Gemcitabine, **322**
    adverse effects, 2263
    for Hodgkin lymphoma, 1616
    for mantle cell lymphoma, 1659*t*
Gemtuzumab ozogamicin
    for acute myelogenous leukemia, 271,
        1395*t*, 1396, 1402*t*, 1403
    ATRA and, 1404
    removal from market, 346, 1403
Gender
    acute lymphoblastic leukemia and, 1506,
        1506*f*
    acute lymphoblastic leukemia prognosis
        and, 1520
    hairy cell leukemia and, 1554
    hemophilia A and, 2116
    lymphoma and, 1570, 1570*f*
    myelodysplastic syndromes and, 1345
    primary myelofibrosis and, 1319
Gene duplication, 147–148
Gene editing, 443–444
Gene expression
    interference with, 153
    macrophage, 1064–1066
    regulation, 165–166
Gene mutations, **146**. *See also individual*
        genes; specific diseases
    in major lymphoid malignancies, 231–237*t*
    in major myeloid malignancies, 226–230*t*
    next-generation sequencing analysis,
        160–161
Gene repair, 453
Gene therapy, **437–444**
    for adenosine deaminase deficiency severe
        combined immunodeficiency, 439
    for brain tumors, 442
    for chronic granulomatous disease, 1032
    for chronic lymphocytic leukemia, 442
    definition and history, 437
    for Diamond-Blackfan anemia, 540
    ex vivo, 437, 438*f*
    for Fanconi anemia, 442
    for Glanzmann thrombasthenia, 2062
    graft-versus-host disease prevention in,
        440, 440*f*
    hematopoietic stem cells in, 437
    for hemophilia, 2129–2130
    for HIV infection, 440–441, 454, 1243
    in vivo, 437, 438*f*
    for leukodystrophies, 439
    MGMT selective method, 442, 443*f*
    principles, 153, 437, 438*f*, 453–454
    for sickle cell disease, 453

targeted-insertion, 443–444, 443*f*
    for thalassemias, 753
    T lymphocytes in, 438
    vectors for, 438–439
    for Wiskott-Aldrich syndrome, 439
    for X-linked severe combined
        immunodeficiency, 437, 439, 453,
        1219
Genetic Information Nondiscrimination Act
        (GINA), 162
Genetics. *See also specific diseases*
    aging and, **130**
    autosomal dominant inheritance, 148, 148*f*
    autosomal recessive inheritance, 149, 149*f*
    chromosomal abnormalities. *See*
        Chromosomal abnormalities
    expressivity, 149
    linkage analysis, 151–152, 151*f*
    Mendelian, 147
    mutations. *See* Gene mutations
    penetrance, 149
    X inactivation, 150, 150*f*
    X-linked inheritance, 149–151
Genitourinary system
    blood loss from, 629
    complications in sickle cell disease,
        770–771
    history of disorders of, 5–6
    primary lymphomas in, 1581–1582
Genome, 145
Genome-wide association studies (GWAS),
        162
Genomics
    history, 155
    next-generation sequencing. *See* Next-
        generation sequencing
Genotype-phenotype correlations, 146
Gentamicin, 387*t*
Geranylgeranyltransferase-1 inhibitors, 1403
Gerbich blood group, 2332*t*, 2337, 2346*t*
Gerbich-negative phenotype, 2342–2343
Germ cell tumors, mediastinal, 1386–1387
Germinal center, lymph node, 1589, 1590*f*
Germinal center B-cell-like diffuse large
        B-cell lymphoma, 234–235*t*, 1495*t*,
        1626, 1627*t*
Germline mosaicism, 148
Gestational thrombocytopenia, 45, 121–122,
        2010
GFI1B, 2061
GH (growth hormone), 561, 1407
Giant cell reticulosis, 1109
Giant cell tumor of the bone, 1110
Giant follicular lymphoma, 1569
Giant metamyelocyte, 593
Giardia lamblia, 1212, 1216

GIG2. *See* CD9
Gilbert syndrome, 565
Gil blood group, 2332*t*
Gingival bleeding, 5, 8, 1987
Ginkgo biloba, 1986
Ginseng, 1986
Givinostat, for polycythemia vera, 1300
Gla (γ-carboxyl glutamic acid) domain,
        1915–1918, 1917*f*, 1918*f*, 1919*f*
Glanzmann thrombasthenia (GT), **2042–2047**
    clinical features, 1985, 2046, 2046*t*
    definition and history, 2042–2043
    etiology and pathogenesis, 1842, 1865,
        1995, **2043–2046**, 2043*f*, 2044*f*,
        2359
    laboratory features, 2046–2047, 2046*t*
    therapy, course, and prognosis, 2047, 2062
Gliomas, 170
Gln506-factor V. *See* Factor V Leiden/factor V
        G1691A
GLOB blood group, 2332*t*, 2334*t*, 2337, 2344*t*
Globin chains, 728, 740, 781
Globin gene clusters, **728–730**, 729*f*
Globin synthesis, disorders of. *See*
        Thalassemias
Globoside, 2340
Gloves-and-socks syndrome, 2104
Glucocerebrosidase, 1121, 1122, 1122*f*
Glucocorticoids
    for acute lymphoblastic leukemia, 1515,
        1516, 1517
    for antiphospholipid syndrome in
        pregnancy, 2245
    for aplastic anemia, 526
    for autoimmune hemolytic anemia, 838,
        840, 1541
    for chronic lymphocytic leukemia,
        1536–1537
    for Diamond-Blackfan anemia, 540
    eosinophilic granulomatosis with angiitis,
        960
    for Erdheim-Chester disease, 1111
    erythropoietin and, 560
    excess, 2107–2108
    for hypereosinophilic syndrome, 959
    for immune thrombocytopenia, 2003–
        2004
    for lymphomatoid papulosis, 1689
    macrophage deactivation and, 1070*t*
    for mastocytosis, 977
    for mononucleosis, 1269
    for mycosis fungoides, 1685
    for neonatal alloimmune
        thrombocytopenia, 2013
    neutrophilia and, 1001
    neutrophil motility and, 1026

for paroxysmal nocturnal hemoglobinuria, 578
for thrombocytopenia in pregnancy, 2010–2011
for thrombotic thrombocytopenic purpura, 2256
in thymic development, 85
for Waldenström macroglobulinemia, 1793
Glucose metabolism
enzymes, 692t, 694–697
pathways, 192–193, 193f, 692–694, 693f
Glucose-6-phosphate, 192, 694
Glucose-6-phosphate dehydrogenase (G6PD)
in chronic myelogenous leukemia, 1470
erythrocyte aging and, 497
gene for, 697, 702
in glucose metabolism, 696–697
structure, 696–697, 697f
variants, 702, 703t
Glucose-6-phosphate dehydrogenase (G6PD) deficiency
clinical features, 700t, 1020t
common forms for, 708–709
course and prognosis, 712
definition and history, 689–690
differential diagnosis, 711
epidemiology, 690, 691f
favism in, 692, 707, 709
genetics, 702
hemolysis/hemolytic anemia in, 707, 708, 708t
laboratory features, 700t, 710–711
malaria resistance and, 690
neonatal icterus/jaundice in, 709
platelet abnormalities in, 2061
sickle cell disease severity and, 690
therapy, 711
Glucose phosphate isomerase (GPI)
activity, 192, 692t
deficiency, 694, 700t, 704
in glucose metabolism, 694
GLUT1 (SLC2A1), 192
GLUT-3, 1836
Glutamate carboxypeptidase II (folate hydrolase), 586–587
Glutamate cysteine ligase (GCL) deficiency, 705
Glutamate cysteine synthetase, 698
Glutamate oxaloacetate transaminase (GOT), 193
Glutamine, 192–193, 193f, 199
γ-Glutamylcysteine synthetase, 688, 692t
γ-D-Glutamyl diaminopimelic acid (DAP), 299, 301f
Glutathione (GSH), 694, 698, 706–707
Glutathione disulfide (GSSG), 698

Glutathione peroxidase, 692t, 701t
Glutathione reductase (GR), 692t, 698
Glutathione reductase (GR) deficiency, 698, 700t, 701t, 705, 1020t, 1033
Glutathione S transferase, 701t
Glutathione synthetase (GS), 692t, 698
Glutathione synthetase (GS) deficiency, 700t, 705, 709, 1020t, 1033
Glutathione-5-transferase, 692t
Glutethimide, megaloblastic anemia and, 606t
GLUTs, 192
Glycation, aging and, 130–131
Glyceraldehyde-3-phosphate, 694, 695
Glyceraldehyde-3-phosphate dehydrogenase, 701t
Glyceraldehyde phosphate dehydrogenase, 692t, 695
Glycine C-succinyl transferase, 892
Glycine N-methyl transferase, 588
Glycocalicin, 1866
Glycocalix, 1834
Glycogen storage diseases, 994
Glycogen storage disease type 1b, 1026
Glycolipids, erythrocyte membrane, 662
Glycolipid storage diseases. See Lipid storage diseases
Glycolysis, 192–193, 193f, 199
in neutrophils, 932, 933t
in platelets, 1839–1840
Glycolytic (Embden-Meyerhof) pathway, 692–694, 693f, 932, 933t
Glycophorin A, 2337, 2338f
Glycophorin B, 2338f
Glycophorin C, 668, 670t
Glycophorins, 663t, 664–665
Glycoprotein (GP)
lymphocyte function-associated, 1184–1185, 1185f
in neutrophils, 2358
in newborn, 108
in platelet membrane, 1838f, 1846–1847t, 1857–1874, 1858–1859t. See also specific proteins
glycosyl phosphatidylinositol-anchored proteins, 571, 1871
immunoglobulin family of cell surface adhesion receptors, 1868–1870
integrins. See Integrins
lectin-containing receptors, 1870–1871
leucine-rich repeat glycoprotein receptors, 1865–1868
scavenger receptors, 1871
tetraspanins, 1871
tyrosine kinase receptors, 1871–1872

β₂Glycoprotein (GP)I (apolipoprotein H), 2234, 2235, 2235f, 2236f, 2237
Glycoprotein (GP)Ia/IIa. See Integrin α₂β₁
Glycoprotein (GP)Ib, 1830–1831f, 1841, 1865, 1866f, 1867f, 1868
Glycoprotein (GP)Ibα (CD42b,c), 1833, 1837, 1865–1868, 1866f, 1867f, 1877. See also Platelet-type (pseudo-) von Willebrand disease
Glycoprotein (GP)Ibβ, 1866–1867
Glycoprotein (GP)Ib/IX complex, 1815–1816, 1831, 1834, 1866f, 1867f, 1877
Glycoprotein (GP)Ib/IX/V complex (CD42), 1839, 1865–1868, 1866f, 1867f, 1875f, 1881. See also Bernard-Soulier syndrome
Glycoprotein (GP)Ic/IIa. See Integrin α₆β₁
Glycoprotein (GP)Ic*/IIa. See Integrin α₅β₁
Glycoprotein (GP)IIb/IIIa. See Integrin αIIbβ₃
Glycoprotein (GP)IIb/IIIa antagonists. See Integrin αIIbβ₃ antagonists
Glycoprotein (GP)IV (CD36, FAT, SCARB3), 1872
deficiency, 2359
in dense bodies, 1843
in fatty acid transport, 1872
in monocytes and macrophages, 1052f, 1055, 1057t
in platelet adhesion, 1833, 1872
in platelet-leukocyte interactions, 1856
in platelet membrane, 1836
thrombosis and, 1856
thrombospondin and, 1845, 1879
Glycoprotein (GP)IV (CD36, FAT, SCARB3) deficiency, 2051
Glycoprotein (GP)V, 1816, 1868, 1881
Glycoprotein (GP)VI, 1833, 1851, 1857, 1869, 1879–1880, 1880f, 2293
Glycoprotein (GP)VI deficiency, 2052
Glycoprotein (GP)IX (CD42a), 1865, 1866, 1866f, 1867f
Glycoprotein (GP)27. See CD151
Glycosaminoglycans (GAGs), 69, 1936, 1936f, 2027f, 2028
Glycosphingolipids, 1956
Glycosylation
abnormalities, in congenital dyserythropoietic anemia type II, 567
in biosynthesis of von Willebrand factor, 2166
in biosynthesis of VWF, 2167f
Glycosyl phosphatidylinositol-anchored proteins (GPI-APs), 571, 1871

Glycosyl phosphatidylinositol (GPI) anchors, 37, 1007

Glycosyl phosphatidylinositol (GPI)-anchor synthesis pathway, 573, 573*f*, 578

Glyoxalase 1, 701*t*

GM11070, for sickle cell disease, 777*t*

GM-CSF. *See* Granulocyte-macrophage colony-stimulating factor (GM-CSF); Granulocyte-monocyte colony-stimulating factor (GM-CSF)

GMP. *See under* Granulocyte-macrophage progenitor (GMP)

GMP140. *See* P-selectin

GNA 12/13, 1627*t*

GNAS/GNB1, 1346*t*, 1348

Gold salts, 2015

Gonadal function, acute myelogenous leukemia treatment and, 1411

Gonadotropins, 561

GOT (glutamate oxaloacetate transaminase), 193

Gout, in polycythemia vera, 1293

Gower-1 hemoglobin, 101, 101*t*, 728

Gower-2 hemoglobin, 101, 101*t*, 728

GP. *See under* Glycoprotein (GP)

gp91^phox (*CYBB*), 1013*t*, 1028*t*, 1029

gp 100, 413

GPI. *See* Glucose phosphate isomerase (GPI); Glycosyl phosphatidylinositol (GPI)

G protein, 1016

G-protein–coupled chemokine receptors, 1878

G-protein–coupled receptors (GPCRs) in monocytes and macrophages, 1059, 1060*t* in neutrophils, 1008 in platelet activation, 1874, 1875*f* structure and function, 248*f*, **250**

G proteins, 1882–1883

GPYA, 2339

GR. *See* Glutathione reductase (GR)

Graft-versus-host disease (GVHD) acute, **370–372** clinical features, 370–371, 1197 pathophysiology, 371 prevention, 357, 371 risk factors, 370 treatment, 371–372, 429*t* after allogenic hematopoietic cell transplantation, 1399–1400, 2374 chronic, 356, **372**, 1197 dendritic cells in, 310 gene therapy and, 440, 440*f*

human leukocyte antigens and, 357–358, 2356 mesenchymal stromal cells for, 449–450 with peripheral blood progenitor cells vs. marrow, 356 prevention, 440, 440*f*, 2374 T-cell therapy and, 410 transfusion-associated, 2377, 2388

Graft-versus-leukemia (GVL) effect, 307, 310, 1400, 1461

Graft-versus-tumor effects, **359**

Granular lymphocytes, 20*f*, 23

Granulocyte colony-stimulating factor (G-CSF), 100 for aplastic anemia, 525*t*, 526 for chemotherapy enhancement, 1396, 1402*t* for evaluation of neutrophil reserves, 943 in hematopoiesis, 264*t* for hematopoietic stem cell mobilization, 73, 355 for hypersplenism, 867 in innate immune response, 303 monocytosis and, 1097 for myelodysplastic syndromes, 1358, 1361 for neutropenia, 993, 994 neutropenia and, 992 neutrophilia and, 985, 1000 in neutrophilic granulopoiesis, 940 in neutrophil protein synthesis, 932 neutrophils and, 66. secondary acute myelogenous leukemia and, 1407

Granulocyte-macrophage colony-stimulating factor (GM-CSF) eosinophils and, 949, 953 in erythropoiesis, 483*f* in hematopoiesis, 258*f*, 264*t*, 268 in innate immune response, 303 in monocyte and macrophage differentiation, 1077–1078 monocytosis and administration of, 1097 for myelodysplastic syndromes, 1358 natural killer cells and, 1191 neutropenia and, 992 neutrophilia and, 1000 neutrophils and, 1008 regulation, 1444 vaccine therapy and, 423, 423*f*, 424*f*

Granulocyte-macrophage progenitor (GMP), 271

Granulocyte-macrophage progenitor (GMP)-33 (thrombospondin N-terminal fragment), 1873

Granulocyte-monocyte colony-stimulating factor (GM-CSF), 100

for chemotherapy enhancement, 1396 eosinophils and, 947 in neutrophilic granulopoiesis, 939–940

Granulocyte-monocyte progenitors, **271**, 1154

Granulocyte progenitors, **271**

Granulocytes in chronic myelogenous leukemia, 1445, 1446*f* defined, 939 differentiation, 65 marrow, 34 precursor cell kinetics, 75*t* release, 71–72

Granulocytic sarcoma. *See* Myeloid (granulocytic) sarcoma

Granulocytopenia, 991. *See also* Neutropenia

Granulocytopoiesis, in newborn, 105

Granulocytosis, 997. *See also* Neutrophilia in Hodgkin lymphoma, 1610 in primary myelofibrosis, 1326

Granulomatous inflammation, 279

Granulomonopoiesis, 105

Granulophysin. *See* CD63

Granulopoiesis, neutrophilic. *See* Neutrophils, granulopoiesis

Granzyme B, 204*f*, 205, 1565*f*, 1567

Granzymes, 1145

Graves disease, 518

Gray platelet syndrome (α-storage pool deficiency), 1850, 1853, 1996, **2054–2055**, 2055*f*

GRB2 (growth factor receptor-bound protein-2), 1443

Green sickness, 628

Griscelli syndrome, 994, 1020, 1229, 1849

Group B streptococcal infection, in newborn, 105–106

Growth, iron deficiency and, 632

Growth arrest-specific 6 (Gas 6) protein, 484, 1845

Growth differentiation factor 15, 622, 641

Growth factor receptor-bound protein-2 (GRB2), 1443

Growth hormone (GH), 561, 1407

GS. *See* Glutathione synthetase (GS)

GSH (glutathione), 694, 698, 706–707

GSSG (glutathione disulfide), 698

GT. *See* Glanzmann thrombasthenia (GT)

GTPases, 1059, 1833*t*

Guanine-nucleotide exchange factor (GEF), 1063*f*

Guanosine triphosphate-binding protein defects, 2057

Guillain-Barré syndrome, 1265

Günther disease. *See* Congenital
    erythropoietic porphyria
Gut-associated lymphoid tissue (GALT),
    93–94, 94*f*
Gut microbiome, 2287
GVD regimen, for Hodgkin lymphoma,
    1616
GVHD. *See* Graft-versus-host disease
    (GVHD)
GVL (graft-versus-leukemia) effect, 307, 310,
    1400, 1461
GWAS (genome-wide association studies),
    162
GX15-070 (obatoclax), 1403
GYPA/B/C, 2339, 2342–2343

H
H3K27me3, 170
5H9. *See* CD9
H60, 515
Haemophilus influenzae
    hemolytic anemia and, 819
    in hyperimmunoglobulin E syndrome,
        1026
    hyposplenism and, 868
    inflammation and, 290
    red cell antigens and, 2340
    vaccination, 869
    X-linked recessive agammaglobulinemia
        and, 1212
Hageman factor. *See* Factor XII
Hair loss, iron deficiency and, 632
Hairy cell leukemia (HCL), **1553–1559**
    chromosomal abnormalities, 1494*t*
    clinical features, **1554–1555**, 2082
    course and prognosis, 1559
    definition and history, 1553–1554
    differential diagnosis, 42, 1327, 1543, 1555,
        1557, 1558*t*
    epidemiology, 1554
    etiology and pathogenesis, 1554
    gene mutations, 232*t*, 1494*t*, 1554
    laboratory features, 1555
        blood, 1089, 1555
        histopathology, 1494*t*
        immunophenotypic profile, 1555, 1556*f*
        marrow, 31–32, 1555, 1557*f*
        monocytopenia, 1098
    treatment, **1557–1559**, 1559*t*
        followup care, 1558–1559
        initiation, 1557
        minimal residual disease, 1558
        at relapse, 1559
        standard approach, 1557–1559
    variant (HCL-v), 1495*t*, 1554, 1555, 1558*t*
    von Willebrand disease and, 2082

Hallervorden-Spatz syndrome. *See*
    Pantothenate kinase-associated
    neurodegeneration (PKAN)
Hallucinations, olfactory, 5
HAMP (hepcidin) mutations, 642
Ham test, 571, 576
Hand-foot syndrome, 771
Hand-Schüller-Christian disease. *See*
    Langerhans cell histiocytosis
Hantavirus, 2104
H antigen, 2330
Haploid, 175*t*
Hapten-drug absorption, 825*f*, 826*t*, 829–830,
    830*t*
Haptocorrin deficiency, 607
Haptocorrins, 583, 591*t*, **592–593**, 593*t*, 1448
Haptoglobin, 293, 499, 500*f*
HARP (hypobetalipoproteinemia,
    acanthocytosis, retinitis
    pigmentosa and pallidal
    degeneration) syndrome, 682
HAS-BLED score, 396, 396*t*
Hashimoto thyroiditis, lymphomas and,
    1575, 1583, 1664
Hassall corpuscles, 85, 86*f*
HAT (hepatic artery thrombosis), 2195
HAT (histone acetyltransferase) enzymes,
    167*f*, 168
HATs (histone acetylases), 240
HAX1, 983, 993
Hb. *See* Hemoglobin (Hb)
H blood group, 2332*t*, 2333*t*
HBV (hepatitis B virus) infection, 1574, 2126
HCAM (lymphocyte homing cell adhesion
    molecule), 68
hCAP-18 (LL-37, CAMP), 1012*t*, 1013
HCDs. *See* Heavy-chain diseases (HCDs)
HCL. *See* Hairy cell leukemia (HCL)
HCP (hematopoietic cell phosphatase), 253,
    485, 486*f*, 1163
Hct. *See* Hematocrit (Hct)
HCT. *See* Hematopoietic cell transplantation
    (HCT)
HCV infection. *See* Hepatitis C virus (HCV)
    infection
HDAC inhibitors. *See* Histone deacetylase
    (HDAC) inhibitors
HDACs (histone deacetylases), **239–240**,
    239*t*, 240*f*
HDFN. *See* Alloimmune hemolytic disease of
    the fetus and newborn (HDFN)
HDL. *See* High-density lipoprotein (HDL)
HDL2 (Huntington disease-like 2) disorder,
    682
HE. *See* Hereditary elliptocytosis (HE)
Headache

history of, 4–5
    iron deficiency and, 632
Health history, **3–7**, 4*t*
Heart disease. *See* Cardiovascular disease
Heart valve hemolysis, **804–806**, 805*f*, 805*t*
Heat-shock protein 70 peptide vaccine, 423
Heat-shock protein inhibitors, 1403
Heat-shock proteins, 2288
Heat stroke, disseminated intravascular
    coagulation and, 2209
Heavy-chain diseases (HCDs), **1803–1810**,
    1804*t*
    α-heavy-chain disease, **1806–1808**, 1807*f*
    γ-heavy-chain disease, **1803–1806**, 1805*f*
    μ-heavy-chain disease, **1809–1810**, 1810*f*
Heavy chains, immunoglobulin, 1159–1163
    allotypes, 1170
    class switching, 1168–1169
    gene complexes, 1165*f*, 1167*f*
Hef2, 1444
Heinz bodies
    characteristics, 467*f*, 468
    in G6PD deficiency, 710, 711
    in hemoglobin H disease, 747, 747*f*
    hemolytic anemia with, 810
    in hyposplenism, 869
Helicobacter pylori
    in extranodal margin zone lymphoma of
        MALT type, 1595, 1664, 1665
    immune thrombocytopenia and, 2009–
        2010
    iron-deficiency anemia and, 629, 630
    lymphomas and, 1573, 1581
    mastocytosis and, 976
    pernicious anemia and, 596
    T-cell response to, 1180
HELLP syndrome, **801–802**
    clinical features, 802
    course and prognosis, 803
    differential diagnosis, 802, 2012
    disseminated intravascular coagulation
        and, 2211
    eclampsia and, 122
    epidemiology, 801, 2211
    etiology and pathophysiology, 801–802,
        2211
    folic acid deficiency and, 599
    laboratory features, 802
    thrombocytopenia in, 2012
    treatment, 802–803, 2012, 2211
Helmet cells. *See* Schizocytes (schistocytes)
Helminths
    as cause of eosinophilia, 956–957, 957*t*
    eosinophils and inactivation of, 952
Helper T cells. *See* CD4+ T cells (helper
    T cells)

Hemangioblasts, 257, 258
Hemangioendothelioma, Kaposi-like, 2014
Hemangiomas, 2209–2210
Hemarthroses, 1988, 2116–2117, 2117*f*,
　　2118*f*, 2119*f*, 2122*t*, 2129
Hematemesis, 5, 1987
Hematochezia, history of, 5
Hematocrit (Hct), **488**, 488*f*
　anemia and, 505*f*
　blood viscosity and, 506, 508*f*
　in chronic renal disease and, 550*f*
　hypervolemia and, 506, 510*f*
　measurement, 13–14
　neonatal, 102–103
　reference ranges, 18*t*
　total-body, **489**
Hematologic consultation, **3**, 4*t*
　advice to referring physicians, 49
　for anemia, 42
　for bleeding, 46
　for erythrocytosis/polycythemia, 44–45
　for immature cells on the blood film,
　　47–48
　for leukocytosis, 43–44
　for leukopenia, 41–42
　for lymphadenopathy, 48
　for monoclonal gammopathy, 48–49
　for pancytopenia, 43
　in pregnancy, 45–46
　for splenomegaly, 48
　for thrombocytopenia, 42–43
　for thrombocytosis, 45
　for thrombosis, 46–47
Hematomas, 2117–2118, 2119*f*, 2122*t*
Hematon, 263
Hematopoiesis
　in acute myelogenous leukemia, 1281*f*
　aging and, **132–134**
　controversies in, **267–268**
　developmental biology of, **257–259**
　dysfunction of, in primary myelofibrosis,
　　1321–1322
　extramedullary, 1323
　fetal, **99–102**, 100*f*, 102*f*, 1149–1150
　hepatic, 100–101
　interplay of clonal and polyclonal, 1284
　marrow, fetal, 101
　murine, 1149
　natural killer cells and, 1191–1192
　neonatal, **102–109**
　overview, **257**, 258*f*, 1282, 1282*f*
　regulation
　　adipocytes in, 59
　　adventitial reticular cells in, 57–59, 58*f*
　　bone cells in, 59–60
　　macrophages in, 61, 1071

marrow endothelial cells in, 56–57
　osteoblasts in, 60
　osteoclasts in, 60–61
　sites of, **54–55**, 54*f*
　stem cell model of, **354–355**
　yolk sac, 99–100
Hematopoietic cell phosphatase (HCP,
　　SHP1), 253, 485, 486*f*, 1163
Hematopoietic cell transplantation (HCT),
　　353–374
　allogeneic, **358–359**
　　cytomegalovirus infection following,
　　　409–410
　　dendritic cell role in, 310
　　graft failure after, 367
　　graft-versus-tumor effects, 359
　　nonmyeloablative, 1400, 1408
　　preparative regimens, 359–360
　　relapse after, 373
　　for tolerance of solid-organ allografts,
　　　373–374
　assays, 259–260
　autologous, **358**
　　graft failure after, 367
　　graft purging strategies, 358
　　preparative regimens, 359–360
　　relapse after, 373
　　secondary acute myelogenous leukemia
　　　and, 1407
　　tumor contamination in, 358
　candidate evaluation and selection, **361–
　　362**, 361*t*
　complications, **366–373**, 367*t*
　　bleeding, 2382
　　cytomegalovirus infection, 1267–1268,
　　　2373–2374
　　graft failure, 366–367
　　graft-versus-host disease. *See* Graft-
　　　versus-host disease (GVHD)
　　infection. *See* Infection, in
　　　immunocompromised host
　　regimen-related organ toxicities,
　　　367–368
　　relapsed malignancy, **373**
　　thrombotic microangiopathy, 2262
　　transfusion-related, 2373–2374, 2373*t*
　future directions, 373–374
　history, **353–354**, 354*t*
　indications, **362–363**
　　acute lymphoblastic leukemia,
　　　1517–1518
　　acute myelogenous leukemia,
　　　1399–1400, 1402, 1407
　　acute promyelocytic leukemia, 1406
　　adult T-cell leukemia/lymphoma, 1701
　　AL amyloidosis, 1780

aplastic anemia, 522–523
　　Burkitt lymphoma, 1676
　　Chédiak-Higashi syndrome, 1020
　　chronic granulomatous disease, 1032
　　chronic lymphocytic leukemia, 1539
　　chronic myelogenous leukemia,
　　　1460–1461, 1466–1467
　　diffuse large B-cell lymphoma,
　　　1631–1632
　　familial hemophagocytic
　　　lymphohistiocytosis, 1228
　　follicular lymphoma, 1648, 1648*f*
　　Hodgkin lymphoma, 1248, 1616
　　inherited platelet disorders, 2062
　　inherited pure red cell aplasia, 540
　　juvenile myelomonocytic leukemia,
　　　1471
　　mantle cell lymphoma, 1656, 1656*f*,
　　　1658*t*
　　myelodysplastic syndromes, 1361–1362
　　myeloma, 1750–1751, 1755–1756
　　Omenn syndrome, 1219
　　paroxysmal nocturnal hemoglobinuria,
　　　579–580, 579*t*
　　peripheral T-cell lymphoma, 1696, 1697
　　polycythemia vera, 1301
　　primary myelofibrosis, 1330–1331
　　severe combined immunodeficiency,
　　　1219
　　sickle cell disease, 775
　　systemic mastocytosis, 977
　　thalassemias, 753–754
　　Waldenström macroglobulinemia, 1796
　　Wiskott-Aldrich syndrome, 1225
　preparative regimens, **359–361**
　　chemotherapy-only, 360
　　reduced-intensity, 360–361, 367
　　total-body irradiation, 359–360
　results, **363–366**, 365*f*. *See also specific
　　diseases*
　sources of stem cells for, **355–358**
　　alternative donors, 356–357
　　blood, 355–356
　　comparison of, 358
　　HLA-haploidentical donors, 357–358
　　marrow, 355
　　umbilical cord blood, 357
　stem cell model of hematopoiesis and,
　　354–355
　syngeneic, 359
　trafficking/homing of hematopoietic stem
　　cells and, 355
　transfusion support, 2372–2374, 2373*t*
Hematopoietic cytokine receptor family,
　　247–249
Hematopoietic dysplasia, 1277, 1343

Hematopoietic lineages, morphologic differentiation of, 33–34
Hematopoietic microenvironment, 263–267
    aging and, 267
    anatomy, 263
    cell adhesion in, 65–68, 67t
    cell proliferation, apoptosis, and maturation in, 74–75
    cellular homing in, 68–71
    cellular release in, 71–74, 72f, 73f
    cytokines, 264–266, 264t
    general considerations, 53–54
    histogenesis of, 55
    matrix proteins, 266–267
    in myeloma, 1712
    in neutrophilic granulopoiesis, 939
    stromal cells, 264
Hematopoietic niche, 56
Hematopoietic progenitors, 258f, 269–272
    assays, 269
    B cells, 1151, 1168
    in chronic myelogenous leukemia, 1440, 1447
    dendritic cell, 310, 1076f, 1081
    in erythropoiesis, 480–481
    lymphoid, 269–270
    macrophage, 1076, 1076f, 1081
    myeloid, 270–272
    in primary myelofibrosis, 1326
Hematopoietic stem cells (HSCs), 259–263
    adhesion, 65–66
    aging and, 132–133, 263
    assays, 259–260
    cell-cycle characteristics, 261
    circulation, 55–56, 56f
    derivation from induced pluripotent stem cells, 449
    differentiation and maturation, 1282, 1282f
    early development, 54, 54f
    expansion, self-renewal, and differentiation, 268–269
    fetal, 100f
    functional definition, 259
    gene expression profile, 261–262
    in gene therapy, 437
    for hematopoietic cell transplantation. See Hematopoietic cell transplantation, sources of stem cells for
    integrins, 260–261
    kinetics, 259
    metabolic characteristics, 196–197, 197f, 261
    microenvironment, 53–54. See also Hematopoietic microenvironment
    ontogeny of, 101
    organization, 64–65

plasticity, 54–55, 269
preleukemic, 1376
proliferation, apoptosis, and maturation, 74–75
release, 71–74
surface phenotype, 260
trafficking and homing, 68–71, 355
transcription factor profile, 262–263
viral transgenesis, 453–454
Hematopoietic stem cell transplantation (HSCT). See Hematopoietic cell transplantation (HCT)
Hematopoietic tissue, 55
Hematuria, 5, 766, 1987, 2119, 2374
Heme
    biosynthesis, 891f, 892–896, 893f
    defects in synthesis, 916
    intravascular destruction of red cells and, 5, 500f
    structure, 761, 761f, 790–791, 791f, 892, 892f
Heme iron, 619
Heme oxygenase (HO), 499
Heme pocket, substitutions near, 781
Heme synthetase (ferrochelatase), 893f, 895, 917
Hemin
    for ALA dehydratase porphyria, 900
    intravenous, for acute intermittent porphyria, 904
    structure, 892, 892f
Hemochromatosis, 639–645
    classification, 640, 640t
    clinical features, 643
    course and prognosis, 644–645
    definition and history, 639–640
    differential diagnosis, 643
    epidemiology, 640
    etiology and pathogenesis, 640–643
        animal models, 642–643
        genetics, 642
        iron overload, 641
        iron toxicity, 640–641
        pathology, 641–642
    hereditary, 429t, 432, 640, 640t, 643
    juvenile, 640, 643
    laboratory features, 643
    neonatal, 640
    secondary, 640, 643
    treatment, 644
Hemochrome, 892, 892f
Hemochromogen, 892
Hemoglobin (Hb), 617
    abnormal, 762, 776–778, 778t
    concentration in pregnancy, 119
    deoxygenation of, 796–797, 796f, 797f

disorders of, 778–782. See also specific types and Sickle cell disease
    in erythropoiesis, 479–480
    fetal, synthesis of, 101, 101t, 102f, 728, 730
    genetic control, 728–730, 729f
    high-oxygen affinity, 782, 872, 876
    intravascular destruction of red cells and, 499, 500f
    low-oxygen affinity, 782, 794–795, 794t
    measurement, 13–14
    neonatal, 102–103
    nitric oxide and, 796–797, 796f, 797f
    polymerization of, 763–764, 765f
    quaternary structures, 761t, 763–764
    red cell viscosity and, 668
    reference ranges, 18t
    structure and function, 759–761, 760f, 761f, 761t
    thresholds for red cell transfusion, 2369–2370, 2370t. See also Red cell transfusion
    unstable, 781–782
Hemoglobin A, 481, 728, 751, 762
Hemoglobin A_2, 728, 750–751
Hemoglobin AS (sickle cell trait), 762, 766
Hemoglobin Bart's, 726
Hemoglobin Bart's hydrops fetalis syndrome
    α-thalassemia and, 739
    clinical features, 745
    laboratory features, 747
    pathophysiology, 740
Hemoglobin C, 762
Hemoglobin C disease
    clinical features, 779
    definition and history, 778
    differential diagnosis, 780
    etiology and pathogenesis, 778–779
    laboratory features, 779, 779f
    therapy, 780
Hemoglobin Constant Spring, 748, 748f
Hemoglobin C thalassemia, 749–750
Hemoglobin D, 762
Hemoglobin D disease, 779f, 781
Hemoglobin D_{Ibadan}, 762, 781
Hemoglobin $D_{Los Angeles}$, 762, 781
Hemoglobin D_{Punjab}, 762, 781
Hemoglobin E, 762
Hemoglobin E disease
    clinical features, 780
    course and prognosis, 781
    definition and history, 780
    etiology and pathogenesis, 780
    laboratory features, 779f, 780
    therapy, 780
Hemoglobin E thalassemia, 749, 779f
Hemoglobin E-β^0-thalassemia, 780

Hemoglobin F. *See also* Hereditary persistence of fetal hemoglobin (HPFH)
  structure, 728
  switch to adult hemoglobin, 730
  synthesis, 101, 101t, 102f
  in thalassemias, 741
  therapy to increase, 753, 774–775, 775t
  types, 101, 101t
Hemoglobin G$_{Philadelphia}$, 778
Hemoglobin G Philadelphia H disease, 751
Hemoglobin H, 726
Hemoglobin Hasharon H disease, 751
Hemoglobin H disease
  clinical features, 745
  differential diagnosis, 637
  laboratory features, 747, 747f
  molecular basis, 739
  in myelodysplastic syndromes, 1353
  treatment, 753
Hemoglobin H inclusions, 467f, 468
Hemoglobin$_{Kansas}$, 789, 794t
Hemoglobin Kenya, 735
Hemoglobin$_{Köln}$, 762
Hemoglobin Köln disease, 637
Hemoglobin Lepore, 733–734, 735f, 748
Hemoglobin Lincoln Park, 734
Hemoglobin M. *See also* Methemoglobinemia
  clinical features, 792
  history, 789
  laboratory features, 792, 793f
  properties, 782, 790–791, 791t
Hemoglobin M$_{Boston}$, 791t
Hemoglobin M$_{Fort Ripley}$, 791t
Hemoglobin M$_{Hyde Park}$, 791t, 792
Hemoglobin M$_{Iwate}$, 791t
Hemoglobin Miyada, 734
Hemoglobin M$_{Milwaukee}$, 791, 791t
Hemoglobin M$_{Osaka}$, 791t
Hemoglobin M$_{Saskatoon}$, 791t, 792
Hemoglobinopathies, 725
  in pregnancy, **125–126**
  sickle cell disease. *See* Sickle cell disease
  thalassemias. *See* Thalassemias
Hemoglobin P-Nilotic, 734
Hemoglobin QH disease, 751
Hemoglobin S, 762, 763–764, 765f. *See also* Sickle cell disease
Hemoglobin SC disease, 779f
Hemoglobin$_{Seattle}$, 794t
Hemoglobinuria, 631
Hemoglobin$_{Zurich}$, 762, 795
Hemojuvelin (HJV), 566, 621, 621t, 642
Hemojuvelin (HJV) mutations, 642
Hemolysins, 823, 829
Hemolysis/hemolytic disease

differential diagnosis, 637
drug-induced, 553
of the fetus and newborn. *See* Alloimmune hemolytic disease of the fetus and newborn (HDFN)
in G6PD deficiency, 706–707, 707t
heart valve, **804–806**, 805f, 805t
in hereditary spherocytosis, 674
intravascular, 631
mechanisms
  chemical and physical agents, **809–810**
  enzyme deficiencies, **706–708**, 707t
megaloblastic anemia and, 597
in sickle cell disease, 764
Hemolytic anemia
  alloimmune, 836
  autoimmune. *See* Autoimmune hemolytic anemia
  cold agglutinin, 1790
  Donath-Landsteiner, 824
  drug-induced immune, 708, 708t, 826t
    classification, 824t, 825
    clinical features, 832
    course and prognosis, 840
    differential diagnosis, 837
    epidemiology, 827
    etiology, 827
    laboratory features, 832
    pathogenesis, 825, 825f, 829–831, 830t
    serologic features, 836
    therapy, 839–840
  folate deficiency in, 598
  fragmentation, **801–806**
    cancer-associated microangiopathic, 803, **803–804**
    heart valve hemolysis, **804–806**
    Kasabach-Merritt phenomenon, 806
    march hemoglobinuria, 806
    preeclampsia/eclampsia and HELLP syndrome, **801–803**. *See also* HELLP syndrome
  hereditary nonspherocytic. *See* Hereditary nonspherocytic hemolytic anemia
  infection-related, **815–820**, 816t
    babesiosis, 429t, 432, 817f, **818–819**
    bartonellosis, **818**, 997
    Clostridium perfringens septicemia, **819**
    in G6PD deficiency, 708–709
    malaria. *See* Malaria
  in newborns, 848. *See also* Alloimmune hemolytic disease of the fetus and newborn (HDFN)
  in paroxysmal nocturnal hemoglobinuria, 571, 573f
  in Rosai-Dorfman disease, 1113

stress reticulocytes in, 482f
unstable hemoglobins and, **781–782**
Hemolytic uremic syndrome (HUS)
  atypical, 1932, 1953, **2259–2261**, 2259t
  differential diagnosis, 837
  Shiga toxin *E. coli*-associated, 132., 2258–2259
  therapy, 429t
Hemopexin, 293, 499, 500f
Hemophagocytic lymphohistiocytosis (HLH)
  Chédiak-Higashi syndrome and, 1018
  clinical features, 1114
  definition and history, 1113
  diagnostic criteria, 1114, 1114t
  differential diagnosis, 1115
  epidemiology, 1113
  etiology and pathogenesis, 1101, 1113–1114
  histopathology, 1102t
  immune deficiencies associated with, 304, 1114
  laboratory features, 1114f, 1115
  macrophage activation syndrome in, 1115–1116
  therapy, 1115
Hemophagocytic syndrome
  Epstein-Barr virus mononucleosis and, 1265
  HIV-associated, 1250–1251, 1251t
Hemophilia A (classic hemophilia, factor VIII deficiency), 1985, **2113–2126**
  acquired, **2183–2186**
  clinical features, **2116–2120**, 2116t
    bleeding following circumcision, 1988
    dental and surgical bleeding, 2120
    gene mutations, 441
    gene therapy, 442
    hemarthroses, 2116–2117, 2117f, 2118f
    hematomas, 2117–2118, 2119f
    hematuria, 2119
    mucous membrane hemorrhage, 2120
    neurologic, 2119–2120
    pseudotumors, 2119, 2120f
  course and prognosis, **2124–2126**, 2124t, 2125t
    anti-factor VIII antibodies and, 2124–2126, 2124t, 2125t, 2126t
    infectious complications, 2126
  definition and history, 2113–2114
  differential diagnosis, 2121
  etiology and pathogenesis, 2114
  gene mutations, 2114–2116, 2114f, 2115f
  laboratory features, 2120–2121
  pregnancy and, 121
  prenatal diagnosis and carrier detection, 121, 2116

special problems associated with, 2130
therapy, **2121–2124**
    antifibrinolytic agents, 2123, 2317*t*, 2318
    desmopressin, 2122–2123
    factor VIII replacement therapy,
        2121–2122, 2121*t*, 2122*t*
    fibrin glue, 2123
    gene therapy, 441–442, 2129–2130
    home therapy, 2124
    liver transplantation, 2129
    of major nonsurgical hemorrhage, 2123
    of minor/moderate hemorrhage, 2123
    prophylactic, 2124
    for surgical procedures, 2123–2124
Hemophilia B (factor IX deficiency,
        Christmas factor deficiency), 1985,
        2126–2130
    clinical features, 1988, 2128–2129
    course and prognosis, 2129
    differential diagnosis, 2128
    etiology and pathogenesis, 1922, 2126
    factor IX inhibitor in, 2129
    gene therapy, 441–442, 2129–2130
    genetics and molecular biology, 441,
        2126–2127, 2127*f*
    laboratory features, 2128
    pregnancy and, 121
    prenatal diagnosis and carrier detection,
        121, 2127
    special problems associated with, 2130
    therapy, 2128–2129, 2128*t*
Hemoptysis, 5, 1987
Hemorrhage. *See* Bleeding
Hemorrhagic fevers, 2086, 2207
Hemosiderin, 42., 618, 633
Hemosiderosis, 639
Hemostasis. *See also under* Coagulation
    disorders. *See also* Platelets, disorders
        in acute promyelocytic leukemia, 1405
        bleeding history, 1985–1986
        classification, 1985, 1986*t*
        clinical manifestations, 1987–1988,
            1987*t*
        evaluation/diagnosis, 1988–1989, 1989*f*,
            2040–2042, 2041*f*
        iron deficiency in, 629
        laboratory features, 1990–1991
        physical examination, 1988
        preoperative assessment of, 1990, 1990*t*
    inflammatory mediators in, 1979*t*
    pathways. *See* Coagulation, pathways;
        Coagulation factors
    platelet function in, 2039
    vascular function in, **1967–1979**
        adhesion molecules, 1976
        eicosanoid pathway, 1969–1970

endothelium, 1968–1969, 1968*f*, 1968*t*,
    1969*f*, 1970*f*
fibrinolysis, 1972–1975, 1973*f*, 1974*t*,
    1975*f*
inhibition of platelet activation and
    recruitment, 1971, 1972*f*
molecular changes in inflammation,
    1976–1979, 1977*t*, 1979*t*
nitric oxide, 1970–1971
protein C pathway, 1971–1972
HEMPAS (hereditary erythroblastic
    multinuclearity with a positive
    acidified serum test), 567, 2340
Henoch-Schönlein purpura (HSP), 1162,
    2103–2104, 2104*f*
Heparan sulfate, 62, **267**
Heparin, **397–398**. *See also* Low-molecular-
    weight heparin (LMWH)
    administration and monitoring, 397
    adverse effects, 397–398, 2099–2100,
        2277. *See also* Heparin-induced
        thrombocytopenia (HIT)
    for antiphospholipid syndrome, 2244, 2245
    antithrombin and, 2202
    binding to von Willebrand factor, 2168
    choice of, 398
    for disseminated intravascular coagulation,
        2213–2214
    during fibrinogen replacement therapy,
        2157
    maternal ingestion of, effect on fetus and
        newborn, 112
    mechanism of action, 1919, 1919*t*, 1959
    for myocardial infarction, 2295–2296
    for paroxysmal nocturnal hemoglobinuria
        during pregnancy, 580
    pharmacology of, **396**
    platelet factor 4 and, 1844, 2026–2028,
        2026*f*, 2027*f*
    platelet function and, 2078
    resistance to, 397
    reversal of therapy, 397
    for unstable angina, 2296
    for venous thromboembolism, 2273–2274
    for venous thromboembolism prophylaxis
        during pregnancy, 123
Heparin-binding protein (azurocidin), 1012*t*,
    1013
Heparin cofactor II, 1952*t*, 1960
Heparin-induced osteoporosis, 2277
Heparin-induced thrombocytopenia (HIT),
    2025–2032
    clinical features, 2028–2029, 2029*t*
    complications, 396, 2277
    differential diagnosis, 2029, 2031
    epidemiology, 2025, 2277

    etiology and pathogenesis, 398,
        2026–2028, 2026*f*, 2026*t*, 2027*f*
    hemodialysis and, 2032
    heparin reexposure following, 2032
    laboratory features, 2029–2030, 2030*t*
    in pregnancy, 2032, 2277
    treatment
        danaparoid, 398, 2030
        duration, 2032
        fondaparinux, 399, 2030
        nonheparin anticoagulants, 2030–2031,
            2031*t*
        plasma exchange, 429*t*
        platelet transfusion, 2032
        warfarin, 396, 2031–2032
Hepatic artery thrombosis (HAT), 2195
Hepatic disease/dysfunction
    acanthocytosis in, **680–681**
    in acute fatty liver of pregnancy, 2012,
        2211
    in AL amyloidosis, 1779, 1781–1782
    in antiphospholipid syndrome, 2240
    bleeding in, 2193
    chronic, 636
    in disseminated intravascular coagulation,
        2204, 2204*t*, 2205*t*
    disseminated intravascular coagulation
        and, 2208
    dose modification in patients with, 316*t*
    drug-related, 1410
    dysfibrinogenemia in, 2159
    in erythropoietic protoporphyria, 898, 899
    in hemochromatosis, 641–642, 643
    hemostatic alterations in, **2191–2195**
        in acute liver failure, 2193
        changes contributing to bleeding/
            thrombosis, 2192, 2193*t*
        fibrinolysis, 2192
        during liver transplantation, 2193
        management, 2193–2194
        primary hemostasis, 2191
        secondary hemostasis, 2192
    in Langerhans cell histiocytosis, 1104, 1106
    in mastocytosis, 974
    multipotential cell therapy for, 452
    platelet dysfunction in, 2086
    vs. primary myelofibrosis, 1327
    in sickle cell disease, 772
    thrombocytopenia and, 2013
    thrombosis in, 2194–2195
Hepatic endoplasmic reticulum retention,
    2155
Hepatic hematopoiesis, 100–101
Hepatic porphyrias, 889. *See also* Porphyria
    cutanea tarda (PCT)
Hepatic stem/progenitor cells, 452

Hepatic vein thrombosis, in polycythemia vera, 1293

Hepatitis, aplastic anemia and, 518

Hepatitis A virus, mononucleosis and, 1268

Hepatitis B virus (HBV) infection, 518, 1410, 1574, 2126, 2370t

Hepatitis C virus (HCV) infection
    antiphospholipid antibodies and, 2234, 2240
    as complication of factor VIII replacement, 2126
    cryoglobulinemia and, 2097
    immune thrombocytopenia and, 2009
    lymphomas and, 1574, 1664, 1666
    porphyria cutanea tarda and, 906, 909
    transfusion-related, 518, 1410, 2370t
    Waldenström macroglobulinemia and, 1711

Hepatocyte growth factor, 1449

Hepatocytes, 551

Hepatocyte transplantation, 452

Hepatoerythropoietic porphyria, 889, 890t, 891t, 905, 906. See also Porphyria cutanea tarda (PCT)

Hepatoma, erythrocytosis and, 879

Hepatosplenic T-cell lymphoma (HSTCL), 185t, 1498t, 1567, **1701**

Hepatosplenomegaly
    in alloimmune hemolytic disease of the fetus and newborn, 848
    in NK-cell leukemia, 1566
    in primary myelofibrosis, 1324

Hepcidin
    in iron regulation, 551, 551f, 552, 620–622, 620f, 621t
    in myeloma, 1740

Hepcidin (*HAMP*) mutations, 642

Hephaestin, 621t

Heptahelical receptors. See G-protein–coupled receptors (GPCRs)

Herald state of leukemia, 1342

Herbicides, lymphomas and, 1571, 1572–1573

Hereditary coproporphyria, 889, 890t, 891t, **904–905**

Hereditary elliptocytosis (HE), **677–680**
    clinical features, 679
    definition and history, 677
    differential diagnosis, 679
    epidemiology, 677
    erythrocyte membrane protein defects, 677–678
    etiology and pathogenesis, 473, 677
    in infancy, 679
    inheritance, 679
    laboratory features, 670f, 679

molecular determinants of clinical severity, 678–679
    therapy and prognosis, 679–680

Hereditary erythroblastic multinuclearity with a positive acidified serum test (HEMPAS), 567, 2340

Hereditary folate malabsorption, **608**

Hereditary hemochromatosis. See Hemochromatosis, hereditary

Hereditary hemorrhagic telangiectasia (HHT), 629, 1986, 1987, 2108–2109, 2109f, 2172

Hereditary hydrocytosis, 682t, **683–684**

Hereditary methemoglobinuria, 793. See also Cytochrome b_5 reductase deficiency

Hereditary nonspherocytic hemolytic anemia, 690
    course and prognosis, 712
    differential diagnosis, 711
    enzyme abnormalities in, 700t
    G6PD variants and, 702
    laboratory features, 710–711
    pyruvate kinase deficiency in, 690, 709
    therapy, 711–712

Hereditary orotic aciduria, 608

Hereditary persistence of fetal hemoglobin (HPFH)
    deletion forms, 726, 734f, 735, 736t
    δβ type, 748–749
    heterocellular, 749
    molecular basis, 735–736, 736t, 737f
    nondeletion forms, 726, 735–736, 736t, 749
    pathophysiology, 741

Hereditary pyropoikilocytosis (HPP), **677–680**
    clinical features, 679
    definition and history, 677
    differential diagnosis, 679
    epidemiology, 677
    erythrocyte membrane protein defects, 677–678
    etiology and pathogenesis, 677
    in infancy, 679
    laboratory features, 677f, 679
    molecular determinants of clinical severity, 678–679
    therapy and prognosis, 679–680

Hereditary spherocytosis (HS), **669–676**
    vs. autoimmune hemolytic anemia, 835
    clinical features/classification, **673–674**, 673t
    complications, **674–675**
    definition and history, 669
    differential diagnosis, 675–676
    epidemiology, 669

erythrocyte membrane protein defects in, **670–672**, 670t
    ankyrin, 671–672
    band 3, 672
    protein 4.2, 672
    spectrin, 672
    etiology and pathogenesis, 669–670, 671f
    genetic counseling, 676
    in infants, 674
    inheritance of, 673
    laboratory features, 670f, **675**
    molecular determinants of severity, 673
    nonerythroid manifestations, 675
    pregnancy and, 674
    secondary membrane defects in, 672–673
    spleen in, 673
    therapy/prognosis, **676**

Hereditary stomatocytosis syndromes, **682–683**, 682t
    cryohydrocytosis, **684**
    familial deficiency of high-density lipoproteins, **684**
    hereditary stomatocytosis/hydrocytosis, **683–684**
    hereditary xerocytosis, **683**
    intermediate syndromes, 682t
    laboratory features, 670f
    pathophysiology, 473
    Rh-deficiency syndrome, **684**

Hereditary thrombophilia, **2221–2229**
    antithrombin deficiency. See Antithrombin (AT) deficiency
    arterial thromboembolic disease risk in, 2226–2227
    cardiovascular disease and, 2221
    classification, 2222
    clinical implications of testing for, 2225, 2227–2229, 2228t
    factor V Leiden. See Factor V Leiden/ factor V G1691A
    history, 2222
    hyperhomocysteinemia. See Hyperhomocysteinemia
    persistent elevated factor VIII. See Factor VIII, increased levels
    pregnancy complications and, 2221, 2225t, 2227, 2228t, 2229
    prevalence, 2222t
    protein C deficiency. See Protein C deficiency
    protein S deficiency. See Protein S deficiency
    prothrombin G20210A. See Prothrombin G20210A

venous thromboembolism risk and,
2221–2222, 2225–2226, 2225t,
2226t, 2268, 2268t
Hereditary xerocytosis, 682t, **683**
Hermansky-Pudlak syndrome (HPS)
clinical features, 1229, 2053
differential diagnosis, 1020
etiology and pathogenesis, 1229, 1818,
1843, 1871, 2052–2053, 2053f
laboratory features, 2053–2054
therapy, course, and prognosis, 2054
Herpes simplex virus (HSV) infections
encephalitis, 304, 1230
after hematopoietic cell transplantation,
370
in immunocompromised host, 384
Herpes simplex virus thymidine kinase
(*HSV-TK*), 440
Herpesviruses. *See under* Human herpes
virus (HHV)
Herpes zoster
idiopathic CD4+ T lymphocytopenia and,
1206
prophylaxis, 1746
15-HETE, 952
HETE1, 1877
Heterogenous nucleation, 763
Heterophile antibody test, 1261
HEVs (high endothelial venules), 68, 93
Hexagonal phase assay, 2243
Hexokinase (HK), 497, 692t, 694
Hexokinase (HK) deficiency, 694, 700t, 704,
2061
L-Hexonate dehydrogenase, 697
Hexose monophosphate shunt, 693f, 694,
694f, 932
HFE, 621, 621t, 623
HFE
epidemiology, 640
hemochromatosis and, 642
porphyria cutanea tarda and, 889, 907
2-HG (2-hydroxyglutarate), 198
HHT (hereditary hemorrhagic
telangiectasia), 629, 1986, 1987,
2108–2109, 2109f, 2172
HHV. *See under* Human herpes virus (HHV)
HIES (hyperimmunoglobulin E syndrome),
1020t, 1026–1027, 1182, **1225**
HIF. *See* Hypoxia-inducible transcription
factor (HIF)
High-affinity folate receptors, 588
High-altitude polycythemia
clinical features, 881
epidemiology, 873
etiology and pathogenesis, 874–875, 874f
treatment, 884

High-density lipoprotein (HDL), 2283
activated protein C and, 1956
atherosclerosis and, 2287–2288
disseminated intravascular coagulation
and, 2203
familial deficiency, 684
High endothelial venules (HEVs), 68, 93
High-mobility group protein-1/2 (HMG1/2),
1167
High-molecular-weight kininogen (HK),
1916t, 1929
High-throughput DNA sequencing
technologies. *See* Next-generation
sequencing
Hill plot, 761
Hip fracture repair, 2370–2371, 2370t
Hirudin, 1919
Hispanic Americans, sickle cell disease and,
763
HIST1H1B-E mutations, 235t
Histamine, 286t, 289, 1448, 1979t
Histidine catabolism, 586t
Histiocytes, 1089, 1101, 1102t, 1446. *See also*
Macrophages
Histiocytic lymphoma, 1569
Histiocytosis(es)
classification, 1090–1091, 1090t, 1101,
1102t
definition, 1089
effects, 1092
Erdheim-Chester disease, 1101, 1102t,
1110–1111
hemophagocytic lymphohistiocytosis.
See Hemophagocytic
lymphohistiocytosis (HLH)
juvenile xanthogranuloma, 1101, 1102t,
1111–1112
Langerhans cell. *See* Langerhans cell
histiocytosis
malignant, 1101, 1102t, **1109–1110**
sinus histiocytosis with massive
lymphadenopathy (Rosai-Dorfman
disease), **1112–1113**
Histiocytosis X. *See* Langerhans cell
histiocytosis
Histone acetylases (HATs), 240
Histone acetyltransferase (HAT) enzymes,
167f, 168
Histone deacetylase (HDAC) inhibitors,
336–337. *See also specific drugs*
for acute myelogenous leukemia,
1403
mechanism of action, 240
for mycosis fungoides, 1686–1687
for myelodysplastic syndromes, 1361
for myeloma, 1754

for polycythemia vera, 1300
for sickle cell disease, 774t, 775
Histone deacetylases (HDACs), **239–240**,
239t, 240f, 1838
Histone modification, **167–168**, 167f, 234t
Histoplasma infection, 384
History taking, **3–7**, 4t
HIT. *See* Heparin-induced thrombocytopenia
(HIT)
HIV. *See under* Human immunodeficiency
virus
HIVEP2, 1787
HJV (hemojuvelin), 566, 621, 621t, 642
HJV (hemojuvelin) mutations, 642
HK. *See* Hexokinase (HK)
HK (high-molecular-weight kininogen),
1916t, 1929
HK1, 694
HLA. *See under* Human leukocyte antigen
(HLA)
HLH. *See* Hemophagocytic
lymphohistiocytosis (HLH)
HMG1/2 (high-mobility group protein-1/2),
1167
HMGA2, 1321
HNAs. *See* Human neutrophil antigens
(HNAs)
HO (heme oxygenase), 499
Hodgkin cells, 1605, 1606
Hodgkin lymphoma, **1603–1618**
anatomic distribution of disease, 1609
classical, 1497t, 1599–1600, 1599f, 1604t
lymphocyte-depletion subtype, 1609
lymphocyte-rich subtype, 1609
mixed cellularity subtype, 1600, 1600f,
1609
nodular sclerosis subtype, 1600, 1600f,
1609
classification, 1493, 1497t, 1604t
clinical features, 1607–1609
course and prognosis, 1613t, 1616–1617
definition and history, 1603–1604
differential diagnosis, 1610
epidemiology, 1571f, 1604–1605, 1604f,
1605f
etiology and pathogenesis
genetic basis, 1605
infectious, 1605
microenvironment, 1607
Reed-Sternberg cell, 1605–1606, 1605f,
1607f
HIV-associated
antiretroviral therapy and chemotherapy
for, 1248
characteristics, 1247, 1248t
chemotherapy for, 1247–1248

Hodgkin lymphoma, HIV-associated (*Cont.*):
  hematopoietic cell transplantation for, 1248
  incidence, 1243, 1247, 1605
  laboratory features, 1610
    histopathology, 1497t, 1599–1601, 1600f, 1601f
    monocytosis, 1097
    radiographic, 1608, 1608f
  nodular lymphocyte-predominant
    differential diagnosis, 1609
    immunophenotype, 1497t, 1604t
    laboratory features, 1497t, 1600–1601, 1600f, 1601f, 1609
    treatment, 1616
  in pregnancy, **123–124**
  staging, 1609–1610, 1610t
  therapy, **1610–1616**
    advanced disease, 1613–1615
    chemotherapy regimens, 1612t
    clinical trials, 1615t
    complications, 1617–1618
    favorable, limited-stage disease, 1611–1613, 1612t
    hematopoietic cell transplantation, 366
    historical perspective, 1610–1611
    nodular lymphocyte predominant disease, 1616
    recurrent disease, 1616
    unfavorable limited-stage disease, 1613
Holotranscobalamin, 593, 603
Holotransferrin, 622, 623f
Homocysteine, 598–599, 603, 1976, 2222
Homocystinuria (cbIE and cbIG), 607, 607t, 2222
Homogenous nucleation, 763
Homologous desensitization, 1877
Homologous recombination (HR), 453
Horn cells. *See* Keratocytes (horn cells)
Host defense
  basophils and mast cells in, 969–970
  iron deficiency and, 631–632
Howell-Jolly bodies
  characteristics, 467–468, 467f
  in hyposplenism, 868–869, 869f
  in megaloblastic anemia, 594
HOX11, 863, 1508t, 1513t
HOX11L2, 1508t
HOXA9, 234t, 266, 268
HOXB4, 266, 268
Hox family of transcription factors, 262
Hoyeraal-Hreidarsson syndrome, 531
HPAs. *See* Human platelet antigens (HPAs)
5-HPETE, 289
12-HPETE, 1877

HPFH. *See* Hereditary persistence of fetal hemoglobin (HPFH)
HPP. *See* Hereditary pyropoikilocytosis (HPP)
HPRT (hypoxanthine phosphoribosyltransferase), 1439
HPS (Hermansky-Pudlak syndrome). *See* Hermansky-Pudlak syndrome (HPS)
HR (homologous recombination), 453
HRE (hypoxia-response element), 484, 486
HS. *See* Hereditary spherocytosis (HS)
HS40, 730
HSCs. *See* Hematopoietic stem cells (HSCs)
HSCT. *See* Hematopoietic cell transplantation (HCT)
HSP (Henoch-Schönlein purpura), 1162, 2103–2104, 2103f
Hsp90, 219, 487
HSTCL (hepatosplenic T-cell lymphoma), 185t, 1498t, 1567, **1701**
HSV. *See under* Herpes simplex virus (HSV)
HSV-TK (herpes simplex virus thymidine kinase), 440
HTLV. *See* Human T lymphotropic virus (human T-cell leukemia/lymphoma virus) (HTLV)-1
HtrA2, 208
huCRIg(L), 1053f
huCRIg(S), 1053f
Human androgen-receptor gene (HUMARA), 883
Human Genome Project, 152
Human herpes virus (HHV)-6
  aplastic anemia and, 518
  mononucleosis syndrome and, 1268
  T-cell therapy, 412
Human herpes virus (HHV)-8
  in Castleman disease, 1249–1250, 1496t
  epidemiology, 1573–1574
  in Kaposi sarcoma, 1573
  in primary effusion lymphoma, 1246–1247, 1574
Human immunodeficiency virus (HIV)-1, 1239
Human immunodeficiency virus (HIV)-2, 1239
Human immunodeficiency virus (HIV)–associated malignancies, 1500t
  Burkitt lymphoma, 187, 1244f, 1245, 1247, 1672, 1676
  Castleman disease, 1249–1250
  diffuse large B-cell lymphoma, 187, 1243–1245, 1244f, 1247, 1571
  etiology, 1573

hematopoietic cell transplantation for, 1248
  hemophagocytic syndrome, 1250–1251, 1250t
  Hodgkin lymphoma. *See* Hodgkin lymphoma, HIV-associated
  incidence, 1243, 1244f, 1571
  Kaposi sarcoma–associated herpesvirus-associated inflammatory cytokine syndrome, 1250
  plasmablastic lymphoma, 1246
  primary central nervous system lymphoma, 1244f, 1246, 1579
  primary effusion lymphoma, 1246–1247, 1496t
  prognosis, 1247
Human immunodeficiency virus (HIV) infection
  anemia in
    causes, 1251–1252, 1251t
    incidence, 1251
    medication-related, 1252
    treatment, 1252
  antiphospholipid antibodies and, 2234, 2241
  aplastic anemia in, 518
  cardiovascular disease and, 2281
  CCR5 expression in, 440, 1240
  clinical features, 1240–1242
  as complication of factor VIII replacement, 2126
  disease progression, 1240–1242
  epidemiology and transmission, 1239–1240
  lymphocytopenia in, 1204
  malignancies in. *See* Human immunodeficiency virus (HIV)–associated malignancies
  mannose-binding lectin deficiency and, 1017
  mast cells in, 970, 972
  megaloblastic anemia in, 605
  mononucleosis syndrome in, 1268
  neutropenia in, 997, 1254
  opportunistic infections in, 1240–1241, 1241t
  pathogenesis, 1240
  persistent B19 parvovirus infection with red cell aplasia in, 543, 544, 545f, 1251–1252
  porphyria cutanea tarda in, 906–907
  in pregnancy, 1269
  prevention and cure, 1242–1243
  primary, 1240, 1268
  staging, 1240–1241, 1240t

thrombocytopenia in, 1252–1254, 1253t, 2009
thrombotic microangiopathy in, 1252
transfusion-related transmission of, 2370t
treatment
    antiretroviral therapy, 1242, 1242t
    gene therapy, 440–441, 454, 1243
Human leukocyte antigen (HLA), **2353–2356.** *See also* Major histocompatibility complex (MHC)
antibodies, 2356, 2385
class I, 2353–2354, 2354t
class II, 2353, 2354t
clinical applications, 2356
definition, 2353
genetics, 2353, 2355, 2355f
nomenclature, 2354–2355
structure and function, 2353–2354, 2354f
tumor-derived molecules, 421
typing, 2355–2356
Human leukocyte antigen (HLA)-A2, 1617, 2354f
Human leukocyte antigen (HLA) class II receptors, 1055–1056
Human leukocyte antigen (HLA)-DP, 1055, 1700
Human leukocyte antigen (HLA)-DQ, 1055, 1700
Human leukocyte antigen (HLA)-DQ2, 1699
Human leukocyte antigen (HLA)-DR, 948, 1055, 1647
    in adult T-cell leukemia/lymphoma, 1700
    in mycosis fungoides, 1682
Human leukocyte antigen (HLA)-DR2, 515
Human leukocyte antigen (HLA)-DR15, 1359
Human neutrophil antigens (HNAs), **2356–2359,** 2357t
antibodies, 2358–2359
HNA-1, 2356–2357
HNA-2, 2357–2358
HNA-3, 2358
HNA-4 and HNA-5, 2358
Human neutrophil peptides. *See* Defensins
Human platelet antigens (HPAs), **2359–2362**
alloantigens, 2359, 2360–2361t
clinical importance, 2362
detection methods, 2361–2362
genetics and structure, 2359
isoantigens, 2359
in newborn, 108
nomenclature, 2359, 2361
Human Reference Genome, 155
Human T lymphotropic virus (human T-cell leukemia/lymphoma virus) (HTLV)-1 infection

adult T-cell leukemia/lymphoma and, 1573, 1694, 1700
epidemiology, 1573
transfusion-related, 2370t
HUMARA (human androgen-receptor gene), 883
Humoral immunity
neonatal, 108–109
primary myelofibrosis and, 1325
in T-cell large granular lymphocytic leukemia, 1563
Humoral mediators, **268**
Huntington disease-like 2 (HDL2) disorder, 682
Hurler syndrome, 22f
HUS. *See* Hemolytic uremic syndrome (HUS)
Hyaladherins, 67t, 68
Hyaluronan, 266–267
Hybrid capture, 159–160, 159f
Hybrid leukemia, 1386
Hydroa aestivale, 890
Hydroa vacciniforme-like lymphoma, 1499t
Hydrocytosis, hereditary, 682t, **683–684**
Hydrogen peroxide, 284t, 286
    in drug-induced hemolysis, 706, 707f
    in erythrocyte metabolism, 698–699
5-Hydroperoxyeicosatetraenoic acid (5-HPETE), 289
12-Hydroperoxyeicosatetraenoic acid (12-HPETE), 1877
15-Hydroperoxyeicosatetraenoic acid (15-HETE), 952
Hydrops fetalis, 849, 851. *See also* Hemoglobin Bart's hydrops fetalis syndrome
Hydroxychloroquine
for antiphospholipid syndrome, 2245
for porphyria cutanea tarda, 908
Hydroxycobalamin, 589
Hydroxyethyl starch, 2079
2-Hydroxyglutarate (2-HG), 198
Hydroxyl radicals, 284t, 286, 2203
Hydroxymethylbilane, 891f
Hydroxymethylbilane synthase. *See* Porphobilinogen deaminase (PBGD)
5-Hydroxytryptamine (serotonin), 286t, 289, 1848, 1878–1879
Hydroxyurea, **325,** 336
adverse effects, 325, 1313–1314
for chronic eosinophilic leukemia, 1470
for chronic myelogenous leukemia, 1459
for chronic myeloproliferative disorders, 2081

for cytoreduction in chronic myelogenous leukemia, 1450
for essential thrombocythemia, 1313–1314, 1313t, 1314t, 2081
for hyperleukocytosis, 1286, 1397
megaloblastic anemia and, 605, 606t
for myelodysplastic syndromes, 1362
pharmacology, 325
for polycythemia vera, 1298–1299, 1298t
for primary myelofibrosis, 1329
for sickle cell disease, 774, 774t, 775f
Hydroxyzine, for mastocytosis, 976
Hyperactivity syndromes, iron deficiency and, 632
Hyperbilirubinemia, 832, 857
Hypercalcemia
in acute myelogenous leukemia, 1287, 1383
in chronic myelogenous leukemia, 1448–1449
in myeloma, 1502, 1744
HyperCVAD regimen
for acute lymphoblastic leukemia, 1516
for Burkitt lymphoma, 1675t, 1676
for hepatosplenic T-cell lymphoma, 1701
for HIV-associated lymphoma, 1245
Hyperdiploidy, 175t, 183, 222t, 224t
Hypereosinophilic syndromes. *See also* Chronic eosinophilic leukemia
eosinophilic fasciitis, 518, 960
eosinophilic granulomatosis with polyangiitis, 959–960
eosinophilorrachia, 960
eosinophiluria, 960
history and definition, 1469
idiopathic, **957–959**
neoplasms and, 959
toxic oil syndrome, 959
Hyperfibrinolysis, 2192, 2194
Hyperglycemia, 1519, 2203
Hyperhemolytic crisis, in sickle cell disease, 767
Hyperhomocysteinemia
acquired causes, 2224, 2224t
arterial thromboembolic disease risk and, 2227
clinical features, 2222
epidemiology, 2222t, 2224
etiology and pathogenesis, 598–599, 2224
venous thromboembolism risk and, 2222, 2224–2225, 2225t, 2226t
Hyperimmunoglobulin E syndrome (HIES), 1020t, 1026–1027, 1182, 1215t, **1225**

Hyperimmunoglobulin M syndromes, **1213–1215**
  autosomal recessive caused by intrinsic B-cell defect, 1215
  autosomal recessive with CD40 mutations, 1215
  clinical and laboratory features, 1214t
  definition, 1213
  genetic abnormalities, 1213
  X-linked, with CD40L deficiency, 993, 1213, 1575t
  X-linked anhydrotic ectodermal dysplasia with immunodeficiency caused by NEMO mutation, 1215
Hyperkalemia
  in acute myelogenous leukemia, 1287
  in chronic myelogenous leukemia, 1448–1449
Hyperleukocytic syndromes, **1285–1286**
  in acute lymphoblastic leukemia, 1514
  in acute myelogenous leukemia, 1285, 1384
  in chronic lymphocytic leukemia, 1540
  in chronic myelogenous leukemia, 1285, 1449
  clinical features, 1286t
  complications, 1285–1286, 1396–1397
  laboratory features, 1285
  pathogenesis, 1092
  treatment, 1286, 1397, 1514
Hyperparathyroidism, anemia and, 561
Hyperplastic granulopoiesis, 983
Hypersensitivity reactions, 1204, 2375
Hypersplenism, **863–867**. *See also* Splenomegaly
  clinical features, 864–865
  definition, 863
  imaging, 866f, 867f
  laboratory features, 866
  pathophysiology, 864, 865t
  therapy, course, and prognosis, 866–867
  thrombocytopenia and, 2013
Hypertension, maternal, neonatal neutropenia and, 994
Hyperthyroidism, anemia and, **559**
Hyperuricemia, 1286, 1448, 1450
Hyperviscosity syndrome, 1746, 1788–1789, 1789f, 1789t, 1792
Hypervolemia, 506, 510f
Hypobetalipoproteinemia, acanthocytosis, retinitis pigmentosa and pallidal degeneration (HARP) syndrome, 682
Hypochondriac, 863
Hypochromia, 21f
Hypodense eosinophils, 950

Hypodiploidy, 175t, 222t
Hypodysfibrinogenemia. *See* Dysfibrinogenemia/ hypodysfibrinogenemia
Hypoferremia, 551
Hypofibrinogenemia. *See* Afibrinogenemia/ hypofibrinogenemia
Hypofibrinogenemic hemorrhage, 1397
Hypogammaglobulinemia
  in chronic lymphocytic leukemia, 1531, 1541
  in myeloma, 1746
Hypohalous acids, 284t
Hypokalemia
  in acute myelogenous leukemia, 1287, 1383
  in chronic myelogenous leukemia, 1448–1449
Hyponatremia, in acute myelogenous leukemia, 1287, 1383
Hypopituitarism, anemia and, 560–561
Hypoplastic anemia, 637
Hypoplastic leukemia, 1384
Hyposplenism, **867–869**, 868t, 869f. *See also* Splenectomy
Hypothermia, 2014
Hypothyroidism
  acanthocytosis and, 680
  anemia of, **559**, 637
Hypotonic lysis, 809
Hypoxanthine-guanine phosphoribosyl transferase, 701t
Hypoxanthine phosphoribosyltransferase (HPRT), 1439
Hypoxia
  chemically induced, 876
  high-altitude. *See* High-altitude polycythemia
  macrophage phenotype and, 1071f
  physiologic processes regulated by, 504, 504f
  in pulmonary disease, 875
Hypoxia-inducible transcription factor (HIF)-1, 486–487, 486f, 1071f
Hypoxia-inducible transcription factor (HIF)-1α, 192, 196, 486–487, 503, 877
Hypoxia-inducible transcription factor (HIF)-2, 486–487, 486f, 503–504, 877, 1071f
Hypoxia-inducible transcription factor (HIF)-2α, 486–487, 486f, 510, 878
Hypoxia-inducible transcription factor (HIF)-2α mutations, 878
Hypoxia-response element (HRE), 484, 486
Hypoxia sensing, disorders of, 510, **876–878**

Chuvash polycythemia. *See* Chuvash polycythemia
  classic von Hippel-Lindau syndrome, 877–878
  EPAS1 gain of function mutations, 878
  proline hydroxylase deficiency, 878
  unexplained, 878

I

IAP (inhibitor of apoptosis) proteins, 207–208, 210, 1858–1859t
Iatrogenic lymphocytopenia, 1205–1206, 1205t
I blood group, 2332t, 2334t, 2339, 2344t
Ibrutinib, **342**
  adverse effects, 1203–1204, 1538
  for chronic lymphocytic leukemia, 1538, 1540
  for mantle cell lymphoma, 1658–1659, 1660t
  mechanism of action, 1529, 1538
  for Waldenström macroglobulinemia, 1795
Ibuprofen, 404, 2075
ICAM, 932, 1007, 1008, 1184, 1185f
ICAM-1 (CD54)
  in eosinophils, 948, 950
  in hemostasis, 1978
  in inflammatory response, 282–283
  in lymphocytes, 1184
  in malaria, 815
  in myeloma, 1712
  in neutrophils, 1008
ICAM-2 (CD102)
  in eosinophils, 950, 1008
  in hemostasis, 1978
  in lymphocytes, 1184
  in platelets, 1856, 1858t, 1859t, 1870
ICAM-4, 462
iCasp9 (inducible caspase-0 protein), 440, 440f
Iccosomes, 93
ICE regimen
  for hepatosplenic T-cell lymphoma, 1701
  for Hodgkin lymphoma, 1616
  for peripheral T-cell lymphoma, 1696
iCOS (CD278), 1184
Icterus, neonatal, 689, 707, 709
ID3, 1672
Idarubicin, **327–328**
  for acute myelogenous leukemia, 1395–1396, 1395t, 1402t
  for acute promyelocytic leukemia, 1404, 1405t
  adverse effects, 328, 1519t
  for myelodysplastic syndromes, 1361

Idelalisib, **1538**
    for chronic lymphocytic leukemia, 1529,
        1540
    for mantle cell lymphoma, 1659
Id family, 270
IDH (isocitrate dehydrogenase), 170, 198,
    199f, 337, 337f
IDH1/2
    in acute myelogenous leukemia, 226t,
        1376, 1378t, 1379
    in myelodysplastic syndromes, 228t, 1346t,
        1351
    in Ph-chromosome negative
        myeloproliferative neoplasms, 229t
IDH (isocitrate dehydrogenase) inhibitors,
    337f
Idiopathic CD4+ T lymphocytopenia, 1206
Idiopathic neutropenia, 995
Idiopathic pneumonia syndrome (IPS), 368
Idiopathic thrombocytopenic purpura. *See*
        Immune thrombocytopenia (ITP)
IFN. *See under* Interferon (IFN)
IFNG, 1573
Ifosfamide. *See also* CODOX-M/IVAC
        regimen
    for acute lymphoblastic leukemia, 1515
    for α-heavy-chain disease, 1808
    for Burkitt lymphoma, 1675, 1675t, 1676
    for diffuse large B-cell lymphoma, 1628
    for enteropathy-associated T-cell
        lymphoma, 1700
    high-dose, 331t, 332t
    for Hodgkin lymphoma, 1616
    for malignant histiocytic diseases, 1110
    mechanism of action, 329
    pharmacology, 330
Ig. *See under* Immunoglobulin (Ig)
IGF-1 (insulin-like growth factor-1), 487
IGH. *See* Immunoglobulin heavy-chain
        (IGH) genes
IGH
    in Burkitt lymphoma, 1598
    in chronic lymphocytic leukemia, 187,
        1592
    in myeloma, 188, 1735
IGHD, 1164f
IGHV
    in chronic lymphocytic leukemia, 231t
    in extranodal marginal zone lymphoma,
        1664, 1664t
    gene complex, 1164f
    in mantle cell lymphoma, 236t
    in nodal marginal zone lymphoma, 1667
    in splenic marginal zone lymphoma,
        1666
IGHV4-34, 828

IGHV (immunoglobulin heavy-chain
        variable) region, 1531, 1531t,
        1532t, 1542
IGJH, 1164f
IGKV, 1165f, 1166
IGLC, 1165f
IH7R, 232t
IHH (Indian hedgehog), 54
Ii (I/i) antigens, 835, 2333t, 2334t, 2337, 2340
I-κB, 209
I-κB-kinase (IKK), 251, 252, 298
Ikaros
    in gene activation, 167
    in hematopoietic stem cell to common
        lymphoid progenitor commitment,
        262
    in lymphopoiesis, 1155
IKBKG, 1215, 1220
IKKγ (inhibitor of κB kinase γ), 298
IKZF1
    in acute lymphoblastic leukemia, 183,
        1507, 1508
    in B-cell acute lymphoblastic leukemia,
        232t
    detection, 177f
    in Philadelphia chromosome-like B-cell
        acute lymphoblastic leukemia, 233t
    in Ph-negative myeloproliferative
        neoplasms, 229t
IL. *See under* Interleukin (IL)
IL2RB, 232t
IL2RG, 453, 1217
IL4, 1573
IL7R, 1217
Illumina sequencing-by-synthesis method,
        156–157, 156f
Imatinib
    for acute lymphoblastic leukemia, 1518
    for acute myelogenous leukemia, 1403
    adverse effects, 339t, 341, 1451t, 1453
    in children and older patients, 1452–1453
    for chronic eosinophilic leukemia, 1470
    for chronic myelogenous leukemia. *See*
        Chronic myelogenous (myeloid)
        leukemia (CML), therapy
    for chronic myelomonocytic leukemia,
        1469
    comparison with other tyrosine kinase
        inhibitors, 1451t
    drug interactions, 339t, 1451t
    gene mutations and response to, 1279,
        1452
    after hematopoietic cell transplantation,
        1461–1462
    for hypereosinophilic syndrome, 959
    for mastocytosis, 977

mechanism of action, 338
pharmacology, 338, 339t, 340–341
during pregnancy, 1459
for primary myelofibrosis, 1329
resistance to, 178, 318, 319t, 340–341,
        1279, 1456–1457, 1457t
structure, 340f
Imerslund-Gräsbeck disease, 607
Imiglucerase, for Gaucher disease, 1127
Imipenem, 384, 387t
Imiquimod, 1686
Imitation SWI- (ISWI-) remodelers, 166,
        166f
Immune antibodies, 2347–2348
Immune cell therapy (adoptive cellular
        therapy)
    future directions, 416
    of malignancy, **412–416**, 412t
        genetic retargeting of T cells for,
            414–416, 414f
        leukemia, **413–414**
        melanoma, **412–413**
    of viral diseases, **409–412**
        cytomegalovirus infection, **409–411**,
            410f, 411f
        Epstein-Barr virus infection, **411–412**
        multispecific T-cell therapy, 412
Immune complex mechanism, 830
Immune dysregulation, polyendocrinopathy,
        enteropathy, X-linked–like
        syndromes, **1223–1224**
Immune dysregulation, polyendocrinopathy,
        enteropathy, X-linked syndrome
        (IPEX syndrome), 1181, 1215t,
        1223
Immune function. *See also* Adaptive
        immunity; Innate immunity
    aging and, **135–136**, 136f
    basophilia and, 971
    eosinophils and, 952
    iron deficiency and, 631–632
    splenic, 91
    T-cell disorders and impaired, 1195–1197
Immune neutropenia, 995
Immune reconstitution inflammatory
        syndrome (IRIS), 1242
Immune-related fibrosis, 1330
Immune senescence, 136
Immune thrombocytopenia (ITP),
        1999–2009
    primary
        bleeding risk in, 2001–2002, 2002t
        in children, 2001, 2002t
        classification, 2001
        clinical features, 2001–2002, 2002t, 2107
        differential diagnosis, 2003

Immune thrombocytopenia (ITP),
     primary (*Cont.*):
   genetic factors, 2001
   history, 1999–2000
   incidence, 2001
   laboratory features, 2002–2003
   pathophysiology, 2000–2001, 2084–2085
   during pregnancy, 121–122, 2010–2011
   therapy
     for acute bleeding, 2003, 2085, 2385
     adjunctive, 2007
     anti-(Rh)D, 2005
     azathioprine, 2006
     cyclophosphamide, 2007
     cyclosporine, 2007
     danazol, 2007
     dapsone, 2007
     glucocorticoids, 2003–2004
     initial management, 2003
     intravenous immunoglobulin,
       2004–2005
     rituximab, 2005
     splenectomy, 2004
     thrombopoietic receptor agonists,
       1825, 2005–2006
     vinca alkaloids, 2007
   types, 1999*t*
   secondary
     in antiphospholipid syndrome, 2008
     in bacterial infections, 1856
     in chronic lymphocytic leukemia,
       1541–1542
     etiology, 2007–2008, 2007*f*
     in hepatitis C infection, 2009
     in HIV infection, 1252–1254, 1253*t*,
       1999
     in *H. pylori* infection, 2009–2010
     incidence, 2007*f*
     in systemic lupus erythematosus,
       2008–2009
     in viral infections, 1513, 2009
Immunization
   antibodies generated in response to,
     2347–2348
   complications, **7**
Immunoadsorption apheresis, 429*t*, 430*t*
Immunobead assay, 2000
Immunodeficiency diseases, **1211–1232**
   cartilage hair hypoplasia, 993, **1226**
   chromosomal instability syndromes
     associated with, **1226–1227**
     ataxia-telangiectasia.
       See Ataxia-telangiectasia
     ataxia-telangiectasia-like disorder,
       1227
     Bloom syndrome, **1227**, 1507, 1575*t*

Nijmegen breakage syndrome, 530*t*,
     1227, 1575*t*
     rare, 1227
   clinical features, 1213*t*, 1214–1215*t*
   combined immunodeficiencies. *See*
     Combined immunodeficiencies
     (CID)
   cytotoxicity disorders, **1227–1229**
     Chédiak-Higashi syndrome. *See*
       Chédiak-Higashi syndrome
     familial hemophagocytic
       lymphohistiocytosis, **1228**, 1849,
       2061
     Griscelli syndrome, 994, 1020, 1229,
       1849
     Hermansky-Pudlak syndrome. *See*
       Hermansky-Pudlak syndrome
       (HPS)
     X-linked lymphoproliferative disease,
       1228–1229, 1266, 1575*t*
   in defective thymic development
     CHARGE syndrome, 1222
     congenital alopecia and absence of
       thymus, 1223
     DiGeorge syndrome, 86–87, **1222**
   genetically determined deficiencies of
     complement system, **1232**
   hyperimmunoglobulin E syndromes,
     1020*t*, 1026–1027, 1182, 1215*t*,
     1225
   laboratory features, 1214–1215*t*
   lymphocytopenia in, 1204
   lymphomas and, 1574, 1575*t*
   neutropenia in, 993
   predominant antibody deficiencies,
     1212–1216
     clinical features, 1213*t*, 1214*t*
     common variable immunodeficiency
       and selective IgA deficiency, 993,
       1214*t*, **1216**
     hyperimmunoglobulin M syndromes.
       See Hyperimmunoglobulin M
       syndromes
     laboratory features, 1214*t*
     lipopolysaccharide responsive beige-like
       anchor deficiency, 1216
     X-linked and autosomal recessive
       agammaglobulinemia, 993,
       1212–1213, 1214*t*
   primary, presenting as autoimmune
     diseases, **1223–1224**
     autoimmune lymphoproliferative
       syndrome, 210, **1224**, 1575*t*
     autoimmune polyendocrinopathy,
       candidiasis, and ectodermal
       dystrophy syndrome, 87, 1181, **1224**

     immune dysregulation,
       polyendocrinopathy, enteropathy,
       X-linked–like syndromes,
       1223–1224
     immune dysregulation,
       polyendocrinopathy, enteropathy,
       X-linked syndrome, 1181, 1215*t*,
       1223
     Schimke syndrome, 1226
   with selective susceptibility to pathogens,
     1230–1231
     impaired signaling through toll-like
       receptors, **1230**
     Mendelian susceptibility to
       mycobacterial disease, **1231**
   severe combined immunodeficiency.
     See Severe combined
     immunodeficiency (SCID)
   WASp-interacting protein deficiency,
     1225
   WHIM syndrome, 994, **1226**
   Wiskott-Aldrich syndrome. *See* Wiskott-
     Aldrich syndrome (WAS)
Immunogenicity, 2336
Immunoglobulin (Ig)
   allotypes, 1170
     heavy-chain, 1170
     light-chain, 1170–1171
   in B-cell development, 1151
   B-cell disorders and defects in, 1195, 1501
   genetics, **1163–1169**
     gene complexes, 1163–1164, 1164*f*,
       1165*f*, 1166*f*
     gene rearrangement, 1166–1168, 1167*f*
     heavy-chain class switching, 1168–1169
     mechanisms for generating antibody
       diversity, 1169
     surrogate λ light chains, 1168
   idiotypes, 1160
   IgA. *See* Immunoglobulin (Ig) A
   IgD. *See* Immunoglobulin (Ig) D
   IgE. *See* Immunoglobulin (Ig) E
   IgG. *See* Immunoglobulin (Ig) G
   IgM. *See* Immunoglobulin (Ig) M
   for immune-related fibrosis, 1330
   oligoclonal, 1725–1726
   structure and function, **1159–1163**
     biologic properties, 1160*t*
     heavy chains, 1161*t*, 1162*f*, 1163
     light chains, 1159
     physical properties, 1159, 1160*f*, 1160*t*
     surface immunoglobulin, 1163
   synthesis and secretion, **1171–1172**
   therapy. *See* Intravenous immunoglobulin
     (IVIg)
   variable-region structure, 1170

Immunoglobulin (Ig) A
  in α-heavy-chain disease, 1806
  in ataxia-telangiectasia, 1226
  blood group activity and, 2347
  in class switching, 1168
  in complement system, 290
  in γ-heavy-chain disease, 1804
  immune antibodies, 2348
  levels in newborns, 108
  in mycosis fungoides, 1680
  in myeloma, 1714
  naturally occurring antibodies, 2347
  selective deficiency, 1214t, **1216**, 2375
  structure and function, 1160t, **1161–1162**,
      1161t
Immunoglobulin (Ig)-α. See CD79a (Ig-α)
Immunoglobulin (Ig) A monoclonal
      gammopathy, 1722, 1722t, 1725,
      1727, 1741. See also Essential
      monoclonal gammopathy
Immunoglobulin (Ig) A nephropathy, 1161
Immunoglobulin (Ig)-β (CD79b), 1162, 1162f
Immunoglobulin (Ig) D
  pre-B cells and, 1168
  structure and function, 1160t, 1161t, 1162
Immunoglobulin (Ig) D+, 863
Immunoglobulin (Ig) E
  in ataxia-telangiectasia, 1226
  in chronic inflammation, 291
  excess levels. See Hyperimmunoglobulin E
      syndrome (HIES)
  in mycosis fungoides, 1680
  structure and function, 1160t, 1161t,
      1162–1163
Immunoglobulin (Ig) E-associated responses,
      932, 969, 971
Immunoglobulin (Ig) family cell adhesion
      molecules, 1858–1859t, 1868–1870
Immunoglobulin (Ig) G
  atherosclerosis and, 2287
  in autoimmune hemolytic anemia, 823,
      834, 834f, 835
  blood group activity and, 2343
  in complement system, 289–290, 289f
  cryoglobulinemia and, 2097
  direct antiglobulin test reaction patterns,
      834t
  eosinophil receptors for, 953
  human body content of, 1171
  immune antibodies, 2348
  immune thrombocytopenia and, 2000
  infusions. See Intravenous
      immunoglobulin (IVIg)
  levels in newborns, 108
  major subclasses, 1161t
  in myeloma, 1714

  naturally occurring antibodies, 2347
  in newborn, 106
  structure and function, **1160–1161**, 1160f,
      1160t, 1161t
Immunoglobulin (Ig) G+ B lymphocytes, 863
Immunoglobulin (Ig) G monoclonal
      gammopathy, 1722, 1722t, 1725,
      1727, 1741. See also Essential
      monoclonal gammopathy
Immunoglobulin heavy-chain (IGH) genes
  in chronic lymphocytic leukemia, 1531,
      1531t, 1532t, 1542
  in myeloma, 1734–1735, 1735f, 1736t
  structure, 1163–1164, 1164f, 1167f
Immunoglobulin light-chain (AL)
      amyloidosis
  chromosomal abnormalities, 1712, 1774
  clinical features, 1744–1745, 1760, 1774–
      1775, 1774f, 1775f, 1775t
    cardiac, 1777–1779, 1778f
    hepatic, 1779
    neurologic, 1779
    renal, 1776–1777
  course and prognosis, 1781–1782
  definition and history, 1773
  diagnosis, 1760, 1779t
  differential diagnosis, 1775–1776, 1776f
  epidemiology, 1773
  etiology and pathogenesis, 1781–1782
  laboratory features, 1775
  treatment, 1760–1761, **1779–1781**
Immunoglobulin (Ig) light chains, 1159
  allotypes, 1170–1171
  in amyloidosis, 1773–1774. See also
      Immunoglobulin light-chain (AL)
      amyloidosis
  in essential monoclonal gammopathy,
      1708, 1721
  gene complexes, 1165f, 1167f
  laboratory evaluation, 1714
  in myeloma, 1714, 1741, 1742f
  surrogate λ, 1168
  vasculopathy, 2099
Immunoglobulin (Ig) M
  atherosclerosis and, 2287
  in autoimmune hemolytic anemia, 2348
  blood group activity and, 2343, 2347
  in complement system, 289, 289f
  excess levels. See Hyperimmunoglobulin
      M syndromes
  immune antibodies, 2348
  naturally occurring antibodies, 2347
  pre-B cells and, 1168
  production, 1151
  structure and function, 1160t, 1161t, **1162**,
      1162f

  synthesis, 1171
  in Waldenström macroglobulinemia, 1714,
      1788–1791, 1789t
Immunoglobulin (Ig) M+ B lymphocytes,
      863
Immunoglobulin (Ig) M monoclonal
      gammopathy, 1722, 1722t, 1725.
      See also Essential monoclonal
      gammopathy
Immunoglobulin (Ig) M myeloma, 1760
Immunoglobulin (Ig) superfamily, **66**, 67t,
      282t
Immunological synapse, 1185–1186
Immunologic theory of aging, 131
Immunomodulation, of macrophage
      phenotype, 1084, 1085f
Immunomodulatory drugs, **333–335**, 333f.
      See also specific drugs
  for myeloma, 1754
  for sickle cell disease, 774t, 775
Immunoosseous dysplasias
  cartilage hair hypoplasia, 993, **1226**
  Schimke syndrome, **1226**
Immunophenotyping, 35
  of abnormal population, **37–38**
  methodology, **36–37**
  of mycosis fungoides, 1682, 1682f
Immunoproliferative small intestinal disease
      (IPSID), 1663, 1665, 1808, 1809
Immunoreceptor tyrosine-based activation
      motifs (ITAMs)
  Fc receptors and, 1053f
  glycoprotein VI and, 1869
  immunoglobulins and, 1162f, 1163
  Src binding and, 1016
  T-cell receptors and, 1176f, 1178
Immunoreceptor tyrosine-based switch motif
      (ITSM), 1868
Immunoreceptor tyrosine inhibitory motif
      (ITIM), 1184, 1190, 1868, 1884
Immunosuppressive therapy
  for acquired hemophilia A, 2186
  for aplastic anemia, 523–526, 524t, 525t
  for autoimmune hemolytic anemia, 839
  lymphoma and, 1574
  for myelodysplastic syndromes, 1359
  for pure red cell aplasia, 544
Immunotherapy
  for acute myelogenous leukemia, 1404
  dendritic cells in, 310
  for hemophagocytic lymphohistiocytosis,
      1115
  natural killer cells in, 1192
Immunothrombosis, 1940–1941, 1941f
Immunotoxins, **345–346**
Impairment of consciousness, history of, 5

IMPDH1/2, 200
Impotence, history of, 5
IMPs (intramembrane particles), 1047
Inborn errors of metabolism, 890
Inclusion body β-thalassemia, 732
Incomplete infarction, 2269
Indian blood group/antigens, 2332t, 2337, 2346t
Indian hedgehog (IHH), 54
Indomethacin
    antiplatelet effects, 404, 2075
    for patent ductus arteriosus, 107
Induced pluripotent stem cells (iPSCs), 448–449
Induced proximity model, 205
Inducible caspase-0 protein (iCasp9), 440, 440f
Induction of hepatic ALASI, 901
I-negative phenotype (i adult), 2343
Infants. *See* Newborns/infants
Infection
    atherosclerosis and, 2288
    bacterial. *See* Bacterial infections
    blood group association, 2341–2342t
    bone marrow infiltration, 33, 33f
    disseminated intravascular coagulation and, 2204t, 2207
    eosinophilia in, 955t
    fungal. *See* Fungal infections
    hemolytic anemia caused by.
        See Hemolytic anemia, infection-related
    in hemophilia A, 2126
    in immunocompromised host, **383–389**
        bacterial, 369, 383, 384–385, 388–389
        cytomegalovirus, 1267–1268
        diagnosis, 384
        fungal, 369, 383, 385–386, 389
        after hematopoietic cell transplantation, 357, **368–370**, 389
        mycobacterial, 384, 386
        prevention, **388–389**
        risk factors, **383**
        treatment, **384–388**
            adjustments, 386
            duration, 386
            of fever after recovery from chemotherapy, 386, 388
            initial, 384–386, 387–388t
            outpatient, 388
            viral, 369–370, 383–384, 386, 389
    lymphocytopenia and, 1204–1205
    lymphocytosis and, 1204
    monocytosis and, 1097
    neutropenia and, 991, 997
    neutrophilia and, 1000–1001, 1000t

parasitic. *See* Parasitic infections
platelet function in, 1855–1856
purpura and, 2104–2105, 2104f, 2105f
recurrent, workup of, 1034f
red cell antigens and susceptibility to, 2340
susceptibility to
    in acute lymphoblastic leukemia, 1514
    in chronic granulomatous disease, 1029–1030, 1031t
    in chronic lymphocytic leukemia, 1528, 1530, 1541
    in Gaucher disease, 1125
    in hairy cell leukemia, 1555–1556, 1559
    in HIV infection, 1240–1241, 1241t
    in immunodeficiency diseases. *See* Immunodeficiency diseases
    in myeloma, 1745–1746
    in sickle cell disease, 773
    in thalassemias, 742
    thrombotic microangiopathy and, 2260–2261
    viral. *See* Viral infections
Infectious mononucleosis. *See* Mononucleosis syndromes
Inferior vena cava filter, 2278
Infertility. *See* Reproductive system disorders
Infiltrative lesions, history of, 6
Inflammasome pathway, **299**, 300f
Inflammasomes, 284, 1063, 1065f, 1066f
Inflammation. *See also* Inflammatory response
    anemia of. *See* Anemia of inflammation (AI)
    in atherosclerosis. *See* Atherosclerosis, inflammation and
    chronic, 279, **290–291**
    in disseminated intravascular coagulation, 2200, 2201
    endothelial, 2283
    frailty and, 137
    hepcidin regulation by, 622
    monocytosis and, 1097
    thrombocytosis in, 2035–2036
Inflammatory bowel disease, 1229
Inflammatory lipids, 288–289
Inflammatory response, **279–291**. *See also* Inflammation
    acute, 279, **280–285**
        acute-phase response, 284–285
        hemodynamic changes in, 280, 281f
        leukocyte adhesion and transmigration in, 280–283, 282f, 282t
        leukocyte chemotaxis and activation in, 283–284
    basophilia and, 971
    characteristics, 279–280

chronic, 279, **290–291**
history, 279
molecular changes in, **1976–1979**
    acute, 1978
    adhesion molecules, 1978
    chronic, 1978
    immediate, 1976–1978
    inflammatory mediators, 1979t
    leukocyte-endothelial cell matrix interactions promoting coagulation, 1979
    leukocyte-platelet and endothelial cell-platelet interactions, 1977t, 1978–1979
monocytes/macrophages in, **1083–1086**
    cytokine-induced priming and, 1085–1086, 1086f
    G-protein–coupled receptors in, 1059, 1060t
    immunomodulation of, 1084, 1084f
    innate activation of, 1084
    recruitment of, 1083–1084, 1084f
natural anticoagulants and, 2202
neutrophilia and, 1000–1001, 1000t
platelets in, 1855–1856
regulation, **286–290**, 286t
    coagulation system in, 290
    complement system in, 289–290
    cytokines and chemokines in, 287–288, 287t, 288t
    inflammatory lipids in, 288–289
    kinins in, 289
    lysosomal granule constituents in, 287
    neutrophil apoptosis in, 285
    proteinase-activated receptors in, 290
    reactive nitrogen intermediates in, 286–287
    reactive oxygen intermediates in, 286
    vasoactive amines in, 289
    repair process and, 280, 290–291
    resolution, **285–286**
    in sickle cell disease, 765
    suppressive effects on erythropoietin precursors, 550
Infliximab, 1359
Influenza, 1064f
Inhibitor of apoptosis (IAP) proteins, 207–208, 210, 1858–1859t
Inhibitor of κB kinase γ (IKKγ), 298
Inhibitory signals, 253
Innate immunity, **293–304**
    activation of adaptive immunity and, 303–304
    vs. adaptive immunity, **293**, 294t
    atherosclerosis and, 2285–2286
    dendritic cells and, 307

effector cytokines in, 303
inappropriate response of, 304
innate defects, 304
platelet coagulant activity and, 1855
sensors of the nucleotide-binding
    oligomerization domain-like
    receptor family in, **298–300**, 299f,
    300f, 301f
sensors of the RIG-I-like helicase pathways
    in, **300–303**, 302f
toll-like receptors in. *See* Toll-like
    receptors (TLRs)
types, 293–294
Innocent bystander mechanism, 830
Inosine triphosphatase, 701t
Inositol 1,4,5-triphosphate (IP$_3$), 935, 1016,
    1836, 1840
INR (international normalized ratio),
    395–396, 396t
Insulin-like growth factor-1 (IGF-1), 487
Insulin receptor substrates, 251
Integral membrane proteins. *See* Membrane
    proteins, integral
Integrin activation deficiency disease (LAD,
    LAD-1 variant), 1019t, 1024, 2060
Integrin α$_2$β$_1$ (GPIa/IIa, CD49b/CD29,
    VLA-2, collagen receptor),
    1864–1865
    characteristics, 1858–1859t
    in collagen activation of platelets,
        1879–1881, 1880f
    gene mutations, 1864
    in platelets, 1833, 1847t, 1851, 1858–1859t,
        1864
    structure, 1847t, 1864
    synthesis, 1847t
Integrin α$_2$β$_1$ (GPIa/IIa, CD49b/CD29,
    VLA-2, collagen receptor)
    deficiency, 2051
Integrin α$_{IIb}$β$_3$ (GPIIb/IIIa, fibrinogen
    receptor, CD41/CD61), **1861–1864**
    abnormalities
        in Glanzmann thrombasthenia. *See*
            Glanzmann thrombasthenia
        select macrothrombocytopenias, 2047
    activation, 1836, 1837, 1838f, 1860f,
        1863–1864
    biogenesis, 2043–2044, 2043f
    in clot retraction, 1842
    fibrinogen binding to, 1861
    immune thrombocytopenia and, 2000
    inside-out activation, 1860f, 1862–1863,
        1863f, 1883–1884
    outside-in signaling by, 1851, 1860f,
        1862–1863, 1863f, 1883–1884
    platelet activation and, 2293

in platelet adhesion, 1834, 1847t, 1979
in platelet aggregation, 1863–1864
in platelet spreading, 1841–1842
prothrombin and, 1854
structure, 1184, 1860f, 1861–1862
in thrombocytopenia, 2008
variants, 1851
von Willebrand factor binding to, 2168
Integrin α$_{IIb}$β$_3$ receptor antagonists, 405–406,
    1855, 1995–1996, 2074t, 2077,
    2296. *See also* Abciximab
Integrin α$_{IIb}$β$_3$ receptors, 1833–1834, 1861,
    2043–2044, 2043f
Integrin α$_4$β$_1$ (VLA-4), 261, 949, 950, 1185,
    1737, 1977t
Integrin α$_4$β$_7$, 1138–1139
Integrin α$_5$β$_1$ (GPIc*/IIa, fibronectin receptor,
    VLA-5, CD49e/CD29), 261, 1847t,
    1858–1859t, **1865**
Integrin α$_6$β$_1$ (GPIc/IIa, laminin receptor,
    VLA-6, CD49f/CD29), 1847t,
    1858–1859t, **1865**
Integrin α$_M$β$_2$. *See* CD11b/CD18 (Mac-1,
    Mo1, CR3, α$_M$β$_2$)
Integrin α$_v$β$_3$ (vitronectin receptor, CD51/
    CD61), 1847t, 1858–1859t, **1865**,
    2043f, 2044
Integrin β$_1$, 282–283, 1007
Integrin β$_2$
    in leukocyte adhesion, 282–283, 282f, 282t
    in lymphocytes, 1138–1139
    in monocyte adhesion, 1059
    in neutrophils, 2358
Integrin β$_3$, 1851, 1885
Integrins, **66**, 67t, 1858–1859t, **1861–1865**
    in cell signaling, **250**, 1015
    in hematopoietic stem cells, **260–261**
    inflammatory response and, 1083
    in leukocyte activation, 284
    in leukocyte adhesion, 282–283, 282f, 282t
    monocytes and, 1059
    in neutrophil adhesion, 1007, 1007f
    neutrophils and, 1007
    in sickle cell disease, 764–765
    in T-cell adhesion, 1184
    trafficking of hematopoietic stem cells and,
        355
Integrin transmembrane complex, 1862f
Intercellular adhesion molecules. *See under*
    ICAM
Interdigitating cells, 309. *See also* Dendritic
    cells (DCs)
Interdigitating dendritic cell sarcoma, 1110
Interferon (IFN)
    in innate immune response, 303
    for primary myelofibrosis, 1329–1330

signaling pathways, 1069f
spleen and production of, 1082
thalidomide and, 334
Interferon (IFN)-α
    adverse effects, 1314, 1459
    for chronic myelogenous leukemia, 1459
    in chronic myelogenous leukemia,
        1440–1441
    with cladribine, for mastocytosis, 977
    for congenital dyserythropoietic anemia
        type I, 566
    for Erdheim-Chester disease, 1111
    for essential thrombocythemia, 1313t,
        1314
    for follicular lymphoma, 1647–1648
    for hairy cell leukemia, 1553
    for lymphomatoid papulosis, 1689
    in macrophages, 1064, 1069f
    in megakaryopoiesis, 1823
    for mycosis fungoides, 1687
    natural killer cells and, 1191
    in neutrophils, 933t
    for polycythemia vera, 1298t, 1299
    during pregnancy, 1459
    for primary myelofibrosis, 1329–1330
    production, 309
    for thrombocytopenia, 1824
Interferon (IFN)-β, 1064, 1069f, 1823
Interferon (IFN)-β promoter stimulator 1
    (IPS-I). *See* Mitochondrial antiviral
    signaling protein (MAVS)
Interferon (IFN)-γ, 291
    in aplastic anemia, 515
    for chronic granulomatous disease, 1012
    in inflammatory response, 1978
    in large granular lymphocytic leukemia,
        1203
    in macrophage activation, 308, 1070t, 1085
    in megakaryopoiesis, 1823
    in natural killer cells, 1189
    in newborn, 107
    in nitrogen metabolism, 1069f
    for primary myelofibrosis, 1329–1330
    in reactive thrombocytosis, 2036
    in Th cells, 1180
    in vaccines, 422
Interferon (IFN)-γR1 deficiency, 1231
Interferon (IFN)-γR2 deficiency, 1231
γ-Interferon (IFN)-inducible protein, 288t
Interferon-regulated factor 8 (IRF8), 235t,
    1231
Interferon regulatory factor 4 (IRF4),
    1171–1172, 1710, 1710f
Interferon (INF) response factor (IRF), 297f,
    298
Interferon-stimulated gene 15 (ISG15), 1231

Interleukin (IL)-1
  aplastic anemia and, 519, 526
  in disseminated intravascular coagulation, 2200, 2202
  in familial Mediterranean fever, 1025
  fibrinolysis and, 2202
  hematopoiesis and, 258f
  in hematopoietic stem cells, 264t
  in inflammation, 287–288, 287t
  in inflammatory response, 1978
  interleukin-6 production and, 2036
  matrix association, 62t
  monocytopenia and, 1091
  in neutrophils, 932, 934
Interleukin (IL)-1α, 303
Interleukin (IL)-1β
  in disseminated intravascular coagulation, 2208
  in inflammation, 281, 282, 284, 287–288
  in innate immune response, 303
  in neutrophils, 932, 933t
  in primary myelofibrosis, 1325
  in sickle cell disease, 765
  Th17 T cells and, 1182
Interleukin-1-β-converting enzyme-protease activating factor (Ipaf), 1066f
Interleukin (IL)-2, 264t
  for acute myelogenous leukemia, 1404
  in aplastic anemia, 515
  in cellular therapy, 412
  in large granular leukocytic leukemia, 1203
  in lymphopoiesis, 1154
  T-cell receptors and, 1178, 1181
  in vaccine therapy, 422
Interleukin (IL)-2R, 1154
Interleukin (IL)-2Rα, 1700
Interleukin (IL)-2 receptor antibody. See Daclizumab
Interleukin (IL)-2 receptor family, 248f, 249
Interleukin (IL)-3
  basophils and, 966
  BCR-ABL1 and, 1441
  BFU-E and, 483f
  for Diamond-Blackfan anemia, 540
  eosinophils and, 947, 949
  hematopoiesis and, 258f
  in hematopoietic stem cells, 264t
  in inflammatory response, 1978
  in megakaryopoiesis, 1817, 1821
  in myeloma, 1713
  neutrophilic granulopoiesis and, 940
Interleukin (IL)-4
  basophil-derived, 968
  in basophils, 932
  in eosinophils, 950, 952
  hematopoiesis and, 258f

  in hematopoietic stem cells, 264t
  in inflammatory response, 1978
  lymphoma and, 1573
  in lymphopoiesis, 1154
  macrophage activation and, 1070t, 1085–1086
  in macrophages, 1064, 1066
  monocytes and, 1046
  in neutrophils, 932
  T_FH cells and, 1182
  Th cells and, 1180
  in vaccine therapy, 422
Interleukin (IL)-5, 264t, 947, 949, 950, 951
Interleukin (IL)-5Rα, 1141
Interleukin (IL)-6
  in Castleman disease, 1249–1250
  in disseminated intravascular coagulation, 2200, 2201, 2208
  in heat stroke, 2209
  in hematopoietic stem cells, 264t
  hepcidin and, 551, 552, 620
  in Hodgkin lymphoma, 1610
  in inflammation, 284, 288
  in innate immune response, 303
  in large granular leukocytic leukemia, 1203
  in megakaryopoiesis, 1821
  monocytopenia and, 1091
  in myeloma, 1709, 1759
  in neutrophils, 933t
  in primary myelofibrosis, 1325
  in sickle cell disease, 765
  in thrombopoiesis, 2035–2036
Interleukin (IL)-6 receptor family, 247–248, 248f
Interleukin (IL)-7
  in hematopoiesis, 258f
  in hematopoietic stem cells, 264t
  in lymphopoiesis, 270, 1154
  in severe combined immune deficiency, 1217
Interleukin (IL)-7Rα, 1154, 1214t
Interleukin (IL)-8 (neutrophil-activating peptide 1)
  in disseminated intravascular coagulation, 2208
  in heat stroke, 2209
  lymphoma and, 1573
  in neutrophils, 288t, 932, 1007, 1007f, 1844
Interleukin (IL)-9, 264t, 950, 1154
Interleukin (IL)-10
  in Hodgkin lymphoma, 1607, 1610, 1617
  lymphoma and, 1573
  macrophage activation and, 1086
  macrophage deactivation and, 1070t
  monocytes and, 1091
  monocytosis and, 1097

  in neutrophils, 932, 1008
  T_FH cells and, 1182
  Th cells and, 1180
  in vaccine therapy, 422
Interleukin (IL)-11
  in hematopoietic stem cells, 264t
  in megakaryopoiesis, 1821
  for thrombocytopenia, 1824
Interleukin (IL)-12
  immunodeficiencies and, 1230
  in innate immune response, 303
  monocytopenia and, 1091
  mycobacterial disease and, 1231
  in neutrophils, 933t
  Th cells and, 1180
Interleukin (IL)-12p40 deficiency, 1231
Interleukin (IL)-12R, 1231
Interleukin (IL)-12Rβ₁ deficiency, 1231
Interleukin (IL)-13
  basophil-derived, 968
  in basophils, 932
  macrophage activation and, 1070t, 1085–1086
Interleukin (IL)-15
  in hematopoietic stem cells, 264t
  in neutrophils, 932, 934
  in vaccine therapy, 422
Interleukin (IL)-15R, 1154
Interleukin (IL)-17, 1182
Interleukin (IL)-21, 264t, 1154, 1172, 1699
Interleukin (IL)-22, 1182, 1699
Interleukin (IL)-23, 1182
Interleukin receptor-associated kinase (IRAK), 298
Interleukin receptor-associated kinase (IRAK)-4 deficiency, 1054, 1230
Interlineal leukemia, 1386
International normalized ratio (INR), 395–396, 396t
Intestinal disorders. See Gastrointestinal tract disorders
Intraarterial thrombolysis, 2315–2316
Intracranial hemorrhage, 2119, 2123, 2315
Intramembrane particles (IMPs), 1047
Intraocular lymphoma, 1580–1581
Intravascular large B-cell lymphoma, 1496t, 1626, 1635–1636
Intravenous immunoglobulin (IVIg)
  for acquired von Willebrand disease, 2082
  for agammaglobulinemia, 1213
  for alloimmune hemolytic disease of the fetus and newborn, 857–858
  for antiphospholipid syndrome in pregnancy, 2245
  for aplastic anemia, 527
  for autoimmune hemolytic anemia, 838

for chronic lymphocytic leukemia, 1541
for immune-related myelofibrosis, 1330
for immune thrombocytopenia, 2000,
    2003, 2004–2005, 2011
for neuropathy, 1724
for persistent B19 parvovirus infection,
    544–545
for X-linked anhydrotic ectodermal
    dysplasia, 1215
Intrinsic factor
    assays of, 603
    in cobalamin absorption, 591, 591t
    congenital deficiency, 605
    in pernicious anemia, 18
Intrinsic mutagenesis theory of aging, 130,
    130t
Introns, 147
Invariant CD3 proteins, 1176, 1176f
Inversions, chromosomal
    in acute myelogenous leukemia, 180–181,
        1377, 1384t, 1414–1415
    definition, 175t
Iodine, radioactive
    in plasma labeling, 488
    in transplant preparation, 360
Ion Torrent platform, 157–158, 157f
IP₃ (inositol 1,4,5-triphosphate), 935, 1016,
    1836, 1840
Ipaf (interleukin-1-β-converting
    enzyme-protease activating factor),
    1066f
IPEX syndrome (immune dysregulation,
    polyendocrinopathy, enteropathy,
    X-linked syndrome), 1181, 1215t,
    1223
IPH2101, 1192
IPS (idiopathic pneumonia syndrome), 368
iPSCs (induced pluripotent stem cells),
    448–449
IPS-I (interferon-β promoter stimulator
    1). See Mitochondrial antiviral
    signaling protein (MAVS)
IPSID (immunoproliferative small intestinal
    disease), 1663, 1665, 1808, 1809
IRAK (interleukin receptor-associated
    kinase), 298, 1230
IRAK (interleukin receptor-associated
    kinase)-4 deficiency, 1054, 1230
IREs (iron-responsive elements), 623, 624f
IRF (interferon response factor), 297f, 298
IRF4 (interferon regulatory factor 4),
    1171–1172, 1710, 1710f
IRF4 (MUM1), 234t
IRF8 (interferon-regulated factor 8), 235t,
    1231
Irinotecan, 326–327

IRIS (immune reconstitution inflammatory
    syndrome), 1242
Iron
    bioavailability, 618–619
    dietary, 618–619, 618t
    distribution, 617–618, 618t
    inhibition of intestinal absorption of, 552
    labile pool, 618
    levels of, in newborn, 104
    malabsorption, 630
    metabolism
        absorption and, 619–622, 619f
        erythrocyte production and, 490–491,
            491f, 491t
        excretion and, 624–625
        homeostasis and, 620–622, 620f, 621t,
            623
        in iron deficiency anemia, 552, 553t
        macrophages in, 1063, 1065f
        regulation by hypoxia, 504f
        in sideroblastic anemia, 918
        in thalassemia, 742
    mitochondrial, 623–624
    in myoglobin, 618
    overload, 641. See also Hemochromatosis
    poisoning, 638–639
    radioactive, in red cell labeling, 488
    recycling, 619
    storage compartments, 617–618, 618t
    therapeutic. See Iron therapy
    toxicity, 640–641
    transport, 622–624, 622f
        erythroblast and, 623–624
        across intestinal mucosa, 619, 620f
        intracellular iron homeostasis and, 623,
            625f
        transferrin endocytosis in, 622–623,
            623f, 624f
    turnover, 490–491, 490f
    unavailability, 551–552, 551f
Iron-binding capacity, 634
Iron chelation therapy
    for congenital dyserythropoietic anemia,
        567
    for hemochromatosis, 644
    for iron overload in sickle cell disease, 776
    monitoring, 752
    for myelodysplastic syndromes, 1358
    for thalassemias, 751–752
Iron cycle, 622f
Iron deficiency, 628–639
    clinical features, 632–633
    course and prognosis, 639
    definition and history, 628
    differential diagnosis, 635–638, 635f, 636t
    epidemiology, 628

etiology, 628
    blood loss, 628–630, 628t
    dietary, 630
    genetic, 631
    hemoglobinuria, 631
    intravascular hemolysis, 631
    malabsorption, 630
    paroxysmal nocturnal hemoglobinuria,
        579
    in pregnancy, 120, 630
    iron metabolism in, 552, 553t
    laboratory features, 633–635, 633f, 634f,
        638
    pathogenesis, 631–633, 631f
    reactive thrombocytosis in, 2036
    thrombocytopenia and, 1997
    treatment, 638–639
Iron dextran, 639
Iron overload
    in congenital dyserythropoietic anemia,
        567
    in myelodysplastic syndromes, 1358
    porphyria cutanea tarda and, 907
    in sickle cell disease, 776
    in sideroblastic anemia, 920
    in thalassemias, 742
Iron protoporphyrin IX. See Heme
Iron-regulatory protein (IRP-1), 623, 624f
Iron-responsive elements (IREs), 623, 624f
Iron storage disease, 639. See also
    Hemochromatosis
Iron stores, marrow, 34–35
Iron therapy, 638
    for anemia of chronic kidney disease, 554t,
        555
    for anemia of inflammation, 554, 554t
    iron overload and, 641
    oral, 638–639
    parenteral, 639
    for paroxysmal nocturnal hemoglobinuria,
        579
IRP-1 (iron-regulatory protein), 623, 624f
Irradiation. See also Radiation therapy
    platelets, 2388
    total-body, 353, 359–360
Irreversibly sickled cells (ISCs), 475, 764
Isavuconazole, 385
Ischemia, protein C activation and, 1954
Ischemia pneumonitis, 2269
Ischemia–reperfusion injury, in sickle cell
    disease, 765
Ischemic stroke. See Stroke
ISCs (irreversibly sickled cells), 475, 764
ISG15 (interferon stimulated gene 15),
    1231
Isochromosome, 175t

Isocitrate dehydrogenase (IDH), 170, 198, 199f, 337, 337f

Isocitrate dehydrogenase (IDH) inhibitors, 337

Isofagomine tartrate, 1128

Isoniazid, for tuberculosis, 386

ISWI-(imitation SWI) remodelers, 166, 166f

ITAMs. See Immunoreceptor tyrosine-based activation motifs (ITAMs)

ITCH E3 ubiquitin protein ligase deficiency, 1224

Itching. See Pruritus/itching

ITF4 (MUM1), 234t

ITGB3, 1851

ITIM (immunoreceptor tyrosine inhibitory motif), 1184, 1190, 1868, 1884

ITK, 1643

ITK-SYK, 1696

131I-tositumomab
  for diffuse large B-cell lymphoma, 1632
  for follicular lymphoma, 1647

ITP. See Immune thrombocytopenia (ITP)

Itraconazole, 387t, 389

ITSM (immunoreceptor tyrosine-based switch motif), 1868

IVIg. See Intravenous immunoglobulin (IVIg)

Ixazomib, 1754

Ixodes dammini, 2311

J

Jagged ligand, 1824

JAK. See under Janus kinase (JAK)

JAK1, 232t, 233t, 235t

JAK2
  in B-cell acute lymphoblastic leukemia, 232t, 1508
  in essential thrombocythemia, 228t, 1278
  in familial thrombocytosis, 1310
  in myelodysplastic syndromes, 228t
  in myelofibrosis, 228t, 1278
  in polycythemia vera, 228t, 1278, 1450
  in primary myelofibrosis, 1319, 1450

JAK2 exon 12 mutations, 1296

JAK2 inhibitors
  for essential thrombocythemia, 1314
  for polycythemia vera, 1300
  for primary myelofibrosis, 1328–1329, 1329t

JAK2^{V617F}
  in acute myelogenous leukemia, 181t
  in chronic neutrophilic leukemia, 1279, 1468t, 1472
  in essential thrombocythemia, 1307, 1308f, 1311, 1312, 1312f, 1315
  in hypereosinophilic syndrome, 958

in myelodysplastic syndromes, 181t, 1352
in polycythemia vera, 178, 1292, 1295–1296, 1312, 1312f, 1313f
in primary myelofibrosis, 1320–1321

JAK3, 232t, 233t

JAK3 deficiency, 1214t, 1217–1218

JAM. See under Junctional adhesion molecule (JAM)

Jamshidi biopsy instrument, 28, 28f, 29

Janus kinase (JAK), 248, 249, 251f, 252

Janus kinase (JAK)-2, 250, 485, 486f, 932

Janus kinase (JAK)-3, 1154, 1217–1218

Janus kinase (JAK) inhibitors, 341–342

Janus kinase (JAK)/STAT pathway, 1606

Jaundice
  in alloimmune hemolytic disease of the fetus and newborn, 848–849
  eye, 8
  history of, 6
  neonatal, 707, 709
  skin, 7–8

JC polyomavirus infection, 1240, 1536

Jk(a–b–) phenotype, 2343

$J_\lambda C_\lambda$ gene segments, 1170

JMH blood group/antigens, 2337, 2346t

JNK (c-Jun N-terminal kinase), 249, 298, 1178

Job syndrome. See Hyperimmunoglobulin E syndrome (HIES)

John Milton Hagen blood group, 2332t

Joints, examination of, 9. See also Hemarthroses

JR blood group, 2332t

Junctional adhesion molecule-3 (JAM-3), 1856

Junctional adhesion molecule-A (JAM-A), 1870

Junctional adhesion molecule-A (JAM-C), 1870, 1977t, 1979

c-Jun N-terminal kinase (JNK), 249, 298, 1178

Juvenile myelomonocytic leukemia, 1096, 1468t, **1470–1471**

Juvenile rheumatoid arthritis, 1090–1091, 1513

Juvenile xanthogranuloma (JXG), 1101, 1102t, **1111–1112**

K

Kallikrein, 286t, 289

Kaolin clotting time, 2243

Kaposi-like hemangioendothelioma, 2014

Kaposi sarcoma, 1239, 1250, 1573

Kaposi sarcoma–associated herpesvirus-associated inflammatory cytokine syndrome (KICS), 1250

κ light-chain (KM) allotypes, 1170, 1741

κ light-chain gene complex, 1165f, 1167f

Karnovsky scale, 4t

Karyotype, 175t

Kasabach-Merritt syndrome (KMS), 806, **2014–2015**, 2317t, 2318

Kawasaki disease, neutropenia and, 997

KEAP1, 196

KEL, 851

Kell blood group
  antibodies, 2345t
  antigens, 2335t, 2337
  characteristics, 2331t, 2334t
  disease association, 2331t, 2340
  fetal expression, 104
  frequency, 2334t
  genetics, 2339
  in hemolytic disease of the fetus and newborn, 851, 851f
  phenotypes, 2334t
  in pregnancy, 853–854
  variation in expression, 2337
  XK protein, 681. See also McLeod phenotype

Keratocytes (horn cells), 473f, 473t, 474f

Kernicterus, 849, 858

Ketanserin, 2079

α-Ketoglutarate. See 2-Oxoglutarate (2OG)

Ketotifen, for mastocytosis, 976

Ketron-Goodman variant, pagetoid reticulosis, 1684

Keyhole limpet hemocyanin (KLH), 423, 423f, 424f, 1648

Ki-67, 1654

KIAA0023, 414

KICS (Kaposi sarcoma–associated herpesvirus-associated inflammatory cytokine syndrome), 1250

Kidd blood group/antigens, 2331t, 2335t, 2337, 2340, 2345t

Kidney disease/dysfunction. See Renal disease/dysfunction

Kidney transplantation. See Renal transplantation

KIF23, 568

Killer cell immunoglobulin-like receptors (KIRs), 1190, 1401, 1461, 1565

Kinases
  cyclin-dependent. See Cyclin-dependent kinases (cdks)
  Janus. See under Janus kinase (JAK)

Kindlin, 1884

Kindlin-3 deficiency (LAD; LAD-1 variant; integrin activation deficiency), 1019t, 1024, 2060

Kininogen, high-molecular-weight, 1916t, 1929, 2121
Kinins, 286t, 289
KIRs (killer cell immunoglobulin-like receptors), 1190, 1401, 1461, 1565
KIT
  in acute myelogenous leukemia, 181, 181t, 227t, 1376
  imatinib sensitivity and, 1279
  in mast cell disorders, 965, 973, 976, 977
  in primary myelofibrosis, 1321
Klebsiella infections, 383, 1030. *See also* Bacterial infections
Kleihauer-Betke test, 859, 859f
KLF1/KLF1, 568, 730, 2337
KLH (keyhole limpet hemocyanin), 423, 423f, 424f, 1648
KLHL6, 1529
KM (κ light-chain) allotypes, 1170, 1741
KMD6A, 1346t
KMS (Kasabach-Merritt syndrome), 806, **2014–2015**, 2317t, 2318
KMT2A, 183
KMT2A/MLL, 176f
KMT2D (MLL2), 1644
KMTA/AFF1 (MLL-AF4), 1507
Knockout animal models, 153
Knops blood group/antigens, 2332t, 2337, 2346t
Koilonychia, 8, 632
Kostmann syndrome, 983, **992–993**, 993f
Kpª/Jsª blood group, 2335t
KRAS (K-RAS)
  in acute myelogenous leukemia, 1376, 1384t
  in chronic myelomonocytic leukemia, 1468
  in juvenile myelomonocytic leukemia, 1468t
  in myelodysplastic syndromes, 1346t
  in myeloma, 188, 233t, 1709, 1737, 1759, 1760
Kruppel-like factor (KLF1), 568, 730, 2337
Ku70, 1167
Ku80, 1167
Kwashiorkor, **654**
Kx blood group/antigens, 2332t, 2337, 2342
Kyphoplasty, 1756

L
L444P, 1123, 1123t
LA (lupus anticoagulants), 2101f, 2186, 2233, 2243
Labile iron pool, 618
Lactate dehydrogenase (LDH)
  abnormalities, 701t

activity, 692t
  in Burkitt lymphoma, 1245
  in chronic lymphocytic leukemia, 1532, 1532t
  in chronic myelogenous leukemia, 1448
  in diffuse large B-cell lymphoma, 1632
  in glucose metabolism, 692, 696
  in HELLP syndrome, 802
  in megaloblastic anemia, 597
  in myeloma, 1716
  in paroxysmal nocturnal hemoglobinuria, 575
Lactoferrin, 284t, 285, 1012t, 1013
Lactoferrin receptors, 1058t
LAD. *See* Leukocyte adhesion deficiency
λ gene, 1168
λ light chains, 1163
Lamellipodium, 1005
Laminin, 63, **267**, 1846t, 1865
Laminin receptor. *See* Integrin α₆β₁
LAMP-1 (CD107a), 1873
LAMP-2 (CD107b), 1873
LAMP-3. *See* CD63
Lan blood group, 2332t
Landsteiner-Wiener blood group, 2331t
Langerhans cell histiocytosis
  adult, **1108–1109**
  clinical features
    multisystem, 1104–1105, 1105f
    single-site, 1103–1104, 1103f
  consequences and late effects of treatment, 1107–1108
  course and prognosis, 1107
  differential diagnosis, 1106
  epidemiology and inheritance, 1102–1103
  etiology and pathogenesis, 1101, 1103
  histopathology, 1102t
  history, 1100
  laboratory features, 1105–1106, 1105f
  treatment, 1106–1107, 1106t
Langerhans cells, 310, 1078, 1078f, 1082, 1101
Langerhans cell sarcomas, 1110
Lansoprazole, megaloblastic anemia and, 606t
Large granular lymphocytic leukemia (LGLL), 1352, 1499t, 1563. *See also* T-cell large granular lymphocytic leukemia (T-LGLL)
Large granular lymphocytosis, 1189, 1202–1203
Larval myeloma, 1725
Lassitude, history of, 4
Lasthénie de Ferjol syndrome, 630
LAT (linker of activation of T cells), 1144, 1178

Late hemorrhagic disease of the newborn, 109
Latent membrane protein 1 (LMP1), 1606
LCAD (long-chain acyl coenzyme A dehydrogenase) deficiency, 2211
LCDD (light chain deposition disease), 1744, 1760
LCMV (lymphocytic choriomeningitis virus), 1192
LCR (locus control region), 730
LDH. *See* Lactate dehydrogenase (LDH)
Lead poisoning, 811
Lectin-containing receptors, 1870–1871
Lectins. *See* Selectins (lectins)
LEF1, 1643
Legionella, 1062, 1064f, 1066f
Legionnaire disease, 304
Leg ulcers, 6, 8, 771–772
Leishmania, 1062, 1064f
Lenalidomide, **333–335**
  for acute myelogenous leukemia, 1404
  adverse effects, 334–335, 1741, 1752, 1756–1757
  for AL amyloidosis, 1761, 1780–1781
  for chronic lymphocytic leukemia, 1538–1539
  clinical use, 334
  for diffuse large B-cell lymphoma, 1631
  for mantle cell lymphoma, 1658, 1659t, 1660t
  mechanism of action, 333–334, 1192
  for myelodysplastic syndromes, 1359
  for myeloma, 364, 365f, 1750–1751, 1752, 1752t, 1753, 1753t, 1754
  pharmacology, 334
  for primary myelofibrosis, 1329
  structure, 333f
Lentiviral vectors, 439, 443
Lepirudin
  for heparin-induced thrombocytopenia, 2030
  pharmacology, 399
  removal from market, 399
  for unstable angina, 2296
Leptocytes, 473t, 474f
Leptomeningeal myelomatosis, 1746
Lesch-Nyhan syndrome, 608
Letterer-Siwe disease. *See* Langerhans cell histiocytosis
LEU7 (CD57), 1528
Leu33Pro, 1851
Leucine-rich repeat glycoprotein receptors, 1858–1859t, **1865–1868**
Leucovorin, 320–321, 584
Leukämie, 1438
Leukapheresis, 1450, 1540, 2368

Leukemia. *See also individual types*
  α-thalassemia and, 739
  associated with basophilia, 971–972, 972*t*
  B-cell, 1494*t*
  cell growth and metabolism in, 197–198, 198*f*
  cellular therapy, **413–414**
  disseminated intravascular coagulation and, 2207
  mast cell, 978
  platelet function and, 2081–2082
  during pregnancy, 124
  T-cell, 1498*t*, 1571, 1573
Leukemia-associated proteins, 414
Leukemia inhibitory factor, 1821
Leukemia stem cell, 1376
Leukemic blast cells
  in acute myelogenous leukemia, 1381
  in clonal myeloid disorder classification, 1277
  extramedullary tumors and, 1285
  hyperleukocytic syndromes and, 1285–1286, 1286*t*
  procoagulant and fibrinolytic activator release and, 1285
Leukemic reticuloendotheliosis, 1553. *See also* Hairy cell leukemia (HCL)
Leukemic transformation
  in clonal myeloid diseases, 1280–1281
  in polycythemia vera, 1295
  in thrombocythemia, 1310
Leukemoid reaction, 999
Leukocytapheresis, 429*t*, 433
Leukocyte adhesion deficiency type 1 (LAD-1)
  clinical features, 1019*t*, 1021*t*, 1022–1023
  definition and history, 1021–1022
  differential diagnosis, 1023–1024
  etiology and pathogenesis, 1019*t*, 1022
  gene mutations, 1021*t*
  laboratory features, 1021*t*, 1023, 1023*f*
  therapy, course, and prognosis, 1024
Leukocyte adhesion deficiency type 2 (LAD-2), 1019*t*, 1021*t*, 1023–1024, 2343
Leukocyte adhesion deficiency type 3 (LAD-3, LAD-1 variant syndrome), 1019*t*, 1024, 2060
Leukocyte antigens, human. *See* Human leukocyte antigens (HLAs)
Leukocyte common antigen. *See* CD45 (T200)
Leukocyte count, 16
  in acute lymphoblastic leukemia, 1510, 1510*t*
  in acute myelogenous leukemia, 1381

  in children, 15*t*
  in chronic myelogenous leukemia, 1445, 1445*f*
  in newborn, 105, 105*t*
  in primary myelofibrosis, 1326
  reference ranges, 18*t*
Leukocyte differential, 16–17
Leukocyte function antigen. *See under* LFA
Leukocyte integrin (β₂) subfamily, 1054
Leukocytes
  in acute inflammation, **280–284**
    adhesion and transmigration, 280–283, 282*f*, 282*t*
    chemotaxis and activation, 283–284, 284*t*
  artifacts, 23
  automated analysis, **16–17**
  cellular homing and, 68–69
  donor infusions of, 1400–1401
  fetal liver, 100
  inclusions, 23
  interactions with endothelial cells, 1977–1978, 1977*t*, 1979
  interactions with platelets, 1829–1834, 1830–1831*f*, 1852*f*, 1855–1856, 1857*f*, 1978–1979
  iron deficiency and, 633
  levels of, in older persons, 134
  in marrow infiltration, 659*f*
  morphology, **22–23**
  in newborn, 105
  nucleotides in, 935*t*
  in polycythemia vera, 1295
  release, 71
  response, 247
  types, 20*f*
Leukocytoclastic vasculitis, 2096*f*
Leukocytosis, 43–44, 997. *See also* Neutrophilia
Leukodystrophies, 439
Leukoerythroblastic reaction, 657, 659*f*
Leukolysin, 1012*t*, 1014
Leukomethylene blue, 793
Leukopenia, 991. *See also* Neutropenia
Leukoreduction, for platelet transfusion, 2388
Leukosialin, 1873
Leukotriene B₄, 283, 952
Leukotrienes, 1830–1831*f*
Levofloxacin, 387*t*
Lewis blood group/antigens, 104, 2331*t*, 2334*t*, 2337, 2340, 2344*t*
LFA-1. *See* CD11a (LFA-1)
LFA-2 (CD2), **1185**, 1185*f*
LFA-3 (CD58), 1184, 1185, 1978
LFA (lymphocyte function-associated) glycoproteins, 1184–1185, 1185*f*

LGLL (large granular lymphocytic leukemia), 1563. *See also* T-cell large granular lymphocytic leukemia (T-LGLL)
LGMN, 1643
LGP2, 300
Lhermitte sign, 1618
Lidocaine, toxic methemoglobinemia and, 789
Life span, 131–132
Li-Fraumeni syndrome, 1575*t*
LIGHT (tumor necrosis factor receptor superfamily member 14), 1873
Light chain deposition disease (LCDD), 1744, 1760
Light chain glomerulonephropathy, 1744
Light chains, immunoglobulin. *See* Immunoglobulin (Ig) light chains
Light-chain vasculopathy, 2099
Lindane, 517
Linezolid, 384, 385, 388*t*
Linkage analysis, 151–152, 151*f*
Linker of activation of T cells (LAT), 1144, 1178
Lipid granulomatosis. *See* Erdheim-Chester disease
Lipid mediators, 952, 1878
Lipid rafts, 662, 1836
Lipids
  disseminated intravascular coagulation and, 2203
  inflammatory, 288–289
  membrane. *See* Membrane lipids
  in neutrophils, 935, 935*t*
  peroxidation, 2287
Lipid storage diseases, **1121–1130**
  catabolic pathways of glycosphingolipids in, 1122*f*
  definition, 1121
  Gaucher disease. *See* Gaucher disease
  Niemann-Pick disease. *See* Niemann-Pick disease
Lipopolysaccharide (LPS), 294, 298, 2203
Lipopolysaccharide responsive beige-like anchor (LRBA) deficiency, 1216
Lipoprotein(a), 1287, 1976
Lipoprotein-associated coagulation inhibitor. *See* Tissue factor pathway inhibitor (TFPI)
Lipoprotein phospholipase A₂, 2286
Liposomal amphotericin-B, 385, 387*t*
Lipoxins, 289, 1857*f*
Lipoxygenases, 2287
Listeria, 1062, 1064*f*
Listeria infection, 383. *See also* Bacterial infections
Livedoid reticularis, 2240, 2298

Livedoid vasculitis, 2101
Liver
   B-cell development in, 1151
   disease/dysfunction. *See* Hepatic disease/
      dysfunction
   examination of, 9
   fetal, hematopoiesis in, 100–101
   heme synthesis in, 895–896
   macrophages in, 1081*f*, 1082
   natural killer cell development in, 1151
   primary lymphomas in, 1581
Liver transplantation
   for acute intermittent porphyria, 904
   for afibrinogenemia, 2157
   antifibrinolytic therapy in, 2317*t*, 2318
   for hemophilia, 2129
   hemostatic alterations during, 2193
   hemostatic management during, 2194
   for hypersplenism, 867
   thrombosis following, 2195
LKB1, 195, 196
LL-37 (hCAP-18, CAMP), 1012*t*, 1013
LMAN1/*LMAN1*, 2135*t*, 2139
LMO2, 1632
LMO2 protooncogene, 437
LMP1 (latent membrane protein 1), 1606
LMPP (lymphoid-myeloid primed
      progenitor), 61, 1152*f*, 1153
LNK (*SH2B3*), 229*t*, 232*t*, 233*t*
Locus, 147
LOH (loss of heterozygosity), 174, 177*f*
Lonafarnib, 1459
Long-chain acyl coenzyme A dehydrogenase
      (LCAD) deficiency, 2211
Long-term culture-initiating cells (LTC-ICs),
      260, 1440
Lorvotuzumab mertansine, for myeloma,
      346*t*
Loss of heterozygosity (LOH), 174, 177*f*
Low-density lipoprotein (LDL)
   accumulation in macrophages, 2287
   accumulation in vascular wall, 2287
   in antiphospholipid syndrome, 2235, 2237
   arterial thrombosis and, 2294
   nitric oxide synthases and, 2283, 2283*f*
   platelet activation and, 1878
Low-density lipoprotein receptor-related
      protein 1 (LRP1), 2309
Low-infiltrate leukemia. *See* Oligoblastic
      myelogenous leukemia (refractory
      anemia with excess blasts)
Low-molecular-weight heparin (LMWH),
      398–399. *See also* Heparin
   argatroban. *See* Argatroban
   bivalirudin. *See* Bivalirudin
   choice of, 398

danaparoid. *See* Danaparoid
fondaparinux. *See* Fondaparinux
lepirudin. *See* Lepirudin
for myocardial infarction, 2295–2296
pharmacology, **398**
in pregnancy, 2277
for unstable angina, 2296
for venous thromboembolism, 2273–2274,
   2274*t*, 2276–2277
5-LOX, 1877
12-LOX, 1877
Loxosceles laeta, 809
Loxosceles reclusa, 809
LPA (lysophosphatidic acid), 1878
LPIN2, 568
LPL. *See* Lymphoplasmacytic lymphoma
   (LPL)
LPS. *See* Lipopolysaccharide (LPS)
LRBA (lipopolysaccharide responsive
      beige-like anchor) deficiency,
      1216
LRP1 (low-density lipoprotein receptor-
      related protein 1), 2309
LRRFIP1, 1853
LRRK2, 233*t*
L-selectin (CD62L)
   activities, 66, 68
   counterreceptor, 282*t*
   in disseminated intravascular coagulation,
      2207
   distribution, 67*t*
   expression, 281, 1870
   hematopoietic stem cell trafficking and,
      355
   in inflammatory response, 1083,
      1976–1977, 1977*t*, 1979
   in leukemic cells, 1440
   ligands, 67*t*
   in lymphocytes, 1139
   in monocytes, 1052*f*
   neutrophils and, 1006
   in T-cells, 1183
LSG15 regimen, for adult T-cell leukemia/
      lymphoma, 1701
LSK CD34+FLT3hi, 1153
*LTA*₄*H*, 2288
LTC₄, 952
LTC-ICs (long-term culture-initiating cells),
      260, 1440
Luᵃ antigens, 104
Luᵇ antigens, 104
LuLu-type null phenotype, 2343
Lumbar puncture, bleeding risk and, 2384
Lung
   disease/dysfunction. *See* Pulmonary
      disease/dysfunction

macrophages in, 1082–1082
stem cell therapy for repair of, 451
Lupus anticoagulant (LA), 2101*f*, 2186, 2233,
   2243
Lutheran blood group
   antibodies, 2341*t*, 2343, 2345*t*
   antigens, 2335*t*, 2337
   characteristics, 2331*t*, 2335*t*
   disease association, 2331*t*
   fetal expression, 104
   frequency, 2335*t*
   genetics, 2339
   null phenotypes, 2342*t*, 2343
LYL1, 1508*t*
Lyme disease, 819, 2104, 2104*f*, 2311
Lymphadenopathy
   in chronic lymphocytic leukemia, 1530
   consultative approach to, 48
   in follicular lymphoma, 1641
   in Langerhans cell histiocytosis, 1104
   in mastocytosis, 973–974
Lymph nodes
   anatomy, 91, 92*f*
   B-cell development in, 1151
   examination of, 8
   function, 93
   germinal centers, 1589, 1590*f*
   macrophages in, 1082
   reactive, 1589*f*, 1590*f*
   structure, 91–93, 92*f*
Lymphoblastic leukemia, 1498*t*
Lymphoblastic lymphoma, 1498*t*
Lymphoblasts, 1511, 1511*f*
Lymphocyte doubling time, 1532, 1532*t*
Lymphocyte function-associated antigens.
   See under LFA
Lymphocyte function-associated (LFA)
      glycoproteins, 1184–1185, 1185*f*
Lymphocyte homing cell adhesion molecule
      (HCAM), 68
Lymphocytes. *See also* B cells; T cells
   antigens
      B-lymphocyte, 1141, 1141*f*
      surface, 1143
      T-lymphocyte and NK cell, 1141–1142,
         1142*f*, 1142*t*
   cell adhesion and homing, 66
   in chronic inflammation, 291
   composition, **1143–1144**, 1144*t*
   in cutaneous T-cell lymphoma, 1681*f*
   cytochemical reactions, 1049*t*
   differentiation, 61
   disorders, **1195–1197**
      B lymphocyte, 1195
      classification, 1195, 1196–1197*t*
      clinical manifestations, 1195–1197

Lymphocytes, disorders (*Cont.*):
　combined T-and B-cell, 1197
　natural killer cell, 1197
　T lymphocyte, 1195–1197
　infants, 108–109, 109*t*
　infusions from donor, in allogenic
　　hematopoietic cell transplantation,
　　359, 373
　large granular, 23
　marrow, 32*t*, **35**
　in mycosis fungoides, 1683*f*
　in myelodysplastic syndromes, 1353
　in newborn, 105*t*
　precursors, increased apoptosis of, 1217
　reactive, 23
　reference ranges, 15*t*, 18*t*
　release, 72
　structure, **1137–1140**
　　changes associated with activation,
　　　1138*f*, 1139–1140, 1140*f*
　　cytomatrix, 1144–1145
　　definition and history, 1137
　　microscopy and histochemistry, 966*f*,
　　　1137–1139, 1138*f*, 1139*f*
　　organelles, 1145
　　types, 20*f*, 23
Lymphocytic choriomeningitis virus
　(LCMV), 1192
Lymphocytopenia, **1204–1206**
　acquired, 1204–1206, 1205*t*
　　iatrogenic, 1205–1206
　　in infectious diseases, 1204–1205
　　nutritional or dietary, 1206
　　in systemic disease, 1206
　definition, 1204
　idiopathic CD4+ T, 1206
　inherited causes, 1204, 1205*t*
Lymphocytosis, **1199–1204**
　causes, 1200*t*
　consultative approach to, 44
　definition, 1199
　primary, **1199–1202**
　　monoclonal B-cell lymphocytosis,
　　　1199–1200, 1201*t*, 1542–1543
　　persistent polyclonal lymphocytosis of B
　　　lymphocytes, 1200–1202, 1201*f*
　secondary (reactive), **1202–1204**
　　acute infection lymphocytosis, 1202,
　　　1203*f*
　　drug-induced lymphocytosis,
　　　1203–1204
　　hypersensitivity reactions, 1204
　　infectious mononucleosis, 1202
　　large granular lymphocytosis,
　　　1202–1203
　　persistent lymphocytosis, 1204

　pertussis, 1202
　stress lymphocytosis, 1204
Lymphoid fibrosis, 1553. *See also* Hairy cell
　leukemia (HCL)
Lymphoid-myeloid primed progenitor
　(LMPP), 61, 1152*f*, 1153
Lymphoid progenitors, **269–270**
　functional characterization, 1154
　human, 1153
　murine, 1153
　thymic, 1154
Lymphoid tissues, **85**
　lymph nodes. *See* Lymph nodes
　mucosa-associated, **93–94**
　Peyer patches, 94, 94*f*
　spleen. *See* Spleen
　thymus. *See* Thymus
　tonsils, 94, 1081*f*
Lymphokines, 208–209
Lymphomas, **1569–1583**. *See also individual
　　types*
　aggressive, 1501*t*
　cell growth and metabolism in, 199–200
　chromosomal abnormalities, 184–185*t*,
　　187–188, 224–225*t*, **1576–1577**
　vs. chronic lymphocytic leukemia, 1543
　classification, **1493–1501**, 1587–1589,
　　1588*t*
　clinical features, 1493, 1577
　　abnormal immunoglobulin production,
　　　1501
　　lymphokine-induced disorders, 1502
　　marrow and tissue infiltration, 1502
　　metabolic signs, 1502
　　systemic symptoms, 1502
　definition and history, 1569–1570
　diagnosis, 1590–1592, 1591*t*
　early precursor lesions, 1501
　epidemiology, 1570–1571, 1570*f*, 1571*f*
　etiology and pathogenesis, **1571–1576**
　　autoimmunity, 1574–1575
　　environmental factors, 1571, 1572–1573
　　histopathologic heterogeneity,
　　　1571–1572, 1572*t*
　　immunosuppression, 1574, 1575*t*
　　infectious agents, 1265, 1573–1574
　　interaction of environment and
　　　genotype, 1573
　extranodal involvement, 1502
　gene mutations, 166, 209–210
　hematopoietic cell transplantation for, 366
　histologic subtypes and frequency of,
　　1571–1572, 1572*t*
　HIV-associated. *See* Human
　　immunodeficiency virus
　　(HIV)–associated malignancies

　Hodgkin lymphoma treatment and, 1617
　indolent, 1501*t*, 1570
　marrow findings, 31–32
　monocytosis and, 1097
　in pregnancy, **124**
　response assessment, 1570, 1578–1579,
　　1579*t*, 1580*t*
　secondary acute myelogenous leukemia
　　and, 1407
　staging, 1570, 1577–1579, 1577*f*, 1578*t*,
　　1579*t*
　vaccine therapy for, 423, 423*f*, 424*f*
Lymphomatoid granulomatosis, **1635**
Lymphomatoid papulosis, 1499*t*, **1688–1689**,
　　1688*t*
Lymphomatous polyposis, 1593, 1593*f*
Lymphopenia, consultative approach to, 42
Lymphoplasmacytic lymphoma (LPL).
　　See also Waldenström
　　macroglobulinemia (WM)
　chromosomal abnormalities, 184*t*, 1494*t*
　definition, 1785
　differential diagnosis, 1667, 1668
　gene mutations, 184*t*, 234*t*, 1494*t*
　laboratory features, 1592–1593, 1593*f*
Lymphopoiesis, **1149–1156**, 1282*f*
　differentiation pathways, **1151–1154**, 1152*f*
　　functional characterization of
　　　progenitors in, 74.
　　human lymphoid progenitors in, 1153
　　murine lymphoid progenitors in, 1153
　　thymic progenitors in, 1154
　fetal, 101
　neonatal, **108–109**
　during prenatal development, **1149–1151**,
　　1150*f*
　regulation, **1154–1156**
Lymphosarcoma, 1569, 1603
Lyso-glucosylsphingosine, 1126
Lysophosphatidic acid (LPA), 1878
Lysosomal granule constituents, 286*t*, 287
Lysosomal proteases, 284*t*
Lysosomal storage diseases. *See* Lipid storage
　　diseases
Lysosome-associated membrane proteins. *See*
　　under LAMP
Lysosomes, 1145, 1843
Lysozyme, 284*t*, 1012*t*, 1014, 1064, 1067*t*
LYST, 994, 1229, 1843
Lytic state, 403

M

mAbs. *See* Monoclonal antibodies (mAbs)
MAC, 234*t*
MAC (membrane attack complex), 572, 572*f*
Mac-1. *See* CD11b/CD18 (Mac-1)

MACOP-B regimen
  for anaplastic large cell lymphoma, 1699
  for diffuse large B-cell lymphoma, 1630
  for primary mediastinal large B-cell
          lymphoma, 1634
Macrocyte, 21
Macrocytic anemia, 506
Macrocytosis, 559, 654, 655
α₂-Macroglobulin, 1960–1961, 2308
Macroglobulinemia. *See* Waldenström
          macroglobulinemia
Macroglossia, 5, 1774, 1775*f*
Macrophage activation syndrome,
          1115–1116, 1539
Macrophage colony-stimulating factor
          (M-CSF), 62*t*, 249, 1077–1078,
          1077*f*
Macrophage inflammatory protein (MIP)-1α,
          288*t*, 1440, 1737–1738, 1738*f*, 1739*f*
Macrophage inflammatory protein (MIP)-1β,
          288*t*
Macrophage receptor with collagenous
          structure (MARCO), 1055, 1057*t*,
          1080, 1082, 1084, 1085*f*
Macrophages
  activation, 283, **1083–1086**
    classical and alternative, 1085–1086,
          1086*f*
    immunomodulation, 1084, 1085*f*
    innate, 1084–1085
    in response to inflammation and
          tumors, 1083–1084, 1084*f*
  in atherothrombosis, 2287
  blood dendritic cells and, 1092
  disorders, 1089, 1090*t*. *See also* Monocytes,
          disorders
  distribution
    in central nervous system, 1083
    in lymph nodes, 1082
    in marrow, 1081–1082, 1082*f*, 1083*f*
    in nonlymphohematopoietic organs,
          1082–1083
    in spleen, 90–91, 1082
  functions
    apoptosis, 1060–1061, 1061*f*
    cell adhesion and homing, 66
    cellular interactions, 1066, 1071, 1071*f*
    in chronic inflammation, 284, 291
    endocytosis, phagocytosis, and killing,
          1061–1063, 1062*f*, 1063*f*, 1064*f*,
          1065*f*
    gene expression, synthesis, and
          secretion, 1064–1066, 1067*t*, 1068*f*,
          1069*f*, 1070*f*, 1070*t*
    G-protein-coupled receptors and, 1060*t*
    inflammasome, 1063, 1065*f*, 1066*f*

interaction with coagulation cascade,
          1059
    motility, 1059
    recognition and clearance, 1060
  hematopoietic functions, 1071
  immunomodulation of phenotype, 1070*t*
  iron released from, 551
  M1 and M2 phenotypes, 284, 285
  markers, 1080*t*
  marrow, 32*t*, 34
  morphology, **1048–1052**, 1050*f*, 1051*f*
  neonatal, 108–109
  production
    development, 1075–1076
    growth, differentiation, and turnover,
          1076, 1076*f*
    in hematopoietic organs, 61
    maturation and differentiation,
          1077–1078, 1077*f*
  receptors
    CD4, 1056–1057
    CD11, 1056
    CD14, 1056
    CD16, 1056
    chemokine, 1057–1058, 1058*t*
    complement, 1054
    Fc, 1053–1054, 1053*f*
    human leukocyte antigen class II,
          1055–1056
    non–toll-like, nonopsonic, 1054–1055,
          1056*f*, 1057*t*
    surface, 1052–1053, 1058*t*
    surface antigens, 1052*f*
    toll-like, 1054, 1055*f*
  resident populations in adult tissues,
          1079–1080, 1080*t*
  secretion products, 1067*t*
  stromal, 1082*f*, 1083*f*
  study methods, **1075**
Macroreticulocytes, 467
MAdCAM-1 (mucosal addressin cell
          adhesion molecule 1), 950, 1977
MAF (MAF), 233*t*, 1713, 1736, 1736*t*
MAG (myelin-associated glycoprotein),
          1790
MAGE-1, 412
Magnesium sulfate, for sickle cell disease,
          777*t*
Magnesium transporter 1 defects, 1221
Magnetic resonance imaging (MRI)
  in cardiac amyloidosis, 1779, 1780*f*
  for marrow evaluation, 659
  in myeloma, 1715, 1748, 1749*f*
  for pulmonary embolism, 2271–2272
  in Waldenström macroglobulinemia,
          1792

MAGT1, 1221
Major basic protein (MBP), 929, 948, 952
Major cytogenic response (MCyR), 1452*t*
Major histocompatibility complex (MHC),
          2353, 2354*f*, 2355. *See also* Human
          leukocyte antigen (HLA)
Major histocompatibility complex (MHC)
          class I, 409, 1141, 1177, 1190
Major histocompatibility complex (MHC)
          class I deficiency, 1215*t*, **1221**
Major histocompatibility complex (MHC)
          class II, 1141, 1177, 1214*t*, 1978
Major histocompatibility complex (MHC)
          class II deficiency, 1215*t*, **1221**
Major molecular response (MMR), 1452*t*
MAL (MyD88 adapter-like), 297*f*, 298
Malaise, history of, 4
Malaria, **815–818**
  alterations in infected red cell, 815–816
  blood antigens associated with resistance
          to, 2340
  Burkitt lymphoma and, 1573, 1672
  clinical features, 817
  course and prognosis, 818
  diagnostic methods, 817–818, 817*f*
  epidemiology, 815
  G6PD deficiency and, 690
  glycoprotein IV deficiency and, 2359
  pathogenesis, 816–817
  Plasmodium spp. and severity of anemia
          in, 816
  prevention, 818
  pyruvate kinase deficiency and, 704
  red cell exchange for, 432
  sickle cell trait and, 763
  Southeast Asian ovalocytosis and, 680
  thalassemias and, 728
  treatment, 818
Malignancy. *See* Cancer
Malignant fibrous histiocytoma, 1110
Malignant hypertension, 2263
Malignant transformation, 132
MALT (mucosa-associated lymphoid tissue),
          93–94
MALT lymphoma. *See* Extranodal marginal
          zone lymphoma of MALT type
Mammalian target of rapamycin (mTOR),
          194, 1654, 2237, 2237*f*
Mammalian target of rapamycin (mTOR)
          inhibitors, 1220, 1403. *See also*
          Temsirolimus
Mannan-binding lectin (MBL) pathway, 289*f*,
          290
Mannose-binding lectin (MBL), 1017
Mannose receptors (MRs), 284, 1054, 1057*t*,
          1080, 1081*f*

Mantle cell lymphoma (MCL)
  blastoid cell variant, 1653, 1654*f*
  clinical features, 1654–1655, 1654*t*
  course prognosis, 1655, 1655*f*, 1659
  definition and history, 1653
  differential diagnosis, 1543, 1655, 1667
  epidemiology, 1571, 1653
  etiology and pathogenesis
    chromosomal abnormalities,
      1653–1654, 1654*f*
      t(11;14), 184*t*, 187, 224*t*, 1577, 1593,
        1654*f*
      translocations, 187, 1494*t*
    gene mutations, **1653–1654**, 1654*f*
      ATM, 236*t*, 1654
      BCL1, 1494*t*
      BIRC3, 237*t*
      CCND1, 236*t*, 1577
      EZH2, 170
      gene expression, 1593–1594
      IGH, 236*t*, 1577
      MEF2B, 236*t*
      MLL2, 236*t*
      NOTCH1/2, 237*t*
      SOX11, 236*t*
      TLR2, 237*t*
      TP53, 236*t*, 1494*t*
      TRAF2, 237*t*
      WHSC1, 236*t*
  laboratory features
    histopathology, 1494*t*, 1593–1594, 1593*f*
    large bowel involvement, 1593, 1593*f*
  small cell variant, 1653
  therapy
    for advanced disease, 1655–1657, 1657*t*,
      1658*t*
    hematopoietic cell transplantation, 366
    for localized disease, 1655
    palbociclib, 218
    recommendations, 1656*f*
    for relapsed or recurrent disease,
      1658–1659, 1659*t*
    watchful waiting, 1655
MAPIPA (monoclonal antibody-specific
    immobilization of platelet antigens)
    assay, 2000
MAPK (mitogen-activated protein kinase),
    237, 266, 1054, 1055*f*, 1178, 1817
Maraviroc, for graft-versus-host disease
    prophylaxis, 371
March hemoglobinuria, 631, 806
MARCKS (myristoylated alanine-rich
    C-kinase substrate), 667, 668*f*
MARCO (macrophage receptor with
    collagenous structure), 1055, 1057*t*,
    1080, 1082, 1084, 1085*f*

Marfan syndrome, 2061
Marginal neutrophil pool (MNP), 942*t*
Marginal zone, spleen, 88–89
Marginal zone B-cell lymphomas, **1663–1668**
  definition and classification, 1595, 1663
  epidemiology, 1663
  extranodal. *See* Extranodal marginal zone
      lymphoma of MALT type
  laboratory features, 1595*f*
  nodal, 1495*t*, 1595, 1595*f*, **1667–1668**,
      1668*f*
  splenic, 1495*t*, 1557, 1558*t*, **1666–1667**
Marginated pool, 941–942
Margination, 280
Maribavir, for cytomegalovirus prophylaxis,
    369–370
Marrow
  aging, 132–134, 133*f*, 136
  B-cell development in, 1151
  cellularity, 31
  dendritic cell development in, 1151
  drug-induced suppression, 553
  examination. *See* Marrow examination
  failure, in paroxysmal nocturnal
      hemoglobinuria, 576–578, 576*t*
  gelatinous transformation, 33
  infections infiltrating, 33
  infiltration, **31–33**, **657–659**
    in amyloidosis, 33
    clinical features, 658
    definition and history, 657
    differential diagnosis, 659
    etiology and pathogenesis, 657–658,
      658*t*
    fibrosis, 32
    laboratory features, 658–659, 659*f*
    by malignant neoplasms, 31–32
    in storage disorders, 33
    therapy, course, prognosis, 659
  iron deficiency and, 633
  iron levels in, 635
  iron stain, 552–553
  lymphocyte differentiation in, 61
  macrophage differentiation in, 61
  macrophages in, 1081–1082, 1082*f*
  microenvironment. *See* Hematopoietic
      microenvironment
  necrosis, 33, 657, 658*f*
    in acute myelogenous leukemia, 1385
    in clonal myeloid diseases, 1287
  neutrophil kinetics, 940–941, 941*t*
  neutrophil reserves, 1000
  precursor development in, 925, 926*f*
  reticulocytes, 482*t*
  as source of hematopoietic stem cells for
      transplantation, **355**, 356

storage pool shift, 1000
structure, **55–65**
  extracellular matrix, **61–64**
  hematopoietic cell organization and,
      64–65
  hematopoietic niches, **56**
  innervation, **56**
  sinus architecture, **56–59**, 57*f*, 58*f*, 59*f*
  vasculature, **55–56**, 56*f*
  transplantation of. *See* Hematopoietic cell
      transplantation
Marrow blast crisis, 1465–1466
Marrow examination, **27–37**
  in acute lymphoblastic leukemia,
      1510–1511
  in acute myelogenous leukemia,
      1381–1383, 1382*f*
  in amyloidosis, 33
  in aplastic anemia, 519–520, 520*f*
  aspiration technique for, 28–29, 28*f*
  in chronic myelogenous leukemia,
      1446–1447, 1446*f*
  in clonal myeloid diseases, 1287
  in congenital dyserythropoietic anemia,
      type I, 565*f*
  differential cell count, 32*t*
  in diffuse large B-cell lymphoma, 1627
  in essential thrombocythemia, 1309*f*, 1310
  flow cytometry for, 35–37, 36*f*
  in hairy cell leukemia, 1555, 1557*f*
  in hemochromatosis, 642
  history, 27, 53
  in immune thrombocytopenia, 2003
  indications for, 27
  in infections, 33
  interpretation, 22*f*, **30–33**, 32*t*, 33*f*
  iron stores, 34–35
  in Langerhans cell histiocytosis, 1104
  in lymphomas, 31–32
  macrophages, 1050*f*
  in mastocytosis, 974–975, 975*f*
  in megaloblastic anemia, 595, 595*f*
  morphologic differentiation of
      hematopoietic lineages, **33–35**
  myeloblasts, 927*f*
  in myelodysplastic syndromes, 1350*f*,
      1353–1354
  in myeloma, 31–32, 1715, 1741–1744,
      1742*f*, 1743*f*, 1744*f*
  needle biopsy technique for, 29
  in pernicious anemia, 595*f*
  polycythemia vera and, 1296
  in primary myelofibrosis, 1323*f*,
      1326–1327
  sample adequacy in, 30–31
  in sideroblastic anemia, 916d

specimen preparation for, 27–28
in storage diseases, 33
in T-cell large granular lymphocytic leukemia, 1565, 1565*f*
in transient aplastic crisis, 541*f*
in Waldenström macroglobulinemia, 1786*f*, 1788*t*, 1791, 1792*f*
MART-1, 412
Masked Ph chromosome, 1447
Masked translocation, 1447
Massively parallel digital sequencing. *See* Next-generation sequencing
Massive transfusion, 2385
Mast cell activation syndrome (MCAS), 978
Mast cell growth factor. *See* Stem cell factor (SCF)
Mast cell knockin mice, 970
Mast cell leukemia, 978
Mast cell nevi, 973
Mast cells
 in asthma, 969
 basophils and, **967–968**
 in chronic inflammation, 291
 disorders
  mast cell activation syndrome, 978
  mast cell leukemia, 978
  mast cell nevi, 978
  mast cell sarcoma, 978
  monoclonal mast cell activation syndrome, 977–978
  systemic mastocytosis. *See* Systemic mastocytosis
 distinguishing features, **966**, 966*f*
 heterogeneity, 966–967
 in host defense, **969–970**
 in IgE-associated immune response, 969
 marrow, 35
 mediators, 967*t*, 968
 natural history, 967*t*
 normal levels, 972
 secondary changes in numbers of, 972–973, 972*t*
 structure, 931*f*, 932, **968**
 surface membrane structures, 967*t*
 in Waldenström macroglobulinemia, 1788, 1791, 1792*f*
Mast cell sarcoma, 978
Mastocytomas, 973
Mastocytosis, 973. *See also* Systemic mastocytosis
Matriptase 2 (Tmprss6), 621, 621*t*
Matrix metalloproteinases (MMPs), 1014, 1874, 1881, 2307, 2311
Matrix modulators, 2284*f*
Matrix proteins, **266–267**. *See also specific types*

Mature neutrophil reserve, 941, 941*t*
Mature T-cell lymphomas
 cutaneous. *See* Cutaneous T-cell lymphoma (CTCL)
 systemic. *See* Peripheral T-cell lymphoma (PTCL)
MAVS (mitochondrial antiviral signaling protein), 302, 302*f*, 303
MAX, 234*t*
May-Hegglin disease/anomaly, 22*f*, 23, 2061
m-BACOD regimen, for diffuse large B-cell lymphoma, 1629–1630
m-*bcr* breakpoints, 1443, 1449
M-*bcr* breakpoints, 1442
MBL (mannose-binding lectin), 1017
MBL (monoclonal B-cell lymphocytosis), **1199–1200**, 1201*t*, 1542–1543
MBL (mannan-binding lectin) pathway, 289*f*, 290
MBP (major basic protein), 929, 948, 952
MCAS (mast cell activation syndrome), 978
MCFD2/*MCFD2*, 2135*t*, 2139
MCH (mean cell hemoglobin), 14
MCHC (mean cell hemoglobin concentration), 14, 766
MCL. *See* Mantle cell lymphoma (MCL)
MCL-1, 1528, 1711
MCL-1 (*MCL1*), 210, 1736
Mcl-1 protein, 206, 216, 218, 231*t*, 237
McLeod phenotype/syndrome, **681**, 2341*t*, 2342
MCP, 2260, 2259*t*
MCP-1 (monocyte chemoattractant protein). *See* CCL2 (monocyte chemoattractant protein, MCP-1)
MCP regimen
 for follicular lymphoma, 1646*t*
 for mantle cell lymphoma, 1657*t*
M-CSF (macrophage colony-stimulating factor), 62*t*, 249, 1077–1078, 1077*f*
M-CSF (monocyte colony-stimulating factor), 264*t*, 1352
MCSs (multispecies conserved sequences), 730
MCV (mean cell volume), 14, 18*t*, 19*f*, 21
MCV (mean corpuscular volume), 634*f*
MCV (mean red cell volume), 102
MCyR (major cytogenic response), 1452*t*
mCyR (minor cytogenic response), 1452*t*
MD2, 1054
MDA5 (melanoma differentiation-associated gene 5), 300–301, 302*f*
MDM2 (murine double minute protein 2), 238
MDP (muramyl dipeptide), 299, 301*f*
MDR, 341

MDR protein-1, 1404
MDSs. *See* Myelodysplastic syndromes (MDSs)
Mean cell hemoglobin (MCH), 14
Mean cell hemoglobin concentration (MCHC), 14, 766
Mean cell volume (MCV), 14, 18*t*, 19*f*, 21
Mean corpuscular hemoglobin concentration (MCHC)
 in hereditary spherocytosis, 675
 iron deficiency and, 634*f*
Mean corpuscular volume (MCV), 634*f*
Mean platelet volume (MPV), 17
Mean red cell volume (MCV), 102
Measles
 lymphocytopenia and, 1204
 purpura and, 2104
Mechlorethamine. *See* Nitrogen mustard
Meckel diverticulum, blood loss and, 629
Mediastinal germ cell tumors, 1386–1387
Mediators
 basophil, 967*t*, 968
 lipid, eosinophils and release of, 952
 mast cells, 967*t*, 968
MEF2B, 235*t*, 236*t*, 1627*t*, 1644
MEFV, 1025
Megakaryoblasts, **1815–1817**, 1816*f*
Megakaryocyte-erythroid progenitor (MEP) cells, 259, 268
Megakaryocytes
 marrow, 32*t*, 35
 in myelodysplastic syndromes, 1350*f*, 1354
 release, 72, 73*f*
Megakaryopoiesis, 64–65, **1815–1824**
 extrinsic regulation, **1821–1823**
 maturation stages, 1816*t*
 precursor cell kinetics, 75*t*
 progenitors, **271**
 stage I (megakaryoblasts), 1815–1817, 1816*f*
 stage II, 1817–1818
 stage III/IV, 1818–1820, 1819*f*, 1820*f*
Megaloblastic anemias, **593–608**
 acute, **604–605**
 autosomal recessive, 605
 clinical features, 594
 definition, 593
 etiology and pathogenesis, 584, **593–594**, 596*t*
  acute erythroid leukemia and, 608
  in childhood, **605**, **607**
  cobalamin deficiency, 583, 590. *See also* Cobalamin deficiency
  congenital dyserythropoietic anemia, 608
  drug-related, 596*t*, **605**, 606*t*

Megaloblastic anemias, etiology and
    pathogenesis (*Cont.*):
  folate deficiency, 583, 590.
      See also Folate deficiency
  hereditary orotic aciduria, 608
  inborn errors of cobalamin metabolism,
      607, 607*t*
  inborn errors of folate metabolism,
      607–608
  Lesch-Nyhan syndrome, 608
  incomplete, 596
  ineffective erythropoiesis and, 597
  iron deficiency and, 637
  laboratory features
    blood cells, 594–595, 594*f*
    in body fluids, 597
    cytokinetics, 597
    in epithelial cells, 597
    marrow, 595, 595*f*
    neutropenia, 994
  with microcytic anemia, 596
  misdiagnosed as acute leukemia, 597
  refractory, 608
  thiamine-responsive, 608, 652
Megaloblastic crisis, in hereditary
    spherocytosis, 674
Megaloblastoid erythropoiesis, 1350*f*, 1354
MEK (mitogen-activated extracellular-
    regulated kinase), 298, 1016
Melanesian elliptocytosis. *See* Southeast
    Asian ovalocytosis (SAO)
Melanocyte growth-stimulating activity, 288*t*
Melanoma
  cellular therapy, **412–413**
  marrow infiltration in, 659*f*
Melanoma differentiation-associated 5
    (MDA5), 300–301, 302*f*
MELAS syndrome, 2108
MELD (model of end-stage liver disease),
    2192
Melena, 5, 1987
Melphalan
  for AL amyloidosis, 1761, 1779–1780
  for γ-heavy-chain disease, 1806
  high-dose, before hematopoietic cell
      transplantation, 331*t*, 364, 365*f*
  for Hodgkin lymphoma, 1616
  mechanism of action, 329
  for myeloma, 1751, 1752*t*
  platelet function and, 2079
Membrane
  basophil, 967*t*
  erythrocyte. *See* Erythrocyte membrane
  lymphocyte, 1143–1144, 1144*t*
  mast cell, 967*t*
  platelet. *See* Platelets

Membrane attack complex (MAC), 572, 572*f*
Membrane folate transporter, 588
Membrane inhibitor of reactive lysis (MIRL),
    572
Membrane lipids
  in abetalipoproteinemia, 681
  erythrocyte, 662
  in hereditary spherocytosis, 672–673
  modification, in cell signaling, 251
Membrane matrix metalloproteinase
    leukolysin, 1010
Membrane proteins, **662–667**, 663*t*
  classification, 664
  defects. *See* Erythrocyte membrane
      disorders
  integral, 664–665
    band 3, **664**, 664*f*
    glycophorins, **664–665**
    Rh-RhAG group, 665
  peripheral, 663*t*, **665–667**
    actin and actin-binding proteins, 667
    adducin, 667
    ankyrin, 666, 666*f*, 670–671
    defects, 670–672, 670*t*
    p55, 667, 667*f*
    protein 4.1R, 666–667, 667*f*, 678
    protein 4.2, 667
    spectrin. *See* Spectrin
Memory B cells, 1172
Memory stem cells (CD62L+ cells), 411
Memory T cells, **1182–1183**
  aging and, 135–136
  in immune cell therapy, 411
  killer cell immunoglobulin-like receptors
      and, 1190
Menatetrenone (vitamin K₂), 1360
Mendelian genetics, 147
Mendelian susceptibility to mycobacterial
    disease, **1231**
Meningococcal disease, 304
Meningococcal vaccine, 773
Menorrhagia, 5–6, 1987, 2007, 2135, 2139
Menstrual bleeding, iron deficiency and, 629
Mental retardation, α-thalassemia and, 739,
    745
MEP (megakaryocyte-erythroid progenitor)
    cells, 259, 268
Meperidine, 767
Mephenytoin, drug-related hemolytic anemia
    and, 824
Mepolizumab, 954
Mer, 1845
MER2. *See* CD151
MER2 antigen, RAPH blood group, 2343
Mercaptoethane sulfonate (MESNA). *See also*
    CODOX-M/IVAC regimen

  for alkylating drug toxicity, 330
  for diffuse large B-cell lymphoma, 1629*t*
  for malignant histiocytic diseases, 1110
6-Mercaptopurine (6-MP)
  for acute lymphoblastic leukemia, 1505,
      1516
  adverse effects, 324, 1519*t*
  for autoimmune hemolytic anemia, 839
  for Langerhans cell histiocytosis, 1106,
      1107
  mechanism of action, 323
  megaloblastic anemia and, 606*t*
  pharmacology, 323–324
  resistance to, 319*t*
  structure, 323*f*
Meropenem, as empiric therapy for
    infections, 384, 387*t*
Mesenchymal cell plasticity, 54–55
Mesenchymal stromal cells (MSCs), 449–450,
    451
MESNA. *See* Mercaptoethane sulfonate
    (MESNA)
Messenger RNA. *See* mRNA (messenger
    RNA)
Metabolic syndrome, 5
Metabolism
  inborn errors. *See* Inborn errors of
      metabolism
  iron deficiency and, 632
  of red cells, in newborn, 104
Metabolites, in erythrocytes, 471*t*
Metacentric centromere, 175*t*
Metachromatic leukodystrophy, 439
Metal ion-dependent adhesion site (MIDAS),
    2044–2045, 2044*f*
Metamyelocytes
  marrow, 34
  maturation, 926*f*, 940–941, 940*f*, 941*t*
  normal values, 32*t*
  structure, 925–926, 927*f*
Metformin, megaloblastic anemia and,
    606*t*
Methemoglobin. *See* Hemoglobin M
Methemoglobinemia, **789–794**
  clinical features, 791*t*, 792
  definition and history, 789
  epidemiology, 789
  etiology and pathogenesis, 789–791, 790*t*,
      791*f*, 791*t*
  laboratory features, 792, 793*f*
  treatment and course, 432, 793
Methicillin-resistant *Staphylococcus aureus*
    (MRSA) infections, 384–385
Methionine synthesis, 586*t*, 589–590
Methotrexate, **318–321**. *See also* CODOX-M/
    IVAC regimen

for acute lymphoblastic leukemia, 1515, 1516, 1517
adverse effects, 321, 368, 599, 1407, 1519*t*
for α-heavy-chain disease, 1809
for Burkitt lymphoma, 1675, 1675*t*, 1676
for diffuse large B-cell lymphoma, 1628
for graft-versus-host disease prophylaxis, 368, 371
for intravascular large B-cell lymphoma, 1636
for Langerhans cell histiocytosis, 1106, 1107
for large granular lymphocytic leukemia, 1567
leucovorin rescue for, 320–321
for lymphomatoid papulosis, 1689
mechanism of action, 318–319, 320*f*
megaloblastic anemia and, 605, 606*t*
for mycosis fungoides, 1687
pharmacology, 319–321
resistance to, 319*t*
structure, 320*f*
6-Methoxy-arabinosylguanine. *See* Nelarabine
Methoxypsoralen, for mastocytosis, 977
Methylcobalamin, 589, 592
α-Methyldopa, 827, 831, 832, 835, 840
Methylene blue, 793
Methylenetetrahydrofolate reductase (MTHFR). *See under* MTHFR
Methylfolate trap hypothesis, 590–591, 590*f*
Methylmalonic acid, 603
Methylmalonic aciduria (cblA, cblB, cblH), 607, 607*t*
Methylmalonic aciduria and homocystinuria (cblC, cblD, cblF), 607, 607*t*
Methylmalonyl coenzyme A mutase, 589, 589*f*
Methylprednisolone. *See also* ESHAP regimen
for autoimmune hemolytic anemia, 838
for chronic lymphocytic leukemia, 1536–1537
for Diamond-Blackfan anemia, 540
for diffuse alveolar hemorrhage, 368
for graft-versus-host disease, 371
for immune thrombocytopenia, 2004
N^5-Methyltetrahydrofolate–homocysteine methyltransferase, 585, 587*f*, 589
N^5-Methyltetrahydrofolate–homocysteine methyltransferase deficiency, 608
Methylthioadenosine phosphorylase (MTAP), 238–239
Metoclopramide, 901
Mevalonate kinase deficiency, 568
MF. *See* Mycosis fungoides (MF)

MGA1 (autosomal recessive megaloblastic anemia), 605
MGC22455. *See* TSSC6
MGCD0103, 1403
MGMT (O^6-methylguanine-DNA methyltransferase), 442
MGUS (monoclonal gammopathy of unknown significance), 1721. *See also* Essential monoclonal gammopathy
mHAgs (minor histocompatibility antigens), 413–414
MHC. *See under* Major histocompatibility complex (MHC)
MI. *See* Myocardial infarction (MI)
MIC3. *See* CD9
Micafungin, 388*t*, 389
Miconazole, 2078
Microangiopathic hemolytic anemia, **803–804**, 803*t*
Microarray analysis, 174–175, 177*f*
Micrococcus infection, 2340
Microcyte, 21
Microcytic hypochromic anemia, 506
Microglia, 1083
$β_2$-Microglobulin
in chronic lymphocytic leukemia, 1532
in diffuse large B-cell lymphoma, 1632
in essential monoclonal gammopathy, 1726
in human leukocyte antigen, 2353
infection susceptibility and, 1746
in iron homeostasis, 621*t*
in mantle cell lymphoma, 1655
in myeloma, 1715–1716, 1746, 1747–1748, 1748*t*, 1759
Microgranular leukemia, 1390
Microparticles, platelet, 1854
MicroRNAs
in acute myelogenous leukemia, 1280
in chronic lymphocytic leukemia, 1529, 1532
in erythropoiesis, **487–488**
in gene regulation, 239
in myelodysplastic syndromes, 1347
in neutrophil granule protein expression, 1011
platelet, 1853
Microvilli, neutrophil, 1006
MIDAS (metal ion-dependent adhesion site), 2044–2045, 2044*f*
Midazolam, 28
MIDD (monoclonal immunoglobulin deposition disease), 1497*t*, 1744
Midostaurin, 977, 1403
Migfilin, 1832*t*, 1837
Miglustat, 1128, 1130

Migraines, 2239
Milatuzumab, for myeloma, 346*t*
Milk, folate-binding proteins of, 588
Milk fat globulin, macrophages and, 1054
Miller-Fisher syndrome, 1790
Minimal-deviation myeloid clonal disorders, 1276*t*, **1277–1278**
Minimal residual disease (MRD)
in acute myelogenous leukemia, 1412, 1414
in chronic lymphocytic leukemia, 1540
in chronic myelogenous leukemia, 1463–1464
in hairy cell leukemia, 1554, 1558
in myeloma, 1716–1717, 1758
next-generation sequencing for detection of, 163
Minor-*BCR*-breakpoint-positive chronic myelogenous leukemia, 1449
Minor cytogenic response (mCyR), 1452*t*
Minor histocompatibility antigens (mHAgs), 413–414
MIP (macrophage inflammatory protein)-1α, 288*t*, 1440, 1737–1738, 1738*f*, 1739*f*
MIRL (membrane inhibitor of reactive lysis), 572
miRNAs. *See* MicroRNAs
Missense mutations, 146
Mithramycin, 2079
Mitochondria
in cell death pathways, 205
ferritin in, 624
iron in, 623–624
in platelets, 1840
Mitochondrial antiviral signaling protein (MAVS), 302, 302*f*, 303
Mitochondrial myopathy and sideroblastic anemia (MLASA), 919
Mitochondrial outer membrane permeabilization (MOMP), 206
Mitogen-activated extracellular-regulated kinase (MEK), 298, 1016
Mitogen-activated protein kinase (MAPK), 237, 266, 1054, 1055*f*, 1178., 1817
Mitogen-activated protein kinase (MAPK) pathway, 237, 252
Mitogens, 1139
Mitomycin C, 1824, 2262–2263
Mitosis, 213
Mitoxantrone, **327–328**
for acute lymphoblastic leukemia, 1516
for acute myelogenous leukemia, 1395, 1395*t*, 1402*t*
in children, 1409
in older patients, 1408

Mitoxantrone (*Cont.*):
  adverse effects, 328
  for chronic lymphocytic leukemia, 1535
  for diffuse large B-cell lymphoma, 1631
  for follicular lymphoma, 1645*t*
  secondary acute myelogenous leukemia
      and, 1407
Mixed chimerism, following
      reduced-intensity transplantation,
      360–361
Mixed leukemia, 1386
Mixed-lineage kinase domain-like (MLKL)
      protein, 207
Mixed-lineage leukemia (MLL) protein, 169
MLASA (mitochondrial myopathy and
      sideroblastic anemia), 919
MLKp1, 568
MLL, 170
  in acute lymphoblastic leukemia, 1508,
      1512, 1521
  in acute myelogenous leukemia, 215, 225,
      1376, 1383, 1384*t*
  in follicular lymphoma, 235*t*
  in mantle cell lymphoma, 236*t*
  in myeloma, 234*t*
MLL2 (*KMT2D*), 236*t*, 1644
MLL3, 1347
MLL-AF4 (*KMTA/AFF1*), 1507, 1513*t*
MLL-ENL, 1508*t*
MLL (mixed-lineage leukemia) protein, 169
MLL-PTD, 226*t*, 1378, 1378*t*
MMACHC, 2263
MMAS (monoclonal mast cell activation
      syndrome), 977–978
MML (myelomastocytic leukemia), 978
MMPs (matrix metalloproteinases), 1014,
      1874, 1881, 2307, 2311
MMR (major molecular response),
      1452*t*
MMSET (*WHSC1*), 236*t*, 1735
MNP (marginal neutrophil pool), 942*t*
MNS blood group/antigens, 2331*t*, 2334*t*,
      2339, 2343, 2344*t*
Mo1. *See* CD11b/CD18 (Mac-1, Mo1, CR3,
      α$_M$β$_2$)
Mocetinostat, 240
Model of end-stage liver disease (MELD),
      2192
Moderate-deviation clonal myeloid disorders,
      1276*t*, **1278–1279**
Moderately severe-deviation clonal myeloid
      disorders, 1276*t*, **1279**
Moesin, 1006
Mogamulizumab, for adult T-cell leukemia/
      lymphoma, 1701
Molecular biology, **152–153**

MOMA-1, 1082*f*
MOMP (mitochondrial outer membrane
      permeabilization), 206
MondoA, 197
Monge disease, 875
Monoblasts, 1046
Monoclonal antibodies (mAbs), **343–346**.
      See also specific drugs
  dose and toxicity, 343*t*
  for follicular lymphoma, 1645–1646
  immunotoxins, 345–346
  for mycosis fungoides, 1687
  for myeloma, 345, 345*f*, 346*t*, 1755
  radioimmunoconjugates, 346, 360
Monoclonal antibody-specific
      immobilization of platelet antigens
      (MAPIPA) assay, 2000
Monoclonal B-cell lymphocytosis (MBL),
      1199–1200, 1201*t*, 1542–1543
Monoclonal gammopathy of unknown
      significance (MGUS), 1721.
      See also Essential monoclonal
      gammopathy
Monoclonal gammopathy with a coinciding
      disease, 1724–1725, 1725*t*
Monoclonal immunoglobulin deposition
      disease (MIDD), 1497*t*, 1744
Monoclonal mast cell activation syndrome
      (MMAS), 977–978
Monoclonal proteins. *See* M-proteins
Monocyte chemoattractant protein
      (MCP-1). *See* CCL2 (monocyte
      chemoattractant protein, MCP-1)
Monocyte colony-stimulating factor
      (M-CSF), 264*t*, 1352
Monocyte–macrophage system, 619
Monocytes
  activation, 283
    classical and alternative, 1085–1086,
      1086*f*
    immunomodulation, 1084, 1085*f*
    innate, 1084–1085
    in response to inflammation and
      tumors, 1083–1084, 1084*f*
  blood dendritic cells and, 1092
  cell adhesion and homing, 66
  in children, 15*t*
  cytochemical reactions, 1049*t*
  development, 1075–1076
    growth, differentiation, and turnover,
      1076, 1076*f*
    maturation and differentiation,
      1077–1078, 1077*f*,
      1078*f*
  disorders
    classification, 1089, 1090*t*

clinical manifestations, 1091
    histiocytosis, 1090–1091, 1090*t*. *See also*
      Histiocytosis(es)
    monocytopenia. *See* Monocytopenia
    monocytosis. *See* Monocytosis
    qualitative, 1091
    thromboatherogenesis and, 1092
  distribution
    in marrow, 32*t*, 34, 1081–1082
    in nonlymphohematopoietic organs,
      1082–1083
  functions
    cellular interactions, 1066, 1071, 1071*f*
    G-protein-coupled receptors and, 1060*t*
    inflammasome, 1063–1064, 1065*f*,
      1066*f*
    interaction with coagulation cascade,
      1059
    motility, **1059**, 1060*t*
  heterogeneity, **1078–1081**, 1079*f*, 1080*t*
  histochemistry, 1048, 1049*t*
  inflammatory response in, 1970*f*
  markers, 1080*t*
  in myelodysplastic syndromes, 1353
  in newborn, 105*t*
  normal blood concentration, 1095
  precursors, 1046
  properties, 1095
  receptors
    CD4, 1056–1057
    CD11, 1056
    CD14, 1056
    CD16, 1056
    chemokine, 1057–1058, 1058*t*
    complement, 1054
    Fc, 1053–1054, 1053*f*
    human leukocyte antigen class II,
      1055–1056
    non–toll-like, nonopsonic, 1054–1055,
      1056*f*, 1057*t*
    surface, 1052–1053, 1058*t*
    surface antigens, 1052*f*
    toll-like, 1054, 1055*f*
  reference ranges, 18*t*
  release, 72
  in sickle cell disease, 765
  small immature, 1045
  structure, 20*f*, 23, **1045–1047**, **1046–1047**,
      1046*f*, 1047*f*, 1048*f*, 1049*f*
  subset variations in disease, 1098
Monocytic leukemia
  acute. *See* Acute monocytic leukemia
  chronic. *See* Chronic myelomonocytic
      leukemia
Monocytic progenitors, **271**
Monocytoid B cells, 1595

Monocytoma. *See* Myeloid (granulocytic) sarcoma
Monocytopenia, **1089**
   clinical features, 1091
   consultative approach to, 42
   disorders associated with, 1090t, 1098, 1098t
Monocytopoiesis, in newborn, 105
Monocytosis
   classification, 1089, 1090t
   consultative approach to, 44
   disorders associated with, **1095–1097**, 1096t
   tissue effects, 1092
Monoferric transferrin pool, 491
MonoMAC syndrome, 1089, 1098, 1231, 1351, 1379
Monomethoxypolyethylene glycol (PEG), 332
Mononeuritis multiplex, 959
Mononuclear phagocyte system (MPS), 1045, 1046t. *See also* Macrophages; Monocytes
Mononucleosis syndromes, **1261–1269**
   autoimmune hemolytic anemia and, 824, 835
   cytomegalovirus. *See* Cytomegalovirus (CMV) mononucleosis
   definition and history, 1261
   differential diagnosis, 1269, 1513
   Epstein-Barr virus. *See* Epstein-Barr virus (EBV) mononucleosis
   etiology and pathogenesis, 1261, 1262t
   Hodgkin lymphoma and, 1605
   neutropenia and, 997
   in pregnancy, 1269
   in primary HIV infection, 1268
   therapy, 1269
Monophosphoglyceromutase, 692t
Monosomy 7, 521, 1347
MOPP regimen, for Hodgkin lymphoma, 1604, 1611, 1617, 1618
Morbus caeruleus, 871
Morphine, 767–768
Morula (Mott) cell, 1742, 1743f
Mountain sickness, 875, 881
Mouth
   examination, 8
   history of dryness of, 5
6-MP. *See* 6-Mercaptopurine (6-MP)
MPC (multiparameter flow cytometry), 1716
M-phase promoting factors, 213
MPL, 519
   in acute megakaryoblastic leukemia, 1392
   in essential thrombocythemia, 229t, 1307, 1308f, 1310
   in familial thrombocytosis, 1310

in myelofibrosis, 229t
   in primary myelofibrosis, 1321
   in refractory anemia with ring sideroblasts with thrombocytosis, 1352
MPLV (myeloproliferative leukemia virus), 1822
MPO (myeloperoxidase), 107, 1011, 1012t, 1068f
MPO (myeloperoxidase) deficiency, 1020t, 1033
M-proteins, 1714, 1723, 1741
MPS (mononuclear phagocyte system), 1045, 1046t. *See also* Macrophages; Monocytes
MPV (mean platelet volume), 17
MRD. *See* Minimal residual disease (MRD)
MRI. *See* Magnetic resonance imaging (MRI)
mRNA (messenger RNA)
   globin gene clusters regulation and, 729–730
   mutations causing abnormal translation of, 731–732, 732f
   platelet, 1851–1853, 1852f
   in protein synthesis, 147
   von Willebrand factor, 2164, 2165f
MRP-1. *See* CD9
MRP-14 (S100A9), 1856, 1872
MRPs (multidrug resistance-associated proteins), 318
MRs (mannose receptors), 284, 1054, 1057t, 1080, 1081f
MRSA (methicillin-resistant *Staphylococcus aureus*) infections, 384–385
MSCs (mesenchymal stromal cells), 449–450, 451
MTA (5′-deoxy-5′[methylthio] adenosine), 239
MTA (metastasis-associated), 166
MTA3, 166
MTAP (methylthioadenosine phosphorylase), 238–239
MTHFR
   colon cancer and, 599
   hyperhomocysteinemia and, 599, 2224. *See also* Hyperhomocysteinemia
MTHFR (methylenetetrahydrofolate reductase), 585, 590
MTHFR (methylenetetrahydrofolate reductase) deficiency, 608
mTOR (mammalian target of rapamycin), 194, 1654, 2237, 2237f
mTOR (mammalian target of rapamycin) inhibitors, 1220, 1403. *See also* Temsirolimus
Mucopolysaccharidoses, 23

Mucosa-associated lymphoid tissue (MALT), **93–94**. *See also* Extranodal marginal zone lymphoma of MALT type
Mucosal addressin cell adhesion molecule 1 (MAdCAM-1), 950, 1977
Mucositis, **368**
Mucous membrane hemorrhage, 2120
μ-heavy-chain disease, **1809–1810**, 1810f
Multidrug resistance, 318
Multidrug resistance-associated proteins (MRPs), 318
Multimerin, 1845, 1846t, 1924
Multiparameter flow cytometry (MPC), 1716
Multiple intestinal atresia, 1222
Multiple myeloma. *See* Myeloma
Multiple sclerosis, 1265, 2239
Multipotential cells
   embryonic stem cells, 448–449
   hematopoietic stem cells. *See* Hematopoietic stem cells (HSCs)
   induced pluripotent stem cells, 449
   leukemia stem cell, 1376
   mesenchymal stromal cells, 449–450
   for tissue repair. *See* Multipotential cell therapy
Multipotential cell therapy
   for brain and spinal cord repair, 451–452
   for cardiac repair, 450
   gene edited cells in, 453–454
   for liver and pancreas repair, 452–453
   for lung repair, 451
   principles, 447, 448f
Multispecies conserved sequences (MCSs), 730
Multivesicular bodies (MVBs), 1844
MUNC13-4 (Munc13-4), 1114, 1849
Muramyl dipeptide (MDP), 299, 301f
Murine double minute protein 2 (MDM2), 238
Murine stem cells, assays of, 259
Muscular function, iron deficiency and, 631
Mutasome, 1169
MY01G, 414
MYBL2, 1347–1348
MYC
   activation, 194–195, 194f, 195f
   functions, 187, 192
   in myeloma, 200
MYC/Myc, 1576
   in Burkitt lymphoma, 1245, 1672, 1674
   in diffuse large B-cell lymphoma, 1626, 1627t, 1632–1633
   in "double-hit" lymphoma, 1502, 1596, 1633, 1674
   in myeloma, 1709, 1711, 1735, 1735f, 1736

Mycobacterial infections
    chronic inflammation and, 290, 291
    evasion of phagocytic mechanisms in, 1062, 1064f
    in HIV infection, 1097, 1240, 1241t
    in idiopathic CD4+ lymphocytopenia, 1206
    after hematopoietic cell transplantation, 369
    in immunocompromised host, 384
    Mendelian susceptibility to, **1231**
    monocytosis in, 1097
    treatment, 386
Mycophenolate mofetil
    for autoimmune hemolytic anemia, 839
    in reduced-intensity conditioning, 360
Mycophenolic acid, 200
Mycoplasma pneumoniae
    autoimmune hemolytic anemia and, 824, 828
    hemolytic anemia and, 820
Mycosis fungoides (MF). *See also* Cutaneous T-cell lymphoma (CTCL)
    classification, 1680t
    clinical features, 1680, 1681f
    definition and history, 1679
    differential diagnosis, 1683–1684
    epidemiology, 1679
    erythrodermic subset, 1683, 1684t
    etiology and pathogenesis, 1680
    gene mutations, 1498t
    laboratory features, 1498t, 1680–1682, 1681f, 1682f, 1683f
    prognosis, 1688
    staging, 1682–1683, 1682t, 1683f, 1683t
    treatment, **1684–1688**
        guidelines/algorithm, 1684–1685, 1685f
        skin-directed, 429t, 433, 1684t, 1685–1686
        systemic, 1684t, 1686–1688
MYD88, 231t, 234t, 235t, 1529, 1644, 1712
MyD88 (myeloid differentiation factor/protein 88), 1054, 1084, 1230
MyD88 (myeloid differentiation primary response 88), 297f, 298
MyD88 adapter-like (MAL), 297f, 298
MYD88L265, 1711, 1722
MYD88^{L265P}, 1786–1787, 1787f, 1788, 1791
Myelin-associated glycoprotein (MAG), 1790
Myeloblastoma. *See* Myeloid (granulocytic) sarcoma
Myeloblasts
    in acute myelogenous leukemia, 1381
    acute myelogenous leukemia and, 1375
    marrow, 32t, 34, 927f

maturation, 926f, 940–941, 940f, 941t
structure, 925
Myelocytes
    marrow, 32t, 34
    maturation, 940–941, 940f, 941t
    neutrophilic, 925, 927f
Myelodysplasia
    α-thalassemia and, 739
    aplastic anemia and, 520
    definition, 1277–1278, 1343
    gene mutations, 1308t
Myelodysplastic syndromes (MDSs)
    acute myelogenous leukemia and, 178, 180, 1341–1342
    acute promyelocytic leukemia and, 1406
    vs. aplastic anemia, 520
    classification, 1343–1344, 1343t
    clinical features, 1352–1353, 2081–2082
    definition, 1341–1342
    diagnostic criteria, 1354, 1355t
    epidemiology, 1344–1345, 1344f
    etiology, 1345
    history, 1342–1343
    laboratory features
        blood, 1350f, 1353
        marrow, 37, 1350f, 1353–1354
        plasma, 1353
    monocytosis in, 1096
    paroxysmal nocturnal hemoglobinuria and, 576t, 578
    pathogenesis, **1345–1352**
        chromosomal abnormalities, 178, 180t, 182, 221t, **1346–1348**, 1346t
        epigenetic regulators, 1349–1352
        gene mutations, 180t, 181t, 227–228t, 233–234t, 1346t, 1348–1349
        microenvironmental changes, 1352
    prognosis, 1355–1356, 1355t, 1356t
    sideroblastic anemia and, 918–919
    therapy-related, 182, 182f, 1354
    treatment, **1356–1362**
        demethylating agents, 239, 336
        in higher-risk disease, 1360–1362
        in lower-risk disease, 1357–1360
        prognostic score and, 1356–1357
Myelodysplastic transformation, in polycythemia vera, 1295
Myelofibrosis
    primary. *See* Primary myelofibrosis (PMF)
    secondary, 1325
Myelofibrotic transformation, in thrombocythemia, 1309
Myelogene, 1373, 1438
Myeloid dendritic cells, markers, 1080t
Myeloid differentiation factor/protein 88 (MyD88), 1054, 1084, 1230

Myeloid differentiation primary response 88 (MyD88), 297f, 298
Myeloid leukemia hybrid, 1386
Myeloid-lymphoid leukemias, 1386
Myeloid–natural killer cell hybrid leukemia, 1386
Myeloid progenitors, **270–271**
Myeloid (granulocytic) sarcoma
    in acute myelogenous leukemia, 1285, 1381
    in chronic myelogenous leukemia, 1465
    nonleukemic, 1398
Myeloid series, marrow, 34
Myeloid-to-erythroid (M:E) ratio, marrow, 31
Myelokathexis, 994, 1226
Myeloma
    chronic lymphocytic leukemia and, 1541
    clinical features, 1740t, 1741f
        cast nephropathy, 428, 430t, 1744
        extramedullary disease, 1746
        hematologic abnormalities, 1740–1741
        hypercalcemia, 1744
        hyperviscosity, 1746
        infections, 1745–1746
        neuropathy, 1746
        pain, 1745
        plasma cell leukemia, 1746. *See also* Plasma cell leukemia
        platelet dysfunction, 2082
        renal disease, 1744–1745
        spinal cord compression, 1746–1747
    definition and history, 1733
    differential diagnosis, 1726, 1726t, 1750
    epidemiology, 1734
    essential monoclonal gammopathy and, 1722, 1734, 1734f
    etiology and pathogenesis, 1709
        bone metabolism, 1713, 1737–1738, 1739f
        cell growth and metabolism, 200–201
        chromosomal abnormalities, 185t, **188**
            1q/1p, 188, 223t, 1759
            deletions, 185t, 1736, 1736t, 1744, 1744f, 1745f, 1759
            detection methods, 1711
            hyperdiploidy, 185t, 224t, 1735, 1736t
            karyotype abnormalities, 1735f, 1745f
            prognosis and, 1759–1760
            translocations, 185t, 188, 224t, 225, 1735–1736, 1735f, 1736t, 1744, 1744f
        endogenous factors, 1709
        exogenous factors, 1709, 1734
        gene expression, 1711
        gene mutations, 166, 170, **188**, 233–234t
            BRAF, 233t, 1737

detection methods, 1711
DIS3, 233*t*, 1737
drug resistance and, 1711
early events, 1710
EGR1, 234*t*
FAM46C, 1737
FGFR3, 233*t*
heterogeneity, 1760
IGH, 188
KRAS (*K-RAS*), 188, 233*t*, 1709, 1737, 1759, 1760
late events, 1710–1711
LRRK2, 233*t*
MAF, 233*t*
MYC, 1711
NRAS (*N-RAS*), 188, 233*t*, 1709, 1759
p53, 1710
PRDM1, 234*t*
prognosis and, 1759–1760
RAS, 1710, 1735*f*, 1736*t*, 1737
RB/RB1, 234*t*, 1710
somatic, 1736–1737
TP53, 1735*f*
TP53, 233*t*, 1737
marrow microenvironment, 1712–1713, 1737, 1738*f*
myeloma stem cell, 1713–1714, 1734
occupation, 1709, 1734
plasma cell differentiation, 1710, 1710*f*
preclinical models, 1739–1740, 1739*f*
radiation, 1709
stages, 1734–1735, 1734*f*
Gaucher disease and, 1125
IgM, 1760
initial evaluation, 1747, 1747*t*
laboratory features, 1740*t*
blood, 1740–1741
imaging, 1715, 1748–1749, 1748*f*, 1749*f*
immunoglobulins, 1714, 1741
lactate dehydrogenase levels, 1716
marrow, 31–32, 1715, 1741–1744, 1742*f*, 1743*f*, 1744*f*
β_2-microglobulin, 1715–1716
serum, 1714
urine, 1714
larval, 1726
minimal residual disease assessment, 1716–1717
monocytosis and, 1097
plasmablastic, 1742
prognosis, 1712, 1759–1760
smoldering, 1708–1709, 1726, 1734*f*, 1761
staging, 1747–1748, 1747*t*, 1748*t*
treatment
of bone pain, 1756
of complications, 1756–1757

consolidation therapy, 1752–1753
continuous therapy, 1753
cyclin-dependent kinase inhibitors, 218
hematopoietic cell transplantation, 364–366, 365*f*, 1750, 1755–1756
histone deacetylase inhibitors, 240, 1754
immunomodulatory drugs, 1754
maintenance therapy, 1751–1752, 1752*t*
monoclonal antibodies, 345, 345*f*, 346*t*, 1754–1755
of osteonecrosis of the jaw, 1757
of peripheral neuropathy, 1757
proteasome inhibitors, 342–343, 1749–1750
in relapsed or refractory disease, 1753–1755, 1753*t*
response criteria, 1758, 1758*t*
in transplant-eligible patients, 1748*t*, 1750–1751
in transplant-ineligible patients, 1751, 1752*t*
of venous thromboembolism, 1756–1757
Myeloma stem cell, 1713–1714
Myelomastocytic leukemia (MML), 978
Myelomonocytic leukemia. *See* Acute myelomonocytic leukemia; Chronic myelomonocytic leukemia (CMML)
Myeloperoxidase (MPO), 107, 1011, 1012*t*, 1068*f*
Myeloperoxidase (MPO) deficiency, 1020*t*, 1033
Myelophthisic anemia, 657. *See also* Marrow, infiltration
Myeloproliferative disease, atypical, 1473
Myeloproliferative leukemia virus (MPLV), 1822
Myelosuppression, for polycythemia vera, 1298–1299, 1298*t*
MYH9 (*Myh9*), 1818, 1842
MYH9-related thrombocytopenia syndromes, 1996, 1999*f*, 2061
MYL9, 2058, 2060
Myocardial infarction (MI), **2294–2297**
clinical features, 2295
diagnosis, 2294–2295
factor VIII levels and, 2226–2227
genetic factors, 1850, 1853, 2288
in hemophilia, 2130
laboratory features, 2295
monocytosis and, 1097
therapy, 1855, 2076, **2295–2297**, 2313
Myoglobin, 618
Myosin, 1833*t*, 1842
Myosin II, 1833*t*

Myosin light-chain kinase, 1833*t*
Myristoylated alanine-rich C-kinase substrate (MARCKS), 667, 668*f*

N
N^5-formyl FH$_4$, 584
N^5-methyl FH$_4$–homocysteine methyltransferase, 585, 587*f*, 589–590
N^5-methyl FH$_4$–homocysteine methyltransferase deficiency, 608
N370S, 1122, 1123, 1123*t*
N803, 487
NAD+, in glucose metabolism, 693
NADH, in glucose metabolism, 692
NADH diaphorase. *See* Cytochrome b$_5$
NADH-methemoglobin reductase, 692*t*
NADP
in folate metabolism, 584
in glucose metabolism, 694
NADPH
in folate metabolism, 584, 585
in glucose metabolism, 694
in neurodegenerative disorders, 1840
NADPH diaphorase, 692*t*, 701*t*, 790, 793
NADPH oxidase
in atherothrombosis, 2283
in chronic granulomatous disease, 1027–1029, 1028*f*
in inflammatory response, 286
neutrophil granules and, 927
respiratory burst and, 1068*f*
Nadroparin, 2274*t*
Nails, examination of, 8
NAIT (neonatal alloimmune thrombocytopenia). *See* Newborns/infants, alloimmune thrombocytopenia in
Nalidixic acid, maternal ingestion of, effect on fetus and newborn, 112, 112*t*
NAMPT (nicotinamide phosphoribosyltransferase), 200
Nantucket fever, 819
NAP-1 (neutrophil-activating peptide 1). *See* Interleukin (IL)-8
NAP-2 (neutrophil-activating peptide 2), 1856
NAPc2 (nematode anticoagulant protein c2), 2214
Naproxen
antiplatelet effects, 404, 2075
maternal ingestion of, effect on fetus and newborn, 112
Nasopharynx, history of disorders of, 5
Natural killer (NK) cell antigens, 1142, 1142*t*

Natural killer (NK) cell lymphocytosis, 1202–1203

Natural killer (NK) cell lymphoproliferation, 1265

Natural killer (NK) cell neoplasms. *See also specific types*
  leukemia, 1192, 1499*t*, 1563, 1566
  lymphoma/lymphoproliferative disorders
    chromosomal abnormalities, 185*t*
    extranodal, 1192, 1498*t*
    histologic subtypes and frequency of, 1572*t*

Natural killer (NK) cell progenitors, **270**

Natural killer (NK) cell receptors, 1190–1191, 1190*f*, 1192

Natural killer (NK) cells
  antigens, 1142, 1142*t*
  in cancer treatment, 1192–1193
  in chronic myelogenous leukemia, 1440
  cytoplasmic granules in, 1145
  definition, 1189
  dendritic cells and, 307
  development, 1151
  disorders, 1197. *See also* Chronic lymphoproliferative disorders of NK cells (CLPD-NK); Natural killer (NK) cell neoplasms
  functions, 1190–1191
    cell-mediated cytotoxicity, 1190–1191, 1190*f*
    cytokine production, 1191
  in lymph nodes, 93
  morphology, 1142, 1189
  in mycosis fungoides, 1680
  origin and tissue distribution, 1189
  pathologic alterations in numbers of, 1192
  physiologic roles
    innate resistance, 1191, 1191*f*
    modulation of hematopoiesis, 1191–1192
    regulation of adaptive immunity, 1191

Natural killer (NK)/T-cell lymphoma, 1581, 1694*t*, 1695*t*. *See also* Extranodal natural killer (NK)/T-cell lymphoma, nasal type

NB1 glycoprotein, 2358

NBEAL2, 1850, 1853

NBT (nitroblue tetrazolium), in newborn, 107

NCAM (neuronal cell-adhesion molecule, CD56), 1142, 1189, 1699, 1726, 1737

NCF1 (p47*phox*), 1028*t*, 1029

NCF2 (p67*phox*), 1028*t*, 1029

NCF4 (p40*phox*), 1029

Necator americanus, 949

Neck, history of disorders of, 5

Necrosis, marrow, 33

Necrotic lesions, history of, 6

Neisseria meningitidis, 868, 869, 1017, 2104, 2340

NEK2, 1711, 1712

Nelarabine, 323*f*, **325**, 1518

Nematode anticoagulant protein c2 (NAPc2), 2214

NEMO (NF-κB essential modulator), 298, 1214*t*, 1215

NEM-sensitive fusion protein (NSF), 1016

Neocytolysis, 498, 810–811

Neogenin, 621*t*

Neomycin, megaloblastic anemia and, 606*t*

Neonates/neonatal disease. *See* Newborns/infants

Neoplastic megakaryocytopoiesis, 1321

Neoplastic myeloid disorders. *See* Clonal myeloid disorders

Netosis, 1017

NETs (neutrophil extracellular traps), 1007*f*, 1017, 1856

Neulasta, for diffuse large B-cell lymphoma, 1629*t*

Neural stem cells (NSCs), 451

Neural tube defects, 598

Neuroacanthocytosis, **681**
  abetalipoproteinemia, **681**
  chorea-acanthocytosis syndrome, **681**
  differential diagnosis, 682
  HARP syndrome, 682
  Huntington disease-like 2 disorder, 682
  McLeod syndrome, **681**
  pantothenate kinase-associated neurodegeneration, 682

Neuroendocrine theory of aging, 131

Neurologic disease/symptoms. *See also* Central nervous system
  in acute lymphoblastic leukemia relapse, 1517, 1518
  in acute myelogenous leukemia, 1381, 1397–1398
  in AL amyloidosis, 1760, 1775, 1775*t*, 1779
  in antiphospholipid syndrome, 2238–2239
  brain injury, multipotential cell therapy for, 451–452
  brain tumors, erythrocytosis and, 879
  in cobalamin deficiency, 602, 602*f*
  in disseminated intravascular coagulation, 2204, 2208
  in Erdheim-Chester disease, 1111
  in essential monoclonal gammopathy, 1724
  in Gaucher disease, 1125
  in hemolytic uremic syndrome, 2259
  in hemophilia, 2119–2120

  in iron deficiency, 632
  in Langerhans cell histiocytosis, 1105, 1105*f*, 1106, 1107
  macrophages and, 1083
  in myeloma, 1746, 1757
  red cell transfusion in, 2371
  in sickle cell disease, 769–770
  in thrombotic thrombocytopenic purpura, 2254
  in Waldenström macroglobulinemia, 1789–1790, 1791

Neurologic examination, 4–5, 9

Neuronal cell-adhesion molecule (NCAM, CD56), 1142, 1189, 1699, 1726, 1737

Neuroreticular complex, 56

Neutropenia, **991–997**
  chronic idiopathic, 983, 985, 995
  classification, 41, 983, 984*t*
  clinical approach to, 997
  clinical features, 985
  congenital, 992–993, 993*f*
  consultative approach to, 41–42
  cyclic, 983, 985, 994, 1097
  definition, 985, 991
  etiology, 984*t*, 985
    autoimmune, 995, 996*f*
    disorders affecting neutrophil utilization and turnover, 995–996
    disorders of production, 992–995
    drug-induced, 985, 992, 996–997, 998*t*
    "ethnic," 985
    in HIV infection, 997, 1254
    infectious, 997
  hematopoietic cell transplantation and, 369
  pathophysiologic mechanisms, 991–992, 992*f*
  pseudo-, 985
  severity of, infection risk and, 383

Neutropenic enterocolitis, 1410

Neutrophil actin dysfunction, 1024

Neutrophil-activating peptide-1. *See* Interleukin (IL)-8

Neutrophil-activating peptide-2, 288*t*

Neutrophil alkaline phosphatase activity
  in chronic myelogenous leukemia, 1445
  in myelodysplastic syndromes, 1353
  in primary myelofibrosis, 1326

Neutrophil antigens. *See* Human neutrophil antigens (HNAs)

Neutrophil collagenase, 1012*t*, 1014, 1322

Neutrophil extracellular traps (NETs), 1007*f*, 1017, 1856, 1941, 1941*f*

Neutrophil gelatinase-associated lipocalin (NGAL), 1009, 1012*t*, 1013–1014

Neutrophilia, **997–1001**

acute, 999–1000
chronic, 1000
classification, 984*t*
clinical approach to, 1001
consultative approach to, 44
definition, 997, 999
disorders associated with, 1000–1001
etiology, 985–986, 999–1000, 1000*t*
mechanisms, 999–1000, 999*f*
pseudo-, 999–1000
in sickle cell disease, 765
vascular or tissue damage and, 984*t*, 986
Neutrophilic chronic myelogenous leukemia, 1449
Neutrophilic dermatosis (Sweet syndrome), 1001, 1324, 1380, 2102–2103, 2102*f*
Neutrophilic leukocytosis, 997. *See also* Neutrophilia
Neutrophilic myelocyte, 925, 926*f*
Neutrophils, 22
abnormalities
in megaloblastic anemia, 594*f*, 595
in myelodysplastic syndromes, 1350*f*, 1353
adhesion molecules, 934*t*
amino acids, 935, 935*t*
apoptosis in, 285
biochemical features, 935, 935*t*
chemotactic receptors, 934*t*
cytochemical reactions, 1049*t*
definition and history, 939
disorders, **983–986, 1017–1034**
actin dysfunction, 1024
adhesion abnormalities, 1019*t*, 1021–1024, 1021*t*, 1023*f*
classification, 983, 984*t*, 1017
clinical manifestations, 983–985
degranulation abnormalities
Chédiak-Higashi syndrome. *See* Chédiak-Higashi syndrome
specific granule deficiency, 1019*t*, 1020–1021
diagnostic approach, 1034, 1035*f*
microbicidal activity defects
chronic granulomatous disease. *See* Chronic granulomatous disease
glucose-6-phosphate dehydrogenase (G6PD) deficiency. *See* Glucose-6-phosphate dehydrogenase (G6PD) deficiency
glutathione reductase and glutathione synthetase deficiencies, 698, 700*t*, 701*t*, 705, 709, 1020*t*, 1033
myeloperoxidase deficiency, 1020*t*, 1033
Rac-2 deficiency, 1020*t*

motility disorders, 1019*t*, 1026
drugs and extrinsic agents and, 1026
familial Mediterranean fever, **1024–1026**
hyperimmunoglobulin E syndrome, 1020*t*, 1026–1027, 1182, 1215*t*, **1225**
neutropenia. *See* Neutropenia
neutrophilia. *See* Neutrophilia
qualitative abnormalities, 984*t*, 986
signal mechanism abnormalities, 1017
vascular or tissue damage and, 984*t*, 986
evaluation of reserves, 943
function, **1005–1017**
adhesion, 1006
adhesion and spreading, 1006–1008, 1007*f*
carbohydrate metabolism, 932
chemotaxis and motility, 1005
ingestion, 1005–1006, 1006*f*
microvilli dynamics, 1006
protein synthesis, 932, 933*t*
receptor-ligand interactions, **1014–1017**, 1015*f*
rolling and tethering, 1006
secretory vesicles, 1009
stimulus-response coupling, 1014
surface proteins, 1008–1009
transendothelial migration, 1008
granules, **1009–1011**
abnormal, 23
azurophil. *See* Azurophil granules
biosynthetic timing, 1010, 1010*f*
constitutive and regulated exocytotic pathway, 1010–1011
contents, 927, 930*t*
control of protein expression, 1010*f*, 1011
heterogeneity, 1009–1010
microRNAs and, 1011
nomenclature, 1009
peroxidase-negative, 1013–1014
physical-chemical and functional properties of, **1011–1014**, 1012–1013*t*
structure, 926–927
granulopoiesis, **939**
blood kinetics, 941–942, 942*t*
humoral regulators, 939–940
hyperplastic, 983
marrow kinetics, 940–941, 941*t*
maturation of precursor cells, 940, 941*f*
migration into tissues, 942–943
in inflammation, 289
life span, 943
marrow, 32*t*

nucleotides, 935, 935*t*
opsonic receptors, 934*t*
phenotypic changes, 934–935
recruitment of, in inflammation, 283
reference ranges, 18*t*, 19*f*
release, 71, 71*f*
structure, **925–926**
band, 20*f*, 925–926, 926*f*, 927*f*, 939, 941*t*
inclusions, 23
lipids, 935, 935*t*
mature, 925–926, 926*f*, 927*f*, 929*f*
metamyelocyte, 925–926, 926*f*, 927*f*, 929*f*
myeloblast, 925, 926*f*, 927*f*
neutrophilic myelocyte, 925, 927*f*
promyelocyte, 925, 926*f*, 927*f*, 928*f*
segmented, 20*f*
Neutrophil serine protease 4 (NSP4), 1012*t*
Neutrophil turnover rate (NTR), 941, 942, 942*t*
Newborns/infants
alloimmune hemolytic disease of. *See* Alloimmune hemolytic disease of the fetus and newborn (HDFN)
alloimmune neutropenia in, 995, 2358
alloimmune thrombocytopenia in, **2012–2013**, 2359, 2361, 2362
disseminated intravascular coagulation in, 2211
hematology, **102–112**. *See also specific cell type*
bone marrow, 32*t*
coagulation, **109–111**, 110*t*, 111*t*
erythropoiesis and red cells, **102–105**, 103*t*, 104*f*, 105*t*
lymphopoiesis, **108–109**, 108*t*, 109*t*
maternal drugs and, **112**, 112*t*
thrombopoiesis and platelets, 107–108
white cells, **105–107**
hemochromatosis, 640
hereditary elliptocytosis in, 679
hereditary pyropoikilocytosis in, 679
hereditary spherocytosis in, 674
icterus in, 689, 707, 709
immunoglobulin in, 2347
iron deficiency in, 630, 632
jaundice in, 707, 709
leukemia in, 1379, 1386, 1515
methemoglobinemia susceptibility in, 790
myeloproliferative syndromes in, 1385–1386
neutropenia in, 994, 995
neutrophil motility in, 1026
polycythemia in, 879, 881
red cell transfusion in, 2371, 2372*t*
thrombocytopenia in, 2011

Next-generation sequencing (NGS)
    for chromatin accessibility studies,
        161–162
    for chromatin modification studies, 161
    as clinical tool, 162
    data analysis methods, 160–161
    for DNA methylation and
        hydroxymethylation studies, 162
    overview, 152, 155–156
    by pH change sensing, 157–158, 157f
    for research purposes, 162
    Sanger, 155
    single-molecule, 158–159, 158f
    by synthesis, 156–157, 156f
    targeted, 159–160, 159f
    for transcriptome analysis, 161
NF1, 1444, 1471
NFATs (nuclear factor of activated T cells),
        1178, 1528
NFE-2, 730
NF-E2, 893, 894, 1818, 1820
NFKBIE, 231t
NF-κB (nuclear factor-kappa B)
    apoptosis regulation and, 208f, 209
    in chronic lymphocytic leukemia, 1528
    in extranodal marginal zone lymphoma of
        MALT type, 1663–1664
    impaired activation, 1220
    in inflammation, 2202
    in myeloma, 1710, 1711
    p210^{BCR-ABL} and, 1444
    in splenic marginal zone lymphoma, 1666
    in toll-like receptor signaling, 1054, 1055f
    in Waldenström macroglobulinemia,
        1786–1787
NF-κB essential modulator (NEMO), 298,
        1215
NF-κB inhibitors, for acute myelogenous
        leukemia, 1403
NF-κB pathway, 233t, 1606
NGAL (neutrophil gelatinase-associated
        lipocalin), 1009, 1012t, 1013–1014
NGS. See Next-generation sequencing (NGS)
NHEJ (nonhomologous DNA end joining),
        1166, 1169
NHEJ (nonhomologous end-joining), 453
Niacin deficiency (pellagra), 652
Niclosamide, 604
Nicotinamide, 1193
Nicotinamide adenine dinucleotide. See
        under NAD
Nicotinamide phosphoribosyltransferase
        (NAMPT), 200
Niemann-Pick disease, 1128–1130
    course and prognosis, 1130
    epidemiology, 1129

etiology and pathogenesis, 1122f, 1129
history and classification, 1128–1129
laboratory features and differential
    diagnosis, 1130
pathology and clinical manifestations,
    1129–1130, 1129f
treatment, 1130
types, 1129
Night sweats, history of, 4
Nijmegen breakage syndrome, 530t, 1227,
        1575t
    acute lymphoblastic leukemia and, 1507
Nilotinib
    adverse effects, 339t, 341, 1451t, 1454
    for chronic myelogenous leukemia, 176,
        339t, 1451t, 1454, 1457, 1466
    comparison with other tyrosine kinase
        inhibitors, 1451t, 1454
    drug interactions, 339t, 1451t
    pharmacology, 339t, 340–341
Nippostrongylus, 956
Nippostrongylus brasiliensis, 956
Nitric oxide (NO), 1970–1971
    characteristics, 1967
    in disseminated intravascular coagulation,
        2203
    functions, 1970–1971
    in high-altitude dwellers, 875
    in inflammatory response, 280, 286–287,
        286t
    inhaled, 797
    pathophysiology, 797
    platelet adhesion and, 1834, 1885
    platelet aggregation and, 1971
    platelet function and, 2077, 2078
    red blood cells and, 796–797, 796f, 797f
    scavenging, in sickle cell disease, 764
    synthesis, 1885, 1971
Nitric oxide synthase (NOS)
    endothelial activation and, 1970–1971
    in inflammatory response, 286–287
    platelet effects, 1971
    structure and biochemical properties, 1971
    vascular tone and, 2283, 2283f
Nitrites, toxic methemoglobinemia, 789, 790t
Nitroblue tetrazolium (NBT), in newborn,
        107
Nitrofurantoin
    maternal ingestion of, effect on fetus and
        newborn, 112, 112t
    platelet function and, 2078
Nitrogen mustard, 329, 330, 1106, 1685,
        1687. See also MOPP regimen;
        Stanford V regimen
Nitroglycerin, 790t, 2078, 2295
Nitroprusside, 2078

Nitrosoureas, 319t, 329, 330, 1824
Nitrous oxide, 604–605, 801
Nitrovasodilators, 1968t
Nix, 487
NK. See under Natural killer (NK)
NKG2A, 1190, 1192
NLRs (nucleotide-binding oligomerization
        domain-like receptors), 298–299,
        299f, 1008, 1063, 1065f
NO. See Nitric oxide (NO)
Nocardia infection, 369, 383. See also
        Bacterial infections
Nocturnal enuresis, 770–771
Nodal marginal zone lymphoma, 1495t, 1592,
        1592f, 1667–1668, 1668f
NOD (nucleotide-binding oligomerization
        domain)-like receptors (NLRs),
        298–299, 299f, 1008
NOD (nucleotide-binding oligomerization
        domain) pathways, 299–300, 301f
Nodular lymphocyte-predominant Hodgkin
        lymphoma (NLPHL). See Hodgkin
        lymphoma, nodular lymphocyte-
        predominant
Non-Burkitt (small noncleaved cell)
        lymphoma, 187
Nongerminal center B-cell–like lymphoma,
        1496t
Non-Hodgkin lymphoma. See Lymphomas
Nonhomologous DNA end joining (NHEJ),
        1166, 1169
Nonhomologous end-joining (NHEJ), 453
Nonimmune hydrops, 849
Nonimmunologic protein adsorption,
        drug-induced, 825f, 826t, 830t, 831
Nonopsonic receptors, 1054–1055, 1057t
Nonsense-mediated RNA decay, 733
Nonsense mutations, 146
Non-ST elevation myocardial infarction
        (NSTEMI), 2296. See also
        Myocardial infarction (MI)
Nonsteroidal antiinflammatory agents.
        See NSAIDs
Non–toll-like, nonopsonic receptors,
        1054–1055, 1057t
Nontropical sprue, 597
NOP10, 531f
NOP10, 531
Normocytic anemia, 506
NOS. See Nitric oxide synthase (NOS)
Notch, 1824
Notch 1, 1606
NOTCH1/2
    in chronic lymphocytic leukemia, 231t,
        1529
    in follicular lymphoma, 236t

in mantle cell lymphoma, 237t
in splenic marginal zone lymphoma, 1666
in T-cell acute lymphoblastic leukemia, 186, 233t, 1508, 1508t, 1513t
prognosis and, 1521
Notch activation, 270
Notch ligands, **266**, 1155
Notch signaling, 1155–1156
NPC1/2, 1129
NPM1
in acute myelogenous leukemia, 181, 181t, 226t, 363, 1280, 1377, 1378t, 1383, 1415
detecting mutations in, 1415
in myelodysplastic syndromes, 181t, 1346
NPM-ALK, 1698
NR4A receptors, 2284
Nramp1 (SLC11A1), 621, 1010, 1014
Nramp2. *See* Divalent metal transporter (DMT)-1
NRAS (N-RAS)
in acute myelogenous leukemia, 227t, 1376, 1378t, 1383
in chronic myelogenous leukemia transformation, 1464
in chronic myelomonocytic leukemia, 1468
in myelodysplastic syndromes, 228t, 1346t, 1348, 1352
in myeloma, 188, 233t, 1709, 1759
in pure red cell aplasia, 543
NRF-1 (nuclear regulatory factor-1), 894
NRF2 (nuclear respiratory factor-2), 196
NSAIDs
antiplatelet effects, 404, 2075
for mastocytosis, 977
for polyarteritis nodosa, 2106
for sickle cell disease pain, 767
NSCs (neural stem cells), 451
NSF (NEM-sensitive fusion protein), 1016
NSP4 (neutrophil serine protease 4), 1012t
NSTEMI (non-ST elevation myocardial infarction), 2296. *See also* Myocardial infarction (MI)
NTPDases, 1886
NTR (neutrophil turnover rate), 941, 942, 942t
NTRK3, 233t
NTX, 1738
Nuclear-cytoplasmic asynchrony, 593
Nuclear factor kappa-B. *See* NF-κB
Nuclear factor of activated T cells (NFATs), 1178, 1528
Nuclear receptors, **250**
Nuclear regulatory factor-1 (NRF-1), 894
Nuclear respiratory factor-2 (NRF2), 196

Nuclear translocation, 251
Nucleoid, 1843
Nucleoside phosphorylase, 692t
Nucleosome remodeling and deacetylation factor (NuRD), 166
Nucleosome remodeling factor (NURF), 167
Nucleotide-binding oligomerization domain (NOD)-like receptors (NLRs), **298–299**, 299f, 1063, 1065f
Nucleotide-binding oligomerization domain (NOD) pathway, **299–300**, 301f
Nucleotides
in erythrocytes, 470t, 699
in neutrophils, 935, 935t
Null phenotypes, 2340–2343
Null phenotypes, diseases associated with, 2341–2342t
NuRD (nucleosome remodeling and deacetylation factor), 166
NURF (nucleosome remodeling and factor), 167
Nutritional deficiencies
cobalamin. *See* Cobalamin deficiency
folate. *See* Folate deficiency
history of, **7**
iron. *See* Iron deficiency
lymphocytopenia and, 1206
neutropenia and, 994–995
thrombocytopenia and, 1997–1998
NY-ESO-1, 412

O

O⁶-methylguanine-DNA methyltransferase (MGMT), 442
Obatoclax (GX15-070), 1403
Obesity
acute myelogenous leukemia and, 1374
lymphoma and, 1573
myeloma and, 1734
Obinutuzumab, **344–345**
adverse effects, 343t, 1536
for chronic lymphocytic leukemia, 1536, 1540, 1645
mechanism of action, 343t
Obstetric complications. *See* Pregnancy
Obstructive sleep apnea, 872, 876
OCT-1, 1456
OCT2 (POU2F2), 235t
Ocular disorders
in antiphospholipid syndrome, 2241
in essential monoclonal gammopathy, 1724
history of, 5
primary lymphomas, 1571, 1574, 1579–1581, 1665

retinal hemorrhages, 8
in sickle cell disease, 772
in Waldenström macroglobulinemia, 1791, 1792
ODC (ornithine decarboxylase), 200, 238
Odo-leukemias, 1342
Ofatumumab, **344**
adverse effects, 343t, 1536
for chronic lymphocytic leukemia, 1536, 1540
mechanism of action, 343t
2OG (2-oxoglutarate, α-ketoglutarate), 169, 170
Oil-in-water emulsions, 422
Ok blood group/antigens, 2332t, 2337
Older persons, **129–137**
acute myelogenous leukemia in
biologic features, 1408
incidence, 1375, 1375f
treatment, 1408–1409
coagulant and anticoagulant factors in, 135
coagulation dysregulation and frailty in, 137
C-reactive protein in, 135
endothelial vasodilation in, 2283
erythrocytes in, 134
erythropoietin levels in, 134
functional decline in, **129–130**
hematopoiesis in, **132–134**
hematopoietic cell transplantation in, **361–362**
hematopoietic microenvironment in, 267
immunity and, **135–136**, 136f
inflammation and frailty in, 137
leukocytes in, 134
lymphoma incidence in, 1570, 1570f
neutrophil motility in, 1026
platelets in, 134–135
primary myelofibrosis in, 1319
prothrombotic state in, 135
Olfactomedin 4 (OLFM4), 1012t, 1014
Olfactory hallucinations, history of, 5
Oligoblastic myelogenous leukemia (refractory anemia with excess blasts)
acute myelogenous leukemia and, 1280, 1374–1385
characteristics, 1343, 1343t
chromosomal abnormalities, 178
definition, 1277
history, 1343
vs. primary myelofibrosis, 1327
transition to other clonal myeloid diseases, 1280

Oligoclonal immunoglobulins, 1725–1726
Oligodendrocyte progenitor cells (OPCs), 452
Omacetaxine, 1458, 1466
Omega-3-fatty acids
    for sickle cell disease, 777t
    for stroke prevention, 2297
Omenn syndrome, 1166, **1219–1220**
Omeprazole, megaloblastic anemia and, 605, 606t
Oncogenes, **219**. *See also* Chromosomal abnormalities; Gene mutations
Oncostatin M, 248, 933t, 1978
One-compartment model, 430f
Onion extract, 2079
OPCs (oligodendrocyte progenitor cells), 452
Open canalicular system, 1835f, 1836
OPG (osteoprotegerin), 249, 1713, 1737, 1738f, 1739f
Opioids, for sickle cell disease pain, 767–768
Oprelvekin, 1358
Oprozomib, for myeloma, 1753
Opsonic receptors, 934t, 1054
Opsonins, 106, 284, 1017, 1054
Opsonization, 1160
ORAI1 (Orai1), 1221, 1836
Oral cavity, history of disorders of, 5
Oral contraceptives
    venous thromboembolism risk and, 2226t, 2227
    for von Willebrand disease, 2176
Oral hairy leukoplakia, 1266
Orbital adnexal lymphoma, 1571, 1579
Orbital compression syndrome, 772
Organic acids, in erythrocytes, 471t
Organismal aging, **132**
ORMDL3 (orosomucoid-like 3), 950
Ornithine decarboxylase (ODC), 200, 238
Oropharynx, history of disorders of, 5
Orosomucoid-like 3 (ORMDL3), 950
Oroya fever (*Bartonella* infection), **818**, 997
Orthochromic (orthochromatic) erythroblasts, 34, 463f, 465, 465f
Orthochromic normoblast, 463f
Orthopedic surgery, 2371
Oseltamivir, 386
Osteoblasts, marrow, 35, 60
Osteoclasts
    deficiency, 1091
    development, 1077, 1077f, 1078
    markers, 1080t
    marrow, 35, 60–61
Osteogenesis imperfecta, 2061
Osteomyelitis, 771, 1513
Osteonecrosis
    in Gaucher disease, 1125f

of the jaw, 1757
Osteopenia, 771
Osteopetrosis, 1091
Osteopontin, 64, 1846t
Osteoporosis
    acute lymphoblastic leukemia treatment and, 1520
    heparin-induced, 2277
    mast cell numbers and, 972
    in mastocytosis, 977
    in sickle cell disease, 771
Osteoprotegerin (OPG), 249, 1713, 1737, 1738f, 1739f
Osteosclerosis, 1325, 1330
Osteosclerotic myeloma (POEMS syndrome), 9, 1733, 1746
Ostwald viscosimeter, 506
Ovalocytes. *See* Elliptocytes (ovalocytes)
Ovary, primary lymphomas in, 1582
Owren parahemophilia, 1925
Oxidant damage, hemolysis and, 809–810
2-Oxoglutarate (2OG, α-ketoglutarate), 169, 193, 196
Oxygen dissociation curve, 761
Oxygen gas, hemolytic anemia and, 809–810
Oxygen transport
    anemia and, 504–505, 504f, 505f
    hemoglobin and, 761
    hypervolemia and, 506, 510f
    in red cells in newborn, 104, 104f
Oxymetholone, for anemia of primary myelofibrosis, 1328
Ozone, 809–810

P

P1PK blood group/antigens, 2331t, 2334t, 2337, 2339, 2340, 2344t
P2RY8, 1508
$P2X_1$, 1874, 2056–2057
$P2Y_1$, 1874–1875
$P2Y_{12}$, 1874–1875, 2056–2057
P4P (polyphosphate-4-phosphatase), 1817
$p14^{ARF}$, 218, 238
p15 (*CDKN2B*), 232t
p16 (*CDKN2*), 232t, 236t, 1654, 1734
p16 (*INK4A/ARF*), 230t
$p16^{INK4A}$, 214, 238
$p16^{INK4A}$/cyclin D_1/cdk4/RB/E24 cascade, 215, 217
$p16^{INK4A}$-RB pathway, 214, 225
$p16^{INK4B}$, 218
$p16^{INK4C}$, 218
$p16^{INK4D}$, 218
$p21^{cip1}$, 217–218, 225
$p22^{phox}$ (*CYBA*), 1013t, 1027, 1028t, 1029
P24. *See* CD9

$p27^{kip1}$, 218
p38 kinases, 298, 301f
$p40^{phox}$ (*NCF4*), 1029
$p47^{phox}$ (*NCF1*), 1028t, 1029
p53
    apoptosis and, 208f, 209
    cancer and, 132, 195, 210, 238
    in chronic myelogenous leukemia transformation, 1464
    functions, 195
    vascular tone and, 2283
p53
    in diffuse large B-cell lymphoma, 1626
    in mantle cell lymphoma, 1654
    in myeloma, 1710
p55, 663t, 667, 667f
$p67^{phox}$ (*NCF2*), 1028t, 1029
p107, 217, 238
p130, 238
P140K-MGMT, 442, 443f
p190, 1442
p205 radixin, 1006
$p210^{BCR-ABL}$, 1440–1441, 1442–1443
p230, 1442
PA. *See* Pernicious anemia (PA)
PACAP, 2061
Pacific Biosciences real-time sequencing, 158–159, 158f
Paclitaxel, **326**, 1631, 2297
PAD (peripheral arterial disease), **2297**
PADGEM. *See* P-selectin
PAF. *See* Platelet-activating factor (PAF)
Pagetoid reticulosis, 1683
PAI-1. *See* Plasminogen activator inhibitor (PAI)-1
Pain
    abdominal, history of, 5
    bone, history of, 6
    chest, history of, 5
    shoulder, history of, 6
    in sickle cell disease, 767–768
    in tongue, history of, 5
Palbociclib, 215, 218
Palifermin, 368
Pallor
    eyes, 8
    history of, 6
    mouth, 8
    skin, 7
Palpitations, history of, 5
PALS (periarterial lymphoid sheath), 88, 89f, 90f
Pamidronate, 1756
Pancreas, 452
Pancreatic disease
    cobalamin deficiency and, 602

multipotential cell therapy for, 452–453
primary lymphoma, 1581
Pancytopenia
  in acute lymphoblastic leukemia, 1514
  in clonal myeloid disorders, 1277
  consultative approach to, 43
  differential diagnosis, 1513
  in hairy cell leukemia, 1555
  in HIV infection, 1253t
  with hyperplastic marrow, 1342
Panobinostat, 240, 1754
Pantothenate kinase-associated
        neurodegeneration (PKAN), 682
Pantothenic acid deficiency, 652
Papaverine, cAMP inhibition and, 404
Papillon-Lefèvre syndrome, 1013
Pappenheimer bodies, 468, 868, 869
PAR. See Protease (proteinase)-activated
        receptor (PAR)-1
Paracentric inversion, 175t
Paragangliomas, 560, 872, 878–879
Parahemophilia (factor V deficiency). See
        Factor V deficiency
Paranasal sinuses, primary lymphomas in,
        1581
Paraneoplastic vasculitis, 2106
Parasitic infections
  blood loss from, 629
  eosinophils and, 956–957, 957t
  purpuras and, 2105, 2105f
Paratarg-7, 1708, 1709–1710, 1734
Paresthesias, 5, 632
Paris-Trousseau syndrome, 2061
Parkinson disease, 453, 1125
Paroxetine, 2079
Paroxysmal cold hemoglobinuria (PCH),
        837, 839, 2348
Paroxysmal nocturnal hemoglobinuria
        (PNH), 571–581
  aplastic anemia, 520, 521
  vs. autoimmune hemolytic anemia, 837
  in children, 580
  classification of, 576t
  clinical features, 573, 575, 1286, 2100,
        2100f
  course and prognosis, 580–581
  definition and history, 570
  differential diagnosis, 576–578
  epidemiology, 571–572
  etiology and pathogenesis, 572–573
    complement-mediated, 572, 572f
    GPI-linked protein deficiency, 1871,
        2337
    molecular and genetic basis of, 572–573,
        573f
    phenotypic mosaicism in, 573, 574–575f

laboratory features, 575–576, 575f, 575t,
        576t, 577f, 577t
  pregnancy and, 580
  prognosis, 581
  screening recommendations, 575t
  therapy
    eculizumab, 578
    hematopoietic cell transplantation,
        579–580, 579t
    supportive, 578–579
    thrombophilia management, 580
PARs (proteinase-activated receptors), 290.
        See also Protease (proteinase)-
        activated receptor (PAR)-1
Partial cytogenic response (pCyR), 1452t
Particle film, 29
Parturition, iron deficiency in, 630
Parvovirus B19 infection
  antiphospholipid antibodies and, 2234
  aplastic crisis and, 767
  erythema and, 2104, 2105f
  hereditary spherocytosis and, 674
  immunoglobulins for, 544–545, 545f
  persistent, red cell aplasia and, 543, 544–
        545, 545f, 1251–1252, 1542
  in pregnancy, 849
  red cell antigens and resistance to, 2340
  transient aplastic crisis and, 541
Passenger mutations, 1348
Pasteur effect, 504
Patch, 1680
Paternal zygosity, 852
Patient blood management, 2378
Patient-specific blood donation, 2368
Pattern recognition receptors
  dendritic cells and, 307
  macrophage polarization and, 1085
Pauciblastic leukemia. See Oligoblastic
        myelogenous leukemia (refractory
        anemia with excess blasts)
Pautrier microabscesses, 1681
Pax5, 1141, 1155
PAX5, 1606, 1627, 1710, 1710f
PAX5, 1508, 1626
Paxillin, 251, 266
PBG (porphobilinogen), 889, 891f, 903
PBGD, 901
PBGD (porphobilinogen deaminase), 701t,
        894
PBG (porphobilinogen) synthase, 894, 918
PBPCs (peripheral blood progenitor cells),
        355–356
PCC (prothrombin complex concentrate),
        396, 2135, 2136, 2136t
PCFCL (primary cutaneous follicular center
        lymphoma), 184t

PCH (paroxysmal cold hemoglobinuria),
        837, 839, 2348
PCI (percutaneous coronary intervention),
        2295
PCMZL (primary cutaneous marginal zone
        B-cell lymphoma), 184t, 1581
PCP (pentachlorophenol), 517
PC-TP, 1853
pCyR (partial cytogenic response), 1452t
PD-1 (programmed death-1), 424, 1755
PD-1 (programmed death-1) receptor, 416
PDCD1 (CD279), 1184
PDGF (platelet-derived growth factor), 1322,
        1845, 1848
PDGFR-α, 1279, 1468t
PDGFR-β (PDGFRB), 232t, 1468, 1469
PDW (platelet volume distribution width), 17
PEAR1, 1853
Pearson marrow-pancreas syndrome, 919,
        920
PECAM-1. See Platelet-endothelial cell
        adhesion molecule-1 (PECAM-1,
        CD31)
PEG (monomethoxypolyethylene glycol), 332
Pegaspargase, 1515
PEG-IFN-α. See Interferon (IFN)-α
Pel-Ebstein fever, 1607
Pelger-Huët anomaly, 1350f, 1353, 1465
Pellagra (niacin deficiency), 652
Pemetrexed, megaloblastic anemia and, 605,
        606t
Penetrance, 149
Penicillins
  for bartonellosis, 818
  drug-mediated immune injury and,
        829–830, 832
  platelet function and, 2078
  prophylactic, in sickle cell disease, 773
Pentachlorophenol (PCP), 517
Pentostatin (deoxycoformycin), 325
  for chronic lymphocytic leukemia, 1534,
        1535, 1537
  for hairy cell leukemia, 1553, 1557–1558,
        1559t
  for hepatosplenic T-cell lymphoma, 1701
  mechanism of action, 322
  for mycosis fungoides, 1687
  structure, 323f
  for Waldenström macroglobulinemia, 1794
Pentoxifylline
  antiplatelet effects, 404
  clinical uses, 404t
  dosage, 404t
  for heart valve hemolysis, 805
  for peripheral arterial disease, 2297
  for peripheral vascular disease, 405

Pentraxin-3, 1013*t*, 1014
Peptide vaccines, for myeloid leukemias, 423
Peptidylprolyl isomerase (PIN1), 951
PER-ARNT-SIM (PAS)-domain, 486
Percutaneous coronary intervention (PCI), 2295
Percutaneous umbilical blood sampling, 854
Perforin, 1114, 1145, 1228, 1567
Performance status, 3, 4*t*
Periarterial lymphoid sheath (PALS), 88, 89*f*, 90*f*
Pericentric inversion, 175*t*
Pericytes, 1008
Perifosine, for acute myelogenous leukemia, 1403
Peripheral arterial disease (PAD), **2297**
Peripheral blood progenitor cells (PBPCs), 355–356
Peripheral membrane proteins. *See* Membrane proteins, peripheral
Peripheral T-cell lymphoma (PTCL)
    chromosomal abnormalities, 185*t*
    classification, 1693, 1694*t*
    diagnosis, 1693–1694
    epidemiology, 1693, 1694*t*
    laboratory features, 1498*t*, 1598, 1598*f*
    prognosis, 1694, 1695*t*
    subtypes
        adult T-cell leukemia/lymphoma. *See* Adult T-cell leukemia/lymphoma (ATL/ATLL)
        anaplastic large cell lymphoma. *See* Anaplastic large cell lymphoma (ALCL)
        angioimmunoblastic T-cell lymphoma, 1498*t*, 1598, **1697–1698**
        enteropathy-associated T-cell lymphoma, **1699–1700**
        extranodal NK/T-cell lymphoma, nasal type, 1498*t*, 1500*t*, 1573, **1701–1702**
        hepatosplenic T-cell lymphoma, 185*t*, 1498*t*, 1567, **1701**
        peripheral T-cell lymphoma, not otherwise specified, 1694*t*, 1695*t*, 1697
        subcutaneous panniculitis-like T-cell lymphoma, 1498*t*, **1702**
    treatment
        initial, **1694–1696**, 1695*t*
        for relapsed or refractory disease, 1696–1697, 1696*t*
Peripheral vascular disease, 2240, 2316–2317
Pernicious anemia (PA), **600**. *See also* Cobalamin deficiency
    in adrenal insufficiency, 560

    autoimmune diseases and, 600
    blood films, 594*f*
    gastric disorders in, 600
    in hypothyroidism, 559
    inherited predisposition to, 600
    marrow films, 595*f*
    stomach and intestine in, 583, 600–601, 601*f*
    true juvenile, 607
Peroxidase, promonocytes and, 1046
Peroxidase-negative neutrophil granules, 1009, 1012–1013*t*, 1013–1014. *See also* Neutrophils, granules
Peroxidase-positive neutrophil granules, 1009. *See also* Neutrophils, granules
Peroxiredoxin 2, 699
Peroxisome proliferator-activated receptor (PPAR), 197, 452, 1873–1874
Peroxisomes, platelet, 1840
Peroxynitrite, 284*t*, 2203
Persistent lymphocytosis, 1204
Persistent polyclonal lymphocytosis of B lymphocytes (PPBL), 1200–1202, 1201*f*
Pertussis. *See Bordetella pertussis* infections
Pesticides, lymphoma and, 1571, 1572–1573
PETA-3. *See* CD151
PET-CT. *See* FDG-PET
Petechiae, 6, 8, 1987
Peyer patches, 94, 94*f*
PF4. *See* CXCL4 (platelet factor 4)
PFK. *See* Phosphofructokinase (PFK)
PFKL, 695
PFKM, 695
PGA (polyglandular autoimmune) syndrome, 87
PGK. *See* Phosphoglycerate kinase (PGK)
P-gp, 1404
Phagocytes
    cell surface proteins, 1017
    killing and degradation of microorganisms in, 284*t*
    mononuclear. *See* Macrophages; Monocytes
    in newborn, 105–106
    respiratory burst, 1068*f*
Phagocytosis
    evasion of, 1064*f*
    in inflammatory response, 279, 284
    pathways, 1061–1062, 1061*f*, 1062*f*, 1063*f*
    surface components for, 1008–1009
Pharmacologic chaperones, 1128
pH change sensing, for DNA sequencing, 157–158, 157*f*
Ph chromosome. *See* Philadelphia (Ph) chromosome

PHD2, 510, 875
PHDs (proline hydroxylases), 486, 486*f*
PHEMX. *See* TSSC6
Phenazopyridine, 5
Phenformin, megaloblastic anemia and, 606*t*
Phenobarbital
    maternal ingestion of, effect on fetus and newborn, 112
    megaloblastic anemia and, 606*t*
Phenotype, 147
Phenotypic mosaicism, in paroxysmal nocturnal hemoglobinuria, 573, 574–575*f*
Phenylbutazone, maternal ingestion of, effect on fetus and newborn, 112
Phenytoin
    maternal ingestion of, effect on fetus and newborn, 109, 112, 112*t*
    megaloblastic anemia and, 606*t*
Pheochromocytomas, 560, 879
PHF6, 227*t*, 233*t*, 1346*t*
Philadelphia (Ph) chromosome
    in acute lymphoblastic leukemia, 183, 364, 1517, 1521
    in acute myelogenous leukemia, 1385, 1407
    characteristics, 1441, 1441*f*, 1448*f*
    in chronic myelogenous leukemia, 176, 178, 1278, 1438–1440, 1447, 1452
    in clonal myeloid diseases, 1450
    in eosinophilic chronic myelogenous leukemia, 1445
    masked, 1447
Philadelphia chromosome–like acute lymphoblastic leukemia, 177*f*, 186
Philadelphia chromosome-negative chronic myelogenous leukemia, 1450
Philadelphia chromosome-positive eosinophilic chronic myelogenous leukemia, 1445
Phlebotomy
    for bleeding in chronic myeloproliferative neoplasms, 2081
    for hemochromatosis, 644
    for polycythemia vera, 1298*t*, 1299–1300
    for porphyria cutanea tarda, 908
PHMX. *See* TSSC6
Phorbol myristate acetate (PMA), 1011
Phosphatases, 253
Phosphatidylethanolamine, 1955
Phosphatidylinositol-4,5-bisphosphate, 1016
Phosphatidylinositol-4-monophosphate, 1016
Phosphatidylserine, 1060, 1061*f*
Phosphatidyl serine antibody assay, 2242
Phosphatidylserine exposure model, 498

Phosphodiesterases, 1885
Phosphofructokinase (PFK)
    activity, 692t
    deficiency, 690, 700t, 704
    in glucose metabolism, 694–695
Phosphoglucomutase, 692t, 701t
6-Phosphogluconate dehydrogenase, 692t,
        697, 701t
6-Phosphogluconolactonase, 692t, 697, 701t
3-Phosphoglycerate, in glucose metabolism,
        692–693, 695
Phosphoglycerate kinase (PGK)
    activity, 692t
    deficiency, 700t, 704–705
    in glucose metabolism, 695
Phosphoglycerate mutase, 695
Phosphoglycolate phosphatase, 692t
Phosphoinositide/phosphoinositol/
        phosphatidylinositol 3-kinase
        (PI3K)
    in eosinophils, 951
    in Hodgkin lymphoma, 1606
    inhibitors, 1403
    in mantle cell lymphoma, 1654
    in platelets, 1833t, 1882
Phosphoinositide/phosphoinositol/
        phosphatidylinositol 3-kinase
        (PI3K) inhibitors, 1529, 1538
Phospholipase A, 1970
Phospholipase A_2 (PLA$_2$), 1016, 1876
Phospholipase β, 1874
Phospholipase C (PLC), 1016, 1874, 2057–
        2058
Phospholipase Cβ$_2$ (PLC-β$_2$) deficiency,
        2057–2058
Phospholipase Cγ$_1$ (PLC-γ$_1$), 1178, 1529
Phospholipase Cγ$_2$ (PLCγ$_2$), 1538
Phospholipase δ, 1874
Phospholipase γ, 1874
Phospholipids
    activated protein C and, 1956
    arterial thrombosis and, 2294
    in erythrocyte membrane, 662
    in erythrocytes, 469t
    in neutrophils, 1016
    in platelets, 1836, 1854
Phosphomannose isomerase, 692t
Photochemotherapy/photopheresis,
        extracorporeal, 429t, 433, 1687
Photodynamic therapy, 1686
Photosensitivity, 897, 898
Phototherapy, 857, 1686
Physical examination, 7–9
PI3K. See Phosphoinositide/phosphoinositol/
        phosphatidylinositol 3-kinase
        (PI3K)

PIAS (protein inhibitor of activated STATs),
        253
Pica, 120, 632
Pickwickian syndrome, 876, 882
PIGA, 571, 572–573, 574–575, 577, 1346t
Pim-1, 218
PIM1, 1626
PIN1 (peptidylprolyl isomerase), 951
Piperacillin-tazobactam, 384, 387t
Pipobroman, for essential thrombocythemia,
        1313t, 1314
Piroxicam, 2075
Pituitary gland
    anemia and, 560–561
    in Langerhans cell histiocytosis, 1104,
        1105, 1106
Pituitary gland, primary lymphomas in, 1579
PK. See Pyruvate kinase (PK)
PK (prekallikrein), 1929, 2121
PKC (protein kinase C), 1016, 1178, 1837,
        1841
PKC-β, 235t
PKC-θ deficiency, 2058
PLA$_2$ (phospholipase A$_2$), 1016, 1876
Placental growth factor, 801
Plaque
    atherosclerotic. See Atherosclerosis
    cutaneous, 1680, 1681f
Plasma
    in aplastic anemia, 519
    in myelodysplastic syndromes, 1353
    platelet storage in, 2388–2389, 2388t
    in polycythemia vera, 1295
    in primary myelofibrosis, 1327
Plasmablastic lymphoma, 1246, 1496t
Plasma cell leukemia, 1736t, 1737, 1743f,
        1746
Plasma cell myeloma, 188, 1497t
Plasma cell neoplasms
    classification, 1497t
    cytogenetic assessment techniques,
        1711–1712
    definition and history, 1707
    essential monoclonal gammopathy. See
        Essential monoclonal gammopathy
    etiology and pathogenesis, 1708–1710
    immunoglobulin light-chain amyloidosis.
        See Immunoglobulin light-chain
        (AL) amyloidosis
    light chain deposition disease, 1744,
        1760
    minimal residual disease assessment,
        1716–1717
    myeloma. See Myeloma
    POEMS syndrome (osteosclerotic
        myeloma), 9, 1733, 1746

    smoldering myeloma, 1708–1709, 1725,
        1734f, 1761
    solitary plasmacytoma, 1497t, 1733, 1760
    Waldenström macroglobulinemia. See
        Waldenström macroglobulinemia
        (WM)
Plasma cells
    antigens, 1141, 1141f
    composition, 1145
    development, 61, 1710f
    generation of, 1171–1172
    in immunoglobulin synthesis regulation,
        1171–1172
    marrow, 32t, 35
    structure, 1137, 1138f, 1140
Plasma coagulation factors, in neonate,
        109–111
Plasmacytoid dendritic cells, 309
Plasmacytoid lymphocytes, 1203f
Plasmacytoma, 1497t, 1760
Plasma derivatives, 2366, 2368
Plasma exchange
    adverse effects, 431, 2257
    for atypical hemolytic uremic syndrome,
        2261
    for autoimmune hemolytic anemia, 839
    for cryoglobulinemia, 428
    definition, 427
    for HELLP syndrome, 802–803
    for hyperviscosity, 428
    indications for, 427–428, 428t, 429–430t
    for myeloma cast nephropathy, 428
    for neuropathy, 1724
    principles, 427, 430f, 431f
    for thrombotic microangiopathies, 428,
        431
    for thrombotic thrombocytopenic
        purpura, 2256
Plasma factor concentrations, in older
        persons, 135
Plasma labels, 489
Plasmalyte, 2389, 2389t
Plasmapheresis, 427, 544, 2368. See also
        Plasma exchange
Plasma proteins, in pregnancy, 119–120
Plasma thromboplastin component (PTC),
        2113. See also Factor IX
Plasma tissue-type plasminogen, aging and,
        135
Plasma volume, **488–489**
Plasmin
    disorders of generation of, 2311–2312
    in fibrinolysis and angiogenesis, 2311
    fibrinolytic actions of, 2304f, 2309–2311,
        2310f
    in inflammatory response, 290

Plasmin (*Cont.*):
  inhibitors, 2307–2308
  nonfibrinolytic vascular functions, 1974
  platelet function and, 2078
  as tissue remodeler, 2311
Plasminogen (Plg), **2303**
  activation, 2304f, 2310–2311
  functions, 2303
  properties, 2304–2305t
  structure, 2303
Plasminogen activator inhibitor (PAI)-1,
      1975, **2308**
  activities, 1923, 2308
  characteristics, 2305t, 2308
  in disseminated intravascular coagulation,
      2206, 2208
  in fibrinolysis regulation, 1845, 2202, 2311
  gene expression, 2308
  plasmin generation and, 1973–1974
  in platelets, 1845
Plasminogen activator inhibitor (PAI)-1
      deficiency, 2318
Plasminogen activator inhibitor (PAI)-2,
      2305t, 2308, 2312
Plasminogen activators, **2303–2307**
  accessory, 2307
  comparison, 2304–2305t, 2313t
  fibrinolysins, 2307
  in fibrinolytic therapy. *See* Fibrinolytic
      therapy
  genes, 2306f, 2307t
  physiologic functions, 2307
  tissue-type. *See* Tissue-type plasminogen
      activator (t-PA)
  urokinase. *See* Urokinase plasminogen
      activator (u-PA)
Plasminogen receptors, 2308
Plasmodium falciparum
  glycophorins and, 664, 2340
  life cycle, 815
  malaria and. *See* Malaria
  mannose-binding lectin deficiency and,
      1017
  pyruvate kinase deficiency and, 704
  Southeast Asian ovalocytosis and, 680
  thalassemias and, 728
  TIRAP and, 1054
Plasmodium knowlesi, 2340
Plasmodium ovale, 815
Plasmodium vivax, 728, 815, 817, 817f, 2340
Platelet-activating factor (PAF)
  in inflammatory response, 281, 284t, 286t,
      289, 1979t
  as lipid mediator, **1878**
  neutrophils and, 1007, 1016
  production, 1977

release, 1852f, 1856
  synthesis, 1840
  in thrombosis and hemostasis, 1979t
Platelet-activating factor (PAF) receptor
      defect, 2057
Platelet antigens (human). *See* Human
      platelet antigens (HPAs)
Platelet count, **17–18**
  in acute lymphoblastic leukemia, 1510,
      1510t
  bleeding risk and, 2382–2383
  in chronic myelogenous leukemia, 1445,
      1445f
  in disseminated intravascular coagulation,
      2205t
  in essential thrombocythemia, 1310, 1311t
  in hemostatic disorders, 1988, 1989f
  in heparin-induced thrombocytopenia,
      2028
  in hepatic disease, 2191
  in immune thrombocytopenia, 2002
  normal, 1994, 2035
  platelet destruction and, 2381–2382, 2382f
  during pregnancy, 119, 2010
  in primary myelofibrosis, 1326
  reference ranges, 18t, 19f
  technique, 1994
  transfusion threshold, 2383
Platelet-derived growth factor (PDGF), 1322,
      1845, 1848
Platelet-endothelial cell adhesion molecule-1
      (PECAM-1, CD31)
  in inflammatory response, 1977t, 1978
  in leukocyte adhesion, 283
  in monocytes, 1052f
  in neutrophil function, 2273
  in platelet adhesion and aggregation, 1868
  Src activation and, 1884
  structure, 1858–1859t, 1868
Platelet factor 4. *See* CXCL4 (platelet factor 4)
Plateletpheresis, 2368
Platelet-rich plasma method, 2386, 2386f
Platelets. *See also* Thrombopoiesis
  activation, 2293
  adhesion, aggregation, and thrombus
      formation, 1830–1831f,
      1830–1834, 1852f, 1857f, 1940
  alloimmunization, 2084–2085
  antibody-induced agglutination, 1995
  antiphospholipid antibodies and, 2237
  automated analysis, **16–17**, 18t, 19f
  calcium homeostasis, 1837f
  CD39 inhibition, 1971
  characteristics, 1993
  clearance, 1993
  coagulant activity, 1854

discoid, 1835f
  disorders, 1991. *See also*
      Thrombocythemia;
      Thrombocytopenia; *specific type*
  acquired, **2073–2086**
      in acquired von Willebrand
          syndrome, 2082–2083
      antiplatelet antibodies and,
          2084–2085
      in Bartter syndrome, 2086
      cardiopulmonary bypass and,
          2085–2086
      in chronic myeloproliferative
          neoplasms, 2079–2081
      in disseminated intravascular
          coagulation, 2086, 2200–2201
      drug-induced, 2073–2079
      in dysproteinemias, 2082
      in hemorrhagic fevers, 2086
      in hepatic disease, 2086, 2191
      in iron deficiency, 633
      in leukemias and myelodysplastic
          syndromes, 1353, 2081–2082
      in polycythemia vera, 1295
      in uremia, 2083–2084
  hereditary, **1996–1997, 2039–2062**.
      See also specific disorders
      adhesion receptor abnormalities,
          2040t, **2042–2052**
      approach to, 1996, 2040–2042, 2041f
      classification, 1996, 1998t, 2039–2040
      clinical features, 1996, 2040
      coagulant activity abnormalities,
          2040t, **2058–2059**
      cytoskeletal linking protein
          abnormalities, 2040t, **2059–2060**
      cytoskeletal structural protein
          abnormalities, 2040t, **2059**
      granule abnormalities, 2040t,
          2052–2056, 2052f
      laboratory features, 1996–1997
      in pregnancy, 2062
      signaling and secretion abnormalities,
          2040t, **2056–2058**
      surgical management in, 2062
      therapy, 2061–2062
      transcription factor mutations, 2040t,
          2060–2061
  energy metabolism, **1839–1840**
  formation, 1820–1821. *See also*
      Megakaryopoiesis
  functions
      in hemostasis, 2039
      in inflammation and infection,
          1855–1857, 1857f
      in newborns, 107–108

in thrombolysis, 1855t
in vessel integrity and development, 1857
gene expression
  gene variants associated with disease, 1850
  gene variants associated with platelet traits, 1850–1851, 1850f
  genomics, 1850
  proteomics, 1853–1854
  transcriptomics, 1851–1853, 1852f
granule formation, 1818, 1819f
granule-plasma membrane fusion, 1849
inflammatory response in monocytes and, 1970f
interactions with endothelial cells, 1978–1979
interactions with leukocytes, 1830–1831f, 1852f, 1857f, 1978–1979
interaction with monocytes and macrophages, 1059
life span, 1993, 2381–2382, 2382f
membrane glycoproteins, 1858
  C1q receptors, 1873
  CD40 ligand, 1872–1873
  cell-surface adhesion receptors and membrane proteins, 1868–1870
  Fas ligand, LIGHT, TRAIL, 1873
  glycosylphosphatidylinositol-anchored proteins, 1871
  GMP-33, 1873
  integrins, 1861–1865
  lectin-containing receptors, 1870–1871
  leucine-rich repeat glycoprotein receptors, 1865–1868, 1866f, 1867f
  leukosialin, sialophorin, 1873
  lysosome-associated membrane proteins, 1873
  matrix metalloproteinases, 1874
  peroxisome proliferator-activated receptors, 1873–1874
  scavenger receptors, 1872
  tetraspanins, 1871
  tyrosine kinase receptors, 1871–1872
membranes, 1818
morphology and biochemistry, 21–22, 1834–1839
  cytoskeletal elements, 1836–1839
    actin filaments, 1838–1839, 1839f
    membrane skeleton, 1835f, 1837–1838, 1838f
    microtubules, 1835f, 1838
    proteins, 1832–1833t, 1858–1859t
  dense tubular system/sarcoplasmic reticulum, 1835f, 1836
  lipid rafts, 1836

microscopic appearance, 1834, 1835f
open canalicular system, 1835f, 1836
organelles, 1840
plasma membrane, 1834, 1835f, 1836, 1837f
in newborn, 107–108
in older persons, 134–135
reference ranges, 18t
release, 72
response, 247
ristocetin binding to, 2168, 2173
satellitism, 1995, 1995f
secretory machinery and secretion
  adhesive glycoproteins, 1846–1847t
  α granules, 1843–1845, 1844f, 1848
  dense bodies, 1835f, 1843
  exocytosis, 1849–1850
  exosomes, 1848
  lysosomes, 1843
  secretion, 1849
shape change, spreading, contraction, and clot retraction
  contraction and clot retraction, 1842–1843
  overview, 1832–1833t, 1840
  shape change, 1835f, 1840–1841
  spreading and surface-induced activation, 1841–1842
signaling pathways, 1874–1886, 1875f
  agonist-induced platelet activation, 1874–1881
    adenosine diphosphate, 1874–1876
    angiotensin II, 1879
    chemokines, 1878
    collagen, 1879–1881, 1880f
    epinephrine, 1876
    GpIb/IX/V, 1881
    G-protein–coupled receptors, 1874, 1875f
    lipid mediators, 1878
    serotonin, 1878–1879
    tachykinins, 1878
    thrombin, 1877, 1877f
    thrombospondin, 1879
    thromboxane A₂, 1876–1877
    vasopressin, 1879
  inhibitory
    CD39, 1885–1886
    nitric oxide, 1885
    prostaglandins, 1885
  intermediate signaling molecules
    calcium, 1837f, 1881–1882
    calcium-dependent proteases, 1883
    integrin αIIbβ3, 1883–1885
    phosphoinositide 3′-kinases, 1882
    small G proteins, 1882–1883

thrombolysis and, 1855
for transfusion. See Platelet transfusion
von Willebrand factor binding to, 2168
Platelet satellitism, 22, 22f
Platelet transfusion
  adverse effects, 2381, 2385
  for aplastic anemia, 522
  for bleeding, 2385
  bleeding time and, 2384, 2384f
  for disseminated intravascular coagulation, 2213
  dose and response to, 2383–2384
  for heparin-induced thrombocytopenia, 2032
  human leukocyte antigens typing and, 2356
  incidence, 2381
  indications, 2383
  for inherited platelet disorders, 2061
  for invasive procedures, 2384
  for myelodysplastic syndromes, 1357
  for neonatal alloimmune thrombocytopenia, 2013
  for paroxysmal nocturnal hemoglobinuria during pregnancy, 580
  platelet increments, corrected count increments, and transfusion interval, 2387–2388
  preparation methods
    apheresis, 2386
    concentrates from whole blood, 2386, 2386f
    for extended storage, 2388–2389, 2389t
    irradiation, 2388
    pathogen reduction, 2388
    response and, 2386–2387, 2387f
    volume reduction, 2388
  prophylactic vs. therapeutic, 2383
  refractoriness to, 2385
  response to, 2000, 2381–2382, 2382f, 2387f
  for thrombocytopenic patient on anticoagulant therapy, 2385
  for thrombotic thrombocytopenic purpura, 2256
Platelet-type (pseudo-) von Willebrand disease, 2050–2051, 2165t, 2174
Platelet volume distribution width (PDW), 17
Platinating drugs, resistance to, 319t
Platinum analogues, 329
PLC (phospholipase C), 1016, 1874, 2057–2058
PLC-β2 (phospholipase C-β2) deficiency, 2057–2058
PLC-γ1 (phospholipase Cγ1), 1178, 1529
PLC-γ2 (phospholipase Cγ2), 1538
Pleckstrin, 1841

Plerixafor, 355

Plethora, 8

Plg. *See* Plasminogen (Plg)

PLL. *See* Prolymphocytic (prolymphoblastic) leukemia (PLL)

Pluripotential stem cell lesion, 1439–1440

Pluripotential stem cell pool, 1283

PLZF, 230

PLZF, 1405

PMA (phorbol myristate acetate), 1011

PMF. *See* Primary myelofibrosis (PMF)

PML (progressive multifocal leukoencephalopathy), 1536

PML (promyelocytic leukemia). *See* Acute promyelocytic leukemia (APL)

PML-RARα

in acute myelogenous leukemia, 1377, 1384*t*

in acute promyelocytic leukemia, 181, 225, 230, 240, 1390–1392, 1415

PMN (polymorphonuclear neutrophils), 940*f*

Pneumococcal polysaccharide vaccine (PPV23), 773

Pneumococcal vaccine (PCV7), 773

Pneumococcus infections, 384. *See also* Bacterial infections

Pneumocystis jiroveci (*P. carinii*) infections

cytomegalovirus infection and, 1268

in HIV infection, 1239, 1240, 1241*t*

in hyperimmunoglobulin M syndromes, 1213

idiopathic CD4+ T lymphocytopenia and, 1206

in immunocompromised host, 384

prevention, 389, 524, 1115, 1241*t*, 1514

in severe combined immunodeficiency syndrome, 1218

treatment, 386

PNH. *See* Paroxysmal nocturnal hemoglobinuria (PNH)

Pocked (pitted) red cells, 468

Podoplanin, 1870–1871

Podosomes, 60

POEMS syndrome (osteosclerotic myeloma), 9, 1733, 1746

Poikilocytosis, 21, 21*f*

Poloxamer 188, for sickle cell disease, 777*t*

Polyamines, 200

Polyarteritis nodosa, 2106, 2106*f*

Polychromatophilic cells, 21

Polychromatophilic erythroblasts, 34, 463*f*, 464–465, 465*f*

Polychromatophilic erythrocytes, 34

Polychromatophilic megaloblasts, 595*f*

Polyclonal hematopoiesis, 83.1012

Polycythemia (erythrocytosis), **506–510, 871–884**. *See also* Polycythemia vera

apparent (relative), 872, 880

classification, 509–510, 509*t*, 871–872

clinical features, 506, 508–509, **880–881**

consultative approach to, 44–45

course and prognosis, 884

definition and history, **871–872**

differential diagnosis, **882–884**, 883*f*

epidemiology, **872–873**

etiology and pathogenesis, **873–880**

laboratory features, 505*f*, **881–882**

neonatal, 879–880, 881

pathophysiology, **506**, 508*f*

primary familial and congenital, 509, 509*t*, **871**

Chuvash polycythemia. *See* Chuvash polycythemia

clinical features, 880

definition and history, 871

disorders of hypoxia sensing. *See* Hypoxia sensing, disorders of

epidemiology, 872

etiology and pathogenesis, 873, 873*t*, 874*f*, 877–878

laboratory features, 881

pheochromocytoma and, 879, 881

VHL mutations associated with, 510, 876–877, 877*f*, 878*f*, 882*t*

renal, 879–880. *See also* Renal transplantation, erythrocytosis following

secondary, 509, 509*t*, **871–872**

chemically induced tissue hypoxia and, 876

course and prognosis, 884

definition and history, 871–872

in Eisenmenger syndrome, 872, 876, 881

endocrine disorders and, 872, 879, 880*f*

epidemiology, 872–873

erythrocyte enzyme deficiencies and, 876

etiology and pathogenesis, 874

high altitude. *See* High-altitude polycythemia

high oxygen-affinity hemoglobins and, 782, 872, 876

laboratory features, 882

post–renal transplant. *See* Renal transplantation, erythrocytosis following

pulmonary disease and, 872, 881

sleep apnea-related, 872, 876

smoking-related, 872, 876, 876*t*

testosterone treatment-related, 872, 879, 880*f*

tumors and, 872, 879, 881

spurious, 872, 884

stress, 872

therapy, **884**

Polycythemia hypertonica, 872

Polycythemia vera (PV), **1291–1301**

clinical features, **1293–1295**

leukemic transformation, 178, 1295

signs and symptoms, 1293–1294, 1294*f*

spent phase, 1294–1295, 1294*f*

thrombosis and bleeding, 2079–2081

thrombosis and hemorrhage, 1286, 1293

transition to other clonal myeloid diseases, 1280, 1295

course and prognosis, 1278*t*, **1301**, 1301*f*

definition and history, 1291

differential diagnosis, 1297, 1297*t*, 1449–1450

epidemiology, 1291

etiology and pathogenesis, 1278, 1291–1292

chromosomal abnormalities, 178, 179*t*

gene mutations

frequency, 1308*f*

JAK2, 228*t*, 1278, 1308*f*

JAK2^{V617F}, 178, **1292, 1295–1296**, 1312*f*, 1313*f*

TET2, 229*t*, 1292, 1308*f*

iron deficiency and, 629

laboratory features, **1295–1296**

blood findings, 1295

clonality in female subjects, 1296

erythroid colony cultures, 1296

erythropoietin levels, 883, 1296

JAK2 exon 12 mutations, 1296

JAK2^{V617F} mutations, 1295–1296

marrow findings, 1296

in pregnancy, **125**, 2081

surgical considerations, 1294

treatment, **1297–1301**, 1298*t*

erythrocytapheresis, 429*t*, 432

JAK inhibitors, 341–342

plethoric phase, **1297–1300**

anagrelide, 1300

aspirin, 1300, 2081

epigenetic modulation, 1300

interferon, 1299

JAK2 inhibitors, 1300

myelosuppression, 1298–1299

phlebotomy, 1299–1300

summary, 1300

symptomatic therapy for pruritus, 1300

spent phase, 1301
  hematopoietic cell transplantation, 1301
  splenectomy, 1301
  for thrombosis or bleeding, 2081
Polyglandular autoimmune (PGA) syndrome, 87
Poly-Ig receptor, 1161
Polymerase chain reaction (PCR), **152**, 1716
Polymorphisms, 147
Polymorphonuclear leukocytosis, 997. *See also* Neutrophilia
Polymorphonuclear neutrophils (PMN), 940*f*
Polyphosphate-4-phosphatase (P4P), 1817
Polyposis coli, 1654
Pomalidomide, **333–335**
  adverse effects, 335
  for AL amyloidosis, 1761, 1781
  mechanism of action, 333–334
  for myeloma, 1753*t*, 1754
  pharmacology, 334
  structure, 333*f*
Ponatinib
  adverse effects, 339*t*, 341, 1451*t*, 1458
  for chronic myelogenous leukemia, 339*t*, 1454, 1458, 1466
  comparison with other tyrosine kinase inhibitors, 1451*t*
  drug interactions, 339*t*, 1451*t*
  pharmacology, 339*t*, 340
  structure, 340*f*
Popcorn cells, 1600, 1601*f*
Porcine factor VIII, 2185
Porphobilinogen (PBG), 889, 891*f*, 903
Porphobilinogen deaminase (PBGD), 701*t*, 894
Porphobilinogen (PBG) synthase, 894, 918
Porphyria cutanea tarda (PCT), **905–908**
  clinical features, 643, 890*t*, 907, 907*f*
  definition, 905
  diagnosis, 907–908
  enzymes affected by, 890*t*, 891*f*
  laboratory features, 891*t*
  pathogenesis of clinical findings, 906–907
  pathophysiology, 905–906
  therapy, 908–909
Porphyrias, **889–909**
  δ-aminolevulinate dehydratase (ADP), 894, 900
  congenital. *See* Congenital erythropoietic porphyria (CEP)
  definition and history, **889–890**
  enzyme defects in, 890*t*, 891*f*
  erythropoietic protoporphyria. *See* Erythropoietic protoporphyria (EPP)

etiology and pathogenesis, **892–896**
hepatoerythropoietic, 889, 905, 906, 909. *See also* Porphyria cutanea tarda (PCT)
hereditary coproporphyria, 890*t*, **904–905**
intermittent. *See* Acute intermittent porphyria (AIP)
laboratory features, 890*t*
porphyria cutanea tarda. *See* Porphyria cutanea tarda (PCT)
variegate, **904–905**
X-linked coproporphyria, 889, 890*t*, 891*t*
Porphyrin precursors, 891*t*
Porphyrins, 889, 891*t*
  in congenital erythropoietic porphyria, 897
  in hepatoerythropoietic porphyria, 905–906
  in hereditary coproporphyria, 905–906
  in porphyria cutanea tarda, 905–906
Portal hypertension, in primary myelofibrosis, 1324–1325
Portal-systemic vascular shunt surgery, for primary myelofibrosis, 1330
Portal vein thrombosis, 2195
Portland hemoglobin, 101, 101*t*, 728, 747
Posaconazole, 385, 387*t*, 389, 1397
Positive regulatory domain 1-binding factor-1 (PRDM1), 1171–1172
Positron emission tomography (PET). *See* FDG-PET
Postpartum hemorrhage, 1987, 2137, 2138
Postthrombotic syndrome, 2273
Posttransfusion purpura (PTP), 2359, 2361
Posttranslational effects, aging and, 130–131
Posttransplant lymphoproliferative disorders (PTLD), 1265–1266, 1500*t*, 1574, **1636**
Potassium chlorate, 810
PP1R12C, 444
PPAR (peroxisome proliferator-activated receptor), 197, 452, 1873–1874
PPBL (persistent polyclonal lymphocytosis of B lymphocytes), 1200–1202, 1201*f*
PPO (protoporphyrinogen oxidase), 895
PR1 vaccine, 423
Pracinostat, 240
Pralatrexate, 1687, 1696*t*
Prasugrel
  for acute coronary syndromes, 2076
  antiplatelet effects, 404*t*, 405
  for sickle cell disease, 777*t*
PRAT4A, 296, 296*f*
Praziquantel, 604
PRDM1, 234*t*, 1171, 1737, 1786
PRDM1 (positive regulatory domain 1-binding factor-1), 1171–1172

Pre-B cell, 270
Precursor (immature) B-cell acute lymphoblastic leukemia, 183, 184*t*, 186*f*, 1515–1517, 1521*t*
Precursor (immature) B-cell lymphomas/leukemias, 1494*t*, 1592
Precursor B cells, 1151, 1168
Precursor cells, in erythropoiesis, 482*f*, 482*t*, **483**, 483*f*
Precursor (immature) T-cell lymphomas/leukemias, 1498*t*, 1592, 1592*f*
Precursor thymocytes, 1179
Prednisolone
  for acute lymphoblastic leukemia, 1515
  adverse effects, 1519*t*
  for antiphospholipid syndrome in pregnancy, 2245
  for immune thrombocytopenia, 2004
  for Langerhans cell histiocytosis, 1107
  for NK/T-cell lymphoma, 1702
  for α-heavy-chain disease, 1808
  for μ-heavy-chain disease, 1810
Prednisone. *See also* BEACOPP regimen; CHOP regimen; COPP regimen; EPOCH regimen; MOPP regimen; Stanford V regimen
  for acute lymphoblastic leukemia, 1515
  for adult Langerhans cell histiocytosis, 1108
  adverse effects, 1519*t*
  for AL amyloidosis, 1779–1780
  for α-heavy-chain disease, 1808
  for autoimmune hemolytic anemia, 838
  for chronic lymphocytic leukemia, 1534–1535
  for diffuse large B-cell lymphoma, 1629*t*
  for follicular lymphoma, 1645*t*, 1646
  for γ-heavy-chain disease, 1806
  for graft-versus-host disease, 372
  for immune thrombocytopenia, 2004
  for Langerhans cell histiocytosis, 1107
  for large granular lymphocytic leukemia, 1567
  lenalidomide and, 334
  for mononucleosis, 1269
  for mycosis fungoides, 1688
  for myeloma, 1751, 1752*t*
  for primary myelofibrosis, 1328
  thalidomide and, 334
  for Waldenström macroglobulinemia, 1793, 1794–1795
Preeclampsia, 2011–2012, 2210–2211
Prefibrotic primary myelofibrosis, 1323*t*, 1324
p region, 1166

Pregnancy, **119–126**
  acute fatty liver of, 2012, 2211
  acute intermittent porphyria and, 901
  acute myelogenous leukemia during, 1409
  adaptations to, 119
  alloimmunized, 849, 853f. *See also*
    Alloimmune hemolytic disease of
    the fetus and newborn (HDFN)
  anemia in, **120**
  anticoagulant therapy during, 112, 112t,
    2277
  antiphospholipid syndrome in, 2239, 2244,
    2245
  aplastic anemia and, 518
  blood volume, erythropoietin level, and
    hemoglobin concentration in, 119
  carbon monoxide poisoning in, 796
  chemotherapy during, 124
  chronic myelogenous leukemia during,
    1459–1460
  coagulation factor deficiencies and, 121,
    2135, 2141, 2144
  cobalamin deficiency in, 598
  congenital thrombotic thrombocytopenic
    purpura in, 2257–2258
  disseminated intravascular coagulation
    during, 120–121, 2204t,
    2210–2211
  essential thrombocythemia and, **124–125**,
    1314–1315, 2081
  factor V deficiency in, 2138
  fibrinogen abnormalities in, 2155, 2156,
    2159
  fibrinolytic activity during, 2312
  folate requirements/deficiency in, 120, 584,
    597–598, 599
  HELLP syndrome in. *See* HELLP
    syndrome
  hematologic consultation in, 45–46
  hematologic malignancies in, treatment of,
    123–124
  hemoglobinopathies in, **125–126**
  heparin-induced thrombocytopenia in,
    2032
  hereditary spherocytosis and, 674
  HIV infection in, 1269
  hypertension during, neonatal neutropenia
    and, 994
  inherited platelet disorders in, 2062
  iron deficiency in, **120**, 630
  lymphoma treatment during, 1634
  mononucleosis in, 1269
  paroxysmal nocturnal hemoglobinuria
    and, 580
  parvovirus B19 infection in, 849
  polycythemia vera in, **125**, 2081

  postpartum hemorrhage and, 1987, 2137,
    2138
  preeclampsia in, 2011–2012, 2210–2211
  Rh blood groups and, 2336
  sepsis during, 2211
  sickle cell disease and, 772–773
  thalassemia syndromes in, 126
  thrombocytopenia during, **121–122**,
    2010–2012, 2010t
  thrombophilia in, **122–123**, 2221, 2225t,
    2227
  thrombophilia testing in, 2228t, 2229
  thrombotic microangiopathy in, 2262
  toxoplasmosis in, 1269
  von Willebrand disease and, 121, 2176
  warfarin therapy during, 112, 112t
Pregnane X receptor, 893
Prekallikrein (PK), 1929, 2121
Preleukemic anemia, 1342
Preleukemic stem cells, 1376
Prenatal diagnosis/testing
  for hemophilia A, 2116
  for hemophilia B, 2127
  for thalassemias, 754
  for von Willebrand disease, 2174
Prepromultimerin, 1845
Presenilin, 1013
Preventive hematology, **7**
Priapism, 770
Primary adrenal lymphoma, 1583
Primary autoimmune myelofibrosis, 1327
Primary central nervous system lymphoma,
    1244f, 1246, 1579
Primary cutaneous anaplastic large cell
    lymphoma, 1499t, 1687, **1688**,
    1688f
Primary cutaneous diffuse large B-cell
    lymphoma, leg type, **1637**
Primary cutaneous follicular center
    lymphoma (PCFCL), 184t, 1581
Primary cutaneous marginal zone B-cell
    lymphoma (PCMZL), 184t, 1581
Primary cutaneous peripheral T-cell
    lymphomas, 1499t
Primary effusion lymphoma, 1246–1247,
    1496t
Primary extranodal lymphoma, **1579–1583**
  bone, 1583
  breast, 1583
  central nervous system, 1244f, 1246, 1579
  chest and lung, 1581
  endocrine glands, 1583
  eye, 1574, 1579–1581
  gastrointestinal tract, 1581
  genitourinary, 1246, 1581–1582, 1582f,
    1634

  heart, 1581
  paranasal sinuses, 1581
  skin, 1581
  spleen, 1582
Primary mediastinal large B-cell lymphoma,
    1634–1635
  clinical features, 1634
  definition, 1634
  epidemiology, 1634
  gene mutations, 225t, 1496t, 1597f, 1626
  laboratory features, 1496t, 1596, 1596f,
    1634
  therapy, 1635
Primary myelofibrosis (PMF), **1319–1332**
  clinical features, **1324–1325**
    bone changes, 1325, 1325t
    extramedullary tumors, 1324
    immune and inflammatory, 1325
    portal hypertension and varices and
      pulmonary arterial hypertension,
      1324–1325
    prefibrotic stage, 1323t, 1324
    presenting signs, 1324
    presenting symptoms, 1324
    thrombocytosis, 1311
    thrombosis and bleeding, 2079–2081
    thrombosis and hemorrhage, 1325
  course and prognosis, 1278, **1331–1332**
  definition and history, 1319
  differential diagnosis, 1311, **1327–1328**,
    1449–1450
  epidemiology, 1319–1320
  essential thrombocythemia and, 1312–
    1313
  etiology and pathogenesis, **1320–1323**
    CD34+ cell egress and neoplastic
      megakaryocytopoiesis, 1321
    chromosomal abnormalities, 178, 179t
    clonal myeloid disease, animal models,
      and activating mutations, 1320–
      1321
    enhanced angiogenesis and splenic
      endothelial cells, 1321
    exogenous factors, 1320
    extramedullary hematopoiesis, 1278,
      1323
    fibroplasia, 1322–1323, 1322t
    gene mutations, 228–229t, 1278, 1308t,
      1320–1321
    hematopoietic dysfunction, 1321–1322
    immune mechanisms, 1320
  laboratory features, **1325–1327**
    blood cell counts and morphology,
      1323f, 1323t, 1325–1326
    functional abnormalities of blood cells,
      1326

marrow, 1322t, 1325t, 1326–1327
monocytosis, 1096
plasma and urine chemical, 1322t, 1325, 1327
therapy, **1328–1331**
  androgens and glucocorticoids for anemia, 1328
  bisphosphonates for bone disease, 1330
  decision to treat, 1328
  drug therapy for myeloproliferation, splenomegaly or cytopenias, 1328–1330, 1329t
  hematopoietic cell transplantation, 1330–1331
  intravenous immunoglobulin, 1330
  portal-systemic vascular shunt surgery, 1330
  radiotherapy, 1330
  recombinant human erythropoietin for anemia, 1328
  red cell transfusion, 1328
  ruxolitinib, 341–342
  splenectomy, 1330
  for thrombosis and bleeding, 2081
transitions to and from, 1328
Primary pituitary lymphoma, 1579
Primary polycythemia. *See* Polycythemia (erythrocytosis), primary familial and congenital
Primary testicular lymphoma, 1246, 1581–1582, 1582f, **1634**
Primary thrombocythemia, vs. primary myelofibrosis, 1327
Primary thyroid lymphoma, 1583
Primidone, megaloblastic anemia and, 606t
Prion protein, 1871
Prions, 2126
PRKAR1B, 1853
Proband, 148
Pro-B cell, 270
PROC, 1923, 1923f
Procainamide, 2015
Procarbazine. *See also* BEACOPP regimen; COPP regimen; MOPP regimen
  for α-heavy-chain disease, 1808
  mechanism of action, 329
  pharmacology, 330
  resistance to, 319t
Procoagulants, 1285
PROCR, 1932
Proerythroblasts, 32t, 34, 463–464, 463f, 464f, 482t
Profilin, 1832t, 1841
Progenitor cell leukemia, 1283
Progenitor cells. *See* Hematopoietic progenitors

Progesterone, 901
Programmed cell death, 203. *See also* Apoptosis
Programmed death-1 (PD-1), 424, 1755
Programmed death-1 (PD-1) receptor, 416
Progressive multifocal leukoencephalopathy (PML), 1536
Prolactin, 561
Proline hydroxylase deficiency, 878
Proline hydroxylases (PHDs), 486, 486f
Prolymphocytic (prolymphoblastic) leukemia (PLL)
  chromosomal abnormalities, 187, 223t, 225, 1494t
  chronic lymphocytic leukemia and, 1542
  gene mutations, 1494t
  laboratory features, 1494t
ProMACE/CytaBOM regimen
  for diffuse large B-cell lymphoma, 1629–1630
  for posttransplant lymphoproliferative disorders, 1636
ProMACE/MOPP regimen, for follicular lymphoma, 1644
Promegaloblasts, 595f
Promonocytes, 34, 1046
Promyelocytes
  marrow, 32t, 34
  maturation, 926f, 940–941, 940f, 941t
  structure, 925, 927f
Promyelocytic leukemia, 1390
Proplatelets, 72, 73f, 1815, 1818, 1820f
Propofol, 28
Propranolol, 2078
PROS1, 1926–1927, 1928f
Prostacyclin (prostaglandin I$_2$)
  antiplatelet effects, 404, 1885, 1967, 2074
  as autacoid, 1970
  in HELLP syndrome, 801
  inflammation and, 288–289, 2202
  synthesis, 1834, 1969–1970
Prostacyclin G/H synthase, 1970
Prostaglandin E$_2$, 1182, 1885
Prostaglandin H$_2$ synthase-1 (cyclooxygenase) deficiency, 2058
Prostaglandin I$_2$. *See* Prostacyclin
Prostaglandins, 404, 1885, 2074. *See also* Eicosanoids
Prostate, primary lymphomas in, 1572
Prosthetic heart valves, hemolysis and, **804–806**, 805t
Protamine, for heparin reversal, 397
Protease (proteinase)-activated receptor (PAR)-1, **290**, **1954**
  activation, 1877, 1877f, 1881

  characteristics, 1952t
  in coagulation reactions, 1949, 2201
  in platelets, 1843
  signaling, 1956, 1957f, 2076
Protease (proteinase)-activated receptors (PARs), **290**
Protease–cofactor complexes, 1917–1918, 1918t
Protease inhibitors, 1242, 1249, 1941–1942, 1958–1959. *See also* Antithrombin (AT); Heparin
Proteasome, **240–241**
Proteasome inhibitors, 209, **342–343**, 342f, 1750–1751, 1754. *See also specific drugs*
Protectins, 286
Protein 4.1R, 663t, 666–667, 667f, 670t, 678
Protein 4.2, 663t, 667, 670t, 672
Protein antigens, 2337
Proteinase 3, 283, 414, 1012t, 1013
Proteinase (protease)-activated receptors (PARs), **290**. *See also* Protease (proteinase)-activated receptor (PAR)-1
Protein C, **1951–1952**
  activation, 1923. *See also* Activated protein C (APC)
  antibodies, 2187
  endothelial protein C receptor and, 1953
  functions, 1952t
  gene structure and variations, 1923, 1923f, 1952
  mutations, 1952
  structure, 1854, 1917f, 1923, 1951–1952, 1951f, 1952t
  synthesis, 1951–1952
  therapeutic forms, 1952
  thrombomodulin and, 1953, 1972
Protein C deficiency
  acquired causes, 2224t
  clinical features, 2100, 2223
  clinical implications of testing for, 2228t
  epidemiology, 2222t
  etiology and pathogenesis, 1923, 1952, 2222–2223
  venous thromboembolism risk and, 2225t, 2226t
Protein C pathway
  antiphospholipid antibodies and, 2237
  coagulation pathways and, **1949–1951**, 1950f
  components, **1951–1954**, 1952t
    endothelial protein C receptor. *See* Endothelial protein C receptor (EPCR)

Protein C pathway, components (*Cont.*):
  protease activated receptor-1. *See*
    Protease (proteinase)-activated
    receptor (PAR)-1
  protein C. *See* Protein C
  protein S. *See* Protein S
  thrombomodulin. *See* Thrombomodulin
    (TM)
  in disseminated intravascular coagulation,
    2201*f*, 2202
  in inflammatory response, 1971–1972,
    2202
Protein deficiency, anemia of, **654**
Protein inhibitor of activated STATs (PIAS),
  253
Protein kinase B (Akt), 208*f*, 209, 251, 1882
Protein kinase C (PKC), 1016, 1178, 1837,
  1841
Protein kinase C-θ deficiency, 2058
Proteins
  adaptor, 251–252
  in α-heavy-chain, 1807–1808
  α-heavy-chain disease, 1807, 1807*f*
  cross-presentation, 308
  in erythrocytes, 469*t*
  fibrinolytic, 2304–2305*t*
  fusion, 1015–1016
  in γ-heavy-chain disease, 1803, 1805*f*
  iron-containing, 631
  in iron homeostasis, 621*t*
  leukemia-associated, 414
  membrane. *See* Membrane proteins
  in μ-heavy-chain disease, 1809–1810,
    1810*f*
  in neutrophil granules, 1011–1014
  nonimmunologic adsorption, 825*f*, 826*t*,
    830*t*
  nonimmunologic protein adsorption, 831
  phosphorylation, **250–251**
  prion, 1871
  secretory, 1161
  synthesis
    genes and, 147
    in mature neutrophils, 932, 933*t*
Protein S, 1949, **1952–1953**
  activated protein C and, 1955, 2202
  anticoagulant activity, 1958
  cofactor function, 1926
  gene structure and variations, 1926–1927,
    1928*f*, 1953
  in platelets, 1845
  structure, 1926, 1927*f*, 1951*f*, 1952*t*,
    1953–1954
Protein S deficiency
  acquired causes, 2224*t*
  clinical features, 2100, 2223

clinical implications of testing for, 2228*t*
epidemiology, 2222*t*
etiology and pathogenesis, 1927, 1953,
  2222–2223
venous thromboembolism risk and, 1927,
  1958, 2225*t*, 2226*t*
Protein tyrosine phosphatases (PTPs), 253
Protein Z, 1938, 1952*t*
Protein Z-dependent protease inhibitor
  (ZPI), 1916*t*, 1938, 1952*t*, **1960**
Proteoglycans, 62
Proteomics, platelet, 1853–1854
Proteus infections, 383, 2207. *See also*
  Bacterial infections
Proteus vulgaris, 2340
Prothrombin (factor II)
  activation and activity, 1854, 1918–1919
  characteristics, 1917*t*
  conversion to thrombin, 1918–1919, 1919*f*,
    2136–2137
  gene structure and variations, 1920, 1920*f*,
    2137
  lupus anticoagulant activity and, 2186
  structure, 1917*f*, 1918, 2136
Prothrombin complex concentrate (PCC),
  396, 2135, 2136, 2136*t*
Prothrombin (factor II) deficiency,
  2135–2137
  clinical features, 2137
  definition, 2135–2136
  gene mutations, 2135*t*, 2137
  incidence, 2133, 2134*t*
  therapy, 2136*t*, 2137
Prothrombin G20210A
  arterial thromboembolic disease risk and,
    2226–2227
  clinical implications of testing for,
    2227–2228, 2228*t*
  epidemiology, 2222*t*, 2224
  etiology and pathogenesis, 2224
  venous thromboembolism risk and, 2225,
    2225*t*, 2226*t*, 2268
Prothrombin time (PT)
  in anticoagulant monitoring, 395
  in disseminated intravascular coagulation,
    2205*t*
  in hemostatic disorders, 1988, 1989*f*
Prothymocytes, 87
Protoheme-ferrolyase, 895
Protoporphyrin IX, 891*f*, 892*f*, 893*f*
Protoporphyrinogen oxidase (PPO), 895
Prourokinase. *See* Urokinase plasminogen
  activator (u-PA)
Proximal vein thrombosis, 2268, 2273
PRPS2, 200
Pruritus/itching

history of, 6, 8
in mycosis fungoides, 1680
in polycythemia vera, 1293
symptomatic therapy for, 1300
PSC-833, 1404
PSD95, 1872
P-selectin (GMP140, PADGEM, CD62P),
  1870
  activities, 68
  characteristics, 1858–1859*t*
  in coagulation system, 290
  counterreceptor, 282*t*
  in disseminated intravascular coagulation,
    2207
  distribution, 67*t*
  in eosinophils, 950
  expression, 281
  glycoprotein Ib and, 1868
  hematopoietic stem cell trafficking and,
    355
  in inflammatory response, 1976–1977,
    1978–1979
  ligands, 67*t*
  L-selectin (CD62L), 66
  in neutrophils, 1006, 1007*f*
  platelets expressing, 1830–1831*f*, 1834,
    1852*f*, 1854
  PSGL-1 and, 1854, 1855–1856, 1870
  in sickle cell disease, 765
  von Willebrand factor and, 2166
Pseudoaddiction, 767
Pseudodiploid, 175*t*
Pseudoleukemia, 1393
Pseudolymphoma syndrome, 1097
Pseudomonas exotoxin, 345
Pseudomonas infections. *See also* Bacterial
  infections
  disseminated intravascular coagulation
    and, 2207
  in immunocompromised host, 383
  in leukocyte adhesion deficiency, 1023
  neutropenia and, 985
  neutrophil abnormalities and, 986
  in newborn, 105, 106
  in specific granule deficiency, 1021
Pseudoneutropenia, 985
Pseudoneutrophilia (demargination),
  999–1000
Pseudoscleroderma, 907
Pseudothrombocytopenia (spurious
  thrombocytopenia), 43, **1994–1996**
Pseudotumors (blood cysts), 2119, 2120*f*
Pseudovasculogenesis, 2011
Pseudo- (platelet-type) von Willebrand
  disease, **2050–2051**, 2174
Pseudoxanthoma elasticum, 2108

Pseudo-Zollinger-Ellison syndrome, iron deficiency and, 629
PSGL-1, 1852f, 1854, 1855–1856, 1870, 1976–1977, 1977t, 1979t
PSMD4, 1736
Psoralen plus ultraviolet A (PUVA), 433, 1106, 1686, 1687, 1689
Psoriasis, 1575
Psychotropic drugs, 2079
PT. *See* Prothrombin time (PT)
PTCL. *See* Peripheral T-cell lymphoma (PTCL)
PTEN, 195, 1443
PTEN, 231t, 1626, 1736t
Pteroic acid, 584
Pteroylglutamic acid (folic acid), 584, 585f. *See also* Folate
PTGS1/COX1, 1456
PTLD (posttransplant lymphoproliferative disorders), 1265–1266, 1500t, 1574, **1636**
PTP (posttransfusion purpura), 2359, 2361
PTPN11, 1346t, 1352, 1471
PTPN12, 1699
PTPRD, 234t
PTPs (protein tyrosine phosphatases), 253
PU.1
    in B cell function, 271
    in erythroid differentiation, 272, 483
    GATA1 and, 268, 483
    in hematopoietic stem cell to common lymphoid progenitor commitment, 262
    in lymphopoiesis, 1155
    in myelopoiesis, 1011
    RB and, 217
Pulmonary angiography, 2272
Pulmonary disease/dysfunction
    in acute myelogenous leukemia, 1381
    in adult Langerhans cell histiocytosis, 1108
    anemia and, 505
    in antiphospholipid syndrome, 2240
    in disseminated intravascular coagulation, 2204–2205, 2205t
    erythrocytosis of, 872, 875, 881
    in Gaucher disease, 1124
    Hodgkin lymphoma treatment and lung cancer risk, 1618
    after hematopoietic cell transplantation, 368
    in Langerhans cell histiocytosis, 1104
    primary lymphoma, 1581
    in sickle cell disease, 768–769, 769f
    in Waldenström macroglobulinemia, 1791
Pulmonary embolism. *See also* Venous thrombosis/thromboembolism

clinical features, 2269
complications, 2269
definition and epidemiology, 2267
differential diagnosis, 2270
etiology and pathogenesis, 2268
in hepatic disease, 2194–2195
objective testing for, 2271–2273
therapy. *See* Venous thrombosis/thromboembolism, therapy
Pulmonary eosinophilia, 949–950
Pulmonary hypertension
    chronic thromboembolic, 2273
    in polycythemia vera, 1293
    in primary myelofibrosis, 1324–1325
    vs. primary myelofibrosis, 1327–1328
    sickle cell disease and, 769
    treatment, 797
Punctate basophilia, 468
Pure erythroid leukemia, 1390
Pure red cell aplasia
    acquired, **542–545**
        in chronic lymphocytic leukemia, 1542
        clinical features, 543–544
        definition and history, 542–543
        differential diagnosis, 544
        etiology and pathogenesis, 543
        laboratory features, 544
        in large granular lymphocytic leukemia, 1566
        parvovirus B19 infection and, 1251–1252
        therapy, course, and prognosis, 544–545, 545f, 1542
    classification of, 542t
    inherited (Diamond-Blackfan anemia), **539–540**, 994
    during pregnancy, 120
    transient aplastic crisis and transient erythroblastopenia of childhood, **541–542**, 541f
Pure white cell aplasia, 995
Purine analogues, **322–324**. *See also specific drugs*
    adverse effects, 324
    mechanism of action, 323
    megaloblastic anemia and, 606t
    for mycosis fungoides, 1687
    pharmacology, 323–324
    structure, 323f
Purine nucleoside phosphorylase deficiency, 1214t, 1217
Purine synthesis, 585, 586t, 587f
Purpura
    amyloid, 1774, 1774f
    in immune thrombocytopenia, 2002

posttransfusion, 2359, 2361
    vascular. *See* Vascular purpuras
Purpura fulminans, 2104, 2207
PUVA (psoralen plus ultraviolet A), 433, 1686, 1687, 1689
PV. *See* Polycythemia vera (PV)
PYD (pyridinoline), 1738
Pyoderma gangrenosum, 2100, 2100f, 2102
Pyrazinamide, for tuberculosis, 386
Pyridinoline (PYD), 1738
Pyridoxine, 651, 917–918, 920
Pyrimethamine, 606t, 1269
Pyrimidine 5′-nucleotidase, 692t, 699, 700t, 706, 706f
Pyrimidine analogues, megaloblastic anemia and, 606t
Pyrimidine synthesis, 587f
Pyrin, 298–299
PYRIN, 1025
Pyropoikilocytes, 475
Pyropoikilocytosis, hereditary. *See* Hereditary pyropoikilocytosis
Pyrrole rings, 892f
Pyruvate kinase (PK)
    activity, 692t
    erythrocyte aging and, 497
    in glucose metabolism, 696
    mutants/variants, 702
    structure, 696, 696f
Pyruvate kinase (PK) deficiency
    in animals, 704
    clinical features, 690, 700t
    diagnosis, 700t
    differential diagnosis, 691
    epidemiology, 690
    genetics, 702, 704
    in hereditary nonspherocytic hemolytic anemia, 709
    malaria resistance and, 704
    therapy, 711–712

Q
22q 11.2 deletion syndrome (DiGeorge syndrome), 86–87, 1214t, **1222**
Q43P, 1838
3q abnormalities, 1377
5q-minus syndrome, 1312, 1347, 1347f
Quat Sha, 2107
Quebec platelet syndrome/disorder, 1853, 1854, 2055–2056, 2138
Quinacrine, aplastic anemia and, 515
Quinidine, 2017, 2079
Quinine, 817, 819, 2015, 2017, 2245, 2262
Quinolones, 384, 388–389
Quinupristin/dalfopristin, 385
Quizartinib, 1403

R

R207H, 1838

Rab, 1065*f*, 1849

Rab GTPases, 1883

Rac (Rac), 237, 1841

Rac-2 deficiency, 1020*t*

Rac GTPases, 1883

RACK1 (receptor of activated protein kinase C), 487

R-ACVBP, for diffuse large B-cell lymphoma, 1630

RAD21, 1346*t*, 1352

Rad-57, 792

Radial nuclear segmentation, 23

Radiation exposure

    acute lymphoblastic leukemia and, 1507

    acute myelogenous leukemia and, 1374

    aplastic anemia and, 518

    chronic lymphocytic leukemia and, 1528

    chronic myelogenous leukemia and, 1438

    hemolytic anemia and, 811

    lymphoma and, 1573

    myelodysplastic syndromes and, 1342, 1345

    primary myelofibrosis and, 1319

Radiation therapy

    for acute lymphoblastic leukemia, 1517

    for bone pain in myeloma, 1756

    for chronic lymphocytic leukemia, 1540

    for chronic myelogenous leukemia, 1459

    cranial, 1519*t*, 1520

    for diffuse large B-cell lymphoma

        with CHOP, 1628

        with R-CHOP, 1628

    for follicular lymphoma, 99.

    for Hodgkin lymphoma, 1248, 1611, 1613, 1614

    for mantle cell lymphoma, 1656–1657

    for ocular/intraocular lymphoma, 1581

    for primary myelofibrosis, 1330

Radioactive phosphorus, 1298*t*, 1299, 1313*t*, 1314

Radioimmunoconjugates, **346**, 360

Radioimmunotherapy

    adverse effects, 1647

    for diffuse large B-cell lymphoma, 1632

    for follicular lymphoma, 1647, 1649

Radionuclide lung scanning, 2271

RAEB (refractory anemia with excess blasts). *See* Oligoblastic myelogenous leukemia (refractory anemia with excess blasts)

RAG1/2, 1164, 1214*t*, 1218, 1219

Rag-1/Rag-2 complex, 1164, 1166–1167, 1166*f*, 1168

Rai clinical staging system, 1533*t*

Ral GTPases, 1883

Random-label methods, for red cell life span measurement, 495–496, 496*f*

RANK (receptor activator of NF-κB), 1606, 1713

RANKL (receptor activator of NF-κB ligand), 1077*f*, 1713, 1737, 1738*f*, 1739*f*

RANTES (CCL5), 1607, 1852*f*, 1855, 2286

Rapamycin, 1220

Rap GTPases, 1883

RAPH. *See* CD151

Raph blood group, 2332*t*

RAPH~null~ phenotype, 2343

Rapoport Luebering shunt, 692

Rare bleeding disorders (RBDs), **2133–2145**

    classification, 2134

    combined deficiency of factors V and VIII, **2139–2140**

    factor V deficiency. *See* Factor V deficiency (parahemophilia)

    factor VII deficiency. *See* Factor VII deficiency

    factor X deficiency. *See* Factor X deficiency

    factor XI deficiency. *See* Factor XI deficiency

    factor XIII deficiency. *See* Factor XIII deficiency

    gene mutations, 2134–2135, 2135*t*

    incidence, 2133, 2134*t*

    laboratory features, 2133–2134

    prothrombin deficiency. *See* Prothrombin (factor II) deficiency

    treatment, 2135, 2136*t*

    in women, 2135

RARS (refractory anemia, with ring sideroblasts), 178, 1343, 1343*t*, 1349

RARS-T (refractory anemia, with ring sideroblasts with thrombocytosis), 178, 1343, 1343*t*, 1349, 1352

RAR-α, 1390–1391

Ras, 238

RAS (RAS)

    in acute myelogenous leukemia, 1398

    in cell growth, 192

    in cellular senescence, 132

    in chronic myelogenous leukemia, 1443, 1471

    in myeloma, 1710, 1735, 1736*t*, 1737

    in primary myelofibrosis, 1320, 1321

RAS (renin-angiotensin system), 487

Rasburicase

    in G6PD deficiency, 712

    for hyperuricemia, 1394, 1450, 1514, 1675

Ras family proteins, 230, 237

Ras GTPases, 1882–1883

Ras/Raf/MAPK pathway gene mutations, 232*t*, 233*t*

Ras/Raf/MEK/ERK cascade, 237

RB, 238, 1710

RB1, 232*t*, 234*t*, 1464, 1653, 1736, 1737

RB–E2F complex, 217, 217*f*

R binder. *See* Haptocorrin

RBM8A, 2061

RB (Rb) proteins, 217, 217*f*, 1444

RCF (ristocetin cofactor) activity, 1988, 1991

R-CHOP regimen

    for Castleman disease, 1250

    for diffuse large B-cell lymphoma, 1628, 1628*t*, 1629*t*, 1630

    for follicular lymphoma, 1645*t*, 1646–1647, 1646*t*, 1649

    for HIV-associated lymphoma, 1245

    for intravascular large B-cell lymphoma, 1636

    for mantle cell lymphoma, 1656, 1656*f*, 1657*t*, 1658*t*

    for posttransplant lymphoproliferative disorders, 1636

    for primary testicular lymphoma, 1634

    for T-cell-histiocyte-rich large B-cell lymphoma, 1637

    for Waldenström macroglobulinemia, 1794–1795

R-CP regimen, for Waldenström macroglobulinemia, 1795

R-CVP regimen

    for follicular lymphoma, 1645*t*, 1646–1647, 1646*f*, 1646*t*, 1649

    for mantle cell lymphoma, 1656

    for Waldenström macroglobulinemia, 1795

RDAs. *See* Recommended daily allowances (RDAs)

R-DHAP regimen, for diffuse large B-cell lymphoma, 1631

RDW (red cell distribution width), 14

Reactive hypereosinophilia, 959

Reactive leukocytosis, 1450

Reactive lymphocytes, 23, 1203*f*, 1264, 1264*f*

Reactive nitrogen intermediates, 286–287, 286*t*

Reactive oxygen intermediates, 286, 286*t*

Reactive oxygen species (ROS), 195–196, 1663

Reactive thrombocytosis, 1310, 1312*t*, **2035–2037**

Reaginic antibody, 1162

Receiver operator characteristic curves, 635, 635*f*

Receptor activator of NF-κB (RANK), 1606, 1713

Receptor activator of NF-κB ligand (RANKL), 1077f, 1713, 1737, 1738f, 1739f
Receptor down-modulation, 252–253
Receptor of activated protein kinase C (RACK1), 487
Receptor protein-tyrosine kinases (rPTKs), 230
Receptor tyrosine kinases (RTKs), **249**
Recessiveness, 147, 149
Recombinant factor VIIa. *See* Factor VIIa replacement
Recombinant factor VIII. *See* Factor VIII replacement
Recombinant human erythropoietin. *See* Erythropoiesis-stimulating agents (ESAs)
Recombinant tissue plasminogen activator. *See* Alteplase; Reteplase; Tenecteplase
Recombination signal sequences (RSS), 1164
Recommended daily allowances (RDAs)
    cobalamin, 589
    folate, 584
    iron, 618t
Rectal bleeding, 1987
Recurrence risk, 148, 150
Recurring abnormality, 175t
Red cell antigens, in newborns, 104
Red cell aplasia. *See* Pure red cell aplasia
Red cell clearance, splenic, 90–91
Red cell count, 13–14
Red cell distribution width (RDW), 14
Red cell enzyme disorders. *See* Erythrocyte enzyme disorders
Red cell exchange
    adverse effects, 433
    indications for, 428t, 429t, 432
    principles, 431
    for protozoan disease, 432
    for sickle cell disease, 431–432
Red cell flicker, 469
Red cells. *See* Erythrocytes
Red cell transfusion
    ABO incompatibility and, 2330
    adverse effects. *See* Iron overload; Transfusion reactions
    for anemia of chronic renal disease, 554
    for anemia of inflammation, 554, 554t
    for aplastic anemia, 522
    for autoimmune hemolytic anemia, 837
    for β-thalassemia, 751, 2372
    in cardiovascular patients, 2369–2370
    in children, 2371
    in critically ill patients, 2369–2370, 2370t
    for Diamond-Blackfan anemia, 540

    indications, 2369
    massive, thrombocytopenia associated with, 2014
    for myelodysplastic syndromes, 1357
    in newborns, 2371, 2372t
    in orthopedic patients, 2370
    for paroxysmal nocturnal hemoglobinuria, 579
    patient blood management for avoidance of, 2378
    in preterm infants, 2371, 2372t
    red cell age and outcome of, 2376–2377
    for sickle cell disease, 776, 2371–2372
    in solid-organ transplant patient, 2374
    for thrombocytopenia, 1541
Red marrow, 28
Red pulp, spleen, 89f, 90, 90f
Red thrombi, 2292
Reduced-intensity conditioning, for hematopoietic cell transplantation, **360–361**, 367
Red urine, history of, 5
Reed-Sternberg cells
    antigen receptor rearrangements, 1606
    genetic alterations and signaling pathways, 1606
    histopathology, 1599f, 1605f
    in Hodgkin lymphoma, 1599, 1599f, 1605–1607, 1605f
    microenvironment, 1607
    origin, 1606–1607
    reprogramming, 1606
Reference ranges, **18–19**, 18t, 19f
Refractory anemia
    with excess blasts (RAEB). *See* Oligoblastic myelogenous leukemia (refractory anemia with excess blasts)
    history, 1342
    paroxysmal nocturnal hemoglobinuria and, 575t, 578
    with ring sideroblasts (RARS), 178, 1343, 1343t, 1349
    with ring sideroblasts with thrombocytosis (RARS-T), 178, 1343, 1343t, 1349, 1352
Refractory cytopenia
    of childhood, 178
    with multilineage dysplasia, 1343, 1343t
        paroxysmal nocturnal hemoglobinuria and, 575t, 578
    with unilineage dysplasia, 178, 1343, 1343t
Refractory leukemia, 1401
Refractory megaloblastic anemia, 608
Regadenoson, for sickle cell disease, 777t
Regenerative medicine. *See* Multipotential cell therapy

Regulatory T (T$_{REG}$) cells. *See* CD4+CD25+ regulatory T (T$_{REG}$) cells
Relapsed leukemia, 1401
Relative anemia, 506
Relative erythrocytosis, 872, 880
Remodelers (ATP-dependent chromatin remodeling complexes), 166–168, 166f
Renal disease/dysfunction
    in acute hemolytic transfusion reaction, 2374
    in acute myelogenous leukemia, 1381
    in AL amyloidosis, 1775, 1775t, 1776–1777, 1781
    in antiphospholipid syndrome, 2241
    chronic, anemia of. *See* Anemia of chronic kidney disease
    in disseminated intravascular coagulation, 2204, 2205t
    dose modification in patients with, 316t
    in essential monoclonal gammopathy, 1723–1724
    folate excretion and, 588
    in hemolytic uremic syndrome, 2258–2259
    in myeloma, 1744–1745
    polycythemia and, 878–879, 881
    primary lymphoma, 1582
    in sickle cell disease, 770
    in thrombotic thrombocytopenic purpura, 2254
    in Waldenström macroglobulinemia, 1791
Renal transplantation
    for atypical hemolytic uremic syndrome, 2261
    erythrocytosis following
        clinical features, 881
        epidemiology, 873
        etiology and pathogenesis, 878–879
        therapy, 884
    hematopoietic cell transplantation for tolerance of, 373–374
Rendu-Osler-Weber disease. *See* Hereditary hemorrhagic telangiectasia (HHT)
Renin-angiotensin system (RAS), 487
Reperfusion therapy, 2295
Replicative senescence, 132
R-EPOCH regimen
    for Burkitt lymphoma, 1675t, 1676
    for diffuse large B-cell lymphoma, 1629t, 1630
    for HIV-associated lymphoma, 1245, 1247
    for lymphomatoid granulomatosis, 1635
    for primary mediastinal large B-cell lymphoma, 1635

Reproductive system disorders
   acute myelogenous leukemia treatment
      and, 1411
   history of, 5–6
   Hodgkin lymphoma treatment and, 1618
   testicular lymphoma, 1246, 1581–1582,
      1582f, **1634**
Resolvins, 286
Respiration, regulation by hypoxia, 504f
Respiratory burst reactions, 1068f
Respiratory syncytial virus (RSV) infection,
   384, 386
Respiratory tract. See also Pulmonary
   disease/dysfunction
   iron deficiency and bleeding in, 630
   macrophages in, 1082–1083
Response to injury hypothesis, 2281
Restenosis, 1975, 1975f, 2296–2297
Restriction fragment length polymorphisms
   (RFLPs), 2116
Reteplase, **403**, 2313t
Reticular dysgenesis, 530t, 532, 993, 1214t
Reticulocyte count, 14, 16
Reticulocyte indices, 16
Reticulocytes, 21, 482t
   in autoimmune hemolytic anemia, 832
   automated analysis, 14, 16
   birth, 465–466, 467f
   hemoglobin content, 635
   iron deficiency and, 633
   macro-, 467
   maturation, 466–467, 466f
   pathology, 467
   precursor cell kinetics, 75t
   release, 72, 72f
   RNA content, 14
   in sickle cell disease, 764–765
   stress, 482f, 505
Reticulum cell sarcoma, 1569
Retinal abnormalities, 2241
Retinal hemorrhages, 8
Retinoblastoma protein. See RB (Rb) proteins
all-trans-Retinoic acid. See ATRA (all-trans-
   retinoic acid)
Retinoic acid inducible gene I (RIG-I),
   300–301, 302f
Retinoic acid receptor (RAR), 169
Retinoic acid-related orphan receptor γ
   (RORγt), 1181f, 1182
Retinoic acid syndrome (differentiation
   syndrome), 1405
Retinoic receptor α (RARα), 1714
Retinoids, **335**. See also ATRA (all-trans-
   retinoic acid)
   for lymphomatoid papulosis, 1689
   for mycosis fungoides, 1685–1686

Retinopathy, in sickle cell disease, 772
Retroviral vectors, 439
Reviparin, 2274t
R-FCM regimen, for follicular lymphoma,
   1647
RFLPs (restriction fragment length
   polymorphisms), 2116
R-FND, for follicular lymphoma, 1649
RHAg, 2337, 2339, 2342
RHAMM, 266–267
Rh-associated glycoprotein, 2332t
Rh blood group, **2330, 2336**
   ABO-Rh compatibility guidelines, 2350t
   antibodies, 2344t
   antigens, 2331t, 2333–2334t, 2336, 2337
   autoantibody and, 2340
   disease associations, 2331t
   frequency, 2333–2334t
   genetics, 2339
   membrane structures in, 2330f
   nomenclature, 2336
   serologic detection, 2348–2349
RHCE, 2339
RHD, 850, 2339
Rh-deficiency syndrome, **684**
Rheumatoid arthritis
   aplastic anemia in, 518
   Epstein-Barr virus infection and, 1265
   large granular lymphocytic leukemia and,
      1565
   lymphomas and, 1574
   neutropenia and, 996
Rh hemolytic disease, 849–850, 851f,
   852t, 856f. See also Alloimmune
   hemolytic disease of the fetus and
   newborn (HDFN)
Rh immunoglobulin (RhIg), 858–859
Rh-negative, 2348
Rh_null phenotype, 2340, 2341t, 2342
Rho family, 230, 237, 1444, 1882–1883
RhoH/TTF, 1626
Rh-positive, 2348
Rh proteins, 835
Rh-RhAG proteins, 665
Rh sensitization, 432
R-hyperCVAD regimen, for mantle cell
   lymphoma, 1657, 1657t, 1658t
Ribavirin, 386
Riboflavin (vitamin B_2), 652t, 793, 2388
Riboflavin (vitamin B_2) deficiency, 651–652
Ribonucleotide reductase, 582f
Ribonucleotide reductase inhibitors, **325**,
   606t. See also Hydroxyurea
Ribosephosphate isomerase, 692t, 697
Ribosomal RNA (rRNA), 147, 195
Ribosomes, 147, 192, 195

Ribozymes, 153
Ribulose-phosphate epimerase, 697
R-ICE regimen, for diffuse large B-cell
   lymphoma, 1629t, 1631
Richter syndrome, 1542
Ricin A chain, 345
Rickettsial infections, 997, 2105–2106
Rifampin
   maternal ingestion of, effect on fetus and
      newborn, 112t
   for tuberculosis, 386
RIG-I (retinoic acid inducible gene I),
   300–301, 302f
RIG-I-like helicase (RLH) pathway, 300–303
Rigosertib, for myelodysplastic syndromes,
   1361
Ring sideroblasts, 178, 465, 567, 624, 918,
   1353. See also Sideroblastic
   anemias
Rip1, 207, 207f
RIPA (ristocetin-induced platelet
   agglutination), 2173
RIPK4, 1711
RISC (RNA-induced silencing complex),
   153
Ristocetin, 1867, 2168
Ristocetin cofactor assay/activity, 2164t, 2173
Ristocetin-induced platelet agglutination
   (RIPA), 2173
Ristocetin-induced platelet aggregation test,
   1988–1989
Ritonavir, 1249
Rituximab, **344**
   for acquired hemophilia A, 2186
   adverse effects, 343t, 344, 1250, 1519t,
      1535–1536, 2005, 2256
   for antiphospholipid syndrome, 2245
   for aplastic anemia, 526
   for atypical hemolytic uremic syndrome,
      2261
   for autograft purging, 358
   for autoimmune hemolytic anemia, 838,
      839
   for autoimmune lymphoproliferative
      syndrome, 1224
   for B-cell acute lymphoblastic leukemia,
      1515
   for Burkitt lymphoma, 1676
   for Castleman disease, 1249–1250
   with CHOP. See R-CHOP regimen
   for chronic lymphocytic leukemia,
      1535–1536, 1537
   for diffuse large B-cell lymphoma, 1628,
      1628t, 1629t, 1630, 1631
   dose, 343t, 344
   with EPOCH. See R-EPOCH regimen

for follicular lymphoma, 1644, 1645–1647, 1645t, 1646f, 1646t, 1649
for γ-heavy-chain disease, 1806
for gastric MALT lymphoma, 1666, 1666t
for graft-versus-host disease prophylaxis, 372
for Hodgkin lymphoma, 1616, 1617
for immune thrombocytopenia, 122, 2000, 2005
for intravascular large B-cell lymphoma, 1636
for mantle cell lymphoma, 1655–1656, 1656f, 1657t, 1658, 1658t, 1659t, 1660t
for μ-heavy-chain disease, 1810
for posttransplantation lymphoproliferative disease, 1266, 1636
in pregnancy, 1634
for primary cutaneous diffuse large B-cell lymphoma, leg type, 1637
for primary mediastinal large B-cell lymphoma, 1634
for pure red cell aplasia, 544
in reduced-intensity conditioning, 360
resistance to, 344
for splenic marginal zone lymphoma, 1667
for thrombocytopenia, 2008
for thrombotic thrombocytopenic purpura, 2256
for Waldenström macroglobulinemia, 1794
Rivaroxaban, **401–402**
    adverse effects, 2275t
    for antiphospholipid syndrome, 2245
    clinical studies, 400t
    mechanism of action, 1922
    for venous thromboembolism, 2274–2275, 2274t, 2275t
RLH (RIG-I-like helicase) pathway, 300–303
R-MCP regimen
    for follicular lymphoma, 1646t
    for mantle cell lymphoma, 1657t
RMRP, 1226
RNA, 147, 153. See also mRNA (messenger RNA)
RNA-induced silencing complex (RISC), 153
RNA polymerase, 147
RNA sequencing, 161, 1851, 1852f
ROBO1, 1737
Rocky Mountain spotted fever, 2105, 2105f
Rofecoxib, 2075
Romidepsin, **336–337**
    for acute myelogenous leukemia, 1403
    for mycosis fungoides, 1687
    for peripheral T-cell lymphoma, 1696, 1696t

Romiplostim
    adverse effects, 2006
    for hypersplenism, 867
    for immune thrombocytopenia, 2001, 2006
    for myelodysplastic syndromes, 1358, 2384
RORγt (retinoic acid-related orphan receptor γ), 1181f, 1182
ROS (reactive oxygen species), 195–196, 1663
Rosai-Dorfman disease (sinus histiocytosis with massive lymphadenopathy), 1101, **1112–1113**
Rosette test, 859
Rotational thromboelastography, 2206–2207
Rouleaux, 21
RPS14, 539, 1347
RPS19, 539, 540
rPTKs (receptor protein-tyrosine kinases), 230
rRNA (ribosomal RNA), 147, 195
RSS (recombination signal sequences), 1164
RSV (respiratory syncytial virus) infection, 384, 386
RTKs (receptor tyrosine kinases), **249**
Rubella, mononucleosis and, 1268
Rubor, 508
RUNX1, 1817
RUNX1 (AML1)
    in acute myelogenous leukemia, 181t, 225, 226t, 237, 1376, 1378, 1378t, 1384t, 1415, 2060
    in congenital neutropenia, 993
    in myelodysplastic syndromes, 181t, 228t, 1345, 1346t, 1351
RUNX1-RUNX1T1 rearrangement, 225
RUNXT1 (ETO), 1351, 1384t, 1414
Russell bodies, 1742, 1743f
Ruxolitinib, **341–342**
    for polycythemia vera, 1300
    for primary myelofibrosis, 1329, 1329t

S
S1P (sphingosphine-1-phosphate), 1857, 1878
S100A9 (MRP-14), 1856, 1872
S100A10, 2309
S-adenosylhomocysteine (SAH), 588
S-adenosylmethionine (SAMe), 196, 590
SAGE (serial analysis of gene expression), 421
SAH (S-adenosylhomocysteine), 588
SAHA (suberoylanilide hydroxamic acid), 1403
Salicylates, 112
Saline (direct) agglutinins, 823
Salmonella spp., 819
Salmonella typhimurium, 1066f

Salt bridges, in deoxyhemoglobin, 761, 761f
SAMHD1, 231t
Sanger sequencing, 155
SAO (Southeast Asian ovalocytosis), 670f, **680**
SAP (SLAM-associated protein), 1228
Saposin C, 1122
SARA (SMAD anchor for receptor activation), 251
Sarcoidosis, 1097, 1575
Sarcoma
    dendritic cell, 1110
    extranodal histiocytic, 1110
    Langerhans cell, 1110
    lympho-, 1569, 1603
    mast cell, 978
    myeloid, 1381
    nonleukemic myeloid, 1398
    reticulum cell, 1569
Sarcoplasmic reticulum, 1836
Sarcosine dehydrogenase, 588
Sargramostim, 1358. See also Granulocyte-macrophage colony-stimulating factor (GM-CSF)
SARM (sterile-α and armadillo motif), 298
Saruplase, 2313t
Satellitism, platelet-leukocyte, 1995, 1995f
Satiety, premature, history of, 5
SBDS, 532
Sca1, 260
Scar tissue, 280
Scavenger receptor-B1 (SCARB1, CLA-1), 1872
Scavenger receptor-B3 (SCARB3). See Glycoprotein (GP)IV
Scavenger receptors (SRs), 1054–1055, 1057t, 1872, 2287
SCF. See Stem cell factor (SCF)
Schilling test, 584
Schimke syndrome, **1226**
Schistosoma, 956, 957t, 1180
Schistosomula, killing of, 953
Schizocytes (schistocytes), 21f, 472f, 472t, **475**, 2255–2256
Schnitzler syndrome, 1791
Scianna blood group/antigens, 2331t, 2337, 2346t
SCID. See Severe combined immunodeficiency (SCID)
SCL (stem cell leukemia), 262
SCL40A1, 642
SCL/TAL1 (stem cell leukemia/T-cell acute lymphoblastic leukemia 1), 484
SCNT (somatic cell nuclear transfer), 448
Scorpion bites, 809
Scott syndrome, **2058–2059**

Scramblase, 662
Scurvy (vitamin C deficiency), 652, 1986, 2108, 2108f
SCYA3, 1632
SDF-1. *See* CXCL12 (stromal cell-derived factor-1)
Sea-blue histiocytes, 1446
Sealing zones, 60
Sec1/Munc18 (SM), 1849
SEC23B, 564, 567
Seckel syndrome, 530t, 532
Secondary myelofibrosis, 1325
Secretory protein, 1161
Secretory vesicles, 930t, 1009
Sedormid purpura, 824
Segmented granulocytes, 32t, 34
Segmented neutrophils, 32t
Selectins (lectins), **66**, 67t. *See also* E-selectin; L-selectin; P-selectin
    counterreceptors, 282t
    expression, 281
    functions, 1054
    ligands, 1057t
    structure, 282t
Selenium, 652t
Selenium deficiency, 654
Self-antigens, 2343
Self-inactivating (SIN) viral vectors, 437
Senicapoc, for sickle cell disease, 777t
Senile purpura, 2107, 2108f
Sepsis
    activated protein C and, 1956
    C. perfringens, **819**
    disseminated intravascular coagulation and, 2202, 2207
    hyposplenism and, 868
    postsplenectomy, 2004
    during pregnancy, 2211
    transfusion-related, 2376
    tumor necrosis factor -α in, 285
SEPT10, 1643
Septic arthritis, 771
Sequestration crisis, in sickle cell disease, 767
Serglycin, 1011
Serial analysis by recombinant expression cloning (SEREX), 421
Serial analysis of gene expression (SAGE), 421
Serine hydroxymethyltransferase (SHMT), 584–585
Serine proteases, 1012t, 1013, 1916–1917, 1918t
Serosal implants, for primary myelofibrosis, 1330
Serotonin (5-hydroxytryptamine), 286t, 289, 1848, 1878–1879

Serotonin transporter (SERT), 1879
Serpentine receptors. *See* G-protein–coupled receptors (GPCRs)
SERPIN, 1958
SERPINA1, 1699
SERPINA10, 1938
SERPINC1, 1937
Serpins (serine protease inhibitors), 1145, 1958, 2304t, 2307–2308
Serratia marcescens, 106, 1030, 1033
SERT (serotonin transporter), 1879
Serum sickness, 2103, 2103f
SETBP1, 1348, 1472
Severe combined immunodeficiency (SCID), **1216–1219**
    adenosine deaminase deficiency, 439
    clinical features, 1214t, 1218
    cytokine-mediated signaling defects and, 249, 1217–1218
    defective signaling through T-cell receptor and, 1218
    definition and history, 1216–1217
    gene mutations, 1154, 1575t
    increased lymphocyte precursor apoptosis in, 1217
    laboratory features, 1214t, 1218
    lymphomas and, 1575t
    molecular defects and pathogenesis, 1217, 1217f
    neutropenia in, 993
    therapy, course, and prognosis, **1218–1219**
        gene therapy, 437, 439, 453, 1219
        hematopoietic cell transplantation, 363, 1219
        X-linked, 437, 439
Severe-deviation clonal myeloid disorders, 1276t, **1279–1280**
Sexual history, **7**
Sézary cell, 1683f, 1684f
Sézary syndrome (SS), 1498t, 1679, 1683t, 1684t. *See also* Cutaneous T-cell lymphoma (CTCL); Mycosis fungoides (MF)
SF1, 1348
SF3B1, 227t, 231t, 1346t, 1349, 1529
SFA1. *See* CD151
SGI-110, for myelodysplastic syndromes, 1361
SH2B3 (*LNK*), 229t, 232t, 233t
Shiga toxin *E. coli*-associated hemolytic uremic syndrome (STEC-HUS), 2255, 2258–2259
Shigella dysenteriae, 2340
Shigella flexneri, 1066f
SHIP1, 1443

SHMT (serine hydroxymethyltransferase), 584–585
Shock, in disseminated intravascular coagulation, 2204, 2205t
Short tandem repeats (STRs), 147
Shoulder pain, history of, 6
SHP1 (hematopoietic cell phosphatase), 253, 485, 486f, 1163
Shwachman-Diamond syndrome, **532**, 993–994, 1026
Sialoadhesin (Siglec1), 1054, 1080, 1081f, 1082, 1083f
Sialomucins, 67t, 68
Sialophorin, 1873
Sickle cell β⁰-thalassemia, 762
Sickle cell β+-thalassemia, 762
Sickle cell disease, **762–776**
    clinical features and management, **766–773**, 767t
        in anesthesia and surgery, 773
        aplastic crises, 767
        avascular necrosis, 771, 771f
        cardiac, 769
        dactylitis, 771
        hepatobiliary, 772
        hyperhemolytic crises, 767
        infection, 773
        leg ulcers, 771–772
        nocturnal enuresis, 770–771
        ophthalmic, 772
        osteomyelitis, septic arthritis, and bone infarction, 771
        osteopenia and osteoporosis, 771
        pain control, 767–768
        in pregnancy, 772–773
        priapism, 770
        pulmonary, 768–769, 769f
        renal failure, 770
        sequestration crises, 767
        splenic, 772
        stroke, 769–770
        vasoocclusive crises, 766–767, 768f
    course and prognosis, 766
    epidemiology, 763
    G6PD deficiency and, 690
    history, 762–763, 762f
    hyposplenism and, 868
    i antigen and, 2340
    inheritance, 149, 149f
    laboratory features, 762f, 766, 779f
    modifiers of disease severity, 773–774
    pathophysiology, **763–766**, 764f, 765f
        abnormal cell adhesiveness, 764–765
        activation of coagulation system, 765
        adenosine signaling, 765–766
        cellular dehydration, 764

hemoglobin polymerization, 763–764
hemolysis and nitric oxide scavenging, 764
inflammation and chronic vasculopathy, 765
ischemia–reperfusion injury, 765
in pregnancy, **125–126**
transient aplastic crisis and, 541
treatment, **774–776**
DNA methyltransferase inhibitors, 775
fetal hemoglobin-inducing agents, 774–775
gene therapy, 453
hematopoietic cell transplantation, 362–363, 775
histone deacetylase inhibitors, 775
hydroxyurea, 774, 774t, 775f
investigative, 776, 777t
iron overload associated with, 776
potential targets, 767t
red cell exchange, 430t, 431–432
transfusions, 776, 2371–2372
Sickle cell-Hb C disease, 762
Sickle cells (drepanocytes), 473f, 473t, 474f, **475**
Sickle cell thalassemia, 749
Sickle cell trait (hemoglobin AS), 762, 766
Side-population cells, 450
Sideroachrestic anemia, 1342
Sideroblastic anemias, **915–920**
classification, 916t
clinical and laboratory features, 920
definition and history, 915
differential diagnosis, 637
drugs causing, 916t, 919
epidemiology, 915
hereditary
autosomal, 890–891
Pearson marrow-pancreas syndrome, 919, 920
X-linked, 894, 916–917, 920
X-linked with ataxia, 918
mitochondrial myopathy and, 919
pathogenesis
anemia mechanism, 919
heme synthesis defects, 916
metabolic defects, 918
mitochondrial myopathy, 919
morphology, 915–916, 916f
pyridoxine metabolism, 917–918
ring sideroblast formation, 918
primary acquired (clonal), 918–919
secondary acquired, **919–920**
treatment, **920**
Sideroblasts
absence of, 552

intermediate, 1353
in megaloblastic anemia, 595
morphology, 915–916
normal, 465, 552, 623–624, 916f
pathologic, 465, 466f, 916f
ring, 178, 465, 567, 624, 918, 1353
Siderocyte, 467f
Siderosomes, 465, 468
Siglec1 (sialoadhesin), 1054, 1080, 1081f, 1082, 1083f
Siglec-2. See CD33
Siglec 8, 949
Siglec 10, 949
Signaling lymphocyte activation molecule (SLAM), 54
Signal transduction pathways, **247–253**
apoptosis and, 208–209, 208f
BCR-ABL1 and, 1443–1444, 1444f
coordination and crosstalk, 253
downstream signals, **250–252**, 251f
extinguishing signals in, **252–253**
insulation, 252
metabolism and, 193–196, 194f, 195f
overview, **247**
in platelets. See Platelets, signaling pathways
receptors, **247–250**, 248f. See also specific receptors
specificity within receptor families, 252
Silent alleles, blood group, 2339
Silent β-thalassemia, 733, 750
Siltuximab
for Castleman disease, 1250
for myeloma, 345f, 346t
Single-molecule sequencing, 158–159, 158f
Single nucleotide polymorphism (SNP), 147, 174
Singlet oxygen, 284t, 286
Sinus histiocytosis with massive lymphadenopathy (Rosai-Dorfman disease), 1101, **1112–1113**
Sinusoidal obstructive syndrome (SOS), **368**
SIN (self-inactivating) viral vectors, 437
siRNA, 153
Sirolimus
for APECED syndrome, 1224
in drug-eluting stents, 2297
for Erdheim-Chester disease, 1111
for IPEX syndrome, 1223
Site I, 248
Site II, 248
Sitosterolemia, 1996
Sjögren syndrome
lymphocytopenia in, 1206
lymphomas and, 1574–1575, 1664
neutropenia in, 996

Skeletal survey, in myeloma, 1715, 1748, 1748f
Skin disorders
in acute myelogenous leukemia, 1380, 1410
in adult Langerhans cell histiocytosis, 1108
in antiphospholipid syndrome, 2240
in chronic lymphocytic leukemia, 1541
eosinophils and, 954, 956t
in Erdheim-Chester disease, 1111
hemorrhage, 1987
history of, 6
in juvenile xanthogranuloma, 1112
in Langerhans cell histiocytosis, 1103–1104, 1103f, 1106
in mycosis fungoides. See Mycosis fungoides (MF)
primary lymphomas, 1581, 1665
in Rosai-Dorfman disease, 1113
in systemic mastocytosis, 973–974, 974f
in Waldenström macroglobulinemia, 1791
warfarin-related necrosis, 396, 2100, 2100f, 2223
Skin examination, 7–8
Skp2, 217
Skull lesions, in Langerhans cell histiocytosis, 1104, 1106
SLAM (signaling lymphocyte activation molecule), 54
SLC1A5 (ASCT2), 197, 198
SLC2A1 (GLUT1), 192
SLC4A1, 664
SLC11A1 (Nramp1), 621, 1010, 1014
SLC11A3. See Ferroportin (SLC40A1, SLC11A3)
SLC19A2, 652
SLC25A38, 916
SLC40A1. See Ferroportin (SLC40A1, SLC11A3)
SLE. See Systemic lupus erythematosus (SLE)
SM (Sec1/Munc18), 1849
SMAC, 204f, 208, 1186
SMAD, 251, 1713
SMAD4, 621t
SMAD anchor for receptor activation (SARA), 251
Small G proteins, 1882–1883
Small immature monocyte, 1045
Small lymphocytic lymphoma (SLL), 184t, 1533, 1592–1593, 1592f
Small noncleaved cell (non-Burkitt) lymphoma, 187
Small ubiquitin-like modifier (SUMO), 253
SMARCAL1, 1226
SMC1A, 1346t, 1352
SMC3, 1346t, 1352

SMILE regimen, for NK/T-cell lymphoma, 1702
Smoking. *See* Cigarette smoking
Smoldering leukemia. *See* Oligoblastic myelogenous leukemia (refractory anemia with excess blasts)
Smoldering myeloma, 1708–1709, 1725, 1734f, 1761
Smooth muscle cells, 2283–2284, 2284f
Smudge cells, 23, 1530, 1530f
SMZL (splenic marginal zone lymphoma), 1495t, 1557, 1558t, **1666–1667**
Snake bites, 2209, 2318
Snake venoms, 970
SNAP-23 (soluble N-ethylmaleimide-sensitive factor) attachment protein-23, 926, 1849
SNARE (SNAP receptor), 953, 1016–1017, 1849
S-nitrosohemoglobin (SNO-Hgb), 796, 796f
SNP (single nucleotide polymorphism), 147, 174
SOCS1, 236t
SOCS3 (CIS3), 485, 486f
SOCS (suppressors of cytokine signaling) proteins, 253, 298
SOD (superoxide dismutase), 196, 286, 692t, 698
SOD1, 698
Sodium chlorate, 810
Sodium citrate, 1996
Sodium phenyl butyrate, 775
Solitary plasmacytoma, 1733, 1760
Soluble NSF (N-ethylmaleimide-sensitive factor) attachment protein (SNAP)-23, 926
Somatic cell nuclear transfer (SCNT), 448
Somatic hypermutation, 1169
Somatic mutation, aging and, 130
Sorafenib, for acute myelogenous leukemia, 1403
SOS (sinusoidal obstructive syndrome), **368**
Sotatercept
    for myelodysplastic syndromes, 1360
    for myeloma, 1713
Southeast Asian ovalocytosis (SAO), 670f, **680**
SOX11 (SOX11), 236t, 1653, 1655
SP140, 234t
20S particle, 240
Specific granule deficiency, 1019t, 1020–1021
Spectrin
    defects of
        in erythrocyte membrane disorders, 670t
        in hereditary elliptocytosis, 677–678

in hereditary pyropoikilocytosis, 677–678
in hereditary spherocytosis, 672
in erythrocyte membrane skeleton, 666, 666f
in platelets, 1833t, 1837
structure, **665–666**, 665f
Spent phase, of polycythemia vera, 1294–1295, 1294f
Spermidine, 200
S-phase checkpoint, 219
S-phase promoting factors, 213
Spherocytes, **473**
    abnormal, 671f. *See also* Hereditary spherocytosis (HS)
    in autoimmune hemolytic anemia, 832
    characteristics, 21, 472t, 474f
    diseases associated with, 472t
Spherostomatocyte, 472f, 472t
Sphingomyelin, 662
Sphingomyelinase, 1129
Sphingomyelinase D, 809
Sphingosine, 1956
Sphingosphine-1-phosphate (S1P), 1857, 1878
Spi-1. *See* PU.1
Spider bites, 809, 2102
Spider telangiectasia, 2098f
Spinal cord compression, 1746–1747, 1748, 1749f
Spinal cord injury, 451–452
Spindle-pole body duplication checkpoint, 213
Spleen, **87–91**
    anatomy, 88, 89f, 864
    architecture, 88, 89f, 90, 90f
    B-cell development in, 1151
    disorders
        in hereditary spherocytosis, 673
        hypersplenism. *See* Hypersplenism
        hyposplenism, **867–869**, 868t, 869f
        in Langerhans cell histiocytosis, 1104
        in mastocytosis, 974
        primary lymphomas, 1582
        in sickle cell disease, 772
        in T-cell large granular lymphocytic leukemia, 1566, 1566f
    erythropoiesis in, 480
    examination, 8–9
    function, 90–91, 864
    macrophages in, 1081f, 1082
    ontogeny, 863
Splenectomy
    for aplastic anemia, 527
    atherosclerosis and, 2288

for autoimmune lymphoproliferative syndrome, 1224
for chronic lymphocytic leukemia, 1539
for chronic myelogenous leukemia, 1459, 1467
complications, 2004
for Gaucher disease, 1127
for Hb C disease, 780
for hereditary nonspherocytic hemolytic anemia, 712
for hereditary spherocytosis, 676
for hypersplenism, 866–867
for immune thrombocytopenia, 2003, 2004
lymphocytosis following, 1204
management following, 869
for mastocytosis, 978
minimally invasive, 2004
monocytosis following, 1097
for paroxysmal nocturnal hemoglobinuria, 579
for polycythemia vera, 1301
for primary myelofibrosis, 1330
for sequestration crisis, 767
for splenic marginal zone lymphoma, 1667
for T-cell large granular lymphocytic leukemia, 1567
for thrombocytopenia, 2008
for thrombotic thrombocytopenic purpura, 2256
for warm-antibody autoimmune hemolytic anemia, 838
for Wiskott-Aldrich syndrome, 2060
Splenic diffuse red pulp small B-cell lymphoma, 1495t, 1557, 1558t
Splenic marginal zone lymphoma (SMZL), 1495t, 1557, 1558t, **1666–1667**
Splenomegaly. *See also* Hypersplenism
    in chronic lymphocytic leukemia, 1530
    classification and causes, 863, 864, 865t, 866t
    in clonal myeloid diseases, 1287
    consultative approach to, 48
    in hairy cell leukemia, 1554
    in juvenile myelomonocytic leukemia, 1471
    in Langerhans cell histiocytosis, 1104
    neutropenia and, 996, 997
    platelet transfusion in, 2385
    in primary myelofibrosis, 1324
    in splenic marginal zone lymphoma, 1666
    in thalassemia, 742
    thrombocytopenia and, 2013
Splenoptosis, 865–866
Splice-site mutations, 146
Spontaneous abortions, 1988
Spontaneous mutations, 146

Spooning, purpura and, 2107
Spur cell. *See* Acanthocytes
Spur cell anemia. *See* Acanthocytosis
Spur cell hemolytic anemia, 655
SR-A I/II, 1055, 1057*t*
Src, 1884
SRs (scavenger receptors), 1054–1055, 1057*t*, 1872
SRSF2, 227*t*, 1346*t*, 1349, 1468, 1468*t*
SRT (substrate reduction therapy), 1128, 1130
SS (Sézary syndrome), 1498*t*, 1679, 1683*t*, 1684*t*. *See also* Cutaneous T-cell lymphoma (CTCL)
STAG2, 1346*t*, 1352
Stanford CVP regimen, for follicular lymphoma, 1645*t*
Stanford V regimen, for Hodgkin lymphoma, 1612*t*, 1614, 1615*t*
Staphylococcus aureus
    methicillin-resistant, 384–385
    vancomycin-resistant, 385
Staphylococcus infections
    in Chédiak-Higashi syndrome, 1018
    in chronic granulomatous disease, 1030, 1032
    disseminated intravascular coagulation and, 2207
    in hyperimmunoglobulin E syndrome, 985
    in leukocyte adhesion deficiency, 1023
    neutropenia and, 522, 985
    neutrophil abnormalities and, 986
    in neutrophil motility disorders, 1026
    in newborn, 106
    in specific granule deficiency, 1021
    Th17 T cells and, 1182
    in X-linked agammaglobulinemia, 1030
Staphylokinase, 2313*t*, 2316
Starvation, anemia of, **654**
STAT, 252
STAT1 deficiency, 1231
STAT1 gain-of-function mutations, 1223, 1231
STAT3, 1026, 1181*f*, 1182, 1379, 1528
STAT3, 237*t*, 1215*t*, 1223–1224, 1225, 1564
STAT4, 1643
STAT5, 485, 486*f*, 1180, 1181*f*, 1444, 1606
STAT5b deficiency, 1223
STAT6, 1180
STAT6, 236*t*
Statins
    for acute myelogenous leukemia, 1403
    for antiphospholipid syndrome, 2245
    CD40 expression and, 2288
    for myocardial infarction, 2296
STAT proteins, 932
Stavudine, 1249, 1252

STEAP3, 623
STEC-HUS (*Shiga* toxin *E. coli*-associated hemolytic uremic syndrome), 2255, 2258–2259
Steel factor. *See* Stem cell factor (SCF)
Stem cell factor (SCF)
    aplastic anemia and, 519
    components, 218
    in hematopoiesis, 253, **264–265**, 264*t*, 266
    mast cells and, 966
    in megakaryopoiesis, 1817, 1821
    synthesis, 265
Stem cell leukemia (SCL), 262
Stem cell leukemia/T-cell acute lymphoblastic leukemia 1 (SCL/TAL1), 484
Stem cells. *See* Hematopoietic stem cells (HSCs); Multipotential cells
Stem cell transplantation. *See* Hematopoietic cell transplantation (HCT)
STEMI (ST-segment elevation myocardial infarction). *See* Myocardial infarction (MI)
Sterile inflammation (autoinflammatory disease), 298
Sterile-α and armadillo motif (SARM), 298
Sternum, history of tenderness of, 5
Steroids. *See* Glucocorticoids
Stevens-Johnson syndrome, 2075, 2106
Stibophen, drug-related hemolytic anemia and, 824
Stiff heart syndrome, 1777
STIM1 (stromal interaction molecule 1), 1221, 1836
STING (stimulator of IFN genes), 302, 302*f*
Stoddard solvent, 517
Stomach, primary lymphoma in, 1581
Stomatin, 663*t*
Stomatocytes, 21*f*, 472*f*, 472*t*, **473**, 474*f*, 671*f*
Stomatocytic elliptocytosis. *See* Southeast Asian ovalocytosis (SAO)
Stomatocytosis
    acquired, 684
    hereditary. *See* Hereditary stomatocytosis syndromes
Storage pool disease, 2085
Streptococcus infections
    chronic inflammation and, 290
    cytarabine therapy and, 322
    disseminated intravascular coagulation and, 2207
    hyposplenism and, 868
    in immunocompromised host, 383
    red cell antigens and susceptibility to, 2340
    thrombotic microangiopathy and, 2261–2262
    vaccination, 869

X-linked agammaglobulinemia and, 1212
Streptokinase, **402–403**
    for acute myocardial infarction, 2295
    clinical uses, 403
    comparison to other fibrinolytic agents, 2313*t*
    mechanism of action, 402–403
    for peripheral vascular disease, 2316
    platelet function and, 2078
    for stroke, 2315
Streptomyces pilosus, 644
Streptomyces verticillus, 331
Stress lymphocytosis, 1204
Stress polycythemia, 872
Stress reticulocytes, 467, 482*f*, 505
Stroke
    antiphospholipid syndrome and, 2238–2239
    double platelet blockade and, 2076
    etiology and pathogenesis, 2297
    fibrinolytic therapy for, **2313–2316**
        clinical studies, 2314, 2314*t*
        intraarterial thrombolysis, 2315–2316
        patient selection, 2313*t*
        principles, 2314–2315
        streptokinase, 2315
        tenecteplase, 2315
        tissue-type plasminogen activator, 2314–2315, 2316*t*
    integrin $\alpha_{IIb}\beta_3$ blockers for, 1855
    in sickle cell disease, 769–770
    therapy, 2297
Stroma, histogenesis of, 55
Stromal cell-derived factor-1. *See* CXCL12 (stromal cell-derived factor-1)
Stromal cells, **264**
Stromal interaction molecule 1 (STIM1), 1221, 1836
Stromal microenvironment, aplastic anemia and, 519
Stromatin, 1013
Strongyloides, 956, 957*t*
Strongyloidiasis, 1203, 2105, 2105*f*
STRs (short tandem repeats), 147
ST-segment elevation myocardial infarction (STEMI). *See* Myocardial infarction (MI)
Stuart-Prower factor. *See* Factor X
Stuttering priapism, 770
STXB5/*STXB5*, 1849, 2061
Subacute leukemia. *See* Oligoblastic myelogenous leukemia (refractory anemia with excess blasts)
Subcutaneous fat aspiration, 1776, 1776*f*
Subcutaneous panniculitis-like T-cell lymphoma, 1498*t*, **1702**

Substance P, 1878
Substrate reduction therapy (SRT), 1128, 1130
Succinyl coenzyme A (CoA), 892, 893f
Sugar water test, 571, 576
Suicide genes, 416, 440, 440f
Sulfamethoxazole
    hemolytic anemia and, 708
    methemoglobinemia and, 790t
Sulfasalazine, megaloblastic anemia and, 606t
Sulfhemoglobin/sulfhemoglobinemia, **793–794**
Sulfinpyrazone, 2075
Sulfonamides
    maternal ingestion of, effect on fetus and newborn, 112, 112t
    thrombocytopenia and, 2017
    toxic methemoglobinemia and, 789, 790t
Sulindac, 2075
SUMO (small ubiquitin-like modifier), 253
Sunitinib
    for acute myelogenous leukemia, 1404
    adverse effects, 2263
Superoxide anion, 284t, 286
Superoxide dismutase (SOD), 196, 286, 692t, 698
Superoxides, 809, 2203
Suberoylanilide hydroxamic acid (SAHA), 1403
Suppressors of cytokine signaling (SOCS) proteins, 253, 298
Surface immunoglobulin, 1163
Surgical procedures
    in essential thrombocythemia, 1315
    evaluation of bleeding risk during, 1990, 1990t
    in hemophilia, 2120, 2123–2124
    hemorrhage during, 1988
    in inherited platelet disorders, 2062
    in patients with factor VIII inhibition, 2125
    platelet transfusions for, 2384
    in polycythemia vera, 1294
    in sickle cell disease, 773
Surrogate λ light chains, 1168
SVIL, 1851
Sweet syndrome (neutrophilic dermatosis), 1001, 1324, 1380, 2102–2103, 2102f
Swelling, neck, 5
SWI/SNF (switch and sucrose nonfermenting) remodeler, 166, 166f
Syk, 1054, 1880
Syk, 1016
SYK, 1696–1697
Syndecan 1 (CD138), 1141, 1712, 1714, 1737
Syndecan-4, 2202

Syngeneic hematopoietic cell transplantation, 359
Syntaxins, 926, 1114, 1228, 1849
Systemic amyloidosis, 2108
Systemic inflammatory response syndrome, 2200
Systemic lupus erythematosus (SLE)
    antiphospholipid syndrome and, 2238
    antiplatelet antibodies and, 2084–2085
    aplastic anemia and, 518
    arterial thrombosis and, 2293
    autoimmune hemolytic anemia and, 824
    Epstein-Barr virus infection and, 1265
    lymphocytopenia in, 1206
    lymphomas and, 1574
    monocytosis in, 1097
    neutropenia in, 996
    thrombocytopenia in, 2008–2009
    thrombotic microangiopathy and, 2262
Systemic mastocytosis
    with associated clonal, hematologic non-mast-cell lineage disease, 973, 978
    classification, 973, 973t
    clinical features, 973–976
    course and prognosis, 978
    definition and history, 973
    differential diagnosis, 976
    etiology and pathogenesis, 973
    indolent, 975f, 978
    laboratory features, 974, 975f, 975t, 976
    therapy, 976–978

T
T200 (CD45), 1183
T315I mutation, *ABL1*, 1457, 1457t
Tabalumab, for myeloma, 346t, 1755
TACE (ADAM17), 1144, 1874
Tachykinins, 1878
TACI (transmembrane activator and calcium modulator and cyclophilin ligand interactor), 1606
TACO (transfusion-associated circulatory overload), 2376
Tacrolimus
    adverse effects, 2262
    for graft-verus-host disease prevention, 371
    for IPEX syndrome, 1223
    for mycosis fungoides, 1685
    overdose treatment, 432
TAFI. *See* Thrombin-activatable fibrinolysis inhibitor (TAFI)
TALEN (transcription activator-like effector nuclease), 444
Taliglucerase alfa, for Gaucher disease, 1127
Talin, 1832t, 1837, 1838f, 1884

Tamm-Horsfall mucoprotein (uromodulin), 1744
TAMs (tumor-associated macrophages), 1083
TANK-binding kinase (TBK), 298, 302f
T (Thomsen-Friedenreich) antigen, 2262
TAP1/2, 1221
Tapasin, 1221
Target cells. *See* Codocytes (target cells)
Targeted disruption models of hemochromatosis, 643
Target of rapamycin complex 1 (TORC1), 192
TAR (thrombocytopenia and absent radii) syndrome, 1996, 1997f, 2061
TAT (thrombin-antithrombin) complexes, 2209
Taxanes, 319t, **326**
Taxus brevifolia, 326
TBI (total-body irradiation), 353, **359–360**, 1656–1657
TBK (TANK-binding kinase), 298, 302f
TBNP (total blood neutrophil pool), 942, 942t
TCA (tricarboxylic acid) cycle, 192, 193f
T-cell acute lymphoblastic leukemia (T-ALL). *See also* Acute lymphoblastic (lymphocytic) leukemia (ALL)
    chromosomal abnormalities, 184t, **186–187**, 186f, 222–223t
    gene mutations, 233t
    laboratory features, 1511–1512, 1512t
    prognosis, 1520, 1521
    treatment, 1515–1517
T-cell antigens, 1141–1142, 1142f, 1142t
T-cell-histiocyte-rich large B-cell lymphoma, **1636–1637**
T-cell large granular lymphocytic leukemia (T-LGLL)
    chromosomal abnormalities, 187
    clinical features, 1564t, 1565–1566
    definition and history, 1563
    diagnostic criteria, 1566
    differential diagnosis, 1566–1567
    etiology and pathogenesis, 1563–1564
    gene mutations, 237t, 1498t, 1564
    histologic and immunophenotypic features, 1498t, 1565, 1565f
    laboratory features, 1203, 1565–1566, 1566f
    vs. large granular lymphocytosis, 1202
    therapy, course, and prognosis, 1567
T-cell lymphoproliferation, 1265
T-cell neoplasms. *See also specific types*
    clinical behavior, 1493
    extranodal involvement, 1502
    immature, 1498t
    leukemias, 1498t, 1571, 1573

lymphomas/lymphoproliferative disorders. *See also* Cutaneous T-cell lymphoma (CTCL); Peripheral T-cell lymphoma (PTCL)
  chromosomal abnormalities, 185t
  classification, 1493, 1498–1499t, 1598–1599
  epidemiology, 1571
  etiology, 1573
  histologic subtypes, 1498–1499t, 1572t
T-cell/NK cell progenitors, **270**
T-cell precursors, 438
T-cell progenitors, **270**
T-cell prolymphocytic lymphoma (T-PLL), 1498t, 1542
T-cell receptor (TCR) genes, 414–415
T-cell receptor-interacting molecule 25 (TRIM25), 302, 302f
T-cell receptors (TCRs), **1175–1177**
  CD4. *See* CD4
  CD8. *See* CD8
  composition, 1177–1178
  diversity in, 1177
  heterodimers, 1175–1176, 1176f
    antigen presentation to, 1177
    gene rearrangements in, 1176–1177
  molecular features, 1178
  signaling defects, 1218, 1220
  signal transduction in, 1178–1179
  in thymus, 87
T cells. *See also* Lymphocytes
  adhesion molecules, **1184–1185**, 1185f
  aging and, 135–136
  antigen receptors. *See* T-cell receptors
  antigens, 1141–1142, 1142f, 1142t
  in atherosclerosis, 2286
  autoreactive cytotoxic, in aplastic anemia, 515
  CD4+. *See* CD4+ T cells (helper T cells)
  CD4+CD25+. *See* CD4+CD25+ regulatory T (T$_{REG}$) cells
  CD8+. *See* CD8+ T cells (cytotoxic T lymphocytes, CTLs)
  in chronic inflammation, 291
  commitment, regulation of, 1155–1156
  cytomegalovirus-specific, 409–411, 410f, 411f
  cytotoxic. *See* CD8+ T cells (cytotoxic T lymphocytes, CTLs)
  dendritic cells and, 308
  development, 86–87, 87f
  disorders, 1195–1197, 1196–1197t.
    See also Cutaneous T-cell lymphoma (CTCL); Peripheral T-cell lymphoma (PTCL); T-cell neoplasms

immunodeficiencies with impaired NF-κB activation, 1220
Epstein-Barr virus-specific, 411–412
erythropoietic failure and, 543
fetal, 101
in gene therapy, 438
genetic retargeting, 414–416, 414f, 415f
helper. *See* CD4+ T cells (helper T cells)
Hodgkin lymphoma and, 1607
immune modulatory molecules
  CD28, 415–416, 1183, 1184, 1185f
  CD152 (CTLA-4), 424, 1184
immunological synapse, 1185–1186
in immunologic response, 969
leukemia-specific, 413–414
in lymph nodes, 92–93
melanoma-specific, 412–413
memory. *See* Memory T cells
multispecific, 412
neonatal, 108
regulatory. *See* CD4+CD25+ regulatory T (T$_{REG}$) cells
in spleen, 91
suicide genes, 416
tolerance in, 308
T-cell therapy. *See* Immune cell therapy (adoptive cellular therapy)
TCF-1, 1156
TCF3, 1672
TCF3-PBX1 (E2A-PBX1), 1507, 1516
TCL1, 1529
TCRA, 1218
TCRs. *See* T-cell receptors
TdT (terminal deoxynucleotidyl transferase), 1465–1466
Teardrop cells. *See* Dacryocytes (teardrop cells)
TEL (ETV6), 228t, 230, 1346t, 1351
TEL-AMI1. *See* ETV6-RUNX1
Telangiectasia macularis eruptiva perstans, 973
Telangiectasias, 1988
Telomerase reverse transcriptase (TERT), 1444–1445
Telomere defects
  in acute myelogenous leukemia, 1376
  in aplastic anemia, 515
  in chronic myelogenous leukemia, 1444–1445
  in dyskeratosis congenita, 530–531, 531f
Temozolomide
  for acute myelogenous leukemia, 1408
  mechanism of action, 329
  pharmacology, 330

Temsirolimus, for mantle cell lymphoma, 1658, 1659t, 1660t. *See also* Mammalian target of rapamycin (mTOR) inhibitors
Tenascin, 63, **267**
Tenderness of the sternum, history of, 5
Tenecteplase, **403**
  comparison to other fibrinolytics, 2313t
  for myocardial infarction, 2295
  for pulmonary embolism, 2277–2278
  for stroke, 2315
Teniposide, **328–329**
  adverse effects, 329, 1519t, 1520
  for α-heavy-chain disease, 1808
  secondary acute myelogenous leukemia and, 183
TERC, 531, 531f
Terminal deoxynucleotidyl transferase (TdT), 1465–1466
Ternary complex formation, 825f, 826t, 830–831, 830t
TERT, 531, 531f
TERT (telomerase reverse transcriptase), 1444–1445
TERT/TERC, 1346t
Testicular lymphoma, primary, 1246, 1581–1582, 1582f, **1634**
Testicular relapse, in acute lymphoblastic leukemia, 1518
Testosterone
  for anemia of primary myelofibrosis, 1328
  erythropoietic response to, 872, 879–880, 880f
TET2
  in acute myelogenous leukemia, 198, 226t, 1376, 1378–1379, 1378t
  in chronic myelomonocytic leukemia, 170, 1468
  in myelodysplastic syndromes, 227t, 1346t, 1348, 1351
  in peripheral T-cell lymphoma, 1697
  in Ph-chromosome negative myeloproliferative neoplasms, 229t
  in polycythemia vera, 1292
TET proteins, 169
Tetracyclines, 830
Tetrahydrofolate acid (FH$_4$), 584, 586f
Tetrahydrofolate triglutamate, 584, 585f
Tetraspanins, 1858–1859t, 1871
Textarin/ecarin test, 2243
TF. *See* Tissue factor (TF)
T follicular helper (T$_{FH}$) cells, 1182
TFPI. *See* Tissue factor pathway inhibitor (TFPI)
TFPI, 1937
TfR2, 641, 642
TGF. *See under* Transforming growth factor (TGF)

Thalassemias, **725–754**
 clinical features, **743–745**, 744f, 744t
 definitions and history, 725
 differential diagnosis, 568–569, 748, 749f
 epidemiology and population genetics,
  727–728, 727f
 etiology and pathogenesis, **728–730**, 729f
 forms, 726, 726t
  α. See α-thalassemias
  β. See β-thalassemias
  δ, 726, 736, 751
  δβ. See δβ-thalassemias
  εγδβ, 735, 745, 751
  εωδβ, 726
  hereditary persistence of fetal
   hemoglobin and. See Hereditary
   persistence of fetal hemoglobin
   (HPFH)
 as global health problem, 754
 globin gene clusters and, **728–730**, 729f
 hemoglobin C, 749–750
 hemoglobin E, 750
 hyposplenism and, 868
 i antigen and, 2340
 intermedia, 725, 753
 laboratory features, **745–748**, 746f, 747f
 major, 725
 minima, 725
 minor, 553, 636, 725
 molecular basis, **730–739**. See also specific
  forms
 pathophysiology, **739–743**
  abnormal iron metabolism, 742
  cellular heterogeneity, 741
  clinical heterogeneity, 742–743, 743f
  coagulation defects, 742
  compensatory mechanisms for anemia,
   741
  erythroid precursor damage, 740–741
  imbalance globin-chain synthesis, 740
  infection, 742
  persistent fetal hemoglobin production,
   741
  red cell damage, 740–741
  splenomegaly, 742
 pregnancy and, 126
 prevention of, 753–754
 prognosis, 753
 sickle cell, 749
 treatment, 362–363, **751–753**, 2372
Thalassic anemia, 725
Thalidomide, **333–335**
 for acute myelogenous leukemia, 1404
 for adult Langerhans cell histiocytosis,
  1109
 adverse effects, 334, 1741, 1757

clinical use, 334
 for Langerhans cell histiocytosis, 1106,
  1107
 for malignant histiocytic diseases, 1110
 for mantle cell lymphoma, 1659t, 1660t
 mechanism of action, 334
 for myelodysplastic syndromes, 1359
 for myeloma, 1750, 1752, 1752t, 1754
 pharmacology, 334
 for primary myelofibrosis, 1329
 structure, 333f
THBD, 1931–1932, 1932f
T-helper cells. See CD4+ T cells
  (helper T cells)
T-helper type 1 (Th1) cells, 1180, 1181f
T-helper type 2 (Th2) cells, 1180, 1181f
T-helper type 9 (Th9) cells, 1181f, 1182
T-helper type 17 (Th17) cells, 1182, 2000
Theophylline, cAMP inhibition and, 404
Therapeutic apheresis. See Apheresis
Therapy-related myeloid neoplasms
 acute myelogenous leukemia. See Acute
  myelogenous (myeloid) leukemia
  (AML), therapy-related
 myelodysplastic syndromes. See
  Myelodysplastic syndrome (MDSs),
  therapy-related
Thiamine deficiency, 652
Thiamine-responsive megaloblastic anemia,
  608, 652
Thiazides, maternal ingestion of, effect on
  fetus and newborn, 112, 112t
Thienopyridines, 2074t, 2075–2076
6-Thioguanine
 for acute lymphoblastic leukemia, 1505,
  1516, 1517
 for acute myelogenous leukemia, 1395t,
  1399, 1409
 adverse effects, 324
 for autoimmune hemolytic anemia,
  839
 mechanism of action, 323
 megaloblastic anemia and, 606t
 pharmacology, 323–324
 structure, 323f
Thiopurine methyltransferase, 316, 319t, 323,
  1516
6-Thiopurines, 319t, 323
Thiotepa, 331, 331t, 332t
Thomsen-Friedenreich (T) antigen, 2262
Thorium dioxide, 518
Thrombin, 290, **1877**
 binding to fibrinogen and fibrin, 2154
 in disseminated intravascular coagulation,
  2200–2201
 formation, 1842, 1854

generation, 1918–1919, 1919f, 1940, 1940f,
  1949, 1950f
 in inflammatory response, 1979t, 2201
 inhibitors, 1919, 1919t
 PI3K pathway and, 1841
 in platelet activation, 2293
 platelet activation and, 1834, 1836, 1845,
  1919
 structure, 1919
 in thrombosis and hemostasis, 1979t
 transforming growth factor β and, 1848
Thrombin-activatable fibrinolysis inhibitor
  (TAFI), 1972
 activation, 1935
 aging and, 135
 characteristics, 1916t, 1935, 2308
 in disseminated intravascular coagulation,
  2206
 in fibrinolysis, 2203
 gene structure and variations, 1935–1936
 plasminogen and, 2154
 structure, 1935, 2308
Thrombin-antithrombin (TAT) complexes,
  2209
Thrombin receptor antagonists, 406,
  2076–2077
Thrombin time, 1989
Thromboatherogenesis, 1092
Thrombocythemia, BCR-ABL-positive, 1449
Thrombocytopenia, **1993–2018**
 acquired pure amegakaryocytic, 1999
 in acute myelogenous leukemia, 1381
 alcohol consumption and, 1998
 in alloimmune hemolytic disease of the
  fetus and newborn, 849
 in antiphospholipid syndrome, 2240
 classification, 1994t
 consultative approach to, 42–43
 cyclic, 2015
 definition and history, 1993–1994
 diagnosis, 1740, 1994
 drug-induced, 2015–2018, 2016t, 2017t,
  2077
 etiology and pathogenesis, 1985, 1986t
 gestational, 45, 121–122, 2010
 heparin-induced. See Heparin-induced
  thrombocytopenia (HIT)
 in hepatic disease, 2194
 in Hodgkin lymphoma, 1610
 hypersplenism and, 2014
 hypothermia and, 2014
 immune. See Immune thrombocytopenia
  (ITP)
 in inherited platelet disorders, 1996–1997,
  1998t. See also Platelets, disorders
 interferon-induced, 1825

in Kasabach-Merritt syndrome (KMS), 806, **2014–2015**

in large granular lymphocytic leukemia, 1566

in leukemias, 2081–2082

massive transfusion and, 2014

in myelodysplastic syndromes, 1353, 2081–2082

in myeloma, 1740

neonatal alloimmune, **2012–2013**

nutritional deficiencies and, 1997–1998

in paroxysmal nocturnal hemoglobinuria, 580

from platelet trapping, **2014–2015**

during pregnancy, 121–122, 580, 802, 2010–2012, 2010*t*

purpuras in, 2107

splenomegaly and, 2013

spurious (pseudothrombocytopenia), 43, **1994–1996**

in thrombotic thrombocytopenic purpura, 2255

treatment, 1824–1825, 2213, 2385

in von Willebrand disease, 2172

X-linked, 1224–1225

Thrombocytopenia and absent radii (TAR) syndrome, 1996, 1997*f*, 2061

Thrombocytosis

consultative approach to, 45

etiology, 1312*t*, 2036*t*

reactive, 1310, 1312*t*, **2035–2037**

thrombocytapheresis for, 433

Thromboembolectomy, 2316–2317

Thromboembolism. *See* Venous thrombosis/ thromboembolism

β-Thromboglobulins, 1844–1845

Thrombokinase, 2113

Thrombolytic therapy. *See* Fibrinolytic therapy

Thrombomodulin (TM), **1953**

blood fluidity and, 2285

characteristics, 1916*t*, 1931

functions, 1931, 1952*t*, 1972

gene structure and variations, 1931–1932, 1932*f*, 1953

protein C activation and, 1954, 1972, 2202

structure, 1931, 1951*f*, 1952*t*

Thrombophilia

acquired, 2221, 2224*t*. *See also* Antiphospholipid syndrome (APS)

in clonal myeloid diseases, 1286

definition, 2221

hereditary. *See* Hereditary thrombophilia

in paroxysmal nocturnal hemoglobinuria, 580

during pregnancy and puerperium, **122–123**

Thromboplastin. *See* Tissue factor (TF)

Thrombopoiesis, **1815–1821**

cellular physiology, **1815–1821**

megakaryopoiesis. *See* Megakaryopoiesis

platelet formation, 1820–1821

kinetics, 1815

in newborns, 107–108

regulation, 2035

therapeutic manipulation, 1824–1825

Thrombopoietin (TPO)

actions, 265

in DNA repair, 268

in hematopoietic stem cells, 261, 264*t*, **265**

in immune thrombocytopenia, 2000–2001

in megakaryopoiesis, 64–65, 1817, 1822–1823

in newborn, 107

regulation, 2000

for thrombocytopenia, 1824–1825

Thrombopoietin (TPO) receptor (c-mpl, CD110), 260, 265, 1822, 1872, 2036

Thrombopoietin (TPO) receptor agonists. *See also* Eltrombopag; Romiplostim

adverse effects, 2006

for aplastic anemia, 526

development, 1825, 2001

for hypersplenism, 867

for immune thrombocytopenia, 2005–2006

for myelodysplastic syndromes, 1358

Thromboregulation, 1968

Thromboregulatory molecules, endothelial, 1967–1968, 1968*f*, 1968*t*

Thrombosis. *See also* Arterial thrombosis; Venous thrombosis

acute myelogenous leukemia treatment and, 1410

in disseminated intravascular coagulation, 2204

in essential thrombocythemia, 1308, 1309*f*

fibrinolytic deficiency and, 2311–2312

in hemophilia, 2130

inflammatory mediators in, 1978–1979, 1979*t*

in newborns, 112

in polycythemia vera, 1293

in primary myelofibrosis, 1325

Thrombospondin, 63, 765, 1856, 1879

Thrombospondin-1, 1845, 1846*t*, 1848

Thrombospondin N-terminal fragment (GMP-33), 1873

Thrombotic microangiopathies, **2253–2263**

in autoimmune disorders, 2262

in cancer, 2262

classification, 2255*t*

in cobalamin metabolic defects, 2263

in disseminated intravascular coagulation, 2261

drug-induced, 428, 431, 2262–2263

hemolytic uremic syndrome. *See* Hemolytic uremic syndrome (HUS)

in HIV infection, 1252

in infections, 2261–2262

in malignant hypertension, 2263

mechanical hemolysis and, 2263

in organ transplant recipients, 2262

plasma exchange for, 428, 430*t*, 431

in pregnancy, 2262

thrombotic thrombocytopenic purpura. *See* Thrombotic thrombocytopenic purpura (TTP)

Thrombotic thrombocytopenic purpura (TTP)

clinical features, 2107, 2254–2255

congenital, 2257–2258

course and prognosis, 2257

definition and history, 2253–2254

differential diagnosis, 837, 2255–2256, 2255*t*

epidemiology, 2254

etiology and pathogenesis, 428, 2254

laboratory features, 2255

treatment, 428, 2256–2257

Thromboxane A$_2$ (TXA$_2$), 288, 1830, 1852*f*, 1876–1877, 1968*t*, 2074

Thromboxane A$_2$ (TXA$_2$) receptor defect, 2056

Thromboxane B$_2$ (TXB$_2$), 952

Thromboxane prostanoid receptor, 1876–1877

Thromboxane synthase deficiency, 2058

Thrombus. *See also* Thrombosis

formation, 1829–1834

red, 2292

white, 2291

Thymectomy, for autoimmune hemolytic anemia, 839

Thymic corpuscles, 85

Thymic progenitors, 1154

Thymidine kinase, 1532, 1532*t*

Thymidylate synthesis, 586*t*, 587*f*

Thymocytes, 85–86, 87*f*, 1141, 1142*f*, 1179

Thymoma, 518, 544, 1204

Thymosin β$_4$, 1832*t*, 1839*f*, 1841, 1848

Thymus, **85–87**

aging of, 131, 133, 133*f*

anatomy, 85

architecture, 85–86, 86*f*

Thymus (*Cont.*):
  defective development
    CHARGE syndrome, 1222
    congenital alopecia and absence of
      thymus, 1223
    DiGeorge syndrome, 86–87, 1214*t*, **1222**
  development, 1150–1151
  immune function, 86–87, 87*f*
  in Langerhans cell histiocytosis, 1104
  T-cell development in, 85–86, 87*f*
Thyroid disease/dysfunction
  anemia and, **559**
  Hodgkin lymphoma treatment and, 1618
  primary lymphomas, 1583
TIA-1, 1567
TIBC (total iron-binding capacity), 634
Ticagrelor
  for acute coronary syndromes, 2076
  antiplatelet effects, 404*t*, 405
TICAM1. *See* Toll/interleukin-1 receptor
    domain-containing adaptor
    inducing IFN-β (TRIF)
TICAM2. *See* TRIF-related adaptor molecule
    (TRAM)
Ticlopidine
  adverse effects, 2262
  antiplatelet effects, 404*t*, 405, 2075–2076
Tigecycline, 384–385
TILs (tumor-infiltrating lymphocytes), 412
TIMP-1 (tissue inhibitor of
    metalloproteinase), 1975
Tingible body macrophages, 1596
Tingling in tongue, history of, 5
Tinzaparin, for venous thromboembolism,
    2274*t*
Tipifarnib
  for acute myelogenous leukemia, 1459
  for primary myelofibrosis, 1329
TIR (toll/interleukin-1 receptor), 295–297,
    297*f*
TIRAP. *See* MyD88 adapter-like (MAL)
TIRAP (toll-interleukin receptor adaptor
    protein), 1054, 1230, 1352
Tirofiban, **405**
  antiplatelet effects, 405, 2045, 2077
  clinical uses, 404*t*, 405
  dosage, 404*t*
  thrombocytopenia and, 2015, 2077
  for unstable angina, 2296
Tissue
  hypoxia, anemia and, 506
  perfusion of, anemia and, 504–505, 505*f*
Tissue factor (TF)
  activation and cofactor function,
    1930–1931
  arterial thrombosis and, 2293–2294

characteristics, 1930
  in disseminated intravascular coagulation,
    2200, 2207
  in endothelial cells, 2285
  factor VIIa and, 1930, 1940, 1940*f*
  gene structure and variations, 1931, 1931*f*
  in leukocytes, 2237
  sickle cell disease and, 765
  structure, 1920*f*, 1930
Tissue factor pathway inhibitor (TFPI),
    1959–1960
  characteristics, 1916*t*, 1937
  in disseminated intravascular coagulation,
    2201, 2202
  functions, 1922, 1937, 1960, 1968
  gene structure and variations, 1937, 1960
  recombinant, 2214
  structure, 1937, 1952*t*, 1959–1960, 1959*f*
  synthesis, 1960
Tissue inhibitor of metalloproteinase
    (TIMP-1), 1975
Tissue iron compartment, 618
Tissue macrophages, 291
Tissue plasminogen activator (t-PA), 1973, 1975
Tissue thromboplastin inhibition test, 2243
Tissue-type plasminogen activator (t-PA)
  in fibrinolysis, 2202, 2304*f*, 2306, 2307
  for fibrinolytic therapy. *See* Fibrinolytic
    therapy, agents for
  gene, 2305–2306, 2306*f*
  in plasminogen activation, 2310
  production, 1973
  structure, 2303, 2304–2305*t*, 2305
T-LGLL. *See* T-cell large granular
    lymphocytic leukemia (T-LGLL)
TLI (total lymphoid irradiation), 360
TLR2, 236*t*
TLR4, 1711
TLR5, 1643
TLRs. *See* Toll-like receptors (TLRs)
TLX1, 186
T lymphocytes. *See* T cells
TM. *See* Thrombomodulin (TM)
TMD (transient myeloproliferative disorder),
    1385–1386
Tmprss6 (matriptase 2), 621, 621*t*
TNF. *See* Tumor necrosis factor (TNF)
TNFAIP3 (*A20*), 235*t*, 236*t*, 1644, 1664*t*,
    1786, 1787
TNFRSF14, 1627*t*
TNT (trinitrotoluene), 518
Tobacco. *See* Cigarette smoking
Tobramycin, 387*t*
Tocilizumab
  for Castleman disease, 1250
  for Erdheim-Chester disease, 1111

Toll/interleukin-1 receptor (TIR), 295–297,
    297*f*
Toll/interleukin-1 receptor domain-
    containing adaptor inducing IFN-β
    (TRIF), 297*f*, 298
Toll-interleukin receptor adaptor protein
    (TIRAP), 1054, 1230, 1352
Toll-like receptors (TLRs), 75
  in dendritic cells, 307
  discovery, 294–295
  macrophage activation and, 1084
  microbe recognition by, 294, 294*t*
  in monocytes and macrophages, 1054,
    1055*f*
  in neutrophils, 1008
  in platelets, 1873
  signaling defects, 1230
  signaling pathways, 296–298, 297*f*, 1055*f*
  structure, 295–296, 295*f*, 296*f*
Tomosyn1/syntaxin binding protein 5, 1849
Tongue
  burning, in iron deficiency, 632
  enlarged, in AL amyloidosis, 1774, 1775*f*
  examination of, 8
  hematoma, in hemophilia, 2118, 2119*f*
  history of pain or tingling in, 5
Tonsils, 94, 1081*f*
Tooth extractions. *See* Dental bleeding/
    extractions
Topoisomerase inhibitors, **326–329**
  anthracyclines. *See* Anthracyclines
  camptothecins, **326–328**
  secondary acute myelogenous leukemia
    and, 183, 1407
Topotecan, 326–327
TORC1 (target of rapamycin complex 1),
    192
Torulopsis glabrata infection, 369
Total blood neutrophil pool (TBNP), 942,
    942*t*
Total blood volume, anemia and, 505, 505*f*
Total-body hematocrit, **489**
Total-body irradiation (TBI), 353, **359–360**,
    1656–1657
Total erythropoiesis, **490**
Total iron-binding capacity (TIBC), 634
Total lymphoid irradiation (TLI), 360
Touch imprint, 29
Touch preparations, 30
Toxic granulation, 22*f*, 23
Toxic methemoglobinemia, 789, 790*t*, 792,
    793. *See also* Methemoglobinemia
Toxic oil syndrome, 959
Toxocara canis, 291, 957*t*
Toxoplasmosis
  central nervous system, 1246

idiopathic CD4+ T lymphocytopenia and, 1206

mononucleosis and, 1261, 1262t, 1268

in pregnancy, 1269

prophylaxis, in HIV infection, 1241t

TP53

in acute myelogenous leukemia, 227t

in B-cell acute lymphoblastic leukemia, 232t

in chronic lymphocytic leukemia, 231t, 1529

in chronic myelogenous leukemia, 230t

in mantle cell lymphoma, 236t

in myelodysplastic syndromes, 228t, 1346t, 1347, 1348, 1352

in myeloma, 233t, 1735f, 1736, 1736t, 1737, 1759

in plasma cell leukemia, 1736t

in Waldenström macroglobulinemia, 1788

t-PA. See Tissue plasminogen activator (t-PA)

TPI. See Triosephosphate isomerase (TPI)

T-PLL (T-cell prolymphocytic lymphoma), 1498t, 1542

TPO. See Thrombopoietin (TPO)

Trace metal deficiency, 653–654

TRADD (TNF receptor death domain), 207f, 249, 302, 302f

TRAF, 249, 298, 302, 302f

TRAF2 (TRAF2), 207, 207f, 236t

TRAF3 (TRAF3), 233t, 1711, 1737

TRAF6 (TRAF6), 298, 1220, 1352

TRAIL (TNF-related apoptosis-inducing ligand), 204f, 205, 249, 951, 996, 1193, 1873

Trained immunity, 168

TRALI (transfusion-related acute lung injury), 2359, 2375–2376

TRAM (TRIF-related adaptor molecule), 297f, 298, 1008, 1054

Tranexamic acid

adverse effects, 2318

for bleeding not response to platelet transfusion, 2385

in cardiopulmonary bypass, 2086

for combined deficiency of factors V and VIII, 2140

for disseminated intravascular coagulation, 2214

for epistaxis, 2139

for hemophilia A, 2123

for inherited platelet disorders, 2062

for mucosal bleeding in immune thrombocytopenia, 2007

pharmacology, 2317–2318

for von Willebrand disease, 2176

Transaldolase, 692t, 697, 701t

Transcobalamin, 591, 591t, 592, 593, 593t, 1448

Transcobalamin I and III. See Haptocorrins

Transcobalamin deficiency, 607

Transcription, 147

in hematopoietic stem cells, 262–263

in lymphopoiesis, 1154–1155

Transcription activator-like effector nuclease (TALEN), 444

Transcription factors, 165–166, 267–268

Transcriptome, 161, 1851, 1853–1854

Transcriptomics, platelet, 1851–1853, 1852f

Transdifferentiation, 269

Transferrin, 618

in anemia of chronic inflammation, 552

endocytosis of, 622–623, 623f

iron-binding capacity and, 634

in iron homeostasis, 621t, 917f, 918

levels of, in newborn, 104

Transferrin receptor-1, 621, 621t, 623

Transferrin receptor-2, 621, 621t, 623

Transferrin receptors, 622–623, 623f, 635, 1058t

Transfer RNA (tRNA), 147

Transforming growth factor (TGF) α, 62t

Transforming growth factor (TGF) β, 266

atherosclerosis and, 2288

in chronic myelogenous leukemia, 1440

in fibroplasia, 1322

in macrophages, 1070t

in megakaryopoiesis, 1823

in platelets, 1848

Transforming growth factor (TGF) β family, 249

Transfusion reactions

acute hemolytic, 2374–2375

acute lung injury, 2359, 2375–2376

allergic, 2375

circulatory overload, 2376

delayed hemolytic, 2372, 2377

disseminated intravascular coagulation and, 2210

febrile nonhemolytic, 2375

graft-versus-host disease, 2374, 2377

HNA antibodies and, 2358–2359

pathophysiology, 2348

sepsis, 2376

Transfusions. See also Exchange transfusion; Platelet transfusion; Red cell transfusion

for acquired pure red cell aplasia, 544

for autoimmune hemolytic anemia, 837

for cobalamin deficiency, 584

for G6PD deficiency, 711–712

intrauterine fetal, 854–855

iron overload and, 641

massive, thrombocytopenia associated with, 2014

for sickle cell disease, 776

Transgenic animal models, 153

Transient aplastic crisis, 541–542

Transient erythroblastopenia of childhood, 541–542

Transient ischemic attacks, 2238–2239

Transient myeloproliferative disorder (TMD), 1385–1386

Transitional cells, marrow, 32t

Transketolase, 692t, 697

Translation, 147

Translocations, 173, 174, 175t, 251

Transmembrane activator and calcium modulator and cyclophilin ligand interactor (TACI), 1606

Transplantation

alloimmune hemolytic anemia following, 836

cytomegalovirus infection following, 1267–1268

hematopoietic cell. See Hematopoietic cell transplantation (HCT)

liver. See Liver transplantation

red cell transfusion and, 2374

renal. See Renal transplantation

thrombotic microangiopathy following, 2262

Transport compartment, plasma, 618

Transthyretin (TTR), 1773, 1776, 1777–1778

TRAPS (TNF receptor-associated periodic syndrome), 1025

Trauma

disseminated intravascular coagulation and, 2204t, 2208

vascular purpura and, 2107

T_REG (regulatory T) cells. See CD4+CD25+ regulatory T (T_REG) cells

TREM (triggering receptors expressed on myeloid cells)-like transcript-1 (TLT-1), 1869

Trench fever, 818

Treponema pallidum infections, 290

TRF-1101, for sickle cell disease, 777t

Triamterene, megaloblastic anemia and, 606t

Tricarboxylic acid (TCA) cycle, 192, 193f

Trichinella spiralis, 949, 956, 957t

TRIF (toll/interleukin-1 receptor domain-containing adaptor inducing IFN-β), 297f, 298

TRIF-related adaptor molecule (TRAM), 297f, 298, 1008, 1054

Triggering receptors expressed on myeloid cells (TREM)-like transcript-1 (TLT-1), 1869

TRIM25 (T-cell receptor-interacting molecule 25), 302, 302f
Trimethoprim, megaloblastic anemia and, 605, 606t
Trimethoprim-sulfamethoxazole
  adverse effects, 1252
  as empiric therapy for infections, 386, 387t
  prophylactic, 389, 1213, 1514
Trinitrotoluene (TNT), 518
Triosephosphate isomerase (TPI)
  activity, 692t
  deficiency, 695, 700t, 704
  in glucose metabolism, 695
Trisomy 7, acute myelogenous leukemia and, 1383
Trisomy 8, 220t, 221t, 521, 1347, 1384t, 1466
Trisomy 11, 181
Trisomy 12, chronic lymphocytic leukemia and, 187, 1529, 1531t, 1532t
Trisomy 19, 1466
Trisomy 21
  acute lymphoblastic leukemia and, 1506
  acute myelogenous leukemia and, 1383, 1386
  neonatal leukemia and, 1386
  platelet abnormalities in, 2061
tRNA (transfer RNA), 147
Tropical spastic paraparesis, 1573
Tropical sprue, 597, 599
Tropomodulins, 663t, 1837
Tropomyosin, 663t, 1832t
True juvenile pernicious anemia, 607
Tryptase, serum, 1470
Tryptophan, for sideroblastic anemia, 920
4T score, 2029, 2029t
t-SNARE, 1849
Tspan9, 1871
TSPAN24. See CD151
TSPAN29. See CD9
TSPAN32. See TSSC6
TSSC6, 1871
TTC7A, 1222
TTP. See Thrombotic thrombocytopenic purpura (TTP)
TTR (transthyretin), 1773, 1776, 1777–1778
Tuberculosis
  lymphocytopenia and, 1204
  macrophage-derived giant cells in, 1078, 1078f
  monocytosis in, 1097
  prophylaxis, in HIV infection, 1241t
Tubulin, 1838
β₁-Tubulin abnormalities, 2059
Tufted angioma, 2014
Tumor antigens, 412t

Tumor-associated macrophages (TAMs), 1083
Tumor-infiltrating lymphocytes (TILs), 412
Tumor lysis syndrome, 1287, 1502, 1535, 1539, 1675
Tumor necrosis factor (TNF), monocytes and, 1091
Tumor necrosis factor (TNF)-α
  in aplastic anemia, 515
  basophils and, 969
  in cell membrane, 62t
  in disseminated intravascular coagulation, 2200, 2208
  effects on erythropoiesis, 550
  in fibrinolysis, 2202
  in fibroplasia, 1322
  hematopoiesis and, 258f
  in inflammation, 284, 287–288, 287t
  in inflammatory response, 1978
  in innate immune response, 303
  interleukin-6 production and, 2036
  in leukocyte adhesion, 281, 282
  in myelodysplastic syndromes, 1352
  neutrophils and, 932, 933t, 1008
  in primary myelofibrosis, 1325
  in sepsis and septic shock, 285
  in sickle cell disease, 765
Tumor necrosis factor (TNF)-α receptors, 249
Tumor necrosis factor (TNF) receptor-1 (TNFR1), 207–208, 207f
Tumor necrosis factor (TNF) receptor-associated factors (TRAFs). See under TRAF
Tumor necrosis factor (TNF) receptor-associated periodic syndrome (TRAPS), 1025
Tumor necrosis factor (TNF) receptor death domain (TRADD), 249, 302, 302f
Tumor necrosis factor (TNF) receptor superfamily, 204f, 249, 252
Tumor necrosis factor (TNF) receptor superfamily member 14 (LIGHT), 1873
Tumor necrosis factor (TNF)-related apoptosis-inducing ligand (TRAIL), 204f, 205, 249, 951, 996, 1193, 1873
Tumor necrosis factor (TNF)-RII, in primary myelofibrosis, 1325
Tumors, solid
  disseminated intravascular coagulation and, 803–804, 2207–2208
  hematopoietic cell transplantation for, 362
Tumor-suppressor genes, 219, 237–239
Tumor suppressors, 195

Turmeric, 2079
TXA₂ (thromboxane A₂), 288, 1830, 1852f, 1876–1877, 1968t
TXB₂ (thromboxane B₂), 952
TYK2, 232t
Tyrosine kinase
  activation in neutrophils, 1016
  phosphorylation, 1884
  in platelets, 1833t
Tyrosine kinase inhibitors, 338–341. See also specific drugs
  for acute lymphoblastic leukemia, 1518
  for acute myelogenous leukemia, 1403
  adverse effects, 341
  for chronic eosinophilic leukemia, 1470
  for chronic myelogenous leukemia. See Chronic myelogenous (myeloid) leukemia (CML), therapy
  comparison, 1451t
  after hematopoietic cell transplantation, 1461–1462
  for mastocytosis, 977, 1279
  mechanism of action, 338
  pharmacology, 338, 340–341
  resistance to
    chromosomal abnormalities associated with, 230
    in chronic myelogenous leukemia, 1456–1458, 1457t
    gene mutations associated with, 178, 318, 340–341
    management, 1457–1458
    in mastocytosis, 1279
    mechanisms, 318, 319t, 338, 340, 1456–1457
  response to, 1451–1452, 1452t, 1454–1455
  secondary chromosomal changes with, 1456
  structure, 340f
Tyrosine kinase receptors, 1871–1872

U
U2AF1, 1349
U2AF2, 1348
Ubiquitin, 253
UCM (upregulation of costimulatory molecules), 304
UGT1A1, 565, 567
UIBC (unsaturated or latent iron-binding capacity), 634
Ulceration/ulcers
  gastric, 629
  leg, 6, 8, 771–772
  mouth, 8
  tongue, 5
Ultrasonography

in deep vein thrombosis, 2269–2270
fetal, 854, 855*f*
spleen, 850*f*, 851*f*
Ultraviolet light therapy. *See* Phototherapy;
Psoralen plus ultraviolet A (PUVA)
Umbilical cord blood, 102, **357**, 358
Umbilical stump, bleeding from, 1988
UNC93B1, 296, 296*f*
Unexplained anemia, 136
UNG (uracil DNA glycosylase), 1169, 1214*t*,
1215
Unsaturated or latent iron-binding capacity
(UIBC), 634
Unstable angina, 2296
Unstable hemoglobins, **781–782**
u-PA (urokinase plasminogen activator),
1973, 1973*f*, 1975
Upregulation of costimulatory molecules
(UCM), 304
Upshaw-Schulman syndrome (congenital
thrombotic thrombocytopenic
purpura), 2257–2258
Uracil DNA glycosylase (UNG), 1169, 1214*t*,
1215
URAF1, 1346*t*
Ureaplasma urealyticum, 1212
Uremia, **2083–2084**
Ureter, primary lymphomas in, 1582
Urine
in primary myelofibrosis, 1327
protein electrophoresis, 1714
UROD. *See* Uroporphyrinogen decarboxylase
(UROD)
UROD, 905, 906
Urokinase plasminogen activator (u-PA)
comparison to other fibrinolytic agents,
2291*t*
in fibrinolysis, 1975, 2304*f*, 2307
gene, 2306*f*
in plasmin generation, 2311
production, 1973
structure, 2304–2305*t*, 2306–2307
Urokinase plasminogen activator receptor
(uPAR), 1973, 2305*t*, 2308–2309
Uromodulin (Tamm-Horsfall mucoprotein),
1744
Uroporphyrinogen decarboxylase (UROD)
functions, 895
porphyria cutanea tarda and, 905–906, 908
Uroporphyrinogen I synthase. *See*
Porphobilinogen (PBG) deaminase
Uroporphyrinogens, 891*f*, 893–894, 893*f*
Uroporphyrinogen synthase (UROS), 893,
894–895
UROS, 896
Ursodeoxycholic acid, 806

Urticaria pigmentosa, 973–974, 974*f*, 977
UTAF1, 228*t*
Uterus, primary lymphomas in, 1582
UTX, 1736, 1736*t*
UTY, 414

V
V1-type receptor, 1879
Vaccine therapy
for acute myelogenous leukemia, 1404
advantages, 421
antigen discovery for, 421, 422*t*
assays of efficacy, 422, 423*t*
B-cell antigen-receptor, 423, 423*f*, 424*f*
clinical trial design, 422
components, **421–422**
delivery strategies for, 422
for follicular lymphoma, 1648
future directions, 424
immunostimulants for enhanced efficacy
of, 422
impediments to, 423–424
for myeloid leukemias, 423
VACOP-B regimen, for primary mediastinal
large B-cell lymphoma, 1635
Vacuolization, 23
VAD regimen, for myeloma, 1750
Valacyclovir
as empiric therapy for infections, 386, 387*t*
prophylactic, 369, 389
Valdecoxib, 2075
Valganciclovir
adverse effects, 1252
as empiric therapy for infections, 386, 387*t*
prophylactic, 389
Valproic acid, 240
VAMP, 1849, 1853
Vancomycin, 385, 387*t*
Varicella zoster virus (VZV) infections, 370,
384
Varices, blood loss from, 629
Variegate porphyria, 889, 890*t*, 891*t*, **904–905**
Vasa nervorum, 1746
Vascular anomalies, blood loss from, 629
Vascular cell adhesion molecule (VCAM)-1
atherosclerosis and, 2286
endothelial inflammation and, 2283
in eosinophils, 950
in hematopoietic stem cells, 261
in inflammatory response, 1978
in leukocyte adhesion, 282–283
in sickle cell disease, 765
in T-cell adhesion, 1185
Vascular disease/injury. *See also*
Cardiovascular disease
in antiphospholipid syndrome, 1976, 2237*f*

fibrinolytic assembly and, 1975–1976,
1975*f*
fibrinolytic function in, 1974–1975, 1974*t*,
1975*f*
folic acid deficiency and, 598–599
homocysteine in, 1976
lipoprotein(a) in, 1976
peripheral vascular disease, 2240, 2316–
2317
sickle cell disease and, 765
Vascular endothelial growth factor (VEGF)
in α-granules, 1843, 1844*f*
in chronic myelogenous leukemia, 1449
in platelets, 1848
in preeclampsia, 801, 2011–2012
Vascular endothelial growth factor (VEGF)
inhibitors, 2263
Vascular endothelial growth factor (VEGF)
receptor-1, 801
Vascular fibrinolysis. *See* Fibrinolysis,
vascular
Vascular purpuras, **2097–2109**. *See also*
specific conditions
definition and diagnostic approach, 2097,
2098*f*
nonpalpable, noninflammatory, round,
2098*t*, 2107–2109
palpable and nonpalpable inflammatory,
2098*t*, 2102–2107
palpable noninflammatory, **2097–2102**,
2098*t*
Vasculitis
antineutrophil cytoplasmic antibody-
associated, 2107, 2107*f*
drug-induced, 2106, 2106*f*
paraneoplastic, 2106
Vasoactive amines, 286*t*, 289
Vasoactive intestinal peptide, 952
Vasoactive substances, 2284*f*
Vasoocclusive crisis, in sickle cell disease,
766–767, 768*f*
Vasopressin, 1879. *See also* Desmopressin
(DDAVP)
VASP, 1833*t*, 1875, 1885
VCAM. *See under* Vascular cell adhesion
molecule
V(D)J recombination, 1166*f*, 1168
Vegans, 602
VEGF. *See* Vascular endothelial growth factor
Velaglucerase alfa, for Gaucher disease,
1127
Vel blood group, 104, 2333*t*
Vemurafenib
for Erdheim-Chester disease, 1111
for hairy cell leukemia, 1559
for Langerhans cell histiocytosis, 1107

Venetoclax (ABT-199)
    for chronic lymphocytic leukemia, 1539
    for mantle cell lymphoma, 1660*t*
Venipuncture, 2367
Venography, 2269–2270
Venoms, 970
Venoocclusive disease with
        immunodeficiency (VODI), 1222
Venous thrombosis/thromboembolism,
    2267–2278
    in antiphospholipid syndrome, 2238,
        2238*f*, 2244
    vs. arterial thrombosis, 2291*t*
    in chronic myeloproliferative neoplasms,
        2079–2081
    clinical course, 2273
    clinical features, 2268–2269. *See also*
        Deep vein thrombosis (DVT);
        Pulmonary embolism
    consultative approach to, 46–47
    definition and epidemiology, 2267–2268
    in disseminated intravascular coagulation,
        2204, 2205*t*
    etiology and pathogenesis, 2268
    in heparin-induced thrombocytopenia,
        2028
    in immune thrombocytopenia, 2002
    laboratory features/objective testing,
        2269–2273, 2270*f*, 2272*f*
    in liver disease, 2192, 2193*t*, 2194–2195
    after liver transplantation, 2195
    in myeloma, 1741, 1756–1757
    in paroxysmal nocturnal hemoglobinuria,
        580
    during pregnancy, 123
    prophylaxis, 2268
    risk factors, 2268*t*
    therapy. *See also specific drugs*
        anticoagulants
            adverse effects, 2277
            in cancer patients, 2276–2277
            contraindications, 2273
            duration, 2276
            objective and principles, 2273
            oral, 2274–2276, 2275*t*
            parenteral, 2273–2274
            in pregnancy, 580, 2277
            regimens, 2273, 2274*t*
        fibrinolytic, 2277–2278, 2313*t*
        inferior vena cava filter, 2278
    thrombophilia testing in, 2228. *See also*
        Hereditary thrombophilia
Verapamil, 2079
Verruca peruviana, 818
Vertebroplasty, 1756
Very-late-antigen. *See under* VLA

Vesicle-associated membrane protein-2, 926,
    1010
V genes, 1163, 1167*f*, 1169, 1170, 1177, 1708
VH3/JH4, 1786
VH-34, 1554, 1557
VHL. *See under* Von Hippel-Lindau
VHL, polycythemia and, 510, 876–877, 877*f*,
    878*f*, 882*t*
Vibrio cholerae, 2340
Vibrio parahaemolyticus, 2340
Vimentin, 1837
Vinblastine, **325–326**. *See also* ABVD
    regimen; Stanford V regimen
    for adult Langerhans cell histiocytosis,
        1108
    adverse effects, 326, 1108
    for immune thrombocytopenia, 2007
    for juvenile xanthogranuloma, 1112
    for Langerhans cell histiocytosis, 1107
    mechanism of action, 325
    pharmacology, 325–326
    resistance to, 319*t*
    stomatocytosis and, 684
    for α-heavy-chain disease, 1808
Vinca alkaloids. *See* Vinblastine; Vincristine
Vincristine, **325–326**. *See also* BEACOPP
    regimen; CHOP regimen;
    CODOX-M/IVAC regimen;
    COPP regimen; EPOCH regimen;
    HyperCVAD regimen; MOPP
    regimen; R-CVP regimen; Stanford
    V regimen
    for acute lymphoblastic leukemia, 1515,
        1516, 1517
    adverse effects, 325–326, 1519*t*
    for α-heavy-chain disease, 1808
    for blast crisis in chronic myelogenous
        leukemia, 1466
    for Burkitt lymphoma, 1676
    for diffuse large B-cell lymphoma, 1629*t*
    for follicular lymphoma, 1645*t*, 1646
    for γ-heavy-chain disease, 1806
    for immune thrombocytopenia, 2003,
        2007
    mechanism of action, 325
    for μ-heavy-chain disease, 1810
    for myeloma, 1750, 1752*t*
    for NK/T-cell lymphoma, 1702
    pharmacology, 325–326
    resistance to, 319*t*
    stomatocytosis and, 684
    for thrombotic thrombocytopenic
        purpura, 2256–2257
    for Waldenström macroglobulinemia,
        1794–1795
Vinculin, 1832*t*, 1848

Vindesine, for diffuse large B-cell lymphoma,
    1628
Vinorelbine, for Hodgkin lymphoma, 1616
Viral infections. *See also specific viruses*
    aplastic anemia and, 518
    disseminated intravascular coagulation
        and, 2207
    erythema multiforme and, 2106
    after hematopoietic cell transplantation,
        369–370
    immune cell therapy of. *See* Immune cell
        therapy (adoptive cellular therapy),
        of viral diseases
    immune thrombocytopenic purpura and,
        2009
    in immunocompromised host, **383–384**
    immunodeficiencies with increased
        susceptibility to, 1230
    mast cells/basophils in host response to,
        970
    prevention, 389
    purpura and, 2104, 2105*f*
    transmission in factor VIII products,
        2126
    treatment, 386, 387*t*
Viral vectors, for gene therapy
    adeno-associated, 438–439, 442
    adenoviral, 438
    lentiviral, 439, 443
    retroviral, 439
    self-inactivating, 437
VISA. *See* Mitochondrial antiviral signaling
    protein (MAVS)
Vitamin A, 335, 652*t*
Vitamin A deficiency, **651**
Vitamin B$_2$ (riboflavin), 652*t*, 793, 2388
Vitamin B$_2$ (riboflavin) deficiency, 651–652
Vitamin B$_6$, 652*t*
Vitamin B$_6$ deficiency, 651
Vitamin B$_{12}$ (cyanocobalamin), 588, 588*f*,
    589, 592*f*, 1448. *See also* Cobalamin
Vitamin B$_{12}$ deficiency. *See* Cobalamin
    deficiency
Vitamin C (ascorbic acid)
    blood levels, 652*t*
    for Chédiak-Higashi syndrome, 1020
    for erythropoietic protoporphyria, 899
    hemolytic anemia and, 708
    for hereditary methemoglobinuria, 793
    for TET protein activity enhancement, 170
Vitamin C (ascorbic acid) deficiency
    (scurvy), **652**, 1986, 2108, 2108*f*
Vitamin D, 335, 2245
Vitamin E
    for abetalipoproteinemia, 681
    functions, 653

for G6PD deficiency, 711
normal levels, 652t
Vitamin E deficiency, 653
Vitamin K
neonate and, 109
for warfarin reversal, 396, 396t
Vitamin K$_2$ (menatetrenone), 1360
Vitamin K antagonists, 393. *See also* Warfarin
Vitamin K deficiency, 1986, 1986t, 1988, 1989f
Vitamin K–dependent zymogens, 1915–1918, 1916t, 1917f, 1918f, 1918t
factor VII. *See* Factor VII
factor IX. *See* Factor IX
factor X. *See* Factor X
protein C. *See* Protein C
prothrombin. *See* Prothrombin (factor II)
Vitamin K epoxide reductase complex (VKORC), 395
Vitamins
in erythrocytes, 470t
in neutrophils, 935
Vitronectin, 63–64, 1834, 1845, 1846t, 1865
Vitronectin receptor. *See* Integrin α$_v$β$_3$
VKORC (vitamin K epoxide reductase complex), 395
VLA (very-late-activation antigen), 1185, 1712
VLA-2. *See* Integrin α$_2$β$_1$
VLA-4. *See* Integrin α$_4$β$_1$
VLA-5. *See* Integrin α$_5$β$_1$
VLA-6. *See* Integrin α$_6$β$_1$
VODI (venoocclusive disease with immunodeficiency), 1222
Volasertib, for myelodysplastic syndromes, 1361
Volume expanders, 2079
von Hippel-Lindau (VHL) protein-ubiquitin-proteasome pathway, 486, 486f
von Hippel-Lindau (VHL) syndrome, classic, 877–878
von Willebrand disease (VWD), 2163–2176
acquired, 2082–2083, 2174–2175
classification, 2165t
clinical features, 1987, 2171–2172
definition and history, 2163–2164
differential diagnosis, 2121, 2174–2175
epidemiology, 2171
etiology and pathogenesis, 2164–2171
molecular genetics, 2049f, 2168–2171, 2168f, 2169f
von Willebrand factor binding to platelets, 2168
von Willebrand factor binding to the vessel wall, 2167–2168

von Willebrand factor biosynthesis, 2166–2167, 2167f
von Willebrand factor interaction with factor VIII, 2168
von Willebrand factor role, 2167
VWF and complementary DNA, 2164, 2166
inheritance, 2171
iron deficiency and, 629
laboratory features, 1988, 2172–2174
platelet-type (pseudo-), **2050–2051**, 2165t, 2174
pregnancy and, 121
prenatal diagnosis, 2174
terminology, 2164t
therapy, course, and prognosis, **2175–2176**, 2318
type 1, 2165t, 2169–2170, 2171–2172, 2175–2176
type 2A, 2165t, 2170, 2175–2176
type 2B, 2165t, 2170–2171, 2172, 2175–2176
type 2M, 2165t, 2171, 2175–2176
type 2N, 2165t, 2171, 2172, 2175–2176
type 3, 1985, 2165t, 2170, 2172, 2175–2176
von Willebrand disease (VWD)-Normandy, 2121
von Willebrand factor (VWF)
binding to platelets, 2168
binding to vessel wall, 2167–2168
biosynthesis, 2164, 2166–2167, 2167f
characteristics, 1916t, 1928
collagen-binding activity, 2164t
factor VIII and, 2164, 2168
functions, 1928, 2167
gene structure and variations, 1928
glycoprotein Ib and, 1866–1867
in hepatic disease, 2191–2192
history, 2163
in inflammatory response, 1979
interactions, 1846t
laboratory evaluation, 1988
in liver transplantation, 2193
penicillins and, 2078
in platelets, 1830–1831f, 1831, 1833–1834, 1845, 2164
ristocetin binding to, 2168
structure, 1846t, 1928, 2254f
terminology, 2164t
in thrombotic thrombocytopenic purpura, 2253–2254
von Willebrand factor (VWF) antigen, 2164t, 2173
von Willebrand factor (VWF) multimers, 2173
von Willebrand factor (VWF) propeptide, 2166

von Willebrand factor (VWF) receptor, 1858–1859t
von Willebrand factor (VWF) replacement therapy, 2176
Vorapaxar, 404t, 406, 2076–2077, 2295, 2297
Voriconazole
as empiric therapy for infections, 385, 387t
prophylactic, 389
Vorinostat, **336–337**
for acute myelogenous leukemia, 1403
mechanism of action, 240
for mycosis fungoides, 1686–1687
for myeloma, 1753t, 1754
for primary effusion lymphoma, 1247
Vosaroxin, for myelodysplastic syndromes, 1361
VpreB, 1168
v-SNARE, 1010, 1018, 1849
VTE. *See* Venous thrombosis/thromboembolism
VWD. *See* Von Willebrand disease (VWD)
VWF. *See* Von Willebrand factor (VWF)
VWF, 1928, 2164, 2165f, 2168–2171, 2169f
VZV (varicella zoster virus) infections, 370, 384

W
W515K/L, 1392
Waldenström hyperglobulinemic purpura, 2099, 2099f
Waldenström macroglobulinemia (WM), **1785–1798**
clinical features, 1788–1791, 1788t, 1789t
autoantibody activity, 1789
cold agglutinin anemia, 827, 1790
cryoglobulinemia, 1789, 1790f
hyperviscosity syndrome, 428, 1788–1789, 1789f
immunoglobulin M tissue deposition, 1790–1791
neuropathy, 1789–1790
platelet dysfunction, 2082
tissue infiltration by neoplastic cells, 1791
course and prognosis, 1797–1798, 1797t
definition and history, 1785
differential diagnosis, 827
epidemiology, 1785
etiology and pathogenesis, 1709–1710
gene mutations, 234t, 1712
laboratory features, 1786f, 1788t, **1791–1792**, 1792f
pathogenesis
B-cell clones, 1785–1786
gene mutations, 1786–1788, 1787f
marrow microenvironment, 1787f, 1788

Waldenström macroglobulinemia (WM)
    (*Cont.*):
    platelet dysfunction in, 2082
    treatment, **1792–1797**
        alkylating agents, 1793
        combination therapies, 1794–1795
        everolimus, 1795–1796
        hematopoietic cell transplantation, 1796
        ibrutinib, 1795
        initiation, 1792–1793
        maintenance therapy, 1796
        nucleoside analogues, 1793–1794
        proteasome inhibitors, 1794
        response criteria, 1796–1797, 1796*t*
        rituximab, 1794
Waldeyer ring, 94
Wandering spleen, 865–866
Warburg effect, 504
Warfarin, **393–397**
    administration and monitoring, 394–395
    adverse effects, 396, 2100, 2100*f*, 2223,
        2277
    for antiphospholipid syndrome, 2244
    complications, 395–396, 396*t*
    contraindication during pregnancy, 580
    drug interactions, 394*t*
    in heparin-induced thrombocytopenia,
        2031–2032
    maternal ingestion of
        effect on fetus and newborn, 112, 112*t*
        neonatal hemorrhage and, 109
    for myocardial infarction, 2296
    pharmacology, **394**
    reversal, 396–397, 396*t*
    for venous thromboembolism, 2274
Warm-antibody autoimmune hemolytic
        anemia. *See* Autoimmune
        hemolytic anemia, warm-antibody
WAS. *See* Wiskott-Aldrich syndrome (WAS)
WASP (Wiskott-Aldrich syndrome protein),
    2059–2060
WASp-interacting protein (WIP) deficiency,
    1225
Wasp stings, 809
WASp/WASP (Wiskott-Aldrich syndrome
        protein), 60, 439, 1063*f*, 1224,
        1841
Water
    in erythrocytes, 469*t*
    in lymphocytes, 1143
Waterhouse-Friderichsen syndrome, 2207
WBC. *See* White blood cell count (WBC)
Weakness, history of, 4
Wee1, 219
Wegener granulomatosis, 1013, 2107, 2107*f*
Weibel-Palade bodies, 281, 2166

Weight loss, history of, 3
Weisses Blut, 1438
WGBS (whole-genome bisulfite sequencing),
    162
WHIM syndrome, 994, **1226**, 1787
White blood cell count (WBC)
    fetal, 102
    newborn, 105, 105*t*
    in pregnancy, 119
    reference ranges, 18*t*
White pulp, of spleen, 88, 89*f*, 90*f*
White thrombi, 2291
Whole-genome bisulfite sequencing (WGBS),
    162
WHSC1 (*MMSET*), 236*t*, 1735
Wilms tumor, erythrocytosis and, 879
Wilms tumor antigen-1 (WT-1), 414
Wilson disease, 810*f*, 811
WIP (WASp-interacting protein) deficiency,
    1225
Wiskott-Aldrich syndrome (WAS),
    1224–1225
    clinical and laboratory features, 1215*t*,
        1225, 2059
    definition, 1224–1225
    gene therapy, 439
    hyposplenism and, 868
    lymphocytopenia in, 1204
    lymphomas and, 1575*t*
    macrophages in, 1059
    neutropenia in, 993
    pathogenesis, 2059
    treatment, 2059
Wiskott-Aldrich syndrome protein
        (WASp/WASP), 60, 439, 1063*f*,
        1224, 1841, **2059–2060**
WM. *See* Waldenström macroglobulinemia
        (WM)
Wnt pathway, 232*t*, 237
Wnt proteins, **266**
Women. *See also* Pregnancy
    iron deficiency in, 630
    menorrhagia in, 5–6, 1987, 2007, 2135,
        2139
    rare bleeding disorders in, 2135
Woringer-Kolopp disease, 1683
Work performance, iron deficiency and,
    632
WT1, 227*t*, 863, 1378*t*, 1379, 1465
WT1 vaccine, 423, 1404
WT syndrome, 530*t*

X

X-chromosome–based polymorphism assays,
    883
Xerocytosis, hereditary, 682*t*, **683**

Xg blood group/antigens, 104, 2331*t*, 2337,
        2345*t*
XIAP, 204*f*, 207, 210, 218
ξ-globin chain, 728
X inactivation, 150, 150*f*
XIST, 150
XK protein, 681. *See also* McLeod phenotype
X-linked adrenoleukodystrophy, 439
X-linked agammaglobulinemia (XLA), 993,
        1212–1213, 1214*t*
X-linked anhydrotic ectodermal dysplasia
        with immunodeficiency caused by
        NEMO mutations, 1215
X-linked chronic granulomatous disease,
        1029, 1030–1031, 1031*t*
X-linked hyperimmunoglobulin
        M syndromes. *See*
        Hyperimmunoglobulin M
        syndromes
X-linked inheritance, 149–151
X-linked lymphoproliferative disease,
        1228–1229, 1266, 1575*t*
X-linked protoporphyria (XLP), 889, 890*t*,
        891*t*, 896
X-linked severe combined immune
        deficiency, 437, 439, 1217.
        See also Severe combined
        immunodeficiency (SCID)
X-linked sideroblastic anemia (XLSA), 894,
        916–917, 920
X-linked sideroblastic anemia with ataxia
        (XLSA/A), 918
X-linked thrombocytopenia, 1224–1225,
        2059
XPO1, 231*t*, 1529
X-ray repair complementing defective
        repair in Chinese hamster cells 4
        (XRCC4), 1167

Y

Yellow marrow, 28
Yersinia enterocolitica, 742
⁹⁰Y-ibritumomab tiuxetan, **346**
    adverse effects, 343*t*
    for diffuse large B-cell lymphoma, 1632
    for follicular lymphoma, 1647
    in hematopoietic cell transplantation,
        360
    for MALT lymphoma, 1666
    for mantle cell lymphoma, 1657*t*
    mechanism of action, 343*t*
Yolk sac, hematopoiesis in, 54, 99–100, 100*f*,
        257–258
Yt blood group/antigens, 2331*t*, 2337,
        2345*t*
⁹⁰Yttrium, 360

Z

Zanamivir, 386

ZAP-70 (zeta-associated protein of 70 kDa), 1178, 1214*t*, 1220, 1531–1532

Zellweger syndrome, 1840

Zero-mode waveguides (ZMWs), 158

Zeta-associated protein of 70 kDa (ZAP-70), 1178, 1531–1532

Zidovudine (AZT)

chemotherapy drugs and, 1249

for HIV infection, 1242

macrocytic anemia and, 1252

megaloblastic anemia and, 605, 606*t*

Zieve syndrome, 655

Zinc, 652*t*

Zinc deficiency, **653**

lymphocytopenia in, 1206

senile purpura and, 2107

Zinc finger nucleases (ZFNs), 440, 443–444, 443*f*, 453

Zoledronic acid, 1756

Zollinger-Ellison syndrome, 601, 629

ZPI (protein Z-dependent protease inhibitor), 1916*t*, 1938, 1952*t*, **1960**

ZRSR2, 1346*t*

ZU5-ANK, 666